CLINICAL RADIATION ONCOLOGY

ASSOCIATE EDITORS

K. Kian Ang, MD, PhD
Professor
Gilbert H. Fletcher Memorial Distinguished Chair
Department of Radiation Oncology
University of Texas M.D. Anderson Cancer Center
Houston, Texas
HEAD AND NECK TUMORS

Hak Choy, MD
Professor and Chairman
Nancy B. and Jake L. Hamon Distinguished Chair in Therapeutic Oncology Research
Department of Radiation Oncology
University of Texas Southwestern Medical Center at Dallas
Dallas, Texas
THORACIC NEOPLASMS

Jay R. Harris, MD
Professor and Chair
Department of Radiation Oncology
Dana-Farber Cancer Institute
Brigham and Women's Hospital
Harvard Medical School
Boston, Massachusetts
BREAST CANCER

Larry E. Kun, MD
Professor
Department of Radiology
Department of Pediatrics
University of Tennessee College of Medicine
Chair
Department of Radiological Sciences
St. Jude Children's Research Hospital
Memphis, Tennessee
CHILDHOOD CANCERS

Peter Mauch, MD
Professor
Department of Radiation Oncology
Harvard Medical School
Associate Chair
Department of Radiation Oncology
Dana-Farber Cancer Institute
Brigham and Women's Hospital
Boston, Massachusetts
LYMPHOMA AND HEMATOLOGIC MALIGNANCIES

Edward G. Shaw, MD
Professor and Chair
Department of Radiation Oncology
Wake Forest University School of Medicine
Director, Clinical Research Program
Comprehensive Cancer Center of Wake Forest University
Winston-Salem, North Carolina
CENTRAL NERVOUS SYSTEM TUMORS

Gillian M. Thomas, MD
Professor
Department of Radiation Oncology
Department of Obstetrics and Gynaecology
University of Toronto Faculty of Medicine
Sunnybrook Regional Cancer Centre
Toronto, Ontario
Canada
GYNECOLOGIC TUMORS

Anthony L. Zietman, MD
Professor of Radiation Oncology
Harvard Medical School
Department of Radiation Oncology
Massachusetts General Hospital
Boston, Massachusetts
GENITOURINARY TUMORS

CLINICAL RADIATION ONCOLOGY

Second Edition

Senior Editors

Leonard L. Gunderson, MD, MS
Getz Family Professor and Chair
Department of Radiation Oncology
Mayo Clinic College of Medicine and Mayo Clinic
Deputy Director for Clinical Affairs
Mayo Clinic Cancer Center – Scottsdale
Scottsdale, Arizona

Joel E. Tepper, MD
Hector MacLean Distinguished Professor of Cancer Research
Chairman
Department of Radiation Oncology
UNC/Lineberger Comprehensive Cancer Center
University of North Carolina School of Medicine
Chapel Hill, North Carolina

ELSEVIER
CHURCHILL
LIVINGSTONE

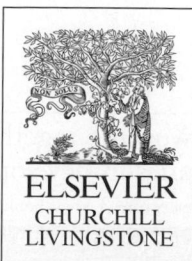

ELSEVIER
CHURCHILL
LIVINGSTONE

1600 John F. Kennedy Blvd.
Suite 1800
Philadelphia, PA 19103-2899

CLINICAL RADIATION ONCOLOGY, SECOND EDITION

ISBN-13: 978-0-443-06840-9
ISBN-10: 0-443-06840-2

Notice

Knowledge and best practice in this field are constantly changing. As new research and experience broaden our knowledge, changes in practice, treatment and drug therapy may become necessary or appropriate. Readers are advised to check the most current information provided (i) on procedures featured or (ii) by the manufacturer of each product to be administered, to verify the recommended dose or formula, the method and duration of administration, and contraindications. It is the responsibility of the practitioner, relying on their own experience and knowledge of the patient, to make diagnoses, to determine the dosages and the best treatment for each individual patient, and to take all appropriate safety precautions. To the fullest extent of the law, neither the Publisher nor the Editors assume any liability for any injury and/or damage to persons or property arising out or related to any use of the material contained in this book.

THE PUBLISHER

ISBN-13: 978-0-443-06840-9
ISBN-10: 0-443-06840-2

Library of Congress Control Number: 2006930289

Acquisitions Editor: Dolores Meloni
Developmental Editor: Agnes Byrne
Publishing Services Manager: Tina Rebane
Project Manager: Mary Anne Folcher
Design Direction: Karen O'Keefe Owens

Printed in China

Last digit is the print number: 9 8 7 6 5 4 3 2 1

To my wife Katheryn, our children and their families, our parents and siblings, for their love and support in relation to our activities as a family and my career in medicine.

To my sister, Robin, who lost a gallant 6-year battle with metastatic breast cancer in June, 2005, but lived to see her son, Josh, graduate from high school in May, 2005; to my sister, Judy, who is wheelchair bound from multiple sclerosis but notes "I have lost use of my legs, not my brain" and "Depression is not in my vocabulary."

To my colleagues in Radiation Oncology, Surgery and Medical Oncology at Mayo Clinic and other institutions where I trained and practiced, for the opportunity to work together as a multidisciplinary team in the diagnosis and care of our patients.

To the Master Healer, for the spiritual component of healing that can be of major importance to the mind and body of both patient and physician.

LEONARD L. GUNDERSON

To my family, including Laurie, Abigail, Miriam, Adam, Zekariah, and Zohar, for the love and support they have given me for many years.

To my parents who taught me the importance of education, learning, and doing that which should be done.

To my many mentors who taught me in the past, and those who continue to teach me.

To my professional colleagues, both at the University of North Carolina and around the country, who have made me a better physician.

JOEL E. TEPPER

CONTRIBUTORS

Ross A. Abrams, MD
Chair
Frank R. Henderson Professor
Department of Radiation Oncology
Rush University Medical Center
Chicago, Illinois
Chapter 45, Pancreatic Cancer

Anesa Ahamad, MD
Department of Radiation Oncology
University of Texas M.D. Anderson Cancer Center
Houston, Texas
Chapter 33, Sinonasal Cancer

Raef S. Ahmed, MD
Research Fellow
Department of Radiation Oncology
University of Alabama at Birmingham
School of Medicine
Birmingham, Alabama
Chapter 24, High-Grade Gliomas

K. Kian Ang, MD
Professor
Department of Radiation Oncology
University of Texas M.D. Anderson Cancer Center
Houston, Texas
Overview, Disease Sites, Part B, Head and Neck Tumors; Chapter 30, Oropharyngeal Cancer; Chapter 32, Larynx and Hypopharynx Cancer; Chapter 33, Sinonasal Cancer; Chapter 38, Cutaneous Carcinoma; Chapter 39, Malignant Melanoma

Douglas W. Arthur, MD
Associate Professor, Interim Chair
Radiation Oncology Department
Virginia Commonwealth University Medical Center
Medical College Virginia Campus
Richmond, Virginia
Chapter 59, Noninvasive Breast Cancer

Matthew T. Ballo, MD
Associate Professor
Department of Radiation Oncology
Associate Clinical Medical Director
Sarcoma Center
EVP, Chief Operating Officer
Associate Medical Director
Melanoma/Skin Center
University of Texas M.D. Anderson Cancer Center
Houston, Texas
Chapter 39, Malignant Melanoma

M. Kevin Barry, MD
Department of Surgery
Mayo Clinic
Rochester, Minnesota
Chapter 7, Surgical Principles

Glenn Bauman, MD
Director of Research
London Regional Cancer Program
London Health Sciences Centre
London, Ontario Canada
Chapter 25, Meningioma, Ependymoma, and Other Adult Brain Tumors

Edgar Ben-Josef, MD
Clinical Associate Professor
Department of Radiation Oncology
University of Michigan
Medical School
Ann Arbor, Michigan
Chapter 46, Hepatobiliary Tumors

Laurie E. Blach
Mt. Sinai Medical Center
Department of Radiation Oncology
Miami Beach, Florida
Chapter 65, Pediatric Soft Tissue Sarcomas

A. William Blackstock, MD
Associate Professor
Department of Radiation Oncology
Wake Forest University School of Medicine
Winston-Salem, North Carolina
Chapter 42, Cancer of the Esophagus

Lawrence S. Blaszkowsky, MD
Instructor
Harvard Medical School
Massachusetts General Hospital
Boston, Massachusetts
Chapter 8, Principles of Chemotherapy

James A. Bonner, MD
Chairman and Merle M. Salter Professor
Department of Radiation Oncology
University of Alabama at Birmingham
School of Medicine
Birmingham, Alabama
Chapter 4, Interaction of Chemotherapy and Radiation; Chapter 31, Nasopharyngeal Carcinoma; Chapter 34, Salivary Gland Cancer

J. Daniel Bourland, PhD
Associate Professor, Head
Physics Research and Education
Department of Radiation Oncology
Wake Forest University School of Medicine
Winston-Salem, North Carolina
Chapter 6, Radiation Oncology Physics

Ian J. Bristol, MD
Radiation Oncology Residency Program
Department of Radiation Oncology
University of Texas M.D. Anderson Cancer Center
Houston, Texas
Chapter 33, Sinonasal Cancer

Paul D. Brown, MD
Associate Professor
Department of Radiation Oncology
Mayo Clinic College of Medicine
Rochester, Minnesota

Chapter 23, Low-Grade Gliomas

John L. Bryant, PhD
Professor of Biostatistics
Graduate School of Public Health
University of Pittsburgh
Associate Director
NASBP Biostatistical Center
Pittsburgh, Pennsylvania

Chapter 12, Statistics and Clinical Trials

Thomas A. Buchholz, MD
Professor
Radiation Oncology
Director
Breast Cancer Radiation Oncology Program
University of Texas M.D. Anderson Cancer Center
Houston, Texas

Chapter 61, Breast Cancer: Stages III and IV

Donald J. Buchsbaum, PhD
Professor
Department of Radiation Oncology
The University of Alabama at Birmingham
School of Medicine
Birmingham, Alabama

Chapter 4, Interaction of Chemotherapy and Radiation

Michael Burke, MD
Department of Radiology
University of North Carolina Hospitals
Chapel Hill, North Carolina

Chapter 9, Imaging in Oncology

Steven J. Buskirk, MD
Associate Professor of Oncology
Mayo Clinic College of Medicine
Consultant
Department of Radiation Oncology
Mayo Clinic
Jacksonville, Florida

Chapter 53, Kidney and Ureteral Carcinoma

Stuart K. Calderwood, PhD
Associate Professor
Harvard Medical School
Director
Molecular and Cellular Biology
Department of Radiation Oncology
Beth Israel Deaconess Medical Center
Boston, Massachusetts

Chapter 2, Molecular and Cellular Biology

Felipe A. Calvo, MD
Professor and Chair
Department of Oncology
Hospital General Universitario
Hospital General Universaro
Gregorio Maranon
Madrid, Spain

Chapter 44, Stomach Cancer

Higinia Cardenes, MD, PhD
Clinical Associate Professor
Department of Radiation Oncology
Indiana University School of Medicine
Indianapolis, Indiana

Chapter 58, Ovarian Cancer

Charles Catton, MD, FRCPC
Associate Professor
Department of Radiation Oncology
Princess Margaret Hospital
University of Toronto Faculty of Medicine
Toronto, Ontario Canada

Chapter 62, Soft Tissue Sarcoma

Bruce A. Chabner, MD
Professor of Medicine
Harvard Medical School
Clinical Director
Dana-Farber Cancer Institute
Massachusetts General Hospital
Boston, Massachusetts

Chapter 8, Principles of Chemotherapy

Michael G. Chen, MD
Professor Emeritus, Consultant
Department of Radiation Oncology
Mayo Clinic College of Medicine
Rochester, Minnesota

Chapter 75, Multiple Myeloma and Other Plasma Cell Neoplasms

L. Chinsoo Cho, MD, MS
Associate Professor
Department of Radiation Oncology
University of Texas Southwestern Medical Center at Dallas
Dallas, Texas

Overview, Disease Sites, Part C, Thoracic Neoplasms

Julia Choo, MD
Associate Physician
Radiation Oncology
Kaiser Permanente
Los Angeles, California

Chapter 45, Pancreatic Cancer

Hak Choy, MD
Professor and Chairman
Department of Radiation Oncology
University of Texas Southwestern Medical Center at Dallas
Dallas, Texas

Overview, Disease Sites, Part C, Thoracic Neoplasms

Peter Chung, MD, FRCPC
Department of Radiation Oncology
Princess Margaret Hospital
University of Toronto
Toronto, Ontario Canada
Chapter 62, Soft Tissue Sarcoma

Louis S. Constine, MD
Professor
Department of Radiation Oncology and Pediatrics
Vice Chair
Department of Radiation Oncology
James P. Wilmot Cancer Center
University of Rochester Medical Center
Rochester, New York
Chapter 71, Pediatric Hodgkin's Lymphoma

Oana Craciunescu, PhD
Assistant Clinical Professor
Department of Radiation Oncology
Duke University Medical Center
Durham, North Carolina
Chapter 20, Hyperthermia

Carien L. Creutzberg, MD, PhD
Associate Professor of Radiation Oncology
Department of Clinical Oncology
Leiden University Medical Center
Leiden, The Netherlands
Chapter 56, Endometrial Cancer

Massimo Cristofanilli, MD
Associate Professor
Department of Breast Medical Oncology
University of Texas M.D. Anderson Cancer Center
Houston, Texas
Chapter 61, Breast Cancer: Stages III and IV

Juanita Crook, MD, FRCPC
Professor
Department of Radiation Oncology
University of Toronto Faculty of Medicine
Head
Department of Brachytherapy
Princess Margaret Hospital
University Health Network
Toronto, Ontario Canada
Chapter 54, Penile Cancer

Walter J. Curran, Jr., MD, FACR
Professor, Chair
Department of Radiation Oncology
Jefferson Medical College of Thomas Jefferson University
Philadelphia, Pennsylvania
Chapter 40, Small Cell Lung Cancer

Brian G. Czito, MD
Assistant Professor
Department of Radiation Oncology
Duke University Medical Center
Durham, North Carolina
Chapter 15, Intraoperative Irradiation; Chapter 47, Colon Cancer

Shiva K. Das, PhD
Associate Research Professor
Department of Radiation Oncology
Duke University Medical Center
Durham, North Carolina
Chapter 20, Hyperthermia

Marc David, MD, FRCPC
Assistant Professor
McGill University Faculty of Medicine
Montreal General Hospital
Montreal, Quebec Canada
Chapter 22, Palliation of Metastases: Bone, Spinal Cord, Brain, Liver

Waldemar Debinski, MD, PhD
Professor
Department of Neurosurgery and Radiation Oncology
Wake Forest University School of Medicine
Director of Brain Tumor Center of Excellence
Comprehensive Cancer Center of Wake Forest University
Winston-Salem, North Carolina
Overview, Disease Sites, Part A, Central Nervous System Tumors

Thomas F. DeLaney, MD
Department of Radiation Oncology
Massachusetts General Hospital
Northeast Proton Therapy Center
Boston, Massachusetts
Chapter 18, Charged Particle Radiotherapy

Mark Dewhirst, DVM, PhD
Gustavo S. Montana Professor of Radiation Oncology
Professor of Pathology and Biomedical Engineering
Duke University Medical Center
Durham, North Carolina
Chapter 20, Hyperthermia

John H. Donohue, MD
Professor of Surgery
Mayo Clinic College of Medicine
Consultant in Surgery
Mayo Clinic
Rochester, Minnesota
Chapter 7, Surgical Principles

Thierry Duprez, MD
Associate Professor
Diagnostic Radiology Department
Head and Neck Oncology Program
Université Catholique de Louvain
Cliniques Universitaires St-Luc
Service de Radiologie, RMN
Brussels, Belgium
Chapter 37, Management of the Neck

Avraham Eisbruch, MD
Professor
Department of Radiation Oncology
University of Michigan Medical School
Ann Arbor, Michigan
Chapter 14, Conformal Therapy: Treatment Planning, Treatment Delivery, and Clinical Results

Tony Y. Eng, MD
Associate Professor, Vice Chair
Department of Radiation Oncology
University of Texas Health Science Center at San Antonio
Cancer Therapy and Research Center
San Antonio, Texas

Chapter 43, Uncommon Thoracic Malignancies

Colleen Euler, BSc MRT(T)
Sarcoma Research Radiation Therapist
Department of Radiation Oncology
Princess Margaret Hospital
University of Toronto
Toronto, Ontario Canada

Chapter 62, Soft Tissue Sarcoma

Matthew G. Ewend, MD
Chief of Neurosurgery
University of North Carolina at Chapel Hill
School of Medicine
Chapel Hill, North Carolina

Chapter 26, Pituitary Tumors

Julia R. Fielding, MD
Associate Professor
Department of Radiology
University of North Carolina at Chapel Hill
School of Medicine
Chapel Hill, North Carolina

Chapter 9, Imaging in Oncology

Barbara Fisher, MD
Associate Professor
Department of Oncology
University of Western Ontario
Consultant
London Regional Cancer Program
London Health Sciences Center
London, Ontario Canada

Chapter 25, Meningioma, Ependymoma, and Other Adult Brain Tumors

John B. Fiveash, MD
Associate Professor
Department of Radiation Oncology
The University of Alabama at Birmingham
School of Medicine
Birmingham, Alabama

Chapter 24, High-Grade Gliomas

Robert L. Foote, MD
Professor of Oncology
Mayo Clinic College of Medicine
Consultant
Department of Radiation Oncology
Mayo Clinic
Rochester, Minnesota

Chapter 29, Oral Cavity; Chapter 31, Nasopharyngeal Carcinoma; Chapter 34, Salivary Gland Cancer

Benedick A. Fraass, PhD
Professor
Department of Radiation Oncology
Director
Radiation Physics Division
University of Michigan Medical Center
Ann Arbor, Michigan

Chapter 14, Conformal Therapy: Treatment Planning, Treatment Delivery, and Clinical Results

Arnold Freedman, MD
Associate Professor
Harvard Medical School
Dana-Farber Cancer Institute
Department of Medical Oncology/Hematologic Malignancies
Boston, Massachusetts

Chapter 73, Hodgkin's Disease

Yolanda I. Garces, MD
Assistant Professor of Oncology
Mayo Clinic College of Medicine
Consultant
Department of Radiation Oncology
Mayo Clinic
Rochester, Minnesota

Chapter 4, Interaction of Chemotherapy and Radiation

Adam S. Garden, MD
Professor
Department of Radiation Oncology
Section Chief Head and Neck Cancer
University of Texas M.D. Anderson Cancer Center
Houston, Texas

Chapter 30, Oropharyngeal Cancer; Chapter 32, Larynx and Hypopharynx Cancer; Chapter 33, Sinonasal Cancer

Morie A. Gertz
Professor of Medicine
Mayo Clinic College of Medicine
Chair
Division of Hematology and Internal Medicine
Mayo Clinic
Rochester, Minnesota

Chapter 75, Multiple Myeloma and Other Plasma Cell Neoplasms

Mary K. Gospodarowicz, MD, FRCPC
Professor, Chair
Department of Radiation Oncology
University of Ontario
Chief
Radiation Medicine Program
Princess Margaret Hospital
Toronto, Ontario Canada

Chapter 52, Testicular Cancer; Chapter 74, Non-Hodgkin's Lymphoma

Cai Grau, MD, DMSc
Professor
Department of Oncology
Aarhus University Hospital
Aarhus, Denmark

Chapter 3, Dose Response Modifiers in Radiation Oncology

Vincent Grégoire, MD, PhD
Professor
Radiation Oncology Department
Head and Neck Oncology Program
Université Catholique de Louvain
Cliniques Universitaires St-Luc
Brussels, Belgium

Chapter 37, Management of the Neck

Craig M. Greven, MD
Professor, Chairman
Department of Ophthalmology
Wake Forest University School of Medicine
Winston-Salem, North Carolina

Chapter 28, Orbital, Ocular, and Optic Nerve Tumors

Kathryn McConnell Greven, MD
Professor
Department of Radiation Oncology
Wake Forest University School of Medicine
Winston-Salem, North Carolina

Chapter 28, Orbital, Ocular, and Optic Nerve Tumors

Leonard L. Gunderson, MD, MS
Getz Family Professor, Chair
Department of Radiation Oncology
Mayo Clinic College of Medicine and Mayo Clinic
Deputy Director for Clinical Affairs
Mayo Clinic Cancer Center-Scottsdale
Scottsdale, Arizona

Overview, Disease Sites, Part D, Gastrointestinal Tumors; Chapter 44, Stomach Cancer

Michael G. Haddock, MD
Associate Professor of Oncology
Mayo Clinic College of Medicine
Consultant
Department of Radiation Oncology
Mayo Clinic
Rochester, Minnesota

Chapter 49, Anal Carcinoma; Chapter 53, Kidney and Ureteral Carcinoma

Marc Hamoir, MD
Professor
Otolaryngology
Department of Head and Neck Surgery
Head and Neck Oncology Program
Université Catholique de Louvain
Cliniques Universitaires St-Luc
Brussels, Belgium

Chapter 37, Management of the Neck

Jay R. Harris, MD
Professor, Chair
Department of Radiation Oncology
Dana-Farber Cancer Institute
Brigham and Women's Hospital
Harvard Medical School
Boston, Massachusetts

Overview, Disease Sites, Part C, Breast Cancer

Ian D. Hay, MD, PhD
Dr. Richard F. Emslander Professor of Endocrinology Research
Professor of Medicine
Mayo Clinic College of Medicine
Consultant
Endocrinology, Internal Medicine
Mayo Clinic
Rochester, Minnesota

Chapter 35, Thyroid Cancer

Russell W. Hinerman, MD
Associate Professor
Department of Radiation Oncology
University of Florida Shands Hospital
University of Florida Health Science Center
Gainesville, Florida

Chapter 29, Oral Cavity

Michael R. Horsman, PhD, DMSc
Associate Professor
Department of Experimental Clinical Oncology
Aarhus University Hospital
Aarhus, Denmark

Chapter 3, Dose Response Modifiers in Radiation Oncology

Melissa M. Hudson, MD
Professor of Pediatrics
University of Tennessee Health Sciences Center
College of Medicine
Department of Hematology-Oncology
St. Jude Children's Research Hospital
Memphis, Tennessee

Chapter 71, Pediatric Hodgkin's Lymphoma

Valerie S. Jewells, DO
Assistant Professor
Department of Radiology
University of North Carolina at Chapel Hill
School of Medicine
Chapel Hill, North Carolina

Chapter 9, Imaging in Oncology

Ellen L. Jones, MD, PhD
Associate Professor
Department of Radiation Oncology
Duke University Medical Center
Durham, North Carolina

Chapter 20, Hyperthermia

Glenn Jones, MD
Associate Professor
Department of Radiation Oncology
McMaster University
Hamilton, Ontario
Radiation Oncologist
Peel Regional Cancer Centre
Credit Valley Hospital
Mississauga, Ontario Canada

Chapter 76, Mycosis Fungoides

John A. Kalapurakal, MD
Associate Professor
Department of Radiation Oncology
Northwestern University Medical School
Northwestern Memorial Hospital
Chicago, Illinois

Chapter 67, Wilms' Tumor

Amir H. Khandani, MD, PhD
Assistant Professor
Department of Radiology
Director
PET Imaging, Division of Nuclear Medicine
Department of Radiology
University of North Carolina School of Medicine
Lineberger Comprehensive Cancer Center
Chapel Hill, North Carolina

Chapter 10, Nuclear Medicine

Deepak Khuntia, MD
Clinical Assistant Professor
Department of Human Oncology
University of Wisconsin School of Medicine
Madison, Wisconsin

Chapter 16, Stereotactic Irradiation: Linear Accelerator and Gamma Knife

Susan J. Knox, PhD, MD
Professor
Department of Radiation Oncology
Stanford University School of Medicine
Stanford, California

Chapter 21, Targeted Radionuclide Therapy

Wui-Jin Koh, MD
Associate Professor
Department of Radiation Oncology
University Cancer Center
University of Washington Medical Center
Seattle, Washington

Chapter 55, Cervical Cancer

Deborah A. Kuban, MD
Professor
Department of Radiation Oncology
University of Texas M.D. Anderson Cancer Center
Houston, Texas

Chapter 50, Prostate Cancer

Larry E. Kun, MD
Professor
Department of Radiology
Department of Pediatrics
University of Tennessee College of Medicine
Chair
Department of Radiological Sciences
St. Jude Children's Research Hospital
Memphis, Tennessee

Overview, Disease Sites, Part I, Childhood Cancers

George E. Laramore, MD, PhD
Professor, Chair
Department of Radiation Oncology
University of Washington School of Medicine
Director
Cancer Center
University of Washington Medical Center
Seattle, Washington

Chapter 19, Neutron Radiotherapy

Robert S. Lavey, MD, MPH
Head
Radiation Oncology Department
Children's Hospital Los Angeles
Los Angeles, California

Chapter 68, Retinoblastoma

Theodore S. Lawrence, MD, PhD
Isadore Lampe Professor, Chair
Department of Radiation Oncology
University of Michigan School of Medicine
Ann Arbor, Michigan

Chapter 46, Hepatobiliary Tumors

Colleen A. Lawton, MD
Professor
Director, Residency Program
Department of Radiation Oncology
Medical College of Wisconsin
Milwaukee, Wisconsin

Chapter 50, Prostate Cancer

Benoît Lengelé, MD, PhD
Professor
Department of Plastic and Reconstructive Surgery
Unit of Human Anatomy and Head and Neck Oncology Program
Université Catholique de Louvain
Cliniques Universitaires St-Luc
Brussels, Belgium

Chapter 37, Management of the Neck

William P. Levin, MD
Clinical Fellow
Department of Radiation Oncology
Massachusetts General Hospital
Northeast Proton Therapy Center
Boston, Massachusetts

Chapter 18, Charged Particle Radiotherapy

Jean E. Lewis, MD
Associate Professor
Department of Laboratory Medicine and Pathology
Mayo Clinic School of Medicine
Rochester, Minnesota

Chapter 34, Salivary Gland Cancer

Chuan-Yuan Li, PhD
Associate Research Professor
Department of Radiation Oncology
Duke University Medical Center
Durham, North Carolina

Chapter 20, Hyperthermia

Jacob C. Lindegaard, MD, DMSc
Consultant
Department of Oncology
Aarhus University Hospital
Aarhus, Denmark

Chapter 3, Dose Response Modifiers in Radiation Oncology

William J. Mackillop, MD
Professor, Chair
Department of Community Health and Epidemiology
Queen's University
Senior Radiation Oncologist
Cancer Centre of Southeastern Ontario
Head
Division of Cancer Care and Epidemiology
Queen's University Cancer Research Institute
Kingston, Ontario Canada

Chapter 11, Health Services Research in Radiation Oncology

Anthony A. Mancuso, MD
Professor, Chairman
Department of Radiology
College of Medicine
University of Florida
Gainesville, Florida

Chapter 36, Unknown Head and Neck Primary Site

Karen J. Marcus, MD
Associate Professor
Department of Radiation Oncology
Harvard Medical School
Children's Hospital
Boston, Massachusetts

Chapter 70, Pediatric Leukemias and Lymphomas

James M. Markert, MD
Professor
Department of Neurosurgery
The University of Alabama at Birmingham
School of Medicine
Birmingham, Alabama

Chapter 24, High-Grade Gliomas

James A. Martenson, Jr., MD
Professor of Oncology
Mayo Clinic College of Medicine
Consultant, Department of Radiation Oncology
Mayo Clinic
Rochester, Minnesota

Chapter 49, Anal Carcinoma

Alvaro A. Martinez, MD, FACR
Corporate Chairman
Department of Radiation Oncology
William Beaumont Hospital
Royal Oak, Michigan

Chapter 13, Brachytherapy

Peter Mauch, MD
Professor
Department of Radiation Oncology
Harvard Medical School
Associate Chair
Department of Radiation Oncology
Brigham and Women's Hospital
Dana-Farber Cancer Institute
Boston, Massachusetts

Overview, Disease Sites, Part J, Lymphoma and Hematologic Malignancies

Jean-Jacques Mazeron, MD, PhD
Head
Department of Radiation Oncology
Groupe Hospitalier Pitié-Salpêtrière
Paris, France

Chapter 54, Penile Cancer

Minesh P. Mehta, MD
Professor, Chair
Department of Human Oncology
University of Wisconsin School of Medicine
Madison, Wisconsin

Chapter 16, Stereotactic Irradiation: Linear Accelerator and Gamma Knife

William M. Mendenhall, MD
Department of Radiation Oncology
University of Florida Shands Hospital
University of Florida Health Science Center
Gainesville, Florida

Chapter 29, Oral Cavity; Chapter 36, Unknown Head and Neck Primary Site

Thomas E. Merchant, DO, PhD
Chief
Division of Radiation Oncology
St. Jude Children's Research Hospital
Memphis, Tennessee

Chapter 64, Central Nervous System Tumors in Children

Ruby F. Meredith, MD, PhD
Professor
Department of Radiation Oncology
The University of Alabama at Birmingham
School of Medicine
Birmingham, Alabama

Chapter 21, Targeted Radionuclide Therapy

Bruce D. Minsky, MD
Vice Chairman
Department of Radiation Oncology
Memorial Sloan-Kettering Cancer Center
New York, New York

Chapter 48, Rectal Cancer

David H. Moore, MD
Professor
Department of Obstetrics and Gynecology
Indiana University School of Medicine
Indianapolis, Indiana

Chapter 55, Cervical Cancer

David E. Morris, MD
Department of Radiation Oncology
University of North Carolina School of Medicine
Chapel Hill, North Carolina

Chapter 26, Pituitary Tumors

William H. Morrison, MD
Associate Professor
Department of Radiation Oncology
University of Texas M.D. Anderson Cancer Center
Houston, Texas

Chapter 30, Oropharyngeal Cancer; Chapter 32, Larynx and Hypopharynx Cancer

Louis B. Nabors, MD
Associate Professor
Department of Neurology
The University of Alabama at Birmingham
School of Medicine
Birmingham, Alabama

Chapter 24, High-Grade Gliomas

Andrea K. Ng, MD, MPH
Associate Professor
Department of Radiation Oncology
Harvard Medical School
Dana-Farber Cancer Institute
Brigham and Women's Hospital
Boston, Massachusetts

Overview, Disease Sites, Part J, Lymphoma and Hematologic Malignancies; Chapter 73, Hodgkin's Disease

Robert S. Nordal, MD
Assistant Professor
Department of Radiation Oncology
The University of Alabama at Birmingham
School of Medicine
Birmingham, Alabama

Chapter 24, High-Grade Gliomas

Marianne Nordsmark, MD, PhD
Staff Specialist
Department of Oncology
Aarhus University Hospital
Aarhus, Denmark

Chapter 3, Dose Response Modifiers in Radiation Oncology

Kerry D. Olsen, MD
Professor
Department of Otolaryngology
Mayo Clinic, College of Medicine and Mayo Clinic
Rochester, Minnesota

Chapter 34, Salivary Gland Cancer

Bert O'Neil, MD
Assistant Professor
Division of Hematology Oncology
Department of Internal Medicine
Lineberger Comprehensive Cancer Center
University of North Carolina at Chapel Hill
Chapel Hill, North Carolina

Chapter 5, Biologics and Interactions with Radiation

Brian O'Sullivan, MD, FRCPC
Professor
Department of Radiation Oncology
Princess Margaret Hospital
University of Toronto
Toronto, Ontario Canada

Chapter 62, Soft Tissue Sarcoma

Roger Ove, MD, PhD
Assistant Professor
Department of Radiation Oncology
The University of Alabama at Birmingham
School of Medicine
Mid-South Imaging and Therapeutics
Memphis, Tennessee

Chapter 31, Nasopharyngeal Carcinoma

Jens Overgaard, MD, DMSc
Professor
Department of Experimental Clinical Oncology
Aarhus University Hospital
Aarhus, Denmark

Chapter 3, Dose Response Modifiers in Radiation Oncology

Alberto S. Pappo, MD
The Hospital for Sick Children
Toronto, Ontario Canada

Chapter 65, Pediatric Soft Tissue Sarcomas

Alexander S. Parker, PhD
Assistant Professor
Epidemiology, Department of Health Sciences Research
Mayo Clinic College of Medicine
Senior Associate Consultant
Mayo Clinic
Jacksonville, Florida

Chapter 53, Kidney and Ureteral Carcinoma

Ivy A. Petersen, MD
Assistant Professor, Consultant
Department of Radiation Oncology
Mayo Clinic
Rochester, Minnesota

Chapter 35, Thyroid Cancer

Thomas M. Pisansky, MD
Professor
Department of Radiation Oncology
Mayo Clinic
Rochester, Minnesota

Chapter 50, Prostate Cancer

Arthur T. Porter, MD, FRCPC
Professor of Oncology
CEO
McGill University Health Center
Montreal, Quebec Canada

Chapter 22, Palliation of Metastases: Bone, Spinal Cord, Brain, Liver

Louis Potters, MD
Medical Director
New York Prostate Institute
Associate Director
Department of Radiation Oncology
South Nassau Communities Hospital
Oceanside, New York

Chapter 50, Prostate Cancer

Leonard Prosnitz, MD
Professor
Department of Radiation Oncology
Duke University Medical Center
Durham, North Carolina
Chapter 20, Hyperthermia

David Raben, MD
Associate Professor
Department of Radiation Oncology
University of Colorado Health Science Center
School of Medicine
Denver, Colorado
Chapter 5, Biologics and Interactions with Radiation

Abram Recht, MD
Professor
Department of Radiation Oncology
Harvard Medical School
Deputy Chief
Department of Radiation Oncology
Beth Israel Deaconess Medical Center
Boston, Massachusetts
Chapter 60, Breast Cancer: Stages I and II

David Rice, MD
Assistant Professor
Division of Thoracic and Cardiovascular Surgery
University of Texas M.D. Anderson Cancer Center
Houston, Texas
Chapter 43, Uncommon Thoracic Malignancies

Mike E. Robbins, PhD
Professor
Department of Radiation Oncology
Head
Section of Radiation Biology
Wake Forest University School of Medicine
Winston-Salem, North Carolina
Overview, Section III, Disease Sites, Part A, Central Nervous System Tumors

Jason K. Rockhill, MD, PhD
Assistant Professor
Department of Radiation Oncology
University of Washington Medical Center
Seattle, Washington
Chapter 19, Neutron Radiotherapy

Claus Rödel, MD
Associate Professor
Attending Physician
Department of Radiation Therapy
University of Erlangen
Erlangen, Germany
Chapter 48, Rectal Cancer

Anthony H. Russell, MD
Associate Professor of Radiation Oncology
Harvard Medical School
Department of Radiation Oncology
Massachusetts General Hospital
Boston, Massachusetts
Chapter 57, Vulvar and Vaginal Carcinoma

Thaddeus V. Samulski, PhD
Assistant Clinical Professor
Department of Radiation Oncology
Duke University Medical Center
Durham, North Carolina
Chapter 20, Hyperthermia

Pamela R. Sandow, DMD
Clinical Associate Professor
Department of Oral and Maxillofacial Surgery and Diagnostic Sciences
University of Florida College of Dentistry
Gainesville, Florida
Chapter 29, Oral Cavity

Carolyn I. Sartor, MD
Associate Professor
Department of Radiation Oncology
University of North Carolina School of Medicine
Chapel Hill, North Carolina
Chapter 5, Biologics and Interactions with Radiation

Steven E. Schild, MD
Professor of Oncology
Mayo Clinic College of Medicine
Vice Chair
Department of Radiation Oncology
Mayo Clinic
Scottsdale, Arizona
Chapter 25, Meningioma, Ependymoma, and Other Adult Brain Tumors; Chapter 40, Small Cell Lung Cancer

Jeanne Schilder, MD
Assistant Professor
Division of Gynecologic Oncology
Indiana University School of Medicine
Indianapolis, Indiana
Chapter 58, Ovarian Cancer

Andreas Schuck, MD, PhD
Department of Radiotherapy
University Hospital of Münster
Münster, Germany
Chapter 66, Pediatric Sarcomas of Bone

Michael Heinrich Seegenschmidt
Klinik für Radioonkologie
Strahlentherapie und Nuklearmedizin
Alfried-Krupp von Bohlen und Halbach
Essen, Germany
Chapter 63, Nonmalignant Diseases

Brenda Shank, MD, PhD, FACR
Medical Director
J.C. Robinson, M.D. Regional Cancer Center
San Pablo, California
Chapter 17, Total Body Irradiation

Julie Sharpless, MD
Clinical Assistant Professor of Medicine
University of North Carolina at Chapel Hill
School of Medicine
Chapel Hill, North Carolina

Chapter 26, Pituitary Tumors

Edward G. Shaw, MD
Professor, Chair
Department of Radiation Oncology
Wake Forest University School of Medicine
Director, Clinical Research Program
Comprehensive Cancer Center of Wake Forest University
Winston-Salem, North Carolina

Overview, Disease Sites, Part A, Central Nervous System Tumors; Chapter 23, Low-Grade Gliomas; Chapter 25, Meningioma, Ependymoma, and Other Adult Brain Tumors; Chapter 27, Spinal Cord Tumors

Arif Sheikh, MD
Assistant Professor
Division of Nuclear Medicine
Department of Radiology
University of North Carolina at Chapel Hill
School of Medicine
Chapel Hill, North Carolina

Chapter 10, Nuclear Medicine

William U. Shipley, MD
Andres Soriano Professor of Radiation Oncology
Harvard Medical School
Department of Radiation Oncology
Massachusetts General Hospital
Boston, Massachusetts

Chapter 51, Bladder Cancer

Benjamin D. Smith, MD
Department of Therapeutic Radiology
Yale University School of Medicine
New Haven, Connecticut
Attending Physician
Wilford Hall Medical Center
Lackland Air Force Base
San Antonio, Texas

Chapter 76, Mycosis Fungoides

Craig W. Stevens, MD, PhD
Associate Professor
Division of Radiation Oncology
University of Texas M.D. Anderson Cancer Center
Houston, Texas

Chapter 43, Uncommon Thoracic Malignancies

Mary Ann Stevenson, MD, PhD
Associate Professor
Harvard Medical School
Chair
Department of Radiation Oncology
Beth Israel Deaconess Medical Center
Boston, Massachusetts

Chapter 2, Molecular and Cellular Biology

Volker W. Stieber, MD
Assistant Professor
Department of Radiation Oncology
Wake Forest University School of Medicine
Winston-Salem, North Carolina

Chapter 27, Spinal Cord Tumors

Ori Shokek, MD
Department of Radiation Oncology and Molecular Radiation Sciences
Johns Hopkins School of Medicine
Baltimore, Maryland

Chapter 72, Rare Pediatric Tumors

Eric A. Strom, MD
Associate Professor
Department of Radiation Oncology
Director
Nellie B. Connally Breast Cancer Center
University of Texas M.D. Anderson Cancer Center
Houston, Texas

Chapter 61, Breast Cancer: Stages III and IV

Jeremy F.G. Sturgeon, MB, FRCPC
Clinical Studies Resource Centre Member
Ontario Cancer Institute
Department of Medical Oncology
Princess Margaret Hospital
Toronto, Ontario Canada

Chapter 52, Testicular Cancer

John H. Suh, MD
Director
Gamma Knife Center
Brain Tumor Institute
Cleveland Clinic Foundation
Cleveland, Ohio

Chapter 16, Stereotactic Irradiation: Linear Accelerator and Gamma Knife

Jeffrey G. Supko, PhD
Division of Hematology/Oncology
Dana-Farber Cancer Institute
Harvard Medical School
Boston, Massachusetts

Chapter 8, Principles of Chemotherapy

Winston W. Tan, MD, FACP
Assistant Professor of Oncology
Mayo Clinic College of Medicine
Consultant, Division of Hematology/Oncology
Jacksonville, Florida

Chapter 53, Kidney and Ureteral Carcinoma

Joel E. Tepper, MD
Hector MacLean Distinguished Professor of Cancer Research
Chairman
Department of Radiation Oncology
UNC Lineberger Comprehensive Cancer Center
University of North Carolina School of Medicine
Chapel Hill, North Carolina

Overview, Disease Sites, Part D, Gastrointestinal Tumors; Chapter 44, Stomach Cancer

Charles Richard Thomas, Jr., MD
Professor, Chair
Department of Radiation Medicine
Professor
Division of Hematology/Oncology
Attending Physician
Oregon Health and Science University Medical Center
Portland, Oregon

Chapter 43, Uncommon Thoracic Malignancies

Gillian M. Thomas
Professor
Department of Radiation Oncology
Department of Obstetrics and Gynecology
University of Toronto Faculty of Medicine
Toronto, Ontario Canada

Overview, Disease Sites, Part F, Gynecologic Tumors

Patrick R.M. Thomas, MD, FACR
Professor
Department of Radiology
Pennsylvania State University School of Medicine
Radiation Oncologist
Penn State Cancer Institute
Milton S. Hershey Medical Center
Hershey, Pennsylvania

Chapter 67, Wilms' Tumor

Wolfgang Tomé, PhD
Associate Professor
Department of Human Oncology
University of Wisconsin School of Medicine
Madison, Wisconsin

Chapter 16, Stereotactic Irradiation: Linear Accelerator and Gamma Knife

Richard W. Tsang, MD, FRCPC
Associate Professor
Department of Radiation Oncology
University of Toronto Faculty of Medicine
Princess Margaret Hospital
Toronto, Ontario Canada

Chapter 74, Non-Hodgkin's Lymphoma

Vincenzo Valentini, MD
Professor
Department of Radiation Therapy
Cattedra di Radioterapia
Dipartimento di Bioimmagine e Scienze Radiologiche
Università Cattolica S. Cuore
Rome, Italy

Chapter 48, Rectal Cancer

Mahesh A. Varia, MD
Professor
Department of Radiation Oncology
Lineberger Comprehensive Cancer Center
University of North Carolina School of Medicine
Chapel Hill, North Carolina

Chapter 26, Pituitary Tumors

Frank A. Vicini, MD
Department of Radiation Oncology
William Beaumont Hospital
Royal Oak, Michigan

Chapter 59, Noninvasive Breast Cancer

Douglas B. Villaret, MD
Assistant Professor
Department of Otolaryngology
University of Florida College of Medicine
Gainesville, Florida

Chapter 36, Unknown Head and Neck Primary Site

Zelijko Vujaskovic, MD, PhD
Associate Clinical Professor
Department of Radiation Oncology
Duke University Medical Center
Durham, North Carolina

Chapter 20, Hyperthermia

Henry Wagner, Jr., MD
Division of Radiation Oncology
Penn State Cancer Institute
Milton S. Hershey Medical Center
Hershey, Pennsylvania

Chapter 41, Non-Small-Cell Lung Cancer

Padraig R. Warde, MB, MRCPI, FRCPC
Professor
Department of Radiation Oncology
University of Toronto Faculty of Medicine
Associate Director
Radiation Medicine Program
Princess Margaret Hospital
Toronto, Ontario Canada

Chapter 52, Testicular Cancer

Randal S. Weber, MD
Professor, Chair
Department of Head and Neck Surgery
University of Texas M.D. Anderson Cancer Center
Houston, Texas

Chapter 38, Cutaneous Carcinoma

Michael J. Wehle, MD
Assistant Professor
Mayo Clinic College of Medicine
Department of Urology
Mayo Clinic
Jacksonville, Florida

Chapter 53, Kidney and Ureteral Carcinoma

Lawrence Weiss, MD
Chair
Department of Pathology
City of Hope National Cancer Center
Duarte, California

Chapter 73, Hodgkin's Disease

Moody D. Wharam, Jr., MD, FACR
Willard and Lillian Hackerman Professor of Radiation Oncology
Professor
Neurological Surgery and Pediatrics
Department of Radiation Oncology and Molecular Radiation Sciences
Johns Hopkins School of Medicine
Baltimore, Maryland

Chapter 72, Rare Pediatric Tumors

Harry Samuel Wieand, MD[†]
Professor of Biostatistics
Graduate School of Public Health
University of Pittsburgh
Director
Biostatistical Center
Pittsburgh, Pennsylvania

Chapter 12, Statistics and Clinical Trials

Christopher G. Willett, MD
Professor, Chair
Department of Radiation Oncology
Duke University Medical Center
Durham, North Carolina

Chapter 15, Intraoperative Irradiation; Chapter 47, Colon Cancer

Lynn D. Wilson, MD, MPH
Associate Professor
Department of Therapeutic Radiology
Department of Dermatology
Yale University School of Medicine
Clinical Director, Vice Chairman
Department of Therapeutic Radiology
Yale University School of Medicine
New Haven, Connecticut

Chapter 76, Mycosis Fungoides

Suzanne Wolden, MD
Associate Member
Department of Radiation Oncology
Memorial Sloan-Kettering Cancer Center
New York, New York

Chapter 69, Neuroblastoma

Jeffrey Y.C. Wong, MD
Professor, Chair
Department of Radiation Oncology
City of Hope Cancer Center
Duarte, California

Chapter 21, Targeted Radionuclide Therapy

William W. Wong, MD
Associate Professor Consultant
Mayo Clinic College of Medicine
Department of Radiation Oncology
Mayo Clinic
Scottsdale, Arizona

Chapter 53, Kidney and Ureteral Carcinoma

Elaine M. Zeman, PhD
Associate Professor
Department of Radiation Oncology
University of North Carolina
School of Medicine
Chapel Hill, North Carolina

Chapter 1, Biologic Basis of Radiation Oncology

Anthony L. Zietman, MD
Professor of Radiation Oncology
Harvard Medical School
Department of Radiation Oncology
Massachusetts General Hospital
Boston, Massachusetts

Overview, Disease Sites, Part E, Genitourinary Tumors; Chapter 51, Bladder Cancer

[†]Deceased

PREFACE

The first edition of *Clinical Radiation Oncology* was very well received by the radiation oncology community for its focus and clear presentation, and it has become the standard radiation oncology textbook for many physicians. For the second edition of *Clinical Radiation Oncology*, the intent is to maintain the many excellent features of the first edition while adding some new features and chapters. The most exciting new feature is that this is a "full-color" textbook with the presence of four colors within each section and chapter. Accordingly, figures pertinent to individual chapters are found within the chapter, instead of in color plates, as in the prior edition and many other textbooks. This feature allows a more complete integration of text, tables, and figures, and a better learning experience for the reader.

The second edition contains separate sections on Scientific Foundations of Radiation Oncology, Techniques and Modalities, and Disease Sites. Within the section on Scientific Foundations of Radiation Oncology, several new chapters are added: Biologics and Interactions with Radiation and Health Services Research in Radiation Oncology. Two imaging chapters, Imaging in Oncology and Nuclear Medicine, are also new. In the Techniques and Modalities section, the chapter in the last edition on Particle Radiation Therapy is split into separate chapters on Charged Particle Radiotherapy and Neutron Radiotherapy with the opportunity for additional perspectives.

The section on Disease Sites now includes some new chapters and authors. In the Central Nervous System Tumors component, a new chapter is added on Meningioma, Ependymoma, and other Adult Brain Tumors. Within the Head and Neck Tumors subsection, there are new chapters on Management of the Neck and Malignant Melanoma. In the Thoracic Neoplasms section, a new chapter is added on Uncommon Thoracic Malignancies, and under Genitourinary Tumors, a chapter on Penile Cancer. A new chapter is also included on Nonmalignant Diseases.

The contributions of Associate Editors for the Disease Sites chapters was an important feature in the success of the first edition and was therefore maintained. Associate Editors are involved in the selection of chapter authors and in editing the chapters for scientific content and accuracy. In addition, for most Disease Sites, the Associate Editors wrote an Overview that allowed them to discuss issues common to various Disease Sites within the section (anatomy, epidemiology/etiology, biology, and so forth) and to give their unique perspective on important issues.

Features that are retained within Disease Sites chapters include an opening page format summarizing some of the most important issues, liberal use of tables and figures, and a closing section that has a treatment algorithm, reflecting the treatment approach of the senior author, along with a discussion of controversies and problems. Chapters are edited not only for scientific accuracy, but also for organization, format, and adequacy of outcome data (disease control, survival, and treatment tolerance). New features include the previously mentioned significant change of four color chapters with self-contained text, figures, and tables and the addition of diagnostic algorithms.

We are again indebted to the many national and international experts who contributed to the second edition of *Clinical Radiation Oncology* as senior authors, co-authors, or Associate Editors. Their outstanding efforts combined with ours will hopefully allow this new edition to be a valuable contribution and resource in the coming years.

Leonard L. Gunderson
Joel E. Tepper

ACKNOWLEDGMENTS

We wish to thank our wives, Katheryn and Laurie, and our secretaries, Carol Heinbockel and Anne Edwards, for their patience and assistance during the many months we were involved in the preparation of the second edition of *Clinical Radiation Oncology*.

And we also thank the Associate Editors and the many contributors for their time, efforts, and outstanding contributions to this edition.

We also wish to acknowledge the editors and production staff at Elsevier, especially Dolores Meloni, Agnes Byrne, Ann Morris, and Mary Anne Folcher, who have done an outstanding job in collating and producing the second edition of *Clinical Radiation Oncology*. Some important features were added as a result of the fruitful collaboration and interaction between ourselves and Dolores Meloni in the planning phase of this second edition.

CONTENTS

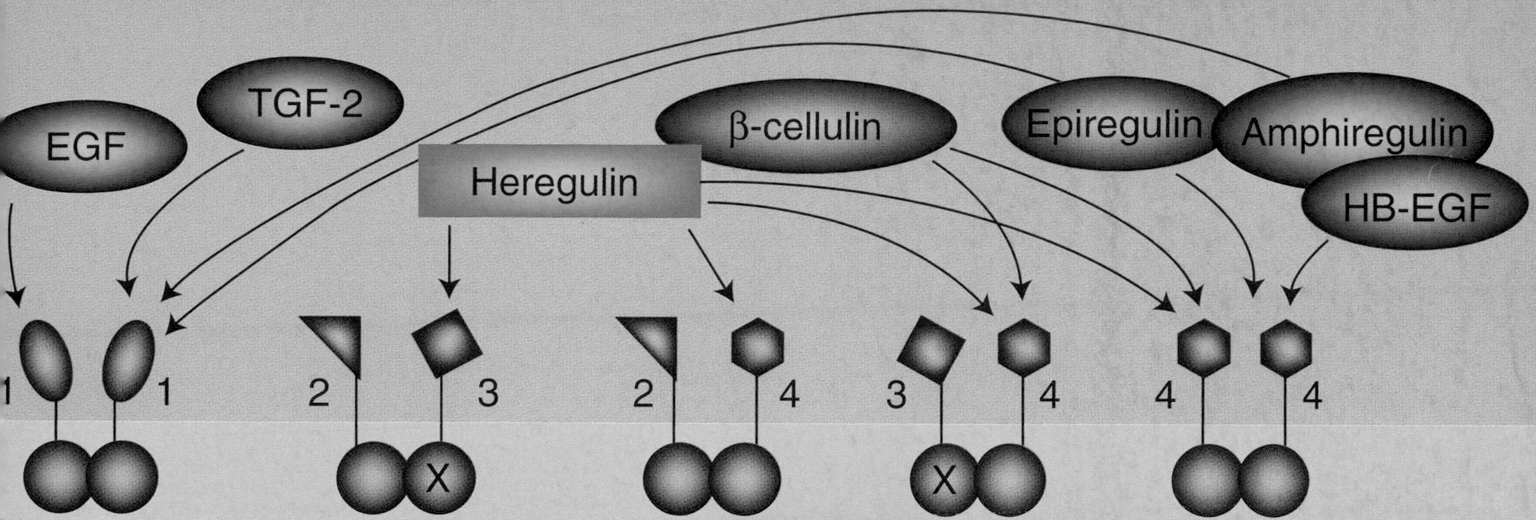

SECTION I

SCIENTIFIC FOUNDATIONS OF RADIATION ONCOLOGY

PART A

RADIOBIOLOGY

CHAPTER 1

BIOLOGIC BASIS OF RADIATION ONCOLOGY

Elaine M. Zeman

WHAT IS RADIATION BIOLOGY?

Radiation biology is the study of the effects of electromagnetic radiation on biologic systems. The effects may include everything from DNA strand breaks to genetic mutations, chromosome aberrations, cell death, disturbed cell proliferation patterns, neoplastic transformation, early and late effects in normal tissues, teratogenesis, cataractogenesis, and carcinogenesis.

Electromagnetic radiation refers to any type of radiant energy in motion with wave or particulate characteristics that has the capacity to impart some or all of its energy to the medium through which it passes. Depending on the type of electromagnetic radiation, the amount of energy deposited can vary by 25 orders of magnitude. For example, 1-kHz radio waves have energies in the range of 10^{-11} to 10^{-12} eV, whereas x-rays or gamma rays (photons) may have energies up to 10 MeV or more. The more energetic forms of electromagnetic radiation, the so-called ionizing radiations, deposit energy as they traverse the medium by setting in motion secondary charged particles that produce further ionizations. Biologic systems may be simple cell-free solutions of biomolecules or increasingly complex, from prokaryotes to single-celled eukaryotes, from DNA to mammalian cells in culture, to tissues and tumors in laboratory rodents (or humans), and to entire ecosystems.

Radiotherapy-oriented radiobiology focuses on the portion of the electromagnetic spectrum energetic enough to cause ionization of atoms. Application of this energy ultimately results in breaking chemical bonds, which can damage important biomolecules. The most significant effect of ionizing radiation in this context is the magnitude of cell kill, which is at the root of most of the normal tissue and tumor responses occurring in patients.

Cytotoxicity is not the only significant biologic effect caused by radiation exposure, although it is the main focus of this chapter. Other important radiation effects, such as carcinogenesis, are mentioned briefly. Carcinogenesis is itself a large discipline involving investigators from fields as diverse as biochemistry, toxicology, epidemiology, environmental sciences, molecular biology, tumor biology, and health and medical physics, as well as radiobiology. Most radiation protection standards are based on minimizing the risks associated with mutagenic and carcinogenic events. Radiologic health professionals therefore are de facto educators of and advocates for the general public when it comes to ionizing radiation, and need to be fully conversant in the potential risks and benefits of medical procedures involving radiation.

Most of this chapter is devoted to classic radiobiology, including studies that largely predate the revolution in molecular biology of the 1980s and 1990s. Although this body of knowledge may be considered primitive by modern standards, relying too heavily on phenomenology, empiricism, and simplistic, descriptive models and theories, the real challenge is to integrate the new biology into the existing framework of classic radiobiology.

RADIOTHERAPY-ORIENTED RADIOBIOLOGY: A CONCEPTUAL FRAMEWORK

Before considering any one aspect of radiobiology in depth, several general concepts should be examined to provide a framework for the information.

Therapeutic Ratio

The most fundamental of these concepts is the *therapeutic ratio,* which provides a risk-benefit approach to planning a radiotherapy regimen. Many of the radiobiologic phenomena discussed in this chapter are thought to play important roles in optimizing or at least fine-tuning the therapeutic ratio. In theory, it should be possible to eradicate all malignant tumors by delivering sufficiently high doses of radiation. In practice, the biologic consequences for normal tissues that are necessarily irradiated along with the tumor limit the total dose that can be safely administered. A balance must be struck between what is deemed an acceptable probability of a radiation-induced complication in a normal tissue and the probability of tumor control. The objective is to achieve the maximum likelihood of tumor control that does not produce unacceptable normal tissue damage.

The concept of therapeutic ratio is best illustrated graphically by directly comparing dose-response curves for tumor control with normal tissue complication rates plotted as a function of dose. Examples of this approach are shown in Figure 1-1 for cases in which the therapeutic ratio is unfavorable, favorable, or optimal, bearing in mind that these are theoretical curves. Actual dose-response curves derived from experimental or clinical data are much more variable, particularly for tumors, which tend to show much shallower dose-response relationships.[1] This underscores how difficult it can

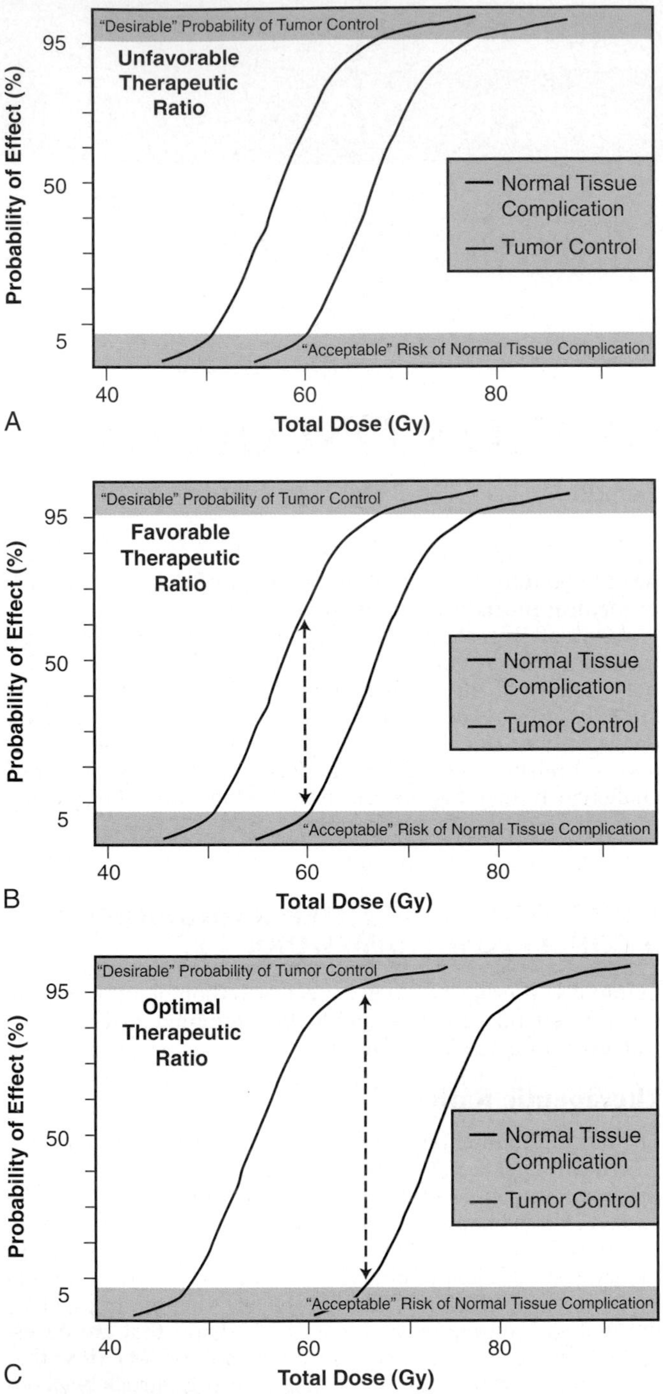

Figure 1-1 The graphs illustrate the concept of therapeutic ratio under conditions in which the relationship between the normal tissue tolerance and tumor control dose-response curves is unfavorable (**A**), favorable (**B**), and optimal (**C**).

be in practice to assign a single numeric value to the therapeutic ratio in any given situation.

Many of the radiobiologic properties of cells (and therefore tissues) can have a favorable or adverse effect on the therapeutic ratio. In planning a course of radiotherapy, the goal should be to optimize the therapeutic ratio as much as possible; using our graphical approach, this means increasing the separation between the tumor control and normal tissue complication curves. This can be accomplished by shifting the tumor control curve to the left with respect to the dose axis (toward lower doses or tumor radiosensitization), by shifting the normal tissue complication curve to the right (toward higher doses or normal tissue radioprotection), or by some combination of both approaches. The key is to shift these curves *differentially*, which is not an easy task because there are few exploitable differences in the radiobiology of cells derived from tumors and those derived from normal tissues.

Radiation Biology Continuum

There is a surprising continuity between the physical events that occur in the first picosecond (or less) after ionizing radiation interacts with biologic material and the ultimate consequences of that interaction on tissues. The consequences themselves may not become apparent until days, weeks, months, or years after the radiation exposure. Some of the important steps in this radiobiology continuum are listed in Table 1-1. The orderly progression from one stage of the continuum to the next—from physical to physicochemical to biochemical to biologic—is particularly noteworthy because of the vastly different time scales over which the critical events occur and because of the increasing biologic complexity associated with each of the end points or outcomes. Each stage of the continuum also offers a unique radiobiologic window of opportunity to intervene in the process and thereby modify all the events and outcomes that follow.

Levels of Complexity in Radiobiologic Systems

Other important considerations in all radiobiologic studies are the nature of the experimental system used to study a particular phenomenon, the assays used, and the end points assessed. For example, an investigator may be interested in studying DNA damage caused by ionizing radiation, particularly the frequency of DNA double-strand breaks (DSBs) produced per unit dose. As an experimental system, DNA extracted from mammalian cells may be chosen. Using a DNA elution assay, the rate at which the irradiated DNA passes through a semipermeable membrane is measured as an end point and compared with the rate of elution of DNA extracted from cells that had not been irradiated. DNA containing more DSBs elutes faster than DNA containing fewer breaks, allowing a calibration curve to be generated that relates the radiation dose received to the elution rate. Another investigator may be interested in improving the control rate of head and neck cancers with radiotherapy by employing a nonstandard fractionation schedule. In this case, the type of experiment is a clinical trial, and the experimental system is a cohort of patients, some of whom are randomized to receive nonstandard fractionation while the rest receive standard fractionation. The end points assessed may include locoregional control, long-term survival, disease-free survival, and normal tissue complication frequency, which are evaluated at specific times after completion of the radiotherapy.

In considering the strengths and weaknesses of these two investigators' studies, any number of questions may be asked. Which is the more complex or heterogeneous system? Which is the more easily manipulated and controlled system? Which is more relevant for the daily practice of radiotherapy? What kinds of results are gleaned from each, and can these results be obtained in a timely manner? In this example, human patients with spontaneously arising tumors represent a far more heterogeneous and complex experimental system than an extract of mammalian DNA. However, the DNA system is much more easily manipulated, possible confounding factors can be more easily controlled, and the measurement of the desired end point (i.e., elution rate) plus the data analysis can

Table 1-1 Stages in the Radiobiology Continuum

Time Scale of Events (Stage)	Initial Event	Final Event	Response Modifiers and Possible Interventions
10^{-16} to 10^{-12} second (physical)	Ionization of atoms	Free radicals formed in biomolecules	Type of ionizing radiation, shielding
10^{-12} to 10^{-2} second (physicochemical)	Free radicals formed in biomolecules	DNA damage	Presence or absence of free radical scavengers, molecular oxygen and/or oxygen-mimetic radiosensitizers
1.0 second to several hours (biochemical)	DNA damage	Unrepaired or mis-rejoined DNA damage	Presence or absence of functioning DNA repair systems, repair-inhibiting drugs, altering the time required to complete repair processes
Hours to years (biologic)	Unrepaired or mis-rejoined DNA damage	Clonogenic cell death, apoptosis, mutagenesis, transformation, carcinogenesis, early and late effects in normal tissues, whole-body radiation syndromes, tumor control	Cell-cell interactions, biologic response modifiers, adaptive mechanisms, structural and functional organization of tissues, cell kinetics

be completed within 1 or 2 days. This is not the case with the human studies because numerous confounding factors influence results, manipulation of the system can be difficult or impossible, and the experimental results typically take years to obtain.

The issue of relevance is an even thornier one. Arguably, both studies are relevant to the practice of radiotherapy insofar as the killing of cells is at the root of all normal tissue and tumor toxicity caused by radiation exposure, and the cell kill is a direct or indirect consequence of irreparable damage to DNA. Any laboratory findings that contribute to the knowledge base of radiation-induced DNA damage are relevant. However, clinical trials with human patients are a more familiar experimental system for clinicians, and efficacy in cancer patients is ultimately the gold standard against which all new therapeutic strategies are judged.

There is a time and place for relatively simple systems and for more complex ones. The relatively simple, homogeneous, and easily manipulated systems are best suited for the study of the mechanisms of radiation action, such as measuring DNA or chromosomal damage, changes in gene expression, perturbations of the cell cycle, or the clonogenic survival of cells maintained in tissue culture. The more complicated and heterogeneous systems, with their unique end points, are more clinically relevant, such as assays of tumor control or normal tissue complication rates. Both types of assay systems have inherent strengths and weaknesses, and both are critically important if we hope to improve the practice of radiotherapy based on sound biologic principles.

Tissue Heterogeneity

Why is radiotherapy successful in controlling one patient's tumor but not that of another, even when the two tumors seem identical? Why are we generally more successful at controlling certain types of cancers than others? The short answer to such questions is that although the tumors may appear identical macroscopically, their component cells may be quite different phenotypically or genotypically. There also may be important differences between the two patients' normal tissues.

Normal tissues are composed of more than one type of cell and are somewhat heterogeneous. Because of the genetic instability of individual tumor cells and microenvironmental differences, tumors are very heterogeneous. Different subpopulations of cells have been isolated from many types of human and experimental cancers, and these may differ in antigenicity, metastatic potential, and sensitivity to radiotherapeutic and chemotherapeutic agents.[1,2] This heterogeneity manifests within a particular patient and, to a much greater extent, between patients with otherwise similar tumors. Both intrinsic and extrinsic factors contribute to this heterogeneity. Intrinsic factors may include inherent radiosensitivity, gene expression, biochemical repair processes, modes of cell death (e.g., clonogenic, apoptotic), genetic instability, cell cycle kinetics, and structural and functional arrangement of the tissue. Extrinsic factors tend to be related to physiologic or epigenetic differences between tissues, such as the degree of vascularity, availability of oxygen and nutrients, pH, energy charge, and the proximity of and degree of contact between normal host tissue and the tumor.

What are the practical implications of normal tissue and tumor heterogeneity? First, if normal tissues are assumed to be the more uniform and predictable in behavior of the two, tumor heterogeneity is directly or indirectly responsible for most radiotherapy failures. If so, this suggests that a valid clinical strategy may be to identify the radioresistant subpopulations of tumor cells and tailor therapy specifically to cope with them. This approach is much easier said than done. Some prospective clinical studies include one or more pretreatment determinations of, for example, extent of tumor hypoxia[3-5] or potential doubling time of tumor clonogens[6] as criteria for assigning patients to different treatment groups.

Another consequence of tissue heterogeneity is that any radiobiologic end point measured in an intact tissue is necessarily related to the radiosensitivities of all the subsets of cells plus all the other intrinsic and extrinsic factors contributing to the overall response of the tissue. Because data on normal tissue tolerances and tumor control probabilities are also averaged among a number of patients, heterogeneity is even more pronounced.

Powers of Ten

Tumor control is achieved only when all clonogenic cells are killed or otherwise rendered unable to sustain tumor growth indefinitely. To estimate the likelihood of cure, it is necessary to know or at least to have an appreciation for approximately how many clonogenic cells the tumor contains, how radiosensitive these cells are (i.e., some measure of killing efficiency per unit radiation dose), and what the relationship is between the number of clonogenic cells remaining after treatment and the probability of recurrence. The latter estimate is perhaps the easiest to ascertain because of our knowledge of the random and discrete nature of radiation damage and the general shape of dose-response curves for mammalian cells and tissues (i.e., approximately exponential for multifraction irradiation). For a given number of surviving cells per tumor, the probability of local control can be derived from Poisson statistics using the equation:

$$P = e^{-n}$$

in which P is the tumor control probability and n is the average number of surviving clonogenic tumor cells. For a large number of tumors, if about two clonogenic cells per tumor remain at the end of radiotherapy, the tumor control rate will be about 10%; 9 of 10 tumors of the same size and relative radiosensitivity will recur. If the treatment reduces clonogenic cell numbers to an average of 0.1 per tumor, the tumor control probability will increase to 90%; for 0.05 per tumor, it will be 95%; and for 0.01 per tumor, it will be 99%.

The tumor control probability for a given fraction of surviving cells is not particularly helpful if the total number of cells at risk is unknown, and this is where an understanding of logarithmic relationships and exponential cell kill is useful. Based on the resolution of existing tools and technology for cancer detection, let us assume that a 1-cm^3 (1-g) tumor mass can be identified reliably. A tumor of this size has been estimated to contain approximately 10^9 cells,[7] a theoretical value that assumes all cells are perfectly arranged and of uniform size and that the tumor contains no stroma. An assumption that all such cells are clonogenic (rarely the case) suggests that at least 9 logs of cell kill would be necessary before any appreciable tumor control (about 37%) would be achieved and that 10 logs of cell kill would be required for a high degree of tumor control (90%).

After the first 1 or 2 logs of cell kill, some tumors respond by shrinking (i.e., partial response). After 2 to 3 logs of cell kill, the tumor may shrink to a size below the current limits of clinical detection (i.e., complete response). Although partial and complete responses are valid clinical end points, a complete response does not necessarily mean cure of disease. At least 6 more logs of cell kill are required before any significant probability of cure would be expected. This explains why radiotherapy is not halted if the tumor disappears during the course of treatment, a concept that is illustrated in Figure 1-2.

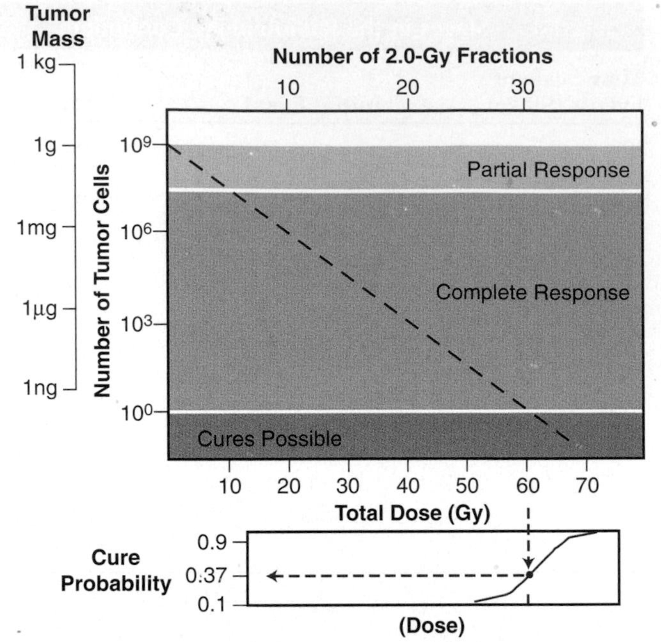

Figure 1-2 The relationship between radiation dose and tumor cell survival during fractionated radiotherapy of a hypothetical, 1-g tumor containing 10^9 clonogenic cells. Although a modest decrease in cell surviving fraction can cause the tumor to shrink (i.e., partial response) or disappear below the limits of clinical detection (i.e., complete response), few cures would be expected until at least 9 logs of clonogenic cells have been killed. In this example, a total dose of at least 60 Gy delivered as daily, 2-Gy fractions is required to produce a tumor control probability of 0.37, assuming each dose reduced the surviving fraction to 0.5. (Adapted from Steel G, Adams G, Peckham M (eds): The Biological Basis of Radiotherapy. New York, Elsevier, 1983.)

Although the goal of curative radiotherapy is to reduce tumor cell survival by at least 9 logs, even for the smallest tumor likely to be encountered, it is much less clear how many logs of cell kill a particular normal tissue can tolerate before it loses its structural or functional integrity. This depends on how the tissue is organized structurally, functionally, and proliferatively; which constituent cells are the most and least radiosensitive; and which cells are the most important to the integrity of the tissue. It is unlikely, however, that many normal tissues could tolerate a depletion of 2 logs (99%) of their cells, let alone 9 or more logs.

RADIATION BIOLOGY AND THERAPY: THE FIRST 50 YEARS

In less than 4 years after the discovery of x-rays by Roentgen,[8] radioactivity by Becquerel,[9] and radium by the Curies,[10] the new modality of cancer treatment known as *radiation therapy* claimed its first apparent cure of skin cancer.[11,12] More than a century later, radiotherapy is most commonly given as a series of daily, small-dose fractions of approximately 1.8 to 2.0 Gy each, given 5 days per week over a period of 5 to 7 weeks to a total dose of 50 to 70 Gy. Although it is true that the historical development of this conventional radiotherapy schedule was empirically based, a number of early radiobiologic experiments also suggested this approach.

In the earliest days of radiotherapy, x-rays and radium were used for cancer treatment. Because of the greater availability and convenience of using x-ray tubes and the higher intensities of radiation output achievable, it was fairly easy to deliver large single doses in short overall treatment times. From about 1900 into the 1920s, this so-called *massive dose technique*[13] was a common way of administering radiotherapy. Unfortunately, normal tissue complications were quite severe. To make matters worse, the rate of local tumor recurrence was still unacceptably high.

Radium therapy was used more extensively in France than in other countries. Because of the low activities available, radium applications involved longer overall treatment times to reach comparable total doses. Although extended treatments were less convenient, clinical results were often superior. Perceiving that the change in overall time was the critical factor, physicians began to experiment with the use of multiple, smaller x-ray doses delivered over extended periods. At that time, there was already a radiobiologic precedent for expecting improvement in tumor control when radiation treatments were protracted.

As early as 1906, Bergonié and Tribondeau observed histologically that the immature, dividing cells of the rat testis showed evidence of damage at lower radiation doses than the mature, nondividing cells.[14] Based on these observations, they concluded that x-rays were more effective on cells that were actively dividing, likely to continue dividing indefinitely, and undifferentiated.[14] Because tumors were known to contain cells that were less differentiated and exhibited greater mitotic activity, they reasoned that several radiation exposures might preferentially kill these tumor cells but not their slowly proliferating, differentiated counterparts in the surrounding normal tissues.

Common use of the single-dose technique in favor of fractionated treatment ended during the 1920s as a consequence of the pioneering experiments of Claude Regaud and colleagues.[15] The testis of the rabbit was used as a model tumor system because the rapid and unlimited proliferation of spermatogenic cells simulated to some extent the pattern of cell proliferation in malignant tumors. Regaud and coworkers showed that only through the use of multiple radiation exposures could animals be completely sterilized without producing severe injury to the scrotum.[15-17] Regaud and Ferroux suggested that the superior results afforded the multifraction irradiation scheme were related to alternating periods of relative radioresistance and sensitivity in the rapidly proliferating germ cells.[18] These principles were soon tested in the clinic by Henri Coutard, who first used fractionated radiotherapy for the treatment of head and neck cancers, with spectacularly improved results.[19,20] Largely as a result of these and related experiments, fractionated treatment became the standard form of radiotherapy.

Time-dose equivalents for skin erythema published by Reisner,[21] Quimby and MacComb,[22,23] and others[24-26] formed the basis for the calculation of equivalents for other tissue and tumor responses. By plotting the total doses required for each of these equivalents for a given level of effect in a particular tissue as a function of a treatment parameter such as overall treatment time, number of fractions, or dose per fraction, an isoeffect curve can be derived. All time-dose combinations that fell along such a curve theoretically would produce tissue responses of equal magnitude. Isoeffect curves, relating the total dose to the overall treatment time, derived in later years from some of these data[27] are shown in Figure 1-3.

The first published isoeffect curves were produced by Strandqvist in 1944[28] (see Fig. 1-3). When transformed on log-log coordinates, isoeffect curves for a variety of skin reactions and for the cure of skin cancer were drawn as parallel lines that had common slopes of 0.33.[28] These results implied that there would be no therapeutic advantage to using prolonged treatment times (i.e., multiple small fractions versus one or a few large doses) for the preferential eradication of tumors while simultaneously sparing normal tissues.[13] It was somewhat ironic that the Strandqvist curves were so popular in the years that followed, because it was already known that the therapeutic ratio did increase (to a point) with prolonged overall treatment times. However, these isoeffect curves were quite reliable at predicting skin reactions, which were the dose-limiting factors at that time.

GOLDEN AGE OF RADIATION BIOLOGY AND THERAPY: THE SECOND 50 YEARS

The golden age of radiation biology was ushered in by the publication of the first survival curve for mammalian cells exposed to graded doses of ionizing radiation.[29] This first report of a quantitative measure of intrinsic radiosensitivity of a human cell line (i.e., HeLa, derived from a cervical carcinoma[30]) was published by Puck and Marcus in 1956.[29] To put this seminal work in proper perspective, it is first necessary to review the physicochemical basis for why ionizing radiation is toxic to biologic materials.

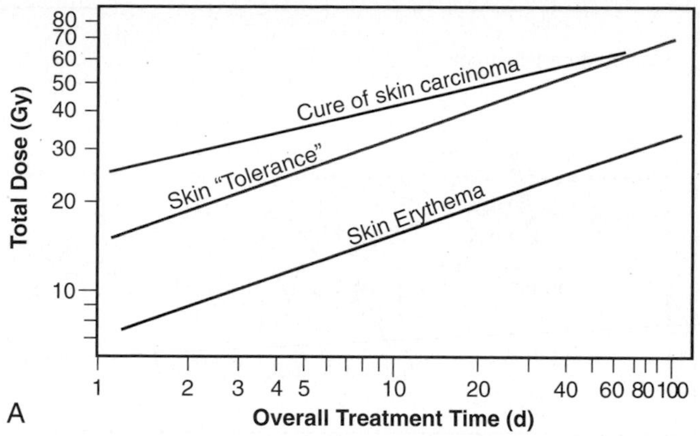

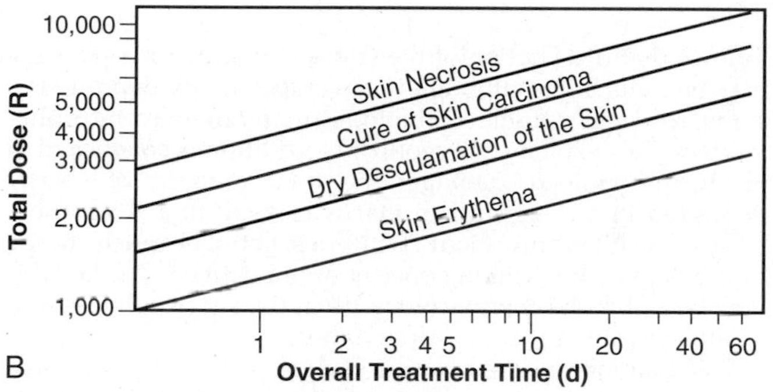

Figure 1-3 Isoeffect curves relating the log of the total dose to the log of the overall treatment time for various levels of skin reaction and the cure of skin cancer. **A,** Isoeffect curves were constructed by Cohen on the basis of a survey of earlier published data on radiotherapy equivalents.[21-26] The slope of the curves for skin complications was 0.33, and the slope for tumor control was 0.22. **B,** The Strandqvist[28] isoeffect curves were first published in 1944. All lines were drawn parallel and had a common slope of 0.33. (**A,** Adapted from Cohen L: Radiation response and recovery: Radiobiological principles and their relation to clinical practice. *In* Schwartz E (ed): The Biological Basis of Radiation Therapy. Philadelphia, JB Lippincott, 1966, p 208; **B,** adapted from Strandqvist M: Studien uber die kumulative Wirkung der Roentgenstrahlen bei Fraktionierung. Acta Radiol Suppl 55:1, 1944.)

Interaction of Ionizing Radiation with Biologic Materials

Ionizing radiation deposits energy as it traverses the absorbing medium through which it passes. The most important feature of the interaction of ionizing radiation with biologic materials is the random and discrete nature of the energy deposition. Energy is deposited in increasingly energetic packets referred to as *spurs* (≤100 eV deposited), *blobs* (100 to 500 eV), or *short tracks* (500 to 5000 eV), each of which can leave approximately three to several dozen ionized atoms in its wake. This is illustrated in Figure 1-4, along with a segment of a double-helical DNA strand shown to scale. The frequency distribution and density of the different types of energy-deposition events along the track of the incident photon or particle are measures of the radiation's linear energy transfer (LET). Because these energy-deposition events are discrete, it

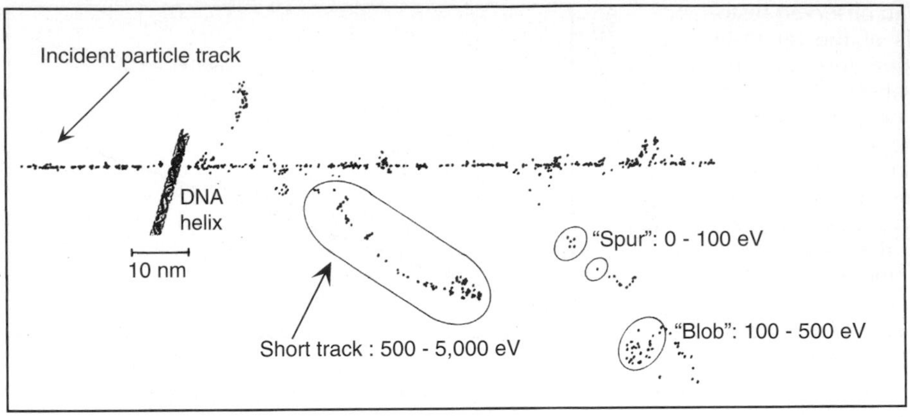

Figure 1-4 Hypothetical alpha particle track through an absorbing medium, illustrating the random and discrete energy-deposition events along the track. Each event can be classified according to the amount of energy deposited locally, which determines how many ionized atoms will be produced. A segment of a DNA double helix is shown approximately to scale. (Adapted from Goodhead D: Physics of radiation action: Microscopic features that determine biological consequences. *In* Hagen U, Harder D, Jung H, et al (eds): Radiation Research 1895-1995, Proceedings of the 10th International Congress of Radiation Research, vol 2. Congress Lectures. Wurzburg, Universitatsdruckerei H Sturtz, 1995, p 43.)

follows that distribution of the energy on a microscopic scale may be quite large, although the average energy deposited in a macroscopic volume of biologic material may be rather modest. This explains why ionizing radiation is so efficient at producing biologic damage; the total amount of energy deposited in a 70-kg human that will result in a 50% probability of death is only about 70 calories, about as much energy as is absorbed by drinking one sip of hot coffee.[31] The key difference is that the energy contained in the sip of coffee is uniformly distributed, not random and discrete.

The biomolecules receiving a direct hit from a spur or blob get a relatively huge radiation dose because of the large deposition of energy in a very small volume. For photons and charged particles, this energy deposition results in the ejection of orbital electrons, causing the target molecule to be converted first into an ion pair and then into a free radical. The ejected electrons, which are themselves energetic charged particles, can produce additional ionizations. For uncharged particles such as neutrons, the interaction is between the incident particles and the nuclei of the atoms in the absorbing medium, causing the ejection of recoil protons (charged) and lower-energy neutrons. The cycle of ionization, free radical production, and release of secondary charged particles continues until all the energy of the incident photon or particle is expended. These interactions are complete within a picosecond after the initial energy transfer. After that time, the chemical reactions of the resulting free radicals predominate the radiation response.

Any and all cellular molecules are potential targets for the localized energy-deposition events that occur in spurs, blobs, or short tracks. Whether the ionization of a particular biomolecule results in a measurable biologic effect depends on a number of factors, including how probable a target the molecule represents from the point of view of the ionizing particle, how important the molecule is to the continued health of the cell, how many copies of the molecule are normally present in the cell and to what extent the cell can react to the loss of working copies, and how important the cell is to the structure or function of its corresponding tissue or organ. DNA, for example, is an important cellular macromolecule, one that is present only as a single, double-stranded copy. Other molecules in the cell may be less crucial to survival but are much more abundant than DNA and therefore have a much higher probability of being hit and ionized. The most abundant molecule in the cell is water, constituting 80% to 90% of the cell by weight. The highly reactive free radicals formed by the radiolysis of water are capable of adding to the DNA damage resulting from direct energy absorption by migrating to the DNA and damaging it indirectly. This mechanism is referred to as *indirect radiation action* to distinguish it from *direct radiation action*.[32] The direct and indirect action pathways for ionizing radiation are delineated:

Direct effect:

$$\text{DNA} \xrightarrow[\text{(irradiate)}]{} \underset{\text{(ion pair)}}{[\text{DNA}^+ + e^-]} \longrightarrow \underset{\text{(DNA free radical)}}{\text{DNA}\bullet}$$

Indirect effect:

$$\underset{\text{(irradiate)}}{H_2O} \longrightarrow \underset{\text{(ion pair)}}{[H_2O^+ + e^-]} \longrightarrow \underset{\text{(other radical reactions)}}{\bullet OH} + \text{DNA} \longrightarrow \underset{\text{(DNA free radical and water)}}{\text{DNA}\bullet + H_2O}$$

The most highly reactive and damaging species produced by the radiolysis of water is the hydroxyl radical (•OH), although other free radical species are also produced in various yields.[33,34] Ultimately, it has been determined that cell killing by indirect action constitutes about 70% of the total damage produced in DNA for low-LET radiation.

How do the free radicals produced by the direct and indirect action of ionizing radiation cause the myriad lesions that have been identified in irradiated DNA? Because they contain unpaired electrons, free radicals are highly reactive chemically, and they undergo any number of reactions in an attempt to acquire new electrons or rid themselves of remaining unpaired ones. These reactions are considered quite slow compared with the time scale of the initial ionization events, but they are quite fast relative to normal enzymatic processes in a typical mammalian cell. For all intents and purposes, free radical reactions are complete in less than a second after irradiation. The •OH radical is capable of abstraction of hydrogen atoms from other molecules and addition across carbon-carbon or other double bonds. More complex macromolecules that have been converted to free radicals can undergo a series of transmutations in an attempt to rid themselves of unpaired electrons, many of which result in the breakage of nearby chemical bonds. In the case of DNA, these broken bonds may result in the loss of a base or an entire nucleotide or a frank scission of the sugar phosphate backbone involving one or both DNA strands. In some cases, chemical bonds are first broken and then rearranged, exchanged, or rejoined in inappropriate ways. Bases in DNA may be modified by the addition of one or more hydroxyl groups (e.g., the base thymine converted to thymine glycol), pyrimidines may become dimerized, and the DNA may become cross-linked to itself or to associated protein components. Because the initial energy-deposition events are discrete, the free radicals produced are clustered and therefore undergo their multiple chemical reactions and produce multiple damages in a highly localized area. This has been called the *multiply damaged site*[35] or *cluster*[36] *hypothesis*. Examples of the types of damage found in irradiated DNA are shown in Figure 1-5.

Biochemical Repair of DNA Damage

DNA is unique insofar as it is the only cellular macromolecule with its own repair system. Until recently, little was known about DNA repair processes in mammalian cells, particularly because of the complexities involved and the relative lack of spontaneously occurring mutants defective in genes involved with DNA repair. As a consequence, most studies of DNA repair were carried out in bacteria or yeasts and usually employed ultraviolet (UV) radiation as the tool for producing DNA damage. Although these were rather simple and relatively clear-cut systems in which to study DNA repair, their relevance to mammalian repair systems and to the broader spectrum of DNA damage produced by ionizing radiation ultimately limited their usefulness.

The study of DNA repair in mammalian cells received a significant boost during the late 1960s with publications by Cleaver[37,38] that identified the molecular defect responsible for the human disease xeroderma pigmentosum (XP). Patients with XP are exquisitely sensitive to sunlight and highly prone to cancer, particularly skin cancers. Cleaver showed that cells derived from such patients were likewise sensitive to UV radiation and defective in the nucleotide excision repair pathway. However, these cells were not especially sensitive to ionizing radiation. Several years later, Taylor and colleagues[39] reported that cells derived from patients with a second cancer-prone disorder called ataxia telangiectasia (AT) were extremely sensitive to ionizing radiation and radiation-mimetic drugs, but not UV. In the years that followed, cell cultures derived from patients with these two conditions were used to help elucidate the complicated processes of DNA repair in mammalian cells.

Many rodent and human genes involved in DNA repair have been cloned.[40] Almost 20 distinct gene products participate in excision repair of base damage,[41,42] and even more are involved in the repair of strand breaks.[43] Many of these proteins function as component parts of larger repair complexes; some of these parts are interchangeable and participate in other DNA repair and replication pathways. Some are not involved directly with the repair process but instead link DNA repair to other cellular functions, including transcription, cell cycle arrest, and apoptosis; these cases demonstrate that the maintenance of genomic integrity results from a complex interplay between the repair proteins themselves and others that serve as damage sensors, signaling intermediates, and regulators. For example, the defect responsible for the disease AT is not in a gene that codes for a repair protein, but rather in a gene that participates in a related pathway that normally prevents cells from entering S phase of the cell cycle and beginning DNA synthesis while residual DNA damage is present. This has been called the *G_1/S checkpoint response*.[44] Because of this genetic defect, AT cells do not experience the normal G_1 arrest after irradiation, and they enter S phase with residual DNA damage. This accounts for the exquisite radiosensitivity of AT cells and the resulting genomic instability that can lead to carcinogenesis. What is known about the various types of DNA repair in mammalian cells is outlined in the following sections.

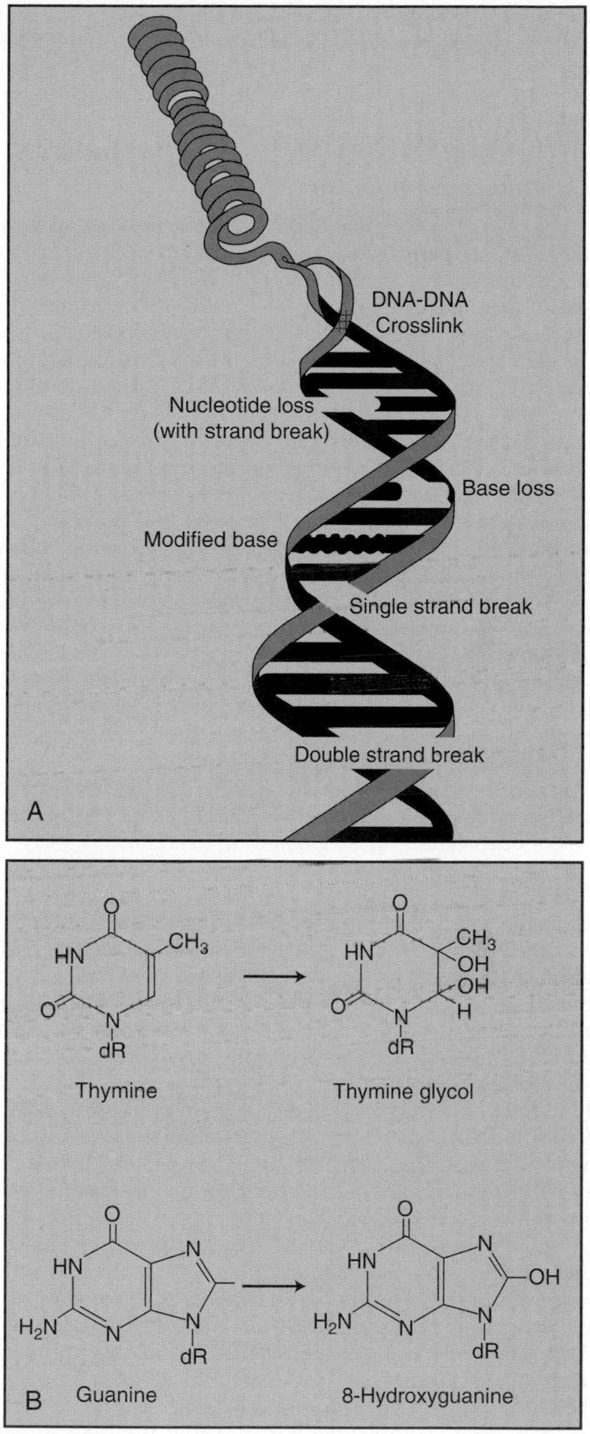

Figure 1-5 Types of DNA damage produced by ionizing radiation. **A,** Segment of irradiated DNA containing single- and double-strand breaks, cross-links, and base damage. **B,** Two types of modified bases observed in irradiated DNA include thymine glycol, which results from the addition of two hydroxyl (OH) groups across the carbon-carbon double bond of thymine, and 8-hydroxyguanine, produced by •OH radical addition to guanine.

Base Excision Repair

The repair of base damage is initiated by DNA repair enzymes called *DNA glycosylases,* which recognize specific types of damaged bases and excise them without otherwise disturbing the DNA strand.[45] The action of the glycosylase itself results in the formation of another type of damage observed in irradiated DNA: an apurinic or apyrimidinic (AP) site. The AP site is then recognized by another repair enzyme, an AP endonuclease, which nicks the DNA adjacent to the lesion. The resulting strand break becomes the substrate for an exonuclease, which removes the abasic site, along with a few additional bases. The small gap that results is patched by DNA polymerase, which uses the opposite, hopefully undamaged, DNA strand as a template. DNA ligase seals the patch in place.

Nucleotide Excision Repair

The DNA glycosylases that begin the process of base excision repair do not recognize all known forms of base damage, particularly bulky or complex lesions.[45] In such cases, another group of enzymes, called *structure-specific endonucleases*, initiate the excision repair process. These repair proteins do not recognize the specific lesion but instead recognize more generalized structural distortions in DNA that necessarily accompany a complex base lesion. The structure-specific endonucleases incise the affected DNA strand on both sides of the lesion, releasing an oligonucleotide fragment made up of the damaged site and several bases on either side of it. Because a longer segment of DNA, including bases and the sugar phosphate backbone, is generated, this type of excision repair is referred to as *nucleotide excision repair* to distinguish it from base excision repair (described earlier), in which the initial step in the repair process is removal of the damaged base only. After this step, the remainder of the nucleotide excision repair process is similar to that of base excision repair; the gap is then filled in by DNA polymerase and sealed by DNA ligase. Overall, nucleotide excision repair is a much slower process, with a half-time of approximately 12 hours.

For both types of excision repair, active genes in the process of transcription are repaired preferentially and more quickly. This has been called *transcription-coupled repair*.[46]

Strand Break Repair

Despite the fact that unrepaired or mis-rejoined strand breaks, particularly double-strand breaks, often have the most catastrophic consequences for the cell in terms of loss of reproductive integrity,[47] how mammalian cells repair strand breaks has been more difficult to elucidate than how they repair base damage. Much of what was originally discovered about these repair processes is derived from studies of x-ray–sensitive rodent cells and microorganisms that were found to harbor specific defects in strand break repair; since then, other human genetic diseases characterized by DNA repair defects have been identified and are used to help probe these fundamental processes.

A genetic technique known as *complementation analysis* allows further characterization of genes involved in DNA repair. Complementation analysis involves the fusion of different strains of cells possessing the same phenotypic defect and subsequently testing the hybrid cell for the presence or absence of this phenotype. If two cell types bearing the defect yield a phenotypically normal hybrid cell, it implies that the defect has been "complemented" and that the defective phenotype must result from mutations in at least two different genes. With respect to DNA strand break repair, eight different genetic complementation groups have been identified in rodent cell mutants. For example, a mutant Chinese hamster cell line designated EM9 appears to be especially radiosensitive because of delayed repair of DNA single-stranded breaks, a process that is normally complete within minutes of irradiation.[48]

With respect to the repair of DNA DSBs, the situation is more complicated because the damage on each strand of DNA may be different, and no intact template would be available to guide the repair process. Under these circumstances, cells depend on genetic recombination (i.e., nonhomologous end joining or homologous recombination[49-52]) to cope with the damage.

Nonhomologous end joining (NHEJ) is a repair mechanism that directly ligates broken ends of DNA DSBs using a heterodimeric enzyme complex consisting of the proteins KU70 (formerly designated XRCC6) and KU80 (formerly XRCC5), the catalytic subunit of DNA protein kinase (DNA-PK_{CS}), and XRCC4/ligase IV. Because no intact complementary strand is available as a template, this process is error prone and generally results in minor deletions in the DNA sequence. NHEJ predominates during the G_1 phase of the cell cycle. Homologous recombination involves digestion and "cleaning up" of the broken DNA ends followed by assembly of a nucleoprotein filament that contains, among others, the proteins RAD51 and RAD52. This filament then invades the homologous DNA sequence of a sister chromatid, which becomes the template for essentially error-free repair of the broken ends by DNA synthesis. Homologous recombination is active during S and G_2 phases of the cell cycle (i.e., after DNA replication) when an identical copy of the DNA strand—the sister chromatid—is available.

The products of the *BRCA1* and *BRCA2* genes are also implicated in homologous recombination (and possibly NHEJ) because they interact with the RAD51 protein. Defects in these genes are associated with hereditary breast and ovarian cancer.[53]

Mismatch Repair

The primary role of mismatch repair is to eliminate from newly synthesized DNA errors such as base-base mismatches and insertion-deletion loops caused by DNA polymerase.[54-56] Descriptively, this process consists of three steps: mismatch recognition and assembly of the repair complex, degradation of the error-containing strand, and repair synthesis. In humans, mismatch repair involves at least five proteins, including hMSH2, hMSH3, hMSH6, hMLH1, and hPMS2, as well as other members of the DNA repair and replication machinery.

One manifestation of a defect in mismatch repair is microsatellite instability, mutations observed in DNA segments containing repeated sequence motifs.[57] Collectively, this causes the cell to assume a hypermutable state (i.e., mutator phenotype) that has been associated with certain cancer predisposition syndromes, particularly hereditary nonpolyposis colon cancer (HNPCC).[58]

Cytogenetic Effects of Ionizing Radiation

When cells divide after radiation exposure, chromosomes frequently contain visible structural aberrations, most of which are lethal to the cell. In some cases, these aberrations physically interfere with the processes of mitosis and cytokinesis, and they result in prompt cell death. In other cases, cell division can occur, but the loss or uneven distribution of genetic material between the cell's progeny is ultimately lethal, although the affected cells may linger for several days before they die, and some may even be able to go through a few more cell divisions in the interim. These aberrations are the result of unrepaired or mis-rejoined DNA damage that persists from the time of irradiation until the time of the next cell division. It is not known how an unrepaired DSB in essentially naked DNA is transformed into such a large lesion (e.g., a broken arm of a chromosome) given that the chromosome has undergone many levels of modification, folding, and packaging; association with chromatin and other proteins; and condensation in preparation for mitosis.

Most chromosomal aberrations result from an interaction between two (or more) damaged sites and can be grouped into three different types of exchange categories. A fourth category is reserved for chromosomal aberrations that are thought to result from a single site of damage.[59] These categories are described as follows, and representative types of aberrations from each category are shown in Figure 1-6:

Intra-arm exchanges: an interaction between lesions on the same arm of a single chromosome (e.g., interstitial deletion)

Interarm exchanges: an interaction between lesions on opposite arms of the same chromosome (e.g., centric ring)

Interchanges: an interaction between lesions on different chromosomes that are homologous or nonhomologous (e.g., dicentric)

Single-hit breaks: complete severance of part of one arm of a single chromosome not obviously associated with any more than a single lesion (e.g., terminal deletion)

These four categories can be further subdivided according to whether the initial radiation damage occurred before or after the DNA is replicated during S phase of the cell cycle (i.e., chromosomal versus chromatid-type aberration), and for the three exchange categories, category subdivision depends on whether the lesion interaction was symmetric or asymmetric. Asymmetric exchanges always lead to the formation of acentric fragments, which are usually lost in subsequent cell divisions and therefore are usually fatal to the cell. These fragments may be retained transiently in the cell's progeny as extranuclear chromatin bodies called *micronuclei.* Symmetric exchanges are more insidious because they do not lead to the formation of acentric fragments and the accompanying loss of genetic material at the next cell division. They are sometimes difficult to detect cytologically, and they are not invariably lethal to the cell. They are transmitted to all the progeny of the original cell. Some types of symmetric exchanges (e.g., reciprocal translocation) have been implicated in radiation-induced carcinogenesis because they have the net effect of bringing new combinations of genes together or separating preexisting groups of genes.[31,59] Depending on where in the genome the translocation takes place, genes can be turned off or on, sometimes with adverse consequences.

Quantification of the types and frequencies of chromosomal aberrations in irradiated cells can be used to probe dose-response relationships for ionizing radiation, and to a first approximation, they can serve as a radiation dosimeter. For example, the dose-response curve for the induction of exchange-type aberrations after exposure to low-LET radiation tends to have a linear-quadratic shape, whereas that for single-hit aberrations tends to be linear. In mathematical terms, the incidence (I) of a particular aberration as a function of radiation dose (D) can be expressed as follows:

$$I = \alpha D + \beta D^2 + c \quad \text{for exchange-type aberrations}$$

$$I = \alpha D + c \quad \text{for single-hit aberrations}$$

In these equations, α and β are proportionality constants related to the yields of the particular type of aberration, and c is the spontaneous frequency of that aberration in unirradiated cells. For fractionated doses of low-LET radiation or continuous low dose rates, the yield of exchange-type aberrations decreases relative to that for acute doses, and the dose-response curve tends to become more linear. For high-LET

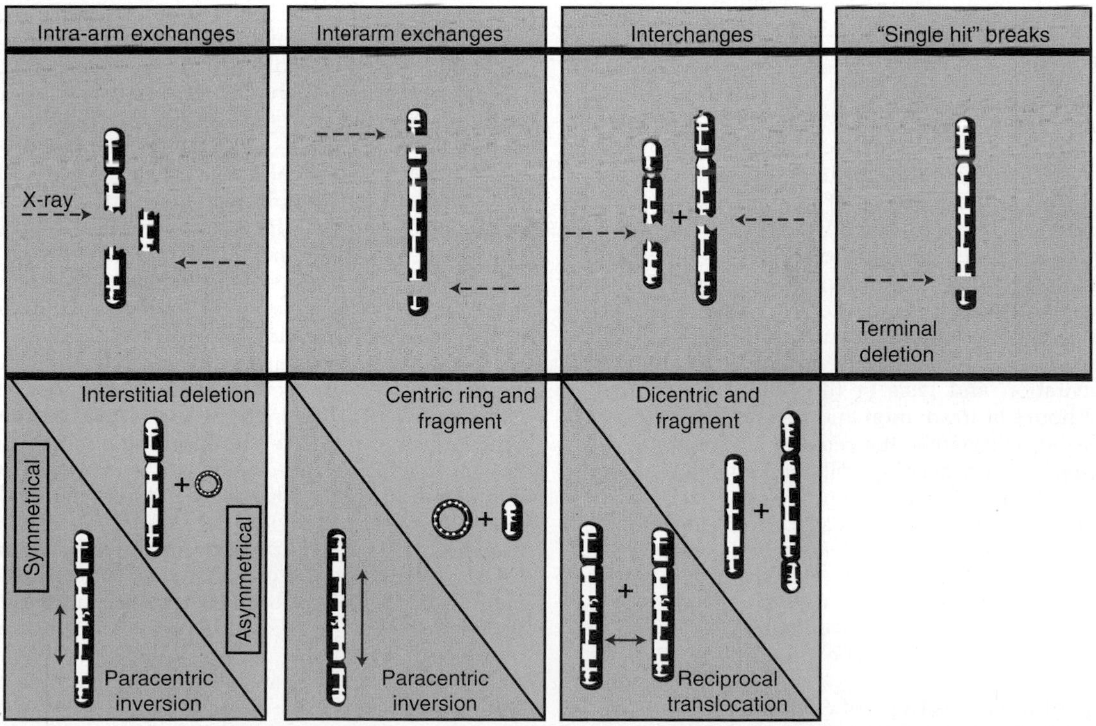

Figure 1-6 Types of radiation-induced chromosome aberrations that are the result of unrepaired or mis-rejoined DNA damage. Aberrations are classified according to whether they involve a single or multiple chromosomes; whether the damage is thought to be caused by the passage of a single charged particle track (i.e., one-hit aberration) or by the interaction of damages produced by two different tracks (i.e., two-hit aberration); and whether the irradiation occurred before or after the chromosomes had replicated (i.e., chromosome- versus chromatid-type aberrations, respectively; only chromosome-type aberrations are shown). The aberrations can be further subdivided according to whether broken pieces of the chromosome rearrange themselves symmetrically (with no net loss of genetic material) or asymmetrically (acentric fragments produced).

radiations, dose-response curves for aberration induction become steeper (i.e., higher aberration yields) and more linear compared with those for low-LET radiations.

Historically, exchange-type chromosomal aberrations had been assumed to involve no more than two breakpoints, which were presumably proximate in space and time. However, the use of fluorescent in situ hybridization (FISH), which employs fluorescent antibody probes to label whole chromosomes,[60-62] has demonstrated that some exchanges are complex in that their formation requires at least three breakpoints in at least two chromosomes. It is hoped that characterization of such complex chromosomal aberrations will provide further insights into mechanisms of radiation-induced clustered damage in DNA, nuclear structure and organization, and DNA repair. Another tantalizing finding is that high-LET radiations tend to produce complex aberrations more readily than low-LET radiations, suggesting that the presence of such aberrations could be a marker for exposure to high LET.[63]

Cell-Survival Curves and Survival Curve Theory

Cell Death

The traditional definition of death as a permanent, irreversible cessation of vital functions is different from that used by the radiation biologist or oncologist. For proliferating cells (including those maintained in vitro), the stem cells of normal tissues, and tumor clonogens, cell death in the radiobiologic sense refers to a loss of reproductive integrity (i.e., inability to sustain proliferation indefinitely). This type of reproductive or clonogenic death does not preclude the possibility that a cell may remain physically intact, be metabolically active, and continue its tissue-specific functions for some time after irradiation. Some reproductively dead cells can even complete a few additional mitoses before death in the more traditional sense.[31,64]

Apoptosis, or programmed cell death, is a type of nonreproductive or interphase death commonly associated with embryonic development and, in amphibians, with metamorphosis and tissue regeneration as well.[31,65] However, certain normal tissue and tumor cells also undergo apoptosis after irradiation, including normal cells of hematopoietic or lymphoid origin, crypt cells of the small intestine, salivary gland cells, and some experimental tumor cell lines of gynecologic and hematologic origin.[66] Cells undergoing apoptosis exhibit a number of characteristic morphologic (e.g., nuclear condensation and fragmentation, membrane blebbing) and biochemical (e.g., DNA degradation) changes that culminate in the fragmentation and lysis of the cell, often occurring within 6 to 12 hours of irradiation and before the first postirradiation division. Ultimately, the remains of apoptotic cells are phagocytized by neighboring cells and therefore do not cause the type of tissue destruction and disorganization characteristic of necrosis. Apoptosis is an active and carefully regulated pathway that involves several genes and gene products and an appropriate signal that activates the pathway. The molecular biology of apoptosis, the apoptosis-resistant phenotype observed for many types of tumor cells, and the role that radiation may play in the process are discussed elsewhere.

Most assays of radiosensitivity of cells and tissues, including those described subsequently, directly or indirectly use reproductive integrity as an end point. Although such assays have served the radiation oncology community well in terms of elucidating dose-response relationships for normal tissues and tumors, reproductive death is not necessarily the whole story. It is not clear whether and to what extent apoptosis contributes to our traditional measures of radiosensitivity based on reproductive integrity and whether pretreatment assessment of apoptotic propensity in tumors or dose-limiting normal tissues has any prognostic significance. The relationships between the different pathways of cell death can be quite complex. For example, Meyn[66] suggested that a tumor with a high spontaneous apoptotic index might be inherently more radiosensitive because cell death might be triggered by lower doses than are usually required to cause reproductive death. Tumors that readily undergo apoptosis may have higher rates of cell loss, the net effect of which would be to partially offset cell production, thereby reducing the number of tumor clonogens. However, not all types of tumor cells undergo apoptosis, and even among those that do, radiotherapy itself may have the undesirable side effect of selecting for subpopulations of cells that are already apoptosis resistant.

Cell-Survival and Dose-Response Curve Models

As had been the case during the early years of radiotherapy, advances in radiation physics, specifically biophysics, preceded advances in radiation biology. Survival curve theory originated in a consideration of the physics of energy deposition in matter by ionizing radiation. Early experiments with macromolecules and prokaryotes established the fact that dose-response relationships could be explained, in principle, by the random and discrete nature of energy absorption, if it was assumed that the response resulted from critical targets receiving random hits.[67] With an increasing number of shouldered survival and dose-response curves being described for cells irradiated in vitro and in vivo, various equations were developed to fit these data. Target theory pioneers studied a number of different end points in the context of target theory, including enzyme inactivation in cell-free systems,[32] cellular lethality, chromosomal damage, and radiation-induced cell cycle perturbations in microorganisms.[67,68] Survival curves, in which the log of the extent of a certain biologic activity was plotted as a function of the radiation dose, were found to have exponential or sigmoid shapes, with the latter usually seen for the survival of more complex organisms.[32]

Exponential survival curves were thought to result from the single-hit, all-or-nothing inactivation of a single target, producing loss of activity. A mathematical expression used to fit this kind of dose-response relationship was $S = e^{-D/D_0}$. In this equation, S is the fraction of cells that survive a given dose (D), and D_0 is the dose increment that reduces the cell survival to 37% (1/e) of some initial value on the exponential portion of the curve (i.e., a measure of the reciprocal of the slope). The sigmoid curves, characterized by a shoulder at low doses, were consistent with target theory if it was assumed that multiple targets or multiple hits in a single target (or a combination of both) were necessary for radiation inactivation. A mathematical expression based on target theory that provided a fairly good fit to survival data was $S = 1 - (1 - e^{-D/D_0})^n$, with n being the back extrapolation of the exponential portion of the survival curve to zero dose (i.e., a measure of the steepness of the shoulder). Implicit in this multitarget model was that damage had to accumulate before the overall effect was registered.

It soon became apparent that some features of this model were inadequate.[69] The most obvious problem was that the single-hit, multitarget equation predicted that survival curves should have initial slopes of zero; for vanishingly small doses (i.e., repeated, small doses per fraction or continuous low dose rates), the probability of killing cells would approach zero. This was *not* observed in practice for mammalian cell survival curves or as inferred from clinical studies in which highly fractionated or low dose rate treatment schedules were compared

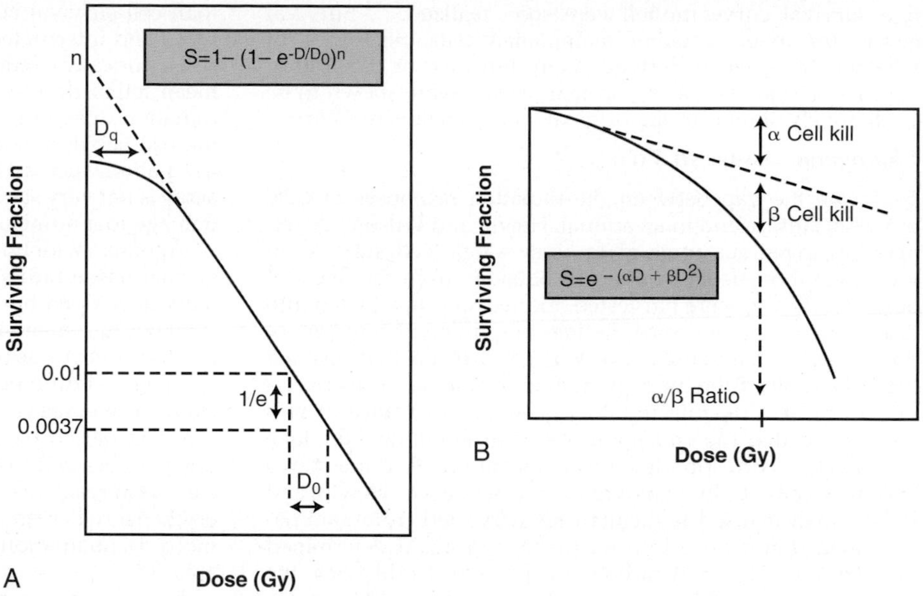

Figure 1-7 Comparison of two mathematical models commonly used to fit cell survival curve data. **A,** The single-hit, multitarget model is shown with its associated parameters, D_0, n, and D_q. Although this model has since been invalidated, values for its parameters are still used for comparative purposes. D_0, dose increment that reduces the cell survival to 37% (1/e) of some initial value on the exponential portion of the curve (i.e., a measure of the reciprocal of the slope); D_q, a measure of the width of the shoulder; n, back extrapolation of the exponential portion of the survival curve to zero dose (i.e., a measure of the steepness of the shoulder). **B,** The linear-quadratic model and its associated parameters, α and β, form the basis for current isoeffect formulas used in radiation therapy treatment planning.

with more conventional fractionation. There was no fractionation schedule that produced essentially no cell kill, all other radiobiologic factors being equal.

A different interpretation of cell survival was proposed by Kellerer and Rossi[70] in the late 1960s and early 1970s. The linear-quadratic or alpha-beta equation, $S = e^{-(\alpha D+\beta D^2)}$, was shown to fit many survival data quite well, particularly in the low-dose region of the curve, and it provided for the negative initial slope investigators had described.[69] In this expression, S is the fractional cell survival after a dose D, α is the rate of cell kill by a single-hit process, and β is the rate of cell kill by a two-hit mechanism. The theoretical derivation of the linear-quadratic equation is based on two very different sorts of observations. Based on microdosimetric considerations, Kellerer and Rossi[70] proposed that a radiation-induced lethal lesion resulted from the interaction of two sublesions. According to this interpretation, the αD term is the probability of these two sublesions being produced by a single event (i.e., the intratrack component), whereas βD^2 is the probability of the two sublesions being produced by two separate events (i.e., the intertrack component). Chadwick and Leenhouts[71] derived the same equation based on a different set of assumptions: that a double-strand break in DNA was a lethal lesion and that such a lesion could be produced by a single energy deposition involving both polynucleotide strands in DNA or by two separate events, each involving a single strand. The features and parameters of the target theory and linear-quadratic survival curve expressions are compared in Figure 1-7.

Clonogenic Assays In Vitro

It was not until the mid-1950s that mammalian cell culture techniques were sufficiently refined to allow quantification of the radiation responses of single cells.[72,73] Puck and Marcus[29] described an acute-dose x-ray survival curve for the human tumor cell line HeLa (Fig. 1-8). After graded x-ray doses, the reproductive integrity of single HeLa cells was measured by their ability to form macroscopic colonies of at least 50 cells (corresponding to approximately six successful cell divisions) on Petri dishes. Several features of this survival curve were of particular interest. First, the shape of the curve was qualitatively similar to those previously determined for many

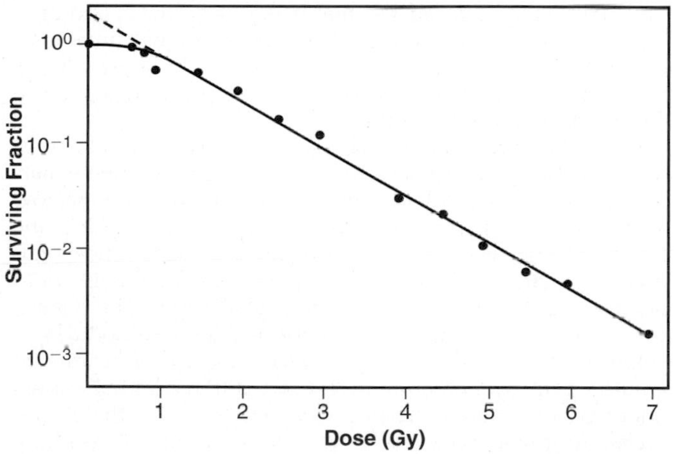

Figure 1-8 Clonogenic survival of HeLa cells in vitro as a function of x-ray dose. Like many mammalian cells of tumorigenic and nontumorigenic origin, the HeLa cell survival curve is characterized by a modest initial shoulder region (n ≈ 2.0) followed by an approximately exponential final slope ($D_0 \approx 1.0$ Gy). (Adapted from Puck TT, Marcus PI: Action of x-rays on mammalian cells. J Exp Med 103:653, 1956; copyright permission of The Rockefeller University Press.)

microorganisms, characterized by a shoulder at low doses and a roughly exponential region at high doses. However, the D_0 for HeLa cells was only 96 R, about 10- to 100-fold less than the D_0 values determined for microorganisms and 1000- to 10,000-fold less than the D_0 values for the inactivation of isolated macromolecules.[64] Cellular reproductive integrity was found to be a much more radiosensitive end point for HeLa cells than for prokaryotes or primitive eukaryotes. The value of the extrapolation number (n) for HeLa cells was approximately 2.0, indicating that the survival curve did have a small shoulder, but it was much smaller than typically observed for microorganisms. Puck and Marcus[29] suggested that the n value was a reflection of the number of critical targets in the cell, each requiring a single hit before the cell would be killed, and they further postulated that the targets were the chromosomes themselves. However, the potential pitfalls of deducing mechanisms of radiation action from parameters of a descriptive survival curve model were soon realized.[74,75] Survival curves for other types of mammalian cells, regardless of whether they were derived from humans or laboratory animals or from tumors or normal tissues, were shown to be qualitatively similar to the original HeLa cell survival curve.

Clonogenic Assays In Vivo

To bridge the gap between the radiation responses of cells grown in culture and in an animal, Hewitt and Wilson[76] developed an ingenious method to assay single cell survival in vivo. Lymphocytic leukemia cells obtained from the livers of donor CBA mice were harvested, diluted, and inoculated into disease-free recipient mice. By injecting different numbers of donor cells, a standard curve was constructed that enabled determination of the average number of injected cells necessary to cause leukemia in 50% of the recipient mice. It was determined that the end point of this titration, the 50% take dose (TD_{50}), corresponded to an inoculum of a mere two leukemia cells. Using this value as a reference, Hewitt and Wilson then injected leukemia cells harvested from gamma-irradiated donor mice into recipients and again determined the TD_{50} after different radiation exposures. In this way, the surviving fraction after a given radiation dose could be calculated from the ratio of the TD_{50} for unirradiated cells to that for the irradiated cells. Using this technique, a complete survival curve was constructed that had a D_0 of 162 R and an n value close to 2.0, which were quite similar to the values generated for cell lines irradiated in vitro. For the most part, in vivo survival curves for a variety of cell types were similar to corresponding in vitro curves.

A similar trend was apparent when in vivo survival curves for nontumorigenic cells were first produced. The first experiments by Till and McCulloch[77,78] using normal bone marrow stem cells were inspired by the knowledge that failure of the hematopoietic system was a major cause of death after total-body irradiation and that lethally irradiated animals could be rescued by bone marrow transplantation. The viable, transplanted bone marrow cells formed discrete nodules or colonies in the otherwise sterilized spleens of irradiated animals. Subsequently, the investigators transplanted known quantities of irradiated donor bone marrow into lethally irradiated recipient mice and were able to count the resulting splenic nodules and then calculate the surviving fraction of the injected cells in much the same way as was done for in vitro experiments. The D_0 for mouse bone marrow was 0.95 Gy.[77] Other in vivo assay systems based on the counting of colonies or nodules included the skin epithelium assay of Withers,[79] the intestinal crypt assays of Withers and Elkind,[80,81] and the lung colony assay of Hill and Bush.[82] During the late 1960s and early 1970s, it became possible to do excision assays, in which tumors irradiated in vivo were removed and enzymatically dissociated, and single cells were plated for clonogenic survival in vitro, thereby allowing more quantitative measurement of survival and avoiding some of the pitfalls of in vivo assays.[83]

Nonclonogenic Assays In Vivo

Unfortunately, some normal tissues and tumors are not amenable to clonogenic assays. New assays were needed that had clinical relevance but did not rely on reproductive integrity as an end point. Use of such assays required one leap of faith, because the end points assessed would have to be a consequence of the killing of clonogenic cells, although not necessarily in a direct, one-to-one manner. Because nonclonogenic assays do not directly measure cell survival as an end point, data derived from them and plotted as a function of radiation dose are properly called dose-response curves rather than cell survival curves, although such data are often analyzed and interpreted in much the same way.

Historically, among the first nonclonogenic assays was the mean lethal dose or LD_{50} assay, in which the (whole-body) radiation dose to produce lethality in approximately 50% of the test subjects is determined, usually at a fixed time after irradiation, such as 30 ($LD_{50/30}$) or 60 days ($LD_{50/60}$). The LD_{50} assay is not very specific in that the cause of death results from damage to a number of different tissues.

Another widely used nonclonogenic method to assess normal tissue radioresponse is the skin reaction assay, originally developed by Fowler and colleagues.[84] Pigs were often used because their skin is similar to that of humans in several key respects. An ordinate scoring system was used to compare and contrast different radiation schedules, and it was derived from the average severity of the skin reaction observed during a certain period (specific to the species and whether the end point occurs early or late) after irradiation. For example, for early skin reactions, a skin score of 1 may correspond to mild erythema, whereas a score of 4 may correspond to confluent moist desquamation over more than one half of the irradiated area.

Two common nonclonogenic assays for tumor response are the growth delay or regrowth delay assay[85] and the tumor control dose assay.[86] Both assays are simple and direct, are applicable to most solid tumors, and are clinically relevant. The growth delay assay involves the periodic measurement of a tumor's dimensions as a function of time after irradiation and a calculation of the tumor's approximate volume. For tumors that regress rapidly during and after radiotherapy, the end point scored is typically the time in days it takes for the tumor to regrow to its original volume at the start of irradiation. For tumors that regress more slowly or not at all, a more appropriate end point may be the time it takes for the tumor to grow or regrow to a specified size, such as three times its original volume. Dose-response curves are generated by plotting the growth delay as a function of radiation dose.

The tumor control assay is a logical extension of the growth delay assay. The end point of this assay is the total radiation dose required to achieve a specified probability of (local) tumor control—usually 50% (TCD_{50})—in a specified period after irradiation. The TCD_{50} value is obtained from a plot of the percentage of tumors locally controlled as a function of total dose. The slope of the resulting dose-response curve may be used for comparative purposes as a measure of the tumor's inherent radiosensitivity or its degree of heterogeneity, or both. More heterogeneous tumors tend to have shallower dose-response curves than more homogeneous ones, as do spontaneous tumors relative to experimental ones maintained in inbred strains of mice.

Cellular Repair: Sublethal and Potentially Lethal Damage Recovery

Taking the cue from target theory that the shoulder region of the radiation survival curve indicated that hits had to accumulate before cell killing occurred, Elkind and Sutton[87,88] sought to better characterize the nature of the damage caused by these hits and how the cell processed this damage. Even in the absence of any detailed information about DNA damage and repair processes at that time, a few things seemed obvious. First, the hits or damages that were registered as part of the accumulation process but did not kill cells were, by definition, sublethal. Second, sublethal damage became lethal only when it interacted with additional sublethal damage, when the total amount of damage had accumulated to a sufficient level to cause cell death.

What would be the result of deliberately interfering with the damage accumulation process by, for example, delivering part of the intended radiation dose, inserting a radiation-free interval, and then delivering the remainder of the dose? The results of such split-dose experiments were crucial to understanding why and how fractionated radiotherapy works as it does. The discovery and characterization of sublethal damage may be the single most important contribution radiation biology has made to the practice of radiation oncology.

By varying the time interval between two doses of approximately 5.0 Gy and plotting the log of the surviving fraction of cells after both doses (i.e., 10-Gy total dose) as a function of the time between the doses, the resulting split-dose recovery curve was observed to rise to a maximum after about 2 hours and then level off. The overall surviving fraction of cells after 10 Gy was higher if the dose was split into two fractions with a time interval between them rather than being delivered as a single dose. Elkind and Sutton[87,88] interpreted these results as indicating that the cells that survived the initial dose fraction had repaired some of the damage during the radiation-free interval and that the damage was no longer available to interact with the damage inflicted by the second dose. The investigators referred to this phenomenon as *sublethal damage repair* (SLDR), although it is perhaps preferable to call it *sublethal damage recovery* because biochemical DNA repair processes were not measured.

The shape of the split-dose recovery curve varied with the temperature during the radiation-free interval (Fig. 1-9). When the cells were kept at room temperature between the split doses, the SLDR curve rose to a maximum after about 2 hours and then leveled off. When the cells were returned to a 37°C incubator for the radiation-free interval, a different pattern emerged. Initially, the split-dose recovery curve rose to a maximum after 2 hours, but then the curve exhibited a series of oscillations, dropping to a second minimum at about 4 to 5 hours and then rising again to a higher maximum for split-dose intervals of 10 hours or more. The interpretation of this pattern of SLDR was that other radiobiologic phenomena operate simultaneously with cellular recovery. In this case, the fine structure of the split-dose recovery curve was not caused by an oscillating repair process, but rather by a superimposed cell cycle effect, the so-called *radiation age response* through the

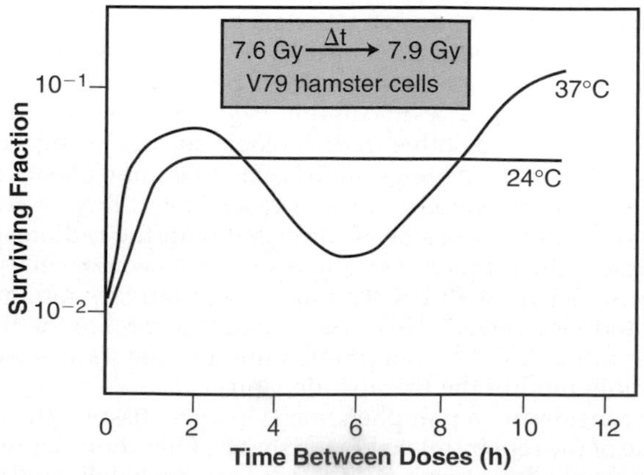

Figure 1-9 Split-dose or sublethal damage recovery demonstrated in cultured hamster V79 cells that received a first x-ray dose at time = 0, followed by a second dose after a variable radiation-free interval. Cells were maintained at room temperature (24°C) or at 37°C during the split time. (Adapted from Elkind M, Sutton-Gilbert H, Moses W, et al: Radiation response of mammalian cells grown in culture. V. Temperature dependence of the repair of x-ray damage in surviving cells (aerobic and hypoxic). Radiat Res 25:359, 1965.)

cell cycle. This topic is discussed later in the "Ionizing Radiation and the Cell Cycle" section of this chapter (see Fig. 1-14).

Since Elkind and Sutton's original work,[87,88] SLDR kinetics have been described for many different types of mammalian cells in culture[64] and for most normal and tumor tissues in vivo.[89,90] Several of their findings are pertinent to this discussion:

1. The amount of sublethal damage capable of being repaired for a given cell type varies with the radiation quality (i.e., less for radiations of increasing LET) and the oxygenation status of the cells (i.e., recovery is reduced or absent at extremely low oxygen tensions).[31]
2. The average half-time for SLDR in mammalian cells in culture is about 1 hour, although it seems to be somewhat longer for late-responding normal tissues in vivo.[31]
3. The survival increase between split doses is a manifestation of the regeneration of the shoulder of the radiation survival curve. After an initial radiation dose and an adequate time interval for SLDR, the response of surviving cells to graded additional doses is almost identical to that obtained from cells without previous radiation exposure. The shoulder of a survival curve (i.e., its extrapolation number, n, using the target theory model or, conversely, the α/β ratio using the linear-quadratic model) came to be associated with the capacity of the cells for recovery from sublethal damage (Fig. 1-10).
4. Cells are able to undergo repeated cycles of damage and recovery without an apparent change in recovery capacity. An equal effect per dose fraction can be predicted during the course of fractionated radiotherapy. Practically, this means that a multifraction survival curve can be generated using the formula $SF_n = (SF_1)^n$, in which SF_1 is the surviving fraction of cells after a single dose fraction (i.e., determined from a single dose-survival curve or comparable assay), and SF_n is the surviving fraction of cells after n dose fractions. Multifraction survival curves are shoulderless and exponential (Fig. 1-11).
5. SLDR is largely responsible for the so-called dose rate effect for low-LET radiation (discussed later). As the dose per fraction (i.e., intermittent irradiation) or dose rate (i.e., continuous irradiation) is decreased and the overall treatment time increased, the biologic effectiveness of a given total dose is reduced. (SLDR also occurs during continuous irradiation; a radiation-free interval is not required.)

A second type of cellular recovery after irradiation is called *potentially lethal damage repair or recovery* (PLDR). It was first described for mammalian cells by Phillips and Tolmach[91] in 1966. PLD is a spectrum of radiation damage that may or may not result in cell lethality depending on the cells' postirradiation conditions. Conditions that favor PLD recovery include maintenance of cells in overcrowded conditions (i.e., plateau phase or contact inhibited[92,93]), incubation after irradiation at reduced temperatures,[94] in the presence of certain metabolic inhibitors,[91] or in balanced salt solutions rather than complete culture medium.[94] All of these treatment conditions are *suboptimal* for the continued growth of cells. Presumably, resting cells (regardless of why they are resting) have more opportunity to repair DNA damage before cell division than cells that continue traversing the cell cycle immediately after irradiation. Phillips and Tolmach[91] were the first to propose this repair-fixation or competition model to explain PLDR.

Although some of these postirradiation conditions are not likely to be encountered in vivo, the slow growth of cells in general, with or without a large fraction of resting cells, is a common characteristic of intact tissues. Tumors and selected

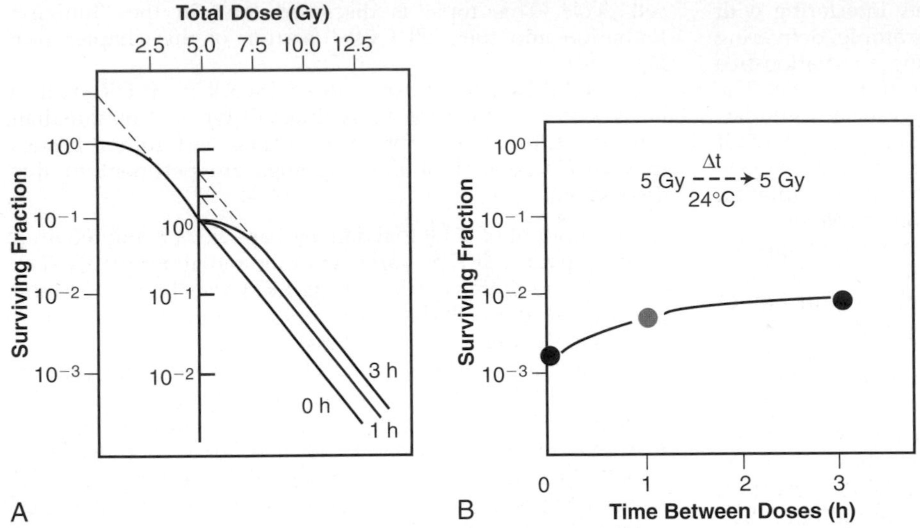

Figure 1-10 Sublethal damage recovery manifests as a return of the shoulder on the radiation survival curve when a total dose is delivered as two fractions separated by a time interval (**A**). If the interfraction interval is shorter than the time it takes for this recovery to occur, the shoulder will only be partially regenerated (compare the shoulder regions of the survival curves for intervals of 1 versus 3 hours). Regeneration of the shoulder (**B**) accounts for the observed survival increase in the corresponding split-dose assay (see Fig. 1-9).

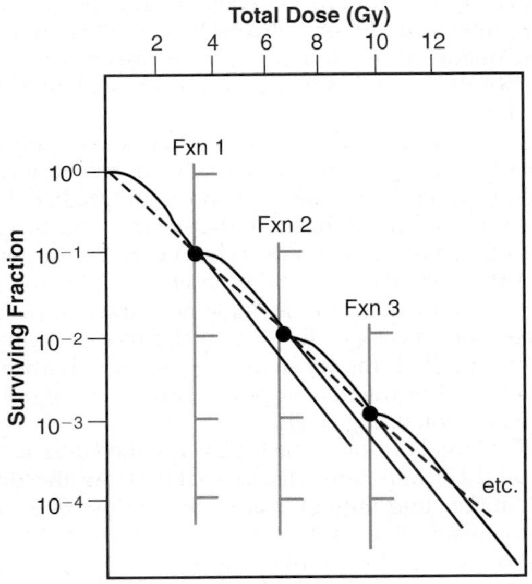

Figure 1-11 Hypothetical multifraction survival curve *(dashed line)* for repeated 3.0-Gy fractions under conditions in which sufficient time between fractions is allowed for full sublethal damage recovery and cell cycle and proliferative effects are negligible. The multifraction survival curve is shallower than its corresponding single dose curve *(solid lines)* and has no shoulder (i.e., the surviving fraction is an exponential function of total dose).

normal tissues amenable to clonogenic assay were shown to repair PLD.[95] Experiments using rodent tumors were modeled after comparable studies using plateau-phase cells in culture; a delayed-plating assay was used. For such an experiment, the protocol involves irradiating the cell culture or animal tumor and then leaving the cells of interest in a confluent state (in the overcrowded cell culture or in the intact tumor in the animal) for various periods before removing them, dissociating them into single-cell suspensions, and plating the cells for clonogenic survival at a low density. The longer the delay between irradiation and the clonogenic assay, the higher the resulting surviving fraction of individual cells, even though the radiation dose is the same. In general, survival rises to a maximum within 4 to 6 hours and levels off thereafter (Fig. 1-12).

The kinetics and extent of recovery from sublethal damage and PLD have been correlated with the molecular repair of DNA and with the rejoining of chromosome breaks.[96,97] What remains to be seen is whether the biochemical repair of a particular DNA lesion or the rejoining of a particular type of chromosomal aberration accounts for one or the other type of cellular recovery. It is difficult to determine whether SLDR and PLDR are independent processes or two manifestations of the same process. For the purposes of radiotherapy, this may be a moot point; the most important consideration is that both processes have the potential to increase the surviving fraction of cells between subsequent dose fractions. Such a survival increase would manifest clinically as increased normal tissue tolerance or decreased tumor control. It is also important to appreciate that small differences in recovery capacity between normal and tumor cells after a single dose fraction are magnified into large differences after 30 or more dose fractions.

Repair in Tissues

The sparing effect of dose fractionation for normal and tumor tissues can be largely explained by SLDR between fractions. However, at sufficiently small doses per fraction, the degree of sparing reaches a maximum below which no further sparing occurs, all other radiobiologic factors being equal. There has also been interest in the role PLDR may play in dose fractionation responses. In some cases, the ability of tumor cells to repair PLD has been correlated with the radioresponsiveness of their tumor of origin, with tumors whose cells were quite proficient at PLDR tending to be relatively radioresistant, and vice versa.[98] This would be detrimental to the therapeutic ratio. PLDR by nonproliferating normal tissues would favorably modify the therapeutic ratio.

In considering repair phenomena in intact tissues, the magnitude of the repair (related to the shape of the shoulder region of the single dose survival curve and the dose delivered) and the rate of the repair can influence how the tissue behaves during a course of radiotherapy. For example, a particular tissue (normal or tumor) may be capable of repairing most damage produced by each dose fraction, but if the interfraction interval is too short to allow all the damage to be repaired before the next dose, the tolerance of that tissue will be less than otherwise anticipated.

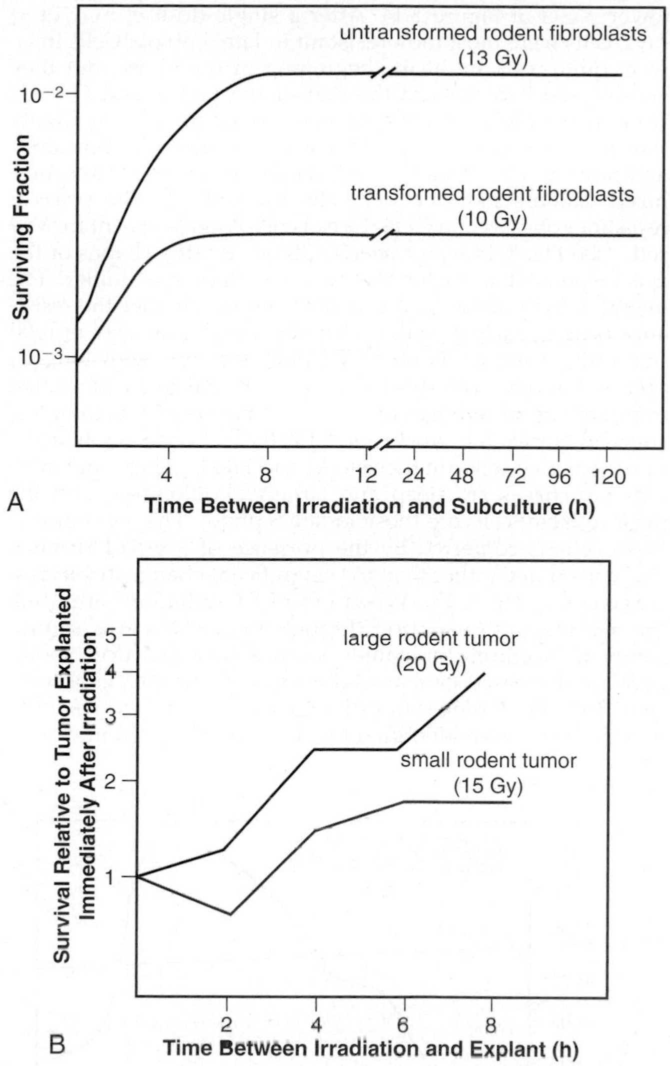

Figure 1-12 Potentially lethal damage recovery can be demonstrated using a delayed-plating assay in which a variable delay time is inserted between exposure to a large, single dose of radiation and the harvesting of the cells for a clonogenic assay. If cells are maintained in overcrowded or nutrient-deprived conditions during the delay period, the surviving fraction increases relative to that obtained when there is no delay. **A,** Potentially lethal damage recovery occurs in vitro in a nontumorigenic rodent fibroblast cell line and its transformed, tumorigenic, counterpart. **B,** Potentially lethal damage recovery occurs in vivo in small and large mouse fibrosarcomas. (**A,** Adapted from Zeman E, Bedford J: Dose-rate effects in mammalian cells. V. Dose fractionation effects in noncycling C3H 10T1/2 cells. Int J Radiat Oncol Biol Phys 10:2089, 1984; **B,** adapted from Little J, Hahn G, Frindel E, et al: Repair of potentially lethal radiation damage in vitro and in vivo. Radiology 106:689, 1973.)

Ionizing Radiation and the Cell Cycle

Another basic feature of the cellular response to ionizing radiation is perturbation of the cell cycle. Such effects can modify the radioresponsiveness of tissues directly or indirectly, depending on the fraction of cycling cells present in the tissue of interest, their proliferation rates, and the kinetic organization of the tissue or tumor as a whole.

Advances in techniques for the study of cell cycle kinetics during the 1950s and 1960s paved the way for the analysis of radiation responses of cells as a function of their age. Using a technique known as autoradiography that involved the incubation of cells with radioactive DNA precursor compounds, followed by the detection of cells that had incorporated such precursors by their ability to expose radiographic film, Howard and Pelc[99,100] were able to identify the DNA synthetic phase of the cell cycle. When combined with the other cytologically obvious cell cycle marker, mitosis, they were able to discern the four phases of the cell cycle for actively growing cells: G_1, S, G_2, and M.

Methodology

Several techniques were developed for the collection of synchronized cells in vitro. One of the most widely used was the mitotic harvest or shake-off technique first described by Terasima and Tolmach.[101,102] By shaking cultures, mitotic cells, which tend to round up and become loosely attached to the culture vessel's surface, can be dislodged, collected along with the overlying medium, and inoculated into new culture flasks. By incubating these flasks at 37°C, cells begin to proceed synchronously into G_1 phase (and semi-synchronously thereafter). By knowing the length of the various phase durations for the cell type being studied and then delivering a radiation dose at a time of interest after the initial synchronization, the survival response of cells in different phases of the cell cycle can be determined.

A second synchronization method involved the use of DNA synthesis inhibitors such as fluorodeoxyuridine[103] and hydroxyurea[104] to selectively kill S-phase cells but allow cells in other phases to continue progression through the cell cycle until they become blocked at the border of the G_1 and S phases. By incubating cells in these inhibitors for times sufficient to collect nearly all cells at the block point, large numbers of cells can be synchronized. The inhibitor technique has two other advantages: that some degree of synchronization is possible in vivo[105] and in vitro; and that by inducing synchrony at the end of G_1 phase, a higher degree of synchrony can be maintained for longer periods than if synchronization had been achieved at the beginning of G_1. However, the mitotic selection method does not rely on the use of agents that could perturb the normal cell cycle kinetics of the population under study. In later years, the mitotic selection and inhibitor methods were combined to achieve even higher degrees of cell synchrony. Developments in the early 1970s provided what is now considered among the most valuable tools for the study of kinetic effects: the flow cytometer and its offshoot, the fluorescence-activated cell sorter.[106]

Using this powerful technique, single cells are stained with a fluorescent probe that binds stoichiometrically to a specific cellular component, which is DNA in the case of cell cycle distribution analysis. The stained cells are then introduced into a pressurized flow cell and forced to flow single file and at a high rate of speed through an intense, focused laser beam that excites the fluorescent dye. The resulting light emission from each cell is collected by photomultiplier tubes, recorded, and output as a frequency histogram of cell number as a function of relative fluorescence, with the amount of fluorescence directly proportional to DNA content. Accordingly, cells with a 1× DNA content correspond to cells in G_1 phase, cells with a 2× DNA content correspond to cells in G_2 or M phase, and cells with DNA contents between 1× and 2× values correspond to those in the S phase of the cell cycle. By performing a mathematical fit to the DNA histogram, the proportion of cells in each phase of the cell cycle can be determined, the phase durations can be derived, and differences in DNA ploidy can be identified. DNA flow cytometry is quite powerful in that a static measure of cell cycle distribution can be obtained for a cell population of interest and because dynamic studies of, for example, transit through the various cell cycle phases or treatment-induced kinetic perturbations can be monitored over time (Fig. 1-13). A flow cytometer can be outfitted to include a cell-sorting feature; in this case, cells analyzed for a property of interest can be collected in separate bins after they pass through the laser beam and, if possible, used for other experiments.

Age Response through the Cell Cycle

Results of an age response experiment of Terasima and Tolmach,[101] using synchronized HeLa cells, are shown in the lower panel of Figure 1-14. After a single dose of 5 Gy of x-rays, cells were most radioresistant in late S phase. Cells in G_1 were quite resistant at the beginning of the phase, but they became sensitive toward the end of the phase, and G_2 cells were increasingly sensitive as they moved toward the highly sensitive M phase. In subsequent experiments by Sinclair[107] and Sinclair and Morton,[108] age response curves for synchronized Chinese hamster V79 cells showed that the peak in resistance observed in G_1 HeLa cells was largely absent for V79 cells (see Fig. 1-14, *upper panel*). Otherwise, the shapes of the age response curves for the two cell lines are similar. The overall length of the G_1 phase determines whether the resistance peak in early G_1 will occur; in general, this peak of relative radioresistance is observed only for cells with long G_1 phases. For cells with short G_1 phases, the entire phase is often intermediate in radiosensitivity. An analysis of the complete survival curves for synchronized cells[107,109] confirms that the most sensitive cells are those in M and late G_2 phase, in which survival curves are steep and largely shoulderless, and the most resistant cells are those in late S phase. The resistance of these cells is conferred by the presence of a broad survival curve shoulder, rather than by a significant change in survival curve slope (Fig. 1-15). When high-LET radiations are used, the age response variation through the cell cycle is significantly reduced or eliminated, because survival curve shoulders are decreased or removed altogether by such exposures (see "Relative Biologic Effectiveness"). Similar age response patterns have been identified for cells synchronized in vivo.[105]

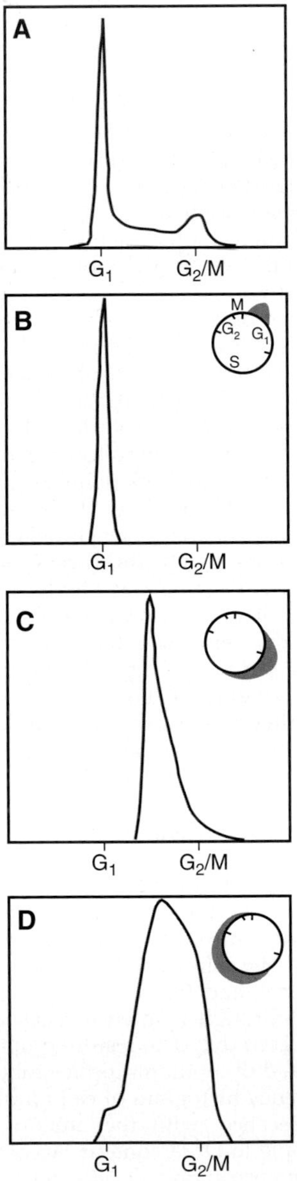

Figure 1-13 The analytic technique of flow cytometry has revolutionized the study of cell cycle kinetics by allowing rapid determination of DNA content in cells stained with a fluorescent dye that binds stoichiometrically to cellular DNA. **A,** Frequency distribution for a population of exponentially growing cells. The large and small peaks correspond to cells with G_1 (1×) and G_2/M (2×) phase DNA content, respectively; the cells in S phase have an intermediate DNA content. **B–D,** DNA histograms for a cell population synchronized initially in mitosis and then allowed to progress into G_1 (**B**), S, and G_2/M (**C** and **D**).

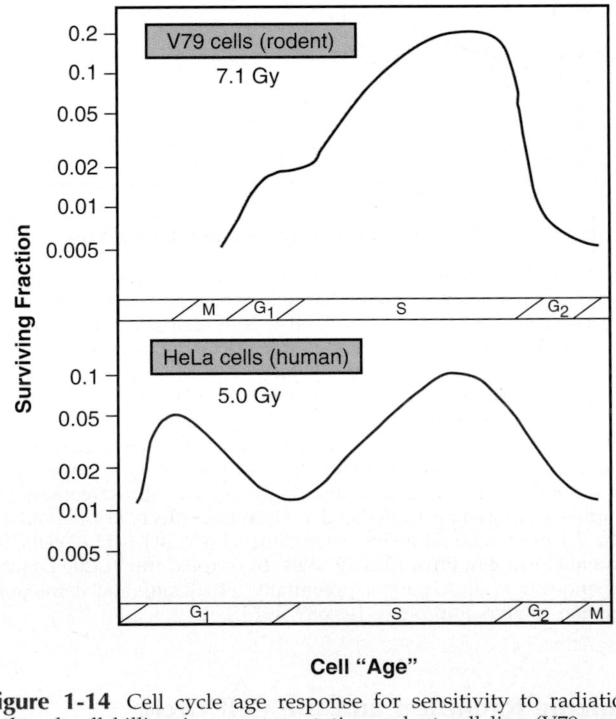

Figure 1-14 Cell cycle age response for sensitivity to radiation-induced cell killing in a representative rodent cell line (V79, *upper panel*) having a short G_1 phase duration and in a representative human cell line (HeLa, *lower panel*) having a long G_1 phase duration. Both cell lines exhibit a peak of radioresistance in late S phase and maximum radiosensitivity in late G_2/M phase. A second trough of radiosensitivity can be discerned near the G_1/S border for cells with long G_1-phase durations. (Adapted from Sinclair W: Dependence of radiosensitivity upon cell age. *In* Proceedings of the Carmel Conference on Time and Dose Relationships in Radiation Biology as Applied to Radiotherapy. BNL Report 50203. Upton, NY, Brookhaven National Laboratory, 1969.)

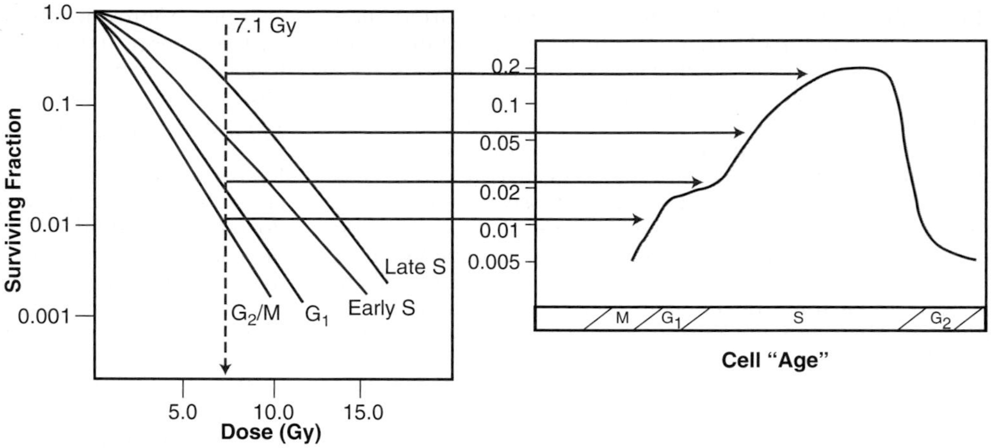

Figure 1-15 Cell survival curves for irradiated populations of Chinese hamster cells synchronized in different phases of the cell cycle *(left panel)*, illustrating how these radiosensitivity differences translate into the age response patterns shown in the *right panel* (see Fig. 1-14).

The existence of a cell cycle age response for ionizing radiation provided an explanation for the unusual pattern of SLDR observed for cells maintained at 37°C (i.e., normal physiologic conditions) during the recovery interval (see Fig. 1-9). In Elkind and Sutton's experiments,[87,88] exponentially growing cells were used; cells were asynchronously distributed across the different phases of the cell cycle: G_1, S, G_2, and M. The cells that survived irradiation tended to be those that were most radioresistant. The remaining population was enriched with the more resistant cells and partially synchronized. For low-LET radiation, cells that were most resistant were the cells that were in S phase at the time of the first radiation dose. However, at 37°C, cells continued to progress through the cell cycle, and the surviving cells in S phase at the time of the first dose might have moved into G_2 phase by the time the second dose was delivered. The observed survival nadir in the SLDR curve did not result from a loss or reversal of repair, but rather because the population of cells became enriched in G_2 phase cells, which are inherently more radiosensitive. For even longer radiation-free intervals, it is possible that the cells surviving the first dose will transit from G_2 to M and back into G_1 phase; these cells will divide and double their numbers. In this case, the SLDR curve shows a surviving fraction increase because the number of cells has increased. None of these cell cycle-related phenomena occurs when the cells are maintained at room temperature during the radiation-free interval, because movement through the cell cycle is inhibited under such conditions; in that case, only the initial survival increase due to prompt SLDR is observed.

Radiation-Induced Cell Cycle Blocks and Delays

Radiation can disrupt the normal proliferation kinetics of cell populations. This effect was recognized by Canti and Spear[110] in 1927 and studied in conjunction with radiation's ability to induce cellular lethality. With the advent of mammalian cell culture and synchronization techniques and of time-lapse cinemicrography, it became possible for investigators to study mitotic and division delay phenomena in greater detail.

Mitotic delay, defined as a delay in the entry of cells into mitosis, is a consequence of transient upstream blocks or delays in the movement of cells from one cell cycle phase to the next. *Division delay,* a delay in the time of appearance of new cells at the completion of mitosis, is caused by the combined effects of mitotic delay and any further lengthening of the mitosis process itself. Division delay increases with dose and is, on average, about 1 to 2 hours per Gy,[101] depending on the cell line.

The cell cycle blocks and delays primarily responsible for mitotic and division delay are, respectively, a block in G_2-to-M phase transition and a block in the G_1-to-S phase transition. The duration of the G_2 delay, like the overall division delay, varies with cell type, but for a given cell type, it is dose and cell cycle age dependent. In general, the length of the G_2 delay increases linearly with dose. For a given dose, the G_2 delay is longest for cells irradiated in S or early G_2 phase and shortest for cells irradiated in G_1 phase.[101] Another factor contributing to mitotic and division delay is a block in the flow of cells from G_1 into S phase. For x-ray doses of about 6 Gy or higher, there is a 50% decrease in the rate of tritiated thymidine uptake in exponentially growing cultures of mouse L cells. Little[111] reached a similar conclusion from G_1 delay studies using human liver LICH cells maintained as confluent cultures.

A possible role for DNA damage and its repair in the cause of division delay was bolstered by the finding that certain cell types that did not exhibit the normal cell cycle delays associated with radiation exposure (e.g., AT cells[44]) or, conversely, that were treated with chemicals (e.g., caffeine) that ameliorated the radiation-induced delays,[112,113] tended to contain higher amounts of residual DNA damage and to show increased radiosensitivity.

It is now understood that the radiation-induced perturbations in cell cycle transit are under the control of cell cycle checkpoint genes, whose protein products normally govern the orderly and unidirectional flow of cells from one phase to the next. The checkpoint genes are responsive to feedback from the cell about its general condition and readiness to transit to the next cell cycle phase. DNA integrity is but one of the criteria used by these genes to help make the decision whether to continue traversing the cell cycle or to pause temporarily or permanently. Cell cycle checkpoint genes are discussed elsewhere.

Redistribution in Tissues

Because of the age response through the cell cycle, an initially asynchronous population of cells surviving a dose of radiation becomes enriched with S-phase cells. However, because of variations in the rate of further cell cycle progression, this partial synchrony decays rapidly. Such cells are said to have redistributed,[114] with the net effect of sensitizing the population as a whole to a subsequent dose fraction (relative to what would have been expected had the cells remained in their resistant phases). A second type of redistribution, in which cells accumulate in G_2 phase (in the absence of cell division)

always seen in the centers of cylindrical tumor cords having a radius in excess of 200 μm. Regardless of how large the central necrotic region was, the sheath of apparently viable cells around the periphery of this central region never had a radius greater than about 180 μm. The investigators calculated the expected maximum diffusion distance of oxygen from blood vessels located in the normal tissue stroma and found that the value of 150 to 200 μm agreed quite well with the radius of the sheath of viable tumor cells observed histologically. Since that time, the average diffusion distance of oxygen has been revised downward to approximately 70 μm.[31] The oxygenation status of tumor cells varied from fully oxic to completely anoxic, depending on where the cells were located in relation to the nearest blood vessels. It was inferred from these studies that cells at intermediate distances from the blood supply would be hypoxic and radioresistant but remain clonogenic.

The first unambiguous demonstration that a solid animal tumor contained viable, radioresistant hypoxic cells was by Powers and Tolmach[124] in 1963; they used the dilution assay to generate an in vivo survival curve for mouse lymphosarcoma cells. The in vivo survival curve for this solid tumor was biphasic, having an initial D_0 of about 1.1 Gy and a final D_0 of 2.6 Gy (Fig. 1-20). Because the survival curve for lymphoid cells is essentially shoulderless, it was simple to back-extrapolate the shallower component of the curve to the surviving fraction axis and determine that the resistant fraction of cells constituted about 1.5% of the total population. This was considered compelling evidence (but did not prove) that this subpopulation of cells was hypoxic and clonogenic.

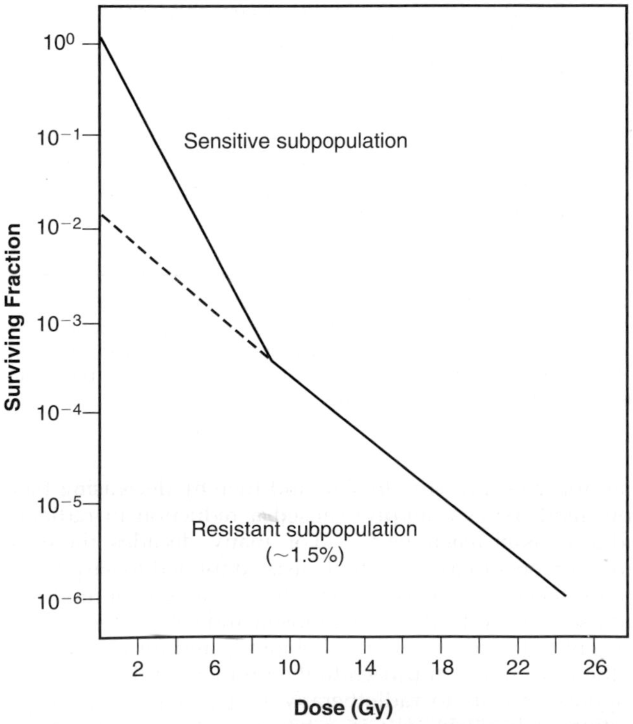

Figure 1-20 Cell survival curve for a murine lymphosarcoma growing subcutaneously and irradiated in vivo. The biphasic curve suggests the presence of a small but relatively radioresistant subpopulation of cells, determined in accompanying experiments to represent the tumor's clonogenic hypoxic fraction. (Adapted from Powers WE, Tolmach LJ: A multicomponent x-ray survival curve for mouse lymphosarcoma cells irradiated. Nature 197:710, 1963.)

The question then became how to prove that this small fraction of tumor cells was radioresistant because of hypoxia rather than other reasons. An elegant if somewhat macabre method was developed to address this dilemma; it was called the *paired survival curve technique*.[124,125] In this assay, laboratory animals bearing tumors were divided into three treatment groups, with one group irradiated while breathing air (approximately 20% oxygen), a second group irradiated while breathing pure oxygen (presumably fully oxic), and a third group killed first by cervical dislocation and then promptly irradiated (presumably fully anoxic). Within each group, animals received graded radiation doses so that complete survival curves were generated for each treatment condition. When completed, the paired survival curve method yielded three different tumor cell survival curves: a fully oxic curve (most radiosensitive), a fully hypoxic curve (most radioresistant), and the survival curve for air-breathing animals that, if the tumor contained viable, hypoxic cells, was biphasic and positioned between the other two curves. It was then possible to mathematically strip the fully aerobic and hypoxic curves from the curve for air-breathing animals and determine the radiobiologically hypoxic fraction.

Across a variety of rodent tumors, the percentage of hypoxic cells was found to vary between 0% and 50%, with an average of about 15%.[125]

Mechanistic Aspects

A more rigorous analysis of the nature of the oxygen effect is possible with cells or bacteria grown in vitro. Historically, oxygen had been called a *dose-modifying agent;* the ratio of doses to achieve a given survival level under hypoxic and aerated conditions was constant, regardless of the survival level chosen for a given type of radiation. This dose ratio to produce the same biologic end point is called the *oxygen enhancement ratio* (OER), and it is used for comparative purposes (Fig. 1-21). The OER typically has a value of between 2.5 and 3.0 for large, single doses of x-rays or gamma rays; 1.5 to 2.0 for radiations of intermediate LET; and 1.0 (i.e., no oxygen effect) for high-LET radiations.

There is evidence that oxygen is not strictly dose modifying; however, several studies have shown that the OER for

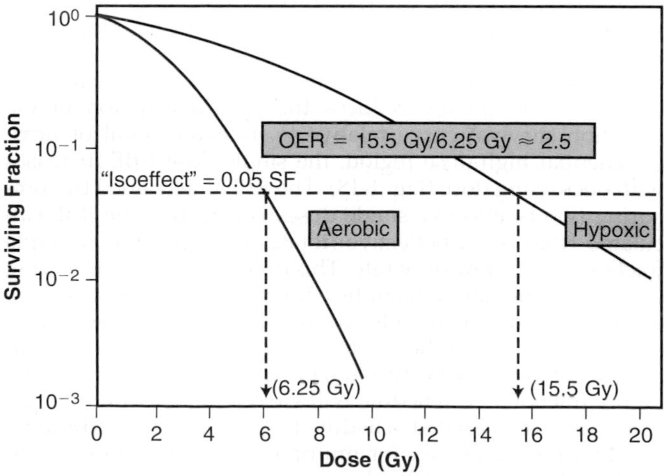

Figure 1-21 Representative survival curves for cells irradiated with x-rays in the presence (aerobic) or virtual absence (hypoxic) of oxygen. The oxygen enhancement ratio (OER) is defined as the ratio of doses under hypoxic-to-aerobic conditions to yield the same biologic effect, which in this case is a cell surviving fraction (SF) of 0.05.

sparsely ionizing radiation is lower at lower doses than at higher doses. This has been observed for exponentially growing cells in culture when the OER was calculated from high-resolution survival determinations in the shoulder region of the survival curve. Lower OERs and decreased effectiveness of hypoxic cell radiosensitizers (see Chapter 3) for doses per fraction in the range commonly used in radiotherapy have also been inferred indirectly from clinical and experimental tumor data plus some laboratory findings for cells in culture.[126,127] It has been suggested that the lower OERs result from an apparent age response for the oxygen effect, not unlike the age responses for inherent radiosensitivity and cell cycle delay.[31] Assuming cells in G_1 phase of the cell cycle have a lower OER than those in S phase and because G_1 cells are also more radiosensitive, they would tend to dominate the low-dose region of the cell survival curve.

Although the exact mechanisms of the oxygen effect are likely complex, a simple model can be used to illustrate our current understanding of this phenomenon (Fig. 1-22). The *radical competition model* holds that oxygen acts as a radiosensitizer by forming peroxides in important biomolecules (including DNA) already damaged by radiation exposure, thereby fixing the radiation damage. In the absence of oxygen, DNA can be restored to its preirradiated condition by hydrogen donation from endogenous reducing species in the cell, such as the free radical scavenger glutathione (a thiol compound). In essence, this can be considered a type of very fast chemical restitution or repair. These two processes, fixation and restitution, are considered to be in a dynamic equilibrium, such that changes in the relative amounts of the radiosensitizer, oxygen, or the radioprotector, glutathione, tip the scales in favor of fixation (i.e., more damage, greater cell kill, and greater radiosensitivity) or restitution (i.e., less damage, less cell kill, and greater radioresistance).

Consistent with this free radical–based interpretation of the oxygen effect is the finding that oxygen needs to be present only during the irradiation (or no more than about 5 ms after irradiation) to produce an aerobic radioresponse.[128,129] The concentration of oxygen necessary to achieve essentially maximum sensitization is quite small, which is evidence for the high efficiency of oxygen as a radiosensitizer. A sensitivity midway between a fully hypoxic and fully aerobic radioresponse is achieved at an oxygen tension of about 3 mm Hg, corresponding to about 0.5% oxygen, more than a factor of 10 lower than partial pressures of oxygen usually encountered in normal tissues. This value of 0.5% has been called the oxygen *k value*, and it is obtained from an oxygen *k curve* of relative radiosensitivity (in which a relative radiosensitivity of 1.0 is consistent with hypoxic conditions and a value of 3.0 with well-aerated conditions) plotted as a function of oxygen tension (Fig. 1-23).[130]

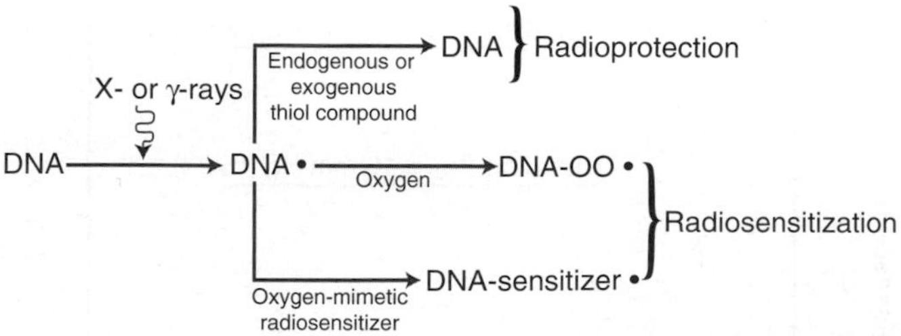

Figure 1-22 Schematic representation of the proposed mechanism of action for the oxygen effect. The radical competition model holds that oxygen acts as a radiosensitizer by forming peroxides in DNA already damaged by radiation, thereby fixing the damage. In the absence of oxygen, DNA can be restored to its preirradiated state by hydrogen donation from endogenous reducing species in the cell, such as the free radical scavenger glutathione. An oxygen-mimetic, hypoxic cell radiosensitizer may be used to substitute for oxygen in these fast, free radical reactions, or an exogenously supplied thiol compound may be used to act as a radioprotector.

Reoxygenation in Tumors

After the convincing demonstration of hypoxic cells in a mouse tumor,[124] it was assumed that human tumors also contained a viable hypoxic fraction. However, if human tumors contained even a small fraction of clonogenic hypoxic cells, simple calculations suggested that tumor control would be almost impossible with radiotherapy.[131] Because therapeutic successes did occur, some form of reoxygenation must take place during the course of multifraction irradiation. This was not an unreasonable idea because the demand for oxygen by sterilized cells would gradually decrease as they were removed from the tumor, and a decrease in tumor size, a restructuring of tumor vasculature, or intermittent changes in blood flow could make oxygen available to these previously hypoxic cells.

The reoxygenation process was extensively studied by van Putten and Kallman,[132] who serially determined the fraction of hypoxic cells in a mouse sarcoma during the course of a typical multifraction irradiation protocol. The fact that the hypoxic fraction was about the same at the end of treatment as at the beginning of treatment was strong evidence for a reoxygenation process. Reoxygenation of hypoxic, clonogenic tumor cells during an extended multifraction treatment would increase the therapeutic ratio, assuming that normal tissues remained well oxygenated. This is thought to be another major factor in the sparing of normal tissues relative to tumors during fractionated radiotherapy.

What physiologic characteristics would lead to tumor reoxygenation during a course of radiotherapy, and at what rate would this be expected to occur? One possible cause of

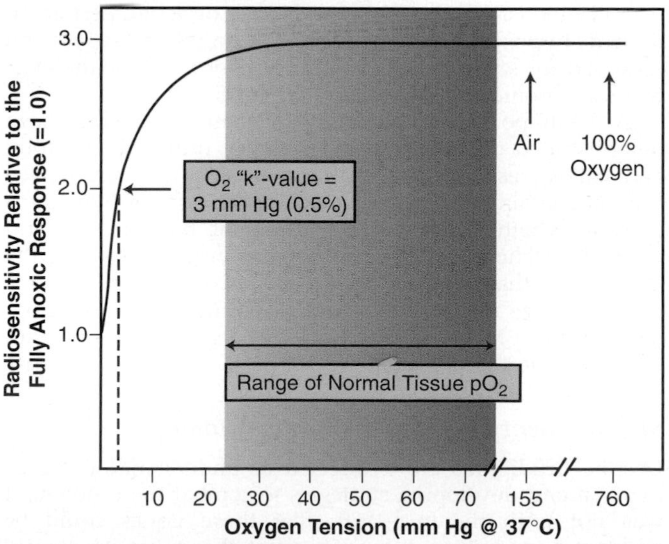

Figure 1-23 An oxygen *k curve* is used to illustrate the dependence of radiosensitivity on oxygen concentration. If a fully anoxic cell culture is assigned a relative radiosensitivity of 1.0, introducing even 0.5% (3 mm Hg) oxygen into the system increases the radiosensitivity of cells to 2.0. By the time the oxygen concentration reaches about 2.0%, cells respond as if they are fully aerated (i.e., radiosensitivity ≈ 3.0). The *green shaded area* represents the approximate range of oxygen concentrations encountered in human normal tissues.

tumor hypoxia and, by extension, a possible mechanism for reoxygenation was suggested by Thomlinson and Gray's pioneering work.[123] The type of hypoxia that they proposed is what is now called chronic or *diffusion-limited hypoxia*. This results from the tendency of tumors to outgrow their blood supply, and given that oxygen is used by tumor cells for oxidative metabolism and energy production, it follows that natural gradients of oxygen tension should develop as a function of distance from blood vessels. Cells situated beyond the diffusion distance of oxygen would be expected to be dead or dying, but in regions of chronically low oxygen tension, clonogenic and radioresistant hypoxic cells may persist. If the tumor shrinks as a result of radiotherapy, or if cells killed by radiation have a decreased demand for oxygen, it is likely that this would allow some of the chronically hypoxic cells to reoxygenate. However, such a reoxygenation process could be quite slow—on the order of days or more—depending on how quickly tumors regress during treatment. The patterns of reoxygenation in some experimental rodent tumors are consistent with this mechanism of reoxygenation, but others are not.

Other rodent tumors reoxygenate very quickly, from about one-half hour upward to several hours or perhaps a day.[133] This occurs in the absence of any measurable tumor shrinkage or change in oxygen use by tumor cells. In such cases, the model of chronic, diffusion-limited hypoxia and slow reoxygenation does not fit the experimental data. During the late 1970s, Brown[134] proposed that a second type of hypoxia might exist in tumors: acute, *perfusion-limited hypoxia*. Based on the knowledge of the vascular physiology of tumors, it was clear that tumor vasculature was often abnormal in structure or function, or both. If tumor vessels were to close transiently from temporary blockage by blood cell components, vascular spasm, or interstitial pressure changes, the tumor cells in the vicinity of those vessels would become acutely hypoxic almost immediately. Assuming blood flow resumed in minutes to hours, the tumor cells would then reoxygenate. Acute hypoxia can also occur in the absence of frank closure or blockage of tumor vessels, such as from changes in red blood cell flux or overall blood flow rate.[135] The existence of acute, perfusion-limited hypoxia would explain the rapid reoxygenation observed for some tumors, but it does not preclude the existence of chronic, diffusion-limited hypoxia.

Acute hypoxia with rapid reoxygenation has since been demonstrated unambiguously for rodent tumors by Chaplin and colleagues.[136,137] It is still not clear how many *human* tumors contain regions of hypoxia, what type of hypoxia is present, whether this varies with tumor type or site, and whether and how rapidly reoxygenation occurs. However, the knowledge that tumor hypoxia is a diverse and dynamic process opens up a number of possibilities for the development of novel interventional strategies designed to cope with or even exploit hypoxia.

Measurement of Hypoxia in Human Tumors

Despite prodigious effort directed at understanding tumor hypoxia and developing strategies to combat the problem, it was not until the mid-1980s that these issues could be addressed for human tumors because there was no way to measure hypoxia in human tumors directly. Before that time, the only way to infer that a human tumor contained treatment-limiting hypoxic cells was by using indirect, nonquantitative methods. Some indirect evidence supporting the notion that human tumors contained clonogenic, radioresistant hypoxic cells (in addition to Thomlinson and Gray's histopathologic study[123]) includes the following:

1. An association between anemia and poor local control rates, which in some cases could be mitigated by blood transfusions before irradiation[138]
2. Success of some clinical trials in which hyperbaric oxygen breathing was used to better oxygenate tumors[139,140]
3. Success of a few clinical trials of oxygen-mimetic hypoxic cell sensitizers combined with radiotherapy[141,142]
4. Variations in vascular density,[143] hemoglobin oxygen load,[144] or specific tumor metabolic functions[145] measured with quantitative histomorphometric techniques, cryospectrophotometry, or ^{31}P nuclear magnetic resonance spectroscopy

In 1988, Gatenby[3] published one of the first studies showing a strong association between directly measured oxygenation status in tumors and clinical outcome. An oxygen-sensing electrode was inserted into the patient's tumor, and multiple readings were taken at different depths along the probe's track. The electrode was also repositioned in different regions of the tumor to assess intertrack variability in oxygen tension. The arithmetic mean Po_2 value for a particular tumor and the tumor volume–weighted Po_2 value directly correlated with local control rate. A high tumor oxygen tension was associated with a high complete response rate, and vice versa. In a similar, prospective study, Höckel and colleagues[4,5] concluded that pretreatment tumor oxygenation was a strong predictor of outcome among patients with intermediate and advanced-stage cervical carcinoma (Fig. 1-24).

Oxygen electrodes are still considered the gold standard against which all other methods for measuring tumor oxygenation are compared. Unfortunately, the method has its limitations. One weakness is that relative to the size of individual tumor cells, the electrode is large, with an average outer diameter of 300 μm, a tip recess of 120 μm, and a sampling area of about 12 μm in diameter.[146] The oxygen tension measurement is regional, and insertions and removals of the probe no doubt perturb the oxygenation status. Another problem is that there is no way to determine whether the tumor cells are viable. If such cells were hypoxic but not clonogenic, they would not be expected to affect the outcome of radiotherapy.

A second direct technique for measuring oxygenation status takes advantage of a serendipitous finding concerning how hypoxic cell radiosensitizers are metabolized. Certain

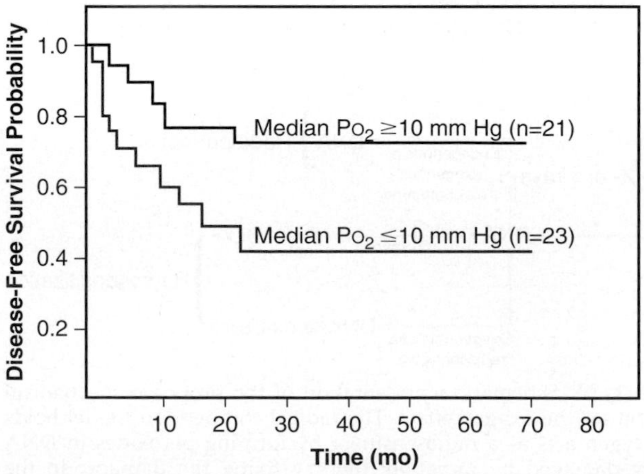

Figure 1-24 The disease-free survival probability of a small cohort of cervical cancer patients stratified according to pretreatment tumor oxygenation measured using an oxygen electrode. (Adapted from Höckel M, Knoop C, Schlenger K, et al: Intratumoral Po_2 predicts survival in advanced cancer of the uterine cervix. Radiother Oncol 26:45, 1993.)

classes of radiosensitizers, including the nitroimidazoles, undergo a bioreductive metabolism in the absence of oxygen that leads to their becoming covalently bound to cellular macromolecules.[147,148] Assuming that the bioreductively bound drug can be quantified by radioactive labeling[149] or tagged with an isotope amenable to detection using positron emission tomography[150] or magnetic resonance spectroscopy,[151] a direct measure of hypoxic fraction can be obtained. Another approach to detecting cells containing bound drug was developed by Raleigh and colleagues.[152-154] This immunohistochemical method involved the development of antibodies specific for the already metabolized, bound nitroimidazoles. After injecting the parent drug, allowing time for the reductive metabolism to occur, taking biopsies of the tumor, and preparing histopathology slides, the specific antibody is then applied to the slides, and regions containing the bound drug are visualized directly. This immunostaining method has the distinct advantages that hypoxia can be studied at the level of individual tumor cells,[155] spatial relationships between regions of hypoxia and other tumor physiologic parameters can be assessed,[156,157] and the drug does not perturb the tumor microenvironment. However, the method remains an invasive procedure, is labor intensive, does not address the issue of the clonogenicity of stained cells (although such cells do have to be metabolically active), and requires multiple samples to be taken because of tumor heterogeneity.

One hypoxia marker (pimonidazole hydrochloride [Hypoxyprobe-1, Chemicon, Temecula, CA]) based on the immunohistologic method is commercially available. It detects reductively bound pimonidazole, and it has been used in experimental and clinical studies around the world.[158-162] Applying Hypoxyprobe-1 to human tumor specimens yields a range of hypoxic fractions similar to that found for experimental rodent tumors and a mean value of approximately 15%.[154,163,164] This marker can also be used to probe disease states other than cancer for which the induction of tissue hypoxia may be part of the cause, such as cirrhosis of the liver[165,166] and ischemia-reperfusion injury in the kidney.[167]

There is also considerable interest in *endogenous* markers of tissue hypoxia[168] that could reduce to some extent the procedural steps involved in and the invasive aspects of detecting hypoxia using exogenous agents. Among the endogenous cellular proteins being investigated in this regard are the hypoxia-inducible factor 1-α (HIF1A, a transcription factor),[169,170] the enzyme carbonic anhydrase IX (CA-9 or CAIX),[171,172] glucose transporter-1 (GLUT1),[173-175] and involucrin, a structural protein found in differentiated squamous epithelial cells.[176,177]

Radiosensitizers, Radioprotectors, and Bioreductive Drugs

The perceived threat that tumor hypoxia posed spawned much research into ways of overcoming the hypoxia problem. One of the earliest proposed solutions was the use of high-LET radiations,[178] which were less dependent on oxygen for their biologic effectiveness. Other agents enlisted to deal with the hypoxia problem included hyperbaric oxygen breathing[139]; artificial blood substitutes with increased oxygen carrying capacity[179]; oxygen-mimetic hypoxic cell radiosensitizers such as misonidazole or etanidazole[141]; hyperthermia[180]; normal tissue radioprotectors, such as amifostine[181]; vasoactive agents thought to modify tumor blood flow, including nicotinamide[182,183]; agents that modify the oxygen-hemoglobin dissociation curve, such as pentoxifylline[184]; and bioreductive drugs designed to be selectively toxic to hypoxic cells, such as tirapazamine.[185,186]

Radiosensitizers

Radiosensitizers are loosely defined as chemical or pharmacologic agents that increase the cytotoxicity of ionizing radiation. *True radiosensitizers* meet the stricter criterion of being relatively nontoxic, acting only as potentiators of radiation toxicity. *Apparent radiosensitizers* still produce the net effect of making the tumor more radioresponsive, but the mechanism is not necessarily synergistic, nor is the agent necessarily nontoxic in and of itself. Ideally, a radiosensitizer is only as good as it is selective for tumors. Agents that show little or no differential effect between tumors and normal tissues do not improve the therapeutic ratio and therefore may not be of much clinical utility. Table 1-2 summarizes some of the classes of radiosensitizers and radioprotectors that have been used in the clinic.

Hypoxic Cell Radiosensitizers

The increased radiosensitivity of cells in the presence of oxygen is believed to result from oxygen's affinity for the electrons produced by the ionization of biomolecules. Molecules other than oxygen also have this chemical property, known as *electron affinity,*[187] including some agents that are not otherwise consumed by the cell. Assuming such an electrophilic compound is not used by the cell, it should diffuse further from capillaries and reach hypoxic regions of a tumor and, acting in an oxygen-mimetic fashion, sensitize hypoxic cells to radiation.

One class of compounds that represented a realistic trade-off between sensitizer efficiency and diffusion effectiveness was the nitroimidazoles, which include such drugs as metronidazole, misonidazole, etanidazole, pimonidazole, and nimorazole. The nitroimidazoles consist of a nitroaromatic imidazole ring, a hydrocarbon side chain that determines the drug's relative lipophilicity, and a nitro group that determines the drug's electron affinity. Misonidazole was extensively characterized in cellular and animal model systems, culminating in its use in clinical trials. Clinical experiences with misonidazole and some of its successor compounds are discussed in Chapter 3.

The relative efficacy of a particular hypoxic cell radiosensitizer is most often described in terms of its sensitizer enhancement ratio (SER), a parameter similar in concept to the OER. Whereas the OER is the ratio of doses to produce the same biologic end point under hypoxic compared with aerobic conditions, the SER is the dose ratio for an isoeffect under hypoxic conditions alone compared with under hypoxic conditions in the presence of the hypoxic cell sensitizer. If a dose of a sensitizer produces an SER of 2.5 to 3.0 for large, single doses of low-LET radiation, it can be considered to a first approximation as effective as oxygen. However, this can be misleading because the dose of the sensitizer required to produce the SER of 3.0 is higher than the comparable amount of oxygen, high enough in some cases to preclude its use clinically. Because the primary mechanism of action of the nitroimidazoles is substitution for oxygen in radiation-induced free radical reactions, these drugs need to be present only in hypoxic regions of the tumor at the time of irradiation.

Unfortunately, the nitroimidazoles also have characteristics that decrease their clinical usefulness. The hydrocarbon side chain of the molecule determines its lipophilicity, and this chemical property affects the drug's pharmacokinetics, which is a primary determinant of drug-induced side effects.[188] The dose-limiting toxicity of the fairly lipophilic agent misonidazole is peripheral neuropathy, an unanticipated and serious side effect.[141,189] Etanidazole was specifically designed to be

Table 1-2 Selected Chemical Modifiers of Radiation Therapy

Chemical Structure	Name (Type of Compound)	Mechanism of Action	Clinical Status	Other Comments
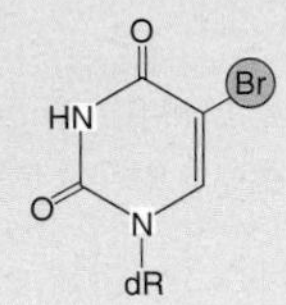	5-Bromodeoxyuridine (halogenated pyrimidine)	Sensitizer of rapidly proliferating cells by incorporation into DNA during S phase of the cell cycle; incorporation results in decrease or removal of shoulder of radiation survival curve	Current laboratory studies focus on ways to increase radiosensitization by altering the method of drug delivery (e.g., longer continuous infusions versus short, repeated exposures)	Requires prolonged exposure before irradiation to be effective; sensitizes rapidly proliferating cells in normal tissues
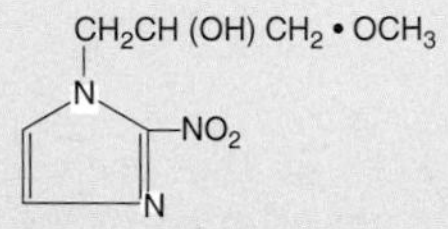	Misonidazole (2-nitroimidazole)	Radiosensitizer of hypoxic cells; principal mechanism of action is mimicry of molecular oxygen's ability to "fix" free radical damage caused by ionizing radiation (and some toxic chemicals)	Disappointing overall, except in selected sites, most notably head and neck tumors; failure ascribed to insufficient tumor levels of drug because of dose-limiting neurologic toxicity	Need only be present at the time of irradiation to be effective; some potential for use as a chemosensitizer and possibly in combination with intraoperative radiation therapy
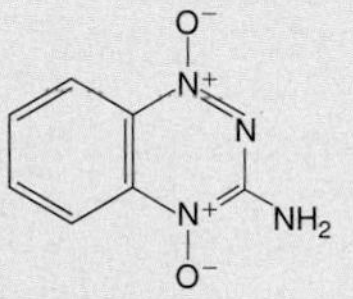	Tirapazamine (organic nitroxide)	Bioreductive drug selectively toxic to hypoxic cells; drug reduced to a toxic intermediate only in the absence of oxygen	In early stages of phase III clinical trials in both North America and Europe as an adjunct to radiation therapy and in phase II trials with platinum compounds	Also called SR 4233; shows overlapping toxicity with ionizing radiation by eliminating an otherwise radioresistant population of (hypoxic) tumor cells; little normal tissue toxicity observed
$NH_2-(CH_2)_3-NH-(CH_2)_2-SH_2PO_3$	Amifostine (thiol compound, free radical scavenger)	Radioprotective compound capable of reversing or "restituting" free radical damage caused by ionizing radiation and some toxic chemicals	Human investigations have focused on the use of amifostine as protection against the nephrotoxicity and ototoxicity of platinum compounds and the hematologic toxicity of cyclophosphamide	Also called WR 2721 (dephosphorylated active metabolite is WR 1065); selectivity for normal tissues achieved due to slow uptake of drug in tumors; need only be present at the time of irradiation to be effective

less lipophilic[190] in the hope of decreasing the neurologic toxicity. Although this goal was accomplished, clinical results with etanidazole were disappointing[191] (see Chapter 3).

In considering the prodigious amount of research and clinical effort that has gone into the investigation of hypoxic cell radiosensitizers over the past 40 years, it is difficult not to be discouraged by the predominantly negative results of the clinical trials. However, these negative results have prompted reevaluation of the hypoxia problem and novel approaches to dealing with it, as well as consideration of other factors that may have contributed to the lack of success of the nitroimidazole radiosensitizers.[189] The following are included among the more obvious issues raised:

1. Did all of the human tumors entered in the clinical trials contain clonogenic hypoxic cells?
2. Do hypoxic cells really matter to the outcome of radiotherapy? If reoxygenation is fairly rapid and complete during radiotherapy, the presence of hypoxic cells before the start of treatment may be of little consequence.
3. Given that the OER is lower for small than for large doses, it follows that the SER would be reduced as well. If so, a benefit in a subgroup of patients might not be readily observed, at least not at a level of statistical significance.

Proliferating Cell Radiosensitizers

Another source of apparent radioresistance is the presence of rapidly proliferating cells. Such cells may not be inherently radioresistant, but instead have the effect of making the tumor seem refractory to treatment because the production of new cells outpaces the cytotoxic action of the therapy.

Analogues of the DNA precursor thymidine, such as bromodeoxyuridine or iododeoxyuridine, can be incorporated into the DNA of actively proliferating cells in place of thymidine because of close structural similarities between the compounds. Cells containing DNA substituted with these halogenated pyrimidines are more radiosensitive than normal cells, with the amount of sensitization directly proportional to the fraction of thymidine replaced.[192] Radiosensitization generally takes the form of a decrease in or elimination of the shoulder region of the radiation survival curve. To be maximally effective, the drug must be present for at least several rounds of DNA replication before irradiation. Although the mechanism by which bromodeoxyuridine and iododeoxyuridine exert their radiosensitizing effect remains somewhat unclear, it is likely that the formation of more complex radiation-induced lesions in the vicinity of the halogenated pyrimidine molecules and interference with DNA damage sensing or repair are involved.[193,194]

The clinical use of halogenated pyrimidines began in the late 1960s, with a major clinical trial in head and neck cancer.[195] In retrospect, the choice of head and neck tumors for this study was far from ideal, because the oral mucosa is also a rapidly proliferating tissue and is similarly radiosensitized, causing severe mucositis.[195] In later years, tumors selected for therapy with halogenated pyrimidines were chosen in the hopes of maximizing a differential radiosensitization between tumors and normal tissues.[196] For example, aggressively growing tumors surrounded by slowly or nonproliferating normal tissues, such as high-grade gliomas, have been targeted.[197-199] Two newer strategies for improving radiosensitization by bromodeoxyuridine and iododeoxyuridine involve changing the schedule of drug delivery in the hope of increasing the therapeutic ratio: giving the drug as a long, continuous infusion before and during radiotherapy[200] and administering the drug as a series of short, repeated exposures.[201]

Bioreductive Drugs

In the wake of the failure of most hypoxic cell radiosensitizers to live up to their clinical potential, a new approach to combating the hypoxia problem emerged: the use of bioreductive drugs that are selectively toxic to hypoxic cells. Although these agents kill rather than sensitize hypoxic cells, the net effect of combining them with radiotherapy is an apparent sensitization of the tumor due to the elimination of an otherwise radioresistant subpopulation. Such drugs have outperformed the nitroimidazole radiosensitizers in experimental studies with clinically relevant fractionated radiotherapy.[202] To the extent that hypoxic cells are also resistant to chemotherapy because of tumor microenvironmental differences in drug delivery, pH, or the cell's proliferative status, complementary tumor cell kill may be anticipated for combinations of bioreductive agents and anticancer drugs.[203]

Most hypoxia-specific cytotoxic drugs fall into three distinct categories: nitroheterocyclics, quinone antibiotics, and organic nitroxides.[204] All require bioreductive activation by nitroreductase enzymes such as cytochrome P450, DT-diaphorase, and the xanthine oxidases to reduce the parent compound to its cytotoxic intermediate, usually an oxidizing free radical capable of damaging DNA and other cellular macromolecules. The active species is not formed or immediately back-oxidized to the parent compound in the presence of oxygen, which accounts for its preferential toxicity under hypoxic conditions. Examples of nitroheterocyclic drugs with bioreductive activity include misonidazole and etanidazole[205,206] and dual-function agents such as RSU 1069[207] and its less systemically toxic pro-drug, RB 6145.[208] The latter drugs are called *dual function* because their bioreduction also activates a bifunctional alkylating moiety capable of introducing crosslinks into DNA. Mitomycin C and several of its analogues (including porfiromycin and EO9) are quinones with bioreductive activity that have been or are being tested in randomized clinical trials of treatment for head and neck tumors.[209]

The lead compound for the third class of bioreductive drugs, the organic nitroxides, is tirapazamine (SR 4233)[185,186,202] (see Table 1-2). The dose-limiting toxicity for single doses of tirapazamine is a reversible hearing loss[210,211]; other effects observed include nausea and vomiting, and muscle cramps.

Tirapazamine is particularly attractive because it retains its hypoxia-selective toxicity over a broader range of (low) oxygen concentrations than the quinones and nitroheterocyclic compounds,[210] and its *hypoxic cytotoxicity ratio,* the ratio of drug doses under hypoxic versus aerobic conditions to yield the same amount of cell kill, averages an order of magnitude higher than for the other classes of bioreductive drugs.[185,186,203] Laboratory and clinical data also support a tumor-sensitizing role for tirapazamine in combination with the chemotherapy agent cisplatinum.[211-214]

Normal Tissue Radioprotectors

Amifostine (WR 2721) is a phosphorothioate compound developed by the U.S. Army for use as a radiation protector (see Table 1-2). Modeled after naturally occurring radioprotective sulfhydryl compounds such as cysteine, cysteamine, and glutathione,[215] amifostine's mechanism of action involves the scavenging of free radicals produced by ionizing radiation, radicals that otherwise could react with oxygen and fix the chemical damage. Amifostine can also detoxify other reactive species through the formation of thioether conjugates, and in part because of this, the drug can also be used as a chemoprotective agent.[181,216] Amifostine is a prodrug that is dephosphorylated by plasma membrane alkaline phosphatase to the free thiol WR 1065, the active metabolite. As is the case with the hypoxic cell radiosensitizers, amifostine need only be present at the time of irradiation to exert its radioprotective effect.

In theory, if normal tissues could be made to tolerate higher total doses of radiation through the use of radioprotectors, the relative radioresistance of hypoxic tumor cells would be negated. However, encouraging preclinical studies demonstrating radioprotection of a variety of cells and tissues notwithstanding,[217-219] radioprotectors such as amifostine would *not* be expected to increase the therapeutic ratio unless they could be introduced selectively into normal tissues but not tumors. The pioneering studies of Yuhas and colleagues[181,220,221] addressed this issue by showing that the drug's active metabolite reached a higher concentration in most normal tissues than in tumors and that this effect mirrored the extent of radioprotection or chemoprotection. The selective protection of normal tissues apparently results from tumors being less able to convert amifostine to WR 1065 and to transport this active metabolite throughout the cell.

Dose-reduction factors (DRFs) (i.e., the ratio of radiation doses to produce an isoeffect in the presence versus the absence of the radioprotector) in the range of 1.5 to 3.5 are achieved for normal tissues, whereas the corresponding DRFs for tumors seldom exceed 1.2. Normal tissues exhibiting the highest DRFs include bone marrow, gastrointestinal tract, liver, testes, and salivary glands.[181] Brain and spinal cord are not protected by amifostine, and oral mucosa is only marginally protected.[181] Comparable protection factors are obtained for some chemotherapy agents, including cyclophosphamide and cisplatin.[222,223] The dose-limiting toxicities associated with the use of amifostine include hypotension, emesis, and generalized weakness or fatigue.[224] Clinical trials with amifostine are described in more detail elsewhere.

Just as there are apparent radiosensitizers, there are apparent radioprotectors that have the net effect of allowing normal tissues to better tolerate higher doses of radiation and chemotherapy, although through mechanisms of action not directly related to the scavenging of free radicals. Various biologic response modifiers, including cytokines, prostaglandins (e.g., misoprostol[225,226]), anticoagulants (e.g., pentoxifylline[227,228]), and protease inhibitors are apparent radioprotectors because they can interfere with the chain of events that normally follows the killing of cells in tissues by, for example, stimulating compensatory repopulation or preventing the development of fibrosis.

CLINICAL RADIOBIOLOGY

Growth Kinetics of Normal Tissues and Tumors

In the simplest sense, normal tissues are normal because the net production of new cells exactly balances the loss of cells from the tissue. In tumors, the production of new cells exceeds cell loss, even if only by a small amount. Although the underlying radiobiology of cells in vitro applies equally to the radiobiology of tissues, the imposition by growth kinetics of this higher level of organizational behavior makes the latter far more complex systems.

Descriptive Classification Systems

Two qualitative classification systems based loosely on the proliferation kinetics of normal tissues are in use. Borrowing heavily from the pioneering work of Bergonié and Tribondeau,[14] Rubin and Casarett's[229] classification system for tissue radiosensitivity has four main categories:

Type I or vegetative intermitotic cells (VIMs) are considered the most radiosensitive and consist of regularly dividing, undifferentiated stem cells, such as those found in the bone marrow, intestinal crypts, and the basal layer of the epidermis of the skin.

Type II or differentiating intermitotic cells (DIMs) are somewhat less radiosensitive and consist of transitional cells that are in the process of developing differentiated characteristics but are still capable of a limited number of cell divisions. Myelocytes of the bone marrow and spermatocytes of the testis are examples of type II cells.

Type III or reverting postmitotic cells (RPMs) are relatively radioresistant and consist of the few types of cells that are fully differentiated and do not divide regularly, but under certain conditions, they can revert to a stem cell–like state and divide as needed. Examples of type III cells include hepatocytes and lymphocytes, although the latter are unique in that they are an exception to the Rubin and Casarett classification system—a reverting postmitotic cell type that is exquisitely radiosensitive.

Type IV or fixed postmitotic cells (FPMs) are the most radioresistant and consist of the terminally differentiated, irreversibly postmitotic cells characteristic of most normal tissue parenchyma, such as neurons and muscle cells. To the best of our current knowledge if these cells are killed by radiation, they cannot be replaced.

A second, simpler classification system, based on anatomic and histologic considerations, has been proposed by Michalowski.[230] Using this system, tissues are categorized on the basis of whether the tissue stem cells, if any, and the functional cells are compartmentalized (i.e., so-called type H or hierarchical tissues, such as skin, gut epithelium, and testis) or intermixed (i.e., type F or flexible tissues, such as lung, liver, kidney, and spinal cord).

Growth Kinetic Parameters and Methodologies

To predict the response of an intact tissue to radiotherapy in a more quantitative way, a number of kinetic parameters have been described that provide a better picture of the proliferative organization of tumors and normal tissues (Table 1-3).

GROWTH FRACTION

Among the first kinetic characteristics described was the growth fraction. The presence of a fraction of slowly cycling or noncycling cells in experimental animal tumors was

Table 1-3 Estimated Cell Cycle Kinetic Parameters for Human Tumors

Parameter	Definition	How Measured	Values for Human Solid Tumors	Comments
T_c	Average cell cycle time	Percent labeled mitosis technique; flow cytometry	0.5-6.5 days (median ≈ 2.5 days)	T_c in vivo usually longer than for comparable cells cultured in vitro
GF	Growth fraction	Estimated from continuous labeling technique	0.05-0.90 (median ≈ 0.40?)	Difficult to measure directly—not much data available
T_{pot}	Potential doubling time	Flow cytometry (relative movement method: $T_{pot} = \lambda T_s/LI$)	2-19 days (median ≈ 5 days)	$T_{pot} \approx T_c$ as GF approaches 1.0
ϕ	Cell loss factor	$1-T_{pot}/T_d$	0.30-0.95 (median ≈ 0.90?)	Thought to be the major cause of long T_d values for human tumors, particularly high in carcinomas
T_d	Volume doubling time	Direct measurement of tumor dimensions over time	5-650 days (median ≈ 90 days)	Increases with increasing tumor size, often because of increases in T_c and ϕ and a decrease in GF
T_{eff}	Effective clonogen doubling time	Estimated from clinical data on the loss of local control with increasing overall treatment time	4-8 days	T_{eff} approaches T_{pot} near the end of a course of fractionated radiation therapy

LI, S-phase pulse labeling index; T_S, duration of S phase; λ, correction factor related to the nonuniform distribution of cell ages in a growing population.
Data from Steel G (ed): Basic Clinical Radiobiology, 3rd ed. London, Arnold, 2002; Steel G: Growth Kinetics of Tumours. Oxford, Clarendon Press, 1977.

first observed by Mendelsohn and colleagues[231,232] and subsequently observed in human tumors by other investigators. Although normal tissues do not "grow" and therefore do not have a growth fraction, some are composed of noncycling cells that have differentiated to carry out tissue-specific functions. Some normal tissues do contain a small fraction of actively proliferating stem cells, and others contain apparently dormant or resting cells that are temporarily out of the traditional four-phase cell cycle but are capable of renewed proliferation in response to appropriate stimuli. Lajtha[233] gave these resting but recruitable cells of normal tissues the designation G_0. A tumor counterpart of the G_0 cell may or may not exist, but most slowly or noncycling tumor cells are thought to be in such a state because of nutrient deprivation, not because of a normal cell cycle regulatory mechanism. Dethlefsen[234] suggested that the term *Q cell* be reserved for quiescent cells in tumors to distinguish them from the G_0 cell of normal tissues.

Measurement of the growth fraction is problematic,[235,236] but an estimate can be obtained with a technique known as *continuous thymidine labeling*. Using this method, the tumor receives a continuous infusion of radiolabeled thymidine for a period long enough for all proliferating cells to have gone through at least one round of DNA synthesis and incorporated the radioactive label. Then, a biopsy of the tumor is obtained and tissue sections prepared for autoradiography. After the slides are processed and scored, the continuous labeling index, which is the fraction of the total population of tumor cells containing tritiated thymidine, is calculated. This value is a rough estimate of the tumor's growth fraction.

Cell Cycle and Volume Doubling Times

The percent labeled mitosis (PLM) technique of Quastler and Sherman[237] was a key development in the study of the cell cycle in vivo, because it provided a unique window into the behavior of that small fraction of cells within a tissue that was actively proliferating. By focusing on cells in mitosis, the assay allowed the overall cell cycle time (T_c) and the durations of the individual cell cycle phases to be determined without the uncertainties introduced by the presence of noncycling cells in the population. Flow cytometric methods have largely replaced the arduous and time-consuming PLM assay.

The PLM technique involves tracking over time a cohort of proliferating cells that initially were in S phase (and exposed briefly to tritiated thymidine) and then proceeded through subsequent mitotic divisions. Serial biopsy samples from the tissue of interest are obtained at regular intervals after labeling, and the fraction of cells in mitosis (identified cytologically) and carrying the radioactive label is determined. A first peak of labeled mitoses is seen within 24 hours after labeling, and as cells pass through their second division, a second wave of labeled mitoses is observed. The average T_c for the population of proliferating cells corresponds to the peak-to-peak interval of the resulting PLM curve, a plot of the fraction of labeled mitoses as a function of time after the radioactive pulse. With sufficiently robust data, the durations of the individual cell cycle phases also can be obtained. The PLM technique is illustrated schematically in Figure 1-25.

Historically, the interpretation of PLM curves was sometimes hampered by technical artifacts and by the fact that proliferating cell populations have distributed cell cycle times.[235,236,238] Despite these limitations, it is known that most cells in vivo proliferate more slowly than their in vitro counterparts. Although the variation in intermitotic times is quite large, a median value for T_c of 2 to 3 days is a reasonable estimate.[140,235]

Even though the cycle times of proliferating cells in vivo are long by cell culture standards, they are quite short compared with the corresponding population or volume doubling times (T_d) for human tumors. Although highly variable from tumor type to tumor type and somewhat difficult to measure, the T_d for human solid tumors averages about 3 to 4 months.[140,235] In many cases, sample calculations further suggest that the discrepancy between T_c for proliferating

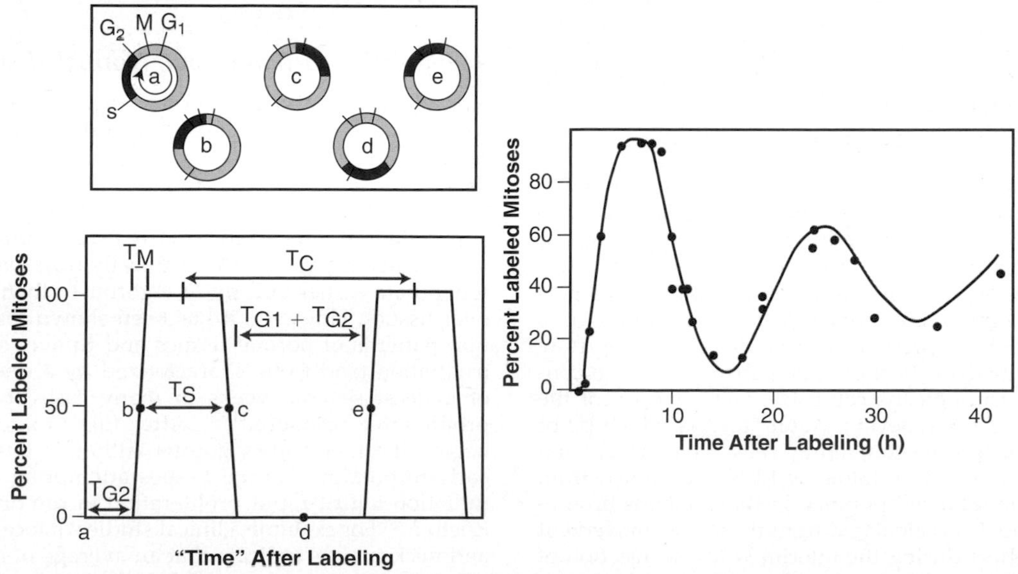

Figure 1-25 The technique of percent labeled mitoses (PLM) for an idealized cell population with identical cell cycle times *(left panels)* and for a representative normal tissue or tumor with a dispersion in cell cycle times *(right panel)*. *Upper left panel,* After a brief exposure to tritiated thymidine or equivalent at time a, the labeled cohort of S-phase cells continues *(dark shading)* around the cell cycle and is sampled at times b, c, d, and e. *Lower left panel,* For each sample, the percentage of cells both in mitosis and containing the thymidine label is determined, and it is plotted as a function of time. From such a graph, individual cell cycle phase durations can be derived. *Right panel,* In this more practical example, a mathematical fit to the PLM data would be needed to calculate the (average) cell cycle phase durations.

tumor cells and T_d for the tumor as a whole cannot be accounted for solely by the tumor having a low growth fraction.

Cell Loss Factor

Cell kineticists initially adhered to the notion that the continued growth of tumors over time necessarily reflected abnormalities in cell production. Pathologists and tumor biologists had ample evidence that tumors routinely lost large numbers of cells as the result of cell death, maturation, or emigration.[235,239] It is now clear that the overall rate of tumor growth, as reflected by its T_d, is governed by the competing processes of cell production and cell loss. The cell loss factor (ϕ), the rate of cell loss expressed as a fraction of the cell production rate, is surprisingly high for experimental and human tumors; it is as high as 0.9 or more for carcinomas and lower, on average, for sarcomas.[240] Cell loss is probably the single most important factor governing the overall volume doubling time of solid tumors.

The clinical implications of tumors having high rates of cell loss are obvious. First, any attempts at making long-term predictions of treatment outcome based on short-term regression rates of tumors during treatment are misleading. Second, although regression rate may not correlate well with eventual outcome, it may be a reasonable indicator of when best to schedule subsequent therapy, on the assumption that a smaller tumor will be more radiosensitive and chemosensitive, as well as easier to remove surgically.

Potential Doubling Time and Effective Doubling Time

With the recognition that cell loss played a major role in the overall growth rate of tumors and that it could mask a high cell production rate, a better measure of the potential repopulation rate of normal tissues and tumors was needed.[241] The best available indicator of regenerative capacity is the potential doubling time, usually referred to as T_{pot}.[235,242] By definition, T_{pot} is an estimate of the time that would be required to double the number of clonogenic cells in the absence of cell loss. It follows that T_d usually is much longer than T_{pot} because of cell loss and that T_c usually is shorter than T_{pot} because of the presence of nonproliferating cells.[238]

T_{pot} can be estimated from a comparison of the S-phase pulse labeling index (LI) and the duration of S phase (T_S) by using the following equation:

$$T_{pot} = \lambda T_S / LI$$

in which λ is a correction factor related to the nonuniform distribution of cell ages in a growing population (usually, $\lambda \approx 0.8$). T_S and LI can be determined by the relative movement method.[242,243] This technique involves an injection of a thymidine analogue, usually bromodeoxyuridine, which is promptly incorporated into newly synthesized DNA of S phase cells and whose presence can be detected using flow cytometry. The labeled cohort of cells is then allowed to continue movement through the cell cycle, and a biopsy of the tissue of interest is taken several hours later, at which point most bromodeoxyuridine-containing cells have progressed into G_2 phase or beyond. A value for LI is determined from the fraction of the total cell population that contains bromodeoxyuridine, and T_S is calculated from the rate of movement of the labeled cohort during the interim between injection of the tracer and biopsy.

Values for T_{pot} for human tumors have been obtained by several investigators, and although quite variable, they typically range between 2 and 20 days.[235,241,244-246] These findings lend support to the idea that slowly growing tumors can contain subpopulations of rapidly proliferating cells; to the extent that these cells retain unlimited reproductive potential, they may be considered the tumor stem cells (to a first approximation), which are capable of causing recurrences after treatment. These cells represent a serious threat to local control of the tumor by conventional therapies, especially protracted therapies.

The use of a cell kinetic parameter such as T_{pot} as a predictor of a tumor's response to therapy or as a means of identifying subsets of patients particularly at risk for recurrence has been attempted, with some positive but mostly negative results.[6,140,247] These negative findings may suggest that proliferation in tumors is not important, but it is unlikely that a pretreatment estimate of T_{pot} or any other single cell kinetic parameter (e.g., LI) would be relevant after treatment commences and the growth kinetics of the tumor are perturbed.

One approach to dealing with this problem is to measure proliferative activity during treatment. Although not without other limitations, the use of an *effective clonogen doubling time* (T_{eff}) has been advocated.[244-246,248] Estimates of T_{eff} can be obtained from two types of experiments. In an experimental setting, T_{eff} can be inferred from the additional dose necessary to keep a certain level of tissue reaction constant as the overall treatment time is increased. (When expressed in terms of dose rather than time, the proper term would be D_{eff}, although the underlying concept is the same.) For example, acute skin reactions usually develop and begin to resolve during the course of radiotherapy, suggesting that the production of new cells in response to injury gradually surpasses the killing of existing cells by each subsequent dose fraction. By intensifying treatment after this repopulation begins, it is theoretically possible to reach a steady state in which the tissue reaction remains constant. In a clinical setting, T_{eff} can be obtained from studies in which a fairly standard fraction size and dose are used to treat a particular type of tumor, but the overall treatment time varies from patient to patient. In some cases, the rate of loss of local control with increasing overall treatment time provides an estimate of T_{eff} and of the delay time before the repopulation begins, sometimes referred to as the repopulation *kickoff time* (T_k).[245,249-251]

Repopulation in Tumors and Normal Tissues

Normal tissues and tumors are capable of increasing their cell production rate in response to depopulation caused by radiation, a process known as *regeneration* or *repopulation*. The time of onset of the regenerative response varies with the turnover rate of the tissue or tumor, because cell death (and depopulation) after irradiation is usually linked to cell division. Generally, tissues that naturally turn over fairly rapidly repopulate earlier and more vigorously than slowly turning over tissues. However, it has been shown that the repopulation patterns of normal tissues and tumors after the start of irradiation tend to be characterized by a delay (i.e., see T_k), of at least several weeks in many cases, before the rapid proliferative response.[248-250] After this proliferative response begins, it can be quite vigorous. Although this is desirable for early-responding normal tissues attempting to recover from radiation injury, rapid proliferation in tumors is counterproductive.[252] For example, clinical studies of local control of head and neck tumors indicate that an average of about 0.6 Gy per day is lost to repopulation.[248] Unfortunately, attempts to counteract this accelerated proliferation by dose intensification during the latter part of a treatment course can be problematic because late-responding normal tissues do not benefit from accelerated repopulation during treatment, and they risk incurring complications.

Increased cell production in response to injury is thought to occur by one or more of three basic mechanisms: a decrease in the cell loss rate, a shortening of the cell cycle time, or an increase in the growth fraction.[59,235] Normal tissues are capable of using at least the latter two strategies to accelerate repopulation. It is still not clear how, when, and to what extent tumors accelerate their proliferation in response to the cell kill. Laboratory and clinical findings suggest that a decrease in cell loss may be a major mechanism, possibly as a consequence of resistance to apoptosis, a hallmark of most types of cancer.[246,253] This is quite a provocative finding in that it suggests that there may be a fundamental—and potentially exploitable—difference in the way normal and tumor tissues respond to ionizing radiation.

Early and Late Effects in Normal Tissues

Early versus Late

Normal tissue complications observed after radiotherapy are the result of killing critical target cells within the tissue, which are crucial to the tissue's continued functional and structural integrity. Loss of these target cells can occur as a direct consequence of the cytotoxic action of the radiation or as a result of killing other cells. In some cases, the tissue's response to the depletion of its component cells can exacerbate the injury, such as when a hyperproliferation of fibroblasts and the resulting collagen deposition replace a tissue's parenchymal cells, resulting in fibrosis.

A particular tissue or organ may contain more than one type of target cell, each with its own radiosensitivity. Accordingly, one tissue may manifest more than one complication after radiotherapy, with the severity of each determined by the radiosensitivity of the particular target cell and the time-dose-fractionation schedule employed. It follows from this that the severity of one complication does not necessarily predict for the severity of another complication, even within the same tissue, although consequential late effects resulting from severe early reactions are possible in some cases.[254] For example, dry or moist desquamation of the skin results from the depletion of the basal cells of the epidermis, fibrosis results from damage to dermal fibroblasts, and telangiectasia results from damage to small blood vessels in the dermis. For many tissues, however, the target cells whose deaths are responsible for a particular normal tissue injury remain unclear.

The radiosensitivity of the putative target cells determines the severity of an early or late effect in a normal tissue, but the timing of the clinical manifestation of that injury is related to the tissue's proliferative organization. This dissociation between radiosensitivity and radioresponsiveness (i.e., the injury's onset time) was a long-standing source of confusion during the first half of the 20th century. For example, Bergonié and Tribondeau's laws,[14] although still roughly applicable, confuse the concepts of radiosensitivity and radioresponsiveness to some extent.

Whole-Body Irradiation Syndromes

Many human beings have been exposed to total-body irradiation, including the survivors of Hiroshima and Nagasaki, Polynesian Islanders and military personnel present during above-ground nuclear tests during the 1950s, and victims of accidental exposures in the workplace (including Chernobyl). Of the latter, about 100 fatalities due to radiation accidents have been documented since the mid-1940s.[255-257]

The *whole-body irradiation syndromes* are considered early effects of radiation exposure because death occurs within weeks after sufficiently high doses of radiation. The clinical syndromes described later occur only when the entire body is irradiated. Although total-body irradiation (TBI) is a prerequisite for the manifestation of these syndromes, neither the dose received nor its biologic consequences are necessarily uniform. The radiosensitivities of the respective target cells determine the effective threshold dose below which the syndrome does not occur, whereas the onset time of individual symptoms is more a function of the proliferative organization of the tissue.

The mean lethal dose (LD_{50}) is defined as the (whole-body) dose that results in mortality for 50% of an irradiated population. The LD_{50} value is often expressed in terms of the time scale over which the deaths occur, such as at 30 or 60 days after irradiation. For humans, the single dose $LD_{50/60}$ is approximately 3.5 Gy in the absence of medical intervention and about twice that with careful medical management.[31,256] The LD_{50} increases with decreasing dose rate of low-LET radiation, and it decreases for radiations of increasing LET.

Prodromal Syndrome

The prodromal syndrome consists of one or more transient, neuromuscular and gastrointestinal symptoms that begin soon after irradiation and persist for up to several hours. The severity and duration of symptoms, which can include anorexia, nausea, vomiting, diarrhea, fatigue, disorientation, and hypotension, increase with increasing dose. Because in many radiation accident situations the dose is unknown, careful attention to the prodromal syndrome can be used as a crude dosimeter.

Cerebrovascular Syndrome

The cerebrovascular syndrome occurs for total-body doses in excess of 50 Gy. Exposure is followed almost immediately by the onset of signs and symptoms consisting of severe gastrointestinal and neuromuscular disturbances, including nausea and vomiting, disorientation, ataxia, and convulsions.[31,256] The cerebrovascular syndrome is invariably fatal, and survival time is seldom longer than about 48 hours. Only a few instances of accidental exposure to such high doses have occurred, two of which—a nuclear criticality accident at Los Alamos National Laboratory in 1958 and a ^{235}U reprocessing plant accident in Rhode Island in 1964—have been extensively documented in the medical literature.[258,259]

The target cells whose deaths are responsible for the cerebrovascular syndrome remain unclear. The immediate cause of death is likely vascular damage leading to some combination of progressive brain edema, hemorrhage, cardiovascular shock, meningitis, myelitis, and encephalitis.[256] After such high doses delivered in a short period, even cells traditionally considered radioresistant, such as neurons and the parenchymal cells of other tissues and organs, can be considered targets, as well as the more radiosensitive vascular endothelial cells and the various glial cells of the central nervous system.

Gastrointestinal Syndrome

For doses of more than 8 Gy, the gastrointestinal syndrome predominates, characterized by lethargy, vomiting, diarrhea, dehydration, electrolyte imbalance, malabsorption, weight loss, and sepsis. These symptoms begin to appear within a few days of irradiation, and they are progressive in nature, culminating in death after 5 to 10 days. The target cells for the gastrointestinal syndrome are the crypt stem cells of the gut epithelium. As mature cells of the villi are lost over several days, no new cells are available to replace them, and the villi begin to shorten and eventually become completely denuded. This greatly increases the risk of bleeding and sepsis, both of which are aggravated by the declining blood counts.

Before the Chernobyl accident, in which approximately a dozen firefighters received total doses sufficient to succumb to the gastrointestinal syndrome, there was only a single documented case of a human dying of gastrointestinal injury.[31,256] No human has survived exposure to 10 Gy or more of low-LET radiation.

HEMATOPOIETIC SYNDROME

Acute doses of approximately 2.5 Gy or more are sufficient to produce the hematopoietic syndrome, a consequence of killing bone marrow stem cells and lymphocytes. This syndrome is characterized by a precipitous (within a day or two) reduction in the peripheral blood lymphocyte count, followed by a more gradual reduction (over a period of several weeks) in the numbers of circulating leukocytes, platelets, and erythrocytes. The granulocytopenia and thrombocytopenia reach a maximum within 30 days after exposure, and death, if it does occur, is usually a result of infection or hemorrhage, or both.[31,256] Theoretically, the use of antibiotics, blood transfusions, and bone marrow transplantation can save the lives of individuals who receive doses at or near the LD_{50}. In practice, however, the exact dose is seldom known, and if it were high enough to reach the threshold for the gastrointestinal syndrome, heroic measures would be in vain. Unfortunately, this was the case for all but 2 of the 13 Chernobyl accident victims who received bone marrow transplants.[31] Of the two survivors, only one can rightfully be claimed as having had his life saved by bone marrow transplantation; the other survivor showed autologous bone marrow repopulation.

Teratogenesis

One of the most anxiety-provoking risks of irradiation in the eyes of the general public is prenatal exposure of the developing embryo or fetus.[255,256] In part, such concern is warranted because teratogenic effects are quite sensitive to induction by ionizing radiation, with readily measurable neurologic abnormalities observed in individuals exposed prenatally to doses as low as approximately 0.06 Gy.[31] The radiation-induced excess relative risk of teratogenesis during the most sensitive phase of gestation is approximately 40% per Gy.[31] For comparative purposes, the spontaneous incidence of a congenital abnormality occurring during an otherwise normal pregnancy is about 5% to 10%.[255]

Information on the teratogenic effects of radiation in humans comes from two major sources: Japanese atomic bomb survivors and patients who underwent diagnostic or therapeutic irradiation before the establishment of modern radiation protection standards or in clinical emergency situations. Although a range of abnormalities have been identified in individuals irradiated in utero (including anecdotal reports of miscarriages and stillbirths, cataracts and other ocular defects, gross malformations, and sterility), the most commonly reported are microcephaly, mental retardation, more subtle neurologic defects, and growth retardation.[31,255,256] Each of these teratogenic effects has a temporal relationship to the stage of gestation at the time of irradiation, as well as a radiation dose and dose rate dependency. Lethality is the most common consequence of irradiation during the preimplantation stage (≤10 days of conception); growth retardation has been identified for irradiation during the implantation stage (10 to 14 days after conception); and during the organogenesis period (15 to 50 days after conception), the embryo is sensitive to lethal, teratogenic, and growth-retarding effects.[256] Radiation-induced gross abnormalities of the major organ systems do not occur during the fetal period (>40 days after conception), although generalized growth retardation and some neurologic defects have been observed for radiation doses in excess of 1 Gy.

Radiation-Induced Cataracts

Late effects resulting from irradiation of the eye were observed within a few years of the discovery of x-rays,[229,256] with cataracts being the most frequent pathologic finding. From a clinical perspective, the induction of a cataract after radiotherapy is a normal tissue complication that can be corrected surgically, and it is not considered as dire as other late effects. Some radiation-induced lens opacities are subtle and do not interfere with vision. From a radiobiologic perspective, however, cataracts are unique among the somatic effects of radiation in several respects. First, although the lens of the eye is a self-renewing tissue complete with a stem cell compartment of epithelial cells that divide and gradually differentiate into mature lens fibers, there appears to be no clear mechanism of cell loss.[31] The primitive cells damaged by radiation (which manifest as abnormal, opaque lens fibers) persist, eventually leading to a cataract. Second, radiation-induced cataracts are among the few lesions that can be distinguished pathologically from their spontaneously occurring counterparts. Radiation-induced cataracts first appear in the posterior pole of the lens, whereas spontaneous cataracts usually begin in the anterior pole of the lens.[260] Third, radiogenic cataracts exhibit a variable latency period (about 1 year to several decades) that decreases with increasing radiation dose. Unlike many other effects of ionizing radiation, cataract formation is a nonstochastic (deterministic) process; there is a threshold dose below which no cataracts occur, but above the threshold, the severity of the cataract increases with increasing dose.[260] For low-LET radiation, the single-dose threshold for cataractogenesis in humans is approximately 2 Gy, and this increases to about 4 Gy for fractionated exposures. Neutrons also are effective at inducing cataracts, with RBEs of about 5 to 10 commonly observed in laboratory rodents.[256]

Radiation Carcinogenesis

Unrepaired or mis-rejoined DNA damage caused by radiation exposure is usually lethal to the cell, although this is not invariably the case, particularly when the genetic material is rearranged rather than deleted. Whether such changes have further implications for the cell (and the organism) bearing them depends on the location of the damage in the genome, the nature and extent of the mutational event, whether working copies of proteins can still be produced from the gene or genes involved, what function these proteins normally have, and the type of cell. There is compelling evidence that some of these radiation-induced genetic rearrangements—particularly ones that activate oncogenes or inactivate tumor suppressor genes—alone or in combination with other such changes, predispose a cell to neoplastic transformation, a necessary early step in the process of tumor induction.[255,261]

LABORATORY STUDIES

Although ionizing radiation is one of the most studied and best understood of carcinogenic agents, it is not a particularly potent carcinogen. This fact hampers studies of radiation carcinogenesis in humans, because the investigator must identify a modest radiogenic increment of excess risk with a long latency period against a high background spontaneous cancer rate and multiple confounding factors. Nevertheless, from a public health perspective, carcinogenesis is the most important somatic effect of radiation for doses of 1.5 Gy or less.[31]

The use of cell culture and laboratory rodent systems to study carcinogenesis avoids some of the pitfalls of human epidemiologic studies, but they have their own inherent limitations. Cell culture systems employ neoplastic transformation as the end point, which is a prerequisite for but by no means equal to carcinogenesis in vivo. Neoplastic transformation is defined as the acquisition of one or more phenotypic traits in nontumorigenic cells that are usually associated with tumor cells, such as immortalization, reduced contact inhibition of growth, increased anchorage-independent growth, reduced need for exogenously supplied nutrients and growth factors, various morphologic and biochemical changes, and in most cases, the ability to form tumors in histocompatible animals.[238] Such systems can be used to study relatively early events in the carcinogenesis process, have much greater sensitivity and statistical resolution than in vivo assays, and can be used to measure dose-response relationships. Laboratory animal studies, however, are considered more relevant in that tumor formation is the end point, latency periods are shorter, statistical variability is reduced, and the carcinogen exposure conditions can be carefully controlled.

Pertinent results from laboratory studies of radiation carcinogenesis include the following:

1. Carcinogenesis is a stochastic effect; it is a probabilistic function of the dose received, with no evidence of a dose threshold. Increasing the radiation dose increases the probability of the effect, although not its severity.[31,255,256,261]
2. The neoplastic transformation frequency increases linearly with dose, at least over the low dose range (≤1.5 Gy).
3. There is a dose rate effect for transformation and carcinogenesis (for low-LET radiations); protracted exposures carry a reduced risk relative to acute exposures.
4. The processes of neoplastic transformation and carcinogenesis are necessarily in competition with the cell-killing effects of ionizing radiation.[31] Dose-response curves for tumor formation in vivo tend to be bell shaped as a function of dose.[262] In vitro, where cytotoxicity can be assessed separately from transformation and appropriate corrections made, dose-response curves tend to be more linear.

Epidemiologic Studies in Humans

In humans, most of the information useful for risk estimation is derived from epidemiologic studies, with the dose almost always exceeding 0.1 Gy and often exceeding 1.0 Gy. However, most of the controversy concerns doses less than 0.1 Gy that are delivered over protracted periods. To infer low-dose effects from high-dose data, epidemiologists make extrapolations and assumptions about dose-response relationships that may or may not be valid in all cases.

Many sources of error can also plague epidemiologic data, including selection bias, small sample size, heterogeneous population characteristics, and dose uncertainties.[256] The human populations that have been and continue to be evaluated for radiation-induced excess cancers include Japanese atomic bomb survivors, persons exposed to fallout from nuclear tests or accidents, radiation workers receiving occupational exposure, populations living in areas characterized by above-average natural background radiation or in proximity to man-made sources of radiation, and patients exposed to repeated diagnostic or therapeutic irradiation. Pertinent findings from these studies include the following:

1. Within the limits of statistical resolution, the shape of the dose-response curve for radiation carcinogenesis is consistent with a linear, no-threshold model.[255,261]
2. Different tissues have different sensitivities to radiation-induced carcinogenesis, with bone marrow (leukemias other than chronic lymphocytic), breast (female), salivary glands, and thyroid the most susceptible, followed by colon, stomach, lung, ovary, and skin.[256]
3. The latency period between irradiation and the clinical presentation of a solid tumor averages 20 years or more and about one-half that for hematologic malignancies. However, the latency period varies with the age of the individual, generally increasing with decreasing age at exposure.
4. Two risk projection models have been used to predict the risk of radiation carcinogenesis in the human population: the absolute risk model and the relative risk model. Using the absolute risk model, excess risk in an irradiated population begins after the latency period has passed and is *added* to the age-adjusted spontaneous cancer risk. After some period, the cancer risk returns to spontaneous levels. The relative risk model predicts that the excess cancer risk is a *multiple* of the spontaneous incidence. Which model is the most appropriate for estimating the excess cancer risk remains debatable.[256] The epidemiologic data tend to support the relative risk model for most solid tumors and the absolute risk model for leukemia.
5. The recommendations of the International Commission on Radiological Protection (ICRP) state that the nominal probability of radiation-induced cancer death is approximately 4% per sievert (Sv) for working adults and about 5% per Sv for the whole population under conditions of chronic, low-dose exposure.[263] These risk estimates double for acute, high-dose exposures. The sievert (Sv) is a unit of dose equivalent used for radiation protection purposes, and it is equal to the radiation dose (in Gy) multiplied by a quality factor specific for the type of radiation (the quality factor is roughly equivalent to the radiation's RBE).

Carcinogenic Risk from Prenatal Irradiation

The risk of carcinogenesis as a result of prenatal radiation exposure is made even more controversial by conflicting results of epidemiologic studies. One major study cohort consisted of several thousand children (plus a demographically similar population of unirradiated children) who received prenatal exposure from diagnostic procedures during the 1950s and 1960s. The Oxford Survey of Childhood Cancer[264] reported nearly twice the incidence of leukemia in children who had received prenatal irradiation. Although other epidemiologic studies lend credence to the Oxford Survey's findings,[256,261] it is still unclear whether factors other than the x-ray exposure may have caused or contributed to the excess cancer risk. Other studies, particularly from the Japanese A-bomb survivors who were pregnant at the time of the bombing, did not support the Oxford Survey's findings of increased risk of childhood malignancy, but they did support an increased risk of malignancy later in life.[31]

On the assumption that it is preferable to overestimate risk than underestimate it, it is prudent to assume that the carcinogenic risk of radiation exposure to the embryo or fetus is about twice that for postnatal exposure.

Early and Late Effects after Radiotherapy

This section of the chapter cannot provide an exhaustive review of the various histopathologic changes observed in irradiated normal tissues of radiotherapy patients, but more information can be found in textbooks and pertinent review articles on the subject.[229,256,265] This section focuses instead on developments that promise to increase our understanding of the causes of normal tissue injuries and provide clues about how to decrease or prevent their occurrence.

Molecular Cascades and Cytokines

The early and late effects that occur in irradiated normal tissues result directly or indirectly from the killing of critical target cells. Although this statement is true in a general sense, it is an oversimplification of what is now known to be a highly complex and dynamic process of cellular signaling cascades, radiation-inducible gene expression, multiple modes of cell death (e.g., clonogenic death, apoptosis, necrosis), and compensatory proliferative responses. Cytokines and growth factors, inducible proteins released by irradiated tissues that stimulate other cells to produce a biologic response, participate in some of these processes. Although produced locally within the irradiated volume and intended to influence the behavior of cells in the same tissue, some cytokines also enter the circulation and can stimulate cells distant from the irradiated site (see Chapter 2).

For example, the radiation-inducible cytokines interleukin-1 (IL-1) and tumor necrosis factor (TNF), released by leukocytes and tumor cells, alter the growth of hematopoietic progenitor cells, stimulate the growth of vascular endothelial cells, and induce collagen deposition.[266,267] These same molecules are involved in the acute inflammatory response often observed in irradiated tissues and, along with intercellular adhesion molecule-1 (ICAM-1, CD54), in the changes in vascular permeability that lead to edema. Lung irradiation results in the expression of several interleukins, transforming growth factor-β (TGF-β), and basic fibroblast growth factor (bFGF), all of which may play roles in acute radiation pneumonitis and in late fibrosis.[268-270] TNF, bFGF, and platelet-derived growth factor (PDGF) are associated with aberrant growth of cells within blood vessels. These proteins are induced in the vascular endothelium to stimulate cell proliferation and minimize radiation-induced apoptosis.[271]

Functional Subunits and Volume Effects

Radiation oncologists traditionally reduce the total dose when the irradiation field involves a large volume of normal tissue. Although this practice evolved empirically, the biologic basis for decreasing normal tissue tolerance with increasing irradiation volume remains unclear. Withers[241,272] proposed a descriptive model for the pathogenesis of radiation injury in normal tissues based on the structural and functional organization of the tissue at risk for a complication. Conceptually, tissues are considered to be organized into functional subunits (FSUs), which can be inactivated by radiation exposure because their constituent target cells are killed. Because each FSU contains a variable number of target cells that theoretically cannot be resupplied by an adjacent FSU, if all such cells are killed, the FSU is permanently inactivated. If some tissue-specific minimum number of such target cells survives—a *tissue rescuing unit*—the FSU will be able to repopulate itself and may resume its normal function. Whether the inactivation of one or more FSUs impacts the overall tissue function (in the form of a radiation-induced complication) depends on how many of the tissue's FSUs are in the irradiation field and how they are structurally arranged in the tissue.

In some tissues, the FSU model reasonably predicts the pattern of changing tolerance with changing irradiation volume, all other treatment parameters being equal. In other tissues, however, it remains unclear what constitutes an FSU in the anatomic sense, how these are organized, or what the critical target cells are. In the kidney, for example, it is likely that the FSU is the nephron and that renal tubule epithelial cells are among the critical targets.[273] In the epidermis of the skin, basal cells are clearly a target cell population, but what constitutes a discrete epidermal FSU is less clear.[79] The spinal cord and nerve bundles in general respond to changing irradiation volume as if their corresponding FSUs are arranged in series. There is a steep reduction in the tolerance dose for white matter necrosis of the rat spinal cord with increasing treatment volume for small radiation fields (up to about 2 cm exposed cord length), but there is little or no volume dependence for larger treatment fields, presumably because inactivation of one FSU inactivates FSUs of the entire spinal cord.[140] However, the FSUs themselves and their target cells have yet to be identified unambiguously.[274,275]

Reirradiation Tolerance

A common problem that radiation oncologists face is whether or not to risk reirradiation of a previously treated site. If a decision is made to treat again, even in the most ideal case in which the previous treatment course is well documented and the treatment fields still identifiable, the clinician is nevertheless left with the uncertainty of what time, dose, and fractionation pattern to use.

Radiobiologic research in this area has been slow in coming (given the very nature of studies involving late effects), but some progress has been made and some of the factors thought to be involved in normal tissue tolerance to retreatment have been identified. These include whether the initial treatment course was given to full tolerance, the likelihood that residual damage from the first treatment course has persisted, the amount of time that has elapsed between the first course and the second, the target volume to be reirradiated compared with the original target volume, and the structural and function makeup of the tissue at risk.

A few general concepts are beginning to emerge from studies with laboratory rodents, and they have been described in several reviews[140,276,277]:

1. For rapidly proliferating tissues such as skin, bone marrow, or testis, recovery after the first course of treatment is rapid, and the tissue can be reirradiated to near the full tolerance dose within about 2 to 3 months.
2. Some slowly proliferating tissues such as spinal cord and lung are capable of a more limited, long-term recovery after the first course of treatment, and they can be treated again to a partial (50% to 75%) tolerance dose, with the dose generally increasing the longer the time between the two treatments (3 to 6 months minimum).
3. Other slowly dividing tissues such as bladder seem to show permanent, residual injury from the first treatment, and the total dose for a second course must be reduced by at least one half, regardless of how much time has elapsed between treatments. There is evidence that complications arising from repeat treatment tend to occur much earlier (relative to the second treatment) than they would have from a single treatment.
4. One apparent exception to this type of classification system is the kidney, for which re-treatment tolerance actually seems to decrease with time between the first and second treatment courses.

A model that is consistent with these observations suggests that target cells that survive the initial treatment course have three possible fates. Some may regenerate their numbers over time, making the tissue as a whole better able to tolerate a second treatment, with the rate of regeneration determining how much time should elapse between the two treatments and what total dose can be delivered safely during the second course. Other target cells may maintain a steady-state number of survivors after the first treatment, and the tissue therefore appears to harbor residual damage and to be unable to tolerate a full second course of radiotherapy. Some target cells may undergo continued depletion after the first treatment, such that tolerance to a second treatment course actually decreases with longer times between treatments. This may be related to a progressive expression of otherwise subclinical residual damage from the initial treatment.

Radiation-Induced Second Malignancies

With increasing numbers of long-term cancer survivors, the risk of second malignancies arising as a consequence of prior treatment is a significant concern. Leukemia is thought to account for about 20% of the second malignancies, with the remainder manifesting as solid tumors in and around the previously irradiated site.[278,279] For example, large epidemiologic studies have assessed the risk of breast and lung cancer in survivors of Hodgkin's disease,[280,281] leukemia and sarcomas in cervical cancer survivors,[282] and bone sarcomas in long-term survivors of childhood retinoblastoma.[283]

Certain subpopulations of previously treated patients may be at an even higher risk and deserve special attention, including children and young adults, those with a known genetic predisposition to cancer, immunocompromised individuals, and those with known exposure to other carcinogens (e.g., chemotherapy).

Another concern with respect to radiation-induced second malignancies is the growing use of conformal, intensity-modulated radiotherapy, which is designed specifically to deliver lower-than-traditional doses to normal tissues surrounding the tumor at the expense of larger treatment volumes.[284] Conditions of large volumes and low doses tend to be those most associated with radiation carcinogenesis.

Dose Rate and Dose Fractionation Effects

The sparing effects of external beam and brachytherapy are assumed to be a result of the repair of sublethal damage, but other factors, particularly repopulation, also may be involved. In the isoeffect relationship derived by Strandqvist,[28] the time factor included the effects of dose fractionation (presumably the result of SLDR) and overall treatment time (presumably the result of repopulation). It was not until 1963 that Fowler and colleagues[84,131,285] attempted to separate the contributions of these two factors by performing fractionation experiments with pig skin. In their experiments, 5 equal fractions were given in overall treatment times of 4 or 28 days, and three different-sized doses per fraction were used to make sure that at least one of them would result in a measurable level of early skin reaction. In changing from an overall time of 4 days to 28 days, only an additional 6 Gy was required to reach the same level of skin response. This was thought to reflect the contribution of overall time (i.e., repopulation) to the isoeffect total dose, because the size and number of fractions was kept constant. In a parallel series of experiments in which the overall time was kept constant (28 days), but the number of fractions was increased from 5 to 21, an additional 13 Gy was required to reach the skin isoeffect level. This increase was almost as great as the additional 16-Gy dose required when changing from a single-dose treatment to a treatment protocol of 5 fractions in 4 days, implying that the change in fraction number was more important than the change in the overall treatment time.

During the 1960s and 1970s, dose rate effects were studied extensively in an attempt to further develop rational explanations for the biologic factors involved in radiotherapeutic response. The clinical community was also becoming more attuned to the biologic underpinnings of radiotherapy, especially the four Rs of radiotherapy: repair, reoxygenation, redistribution, and repopulation.[286] These are considered key radiobiologic phenomena that influence the outcome of multifraction therapy.

Bedford and Hall[287,288] generated in vitro survival curves for HeLa cells irradiated at various dose rates between about 0.1 Gy per hour and 7.3 Gy per minute. The killing effectiveness per unit dose decreased as the dose rate was reduced; however, a limit to this dose rate or dose fractionation effect was reached under conditions in which cell cycle and proliferative effects were eliminated by the use of lower temperatures[289] or by growing cells to plateau phase before irradiation[290-292] (Fig. 1-26).

Similar conclusions about the nature of dose rate and dose fractionation effects were reached from clinical studies. Dutreix and associates[293] studied dose fractionation effects in human skin under conditions in which cell cycle and proliferative effects were minimized (i.e., short interfraction intervals and overall treatment times). Their data indicated that the incremental dose recovered due to SLDR when a single dose was replaced by two equal fractions became very small when the size of the dose per fraction dropped below approximately 2 Gy (Table 1-4). This finding is consistent with the hypothesis that survival curves have negative (rather than zero) initial slopes and that a limit to the repair-dependent dose fractionation effect should be reached for smaller and smaller sized dose fractions (or dose rates). These investigators cautioned that isoeffect equations in common clinical use at the time (the NSD model, discussed later) would be inaccurate for predicting tolerances when doses per fraction were quite small. Small differences in the initial slopes of acute dose survival curves for different cell types could be magnified into large differences in the limiting slopes for continuous or multifraction survival curves.

Time-Dose-Fractionation Relationships

NSD Model

Based on Strandqvist's isoeffect curves,[28] Fowler and Stern's pig skin experiments,[84,131] and other laboratory and clinical

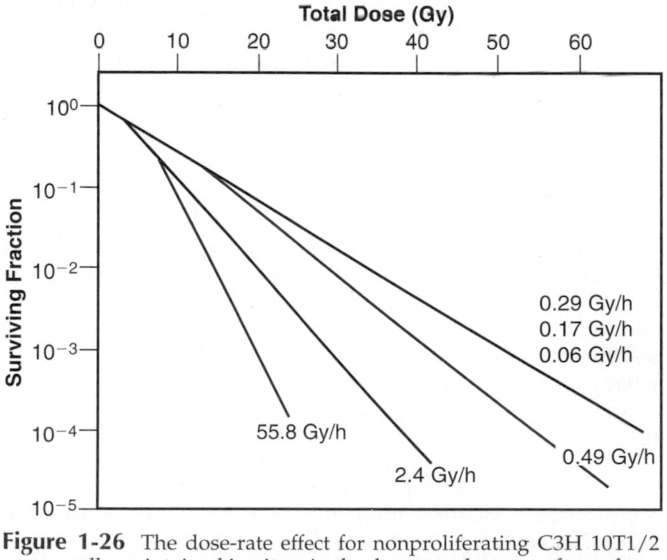

Figure 1-26 The dose-rate effect for nonproliferating C3H 10T1/2 mouse cells maintained in vitro. As the dose rate decreases from about 56 to 0.3 Gy/h, survival curves become progressively shallower, reflecting the repair of radiation damage during the continuous irradiation interval. For dose rates less than about 0.3 Gy/h, no further sparing effect of dose protraction is observed, suggesting that there is an effective limit to the repair-dependent dose rate effect. This is considered compelling evidence that cell survival curves have nonzero initial slopes. (Adapted from Wells R, Bedford J: Dose-rate effects in mammalian cells. IV. Repairable and nonrepairable damage in noncycling C3H 10T1/2 cells. Radiat Res 94:105, 1983.)

Table 1-4 Recovered Dose as a Function of Dose per Fraction for Skin Reactions in Human Radiotherapy Patients

Single Dose, D_s (Gy)	Split Dose,* $2\ D_i$ (Gy)	Recovered Dose,† D_r (Gy)
15	2 × 8.5	2
13	2 × 7.5	2
8	2 × 5.5	3
6	2 × 4	2
3.5	2 × 2	≤0.5

*The interfraction interval (i) was 6 hours.
†$D_r = 2\ D_i - D_s$, in which D_r is the recovered dose, $2\ D_i$ is the split dose, and D_s is the single dose.
Data from Dutreix J, Wambersie A, Bounik C: Cellular recovery in human skin reactions: application to dose fraction number overall time relationship in radiotherapy. Eur J Cancer 9:159, 1973.

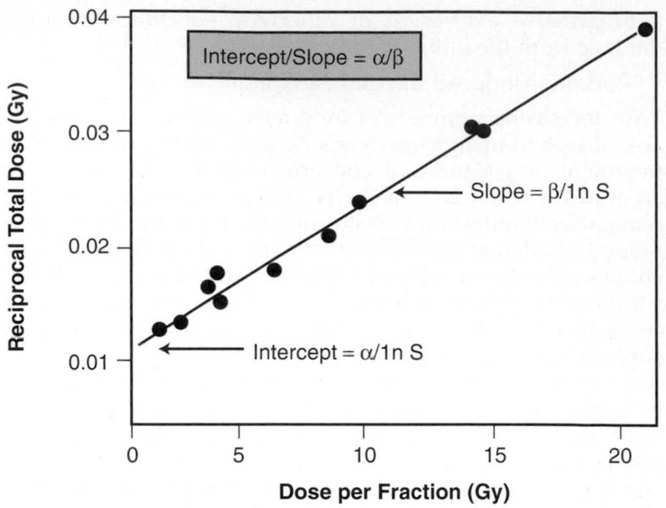

Figure 1-27 The reciprocal dose or Fe plot technique of Douglas and Fowler[299] is used to determine a normal tissue or tumor's α/β ratio. Using this method, the reciprocal of the total dose necessary to reach a given isoeffect is plotted as a function of the dose per fraction. Assuming that the killing of target cells responsible for the tissue effect can be modeled using the linear-quadratic cell survival expression, $S = e^{-(\alpha D+\beta D^2)}$, the α/β ratio can be obtained from the ratio of the isoeffect curve's intercept to slope. (Adapted from Douglas B, Fowler J: The effect of multiple small doses of x-rays on skin reactions in the mouse and a basic interpretation. Radiat Res 66:401, 1976.)

findings,[27] Ellis[294,295] formulated the NSD concept in 1969. The NSD equation is

$$D = (NSD)N^{0.24}T^{0.11}$$

in which D is the total dose delivered, N is the number of fractions used, T is the overall treatment time, and NSD is the nominal standard dose (a proportionality constant thought to be related to the tolerance of the tissue being irradiated). The equation became widely used for the design of biologically equivalent treatment schedules, particularly when its more mathematically convenient derivatives, such as the TDF[296] or CRE[297] equations, became available.

The introduction of the NSD equation theoretically allowed radiotherapy practices worldwide to be compared with respect to putative *biologic equivalence*. It also permitted the calculation of dose equivalents for split-course treatments and brachytherapy and provided a means of revising treatment prescriptions in the event of unforeseen treatment interruptions. Because the NSD formula was based on observations of early-onset radiation effects, it was quite useful as a predictor of some tissue tolerances, as long as it was not used for treatments involving extremes of fraction number or overall time.

The NSD formula was ill-equipped to deal with some clinical problems, particularly the prediction of late effects in normal tissues (especially at nonstandard doses per fraction) and the patterns of repopulation in normal tissues and tumors.[244] The use of a fixed exponent for the overall time component (T) gave the false impression that an extra dose to counteract proliferation would be needed from the outset of treatment, rather than after a delay of several weeks, which is what is observed in practice.[140,298]

In light of the growing frustration with the NSD model and research at the time focusing on the shape of the shoulder region of cell survival curves and the nature of dose rate and dose fractionation effects, newer, radiobiologically based approaches to isoeffect modeling were developed during the late 1970s and early 1980s.

Linear-Quadratic Isoeffect Model

In ambitious multifraction experiments using laboratory rodents in which a broad range of fraction sizes and interfraction intervals was used, Douglas and Fowler[299] developed a novel method of data analysis in which they interpreted their resulting isoeffect curves in terms of the shape of the underlying dose-response curves for the putative target cells. Because overall treatment times were kept quite short, proliferative effects were assumed to be negligible, and repair was thought to be the only factor involved. The shapes of the underlying dose-response curves were deduced by plotting 1/D, in which D was the total dose delivered (D = n × d), as a function of d, the dose per fraction. This *reciprocal dose plot* is used to obtain values for the ratio α/β, parameters of the linear-quadratic survival curve formula,[70,71] which provides good fits to experimental survival data, at least over the first 2 decades of killing cells. A representative reciprocal dose plot is shown in Figure 1-27. However, the curves obtained using this technique are not true cell survival curves, but rather effective dose-response curves derived from isoeffect data for different combinations of time, dose, and fractionation.

This new approach to isoeffect analysis, in which attention is focused on repair parameters and dose-response curve shapes, emphasizes that the critical parameter in radiotherapy is the size of the dose per fraction, more so than the overall treatment time. During the course of experimental and clinical fractionation studies, it became clear that there was a systematic difference between early- and late-responding tissues and tumors in their responses to altered fractionation patterns. In other words, the capacity for repair of radiation damage was somehow related to the proliferative state of the tissues being irradiated (Fig. 1-28).[300,301]

Isoeffect curves for the slowly proliferating or nonproliferating normal tissues, such as kidney and spinal cord, usually are steeper than those for more rapidly proliferating, early-responding tissues, such as skin, gut epithelium, and many tumors.[300,301] A steep isoeffect curve implies that late-effects tissues are more sensitive to changes in the size of the dose per fraction, experiencing greater sparing with decreasing fraction size than their early-effects counterparts (Fig. 1-29). This difference is also reflected in the α/β ratios derived for these tissues, which are usually low for late-responding tissues (on the order of 1 to 6 Gy, with an average of about 3 Gy) and high

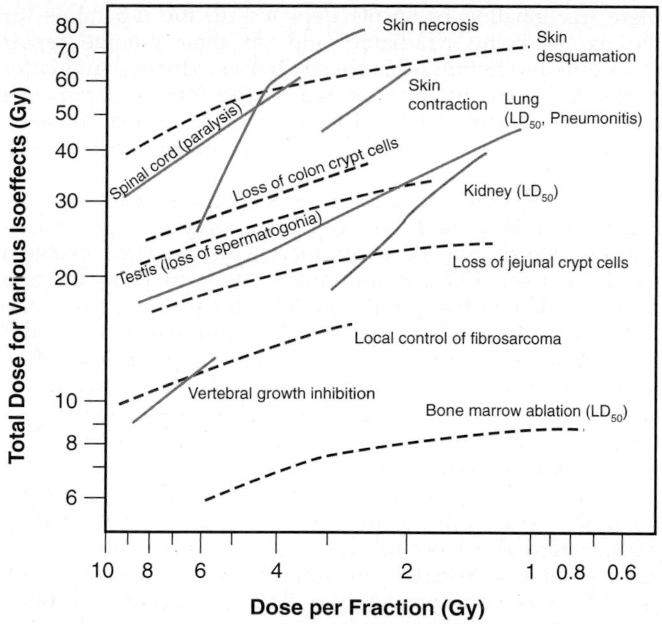

Figure 1-28 Isoeffect curves in which the total dose necessary to produce a certain normal tissue or tumor end point (indicated on the graph) is plotted as a function of the dose per fraction under conditions in which cell proliferation is negligible. Isoeffect curves for late-responding normal tissues *(solid lines)* tend to be steeper than those for early-responding normal tissues and tumors *(dashed lines)*. This suggests that for the same total dose, late reactions may be spared by decreasing the size of the dose per fraction used. It also follows that by using smaller dose fractions, a somewhat higher total dose could be given for the same probability of a late reaction but with the hope of higher tumor control probability. (Adapted from Withers H, Thames H, Peters L, et al: Normal tissue radioresistance in clinical radiotherapy. *In* Withers H, Thames H, Peters L (eds): Biological Basis and Clinical Implications of Tumor Radioresistance. New York, Masson, 1983, p 139.)

for early-responding tissues and tumors (usually 7 to 20 Gy, with an average of about 10 Gy) (Tables 1-5 and 1-6).

Clinical Applications of the Linear-Quadratic Isoeffect Model

The following are the most important assumptions of the linear-quadratic (LQ) model[300-302]:

1. An isoeffect in a tissue is a reflection of isosurvival in the appropriate target cells.
2. The turnover kinetics of target cells determines the time of expression of radiation injury.
3. Radiation damage can be classified as reparable or irreparable, with the reparable damage accounting for the sparing effect of dose fractionation.
4. Sufficient time is allowed between dose fractions for the reparable damage to be completely repaired.
5. Repopulation during the course of treatment is negligible.
6. The damage caused by each successive dose fraction is the same as that produced by the prior dose fraction; there is an equal effect per fraction.

Within this conceptual framework, the shapes of tissue and tumor isoeffect curves and their calculated α/β ratios have a number of clinical applications. One possible application is to custom-design radiotherapy treatments for which the α/β ratios for the dose-limiting tissues are known reasonably well.[249] Using α/β ratios, it is possible to equate treatment schedules employing different-sized doses per fraction to

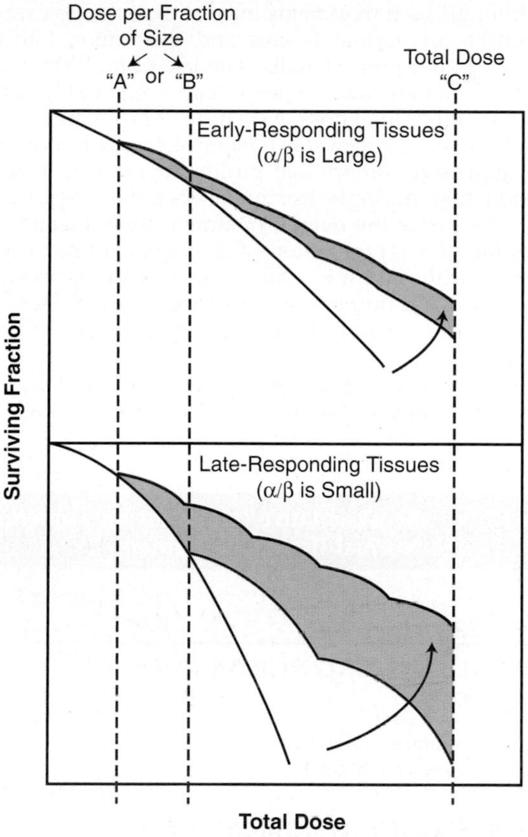

Figure 1-29 Hypothetical survival curves for target cells whose deaths are responsible for an acute *(upper panel)* or late *(lower panel)* effect in an irradiated normal tissue, depending on whether the total dose C is delivered using dose fractions of size A or B. Because of the difference in the initial slopes of the corresponding single dose survival curves for these cell types, reducing the fraction size from B to A preferentially spares late-responding normal tissues *(green shaded areas)*. (Adapted from Withers H, Thames H, Peters L: Differences in the fractionation response of acutely and late-responding tissues. *In* Karcher K, Kogelnik H, Reinartz G (eds): Progress in Radio-Oncology II. New York, Raven Press, 1982, p 287.)

match the probability of causing a tissue injury, assuming the overall treatment times are similar or the tissue at risk of a complication is relatively insensitive to treatment duration.[249] The following equation

$$D_2/D_1 = (\alpha/\beta + d_1)/(\alpha/\beta + d_2)$$

can be used for this purpose. D_1 and d_1 are, respectively, the total dose and dose per fraction (in Gy) of one radiation treatment plan; D_2 and d_2 are the total dose and dose per fraction for an alternate treatment plan designed to be biologically equivalent for a particular tissue effect, and with the fractionation sensitivity of that tissue defined by its unique α/β ratio. Avoiding a normal tissue complication is not the sole criterion used in treatment planning; in considering a particular time, dose, and fraction size combination, the responses of the tumor and *all* incidentally irradiated normal tissues should be taken into account simultaneously.

An important implication of the steeper isoeffect curves for late-effects tissues compared with those for tumors is that it might be possible to increase the therapeutic ratio by using larger numbers of smaller fractions to a somewhat higher total dose than traditionally used.[249-251] There has been increasing interest in the use of nonstandard fractionation in radiotherapy. Although such treatments may be expected to exacerbate acute effects in normal tissues and the tumor, late effects would be spared preferentially. The use of multiple fractions per day of smaller than conventional size (<1.8 Gy) but to a somewhat higher total dose, with little or no change in overall treatment time, has been called *hyperfractionation*. With particularly aggressive tumors that proliferate rapidly, it has been suggested that multiple treatments per day might also be useful to decrease the overall treatment time, thereby allowing less time for repopulation of clonogenic tumor cells.[303,304] Treatment with multiple daily fractions of approximately standard size and number (and to about the same total dose) but in shorter overall times has been called *accelerated fractionation*.

In practice, a combination of accelerated and hyperfractionated treatment is often used.[304] The decision to use one of these fractionation protocols depends on the α/β ratios for the tissues being irradiated and on their relative repair rates and proliferative responses before, during, and after exposure. Although data related to the former parameters continue to accumulate and become more reliable, data on proliferation characteristics, especially for tumors, are still lacking.[244,303]

Assuming that nonstandard fractionation will someday become standard (as it already has in many respects), radiation oncologists will be confronted with the same problem faced by their 1930s counterparts: how to compare and contrast different treatment schedules for presumptive isoeffectiveness. The *biologically equivalent dose* (BED) method[245] (sometimes referred to as the *extrapolated response dose* [ERD] technique[305]), another variation of the LQ model, attempts to address this issue. Although this method is somewhat confusing to use in practice, conceptually the ideas are fairly straightforward. Knowing that cell survival curves have negative initial slopes and that for a sufficiently low dose per fraction or dose rate, a limit to the repair-dependent dose fractionation effect occurs that "traces" this initial slope, a question may be asked: In the limit, for an infinite number of small dose fractions, what total radiation dose will correspond to normal tissue tolerance, tumor control, or any other end point of interest? This theoretical dose will be quite large for a tissue characterized by a dose-response curve or target cell survival curve with a shallow initial slope (e.g., many late-responding normal tissues) and appreciably lower for a tissue characterized by a dose-response curve with a steep initial slope (e.g., many tumors and early-responding normal tissues).

BEDs are not real doses, but rather extrapolated values based on the limiting slope of the multifraction dose-response curves for the tissues at risk, which depend on the α/β ratio. For this reason, the units used to describe these doses are, for example, Gy_3 and Gy_{10}, in which the subscripts 3 and 10 refer to the assumed α/β ratio of the tissue at risk. Another caveat is that, whereas two different radiotherapy treatment schedules can be compared qualitatively on the basis of their respective Gy_3 *or* Gy_{10} "doses," those with Gy_3 *and* Gy_{10} values cannot be compared.

A mathematical rearrangement of the linear-quadratic survival expression, $S = e^{-(\alpha D + \beta D^2)}$, yields the following:

$$BED = E/\alpha = nd(1 + d/\alpha/\beta)$$

in which E is the (iso)effect being measured (i.e., E is divided by α to obtain the BED value in units of dose), n is the number of fractions, d is the dose per fraction, and the α/β ratio is specific for the tissue at risk. The factor $1 + d/\alpha/\beta$ has been called the *relative effectiveness term* because it is a correction factor for the fact that treatment is not really given as an infinite number of infinitely small dose fractions, but rather as a finite number of fractions of a finite size.

Table 1-5 Representative α/β Ratios for Human Normal Tissues and Tumors

Tissue Type (End Point)	α/β Ratio (±95% CI) (Gy)
EARLY-RESPONDING NORMAL TISSUES	
Skin (erythema)	10.6 (1.8 to 22.8)
Skin (desquamation)	11.2 (8.5 to 17.6)
Lung (pneumonitis within 90 days after radiotherapy, esophagitis)	>8.8
Oral mucosa (mucositis)	≈10.8 (5.8 to 18.0)
LATE-RESPONDING NORMAL TISSUES	
Skin (telangiectasia)	2.7 (−0.1 to 8.1)
Skin (fibrosis)	1.7 (0.6 to 3.0)
Lung (pneumonitis more than 90 days after radiotherapy, atelectasis, fibrosis, pulmonary edema)	<3.8
Bowel (perforation or stricture)	3.9 (2.2 to 8.0)
Spinal cord (myelopathy)	<3.3
Cartilage or bone (necrosis)	4.5 (3.4 to 10.6)
Nerve (brachial plexopathy, optic neuropathy)	1.6 to 3.5
TUMORS	
Nasopharynx	16 (−11 to 43)
Vocal cord	≈13
Oropharynx	≈16
Tonsil	>7.2
Larynx	14.5 (9.5 to 19.5)
Lung (squamous cell carcinoma)	≈50 to 90
Cervix (squamous cell carcinoma)	>13.9
Skin (squamous cell carcinoma)	8.5 (4.5 to 11.3)
Skin (melanoma)	0.6 (−1.1 to 2.5)
Liposarcoma	0.4 (−1.4 to 5.4)

Data from references 140, 177, 303.

Table 1-6 Summary of Linear-Quadratic Isoeffect Model Parameters and Concepts

Tissue Type	α/β Ratio*	Dose-Response Curve Shape†	Isoeffect Curve Shape‡
Early-responding normal tissues and most tumors	High (6-30 Gy)	Steep initial slope (α is large)	Shallow
Late-responding normal tissues	Low (1-6 Gy)	Shallow initial slope (α is small)	Steep

*Determined from the reciprocal dose plot technique of Douglas and Fowler.[299]
†Based on the assumption that differences in the calculated α/β ratio are usually caused by differences in α rather than β.
‡Using the isoeffect curve plot (see Fig. 1-28) of Thames and associates.[300]

Table 1-7 **Status of Existing and Proposed Parameters of the LQ Isoeffect Model for Human Normal Tissues and Tumors**

		Availability of Data		
Parameter	**Property Governed**	*Early Effects*	*Late Effects*	*Tumors*
α/β Ratio	Fractionation sensitivity	Poor/fair	Fair	Poor/fair
$T_{[1/2]}$ (repair half-time)	Repair kinetics	Poor	Poor	None
T_{eff} (effective clonogen doubling time) and/or T_k (kickoff time: time proliferation begins relative to the start of treatment)	Dose lost to accelerated proliferation during radiotherapy	Poor/fair	Poor	Poor/fair
Volume effect	Variation in tissue tolerance with increasing target volume	None/poor	None/poor	Poor
γ (normalized dose-response gradient)	Steepness of dose-response curve for effect; can be used to estimate the normal tissue complication probability	Poor	Fair	Fair

Adapted from Bentzen S: Estimation of radiobiological parameters from clinical data. *In* Hagen U, Jung H, Streffer C (eds): Radiation Research 1895-1995, vol 2. Congress Lectures. Wurzburg, Universitatsdruckerei H. Sturtz, 1995, p 833.

Perhaps the best way to illustrate the use of the BED equation is by example. Suppose that a radiation oncologist is considering initiating a clinical protocol in head and neck cancer comparing standard fractionation (30 fractions of 2 Gy to a total dose of 60 Gy in an overall treatment time of about 6 weeks) with a schedule of 50 fractions of 1.4 Gy to a total dose of 70 Gy in approximately the same overall treatment time. The tissues at risk for radiation injury are the tumor, the oral mucosa, and the spinal cord (i.e., two early- and one late-responding tissues). Assume an α/β ratio of 10 Gy is appropriate for the tumor and oral mucosa, and an α/β ratio of 3 Gy is appropriate for the spinal cord. For the standard fractionation schedule, the following equations apply.

For tumor and mucosa:

$$E/\alpha = 60\,\text{Gy}\ (1 + 2\,\text{Gy}/10\,\text{Gy}) = 72\,\text{Gy}_{10}$$

For the spinal cord:

$$E/\alpha = 60\,\text{Gy}\ (1 + 2\,\text{Gy}/3\,\text{Gy}) = 100\,\text{Gy}_3$$

For the more highly fractionated schedule (rounded off to the nearest whole number), the following equations apply.

For tumor and mucosa:

$$E/\alpha = 70\,\text{Gy}\ (1 + 1.4\,\text{Gy}/10\,\text{Gy}) = 80\,\text{Gy}_{10}$$

For the spinal cord:

$$E/\alpha = 70\,\text{Gy}\ (1 + 1.4\,\text{Gy}/3\,\text{Gy}) = 103\,\text{Gy}_3$$

Although little quantitative information can be gleaned from this exercise, a few qualitative statements can be made. First, a comparison of the Gy_{10} values for the two treatment schedules suggests that the more highly fractionated schedule should result in somewhat better tumor control, albeit at the expense of more vigorous mucosal reactions (i.e., 72 Gy_{10} compared with 80 Gy_{10}). However, the comparison of the Gy_3 values for the two schedules suggests that the spinal cord tolerance would be essentially unchanged (i.e., 100 Gy_3 compared with 103 Gy_3).

Although the BED concept is only semiquantitative at best, its use for treatment planning purposes over the past 2 decades has provided a wealth of clinical data that has allowed a better definition of what is or is not tolerable for a particular normal tissue in terms of Gy_3 or Gy_{10} values. Using head and neck cancer as an example, Fowler and colleagues[306,307] suggested that the tolerance dose for acute mucosal reactions was about 59 to 61 Gy_{10}, and for temporal lobe necrosis, it was approximately 110 to 115 Gy_3.

Another way of using the BED equation would be to design schedules to match an acceptable probability of a complication such as radiation myelitis and then calculate the expected benefit (or lack thereof) with respect to tumor control.

It would be remiss to conclude any discussion of the LQ isoeffect model or any biologically based model with potential clinical application without a few words of warning. This model, although certainly more robust than the NSD model and much better grounded in biologic principles, is still a theoretical model. Some limitations of the basic model are obvious: no provision for the influence of cell cycle, proliferative or microenvironmental effects in the overall dose-response relationship; no way to account for differences in repair rates between different tissues (particularly important for fractionated therapy using short interfraction intervals and for continuous, low dose rate or pulsed, high dose rate brachytherapy[140]); no consideration of radiation volume effects; and scant knowledge of how to apply this model to patients receiving both radiation and chemotherapy.

Various amendments to the LQ model have been proposed,[308-310] especially with respect to compensating for tumor cell repopulation and differing repair rates between different tissues. However, the lack of robust values at present for the parameters introduced in such calculations (e.g., potential doubling times, half-times for repair, repopulation kick-off times) ultimately limits their usefulness beyond rough approximations or proofs-of-concept. The current status of some of the existing and proposed parameters of the LQ model for human tumors and normal tissues is summarized in Table 1-7.

RADIATION BIOLOGY IN THE 21ST CENTURY

Since the mid-1980s, most graduate students pursuing careers in oncology necessarily have trained as molecular, cellular, or tumor biologists, not as radiation biologists, although a few may have worked with ionizing radiation as a tool for probing fundamental cellular processes or as part of translational research designed to develop new cancer therapies. Even fewer have ever taken a formal course on the principles of radiation biology, let alone in its more clinical aspects. This shift in focus and training is part of the natural evolution of the oncologic sciences over the years and not an unexpected or unwarranted one, but the fact remains that the field of radiation biology as a distinct entity, with its rich, 110-year history that has contributed in major ways to fields as diverse as carcinogenesis, epidemiology, toxicology, DNA damage and repair, genetics and cytogenetics, cell cycle biology, and radiation oncology, is threatened with extinction.

This could be viewed as a necessary price of scientific progress if it were not for the fact that there remains a need for all radiologic science professionals (including radiologic technologists, radiation therapists, medical physicists and dosimetrists, radiologists, and radiation oncologists) to be reasonably well versed in the basic principles of radiation biology. Physicians in particular need to be familiar with the classic and modern aspects of the field, in keeping with the close relationship between the histories of ionizing radiation itself, radiation biology, and the medical specialties of radiology and radiation oncology. Since the events of September 11, 2001, a new mandate has emerged: the need to provide expertise in the basics of radiation biology and radiation protection to emergency responders, civic leaders, and even the general public in the event of a radiologic or nuclear terrorist attack.

Nevertheless, 21st century radiation biology continues to flourish and remains cutting edge in many respects. Fundamental studies of genomic instability, a hallmark of malignant transformation and carcinogenesis,[311,312] and cell signaling as it applies to radiation response[313,314] continue to be active areas of research. Our growing understanding of the complex roles played by cytokines in the cause of normal tissue complications after radiation exposure[315-318] promises to someday deliver novel, molecularly based radioprotectors that may benefit radiation accident victims, first responders during radiation emergencies, and astronauts on deep-space missions. Radiation cytogeneticists study complex chromosomal aberrations[62,63] and the roles telomeres and telomerase play in cellular aging and neoplastic transformation.[319-321] Radiation scientists have also been important contributors to the field of functional and molecular imaging and to the search for tumor-specific biomarkers that can aid in cancer diagnosis and staging and in the monitoring of treatment progress.

A relatively new area of research is the *radiation bystander effect*.[322,323] The bystander effect—the appearance of radiation injury, including death and mutagenesis, in unirradiated cells proximate to those directly irradiated—challenges the long-held belief in radiation biology that irreparable DNA damage caused by a direct or indirect energy-deposition event is the principal cause of radiation-induced cellular injury. That unirradiated, bystander cells may also be damaged or killed may have profound implications for risk assessment and radiation protection standards for workers and the general public, and it may provide insights into how damage to DNA is identified and processed by the cell and how cell-cell communication occurs at the molecular level.[323]

To the extent that the molecular underpinnings of processes such as the bystander effect and genomic instability are still poorly understood and that a more comprehensive picture of the full range of radiation-induced gene expression and signaling remains elusive, there will always be a role for radiation biology research.

REFERENCES

1. Heppner G, Miller B: Tumor heterogeneity: biological implications and therapeutic consequences. Cancer Metastasis Rev 2:5, 1983.
2. Heppner GH: Tumor heterogeneity. Perspect Cancer Res 44:2259, 1984.
3. Gatenby R, Kessler H, Rosenblum J, et al: Oxygen distribution in squamous cell carcinoma metastases and its relationship to outcome of radiation therapy. Int J Radiat Oncol Biol Phys 14:831, 1988.
4. Höckel M, Knoop C, Schlenger K, et al: Intratumoral PO_2 predicts survival in advanced cancer of the uterine cervix. Radiother Oncol 26:45, 1993.
5. Höckel M, Schlenger K, Mitze M, et al: Hypoxia and radiation response in human tumors. Semin Radiat Oncol 6:3, 1996.
6. Begg A, Hofland I, Van Glabekke M: Predictive value of potential doubling time for radiotherapy of head and neck tumour patients: results from the EORTC Cooperative Trial 22857. Semin Radiat Oncol 2:22, 1992.
7. Norton L, Simon R: Growth curve of an experimental solid tumor following radiotherapy. J Natl Cancer Inst 58:1735, 1977.
8. Roentgen WC: Über eine neue Art von Strahlen. Sitzgsber Physik Med Ges Wuerzburg 137:132, 1895.
9. Becquerel H: Emission of the new radiations by metallic uranium. C R Acad Sci 122:1086, 1896.
10. Curie P, Curie M: Sur une substance nouvelle radioactive, contenue dans la pechblende. C R Acad Sci 127:175, 1898.
11. Stenbeck T: Ein Fall von Hautkrebs geheilt durch Rontgenbestrahlung. Mitteil Grenzgeb Med Chir 6:347, 1900.
12. Sjogren T: Die Rontgenbehandlung des Ulcus rodens. Fortschr Rontgenstr 5:37, 1901.
13. Fletcher G: Keynote address: the scientific basis of the present and future practice of clinical radiotherapy. Int J Radiat Oncol Biol Phys 9:1073, 1983.
14. Bergonié J, Tribondeau L: Interpretation de quelques resultats de la radiotherapie. C R Acad Sci 143:983, 1906.
15. Regaud C: Influence de la duree d'irradiation sur les effete determine's dans le testicule par le radium. C R Soc Biol 86:787, 1922.
16. Regaud C: Sur les principles radiophysiologiques de la radio therapie des cancers. Acta Radiol 86:456, 1930.
17. Regaud C, Ferroux R: Discordance des effets de rayons X, d'une part dans le testicule, par le peau, d'autre part dans la fractionnement de la dose. C R Soc Biol 97:431, 1927.
18. Regaud C, Ferroux R: Uber den einflub des zeitfaktors auf die sterilisation des normalen und des neoplastischen zellnachwuchees durch radiotherapie. Strahlentherapie 31:495, 1929.
19. Coutard H: Roentgen therapy of epitheliomas of the tonsillar region, hypopharynx and larynx from 1920 to 1926. AJR Am J Roentgenol 28:313, 1932.
20. Coutard H: Present conception of treatment of cancer of the larynx. Radiology 34:136, 1940.
21. Reisner A: Untersuchungen uber die veranderungen der Hauttoleranz bei verschiedener Unterterlung. Strahlentherapie 37:779, 1930.
22. MacComb W, Quimby E: The rate of recovery of human skin from effects of hard or soft roentgen or gamma rays. Radiology 27:196, 1936.
23. Quimby E, MacComb W: Further studies on the rate of recovery of human skin from the effects of roentgen or gamma rays. Radiology 29:305, 1937.
24. Paterson R: The value of assessing and prescribing dosage in radiation therapy in simple terms. Radiology 32:221, 1939.
25. Ellis F: Tolerance dose in radiotherapy with 200 keV x-rays. Br J Radiol 15:348, 1942.
26. Jolles B, Mitchell R: Optimal skin tolerance dose levels. Br J Radiol 20:405, 1947.
27. Cohen L: Radiation response and recovery: radiobiological principles and their relation to clinical practice. *In* Schwartz E (ed): The Biological Basis of Radiation Therapy. Philadelphia, JB Lippincott, 1966, p 208.
28. Strandqvist M: Studien uber die kumulative Wirkung der Roentgenstrahlen bei Fraktionierung. Acta Radiol Suppl 55:1, 1944.
29. Puck TT, Marcus PI: Action of x-rays on mammalian cells. J Exp Med 103:653, 1956.
30. Puck T, Marcus P: A rapid method for viable cell titration and clone production with HeLa cells in tissue culture: the use of x-

irradiated cells to supply conditioning factors. Proc Natl Acad Sci U S A 41:432, 1955.
31. Hall E: Radiobiology for the Radiologist, 5th ed. Philadelphia, JB Lippincott, 2000.
32. Hutchinson F: Molecular basis for action of ionizing radiations. Science 134:533, 1961.
33. Johansen I, Howard-Flanders P: Macromolecular repair and free radical scavenging in the protection of bacteria against x-rays. Radiat Res 24:184, 1965.
34. Chapman J, Dugle D, Reuvers C, et al: Chemical radiosensitization studies with mammalian cells growing in vitro. *In* Nygaard O, Adler H, Sinclair W (eds): Radiation Research: Biomedical, Chemical, and Physical Perspectives. New York, Academic Press, 1976, p 752.
35. Ward J: Biochemistry of DNA lesions. Radiat Res Suppl 104:103, 1985.
36. Goodhead D: Physics of radiation action: microscopic features that determine biological consequences. *In* Hagen U, Harder D, Jung H, et al (eds): Radiation Research 1895-1995, Proceedings of the Tenth International Congress of Radiation Research, vol 2. Congress Lectures. Wurzburg, Universitatsdruckerei H Stürtz, 1995, p 43.
37. Cleaver J: Defective repair replication of DNA in xeroderma pigmentosum. Nature 218:652, 1968.
38. Cleaver J: Xeroderma pigmentosum: a human disease in which an initial stage of DNA repair is defective. Proc Natl Acad Sci U S A 63:428, 1969.
39. Taylor A, Harnden D, Arlett C, et al: Ataxia telangiectasia: a human mutation with abnormal radiation sensitivity. Nature 258:427, 1975.
40. Whitmore G: One hundred years of x-rays in biological research. Radiat Res 144:148, 1995.
41. Sancar A: Mechanisms of DNA excision repair. Science 266:1954, 1994.
42. Lehmann A: Workshop on eukaryotic DNA repair genes and gene products. Cancer Res 55:968, 1995.
43. Collins A: Mutant rodent cell lines sensitive to ultraviolet light, ionizing radiation and cross-linking agents: a comprehensive survey of genetic and biochemical characteristics. Mutat Res 293:99, 1993.
44. Painter R, Young B: Radiosensitivity in ataxia-telangiectasia: a new explanation. Proc Natl Acad Sci U S A 77:7315, 1980.
45. Friedberg E, Walker G, Siede W: DNA Repair and Mutagenesis. Washington, DC, American Society for Microbiology, 1995.
46. Tornaletti S, Hanawalt PC: Effect of DNA lesions on transcription elongation. Biochimie 81:139, 1999.
47. Powell S, McMillan T: DNA damage and repair following treatment with ionizing radiation. Radiother Oncol 19:95, 1990.
48. Thompson L, Brookman K, Jones N, et al: Molecular cloning of the human XRCC1 gene, which corrects defective DNA strand break repair and sister chromatid exchange. Mol Cell Biol 10:6160, 1990.
49. Kirchgessner C, Patil C, Evans J, et al: DNA-dependent kinase (p350) as a candidate gene for the murine SCID defect. Science 267:1178, 1995.
50. Lees-Miller S, Godbout R, Chan D, et al: Absence of p350 subunit of DNA-activated protein kinase from a radiosensitive human cell line. Science 267:1183, 1995.
51. Jackson S: Detecting, signalling and repairing DNA double-strand breaks. Biochem Soc Trans 29:655, 2001.
52. Thompson LH, Schild D: Recombinational DNA repair and human disease. Mutat Res 509:49, 2002.
53. Narod SA, Foulkes W: BRCA1 and BRCA2: 1994 and beyond. Nat Rev Cancer 4:665, 2004.
54. Parsons R, Li G, Longley M, et al: Mismatch repair deficiency in phenotypically normal human cells. Science 268:738, 1995.
55. Modrich P, Lahue R: Mismatch repair in replication fidelity, genetic recombination, and cancer biology. Annu Rev Biochem 65:101, 1996.
56. Modrich P: Strand-specific mismatch repair in mammalian cells. J Biol Chem 272:24727, 1997.
57. Lipkin SM, Wang V, Jacoby R, et al: MLH3: a novel DNA mismatch repair gene associated with mammalian microsatellite instability. Nat Genet 24:27, 2000.
58. Peltomaki P, Vasen HF: Mutations predisposing to hereditary nonpolyposis colorectal cancer: database and results of a collaborative study. The International Collaborative Group on Hereditary Nonpolyposis Colorectal Cancer. Gastroenterology 113:1146, 1997.
59. Steel G, Adams G, Peckham M (eds): The Biological Basis of Radiotherapy. New York, Elsevier, 1983.
60. Lucas J, Tenjin T, Straume T, et al: Rapid human chromosome aberration analysis using fluorescence in situ hybridization. Int J Radiat Biol 56:35, 1989.
61. Brown J, Kovacs M: Visualization of non-reciprocal chromosome exchanges in irradiated human fibroblasts by fluorescence in situ hybridization. Radiat Res 136:71, 1993.
62. Cornforth M: Analyzing radiation-induced complex chromosome rearrangements by combinatorial painting. Radiat Res 155:643, 2001.
63. Anderson R, Marsden S, Wright E, et al: Complex chromosome aberrations in peripheral blood lymphocytes as a potential biomarker of exposure to high-LET alpha-particles. Int J Radiat Biol 76:31, 2000.
64. Elkind M, Whitmore G: The Radiobiology of Cultured Mammalian Cells. New York, Gordon & Breach Science Publishers, 1967.
65. Kerr J, Wyllie A, Currie A: Apoptosis: a basic biological phenomenon with wide ranging implications in tissue kinetics. Br J Cancer 26:239, 1972.
66. Meyn R: Apoptosis and response to radiation: implications for radiation therapy. Oncology 11:349, 1997.
67. Lea D: Actions of Radiation on Living Cells. Cambridge, Cambridge University Press, 1946.
68. Zimmer K: That was the radiobiology that was: a selected bibliography and some comments. *In* Lett J, Adler H (eds): Advances in Radiation Biology, vol 9. New York, Academic Press, 1981, p 411.
69. Alper T: Keynote address: survival curve models. *In* Meyn R, Withers H (eds): Radiation Biology in Cancer Research. New York, Raven Press, 1980, p 3.
70. Kellerer A, Rossi H: The theory of dual radiation action. Curr Top Radiat Res Q 8:85, 1972.
71. Chadwick K, Leenhouts H: A molecular theory of cell survival. Phys Med Biol 18:78, 1973.
72. Puck T, Morkovin D, Marcus P, et al: Action of x-rays on mammalian cells. II. Survival curves of cells from normal tissues. J Exp Med 106:485, 1957.
73. Puck T, Marcus P, Cieciura S: Clonal growth of mammalian cells in vitro. Growth characteristics of colonies from single HeLa cells with and without a "feeder" layer. J Exp Med 103:273, 1956.
74. Alper T, Gillies N, Elkind M: The sigmoid survival curve in radiobiology. Nature 186:1062, 1960.
75. Alper T, Fowler J, Morgan R, et al: The characterization of the "type C" survival curve. Br J Radiol 35:722, 1962.
76. Hewitt H, Wilson C: A survival curve for cells irradiated in vivo. Nature 183:1060, 1959.
77. McCulloch EA, Till JE: The sensitivity of cells from normal mouse bone marrow to gamma radiation in vitro and in vivo. Radiat Res 16:822, 1962.
78. Till JE, McCulloch EA: A direct measurement of the radiation sensitivity of normal mouse bone marrow cells. Radiat Res 14:213, 1961.
79. Withers H: The dose-survival relationship for irradiation of epithelial cells of mouse skin. Br J Radiol 40:187, 1967.
80. Withers H, Elkind M: Radiosensitivity and fractionation response of crypt cells of mouse jejunum. Radiat Res 38:598, 1969.
81. Withers H, Elkind M: Microcolony survival assay for cells of mouse intestinal mucosa exposed to radiations. Int J Radiat Biol 17:261, 1970.
82. Hill R, Bush R: A lung-colony assay to determine the radiosensitivity of cells of a solid tumor. Int J Radiat Biol 15:435, 1969.
83. Rockwell S, Kallman R: Cellular radiosensitivity and tumor radiation response in the EMT6 tumor cell system. Radiat Res 53:281, 1973.
84. Fowler J, Morgan R, Silvester J, et al: Experiments with fractionated x-ray treatment of the skin of pigs. I. Fractionation up to 28 days. Br J Radiol 36:188, 1963.

85. Thomlinson R: An experimental method for comparing treatments of intact malignant tumours in animals and its application to the use of oxygen in radiotherapy. Br J Cancer 14:555, 1960.
86. Suit H, Shalek R: Response of spontaneous mammary carcinoma of the C3H mouse to x-irradiation given under conditions of local tissue anoxia. J Natl Cancer Inst 31:497, 1963.
87. Elkind M, Sutton H: X-ray damage and recovery in mammalian cells. Nature 184:1293, 1959.
88. Elkind M, Sutton H: Radiation response of mammalian cells grown in culture. I. Repair of x-ray damage in surviving Chinese hamster cells. Radiat Res 13:556, 1960.
89. Belli J, Dicus G, Bonte F: Radiation response of mammalian tumor cells. I. Repair of sublethal damage in vivo. J Natl Cancer Inst 38:673, 1967.
90. Emery E, Denekamp J, Ball M: Survival of mouse skin epithelial cells following single and divided doses of x-rays. Radiat Res 41:450, 1970.
91. Phillips R, Tolmach L: Repair of potentially lethal damage in x-irradiated HeLa cells. Radiat Res 29:413, 1966.
92. Little J: Repair of sublethal and potentially lethal radiation damage in plateau phase cultures of human cells. Nature 224:804, 1969.
93. Hahn G, Little J: Plateau phase cultures of mammalian cells: an in vitro model for human cancer. Curr Top Radiat Res Q 8:39, 1972.
94. Belli J, Shelton M: Potentially lethal radiation damage: repair by mammalian cells in culture. Science 165:490, 1969.
95. Little J, Hahn G, Frindel E, et al: Repair of potentially lethal radiation damage in vitro and in vivo. Radiology 106:689, 1973.
96. Nagasawa H, Little J: Induction of chromosome aberrations and sister chromatid exchanges by x-rays in density inhibited cultures of mouse 10T1/2 cells. Radiat Res 87:538, 1981.
97. Cornforth M, Bedford J: X-ray-induced breakage and rejoining of human interphase chromosomes. Science 222:1141, 1983.
98. Weichselbaum R, Little J: Radiation response of human tumor cells in vitro. *In* Meyn R, Withers H (eds): Radiation Biology in Cancer Research. New York, Raven Press, 1980, p 345.
99. Howard A, Pelc SR: Nuclear incorporation of P32 as demonstrated by autoradiographs. Exp Cell Res 2:178, 1951.
100. Howard A, Pelc SR: Synthesis of desoxyribonucleic acid in normal and irradiated cells and its relation to chromosome breakage. Heredity 6(Suppl):261, 1953.
101. Terasima T, Tolmach L: Variations in several responses of HeLa cells to x-irradiation during the division cycle. Biophys J 3:11, 1963.
102. Terasima T, Tolmach L: Changes in x-ray sensitivity of HeLa cells during the division cycle. Nature 190:1210, 1961.
103. Eidinoff M, Rich M: Growth inhibition of a human tumor cell strain by 5-fluoro-2′-deoxyuridine: time parameters for subsequent reversal by thymidine. Cancer Res 19:521, 1959.
104. Sinclair W: The combined effect of hydroxyurea and x-rays on Chinese hamster cells in vitro. Cancer Res 28:190, 1968.
105. Withers H, Mason K, Reid B, et al: Response of mouse intestine to neutrons and gamma rays in relation to dose fractionation and division cycle. Cancer 34:39, 1974.
106. Crissman H, Mullaney P, Steinkamp J: Methods and applications of flow systems for analysis and sorting of mammalian cells. *In* Prescott D (ed): Methods in Cell Biology, vol 9. New York, Academic Press, 1975, p 179.
107. Sinclair W: Cyclic x-ray responses in mammalian cells in vitro. Radiat Res 33:620, 1968.
108. Sinclair W, Morton R: X-ray sensitivity during the cell generation cycle of cultured Chinese hamster cells. Radiat Res 29:450, 1966.
109. Dewey W, Stone L, Miller H, et al: Radiosensitization with 5-bromodeoxyuridine of Chinese hamster cells x-irradiated during different phases of the cell cycle. Radiat Res 47:672, 1971.
110. Canti R, Spear F: The effect of gamma irradiation on cell division in tissue culture in vitro. Proc R Soc Biol 102:92, 1927.
111. Little J: Differential response of rapidly and slowly proliferating human cells to x-irradiation. Radiology 97:303, 1969.
112. Tolmach L, Jones R, Busse P: The action of caffeine on x-irradiated HeLa cells. Radiat Res 71:653, 1977.
113. Walters R, Gurley L, Tobey R: Effects of caffeine on radiation-induced phenomena associated with cell cycle traverse of mammalian cells. Biophys J 14:99, 1974.
114. Withers H: Cell cycle redistribution as a factor in multifraction irradiation. Radiology 114:199, 1975.
115. Bedford J, Mitchell J: Dose-rate effects in synchronous mammalian cells in culture. Radiat Res 54:316, 1973.
116. Szechter A, Schwarz G: Cell redistribution during continuous irradiation. Radiat Res 74:493, 1978.
117. Bedford J, Mitchell J, Fox M: Variations in responses of several mammalian cell lines to low dose-rate irradiation. *In* Meyn R, Withers H (eds): Radiation Biology in Cancer Research. New York, Raven Press, 1980, p 251.
118. Blakely E, Chang P, Lommel L: Cell-cycle-dependent recovery from heavy-ion damage in G_1-phase cells. Radiat Res Suppl 104:5145, 1985.
119. Withers H, Thames H, Peters L: Biological bases for high RBE values for late effects of neutron irradiation. Int J Radiat Oncol Biol Phys 8:2071, 1982.
120. Barendsen G: Responses of cultured cells, tumors and normal tissues to radiations of different linear energy transfer. Curr Top Radiat Res 4:295, 1968.
121. Kaplan H: Radiobiology's contribution to radiotherapy: promise or mirage? Radiat Res 43:460, 1970.
122. Kaplan H: Historic milestones in radiobiology and radiation therapy. Semin Oncol 6:479, 1979.
123. Thomlinson R, Gray L: The histological structure of some human lung cancers and the possible implications for radiotherapy. Br J Cancer 9:539, 1955.
124. Powers WE, Tolmach LJ: A multicomponent x-ray survival curve for mouse lymphosarcoma cells irradiated. Nature 197:710, 1963.
125. Moulder J, Rockwell S: Hypoxic fractions of solid tumors: experimental techniques, methods of analysis and a survey of existing data. Int J Radiat Oncol Biol Phys 10:695, 1984.
126. Palcic B, Skarsgard LD: Reduced oxygen enhancement ratio at low doses of ionizing radiation. Radiat Res 100:328, 1984.
127. Brown J, Yu N: Radiosensitization of hypoxic cells in vivo by SR 2508 at low radiation doses: a preliminary report. Int J Radiat Oncol Biol Phys 10:1207, 1984.
128. Howard-Flanders P, Moore D: The time interval after pulsed irradiation within which injury to bacteria can be modified by dissolved oxygen. I. A search for an effect of oxygen 0.02 second after pulsed irradiation. Radiat Res 9:422, 1958.
129. Michael B, Adams G, Hewitt H, et al: A posteffect of oxygen in irradiated bacteria: a submillisecond fast mixing study. Radiat Res 54:239, 1973.
130. Alper T, Howard-Flanders P: The role of oxygen in modifying the radiosensitivity of *E. coli* B. Nature 178:978, 1956.
131. Fowler J, Morgan R, Wood C: Pretherapeutic experiments with the fast neutron beam from the Medical Research Council cyclotron. I. The biological and physical advantages and problems of neutron therapy. Br J Radiol 36:163, 1963.
132. van Putten L, Kallman R: Oxygenation status of a transplantable tumor during fractionated radiotherapy. J Natl Cancer Inst 40:441, 1968.
133. Kallman RF: The phenomenon of reoxygenation and its implications for fractionated radiotherapy. Radiology 105:135, 1972.
134. Brown J: Evidence for acutely hypoxic cells in mouse tumours, and a possible mechanism of reoxygenation. Br J Radiol 52:650, 1979.
135. Kimura H, Braun R, Ong E, et al: Fluctuations in red cell flux in tumor microvessels can lead to transient hypoxia and reoxygenation in tumor parenchyma. Cancer Res 56:5522, 1996.
136. Chaplin D, Durand R, Olive P: Acute hypoxia in tumors: implication for modifiers of radiation effects. Int J Radiat Oncol Biol Phys 12:1279, 1986.
137. Chaplin D, Olive P, Durand R: Intermittent blood flow in a murine tumor: radiobiological effects. Cancer Res 47:597, 1987.
138. Dische S: Radiotherapy and anemia—the clinical experience. Radiother Oncol 20(Suppl 1):35, 1991.
139. Dische S: What have we learnt from hyperbaric oxygen? Radiother Oncol 20(Suppl 1):71, 1991.
140. Steel G (ed): Basic Clinical Radiobiology, 3rd ed. London, Arnold, 2002.

141. Dische S: Chemical sensitizers for hypoxic cells: a decade of experience in clinical radiotherapy. Radiother Oncol 3:97, 1985.
142. Overgaard J, Hansen H, Anderson A, et al: Misonidazole combined with split course radiotherapy in the treatment of invasive carcinoma of larynx and pharynx: report from the DAHANCA 2 study. Int J Radiat Oncol Biol Phys 16:1065, 1989.
143. Awwad H, El Naggar M, Mocktar N, et al: Intercapillary distance measurements as an indicator of hypoxia in carcinoma of the cervix uteri. Int J Radiat Oncol Biol Phys 12:1329, 1986.
144. Fenton B, Rofstad E, Degner F, et al: Cryospectrophotometric determination of tumor intravascular oxyhemoglobin saturations: dependence on vascular geometry and tumor growth. J Natl Cancer Inst 80:1612, 1988.
145. Okunieff P, McFarland E, Rummeny E, et al: Effects of oxygen on the metabolism of murine tumors using in vivo phosphorus-31 NMR. Am J Clin Oncol 10:475, 1987.
146. Schneiderman G, Goldstick T: Oxygen electrode design criteria and performance characteristics: recessed cathode. J Appl Physiol 45:145, 1978.
147. Varghese A, Whitmore G: Binding to cellular macromolecules as a possible mechanism for the cytotoxicity of misonidazole. Cancer Res 40:2165, 1980.
148. Chapman J, Franko A, Sharplin J: A marker for hypoxic cells in tumours with potential clinical applicability. Br J Cancer 43:546, 1981.
149. Urtasun R, Koch C, Franko A, et al: A novel technique for measuring human tissue pO2 at the cellular level. Br J Cancer 54:453, 1986.
150. Koh W, Bergman K, Rasey J, et al: Evaluation of oxygenation status during fractionated radiotherapy in human non-small cell lung cancers using F-18 fluoromisonidazole positron emission tomography. Int J Radiat Oncol Biol Phys 32:391, 1995.
151. Jin G, Li S, Moulder J, et al: Dynamic measurements of hexafluoromisonidazole (CCI-103F) retention in mouse tumours by $^{1}H/^{19}F$ magnetic resonance spectroscopy. Int J Radiat Biol 58:1025, 1990.
152. Cline J, Thrall D, Rosner G, et al: Distribution of the hypoxia marker CCI-103F in canine tumors. Int J Radiat Oncol Biol Phys 28:921, 1994.
153. Raleigh J, La Dine J, Cline J, et al: An enzyme-linked immunosorbent assay for hypoxia marker binding in tumours. Br J Cancer 69:66, 1994.
154. Kennedy A, Raleigh J, Perez G, et al: Proliferation and hypoxia in human squamous cell carcinoma of the cervix: first report of combined immunohistochemical assays. Int J Radiat Oncol Biol Phys 37:897-905, 1997.
155. Raleigh J, Dewhirst M, Thrall D: Measuring tumor hypoxia. Semin Radiat Oncol 6:37, 1996.
156. Zeman E, Calkins D, Cline J, et al: The relationship between proliferative and oxygenation status in spontaneous canine tumors. Int J Radiat Oncol Biol Phys 27:891, 1993.
157. Raleigh J, Zeman E, Calkins D, et al: Distribution of hypoxia and proliferation associated markers in spontaneous canine tumors. Acta Oncol 34:345, 1995.
158. Murphy B, Andrews G, Bittel D, et al: Activation of metallothionein gene expression by hypoxia involves metal response elements and MTF-1. Cancer Res 59:1315, 1999.
159. Bussink J, Kaanders J, Rijken P, et al: Changes in blood perfusion and hypoxia after irradiation of a human squamous cell carcinoma xenograft tumor line. Radiat Res 153:398, 2000.
160. Ljungkvist A, Bussink J, Raleigh J, et al: Changes in tumor hypoxia measured with a double hypoxic marker technique. Int J Radiat Oncol Biol Phys 48:1529, 2000.
161. Nordsmark M, Loncaster J, Chou S-C, et al: Invasive oxygen measurements and pimonidazole labelling in human cervix carcinomas. Int J Radiat Oncol Biol Phys 49:581, 2001.
162. Olive P, Banath J, Aquino-Parsons C: Measuring hypoxia in solid tumors. Is there a gold standard? Acta Oncol 40:917, 2001.
163. Janssen H, Haustermans KM, Sprong D, et al: HIF-1A, pimonidazole, and iododeoxyuridine to estimate hypoxia and perfusion in human head-and-neck tumors. Int J Radiat Oncol Biol Phys 54:1537, 2002.
164. Varia M, Calkins-Adams D, Rinker L, et al: Pimonidazole: a novel hypoxia marker for complementary study of tumor hypoxia and cell proliferation in cervical carcinoma. Gynecol Oncol 71:270, 1998.
165. Arteel G, Thurman R, Raleigh J: Reductive metabolism of the hypoxia marker pimonidazole is regulated by oxygen tension independent of the pyridine nucleotide redox state. Eur J Biochem 253:743, 1998.
166. Arteel G, Thurman R, Yates J, et al: Evidence that hypoxia markers detect oxygen gradients in liver: pimonidazole and retrograde perfusion of rat liver. Br J Cancer 73:889, 1995.
167. Yin M, Zhong Z, Connor H, et al: Protective effect of glycine on renal injury induced by ischemia-reperfusion in vivo. Am J Physiol Renal Physiol 282:417, 2002.
168. Vordermark D, Brown J: Endogenous markers of tumor hypoxia predictors of clinical radiation resistance? Strahlenther Onkol 179:801, 2003.
169. Vukovic V, Haugland H, Nicklee T, et al: Hypoxia-inducible factor-1 alpha is an intrinsic marker for hypoxia in cervical cancer xenografts. Cancer Res 61:7394, 2001.
170. Vordermark D, Katzer A, Baier D, et al: Cell type-specific association of hypoxia-inducible factor-1 alpha (HIF-1α) protein accumulation and radiobiologic tumor hypoxia. Int J Radiat Oncol Biol Phys 58:1242, 2004.
171. Wykoff C, Beasley N, Watson P, et al: Hypoxia-inducible expression of tumor-associated carbonic anhydrases. Cancer Res 60:7075, 2000.
172. Olive P, Aquino-Parsons C, MacPhail S, et al: Carbonic anhydrase 9 as an endogenous marker for hypoxic cells in cervical cancer. Cancer Res 61:8924, 2001.
173. Airley R, Loncaster J, Davidson S, et al: Glucose transporter glut-1 expression correlates with tumor hypoxia and predicts metastasis-free survival in advanced carcinoma of the cervix. Clin Cancer Res 7:928, 2001.
174. Cooper R, Sarioglu S, Sokmen S, et al: Glucose transporter-1 (GLUT-1): a potential marker of prognosis in rectal carcinoma? Br J Cancer 89:870, 2003.
175. Airley R, Loncaster J, Raleigh J, et al: GLUT-1 and CAIX as intrinsic markers of hypoxia in carcinoma of the cervix: relationship to pimonidazole binding. Int J Cancer 104:85, 2003.
176. Azuma Y, Chou S-C, Lininger R, et al: Hypoxia and differentiation in squamous cell carcinomas of the uterine cervix. Clin Cancer Res 9:4944, 2003.
177. Chou S-C, Azuma Y, Varia M, et al: Evidence that involucrin, a marker for differentiation, is oxygen regulated in human squamous cell carcinomas. Br J Cancer 90:728, 2004.
178. Hall E: High-LET radiations. *In* Becker F (ed): Cancer: a Comprehensive Treatise, vol 6. New York, Plenum Press, 1977, p 281.
179. Rockwell S, Baserga S, Knisely J: Artificial blood substitutes in radiotherapy. *In* Hagen U, Harder D, Jung H, et al (eds): Radiation Research 1895-1995: Proceedings of the Tenth International Congress of Radiation Research, vol 2. Wurzburg, Universitatsdruckerei H Stürtz, 1996, p 795.
180. Gerweck L, Gillette E, Dewey W: Killing of Chinese hamster cells in vitro by heating under hypoxic or aerobic conditions. Eur J Cancer 10:691, 1974.
181. Yuhas J, Spellman J, Culo F: The role of WR 2721 in radiotherapy and/or chemotherapy. *In* Brady L (ed): Radiation Sensitizers. New York, Masson, 1980, p 303.
182. Horsman M, Chaplin D, Overgaard J: The use of blood flow modifiers to improve the treatment response of solid tumors. Radiother Oncol 20(Suppl 1):47, 1991.
183. Laurence V, Ward R, Dennis I, et al: Carbogen breathing with nicotinamide improves the oxygen status of tumours in patients. Br J Cancer 72:198, 1995.
184. Lee I, Kim J, Levitt S, et al: Increases in tumor response by pentoxifylline alone or in combination with nicotinamide. Int J Radiat Oncol Biol Phys 22:425, 1992.
185. Zeman E, Brown J, Lemmon M, et al: SR 4233: a new bioreductive agent with high selective toxicity for hypoxic mammalian cells. Int J Radiat Oncol Biol Phys 12:1239, 1986.
186. Brown J: SR 4233 (tirapazamine): a new anticancer drug exploiting hypoxia in solid tumors. Br J Cancer 67:1163, 1993.
187. Adams G, Dewey D: Hydrated electrons and radiobiological sensitization. Biochem Biophys Res Commun 12:473, 1963.

188. Brown J, Workman P: Partition coefficient as a guide to the development of radiosensitizers which are less toxic than misonidazole. Radiat Res 82:171, 1980.
189. Brown J: Clinical trials of radiosensitizers: what should we expect? Int J Radiat Oncol Biol Phys 10:425, 1984.
190. Brown J, Yu N, Brown D, et al: SR 2508: a 2-nitroimidazole amide which should be superior to misonidazole as a radiosensitizer for clinical use. Int J Radiat Oncol Biol Phys 7:695, 1981.
191. Lee D, Cosmatos D, Marcial V, et al: Results of an RTOG phase III trial (RTOG 85-27) comparing radiotherapy plus etanidazole with radiotherapy alone for locally advanced head and neck carcinomas. Int J Radiat Oncol Biol Phys 32:567, 1995.
192. Szybalski W: Properties and applications of halogenated deoxyribonucleic acids. *In* The Molecular Basis of Neoplasia. Austin, University of Texas Press, 1962, p 147.
193. Kaplan H: Radiosensitization by the halogenated pyrimidine analogues: laboratory and clinical investigations. *In* Moroson H, Quintilliani M (eds): Radiation Protection and Sensitization. London, Taylor & Francis, 1970, p 35.
194. Cecchini S, Girouard S, Huels M, et al: Single-strand-specific radiosensitization of DNA by bromodeoxyuridine. Radiat Res 162:604, 2004.
195. Bagshaw M, Doggett R, Smith K: Intra-arterial 5-bromodeoxyuridine and x-ray therapy. AJR Am J Roentgenol 99:889, 1967.
196. Kinsella T, Mitchell J, Russo A, et al: The use of halogenated thymidine analogs as clinical radiosensitizers: rationale, current status, and future prospects. Int J Radiat Oncol Biol Phys 10:139, 1984.
197. Mitchell J, Kinsella T, Russo A, et al: Radiosensitization of hematopoietic precursor cells (CFUc) in glioblastoma patients receiving intermittent intravenous infusions of bromodeoxyuridine (BUdR). Int J Radiat Oncol Biol Phys 9:457, 1983.
198. Epstein H, Cook J, Goffman T, et al: Tumour radiosensitization with the halogenated pyrimidines 5′-bromo- and 5′-iododeoxyuridine. Br J Radiol 24(Suppl):209, 1992.
199. Prados M, Scott C, Sandler H, et al: A phase III randomized study of radiotherapy plus procarbazine, CCNU, and vincristine (PCV) with or without BUdR for the treatment of anaplastic astrocytoma: a preliminary report of RTOG 9404. Int J Radiat Oncol Biol Phys 45:1109, 1999.
200. Rodriguez R, Ritter M, Fowler J, et al: Kinetics of cell labeling and thymidine replacement after continuous infusion of halogenated pyrimidines in vivo. Int J Radiat Oncol Biol Phys 29:105, 1994.
201. Lawrence T, Davis M, Mayburn J, et al: The dependence of halogenated pyrimidine incorporation and radiosensitization on the duration of drug exposure. Int J Radiat Oncol Biol Phys 18:1393, 1990.
202. Brown J, Lemmon M: Potentiation by the hypoxic cytotoxin SR 4233 of cell killing produced by fractionated irradiation of mouse tumors. Cancer Res 50:7745, 1990.
203. Brown J, Siim B: Hypoxia-specific cytotoxins in cancer therapy. Semin Radiat Oncol 6:22, 1996.
204. Adams G: The Henry S. Kaplan Award Lecture: the search for specificity. *In* Hagen U, Harder D, Jung H, et al (eds): Radiation Research 1895-1995, vol 2. Congress Lectures. Wurzburg, Universitatsdruckerei H Stürtz, 1995, p 33.
205. Brown J: Cytotoxic effects of the hypoxic cell radiosensitizer Ro 07-0582 to tumor cells in vivo. Radiat Res 72:469, 1977.
206. Denekamp J, McNally N: The magnitude of hypoxic cell cytotoxicity of misonidazole in human tumours. Br J Radiol 51:747, 1978.
207. Adams G, Ahmed I, Sheldon P, et al: Radiation sensitization and chemopotentiation: RSU 1069, a compound more efficient than misonidazole in vitro and in vivo. Br J Cancer 49:571, 1984.
208. Jenkins T, Naylor M, O'Neill P, et al: Synthesis and evaluation of 1-(3-(2-haloethylamino)propyl)-2-nitroimidazoles as pro-drugs of RSU 1069 and its analogs, which are radiosensitizers and bioreductively activated cytotoxins. J Med Chem 33:2603, 1990.
209. Haffty B, Son Y, Sasaki C, et al: Mitomycin C as an adjunct to postoperative radiation therapy in squamous cell carcinoma of the head and neck: results from two randomized clinical trials. Int J Radiat Oncol Biol Phys 27:241, 1993.
210. Koch C: Unusual oxygen concentration dependence of toxicity of SR 4233, a hypoxic cell toxin. Cancer Res 53:3992, 1993.
211. Dorie M, Brown J: Tumor-specific, schedule-dependent interaction between tirapazamine (SR 4233) and cisplatin. Cancer Res 53:4633, 1993.
212. Lartigau E, Guichard M: The effect of tirapazamine (SR-4233) alone or combined with chemotherapeutic agents on xenografted human tumours. Br J Cancer 73:1480, 1996.
213. Reck M, von Pawel J, Nimmermann C, et al: Phase II trial of tirapazamine in combination with cisplatin and gemcitabine in patients with advanced non-small-cell-lung-cancer (NSCLC). Pneumologie 58:845, 2004.
214. Rischin D, Peters L, Fisher R, et al: Tirapazamine, cisplatin, and radiation versus fluorouracil, cisplatin, and radiation in patients with locally advanced head and neck cancer: a randomized phase II trial of the Trans-Tasman Radiation Oncology Group (TROG 98.02). J Clin Oncol 23:79, 2005.
215. Patt H: Cysteine protection against x-irradiation. Science 110:213, 1949.
216. Schuchter L, Glick J: The current status of WR-2721 (amifostine): a chemotherapy and radiation therapy protector. Biol Ther Cancer 3:1, 1993.
217. Bacq Z: The amines and particularly cysteamine as protectors against roentgen rays. Acta Radiol 41:47, 1954.
218. Rasey J, Nelson N, Mahler P, et al: Radioprotection of normal tissues against gamma rays and cyclotron neutrons with WR 2721: LD_{50} studies and ^{35}S-WR 2721 biodistribution. Radiat Res 97:598, 1984.
219. Rojas A, Stewart F, Soranson J, et al: Fractionation studies with WR 2721: normal tissues and tumor. Radiother Oncol 6:51, 1987.
220. Yuhas J: Improvement of lung tumor radiotherapy through differential chemoprotection of normal and tumor tissue. J Natl Cancer Inst 48:1255, 1972.
221. Yuhas J, Storer J: Differential chemoprotection of normal and malignant tissues. J Natl Cancer Inst 42:331, 1969.
222. Glover D, Glick J, Weiler C, et al: Phase I/II trials of WR 2721 and *cis*-platinum. Int J Radiat Oncol Biol Phys 12:1509, 1986.
223. Glover D, Glick J, Weiler C, et al: WR 2721 protects against the hematologic toxicity of cyclophosphamide: a controlled phase II trial. J Clin Oncol 4:584, 1986.
224. Kligerman M, Turrisi A, Urtasun R, et al: Final report on phase I trial of WR-2721 before protracted fractionated radiation therapy. Int J Radiat Oncol Biol Phys 14:1119, 1988.
225. Delaney J, Bonsack M, Felemovicius I: Misoprostol in the intestinal lumen protects against radiation injury of the mucosa of the small bowel. Radiat Res 137:405, 1994.
226. Hanson W, Marks J, Reddy S, et al: Protection from radiation-induced oral mucositis by misoprostol, a prostaglandin E(1) analog: a placebo-controlled, double-blind clinical trial. Am J Ther 2:850, 1995.
227. Moulder J: Pharmacological intervention to prevent or ameliorate chronic radiation injuries. Semin Radiat Oncol 13:73, 2003.
228. Delanian S, Lefaix J: The radiation-induced fibroatrophic process: therapeutic perspective via the antioxidant pathway. Radiother Oncol 73:119, 2004.
229. Rubin P, Casarett G: Clinical Radiation Pathology. Philadelphia, WB Saunders, 1968.
230. Michalowski A: Effects of radiation on normal tissues: hypothetical mechanisms and limitations of in situ assays of clonogenicity. Radiat Environ Biophys 19:157, 1981.
231. Mendelsohn M: The growth fraction: a new concept applied to tumors. Science 132:1496, 1960.
232. Mendelsohn M, Dohan F, Moore H: Autoradiographic analysis of cell proliferation in spontaneous breast cancer of C3H mouse. J Natl Cancer Inst 25:477, 1960.
233. Lajtha L: On the concepts of the cell cycle. Cell Comp Physiol 62:143, 1963.
234. Dethlefsen L: In quest of the quaint quiescent cells. *In* Meyn R, Withers H (eds): Radiation Biology in Cancer Research. New York, Raven Press, 1980, p 415.
235. Steel G: Growth Kinetics of Tumours. Oxford, Clarendon Press, 1977.
236. Steel G: The heyday of cell population kinetics: insights from the 1960s and 1970s. Semin Radiat Oncol 3:78, 1993.

237. Quastler H, Sherman F: Cell population kinetics in the intestinal epithelium of the mouse. Exp Cell Res 17:420, 1959.
238. Tannock I, Hill R: The Basic Science of Oncology, 3rd ed. New York, McGraw-Hill Health Professions, 1998.
239. Tannock I: The relation between cell proliferation and the vascular system in a transplanted mouse mammary tumor. Br J Cancer 22:258, 1968.
240. Steel G: Cell loss from experimental tumors. Cell Tissue Kinet 1:193, 1968.
241. McBride W, Withers H: Biological basis of radiation therapy. *In* Perez C, Brady L, Halperin E, et al (eds): Principles and Practice of Radiation Oncology, 4th ed. Philadelphia, Lippincott Williams & Wilkins, 2003.
242. Begg A, McNally N, Shrieve D, et al: A method to measure the duration of DNA synthesis and the potential doubling time from a single sample. Cytometry 6:620, 1985.
243. Wilson G, McNally N, Dische S: Measurement of cell kinetics in human tumors in vivo using bromodeoxyuridine incorporation and flow cytometry. Br J Cancer 58:423, 1988.
244. Bentzen S: Estimation of radiobiological parameters from clinical data. *In* Hagen U, Jung H, Streffer C (eds): Radiation Research 1895-1995, vol 2. Congress Lectures. Wurzburg, Universitatsdruckerei H Stürtz, 1995, p 833.
245. Fowler J: The linear-quadratic formula and progress in fractionated radiotherapy. Br J Radiol 62:679, 1989.
246. Thames H, Ruifrok A, Milas L, et al: Accelerated repopulation during fractionated irradiation of a murine ovarian carcinoma: downregulation of apoptosis as a possible mechanism. Int J Radiat Oncol Biol Phys 35:951, 1996.
247. Begg A, Haustermans K, Hart A, et al: The value of pretreatment cell kinetic parameters as predictors of radiotherapy outcome in head and neck cancer: a multicenter analysis. Radiother Oncol 50:13, 1999.
248. Withers H, Taylor J, Maciejewski B: The hazard of accelerated tumor clonogen repopulation during radiotherapy. Acta Oncol 27:131, 1988.
249. Fowler J: The James Kirk Memorial Lecture. What next in fractionated radiotherapy? Br J Cancer Suppl 46:285, 1984.
250. Fowler J: Non-standard fractionation in radiotherapy. Int J Radiat Oncol Biol Phys 10:755, 1984.
251. Fowler J: Review: total doses in fractionated radiotherapy—implications of the new radiobiological data. Int J Radiat Oncol Biol 46:103, 1984.
252. Hermens A, Barendsen G: Changes of cell proliferation characteristics in a rat rhabdomyosarcoma before and after x-irradiation. Eur J Cancer 5:173, 1969.
253. Hanahan D, Weinberg R: The hallmarks of cancer. Cell 100:57, 2000.
254. Dorr W, Hendry J: Consequential late effects in normal tissues. Radiother Oncol 61:223, 2001.
255. United Nations Scientific Committee on the Effects of Atomic Radiation: Sources and Effects of Ionizing Radiation. Report to the General Assembly, with Annexes. Vienna, United Nations Publications, 1994.
256. Mettler F, Upton A: Medical Effects of Ionizing Radiation, 2nd ed. Philadelphia, WB Saunders Company, 1995.
257. Hemplemann L, Lisco H, Hoffman J: The acute radiation syndrome: a study of nine cases and a review of the problem. Ann Intern Med 36:279, 1952.
258. Shipman T, Lushbaugh C, Peterson D, et al: Acute radiation death resulting from an accidental nuclear critical excursion. J Occup Med Suppl 3:146, 1961.
259. Karas J, Stanbury J: Fatal radiation syndrome from an accidental nuclear excursion. N Engl J Med 272:755, 1965.
260. Cogan C, Donaldson D, Reese A: Clinical and pathological characteristics of the radiation cataract. Arch Ophthalmol 47:55, 1952.
261. Committee on the Biological Effects of Ionizing Radiation: Health effects of exposure to low levels of ionizing radiation. Washington, DC, National Academy Press, 1990.
262. Upton A: The dose-response relation in radiation-induced cancer. Cancer Res 21:717, 1961.
263. International Commission on Radiological Protection: 1990 Recommendations, no. 60, vol 21. Oxford, UK, Pergamon Press, 1991.
264. Stewart A, Webb D, Hewitt B: A survey of childhood malignancies. Br Med J 1:1495, 1958.
265. Fajardo L: Pathology of Radiation Injury. New York, Masson Publishing, 1982.
266. Hallahan D: Radiation-mediated gene expression in the pathogenesis of the clinical radiation response. Semin Radiat Oncol 6:250, 1996.
267. Hallahan D, Haimovitz-Friedman A, Kufe D, et al: The role of cytokines in radiation oncology. Important Adv Oncol (no vol):71, 1993.
268. Anscher M, Murase T, Prescott D, et al: Changes in plasma TGF beta levels during pulmonary radiotherapy as a predictor of the risk of developing radiation pneumonitis. Int J Radiat Oncol Biol Phys 30:671, 1994.
269. Brizel D: Future directions in toxicity prevention. Semin Radiat Oncol 8:17, 1998.
270. Chen L, Brizel D, Rabbani Z, et al: The protective effect of recombinant human keratinocyte growth factor on radiation-induced pulmonary toxicity in rats. In J Radiat Oncol Biol Phys 60:1520, 2004.
271. Haimovitz-Friedman A, Kolesnick R, Fuks Z: Modulation of the apoptotic response: potential for improving the outcome in clinical radiotherapy. Semin Radiat Oncol 6:273, 1996.
272. Withers H, Taylor J, Maciejewski B: Treatment volume and tissue tolerance. Int J Radiat Oncol Biol Phys 14:751, 1988.
273. Withers H, Mason K, Thames H: Late radiation response of kidney assayed by tubule cell survival. Br J Radiol 59:587, 1986.
274. van der Kogel A: Effect of volume and localization on rat spinal cord. *In* Fielden E, Fowler J, Hendry J, et al (eds): Proceedings of the Eighth International Congress of Radiation Research. London, Taylor & Francis, 1987, p 352.
275. Hopewell J, Morris A, Dixon-Brown A: The influence of field size on the late tolerance of the rat spinal cord to single doses of x-rays. Br J Radiol 60:1099, 1987.
276. Travis E, Terry N: Cell depletion and initial and chronic responses in normal tissues. *In* Vaeth J, Meyer J (eds): Radiation Tolerance of Normal Tissues. Frontiers of Radiation Therapy and Oncology, vol 23. Basel, Karger, 1989, p 41.
277. Thames H, Hendry J: Fractionation in Radiotherapy. Philadelphia, Taylor & Francis, 1987.
278. Inskip P: Second cancers following radiotherapy. *In* Inskip P (ed): Multiple Primary Cancers. Philadelphia, Lippincott Williams & Wilkins, 1999, p 91.
279. Boice JD, Storm HH, Curtis RE, et al: Introduction to the study of multiple primary cancers. Natl Cancer Inst Monogr 68:3, 1985.
280. Travis L, Gospodarowicz M, Curtis R, et al: Lung cancer following chemotherapy and radiotherapy for Hodgkin's Disease. J Natl Cancer Inst 94:182, 2002.
281. Travis L, Hill D, Dores G, et al: Breast cancer following radiotherapy and chemotherapy among young women with Hodgkin's disease. JAMA 290:465, 2003.
282. Kleinerman R, Boice J, Storm H, et al: Second primary cancer after treatment for cervical cancer. Cancer 76:442, 1995.
283. Wong F, Boice J, Abramson D, et al: Cancer incidence after retinoblastoma: radiation dose and sarcoma risk. JAMA 278:1262, 1997.
284. Hall E, Wuu C: Radiation-induced second cancers: the impact of 3D-CRT and IMRT. Int J Radiat Oncol Biol Phys 56:83, 2004.
285. Fowler J, Stern B: Dose-time relationships in radiotherapy and the validity of cell survival curve models. Br J Radiol 36:163, 1963.
286. Withers H: The four R's of radiotherapy. *In* Adler H, Lett J, Zelle M (eds): Advances in Radiation Biology, vol 5. New York, Academic Press, 1975, p 241.
287. Bedford J, Hall E: Survival of HeLa cells cultured in vitro and exposed to protracted gamma irradiation. Br J Radiol 39:896, 1964.
288. Hall E, Bedford J: Dose-rate: its effect on the survival of HeLa cells irradiated with gamma-rays. Radiat Res 22:305, 1964.
289. Szechter A, Schwarz G: Dose-rate effects, fractionation and cell survival at lower temperatures. Radiat Res 71:593, 1977.
290. Mitchell J, Bedford J, Bailey S: Dose-rate effects in plateau-phase cultures of S3 HeLa and V79 cells. Radiat Res 79:552, 1979.

291. Wells R, Bedford J: Dose-rate effects in mammalian cells. IV. Repairable and nonrepairable damage in noncycling C3H 10T1/2 cells. Radiat Res 94:105, 1983.
292. Zeman E, Bedford J: Dose-rate effects in mammalian cells. V. Dose fractionation effects in noncycling C3H 10T1/2 cells. Int J Radiat Oncol Biol Phys 10:2089, 1984.
293. Dutreix J, Wambersie A, Bounik C: Cellular recovery in human skin reactions: application to dose fraction number overall time relationship in radiotherapy. Eur J Cancer 9:159, 1973.
294. Ellis F: Dose, time and fractionation: a clinical hypothesis. Clin Radiol 20:1, 1969.
295. Ellis F: Relationship of biological effect to dose-time-fractionation factors in radiotherapy. *In* Ebert M, Howard M (eds): Current Topics in Radiation Research. Amsterdam, North Holland Publishing, 1968, p 357.
296. Orton C, Ellis F: A simplification in the use of the NSD concept in practical radiotherapy. Br J Radiol 46:529, 1973.
297. Kirk J, Gray W, Watson R: Cumulative radiation effect. Part I. Fractionated treatment regimes. Clin Radiol 22:145, 1971.
298. Denekamp J: Changes in the rate of proliferation in normal tissues after irradiation. *In* Nygaard O, Adler H, Sinclair W (eds): Radiation Research: Biomedical, Chemical and Physical Perspectives. New York, Academic Press,1975.
299. Douglas B, Fowler J: The effect of multiple small doses of x-rays on skin reactions in the mouse and a basic interpretation. Radiat Res 66:401, 1976.
300. Thames H, Withers H, Peters L, et al: Changes in early and late radiation responses with altered dose fractionation: implications for dose-survival relationships. Int J Radiat Oncol Biol Phys 8:219, 1982.
301. Withers H, Thames H, Peters L: Differences in the fractionation response of acutely and late-responding tissues. *In* Karcher K, Kogelnik H, Reinartz G (eds): Progress in Radio-Oncology II. New York, Raven Press, 1982, p 287.
302. Withers H: Biology of altered fractionation. *In* Karcher K, Kogelnik H, Stadler B, et al (eds): Progress in Radio-Oncology IV. New York, Raven Press, 1988, p 181.
303. Thames H, Bentzen S, Turesson I, et al: Time-dose factors in radiotherapy: a review of human data. Radiother Oncol 19:219, 1990.
304. Thames H, Peters L, Withers H, et al: Accelerated fractionation vs. hyperfractionation: rationale for several treatments per day. Int J Radiat Oncol Biol Phys 9:127, 1983.
305. Barendsen G: Dose fractionation, dose rate and iso-effect relationships for normal tissue responses. Int J Radiat Oncol Biol Phys 8:1981, 1982.
306. Lee A, Sze W-M, Fowler J, et al: Caution on the use of altered fractionation for nasopharyngeal carcinoma. Radiother Oncol 52:201, 1999.
307. Fowler J, Harari P, Leborgne F, et al: Acute radiation reactions in oral and pharyngeal mucosa: tolerable levels in altered fractionation schedules. Radiother Oncol 69:161, 2003.
308. Fowler J: Repair between dose fractions: a simpler method of analyzing and reporting apparently bioexponential repair. Radiat Res 158:141, 2002.
309. Gasinska A, Fowler J, Lind B, et al: Influence of overall treatment time and radiobiological parameters on biologically effective doses in cervical cancer patients treated with radiation alone. Acta Oncol 43:657, 2004.
310. Fowler J, Welsh J, Howard S: Loss of biological effect in prolonged fraction delivery. Int J Radiat Oncol Biol Phys 59:242, 2004.
311. Ellsworth D, Ellsworth R, Liebman M, et al: Genomic instability in histologically normal breast tissues: implications for carcinogenesis. Lancet Oncol 5:753, 2004.
312. Streffer C: Bystander effects, adaptive response and genomic instability induced by prenatal irradiation. Mutat Res 568:79, 2004.
313. McBride W, Chiang C, Olson J, et al: A sense of danger from radiation. Radiat Res 162:1, 2004.
314. Karagiannis T, El-Osta A: Double-strand breaks: signaling pathways and repair mechanisms. Cell Mol Life Sci 61:2137, 2004.
315. Coleman C, Stone H, Moulder J, et al: Medicine. Modulation of radiation injury. Science 304:693, 2004.
316. Okunieff P, Augustine E, Hicks J, et al: Pentoxifylline in the treatment of radiation-induced fibrosis. J Clin Oncol 22:2207, 2004.
317. van der Meeren A, Mouthon M, Vandamme M, et al: Combinations of cytokines promote survival of mice and limit acute radiation damage in concert with amelioration of vascular damage. Radiat Res 161:549, 2004.
318. Hayashi T, Morishita Y, Kubo Y, et al: Long-term effects of radiation dose on inflammatory markers in atomic bomb survivors. Am J Med 118:83, 2005.
319. Greider C, Blackburn E: Telomeres, telomerase and cancer. Sci Am 274:92, 1996.
320. Shay J, Wright W: Telomeres and telomerase: implications for cancer and aging. Radiat Res 155:188, 2001.
321. Neumann A, Reddel R: Telomere maintenance and cancer—look, no telomerase. Nature Rev Cancer 2:879, 2002.
322. Mothersill C, Seymour C: Radiation-induced bystander effects: past history and future directions. Radiat Res 155:759, 2001.
323. Prise K, Folkard M, Michael B: Bystander responses induced by low LET radiation. Oncogene 22:7043, 2003.
324. Elkind M, Sutton-Gilbert H, Moses W, et al: Radiation response of mammalian cells grown in culture. V. Temperature dependence of the repair of x-ray damage in surviving cells (aerobic and hypoxic). Radiat Res 25:359, 1965.
325. Sinclair W: Dependence of radiosensitivity upon cell age. *In* Proceedings of the Carmel Conference on Time and Dose Relationships in Radiation Biology as Applied to Radiotherapy. BNL Report 50203. Upton, NY, Brookhaven National Laboratory, 1969.
326. Nias A: Clinical Radiobiology, 2nd ed. New York, Churchill Livingstone, 1988.
327. Withers H, Thames H, Peters L, et al: Normal tissue radioresistance in clinical radiotherapy. *In* Withers H, Thames H, Peters L (eds): Biological Basis and Clinical Implications of Tumor Radioresistance. New York, Masson, 1983, p 139.

CHAPTER 2

MOLECULAR AND CELLULAR BIOLOGY

Mary Ann Stevenson and Stuart K. Calderwood

The past decade has seen a revolution in two areas of cell and molecular biology closely related to radiation therapy. The pathways involved in response to genomic stress, including mechanisms for sensing DNA damage and responding to cell cycle changes and DNA repair, have been elucidated by studies of model organisms, particularly the yeast *Saccharomyces cerevisiae*.[1,2] In the second major area, understanding pathways of programmed cell death (PCD), which may play a major role in treatment response, studies of *Caenorhabditis elegans* were the most informative in demonstrating the significance of individual death genes.[3] The challenge is to combine these two areas of knowledge to provide a rational understanding of how tumor cells can be made to enter the death pathways after processing DNA damage using the genomic stress response. Considerable technologic improvements also have enabled significant progress in translational work, including rational, in silico drug design and high-throughput screening of chemical libraries, which may permit the application of advances in molecular biologic knowledge to the development of drugs for use in combination with radiation therapy.

ESSENTIAL STEPS IN TUMOR PROGRESSION

Most evidence suggests that tumors are formed by stepwise progression of cells from a minimally altered state, where they are able to grow and form nodules or polyps (e.g., solid tumors) to a state of maximal transformation, characterized by multiply deviated cells that are capable of unlimited growth, manipulation of their local environment, invasion of surrounding tissues, and escape into the circulation to establish new colonies of secondary tumors, or metastases.[4] Such phenotypic and genotypic progression involves a vast array of molecular and morphologic changes. In their landmark review, Hanahan and Weinberg[5] suggested organizing these traits into six essential alterations in cell physiology: self-sufficiency in growth signals, insensitivity to growth inhibition, evasion of PCD, limitless replicative potential, sustained angiogenesis, and tissue invasion and metastasis. Although the initial steps are believed to occur earlier in tumor progression, the exact order of occurrence varies among different malignancies, and some phenotypic transformations appear to require more than one molecular change.[5] The occurrence in tumor cells of this series of radical, primarily genetic alterations in physiology is in part the result of an evolving instability of the tumor genome due to a breakdown in the DNA repair pathways that accompanies tumor progression.[6,7] In addition to progressing and acquiring enhanced malignant capabilities, most human tumors undergo further selections through exposure to various forms of cytotoxic therapy such as irradiation and chemotherapy, leading to the development of resistant phenotypes in the cells that survive the toxic insult.

All cancer treatments are aimed at reversing these hallmarks of neoplastic transformation and tipping the balance toward tumor cell death. Ionizing radiation kills cells almost exclusively through the generation of DNA double-strand breaks (DSBs).[8] The evolving modification of the cellular phenotype during tumorigenesis leads to the development of resistance to therapy. Our major task is to explore the links among DSB response pathways, engagement of cell death mechanisms, and the outcome of radiation therapy.

RADIATION THERAPY AND RADIATION BIOLOGY

Application of ionizing radiation has long been known to be a potent modality in cancer therapy, one that can kill cells and lead to tumor regression.[9] Early studies showed that killing by ionizing radiation involves the oxygen-dependent generation of free radicals and subsequent damage to multiple molecular structures within the cell.[8] The generation of DSBs in DNA is the dominant form of direct lethality.[10] It has been estimated that the existence of even one unrepaired DSB can lead to cell death. Within whole organisms, direct and indirect forms of lethality occur. Radiation can cause the death of hematopoietic stem cells in the bone marrow and stem cells in crypts of the small intestine, which leads to secondary damage caused by immunosuppression and gross infection, as the gastrointestinal lining is lost.[8,11,12] The challenge facing radiation therapy is to enhance cell kill within tumors while avoiding dose-related complications in organs containing rapidly renewing stem cell populations. Early studies using the clonogenic cell survival assay established the notion of optimizing radiobiologic parameters such as dose, fractionation, and cell cycle inhibition as a means of inhibiting reproductive cell death in critical normal tissues.[13] The clonogenic cell survival assay is a useful measure of cell inactivation because the effects of ionizing radiation seen in vitro often mirror the responses of tumors in vivo.[8] However, its critical weakness is that it does not allow for discrimination or elucidation of the various mechanisms leading to cell death. That kind of detailed information is essential for the successful combination of radiation therapy with other modalities, which may result in sensitization or protection, or both. Irradiation activates a number of pathways that mediate reproductive death, including various forms of PCD (e.g., apoptosis, autophagy), replicative senescence, and necrosis, the default pathway that often dominates when other types of cell death are inhibited.[14-16] Susceptibility to each of these forms of cell death changes over the course of tumor progression, and the tumor cell response to ionizing radiation is likely to reflect the aggregate of genetic changes that accompany tumor progression. The task of modern radiation biology is to examine the mechanisms by which ionizing radiation gives rise to unrepaired DNA DSBs and how such damage is coupled to the pathways of cell killing within the moving target of the evolving cancer cell.

DNA DOUBLE-STRAND BREAK RESPONSE

All cells have evolved to live in an environment that is more or less mutagenic, and they have evolved responses to permit survival when the genome is damaged.[17] DNA may be damaged during the normal processes of DNA replication and segregation.[17] Within tumor cells, these initial changes become progressively altered as cells compete for survival in the tumor milieu and are subjected to selection by various forms of cytotoxic therapy.[4] The response to DSB appears to involve two principal components: arrest of cell proliferation to prevent replication and segregation of the damaged DNA and, when possible, repair of the lesion.[18] A third component in the DSB response in multicellular organisms may be altruistic entry of irreversibly damaged cells into the PCD pathways.[19,20] The latter effect is the desired response to cytotoxic therapy. Understanding how the DSB response is regulated at the molecular level may be one of the keys to understanding the differential response to irradiation in individual tumors and the rational design of radiosensitizing drugs. There are several basic questions regarding regulation of this response. By which mechanism do tumor cells arrest in the cell cycle? How is the presence of DNA DSB detected in such cells? What are the major pathways for repair of DSB? How does the deployment of these pathways affect tumor response to therapy?

Mechanisms of Cell Cycle Arrest: The Cell Cycle and Checkpoints

The cell cycle is a series of molecular programs that read out in an invariant order that leads to the duplication of the genome and other cellular components and permits division into two cells, each with a full set of chromosomes and the organelles required for life.[21] Orderly, high-fidelity, and complete duplication of the genome is required for progression through the cell cycle. This is achieved through a surveillance system that detects DNA damage or unreplicated DNA and imposes cell cycle arrest at designated *checkpoints*, blocking the forward progress of the cell cycle engine (Fig. 2-1). Because ionizing radiation produces severe damage to DNA, cell cycle checkpoints are essential for facilitating repair and subsequent cell survival after radiation exposure, and they provide an ultimate target for strategies aimed at sensitizing cells to radiation therapy.

Much accumulated evidence indicates that the cell cycle is driven at the fundamental level by sequential activation of a series of protein kinases that determine the order and rate of the metabolic events required in each stage. These cell division kinases, or cyclin-dependent kinases (CDKs) are activated by binding proteins originally designated as cell division cycle (CDC) molecules, now known as cyclins.[21] The cyclin-CDK complexes are master regulators that determine the rates of the individual component reactions that mediate the events at each stage of the cell cycle.[22] Phosphorylation of cell cycle effector proteins by the cyclin-CDK complexes acts as a switch, turning them on in orderly fashion. In mammalian cells, many cyclins regulate individual stages of the cell cycle, including G_1 cyclins (cyclins D and E), S phase–specific cyclins, and G_2-specific cyclins (cyclins A and B), which associate, respectively, with G_1-specific (CDK2, CDK4, and CDK6), S-specific, and G_2-specific (CDC2) cyclin-dependent kinases. The events of G_1 (i.e., synthesis of enzymes and other molecules involved in DNA replication), S phase (i.e., DNA replication), and G_2/M (i.e., chromosome condensation, disappearance of the nuclear envelope, and mitosis) are regulated by the transient accumulation and subsequent degradation of the cyclins.[21-23] Switching off involves the targeted degradation of the cyclins by a protein destruction machine called the *proteasome*.[24] Targeted destruction of the cyclins after they have carried out their function ensures unidirectional, irreversible progression around the cell cycle.[23] The timing of the various cell cycle phases under normal conditions appears to be related to the time required for cyclin-CDK complexes to reach appropriate, critical concentrations and for the phosphorylation of key substrates.[23]

Irradiation leads to prolongation of the cell cycle and arrests in G_1, G_2, and S phases because of DNA damage–induced activation of cell cycle checkpoints (see Fig. 2-1).[25] Although this phenomenon was observed many years ago, it has only recently been understood at the biochemical and genetic levels. Arrest of cells at the G_1 checkpoint has been particularly well studied (see Fig. 2-1A). G_1 arrest is caused by the accumulation of a CDK inhibitory protein, CDKN1A (formerly designated p21 or Cip1), in the irradiated cells, which prevents

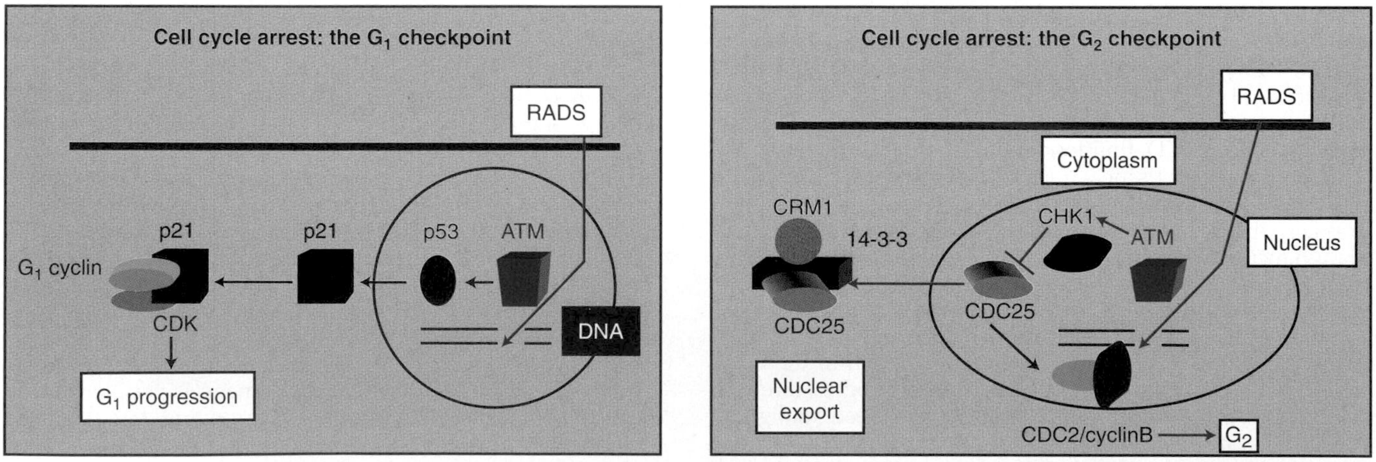

A B

Figure 2-1 Cell cycle checkpoints. **A,** To progress through G_1 to the replication (S) phase, cells require the activity of G_1 cyclins (D, E) and cyclin-dependent kinases (CDK2, CDK4, and CDK6) to phosphorylate substrates such as the retinoblastoma protein (RB1). DNA damage is sensed by the protein kinase ATM, which activates TP53 (p53), leading to transcription of the CDKN1A (p21) protein, a powerful inhibitor of cyclin-CDK complex kinase activity, and to arrest in G_1. DNA damage may be repaired, leading to deactivation of the checkpoint block and progression into S phase. If it is unrepaired, TP53-dependent programmed cell death may occur. **B,** To progress through G_2 into M, the activity of the protein phosphatase CDC25 is required. DNA damage *(red arrows)* also leads to ATM activation, which causes a cascade response as ATM kinase activates the CHK kinases and CHK1 phosphorylates CDC25, leading to recruitment of the activation protein YWHA (formerly designated 14-3-3) and an adapter protein that couples CDC25 to the nuclear export machinery of the cell. Exported from the nucleus, CDC25 is no longer able to mediate dephosphorylation of CDC2 at the G_2/M transition and progression through G_2.

key events that are required for transit through G_1, including phosphorylation of the retinoblastoma (RB1) protein and activation of the E2F transcription factors (e.g., E2F1, E2F2, E2F4, E2F6) necessary for accumulation of enzymes required to traverse S phase.[26-28] CDKN1A is induced at the transcriptional level by TP53 (also known as p53), which accumulates in irradiated cells and binds to the *CDKN1A* promoter, thereby activating transcription.[27,28] TP53 accumulation appears to be at least partially caused by the activation of a DSB sensor molecule, the protein kinase ATM (ataxia-telangiectasia, mutated).[27-30] The exact mechanism involved in sensing DSBs and activation of ATM is unclear, although it appears to involve ATM autophosphorylation.[30] The common mechanism for regulating the G_1 and G_2 checkpoints is inhibition of the CDK components of the interphase cell cycle engine, which inhibits phosphorylation and switching on of the effector molecules (see Fig. 2-1).[23,31] A variation on this theme is seen at the mitotic spindle checkpoint. Progression through mitosis requires switching off CDK activity through targeted degradation of cyclin B.[32] Arrest in M phase, when the mitotic spindle is compromised, involves the TP53-dependent stabilization of cyclin B. The mitotic spindle checkpoint guarantees that replication is followed by cell division, ensuring prevention of aneuploidy. Not surprisingly, the polyploidy nature of many tumor cells appears to be related to TP53 inactivation.[32] Most evidence indicates that ATM (and its homologues in other organisms) functions as a sensor for DNA damage through a complex series of interactions with the damaged DNA. This ultimately leads to ATM activation and downstream signaling cascades involving the kinases CHK1 and CHK2 (also called CHEK1 and CHEK2), which couple to the cell cycle engine at the level of individual cyclin-CDK complex molecules (see Fig. 2-1B).[1,2,18,29,31] The molecular details of these processes are evolving rapidly, and referenced reviews can provide more detailed insight into the mechanisms of DNA damage, sensing, and checkpoint engagement.

TP53: Cellular Triage after Ionizing Radiation Exposure

TP53 is a nuclear phosphoprotein that possesses sequence-specific DNA binding activity. It functions as a transcriptional activator and appears to play a triage role in the decision to undergo cell cycle arrest and repair or to enter the pathways of PCD or replicative senescence (Fig. 2-2).[27,28,33,34] When cells are exposed to ionizing radiation or chemotherapeutic agents, the levels of wild-type TP53 protein are increased. TP53 then transcriptionally activates a number of genes, most notably *CDKN1A*, the CDK inhibitor that mediates many of the properties of TP53.[35] In addition to G_1 arrest, genotoxic stress and ionizing radiation can induce TP53-dependent PCD pathways, including caspase-dependent apoptosis.[27,33] TP53 can transcriptionally activate the proapoptotic *BAX* gene, induce synthesis of JUN kinase, and repress transcription of the antiapoptotic gene *BCL2*, suggesting that TP53 is a central mediator of PCD processes.[27,33] DNA damage in the presence of wild-type TP53 causes G_1 arrest, followed by a period of DNA repair; if the damage is too great to be easily repaired, the cell is eliminated through TP53-dependent PCD pathways. However, approximately 50% of human tumors possess inactivating mutations in the *TP53* gene.[36] TP53 becomes inactivated in many tumors due to selection against its proapoptotic properties. The resultant loss of its central function as "sentinel of the genome" may be a type of collateral damage incurred in cells due to the selection advantage for survival that accrues from the loss of *TP53* apoptotic function.[34,37] The loss of *TP53* function is linked to poorer prognosis in malignancies such as lung, breast, colorectal, and hematopoietic tumors.[28] Many tumor cell lines containing mutant TP53, including breast, glioma, and lymphoma cell lines, are more resistant to therapy than their wild-type *TP53* counterparts.[38,39]

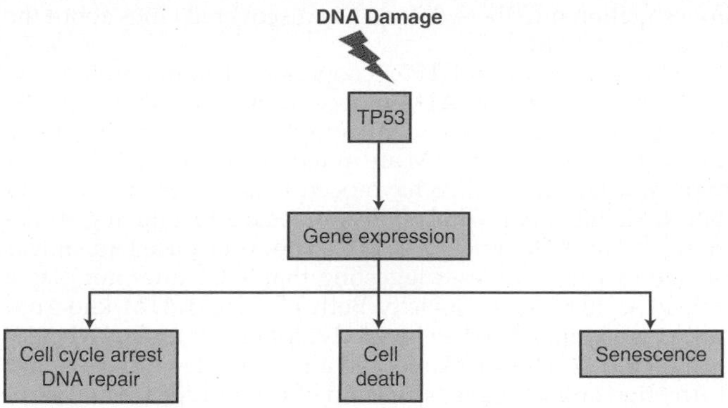

Figure 2-2 TP53 plays a triage role in deciding a cell's fate after exposure to ionizing radiation. TP53 is activated after irradiation, largely through protein stabilization that results from phosphorylation by the protein kinase ATM. Most effects of TP53 are mediated through its transcriptional activity, with some gene products (e.g., CDKN1A [p21]) leading to cell cycle arrest and others (e.g., BID, BBC3 [formerly designated PUMA], PMAIP1 [formerly NOXA]) to programmed cell death. A third fate appears to be senescence, which is mediated largely through CDKN1A. The triage decision appears to be related to radiation dose (i.e., degree of DNA damage), with greater damage favoring the death and senescence pathways.

The loss of wild-type *TP53* function in human malignancies may be a key step in the progression of human cancer, and the *TP53* status of cells may control the outcome of many tumor types in response to chemotherapy or radiation therapy.[37] Although most of the other DSB response genes have molecular equivalents in yeast, *TP53* does not. The *TP53* gene appears to be required to determine the fate of damaged cells, which in mammalian cells may be PCD, a sacrifice that contributes to the well-being of the whole organism. The TP53 protein may monitor the degree of damage and act as a master switch, moving the cells from a state of cycle arrest and DNA repair to death or senescence pathways. Loss of TP53 in tumors compromises this critical surveillance and triage function. With the loss of this critical decision-point molecule, damaged and mutated tumor cells may survive to generate new and more malignant phenotypes (see Fig. 2-2).

ATM Gene: Master Regulator of the DNA Double-Strand Break Response

One of the many defects in ataxia-telangiectasia (AT) cells is increased chromosomal instability. Exposure to ionizing radiation also produces an increased number of chromosomal aberrations in AT cells compared with normal cells. This effect and the *ATM* gene's homology[40,41] with the DNA repair protein DNA-PK suggested that AT cells might have deficient DNA repair. However, many investigations have revealed that AT cells do not have gross abnormalities in their ability to repair DNA damage. In general, it does not appear that the radiosensitivity of AT cells is caused by faulty DNA repair; it more likely results from an inability to detect the presence of DNA damage. Exposure to ionizing radiation causes normal cells to delay at the G_1/S and G_2/M transition phases of the cell cycle, and these checkpoints are thought to allow the cells to repair DNA damage before DNA synthesis or mitosis occurs.[31] Both of these checkpoints are absent in AT cells, and investigation into these defects has discovered clues about the function of ATM.[31]

Although ATM and TP53 cooperate in radiation-induced apoptosis, there are ATM-independent pathways for the induction of TP53-dependent apoptosis, and many of the downstream effects of ATM are independent of TP53.[29,31] Wild-type and knockout mice have been evaluated for acute and late toxicities after whole-body exposure to ionizing radiation.[29,31] The *ATM*- and *ATM/TP53*-knockout mice had similar severe toxicity profiles, suggesting that TP53 does not play a role in acute radiation toxicity. Both *TP53*- and *ATM*-knockout mice preferentially developed lymphoid tumors, whereas *ATM/TP53* double knockouts had an accelerated time to tumor formation and a broader spectrum of tumor types. Analysis of the acquired tumors in *ATM*-null/*TP53*-heterozygous mice revealed that three of seven had loss of the remaining *TP53* allele. These studies showed that ATM and TP53 interact in a complex manner that is specific to cell type and outcome. This interaction most likely relies on a variety of other pathways (discussed later) and will require much additional work before a complete understanding of the ATM/TP53 relationship is obtained.

With isolation of the *ATM* gene, it became possible to attempt correction of the cellular defects of the AT phenotype using gene transduction techniques. Several groups have reported that the introduction of ATM into AT cells resulted in reversal of AT defects.[31,40] The transfection of full-length ATM into AT cells reversed DSB, restored normal sensitivity to ionizing radiation, and decreased the number of chromosomal abnormalities. Transfection of full-length ATM also reversed the defective activation of CDKN1A (p21) and JUN kinase in response to ionizing radiation.[42,43]

Histones and Chromatin Structure

Native DNA exists in the cell in the form of chromatin complexed with a family of proteins called *histones*. The histones are involved in packaging DNA in the nucleus into a compact, metabolically inert form. For processes such as transcription or DNA repair to occur, the histones must be altered by post-translational modifications, most notably acetylation, that permit decondensation and access to the DNA.[44] For effective DNA repair, acetylation of histones by histone acetylases must occur to permit access of repair proteins to the sites of DSB.[45] A novel histone, H2AX, found in low concentrations on chromatin, has been shown to play a crucial signaling role in the response to genomic stresses such as ionizing radiation. H2AX phosphorylation is one of the earliest events occurring after exposure to ionizing radiation, and ATM-dependent phosphorylation of H2AX may be involved in signaling to cell cycle checkpoints and DNA repair enzymes involved in recombination repair.[46,47]

Mechanisms of DNA Repair after Ionizing Radiation

Because maintaining undamaged DNA is essential to cell survival, cells have evolved a wide range of mechanisms to halt cell cycle progression, survey DNA, and repair damage. Radiation can induce a range of lesions by direct interaction with DNA or indirectly through damage induced in nearby water molecules by free radicals. The products of radiation damage include DNA base damage, damage to the deoxyribose sugar backbone, and physical breaks in one or both strands of the DNA. DNA damage induced by ionizing radiation tends to be clustered so that there is more than one damaged site in proximity along the double helix, known as *locally multiply damaged sites*.[48]

Among the less catastrophic forms of DNA damage induced by ionizing radiation are the singly damaged bases, which can be repaired by a process called *base excision repair*. This is a procedure by which the damaged base is recognized and removed by an *N*-glycosylase, the apurinic or apyrimidinic (AP) site is cleaved by an AP endonuclease, a patch of DNA is excised, DNA is then resynthesized using the other strand as the template, and the repaired strand is ligated.[49,50] In settings in which the base damage is not recognized by the *N*-glycosylase, another mechanism for repair exists, called *nucleotide excision repair*. In a manner somewhat similar to base excision repair, a damaged section of DNA is removed by incision and excision, a patch is resynthesized using the remaining strand, and the repaired strand is then ligated. Although no naturally occurring mammalian mutants have been identified that are defective in base excision repair, there are a number of different excision repair mutants, which are exemplified by xeroderma pigmentosum and Cockayne's syndrome. They are characterized by abnormalities in the repair of damage caused by ultraviolet light, although the clinical spectrum of these repair-deficiency syndromes varies. The abnormal genes are identified by finding the human gene that corrects rodent cell defects, called *excision repair cross-complementing* (ERCC) groups. Several reviews offer more details on ionizing radiation and DNA repair.[17,49,50]

DNA Strand Breaks

The essential DNA lesion for cellular lethality is the DSB.[51-53] Misjoined or unrepaired DSBs can produce deletions, translocations, and acentric or dicentric chromosomes, all of which have serious consequences for the cell. As with the excision repair defects (e.g., ERCCs), there are several x-ray repair defects in the x-ray cross-complementation (XRCC) groups involved in the repair of DSBs. Single-strand repair is carried out in a manner similar to base damage repair, with the undamaged DNA strand serving as a template. DSB repair is more complicated, because there is no adjacent, undamaged template available to repair the broken strands. The ends of the broken DNA must be protected, and the damaged site must be reconstituted by the processes of *homologous recombination* and *nonhomologous end joining* (NHEJ) .

The processes involved in DNA DSB repair have much in common with the recombinatorial processes involved in immunoglobulin and T-cell receptor gene rearrangement. The XRCC groups that have been identified and are involved in DNA DSB repair include genes that produce DNA end-binding proteins XRCC6 (formerly designated KU70 or Ku70) and XRCC5 (formerly designated KU80 or Ku80) and a DNA-dependent protein kinase (DNA-PK). Defects in DNA repair genes are seen in severe combined immunodeficiency (SCID) mice, indicating the importance of recombination in the restoration of DNA integrity after DSBs and in the immune response.[17,51]

Double-Strand Break Damage and Repair

Experiments in yeast and human cells indicate that the accumulation of a single DSB in irradiated cells can lead to cell death.[31,51,53] Accumulating evidence points to the existence of a system in eukaryotes that recognizes DSBs and leads to DSB repair and other processes. Such a system would be predicted to include three functional components: a mechanism for detecting and gauging DNA damage, a signal transduction system, and an effector system for DNA repair. These components are discussed in the following paragraphs, commencing with the repair component. DSBs can be repaired by a number of mechanisms, but the most prevalent are homologous recombination and NHEJ. Human cells appear to differ from yeast in that NHEJ appears to predominate in yeast.[17,51]

Genetic analysis has revealed the existence of a large number of genes that regulate DSB repair. One essential gene, involved in resistance to cell killing by ionizing radiation and the repair of DSB, is *XRCC5*, which encodes XRCC5, a protein that binds with high affinity to the ends of the double strands in a complex that includes another protein, XRCC6 (Fig. 2-3A).[1,5,17] XRCC5 functions in normal cellular processes that require DSB rejoining, most notably V(D)J rejoining in the immunoglobulin and T-cell receptor genes of immature B and T lymphocytes. XRCC5 exists in cells in a heterodimeric complex with XRCC6, the product of the *XRCC6* gene. The XRCC5/XRCC6 heterodimer is required for the end-binding and repair functions.[54] The XRCC (formerly designated KU) proteins carry out the important function of recognizing the ends of DSBs and protecting them from further degradation before initiation of the end-joining reactions that mediate DSB repair. An associated protein in the complex with important functions in DNA repair is DNA-PK, which is the product of the *XRCC7* gene.

The double-strand DNA-PK is a serine/threonine kinase involved in regulating the cellular response to DNA damage.[54,55] DNA-PK is a member of the phosphatidylinositol-3-kinase gene family *(PIK)* that produce a group of high-molecular-weight proteins that contain a conserved kinase domain at the carboxyl-terminal end. PIK proteins have been identified in yeast, *Drosophila*, and in mammalian cells, and the PIK family includes the human ataxia-telangiectasia gene *(XRCC7)* for DNA-PK and the yeast genes *TEL1* and *MEC1*.[54,55] Homology with genes of other organisms can provide a clue to the function of the family of genes in mammalian systems. For example, the *S. cerevisiae TEL1* gene is a homologue of the human *ATM* gene. *TEL1* mutants have shortened telomeres and exhibit chromosome instability. In mice, the SCID mutation results in the loss of expression of functional DNA-PK.[56] SCID mice are deficient in the repair of DNA DSBs, have faulty V(D)J recombination, and are extremely sensitive to radiation.[56] The binding of the XRCC (formerly KU) complex (XRCC5 and XRCC6) to DNA-PK activates the serine/threonine kinase of the catalytic subunit of DNA-PK. The DNA-PK/XRCC complex is involved in recognition of DNA DSBs. In SCID cells, the catalytic subunit for DNA-PK is absent, and the loss of DNA-PK activity may account for the increased sensitivity to ionizing radiation, the inability to repair DNA DSBs, and the immune defects.

Genetic evidence indicates the existence of numerous other factors required for efficient DSB repair in human cells.[18,51,53] Among the genes are homologues of the yeast *RAD52* epistasis group, *RAD50* and *MRE11*.[57-59] RAD50 and MRE11, together with the product of the *XRS2* gene, form a complex in *S. cerevisiae* that is involved in nonhomologous recombination (see Fig. 2-3B). RAD50 has been suggested to bind to DNA at the site of DSBs and mark them for repair or recombination. Such a signaling role for RAD50/MRE11 complexes is suggested by studies indicating the formation of nuclear foci containing these proteins in cells after irradiation. The RAD50/MRE11 complexes also contain another important protein, NBN (nibrin; formerly NBS1 or p95), which is inactivated in the Nijmegen breakage syndrome.[57-59] The RAD50/MRE11 foci failed to form in ATM-deficient cells, suggesting a position for this complex downstream of the ATM protein. Numerous molecules are involved in double-strand DNA damage recognition, response, and repair. DSB repair can also be carried out in human cells by homologous recombination, an alternative pathway that involves a different group of genes, including *RAD51* through *RAD57*. RAD51, the eukaryotic homologue of

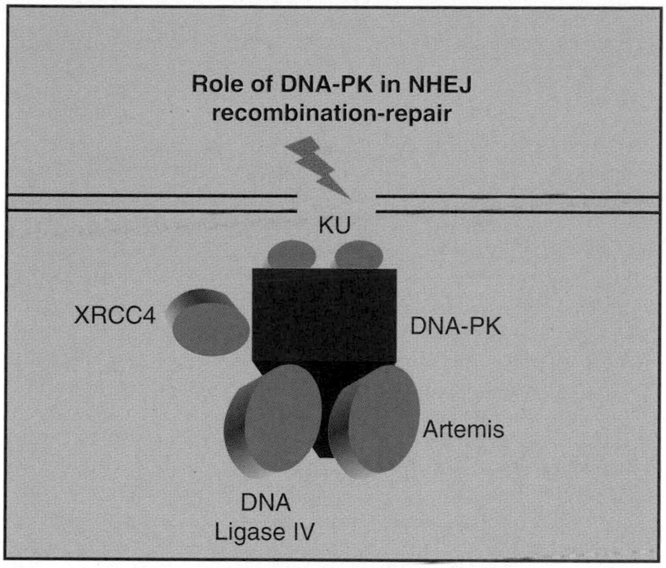

A

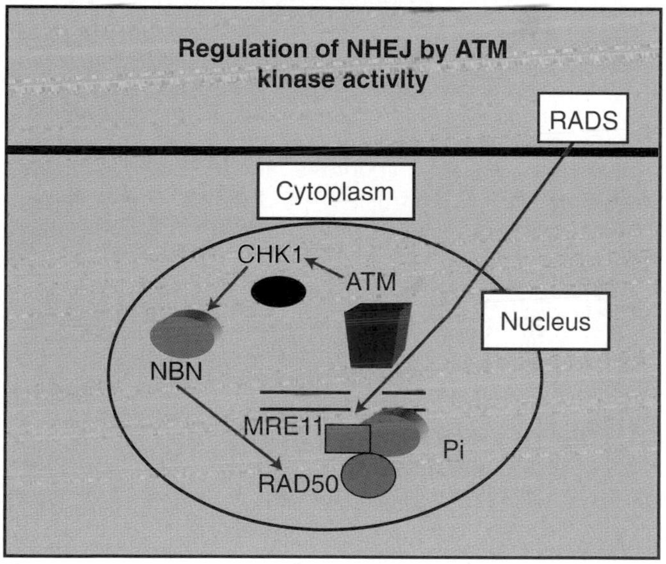

B

Figure 2-3 **A,** Formation of DNA repair complexes on damaged DNA. Radiation-induced DNA damage causes immediate changes in the vicinity of double-strand breaks (DSBs). These include rapid phosphorylation of the atypical histone H2AFX and activation of ATM. Protein complexes then begin to assemble on DNA, including the DNA-dependent protein kinase (DNA-PK) complex shown here. This complex is a molecular machine for DNA repair that includes DNA end-binding proteins XRCC6 (formerly KU70) and XRCC5 (formerly KU80); DNA-PK itself, which appears to be a signaling and scaffold protein; and proteins involved in the effector stages of repair. **B,** Another important protein complex mediating DNA DSB repair by the nonhomologous end joining (NHEJ) pathway is the RAD50 complex. The diagram shows the signal transduction pathway leading from ATM, the sensor of DNA DSB, to the phosphorylation of NBN (nibrin, formerly designated NBS1), which induces recruitment of RAD50 and MRE11 into a DNA repair complex at the site of the DNA DSB.

the bacterial RecA protein, forms structures in meiotic chromosomes that contain the ATM protein, suggesting functional coupling between these proteins. The complex also contains TP53 and may be involved in coupling of DNA DSB formation sensing to cell cycle arrest, as well as in carrying out recombination and repair. The formation of DSBs is coupled to cell cycle arrest by ATM during pathologic processes that lead to DSBs and normal processes that involve DSBs, including meiosis, mitosis, and V(D)J recombination.

The tumor suppressor genes *BRCA1* and *BRCA2* also may function in DNA repair processes. Although the roles of these gene products appear to be multifactorial, it has been shown that *BRCA1* interacts with the recombination and repair protein RAD51 and that one function of *BRCA1* is to assist in cell cycle arrest through activation of *CDKN1A,* a gene that is normally activated by TP53.[60] RAD51 is targeted by three major gene products: ATM, TP53, and BRCA1. The loss of RAD51 can lead to cancer development, suggesting that this pathway of DNA repair and replication is crucial in protection of cells from genotoxic stress. That this RAD51 pathway of DSB repair is separate from the RAD50 end-joining pathway is indicated by findings that ionizing radiation causes the formation of nuclear foci containing RAD50 or RAD51 but never both complexes. However, further studies are required to understand the relative contributions of the two pathways to cell survival after exposure to ionizing radiation. As with the RAD50 pathway, understanding of the regulation of recombination repair is still at an early stage of development and cannot be assembled into a fully coherent molecular pathway. It has been shown that *BRCA2* mutant cancer cells are deficient in DNA DSB repair and have increased radiosensitivity.[60] The field of DNA damage recognition and repair is complex, involving interaction among molecules that can cause cell cycle arrest, apoptosis, and signal transduction. Defects in any of these pathways could lead to radiation sensitivity in normal tissues (and perhaps the corresponding tumor) or to the development of secondary mutations and the mutator phenotype, as with mismatch repair defects. For radiation therapy, the DNA DSB is a key determinant of cell survival, and the relationship between DSB repair and recombination in immune cells has opened up a new line of investigation.

PATHWAYS OF IONIZING RADIATION–INDUCED PROGRAMMED CELL DEATH

Because the desired outcome of radiation therapy is tumor cell destruction, it is crucial to understand how cells die. The ability of cells to inhibit the normal pathways of cell death appears to be a key step in the origin of cancer cells, with the small percentage of cells that are able to evade PCD being the ones most capable of forming tumors.[5,15] Multiple genetic alterations are involved in the escape from PCD, most notably in the *TP53* and *BCL2* families of genes.[15] Radiation oncology is faced with the undesirable situation in which tumor cells are selected for resistance to PCD while normal cells retain these altruistic pathways.[34] Apoptosis and autophagy are key PCD pathways with a potential role in cancer induction and resistance to therapy. Excellent reviews have been provided by Edinger and Thompson[15] and Danial and Korsmeyer.[61]

Apoptosis is a normal physiologic process that is a biochemically regulated mode of cell death. Apoptosis is characterized morphologically by cell shrinkage, membrane blebbing, chromatin condensation, and ultimate fragmentation of the cell into apoptotic bodies. Several biochemical characteristics commonly observed include activation of enzymes that degrade proteins, called *caspases,* which are involved in intracellular death signaling; activation of enzymes that degrade DNA (endonucleases); and alteration of the cell surface (including expression of annexin V binding sites on the plasma membrane) so that neighboring cells can remove the apoptotic bodies without the induction of an inflammatory reaction. Apoptosis appears to be mediated by changes in the outer mitochondrial membrane that lead to the release of death signals such as cytochrome *c.* BCL2 and related family members function as antiapoptotic factors by blocking prodeath changes in mitochondrial membrane potential or as antiapoptotic factors by antagonizing the proapoptotic factor BAX. The terminal stages involve DNA degradation, which cleaves DNA into 50- to 300-kb fragments and later into smaller fragments by cleavage of the exposed regions of DNA between nucleosomes.

Autophagy, another form of cell death, also involves autodigestion, this time through a specialized organelle, the lysosome, which is a dedicated digestive organelle containing key proteases (i.e., cathepsins) that participate in killing cells.[15] Many of the upstream signals of caspase-dependent apoptosis may be shared by the autophagic pathway.[15] Because TP53 plays a key role in both processes, its loss in many cancers may inhibit the activation of these processes by ionizing radiation. Inhibition of cell death through these more regulated forms of PCD can lead to death by necrosis in a proportion of targeted cells.[62] This form of death may be less efficient than other death pathways, permitting continued survival of deranged or damaged cells that would otherwise have been targeted for PCD. Necrosis that occurs as a result of inhibition of PCD pathways or of ischemia in the poorly perfused tumor core leads to release of cell contents into the tumor milieu; this initiates the formation of an inflammatory response and environment in the vicinity of the tumor, facilitating unwanted secondary effects such as angiogenesis, tumor cell invasion, and metastasis.[15]

REPLICATIVE SENESCENCE

In addition to vulnerability to overt killing, all somatic cells possess replicative checkpoints that place limits on the number of permitted cell divisions over the lifetime of the cell. For unlimited growth, cells must bypass *crisis,* the point at which the telomeres on chromosomes have shortened enough to prevent successful future cell divisions. TP53-sensitive (and CDKN1A-sensitive) expression of the enzyme telomerase in tumor cells is sufficient to bypass crisis and permit unlimited growth in some cells (see Fig. 2-2). In addition to crisis, cells undergo telomerase-independent forms of senescence, regulated in many cases by the retinoblastoma protein RB1 and the CDK inhibitory protein CDKN2A (formerly designated p16). However, TP53 appears to be the primary regulator of senescence; it can induce senescence downstream of DNA damage detected by ATM activation or through other pathways.[14] Few experiments have been carried out to examine the role of senescence in responses to ionizing radiation, although in one study, ionizing radiation induced premature senescence that occurred independently of ATM expression.[63] A large increase in the volume of experiments dealing with this subject is anticipated.

ACTIVATION OF ANABOLIC SIGNALING PATHWAYS BY IONIZING RADIATION

One of the primary features of cancer is its autonomy in terms of growth signals.[5] There are three operationally defined steps in growth signaling: (1) transmembrane receptor occupation by growth factors and transmembrane signaling, (2) stimulation of cytoplasmic cascades that amplify primary signals, and (3) activation of downstream effector proteins. Step 1 classically involves receptor dimerization and autophosphorylation

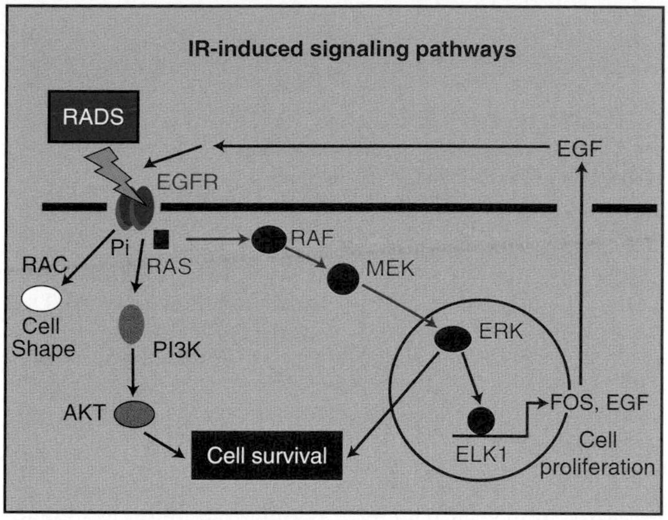

Figure 2-4 Induction of transmembrane signals by ionizing radiation (IR), which directly activates several transmembrane receptors. Free radicals induced in cells by ionizing radiation can activate transmembrane tyrosine kinase receptors such as the epidermal growth factor (EGFR) and HER2, HER3, and HER4 (not shown). Receptor activation gives rise to a network of signals that lead to activation of the powerful prosurvival PI3K/AKT pathway and the growth-mediating RAF/MEK/ERK cascade. Further amplification may take place as a result of transcriptional induction and the release from cells of cytokines with growth factors such as EGF and transforming growth factor-α, which give rise to secondary activation of receptors.

of receptor tyrosine kinases (RTKs) or recruitment of nonreceptor tyrosine kinases (NRTKs). Such events occur commonly after ionizing radiation, and a generalized activation of the HER1 through HER4 RTKs occurs in irradiated cells (Fig. 2-4).[64] Studies show that ionizing radiation can induce the release of growth factors such as epidermal growth factor (EGF) and paracrine activation of growth in adjacent cells.[64] Increases in cellular phosphotyrosine levels were observed after exposure to x-rays in a number of cells, and activation of NRTKs has been observed.[64] Of particular importance in step 2 processes are members of the mitogen-activated protein kinase (MAPK) family, which play a crucial role in cell growth and survival. Ionizing radiation stimulates the activity of MAPK members that carry the mitogenic signal (e.g., MAPK1 [formerly ERK2], MAPK3 [formerly ERK1]).[65] The paradigm for step 3 is the activation of factors that bind the promoters of mammalian immediate early genes such as *FOS* and *EGR1* through receptor activation, tyrosine phosphorylation, and MAPK activation. Such transcription factors include serum response factor, ETS domain factors such as TCF62, ELK-1, activating protein-1 (AP1), and cyclic adenosine monophosphate–binding protein (i.e., cAMP response element binding [CREB]).[66] Each of these factors is activated by ionizing radiation, and the promoter of at least one immediate early gene *(EGR1)* is induced by radiation treatment. Exposure to ionizing radiation may amplify the growth signals already active in cancer cells, suggesting that the RTK-MAPK pathway may be a fruitful target in the selection of radiation sensitizers.[64,67]

A clue to the physiologic significance of radiation-induced signaling may be afforded by understanding the molecular changes that initiate radiation-induced signaling. Radiation produces two main species that combine to kill cells in a clinical setting and that may also double as primary stress signals involved in triggering cell survival responses.[8] These signals are reactive oxygen species (ROS) and DNA DSBs.[8] ROS play a role in signal transduction events after stimulation by platelet-derived growth factor (PDGF) and phorbol esters.[8,65,68] ROS produced by cellular stress, such as peroxide, superoxide, hydroxyl radicals, and nitrous oxide, may feed into this ROS-transduced pathway at a number of places.[69] Cell kill by radiation is closely correlated with the accumulation of DNA DSBs. The dictates of logic and much preliminary evidence strongly suggest a role for DSBs in the sensing and response to ionizing radiation. Cells evidently possess at least one system to sense and respond to radiation; this system involves the ATM family of protein kinases, which appear to be situated close to the primary event in DSB-induced signaling.[1,30,31,51,70] ATM activation leads to phosphorylation of the TP53 tumor antigen, coupling DSB accumulation to cell cycle arrest in G_1; vectorial signaling is then coupled to the cyclic events of the cell division cycle.[29] ATM belongs to the lipid kinase family that includes PIK and DNA-PK.[31,41] PIK is activated by ionizing radiation and is required for cell survival during irradiation. DNA-PK is intimately involved in cell responses to radiation, and its ability to sense DSBs in combination with DNA end-binding proteins XRCC6 and XRCC5 suggests that it may be able to function independently of ATM in cell signaling after exposure to ionizing radiation.[54]

Regulatory changes in cells after irradiation may be caused by the aggregate and combinatorial interactions of three distinct types of signaling pathways: classic signal transduction, signaling pathways mediated by ROS, and those initiated in the nucleus by DSBs.

TUMOR MICROENVIRONMENT AND RESPONSES TO IONIZING RADIATION IN VIVO

In addition to malignant cells, tumors contain many normal cells and structural elements, including endothelial cells, fibroblasts, extracellular matrix, inflammatory cells, blood vessels, cytokines, growth factors, and biochemical metabolites. The tumor microenvironment is abnormal, is largely deficient in nutrients such as oxygen and glucose, and contains increased levels of waste products such as lactic acid and carbon dioxide.[71,72] The concentrations of nutrients and cell-cell and cell-matrix contacts are abnormal, and they may be in a constant state of flux because of intermittent perfusion.[8] The tumor microenvironment is a key determinant of the response to ionizing radiation. Hypoxic cells are markedly resistant to radiation because of the requirement for oxygen in the formation of destructive free radical species (e.g., ROS) that mediate radiation-induced DSB formation.[8] Defining the tumor milieu and how it is regulated is of central importance to the understanding of radiation effects at the tissue and organ levels.

Hypoxia, Microenvironment, and Radiation Response

The role of cellular hypoxia in producing radioresistance is well known.[73] Cell killing by radiation therapy is decreased at intermediate and low oxygen conditions, and a number of studies have correlated low pretreatment tumor oxygenation with a worse disease outcome.[74,75] Whether there is a direct cause-and-effect relationship between low oxygen concentration and outcome or the low oxygen concentration indicates a more malignant tumor phenotype remains to be resolved, primarily through clinical trials that deliberately attempt to correct the poor oxygenation status of the tumors. Hypoxia can, for instance, induce growth arrest by inhibiting

DNA synthesis.[74,75] In addition to directly inhibiting cell killing by ionizing radiation, hypoxia may amplify the mutator phenotype in the severely hypoxic cells in the central cores of tumors, increasing the rate of evolution of resistant clones and amplifying the malignant phenotype.[76] Targeting of hypoxic cells in radiation therapy is indicated for many reasons. The role of hypoxia in promoting angiogenesis has been described previously. An exciting discovery is that of hypoxia-inducible factor-1 (HIF1), which induces hypoxia-responsive genes.[77,78]

Many genes are induced or repressed within the acutely hostile tumor microenvironment.[77,78] The largely unregulated environment found in poorly vascularized tumors can be thought of as resembling the conditions under which many unicellular organisms grow. Survival for these organisms depends on their ability to withstand environmental stresses such as nutritional deprivation, temperature and pH changes, radiation exposure (e.g., ultraviolet light, x-rays), and xenobiotics. Among the molecules induced by hypoxia are members of the unfolded protein response family stress proteins (e.g., glucose-regulated proteins [GRPs], redox enzymes such as heme oxygenase, metallothionien IIA, DT-diaphorase; transcription factors such as JUN, FOS, AP1, TP53, nuclear factor-κB [NF-κB], HIF1) and growth factors or cytokines (e.g., erythropoietin, vascular endothelial cell growth factor [VEGF], EGF receptor, interleukin-1α [IL-1α]). However, the key molecule in the response of cells to the microenvironment at the molecular level is the transcription factor HIF1A, which regulates expression of many of the factors that mediate angiogenesis.[77,78]

Tumor Angiogenesis

One of the hallmarks of cancer is the ability of cancer cells to induce de novo angiogenesis to sustain tumor cell growth.[5] Numerous reviews on the subject have emphasized the critical importance of angiogenesis in tumor progression.[79,80] Given the importance of cellular hypoxia for cell killing by ionizing radiation, tumor vascularity, perfusion, and the microenvironment are likely to be critical to clinical outcomes with radiation therapy.[8]

There is a long list of stimulatory factors, including angiopoietin, acidic fibroblast growth factor (FGF), basic FGF, angiogenin, PDGF, prostaglandins E_1 and E_2, transforming growth factor-β, tumor necrosis factor-α, and VEGF (also known as vascular permeability factor). The VEGF family includes angiogenic factors and is receiving attention as a potential therapeutic target. Among the receptors for VEGF are FLT1 and FLK1. Inhibitory factors include angiostatin, endostatin, interferon-α and interferon-β, thrombospondin, and tissue inhibitor of metalloproteinase. These topics are more extensively reviewed elsewhere.[79,81]

The use of antiangiogenic therapy with local radiation has been investigated in several laboratories.[82,83] One important aspect for radiation therapy and probably also for systemic agents is whether antiangiogenic therapy increases or decreases tumor oxygenation. The relationships among angiogenesis, antiangiogenic therapy, and the more conventional cancer therapies remain to be elucidated but offer some exciting areas of investigation. The ability to suppress metastases and hold local tumor growth in check may greatly increase the potential role for radiation therapy. However, if antiangiogenic therapy leads to hypoxia or decreased perfusion of therapeutic molecules, there may be a need to counter this effect by the addition of appropriate pharmacologic agents or modifiers to treatment regimens involving antiangiogenesis agents and radiation therapy. Given the role of blood vessels in late radiation injury, the use of antiangiogenic therapy with radiation in clinical treatment will require careful study and assessment of long-term toxicities and late effects.

TARGETING MOLECULAR PATHWAYS IN THE RADIATION RESPONSE: DISCOVERY OF NEW DRUGS

The accumulation of data regarding the signaling circuitry that underlies the response of cells to DSBs suggests a great opportunity for the development of novel adjuvant therapies based on understanding of the molecular biology of the DSB response. Approaches based on small-molecule inhibitors of specific reactions, RNA interference (small interfering RNAs), and antisense and gene therapy are attractive and follow directly from the basic research available. There is much excitement regarding the potential use of kinase inhibitors in cancer treatment, based on the idea that they work catalytically, are present in small amounts, and often regulate key processes in the cell. The most popular paradigm is a kinase inhibitor, known as imatinib (Gleevec), which has greatly influenced the treatment of hematologic malignancies. Given that the cell cycle checkpoint component of the DNA DSB response is regulated largely at the posttranscriptional level by batteries of protein kinases and phosphatases, many inviting targets are available.[1,18,23,31,58,64] Proof of principle that such an approach may work is suggested by studies using agents that inhibit the RAS signal transduction pathway, protein kinase C, or the PIK pathway, which were shown to enhance radiation-induced cell killing.[84-89] Members of the PIK family may be feasible targets for pharmacologic intervention in the clinic. Loss of function of PIK proteins is usually associated with increased radiosensitivity. Compounds that block the function of these proteins would greatly enhance the efficacy of agents that cause DNA damage, such as radiation therapy, and allow for the treatment of tumors that are particularly radioresistant. The fungal metabolite wortmannin is a specific inhibitor of the p110 PIK, now designated PIK3CD. Wortmannin forms a covalent adduct with Lys802 of PIK3CD, inactivating the kinase activity. This Lys802 is conserved in DNA-PK and AT proteins, suggesting that both would be sensitive to wortmannin. In vitro studies with a wide range of tumor-derived cells, including those of the breast, colon, and prostate, indicate that wortmannin is an effective radiosensitizer of human cells. Wortmannin can inhibit the kinase activity of DNA-PK in vitro and in vivo. DNA-PK also is involved in the activation of TP53 after irradiation of cells, and wortmannin suppresses the activation of TP53 after irradiation. Other studies have shown that wortmannin may exert its primary effect by inhibiting the repair of DNA strand breaks in cells.

In addition to drugs, the development of small interfering RNA approaches offers the promising possibility of "knocking down" selective genes that may mediate resistance.[90,91] There has been much excitement regarding the use of targeted gene therapy to introduce genes of interest or their antisense partners within viral vectors.[92] Some of the enthusiasm about these approaches has waned due to the potential toxicity of the viral vectors and a number of other operational problems, such as accurately reaching the target site, achieving sufficient gene production in situ (i.e., drug, enzyme, or toxic molecule) to alter the radiation response, altering the radiation response sufficiently to show an impact on local tumor control, having a positive therapeutic ratio in that tumor cell killing is enhanced more than normal tissue injury, and ideally, having an impact on survival in addition to enhanced local control. Despite these problems, the approach remains popular, particularly for local expression of products that diffuse from cells, such as cytokines.

Radiation modifiers in clinical use[92,93] have been developed based on conventional radiation biology models, such as hypoxia (e.g., radiation sensitizers and enhancers, altered oxygen delivery), the competition model (e.g., thiol depletion and radioprotectors), and increasing susceptibility of DNA to radiation damage (e.g., halopyrimidines). Although such therapies were not based on the new molecular targets that have more recently been elucidated, much can be learned by studying the relationships between these therapies and the molecular processes. For example, it may be possible to understand how better to use the halopyrimidines in relation to cell cycle checkpoints, hypoxic sensitizers in relation to hypoxia-induced processes, and protectors in terms of specific DNA lesions or activity of repair enzymes.

Tumors exist in a unique microenvironment that is depleted of oxygen and glucose and rich in carbon dioxide and lactate.[71,72] Drugs may be designed to interact with this altered microenvironment and enhance treatment efficacy. Among these more conventional approaches, the bioreductive agents, such as mitomycin C and tirapazamine, require enzymatic activation that occurs preferentially in hypoxic environments.[94]

NORMAL TISSUES

Radiation therapy depends for its selective treatment of cancer on tight control of delivery to tumors and avoidance of normal tissues. Many normal tissues that express wild-type TP53 are sensitive to TP53-induced PCD.[95] Renewable tissues such as hematopoietic stem cells and crypt cells in the gastrointestinal tract may be particularly vulnerable.[35] Indirect forms of lethality may occur in whole-body irradiation, leading to the death of hematopoietic stem cells in the bone marrow, or depletion of mature tissues can lead to secondary damage caused by red blood cell depletion, immunosuppression, and gross infection as the gastrointestinal lining is lost.[8,11,12]

Additional changes occur that are thought to be the result of a persistent oxidative state in tissues such as lung, which may lead to chronic inflammatory changes and induction of cytokines and adhesion molecules.[96,97] Changes may result from induction of the factor NF-κB by ionizing radiation in an ATM-dependent manner (Fig. 2-5).[70,98] NF-κB, in addition to its role in cytoprotection, plays a broader part in the acute inflammatory response through transcription of a wide range of proinflammatory cytokines and adhesion molecules.[99] Induction of an inflammatory environment in normal tissues may be a side effect of activation of NF-κB in a cytoprotective reaction (see Fig. 2-5).

BASIC CONCEPTS AND TECHNIQUES OF RADIATION SCIENCES

Techniques and approaches to molecular and cellular biology in humans and other model organisms, largely developed in the 1960s and 1970s, continue to revolutionize knowledge of basic cancer biology and radiation sciences. The ability to inactivate genes by homologous recombination, which came into frequent use in the 1980s, has permitted the movement of this approach into animal models, allowing study of molecular genetics in vivo. This led to the identification of the key genes involved in the cell cycle, DNA repair, and PCD, which mediate the sensitivity of cells to ionizing radiation and define their exact significance to the host. The big biology approaches, including genomic techniques such as microarray technology, permit the screening of the expression of multiple

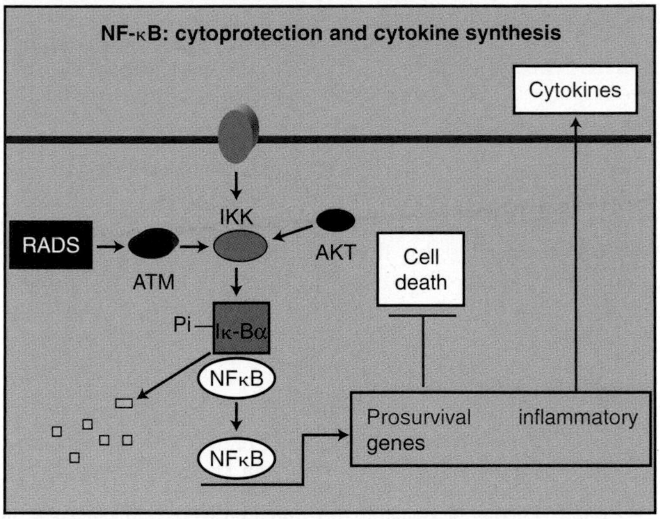

Figure 2-5 Ionizing radiation activates the NF-κB pathway. NF-κB is induced by inflammatory ligands such as bacterial products that stimulate the IKK kinase complex and activate NF-κB through destruction of the inhibitor Iκ-Bα. This pathway also can be activated by ionizing radiation through a number of mechanisms, particularly IKK activation by the DNA double-strand break sensor molecule ATM. NF-κB activation has at least two known consequences: increased cell survival through synthesis of death-antagonizing NF-κB products and proinflammatory effects caused by increased expression of cytokines and adhesion factors.

genes using microchip-based approaches.[100] Because of the progress in deciphering human and other genomes in the 1990s, a total readout of expression of all human genes can be undertaken. This has opened the way for identification of signature genes in human cancers that correspond to poor prognosis, treatment resistance, and metastasis.[101,102] The impact of this approach on radiation biology is perhaps less than in general cancer biology, because most responses to genomic stress occur at the posttranscriptional level. An allied approach of proteomics is being developed, based on advances in the field of mass spectrometry, and this may permit the rapid study of critical changes in posttranslational modification, such as phosphorylation, acetylation, and ubiquitination, that mediate many of the regulatory responses to genomic stress. The increased speed and accuracy of drug development, based on robotic approaches to assaying chemical libraries and in silico design, should increase the rate of drug discovery and hasten the translation of molecular findings into the clinic.

SUMMARY

The past 10 years have seen an almost complete transformation in understanding of the genes that determine the development of the cancer cell, its subsequent response to radiation and chemotherapy, and the signaling circuitry that links the products of such genes to DNA damage response pathways. The rate of accumulation of new knowledge, particularly in the field of DNA sensing and repair, has been so rapid that its future impact on the practice of radiation oncology is difficult to predict. One area of incomplete knowledge is the exact molecular mechanisms of radiation cell death, their link to the DNA damage response pathways, and how they might be altered by the evolving patterns of gene expression in tumor progression. This dilemma is well illustrated by TP53, the factor that in normal cells links the accumulation of genomic damage to cell death by apoptosis, autophagy, and senescence but that is inactivated in most cancers. In contrast, identification of ATM as the master regulator of the response to genomic stress suggests this pathway as one that can be targeted for radiation sensitization. Another interesting possibility for targeting new treatment approaches is that of necrosis, particularly in tumor cells, in which the pathways of PCD have been closed off through alterations in the TP53 and BCL2 pathways. The success of future approaches to cancer treatment and cure will be determined by their ability to inhibit or facilitate normal and adaptive changes in cell physiology to maximize the deleterious effects on the tumor while preserving viability of the surrounding normal tissues.

REFERENCES

1. Sanchez Y, Bachant J, Wang H, et al: Control of the DNA damage checkpoint by chk1 and rad53 protein kinases through distinct mechanisms. Science 286:1166-1171, 1999.
2. Zou L, Elledge SJ: Sensing and signaling DNA damage: roles of Rad17 and Rad9 complexes in the cellular response to DNA damage. Harvey Lect 97:1-15, 2001.
3. Metzstein MM, Stanfield GM, Horvitz HR: Genetics of programmed cell death in *C. elegans:* past, present and future. Trends Genet 14:410-416, 1998.
4. Vogelstein B, Kinzler KW: The multistep nature of cancer. Trends Genet 9:138-141, 1993.
5. Hanahan D, Weinberg RA: The hallmarks of cancer. Cell 100:57-70, 2000.
6. Fishel R, Kolodner RD: Identification of mismatch repair genes and their role in the development of cancer. Curr Opin Genet Dev 5:382-395, 1995.
7. Fishel R, Lescoe MK, Rao MR, et al: The human mutator gene homolog MSH2 and its association with hereditary nonpolyposis colon cancer. Cell 75:1027-1038, 1993.
8. Hall EJ: Radiobiology for the Radiologist. Philadelphia, Lippincott-Raven, 1993, pp. 15-29.
9. Fowler J: Biological foundations of radiotherapy. Amsterdam, Excerpta Medica, 1967.
10. Revell SH: Relationship between chromosome damage and cell death. New York, Alan Liss, 1983, pp. 215-233.
11. Dubois A, Walker RI: Prospects for management of gastrointestinal injury associated with the acute radiation syndrome. Gastroenterology 95:500-507, 1988.
12. Dainiak N, Ricks RC: The evolving role of haematopoietic cell transplantation in radiation injury: potentials and limitations. BJR 27(Suppl):169-174, 2005.
13. Alper T, Gillies NE, Elkind MM: The sigmoid survival curve in radiobiology. Nature 186:1062-1063, 1960.
14. Lombard DB, Chua KF, Mostoslavsky R, et al: DNA repair, genome stability, and aging. Cell 120:497-512, 2005.
15. Edinger AL, Thompson CB: Death by design: apoptosis, necrosis and autophagy. Curr Opin Cell Biol 16:663-669, 2004.
16. Campisi J: Senescent cells, tumor suppression, and organismal aging: good citizens, bad neighbors. Cell 120:513-522, 2005.
17. Friedberg EC, Walker GC, Siede W: DNA repair and mutagenesis. Washington, DC, ASM Press, 1995.
18. McGowan CH, Russell P: The DNA damage response: sensing and signaling. Curr Opin Cell Biol 16:629-633, 2004.
19. Sancar A, Lindsey-Boltz LA, Unsal-Kacmaz K, Linn S: Molecular mechanisms of mammalian DNA repair and the DNA damage checkpoints. Annu Rev Biochem 73:39-85, 2004.
20. Stergiou L, Hengartner MO: Death and more: DNA damage response pathways in the nematode *C. elegans.* Cell Death Differ 11:21-28, 2004.
21. Murray AW, Kirschner MW: What controls the cell cycle? Sci Am 264:56-63, 1991.
22. Sherr CJ: Cancer cell cycles. Science 274:1672-1677, 1996.
23. Murray AW: Recycling the cell cycle: cyclins revisited. Cell 116:221-234, 2004.
24. Lim HH, Surana U: Tome-1, weel, and the onset of mitosis: coupled destruction for timely entry. Mol Cell 11:845-846, 2003.
25. Rudoltz MS, Kao G, Blank KR, et al: Molecular biology of the cell cycle: potential for therapeutic applications in radiation oncology. Semin Radiat Oncol 6:284-294, 1996.
26. Chin PL, Momand J, Pfeifer GP: In vivo evidence for binding of p53 to consensus binding sites in the p21 and GADD45 genes in response to ionizing radiation. Oncogene 15:87-99, 1997.
27. Fei P, El-Deiry WS: P53 and radiation responses. Oncogene 22:5774-5783, 2003.
28. Wahl GM, Carr AM: The evolution of diverse biological responses to DNA damage: insights from yeast and p53. Nat Cell Biol 3:E277-E286, 2001.
29. Morgan SE, Kastan MB: P53 and ATM: cell cycle, cell death, and cancer. Adv Cancer Res 71:1-25, 1997.
30. Bakkenist CJ, Kastan MB: DNA damage activates ATM through intermolecular autophosphorylation and dimer dissociation. Nature 421:499-506, 2003.
31. Kastan MB, Bartek J: Cell-cycle checkpoints and cancer. Nature 432:316-323, 2004.
32. Andreassen PR, Lohez OD, Margolis RL: G2 and spindle assembly checkpoint adaptation, and tetraploidy arrest: implications for intrinsic and chemically induced genomic instability. Mutat Res 532:245-253, 2003.
33. Polyak K, Xia Y, Zweier JL, et al: A model for p53-induced apoptosis. Nature 389:300-305, 1997.
34. Schmitt CA, Fridman JS, Yang M, et al: Dissecting p53 tumor suppressor functions in vivo. Cancer Cell 1:289-298, 2002.
35. Komarova EA, Christov K, Faerman AI, Gudkov AV: Different impact of p53 and p21 on the radiation response of mouse tissues. Oncogene 19:3791-3798, 2000.
36. Paulovich AG, Toczyski DP, Hartwell LH: When checkpoints fail. Cell 88:315-321, 1997.
37. Fridman JS, Lowe SW: Control of apoptosis by p53. Oncogene 22:9030-9040, 2003.
38. Feki A, Irminger-Finger I: Mutational spectrum of p53 mutations in primary breast and ovarian tumors. Crit Rev Oncol Hematol 52:103-116, 2004.
39. Munro AJ, Lain S, Lane DP: P53 abnormalities and outcomes in colorectal cancer: a systematic review. Br J Cancer 92:434-444, 2005.
40. Ting NS, Lee WH: The DNA double-strand break response pathway: becoming more BRCAish than ever. DNA Repair (Amst) 3:935-944, 2004.
41. Lavin MF, Shiloh Y: The genetic defect in ataxia-telangiectasia. Annu Rev Immunol 15:177-202, 1997.
42. Morgan SE, Lovly C, Pandita TK, et al: Fragments of ATM which have dominant-negative or complementing activity. Mol Cell Biol 17:2020-2029, 1997.
43. Zhang N, Chen P, Khanna KK, et al: Isolation of full-length ATM cDNA and correction of the ataxia-telangiectasia cellular phenotype. Proc Natl Acad Sci U S A 94:8021-8026, 1997.
44. Luger K, Rechsteiner TJ, Richmond TJ: Expression and purification of recombinant histones and nucleosome reconstitution. Methods Mol Biol 119:1-16, 1999.
45. Tamburini BA, Tyler JK: Localized histone acetylation and deacetylation triggered by the homologous recombination pathway of double-strand DNA repair. Mol Cell Biol 25:4903-4913, 2005.
46. Morrison AJ, Highland J, Krogan NJ, et al: INO80 and gamma-H2AX interaction links ATP-dependent chromatin remodeling to DNA damage repair. Cell 119:767-775, 2004.
47. Morrison AJ, Shen X: DNA repair in the context of chromatin. Cell Cycle 4:568-571, 2005.
48. Ward JF: Complexity of damage produced by ionizing radiation. Cold Spring Harb Symp Quant Biol 65:377-382, 2000.
49. Leadon SA: Production and repair of DNA damage in mammalian cells. Health Phys 59:15-22, 1990.
50. Leadon SA: Repair of DNA damage produced by ionizing radiation: a minireview. Semin Radiat Oncol 6:295-305, 1996.
51. Bassing CH, Alt FW: The cellular response to general and programmed DNA double strand breaks. DNA Repair (Amst) 3:781-796, 2004.
52. Collis SJ, DeWeese TL, Jeggo PA, Parker AR: The life and death of DNA-PK. Oncogene 24:949-961, 2005.

53. Lisby M, Rothstein R: DNA repair: keeping it together. Curr Biol 14:R994-R996, 2004.
54. Burma S, Chen DJ: Role of DNA-PK in the cellular response to DNA double-strand breaks. DNA Repair (Amst) 3:909-918, 2004.
55. Abraham RT: PI 3-kinase related kinases: "big" players in stress-induced signaling pathways. DNA Repair (Amst) 3:883-887, 2004.
56. Jackson SP, Jeggo PA: DNA double-strand break repair and V(D)J recombination: involvement of DNA-PK. Trends Biochem Sci 20:412-415, 1995.
57. Maser RS, Monsen KJ, Nelms BE, Petrini JH: hMre11 and hRad50 nuclear foci are induced during the normal cellular response to DNA double-strand breaks. Mol Cell Biol 17:6087-6096, 1997.
58. Petrini JH, Stracker TH: The cellular response to DNA double-strand breaks: defining the sensors and mediators. Trends Cell Biol 13:458-462, 2003.
59. Petrini JH: S-phase functions of the Mre11 complex. Cold Spring Harb Symp Quant Biol 65:405-411, 2000.
60. Scully R, Xie A, Nagaraju G: Molecular functions of BRCA1 in the DNA damage response. Cancer Biol Ther 3:521-527, 2004.
61. Danial NN, Korsmeyer SJ: Cell death: critical control points. Cell 116:205-219, 2004.
62. Proskuryakov SY, Konoplyannikov AG, Gabai VL: Necrosis: a specific form of programmed cell death? Exp Cell Res 283:1-16, 2003.
63. Naka K, Tachibana A, Ikeda K, Motoyama N: Stress-induced premature senescence in hTERT-expressing ataxia telangiectasia fibroblasts. J Biol Chem 279:2030-2037, 2004.
64. Schmidt-Ullrich RK, Contessa JN, Lammering G, et al: ERBB receptor tyrosine kinases and cellular radiation responses. Oncogene 22:5855-5865, 2003.
65. Stevenson MA, Pollock SS, Coleman CN, Calderwood SK: X-irradiation, phorbol esters, and H2O2 stimulate mitogen-activated protein kinase activity in NIH-3T3 cells through the formation of reactive oxygen intermediates. Cancer Res 54: 12-15, 1994.
66. Treisman R: The serum response element. Trends Biochem Sci 17:423-426, 1992.
67. Lammering G, Hewit TH, Valerie K, et al: Anti-erbB receptor strategy as a gene therapeutic intervention to improve radiotherapy in malignant human tumours. Int J Radiat Biol 79:561-568, 2003.
68. Chen Q, Olashaw N, Wu J: Participation of reactive oxygen species in the lysophosphatidic acid-stimulated mitogen-activated protein kinase kinase activation pathway. J Biol Chem 270:28499-28502, 1995.
69. Schmidt-Ullrich RK, Dent P, Grant S, et al: Signal transduction and cellular radiation responses. Radiat Res 153:245-257, 2000.
70. Piret B, Schoonbroodt S, Piette J: The ATM protein is required for sustained activation of NF-kappaB following DNA damage. Oncogene 18:2261-2271, 1999.
71. Gullino PM: The internal milieu of tumors. Prog Exp Tumor Res 8:1-25, 1966.
72. Gullino PM: Tumor pathophysiology: the perfusion model. Antibiot Chemother 28:35-42, 1980.
73. Weinmann M, Welz S, Bamberg M: Hypoxic radiosensitizers and hypoxic cytotoxins in radiation oncology. Curr Med Chem Anticaner Agents 3:364-374, 2003.
74. Hockel M, Schlenger K, Aral B, et al: Association between tumor hypoxia and malignant progression in advanced cancer of the uterine cervix. Cancer Res 56:4509-4515, 1996.
75. Vaupel P, Mayer A, Hockel M: Tumor hypoxia and malignant progression. Methods Enzymol 381:335-354, 2004.
76. Bindra RS, Glazer PM: Genetic instability and the tumor microenvironment: towards the concept of microenvironment-induced mutagenesis. Mutat Res 569:75-85, 2005.
77. Semenza GL: HIF-1 and tumor progression: pathophysiology and therapeutics. Trends Mol Med 8:S62-S67, 2002.
78. Pugh CW, Ratcliffe PJ: The von Hippel-Lindau tumor suppressor, hypoxia-inducible factor-1 (HIF-1) degradation, and cancer pathogenesis. Semin Cancer Biol 13:83-39, 2003.
79. Folkman J: Role of angiogenesis in tumor growth and metastasis. Semin Oncol 29:15-18, 2002.
80. Folkman J: Angiogenesis and apoptosis. Semin Cancer Biol 13:159-167, 2003.
81. Gupta MK, Qin RY: Mechanism and its regulation of tumor-induced angiogenesis. World J Gastroenterol 9:1144-1155, 2003.
82. Koukourakis MI: Tumour angiogenesis and response to radiotherapy. Anticancer Res 21:4285-4300, 2001.
83. Chan LW, Camphausen K: Angiogenic tumor markers, antiangiogenic agents and radiation therapy. Expert Rev Anticancer Ther 3:357-366, 2003.
84. Rudoltz MS, Kao G, Blank KR, et al: Molecular biology of the cell cycle: potential for therapeutic applications in radiation oncology. Semin Radiat Oncol 6:284-294, 1996.
85. Bernhard EJ, McKenna WG, Hamilton AD, et al: Inhibiting Ras prenylation increases the radiosensitivity of human tumor cell lines with activating mutations of ras oncogenes. Cancer Res 58:1754-1761, 1998.
86. Chmura SJ, Mauceri HJ, Advani S, et al: Decreasing the apoptotic threshold of tumor cells through protein kinase C inhibition and sphingomyelinase activation increases tumor killing by ionizing radiation. Cancer Res 57:4340-4347, 1997.
87. Tsuchida E, Urano M: The effect of UCN-01 (7-hydroxystaurosporine), a potent inhibitor of protein kinase C, on fractionated radiotherapy or daily chemotherapy of a murine fibrosarcoma. Int J Radiat Oncol Biol Phys 39:1153-1161, 1997.
88. Price BD, Youmell M: The phosphatidylinositol 3-kinase inhibitor wortmannin sensitizes murine fibroblasts and human tumor cells to radiation and blocks induction of p53 following DNA damage. Cancer Res 56:246-250, 1996.
89. Rosenzweig KE, Youmell MB, Palayoor ST, Price BD: Radiosensitization of human tumor cells by the phosphatidylinositol3-kinase inhibitors wortmannin and LY294002 correlates with inhibition of DNA-dependent protein kinase and prolonged G2-M delay. Clin Cancer Res 3:1149-1156, 1997.
90. Duursma AM, Agami R: Ras interference as cancer therapy. Semin Cancer Biol 13:267-273, 2003.
91. Rye PD, Stigbrand T: Interfering with cancer: a brief outline of advances in RNA interference in oncology. Tumour Biol 25:329-336, 2004.
92. Coleman CN: Modulating the radiation response. Stem Cells 14:10-15, 1996.
93. Coleman CN: Chemical sensitizers and protectors. Int J Radiat Oncol Biol Phys 42:781-783, 1998.
94. Brown JM, Wilson WR: Exploiting tumour hypoxia in cancer treatment. Nat Rev Cancer 4:437-447, 2004.
95. Rosen EM, Fan S, Rockwell S, Goldberg ID: The molecular and cellular basis of radiosensitivity: implications for understanding how normal tissues and tumors respond to therapeutic radiation. Cancer Invest 17:56-72, 1999.
96. Robbins ME, Zhao W: Chronic oxidative stress and radiation-induced late normal tissue injury: a review. Int J Radiat Biol 80:251-259, 2004.
97. Epperly MW, Guo H, Shields D, et al: Correlation of ionizing irradiation-induced late pulmonary fibrosis with long-term bone marrow culture fibroblast progenitor cell biology in mice homozygous deletion recombinant negative for endothelial cell adhesion molecules. In Vivo 18:1-14, 2004.
98. Huang TT, Wuerzberger-Davis SM, Wu ZH, Miyamoto S: Sequential modification of NEMO/IKKgamma by SUMO-1 and ubiquitin mediates NF-kappaB activation by genotoxic stress. Cell 115:565-576, 2003.
99. Ghosh S, Karin M: Missing pieces in the NF-κB puzzle. Cell 109:S81-S96, 2002.
100. Eisen MB, Spellman PT, Brown PO, Botstein D: Clustering analysis and display of genome-wide expression patterns. Proc Natl Acad Sci U S A 95:14863-14868, 1998.
101. van't Veer LJ, Dai H, van de Vijver MJ, et al: Gene expression profiling predicts clinical outcome of breast cancer. Nature 415:530-536, 2002.
102. van de Vijver MJ, He YD, Vant Ver JL, et al: A gene-expression signature as a predictor of survival in breast cancer. N Engl J Med 347:1999-2009, 2002.

CHAPTER 3

DOSE-RESPONSE MODIFIERS IN RADIATION THERAPY

Michael R. Horsman, Jacob C. Lindegaard, Cai Grau, Marianne Nordsmark, and Jens Overgaard

When cancer patients undergo radiation therapy, there is a clear relationship between the dose delivered and the response of the tumor to the radiation. This is illustrated in Figure 3-1. Unfortunately, there is also an increase in normal tissue damage with increasing radiation dose, and this complication limits the total radiation dose that can be given. Substantial effort has been made to modify these dose-response relationships and increase the separation between the tumor and normal tissue dose-response curves. The approach has been to either selectively increase the radiation damage in tumors without affecting the normal tissues or protect the normal tissues without protecting the tumors.

Agents that can enhance the radiation response include certain conventional chemotherapeutic drugs, the halogenated pyrimidines, and treatments that specifically overcome radioresistance resulting from the presence of hypoxic cells that occur because of the environmental conditions within most solid tumors. The most widely investigated method applied to the hypoxia problem is radiosensitization of the hypoxic cells with electron-affinic sensitizing drugs or hyperthermia. Another approach often used to reduce hypoxia, especially in experimental systems, involves increasing oxygen availability by the subject breathing gas with a high oxygen content, introducing perfluorochemical emulsions into the vascular system to increase the oxygen carrying capacity of the blood, using agents that affect hemoglobin, or using drugs that increase tumor blood perfusion. Many experimental studies have demonstrated that hypoxic cells can be preferentially killed by means of bioreductive drugs that are active under reduced oxygen conditions or by using hyperthermia, and all these hypoxic cell cytotoxins can improve the radiation response of tumors.

Preliminary data suggest that vascular-targeting agents have the potential to enhance radiation damage. These include drugs that inhibit angiogenesis, the process by which tumors develop their own vascular supply, or agents that preferentially damage the already established tumor vessels.

Radiation protectors fall into several categories. True radiation protectors, particularly sulfhydryl compounds, primarily appear to interact with radicals that are formed after radiation exposure. Another group consists of agents that decrease oxygen delivery to tissues, which should reduce the amount of radiation damage induced. Additional agents, such as various cytokines, growth factors, prostaglandins, and essential fatty acids, have been shown to be capable of radioprotection, but their mechanisms of action are not entirely clear.

Because radiosensitization by conventional chemotherapeutic agents (e.g., cisplatin, 5-fluorouracil, mitomycin C), halogenated pyrimidines (e.g., 5-bromodeoxyuridine, 5-iododeoxyuridine), and hyperthermia are discussed in detail elsewhere in this book, they are not considered in this chapter. Instead, we focus on studies that involve the use of hypoxic cell modifiers, vascular-targeting drugs, and radioprotectors.

HYPOXIA PROBLEM

Importance of Oxygen

In 1909, Gottwald Schwarz, in a simple but elegant experiment, demonstrated that the radiation response of skin was markedly decreased if the blood flow in the irradiated area was reduced by compression.[1] Although he did not acknowledge that the phenomenon was the result of a lack of oxygen, it was probably the first radiobiologically oriented clinical study implicating the importance of environmental parameters on the outcome of radiotherapy. This finding of Gottwald Schwarz was used to introduce the concept of *kompressionsanämie*, by which the skin was made anemic, thereby allowing a higher dose to be given to deeply situated tumors. Continuing from the work of Schwarz, Müller reported in 1910 that tissues in which the blood flow was stimulated by diathermia showed a more prominent response to irradiation.[2] This early study demonstrated the importance of oxygen supply in radiotherapy and was the first clinical approach to assessing how resistance could be overcome by using hyperthermia. During the first half of the century, there were sporadic clinical and experimental observations indicating the importance of sufficient blood supply in securing an adequate radiation response. These observations led Gray and coworkers in the early 1950s to postulate the role of oxygen deficiency or hypoxia as a major source of radiation resistance.[3]

The first clinical indication that hypoxia existed in tumors was made around this time by Thomlinson and Gray. From histologic observations in carcinoma of the bronchus, they reported seeing viable tumor regions surrounded by vascular stroma from which the tumor cells obtained their nutrient and oxygen requirements.[4] As the tumors grew, the viable regions expanded, and areas of necrosis appeared at the center. The thickness of the resulting shell of viable tissue was between 100 and 180 µm, which was within the same range as their calculated diffusion distance for oxygen in respiring tissues. It was suggested that as oxygen diffused from the stroma, it was consumed by the cells, and although those beyond the diffusion distance were unable to survive, the cells immediately bordering the necrosis might be viable yet hypoxic. In 1968, Tannock described an inverted version of the Thomlinson and Gray picture, with functional blood vessels surrounded by cords of viable tumor cells, outside of which were areas of necrosis.[5] This "corded" structure is illustrated in Figure 3-2, and it is the typical picture found in most solid tumors.[6]

The corded structure arises because the tumor blood vessels, which are derived from the normal tissue vessels by a process of angiogenesis, are inadequate to meet the needs of the rapidly growing tumor cells. This hypoxia is more commonly referred to as chronic. It was also suggested that hypoxia in tumors could be acute in nature.[7] Later, Chaplin and colleagues[8] were able to confirm the existence of acutely hypoxic cells in tumors and demonstrate that these cells were the result of transient stoppages in tumor blood flow (see

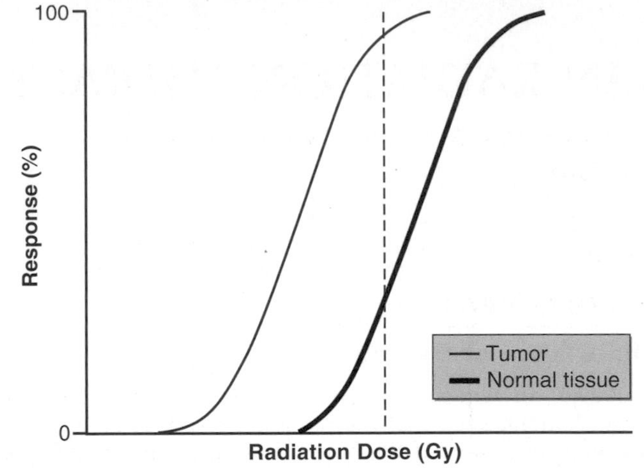

Figure 3-1 Schematic illustration of the proportion of patients cured and patients with normal tissue complications as a function of the total radiation dose received.

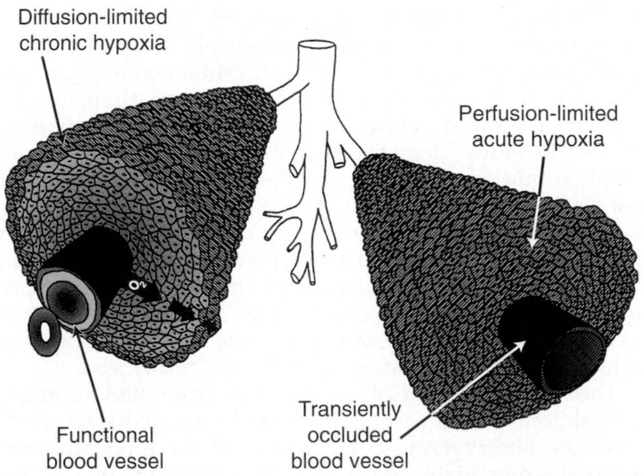

Figure 3-2 Schematic representation of the relationship between tumor cells and the vascular supply. Cells are seen *(left)* growing as a corded structure around a functional vessel from which the cells receive their oxygen supply. As oxygen diffuses out from the vessel, it is used up, and the outermost viable cells *(shaded)* are oxygen deprived or chronically hypoxic. A similar arrangement is seen on the *right*, but flow through the vessel is transiently stopped, making all the cells oxygen deprived. (From Horsman MR: Measurement of tumor oxygenation. Int J Radiat Oncol Biol Phys 42:701-714, 1998.)

Fig. 3-2). These temporary cessations in blood flow have been observed in mouse and rat tumors, as well as in human tumor xenografts, with about 4% to 8% of the total functional vessels involved,[9] although the exact causes of these stoppages are not known. The use of *chronic* and *acute* to explain hypoxia in tumors is probably an oversimplification of the real situation. Chronic hypoxia generally refers to prolonged and reduced oxygen concentrations that influence radiation response, but there is evidence that oxygen concentrations that are higher but below normal physiologic levels are often found.[10] Perfusion reduction can be partial or total,[11] and although cells under the former condition would be oxygen deprived, with a total lack of perfusion they would be starved of oxygen and nutrients, and their survival and response to therapy would be expected to be different.

Evidence for Hypoxia in Tumors

In experimental tumors, it is relatively easy to identify hypoxia and to quantitatively estimate the percentage of cells that are hypoxic. Three major techniques are routinely used.[12] These are the paired survival curve, the clamped tumor growth delay, and the clamped tumor control assays. All involve a comparison of the response of tumors when irradiated under normal air-breathing conditions or when tumors are artificially made hypoxic by clamping. Using these procedures, hypoxia has been directly identified in most animal solid tumors, with the values ranging from less than 1% to more than 50% of the total viable cell population.[12] Unfortunately, none of these procedures can be applied to the clinical situation, and investigation therefore must rely on indirect techniques.

Tumor hypoxia has previously been estimated clinically by measurements of tumor vascularization, using such end points as intercapillary distance, vascular density, and the distance from tumor cells to the nearest blood vessel[13-15]; by measuring tumor metabolic activity, using biochemical, high-performance liquid chromatography, and bioluminescent and magnetic resonance techniques[16]; and by estimating the degree of DNA damage, as with the Comet assay.[17] The more popular techniques being investigated include measuring the binding of exogenous markers that can be identified immunohistochemically from histologic sections (e.g., pimonidazole or fluorinated ethanidazole)[18,19] or noninvasively using positron emission tomography (e.g., ^{18}F-labeled misonidazole or azomycin arabinoside),[20,21] single-photon emission computed tomography (e.g., ^{123}I-labeled azomycin arabinoside)[22] or magnetic resonance spectroscopy (e.g., SR4554)[23]; by the upregulation of endogenous proteins immunohistochemically (e.g., carbonic anhydrase IX, GLUT1 or HIF1)[24,25] or from blood samples (e.g., osteopontin)[26]; and by measurement of oxygen partial pressure (pO_2) distributions with polarographic electrodes.[13,27-32] The latter method has become by far the most popular, and the latest results from an international multicenter study in head and neck cancer patients are illustrated in Figure 3-3. In that study, tumor pO_2 was measured before radiation therapy and found to correlate with overall survival; patients with lower tumor oxygenation status did significantly worse.[33]

Probably the best evidence for the existence of hypoxia in human tumors comes from the large number of clinical trials in which hypoxic modification has shown some benefit.[34] The latter situation constitutes a circular argument; if hypoxic modification shows an improvement, hypoxic clonogenic cells must have been present in tumors. It is, however, likely that even within the same histology and tumor type, there exists a substantial heterogeneity with respect to the extent of hypoxia, and almost a century after the first clinical description, the importance of hypoxia and its influence on the outcome of radiotherapy are still subjects of substantial debate. In the following sections, we discuss how different hypoxic modifiers have been used to modify the radiation dose-response relationship of tumors.

OVERCOMING TUMOR HYPOXIA

Breathing High-Oxygen-Content Gas

Because the oxygen supply to tumors is insufficient to meet the needs of all the tumor cells, giving rise to radiation-resistant hypoxia, one solution to improving the radiation response of tumors would be to increase the oxygen supply. This has been tried experimentally and clinically by allowing the tumor-bearing host to breathe gas mixtures with high oxygen contents before and during irradiation.

Early experimental studies reported that oxygen and carbogen (95% O_2 + 5% CO_2) breathing could substantially enhance the response of murine tumors to radiation and that the best effect was generally seen when the gasses were inspired under hyperbaric (typically 3 atmospheres) rather than normobaric conditions.[35,36] This is not surprising, because hyperbaric conditions would be expected to saturate the blood with oxygen more than normobaric conditions. However, later studies indicated that the radiosensitizations produced by normobaric oxygen or carbogen were quite substantial,[37-39] and because it is quicker and easier to breathe gas under normobaric conditions, the use of cumbersome, expensive, and complex hyperbaric chambers is probably unnecessary.

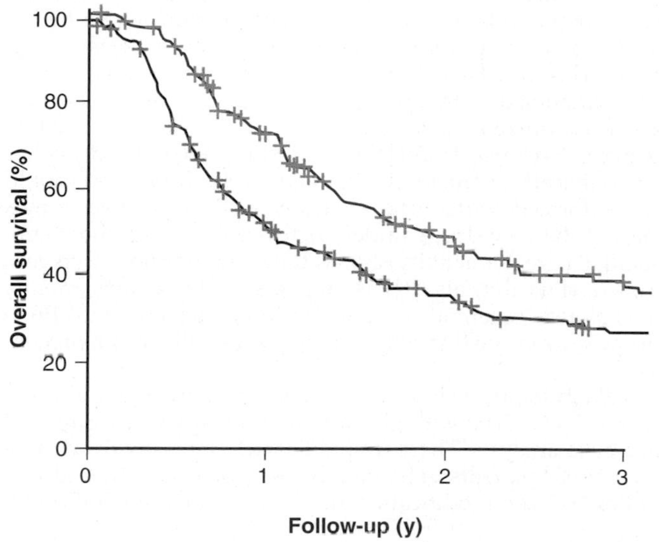

Figure 3-3 Oxygen levels were measured with Eppendorf electrodes before radiation therapy in 397 patients with squamous cell carcinomas of the head and neck. Tumors were stratified by whether the fraction of pO_2 values less than 2.5 mm Hg (HP2.5) was above or below the median value for the whole group (i.e., 19%). The lines show Kaplan-Meier estimates of actuarial overall survival probability for patients with less hypoxic tumors (HP2.5 < 19%, *red line*) compared with more hypoxic tumors (HP2.5 > 19%, *blue line*); P = .006. (From Nordsmark M, Bentzen SM, Rudat V, et al: Prognostic value of tumor oxygenation in 397 head and neck tumors after primary radiation therapy. An international multi-center study. Radiother Oncol 77:18-24, 2005)

Clinically, the use of high-oxygen-content gas breathing, specifically under hyperbaric conditions, was introduced relatively early by Churchill-Davidson and colleagues.[40] Most trials were fairly small and suffered from the applications of unconventional fractionation schemes, but it appeared that the effect of hyperbaric oxygen was superior to radiotherapy given in air, especially when few and large fractions were applied.[40-42] In the large multicenter clinical trials conducted by the Medical Research Council (Table 3-1), the results from treating uterine cervix and advanced head and neck cancers showed a significant benefit in local tumor control and subsequent survival.[41,43-46] The same was not observed in cases of bladder cancer, nor was it repeated in a number of smaller studies.[46] In retrospect, the use of hyperbaric oxygen was stopped somewhat prematurely, partly because of the introduction of hypoxic radiosensitizers and partly because of problems with patients' compliance. It has been claimed that hyperbaric treatment caused significant suffering, but the discomfort associated with such a treatment must be considered minor compared with the often life-threatening complications associated with chemotherapy, which is used with a less restrictive indication.

The use of high-oxygen-content gas breathing under normobaric conditions to radiosensitize human tumors has also been tried clinically, but it failed to show any dramatic improvement.[47,48] One possible explanation may be the failure to achieve the optimal time for preirradiation gas breathing, because a number of experimental studies have shown that this is critical for the enhancement of radiation damage and that it can vary from tumor to tumor.[36-38,49]

Hypoxic Cell Radiosensitizers

An alternative approach to the hypoxia problem is the use of chemical agents that mimic oxygen and preferentially sensitize the resistant population to radiation. The advantages of these drugs over oxygen are that they are not rapidly metabolized by the tumor cells through which they diffuse and that they can penetrate further than oxygen and so reach all the tumor cells. In the early 1960s, it was found that the efficiency of radiosensitization was directly related to electron affinity,[50] and this ultimately led to in vitro studies demonstrating preferential radiosensitization of hypoxic cells by highly electron-affinic nitroaromatic compounds.[51,52] Several of these compounds were later shown to be effective at enhancing radiation damage in tumors in vivo,[53] and as a result, they underwent clinical testing.

Table 3-1 Multicenter, Randomized Trials with Hyperbaric Oxygen

Anatomic Site and Study	No. of Patients	End Point*	Hyperbaric Oxygen	Air
HEAD AND NECK CARCINOMA				
MRC 1st trial (1977)	294	Control (5 y)	53%	30% (P < .01)
MRC 2nd trial (1986)	106	Control (5 y)	60%	41% (P < .05)
UTERINE CERVIX CARCINOMA				
MRC (1978)	320	Control (5 y)	67%	47% (P < .001)
BRONCHOGENIC CARCINOMA				
MRC; 60 Gy/40 fx (1978)	51	Survival (2 y)	15%	8% (NS)
MRC; 36 Gy/6 fx (1978)	123	Survival (2 y)	25%	12% (P < .05)
CARCINOMA OF THE BLADDER				
MRC (1978)	241	Survival (5 y)	28%	30% (NS)

*End points were control (locoregional control) or survival. See Overgaard[46] for additional details.
fx, fractions; NS, not significant.

Nine drugs—metronidazole, misonidazole, benznidazole, desmethylmisonidazole, etanidazole, pimonidazole, nimorazole, ornidazole, and RSU 1069—reached clinical evaluation. The initial clinical studies were with metronidazole in brain tumors and were followed in the latter part of the 1970s by a boom in clinical trials exploring the potential of misonidazole as a radiosensitizer.[46,53,54] The results from the multicenter, randomized trials are summarized in Table 3-2. Most of the trials with misonidazole were unable to generate any significant improvement in radiation response, although a benefit was seen in some trials, especially the Danish Head and Neck Cancer study (DAHANCA 2), which found highly significant improvement in the stratification subgroup of pharyngeal tumors, but not in the prognostically better glottic carcinomas.[55] The overall impression of the "misonidazole era" was a prolongation of the inconclusive experience from the hyperbaric oxygen trials; the problems related to hypoxia had not been finally excluded.[53] The search for more efficient or less toxic hypoxic sensitizers has continued. The experience from the misonidazole trials has been taken into account to select a more homogeneous tumor population in which hypoxia is more likely to exist. Subsequent trials have evaluated pimonidazole, etanidazole, and nimorazole. The European pimonidazole trial enrolling patients with uterine cervix carcinomal was very disappointing,[56] and the two other multicenter trials using etanidazole in head and neck cancer showed no benefit.[53,57] Studies with the low toxic drug nimorazole given to patients with supraglottic and pharyngeal carcinomas (DAHANCA 5) showed a highly significant benefit in terms of improved locoregional tumor control and disease-free survival (Fig. 3-4),[58] confirming the result of the DAHANCA 2 study.

The clinical evaluation of nitroimidazoles has been difficult, and many of the drugs that were the more promising in preclinical testing did not achieve the expected clinical outcome. Although this may be caused by clinical evaluation in the wrong tumor sites and the small number of patients in many of the trials, a more likely explanation is that the drugs that were thought to be the most effective against hypoxia have shown substantial dose-limiting clinical toxicity. Figure 3-5 summarizes the peak plasma and tumor levels measured after administration of the maximum tolerable doses in patients after single doses or when given with a 30-fraction schedule. For the 5-nitroimidazoles (i.e., metronidazole and nimorazole), the peak levels are as good as and sometimes better than the 2-nitroimidazoles (i.e., misonidazole, etanidazole, and pimonidazole). Although preclinical studies suggest that the 2-nitroimidazoles are more efficient sensitizers than 5-nitroimidazoles on a concentration basis,[59] the fact that the latter compounds are less toxic in humans, allowing for higher levels to be achieved, may make them more efficient in the clinic. This may go a long way to explaining the success seen with nimorazole. In retrospect, the studies with electron-affinic sensitizers have demonstrated a lack of interaction between preclinical and clinical testing; after the drug has been clinically evaluated, additional preclinical studies should be performed within the clinically achievable dose range. Only if the new drugs under such circumstances show substantially greater activity should they be introduced into controlled clinical trials. There appears to be a substantially unexplored potential in the 5-nitroimidazoles, and these drugs warrant further investigation, especially at the preclinical level.

All randomized clinical studies in which hypoxic radiosensitizers were given with primary radiotherapy were combined in a meta-analysis. These (unpublished) results involved more than 11,000 patients in 91 randomized trials and showed that radiosensitizer modification of tumor hypoxia significantly

Table 3-2 Multicenter, Randomized Trials with Nitroimidazoles

Anatomic Site and Study	No. of Patients	Sensitizer	Rafterconex End Point*	RT and Sensitizer	RT Alone
HEAD AND NECK CARCINOMA					
DAHANCA 2 (1989)	626	MISO	Control (5 y)	41%	34% ($P < .05$)
MRC (1984)	267	MISO	Control (>2 y)	40%	36% NS
EORTC (1986)	163	MISO	Control (3 y)	52%	44% NS
RTOG (1987)	306	MISO	Control (3 y)	19%	24% NS
RTOG 79-04 (1987)	42	MISO	Control (2 y)	17%	10% NS
DAHANCA 5 (1992)	414	NIM	Control (5 y)	49%	34% ($P < .002$)
RTOG 85-27 (1995)	500	ETA	Control (2 y)	39%	38% NS
European multicenter (1991)	374	ETA	Control (2 y)	57%	58% NS
UTERINE CERVIX CARCINOMA					
Scandinavian study (1989)	331	MISO	Control (5 y)	50%	54% NS
MRC (1984)	153	MISO	Control (>2 y)	59%	58% NS
RTOG (1987)	119	MISO	Control (3 y)	53%	54% NS
MRC (1993)	183	PIM	Control (4 y)	64%	80% ($P < .01$)
GLIOBLASTOMA					
Scandinavian study (1985)	244	MISO	Survival	10	10 NS
MRC (1983)	384	MISO	Survival	8	9 NS
EORTC (1983)	163	MISO	Survival	11	12 NS
RTOG (1986)	318	MISO	Survival	11	13 NS
BRONCHOGENIC CARCINOMA					
RTOG (1987)	117	MISO	Survival	7	7 NS
RTOG (1989)	268	MISO	Survival	7	8 NS

*End points were control (locoregional control) and survival (median survival in months). See Overgaard and colleagues[53] for additional information.

DAHANCA, Danish Head and Neck Cancer study; EORTC, European Organization for Research and Treatment of Cancer; ETA, etanidazole; MISO, misonidazole; MRC, Medical Research Council; NIM, nimorazole; NS, not significant; PIM, pimonidazole; RT, radiation therapy; RTOG, Radiation Therapy Oncology Group.

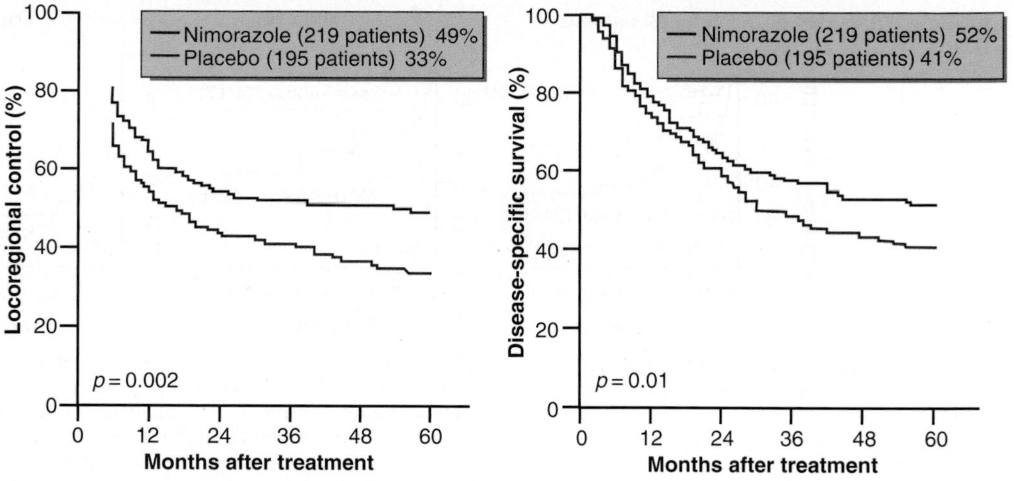

Figure 3-4 Actuarial estimated locoregional tumor control and disease-specific survival rate in patients randomized to receive nimorazole or placebo in conjunction with conventional radiotherapy for carcinoma of the pharynx and supraglottic larynx. (From Overgaard J, Sand Hansen H, Overgaard M, et al: A randomised double-blind phase III study of nimorazole as a hypoxic radiosensitizer of primary radiotherapy in supraglottic larynx and pharynx carcinoma. Results of the Danish head and neck cancer study [DAHANCA] protocol 5-85. Radiother Oncol 46:135-146, 1998.)

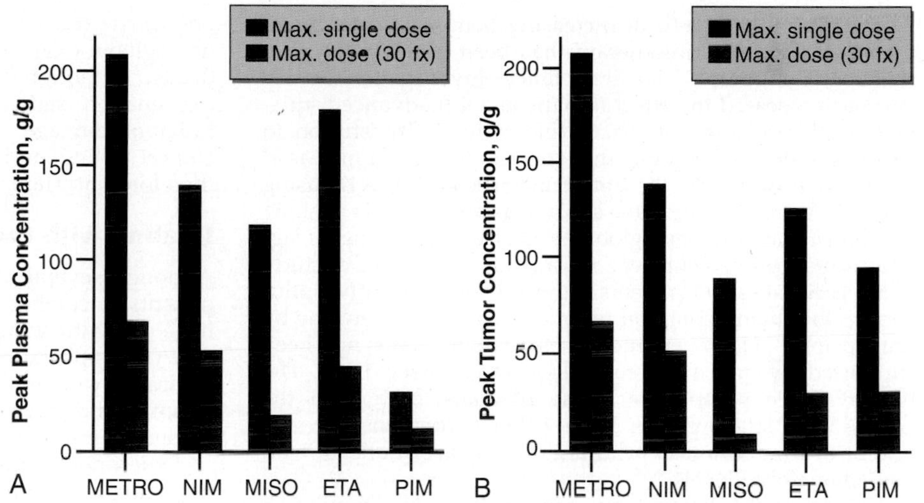

Figure 3-5 Peak plasma (**A**) and tumor (**B**) concentrations after the maximal tolerable single dose and when given in 30 fractions. The data are based on the tolerance doses, peak plasma concentrations, and tumor plasma ratios previously described by Overgaard.[55] ETA, etanidazole; METRO, metronidazole; MISO, misonidazole; NIM, nimorazole; PIM, pimonidazole.

improved the locoregional tumor control after radiotherapy, with an odds ratio of 0.78 (95% CI, 0.72 to 0.85). This treatment benefit was mostly the result of an improved response in head and neck tumors, with an odds ratio of 0.74 (95% CI, 0.65 to 0.83), and to a lesser extent, in bladder tumors. No significant effect was observed in other tumor sites (i.e., cervix, lung, central nervous system, and esophagus). The overall survival rate was also improved, with an overall odds ratio of 0.83 (95% CI, 0.77 to 0.90).

Hypoxic radiosensitizers have demonstrated significant benefit of local control and survival in certain tumor sites. The overall observed gain was in the order of a 5% to 10% improvement in local control. Although small, such gains should be pursued, especially because they are associated with a similar improvement in survival. There is no need for disappointment about the apparent lack of a major clinical benefit. The nonsignificant outcome of most clinical trials may not result from a biologic lack of importance of hypoxia, but in most cases, it may be considered a consequence of poor clinical trials methodology with a too optimistic study design and an expected treatment gain that goes far beyond what is reasonable. Overall, the results with nitroimidazoles add to the general consensus that nontoxic hypoxic modifications may be relevant as a baseline therapy together with radiotherapy for cancers such as advanced head and neck tumors. Such a strategy has been adopted in Denmark, where nimorazole has become part of the standard radiotherapy treatment for head and neck cancers.

Dose Modification Based on Hemoglobin

One of the major factors influencing the delivery of oxygen to tumors is the concentration of hemoglobin. Low hemoglobin concentration reduces the radiation response of tumors. In a review of 51 studies involving 17,272 patients, the prognostic relationship between hemoglobin concentration and local tumor control was analyzed; 39 of these studies (14,482 patients) showed a correlation, and only 12 studies (2790 patients) did not.[60] This is illustrated in Figure 3-6 for 67 head and neck cancer patients treated with radiotherapy. Separating the patients into two groups based on the median hemoglobin concentration had a significant impact on local tumor control. However, subgroup analysis using pretreatment pO_2 measurements showed that hypoxia was a significant factor only in the higher hemoglobin group, questioning the relationship between hemoglobin concentration and tumor oxygenation status. This lack of a correlation has been confirmed in an international multicenter study of 357 patients with head and neck cancers.[33]

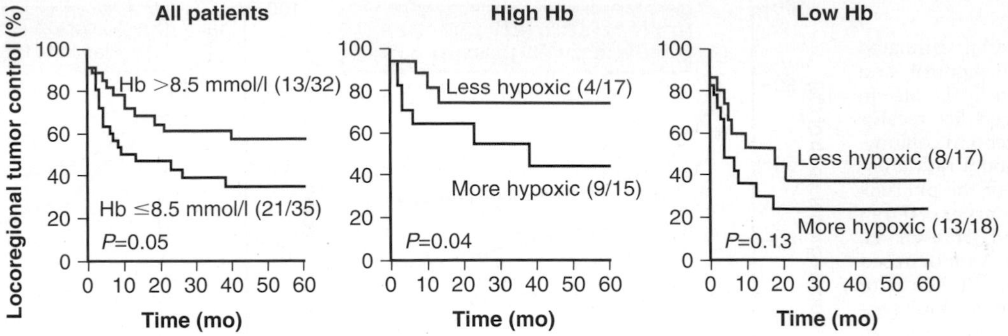

Figure 3-6 Kaplan-Meier analysis showing locoregional control after radiation therapy in patients with advanced head and neck cancer. All patients ($N = 67$) were stratified according to whether the pretreatment hemoglobin (Hb) concentration was above or below the median value (8.5 mmol/L) or subdivided into high (>8.5 mmol/L; $n = 32$) or low (<8.5 mmol/L; $n = 35$) hemoglobin and then stratified based on whether the fraction of pretreatment pO_2 values less than 2.5 mm Hg, as measured with an Eppendorf electrode, was above (more hypoxic) or below (less hypoxic) the median value (i.e., 22%) for the whole group. (Adapted from Nordsmark M, Overgaard J: Tumor hypoxia is independent of hemoglobin and prognostic for loco-regional tumor control after primary radiotherapy in advanced head and neck cancer. Acta Oncol 43:396-403, 2004.)

The potential benefit of increasing hemoglobin by blood transfusion before radiotherapy has been investigated in a number of studies.[61] The first clinical investigation of this approach assessed the effect in patients with advanced squamous cell carcinoma of the uterine cervix.[62] Transfusion to patients with low hemoglobin levels resulted in an increased oxygen tension within the tumor, as measured directly using oxygen electrodes. The same study was also the first to show that transfusion to a hemoglobin level of 11 g/dL or higher significantly improved survival. A Canadian retrospective study of 605 cervical cancer patients showed that the negative influence of low hemoglobin on prognosis could be overcome by transfusion.[63] However, these observations have not been supported by data from controlled, randomized trials. The two available prospective phase III trials, both from the DAHANCA study group, have failed to demonstrate any benefit of transfusion in head and neck cancer patients with low hemoglobin levels.[58,64]

Increasing the hemoglobin concentration by stimulation with the hormone erythropoietin has been investigated. Several preclinical studies have shown that the induction of anemia in animals could be corrected by serial injection with erythropoietin and that this treatment overcame the anemia-induced radiation resistance.[65,66] The concept of using erythropoietin to correct for anemia has been tested in a few clinical trials. However, although low hemoglobin can be effectively and safely improved by erythropoietin treatment,[67] two studies of patients undergoing treatment for head and neck cancer failed to show any benefit.[68,69] In one of those studies, the patients who received erythropoietin had a significantly poorer outcome than those that did not.[68] Although that study has come under some criticism, the results may indicate that erythropoietin stimulates tumor growth. Such a possibility is not entirely surprising, because erythropoietin is a growth hormone. However, an erythropoietin-induced increase in tumor growth has not been seen in preclinical studies,[66] and additional investigations are warranted.

Other hemoglobin-related methods for improving tumor oxygenation have been investigated. These include the use of artificial blood substances, such as perfluorocarbons,[70] which are small particles capable of carrying more oxygen than hemoglobin, or manipulating the oxygen unloading capacity of blood by modifying the oxyhemoglobin dissociation curve. This can be achieved by increasing the red blood cell content of 2,3-diphosphoglycerate (2,3-DPG),[71] with 2,3-DPG being one of the most important allosteric factors controlling the hemoglobin-oxygen dissociation curve, or using antilipidemic drugs.[72] Although each of these approaches has improved the oxygenation status of experimental tumors or enhanced radiation damage, none of them has yet reached controlled clinical testing, and their potential usefulness in the clinic is therefore uncertain.

Dealing with the Problem of Acute Hypoxia

Although several of the procedures that have been used in patients to combat radiation resistance due to hypoxic cells have met with some success, the results are far from satisfactory. One explanation may be that most of the procedures used clinically operate primarily against diffusion-limited chronic hypoxia and have little or no influence on acute hypoxia caused by transient variations in tumor blood flow.[9,16]

Experimental studies have demonstrated that the vitamin B_3 analogue, nicotinamide, can enhance radiation damage in a variety of murine tumor models using single-dose and fractionated schedules (Fig. 3-7).[9] The enhancement of radiation damage appears to depend on the tumor type, drug dose, and time of irradiation after drug administration.[9] This drug can also enhance radiation damage in certain normal tissues, but in general, the effects are less than those seen in tumors.[9] Nicotinamide primarily prevents or reduces the transient fluctuations in tumor blood flow that normally lead to the development of acute hypoxia.[9] This finding suggested that the optimal approach would be to combine nicotinamide with treatments that specifically overcome chronic hypoxia. This effect was subsequently demonstrated with hyperthermia,[73] perfluorochemical emulsions,[74] and carbogen breathing.[49,75,76] The combination of nicotinamide and carbogen is being tested in a number of European clinical studies, and the preliminary results for at least two studies (bladder[77] and head and neck[78] cancers) suggest that such an approach can improve the radiation response.

Bioreductive Drugs

No discussion of methods used to preferentially enhance radiation damage in tumors by overcoming radiation-resistant hypoxia would be complete without mentioning bioreductive drugs. These compounds undergo intracellular reduction to form active cytotoxic species. Much of the development of these agents arose after it was discovered that the electron-

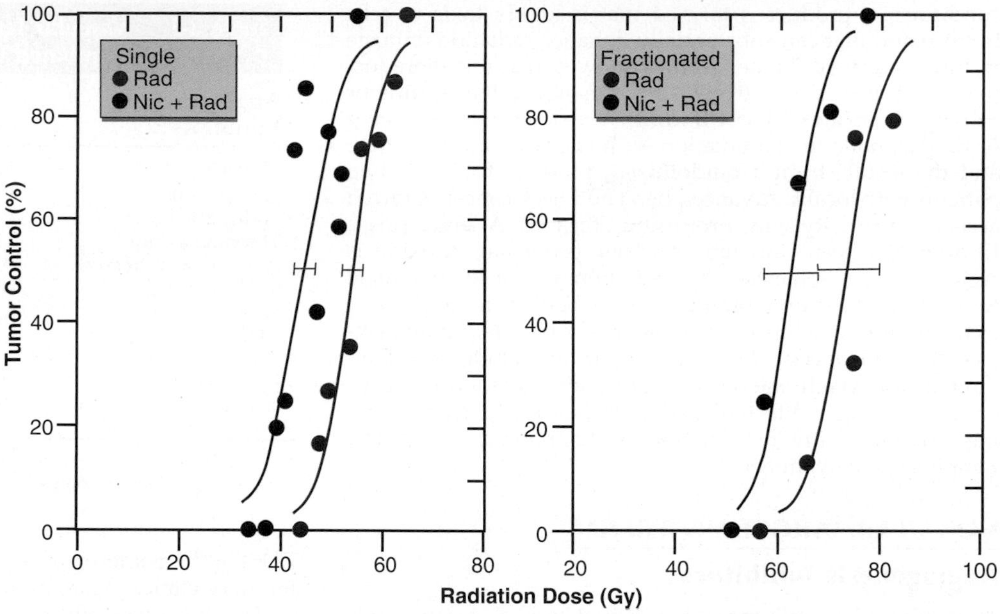

Figure 3-7 Effect of nicotinamide (500 to 1000 mg/kg) on local tumor control measured as a function of the total radiation dose given as a single treatment to C3H mammary carcinomas or in a fractionated schedule to the carcinoma NT. The drug was injected intraperitoneally 30 to 60 minutes before irradiation. (Adapted from Horsman MR, Chaplin DJ, Overgaard J: Combination of nicotinamide and hyperthermia to eliminate radioresistant chronically and acutely hypoxic tumor cells. Cancer Res 50:7430-7436, 1990; Kjellen E, Joiner MC, Collier JM, et al: A therapeutic benefit from combining normobaric carbogen or oxygen with nicotinamide in fractionated x-ray treatments. Radiother Oncol 22:81-91, 1991.)

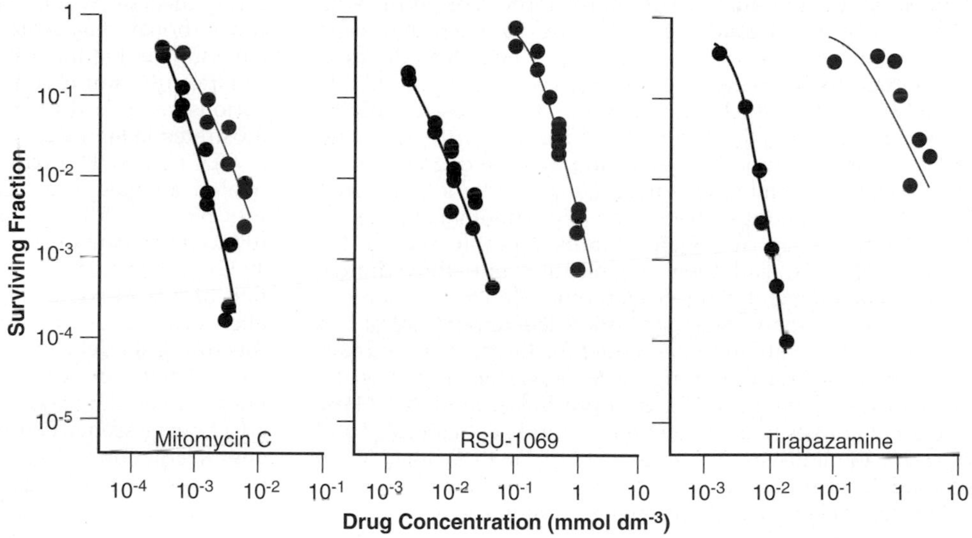

Figure 3-8 Survival of mammalian cells exposed to mitomycin C, RSU 1069, or tirapazamine under aerobic *(red)* of hypoxic *(blue)* conditions. (Adapted from Stratford IJ, Stephens MA: The differential hypoxic cytotoxicity of bioreductive agents determined in vitro by the MTT assay. Int J Radiat Oncol Biol Phys 16:973-976, 1989; Hall EJ: Radiobiology for the Radiobiologist, 4th ed. Philadelphia, JB Lippincott, 1994.)

affinic radiosensitizers discussed earlier, which were relatively nontoxic to cells under normal oxygenated conditions, were reduced to a more toxic form under hypoxic conditions.[79] This ability to preferentially kill the radiation-resistant tumor cell population makes bioreductive drugs an excellent choice for improving radiation response.

The prototype bioreductive drug is mitomycin C,[80] which is activated by bioreduction to form products that cross-link DNA. It has been used for many years in patients as a chemoradiosensitizer. In several studies, it has been used to specifically overcome hypoxic cell radioresistance. In two randomized clinical trials enrolling patients with squamous cell carcinoma of the head and neck, mitomycin C improved radiation-induced local tumor control without any enhancement of radiation reactions in normal tissues.[81,82] However, in two other trials, no major influence on response or survival was seen.[83,84] This absence of any improved response is perhaps not surprising because the drug was only given once during the radiation schedule and showed little difference between aerobic and hypoxic cell killing (Fig. 3-8).

The finding that misonidazole showed preferential toxicity toward hypoxic cells led to numerous efforts to find other nitroimidazole radiosensitizers that were effective as hypoxic cell cytotoxins. RSU 1069 (see Fig. 3-8) has the classic 2-nitroimidazole radiosensitizing properties, but an aziridine ring at the terminal end of the chain gives the molecule substantial potency as a hypoxic cell cytotoxin. Although the drug was found to have substantial activity in hypoxic cells in vitro and in tumors in vivo,[85] preliminary clinical studies indicated dose-limiting gastrointestinal toxicity. A less toxic pro-drug, RB 6145, was then developed, which in vivo is reduced to RSU 1069. Although this drug was shown to have potent antitumor activity in experimental systems, large-animal toxicity
revealed the potential of this agent to caus
Further development of this drug has bee

Another group of bioreductive compou
siderable promise are the organic nitroxi
benzotriazene di-*N*-oxide, tirapazamine, is
pound (see Fig. 3-8). The parent moiety sh
ity toward aerobic cells, but after reductio

th
dru

conditions, a product is formed that is highly toxic to cells in vitro and that can substantially enhance radiation damage in tumors in vivo.[86] Later studies showed that this bioreductive drug was very effective at enhancing the antitumor activity of cisplatin.[87] These findings have led to clinical testing of tirapazamine in combination with cisplatin and radiation, and the results from a randomized, phase II trial enrolling patients with locally advanced head and neck cancers showed acceptable toxicity with promising efficacy.[88] A larger phase III trial has been initiated. Another promising *N*-oxide is AQ4N, which enhances the radiation response in animal tumors[89] and is undergoing clinical testing in a phase I trial enrolling patients with refractory or recurrent malignancies (i.e., advanced solid tumors or non-Hodgkin's lymphoma) for which standard curative measures do not exist or are no longer effective and in a phase I/II trial enrolling patients with non-Hodgkin's lymphoma or chronic lymphocytic leukemia.

Table 3-3 Vascular Targeting Agents That Have Been Combined with Radiation

Angiogenesis Inhibitors	Vascular Disrupting Agents
TNP-470	Hyperthermia
Angiostatin	Photodynamic therapy
Endostatin	Colchicine
Thrombospondin	Tumor necrosis factor
Anti-VEGF antibodies	Arsenic trioxide
SU 5416	Flavone acetic acid
SU 6668	5,6-Dimethylxanthenone-4-acetic acid
PTK 787	Combretastatin A-4 disodium phosphate
SU 11248	AVE 8062
ZD 6474	ZD 6126

VEGF, vascular endothelial growth factor.
Additional information is available in references 96 through 100.

VASCULAR TARGETING AGENTS

Angiogenesis Inhibitors

The tumor microenvironment, which plays such a critical role in determining the tumor's response to radiation, is strongly influenced by the tumor vascular supply. For most solid tumors to grow beyond 1 to 2 mm in diameter, they need to develop their own blood supply, which they do from the normal tissue vessels by angiogenesis.[90] This is a highly complex process, which is triggered by the release of specific growth factors from the tumor cells.[91] These growth factors initiate a series of physical steps, including local degradation of the basement membrane surrounding capillaries, invasion into the surrounding stroma by the endothelial cells in the direction of the angiogenic stimulus, proliferation of the endothelial cells, and their organization into three-dimensional structures that connect with other similar structures to form the new blood vessel network.[91] The importance of this process makes it an attractive target for therapy, and numerous approaches for inhibiting the various steps in the angiogenic process have been tested in preclinical models.[92] Many of these therapies have moved into clinical evaluation,[93,94] and of these, the anti-vascular endothelial growth factor (VEGF) antibody Avastin has been shown to improve the response of colorectal cancer patients receiving chemotherapy.[95] Preclinical studies using rodent and human tumor xenografts have shown that certain angiogenesis inhibitors can be effectively combined with radiation to improve tumor response (Table 3-3).[96] As a result, a limited number of clinical studies have combined certain angiogenesis inhibitors, especially Avastin and thalidomide, with radiation therapy.[94]

Vascular Disrupting Agents

An alternative approach for targeting tumor vasculature involves the use of agents that can damage established tumor vessels.[92] This is not a new concept; it was first demonstrated with the tubulin binding agent colchicine in the 1940s.[97] Since then, a number of agents have been shown to be capable of preferentially damaging tumor vessels, leading to a reduction in tumor perfusion that results in an increase in tumor ischemia and necrosis, producing an inhibitory effect on tumor growth. These include physical treatments such as hyperthermia, photodynamic therapy, and irradiation,[98] but they more commonly include tumor necrosis factor, the flavanoid derivatives flavone acetic acid and 5,6-dimethylxanthenone-4-acetic acid (DMXAA), and the tubulin-binding drugs combretastatin A-4 disodium phosphate (CA4DP) and ZD6126.[98,99] Some of these small-molecule drugs are in preliminary clinical evaluations.[99]

The antitumor effects of these agents when used on their own are not substantial, suggesting that their potential clinical application would be better when combined with more conventional treatments, especially radiation. Several studies have shown that the response of tumors to radiation could be significantly improved when animals were treated with various vascular disrupting agents (see Table 3-3).[99,100] This is illustrated in Figure 3-9 for a C3H mammary carcinoma grown in CDF1 mice. The radiation dose needed to control 50% of treated animals after single-dose radiation treatment alone was 53 Gy (95% CI, 51 to 56 Gy). This was significantly reduced (chi-square test, $P < .05$) to 46 Gy (95% CI, 42 to 49 Gy) when mice were given a single intraperitoneal injection of a nontoxic dose of CA4DP (250 mg/kg) 30 minutes after local tumor irradiation. Such a drug dose on its own in this tumor model can slow the growth of the tumors by only about 2 days. This enhancement of tumor radiation damage is known to be time and schedule dependent, with the greatest effect being seen when the drug is given within a few hours after irradiation.[99,100] It is also tumor specific, with no enhancement of radiation response seen in normal tissues. This has been shown for CA4DP in early-responding normal skin (see Fig. 3-9) or late-responding bladder and lung.[101] These differences between the tumor and normal tissue results are entirely consistent with the drugs' ability to induce damage in tumor but not normal tissue vessels.[102]

RADIATION PROTECTORS

Sulfhydryl-Containing Compounds

More than 50 years ago, it was realized that certain amino acids, glutathione, and ascorbic acid were able to modulate radiation-induced inactivation of biologic material. Based on those observations, Patt and colleagues investigated the effect of treating mice with the thiol-containing amino acid cysteine.[103] They found that administering this compound to mice before whole-body irradiation resulted in a remarkable increase in animal survival (Fig. 3-10). In contrast, no effect was observed when cysteine was given after irradiation. During the Cold War, this finding led to a large research program at the Walter Reed Army Institute of Research, which was aimed at developing a drug that could protect soldiers from nuclear weapons.[59] Numerous sulfhydryl-containing substances with substantial radioprotective properties were

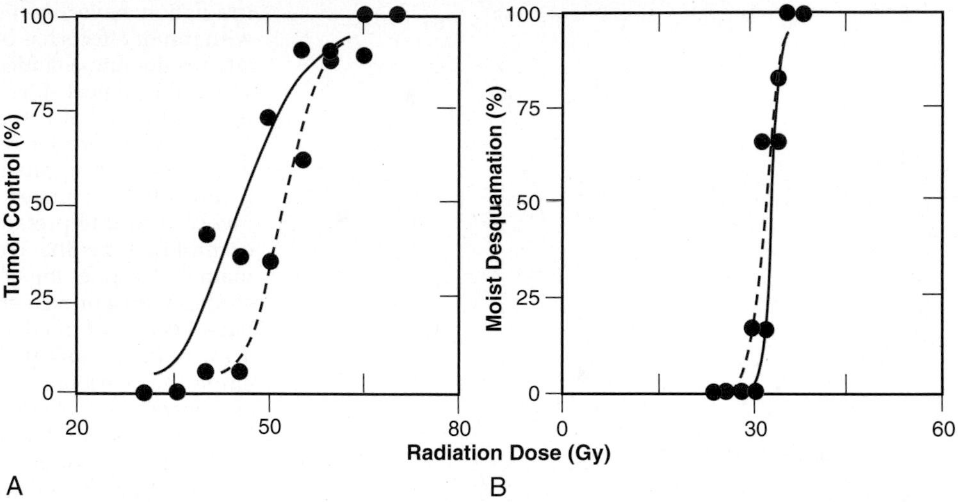

Figure 3-9 Effect of combretastatin A-4 disodium phosphate (250 mg/kg) on local control of a C3H mammary carcinoma (**A**) or the development of moist desquamation in the foot skin of CDF1 mice (**B**) after radiation treatment. Radiation was given alone *(red)* or 30 minutes before intraperitoneal injection of the drug *(blue)*. (Adapted from Murata R, Siemann DW, Overgaard J, Horsman MR: Interaction between combretastatin A-4 disodium phosphate and radiation in murine tumours. Radiother Oncol 60:155-161, 2001.)

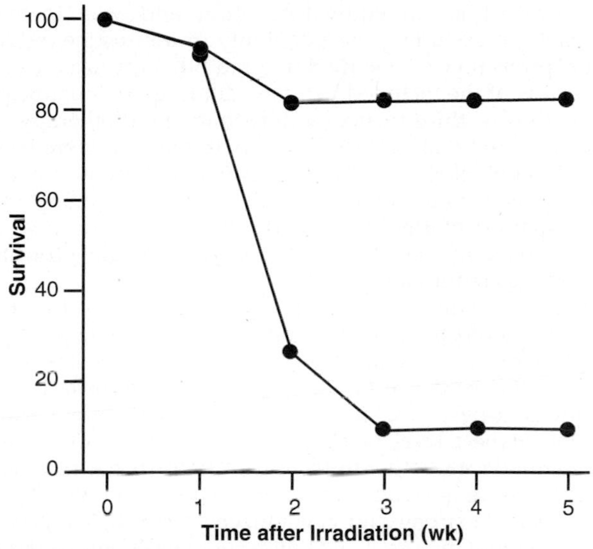

Figure 3-10 Percentage of rodents surviving after whole-body irradiation with 8 Gy. Animals were control irradiated *(blue)* or given radiation after injection with 575 mg of cysteine *(red)*. (Adapted from Patt HM, Tyree EB, Straub RL, Smith DE: Cysteine protection against X irradiation. Science 110:213-214, 1949.)

detected, but only WR-2771 (amifostine) was found to exhibit acceptable toxicity. The idea of using amifostine in oncology arose when preclinical studies, performed mainly in the 1970s and 1980s, suggested a selective protection of normal tissue from damage induced by irradiation and by chemotherapy.[104,105] Despite these findings, the interest in amifostine over the years has waxed and waned, although it has recently been boosted by the commercialization of the drug primarily for use in combination with chemotherapy, by U.S. Food and Drug Administration (FDA) approval, and by establishment of authoritative guidelines.[106] The lack of interest was probably related to the fact that there was no fail-safe modification of traditional radiotherapy.[107] Numerous normal tissues are dose limiting, and the evaluation of therapeutic benefit when using a radioprotector requires that the protector can ensure absolute normal tissue selectivity and fewer complications with an unchanged rate of tumor control for a given radiation dose, or if selectivity is uncertain, an increase in radiation dose may be needed to maintain the same rate of tumor control. However, this scenario requires that the protective effect on tumor tissues is predictable and exceeded by the protection offered to all relevant normal tissues. The "perfect" radioprotector must have an acceptable toxicity profile and must be easy to handle if general clinical use is to be expected with routine fractionated radiotherapy.[108-110]

It is not clear how amifostine induces radioprotection. The drug must first undergo dephosphorylation to its active metabolite, WR-1065. WR-1065 is further metabolized to the disulfide WR-33278; the latter metabolite may also afford some protection, although to a lesser extent.[111] Several mechanisms are involved in radioprotection, depending on the quality of the radiation. Protection against sparsely ionizing radiation, such as x-rays, is mainly obtained by scavenging of free radicals.[59,112,113] Because WR-1065 and WR-33278 react with free radicals in competition with oxygen, the protection obtained by scavenging is highly influenced by oxygen tension (Fig. 3-11). The protection is maximal at intermediate levels of oxygen (20% to 50% oxygen in the inspired air). At higher oxygen tensions, WR-1065 is outbalanced by excess oxygen, and the protection is gradually lost. The degree of protection is also diminished at low oxygen tensions, at which levels scavenging of free radicals is no longer important because the lack of oxygen by itself provides radioprotection. Additional and complex mechanisms are undoubtedly involved. Some of these may involve hypoxia created locally by direct interaction of thiols with oxygen, chemical repair by thiol donation of hydrogen, or decreased accessibility of radiolytic attack sites by induction of DNA packaging.[108]

Preclinical studies have shown that many tissues can be protected from radiation damage by amifostine (Table 3-4). However, the protection observed in different normal tissues is unfortunately very heterogeneous. Some normal tissue such as the central nervous system, which often is dose limiting in radiotherapy, is not protected, because amifostine probably does not cross the blood-brain barrier.[114] In other normal tissues such as salivary glands and hematopoietic system, amifostine affords very significant radioprotection. These variations are probably explained by tissue variations in oxygen concentration, dephosphorylation activity, and distribution of amifostine and its metabolites.[111,113,115] To make things even more complicated, tumor protection has been impossible to exclude by preclinical experiments.[107] Large, single doses of

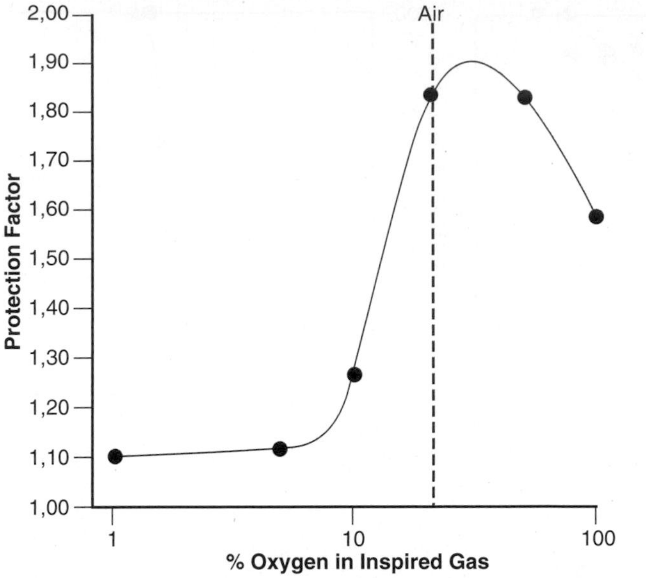

Figure 3-11 The variation in normal skin protection in mice that breathed various oxygen concentrations and were given 400 mg/kg of WR-2721, 30 to 45 minutes before irradiation. (Adapted from Denekamp J, Michael BD, Rojas A, Stewart FA: Radioprotection of mouse skin by WR-2721: the critical influence of oxygen tension. Int J Radiat Oncol Biol Phys 8:531-534, 1982.)

Table 3-4 Protection Factors Achieved by Amifostine in Normal Tissues and Tumors

Tissue	Protection Factor
Salivary gland	2.3-3.3
Bone marrow	1.8-3.0
Jejunum	1.5-2.1
Skin	1.4-2.1
Testis	1.5-1.6
Kidney	1.3-1.5
Bladder	1.3-1.5
Lung	1.2-1.4
Heart	>1.0
Tumor	1.0-2.8

Data from references 107, 113, 115, 121-124.

irradiation have often been used, and relevant comparison with tumor effects has been absent, making it difficult to translate results into a clinically meaningful context.[108]

On the clinical side, there have been far too many publications of phase I or II studies with limited numbers of patients and a few underpowered randomized studies. Chemotherapy has often been applied together with radiotherapy, making it difficult to evaluate the results (Table 3-5). The problems involved in interpretation of the results from such trials are exemplified by the correspondence of Dubray and Dhermain.[116] Despite the long list of preclinical normal tissue studies with a proven effect of amifostine, disappointingly few have been confirmed in the clinical setting. Amelioration of acute radiation toxicity has been observed in studies that often employed various types of treatment intensification such as concomitant chemotherapy or accelerated radiotherapy. However, definite confirmation regarding late morbidity such as fibrosis has not been obtained. Hopes rose with the publication of the pivotal trial by Brizel and coworkers,[117] which showed that amifostine significantly protected against radiation-induced xerostomia with no apparent loss of tumor control in head and neck cancers. Unfortunately, the study was not powered as an equivalence trial and was therefore incapable of excluding the possibility of amifostine-induced tumor protection.[110] Postoperative radiotherapy was used in two thirds of the included patients, diluting potential protection in the one third treated with definitive radiotherapy. The study required that at least 75% of both parotids were irradiated. Modern three-dimensional target definition and dose delivery, such as by intensity-modulated radiotherapy, often allow sparing of significant parts of the parotids possible, thereby making the attempt for pharmacologic protection more or less redundant.

After the study by Brizel and colleagues,[117] the FDA approved amifostine for use in patients undergoing postoperative fractionated radiotherapy in the head and neck region to decrease the incidence of acute and chronic xerostomia. The American Society of Clinical Oncology has awarded amifostine the highest level of recommendation for postoperative and definitive radiotherapy,[106] but in light of the paucity of clinical data, this recommendation seems premature.[110,118] To sustain such a strong and generalized approval, a reproduction of the trial by Brizel and colleagues employing definitive irradiation of head and neck cancer in an adequate number of patients to rule out significant tumor protection is the least evidence that should be required. Nonetheless, reduction of treatment toxicity is as important as ever. Traditionally, late-

Table 3-5 Randomized Clinical Trials Investigating the Effect of Amifostine on Outcome in Radiotherapy Administered Alone or with Chemotherapy

Study	Year	Anatomic Site	Treatment	No. of Patients
Komaki et al[125]	2004	Lung	RT + Chemo	62
Leong et al[126]	2003	Lung	RT + Chemo	60
Antonadou et al[127]	2003	Lung	RT + Chemo	73
Antonadou et al[128]	2001	Lung	RT	146
Athanassiou et al[129]	2003	Pelvis	RT	205
Momm et al[130]	2001	Head and neck	RT	73
Brizel et al[117]	2000	Head and neck	RT	315
Bourhis et al[131]	1999	Head and neck	RT	26
Buntzel et al[132]	1998	Head and neck	RT + Chemo	39
Bohouslavizki et al[133]	1998	Thyroid	RT (^{131}I)	50
Liu et al[134]	1992	Rectum	RT	100

Chemo, chemotherapy; RT, radiotherapy.

reacting tissues have been dose limiting in radiotherapy. However, treatment intensification using alternative fractionation schedules, concomitant chemotherapy, and biologic modifiers is increasingly being explored. It is therefore foreseeable that radiation dose will increasingly be limited by acute toxicity. Whether sufficient and tolerable doses of amifostine can be applied in this scenario even by the subcutaneous route is unknown.[109,119] Even though amifostine may show evidence of protective activity in the setting of intensified radiotherapy, it does not imply therapeutic benefit. It is therefore important that future trials do not expose the control arm to a treatment intensification that places them at greater risk of the toxicity that the protective agent is designed to prevent.[120]

Modifiers of the Oxygen Supply

Hypoxia reduces radiation sensitivity, and decreasing oxygen availability to tissues may be a viable approach for achieving radiation protection. This may be achieved by modification of hemoglobin-oxygen affinity. The most widely studied agents in this context are the substituted benzaldehyde (BW12C) and its derivatives.[135,136] These agents preferentially bind to oxyhemoglobin and increase the affinity of the hemoglobin for oxygen.[137,138] This shift decreases the amount of oxygen available to the tissues. Although this has been shown to protect some normal tissues from radiation,[135,139] there is limited evidence that BW12C can increase perfusion in certain normal tissues,[140] which should increase oxygen delivery. Evidence from experimental studies indicates that BW12C also can significantly protect tumors from radiation.[135,136]

Carbon monoxide reduces oxygen transport to tissues by binding to hemoglobin, decreasing the molecular sites available for oxygen transport and causing a left shift of the hemoglobin-oxygen dissociation curve; any oxygen that binds to the hemoglobin does so more strongly.[141] The ability of this approach to increase hypoxia and reduce the radiation response has been well documented in experimental systems.[142,143] Unfortunately, this effect was demonstrated in tumors, not normal tissues. The effect of carbon monoxide in patients has also been observed. Figure 3-12 shows patients with head and neck carcinomas who were smokers and therefore had higher carboxyhemoglobin levels. They had a poorer response to radiation therapy than nonsmokers.

Because most modifiers of the oxygen supply protect tumors as well as normal tissues from radiation, their use in this context is limited. However, this may not be true for pentoxifylline, a drug that alters red blood cell deformability, inhibits platelet aggregation, and reduces fibrinolytic activity.[144] Because of these effects, red blood cells are better able to traverse narrowed arterioles and capillaries. When given before irradiation, pentoxifylline enhances radiation damage in tumors,[145] presumably because of improved oxygen delivery,[146,147] but it has no effect on the response of normal tissues.[145] When administered on a daily basis after irradiation, pentoxifylline had no effect on early skin reactions in mice, but it did significantly reduce the incidence of late reactions.[148]

Other Radioprotectors

Various cytokines have also been reported to be capable of radioprotecting certain normal tissues, although the radioprotective role is somewhat controversial. Injection of granulocyte-macrophage colony-stimulating factor has been shown to rescue mice, dogs, and monkeys from radiation injury.[149] Radioprotection has also been seen with interleukin-1 (IL-1), tumor necrosis factor-α (TNF-α), and transforming growth factor-β (TGF-β).[150-152] However, the effects of IL-1 and TNF-α were time dependent; although survival of intestinal crypt cells was increased when either agent was administered 20 hours before irradiation, radiosensitization was observed with only a 4-hour interval.[151,152] Moreover, production of IL-1, TNF-α, and TGF-β has been elevated after irradiation of normal tissue, and this may be one of the important steps in the development of fibrosis.[153-155] Radioprotection has also been seen in lung and bone after treatment with basic fibroblast growth factor,[156,157] but more significantly, such treatment had no effect on the radiation response of at least one murine tumor model.[156]

Other agents that are capable of reducing radiation injury in normal tissues include the angiotensin-converting enzyme inhibitor captopril,[158,159] corticosteroids,[160] prostaglandins,[161,162] and essential fatty acids.[163] However, the mechanisms of action are not entirely clear, nor is there evidence that these agents do not also protect tumors from radiation.

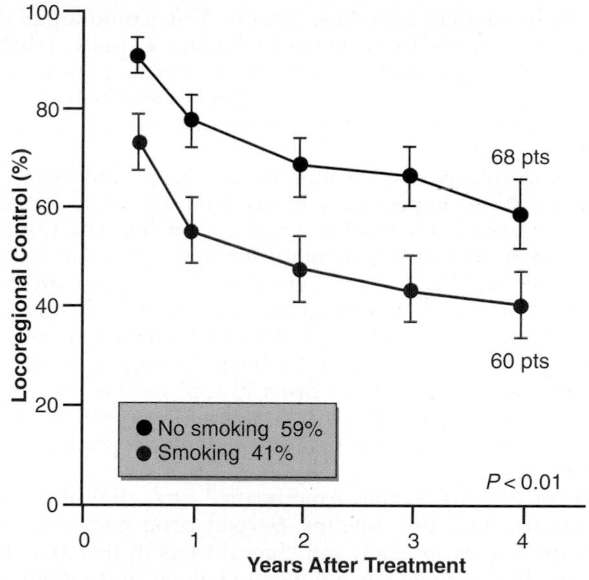

Figure 3-12 Influence of smoking during treatment on the outcome of radiotherapy in 128 patients (pts) with advanced head and neck carcinoma. (From Overgaard J, Horsman MR: Modification of hypoxia-induced radioresistance in tumors by the use of oxygen and sensitizers. Semin Radiat Oncol 6:10-21, 1996.)

SUMMARY

The use of radiation to treat certain types of cancer with curative intent is a well-established and effective therapy, but there is room for improvement. The use of additional treatments that can increase radiation damage in tumors without affecting normal tissues or protect normal tissues without having a similar protective effect in tumors is clearly warranted.

Many agents have been shown to modify hypoxia experimentally, but for those that have progressed to the clinic, the results have been far from satisfactory; the reason for this is not clear. One argument is that the animal models used were inappropriate for demonstrating potential effects in humans, but because hyperbaric oxygen and nimorazole were shown to work in animal models and humans, this is unlikely to be the explanation. Poor design of clinical trials has also been proposed, but it is hard to imagine that this accounts for all of the failures in humans. It is known that hypoxia is important only in certain tumor types and that there is substantial heterogeneity in patients with those tumors. This would argue that more effort needs to be made in finding a quick, reliable, and routinely applicable method for identifying patients with hypoxic tumors who would most likely benefit from some form of modification. What that modifier should be is not clear.

Nimorazole is easy to administer, cheap, and relatively nontoxic. More importantly, it has been shown to work in certain tumors of the head and neck region, and as a result, it has become part of the standard therapy with radiation for head and neck tumors in Denmark. Why it has not been adopted elsewhere remains a mystery. Hyperbaric oxygen was also proved to be beneficial, but that treatment was difficult to apply on a routine basis. Carbogen breathing (with and without nicotinamide) is far easier to apply and is under clinical investigation, and if the results from those studies prove effective, we may see this treatment being adopted by more institutions.

There is considerable experimental and clinical interest in vascular targeting therapy. Several drug companies are keen to support research and clinical trials in this area. It is unlikely that such agents will be used alone, and radiation is potentially the best adjuvant treatment with which these drugs should be combined. If the preclinical results can be translated into the clinical setting, such combination therapy could have a substantial impact on the benefits seen with radiotherapy.

The use of radioprotectors is more controversial. There is good experimental evidence that a number of agents can protect certain normal tissues from radiation, but data also show that some of these agents are capable of inducing protection against radiation damage in tumors. The results from clinical studies that have investigated the potential of radioprotectors have been inconclusive, and until good human data demonstrating the ability of such agents to protect normal tissues, but not tumors, from radiation become available, the use of radioprotectors must be considered experimental.

REFERENCES

1. Schwarz G: Über Desensibiliserung gegen Röntgen- und Radiumstrahlen. Munch Med Wochenschr 24:1-2, 1909.
2. Müller C: Eine neue Behandlungsmethode bösartiger Geschwülste. Munch Med Wochenschr 28:1490-1493, 1910.
3. Gray LH, Conger AD, Ebert M, et al: The concentration of oxygen dissolved in tissues at the time of irradiation as a factor in radiotherapy. Br J Radiol 26:638-648, 1953.
4. Thomlinson RH, Gray LH: The histological structure of some human lung cancers and the possible implications for radiotherapy. Br J Cancer 9:539-549, 1955.
5. Tannock IF: The relationship between cell proliferation and the vascular system in a transplanted mouse mammary tumour. Br J Cancer 22:258-273, 1968.
6. Horsman MR, Overgaard J: Overcoming tumour radiation resistance resulting from acute hypoxia. Eur J Cancer 28A:717-718, 1992.
7. Brown JM: Evidence for acutely hypoxic cells in mouse tumours, and a possible mechanism of reoxygenation. Br J Radiol 52:650-656, 1979.
8. Chaplin DJ, Olive PL, Durand RE: Intermittent blood flow in a murine tumor: radiobiological effects. Cancer Res 47:597-601, 1987.
9. Horsman MR: Nicotinamide and other benzamide analogs as agents for overcoming hypoxic cell radiation resistance in tumours. Acta Oncol 34:571-587, 1995.
10. Helmlinger G, Yuan F, Dellian M, Jain RK: Interstitial pH and pO_2 gradients in solid tumors in vivo: high-resolution measurements reveal a lack of correlation. Nat Med 3:177-182, 1997.
11. Kimura H, Braun RD, Ong ET, et al: Fluctuations in red cell flux in tumor microvessels can lead to transient hypoxia and reoxygenation in tumor parenchyma. Cancer Res 56:5522-5528, 1996.
12. Moulder JE, Rockwell S: Hypoxic fractions of solid tumour. Int J Radiat Oncol Biol Phys 10:695-712, 1984.
13. Kolstad P: Intercapillary distance, oxygen tension and local recurrence in cervix cancer. Scand J Clin Lab Invest 106:145-157, 1968.
14. Lauk S, Skates S, Goodman M, Suit HD: Morphometric study of the vascularity of oral squamous cell carcinomas and its relation to outcome of radiation therapy. Eur J Cancer Clin Oncol 25:1431-1440, 1989.
15. Révész L, Siracka E, Siracky J, et al: Variation of vascular density within and between tumors of the uterine cervix and its predictive value for radiotherapy. Int J Radiat Oncol Biol Phys 11:97-103, 1989.
16. Horsman MR: Hypoxia in tumours: its relevance, identification and modification. *In* Beck-Bornholdt HP (ed): Current Topics in Clinical Radiobiology of Tumours. Berlin, Springer-Verlag, 1993, pp 99-112.
17. Olive P, Durand RE, LeRiche J, et al: Gel electrophoresis of individual cells to quantify hypoxic fraction in human breast cancers. Cancer Res 53:733-736, 1993.
18. Raleigh JA, Dewhirst MW, Thrall DE: Measuring tumor hypoxia. Semin Radiat Oncol 6:37-45, 1996.
19. Olive PL, Aquino-Parsons C: Measurement of tumor hypoxia using single cell methods. Semin Radiat Oncol 14:241-248, 2004.
20. Rasey JS, Koh WJ, Evans ML, et al: Quantifying regional hypoxia in human tumors with positron emission tomography of ^{18}F-fluoromisonidazole: a pretherapy study of 37 patients. Int J Radiat Oncol Biol Phys 36:417-428, 1996.
21. Piert M, Machulla HJ, Picchio M, et al: Hypoxia-specific tumor imaging with ^{18}F-fluoroazomycin arabinoside. J Nucl Med 46:106-113, 2005.
22. Urtasun RC, Parliament MB, McEwan AJ, et al: Measurement of hypoxia in human tumours by non-invasive SPECT imaging of iodoazomycin arabinoside. Br J Cancer 74(Suppl):S209-S212, 1996.
23. Seddon BM, Payne GS, Simmons L, et al: A phase I study of SR-4554 via intravenous administration for noninvasive investigation of tumor hypoxia by magnetic resonance spectroscopy in patients with malignancy. Clin Cancer Res 9:5101-5112, 2003.
24. Hui EP, Chan ATC, Pezzella F, et al: Coexpression of hypoxia-inducible factors 1α and 2α, carbonic anhydrase IX, and vascular endothelial growth factor in nasopharyngeal carcinoma and relationship to survival. Clin Cancer Res 8:2595-2604, 2002.
25. Airley RE, Loncaster J, Raleigh J, et al: GLUT-1 and CAIX as intrinsic markers of hypoxia in carcinoma of the cervix: relationship to pimonidazole binding. Int J Cancer 104:85-91, 2003.
26. Le QT, Sutpin PD, Raychaudhuri S, et al: Identification of osteopontin as a prognostic plasma marker for head and neck squamous cell carcinomas. Clin Cancer Res 9:59-67, 2003.
27. Gatenby RA, Kessler HB, Rosenblum JS, et al: Oxygen distribution in squamous cell carcinoma metastases and its relationship to outcome of radiation therapy. Int J Radiat Oncol Biol Phys 14:831-838, 1988.
28. Hoeckel M, Schlenger K, Aral B, et al: Association between tumor hypoxia and malignant progression in advanced cancer of the uterine cervix. Cancer Res 56:4509-4515, 1996.
29. Brizel DM, Scully SP, Harrelson JM, et al: Tumor oxygenation predicts for the likelihood of distant metastasis in human soft tissue sarcoma. Cancer Res 56:941-943, 1996.
30. Brizel DM, Sibley GS, Prosnitz LR, et al: Tumor hypoxia adversely affects the prognosis of carcinoma of the head and neck. Int J Radiat Oncol Biol Phys 38:285-289, 1997.
31. Nordsmark M, Overgaard M, Overgaard J: Pretreatment oxygenation predicts radiation response in advanced squamous cell carcinoma of the head and neck. Radiother Oncol 41:31-39, 1996.
32. Nordsmark M, Alsner J, Keller J, et al: Hypoxia in soft tissue sarcomas: adverse impact on survival and no association with p53 mutations. Br J Cancer 84:1070-1075, 2001.
33. Nordsmark M, Bentzen SM, Rudat V, et al: Prognostic value of tumor oxygenation in 397 head and neck tumors after primary

radiation therapy: an international multi-center study. Eur J Cancer 37:37, 2001.
34. Overgaard J, Horsman MR: Modification of hypoxia-induced radioresistance in tumors by the use of oxygen and sensitizers. Semin Radiat Oncol 6:10-21, 1996.
35. Du Sault LA: The effect of oxygen on the response of spontaneous tumours in mice to radiotherapy. Br J Radiol 36:749-754, 1963.
36. Suit HD, Marshall N, Woerner D: Oxygen, oxygen plus carbon dioxide, and radiation therapy of a mouse mammary carcinoma. Cancer 30:1154-1158, 1972.
37. Siemann DW, Hill RP, Bush RS: Smoking: The influence of carboxyhemoglobin (HbCO) on tumor oxygenation and response to radiation. Int J Radiat Oncol Biol Phys 40:657-662, 1978.
38. Rojas A: Radiosensitization with normobaric oxygen and carbogen. Radiother Oncol 20(Suppl 1):65-70, 1991.
39. Grau C, Horsman MR, Overgaard J: Improving the radiation response in a C3H mouse mammary carcinoma by normobaric oxygen and carbogen breathing. Int J Radiat Oncol Biol Phys 22:415-419, 1992.
40. Churchill-Davidson I: The oxygen effect in radiotherapy—historical review. Front Radiat Ther Oncol 1:1-15, 1968.
41. Dische S: Hyperbaric oxygen: the Medical Research Council trials and their clinical significance. Br J Radiol 51:888-894, 1979.
42. Dische S, Anderson PJ, Sealy R, et al: Carcinoma of the cervix—anaemia, radiotherapy and hyperbaric oxygen. Br J Radiol 56:251-255, 1983.
43. Henk JM, Kunkler PB, Smith CW: Radiotherapy and hyperbaric oxygen in head and neck cancer. Final report of first controlled clinical trial. Lancet 2:101-103, 1977.
44. Henk JM, Smith CW: Radiotherapy and hyperbaric oxygen in head and neck cancer. Interim report of second clinical trial. Lancet 2:104-105, 1977.
45. Watson ER, Halnan KE, Dische S, et al: Hyperbaric oxygen and radiotherapy: a medical research council trial in carcinoma of the cervix. Br J Radiol 51:879-887, 1978.
46. Overgaard J: Sensitization of hypoxic tumour cells—clinical experience. Int J Radiat Biol 56:801-811, 1989.
47. Bergsjø P, Kolstad P: Clinical trial with atmospheric oxygen breathing during radiotherapy of cancer of the cervix. Scand J Clin Lab Invest 106(Suppl):167-171, 1968.
48. Rubin P, Hanley J, Keys HM, et al: Carbogen breathing during radiation therapy. The RTOG study. Int J Radiat Oncol Biol Phys 5:1963-1970, 1979.
49. Chaplin DJ, Horsman MR, Siemann DW: Further evaluation of nicotinamide and carbogen as a strategy to reoxygenate hypoxic cells in vivo: importance of nicotinamide dose and pre-irradiation breathing time. Br J Cancer 68:269-273, 1993.
50. Adams GE, Cooke MS: Electron-affinic sensitization. I. A structural basis for chemical radiosensitizers in bacteria. Int J Radiat Biol 15:457-471, 1969.
51. Asquith JC, Watts ME, Patel K, et al: Electron-affinic sensitization. V. Radiosensitization of hypoxic bacteria and mammalian cells in vitro by some nitroimidazoles and nitropyrazoles. Radiat Res 60:108-118, 1974.
52. Adams GE, Flockhart IR, Smithen CE, et al: Electron-affinic sensitization. VII. A correlation between structures, one-electron reduction potentials and efficiencies of some nitroimidazoles as hypoxic cell radiosensitizers. Radiat Res 67:9-20, 1976.
53. Overgaard J: Clinical evaluation of nitroimidazoles as modifiers of hypoxia in solid tumors. Oncol Res 6:509-518, 1994.
54. Dische S: Chemical sensitizers for hypoxic cells: a decade of experience in clinical radiotherapy. Radiother Oncol 3:97-115, 1985.
55. Overgaard J, Sand Hansen H, Overgaard M, et al: The Danish Head and Neck Cancer study group (DAHANCA) randomized trials with hypoxic radiosensitizers in carcinoma of the larynx and pharynx. *In* Dewey WC, Edington M, Fry RJM, et al (eds): Radiation Research. A Twentieth-Century Perspective, vol II. Congress Proceedings. Toronto, ICRR, 1991, pp 573-577.
56. Dische S, Machin D, Chassagne D: A trial of Ro 03-8799 (pimonidazole) in carcinoma of the uterine cervix: an interim report from the Medical Research Council Working Party on advanced carcinoma of the cervix. Radiother Oncol 26:93-103, 1993.
57. Lee D-J, Cosmatos D, Marcial VA, et al: Results of an RTOG phase III trial (RTOG 85-27) comparing radiotherapy plus etanidazole (SR-2508) with radiotherapy alone for locally advanced head and neck carcinomas. Int J Radiat Oncol Biol Phys 32:567-576, 1995.
58. Overgaard J, Sand Hansen H, Overgaard M, et al: A randomised double-blind phase III study of nimorazole as a hypoxic radiosensitizer of primary radiotherapy in supraglottic larynx and pharynx carcinoma. Results of the Danish head and neck cancer study (DAHANCA) protocol 5-85. Radiother Oncol 46:135-146, 1998.
59. Hall EJ: Radiobiology for the Radiobiologist, 4th ed. Philadelphia, JB Lippincott, 1994.
60. Grau C, Overgaard J: Significance of haemoglobin concentration for treatment outcome. *In* Molls M, Vaupel P (eds): Medical Radiology: Blood Perfusion and Microenvironment of Human Tumours. Heidelberg, Springer-Verlag, 1998, pp 101-112.
61. Thomas GM: Raising hemoglobin: an opportunity for increasing survival? Oncology 63:19-28, 2002.
62. Evans JC, Bergsjø P: The influence of anemia on the results of radiotherapy in carcinoma of the cervix. Radiology 84:709-717, 1965.
63. Grogan M, Thomas GM, Melamed I, et al: The importance of hemoglobin levels during radiotherapy for carcinoma of the cervix. Cancer 86:1528-1536, 1999.
64. Overgaard J, Hansen HS, Overgaard M, et al: Randomized trial evaluating the role of blood transfusion before radiotherapy in 414 patients with head and neck carcinoma. Eur J Cancer 35:S601, 1999.
65. Stuben G, Pottgen C, Knuhmann K, et al: Erythropoietin restores the anemia-induced reduction in radiosensitivity of experimental human tumors in nude mice. Int J Radiat Oncol Biol Phys 55:1358-1362, 2003.
66. Thews O, Koenig R, Kelleher DK, et al: Enhanced radiosensitivity in experimental tumours following erythropoietin treatment of chemotherapy-induced anaemia. Br J Cancer 78:752-756, 1998.
67. Lavey RS, Dempsey WH: Erythropoietin increases hemoglobin in cancer patients during radiotherapy. Int J Radiat Oncol Biol Phys 27:1147-1152, 1993.
68. Henke M, Laszig R, Rube C, et al: Erythropoietin to treat head and neck cancer patients with anaemia undergoing radiotherapy: randomized, double-blind, placebo-controlled trial. Lancet 362:1255-1260, 2003.
69. Machtay M, Pajak T, Suntharalingam M, et al: Definitive radiotherapy + erythropoietin for squamous cell carcinoma of the head and neck: preliminary report of RTOG 99-03. Int J Radiat Oncol Biol Phys 60:S132, 2004.
70. Rockwell S: Use of a perfluorochemical emulsion to improve oxygenation in a solid tumor. Int J Radiat Oncol Biol Phys 11:97-103, 1985.
71. Siemann DW, Macler LM: Tumor radiosensitization through reductions in hemoglobin affinity. Int J Radiat Oncol Biol Phys 12:1295-1297, 1986.
72. Hirst DG, Wood PJ: Could manipulation of the binding affinity of haemoglobin for oxygen be used clinically to sensitize tumours to radiation? Radiother Oncol 20(Suppl 1):53-57, 1991.
73. Horsman MR, Chaplin DJ, Overgaard J: Combination of nicotinamide and hyperthermia to eliminate radioresistant chronically and acutely hypoxic tumor cells. Cancer Res 50:7430-7436, 1990.
74. Chaplin DJ, Horsman MR, Aoki DS: Nicotinamide, fluosol DA and carbogen: a strategy to reoxygenate acutely and chronically hypoxic cells in vivo. Br J Cancer 63:109-113, 1991.
75. Kjellen E, Joiner MC, Collier JM, et al: A therapeutic benefit from combining normobaric carbogen or oxygen with nicotinamide in fractionated x-ray treatments. Radiother Oncol 22:81-91, 1991.
76. Horsman MR, Nordsmark M, Khalil AA, et al: Reducing chronic and acute hypoxia in tumours by combining nicotinamide with carbogen breathing. Acta Oncol 33:371-376, 1994.
77. Hoskin PJ, Saunders MI, Dische S: Hypoxic radiosensitizers in radical radiotherapy for patients with bladder cancer: hyperbaric oxygen, misonidazole, and accelerated radiotherapy, carbogen and nicotinamide. Cancer 86:1322-1328, 1999.
78. Kaanders JHAM, Pop LAM, Marres HAM, et al: ARCON: experience in 215 patients with advanced head-and-neck cancer. Int J Radiat Oncol Biol Phys 52:769-778, 2002.

79. Hall EJ, Roizin-Towle L: Hypoxic sensitizers: radiobiological studies at the cellular level. Radiology 117:453-457, 1975.
80. Kennedy KA, Rockwell S, Sartorelli AC: Preferential activation of mitomycin C to cytotoxic metabolites by hypoxic tumor cells. Cancer Res 40:2356-2360, 1980.
81. Weissberg JB, Son YH, Papac RJ, et al: Randomized clinical trial of mitomycin C as an adjunct to radiotherapy in head and neck cancer. Int J Radiat Oncol Biol Phys 17:3-9, 1989.
82. Haffty BG, Son YH, Sasaki CT, et al: Mitomycin C as an adjunct to postoperative radiation therapy in squamous cell carcinoma of the head and neck: results from two randomized clinical trials. Int J Radiat Oncol Biol Phys 27:241-250, 1993.
83. Dobrowsky W, Naude J, Dobrowsky E, et al: Mitomycin C (MMC) and unconventional fractionation (V-CHART) in advanced head and neck cancer. Acta Oncol 34:270-272, 1995.
84. Grau C, Agarwal JP, Jabeen K, et al: Radiotherapy with or without mitomycin C in the treatment of locally advanced head and neck cancer: results of the IAEA multicentre randomized trial. Radiother Oncol 67:17-27, 2003.
85. Stratford IJ, O'Neill P, Sheldon PW, et al: RSU 1069, a nitroimidazole containing an aziridine group: bioreduction greatly increases cytotoxicity under hypoxic conditions. Biochem Pharmacol 35:105-109, 1986.
86. Zeman EM, Hirst VK, Lemmon MJ, Brown JM: Enhancement of radiation-induced tumor cell killing by the hypoxic cell toxin SR 4233. Radiother Oncol 12:209-218, 1988.
87. Dorie MJ, Brown JM: Tumor-specific, schedule dependent interaction between tirapazamine (SR 4233) and cisplatin. Cancer Res 53:4633-4636, 1993.
88. Rischin D, Peters L, Fisher R, et al: Tirapazamine, cisplatin, and radiation versus fluorouracil, cisplatin, and radiation in patients with locally advanced head and neck cancer: a randomized phase II trial of the Trans-Tasman Radiation Oncology Group (TROG 98.02). J Clin Oncol 23:79-87, 2005.
89. McKeown SR, Friery OP, McIntyre IA, et al: Evidence for a therapeutic gain when AQ4N or tirapazamine is combined with radiation. Br J Cancer 74:S39-S42, 1996.
90. Folkman J: What is the evidence that tumors are angiogenesis dependent? J Natl Cancer Inst 82:4-6, 1990.
91. Fidler IJ, Langley RR, Kerbel RS, Ellis LM: Angiogenesis. *In* DeVita VT, Hellman S, Rosenberg SA (eds): Cancer: Principles and Practice of Oncology, 7th ed. Philadelphia, Lippincott Williams & Wilkins, 2005, pp 129-137.
92. Denekamp J: Inadequate vasculature in solid tumours: consequences for cancer research strategies. Br J Radiol 24(Suppl):111-117, 1992.
93. Brower V: Tumor angiogenesis—new drugs on the block. Nat Biotechnol 17:963-968, 1999.
94. National Cancer Institute: Available at the web site: www.cancer.gov/clinicaltrials
95. Kabbinavar F, Hurwitz HI, Fehrenbacher L, et al: Phase II, randomized trial comparing bevacizumab plus fluorouracil (FU)/leucovorin (LV) with FU/LV alone in patients with metastatic colorectal cancer. J Clin Oncol 21:60-65, 2003.
96. Wachsberger P, Burd R, Dicker AP: Tumor response to ionizing radiation combined with antiangiogenesis or vascular targeting agents: exploring mechanisms of interaction. Clin Cancer Res 9:1957-1971, 2003.
97. Ludford RJ: Colchicine in the experimental chemotherapy of cancer. J Natl Cancer Inst 6:89-101, 1945.
98. Denekamp J, Hill S: Angiogenic attack as a therapeutic strategy for cancer. Radiother Oncol 20(Suppl):103-112, 1991.
99. Siemann DW, Chaplin DJ, Horsman MR: Vascular-targeting therapies for treatment of malignant disease. Cancer 100:2491-2499, 2004.
100. Horsman MR, Murata R: Combination of vascular targeting agents with thermal or radiation therapy. Int J Radiat Oncol Biol Phys 54:1518-1523, 2002.
101. Horsman MR, Murata R, Overgaard J: Combination studies with combretastatin and radiation: effects in early and late responding normal tissues. Radiother Oncol 64:S50, 2002.
102. Murata R, Overgaard J, Horsman MR: Comparative effects of combretastatin A-4 disodium phosphate and 5,6-dimethylxanthenone-4-acetic acid on blood perfusion in a murine tumour and normal tissues. Int J Radiat Biol 77:195-204, 2001.
103. Patt HM, Tyree EB, Straub RL, Smith DE: Cysteine protection against X irradiation. Science 110:213-214, 1949.
104. Yuhas JM: Active versus passive absorption kinetics as the basis for selective protection of normal tissues by S-2(3-aminopropylamino)-ethylphosphorothioic acid. Cancer Res 40: 1519-1524, 1980.
105. Yuhas JM: Protective drugs in cancer therapy: optimal clinical testing and future directions. Int J Radiat Oncol Biol Phys 8:513-517, 1982.
106. Schuchter LM, Hensley ML, Meropol NJ, Winer EP: 2002 Update of recommendations for the use of chemotherapy and radiotherapy protectants: clinical practice guidelines of the American Society of Clinical Oncology. J Clin Oncol 20:2895-2903, 2002.
107. Denekamp J, Stewart FA, Rojas A: Is the outlook grey for WR-2721 as a clinical radioprotector. Int J Radiat Oncol Biol Phys 9:595-598, 1983.
108. Lindegaard JC, Grau C: Has the outlook improved for amifostine as a clinical radioprotector? Radiother Oncol 57:113-118, 2000.
109. Rades D, Fehlauer F, Bajrovic A, et al: Serious adverse effects of amifostine during radiotherapy in head and neck cancer patients. Radiother Oncol 70:261-264, 2004.
110. Brizel DM, Overgaard J: Does amifostine have a role in chemoradiation treatment? Lancet Oncol 4:378-381, 2003.
111. Savoye C, Swenberg C, Hugot S, et al: Thiol WR-1065 and disulphide WR-33278, two metabolites of the drug Ethyol (WR-2721), protect DNA against fast neutron-induced strand breakage. Int J Radiat Biol 71:193-202, 1997.
112. Denekamp J, Michael BD, Rojas A, Stewart FA: Radioprotection of mouse skin by WR-2721: the critical influence of oxygen tension. Int J Radiat Oncol Biol Phys 8:531-534, 1982.
113. Travis EL: The oxygen dependence of protection by aminothiols: implications for normal tissues and solid tumors. Int J Radiat Oncol Biol Phys 10:1495-1501, 1984.
114. Washburn LC, Rafter JJ, Hayes RL: Prediction of the effective radioprotective dose of WR-2721 in humans through an interspecies tissue distribution study. Radiat Res 66:100-105, 1976.
115. Yuhas JM, Afzal SMF, Afzal V: Variation in normal tissue responsiveness to WR-2721. Int J Radiat Oncol Biol Phys 10:1537-1539, 1984.
116. Dubray B, Dhermain F: In regard to Antonadou et al. Randomized trial investigating the effects of daily amifostine in addition to radiation therapy in 146 patients with advanced lung cancers [author reply 1396]. Int J Radiat Oncol Biol Phys 53:1395-1396, 2002.
117. Brizel DM, Wasserman TH, Henke M, et al: Phase III randomized trial of amifostine as a radioprotector in head and neck cancer. J Clin Oncol 18:3339-3345, 2000.
118. Lindegaard JC: Has the time come for routine use of amifostine in clinical radiotherapy practice? Acta Oncol 42:2-3, 2003.
119. Koukourakis MI, Kyrias G, Kakolyris S, et al: Subcutaneous administration of amifostine during fractionated radiotherapy: a randomized phase II study. J Clin Oncol 18:2226-2233, 2000.
120. Phillips KA, Tannock IF: Design and interpretation of clinical trials that evaluate agents that may offer protection from the toxic effects of cancer chemotherapy. J Clin Oncol 16:3179-3190, 1998.
121. Kruse JJ, Strootman EG, Wondergem J: Effects of amifostine on radiation-induced cardiac damage. Acta Oncol 42:4-9, 2003.
122. Bohuslavizki KH, Klutmann S, Jenicke L, et al: Radioprotection of salivary glands by S-2-(3-aminopropylamin)-ethylphosphorothioic (amifostine) obtained in a rabbit animal model. Int J Radiat Oncol Biol Phys 45:181-186, 1999.
123. Rojas A, Denekamp J: The influence of x-ray dose level on normal tissue radioprotection by WR-2721. Int J Radiat Oncol Biol Phys 10:2351-2356, 1984.
124. Rojas A, Stewart FA, Soranson JA, Denekamp J: Fractionated studies with WR-2721: normal tissues and tumour. Radiother Oncol 6:51-60, 1986.
125. Komaki R, Lee JS, Milas L, et al: Effects of amifostine on acute toxicity from concurrent chemotherapy and radiotherapy for inoperable non–small-cell lung cancer: report of a randomized comparative trial. Int J Radiat Oncol Biol Phys 58:1369-1377, 2004.

126. Leong SS, Tan EH, Fong KW, et al: Randomized double-blind trial of combined modality treatment with or without amifostine in unresectable stage III non–small-cell lung cancer. J Clin Oncol 2003:1767-1774, 2003.
127. Antonadou D, Throuvalas N, Petridis A, et al: Effect of amifostine on toxicities associated with radiochemotherapy in patients with locally advanced non–small-cell lung cancer. Int J Radiat Oncol Biol Phys 57:402-408, 2003.
128. Antonadou D, Coliarakis N, Synodinou M, et al: Randomized phase III trial of radiation treatment +/− amifostine in patients with advanced-stage lung cancer. Int J Radiat Oncol Biol Phys 51:915-922, 2001.
129. Athanassiou H, Antonadou D, Coliarakis N, et al: Protective effect of amifostine during fractionated radiotherapy in patients with pelvic carcinomas: results of a randomized trial. Int J Radiat Oncol Biol Phys 56:1154-1160, 2003.
130. Momm F, Bechtold C, Rudat V, et al: Alteration of radiation-induced hematotoxicity by amifostine. Int J Radiat Oncol Biol Phys 51:947-951, 2001.
131. Bourhis J, De Crevoisier R, Abdulkarim B, et al: A randomized study of very accelerated radiotherapy with and without amifostine in advanced head and neck squamous cell carcinoma. Int J Radiat Oncol Biol Phys 46:1105-1108, 1999.
132. Buntzel J, Kuttner K, Frohlich D, Glatzel M: Selective cytoprotection with amifostine in concurrent radiochemotherapy for head and neck cancer. Ann Oncol 9:505-509, 1998.
133. Bohuslavizki KH, Klutmann S, Bleckmann C, et al: Salivary gland protection by amifostine in high-dose radioiodine therapy of differentiated thyroid cancer. Strahlenther Onkol 175:57-61, 1999.
134. Liu T, Liu Y, He S, et al: Use of radiation with or without WR-2721 in advanced rectal cancer. Cancer 69:2820-2825, 1992.
135. Adams GE, Barnes DW, du-Boulay C, et al: Induction of hypoxia in normal and malignant tissues by changing the oxygen affinity of hemoglobin—implications for therapy. Int J Radiat Oncol Biol Phys 12:1299-1302, 1986.
136. Adams GE, Stratford IJ, Nethersell AB, White RD: Induction of severe tumor hypoxia by modifiers of the oxygen affinity of hemoglobin. Int J Radiat Oncol Biol Phys 16:1179-1182, 1989.
137. Beddell CR, Goodford PJ, Kneen G, et al: Substituted benzaldehydes designed to increase the oxygen affinity of human haemoglobin and inhibit the sickling of sickle erythrocytes. Br J Pharm 82:397-407, 1984.
138. Keidan AJ, Franklin IM, White RD: Effect of BW12C on oxygen affinity of haemoglobin in sickle cell disease. Lancet 1:831-834, 1986.
139. Van den Aardweg GJMJ, Hopewell JW, Barnes DWH, et al: Modification of the radiation response of pig skin by manipulation of tissue oxygen tension using anaesthetics and administration of BW12C. Int J Radiat Oncol Biol Phys 16:1191-1194, 1989.
140. Honess DJ, Hu DE, Bleehen NM: BW12C: effects on tumour hypoxia, tumour radiosensitivity and relative tumour and normal tissue perfusion in C3H mice. Br J Cancer 64:715-722, 1991.
141. Roughton FJW, Darling RC: The effect of carbon monoxide on the oxyhemoglobin dissociation curve. Am J Phys 141:17-31, 1944.
142. Siemann DW, Hill RP, Bush RA: The importance of the pre-irradiation breathing times of oxygen and carbogen (5% CO_2; 95% O_2) on the in vivo radiation response of a murine sarcoma. Int J Radiat Oncol Biol Phys 2:903-911, 1977.
143. Grau C, Khalil AA, Nordsmark M, et al: The relationship between carbon monoxide breathing, tumour oxygenation and local tumour control in the C3H mammary carcinoma in vivo. Br J Cancer 69:50-57, 1994.
144. Ward A, Clissold SP: Pentoxifylline: a review of its pharmacodynamic and pharmacokinetic properties, and its therapeutic efficacy. Drugs 34:50-97,1987.
145. Lee I, Kim JH, Levitt SH, Song CW: Increases in tumor response by pentoxifylline alone or in combination with nicotinamide. Int J Radiat Oncol Biol Phys 22:425-429, 1992.
146. Honess DJ, Andrews MS, Ward R, Bleehen NM: Pentoxifylline increases RIF-1 tumour pO_2 in a manner compatible with its ability to increase relative tumour perfusion. Acta Oncol 34:385-389, 1995.
147. Price MJ, Li LT, Tward JD, et al: Effect of nicotinamide and pentoxifylline on normal tissue and FSA tumor oxygenation. Acta Oncol 34:391-395, 1995.
148. Dion MW, Hussey DH, Osborne JW: The effect of pentoxifylline on early and late radiation injury following fractionated irradiation in C3H mice. Int J Radiat Oncol Biol Phys 17:101-107, 1989.
149. Hendry JH: Biological response modifiers and normal tissue injury after irradiation. Semin Radiat Oncol 4:123-132, 1994.
150. Bernstein EF, Harisiadis L, Salomon G, et al: Transforming growth factor-β improves healing of radiation-impaired wounds. J Invest Dermatol 97:430-434, 1991.
151. Hancock SL: Effects of tumor necrosis factor α on the radiation response of murine intestinal stem cells and lung [abstract P-06-5]. Radiation Research Society Meeting, March 1992, Salt Lake City, Utah.
152. Hancock SL, Chung RT, Cox RS, Kallman RF: Interleukin 1β initially sensitizes and subsequently protects murine intestinal stem cells exposed to photon radiation. Cancer Res 51:2280-2285, 1991.
153. Barcellos-Hoff MH: Radiation-induced transforming growth factor β and subsequent extracellular matrix reorganisation in murine mammary gland. Cancer Res 53:3880-3886, 1993.
154. Anscher MS, Kong F-M, Murase T, Jirtle RL: Normal tissue injury after cancer therapy is a local response exacerbated by an endocrine effect of TGFβ. Br J Radiol 68:331-333, 1995.
155. Rubin P, Johnston CJ, Williams JP, et al: A perpetual cascade of cytokines postirradiation leads to pulmonary fibrosis. Int J Radiat Oncol Biol Phys 33:99-109, 1995.
156. Okunieff P, Abraham EH, Moini M, et al: Basic fibroblast growth factor radioprotects bone marrow and not RIF-1 tumor. Acta Oncol 34:435-438, 1995.
157. Okunieff P, Wang X, Rubin P, et al: Radiation-induced changes in bone perfusion and angiogenesis. Int J Radiat Oncol Biol Phys 42:885-889, 1998.
158. Robbins MEC, Hopewell JW: Physiological factors affecting renal radiation tolerance: a guide to the treatment of late effects. Br J Cancer 53:265-267, 1986.
159. Ward WF, Molteni A, Tsao CH, et al: Radiation pneumotoxicity in rats: modification by inhibition of angiotensin converting enzyme. Int J Radiat Oncol Biol Phys 22:623-625, 1992.
160. Halnan KE: The effect of corticosteroids on the radiation skin reaction. Br J Radiol 35:403-408, 1962.
161. Walden TL, Patchen M, Snyder SL: 16,16-Dimethyl prostaglandin-E_2 increases survival in mice following irradiation. Radiat Res 109:540-549, 1987.
162. Hansen WR, Pelka AE, Nelson AK, et al: Subcutaneous or topical administration of 16,16-dimethyl prostaglandin-E_2 protects from radiation-induced alopecia in mice. Int J Radiat Oncol Biol Phys 23:333-337, 1992.
163. Hopewell JW, Robbins MEC, van den Aardweg GJMJ: The modulation of radiation-induced damage to pig skin by essential fatty acids. Br J Cancer 68:1-7, 1993.

CHAPTER 4

INTERACTION OF CHEMOTHERAPY AND RADIATION

James A. Bonner, Yolanda I. Garces, and Donald J. Buchsbaum

The interaction of radiotherapy and chemotherapy is a broad topic, and the concepts involved are best illustrated by examples of in vitro or in vivo experiments and clinical trials. The interactions of radiation with chemotherapeutic agents or of nontoxic agents with radiation or chemotherapeutic drugs are being investigated to discover combinations that may be more lethal to tumor cells but still have an acceptable level of toxicity for normal cells. The various interactions may be synergistic, and this chapter explores their significance—or lack of significance—and the terms used to describe them.[1-7]

Many of the exciting explorations of radiation and chemotherapy interactions have been the result of trial and error. Serendipity also has had a role in many of the advances in this area. However, increased understanding of the molecular mechanisms involved in the interactions of radiation and pharmacologic agents is elucidating possible exploitable interactions.

This chapter reviews the historical aspects of the concepts of integrating chemotherapy and radiation and the concepts of subadditive, additive, and synergistic interactions. Several recent efforts are presented as models, and directions for future investigation are explored.

HISTORICAL BACKGROUND

Radiosensitization and chemosensitization are complex concepts because they have many different interpretations and, during the past 40 years, have been used to describe many different interactions.[1-7] The use of radiation and chemotherapy for mutual or even simultaneous sensitization adds to the intricacies of these interactions. Although radiosensitization is considered first, the same issues are involved in chemosensitization.

In the simplest terms, *radiosensitization* can be defined as the application of an agent that, when given concomitantly with ionizing radiation, increases the lethal effects of ionizing radiation.[5] This definition is useful in describing various interactions of radiation with other agents. However, it becomes confusing if it is used to describe combinations of radiation and agents that cause cytotoxicity in the absence of radiation (e.g., chemotherapeutic agents). The proper definition of radiosensitization has been debated for many years. This chapter describes some of the issues involved, as well as methods of analyzing radiation and chemotherapeutic interactions.

The importance of the simplistic definition of radiosensitization is considered, and the variations of this definition are described. The role of oxygen in radiosensitization is explored, because oxygen was one of the first identified modulators of the radiation response and because oxygen mimetics, like some other radiosensitizers, have evolved into cytotoxic chemotherapeutic agents (e.g., tirapazamine). Much effort and many resources have been expended in investigating combinations of radiation, chemotherapeutic agents, and pharmacologic agents that mimic oxygen.

Oxygen Effect on Radiation Response

The effect of oxygen on the radiation response can be described by the simple definition of radiosensitization already given. The effects of oxygen have been known since 1921, when Holthusen[8] discovered that *Ascaris* eggs were more sensitive to radiation in the presence of oxygen than in its absence. The enhancement of radiation sensitivity by oxygen has been one of the most studied effects in radiobiology, and investigations are seeking to better define the interaction of oxygen and irradiation at the molecular level and to find methods of increasing the radiosensitivity of hypoxic cells.

After the discovery that oxygen exposure, compared with oxygen deprivation, sensitized cells to the effects of radiation, the mechanism of this interaction was studied intensely. Investigations in the early 1940s showed that more chromosomal rearrangements were detected after irradiation of *Drosophila* sperm at high oxygen concentrations than under anoxic conditions.[9] However, in the early 1950s, the mechanism of these increased chromosomal rearrangements was debated.[10-14] Several investigators believed that well-oxygenated conditions, compared with anoxic conditions, led to an increased number of radiation-induced DNA double-strand breaks.[10,14] However, others believed that the increased number of chromosomal rearrangements was a result of prolonged rejoining of DNA double-strand breaks.[10,14]

This debate was partially resolved in the 1980s and 1990s as improved methods of detecting DNA damage and associated repair rates were developed. It became evident that well-oxygenated cells sustained approximately three times as many radiation-induced DNA double-strand breaks as anoxic cells and that anoxia slowed the rate of repair of DNA damage.[15] The increased DNA damage under well-oxygenated conditions was believed to be associated with the stabilization of radiation-induced free radical species, which can cause increased DNA damage. The attachment of an electron to a molecule of high electron affinity, such as oxygen, was believed to increase the diffusion radius of this potentially DNA-damaging species before a neutralization reaction could occur.[16] Compared with anoxic conditions, when oxygen is present in proximity to the ionizations created by radiation-induced energy deposition, free radical species may be able to cause more damage to DNA and to other central structures over a longer period.

Hypoxic Cell Sensitizers

Because oxygen was one of the first agents found to modulate the response of cells to radiation, considerable investigation centered on developing pharmacologic agents that might mimic the radiosensitizing properties of oxygen while having better diffusion capacity into potentially anoxic tissue (tumor tissue) than oxygen has. Research focused on potential radiosensitizers that were "molecules of very high electron affinity arising from resonant interaction between two or more electron-acceptor groups in the molecule."[16] Adams and Cooke[16] systematically tested many organic compounds with high electron affinity: unsaturated diesters, indanediones, and derivatives of pyruvic acid, quinones, and several other compounds. As hypothesized, these compounds caused radiosensitization (by the simple definition) under anoxic conditions but not under well-oxygenated conditions using a bacterial model system (*Serratia marcescens*).

At approximately the same time, other investigators were examining various clinical agents to identify those with high electron affinities that could be used in combination with radiation. These studies showed that metronidazole (an antitrichomonal agent) sensitized hypoxic cells in vitro and in vivo to the effects of radiation.[17-19] Metronidazole is a member of the 2-nitroimidazole class of pharmacologic agents. Subsequently, other agents of this class were found to be radiosensitizers. Similar to metronidazole, misonidazole produced radiosensitization of hypoxic cells but at lower molar concentrations.[20-33]

Clinical studies were performed in the 1970s using combinations of misonidazole or metronidazole with radiation.[33-41] The results of initial clinical trials were somewhat disappointing (Table 4-1). A meta-analysis of studies (1970 to 1996) examining radiation with and without misonidazole in patients with astrocytomas indicated a Peto odds ratio of 0.92 in favor of the treatment with misonidazole, but the difference in odds ratios was not statistically significant.[41] The lack of definite benefit from the use of hypoxic radiation sensitizers was attributed to reoxygenation of hypoxic portions of tumors that occurred because the radiation treatment was protracted over several days.

During this same period (1970 to 1996), it became clear that the 2-nitroimidazole compounds could be used to sensitize cells to the effects of chemotherapy under poorly oxygenated conditions.[5,20,32,33] In early investigations, in vitro chemosensitization under hypoxic conditions was most pronounced for the bifunctional alkylating agents.[5,21,22,25] As with the trials involving radiation and 2-nitroimidazole compounds, results of few trials suggested a benefit for the use of chemotherapy in combination with 2-nitroimidazole compounds (Table 4-2).

Table 4-1 Randomized Trials of Standard Irradiation Versus Standard Treatment with Misonidazole or Other 2-Nitroimidazole Compounds

Study	Treatment	Outcome
Overgaard et al[34] (1979-1982), 331 patients with uterine cervix carcinoma (stages IIB, III, IVA)	Randomized to RT alone vs RT and MISO (total dose of 12 g/m², generally given in daily fractions)	No difference in LC or SR; Hgb <7 mmol/L vs ≥7 mmol/L, 24% vs 47% LC, respectively
Overgaard et al[35] (1979-1985), 626 patients with pharyngeal and laryngeal malignant tumors (stage II-V laryngeal and I-IV pharyngeal cancer, UICC, 1978)	Randomized to RT alone vs RT and MISO (total dose of 11 g/m², generally given in daily fractions)	Overall LC equal; improved LC with MISO in pharyngeal subgroup (38% vs 27%, *P* < .05)
Leibel et al[36] (1980-1984), 119 patients with uterine cervix carcinoma (stages IIIB, IVA)	Randomized to RT alone (external beam, generally with intracavitary boost) vs RT and MISO (400 mg/m² daily, 2-4 h before RT)	Peripheral neuropathy in 26% of MISO patients. No difference in SR between arms (median, 1.9 and 1.6 y, respectively)
Van den Bogaert et al[37] (1981-1984), 523 patients with advanced head and neck malignancies	Randomized to once-daily RT (70 Gy), 3 × daily RT (67.2-72 Gy), or 3 × daily RT with MISO (1 g/m² daily)	No difference in LC or SR for the three arms
Simpson et al[38] (1979-1983), 268 patients with unresectable, locally advanced non–small cell lung cancer (stages IIIA, IIIB)	Randomized to RT alone (60 Gy) vs RT and MISO (400 mg/m² 2-4 h before RT)	CR, 27% vs 21%; median SR, 8 vs 7.4 mo; no difference between arms
Huncharek[41] (1970-1996), meta-analysis of nine RCTs (*N* = 711), high-grade astrocytoma	Randomized studies of RT (43.5-66.5 Gy) vs RT (39-66.5 Gy) and MISO (0.6-3.0 g/m²)	Peto odds ratio of 0.92 (95% CI, 0.77-1.09) for RT and MISO

CI, confidence interval; CR, complete response; Hgb, hemoglobin; LC, local control; MISO, misonidazole; *N*, total number of patients; RCT, randomized clinical trial; RT, irradiation; SR, survival; UICC, Union Internationale Contre Le Cancer (International Union Against Cancer).

Table 4-2 Trials Including Combinations of Standard Treatment, Chemotherapy, and Misonidazole or Benznidazole

Study	Treatment	Outcome
Glover et al[42] (1986), 30 patients with metastatic renal cell carcinoma	Cyclophosphamide (1000-1200 mg/m²) + MISO (5 g/m²) 2 h before cyclophosphamide	One of 30 patients had partial response, 29 of 30 had stable or progressive disease, 3/30 had severe neurotoxicity
Bleehen et al[43] (1983-1986), 44 patients with high-grade malignant glioma	Randomized to CCNU alone vs CCNU with benznidazole (20 mg/kg orally 3.5 h before CCNU)	Benznidazole-treated patients had median survival of 25 weeks vs 30 weeks for CCNU alone; no advantage for either treatment
Coleman et al[44] (1988), 100 patients (84 evaluable) with metastatic non–small cell lung cancer	Melphalan vs melphalan with MISO	Melphalan vs melphalan with MISO, response of 0% vs 14% (*P* = .02)

CCNU, chloroethylcyclohexylnitrosourea; MISO, misonidazole.

The disappointing results of trials that used the early 2-nitroimidazole compounds[42-46] led to the synthesis of new compounds with greater electron affinity and a superior lipophilic profile compared with earlier compounds.[47,48] As indicated by its lipophilic profile, misonidazole had good penetration into tumor cells and neural tissue; neurotoxicity was the limiting factor of the early 2-nitroimidazole compounds. Brown[32] characterized a new 2-nitroimidazole compound, etanidazole (SR-2508), with a reduced octanol-to-water partition coefficient but an increased drug efficiency ratio (i.e., ratio of median lethal dose in mice to drug dose to produce a sensitizer enhancement: 1.6 in vitro) compared with misonidazole. However, the clinical results of trials with etanidazole as a radiosensitizer or chemosensitizer also were disappointing.[49-51] Examples of such results are illustrated by two large trials of patients with stage III and IV head and neck cancer (Table 4-3).[49,50]

Although the clinical results of the 2-nitroimidazole compounds were disappointing, continued in vitro experimentation with new compounds provided greater insight about possible methods of exploiting tumor hypoxia with pharmacologic agents. It was hypothesized that reoxygenation of hypoxic portions of tumors occurred during the course of protracted radiation treatment, and the initial treatments with radiation (or chemotherapy) were believed to kill mostly well-oxygenated tumor cells, allowing poorly oxygenated tumor cells to gain access to the often tenuous blood supply of the tumor. The concept developed that agents causing radiosensitization primarily in poorly oxygenated tumor cells might not create the necessary clinical impact and that the increased radiosensitivity might not be sufficient to kill the most resistant poorly oxygenated tissue. Agents were synthesized that caused radiosensitization in poorly oxygenated tissue and significant selective cytotoxicity of poorly oxygenated cells (at concentrations that could be achieved in the plasma) in the absence of radiation.

One of these agents is tirapazamine (SR-4233), a benzotriazine di-*N*-oxide.[52] Tirapazamine shows marked selective toxicity for anoxic cells compared with well-oxygenated cells. Tirapazamine causes cytotoxicity of anoxic cells at concentrations 150 times lower than that required for cytotoxicity of well-oxygenated cells. The mechanism of this anoxic-selective toxicity is related to the reduction of tirapazamine to various reactive intermediates under anoxic conditions.[53] Olive[15] demonstrated that exposure of SCCVII squamous cell carcinoma cells (transplanted subcutaneously in mice) to 20 mg/kg of tirapazamine resulted in 20 times more single-strand breaks under fully anoxic, compared with fully aerobic, conditions.

Rehypoxiation

The development of agents such as tirapazamine gave rise to the concept of rehypoxiation. Just as changes in the distribution of blood flow after initial radiation treatment of a tumor appeared to account for reoxygenation of cells that were once poorly oxygenated, experiments demonstrated that the surviving well-oxygenated tumor cells developed new areas of hypoxia after initial treatment with pharmacologic agents having selective toxicity for poorly oxygenated tissue.[33] Brown and Giaccia[33] performed experiments in a xenograft setting with the same cell line (SCCVII) used by Olive.[15] In these in vivo experiments, the time course for rehypoxiation was similar to that for reoxygenation, occurring several hours after the initial treatment (Fig. 4-1). Rehypoxiation and reoxygenation may occur in human tumors before a second treatment is delivered at 1 to 7 days after the first treatment.

Because of the findings of Brown and others,[15,33] it may be beneficial to use an anoxic cytotoxin concomitantly with fractionated radiotherapy. During the course of fractionated treatment, reoxygenation will occur and allow subsequent irradiation to kill cells that previously were hypoxic. However, if rehypoxiation occurs during fractionated irradiation, the addition of an anoxic cytotoxin may obliterate the deleterious effects of hypoxia over the entire course of treatment. To determine whether the findings in murine systems are appli-

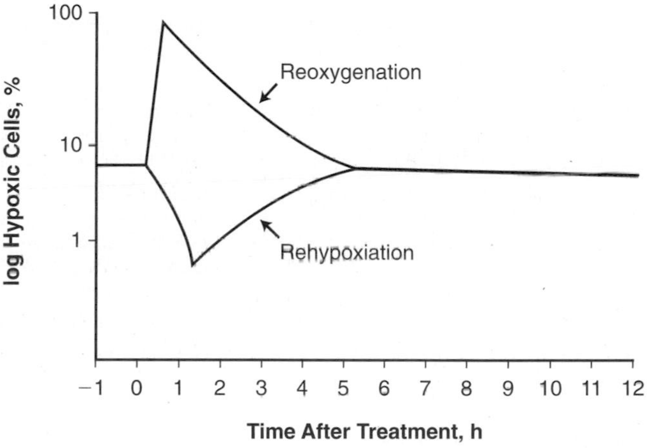

Figure 4-1 Graph of the course of rehypoxiation and reoxygenation in a tumor after irradiation. (Adapted from Brown JM, Giaccia AJ: Tumour hypoxia: the picture has changed in the 1990s. Int J Radiat Biol 65:95-102, 1994.) With permission from Taylor & Francis Ltd. http://www.tandf.co.uk/journals

Table 4-3 Phase III Randomized Trials Involving Etanidazole and Radiation Therapy

Study	Treatment	Outcome
Lee et al[49] (1988-1991), stage III or IV head and neck cancer (*N* = 521)	Phase III randomized trial	No statistically significant differences in local control or survival
	Arm A: RT alone (66 Gy/33 Fx, 74 Gy/37 Fx)	2-year survival: 41%
	Arm B: RT + etanidazole (2 g/m² 3 × weekly for 17 doses)	2-year survival: 43%
Chassagne et al[50] (1987-1990), advanced head and neck cancer (*N* = 374)	Phase III randomized trial	No statistically significant differences in local control or survival
	Arm A: RT alone (66 Gy/33 Fx, 74 Gy/37 Fx)	Complete response: 75.3%
	Arm B: RT + etanidazole (2 g/m² 3 × weekly for 17 doses)	Complete response: 77.6%

Fx, fractions; *N*, total number of patients; RT, radiation therapy.

cable to actual clinical phenomena, clinical trials have been performed with tirapazamine.

Trials of Hypoxic Cell Radiosensitizers

Tirapazamine has been tested as a radiosensitizer in several clinical trials (Table 4-4). Tirapazamine sensitizes cells to radiation and sensitizes tumor cells (in a model system) to the effects of cisplatin. One study showed sensitization to cisplatin when tirapazamine preceded cisplatin treatment by 2 to 3 hours.[62] Grau and Overgaard[63] showed that cisplatin was a potent cytotoxic agent for well-oxygenated cells (in a model system) but was not effective in the treatment of anoxic cells. The combination of cisplatin (with and without radiation) and tirapazamine is being studied. The hypoxia-specific cytotoxic properties of tirapazamine may complement cisplatin by enhancing tumor kill of cisplatin-treated cells through chemosensitization and through treatment of a population of cells not well treated by cisplatin alone[54-61] (see Table 4-4). The combination of tirapazamine, cisplatin, and radiation is being studied in head and neck cancer (Peters L, personal communication, April 2005).[64]

Previous studies combining conventional cancer therapeutics with tirapazamine have produced mixed results. This was the case for patients with non–small cell lung cancer (NSCLC)[56,57] and head and neck cancer.[60,61] One trial enrolling patients with advanced NSCLC indicated an improvement in median survival (34.6 versus 27.7 weeks) for the combination of cisplatin and tirapazamine versus cisplatin alone.[56] However, investigation continues as researchers explore tirapazamine in combination with multiagent chemotherapy regimens (Peters L, personal communication, April 2005). A randomized trial of tirapazamine in combination with paclitaxel and carboplatin versus paclitaxel and carboplatin alone showed no difference in survival (see Table 4-4).[57] A pilot investigation by the Southwest Oncology Group explored tira-

Table 4-4 Trials of Tirapazamine Plus Another Cytotoxic Agent

Study	Treatment	Outcome
Del Rowe et al[54] (2000), glioblastoma multiforme (*N* = 124), phase II study: RTOG 9417	RT (60 Gy/30 Fx) and tirapazamine (159 mg/m^2 or 260 mg/m^2 3 × weekly during RT for 12 treatments)	No improved median survival (9.5-10.8 mo); no difference when compared with RTOG database per RPA class
Aghajanian et al[55] (1997), recurrent cervical carcinoma	Cisplatin (75 mg/m^2 every 21 days), tirapazamine (195, 260, 330, or 390 mg/m^2) given 1 h before cisplatin	MTD of 330 mg/m^2; major or minor responses were seen at this dose
von Pawel et al[56] (2000), non–small cell lung cancer (*N* = 446), CATAPULT I Study Group	Randomized phase III of cisplatin (75 mg/m^2 every 3 wk) vs tirapazamine (390 mg/m^2) and cisplatin	Improved median survival with addition of tirapazamine (34.6 vs 27.7 wk, *P* = .008)
Williamson et al[57] (2003), non–small cell lung cancer (*N* = 377), CATAPULT II Study Group	Randomized phase III of paclitaxel/carboplatin (P, 225 mg/m^2; C, AUC = 6) vs P/C + tirapazamine (T, 260 mg/m^2 with escalation to 330 mg/m^2 all on day 1, every 3 wk)	Closed early after interim analysis demonstrated no attainable difference in survival. Median survival, 7 to 9 mo.
Le et al[58] (2004), limited-stage small cell lung cancer, phase I study (*N* = 30)	RT (61 Gy/33 Fx) with tirapazamine (260-330 mg/m^2) + cisplatin (50 mg/m^2) × 4 with etoposide (50 mg/m^2) × 2, then consolidation	MTD of 260 mg/m^2, toxicity increased, but acceptable, led to ongoing phase II trial
Lara et al[59] (2003), advanced malignant solid tumors, phase I study (*N* = 42)	Tirapazamine (260-390 mg/m^2) + carboplatin (AUC = 6) + paclitaxel (200-225 mg/m^2)	MTD in chemotherapy naïve of 330 mg/m^2, 260 mg/m^2 for previously treated patients
Horst et al[60] (2003), advanced head and neck cancer, randomized phase II study (*N* = 59)	Induction chemotherapy followed by RT (median dose, 66 Gy) + 5-FU + cisplatin ± tirapazamine (160-260 mg/m^2 × 6)	No difference in response rate or OS. QOL better in the no tirapazamine arm for the physical and emotional domains
Rischin et al[61] (2001), advanced head and neck cancer T3/4 and/or N2/N3 and M0 (*N* = 17)	Phase I study of RT (70 Gy/35 Fx) with tirapazamine (290 mg/m^2 on day 2 for weeks 1, 4, 7 and 160 mg/m^2 on day 1, 3, 5 for weeks 2, 3, 5, 6) + cisplatin (75 mg/m^2 on day 1 for weeks 1, 4, 7)	MTD established by omitting tirapazamine during wk 5 and 6 leading to phase III study below
Peters (2002–ongoing),* advanced head and neck cancer, stage III or IV (*N* = 550)	Randomized phase III of RT (70 Gy/35 Fx) with cisplatin (100 mg/m^2 every 3 wk) vs RT with tirapazamine (290 mg/m^2 on day 1 for weeks 1, 4, 7 and 160 mg/m^2 on day 1, 3, 5 for weeks 2, 3) + cisplatin (75 mg/m^2 on day 1 for weeks 1, 4, 7)	Ongoing multicenter study

*Peters L, personal communication, April 2005.

AUC, area under the curve; C, cisplatin; CATAPULT, Cisplatin and Tirapazamine in Subjects with Advanced Previously Untreated Non–Small Cell Lung Tumors; 5-FU, 5-fluorouracil; Fx, fractions; MTD, maximum tolerated dose; *N*, total number of patients; OS, overall survival; P, paclitaxel; QOL, quality of life; RPA, recursive partitioning analysis; RT, irradiation; RTOG, Radiation Therapy Oncology Group; T, tirapazamine.

pazamine in combination with etoposide and cisplatin in limited-stage small cell lung cancer (SCLC) with intriguing initial results.[58] The investigators concluded that the survival results warranted further study. In head and neck cancer, there is interest in combining tirapazamine, cisplatin, and radiation because of the sensitization issues discussed previously. A pilot trial using a regimen of this nature[64] produced intriguing results that led to a phase III trial (see Table 4-4).[61]

Although many of the trials attempting to exploit tirapazamine's radiosensitizing properties have been disappointing, the results of ongoing clinical studies will provide further clarity to this avenue of research. Likewise, gene therapy approaches have been implemented to augment the effectiveness of tirapazamine (see "Future Directions"). Better localization of tumor hypoxia may provide improved means of killing tumor cells in these areas.

COMBINING CYTOTOXIC AGENTS

Definitions

The concept of radiosensitization originated many years ago, and classic radiosensitization has been defined as an increased amount of radiation-induced cell death resulting from exposure to a second agent after correction for the cytotoxicity of the second agent. According to this definition, radiation causes radiosensitization. For example, if human cells are exposed to a small dose (2 Gy) of radiation in vitro, the cell death that occurs usually is less than the difference in cell death between a 4-Gy and a 2-Gy dose. If cells are exposed to 2 Gy and immediately treated with a second dose of 2 Gy, the second dose is more lethal than it would have been without the initial 2 Gy (Fig. 4-2). This phenomenon occurs because the cells have not had time to repair radiation-induced sublethal damage after the first 2-Gy dose. This example illustrates that the classic definition of radiosensitization is occasionally difficult to interpret.

Although the phenomenon described may qualify as an example of radiosensitization, it does not represent a synergistic interaction according to most definitions of synergy. Synergy, like radiosensitization, has many definitions. Classically, synergy implies that the cytotoxicity caused by two agents given together is more than additive, taking into account the kinetics of cytotoxicity for both agents. With this definition, radiation cannot cause radiosensitization. It is important not to minimize the classic definition of radiosensitization, because it serves a purpose, which will become clear as this chapter unfolds. The classic definition describes a type of interaction: If exposure to one agent makes radiation more toxic after correction for cytotoxicity of the agent, there is an interaction between the agents. Much must be learned about the interactions of various agents at the molecular level, even though they may not be synergistic.

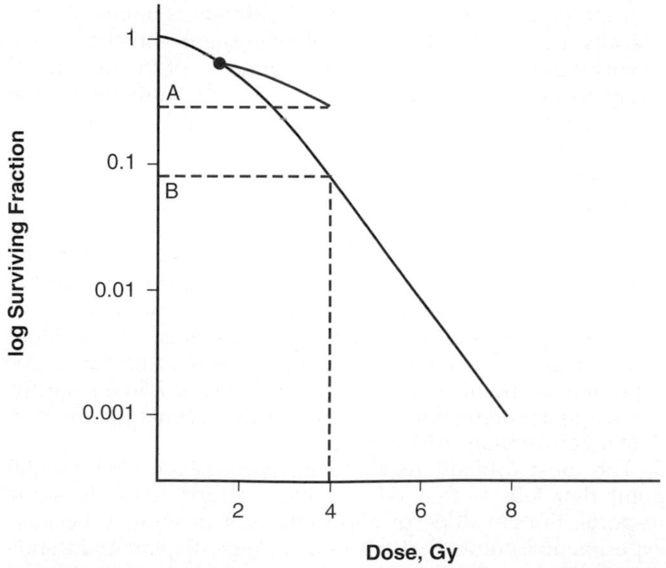

Figure 4-2 Graph of the concept of an immediate second treatment with radiation as a radiosensitizer compared with a delayed second radiation treatment. *Point A* indicates the surviving fraction of tumor cells for two 2-Gy doses given 6 to 8 hours apart. *Point B* indicates the surviving fraction for a 2-Gy dose followed immediately by another 2-Gy dose.

Although this discussion may seem like an exercise in semantics, it illustrates some of the difficulties that have been encountered when investigators have tried to quantify the interaction of various agents given together. Many investigators have sought to improve the descriptions of interactions between irradiation and chemotherapy. Tyrrell[1] developed the following descriptive system, which is a starting point for describing various interactions:

Antagonism: used in all cases in which the action of two treatments is less than would be expected from the addition of the two treatments given independently

Zero interaction: used when two treatments lead to the effect expected from the addition of the two treatments given independently

Positive interaction: used in all cases in which the action of two treatments is greater than would be expected from the addition of the two treatments given independently

Synergism: a special case of a positive interaction; strictly, used when kinetic data are available

Many systems have been developed to assess whether an interaction is synergistic. Two common systems are isobologram analysis, described by Steel and Peckham,[65] and median effect principle analysis, described by Chou and Talalay.[66]

Isobologram Analysis

Isobologram analysis, as a method to evaluate the interaction of two treatments, requires the construction of an *envelope of additivity* that is bordered by mode 1 and mode 2 lines (Fig. 4-3). The mode 1 line assumes that the two agents have completely independent mechanisms of action. The mode 2 line assumes that the two agents have exactly the same mechanism of action. To begin construction of these lines and the envelope of additivity they border, it is important to collect a complete set of dose-response data for each agent given separately. The following is a step-by-step procedure for calculating isobolograms using Steel and Peckham's method[65,67] (see Fig. 4-3).

Step 1. The investigator must choose to make the assessments at one level of cytotoxicity (e.g., construct an isobologram that represents the interaction of the agents for a cumulative cytotoxicity of 50%, 10%, or 1%). The example in Figure 4-3 depicts the chosen level of cytotoxicity as horizontal line Z: 1% cytotoxicity (0.01 surviving fraction) in this case.

Step 2. Plots are made of dose-response data for both agents. In Figure 4-3, the dose-response data for the two agents are represented by curves A and B.

Step 3. The extreme points of the envelope of additivity are determined. Initially, a separate cartesian graph is created. The y-axis represents the dose of agent B, and the x-axis the dose of agent A. The first extreme point of the envelope is placed on the y-axis at the dose of agent B alone that causes

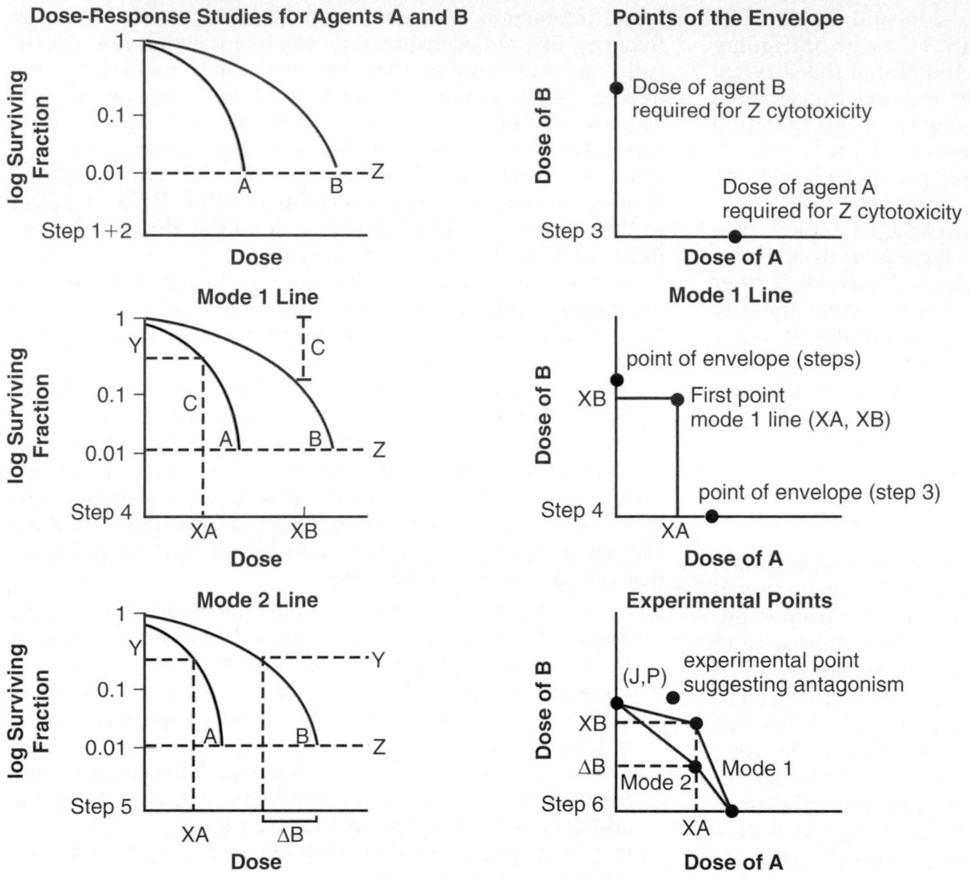

Figure 4-3 Step-by-step construction of an isobologram to define an envelope of additivity for two cancer treatments. Isobologram analysis is used to evaluate the interaction of two treatments, and it requires the construction of an envelope of additivity that is bordered by mode 1 and mode 2 lines. The mode 1 line assumes that the two agents have completely independent mechanisms of action, whereas the mode 2 line assumes that the two agents have the same mechanism of action.

a specific level of cytotoxicity, as determined by the dose-response curve of agent B, at the intersection of line Z (see Fig. 4-3). The second extreme point of the envelope is placed on the x-axis, at the dose of agent A alone that results in that level of cytotoxicity at the intersection of the dose-response curve with line Z (see Fig. 4-3).

Step 4. The mode 1 line is constructed assuming that the agents function independently. The individual dose-response curves are used for this construction. After exposure to dose X of agent A (XA), a level of cytotoxicity is obtained at a point on the dose-response curve that is above line Z. This level of cytotoxicity is identified as Y. Next, the dose of agent B (XB) that is required to produce cytotoxicity equal to the difference in cytotoxicity at line Z and point Y (identified as C) is determined. The cartesian coordinate (XA, XB) is plotted and becomes a point on the mode 1 line. The entire mode 1 line is constructed in this manner by varying the dose of agent A (for a resulting level of cytotoxicity that falls above line Z) and subsequently calculating the appropriate complementary dose of agent B as described.

Step 5. The mode 2 line is constructed assuming that the two agents have the same mechanism of action. As for mode 1 line construction, exposure to dose X of agent A (XA) results in a level of cytotoxicity identified as Y. The dose-response curve for agent B is then examined. The dose of agent B required for cytotoxicity equivalent to Y is determined and identified as YB. The change in dose of agent B that is required to increase cytotoxicity from YB to line Z is determined and labeled ΔB. The cartesian coordinate (XA, ΔB) is plotted. Similar points are calculated for various initial doses of agent A, and the mode 2 line is formed. The mode 2 line varies in shape depending on whether agent A or agent B is selected first for step 5. Generally, the mode 2 line that results in the greatest separation from the mode 1 line is chosen for the envelope of additivity.

Step 6. The two agents are given concomitantly, and a dose-response curve for concomitant treatment is obtained (typically by holding the dose of one agent constant while varying the dose of the other). The doses of the individual agents that result in combined cytotoxicity equivalent to the level represented by line Z are plotted (J,P).

This procedure allows for characterization of experimental data. The experimental point (J,P) represents an antagonistic interaction if the point falls above the envelope of additivity. The effect of the combination treatment is less than would be expected if the agents had completely independent mechanisms of action. An experimental point that falls directly on the mode 1 line suggests that the agents have independent mechanisms of action and the interaction is additive. An experimental point that falls below the mode 2 line suggests a synergistic interaction between the two agents for the particular concomitant treatment used.

The most difficult result to interpret is an experimental point that falls within the envelope of additivity. In some respects, the envelope of additivity is a misnomer, because experimental points that fall in this range display an interaction that is greater than the additive effect that is achieved if the agents function by completely independent mechanisms. The interaction between the agents may be positive if the agents have independent mechanisms of action, or it may be negative if they have identical mechanisms of action.

Although the isobologram analysis is useful, it is somewhat limited because interactions in each analysis are investigated at a single level of cytotoxicity. The investigation of interactions at several levels of cytotoxicity requires the construction of several envelopes of additivity. The ambiguity associated with experimental points that fall within the envelope can be disconcerting and may lead to erroneous conclusions, especially if several levels of cytotoxicity are not investigated. Other mathematical modeling systems have been developed to assess the interaction of agents that cause cytotoxicity. These assessments aim to account for the kinetics of cytotoxicity of the involved agents and to assess multiple levels of cytotoxicity.

Median Effect Principle Analysis

A mathematical modeling system that has gained widespread use for interactions of cytotoxic agents is the median effect principle of Chou and Talalay.[66-68] This system was derived from Michaelis-Menten equations and basic mass-action law considerations. This system has been useful for describing competitive enzyme interactions and interactions of cytotoxic agents. The primary relationship of the median effect principle is described by the following equation: $f_a/f_u = (D/D_m)^m$, in which D is dose, f_a is the fraction affected, f_u is the fraction unaffected, D_m is the dose required to produce the median effect (50%), and m is a Hill-type coefficient used to describe the sigmoid nature of the curve. For first-order Michaelis-Menten kinetics, m = 1.

The following manipulation of this equation can be performed, with surviving fraction (SF) substituted for fraction unaffected in the last step:

$$\log(f_a/f_u) = \log[(D/D_m)^m]$$

$$\log(f_a/f_u) = m\log(D) - m\log(D_m)$$

$$\log[(1/SF) - 1] = m\log(D) - m\log(D_m)$$

The general equation is $y = mx + b$.

A plot of $\log[(1/SF) - 1]$ on the y-axis and log(D) on the x-axis results in a line with a slope of m and a y-intercept of $m\log(D_m)$. The survival curves for the individual agents and for the combination treatment (the individual agents given together in some fashion) can be fitted to the equation for a line by linear regression. If the interaction of two agents is assessed, three lines (i.e., median effect plots) are produced: one for each agent and one for the combination treatment. A graph of the median effect plots for mock individual agents A and B and for the combination of A and B is shown in Figure 4-4. For the combination treatment, D is the sum of the doses of the two agents given concomitantly; it is helpful to perform the experiments with the two agents given together in a fixed ratio of doses (e.g., 1:2). By using various total doses (i.e., the sum), with the agents given in the same ratio, it is possible to determine the contribution of the individual agents to the combination treatment in a later calculation.

This concept can be visualized in Figure 4-4. For instance, in the case of $\log[(1/SF) - 1] = 0$, where SF is surviving fraction, the corresponding log(D), D indicating the sum of the doses of the two agents, can be calculated from the median effect plot for the combination treatment. An example of an actual combination treatment that has been assessed in this manner is radiation followed by a 24-hour exposure to etoposide.[67] In this example, a set of experiments was performed with the dose ratio fixed as 32 Gy to 1 μg/mL of etoposide. In this example, the dose D that resulted in $\log[(1/SF) - 1]$ equaling a given value was a combination of radiation and etoposide given in the ratio of 32:1. The radiation and etoposide components could be discerned, from the median effect plot of the combination treatment, by dividing the resulting dose into the appropriate components based on the ratio of delivery of the two agents.

Definitions used in the median effect principle include the following:

Mutually exclusive: the agents of interest have similar modes of action and do not act independently.

Mutually nonexclusive: the agents of interest have different modes of action or act independently.

Combination index (CI): the derivation of this index is beyond the scope of this chapter. Calculation of CI allows characterization of an interaction as synergistic (CI < 1), antagonistic (CI > 1), or a summation (CI = 1). Chou and Talalay[66] provide a full description.

CI can be calculated for any surviving fraction and for mutually exclusive or mutually nonexclusive interactions. For a mutually exclusive interaction,

$$CI = [D_1/(Dx)_1] + [D_2/(Dx)_2]$$

For a mutually nonexclusive interaction,

$$CI = [D_1/(Dx)_1] + [D_2/(Dx)_2] + [D_1D_2/(Dx)_1(Dx)_2]$$

in which

$(Dx)_1 = D_m[(1/SF) - 1]^{1/m}$, solving the general equation for agent 1 given alone in a dose x.

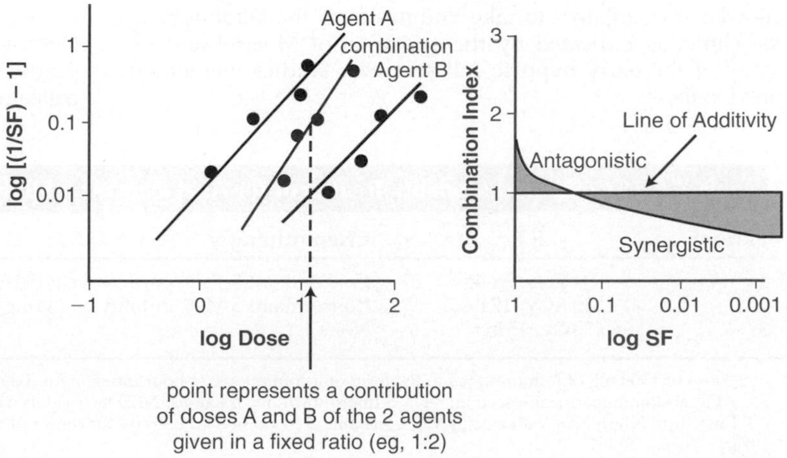

Figure 4-4 The hypothetical graph *(left)* demonstrates the median effect principle analysis for agents A and B given alone or in combination. The combination treatments are given in a fixed ratio so that the individual contribution of each agent to the combined effect can be calculated. The combination index *(right)* is then calculated at various levels of cytotoxicity as measured by surviving fraction (SF). The areas of antagonism, additivity, and synergism are indicated.

$(Dx)_2 = D_m[(1/SF) - 1]^{1/m}$, solving the general equation for agent 2 given alone in a dose x.

$(Dx)_{1,2} = D_m[(1/SF) - 1]^{1/m1,2}$, solving the general equation for the agents given in combination for dose x, which represents the sum of the doses of the agents given in a fixed combination.

$D_1 = (Dx)_{1,2} \times$ (fraction of the mixture that is agent 1).

$D_2 = (Dx)_{1,2} \times$ (fraction of the mixture that is agent 2).

CI represents the doses of the agents required for a given effect when they are given together, divided by the doses required when the agents are given alone; in this way, CI less than 1 represents a synergistic interaction. A diagram of a CI plot for various levels of surviving fraction is shown in Figure 4-4.

CHEMOTHERAPY WITH IRRADIATION AND COMBINATIONS OF CYTOTOXIC AGENTS

General Concepts

From the Bench to the Clinic

Occasionally, the process of quantifying interactions of chemotherapy and radiation has frustrated clinicians attempting to interpret in vitro and in vivo laboratory information, as exemplified by Charles Moertel (quoted by Tannock[69]) in his keynote speech at the first International Conference on Combined-Modality Therapy in 1978:

> Based on the results of various individual studies, I could conclude that it is most ideal to administer the nitrosourea 15 hours before irradiation, 2 hours before irradiation, simultaneously with irradiation, or 6 hours after irradiation. While we will continue to cheer our radiation biology colleagues on from the sidelines, I am afraid that we are not yet at the stage where we can comfortably incorporate their results into our clinical practice.

This was not meant as disrespect for the radiobiology community but to point out that, at that time, the laboratory models were potentially quite different from the clinical setting. Because it has been difficult to extrapolate from laboratory results to clinical results, many clinicians have used combination treatments on a trial-and-error basis. However, the reverse order of study has occasionally been fruitful, and efficacious combinations of treatment demonstrated in clinical studies have inspired laboratory investigations that revealed interesting molecular bases of interaction.[67,68] Translational research ideally occurs with a concept that arises from laboratory findings and subsequently is shown to have clinical efficacy. However, preclinical model systems have not always allowed investigators to take findings from the laboratory to the clinic, as indicated by the quotation of Moertel and by many of the early hypoxic cell sensitizer studies mentioned previously.

Therapeutic Benefits

Tannock[69] mentioned another problem with translating findings from the laboratory to the clinical setting, emphasizing that investigators must not merely explore combinations of therapeutic agents to find synergistic interactions but must also find interactions that will produce a therapeutic benefit (e.g., provide greater cytotoxicity in tumor cells than in normal cells). To categorize potentially exploitable differences, Tannock[69] described three main categories of biologic diversity between tumor cells and normal cells: tumor cells may display genetic instability compared with normal tissues; tumor cells and normal cells may be different with respect to cellular proliferation or proliferation that occurs after treatment; and environmental factors such as oxygenation and pH may affect tumor cells and normal cells differently. As findings are translated from the laboratory to the clinical setting, it is important to consider the effects of the host mechanisms on these three areas.

Evolution of Combined-Modality Treatment for Anal Cancer

Clinical and Laboratory Investigations

A classic example of the evolution of an efficacious interaction of chemotherapy and radiotherapy is combined-modality treatment for anal cancer. In the early 1970s, it was discovered that anal cancer could be treated successfully with a combination of 5-fluorouracil (5-FU), mitomycin C, and irradiation.[70] In 1974, Nigro and colleagues[70] reported on three patients who received variations of these three treatments, with excellent responses to the preoperative therapy (Table 4-5). This article became a classic in the oncology literature, and the regimen became prominent in the treatment of anal cancer. Because of this regimen, many patients were spared abdominal perineal resection.

After the initial report of Nigro and colleagues,[70] several other groups confirmed the efficacy of chemotherapy and irradiation (without surgery) as the standard treatment for primary anal cancer (Table 4-6).[71-74] Subsequently, an intergroup effort was undertaken to determine whether mitomycin C could be removed from the regimen, because its inclusion resulted in increased toxicity compared with that of 5-FU and radiation without mitomycin C. With the exclusion of mitomycin C, however, fewer patients were able to avoid colostomy (see Table 4-6). Presently, the combination of 5-FU, mitomycin C, and irradiation remains the standard regimen for anal cancer, although ongoing investigations may produce improvements in this regimen (see Table 4-6).

The clinical finding of the efficacious combination of 5-FU, mitomycin C, and irradiation led to laboratory studies. Dobrowsky and associates[75] performed a complex isobologram analysis using the same agents reported by Nigro and colleagues.[70] The assessment by Dobrowsky and colleagues,[75]

Table 4-5 Combined-Modality Treatment for Anal Cancer: a Study of Three Patients

Patient	RT	Chemotherapy	Results
1	34.7 Gy/5 wk	Concomitant 5-FU*/porfiromycin (50 mg)	APR 9 wk after RT, NED
2	30.6 Gy/17 Fx	Concomitant 5-FU*/mitomycin (30 mg)	Clinically free of disease, patient refused APR
3	30 Gy/15 Fx	None	APR 8 wk after RT, NED

*Dose of 1500 mg of 5-fluorouracil in the form of a continuous 24-hour infusion for 5 days.

APR, abdominoperineal resection; 5-FU, 5-fluorouracil; Fx, fractions; NED, no evidence of disease; RT, irradiation.

Data from Nigro ND, Vaitkevicius VK, Considine B Jr: Combined therapy for cancer of the anal canal: a preliminary report. Dis Colon Rectum 17:354-356, 1974.

Table 4-6 **Concomitant Radiation and Chemotherapy for Anal Cancer**

Study	Regimen	Outcome
Nigro[71] (1987), Wayne State University	RT (30 Gy/15 Fx) with CI 5-FU (1000 mg/m^2) for 4 days × 2 cycles and mitomycin C (15 mg/m^2) on day 1	Of 104 patients, 31 required APR
Sischy et al[72] (1989), RTOG/ECOG	RT (40 Gy/20 Fx) with CI 5-FU (1,000 mg/m^2) for 4 days × 2 cycles and mitomycin C (10 mg/m^2) on day 2	Of 79 patients, 8 required APR
Flam et al[73] (1995), RTOG/ECOG	RT (45 Gy/25 Fx) with CI 5-FU as above during weeks 1 and 4, with randomization to mitomycin C (10 mg/m^2) on days 1 and 29 vs no mitomycin C	Colostomy-free survival improved with mitomycin C, 71% vs 59% (P = .02)
Bartelink et al[74] (1997), EORTC	RT (60-65 Gy*) alone vs RT plus 5-FU (750 mg/m^2 on days 1-5, 29-33) and mitomycin C (15 mg/m^2) on day 1	Improved event-free survival with RT and chemotherapy compared with RT alone (P = .03)
Intergroup Study (opened in 1998), principal investigators: Ajani, Pederson, and Gunderson; coordinated by RTOG (98-11)	RT (55-59 Gy) with CI 5-FU (1000 mg/m^2) and mitomycin C (10 mg/m^2) on days 1 and 29 vs CI 5-FU (1000 mg/m^2) + cisplatin (75 mg/m^2 on days 1 and 29) with induction chemotherapy	Ongoing multicenter trial; required sample size (N = 650); completed accrual in 2005

*Surgery 6 weeks after initial 45 Gy if no response.
APR, abdominoperineal resection; CI, continuous infusion; ECOG, Eastern Cooperative Oncology Group; EORTC, European Organization for Research and Treatment of Cancer; 5-FU, 5-fluorouracil; Fx, fractions; *N*, total number of patients; RT, radiation therapy; RTOG, Radiation Therapy Oncology Group.

using an in vitro system of a squamous tumor cell line, illustrated some of the difficulties with the ideal progression of taking laboratory discoveries to the clinic. Two different end points were used: colony formation (i.e., cells plated after treatment and allowed to form colonies) and viable cells per flask (i.e., obtained by multiplying the number of cells per flask at 96 hours by the surviving fraction, as stipulated by a standard colony formation assay). In an attempt to duplicate the clinical treatment of Nigro and colleagues,[70] mitomycin C was given as a 1-hour exposure and 5-FU as a 4-day exposure after initial irradiation.

The first experiments assessed the interaction of 5-FU and mitomycin C without irradiation. Initially, a single dose of mitomycin C (0.5 µg/mL for 1 hour) was combined with various doses of 5-FU. Isobolograms were constructed for the colony formation end point at a surviving fraction of 0.04. The combination treatment resulted in an experimental point below the envelope of additivity at this level of cytotoxic assessment. Isobolograms also were constructed for the viable cells per flask end point at the 1% viability level; the experimental point for combined 5-FU and mitomycin C was directly on the mode 2 line. This end point was included because it was believed to account for the cytotoxic and cytostatic effects of the treatment.

Because the results of this synergy analysis varied with the end point used, the optimal end point, whether colony formation or viable cells per flask, is not known. The use of these slightly different end points produced slightly different isobologram results, illustrating one of the problems in interpreting in vitro data and attempting to extrapolate this information to the clinical setting. In the future, it may be possible to assess which end points are most useful for various cytotoxic agents and tumors based on the relative contribution of cytotoxic and cytostatic effects for a given situation.

On the basis of the experiments without irradiation, specific concentrations of mitomycin C (0.5 µg/mL) and 5-FU (0.15 µg/mL) were selected for subsequent experiments involving radiation[75]; these concentrations resulted in 60% and 80% surviving fractions, respectively. With colony formation as the end point, it was discovered that the interaction of radiation and 5-FU or radiation and mitomycin C (at the levels of cytotoxicity assessed) produced experimental points below the envelope of additivity. These results corroborated those reported previously by Byfield and colleagues,[76] in which some level of 5-FU cytotoxicity was required for a positive interaction with radiation. However, the results of radiation in conjunction with mitomycin C were not entirely consistent with those of previous reports, which had suggested that a positive interaction of these agents did not exist.[77]

This example illustrates some of the challenges of using interpretation of in vitro or in vivo experimental data to guide the design of clinical trials. An investigator using these laboratory data would first need to decide which in vitro end point (viable cells per flask or colony formation) is most relevant to anal cancer, and this decision would affect whether 5-FU and mitomycin C are considered to interact synergistically. Second, the investigator would need to decide which assessment of mitomycin C and radiation is most relevant to the treatment of anal cancer, because authors have disagreed about whether this interaction is synergistic. Such challenges can be exciting as we learn more about the significance of various end points at the molecular level and how these molecular events may be manipulated in a particular tumor.

Investigations in Anal Cancer

Although anal sphincter preservation rates for primary radiotherapy can be as high as 65% to 85%, additional improvements in local control and overall survival should be sought. The use of mitomycin C has been questioned because of its toxicity profile. The ongoing Intergroup study coordinated by the Radiation Therapy Oncology Group (RTOG) (see Table 4-6) seeks to study induction chemotherapy (5-FU and cisplatin) followed by the same chemotherapy concurrently with irradiation versus standard concurrent chemotherapy (5-FU and mitomycin C) with irradiation. The hypothesis is that the induction chemotherapy will decrease tumor bulk, making radiotherapy more effective and improving local control. The additional cycles of induction chemotherapy may improve overall survival by decreasing distant metastases.

In the future, understanding the molecular basis of anal cancer may contribute to the advancement of treatments. For example, the etiologic association of human papillomavirus with anal cancer is an area that requires further study regarding its interaction with treatment and prognosis.[78]

Evolution of Chemoradiotherapy in Lung Cancer

Selection of the Chemotherapy Regimen

Until enthusiasm developed for new agents (e.g., paclitaxel-based chemotherapy, topoisomerase I inhibitor–based regimens) in the treatment of lung cancers, the use of etoposide in combination with cisplatin (a platinum-based drug) was a standard approach to extensive-stage and limited-stage SCLC (ESSCLC and LSSCLC) and NSCLC. In the late 1980s, the North Central Cancer Treatment Group (NCCTG) designed a trial to assess the efficacy of several reported methods of delivering etoposide and cisplatin in combination for ESSCLC.[79] A phase III randomized trial was performed that included 452 patients with LSSCLC or ESSCLC. Patients were randomly assigned to one of the following four treatment arms: A, cisplatin bolus followed by etoposide bolus; B, etoposide bolus followed by cisplatin bolus; C, etoposide 24-hour infusion with a cisplatin bolus at the end of etoposide; and D, etoposide 24-hour infusion followed by a 48-hour infusion of cisplatin. Arm A produced the best rate of complete response and overall survival, and cisplatin bolus followed by etoposide bolus became the standard method of delivery of these agents for many of the NCCTG facilities and other groups across the United States.

Before the NCCTG trial, laboratory investigations directed at the interaction of cisplatin and etoposide did not provide information about optimal scheduling or doses of the agent. Primarily, these studies had merely suggested a possible synergistic interaction between the two agents. One of these studies used a mouse tumor xenograft model system.[80] A crude addition of the mouse cure rates with cisplatin alone, etoposide alone, or the combination suggested a positive interaction between the agents.[75]

Because the combination of etoposide and cisplatin became a prominent regimen against lung cancer after 1980, other in vitro analyses of this drug combination were performed. Tsai and colleagues,[81] of the National Cancer Institute, investigated four SCLC and four NSCLC cell lines for potential synergistic interactions of etoposide and cisplatin. In these studies, the agents were given concomitantly and the concentration of one agent was varied. The tetrazolium-based colorimetric assay was used to assess cellular viability, and isobologram analysis was used to assess synergy. With these multiple tumor cell lines and multiple media, the investigators found no clear evidence that etoposide and cisplatin functioned synergistically at the cellular level. In one NSCLC cell line (NCI-H23), there was suggestion of synergy when a low concentration of etoposide (relative to cisplatin) was compared with a high concentration of etoposide (relative to cisplatin). However, after numerous interactions were studied, the investigators believed that they were unable to show consistent synergy.

The study of Tsai and colleagues[81] illustrates several concepts. In their isobologram analyses, the experimental points frequently fell within the so-called envelope of additivity; if the agents have independent mechanisms of action, these points may represent a positive interaction, but one that is not strictly synergistic. The authors mentioned that the in vitro analysis was limited when translations to the clinic were attempted. Isobolograms were constructed for various levels of cytotoxicity, but not for all potential levels. It is difficult to determine the effect that combinations of agents may display in vivo, where drug half-lives and drug metabolism are factors; additional work is necessary to determine the clinical implications of these factors. Although the laboratory work of Tsai and colleagues[81] did not provide a firm foundation for new methods of integrating etoposide and cisplatin, the regimen became popular because of its clinical activity. The clinical efficacy of cisplatin and etoposide may represent an example of potential problems with translational research, as reviewed by Tannock.[69] It is possible that this regimen was more efficacious in tumors proliferating in patients than in surrounding normal cells (i.e., improved therapeutic index). This therapeutic benefit may not have been detectable in the laboratory.

Clinical Progression of Chemoradiotherapy Regimens in Non–Small Cell Lung Cancer

Studies conducted in the late 1980s and early 1990s showed that the addition of cisplatin with or without etoposide chemotherapy to irradiation led to improved local control[82-84] and survival for patients with locally advanced (stage III) NSCLC.[82-87] Five-year survival rates with the combination of irradiation and platinum-based chemotherapy were still only 8% to 17%,[86,87] and locoregional recurrence rates approached 90%.[85] Investigators explored additional methods of sequencing treatments and the use of new agents in combination with irradiation.

Controversy exists regarding the optimal sequencing of irradiation and chemotherapy. Although some of the best results in the literature were obtained using two cycles of cisplatin and vinblastine followed by 60 Gy administered in fractions of 2 Gy daily,[87] a contemporary study using the same regimen suggested a more modest 5-year survival rate of 8%.[86] However, a Japanese study and an RTOG study provided strong evidence that concurrent administration of chemotherapy and irradiation led to a better outcome than did sequential administration.[88,89] Because the median survival time increased only from approximately 12 months (with sequential chemotherapy) to 17 months with concurrent chemotherapy, continued focus on new agents and novel combinations is warranted.

One promising agent is topotecan. It is in a class of tumoricidal chemotherapeutic agents called *camptothecins*, which showed substantial activity in several malignancies in laboratory and early clinical studies. Two of the cancers against which topotecan appears to be active in the clinical setting are SCLC (response rates in previously untreated patients of 10% to 39%)[90-93] and NSCLC (response rates in previously untreated patients of 0% to 15%).[94-96] Topotecan has been shown to be active as a cytotoxin and a radiosensitizer.

Topotecan's cytotoxic effects appear to be preferentially S-phase selective. Its mechanism of action is related to the inhibition of topoisomerase I, a nuclear enzyme involved in allowing DNA to relax and thereby facilitate replication, transcription, and repair. Topotecan binds noncovalently to the topoisomerase I/DNA (cleavable) complex, preventing the cleaved strand of DNA from repairing. When the cleavable complex, stabilized by topotecan, meets a DNA replication fork (particularly during S phase), it can lead to cell death. Radiation-induced cytotoxicity occurs during the G_2 and M phases. This combination may also result in clinically significant synergy.

Laboratory-based studies have supported the idea of topotecan-associated radiosensitization. In vitro radiosensitization has been consistently demonstrated in tumor cell lines, including melanoma,[97] NSCLC,[98] and glioma.[98] In vivo animal studies have yielded similar results.[99,100] The interaction of radiation and topotecan has shown potential in early clinical trials of NSCLC. Chachoua and associates[101] administered continuous-infusion topotecan in combination with radiation (60 Gy) to 22 patients with NSCLC, establishing this as a tolerable regimen. Additional work is required to determine whether the topoisomerase I inhibitors will have a substantive role in chemoradiotherapeutic approaches (with or without biologic agents) for locally advanced NSCLC.

Paclitaxel is another example of a promising radiosensitizing agent that has been studied for the treatment of locally advanced NSCLC. It has shown substantial activity in lung cancer.[102-104] Several studies have suggested that more protracted infusions (>24 hours) of paclitaxel may lead to better responses in various tumors.[104-106] These protracted treatments may be most appropriate for chemoradiotherapy regimens involving paclitaxel. In in vivo animal studies, paclitaxel increased the effect of radiation by 1.2 to 2.0 times, and the maximal effect occurred when radiation was delivered approximately 24 to 96 hours after paclitaxel administration.[107-110] Studies of this nature also have suggested that the use of paclitaxel as a radiosensitizer may be most effective when it is given weekly rather than every 3 weeks.

Several studies have investigated the use of concurrent weekly paclitaxel and radiotherapy in the setting of locally advanced NSCLC. Most of these trials have also included concurrent carboplatin. In a study by Belani and coworkers,[111] 38 patients with locally advanced NSCLC were treated with weekly paclitaxel (45 mg/m^2 as a 3-hour infusion), weekly carboplatin (100 mg/m^2), and standard fractionated radiotherapy (1.8 Gy/fraction to a total dose of 60 to 65 Gy). The regimen was reasonably well tolerated, with 24% of patients having grade 3 leukopenia and 8% having grade 3 mucositis or esophagitis. In a separate study by Choy and associates,[112] 40 patients with inoperable, locally advanced NSCLC were treated with weekly paclitaxel (50 mg/m^2 weekly as a 1-hour infusion) and concurrent weekly carboplatin and radiotherapy. The radiation regimen was somewhat more aggressive than in the former study, with all patients assigned to receive 66 Gy at 2 Gy/fraction. The regimen was reasonably well tolerated. Grade 4 neutropenia and lymphopenia developed in 5% and 48% of patients, respectively. Although grade 3 or 4 esophagitis developed in 46% of patients, late esophageal toxicity (stricture) developed in only 5% of patients. The 2-year survival rates in both studies were impressive, at 54% and 38%, respectively.

Other new agents are being studied in chemoradiotherapy regimens for lung cancer.[113] The examples given earlier provide insight into the interplay between laboratory investigations and clinical findings. Even when direct translational research does not occur, the laboratory and clinical findings frequently complement each other and lead to additional investigation.

ADDITIONAL TUMOR FACTORS INVOLVED IN CHEMOTHERAPY AND IRRADIATION INTERACTIONS

The discussion to this point has focused on the interaction of chemotherapy and irradiation at the clinical and cellular levels and how positive interactions at the cellular level may eventually be used to guide clinical studies as more is learned about cytostatic versus cytotoxic interactions, pharmacokinetics, and patients' metabolic processes with respect to various agents. The concept of therapeutic benefit was also introduced. Tannock[2,69] made the important point that one of the main goals must be to find interactions that maximize control of tumor tissue while minimizing harm to normal tissue. He emphasized that positive interactions may use combinations of agents that exploit the differences between tumors and normal tissues with respect to genetic instability, proliferation rate, and environmental factors.

If tumor tissue is considered (rather than the tumor cells themselves), two other important concepts arise. First is the concept of spatial cooperation of agents. Various agents may be used together to target tumor tissue in spatially different areas (metastatic versus local) or within the same tumor mass but in areas with different environmental factors. The second concept, related to the Goldie-Coldman hypothesis (discussed later), is that certain tumors are composed of some cells that are sensitive and other cells that are resistant to a given agent and that this resistance may be circumvented by the application of non–cross-resistant agents that have activity for the different populations of cells in the tumor.

Spatial Cooperation

A classic example of spatial cooperation between chemotherapy and irradiation is the treatment of LSSCLC. By definition, LSSCLC is limited at the outset to the thorax, but it is known that local treatment of thoracic disease alone is not effective and that most patients die of systemic disease.[114] It is believed that patients with LSSCLC harbor microscopic metastatic disease at the outset. For this reason, patients require systemic chemotherapy as a component of the initial therapy. However, an important question arose in the late 1980s and 1990s regarding whether these patients require local thoracic radiotherapy (TRT). Initially, retrospective reviews of patients with LSSCLC who were treated with chemotherapy alone reported thoracic recurrence rates of 60% to 100%.[115,116] Several prospective phase III randomized trials were undertaken to investigate whether the addition of TRT to chemotherapy improved survival of patients with LSSCLC.[117-120] Three noteworthy trials showed an advantage for the use of TRT with chemotherapy compared with chemotherapy alone (Table 4-7)[117-119]; other trials,[120] however, did not show a beneficial effect of TRT. Pignon and associates[120] performed a meta-analysis of the 13 published and unpublished trials of chemotherapy and TRT. There was a statistically significant improvement in overall

Table 4-7 Chemotherapy with or without Thoracic Irradiation in Trials of Limited-Stage Small Cell Lung Cancer

Study	RT Start	Continuous RT vs Split Course	RT Concomitant with Chemotherapy	RT Volume before or after Chemotherapy	RT Dose
Bunn et al[117] (1987)	Day 1	C	Yes	Before chemotherapy	40 Gy/15 Fx
Perry et al[118] (1987)	Day 1 or day 63	C	Yes	Before chemotherapy	50 Gy/25 Fx
Perez et al[119] (1984)	Day 28	S	No (alternating)	Before chemotherapy	40 Gy/15 Fx

C, continuous; Fx, fractions; S, split; RT, radiation therapy.

survival associated with the use of TRT in addition to chemotherapy, and the associated 3-year survival rate increased from 10% to 16%.

The three trials in Table 4-7 illustrate an important point about spatial cooperation of chemotherapy and irradiation. All three showed a survival advantage with the use of chemotherapy (to address the systemic disease) in combination with TRT (to address the local disease) compared with chemotherapy alone; however, each trial used a different method of spatial cooperation. The integration, doses, and scheduling of treatments were completely different among the trials, but they all resulted in positive interactions between chemotherapy and irradiation. The challenge that faces current investigators of SCLC is to determine the optimal integration, doses, and schedules for the interaction of chemotherapy and irradiation and how these factors may change with the introduction of new chemotherapeutic agents and new methods of delivering TRT.

Non–cross-resistant Regimens

In the latter half of the 20th century, the concept of non–cross-resistant agents became important in the design of many clinical trials. Although this concept has often been used for selecting combinations of chemotherapeutic agents[121-125] that may target different populations of tumor cells (with variable sensitivity to chemotherapeutic agents) in the same tumor, it is also relevant to the combination of irradiation and chemotherapy.[126-128]

The idea that tumor masses could be composed of tumor cells with several intrinsic sensitivities to a given cytotoxic agent developed in the 1970s; however, the origin of this idea is often credited to a similar finding made in studying bacteria in 1943.[129] It was discovered that as *Escherichia coli* grew and developed daughter cells, the daughter cells had resistance to bacteriophages (i.e., bacterial viruses). This resistance was a result of the increasing population of the bacterial colony, not of previous exposure to the bacteriophage.[130] Goldie and Coldman[121-124] applied this concept to a growing tumor mass and hypothesized that even small tumor masses may contain mutated cells (compared with the original population) that display variable resistance to a cytotoxic agent. As the tumor mass grows, the number of mutations increases, and the spectrum of sensitivity to a chemotherapeutic agent increases. This led to the hypothesis that tumors should be treated with multiple non–cross-resistant agents.

This hypothesis was hampered by the difficulty of finding truly non–cross-resistant agents and by the fact that individual doses of agents must often be decreased when they are given in combination, thereby decreasing their effectiveness. Considering these limitations, investigators theorized that rapidly alternating delivery of non–cross-resistant agents may permit adequate dosing of individual agents while still addressing the problem that tumors may be composed of cells with different intrinsic sensitivities to a given cytotoxic agent.

On the basis of this principle, several clinical trials of rapidly alternating chemotherapeutic regimens have been undertaken.[131,132] The results of some of these trials were disappointing, although the agents may not have been truly non–cross-resistant. An example is the trial performed by the Southeastern Cancer Study Group in patients with ESSCLC.[133] Patients were randomly assigned to treatment with cyclophosphamide, doxorubicin, and vincristine; etoposide and cisplatin; or cyclophosphamide, doxorubicin, and vincristine alternating with etoposide and cisplatin. No survival advantage was observed for the alternating regimens.

In contrast, rapidly alternating non–cross-resistant chemotherapeutic regimens have shown promise in other disease sites. For example, the National Cancer Institute of Milan conducted a trial for patients with advanced Hodgkin's disease who were randomly assigned to treatment consisting of a standard MOPP regimen (mechlorethamine, vincristine, procarbazine, and prednisone) versus MOPP alternating with ABVD (doxorubicin, bleomycin, vinblastine, and dacarbazine). The patients treated with the alternating regimen had a statistically significant improvement in relapse-free survival compared with those receiving the standard treatment.[134] The conflicting results of the two trials suggest that further work is needed to determine the tumor histopathologic types that may benefit from the non–cross-resistant treatment approach.

Rapidly alternating regimens of cytotoxic therapy have also been adapted to the treatment of local disease (as opposed to systemic disease) and have incorporated irradiation as a potentially non–cross-resistant treatment.[126,127] The concept of alternating chemotherapy and radiotherapy as a potential non–cross-resistant regimen was tested experimentally in a rat hepatoma model by Looney and Hopkins (Table 4-8).[126] Cyclophosphamide alternating with three interrupted courses of accelerated fractionated radiotherapy produced a 70% cure rate, but concomitant treatment resulted in no cures (see Table 4-8).

These experimental results stimulated many investigators to explore alternating treatments of chemotherapy and irradiation as a method of delivering these potentially non–cross-resistant agents at full dose compared with a concomitant regimen that may require dose reduction.[135,136] One tumor in

Table 4-8 Interaction of Radiation and Cyclophosphamide (CTX) in Rat Hepatoma Model (Alternating Approach)

Total Radiation Dose (Gy)	Radiation Treatment*	CTX (150 mg/kg)	Complete Response (%)	Cure (%)
75	A	None	0	0
75	B	None	0	0
75	A	Days 2, 13, and 24	60	60
75	A	Days 8, 19, and 30	70	70
75	A	Days 0, 11, and 22	0	0
75	B	Days 10, 21, and 32	0	0
0	—	Days 0, 11, and 22	0	0

*Treatment A: 2.5 Gy given 5 × daily on days 0, 1, 11, 12, 22, and 23. Treatment B: 2.5 Gy given once each day on days 0-9, 11-20, and 22-31.

Data from Looney WB, Hopkins HA, Carter WH Jr: Solid tumor models for the assessment of different treatment modalities. XXII. The alternate utilization of radiotherapy and chemotherapy. Cancer 54:416-425, 1984; Looney WB, Hopkins HA, Carter WH Jr: Solid tumor models for the assessment of different treatment modalities. XXIII. A new approach to the more effective utilization of radiotherapy alternated with chemotherapy. Int J Radiat Oncol Biol Phys 11:2105-2117, 1985.

which the alternating approach seemed attractive was SCLC; delivery of the agents in an alternating manner may decrease pulmonary and esophageal toxicity. The Southeastern Cancer Study Group demonstrated a survival advantage for patients treated with alternating chemotherapy and TRT compared with chemotherapy alone,[119] and toxicity was acceptable for the alternating approach (see Table 4-7). Other groups also had promising results from pilot trials of alternating chemotherapy and TRT for SCLC (Table 4-9).[137-141] These studies resulted in the investigation of this treatment in phase III studies (Tables 4-9 and 4-10).[137-146] The use of alternating TRT with chemotherapy for patients with LSSCLC has not proved to be superior to nonalternating regimens of these agents (see Table 4-9).[98,141] However, one study of alternating chemoradiotherapy suggested that the alternating approach may be more tolerable without resulting in a decrement in survival compared with concurrent chemoradiotherapy.[141]

Improvement has been suggested in the outcome of patients with advanced head and neck malignancies with the use of alternating chemotherapy and local irradiation (see Table 4-10).[142-146] Two trials from a group in Genoa, Italy, demonstrated survival advantages for patients with inoperable head and neck cancer treated with an alternating approach compared with sequential chemotherapy and radiation or with radiation alone (see Table 4-10).[143,144] The subsequent studies in Table 4-10 were not randomized. The first was a phase I study that determined the maximum tolerated dose of gemcitabine in combination with 5-FU, paclitaxel, and radiotherapy.[145] The second study determined the response rate for gemcitabine in combination with cisplatin alternating with gemcitabine given with radiotherapy.[146]

Large-Field Radiation as a Systemic Non–cross-resistant Cytotoxic Agent

Local radiation may be used as a non–cross-resistant agent in combination with alternating chemotherapy, or it may be integrated with chemotherapy in other ways. Large-field irradiation also may add to the systemic benefit of chemotherapy, because it may act as a non–cross-resistant agent in the treatment of systemic disease. This has been the hypothesis for bone marrow transplantation induction regimens that use total-body irradiation (TBI) as a portion of the induction therapy. A typical regimen of this type was reported by the Southwest Oncology Group for the preparative regimen in autologous bone marrow transplantation in patients with relapse or refractory diffuse aggressive non-Hodgkin's lymphoma (NHL). The regimen used high-dose cyclophosphamide and etoposide with TBI consisting of 12 Gy in 8 fractions, twice daily over 4 days (days 5, 6, 7, and 8).[147] Although the doses of TBI used in bone marrow transplantation are much lower than those for curative treatment of a localized solid tumor, they are still very effective for bone marrow suppression. Laboratory and clinical evidence suggest that the volume of the field is paramount in the effect on bone marrow and is more important than dose.[148] Whether this concept can be extrapolated from bone marrow suppression to systemic tumor burden is controversial.

Considering the uses described previously and the theoretical aspects of TBI, the question has been posed whether large-field radiation could be used as a systemic non–cross-resistant complementary agent for patients undergoing systemic chemotherapy without bone marrow transplanta-

Table 4-9 Chemotherapy and Irradiation: Alternating Approaches in Small Cell Lung Cancer

Study	Treatment	Outcome
Arriagada et al[137] (1994)		
Limited-stage disease, protocol 1	Chemo: doxorubicin, etoposide, cyclophosphamide, and methotrexate × 6 TRT: 3 courses of 15 Gy/6 Fx 10 days after chemo cycles 2, 3, and 4	CR: 86% MS: 14 mo
Limited-stage disease, protocol 2	Chemo: protocol 1 with cisplatin TRT: 3 courses of TRT (20 Gy/8 Fx, 20 Gy/8 Fx, and 15 Gy/6 Fx) 10 days after chemo cycles 2, 3, and 4	CR: 91% MS: 20 mo
Gregor et al[138] (1997) Limited-stage disease (*N* = 335)	Randomized phase III Arm A: chemo (cyclophosphamide, doxorubicin, and etoposide) × 5 followed by TRT (50 Gy/20 Fx) Arm B: same chemo with TRT given as 12.5 Gy/5 Fx 14 days after chemo cycles 2, 3, 4, and 5	No difference between A and B MS (A): 15 mo; 3-year survival: 15% MS (B): 14 mo; 3-year survival: 12%
Johnson et al[139] (2003) Limited and extensive stage (*N* = 18)	Phase I study Alternating cycles of irinotecan (80-100 mg/m^2) + cisplatin (20 mg/m^2) with etoposide (60 mg/m^2) + cisplatin, weekly TRT for limited stage (45 Gy/30 Fx bid) on weeks 4-6 with EP	MTD of irinotecan: 100 mg/m^2 Overall response: 15/16 (1 CR)
Garces et al[140] (2005) Limited-stage disease (*N* = 15)	Phase I study (escalating radiotherapy) Induction topotecan and paclitaxel every 21 d × 2, followed by concurrent etoposide (50 mg/m^2/d) + cisplatin (mg/m^2/d) with TRT (48-66 Gy/40-55 Fx bid) with SQ amifostine given before PM Fx	MTD: 60 Gy/50 Fx bid with etoposide, cisplatin, and SQ amifostine MS: 14.5 mo
Lebeau et al[141] (1999) Limited-stage disease (*N* = 104)	Phase III concurrent chemoradiotherapy (at cycle 2) vs alternating chemoradiotherapy with TRT in 3 separate courses after cycles 2, 3, and 4 of chemo	No survival difference but better tolerability of the alternating regimen

bid, twice daily; chemo, chemotherapy; CR, complete response; EP, etoposide and cisplatin; Fx, fractions; MS, median survival; MTD, maximum tolerated dose; *N*, total number of patients; SQ, subcutaneous; TRT, thoracic radiation therapy.

Table 4-10 **Chemotherapy and Radiation: Alternating Approaches in Head and Neck Cancer**

Study	Treatment	Outcome
Yu et al[142] (1995), 23 patients with advanced hypopharyngeal lesions	Chemo: 5-FU and cisplatin RT: 1.8-2.0 Gy 2 × daily to 20 Gy × 3 on wk 2, 5, and 8 (the week after chemo)	CR: 83% Local control at 2 y: 52%
Merlano et al[143] (1991), inoperable HNC (*N* = 116)	Randomized phase III Arm A: chemo (vinblastine, bleomycin, and methotrexate) × 4 followed by 70 Gy RT Arm B: same chemo as in arm A with 20 Gy/10 Fx RT after each of first 3 cycles of chemo	Statistically significant improvement in CR and survival for arm B CR: 7/48 4-year survival: 10% CR, 19/57 4-year survival: 22%
Merlano et al[144] (1996), inoperable HNC (*N* = 157)	Randomized phase III Arm A: chemo (cisplatin, 5-FU) on wk 1, 4, 7, and 10, with 20 Gy/10 Fx RT during wk 2-3, 5-6, and 8-9 for total of 60 Gy Arm B: RT alone, 70 Gy	Statistically significant improvement in CR and survival for arm A CR, 43% 5-year survival: 24% CR: 22% 5-year survival: 10%
Milano et al[145] (2004), recurrent or inoperable HNC (*N* = 72)	Phase I study 5-FU (600 mg/m²/d × 5 d), paclitaxel (100 mg/m² on day 1) and gemcitabine (50-300 mg/m² on day 1) + RT (1.5 Gy/Fx, bid); all given every other week; RT total dose = 70-76 Gy	MTD: gemcitabine, 100 mg/m² or 200 mg/m² if given cycles 1-5 or 3-5, respectively Local control at 5 y: 61.4%
Benasso et al[146] (2004), inoperable HNC (*N* = 47)	Phase II study Gemcitabine 800 mg/m² on day 1 + cisplatin (20 mg/m² on days 2-5) for weeks 1, 4, 7, and 10, alternated with gemcitabine (300 mg/m² on day 1); 60 Gy RT (weeks 2-3, 5-6, and 8-9)	CR, 72%; 3-year survival, 43%

chemo, chemotherapy; CR, complete response; 5-FU, 5-fluorouracil; Fx, fractions; HNC, head and neck cancer; MTD, maximum tolerated dose; *N*, total number of patients; RT, radiation therapy.

tion. Initially, investigators hypothesized that large-field irradiation may have non–cross-resistant potential for malignancies that traditionally were very sensitive to radiation, because the doses that can be delivered with large-field irradiation are low compared with more conventional radiation doses. SCLC is very sensitive to radiation in vitro (lack of shoulder on the radiation survival curve) and in the clinical setting.[149] SCLC was targeted initially as a disease for which large-field irradiation and chemotherapy could potentially be used as a non–cross-resistant systemic regimen. Initial studies were performed to determine the tolerance and response of patients to TBI.[150]

A group from Rotterdam also used TBI during initial therapy for patients with LSSCLC.[150] Eighteen patients with limited disease received TBI consisting of 1 Gy given in 10 fractions during the first 2 weeks of therapy. Next, the patients received TRT consisting of 40 Gy in 20 fractions over 4 weeks. The liver was treated to a dose of 20 Gy in 10 fractions. Of the 18 patients, 16 had complete responses, and 1 was still in remission at 24 months. Nine patients remained in remission for 11 to 15 months before distant metastases developed. The investigators concluded that TBI seemed to be as effective as extensive chemotherapy for induction therapy of SCLC, but this conclusion appeared to be more of an impression than a comparison based on data.[150]

The results of this study and others suggest that TBI alone may be effective in SCLC. Because of the suggested efficacy of large-field irradiation in SCLC, other investigators have explored the use of large-field irradiation in combination with chemotherapy to treat patients with possible non–cross-resistant systemic agents. An early study of sequential hemibody irradiation in combination with chemotherapy suggested that this treatment regimen was tolerable and might improve on the results of standard treatment.[151] Treatment consisted of integrating sequential hemibody irradiation (6 Gy of upper hemibody irradiation during week 6 and 6 Gy of lower hemibody irradiation during week 17) during the induction phase and the consolidation phase of treatment for LSSCLC and ESSCLC.[151] Sequential hemibody irradiation was given during weeks when chemotherapy was not planned. This phase I/II trial of 41 patients demonstrated the feasibility of this type of regimen.

A trial performed at Mayo Clinic also suggested that sequential hemibody irradiation may be efficacious in ESSCLC.[152] Nineteen patients were enrolled in a phase I/II trial of aggressive chemotherapy, TRT, and prophylactic cranial irradiation. After these treatments, patients were to receive 6 Gy of upper hemibody irradiation followed by 8 Gy of lower hemibody irradiation. Of the 19 patients, 13 remained in the study and completed the upper hemibody irradiation, and 8 completed upper and lower hemibody irradiation. The 5-year progression-free survival and 5-year overall survival rates were 27% and 15%, respectively. Seven patients had long-term survival times (>5 years) or died without evidence of disease. More work is warranted to determine whether large-field irradiation can be used as a non–cross-resistant systemic agent in combination with chemotherapy for various malignancies such as SCLC.

Systemic Radiation and Chemotherapy: Lymphoma as an Example for Future Study

The increasing use of radiolabeled antibodies or other radiolabeled conjugates has brought interest to a new group of potential interactions between chemotherapy and these methods of delivering radiation treatment. Several excellent reviews of these new treatments have been published.[153,154] Hematologic malignancies are sensitive to low doses of radiotherapy, which makes them an ideal target for radiolabeled monoclonal antibodies. Much of the pioneering work in this area has been done in patients with NHL.

The use of unlabeled and radiolabeled antibodies to target relapsed or refractory B-cell NHL has been established as a treatment option. In 1997, rituximab (Rituxan) was the first therapeutic monoclonal antibody to be approved by the U.S. Food and Drug Administration (FDA). The approval of another antibody, yttrium 90–labeled ibritumomab tiuxetan (Zevalin), followed in 2002. Both monoclonal antibodies specifically target the CD20 receptor, which is found on more than 90% of B-cell NHL cells and is not found on stem cells, plasma cells, or nonhematologic tissue.[153] Yttrium 90 has a physical half-life of 2.7 days; it is a beta emitter with a maximum energy of 2.27 MeV, and it has a maximal penetration of 11.9 mm.[154]

One study explored the use of radioimmunotherapy in combination with unlabeled systemic immunotherapy.[155] Patients with recurrent or refractory low-grade, follicular, or transformed NHL were randomly assigned to receive rituximab with or without ^{90}Y-labeled ibritumomab tiuxetan. This study found an improvement in overall response rate from 56% to 80% for those patients who received ^{90}Y-labeled ibritumomab tiuxetan (P = .002).[155]

Building on experiences of this nature, combinations of ^{90}Y-labeled ibritumomab tiuxetan with chemotherapy have shown potential as novel treatments of NHL and as preparatory regimens for bone marrow transplantation.[156,157] A report described use of ZBEAM (carmustine, cytarabine, etoposide, melphalan, and ^{90}Y-ibritumomab tiuxetan) in preparation for autologous stem cell transplantation in elderly patients with NHL. The regimen showed tolerability similar to that of chemotherapy alone, and initial results were encouraging.[157] It will be important to refine the combinations of radioimmunotherapy and chemotherapy on the basis of these initial observations.

As advances in radioimmunotherapy bring more of these treatments to daily clinical practice, it will be important to evaluate them with respect to general radiation principles. Those evaluations will include addressing the combination of these systemic radiotherapy treatments with anoxic or hypoxic cytotoxins (conceptually, chemotherapeutic agents with hypoxic cell radiosensitizing properties) such as tirapazamine. Blumenthal and colleagues[158] have studied tumor hypoxia after radioimmunotherapy using a radioiodinated anti-carcinoembryonic antigen murine monoclonal antibody in the treatment of human GW-39 colonic xenografts. Through the use of oxygen microelectrodes and radiolabeled misonidazole injections (detection of hypoxia), it was determined that the colon carcinomas were maximally hypoxic at 14 days or more after radioimmunotherapy. These oxygen measurements were corroborated by tumor toxicity studies. Tirapazamine was more effective when delivered 2 weeks or longer after radioimmunotherapy, compared with simultaneous delivery. These results suggest that novel radioimmunotherapy approaches may be enhanced by the appropriate delivery of more traditional hypoxic cytotoxins or hypoxic cell radiosensitizers. The latest innovations in systemic radiotherapy may benefit from studies based on years of traditional investigation into methods of radiosensitization.

The study of radioimmunotherapy with solid tumors is also underway. Because solid tumors are less responsive than lymphomas to radiotherapy, the challenges have been different and more difficult. Some of the tumors being studied are prostate, ovarian, colorectal, and thyroid cancers.[159] Combinations of radioimmunotherapy and chemotherapy will be the subject of future studies. Such combinations may lead to exciting new concepts in systemic irradiation.

FUTURE DIRECTIONS

Manipulation of Hypoxia Incorporates Gene Therapy

The possibility of exploiting tumor hypoxia has been explored from the perspective of gene therapy.[160-165] The outgrowths of this new direction of research will call on the earlier efforts to create clinically useful combinations of chemotherapy and irradiation that exploit tumor hypoxia. Because hypoxia generally is a characteristic of tumor cells with inadequate blood supply (similar situations are much less common in normal tissue), the delivery of genetic material for selective cytotoxicity of hypoxic cells would have the advantage of being tumor specific. If genetic material could be delivered to hypoxic cells to make them more susceptible to chemotherapy or radiation, the associated increase in cytotoxicity of chemotherapy or irradiation, or both, would generally occur in tumor tissue and not normal tissue. The latter concept can be summarized as selectively enhancing chemotherapy and irradiation interactions in tumor cells.

Dachs and colleagues[165] explored an in vitro example of this procedure. They investigated the transfection of a human fibrosarcoma cell line with a hypoxia-responsive element coupled to sequences encoding cytosine deaminase, an enzyme responsible for the conversion of 5-fluorocytosine (5-FC) to its active chemotherapeutic form, 5-FU. The transfectants were more sensitive to 5-FC after anoxia (5.4-fold factor) compared with the parental cells. Because 5-FU causes radiosensitization, the ramifications of this type of therapy are important for potentially enhancing chemotherapy-induced cytotoxicity of hypoxic cells and for chemotherapy and irradiation interactions in hypoxic cells.

Because tirapazamine has been shown to be a radiosensitizer, other investigators have focused on gene therapy approaches that may augment tirapazamine-induced effects.[166,167] Cowen and colleagues,[167] using a novel gene therapy approach, showed enhanced expression of NADPH-cytochrome P450 reductase (P450R) in fibrosarcoma cells with known low P450R levels. The overexpressed P450R resulted in enhanced metabolic activation of tirapazamine under hypoxic conditions.[167] When mice bearing tumor xenografts were treated with 10 Gy, the time to tumor growth amounting to four times that at initiation of treatment was increased from 9 ± 4 days to 32 ± 4 days. Tirapazamine alone did not increase this radiation response. However, gene therapy–induced P450R treatment (2 days before tirapazamine and 10 Gy) resulted in a complete regression rate of 85%, and these mice were free of tumor at 90 days after therapy.[167] The study of gene therapy approaches that may enhance the effects of radiation or chemotherapy holds much promise because of the diversity of chemotherapy and radiotherapy interactions that may be modified by these approaches.

Molecular Manipulation of Chemotherapy and Irradiation Interactions

Pederson and associates[168] explored the implications, in the nonhypoxic context, of the studies outlined previously. An adenoviral vector system was used to transfect human cholangiocarcinoma cells with *E. coli* cytosine deaminase, according to published techniques. After it was confirmed that the transfected cells overexpressed cytosine deaminase, the transfected cells were found to be more sensitive to 5-FC than the control cells. Subsequently, an interactive effect of radiation and 5-FC was confirmed in vitro and in vivo for the transfected cells.

This same concept was investigated in an animal model study with fractionated radiotherapy.[169] A cholangiocarcinoma xenograft model was used with an adenoviral gene therapy approach to enhance cytosine deaminase expression. The gene therapy–treated tumors showed a response to treatment with 5-FC and radiotherapy similar to that for treatment with 5-FU and radiotherapy without gene therapy–induced cytosine deaminase. This gene therapy approach demonstrated that it is possible to selectively enhance metabolic conversion of a radiosensitizer in tumor tissue and spare normal tissue.

This paradigm is moving forward with other radiosensitizing gene therapy approaches. Better delivery systems for these gene therapy approaches will advance the clinical study of molecular chemotherapy.

Interactions of Antibodies, Drugs, and Radiation

Cetuximab with Chemotherapy and Irradiation

The use of monoclonal antibodies in cancer therapeutics has progressed from investigational studies to standard practice for certain tumors in the past several years. The use of rituximab in NHL has already been characterized (see "Systemic Radiation and Chemotherapy").

Cetuximab (Erbitux) is a monoclonal antibody that has gained FDA approval and is particularly relevant to the topic of interactions of chemotherapy and irradiation. Cetuximab targets the external binding domain of the epidermal growth factor receptor (EGFR). Laboratory studies have shown radiosensitizing and chemosensitizing properties of cetuximab in various tumors and have served as the nidus for multiple clinical studies exploring combinations of cetuximab with irradiation or chemotherapy.

Cetuximab is FDA approved for use in patients with metastatic colon carcinoma refractory to irinotecan-based chemotherapy. It was approved for use in combination with irinotecan after studies showed an improvement in response for the combination treatment compared with cetuximab alone for patients with irinotecan-refractory tumors.[170]

A study of cetuximab in combination with radiation in patients with locoregionally advanced head and neck cancer showed a locoregional control and survival advantage (Fig. 4-5A).[171] Cetuximab has demonstrated preclinical and clinical properties of a radiosensitizer and chemosensitizer.

On the basis of these properties, interest has grown in combining chemotherapy, radiation, and cetuximab for the treatment of various malignancies. For instance, the Eastern Cooperative Oncology Group has initiated a trial of cetuximab, cisplatin, and radiation for patients with locoregionally advanced head and neck cancer, building on the experience of cetuximab and radiotherapy (see Fig. 4-5B).

The potential exists to combine cetuximab (as well as other antibodies) with multiple chemoradiotherapy regimens in several different tumors in which EGFR may have a substantial role in tumor growth. There is evidence that EGFR is over-

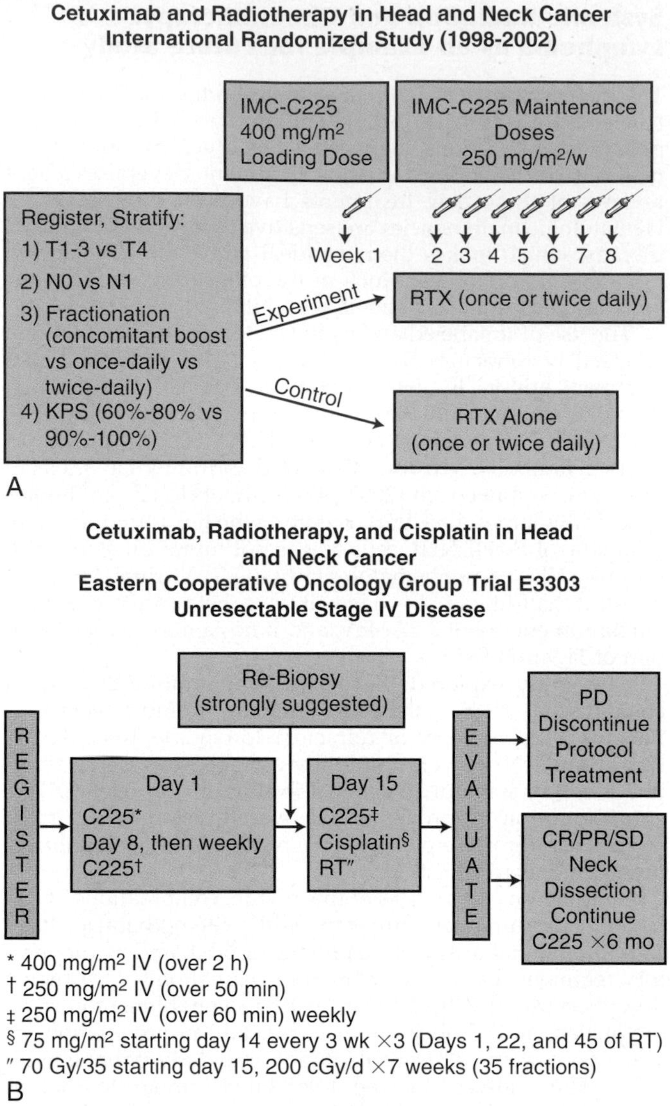

Figure 4-5 **A,** Study design of a randomized trial that found a survival advantage for the use of the monoclonal antibody cetuximab (IMC-C225) and radiotherapy (RTX) compared with radiotherapy alone.[171] **B,** Study design of a subsequent trial combining cetuximab (C225), radiotherapy (RT), and chemotherapy. CR, complete response; IV, intravenous; KPS, Karnofsky performance score; PD, progressive disease; PR, partial response; SD, stable disease.

expressed in human pancreatic carcinomas[172,173] and may be important in their growth. A correlation was found between the coexpression of EGFR, EGF, or transforming growth factor-α and survival in pancreatic cancer,[174,175] suggesting that EGFR may be a target for therapy of pancreatic cancer.[176] Cetuximab was found to inhibit growth of pancreatic carcinoma cell lines.

The potential mechanisms involved in cetuximab-induced inhibition of tumor growth (in vitro and in vivo) include arrest of cell cycle progression, activation of apoptosis, inhibition of angiogenesis, inhibition of invasion or metastasis, and an immune or inflammatory response mediated by the Fc portion of the monoclonal antibody.[177-187] In preclinical and clinical studies, cetuximab was shown to enhance the antitumor effects of several chemotherapeutic agents.[177,179,188-190] Interaction between anti-EGFR antibodies and chemotherapy may be based on several mechanisms, including inhibition of DNA repair mechanisms, alteration in paracrine growth factor production, and promotion of apoptotic cell death.[188,191]

Studies of cetuximab and 5-FU or gemcitabine have shown regression of human pancreatic cancer xenografts (growing subcutaneously or orthotopically in nude mice) and abrogation of metastases.[176,187] Gemcitabine has been shown to cause radiosensitization in human pancreatic cancer cells.[192-196] A phase II clinical trial using cetuximab in combination with gemcitabine for patients with pancreatic cancer showed promising activity.[192] On the basis of previous studies demonstrating the radiosensitizing property of cetuximab,[184] investigators hypothesized that cetuximab in combination with gemcitabine chemotherapy and irradiation may have pronounced efficacy against human pancreatic cancer cells and tumor xenografts compared with chemoradiotherapy alone.

Athymic nude mice bearing MIA PaCa-2 human pancreatic carcinoma cells as subcutaneous xenografts were treated with cetuximab (IMC-C225), gemcitabine, and radiation.[197] The ability of various combinations of treatment to inhibit the growth of MIA PaCa-2 xenografts is shown in Figure 4-6. Of the eight tumors in each treatment group, eight (100%) regressed in the triple-therapy group (i.e., cetuximab, gemcitabine, and radiation), compared with none (0%) in the single-therapy groups. Regression in the triple-therapy group was also significantly greater than in the double-therapy groups, except for the combination of cetuximab and irradiation, which produced regression in five (63%) of eight tumors.[197] These results suggest that the combination of cetuximab, gemcitabine, and irradiation may be efficacious for treatment of locally advanced pancreatic cancer. Trials of this nature are moving forward into the clinic.

Monoclonal Antibodies That Target TRAIL Death Receptors in Combination with Chemotherapy and Irradiation

Extensive molecular and tumor biologic research has focused on tumor necrosis factor (TNF)–related apoptosis-inducing ligand (TRAIL/Apo2L) since its discovery in 1995.[198-201] TRAIL is a TNF family member that is expressed constitutively in many normal tissues. It is a type 2 transmembrane protein that can be cleaved by specific proteases to release a soluble form of the molecule. The monomer has minimal biologic activity but can form a homotrimer of about 60 kd that has powerful cytotoxicity to tumor cells. An array of membrane receptors have been described that are capable of binding to TRAIL, two of which (DR4 and DR5) have cytoplasmic death domains capable of signaling downstream caspase activation with apoptosis induction. At least three "decoy" receptors lacking cytoplasmic death domains are thought to modulate (i.e., inhibit) TRAIL effects.

TRAIL induces apoptosis and cytotoxicity in tumor cells with little or no adverse effects on normal cells. Approximately 75% to 80% of tumor cell lines can be lysed by TRAIL to varying degrees (some are highly sensitive and others less so), and the rest are TRAIL resistant. Pancreatic cancer cells have been shown to undergo apoptosis after treatment with TRAIL.[202,203] Several chemotherapy agents, such as actinomycin D,[203] cisplatin,[204,205] adriamycin,[205] taxanes,[206] 5-FU,[207] CPT-11 (irinotecan),[199,208] and gemcitabine,[209] can transform TRAIL-resistant cells to a TRAIL-sensitive state or can enhance the TRAIL-induced cytotoxicity of sensitive cell lines. In some instances, the drug induced upregulation of death receptors[205]; in others, signal transduction in the apoptotic pathways was enhanced or cofactors were modulated. It has been reported that the combination of radiation and TRAIL is synergistic in breast cancer cell lines.[210]

Griffith and coworkers[211] first described the effects of monoclonal antibodies specific for the TRAIL receptors and their biologic behavior. He reported the need for antibodies to DR4 and DR5 to be crosslinked or immobilized in order to mediate cytotoxicity. Tumor cells' sensitivity to DR4 and DR5 cytotoxicity correlated with their sensitivity to TRAIL. The decoy receptors showed no evidence of cytotoxicity or modulation. TRAIL and anti-DR4 or anti-DR5 had similar levels of caspase activation. Actinomycin D may transform cell lines from a TRAIL-resistant to an anti-DR4– and anti-DR5–sensitive state.

An immunoglobulin G (IgG1k) agonistic antibody, TRA-8, was discovered by screening murine monoclonal antibodies from DR5 fusion protein–immunized mice.[212] This antibody has shown a high affinity for DR5 (3 nM) and competes with TRAIL for binding to DR5. It has shown potent cytotoxicity in vitro for various tumor cells without crosslinking.[212] After BALB/c mice were immunized with purified human DR4-Fc fusion protein,[212] the hybridomas that reacted with DR4-Fc but

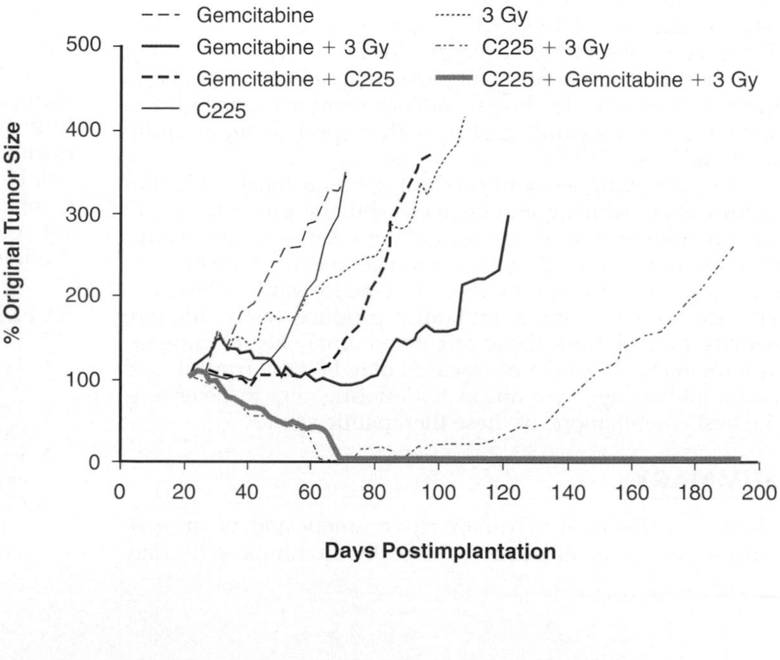

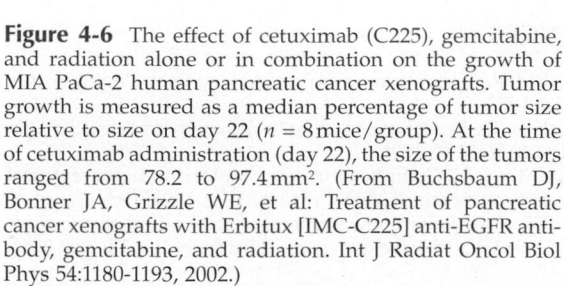

Figure 4-6 The effect of cetuximab (C225), gemcitabine, and radiation alone or in combination on the growth of MIA PaCa-2 human pancreatic cancer xenografts. Tumor growth is measured as a median percentage of tumor size relative to size on day 22 (n = 8 mice/group). At the time of cetuximab administration (day 22), the size of the tumors ranged from 78.2 to 97.4 mm². (From Buchsbaum DJ, Bonner JA, Grizzle WE, et al: Treatment of pancreatic cancer xenografts with Erbitux [IMC-C225] anti-EGFR antibody, gemcitabine, and radiation. Int J Radiat Oncol Biol Phys 54:1180-1193, 2002.)

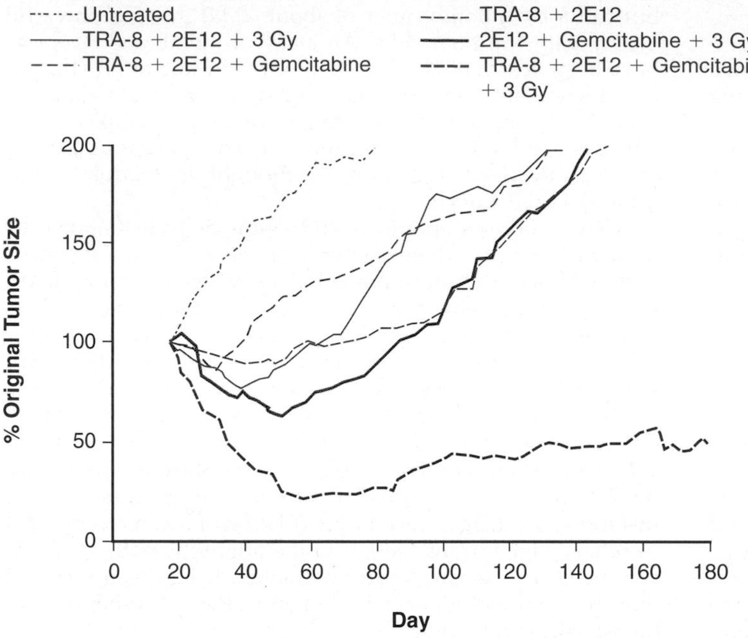

Figure 4-7 The effect of monoclonal antibodies TRA-8 and 2E12, gemcitabine, and radiation in athymic nude mice bearing pancreatic cancer xenografts. MIA PaCa-2 cells (2×10^7) were injected subcutaneously into athymic nude mice on day 0. Groups of mice were injected intraperitoneally with 200 μg of TRA-8 or 2E12, or both, on days 17, 21, 24, 28, 31, 38, and 42. Groups of mice received intraperitoneal gemcitabine (120 mg/kg) on days 18, 25, and 39. Groups of mice received 3 Gy of cobalt 60 (^{60}Co) to the tumor on days 19, 26, and 40. One group of mice was untreated. Data are expressed as the average percentage of tumor size relative to size on day 17 (n = 8 mice/group).

not with the Fc of human IgG1 were selected and subcloned. The specificity of five established hybridoma clones to human DR4 was determined by enzyme-linked immunosorbent assay. The 2E12 anti-DR4 antibody was selected because of its specificity and IgG1 subtype. In this way, monoclonal antibodies to DR5 (TRA-8) and DR4 (2E12) were produced.

Using pancreatic carcinoma as one model, investigators became interested in combining these antibodies with relevant chemotherapy and irradiation regimens, similar to the previous preclinical work with cetuximab described earlier. Initial studies examined the effect of combining TRA-8 and 2E12 with or without gemcitabine and radiation in the BxPC-3 (human pancreatic cells) xenograft model, which has intermediate sensitivity in vitro. The combination of antibodies, gemcitabine, and radiation produced the greatest inhibition of tumor growth compared with single agents and two-agent combinations (Fig. 4-7). The mean time to tumor doubling was 30 days for TRA-8 alone; 39 days for TRA-8, 2E12, and gemcitabine; 45 days for TRA-8, 2E12, and radiation; 47 days for TRA-8 and 2E12; 50 days for TRA-8, 2E12, and gemcitabine; and 54 days for TRA-8, 2E12, gemcitabine, and radiation. These early observations require further corroboration, but even this moderately resistant pancreatic cell line appeared to behave similarly to breast adenocarcinoma and glioma xenografts in previous studies with respect to these multimodality effects.[213,214]

This intriguing work of combining monoclonal antibodies (with radiosensitizing and chemosensitizing properties) with chemoradiotherapy is advancing the science of interactive therapeutics. The work with cetuximab and with the humanized death receptor antibodies is moving forward in the clinic. Because the monoclonal antibodies produce vastly different toxicity profiles from those of conventional chemoradiotherapy regimens, this area of research may be very fruitful, and exciting challenges are ahead for investigators to determine the best combinations of these therapeutic agents.

SUMMARY

Molecular alteration of tumor environment and of drug or radiosensitizer metabolism specifically in tumor cells may lead to promising avenues of clinical research in the area of chemotherapy and irradiation interactions. The new techniques may be applied in many other ways to enhance chemotherapy and irradiation interactions. Investigations are determining whether the response of a tumor to irradiation and chemotherapy may be enhanced by increasing the expression of proapoptotic genes versus antiapoptotic genes (Table 4-11). Chemotherapy and irradiation interactions may be manipulated by genetically altering normal tissue to protect it from cytotoxic agents. In future investigations into molecular manipulation of irradiation and chemotherapy responses, it will be important to focus on the three factors that Tannock[69] emphasized as possible areas of exploitable differences between tumor tissue and normal tissue: genetic instability, proliferation rates, and environmental factors.

Table 4-11 Proapoptotic and Antiapoptotic Factors That May Be Used in the Future to Influence Chemotherapy and Irradiation Interactions

Proapoptotic	Antiapoptotic
TP53	BCL2
BCL-x5	BCL2L1 (BCL-xL)
E1A	E1B
HRAS	BIRC5 (survivin)
TNFSF10 (TRAIL)	STAT3

REFERENCES

1. Tyrrell RM: Radiation synergism and antagonism. Photobiol Rev 3:35-113, 1978.
2. Tannock IF: Treatment of cancer with radiation and drugs. J Clin Oncol 14:3156-3174, 1996.
3. von der Maase H: Complications of combined radiotherapy and chemotherapy. Semin Radiat Oncol 4:81-94, 1994.
4. Colin PH: Concomitant chemotherapy and radiotherapy: theoretical basis and clinical experience. Anticancer Res 14:2357-2361, 1994.

5. Shenoy MA, Singh BB: Chemical radiosensitizers in cancer therapy. Cancer Invest 10:533-551, 1992.
6. Berenbaum MC: What is synergy? Pharmacol Rev 41:93-141, 1989. Erratum in: Pharmacol Rev 41:422, 1990.
7. Greco WR, Bravo G, Parsons JC: The search for synergy: a critical review from a response surface perspective. Pharmacol Rev 47:331-385, 1995.
8. Holthusen H: Beiträge zur biologie der strahlenwirkung. Untersuchungenen an Askarideneiern [German]. Arch Ges Physiol 187:1-24, 1921.
9. Muller HJ: Radiation treatment under anoxic conditions. J Genet 40:1-66, 1940.
10. Baker WK, Von Halle ES: The basis of the oxygen effect on x-irradiated *Drosophila* sperm. Proc Natl Acad Sci U S A 39:152-161, 1953.
11. Gray LH, Conger AD, Ebert M, et al: The concentration of oxygen dissolved in tissues at the time of irradiation as a factor in radiotherapy. Br J Radiol 26:638-648, 1953.
12. Giles NH Jr, Beatty AV: The effect of x-irradiation in oxygen and in hydrogen at normal and positive pressures on chromosome aberration frequency in *Tradescantia* microspores. Science 112: 643-645, 1950.
13. Alper T: The modification of damage caused by primary ionization of biological targets. Radiat Res 5:573-586, 1956.
14. Schwartz D: The effect of oxygen concentration on x-ray-induced chromosome breakage in maize. Proc Natl Acad Sci U S A 38:490-494, 1952.
15. Olive PL: Detection of hypoxia by measurement of DNA damage in individual cells from spheroids and murine tumours exposed to bioreductive drugs. I. tirapazamine. Br J Cancer 71:529-536, 1995.
16. Adams GE, Cooke MS: Electron-affinic sensitization. I. A structural basis for chemical radiosensitizers in bacteria. Int J Radiat Biol Relat Stud Phys Chem Med 15:457-471, 1969.
17. Stone HB, Withers HR: Tumor and normal tissue response to metronidazole and irradiation in mice. Radiology 113:441-444, 1974.
18. Begg AC, Sheldon PW, Foster JL: Demonstration of radiosensitization of hypoxic cells in solid tumours by metronidazole. Br J Radiol 47:399-404, 1974.
19. Rauth AM, Kaufman K: In vivo testing of hypoxic radiosensitizers using the KHT murine tumour assayed by the lung-colony technique. Br J Radiol 48:209-220, 1975.
20. Adams GE: Chemical radiosensitization of hypoxic cells. Br Med Bull 29:48-53, 1973.
21. Mulcahy RT, Siemann DW: In vivo chemosensitization by misonidazole in sensitive and resistant tumor lines. Cancer Res 43:4709-4713, 1983.
22. Tannock IF: In vivo interaction of anti-cancer drugs with misonidazole or metronidazole: methotrexate, 5-fluorouracil and adriamycin. Br J Cancer 42:861-870, 1980.
23. Siemann DW, Chapman M, Beikirch A: Effects of oxygenation and pH on tumor cell response to alkylating chemotherapy. Int J Radiat Oncol Biol Phys 20:287-289, 1991.
24. Siemann DW, Hill SA: Increased therapeutic benefit through the addition of misonidazole to a nitrosourea-radiation combination. Cancer Res 46:629-632, 1986.
25. Roizin-Towle L, Hall EJ, Flynn M, et al: Enhanced cytotoxicity of melphalan by prolonged exposure to nitroimidazoles: the role of endogenous thiols. Int J Radiat Oncol Biol Phys 8:757-760, 1982.
26. Siemann DW, Hill SA: Enhanced tumor responses through therapies combining CCNU, MISO and radiation. Int J Radiat Oncol Biol Phys 10:1623-1626, 1984.
27. McNally NJ, Soranson JA: Radiosensitization by misonidazole during recovery of cellular thiols following depletion by BSO or DEM. Int J Radiat Oncol Biol Phys 16:1331-1334, 1989.
28. Guichard M: Chemical manipulations of tissue oxygenation for therapeutic benefit. Int J Radiat Oncol Biol Phys 16:1125-1130, 1989. Erratum in: Int J Radiat Oncol Biol Phys 17:1365, 1989.
29. Stratford IJ, Hickson ID, Robson CN, et al: Radiosensitizing and cytotoxic effects of nitroimidazoles in CHO cells expressing elevated levels of glutathione-*S*-transferase. Int J Radiat Oncol Biol Phys 16:1307-1310, 1989.
30. Siemann DW, Flaherty AA, Penney DP: Effect of thiol manipulation on chemopotentiation by nitroimidazoles. Int J Radiat Oncol Biol Phys 16:1341-1345, 1989.
31. Stewart FA: Modification of normal tissue response to radiotherapy and chemotherapy. Int J Radiat Oncol Biol Phys 16:1195-1200, 1989.
32. Brown JM: Keynote address. Hypoxic cell radiosensitizers: where next? Int J Radiat Oncol Biol Phys 16:987-993, 1989.
33. Brown JM, Giaccia AJ: Tumour hypoxia: the picture has changed in the 1990s. Int J Radiat Biol 65:95-102, 1994.
34. Overgaard J, Bentzen SM, Kolstad P, et al: Misonidazole combined with radiotherapy in the treatment of carcinoma of the uterine cervix. Int J Radiat Oncol Biol Phys 16:1069-1072, 1989.
35. Overgaard J, Hansen HS, Andersen AP, et al: Misonidazole combined with split-course radiotherapy in the treatment of invasive carcinoma of larynx and pharynx: report from the DAHANCA 2 study. Int J Radiat Oncol Biol Phys 16:1065-1068, 1989.
36. Leibel S, Bauer M, Wasserman T, et al: Radiotherapy with or without misonidazole for patients with stage IIIB or stage IVA squamous cell carcinoma of the uterine cervix: preliminary report of a Radiation Therapy Oncology Group randomized trial. Int J Radiat Oncol Biol Phys 13:541-549, 1987.
37. Van den Bogaert W, van der Schueren E, Horiot JC, et al: The EORTC randomized trial on three fractions per day and misonidazole (trial no. 22811) in advanced head and neck cancer: long-term results and side effects. Radiother Oncol 35:91-99, 1995.
38. Simpson JR, Bauer M, Perez CA, et al: Radiation therapy alone or combined with misonidazole in the treatment of locally advanced non-oat cell lung cancer: report of an RTOG prospective randomized trial. Int J Radiat Oncol Biol Phys 16:1483-1491, 1989.
39. Fischbach AJ, Martz KL, Nelson JS, et al: Long-term survival in treated anaplastic astrocytomas: a report of combined RTOG/ECOG studies. Am J Clin Oncol 14:365-370, 1991.
40. Lee DJ, Pajak TF, Stetz J, et al: A phase I/II study of the hypoxic cell sensitizer misonidazole as an adjunct to high fractional dose radiotherapy in patients with unresectable squamous cell carcinoma of the head and neck: a RTOG randomized study (#79-04). Int J Radiat Oncol Biol Phys 16:465-470, 1989.
41. Huncharek M: Meta-analytic re-evaluation of misonidazole in the treatment of high grade astrocytoma. Anticancer Res 18:1935-1939, 1998.
42. Glover D, Trump D, Kvols L, et al: Phase II trial of misonidazole (MISO) and cyclophosphamide (CYC) in metastatic renal cell carcinoma. Int J Radiat Oncol Biol Phys 12:1405-1408, 1986.
43. Bleehen NM, Freedman LS, Stenning SP: A randomized study of CCNU with and without benznidazole in the treatment of recurrent grades 3 and 4 astrocytoma: report to the Medical Research Council by the Brain Tumor Working Party. Int J Radiat Oncol Biol Phys 16:1077-1081, 1989.
44. Coleman CN, Carlson RW, Artim RA, et al: Enhancement of the clinical activity of melphalan by the hypoxic cell sensitizer misonidazole. Cancer Res 48:3528-3532, 1988. Erratum in: Cancer Res 49:256, 1989.
45. Deutsch M, Green SB, Strike TA, et al: Results of a randomized trial comparing BCNU plus radiotherapy, streptozotocin plus radiotherapy, BCNU plus hyperfractionated radiotherapy, and BCNU following misonidazole plus radiotherapy in the postoperative treatment of malignant glioma. Int J Radiat Oncol Biol Phys 16:1389-1396, 1989.
46. Hatlevoll R, Lindegaard KF, Hagen S, et al: Combined modality treatment of operated astrocytomas grade 3 and 4: a prospective and randomized study of misonidazole and radiotherapy with two different radiation schedules and subsequent CCNU chemotherapy. Stage II of a prospective multicenter trial of the Scandinavian Glioblastoma Study Group. Cancer 56:41-47, 1985.
47. Hurwitz SJ, Coleman CN, Riese N, et al: Distribution of etanidazole into human brain tumors: implications for treating high grade gliomas. Int J Radiat Oncol Biol Phys 22:573-576, 1992.
48. Coleman CN, Noll L, Riese N, et al: Final report of the phase I trial of continuous infusion etanidazole (SR 2508): a Radiation Therapy Oncology Group study. Int J Radiat Oncol Biol Phys 22:577-580, 1992.

49. Lee DJ, Cosmatos D, Marcial VA, et al: Results of an RTOG phase III trial (RTOG 85-27) comparing radiotherapy plus etanidazole with radiotherapy alone for locally advanced head and neck carcinomas. Int J Radiat Oncol Biol Phys 32:567-576, 1995.
50. Chassagne D, Charreau I, Sancho-Garnier H, et al: First analysis of tumor regression for the European randomized trial of etanidazole combined with radiotherapy in head and neck carcinomas. Int J Radiat Oncol Biol Phys 22:581-584, 1992.
51. Brown JM: Hypoxic cell radiosensitizers: the end of an era? Regarding Lee et al., IJROBP 32:567-576, 1995 [editorial]. Int J Radiat Oncol Biol Phys 32:883-885, 1995.
52. Zeman EM, Brown JM, Lemmon MJ, et al: SR-4233: a new bioreductive agent with high selective toxicity for hypoxic mammalian cells. Int J Radiat Oncol Biol Phys 12:1239-1242, 1986.
53. Walton MI, Workman P: Pharmacokinetics and bioreductive metabolism of the novel benzotriazine di-*N*-oxide hypoxic cell cytotoxin tirapazamine (WIN 59075; SR 4233; NSC 130181) in mice. J Pharmacol Exp Ther 265:938-947, 1993.
54. Del Rowe J, Scott C, Werner-Wasik M, et al: Single-arm, open-label phase II study of intravenously administered tirapazamine and radiation therapy for glioblastoma multiforme. J Clin Oncol 18:1254-1259, 2000.
55. Aghajanian C, Brown C, O'Flaherty C, et al: Phase I study of tirapazamine and cisplatin in patients with recurrent cervical cancer. Gynecol Oncol 67:127-130, 1997.
56. von Pawel J, von Roemeling R, Gatzemeier U, et al: Tirapazamine plus cisplatin versus cisplatin in advanced non-small-cell lung cancer: a report of the international CATAPULT I study group. J Clin Oncol 18:1351-1359, 2000.
57. Williamson SK, Crowley JJ, Lara PN, et al, for the Southwest Oncology Group: Paclitaxel/carboplatin (PC) v PC + tirapazamine (PCT) in advanced non-small cell lung cancer (NSCLC): a phase III Southwest Oncology Group (SWOG) Trial [abstract]. Prog Proc Am Soc Clin Oncol 22:622, 2003.
58. Le Q-T, McCoy J, Williamson S, et al: Phase I study of tirapazamine plus cisplatin/etoposide and concurrent thoracic radiotherapy in limited-stage small cell lung cancer (S0004): a Southwest Oncology Group study. Clin Cancer Res 10:5418-5424, 2004.
59. Lara PN Jr, Frankel P, Mack PC, et al: Tirapazamine plus carboplatin and paclitaxel in advanced malignant solid tumors: a California cancer consortium phase I and molecular correlative study. Clin Cancer Res 9:4356-4362, 2003.
60. Horst KC, Su CK, Budenz S, et al: Quality-of-life assessment in a phase II randomized trial of tirapazamine in advanced squamous cell carcinomas of the head and neck [abstract]. Int J Radiat Oncol Biol Phys 57(Suppl):S223-S224, 2003.
61. Rischin D, Peters L, Hicks R, et al: Phase I trial of concurrent tirapazamine, cisplatin, and radiotherapy in patients with advanced head and neck cancer. J Clin Oncol 19:535-542, 2001.
62. Dorie MJ, Brown JM: Tumor-specific, schedule-dependent interaction between tirapazamine (SR 4233) and cisplatin. Cancer Res 53:4633-4636, 1993.
63. Grau C, Overgaard J: Effect of cancer chemotherapy on the hypoxic fraction of a solid tumor measured using a local tumor control assay. Radiother Oncol 13:301-309, 1988.
64. Rischin D, Peters L, Fisher R, et al: Tirapazamine, cisplatin, and radiation versus fluorouracil, cisplatin, and radiation in patients with locally advanced head and neck cancer: a randomized phase II trial of the Trans-Tasman Radiation Oncology Group (TROG 98.02). J Clin Oncol 23:79-87, 2005.
65. Steel GG, Peckham MJ: Exploitable mechanisms in combined radiotherapy-chemotherapy: the concept of additivity. Int J Radiat Oncol Biol Phys 5:85-91, 1979.
66. Chou TC, Talalay P: Quantitative analysis of dose-effect relationships: the combined effects of multiple drugs or enzyme inhibitors. Adv Enzyme Regul 22:27-55, 1984.
67. Haddock MG, Ames MM, Bonner JA: Assessing the interaction of irradiation with etoposide or idarubicin. Mayo Clin Proc 70:1053-1060, 1995.
68. Bonner JA, Kozelsky TF: The significance of the sequence of administration of topotecan and etoposide. Cancer Chemother Pharmacol 39:109-112, 1996.
69. Tannock IF: Potential for therapeutic gain from combined-modality treatment. Front Radiat Ther Oncol 26:1-15, 1992.
70. Nigro ND, Vaitkevicius VK, Considine B Jr: Combined therapy for cancer of the anal canal: a preliminary report. Dis Colon Rectum 17:354-356, 1974.
71. Nigro ND: Multidisciplinary management of cancer of the anus. World J Surg 11:446-451, 1987.
72. Sischy B, Doggett RL, Krall JM, et al: Definitive irradiation and chemotherapy for radiosensitization in management of anal carcinoma: interim report on Radiation Therapy Oncology Group study no. 8314. J Natl Cancer Inst 81:850-856, 1989.
73. Flam MS, John M, Pajak T, et al: Radiation (RT) and 5-fluorouracil (5FU) vs. radiation, 5FU, mitomycin-C (MMC) in the treatment of anal carcinoma: results of a phase III randomized RTOG/ECOG intergroup trial [abstract]. Prog Proc Am Soc Clin Oncol 14:191, 1995.
74. Bartelink H, Roelofsen F, Eschwege F, et al: Concomitant radiotherapy and chemotherapy is superior to radiotherapy alone in the treatment of locally advanced anal cancer: results of a phase III randomized trial of the European Organization for Research and Treatment of Cancer Radiotherapy and Gastrointestinal Cooperative Groups. J Clin Oncol 15:2040-2049, 1997.
75. Dobrowsky W, Dobrowsky E, Rauth AM: Mode of interaction of 5-fluorouracil, radiation, and mitomycin C: in vitro studies. Int J Radiat Oncol Biol Phys 22:875-880, 1992.
76. Byfield JE, Calabro-Jones P, Klisak I, et al: Pharmacologic requirements for obtaining sensitization of human tumor cells in vitro to combined 5-fluorouracil or ftorafur and x rays. Int J Radiat Oncol Biol Phys 8:1923-1933, 1982.
77. Rockwell S: Cytotoxicities of mitomycin C and x rays to aerobic and hypoxic cells in vitro. Int J Radiat Oncol Biol Phys 8:1035-1039, 1982.
78. Daling JR, Madeleine MM, Johnson LG, et al: Human papillomavirus, smoking, and sexual practices in the etiology of anal cancer. Cancer 101:270-280, 2004.
79. Maksymiuk AW, Jett JR, Earle JD, et al: Sequencing and schedule effects of cisplatin plus etoposide in small-cell lung cancer: results of a North Central Cancer Treatment Group randomized clinical trial. J Clin Oncol 12:70-76, 1994.
80. Schabel FM Jr, Trader MW, Laster WR Jr, et al: *cis*-Dichlorodiammineplatinum(II): combination chemotherapy and cross-resistance studies with tumors of mice. Cancer Treat Rep 63:1459-1473, 1979.
81. Tsai C-M, Gazdar AF, Venzon DJ, et al: Lack of in vitro synergy between etoposide and *cis*-Diammine dichloroplatinum(II). Cancer Res 49:2390-2397, 1989.
82. Schaake-Koning C, van den Bogaert W, Dalesio O, et al: Effects of concomitant cisplatin and radiotherapy on inoperable non-small-cell lung cancer. N Engl J Med 326:524-530, 1992.
83. Jeremic B, Shibamoto Y, Acimovic L, et al: Hyperfractionated radiation therapy with or without concurrent low-dose daily carboplatin/etoposide for stage III non-small-cell lung cancer: a randomized study. J Clin Oncol 14:1065-1070, 1996.
84. Bonner JA, McGinnis WL, Stella PJ, et al: The possible advantage of hyperfractionated thoracic radiotherapy in the treatment of locally advanced nonsmall cell lung carcinoma: results of a North Central Cancer Treatment Group phase III study. Cancer 82:1037-1048, 1998.
85. Arriagada R, Le Chevalier T, Rekacewicz C, et al: Cisplatin-based chemotherapy (CT) in patients with locally advanced non-small cell lung cancer (NSCLC): late analysis of a French randomized trial [abstract]. Prog Proc Am Soc Clin Oncol 16:446a, 1997.
86. Sause WT, Scott C, Taylor S, et al: Radiation Therapy Oncology Group (RTOG) 88-08 and Eastern Cooperative Oncology Group (ECOG) 4588: preliminary results of a phase III trial in regionally advanced, unresectable non-small-cell lung cancer. J Natl Cancer Inst 87:198-205, 1995.
87. Dillman RO, Herndon J, Seagren SL, et al: Improved survival in stage III non-small-cell lung cancer: seven-year follow-up of cancer and leukemia group B (CALGB) 8433 trial. J Natl Cancer Inst 88:1210-1215, 1996.
88. Furuse K, Fukuoka M, Kawahara M, et al: Phase III study of concurrent versus sequential thoracic radiotherapy in combination

with mitomycin, vindesine, and cisplatin in unresectable stage III non-small-cell lung cancer. J Clin Oncol 17:2692-2699, 1999.
89. Curran WJ Jr, Scott C, Langer C, et al: Phase III comparison of sequential vs concurrent chemoradiation for PTS with unresected stage III non-small cell lung cancer (NSCLC): initial report of Radiation Therapy Oncology Group (RTOG) 9410 [abstract]. Prog Proc Am Soc Clin Oncol 19:484a, 2000.
90. Perez-Soler R, Glisson BS, Lee JS, et al: Phase II study of topotecan in patients with small cell lung cancer (SCLC) refractory to etoposide [abstract]. Prog Proc Am Soc Clin Oncol 14:355, 1995.
91. Wanders J, Ardizzoni A, Hansen HH, et al, for the EORTC-ECTG and EORTC-LCCG: Phase II study of topotecan in refractory and sensitive small cell lung cancer (SCLC) [abstract]. Prog Proc Am Assoc Cancer Res 36:237, 1995.
92. Schiller JH, Kim K, Hutson P, et al: Phase II study of topotecan in patients with extensive-stage small-cell carcinoma of the lung: an Eastern Cooperative Oncology Group trial. J Clin Oncol 14:2345-2352, 1996.
93. Ardizzoni A, Hansen H, Dombernowsky P, et al, for the European Organization for Research and Treatment of Cancer Early Clinical Studies Group and New Drug Development Office, and the Lung Cancer Cooperative Group: Topotecan, a new active drug in the second-line treatment of small-cell lung cancer: a phase II study in patients with refractory and sensitive disease. J Clin Oncol 15:2090-2096, 1997.
94. Lynch TJ Jr, Kalish L, Strauss G, et al: Phase II study of topotecan in metastatic non-small-cell lung cancer. J Clin Oncol 12:347-352, 1994.
95. Weitz JJ, Jung S-H, Marschke RF Jr, et al: Randomized phase II trial of two schedules of topotecan for the treatment of advanced stage non-small cell lung carcinoma (NSCLC): a North Central Cancer Treatment Group (NCCTG) trial [abstract]. Prog Proc Am Soc Clin Oncol 14:348, 1995.
96. Perez-Soler R, Fossella FV, Glisson BS, et al: Phase II study of topotecan in patients with advanced non-small-cell lung cancer previously untreated with chemotherapy. J Clin Oncol 14:503-513, 1996.
97. Lamond JP, Wang M, Kinsella TJ, et al: Concentration and timing dependence of lethality enhancement between topotecan, a topoisomerase I inhibitor, and ionizing radiation. Int J Radiat Oncol Biol Phys 36:361-368, 1996.
98. Marchesini R, Colombo A, Caserini C, et al: Interaction of ionizing radiation with topotecan in two human tumor cell lines. Int J Cancer 66:342-346, 1996.
99. Kim JH, Kim SH, Kolozsvary A, et al: Potentiation of radiation response in human carcinoma cells in vitro and murine fibrosarcoma in vivo by topotecan, an inhibitor of DNA topoisomerase I. Int J Radiat Oncol Biol Phys 22:515-518, 1992.
100. Boscia RE, Korbut T, Holden SA, et al: Interaction of topoisomerase I inhibitors with radiation in *cis*-diamminedichloroplatinum (II)-sensitive and -resistant cells in vitro and in the FSAIIC fibrosarcoma in vivo. Int J Cancer 53:118-123, 1993.
101. Chachoua A, Hochster H, Steinfeld A, et al: Feasibility of seven weeks concomitant topotecan (T) continuous infusion with thoracic radiation [abstract]. Prog Proc Am Soc Clin Oncol 18:485a, 1999.
102. Chang AY, Kim K, Glick J, et al: Phase II study of Taxol, merbarone, and piroxantrone in stage IV non-small-cell lung cancer: the Eastern Cooperative Oncology Group results. J Natl Cancer Inst 85:388-394, 1993.
103. Murphy WK, Fossella FV, Winn RJ, et al: Phase II study of Taxol in patients with untreated advanced non-small-cell lung cancer. J Natl Cancer Inst 85:384-388, 1993.
104. Akerley W, Choy H, Glantz M, et al: Phase II trial of weekly paclitaxel for advanced non-small cell lung cancer (NSCLC) [abstract]. Prog Proc Am Soc Clin Oncol 16:450a, 1997.
105. Eisenhauer EA, ten Bokkel Huinink WW, Swenerton KD, et al: European-Canadian randomized trial of paclitaxel in relapsed ovarian cancer: high-dose versus low-dose and long versus short infusion. J Clin Oncol 12:2654-2666, 1994.
106. Fennelly D, Aghajanian C, Shapiro F, et al: Phase I and pharmacologic study of paclitaxel administered weekly in patients with relapsed ovarian cancer. J Clin Oncol 15:187-192, 1997.
107. Milas L, Hunter NR, Mason KA, et al: Role of reoxygenation in induction of enhancement of tumor radioresponse by paclitaxel. Cancer Res 55:3564-3568, 1995.
108. Milas L, Hunter NR, Mason KA, et al: Enhancement of tumor radioresponse of a murine mammary carcinoma by paclitaxel. Cancer Res 54:3506-3510, 1994.
109. Milas L, Saito Y, Hunter N, et al. Therapeutic potential of paclitaxel-radiation treatment of a murine ovarian carcinoma. Radiother Oncol 40:163-170, 1996.
110. Milross CG, Mason KA, Hunter NR, et al: Enhanced radioresponse of paclitaxel-sensitive and -resistant tumours in vivo. Eur J Cancer 33:1299-1308, 1997.
111. Belani CP, Aisner J, Day R, et al: Weekly paclitaxel and carboplatin with simultaneous thoracic radiotherapy (TRT) for locally advanced non-small cell lung cancer (NSCLC): three year follow-up [abstract]. Prog Proc Am Soc Clin Oncol 16:448a, 1997.
112. Choy H, Akerley W, Safran H, et al: Multiinstitutional phase II trial of paclitaxel, carboplatin, and concurrent radiation therapy for locally advanced non-small-cell lung cancer. J Clin Oncol 16:3316-3322, 1998.
113. Reboul FL: Radiotherapy and chemotherapy in locally advanced non-small cell lung cancer: preclinical and early clinical data. Hematol Oncol Clin North Am 18:41-53, 2004.
114. Seydel HG, Creech R, Pagano M, et al: Combined modality treatment of regional small cell undifferentiated carcinoma of the lung: a cooperative study of the RTOG and ECOG. Int J Radiat Oncol Biol Phys 9:1135-1141, 1983.
115. Salazar OM, Creech RH: "The state of the art" toward defining the role of radiation therapy in the management of small cell bronchogenic carcinoma. Int J Radiat Oncol Biol Phys 6:1103-1117, 1980.
116. Warde P, Payne D: Does thoracic irradiation improve survival and local control in limited-stage small-cell carcinoma of the lung? A meta-analysis. J Clin Oncol 10:890-895, 1992.
117. Bunn PA Jr, Lichter AS, Makuch RW, et al: Chemotherapy alone or chemotherapy with chest radiation therapy in limited stage small cell lung cancer: a prospective, randomized trial. Ann Intern Med 106:655-662, 1987.
118. Perry MC, Eaton WL, Propert KJ, et al: Chemotherapy with or without radiation therapy in limited small-cell carcinoma of the lung. N Engl J Med 316:912-918, 1987.
119. Perez CA, Einhorn L, Oldham RK, et al, Southeastern Cancer Study Group: Randomized trial of radiotherapy to the thorax in limited small-cell carcinoma of the lung treated with multiagent chemotherapy and elective brain irradiation: a preliminary report. J Clin Oncol 2:1200-1208, 1984.
120. Pignon JP, Arriagada R, Ihde DC, et al: A meta-analysis of thoracic radiotherapy for small-cell lung cancer. N Engl J Med 327:1618-1624, 1992.
121. Goldie JH, Coldman AJ, Gudauskas GA: Rationale for the use of alternating non-cross-resistant chemotherapy. Cancer Treat Rep 66:439-449, 1982.
122. Goldie JH, Coldman AJ: Quantitative model for multiple levels of drug resistance in clinical tumors. Cancer Treat Rep 67:923-931, 1983.
123. Goldie JH, Coldman AJ: Application of theoretical models to chemotherapy protocol design. Cancer Treat Rep 70:127-131, 1986.
124. Goldie JH: Arguments supporting the concept of non-cross-resistant combinations of chemotherapy. Cancer Invest 12:324-328, 1994.
125. Vokes EE, Panje WR, Mick R, et al: A randomized study comparing two regimens of neoadjuvant and adjuvant chemotherapy in multimodal therapy for locally advanced head and neck cancer. Cancer 66:206-213, 1990.
126. Looney WB, Hopkins HA: Solid tumor models for the assessment of different treatment modalities: XXV. Comparison of the effect of one radiation fraction per day with multiple fractions per day (MFD) given either continuously or intermittently on tumor response and normal tissue reaction. Int J Radiat Oncol Biol Phys 12:203-210, 1986.
127. Goldie JH, Coldman AJ, Ng V, et al: A mathematical and computer-based model of alternating chemotherapy and radiation

therapy in experimental neoplasms. Antibiot Chemother 41:11-20, 1988.
128. Arriagada R, Bertino JR, Bleehen NM, et al: Consensus report on combined radiotherapy and chemotherapy modalities in lung cancer. Antibiot Chemother 41:232-241, 1988.
129. DeVita VT Jr: Principles of cancer management: chemotherapy. *In* DeVita VT Jr, Hellman S, Rosenberg SA (eds): Cancer Principles and Practice of Oncology, 5th ed. Philadelphia, Lippincott-Raven, 1997, pp 336-337.
130. Luria SE, Delbrück M: Mutations of bacteria from virus sensitivity to virus resistance. Genetics 28:491-511, 1943.
131. Ensley J, Kish J, Tapazoglou E, et al: An intensive, five course, alternating combination chemotherapy induction regimen used in patients with advanced, unresectable head and neck cancer. J Clin Oncol 6:1147-1153, 1988.
132. Joss RA, Bacchi M, Hurny C, et al, Swiss Group for Clinical Cancer Research (SAKK): Early versus late alternating chemotherapy in small-cell lung cancer. Ann Oncol 6:157-166, 1995.
133. Roth BJ, Johnson DH, Einhorn LH, et al: Randomized study of cyclophosphamide, doxorubicin, and vincristine versus etoposide and cisplatin versus alternation of these two regimens in extensive small-cell lung cancer: a phase III trial of the Southeastern Cancer Study Group. J Clin Oncol 10:282-291, 1992.
134. Bonadonna G, Valagussa P, Santoro A: Alternating non-cross-resistant combination chemotherapy or MOPP in stage IV Hodgkin's disease: a report of 8-year results. Ann Intern Med 104:739-746, 1986.
135. Merlano M, Grimaldi A, Benasso M, et al: Alternating cisplatin-5-fluorouracil and radiotherapy in head and neck cancer. Am J Clin Oncol 11:538-542, 1988.
136. Johnson DH, Turrisi AT, Chang AY, et al: Alternating chemotherapy and twice-daily thoracic radiotherapy in limited-stage small-cell lung cancer: a pilot study of the Eastern Cooperative Oncology Group. J Clin Oncol 11:879-884, 1993.
137. Arriagada R, Le Chevalier T, Ruffie P, et al, French FNCLCC Lung Cancer Study Group: Alternating radiotherapy and chemotherapy in limited small cell lung cancer: the IGR protocols. Lung Cancer 10(Suppl 1):S289-S298, 1994.
138. Gregor A, Drings P, Burghouts J, et al: Randomized trial of alternating versus sequential radiotherapy/chemotherapy in limited-disease patients with small-cell lung cancer: a European Organization for Research and Treatment of Cancer Lung Cancer Cooperative Group study. J Clin Oncol 15:2840-2849, 1997.
139. Johnson FM, Kurie JM, Peeples BO, et al: Phase I study of weekly alternating therapy with irinotecan/cisplatin and etoposide/cisplatin for patients with small-cell lung cancer. Clin Lung Cancer 5:40-45, 2003.
140. Garces YI, Okuno SH, Schild SE, et al: A phase I/II NCCTG trial of escalating doses of twice daily thoracic radiation therapy (TRT) in limited-stage small cell lung cancer (LSCLC) [abstract]. J Clin Oncol 23(Suppl):661s, 2005.
141. Lebeau B, Urban T, Bréchot J-M, et al, for the Petites Cellules Group: A randomized clinical trial comparing concurrent and alternating thoracic irradiation for patients with limited small cell lung carcinoma. Cancer 86:1480-1487, 1999.
142. Yu L, Vikram B, Malamud S, et al: Chemotherapy rapidly alternating with twice-a-day accelerated radiation therapy in carcinomas involving the hypopharynx or esophagus: an update. Cancer Invest 13:567-572, 1995.
143. Merlano M, Corvo R, Margarino G, et al: Combined chemotherapy and radiation therapy in advanced inoperable squamous cell carcinoma of the head and neck: the final report of a randomized trial. Cancer 67:915-921, 1991.
144. Merlano M, Benasso M, Corvo R, et al: Five-year update of a randomized trial of alternating radiotherapy and chemotherapy compared with radiotherapy alone in treatment of unresectable squamous cell carcinoma of the head and neck. J Natl Cancer Inst 88:583-589, 1996.
145. Milano MT, Haraf DJ, Stenson KM, et al: Phase I study of concomitant chemoradiotherapy with paclitaxel, fluorouracil, gemcitabine, and twice-daily radiation in patients with poor-prognosis cancer of the head and neck. Clin Cancer Res 10:4922-4932, 2004.
146. Benasso M, Corvo R, Ponzanelli A, et al: Alternating gemcitabine and cisplatin with gemcitabine and radiation in stage IV squamous cell carcinoma of the head and neck. Ann Oncol 15:646-652, 2004.
147. Stiff PJ, Dahlberg S, Forman SJ, et al: Autologous bone marrow transplantation for patients with relapsed or refractory diffuse aggressive non-Hodgkin's lymphoma: value of augmented preparative regimens. A Southwest Oncology Group trial. J Clin Oncol 16:48-55, 1998.
148. Scarantino CW, Rubin P, Constine LS III: The paradoxes in patterns and mechanism of bone marrow regeneration after irradiation. 1. Different volumes and doses. Radiother Oncol 2:215-225, 1984.
149. Johnson RE, Canellos GP, Young RC, et al: Chemotherapy (cyclophosphamide, vincristine, and prednisone) versus radiotherapy (total body irradiation) for stage III-IV poorly differentiated lymphocytic lymphoma. Cancer Treat Rep 62:321-325, 1978.
150. Qasim MM: Total body irradiation in oat cell carcinoma of the bronchus. Clin Radiol 32:37-39, 1981.
151. Powell BL, Jackson DV Jr, Scarantino CW, et al: Sequential hemibody and local irradiation with combination chemotherapy for small cell lung carcinoma: a preliminary analysis. Int J Radiat Oncol Biol Phys 11:457-462, 1985.
152. Bonner JA, Eagan RT, Liengswangwong V, et al: Long term results of a phase I/II study of aggressive chemotherapy and sequential upper and lower hemibody radiation for patients with extensive stage small cell lung cancer. Cancer 76:406-412, 1995.
153. Hernandez MC, Knox SJ: Radiobiology of radioimmunotherapy: targeting CD20 B-cell antigen in non-Hodgkin's lymphoma. Int J Radiat Oncol Biol Phys 59:1274-1287, 2004.
154. Chinn P, Braslawsky G, White C, et al: Antibody therapy of non-Hodgkin's B-cell lymphoma. Cancer Immunol Immunother 52:257-280, 2003 May.
155. Witzig TE, Gordon LI, Cabanillas F, et al: Randomized controlled trial of yttrium-90-labeled ibritumomab tiuxetan radioimmunotherapy versus rituximab immunotherapy for patients with relapsed or refractory low-grade, follicular, or transformed B-cell non-Hodgkin's lymphoma. J Clin Oncol 20:2453-2463, 2002.
156. Micallef IN: Ongoing trials with yttrium 90-labeled ibritumomab tiuxetan in patients with non-Hodgkin's lymphoma. Clin Lymphoma 5(Suppl 1):S27-S32, 2004.
157. Krishnan AY, Nademanee A, Forman SJ, et al: The outcome of ZBEAM, a regimen combining ^{90}Y ibritumomab tiuxetan with high dose chemotherapy in elderly patients with non-Hodgkin's lymphoma (NHL) [abstract]. J Clin Oncol 23(Suppl):576s, 2005.
158. Blumenthal RD, Taylor A, Osorio L, et al: Optimizing the use of combined radioimmunotherapy and hypoxic cytotoxin therapy as a function of tumor hypoxia. Int J Cancer 94:564-571, 2001.
159. Goldenberg DM: Advancing role of radiolabeled antibodies in the therapy of cancer. Cancer Immunol Immunother 52:281-296, 2003 May.
160. Hallahan DE, Mauceri HJ, Seung LP, et al: Spatial and temporal control of gene therapy using ionizing radiation. Nat Med 1:786-791, 1995.
161. Wang GL, Semenza GL: General involvement of hypoxia-inducible factor 1 in transcriptional response to hypoxia. Proc Natl Acad Sci U S A 90:4304-4308, 1993.
162. Connors TA: The choice of prodrugs for gene directed enzyme prodrug therapy of cancer. Gene Ther 2:702-709, 1995.
163. Levy AP, Levy NS, Wegner S, et al: Transcriptional regulation of the rat vascular endothelial growth factor gene by hypoxia. J Biol Chem 270:13333-13340, 1995.
164. Stein I, Neeman M, Shweiki D, et al: Stabilization of vascular endothelial growth factor mRNA by hypoxia and hypoglycemia and coregulation with other ischemia-induced genes. Mol Cell Biol 15:5363-5368, 1995.
165. Dachs GU, Patterson AV, Firth JD, et al: Targeting gene expression to hypoxic tumor cells. Nat Med 3:515-520, 1997.
166. Shannon AM, Bouchier-Hayes DJ, Condron CM, et al: Tumour hypoxia, chemotherapeutic resistance and hypoxia-related therapies. Cancer Treat Rev 29:297-307, 2003.

167. Cowen RL, Williams KJ, Chinje EC, et al: Hypoxia targeted gene therapy to increase the efficacy of tirapazamine as an adjuvant to radiotherapy: reversing tumor radioresistance and effecting cure. Cancer Res 64:1396-1402, 2004.
168. Pederson LC, Buchsbaum DJ, Vickers SM, et al: Molecular chemotherapy combined with radiation therapy enhances killing of cholangiocarcinoma cells in vitro and in vivo. Cancer Res 57:4325-4332, 1997.
169. Stackhouse MA, Pederson LC, Grizzle WE, et al: Fractionated radiation therapy in combination with adenoviral delivery of the cytosine deaminase gene and 5-fluorocytosine enhances cytotoxic and antitumor effects in human colorectal and cholangiocarcinoma models. Gene Ther 7:1019-1026, 2000.
170. Cunningham D, Humblet Y, Siena S, et al: Cetuximab monotherapy and cetuximab plus irinotecan in irinotecan-refractory metastatic colorectal cancer. N Engl J Med 351:337-345, 2004.
171. Bonner JA, Harari PM, Giralt J, et al: Cetuximab prolongs survival in patients with locoregionally advanced squamous cell carcinoma of head and neck: a phase III study of high dose radiation therapy with or without cetuximab [abstract]. J Clin Oncol 22(Suppl):489s, 2004.
172. Korc M, Chandrasekar B, Yamanaka Y, et al: Overexpression of the epidermal growth factor receptor in human pancreatic cancer is associated with concomitant increases in the levels of epidermal growth factor and transforming growth factor alpha. J Clin Invest 90:1352-1360, 1992.
173. Friess H, Wang L, Zhu Z, et al: Growth factor receptors are differentially expressed in cancers of the papilla of Vater and pancreas. Ann Surg 230:767-774, 1999.
174. Uegaki K, Nio Y, Inoue Y, et al: Clinicopathological significance of epidermal growth factor and its receptor in human pancreatic cancer. Anticancer Res 17:3841-3847, 1997.
175. Dong M, Nio Y, Guo KJ, et al: Epidermal growth factor and its receptor as prognostic indicators in Chinese patients with pancreatic cancer. Anticancer Res 18:4613-4619, 1998.
176. Overholser JP, Prewett MC, Hooper AT, et al: Epidermal growth factor receptor blockade by antibody IMC-C225 inhibits growth of a human pancreatic carcinoma xenograft in nude mice. Cancer 89:74-82, 2000.
177. Mendelsohn J: Epidermal growth factor receptor inhibition by a monoclonal antibody as anticancer therapy. Clin Cancer Res 3(Pt 2):2703-2707, 1997.
178. Mendelsohn J: Blockade of receptors for growth factors: an anticancer therapy. The fourth annual Joseph H Burchenal American Association of Cancer Research Clinical Research Award Lecture. Clin Cancer Res 6:747-753, 2000.
179. Prewett M, Rockwell P, Rockwell RF, et al: The biologic effects of C225, a chimeric monoclonal antibody to the EGFR, on human prostate carcinoma. J Immunother Emphasis Tumor Immunol 19:419-427, 1996.
180. Fan Z, Lu Y, Wu X, et al: Antibody-induced epidermal growth factor receptor dimerization mediates inhibition of autocrine proliferation of A431 squamous carcinoma cells. J Biol Chem 269:27595-27602, 1994.
181. Wu X, Fan Z, Masui H, et al: Apoptosis induced by an anti-epidermal growth factor receptor monoclonal antibody in a human colorectal carcinoma cell line and its delay by insulin. J Clin Invest 95:1897-1905, 1995.
182. Peng D, Fan Z, Lu Y, et al: Anti-epidermal growth factor receptor monoclonal antibody 225 up-regulates p27KIP1 and induces G1 arrest in prostatic cancer cell line DU145. Cancer Res 56:3666-3669, 1996.
183. Prewett M, Rothman M, Waksal H, et al: Mouse-human chimeric anti-epidermal growth factor receptor antibody C225 inhibits the growth of human renal cell carcinoma xenografts in nude mice. Clin Cancer Res 4:2957-2966, 1998.
184. Saleh MN, Raisch KP, Stackhouse MA, et al: Combined modality therapy of A431 human epidermoid cancer using anti-EGFr antibody C225 and radiation. Cancer Biother Radiopharm 14:451-463, 1999.
185. Perrotte P, Matsumoto T, Inoue K, et al: Anti-epidermal growth factor receptor antibody C225 inhibits angiogenesis in human transitional cell carcinoma growing orthotopically in nude mice. Clin Cancer Res 5:257-265, 1999.
186. Milas L, Mason K, Hunter N, et al: In vivo enhancement of tumor radioresponse by C225 antiepidermal growth factor receptor antibody. Clin Cancer Res 6:701-708, 2000.
187. Bruns CJ, Harbison MT, Davis DW, et al: Epidermal growth factor receptor blockade with C225 plus gemcitabine results in regression of human pancreatic carcinoma growing orthotopically in nude mice by antiangiogenic mechanisms. Clin Cancer Res 6:1936-1948, 2000.
188. Mendelsohn J, Fan Z: Epidermal growth factor receptor family and chemosensitization. J Natl Cancer Inst 89:341-343, 1997.
189. Ciardiello F, Bianco R, Damiano V, et al: Antitumor activity of sequential treatment with topotecan and anti-epidermal growth factor receptor monoclonal antibody C225. Clin Cancer Res 5:909-916, 1999.
190. Inoue K, Slaton JW, Perrotte P, et al: Paclitaxel enhances the effects of the anti-epidermal growth factor receptor monoclonal antibody ImClone C225 in mice with metastatic human bladder transitional cell carcinoma. Clin Cancer Res 6:4874-4884, 2000.
191. Fan Z, Mendelsohn J: Therapeutic application of anti-growth factor receptor antibodies. Curr Opin Oncol 10:67-73, 1998.
192. Abbruzzese JL, Rosenberg A, Xiong Q, et al: Phase II study of anti-epidermal growth factor receptor (EGFR) antibody cetuximab (IMC-C225) in combination with gemcitabine in patients with advanced pancreatic cancer [abstract]. Prog Proc Am Soc Clin Oncol 20:130a, 2001.
193. Lawrence TS, Chang EY, Hahn TM, et al: Radiosensitization of pancreatic cancer cells by 2′,2′-difluoro-2′-deoxycytidine. Int J Radiat Oncol Biol Phys 34:867-872, 1996.
194. Lawrence TS, Eisbruch A, McGinn CJ, et al: Radiosensitization by gemcitabine. Oncology (Huntingt) 13(Suppl 5):55-60, 1999.
195. Kroep JR, Pinedo HM, van Groeningen CJ, et al: Experimental drugs and drug combinations in pancreatic cancer. Ann Oncol 10(Suppl 4):234-238, 1999.
196. Pipas JM, Mitchell SE, Barth RJ Jr, et al: Phase I study of twice-weekly gemcitabine and concomitant external-beam radiotherapy in patients with adenocarcinoma of the pancreas. Int J Radiat Oncol Biol Phys 50:1317-1322, 2001.
197. Buchsbaum DJ, Bonner JA, Grizzle WE, et al: Treatment of pancreatic cancer xenografts with Erbitux (IMC-C225) anti-EGFR antibody, gemcitabine, and radiation. Int J Radiat Oncol Biol Phys 54:1180-1193, 2002.
198. Rowinsky EK: Targeted induction of apoptosis in cancer management: the emerging role of tumor necrosis factor-related apoptosis-inducing ligand receptor activating agents. J Clin Oncol 23:9394-9407, 2005.
199. Ashkenazi A, Pai RC, Fong S, et al: Safety and antitumor activity of recombinant soluble Apo2 ligand. J Clin Invest 104:155-162, 1999.
200. Nicholson DW: From bench to clinic with apoptosis-based therapeutic agents. Nature 407:810-816, 2000.
201. Kim K, Fisher MJ, Xu SQ, et al: Molecular determinants of response to TRAIL in killing of normal and cancer cells. Clin Cancer Res 6:335-346, 2000.
202. Ozawa F, Friess H, Kleeff J, et al: Effects and expression of TRAIL and its apoptosis-promoting receptors in human pancreatic cancer. Cancer Lett 163:71-81, 2001.
203. Matsuzaki H, Schmied BM, Ulrich A, et al: Combination of tumor necrosis factor-related apoptosis-inducing ligand (TRAIL) and actinomycin D induces apoptosis even in TRAIL-resistant human pancreatic cancer cells. Clin Cancer Res 7:407-414, 2001.
204. Nagane M, Pan G, Weddle JJ, et al: Increased death receptor 5 expression by chemotherapeutic agents in human gliomas causes synergistic cytotoxicity with tumor necrosis factor-related apoptosis-inducing ligand in vitro and in vivo. Cancer Res 60:847-853, 2000.
205. Lacour S, Hammann A, Wotawa A, et al: Anticancer agents sensitize tumor cells to tumor necrosis factor-related apoptosis-inducing ligand-mediated caspase-8 activation and apoptosis. Cancer Res 61:1645-1651, 2001.
206. Nimmanapalli R, Perkins CL, Orlando M, et al: Pretreatment with paclitaxel enhances apo-2 ligand/tumor necrosis factor-related apoptosis-inducing ligand-induced apoptosis of prostate cancer cells by inducing death receptors 4 and 5 protein levels. Cancer Res 61:759-763, 2001.

207. Keane MM, Ettenberg SA, Nau MM, et al: Chemotherapy augments TRAIL-induced apoptosis in breast cell lines. Cancer Res 59:734-741, 1999.
208. Gliniak B, Le T: Tumor necrosis factor-related apoptosis-inducing ligand's antitumor activity in vivo is enhanced by the chemotherapeutic agent CPT-11. Cancer Res 59:6153-6158, 1999.
209. Zisman A, Ng C-P, Pantuck AJ, et al: Actinomycin D and gemcitabine synergistically sensitize androgen-independent prostate cancer cells to Apo2L/TRAIL-mediated apoptosis. J Immunother 24:459-471, 2001.
210. Chinnaiyan AM, Prasad U, Shankar S, et al: Combined effect of tumor necrosis factor-related apoptosis-inducing ligand and ionizing radiation in breast cancer therapy. Proc Natl Acad Sci U S A 97:1754-1759, 2000.
211. Griffith TS, Rauch CT, Smolak PJ, et al: Functional analysis of TRAIL receptors using monoclonal antibodies. J Immunol 162:2597-2605, 1999.
212. Ichikawa K, Liu W, Zhao L, et al: Tumoricidal activity of a novel anti-human DR5 monoclonal antibody without hepatocyte cytotoxicity. Nat Med 7:954-960, 2001.
213. Buchsbaum DJ, Zhou T, Grizzle WE, et al: Antitumor efficacy of TRA-8 anti-DR5 monoclonal antibody alone or in combination with chemotherapy and/or radiation therapy in a human breast cancer model. Clin Cancer Res 9(Pt 1):3731-3741, 2003.
214. Fiveash JB, Gillespie GY, Buchsbaum DJ: Enhancement of glioma radiation therapy and chemotherapy response with targeted antibody therapy against death receptor 5 [abstract]. Int J Radiat Oncol Biol Phys 60(Suppl):S174, 2004.

CHAPTER 5

BIOLOGICALS AND THEIR INTERACTIONS WITH RADIATION

Carolyn I. Sartor, David Raben, and Bert O'Neil

Advances in oncology during the past decade have generated an era of molecularly targeted therapeutics. Improved understanding of the molecular mechanisms underlying malignant processes has allowed the development of novel therapeutic agents that target specific cellular processes. Molecularly targeted therapeutic agents, or *biologicals,* encompass a class of agents that have been developed to specifically interfere with functions central to the pathophysiology of the malignant phenotype. Several biologic modifiers have now been approved for clinical use, and more are in the final stages of testing (Table 5-1).

Although initially targeted in the single-agent setting and then in combination with chemotherapy, many of these biologic pathways also are central to radiation response, which raises the likelihood that some of these agents may be effective radiosensitizers. This has been shown to be the case in model systems, and it has been demonstrated clinically with cetuximab. Radiation oncologists should become familiar with therapies that their patients are likely to be receiving. The potential for radiosensitization mandates awareness of the potential for these agents to exacerbate toxicity or improve efficacy in the standard radiotherapy setting. The potential to take advantage of the new biologicals as radiosensitizers offers an exciting opportunity to improve local control for many tumor types treated with primary or adjuvant radiotherapy. In this chapter, we discuss a few representative biologicals that appear most promising for development in the context of radiation therapy.

EPIDERMAL GROWTH FACTOR RECEPTOR FAMILY INHIBITORS

Epidermal Growth Factor Receptor Family Biology

The epidermal growth factor receptor (EGFR) family of receptors regulates mesenchymal-epithelial interactions during growth and development, transmitting extracellular cues to intracellular signaling cascades.[8-10] The family has four known members: EGFR, HER2 (ERBB2), HER3 (ERBB3), and HER4 (ERBB4). These membrane-spanning tyrosine kinase receptors contain an extracellular ligand-binding domain, a transmembrane domain, and an intracellular tyrosine kinase domain. The receptors are normally quiescent, but they are activated when ligand binds to the extracellular domain of a receptor monomer. Ligand-binding induces a structural change that favors dimerization with a same (homodimer) or different (heterodimer) member of the family. When dimerized, the tyrosine kinase domains are activated and phosphorylate key tyrosine residues in the intracellular domain. Phosphorylation induces recruitment of scaffolding and signaling proteins to the cytoplasmic domain of the receptors, resulting in activation of several signaling cascades.

The end result of receptor activation—proliferation, differentiation, migration, or survival signaling—depends on many factors, including which receptor pairs are formed and for how long they are activated.[11] This, in turn, depends on which receptors are predominantly present in the cell and which ligand is involved in activation. Two complicated ligand families can activate the EGFR family receptors: the epidermal growth factor (EGF)–like and heregulin (neuregulin) families.[12,13] The EGF-like family includes EGF, transforming growth factor-α (TGF-α), amphiregulin, betacellulin, and heparin-binding epidermal growth factor–like growth factor (HB-EGF). The heregulin family includes many proteins resulting from splice variations of two different genes, all designated as heregulin with different subtypes. The ligands exhibit preference for particular receptors and induce different receptor combinations (Fig. 5-1A). For instance, EGF activates predominantly EGFR:EGFR homodimers, particularly if HER2 is not highly expressed, whereas heregulin B1 activates preferentially HER2:HER3 heterodimers. Different tissue environments may influence different outcomes, depending on the ligand milieu. HER2 has no known ligand. Instead, HER2 is the favored partner of the other receptors when ligand binds to EGFR, HER3, or HER4.[14] This complex interplay of receptors is important for understanding and interpreting the effect of an inhibitor of a single member of the family.

The effect of receptor activation also depends on which downstream signals are activated. EGFR family members signal by a diverse network of signal transduction pathways, including the protein kinase C (PKC), RAS-RAF-ERK, PI3K-AKT, and STAT pathways (see Fig. 5-1B).[15] Different receptor pairs recruit different downstream effectors. For instance, HER3 contains multiple phosphatidylinositol-3-kinase (PI3K)–binding motifs, resulting in strong signaling by means of PI3K, which plays a role in cell survival, invasion, and proliferation. HER3 alone among the receptors has an inefficient kinase domain, requiring heterodimerization with other family members to become phosphorylated. The need for heterodimerization juxtaposes the PI3K signal emanating from HER3 with the RAS-RAF-ERK or STAT signal emanating from EGFR, HER2, or HER4.

Epidermal Growth Factor Receptor Family and Tumor Pathogenesis

In 1986, the Nobel Prize was awarded to Stanley Cohen for the discovery of growth factors, resulting from his work identifying EGF and its receptor.[16] EGFR was first identified as a proto-oncogene due to homology to the avian erythroblastosis (*ERB*) oncogene.[17] Aberrant function of EGFR or HER2 occurs frequently in human tumors; gene amplification results in massive overexpression in a proportion of gliomas and breast cancers.[18-20] Alternatively, dysregulation also occurs at more modest levels of expression when the receptor is activated due to autocrine stimulation, by which the tumor produces its own ligand to activate the receptor. This type of dysregulation occurs frequently in head and neck cancer, gastrointestinal malignancies, and prostate cancer.[21-24] Another mechanism of dysregulation is the development of mutations in the kinase domain that render the kinase activity more potent, as has been evidenced in lung cancer.[25] Likewise, mutations in the ligand binding domain can cause the receptor to be constitu-

Table 5-1 FDA-Approved Biologic Modifiers

Agent	Class	Approved Indication	Toxicity	Reference
Herceptin (trastuzumab)	HER2 MAb	HER2-overexpressing metastatic breast cancer	Cardiac	1
Erbitux (cetuximab)	EGFR MAb	Irinotecan-refractory metastatic colorectal cancer	Anaphylaxis, rash	2
Iressa (gefitinib)	EGFR TKI	Chemotherapy-refractory NSCLC	Rash, diarrhea	3
Tarceva (erlotinib)	EGFR TKI	Chemotherapy-refractory NSCLC	Rash, diarrhea	Unpublished data
Avastin (bevacizumab)	VEGFR MAb	Colon cancer	Hemorrhage	4
Velcade (bortezomib)	Proteasome inhibitor	Chemotherapy-refractory multiple myeloma	Neutropenia, neuropathy	5
Gleevec (imatinib)	*BCR-ABL* TKI	First-line and interferon-refractory CML	Myelosuppression	6, 7

BCR-ABL, tyrosine kinase oncogene, the product of the t(9;22) Philadelphia translocation; CML, chronic myeloid leukemia; EGFR, epidermal growth factor receptor; MAb, monoclonal antibody; NSCLC, non–small cell lung cancer; TKI, tyrosine kinase inhibitor; VEGFR, vascular endothelial growth factor receptor.

Table 5-2 Epidermal Growth Factor Receptor Family Inhibitors in Clinical Development

Generic and Trade Names of Inhibitors	Type of Inhibitor	EGFR Targets
Cetuximab (Erbitux, C225)	Antibody	EGFR
Trastuzumab (Herceptin)	Antibody	HER2
2C4	Antibody	HER2
ABX-EGF	Antibody	EGFR
h-R3	Antibody	EGFR
EMD-7200	Antibody	EGFR
Gefitinib (Iressa, ZD1839)	TKI	EGFR
Erlotinib HCl (Tarceva, OSI-774)	TKI	EGFR
Lapatinib (GW572106)	TKI	EGFR/HER2
PKI-166	TKI	EGFR/HER2
CI-1033	TKI	EGFR/HER2/HER3/HER4

EGFR, epidermal growth factor receptor; TKI, tyrosine kinase inhibitor.

tively active even in the absence of ligand, as occurs in a significant proportion of gliomas.[26] Dysregulation by mechanisms other than amplification may not always result in overexpression as detected by standard immunohistochemistry, raising the issue of how best to identify all tumors in which EGFR dysregulation promotes tumor proliferation and resistance to therapy.

Epidermal Growth Factor Receptor Family Inhibitors

Frequent dysregulation of the EGFR family in tumors makes it an attractive target, promoting remarkable progress in the development of EGFR family inhibitors.[27] Both antibodies directed against the extracellular domains of EGFR and HER2 and small molecular tyrosine kinase inhibitors are in various stages of development.[28] Table 5-2 lists the primary EGFR family inhibitors undergoing clinical testing.

The first EGFR family targeted agent to be approved for clinical use was the HER2-specific antibody, trastuzumab (Herceptin, Genentech, Inc., South San Francisco, CA). Herceptin binds to the extracellular domain of HER2, enhancing receptor downregulation, but its major efficacy may result from immune-mediated cytotoxicity, perhaps by "tagging" HER2 overexpressing cells.[29,30] Herceptin is approved as a single agent or in combination with paclitaxel for metastatic, HER2-overexpressing breast cancer, and it is being investigated for approval for use in the adjuvant setting. Herceptin is only effective when HER2 is highly overexpressed due to gene amplification (20% to 25% of breast cancers); Herceptin is not indicated for treatment of tumors that do not overexpress HER2. The primary toxicity of Herceptin was unanticipated. Initial studies demonstrated low toxicity rates, but when Herceptin was investigated in combination with anthracycline-based chemotherapy, an unexpectedly high incidence of congestive heart failure was observed.[31] Subsequent studies have not clearly elucidated the mechanism, but one hypothesis is that HER2 may be involved in recovery from anthracycline-induced cardiac stress. HER2-knockout mice have defects in cardiac and neural development.[32] Although neurotoxicity has not been reported with Herceptin, there is a distinct possibility that addition of Herceptin to radiotherapy may increase cardiac or central nervous system toxicity. While the effects of radiation and Herceptin on cardiotoxicity are being evaluated to some extent in the ongoing adjuvant breast cancer trials, many patients are receiving concurrent Herceptin and palliative radiotherapy in an unmonitored setting. An ongoing registry may help to evaluate toxicity in patients receiving Herceptin and radiotherapy in nontrial settings.

Cetuximab (Erbitux, ImClone Systems, Inc., New York, NY) is an anti-EGFR monoclonal antibody that binds to the extracellular domain of EGFR, interfering with ligand binding and therefore dimerization and activation.[33] Like Herceptin, Erbitux has modest activity as a single agent, but it is more impressive when combined with cytotoxic therapy. Erbitux is

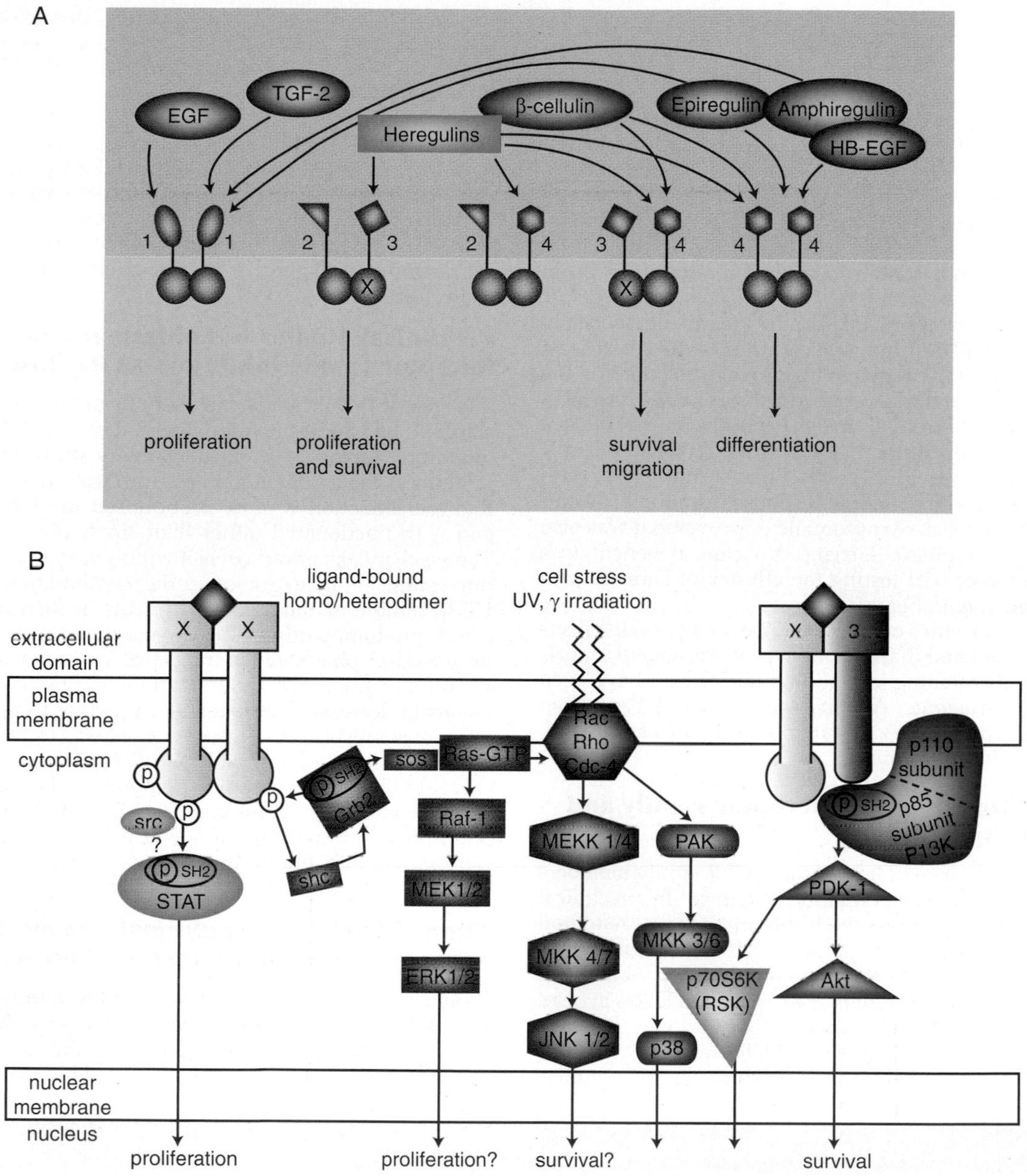

Figure 5-1 Epidermal growth factor receptor (EGFR) family activation and signaling. The receptors are activated when ligand binds to the extracellular domain, inducing dimerization. Two large ligand families (i.e., EGF and heregulin) elicit specificity due to the preference of individual ligands to bind to one or more of the receptors, inducing various dimer combinations and durations of activation (**A**). Depending on the composition of the receptor dimer, activation of the tyrosine kinase phosphorylates and activates signaling intermediaries, resulting in complex signaling cascades and diverse outcomes (**B**).

delivered intravenously on a weekly schedule. On the basis of a trial enrolling 329 patients randomized to receive cetuximab plus irinotecan or cetuximab alone, Erbitux is approved for use in irinotecan-refractory metastatic colorectal cancer as a single agent or in combination with irinotecan.[2] The response rates were higher with combination therapy than with monotherapy, as was median time to progression (4.1 versus 1.5 months) and median survival (8.6 versus 6.9 months). Unlike Herceptin, Erbitux demonstrates no cardiotoxicity. The primary toxicity of Erbitux is a skin reaction, which occasionally can limit treatment. As with Herceptin, this toxicity was not anticipated from animal studies; however, because EGFR was known to be expressed in the epidermis and hair follicles, this toxicity was not entirely unexpected.

Two small-molecule tyrosine kinase inhibitors have been approved. Gefitinib (Iressa, AstraZeneca, Wilmington, DE) and erlotinib (Tarceva, OSI Pharmaceuticals/Genentech, South San Francisco, CA) specifically inhibit the tyrosine kinase activity of EGFR, while relatively sparing the other EGFR family members and related tyrosine kinases. Iressa is approved for use in locally advanced or metastatic non–small cell lung cancer after failure of platinum-based and docetaxel chemotherapy. Its use is based on an objective response rate of 10.6%, with a median response duration of 7 months in a setting in which no other drug demonstrated efficacy.[3] The expedited approval requires additional evaluation of efficacy and evidence of clinically meaningful improvement. Combined treatment with cytotoxic chemotherapy has not shown to be better than monotherapy.[34,35] The decision to approve Iressa was based in part on significant response rates in a small subset of patients. Further investigation revealed that these patients' tumors contained mutations in the kinase domain of the EGFR, rendering it highly susceptible to inhibition by Iressa.[25,36] The mutations were found predominantly in female nonsmokers with adenocarcinoma. Whether screening for kinase domain mutations will be an effective means of selecting patients likely to benefit from Iressa remains to be proved. A more controversial question is whether patients whose tumors do not contain a mutation should be given Iressa.

Tarceva has been approved for the treatment of locally advanced non–small cell lung cancer after failure of at least one prior chemotherapy regimen. Approval was based on the results of a randomized trial comparing Tarceva with placebo. The median overall survival was 6.7 months in the Tarceva group and 4.7 months in the placebo group ($P < .001$). The 1-year survival rate was 31.2% with Tarceva and 21.5% with placebo ($P < .001$), with a median response duration of 34 and 16 weeks, respectively.[37] Symptomatic improvement was also demonstrated in a phase II trial.[36] No clinical benefit was observed in another trial testing the efficacy of Tarceva with platinum-based chemotherapy.

The primary toxicities of Iressa and Tarceva are skin effects (similar to Erbitux) and diarrhea. However, infrequent reports of serious, life-threatening interstitial lung disease have been reported for both agents. Anaphylactic reactions have been reported with Erbitux in 3% of patients, and they can be fatal. Careful monitoring is required.

Epidermal Growth Factor Receptor Family and Radiation Response

Several lines of evidence indicated that EGFR family members play an important role in radiation response. In preclinical studies, cells made to express the ERBB protein were rendered radioresistant.[38] Similarly, breast cancer cell lines become more radioresistant when made to overexpress HER2.[39] Likewise, radioresistance correlates with EGFR expression levels in head and neck cancer cells.[40-42]

Clinical studies also suggest that EGFR family dysregulation influences radiation response. A study of 170 gliomas treated with primary radiotherapy demonstrated lower response rates in tumors that overexpressed EGFR; the response rate was 33% for patients with EGFR-negative tumors, 18% for those with EGFR-intermediate tumors, and 9% for those with EGFR-positive tumors.[43] In smaller series of head and neck cancer patients, locoregional recurrence after radiotherapy was associated with EGFR overexpression.[44,45] A case-control series of breast cancer patients with in-breast tumor recurrence after breast-conserving surgery and radiotherapy found that the proportion of patients with HER2 overexpression was higher in the recurrence group than in the control group.[46]

Preclinical Studies of Epidermal Growth Factor Receptor Family Inhibitors as Radiosensitizers

The role of EGFR family members in radiation response was clarified by studies using newly developed EGFR family inhibitors (Table 5-3). In virtually every study, EGFR or HER2 inhibitors have demonstrated modest radiosensitization. Radiosensitization is more pronounced in vivo than in vitro and with fractionated rather than single-dose irradiation.[47-50] The mechanisms of radiosensitization are proving to be quite interesting.[51-53] In every case, the combination of EGFR or HER2 inhibitors and radiation results in increased cell cycle arrest, predominantly in the G_1 phase, but with a substantial decrease in S phase, which translates in vivo to decreased proliferation. Radiosensitization with EGFR family inhibitors also results in decreased angiogenesis. Whether this is an additive effect of combined antiangiogenesis effects from radiation and EGFR inhibitors or the EGFR inhibitors further increase the susceptibility of the vascular elements of the tumor to radiation is not clear. The combination of EGFR inhibitors and radiation increases apoptosis in some models. Intriguing results indicate that EGFR inhibitors may directly interfere with repair of radiation-induced DNA damage.

Clinical Studies of Epidermal Growth Factor Receptor Family Inhibitors as Radiosensitizers

Promising preclinical studies with EGFR family inhibitors as radiosensitizers have prompted a number of clinical studies, many of which are ongoing. The most mature is a phase III trial that compared the efficacy of standard radiotherapy

Table 5-3 Preclinical Studies of Epidermal Growth Factor Receptor Family Inhibitors

Agent	Model	Result	Reference
Iressa	Colorectal cancer (LoVo) xenografts	Significantly better growth inhibition with combination	54
Iressa	Glioblastoma (U251) cell line	In vitro radiosensitization	55
Iressa	Colon cancer (GEO) xenografts	Durable tumor regression; significantly improved survival	56
Iressa	Vulvar cancer (A431) xenograft	Greater than additive effects on tumor growth delay	57
Iressa	NSCLC (A549) xenografts	Additive tumor growth delay with Iressa plus radiation therapy; significantly improved with addition of antiangiogenic agent	58
Iressa	HNSCC (SCC-1, SCC-6) xenografts	Tumor regression and regrowth delay	59
Iressa	HNSCC (HSC2, HSC3) xenografts	Tumor regression and regrowth delay	60
Erbitux	Pancreatic cancer (MiaPaCa-2, BxPC-3) xenografts	Complete regression of MiaPaCa-2 with combined Erbitux, gemcitabine, and radiation therapy	61
Erbitux	Vulvar cancer (A431) xenografts	Tumor growth delay	62, 63
Erbitux	HNSCC cell lines and xenografts	In vitro radiosensitization; tumor regression	64, 65
Lapatinab	Breast cancer cell lines (SUM149, SUM102, SUM225)	In vitro radiosensitization	66
Herceptin	Breast cancer cell lines and xenografts (MCF7-HER2, SKBR3)	Tumor regression with combination	39
CI-1033	Colorectal (LoVo, Caco-2) xenografts	Significantly prolonged regrowth delay	67
CI-1033	Cholangiocarcinoma (HuCCT-1) cell line	Increased apoptosis	68

HNSCC, head and neck squamous cell carcinoma; NSCLC, non–small cell lung cancer.

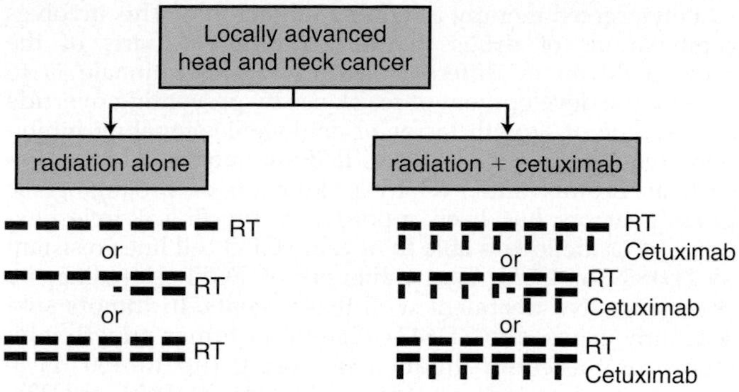

Figure 5-2 Schema of a radiosensitization trial. Patients with locally advanced head and neck cancer were randomly assigned to receive radiation alone or radiation plus weekly cetuximab. Daily, concurrent boost, or twice-daily radiation schedules were allowed but concurrent chemotherapy was not.

with standard radiotherapy plus the anti-EGFR antibody, cetuximab (Fig. 5-2). A total of 424 patients with stage III or IV squamous cell carcinoma of the oropharynx, hypopharynx, or larynx were stratified by T stage, nodal status, and performance score, and they were then randomly assigned to receive radiotherapy alone or radiotherapy plus weekly, concurrent Erbitux. Radiotherapy was delivered using one of three fractionation regimens (stratified): once daily (2 Gy × 35 fractions over 7 weeks), twice daily (1.2 Gy × 60 to 64 fractions over 5 to 5.5 weeks), or concomitant boost (1.8 Gy × 30 fractions, with a second daily fraction of 1.5 Gy for the last 12 treatment days over 6 weeks). Concurrent chemotherapy was not allowed. The 2-year local control rate was 56% in the radiotherapy plus Erbitux arm, compared with 48% in the radiotherapy-alone arm, with a median duration of local control of 36 versus 19 months, respectively (P = .02). Remarkably, overall survival was also significantly enhanced with the combined therapy; the 3-year survival rate was 57% for the radiotherapy plus Erbitux arm, compared with 44% for the radiotherapy-alone arm, with a median survival of 54 versus 28 months, respectively (P = .02). The improvement in outcome was associated with an increase in acute skin toxicity, but not mucosal toxicity. Although not necessarily defining the appropriateness of addition of Erbitux to the current standard of chemoradiotherapy for head and neck cancer, the results of this trial prove that EGFR inhibitors can effectively radiosensitize at least a subset of head and neck cancers. The results of ongoing trials testing EGFR family inhibitors as radiosensitizers for other disease sites are eagerly awaited.

ANGIOGENESIS INHIBITORS

Angiogenesis and Tumor Pathogenesis

All tumors require development or expansion of blood vessels to promote further tumor growth and nutritional support beyond the initial 2 mm diameter.[69] Molecules such as vascular endothelial growth factor (VEGF) mediate stimulation of angiogenic signaling and neovascularization. Elevated levels of specific isoforms of VEGF and other indirect markers predict for a worse prognosis in many different types of cancers, including those of the gastrointestinal tract such as pancreas and esophageal cancer.[70,71] VEGF expression is affected by the genetic aberrancies of the particular cancer and by microenvironment changes, including hypoxia.

After VEGF binding activates VEGF receptor signaling, a cascade of transcriptional signals to promote blood vessel formation is set in motion. Tumors develop a nutritional support system by borrowing existing blood vessels, growing new vessels from surrounding endothelium, and entrapping circulating endothelial stem cells. In contrast to mature vessels, developing tumors display vessels that are immature and chaotic, with a resultant lack of cohesion within the vessel matrix. As a result of increased permeability, blood perfusion through the tumor can be heterogeneous. This can lead to areas of hypoxia, which results in activation of proangiogenic molecules such as HIF1A and NF-κB. Transcriptional activation occurs with further production of VEGF and additional proangiogenic proteins such as cyclooxygenase-2 (COX-2), TEK (formerly designated TIE2), osteopontin, histone deacetylase, and hepatocyte growth factor. An autocrine and paracrine cascade is created to further tumor growth and invasion.

Angiogenesis Inhibitors

A variety of approaches can interfere with angiogenic signaling. Under scrutiny in preclinical and clinical studies are agents that target VEGF or its associated receptors (VEGFR), endothelial cell–related integrins, angiostatin, COX-2 interference, and the tumor-related vasculature.

Three main strategies that are being considered in preclinical or clinical investigations and that provide examples of the important concepts underlying angiogenic inhibition include the use of small-molecule tyrosine kinase inhibitors (TKIs) to target VEGFR signaling, agents that directly target the tumor vasculature, or vascular-targeting agents (VTAs) that inhibit VEGF.

Zactima (ZD6474, AstraZeneca) is one of several VEGFR TKIs that hold promise, and it is in phase II clinical trials. Zactima has dual anti-EGFR and anti-VEGFR properties, making it attractive to study alone or in combination with ionizing radiation. Examples of other VEGFR TKIs in clinical trials are PTK787/ZK 222584 (orally bioavailable) and SU6668. SU6668, a broad-spectrum receptor TKI, inhibits VEGFR, fibroblast growth factor (FGF) receptor, and platelet-derived growth factor (PDGF) receptor, and it has wide activity against many epidermoid human xenograft cancer models, including glioma, melanoma, and lung, colon, and ovarian cancers.[72]

Agents are being studied that target the microtubule formation of intratumoral vasculature, destabilizing these vessels and causing a rapid necrosis within the central part of a tumor. The rationale for pursuing agents that attack intratumoral vessels is based on the premise that endothelial cells in tumors display a chaotic and rapidly expanding growth pattern that is quite different from that of normal tissues. VTAs were developed to take advantage of this difference to selectively occlude or destroy tumor blood vessels. The validity of this approach was demonstrated a decade ago.[73] In general, two classes of agents are used to target the tumor vasculature: VTAs, which use ligand-directed strategies to deliver toxins, such as to the intratumoral vasculature, and the small-molecule VTAs, which exploit the differences between the disorganized immature vessels within the tumors and the surrounding mature endothelial matrix. Either approach is designed to establish an occlusive, ischemic pattern within tumors within a short period (<24 hours), resulting in extensive necrosis within the central core of the tumor. Several studies have confirmed the validity of this targeting strategy. ZD6126, a pro-drug of *N*-acetylcolchinol, binds beta tubulin, resulting in tumor vessel occlusion and central necrosis in a variety of human tumor models.[74,75]

As an alternative, inhibiting VEGF using an anti-VEGF monoclonal antibody is akin to scooping up the keys rather than blocking the lock. Antibodies against VEGF have shown anticancer activity in preclinical colorectal cancer models.[76] Bevacizumab (Avastin, Genentech, Inc.), a recombinant humanized version of a murine antihuman VEGF monoclonal antibody (rhuMAb VEGF), demonstrated efficacy in patients treated with concurrent bevacizumab and irinotecan/5-fluorouracil/leucovorin for refractory colon cancer and was approved by the U.S. Food and Drug Administration (FDA).[4]

Angiogenesis Inhibitors as Radiosensitizers

Intuitively, blocking angiogenesis from a radiation oncology perspective may appear counterproductive. If angiogenesis is inhibited, will it cause diminished blood perfusion to the tumor and resultant hypoxia? If tumors become more hypoxic, will radioresistance result? The past 10 years have demonstrated the opposite effect—enhanced radiation sensitivity.

Because hypoxia induces proangiogenic factors contributing in part to radioresistance, is it rational to inhibit angiogenic signaling to enhance radiotherapeutic response? Early work by Teicher and colleagues demonstrated enhanced radiation response to TNP-470, an antiangiogenic compound.[77] Later studies designed to inhibit angiogenic signaling in the surrounding endothelium confirmed the earlier results by Teicher, improving radiation cytotoxic effects in a variety of models.[78-82] Comprehensive reviews of combination antiangiogenic inhibitors and radiation provide pertinent information regarding the different strategies under investigation.[83,84] Improved oxygenation through stabilization of tumor vessels contributes to the cooperative effects between antiangiogenic agents and radiation.[85] Reduced hypoxia is a result. By inhibiting proangiogenic signaling, regulation of antiapoptotic proteins such as amplified NF-κB can be improved. Because many of these molecules, including VEGF, are activated by radiation, it would seem logical to reverse this process. This may prevent development of radioresistance.

The VTAs leave a viable, oxic rim of tumor remaining in the periphery. This surviving rim of tumor provides a rationale for combining these types of agents with radiation. In combination with radiation, cooperative effects were reported.[58,86,87] PTK787/ZK 222584 induced marked tumor growth inhibition in radiation-resistant TP53-dysfunctional SW480 colon adenocarcinoma xenografts when combined with ionizing radiation.[88] SU6668 inhibited tumor growth alone in C3H mice bearing SCC VII carcinomas known to express VEGF, FGF, PDGF, and their cognate receptors, and it enhanced the efficacy of irradiation.[82] ZD6474 sequencing with radiation was investigated in a xenograft model bearing EGFR TKI–insensitive NSCLC Calu-6 tumors.[89] Of the two combined treatment schedules examined—a concurrent schedule, with ZD6474 (50 mg/kg) dosing given 2 hours before the first dose of radiation, or a sequential schedule, with ZD6474 dosing given 30 minutes after the last dose of radiotherapy—the sequential approach was superior in terms of the time for treated tumors to quadruple in volume (RTV_4) from their pretreatment size ($P < .0001$). The reduced RTV_4 (30 ± 1 day) in the concurrent schedule was also significantly better than ZD6474 or radiation alone ($P < .02$).

Similar to studies showing enhanced radiation effects with VEGFR signaling interference, studies combining anti-VEGF antibodies with radiation confirmed that although exposure of human tumor xenografts to radiation promoted induction of VEGF expression, inhibiting VEGF with anti-VEGF antibodies supplanted this effect and resulted in increased endothelial cell killing and synergized antitumor effects in murine tumor model systems.[90]

Polytargeted therapy is gaining momentum. This involves combinations of drugs that target different parts of the same pathway or different pathways. The rationale is to prevent the development of resistance by preventing override of one type of growth factor or angiogenic signaling inhibition. Acquired resistance to anti-EGFR monoclonal antibodies such as Erbitux and hR3 by production of proangiogenic growth factors has been reported in preclinical investigations.[91] Ciardiello was able to develop GEO cell lines resistant to ZD1839 or C225, both inhibitors of EGFR signaling, by chronic in vivo treatment with these agents. In tumors subsequently exposed to ZD6474, significant tumor growth inhibition for the entire duration of dosing (up to 150 days) was observed; in contrast, animals bearing ZD1839- or C225-resistant tumors failed to respond after breaking animals from treatment and then again treating with ZD1839 or C225.[92] Combinations of Iressa and ZD6126, a VTA, in a human lung tumor mouse model resulted in greater tumor growth delay than either agent alone.[58] Moreover, when both agents were combined with radiation (i.e., triple therapy), tumor growth delay was optimized and was greater than with ZD1839 or ZD6126 with radiation (i.e., doublet therapy). Phase I/II clinical trials are testing this concept in head and neck and lung cancer, combining bevacizumab with Tarceva, one of the small-molecule EGFR TKIs. Siemann and colleagues provided evidence that combining ZD6474, a VEGFR TKI, with ZD6126 provided greater tumor growth delay than either agent alone in human renal cell and Kaposi sarcoma models.[93] This suggests that targeting two different parts of the angiogenic pathway may be worth testing in human clinical trials.

SURVIVAL FACTOR INHIBITORS: FOCUS ON NUCLEAR FACTOR-κB

NF-κB Biology

NF-κB is a potentially antiapoptotic transcription regulator that is constitutively active in many cancers and that may be a principal cause of de novo treatment resistance. NF-κB was first described as an important controller of immune and inflammatory responses, a property that likely stems from the ability of NF-κB to inhibit apoptosis. This finding led to study of NF-κB in malignancy, and it was found to be a potentially important inhibitor of apoptosis initiated by cancer therapies, including radiation. NF-κB is a collection of homodimers and heterodimers comprising a family of five subunits: RELA (p65), RELB, REL, p50, and p52.[94] The heterodimer made of the p50 and p65 subunits has been implicated in the ability of NF-κB to inhibit apoptosis resultant from therapeutic damage to cancer cells.

The pathway that regulates NF-κB, not NF-κB itself, constitutes the potential therapeutic target. NF-κB is likely present in all cells, but it is activated when released from a constitutively expressed repressor protein known as I-κB (Fig. 5-3). I-κB is targeted for degradation by the proteasome (i.e., proteinase complex through which most cellular proteins are "recycled" into amino acids) on specific phosphorylation and subsequent polyubiquitylation.[95] The phosphorylation of I-κB is in part accomplished by a kinase complex, I-κB kinase (IKK), which has three subunits. On release from I-κB, NF-κB dimers translocate from the cytoplasm to the nucleus, where they bind a large number of promoter elements. Important gene products that are upregulated by NF-κB are antiapoptotic effectors, including BCL2 family members BCL2L1 (BCL-XL) and BCL2A1 (BFL1[A1]); the inhibitors of apoptosis BIRC4

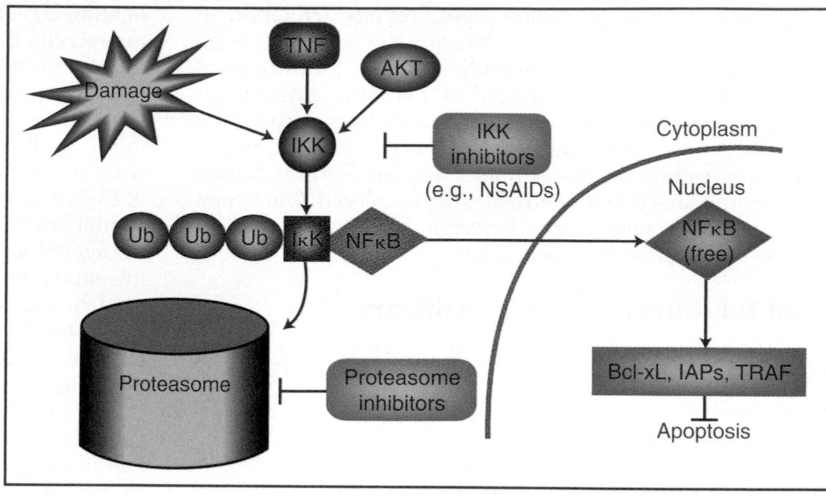

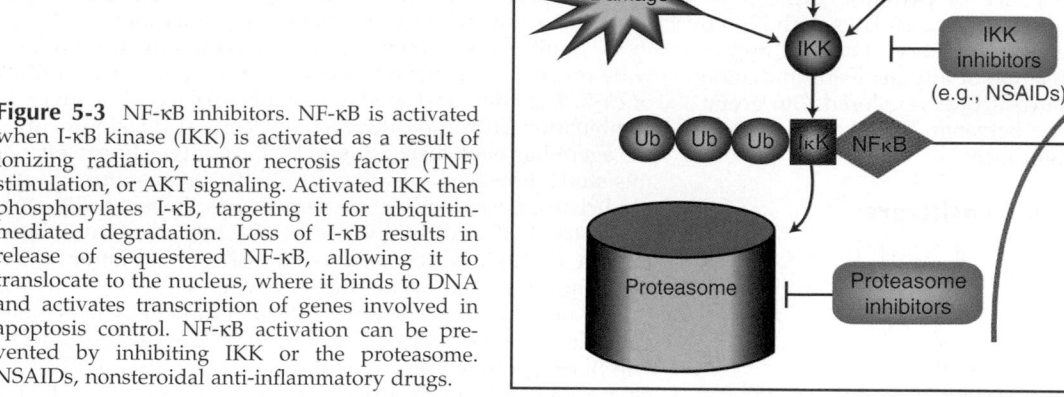

Figure 5-3 NF-κB inhibitors. NF-κB is activated when I-κB kinase (IKK) is activated as a result of ionizing radiation, tumor necrosis factor (TNF) stimulation, or AKT signaling. Activated IKK then phosphorylates I-κB, targeting it for ubiquitin-mediated degradation. Loss of I-κB results in release of sequestered NF-κB, allowing it to translocate to the nucleus, where it binds to DNA and activates transcription of genes involved in apoptosis control. NF-κB activation can be prevented by inhibiting IKK or the proteasome. NSAIDs, nonsteroidal anti-inflammatory drugs.

(XIAP), BIRC2 (IAP1), and BIRC3 (IAP2); and the apical caspase inhibitors TRAF1 and TRAF2.[96]

Various stimuli can activate IKK to phosphorylate I-κB and thereby activate NF-κB, but the mechanisms by which these stimuli activate IKK are still mostly coming to light. Adding additional complexity to the system, some signals may activate NF-κB independently of IKK, a finding with significant relevance in the development of NF-κB–inhibiting drugs.[97,98] Stimuli that can cause NF-κB activation classically involve exposure to tumor necrosis factor-α (TNF-α) but also include DNA damage (by ionizing radiation or chemotherapeutic agents) and signaling through the TNF-related apoptosis-inducing ligand (TRAIL) pathway.

NF-κB Biology and Tumor Pathogenesis

Although there are no known mutations of members of the NF-κB pathway in cancer, certain malignancies appear to be exquisitely dependent on NF-κB activity, including multiple myeloma. Myeloma and some other lymphoid malignancies are dozens to hundreds of times more sensitive to loss of NF-κB function than their normal cellular counterparts.[99-101] The reason for this dependence on NF-κB activity is unclear, but it appears to reflect a distinction between normal and tumor cells.

Solid tumors may partially depend on NF-κB activation (particularly compared with most normal tissues) due to constitutive activation of signaling pathways that activate NF-κB, such as AKT, which directly phosphorylates IKK. In a study of human gliomas, the activation status of AKT and NF-κB strongly correlated.[102] AKT is frequently dysregulated in tumors by a variety of mechanisms. Chief among these is PTEN, a tumor suppressor that acts by preventing AKT activation by means of the phosphatidylinositol-3-kinase (PI3K) pathway. PTEN loss is common in malignancy, and it is seen frequently in gliomas and in prostate, breast, and colorectal cancers. AKT activation also occurs in cancers that contain RAS mutations or contain deregulated EGFR. PI3K has been described as being mutated in a potentially activating way in almost one third of colorectal cancers.[103] It would therefore be predicted that tumors expressing active AKT would potentially be the most sensitive to NF-κB inhibition, a hypothesis that has yet to be studied in the clinical setting.

Evidence that NF-κB activation is prognostically important in patients is accumulating. NF-κB expression (determined by immunohistochemistry or DNA-binding assays) has been negatively correlated with prognosis in studies of breast cancer,[104] colorectal cancer,[105] gastric cancer,[106] glioma,[102] and prostate cancer.[107] These studies are small, however, and confirmation is warranted.

NF-κB Inhibitors

Specific inhibition of NF-κB can be achieved by the introduction of an altered, nondegradable I-κB molecule known as a *super-repressor* of NF-κB. Introduction of super-repressor I-κB into myeloma cells results in massive apoptosis. Proteasome inhibitors are another, albeit less selective, means of inhibiting NF-κB. Inhibition of the proteasome by molecule inhibitors results in cellular accumulation of I-κB by preventing its targeted degradation (see Fig. 5-3). The response of myeloma cells to proteasome inhibitors mimics that achieved with super-repressor I-κB.[99,108,109] COX inhibitors, thalidomide, and curcumin also are potential NF-κB inhibitors.[110-112]

The proteasome inhibitor bortezomib (PS-341 [Velcade], Millenium Pharmaceuticals, Cambridge, MA) was approved as single-agent therapy for multiple myeloma based on striking activity in chemotherapy-refractory disease.[113,114] Toxicities include modest cytopenias, diarrhea (or constipation), mild nausea, and occasionally significant neuropathy, particularly in patients with myeloma who have some neuropathy at baseline.[114] Several trials are investigating Velcade in combination with cytotoxic chemotherapy for a variety of solid tumors, including lung, breast, and ovarian cancers. As expected from the preclinical data, single-agent activity with bortezomib in solid tumors has been modest, although clear tumor regression has occurred.[115] The ongoing studies will indicate whether combination therapy will be more effective.

NF-κB and Radiation Response

Ionizing radiation is a classic inducer of NF-κB activity as a result of radiation-induced activation of the ataxia-telangiectasia mutation (ATM) repair protein.[116-119] It is speculated that lack of NF-κB activation in ATM deficient cells may in large part explain the radiosensitivity of ATM patients by allowing excessive abnormal apoptosis in radiation or ultraviolet (UV) light–exposed cells.

NF-κB expression in cell lines correlates with radioresistance in a number of models, including head and neck cancer cells, Hodgkin's lymphoma cells, and melanoma cells.[120-122] There is also early clinical evidence for a role for NF-κB in the radioresistance of some tumor types. NF-κB activation in esophageal adenocarcinoma has negatively correlated with response to neoadjuvant chemoradiation.[123] It has also been demonstrated that radioresistance of pediatric B-precursor acute lymphoblastic leukemia strongly correlates with NF-κB pathway activity.[124] Although this evidence of clinical importance is interesting, the correlation of any gene and radiation response is an area that is relatively underexplored. Our group is exploring the relationship between NF-κB activity and response to radiation in rectal cancer.

NF-κB Inhibitors as Radiosensitizers

In solid tumor models, inhibition of NF-κB (or the proteasome) alone results in little effect in many cell types; however, NF-κB is strongly activated by certain therapeutic stimuli, including ionizing radiation. Inhibition of NF-κB in conjunction with radiation has been shown preclinically to sometimes result in a dramatic increase in apoptosis in tumors that are relatively resistant to therapy. For example, glioma cells transfected with super-repressor I-κB were more radiosensitive than parental cell lines.[125] Similarly, transfection of a super-repressor I-κB is able to radiosensitize HT29 and HCT15 colorectal cancer cells.[126] The human immunodeficiency virus (HIV) protease inhibitor saquinavir, which also inhibits the proteasome, has been shown to radiosensitize cancer cell lines, with demonstration of NF-κB inhibition.[127] In a LoVo colorectal cancer xenograft model, proteasome inhibition by bortezomib dramatically radiosensitized tumors.[128]

Trials are assessing the radiosensitization potential of Velcade. Van Waes and coworkers at the National Cancer Institute have completed a phase I trial of bortezomib in conjunction with external beam radiation therapy for squamous cell cancers of the head and neck. In that trial, patients were treated with doses of bortezomib ranging from 0.6 mg/m^2 up to an maximum tolerated dose of 0.9 mg/m^2 (Carter Van Waes, personal communication, 2005). In that study, increases in mucositis were not observed, but hyponatremia and dehydration were dose-limiting factors, possibly reflecting the patient population. At the University of North Carolina School of Medicine, we are conducting a trial of bortezomib in combination with 5-fluorouracil and radiotherapy.

An important question pertinent to the utility of NF-κB as a radiosensitizing strategy is whether NF-κB activation is specifically protective of cancer cells compared with normal tissues. It appears that tumors may depend more on NF-κB than normal tissues, but some data indicate a need for caution. Although proteasome inhibition by bortezomib is relatively well tolerated, the drug does have the relatively narrow therapeutic index of a chemotherapeutic agent, unlike the other biologic agents previously discussed. In mice, whole-body ionizing radiation results in NF-κB activation in a variety of tissues, including nodal tissues and spleen, but no other normal tissues. However, NF-κB may play a role in normal tissue radioprotection, as evidenced by studies indicating that normal intestinal mucosa is protected from radiation damage by NF-κB[129] and that NF-κB inhibition markedly increases epithelial cell apoptosis. In the case of the head and neck trial carried out at the National Cancer Institute, there did not appear to be a significant increase in mucositis.

FUTURE DIRECTIONS

Several other classes of agents have not yet received FDA approval but have significant potential as radiosensitizers. The central role of signal transduction, DNA repair, and cell cycle control in radiation response has prompted interest in investigating agents that selectively perturb these processes in tumor cells as radiosensitizers.[130,131] For instance, the farnesyl transferase inhibitors, which block a step in the activation of RAS, are promising radiosensitizers.[132,133] Expression of activated RAS induces radioresistance, whereas farnesyl transferase inhibitor treatment results in radiosensitization in a wide range of preclinical human tumor models. Phase I trials of LY-778,123 demonstrated acceptable toxicity when given in combination with radiotherapy, but clinical development of the agent has been discontinued.[134,135] An interesting aspect of this study, however, was that RAS mutational status did not predict response, lending support to preclinical studies that suggested that RAS might not be the relevant farnesylated protein through which farnesyl transferase inhibitors exert their antitumor and radiosensitizing effects.

The next few years will see a proliferation of available targeted therapeutic agents. Maturing data from ongoing trials will likely promote the use of these agents with radiotherapy as convenient combinations or as frank radiosensitizers. However, many questions remain to be answered as we begin to embrace the potential of biologic modifiers. How do we best select patients whose tumors are likely to respond to a specific intervention? We still have much to learn with regard to accurately predicting which tumors are amenable to which agent. How do we best combine biologic modifiers with radiotherapy? In some instances, the combination may radiosensitize normal tissues, whereas in others, the radiosensitization may be quite specific to tumors. In some instances, interference with a particular radiation response pathway may result in tumor sensitivity. In others, it may protect tumor or normal cells from radiation-induced cytotoxicity. How do we best sequence chemotherapy, radiotherapy, and biologic therapy? How do we evaluate efficacy in settings where chronic inhibitor use leads to clinically meaningful stable disease but little overt evidence of response? How do we select from among the plethora of available options? How do we manage resources to make room for these expensive designer drugs? There is significant potential for these new agents to alter the practice of radiation oncology, presenting exciting opportunities to improve treatment results.

REFERENCES

1. Slamon DJ, Leyland-Jones B, Shak S, et al: Use of chemotherapy plus a monoclonal antibody against HER2 for metastatic breast cancer that overexpresses HER2. N Engl J Med 344:783-792, 2001.
2. Cunningham D, Humblet Y, Siena S, et al: Cetuximab monotherapy and cetuximab plus irinotecan in irinotecan-refractory metastatic colorectal cancer. N Engl J Med 351:337-345, 2004.
3. Cohen MH, Williams GA, Sridhara R, et al: United States Food and Drug Administration drug approval summary: gefitinib (ZD1839; Iressa) tablets. Clin Cancer Res 10:1212-1218, 2004.
4. Hurwitz H, Fehrenbacher L, Novotny W, et al: Bevacizumab plus irinotecan, fluorouracil, and leucovorin for metastatic colorectal cancer. N Engl J Med 350:2335-2342, 2004.
5. Richardson PG, Barlogie B, Berenson J, et al: A phase 2 study of bortezomib in relapsed, refractory myeloma. N Engl J Med 348:2609-2617, 2003.
6. Kantarjian H, Sawyers C, Hochhaus A, et al: Hematologic and cytogenetic responses to imatinib mesylate in chronic myelogenous leukemia. N Engl J Med 346:645-652, 2002.
7. O'Brien SG, Guilhot F, Larson RA, et al: Imatinib compared with interferon and low-dose cytarabine for newly diagnosed chronic-phase chronic myeloid leukemia. N Engl J Med 348:994-1004, 2003.
8. Earp HS 3rd, Calvo BF, Sartor CI: The EGF receptor family—multiple roles in proliferation, differentiation, and neoplasia with an emphasis on HER4. Trans Am Clin Climatol Assoc 114:315-333; discussion 333-334, 2003.

9. Yarden Y: The EGFR family and its ligands in human cancer signalling mechanisms and therapeutic opportunities. Eur J Cancer 37(Suppl 4):S3-S8, 2001.
10. Ullrich A, Schlessinger J: Signal transduction by receptors with tyrosine kinase activity. Cell 61:203-212, 1990.
11. Klapper LN, Kirschbaum MH, Sela M, et al: Biochemical and clinical implications of the ErbB/HER signaling network of growth factor receptors. Adv Cancer Res 77:35-79, 2000.
12. Olayioye MA, Neve RM, Lane HA, et al: The ErbB signaling network: receptor heterodimerization in development and cancer. EMBO J 19:3159-3167, 2000.
13. Riese DJ, 2nd, Stern DF: Specificity within the EGF family/ErbB receptor family signaling network. Bioessays 20:41-48, 1998.
14. Klapper LN, Glathe S, Vaisman N, et al: The ErbB-2/HER2 oncoprotein of human carcinomas may function solely as a shared coreceptor for multiple stroma-derived growth factors. Proc Natl Acad Sci U S A 96:4995-5000, 1999.
15. Schlessinger J: Cell signaling by receptor tyrosine kinases. Cell 103:211-225, 2000.
16. Cohen S, Carpenter G, King L Jr: Epidermal growth factor-receptor-protein kinase interactions. Co-purification of receptor and epidermal growth factor-enhanced phosphorylation activity. J Biol Chem 255:4834-4842, 1980.
17. Downward J, Yarden Y, Mayes E, et al: Close similarity of epidermal growth factor receptor and v-erb-B oncogene protein sequences. Nature 307:521-527, 1984.
18. Ekstrand AJ, Sugawa N, James CD, et al: Amplified and rearranged epidermal growth factor receptor genes in human glioblastomas reveal deletions of sequences encoding portions of the N- and/or C-terminal tails. Proc Natl Acad Sci U S A 89:4309-4313, 1992.
19. Slamon DJ, Clark GM, Wong SG, et al: Human breast cancer: correlation of relapse and survival with amplification of the HER-2/neu oncogene. Science 235:177-182, 1987.
20. Ohgaki H, Dessen P, Jourde B, et al: Genetic pathways to glioblastoma: a population-based study. Cancer Res 64:6892-6899, 2004.
21. Grandis JR, Tweardy DJ: Elevated levels of transforming growth factor alpha and epidermal growth factor receptor messenger RNA are early markers of carcinogenesis in head and neck cancer. Cancer Res 53:3579-3584, 1993.
22. Yamanaka Y, Friess H, Kobrin MS, et al: Coexpression of epidermal growth factor receptor and ligands in human pancreatic cancer is associated with enhanced tumor aggressiveness. Anticancer Res 13:565-569, 1993.
23. Spano JP, Lagorce C, Atlan D, et al: Impact of EGFR expression on colorectal cancer patient prognosis and survival. Ann Oncol 16:102-108, 2005.
24. Scher HI, Sarkis A, Reuter V, et al: Changing pattern of expression of the epidermal growth factor receptor and transforming growth factor alpha in the progression of prostatic neoplasms. Clin Cancer Res 1:545-550, 1995.
25. Lynch TJ, Bell DW, Sordella R, et al: Activating mutations in the epidermal growth factor receptor underlying responsiveness of non–small-cell lung cancer to gefitinib. N Engl J Med 350:2129-2139, 2004.
26. Wong AJ, Ruppert JM, Bigner SH, et al: Structural alterations of the epidermal growth factor receptor gene in human gliomas. Proc Natl Acad Sci U S A 89:2965-2969, 1992.
27. Arteaga C: Targeting HER1/EGFR: a molecular approach to cancer therapy. Semin Oncol 30:3-14, 2003.
28. Fry DW: Mechanism of action of erbB tyrosine kinase inhibitors. Exp Cell Res 284:131-139, 2003.
29. Sliwkowski MX, Lofgren JA, Lewis GD, et al: Nonclinical studies addressing the mechanism of action of trastuzumab (Herceptin). Semin Oncol 26:60-70, 1999.
30. Clynes RA, Towers TL, Presta LG, et al: Inhibitory Fc receptors modulate in vivo cytoxicity against tumor targets. Nat Med 6:443-446, 2000.
31. Perez EA, Rodeheffer R: Clinical cardiac tolerability of trastuzumab. J Clin Oncol 22:322-329, 2004.
32. Morris JK, Lin W, Hauser C, et al: Rescue of the cardiac defect in ErbB2 mutant mice reveals essential roles of ErbB2 in peripheral nervous system development. Neuron 23:273-283, 1999.
33. Mendelsohn J: Epidermal growth factor receptor inhibition by a monoclonal antibody as anticancer therapy. Clin Cancer Res 3:2703-2707, 1997.
34. Herbst RS, Giaccone G, Schiller JH, et al: Gefitinib in combination with paclitaxel and carboplatin in advanced non–small-cell lung cancer: a phase III trial—INTACT 2. J Clin Oncol 22:785-794, 2004.
35. Giaccone G, Herbst RS, Manegold C, et al: Gefitinib in combination with gemcitabine and cisplatin in advanced non–small-cell lung cancer: a phase III trial—INTACT 1. J Clin Oncol 22:777-784, 2004.
36. Perez-Soler R, Chachoua A, Hammond LA, et al: Determinants of tumor response and survival with erlotinib in patients with non–small cell lung cancer. J Clin Oncol 22:3238-3247, 2004.
37. Package insert Tarceva tablets. http://www.fda.gov/medwatch/safety/2005/Nov_PI/tarceva2.pdf
38. FitzGerald TJ, Henault S, Sakakeeny M, et al: Expression of transfected recombinant oncogenes increases radiation resistance of clonal hematopoietic and fibroblast cell lines selectively at clinical low dose rate. Radiat Res 122:44-52, 1990.
39. Pietras RJ, Poen JC, Gallardo D, et al: Monoclonal antibody to HER-2/neureceptor modulates repair of radiation-induced DNA damage and enhances radiosensitivity of human breast cancer cells overexpressing this oncogene. Cancer Res 59:1347-1355, 1999.
40. Miyaguchi M, Takeuchi T, Morimoto K, et al: Correlation of epidermal growth factor receptor and radiosensitivity in human maxillary carcinoma cell lines. Acta Otolaryngol (Stockh) 118:428-431, 1998.
41. Sheridan MT, West CM: Ability to undergo apoptosis does not correlate with the intrinsic radiosensitivity (SF2) of human cervix tumor cell lines. Int J Radiat Oncol Biol Phys 50:503-509, 2001.
42. Akimoto T, Hunter NR, Buchmiller L, et al: Inverse relationship between epidermal growth factor receptor expression and radiocurability of murine carcinomas. Clin Cancer Res 5:2884-2890, 1999.
43. Barker FG 2nd, Simmons ML, Chang SM, et al: EGFR overexpression and radiation response in glioblastoma multiforme. Int J Radiat Oncol Biol Phys 51:410-418, 2001.
44. Gupta AK, McKenna WG, Weber CN, et al: Local recurrence in head and neck cancer: relationship to radiation resistance and signal transduction. Clin Cancer Res 8:885-892, 2002.
45. Ang KK, Berkey BA, Tu X, et al: Impact of epidermal growth factor receptor expression on survival and pattern of relapse in patients with advanced head and neck carcinoma. Cancer Res 62:7350-7356, 2002.
46. Haffty BG, Brown F, Carter D, et al: Evaluation of HER-2 neu oncoprotein expression as a prognostic indicator of local recurrence in conservatively treated breast cancer: a case-control study. Int J Radiat Oncol Biol Phys 35:751-757, 1996.
47. Sartor CI: Epidermal growth factor family receptors and inhibitors: radiation response modulators. Semin Radiat Oncol 13:22-30, 2003.
48. Harari PM, Huang SM: Radiation response modification following molecular inhibition of epidermal growth factor receptor signaling. Semin Radiat Oncol 11:281-289, 2001.
49. Raben D, Helfrich B, Bunn PA Jr: Targeted therapies for non–small-cell lung cancer: biology, rationale, and preclinical results from a radiation oncology perspective. Int J Radiat Oncol Biol Phys 59:27-38, 2004.
50. Milas L, Fan Z, Mason K, et al: Role of epidermal growth factor receptor (EGFR) and its inhibition in radiotherapy. Heidelberg, Germany, Springer-Verlag, 2002.
51. Sartor CI: Mechanisms of disease: Radiosensitization by epidermal growth factor receptor inhibitors. Nat Clin Pract Oncol 1:80-87, 2004.
52. Raben D, Helfrich B, Ciardiello F, et al: Understanding the mechanisms of action of EGFR inhibitors in NSCLC: what we know and what we do not know. Lung Cancer 41(Suppl 1):S15-S22, 2003.
53. Schmidt-Ullrich RK, Contessa JN, Lammering G, et al: ERBB receptor tyrosine kinases and cellular radiation responses. Oncogene 22:5855-5865, 2003.

54. Williams K, Telfer B, Stratford I, et al: Combination of ZD1839 (Iressa), and EGFR-TKI, and radiotherapy increases antitumor efficacy in a human colon cancer xenograft. Presented at the American Association for Cancer Research 92nd Annual Meeting, New Orleans, LA, 2001, pp A3480.
55. Stea B, Falsey R, Carey S, et al: Growth inhibition and radiosensitization of glioblastoma multiforme by the tyrosine kinase inhibitor ZD1839 (Iressa). Presented at the American Association for Cancer Research 93rd Annual Meeting, San Francisco, CA, 2002, pp A3899.
56. Bianco C, Tortora G, Bianco R, et al: Enhancement of antitumor activity of ionizing radiation by combined treatment with the selective epidermal growth factor receptor-tyrosine kinase inhibitor ZD1839 (Iressa). Clin Cancer Res 8:3250-3258, 2002.
57. Solomon B, Hagekyriakou J, Trivett MK, et al: EGFR blockade with ZD1839 ("Iressa") potentiates the antitumor effects of single and multiple fractions of ionizing radiation in human A431 squamous cell carcinoma. Epidermal growth factor receptor. Int J Radiat Oncol Biol Phys 55:713-723, 2003.
58. Raben D, Bianco C, Damiano V, et al: Antitumor activity of ZD6126, a novel vascular-targeting agent, is enhanced when combined with ZD1839, an epidermal growth factor receptor tyrosine kinase inhibitor, and potentiates the effects of radiation in a human non–small cell lung cancer xenograft model. Mol Cancer Ther 3:977-983, 2004.
59. Huang SM, Li J, Armstrong EA, et al: Modulation of radiation response and tumor-induced angiogenesis after epidermal growth factor receptor inhibition by ZD1839 (Iressa). Cancer Res 62:4300-4306, 2002.
60. Shintani S, Li C, Mihara M, et al: Enhancement of tumor radioresponse by combined treatment with gefitinib (Iressa, ZD1839), an epidermal growth factor receptor tyrosine kinase inhibitor, is accompanied by inhibition of DNA damage repair and cell growth in oral cancer. Int J Cancer 107:1030-1037, 2003.
61. Buchsbaum DJ, Bonner JA, Grizzle WE, et al: Treatment of pancreatic cancer xenografts with Erbitux (IMC-C225) anti-EGFR antibody, gemcitabine, and radiation. Int J Radiat Oncol Biol Phys 54:1180-1193, 2002.
62. Milas L, Mason K, Hunter N, et al: In vivo enhancement of tumor radioresponse by C225 antiepidermal growth factor receptor antibody [see comments]. Clin Cancer Res 6:701-708, 2000.
63. Milas L, Fan Z, Andratschke NH, et al: Epidermal growth factor receptor and tumor response to radiation: in vivo preclinical studies. Int J Radiat Oncol Biol Phys 58:966-971, 2004.
64. Harari PM, Huang SM: Head and neck cancer as a clinical model for molecular targeting of therapy: combining EGFR blockade with radiation. Int J Radiat Oncol Biol Phys 49:427-433, 2001.
65. Huang SM, Harari PM: Modulation of radiation response after epidermal growth factor receptor blockade in squamous cell carcinomas: inhibition of damage repair, cell cycle kinetics, and tumor angiogenesis. Clin Cancer Res 6:2166-2174, 2000.
66. Zhou H, Kim YS, Peletier A, et al: Effects of the EGFR/HER2 kinase inhibitor GW572016 on EGFR- and HER2-overexpressing breast cancer cell line proliferation, radiosensitization, and resistance. Int J Radiat Oncol Biol Phys 58:344-352, 2004.
67. Nyati MK, Maheshwari D, Hanasoge S, et al: Radiosensitization by pan ErbB inhibitor CI-1033 in vitro and in vivo. Clin Cancer Res 10:691-700, 2004.
68. Murakami M, Sasaki T, Yamasaki S, et al: Induction of apoptosis by ionizing radiation and CI-1033 in HuCCT-1 cells. Biochem Biophys Res Commun 319:114-119, 2004.
69. Folkman J: What is the evidence that tumors are angiogenesis dependent? J Natl Cancer Inst 82:4-6, 1990.
70. Millikan KW, Mall JW, Myers JA, et al: Do angiogenesis and growth factor expression predict prognosis of esophageal cancer? Am Surg 66:401-405; discussion 405-406, 2000.
71. Niedergethmann M, Hildenbrand R, Wostbrock B, et al: High expression of vascular endothelial growth factor predicts early recurrence and poor prognosis after curative resection for ductal adenocarcinoma of the pancreas. Pancreas 25:122-129, 2002.
72. Laird AD, Vajkoczy P, Shawver LK, et al: SU6668 is a potent antiangiogenic and antitumor agent that induces regression of established tumors. Cancer Res 60:4152-4160, 2000.
73. Burrows FJ, Thorpe PE: Vascular targeting—a new approach to the therapy of solid tumors. Pharmacol Ther 64:155-174, 1994.
74. Blakey DC, Westwood FR, Walker M, et al: Antitumor activity of the novel vascular targeting agent ZD6126 in a panel of tumor models. Clin Cancer Res 8:1974-1983, 2002.
75. Thorpe PE: Vascular targeting agents as cancer therapeutics. Clin Cancer Res 10:415-427, 2004.
76. Ferrara N, Davis-Smyth T: The biology of vascular endothelial growth factor. Endocr Rev 18:4-25, 1997.
77. Teicher BA, Emi Y, Kakeji Y, et al: TNP-470/minocycline/cytotoxic therapy: a systems approach to cancer therapy. Eur J Cancer 32A:2461-2466, 1996.
78. Mauceri HJ, Hanna NN, Beckett MA, et al: Combined effects of angiostatin and ionizing radiation in antitumour therapy. Nature 394:287-291, 1998.
79. Gorski DH, Mauceri HJ, Salloum RM, et al: Potentiation of the antitumor effect of ionizing radiation by brief concomitant exposures to angiostatin. Cancer Res 58:5686-5689, 1998.
80. Gorski DH, Mauceri HJ, Salloum RM, et al: Prolonged treatment with angiostatin reduces metastatic burden during radiation therapy. Cancer Res 63:308-311, 2003.
81. Kozin SV, Boucher Y, Hicklin DJ, et al: Vascular endothelial growth factor receptor-2-blocking antibody potentiates radiation-induced long-term control of human tumor xenografts. Cancer Res 61:39-44, 2001.
82. Ning S, Laird D, Cherrington JM, et al: The antiangiogenic agents SU5416 and SU6668 increase the antitumor effects of fractionated irradiation. Radiat Res 157:45-51, 2002.
83. Wachsberger P, Burd R, Dicker AP: Tumor response to ionizing radiation combined with antiangiogenesis or vascular targeting agents: exploring mechanisms of interaction. Clin Cancer Res 9:1957-1971, 2003.
84. Raben D, Helfrich B: Angiogenesis inhibitors: a rational strategy for radiosensitization in the treatment of non–small-cell lung cancer? Clin Lung Cancer 6:48-57, 2004.
85. Lee CG, Heijn M, di Tomaso E, et al: Anti-vascular endothelial growth factor treatment augments tumor radiation response under normoxic or hypoxic conditions. Cancer Res 60:5565-5570, 2000.
86. Horsman MR, Murata R: Vascular targeting effects of ZD6126 in a C3H mouse mammary carcinoma and the enhancement of radiation response. Int J Radiat Oncol Biol Phys 57:1047-1055, 2003.
87. Siemann DW, Rojiani AM: Enhancement of radiation therapy by the novel vascular targeting agent ZD6126. Int J Radiat Oncol Biol Phys 53:164-171, 2002.
88. Hess C, Vuong V, Hegyi I, et al: Effect of VEGF receptor inhibitor PTK787/ZK222584 [correction of ZK222548] combined with ionizing radiation on endothelial cells and tumour growth. Br J Cancer 85:2010-2016, 2001.
89. Williams KJ, Telfer BA, Brave S, et al: ZD6474, a potent inhibitor of vascular endothelial growth factor signaling, combined with radiotherapy: schedule-dependent enhancement of antitumor activity. Clin Cancer Res 10:8587-8593, 2004.
90. Gorski DH, Beckett MA, Jaskowiak NT, et al: Blockage of the vascular endothelial growth factor stress response increases the antitumor effects of ionizing radiation. Cancer Res 59:3374-3378, 1999.
91. Viloria-Petit A, Crombet T, Jothy S, et al: Acquired resistance to the antitumor effect of epidermal growth factor receptor-blocking antibodies in vivo: a role for altered tumor angiogenesis. Cancer Res 61:5090-5101, 2001.
92. Ciardiello F, Bianco R, Caputo R, et al: Antitumor activity of ZD6474, a vascular endothelial growth factor receptor tyrosine kinase inhibitor, in human cancer cells with acquired resistance to antiepidermal growth factor receptor therapy. Clin Cancer Res 10:784-793, 2004.
93. Siemann DW, Shi W: Efficacy of combined antiangiogenic and vascular disrupting agents in treatment of solid tumors. Int J Radiat Oncol Biol Phys 60:1233-1240, 2004.
94. Orlowski RZ, Baldwin J, Albert S: NF-κB as a therapeutic target in cancer. Trends Mol Med 8:385-389, 2002.
95. Voorhees PM, Dees EC, O'Neil B, et al: The proteasome as a target for cancer therapy. Clin Cancer Res 9:6316-6325, 2003.

96. Baldwin AS: Control of oncogenesis and cancer therapy resistance by the transcription factor NF-kappaB. J Clin Invest 107:241-246, 2001.
97. Russell JS, Tofilon PJ: Radiation-induced activation of nuclear factor-kappaB involves selective degradation of plasma membrane-associated IκBα. Mol Biol Cell 13:3431-3440, 2002.
98. Lin YC, Brown K, Siebenlist U: Activation of NF-kappaB requires proteolysis of the inhibitor I αB-α: signal-induced phosphorylation of I kappaB-alpha alone does not release active NF-kappaB. Proc Natl Acad Sci U S A 92:552-556, 1995.
99. Hideshima T, Richardson P, Chauhan D, et al: The proteasome inhibitor PS-341 inhibits growth, induces apoptosis, and overcomes drug resistance in human multiple myeloma cells. Cancer Res 61:3071-3076, 2001.
100. Masdehors P, Omura S, Merle-Beral H, et al: Increased sensitivity of CLL-derived lymphocytes to apoptotic death activation by the proteasome-specific inhibitor lactacystin. Br J Haematol 105:752-757, 1999.
101. Guzman ML, Swiderski CF, Howard DS, et al: Preferential induction of apoptosis for primary human leukemic stem cells. Proc Natl Acad Sci U S A 99:16220-16225, 2002.
102. Wang H, Zhang W, Huang HJ, et al: Analysis of the activation status of Akt, NF kappaB, and Stat3 in human diffuse gliomas. Lab Invest 84:941-951, 2004.
103. Samuels Y, Velculescu VE: Oncogenic mutations of PIK3CA in human cancers. Cell Cycle 3:1221-1224, 2004.
104. Hou M-F, Lin S-B, Yuan S-SF, et al: The clinical significance between activation of nuclear factor kappaB transcription factor and overexpression of HER-2/neu oncoprotein in Taiwanese patients with breast cancer. Clin Chim Acta 334:137-144, 2003.
105. Kojima M, Morisaki T, Sasaki N, et al: Increased nuclear factor-kB activation in human colorectal carcinoma and its correlation with tumor progression. Anticancer Res 24:675-681, 2004.
106. Yamanaka N, Sasaki N, Tasaki A, et al: Nuclear factor-kappaB p65 is a prognostic indicator in gastric carcinoma. Anticancer Res 24:1071-1075, 2004.
107. Lessard L, Mes-Masson A-M, Lamarre L, et al: NF kappaB nuclear localization and its prognostic significance in prostate cancer. BJU Int 91:417-420, 2003.
108. Ni H, Ergin M, Huang Q, et al: Analysis of expression of nuclear factor kappaB in multiple myeloma: downregulation of NF kappaB induces apoptosis. Br J Haematol 115:279-286, 2001.
109. Feinman R, Koury J, Thames M, et al: Role of NF-kappaB in the rescue of multiple myeloma cells from glucocorticoid-induced apoptosis by Bcl-2. Blood 93:3044-3052, 1999.
110. Kopp E, Ghosh S: Inhibition of NF-kappaB by sodium salicylate and aspirin. Science 265:956-959, 1994.
111. Keifer JA, Guttridge DC, Ashburner BP, et al: Inhibition of NF-kappaB activity by thalidomide through suppression of I kappaB kinase activity. J Biol Chem 276:22382-22387, 2001.
112. Chendil D, Ranga RS, Meigooni D, et al: Curcumin confers radiosensitizing effect in prostate cancer cell line PC-3. Oncogene 23:1599-1607, 2004.
113. Orlowski RZ, Stinchcombe TE, Mitchell BS, et al: Phase I trial of the proteasome inhibitor PS-341 in patients with refractory hematologic malignancies. J Clin Oncol 20:4420-4427, 2002.
114. Richardson PG, Barlogie B, Berenson J, et al: A phase 2 study of bortezomib in relapsed, refractory myeloma. N Engl J Med 348:2609-2617, 2003.
115. Aghajanian C, Soignet S, Dizon DS, et al: A phase I trial of the novel proteasome inhibitor PS341 in advanced solid tumor malignancies. Clin Cancer Res 8:2505-2511, 2002.
116. Jung M, Zhang Y, Lee S, et al: Correction of radiation sensitivity in ataxia telangiectasia cells by a truncated I kappaB-alpha. Science 268:1619-1621, 1995.
117. Jung M, Kondratyev A, Lee SA, et al: ATM gene product phosphorylates I kappaB-alpha. Cancer Res 57:24-27, 1997.
118. Lee SJ, Dimtchev A, Lavin MF, et al: A novel ionizing radiation-induced signaling pathway that activates the transcription factor NF-kappaB. Oncogene 17:1821-1826, 1998.
119. Panta GR, Kaur S, Cavin LG, et al: ATM and the catalytic subunit of DNA-dependent protein kinase activate NF-kappaB through a common MEK/extracellular signal-regulated kinase/p90(rsk) signaling pathway in response to distinct forms of DNA damage. Mol Cell Biol 24:1823-1835, 2004.
120. Sahijdak WM, Yang CR, Zuckerman JS, et al: Alterations in transcription factor binding in radioresistant human melanoma cells after ionizing radiation. Radiat Res 138:S47-S51, 1994.
121. Didelot C, Barberi-Heyob M, Bianchi A, et al: Constitutive NF-kappaB activity influences basal apoptosis and radiosensitivity of head-and-neck carcinoma cell lines. Int J Radiat Oncol Biol Phys 51:1354-1360, 2001.
122. Pajonk F, Pajonk K, McBride WH: Apoptosis and radiosensitization of Hodgkin cells by proteasome inhibition. Int J Radiat Oncol Biol Phys 47:1025-1032, 2000.
123. Abdel-Latif MM, O'Riordan J, Windle HJ, et al: NF-kappaB activation in esophageal adenocarcinoma: relationship to Barrett's metaplasia, survival, and response to neoadjuvant chemoradiotherapy. Ann Surg 239:491-500, 2004.
124. Weston VJ, Austen B, Wei W, et al: Apoptotic resistance to ionizing radiation in pediatric B-precursor acute lymphoblastic leukemia frequently involves increased NF-κB survival pathway signaling. Blood 104:1465-1473, 2004.
125. Yamagishi N, Miyakoshi J, Takebe H: Enhanced radiosensitivity by inhibition of nuclear factor kappaB activation in human malignant glioma cells. Int J Radiat Biol 72:157-162, 1997.
126. Mukogawa T, Koyama F, Tachibana M, et al: Adenovirus-mediated gene transduction of truncated I kappaB alpha enhances radiosensitivity in human colon cancer cells. Cancer Sci 94:745-750, 2003.
127. Pajonk F, Pajonk K, McBride WH: Inhibition of NF-kappaB, clonogenicity, and radiosensitivity of human cancer cells. J Natl Cancer Inst 91:1956-1960, 1999.
128. Russo SM, Tepper JE, Baldwin AS Jr, et al: Enhancement of radiosensitivity by proteasome inhibition: implications for a role of NF-kappaB. Int J Radiat Oncol Biol Phys 50:183-193, 2001.
129. Egan LJ, Eckmann L, Greten FR, et al: I kappaB-kinase beta–dependent NF-kappaB activation provides radioprotection to the intestinal epithelium. Proc Natl Acad Sci U S A 101:2452-2457, 2004.
130. Ma BB, Bristow RG, Kim J, et al: Combined-modality treatment of solid tumors using radiotherapy and molecular targeted agents. J Clin Oncol 21:2760-2776, 2003.
131. Maity A, Kao GD, Muschel RJ, et al: Potential molecular targets for manipulating the radiation response. Int J Radiat Oncol Biol Phys 37:639-653, 1997.
132. Brunner TB, Gupta AK, Shi Y, et al: Farnesyltransferase inhibitors as radiation sensitizers. Int J Radiat Biol 79:569-576, 2003.
133. McKenna WG, Muschel RJ, Gupta AK, et al: The RAS signal transduction pathway and its role in radiation sensitivity. Oncogene 22:5866-5875, 2003.
134. Martin NE, Brunner TB, Kiel KD, et al: A phase I trial of the dual farnesyltransferase and geranylgeranyltransferase inhibitor L-778,123 and radiotherapy for locally advanced pancreatic cancer. Clin Cancer Res 10:5447-5454, 2004.
135. Hahn SM, Bernhard EJ, Regine W, et al: A Phase I trial of the farnesyltransferase inhibitor L-778,123 and radiotherapy for locally advanced lung and head and neck cancer. Clin Cancer Res 8:1065-1072, 2002.

PART B

PHYSICS

CHAPTER 6

RADIATION ONCOLOGY PHYSICS

J. Daniel Bourland

Radiation oncology is a physical medical modality by which radiative energy is delivered to a target volume to effect palliation or cure. An understanding of the particles and processes involved in imparting radiation energy to matter is fundamental to the clinical application of radiation to patients.

In the irradiation of a biologic system, physical and biologic events occur in the following order:

1. Physical events: Physical interactions (e.g., photoelectric, Compton, collisional) result in ionizations and radiation dose.
2. Chemical events: Ionizations result in broken atomic and molecular bonds, or chemical changes.
3. Biologic events: Changes in the chemistry of molecules mean that there are changes in biologic function (i.e., cells have improper or changed function).
4. Clinical events: Biologic alteration may result in clinical changes such as tumor regression, cancer induction, and tissue fibrosis.

MATTER AND PHYSICAL DEFINITIONS

Atomic and Nuclear Structure, Particles, and Nomenclature

Matter is made up of atomic and nuclear particles that have interaction and binding energies from 1 to 10 million electron volts (MeV). The largest subunit of an element, the atom, has a nucleus consisting of one or more protons and zero or more neutrons and a surrounding cloud of orbiting electrons. In an atom with zero net electrical charge, the number of orbital electrons equals the number of protons. A simplistic representation shows the atom to be neatly arranged with neutrons and protons in the nucleus and electrons in uniform orbits (Fig. 6-1). In reality, the atom is a dynamic structure with defined energy states for the electron orbits and the nucleus. Detailed atomic and nuclear models have been formalized.[1,2]

Neutrons and protons are the building blocks of the nucleus; hence, they are called *nucleons.* The two particles have similar rest masses (the mass of the particle at rest, when kinetic energy is zero), but different electrical charges. The neutron, symbolized by n, has no charge (neutron for neutral) and the proton, p, has a charge of +1. The electron, e, has an atomic mass about $^1/_{2000}$ that of a proton or neutron and has a charge of −1. Besides the neutron, proton, and electron, other particles exist with unique masses and properties (such as spin). These include neutrinos, pions, muons, and others. The neutrino was first proposed as the neutral accompanying particle emitted in beta decay. There has been great interest in whether the neutrino has mass. If nonzero mass is found, the cumulative neutrino mass may account for the "missing mass" in the universe, with great cosmologic implications. Some research claims to have measured nonzero neutrino mass,[3] inferred through observed oscillations in the neutron state, a significant discovery if found to be valid.

Particles are classified by their mass as leptons or hadrons. Leptons, which include the electron and neutrino, are "lightweight" particles with mass comparable to that of the electron and spin of $^1/_2$. Hadrons are heavy particles with two subclasses called *mesons* (middleweight, spin 0 or 1) and *baryons* (heavyweight, spin $^1/_2$ or $^3/_2$). Fundamental, or elementary, particles are those that have no subparts and cannot be divided. All leptons are elementary particles; however, the neutron and proton are not and are instead made up of three fundamental particles each, called *quarks,* which have been observed through high-energy physics experiments. They have positive or negative charge in integer increments of $^1/_3$, spin of $^1/_2$, and other properties with whimsical, quark-deserving names.[1] Combinations of quarks yield the neutron, proton, and all other hadrons. For instance, a proton is made of two up quarks and one down quark, whereas a neutron is made of one up and two down quarks, which explains their similar mass but difference in charge. Antimatter is real, and an *antiparticle* is defined as a particle with identical mass but opposite charge to the particle. An antiparticle for a neutral particle has opposite spin or internal charge (i.e., quark) from the particle.

Matter is held together by four fundamental forces that operate over certain ranges and with certain particles. They are the strong, electromagnetic (coulomb [C]), weak, and gravitational forces, with respective relative strengths of 10^1, 10^{-2}, 10^{-13}, and 10^{-42}.[1] Each force acts by exchange of its respective mediator particle: the gluon, the photon, the W and Z particles, and the graviton. Counting mediators, leptons, hadrons, and their antiparticles, there are about 170 fundamental and composite particles that make up matter.[1] The model in which matter consists of fundamental particles as described earlier is called the *standard model.*[1] Table 6-1 summarizes the fundamental particles in the standard model. A new theory called *string theory* is a descriptor of how quarks and other fundamental particles are assembled. Vibration (energy) states for stringlike entities give each fundamental particle its unique character.[4]

Particle mass can be expressed as the atomic mass unit (amu, $^{1}/_{12}$ of the mass of the carbon nucleus) or in units of energy by conversion with Einstein's formula, $E = mc^2$. Table 6-2 gives the symbol, charge, mass, and stability for the electron, proton, neutron, and other particles of interest.

Combinations of nucleons form a variety of nuclei and determine the physical character of an atom. The number of protons in the nucleus, Z, is called the *atomic number* and determines the chemical properties of an atom and the atom's identity as an element. The atomic number also equals the number of electrons in the neutral atom, with one electron per proton. The number of neutrons in the nucleus, N, is called the *neutron number*. Whole protons and neutrons constitute the nucleus, and Z and N have integer values. An atom's mass number, A, is the sum of its neutrons and protons. The mass number (an integer) does not equal the actual nuclear mass. Their values are similar but must not be confused. Nuclear mass is the sum of the masses of the individual particles minus their binding energies. Definitions for Z, N, and A are summarized in Table 6-3.

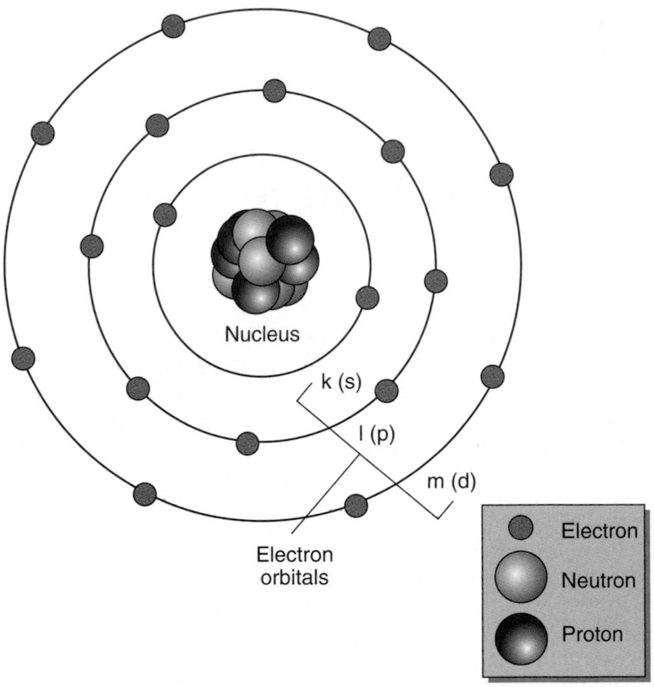

Figure 6-1 The atom has a nucleus composed of protons and neutrons. The nucleus is surrounded by a cloud of electrons in distinct energy levels called *orbitals* named s, p, d, and so on by chemists or called *shells* named k, l, m, and so on by physicists.

Nuclides and Radionuclides

Nuclides are atomic species made of different combinations of nucleons, and they may be classified by their number of protons, neutrons, or nucleons (Z, N, or A) and by their energy state. Nuclei with the same Z but different N are called *isotopes* (p for proton), and they exhibit identical chemical characteristics (they are the same elements). Nuclei with the same N but different Z are called *isotones* (n for neutron). Nuclei with the same A but different Z and N are called *isobars*. In a

Table 6-1 The Standard Model of Matter: Fundamental Particles and Mediators

	GENERATIONS I	II	III	Mediator (Force)
Quarks	Up	Charm	Top	Photon (electromagnetic)
	Down	Strange	Bottom	Gluons (strong)
Leptons	ν_e	ν_μ	ν_τ	Z (weak)
	e	μ	τ	W+, W− (weak)

Table 6-3 Atomic Nomenclature

Symbol	Item	Definition
Z	Atomic number	Number of protons in the nucleus and the amount of nuclear charge (+Z); also equal to the number of electrons in the neutral atom
N	Neutron number	Number of neutrons in the nucleus
A	Mass number	Total number of nucleons: A = Z + N

Class	Z	N	A	Examples
Isotopes	Same	Different	Different	^{1}H, ^{2}H, ^{3}H; ^{125}I, ^{131}I
Isotones	Different	Same	Different	$^{8}He_{6}$, $^{9}Li_{6}$; $^{137}Cs_{82}$, $^{138}Ba_{82}$
Isobars	Different	Different	Same	^{60}Ni, ^{60}Co; ^{137}La, ^{137}Ba, ^{137}Cs
Isomers	Same	Same	Same	^{99}Tc, ^{99m}Tc (Δ energy state)

Table 6-2 Physical Characteristics of Selected Atomic and Nuclear Particles

Name	Symbol	amu	MeV	m_e	Charge	Lifetime
Electron	e^-	.000549	.511	1	−1	Stable
Positron	e^+	.000549	.511	1	+1	10^{-6} s
Proton	p	1.007276	938.256	1836.1	+1	Stable
Neutron	n	1.008665	939.550	1838.6	0	12 min
Neutrino	ν, $\bar{\nu}$	.000000?	.000?	0	0	?
Muon	μ	.11320	105.659	206.4	−1	Unstable
Pion	±π	.14990	139.578	273.2	±1	Unstable

amu, atomic mass unit.

last category, nuclei with the same Z and N, and therefore A, but different nuclear energy states (i.e., excited vs. ground) are called *isomers*. Table 6-3 shows these classifications and example nuclides. A nuclide, or nuclear species, X, is denoted as

$$^{A}_{Z}X_{N}$$

in which X is the chemical symbol for the element with atomic number Z, N is the neutron number, and A is the mass number. Because A = Z + N, the N value is often dropped to give the following form:

$$^{A}_{Z}X$$

Because the atomic number determines the element's name, represented by the chemical symbol X, the Z is also dropped to give the form ^{A}X. An alternative nomenclature uses the nuclide's name followed by the mass number, such as hydrogen 3 and iridium 192.

Not all combinations of Z and N exist in nature or can be manufactured. Instead, certain combinations are possible, whereas other combinations cannot occur. Figure 6-2 shows the distribution of stable nuclides as a function of the number of neutrons and protons. Notice that at low Z, the ratio of neutrons to protons (N:Z) is about 1.0. Above Z = 20, stable nuclides have more neutrons than protons (N:Z > 1.0). At higher Zs, the stability of nuclei tends toward neutron-rich nuclides. It has been observed that nuclei with 2, 8, 20, 28, 50, 82, or 126 nucleons (protons and neutrons combined) are stable. These "magic numbers" relate to the filling of nuclear energy levels. Pairing of like nucleons also results in increased nuclear stability. There are 165 stable nuclei with an even number of both protons and neutrons, 57 stable nuclei with an even number of protons and odd number of neutrons, 53 stable nuclei with an odd number of protons and even number of neutrons, but only 6 stable nuclei with an odd number of both protons and neutrons.

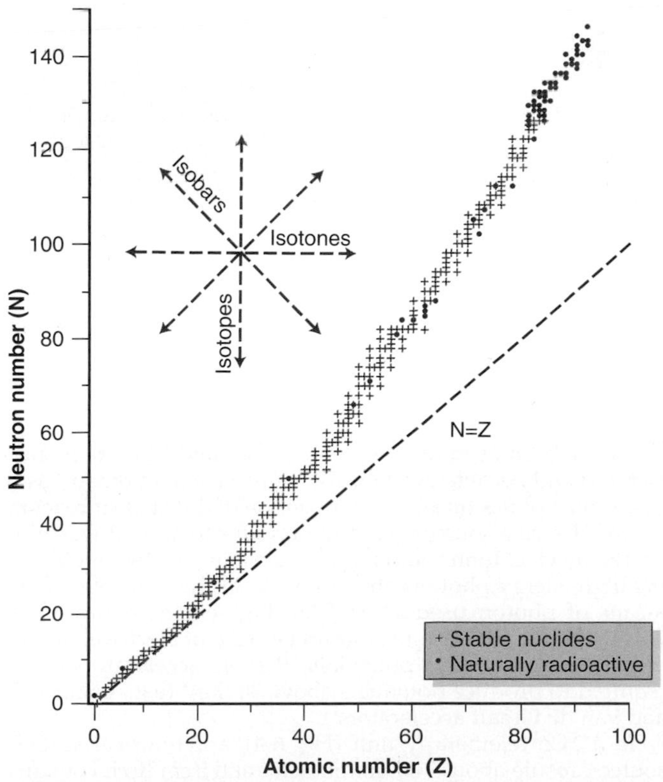

Figure 6-2 Distribution of stable and naturally radioactive nuclides. (Data from Radiological Health Handbook. Bethesda, MD, U.S. Department of Health, Education, and Welfare, 1970.)

Some nuclides are unstable and eventually transform to stable states by the emission of particles or energy. These nuclides are called *radionuclides* or *radioactive species,* because a particle or energy is given off during the nuclear transition. Unstable nuclides lie off the line of stability and will have a neutron or proton excess relative to the stable nuclide. In Figure 6-2, isotopes lie along a vertical axis, isotones lie along a horizontal axis, and isobars lie at 45 degrees to either axis, perpendicular to the line of N = Z. Modes of radioactive decay depend on the type of nucleon excess, whether neutron or proton, and are discussed later in more detail.

Stable nuclides include ^{1}H, ^{12}C, ^{33}P, ^{34}S, and ^{59}Co. Radioactive nuclides for these elements include ^{3}H, ^{14}C, ^{32}P, ^{35}S, and ^{60}Co. Other radionuclides of interest to the medical field include ^{99m}Tc, ^{125}I, ^{131}I, ^{137}Cs, and ^{226}Ra.

Photons and Other Definitions

Interactions of ionizing radiation occur at the atomic and nuclear level, where binding energies are small compared with macroscopic realms. Electromagnetic radiation, or photons, are particles that have wavelike qualities with zero mass, which transfer energy from one location to another by propagation of an electromagnetic wave at the speed of light, c ($c = 3 \times 10^{8}$ m/s). Photons are also the mediators of charged particle bonds. A photon has wavelength λ, frequency ν, speed $c = \lambda\nu$, and energy $E = h\nu$; c is the speed of light, and h is Planck's constant. The electromagnetic spectrum consists of photons with wavelength, frequency, and energy ranges over 10 orders of magnitude (the range is really infinite). From low to high energy, there are radar waves, microwaves, infrared, light (visible photons), ultraviolet, x-rays, and gamma rays. Photons are named by their wavelength (e.g., radar waves, microwaves), character (e.g., "purple"), and origins (e.g., x-rays from the atom, gamma rays from the nucleus) (Table 6-4).

RADIATION PRODUCTION AND TREATMENT MACHINES

External beam radiation treatment machines produce ionizing radiation by radioactive decay of a nuclide or electronically by the acceleration of electrons or other charged particles like protons. The most commonly used radionuclide has been ^{60}Co. Although once quite common, ^{60}Co teletherapy machines in the United States have been mostly replaced over the past 10 to 20 years by linear accelerators, which produce high-energy x-rays and electrons by electronic means. Basic components of all external beam treatment machines include a radiation source, a collimating system to form and direct a radiation beam, inherent or added shielding for protection, a control system to turn the beam on and off, a light field to delineate visibly the radiation field to be treated, a means to rotate the beam or otherwise change its direction, and a support assembly for the patient. These components are assembled for modern treatment machines in an isocentric geometry (Fig. 6-3). The isocenter is a point in space at which the treatment machine rotational axes all intersect. Any mechanical rotation is about an axis that passes through the isocenter. With many common components, ^{60}Co teletherapy units and linear accelerators differ primarily in the method of photon production: radioactive source versus electronic source.

Table 6-4 Physical Definitions

Item	Symbol	Definition
Atom	a	Smallest subunit of an element retaining the character of that element; composed of a nucleus of protons and neutrons and orbital electrons
Electron	e^-	Particle with a charge of −1 and mass of .511 MeV; used for radiation treatment when accelerated to energies capable of ionization
Photon	hν, γ, x	Particle with zero charge and mass consisting of electromagnetic radiation; used for radiation treatment at energies capable of ionizing matter
Gamma ray	γ	Photon (electromagnetic radiation) originating from within the nucleus due to nuclear transformations
X-ray	x	Photon (electromagnetic radiation) originating from within the atom due to atomic transformations
Ionization		Removal of an electron from an atomic shell, leaving the atom with a charge of −1
Ionizing radiation		Radiation of sufficient energy to cause ionization upon interaction
Ion	X^-, X^+	Atom of element X with an electron deficit, as is formed after ionization, or an electron excess
Nonionizing radiation		Radiation of insufficient energy to cause ionization on interaction
Electron volt	eV	The energy gained by 1 electron when it is accelerated through a potential of 1 V
Kiloelectron volts	keV	1000 electron volts; used to denote the energy of a monoenergetic particle or photon, as in "100-keV photons" or "10-keV electrons"
Million electron volts	MeV	1 million electron volts; used to denote the energy of a monoenergetic particle or photon, as in "1.17-MeV gamma rays" or "7-MeV electrons"
Million volts	MV	Million volts; used to denote a spectrum of polyenergetic particles or photons with a maximum energy, as in "18-MV x-rays." In this case, the x-rays have a maximum energy of 18 MeV and a continuous energy distribution for 18 to 0 MeV.

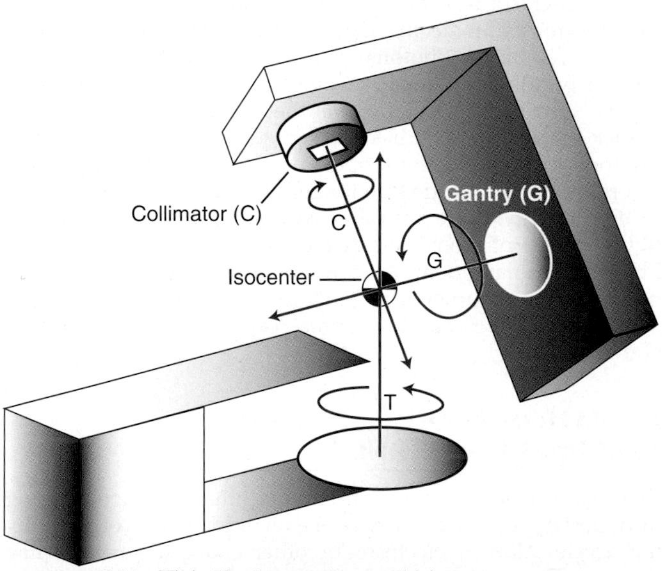

Figure 6-3 Machine geometry for treatment. Three rotational axes intersect at a point called the *isocenter*. The table surface can translate three directions for a total of 6 degrees of freedom.

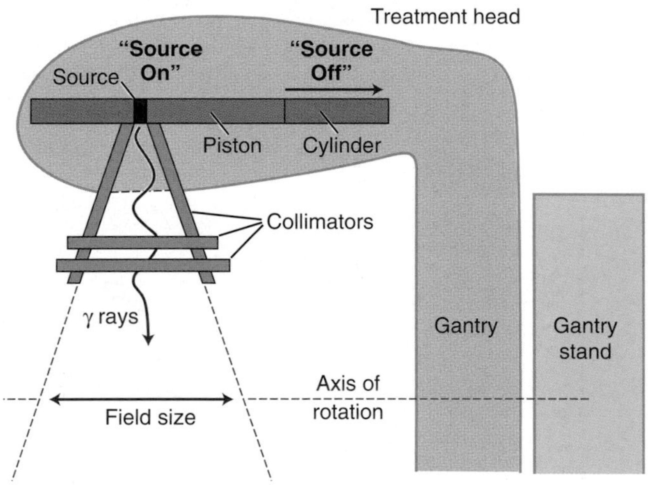

Figure 6-4 In a typical ^{60}Co unit, the source moves from the shielded position (Off) into an unshielded position (On) to produce a treatment beam.

Radiation Production by Radioactive Decay

Teletherapy is the use of radioactive material for production of a beam of gamma rays for treatment at a distance from the radioactive source (*tele,* meaning "at a distance"). The term is historical and is in contrast to brachytherapy, where the radioactive source is placed in or on the treatment volume (*brachy*, meaning "close"). Gamma rays are emitted from a daughter nucleus formed after radioactive decay of an unstable parent nucleus. Each gamma ray has a unique energy that relates to the immediately preceding nuclear transformation, and this unique energy can be used to identify the daughter (and therefore the parent). ^{226}Ra, ^{137}Cs, and most commonly ^{60}Co have been used for teletherapy. ^{137}Cs and ^{60}Co are manufactured and became available by neutron activation and as a by-product of fission after the invention of the nuclear reactor. Use of ^{60}Co as a source of gamma rays for treatment was pioneered by H.E. Johns[5] and represented a major step in obtaining high-energy photons above 1 MeV. At the time, electronic means of photon production from high-energy x-ray tubes was limited to 300 keV maximum because of electrical arcing at higher accelerating potentials. Particle accelerators were required to produce potentials above 300 keV (e.g., betatrons[6] and van de Graaff accelerators[7]).

In a ^{60}Co teletherapy unit (Fig. 6-4), a cylindrical sealed-source capsule about 3 cm in diameter and 5 cm high contains pellets of ^{60}Co. In each transformation a ^{60}Co nucleus decays to ^{60}Ni, with the prompt emission of two gamma rays at 1.17 and 1.33 MeV each (1.25 MeV average). Typical activity is 9000

Ci (3.33×10^{14} Bq) for a dose rate of approximately 300 cGy/min at 80 cm from the source (200 cGy/min at 100 cm from the source). The source decays with a half-life of 5.263 years and is replaced every 5 to 7 years when the dose rate becomes "too low."

The source is stored in a shielded head of the machine and in one configuration is mounted on the end of a movable piston in a horizontal cylinder (see Fig. 6-4). On the initiation of treatment, the source is moved pneumatically to a position over an opening in the shield that allows a treatment beam to exit. A collimator consisting of interleaved bars of a high Z material is used to define the field size as the beam exits the shield port. Trimmer bars can be used to reduce the beam penumbra, which is large because of the relatively large source size of approximately 1.5 inches. Maximum field size is $32 \times 32\,cm^2$ at 80 cm from the source. Irradiation time is measured and controlled by two independent timers. An end effect due to the mechanical movement of the source, for which the effective irradiation time is less than the timer setting, is inherent and can be measured. Cross-hairs and a field light are used to delineate the central ray and field dimensions. There is a source-to-surface indicator. Source movement is designed so that in the event of treatment termination or device failure, the source is automatically returned to the shielded condition. An emergency pushbar (T-bar) can be used to manually return the source to the shielded position, if necessary.

The machine has a rotatable gantry allowing 360-degree rotation of the source and an isocenter position of 80 cm from the source. Later models have a 100-cm isocenter. An additional degree of freedom is provided by a head swivel mechanism that allows the beam direction to be rotated away from isocenter, if desired. A beam stopper may be used to intercept the beam for additional shielding of the exit beam. The beam stop also acts as a counterweight for the head of the machine. There is a patient support assembly (treatment table) with vertical, longitudinal, lateral, and rotation motions. Beam modifiers include custom or standard field blocks and mechanical wedges for producing angled isodose distributions or tissue compensation.

Radiation Production by Linear Accelerators

In a linear accelerator, electrons are accelerated to high energy and are allowed to exit the machine as an electron beam or are directed into a target to produce x-rays by the bremsstrahlung interaction. The linear accelerator enables convenient production of megavoltage x-rays in a relatively small device, and its existence is directly related to the invention of the magnetron and the klystron during the development of radar in World War II. Linear accelerators are quite versatile, with x-ray and electron modes, multiple energies, and computer controls. These capabilities have led to the replacement of most ^{60}Co teletherapy machines in the United States with linear accelerators.

The principle of operation for linear accelerators is to accelerate electrons down a waveguide by use of alternating microwave fields.[8] Two waveguide designs exist: standing wave and traveling wave. Major electronic components are described in Table 6-5 and are shown in Figure 6-5.

Major mechanical components are similar to those for teletherapy. A rotatable gantry allows 360-degree rotation of the source at an isocenter of 100 cm to enable multiple beam directions. A set of two pairs of high Z collimators ("jaws") provides at least 99.9% attenuation of the primary beam (.1% transmission) and defines the length and width of the rectangular x-ray radiation field. A maximum field size of $40 \times 40\,cm^2$ at 100 cm (isocenter) is common, with 180-degree rotation of the entire collimator assembly about the isocenter. Collimator settings are continuously variable, and jaw pairs can be operated in coupled mode to produce symmetric, rectangular fields, or, in some machines, independently to produce asymmetric fields. Asymmetric operation may include travel of one jaw across the central axis. Cross-hairs and a field light are used to delineate the central ray and field dimensions, and there is a source-to-surface indicator.

A beam stopper may be used to intercept the beam for additional shielding of the exit beam when facility shielding is limited. Otherwise, internal counterweights provide balance to the gantry. There is an isocentric patient support assembly

Table 6-5 Major Electronic Components of Linear Accelerators

Component*	Purpose
Electron gun	Source of electrons to be accelerated
Microwave source	Provides accelerating potential and amplitude (power). Typically, magnetrons are used for ≤10 MV; klystrons are used for >10 MV and for most dual-energy machines.
Pulse-forming network	Synchronizes electron bunches with microwave phase
Transmission waveguide	Carries microwave power from its source to the accelerating waveguide
Injector	Injects pulses of current to the electron gun (i.e., drives electron gun)
Accelerating waveguide	Location of electron acceleration through multiple coupled cavities in a linear geometry (i.e., the linear accelerator)
Bending magnet	Used in horizontally oriented accelerating waveguides to redirect the electron beam, for electron energy selection, and for beam focusing
Target (for x-rays)	Placed in electron beam for x-ray production on electron impact
Scattering foils (for electrons)	Scatter electrons to produce a uniform beam of electrons for treatment
Flattening filter (for x-rays)	Flattens the highly peaked x-ray beam exiting the target to produce a uniform beam of x-rays for treatment
Monitor chambers	Ionization chambers that monitor the amount of radiation in the beam; count dose and turn machine off when set dose is reached; monitor beam flatness and symmetry
Collimators (secondary)	Provide rectangular field shaping for x-rays and set field sizes for electrons
Accessories and beam modifiers†	Define or modify beam shape or intensity
Interlocks†	With other control systems, ensure proper operation of linear accelerator for dose assurance and safety

*Components are shown in Figure 6-5.
†Components are not shown in Figure 6-5.

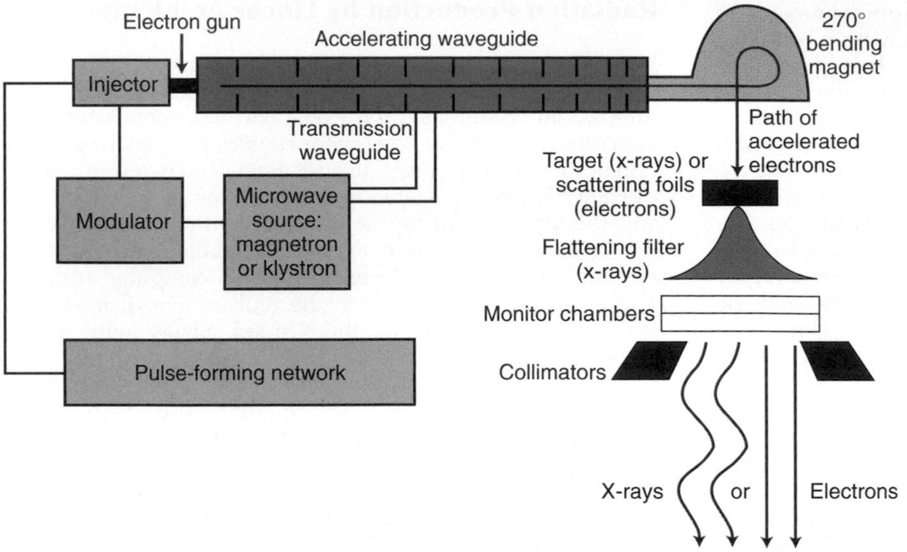

Figure 6-5 Electron linear accelerator schematic. Key components are shown that allow a beam of electrons to be accelerated, producing a treatment beam of electrons or x-rays.

(treatment table) with vertical, longitudinal, lateral, and rotational motions. Fine tolerances for the rotational axes and isocentricity of the gantry, collimator, and table are important for accuracy in patient treatments. The combined variation in rotation and coincidence of the three axes is typically maintained within a 1 mm diameter sphere. The patient support assembly is usually the most difficult rotational axis to set for isocentricity.

Accessories and beam modifiers for linear accelerators are important for customizing the external beam field to an individual patient and include custom or standard shielding blocks to shape a patient's treatment fields to minimize the amount of normal tissue treated or protect critical structures; electron applicators for defining electron fields at the patient surface; physical and "virtual" or "dynamic" wedges for producing angled isodose distributions; and compensators for shaping the dose distribution within a patient for desired dose uniformity. High Z alloys are used for custom block manufacturing, and primary beam attenuation is at least 97% (five half-valve layers [HVLs]). A newer collimator design called the *multileaf collimator* (MLC) is now available for certain machines (Fig. 6-6). MLC provides field-shaping capabilities, replacing standard hand or custom blocks by the use of a large number of adjustable high Z vanes, or leaves. The desired beam outline is shaped as a series of steps by positioning each leaf to approximate a continuous field edge (see Fig. 6-6B). MLCs also have capabilities for dynamic treatment, as discussed later for intensity-modulated treatment. Linear accelerators are becoming more computer controlled, enabling rapid setup and better-optimized dose distributions.

Three differences in radiation sources for teletherapy and linear accelerator devices are fundamental. First, a ^{60}Co source is always "on" in that radioactive decay always occurs; the source must be moved to an unshielded condition to initiate an irradiation. With a linear accelerator, no source is present until the unit is energized; the irradiation is on or off with the flip of an electronic switch. Second, their photon spectra are different (Fig. 6-7). In a ^{60}Co unit, two monoenergetic gamma rays are emitted with each decay to produce a discrete spectrum with peaks at 1.17 and 1.33 MeV. In contrast, a linear accelerator produces a continuous x-ray spectrum through the bremsstrahlung interaction. The spectrum has a maximum energy of E_{max} (i.e., accelerating potential) and all other photon energies down to zero. An average x-ray energy of approximately one-third E_{max} can be determined and is consistent with theoretical predictions for the continuous bremsstrahlung spectrum (see Fig. 6-7). Third, a linear accelerator can produce a treatment beam of electrons as well as photons. The accelerated electron beam is allowed to exit the machine under controlled conditions of scatter. Although ^{60}Co gamma rays occur because of a priori beta decay, the beta particles (electrons) are stopped by the source capsule and cannot be otherwise harnessed for treatment.

Radiation Production by Other Accelerators

Other accelerator techniques have been used to produce a variety of high-energy particles such as electrons, protons, neutrons, and higher Z ions. These techniques include the betatron,[6] van de Graaff accelerators,[7] cyclotrons,[9] the racetrack microtron,[10] and accelerators[11] used for high-energy physics experiments.

INTERACTIONS OF IONIZING RADIATION WITH MATTER

Photon Interactions

Attenuation and Transmission

When incident on matter, ionizing photon radiation undergoes interactions with atomic electrons or nuclei. Interacting photons are removed from the primary beam, an effect called *attenuation*. Photons that do not interact and instead exit the material are called *transmitted photons*. Attenuation and transmission are illustrated in Figure 6-8. A number, N_0, of monoenergetic x-rays or gamma rays is incident to a slab of material, and a smaller number, N, is transmitted. The attenuated photons, $N_0 - N$, are absorbed in the material or scattered in other directions. In narrow-beam geometry, N transmitted photons alone reach a detector as shown. In broad-beam geometry, scattered photons also reach the detector.

Megavoltage photon interaction probabilities are less than 1 and vary with incident photon energy and the atomic number of the interaction material, depending on the interaction type. By physical law, the fractional number of unattenuated photons interacting per unit thickness of a material is constant, such that

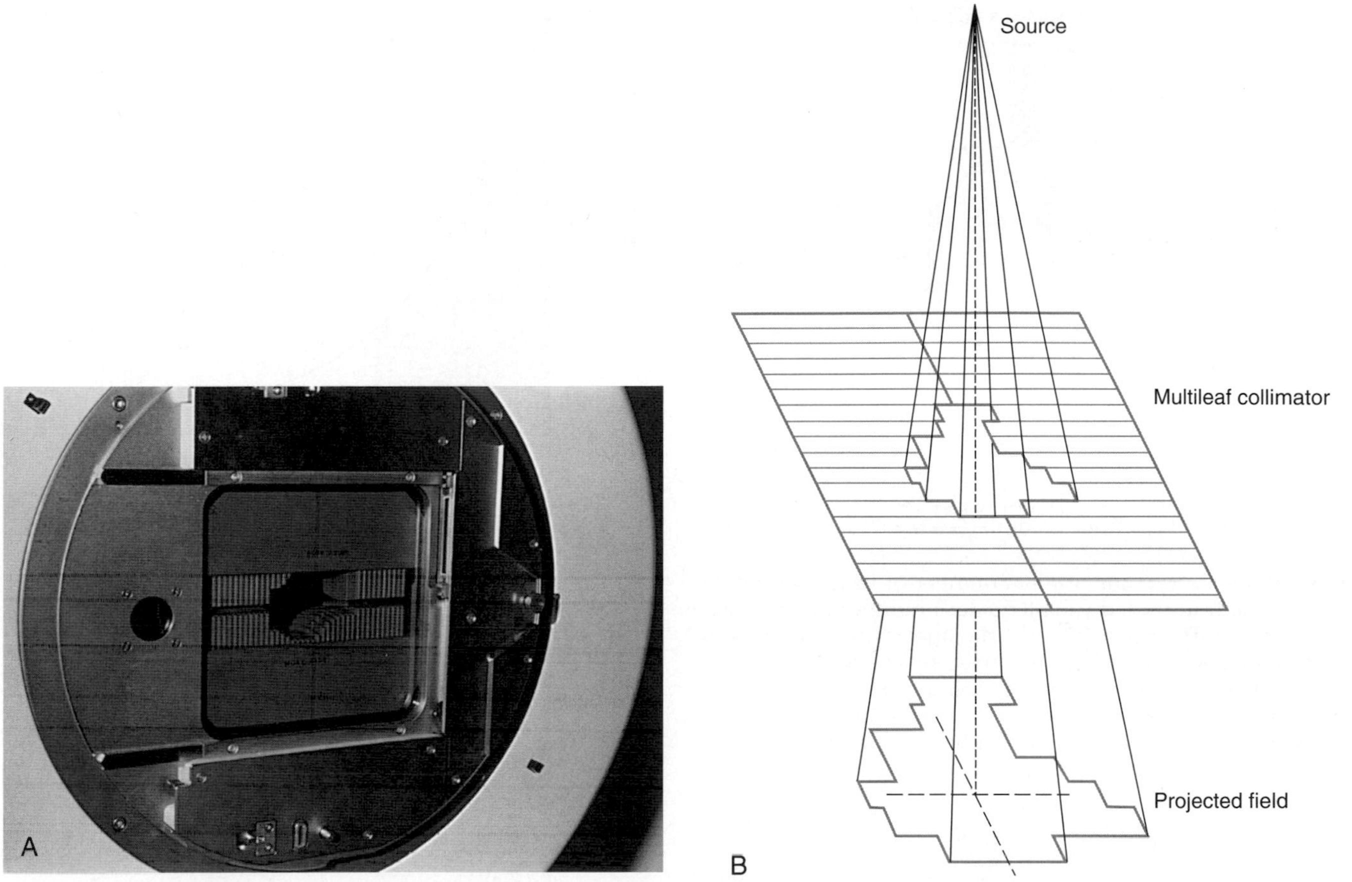

Figure 6-6 The multileaf collimator. **A,** Installed 80-leaf device for a Varian 2100C linear accelerator. **B,** Schematic of beam definition.

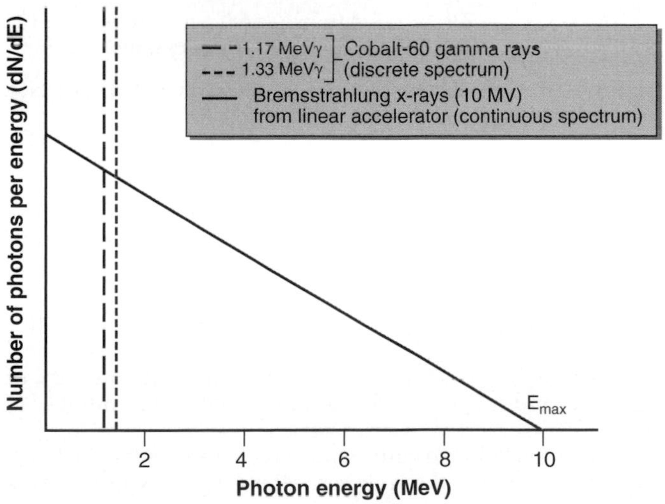

Figure 6-7 Discrete and continuous photon spectra. The discrete spectrum is characteristic of photons emitted by radioactive material. The continuous spectrum is characteristic of bremsstrahlung x-rays emitted by a linear accelerator. E_{max}, 10 MeV.

$$\frac{\Delta N/N}{\Delta x} = -\mu \quad \text{or} \quad \frac{\Delta N}{N} = -\mu \Delta x \qquad \text{Eq. 1}$$

In the equation, ΔN is the change in the number of photons due to attenuation, N is the number of incident photons, μ is a constant that represents the constant fractional attenuation per thickness (called the *linear attenuation coefficient*, with units of length^{-1} [cm^{-1}]), Δx is the thickness traversed by the photons for attenuation ΔN, and the minus sign indicates that the effect is negative, resulting in fewer photons.

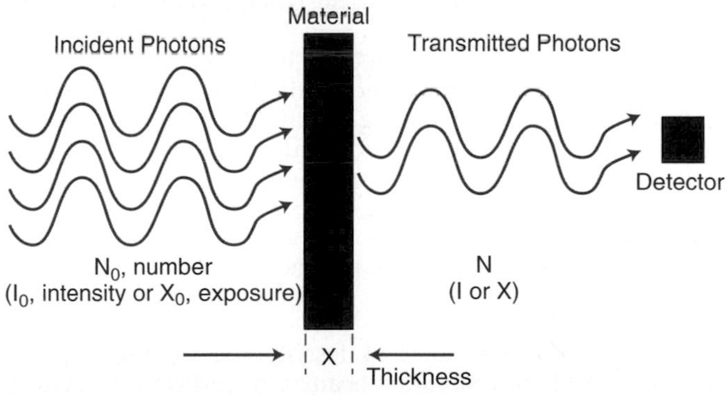

Figure 6-8 Attenuation and transmission. A number, N_0, of monoenergetic x-rays or gamma rays is incident to a slab of material, and a smaller number, N, is transmitted. The attenuated photons, $N_0 - N$, are absorbed in the material or scattered in another direction.

Constant fractional attenuation per unit thickness compounds over successive thicknesses, illustrated in Figure 6-9. This "fraction of a fraction" effect is nonlinear, and the integrated form of Equation 1 yields an important relationship: attenuation in a continuous material is an exponential process:

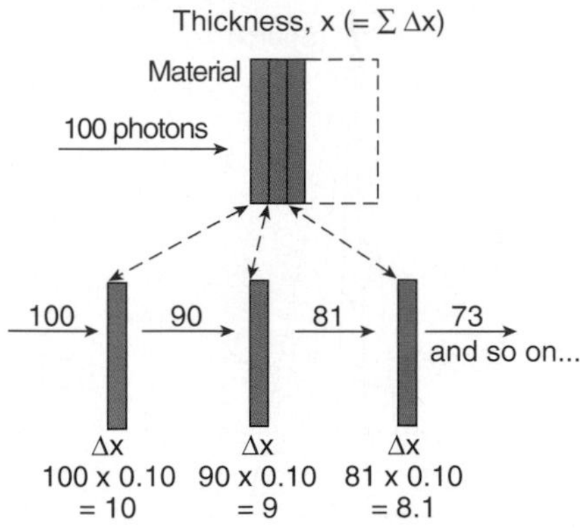

Figure 6-9 Attenuation through successive slabs of material.

$$N(x) = N_0 e^{-\mu x} \quad \text{or} \quad \frac{N(x)}{N_0} = e^{-\mu x} \qquad \text{Eq. 2}$$

In Equation 2, N_0 is the original number of incident photons, N(x) is the transmitted (unattenuated) number of photons, e is Euler's constant ($e \approx 2.7$), μ is the linear attenuation coefficient, and x is the thickness traversed by the photons.

Exponential attenuation is valid for monoenergetic photons and all homogeneous materials in narrow beam geometry and applies to other radiation quantities such as intensity (I) and exposure (X):

$$I = I_0 e^{-\mu x} \quad \text{or} \quad \frac{I}{I_0} = e^{-\mu x} \quad \text{and} \quad X = X_0 e^{-\mu x} \quad \text{or} \quad \frac{X}{X_0} = e^{-\mu x} \qquad \text{Eq. 3}$$

The linear attenuation coefficient is unique for each photon energy and element or material but varies with absorber density. Attenuation coefficients are discussed more fully with radiation interactions.

Equation 2 can be graphed in linear or semi-log form (Fig. 6-10). In semi-log form, the attenuation curve is a straight line with a slope of $-\mu$ (see Fig. 6-10B). A smaller attenuation coefficient means less attenuation and a shallower attenuation curve. Different attenuation coefficients result in a different amount of attenuation for the same thickness traversed and attenuation curves that differ in their slopes (Fig. 6-11). A smaller attenuation coefficient results in less attenuation.

Beam Quality

Beam quality is a term used to describe the amount of penetration by a photon radiation beam. One indicator of quality is beam energy, defined by accelerating potential, effective energy, or gamma ray energy. Another indicator is the half-value layer (HVL). HVL is the thickness of a material that reduces the transmitted intensity to one half of the original intensity. When $I/I_0 = \frac{1}{2}$, the thickness, x, is the HVL, and the attenuation equation becomes

$$\frac{I}{I_0} = \frac{1}{2} = e^{-\mu HVL} \qquad \text{Eq. 4}$$

Two important relationships come from this equation:

$$\mu = .693/HVL \text{ and } HVL = .693/\mu$$

Given the linear attenuation coefficient, the HVL can be computed, and vice versa. For example, if $\mu = .10\ cm^{-1}$, the $HVL = .693/.10\,cm^{-1} = 6.93$ cm, and if HVL = 10 cm, $\mu = .693/10\ cm = .0693\ cm^{-1}$. Notice that the units for HVL are the reciprocal of the units for μ.

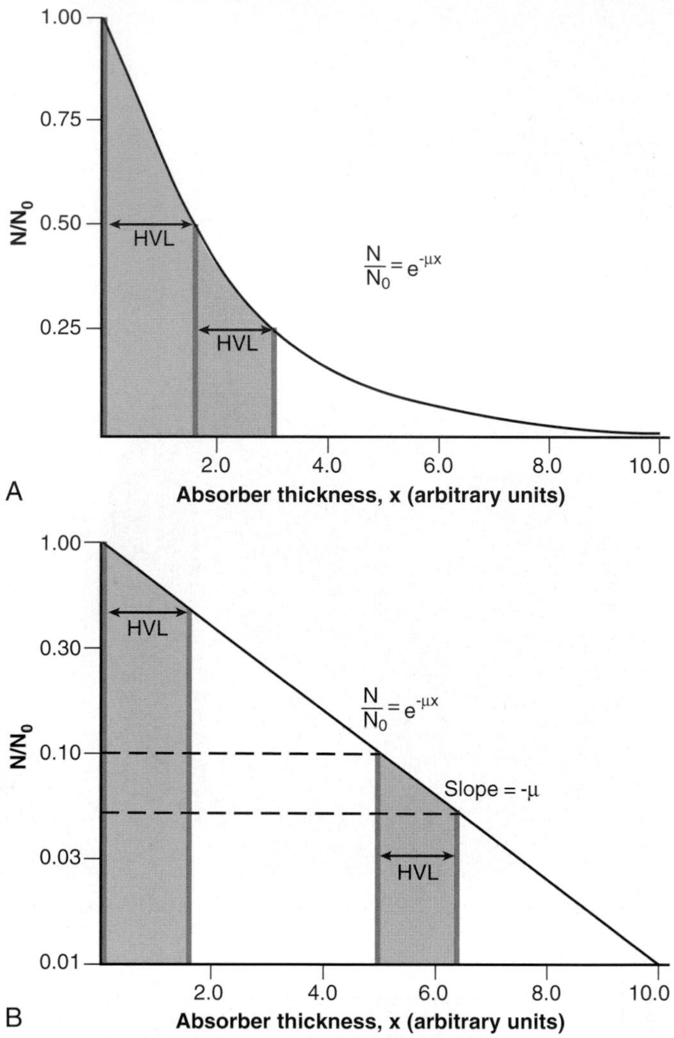

Figure 6-10 Graphic representation of attenuation. **A,** Linear plot. **B,** Semi-log plot. HVL, half-value layer.

Because $e^{-\mu HVL} = \frac{1}{2}$, and given a thickness of material in units of HVL (x = n HVL), the amount of attenuation can be computed by

$$\frac{I}{I_0} = \left(\frac{1}{2}\right)^n \qquad \text{Eq. 5}$$

In Equation 5, I/I_0 is the fractional transmission, intensity, or exposure, and n is the thickness of the material in number of HVLs.

Similar to HVL, the tenth-value layer (TVL) is the thickness required to reduce the number, intensity, or exposure by a factor of 10:

$$\frac{I}{I_0} = \frac{1}{10} = e^{-\mu TVL} \quad \text{and} \quad \frac{I}{I_0} = \left(\frac{1}{10}\right)^m \qquad \text{Eq. 6}$$

In Equation 6, m is the thickness of the material given in number of TVLs.

HVL can be found graphically from the attenuation curve, whether on a linear or log plot (see Fig. 6-10), and for monoenergetic photons can be determined anywhere along the curve because μ is constant; the ratio of the two intensities must be $\frac{1}{2}$. For polyenergetic photons, μ is not constant but instead decreases with increasing depth (Fig. 6-12A). The low-

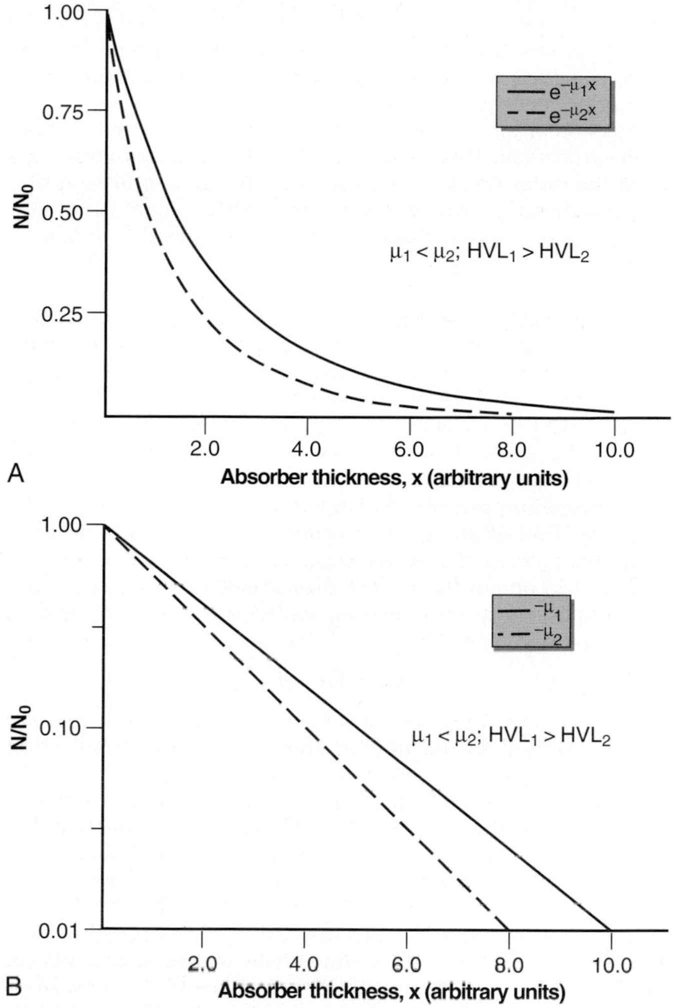

Figure 6-11 Attenuation for two different materials. **A,** Linear plot. **B,** Semi-log plot. HVL, half-value layer.

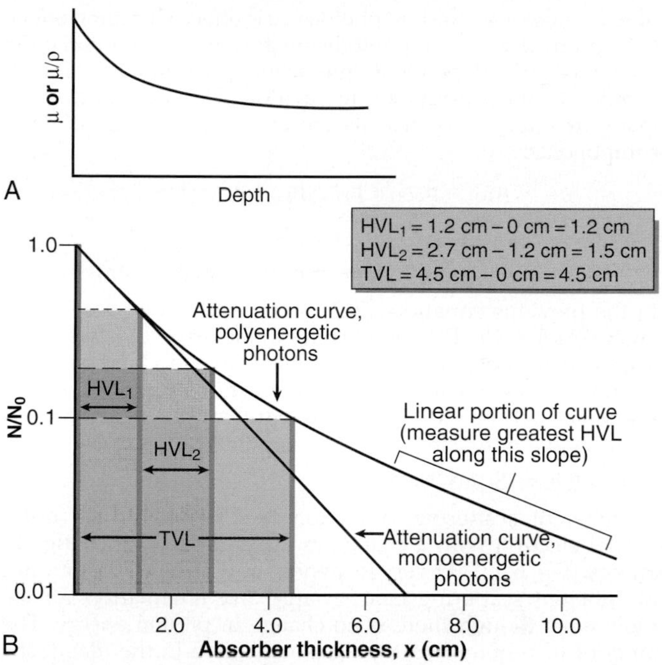

Figure 6-12 Attenuation for polyenergetic photons. **A,** Variation in attenuation coefficient as a function of depth for polyenergetic photons. **B,** Attenuation curve for polyenergetic photons. HVL, half-value layer; TVL, tenth-value layer.

energy component of the beam spectrum is attenuated preferentially, compared with high-energy photons, because of increased attenuation at low energies. As depth increases, the ratio of high-energy to low-energy photons increases, resulting in increased beam penetration, or "beam hardening." After a large number of low-energy photons are attenuated at depth, beam hardening is minimal and μ is essentially constant. The log attenuation curve begins steeply, has curvature, and then becomes linear at depth (see Fig. 6-12B). Because μ changes with depth, HVL also changes, yielding different first and second HVLs, as defined in Figure 6-12B. The monoenergetic case is shown for comparison. HVL_1 is always less than HVL_2 because photons incident on HVL_2 have a higher average energy:

$$HVL_1 < HVL_2$$

The greatest HVL is found at maximum depth, on the linear portion of the curve. For polyenergetic photon beams, an effective attenuation coefficient (μ_{eff},) can be calculated. First, an effective HVL is found over a region of interest, and then μ_{eff} is calculated:

$$\mu_{eff} = .693/HVL_{eff}$$

Characteristics of attenuation curves for monoenergetic and polyenergetic photons are summarized in Table 6-6.

Table 6-6 Characteristics of Attenuation Curves

Monoenergetic	Polyenergetic
1. Exponential curve on linear paper	1. Complex exponential curve on linear paper
2. Linear curve on semi-log paper	2. Curved on semi-log paper
3. Constant μ	3. Varying μ: μ_{eff} can be determined
4. Constant HVL	4. Varying HVL: HVL_1, HVL_2, TVL, and greatest HVL can be determined

HVL, half-value layer; TVL, tenth-value layer. See text for other terms.

Attenuation Coefficients

The linear attenuation coefficient is one representation of photon interaction probabilities. Another form, the mass attenuation coefficient, μ/ρ, is the linear attenuation coefficient divided by the material's density, ρ, and has units of cm^2/g. It is independent of material density and is the form of attenuation coefficient commonly found in physics data tables, presented according to incident photon energy and the attenuating element or material. Its use in attenuation computations requires the density of the material according to

$$\frac{I}{I_0} = e^{-\frac{\mu}{\rho}\rho x} \qquad \text{Eq. 7}$$

Attenuation coefficients can also be expressed in other forms and can be converted from one form to another.[12]

Photon Interactions: X-Rays and Gamma Rays

Attenuation of photon beams is the result of interactions in the intercepting material. There are five possible photon interactions: coherent scattering, photoelectric effect, Compton effect, pair production, and photodisintegration. Each interaction type has an independent interaction probability and contributes to the amount of attenuation. The total linear and mass attenuation coefficients are given by the sum of their components:

$$\mu_{TOT} = \mu_{COH} + \mu_{PE} + \mu_{CE} + \mu_{PP} + \mu_{PD}$$

and

$$\mu/\rho_{TOT} = \mu/\rho_{COH} + \mu/\rho_{PE} + \mu/\rho_{CE} + \mu/\rho_{PP} + \mu/\rho_{PD}$$

In the previous equations, TOT signifies the total coefficient, and COH, PE, CE, PP, and PD refer to the respective five interactions. The photoelectric effect, Compton effect, and pair production are the most important interactions for megavoltage photons used for radiation treatment. Detailed presentations of these five interactions have been published.[2,12,13]

Coherent Scattering

In coherent scattering, a photon is scattered off an outer orbital electron with a change in direction and no change in energy (Fig. 6-13). At very low energies (<10 keV), the amount of coherent scattering can be large and attenuation can be high, even though there is no change in photon energy. The amount of coherent scattering is negligible in the diagnostic and therapy energy ranges compared with other principal interactions.

Photoelectric Effect

The following actions occur in the photoelectric effect (Fig. 6-14):

1. An incident photon with energy, $E_\gamma = h\nu$, interacts with the inner orbital electron with binding energy E_B (most tightly bound). The interaction can occur with other orbital electrons, but the most probable interaction is with the innermost electron.
2. The photon is completely absorbed and no longer exists.
3. The orbital electron, now called the *photoelectron,* is ejected with kinetic energy, E_{pe}, equal to the photon energy minus the binding energy:

$$E_{pe} = E_\gamma - E_B$$

If E_γ is less than E_B, the interaction cannot occur, but the interaction may occur with another orbital electron with a binding energy less than E_γ.

4. Ejection of the orbital electron leaves a vacancy in the inner electron shell. This vacancy is filled by an electron from one of the outer orbitals, with the simultaneous emission of a characteristic x-ray with an energy of E_{CX} equal to the difference of the two electron binding energies (Fig. 6-15):

$$E_{CX} = E_{B1} - E_{B2}$$

5. This process leaves a new vacancy in an outer orbital shell, which is filled by an electron from an orbital beyond, with emission of a second characteristic x-ray of lower energy than the first. This cascade of vacancy creation, filling, and characteristic x-ray emission continues until the most outer orbital electron shell has a vacancy that is filled by a "free," or unbound, electron.
6. A competing process to characteristic x-ray emission is the production of an Auger (pronounced "oh-jhay") electron. In this process, the characteristic x-ray energy, E_{CX}, is transferred to one of the nearby orbital electrons with no x-ray emission, and the electron, called an *Auger electron,* is ejected with energy:

$$E_{AU} = E_{CX} - E_B$$

Characteristic x-rays are so named because their energies are directly related to the unique energy levels of the electron orbits for an element. A material's elemental composition can be determined by detecting its characteristic x-rays. Characteristic x-rays are named for the orbital electron transition that occurred. For instance, a K_α x-ray results in the L shell electron filling the K shell vacancy, an $M \rightarrow K$ transition yields a K_β x-ray, and an $M \rightarrow L$ transition yields an L_α x-ray.

For an atom with five electron orbitals, the possible electron transitions and their characteristic x-rays after a photoelectric interaction are $L \rightarrow K$, $M \rightarrow L$, $N \rightarrow M$, $O \rightarrow N$, $M \rightarrow K$, $N \rightarrow K$, $O \rightarrow K$, $N \rightarrow L$, $O \rightarrow L$, and $O \rightarrow M$. The most probable transitions are those between adjacent orbitals: $L \rightarrow K$,

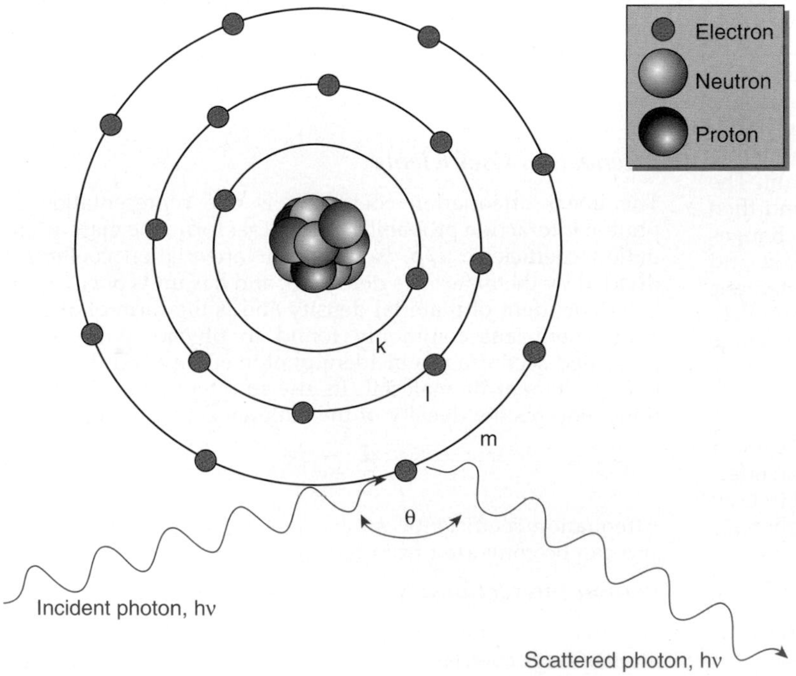

Figure 6-13 Coherent scattering.

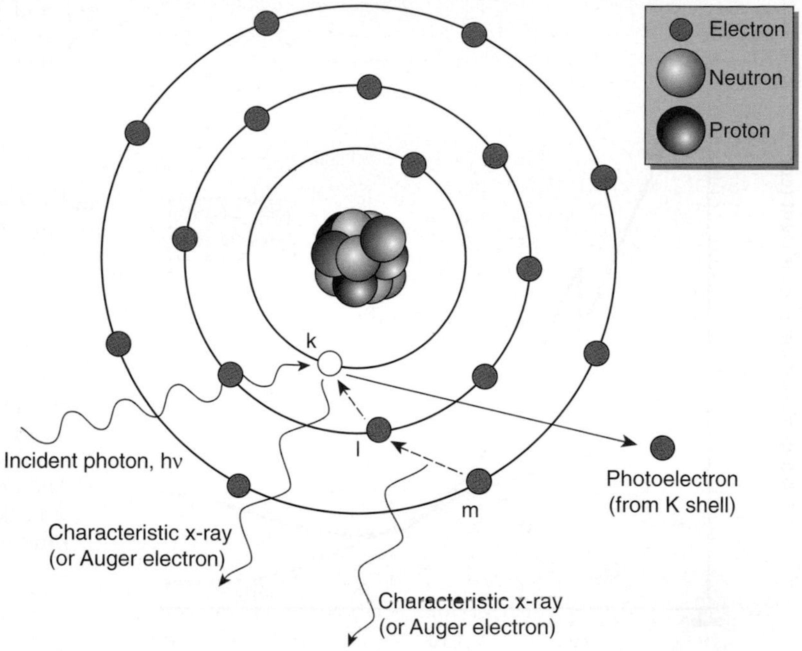

Figure 6-14 Photoelectric effect.

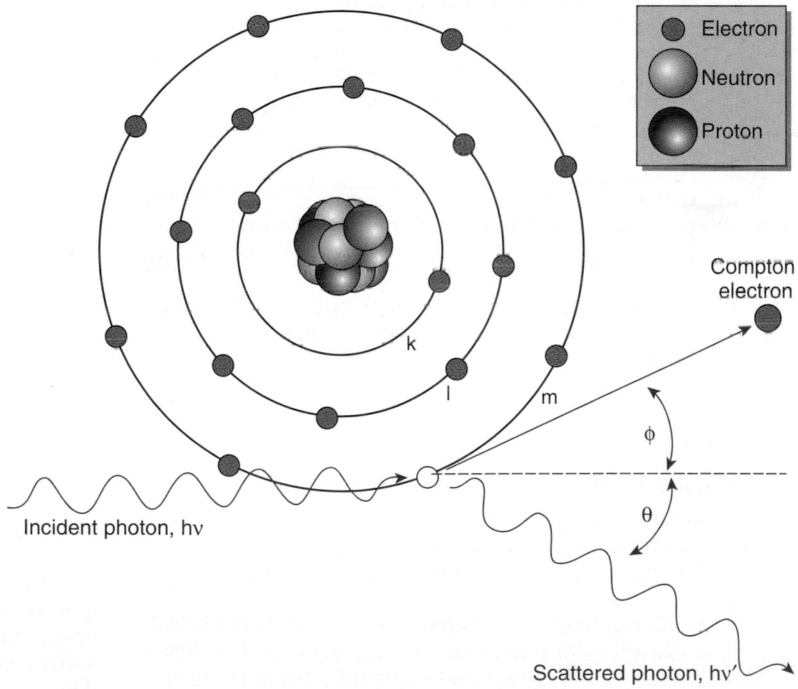

Figure 6-15 Compton effect.

M → L, N → M, and so forth. At the same time, Auger electron emission competes with characteristic x-ray emission, at a rate given by w, the fluorescence coefficient.

The photoelectric effect has a strong dependency on photon energy and atomic number of the material. The mass attenuation coefficient varies as $(1/E_\gamma)^3$ and Z^3, respectively. Mathematically, this is shown as follows, where C_{PE} is a proportionality constant:

$$\mu/\rho_{PE} = C_{PE}Z^3/(E_\gamma)^3 \quad \text{Eq. 8}$$

These dependencies for water are shown graphically in Figure 6-16. In the photoelectric effect, no interaction is possible until the photon energy is greater than the electron binding energy. After the binding energy is barely exceeded, the probability for interaction increases greatly, leading to a sharp increase in μ/ρ_{PE}, called an *absorption edge*. In Figure 6-16, the K and L edge for lead are seen, corresponding to photoelectric interactions for the K and L shell electrons. No absorption edges are shown for water; the binding energies are less than 1 keV and do not show up on the plot.

The dependence on Z and E_γ can be used to approximate the photoelectric contribution in a different material, using the formula:

$$\mu/\rho_{PE,2} = \mu/\rho_{PE,1}(E_{\gamma,1}/E_{\gamma,2})^3(Z_2/Z_1)^3 \quad \text{Eq. 9}$$

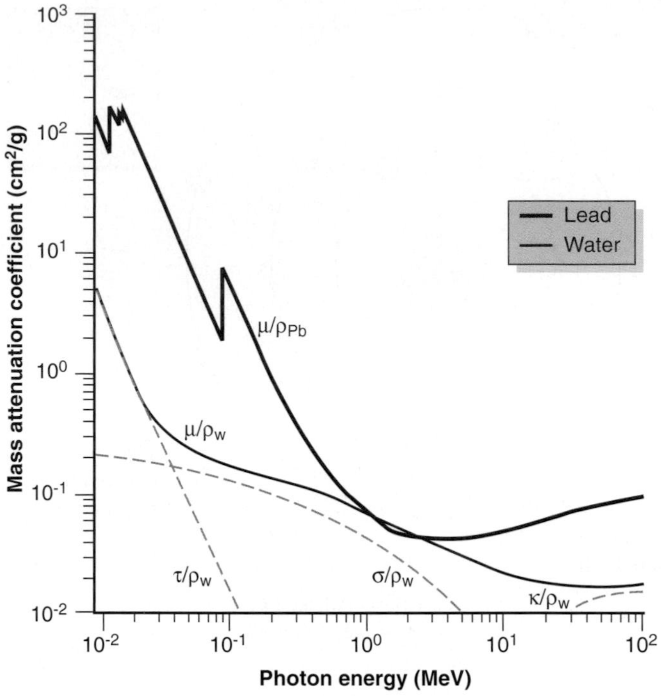

Figure 6-16 Total mass attenuation coefficients for lead and water. Individual interaction coefficients for water *(dashed lines)* also are shown. (Data from Radiological Health Handbook. Bethesda, MD, U.S. Department of Health, Education, and Welfare, 1970; Evans RD: The Atomic Nucleus. Malabar, FL, Robert E. Krieger Publishing, 1955.)

If the material (Z) is constant but energy is changed, the new photoelectric mass attenuation coefficient is found by:

$$\mu/\rho_{PE,2} = \mu/\rho_{PE,1}(E_{\gamma,1}/E_{\gamma,2})^3 \qquad \text{Eq. 10}$$

If the photon energy (E_γ) is constant but the attenuating material is changed, the new photoelectric mass attenuation coefficient is found by:

$$\mu/\rho_{PE,2} = \mu/\rho_{PE,1}(Z_2/Z_1)^3 \qquad \text{Eq. 11}$$

COMPTON EFFECT

In the Compton effect (see Fig. 6-15), several things occur:

1. An incident photon with energy, $E_\gamma = h\nu$ interacts with a loosely bound, outer orbit electron.
2. The photon is scattered at some angle with reduced energy $E'_\gamma = h\nu'$.
3. The orbital electron, now called the *recoil* or *Compton electron,* is ejected with kinetic energy, E_{ce}, equal to the difference between the incident and scattered photon energies:

$$E_{ce} = E_\gamma - E'_\gamma$$

4. Because the interaction is with the outer shell electron, which has negligible binding energy, there are no characteristic x-rays or Auger electrons produced.

The distribution of energies and scattering angles for the Compton photon and electron can be described mathematically. The scattered photon has energy $E'_\gamma = h\nu'$ given by

$$h\nu' = \frac{h\nu}{1+\alpha(1-\cos\theta)} = \frac{m_o c^2}{1+\left(\frac{1}{\alpha}-\cos\theta\right)} \qquad \text{Eq. 12}$$

In Equation 12, $\alpha = h\nu/m_oc^2$ and represents the ratio of the incident photon energy to the rest mass of the electron, m_o, and θ is the angle of photon scattering as defined in Figure 6-15.

The Compton electron has energy E_{ce} given by the following equation:

$$E_{ce} = h\nu\frac{\alpha(1-\cos\theta)}{1+\alpha(1-\cos\theta)} \qquad \text{Eq. 13}$$

and a scattering angle ϕ that depends on the incident photon's energy and its scattering angle, θ:

$$\cos\phi = (1+\alpha)\tan\frac{\theta}{2} \qquad \text{Eq. 14}$$

A few scattering cases can be considered:

1. The minimum energy transfer occurs for a 0-degree photon scatter; there is no interaction, and the "scattered" photon has the same energy as the incident photon. The electron is scattered at 90 degrees (ϕ = 90 degrees) with zero energy.
2. The maximum energy transfer occurs for a direct hit with a backscattered photon (θ = 180 degrees) and yields a (minimum) scattered photon energy of

$$h\nu' = \frac{h\nu}{1+2\alpha} \qquad \text{Eq. 15}$$

The backscattered Compton photon energy will always be less than and will approach 0.25 MeV (which equals $\frac{1}{2}$ m_oc^2) even as the incident photon energy becomes very large. The electron has maximum energy of $E_{ce} = h\nu - h\nu' = h\nu\,(2\alpha/(1+2\alpha))$ and travels in the forward direction.

3. A 90-degree Compton scattered photon has energy:

$$h\nu' = \frac{h\nu}{1+\alpha} \qquad \text{Eq. 16}$$

The 90-degree scattered Compton photon energy will always be less than and will approach 0.511 MeV (which equals m_oc^2) even as the incident photon energy becomes very large. The electron has energy of $E_{ce} = h\nu - h\nu' = h\nu\,(\alpha/(1+\alpha))$, and it travels in a direction that depends on the incident photon energy.

Although isotopically distributed for lower-energy photons, Compton electrons scatter more and more in the forward direction as incident photon energy increases. Their average energy also increases from about 10 keV to 7 MeV as incident photon energy increases from about 100 keV to 10 MeV.[11] The forward-peaked distribution is responsible for the buildup region for megavoltage photon beams, as explained later.

The Compton effect has a slight dependency on incident photon energy, decreasing as energy increases through the megavoltage range, but the interaction probability is essentially constant over most of the megavoltage energy range (see Fig. 6-16). Compton scattering is independent of atomic number and is dependent on the number of electrons available, or electron density (electrons per gram). The electron density for almost all materials is constant at approximately 3 × 10^{23} electrons per gram because N:Z is almost constant. The exception is hydrogen, which with one proton in the nucleus has an electron density of around 6 × 10^{23} electrons per gram. Except for a small energy dependency and increased interaction probabilities for hydrogen-laden materials, the Compton mass attenuation coefficient is remarkably constant across energy and atomic number, especially for low Z biologic materials such as tissues. Mathematically, this relationship is

$$\mu/\rho_{CE} = C_{CE} \qquad \text{Eq. 17}$$

In Equation 17, C_{CE} is almost a constant.

Attenuation by the Compton effect reduces to the following expression:

$$\left.\frac{I}{I_0}\right|_{CE} = e^{-C_{CE}\rho x} \qquad \text{Eq. 18}$$

For unit thickness, the transmitted amount depends only on material density, not atomic number and photon energy, as with the photoelectric effect.

Pair Production

In pair production (Fig. 6-17), the following steps occur:

1. An incident photon with energy $E_\gamma = h\nu$ and E_γ greater than 1.022 MeV passes near a heavy nucleus and spontaneously disappears, creating an electron, e^-, and a positron, e^+, in its place. These two particles are called an *electron-positron pair*. The total kinetic energy of the electron-positron pair, E_{ep}, is equal to the photon energy minus the energy needed to create two electrons, or 1.022 MeV (the rest energy of an electron is 0.511 MeV):

$$E_{ep} = E_\gamma - 1.022\,\text{MeV}$$

The electron and positron travel off in no particular directions and do not have equal energies.

2. The electron gradually slows down and is stopped in the material.
3. The positron, the antiparticle of an electron, slows down very quickly and annihilates with a free electron, giving off two .511-MeV photons (called *annihilation radiation*) that travel in opposite directions (i.e., at 180 degrees).

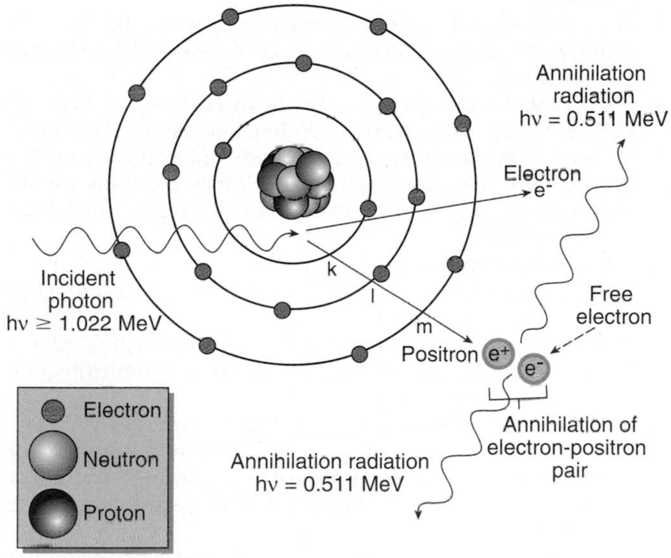

Figure 6-17 Pair production.

The mass attenuation coefficient for pair production varies linearly with atomic number and incident photon energy (when the photon energy is above the threshold of 1.022 MeV):

$$\mu/\rho_{PP} = C_{PP}Z(E_\gamma - 1.022\,\text{MeV}) \qquad \text{Eq. 19}$$

Photodisintegration

Several steps occur in photodisintegration (Fig. 6-18):

1. A very energetic photon of E_γ greater than 8 to 10 MeV interacts with the atomic nucleus.
2. The photon penetrates the nucleus and is absorbed, resulting in the emission of a neutron.
3. Neutron emission leaves a fragmented, possibly unstable nucleus (i.e., radioactive), prompting the name *photodisintegration*.

An energy of greater than 8 to 10 MeV is required because the nuclear binding energies for nucleons are 8 to 10 MeV for most materials. Photodisintegration is the interaction responsible for neutron production for photon energies at 10 MeV and greater and can be an important consideration for facility shielding for photon beams of 15 MeV and greater.

Distribution of Secondary Electrons

Electrons released by ionizing photon interactions can travel in any direction from the interaction point and in general have a complex probability for angular spread, depending on incident photon energy and the interaction that occurs. The probability for forward directions increases with photon energy and is a likely direction for megavoltage photon interactions.[2] As seen later, angular scattering of electrons is responsible for a number of characteristics for megavoltage photon beams,

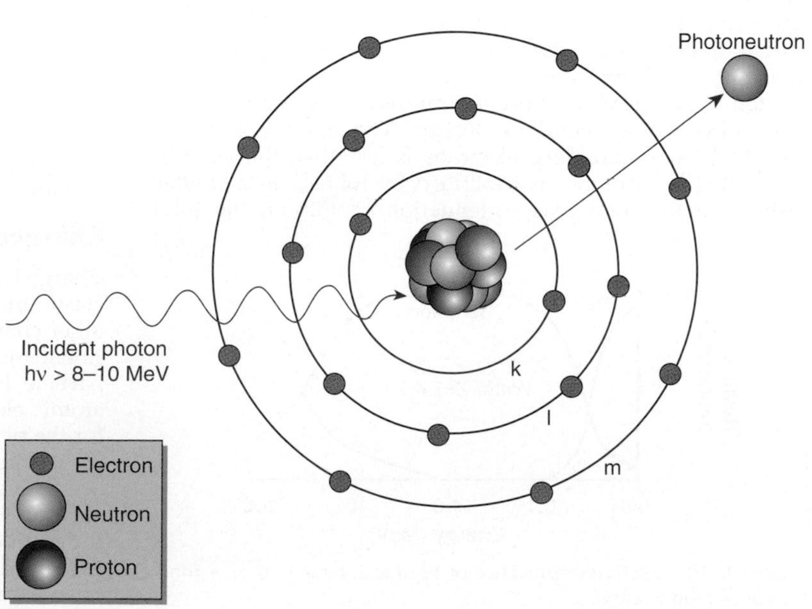

Figure 6-18 Photodisintegration.

including surface dose, the buildup region, the depth of maximum dose, and the penumbra region.

Total Attenuation Coefficient

Each radiation interaction contributes its part to the total attenuation coefficient. Photons having the same energy can undergo any one of the five interactions when energetically possible. However, the probability for each interaction is different and in a particular energy range a particular interaction will dominate.

In Figure 6-16, the individual interaction and total mass attenuation coefficients are shown as a function of energy for lead and water. Notice the K edge in the curve for lead. It can be seen that different energy regions are dominated by particular interactions. For water, the photoelectric effect dominates for photon energies up to 60 keV, the Compton dominates from 60 keV to 10 MeV, and pair production dominates approximately above 10 MeV. For lead, the photoelectric effect dominates up to 700 keV, the Compton effect from 700 keV to 3 MeV, and pair production at 3 MeV and higher. An interaction's region of dominance can be represented graphically to show relative importance as a function of energy (Fig. 6-19).

Comparison of interaction dependencies shows why diagnostic energy photons give good contrast for imaging: the photoelectric effect dominates and is quite sensitive to the atomic numbers of the materials being imaged. Materials with even slightly different Zs have good subject contrast (and image contrast) because attenuation depends on the cube of the atomic numbers. Radiation therapy port films, however, have poor contrast because the dominant interaction is the Compton effect. There is no dependence on atomic number, and the effect is constant for most biologic materials (except for hydrogenous materials). Instead of imaging atomic number, the Compton effect images the density of a material, and subject contrast is essentially density differences. A comparison of simulator and port films is given later (see Fig. 6-49).

Total Absorption Coefficient

Radiation dose relates directly to the amount of energy absorbed at a point, not the amount attenuated, although the two are intimately related. This transfer of energy is done by secondary electrons (photoelectrons, Compton electrons, and the electron-positron pair) that produce ionizations along their paths until their energy is expended. A portion of the photon energy that is attenuated may escape to other regions as a coherent or Compton scattered photon, an annihilation photon (0.511 MeV), or a bremsstrahlung photon after radiative collision of a secondary electron. The amount of energy absorbed from secondary electrons is less than the amount attenuated as photons, as described by Johns[12]. In a similar fashion to the total mass attenuation coefficient, the total mass *energy absorption* coefficient, μ_{en}/ρ, or simply the mass *absorption* coefficient, describes the energy absorbed due to each interaction and is used for computing dose. The value of μ_{en}/ρ is first equal to μ_{TOT}/ρ in the photoelectric region (because all photon energy is transferred to the photoelectron), and then μ_{en}/ρ is less than μ_{TOT}/ρ in the region where the Compton effect dominates (because the Compton scattered photon carries energy away). At very high energies where pair production dominates, μ_{en}/ρ and μ_{TOT}/ρ are almost equal because the fraction of incident photon energy carried off as annihilation photons is negligible compared with the amount transferred to kinetic energy of the electron-positron pair. Over the energy range used for radiation treatment, the amount of absorbed energy at a point in water (tissue) is about one half the amount attenuated at the point. The mass absorption coefficient and dose are discussed more in the next section.

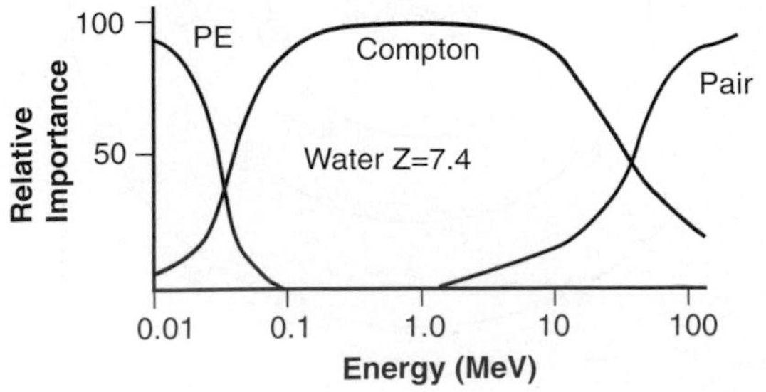

Figure 6-19 Relative importance of photon interactions as a function of photon energy.

Summary of Photon Interactions

1. Coherent scattering occurs at very low photon energies (<10 keV).
2. The photoelectric effect dominates up to 60 keV in water, with strong dependencies of Z^3 and $1/E^3_\gamma$ for other materials.
3. The Compton effect dominates from 60 keV to about 10 MeV in water, with some dependence on energy or atomic number. Compton scattering depends only on the number of electrons per gram, which is almost constant for all materials ($N_g \approx 3.0 \times 10^{23}$, except for hydrogen, for which $N_g \approx 6.0 \times 10^{23}$).
4. Pair production occurs for photon energies only above 1.022 MeV, dominates above 10 MeV in water, and linearly depends on Z and photon energy.
5. Photodisintegration occurs at photon energies above 10 MeV and is responsible for the creation of neutrons in a linear accelerator facility.
6. At diagnostic photon energies, image contrast is determined primarily by differences in atomic numbers of materials being imaged, because the photoelectric effect depends strongly on Z. Material thickness and density are secondary determinants.
7. At therapeutic photon energies, image contrast is provided by the densities of materials being imaged, because the Compton effect depends on the number of electrons per gram, not the atomic number, of a material.
8. The total mass attenuation coefficient describes the amount of attenuation from all processes. A portion of the energy attenuated from the beam is deposited by secondary electrons as dose. The amount of energy absorbed as dose is described by the total mass absorption coefficient, which tracks the total mass attenuation coefficient and is numerically less.

Charged Particle Interactions

Charged particles incident on matter undergo inelastic and elastic interactions with atomic electrons and nuclei, that is, other charged entities.[2,12,13] Inelastic interactions include collisional and radiative processes and result in energy loss by the particle. In an elastic interaction the particle is scattered by an atomic electron or nucleus, resulting in a change of direction for the particle but no energy loss. The interaction probability for charged particles is effectively 1; an incident particle interacts at every opportunity. The quotient dE/dx (units of million electron volts per centimeter) is called the *stopping power*, and it describes the rate of energy loss, dE, that occurs over distance traveled, dx, for inelastic collisions. Stopping power is often expressed as the mass stopping power, dE/ρdx (units of million electron volts per gram per square centimeter), which is independent of the absorber density. Because energy loss is almost continuous and a particle has a particular kinetic energy, E_{KE}, the particle loses this amount of energy and then stops. The distance traveled is finite and is called the *particle range*; the particle can go no farther, and its kinetic energy is zero. For an absorber of density ρ, the particle range, r, can be calculated as follows:

$$r = E_{kE}\frac{1}{\frac{dE}{\rho dx}}\frac{1}{\rho} \qquad \text{Eq. 20}$$

The energy lost through inelastic collisions depends on the particle mass, charge, and kinetic energy, and the mass and charge of the target atom, according to the formula:

$$\frac{dE}{dx} = \frac{2\pi z^2 e^4}{m_o V^2} NZF_Q \qquad \text{Eq. 21}$$

In Equation 21, z is the atomic number of the incident particle of mass M, V is its velocity, e is the electron charge, m_o is the electron mass, NZ is the number of electrons per cubic centimeter in the absorber, and F_Q is a complex function describing energy transfer per interaction.

Collisional energy losses increase by the square of the particle's atomic number and as the incident particle velocity decreases. Increased atomic number results in a greater coulomb force, and decreased velocity increases the amount of interaction time, both leading to increased dE/dx. The energy transfer function, F_Q, is complex and varies with the type of interaction.[2] It accounts for the atomic mass of the absorber, ionization potential, and relativistic effects as V approaches the speed of light.

Light Charged Particle Interactions: Electrons

The electron mass is small compared with any atomic mass, and incident electrons undergo four types of particle interactions with a large amount of scattering.[8] Collisional interactions result in energy loss of dE_{COL}/dx, causing ionizations or excited states (higher electron orbits) (Fig. 6-20). Collisional losses increase as the electron velocity decreases, as stated earlier, and decrease as the absorber atomic number increases. The decrease with absorber atomic number results from the decrease in the number of electrons per gram (NZ/ρ) as Z increases. For equivalent mass thicknesses (mass thickness is thickness divided by density, with units of square centimeters per gram), electrons are stopped sooner in low Z than in high Z materials. Figure 6-21 shows these relationships for water and lead.

Radiative interactions result in x-ray emissions. The incident electron penetrates the electron cloud and interacts with the nucleus's positive electrical field, undergoing an abrupt deceleration with energy loss dE_{RAD}/dx and a change in direction (see Fig. 6-20D). The energy change, dE_{RAD}/dx, is released in the form of x-rays, called *bremsstrahlung* (or braking) *radiation*. With an incident monoenergetic electron fluence, a continuous x-ray spectrum is emitted because the probability of any energy loss, large or small, is equal per interaction. Successive bremsstrahlung interactions may occur as the electron loses its energy; a bremsstrahlung spectrum has a maximum energy equal to the initial electron energy and energies below

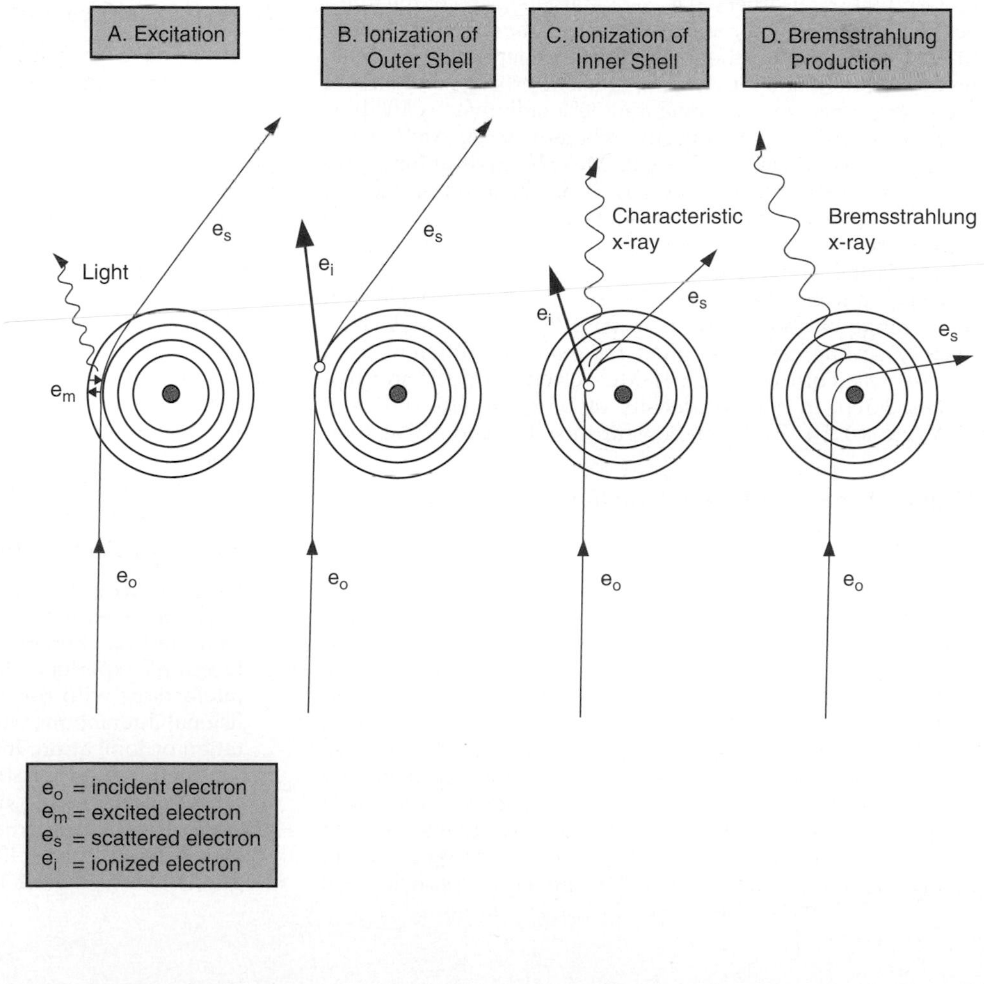

Figure 6-20 Electron interactions. **A,** Excitation. **B,** Ionization of outer shell. **C,** Ionization of inner shell. **D,** Bremsstrahlung production. (Adapted from Johns HE, Cunningham JR: The Physics of Radiology, 3rd ed. Springfield, IL, Charles C Thomas, 1978.)

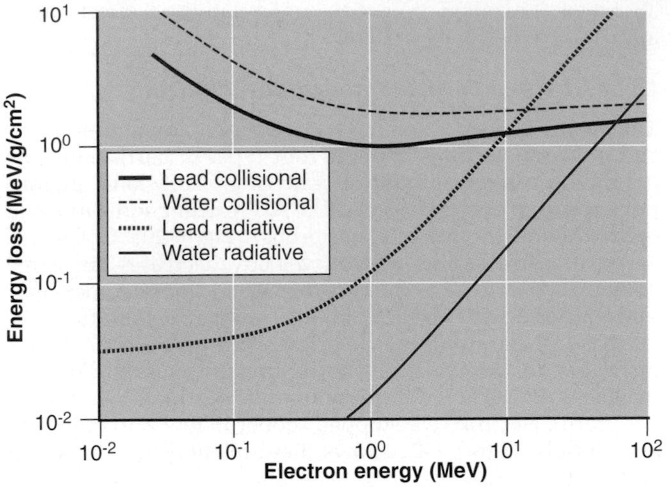

Figure 6-21 Collisional and radiative electron losses as a function of incident electron energy. (Adapted from Johns HE, Cunningham JR: The Physics of Radiology, 3rd ed. Springfield, IL, Charles C Thomas, 1978.)

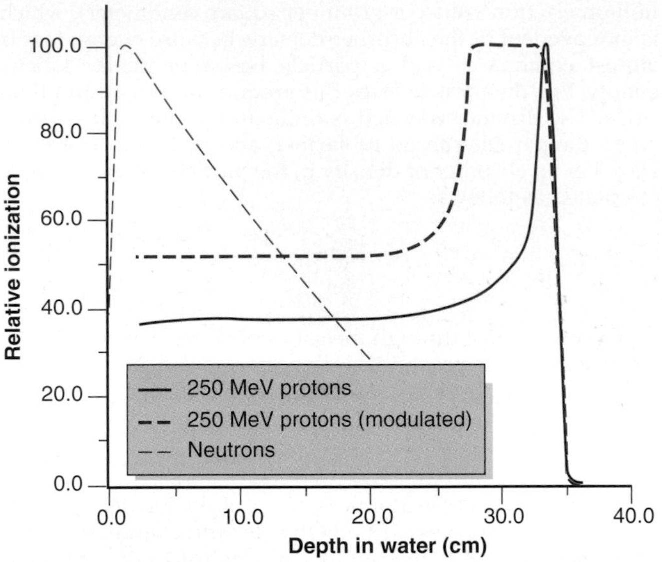

Figure 6-22 Ionization curves for heavy particles. Protons are charged and exhibit a Bragg peak at the end of their range. Neutrons are uncharged and are exponentially attenuated. (Data for protons from Miller DW: Update on proton radiotherapy. *In* Mackie TR, Palta JR [eds]: Teletherapy: Present and Future. Madison, WI, Advanced Medical Publishing, 1996.)

to zero (see Fig. 6-7). Radiative interactions are important; they are the mechanism by which bremsstrahlung x-rays are produced in diagnostic x-ray tubes and linear accelerators. Bremsstrahlung production increases with incident electron energy and the Z of the absorber (see Fig. 6-21).

The probability for collisional and radiative interactions depends on electron energy and the atomic number of the incident material (see Fig. 6-21). At electron energies of 100 keV and for high Z absorbers (e.g., x-ray targets), 99% of the interactions are collisional, and 1% are radiative, resulting ultimately in heat deposition. At electron energies of 10 MeV, bremsstrahlung is a much more efficient process, and 50% of the interactions are collisional and 50% radiative. At 100 keV, x-ray production is inefficient, whereas at 10 MeV, x-ray production is efficient. Above 10 MeV, bremsstrahlung production exceeds collisional losses. It has been observed that dE_{COL}/dx increases as electron kinetic energy decreases below 1 MeV (see Fig. 6-21). As the electron slows down, it loses energy faster. Above 1 MeV, electrons lose about 2 MeV/cm traveling in water ($dE_{COL}/dx \approx 2$ MeV/cm). A 10-MeV electron has a range of about 5 cm in water (10 MeV ÷ 2 MeV/cm). Density scaling can be applied for materials different from unit density. For example, a 10-MeV electron travels approximately 3.3 cm in bone of density of 1.5 g/cm^3 (10 MeV ÷ [2 MeV/cm × 1.5]). These relationships use Equation 20 as their basis.

Heavy Charged Particle Interactions

Heavy charged particles, such as protons and alpha particles, experience mainly inelastic collisions. The rate of energy loss is high, resulting in short ranges. Trajectories in water or tissue are in the forward direction with little scattering; the particle mass is similar to that of the interacting material, and very few large angle direction changes occur, in contrast to the large amount of scattering experienced by electrons. Heavy charged particles exhibit rapidly increasing and large energy losses near the end of their ranges, because of the dependency on Z^2 and $1/V^2$ discussed earlier (see Eq. 21). This increase in energy loss results in a dramatic increase in ionization at the tail of the particle track length after a length of relatively constant loss, a phenomenon called the *Bragg peak*.[2,12,13] Bragg peaks are observable for protons (Fig. 6-22) and alpha particles. All charged particles exhibit a Bragg peak, including electrons; however, electrons are light enough such that multiple scatters occur and ionization paths are randomly oriented, blurring any observable effect.

Heavy Uncharged Particle Interactions: the Neutron

Neutrons have no charge and do not undergo coulomb interactions like charged particles. Instead, neutrons interact by inelastic and elastic collisions with nuclei through the strong force. Commonly for lower and middle Z materials, a neutron penetrates the nucleus and is absorbed, followed by the ejection of a proton (the [n,p] reaction). The new nucleus may be radioactive, a process called *neutron activation*. Neutrons may also cause nuclear disintegrations, similar to photodisintegration. For very heavy nuclei, neutrons may cause fission, a reaction harnessed for power production in nuclear reactors. Elastic scattering of neutrons is also common. The type of collision, inelastic or elastic, that a neutron experiences depends on the neutron energy and the absorber atomic number with complex reaction probabilities.[12,13] Neutrons lack charge, and their interactions with nuclei are exponential in nature, like photons (see Fig. 6-22). Their range is not finite; however, they have a mean path length equal to the inverse of the neutron attenuation coefficient.

Summary of Particle Interactions

1. Particles with kinetic energy have inelastic and elastic interactions with an absorbing material. Inelastic collisions result in loss of energy, whereas elastic collisions do not.
2. Electrons experience inelastic collisions through coulomb interactions with the atomic electrons or the nucleus. Collisional interactions with the atomic electrons result in excitation or ionization. Interactions with the nucleus result in production of bremsstrahlung x-rays.
3. For electrons, collisional energy losses dominate at lower energies, whereas radiative losses dominate at higher energies. Interestingly, collisional energy losses are greater per gram of low Z material than for high Z materials. The mate-

rial of choice for electron shielding is a low Z material because the stopping power per gram is higher and bremsstrahlung production is minimized.

4. In water or tissue, megavoltage electrons lose about 2 MeV/cm traveled. The electron range is finite, and its length in centimeters is found by dividing the energy (in MeV) by 2.
5. Electron interactions result in a large amount of scattering, caused by the light mass of the electron relative to the nuclear mass of any absorber.
6. Charged heavy particles undergo inelastic collisions mainly through coulomb interactions with the atomic electrons, resulting in excitation or ionization. Nuclear interactions occur only at very high energies and do not include bremsstrahlung production.
7. Charged heavy particles have a finite range and experience a rapid increase in energy loss near the end of their track, dumping much of their remaining energy quickly and producing an ionization curve with a Bragg peak.
8. Neutrons experience inelastic and elastic collisions with nuclei, resulting in nuclear rearrangements that are followed by ionization events. Neutrons do not have a finite range.

RADIATION QUANTITIES AND MEASUREMENT

Ionization and Its Fate

Ionizing radiation is quantified by measuring the amount of ionization produced. The number of ions is directly proportional to the amount of energy imparted to a material. An average of 33.92 eV is required to produce one ion pair (ip) in air.[14] This number is called the *W value* (W = 33.92 eV/ip for air), and it is almost independent of the radiation energy. W for other gases is quite similar to that of air, and its uniformity from material to material relates to atomic energy levels and capabilities for transfer of excitation energy.[2]

In four of the five photon interactions, energy is transferred from incident photons to produce ionization or secondary processes. This energy transfer results in radiation dose, and for each interaction, it has origins as follows:

1. In coherent scattering, there is no ionization. However, the scattered photon might be able to undergo an ionizing interaction.
2. In the photoelectric effect, the inner shell electrons are ionized. The photoelectron is ejected and loses its energy by excitation and ionizations. Characteristic x-rays and Auger electrons are energetic enough to cause ionizations.
3. In the Compton effect, the outer shell electrons are ionized. The scattered photons and the Compton (recoil) electrons may be energetic enough to cause ionizations.
4. In pair production, there is no direct ionization of the atom. However, the electron and positron each have enough energy to cause ionizations, and annihilation radiation is energetic enough to cause ionizations.
5. In photodisintegration, there is no direct ionization of the atom. However, the remaining atom (with one fewer neutron) may be unstable and decay by emission of ionizing particles, and the ejected neutron may cause activation of other atoms, resulting in nuclear decay and ionizations.

If these ions are collected and measured, the amount of energy deposited can be determined.

Radiation Quantities and Units

Ionizing radiation is quantified using two important quantities: exposure and dose. A third quantity, kerma, is an important concept that relates to exposure and dose.

Exposure

Exposure, X, is the measurement of the amount of ionization produced by photon interactions per mass of air (charge per mass of air). The unit of exposure is the roentgen (R), named after the discoverer of x-rays, Wilhelm Conrad Roentgen:

$$1\text{R} = 2.58 \times 10^{-4}\,\text{C/kg of air } (= 1\,\text{esu/cm}^3 \text{ in air})$$

In the previous expression, C (coulomb) is a unit of charge (or ionization) such that 1 ip = 1.6×10^{-19} C. The original definition of charge per volume, 1 R = 1 esu/cm^3, was based on the *e*lectrostatic *u*nit and is responsible for the odd units of the roentgen as now defined.

Several important concepts characterize the roentgen:

1. It is defined for all ionizations, primary and secondary, when produced and measured in air.
2. It is defined only for ionizing photons (x-rays and gamma rays), not electrons.
3. It is properly measured only under conditions of electronic equilibrium, and it is difficult to measure for photon energies higher than 3 MeV. Above this energy, the electron range in air becomes too large for electronic equilibrium to be achieved practically.

ELECTRONIC EQUILIBRIUM

With electronic equilibrium, ionization lost downstream from a volume of interest is replaced by an equal amount from upstream, producing an equilibrium and an accurate ionization measurement. The concept is illustrated in Figure 6-23. After interaction, ionization (electrons) travels away from the interaction point in the direction of the incident photons and a portion actually leaves the volume. To accurately measure the amount of ionization produced, the lost kinetic energy of the escaping electrons must be replaced by an equal amount that enters the volume from upstream (see Fig. 6-23). This equilibrium is called *electronic equilibrium* or *charged-particle equilibrium* and is a required condition for measurement of exposure.

Dose

Dose, D, is the measurement of the amount of energy imparted per mass of material (energy per mass).[11] The unit of dose is the gray (Gy): 1 Gy = 1 J/kg. An earlier dose unit is the rad (rad): 1 rad = 100 erg/g = 0.01 Gy = 1 cGy; 1 Gy = 100 rad.

Dose does not have the restrictions of exposure, and the following two statements therefore apply:

1. Dose is valid for any ionizing radiation at any energy (e.g., x-rays, γ-rays, e^-, e^+, n, p, α, π).
2. Dose is valid for any material and phase: solid, liquid, or gas.

In practice, dose to a medium is determined by measuring exposure and converting it to dose using the W value and the mass energy absorption coefficient, μ_{en}/ρ. The mass energy absorption coefficient is similar to the mass attenuation coefficient, except it describes energy absorbed, not attenuated.

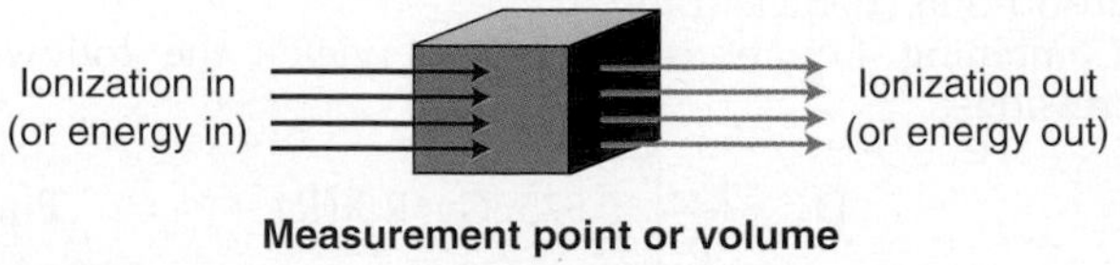

Figure 6-23 Ionization lost downstream from a volume of interest is replaced by an equal amount from upstream, producing electronic equilibrium and an accurate ionization measurement.

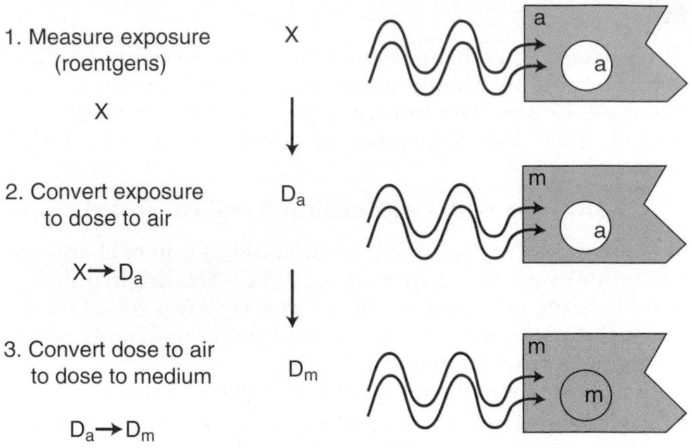

Figure 6-24 The dose measurement process. Exposure to a small mass of air is converted to the dose to medium.

The process is illustrated in Figure 6-24 for the following steps:

1. Exposure, X, of 1 R is given to a small air-filled cavity contained in a material:

$$X = 1\text{R}$$

2. Dose to air in the cavity is computed using the W value and the definition of the roentgen, converting energy units as needed:

$$\begin{aligned} D_a &= WX = 33.92\,\text{eV/ip} \times 1\text{R} \\ (\text{converting units}) &= (33.92\,\text{eV/ip})(1\,\text{ip}/1.6\times10^{-19}\,\text{coul}) \\ &\quad \times (2.58\times10^{-4}\,\text{C/kg/1R}) \\ &\quad \times (1.6\times10^{-12}\,\text{erg/eV}) \\ &\quad \times (1\,\text{kg}/1000\,\text{g}) \\ (\text{converting to cGy}) &= (87.5\,\text{erg/g/R})(1\,\text{cGy}/100\,\text{erg/g}) \\ \text{so} \quad D_a &= 0.875\,\text{cGy/R for an exposure of 1R} \end{aligned}$$

Eq. 22

For X number of roentgens, the dose to air is calculated as follows:

$$D_a = 0.875\,\text{cGy/R}\;X(\text{R}) \qquad \text{Eq. 23}$$

3. Dose to the material is calculated by converting dose to air, D_a, to D_m. Conceptually, this step replaces the air cavity with an identical volume of the material. It can be shown[12,13] that

$$D_m = D_a \left.\frac{\mu_{en}}{\rho}\right|_a^m \qquad \text{Eq. 24}$$

in which $\left.\frac{\mu_{en}}{\rho}\right|_a^m$ is the mass energy absorption coefficient for the material, $\left.\frac{\mu_{en}}{\rho}\right|_m$, divided by $\left.\frac{\mu_{en}}{\rho}\right|_a$, the mass energy absorption coefficient for air.

Combining Equations 23 and 24 yields the following expressions:

$$D_m = \left.\frac{\mu_{en}}{\rho}\right|_a^m 0.875\,\text{cGy/R}\;X(\text{R}) \qquad \text{Eq. 25}$$

and

$$D_m = fX(\text{R}) \qquad \text{Eq. 26}$$

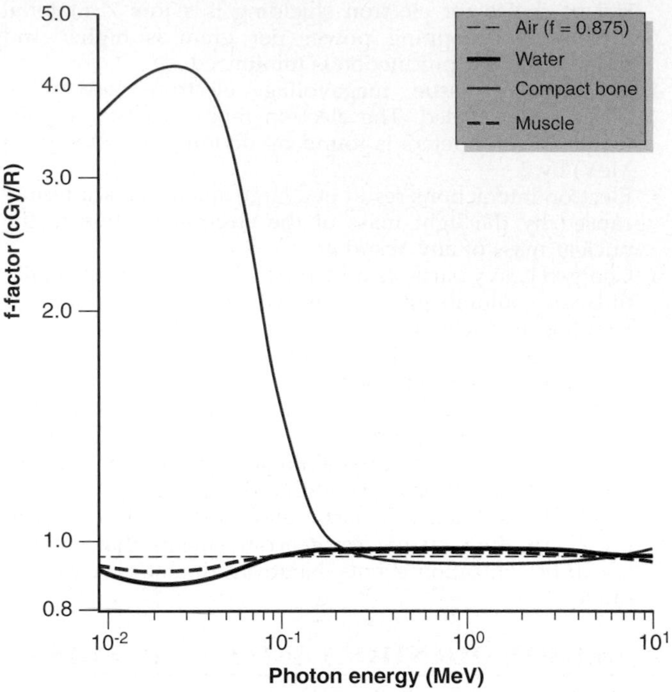

Figure 6-25 The f factor varies as a function of the material and the photon energy. (Data from Radiological Health Handbook. Bethesda, MD, U.S. Department of Health, Education, and Welfare, 1970.)

in which the f factor, f, is calculated as follows:

$$f = \left.\frac{\mu_{en}}{\rho}\right|_a^m 0.875\,\text{cGy/R} \qquad \text{Eq. 27}$$

For any exposure, X(R), measured in air, the dose to a material substituted at that point can be found by multiplying the f factor by the exposure. In practice, the air-filled cavity is an ionization chamber. Ionization collected is converted to exposure and then dose, usually through a calibration procedure.

The f factor is an important parameter, and it varies as a function of the material and the photon energy, as shown for water, muscle, and bone in Figure 6-25. By its definition, the f factor for air is always 0.875. Water, muscle, and air have similar f factors because their effective atomic numbers are similar. Bone has a higher atomic number (by a factor of 2) and receives up to four times the dose that soft tissue would receive in the photoelectric region. This effect is responsible for high bone doses received during orthovoltage treatment as well as the contrast seen in diagnostic x-ray films. Notice the decrease in the f factor for fat in the photoelectric region due to its lower Z because of its high hydrogen content.

For treatment with ionizing radiation, the amount of energy deposited is quite small. It takes about 1 million cGy to raise the temperature of 1 cm^3 of water by 1°C. Conversely, for a daily treatment dose of 200 rad (2 Gy, or 200 cGy), the increase in temperature per gram is only 0.0002°C.

Kerma

When photon radiation interacts with a material, energy is transferred to secondary electrons (the photoelectron, Compton electron, pair production electrons) and results in their kinetic energy. This transferred energy is called *kerma* (*k*inetic *e*nergy *r*eleased in *m*edium). Kerma, K, is expressed as the amount of energy released per mass of irradiated material and has the same unit as for dose, the gray (J/kg). Kerma differs from dose in that kerma is the energy *released* per mass, and dose is the energy *absorbed* per mass. These two quantities may be numerically quite similar, but there are three important aspects to their relationship:

1. The kerma at a point travels (primarily) in the forward direction for megavoltage photons. Secondary particles released at the point deliver their dose downstream from the point, not at the point. Kerma may result in a numerically equal dose but not at the same point of interaction.
2. Even if at the same point of interest, kerma will be greater than dose, because secondary electrons may lose some of their energy by the bremsstrahlung process. The bremsstrahlung x-rays carry energy away from the point of interest. $D = K(1 - g)$, in which g is the fraction of energy lost to bremsstrahlung.
3. If electronic equilibrium is satisfied, and bremsstrahlung is negligible ($g << 1$), dose equals kerma.

Thorough treatments of exposure, dose, kerma, and their relationships are available.[12-14] Much has been studied and written about these and other dosimetric concepts to establish meaningful and consistent definitions. A summary is presented in Table 6-7.

Radiation Detection and Measurement

There are different types of radiation detection and measurement instruments with particular characteristics that enable measurements of a certain kind to be performed. General classes of instruments are gas-filled detectors, scintillation detectors, other solid-state detectors, absolute dosimeters, and personnel dosimeters.

Gas-Filled Detectors

Gas-filled detectors operate on the basic principle of measuring exposure, that is, collecting ionization in air or a substitute gas. A gas-filled volume is defined as one that contains two oppositely charged plates or wires to collect the charge resulting from ionization in the gas. The reading is in units of charge (coulombs), exposure, or exposure rate. Figure 6-26A shows a simple parallel plate gas-filled detector and its components. As the voltage applied to the electrodes is increased from zero, the amount of charge collected increases (see Fig. 6-26B). The distinct voltage regions are expanded in Table 6-8. In general, gas-filled detectors require calibration before making radiation measurements.

IONIZATION CHAMBERS

Ionization chambers operate in region II (see Fig. 6-26B) and are an important type of radiation dosimeter as the principal device used for calibration of radiation therapy beams. The design most commonly used for photon beams is the thimble chamber, also called a *Farmer chamber,* which has a cylindrical geometry with central linear and outer cylindrical electrodes (Fig. 6-27A). An active volume of .6 cc is convention, although chambers with smaller or larger volumes are available for specialized purposes such as small field dosimetry or low dose rate measurements. Parallel-plate chambers are also used and are the recommended chamber geometry for electron beam dosimetry (see Fig. 6-27B). In general, ionization chambers require calibration before use. Ionization currents produced by radiation beams are very small, on the order of 10^{-9} amperes (A), and require a high-precision device called an *electrometer* for accurate measurement. An ionization chamber and electrometer require calibration before use and with a triaxial connecting cable are required tools for radiation beam calibration. Conditions for radiation beam calibrations are set by national protocols such as the Task Group (TG)-51 from the American Association of Physicists in Medicine[15] and by national or state

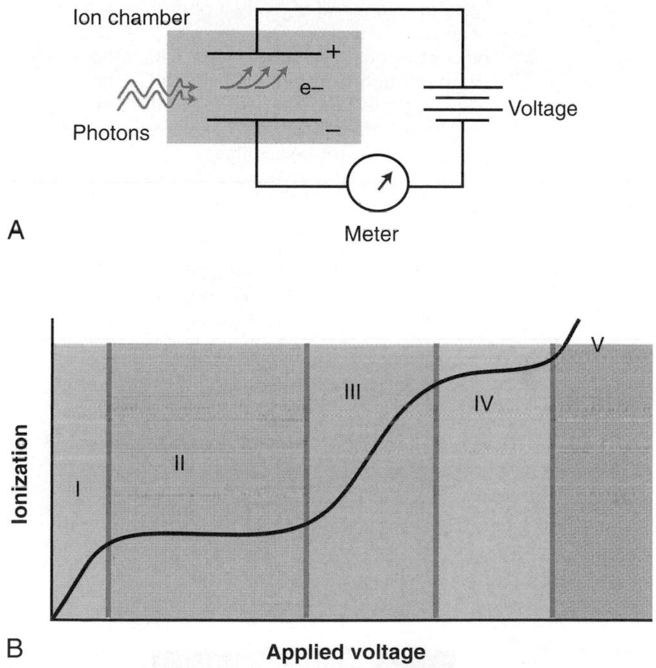

Figure 6-26 Response of a gas-filled detector. **A,** A gas-filled detector collects ionizations from an irradiated volume. **B,** Variation of collected ionization as bias voltage is increased. Regions are explained in Table 6-8.

Table 6-7 Radiologic Units

Quantity	What Is Measured	Unit (Symbol)	Value
Exposure	Ionization in air	Roentgen (R)	2.58×10^{4} C/kg$\|_{air}$
Dose	Energy absorbed in matter	rad (rad)	100 erg/g
Dose (SI)	Energy absorbed in matter	Gray (Gy)	1 J/kg
Kerma	Kinetic energy released in matter	Gray (Gy)	1 J/kg
Dose equivalent	Biologic effect of energy absorbed	rem (rem)	QF × 100 erg/g
Dose equivalent (SI)	Biologic effect of energy absorbed	Sievert (Sv)	QF × 1 J/kg
Activity	Disintegrations per time	Curie (Ci)	3.7×10^{10} d/s
Activity (SI)	Disintegrations per time	Becquerel (Bq)	1 d/s
Exposure rate constant	Exposure rate per activity	Gamma Γ	$R \cdot m^2 \cdot h^{-1} \cdot Ci^{-1}$
Exposure rate constant (SI)	Exposure rate per activity	Gamma Γ	$Gy \cdot m^2 \cdot s^{-1} \cdot Bq^{-1}$
Air kerma strength	Air kerma in free space	S_k	$\mu Gy \cdot m^2 \cdot h^{-1}$

Table 6-8 Voltage Regions of Gas-Filled Detectors

Region	Description
I	The recombination region. The voltage is not high enough to separate the ion pairs and recombination occurs.
II	The saturation region. The voltage is high enough to collect almost 100% of the ionization (hence, "saturation"). Also called the ionization region.
III	The proportional, or gas amplification, region. The voltage is high enough to accelerate the ionized electrons to an energy that causes additional ionization, amplifying the actual amount of initial ionization by a factor M.
IV	The Geiger-Muller, or GM, region. The voltage is high enough that amplification by accelerated ions proceeds so that the entire gas in the detector is ionized each time a photon hits the detector. Whether low or high energy, the amount of ionization that occurs is the same. Thus, a GM counter emits a "click" for each photon seen, and is really a photon counting device.
V	The continuous discharge region. The voltage is high enough to spontaneously ionize the detector gas. Once started, the ionization continues and continues. The detector is not useful at this applied voltage.

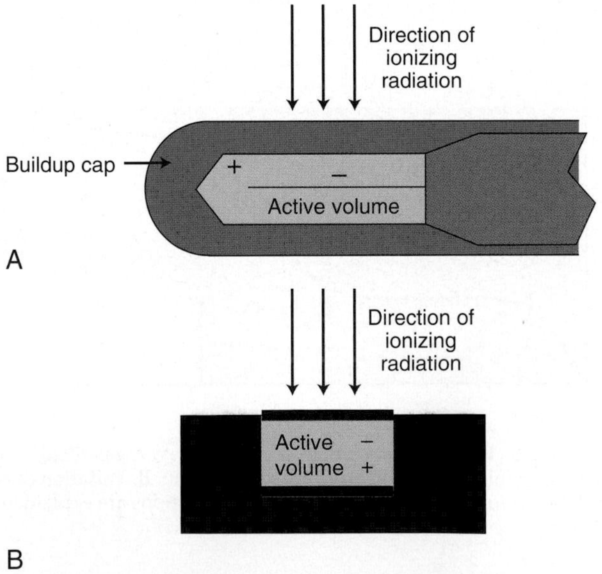

Figure 6-27 Ionization chamber designs. **A,** Thimble chamber. **B,** Parallel-plate chamber. A buildup cap may be added to either chamber to ensure electronic equilibrium, depending on the measurement being performed.

regulatory bodies. A requirement for operation of all ionization chambers is that the chamber be operated under conditions of electronic equilibrium. In disequilibrium conditions, the amount of ionization measured is incorrect, as will be the exposure or dose calculation.

Solid-State Detectors

Thermoluminescent Dosimeters

In a simple model, crystalline solids have two electron energy levels, called the *valence* and *conduction bands.* The valence

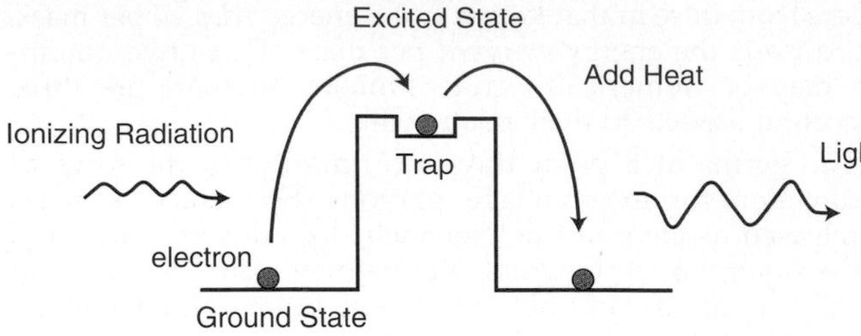

Figure 6-28 Thermoluminescence. Ionizing radiation raises an electron-hole pair to an excited but trapped state. Addition of heat allows de-excitation, which occurs with the emission of light.

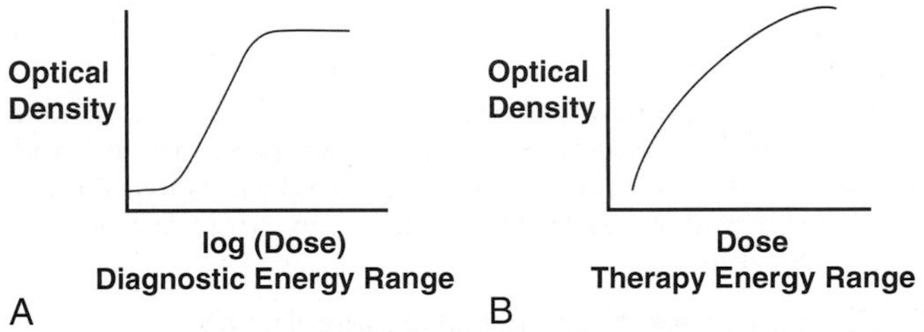

Figure 6-29 Film radiation response varies with film type, photon energy, and dose. **A,** Diagnostic photon energy response. **B,** Therapeutic photon energy response.

band holds bound electrons, whereas the conduction band consists of free electrons. Energy states between these two bands are forbidden. When ionized, a bound electron may gain sufficient energy to jump to the conduction band, leaving a positive "hole" in the valence band. The conduction band electron and the hole can move through the lattice and eventually recombine, with the emission of light on recombination. Because of impurities in the lattice, some crystalline materials have the property of having long-lived "traps" that can hold an electron-hole pair in an excited (or unfilled) state. The electron-hole pair is created and excited into the trap by the absorption of ionizing radiation, which provides the energy to push the pair into the trap (Fig. 6-28). Heating the crystal enables the electron-hole pair to leave the trap and return to the de-excited state. With this transition, an amount of light is emitted that is proportional to the amount of radiation dose. Dose is measured by measuring the amount of light emitted. The two most common types of thermoluminescent dosimeter (TLD) are lithium fluoride (LiF, almost tissue equivalent) and calcium fluoride (CaF, not tissue equivalent). A calibration factor must be obtained before use as a dosimeter. TLD is used for in vivo patient dose monitoring during treatment and for personnel monitoring for radiation safety purposes.

Film

Film is a solid-state detector. The amount of optical density is proportional to the dose. The response is energy sensitive because film is relatively high Z (the silver content). Response curves are shown in Figure 6-29. Film is used to obtain relative dose distributions (i.e., isodose distributions), for treatment machine quality-assurance tests for flatness, symmetry, radiation-light field congruence, and imaging.[16] A dose-response curve must be carefully measured, including constant processor control, to enable film to be used to measure actual (not relative) doses. A new type of tissue-equivalent film, called *radiochromic film,* uses opacity changes from radiation-induced polymerization to indicate dose.[17] This film does not require developing but does have an optimal wave-

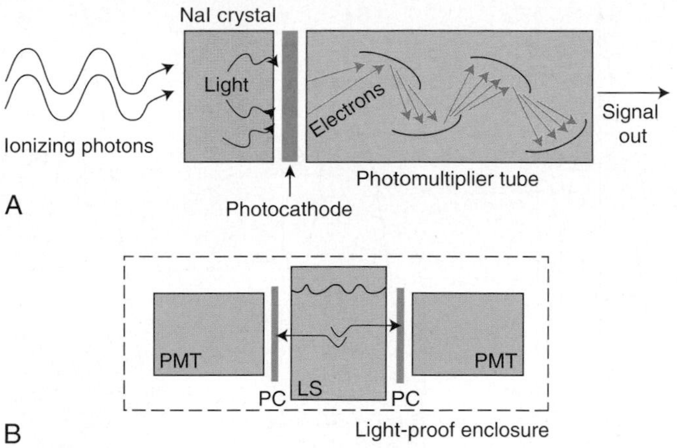

Figure 6-30 Scintillation detectors. Ionizing radiation creates light photons that are converted to electrons and amplified. **A,** Sodium iodine crystal and photomultiplier tube. **B,** Liquid scintillation detection.

length of light for reading. Its primary use is for therapy beam quality assurance and dosimetry, and it is not an imaging device.

SCINTILLATION DETECTORS

Scintillation (light) detectors detect radiation by measuring the amount of light produced in special crystalline materials by the ionizing radiation. The most common material used is sodium iodine (NaI). The NaI crystal is coupled to a photomultiplier tube that amplifies the detection signal coming from the crystal (Fig. 6-30A). NaI detectors are extremely sensitive and detect background radiation easily. They are used to detect low-energy or low-activity (dose rate) sources. They are used in uncalibrated form; a pulse indicates a photon has been detected.

Scintillation materials can also be made in liquid form. With this technique a radiation source (i.e., a sample of radioactive material) is put in direct contact with a liquid scintillator by immersion (see Fig. 6-30B). This intimate contact enables extremely small activities to be detected. Detection limits are in the microcurie and picocurie ranges. This method is used most for detection of very-low-energy beta particles for radioisotope tracer studies, environmental sampling, and isotope analysis of waste or other materials. The liquid scintillator is called a *cocktail* and includes a solvent and the scintillation material. Liquid scintillation detectors require calibration before use, including determination of background count rates.

SEMICONDUCTOR DETECTORS: GERMANIUM AND SILICON

Germanium (GeLi) and silicon (SiLi) detectors are semiconductor materials that can be used to detect the energies of photons. These detectors are useful only at very low dose rates (i.e., small sample activities or low fluence rates) and are used to measure the photon energy spectrum, not dose.

Absolute Dosimeters

Most dosimeters require calibration in the form of the dose or exposure per reading. Absolute dosimeters *do not* require calibration and instead measure the amount of dose directly.

CALORIMETRY

All radiation dose, which is energy imparted per mass, eventually becomes heat. If the change in temperature is measured, the amount of dose is known. Temperature changes per centigray are quite small; a very sensitive device called a *calorimeter* is used. Standard-setting bodies, such as the National Institute of Science and Technology, have calorimeters to set the exact calibration factors for radiation beams and instrumentation.

CHEMICAL OR FRICKE DOSIMETER

The Fricke dosimeter measures chemical changes that are catalyzed by ionizing radiation. The chemical yield of the new product is directly proportional to the radiation dose. The most common reaction used is ferric to ferrous sulfide, such that the amount of Fe^{3+} produced is proportional to the dose delivered.

Personnel Dosimetry

Monitoring of dose for radiation safety purposes is required for occupational workers. Both TLD and film are used, assembled with other components into a radiation "badge" that is worn at the waist or neck during work. Filters that overlay the dosimeter enable discrimination between electrons or low-energy photons and high-energy photons. In high dose rate environments, direct-read dosimeters can be used for instant readout. Personnel dosimeters are made in holders to enable whole-body and extremity monitoring.

References on radiation instrumentation and measurement are available that give detailed theory, design parameters, and operational characteristics for different classes of detectors.[12,13,18]

BUILDUP PHENOMENON

Megavoltage photon beams used for radiation treatment exhibit a phenomenon in which the dose in an absorber is relatively low at the surface but rapidly increases to a maximum during the next few millimeters or tens of millimeters. This region of rapidly increasing dose is called the *buildup region* and is explained as follows (Fig. 6-31). The secondary electrons produced by megavoltage photon interactions travel primarily in the forward direction from the interaction point. The direction and range are represented by the groups of arrows in Figure 6-31. The surface is the first point of interaction, and dose from these interactions is delivered in the forward direction (point A). Because there are no interaction points upstream from the surface to produce secondary electrons, the surface dose is low. Ignoring attenuation and other small changes to the photon fluence with depth, interactions occur in the next layer of material beneath the surface, with a similar forward dose distribution. These electron tracks overlap (sum) with those from the surface. Additional layers at depth have similar interactions and resulting secondary electron distributions that sum with previous ones. The amount of dose increases rapidly and nonlinearly as successive electron tracks overlap (point B). Given an average, finite secondary electron range, a point is eventually reached where full electron overlap occurs (point D). At this point, the number of summed electron tracks is constant because the electrons being produced match those being lost. A maximum dose, D_m, is reached at a depth called d_m (see Fig. 6-31), and d_m indicates the average secondary electron range and is the point at which electronic equilibrium is obtained. Because photon attenuation occurs, the number of interactions and resulting secondary electrons decreases with depth from the surface. Attenuation competes with the buildup process; however, buildup is more rapid than attenuation, resulting in a net gain of dose. The presence and steepness of a buildup region depend on incident photon energy, which governs the type of interaction and the range and distribution of second-

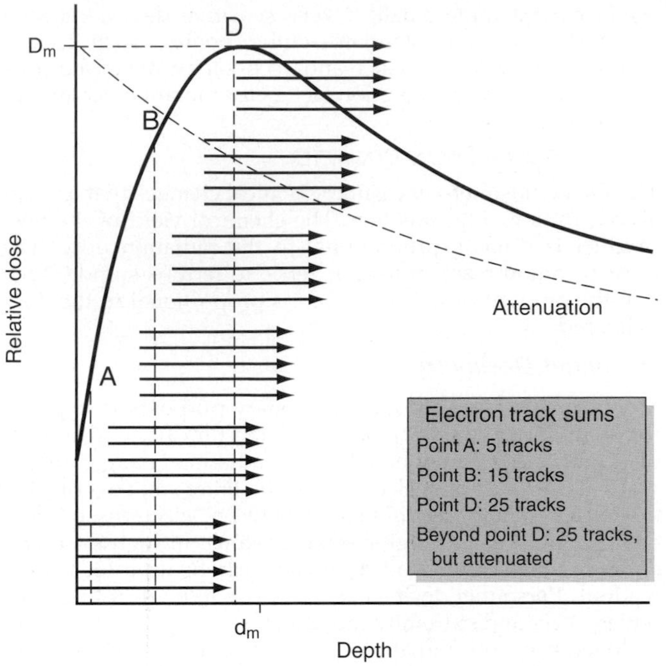

Figure 6-31 Radiation dose buildup. With secondary electrons primarily in the downstream direction, successive electron tracts overlap to produce a rapidly increasing region of dose, called *buildup*. A maximum dose, D_m, is reached at a depth called d_m, indicates the average secondary electron range, and is the point at which electronic equilibrium is obtained. Because photon attenuation occurs, the number of interactions *(dotted line)* and resulting secondary electrons decreases with the depth from the surface. Attenuation competes with the buildup process, but because buildup occurs more rapidly than attenuation, a net gain of dose results.

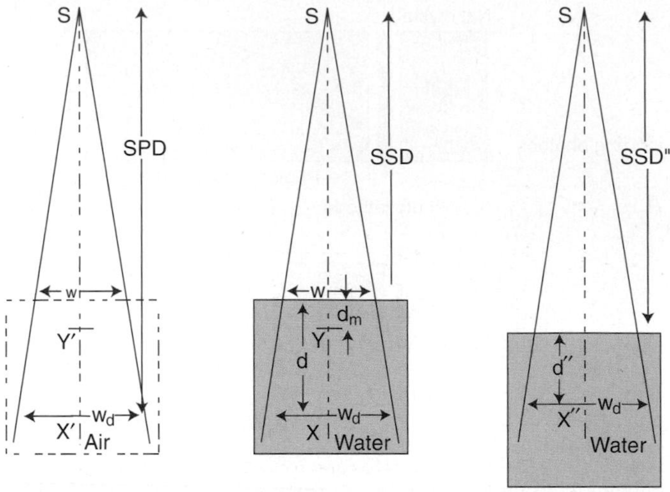

Figure 6-32 Reference irradiation geometries used for measurement of percent depth dose, tissue-air ratio, and tissue-phantom ratio. (Adapted from ICRU Report 24: Determination of Absorbed Dose in a Patient Irradiated by Beams of X and Gamma Rays in Radiotherapy Procedures. Washington, DC, International Commission on Radiation Units and Measurements, 1976.)

ary electrons. At higher photon energies, d_m is larger because the average secondary electron range is greater. Beyond d_m, photon attenuation results in transient electronic equilibrium (i.e., energy in is slightly greater than energy out) and a decrease in dose with depth (shown as the dotted line; the difference is exaggerated).

DOSE RELATIONSHIPS FOR EXTERNAL BEAMS

Three mathematical functions are used to describe the dose characteristics for external radiation beams: percent depth dose (PDD), tissue-air ratio (TAR), and tissue-phantom ratio (TPR).[12,13] These dose functions relate the dose at any point to the dose at a reference point. The irradiation geometry shown in Figure 6-32 illustrates the measurement conditions for the following discussions.[19]

Percent Depth Dose

PDD is the ratio of the dose at depth, D_d, to the maximum dose, D_m, measured along the central axis of the beam and expressed as a percent. Points X and Y are the locations at depth, D_d and D_m, respectively, in Figure 6-32B. PDD is dependent on the depth, d, reference depth, d_m (the point of maximum dose), beam quality (or energy), E, source-to-surface distance, SSD, and field size at the surface, w. Mathematically,

$$\mathrm{PDD}(d, d_m, E, \mathrm{SSD}, w) = \frac{D_d}{D_m} \times 100\% = \frac{D_X}{D_Y} \times 100\% \qquad \text{Eq. 28}$$

PDD is often expressed as a fraction rather than as a percent. PDD was the dose function first measured for diagnostic and therapy radiation beams because of the simplicity of measurement, and it remains a basic dose measurement for beam characterization. Inherent in a PDD measurement are the effects of attenuation by the material and the inverse square effect as the distance from the source is changed. PDD is used for photon and electron beams and is often used in tabular form for monitor unit calculations.

Tissue-Air Ratio

Given a fixed irradiation point in space, the ratio of the dose in phantom, D_X, to the dose in air, D_X', at the same point is called the *TAR* (see Fig.6-32A and B). TAR indicates how dose in air is affected when the air is replaced by tissue. The field size at the point and source-to-point distance are constant; the only variable is the depth in phantom:

$$\mathrm{TAR}(d, w_d, E) = \frac{D_X(d, w_d, E)}{D_X'(w_d, E)} \qquad \text{Eq. 29}$$

TAR is essentially independent of SSD because scatter contributions are almost constant for fixed field sizes, regardless of SSD. This independence enables the use of the TAR over a wide range of clinically used SSDs without correction. TAR is used for photon beams only and is not valid for electron beams.

A special case of the TAR, called the *backscatter factor* (BSF), exists when the point of interest is the depth of maximum dose (when $d = d_m$). In this case, the TAR has a maximum value, and

$$\mathrm{BSF}(w_{d_m}, E) = \mathrm{TAR}(d_m, w_{d_m}, E) = \frac{D_Y}{D_{Y'}} \qquad \text{Eq. 30}$$

The BSF takes its name for historical reasons, from a time when low-energy photons were used and the point of maximum dose was on the surface. Any dose scattered to the surface from the phantom or patient was truly backscattered dose.

To determine the TAR and BSF, dose data are acquired at sampled points in phantom and air across and along the radiation beam central axis for the range of field sizes, depths, and SSDs or source-to-axis distances (SADs) clinically relevant.

Tissue-Phantom Ratio

TPR must be used for photon energies above about 4 MV, when in-air measurements required for the TAR are impractical. As with PDD and the TAR, the TPR is the ratio of two doses; however, both doses are made in phantom. The TPR is the ratio of dose D_X, measured at depth d, to dose $D_{X''}$, measured at a reference depth d″ (see Fig. 6-32B and C):

$$TPR(d, W_d, E, d'') = D_{X''} \frac{D_X(d, W_d, E)}{(d'', W_{d''}, E)} \quad \text{Eq. 31}$$

Both measurement points are fixed in space such that the source-to-point distance and field size are the same at each point. The depth of point X is varied to generate TPRs over a range of depths for a particular field size. TPR is essentially independent of SSD because scatter contributions are almost constant for fixed field sizes, regardless of SSD. This independence enables the use of the TPR over a wide range of clinically used SSDs without correction. TPR is used for photon beams only and is not valid for electron beams.

When d″ is the depth of maximum dose, the TPR is called the *tissue-maximum ratio* (TMR). The TPR and the TMR are used in the same manner as the TAR in dose calculations. TMR is the most common data format used for monitor unit calculations in simple computer programs and manual (hand) calculations.

Primary and Scatter Dose: The Scatter-Air Ratio

Mayneord first proposed that PDD could be separated into primary and secondary (or scatter) components.[11] Later, Clarkson[20] proposed sector integration of scatter components in calculating the PDD at any point inside or outside an irregular field. This concept was later applied by Gupta and Cunningham to the TAR.[21] The concept states that dose at a point is the sum of primary and scatter components. The primary dose results from photons that have interactions at the point of interest. The secondary dose results from photons and electrons that scatter to the point of interest from other interaction points. With this concept, TAR is given by the following expression:

$$TAR = TAR_0 + SAR \quad \text{Eq. 32}$$

In the equation, TAR_0 is the TAR for zero field size, representing primary dose, and SAR is the scatter-air ratio, representing secondary dose. The TAR_0 is found by extrapolation of circular field TARs to zero field size. The SAR is calculated as the difference between the TAR and the TAR_0. For an irregular field, an effective TAR can be found that is the sum of the TAR_0 and an effective SAR for the irregular field:

$$TAR_{irreg}(d, W_d, E) = TAR_0(d, E) + SAR_{irreg}(d, W_d, E) \quad \text{Eq. 33}$$

The irregular field SAR is found by sector integration:

$$SAR_{irreg}(d, W_d, E) = \frac{1}{2\pi} \sum SAR_i(d, W_{d_i}, E) \times \Delta\Theta \quad \text{Eq. 34}$$

in which $\Delta\theta$ is the angular increment in radians for each sector. Separation of primary and secondary dose can be applied to any of the dose functions in a similar fashion. For instance, the TMR can be represented as $TMR = TMR_0 + SMR$.

The TAR/SAR and TMR/SMR functions are more commonly used than PDD in dose computation algorithms because fewer inverse square corrections are needed. The TAR and TMR are easily found for isocentric treatment geometries where the size of the treatment field at the isocenter is equal to the treatment field size at the center of the target volume, which simplifies hand (noncomputer) calculations.

Although PDD can be measured with an ionization chamber beyond d_m over the wide range of clinically used photon energies, the TAR cannot be measured when the photon energy exceeds about 3 MV because the range of secondary electrons exceeds the thickness of the buildup cap for the ionization chamber. At these energies, PDD is measured and converted to TPR and TMR by well-known relationships.[12,13]

CHARACTERISTICS OF RADIATION THERAPY PHOTON BEAMS

Dose Characteristics

Photon beams used in radiation therapy have dose characteristics that vary primarily as a function of beam energy and treatment machine design. In the standard irradiation geometry (see Fig. 6-32B and C), PDD measurements are obtained along the central axis, beginning at the surface and proceeding to depth. A typical PDD curve shown in Figure 6-33 for megavoltage beams has the characteristics listed in Table 6-9.

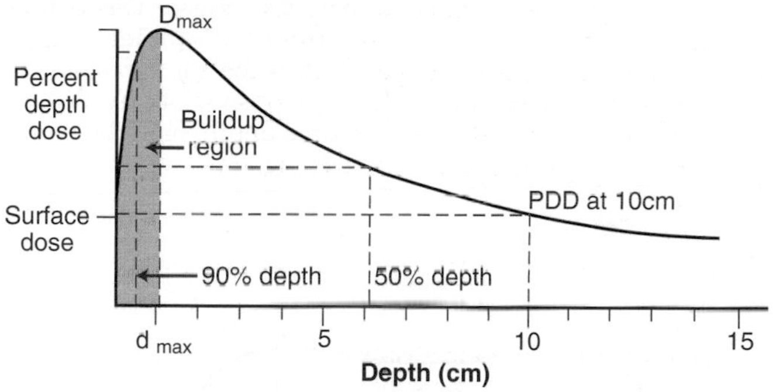

Figure 6-33 A typical photon percent depth dose (PDD) curve is characterized by surface dose, a buildup region, a point of maximum dose, and an exponentially attenuated region. Standard PDD measurements are obtained along the central axis *(dotted line)*, beginning at the surface and proceeding to depth.

Table 6-9 Characteristics of a Typical Percent Depth Dose Curve for Megavoltage Beams

Characteristic	Definition
Surface dose	Nonzero dose at the incident surface
Buildup region	Region between the incident surface and d_{max} where the dose rapidly increases
D_{max}	Maximum dose along the central axis; often used as a reference dose
d_{max}	Depth of maximum dose; often used as a reference point
Percent depth dose	Dose along the central axis of the beam, as a percentage of the d_{max} dose
90% dose depth	Depth from the surface where the dose in the buildup region reaches 90% of D_{max}
50% dose depth	Depth from the surface beyond d_{max}, where the dose falls to 50% of D_{max}
10-cm percent dose	The percent depth dose at 10 cm from the surface, a value often quoted as an indicator of beam penetration

Other important descriptors include an effective attenuation coefficient for depths beyond the maximum depth (d_{max}) and the HVL. The 10 cm PDD in water is most used as an indicator of beam quality, in place of the HVL, because the 10 cm PDD has clinical relevance and the HVL is a better indicator for shielding purposes.

Field size, flatness, symmetry, and sharpness of the beam edge can be measured with a dose profile (Fig. 6-34), which is a scanned dose measurement perpendicular to the central axis, across a beam (at a fixed depth, occurring along the horizontal line w_d in Fig. 6-32B and C). Dose profiles are normally made at several depths of interest (i.e., d_m, 5 cm, 10 cm, and 25 cm). Beam characteristics from a dose profile are listed in Table 6-10.

The flattening filter and beam steering determine flatness and symmetry in a linear accelerator. Flatness is defined at a reference depth, for instance at a 10-cm depth at the isocenter (SSD = 90 cm). A typical specification is for no more than 3% dose variation across the useful 80% of the field width (see Fig. 6-34). A radiation beam does not have a perfectly sharp edge but instead has a gradient from high to low dose with a rounded "shoulder" and "toe." This penumbra region is named for geometric shadowing of part of the source, as is the case for ^{60}Co teletherapy beams, which have a large (2 cm) physical source size. However, the penumbra region for linear accelerator beams is mostly a radiation component of secondary electrons and photons scattered from within the field and from the collimators to outside the beam edges. This scatter degrades the beam edge; the dose from the shoulder region scatters outside the beam edge to form the toe. *Penumbra* is defined as the distance over which the dose falls from 80% to 20% of the central axis dose at the same depth, or at the width of the 90% to 10% dose gradient (see Fig. 6-34).

Various methods exist to measure a radiation beam along lines of equal dose, called *isodose lines.* A certain dose level is identified in the standard geometry and then tracked to obtain a drawing of the dosimetric shape of the beam. Figure 6-35 shows sample isodose curves for a plane containing the central ray of a beam and a plane perpendicular to the central ray.

Effect of Energy

Photon beam characteristics change with beam energy. Representative beam data are presented in Table 6-11, PDDs in Figure 6-36, and isodose curves in Figure 6-37. Several key observations should be considered:

- PDD increases as energy increases. This effect can be represented by the depth of the 50% dose or the PDD at 10 cm and is consistent with the change in the effective attenuation coefficient.
- Surface dose decreases as energy increases. Scattered radiation is more forwardly directed, away from the surface, as energy increases, reducing the dose contribution at the surface. The breakthrough in achieving megavoltage energies is that surface dose decreased from 100% and d_m moved away from the surface, providing "sparing" of skin and superficial tissues.
- The buildup region has a very steep climb of PDD to D_m. Most therapy beams have reached at least 90% of their D_m dose within 1 cm of the surface.
- The d_m is at or near the surface for low energy beams and increases in depth as energy increases. As incident photon energy increases, the effective electron range (photoelectrons and Compton electrons) increases and the scatter component (secondary electrons and Compton scattered

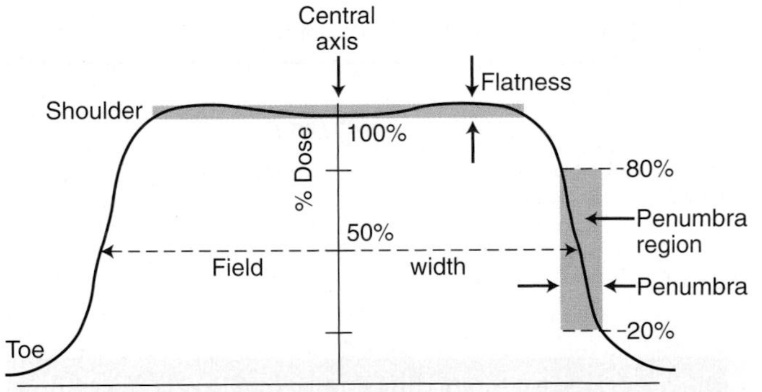

Figure 6-34 The dose profiles of a typical photon beam are characterized by shoulder and toe regions, with definitions for field width, flatness, and penumbra as indicated.

Table 6-10 Beam Characteristics from a Dose Profile

Characteristic	Definition
Field size	Distance from field edge to opposite edge at the 50% dose level, with normalization to 100% on the central axis (basically, full-width at half-maximum [FWHM])
Flatness	Deviation in dose level across the width of the field
Symmetry	Deviation in dose level for points symmetric about the central axis
Penumbra	Dose gradient regions from high to low dose at the beam edge

Table 6-11 Photon Beam Characteristics in Water

Beam Energy	Surface Dose (%)	90% Buildup Depth (cm)	d_{max} (cm)	50% Dose Depth (cm)	10 cm PDD	HVL and Material
60 kVp	100	None	.0	2	10	1.9 mm Al
120 kVp	100	None	.0	4	21	5.0 mm Al
300 kVp	100	None	.0	7	35	3.17 mm Cu
^{60}Co	40-90	.4	.5	12	55	11.9 mm Pb
4 MV x-rays	20-40	.3-.6	1.2	15	63	14.8 mm Pb
6 MV x-rays	10-30	.4-.7	1.5	15	67	15.4 mm Pb
10 MV x-rays	6-30	.7-1.0	2.5	19	74	16.9 mm Pb
18 MV x-rays	6-30	1.0-1.5	3.2	22	80	16.2 mm Pb

HVL, half-value layer; PDD, percent depth dose.

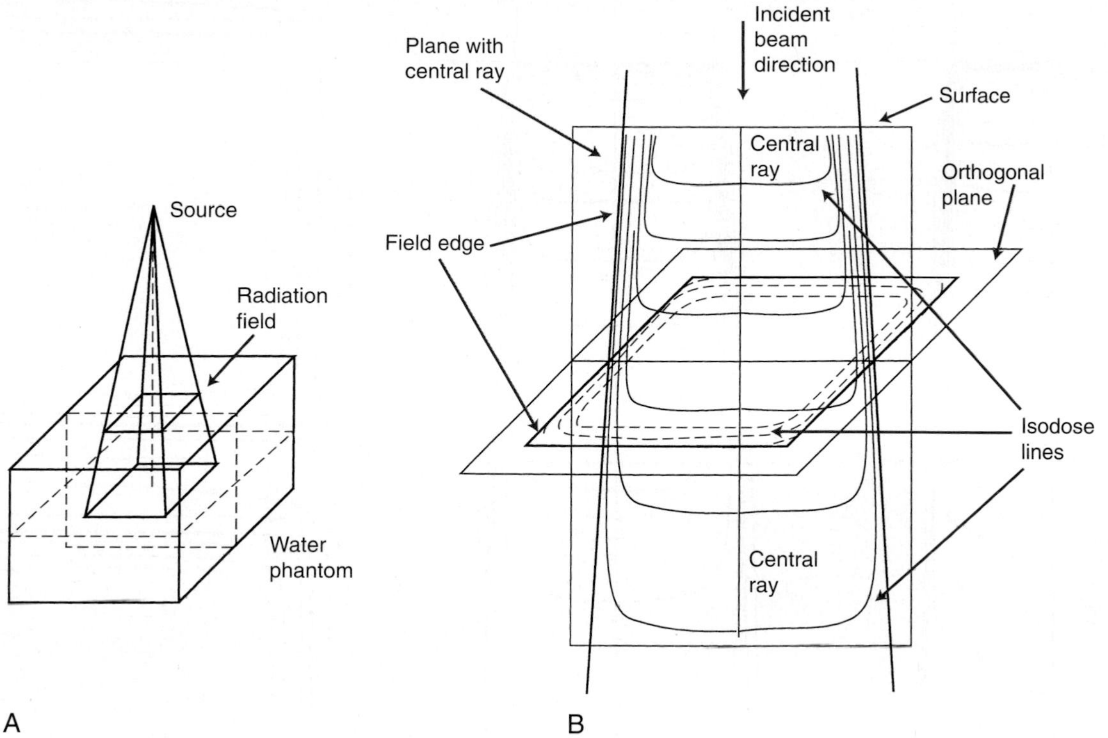

Figure 6-35 Irradiation geometries for isodose measurements. **A,** Beam orientation with phantom. **B,** Planes orthogonal to the central axis and isodose curves.

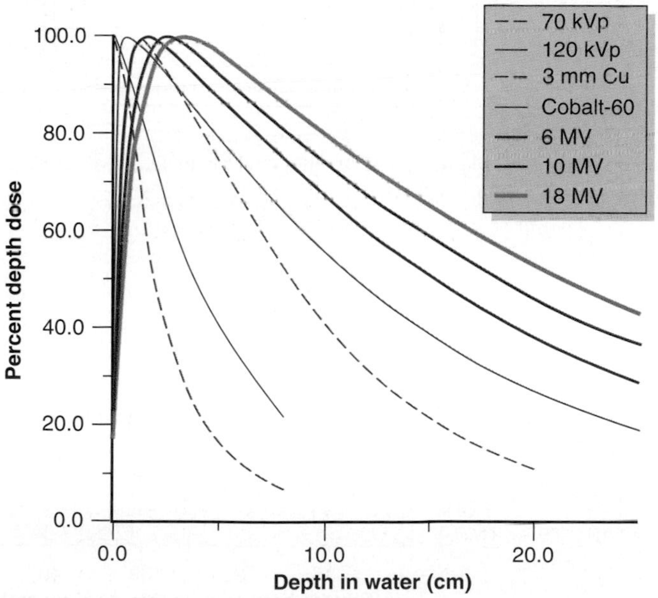

Figure 6-36 Photon percent depth dose curves. (Data courtesy of Wake Forest University Baptist Medical Center, Winston-Salem, NC; and data from Radiological Health Handbook. Bethesda, MD, U.S. Department of Health, Education, and Welfare, 1970.)

photons) is more forwardly directed. The d_m value is directly related to the average energy of secondary electrons produced in photoelectric and Compton interactions; d_m increases with energy.

- D_m is defined as a point, but as energy increases the PDD curve becomes very broad because of a broader spectrum for the scattered electrons. Strictly speaking, D_m is the one point where electronic equilibrium occurs.
- An effective attenuation coefficient can be found that describes the exponential fall-off in dose with depth.
- HVL, measured in lead at megavoltage energies, increases as peak energy is increased until about 6 MV, and it then falls slightly (see Table 6-11). HVL decreases because an increased amount of pair production increases the attenuation coefficient for photon energies above 6 MV (see Fig. 6-16). In tissue or water the attenuation coefficient decreases monotonically and the minimum is reached at very high energies, to the far right in Figure 6-16.
- Linear accelerator photon beams have an effective photon energy of approximately one third of the accelerating potential. For example, an 18-MV photon beam (polyenergetic, bremsstrahlung spectrum) has an effective monoenergetic value of 6-MeV photons.
- The central axis portion of a megavoltage beam from a linear accelerator is "harder" than the off-axis region because of the use of a flattening filter that is thicker in the central ray than off-axis (see Fig. 6-5). Because the flattening filter is designed to produce a flat field at a depth of 10 cm, not d_m, and the off-axis beam is softer than the central axis, a greater beam intensity off-axis is allowed at the depth of d_m to compensate for the increased attenuation of the off-axis beam component. This greater intensity is exhibited as "horns" in the isodose distribution for off-axis regions near d_m (see Fig. 6-37A). This effect is greater for lower energy megavoltage photons than for higher energies.

Effect of Field Size

Field size determines the amount of scatter present in the beam, with the following observations:

- PDD increases as the field size is increased. The effect results from a differential increase in scatter such that points

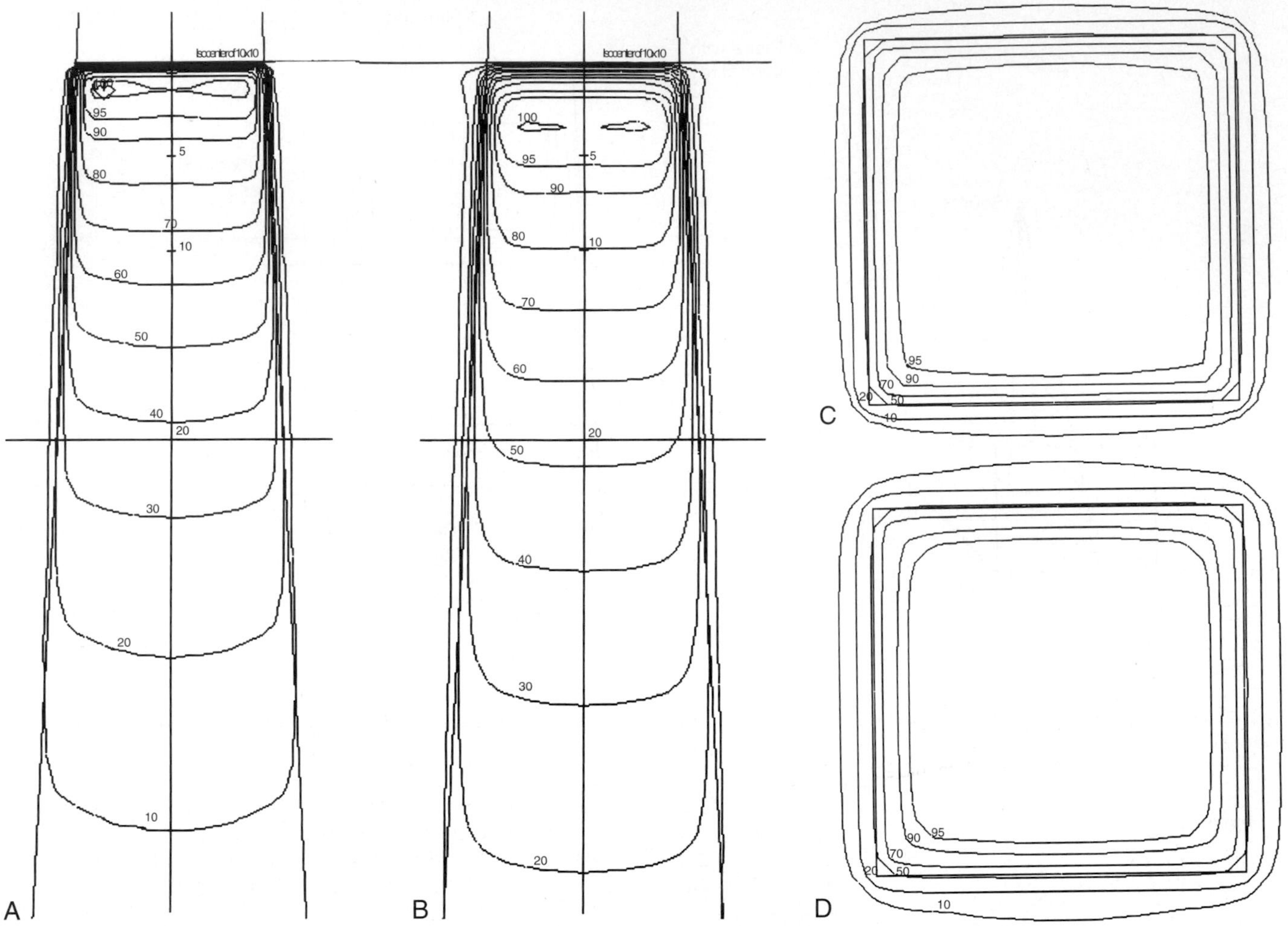

Figure 6-37 Photon isodose curves, 10 × 10 cm² fields. **A,** 6 MV, cross plane. **B,** 18 MV, cross plane. **C,** 6 MV, orthogonal plane. **D,** 18 MV, orthogonal plane. (Data courtesy of Wake Forest University Baptist Medical Center, Winston-Salem, NC.)

at depth receive a greater relative amount of scatter than does d_m, leading to an increase in PDD. The increased scatter at depth comes from interactions that occur in the increased irradiation volume.

- Surface dose increases as the field size is increased because the amount of scattered radiation from the collimator faces is increased. This scattered radiation includes secondary electrons and scattered photons of lower energy.
- Absolute dose rate, or beam output, increases as field size increases (Fig. 6-38). Output increases because there is increased scatter at d_m from the collimator faces as well as from interactions that occur in the increased volume of irradiated material. Figure 6-38 also illustrates the separation of dose into primary and secondary components.
- In a more subtle effect, d_m decreases as the field size increases because of the presence of an increased amount of lower energy photon and electron scatter.

Penumbra

Beam edge sharpness, or penumbra, is typically 7 to 12 mm in width and varies with the amount and energy of secondary electrons and scattered photons. As the amount of scatter increases, penumbra does likewise:

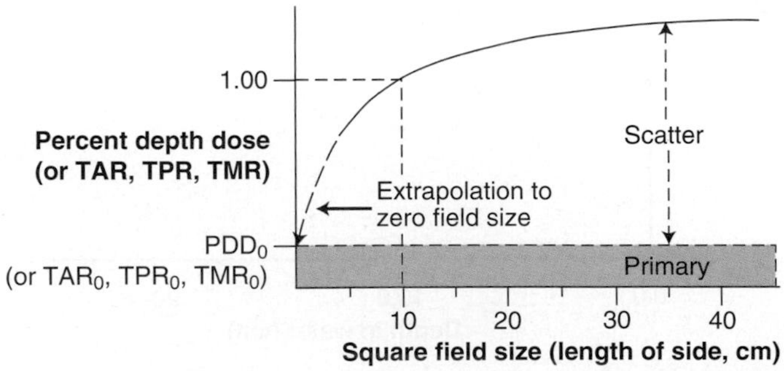

Figure 6-38 Relative dose as a function of photon field size.

- Penumbra increases as depth increases. At depth there is more scatter from the larger irradiated volume upstream, so the penumbra is wider.
- Penumbra increases with field size because of increased scatter from the increased volume of irradiated material and because there is a slight increase in beam divergence (a geometric effect).
- Penumbra increases as SSD increases.

- ^{60}Co has a wide penumbra because the source size is large and the geometric penumbra is large. However, some units have "trimmer" bars that greatly reduce the geometric penumbra component, yielding penumbrae comparable to those of linear accelerations.
- Penumbra increases with energy. Scattered electrons and photons that have a higher effective energy have a corresponding higher lateral range of scatter outside the beam edge. This effect is seen as a degradation of the profile (more pronounced shoulder and toe). This comparison is shown in Figure 6-37A and B.

Beam Modifiers

Various devices can be put into a photon beam to modify the shape of the beam and its dose distribution. Collimators and custom blocks are used to shape the field, as previously discussed. Their dosimetric effect is to change the irradiated volume and therefore the amount of scatter.

Physical wedges produce skewed isodose lines at fixed angles across the central ray (Fig. 6-39) to compensate for beam angle of incidence, tissue shape, or the trajectory of other treatment beams. Historically, wedge angles of 15, 30, 45, and 60 degrees have been available using physical wedges made of steel or lead. Isodoses show the wedge angle is measured from a perpendicular to the central ray, typically at a depth of 10 cm. A physical wedge produces an attenuated beam that is decreased in absolute dose rate and slightly more penetrating due to beam hardening by the wedge. An alternative wedging system uses no physical wedge and produces angled isodose lines by scanning one of the independent collimator jaws across the field while the beam is on. This dynamic method does not result in hardening or attenuation of the beam and is called a *dynamic*, *virtual*, or *soft wedge*.

Compensators attenuate the beam in desired locations to provide dosimetric shaping. A variety of methods exist that include simple and complex approaches.[13] Compensators have an important role in dose optimization schemes that include static applications[22] as an alternative to dynamic techniques.

CHARACTERISTICS OF RADIATION THERAPY ELECTRON BEAMS

Dose Characteristics

Electrons differ from photons in that electrons have a *finite range*; electrons travel a certain distance and then stop, and their kinetic energy is zero. PDD measurements are obtained along the central axis in the standard irradiation geometry as for photons (see Fig. 6-32). The one difference in the geometry is that an electron cone is used that requires fixed collimator positions in length and width. A typical PDD curve for megavoltage electrons (Fig. 6-40) has many of the same characteristics as do photons, including surface dose, a "buildup region," D_m, and d_m. An electron PDD curve also has the characteristics listed in Table 6-12.

Table 6-13 gives several characteristics for megavoltage electron beams as a function of energy. Although electron beams have some of the same features as photon beams, their finite range and the presence of bremsstrahlung contamination are unique.

Field size, flatness and symmetry, and sharpness of the beam edge for electrons can be measured similarly as for photon beams (see Fig. 6-34); however, the measurement depth is typically at d_m or at the 95% dose level beyond d_m. Beam steering, scattering foils, monitor chambers, collimator

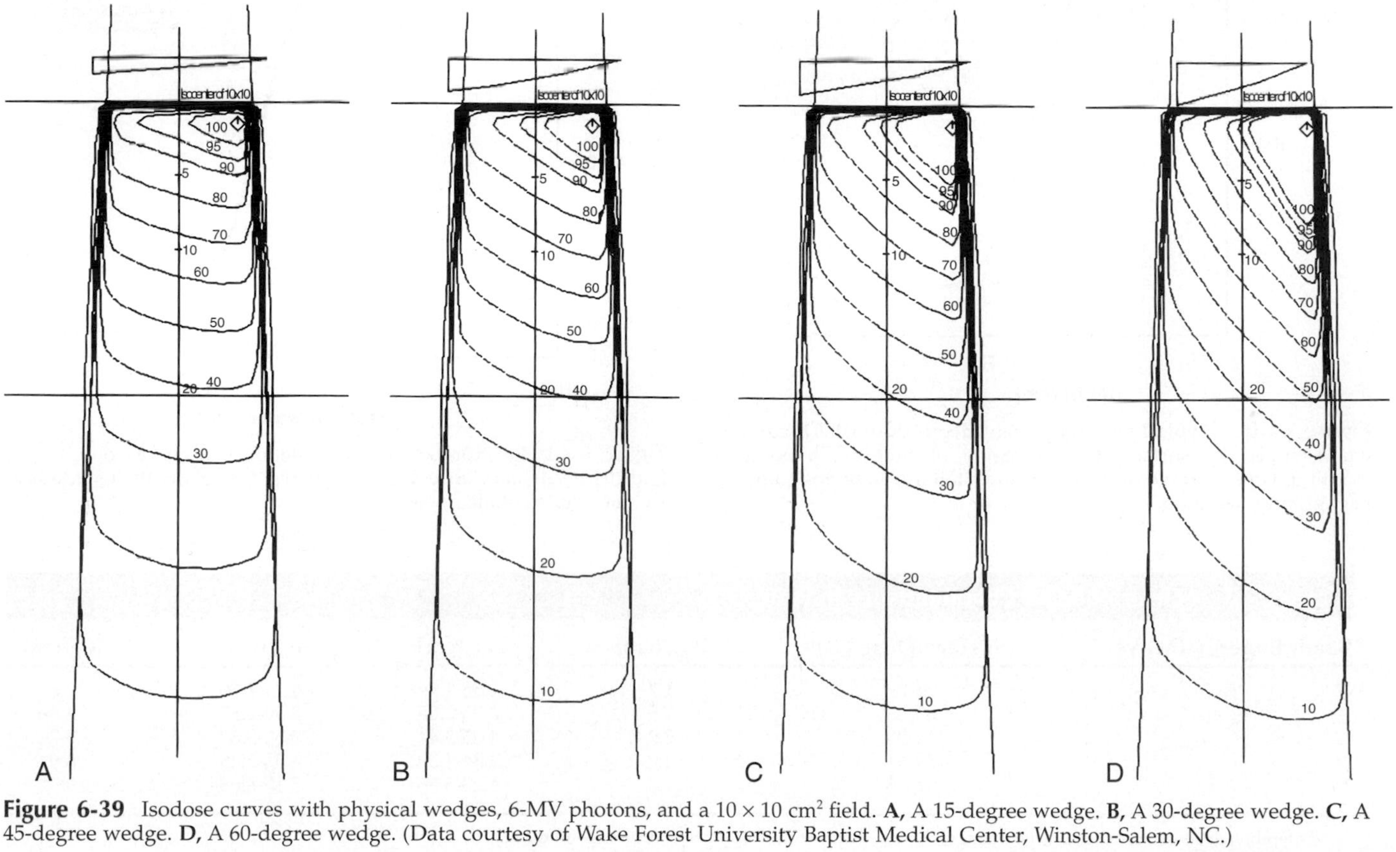

Figure 6-39 Isodose curves with physical wedges, 6-MV photons, and a 10 × 10 cm^2 field. **A,** A 15-degree wedge. **B,** A 30-degree wedge. **C,** A 45-degree wedge. **D,** A 60-degree wedge. (Data courtesy of Wake Forest University Baptist Medical Center, Winston-Salem, NC.)

length and width, and electron applicator design all determine flatness and symmetry for electron beams.[23] These design parameters are important for controlling the distribution and amount of electron scatter. Penumbra is due wholly to electron scattering and is defined similarly as for photons.

Table 6-12 Characteristics of an Electron PDD Curve

Characteristic	Definition
Dose fall-off	Region beyond where the dose falls steeply and almost linearly
d_{90}	Depth of the 90% dose beyond d_m—a clinically relevant point beyond which dose is not therapeutic
d_{80}	Depth of the 80% dose beyond d_m
d_{50}	Depth of the 50% dose beyond d_m
R_p	Practical range—the maximum depth to which electrons penetrate; determined by the intersection of the linear part of the dose fall-off curve and the bremsstrahlung background
Bremsstrahlung background	Contamination of the electron beam by bremsstrahlung x-rays created by collisions of the electrons with parts of the machine and with the patient; prevents the dose from going to zero at depth

PDD, percent depth dose.

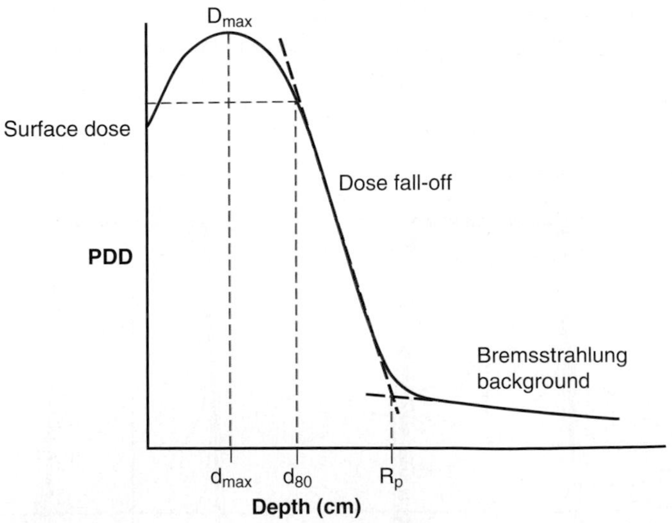

Figure 6-40 A typical electron percent depth dose (PDD) curve is characterized by surface dose, a region of buildup, a point of maximum dose, a rapid dose fall-off, and a tail due to Bremsstrahlung background radiation.

Effect of Energy

Electron beam characteristics change with beam energy. Representative beam data are presented in Table 6-13, central axis PDD in Figure 6-41, and isodose curves in Figure 6-42. Several key observations apply:

- PDD increases as energy increases because the electron range increases with energy. The values for d_{90}, d_{80}, and R_p (see Table 6-12) all increase with energy.
- Surface dose is high, usually in the 70% to 90% range (see Table 6-13), and it *increases* as energy increases (an opposite effect from photon beams) due to changes in the amount of lateral electron scattering and its dose contribution at d_m.
- In general, d_m starts at shallow depths and increases as energy increases because the electron range increases with energy.
- As energy increases, the region around D_m becomes quite broad. In this case d_m is defined at a selected point.
- The steepness of the dose fall-off region lessens with increasing energy. Increased scattering occurs, and a wider energy spectrum is created with a distribution of electron ranges. The originally monoenergetic electron beam is degraded into a wide spectrum beam with varied practical range.
- The amount of bremsstrahlung contamination increases with energy because the probability for radiative interaction increases with electron energy. Bremsstrahlung contamina-

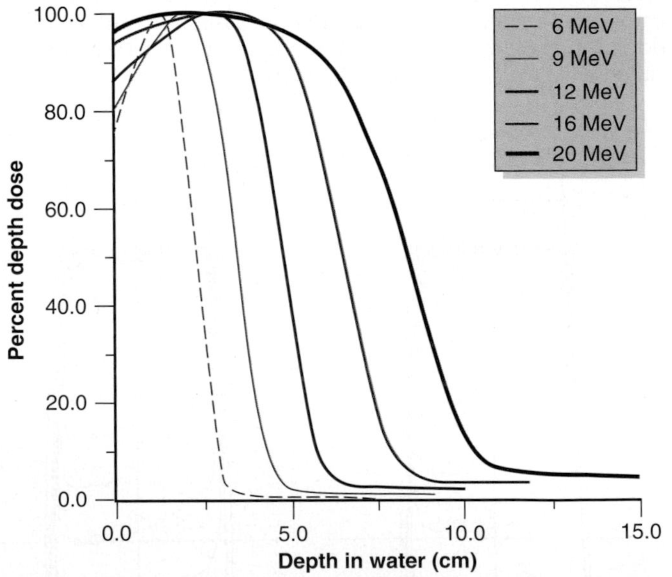

Figure 6-41 Electron beam percent depth dose curves: 6, 9, 12, 16, and 20 MeV. (Data courtesy of Wake Forest University Baptist Medical Center, Winston-Salem, NC.)

Table 6-13 Electron Beam Characteristics in Water

Beam Engergy (MeV)	Surface Dose (%)	d_{max} (cm)	d_{90} (cm)	d_{80} (cm)	R_p (cm)
6	78-79	1.2	1.55-1.59	1.74-1.78	2.8
9	83-86	1.5	2.25-2.58	2.59-2.87	4.4
12	84-88	2.0	3.05-3.44	3.50-3.82	5.7
16	89-91	2.0	3.84-4.89	4.53-5.49	8.0
20	91-95	2.0	4.28-5.86	5.15-6.68	9.9

d, depth; max, maximum; R_p, practical range; d_{90}, d_{80}, depth of the 90% or 80% dose beyond d_{max}.

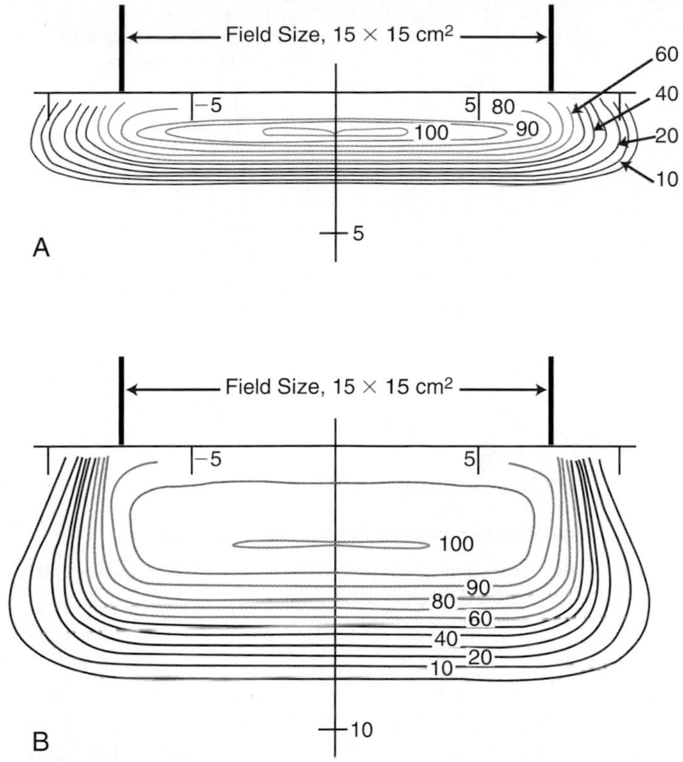

Figure 6-42 Electron beam isodose curves for a field size of 15 × 15 cm^2. **A,** 6 MeV. **B,** 20 MeV. (Data from Hogstrom KR, Steadham RE: Electron beam dose computation. *In* Mackie TR, Palta JR [eds]: Teletherapy: Present and Future. Madison, WI, Advanced Medical Publishing, 1996, pp 137-174.)

tion can be minimized but not eliminated totally. Structures lying beyond the electron range still receive dose from bremsstrahlung x-rays.

- The approximate d_{80} (in centimeters) in tissue can be found by dividing the nominal electron energy (in million electron volts) by 3. The d_{80} of a 9-MeV electron beam is 9/3, or about 3 cm. This number is useful for indicating the largest therapeutic depth, although many clinicians consider the d_{90} as the maximum effective range.

Effect of Field Size

Electron field sizes are changed by using fixed-size applicators to produce square field sizes from approximately 6 × 6 cm^2 up to 35 × 35 cm^2. Custom cutouts can be used that are inserted into an applicator to provide a shaped field to match a target outline.

- PDD increases only slightly as field size is increased. Scattered electrons have a finite range that is much less than R_p; therefore, for increasing field sizes above 10 × 10 cm^2 or greater, the contribution to the central axis is small. This effect is different from photon beams where scattered photons still have a relatively large mean path length.
- Surface dose increases slightly as field size is increased because the amount of scattered electrons from the beam path is increased.
- The d_m decreases as field size increases because the amount of lateral electron scatter increases near the surface.
- Absolute dose rate, or beam output, measured at d_m, usually increases as field size increases, but can decrease depending on collimator design.

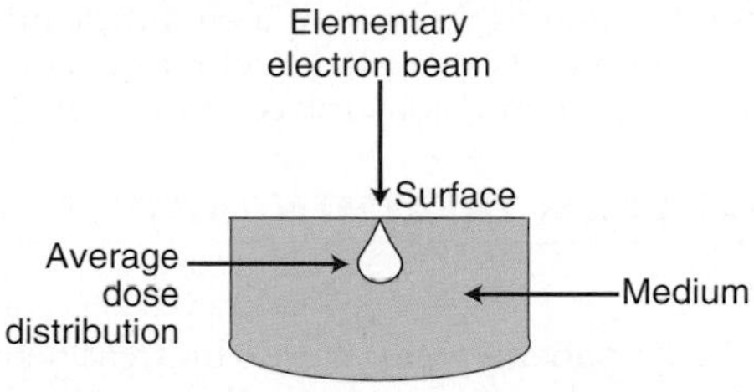

Figure 6-43 Elementary electron scattering kernel. (Adapted from Khan F: The Physics of Radiation Therapy, 2nd ed. Baltimore, Williams & Wilkins, 1994.)

Penumbra

Beam edge sharpness for electron beams varies with measurement depth due to the nature of electron scattering.[13] On interaction at a point, an elementary line of electrons produces a scattering envelope that is teardrop shaped in the forward direction of the beam (Fig. 6-43). Electron scattering angles, which initially are primarily in the forward direction, become more randomly oriented at depth.

- Penumbra increases with energy because scattered electrons have a higher effective energy and a corresponding increased range. This effect is seen as a degradation of the profile (enhanced shoulder and toe).
- Penumbra increases as depth increases because of the teardrop shape of electron scattering (see Fig. 6-43).
- The field width corresponds to the 50% dose width at d_m, but the shape of the isodose curves changes with increased depth. This effect should be considered during treatment planning.
- Penumbra increases with field size because of increased scatter from the increased volume of irradiated material.
- Penumbra increases as the distance increases from the end of the applicator to the surface. An increased gap allows electrons to scatter laterally before reaching the surface, degrading the field edge.

Other Effects

- Electrons scatter easily, and regions of bone and air greatly change the dose distribution.
- Density scaling can be applied to approximate the electron range in nonunit density materials (see Eq. 20). R_m, the approximate electron range for a material of density ρ_m, is given by the following equation, in which R_w is the range in water and ρ_W is the density of water (1 g/cm^2). For instance, the electron range for a material with a density of 2 g/cm^3 is 0.5 times the range in water.

$$R_m = R_w \times \frac{\rho_W}{\rho_m} \qquad \text{Eq. 35}$$

- Electron beams follow the inverse square law, but the reference distance is not the actual source location (that is, the scattering foil) but instead a virtual source point that is located along the beam path. This distance is called the *effective source-to-skin distance* (effective SSD) and is usually less than the SAD. Effective SSD is measured for each energy and applicator and occurs because of multiple electron scatterings along the beam path.
- Use of electron cutouts for field shaping affects scattering conditions and changes output, penumbra, the position of d_{max}, and field homogeneity. These effects are most pronounced when the cutout size is less than one fourth of the applicator dimension or on the order of the electron

range.[13] Individual calibration of a cutout or other procedures are required to establish the cutout's dosimetric character when these poor geometric conditions exist.

EXTERNAL BEAM TREATMENT SIMULATION

Purpose

In the "old" days patients were taken to the treatment machine and fields were chosen based on the clinician's general anatomic knowledge and the patient's disease. Diagnostic radiographs were available to help localization. This process is called *clinical setup* because the treatment machine is used with various aids to decide on the beam geometry. Simple fields and hand blocking are used. Clinical setup is no longer commonly done. Instead, *simulation* is performed on a special x-ray machine, called a *simulator,* also called a *conventional simulator* (in contrast to a CT simulator). A conventional simulator reproduces all the geometric parameters of the radiation treatment machine and its use has the following advantages:

1. Clinical setup competes with treatment for time on the treatment machine. Simulation on a dedicated simulator does not.
2. Simulators are diagnostic machines with radiographic and fluoroscopic capabilities. Images are of diagnostic quality instead of poor port film quality.
3. The machine can simulate different treatment machine geometries with regard to SSD, SAD, block position, and field size.
4. Simulators are dedicated to the simulation process. Different treatment geometries can be explored without the pressure to turn the room back over for treatment.
5. Simulators can be used to localize and verify brachytherapy implants within the confines of the radiation oncology department (no exposure to outside individuals) and under controlled conditions.

Treatment Setup

There are two basic methods for patient setup: SSD and SAD (Fig. 6-44).

SSD Treatment

If a treatment technique is set up as an SSD treatment, the distance to the patient's skin is recorded in the chart and used as a reference distance for each treatment. The SSD is measured and set to the same point on the patient's surface each time the field is treated. When a different field is treated, the new SSD is set as required before the patient is treated. Each field is independently set and treated. The SSD is standardized to equal the SAD for isocentric machines, so a normal SSD treatment is at 100 cm (80 cm on older machines). The standard SSD is also the distance used for machine calibration. Occasionally, alternative SSDs are used to allow larger field sizes to be used.

Compared with SAD treatments, SSD treatments place the target further away from the source. Because the inverse square effect is less, PDDs are greater, and larger field sizes may be possible. The disadvantage is that each treatment field has to be individually set, requiring movements of the treatment couch and patient between successive fields.

SAD Treatment

An alternative to setting the SSD is to set the target volume at the SAD (the isocenter of rotation of the machine). This isocenter is a point in space in the treatment room about which the gantry, collimator, and table all rotate (see Fig. 6-3). In this case

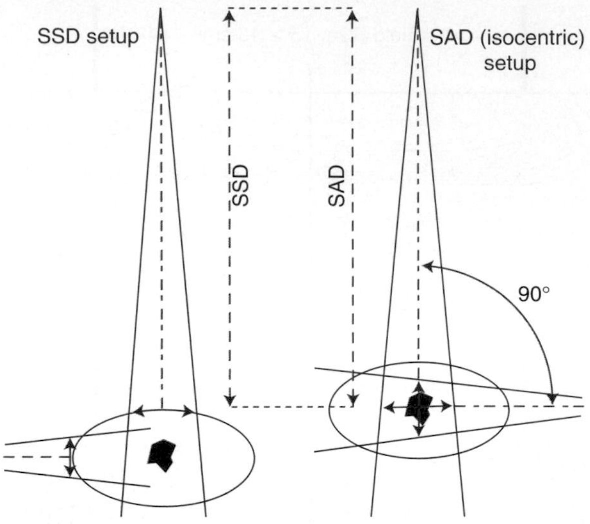

Figure 6-44 Treatment geometries: source-to-skin distance (SSD) and source-to-axis (SAD) approaches.

the SSD is always less than the SAD (SSD < 100 cm). In SAD treatments the target volume always intercepts the beam regardless of gantry, table, or collimator angles.

An advantage is that after one field is set properly, the target is at the isocenter and subsequent treatment fields can be set up rapidly without having to set multiple SSDs. Treatment of a multifield plan therefore is more quickly done because of less set-up time, and the target cannot be missed. The disadvantage is that field sizes may occasionally be limited, and there is slightly more inverse square effect.

The advantages of rapid setup and targeting for SAD treatment outweigh those of larger field size and increased PDD for SSD treatments in most cases, and SAD treatments are performed for most patients. This has been especially true because isocenters changed from 80 to 100 cm, providing larger field sizes and less PDD effect.

Simulator Description and Components

A conventional simulator unit has the following components in the geometry shown in Figure 6-3:

1. The gantry is the structure that contains the x-ray tube and collimator at one end and the image intensifier (for fluoroscopy) on the other. The gantry is mounted isocentrically, and the x-ray tube can be positioned to a wide range of SADs or SSDs.
2. The x-ray tube is a diagnostic energy x-ray tube that rides at the top of the gantry. Kilovoltage ranges from 60 to 120 kV(p), and tube current is as much as 1000 mA.
3. The collimator is an assembly that defines the radiographic (image) field size at a given SAD (usually 100 cm). The collimator is isocentric and has field size and rotation capabilities like the treatment machines.
4. Two pairs of field-defining wires are in the collimator, one positioned in the x direction and one in the y direction. They are used to indicate the size of the treatment field as would be defined by the collimator jaws on the treatment machine. A simulator radiograph shows two radiation fields. The larger field is the actual field imaged as defined by the collimator. The smaller field is the treatment field, indicated by images of the delineator wires. A simulator

film shows the treatment field and nearby contextual region.

5. The simulator table is isocentric and has vertical, lateral, longitudinal, and rotational motions. It can be remotely operated from the console, so as to move the patient during fluoroscopy.
6. Hand and console controls allow operation of all of the machine motions from a hand-control unit or the table pedestal in the room, and some of these are duplicated at the control console. All radiographic technique settings are done at the console.

Conventional Simulation Procedures

A patient to be simulated is placed on the conventional simulator in the treatment position. The supine position is most common, but prone positioning and other geometries are also used. Immobilization devices of various functions and rigidity may be used to maintain patient position, including head holders, thermoplastic face masks, foam molds, cushions and pillows, bite blocks, and vacuum bags. The patient is moved in the treatment position to align the target region or other reference anatomy with the simulator's isocenter. This location is chosen based on available information on the target volume and nearby structures (from film, computed tomography [CT], magnetic resonance imaging [MRI], clinical examination, surgical reports) or in anticipation of imaging studies for treatment planning. Fluoroscopic imaging or static films are used to determine the location of the isocenter or other reference point in the patient coordinate system. An SSD or SAD setup is chosen, and orthogonal films are usually taken to record the patient's position. All geometric information (gantry angle, collimator angle, table position, field size, SSD, SAD) is recorded for each film. Marks are placed on the patient's skin or the immobilization device to indicate the reference field axes.

In conventional simulation, individual treatment field geometries are determined at the time of simulation. All field data are recorded, and simulator films are taken for each field as a record of the intended treatment and for use in designing field shapes. Target and other data are often drawn on each film. Films with added contrast agents show certain structures (bladder, rectum). Other data are the clinical examination, surgical reports, surgical clips, markers placed during simulation, and manually transferred contours from CT or MRI scans. After the desired data are on the film, a treatment field is drawn that will later be defined by a custom block or MLC.

Additional geometric information on the patient is needed if treatment planning is to be performed, such as an external contour and the locations of important internal anatomy, including the target, landmarks, and critical structures. For simple two-dimensional (2D) planning, at least one transverse contour is obtained; however, sagittal and coronal slices (or obliques) can also be obtained. Sources for patient contours include mechanical methods (e.g., solder wire, tracer device), optical methods (e.g., laser grid, light grid, stereo-shift camera), and CT or ultrasound acquisition.[13]

Computer-Aided Simulation

Computer-aided simulation, also called *virtual simulation*[24] or *CT simulation,* uses a volumetric image of the patient in treatment position and computer software to perform patient simulation without a conventional simulator. This alternative procedure to conventional simulation, in this definition, includes simulation only and does *not* include dose calculations. The simulation is performed on a volumetric image of the patient (usually a CT image), not the patient, hence the name *virtual* simulation. Initially, treatment position and the isocenter location within the patient can be determined on a conventional simulator and confirmed with orthogonal projection radiographs. The patient and any immobilization device are marked with the isocenter location. CT scans or other digital imaging (e.g., MRI) is then obtained with the patient in the treatment position. The virtual simulation process then takes place within the computer where the proposed treatment geometry is designed and viewed on screen. Software tools are used to identify and segment anatomic information within the image set (external contour, and volumes such as lung, kidney, cord, and tumor). This information is displayed and the treatment beam geometry is reviewed and selected. Dedicated CT simulators as turnkey devices, including a CT scanner and simulation software, exist in commercial form[25] and are in clinical use.[26] Moving simulation to a digital format allows a variety of image processing tools to be applied to the process. An alternative and less commonly used approach to the CT simulator is the simulator CT, which uses a conventional simulator as a fan-beam CT scanner, along with digital imaging capabilities. In either case of CT simulation or simulation CT, isodose calculations are performed later to complete the planning process. Treatment planning techniques are discussed in the next section.

EXTERNAL BEAM TREATMENT PLANNING AND DOSIMETRY

Purpose and Procedures

After conventional or computer-aided simulation, the simulator films; CT, MRI, and other digital images; beam geometries; and other patient data are transferred to dosimetry for further treatment planning. During treatment planning, possible beam geometries and combinations are investigated. Simulated beams may be fine tuned, or new beams may be created—the beam weights may be adjusted, wedges added, beam energy changed, field sizes adjusted, different normalizations used, and compensation checked. The intent is to produce a treatment plan in the form of an isodose distribution through one or many transverse or other planes that can be evaluated by the physician and approved or modified. Treatment plans describe the following characteristics about the patient's treatment, as illustrated in Figure 6-45:

1. Prescription isodose or depth (i.e., the 97% line or at 3 cm deep) gives the location where the prescribed dose is to be given.
2. Various tumor, target, and normal tissue volumes as specified according to the International Commission on Radiation Units and Measurement Reports 50 and 62 (ICRU 50 and ICRU 62) recommendations for volumes of interest. This information must be represented in some manner to enable plan evaluation (discussed later). These volumes may be three-dimensional (3D) contours or isodose lines or surfaces.
3. Beam weights indicate the relative dose delivered to the prescription or normalization point by each beam.
4. The presence of beam modifiers (i.e., wedge, custom block, compensation filter, dynamic field shaping, or intensity modulation) is specified.
5. The size and shape of each field (i.e., collimator settings) are specified.
6. The SSD is specified for each field.
7. "Inhomogeneities" are identified. These are volumes that are not water or soft tissue equivalents (e.g., lung, bone, metal prosthesis) for which dose may need to be corrected.

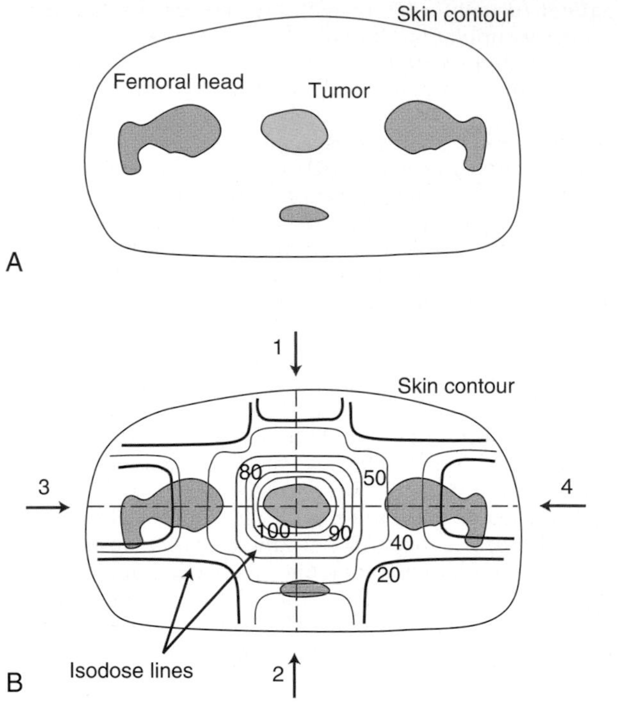

Beam Data
1. AP:18MV x-rays, SSD=92.5 cm, weight=1.0, field size=8×10, G:0 C:0 T:0
2. PA:18MV x-rays, SSD=90.5 cm, weight=1.0, field size=8×10, G:180 C:0 T:0
3. RLAT:18MV x-rays, SSD=87.5 cm, weight=1.2, field size=8×8, G:270 C:0 T:0
4. LLAT:18MV x-rays, SSD=87.5 cm, weight=1.2, field size=8×8, G:90 C:0 T:0

Figure 6-45 Typical treatment plan information. **A,** The patient contour and segmented regions of interest. **B,** A treatment plan with superimposed isodose lines. Beam data are shown. AP, anteroposterior; LLAT, left lateral; PA, posteroanterior; RLAT, right lateral; SSD, source-to-skin distance.

8. Number of monitor units, or amount of exposure time, that must be set on the machine for each beam.

Dose Specification

Components of a dose prescription for a patient treatment course include the patient's name, clinic identification number, treatment site, radiation energy and modality (photons or electrons), prescription point location, dose per fraction, number of fractions, and total dose. These components are recognized standards[27] and are required by most regulatory bodies.[28] The point of prescription defines the location within the patient where dose is to be delivered and therefore defines the geometric point for dose computation. Prescription point selection and additional recommendations for prescribing, recording, and reporting volumes of interest and dosimetric parameters for photon beam treatment are specified by ICRU 50 and ICRU 62.[29,30]

Volumes of Interest

ICRU 50 defines five volumes of interest related to treatment. The following definitions are illustrated in Figure 6-46 for an idealized case:

Gross tumor volume (GTV): The GTV is the volume that contains the gross palpable or visible extent and location of malignant growth. The GTV may be identified on a simple contour, a radiograph, or sectional images.

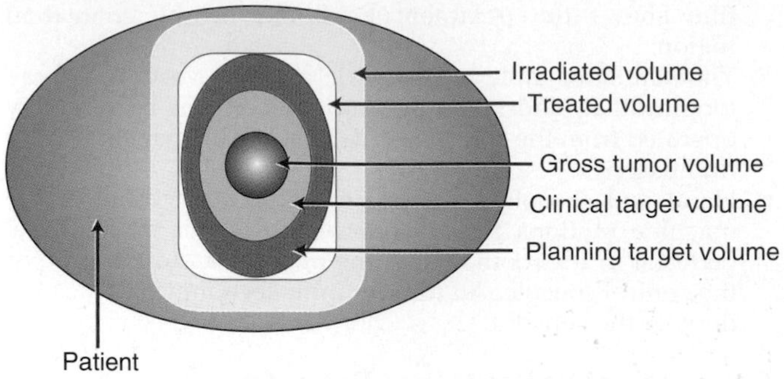

Figure 6-46 The International Commission on Radiation Units and Measurement Report 50 (ICRU 50) defines five volumes of interest related to treatment. (From ICRU Report 50: Prescribing, Recording, and Reporting Photon Beam Therapy. International Commission on Radiation Units and Measurements, 1993.)

Clinical target volume (CTV): The CTV is the volume that contains the GTV and any suspected microscopic disease. The CTV is the volume that must receive the prescribed dose to effect cure or palliation.

Planning target volume (PTV): The PTV is a volume that contains the GTV and CTV and that is defined to account for the irradiation geometry and all uncertainties in treatment, such as organ and patient motions and set-up errors. The PTV is a volume that, when covered by the prescription dose, will ensure the delivery of the prescription dose to the CTV. The PTV includes a margin for motion and set-up error but not for microscopic disease. The PTV is a function of treatment geometry, because the number of beams and their orientations may impose limitations on the PTV's shape or scope.

Treated volume (TV): The TV is the volume enclosed by a selected (prescribed) isodose surface and is a function of the treatment geometry required for planning the PTV. For an acceptable plan, the TV is greater than the PTV, although an ideal TV/PTV ratio would be 1.0, indicating perfect conformation (assuming the locations of the volumes were identical).

Irradiated volume (IV): The IV is a volume that receives a significant dose; significance is determined by morbidity or other measures.

Dose Recording and Reporting

The ICRU recommendations for dose include a point for dose computation and indicators of dose homogeneity. The *reference point* is a point within the PTV at which dose is specified. There are several criteria for selecting the reference point:

- The dose at the point is clinically relevant and representative of dose in PTV.
- The point is easily defined by anatomy or geometry.
- The point is a location where dose can be accurately determined.
- The dose gradient at the point is not steep.

With these criteria, suitable point locations include the center of PTV, near the central axis, or where tumor cell density is a maximum. In many cases, the isocenter has these characteristics and serves as the reference point.

Dose homogeneity is also to be reported and is represented by the maximum and minimum doses in the PTV. Together, the reference, maximum, and minimum point doses represent the dose to the PTV as well as the variation in that dose.

Dose Reporting for Different Techniques

ICRU 50 demonstrates its recommendations for three levels of complexity: single plane plans, multiple planes, and 3D volume studies. In each case the reference point dose is computed and the maximum and minimum point doses are estimated or computed. Isodose distributions are computed if a contour plane or multiple planes are acquired. In the highest complexity, dose evaluation tools such as dose-volume histograms are recommended.

ICRU 50 considered radiation target volumes only, and did not specify normal tissue volumes that might be relevant for morbidity and avoidance. ICRU 62 addresses this deficiency by specifying organs at risk (OARs) and the planning organs at risk values (PRVs).[30] Tissue physiologic organization of OARs as serial or parallel units, or combinations of the two, are considered to aid risk assessment.

The ICRU 50/62 recommendations create a standard to enable the comparison of treatment plans across institutional and international boundaries. Institutions use the ICRU 50/62 recommendations, and they have been adopted by national protocol groups.

Beam Nomenclature

When using complex field arrangements, it can be difficult to describe the precise beam orientation. A system has been developed to allow this description to be done simply.[31,32] The suggested nomenclature defines a coordinate system that corresponds to the patient's anatomic position (Fig. 6-47). The axes are labeled A, L, and S (for anterior, left, and superior) and P, R, and I (for posterior, right, and inferior). A beam name begins with the closest cardinal axis and then gives the angle of rotation from that axis to the beam central axis. Simple beams with no off-axis rotation are named after their anatomic positions. Examples include A, P, R, and L for the beam orientations commonly called AP, PA, right lateral, and left lateral, respectively. Beams with off-axis rotations include the angle of rotation. For instance, A30S indicates an anterior beam that is angled 30 degrees to the superior, and A60L30S indicates an anterior beam that is angled 60 degrees to the left then angled 30 degrees superior (see Fig. 6-47). This nomenclature is in clinical use in several institutions, and its use removes ambiguities in beam identification. An advantage over naming conventions based on machine coordinates (i.e., the GTC system, for gantry, table, and collimator) is that beam names are reported in the patient coordinate system and can be readily interpreted with respect to the patient position.

Radiation Treatment Planning

Two-Dimensional Treatment Planning

Treatment plans such as those shown in Figure 6-45 are the results of 2D treatment planning. The patient contour, whether manually obtained at the time of simulation or obtained from a single CT slice, must contain the central ray and one collimator axis of the beam; the beam must be coplanar with the contour plane. Beam orientations with central rays outside the contour plane are not permitted. Uses and limitations of 2D treatment planning have been thoroughly discussed.[33,34]

Three-Dimensional Treatment Planning

With 3D treatment planning, radiation beam geometries are not constrained to lie in an image plane. Instead, beam trajectories are possible over all solid angles, greatly increasing the number of potential beam paths (see Fig. 6-47). Software tools enable target and volume of interest localization/segmentation, image reconstructions, automatic and beam's eye view field designs, 3D dose calculations, and visualization techniques and metrics for plan evaluation. Possible advantages of 3D treatment include better target localization due to image-based planning, more accurate field delineation to include target and exclude critical and normal structures, and improved dose calculation models that consider the 3D shape of the patient and composition. Chapter 14 presents 3D treatment planning in detail, and comprehensive reviews are available.[35-38]

Dose Computation Algorithms

Photon dose calculation methods can be classified as one of three types: (1) empirical or semi-empirical models (e.g., broad beam methods based on the TMR and SMR), (2) analytic models based on first principles, and (3) random sampling or Monte Carlo models. Advances include convolution pencil beams and full Monte Carlo methods, which account for the 3D electron density distribution of the irradiated volume, radiation transport, and the spectral components of megavoltage

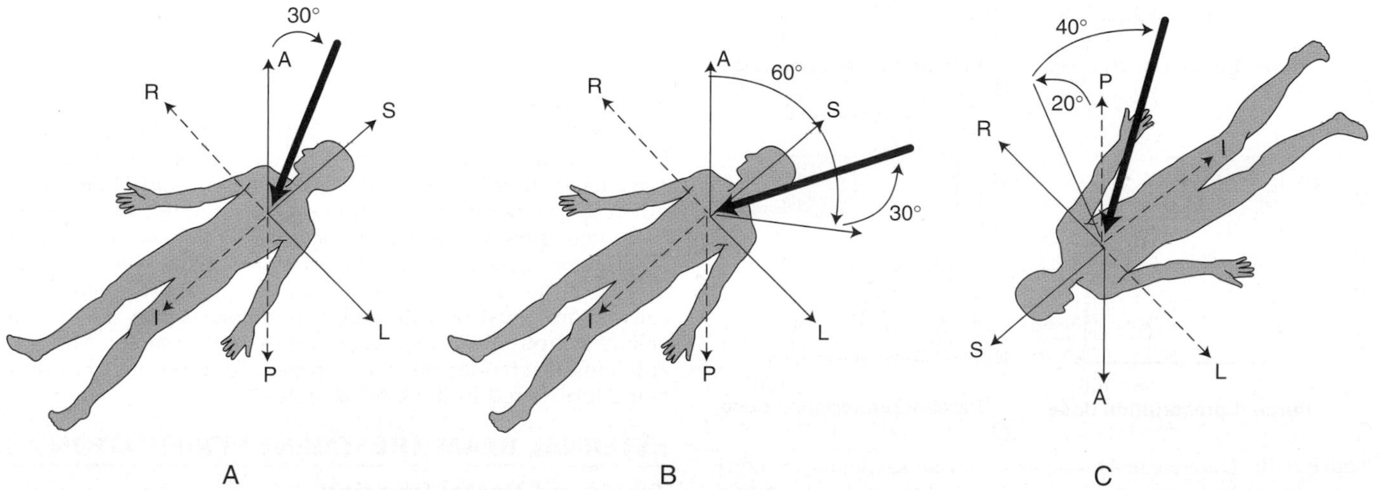

Figure 6-47 Three-dimensional beam nomenclature. Beams are named in reference to the patient coordinate system. **A,** The A30S beam is 30 degrees superior from the anterior axis. **B,** The A60L30S beam is 60 degrees left from the anterior axis and 30 degrees superior. **C,** The P20R40I beam is 20 degrees right from the posterior axis and 40 degrees inferior.

photon and electron beams. Broad beam methods have been reviewed,[34] and work continues on higher fidelity models.[35,36,39-41] A clinically implemented electron calculation model with acceptable accuracy has been published.[42] In the relatively near future photon and electron doses will be computed rapidly with great accuracy, accounting for all unique aspects of the patient data set, without needing any inhomogeneity or other "corrections" to compensate for inadequacies in the computation model.

Treatment Plan Evaluation and Optimization

Evaluation of a treatment plan to determine clinical acceptability is a process that depends on the patient geometry, target dose coverage, protection of normal structures, and other clinical criteria. A treatment planner (dosimetrist) can provide several "reasonable" plans under physician guidance, but acceptability is a clinical decision by the radiation oncologist. One tool that aids quantitative plan evaluation is the dose-volume histogram (DVH).[43] A DVH represents a treatment plan by graphically indicating the fractional amount of a volume of interest that receives a specified dose (or more). Two histograms are possible. The differential DVH (dDVH) shows the fractional volume receiving a specified dose. The cumulative DVH (cDVH) is the integral form and shows the fractional volume receiving a specified dose or more. Both forms are shown in Figure 6-48 for hypothetical target and normal tissue volumes. The cDVH is the form most commonly used. Although DVHs show dose coverage of a volume, a disadvantage is that spatial information of the dose distribution is lost. For instance, inadequate coverage of a target volume may be indicated by the shape of the DVH, but the location of the poorly covered region is not indicated; the treatment plan must be viewed to determine the location.

Optimization of treatment plans depends on quantification of optimization criteria and may include dosimetrics (dose constraints at points or regions), permitted and prohibitive beam geometries, DVH indices, and approximations to biologic response functions such as tumor control probability (TCP) and normal tissue complication probability (NTCP), or other indices.[39,40] Mathematical optimization does not necessarily equate with clinical acceptability—optimization criteria may be improperly selected or otherwise limited. Similarly, rank-ordered, mathematically optimized plans may yield numerous clinically equivalent plans. Continuing work in treatment planning, research, and development requires clinical trials to show efficacy of the techniques. Various trials are underway, as discussed in Chapter 14.

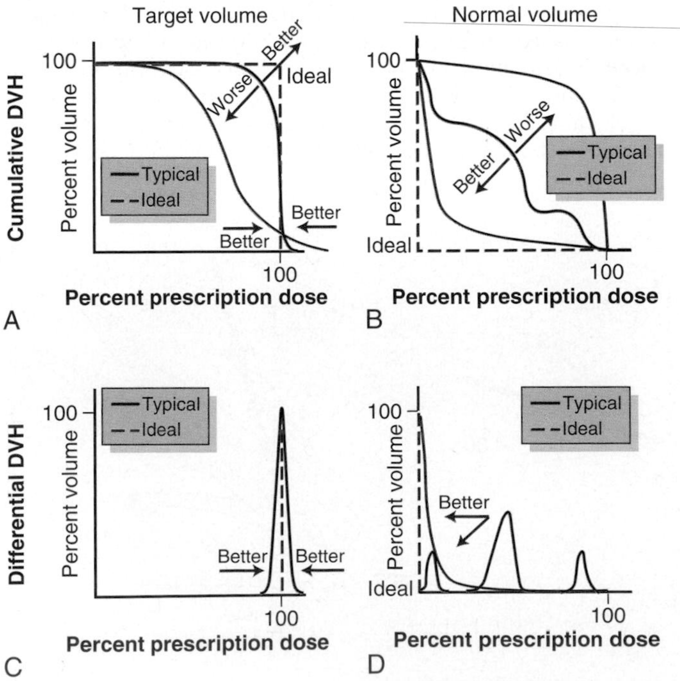

Figure 6-48 Dose-volume histograms (DVHs). **A,** Cumulative DVH for the target. **B,** Cumulative DVH for normal tissue. **C,** Differential DVH for the target. **D,** Differential DVH for normal tissue. Ideal DVHs are shown by the *dashed lines*. Indications for better or worse DVHs are shown.

Monitor Unit Calculations

Treatment planning data include beam parameters and weights that indicate the dose contribution of each beam to the prescription point. The setting on the treatment machine that controls dose delivery, either monitor units (MUs) or timer setting, must be computed so that the proper dose for each beam will be delivered.

The MU or timer setting can be calculated with the basic equation:

$$\text{Setting} = \frac{\text{Dose}}{\text{Dose rate}} = \frac{D}{\dot{D}} \qquad \text{Eq. 36}$$

in which the dose, D, is the desired dose (in centigrays) to the prescription point from the beam (target dose), and the dose rate, $\dot{D}$, is the dose per MU (centigrays per MU), or dose per time (centigrays per minute), that the beam delivers to the prescription point. Dose rate is relative to the calibrated dose rate of the treatment unit.

Equation 37 is used for calculation of monitor units:

$$\text{MU} = \frac{D(\text{cGy})}{\dot{D}(\text{cGy/MU})} \qquad \text{Eq. 37}$$

Equation 38 is used for timer calculations:

$$T(\text{min}) = \frac{D(\text{cGy})}{\dot{D}(\text{cGy/min})} \qquad \text{Eq. 38}$$

The real work comes in determining the dose rate for the particular treatment geometry being calculated. $\dot{D}$ (centigray per MU or centigray per minute) can be found from the reference dose rate, $\dot{D}_0$, by the following equation:

$$\dot{D} = \dot{D}_0 \times \text{PDD(or TMR or TAR)} \times \text{OF} \qquad \text{Eq. 39}$$

The term *OF* represents *other factors* such as attenuation factors for beam modifiers (blocks, wedges, and compensators), output factors for field sizes, an inverse square term if needed, transmission and buildup factors for immobilization devices (sponges, Aquaplast, head holder, boards, table inserts), and any other devices or parameters that must be considered. In some cases the beam weight and $\dot{D}$ are computed by the treatment planning system, yielding a completed MU calculation. In most cases beam weights and other treatment planning data are combined in an independent calculation to determine MU. Although simply performed, MU calculations must be thoroughly understood and defined to ensure computation of the correct dose to the patient. MU calculations are standardized in Europe, and the nomenclature is being formalized in the United States.[44]

EXTERNAL BEAM TREATMENT VERIFICATION

Treatment Portal Imaging

External beam treatments are verified by validating set-up data such as beam geometries, including SSD measurements,

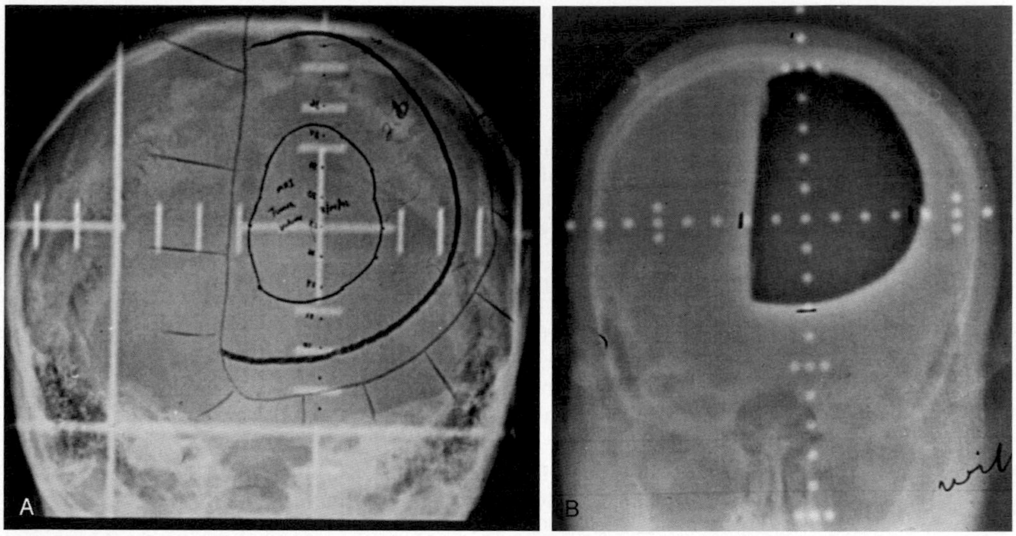

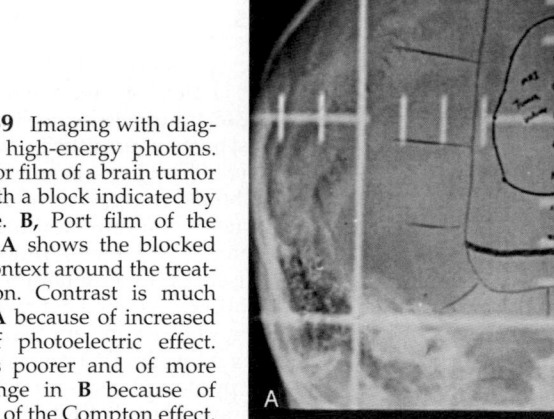

Figure 6-49 Imaging with diagnostic and high-energy photons. **A,** Simulator film of a brain tumor patient, with a block indicated by the outline. **B,** Port film of the patient in **A** shows the blocked area and context around the treatment region. Contrast is much higher in **A** because of increased amount of photoelectric effect. Contrast is poorer and of more limited range in **B** because of dominance of the Compton effect.

and through comparison of simulator and treatment portal films. The use of portal films has been shown to have a positive impact on treatment,[45] and common practice is to obtain ports at the beginning of treatment and for each week thereafter. The image quality of megavoltage port films is poor compared with the quality for companion simulator film (Fig. 6-49) because of poor subject contrast[46] caused by the dominance of the Compton effect. Improvements to portal image quality have included design of more sensitive films; enhancement of image capture by the use of specifically designed screens, cassettes, or film-screen-cassette systems; combination diagnostic and therapy imaging; image enhancement of digitized portal films; and digital acquisition of the portal image.[47] This latter category is an active area of work, and digital portal imaging systems are now referred to as *electronic portal imaging devices* (EPIDs). There are at least five types of EPIDs,[46] depicted schematically in Figure 6-50: mirror-based video systems, fiberoptic video systems, liquid ionization chamber systems, scanning ionization chamber systems, and static solid-state systems. The role of EPIDs in clinical practice is being determined and includes simple replacement of film, treatment verification by manual comparison with digital reference films, image enhancement by digital techniques for improved structure recognition, automatic determination of patient positioning to permit or prohibit treatment, dynamic monitoring of conventional treatment, and dynamic monitoring of dynamic treatment (e.g., intensity-modulated treatment). These applications depend on the design and operational characteristics of the devices, such as image sampling and refresh rates, signal-to-noise ratio, detector resolution, detector radiation sensitivity, size of the active imaging area, software for image processing, physical size, and ease of use.

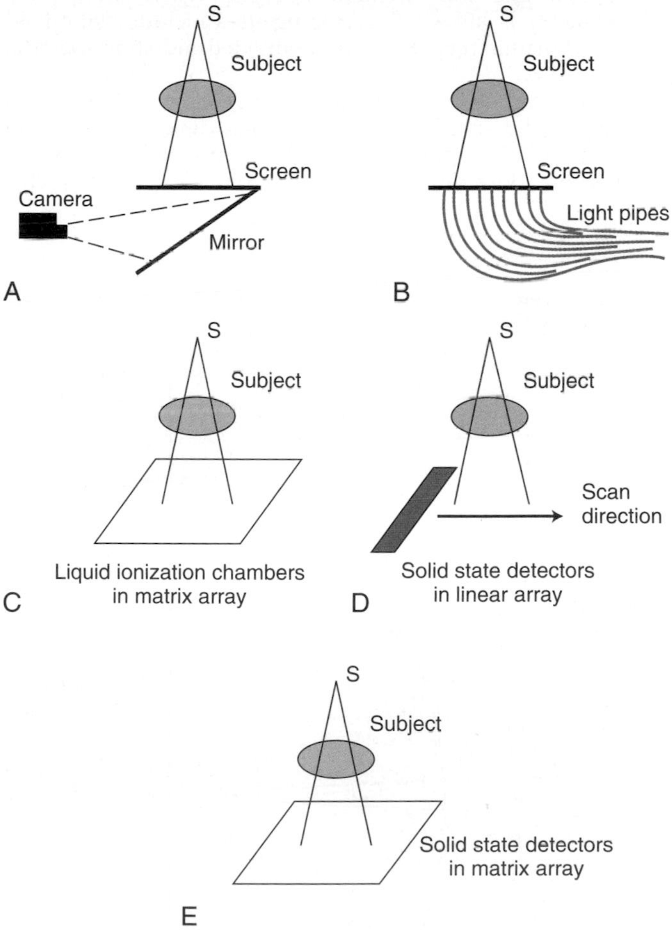

Figure 6-50 Five methods for electronic portal imaging. **A,** Fluorescent screen, mirror, and camera. **B,** Fluorescent screen and light pipe carrier. **C,** Direct irradiation of the matrix array of liquid ionization chambers. **D,** Direct irradiation of the linear array of solid-state detectors, with scanning. **E,** Direct irradiation of the matrix array of solid-state detectors.

In Vivo Dosimetry

Dosimetric verification of treatment is sometimes required for unique patient geometries or critical situations such as total-body irradiation. Techniques for in vivo dose measurements include the following:

1. TLD can be packaged in capsules or protective bags and placed in cavities, on the skin surface, and under extremities or bolus. Evaluation of results can be challenging for geometries where buildup is not complete. TLD is a commonly used method for in vivo dosimetry.

2. Diode detectors with integral buildup may be placed superficially or intracavitarily. Diode systems can be set up rapidly and results are immediately available. They have gained popularity because of their ease of use compared with TLD.
3. Film can be used in a patient-equivalent phantom in the replicated patient treatment geometry. Film density is read with an automated densitometer as isodensity lines and yields a qualitative indicator of the dose distribution delivered.
4. A patient-equivalent phantom is tissue equivalent and includes internal structures such as bone, lung, and airways. Some phantoms are sectioned into transverse slabs and can accept film or TLD at a particular anatomic level. Anatomic phantoms differ in shape or anatomy from the real patient but are useful for studying treatment geometries.
5. Ionization chambers rarely are used for in vivo dosimetry but may be placed superficially or in intracavitary locations, such as for monitoring a high dose rate brachytherapy procedure.
6. EPID can be used for transmission dosimetry for integrated or real-time measurement of dose when the patient geometry is known. Developing uses include static field and dynamic (i.e., intensity-modulated radiation therapy) dosimetry.
7. Remote reporting detectors are available. A variety of small, solid-state detectors are being developed that can be interstitially implanted and interrogated remotely to measure dose in situ. Such devices are biocompatible, relatively small, and can be visualized with kilovoltage imaging.

EXTERNAL BEAM TREATMENTS: GENERAL TECHNIQUES

Target depth, size, anatomic site, and proximity of critical structures all influence the choice of treatment modality (photons or electrons) and the technique to be used. Technique includes the number of beams; beam energy; beam weight (the relative amount of dose delivered by a beam); field shape; irradiation geometry; and use of bolus, wedges, compensators, or other special devices. Treatment planning techniques have been well studied and presented.[12,13,48] General practice is that photons are almost always used in a combination of two or more fields (i.e., parallel opposed, wedged pair, three field, four field, more field, or arc) and electrons are used as single en face fields (perhaps junctioned with other electron fields to cover a larger area). Example photon plans demonstrate these principles for the parallel-opposed, wedged-pair, three-field, four-field, and arc techniques in Figures 6-51 through 6-56. As the number of fields increases, there are two observations: The high-dose region becomes more conformal to the target, and the peripheral dose decreases but the volume of tissue covered by peripheral dose increases.[12] Electron treatment planning is less mature than photon planning and is often not performed at all, although new calculation algorithms are available with accuracies that are clinically acceptable.[42] Typically, electron treatment plans are based on graphical or tabulated measured data as previously shown (see Figs. 6-42 and 6-43).

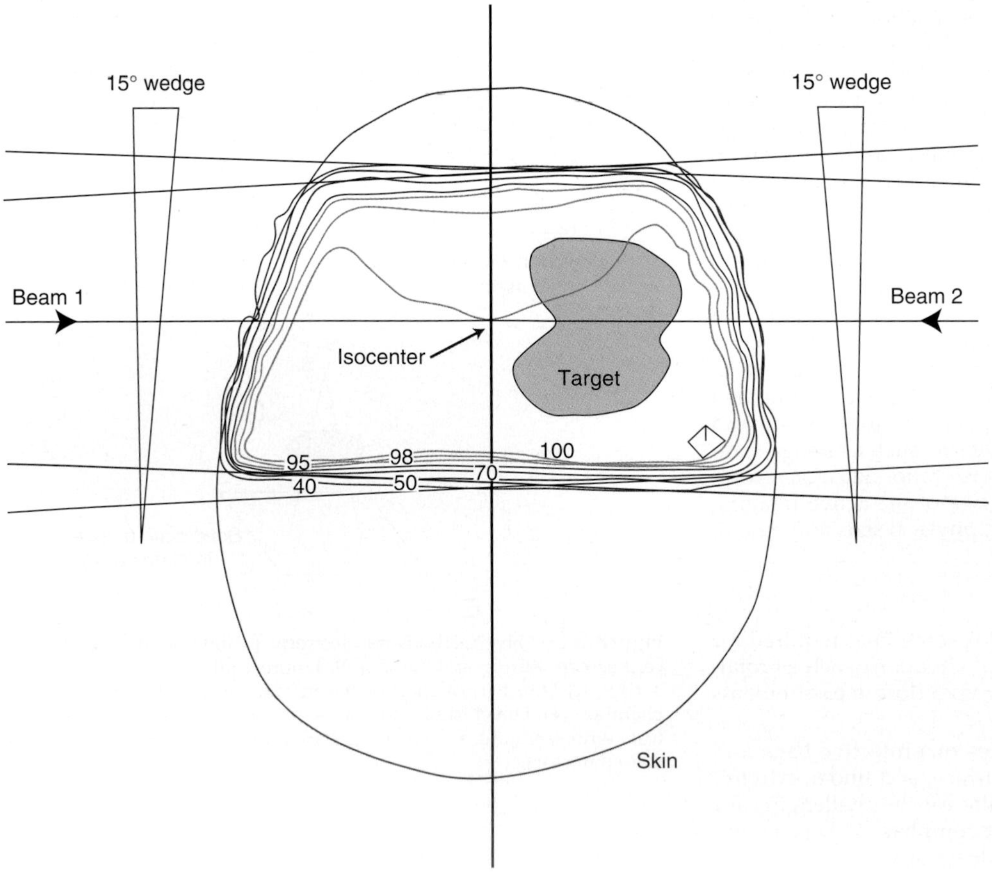

Figure 6-51 Parallel-opposed plan for treatment of a target in the head or neck.

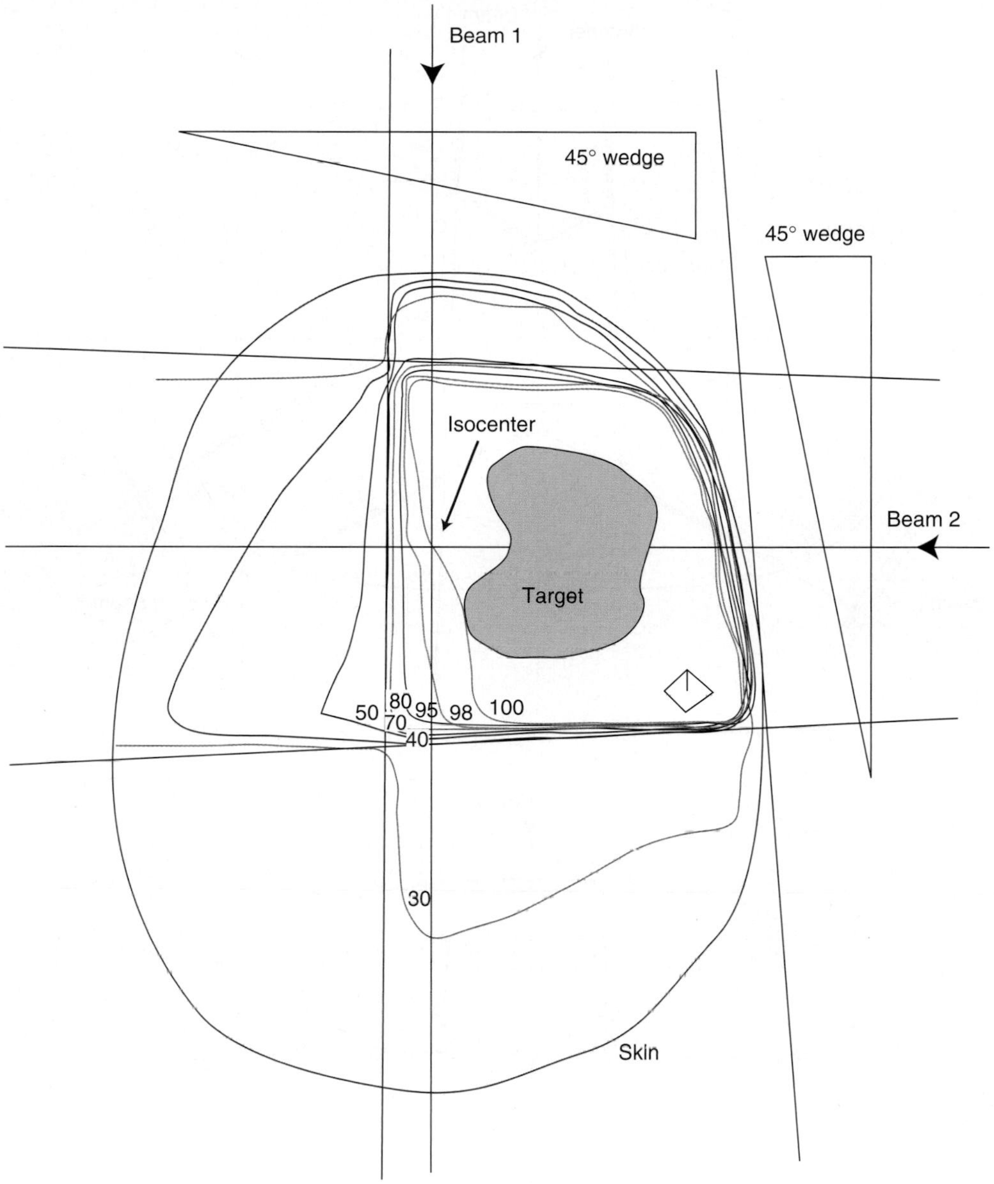

Figure 6-52 Wedged-field plan for treatment of a target in the head or neck.

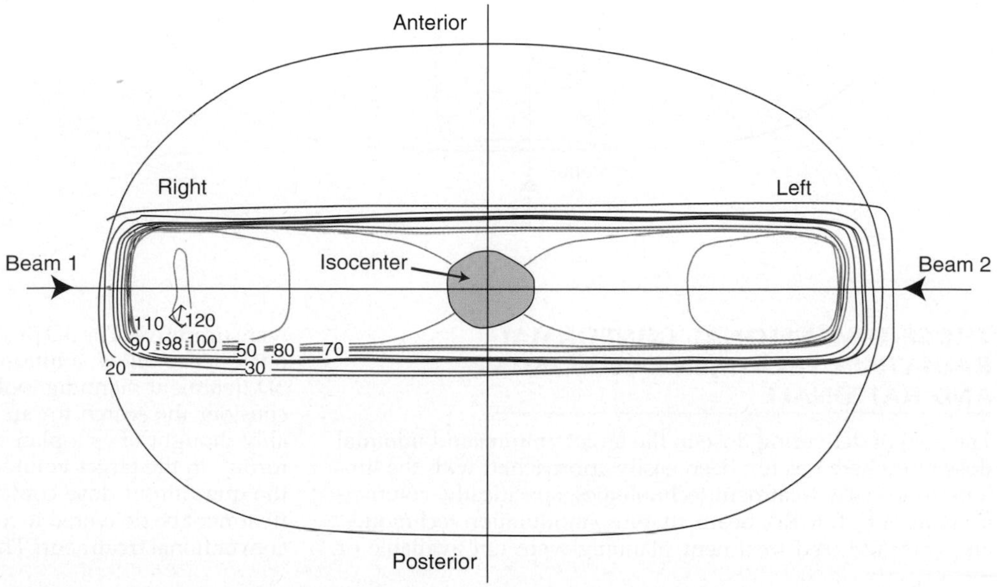

Figure 6-53 Parallel-opposed plan for treatment of a target in the pelvis.

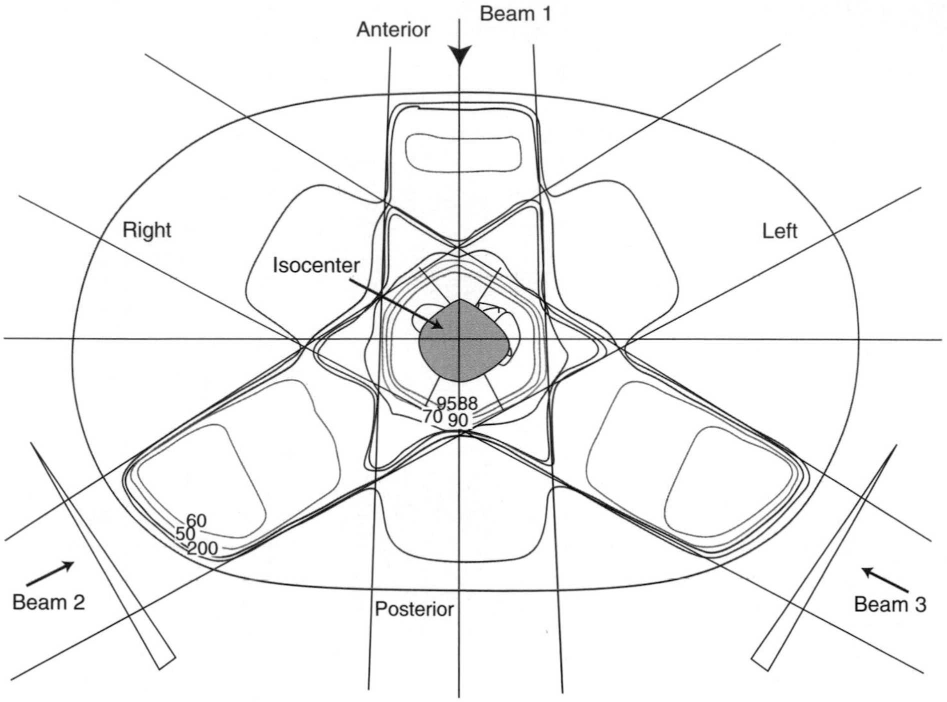

Figure 6-54 Three-field plan for treatment of a target in the pelvis.

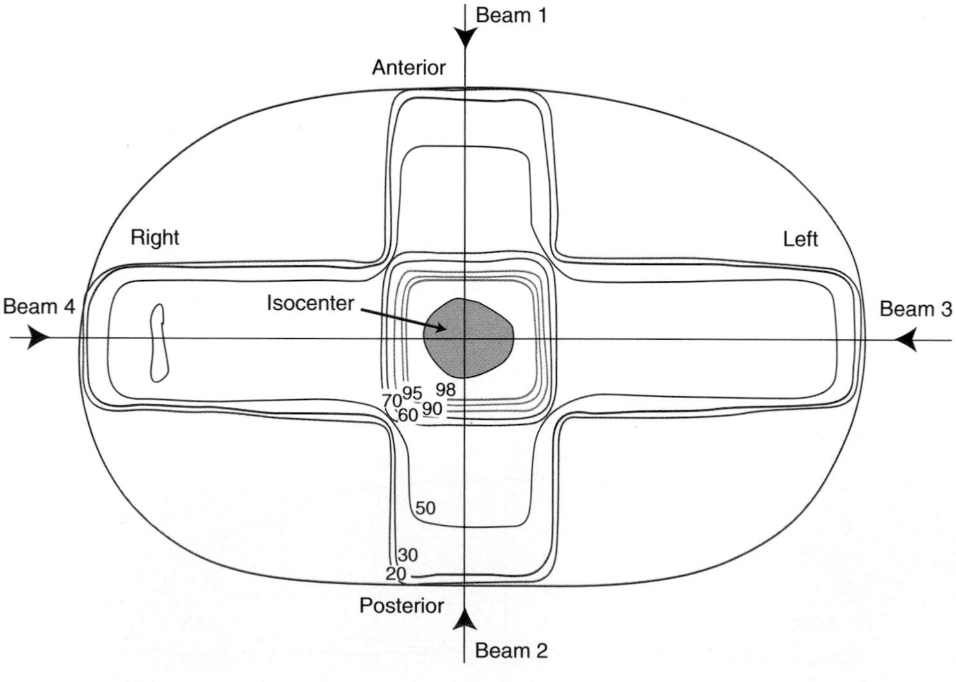

Figure 6-55 Four-field plan for treatment of a target in the pelvis.

THREE-DIMENSIONAL CONFORMAL RADIATION TREATMENT: CONCEPTS AND RATIONALE

The goal of delivering dose to the target volume and minimal dose elsewhere has not been easily approached with the limitations of early treatment technologies; specifically, volumetric images (CT, MRI), beam shaping/modulation techniques, and computerized treatment planning were not available or were primitive. The 3D problem was understood, but tools did not exist to allow solution. Development and maturation of 3D treatment planning tools have rapidly enabled workers to consider the search for an "optimal" treatment plan, reasonably thought of as a plan with a dose distribution that "conforms" to the target volume (Fig. 6-57). This search has led to the question of dose conformation: Can conformal radiation treatment be delivered to a target volume, and is it better than conventional treatment? The first part of this question is under

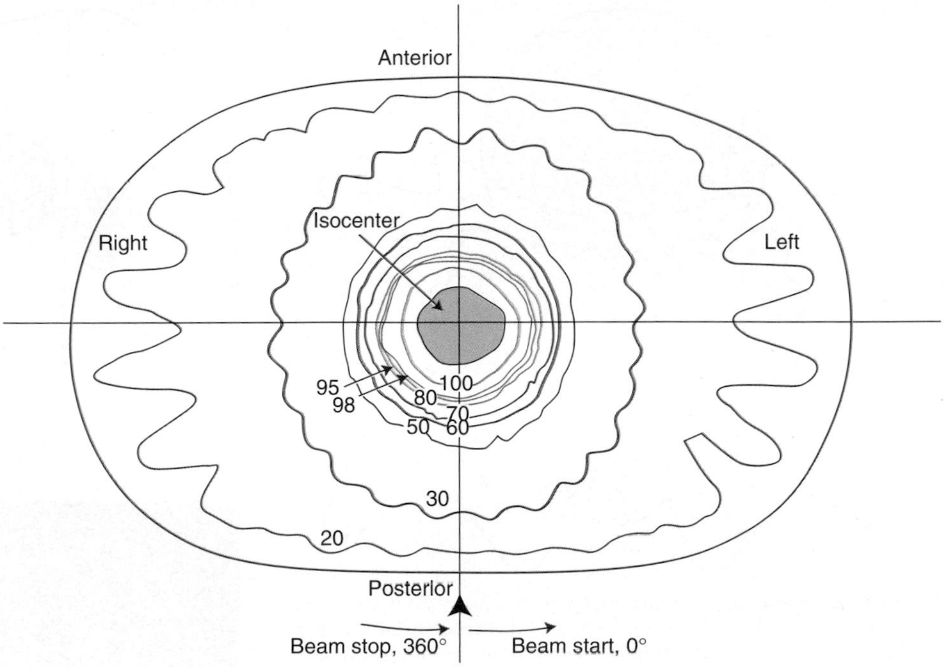

Figure 6-56 Arc plan for treatment of a target in the pelvis.

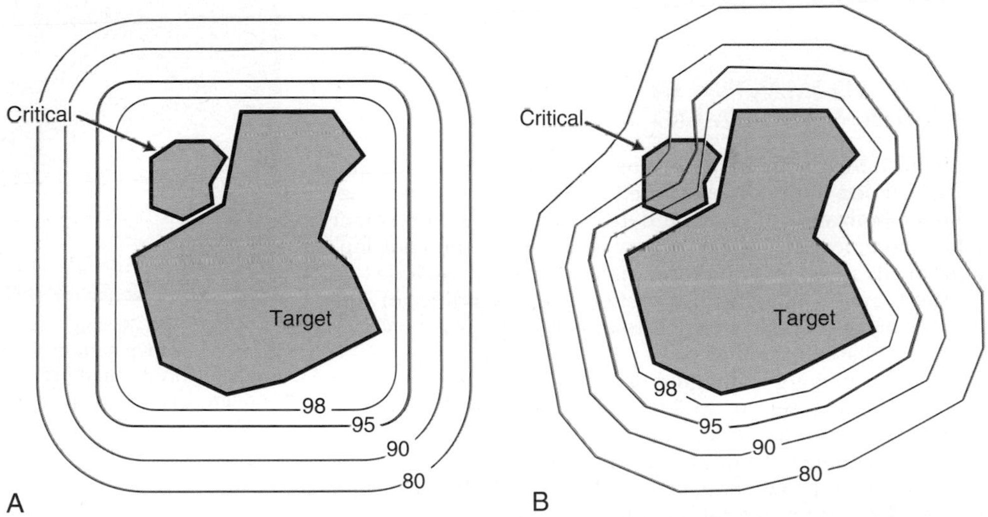

Figure 6-57 The conformal problem. A conventional plan (**A**) treats the target quite well but also treats a nearby critical structure. A conformal plan (**B**) treats the target well and spares part of the critical structure. Is the conformal plan better than the conventional plan?

active investigation and is now reviewed. Clinical trials to test the efficacy of conformal treatment are being devised and are reviewed in Chapter 14.

Conformal radiation treatment plans are realized by using a large number of beams of various weights, sizes or shapes, and orientations to hit the target. If enough beams of the proper kind are used, a dose distribution can be created with a shape that conforms to the target volume. This technique was recognized early[12] and is the reason multiple fields are used. In this regard, all radiation therapy treatment plans are conformal; however, the degree of conformation greatly varies based on the irradiation technique.

Conformal delivery techniques include a variety of approaches. Multiple static fields can be shaped by custom blocks, MLCs, miniature MLCs,[49] and custom stereotactic collimators.[50] Dynamic fields can be delivered using fixed field shapes[51] or variable field shapes[52] for each arc path. Intensity-modulated fields can be delivered using static fields with 3D compensators[22] or by dynamic techniques using a binary collimator[53] or MLCs.[54,55] Some of these approaches are used for single-fraction radiosurgery techniques and others for fractionated treatment.

The reconstruction of a conformal dose distribution by designing intensity-modulated beams is the same process as CT image reconstruction from transmission profiles.[47] If an optimized plan is one that is conformal, solving the inverse radon transform will provide a solution that is optimal. However, it can be shown that a solution cannot be found that will give an exactly conforming distribution because negative beam weights (use of negative energy) are required but are not possible. The approach is to find an approximate solution to the inverse radon transform through iterative techniques. A thorough review of the conformal problem and its solutions is published,[40] and the field continues to develop. An intensity-modulated conformal plan is shown in Figure 6-58, and Chapter 14 gives additional information.

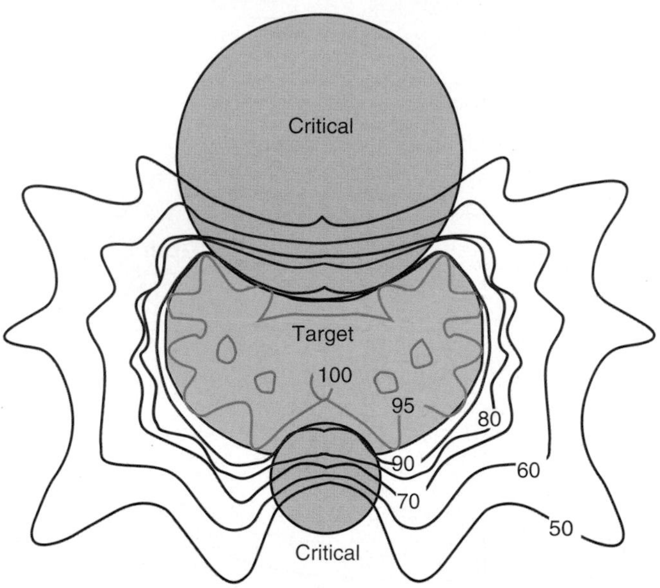

Figure 6-58 Example of a conformal plan. Intensity-modulated plan for a target located between two critical structures. (Adapted from Oldham M, Webb S: A 9-field static tomotherapy planning and delivery study. *In* Proceedings of the XIIth International Conference on the Use of Computers in Radiation Therapy, Salt Lake City, UT. Madison, WI, Medical Physics Publishing, 1997.)

ADVANCED IMAGING IN RADIATION TREATMENT

Radiation treatment is becoming more image based, and image-guided interventions, whether for surgery, lesion ablations, embolization of vascular defects, radiation treatment, or other therapies, are increasing in number.[56-58] The contributions of advanced imaging for radiation treatment include two primary areas: imaging for better understanding of the biology of cancers and normal tissues and imaging for verification of treatment delivery.

Biologic imaging is imaging of physiologic, metabolic, and functional processes to noninvasively measure the biologic character of tumors or normal tissues. Important biologic aspects of tumors to be imaged include metabolite content, the presence of hypoxia, and cell proliferation. Methods with biologic imaging potential include positron emission tomography (PET) and PET/CT with novel radionuclides and ligands for specific receptor targeting, MR spectroscopic imaging (MRSI), functional MR (fMR), MR diffusion and perfusion imaging, ultrasound, and optical methods for targeted receptors.[58]

Brain tumors have been studied using MRSI to measure the spatial distribution of metabolites that correlate with tumor grade.[59,60] Choline, creatine, *N*-acetyl-aspartate (NAA), lactate, and other metabolites relevant to the type of tumor (in this case, brain tumors) are determined by MRSI. The ratio of choline to NAA is determined by spectroscopic peak height analysis and mapped on a contrast-enhanced MR image (Fig. 6-59B). A key observation is that the spatial distribution of metabolite values and ratios for brain tumors differs in size and shape from that of (conventional) contrast-enhanced MR.[59,60] Figure 6-59 shows the problem for targeting with radiation—metabolite ratios or other tumor-specific information from biologic imaging modes will re-define how oncologic targets are determined. Anatomic methods that image endogenous contrast or contrast-enhanced regions will be complemented with advanced biologically based imaging techniques. These multimodality images will be used for targeting. The information is more than having two different imaging modalities such as CT and MR—it is the addition of patient-specific imaging to determine tumor character and environment. The validation of these new imaging techniques is important to ensure the understanding of the image information content, that is, the meaning of an intensity value for a voxel and how the image should be used as part of the radiation planning process.[58,61]

Imaging for validation and verification of treatment delivery is developing as image-guided treatment where the

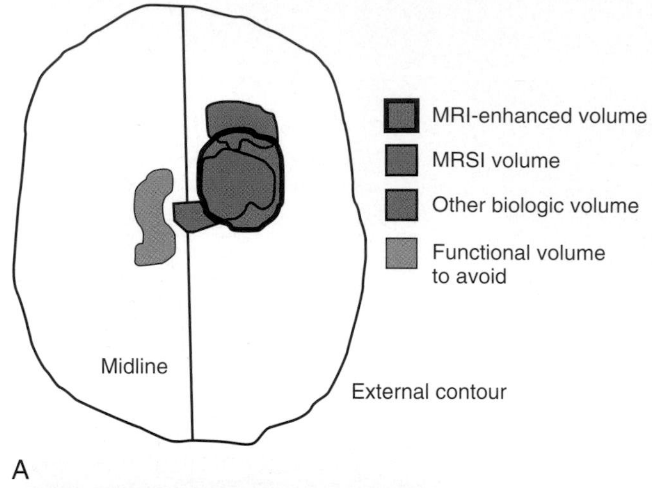

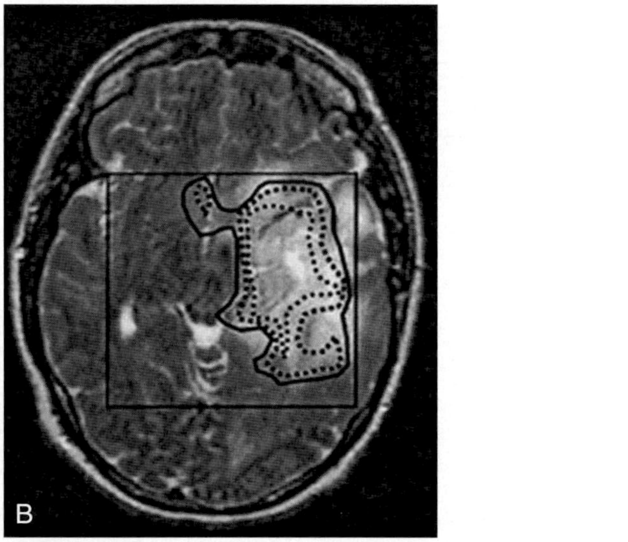

Figure 6-59 Biologic target volumes. **A,** Schematic shows the possible arrangement of three representations of a brain tumor: contrast-enhanced magnetic resonance imaging (MRI, *green*), magnetic resonance spectroscopic image (MRSI, *purple*), and other biologic volume *(violet)*, such as proliferation and receptor density. A region of avoidance *(blue)* is represented as may be obtained by functional MRI. **B,** From inner to outer shells, successive iso-ratio lines for choline–*N*-acetyl-aspartate (NAA) metabolite ratios (cho:NAA) of 6 *(dotted line)*, 4 *(dotted line)*, and 2 *(solid line)*. Distribution of the metabolite map crosses the midline and differs in size and shape from the (conventional) contrast-enhanced region. (**A,** From Bourland JD, Shaw EG: The evolving role of biological imaging in stereotactic radiosurgery. Tech Cancer Treat Res 2:135-140, 2003; **B,** from Pirzkall A, McKnight TR, Graves EE, et al: MR-spectroscopy guided target delineation for high-grade gliomas. Int J Radiat Oncol Biol Phys 50:915-928, 2001.)

imaging is performed in real-time or near real-time relative to the treatment process. Examples include uses of a CT unit in the treatment room with common patient couch for treatment; tomotherapy, which is a hybrid imaging-treatment device that performs CT imaging at the same time as the radiation treatment; and accelerated-mounted cone-beam CT, used to confirm proper patient and target positioning immediately before treatment. Combined with respiratory-gated imaging and subsequent radiation treatment, these advanced, image-guided capabilities will allow more frequent and possibly daily imaging to confirm precise and accurate radiation treatment.

Biologic imaging and methods for image-guided radiation treatment will continue to mature over the next decade. Biologic imaging will contribute especially to the understanding of cancer and normal tissue biology. Costs, technologic aspects of implementation, and clinical benefits of multimodality imaging remain to be solved for biologic imaging and imaging for verification and evaluation of patient response to treatment.[58]

STEREOTACTIC RADIOSURGERY

Radiosurgery refers to the use of single-fraction, small-field, high-dose, focal radiation for treatment of small tumors. By various means, discussed later, each radiation field is aimed accurately to intersect a common point at which a target is positioned. Typical minimum target doses are 12 to 20 Gy (1200 to 2000 rad) in a single fraction, compared with 2 Gy (200 rad) per day for 30 fractions in conventional radiation treatment. Radiosurgery doses can be high because the total irradiated volume is small (usually much less than 20 cc) and the peripheral dose is spread over a large volume. The radiobiologic aspects of radiosurgery are under investigation, and the technique has been studied at institutions and in one national group protocol.[62]

The *stereotactic* component of treatment refers to immobilization or fixation of the patient with a rigid or otherwise stable head frame system that establishes a patient-specific coordinate system for the entire treatment process. After placement of the head frame, typically by use of four pins that penetrate the scalp and impinge the outer table of the skull, imaging studies (e.g., CT, MRI, angiography) are performed to localize the target volume within the head frame coordinates. Fiducial markers attached to the head frame and built-in scales indicate the coordinate system on resulting images. (Stereoscopic or orthogonal radiographic films were used before the invention of CT and MRI.) The target is viewed and its position is determined in the head frame coordinates. Treatment planning consists of determining the field sizes, coordinates, and relative weights of radiation dose to be delivered for target coverage. The head frame and rigidly coupled patient are attached to mounting points on the treatment unit that enable the target coordinates to be registered with the point of irradiation. Often, multiple coordinates are irradiated successively to build a cumulative dose distribution that covers the entire target, as would be needed for large or irregularly shaped targets. Stereotactic radiosurgery is completed in around 4 hours, depending on case complexity. Two basic techniques exist for delivering radiosurgery, one using multiple radioactive sources and one using a modified linear accelerator. These techniques are discussed in the following sections.

Gamma Units

The Gamma Knife invented by Lars Leksell in the 1950s, is a radiation treatment machine used for stereotactic radiosurgery of intracranial lesions.[63,64] Gamma rays from 201 ^{60}Co sources arranged in a torus (Models B and C) or hemisphere (Model U) within a shielded source body are focused at a common point called the *focus*, or *isocenter*, with high accuracy (error < 0.3 mm) (Fig. 6-60). The source-to-focus distance is 40 cm. The nominal dose rate is 300 cGy/min at 40 cm for the 18-mm collimator at an 8-cm depth in tissue. The patient head frame carries scale assemblies to set the y- and z-coordinates. An intracranial target is positioned for treatment by attaching the head frame and patient within a "helmet" that contains 201 circular collimators, one for each source. The trunnions that attach the head frame to the helmet also define the x-coordinate. The helmet and attached patient are moved into the shielded portion of the gamma unit, where the helmet docks with the source body containing the 201 ^{60}Co sources.

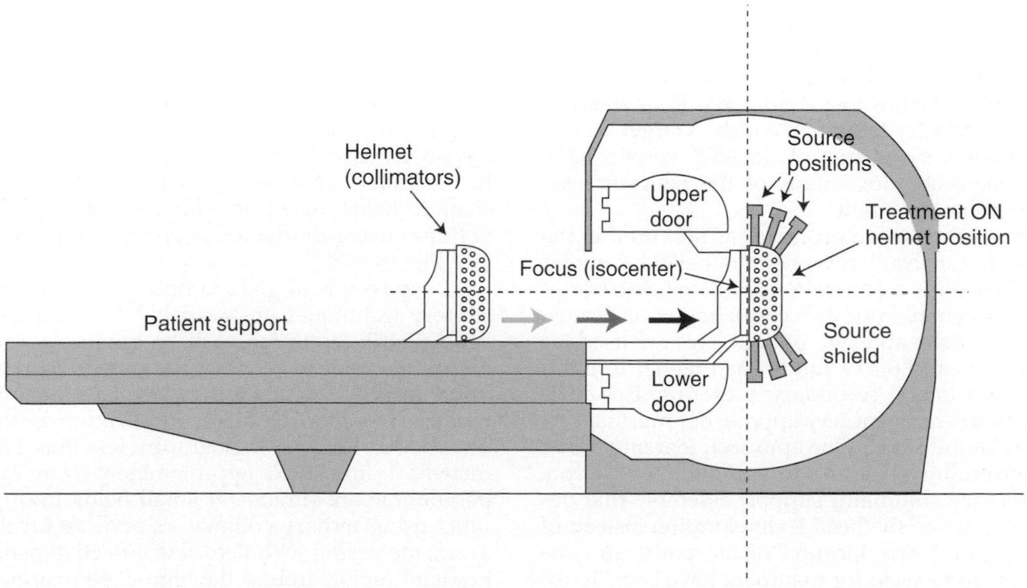

Figure 6-60 The Elekta Leksell Gamma Knife, Model B or C. (Based on a schematic courtesy of Elekta Instruments, AB, Stockholm, Sweden.)

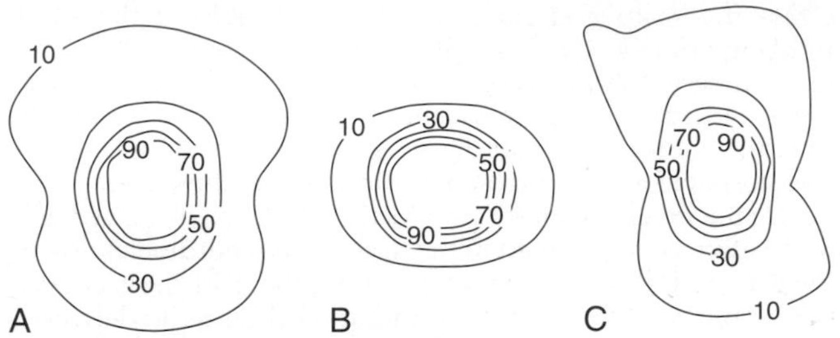

Figure 6-61 Gamma Knife dose distribution. **A,** Coronal plane. **B,** Axial plane. **C,** Sagittal plane. Distributions are for a Leksell Model U unit, 18-mm collimator, and single irradiation (or shot).

When docked, each of the 201 sources and matching collimators is aligned and irradiation at the focus is initiated. The size of the treated volume from an individual "shot" of 201 gamma ray beams is 4, 8, 14, or 18 mm in diameter and is chosen by selecting one of four helmets holding the desired collimator size. The resulting dose distribution from one irradiation is approximately spherical at the 50% isodose level, with some variation in the three orthogonal planes (Fig. 6-61). For large or irregular targets, multiple shot locations and shot sizes can be used to treat the entire target volume with a conformal distribution. Treatment planning capabilities include MRI- and CT-based planning, rapid dose computation, and dose distribution evaluation tools. An automatic positioning system (APS) is available that motorizes the x-, y-, and z-axis movements of the patient to multiple coordinates in succession, allowing more rapid execution of multiple shot treatment plans.

A new gamma unit has been designed in China that uses 30 ^{60}Co sources and source rotation to deliver 4-, 8-, 14-, and 18-mm diameter dose distributions in the stereotactic setting.[65] The nominal dose rate is 300 cGy/min at a source-to-focus distance of 40 cm. The device has been introduced to the United States, with one clinical facility in operation.

Linear Accelerator Units

Stereotactic radiosurgery performed using a linear accelerator is called *linac radiosurgery.* The linear accelerator is modified to accept a tertiary collimator assembly to accurately position circular collimators to form small, circular fields of 4 to 40 mm in diameter. The peripheral dose is spread over a large volume by using radiation paths that follow arcs or other paths. The head frame assembly attaches to a rigid, fixed floor stand or to the end of a high accuracy treatment couch. A target is positioned at the isocenter by means of an XYZ vernier slide assembly or by precision movements of the table that are tracked to ensure proper position.

Figure 6-62 shows the device geometry as first used in the United States,[66] with a specially designed floor stand. Circular collimators are used with a source-to-collimator distance of 77 cm and 100 cm isocenter. Four arcs consisting of one transverse arc, one sagittal arc, and two oblique arcs are used, as shown. Energy is typically 6 MV rather than higher to minimize penumbra from lateral secondary scattering. Isocentric accuracy of linac-based radiosurgery approaches must be verified and routinely monitored.[67] One approach that minimizes linac isocenter uncertainty heading to sub-millimeter errors uses a separate tertiary collimator support assembly that ties the collimator trajectory to the head frame location instead of that of the accelerator.[68] The location of arc paths and the amount of arc angle to be used for treatment have been investigated, with the result that multiple arcs distributed over

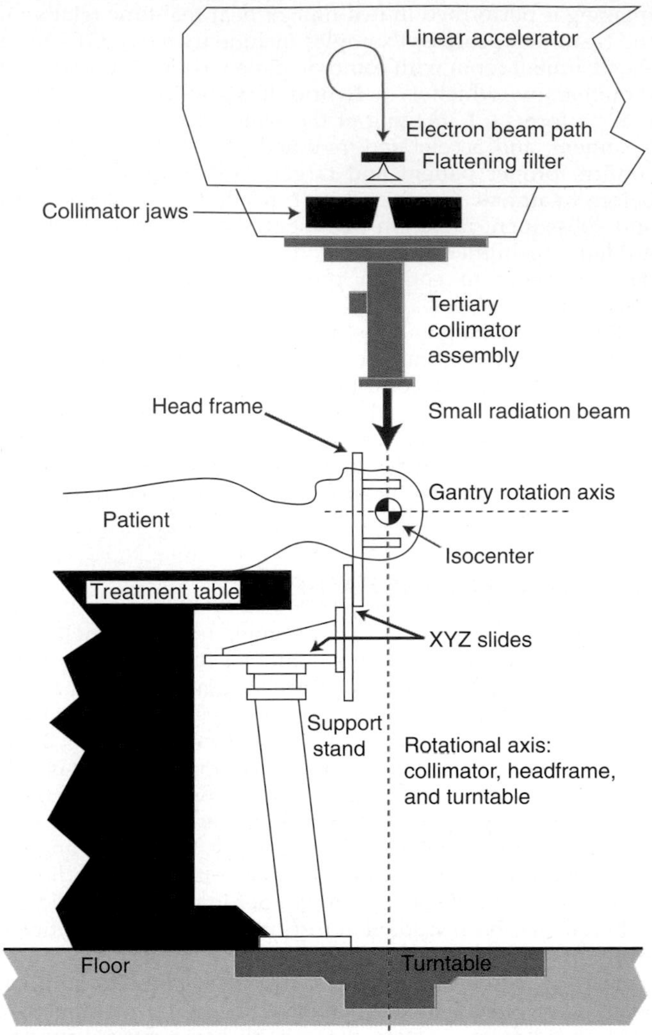

Figure 6-62 The linear accelerator radiosurgery treatment geometry. (From Bourland JD, McCollough KP: Static field conformal stereotactic radiosurgery: physical techniques. Int J Radiat Oncol Biol Phys 28:471-479, 1994, with permission.)

approximately 2π in a solid angle provide an adequate high-dose volume and low peripheral doses (Fig. 6-63). Static arc (gantry only) and dynamic arc (gantry and table) techniques have been used.[69] Field shaping for better target conformation has included small MLCs and shaped collimators.[49,50] Static, shaped fields result in suitable DVHs for sample target volumes using irradiation geometries with 5 to 11 static fields (see Fig. 6-63).[50,70]

Comparisons of gamma unit and linear accelerator radiosurgery techniques are available[50,69,70] and show comparable dose distributions for each technique. Gamma units have higher mechanical accuracy, in general, compared with linac units, but this accuracy may be of little clinical significance because imaging for target localization is the limitation on accuracy, as follows: angiography, less than 1 mm; CT, approximately 1 mm; MR, approximately 1 to 2 mm. Radiologic penumbrae are similar for small fields from gamma or linac units using tertiary collimators and are on the order of 1 to 3 mm, increasing with field size. Effective penumbra, the dose gradient region around the high-dose treatment volume for a target, is larger than 1 to 3 mm and varies with treatment plan

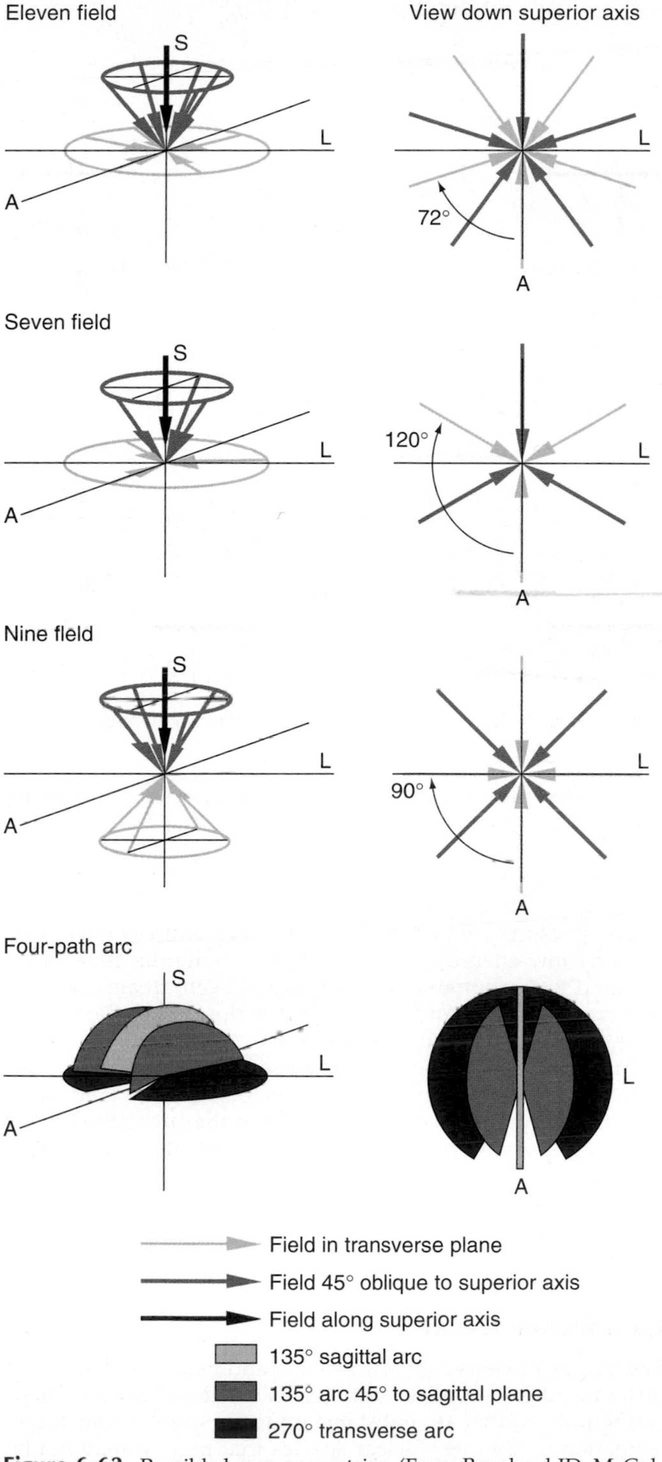

Figure 6-63 Possible beam geometries. (From Bourland JD, McCollough KP: Static field conformal stereotactic radiosurgery: physical techniques. Int J Radiat Oncol Biol Phys 28:471-479, 1994, with permission.)

parameters such as the number of shots, isocenters or arcs, and beam weights.

Radiosurgery remains a growing field, and its techniques are beginning to merge with conformal fractionated approaches for certain classes of patients. New or alternative techniques to be evaluated include noninvasive and replaceable patient fixation, fractionated treatment, extracranial treatment, static or shaped fields, intensity-modulated treatment with large- or small-width collimators, treatment with robot-controlled x-ray units,[71] shape-based planning,[72] and optimization algorithms. With conformal dose plans possible with each technique, treatment planning capabilities (degree of automation), patient morbidity (as governed by the dose gradient or penumbra), and treatment delivery efficiencies for the patient and personnel may be the parameters that most affect the choice of treatment. Parameters likely to affect treatment outcome are target localization accuracy, choice of prescription dose, target volume, and amount of normal tissue volume treated to high dose.

TOTAL-BODY PROCEDURES

Total-body irradiation (TBI) is an irradiation procedure performed as part of bone marrow transplantation and requires special physics measurements for implementation of treatment.[73] The patient is irradiated in the anteroposterior-posteroanterior or lateral-opposed directions at an extended distance from the treatment machine using large photon fields to encompass the whole body (Fig. 6-64). The goal is to provide dose homogeneity within ±10% of the prescription dose at the patient's midline. Dose compensation for narrow-width regions of the body and protection of the lungs with shielding blocks is required, depending on the technique used. Radiation beam data, such as beam profiles, depth dose or tissue-maximum ratios, and reference dose rates, must be obtained at the extended distance used. Data obtained for conventional treatment at the isocenter may not apply to large fields at extended distances, because of changes in scattering conditions. Higher beam energies are used for lateral techniques, matching the increase in patient thickness compared with anteroposterior geometries.

Total-skin electron treatment (TSET) is similar to TBI, except that electrons are used instead of photons. Considerations for this technique, which is used for skin cancers such as mycosis fungoides, have been delineated and include measurement of beam data (e.g., beam profiles, depth dose, and reference dose rate), measurement and any required reduction of bremsstrahlung contamination, and methods for ensuring relatively homogeneous irradiation of the patient surface. In particular, the irradiation geometry must avoid overdoses to thin anatomic regions such as the hands and fingers and prevent underdoses to anatomic regions that might be shielded by skin folds or extremities.[74] Typically, a six-field approach with six different patient positions is recommended.

BRACHYTHERAPY

Brachytherapy is a term that comes from *brachy* ("short"), combined with *therapy,* meaning short-distance therapy. The contrast is *teletherapy,* meaning therapy at a distance, as with ^{60}Co or linear accelerator machines, where the radiation source is 80 to 100 cm from the patient. In brachytherapy radioactive sources of small physical size are placed very close to or in the tumor for surface mold, interstitial, or intracavitary treatment. Several terms are defined:

1. Surface mold: Sources are fixed to an applicator, or mold, that conforms to the patient surface. The surface applicator positions the sources in the desired geometry and is placed on the skin surface to irradiate a superficial target.
2. Interstitial treatment: Sources are implanted in tissues directly or within catheters that are first implanted within the target volume.
3. Intracavitary or intraluminal treatment: Sources are inserted into body cavities by means of applicator devices.

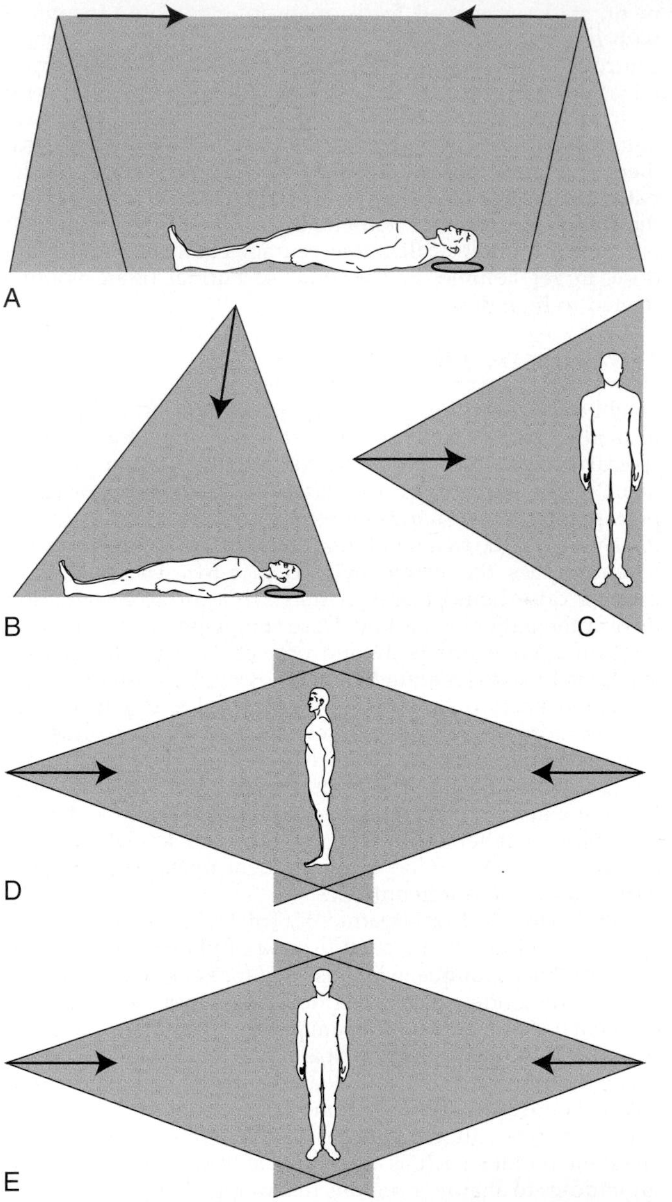

Figure 6-64 Irradiation geometries for total-body irradiation. **A,** Moving-source technique, with the patient on the floor. **B,** Large-field irradiation, with the patient on the floor. **C,** Single, large, lateral field, with the patient erect. **D,** Opposed, large, anterior and posterior fields, with the patient erect. **E,** Opposed, large, lateral fields, with patient erect. (**A–C,** From AAPM RTC Task Group 29: Report 17: The Physical Aspects of Total and Half Body Photon Irradiation. College Park, MD, American Association of Physicists in Medicine, 1986.)

Sites include the oral, rectal, vaginal, and uterine cavities and the tracheal and bronchial lumina.

Brachytherapy has several advantages compared with external beam treatment:

1. The inverse square law dominates the decrease in dose rate and dose as the distance from a source increases. The dose fall-off is very steep so that the dose delivered near a source is quite high (thousands of centigrays), whereas a few centimeters away the dose is low (tens of centigrays). The steep dose gradient confines the high-dose region to a small volume.

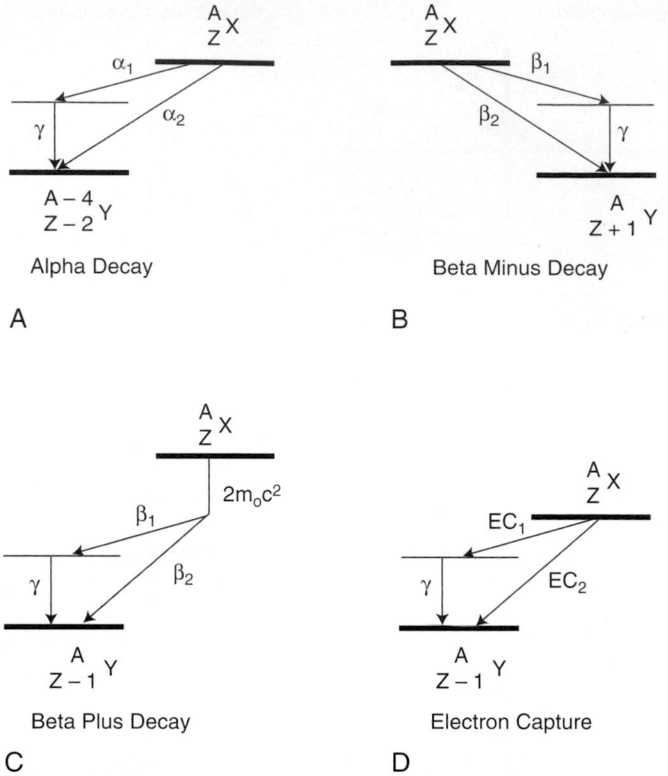

Figure 6-65 Modes of radioactive decay: α decay (**A**), β^- decay (**B**), β^+ decay (**C**), and electron capture (**D**).

2. The photons emitted by brachytherapy sources have relatively low energies and greater attenuation in tissue compared with photons used for external beam treatment. This increased attenuation concentrates dose near the source and minimizes dose at a distance.
3. In conventional brachytherapy prescription dose rates are relatively low, about 40 cGy/hr up to 80 cGy/hr, and treatment is over several days to deliver the prescribed dose. This approach may allow treatment of all cells in each phase of the cell cycle for a radiobiologic advantage. High dose rate remote afterloading brachytherapy has been used, with dose rates of approximately 200 cGy/min at the prescription point, comparable to external beam dose rates.

Radioactive Decay

The atomic nucleus contains protons and neutrons that prefer certain configurations for stability, as discussed earlier. Those configurations that are not stable undergo spontaneous transformation to another nuclear species that may or may not be stable. This spontaneous transformation is called *radioactive decay*. The mode of radioactive decay, meaning the type of transformation and emitted particles, depends on the parent species' nuclear composition. For a particular parent nuclide, a decay mode is allowed or prohibited, and it is one of the following types[2,12,13] (nomenclature is as defined previously, and particles are defined in Table 6-2):

1. In alpha decay (Fig. 6-65A), the nucleus gives off an alpha particle, $^4\alpha^{2+}$ (2 protons and 2 neutrons—a helium nucleus), resulting in a daughter nucleus of mass A − 4 and atomic number Z − 2. Alpha particles are monoenergetic and tend to have 4 to 8 MeV in kinetic energy.

$$^{A}_{Z}X \rightarrow ^{A-4}_{Z-2}Y + ^{4}\alpha^{2+} + Q \qquad 2n + 2p \rightarrow ^{4}\alpha^{2+} + Q$$

Secondary processes after alpha decay include gamma ray emission (or internal conversion, yielding characteristic x-rays or Auger electrons), which may occur after alpha decay as the daughter de-excites to the ground state. Radionuclides undergoing alpha decay tend to have high Zs and include ^{216}Ra, ^{222}Rn, ^{218}Po, ^{235}U, ^{239}Pu, and ^{241}Am.

2. For β decay, a single nucleon (neutron or proton) transforms from one type to the other in the nucleus. The nucleus gives off an electron, called a β particle because of its nuclear origin, and a neutrino. There are two types of β particles, one with negative charge, β^-, which is a "regular" electron, also called a *negatron*, and one with positive charge, β^+, the antiparticle to the electron, also called a *positron*. Radioactive decay modes with emission of a β^- or β^+ are possible.
   a. For β^- decay (i.e., negatron decay) (see Fig. 6-65B), a neutron transforms into a proton in the nucleus. The nucleus gives off a β^- particle and an antineutrino. The resulting daughter nucleus has the same mass A and increased atomic number of Z + 1. The β^- particles have a distribution of energies less than or equal to Q (the antineutrino carries off the remainder). The average β^- energy is about one-third Q.

$$^{A}_{Z}X \rightarrow {}_{Z+1}^{A}Y + \beta^- + \bar{\nu} + Q \qquad n \rightarrow p + \beta^- + \bar{\nu} + Q$$

   Secondary processes after β^- decay include gamma ray emission (or internal conversion, yielding characteristic x-rays or Auger electrons), which may occur after β^- decay as the daughter de-excites to the ground state. The β^- decay occurs for neutron-rich nuclides over all Zs. Example nuclides include ^{3}H, ^{14}C, ^{32}P, ^{60}Co, ^{89}Sr, ^{99}Mo, ^{131}I, ^{137}Cs, and ^{198}Au.
   b. For β^+decay (i.e., positron decay) (see Fig. 6-65C), a proton transforms into a neutron in the nucleus. The nucleus gives off a β^+ particle and a neutrino. The resulting daughter nucleus has the same mass A and decreased atomic number of Z – 1. The β^+ decay requires that 2 m_oc^2, or 1.022 MeV, be available between the parent and initial daughter energy states to be possible. If this energy difference is not available, β^+ decay is prohibited and electron capture may occur. The β^+ particles have a distribution of energies less than or equal to Q (the neutrino carries off the remainder). The average β^+ energy is about one-third Q but is higher than the average β^- energy for the same Q because of repulsion by the nucleus.

$$^{A}_{Z}X \rightarrow {}_{Z-1}^{A}Y + \beta^+ + \nu \qquad p \rightarrow n + \beta^+ + \nu + Q$$

   Secondary processes occur after β^+ decay. The positron, β^+, has a very short lifetime before annihilation. There is a small chance that the β^+ will hit an electron and annihilate in flight. The greater probability is that the β^+ slows down (through coulomb interactions) and combines with a free electron. The combined β^+:e^- (or e^+:e^-) species is called *positronium*. Positronium exists for about 10^{-10} seconds before annihilation and the creation of two 0.511-MeV photons (i.e., one photon for each electron mass). A longer-lived state of positronium (10^{-7} seconds) yields three simultaneous annihilation photons. Gamma ray emission (or internal conversion, yielding characteristic x-rays or Auger electrons) may also occur after β^+ decay as the daughter de-excites to the ground state. The β^+ decay occurs for proton-rich nuclides over lower and intermediate Zs. Example nuclides include ^{11}C, ^{15}O (used in positron emission tomography), and ^{22}Na.

3. In electron capture (see Fig. 6-65D), the nucleus captures an orbiting electron, increasing the nuclear mass by 0.511 MeV and transforming a proton into a neutron. Electron capture is similar to β^+ decay because the daughter has mass Z – 1 and a neutrino is emitted. Most often, the K shell electron is captured. Electron capture occurs for proton-rich nuclides over lower and intermediate Zs when there is not sufficient energy (2 m_0c^2, or 1.022 MeV) for β^+ decay to occur.

$$^{A}_{Z}X + e^- \rightarrow {}_{Z-1}^{A}Y + \nu + Q \qquad p + e^- \rightarrow n + \nu + Q$$

Secondary processes occur after electron capture. Because an orbital electron is captured, subsequent filling of the electron shell results in the emission of characteristic x-rays after an electron capture event. Gamma ray emission (or internal conversion, yielding characteristic x-rays or Auger electrons) may occur after electron capture as the daughter de-excites to the ground state. Nuclides decaying by electron capture include ^{22}Na, ^{40}K, ^{51}Cr, ^{57}Co, and ^{192}Ir (also with β^-).

The term Q in each decay equation represents the total energy given off as kinetic energy of the ejected particles (α, β^-, β^+, $\bar{\nu}$, ν) or the remaining nucleus, or both. The neutrino, with a mass of almost zero, was first postulated for existence because of the observed continuous energy distribution for β^- and β^+ energies in β decay. Without a third reaction product, the β^- or β^+ energies would be monoenergetic and almost equal to Q, reflecting the discrete energy levels in the nucleus.

Secondary Decay Processes

Each of the primary decay modes can leave the daughter nucleus or atom in the ground state or excited state. If an excited state exists, the additional energy is given off in various ways to yield a ground-state daughter.

1. Isomeric transition by fast gamma emission: With an excited daughter nucleus, the excitation energy may be given off by photons called *gamma rays*. The gamma ray energy is equal to the difference between the initial and next energy state of the nucleus. Because energy states are fixed for particular nuclei, gamma emissions are fixed and unique for a particular nucleus. Gamma rays identify their nucleus of origin in the same way characteristic x-rays identify their atom. Gamma emission may result in a ground state nucleus by a single gamma emission or by successive gamma emissions through several energy states. The release of energy by gamma emission is very fast—the excited state exists for no longer than 10^{-6} seconds—gamma emission is immediate after α, β^-, β^+, or electron capture decay. Although the phrases "^{60}Co gamma rays" and "^{137}Cs gamma rays" are used, these gamma rays are really from the daughter nuclei. Gamma rays from ^{60}Co are really ^{60}Ni gamma rays and gamma rays from ^{137}Cs are really ^{137}Ba gamma rays. However, the terminology is based on the parent nuclide's name.
2. Isomeric transition from a metastable state: When an excited nuclear state exists for greater than 10^{-6} seconds before gamma emission, the state is called a *metastable state*. Metastable states sometimes exist long enough to enable the separation of the metastable species from the parent, as is the case for ^{99m}Tc, with a half-life of 6 hours. The "m" refers to metastable. ^{99m}Tc decays to ^{99}Tc (an isomeric transition) by the emission of two gamma rays in succession.
3. Internal conversion: An excited nucleus can de-excite without gamma emission by the process of internal conversion. Instead of a gamma ray, the excitation energy is

used to eject an orbital electron, usually from the K shell. The ejected electron is called a *conversion electron* and has energy equal to the gamma energy minus the electron binding energy. The usual cascade of characteristic x-rays and Auger electrons follows. Internal conversion competes more with gamma emission as Z increases. The pathways of gamma emission and internal conversion are parallel to the competing processes of characteristic x-ray and Auger electron emission—a photon carries off the excitation energy, or the energy is transferred to an electron that is then ejected.

Radioactive decay is characterized by the following observations:

- All nuclei above $Z = 82$ are radioactive.
- For nuclei below $Z = 82$ some are naturally radioactive (e.g., ^{14}C and ^{40}K).
- High Z nuclei tend to undergo alpha decay; their nuclei have an abundance of protons and neutrons that may be emitted as coupled pairs (i.e., an alpha particle).
- Alpha particles tend to have 4 to 8 MeV in kinetic energy.
- Middle-range Z nuclei tend to undergo β^- (i.e., negatron) decay.
- Low Z nuclei tend to undergo β^+ (i.e., positron) decay.
- In general, if the decay rate is high (i.e., short half-life), the decay particles are energetic.
- In general, if the decay rate is low (i.e., long half-life), the decay particles are low energy.

Radioactive Decay Mathematics

Radioactive decay occurs spontaneously but also with a distinct probability for each radioactive nuclide. The number of transformations occurring per unit time, A(t), is called *activity* and is given by the following equation.

$$A(t) = \lambda N(t) \qquad \text{Eq. 40}$$

in which N(t) is the number of atoms of the radioactive species at time t and λ is a proportionality constant called the *decay constant.* The SI unit for activity is the becquerel, equal to one transformation per second. The original unit of activity is the curie, which is 3.7×10^{10} transformations per second ($3.7 \times 10^{10} s^{-1}$), an amount equal to the number of disintegrations occurring in 1 g of ^{226}Ra. λ is called the *decay constant,* which is unique for a nuclide and is equal to ln(2) divided by the half-life, $t_{1/2}$:

$$\lambda = \frac{\ln(2)}{t_{1/2}} = \frac{0.693}{t_{1/2}} \qquad \text{Eq. 41}$$

in which $t_{1/2}$, the half-life, is the amount of time required for the activity or the number of nuclei to decay to one half of the original value. The relationship between λ and $t_{1/2}$ looks like the relationship between HVL and μ.

The half-life, and hence, the decay constant, is constant and unique for a nuclide, and its measurement can be a means for identifying a species. Depending on the species, the half-life can be large or small and governs the lifetime over which decay occurs. The equation that radioactive decay obeys is:

$$N(t) = N_0 e^{-\lambda t} \quad \text{or} \quad A(t) = A_0 e^{-\lambda t} \qquad \text{Eq. 42}$$

where N(t) and N_0 are the number of nuclei at time t and t = 0, respectively, and A(t) and A_0 are the activities (in becquerels or curies) at time t and t = 0, respectively. Decay is exponential and can be represented in linear or semi-log form (Fig. 6-66).

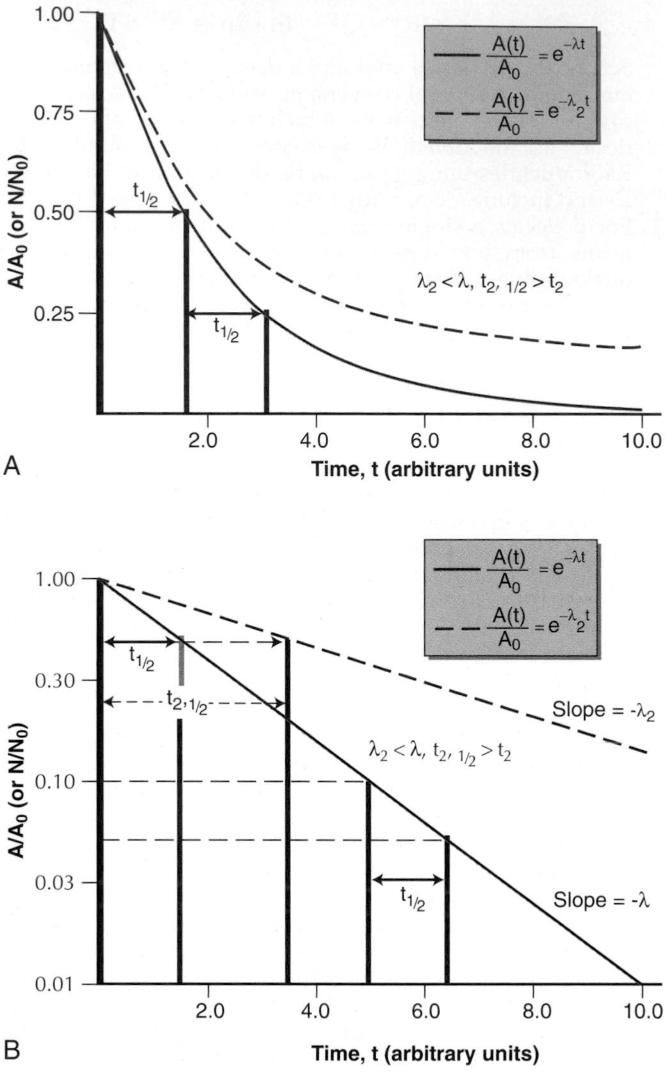

Figure 6-66 Graphic representation of radioactive decay: linear plot (**A**) and semi-log plot (**B**).

Properties and Applications of Isotopes

Table 6-14 lists isotopes, their properties, their physical forms, and their therapeutic applications. As seen, brachytherapy sources may be constructed as sealed sources in the forms of needles, tubes, or seeds. The solid radioactive material, in a stable inorganic or organic chemical form, adsorbed onto a material, or possibly as a liquid or gas, is sealed into a metal source capsule by welds or other means that prevent leakage of the material. Most radioactive sources are beta emitters, and the useful radiations for treatment are the gamma rays or characteristic x-rays emitted after β decay. Besides containment of the source material, the metal encapsulation stops all beta (or alpha) emissions and allows only the gamma or x-rays to be transmitted. Sources can also be used for their beta emissions (i.e., ^{90}Sr) or in unsealed (liquid) form.

Dose distributions from sealed sources have a shape that reflects the rapid fall-off with dose due to the inverse square law, the source energy, the distribution and amount of activity within the source, and the source encapsulation. Source

Table 6-14 Properties and Applications of Isotopes

Nuclide	Half-Life	Decay Mode	Decay Products*	Physical Form	Γ (R·cm²·mCi⁻¹·h⁻¹)	HVL (mm Pb)	Clinical Application
^{60}Co	5.263 yr	β	β, γ	SSS tubes	13.07	11.9	RA, gyn, H/N
^{103}Pd	17 d	EC	γ, .021 $\bar{x}$	SSS seeds	1.48	.008	IS, prostate
^{125}I	60.2 d	EC	.027 $\bar{x}$	SSS seeds	1.46	.025	IS, prostate, H/N, pancreas, sarcoma
^{137}Cs	30.2 yr	β	β, .662 γ	SSS tubes	3.26	5.5	IC, RA, gyn, H/N
^{192}Ir	74.2 d	EC, β	β, γ, .38 $\bar{\gamma}$	SSS, seeds, wire	4.69	2.5	IC, IS, RA, gyn, H/N, breast, sarcoma
^{226}Ra	1602 yr	α	α, β, γ, .83 $\bar{\gamma}$	SSS tubes, needles	8.25	8.0	IC, IS, gyn, H/N, breast
OTHER ISOTOPES							
^{32}P	14.28 d	β	β	LQ	—	—	IC (peritoneal)
^{131}I	8.05 d	β	β, γ	LQ	2.2	2.5	OR, thyroid and mets
^{198}Au	2.7 d	β	β, γ	LQ, seeds	2.38	2.5	IC (peritoneal), IS
^{222}Ra	3.83 d	α	α, β, γ	GSS, seeds	10.15	8.0	IS, breast

*Where a number is given, the units are in MeV. An overlined particle, $\bar{\gamma}$ or $\bar{x}$, indicates that the energy given is an average energy.

SSS, solid sealed source; LQ, liquid pharmaceutical; GSS, glass sealed source; IC, intracavitary; IS, interstitial; RA, remote afterloading; OR, taken orally; HVL, half-value layer; H/N, head and neck; gyn, gynecologic; α, alpha decay; β, beta decay; EC, electron capture; mets, metastatic.

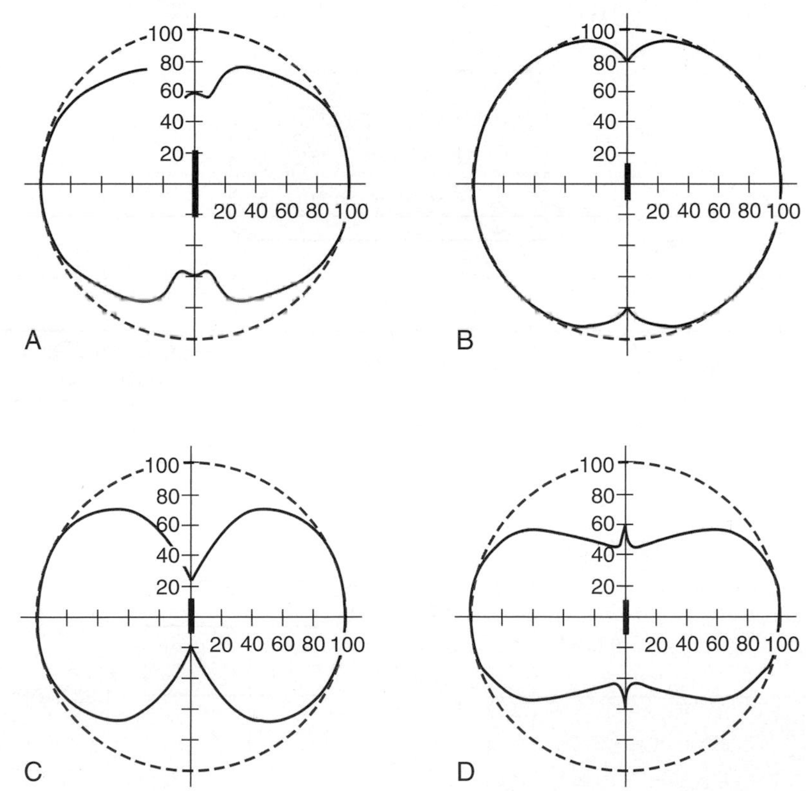

Figure 6-67 Brachytherapy source anisotropy. **A,** Relative dose rate using a 2-cm radius, ^{226}Ra tube, and 1.35 active length. **B,** Relative in-air fluence for ^{192}Ir seed. **C,** Relative in-air fluence for ^{125}I seed, model 6711. **D,** Relative in-air fluence for ^{103}Pd. (**A,** Data from Johns HE, Cunningham JR: The Physics of Radiology, 3rd ed. Spring Field, IL, Charles C Thomas, 1978; **B–D,** data from Interstitial Collaborative Working Group: Interstitial Brachytherapy: Physical, Biological, and Clinical Considerations. New York, Raven Press, 1990.)

encapsulation in particular affects the apparent activity, active length, and shape of the dose distribution through attenuation by the source capsule walls and ends. Sealed-source dose distributions are anisotropic, not uniform, because of increased encapsulation thickness and self-absorption along the length of the source (Fig. 6-67). Investigators have performed measurements and applied Monte Carlo techniques and other models to determine brachytherapy source dose characteristics.[75,76]

Radioactive decay and its energetics are represented by decay schematics (see Fig. 6-65). Horizontal lines represent the relative nuclear energy levels of the parent and daughters. Branches from the parent to the daughter represent the type of decay, whereas the horizontal spacing of each species represents the atomic number, Z. A branch to the left indicates a transition where Z decreases (α, β^+, or electron capture) (see Fig. 6-65A to D). A branch to the right indicates a transition where Z increases (β^- decay) (see Fig. 6-65B). Elevated horizontal lines above the ground state indicate excited nuclear levels. Vertical arrows from one excited level to a lower one or the ground state indicate gamma emission. Fractional or percentage amount of time a transition occurs is indicated, as are the absolute energies of levels, particles, and photons. Decay schemes for the medical isotopes listed in Table 6-14 are presented in Figures 6-68 through 6-76. It is observed that the nuclear configurations and transitions for these isotopes are simple for some and complex for others. For instance, ^{60}Co decays by β^- decay to ^{60}Ni, which de-excites by the emission of two gamma rays, one at 1.17 MeV and one at 1.33 MeV (see Fig. 6-69). ^{125}I decays by electron capture to ^{125}Te, with the emission of one gamma ray (35 keV) and two characteristic x-rays (27.3 keV, 31.4 keV) (see Fig. 6-72). After decay, the resulting daughter nucleus itself may be radioactive, resulting in an additional decay or decays. The decay chain for ^{226}Ra has nine decays (and daughters) until stable ^{206}Pb is reached (Fig. 6-77).

Source Strength

Source strength, that is, the amount of radiation or dose given off per unit time, is an important physical and clinical parameter, because dose rate must be known to enable a prescribed dose to be delivered. Source strength has been specified as the amount of milligrams of ^{226}Ra (mg-Ra), the equivalent amount of milligrams of ^{226}Ra (mg-Ra eq, for ^{226}Ra substitutes such as ^{137}Cs or ^{192}Ir), the actual activity encapsulated, the apparent activity, and the exposure rate at a distance, the most commonly used specification for strength. However, because dose rate is the important quantity, the recommended source strength specification is now air kerma strength[77] (S_K) with units of $\mu Gy/m^2/h$. S_K is based on the air kerma rate in free space, $\dot{K}_1$, which gives the kerma rate in air in micrograys per hour at a fixed distance from the source, measured radially from a point source or along the perpendicular bisector for a linear source. Kerma equals dose with less than 1%

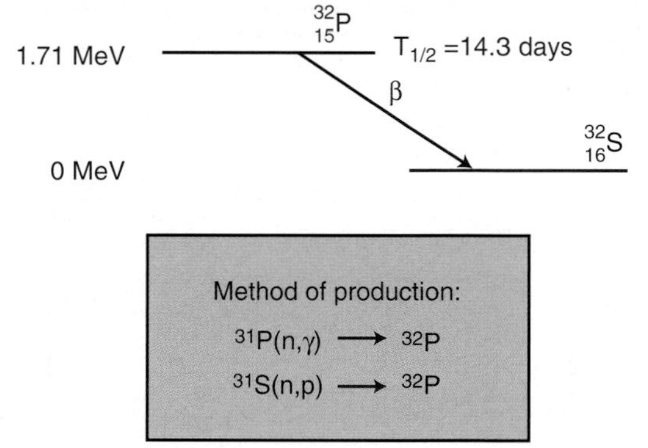

Emitted Radiation	Energy (MeV)	Mean Number per Disintegration
β⁻(Phosphorus-32 βs)	1.710 max, 0.70 average	1.0

Figure 6-68 A ^{32}P decay scheme. (Data from Lederer CM, Hollander JM, Perlman I: Table of Isotopes, 6th ed. New York, Wiley & Sons, 1967; schematic courtesy of E.L. Chaney.)

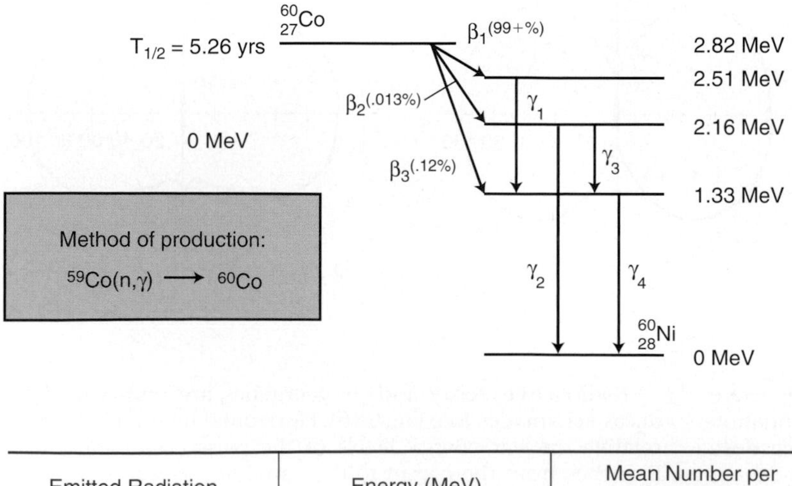

Emitted Radiation	Energy (MeV)	Mean Number per Disintegration
γ ray (Nickel-60 γ rays)	1.173	0.998
"	1.332	1.0

Figure 6-69 A ^{60}Co decay scheme. (Data from Lederer CM, Hollander JM, Perlman I: Table of Isotopes, 6th ed. New York, Wiley & Sons, 1967; schematic courtesy of E.L. Chaney.)

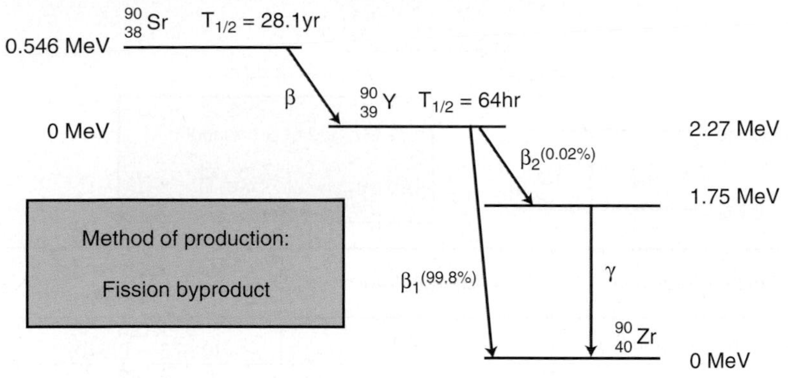

Emitted Radiation	Energy (MeV)	Mean Number per Disintegration
β^- (Strontium-90 βs)	0.546 max	1.0
β^- (Yttrium-90 βs)	2.268 max, 0.90 average	1.0

Figure 6-70 A ^{90}Sr decay scheme. (Data from Lederer CM, Hollander JM, Perlman I: Table of Isotopes, 6th ed. New York, Wiley & Sons, 1967; schematic courtesy of E.L. Chaney.)

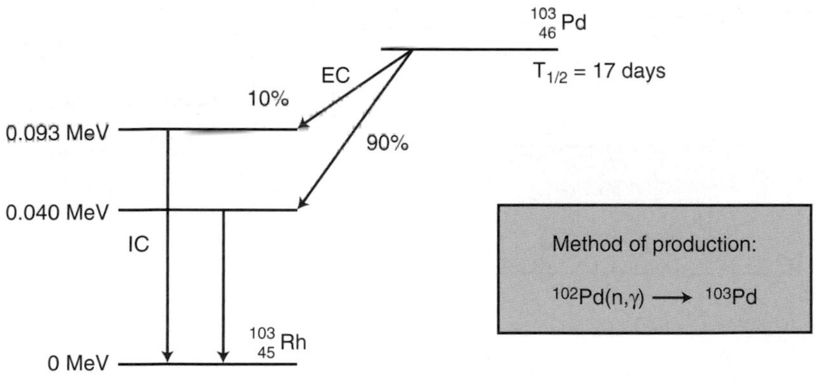

Emitted Radiation	Energy (MeV)	Mean Number per Disintegration
γ ray (Rhenium-103 γ rays)	0.0397	0.001
"	0.357	0.001
x ray, K_α (EC and IC)	0.201	0.656
x ray, K_β (EC and IC)	0.230	0.125

Figure 6-71 A ^{103}Pd decay scheme. (Data from Lederer CM, Hollander JM, Perlman I: Table of Isotopes, 6th ed. New York, Wiley & Sons, 1967; schematic courtesy of E.L. Chaney.)

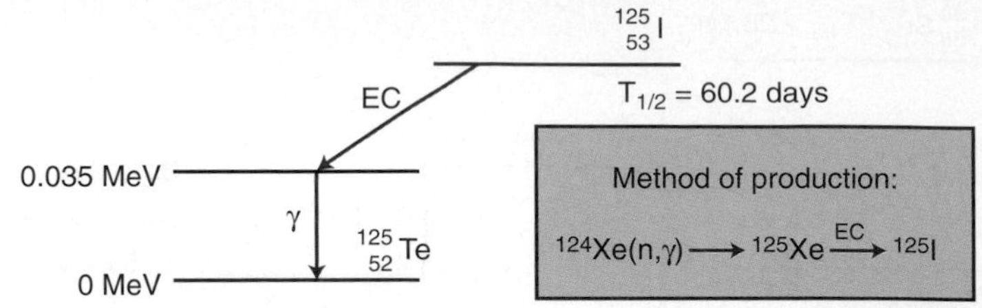

Emitted Radiation	Energy (MeV)	Mean Number per Disintegration
x ray, K_{α} (EC and IC)	27.3	1.126 (0.576 + 0.540)
x ray, K_{β} (EC and IC)	31.4	0.240 (0.124 + 0.116)
γ ray (Tellurium-125 γ rays)	35.5	0.068
"	Average of ~ 28.5 keV	Average of ~ 1.47

Figure 6-72 A ^{125}I decay scheme. (Data from Lederer CM, Hollander JM, Perlman I: Table of Isotopes, 6th ed. New York, Wiley & Sons, 1967; schematic courtesy of E.L. Chaney.)

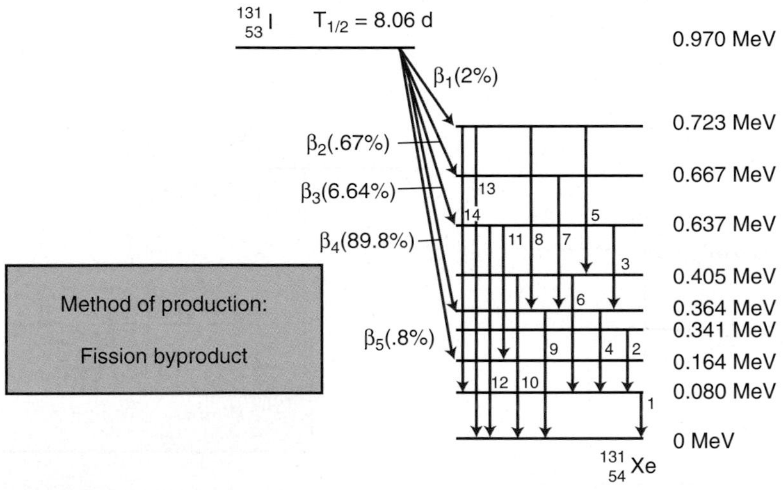

Emitted Radiation	Energy (MeV)	Mean Number per Disintegration
γ rays (Xenon-131 γ rays)	0.080	0.026
"	0.284	0.054
"	0.364	0.820
"	0.637	0.068
"	0.732	0.016

Figure 6-73 A ^{131}I decay scheme. (Data from Lederer CM, Hollander JM, Perlman I: Table of Isotopes, 6th ed. New York, Wiley & Sons, 1967; schematic courtesy of E.L. Chaney.)

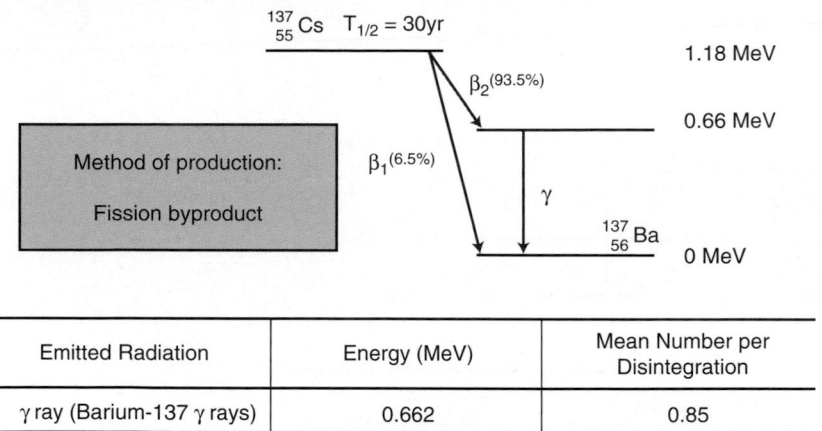

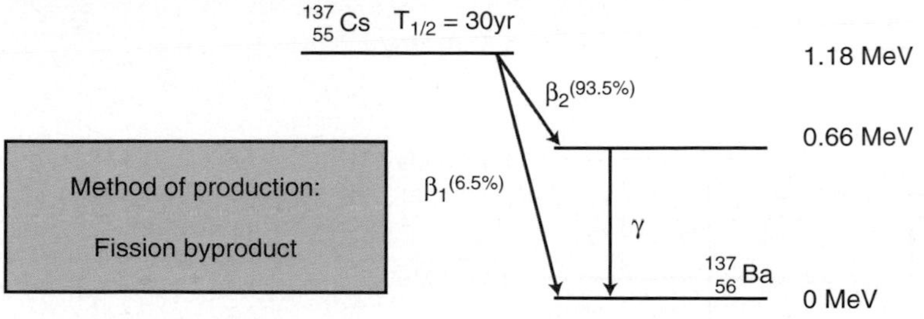

Emitted Radiation	Energy (MeV)	Mean Number per Disintegration
γ ray (Barium-137 γ rays)	0.662	0.85

Figure 6-74 A ^{137}Cs decay scheme. (Data from Lederer CM, Hollander JM, Perlman I: Table of Isotopes, 6th ed. New York, Wiley & Sons, 1967; schematic courtesy of E.L. Chaney.)

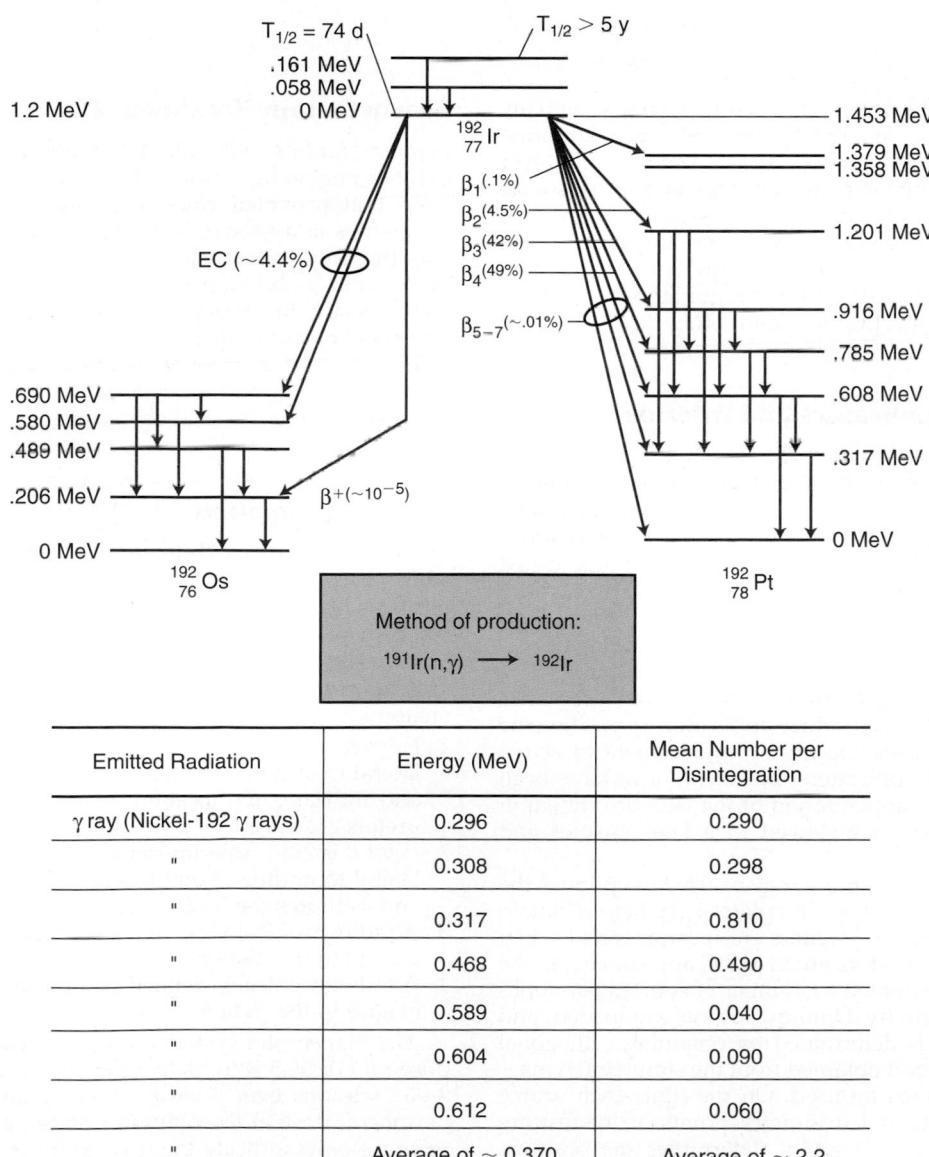

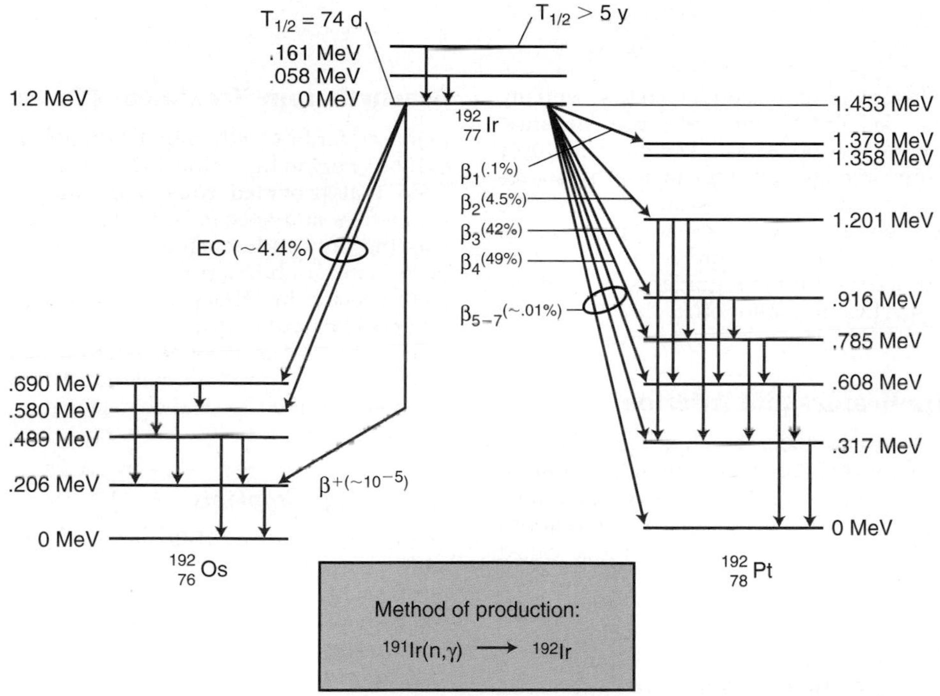

Emitted Radiation	Energy (MeV)	Mean Number per Disintegration
γ ray (Nickel-192 γ rays)	0.296	0.290
"	0.308	0.298
"	0.317	0.810
"	0.468	0.490
"	0.589	0.040
"	0.604	0.090
"	0.612	0.060
"	Average of ~ 0.370	Average of ~ 2.2

Figure 6-75 A ^{192}Ir decay scheme. (Data from Lederer CM, Hollander JM, Perlman I: Table of Isotopes, 6th ed. New York Wiley & Sons, 1967; schematic courtesy of E.L. Chaney.)

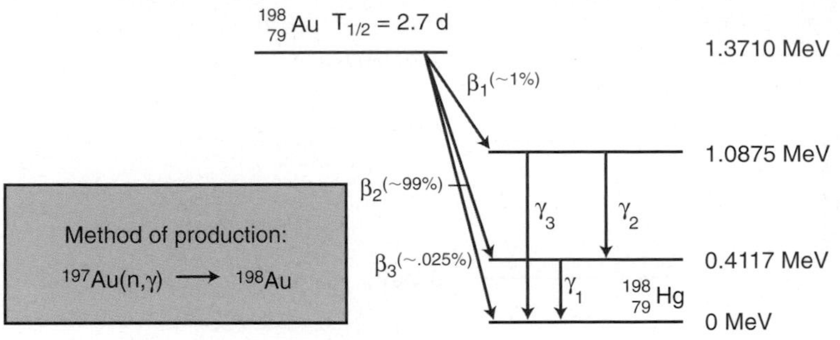

Emitted Radiation	Energy (MeV)	Mean Number per Disintegration
β^- (Gold-198 βs)	0.962 max, 0.30 average	1.0
γ ray (Mercury-198 γ rays)	0.4117	0.95

Figure 6-76 A ^{198}Au decay scheme. (Data from Lederer CM, Hollander JM, Perlman I: Table of Isotopes, 6th ed. New York, Wiley & Sons, 1967; schematic courtesy of E.L. Chaney.)

difference for brachytherapy photon energies, so $\dot{K}_1$ essentially gives the dose rate in air at the reference distance. While air kerma strength is adopted as a standard, multiple specifications for source strength are still in use by source manufacturers and treatment planning systems. The same convention of source strength must be used for the radiation source and the planning system to ensure correct computations of dose rate and dose. Additional guidance is available on source strength specification and other brachytherapy planning issues.[77-79]

Brachytherapy Applicators and Afterloading

When first used in the early 1900s brachytherapy sources were directly implanted into the patient for interstitial or intracavitary treatment. To reduce personnel doses and allow greater flexibility in determining source configurations without having to handle "hot" sources, a technique called *afterloading* was developed in the 1950s, first for intracavitary treatments and later for interstitial applications. With afterloading the source configuration is determined using nonradioactive "dummy" sources and the actual sources are efficiently loaded at a later time. Afterloading techniques require the use of specialized source applicators to position the dummy sources and allow accurate (re)placement of actual sources. A variety of applicators and techniques have been developed to facilitate implantation of the isotopes shown in Table 6-14, and these are reviewed in a later chapter and elsewhere.[12,13,80,81]

In brachytherapy preplanning may be used to optimize the source locations and activities. Templates may help maintain the intended source geometry and are recommended when possible. Once the applicators are in place, adjustments to the implant geometry are limited to number of sources per applicator, spacing, and activity. Dummy sources are loaded, and each source location is determined by obtaining orthogonal films. These films are best obtained from the simulator. A magnification indicator must be used. On the films each source location and anatomic and dosimetry points of interest are identified and digitized. Planning determines the position, activity, and insertion time for each source based on the chosen point of prescription. A plan is represented by isodose distributions that show dose rate in centigrays per hour.

Brachytherapy Treatment Planning

Planning for brachytherapy treatments initially was nonexistent, but beginning in the 1920s various systems were developed that provided rules and guidelines for implantation geometries and specifications for prescription. Initially, ^{226}Ra was the only radionuclide used for brachytherapy because of its natural abundance, and systems were developed that were specific to ^{226}Ra source configurations of needles and tubes. Other radionuclides for brachytherapy became available in the 1950s through neutron activation in a nuclear reactor or as by-product material. The radium systems were modified for the physical characteristics of these nuclear-age radionuclides.

Gynecologic Implants

Three systems using different applicators, source strengths, and treatment times were developed for intracavitary implants of the cervix and uterus.[80] The first two, the Paris and Swedish systems, were modified and became known as the Manchester system, the most widely used brachytherapy system. In the Manchester system, four points of interest are anatomically defined (Fig. 6-78):

1. *Point A* is 2 cm superior to the external cervical os, and 2 cm lateral to midline. Point A is specified on the right and left and indicates the location where the uterine vessels and ureters cross.
2. *Point B* is 2 cm superior to the external cervical os and 5 cm lateral to midline. Point B is specified on the right and left and indicates the location of the obturator lymph nodes.
3. A radiographically defined point indicates the dose of relevance to the *bladder*.
4. A radiographically defined point indicates the dose of relevance to the *rectum*.

The Manchester system prescribes dose to point A using a dose rate of 55.5 R/h, delivering 8000 R in 144 hours in two 3-day sessions over 2 weeks. Point B gives an indication of peripheral dose at the obturator nodes, and the bladder and rectum points indicate the dose at these dose-limiting structures. The classic gynecologic implant uses three 2-cm sources in a line, or *tandem*, in the uterus and two 2-cm sources, one on either side of the cervix, as shown in Figure 6-79. With

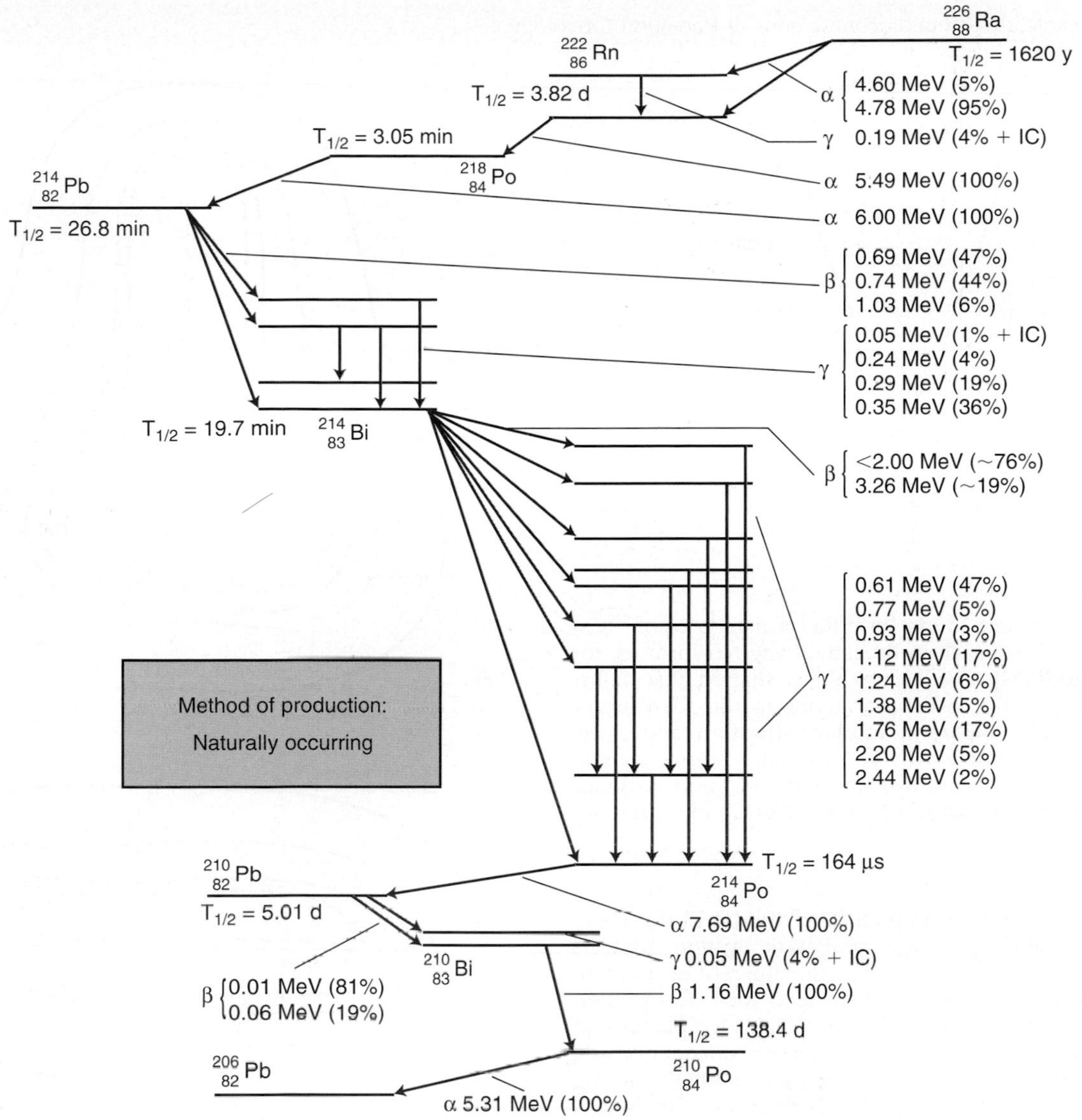

Emitted Radiation	Energy (MeV)	Mean Number per Disintegration
γ ray (Radon-222 γ rays)	0.186	0.040
γ ray (Bismuth-214 γ rays)	0.053	0.020
"	0.242	0.075
"	0.295	0.210
"	0.352	0.380
γ ray (Polonium-214 γ rays)	0.609	0.470
"	0.769	0.053
"	0.935	0.033
"	1.120	0.160
"	1.238	0.060
"	1.379	0.048
"	1.400	0.040
"	1.728	0.032
"	1.764	0.170
"	2.204	0.060
"	2.435	0.020

Figure 6-77 A ^{226}Ra decay scheme. (Data from Lederer CM, Hollander JM, Perlman I: Table of Isotopes, 6th ed. New York, Wiley & Sons, 1967; schematic courtesy of E.L. Chaney.)

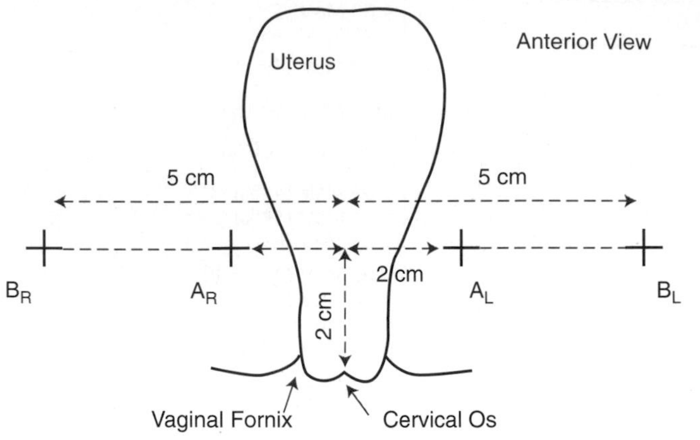

Figure 6-78 Gynecologic anatomy and definitions for points A and B.

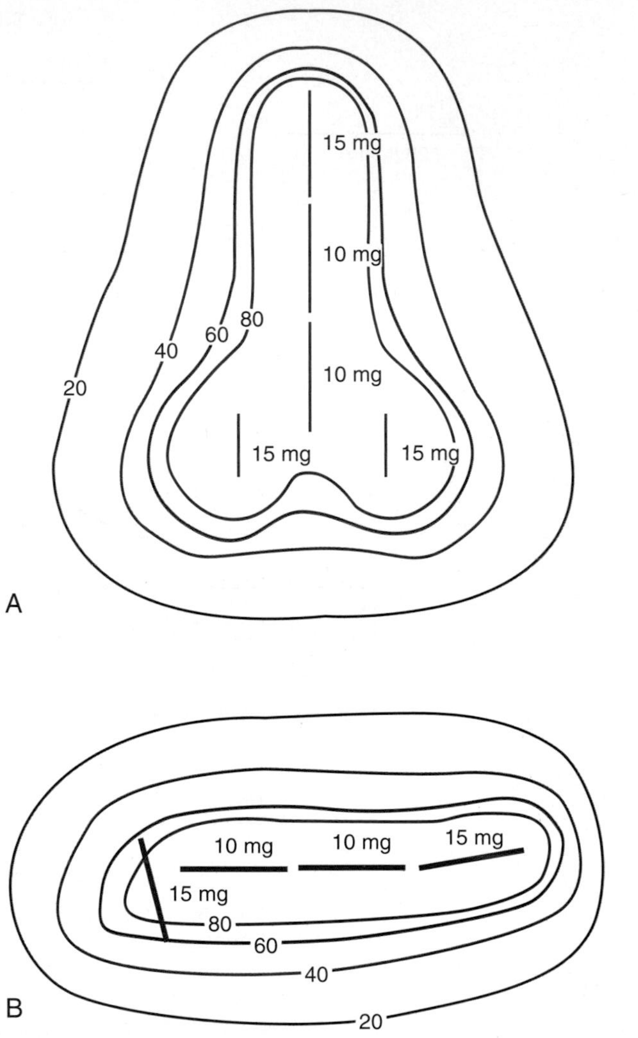

Figure 6-79 Typical gynecologic implant. **A,** Coronal plane. **B,** Sagittal plane. Source arrangement coincides with anatomy shown in Figure 6-77. Isodose values are in units of centigrays per hour.

activities of 15, 10, and 10 mg (of ^{226}Ra, or mg-Ra eq of ^{137}Cs) in tandem and 15 mg each in the lateral vaginal fornices, for a total of 65 mg-Ra eq, a well-known pear-shaped dose distribution results (see Fig. 6-79). Variations to the Manchester system are readily apparent. Implant duration and dose, number of sources, source activity (dose rate), source geometry, applicator design, number of implants, and primary versus boost treatment can all be varied. Gynecologic implant approaches have been reviewed.[12,80,82]

Interstitial Implants

The Manchester system of implantation rules and dose prescription, also called the Paterson-Parker system after its authors,[83,84] has formed the basis for interstitial implant approaches and was originally developed for ^{226}Ra needles. This system specifies source distribution rules for planar and volume implants. The system is based on the concept of using a relatively uniform distribution of sources having differing linear activities to deliver a dose distribution with homogeneity of ±10% of prescription. Rules include the distribution of activity, that is, the percentage of activity to load in the implant center versus the periphery, for planar targets, and cylindrical, spherical, and cubical implant volumes. A fixed source spacing of 1 cm is specified. The Quimby system was developed and used in the United States and is based on the concept of using a uniform distribution of sources of the same linear activity throughout the implant volume (^{226}Ra needles were available in the United States with constant linear activity). Source spacing is uniform, with 1 to 2 cm source intervals. The modern Paris system is based on the use of ^{192}Ir wire. Sources are arranged in parallel fashion in planes, the linear activity is constant for all sources, and source spacing is uniform.[85] Target coverage is by the 85% isodose surface. An example of a single-plane implant is shown in Figure 6-80. Table 6-15 summarizes some of the rules for the Manchester, Quimby, and Paris systems. More complete reviews are available and required for complete details for each system.[12,80,85,86]

Computerized systems have facilitated customized planning for brachytherapy treatments. Planning systems now perform image-based planning and include tools for automated source localization and optimization of the dose distribution. High dose rate planning systems, in particular, have provided optimization schemes to determine source dwell times to provide a desired dose distribution. A planning system must use the source strength convention for the source being applied (i.e., apparent activity or air kerma strength) and must account for radial and axial anisotropies in the dose distribution,[87] such as the anisotropies shown earlier (see Fig. 6-67).

Dose Specification

An implant system specifies dose or dose rate at a point or points (i.e., Point A) or possibly to a plane or volume of interest that contains the implant. The ICRU has recommended that dose be reported to a reference volume and points of interest for gynecologic implants and for mean central and peripheral dose for interstitial implants.[88,89] The recommendations follow similarly to the ICRU's specification of volumes for use in external beam therapy in ICRU 50 and ICRU 62,[29,30] and it is recommended that ICRU's nomenclature be used in clinical practice.[90]

Other Brachytherapy Techniques

Brachytherapy applications also include molds for ocular melanoma using ^{125}I seeds, biliary stent implantation with ^{192}Ir, endovascular brachytherapy for prevention of arterial restenosis with ^{90}Sr, ^{192}Ir, and other nuclides, treatment of pterygium with ^{90}Sr applicators, and ultrasound-guided prostate

Table 6-15 Manchester, Quimby, and Paris Systems

Parameter	SYSTEM *Manchester*	*Quimby*	*Paris*
Dose	6000-8000 R	5000-6000 R	6000-7000 R
Dose rate	40-60 R/hr	60-70 R/hr	25-90 cGy/hr
Prescription point	10% above absolute minimum	On bisector (planar) or periphery (volume)	85% of minimum central dose
Linear activity	Variable	Constant	Constant
Activity distribution			
Single plane	Varies with area	Uniform	Uniform
Volume implant	Varies with shape	Uniform	Multiple, uniform planes
Source spacing	Constant at 1 cm	Constant, 1-2 cm	Constant, .5-2 cm
Crossing needles	Yes	Yes	No

Adapted from Glasgow GP, Perez CA: Physics of brachytherapy. *In* Perez CA, Brady LW (eds): Principles and Practice of Radiation Oncology, 2nd ed. Philadelphia, JB Lippincott, 1987, pp 213-251.

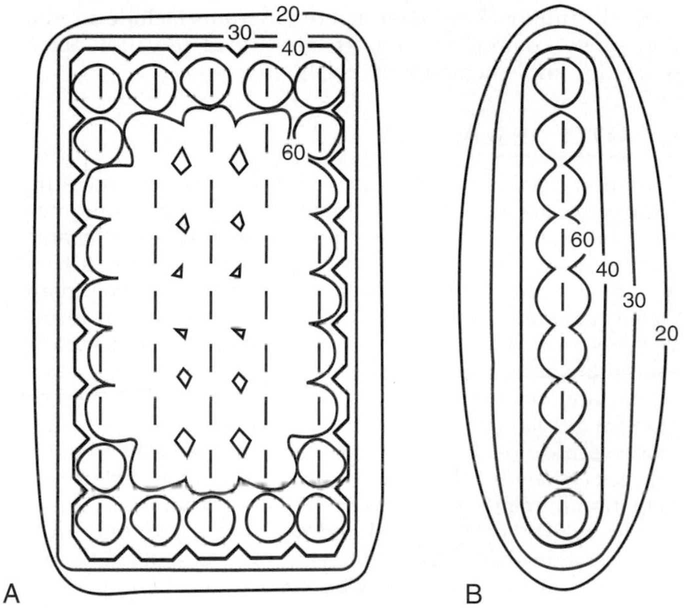

Figure 6-80 Single-plane interstitial implant. **A,** Source plane. **B,** Plane orthogonal to the source plane. Isodose values are in centigrays per hour. (Data from Interstitial Collaborative Working Group: Interstitial Brachytherapy: Physical, Biological, and Clinical Considerations. New York, Raven Press, 1990.)

brachytherapy using ^{103}Pd or ^{125}I.[79,91] Remote afterloading with high dose rate sources (typically, 10 Ci of ^{192}Ir) has become a commonly used technique for gynecologic and interstitial treatment.[92,93] Development of new radionuclides for specific applications is an active field, particularly for endovascular treatment and for liquid forms of radionuclides.

RADIATION PROTECTION

Radiation protection practices are important in the radiation oncology clinic for protection of the patient, radiation oncology personnel, ancillary staff, and the general public. Recommendations by international bodies are enacted into law and serve as dose limits for occupationally exposed individuals and the general public.[94] The dose-related quantity of interest for radiation protection purposes is called the *dose equivalent*, H:

Table 6-16 Quality Factors for Radiation Protection

Radiation	Quality Factor
X-rays, γ rays, and electrons	1
Thermal neutrons	5
Neutrons and heavy particles	20

$$H = D \bullet QF \qquad \text{Eq. 42}$$

In the equation, H is the dose equivalent (in sieverts (Sv), with units of J/kg), D is the dose received (in grays, with units of J/kg), and QF is the quality factor (unitless) of the exposing radiation.

The quality factor indicates the biologic effect of the radiation type, relative to x-rays, and varies with linear energy transfer. High linear energy transfer radiations, such as particle radiations, have a high quality factor (Table 6-16). The units of the sievert are still joules per kilogram, as for the gray; however, the meaning of the sievert is different than that of the gray. Given photon and fast neutron exposures of 1 cGy each, the dose equivalent (meaning the biologic effect) for each is different: The photons deliver 1 cSv; the fast neutrons deliver 20 cSv.

Exposure limits for occupational exposure and the general public are given in Table 6-17. A safety factor of 10 is applied to the general public limits compared with the occupational limits for whole-body exposures. However, for annual whole-body exposures the general public is limited to $^1/_{20}$ the occupational limit if exposure is frequent. This lower limit (.1 rem or .001 Sv) is the regulatory limit for exposure of the general public in the United States. Exposure limits for occupational radiation protection are based on laboratory studies and observed effects for irradiated human populations and are believed to give equivalent risk as in other safe occupations.

Radiation protection principles are based on three factors: time, distance, and shielding. To reduce any dose, minimize the time of exposure, maximize the distance away from the sources, and maximize the shielding between the sources and the point of exposure. The degree to which each of these principles is exercised for a particular exposure scenario depends on the type of radiation source; its physical properties such as energy, intensity, collimation, and beam orientation; the presence of barriers; distances to points of interest; the potential

Table 6-17 Exposure Limits for Radiation Protection

Exposed Region or Site	Occupational (rem)	General Public (rem)
ANNUAL EXPOSURE LIMITS		
Whole body; head and trunk; active blood-forming organs; lens of eyes; gonads	5	.5 (infrequent exposure) .1 (frequent exposure)
Hands/forearms; feet and ankles	75	7.5
Skin of whole body	30	3.0
ADDITIONAL EXPOSURE LIMITS		
Nonoccupational areas		
<2 mrem/h (2 mrem/h ≈ 5 rem/yr if exposed year round)		
<100 mrem/wk (≈ .6 mrem/h)		
Fetal dose		
<500 mrem during the gestation period		
MORTALITY RISK		
Risk from exposure: risk is approximately 2.5×10^{-4} deaths/person/rem, or 2.5×10^{-2} deaths/person/Sv; there are approximately 2.5 deaths if 10,000 people receive 1 rem each		

time of exposure; and the category of individual exposed (occupational or general public). Common protection practices in radiation oncology include the use of heavily shielded vaults for protection of linear accelerator operators and the public, administrative controls that limit access to radiation sources, physical barriers to room entry during exposure, interlocks that prevent irradiation during unsafe conditions, use of long-handled tools when handling brachytherapy sources, afterloading equipment such as source applicators and dummy sources to negate the need to load sources "hot," remote afterloading devices operated under remote control, and the use of lead aprons and shielded control consoles during radiographic or fluoroscopic procedures. A body of literature addresses specific situations that may be encountered.[94-96]

Even though radiation protection exposure limits exist, in general, radiation protection philosophy incorporates the ALARA principle: *a*s *l*ow *a*s *r*eadily *a*chievable. This philosophy holds that although dose rates may be within the legal (acceptable) limits given earlier, all exposures should be reduced as much as possible, given practical constraints of money, time, and human and material resources. Examples of ALARA in practice might be the relocation of clerical personnel away from a radiation source storage area, developing a more efficient method for source handling in a busy brachytherapy practice, or the addition of another HVL of shielding to a linear accelerator room ceiling during a time of renovations to further reduce doses to an upstairs pediatric playroom.

Ownership, use, receipt, and transfer of radiation sources are governed by national or state laws and are authorized or licensed under the supervision of institutional committees and state and national regulatory agencies. The Nuclear Regulatory Commission (NRC) regulates radioactive materials only (such as ^{60}Co, ^{137}Cs), and its laws are published in the Code of Federal Register.[97] These rules apply to all states and U.S. territories. However, the NRC does not regulate electronically produced radiation sources (x-ray tubes and linear accelerators). Some states have agreed to implement the NRC rules as part of their state radiation control program, and these states are called *Agreement states.* Radiation users in Agreement states are inspected by the state, not the NRC. Radiation users in Nonagreement states are inspected directly by the NRC for their radioactive materials. Nonagreement states may have their own state radiation control programs for electronically produced radiation sources. About 75% of U.S. states are Agreement states, and the remaining 25% are Nonagreement states. Other regulatory agencies with radiation-related regulations include the U.S. Department of Transportation, the U.S. Environmental Protection Agency, and possibly other state or local agencies.

General provisions for radiation sources are specified in a license that is granted to an individual or institution by the appropriate regulatory authority. Radiation source licenses cover a variety of classes of sources and generally require adequate administrative controls by the user. For instance, academic institutions with medical and research uses of radiation sources must have a radiation safety program that specifies items such as educational and experience requirements for users, radiation control procedures, and the administrative chain. Institutional radiation safety programs include a radiation safety committee for oversight and a radiation safety officer for implementation of policy.

QUALITY ASSURANCE

Radiation machines and sources, beam modifiers, measurement instrumentation, and treatment planning computers must be regularly verified for proper operation and characteristics to ensure quality and consistency of dose. A basic quality-assurance program for dose-related items entails daily, weekly, monthly, and annual tests with satisfactory results within specified tolerances. Recommendations and standards for quality assurance exist for machines, sources, instrumentation, and treatment planning computers.[27,98-100] References also are available on the general quality-assurance process.[101] Dose verification by an independent, accredited radiologic physics center is a desirable service and is required for participation in many cooperative protocol groups.

The age of computerized and automated radiation treatment planning, delivery, and verification presents new challenges for quality assurance of treatment. Treatment processes may now be wholly contained within commercially provided "black boxes" of computer software and automated treatment machines, such that important quality-assurance tests may be difficult to design and perform, or provide results that are difficult to readily interpret. The implication is that high technology approaches to quality assurance will also be needed with redundant methods for insuring and proving the correct delivery of treatment.

REFERENCES

1. Griffiths D: Introduction to Elementary Particles. New York, John Wiley & Sons, 1987.
2. Evans RD: The Atomic Nucleus. Malabar, FL, Robert E Krieger Publishing, 1955.
3. Fukuda F, Hayakawa T, Ichihara E, et al: Evidence for oscillation of atmospheric neutrinos. Phys Rev Lett 81:8, 1998.
4. Greene B: The Fabric of the Cosmos: Space, Time, and the Texture of Reality. New York, Alfred A Knopf , 2004.
5. Johns HE, Bates LM, Watson GA: 1,000 Curie cobalt units for radiation therapy. I. The Saskatchewan cobalt 60 unit. Br J Radiol 25:296, 1952.
6. Kerst DW: The betatron. Radiology 40:115, 1943.
7. Trump JG, Moster CR, Cloud RW: Efficient deep-tumor irradiation with roentgen rays of several million volts. AJR Am J Roentgenol 57:703, 1947.

8. Karzmark CJ, Morton RJ: A Primer on Theory and Operation of Linear Accelerators in Radiation Therapy, 2nd ed. Madison, WI, Medical Physics Publishing, 1998.
9. Wilson RR: Radiological use of fast protons. Radiology 47:487, 1946.
10. Svensson H, Johnsson L, Larsson LG, et al: A 22 MeV microtron for radiation therapy. Acta Radiol Ther Phys Biol 16:145, 1977.
11. Blosser HG: Compact superconducting synchrocyclotron systems for proton therapy. Nucl Instrum Methods Phys Res B40/41:1326, 1989.
12. Johns HE, Cunningham JR: The Physics of Radiology, 3rd ed. Springfield, IL, Charles C Thomas, 1978.
13. Khan F: The Physics of Radiation Therapy, 3rd ed. Baltimore, Williams & Wilkins, 2003.
14. ICRU Report 33: Radiation Quantities and Units. Washington, DC, International Commission on Radiation Units and Measurements, 1980.
15. Almond PR, Biggs PJ, Coursey BM, et al: AAPM's TG-51 protocol for clinical reference dosimetry of high-energy photon and electron beams. Med Phys 26:1847, 1999.
16. Haus AG, Marks JE: Detection and evaluation of localization errors in patient radiation therapy. Invest Radiol 8:384, 1973.
17. McLaughlin WL, Soares CG, Sayeg JA, et al: The use of a radiochromic detector for the determination of stereotactic radiosurgery dose characteristics. Med Phys 21:379, 1994.
18. Knoll GF: Radiation Detection and Measurement, 2nd ed. New York, John Wiley & Sons, 1989.
19. ICRU Report 24: Determination of Absorbed Dose in a Patient Irradiated by Beams of X and Gamma Rays in Radiotherapy Procedures. Washington, DC, International Commission on Radiation Units and Measurements, 1976.
20. Clarkson JR: A note on depth doses in fields of irregular shape. Br J Radiol 14:265, 1941.
21. Gupta SK, Cunningham JR: Measurement of tissue-air ratios and scatter functions for large field sizes for cobalt 60 gamma radiation. Br J Radiol 39:7, 1966.
22. Chang SX, Cullip T, Miller EP, et al: Dose gradient optimization [abstract]. Med Phys 23:1072, 1996.
23. AAPM RTC Task Group 25: Report 32: Clinical Electron-Beam Dosimetry. College Park, MD, American Association of Physicists in Medicine, 1991.
24. Sherouse GW, Bourland JD, Reynolds K, et al: Virtual simulation in the clinical setting: some practical considerations. Int J Radiat Oncol Biol Phys 19:1059, 1990.
25. AcQSim CT Simulator. Cleveland, OH, Picker International, 1996.
26. Purdy JA: 3-D radiation treatment planning: a new era. *In* Meyer J, Purdy JA (eds): 3-D Conformal Radiotherapy. Basel, Karger, 1996.
27. ACR Standards for the Performance of Radiation Oncology Physics for External Beam Therapy, res 15. Reston, VA, American College of Radiology, 1994.
28. North Carolina Regulations for Protection Against Radiation, 15A NCAC II, NC Department of Environment and Natural Resources, Raleigh, NC, August 1, 2002.
29. ICRU Report 50: Prescribing, Recording, and Reporting Photon Beam Therapy. International Commission on Radiation Units and Measurements, 1993.
30. ICRU Report 62: Prescribing, Recording, and Reporting Photon Beam Therapy (Supplement to ICRU 50). Washington, DC, International Commission on Radiation Units and Measurements, 1999.
31. Sailer SL, Bourland JD, Rosenman JG, et al: 3D beams need 3D names. Int J Radiat Oncol Biol Phys 19:797, 1990.
32. Sailer SL, Rosenman J, Sherouse G, et al: Response to 3D beams need unambiguous 3D names [letter]. Int J Radiat Oncol Biol Phys 21:1105, 1991.
33. Goitein M: Limitations of two-dimensional treatment planning programs. Med Phys 9:580, 1982.
34. Wood RG: Computers in Radiotherapy. New York, John Wiley & Sons, 1981.
35. Int J Radiat Oncol Biol Phys 21, 1991.
36. Proceedings of the IXth International Conference on the Use of Computers in Radiation Therapy. Scheveningen, The Netherlands, 1987, whole issue.
37. Purdy JA, Emami B (eds): 3-D Radiation Treatment Planning and Conformal Therapy. Madison WI, Medical Physics Publishing, 1995.
38. Tepper JE (ed): Semin Radiat Oncol 2, 1992.
39. Oldham M, Webb S: A 9-field static tomotherapy planning and delivery study. *In* Proceedings of the XIIth International Conference on the Use of Computers in Radiation Therapy, Salt Lake City, UT. Madison, WI, Medical Physics Publishing, 1997.
40. Webb S: The Physics of Three-Dimensional Radiation Therapy: Conformal Radiotherapy, Radiosurgery and Treatment Planning. Medical Science Series. Bristol, UK, IOP Publishing, 1993.
41. Mackie TR, Liu HH, McCullough EC: Treatment planning algorithms: Model-based photon dose calculation algorithms. *In* Khan FM, Potish RA (eds): Treatment Planning in Radiation Oncology. Baltimore, Williams & Wilkins, 1998.
42. Hogstrom KR, Steadham RE: Electron beam dose computation. *In* Mackie TR, Palta JR (eds): Teletherapy: Present and Future. Madison, WI, Advanced Medical Publishing, 1996, pp 137-174.
43. Drzymala RE, Mohan R, Brewster L, et al: Dose-volume histograms. Int J Radiat Oncol Biol Phys 21:71, 1991.
44. Bjarngard B: Meter-set calculations. *In* Mackie TR, Palta JR (eds): Teletherapy: Present and Future. Madison, WI, Advanced Medical Publishing, 1996.
45. Marks JD, Haus AG, Sutton GH: Localization error in the radiotherapy of Hodgkin's disease and malignant lymphoma with extended mantle fields. Cancer 34:83, 1974.
46. Boyer A, Antonuk L, Fenster A, et al: A review of electronic portal imaging devices (EPIDs). Med Phys 19:1, 1992.
47. American Association of Physicists in Medicine: Monograph No. 24. *In* Hazle JD, Boyer AL (eds): Imaging in Radiation Therapy. Salt Lake City, UT, Medical Physics Publishing, 1998.
48. Khan FM, Potish RA (eds): Treatment Planning in Radiation Oncology. Baltimore, Williams & Wilkins, 1998.
49. Schlegel W, Pastyr O, Bortfeld T, et al: Computer systems and mechanical tools for stereotactically guided conformation therapy with linear accelerator. Int J Radiat Oncol Biol Phys 24:781, 1992.
50. Bourland JD, McCollough KP: Static field conformal stereotactic radiosurgery: physical techniques. Int J Radiat Oncol Biol Phys 28:471, 1994.
51. Serago CF, Lewin AA, Houdek PV, et al: Improved linac dose distributions for radiosurgery with elliptically shaped fields. Int J Radiat Oncol Biol Phys 21:1321, 1991.
52. Morse R, Varian Oncology Systems: Personal communication, 1995.
53. Carol MP: PEACOCK: a system for planning and rotational delivery of intensity-modulated fields. Int J Imag Syst Tech 6:56, 1995.
54. Spirou S, Chui C: Generation of arbitrary intensity profiles by dynamic jaws or multileaf collimators. Med Phys 21:1031, 1994.
55. Bortfeld T, Kahler D, Waldron T, et al: X-ray field compensation with multileaf collimators. Int J Radiat Oncol Biol Phys 28:723, 1994.
56. Hendee WR, Bourland JD. Image-guided intervention. Acad Radiol 10:896, 2003.
57. Carson PL, Giger M, Welch MJ, et al: Biomedical imaging research opportunities workshop: report and recommendations. Radiology 229:328, 2003.
58. *Ibid.*
59. Pirzkall A, McKnight TR, Graves EE, et al: MR-spectroscopy guided target delineation for high-grade gliomas, Int J Radiat Oncol Biol Phys 50:915, 2001.
60. Pirzkall A, Nelson SJ, McKnight TR, et al: Metabolic imaging of low grade gliomas with three dimensional magnetic resonance spectroscopy. Int J Radiat Oncol Biol Phys 53:1254, 2002.
61. Bourland JD, Shaw EG: The evolving role of biological imaging in stereotactic radiosurgery. Tech Cancer Treat Res 2:135, 2003.
62. Radiation Therapy Oncology Group: RTOG Protocol 90-05: Phase I Study of Small-Field Stereotactic External Beam Irradiation for the Treatment of Recurrent Primary Brain Tumors and

CNS Metastases. Philadelphia, Radiation Therapy Oncology Group, 1990.
63. Elekta Instruments, AB. Stockholm, Sweden, 1999.
64. Goetsch SJ: Stereotactic radiosurgery using the Gamma Knife. *In* Mackie TR, Palta JR (eds): Teletherapy: Present and Future. Madison, WI, Advanced Medical Publishing, 1996, pp 611-642.
65. Rotating Gamma System. San Diego, CA, American Radiosurgery, Inc., 2003.
66. Lutz W, Winston KR, Maleki N: A system for stereotactic radiosurgery with a linear accelerator. Int J Radiat Oncol Biol Phys 14:373, 1988.
67. AAPM RTC Task Group 42: Report 54: Stereotactic Radiosurgery. College Park, MD, American Association of Physicists in Medicine, 1995.
68. Friedman WA, Bova FJ: The University of Florida radiosurgery system. Surg Neurol 32:334, 1989.
69. Podgorsak EB, Pike GB, Olivier A, et al: Radiosurgery with high-energy photon beams: a comparison among techniques. Int J Radiat Oncol Biol Phys 16:857, 1989.
70. Graham JD, Nahum AE, Brada M: A comparison of techniques for stereotactic radiotherapy by linear accelerator based on 3-dimensional dose distributions. Radiother Oncol 22:29, 1991.
71. Adler JR, Cox RS: Preliminary clinical experience with the cyberknife: image-guided stereotactic radiosurgery. *In* Kondziolka D (ed): Radiosurgery 1995. Basel, Karger, 1996, pp 316-326.
72. Wu QJ, Bourland JD: Morphology-guided radiosurgery treatment planning and optimization for multiple isocenters. Med Phys 26:2151, 1999.
73. AAPM RTC Task Group 29: Report 17: The Physical Aspects of Total and Half Body Photon Irradiation. College Park, MD, American Association of Physicists in Medicine, 1986.
74. AAPM RTC Task Group 30: Report 23: Total Skin Electron Therapy: Technique and Dosimetry. College Park, MD, American Association of Physicists in Medicine, 1987.
75. Williamson JF, Meigooni AS: Quantitative dosimetry methods in brachytherapy. *In* Williamson JF, Thomadsen BR, Nath R (eds): Brachytherapy Physics. Madison, WI, Medical Physics Publishing, 1995, pp 87-133.
76. Weaver K: Dose calculation models in brachytherapy. *In* Williamson JF, Thomadsen BR, Nath R (eds): Brachytherapy Physics. Madison, WI, Medical Physics Publishing, 1995, pp 135-147.
77. AAPM RTC Task Group 32: Report 21: Specification of Brachytherapy Source Strength. College Park, MD, American Association of Physicists in Medicine, 1987.
78. Hanson WF: Brachytherapy source strength: Quantities, units, and standards. *In* Williamson JF, Thomadsen BR, Nath R (eds): Brachytherapy Physics. Madison, WI, Medical Physics Publishing, 1995, pp 71-85.
79. Williamson JF, Thomadsen BR, Nath R (eds): Brachytherapy Physics. Madison, WI, Medical Physics Publishing, 1995.
80. Glasgow GP, Perez CA: Physics of brachytherapy. *In* Perez CA, Brady LW (eds): Principles and Practice of Radiation Oncology, 2nd ed. Philadelphia, JB Lippincott, 1987, pp 213-251.
81. Perez CA, Glasgow GP: Clinical applications of brachytherapy. *In* Perez CA, Brady LW (eds): Principles and Practice of Radiation Oncology, 2nd ed. Philadelphia, JB Lippincott, 1987, pp 252-290.
82. Fletcher GH: Textbook of Radiotherapy. Philadelphia, Lea & Febiger, 1973.
83. Paterson R, Parker AM: A dosage system for gamma ray therapy. Br J Radiol 7:592, 1934.
84. Paterson R, Parker AM: A dosage system for interstitial radium therapy. Br J Radiol 11:252, 313, 1938.
85. Gillin MT, Albano KS, Erickson B: Classical systems II for planar and volume temporary interstitial implants: the Paris and other systems. *In* Williamson JF, Thomadsen BR, Nath R (eds): Brachytherapy Physics. Madison, WI, Medical Physics Publishing, 1995, pp 323-342.
86. Anderson LL, Presser JL: Classical systems I for temporary interstitial implants: Manchester Quimby systems. *In* Williamson JF, Thomadsen BR, Nath R (eds): Brachytherapy Physics. Madison, WI, Medical Physics Publishing, 1995, pp 301-321.
87. Meigooni AS, Williamson JF, Nath R: Single-source dosimetry for interstitial brachytherapy. *In* Williamson JF, Thomadsen BR, Nath R (eds): Brachytherapy Physics. Madison, WI, Medical Physics Publishing, 1995, pp 209-233.
88. ICRU Report 38: Dose and Volume Specification for Reporting Intracavitary Therapy in Gynecology. Washington, DC, International Commission on Radiation Units and Measurements, 1985.
89. ICRU Report 58: Dose and Volume Specification for Reporting Interstitial Therapy. Washington, DC, International Commission on Radiation Units and Measurements, 1997.
90. Hanson WF, Graves M: ICRU recommendations on dose specification for brachytherapy. *In* Williamson JF, Thomadsen BR, Nath R (eds): Brachytherapy Physics. Madison, WI, Medical Physics Publishing, 1995, pp 361-378.
91. Interstitial Collaborative Working Group: Interstitial Brachytherapy: Physical, Biological, and Clinical Considerations. New York, Raven Press, 1990.
92. AAPM RTC Task Group 41: Report 41: Remote Afterloading Technology. College Park, MD, American Association of Physicists in Medicine, 1992.
93. Glasgow GP: Principles of remote afterloading devices. *In* Williamson JF, Thomadsen BR, Nath R (eds): Brachytherapy Physics. Madison, WI, Medical Physics Publishing, 1995.
94. NCRP: Report 116: Limitation of Exposure to Ionizing Radiation. Bethesda, MD, National Council on Radiation Protection, 1993.
95. NCRP: Report 49: Structural Shielding Design and Evaluation for Medical Use of X-Rays and Gamma Rays of Energies up to 10 MeV. Bethesda, MD, National Council on Radiation Protection, 1976.
96. NCRP: Report 102: Medical X-Ray, Electron Beam, and Gamma-Ray Protection for Energies up to 50 MeV (Equipment Design, Performance and Use). Bethesda, MD, National Council on Radiation Protection, 1989.
97. United States Nuclear Regulatory Commission: The Code of Federal Regulations, Title 10, Part 20 (10 CFR-20). Washington, DC, U.S. Nuclear Regulatory Commission, 1991.
98. AAPM RTC Task Group 40: Report 46: Comprehensive Quality Assurance for Radiation Oncology. College Park, MD, American Association of Physicists in Medicine, 1994.
99. AAPM RTC Task Group 45: Report 47: AAPM Code of Practice for Radiotherapy Accelerators. College Park, MD, American Association of Physicists in Medicine, 1994.
100. JCAHO Comprehensive Accreditation Manual for Hospitals. Oakbrook Terrace, IL, Joint Commission on Accreditation of Healthcare Organizations, 1996.
101. Starkschall G, Horton JL (eds): Quality Assurance in Radiotherapy Physics. Madison, WI, Medical Physics Publishing, 1991.

PART C

RELATED CANCER DISCIPLINES

CHAPTER 7

SURGICAL PRINCIPLES

M. Kevin Barry and John H. Donohue

The surgeon continues to play a central role in the management of malignant diseases. Surgical involvement includes diagnostic, therapeutic, and follow-up care of the oncologic patient. The surgeon never acts in isolation; instead, interaction with colleagues from other specialties is routine. Because many of the common solid tumors are treated with a combination of therapies, the surgeon usually provides treatment in collaboration with medical and radiation oncologists. This interaction among specialists provides the best chance for patient cure and effective palliation.

Preoperatively, the surgeon follows the routine practice of obtaining an accurate history and relevant physical examination. This is complemented by laboratory investigation and, when indicated, more specialized testing. Surgical goals include providing a histologic diagnosis, staging the disease, and deciding on the intent of treatment: potential cure or palliation. The surgeon's contribution to the relief of patient suffering is particularly beneficial for the tumor complications of visceral obstruction, hemorrhage, perforation, and pain. High-quality radiologic imaging studies such as ultrasonography, computed tomography (CT), and magnetic resonance imaging (MRI) provide fundamental data for planning the appropriate operative procedure. Radiologic biopsies of deep-seated tumors for diagnosis are indicated in selected patients, usually when preoperative (neoadjuvant) or nonoperative therapy is indicated.

This chapter provides an outline of the role of the surgical oncologist in the multidisciplinary management of the cancer patient. Specific examples of the surgical approach are given using malignancies of the breast, pancreas, rectum, and retroperitoneum to illustrate specialist interaction.

HISTOLOGIC DIAGNOSIS

For some patients, a pathologic diagnosis should be secured before performing a definitive surgical procedure. An adequate diagnostic specimen must be obtained with minimal patient morbidity. The biopsy tract should be positioned to allow inclusion with the proposed surgical resection. Although cytologic or histologic samples can be taken, histologic diagnosis usually is preferable. False-negative cytologic results occur for 10% to 20% of cancers, and rare false-positive cytologic diagnoses are well recognized for tumors such as breast cancer. The four most common diagnostic biopsy techniques are aspiration cytology, core-needle biopsy, incisional biopsy, and excisional biopsy. A separate biopsy procedure should be performed only when it affects preoperative treatment planning. Laparoscopically directed biopsies provide another method to evaluate intra-abdominal cancer stage and provide diagnostic biopsies.

Fine-needle aspiration cytology (FNAC) is widely used to evaluate solitary thyroid nodules. Using a 21-gauge needle and syringe, an aspirate of cellular material or fluid is obtained, differentiating between solid and cystic masses. If a cyst does not completely disappear with aspiration, FNAC examination of any residual solid component is necessary. The success of FNAC depends on the experience of the clinician performing the aspiration and on the interpretation of a skilled cytologist. FNAC of the thyroid enables the pathologist to differentiate most benign from malignant tumors. Papillary, medullary, and anaplastic carcinomas have a typical cytologic appearance. Cytologic studies cannot differentiate benign from malignant follicular or Hürthle cell neoplasms. Definitive diagnosis of these thyroid neoplasms depends on histologic examination of the entire excised tumor. The introduction of routine FNAC has dramatically reduced the number of diagnostic surgical operations for benign thyroid lesions.

Percutaneous radiograph-directed FNAC has gained great popularity over the past 15 years.[1] Ultrasonography or CT is routinely used to obtain hepatic, renal, pancreatic, and retroperitoneal biopsies. Percutaneous biopsy techniques are particularly useful to confirm the presence of metastases in a patient with prior malignancy. However, if curable metastases (e.g., limited hepatic metastases from colorectal cancer) are present, this diagnostic test is unwarranted and potentially dangerous because it rarely can cause tumor seeding. If unresectable disease is present at the time of exploratory laparotomy, a confirmatory biopsy should be undertaken.

The choice of ultrasound or CT guidance depends on several factors. In general, ultrasonography is used for superficial lesions. Ultrasonography possesses other advantages, including real-time imaging, which allows constant monitoring of the needle position and lower costs compared with CT. Ultrasonography is limited by overlying bone and gas. CT guidance is more beneficial for deeper tumors, particularly in the retroperitoneum. Advantages of CT-guided biopsy include better spatial resolution and lack of interference from air or bone. Intravenous contrast allows assessment of tumor vascularity.

Core-needle biopsy can be performed by hand if a lesion is easily palpable and can be stabilized by the operator.

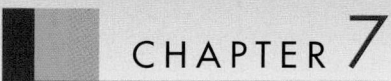

Radiograph-directed core biopsies, particularly of breast lesions, have gained great popularity. The advantage of this method over FNA is that a core of tissue is provided for histologic analysis. This procedure is useful in the evaluation of a palpable solid breast lump. Using local anesthesia, a small (3-mm) incision is made in the skin through which a coring biopsy needle is directed into the center of the lesion. Typically, a 1 × 10 to 20 mm tissue sample is obtained. Core-needle biopsy may also be performed with stereotactic imaging or ultrasonography for nonpalpable breast lesions.

Core-needle biopsies of intra-abdominal and thoracic tumors offer the advantages of histologic diagnosis and greater accuracy than the FNAC. Larger-bore needles, however, can result in more problems, most commonly hemorrhage, and some sites are not safely accessible percutaneously. Core-needle biopsy should not be used routinely for potentially resectable, deep-seated malignancies because of a higher risk of needle track seeding than with FNAC. Core biopsies are preferable to incisional biopsies intraoperatively; however, the decision to resect or not, as in a pancreaticoduodenectomy for painless jaundice, should be based on clinical and operative findings and does not require histologic confirmation.

Incisional biopsy involves removal of a larger portion of a tumor mass. Examples of this method include a full-thickness skin biopsy obtained using a scalpel or punch biopsy tool. The thickest portion of the lesion should be sampled, and the specimen should consist of full-thickness skin plus subcutaneous tissue to allow accurate tumor staging. Incisional biopsy of an extremity sarcoma is performed for large tumors if the diagnosis needs to be confirmed before proceeding with definitive treatment (e.g., amputation, preoperative chemotherapy or radiation). Incisional biopsy of an extremity tumor is preferable through a longitudinal rather than transverse incision, because the longitudinal incision can be more readily incorporated in a wide local excision procedure.[2] Intraoperative incisional biopsies during thoracotomy and laparotomy are rarely indicated and have greater potential to spill tumor cells than FNAC or core-needle biopsies.

Excisional biopsy of a breast mass aptly illustrates the key principles in performing a diagnostic surgical biopsy. This procedure is used for small, palpable lesions that are easily excised completely. If possible, the biopsy incision should be situated within the ellipse of skin that would be used for a mastectomy in case that procedure becomes necessary (Fig. 7-1). If the breast mass is believed to be malignant, it is completely excised with a 1-cm margin of normal tissue, keeping the suspicious lesion centered within the specimen (Fig. 7-2A). The biopsy specimen should be oriented to allow the pathologist to determine which, if any, of the resection margins are microscopically involved by tumor. This is easily achieved with two sutures. A short suture denotes the superior margin, and a long suture indicates the lateral margin (see Fig. 7-2B). If frozen-section evaluation of the resection margins is available, selective additional re-excisions can be performed immediately when tumor clearance is incomplete with the first specimen. When frozen-section evaluation is unavailable, a similar, selective, repeat excision can be performed later if the specimen has been properly oriented with sutures, clips, or multicolored inks. Surgical clips left at the base of the biopsy cavity facilitate accurate partial breast or boost field radiation therapy after breast-conservation surgery. Use of small titanium clips provides accurate information to the radiation oncologist and minimal interference with future imaging studies.

STAGING

Staging of malignancy is critical in determining the goal of intervention. Historic symptoms or physical signs often alert the clinician to likely metastatic disease, but diagnostic studies usually are required to confirm the presence of distant disease spread. Accurate preoperative staging results in optimal patient treatment, because tumor extent remains the single most important determinant of patient prognosis.

Clinical and pathologic stages of disease should be described using the American Joint Committee for Cancer (AJCC) TNM system.[3] In this nomenclature, T refers to the primary tumor, N indicates the status of regional lymph nodes, and M denotes the presence or absence of metastatic disease. For many tumors (e.g., lung, liver, breast) the size of the primary tumor correlates with the probability of metastases.

Clinical tumor staging is normally achieved using a variety of radiologic tests, including a chest radiograph, ultrasonography, CT, and MRI; laparoscopy has been used for a variety of intra-abdominal and some intrathoracic neoplasms to provide more sensitive staging than noninvasive techniques. Positron emission tomography (PET)–CT imaging gives additive information to other imaging studies in a number of disease sites. PET-CT can be especially helpful with regard to diagnosing previously unsuspected metastatic disease (e.g.,

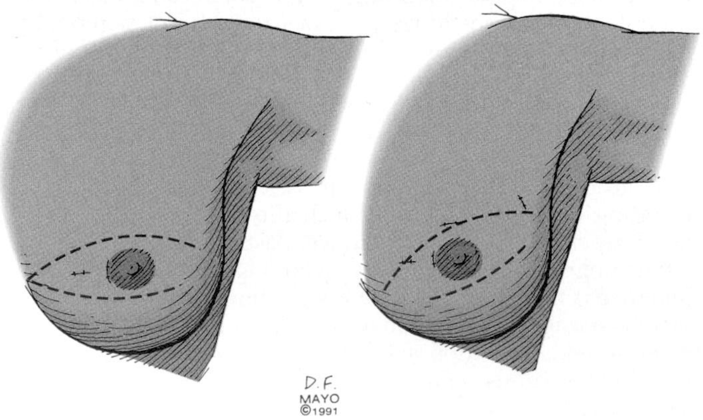

Figure 7-1 Excisional breast biopsy performed within the confines of a mastectomy incision. (Courtesy of the Mayo Foundation.)

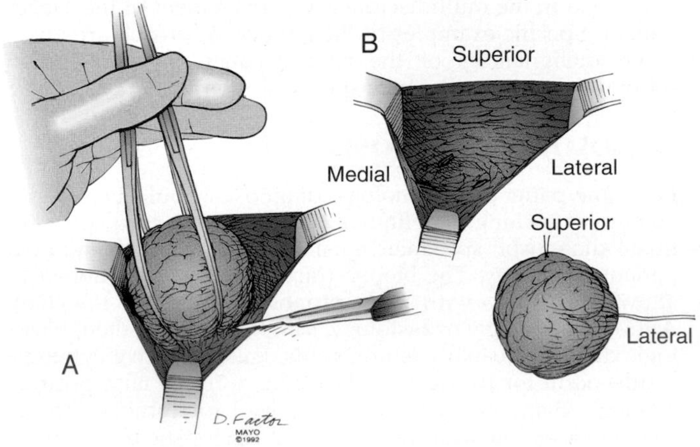

Figure 7-2 **A,** Excisional breast biopsy. **B,** Specimen orientation. (Courtesy of the Mayo Foundation.)

esophagus cancer) and in evaluating patients with possible disease relapse in a prior surgical bed (e.g., locally recurrent rectal cancer). In symptomatic patients, skeletal metastases are usually diagnosed by radioisotope bone scan and correlative plain radiographs.

Role of Laparoscopy

The widespread introduction of laparoscopic techniques in general surgical practice has greatly facilitated the staging of intra-abdominal malignancies, particularly gastric,[4] pancreatic,[5] and some hepatobiliary tumors.[6,7] Thoracoscopy allows inspection of the pleural cavity and biopsy to determine intrathoracic spread of some tumors. When used for diagnostic purposes, laparoscopy allows visualization of peritoneal surfaces, sampling of suspected omental or hepatic tumor deposits, biopsy of lymph nodes, and sampling of ascitic fluid for peritoneal cytology. Laparoscopic ultrasonography further improves the staging of pancreatic and hepatobiliary malignancies.[8-10] With laparoscopic confirmation of advanced malignancy, formal celiotomy and its attendant morbidity can be avoided. Laparoscopy may also be used in a therapeutic fashion to palliate some patients with advanced malignancy.[11] Palliative laparoscopic procedures for malignancy include gastrojejunostomy for gastric outlet obstruction, cholecystojejunostomy for obstructive jaundice, and colostomy formation or segmental resection for colonic obstruction.[11]

Staging of Pancreatic Malignancy

Laparoscopy is frequently used for staging pancreatic and periampullary carcinomas, because hepatic or peritoneal metastases undetectable by radiographic means occur in more than 30% of patients believed to have resectable carcinoma preoperatively.[5,12,13] A complete laparoscopic inspection of the abdominal cavity is undertaken using a 5- or 10-mm port at the umbilicus (Fig. 7-3). An additional subcostal cannula allows retraction of the liver, omentum, and loops of intestine. With this method, it is possible to inspect the upper abdomen, looking for small hepatic metastases or drop metastases of the parietal and visceral peritoneum or the greater omentum. Any suspicious lesions should be sampled using biopsy forceps or coring needle. The left upper quadrant can be examined, as can the peritoneal surfaces of the colon and small bowel. Evidence of direct spread of pancreatic carcinoma into the small bowel mesentery should be evaluated. The pelvis is also examined for peritoneal drop metastases.

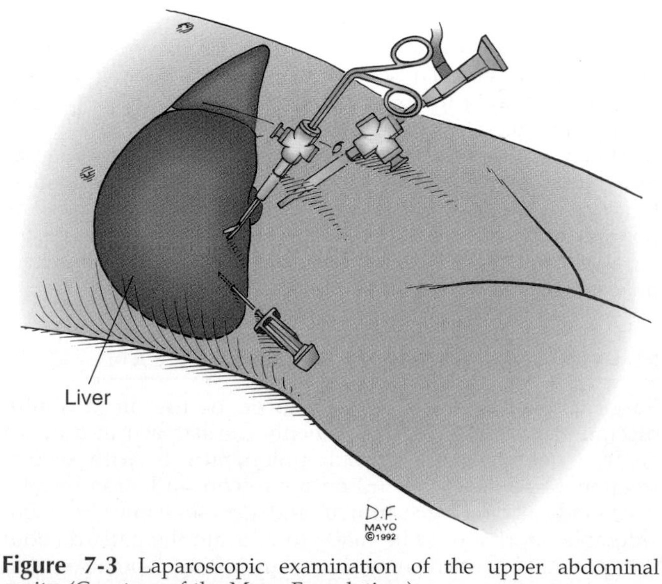

Figure 7-3 Laparoscopic examination of the upper abdominal cavity. (Courtesy of the Mayo Foundation.)

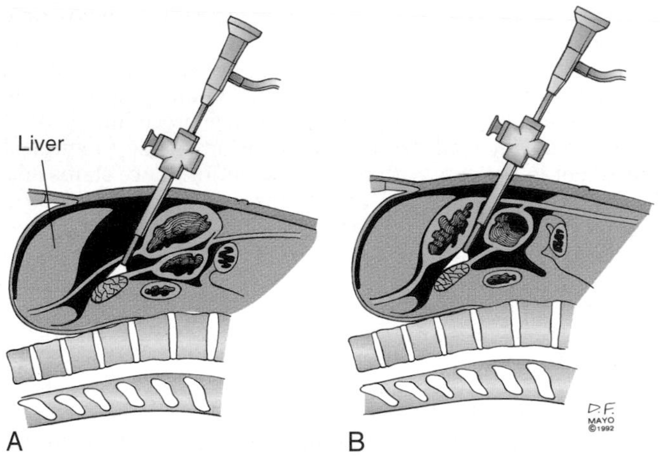

Figure 7-4 Laparoscopic examination of the pancreas: supragastric (**A**) and infragastric (**B**) approaches. (Courtesy of the Mayo Foundation.)

By placing the patient in the reverse Trendelenburg position, limited visualization of the anterior surface of the pancreas may be performed using a supragastric approach after division of the lesser omentum (Fig. 7-4A) or an infragastric approach, entering the lesser sac through the gastrocolic omentum (see Fig. 7-4B). Biopsies of any visible peritoneal implants within the lesser sac should be obtained. Laparoscopic ultrasonography provides a more accurate assessment of visceral vascular involvement and deep hepatic metastases than noninvasive methods.[10]

GOALS OF SURGICAL INTERVENTION

The primary intent of surgical intervention is curative resection when no evidence of metastatic disease exists. The surgeon must be familiar with the biology of the tumor and its modes of spread, whether hematogenous, lymphatic, intracavitary, or by direct extension. En bloc excision of the tumor is performed to provide for the highest probability of cure. This involves complete extirpation of the primary tumor with a margin of normal tissue and in continuity regional lymph node dissection. For tumors such as colon cancers or retroperitoneal sarcomas, it is often necessary to remove normal adjacent structures that are directly invaded or adherent to the malignancy. Lysis of adhesions to adjacent structures may result in residual cancer and intraperitoneal tumor spillage. When the local extent of a nonmetastatic malignancy prevents a gross total resection with negative margins, the surgeon should facilitate the planning for postoperative irradiation by placing metallic clips at the site of residual disease or areas of adherence.

Certain malignancies are appropriately treated by surgical debulking plus perioperative therapy. Examples include ovarian and testicular carcinomas. Pseudomyxoma peritonei, a rare mucinous adenocarcinoma usually of appendiceal origin, can also be managed in this fashion. The goal of operative therapy is to remove all macroscopic intra-abdominal disease. In pseudomyxoma patients in whom all visible tumor is excised or nodules 3 mm or smaller remain, intraperitoneal chemotherapy alone[14] or with radioisotope treatment[15] in the perioperative period may sterilize residual microscopic tumor.

For patients with known metastatic disease who are at risk for complications as a result of locally advanced disease, the surgeon can alleviate symptoms. Operative procedures should be reserved for well-defined problems amenable to surgical treatment in patients with reasonable performance status and life expectancy. Intestinal obstruction can be corrected by a resection, bypass, or proximal diversion (i.e., ostomy formation). When technically feasible (i.e., limited adhesions with access to obstructed bowel), laparoscopic or laparoscopically assisted (i.e., mobilization using laparoscopic technique and a portion of procedure performed through a limited celiotomy) techniques are suitable and often preferable to formal laparotomy. Diffuse peritoneal implantation limits the beneficial effects of palliative surgery and increases the risk of postoperative complications, including infection and bowel fistula formation. The surgeon may prevent life-threatening hemorrhage or pain by removal of the offending tumor. Pain can also be improved by nerve transection or blockade, such as intraoperative celiac plexus block for pancreatic carcinoma.

PERIOPERATIVE CARE OF THE ONCOLOGY PATIENT

The patient with malignancy may present special problems for the surgeon that must be taken into account perioperatively to minimize morbidity and prepare the patient for adjuvant therapy.[16] Patients with malignancy are at increased risk for postoperative complications because of their underlying disease, the magnitude of the operation, and the use of immunosuppressive adjuvant therapy. Patients with gastrointestinal obstruction frequently suffer from malnutrition and associated immunodeficiency. The hematologic, gastrointestinal, pulmonary, and cardiac toxicities associated with chemotherapy further stress the postoperative oncologic patient. The surgical wound must be well healed before initiating adjuvant therapy. This is a particular problem when dealing with malnourished patients.

The surgeon's plan for operative intervention must account for preexisting and malignancy-induced comorbidities. A common tumor-associated complication is cancer cachexia, which results in progressive anorexia and weight loss.[17] Lean tissue wasting and immunodeficiency result from this cachexia. Because malnutrition is a significant risk factor for perioperative morbidity, the surgeon must carefully evaluate the degree of malnutrition present. Although there is evidence from retrospective clinical studies that nutritional support reduces the incidence of postoperative complications in patients with severe malnutrition,[18,19] prospective trials and a meta-analysis do not support the routine use of preoperative nutritional support in the oncologic patient.[20] Total parenteral nutrition is reserved for patients who cannot be nourished enterally, who cannot maintain adequate nutritional status by oral or enteric input during therapy, or who are not treatment candidates until their nutritional status has improved. The gastrointestinal tract should be used for supplemental nutrition whenever possible. Postoperative nutritional support should be routinely considered, especially in the treatment of upper gastrointestinal malignancies such as esophageal, stomach, and pancreatic cancers. The use of a feeding jejunostomy catheter placed at the time of surgery facilitates postoperative nutritional supplementation.

The oncologic patient is at an increased risk for infection. Patients with malignancy may have a compromised immune system as a result of older age, the surgical stress, malnutrition, and impaired host defense mechanisms. A combination of neutropenia and defective cell-mediated immune responses render malnourished patients especially prone to the development of postoperative complications and reduce the patient's ability to respond to sepsis. Patients should receive appropriate perioperative antibiotic therapy and be vigilantly observed postoperatively for potential infection.

Another consideration for the surgical oncologist is the potential for thrombotic complications. Hypercoagulable states are common in patients with pancreatic, prostate, lung, breast, or gastric cancers. Increased clotting factors such as fibrinogen or factors V, VIII, IX, and XI and decreased protein C, protein S, and antithrombin III levels have been implicated as causes of thromboembolic events in cancer patients. Perioperative subcutaneous heparin, thromboembolic stockings, and sequential compression devices should be routinely used for the oncologic patient.

Anemia is frequently encountered in patients with malignancy. Blood transfusion has been associated with immunosuppression, including depression of specific cellular immunity, and with nonspecific immune response, including natural killer cell toxicity and macrophage bactericidal activity. Although some retrospective studies have indicated reduced recurrent-free survival in colorectal carcinoma patients after blood transfusions, controlled trials have not found a definitive adverse effect on tumor control related to perioperative transfusions.[21,22] Blood transfusion should be used as appropriate in the oncologic patient (i.e., a symptomatic patient or a hemoglobin below 8 g/dL in an otherwise healthy patient).

RADIATION THERAPY AND WOUND HEALING

Radiation causes acute inflammatory changes in exposed tissues that are in proportion to the total dose and more profound with larger fraction size. Acute radiation changes are manifested by vasodilation (erythema) and tissue edema.[23] It is best to delay an operation 3 to 6 weeks after moderate-dose preoperative radiation (45 to 50 Gy in 1.8- to 2.0-Gy fractions or the equivalent thereof) to allow partial resolution of these effects.[24] Late radiation changes may include atrophy, fibrosis, and decreased vascularity.

Wound healing is impaired by several factors, including diminished blood supply, impaired collagen formation, and the increased risk of infection resulting in part from decreased leukocyte function. Nonhealing wounds are common in severely injured tissues after high-dose irradiation, and nonirradiated tissues such as vascularized myocutaneous flaps should be brought to the radiation field at the time of tumor resection to allow proper wound healing.[25]

When an irradiated hollow organ (e.g., bowel, esophagus, bile duct, trachea) needs to be partially resected and reanastomosed, it is preferable for one side of the anastomosis to be nonirradiated tissue, if possible. This policy ensures better blood supply to the healing anastomosis and reduces the incidence of postoperative leakage and fistula formation.

SURGICAL TREATMENT OF BREAST CANCER

Surgical treatment of breast cancer occurs in a multidisciplinary setting. Ideally, patients can be seen in a breast clinic, where they can consult preoperatively with several treatment specialists, including a surgeon, radiation oncologist, medical oncologist, nurse, and genetic counselor. Considerable effort should be made to educate the patient about the potential treatment options, including operative and adjuvant therapies.

Surgical treatment of breast cancer has evolved to the point that most patients undergoing surgery for early breast cancers can choose breast conservation. Data from multiple mature controlled trials[26-28] have demonstrated no significant difference in disease control or survival between patients who elect breast-conservation therapy and those who choose mastectomy. Mastectomy is a suitable option if a woman desires this form of treatment.

Mastectomy is preferable for the management of multicentric disease and most large primary tumors (neoadjuvant chemotherapy may be tried in an attempt to allow breast conservation at a later date) or in patients who cannot have therapeutic radiation (e.g., previous chest wall radiation, certain collagen vascular diseases). Most patients undergoing mastectomy are suitable candidates for immediate breast reconstruction. When indicated, preoperative plastic surgical consultation should be obtained to allow the patient to assess the option of immediate reconstruction after mastectomy. The timing of breast reconstruction usually depends on the patient's preference; however, reconstruction is best delayed if chest wall irradiation is indicated by tumor stage.

Early Breast Cancer

Most women with early stage breast cancer (i.e., stage 0, I, or II breast cancers) are suitable candidates for breast-conservation surgery. The goals of breast-conservation surgery are optimal locoregional control of the breast cancer and preservation of the natural appearance of the breast. From a surgeon's perspective, all known breast cancer must be excised from the breast and axilla. (It is not necessary to pathologically stage the axilla for most ductal carcinomas in situ.) Radiation therapy must be administered postoperatively to reduce the risk of local recurrence of disease, given the high incidence of residual microscopic disease, even with pathologically clear margins. Because radiation therapy is an integral component of breast conservation, patients who are unsuitable for radiotherapy should not undergo this form of surgery. Contraindications to breast-conservation surgery include a history of certain collagen vascular diseases (e.g., scleroderma, polymyositis), the presence of diffuse indeterminate or suspicious calcifications on mammography, a history of therapeutic irradiation to the breast, and positive margins of resection despite wide excision.

Breast-conserving surgery is performed through an incision as close to the primary tumor as possible, whether the lesion is a palpable abnormality or a mammographic abnormality that has been localized. It is best to remove the entire abnormality with a gross margin of 1 cm of normal tissue. A curvilinear incision in Langer's lines optimizes the cosmetic result in most locations; a radial incision is often preferable in the lower quadrants. Incisions should be placed so they are encompassed by a standard mastectomy incision wherever possible. After specimen excision, markers (e.g., sutures, clips, dyes) should be placed to provide orientation. If frozen-section pathologic analysis is available, evaluation of margins can be obtained intraoperatively. If margin evaluation is performed later, specimen orientation will result in less tissue removal when the original specimen has tumor involvement of one or more margins. Titanium clips are placed at the base of the biopsy cavity to direct boost field irradiation. The wound is closed without approximation of the breast parenchyma. Sentinel lymph node biopsy or axillary lymph node dissection is best performed through a separate incision. The axillary incision should be placed between the axillary folds and not cross the lateral border of the pectoralis major muscle (Fig. 7-5). Axillary staging aids patient management in

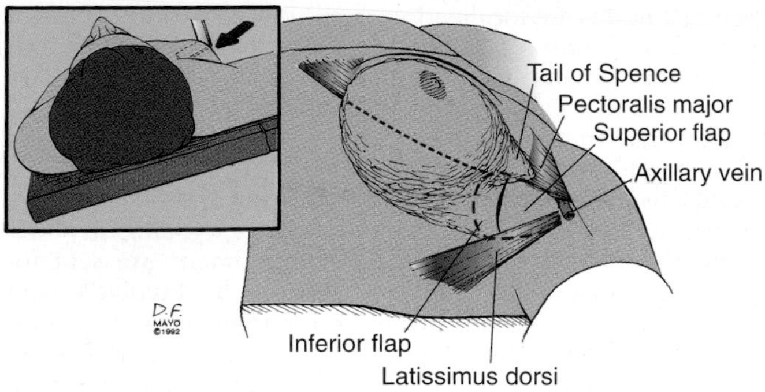

Figure 7-5 Incision of axillary dissection. (Courtesy of the Mayo Foundation.)

determining prognosis and systemic adjuvant treatment. Patients with positive axillary nodes are almost routinely advised to receive systemic treatment, usually combination chemotherapy. Postoperative therapy commences after sufficient wound healing has occurred, usually within 3 to 4 weeks.

Sentinel Lymph Node Biopsy

Until recently, axillary lymph node dissection was routinely performed in women with invasive carcinoma of the breast. The rationale for routine lymphadenectomy has shifted from enhancement of disease cure and regional control to improved disease staging and the determination of systemic therapy. The practice of routine axillary nodal excision for early breast cancer has been increasingly questioned. Because lymph node metastasis is the single most important prognostic variable for breast cancer patients and nodal involvement cannot be accurately predicted other than by histologic evaluation, axillary nodal evaluation remains an important issue.

Formal axillary dissection may produce numerous complications, mostly minor in nature, such as seroma formation, wound infection, prolongation of postoperative care, and sensory nerve interruption. Some women experience more severe and permanent disabilities related to axillary dissection: upper extremity lymphedema and sensory neuropathy. If a limited sampling of the axillary nodes allows an accurate determination of regional metastasis, the prevalence of these side effects should be less. Accurate staging would allow selective completion lymphadenectomy in patients with documented nodal metastasis, thereby maximizing the surgical regional disease control.

Sentinel lymph node biopsy (i.e., removal of the first draining regional node) was first used for predicting nodal metastases in cutaneous malignant melanoma. Guiliano and colleagues[29] presented their experience with similar techniques for breast cancer patients. With their initial 400 patients, using isosulfan blue to isolate the sentinel lymph node, the sentinel node could be localized in 93% of patients and was accurate in detecting axillary metastases. Because of the reliability of this test, Giuliano and associates stopped performing axillary dissection for clinically negative axillae in patients with a negative sentinel node biopsy.[29-31] Multiple other reports[32-35] have confirmed these findings.

The technique of sentinel lymph node is based on the orderly progression of tumor cells within the lymphatic system. Metastasis to regional lymph nodes is not a random event; the primary draining or sentinel lymph node is the first to contain metastases. Sentinel lymph node biopsy has become standard in most medical centers for women without clinical evidence of axillary metastases from early-stage breast cancer.

Sentinel nodes are localized with a dye (i.e., isosulfan blue or methylene blue) or a radiolabeled colloid (usually sulfur colloid or human serum albumin), or both. A limited axillary incision (2 to 3 cm) is made and the blue-stained lymphatics sought near the lateral border of the pectoralis major muscle or a hand-held gamma probe can be used to localize the radioactivity labeled nodes. After tracing the stained lymphatics and removing the draining node or excising all nodes with high radioactivity counts, the specimens are sent for pathologic evaluation. Nodes found to be involved with cancer on frozen-section evaluation normally result in completion axillary dissection. The biologic importance of minimal sentinel node involvement with cancer (detection by immunohistochemical staining only (i.e., N0[i+] and micrometastases defined as a tumor deposit less than 2 mm in diameter) remains controversial, as does the need to routinely complete the axillary dissection for sentinel node involvement.

MULTIMODALITY THERAPY FOR PANCREATIC ADENOCARCINOMA

Carcinoma of the pancreas is the fifth leading cause of cancer-related deaths in the United States. Advances in the past decade have led to some improvement in the overall management of this disease. Resection for curative intent is accomplished in major centers with minimal perioperative mortality.[36] Significant improvements have also taken place in the preoperative evaluation and palliation of advanced disease. Early diagnosis of pancreatic cancer is the only means of improving long-term patient survival. However, because the early symptoms of pancreatic carcinoma are nonspecific, delay in diagnosis is common. Specific symptoms do not occur until there is invasion or obstruction of nearby structures. Because most pancreatic cancers arise in the head of the gland, obstruction of the biliary tree resulting in jaundice is the hallmark presentation. Back pain, when present, is an indicator of locally advanced disease caused by invasion of tumor into the splanchnic plexus and retroperitoneum. Duodenal obstruction with nausea and vomiting is usually a late manifestation of disease progression.

The goal of preoperative staging of pancreatic carcinoma is to determine the feasibility of curative surgery and the optimal treatment for each patient. For many patients, good-quality, thin-cut, spiral CT using oral and intravenous contrast is sufficient to delineate the presence of a pancreatic mass, local vascular invasion, and liver metastasis. Further staging procedures depend on the individual patient and on the surgeon's practice. Additional sensitive staging procedures include endoscopic ultrasonography[37,38] and laparoscopy with or without ultrasonography.[8-13] Endoscopic ultrasonography (EUS) is a minimally invasive technique in which a high-frequency transducer is placed in the gastric and duodenal lumen close to the pancreas to image the gland and adjacent organs. This technique can detect small pancreatic masses (<1 cm), identify enlarged regional lymph nodes, and better define visceral vascular involvement. Some institutions prefer to obtain tissue diagnosis of pancreatic carcinoma at the time of EUS. The use of laparoscopy in staging pancreatic carcinoma was discussed earlier in this chapter. The main role of laparoscopy is the detection of peritoneal or liver metastases that are not detectable with preoperative imaging.

Because only 10% to 20% of patients with carcinoma of the pancreas are suitable for resection, the optimal palliation of symptoms to maximize quality of life is of primary importance for most patients. Palliation can be performed operatively or nonoperatively. Obstructive jaundice can be palliated non-operatively by the use of biliary stenting. A number of prospective, randomized studies have shown that non-operative biliary stenting is equally effective in the relief of jaundice compared with surgical biliary bypass.[39-41] Pain may be alleviated using a combination of oral analgesics and a celiac plexus block. An operative (open or laparoscopic) gastrojejunostomy can treat or prevent gastric outlet obstruction. Expanding metal endoluminal stents placed endoscopically can also treat duodenal obstruction caused by tumor invasion. Stenting generally is less durable than surgical bypass, and multiple treatment procedures are needed with longer patient survival.

Potentially curable pancreatic cancers are typically confined to the head of the gland. Much of the improvement in operative results and long-term survival after pancreaticoduodenectomy has come from centers with extensive patient experience.[42-44] Operative management consists of assessment of tumor resectability and, if the tumor is resectable, completing a pancreaticoduodenectomy with gastrointestinal reconstruction. A diligent search for tumor outside the limits of a standard resection is first performed, including inspection of the liver, peritoneal, and omental surfaces for evidence of carcinomatosis. The regional lymph nodes are also evaluated for the presence of tumor involvement. Metastases in the periaortic lymph nodes, porta hepatis, superior mesenteric artery, or the celiac axis indicate that the tumor is beyond the limits of normal resection. Japanese surgeons advocate radical lymphadenectomy in an attempt to improve patient outcome,[45,46] but two randomized trials testing the value of extended lymph node dissection have not demonstrated improvements in survival.[47,48]

After distant metastases have been excluded, an assessment is made about whether the primary tumor is resectable. Local factors that generally prevent resection include retroperitoneal extension of the tumor to involve the inferior vena cava or aorta or direct involvement or encasement of the superior mesenteric artery, superior mesenteric vein, or portal vein. After excluding regional and distant metastases and proving no tumor involvement of major vascular structures (limited portal venous involvement is not a contraindication to resection if the surgeon is prepared to carry out a vascular reconstruction), the surgeon can proceed with pancreaticoduodenectomy. The surgeon may choose between the classic Whipple procedure, which includes the antrum of the stomach with the resection specimen, or the pylorus-preserving modification. The entire specimen consists of the gallbladder and common bile duct; head, neck, and uncinate process of the pancreas; the entire duodenum and proximal jejunum; and the distal stomach for a traditional Whipple procedure.

Of the patients with clinically resectable disease who undergo curative resection, no more than 25% will survive 5 years. Long-term survival rates improve when patients have complete resection, no lymph node metastases, tumor diameter no larger than 2 cm, and no evidence of perineural or duodenal invasion.[43] Given the overall poor prognosis of patients with pancreatic cancer, even after curative resection, non-surgical therapies have been extensively investigated.

Because approximately 50% of patients experience locoregional recurrence without apparent distant metastases after curative resection, adjuvant irradiation could have beneficial effects on patient survival.[49] In 1985, the Gastrointestinal Tumor Study Group reported encouraging results from a prospective, randomized trial studying the efficacy of adjuvant postoperative irradiation and chemotherapy for adenocarcinoma of the head of the pancreas.[50] Forty-three patients were randomized to receive adjuvant therapy with radiation and 5-fluorouracil (5-FU) or no adjuvant therapy. Median survival for the 21 patients who received adjuvant therapy was 20 months, and 3 (14%) survived at least 5 years. Among the 22 patients who received no adjuvant therapy, median survival was 11 months, and only 1 patient (4.5%) survived 5 years.[51] These results have been duplicated in uncontrolled protocols, providing stronger support for the use of postoperative combined adjuvant therapy.[52,53] In contrast, a European trial[54] showed benefit of adjuvant chemotherapy but a deleterious impact of concurrent chemotherapy and irradiation postoperatively. A meta-analyses[55] did not support adjuvant therapy as a standard of care. Major flaws in the European Study Group for Pancreatic Cancer (ESPAC) trial (ESPAC-1) are discussed in Chapter 45.

Adjuvant chemotherapy and irradiation are still used in many major treatment centers for resectable and locally advanced, unresectable pancreatic tumors. A multidisciplinary team of surgeons, pathologists, medical oncologists, and radiation oncologists should evaluate all patients considered for this therapy. Nonrandomized studies from Johns Hopkins Hospital and Mayo Clinic have confirmed a survival benefit when adjuvant postoperative irradiation plus 5-FU is used in patients with completely resected disease.[43,54,55] Despite improved local control of disease, most patients still succumb to liver metastases or peritoneal spread. These data suggest that pancreatic cancer is usually a systemic disease at diagnosis and that death occurs even with local disease control.

For locally advanced unresectable pancreatic carcinoma, the use of external beam irradiation plus chemotherapy has been reported to result in a doubling of median survival compared with surgical bypass or biliary stenting. The 2-year survival range increases from 0% to 5% up to 10% to 20% with palliative chemoirradiation. Five-year survivors are rare, and nonprogression of the primary tumor is uncommon. Addition of intraoperative radiation to external beam irradiation with or without 5-FU improves local control, as shown by physicians at Mayo Clinic and Massachusetts General Hospital.[56,57] This benefit did not translate into an improved patient survival because of liver and peritoneal metastasis development. If the full course of external beam irradiation, with or without 5-FU, is delivered preoperatively, this sequence allows restaging 2 to 3 months after treatment initiation. The 2-year survival rate appeared to be improved with this sequence of treatment followed by intraoperative radiotherapy.[58] Improvement presumably resulted from altered patient selection, because the incidence of liver plus peritoneal failure was not different. Until better systemic or abdominal therapy is developed, the improved local control of unresectable pancreatic adenocarcinoma observed with intraoperative radiotherapy will not translate into improved survival for patients with advanced disease.

THERAPY FOR ADENOCARCINOMA OF THE RECTUM

Surgical resection continues to be the primary curative modality for patients with adenocarcinoma of the rectum. The goals of surgery are to resect all known malignant tissue from the pelvis and to preserve anal sphincter function whenever possible. Factors determining the choice of operation for cancer of the rectum include the level of the tumor as measured from the anal verge, the microscopic appearance of the tumor, the extent of circumferential involvement, tumor mobility, histologic grade, body habitus, fecal continence, the presence of metastatic disease, and the presence of conditions that may contraindicate the creation of a colostomy, such as blindness, severe arthritis, or mental incapacity.

The distance of the lower edge of the tumor from the anal verge is the single most important factor that aids the surgeon in determining the choice of operation. Abdominal perineal resection has been advised for most tumors less than 6 cm from the anal margin, and anterior resection is performed for lesions located above this level. The choice of operation is ultimately decided only at the time of operation, after complete rectal mobilization has been achieved. All patients with tumors of the middle and low rectum should be advised that abdominal perineal resection with a permanent colostomy may be necessary, depending on intraoperative findings.

Accurate staging of rectal carcinoma is of central importance for surgical strategy and determining the need for adjuvant therapy. The surgeon should be confident preoperatively about the exact location of the tumor and ideally should personally perform digital examination and proctosigmoidoscopy. Preoperative staging should include the use of CT or MRI if locally advanced or metastatic disease is suspected.[59,60] Although CT and MRI are sensitive in the detection of metastatic disease and extrarectal disease extension with fixation, local staging of rectal cancer with these techniques has been disappointing with regard to whether disease extends beyond the muscularis propria. The value of both techniques for postoperative follow-up of rectal cancer can be limited by the inability to distinguish recurrent rectal cancer from fibrotic postoperative changes on a single study.[61] However, the use of serial CT scans can usually establish the diagnosis of recurrent disease; a baseline scan is obtained at 3 months postoperatively and then at 6-month intervals for 2 to 3 years. PET-CT imaging has also been a useful diagnostic tool in distinguishing disease relapse from postoperative changes.

Transrectal ultrasonography is the most sensitive method for preoperative local staging of primary rectal carcinomas.[62,63] Each layer of the rectal wall is sonographically visualized. A cancer appears as a hypoechoic disruption of the rectum. Several investigators have reported accuracy rates of more than 85% in assessing the depth of tumor infiltration and 65% to 75% accuracy in the detecting of lymph node involvement using transrectal ultrasonography.[62-64] The introduction of three-dimensional image analysis has enhanced the diagnostic value of transrectal ultrasonography for preoperative staging and guided needle biopsy.[65]

Low anterior resection is generally performed for cancers that are located at or higher than 6 cm from the anal margin. This operation involves complete mobilization of the rectum with division of the lateral ligaments and middle hemorrhoidal arteries. The anastomosis is performed between the extraperitoneal rectum (i.e., distal to the visceral peritoneal reflection) and the left colon. The anastomosis may be performed using a hand-sewn or stapled technique. The stapled anastomosis is an effective alternative, particularly in the narrow male pelvis. The gradual replacement of the abdominoperineal resection by low-stapled anterior reconstruction is among the most important advances in the management of rectal cancer over the past 2 decades. Despite an increase in the number of sphincter-saving operations, concern has been repeatedly expressed about variability in local recurrence rates and patient survival among surgeons.

The introduction of total mesorectal excision (TME) is a consequence of the variability in local relapse rates. Circumferential margin involvement is a key determinant of outcome after conventional surgery. TME resection results in a specimen less likely to have involved margins than less radical resection.[66] Combined examination of a TME specimen by an experienced surgeon and pathologist provides immediate assessment of the two principal prognostic variables: tumor stage and the adequacy of the surgical margins. The theoretical basis for the TME technique is based on two suppositions. The surgical planes between the integral visceral mesentery of the hindgut and the surrounding tissues provide a unique opportunity for defining a surgically achievable "tumor package," and serendipitously, the field of spread of rectal cancer is commonly limited within this package, or mesorectum.[67] Its total removal encompasses virtually every tumor satellite except in cases in which the tumor is widely disseminated. Meticulous, sharp dissection of the avascular plane between mesorectum and parietes is completed under direct vision. The excised specimen includes the entire posterior, distal, and lateral mesorectum to the plane of the inferior hypogastric nerve plexus, which is carefully preserved whenever possible. Anteriorly, the specimen includes the intact Denonvilliers fascia and the peritoneal reflection. The characteristic smooth bilobed encapsulated appearance posteriorly and distally reflects the contours of the pelvic floor and the midline anococcygeal raphe. Local recurrence rates of less than 5% and 5-year disease-free survival rates approaching 80% have been reported with mesorectal excision alone.[68] No randomized trials have been performed to test TME resection versus standard resection, with or without adjuvant chemotherapy and irradiation. Adjuvant radiotherapy significantly improves local control when combined with TME (97.6% versus 91.8% local control at 2 years) in a large, randomized trial.[69]

Although potentially curative laparoscopic operations for rectal cancer are technically feasible, they have not proved to be as efficacious as open surgery and should be reserved for selected patients or research protocols.[70] Laparoscopic abdominoperineal operations can be performed without a major abdominal incision and anterior resection with only a limited wound. Patients have reduced analgesia requirements, ambulate more readily, and appear to suffer less paralytic ileus. Local recurrence and long-term outcomes depend on strict adherence to established surgical oncology principles. The proximal and distal extent of vascular and lymphatic clearance should be the same as that achieved with open surgery. Spillage of luminal contents must be avoided, and careful handling of the tumor specimen is mandatory to avoid implantation of tumor cells in the pelvis or the potential for port-site recurrence.

Despite curative surgical resection of rectal malignancy, patients are at significant risk for local and distant disease relapse if treated with surgery alone. The risk of locoregional recurrence after complete surgical resection correlates with the degree of disease extension beyond the rectal wall and with nodal involvement. The incidence of locoregional failure for cancer of the rectum by TNM[3] and modified Astler-Coller stages[71] in patients undergoing complete surgical resection is outlined in Table 7-1. The incidence of local recurrence for lesions with involved nodes but with tumor confined to the rectal wall (TNM staging: T1-2N1-2; modified Astler-Coller staging: C1) varies from 20% to 40%. Lesions that have nodal involvement and extension beyond the rectal wall (TNM staging: T3-4N1-2; modified Astler-Coller staging: C2-3) usually have an incidence of locoregional recurrence of between 40% and 65%, but some series have reported recurrence rates of up to 70%. Surgical treatment alone has been found inadequate for more locally advanced rectal cancers, and adjuvant therapy has evolved in response to this problem.

The goals of adjuvant therapy are to prevent symptomatic local tumor recurrence and to eliminate distant metastases.[72] The efficacy of adjuvant therapy in the treatment of adenocarcinoma of the rectum can be evaluated in terms of local recurrence, disease-free survival, and overall survival. Adjuvant therapy has evolved over the past 2 decades, and combined modality therapy is now used routinely for the management of patients with AJCC stages II or III (modified Astler-Coller staging: B2-3 or C1-3) rectal cancer. The first trial to show improved outcomes (e.g., local recurrence rates, disease-free and overall survivals) with adjuvant chemotherapy and radiation after curative rectal resection was published in 1985.[73,74] A second trial[75] confirmed these findings and led to the National Institutes of Health Consensus Conference conclusion that all AJCC stage II and III rectal cancer patients should receive postoperative adjuvant chemotherapy and irradiation.[76] In Europe, preoperative radiation therapy, alone or in conjunction with chemotherapy, has been preferred. A meta-analysis[77] revealed significant reductions in local recurrence, cancer-related death, and overall mortality with combined treatment including preoperative radiation, but no reduction in distant metastases. In a systemic overview of preoperative versus postoperative adjuvant radiation therapy,[78] both combined treatments were found to be effective in reducing local cancer relapse and the probability of death from rectal cancer. A pooled analysis of five phase III North American rectal adjuvant trials[79] found disease-free and overall survival depended on T stage, TN stage, and the type of treatment. The investigators concluded that select patients with intermediate risk rectal cancer (T1-2N1 and T3N0) might not need radiation therapy as a component of adjuvant treatment.[79] Adjuvant chemoradiation therapy administered preoperatively or postoperatively is the standard of care for all T3-4 and node-positive rectal cancer patients. The potential advantage of preoperative versus postoperative chemoradiation was tested in a phase III trial conducted by the German Rectal Cancer Study Group.[80] Patients randomized to receive preoperative chemoradiation (N = 421) had less local relapse and less grade 3 or 4 toxicity compared with patients ran-

Table 7-1 Cancer of the Rectum: Combined Series Survival and Risk of Locoregional Failure by Stage after Complete Surgical Resection

TNM Stage	AJCC Stage	Modified Astler-Coller Stage	Incidence (%)	Survival (%)	Incidence of LF or RF (%)
Tis N0 M0			1-10	90-100	0-17
T1-2 N0 M0	I	A/B1	10-20	75-90	0-22
T3 N0 M0	II	B2	25-45	40-70	15-30
T4 N0 M0	II	B3	25-45	40-70	30-50
T1-2 N1-2	III	C1	5-15	40-70	20-40
T3 N1-2	III	C2	30-45	15-30	30-60
T4 N1-2	III	C3	30-45	15-30	50-70

LF, local failure; RF, regional failure.

domized to receive postoperative chemoradiation (N = 402), but there was no difference in overall survival.

MANAGEMENT OF RETROPERITONEAL SOFT TISSUE SARCOMA

Soft tissue sarcomas constitute less than 1% of all malignant tumors, and approximately 15% of these tumors are located in the retroperitoneum.[81] Retroperitoneal sarcomas present a difficult management problem for the surgical oncologist. Although most patients die of their cancer, many never develop disease outside the abdomen. Because of the locally invasive growth pattern of these tumors, the lack of anatomic boundaries within the retroperitoneum, and absence of specific symptoms, sarcomas are usually of a large size and involve multiple anatomic areas at presentation. The rate of complete surgical resectability had been about 50%,[81] but in some reports, it has increased to 67% to 75%.[82,83] The local recurrence rate after complete surgical resection ranges from 40% to 50% at 5 years after complete resection.[82-85] Of the patients who were disease free at 5 years, 40% have recurrences by 10 years after treatment.[86] Local recurrence is the most common cause of death from retroperitoneal sarcoma. Retrospective analysis in a study of more than 1000 patients indicated the following factors affected survival: primary tumor size; tumor fixation to nerve, vessels, or bones; regional lymph node involvement; presence of metastatic disease; and primary tumor grade.[87] The goal of surgical intervention is extirpation of all malignant tissue, but microscopic tumor remains in most patients.

Patients with retroperitoneal sarcoma most commonly present with an abdominal mass and pain. The single most definitive radiographic study is abdominal CT. CT can establish the extent of tumor, the presence or absence of necrosis, and evidence of liver metastases and define the retroperitoneal location. After the diagnosis of a retroperitoneal sarcoma is made by needle or incisional biopsy, CT of the chest should be obtained to rule out pulmonary metastasis. Percutaneous needle biopsy of a resectable retroperitoneal tumor is indicated to document the tumor type if preoperative radiation or other neoadjuvant therapy is planned. If resection is to be undertaken first, after exclusion of testicular cancer and lymphoma, needle biopsy provides no useful therapeutic information.

Surgical treatment of retroperitoneal sarcomas consists of en bloc resection of the entire tumor mass and any adjacent organs that are invaded or attached to the main tumor. For this reason, patients undergoing resection of the retroperitoneal sarcomas routinely receive a mechanical bowel preparation because of frequent requirement for intestinal resection. Retroperitoneal sarcomas tend to be right sided or left sided, with few actually arising from midline structures. Because retroperitoneal sarcomas commonly reach massive dimensions, en bloc resection often requires removal of the ipsilateral kidney and colon, part of the small bowel, the distal pancreas, and the spleen. Less frequently, partial gastrectomy, pancreaticoduodenectomy, or major hepatic resection may be indicated. If there is any adherence of the sarcoma to adjacent structures or organs, such involvement must be assumed to be malignant in nature, and every effort must be made to include these structures en bloc with the resected specimen. With extensive venous collaterals from vena cava occlusion, the inferior vena cava can be resected without reconstruction in some patients; in others, a prosthetic graft reconstruction is indicated. On rare occasions, aortic resection and replacement may be considered for a sarcoma that arises from or encases this structure, if the sarcoma can be entirely excised. Great care must be used throughout any surgical procedure to avoid tumor spillage. Retroperitoneal sarcomas may contain extensive areas of necrosis, making tumor rupture more likely with manipulation.

An example to illustrate the surgical principles involved in the resection of a retroperitoneal sarcoma and highlight the importance of en bloc resection is presented in Figures 7-6 and 7-7. This patient presented with a painful abdominal mass, and the sarcoma was demonstrated on the CT scan drawn in Figure 7-6. This mass occupied the left upper quadrant and displaced the spleen and distal pancreas anteriorly. The abdomen was explored through a midline incision, and the tumor was found to be confined to the left retroperitoneum. The stomach was mobilized along its greater curvature, and because it was not involved by tumor, it was reflected cephalad. The transverse colon was displaced caudad, permitting excellent exposure of the distal pancreas, spleen, left kidney, and anterior surface of the sarcoma (see Fig. 7-7A). The neck of the pancreas was divided, and the splenic artery and vein were ligated (see Fig. 7-7B). To minimize intraoperative bleeding, the vascular supply to the tumor mass originating along the medial aspect of the sarcoma was ligated before en bloc resection. The superior mesenteric artery and vein were retracted to the right, allowing division and ligation of the left renal artery and vein (see Fig. 7-7C). In this particular case, resection of the retroperitoneal sarcoma required concomitant resection of the spleen, left kidney, and distal pancreas (see Fig. 7-7D).

Data from some retrospective series have suggested an improvement in disease control and survival with radiotherapy after complete surgical resection.[88,89] However, the large-field radiotherapy necessary to treat the resection bed of retroperitoneal sarcomas can result in complications. Intraoperative plus external beam irradiation has been considered as a better alternative to a full course of external beam irradiation because it reduces the toxic effects of radiation by allowing normal tissues to be shielded from a large fraction of radiation delivered to the tumor bed at the time of laparotomy. In a prospective, randomized clinical trial carried out at the National Cancer Institute, intraoperative radiotherapy in combination with postoperative low-dose external beam radiation therapy was compared with postoperative high-dose external beam radiation therapy alone.[90] The results of this study showed no statistically significant difference in survival

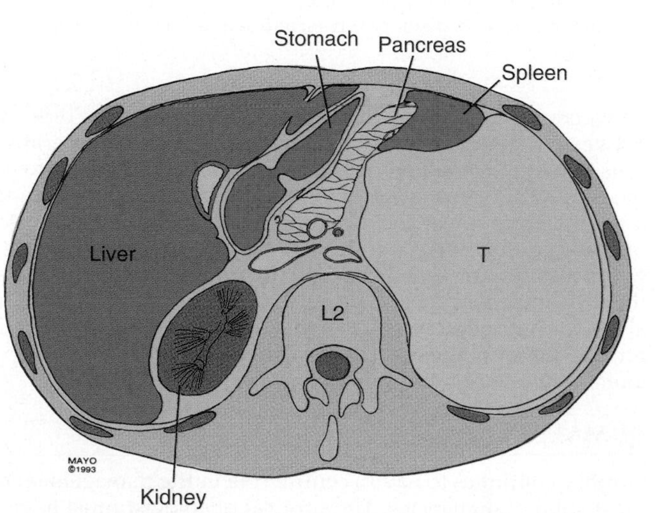

Figure 7-6 Appearance of left upper quadrant mass on CT scan. T, tumor. (Courtesy of the Mayo Foundation.)

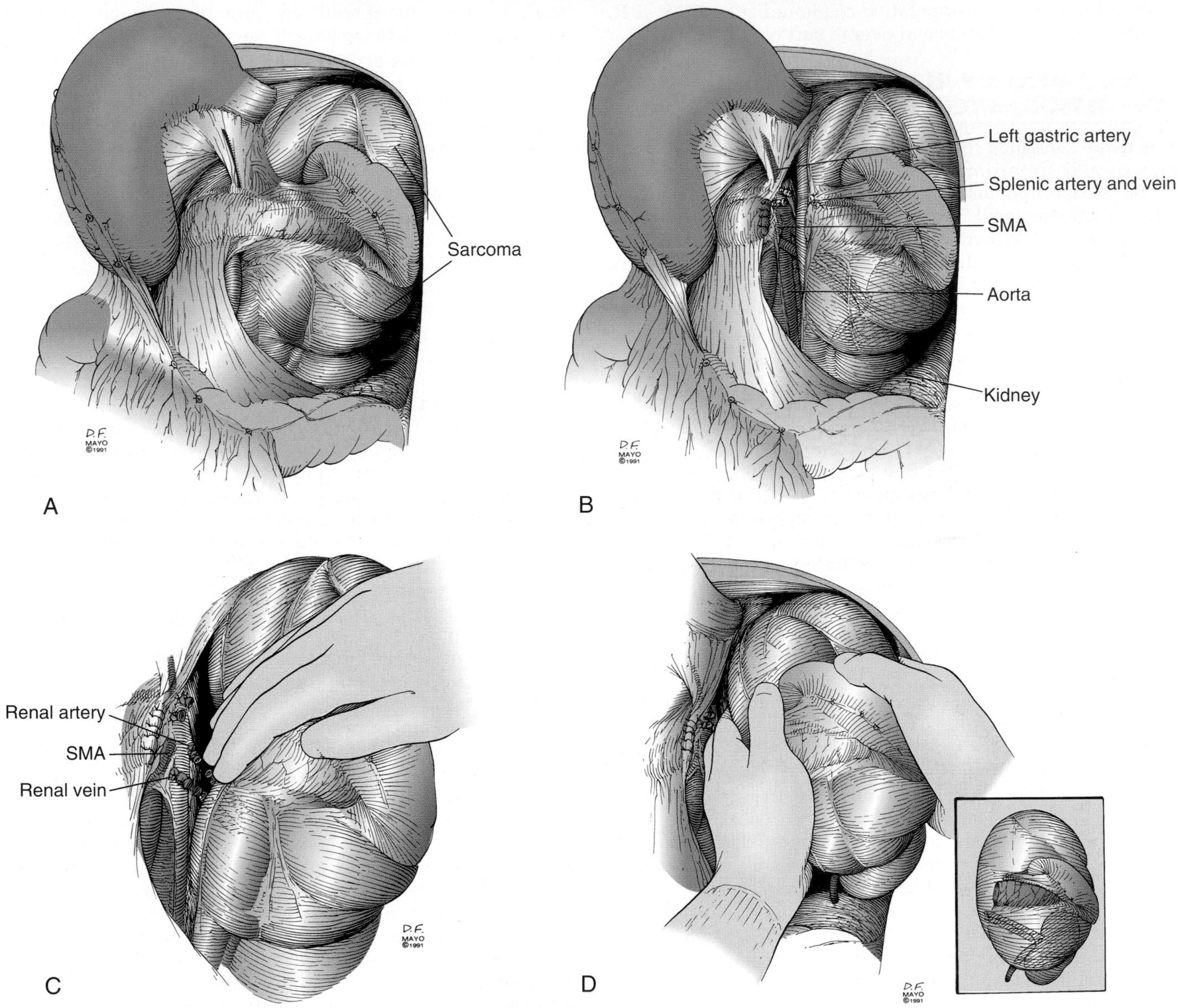

Figure 7-7 **A,** Mobilization of the transverse colon and stomach with exposure of retroperitoneal structures. **B,** Division of the neck of the pancreas and ligation of the splenic artery and vein. **C,** Ligation of the left renal artery and vein. **D,** En bloc resection. *Inset,* Specimen consisting of the sarcoma, spleen, distal pancreas, and left kidney. SMA, superior mesenteric artery. (Courtesy of the Mayo Foundation.)

between patient groups. The pattern of disease failure differed between the two groups; patients receiving intraoperative plus external irradiation demonstrated a significant improvement in local disease control within the irradiation fields and a significantly lower incidence of small bowel toxicity.[90] An ongoing trial by the American College of Surgeons Oncology group is studying whether adjuvant external beam radiation therapy improves local control and survival over resection alone for retroperitoneal sarcomas. There is no proven benefit for the use of adjuvant radiation therapy[91] or chemotherapy after complete retroperitoneal sarcoma resection.

SUMMARY

Surgery continues to have a central role in the management of most solid malignancies. The surgical oncologist must have a full understanding of the biology of the tumor in question and seek complete tumor staging information. The goal of surgical intervention must be defined, and adjuvant radiotherapy and chemotherapy should be used when these modalities are likely to confer additional survival or palliation benefit. The preoperative physiologic status of the patient must be reviewed and appropriate measures taken to provide for surgical care with minimal morbidity or mortality. Surgeons should adhere to strict principles of surgical oncology, including en bloc tumor resection whenever possible. Adequate time must be allowed postoperatively for wound healing to take place before commencing adjuvant therapy. For many solid tumors, further survival improvement will likely be the result of improved nonsurgical treatments rather than more radical surgical procedures.

REFERENCES

1. Gazelle GS, Haaga JR: Guided percutaneous biopsy of intra-abdominal lesions. Am J Radiol 153:929, 1989.

2. Karakousis CP: Principles of surgical resection for soft tissue sarcomas of the extremities. Surg Oncol Clin North Am 2:547, 1993.
3. Greene FL, Page DL, Fleming ID, et al (eds): AJCC Cancer Staging Manual, 6th ed. New York, Springer-Verlag, 2002.
4. D'Ugo DM, Pende V, Persiani R, et al: Laparoscopic staging of gastric cancer: an overview. J Am Coll Surg 196:965, 2003.
5. Jimenez RE, Warshaw AL, Rattner DW, et al: Impact of laparoscopic staging in the treatment of pancreatic cancer. Arch Surg 135:409, 2000.
6. Weber SM, DeMatteo RP, Fong Y, et al: Staging laparoscopy in patients with extrahepatic biliary carcinoma: analysis of 100 patients. Ann Surg 235:392, 200.
7. D'Angelica M, Fong Y, Weber S, et al: The role of staging laparoscopy in hepatobiliary malignancy: prospective analysis of 401 cases. Ann Surg Oncol 10:183, 2003.
8. Schirmer B: Laparoscopic ultrasonography: enhancing minimally invasive surgery. Ann Surg 220:709, 1994.
9. John TG, Greig JD, Carter DC, Garden OJ: Carcinoma of the pancreatic head and periampullary region. Tumor staging with laparoscopy and laparoscopic ultrasonography. Ann Surg 221:156, 1995.
10. John TG, Greig JD, Corsbie JL, et al: Superior staging of liver tumors with laparoscopy and laparoscopic ultrasound. Ann Surg 220:711, 1994.
11. Bogen GL, Mancino AT, Scott-Conner CEH: Laparoscopy for staging and palliation of gastrointestinal malignancy. Surg Clin North Am 76:557, 1996.
12. Conlon KC, Dougherty E, Klimstra DS, et al: The value of minimal access surgery in the staging of patients with potentially resectable peripancreatic malignancy. Ann Surg 223:134, 1996.
13. Pisters PWT, Lee JE, Vauthey JN, et al: Laparoscopy in the staging of pancreatic cancer. Br J Surg 88:325, 2001.
14. Sugarbaker PH: Cytoreductive surgery and peri-operative intraperitoneal chemotherapy as a curative approach to pseudomyxoma peritonei syndrome. Eur J Surg Oncol 27:239, 2001.
15. Gough DB, Donohue JH, Schutt AJ, et al: Pseudomyxoma peritonei: long-term patient survival with an aggressive regional approach. Ann Surg 219:112, 1994.
16. Kelly CJ, Daly DM: Perioperative care of the oncology patient. World J Surg 17:199, 1993.
17. Chen MK, Souba WW, Copeland EM III: Nutritional support of the surgical oncology patient. Hematol Oncol Clin North Am 5:125, 1991.
18. Mullen JL, Buzby GP, Mathews DC, et al: Reduction of operative morbidity and mortality by combined preoperative and postoperative nutritional support. Ann Surg 192:604, 1980.
19. Daly JM, Massar E, Giacco G, et al: Parenteral nutrition in esophageal cancer patients. Ann Surg 196:203, 1982.
20. Detsky AS, Baker JP, O'Rourke K, Goel V: Perioperative parenteral nutrition: a meta-analysis. Ann Intern Med 107:195, 1987.
21. Busch ORC, Hop WCJ, van Papendrecht MAW, et al: Blood transfusions and prognosis in colorectal cancer. N Engl J Med 328:1372, 1993.
22. Houbiers JGA, Brand A, van de Watering LMG, et al: Randomized controlled trial comparing transfusion of leukocyte-depleted or buffy-coat-depleted blood in surgery for colorectal cancer. Lancet 344:573, 1994.
23. Tibbs MK: Wound healing following radiation therapy: a review. Radiother Oncol 42:99, 1997.
24. Bernstein EF, Sullivan FJ, Mitchell JB, et al: Biology of chronic radiation effect on tissues and wound healing. Clin Plast Surg 20:435, 1993.
25. Mathes SJ, Alexander J: Radiation injury. Surg Oncol Clin North Am 5:809, 1996.
26. van Dongen JA, Voogd AC, Fentiman IS, et al: Long-term results of a randomized trial comparing breast-conserving therapy with mastectomy: European Organization for Research and Treatment of Cancer 10801 trial. J Natl Cancer Inst 92:1143, 2000.
27. Fisher B, Anderson S, Bryant J, et al: Twenty-year follow-up of a randomized trial comparing total mastectomy, lumpectomy, and lumpectomy plus irradiation for the treatment of invasive breast cancer. N Engl J Med 347:1233, 2003.
28. Poggi MM, Danforth DN, Sciuto LC, et al: Eighteen-year results in the treatment of early breast carcinoma with mastectomy versus breast conservation therapy. The National Cancer Institute randomized trial. Cancer 98:697, 2003.
29. Giuliano AE, Kirgan DM, Guenther JM, Morton DL: Lymphatic mapping and sentinel lymphadenectomy for breast cancer. Ann Surg 220:391, 1994.
30. Giuliano AE, Dale PS, Turner RR, et al: Improved axillary staging of breast cancer with sentinel lymphadenectomy. Ann Surg 222:394, 1995.
31. Giuliano AE: Lymphatic mapping and sentinel node biopsy in breast cancer. JAMA 277:791, 1997.
32. Krag D, Weaver D, Ashikaga T, et al: The sentinel node in breast cancer: a multicenter validation study. N Engl J Med 339:941, 1998.
33. Derossis AM, Fey J, Yeung H, et al: A trend analysis of the relative value of blue dye and isotope localization in 2,000 consecutive cases of sentinel node biopsy for breast cancer. J Am Coll Surg 193:473, 2001.
34. Schwartz GF, Giuliano AE, Veronesi U, for the Consensus Conference Committee: Proceedings of the consensus conference on the role of sentinel lymph node biopsy in carcinoma of the breast, April 19-22, 2001, Philadelphia, Pennsylvania. Cancer 94:2542, 2002.
35. Veronesi U, Paganelli G, Viale G, et al: A randomized comparison of sentinel-node biopsy with routine axillary dissection in breast cancer. N Engl J Med 349:546, 2003.
36. Lillemoe KD: Current management of pancreatic carcinoma. Ann Surg 221:133, 1995.
37. Legman P, Vignaux O, Dousset B, et al: Pancreatic tumors: Comparison of dual-phase helical CT and endoscopic sonography. AJR Am J Roentgenol 170:1315, 1998.
38. Ahmad NA, Lewis JD, Siegelman ES, et al: Role of endoscopic ultrasound and magnetic resonance imaging in the preoperative staging of pancreatic adenocarcinoma. Am J Gastroenterol 95:1926, 2000.
39. Shepherd AH, Royle G, Ross APR, et al: Endoscopic biliary endoprosthesis in the palliation of malignant obstruction of the distal common bile duct: a randomized trial. Br J Surg 75:1166, 1988.
40. Andersen JR, Sorensen SM, Kruse A, et al: Randomised trial of endoscopic endoprosthesis versus operative bypass in malignant obstructive jaundice. Gut 30:1132, 1989.
41. Smith AC, Dowsett JF, Russell RCG, et al: Randomised trial of endoscopic stenting versus surgical bypass in malignant low bile duct obstructions. Lancet 344:1655, 1994.
42. Trede M, Schwall G, Saeger HD: Survival after pancreatoduodenectomy. Ann Surg 211:447, 1990.
43. Yeo CJ, Cameron JL, Lillemoe KD, et al: Pancreaticoduodenectomy for cancer of the head of the pancreas: 201 patients. Ann Surg 221:721, 1995.
44. Nitecki SS, Sarr MG, Colby TV, van Heerden JA: Long-term survival after resection for ductal adenocarcinoma of the pancreas: is it really improving? Ann Surg 221:59, 1995.
45. Ttakahashi S, Ogata Y, Miyazaki H, et al: Aggressive surgery for pancreatic duct cell cancer: feasibility, validity, limitations. World J Surg 19:643, 1995.
46. Nagakawa T, Nagamori M, Futakami F, et al: Results of extensive surgery for pancreatic carcinoma. Cancer 77:640, 1996.
47. Pedrazolli S, DiCarlo V, Dionigi R, et al: Standard versus extended lymphadenectomy associated with pancreatoduodenectomy in the surgical treatment of adenocarcinoma of the head of the pancreas: a multicenter, prospective randomized study. Lymphadenectomy Study Group. Ann Surg 228:508, 1998.
48. Yeo CJ, Cameron JL, Lillimoe KD, et al: Pancreaticoduodenectomy with or without distal gastrectomy and extended retroperitoneal lymphadenectomy for periampullary adenocarcinoma. Part 2. Randomized controlled trial evaluating survival, morbidity and mortality. Ann Surg 236: 355, 2002.
49. Tepper J, Nardi G, Suit H: Carcinoma of the pancreas: review of MGH experience from 1963 to 1973. Analysis of surgical failure and implications for radiation therapy. Cancer 37:1519, 1977.
50. Kalser MH, Ellenberg SS: Pancreatic cancer: adjuvant combined radiation and chemotherapy following curative resection. Arch Surg 97:28, 1985.

51. Gastrointestinal Tumor Study Group: Further evidence of effective adjuvant combined radiation and chemotherapy following curative resection of pancreatic cancer. Cancer 59:2006, 1987.
52. Foo ML, Gunderson LL, Nagorney DM, et al: Patterns of failure in grossly resected pancreatic ductal adenocarcinoma treated with adjuvant irradiation +/− 5 fluorouracil. Int J Radiat Oncol Biol Phys 26:483, 1993.
53. Yeo CJ, Abrams RA, Grochow LB, et al: Pancreaticoduodenectomy for pancreatic adenocarcinoma: postoperative adjuvant chemoradiation improves survival. A prospective, single-institution experience. Ann Surg 225:621, 1997.
54. Neoptolemas JP, Stocken DD, Friess H, et al: A randomized trial of chemoradiotherapy and chemotherapy after resection of pancreatic cancer. N Engl J Med 350:1200, 2004.
55. Chu QD, Khushalani N, Javle MM, et al: Should adjuvant therapy remain the standard of care for patients with resected adenocarcinoma of the pancreas? Ann Surg Oncol 10:539, 2003.
56. Shipley WU, Wood WC, Tepper JE, et al: Intraoperative irradiation for patients with unresectable pancreatic carcinoma. Ann Surg 200:289, 1984.
57. Gunderson LL, Nagorney DM, Martenson JA, et al: External beam plus intraoperative irradiation for gastrointestinal cancers. World J Surg 19:191, 1995.
58. Garton GR, Gunderson LL, Nagorney DM, et al: High-dose preoperative external beam and intraoperative irradiation for locally advanced pancreatic cancer. In J Radiat Oncol Biol Phys 27:1153, 1993.
59. Freeny PC, Marks WM, Ryan JA, Bolen JW: Colorectal carcinoma evaluation with CT: preoperative staging and detection of postoperative recurrence. Radiology 158:347, 1986.
60. Kusonoki M, Yanagi H, Kamikonya N, et al: Preoperative detection of local extension of carcinoma of the rectum using magnetic resonance imaging. J Am Col Surg 179:653, 1994.
61. Schlag P, Lehner B, Strauss LG, et al: Scar or recurrent rectal cancer. Positron emission tomography is more helpful for diagnosis than immunoscintigraphy. Arch Surg 124:197, 1989.
62. Solomon MJ, McLeod RS: Endoluminal transrectal ultrasonography: accuracy, reliability, and validity. Dis Colon Rectum 36:200, 1993.
63. Mackay SG, Pager CK, Joseph D, et al: Assessment of the accuracy of transrectal ultrasonography in anorectal neoplasia. Br J Surg 90:346, 2003.
64. Hildebrandt U, Klein T, Feifel G, et al: Endoscopy of pararectal lymph nodes: in vitro and in vivo evaluation. Dis Colon Rectum 33:863, 1990.
65. Hunerbein M, Schlag PM: Three-dimensional endosonography for staging of rectal cancer. Ann Surg 225:432, 1997.
66. Heald RJ: Total mesorectal excision is optimal surgery for rectal cancer: a Scandinavian consensus. Br J Surg 82:1297, 1995.
67. Heald RJ: Rectal cancer: the surgical options. Eur J Cancer 31A:1189, 1995.
68. MacFarlane JK, Ryall RDH, Heald RJ: Mesorectal excision for rectal cancer. Lancet 341:457, 1993.
69. Kapiteijn E, Marijnen CAM, Nagtegaal ID, et al: Preoperative radiotherapy combined with total mesorectal excision for resectable rectal cancer. N Engl J Med 345:638, 2001.
70. O'Rourke NA, Heald RJ: Laparoscopic surgery for colorectal cancer. Br J Surg 80:1229, 1993.
71. Gunderson LL, Martenson JA, Smalley SR, Garton GR: Lower gastrointestinal cancers: rationale, results, and techniques of treatment. Front Radiat Ther Oncol 28:140, 1994.
72. O'Connell MJ, Gunderson LL: Adjuvant therapy for adenocarcinoma of the rectum. World J Surg 16:510, 1992.
73. Gastrointestinal Tumor Study Group: Prolongation of the disease-free interval in surgically resected rectal cancer. N Engl J Med 312:1465, 1985.
74. Gastrointestinal Tumor Study Group: Survival after postoperative combination treatment of rectal cancer. N Engl J Med 315:1294, 1986.
75. Krook J, Moertel CG, Gunderson LL, et al: Effective surgical adjuvant therapy for high risk rectal carcinoma. N Engl J Med 324:709, 1991.
76. NIH Consensus Conference: Adjuvant therapy for patients with colon and rectal cancer. JAMA 264:1444, 1990.
77. Cammà C, Giunta M, Fiorica F, et al: Preoperative radiotherapy for resectable rectal cancer: a meta-analysis. JAMA 284:1008, 2000.
78. Colorectal Cancer Collaborative Group: Adjuvant radiotherapy for rectal cancer: a systemic overview of 8507 patients from 22 randomised trials. Lancet 358:1291, 2001.
79. Gunderson LL, Sargent DJ, Tepper JE, et al: Impact of T and N stage and treatment on survival and relapse in adjuvant rectal cancer: a pooled analysis. J Clin Oncol 22:1785, 2004.
80. Sauer R, Becker H, Hohenberger W et al: Preoperative versus postoperative chemoradiotherapy for rectal cancer. N Engl J Med 351:1731, 2004.
81. Dalton RR, Donohue JH, Mucha J Jr, et al: Management of retroperitoneal sarcomas. Surgery 106:725, 1989.
82. Lewis JJ, Leung D, Woodruff JM, Brennan MF: Retroperitoneal soft-tissue sarcoma: analysis of 500 patients treated and followed at a single institution. Ann Surg 228:355, 1998.
83. Hassan I, Park SZ, Donohue JH, et al: Operative management of primary retroperitoneal sarcomas: a reappraisal of an institutional experience. Ann Surg 239:244, 2004.
84. Ferrario T, Karakousis CP: Retroperitoneal sarcomas: grade and survival. Arch Surg 138:248, 2003.
85. Stoeckle E, Coindre J-M, Bonvalot S, et al: Prognostic factors in retroperitoneal sarcoma: a multivariate analysis of a series of 165 patients of the French Cancer Center Federation Sarcoma Group. Cancer 92:359, 2001.
86. Heslin MJ, Lewis JJ, Nadler E, et al: Prognostic factors associated with long-term survival for retroperitoneal sarcoma: implications for management. J Clin Oncol 15:2832, 1997.
87. Russell WO, Cohen J, Enzinger F, et al: A clinical and pathological staging system for soft tissue sarcomas. Cancer 40:1562, 1977.
88. Tepper JR, Suit HD, Wood WC, et al: Radiation therapy of retroperitoneal soft-tissue sarcomas. J Radiat Oncol Biol Phys 10:825,1984.
89. van Doorn RC, Gallee MPW, Hart AAM, et al: Resectable retroperitoneal soft tissue sarcomas: the effect of extent of resection and postoperative radiation therapy on local tumor control. Cancer 73:637, 1994.
90. Sindelar WF, Kinsella TJ, Chen PW, et al: Intraoperative radiotherapy in retroperitoneal sarcomas: final results of a prospective, randomized clinical trial. Arch Surg 128:402, 1993.
91. McGinn CJ: The role of radiation therapy in resectable retroperitoneal sarcomas. Surg Oncol 9:61, 2000.

CHAPTER 8

PRINCIPLES OF CHEMOTHERAPY

Lawrence S. Blaszkowsky, Jeffrey G. Supko, and Bruce A. Chabner

Although the earliest clinical manifestation of cancer is a mass or tumor, in many patients, cancer is often not a localized disease at the time of its discovery. In most patients, the disease has already spread to lymph nodes and other distant sites, even though clinical imaging and random biopsies may fail to disclose its presence. For more than a century, thoughtful investigators have sought systemic treatments for cancer, often using as their paradigms the lessons of infectious illnesses and nutritional disease. Vaccines, natural extracts, vitamins, and synthetic chemicals were touted as cures. However, not until the initial trials of alkylating agents by scientists and clinicians at Yale University, first described in 1946, was there proof that a systemically administered agent could cause regression of a human tumor, which in this case was a mediastinal mass in a patient with Hodgkin's disease.[1] The clinical studies of nitrogen mustard, based on observations of the toxicity of mustard gases in World War II, lacked a clear conceptual basis. Although it was known at the time that these compounds were highly reactive with proteins, nucleic acids, and other electron-rich molecules, the specific intracellular target was not identified until more than a decade later, and we are only now beginning to understand the reasons for the selective action of alkylating agents on tumor cells.

This early experience with alkylating agents led a number of bold investigators to undertake an alternative approach, the synthesis of compounds that would act as fraudulent counterparts of natural metabolites known to stimulate cancer cell growth. Among these metabolic targets, vitamins and nucleic acid bases proved to be most vulnerable (Fig. 8-1). In the late 1940s, scientists from American Cyanamid synthesized analogues of folic acid, a vitamin known to stimulate the proliferation of cancer cells in culture and in humans. Sidney Farber tested these analogues and found striking but short-lived responses to aminopterin, and to the closely related compound, methotrexate, in children with acute lymphoblastic leukemia (ALL).[2] Prospects for the treatment of cancer with drugs dramatically escalated in the following decade. Hitchings, Elion, and others at Burroughs Wellcome experimented with a series of purine analogues and found antitumor effects in animals, leading to the successful development of 6-thioguanine and 6-mercaptopurine. Soon afterward, corticosteroids were discovered as anti-inflammatory agents and were found to kill malignant lymphocytes in children with leukemia and lymphoma.[3]

Equally rewarding efforts in the field of natural product chemistry yielded additional new anticancer drugs with unique mechanisms of action. In the course of their search for natural products for the treatment of diabetes, scientists at Eli Lilly discovered the antimitotic and antitumor properties of the vinca alkaloids.[4] Shortly thereafter, analysis of fermentation broths led to the discovery of mitomycin C, a novel alkylating agent[5]; bleomycin, a DNA-cleaving peptide[6]; and the anthracyclines, which inhibit topoisomerase II,[7] an enzyme that relaxes DNA supercoils during transcription and replication. In the 1960s, further efforts in plant chemistry led to the isolation of paclitaxel,[8] a drug that inhibits formation of the mitotic spindle, and the camptothecins, which block the action of topoisomerase I.[9] However, paclitaxel and the camptothecins did not reach the clinic until 10 to 20 years later.

The beginning of the 21st century has seen the arrival of targeted therapy. The goal of this therapy is not necessarily to induce DNA damage, but to inhibit various signaling pathways that control cell proliferation, cell death, invasion, metastases, and angiogenesis. Although several of these agents are available, we are just learning how to use them. It is unclear if and to what extent they will modulate the effect of chemotherapy and whether they will be best used as an aid in cytoreduction or as maintenance therapy. The role of these agents in combination with radiation, as radiation sensitizers, is also evolving.

MODELS FOR CHEMOTHERAPY

In parallel with the work that led to cytotoxic chemotherapy, Skipper and Perry[10] at the Southern Research Institute characterized murine tumor models, notably the L1210 and P388 leukemias, as well as murine solid tumors such as sarcoma 180. Their model systems allowed reproducible, quantitative chemotherapy experiments to be performed in mice.[10] They tested various strategies for treatment and established a rational basis for understanding the kinetics of cell kill, the evaluation of drug combinations, and the mechanisms of drug resistance. Important concepts of cancer chemotherapy came from their experiments, which established the theoretical basis for rational combination chemotherapy and the cure of ALL in children. Skipper's experiments with murine leukemias established the following principles:

1. *Fractional cell kill.* Each dose of chemotherapy kills a constant fraction of the tumor cell population. Cell kill is a function of the dose (for alkylating agents, kill increases linearly with dose) and the schedule of drug administration. For most cancer drugs, cell kill correlates with a specific pharmacokinetic parameter, the area under the drug concentration × time curve (C × T, or AUC) (Fig. 8-2). For some drugs, the time above a threshold concentration or the peak drug concentration determines the cytotoxicity for tumor and for normal target tissues.
2. *Importance of dose intensity (dose per unit time).* During the time period between cycles of treatment, tumor cells resume proliferation. Short rest periods and high doses of drug produce the best results.
3. *Drug resistance.* Exposure of tumors to single-agent chemotherapy rapidly results in outgrowth of drug-resistant cells. Biochemical studies of these drug-resistant cells disclosed alterations in the drug target, drug transport or activation pathways, or other aspects of drug action. Drug combinations discourage the outgrowth of resistant cells and produce cures where single agents fail.
4. *Cell cycle dependency of cell kill.* Most anticancer drugs, particularly the antimetabolites, have their greatest effect on actively proliferating cells. Drugs that act on DNA synthesis damage cells during periods of DNA synthesis (S phase), whereas mitotic inhibitors produce cell kill through exposure of cells during mitosis (M phase) (Fig. 8-3). The rate of cell proliferation slows and the number of nonpro-

Normal Metabolite	Analogue	Site(s) of Action
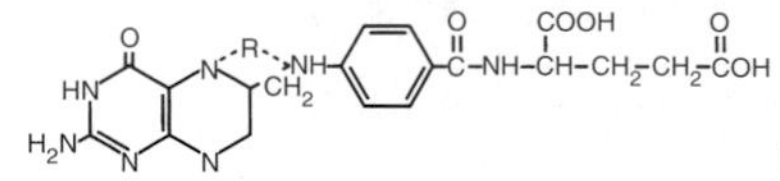 Tetrahydrofolate	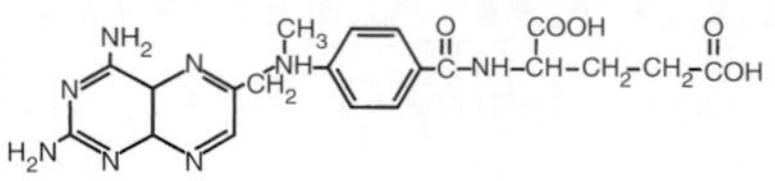 Methotrexate	1. Inhibits dihydrofolate reductase 2. Polyglutamates inhibit thymidylate synthase and purine synthesis
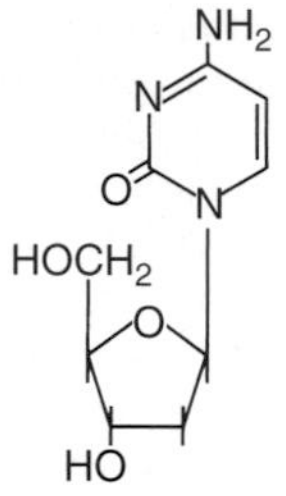 Deoxycytidine	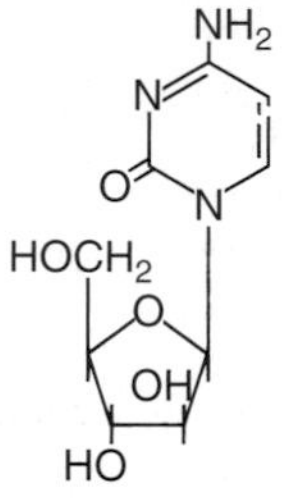 Cytosine arabinoside	1. Blocks DNA polymerization
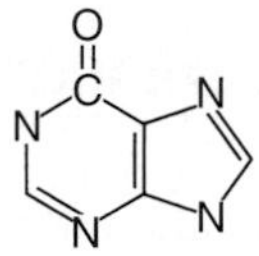 Hypoxanthine	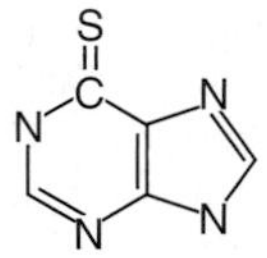 6-Mercaptopurine	1. Blocks *de novo* purine synthesis 2. Incorporated into nucleic acids

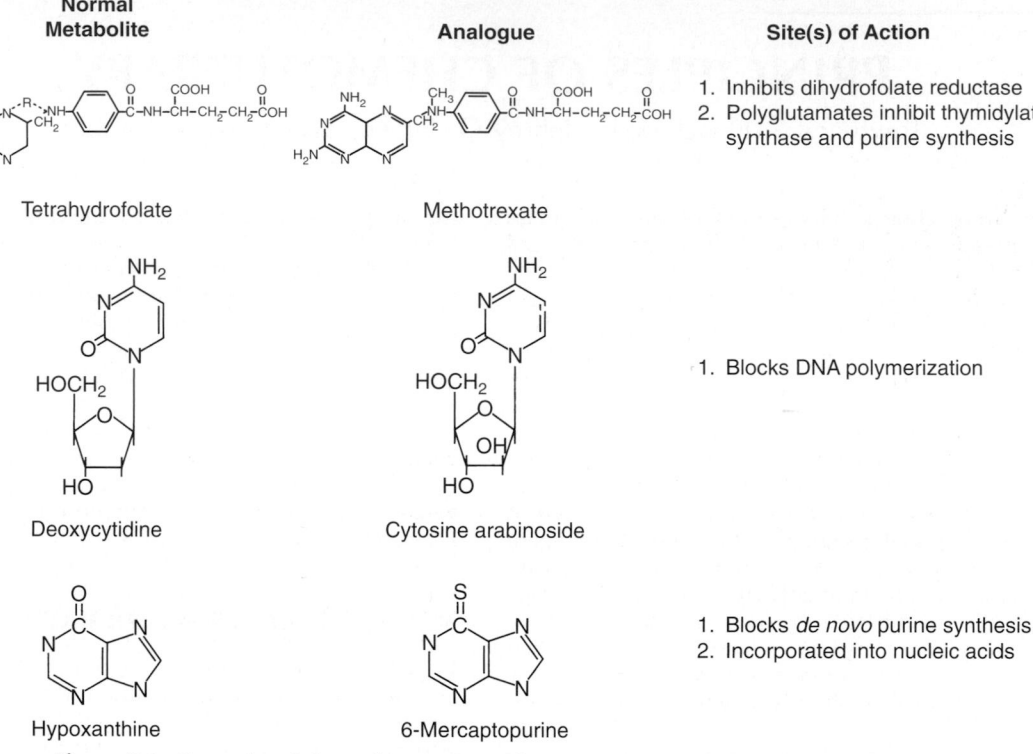

Figure 8-1 Examples of chemotherapy drugs that are analogues of natural metabolites.

liferating cells increases with expansion of the tumor mass. Chemotherapy is most effective when the tumor burden is lowest and cell proliferation is most active.

These principles profoundly influenced all aspects of clinical chemotherapy, including regimen design, the use of drugs in combination, adjuvant chemotherapy, and high-dose chemotherapy. Relying on the these principles, the cure of ALL was accomplished through the efforts of Frei and Freireich at the National Cancer Institute and Holland at Roswell Park, who developed effective combination therapy; Pinkel and colleagues at St. Jude Hospital in Memphis, who identified the central nervous system as a sanctuary for leukemic cells; and the national pediatric cooperative groups, which tested these insights in randomized clinical trials.[11] These investigators combined a knowledge of the drugs and the disease to establish principles for leukemia therapy that persist to this day: intensive, marrow-ablative induction therapy, followed by consolidation to further reduce the leukemic cell population; central nervous system prophylaxis with irradiation and methotrexate; and maintenance chemotherapy to eliminate the last logs of tumor cells. In the course of their work, they identified the importance of supportive care measures, including aggressive broad-spectrum antibiotic treatment of febrile episodes in neutropenic patients, platelet support to prevent bleeding due to thrombocytopenia, and management of opportunistic infection. Each of these insights, further refined by the use of new antibiotics and bone marrow colony-stimulating factors, has become a basic component of modern chemotherapy.

SOLID TUMOR CHEMOTHERAPY

The principles enumerated earlier have been applied with greatest success to the treatment of aggressive and rapidly proliferating tumors such as leukemias, lymphomas, and testicular cancer. The development of drug therapy for the more common solid tumors has taken a slower and more tortuous course. Drugs identified in mouse leukemia screening systems have been less effective against most solid tumors; notable exceptions are choriocarcinoma, testicular cancer, and the lymphomas, all of which can be cured with cycles of intensive chemotherapy. However, chemotherapy has had only limited impact on the common solid tumors in humans, particularly in widely metastatic, end-stage disease. Rational synthesis of 5-fluorouracil by Heidelberger and associates led to the first modestly effective antimetabolite for colon and breast cancers.[12] Other important clinically effective drugs were identified through random screening efforts and serendipity: doxorubicin and cisplatin in the early 1970s, etoposide and paclitaxel in the late 1980s, and the camptothecin analogues and gemcitabine in the 1990s.[13]

An important conceptual breakthrough in solid tumor chemotherapy was the proposal to employ drugs in the adjuvant setting, after removal of the primary tumor in patients at high risk for relapse. The work of Fisher, Bonnadonna, and others established that drugs capable of producing partial responses in advanced disease could cure one third of women with stage II breast cancer, who were otherwise destined to suffer distant recurrence and death.[14] The conceptual basis for this strategy is the increased probability of curing metastatic disease when the tumor burden is small and tumor cells are actively proliferating and therefore more susceptible to cytotoxic drugs. Drugs have a firmly established role in the treatment of lung, breast, and colorectal cancer after or before surgery.

Newer concepts aimed at improving local control of otherwise inoperable tumors have led to so-called neoadjuvant or induction therapy.[15] In this strategy, drugs are used alone or in combination with radiation therapy, before surgery, in the

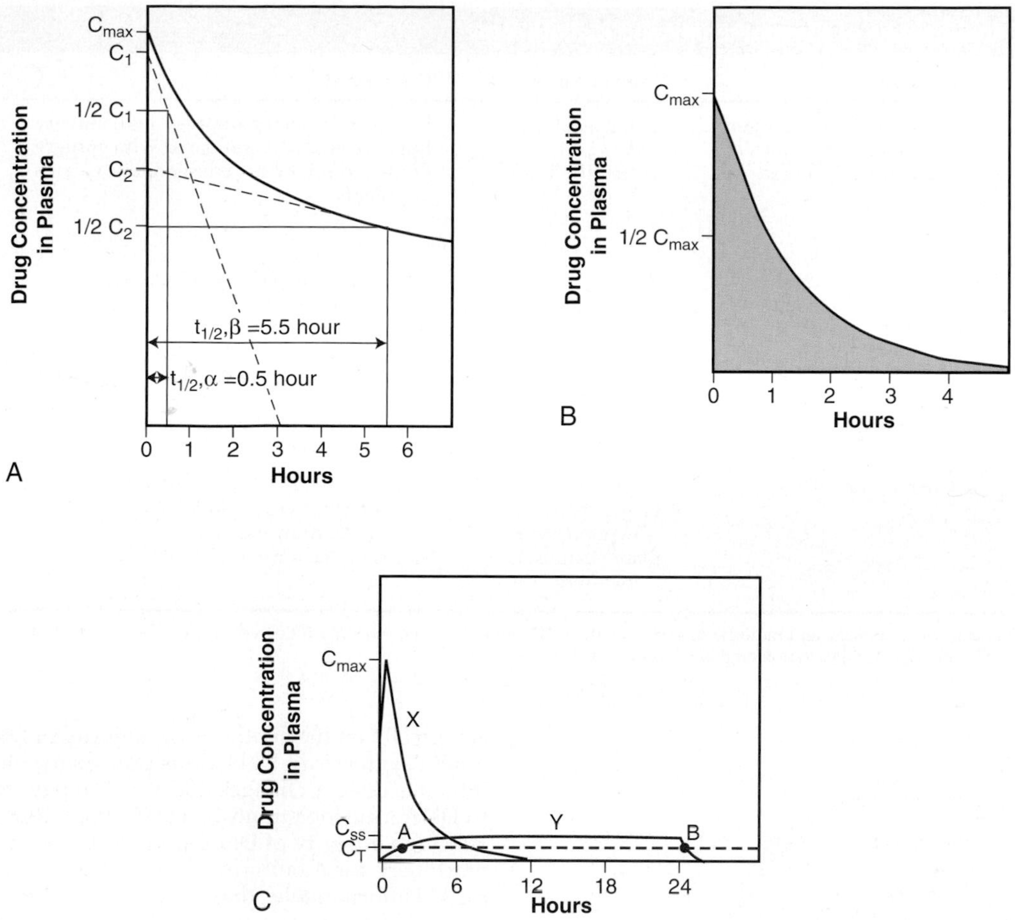

Figure 8-2 Drug elimination from plasma. **A,** The *solid blue curve* illustrates a semi-logarithmic plot of drug concentration versus time after a rapid intravenous injection. The *dashed red line* intercepting the y-axis at C_2 represents an extrapolation of the log-linear terminal phase. The *dashed red line* that intersects the y-axis at C_1 is obtained by subtracting the extrapolated values of the log-linear terminal phase from the observed drug concentrations. Maximum drug concentration in plasma (C_{max}) = $C_1 + C_2$. The initial (α) phase half-life ($t_{1/2,\alpha}$) is the time for C_1 to decay to ½ C_1. The terminal (β) phase half-life ($t_{(1/2),\beta}$) is the time for C_2 to decay to ½ C_2. This biphasic behavior results from distribution of the drug among rapidly and slowly perfused regions of the body, as well as its elimination. **B,** Drug concentration in plasma versus time is plotted on linear axes. The *blue shaded area* is the area under the curve (AUC); it represents the integral of drug concentration over time. The AUC is a measure of total systemic exposure to the drug. **C,** Linear plots of drug concentration versus time are illustrated for a rapid intravenous injection (X) and a 24-hour continuous infusion (Y) of the same total dose of drug (the AUCs are equivalent). Notice that the duration of drug concentrations above the threshold for cytotoxicity (C_T) is much longer with the continuous infusion (represented as B − A) than with the bolus administration. Conversely, the maximum plasma concentration achieved by bolus administration (C_{max}) is much larger than that of the continuous infusion (C_{SS}).

initial treatment of locally advanced breast, head and neck, bladder, and lung (Table 8-1). This preoperative therapy reduces the size of otherwise unresectable tumors to a point where surgical removal is feasible or, in some cases, unnecessary.

At the same time, advances in bone marrow stem cell harvesting, storage, and reinfusion have allowed the introduction of high-dose regimens with stem cell rescue as a basic technique for escalating drug dosage and increasing dose intensity. In this setting, high-dose chemotherapy is remarkably safe and reliably cures a significant minority of patients with relapsed lymphomas and leukemia and probably certain subgroups of patients with breast cancer. As they become safer to use, high-dose regimens are being employed in earlier stages of disease to enhance the cure rate of otherwise incurable patients, such as lymphoma or Hodgkin's disease. The role of such therapy in node-positive breast cancer, however, remains controversial.

Because drugs have become an integral part of the initial therapy of many patients with cancer, it is essential that the medical oncologist, surgeon, and radiation oncologist understand the principles of chemotherapy and the specific features of the commonly used agents. This chapter explains the conceptual basis for the use of cancer chemotherapeutic drugs and provides detailed information for understanding their actions, toxicities, and late side effects.

BASIS OF CANCER CHEMOTHERAPY: CANCER CELL BIOLOGY

Every phase of chemotherapeutic research, from discovery to clinical application, is based on the concepts of cancer cell biology, and drug research has evolved as our knowledge of biology has progressed. The essential properties of the cancer cell, properties that distinguish the cell from its normal counterpart and that form the basis for treatment are excess proliferation, reduced rates of apoptosis (i.e., programmed cell death), invasive capacity, ability to induce nutrient vessels, ability to escape immune surveillance, and ability to metastasize. Each of these properties has been the starting point for

Table 8-1 Combinations of Chemotherapy and Radiotherapy

Objective	Strategy	Malignancy	Comments	References
Control distant disease, improve local control, increase resectability	Chemo/RT, then surgery	Esophageal	Improve survival compared with surgery	54,55
	Various combinations of chemo, RT, surgery	NSCLC, IIIA	Improve survival compared with surgery	56
		Breast, III (T3-4)	Local control, breast conservation in some patients	57,58
Control local and distant disease	Pretoperative chemo/RT	Rectal	Decrease local and distant relapse	59,60
	Postoperative chemo/RT	Breast, I-II	Improve local control and survival	61,62
		NSCLC, IIIA-B	Improve local control and survival	63
	Chemo/RT, no surgery	SCLC	Improve local control and survival	64
		Nasopharyngeal	Improve local control and survival	65
	Chemo, then RT, no surgery	Bulky lymphomas	Improve disease-free survival	66,67
		NHL, stage I	Reduce treatment toxicity, improve distant control	68,69
Preserve organs	Chemo, then RT	Anal	Cure disease, avoid anal resection	70,71
		Larynx and hypopharynx	Avoid laryngectomy in 50-60% of patients, reduce distant relapse	72,73
		Bladder (muscle invasive)	Avoid cystectomy in 60% of patients	74

Chemo/RT, concurrent chemotherapy and radiotherapy; chemo, then RT, sequential chemotherapy followed by radiotherapy; NSCLC, non–small cell lung cancer; SCLC, small cell lung cancer; NHL, non-Hodgkin's lymphoma.

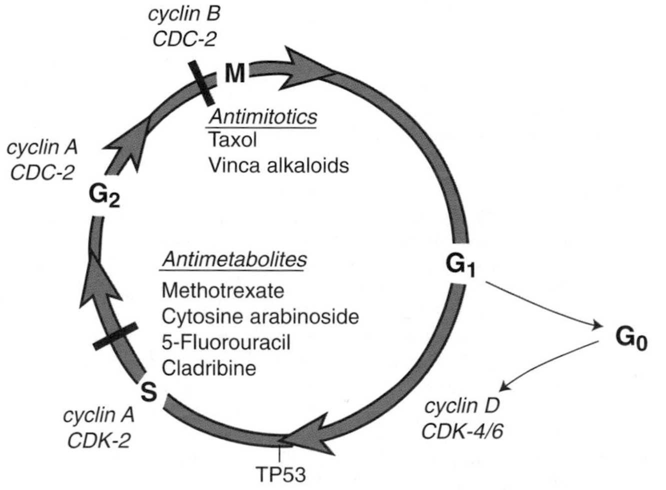

Figure 8-3 The cell cycle, its controls and checkpoints, and the site of action of cell cycle phase–specific drugs. The cell cycle phases are G_0 (nondividing cells), G_1 (resting phase), S (DNA synthesis), G_2 (gap between S and M), and M (mitosis). Transitions between phases are controlled by the appearance of specific cyclin proteins that complex with and activate cyclin-dependent kinases. The G_1/S transition is also controlled at a checkpoint by proteins such as TP53, which monitor DNA integrity. Other proteins monitor the G_2/M checkpoint.

drug discovery efforts, as illustrated in Table 8-2.[17] Most cancer cells display defects in DNA repair that generate a diversity of subclones and increase the probability of drug resistance. However, with few exceptions, the successful drugs have attacked only the first of these properties, proliferation.

DRUGS THAT TARGET DNA SYNTHESIS AND MITOSIS

Although much of the effort in modern cancer drug development is directed at targets that regulate growth signal transmission, most of the successful drugs in current clinical use act directly on the synthesis or integrity of DNA. These drugs inhibit synthesis of DNA or its precursors, block cell division, inhibit necessary changes in DNA topology, or covalently bind to DNA, causing strand breaks or miscoding. All such drugs affect the integrity of DNA, and in the presence of the normal machinery for monitoring DNA integrity, they induce apoptosis. Unfortunately, they also tend to be cytotoxic toward normal cells. The reasons for selectively greater effects of cytotoxic drugs on malignant versus normal cells, as apparent in the cure of certain malignancies, are poorly understood, although the process of malignant transformation may enhance sensitivity to DNA damage.[18] In designing clinical regimens, the relationship of drug action to the cell cycle is of particular importance, because this knowledge serves as the basis for developing drug combinations and sequences in clinical practice and influences their use in combination with radiation therapy.

The cell cycle and its primary controls are shown in Figure 8-3. Antimetabolites such as methotrexate, 5-fluorouracil, cytosine arabinoside, gemcitabine, and the purine antagonists require cells to be actively proliferating to kill them; therefore, they are cell cycle dependent. Many of these agents, including cytosine arabinoside, fludarabine phosphate, and cladribine, must be incorporated into DNA to be cytotoxic. Alternately, agents such as etoposide and doxorubicin produce irreparable DNA strand breaks at any stage of the cell cycle, although these breaks become lethal only as the cell enters DNA synthesis. Still others, such as alkylating agents and platinum compounds, bind covalently to DNA and produce strand cross-links and strand breaks. Their toxicity seems less dependent on stage of the cell cycle; some agents of this class, such as the nitrosoureas, are equally capable of killing nondividing and dividing cells. Antimitotic agents, constituting a separate class of drugs, block the formation or dissociation of the mitotic spindle through their effects on microtubules and thereby prevent separation of chromosomes to the daughter cells. Drugs of this class are therefore most effective against cells that enter the mitotic phase of the cell cycle.

Once damaged through its encounter with a cytotoxic drug, the cancer cell has several options, and its eventual via-

Table 8-2 **Drug Discovery Strategies**

Strategy	Target	Test System for Identifying Lead Compound	Drug	References
Random screening of natural products, chemical libraries	No specific target	Cell culture cytotoxicity	Paclitaxel, BCNU	75
Rationally design antimetabolites	Nucleic acid synthesis	Cell culture cytotoxicity	Fludarabine	76
Inhibit oncogene	Farnesyl transferase	Inhibit protein function	Ras farnesylation inhibitors	77
	RAF message	Inhibit gene expression	RAF antisense oligonucleotide	78
Inhibit growth factor function	HER2/NEU, EGF receptor	Cell culture systems	Anti-HER2 antibody	79
Inhibit angiogenesis	VEGF	Human tumor xenografts	Anti-VEGF antibody	80
	Normal endothelial cells	Corneal vascular assays	Angiostatin, endostatin	81,82
Inhibit metastasis	Metalloproteinase	Enzyme inhibition	Marimastat	83

BCNU, carmustine; EGF, epidermal growth factor; VEGF, vascular endothelial growth factor.

bility depends on which pathway it takes. If the normal monitors for genomic integrity (including most prominently the product of the *TP53* gene) are intact, the cell may halt further progression in the cell cycle while its DNA is repaired. If the damage is sufficiently severe, intact TP53 may initiate apoptosis. If, however, the TP53 function is absent, cell cycle progression may continue despite drug-induced DNA damage, and the cell may prove viable. In most experimental settings, lack of wild-type TP53 is associated with drug and radiation resistance, but with certain drugs (e.g., paclitaxel), loss of the checkpoint function does not interfere with response.[19] Certain DNA repair defects, such as commonly found in mismatch repair (colon cancer), excision repair (ovarian cancer), or alkylation repair (gliomas), may be associated with resistance to drug action, perhaps by preventing recognition of DNA adducts and failing to initiate apoptosis.

From a theoretical viewpoint, it is understandable that rapidly dividing tumor cells, as found in leukemias, lymphomas, and choriocarcinomas, may be exquisitely sensitive to antimetabolites and cell cycle–specific drugs. How do these drugs kill the more slowly dividing solid tumors? Many of these tumors have long cell cycles (4 to 5 days). Many cells are in G_0 (nondividing state), and at any moment, only 1% to 3% of cells are in S phase. Cell kinetic factors diminish the effectiveness of chemotherapy, and the disordered vascularization of tumors may also contribute. Bulky tumors have chronically hypoxic regions, a low nutrient supply, and a leaking capillary vasculature that builds oncotic pressure and discourages the entry of small molecules into the extravascular space. In some tumors, blood flow sometimes may cease or even reverse due to the extravascular fluid pressure. Despite these disadvantages, solid tumor chemotherapy produces meaningful responses. Several factors, including pharmacologic, pharmacokinetic, and tumor cell specific, likely contribute to solid tumor killing:

1. Drugs such as paclitaxel persist in the extracellular fluid for several days after administration. Alternative regimens, such as prolonged drug infusion, seem to increase the activity of 5-fluorouracil, paclitaxel, and other drugs compared with the results of bolus administration.[20]
2. Other drugs, such as methotrexate, which forms intracellular polyglutamated species, and gemcitabine, which forms a long-lived intracellular triphosphate, persist inside the cell long after their disappearance from plasma.[21]
3. Tumor cells may be less able to repair DNA and more susceptible to cell death induced by DNA damage than their normal counterparts. For example, transformed mouse embryo fibroblasts have a heightened sensitivity to cancer drugs compared with their nontransformed parent, provided they have wild-type *TP53* genes.[18]
4. Underlying solid tumor proliferation is a significant cell death rate that results from a number of factors, such as hypoxia, nutrient deprivation, disordered DNA synthesis and mitosis, and in general, a high background rate of mutation that affects genes essential for cell integrity. A small shift in the balance between cell proliferation and cell death may lead to regression of a tumor, despite its low growth fraction.

DRUGS THAT TARGET THE CONTROLS OF CELL PROLIFERATION

Excessive proliferation of tumor cells has many causes, and from observations of tumor biology in model systems and in well-studied human cancers, the proliferative drive may result from sequential mutations that have several distinct effects. Some stimulate cell division (i.e., positive growth signals), whereas others free the cancer cell from normal cell cycle controls (i.e., loss of suppressor functions) or inactivate cell death pathways. Other cancer-causing mutations such as the DNA repair defects associated with familial nonpolyposis colon cancer and the loss of TP53 (previously designated p53 or P53) function increase the basic mutability of the genome; this mutability allows the generation of clones with inherent growth advantages. In the past few years, drug discovery efforts have targeted specific genetic defects (see Table 8-2). Among these mutations, a number of pharmaceutical companies have focused attention on dominant mutations, such as the activation of RAS in pancreatic, colon, and bladder cancer or the activation of cell surface growth factor pathways in epithelial tumors. Their choice of targets is largely driven by the fact that it is exceedingly ambitious if not impossible to develop a product that replaces a missing suppressor gene product such as TP53 or CDKN2A (previously designated p16).

Inhibiting the function of a dominant gene product is a classic problem in drug discovery. The first efforts at targeted inhibition of a signaling pathway led to development of inhibitors of the KRAS protein, a signal transducer that links growth factor receptors to downstream molecules. KRAS is mutated in 80% to 90% of pancreatic cancers and provides the proliferative drive in a number of human cancers.[18] The RAS protein is activated by a series of enzymatic steps that attach a lipid tail, a farnesyl group, to its near-terminal cysteine; methylate the cysteine; and cleave off the three terminal amino acids (Fig. 8-4). In this case, drug design is a relatively straightforward task in which a key enzymatic process or receptor is identified and a potent and specific inhibitor is developed. Several companies have focused on the farnesylation step in RAS processing as a necessary step in activating RAS and have found that inhibitors of farnesylation cause regression of experimental tumors. It is uncertain whether the antitumor effect of these compounds can be ascribed to their action on farnesylation of the RAS protein or on the farnesylation of other proteins. The first farnesylation inhibitors entered clinical trials in late 1997. They have shown some activity in the management of hematologic malignancies, but they have little activity in solid tumors.

A second pathway of great interest in modern cancer drug development is the RB pathway. Mutations may affect any one of the several genes and their proteins (e.g., CDKN2A, CDK4, CCND [cyclin D], RB1) constituting this pathway. These mutations have been found in a variety of human tumors and seem to be an essential step in converting tumors to a highly malignant phenotype. Several pharmaceutical firms have identified candidate inhibitors of cyclin-dependent kinases (CDKs), including CDK4, although most such compounds lack exquisite specificity for their target. One such compound, flavopiridol, an inhibitor of several CDKs, has shown promising activity in chronic lymphocytic leukemia.[23]

Other regulatory pathways have attracted the interest of drug discovery programs. The phosphatidylinositol-3-kinase (PI3K) pathway activates proliferation and downregulates the activity of the intrinsic pathway of apoptosis. Inhibitors of components of this pathway display antitumor activity in early trials, as in the early studies of rapamycin, an inhibitor of FRAP1 (previously designated MTOR) kinase.

In 2003, the U.S. Food and Drug Administration (FDA) approved bortezomib, a proteosome inhibitor, for patients who have progressed on prior therapy for multiple myeloma. Although the exact mechanism of action for this drug is unclear, it acts in part by downregulating nuclear factor-κB (NF-κB).[24] It is being tested in other hematologic malignancies and solid tumors by itself and in combination with cytotoxic chemotherapy and radiation therapy.

AREAS OF DRUG DISCOVERY: ANGIOGENESIS, METASTASIS, AND TARGETED THERAPY

Although most drug discovery efforts are aimed at pathways and targets that govern the balance of cell proliferation and cell death, other unique aspects of cancer biology have attracted notice, particularly the processes of angiogenesis and metastasis. Work has delineated the molecular mechanisms that allow tumor epithelial cells to metastasize. These cells are able to digest their basement membrane, move through interstitial spaces into capillaries, penetrate vessel walls, and adhere to the extracellular matrix at a distant site. Key to tissue penetration is the elaboration by tumors of metalloproteinases that digest collagen and elastin. Inhibitors of matrix metalloproteinases have entered clinical trials as antimetastatic and antiangiogenic agents, but as a class, the antimetastatic drugs

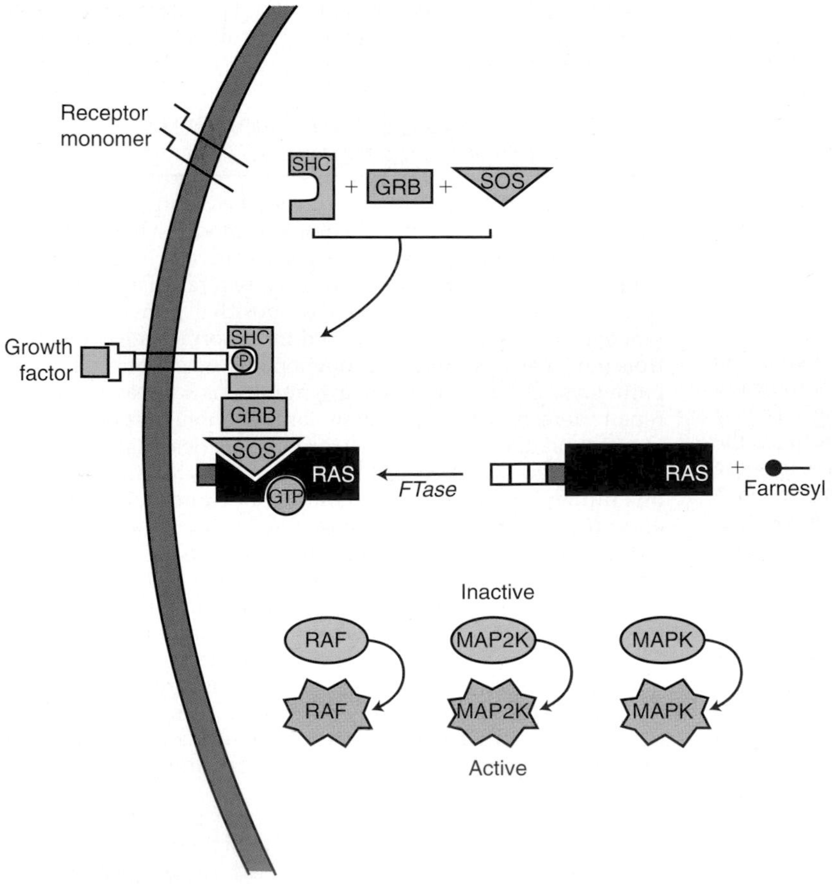

Figure 8-4 The signal transduction pathway is mediated by RAS. With the binding of a specific ligand, the growth factor receptor monomers dimerize. This dimerization induces autophosphorylation of tyrosine residues on the cytoplasmic side of the receptor dimer and subsequent binding of the SHC, GRB, and SOS molecules, which mediate the interactions between the tyrosine kinase, activity of the growth factor receptor, and membrane-bound RAS. Binding of SOS to RAS is thought to provoke a conformational change that allows RAS to bind guanosine triphosphate and become activated. Activated RAS interacts with and activates RAF, which induces a phosphorylation cascade of mitogen-activated protein kinase kinase (MAP2K, formerly designated MEK), mitogen-activated protein kinase (MAPK), and additional downstream transcriptional regulators. To be active, RAS must be modified posttranslationally by the addition of a lipophilic farnesyl group, which serves as its anchor in the plasma membrane. The farnesyl group is linked covalently to the cysteine residue, which is the fourth amino acid residue from the RAS carboxyl terminus, by the enzyme farnesyl transferase (FTase). This is followed by methylation of the cysteine residue and cleavage of the three carboxyl-terminal amino acids.

have been disappointing. The process of tumor angiogenesis has been traced to tumor cell secretion of angiogenic factors such as basic fibroblast growth factor and vascular endothelial growth factor (VEGF), and specific inhibitors of this process, such as anti-VEGF antibody, are now commercially available.[25]

In 2004, the humanized monoclonal antibody bevacizumab was approved by the FDA for the first-line treatment of metastatic colorectal cancer. Compared with chemotherapy alone, the addition of bevacizumab improved the response rate, progression-free survival, and overall survival.[26] Bevacizumab has demonstrated activity as a single agent in renal cell carcinoma, but in many solid tumors, it has little or no effect when used alone. Early results of a study of neoadjuvant 5-fluorouracil combined with radiation therapy for T3 rectal cancer demonstrated decrease in tumor perfusion, vascular volume, microvascular density, interstitial fluid pressure, and the number of viable circulating endothelial cells and progenitor cells after a single administration of bevacizumab.[27] It is anticipated that a reduction in interstitial pressure can improve oxygenation and delivery of the chemotherapy to the tumor, enhancing the radiosensitization properties of the chemotherapy. Bevacizumab targets the ligand VEGF (formerly designated VEGFA) (Table 8-3).

Other antibodies target the extracellular portion of the VEGF receptors and small molecules that inhibit the intracellular tyrosine kinase functions of these receptors. Some of these compounds have multiple targets, affecting more than one tyrosine kinase. One such example is Sunitinib (SU11248), a multitargeted tyrosine kinase inhibitor. Sunitinib (SU11248) inhibits KDR (formerly designated VEGFR or VEGFR2), KIT, and platelet-derived growth factor receptor (PDGFR). Preliminary studies have suggested activity in renal cell carcinoma and gastrointestinal stromal tumors. Another drug designed to target angiogenesis is Sorafenib (BAY 43-9006), an inhibitor of RAF kinase and KDR.

Epidermal growth factor receptor (EGFR) inhibitors constitute another class of agents that have proved useful in non–small cell lung cancer. EGFR is overexpressed in many solid tumors. It plays a critical role in cell cycle progression, proliferation, and survival. Its effects are mediated through RAS. Activation of EGFR is also associated with production of VEGF, leading to angiogenesis and facilitating metastasis. In 2003, the FDA approved the small-molecule tyrosine kinase inhibitor gefitinib as a single agent for the third-line treatment of non–small cell lung cancer (see Table 8-3).

Although 40% to 80% of non–small cell lung cancers overexpress EGFR, only about 10% to 19% of patients with chemotherapy-refractory non–small cell lung cancer respond to this therapy.[28-30] Responses are more frequent in women, nonsmokers, and patients with bronchoalveolar carcinoma or adenocarcinoma with bronchoalveolar features.[31] Mutations due to in-frame deletions or amino acid substitutions clustered around the ATP-binding pocket of the tyrosine kinase domain have been shown to predict response to gefitinib, suggesting a gain of function and increased sensitivity to gefitinib.[32,33]

In 2004, the FDA approved cetuximab, a chimeric monoclonal antibody targeting the extracellular portion of the EGFR, for the treatment of irinotecan-refractory colorectal cancer. The addition of irinotecan to cetuximab in this population results in almost doubling of the response rate, suggesting reversal of resistance. Surprisingly, however, when gefitinib or the related EGFR tyrosine kinase inhibitor erlotinib was added to standard chemotherapy in the first-line management of patients with advanced non–small cell lung cancer, there was no improvement in response or survival. Cetuximab has also proved to be an active agent in the management of squamous cell carcinoma of the head and neck, with or without radiation.[34,35]

Another tyrosine kinase inhibitor, imatinib, was designed to target the BCR/ABL mutation that causes chronic myelogenous leukemia. It was also found to inhibit the KIT (CD117) receptor, and it has proved to be a powerful agent in the management of gastrointestinal stromal tumors. Overexpression of KIT is not the sole predictor of response to imatinib, because this agent has been shown to be ineffective in small cell lung cancer, a tumor that overexpresses KIT. Identification of specific activating mutations within the *KIT* gene predicts for response in patients with gastrointestinal stromal tumors (see Table 8-3).[36] The multitargeted tyrosine kinase inhibitor Sunitinib (SU11248) has demonstrated benefit in imatinib-refractory patients, even in those with mutations that are typically associated with a low response rate to imatinib.[37]

Thalidomide was initially developed as a sedative, but it was taken off the market in the early 1960s when it was found to cause congenital birth defects. These congenital defects led investigators to postulate that the drug interfered with vasculogenesis. It has long been used in the treatment of erythema nodosum leprosum. Its role in angiogenesis was confirmed in a rabbit cornea micropocket assay. The exact mechanisms of action remain unclear. Thalidomide and its metabolites modulate inflammatory cytokines such as tumor necrosis factor-α, γ-interferon, interleukin-12, cyclooxygenase-2, and possibly NF-κB. It also inhibits interleukin-6 and the stimulating effects of insulin-like growth factor-1. Thalidomide is an important

Table 8-3 Approved Targeted Therapies

Drug	Class	Target	Application
Imatinib (Gleevec)	Benzamide	BCR/ABL	CML, GIST
Gefitinib (Iressa)	Quinazolinamine	EGFR-TKI	NSCLC
Cetuximab (Erbitux)	Chimeric monoclonal antibody	EGFR extracellular domain	Colorectal, ENT
Trastuzumab (Herceptin)	Humanized monoclonal antibody	HER2 extracellular domain	Breast
Bevacizumab (Avastin)	Humanized monoclonal antibody	VEGF (formerly VEGFA)	Colorectal
Bortezomib (Velcade)	Modified boronic acid	Proteosome	Myeloma
Rituximab (Rituxan)	Chimeric monoclonal antibody	CD20	Lymphoma
Tositumomab (Bexxar)	^{131}I murine monoclonal antibody	CD20	Lymphoma
Ibritumomab (Zevalin)	^{111}In murine monoclonal antibody	CD20	Lymphoma
Alemtuzumab (Campath)	Humanized monoclonal antibody	CD52	B-CLL
Gemtuzumab (Mylotarg)	Calicheamicin linked to human monoclonal antibody	CD33	AML (CD33$^+$)

AML, acute myelocytic leukemia; B-CLL, B-cell chronic lymphocytic leukemia; CML, chronic myelogenous leukemia; GIST, gastrointestinal stromal tumor; NSCLC, non–small cell lung cancer.

secondary therapy for multiple myeloma, and it is being investigated in several other malignant diseases. Less toxic and potentially more effective thalidomide analogues have been developed and are now commercially available.[38]

Arsenic trioxide is another rediscovered drug and is approved for the management of acute promyelocytic leukemia. Similar to thalidomide, the exact mechanisms of action responsible for its efficacy are unclear. It appears to be antiproliferative and antiangiogenic. Its antiproliferative effects are mediated through the inactivation of cyclins and cyclin-dependent kinases.[39] Exposure of human xenograft models has been shown to induce apoptosis of endothelial cells in new blood vessels. Arsenic trioxide has been shown to inhibit production of VEGF in a leukemic cell line.[40]

PHARMACOKINETICS AND PHARMACODYNAMICS

In the treatment of cancer patients, the ultimate effectiveness of therapy is determined by three factors: the inherent sensitivity of the tumor, the ability to deliver drug to its site of action in therapeutic concentrations, and the limitations of host toxicity. It is generally not possible, except in hematologic malignancies, to measure drug concentrations in tumor, although new imaging techniques such as positron emission tomography and nuclear magnetic resonance do allow the pharmacologist to follow the distribution and transformations of some drugs noninvasively in humans. The pharmacokinetic profile of drug in plasma, or change in drug concentration over time, represents the closest correlate of tumor exposure accessible to measurement in the usual clinical setting. In the initial clinical trials of new agents, pharmacokinetic studies are critical for determining whether cytotoxic drug concentrations are achieved and for adjusting the route and schedule of drug administration to achieve an optimal profile, as suggested by preclinical models. In phase II and III trials, pharmacokinetics can yield important additional information on the effects of age, gender, and organ dysfunction on drug clearance. Pharmacokinetic studies can reveal the existence of drug interactions. Correlations between pharmacokinetic and pharmacodynamic end points, such as organ toxicity and therapeutic outcome, are more difficult to establish, but some important insights into these relationships have been identified for several anticancer drugs (Table 8-4).

For antimetabolites, most natural product drugs, and platinum compounds, pharmacodynamic end points such as antitumor effects and toxicity to bone marrow and intestinal epithelium correlate best with the area under the plasma concentration time curve (see Fig. 8-2). For other drugs, such as paclitaxel, the duration of time above a threshold plasma concentration (0.05 to 0.1 μM) correlates best with toxicity to marrow, and there is preliminary evidence that duration above a threshold level also correlates with clinical effectiveness (see Fig. 8-2).[41] Only for alkylating agents, which display a relatively simple relationship between peak plasma concentration and toxicity, has the duration of systemic exposure had little correlation with the pharmacologic effect. In this instance, dose rather than drug concentration over time correlates best with toxicity and tumor cell kill.

DETERMINANTS OF DRUG CLEARANCE

Anticancer drugs are cleared from the body by one or a combination of several mechanisms, including renal excretion, hepatic metabolism, chemical decomposition, or metabolic alteration at extrahepatic sites (Table 8-5). Considerable variation is often found among individuals in their ability to clear anticancer drugs, which may necessitate dose adjustment for patients presenting with renal or hepatic dysfunction. Other factors, such as gender, age, serum albumin concentration, lean body mass, nutritional status, and performance status, can influence the pharmacokinetic behavior and pharmacologic effect of a drug, but their quantitative impact on drug disposition is difficult to predict. Inherited defects in metabolic capability may lead to severe unexpected toxicity for drugs such as 5-fluorouracil (i.e., dihydropyrimidine dehydrogenase deficiency)[42] and 6-mercaptopurine (i.e., thiopurine methyltransferase deficiency).[43] Genetic variation in the UDP-glucuronosyltransferase 1A1 gene *(UGT1A)*, which is associated with Gilbert's syndrome, results in severe toxicity, primarily neutropenia, in patients receiving irinotecan because of the inability to adequately glucuronidate the active compound, SN-38.[44]

When drugs are used in combination, the potential for interactions that enhance or inhibit antitumor effects becomes an important consideration. Synergistic effects have been convincingly demonstrated for a number of combinations in experimental systems, but clinical results are difficult to interpret. The success of drug combinations against acute leukemia, lymphomas, testicular cancer, and breast cancer (in the adjuvant setting), when single drugs have only temporary effects, probably represents clinical synergy. In other circumstances, drug action may be enhanced by the concurrent administration of a second agent that increases drug binding to its target, such as leucovorin (5-formyl tetrahydrofolate) enhancement of 5-fluorouracil binding to thymidylate synthase. Purely pharmacokinetic interactions of cancer drugs with antibiotics, anti-inflammatory agents, and psychotropic

Table 8-4 Pharmacodynamic Relationships of Chemotherapeutic Agents in Cancer Patients

Drug	Clinical Effect	Pharmacokinetic Correlate	References
Busulfan	Hepatotoxicity	AUC	84
Buthionine sulfoximine	Intracellular GSH depletion	C_p profile (indirect response model)	85
Carboplatin	Thrombocytopenia	AUC	86
Cisplatin	Nephrotoxicity	C_{max} (unchanged drug)	87
Doxorubicin	Cardiotoxicity	C_{max}	88
Etoposide phosphate	Myelosuppression	AUC (etoposide)	89
Fludarabine phosphate	Leukopenia	AUC	90
5-Fluorouracil	Risk of toxicity	AUC	91
Methotrexate	Response	C_{max}	92
Paclitaxel	Neutopenia	Time above threshold C_p	93
Topotecan	Neutropenia	AUC (total drug)	94

AUC, area under the plasma concentration-time profile; C_{max} maximum plasma concentration; C_p plasma concentration; GSH, glutathione.

Table 8-5 Clearance Mechanisms of Anticancer Drugs

Primary Clearance Mechanism	Drug	Dose Modification for Organ Dysfunction
Hepatic metabolism		
CYP450-mediated oxidation	Busulfan	Y
	Chlorambucil	N
	Cyclophosphamide*	N
	Ifosfamide*	N
	Paclitaxel	Y
	Thiotepa	N
	Vinca alkaloids	Y
Reduction	Mitomycin C*	N
Conjugation	Etoposide	N
	6-Mercaptopurine	Y†
Soluble enzymes	Ara-C	N
	5-Fluorouracil	Y‡
	Gemcitabine	N
Nonenzymatic hydrolysis	Camptothecins	N
	BCNU*	N
	Mechlorethamine	N
	Melphalan	N
Biliary excretion	Doxorubicin	P
	Irinotecan	N
	Vinca alkaloids	Y
Renal excretion	Bleomycin	Y
	Carboplatin	Y
	Deoxycoformycin	Y
	Etoposide	Y
	Fludarabine	Y
	Hydroxyurea	Y
	Methotrexate	Y
	Topotecan	Y

*Enzymatic or spontaneous chemical reactions required for drug activation.
†S-methyltransferase deficiency.
‡Dihydropyrimidine dehydrogenase deficiency.
Y, yes; N, no; P, probably.

drugs may lead to unexpected complications or a lack of drug effect; the more important examples are shown in Table 8-6.

PREDICTING TUMOR RESPONSE

Pharmacogenomics may enable the clinician to determine which drugs will be poorly tolerated by an individual and may allow more rational selection of a particular antineoplastic agent in the individual patient. For example, a high level of thymidylate synthase (TYMS), the result of a polymorphism in tandem repeats in the gene's promoter region, predicts for resistance to 5-fluorouracil in patients with colorectal cancer.[45] Although it is tempting to rely on such information from the primary tumor, TYMS levels within metastases of various locations may be very different. Genomic polymorphisms in the DNA repair genes *ERCC2* (formerly designated *XPD*) and *XRCC1* may be prognostic factors in patients with non–small cell lung cancer treated with cisplatin.[46] Genomic polymorphisms in *ERCC1*, *GSTP1*, and the *TYMS* 3′ untranslated region also may be helpful in predicting prognosis in patients with colorectal cancer receiving 5-fluorouracil and oxaliplatin.[47]

SCHEDULES OF DRUG ADMINISTRATION

Cancer drugs are given in repetitive cycles of administration interrupted by rest periods that facilitate the recovery of normal tissues, particularly bone marrow and gastrointestinal mucosa. With the availability of myeloid stimulatory factors such as granulocyte colony-stimulating factor, it is possible to dramatically shorten the period between cycles. The ability to provide such dose-dense therapy with the aid of growth colony-stimulating factor may result in improved outcome without increase in toxicity.[48] The theoretical basis for cyclic chemotherapy was established by the work of Skipper and Schabel, who showed in animal models that for any given drug schedule and dose, a specific fraction of tumor cells is killed. Repeated cycles of treatment are therefore required for curative therapy. Whether it is necessary to eliminate the last tumor cell to cure the disease is still in doubt. Molecular markers for residual disease may continue to show the presence of tumor-related sequences years after remission induction in children with acute leukemia, although in diseases such as breast cancer and other solid tumors, such findings are usually the harbinger of relapse.[49]

Although peak drug plasma concentration, AUC, and time over a threshold level have been correlated with response and toxicity for selected agents, clinical investigators lack pharmacokinetic data for most combination therapy regimens. The end point in combination clinical studies is typically to maximize dose intensity, which is the amount of drug administered per unit of time. Clinical data support a strong relationship between dose intensity and response in the treatment of breast, ovarian, and colon tumors.[50] Taken to its extreme, high-dose chemotherapy with bone marrow stem cell replacement yields the highest dose intensity and the highest response rates in otherwise refractory tumors, but at a high dollar cost and at the risk of fatal toxicity. In practice, most oncologists believe that it is important to administer full doses of drug, using completely reversible and readily tolerated toxicity as their end point.

DRUG RESISTANCE

The fractional cell kill hypothesis must be modified to incorporate concepts of drug resistance. In practice, the response to an initial cycle of chemotherapy may be much greater than to subsequent doses, and in many solid tumors, such as breast cancer and lung cancer, tumors may again grow rapidly after an initial response. The explanation for this finding lies in the problem of drug resistance and the ability of cancer drugs to select for drug-resistant cells. Mechanisms of resistance may affect any of the steps necessary for drug action: entry of drug into tumor cells by means of active transporters, enzymatic drug activation, action at a molecular target within cells, and even the processes in the cell that trigger cell death. Although many examples of drug resistance have been characterized in model systems, the understanding of resistance in clinical practice remains incomplete. Some of the more common mechanisms in model systems and the evidence for their presence in human tumors are given in Table 8-6.

With few exceptions, single-agent treatment of cancer produces only temporary responses. Exceptions may include the use of methotrexate for treating choriocarcinoma and cyclophosphamide for treating Burkitt's lymphoma. The reason for the development of resistance is that at the time of clinical recognition, tumors are significantly heterogeneous because of their underlying genetic instability. Only the sensitive fraction of cells is killed with each dose of drug. Drug-resistant mutants already exist at the time of initial treatment,

Table 8-6 **Drug Resistance Mechanisms in Cancer Chemotherapy**

Molecular Mechanism	Example	Drugs Affected
Decrease in cellular uptake	Deletion of folate transporter Deletion of nucleoside transporter	Methotrexate Ara-C
Increase in cellular efflux	Multidrug resistance (CD116)	Vinca alkaloids Anthracyclines Paclitaxel
Alteration of target protein	Mutant dihydrofolate reductase Mutant topoisomerase I Mutant tubulin	Methotrexate Topotecan Vinca alkaloids Paclitaxel
Deletion of target protein	Deletion of topoisomerase I Deletion of topoisomerase II	Topotecan Anthracyclines Etoposide
Deletion of activating enzyme	Deoxycytidine kinase	Ara-C
Alteration of apoptosis pathways	Mutant TP53, BCL2	Alkylating agents Antimetabolites

From Chabner BA, Longo DL (eds): Cancer Chemotherapy and Biotherapy: Principles and Practice, 2nd ed. Philadelphia, Lippincott-Raven, 1996.

and under the selective pressure of therapy, they expand in number in the presence of the drug. Based on the experience of antibiotic treatment of bacterial infections, it was logical to combine drugs that had different mechanisms of resistance. If the frequency of mutation to resistance is 1 cell of 10^6, the chances of any cell being simultaneously resistant to two drugs would be the product of these probabilities, or 10^{-12}. Goldie and colleagues have argued convincingly that the best strategy for chemotherapy is to employ as many non–cross-resistant agents as early as possible in the treatment regimen.[51] Certain qualifying considerations include the following:

1. Drug resistance, such as the overexpression of the multidrug resistance drug transport system, may confer resistance to broad categories of drugs rather than to single agents, as may defects in cell death pathways, enhanced DNA repair, poor tumor blood flow, or other biologic factors.[52]
2. Simultaneous administration of multiple agents may lead to overwhelming toxicity, inhibitory drug interactions at the molecular target, or unwanted pharmacokinetic interactions. Because of negative interactions, multiple agents may be given sequentially, rather than simultaneously, with more favorable outcome.[53]

COMBINATION CHEMOTHERAPY

With few exceptions, multiagent therapy has proved more effective than single-agent therapy in the treatment of most human cancers. In general, the choice of drugs for combination therapy is made on the basis of mechanistic, pharmacokinetic, and toxicologic considerations. The most important criteria for including drugs in a combination regimen are the following:

1. Single-agent activity in the disease to be treated
2. Nonoverlapping toxicities, allowing full doses of each drug to be used
3. Different mechanisms of action
4. Nonoverlapping mechanisms of resistance

These are not hard and fast rules. There are numerous examples of clinical regimens that employ multiple alkylating agents, multiple natural products (despite their shared cross-resistance), or combinations of myelotoxic drugs. Often, these choices are dictated by impressive single-agent activity in the tumor being treated and the uncertainty of knowledge about clinical mechanisms of drug resistance. For example, individual alkylating agents differ in their mechanisms of activation, transport, and adduct formation. Their DNA adducts are repaired by a variety of enzymatic pathways. It is not clear which of these factors contributes to clinical drug resistance (see Table 8-6). Although these agents belong to the same class of drugs, in the absence of more complete knowledge about resistance, it is possible to construct a reasonable argument for combining different alkylating agents.

CLINICAL SCHEDULES OF DRUG ADMINISTRATION

In developing a chemotherapy regimen, the clinical investigator must choose from a wide range of options regarding route, schedule, and sequence of drug administration. A number of factors determine the final choice of schedule of administration, including the following:

1. *Pharmacokinetics of the individual agents in humans.* Specific factors, such as peak drug concentration and clearance from plasma, desired AUC, and duration of drug concentration above a threshold, are central considerations (see Fig. 8-2). In general, clinical investigators attempt to reproduce a profile of drug concentration and duration of exposure that mimics optimal conditions in experimental systems.
2. *Cell cycle kinetics and cell cycle phase specificity of the agent.* If the agent in question exerts its effects only against cells in a specific phase of the cell cycle, the schedule must be planned to ensure a maximum duration of drug concentration above the threshold. In practice, the best example is the prolonged infusion of antimetabolites (i.e., 5-fluorouracil or cytosine arabinoside given by continuous infusion). Most dividing cells in a relatively rapid growing tumor such as acute myelocytic leukemia are exposed to drug during their DNA synthetic phase if the infusion of cytosine arabinoside lasts for 7 days.

Table 8-7 **Pharmacokinetic Drug Interactions Involving Anticancer Agents**

Chemotherapeutic Agent	Interacting Drugs	Effect on Anticancer Drug Clearance	Probable Mechanism	References
Cyclophosphamide	Phenobarbital	↑	CYP450 enzyme induction	95,96
Doxorubicin	Cyclosporine	↓	Inhibit P-glycoprotein–mediated biliary excretion	97,98
Methotrexate	Aspirin, penicillins	↓	Inhibit tubular secretion	99-101
	Cephalosporins	↑	Inhibit tubular resorption	
Paclitaxel	Verapamil	↓	Inhibit CYP450 metabolism or biliary excretion	102
Vidarabine	Deoxycoformycin	↓	Inhibit adenosine deaminase	103
Vinblastine	Erythromycin	↓	Inhibit CYP450 metabolism	104

3. *Drug interactions*. Interactions that alter pharmacokinetic behavior or enhance or inhibit cytotoxicity (Table 8-7) may dictate the use of a specific schedule or sequence of drug administration.
4. *Drug interactions with irradiation*. The growing interest in combined-modality treatment for solid tumors stems from the expectation that many cancer drugs act as radiosensitizers. In most instances, the maximum radiosensitization is realized if the drug is present during the exposure of tumor to irradiation. Continuous drug infusion or daily administration is favored, although rigorous proof that one schedule is better than another is often lacking. Paclitaxel, 5-fluorouracil, cisplatin, carboplatin, and mitomycin C are potent radiosensitizers.
5. *Toxicity*. Most chemotherapy regimens are developed to allow rapid and complete recovery of normal tissues between cycles of treatment. Ultimately, toxicity limits the dose of drug employed and the duration of administration. If drugs are used in combination with other treatment modalities, further limitations of schedule and dose may be imposed. For example, the radiosensitizing effect of cisplatin-based chemotherapy on mucosa or bone marrow may limit the dose of radiation therapy and chemotherapy if the two are given concurrently and if the field of irradiation includes the marrow, gut, or other epithelial surfaces.
6. *Convenience and cost*. Oral drug administration is the easiest and least expensive way to give drugs. However, because of variable and often limited oral bioavailability of cancer drugs, only a few agents are given by the oral route. Intravenous administration guarantees entry of the full dose into the bloodstream. Intermittent bolus schedules are usually favored, although pharmacokinetic or cell cycle kinetic considerations can pose strong arguments for prolonged infusion schedules. An example of such a phase-specific drug is the antimetabolite 5-fluorouracil. Several studies have demonstrated improved response and reduced toxicity when 5-fluorouracil is administered as a continuous infusion. Reluctance to adopt this method of administration can be attributed to difficulties in reimbursement and the need for patients to have a chronic indwelling venous catheter. This therapy may be administered on an outpatient basis by means of small ambulatory pumps.

SUMMARY

The potential for cancer chemotherapy to aid in the cure of cancer has been fully realized in only a few clinical circumstances, primarily those in which a rapidly proliferating hematologic malignancy has been treated aggressively with a multiagent regimen. Solid tumor chemotherapy, if it is to be employed with curative intent, must be given early in the course of disease, carefully interdigitated with irradiation and surgery, and given in maximal doses. Because of the likelihood of serious side effects and drug-radiation interactions, such regimens are difficult to design and implement. The development of optimal chemoradiotherapy regimens must take into account the advantages and disadvantages of sequential versus concurrent combined-modality approaches. To maximize therapeutic synergy and minimize toxicity, protocol planning must pay careful attention to potential drug-radiation interaction, drug pharmacokinetics, and drug-drug interactions. The patient population being treated (often elderly patients with comorbidity due to heart disease, hypertension, and other evidence of organ dysfunction) may have limited ability to tolerate the rigors of combined-modality treatment. Our hopes and expectations are that advances in cancer biology, particularly in the areas of angiogenesis and metastasis, will lead to newer, more tumor-specific, and less toxic approaches to cancer control.

REFERENCES

1. Goodman LS, Wintrobe MM, Dameshek W, et al: Use of methyl-bis(beta-chloroethyl)amine hydrochloride for Hodgkin's disease, lymphosarcoma, leukemia. JAMA 132:126, 1946.
2. DeVita VT, Hellman S, Rosenberg SA (eds): Cancer: Principles and Practice of Oncology, 4th ed. Philadelphia, JB Lippincott, 1993.
3. Elion GB: Biochemistry and pharmacology of purine analogs. Fed Proc 26:898, 1967.
4. Johnson IS: Historical background of *Vinca* alkaloid research and areas of future interest. Cancer Chemother Rep 52:455, 1968.
5. Wakaki S, Marumo H, Tomioka K: Isolation of new fractions of antitumor mitomycins. Antibiot Chemother 8:228, 1958.
6. Umezawa H, Maeda K, Takeuchi T, et al: New antibiotics, bleomycin A and B. J Antibiot (Tokyo) 19:200, 1966.
7. Arcamone F, Cassinelli G, Fantini G, et al: Adriamycin, 14-hydroxydaunomycin, a new antitumor antibiotic from *S. peucetius* var. *caesius*. Biotechnol Bioeng 11:1101, 1969.
8. Wani MC, Taylor HL, Wall ME, et al: Plant antitumor agents. VI. The isolation and structure of Taxol, a novel antileukemic and antitumor agent from *Taxus brevifolia*. J Am Chem Soc 93:2325, 1971.
9. Wall ME, Wani MC, Cook CE, et al: Plant antitumor agents. I. The isolation and structure of camptothecin, a novel alkaloidal leukemia and tumor inhibitor from *Camptotheca acuminata*. J Am Chem Soc 88:3888, 1966.
10. Skipper HE, Perry S: Kinetics of normal and leukemic leukocyte populations and relevance to chemotherapy. Cancer Res 30:1883, 1970.
11. Reiter A, Schrappe M, Ludwig WD, et al: Chemotherapy in 998 unselected childhood acute lymphoblastic leukemia patients:

results and conclusions of the multicenter trial ALL-BFM 86. Blood 84:3122, 1994.
12. Heidelberger C, Chaudhuari NK, Daneberg P, et al: Fluorinated pyrimidines: a new class of tumor inhibitory compounds. Nature 179:663, 1957.
13. Huang P, Chubb S, Hertel LW, et al: Action of 2′,2′-difluorodeoxycytidine on DNA synthesis. Cancer Res 51:6110, 1991.
14. Fisher B, Dignam J, Wolmark N, et al: Tamoxifen and chemotherapy for lymph node–negative, estrogen receptor-positive breast cancer. J Natl Cancer Inst 89:1673, 1997.
15. Series: Multimodality treatment of cancer. Oncology 11(Suppl 9):9, 1997.
16. Hanahan D, Weinberg RA: The hallmarks of cancer. Cell 100:57, 2000.
17. Barinaga M: From bench top to bedside. Science 278:1036, 1997.
18. Lowe SW, Ruley HE, Jacks T, et al: *P53*-dependent apoptosis modulates the cytotoxicity of anticancer agents. Cell 74:957, 1993.
19. Li Y, Benzera R: Identification of a human mitotic checkpoint gene: *hsMAD2.* Science 274:246, 1996.
20. Koc ON, Phillips WP Jr, Lee K, et al: Role of DNA repair in resistance to drugs that alkylate O^6 of guanine. Cancer Treat Res 87:123, 1996.
21. Gorlick R, Goker E, Trippett T, et al: Defective transport is a common mechanism of acquired methotrexate resistance in acute lymphocytic leukemia and is associated with decreased reduced folate carrier expression. Blood 89:1013, 1997.
22. Gibbs JB, Oliff A, Kohl NE: Farnesyltransferase inhibitors: Ras research yields a potential cancer therapeutic. Cell 77:175, 1994.
23. Lin TS, Dalton JT, Wu D, et al: Flavopiridol given as a 30 minute intravenous bolus followed by 4-hr continuous IV infusion results in clinical activity and tumor lysis in refractory chronic lymphocytic leukemia [abstract 6564]. Proceedings of the American Society of Clinical Oncology, Chicago, 2004.
24. Voorhees PM, Dees EC, O'Neil B, et al: The proteosome as a target for cancer therapy. Clin Cancer Res 9:6316, 2003.
25. Folkman J: Angiogenic therapy. *In* Devita VT, Rosenberg SA, Hellman S (eds): Cancer: Principles and Practice of Oncology, 5th ed. Philadelphia, Lippincott-Raven, 1997, p 3075.
26. Hurwitz H, Fehrenbacher L, Novotny W, et al: Bevacizumab plus irinotecan, fluorouracil and leucovorin for metastatic colorectal cancer. N Engl J Med 350:2335, 2004.
27. Willett C, Boucher Y, di Tomaso E, et al: Direct evidence that the VEGF-specific antibody bevacizumab has antivascular effects in human rectal cancer. Nat Med 10:145, 2004.
28. Artega CL: Erb-B targeted therapeutic approaches in human cancer. Exp Cell Res 284:122, 2003.
29. Kris MG, Natale RB, Herbst RB, et al: Efficacy of gefitinib, an inhibitor of the epidermal growth factor receptor tyrosine kinase, in symptomatic patients with non–small cell lung cancer: a randomized trial. JAMA 290:2149, 2003.
30. Fukuoka M, Yano S, Giaccone G, et al: Randomized Multi-institutional phase II trial of gefitinib for previously treated patients with advanced non–small-cell lung cancer. J Clin Oncol 21:2237, 2003.
31. Shah NT, Miller VA, et al: Bronchoalveolar histology and smoking history predict response to gefitinib [abstract 2524]. Proceedings of the American Association of Clinical Oncology, Orlando, Florida, 2003.
32. Lynch TJ, Bell DW, Sordella R, et al: Activating mutations in the epidermal growth factor receptor underlying responsiveness of non–small cell lung cancer to gefitinib. N Engl J Med 35:2129, 2003.
33. Paez JG, Janne PA, Lee JC, et al: EGFR mutations in lung cancer: correlation with clinical response to gefitinib therapy. Science 304:1497, 2004.
34. Bonner JA, Giralt J, Harari PM, et al: Cetuximab prolongs survival in patients with locoregionally advanced squamous cell carcinoma of the head and neck: a phase III study of high dose radiation therapy with or without cetuximab [abstract 5507]. Proceedings of the American Society of Clinical Oncology, Chicago, 2004.
35. Trigo J, Hitt R, Koralewski P, et al: Cetuximab monotherapy is active in patients with platinum-refractory recurrent/metastatic squamous cell carcinoma of the head and neck: results of a phase II study [abstract 5502]. Proceedings of the American Society of Clinical Oncology, Chicago, 2004.
36. Heinrich MC, Corless CL, Demetri GD, et al: Kinase mutations and imatinib response in patients with metastatic gastrointestinal stromal tumor. J Clin Oncol 21:4342, 2003.
37. Demetri GD, Desai J, Fletcher JA, et al: SU11248, a multi-targeted tyrosine kinase inhibitor, can overcome imatinib resistance caused by diverse genomic mechanisms in patients with metastatic gastrointestinal stromal tumor [abstract 3001]. Proceedings of the American Association of Clinical Oncology, Chicago, 2004.
38. Franks ME, Macpherson GR, Figg WD: Thalidomide. Lancet 363:1802, 2004.
39. Lew YS, Brown SL, Griffin RJ, et al: Arsenic trioxide causes selective necrosis in solid murine tumors by vascular shutdown. Cancer Res 59:6033, 1999.
40. Roboz GJ, Dias S, Lam G, et al: Arsenic trioxide induces dose- and time-dependent apoptosis of endothelium and may exert an antileukemic effect via inhibition of angiogenesis. Blood 96:1525, 2000.
41. Wilson WH, Berg S, Bryant G, et al: Paclitaxel in doxorubicin-refractory or mitoxantrone-refractory breast cancer: a phase I/II trial of 96-hour infusion. J Clin Oncol 12:1621, 1994.
42. Diasio RB, Beavers TL, Carpenter T: Familial deficiency of dihydropyrimidine dehydrogenase: biochemical basis for familial pyrimidinemia and severe 5-fluorouracil–induced toxicity. J Clin Invest 81:47, 1988.
43. Lennard L, VanLoon JA, Weinshilboum RM: Pharmacogenetics of acute azathioprine toxicity: relationship to thiopurine methyltransferase genetic polymorphism. Clin Pharmacol Ther 46:149, 1989.
44. Innocenti F, Undevia SD, Iyer L, et al: Genetic variants in the UDP-glucuronyltransferase 1A1 gene predict the risk of severe neutropenia of irinotecan. J Clin Oncol 22:1382, 2004.
45. Marsh S, McLeod HL: Cancer pharmacogenetics. Br J Cancer 90:8, 2004.
46. Gurubhagavatula S, Liu G, Park S, et al: XPD and XRCC1 genetic polymorphisms are prognostic factors in advanced non–small-cell lung cancer patients treated with platinum chemotherapy. J Clin Oncol 22:2594, 2004.
47. Stoehlmacher J, Park DJ, Zhang W, et al: A multivariate analysis of genomic polymorphisms: prediction of clinical outcome to 5-FU/oxaliplatin combination chemotherapy in refractory colorectal cancer. Br J Cancer 91:344, 2004.
48. Citron ML, Berry DA, Cirrincione C, et al: Randomized trial of dose-dense versus conventionally scheduled and sequential versus concurrent combination chemotherapy as postoperative adjuvant treatment of node-positive primary breast cancer: first report of Intergroup C9741/Cancer and Leukemia Group B Trial 9741. J Clin Oncol 21:2226, 2003.
49. Cote RJ, Taylor C, Neville AM: Detection of occult metastases. Cancer J 8:49, 1997.
50. Hryniuk WM, Levine MN, Levin L: Analysis of dose intensity for chemotherapy in early stage (stage II) and advanced breast cancer. Natl Cancer Inst Monogr 1:87, 1986.
51. Goldie JH, Coldman AJ, Gudanskas GA: Rationale for the use of alternating non–cross-resistant chemotherapy. Cancer Treat Rep 65:439, 1982.
52. Sidransky D, Hollstein M: Clinical implications of the *p53* gene. Annu Rev Med 47:285, 1996.
53. Gianni L, Munzone E, Capri G, et al: Paclitaxel by 3-hour infusion in combination with bolus doxorubicin in women with untreated metastatic breast cancer: high antitumor efficacy and cardiac effects in a dose-finding and sequence-finding study. J Clin Oncol 13:2688, 1995.
54. Al-Sarraf M, Martz K, Herskovic A, et al: Progress report of combined chemoradiotherapy versus radiotherapy alone in patients with esophageal cancer: an intergroup study. J Clin Oncol 15:277, 1997.
55. Walsh TN, Noonan N, Hollywood D, et al: A comparison of multimodal therapy and surgery for esophageal adenocarcinoma. N Engl J Med 335:462, 1996.
56. Rosell R, Gomez-Codina J, Camps C, et al: A randomized trial comparing preoperative chemotherapy plus surgery with

surgery alone in patients with non–small cell lung cancer. N Engl J Med 330:153, 1994.

57. Piccart MJ, de Valeriola D, Paridaens R, et al: Six-year results of a multimodality treatment strategy for locally advanced breast cancer. Cancer 62:2501, 1988.
58. Scholl SM, Fourquet A, Asselain B, et al: Neoadjuvant versus adjuvant chemotherapy in premenopausal patients with tumours considered too large for breast-conserving surgery: preliminary results of a randomized trial-S6. Eur J Cancer 30A:645, 1994.
59. Krook JE, Moertel CG, Gunderson LL, et al: Effective surgical adjuvant therapy for high-risk rectal carcinoma. N Engl J Med 324:709, 1991.
60. Tepper JE, O'Connell MJ, Petroni GR, et al: Adjuvant postoperative fluorouracil-modulated chemotherapy combined with pelvic radiation therapy for rectal cancer: initial results of intergroup 0114. J Clin Oncol 15:2030, 1997.
61. Overgaard M, Hansen PS, Overgaard J, et al: Postoperative radiotherapy in high-risk premenopausal women with breast cancer who receive adjuvant chemotherapy. Danish Breast Cancer Cooperative Group 82b trial. N Engl J Med 337:949, 1997.
62. Ragaz J, Jackson SM, Le N, et al: Adjuvant radiotherapy and chemotherapy in node-positive premenopausal women with breast cancer. N Engl J Med 337:956, 1997.
63. Dillman RO, Herndon J, Seagren SL, et al: Improved survival in stage III non–small cell lung cancer: seven-year follow-up of cancer and leukemia group B (CALGB) 8433 trial. J Natl Cancer Inst 88:1210, 1996.
64. Pignon JP, Arriagada R, Ihde DC, et al: A meta-analysis of thoracic radiotherapy for small cell lung cancer. N Engl J Med 327:1618, 1992.
65. Al-Sarraf M, LeBlanc M, Giri PGS, et al: Superiority of chemoradiotherapy (CT-RT) versus radiotherapy (RT) in patients (PTS) with locally advanced nasopharyngeal cancer (NPC): preliminary results of intergroup (0099) (SWOG 8892, RTOG 8817, ECOG 2388) randomized study [abstract 882]. Proceedings of the American Society of Clinical Oncology, Philadelphia, 1996.
66. Fabian CJ, Mansfield CM, Dahlberg S, et al: Low-dose involved field radiation after chemotherapy in advanced Hodgkin disease: a Southwest Oncology Group randomized study. Ann Intern Med 120:903, 1994.
67. Glick JH, Kim K, Earle J, O'Connell MJ: An ECOG randomized phase III trial of CHOP vs. CHOP + radiotherapy (XRT) for intermediate-grade early-stage non-Hodgkin's lymphoma (NHL) [abstract 1221]. Proceedings of the American Society of Clinical Oncology, Los Angeles, 1995.
68. Connors JM, Klimo P, Fairey RN, Voss N: Brief chemotherapy and involved field radiation therapy for limited-stage, histologically aggressive lymphoma. Ann Intern Med 107:25, 1987.
69. Longo DL, Glatstein E, Duffey PL, et al: Treatment of localized aggressive lymphomas with combination chemotherapy followed by involved-field radiation therapy. J Clin Oncol 7:1295, 1989.
70. Epidermoid anal cancer: Results from the UKCCCR randomised trial of radiotherapy alone versus radiotherapy, 5-fluorouracil, and mitomycin. UKCCCR Anal Cancer Trial Working Party. UK Co-ordinating Committee on Cancer Research. Lancet 348:1049, 1996.
71. Bartelink H, Roelofsen F, Eschwege F, et al: Concomitant radiotherapy and chemotherapy is superior to radiotherapy alone in the treatment of locally advanced anal cancer: results of a phase III randomized trial of the European Organization for Research and Treatment of Cancer Radiotherapy and Gastrointestinal Cooperative Groups. J Clin Oncol 15:2040, 1997.
72. Induction chemotherapy plus radiation compared with surgery plus radiation in patients with advanced laryngeal cancer. The Department of Veterans Affairs Laryngeal Cancer Study Group. N Engl J Med 324:1685, 1991.
73. Lefebvre JL, Chevalier D, Luboinski B, et al: Larynx preservation in pyriform sinus cancer: preliminary results of a European Organization for Research and Treatment of Cancer phase III trial. EORTC Head and Neck Cancer Cooperative Group. J Natl Cancer Inst 88:890, 1996.
74. Kachnic LA, Kaufman DS, Heney NM, et al: Bladder preservation by combined modality therapy for invasive bladder cancer. J Clin Oncol 15:1022, 1997.
75. Wani MC, Taylor HL, Wall ME, et al: Plant antitumor agents. VI. The isolation and structure of taxol, a novel antileukemic and antitumor agent from *Taxus brevifolia.* J Am Chem Soc 93:2325, 1997.
76. Brockman RW, Schabel FM Jr, Montgomery JA: Biologic activity of 9-beta-D-arabinofuranosyl-2-fluoroadenine, a metabolically stable analog of 9-beta-D-arabinofuranosyladenine. Biochem Pharmacol 26:2193, 1977.
77. Kohl NE, Mosser SD, deSolms SJ, et al: Selective inhibition of ras-dependent transformation by a farnesyltransferase inhibitor. Science 260:1934, 1993.
78. Monia BP, Johnston JF, Geiger T, et al: Antitumor activity of a phosphorothioate antisense oligodeoxynucleotide targeted against C-raf kinase. Nat Med 2:668, 1996.
79. Pegram MD, Baly D, Wirth C, et al: Antibody-dependent cell-mediated cytotoxicity in breast cancer patients in phase III clinical trials of a humanized anti-*HER2* antibody [abstract 4044]. Proceedings of the American Association for Cancer Research, San Diego, 1997.
80. Yuan F, Chen Y, Dellian M, et al: Time-dependent vascular regression and permeability changes in established human tumor xenografts induced by an antivascular endothelial growth factor/vascular permeability factor antibody. Proc Natl Acad Sci U S A 93:14765, 1996.
81. O'Reilly M, Boehm T, Shing Y, et al: Endostatin: an endogenous inhibitor of angiogenesis and tumor growth. Cell 88:277, 1997.
82. O'Reilly M, Holmgren L, Chen C, Folkman J: Angiostatin induces and sustains dormancy of human primary tumors in mice. Nat Med 2:689, 1996.
83. Chambers AF, Matrisian LM: Changing views of the role of matrix metalloproteinases in metastasis. J Natl Cancer Inst 89:1260, 1997.
84. Vassal G: Pharmacologically guided dose adjustment of busulfan in high-dose chemotherapy regimens: rationale and pitfalls [review]. Anticancer Res 14:2363, 1994.
85. Gallo JM, Brennan J, Hamilton TC, et al: Time-dependent pharmacodynamic models in cancer chemotherapy: population pharmacodynamic model for glutathione depletion following modulation by buthionine sulfoximine (BSO) in a phase I trial of melphalan and BSO. Cancer Res 55:4507, 1995.
86. Egorin MJ, Van Echo DA, Olman EA, et al: Prospective validation of a pharmacologically based dosing scheme for the *cis*-diamminedichloroplatinum(II) analogue diamminecyclobutanedicarboxylatoplatinum. Cancer Res 45:6502, 1985.
87. Nagai N, Kinoshita M, Ogata H, et al: Relationship between pharmacokinetics of unchanged cisplatin and nephrotoxicity after intravenous infusions of cisplatin to cancer patients. Cancer Chemother Pharmacol 39:131, 1996.
88. Cummings J, Smyth JF: Pharmacology of Adriamycin: the message to the clinician. Eur J Cancer Clin Oncol 24:579, 1988.
89. Kaul S, Srinivas NR, Igwemezie LN, Barbhaiya RH: A pharmacodynamic evaluation of hematologic toxicity observed with etoposide phosphate in the treatment of cancer patients. Semin Oncol 23:15, 1996.
90. Malspeis L, Grever MR, Staubus AE, Young D: Pharmacokinetics of 2-F-ara-A (9-β-D-arabinofuranosyl-2-fluoroadenine) in cancer patients during the phase I clinical investigation of fludarabine phosphate. Semin Oncol 17:18, 1990.
91. van Groeningen CJ, Pinedo HM, Heddes J, et al: Pharmacokinetics of 5-fluorouracil assessed with a sensitive mass spectrometric method in patients on a dose escalation schedule. Cancer Res 48:6956, 1988.
92. Graf N, Winkler K, Betlemovic M, et al: Methotrexate pharmacokinetics and prognosis in osteosarcoma. J Clin Oncol 12:1443, 1994.
93. Gianni L, Kearns CM, Giani A, et al: Nonlinear pharmacokinetics and metabolism of paclitaxel and its pharmacokinetic/pharmacodynamic relationships in humans. J Clin Oncol 13:180, 1995.

94. Grochow LB, Rowinsky EK, Johnson R, et al: Pharmacokinetics and pharmacodynamics of topotecan in patients with advanced cancer. Drug Metab Dispos 20:706, 1992.
95. Jao JY, Jusko WJ, Cohen JL: Phenobarbital effects on cyclophosphamide pharmacokinetics in man. Cancer Res 32:2761, 1972.
96. Chen TL, Passos-Coelho JL, Noe DA, et al: Nonlinear pharmacokinetics of cyclophosphamide in patients with metastatic breast cancer receiving high-dose chemotherapy followed by autologous bone marrow transplantation. Cancer Res 55:810, 1995.
97. Rushing DA, Raber SR, Rodvold KA, et al: The effects of cyclosporine on the pharmacokinetics of doxorubicin in patients with small cell lung cancer. Cancer 74:834, 1994.
98. Kivisto KT, Kroemer HK, Eichelbaum M: The role of human cytochrome P450 enzymes in the metabolism of anticancer agents: implications for drug interactions. Br J Clin Pharmacol 40:523, 1995.
99. Bannwarth B, Pehourcq F, Schaeverbeke T, Dehais J: Clinical pharmacokinetics of low-dose pulse methotrexate in rheumatoid arthritis. Clin Pharmacokinet 30:194, 1996.
100. Ronchera CL, Hernandez T, Peris JE, et al: Pharmacokinetic interaction between high-dose methotrexate and amoxicillin. Ther Drug Monit 15:375, 1993.
101. Iven I, Brasch H: Cephalosporins increase the renal clearance of methotrexate and 7-hydroxymethotrexate in rabbits. Cancer Chemother Pharmacol 26:139, 1990.
102. Berg SL, Tolcher A, O'Shaughnessy JA, et al: Effect of R-verapamil on the pharmacokinetics of paclitaxel in women with breast cancer. J Clin Oncol 13:2039, 1995.
103. Major PP, Agarwal RP, Kufe DW: Clinical pharmacology of arabinofuranosyladenine in combination with deoxycoformycin. Cancer Chemother Pharmacol 10:125, 1983.
104. Tobe SW, Siu LL, Jamal SA, et al: Vinblastine and erythromycin: an unrecognized serious drug interaction. Cancer Chemother Pharmacol 35:188, 1995.

BIBLIOGRAPHY

Chabner BA, Ryan DP, Paz-Ares L, et al: Antineoplastic agents. *In* Handman JG, Limbird LL (eds): Goodman and Gilman's: The Pharmacologic Basis of Therapeutics, 11th ed. New York, McGraw-Hill, 2006.

Chabner BA, Longo DL (eds): Cancer Chemotherapy and Biotherapy: Principles and Practice, 4th ed. Philadelphia, Lippincott-Raven, 2006.

CHAPTER 9

IMAGING IN ONCOLOGY

Julia R. Fielding, Michael Burke, and Valerie L. Jewells

OVERVIEW OF IMAGING MODALITIES

Diagnostic imaging is an essential part of the pretherapy evaluation of the cancer patient and of follow-up evaluation after therapy. For many years, plain radiographs, often with contrast enhancement, represented the standard for radiographic staging, but they have been largely supplanted by computed tomography (CT) and magnetic resonance imaging (MRI). Positron emission tomography (PET) also is commonly used to evaluate the extent of disease and the presence of metastatic tumor. In this chapter, we discuss primarily cross-sectional imaging and its application in specific diseases.

CT has been the mainstay for detection of metastatic disease for the past decade. Advantages include speed, patient comfort, excellent spatial resolution, and high-quality imaging of the abdomen. The current generation of scanners obtains 64 slices for each turn of the gantry, allowing image acquisition of the entire chest, abdomen, and pelvis in less than 1 minute. Three-dimensional, reformatted images in the coronal and sagittal planes are immediately available, and picture archiving and communications systems allow the images to be viewed at multiple sites simultaneously.

Disadvantages include exposure to ionizing radiation (an approximately 0.04-Gy skin dose for a scan of the abdomen and pelvis) and the requirement of relatively large volumes (100 to 150 mL) of iodine-based intravenous contrast agents that are hyperosmolar to serum. In general, CT studies of all regions of the body are performed after administration of intravenous contrast material. Most tumors are hypodense compared with adjacent normal tissue. Oral iodine- or barium-based contrast material is required for most abdominal and pelvic CT. The exception to this is the fused PET/CT scans that are usually performed without the addition of oral contrast material. Although intravenous agents make tumors more conspicuous and allow for vascular mapping for tumor resection, there is also the possibility of allergic-type reactions, ranging from urticaria (2 in 100 cases) to shock (1 in 60,0000 cases).[1-5] These rates are similar to those for the antibiotic penicillin. Active asthma or a history of multiple allergies to food, drugs, or the environment increases the risk of an allergic reaction to iodine-based intravenous contrast by a factor of 20.[1] These patients can be premedicated with steroids to decrease the risk of an adverse reaction. A second possible adverse outcome is that of contrast media–induced nephropathy. Patients with a serum creatinine level less than 2.0 mg/dL usually can undergo intravenous contrast–enhanced CT without significant risk of nephropathy.[5] For patients with elevated serum creatinine levels, vigorous oral and intravenous hydration for several hours after the examination can significantly decrease the risk of renal damage.

CT scans are taken with various slice thicknesses, which impacts the spatial resolution of the study in the craniocaudal direction. Visualization depends on the width of the imaging window and on the midpoint of that window, with different parameters used for viewing different structures (i.e., lung, soft tissue, and bone). The apparent size of a given structure depends on the exact window parameters during visualization.

Technologic development has enabled the fusion of CT with PET images enhanced with ^{18}F-fluorodeoxyglucose (FDG). These fused images have been extremely useful in the localization of active sites of disease, particularly for primary lung and esophageal cancers and lymphoma.

Over the past 10 years, MRI has become more important in staging cancers and has become the preeminent tool for evaluation of the central nervous system. In certain centers, it is also used extensively for head and neck cancers and for detection of liver metastases. Its sensitivity is similar to that of CT, although the spatial resolution of MR is decreased, and breathing and motion artifacts can be problematic. Advantages of MRI include improved lesion characterization because of the wide shades of gray available for depiction of organs and improved identification of normal anatomy, particularly within the central nervous system and bones. The paucity of available protons in the air-filled lungs makes MRI of limited value in the detection of pulmonary nodules.

Most MRI oncology studies are done using an intravenous contrast material composed of a rare earth metal, gadolinium, chelated to diethylenetriaminepentaacetate (DTPA). The risk of anaphylaxis is very low, and the risk of nephrotoxicity is virtually zero. Intravenous contrast volumes are in the range of 10 to 20 mL. Patients must be cooperative, able to lie supine for 20 minutes, and able to tolerate the claustrophobia that can occur in the scanner. The presence of ferromagnetic implants, including cardiac pacemakers, ocular implants, and aneurysm clips, prohibits performance of MRI.[6] Surgical clips, artificial joints, and heart valves can be safely imaged. MRI of the central nervous system, abdomen, and pelvis usually consists of T1-weighted (black fluid), T2-weighted (bright fluid), and contrast-enhanced images obtained sequentially using T1-weighted images in multiple planes. Surface coils are available for each part of the body, increasing signal-to-noise ratio and spatial resolution. T1 and T2 weighting is determined by the time to repetition (TR) of the radiofrequency pulse and the time to echo (TE) signal. Pulse sequences with long TR values (>1000 ms) yield T2-weighted images, whereas those with short TR values (<800 ms) yield T1-weighted images. Most tumors are of increased T2 signal compared with adjacent normal tissue, and they demonstrate characteristic enhancement patterns. Bone imaging often requires fat saturation to demonstrate marrow changes, as well as comparison with plain radiographs.

In the following sections, the imaging appearances of common primary and metastatic cancers in the head, neck, chest, abdomen, and pelvis are demonstrated using CT, MRI, and in some cases, fused PET/CT images obtained with standard imaging protocols. Imaging of primary breast cancer is omitted from this section.

IMAGING OF THE BRAIN, HEAD, AND NECK

Brain Tumors

Imaging is necessary in all brain and head and neck cancer patients to evaluate the extent of disease, determine surgical and therapeutic options, and aid surgical planning to shorten procedure times.[7] Primary brain tumors and metastatic disease can be imaged with CT or MRI. With CT, contrast enhancement (96%) and increasing volume (92%) are the most sensitive criteria for evaluating brain tumors, but these criteria lack specificity (83.3%).[8] The differential diagnosis includes inflammatory and infectious causes. Our preference is to use MRI for all staging of primary and metastatic disease of the brain because of increased conspicuity of lesions, better tumor grading, and improved accuracy of disease extent compared with CT.[9-11]

Primary brain tumors are graded by the World Health Organization (WHO) staging criteria based on cell density, nuclear and cytoplasmic pleomorphism, mitoses, necrosis, and vascular endothelial proliferation. Because enhancement suggesting vascular proliferation and necrosis can be seen on MRI, an estimate of the WHO grade can be inferred from imaging. Grade I (noninfiltrative) tumors are the least malignant, and they do not enhance or demonstrate necrosis on MRI. Grade II tumors infiltrate and may enhance at least heterogeneously, but they do not show necrosis. Grade III and IV lesions enhance and demonstrate necrosis.

The most common adult primary intra-axial brain tumors are, in descending frequency, glioblastoma multiforme (GBM) (WHO grade III-IV), astrocytomas other than GBM (WHO grades I-II), oligodendrogliomas (WHO grade II-III), lymphomas, gliomatosis cerebri (diffuse tumor with cortical involvement and prognosis equal to GBM), and hemangioblastomas.[12-14] Lymphomas are most commonly seen in human immunodeficiency virus (HIV)–positive patients.[15] GBM and lymphoma have a tendency to involve the corpus callosum; metastatic disease is less likely to do so. In general, the size, area of T2 signal abnormality, and contrast enhancement are the three MRI changes to focus on with regard to tumor response. Subependymal spread, necrosis, and dural involvement are poor prognostic signs for primary brain tumors. With CT, size, necrosis, and enhancement are the important findings. Contrast enhancement with CT and MRI is decreased after steroid administration.

Postirradiation changes can be seen after therapy for brain tumors and for head and neck carcinomas, and they can mimic other abnormalities and complicate radiologic assessment of residual disease.[16,17] Within weeks of radiation therapy, early, reversible, T2-weighted white matter signal may be seen within the brain, and within 3 months of therapy, delayed, reversible, increased T2-weighted white matter signal is identified. Late changes, defined as those occurring more than 3 months after treatment, can demonstrate irreversible, increased T2-weighted white matter signal, atrophy, calcification, and contrast enhancement, and they can mimic tumor.[18] In these cases, MR spectroscopy and MR perfusion may be helpful for exclusion of residual tumor.

Disease Metastatic to the Brain

In adults, disease metastatic to the brain occurs as frequently as primary brain tumors, and it is best demonstrated with MRI. The appearance of metastatic disease mimics that of primary brain tumors (Fig. 9-1). The most common sites of origin for brain metastases are bronchial carcinoma (30%), breast carcinoma (15% to 30%), melanoma, prostate carcinoma, renal cell carcinoma, and thyroid carcinoma. In adults, metastases are more common in the posterior fossa than are primary brain tumors. PET scanning can detect metastatic lesions to brain, but it is less sensitive than MRI.[19] Dural-based metastases are more common in cases of breast carcinoma, lymphoma, lung cancer, prostate cancer, and melanoma. Metastases that are likely to hemorrhage include breast carcinoma, choriocarcinoma, lung carcinoma, melanoma, renal cell carcinoma, retinoblastoma, and thyroid carcinoma. Metastatic seeding of primary brain tumors is uncommon in adults, but it does occur with GBM, astrocytomas, and oligodendrogliomas.[15]

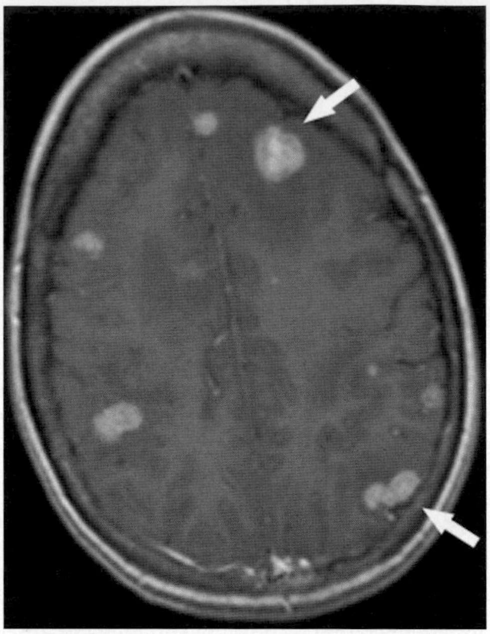

Figure 9-1 A 47-year-old man with known lung cancer. Axial-view, contrast-enhanced MRI of the head shows multiple, rim-enhancing, high-signal nodules *(arrows)* indicative of metastatic disease.

Head and Neck Cancer

Imaging for carcinomas of the sinuses, nasopharynx, and parotid glands is preferentially performed with MRI because of the propensity for these tumors to spread perineurally along cranial nerves V and VII.[20] Nasopharyngeal carcinoma is also likely to spread by deep tissue infiltration into the pharyngobasilar fascia, sinus of Morgagni, cartilaginous eustachian tube, levator veli palatine muscles, and skull base. All of these areas are better imaged with MRI than CT. In some cases, CT may be useful for detection of skull base involvement, and this must be a consideration for surgical planning.

For tumors arising in and around the vocal cords, CT is preferred because of less motion artifact, faster imaging, and extension of imaging into the chest. Imaging to the level of the hila allows assessment for synchronous lung carcinomas and for enlarged hilar and mediastinal nodes (Fig. 9-2).[21,22] This inferior extent of imaging also allows assessment of the course of the entire recurrent laryngeal nerve. MRI may be preferable if multidetector CT with coronal imaging is not available.

PET imaging of the head and neck is being performed more frequently.[23,24] Performing PET without CT or at least CT registration leads to errors in location of the abnormality, and it is therefore limited. PET shows increased uptake based on metabolism of glucose, and results are therefore positive in cases of tumor and infection. Negative PET findings can occur for necrotic nodes that are positive at histology, but this appears to be less of a problem with fused PET/CT.[25] Because fused PET/CT is expensive and time-consuming, it is not the first-line study for tumor detection at our institution, but we use it when the results of CT or MRI are indeterminate. In patients with neck nodes positive for cancer but with an

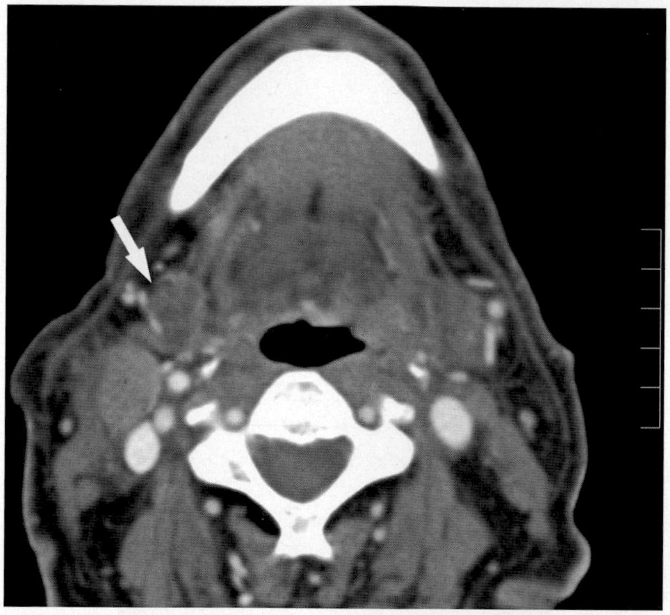

Figure 9-2 A 68-year-old man with known base of tongue cancer. An enlarged node adjacent to the internal jugular vein is seen on the right *(arrow)*.

unknown primary, fused PET/CT has a detection rate of 20%.[26] Some investigators express disappointment with this detection rate because it is less than for unilateral tonsillectomy. PET imaging has also been reported to be of value in the detection of residual disease.

Disease Metastatic to the Neck

Detection of metastatic nodes with ultrasound, particularly with color flow Doppler, may be more sensitive for differentiating benign and malignant cervical adenopathy than CT and MRI.[27,28] When ultrasound reveals no increased blood flow in neck nodes contralateral to the known primary, a unilateral neck dissection is performed. Iron oxide particles, MR spectroscopy, sentinel node mapping, and CT perfusion are newer investigational techniques for improved lesion detection. Quantification of CT perfusion has been shown to accurately differentiate normal adjacent tissue from tumor. This is important because poorly perfused tumors respond poorly to radiotherapy and have increased rates of local recurrence.

IMAGING OF THE CHEST

Lung Cancer

Lung cancer is most commonly discovered on chest radiographs, where it appears as a central or peripheral mass, often with deformation of the mediastinum due to enlarged lymph nodes. A pleural effusion may veil the lucency of the lung. When there is a suspicion of lung cancer clinically or on the basis of a chest radiograph, contrast-enhanced CT is the modality of choice for characterization of the primary mass, identification of additional nodules, and assessment of size and location of lymphadenopathy. Lymph nodes larger than 1 cm in the short axis are considered pathologic.[29] Fused PET/CT images can be useful in determining the avidity of mediastinal and hilar nodes. In most cases, CT or fused PET/CT is used to follow response to therapy (Fig. 9-3).

Histologically, primary lung cancers can be divided into two broad categories: non–small cell lung cancer (NSCLC) and small cell lung cancer. NSCLC is further divided into several histologic subtypes, including adenocarcinoma, squamous cell carcinoma, and large cell carcinoma. Most primary lung cancers (80%) are NSCLCs.[30] For imaging purposes, lung cancer can be divided based on predilection for a peripheral or central location.

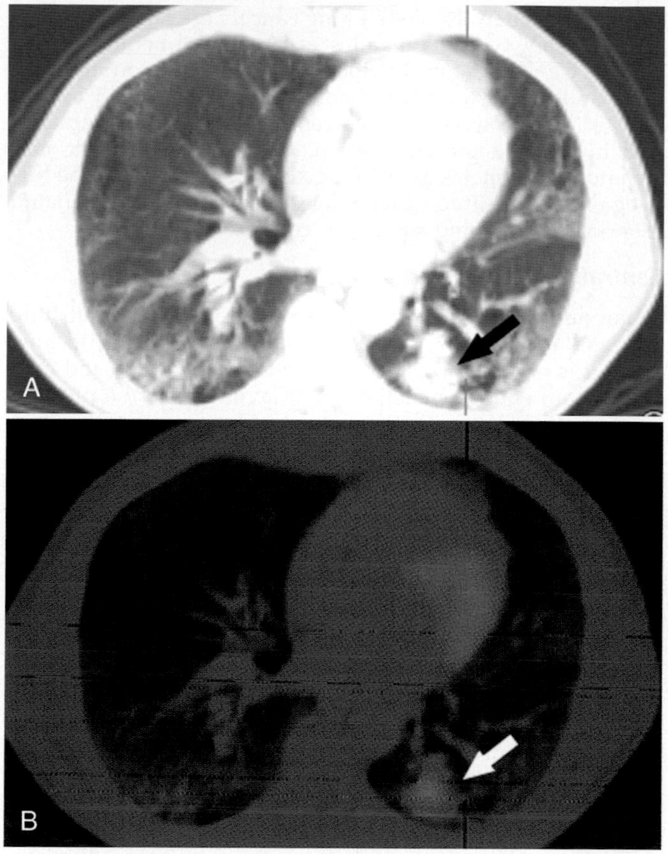

Figure 9-3 A 56-year-old man with treated lung cancer. **A,** Axial CT demonstrates a residual mass within the left lower lobe *(arrow)*. **B,** Corresponding fused PET/CT image reveals increased avidity for fluorodeoxyglucose, similar to the heart and indicative of residual disease *(arrow)*. PET imaging should be performed approximately 8 weeks after radiation therapy to minimize false-positive results due to inflammation of the targeted tissues.

Peripherally Located Tumors

Adenocarcinoma accounts for 40% of all lung cancers.[30] These tumors are typically small, round, smoothly marginated, and peripherally located. Calcifications are present in only 6% of primary lung adenocarcinoma. However, central location does not exclude the diagnosis of adenocarcinoma.[31] When the primary mass is located peripherally, hilar and mediastinal lymph node metastases are present at diagnosis in 18% and 2% of cases, respectively. When the primary mass is located more centrally, hilar and mediastinal lymphadenopathy is present in 40% and 27%, respectively.[31]

Bronchoalveolar carcinoma (BAC) is considered a subtype of adenocarcinoma. Approximately 60% of BACs manifest as a peripheral, solitary pulmonary nodule.[32] Other common forms include multiple nodules (15%) and an alveolar filling pattern that mimics pneumonia (10%).[33] These opacities may present a diagnostic challenge, because they can remain unchanged in size for several years. Mediastinal lymphadenopathy is present at diagnosis in 18% of cases.[33]

Approximately 10% of all lung cancers are large cell carcinomas.[30] They typically manifest as large, peripherally located masses. Cavitation and calcification are uncommon findings. Hilar and mediastinal lymphadenopathies are found in 30% and 10%, respectively.[32] Large cell carcinomas are characterized by a rapid growth pattern, with early lymphatic and hematogenous metastases.[34] Large cell carcinomas can be histologically difficult to differentiate from poorly differentiated adenocarcinomas and squamous cell carcinomas.[30]

Centrally Located Tumors

Squamous cell carcinoma (SCC) constitutes 30% of all lung cancers.[30] Although SCC often manifests as a centrally located mass, it is peripherally located in one third of cases and may occur as an endobronchial mass.[32] Cavitation of the primary mass occurs in 10% to 20% of patients. Most apical or Pancoast tumors are SCCs.[33] Pancoast tumors may extend superiorly and invade the subclavian artery and brachial plexus. Brachial plexus involvement is best examined with MRI.

Small cell lung cancer accounts for 20% of all primary lung cancers.[30] This histologic subtype is composed of neoplasms arising from neuroendocrine cells. Small cell lung neoplasms are commonly central lesions, and they may encase mediastinal structures at diagnosis. Metastases to the bone marrow, liver, adrenals, and brain occur early.[32]

Nodal Involvement of Lung Cancer

Assessing the mediastinum for nodal metastases is important for cancer staging. Contrast-enhanced CT is routinely used for the detection of abnormal lymph nodes. Differentiation between benign and malignant lymph nodes is made using size criteria alone. Lymph nodes with a short-axis diameter greater than 1 cm are defined as pathologically enlarged and prompt concern for metastatic involvement.[29] Unfortunately, morphologic criteria on MRI and CT are not effective in characterizing lymph nodes. Using the 1-cm short-axis criterion, CT has been reported to be 41% to 67% sensitive and 79% to 86% specific for detection of nodal metastases.[35] Often, enlarged nodes are hyperplastic because of infection or inflammation, particularly in the setting of postobstructive pneumonia.

PET is useful in differentiating benign from malignant lymphadenopathy. If an enlarged node discovered by CT is shown not to be avid for FDG, it can be considered to be free of metastases with almost 100% certainty.[36] PET has a reported sensitivity of 76% to 100% and specificity of 82% to 100% for the detection of lymph node metastases.[35] Problems remain with detection of lung nodules less than 5 mm in diameter and with superimposed or concurrent infections, which also show increased uptake.

Lymphoma

Although lymphoma is primarily a disease of nodal origin, more than 80% of patients with Hodgkin's disease have intrathoracic involvement at presentation consisting of enlarged anterior mediastinal and paratracheal lymph nodes.[37] Non-Hodgkin's lymphoma is a more heterogeneous group of diseases, and thoracic lymph node involvement occurs in 45% of cases (Fig. 9-4).[38] The paratracheal and anterior mediastinal lymph nodes remain the most commonly involved sites. Large mediastinal lymphadenopathy (>10 cm) is associated with an increased risk of relapse, and it usually requires aggressive combination therapy.[39] Treated lymph nodes tend to calcify in a rimlike fashion or as a coarse, dense mass. Lung nodules are uncommon in Hodgkin's disease and non-Hodgkin's lymphoma. Non-Hodgkin's lymphoma occurs in 2% to 6% of the post–cardiac transplantation population.[40] It is the third most common cause of death beyond the perioperative period. There is a strong association with the antirejection drug cyclosporine and with Epstein-Barr virus infection. This is the only variety of lymphoma to manifest primarily as a pulmonary mass or nodules.[41,42]

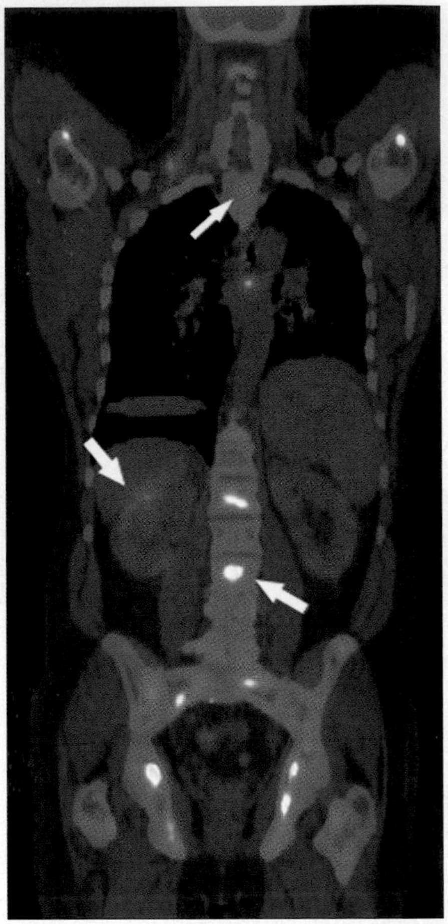

Figure 9-4 A 44-year-old man with known non-Hodgkin's lymphoma. Coronal fused PET/CT image shows multiple regions of increased uptake, including bones, kidneys, and thyroid *(arrows)*.

Disease Metastatic to the Chest

CT scan is the modality of choice for identification of metastatic disease and response to therapy. Many cancers involving the lungs manifest with multiple nodules, although solitary metastatic disease is important to distinguish because surgical resection is often employed. In the case of SCC, nodules are often cavitary. Response to therapy is often determined based on an increase or decrease in size and number of nodules. Even when careful attention is paid to reference nodules that are followed at intervals, it may be difficult to detect a few millimeters of increase in diameter. It is prudent to compare the current scan with the most recent and the most remote scan to avoid overlooking very slowly growing disease. Other manifestations of metastatic disease include enlarged mediastinal, hilar, and axillary lymph nodes; nodular pleural thickening; pleural effusion; and particularly in the case of lung or breast cancer, chest wall invasion. Osteolytic or osteoblastic bone metastases can be identified by changing the window and viewing levels to center on the high calcific density of normal bone. Three-dimensional reconstructions can be of particular value in identifying central lung nodules abutting vessels, chest wall masses, and rib or spine lesions.

IMAGING OF THE ABDOMEN

Esophageal Cancer

In North America, there has been a shift of esophageal cancers toward the gastroesophageal junction over the past few decades. The cell type now seen most often is adenocarcinoma, probably because of reflux disease.[43,44] Although a fluoroscopic examination such as a barium swallow performed in a patient with dysphagia can identify an advanced cancer, most smaller tumors are identified at endoscopy. Enlarged nodes can be sampled during endoscopy to determine involvement and prognosis. Involvement of the chest and liver is best assessed using contrast-enhanced CT. Staging accuracy using combined endoscopic ultrasound and contrast-enhanced CT ranges from 62% to 90%.[45] Fused PET/CT images are used routinely in many centers to follow therapy with diminished uptake indicative of successful cell killing (Fig. 9-5).[45,46]

Stomach Cancer

Gastric adenocarcinoma, similar to distal esophageal cancer, is usually identified at endoscopy and staged using contrast-enhanced CT scan. Endoscopy is superior to CT at depicting the depth of invasion into gastric wall, whereas CT is superior in the identification of lymph nodes that have increased in size and number, ascites, and distant disease.[47,48] Gas-releasing crystals are given orally before CT to distend the stomach. The gastric wall may be focally or diffusely thickened. Ulceration is common. Differential diagnosis includes leiomyosarcoma, gastrointestinal stromal tumor, and lymphoma. For tumors located in the gastric cardia or fundus, lymph node patterns are similar to those of distal esophageal tumors and include the gastrohepatic ligament and periaortic spaces. Distal cancers often drain along the lesser curvature of the stomach. This can be a particularly difficult area to survey on axial images alone, and coronal reformatted images are often helpful.[49]

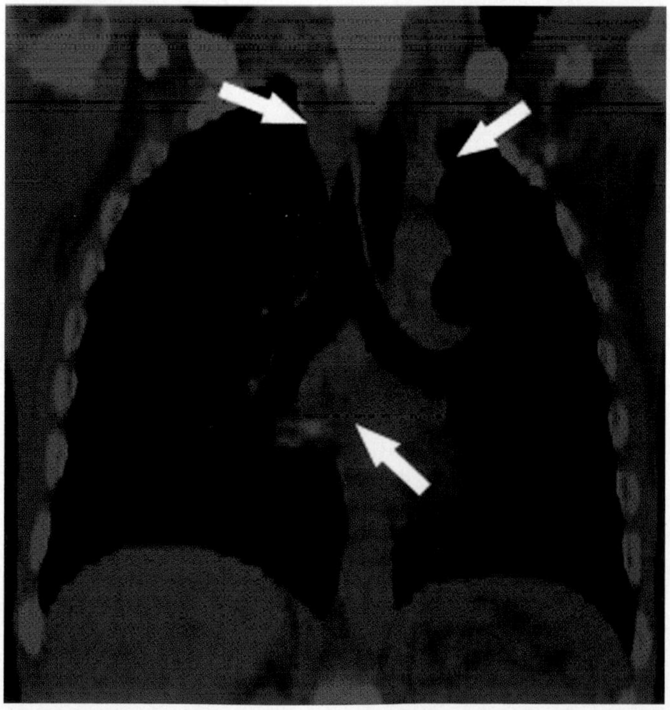

Figure 9-5 A 67-year-old man with known esophageal cancer. Multiple, enlarged nodes involving most mediastinal sites were identified on CT. The coronal fused PET/CT image shows increased avidity in the paratracheal and subcarinal lymph nodes *(arrows)*, indicative of carcinoma.

Small-Bowel Cancer

The two most common primary small-bowel tumors are adenocarcinoma and carcinoid. Adenocarcinoma occurs most commonly at the ligament of Treitz, whereas carcinoid originates most often in the ileum. On small-bowel series, adenocarcinoma usually manifests as a mass, whereas carcinoid has a characteristic tethering of adjacent loops. The differential diagnosis includes metastatic disease, gastrointestinal stromal tumor, and lymphoma. Staging is performed with oral and intravenous contrast-enhanced CT, which often demonstrates extension to mesenteric lymph nodes and the liver.[50,51]

Colon and Rectal Tumors

Primary colorectal tumors are usually discovered during colonoscopy. Occasionally, an obstructing colonic cancer is identified on a CT scan of the abdomen. Wall thickening exists in approximately 20%, and it is often associated with colonic obstruction and advanced disease.[52] The primary use of cross-sectional imaging is identification of locoregional and distant metastatic disease. Patterns of spread are primarily lymphatic and hematogenous. Direct extension occurs when a tumor perforates the serosa and invades adjacent tissue. Depending on the location of the primary tumor, lymphatic disease may spread into the ischiorectal fossa and perianal space (rectum or anus) or along the mesenteric vessels (left and right colon). A common final pathway for many tumors is the retroperitoneum adjacent to the origin of the inferior mesenteric artery. Enlarged nodes may also be seen in the porta hepatis. Lymph nodes larger than 1 cm in the short-axis diameter can contain metastatic disease. Unfortunately, size is not a good indicator of tumor involvement. Lymph nodes larger than 1 cm in diameter harbor cancer in only 65% of cases.[53] Hematogenous spread yields liver metastases. Advanced disease may consist of pulmonary nodules, widespread lymphadenopathy, and solid tumor masses within the mesentery and pelvis due to direct extension of disease.

A particularly valuable use of fused PET/CT and MRI is the identification of recurrent disease after abdominoperineal resection for rectal cancer. These same images can be used to identify complications of therapy such as fistulas. After surgery, it is expected that the bladder and reproductive organs rotate posteriorly to fill the surgical bed and that flat, fibrous tissue borders the anterior wall of the sacrum. The presence of an ovoid, enhancing mass at this site on CT or MRI may indicate tumor. Confirmation of recurrent disease can be made using CT-guided needle biopsy or PET scanning (Fig. 9-6).

Disease Metastatic to the Gastrointestinal Tract

Most serosal metastatic implants tend to distort and narrow the small and large bowel, sometimes leading to obstruction. Although this can be identified on contrast-enhanced CT scans, water-soluble barium enema may be necessary to determine exact locations of disease when planning for colostomy.

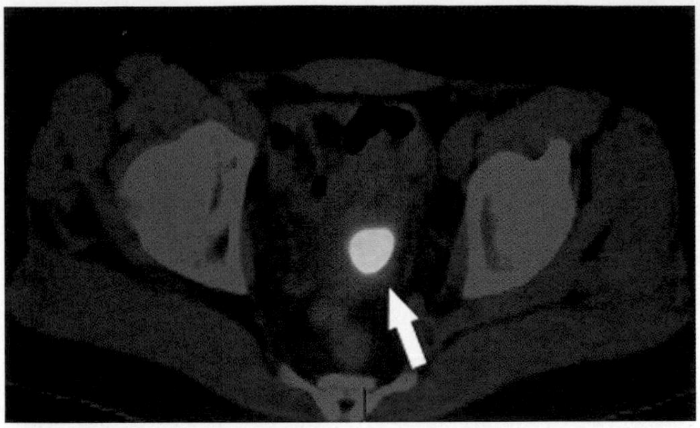

Figure 9-6 A 72-year-old man after resection of sigmoid carcinoma. The fused PET/CT image reveals a region of increased uptake at the anastomotic site *(arrow)*. Biopsy showed this to be recurrent disease.

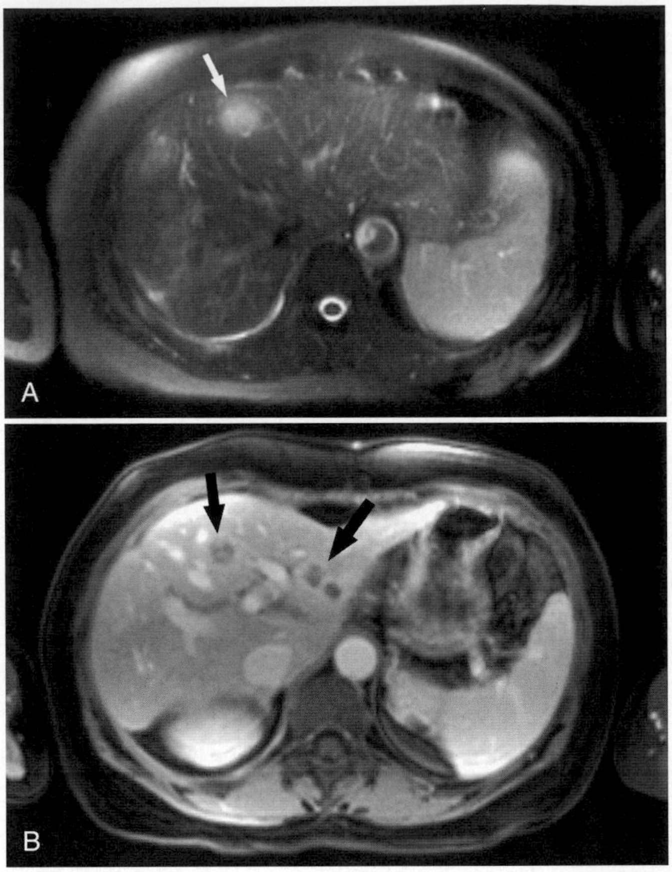

Figure 9-7 A 56-year-old man with a history of colon cancer and known metastatic disease. Axial-view, T2-weighted (**A**) and contrast-enhanced (**B**) MR images of the liver show a high-signal, rim-enhancing mass *(arrows)* with lobulated borders diagnostic of metastatic adenocarcinoma.

Primary Tumors of the Liver

Hepatoma occurs primarily in patients with cirrhosis. The distorted anatomy and scarring of this disease make detection of dysplastic nodules difficult. Dual-phase (arterial and venous) CT and MRI have proved successful in identifying these tumors. On CT, the tumors are often hyperintense on the arterial-phase images, with rapid washout on the portal venous–phase images. On T2-weighted MRI, hepatoma may have a variety of appearances, ranging from low to high signal intensity.[54] Contrast-enhanced MRI demonstrates high-signal-intensity nodules on T1-weighted images, with rapid washin and washout of contrast material.[55] A common association is invasion of the portal vein.

Disease Metastatic to the Liver

Most published studies demonstrate that CT and MRI are of equal sensitivity, with MRI being somewhat more specific for the identification of liver metastases.[53,56-58] A characteristic and specific appearance of adenocarcinoma liver metastasis on CT and MRI is that of a lobulated mass with intensely enhancing borders and minimal central enhancement (Fig. 9-7). Adenocarcinoma metastases have increased signal intensity on T2-weighted images, but they are less bright than cysts or hemangiomas. Another common pattern of metastatic disease is rapid and complete enhancement. Cystic metastases are uncommon. Using CT or MRI, it is usually possible to identify benign lesions with confidence when they exceed 1 cm in diameter.[59]

As resection of liver metastases and radiofrequency ablation become more common treatments for liver metastases, serial imaging is being performed to look for recurrent disease. CT or MRI may be used. After successful ablations, a nonenhancing, spherical defect is seen at the targeted site. After administration of intravenous contrast material, an increase in size of the postablation defect or nodular enhancement of the wall usually indicates recurrent disease.[60,61]

Pancreatic Cancer

The most common pancreatic tumor, adenocarcinoma, usually occurs in the head and may occlude the pancreatic duct or common bile duct, or both. This leads to the classic presentation of painless jaundice with a distended, palpable gallbladder. The first modality used for assessing jaundice is usually ultrasound scanning, which excels at depiction of the biliary system. Stones can be excluded and pancreatic head enlargement identified in most cases.

Biopsy is usually performed using an endoscopic approach. Diagnostic accuracy is high, ranging from 88% to 94%.[62,63] Staging is best done using dual-phase CT on a helical scanner. The arterial and venous phases depict vascular encasement and invasion with a high degree of accuracy and are useful in determining resectability of the tumor. Three-dimensional reconstructions in the sagittal and coronal planes have been shown to add to diagnostic accuracy.[64] Local lymph node enlargement and liver metastases can also be identified. There have been few studies comparing MRI with contrast-enhanced CT; however, it seems likely that both tests are comparable in determining resectability, with an accuracy of approximately 80% (Fig. 9-8).[63] Unfortunately, identification of very small (<1 cm) pancreatic cancers remains difficult. On CT scan, hypodense masses can be reliably identified at 2 cm in diameter. Pancreatic ductal dilation with an abrupt cutoff has been reported as a sign of a small neoplasm.[64]

Kidney Cancer

Renal cell carcinoma is most often identified serendipitously, usually on a CT or ultrasound scan performed for symptoms unrelated to the genitourinary tract. After a solid, vascular mass is identified, treatment is surgical removal or ablation, barring significant medical comorbidities. Staging is per-

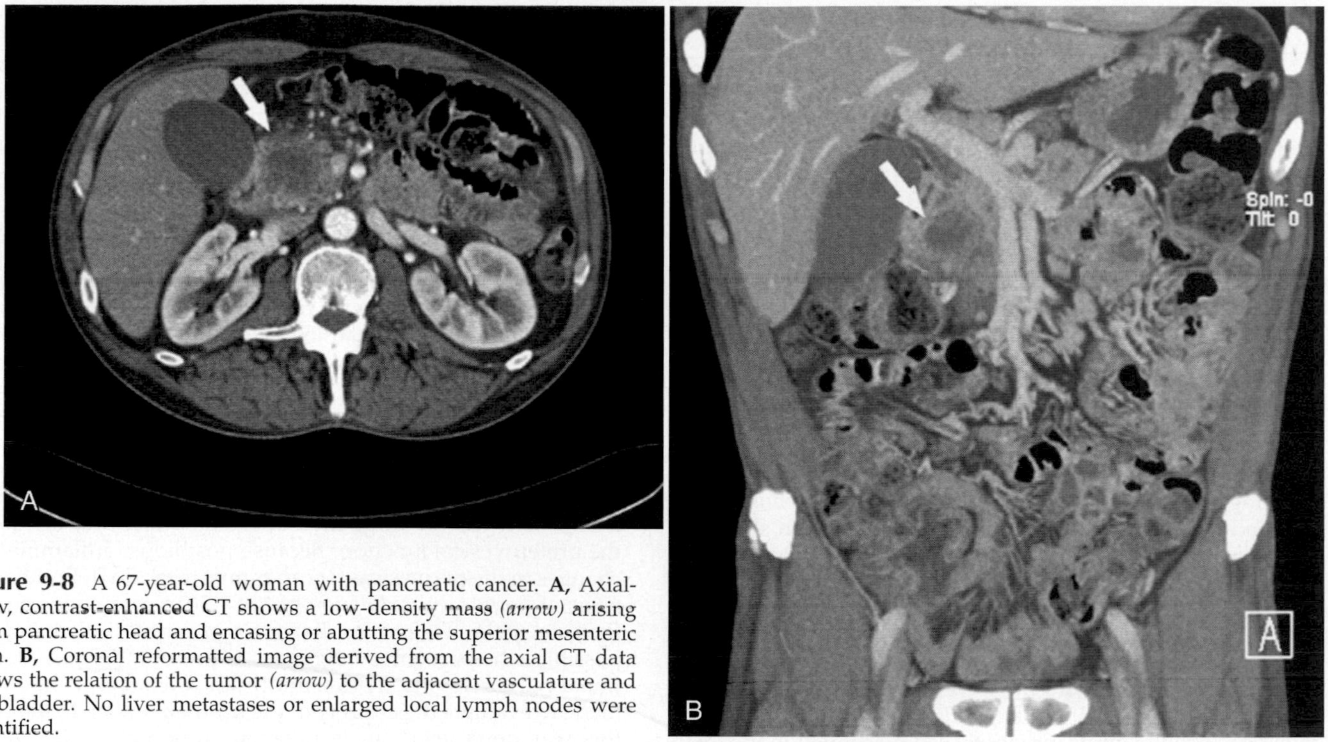

Figure 9-8 A 67-year-old woman with pancreatic cancer. **A,** Axial-view, contrast-enhanced CT shows a low-density mass *(arrow)* arising from pancreatic head and encasing or abutting the superior mesenteric vein. **B,** Coronal reformatted image derived from the axial CT data shows the relation of the tumor *(arrow)* to the adjacent vasculature and gallbladder. No liver metastases or enlarged local lymph nodes were identified.

formed using helical contrast-enhanced CT. MRI can be substituted in the case of an elevated creatinine level. Tumor size, location, and vascular supply are critical in determining whether the patient is a candidate for laparoscopic or partial nephrectomy.[65] Reformatted, three-dimensional images fully depict the vascular anatomy.[66] Extension into the renal vein, presence of enlarged perihilar lymph nodes, involvement of the ipsilateral adrenal gland, and invasion of adjacent organs can also be assessed. Urothelial lesions are now imaged primarily using CT urography, in which delayed axial images are reformatted to produce an image similar to the intravenous urogram.[67,68] Using this same set of data, a bladder or upper tract lesion can be staged, eliminating the need for an additional test.

Cancer of Other Organs

Large masses of the retroperitoneum are often sarcomas. They may arise from the inferior vena cava, renal capsule, muscle, or fat. They are best imaged using contrast-enhanced CT. The high spatial resolution allows determination of the full extent of these soft but relentless tumors. The more common liposarcoma often contains large amounts of fat, which are well depicted on CT. Encasement or displacement of adjacent bowel is critical to treatment planning and is an advantage of CT over MRI.

Disease Metastatic to the Retroperitoneum: Adrenals, Kidneys, and Pancreas

Enlargement of the adrenal gland is a vexing clinical problem for physicians treating oncology patients. Adenomas and hyperplasia are common findings, but they must be accurately identified to avoid overstaging of a primary neoplasm, particularly lung cancer. There are several ways that this can be done, although all techniques work best for lesions 1 cm in diameter or larger.

Unenhanced CT is the most thoroughly tested method. When an adrenal lesion measures less than 10 Hounsfield units (HU) on a non–contrast-enhanced CT, it contains intracytoplasmic lipid and is reliably benign. A second contrast washout method has been developed for lipid-poor adenomas. Adrenal masses that lose 60% of more of contrast enhancement at 15 minutes after injection are also reliably benign.[69-71] At many institutions, MRI is the primary tool for determination of the nature of adrenal masses. Using T1-weighted images, lesions that demonstrate loss of signal compared with the spleen on images in which water and lipid are out of phase are reliably benign.[72] This technique relies on the presence of intracytoplasmic lipid. If CT or MRI fails to characterize a lesion, it is probably best to employ needle biopsy.[73]

A new technique has proved particularly useful for larger adrenal lesions. PET is a reliable technique for the identification of hypermetabolic disease lesions metastatic to the adrenal gland that are larger than 1 cm in diameter. Unfortunately, some adenomas are mildly hypermetabolic with respect to the adjacent liver, and they may require biopsy for final diagnosis.

Disease metastatic to the kidney or pancreas usually manifests as a hypodense mass, which is best imaged using ultrasound or contrast-enhanced CT. Because there are no findings specific for cell type, image-guided biopsy is usually necessary to determine with certainty that the lesion is a metastasis rather than a primary tumor.

IMAGING OF THE PELVIC ORGANS

Testicular Cancer

After the standard treatment of orchiectomy, contrast-enhanced CT scans of the abdomen and pelvis are performed to search for metastatic disease. The lymphatic drainage of the testicles flows to the renal hila. Secondary drainage to the aortoiliac bifurcation also occurs, particularly on the right. Involved lymph nodes are of soft tissue density with dense enhancement. The enlarged nodes may encase the renal vessels and compress and occasionally invade the inferior vena cava. Particularly large and low-density nodes indicate the presence of a teratoma. Unfortunately, node density does not correlate with the degree of cell kill after chemotherapy. Residual, cystic-appearing nodes often undergo surgical débridement to maximize potential for cure. On follow-up scans, all nodes larger than 5 mm in diameter are considered possible metastases.[74] Imaging findings should be correlated with biochemical tumor markers to further direct therapy.

Prostate Cancer

In most institutions, no pelvic imaging is performed before radical prostatectomy. CT scans of the abdomen and pelvis are ordered before the onset of radiation therapy for treatment planning. At the same time, the abdomen and pelvis can be screened for comorbidities, although this has been shown to be an extremely low yield procedure. In advanced disease (prostate-specific antigen [PSA] level > 20), CT is the modality of choice to identify enlarged pelvic and retroperitoneal lymph nodes and hydronephrosis. Images should be examined using bone windows for the presence of osteoblastic metastases, particularly in the lower lumbar spine. Although ultrasonography remains the standard method, CT and MR have been used to guide radiation seed placement in the treatment of prostate cancer.

Small field-of-view, T2-weighted MRI, using a multicoil array or an endorectal coil, or both, can be of value in evaluating the patient with conflicting signs and symptoms, such as a high PSA value and a small, smooth prostate.[75] On T2-weighted images, prostate cancer usually appears as a region of low to intermediate signal intensity. Direct extension of disease through the low T2-signal capsule is indicative of extracapsular extension and poor-prognosis disease. An experienced radiologist can accurately stage prostate carcinoma in approximately 70% of cases.[76] After radical prostatectomy, patients with elevated PSA levels should be examined using MRI. Similar to the patient after abdominoperineal resection, viewing the pelvic floor with high-contrast, T2-weighted or contrast-enhanced images makes it much easier to separate tumor from normal tissue.[77]

Bladder Cancer

Seventy percent of bladder cancers are superficial in origin. Patients do not usually require imaging, because disease is treated cystoscopically with fulguration, snaring, and topical chemotherapy. The remaining 30% of bladder cancers are invasive when discovered.

To determine whether a potentially curative cystectomy should be attempted, the surgeon needs to know if the disease is confined to the bladder wall or extends into the perivesical fat. This is done using a combination of cystoscopic biopsy and CT or MRI. Tumors may be polypoid or sessile, and they often extend to involve a large area of the bladder wall, including the ureterovesical junction. Because postbiopsy inflammatory changes in the perivesical fat can mimic tumor, a definite diagnosis of perivesical extension of tumor can sometimes be difficult to make. Definitive diagnosis of perivesical disease is possible when an enhancing mass is present. Because transitional cell carcinoma is often multifocal, an attempt should be made to evaluate the entirety of the urothelial tract. In the past, this was done using an intravenous urogram. Today, using multidetector CT scans with rapid reformatting, coronal images can be used to check the renal pelves and ureters for the presence of strictures and masses while simultaneously staging the bladder cancer. On T2-weighted MRI, the muscular wall of the bladder has a homogeneously dark signal. Extension into but not through the muscular wall is stage II disease (Fig. 9-9). Extension of a high-signal-intensity mass through the wall indicates stage III disease. Using 1.5-T systems and Gd-DTPA intravenous contrast agent, overall

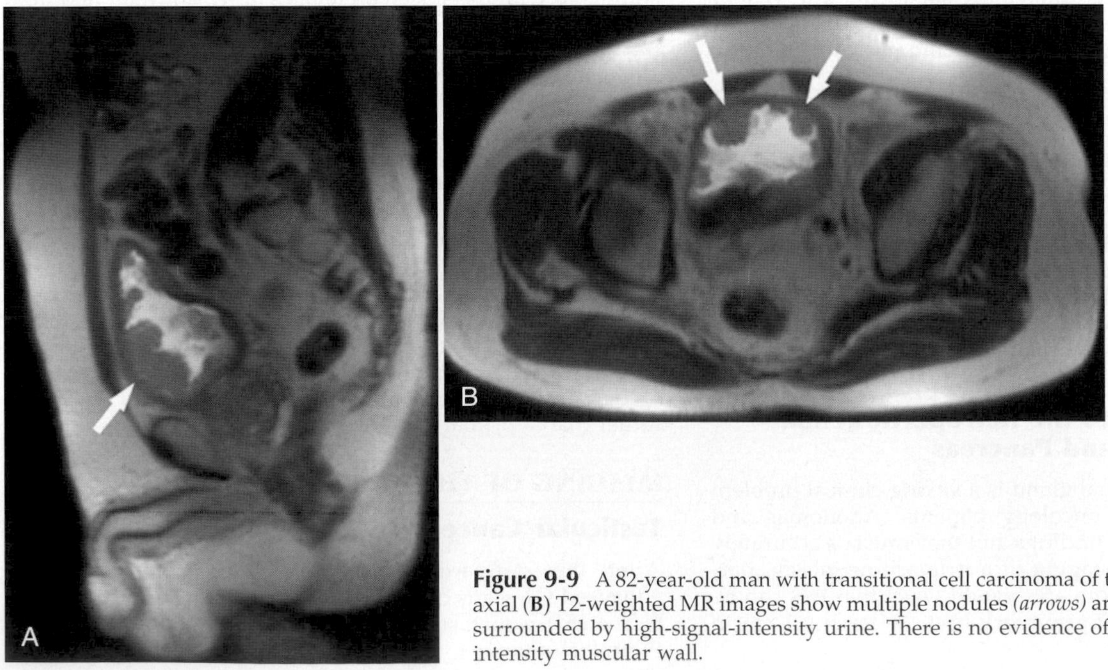

Figure 9-9 A 82-year-old man with transitional cell carcinoma of the bladder. Sagittal (**A**) and axial (**B**) T2-weighted MR images show multiple nodules *(arrows)* arising from the bladder wall, surrounded by high-signal-intensity urine. There is no evidence of invasion of the low-signal-intensity muscular wall.

staging accuracy is approximately 85%.[78] For local extension, T1-weighted, dynamic, post-Gd-DTPA–enhanced images may help in differentiating a mass from adjacent inflammatory stranding. Coronal images of the upper urinary tract, similar to CT or intravenous urography (IVU), can be obtained using a heavily T2-weighted coronal series obtained as a volume or composed of multiple slices. MRI has also been advocated for assessing response to chemotherapy, with delayed enhancement of responding lymph nodes identified after four cycles of methotrexate, vinblastine, doxorubicin (Adriamycin), and cisplatin.[79]

Using CT or MRI, it is best to approach gynecologic malignancies in a systematic way. The goals of abdominal and pelvic imaging are to identify the source of the mass whenever possible; locate findings indicative of direct extension, such as peritoneal implants and ascites; assess lymph nodes for increased size and number; and determine whether there is renal compromise. Hydronephrosis may indicate involvement of the tumor, and it often needs to be treated before chemotherapy can begin.

Cervical Cancer

Any cervical mass that is larger than 1.5 cm in diameter or extends beyond the cervix should be examined using MRI. CT lacks the contrast resolution necessary to be the primary staging procedure for patients with relatively low-volume disease, with overall staging accuracy ranging from 60% to 80%.[80,81] On MRI, cervical cancer usually is usually hyperintense compared with the dark cervical stroma on T2-weighted images. Preservation of the black ring of the cervical stroma, no matter how thin, virtually excludes parametrial extension. These patients are candidates for surgical cure. Those in whom the black line is broken and a mass extends beyond the expected confines of the cervix have an 85% likelihood of parametrial invasion and are usually treated primarily with radiation therapy.[82] It is generally agreed that the administration of intravenous Gd-DTPA improves staging accuracy to between 85% and 90%.[82]

In cases of advanced disease, CT is preferred. It is quick to perform and read, and it has a higher spatial resolution than MRI. The cervix is often enlarged in the anteroposterior direction, and it may contain gas. Images should be scrutinized for extension into the pelvic sidewall manifested by encasement of the iliac vessels or separation of the vessels from the mass by a fat plane that is less than 3 mm wide. CT and MRI are equivalent in the detection of involved lymph nodes. Extension of disease also manifests by thickening of the uterosacral ligaments, although this can be a result of irradiation. Hydronephrosis often develops because of bladder wall or ureteric invasion, and this finding upstages the disease to stage IIIB. Using CT, a survey of the other abdominal organs for the presence of metastases can be accomplished without requiring extra scanning time.

Uterine Cancer

On ultrasound examinations, the endometrial thickness of a postmenopausal woman should not exceed 5 mm. Thickened endometrial linings identified on ultrasound examination may merit biopsy. Even in the presence of vaginal bleeding, endometrial thickness of less than 5 mm excludes endometrial cancer.[83]

Most women with endometrial carcinoma do not require further imaging. Treatment is predicated on physical examination results and low-stage disease confined to the endometrium. Gynecologic oncologists rely heavily on clinical staging; however, enlarged lymph nodes and the depth of primary tumor invasion may not be appreciated. Using clinical staging, Creasman and colleagues reported that only 35 (24%) of 148 patients with presumed stage II endometrial cancer had disease confined to the uterus.[84] MRI is recommended when locally advanced disease is expected based on physical examination findings and in the patient with a difficult physical examination due to obesity or prior irradiation or surgery. Sagittal and axial view, T2-weighted images, as well as contrast-enhanced images, should be obtained and scrutinized for extension of hyperintense tumor into or through the myometrium. Invasion of more than 50% of the myometrium increases the likelihood of involved lymph nodes and connotes a poorer overall prognosis.

On contrast-enhanced CT scans, the nodules of tumor usually rim the dilated endometrial canal and completely fill the lower uterine segment. Metastases can extend by the fallopian tubes to the ovaries, causing development of an adnexal mass. Findings of advanced disease are similar to those of cervical cancer and consist of extension of lymphatic disease to the pelvic sidewall chains and retroperitoneum. When these pathways are blocked by tumor, extension by the processus vaginalis to the inguinal nodes may occur. There is a paucity of data on the accuracy of helical CT for the staging of endometrial cancer. In the sole published study of 25 patients, single-detector-row helical CT was less sensitive than MRI for the detection of deep myometrial invasion (83% and 42%, respectively).[85] However, in a meta-analysis conducted by Kinkel and colleagues, CT, MRI, and ultrasonography were found to perform equally well in the overall staging of endometrial cancer.[86] Sarcomas of the uterus usually mimic endometrial carcinoma (67%) or degenerating fibroids (33%).

Ovarian Cancer

A radiologic diagnostic oncologic trial showed that ultrasonography, CT, and MRI are equal (approximately 87% to 95%) in the overall staging of ovarian cancer.[87] CT and MRI have excellent positive and negative predictive values for tumor resectability (>90%). MRI has a slightly higher detection rate for peritoneal metastases. In routine practice, CT is usually preferred because it is well accepted by the patient and gives an overall view of the abdomen and pelvis that is well understood by referring physicians. MRI is particularly useful in the detection of recurrent disease because its tremendous contrast sensitivity yields excellent identification of even very small, high-signal-intensity cystic implants on T2-weighted images.[88]

Cystadenocarcinoma usually appears on contrast-enhanced CT images as a large, predominantly cystic mass with a nodular, enhancing wall and thick, enhancing septa (Fig. 9-10). Ascites, hydronephrosis, and omental and peritoneal implants are common accompaniments. Enlarged lymph nodes are less common but do occur. On imaging examinations, it is important to identify solid implants before therapy, because a large, solid tumor burden may be treated with chemotherapy rather than primary debulking surgery.

Disease Metastatic to the Pelvis

CT and MR are equivalent for evaluating metastatic or recurrent disease to the pelvis. Using either method, it can be difficult to separate enhancement due to inflammation caused by irradiation or surgical therapy from that due to recurrent disease. The presence of a mass lesion abutting the peritoneal surface generally indicates a metastasis. Enlarged lymph nodes are usually an ominous sign.

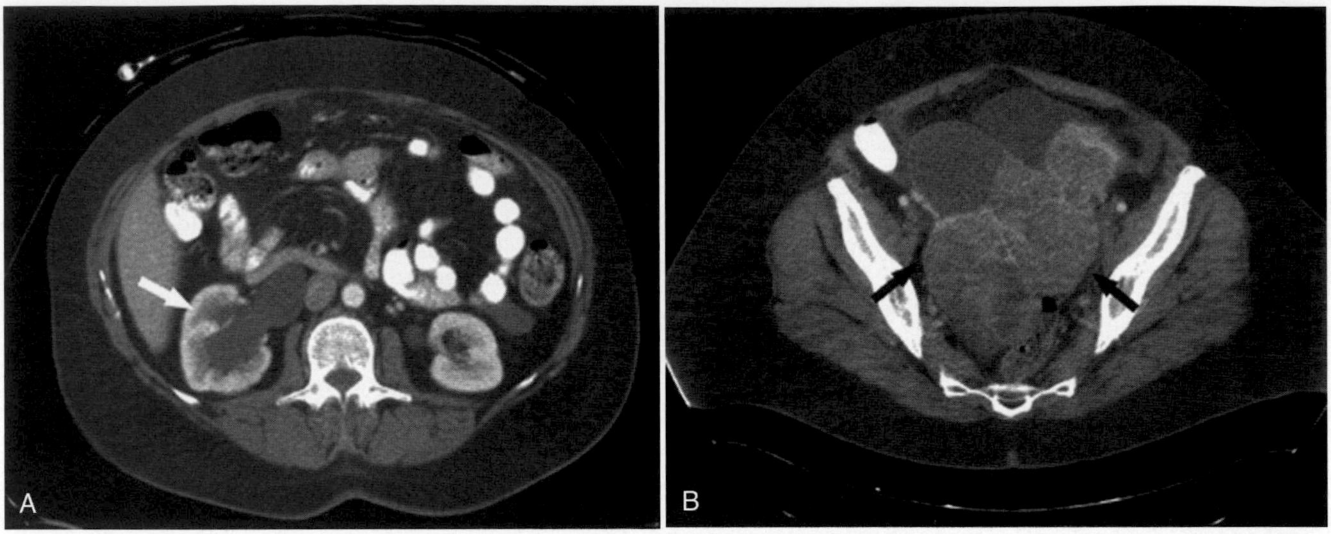

Figure 9-10 A 57-year-old woman with a pelvic mass. Axial-view, contrast-enhanced images at the level of the kidneys (**A**) and pelvis (**B**) show an obstructed right kidney *(white arrow)* and bilateral pelvic masses with cystic and solid components *(black arrows)*. On resection, this mass was found to consist of bilateral ovarian cystadenocarcinomas.

REFERENCES

1. Katayama H, Yamaguchi K, Kozuka T, et al: Adverse reactions to ionic and nonionic contrast media: a report from the Japanese Committee on the Safety of Contrast Media. Radiology 175:621-628, 1990.
2. Tublin ME, Murphy ME, Tessler FN: Current concepts in contrast media-induced nephropathy. AJR Am J Roentgenol 171:933-939, 1998.
3. Lasser EC, Berry CC, Talner LB, et al: Pre-treatment with corticosteroids to alleviate reactions to intravenous contrast material. N Engl J Med 317:845-849, 1987.
4. Bettmann MA, Heeren T, Greenfield A, et al: Adverse events with radiographic contrast agents: results of the SCVIR Contrast Agent Registry. Radiology 203:611-620, 1997.
5. Bettmann MA: Frequently asked questions: iodinated contrast agents. Radiographics 24:S3-S10, 2004.
6. Shellock FG, Crues JV: MR procedures: biologic effects, safety, and patient care. Radiology 232:635-652, 2004.
7. Albercio RA, Husain SH, Sirotkin I: Imaging in head and neck oncology. Surg Oncol Clin North Am 13:13-35, 2004.
8. Schaible R, Hortling N, Stein M, et al: Follow-up in patients with head and neck tumors: evaluation of CT criteria for local tumor recurrence. Laryngorhinootologie 80:563-568, 2001.
9. Galanis E, Buckner JC, Novotny P, et al: Efficacy of neuroradiological imaging, neurological examination, and symptom status in follow-up assessment of patients with high-grade gliomas. J Neurosurg 93:201-207, 2000.
10. Lacroix M, Abi-Said D, Fourney DR, et al: A multi-variate analysis of 416 patients with glioblastoma multiforme: prognosis, extent of resection, and survival. J Neurosurg 95:190-198, 2001.
11. Yokoi K, Kamiya N, Matsuguma H, et al: Detection of brain metastasis in potentially operable non-small cell lung cancer: a comparison of CT and MRI. Chest 115:714-719, 1999.
12. Lebrun C, Fontaine D, Ramaioli A, et al: Long-term outcome of oligodendrogliomas. Neurology 62:1783-1787, 2004.
13. Wierzba-Borowics T, Schmidt-Sidor B, Szpak GM, et al: Haemangioblastoma of the posterior cranial fossa: clinco-neuropathological study. Neuropathology 41:245-249, 2003.
14. Slater A, Moore NR, Huson SM: The natural history of cerebellar hemangioblastomas in von Hippel-Lindau disease. AJNR Am J Neuroradiol 24:1570-1574, 2003.
15. Guinto G, Felix I, Arechiga N, et al: Primary central nervous system lymphomas in immunocompetent patients. Histol Histopathol 19:963-972, 2003.
16. Pekala JS, Mamourian AC, Wishart HA, et al: Focal lesion in the splenium of the corpus callosum on FLAIR images: a common finding with aging and after brain radiation therapy. AJNR Am J Neuroradiol 24:664-665, 2003.
17. Steen RG, Spence D, Wu S, et al: Effect of therapeutic ionizing radiation on the human brain. Ann Neurol 50:787-795, 2001.
18. Kaufman LM, Mafee MF, Song CD, et al: Retinoblastoma and simulating lesions: role of CT, MR imaging and use of Gd-DTPA contrast enhancement. Radiol Clin North Am 36:1101-1117, 1998.
19. Rohen EM, Provenzale JM, Barboriak DP, et al: Screening for cerebral metastasis with FDG PET in patients undergoing whole-body staging of non-central nervous system malignancy. Radiology 226:181-187, 2003.
20. Nemzek WR, Hecht S, Gandour-Edwards R, et al: Perineural spread of head and neck tumors: how accurate is MR imaging? AJNR Am J Neuroradiol 19:701-706, 1998.
21. Mercader VP, Gatenbury RA, Mohr RM, et al: CT surveillance of the thorax in patients with squamous cell carcinoma of the head and neck: a preliminary experience. J Comput Assist Tomogr 21:412-417, 1997.
22. Douglas WG, Rigual NR, Loree TR, et al: Current concepts in the management of a second malignancy of the lung in patients with head and neck cancer. Curr Opin Otolaryngol Head Neck Surg 11:85-88, 2003.
23. Schwartz DL, Rajendran J, Yeuh B, et al: Staging of head and neck squamous cell cancer with extended fluorodeoxyglucose FDG-PET. Arch Otolaryngol Head Neck Surg 129:1173-1178, 2003.
24. Beyer T, Townsend DW, Brun T, et al: A combined PET/CT scanner for clinical oncology. J Nucl Med 41:1369-1379, 2000.
25. Dresel S, Grammerstorff J, Schwenzer K, et al: (18F) FDG imaging of head and neck tumors: comparison of hybrid PET and morphological methods. Eur J Nucl Med Mol Imaging 30:995-1003, 2003.
26. Joshi U, van der Hoeven JJ, Comans EF, et al: In search of an unknown primary tumor presenting with extra-cervical metastases: the diagnostic performance of FDG-PET. Br J Radiol 77:1000-1006, 2004.
27. Yonestu K, Sumi M, Izumi M, et al: Contribution of Doppler sonography blood flow information to the diagnosis of metastatic cervical nodes in patients with head and neck cancer: assessment in relation to anatomic levels of the neck. AJNR Am J Neuroradiol 22:163-169, 2001.
28. Sumi M, Ohki M, Nakamura T: Comparison of sonography and CT for differentiating benign from malignant cervical lymph

nodes in patients with squamous cell carcinoma of the head and neck. AJR Am J Roentgenol 176:1019-1024, 2001.
29. Glazer GM, Gross BH, Quint LE, et al: Normal mediastinal lymph nodes: number and size according to American Thoracic Society Mapping. AJR Am J Roentgenol 144:261-265, 1985.
30. Smith RA, Glynn TJ: Lung cancer: epidemiology of lung cancer. Radiol Clin North Am 38:453-470, 2000.
31. Woodring JH, Stelling CB: Adenocarcinoma of the lung: a tumor with a changing pleomorphic character. AJR Am J Roentgenol 140:657-664, 1983.
32. Patz EF: Diagnosis and staging of lung cancer: imaging bronchogenic carcinoma. Chest 117(Suppl):905-955, 2000.
33. Sider L: Radiographic manifestations of primary bronchogenic carcinoma. Radiol Clin North Am 28:583-597, 1990.
34. Shin MS, Jackson LK, Shelton RW, et al: Giant cell carcinoma of the lung. Chest 89:366-369, 1986.
35. McLoud TC: Imaging techniques for diagnosis and staging of lung cancer. Clin Chest Med 223:123-136, 2002.
36. Wahl RL, Quint LE, Greenough RL, et al: Staging of mediastinal non-small cell lung cancer with FDG PET, CT, and fusion images: preliminary prospective evaluation. Radiology 191:371-377, 1994.
37. Castellino RA, Blank N, Hoppe RT, et al: Hodgkin disease: contributions of chest CT in the initial staging evaluation. Radiology 160:603-605, 1986.
38. Castellino RA, Hilton S, O'Brien JP, et al: Non-Hodgkin lymphoma: contribution of chest CT in the initial staging evaluation. Radiology 199:129-132, 1996.
39. Lymphoid neoplasms. *In* Greene FL, Page DL, Fleming ID (eds): AJCC Cancer Staging Handbook, 6th ed. Chicago, Springer-Verlag, 2002, pp 427-448.
40. McGriffin DC, Kirklin JK, Naftel DC, et al: Competing outcomes after heart transplantation: a comparison of eras and outcomes. J Heart Lung Transplant 16:190-198, 1997.
41. Harris KM, Schwartz ML, Slasky BS, et al: Posttransplantation cyclosporine-induced lymphoproliferative disorders: clinical and radiologic manifestations. Radiology 162:697-700, 1987.
42. Dodd GD III, Ledesma-Medina J, Baron RL, et al: Posttransplant lymphoproliferative disorders: intrathoracic manifestations. Radiology 184:65-69, 1992.
43. Devesa S, Blot W, Fraumeni J: Changing patterns in the incidence of esophageal and gastric carcinoma in the United States. Cancer 83:2049-2053, 1983.
44. Daly J, Fry W, Little AG, et al: Esophageal cancer: results of an American College of Surgeons patient care evaluation study. J Am Coll Surg 190:562-572, 2000.
45. Iyer R, Silverman P, Tamm E, et al: Imaging in oncology from the University of Texas M.D. Anderson Cancer Center—diagnosis, staging, and follow-up of esophageal cancer. AJR Am J Roentgenol 181:785-793, 2003.
46. Lerut T, Flamen P, Ectors N, et al: Histopathologic validation of lymph node staging with FDG-PET scan in cancer of the esophagus and gastroesophageal junction—a prospective study based on primary surgery with extensive lymphadenectomy. Ann Surg 232:743-751, 2000.
47. Polkowski M, Palucki J, Wronska E, et al: Endosonography versus helical computed tomography for locoregional staging of gastric cancer. Endoscopy 36:617-623, 2004.
48. Abdalla EK, Pisters PWT: Staging and preoperative evaluation of upper gastrointestinal malignancies. Semin Oncol 31:513-529, 2004.
49. Matsuki M, Kani H, Tatsugami F, et al: Preoperative assessment of vascular anatomy around the stomach by 3D imaging using MDCT before laparoscopy-assisted gastrectomy. AJR Am J Roentgenol 183:145-151, 2004.
50. Horton KM, Fishman EK: Multidetector-row computed tomography and 3-dimensional computed tomography imaging of small bowel neoplasms: current concept in diagnosis. J Comput Assist Tomogr 28:106-116, 2004.
51. Horton KM, Kamel I, Hofmann L, et al: Carcinoid tumors of the small bowel: a multitechnique imaging approach. AJR Am J Roentgenol 182:559-567, 2004.
52. Xiong L, Chintapalli KN, Dodd GD III, et al: Frequency and CT patterns of bowel wall thickening proximal to cancer of the colon. AJR Am J Roentgenol 182:905-909, 2004.
53. Low RN, McCue M, Barone R, et al: MR staging of primary colorectal carcinoma: comparison with surgical and histopathologic findings. Abdom Imaging 28:784-793, 2003.
54. Hussain HK, Syed I, Nghiem HV, Johnson TD, et al: T2-weighted MR imaging in the assessment of cirrhotic liver. Radiology 230:637-644, 2004.
55. Jeong YY, Mitchell DG, Kamishima T, et al: Small (<20 mm) enhancing hepatic nodules seen on arterial phase MR imaging of the cirrhotic liver: clinical implications. AJR Am J Roentgenol 178:1327-1334, 2002.
56. Braga HJV, Choti MA, Lee VS, et al: Liver lesions: manganese-enhanced MR and dual-phase helical CT for preoperative detection and characterization—comparison with receiver operating characteristic analysis. Radiology 223:525-531, 2002.
57. Bluemke DA, Paulson EK, Choti MA, et al: Detection of hepatic lesions in candidates for surgery: comparison of ferumoxides-enhanced MR imaging and dual-phase helical CT. AJR Am J Roentgenol 175:1653-1658, 2000.
58. Semelka RC, Martin DR, Balci C, et al: Focal liver lesions: comparison of dual-phase CT and multisequence multiplanar MR imaging including dynamic gadolinium enhancement. J Magn Reson Imaging 13:397-401, 2001.
59. Robinson PJ, Arnold P, Wilson D: Small "indeterminate" lesions on CT of the liver: a follow-up study of stability. Br J Radiol 76:866-874, 2003.
60. Catalano O, Esposito M, Nunziata A, et al: Multiphase helical CT findings after percutaneous ablation procedures for hepatocellular carcinoma. Abdom Imaging 25:607-614, 2000.
61. Chopra S, Dodd GD III, Chintapalli KN, et al: Tumor recurrence after radiofrequency thermal ablation of hepatic tumors: spectrum of findings on dual-phase contrast-enhanced CT. AJR Am J Roentgenol 177:381-387, 2001.
62. Agarwal B, Abu-Hamda E, Molke KL, et al: Endoscopic ultrasound-guided fine needle aspiration and multidetector spiral CT in the diagnosis of pancreatic cancer. Am J Gastroenterol 99:844-850, 2004.
63. Soriano A, Castells A, Ayuso C, et al: Preoperative staging and tumor resectability assessment of pancreatic cancer: prospective study comparing endoscopic ultrasonography, helical computed tomography, magnetic resonance imaging, and angiography. Am J Gastroenterol 99:492-501, 2004.
64. Brügel M, Link TM, Rummeny EJ, et al: Assessment of vascular invasion in pancreatic head cancer with multislice spiral CT: value of multiplanar reconstructions. Eur Radiol 14:1188-1195, 2004.
65. Neider AM, Tarneja SS: The role of partial nephrectomy for renal cell carcinoma in contemporary practice. Urol Clin North Am 30:529-542, 2003.
66. Urban BA, Ratner LE, Fishman EK: Three-dimensional volume-rendered CT angiography of the renal arteries and veins: normal anatomy, variants, and clinical applications. Radiographics 21: 373-386, 2001.
67. Lang EK, Macchia RJ, Thomas R, et al: Improved detection of renal pathologic features on multiphasic helical CT compared with IVU in patients presenting with microscopic hematuria. Urology 61:528-532, 2003.
68. Caoili EM, Cohan RH, Korobkin M, et al: Urinary tract abnormalities: initial experience with multi-detector row CT urography. Radiology 222:353-360, 2002.
69. Caoili EM, Korobkin M, Francis IR, et al: Adrenal masses: characterization with combined unenhanced and delayed enhanced CT. Radiology 222:629-633, 2002.
70. Caoili EM, Korobkin M, Francis IR, et al: Delayed enhanced CT of lipid-poor adrenal adenomas. AJR Am J Roentgenol 175:1411-1415, 2000.
71. Korobkin M, Brodeur FJ, Francis IR, et al: CT time-attenuation washout curves of adrenal adenomas and nonadenomas. AJR Am J Roentgenol 170:747-752, 1998.
72. Outwater EK, Siegelman ES, Radecki PD, et al: Distinction between benign and malignant adrenal masses: value of T1-

weighted chemical-shift MR imaging. AJR Am J Roentgenol 165:579-583, 1995.
73. Paulsen SD, Nghiem HV, Korobkin M, et al: Changing role of imaging-guided percutaneous biopsy of adrenal masses: evaluation of 50 adrenal biopsies. AJR Am J Roentgenol 182:1033-1037, 2004.
74. Hilton S, Herr HW, Teitcher JB, et al: CT detection of retroperitoneal lymph node metastases in patients with clinical stage I testicular nonseminomatous germ cell cancer: assessment of size and distribution criteria. AJR Am J Roentgenol 169:521-525, 1997.
75. Cornud F, Flam T, Chauveinc L, et al: Extraprostatic spread of clinically localized prostate cancer: factors predictive of pT3 tumor and of positive endorectal MR imaging examination results. Radiology 224:203-210, 2002.
76. Tempany CM, Zhou X, Zerhouni EA, et al: Staging of prostate cancer: results of Radiology Diagnostic Oncology Group project comparison of three MR imaging techniques. Radiology 192:47-54, 1994.
77. Silverman JM, Krebs TL: MR imaging evaluation with a transrectal surface coil of local recurrence of prostatic cancer in men who have undergone radical prostatectomy. AJR Am J Roentgenol 168:379-385, 1997.
78. Barentsz JO, Jager GJ, van Vierzen PBJ, et al: Staging urinary bladder cancer after transurethral biopsy: value of fast dynamic contrast-enhanced MR imaging. Radiology 201:185-193, 1996.
79. Barentsz JO, Berger-Hartog O, Witjes JA, et al: Evaluation of chemotherapy in advanced urinary bladder cancer with fast dynamic contrast-enhanced MR imaging. Radiology 207:791-797, 1998.
80. Kim SH, Choi BI, Lee HP, et al: Uterine cervical carcinoma: comparison of CT and MR findings. Radiology 175:45-51, 1990.
81. Cobby M, Browning J, Jones A, et al: Magnetic resonance imaging, computed tomography and endosonography in the local staging of carcinoma of the cervix. Br J Radiol 63:673-679, 1990.
82. Scheidler J, Heuck AF: Imaging of cancer of the cervix. Radiol Clin North Am 40:577-590, 2002.
83. Bree RL, Carlos RC: US for postmenopausal bleeding: consensus development and patient-centered outcomes. Radiology 222:595-598, 2002.
84. Creasman WT, DeGeest K, diSaia PJ, et al: Significance of true surgical pathologic staging: a Gynecologic Oncology Group study. Am J Obstet Gynecol 181:31-34, 1999.
85. Hardesty LA, Sumkin JH, Hankim C, et al: The ability of helical CT to preoperatively stage endometrial carcinoma. AJR Am J Roentgenol 176:603-606, 2001.
86. Kinkel K, Kaji Y, Yu KK, et al: Radiologic staging in patients with endometrial cancer: a meta-analysis. Radiology 212:711-718, 1999.
87. Kurtz AB, Tsimikas JV, Tempany CMC, et al: Diagnosis and staging of ovarian cancer: comparative values of Doppler and conventional US, CT, and MR imaging correlated with surgery and histopathologic analysis—report of the Radiology Diagnostic Oncology Group. Radiology 212:19-27, 1999.
88. Forstner R, Hricak H, Occhipinti KA, et al: Ovarian cancer: staging with CT and MR imaging. Radiology 197:619-626, 1995.

CHAPTER 10

NUCLEAR MEDICINE

Amir H. Khandani and Arif Sheikh

POSITRON EMISSION TOMOGRAPHY

Despite the exquisite resolution of computed tomography (CT) and magnetic resonance imaging (MRI), some disease processes may go undetected by these anatomically based modalities. The anatomic modalities also have shortcomings in assessing the response to treatment and in distinguishing responders from nonresponders.

Over the past half-century, a variety of nuclear medicine probes have been used to evaluate disease processes at the cellular level. Nuclear medicine is the only clinical discipline using intracellular contrast agents in imaging, and it is therefore more sensitive than anatomic modalities in detecting disease processes. Some of these probes, such as radioiodine, have been very successful and are heavily used. Nevertheless, most nuclear medicine imaging techniques have suffered from low specificity and low spatial resolution, with the latter being associated with the physics of single-photon–emitting radiotracers. Synthesis of biologically important radiopharmaceuticals with single-photon–emitting radiotracers has been a major challenge.

Positron emission tomography (PET) is a nuclear medicine modality that uses positron emitters such as fluorine 18, oxygen 15, nitrogen 13, and carbon 11. The fact that these nuclides are components of common biologic molecules makes PET particularly suitable for visually capturing different biologic pathways. Although PET has been used for several decades in the research setting, its clinical use has grown substantially in the past decade. PET with ^{18}F-fluorodeoxyglucose (FDG), "radioactive sugar," as its workhorse has substantially influenced clinical oncology practice by refining the processes of diagnosis, staging, and restaging. Although the strengths and limitations of FDG-PET in diagnosing cancer are well known, its role in staging and restaging is evolving. The data indicate that FDG-PET will likely play an important role in monitoring therapy and predicting the course of the disease.

Basic Physics of Positron Emission Tomography

The radioisotope portion of the molecule used in PET imaging emits a positron (i.e., positively charged electron), which travels a distance of a few millimeters in tissue before it collides with a negatively charged electron. This collision annihilates the entire mass of the positron and electron, generating two photons with energy of 511 KeV each. These two photons travel at the speed of light in exactly opposite directions (i.e., 180 degrees apart). Coincident detection of these two photons by two oppositely positioned detectors in the PET scanner results in images with a much higher resolution compared with the conventional, single-photon nuclear medicine studies and produces the possibility of quantitative measurement of the tracer uptake in a lesion of interest.

PET/CT allows the fusion of the metabolic information from PET with the anatomic information from CT. PET/CT increases the diagnostic accuracy compared with stand-alone PET. In PET/CT, the patient undergoes a CT scan, followed by a PET scan, without changing the patient's position. PET for most oncologic indications (whole-body PET) is acquired from the base of the skull through the upper thighs. In some instances, such as in melanoma patients, PET is acquired from the vertex of the skull through the toes. The CT portion (i.e., transmission scan) of PET/CT is acquired within seconds to minutes, whereas the PET acquisition time for each bed position (about 15 cm) is several minutes; the total PET acquisition time in newer machines is 15 to 25 minutes.

In addition to delivering anatomic information, the CT portion of PET/CT is used to measure the attenuation of the x-ray photons traveling through the patient to produce the so-called attenuation map and correct the PET data for tissue attenuation. During PET acquisition, photons from structures deep in the abdomen or pelvis are more strongly attenuated than those from superficial structures and the chest. The intensity of uptake in deeper structures is underestimated on non–attenuation-corrected PET images; the intensity of uptake in the deeper structures is normalized to the intensity of uptake in the superficial structures on the attenuation-corrected PET images (Fig. 10-1). Although correction of the PET data for tissue attenuation is indispensable, misalignment between PET and CT can cause mislocalization of lesions on the fused PET/CT images. This may be caused by the changed position of a body part (e.g., neck, legs) or physiologic changes in the position of an organ (e.g., respiratory movement) between the transmission (CT) and the emission scan (non–attenuation-corrected PET). Because the degree of misalignment and resulting mislocalization can be significant, the radiologist must be cautious when interpreting the attenuation-corrected PET/CT images or using PET/CT images for radiation therapy planning. The magnitude of this misalignment can be assessed by fusing the non–attenuation-corrected PET images with CT, which can be performed on any PET review station. In case of significant misalignment, the non–attenuation-corrected PET images should be reviewed without fusion with CT, and the metabolic findings on PET should be correlated side by side with the anatomic findings on CT (Fig. 10-2).

At its introduction, the CT portion of the PET/CT was acquired without contrast and used solely for attenuation correction and anatomic localization of the PET findings. However, with the development of multislice CT machines and their introduction to PET/CT scanners, an increasing number of institutions are performing the CT portion of the PET/CT studies with diagnostic quality CT, using intravenous and oral contrast as needed. However, because the density of intravenous and oral contrast used in CT can produce artifacts, with overestimation of FDG uptake in areas of high-contrast density, the protocol for CT has to be modified with the general approach of dilution of the contrast medium.

General Aspects of Tumor Visualization on ^{18}F-Fluorodeoxyglucose Positron Emission Tomography

FDG (2-[^{18}F] fluoro-2-deoxy-D-glucose) is the most commonly used radiotracer in clinical PET imaging. Tumor imaging with FDG is based on the principle of increased glucose

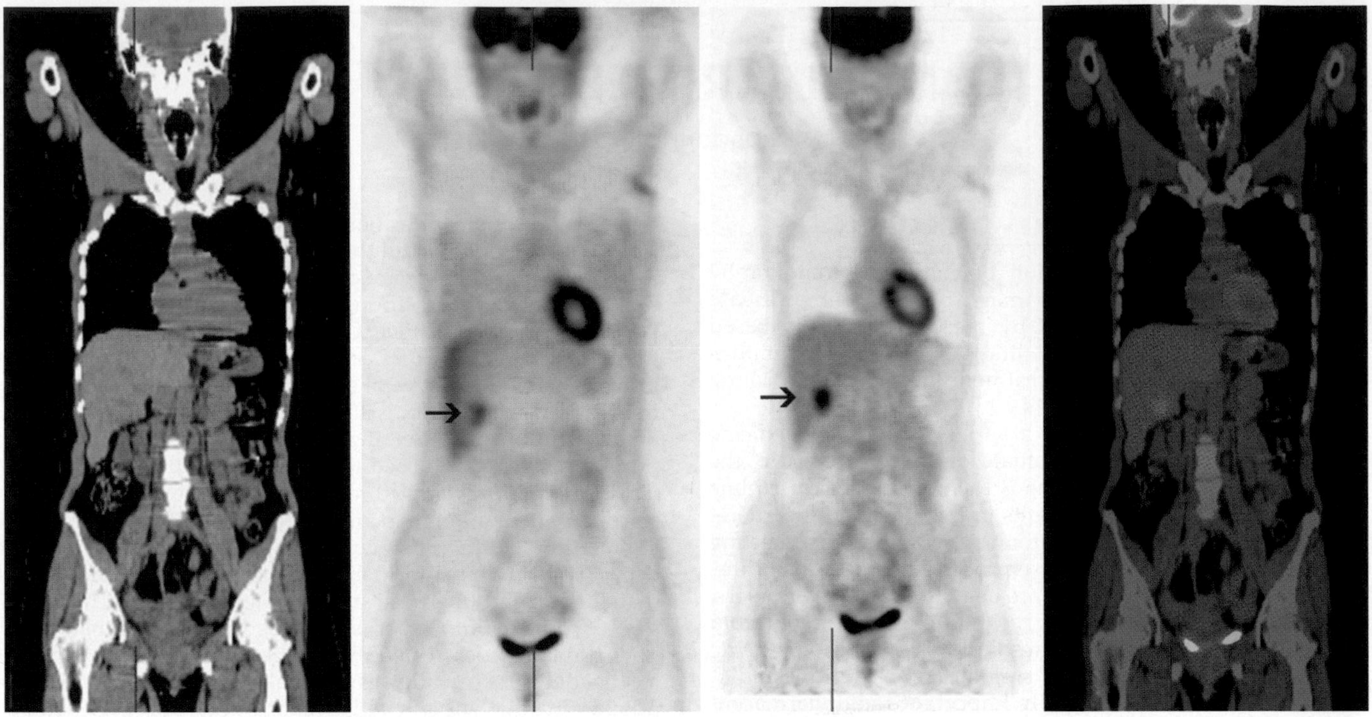

A B C D

Figure 10-1 Computed tomography (CT) (**A**) is used for anatomic localization and as an "attenuation map" to normalize the intensity of uptake in the deeper structures compared with that of the superficial structures. The metastatic liver lesion *(arrow)* is better appreciated on the attenuation-corrected positron emission tomography (PET) image (**C**) or fused attenuation-corrected PET/CT image (**D**) than on the non–attenuation-corrected PET image (**B**).

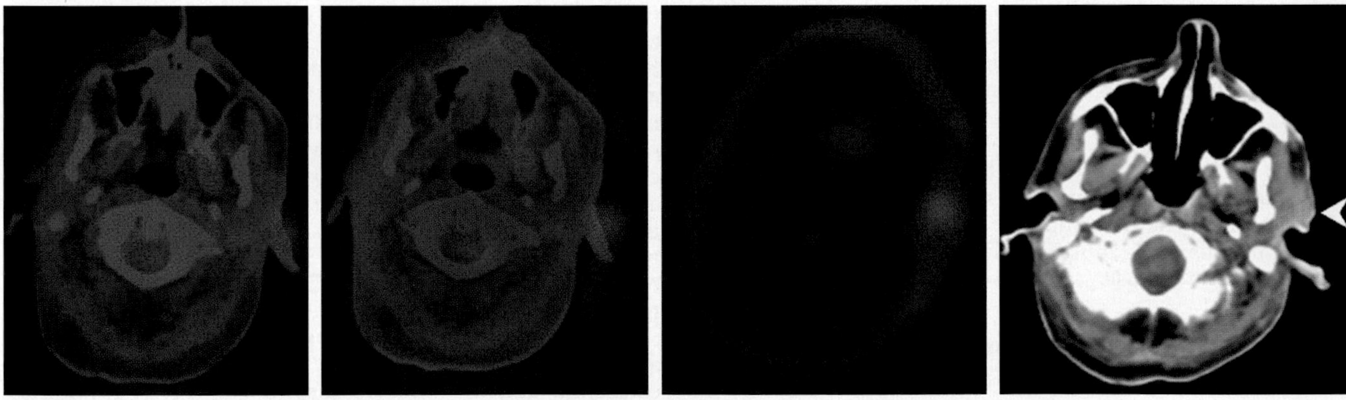

A B C D

Figure 10-2 Lesions can be mislocalized because of movement of the head between computed tomography (CT) and positron emission tomography (PET) acquisition. In a patient with recurrent squamous cell cancer of the left cheek, PET was requested for staging. Fused attenuation-corrected PET/CT images indicated an abnormal focus in the left external auditory canal (**A**). Review of the fused non–attenuation-corrected PET/CT images (**B**) revealed misalignment between CT and PET. Side-by-side review of the non–attenuation-corrected PET (**C**) and CT (**D**) was most useful and could localize the area of abnormal uptake anterior to the left ear *(arrowhead)*.

metabolism of cancer cells. Like glucose, FDG is taken up by the cancer cells through facilitative glucose transporters (GLUTs). GLUTs are glycoproteins; 12 isoforms have been identified. Once in the cell, glucose or FDG is phosphorylated by hexokinase to glucose-6-phospate or FDG-6-phosphate, respectively. Expression of GLUTs and hexokinase, as well as the affinity of hexokinase for phosphorylation of glucose or FDG, is generally higher in cancer cells than in normal cells. Glucose-6-phosphate travels farther down the glycolytic or oxidative pathways to be metabolized, in contrast to FDG-6-phosphate, which cannot be metabolized. In normal cells, glucose-6-phosphate or FDG-6-phosphate can be dephosphorylated and exit the cells. In cancer cells, however, expression of glucose-6-phosphatase is usually significantly decreased, and glucose-6-phosphate or FDG-6-phosphate therefore can become only minimally dephosphorylated and remains in large part within the cell. Because FDG-6-phosphate cannot be metabolized, it is trapped in the cancer cell as a polar metabolite, and it constitutes the basis for tumor visualization on PET.

The intensity of a malignant tumor on PET correlates with the number of malignant cells in the tumor mass. Although most malignant tumors are markedly intense on PET, tumors such as bronchioloalveolar lung cancer may be only moderately or mildly intense or may not be visualized on PET at all. Likewise, the intensity of a tumor decreases as soon as after only one cycle of an effective chemotherapy, possibly because of a decreased number of viable cells or the decreasing metabolic activity of those cells. Although this constitutes the basis for monitoring therapy by PET, the effect can also cause false-negative PET findings.

The intensity of malignant lesions on PET also depends on their location in the body. For example, the FDG avidity of a lung or liver lesion may be underestimated, or the lesion may even go undetected on PET; because of the repetitive craniocaudal movement of the lung and liver lesions during PET acquisition, the effective acquisition time is decreased. Detectability of lung and liver lesions can be improved by *respiratory gating*, in which only emission data collected in certain parts of the respiratory cycle are used for image reconstruction, resulting in better visualization of small lesions with the disadvantage of longer acquisition time. A practical approach in systems not equipped with respiratory gating is to increase the PET acquisition time and view the non–attenuation-corrected images; the latter eliminate any underestimation of uptake due to misalignment between PET and CT.

FDG is also taken up in benign processes such as infection and inflammation because white blood cells and fibroblasts are highly avid for FDG. This is probably the most common reason for false-positive findings on PET scans obtained for oncologic indications. A false-positive reading on PET can partly be avoided by obtaining the patient's medical history and determining the pretest likelihood of an infectious or inflammatory process. There are no published data on the time interval after an invasive procedure or radiation therapy in which a PET scan can be falsely positive, and the inflammatory cell reaction after such a procedure varies among organs. For example, there is evidence that only minimal reactive cell accumulation occurs in the liver within the first 3 days after radiofrequency ablation and that the reactive cells do not cause false-positive PET findings at least in the first 7 days after radiofrequency ablation.[1]

To minimize FDG uptake in the muscle while maximizing its uptake in tumor, patients are instructed to fast for at least 4 hours and avoid excessive physical activity for 24 hours before the PET appointment. Glucose-containing drinks and intravenous glucose must be avoided at least 4 hours before FDG injection. The fasting state lowers the serum level of glucose so that FDG has less competition for uptake by the tumor, whereas muscle uptake is minimized by fasting (by lowering the serum insulin level) and by avoiding excessive physical activity; low FDG uptake in the muscles improves the tumor-to-background ratio and the image quality.

High glucose levels in diabetic patients can decrease the image quality. Although a normal glucose level in diabetic patients before FDG injection is desirable, it often cannot be achieved. Most institutions perform PET for diabetics after one or two attempts to reduce the serum glucose level below an empirically set level of 200 to 250 mg/dL. Although the positive predictive value of the findings on such a scan remains high, the negative predictive value may be reduced. In diabetic patients, the image quality (i.e., muscle and soft tissue uptake) should be assessed before interpretation and mentioned in the report.

FDG uptake in the brown fat in the neck and supraclavicular regions may obscure pathologic findings in these areas. FDG uptake in brown fat is even more extensive in pediatric patients, and it can be seen in the mediastinum, paraspinal region, and upper abdomen. Diazepam administration can reduce the FDG uptake in brown fat.

The standardized uptake value (SUV) is a semiquantitative measure of the tracer uptake in a region of interest that normalizes the lesion activity to the injected dose and body weight; the SUV does not have a unit. Despite initial enthusiasm, it is generally accepted that SUV should not be used to differentiate malignant from benign processes and that the visual interpretation of PET studies by an experienced reader provides the highest accuracy. There are many factors influencing the calculation of SUV, such as the body weight and composition, the time between tracer injection and image acquisition, the spatial resolution of the PET scanner, and the image reconstruction algorithm. Nonetheless, SUV may be useful as a measure to follow the metabolic activity of a tumor over time within the same patient and to compare different subjects within a research study under defined conditions. For example, the SUV of an individual tumor can be measured before and at different time points after therapy, and any change can be used as an index of therapeutic response. However, it is unclear whether this measure can be used for clinical decision-making. Some indicate that the intensity of FDG uptake by itself can assess the aggressiveness of a tumor and therefore correlate with prognosis, regardless of the treatment modality. However, there is no firm evidence that patient management should be modified on the basis of intensity of uptake.[2]

Most Common Indications for ^{18}F-Fluorodeoxyglucose Positron Emission Tomography in Oncology

Lung Cancer

PET has an overall sensitivity higher than 90% and specificity of about 85% for diagnosing malignancy in primary and metastatic lung lesions; the sensitivity and specificity of PET for small cell lung cancer are similar. The sensitivity of PET for bronchioloalveolar lung cancer and carcinoid of the lung is about 60%, and the specificity of PET for lung cancer is lower in areas with a high prevalence of granulomatous lung disease. PET is particularly useful in patients with a low (5% to 20%) or intermediate (20% to 70%) risk of lung cancer, as determined by an evaluation of symptoms, risk factors, and radiographic appearance. In these cases, PET is helpful in moving the patient to the very-low-risk (<5%) or high-risk (>70%) category.[3] It is expected that the use of PET for diagnosing malignancy in indeterminate lung nodules will continue to grow as more patients are diagnosed with nodules on CT performed for other indications or as a screening test. Most of the current PET scanners are capable of detecting lung lesions as small as 6 mm, and the resolution of PET is likely to improve. Most of the literature in this regard is based on data from the 1990s, when the resolution of PET was above 1 cm; studies are being conducted to systematically assess the sensitivity and specificity of PET for detecting malignancy in subcentimeter lung lesions.

In mediastinal staging of non–small cell lung cancer (NSCLC), patients with clinical stage I and II disease have by definition a radiographically negative mediastinum. However, in patients with central tumors, adenocarcinoma, or N1 lymph node enlargement, the false-negative rate of CT for mediastinal involvement is 20% to 25%. It is unclear whether PET should be used instead of mediastinoscopy in staging the disease of these patients. In mediastinal staging of clinical stage III tumors, positive results of PET need to be confirmed by tissue diagnosis because of a relatively high false-positive rate

(15% to 20%). The false-negative rate of PET and mediastinoscopy in assessing enlarged mediastinal lymph nodes is 5% to 10%, and some authorities therefore do not pursue biopsy in the case of a negative PET result for disease in the mediastinum, whereas others argue that mediastinoscopy can detect microscopic metastases, and they are not comfortable accepting a negative PET result.[4] Practically, in larger centers, patients with stage III tumors undergo both PET to assess for distant metastases and mediastinoscopy, but a strong argument for staging of the mediastinum with PET can be made in communities without an experienced mediastinoscopy service.

For patients with clinical stage I peripheral tumors, most authorities do not request mediastinoscopy before surgery because the rate of mediastinal or systemic involvement is very low (about 5%); however, this detection rate is based on investigations before implementation of PET, and PET may increase the detection rate. Among patients with clinical stage II tumors, the rate of metastatic disease is higher, and there is a debate about whether PET is warranted in these patients to assess for systemic disease. For stage III tumors, the false-negative rate of clinical evaluation for systemic disease is about 15% to 30%, and PET therefore is justified instead of a battery of other tests (e.g., bone scan, CT, MRI) to assess for distant metastases.[4] PET is more sensitive (90% versus 80%) and more specific (90% versus 70%) than bone scan in detecting bone metastases from NSCLC; PET has a sensitivity and specificity of greater than 90% in detecting adrenal metastases from NSCLC. Brain CT or MRI is still needed because PET cannot reliably detect brain metastases due to physiologically intense brain uptake of FDG. For patients with stage IV tumors, PET can potentially indicate the best accessible site for biopsy.

PET is also useful in restaging NSCLC. In particular, PET appears to be more sensitive than CT in differentiating postirradiation change from local recurrence, although differentiating these two entities remains a challenge. The postirradiation change in the chest can remain intense on PET for up to several years. In differentiating local recurrence from postirradiation change, the intensity of uptake and its shape should be taken into account (Fig. 10-3).

Head and Neck Cancer

Most patients with head and neck cancer present for PET with a known diagnosis. However, cervical lymph node metastases from an unknown primary constitute about 2% of newly diagnosed head and neck cancer cases; CT and MRI can identify up to 50% of the primary tumors in patients with no findings on physical examination. The overall PET detection rate in patients with negative results of physical examination, CT or MRI, and endoscopy is about 25%. This detection rate is based on studies in which stand-alone PET was used, and it is expected to be higher with fused PET/CT. PET/CT should probably be performed instead of CT or MRI before endoscopy.[5] Knowledge of the variable physiologic uptake patterns in the head and neck region is essential to minimize false-positive interpretations.

In initial staging of head and neck tumors, PET has a sensitivity and specificity of about 90% for nodal staging, and PET therefore is more sensitive and specific than CT or MRI. A weakness of PET is its low sensitivity (30%) for nodal disease in patients with clinically N0 necks. Given the high specificity of PET in nodal staging, it appears reasonable to perform neck dissection in patients with a positive PET result, whereas those with a negative PET result may be able to undergo sentinel node localization and biopsy.[5] In addition to local staging, PET can detect synchronous malignancies and distant metastases. In initial staging of head and neck malignancies, a PET scan is overall most helpful in patients with locally advanced disease, because these patients have a risk of 10% or greater for distant disease.

For restaging of head and neck tumors after radiation therapy, PET is highly sensitive; however, the optimal time to perform PET is a matter of debate. There is a higher likelihood of false-positive findings when PET is performed earlier than 3 months after irradiation. Based on recommendations from large institutions in the United States, PET should be performed 3 months after radiation therapy; patients with a negative scan can be followed without intervention (i.e., high negative predictive value), but those with a positive scan need to undergo further evaluation.[5]

Lymphoma

PET (especially fused PET/CT) is superior to conventional CT in staging of Hodgkin's disease and non-Hodgkin's lymphoma; however, there is no definite evidence that PET changes the initial management of lymphoma patients. Nonetheless, because most recurrences occur at the sites of the primary disease, pretreatment PET appears helpful in identifying recurrence.

Hodgkin's disease and high-grade non-Hodgkin's lymphoma are mostly markedly avid for FDG and almost always visible on PET, whereas low-grade non-Hodgkin's lymphoma can be only mildly intense and, in rare cases, completely invisible on PET. The normal spleen shows mild uptake, whereas the uptake of the normal bone marrow can be variably intense. Intense spleen uptake (i.e., more intense than the liver) before

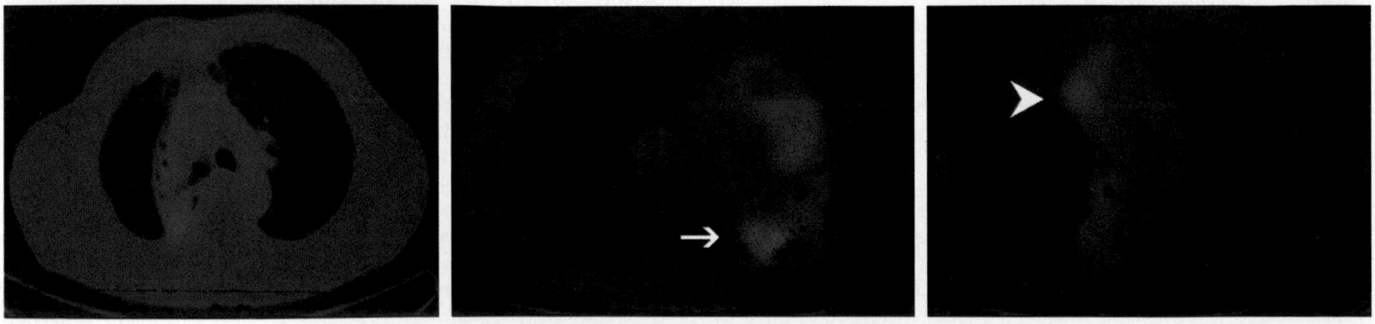

A B C

Figure 10-3 Postirradiation change versus active tumor. **A,** An elongated area of mild uptake strongly suggests postirradiation change. **B,** A focal area of intense uptake *(arrow)* indicates malignancy. **C,** The elongated area suggests postirradiation change, but the more focal area anteriorly *(arrowhead)* may be malignancy, and biopsy or imaging follow-up is warranted.

chemotherapy is a reliable indicator of its involvement, but spleen involvement by lymphoma cannot be excluded with normal uptake. PET cannot be used to reliably evaluate bone marrow involvement. Activation of hematopoiesis after chemotherapy or by bone marrow stimulating factors can cause intense uptake in the bone marrow, spleen, or thymus, which can persist after the termination of the chemotherapy or stimulating factors.

The most promising role of PET in lymphoma management appears to be in therapy monitoring: early prediction of response to chemotherapy (i.e., interim or midway PET) and evaluation of a residual mass for active lymphoma at the completion of chemotherapy (i.e., end-of-treatment PET). The decrease of uptake associated with effective chemotherapy seen on interim PET precedes the anatomic changes seen on CT by weeks to months. Overall, metabolic changes on interim PET after one or a few cycles of chemotherapy are reliable predictors of response, progression-free survival, and overall survival. However, it is unclear how the findings on interim PET should be used in patient care.

End-of-treatment PET has proven impact in patient care. At the completion of chemotherapy, CT demonstrates a residual mass at the initial site of disease in as many as 50% of patients. On the end-of-treatment PET, these patients demonstrate increased FDG uptake in the area of residual lymphoma in contrast to those without active lymphoma. The positive predictive value of residual uptake at the completion of chemotherapy is more than 90%. The negative predictive value is likely lower and associated with microscopic remnant disease. Generally, patients with non-Hodgkin's lymphoma and stages III and IV Hodgkin's disease and negative PET results at the completion of chemotherapy should undergo repeat PET at least once at about 6 weeks after the last cycle of chemotherapy.

In follow-up of patients in remission, PET is more sensitive than CT in detecting recurrent disease. There are no guidelines about how often follow-up PET scans should be performed. Follow-up PET scans often are performed as frequently as every 3 months. PET (especially PET/CT) is superior to gallium scan in all of the previous indications.

Colorectal Cancer

PET plays no role in the screening or diagnosing of colorectal cancer, and neither the depth of the tumor nor the local lymph nodes status can be assessed by PET. However, PET is highly sensitive in detecting distant hepatic and extrahepatic metastases. A meta-analysis of the literature on detection of hepatic metastases from colorectal, gastric, and esophageal cancers by ultrasound, CT, MRI, and PET found that in studies with a specificity higher than 85%, the mean weighted sensitivity was 55% for ultrasound, 72% for CT, 76% for MRI, and 90% for PET. Results of pairwise comparison between imaging modalities demonstrated a greater sensitivity of PET than ultrasound (P = .001), CT (P = .017), and MRI (P = .055). The conclusion was that at equivalent specificity, PET is the most sensitive noninvasive imaging modality for the diagnosis of hepatic metastases from colorectal, gastric, and esophageal cancers.[6] Considering the higher sensitivity of PET in detecting distant metastases and the introduction of intravenous contrast to the CT portion of fused PET/CT, it is conceivable that PET/CT will be increasingly employed in preoperative staging of colorectal cancer; the contrast-enhanced CT portion of PET/CT can be used instead of conventional CT or MRI for evaluation of anatomic resectability of liver metastases. PET plays an important role in restaging of colorectal cancer. PET can visualize the site of the local and distant disease when recurrence is suspected based on the clinical findings, findings on other imaging modalities, or an increasing carcinoembryonic antigen level with sensitivity and specificity higher than 90% (Fig. 10-4).

Breast Cancer

PET can increase the detectability of small primary breast cancers and may be useful especially in evaluating patients with dense breasts. Its role in routine patient care is under investigation. In evaluating the axillary lymph nodes, PET does not play any role because of its low sensitivity (60%) despite relatively high specificity (80%).[7] In contrast, PET is relatively sensitive (85%) and specific (90%), and it is superior to CT (sensitivity of 54%, specificity of 85%) in evaluation of the internal mammary chain lymph node for metastases. The main role of PET in breast cancer lies in the investigation of distant metastases and response monitoring. Compared with CT, PET has a higher sensitivity (90% versus 40%) but lower specificity (80% versus 95%) in detecting metastatic disease. Overall, PET has the same sensitivity as bone scan in detecting bone metastases (both about 90%), but PET appears to be somewhat more sensitive than bone scan for osteolytic lesions and somewhat less sensitive than bone scan for osteoblastic lesions. PET has a higher specificity than bone scan in detecting bone metastases (95% versus 80%). This may be explained by the fact that PET captures the metabolic activity of the

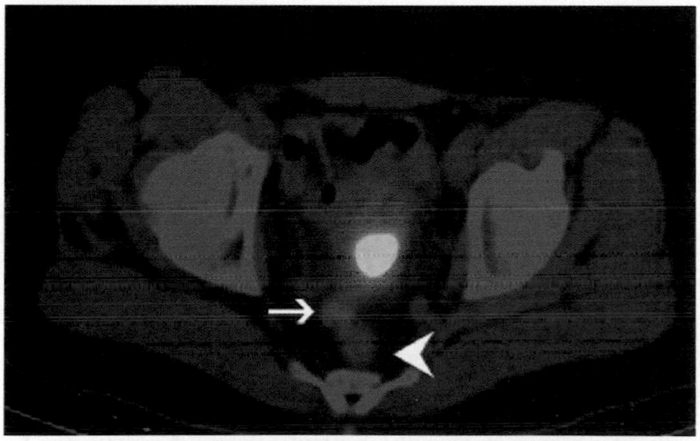

A

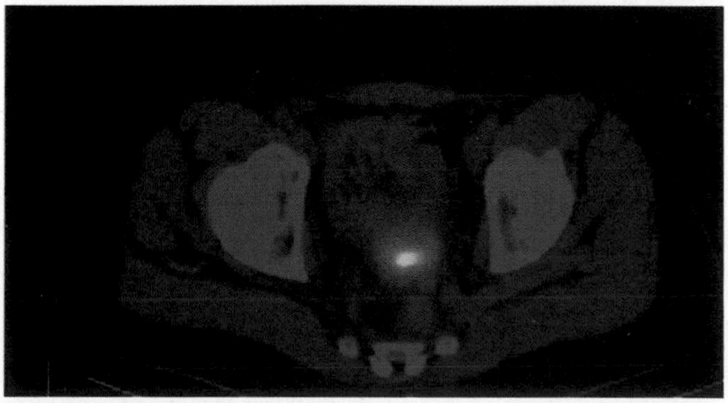

B

Figure 10-4 Positron emission tomography (PET) is used in differentiating local recurrence from scar in a patient with colon cancer after low anterior resection. Recurrent disease was suspected based on the increasing carcinoembryonic antigen level. Computed tomography could not differentiate between scar and local recurrence. **A,** PET indicated an intense focus *(arrow)* suspicious for malignancy, and a second mild focus *(arrowhead)* was interpreted as scar. **B,** The diagnosis was confirmed surgically, and the recurrent tumor was removed.

tumor cells independently of changes in the bone, whereas bone remodeling seen on bone scan can result from metastatic disease and benign causes.

In patients with advanced breast cancer undergoing neoadjuvant chemotherapy, PET differentiates responders from nonresponders as early as after the first cycle of therapy. This may help improve patient management by avoiding ineffective chemotherapy and supporting the decision to continue dose-intensive preoperative chemotherapy in responding patients.

Positron Emission Tomography Applications in Other Malignancies

In esophageal and gastric cancer, PET is useful to assess for distant disease. In esophageal cancer, PET has the potential to be used for monitoring the effect of neoadjuvant therapy. In ovarian, uterine, and cervical cancer, PET is used to assess for recurrent disease. In cases of cervical cancer, PET plays an important role in nodal staging and radiotherapy planning. In malignant melanoma, PET is used to evaluate the presence of distant metastases. In sarcoma, the most intense areas on PET have usually the highest grade and should be considered for biopsy.

TARGETED IMAGING IN NUCLEAR MEDICINE

From its inception, nuclear medicine has used specific physiologic and biophysical targets for imaging and therapy. Many of these targets hold promise for the future, but a few are being used routinely and are expanding the boundaries of research.

Because nuclear imaging techniques have had high sensitivities with known lesser specificities, other agents with greater specificity are being developed. Even though there may be some trade-off in sensitivity compared with other nuclear modalities, they have proved to be better than general radiologic modalities for many indications, and in some cases, they can be used for targeted radionuclide therapies.

Apart from the radiopharmaceuticals, many newer agents rely on targeting using antibodies or their fragments and peptides, or they are receptor or even gene specific. Although established procedures such as FDG-PET imaging are clearly superior to most of these newer methods, they remain clinically important in medical centers where PET may not be available. Other advances have made traditional imaging preparation easier, such as the introduction of Thyrogen (recombinant humanized thyroid-stimulating hormone [rhTSH]).

Advances in Thyroid Cancer Evaluation

Thyroid cancer patients undergo 4 to 6 weeks of L-thyroxine withdrawal to stimulate tumors to take up iodine. The use of rhTSH exogenously stimulates residual thyroid cells to take up radioiodine, and thyroid malignancy evaluation has been revolutionized since its introduction. Results are available within a few days, avoiding the prolonged hypothyroid state that patients traditionally had to go through to get diagnostic studies. Although rhTSH also has been used to deliver therapeutic doses, it is unknown whether long-term outcomes are different for such patients compared with the standard hormone withdrawal method.[8]

Antibody-Based Imaging Agents

One of the more successful agents is ProstaScint (capromab pendetide), an antibody against prostate membrane surface antigen, a type II membrane glycoprotein strongly associated with prostate cancer. The usual indication is a rising PSA level in a patient who has had a prostatectomy but who has no obvious location for a metastatic focus as determined by CT or MRI. These modalities have sensitivities of disease detection of only 5% to 20%, although they have much higher specificities. The accuracies for capromab imaging are about 70%, although it is much less sensitive than bone scan for skeletal metastases. Absence of extrapelvic disease on capromab and other studies may allow for radiotherapy to the pelvis. Because of the limited success for FDG-PET in detection of metastatic prostate cancer, capromab still has utility because it is unclear whether the development of positron labeled agents such as choline or methionine will surpass its performance.

Carcinoembryonic antigen scans use a labeled murine antibody fragment (^{99m}Tc-arcitumomab) to detect recurrent colorectal carcinoma, and the scans can also be used for detecting breast cancer. OncoScint (^{111}In-satumomab pendetide) is another antibody also used for detection of recurrent colorectal and ovarian carcinomas. The sensitivity, specificity, and accuracy of extrahepatic disease recurrence detection for satumomab are 97%, 78%, and 92%, respectively, whereas those for CT scans are 72%, 89%, and 76%, respectively, for colorectal malignancy. For liver metastases, CT is better, with sensitivity, specificity, and accuracy values all about 92%, and those for satumomab are 85%, 92%, and 89%, respectively. When the two modalities are combined, the sensitivity is approximately 90%.[9] Nevertheless, FDG-PET outperforms these modalities and is the scan of choice, although the antibodies are still of great clinical value where FDG-PET is not easily available.

Cellular Imaging

Various agents being developed build on the newer understanding of cellular physiology, including angiogenesis, apoptosis, and other ideas. Some are routinely used clinically, but others show potential for future development and may revolutionize the way cancer is approached.

^{18}F-fluorothymidine (^{18}F-FLT) is a thymidine analogue and a PET tracer, which is phosphorylated by thymidine kinase-1 (TK1) to FLT-monophosphate. FLT uptake correlates with TK1 activity and cellular proliferation. FLT is likely more suitable than FDG to monitor the effect of chemotherapy and radiation therapy. Another important area of current PET tracer research concerns cell-cell and cell-matrix interaction. Tracers such as ^{18}F-galacto-GRD (glycosylated Arg-Gly-Asp) enable the noninvasive determination of integrin $\alpha_v\beta_3$ expression and are expected to be used in assessing angiogenesis and metastatic potential of tumors.

Annexin-V shows great promise for evaluating apoptosis, and it is available as a single-photon and PET agent. Highly apoptotic areas in tumors are likely to be sensitive to irradiation or chemotherapy, and there is the potential for evaluating therapy response or overall disease prognosis with such agents. Similarly, the field of tumor hypoxia is central to the understanding of tumor response to irradiation. PET agents such as ^{18}F-fluoromisonidazole (^{18}F-MISO) and Cu-labeled diacetyl-bis (*N*(4)-methylthiosemicarbazone (Cu-ATSM) can be used to detect intratumoral hypoxia. Although these agents are still in the early evaluation phase, they could be used in the future to evaluate areas of hypoxia for targeting radiation delivery.

Receptor Imaging

^{111}In-octreotide is a peptide that is routinely indicated for neuroendocrine tumors, including carcinoids, tumors associated with the multiple endocrine neoplasias, meningiomas, and lymphomas (i.e., Hodgkin's disease and non-Hodgkin's lymphoma). Increased activity can be seen in benign disease such as sarcoidosis and other inflammatory processes. ^{111}In-octreotide has the highest affinity for somatostatin receptor (SSTR) subtypes 2 and 5, with weaker affinities for others. This agent is considered the gold standard when evaluating neuroendocrine tumors, and it is still relevant in the era of PET because many of the well-differentiated lesions will not take up FDG. Even so, many diseases do not have appropriate receptor expression and therefore have limited detection on such scans. A similar agent, ^{99m}Tc-depreotide, has greater affinities for SSTR 2, 3, and 5 and therefore has the potential for greater sensitivities for tumors with various SSTR expressions and uptake in a broader number of malignancies, including lung cancers. Nonetheless, ^{111}In-octreotide is more widely used, and FDG-PET remains the modality of choice in detecting lung cancers where available.

Routine imaging of neuroblastoma and pheochromocytomas involves metaiodobenzylguanidine (MIBG), a norepinephrine analogue taken up by the uptake 1 mechanism in receptors. Like octreotide, it has uptake in many similar malignancies, although not with the same frequency. For imaging, MIBG may be labeled with ^{131}I, ^{123}I, or ^{124}I, a positron emitter. The sensitivity for lesion detection can exceed 90%, and specificity approaches almost 100% for single-photon imaging.[10] Nevertheless, as tumors de-differentiate or metastasize to other sites, specifically the bones, MIBG becomes less sensitive in detecting disease, in which case a bone scan is useful. With the advent of ^{124}I-MIBG used in PET/CT, it is unknown whether the increased resolution will allow better detection of disease, obviating the need for bone scans.

TARGETED RADIONUCLIDE THERAPY

Imaging agents are valued more for their sensitivity, but for targeted therapy, it is the specificity that is essential. Many imaging agents are specific enough for therapeutic purposes. (Treatment of well-differentiated thyroid cancer, radioimmunotherapy, and bone metastases pain palliation are discussed elsewhere.) The following sections provide examples of assorted therapies used in other clinical settings that show promise for development in the near future.

Benign Thyroid Disease

Thyroid diseases have the most successful application of targeted therapy that is clinically relevant. The thyroid's unique ability to metabolize elemental iodine to synthesize thyroid hormones is fortuitous, because it is a highly specific but easily targeted process with radioactive iodine. Treatment is effective, is virtually definitive, and has minimal side effects. There are practically no long-term sequelae from radioactive iodine administration for benign thyroid disease. Generally, radioactive iodine treatment in benign disease is reserved for hyperthyroid conditions, such as Graves' disease or toxic and multinodular goiters. Radioactive iodine is used when the disease cannot be controlled medically, and it is often a first-line option in clinically hyperthyroid patients. Surgery is reserved for instances in which radioactive iodine may be contraindicated (e.g., pregnancy, marrow suppression) or when there may be compressive findings of the enlarged thyroid on critical structures, such as the trachea.

Octreotide Derivatives in Neuroendocrine Malignancies

A novel application is to use octreotide in targeted radionuclide therapy. ^{111}In-octreotide has been used in clinical trials and initial results were encouraging, although objective response rates were a meager 0% to 8%, with 42% to 81% with stable disease and 12% to 38% showing disease progression. The octreotide molecule has subsequently been modified to increase its specificity for tumor targeting, decrease its affinity for nontargeting areas in other organs, and try to improve its toxicity profile. ^{111}In-octreotide has been altered to create [^{90}Y-DOTA^{0}]- Tyr^{3}-octreotide (DOTATOC) and [^{177}Lu-DOTA^{0}]-Tyr^{3}-otreotate (DOTATATE), with some improvement in their target to nontarget ratios. The DOTATOC trials showed improved objective responses ranging from 7% to 33%, stable disease in 52% to 81%, and disease progression in 9% to 19%. Trials with DOTATATE also showed similar objective response rates. Aside from marrow toxicity and myelodysplasia, nephrotoxicity was the other most significant long-term sequela, which could be decreased with infusion of amino acids before therapy. As in all targeted therapies for solid tumors, hematotoxicity was seen in these patients.[11]

The success of DOTATOC and DOTATATE likely results from their better targeting of tumor compared with octreotide. The radiobiology of the beta emitters ^{90}Y and ^{177}Lu appears to be superior to the Auger emitter ^{111}In. The newer trifunctional, somatostatin-based derivatives have prolonged cell retention, and they are internalized into the cell nucleus, making them optimal for Auger therapy, such as ^{111}In.[12] Future trials with such compounds are of great interest in developing targeted radionuclide modalities.

Metaiodobenzylguanidine Therapy in Neuroendocrine Malignancies

MIBG has been used therapeutically as ^{131}I-MIBG in neuroblastomas in children and pheochromocytomas. Objective responses have ranged from 47% to 80% as a single agent in neuroblastoma. The main toxicity was hematologic, and subsequent trials are being conducted with autologous stem cell reconstitution. Studies have also been conducted combining MIBG with chemoradiotherapy, with various responses.[13]

Other Uses of Targeted Radionuclide Therapies

Polycythemia vera was frequently treated with ^{32}P in the past, but with the advent of modern chemotherapy, this has become uncommon. Although the median survival was improved, there was an increase in the incidence of secondary blood dyscrasias. This therapy is used in patients who cannot tolerate hydroxyurea and other treatments or who have symptoms that do not respond to other therapeutic maneuvers.

Radiocolloids such as ^{198}Au-colloid or chromic phosphates labeled with ^{32}P or ^{90}Y have been used as palliative regimens in malignant ascites in ovarian carcinoma, pleurodesis for pleural effusions, intracavitary injections for cystic brain tumors, and even for radiosynovectomies in benign arthritic diseases. Other therapies have included using ^{35}S-thiouracil for ocular melanoma. Despite being effective treatments, they have been replaced by modern medical management, although they are still rarely used when other therapies fail.

Some of the newer therapies involve using microspheres embedded with ^{90}Y for palliation in hepatocellular carcinoma. They are injected into the hepatic artery directly to the site of diseased liver, where they will reside in the vascular space as the nuclides decay, delivering lethal radiation doses locally. Because the product is not systemically delivered, there are only minimal toxic effects. Although palliative benefits are clear, long-term survival data have not been established. Similarly, ^{131}I-lipiodol is emerging as a candidate for similar indications and has undergone phase II trials with cisplatin, demonstrating a well-tolerated toxicity profile.[14] On the horizon, newer therapies may use liposomes to deliver therapeutic radionuclides to micrometastases in various malignancies to complement antibody-mediated therapies.[15]

Therapy-Enhancing Strategies

Therapy enhancement tries to boost radionuclide uptake and prolong its cellular retention for improving efficacy. In thyroid cancer, lithium has produced a modest increase in free iodine retention and raised the dose delivery to tissue.[16]

Some of the newer antibody therapies use genetically engineered antibodies or altered pharmaceuticals and attach radionuclides with more favorable characteristics to improve tumor-specific targeting and possibly therapeutic efficacy. Other methods employ multistep targeting, all of which are experimental, but they hold promise. Such results have prompted their use in conjunction with external beam therapy and chemotherapy. This could help to develop targeted radionuclide therapy into a clinically relevant option.

REFERENCES

1. Donckier V, Van Laethem JL, Goldman S, et al: [F-18] fluorodeoxyglucose positron emission tomography as a tool for early recognition of incomplete tumor destruction after radiofrequency ablation for liver metastases. J Surg Oncol 84:215-223, 2003.
2. Keyes JW Jr: SUV: standard uptake or silly useless value? J Nucl Med 36:1836-1839, 1995.
3. Detterbeck FC, Falen S, Rivera MP, et al: Seeking a home for a PET. Part 1. Defining the appropriate place for positron emission tomography imaging in the diagnosis of pulmonary nodules or masses. Chest 125:2294-2299, 2004.
4. Detterbeck FC, Falen S, Rivera MP et al: Seeking a home for a PET. Part 2. Defining the appropriate place for positron emission tomography imaging in the staging of patients with suspected lung cancer. Chest 125:2300-2308, 2004.
5. Menda Y, Graham MM: Update on 18F-fluorodeoxyglucose/positron emission tomography and positron emission tomography/computed tomography imaging of squamous head and neck cancers. Semin Nucl Med 35:214-219, 2005.
6. Kinkel K, Lu Y, Both M, et al: Detection of hepatic metastases from cancers of the gastrointestinal tract by using noninvasive imaging methods (US, CT, MR imaging, PET): a meta-analysis. Radiology 224:748-756, 2002.
7. Wahl RL, Siegel BA, Coleman RE, et al: PET Study Group. Prospective multicenter study of axillary nodal staging by positron emission tomography in breast cancer: a report of the Staging Breast Cancer with PET Study Group. J Clin Oncol 22:277-285, 2004.
8. Robbins RJ, Larson SM, Sinha N, et al: A retrospective review of the effectiveness of recombinant human TSH as a preparation for radioiodine thyroid remnant ablation. J Nucl Med 43:1482-1488, 2002.
9. Garcia-Fernandez R, Luna-Perez P, Hernandez-Hernandez DM, et al: Usefulness of scintigraphy images with ^{111}In-CYT-103 in the diagnosis of colonic and rectal recurrence. Gac Med Mex 138:139-144, 2002.
10. Lumbroso JD, Guermazi F, Hartmann O, et al: Meta-iodobenzylguanidine (mIBG) scans in neuroblastoma: sensitivity and specificity: a review of 115 scans. Prog Clin Biol Res 271:689-705, 1988.
11. Kwekkeboom DJ, Mueller-Brand J, Paganelli G, et al: Overview of results of peptide receptor radionuclide therapy with 3 radiolabeled somatostatin analogs. J Nucl Med 46(Suppl 1):62S-66S, 2005.
12. Ginj M, Hinni K, Tschumi S, et al: Trifunctional somatostatin-based derivatives designed for targeted radiotherapy using auger electron emitters. J Nucl Med 46:2097-2103, 2005.
13. Gaze MN, Wheldon TE, O'Donoghue JA, et al: Multi-modality megatherapy with ^{131}I-metaiodobenzylguanidine, high-dose melphalan and total body irradiation with bone marrow rescue: feasibility study of a new strategy for advanced neuroblastoma. Eur J Cancer 31A:252-256, 1995.
14. Raoul JL, Boucher E, Olivie D, et al: Association of cisplatin and intra-arterial injection of (131)I-lipiodol in treatment of hepatocellular carcinoma: results of phase II trial. Int J Radiat Oncol Biol Phys 64:745-750, 2006.
15. Emfietzoglou D, Kostarelos K, Papakostas A, et al: Liposome-mediated radiotherapeutics within avascular tumor spheroids: comparative dosimetry study for various radionuclides, liposome systems, and a targeting antibody. J Nucl Med 46:89-97, 2005.
16. Koong SS, Reynolds JC, Movius EG, et al: Lithium as a potential adjuvant to ^{131}I therapy of metastatic, well differentiated thyroid carcinoma. J Clin Endocrinol Metab 84:912-916, 1999.

CHAPTER 11

HEALTH SERVICES RESEARCH IN RADIATION ONCOLOGY: TOWARD ACHIEVING THE ACHIEVABLE FOR PATIENTS WITH CANCER

William J. Mackillop

WHAT IS HEALTH SERVICES RESEARCH?

Medical research may be considered as a continuum of four overlapping domains: basic or biomedical research, clinical research, health services research (HSR), and population health research. HSR aims to create the knowledge required to improve population health by improving the delivery of health services.[1-7] Although there is some overlap between the domains of clinical research and HSR, their purposes are distinct. *Clinical research* describes the natural history of diseases, it investigates their pathophysiology, and it seeks to discover more effective treatments. *HSR* describes how health systems work, it investigates how they go wrong, and it seeks to discover better ways to deliver health services. The results of clinical research are primarily intended to guide physicians' decisions about the care of individual patients, whereas the results of HSR are intended to guide the decisions of managers and policy makers about the design and implementation of health care programs.[1-7]

Need for Health Services Research in Radiation Oncology

Clinical radiation oncology is a mature science. It has a sound theoretical basis, in both biology and physics. We have a universal language for describing the diseases we treat, the treatments we use, and the outcomes we achieve.[8-10] Much is now known about the factors that influence outcomes in the individual case.[11] We have a well-established process for evaluating the efficacy of treatment,[12] and a large body of empirical information now permits evidence-based decisions about the use of radiotherapy (RT) in the majority of cases.

In contrast, the science of HSR in radiation oncology is at a very much earlier stage of development. There is no comparable universal language for describing the performance of RT programs. There is only limited information available about the factors that influence the performance of RT programs in the population at large. There is no well-established process for measuring the effectiveness of RT programs at the population level. In the absence of empirical evidence, most decisions about the design and management of RT services are guided only by theory and expert opinion, and their consequences are unpredictable. Given that we would no longer tolerate this unscientific approach to decision making in the care of individual patients, it is anomalous that it should still be used in making decisions about health systems that may affect tens of thousands of patients.

The challenges for the HSR community in radiation oncology are to create the knowledge required for evidence-based management of RT programs and to promote the use of evidence in the design and management of RT programs.

How Can Health Services Research Help to Improve the Outcomes of Cancer?

At any point in time, our state of scientific knowledge and technological development sets an upper limit on what is *achievable* for patients with cancer. What is achievable in any particular society is also limited by how much that society is able and willing to spend on cancer care. However, what is actually *achieved* depends not only on what would be achievable if we made optimal use of the available knowledge, technology, and resources, but also on how close we get to attaining the achievable, a quantity we have termed *attainment.*

$$\text{Attainment} = \text{Achieved outcome}/\text{Achievable outcome}$$

The achieved and the achievable outcomes are measured in units that correspond to the outcome of interest. Attainment can have any value between 0 and 1, or may be multiplied by 100 and expressed as a percentage. The equation may be rewritten as

$$\text{Achieved outcome} = \text{Achievable outcome} \times \text{Attainment}$$

Cancer outcomes can be improved by increasing the *achievable* or by increasing *attainment*. Biomedical and clinical research aim to improve outcomes by increasing the achievable. HSR aims to improve outcomes by increasing the attainment of what is already potentially achievable within the limits of existing knowledge, technology, and resources.

What Is the Scope of Health Services Research?

Health system performance has three dimensions: accessibility, quality, and efficiency. Together these determine the extent to which we attain the achievable in health care. *Accessibility* describes the extent to which patients are able to get care they need, when they need it. *Quality* describes the extent to which the right care is delivered in the right way. *Efficiency* describes the extent to which accessibility and effectiveness are optimized in relation to the resources expended. HSR is concerned with measuring these quantities, understanding the factors that influence them, and discovering and evaluating ways of enhancing them. The remainder of this chapter is devoted to describing how HSR has contributed to our understanding of accessibility, quality, and efficiency in radiation oncology.

STUDYING THE ACCESSIBILITY OF RADIOTHERAPY

Concept of Health Care Accessibility

The term *accessibility* was originally used narrowly to describe the ability of patients to obtain entry into the health system.[13] Today, it is usually used more broadly to encompass all the factors that influence the level of use of a service in relation to the level of need for the service in a population.[2] The term *need* is used here as defined by Cuyler,[14] who states that "the need for medical care exists when an individual has an illness for which there is effective and acceptable treatment." The concept of access has been described as representing the overall "degree of fit between the clients and the system."[15] Access can be seen as having a number of dimensions that

Table 11-1 The Dimensions of Health Care Accessibility

AVAILABILITY
Total system capacity in relation to total needs
Total resources, efficiency, flexibility
SPATIAL ACCESSIBILITY
Distance, travel times, costs of transportation
ACCOMMODATION
Hours of operation
Transportation services
Lodges/hostels
AFFORDABILITY
Prices in relation to clients' ability and willingness to pay
Indirect costs
AWARENESS
Physicians' awareness of clients' needs and of potentially useful services
Patients' awareness of needs and services

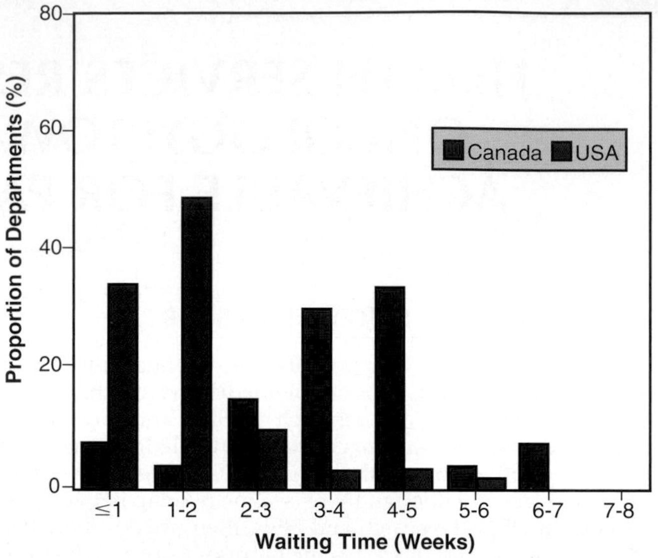

Figure 11-1 Waiting times for RT for carcinoma of the larynx in Canada and the United States. The frequency distributions illustrate the time from referral to initiation of RT for a T2N0M0 carcinoma of the larynx in Canada and the United States based on the results of a mail survey. (Adapted from Mackillop WJ, Zhoou Y, Quirt CF: A comparison of delays in the treatment of cancer with radiation in Canada and the United States. Int J Radiat Oncol Biol Phys 32:531-539, 1995.)

determine that overall degree of fit (Table 11-1). *Availability* describes the volume and type of services available in relation to the number of clients and their needs. Availability encompasses the adequacy of supply of physicians and other personnel and the adequacy of facilities and equipment. For a given level of resources, availability also depends on the degree of efficiency in production of services. *Spatial accessibility* describes the relationship between the location of supply of service and the location of the clients who need the service, taking into account travel times and costs. The term *accommodation* describes the extent to which the system is designed and operated to facilitate clients' access to service,[15] for example, by operating at hours that are convenient to clients or by providing bed and board for those who cannot readily travel for daily treatments. *Affordability* describes the relationship between prices and clients' ability to pay. It also encompasses indirect costs, for example, loss of earnings during treatment that may deter use of the service. *Awareness* describes the extent to which those who need the service are aware that it is available and that they might benefit from it. In the context of a specialized service like RT, the patients' awareness of the potential benefits of RT depends largely on their attending physician's awareness of the indications for RT.

Need for Studies of Access to Radiotherapy

There are several compelling reasons to study access to RT. First, there is strong evidence of the effectiveness of RT in many situations, and to achieve optimal outcomes at the population level, effective treatments have to be accessible to every eligible patient. Second, many societies place a high value on providing adequate and equitable access to health care for all of the citizens. Third, there have been reports of widespread waiting lists for RT that suggest access to RT is less than optimum in many parts of the world.

Waiting Lists for Radiotherapy

In certain countries with publicly funded health systems, most notably the United Kingdom, waiting lists for health care have been in the news for many years. The term "waiting list" has been listed as a key word in Index Medicus since 1975. However, the medical literature was essentially silent on the issue of waiting lists for cancer treatment until the early 1990s, when a report from Ontario demonstrated that waiting times for RT had increased dramatically over the preceding decade and that there were long waiting lists at many cancer centers in the province.[16] Since then, there have been numerous publications about waiting lists for RT, principally from countries with publicly funded health systems, including Canada,[16,17] the United Kingdom,[18,19] and Australia.[20,21] There have been no reports of similar problems in the United States, where the private sector is largely responsible for the provision of health care. In the countries affected, the problem of waiting lists for RT has been one of the dominant concerns of radiation oncologists for the past decade. The HSR community in radiation oncology has been active in measuring waiting times for RT, in investigating the causes and consequences of waiting lists for RT, and in developing methods for setting standards for acceptable waiting times.

Measuring Waiting Times for Radiotherapy

Several different methods have been used to quantify the problem of waiting lists for RT, including the use of mail surveys, retrospective review of preexisting administrative data, and prospective collection of data as patients pass through the system.

Mail surveys can provide a lot of information about waiting times from multiple institutions at modest expense. Surveys can be structured to elicit information about delays in a number of different clinical situations. A survey of heads of radiation oncology at all International Union Against Cancer (UICC, Union Internationale Contre Le Cancer)–listed cancer centers in the United States and Canada conducted in the 1990s confirmed that waiting lists for RT were widespread across Canada but revealed no evidence of similar problems in the United States. Median waiting times for a range of indications for RT were two to three times longer in Canada than in the United States.[22] Figure 11-1 shows, for example, that at almost every Canadian center, patients with laryngeal cancer waited longer for RT than they did at almost any U.S. center.

The results of such surveys are based on the responses of many different individuals who may rely on different sources of information in providing their answers. Survey results therefore may be criticized as lacking objectivity.

Waiting times for RT can often be measured directly by retrospective analysis of data that have been gathered for other purposes. Administrative databases can usually provide information about some of the key milestones in the patient's trajectory through the system, such as date of diagnosis, date of referral for RT, date of first visit to the RT center, and date of start of RT. Durations of delay between these milestones are easy to calculate and provide some information about where the rate-limiting steps in the process were located. Figure 11-2A illustrates waiting times for RT for laryngeal cancer in Ontario. The graphs are reproduced from the first report of the application of this method in Ontario in the 1990s.[16] It shows how waiting times for RT increased dramatically through the late 1980s and early 1990s. It illustrates that there was no increase in the interval between diagnosis and referral to radiation oncology or between referral and consultation. The increases in overall delay between diagnosis and treatment were entirely due to increased waiting times between the consultation with a radiation oncologist and the start of RT, consistent with rate-limiting problems in access to planning and treatment machines. Note that average waiting times are described here in terms of the median because it is less sensitive than the mean to the impact of outlying values. If standards have been set for maximum acceptable waiting times, prevailing waiting times can be described in relation to those standards. The Canadian Association of Radiation Oncologists accepts 2 weeks as the maximum acceptable delay between referral and consultation and 2 weeks as the maximum acceptable delay between consultation and the start of RT. Figure 11-2B shows trends in compliance with those standards over time. While most patients met both standards until the mid 1980s, by 1990 very few patients started treatment within 2 weeks of consultation.

There are limitations to the usefulness of retrospective approaches for monitoring waiting times. The retrospective approach starts by identifying patients treated with RT and then follows them backward to find out how long they waited. This approach is blind to patients who dropped off the waiting list before they were treated. Second, it is unlikely that any database created for other purposes will provide all the information necessary to identify the rate-limiting step in the process. The date of the decision to treat with RT, for example, is an important milestone that signals the transition from pretreatment assessment to planning, and this is collected only in systems designed specifically to monitor flow through the RT process. Administrative databases may also lack information about other elements of the patient's care that are necessary to interpret waiting times for RT. For example, planned deferral of the start of postoperative RT, until after completion of chemotherapy, is indistinguishable from unscheduled delay if information about chemotherapy is not available. Third, this approach does not provide the real-time information needed to fine-tune the performance of an RT program. Prospective collection of the pertinent information is the preferred approach for tracking patients through the system.

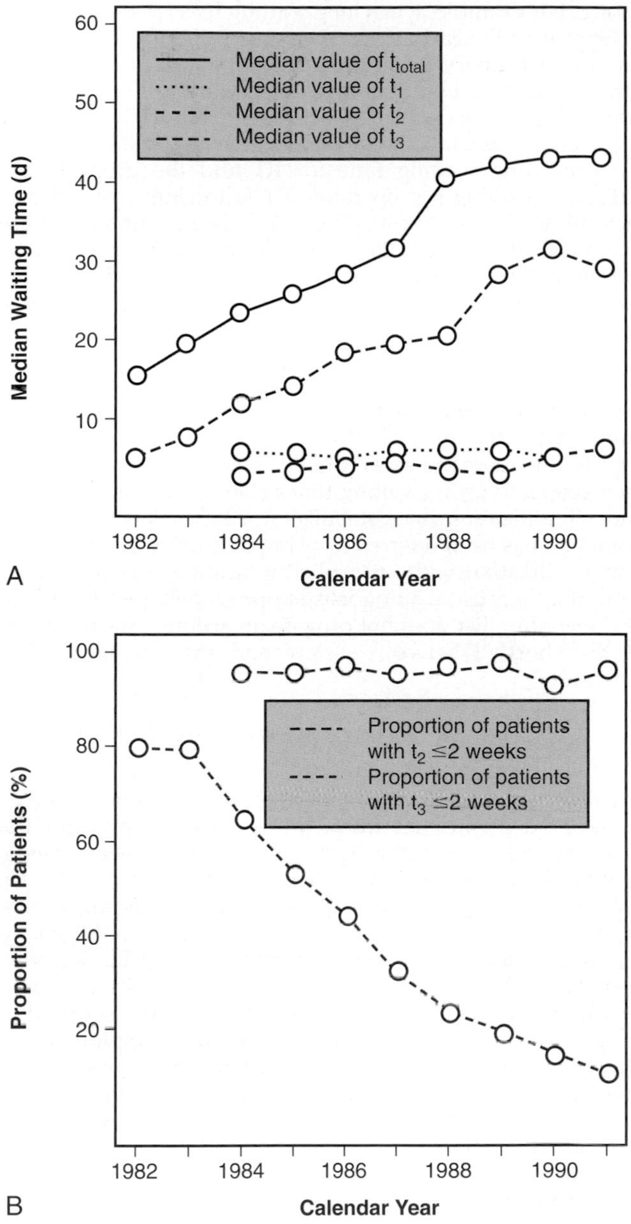

Figure 11-2 Waiting times for RT for carcinoma of the larynx in Ontario. **A,** Temporal trends in median waiting time for RT in Ontario, for which t_{total} is the interval between diagnosis and start of RT, t_1 is the interval between diagnosis and referral to RT, t_2 is the interval between referral and consultation, and t_3 is consultation and start of RT. Data needed to measure t_1 and t_2 were available only from 1984. **B,** The proportion of patients meeting the standards of the Canadian Association of Radiation Oncologists, which states that patients are to be seen in consultation within 2 weeks of referral (i.e., $t_2 < 2$ weeks) and started on RT within 2 weeks of consultation (i.e., $t_3 < 2$ weeks). (Adapted from Mackillop WJ, Fu H, Quirt CF, et al: Waiting for radiotherapy in Ontario. Int J Radiat Oncol Biol Phys 30:221-228, 1994.)

Causes of Waiting Lists for Radiotherapy

Theoretical concepts are introduced before reviewing empirical evidence about the causes of waiting lists for RT.

KINETICS OF WAITING LISTS

When demand for RT exceeds supply, waiting times inevitably increase and a waiting list for RT starts to grow. In theory the waiting list will then continue to grow for as long as demand continues to exceed supply. In reality, waiting lists for RT do not grow indefinitely. When waiting times for RT become longer than the referring physicians believe is acceptable, they may begin to offer their patients alternative treatments, in circumstances in which RT would normally have been their first choice. For example, when long waiting lists for RT developed in Ontario in the early 1990s, there was a significant decline in the use of primary RT in the management of head and neck cancer, followed by a rebound when waiting lists decreased after a major reinvestment in facilities.[23,24] Similarly, it has been shown that there is a significant negative association between the prevailing waiting time for RT and the proportion of patients receiving postoperative RT following a partial mastectomy for breast cancer.[25] This suggests that surgeons prefer to omit RT altogether rather than expose their patients to a distressingly long wait for a treatment that may not be necessary. Furthermore, tumor progression or general deterioration in the patient's condition during the delay may render him or her ineligible for RT that would initially have been appropriate, and these cases drop off the list. Decreasing referrals and increasing dropoffs from the waiting list serve to reduce demand for RT. As demand declines, the balance between supply and demand is eventually restored; the waiting list then ceases to grow, waiting times stabilize at a higher level, and RT utilization rates stabilize at a lower level. This phenomenon has been referred to as implicit rationing, because it limits utilization without explicitly limiting access to care.[26] Note that because waiting lists suppress demand, the length of the waiting list does not provide an accurate measurement of the shortfall between supply and the natural level of demand.

Applications of Queuing Theory to Waiting Lists for Radiotherapy

It is recognized that fluctuations in referral rates may produce peaks in demand that transiently exceed supply and that this may cause a waiting list to develop even when average supply is equal to, or slightly exceeds, average demand.[27] The risk of this happening can be reduced by building reserve capacity, or flexibility in capacity, into the system. The smaller the functional unit, the greater is the impact of random fluctuations, and the more reserve capacity is required to avoid a waiting list.[27] Even in the absence of any shortfall in supply, quite long delays may develop in a complex process like RT planning, simply because of the many serial steps involved.[27] Process mapping and redesign can be useful in streamlining health systems and can reduce delays in some such situations. However, no amount of fine-tuning will have any impact on waiting times for RT if total demand exceeds total supply.[18]

Causes of the Waiting List "Crisis" in Radiotherapy

Although there was no routine surveillance of waiting times for RT anywhere in the world before the early 1990s, there is little doubt that the problem of waiting lists for RT was relatively new when it was first widely reported in the media in the late 1980s. Figure 11-2 shows that even in the mid 1980s, median waiting times were not excessive in Ontario. Why, then, did long waiting lists become so pervasive soon after that? Was there an increase in demand or a decrease in supply or both?

The Ontario experience serves as a useful case study. Analysis of historical data demonstrated that Ontario's problem was multifactorial in origin.[24] Three major factors were identified. First, over the critical period of 1984 through 1993, the incidence of cancer increased by approximately 3% per year, largely due to the aging of the Ontario population. Second, there was a dramatic increase in the proportion of patients referred for RT in three very common cancers. The proportion of new breast cancer cases referred for RT increased, consistent with the evidence-based trend toward breast conservation surgery. The proportion of new cases of rectal cancer referred for RT increased, consistent with the evidence-based adoption of postoperative RT and chemotherapy. The proportion of prostate cancer patients treated with RT increased due to an increase in the proportion of early stage cases detected following the widespread adoption of PSA screening. Third, there was a significant increase in the average number of fractions prescribed per course of RT. This was driven by an increase in the number of fractions per curative or adjuvant course, which outweighed a concomitant but smaller decrease in the number of fractions per palliative course of RT. There was no decrease in treatment capacity. In fact, the number of treatment machines in the province increased faster than the incidence of cancer.[24]

The demographic trends responsible for increasing cancer incidence and the changing indications for RT are international phenomena, which explains why waiting lists developed in several different countries at the about same time. The fact that the United States did not experience similar problems probably reflects the much greater reserve capacity available in the U.S. system and its ability to increase capacity much more rapidly in response to increased demand. In the private sector, increased demand represents a desirable opportunity to increase revenues and providers will strive to put the capacity in place to exploit such opportunities. If demand begins to outgrow supply, the free market system ensures that additional resources will rapidly be titrated into the system until supply once more balances demand. In contrast, in a publicly funded system operating on a fixed budget, increased demand represents a financial liability and management often lacks the authority to put in place any reserve capacity or to respond rapidly when faced with increased demand. Furthermore, government approval processes for new capital projects in publicly funded systems often follow a labyrinthine path that may take years to complete. These built-in delays may make it impossible ever to catch up on a growing problem once it becomes established. Only accurate forecasting of need, linked to a proactive planning process for facilities, equipment, and personnel, can provide a way of avoiding similar problems in the future in a slow-to-react public system.

Consequences of Waiting Lists for Radiotherapy

Delays in starting RT are a source of great concern both to the patients and to those involved in their care. Delays have both direct and indirect effects on the well-being of patients, and waiting lists also have broader economic and social consequences. Some of these are listed in Table 11-2. We have found it useful to classify the direct effects of delay on the well-being of individual patients as *nonstochastic* or *stochastic*.[28] We use these terms as they have been used in the field of radiation protection, where they provide a useful distinction between the effects of radiation that depend on chance and those that do not. The nonstochastic effects of delay include the psychological distress due to the delay and the physical symptoms due to the untreated cancer. They occur in most cases, and often increase in intensity with time, although they may not occur at all before some initial threshold period has been exceeded. The stochastic effects of treatment delay include the development of metastases and failure to achieve local control with radiation. These are all-or-nothing phenomena. Their probability increases as a function of time, but their severity is independent of time, and there is no lower limit of waiting time below which they will not occur. Waiting lists may also have indirect adverse effects on patient care, mediated by changes in medical practice.[28] In addition to their effects on

Table 11-2 The Effects of Waiting Lists for Radiotherapy

DIRECT EFFECTS OF DELAY IN RT ON THE WELL-BEING OF PATIENTS

1.0 Nonstochastic effects
- 1.1 Persistence or worsening of symptoms while waiting for treatment
- 1.2 Psychological distress

2.0 Stochastic effects
- 2.1 Decreased probability of local control
- 2.2 Increased probability of spread beyond the irradiated field
- 2.3 Decreased probability of cure because of 2.1 and 2.2
- 2.4 Increased probability of complications due to compensatory increases in dose and/or volume

INDIRECT EFFECTS OF WAITING LISTS FOR RT ON THE WELL-BEING OF PATIENTS

3.0 Decreased probability of being referred for RT when it is appropriate
- 3.1 Omission of necessary RT
- 3.2 Exposure to less effective and/or more toxic alternatives to RT

4.0 Re-referral to a distant center for RT, with loss of continuity of care

5.0 Decreased quality of practice of radiation oncology
- 5.1 Risk of cutting corners to treat more patients, e.g., hypofractionation
- 5.2 Decreased quality of personal care because of the imperative to maximize technical productivity
- 5.3 Decreased scope for innovation

ECONOMIC EFFECTS OF WAITING LISTS

6.0 Decreased efficiency of RT programs
- 6.1 Decreased net benefits of RT (see 1.0 and 2.0 above)
- 6.2 Increased costs associated with care for patients during delay

7.0 Decreased overall efficiency of cancer treatment programs
- 7.1 Decreased benefits of RT, because of treatment delayed or denied
- 7.2 Increased costs because of the requirement for additional care during delay and/or use of more expensive alternatives to RT

OTHER SOCIETAL EFFECTS OF WAITING LISTS

8.0 Legal liability of providers for failure to provide adequate access to care

9.0 Decreased public confidence in the health care system

health outcomes, waiting lists have important economic and societal implications.

Problems in Measuring the Direct Effects of Delays in Radiotherapy

Some of the direct effects of delays in RT are self-evident. Delays in cancer treatment cause psychological distress and patients who are symptomatic wait longer for relief. There are also good reasons to believe that delays may adversely affect the long-term outcomes of RT. Delay provides an opportunity for tumor progression. There is abundant evidence that the probability of local control decreases as tumor volume increases and that the risk of metastasis increases over time.[28] These arguments are probably sufficient to persuade most radiation oncologists that unnecessary delays in RT should be avoided. However, in health systems like that in Canada, where waiting lists are endemic and widespread, every sector of the health system uses its own waiting list problem to try to lever additional funding from a limited overall pool.

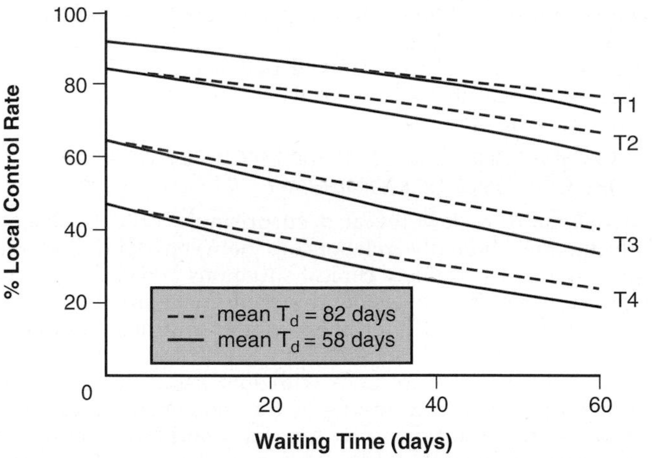

Figure 11-3 The effect of treatment delay on local control in carcinoma of the tonsil. The graph shows the predicted effects of treatment delay on local control rates in carcinoma of the tonsil by T category. The decrease in local control rate associated with delay in each T category was estimated by Monte Carlo simulation. The *dashed red lines* came from a simulation that used a mean T_d of 82 days, and the *solid blue lines* came from a simulation that used a mean T_d of 58 days. (Adapted from Mackillop WJ, Bates JHT, O'Sullivan B, et al: The effect of delay in treatment on local control by radiotherapy. Int J Radiat Oncol Biol Phys 34:243-250, 1996.)

Under these circumstances, expert opinion that delays in RT are dangerous has not been persuasive with the politicians and health system managers who hold the key to additional resources.

The HSR community in radiation oncology community has therefore been challenged to provide more direct evidence that delays in RT have an adverse effect on clinical outcomes. Measuring the magnitude of the stochastic effects of treatment delay is not straightforward. A randomized trial comparing timely RT with delayed RT would be unethical because there is no conceivable benefit in delay. Analysis of the outcome of RT in nonrandomized groups of patients who, in the past, have waited longer or shorter periods of time for treatment is ethical, but it is subject to all the hazards of any retrospective observational study (see Limitations of "Outcomes Research" in Determining the Efficacy of Treatment).

Apart from the specific methodologic problems outlined earlier, it is inherently difficult to measure the risk of treatment failure due to delay, because treatment failures caused by delay are absolutely indistinguishable from treatment failures due to other causes. The problem is analogous to that of defining the risk of carcinogenesis associated with low-dose radiation. One cannot simply count the cancers due to radiation because they are indistinguishable from the many other cancers arising in the population due to causes other than radiation.

Modeling the Effects of Delay on the Outcomes of Radiotherapy

The risk of carcinogenesis has been estimated by mathematical modeling using the best available clinical data combined with principles derived from laboratory studies. A similar approach has been used to estimate the risks of treatment delay. Figure 11-3 shows the effects of delay in RT on local control in cancer of the oropharynx, predicted by a mathematical model. The model was based on radiobiological principles that had been validated in experimental systems, and it incorporated the best available clinical information about tumor doubling times and the relationship between tumor volume and local control.[28] The model predicted a decrease in local control rates of between 5% and 10% per month of delay in the start of RT. Others have since made similar predictions.[29]

Observational Studies of the Effects of Delay on the Outcomes of Radiotherapy

A systematic review revealed surprisingly little published information about the relationship between delay and the outcomes of RT in many clinical situations.[30] However, there were sufficient data available to permit meta-analyses in the context of adjuvant RT for breast cancer and head and neck cancer. In both of these situations, there was a significant increase in local failure rates with increasing delays in RT. Figure 11-4 shows the results of the meta-analysis of eight studies of the association between delay and local recurrence after postoperative RT for breast cancer. Patients who waited between 9 and 16 weeks had a recurrence rate of 9.1%, while those treated within 8 weeks had a local recurrence rate of 5.8%. Assuming that the patients in the delayed group waited on average about 2 months longer than the promptly treated controls, this translates into an increase in risk of recurrence of approximately 1.5% per month of delay. In a subsequent report from McGill University, in which waiting times were entered into a regression analysis as a continuous variable, Benck and colleagues[31] found an increase in local recurrence of approximately 1% per month of delay in this situation.

Indirect Effects of Waiting Lists for Radiotherapy on Patient Care

Table 11-2 summarizes the indirect effects of waiting lists on patient care and population health. The phenomenon of implicit rationing by which waiting lists reduce the use of RT has already been described (see Kinetics of Waiting Lists). Waiting lists may also increase the use of alternative treatments that may be less effective, more morbid, and more expensive than RT. There is also evidence that long waiting lists may cause radiation oncologists to modify the way they prescribe RT. A study from the Queensland Radium Institute shows a significant negative correlation between waiting times and the number of fractions prescribed per course. This was due primarily to decreases in palliative fractionation as waiting times increased.[32] Similar trends have been observed in Ontario.[24] There is obviously a grave risk in modifying the practice of radiation oncology because of pressure of workload. The message here is that problems in accessibility of RT have the potential to generate secondary problems in quality of RT. That being said, the use of single fractions for bone metastases and short courses or single fractions for palliation of advanced lung cancer does have the potential to reduce overall workload and greatly increase the availability of RT without adversely affecting outcomes.[33] The challenge is to ensure that shorter-than-standard courses of RT are used only in circumstances in which it has been shown to be medically appropriate. Under conditions of scarcity of resources, it is particularly important to have explicit standards of care to prevent deterioration of quality in the attempt to maintain access.

Societal Effects of Waiting Lists for Radiotherapy

Waiting lists for RT are potentially costly (Table 11-3). Patients require both care and counseling during delays and the costs of alternative treatments may be considerably higher than those of RT. Waiting lists have also intermittently caused patients to be referred to remote centers for RT with greatly added costs to the health system, as well as loss of continuity of care and support for patients. The inability to provide timely RT has been profoundly distressing for the staff of RT programs. The problems of providing care without adequate resources have been so consuming that many of the affected RT programs have been unable to keep up to date with developments in radiation oncology. Waiting lists also expose RT providers to legal liability. This has been a concern for some provider agencies in Canada for several years, and it has surfaced as a major issue with the commencement of a class action suit on behalf of several thousand women in Quebec who had to wait long periods for adjuvant RT following surgery for breast cancer.[34] Waiting lists in Canada have been used as an argument for reforming the Canadian health system and as an argument against adopting a similar model in the United States.[35]

Setting Standards for Acceptable Waiting Times

There is no established scientific process for setting standards for acceptable waiting times for medical treatment. The "guidelines," "targets," and "standards" that have been adopted around the world have generally been based on expert opinion. However, expert opinions are heterogeneous and unstable. In the mail survey of heads of radiation oncol-

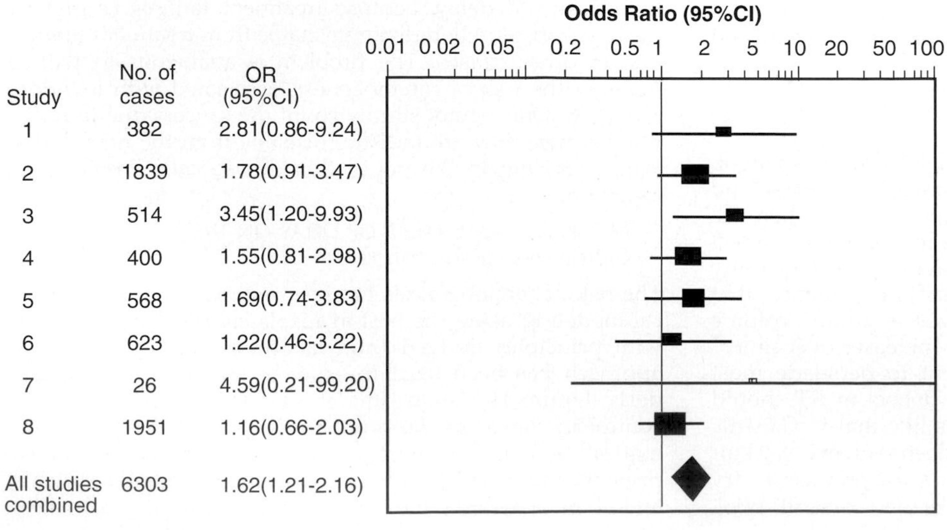

Figure 11-4 The association between delay in postoperative RT for breast cancer and the rate of local recurrence. The plot shows the results of a meta-analysis that included seven studies that compared rates of local recurrence in women with breast cancer who started postoperative RT more than 8 weeks after surgery with the rates observed in those treated within 8 weeks of surgery. (Adapted from Huang J, Barbera L, Brouwers M, et al: Does delay in starting treatment affect the outcomes of radiotherapy? A systematic review. J Clin Oncol 21:555-563, 2003.)

Table 11-3 Factors Affecting the Use of Palliative Radiotherapy in Ontario*

	Odds Ratio	95% Confidence Interval
MEDIAN HOUSEHOLD INCOME		
Low, <Can $20,000.	1.00	—
Medium, Can $20,000-$50,000.	1.09	1.04-1.15
High, >Can $50,000.	1.17	1.11-1.24
RT DEPARTMENT IN DIAGNOSING HOSPITAL		
No	1.00	—
Yes	1.35	1.30-1.40
PROXIMITY OF PATIENT'S HOME TO NEAREST RT CENTER		
No RT center in county of residence	1.00	—
RT center in county of residence	1.24	1.21-1.27
REGION		
Northeast Ontario	0.84	0.79-0.90
Toronto	0.88	0.84-0.92
Windsor	0.90	0.84-0.97
Ottawa	1.00	—
London	1.02	0.97-1.07
Northwest Ontario	1.04	0.96-1.13
Kingston	1.17	1.11-1.26
Hamilton	1.20	1.14-1.26

*From a logistic regression that controlled for age, sex, and primary site.

ogy programs across the United States and Canada cited earlier,[22] respondents were asked what they believed was "the maximum medically acceptable interval" between referral and the start of RT in a number of different clinical situations. There was considerable variation of opinion in both the United States and in Canada, but the Canadians whose departments had much longer waiting times were willing to accept significantly longer delays than were their American counterparts.[22] In Canada, there was a significant correlation between the duration of the prevailing delay in a department and the department head's perception of the maximum acceptable delay.[22] The observed diversity of expert opinion about acceptable waiting times and its apparent susceptibility to drift in response to prevailing conditions both indicate the need for a more explicit and objective process for setting this type of standard. There is a well-developed framework for environmental risk assessment and risk management, which appears well suited to the task of setting standards for exposure to clinical hazards such as delay in treatment. We have begun to apply this process to set waiting time standards for RT in Canada.[36]

Measuring Access to Radiotherapy

Limitations of Waiting Times as an Indicator of Access to Radiotherapy

The existence of a long waiting list for RT is a symptom of inadequate access to RT. The duration of the waiting time for RT may be directly related to the probability of an adverse outcome, and waiting times may therefore serve as a quantitative measure of the quality of care. The length of a waiting list, however, provides no information about the magnitude of the shortfall between supply and demand, and waiting times cannot, therefore, serve as a quantitative measure of accessibility (see Kinetics of Waiting Lists). The absence of a waiting list does not mean that access is optimal. Waiting lists develop only in response to supply-side problems in the availability of services. Waiting times are entirely insensitive to demand-side problems with respect to spatial accessibility, accommodation, affordability, or awareness (see Table 11-2).

Problems in those dimensions of accessibility reduce demand and may actually serve to prevent waiting lists. The absence of a waiting list does not imply that access is optimal. To ensure appropriate access to RT, it is also necessary to monitor RT utilization rate.

Defining Access to Radiotherapy

The best quantitative measure of the accessibility of any service is the rate of its appropriate utilization, that is, the proportion of patients that need a service who actually receive it.

$$\text{Access} = \text{Use}/\text{Need}$$

Access can have any value between 0 and 1, where 1 corresponds to optimal access. These values can also be multiplied by 100 and expressed as a percentage. The measurement of access requires methods for measuring both utilization and need in the general population.

Measuring Radiation Therapy Use

The use of RT may be described as the proportion of cases treated with RT in the population of interest. Comprehensive information about all of the RT provided for that population is required to establish the numerator, and a population-based cancer registry is required to establish the denominator. Some cancer registries actively compile information about treatment and may be able to provide all the necessary information. Alternatively, if all the necessary RT records are available in electronic form, it may be quite simple to link them to individual cases in the registry.[23] It is important to ensure that the numerator is properly matched to the denominator—that is, there should be information available from all the facilities that provide RT for the population of interest, regardless of the location of those facilities. This is probably easier to accomplish in countries with publicly funded systems that typically operate a small number of large RT centers with more or less exclusive responsibility for a given geographic region. The approach was first used in the Netherlands,[37] and we subsequently used it to describe the use of RT in Ontario.[23]

MEASURING THE USE OF RADIOTHERAPY IN THE INITIAL MANAGEMENT OF CANCER

The *incidence* of cancer (i.e., number of new cases diagnosed in the population of interest, over the period of interest) is the appropriate denominator for describing the use of RT in the initial management of the disease. The best way to establish the proportion of cases that are treated with RT is to follow all of them forward in time from the date of diagnosis and find out if and when the patient received RT. The estimated rate of use of RT in the initial management of cancer depends on the cutoff point in time used to define initial RT. If a short cutoff point is chosen to define initial RT (e.g., RT within 3 months of diagnosis), the indicator will miss some patients who receive adjuvant RT following surgery. If a longer cutoff point is chosen (e.g., RT within 1 year), the indicator will include almost all patients who receive RT as part of their initial management, but it will also wrongly include some patients who are actually receiving RT for an early recurrence following primary surgery. The best cutoff point depends on the specific disease under consideration. For practical purposes, we have chosen to use the proportion of incident cases treated within 1 year of diagnosis to describe the initial use of RT in the

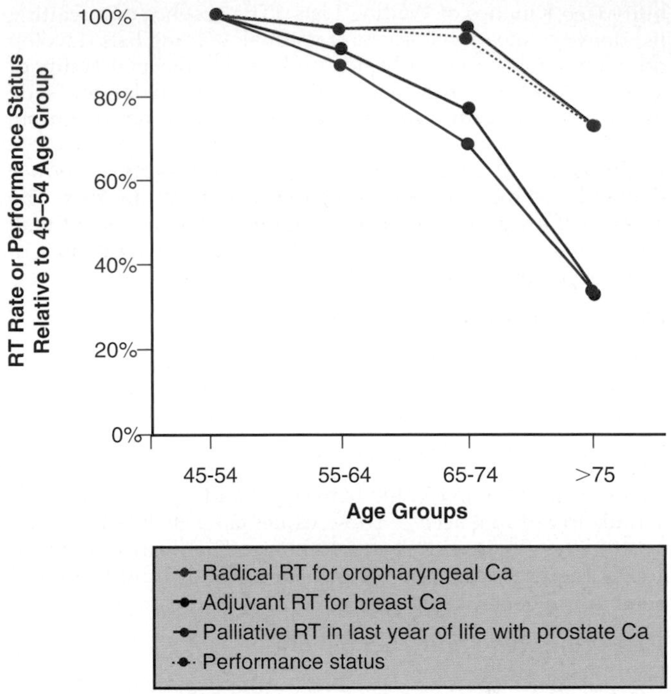

Figure 11-5 The effect of age on the use of RT. The proportion of patients who received RT for specified indications is shown for older age groups and compared with the rate observed in patients between 45 and 54 years old. The expected decline in performance status with increasing age is shown for comparison. (Adapted from Tyldesley S, Zhang-Salomons J, Groome P, et al: Association between age and the utilization of radiotherapy in Ontario. Int J Radiat Oncol Biol Phys 47:469-480, 2000.)

general cancer population. Figure 11-5A describes variations in the use of RT in the initial management of cancer in Ontario in terms of this indicator (R_{1year}).

MEASURING THE USE OF PALLIATIVE RADIATION THERAPY

The incidence of cancer is not the best denominator for describing the utilization of palliative RT, because a high proportion of incident cases will never develop indications for palliative RT. Many of those who do ultimately need palliative RT do not require it until years after the diagnosis. It is preferable to describe the use of palliative RT among patients who die of their cancer. This can be accomplished by identifying patients who died of their disease in a population-based cancer registry and following them back in time to identify those who received RT within a defined interval before death.[38] Figure 11-5B describes variations in the use of palliative RT in the last 2 years of life among patients who died of their disease in Ontario. The same approach lends itself well to the description of the rates of use of other types of care in the terminal phase of the illness.[39]

WHAT FACTORS AFFECT RADIATION THERAPY USE RATES IN THE GENERAL CANCER POPULATION?

Measurements of RT utilization rates have provided information that is important to the design of RT programs. It has been estimated that 50% of cancer patients require RT,[40] but RT utilization among different countries varies.[23,41-44] Caution is required in comparing RT rates because of differences in the specific definitions used to define rates of use of RT.[23] It has also been shown that the use of RT may vary widely among different parts of the same country. It has generally been found that rates of RT use are higher in urban than in rural areas[41,42] and that proximity to an RT facility is associated with higher utilization rates.[23] Figure 11-5 show that the rates of use of RT vary widely across Ontario. Rates of RT utilization are almost twice as high in some parts of the province than in others, with the highest rates being observed in the counties where RT facilities are located. It was also found that the geographic patterns of variation in the use of RT are very similar for several different groups of malignant diseases that are primarily managed by disparate groups of specialists.[23] This phenomenon is more readily explained by some structural aspect of the health system that affects access to RT than by an unlikely series of coincidences about surgical opinions regarding the value of RT.[23] Taken together, these observations suggest that spatial accessibility is an important determinant of the accessibility of RT.

In studying geographic variations in practice, it is obviously important to be able to distinguish systematic variation from variations due to chance alone. This presents some challenges when comparing rates across a number of different geographic regions each with a different population, but modeling techniques have been developed that allow one to identify the systematic component of variation.[23] Multiple factors are involved in determining eligibility for RT in the individual case, and multivariate analysis is helpful in distinguishing the impact of health system–related factors from patient-related factors on the use of RT. Table 11-3 shows the results of a multivariate analysis that examined factors associated with use of palliative RT among patients who died of their cancer in Ontario. Rates of use of palliative RT proved to be significantly lower among patients in whom the diagnosis was made in a hospital without an RT facility, suggesting that awareness of the indications for RT may also be a significant factor in determining accessibility.[38,45] Table 11-3 also illustrates that, even in the context of a publicly funded health system, the socioeconomic status of the patient influences the likelihood of receiving palliative RT.[38]

Measurements of RT use have revealed unexpected inequities in access to care. Figure 11-6 shows that rates of use of palliative and adjuvant RT decrease with increasing age and that this decrease is far greater than can be explained due to declining performance status.[46]

Measuring the Need for Radiotherapy

The observed variation in RT rates begs the question: What proportion of patients with cancer really need RT? It is often stated that approximately 50% of patients with cancer should receive RT at some point in the course of the illness, but that recommendation is based almost entirely on expert opinion.[40,47,48] Two more objective methods have been developed for estimating the need for RT and these are described next.

EVIDENCE-BASED REQUIREMENTS ANALYSIS

Evidence-based requirements analysis (EBRA) is an objective method that can be used to estimate the need for any type of health service, where *need* is defined as existing "when an individual has an illness for which there is effective and acceptable treatment."[14] The process is straightforward. The indications for RT are first identified by systematic review. Next, an epidemiologic approach is used to estimate how frequently each indication for RT occurs in the population of interest. Finally, the results of the systematic review and the epidemiologic analysis are combined to estimate the overall need for RT. In this context, the term *need* can be equated with the *appropriate rate* of utilization of RT, and the two terms

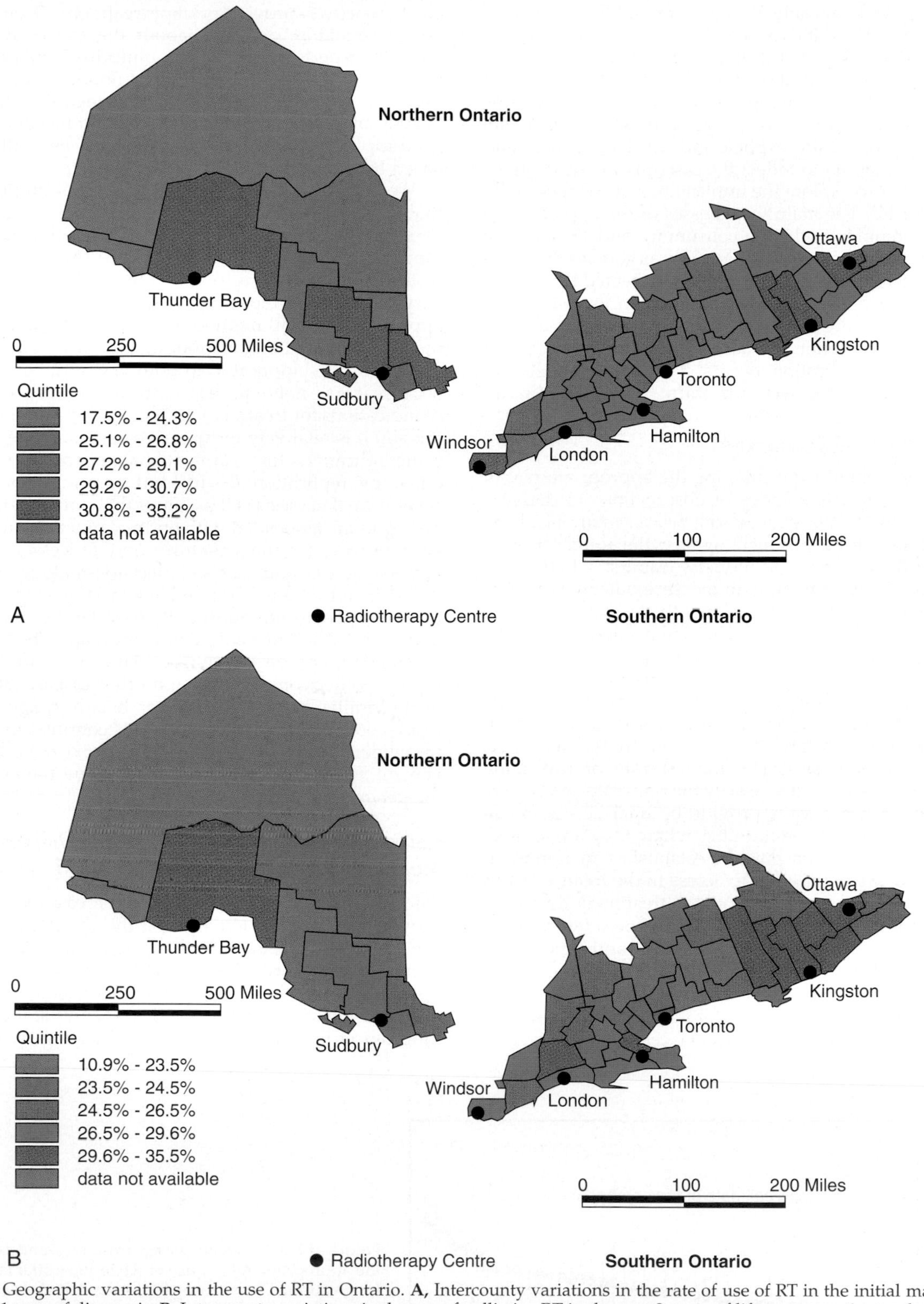

Figure 11-6 Geographic variations in the use of RT in Ontario. **A,** Intercounty variations in the rate of use of RT in the initial management of cancer within 1 year of diagnosis. **B,** Intercounty variations in the use of palliative RT in the past 2 years of life among patients who died of their cancer. The location of the provincial RT centers is shown for comparison. (**A,** Adapted from Mackillop WJ, Groome PA, Zhou Y, et al: Does a centralized radiotherapy system provide adequate access to care? J Clin Oncol 15:1261-1271, 1997; **B,** adapted from Huang J, Zhou S, Groome P, et al: Factors affecting the use of palliative radiotherapy in Ontario. J Clin Oncol 19:137-144, 2001.)

may be used interchangeably. We have applied this method to estimate the need for RT in several major cancer sites.[49-52] Others have since extended it across the whole spectrum of malignant disease,[53] and it is now being used to predict requirements for RT equipment across Europe.[54] The strengths of the method are that (1) it is transparent in that all the assumptions involved are explicit and (2) it is flexible, and models can be adapted to reflect the case mix in any community of interest or to explore the implications of changes in the indications for RT. The main weaknesses of the approach are that (1) it is complex and time consuming and (2) like any other type of modeling, its results are only as good as the information on which it is based. EBRA can be expected to produce valid results when it is applied to major cancers where the indications for RT are well defined and there is sufficient epidemiologic information available to estimate the frequency with which each indication occurs. Published models are available for use on the web site (http://www.krcc.on.ca/estimatingRT).

CRITERION-BASED BENCHMARKING

An alternative method for estimating the appropriate rate of the use of RT is to use a series of observations to derive a "benchmark." In the business world, *benchmarking* has been defined as "measuring products against the toughest competitors or those recognized as industry leaders."[55] In the field of health care, the equivalent is to measure outcomes against the best achieved anywhere or against those achieved in recognized centers of excellence. The same concept may be applied in setting benchmarks for the appropriate rate of utilization of any given treatment. The rate observed under certain very specific conditions may be equated with the appropriate rate of utilization—in other words, with the need for treatment. The rules are different from those used to set benchmarks for outcomes. The highest rate of utilization observed anywhere is not necessarily the right rate and centers of excellence do not always provide optimal access for all those who reside in the communities where they are located. Benchmarks for utilization must be established in communities where there are no barriers to access to the treatment and where circumstances support optimal treatment decisions. Benchmarks for the utilization of RT should be set in communities where there is unimpeded access to RT and expert decision-making about the use of RT. To ensure unimpeded access, there should be no financial barriers, referring physicians should be aware of the indications for RT, and patients should have convenient access to a nearby RT center that has sufficient capacity to provide prompt treatment. To ensure optimal decision-making, decisions about the use of RT should be made by experts practicing in a multidisciplinary setting, and ideally the decision to treat should not affect their remuneration. If these criteria are met, it is reasoned that the rate of utilization of RT should be correct and can be equated with the need for RT. This method has therefore been called criterion-based benchmarking (CBB).

We have been able to select a few communities in Ontario that meet most of the listed criteria and have used them to set benchmarks for the appropriate rate of utilization of RT for lung cancer. Figure 11-7 shows that in this context, estimates of the appropriate rate of RT generated by this method are very similar to those derived from the evidence-based approach. The CBB method has several strengths: (1) It is an inductive method that is grounded in observations in the real world; (2) it is applicable to both rare and common cancers because it does not require an accurate, comprehensive catalog of indications for treatment or detailed information about case mix; (3) it is relatively inexpensive and can be repeated easily if the indications for treatment change; and (4) it can be validated by replication in different communities. It also has several weaknesses: (1) It assumes that optimal structures and processes are associated with optimal practice and this has not been proved; (2) the structures and processes that support optimal access and optimal decision-making are not well defined; and (3) it requires a detailed knowledge of the structures in place in communities that are candidates to be benchmarks and this information may not readily be available.

The CBB approach requires further validation by extending it to other communities and other disease sites. If it produces similar results in different health systems and if the results obtained in other cancer sites continue to converge on the evidence-based estimates, it may prove to be the most convenient and robust method for estimating the need for RT in the general population.

Calculating the Accessibility to Radiotherapy from Measurements of Utilization and Need

Once utilization and need have been measured, it is straightforward to calculate access using the equation. For example, consider the data shown for lung cancer in Figure 11-7. It was estimated that approximately 41.5% of cases of lung cancer need RT as part of their initial management. The overall observed rate of utilization of RT in the initial management of lung cancer in Ontario was 32.5%. Applying the equation,

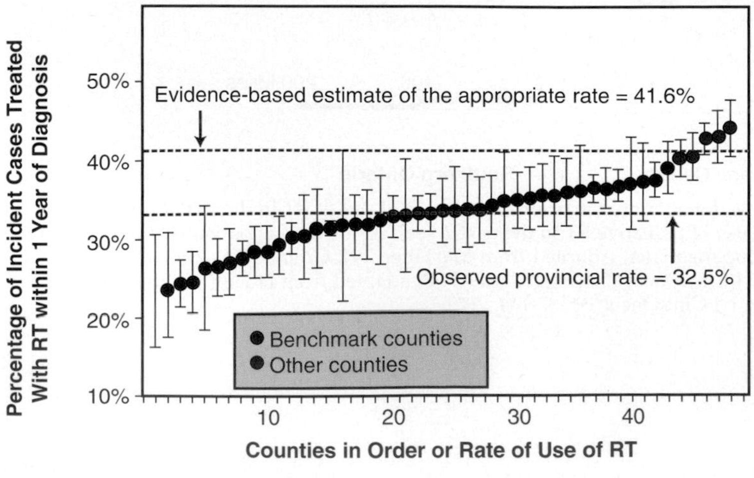

Figure 11-7 Evidence-based estimates and benchmarks of the appropriate rate of use of RT in the initial management of lung cancer. The rates of RT in the initial treatment of lung cancer are shown for each county in Ontario. The *error bars* represent the 95% confidence limits for these observations. Benchmark counties are those where cancer centers with relatively short waiting lists were located. The evidence-based estimate of the appropriate rate and the overall provincial rate are shown as *horizontal lines*; the distance between the lines represents the unmet need for RT. (Adapted from Barbera L, Zhang-Salomons J, Huang J, et al: Defining the need for radiotherapy for lung cancer in the general population: a criterion-based, benchmarking approach. Med Care 41:1074-1085, 2003.)

% Accessibility = 32.5/41.5 × 100% = 78.3%

Thus, less than 80% of cases that need RT in this context actually receive it. This indicates that we may fall more than 20% short of achieving what is readily achievable for patients with lung cancer simply because of inadequate access to RT. In more positive terms, this large defect in attainment of the achievable represents an important opportunity for improving outcomes of lung cancer without having to wait for the discovery of new drugs and new technologies.

STUDYING THE QUALITY OF RADIOTHERAPY

We first discuss the concept of quality in health care and introduce indicators of quality and then describe what HSR has taught us about optimizing the quality of RT and identify what we still need to learn.

Concepts of Quality and Effectiveness in Health Care

In the field of HSR, the term *efficacy* is used to describe the extent to which a treatment achieves its objectives in the controlled setting of a clinical trial. The term *effectiveness* is reserved for describing the extent to which a health program meets its stated objectives in the real world. The term *quality* is used to describe the effectiveness of the care provided, relative to the effectiveness of the best possible care. In this context, the term *quality* is therefore synonymous with attainment as defined earlier in How Can Health Services Research Help to Improve the Outcomes of Cancer?

Almost 40 years ago, Donabedian[57-60] defined *quality* as "a property of, and a judgement upon, some definable unit of health care, and that care is divisible into at least two parts: technical and interpersonal." The quality of technical care is measured by the extent to which "the application of medical science and technology maximizes its health benefits without correspondingly increasing its risks." The quality of interpersonal care is measured by "how well the physician-patient interaction meets the socially defined norms of the relationship."[57,58] Although others may define it somewhat differently today, there is universal agreement that quality is a multidimensional concept that embraces both the technical and personal elements of care.[61]

Donabedian[57-60] also provided an approach for evaluating and improving quality, which Kramer and Herring[62,63] soon astutely recognized as being appropriate for use in radiation oncology. Donabedian's approach was to analyze the quality of programs in terms of *structure, process,* and *outcome*. The term *process* is used here to describe the way that care is delivered. In the context of radiation oncology, it includes pretreatment assessment, medical decision-making, planning, delivery of RT, and supportive care during RT, etc. The term *structure* is used broadly to include facilities, equipment, manpower, and organizational structures. The term *outcome* is used here, as in clinical practice, to describe the consequences of the care that has been provided. It is reasoned that: (1) optimal *process* is necessary for optimal *outcome;* (2) adequate *structure* is necessary, though not sufficient, for optimal *process*; and (3) *outcomes* may be enhanced by identifying and correcting deficiencies in structure, and/or deficiencies in process. This became the philosophy of the U.S. Patterns of Care Study (PCS), administered by the American College of Radiology and funded by the National Cancer Institute, established by Kramer in 1970, which operates on the premise that "practice patterns exist, these differences can be measured, and deficiencies can be corrected."[64]

Methods for Studying Quality in Radiation Oncology

Diverse methods have been used to study structure, process, and outcomes in radiation oncology. Mail surveys have frequently been used to elicit information about the structures in place in radiation oncology programs. Surveys can also be used to discover physicians' opinions about the appropriateness of RT in different situations and to explore the basis of differences of opinion regarding treatment. Surveys are attractive because they can provide information about a large number of different departments or physicians at relatively low cost. Unfortunately, survey methods are rarely appropriate for studying the technical quality of RT processes or the outcomes achieved by RT. These elements of quality require direct observation or review of technical notes and records. This has traditionally been done on site, and it is time consuming and relatively expensive. When studies of process and outcomes involve multiple centers across a large region, careful sampling is needed to permit investigators to obtain generalizable results at reasonable cost. There are increasing opportunities today to use administrative data to learn something about the quality of cancer treatment programs in the general population. Cancer registries can serve to identify all cases of the disease of interest in the region of interest over the study period. The registry may be able provide some of the necessary information about treatment, and it may be possible to link additional information about treatment to the registry from other computerized sources including hospitalization records or billing files. We provide examples of each of these methods in the following sections as we review what has been learned about quality in radiation oncology. Nearly all the studies of quality that have been undertaken so far in radiation oncology are observational rather than experimental. Intervention studies can be done to compare different ways of delivering care, but that approach has not yet been widely adopted in this field.

Quality in Radiotherapy

Studies of the Structure of Radiotherapy Programs

Two different types of research are being undertaken in this area. First, there are descriptive studies of the physical and organizational structures that prevail in RT programs around the world. In some instances, the observed structures are compared with predetermined standards. In others, the description of structures has been linked to studies of process and outcome with the goal of establishing which types of structure are associated with the best results. These studies may rely on mail surveys or involve on-site visits, but they are all cross-sectional or retrospective in design. Second, there is the field of technology evaluation, which is essentially prescriptive rather than descriptive in intent. It seeks to establish prospectively the usefulness of new technologies in patient care and thus contributes information that is important in setting standards for equipment in an RT program.

Describing Structure: Surveys of the Structure of Radiotherapy Programs

In a highly technical specialty like radiation oncology, optimal care can be provided only when the necessary technological infrastructure is in place, including the correct mix and quantity of equipment and the correct mix and quantity of personnel. Nationwide surveys of RT facilities have now been done in many different countries. In the United States, the PCS has taken the lead in describing the basic structural characteristics of radiation oncology facilities for the entire country. Its comprehensive survey of the structure of U.S. facilities serves as the starting point for national surveys of treatment processes and outcomes and permits stratified sampling of different types of facilities.[65-67] In addition to evaluating equipment and personnel, the PCS has described the structure of RT facilities in the following terms: (1) whether they have resident training programs or not, (2) volume of new cases treated per annum, (3) whether they were headed by a full-time or part-time radiation oncologist, and (4) participation in clinical trials.

In Europe, a variety of government[68] and nongovernment agencies[69] and individual investigators[70] have conducted national surveys of RT program infrastructure, primarily as a basis for planning. Most national surveys reveal considerable diversity with respect to the level of technology and expertise that is available in different RT centers. This is particularly true of brachytherapy.[71] The European Society for Therapeutic Radiology (ESTRO) is leading an international initiative to describe and compare the infrastructure of RT programs across Europe in a project called QUARTS (Quantification of Radiation Therapy Infrastructure and Staffing), which has been funded by the European Commission.[72] QUARTS involves an international survey of equipment and personnel,[72] the establishment of guidelines for levels of staffing and equipment,[73] and the estimation of future needs based on projected incidence and estimates of need derived by EBRA.[49,54] In the long term, ESTRO has plans to use this international facilities survey as the starting point for its own pan-European studies of patterns of referral and patterns of care.[74]

The concept of program structure embraces not only physical infrastructure but also organizational structures including systems of funding, management, and governance. These elements of structure in radiation oncology may also have important effects on processes, but they have generally received less attention than the physical elements of structure. Funding arrangements at European RT centers listed in the ESTRO directory were investigated as part of an international study of palliative RT.[75] A broad range of funding mechanisms for RT departments is described, including a global budget, per case payments, fee for service, and all possible combinations thereof. RT centers in Spain, the United Kingdom, and the Netherlands were mainly funded by a global budget plus or minus per case payments, while the majority of centers in Germany and Switzerland received most of their funding through a fee-for-service arrangement.[75] The observed associations between funding mechanisms and patterns of practice are discussed in Impact of Financial Incentives and Disincentives on the Practice of Radiotherapy.

Prescribing Structures: Technology Assessment

New technologies are being developed rapidly, and our specialty needs to develop better ways of evaluating them and of determining their appropriate place in routine clinical practice.[76,77] Wherever possible, new treatment techniques should be evaluated in randomized clinical trials, but it is clear that this approach only lends itself to the study of relatively common presentations of relatively common diseases. A large component of the practice of radiation oncology, however, is directed toward patients who have one of the many less common cancers or one of the infinite range of unusual presentations of a common cancer. In neither of these situations is there ever going to be "level I evidence" to guide our practice. For this reason, it would be impossible for a new approach to treatment such as intensity-modulated radiation therapy to achieve its full potential if we demanded level I evidence for its use in every situation. On the other hand, if we choose to make our decisions about the acquisition and use of new technologies based only on the manufacturers' claims of enhanced precision, we may expose our patients to added risks and added costs without real benefits.[78]

Studies of Process in Radiotherapy

Some processes in an RT program have the potential to affect every patient, while others concern specific groups of patients. We deal first with research in the first area of general quality assurance before considering the process of care for specific groups of cancer patients.

Research on Quality Assurance Processes in Radiotherapy

The RT community has long recognized the importance of routine quality assurance because of the potential for a malfunctioning or wrongly calibrated machine to cause systematic errors in the treatment of a large number of patients. Detailed guidelines and protocols have therefore been developed for commissioning, maintenance, and calibration of treatment machines.[79] However, neither the existence of such guidelines nor an organizational commitment to adhere to them is sufficient to guarantee patient safety. An important survey undertaken some years ago by Horiot and coworkers[80] on behalf of the European Organization for Research and Treatment of Cancer (EORTC) revealed that some centers made systematic errors in radiation dosimetry. It also showed that feedback of the results of the initial survey diminished the frequency of such errors when the study was later repeated.[81]

Although quality assurance on equipment reduces the chance of systematic error, the requirement for individualization of treatment plans creates the added risk of random error caused, for example, by lapses in human judgment or miscommunication. It has been shown that although well-defined care paths or intervention-specific guidelines can minimize the frequency of this type of error, it does not eliminate them.[82] Real-time audit is necessary to avoid rare but potentially serious errors in the context of routine practice[82] and even in the controlled setting of clinical trials.[83] The general rule that emerges from these analyses is that human errors cannot all be avoided, but the vast majority can be detected before they have any adverse impact on the patient.

Research on Practice Patterns in Radiotherapy

During the past 30 years, there have been numerous studies of patterns of care in radiation oncology using methods primarily developed by the PCS.[84-86] Although many different clinical situations have been studied, most work has been done on the major sites in which RT plays an important role in curative treatment, including breast,[87-107] genitourinary,[108-123] gynecologic,[124-132] lung,[133-140] gastrointestinal,[141-148] head and neck,[149-156] and lymphoma.[157-159] There have also been a number of studies of the practice of palliative RT, particularly in the context of bone metastasis.[160-170] Striking variations in practice have been discovered in every situation that has been studied in detail. Practice has been shown to vary at many different points in the pathway of care: in pretreatment assessment[66,124]; in fundamental aspects of the RT prescription, including target volumes,[122,124,161] treatment techniques,[103,104] and dose and fractionation[33,105]; in decisions about adjunctive systemic treatment[118,124,129]; in the planning process[124]; in treatment delivery[155]; in the way that treatment details are recorded[128]; in supportive care during and after treatment[127]; and in arrangements for long-term follow-up.[148]

Why Study Practice Variations in RT? Practice variations have been identified in every field of medicine where anyone has taken the trouble to look for them. As we have seen above, radiation oncology is no exception. In the era of evidence-based medicine, practice variations represent a threat to the credibility of any medical specialty; it is difficult to defend variations in patient care except insofar they reflect variations in the needs of individual patients or unavoidable variations in the availability of resources. Practice variations in radiation oncology represent not only a threat but also an opportunity for improving practice and outcomes. The opportunities to improve the quality of care depend on the state of knowledge in the particular clinical situation under study. If optimal practice has already been established or can be established for the purposes of the study, deviations from the optimal represent opportunities for improving quality of care.[84-86] It then becomes important to understand why practice deviates from the optimal, in order to design interventions that will improve practice. If, on the other hand, optimal practice has not yet been established, practice variations represent an opportunity for learning. Studies of practice patterns may identify controversies that should be addressed in clinical trials. In certain very specific circumstances, it may be possible to explore the relationship between treatments and outcomes in order to determine which approach is superior. The scope and limitations of this type of study are discussed in Relating Structure and Process to Outcomes.

Why Does Practice Vary in Radiation Oncology? In an ideal world, cancer treatment would be guided only by precise classification of the case and the application of scientific knowledge about the optimal treatment of that class of cases, taking into account the patient's personal values and preferences. In the real world, however, other environmental factors may influence patient care. Treatment options are often constrained by the resources available. Scientific knowledge is variably disseminated and may be interpreted differently by individual physicians, depending on their training, experience, and work environment. Moreover, financial considerations have the potential to influence medical decisions, whenever there is more than one defensible treatment option available. We now review what is known about the impact of each of these factors on the practice of RT.

Impact of Program Structure on the Practice of Radiotherapy. Consistent with Donabedian's concept, there is abundant evidence that physical and organizational structures determine processes in RT (see Fig. 11-12). If the total availability of personnel and equipment is not adequate to permit prompt access to RT, referring physicians may choose alternative forms of treatment. Many studies have revealed that radiation oncologists' choices of investigations, treatment techniques, and fractionation schemes are influenced by the resources available.[92,139] The PCS has consistently found significant associations between the structural characteristics of facilities and the quality of processes involved in patient care.[64] For example, in a now classic study of work-up and treatment procedures in head and neck cancer,[66] the PCS found significantly poorer compliance with its criteria of appropriateness of assessment, treatment, and other aspects of care among patients treated at nontraining facilities compared with training facilities (Fig. 11-8A) and at facilities headed by a part-time, rather than full-time, radiation oncologist (see Fig. 11-8B).

Impact of Scientific Evidence on the Practice of Radiotherapy. Practice varies most where there is least evidence available. Decision-making about the use of RT has been shown to be highly variable in the context of adjuvant RT. This is most evident where the value has not been confirmed in randomized trials.[118,131] Although many indications for RT are supported by the results of randomized trials, there have been far fewer formal comparative studies of the details of RT prescriptions and techniques. Not surprisingly, technical practice of RT is even more variable than clinical decision-making in radiation oncology. Even in situations in which there have been several consistent published reports that appear to indicate that one approach is superior to another, it has been shown that physicians may interpret these data very differently and therefore may still vary widely in their treatment recommendations.[135,140]

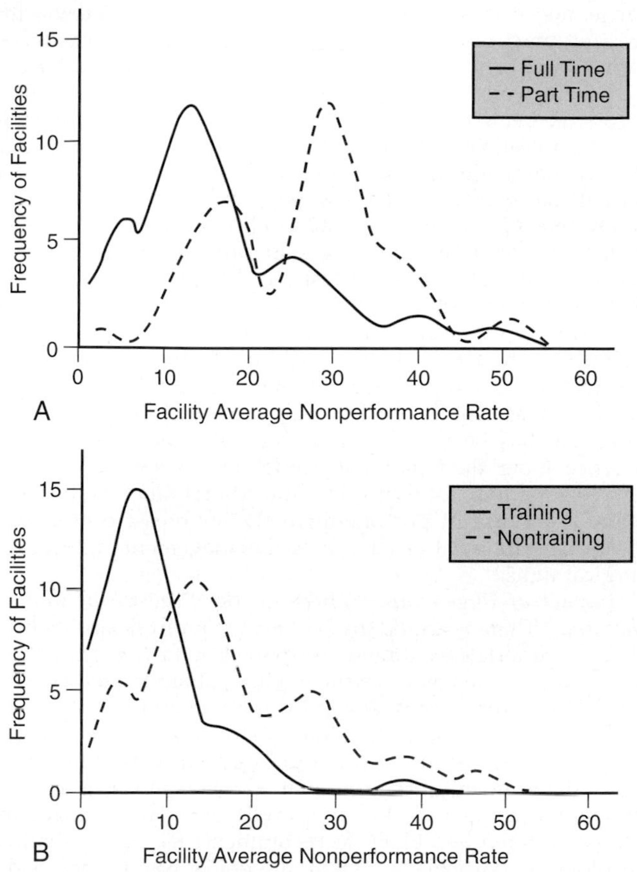

Figure 11-8 Relationships between the structural characteristics of RT programs and quality of practice. **A,** Nonperformance rates for part-time and full-time facilities. **B,** Frequency polygons of nonperformance scores for training and nontraining facilities. (Adapted from MacLean CJ, Davis LW, Herring DF, et al: Variation in work-up and treatment procedures among types of radiation therapy facilities: the Patterns of Care Process Survey for three head and neck sites. Cancer 48:1346-1352, 1981.)

There has been much interest in enhancing the practice of medicine through the synthesis and dissemination of scientific knowledge in the form of treatment guidelines. Guidelines are clearly valuable for reference purposes, but it is not clear to what extent they have actually succeeded in modifying practice in the general population. Changes in practice have sometimes been reported after the introduction of treatment guidelines, but it is usually impossible to conclude that the guidelines themselves were responsible for those changes.[89]

Scientific evidence appears to vary in its impact depending on the practice environment and also on the demographic characteristics of the patients. In 2001, the U.S. Commission on Cancer reported that breast-conserving surgery was still used in less than 50% of U.S. patients with stage 1 and 2 breast cancer and that variations in its use were not consistent with existing practice guidelines.[100] Breast conservation was more rapidly and completely adopted in urban than in rural areas and there were large geographic variations in its adoption across the United States, with much higher rates in the northeast than elsewhere. Older patients and patients from lower socioeconomic groups were less likely than others to have a partial mastectomy, and those who did were less likely to receive postoperative RT. As rates of breast conservation have increased over time, differences in care related to age and socioeconomic status have persisted.[99] There is also evidence that the characteristics of physicians and their type of practice influence the extent to which they rely on guidelines or other published information in reaching treatment decisions. Reliance on published information in decision-making is greater in academic centers and decreases the longer the physician has been in practice.[132] Local policies may affect practice more than national guidelines. A study from the United Kingdom, for example, showed that much of the variation in the use of postoperative RT for breast cancer was attributable to variations in the local management protocols of surgical units.[94]

Impact of Physicians' Beliefs on the Practice of Radiotherapy. There is abundant evidence that physicians' beliefs about appropriate treatment are shaped by factors other than universal knowledge. Physicians' views about the indications for RT are strongly influenced by their training and experience. Because the key decisions about referral are usually made by surgeons, the views of the surgical community are a major determinant of the role that RT plays in cancer care at the population level. It has repeatedly been shown that surgeons are often less likely to recommend RT than radiation oncologists, particularly when a choice has to be made between primary RT and primary surgery. For example, in comparison to radiation oncologists, urologists are less likely to recommend primary RT for prostate cancer[108,109] and otolaryngologists are less likely to recommend RT for laryngeal cancer.[122,152] Medical oncologists today have acquired a significant role in initiating referrals to radiation oncology, but their views about the indications for RT also differ significantly from ours.[134,140]

Impact of Financial Incentives and Disincentives on the Practice of Radiotherapy. There is evidence that funding mechanisms may affect case selection for RT. For example, a study based on administrative claims data from Pennsylvania showed that the patient's health insurance status was associated with the chance of receiving RT following partial mastectomy. Postoperative RT was given in only 45% of Medicaid patients compared with greater than 75% of privately insured and Medicare patients.[90] Similar observations have been made elsewhere.[97] Funding arrangements have also been shown to influence choices of fractionation in some studies. Lievens has explored the effects of funding on patterns of palliative RT in Belgium.[75] She found that fractionated courses of RT were prescribed more frequently than single treatments for bone metastases, at least in part because the funding mechanism in place at that time penalized the use of single fractions. In 2001, a new mechanism of funding of palliative RT was introduced in Belgium, which removed the disincentive to single treatments. Since that time, there has been a trend to reduce the number of fractions prescribed in all except 3 of the 23 centers that responded to her most recent survey. Many of those centers reported that the change in the fee schedule was a significant factor in their decision to change practice.[170] Lievens and coworkers[75] have also shown significant associations between funding models and the practice of palliative RT in an international survey of RT centers across Europe. They found that centers funded by a global budget or per-case payment used a significantly lower number of fractions per course and were less likely to use shielding blocks than were centers funded by fee for service. The growing evidence that funding may shape the way that RT is practiced suggests that it may be possible to improve practice by appropriately manipulating reimbursement systems. However, there is also a high risk that poorly designed fee schedules may compromise quality of care.[171] It has also been pointed out that, under per-case funding arrangements, profits may be inversely related to quality, making it very important to set clear baseline quality standards.[172]

Studies of Outcomes in Radiotherapy Programs

It is important to appreciate that although outcomes may seem to be the ultimate measure of quality, one cannot fine-tune the operation of a cancer program by measuring the long-term outcomes by which we usually judge the success of cancer treatment. It may take a decade to measure the 5-year recurrence-free rates associated with a particular pattern of practice. Any feedback from audit of outcome comes far too slowly to permit optimization of the program performance. Quality improvement programs in oncology largely have to operate on the principle that if you get the structure and the process right, the outcomes will look after themselves. That being said, there is some value in measuring outcomes and the opportunity to do this should not be overlooked.

Surprisingly, it may be easier to measure outcomes than processes in the general population. Accurate information about vital status is usually available in cancer registries, and it may be quite straightforward to measure survival at the population level. Hospital records and billing files may provide information about subsequent surgical procedures that can sometimes provide surrogate measures of local control by RT. For example, survival without subsequent laryngectomy has been used as a surrogate for local control in measuring the success of radical RT for laryngeal cancer, and survival without subsequent cystectomy has been used as a surrogate for local control after radical RT for bladder cancer (Fig. 11-9). The high statistical power of population-based studies also makes it possible to detect and quantify rare but serious late effects that it might be impossible to detect based on the analysis of experience of any individual institution.[173-178]

Large variations in outcome have been observed among different countries and among different regions, demographic groups, and institutions within the same country. The challenge lies in distinguishing the component of variation in outcome attributable to differences in quality from the inevitable variations in outcome due to differences in case mix.

International variations in cancer outcomes are inevitably multifactorial in origin, and it is difficult to attribute them to any individual aspect of health system performance. Nonetheless, such comparisons have proved to be useful.[179,180] Figure 11-10 shows international variations in cancer survival as a function of proportion of gross domestic product spent on health care. It demonstrates a remarkably clear relationship between investment in health care and cancer survival. It is impossible to determine whether the worse outcome observed in countries that spent less on health care was due to more advanced stage of disease at diagnosis, higher levels of comorbidity, poorer access to care, or poorer quality of care. However, despite these uncertainties the message is clear that you get what you pay for. These results had a direct influence on public policy in the United Kingdom and were used to justify an expansion in the budget of the national health service's cancer programs by almost $1 billion, permitting a

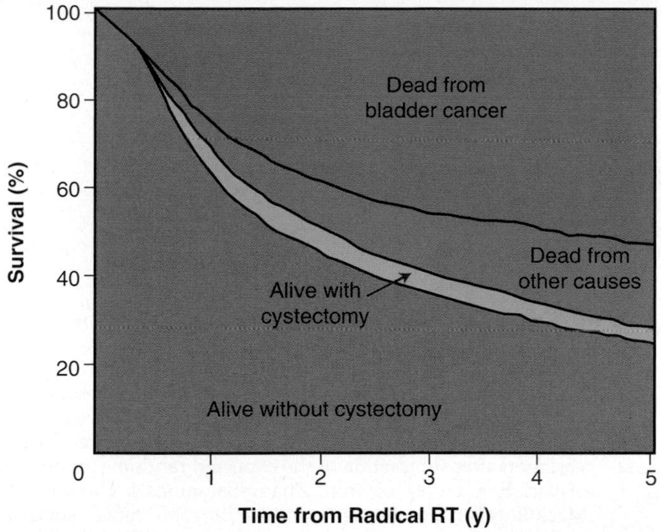

Figure 11-9 Outcome of radical RT for bladder cancer in Ontario. The graph illustrates the results of a population-based study of the outcome of radical RT for bladder cancer in Ontario. The curves show the probability of survival and cystectomy-free survival in 1370 patients who received radical RT for bladder cancer between 1982 and 1984. Deaths from cancer are differentiated from deaths from other causes. (Adapted from Hayter CRR, Paszat LF, Groome PA, et al: A population-based study of the use and outcome of radical radiotherapy for invasive bladder cancer. Int J Radiat Oncol Biol Phys 45:1239-1245, 1999.)

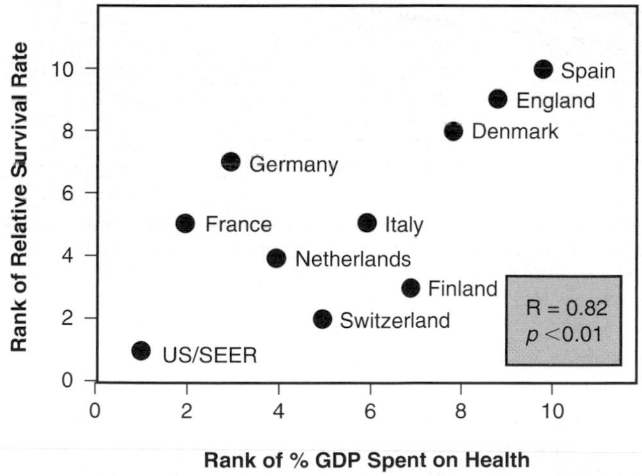

Figure 11-10 Correlation between relative survival and expenditure on health care. The scatter plot shows the relationship between relative survival for all cancer in female patients, and the percentage of gross domestic product (GDP) spent on health care in 10 developed countries. (Adapted from Evans BT, Pritchard C: Cancer survival rates and GDP expenditure on health: a comparison of England and Wales and the USA, Denmark, Netherlands, Finland, France, Germany, Italy, Spain, and Switzerland in the 1990s. Public Health 114:336-339, 2000.)

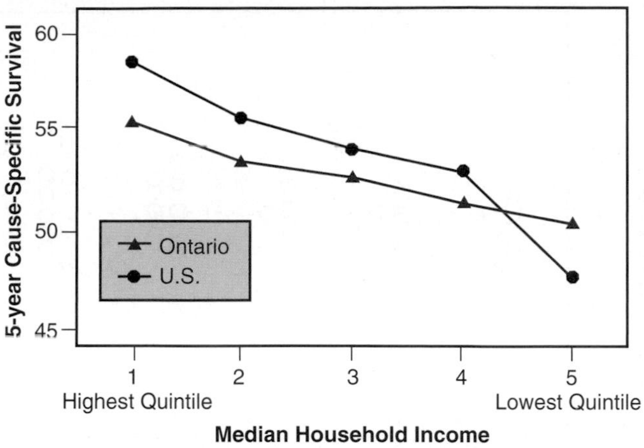

Figure 11-11 Associations between socioeconomic status (SES) and cancer survival in the United States and Canada. The graph shows 5-year, cause-specific cancer survival as a function of SES for all cancers combined (excluding prostate) in the Canadian province of Ontario and in the regions of the United States covered by the Surveillance, Epidemiology, and End Results (SEER) cancer registries. (Data from Boyd CJ, Zhang-Salomons J, Groome PA, et al: Associations between community income and cancer survival in Ontario and the United States. J Clin Oncol 17:2244-2255, 1999.)

massive expansion in the equipment and staffing of its radiation oncology programs.

It has also been shown that cancer outcomes are worse in residents of poorer communities than in residents of richer communities within the same country.[179] Figure 11-11 shows variations in 5-year survival among patients from richer and poorer communities in Canada and the United States. There is a clear gradient in survival across socioeconomic strata in both countries. Some, but not all, of the observed variation is due to more advanced stage at diagnosis among the poorer groups, probably reflecting differences in access to care.[179] Differences in quality of care may be responsible for some of the observed differences in survival not explained by differences in stage mix. These differences in outcome represent potential opportunities for improving overall outcomes at the population level. Before we can develop strategies for reducing these disparities, further studies are needed to explore their causes. Although the socioeconomic status–survival gradient is steeper in the United States, there is still a significant difference in outcome among residents of richer and poorer communities in Canada. This may seem somewhat surprising because Ontario has a single-payer, universal health care system with no parallel private health care sector, and in theory the rich do not have better access to care or quality of care than the poor. Clearly, however, the removal of financial barriers to access to care does not in itself abolish differences in outcome between rich and poor.[179]

Interregional comparisons within the same country may also be informative. When dissimilar populations are compared, it is necessary to control for differences in case mix, but in the absence of any major interregional variations in socioeconomic status, systematic variations in case mix are unlikely. Under these circumstances, variations in outcome, which exceed those expected due to chance alone, may reasonably be attributed to variations in access or quality.[181] Figure 11-12 shows the observed 5-year survival for several major cancer sites in eight different regions of Ontario. Once the observed variations are reduced to take account of the expected variation due to chance alone, the best observed outcomes may be used as a benchmark for the achievable outcome. Figure 11-12 shows that, after adjusting for variation due to chance alone, there were no residual geographic variations in the outcome of cancers of the pancreas, colon, or cervix, but there remained important geographic variations of survival for head and neck cancer, Hodgkin's disease, and testicular cancer. Table 11-4 shows the observed 5-year survival for the province as a whole compared with the estimated

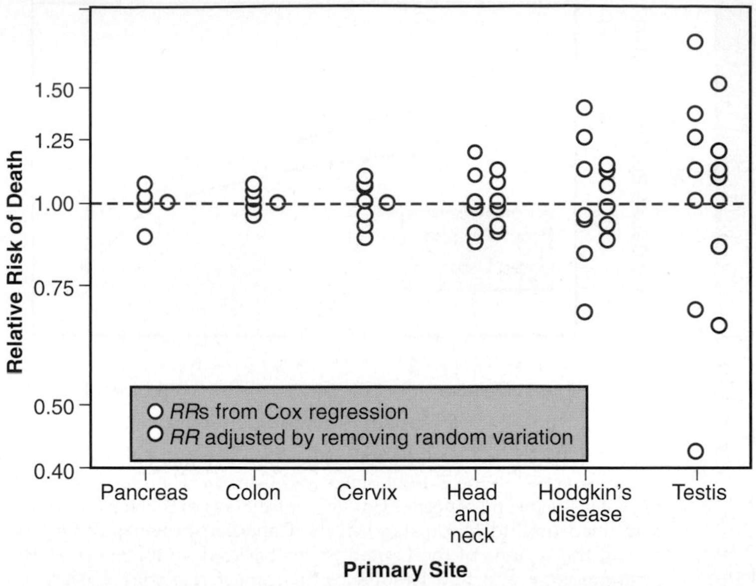

Figure 11-12 Interregional variations in cancer survival in Ontario. The scatter plot shows the relative risk of death from cancer in seven geographic regions of Ontario derived from a Cox regression that controlled for age, sex, and socioeconomic status. The *purple circles* represent the observed variations in survival. The *blue circles* represent the remaining variation after subtraction of the expected random component of variation. (Adapted from Zhang-Salomons J, Groome PA, Mackillop WJ: Estimating the best achievable cancer survival by eliminating regional variations in Ontario. Clin Invest Med 363(Suppl 22): , 1999.)

Table 11-4 Observed Versus Achievable Five-Year Survival for Selected Cancer Sites in Ontario*

Primary Site	Achievable 5-Year Survival Rate (95% Confidence Interval)	Observed 5-Year Survival Rate (95% Confidence Interval) All Ontario	Worst Region
Head and neck	64% (63-65)	60% (59-61)	54% (49-59)
Hodgkin's	88% (86-90)	86% (84-87)	81% (73-89)
Testis	97% (97-98)	95% (94-96)	92% (89-95)
Central nervous system	32% (31-34)	28% (27-29)	27% (24-30)
Rectum	52% (51-54)	50% (49-51)	48% (45-51)
Stomach	21% (20-22)	20% (19-21)	15% (12-17)
Lung	18% (18-19)	15% (15-16)	12% (11-13)
Ovary	49% (47-51)	46% (44-47)	40% (33-48)
Prostate	77% (76-77)	75% (74-75)	71% (69-72)
Bladder	74% (72-75)	73% (72-74)	68% (65-71)

*The best achievable survival was estimated from the highest observed survival in any of the seven regions in Ontario, by subtracting deviations from the provincial average that are expected, due to random variation. Cox regression was used to control for age, sex, and socioeconomic status. This model assumes that there are no systematic variations in case mix among the regions.

achievable survival for several diseases in which geographic variation in outcome exceeded that expected due to chance alone. Although such studies can demonstrate the potential to improve outcome by improving quality, they do not reveal where the defects in quality lie. Further studies are required to identify specific defects in the underlying processes and structures.

Relating Structure and Process to Outcomes

Whether you begin with variations in outcome and work back to try to find their causes or begin with variations in process and work forward to try to identify their consequences, there are significant problems that must be addressed before a causal relationship can be established. We discuss these problems and describe how they should be addressed in the context of outcomes research.

Limitations of "Outcomes Research" in Determining the Efficacy of Treatment

Studies that examine treatment and outcome in the context of routine care are often today referred as "outcomes research." This type of study should *not* generally be used to try to evaluate the efficacy of treatment. It is notoriously difficult to control for bias in retrospective reviews of institutional experience. Comparisons of outcomes achieved in contemporaneous groups of patients who have received different types of treatment at the same institution are inevitably confounded by "treatment selection bias."[182,183] Comparisons of outcomes between groups of patients who received different treatments more or less contemporaneously at different institutions are less subject to treatment selection bias but are vulnerable to "referral bias" due to interinstitutional differences in case mix.[182,183] The use of "historical controls" (i.e., the comparison of outcomes between patient groups who have received different treatment, at different points in time) is also fraught with hazard.[184] Case mix may change systematically over time; investigations may change, resulting in "stage migration"; and collateral aspects of care may also change.[184] It is possible to reduce the impact of these types of bias by controlling for known prognostic factors, but these usually leave much of the variance in outcome unaccounted for. For these reasons, none of these types of retrospective, observational study can substitute for prospective, experimental studies (i.e., randomized controlled trials) in the evaluation of efficacy of treatment.[12] The credibility of our discipline is weakened to the extent that we rely on these less valid methods in situations in which a randomized trial is possible.

Legitimate Roles of "Outcomes Research" in Evaluating Effectiveness

It is important to recognize that there are some aspects of medical practice that cannot be evaluated in randomized trials and must be explored using observational methods.

When a Randomized Trial Is Not Ethical. There are some important aspects of treatment that cannot and should not be studied in a randomized trial. It may be important, for example, to know how much outcomes are affected by deviation from standard practice, such as by delay in initiation of RT, protraction of overall treatment time, the use of lower-than standard doses, or reliance on antiquated equipment. However, one cannot ethically randomize patients to receive nonstandard versus standard treatment when the only real purpose of the exercise is to measure the adverse consequences of the nonstandard approach. We can therefore only learn about this type of issue by investigating the impact of inadvertent or unavoidable deviations from standard practice in retrospective, observational studies of the type discussed earlier.

Some important findings have emerged from this type of study. The PCS found, for example, that after adjusting for stage, recurrence rates were significantly higher in Hodgkin's disease and in cancers of the cervix and prostate in patients treated at facilities with only a cobalt machine compared with facilities with a linear accelerator or a betatron.[82] While it is impossible to attribute changes in the structure of RT programs to the results of any one particular publication or event, it is reasonable to assume that the results of these PCS studies improved the practice of RT in the United States by promoting the dissemination of high-energy treatment machines and discouraging the use of other equipment in this setting. Studies that have identified the adverse consequences of treatment interruptions and delays are in the same category. These issues could not, and should not, and did not have to be addressed in a randomized trial.

It is important to be very cautious in the interpretation of "negative findings" in studies that attempt to explore the consequences of deviations from standard practice. Studies that fail to show a statistically significant difference in outcome between nonstandard and standard treatments often lack the statistical power that would be necessary to rule out small but clinically important adverse effects. When patient safety is on the table, the absence of evidence of adverse effects should never be misconstrued as evidence of their absence.

When a Randomized Trial Is Not Feasible. There are also issues that should ideally be addressed in a randomized trial, but either cannot, or will not, be addressed in this way. Rare clinical problems are often impossible to study in randomized trials. It is impossible to sustain enthusiasm for any trial, or maintain the infrastructure necessary to support it, over a very protracted period of slow accrual. Large well-organized, multicenter clinical trial groups have a greater chance of success in this situation than any individual institution, but there are limits to what any group can do. Nearly all of what we know about the relationship between treatment and outcome in rare situations has to come from observational studies. In other situations, a clinical trial may be theoretically feasible but is rendered impossible by entrenched opposing views about treatment that effectively preclude recruitment to any trial. One such example was the controversy regarding the primary management of more advanced cancers of the larynx. The issue was hotly debated for decades and opinions were highly polarized. The depth of the controversy is clearly illustrated in the results of an international mail survey of patterns of care in laryngeal cancer done in the early 1990s.[152] This showed, for example, that most otolaryngologists in Canada, the United Kingdom, and Scandinavia regarded primary RT, reserving surgery for salvage, as the standard approach for T3 glottic cancer, while most of their counterparts in the United States and Australia favored primary laryngectomy.

Under these circumstances, it may be possible to learn about the relative effectiveness of the competing approaches by comparing the outcome they achieve at the population level. The rationale for this approach is that variations in practice driven by differences in physicians' beliefs, or any other factors unrelated to the characteristics of the patients, can be treated as a natural experiment. If outcomes are compared at the population level and not at the level of the individual patient, the problem of treatment selection bias is avoided. To validate such a comparison, it is necessary either to demonstrate that the case mix in each of the populations that are compared is similar or to control for any observed variations in case mix. This method is sometimes referred to as the *instrumental variable approach*.[185,186] Groome and colleagues have used it to compare the outcomes of treatment for locally advanced laryngeal cancer between Ontario, Canada and the United States. They found that primary laryngectomy was used much more frequently in the United States than in Ontario, consistent with the results of the previous mail survey.[153] Survival at 5 years proved to be identical in the two populations while laryngectomy-free survival was significantly higher in Ontario than in the United States. These observations lend support to the position that primary RT, reserving surgery for salvage, permits retention of natural voice without compromising survival.

STUDYING THE EFFICIENCY OF RADIOTHERAPY

Health economics is the area of specialization within the field of economics that concerns itself with all economic aspects of health and health care. Much of health economics deals with health-related issues on a higher plane than HSR. Macroeconomic analysis of the societal impact of health and health care at the national and international levels lies well beyond the scope of HSR as defined in What Is Health Services Research? On the other hand, microeconomic analysis of the costs and benefits of specific health care programs lies squarely within the domain of HSR. We briefly describe how health economic analysis fits into HSR, introduce the methods that are commonly used, and illustrate their relevance to radiation oncology.

The resources available for health care in any society are finite. What is achievable for cancer patients depends on the size of the total health care budget, on how much of that total budget is directed to cancer care, and on how efficiently the available resources are used in providing cancer care. Health economics aims to provide the information necessary to make rational choices about how to deploy funding for health care and how to make the best possible use of the funds available. Economic analyses are useful at many levels in the health system. High-level decisions about allocation of resources to different health care programs are increasingly based on a comparison of their impact on health in relation to their cost. These decisions are most clearly visible in publicly funded systems, but in the private sector, decisions made by insurers about which services will be reimbursed are based on similar considerations and have a similar effect. Information about the benefits of RT in relation to its costs is therefore required to ensure that an appropriate slice of the cancer budget is allocated to radiation oncology. Economic analyses are also needed to optimize the internal efficiency of RT programs. To ensure that we get the maximum value per dollar invested in RT, it is important that we should be aware of the relative costs of alternative approaches for providing RT.

Measurement Issues in Economic Analyses

Health economics involves much more than the measurement of health care costs, which most economists would regard as no more than accounting. However, economic analysis does require the measurement of costs, and a number of useful studies have been done in comparing alternative approaches for measuring the cost of RT[187-189] and in defining units of workload to which costs can be assigned.[190,191] In assessing the overall costs of RT, it is important to consider not only the direct costs of providing treatment but also the indirect costs of supportive care for complications of RT. It is important to specify the perspective from which an economic analysis is carried out. If the analysis is being conducted from the perspective of the RT provider, it may be appropriate to focus primarily on direct costs, whereas if the perspective is that of the health system as a whole, indirect costs incurred in other sectors must also be considered. If the analysis is being conducted from the societal perspective, loss of productivity as a consequence of the treatment needs to be included and balanced against loss of productivity due to the untreated disease.

Economic analyses typically consider the benefits of health care as well its costs. Four different types of study are usually distinguished: cost minimization studies, cost-benefit studies, cost-effectiveness studies, and cost-utility studies. We briefly outline what is involved in each of these, but for a more complete review of methods for the economic evaluation of health care programs, readers are referred to the useful introductory textbook by Drummond and colleagues.[7]

Cost Minimization Studies

Cost minimization studies, often simply called cost studies, compare the costs of alternative treatments or processes, on the explicit or implicit assumption that each produces similar health outcomes. In RT, this type of study has provided information pertinent to decisions about the acquisition of new equipment,[192,193] about the decision to purchase or lease equipment,[194] about service contracts,[195] and so on. In some instances, simple cost comparisons have been done between slightly different approaches to treatment, such as high-dose rate versus low-dose rate brachytherapy.[196] The assumption that the two approaches are medically equivalent is not entirely valid because they do differ from the patient's perspective, at least in terms of convenience. Nonetheless, their health outcomes are sufficiently similar that their relative cost may be the critical factor in deciding which to adopt. Comparisons of the cost of RT and the cost of alternatives to RT that are associated with a different profile of toxicities, however, do not provide a valid basis for decision-making without concurrent consideration of differences in those health outcomes.[192-199]

Cost-Benefit Analysis

In cost-benefit analysis, the health benefits of treatment are described only in terms of their dollar value; health outcomes are considered only insofar as they have an impact on costs or affect the productivity of those affected. This type of analysis may be useful in some circumstances in demonstrating to policy makers that apparently expensive programs of treatment or prevention may in fact be cost neutral or even save money when the overall financial consequences of providing the program are compared to those of not providing it. However, the idea that the benefits of health care can be adequately described in terms of the money they save is counterintuitive to most clinicians, and this type of analysis has not been widely used in the field of radiation oncology.

Cost-Effectiveness Studies

Cost-effectiveness studies compare alternative treatments or processes with respect to their effectiveness, as well as their cost. Effectiveness is usually described in terms of a single objective outcome measure, such as survival. This is useful in that it enables us to put a dollar value on the outcomes achieved by RT, and it has revealed that RT is relatively inexpensive in relation to the benefits it delivers.[200-203]

Cost-Utility Analysis

Because cost-effectiveness analysis describes the benefits of treatment in terms of a single measure of outcome, it does not provide a satisfactory way of describing and comparing the value of treatments that are associated with different types of health benefit, such as radical RT for cervical cancer and palliative RT for bone metastases. Survival alone is an inadequate measure of palliative RT, and quality of life is an inadequate measure of the effectiveness of curative treatment. The concept of utility, a measure of the relative value of different life states, is useful in reducing the benefits of treatment to a common currency.[7] If utility can be measured, and there is still some question as to whether this is really possible, years of survival can be adjusted for relative value and outcomes expressed as quality-adjusted years of life (QALYs). This measure is sensitive to both duration of survival and quality of life. Cost per QALY can be used to compare the value of treatment in curative and palliative contexts. The value of other forms of medical care has been measured in cost per QALY, and this permits comparison of the value of RT with the value of other treatments both in oncology and in other spheres of medicine.[204-209]

Explicit Rationing

Information about the relative benefits of RT in different clinical contexts could be used as a basis for assigning priorities to one type of case over another in circumstances in which resources are insufficient to provide RT for everyone who needs it. This type of explicit rationing has not, to our knowledge, been used to control access to RT in any of the countries where access to RT is constrained by inadequate supply. Although this approach would serve to mitigate the adverse effects of inadequate access to RT and maximize the societal benefits of the available resources, it seems to have little appeal to policy makers. It has, however, been proposed that cost-effectiveness or cost-utility analysis be used as the basis for selecting the most effective components of care for inclusion in a health benefits package for the uninsured in the United States.[202] In the future, as both the demand for health services and the cost of care continue to increase across the developed world, we anticipate that decisions about which services will be provided within publicly funded systems or managed care programs will increasingly be based on these types of economic analysis. Research in the economics of radiation oncology is likely to be of increasing practical importance in optimizing the effectiveness of RT programs in the future.

SUMMARY

In the past, radiation oncologists and their traditional partners in physics and radiobiology have devoted most research efforts to creating the knowledge necessary to optimize the outcomes of RT in the individual patient. There is a lot of evidence to suggest that we currently fall far short of making the benefits of that research available to all the patients who might benefit from it. It has been demonstrated that in many parts of the world, access to RT is both inadequate and inequitable and that the quality of RT is variable and often suboptimal. These deviations from optimal practice cause us to fall far short of achieving what is theoretically achievable for cancer patients today within the limits of existing scientific knowledge and technology. Deviations from optimal practice represent real opportunities for enhancing the results of RT, without placing reliance on the uncertain outcome of the slow process of basic research, which frequently promises much but delivers little. While fundamental and clinical research must continue, a greater proportion of our efforts should be devoted to enhancing our understanding of the factors that influence access to RT and determine the effectiveness and efficiency of RT programs. RT provides major health benefits for a large proportion of cancer patients, and even a small incremental gain in health system performance would be expected to translate itself into large societal benefits.

HSR in radiation oncology is still a relatively new field, and it offers new investigators a great opportunity to make a real difference. There are a number of good opportunities for training in health services and policy research, and the funding for HSR has greatly increased in recent years. There is real need for radiation oncologists to become involved in leadership roles in HSR because the clinician's insights are vital in choosing the right research questions. Getting the right answers, however, may require a high level of methodologic expertise in areas that are unfamiliar to most radiation oncologists. Success in HSR often depends on building effective collaborations with scientists in other fields such as epidemiology, health economics, and the social sciences. Those who enter the field should also be aware that getting the most out of HSR requires a degree of diplomacy and academic ability. Clinicians involved in HSR need to remember that in the pursuit of the goal of evidence-based management of health care programs, they need to influence health system managers as well as their peers. Investigators need to learn the skill of working collaboratively with the health system managers and policy makers who hold the power to implement some of the changes necessary to optimize outcomes, while keeping some control of the research agenda.

REFERENCES

1. Crombie IK Davies HTO: Research in Health Care: Design, Conduct, and Interpretation of Health Services Research. Department of Epidemiology and Public Health, Ninewells Hospital and Medical School, University of Dundee, UK, 1996.
2. Aday LA, Begley C, Larson DR, Slater CH: Evaluating the Health Care System: Effectiveness, Efficiency, and Equity. Chicago, Health Administration Press, 1998.
3. Shi L: Health Services Research Methods. Albany, NY, Delmar Publishers, 1997.
4. Veney JE, Kaluyzny AD: Evaluation and Decision Making for Health Services, Chicago, Health Administration Press, 1998.
5. Wan TTH: Analysis and Evaluation of Health Care Systems: An Integrated Approach to Managerial Decision Making. Baltimore, MD, Health Professions, 1997.
6. Peckham M, Smith R (eds): The Scientific Basis of Health Services. London, BMJ Publishers, 1996.
7. Drummond ME, O'Brien B, Stoddart GL, et al: Methods for the Economic Evaluation of Health Care Programmes, 2nd ed. Oxford, Oxford University Press, 1997.
8. Percy C, VanHoltan V, Muir C (eds): International Classification of Diseases for Oncology, 2nd ed. Geneva, World Health Organization, 1990.
9. Sobin LH, Wittekind CH (eds): UICC TNM Classification of Malignant Tumors, 6th ed. New York, John Wiley, 2002.
10. International Commission on Radiation Units and Measurements: Prescribing, Recording and Reporting Photon Beam Therapy: Report No. 50. Bethesda, MD, International Commission on Radiation Units and Measurements, 1993.
11. Gospodarowicz MK, Henson DE, Hutter RVP, et al (eds): Prognostic Factors in Cancer, 2nd ed. New York, Wiley-Liss, A. John Wiley & Sons, 2001.
12. Sackett DL: Rules of evidence and clinical recommendations on the use of antithrombotic agents. Chest 95(Suppl 2):2-4, 1989.
13. Salkever DS: Economic class and differential access to care; comparisons among health systems. Int J Health Serv 5:373, 1975.
14. Cuyler AJ: Need and the National Health Service: Economics and Social Choice. Lanham, MD, Rowman and Littlefield, 1976.
15. Penchansky R, Thomas JW: The concept of access: definition and relationship to consumer satisfaction. Med Care 19:127-140, 1981.
16. Mackillop WJ, Fu H, Quirt CF, et al: Waiting for radiotherapy in Ontario. Int J Radiat Oncol Biol Phys 30:221-228, 1994.
17. Cormack DV, Fisher PM, Till JE: A study of waiting times and waiting lists for radiation therapy patients. Can J Oncol 6:427-434, 1996.
18. Munro AJ, Porter S: Waiting times for radiotherapy treatment: Not all that mysterious and certainly preventable. Clin Oncol 6:314-318, 1994.
19. Junor EJ, Macbeth FR, Barrett A: An audit of travel and waiting times for outpatient radiotherapy. Clin Oncol 4:174-276, 1992.
20. Martin J, Ryan G, Duchesne G: Clinical prioritization for curative radiotherapy: a local waiting list initiative. Clin Oncol 16:299-306, 2004.
21. Denham JW, Hamilton CS, Joseph DJ: How should a waiting list for treatment be managed? Austral Radiol 36:274-275, 1992.
22. Mackillop WJ, Zhou Y, Quirt CF: A comparison of delays in the treatment of cancer with radiation in Canada and the United States. Int J Radiat Oncol Biol Phys 32:531-539, 1995.
23. Mackillop WJ, Groome PA, Zhou Y, et al: Does a centralized radiotherapy system provide adequate access to care? J Clin Oncol 15:1261-1271, 1997.
24. Mackillop WJ, Zhou S, Groome PA, et al: Changes in the use of radiotherapy in Ontario: 1984-1995. Int J Radiat Oncol Biol Phys 44:355-362, 1999.
25. Zhang-Salomons J, Huang J, Mackillop WJ: Health system effects on the use of post-lumpectomy radiotherapy. Int J Radiat Oncol Biol Phys 50:1385, 2001.
26. Mechanic D: Dilemmas in rationing health care services: The case for implicit rationing. BMJ 310:1655-1659, 1995.
27. Thomas SJ, Williams MV, Burnet NG, et al: How much surplus capacity is required to maintain low waiting times? Clin Oncol 13:24-28, 2001.
28. Mackillop WJ, Bates JHT, O'Sullivan B, et al: The effect of delay in treatment on local control by radiotherapy. Int J Radiat Oncol Biol Phys 34:243-250, 1996.
29. Waaijer A, Terhaard CH, Dehnad H, et al: Waiting times for radiotherapy: consequences of volume increase for the TCP in oropharyngeal carcinoma. Radiother Oncol 66:271-276, 2003.
30. Huang J, Barbera L, Brouwers M, et al: Does delay in starting treatment affect the outcomes of radiotherapy? A systematic review. J Clin Oncol 21:555-563, 2003.
31. Benck V, Joseph L, Fortin P, et al: Effect of delay in initiating radiotherapy for patients with early stage breast cancer. Clin Oncol 16:6-11, 2004.
32. Franklin CI, Poulsen M. How do waiting times affect radiation dose fractionation schedules? Austral Radiol 44:428-432, 2000.
33. Dixon PF, Mackillop WJ. Could changes in clinical practice reduce waiting lists for radiotherapy? J Health Serv Res Policy 6:70-77, 2001.

34. Pengelley H: Breast cancer patients sue over radiotherapy wait times. CMAJ 170:1655, 2004.
35. Mackillop WJ: The radiotherapy system in Canada. In: Health Care Reform: Hearings Before the Subcommittee on Health of the Committee on Ways and Means. House of Representatives 103 Congress. Second Session, Volume 8, pp 287–298. Washington, DC, US Government Printing Office, 1994.
36. Ashbury F, Angus H, Mackillop WJ: Cancer Quality Council of Ontario Roundtable on Waiting Times Measurement: Final Report: Available at htttp://www.cancercare.on.ca/pdf/CQCOWaitTimesRoundtableReport2004.pdf. Accessed November 2005
37. de Jong B, Crommelian M, Heijden LH, et al: Patterns of radiotherapy for cancer patients in the south eastern Netherlands, 1975-1989. Radiother Oncol 31:213-221, 1994.
38. Huang J, Zhou S, Groome P, et al: Factors affecting the use of palliative radiotherapy in Ontario. J Clin Oncol 19:137-144, 2001.
39. Huang J, Boyd C, Tyldesley S, et al: Time spent in hospital in the last six months of life in patients who died of cancer in Ontario. J Clin Oncol 20:1584-1592, 2002.
40. Intersociety Council for Radiation Oncology: Radiation Oncology in Integrated Cancer Management. Report to the Director of NCI. Washington, DC, NCI, 1991.
41. Denham JW: How do we bring an acceptable level of radiotherapy services to a dispersed population? Austral Radiol 39:171-173, 1995.
42. Lote K, Moller T, Nordman E, et al: Resources and productivity in radiation oncology in Denmark, Finland, Iceland, Norway and Sweden during 1987. Acta Oncol 30:555-561, 1990.
43. Moller TR, Torgil R, Brorsson B, et al, for the SBU Survey Group: A prospective survey of radiotherapy practice 2001 in Sweden. Acta Oncol 42:387-410, 2003.
44. Lindholm C, Cavalin-Stahl E, Ceberg J, et al, for the SBU Survey Group: Radiotherapy practices in Sweden compared to the scientific evidence. Acta Oncol 42:416-429, 2003.
45. Skolnick AA: New study suggests radiation often underused for palliation. JAMA 279:343-344, 1998.
46. Tyldesley S, Zhang-Salomons J, Groome P, et al: Association between age and the utilization of radiotherapy in Ontario. Int J Radiat Oncol Biol Phys 47:469-480, 2000.
47. Duncan W, Jenkin D: The Radiation Oncology Commission. A Report to the Ontario Treatment and Research Foundation and the Ontario Cancer Institute. Toronto, OCTRF, 1990.
48. Cleton FJ, Coebergh JWW, eds, for Steering Committee on Future Health Scenarios: Cancer in the Netherlands. Dordrecht, the Netherlands, Kluwer Academic, 1991.
49. Tyldesley S, Boyd C, Schulze K, et al: Estimating the need for radiotherapy for lung cancer: an evidence-based, epidemiological approach. Int J Radiat Oncol Biol Phys 49:973-985, 2001.
50. Foroudi F, Tyldesley S, Barbera L, et al: Evidence-based estimate of appropriate radiotherapy utilization rate for prostate cancer. Int J Radiat Oncol Biol Phys 55:51-63, 2003.
51. Tyldesley S, Foroudi F, Barbera L, et al: The appropriate rate of breast conserving surgery: an evidence-based estimate. Clin Oncol 15:144-155, 2003
52. Foroudi F, Tyldesley S, Barbera L, et al: An evidence-based estimate of the appropriate radiotherapy utilization rate for colorectal cancer. Int J Radiat Oncol Biol Phys 56:1295-1307, 2003.
53. Featherstone C, Delaney G, Jacob S, et al: Estimating the optimal utilization rates of radiotherapy for hematologic malignancies from a review of the evidence: part I. Lymphoma. Cancer 103:383-392, 2005.
54. Bentzen SM, Heeren G, Cottier B, et al: Towards evidence-based estimates of radiotherapy infrastructure and staffing needs in Europe. Radiother Oncol 73(Suppl 1):146, 2004.
55. Bogan CE, English MJ: Benchmarking for best practices: winning through innovative adaptation. New York, McGraw-Hill, 1994.
56. Barbera L, Zhang-Salomons J, Huang J, et al: Defining the need for radiotherapy for lung cancer in the general population: a criterion-based, benchmarking approach. Med Care 41:1074-1085, 2003.
57. Donabedian A: Evaluating the quality of medical care. Milbank Memorial Fund Q 44:166-206, 1966.
58. Donabedian A: Explorations in quality of care and monitoring: volume 1. The definition of quality and approaches to its assessment. Ann Arbor, MI, Health Administration Press, 1980.
59. Donabedian A: Advantages and limitations of explicit criteria for measuring the quality of health care. Milbank Memorial Fund Q 59:99-106, 1981.
60. Donabedian A: The evaluation of medical care programs. Bull N Y Acad Med 44:117-124, 1968.
61. Lohr KN, Yordy KD, Their SO: Current issues in quality of care. Health Affairs 7:5-18, 1988.
62. Kramer S, Herring D: The patterns of care study: a nation-wide evaluation of the practice of radiation therapy in cancer management. Int J Radiat Oncol Biol Phys 1:1231-1236, 1976.
63. Kramer S: The study of patterns of care in radiation therapy. Cancer 39:780-787, 1997.
64. Coia LR, Hanks GE: Quality assessment in the USA: how the patterns of care study has made a difference. Semin Radiat Oncol 7:146-156, 1997.
65. Owen JB, Coia LR, Hanks GE: The structure of radiation oncology in the United States in 1994. Int J Radiat Oncol Biol Phys 39:179-185, 1997.
66. MacLean CJ, Davis LW, Herring DF, et al: Variation in work-up and treatment procedures among types of radiation therapy facilities: the patterns of care process survey for three head and neck sites. Cancer 48:1346-1352, 1981.
67. Hanks G, Diamond J, Kramer S: The need for complex technology in radiation therapy: correlation of facility characteristics and structure with outcome. Cancer 55:2198-2201, 1985.
68. Moller TR, Einhorn N, Lindholm C, et al, for the SBU Survey Group: Radiotherapy and cancer care in Sweden. Acta Oncol 42:366-375, 2003.
69. Esco R, Palacios A, Pardo J, et al: Infrastructure of radiotherapy in Spain: a minimal standard of radiotherapy resources. Int J Radiat Oncol Biol Phys 56:319-327, 2003.
70. Slotman BJ, Leer JW: Infrastructure of radiotherapy in the Netherlands: evaluation of prognoses and introduction of a new model for determining needs. Radiother Oncol 66:345-349, 2003.
71. Peiffert D, Simon JM, Baillet F: Brachytherapy in France in 1995: final results of the national survey. Cancer Radiother 2:304-309, 1998.
72. Van den Bogaert W: QUARTS: an ESTRO project. Radiother Oncol 73(Suppl 1):145, 2004.
73. Slotman B, Cottier B, Bentzen SM, et al: Guidelines for infrastructure and staffing of radiotherapy ESTRO: QUARTS: Work package 1. Radiother Oncol 73(Suppl 1):322, 2004.
74. The QUARTS Project: A stepping-stone towards a health services research infrastructure for radiotherapy. Radiother Oncol 73(Suppl 1):323, 2004.
75. Lievens Y, Van den Bogaert W, Rijnders A, et al: Palliative radiotherapy practice within western European countries: impact of the radiotherapy financing system. Radiother Oncol 56:289-295, 2000.
76. Battista RN: Towards a paradigm for technology assessment. *In* Peckham M, Smith R (eds): The Scientific Basis of Health Services. London, BMJ Publishers, 1996, pp 11-18.
77. Lagrange H, Lipinski F: The place of conformal radiotherapy in routine practice: national survey of SERO members. Cancer Radiother 5(Suppl 1):44-48, 2001.
78. Glatstein E: The return of the snake oil salesmen. Int J Radiat Oncol Biol Phys 55:561-562, 2003.
79. Mackillop WJ, O'Brien P, Brundage M, et al: Radiotherapy quality and access issues. *In* Sullivan T, Evans W, Angus H, Hudson A: Strengthening the Quality of Cancer Services in Ontario. Ottawa, Ontario, CHA Press, 2003, pp 95-124.
80. Horiot JC, Johansson KA, Gonzalez DG, et al: Quality assurance control in the EORTC Cooperative Group of Radiotherapy. 1. Assessment of radiotherapy staff and equipment. European Organization for Research and Treatment of Cancer. Radiother Oncol 6:275-284, 1986.
81. Horiot JC, van der Schueren E, Johansson KA, et al: The program of quality assurance of the EORTC radiotherapy group: a historical overview. Radiother Oncol 29:81-84, 1993.

82. Brundage MD, Dixon PF, Mackillop WJ, et al: A real-time audit of radiation therapy in a regional cancer center. Radiat Oncol Biol Phys 43:115-124, 1999.
83. Dixon P, O'Sullivan B: Radiotherapy quality assurance: time for everyone to take it seriously. Eur J Cancer 39:423-429, 2003.
84. Owen JB, Sedransk J, Pajak TF: National averages for process and outcome in radiation oncology: methodology of the PCS. Semin Radiat Oncol 7:101-107, 1997.
85. Hanks G, Diamond J, Kramer S: Consensus of best current management; the starting point for clinical quality assessment. Int J Radiat Oncol Biol Phys 10:87-97, 1984.
86. PCS Consensus Committee: 1996 Decision trees and management guidelines. Semin Radiat Oncol 7:163-181, 1997.
87. Shank B, Moughan J, Owen J, et al: The 1993-94 patterns of care process survey for breast irradiation after breast-conserving surgery: Comparison with the 1992 standard for breast conservation treatment. The Patterns of Care Study. American College of Radiology. Int J Radiat Oncol Biol Phys 48:1291-1299, 2000.
88. Fredriksson J, Liljegren G, Arnesson LG, et al: Time trends in the results of breast conservation in 4,694 women. Eur J Cancer 37:1537-1544, 2001.
89. White V, Pruden M, Giles G, et al: The management of early breast carcinoma before and after the introduction of clinical practice guidelines. Cancer 101:476-485, 2004.
90. Young WW, Marks SM, Kohler SA, et al: Dissemination of clinical results: mastectomy versus lumpectomy and radiation therapy. Med Care 34:1003-1017, 1996.
91. Athas WF, Adams-Cameron M, Hunt WC, et al: Travel distance to radiation therapy and receipt of radiotherapy following breast-conserving surgery. J Natl Cancer Inst 92:269-271, 2000.
92. Bickell NA, McEvoy MD: Physicians' reasons for failing to deliver effective breast cancer care: A framework for underuse. Med Care 41:442-446, 2003.
93. Goy JC, Dobbs HJ: Variation in postoperative radiotherapy delivery for patients with screen-detected breast cancer in the south Thames (east) region. Clin Oncol 10:30-34, 1998.
94. Goy JC, Dobbs HJ, Henderson S, et al: Variations in referral patterns for postoperative radiotherapy of patients with screen-detected breast cancer in the south Thames (east region). Clin Oncol 10:24-29, 1998.
95. Athas WF, Adams-Cameron M, Hunt WC, et al: Travel distance to radiation therapy and receipt of radiotherapy following breast-conserving surgery. J Natl Cancer Inst 92:269-271, 2000.
96. Moritz S, Bates T, Henderson SM, et al: Variation in management of small invasive breast cancers detected on screening in the former southeast Thames region: observational study. BMJ 315:1266-1272, 1997.
97. Richardson LC, Schulman J, Sever LE, et al: Early-stage breast cancer treatment among medically underserved women diagnosed in a national screening program, 1992-1995. Breast Cancer Res Treat 69:133-142, 2001.
98. Prehn AW, Topol B, Stewart S, et al: Differences in treatment patterns for localized breast carcinoma among Asian/Pacific Islander women. Cancer 95:2268-2275, 2002.
99. Gilligan MA, Kneusel RT, Hoffman RG, et al: Persistent differences in sociodemographic determinants of breast conserving treatment despite overall increased adoption. Med Care 40:181-189, 2002.
100. Morrow M, White J, Moughan J, et al: Factors predicting the use of breast-conserving therapy in stage I and II breast carcinoma. J Clin Oncol 19:2254-2262, 2001.
101. Veness MJ, Delaney G: Variations in breast tangent radiotherapy: A survey of practice in New South Wales and the Australian Capital Territory. Austral Radiol 43:334-338, 1999.
102. Delaney G, Blakey D, Drummond R, et al: Breast radiotherapy: An Australasian survey of current treatment techniques. Austral Radiol 45:170-178, 2001.
103. Winfield EA, Deighton A, Venables K, et al, START Trial Working Party: Survey of tangential field planning and dose distribution in the UK: background to the introduction of the quality assurance program for the START trial in early breast cancer. B J Radiol, 76:254-259, 2003.
104. Price P, Yarnold JR: Non-surgical management of early breast cancer in the United Kingdom: the role and practice of radiotherapy. Clinical Audit Subcommittee of the Faculty of Clinical Oncology, Royal College of Radiologists, and the Joint Council for Clinical Oncology. Clin Oncol 7:219-222, 1995.
105. Yarnold JR, Price P, Steel GG: Non-surgical management of early breast cancer in the United Kingdom: Radiotherapy fractionation practices. Clinical Audit Subcommittee of the Faculty of Clinical Oncology, Royal College of Radiologists, and the Joint Council for Clinical Oncology. Clin Oncol 7:223-226, 1995.
106. Paszat LP, Groome PA, Schulze K, et al: A population-based study of the effectiveness of breast conservation for newly diagnosed breast cancer. Int J Radiat Oncol Biol Phys 46:345-353, 2000.
107. White J, Moughan J, Pierce LJ, et al: Status of postmastectomy radiotherapy in the United States: A Patterns of Care Study. Int J Radiat Oncol Biol Phys 60:77-85, 2004.
108. Fowler FJ Jr, McNaughton CM, Albertsen PC, et al: Comparison of recommendations by urologists and radiation oncologists for treatment of clinically localized prostate cancer. JAMA 283:3217-3222, 2000.
109. Hanna CL, Mason MD, Donovan H, et al: Clinical oncologists favor radical radiotherapy for localized prostate cancer: a questionnaire survey. BJI Int 90:558-560, 2002.
110. Klabunde CN, Potosky AL, Harlan LC, et al: Trends and black/white differences in treatment for nonmetastatic prostate cancer. Med Care 36:1337-1348, 1998.
111. Meltzer D, Egleston B, Abdalla I: Patterns of prostate cancer treatment by clinical state and age. Am J Public Health 91:126-128, 2001.
112. Feldman-Stewart D, Brundage MD, et al: What questions do patients with curable prostate cancer want answered? Med Decis Making 20:7-19, 2000.
113. Feldman-Stewart D, Brundage MD, Nickel JC, et al: The information required by patients with early-stage prostate cancer in choosing their treatment. BJU Int 87:218-223, 2001.
114. Prestidge BR, Prete JJ, Buchholz TA, et al: A survey of current clinical practice of permanent prostate brachytherapy in the United States. Int J Radiat Oncol Biol Phys 40:461-465, 1998.
115. Prete JJ, Prestidge BR, Bice WS, et al: A survey of physics and dosimetry: Practice of permanent prostate brachytherapy in the United States. Int J Radiat Oncol Biol Phys 40:1001-1015, 1998.
116. Nakamura K, Teshima T, Takahashi Y, et al, Japanese PCS Working Subgroup of Prostate Cancer: Radical radiation therapy for prostate cancer in Japan: a patterns of care study report. Jpn J Clin Oncol 33:122-126, 2003.
117. Nakamura K, Ogawa K, Yamamoto T, et al, Japanese PCS Working Subgroup of Prostate Cancer: Trends in the practice of radiotherapy for localized prostate cancer in Japan: a preliminary patterns of care study report. Jpn J Clin Oncol 33:527-532, 2003.
118. Rodrigues G, D'Souza D, Crook J, et al: Contemporary management of prostate cancer: a practice survey of Ontario genitourinary radiation oncologists. Radiother Oncol 69:63-72, 2003.
119. Chuba PJ, Moughan J, Forman JD, et al: The 1989 Patterns of Care Study for prostate cancer: five-year outcomes. Int J Radiat Oncol Biol Phys 50:325-333, 2001.
120. Lee WR, Moughan J, Owen JB, et al: The 1999 Patterns of Care Study of RT in localized prostate cancer. Cancer 98:1987-1994, 2003.
121. Hayter CRR, Paszat LF, Groome PA, et al: A population-based study of the use and outcome of radical radiotherapy for invasive bladder cancer. Int J Radiat Oncol Biol Phys 45:1239-1245, 1999.
122. Moore MJ, O'Sullivan B, Tannock IF: How expert physicians would wish to be treated if they had genitourinary cancer. J Clin Oncol 6:1736-1745, 1988.
123. Choo R, Sandler H, Warde P, et al: Survey of radiation oncologists: practice patterns of the management of stage I seminoma of the testis in Canada, and a selected group in the United States. Can J Urol 9:1479-1485, 2002.
124. Eifel PJ, Moughan J, Owen J, et al: Patterns of radiotherapy practice for patients with squamous carcinoma of the uterine cervix. Int J Radiat Oncol Biol Phys 43:351-358, 1999.
125. Teshima T, Abe M, Ikeda H, et al: Patterns of Care Study of radiation therapy for cervix cancer in Japan: the influence of the strat-

ification of institution on the process. Jpn J Clin Oncol 28:388-395, 1998.
126. Jones B, Tan LT, Blake PR, et al: Results of a questionnaire regarding the practice of radiotherapy for carcinoma of the cervix in the UK. Br J Radiol 67:1226-1230, 1994.
127. Lancaster L: Preventing vaginal stenosis after brachytherapy for gynaecological cancer: an overview of Australian practices. Eur J Oncol Nursing 8:30-39, 2004.
128. Potter R, Van Limbergen E, Gerstner N, et al: Survey of the use of the ICRU 38 in recording and reporting cervical cancer brachytherapy. Radiother Oncol 58:11-18, 2001.
129. Russell AH, Shingleton HM, Jones WB, et al: Trends in the use of radiation and chemotherapy in the initial management of patients with carcinoma of the uterine cervix. Int J Radiat Oncol Biol Phys 40:605-613, 1998.
130. Naumann RW, Higgins RV, Hall JB: The use of adjuvant radiation therapy by members of the Society of Gynecologic Oncologists. Gynecologic Oncology 75:5-9, 1999.
131. Usmani N, Foroudi F, Du J, et al: An evidence-based estimate of the appropriate radiotherapy utilization rate for cervical cancer. Int J Radiat Oncol Biol Phys 63:812-827, 2005.
132. Maggino T, Romagnolo C, Zola P, et al: An analysis of approaches to the treatment of endometrial cancer in western Europe: a CTF study. Eur J Cancer 31:1993-1997, 1995.
133. Choy H, Shyr Y, Cmelak AJ, et al: Patterns of practice survey for non-small cell lung carcinoma in the U.S. Cancer 88:1336-1346, 2000.
134. Palmer MJ, O'Sullivan B, Steele R, et al: Controversies in the management of non-small-cell lung cancer: the results of an expert surrogate study. Radiother Oncol 19:17-28, 1990.
135. Raby B, Pater J, Mackillop WJ: Does knowledge guide practice? Another look at the management of non-small cell-lung cancer. J Clin Oncol 13:1904-1911, 1995.
136. Mackillop WJ, Dixon P, Zhou Y, et al: Variations in the management and outcome of non-small cell lung cancer in Ontario. Radiother Oncol 32:106-115, 1994.
137. Quirt CF, Mackillop WJ, Ginsburg AD, et al: Do doctors know when their patients don't? A survey of doctor-patient communication in lung cancer. Lung Cancer 18:1-20, 1997.
138. Brundage MD, Davidson JR, Mackillop WJ, et al: Using a treatment trade-off method to elicit preferences for the treatment of locally advanced non-small cell lung cancer. Med Decis Making 18:256-267, 1998.
139. Tai P, Yu E, Battista J, et al: Radiation treatment of lung cancer: patterns of practice in Canada. Radiother Oncol 7:167-174, 2004.
140. Cmelak AJ, Choy H, Shyr Y, et al: National survey on prophylactic cranial irradiation: differences in practice patterns between medical and radiation oncologists. Int J Radiat Oncol Biol Phys 44:157-162, 1999.
141. Coia LR, Minsky BD, John MJ, et al: The evaluation and treatment of patients receiving radiation therapy for carcinoma of the esophagus: results of the 1992-1994 Patterns of Care Survey. J Clin Oncol 18:1475-1480, 2000.
142. Suntharalingam M, Moughan J, Coia LR, et al: The national practice for patients receiving radiation therapy for carcinoma of the esophagus: results of the 1996-1999 Patterns of Care Study. Int J Radiat Oncol Biol Phys 36:981-987, 2003.
143. Tai P, Van Dyk J, Yu E, et al: Variability of target volume delineation in cervical esophageal cancer. Int J Radiat Oncol Biol Phys 42:227-288, 1998.
144. Dominitz JA, Maynard C, Billingsley KG, et al: Race, treatment, and survival of veterans with cancer of the distal esophagus and gastric cardia. Med Care 40(Suppl 1):1114-1126, 2002.
145. Schrag D, Gelfand SE, Bach PB, et al: Who gets adjuvant treatment for stage II and III rectal cancer? Insight from Surveillance, Epidemiology, and End Results—Medicare. J Clin Oncol 19:3712-3718, 2001.
146. Farmer KC, Penfold C, Millar H, et al, Gastrointestinal Committee of the Victorian Cooperative Oncology Group, Cancer Council of Victoria: Rectal cancer in Victoria in 1994: patterns of reported management. ANZ J Surg 72:265-270, 2002.
147. Paszat LF, Brundage MD, Groome PA, et al: A population-based study of rectal cancer: permanent colostomy as an outcome. Int J Radiat Oncol Biol Phys 45:1185-1191, 1999.
148. Earle CC, Grunfeld E, Coyle D, et al: Cancer physicians' attitudes toward colorectal cancer follow-up. Ann Oncol 14:400-405, 2003.
149. James ND, Robertson G, Squire CJ, et al, RCR Clinical Oncology Audit Subcommittee: A national audit of radiotherapy in head and neck cancer. Clin Oncol 15:41-46, 2003.
150. Skarsgard D, Groome P, Mackillop WJ, et al: Cancers of the upper aerodigestive tract in Ontario, Canada, and the United States. Cancer 88:1728-1738, 2000.
151. Hall SF, Boysen M, Groome PA, et al: Squamous cell carcinoma of the head and neck in Ontario, Canada and in South Eastern Norway. Head Neck 113:695-701, 2003.
152. O'Sullivan B, Mackillop WJ, Gilbert R, et al: Controversies in the management of laryngeal cancer: results of an international survey of patterns of care. Radiother Oncol 31:23-32, 1994.
153. Groome PA, O'Sullivan B, Irish JC, et al: Glottic cancer in Ontario, Canada and the SEER areas of the United States: do different management philosophies produce different outcome profiles? J Clin Epidemiol 54:301-315, 2001.
154. Groome PA, O'Sullivan B, Irish JC, et al: Management and outcome differences in supraglottic cancer between Ontario, Canada, and the Surveillance, Epidemiology, and End Results in areas of the United States. J Clin Oncol 21:496-505, 2003.
155. Jackson LD, Groome PA, Schulze K, et al: Radiotherapy patterns of practice: T1N0 glottic cancer in Ontario, Canada. Clin Oncol 15:266-279, 2003.
156. Holzer S, Reiners C, Mann K, et al: Patterns of care for patients with primary differentiated carcinoma of the thyroid gland treated in Germany during 1996. US and German Thyroid Cancer Group. Cancer 89:192-201, 2000.
157. Smitt MC, Stouffer N, Owen JB, et al: Results of the 1988-1989 Patterns of Care Study process survey for Hodgkin's disease. Int J Radiat Oncol Biol Phys 43:335-339, 1999.
158. Ng AK, Li S, Neuberg D, et al: Factors influencing treatment recommendations in early-stage Hodgkin's disease: a survey of physicians. Ann Oncol 15:261-269, 2004.
159. Hodgson DC, Zhang-Salomons J, Rothwell D, et al: The evolution of treatment for Hodgkin's disease: a population-based study of radiotherapy use and outcome. Clin Oncol 15:255-263, 2003.
160. Roos DE: Continuing reluctance to use single fractions of radiotherapy for metastatic bone pain: an Australian and New Zealand practice survey and literature review. Radiother Oncol 56:315-322, 2000.
161. Lutz S, Spence C, Chow E, et al: Survey on use of palliative radiotherapy in hospice care. J Clin Oncol 22:3581-3586, 2004.
162. Chow E, Danjoux C, Wong R, et al: Palliation of bone metastases: a survey of patterns of practice among Canadian radiation oncologists. Radiother Oncol 56:305-314, 2000.
163. Lievens Y, Kesteloot K, Rijnders A, et al: Differences in palliative radiotherapy for bone metastases within western European countries. Radiother Oncol 56:297-303, 2000.
164. Coia LR, Owen JB, Maher EJ, et al: Factors affecting treatment patterns of radiation oncologists in the United States in the palliative treatment of cancer. Clin Oncol 4:6-10, 1992.
165. Ben-Josef E, Shamsa F, Williams AO, et al: Radiotherapeutic management of osseous metastases: a survey of current patterns of care. Int J Radiat Oncol Biol Phys 40:915-921, 1998.
166. Adamietz IA, Schneider O, Muller RP: Results of a nationwide survey on radiotherapy of bone metastases in Germany. Stralentherapie Onkologie 178:531-536, 2002.
167. Roos DE: Continuing reluctance to use single fractions of radiotherapy for metastatic bone pain: an Australian and New Zealand practice survey and literature review. Radiother Oncol 56:315-322, 2000.
168. van der Linden YM, Leer JW: Impact of randomized trial-outcome in the treatment of painful bone metastases: Patterns of practice among radiation oncologists. A matter of believers vs non-believers. Radiother Oncol 56:279-281, 2000.
169. Dodwell D, Bond M, Elwell C, et al: Effect of medical audit on prescription of palliative radiotherapy. BMJ 307:24-25, 1993.
170. Lievens Y, van den Bogaert W, Kesteloo K: The palliative treatment of bone metastases: an update on practice patterns and incentives in Belgium. Radiother Oncol 73(Suppl):324, 2004.

171. Borgelt BB, Stone C: Ambulatory patient classifications and the regressive nature of Medicare reform: is the reduction in outpatient health care reimbursement worth the price? Int J Radiat Oncol Biol Phys 45:729-734, 1999.
172. Schulz U, Schroder M: Quality and the profit situation in ambulatory radiotherapy. Strahlentherapie Onkologie 172:121-127, 1996.
173. Potosky AL, Warren H, Riedel ER, et al: Measuring complications of cancer treatment using the SEER-Medicare data. Med Care 40(Suppl 8):62-68, 2002.
174. Virnig BA, Warren H, Cooper GS, et al: Studying radiation therapy using SEER-Medicare-linked data. Med Care 40:49-54, 2002.
175. Huang J, Mackillop WJ: Increased risk of soft tissue sarcoma after radiotherapy in women with breast carcinoma. Cancer 92:172-180, 2001
176. Huang J, Walker R, Groome PA, et al: Risk of thyroid carcinoma in a female population after radiotherapy for breast carcinoma. Cancer 92:1411-1418, 2001.
177. Paszat LF, Mackillop WJ, Groome PA, et al: Mortality from myocardial infarction following postlumpectomy radiotherapy for breast cancer: a population-based study in Ontario, Canada. Int J Radiat Oncol Biol Phys 43:755-762, 1999.
178. Paszat L, Mackillop WJ, Groome PA, et al: Mortality from myocardial infarction following adjuvant radiotherapy for breast cancer in the SEER Cancer Registries. J Clin Oncol 16:2625-2631, 1998.
179. Boyd CJ, Zhang-Salomons J, Groome PA, et al: Associations between community income and cancer survival in Ontario and the United States. J Clin Oncol 17:2244-2255, 1999.
180. Evans BT, Pritchard C: Cancer survival rates and GDP expenditure on health: a comparison of England and Wales and the USA, Denmark, Netherlands, Finland, France, Germany, Italy, Spain, and Switzerland in the 1990's. Public Health 114:336-339, 2000.
181. Zhang-Salomons J, Groome PA, Mackillop WJ: Estimating the best achievable cancer survival by eliminating regional variations in Ontario. Clin Invest Med 363(Suppl 22), 1999.
182. Feinstein AR: Clinical Epidemiology: The Architecture of Clinical Research. Philadelphia, WB Saunders, 1985.
183. Sackett DI, Haynes RB, Guyatt GH, et al: Clinical Epidemiology: A Basic Science for Clinical Medicine, 2nd ed. Boston, Little, Brown and Company, 1991.
184. Mackillop WJ, Dixon PD: Oesophageal carcinoma: the problems of historical controls. Radiother Oncol 6:327-328, 1986.
185. Groome PA, Mackillop WJ: Uses of ecologic studies in the assessment of intended treatment effects [letters to the editor]. J Clin Epidemiol 52:903-904, 1999.
186. Newhouse JP, McClellan M: Econometrics in outcomes research: the use of instrumental variables. Annu Rev Public Health 19:17-34, 1998.
187. Hayman JA, Lash KA, Tao ML, et al: A comparison of two methods for estimating the technical costs of external beam radiation therapy. Int J Radiat Oncol Biol Phys 47:461-467, 2000.
188. Read G: Estimating the cost of radiotherapy. Clin Oncol 6:35-39, 1994.
189. Goddard M, Maher EJ, Hutton J, et al: Palliative radiotherapy—counting the costs of changing practice. Health Policy 17:243-256, 1991.
190. Griffiths S, Delaney G, Jalaludin B: An assessment of basic treatment equivalent at Cookridge Hospital. Clin Oncol 14:399-405, 2002.
191. Barbera L, Jackson L, Schulze K, et al: Performance of different radiotherapy workload models. Int J Radiat Oncol Biol Phys 55:1143-1149, 2003.
192. Dobson J: The impact of health care economics on the selection of new radiation therapy equipment. Progr Clin Biol Res 216:175-182, 1986.
193. Foroudi F, Lapsley H, Manderson C, et al: Cost-minimization analysis radiation treatment with and without a multi-leaf collimator. Int J Radiat Oncol Biol Phys 47:1443-1448, 2000.
194. Nisbet A, Ward A: Radiotherapy equipment—purchase or lease? Br J Radiol 74:735-744, 2001.
195. Rhine K, Fodor J 3rd: Assessing equipment repair and asset management. Admin Radiol J 17:22-25, 1998.
196. Bastin K, Buchler D, Stitt J, et al: Resource utilization: high dose rate versus low dose rate brachytherapy for gynecologic cancer. Am J Clin Oncol 16:256-263, 1993.
197. Konski AA, Bracy PM, Jurs SG, et al: Cost minimization analysis of various treatment options for surgical stage I endometrial carcinoma. Int J Radiat Oncol Biol Phys 37:367-373, 1997.
198. Macklis RM, Cornelli H, Lasher J: Brief courses of palliative radiotherapy for metastatic bone pain: a pilot cost-minimization comparison with narcotic analgesics. Am J Clin Oncol 2:617-622, 1998.
199. Gregoire V, Harnoir M, Rosier JF, et al: Cost-minimization analysis of treatment options for T1N0 glottic squamous cell carcinoma: comparison between external radiotherapy, laser microsurgery, and partial laryngectomy. Radiother Oncol 53:1-13, 1999.
200. Glazebrook GA: Radiation therapy: a long term cost benefit analysis in a North American region. Clin Oncol 4:302-305, 1992.
201. Lee JH, Glick HA, Hayman JA, et al: Decision-analysis model and cost-effectiveness evaluation of postmastectomy radiation therapy in high-risk premenopausal breast cancer patients. J Clin Oncol 20:2713-2725, 2002.
202. Malin JL, Keeler E, Wang C, et al: Using cost-effectiveness analysis to define a breast cancer benefits package for the uninsured. Breast Cancer Res Treat 74:143-153, 2002.
203. Barbera L, Walker H, Foroudi F, et al: Estimating the benefit and cost of radiotherapy for lung cancer. Int J Technol Assessment Health Care 20:1-7, 2004.
204. van den Hout WB, van der Linden YM, Steenland E, et al: Single-versus multiple-fraction radiotherapy in patients with painful bone metastases: cost-utility analysis based on a randomized trial. J Natl Cancer Inst 95:222-229, 2003.
205. Mehta M, Noyes W, Craig B, et al: A cost-effectiveness and cost-utility analysis of radiosurgery vs resection for single-beam metastases. Int J Radiat Oncol Biol Phys 39:445-454, 1997.
206. Marks LB, Hardenbergh PH, Winer ET, et al: Assessing the cost-effectiveness of post-mastectomy radiation therapy. Int J Radiat Oncol Biol Phys 44:91-98, 1999.
207. Coy P, Schaafsma J, Schofield JA: The cost-effectiveness and cost-utility of high-dose palliative radiotherapy for advanced non-small cell lung cancer. Int J Radiat Oncol Biol Phys 48:1025-1033, 2000.
208. Polsky D, Mandelblatt JS, Weeks JC, et al: Economic evaluation of breast cancer treatment: considering the value of patient choice. J Clin Oncol 2:1139-1146, 2003.
209. Schwartz WB, Joskow PL: Duplicated hospital facilities: how much can we save by consolidating them? N Engl J Med 303:1449-1457, 1980.

CHAPTER 12

STATISTICS AND CLINICAL TRIALS

Sam Wieand† and John Bryant

In this chapter, we address some of the statistical issues associated with clinical trials. We begin with a short description of the basic role of statistics and statisticians and illustrate (with an example) the importance of good communication between investigators and statisticians. We provide an overview of the types of clinical trials (phases I, II, and III) and consider some aspects of the design of phase II trials having to do with sample size determination and early termination. We then discuss some of the unique aspects of phase III trials. We are particularly interested in the essential role of randomization in comparing new and standard therapies. We also discuss the important *intent to treat principle,* which is fundamental in analyzing phase III trials. Finally, we consider some of the special problems that arise in the analysis of survival data that are caused by the phenomenon of *censoring*, which occurs when a patient's time to death cannot be completely determined either because he or she becomes lost to follow-up before death or is still alive when the data are to be analyzed.

Our intent in this chapter is to provide the reader with insight regarding the use of statistics (and statisticians) in the design and analysis of clinical trials rather than to provide all of the details required for an investigator to perform his or her own analyses. Several excellent texts provide the details required to perform analyses, and we cite several such references. In Stratified Randomization Tests, we provide some mathematical details regarding the Mantel-Haenszel[1] approach for stratified treatment comparisons, but a reader can follow the remainder of the chapter without mastering the details of that section.

We define a clinical trial as a designed study involving the treatment of prospectively accrued humans that is specified by a document (protocol) with specific goals and analysis plans. Meinert[2] described some of the unique aspects of clinical trials that distinguish them from other medical research studies, including, among others, observational studies and case-control studies, and enumerates the requirements of a good protocol document.

WHY ARE STATISTICS AND STATISTICIANS USEFUL?

Collaboration between statisticians and clinical investigators can be extremely fruitful, and we hope that by the time a reader finishes this chapter, several advantages of such collaborations will have become apparent. However, at the most basic level, statisticians are interested in two properties of data: variance and bias. Any investigator involved with clinical research data quickly becomes aware of the tremendous variation between individuals. Two patients who present with cancer may have nearly identical clinical (and pathologic) characteristics and receive the same treatment, but one may fail (experience relapse or die) within months while the other may be cured. In fact, in many oncology clinical studies, particularly those involving the effect of treatment on the time to failure, we are still unable to "explain" as much as half the variation between patients when we fit a model using the known prognostic variables. This is often quite different from the experience of laboratory researchers, who may be accustomed to seeing little variation between sampling units relative to the size of the treatment effects they are trying to measure.

If one looks at two sets of 15 patients who differ in one characteristic (possibly treatment) and notices that one group has a median survival that is 2 months longer than the other group, one cannot immediately conclude that the characteristic is truly associated with survival difference. Statistical techniques will be required to determine whether a median survival difference of 2 months was quite likely to occur even if two sets of 15 patients who did not differ in the characteristic had been compared.

Bias can occur in medical research studies if treatments are compared between groups of patients who are not equivalent in terms of characteristics that are associated with prognosis. The fundamental strategy used in clinical trials to avoid biased treatment comparisons is randomization of treatment assignments, which guarantees that the treatment assigned to a patient is not related to her prognosis. In observational studies, this is not possible, although it may be feasible to adjust for potential sources of bias at the data analysis stage. Because it is difficult to identify or quantify all sources of bias, results obtained from randomized clinical trials are generally accepted to be more reliable than those obtained from observational studies. Thus, the role of the statistician in controlling bias is twofold: ensuring patient comparability between treatment groups at the study design stage and using appropriate statistical methodology in an attempt to eliminate biases at the analysis stage.

INTERACTION BETWEEN AN INVESTIGATOR AND A STATISTICIAN

Inadequate communication between an investigator and a statistician might be the most frequent cause of inappropriate designs or analyses in clinical papers. This may occur because the investigator does not explicitly state what he or she is trying to learn from a particular study or because the statistician relies on standard methods that do not satisfactorily address the real question. An example helps to illustrate the point:

Example 1. Suppose an investigator were interested in evaluating a new marker for breast cancer, such as carcinoembryonic antigen or CA-125. He tells the statistician that a useful marker should have larger values in patients with cancer than in patients with benign disease. The investigator has assembled a data set containing the value of the marker for each of 200 patients who have had a biopsy of a lesion identified by a mammogram, 100 of whom were determined to have benign disease and 100 of whom were determined to have cancer after biopsy. The statistician determines that the mean value of the marker among the cancer patients is 10 units higher than that among the patients with benign disease. He or she computes the corresponding statistic (the t test), notes a highly significant difference ($P < .00003$), and concludes that the marker is useful.

Suppose that in the investigator's practice, the large majority of lesions that underwent biopsy turn out to be benign. The investigator, therefore, believes it to be important that patients with benign disease not be misclassified more than 5% of the

†Deceased.

Table 12-1 Distribution of Markers

Range of Marker Values	No. of Patients With Benign Lesions Having Marker Values in the Range	No. of Cancer Patients Having Marker Values in the Range
0-10	5	5
10-20	50	5
20-30	20	10
30-40	10	65
40-50	10	10
50-60	5	5
Mean marker value	23.5	33.5

time (a fact not conveyed to the statistician). Assume that the distribution of the marker is as shown in Table 12-1.

If one did not want to misclassify a benign disease more than 5% of the time and knew that the marker was "on average" higher in cancer patients, he or she would classify patients as having cancer when the marker value exceeded 50. This would be a poor way to use the marker, because the data indicate that such an approach would lead to the correct classification of a case only 5% of the time (i.e., the probability of being classified as having cancer is the same for a patient with benign disease as for a patient with cancer). In fact, even though there is a large (and statistically significant) difference in the average marker value in the two groups of patients, there is no cutoff value that results in levels of sensitivity (proportion of cases that are correctly classified) and specificity (proportion of patients having benign disease that are correctly classified) that are high enough to indicate that the marker would be potentially clinically useful.

The statistician's computations were correct but were nearly irrelevant. The investigator provided the appropriate data to the statistician but received a misleading answer. What went wrong? The investigator correctly indicated that he wanted to know whether values were larger among cancer patients than among patients with benign lesions, but this, by itself, was not enough information for the statistician to choose an appropriate method of analysis. The statistician used a common method to determine whether values were larger in one group than another but did not make sure that he understood the investigator's real goal, which was to determine whether the marker might be clinically useful, with a suitably high level of specificity and sensitivity. These and other potential problems would have been avoided if the statistician had asked the investigator the following questions, among others:

1. What is the ultimate clinical goal?
2. How will the marker be used in practice?
3. What criteria distinguish a useful marker from an unacceptable one?
4. How were the data collected?
5. Will the marker be obtained under the same circumstances in practice?

The investigator should have asked the statistician the following types of questions:

1. What statistics are you thinking of using?
2. Can you explain how these statistics address the aim of the study?
3. Should we look at summary tables together?

We emphasize the prior example because it has been our experience that most bad collaborations are not caused by technically incompetent investigators or statisticians. They are nearly always the result of a failure to communicate with each other.

CLINICAL TRIALS

Clinical trials performed to develop and test new agents or modalities in oncology are often categorized as phase I, phase II, or phase III trials according to their primary aims:

Phase I Trials. These are generally the first trials involving human subjects in which a new treatment is tested. In phase I trials, the goal is to determine the maximum tolerated dose (MTD) of the treatment and to ascertain the profile of toxicities or adverse effects that may be associated with its use. In cancer research, phase I trials generally are offered to patients with advanced disease who have previously failed standard therapy and most often are based on a cautious dose-escalation strategy. The trial starts at a treatment dose low enough to have little probability of resulting in serious toxicity. Patients are then treated in groups (generally including three patients or more) at a common dose. After the observation of patients treated at a given dose level, an additional group of patients is accrued and treated at a higher dose tier only if the resulting toxicity levels are considered to be within acceptable limits. In addition to determining the toxicity profile of the treatment, phase I trials are often used to study the pharmacokinetics associated with new drugs and sometimes to estimate roughly dose-response curves associated with biological or immunologic markers (so-called phase Ib trials).

Phase II Trials. In these trials, the goal is to establish clinical activity and estimate roughly the clinical response rate. Unlike phase I trials, which commonly accrue patients with a variety of cancers, a phase II trial should restrict accrual to a reasonably well-defined patient population. Usually, phase II trials are not comparative (i.e., do not make use of a control group). Instead, patients are accrued to a single arm and are treated at a single dose level that has been suggested by earlier phase I trials. If the treatment appears sufficiently active in comparison to historic response rates in patients with disease and prognosis similar to those accrued to the phase II trial, the treatment may be considered a viable candidate for the phase III setting. Toxicities, expense, and other considerations will often influence whether the drug must be more active or simply as active as standard regimens to warrant further interest.

Phase III Trials. In phase III trials, a new agent or modality is compared with a currently accepted standard treatment by randomly assigning patients accrued from a well-defined patient population to receive either the new treatment or the control treatment. In trials that compare treatments for early-stage disease, the primary end points for comparison are usually survival and disease-free survival. In advanced-disease trials, other end points such as clinical response rate or time to progression may be chosen to be primary.

PHASE II TRIALS

The majority of phase II trials assign the treatment of interest to all patients and compare the response rate to the response rates from previous trials. Suppose in recent treatment trials for a given disease at an institution, the response rate has ranged between 15% and 20%. The new trial might be designed to ensure a high probability of concluding that the new treatment is not worth carrying forward if the true response rate were 10%, as well as to ensure a high probability of carrying the treatment forward if the true response rate were as high as 25%. Such a design would, by default, imply that if the response rate were in the 15% to 20% range, either decision (choosing to abandon the new therapy or to bring it to phase III testing) may be made with nearly equal probability. An important consideration is to ensure that patients entered on the new study are comparable to those enrolled in the earlier studies.

As just indicated, the typical phase II trial is structured to provide the basis for a recommendation either to abandon the therapy or to consider it for further testing. Working in conjunction, the investigator and the statistician together choose an "unacceptable" response rate, p_0 (10% in our example), and an "acceptable" response rate, p_1 (25% in our example). The study is then designed so that if the response rate is as low as p_0 there will be little chance that the treatment will be recommended, whereas if the response rate is as high as p_1 the treatment will be recommended with high probability. These benchmark response rates should in no case be chosen arbitrarily; considerable thought must be given to their selection, and they should be fully justified by comparison to historic data in patients with comparable disease and prognosis.

For example, the considerations just given might lead to the following study design criteria:

1. If the true response rate is $p_0 = 10\%$, there should be no more than a probability of .05 (significance level) of erroneously concluding that the treatment should be carried forward.
2. If the true response rate is 15% to 20%, it will not be harmful to have a fairly high probability of reaching either conclusion.
3. If the true response rate is $p_1 = 25\%$, there should be a probability of at least .8 (power = .80) of concluding the treatment is effective enough to be carried forward.

Using well-known methods, the statistician could determine that each of these criteria would be satisfied if 40 patients were accrued and the treatment recommended for further consideration if and only if at least 8 of the 40 patients responded. In that case, Table 12-2 gives the probabilities that the treatment will be carried forward for various hypothetical response rates.

It is worth noting that the formal decision rule is to conclude the treatment is worth carrying forward if the estimated response rate is at least 8/40 = 20% but not if the response rate is less than or equal to 7/40 = 17.5%. As Table 12-2 indicates, the probability of observing a response rate of at least 20% in our trial if the true response rate is 10% is only .042. In contrast, the probability of observing a response rate of at least 20% is .82 if the true response rate is 25%, and a positive recommendation is extremely likely (probability = .94) if the true response rate is as high as 30%. Other factors may enter into the final decision, particularly if the observed response rate is close to 15% or 20%.

Table 12-2 **Operating Characteristics of a One-Stage Phase II Study Design**

	True Response Rate					
	5%	10%	15%	20%	25%	30%
Probability of recommending treatment for further consideration	.0007	.042	.24	.56	.82	.94

Other issues may arise during the trial. For example, suppose that the first 15 patients who are accrued do not respond to the therapy. At that point, an investigator might begin to believe that the treatment is no better than standard therapy and might even be worse. This raises the question of whether the trial should be terminated. On the one hand, there is some probability that 8 of the next 25 patients will respond, resulting in a recommendation for continued consideration of the treatment. On the other hand, 15 straight failures provides some evidence that the treatment has a low response rate, and one might question the ethics of continuing a trial in the face of such evidence.

More generally, the issue of early stopping rules is as follows: When designing a trial, it may be appropriate to introduce the possibility of stopping early if there is strong evidence that the treatment is no more and possibly less effective than the standard treatment, as long as doing so would not substantially reduce the probability of detecting a true beneficial effect (power). Of course, one might also want to stop early if the treatment appears to be extremely effective, although there is no ethical constraint against assigning patients to an apparently effective treatment, unless doing so would unduly prolong the further development of a very promising therapy.

Consider the following modification of the phase II study design just described. Accrual will proceed in two stages. In the first stage, 15 patients will be accrued, treated, and observed for clinical response. If no patients respond, the trial will be terminated, and the candidate treatment will not be recommended for further consideration; otherwise, an additional 25 patients will be accrued. If in total at least eight responses are observed, the treatment will be recommended for further consideration; otherwise, it will not be so recommended.

This new design has some nice properties. The maximum number of patients required is the same as before, and, as shown in Table 12-3, the new design still satisfies each of the desired criteria 1 to 3 listed previously. However, in addition, if the new treatment has a true response rate of 5% or less, the study has a 46% chance of stopping after 15 patients are accrued, thus sparing 25 patients from treatment with an inactive regimen.

Now consider a design that requires early stopping if only 0 or 1 of the first 15 patients responds; otherwise, 25 more patients are accrued, and the treatment is recommended for further consideration if at least 8 patients respond. This design provides much better protection against the possibility of

Table 12-3 **Operating Characteristics of a Two-Stage Phase II Study Design Allowing Early Stopping for Zero Responses in the First 15 Patients**

	True Response Rate					
	5%	10%	15%	20%	25%	30%
Probability of recommending treatment for further consideration	.0007	.041	.24	.56	.82	.94
Probability of stopping after first stage of accrual	.46	.21	.09	.04	.01	.002

Table 12-4 Operating Characteristics of a Two-Stage Phase II Study Design Allowing Early Stopping for ≤ Response or None in the First 15 Patients

	TRUE RESPONSE RATE					
	5%	10%	15%	20%	25%	30%
Probability of recommending treatment for further consideration	.0006	.038	.23	.53	.78	.92
Probability of stopping after first stage of accrual	.83	.55	.32	.17	.08	.01

accruing an excessive number of patients to an ineffective regimen. However, if this design is used, it would be slightly less likely that a truly effective regimen would be recommended for further consideration. Table 12-4 shows the properties of this design.

Notice that with this design there is an .83 probability that the study will terminate after 15 patients are entered if the regimen has only a 5% response rate. However, the probability of recommending the treatment is now only .78 if there is a 25% response rate.

Numerous authors discussed optimal strategies for choosing phase II designs, including Gehan,[3] Herson,[4] Lee, Staquet, and Simon,[5] Fleming,[6] Chang and associates,[7] Simon,[8] Therneau, Wieand, and Chang,[9] Bryant and Day,[10] and Thall, Simon, and Estey.[11]

PHASE III TRIALS

It is generally recognized that judging the value of a new therapy by comparison to historic data may give an erroneous impression of its efficacy. Pocock and Simon[12] related a number of illuminating examples of this phenomenon. Thus, the phase III trial, in which a new agent or modality is tested against an accepted standard treatment in a randomized comparison, is considered the most satisfactory method of establishing the value of the proposed treatment. In this section, we discuss the rationale for requiring randomized treatment assignments in a phase III trial. We show how such randomization eliminates the possibility for biases caused by patient selection and also how it provides a basis for making statistical inferences about the data obtained from the trial. We then consider methods of restricted randomization, which can be used to balance important patient characteristics across treatment arms more effectively than can be achieved by simple or unrestricted randomization. Finally, we discuss the importance of the intent to treat principle.

Randomized Treatment Assignment

Suppose that two treatments, A and B, are to be assigned to eight patients, with four patients assigned to treatment A and four assigned to treatment B. A (simple) random assignment is defined to be any assignment resulting from a mechanism ensuring an equal probability to all possible assignments. If the patients are assigned identification numbers 1, 2, . . . , 8, then with some patience it is possible to enumerate all possible assignments. These are summarized in Table 12-5.

Table 12-5 Possible Assignments of Two Treatments (A and B) to Eight Patients, with Each Treatment Assigned to Four Patients

	PATIENT IDENTIFICATION		
12345678	12345678	12345678	12345678
AAAABBBB	ABABABBA	BAABBABA	BBABBAAA
AAABABBB	ABABBAAB	BAABBBAA	BBBAAAAB
AAABBABB	ABABBABA	BABAAABB	BBBAAABA
AAABBBAB	ABABBBAA	BABAABAB	BBBAABAA
AAABBBBA	ABBAAABB	BABAABBA	BBBABAAA
AABAABBB	ABBAABAB	BABABAAB	BBBBAAAA
AABABABB	ABBAABBA	BABABABA	
AABABBAB	ABBABAAB	BABABBAA	
AABABBBA	ABBABABA	BABBAAAB	
AABBAABB	ABBABBAA	BABBAABA	
AABBABAB	ABBBAAAB	BABBABAA	
AABBABBA	ABBBAABA	BABBBAAA	
AABBBAAB	ABBBABAA	BBAAAABB	
AABBBABA	ABBBBAAA	BBAAABAB	
AABBBBAA	BAAAABBB	BBAAABBA	
ABAAABBB	BAAABABB	BBAABAAB	
ABAABABB	BAAABBAB	BBAABABA	
ABAABBAB	BAAABBBA	BBAABBAA	
ABAABBBA	BAABAABB	BBABAAAB	
ABABAABB	BAABABAB	BBABAABA	
ABABABAB	BAABABBA	BBABABAA	
	BAABBAAB		

It can be seen from Table 12-5 that there are exactly 70 different ways in which the two treatments can be assigned to the eight patients. If all of the 70 possibilities are equally likely, then the assignment is said to be random. One way that this could be done is to write identification numbers 1 through 8 on slips of paper, place them in a hat, mix them up thoroughly, and then draw four of the slips from the hat without looking. Treatment A is then assigned to the four numbers drawn, and treatment B is assigned to the remaining four numbers. As patients are accrued, they are given identification numbers sequentially and assigned to treatments accordingly.

In practice, phase III clinical trials usually accrue hundreds or thousands of patients, so using slips of paper and a hat to generate a random treatment assignment is not very practical. Instead, the assignment of treatments to sequence numbers is accomplished using a random number generation program on a computer, but the general principle is the same as in our simple example.

Rationale for Randomization

The most obvious reason for randomized assignment is to eliminate the possibility of bias, that is, the intentional or inadvertent assignment of treatments by means of procedures that allow patient characteristics to influence the assignments in a way that may promote an imbalance in patient characteristics between the two treatment arms. The basic idea is very simple. If chance alone determines the assignments and enough patients are accrued, the law of averages will ensure that the characteristics of patients on the two treatment arms will be very nearly identical.

Treatment assignments must be performed in such a way that the accruing physician or coordinator will have no reasonable basis for predicting the arm to which the patient will be assigned. For example, if at some point an accruing physician suspects that assignment to the new treatment is likely, he or she may recruit more favorable patients to the study, thereby allowing subtle differences in patient characteristics to bias the treatment comparison. For this reason, it is common that the randomization of patients is permitted only through contact with a centralized randomization coordinator.

It should be recognized that other potential sources of bias exist that cannot be eliminated by randomized treatment assignment. For some diseases, the application of a treatment may convey psychological effects or promote expectations that impact some end points of interest. In cancer research, the most obvious example is that treatment with chemotherapy or other agents gives rise to expectations of toxicity. Thus, whenever it is feasible without undue hardship to the patients, treatment assignments should be masked by use of placebos. Perhaps even more important is the need to also keep medical personnel unaware of the actual treatment assignments whenever possible to eliminate possible biases in assessing response, relapse, or attribution of causality to adverse events.

Stratification of Treatment Assignments

For large sample sizes, randomized treatment assignment, together with the law of averages, will result in nearly balanced patient characteristics across treatment arms. However, if there are patient characteristics that are known to be strongly prognostic of patient outcome, it is possible to achieve even more complete balance by allowing for separate randomization of treatments to patients within patient subpopulations defined by the various levels of the prognostic variables. Such a restricted randomization scheme is referred to as a *stratified random assignment,* and the prognostic variables are referred to as *stratification variables.* For example, in clinical trials of adjuvant therapy for breast cancer, it is known that rates of relapse are strongly related to the number of axillary nodes found to be positive for tumor on histologic examination and are (less strongly) related to the age of the patient. Thus, the assignment of treatments to patients might be stratified within eight subpopulations, defined by combinations of nodal status (node negative, 1 to 3 positive nodes, 4 to 9 positive nodes, 10+ positive nodes) and age at randomization (≤49 years, ≥50 years). In this way, stratification (to balance the effects of strongly prognostic characteristics) and randomization (to prohibit bias resulting from less obvious or even unforeseen factors) may be used together to promote an unbiased comparison of treatments.

In some cases, it is difficult or even impossible to achieve completely balanced treatment assignments within every combination of the levels of all potential stratification variables. For example, in multicenter cancer clinical trials, it is generally thought to be good practice to balance treatment assignments within each accruing institution, because patient selection may very well differ from institution to institution. However, it is not unusual for cooperative groups in oncology to conduct phase III clinical trials using several hundred accrual sites. Clearly, it would be difficult to stratify completely on the accruing institutions together with other potentially prognostic variables, because the number of resulting combinations of levels of all the stratification variables would be excessive. To circumvent this problem, cooperative groups commonly use algorithms that dynamically maintain nearly balanced assignment of treatments across the levels of all stratification variables marginally but that do not guarantee balance within all combinations of the levels of all of the stratification variables. This approach also results in nearly balanced treatment assignments at all times; this will be beneficial if, as often happens, the characteristics of patients for whom the trial is considered most appropriate in the judgment of accruing physicians tend to change as the trial matures. Details of several such dynamic balancing algorithms may be found in Taves,[13] Pocock and Simon,[14] Freedman and White,[15] and Begg and Iglewicz.[16]

Randomization as a Basis for Inference

Although the most obvious benefit for randomization is the elimination of unforeseen sources of bias, it is also the case that randomizing the assignment of treatments to patients forms a basis for the statistical analysis of data that result from a clinical trial. To illustrate this, we return to our simple example, found in Randomized Treatment Assignment, of a clinical trial in which two treatments A and B are assigned at random to eight patients, identified by the sequence numbers 1 through 8 (of course a randomized clinical trial would be much larger than this example).

Suppose that this trial were an advanced-disease trial and that clinical response was the primary end point. Suppose, in addition, that patients 1, 2, 5, and 8 were randomly assigned to treatment A and patients 3, 4, 6, and 7 to treatment B. (In Table 12-5, the randomly selected treatment assignment is denoted by AABBABBA, the 12th listed assignment of the 70 possibilities, each equally likely to have been selected.) Suppose that patients 1, 2, 6, and 8 responded to their treatment while the remaining four patients did not. Three of four patients receiving treatment A responded, but only one of four patients receiving treatment B did so. The question to be addressed is whether or not this outcome constitutes a reasonably strong basis for claiming that treatment A has a greater response rate than does treatment B.

The classic statistical approach to such problems is to assume tentatively that the two treatments are equivalent (i.e., that patients 1, 2, 6, and 8 would have responded to either treatment A or B and that patients 3, 4, 5, and 7 would have responded to neither) and then to determine whether the data that actually resulted (3/4 responses to treatment A and 1/4 responses to treatment B) are so unlikely under this presumption that we are compelled to discard it. However, this question can be answered directly on realizing that, because treatment assignments are randomized, each of the 70 possible assignments in Table 12-5 were equally likely to have been chosen.

Now if the assignment AAAABBBB had been chosen, the response rate would be 2/4 for treatment A and 2/4 for treatment B under the tentative assumption that the identity of the patients who were observed to be responders (i.e., patients 1, 2, 6, and 8) had nothing to do with which of the two treatments they happened to receive. In the same way, the treatment assignment ABAAABBB would lead to a 1/4 response rate for treatment A and a 3/4 response rate for treatment B. Reasoning in this way for every possible treatment assignment in Table 12-5 leads to the following observation:

One of the 70 possible treatment assignments would lead to zero responses to treatment A.
Sixteen of the possible treatment assignments would lead to exactly one response to treatment A.
Thirty-six of the possible treatment assignments would lead to exactly two responses to treatment A.
Sixteen of the possible treatment assignments would lead to exactly three responses to treatment A.
One of the 70 possible treatment assignments would lead to four responses to treatment A.

Thus, if all possible assignments are equally likely (as is guaranteed by randomizing the treatment assignments) and the two treatments are totally equivalent (so that patients 1, 2, 6, and 8 would have responded in any cases, whereas patients 3, 4, 5, and 7 would not), then

The probability of observing no responses to treatment A is 1/70.
The probability of observing exactly one response to treatment A is 16/70.
The probability of observing exactly two responses to treatment A is 36/70.
The probability of observing exactly three responses to treatment A is 16/70.
The probability of observing exactly four responses to treatment A is 1/70.

If we think of the number of responses to treatment A as a *test statistic*, the set of probabilities just listed is called the *null sampling distribution* of the statistic (i.e., the distribution of the statistic under the null hypothesis that the two treatments are equivalent). From this null distribution, we can conclude that the trial results that we actually observed in our hypothetical example (three responses to treatment A) are not strongly inconsistent with a belief that the null hypothesis is true. Indeed, if the null hypothesis is true, 17 of 70 possible treatment assignments, or a proportion of .24 of all possible assignments, would have led to three or more responses to treatment A. This proportion is referred to as a one-sided P value for a test of the null hypothesis that treatments A and B are equivalent against the alternative hypothesis that A is preferable to B. If, as is usually the case, we wished to test the equivalence hypothesis against a two-sided hypothesis, this P value would be doubled.

The example just given shows that a test of the null hypothesis of treatment equality can be performed just by counting the number of different ways the treatments can be assigned and then determining the proportion of assignments leading to a result at least as discordant with the null hypothesis as the one actually observed. This proportion gives the P value associated with the hypothesis test. Although the example we have presented considers a trial whose size is too small to be very interesting, the principles are exactly the same for larger trials. Suppose, for example, that 200 patients had been accrued to an advanced-disease trial comparing treatments A and B, with 100 patients assigned to each arm. Suppose that altogether 40 patients responded to their therapy, 28 to treatment A and 12 to treatment B. The results can be summarized as in Table 12-6.

It can be shown that of all possible treatment assignments of 200 patients to two treatments, 40 of whom are responders and 160 of whom are not, a proportion of only .0012 of the assignments have 28 or more of the responding patients assigned to treatment A and 12 or fewer assigned to treatment B. A test of the hypothesis of equivalent treatments would, therefore, have a two-sided P value of 2(.0012) = .0024, which would be considered to be strong support in favor of the conclusion that the treatments are, in fact, not equivalent but rather that treatment A is superior to treatment B.

As a practical matter, the number of possible treatment assignments in the previous example is extremely large, so that complete enumeration of all possibilities is not practically feasible. However, mathematical statisticians have been able to show that the proportion of such assignments leading to any given number of responses in one specified treatment arm follows a certain probability distribution known as the *hypergeometric distribution*. This fact was used in the example to compute the required P value. This result also leads to the well-known statistical procedure known as *Fisher's exact test*. However, it is worthwhile to remember that conceptually this larger example is completely analogous to the earlier one involving only eight patients.

Table 12-6 **Results of a Hypothetical Phase III Advanced-Disease Trial**

Treatment	Responder	Nonresponder	Total
A	28	72	100
B	12	88	100
Total	40	160	200

Stratified Randomization Tests

Refer again to the set of possible treatment assignments shown in Table 12-5, and suppose, as before, that patients 1, 2, 6, and 8 are responders, whereas patients 3, 4, 5, and 7 are not. We arrived at the null sampling distribution for the number of responders assigned to treatment A by determining the number of such responders for each possible assignment in Table 12-5. The resulting distribution looked like this:

X = No. of Responses to Treatment A	Probability
0	1/70
1	16/70
2	36/70
3	16/70
4	1/70

It is easy to verify that the average value of X over all 70 possible treatment assignments is 2 and that the average squared difference between X and its average is

$$(0-2)^2 + 16 \cdot (1-2)^2 + 36 \cdot (2-2)^2 + 16 \cdot (3-2)^2 + (4-2)^2/70 = 4/7$$

The average of X over all possible samples is referred to as its expected value, and the averaged squared deviation is its variance. It can be shown more generally that if N patients are randomly assigned to treatments A and B with N_A patients assigned to treatment A and N_B to treatment B ($N_A + N_B = N$), and if altogether M_R of the N patients respond whereas M_N do not ($M_R + M_N = N$), then the expected value of X is equal to $N_A M_R/N$ and the variance of X is $N_A N_B M_R M_N/N^2(N-1)$.

These formulas allow a convenient extension of tests for the equality of treatments to clinical trials that control for the effects of stratification variables. To illustrate, consider a metastatic breast cancer trial comparing treatments A and B in which patients have been stratified according to the site of metastasis (bone, visceral, or other); suppose the following response frequencies had resulted:

	Stratum #1 Bone			Stratum #2 Visceral			Stratum #3 Other Sites		
	Resp	Nonresp	Total	Resp	Nonresp	Total	Resp	Nonresp	Total
Trt A	20	40	60	10	40	50	10	20	30
Trt B	25	35	60	9	41	50	15	15	30
Total	45	75	120	19	81	100	25	35	60

If it is believed that the relative efficacy of the two treatments should be similar at the various sites of metastases, these data should be pooled across strata to arrive at a single test of treatment equivalence that is more powerful than the individual within-strata comparisons. This can be done by aggregating responses to treatment A across strata ($X = X_{Bone} + X_{Visceral} + X_{Other}$) and similarly aggregating expected values and variances ($E = E_{Bone} + E_{Visceral} + E_{Other}$; $V = V_{Bone} + V_{Visceral} + V_{Other}$). The required computations are summarized next:

Stratum	# Responses (X)	Expected Value (E)	Variance (V)
Bone	20	22.5	7.09
Visceral	10	9.5	3.89
Other	10	12.5	3.71
Total	40	44.5	14.69

It can be shown that the standardized total $Z = (X - E)/\sqrt{V}$ is approximately normal under the hypothesis of equivalent treatments. Using this result leads to a two-sided *P* value of about .24, so there appears to be little evidence of any difference in the efficacy of the two treatments. This statistical procedure for stratified treatment comparisons is known as the Mantel-Haenszel test.

INTENT TO TREAT

If treatment assignments are randomized as described earlier, one can be reasonably confident that important prognostic factors will be balanced across treatment arms. However, if any patients are excluded at the time the data are analyzed, the possibility of bias arises once again. An analysis that includes all randomized patients, regarded as though each had received precisely the treatment to which he or she had been randomized, is an intent to treat analysis. In this section, we show how treatment comparisons may be seriously biased by excluding patients from an analysis, even for apparently valid reasons. We then show how an intent to treat analysis may effectively reduce biases that can creep into analyses when not all patients actually receive the treatments to which they have been randomized. We discuss these issues in the context of the following example:

Example 2. A clinical trial was designed to compare the effect of radiation therapy relative to observation in patients with rectal cancer. Three hundred patients were randomized between radiation therapy (arm A) and observation (arm B), 150 to each arm. Suppose all patients actually received all of their intended therapy, and after 7 years of follow-up survival curves were as shown in Figure 12-1. Although the survival curve for patients receiving radiation therapy lies above that for patients on the observation-only arm, suggestive of a benefit from radiation therapy, the difference is not quite statistically significant ($P = .058$).

In any clinical trial, the patients who are accrued exhibit considerable variation in their prognoses. Suppose that we could make use of certain prognostic patient characteristics, which were unavailable in the analysis summarized previously. Suppose further that by using this new information, we could identify the 10% of patients with the worst prognoses. Then we might redraw the survival curves after stratifying on risk, resulting in the plots shown in Figure 12-1B. An analysis of these data that takes this stratification into account again yields a *P* value of .058, which agrees with the *P* value from the unstratified analysis to three decimal places. This insensitivity of analysis to stratification is a direct consequence of the randomization used in the design of the trial, which tends to balance the poor-prognosis patients equally across the two arms of the trial.

Returning to the original analysis of these data, suppose that not all patients in arm A had actually received the radiation therapy to which they had been randomized. The statistician must decide what to do with these noncompliant cases. There are at least three ways to proceed: (1) It may seem logical to discard data corresponding to the noncompliant patients because they did not receive the radiation therapy that was assigned to them; (2) it might even seem reasonable to analyze the noncompliant patients as though they had been randomized to arm B rather than arm A because, in fact, they received no adjuvant therapy, similar to those patients who were randomized to observation; (3) the intent to treat principle states that the noncompliers should be analyzed just as though they had received radiation therapy, even though in actuality they did not.

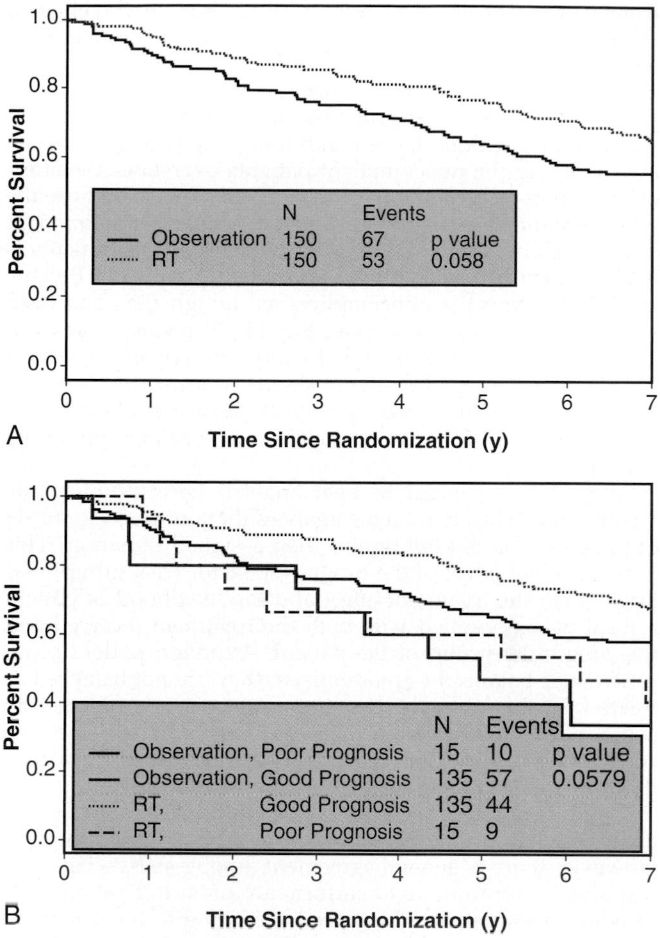

Figure 12-1 **A,** Survival curves that would be observed if all patients receive the prescribed therapy (percent survival versus years from randomization). **B,** Survival curves that would be observed if all patients receive the prescribed therapy, stratified by risk group (percent survival versus years from randomization). RT, radiation therapy.

We now consider the possible consequences associated with these three possibilities. Under the assumption that patients' reasons for refusal of treatment are completely unassociated with prognosis, methods 1 and 2 just presented should lead to estimated treatment differences that are essentially identical to the analysis of Figure 12-1A. If there is a treatment difference, the intent to treat analysis will tend to underestimate this difference, because some of the patients who were not irradiated are counted as having received that therapy. The differences in the three analyses should be rather small under this assumption of no association between refusal of treatment and prognosis.

Alternatively, it is rather likely that reasons for refusal of treatment will be associated with patient prognosis. For example, patients with poorer performance status, or their physicians, may be less liable to accept assignment to a treatment that is known to be associated with significant toxicity.

Deteriorating health may lead to difficulties in traveling to receive treatment; advancing disease may correlate with patients' levels of depression or anxiety, which, in turn, may correlate with compliance. Suppose that it is the 10% of patients with the worst prognosis who refuse to accept their radiotherapy. Under these conditions, analysis of the data after deleting the noncompliant patients overstates the effect of radiotherapy, as shown in Figure 12-2A. This is because the worst-prognosis patients are deleted from consideration in arm A, but no similar deletion of poor-prognosis patients is made in arm B. The result is a spuriously significant *P* value of .021. Treating the noncompliers as though they had been randomized to observation (see Fig. 12-2B) results in an even more serious overstatement of the radiotherapy effect, associated with a *P* value less than .009. In contrast, the intent to treat analysis yields a slightly attenuated treatment effect (P = .065) (see Fig. 12-2C), but no serious misrepresentation of the true effect.

Why did the intent to treat analysis correspond to the "truth" more closely than the analysis that omitted the subset of patients who did not receive their assigned radiation? This is because the effect of the prognostic factor (risk group) was larger than the treatment effect and the likelihood of patient refusal was associated with both the treatment received and the prognostic group of the patient. Although patient prognoses were balanced as randomized, they are not balanced as treated. In this case, the baseline prognosis of patients who actually received radiation was better than among those who were under observation. It is precisely this type of imbalance that the intent to treat analysis is designed to prevent.

There is no one correct answer as to the best approach to analysis when not all patients receive their assigned therapy. However, there is general agreement among statisticians that it is always appropriate to perform an intent to treat analysis in which each patient is analyzed according to the treatment assigned at randomization, regardless of what treatment was actually received. Results of any other analysis should be compared with the results of the intent to treat analysis, and if the results differ substantively, the interpretability of the data must be questioned.

The prior examples illustrated only one type of problem that may be addressed by an intent to treat analysis. Biases similar to those just described can occur if patients elect to cross over study arms, accept a nonstudy therapy, receive only a portion of assigned therapy, or are determined to be ineligible. Thus, we advocate attempting to obtain complete follow-up for all such patients and performing an intent to treat analysis. Sometimes this may not be possible because patients who refuse protocol therapy may also refuse to be followed. If only 1% or 2% of patients fall into this category, there is little danger of important bias; but if this number is larger, say 5% to 10%, there is a real danger that the study may be biased. One might then want to perform what are called sensitivity analyses to examine the possible effect of having so many patients without follow-up. In its simplest form, one might perform one analysis assuming that all of the patients without outcome data on arm A failed early on, whereas those on arm B survived; and then perform an analysis assuming that all of the patients without outcome data on arm A survived, whereas those on arm B failed. If one reaches the same conclusion about treatment effect in either analysis, then the exclusions do not represent a serious problem.

There is often disagreement concerning the inclusion of ineligible patients in analyses, particularly in analyses dependent on patient covariates because ineligible patients may not fit any reasonable classification. The decision as to whether it is appropriate to exclude ineligibles is dependent on the methods used for determining ineligibility. For example, in some studies, each patient is reviewed for eligibility in a uniform way by a reviewer (or review committee) who is unaware of the assigned treatment and uses only information

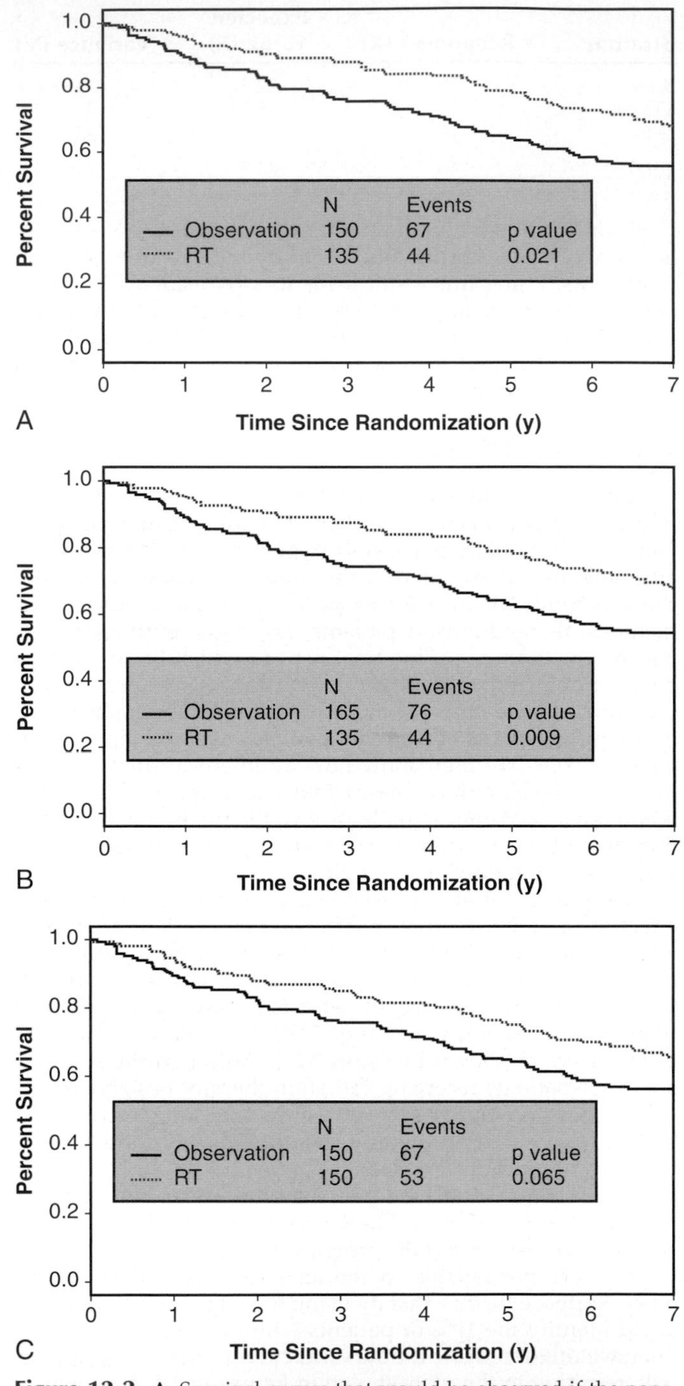

Figure 12-2 **A,** Survival curves that would be observed if the poor-risk patients who refuse radiation therapy (RT) are excluded from the analyses (percent survival versus years from randomization). **B,** Survival curves that would be observed if the poor-risk patients who refuse radiation therapy are included as untreated patients (percent survival versus years from randomization). **C,** Survival curves that would be observed if the poor-risk patients who refuse radiation therapy are included as radiation therapy patients (i.e., the results that would be obtained using an intent to treat analysis [percent survival versus years from randomization]).

that was obtained before randomization. If that is the only mechanism for classifying patients as ineligible, one could reasonably exclude such patients from analyses. However, any less stringent approach that allows patients to be classified as ineligible after randomization could introduce subtle biases. For example, in a trial of radiation versus observation, one might routinely perform a pretreatment examination immediately after a patient is assigned to radiation therapy. If, during that examination, it is determined that the patient had not met an eligibility requirement, exclusion would cause a bias because a similar patient not assigned to radiation would not have had the pretreatment examination and would, therefore, not have been determined to be ineligible.

To summarize, we recommend always performing an intent to treat analysis using all patients as randomized and reporting the results of that analysis in any publication. Further analyses may be performed, but one should be aware of potential biases similar to those described previously. Further discussion of these issues can be found in Pocock[12] and Gail.[17]

The data used in Example 2 were generated using the following assumptions. The expected 5-year survival rate for an untreated good-risk patient was .73, and for an untreated bad-risk patient, .54. The reduction in the death rate associated with radiation treatment was assumed to be 20% in each group. For Figure 12-2, we assumed that all the poor-risk patients had an expected 5-year survival rate of .54 because none received treatment.

SURVIVAL ANALYSIS

Survival analysis differs from other types of statistical analysis in that the analysis of time to an event often is complicated by the lack of complete follow-up for every patient (i.e., there is censored data). An example illustrates why this is important. The example uses hypothetical data chosen to illustrate clearly the problem that censoring can cause.

Example 3. Suppose a radiation oncologist decides to review the outcomes of rectal cancer patients treated with radiation therapy. Of primary interest is the determination of the proportion of patients who remain relapse free through 5 years. Suppose patients have been accrued over the past $7^{1}/_{2}$ years, and by chance the patients have started treatment in pairs at intervals of 1 year. Suppose, furthermore, that if no more patients were accrued and the oncologist could wait 5 more years to obtain 5-year follow-up for every patient, he or she would find that half of them were relapse free for more than 5 years. This (unobserved) relapse pattern is shown in Figure 12-3.

Twelve years after the first patient was entered, the 5-year relapse-free pattern would be as shown in Figure 12-4 (time 0 is the date of entry for each patient). If the investigator had waited 12 years (i.e., until 5-year data for all 16 patients were complete), he or she would have observed that half of the patients were relapse free 5 years after entry (i.e., the 5-year relapse free rate is .50). Suppose, in fact, the investigator decided to look at the patients' experience $7^{1}/_{2}$ years after the first patient had entered. Then the investigator would have observed everything to the left of the vertical line in Figure 12-5. Translated into time from entry, this would be represented as shown in Figure 12-6. In that case, the investigator would have complete 5-year data for 7 of the 8 patients who relapsed and for 3 patients who were relapse free at 5 years (those who were entered at year 0, 1, or 2). For the other 6 patients, his or her knowledge would be that they were relapse free for some amount less than 5 years. The investigator's first

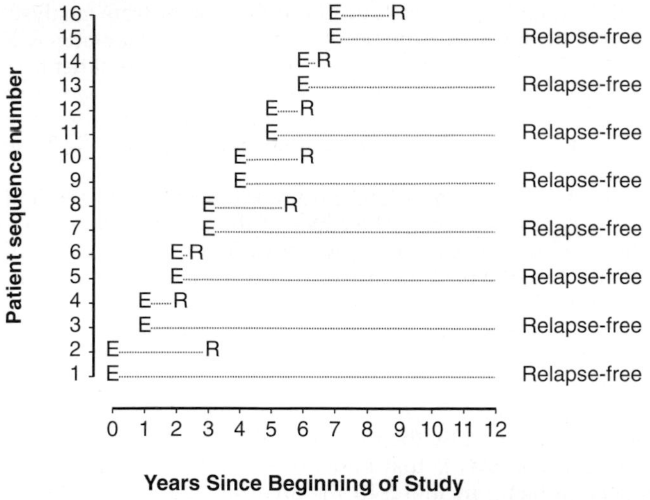

Figure 12-3 Date of entry (E) and relapse (R) of 16 patients monitored over a 12-year period; 8 did not experience relapse.

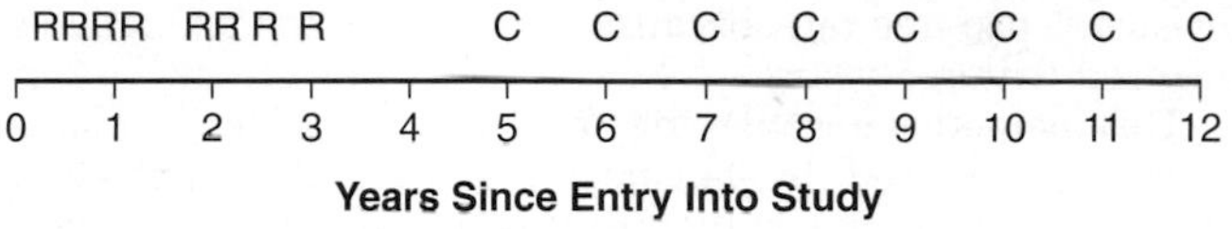

Figure 12-4 Relapse history of 16 patients seen 12 years after beginning of the study: time from entry into the study until relapse or last follow-up. C, censored; R, relapsed.

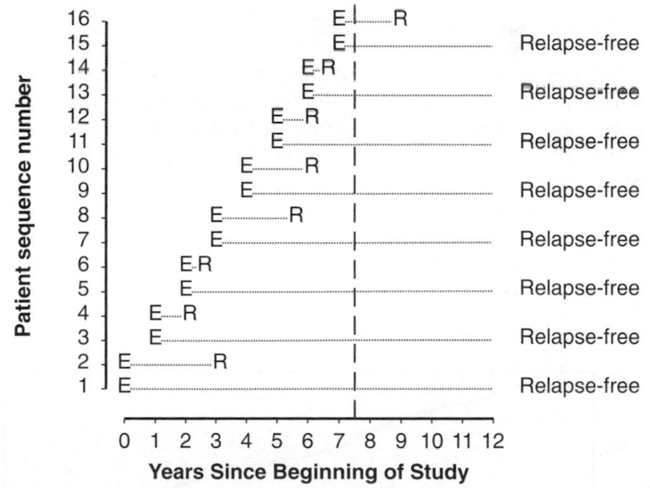

Figure 12-5 Status of follow-up 7.5 years after the first patient was entered in the trial. E, entry; R, relapse.

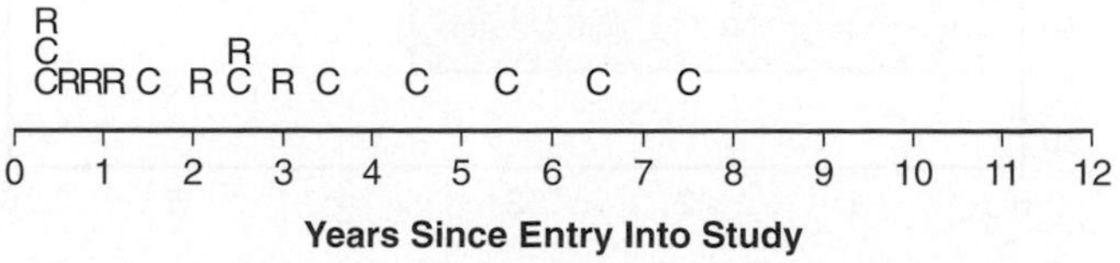

Figure 12-6 Relapse history of 16 patients seen 7.5 years after the beginning of the study: time from entry into the study until relapse or last follow-up. C, censored; R, relapsed.

instinct might be to exclude these 6 patients from analysis because he or she does not know what their relapse status will be after 5 years of follow-up. Of the remaining 10 patients, 7 are known to have relapsed and 3 are known to be disease free for more than 5 years, so that the estimated relapse-free rate at 5 years is 0.30. This estimate does not seem to reflect the data accurately.

The estimate is so different from 0.50 because our method of calculation is biased. The cause of the bias can be seen by studying the seventh and eighth patients in the series of patients (i.e., the patients entered 3 years after the first patient entered). Notice that the seventh patient entered was still relapse free when the radiation oncologist performed his or her analysis but had only been followed for 4½ years (i.e., did not have a known status at 5 years) and hence was excluded. However, the eighth patient (who was entered on the same day) had relapsed by the time of analysis and, therefore, was included. The bias is that patients who relapse have a better chance of being included in the analysis than those who do not relapse. One way to avoid a biased estimate would be to exclude all patients who did not have the potential to be monitored 5 years. Thus, the oncologist would only be able to use the information from the first six patients entered. In this artificial example, this would have led to a correct estimate of the 5-year relapse-free rate, because three of the first six patients relapsed within 5 years.

This method is unsatisfying because not all of the available information is used. In statistical terms, the disadvantage of our proposed solution is that there is considerably more variance associated with an estimate that uses the data from only six patients than one that uses all of the available data. For example, if patients 6 and 7 had entered the study in the opposite order, the relapse-free estimate would jump from 50% to 67%. A better method is described in the next section.

KAPLAN-MEIER METHOD

A common way to summarize survival data is to estimate the "survival curve," which shows, for each value of time, the proportion of subjects who survive at least that length of time. Figure 12-7 shows survival curves for patients with operable breast cancer who have been treated with either pre- or postoperative chemotherapy (doxorubicin and cyclophosphamide) in a large clinical trial. In this section, we discuss the estimation of survival curves using a method proposed by Kaplan and Meier.[18]

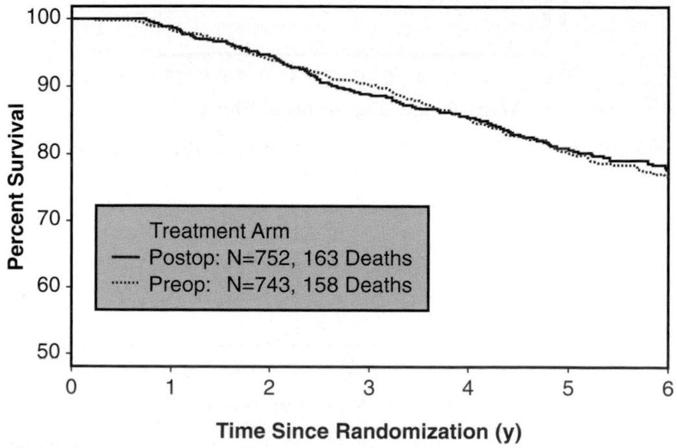

Figure 12-7 Survival of patients with operable breast cancer treated with doxorubicin and cyclophosphamide.

Several excellent references are available that show exactly how a Kaplan-Meier estimate is computed and describe other properties such as the variance of the estimator. A nice summary with formulas for computations can be found in Chapter 2 of Parmar and Machin's text.[19] Here, we provide two examples that provide some insight regarding the Kaplan-Meier method. The first example concerns a data set having no censored observations; the second example extends these ideas to accommodate censored observations.

Example 4. Suppose four patients are entered into a study, possibly at different times, and all four die, with death times of 10 months, 20 months, 25 months, and 40 months, respectively, from time of entry. We want to estimate the 3-year survival rate. Three of the four patients died within 3 years from entry, and one patient remained alive more than 3 years from entry (i.e., one fourth of the patients entered lived at least 3 years). Thus, a reasonable estimate of the 3-year survival rate is $S(3) = .25$. This estimate (the proportion of patients who remained alive at 3 years) is referred to as the empirical survival estimate, and the graph of estimates obtained this way at all time points is called the *empirical survival curve.*

Example 5. Suppose that in the previous example three of the patients have died at 10 months, 25 months, and 40 months, respectively. The fourth patient is still alive but only has been monitored for 20 months. We want to estimate the 3-year survival rate. Notice that if we could wait another 16 months to obtain the estimate (so that we would have 3-year data for all patients), we would obtain an estimate of either one fourth (if the fourth patient dies soon) or one half (if the patient remains alive for another 16 months). The rather intuitive approach we used in Example 3 to estimate the 3-year survival does not work here because we do not know whether there will be two or three survivors when all the patients have died or have been monitored for 3 years (i.e., we do not know how to handle the patient whose follow-up was censored at 20 months). Kaplan and Meier proposed an approach that updates the survival estimate at the time of each death using only those patients who are at risk of failing at each update.

Because none of the patients died during the first 10 months, the Kaplan-Meier estimate of the probability of surviving to any time point less than 10 months is equal to 1. Because four patients are alive at 10 months but only three quarters of them survive beyond 10 months, the Kaplan-Meier estimate changes to three quarters for time points beyond 10 months but before the next death. Although one patient is censored at 20 months, this gives no information regarding the likelihood of a death, so the Kaplan-Meier estimate remains at three quarters for all time points between 10 months and 25 months. One of the two patients who are still at risk just before 25 months dies at that time. Thus, the estimate of the probability of a patient surviving beyond 25 months, given that the patient survived at least 25 months, is one half. The Kaplan-Meier estimate of surviving more than 25 months is the product of three quarters (the estimated probability a patient will survive until 25 months) times one half (the estimated probability that a patient will survive more than 25 months given that the patient was alive at 25 months), which is three eighths. There are no other deaths before 3 years, so the Kaplan-Meier estimate of the 3-year survival rate is three eighths. The Kaplan-Meier method uses all the relevant available data from each patient but excludes the patient who was censored at 20 months from all computations beyond that time.

If the Kaplan-Meier approach is applied to the data in Example 3, the estimate S(3) is equal to the (probability of surviving 10 months) × (probability of surviving more than 10 months given survival of 10 months) × (probability of surviving more than 20 months given survival of 20 months) × (probability of surviving more than 25 months given survival of 25 months) or $1 \times \frac{3}{4} \times \frac{2}{3} \times \frac{1}{2} = \frac{1}{4}$, which matches the empirical survival estimate. In fact, the Kaplan-Meier estimate and the empirical estimate always match when applied to uncensored data.

The reader may verify that application of the Kaplan-Meier approach to the data in Figure 12-6 will result in an estimate of 0.45 for the probability of remaining relapse free through 5 years.

LOG-RANK STATISTIC

Perhaps the most common application of survival analysis techniques is the comparison of survival times (or other waiting times, such as time to disease relapse), between two or more groups of patients that differ in some aspect (e.g., male versus female or treated versus untreated). We discuss the log-rank statistic and the stratified log-rank statistic in some detail. These statistics are commonly used to compare survival times between groups. We avoid excessive mathematical detail; instead, we concentrate on showing how these methods accommodate censored survival times and, in the case of the stratified log-rank statistic, how differences in individual patient characteristics may be controlled to avoid biased group comparisons.

The log-rank statistic deals with the problem of censoring by comparing the groups only when a patient within any of the groups experiences an "event" (if survival times are to be compared across groups, an event would be a death; if times to relapse are to be compared, an event would be a relapse, and so on). This idea is most easily explained in the context of a simple example. Suppose we monitored three patients receiving a standard treatment regimen (this might even be no treatment), which we refer to as treatment A, and three other patients receiving an experimental regimen, which we refer to as treatment B. Suppose, furthermore, that the survival times for the patients receiving treatment A are 10, 40+, and 55 days, respectively, and for the patients receiving treatment B, 15, 50, and 60, respectively (a plus sign after a value refers to a censored time, i.e., a patient with a time of 40+ was last known to be alive at 40 days and no further follow-up is available). These data are represented graphically in Figure 12-8; the three patients receiving treatment A are labeled A1, A2, and A3, and those receiving treatment B are labeled B1, B2, and B3. Deaths are denoted by the letter D, and censored survival times are labeled with the letter C.

When evaluating the log-rank statistic, the first computation occurs at time t = 10, the time at which the first death is observed. Just before this point in time, all six patients are known to be alive (and hence are "at risk" to die at time t = 10). Three of these patients received treatment A and three received treatment B. Exactly one of these six patients is known to have died at time t = 10, and he or she received treatment A. Table 12-7 summarizes the status of patients at this time point. Notice that, at the time of this computation, there are three patients on each arm. Thus, if treatment B was equivalent to treatment A and only one death occurred on one arm or the other, there would be a one-half chance that the death is on arm A. In fact, the death is on arm A; hence, we observe one death when the probability of observing a death on arm A is one half (i.e., there is one half more death on arm A than is expected).

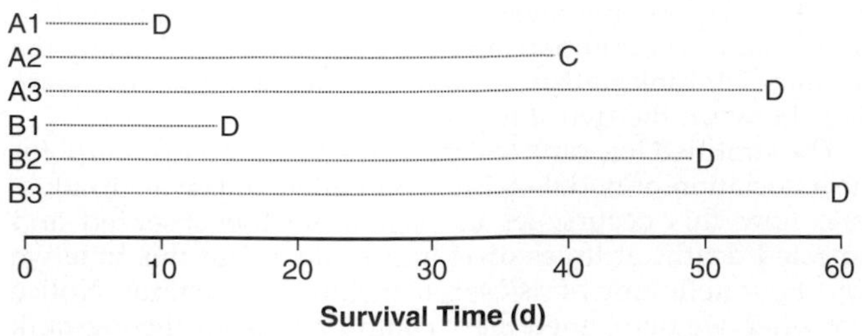

Figure 12-8 Survival times of six patients treated with one of two regimens. C, censored; D, death.

Observations at time t = 15 are listed in Table 12-8. At this point there would be a two-fifths probability that the death would occur on treatment A (if the treatments were equivalent), but the death did not occur on treatment A, so there were two-fifths less deaths on arm A than expected (i.e., the observed deaths minus the expected number is $0 - \frac{2}{5} = -.4$).

The next computation occurs at t = 50; observations are listed in Table 12-9. Notice that patient A2 is not included in this table, even though she is not known to have died at any time before t = 50. Because she was lost to follow-up (censored) at time 40, she is no longer "at risk" at time 50. At this time, there would be a one-third probability that the death would occur on treatment A (if the treatments were equivalent), but the death does not occur on treatment A, so there are one third fewer deaths on arm A than expected (i.e., the observed deaths minus the expected number is $0 - \frac{1}{3} = -.33$).

One may go through the same computations at time = 55 (Table 12-10) and will determine that the number of deaths minus expected deaths on treatment A is $1 - \frac{1}{2} = .5$. At time 60, all remaining patients are on the same arm, so the observed minus the expected number of deaths must be 0. Adding up the observed minus expected number of deaths at times 10, 15, 50, and 55, one obtains 2 observed deaths minus 1.733 expected deaths, so that there were 0.27 deaths more than

Table 12-7 Observed Deaths (t = 10)

Treatment	Dead	Alive	Total
A	1	2	3
B	0	3	3
Total	1	5	6

Table 12-8 Observed Deaths (t = 15)

Treatment	Dead	Alive	Total
A	0	2	2
B	1	2	3
Total	1	4	5

Table 12-9 Observed Deaths (t = 50)

Treatment	Dead	Alive	Total
A	0	1	1
B	1	1	2
Total	1	2	3

Table 12-10 Observed Deaths (t = 55)

Treatment	Dead	Alive	Total
A	1	0	1
B	0	1	1
Total	1	1	2

Table 12-11 Log-Rank (Mantel-Haenszel) Test

Stratum (Event Time)	No. of Deaths on Treatment A (X)	Expected Value (X)	Variance (V)
t = 10	1	$3 \cdot 1/6 = 1/2$	$3 \cdot 3 \cdot 1 \cdot 5/6^2 \cdot 5 = 1/4$
t = 15	0	$2 \cdot 1/5 = 2/5$	$2 \cdot 3 \cdot 1 \cdot 4/3^2 \cdot 4 = 6/25$
t = 50	0	$1 \cdot 1/3 = 1/3$	$1 \cdot 2 \cdot 1 \cdot 2/3^2 \cdot 2 = 2/9$
t = 55	1	$1 \cdot 1/2 = 1/2$	$1 \cdot 1 \cdot 1 \cdot 1/2^2 \cdot 1 = 1/4$
Total	2	1.733	0.9622

expected on arm A, indicating that this treatment might be harmful. However, one's intuition is that this is not a significant difference (i.e., such a small difference could easily be attributed to the play of chance), and in fact this is true. Thus, there is no strong evidence in this example that treatments A and B differ.

More formally, the log-rank statistic is defined to be the difference in observed and expected numbers of deaths on one of the two treatment arms. The statistic may be standardized by dividing by the square root of its variance, yielding a score that, under the hypothesis of equivalent treatments, is approximately standard normal. In the present example, the variance of the log-rank statistic can be shown to equal .9622, so the standardized test statistic is (2 − 1.733)/.9622 = .27, corresponding to a two-sided *P* value of about .79.

In Stratified Randomization Tests, we discussed the use of the Mantel-Haenszel method to provide a test for the equivalence of the response rates of two treatments in a metastatic breast cancer trial, in which patients had been stratified according to the site of metastasis. In that example, we saw that the Mantel-Haenszel test aggregated the treatment comparison over several two-by-two tables. The same idea can be applied to the present survival comparison by considering a Mantel-Haenszel test that treats the set of all patients at risk just before each event as a separate stratum and, therefore, aggregates the treatment comparison over Tables 12-7 to 12-10. The computations are exactly like those in Stratified Randomization Tests and are summarized in Table 12-11.

Notice that our earlier calculations of the observed and expected numbers of deaths on treatment A are exactly the same calculations that are summarized in columns 2 and 3 of Table 12-11. Column 4 summarizes the computation of the variance of the difference in observed and expected numbers of deaths on treatment A, yielding a variance of .9622. The standardized statistic corresponding to the Mantel-Haenszel test is, therefore, $Z = (X - E)/V = .27$, with two-sided *P* value of .79, a result that is identical to the one derived earlier. In fact, this example illustrates that the log-rank comparison of survival times is the Mantel-Haenszel analysis, which results by treating each set of patients at risk just before every event as a separate stratum.

Table 12-12 Observed Deaths (t = 11)

Treatment	Dead	Alive	Total
A	1	14	15
B	0	10	10
Total	1	24	25

Observed − expected deaths on treatment A = 1 − 0.6 = 0.4.

Table 12-13 Observed Deaths (t = 91)

Treatment	Dead	Alive	Total
A	1	9	10
B	0	7	7
Total	1	16	17

Observed − expected deaths on treatment A = 1 − 0.588 = 0.412.

STRATIFIED LOG-RANK STATISTIC

The log-rank test as defined previously uses only survival information and group membership. Other patient characteristics are not taken into account. We now introduce a method to adjust for the possible effects of other covariates. Suppose that we had the following survival times (in days) for a group of breast cancer patients who had differing numbers of positive lymph nodes and who received either treatment A or treatment B:

	1-3 nodes
Treatment A	91, 160+, 230+
Treatment B	32, 101, 131+, 155+, 190+, 210+
	4 or more nodes
Treatment A	11, 22, 42, 63, 72, 110, 120, 141, 155, 180+, 200+, 220+
Treatment B	51, 83, 110, 170+

If we were to ignore our knowledge of the patients' lymph node status and compute a log-rank statistic as we did before, our computations at times 11 and 91 would be as shown in Tables 12-12 and 12-13. If one completes these computations at each time of death, the total for arm A is 10 observed deaths when 8.85 were expected. This translates to 1.15 excess events on arm A.

However, when one examines the distribution of patients, it is not surprising that there is an excess number of events on arm A. After all, 12 of 15 patients on arm A had four or more positive nodes, whereas only 4 of 10 patients on arm B had four or more positive nodes. Given that one would expect patients with four or more positive nodes to be at greater risk than those with one to three positive nodes, it is not clear whether the observation of 1.15 excess deaths on arm A represents a possible treatment effect or reflects the nodal imbalance. That is, the comparison of treatments A and B using the ordinary log-rank statistic is biased by an imbalance of disease stage between the two study arms.

The stratified log-rank test provides a method to control for the association of nodal status with patient survival. To illustrate how this occurs, let us recompute the observed and expected deaths at times of 11 and 91 days, but this time we adjust our definition of risk sets to include nodal status. Notice that when we performed these computations for the log-rank test at time = 11 (as shown previously), we estimated the likelihood that the death that occurred was on arm A to be 15/25,

Table 12-14 Observed Deaths (t = 11, 4 Positive Nodes)

Treatment	Dead	Alive	Total
A	1	11	12
B	0	4	4
Total	1	15	16

Observed − expected deaths = 1 − 0.75 = 0.25.

Table 12-15 Observed Deaths (t = 91, 1 to 3 Positive Nodes)

Treatment	Dead	Alive	Total
A	1	2	3
B	0	5	5
Total	1	7	8

Observed − expected deaths = 1 − 0.375 = 0.625.

based on the fact that 15 of the 25 patients at risk at that time were on arm A. This implicitly assumed that in the absence of a treatment effect, all patients are at the same risk of dying regardless of nodal status. However, the first patient who died was one who had four or more positive nodes. The patients who would be at the same risk of dying as that patient are the other patients with four or more nodes. Because we knew there were 16 patients with four or more nodes who were at risk of dying at t = 11 and that 12 of these patients were on arm A, perhaps we should have estimated the probability to be three quarters that if a patient with four or more nodes died at time t = 11, the patient would be on arm A (given no treatment effect). This is the method used when computing the stratified log-rank test. We now examine the computations at times of 11 and 91 days using this stratified approach (Tables 12-14 and 12-15).

If one restricts these computations only to the patients with four or more positive nodes, the sum of the observed deaths on treatment A minus the expected is 9 − 9.11 = −.11. In the patients with one to three positive nodes, similar computations yield 1 observed death and 0.99 expected death. Summing these values across both strata gives 10 observed deaths on treatment A compared with 10.10 expected deaths for a difference of −.10. Thus, the stratified approach leads to almost no difference between the number of observed and expected deaths, indicating that there is essentially no estimated treatment difference after adjusting for nodal status.

Notice that the difference between the two approaches is seen in the computation of the probability of a death occurring on treatment A at each time point. If one understands the method of computing these probabilities (expected values), one can begin to understand the possible biases of different approaches.

In the prior example, the (unstratified) log-rank test had a potential bias because no adjustment was made for the probable increased risk associated with having four or more positive nodes. This was important because there was a large imbalance in the proportion of such patients by treatment. If this characteristic had been in balance across treatments, the stratified and unstratified approaches would have given much closer results.

Computationally, a stratified log-rank test that controls for specified patient characteristics can be computed by the Mantel-Haenszel approach. First, one jointly stratifies on event times (as in Log-Rank Statistic) and patient characteristics of interest (e.g., nodal status). Computations analogous to those of Table 12-11 are then required to calculate the stratified log-rank statistic, its variance, and the corresponding standardized statistic.

REFERENCES

1. Mantel N, Haenszel W: Statistical aspects of the analysis of data from retrospective studies of disease. J Natl Cancer Inst 2:719-748, 1959.
2. Meinert CL: Clinical Trials: Design, Conduct, and Analysis. Oxford, Oxford University Press, 1989.
3. Gehan A: The determination of the number of patients required in a follow-up trial of new chemotherapeutic agent. J Chronic Dis 13:346-353, 1961.
4. Herson J: Predictive probability early termination plans for phase II clinical trials. Biometrics 35:775-783, 1979.
5. Lee YJ, Staquet M, Simon R: Two-stage plans for patient accrual in phase II cancer clinical trials. Cancer Treat Rep 63:1721-1726, 1979.
6. Fleming TR: One-sample multiple testing procedure for phase II clinical trials. Biometrics 38:143-152, 1982.
7. Chang MN, Therneau TM, Wieand HS, Cha S: Designs for group sequential phase II clinical trials. Biometrics 43:865-874, 1987.
8. Simon R: Optimal two-stage designs for phase II clinical trials. Control Clin Trials 10:1-10, 1989.
9. Therneau TM, Wieand HS, Chang M: Optimal designs for a grouped sequential binomial trial. Biometrics 46:771-781, 1990.
10. Bryant J, Day R: Incorporating toxicity considerations into the design of two-stage phase II clinical trials. Biometrics 51:1372-1383, 1995.
11. Thall PF, Simon RM, Estey EH: Bayesian sequential monitoring designs for single-arm clinical trials with multiple outcomes. Stat Med 14:357-379, 1995.
12. Pocock SJ: Clinical Trials: A Practical Approach. New York, Wiley, 1984, pp 182-186.
13. Taves DR: Minimization: a new method of assigning patients to treatment and control groups. Clin Pharmacol Ther 15:443-453, 1974.
14. Pocock SJ, Simon R: Sequential treatment assignment with balancing for prognostic factors in the controlled clinical trial. Biometrics 31:103-115, 1975.
15. Freedman LS, White SJ: On the use of Pocock and Simon's method for balancing treatment numbers over prognostic factors in the controlled clinical trial. Biometrics 32:691-694, 1976.
16. Begg CB, Iglewicz B: A treatment allocation procedure for sequential clinical trials. Biometrics 36:81-90, 1980.
17. Gail MH: Eligibility exclusions, losses to follow-up, removal of randomized patients, and uncounted events in cancer clinical trials. Cancer Treat Rep 69:1107-1113, 1985.
18. Kaplan EL, Meier P: Nonparametric estimation from incomplete observations. J Am Statist Assoc 53:457-481, 1958.
19. Parmar KB, Machin D: Survival Analysis: A Practical Approach. New York, Wiley, 1995.

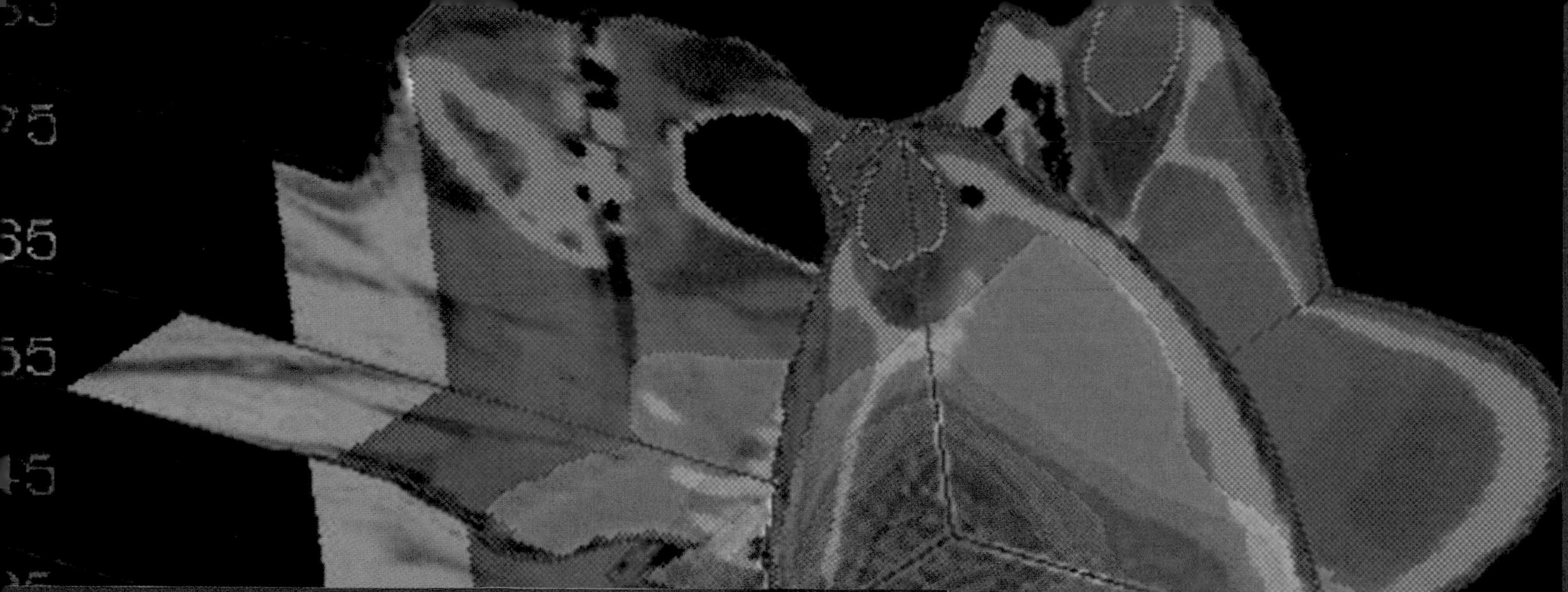

SECTION II

TECHNIQUES AND MODALITIES

CHAPTER 13

BRACHYTHERAPY

Alvaro A. Martinez

Brachytherapy, a term from the Greek language, means "therapy at a short distance." It was increasingly used in the treatment of malignant tumors shortly after the discovery of radium 226 by Marie Curie. In 1960, Henschke[1] published the first paper on afterloading low-dose-rate (LDR) brachytherapy in gynecologic malignancies and later in other tumors. Following soon was a publication describing the Fletcher-Suite afterloading applicators.[2]

Brachytherapy, used as an integral part of cancer treatment for almost a century, sustained a rapid growth with the development of afterloading devices and the introduction of artificial radionuclides.[3,4] In 1961, Henschke[5] developed the first high-dose-rate (HDR) machine using small cobalt sources of high activity. He and his associates stated, "On the basis of our limited experience with such short treatment times in the last 3 years, we feel that they may be used with impunity if the total dose is divided into more fractions."[6] In later reports, they reasoned that moving source remote afterloaders could be used with all gamma-emitting radioisotopes, but ^{137}Cs appeared most suitable, except in the case of short treatment times, for which ^{60}Co and ^{192}Ir would be preferable because of their higher specific activities. New isotopes were available for brachytherapy, including ^{198}Au, ^{60}Co, ^{137}Cs, and ^{192}Ir; a few years later ^{125}I and ^{252}Cf, and more recently, ^{241}Am, ^{103}Pd, ^{169}Yb, ^{75}Se, and ^{145}Sm have been added to our armamentarium. The widespread use of remote afterloading devices has enhanced the clinical applications of brachytherapy and has practically eliminated radiation exposure to the operators. Furthermore, in many parts of the world, HDR brachytherapy has supplanted LDR brachytherapy with equivalent clinical results. According to International Commission on Radiation Units (ICRU) Report No. 38,[7] dose rates of .4 to 2 Gy/h are referred to as LDR, those in the range of 2 to 12 Gy/h are medium-dose rate (MDR), and those greater than 12 Gy/h are HDR.

The distribution of dose around radioactive sources depends on the physical properties of the isotopes, including the encapsulation and activity of the sources, and the inverse-square law. At distances greater than three times the physical length of a source, the inverse-square law applies within practical approximation; at closer distances, the dosimetry is more complex.

To meet all clinical situations, a variety of radioisotopes must be available. However, the most commonly used are ^{226}Ra or ^{137}Cs for intracavitary and ^{192}Ir for interstitial LDR implants. Iodine 125 seeds are widely used for permanent implants in less accessible areas and for tumors that require surgical exposure at laparotomy or thoracotomy, such as lung, head and neck, pancreas, or prostate. Other isotopes, such as ^{103}Pd, ^{241}Am, and ^{152}Cf, have been introduced in clinical practice.

INTERSTITIAL BRACHYTHERAPY

Afterloading

The flexible carrier method was first used with radon seeds by Hames[8] in 1937 and later by Morton and associates,[9] who used cobalt sources. Afterloading was systematized by Henschke and colleagues at Memorial Sloan-Kettering Cancer Center (MSKCC) in New York City. Since the early 1960s, Pierquin and colleagues[10] in Europe popularized the afterloading Henschke techniques with personal modifications and contributed the use of "hairpins" for afterloading with thicker iridium wires mainly for lesions of the oral cavity and oropharynx. Several reports in the literature describe techniques and instrumentation for the use of afterloading interstitial therapy with radium and other isotopes such as tantalum wires, ^{192}Ir, and ^{125}I seeds.[11-19]

Removable implants are performed with either stainless-steel needles or semiflexible Teflon or nylon catheters with metallic guides. Using the one-end implant technique, stainless steel or Teflon 16-gauge tubing is cut to the desired length. The distal end of the tubing is crimped but not closed to hold the afterloaded iridium insert in place, still allowing repositioning should it be required. A barium-impregnated plastic button or a metallic button is fitted snugly at the end. This technique is used in head and neck, breast, female urethra, and anal canal sites and for sarcomas.

Through-and-Through Plastic Tubing Technique

Through-and-through plastic tubing technique is used when a tumor can be transfixed from either of two sides (e.g., tongue, lip, buccal mucosa, extremity sarcomas, breast, or neck masses). In locations in which the guide can be placed through the tumor or normal tissues, the 16-gauge metallic guides are inserted at the appropriate distances to achieve the desired placement. After this, the lead of the nylon tube that will contain the ^{192}Ir nylon thread is inserted through the metallic guide and progressively pushed all the way through along with the nylon tube. When the nylon tube is in place, either a barium-impregnated button or a metallic button is crimped or a Teflon ball is placed at the distal end to secure it. When all of the nylon tubing has been implanted, the desired length of the active wire is measured by using dummy seeds, and the wire is cut a few centimeters longer so that it will protrude beyond the skin and be easier to manipulate. After localization x-ray films are taken with inactive wires or seeds (used to determine the length and position of the radioactive material), the ^{192}Ir active sources are prepared and inserted, and the proximal end of the tubing is crimped with a metallic button. Each dummy and corresponding active source or wire can be identified with different color threads and buttons and specific radiopaque patterns to identify each tube or loading on the patient or the implant radiographs. Afterloading of the active sources with either stainless-steel needles or flexible guides is done after the patient is back in the hospital room. Radiation exposure within the operating and recovery rooms is thereby totally avoided.

Removable Iridium 192 Hairpin Technique

The physical characteristics of the Paris technique were described by Pierquin and coworkers in 1964.[10] Metallic gutter guides have been constructed to facilitate insertion of the iridium wires. The usual separation of the legs is 1.2 cm, although .9- or 1.5-cm separation can be used. The standard gutter length is 2.5, 3, 4, or 5 cm. Iridium wire ends are inserted along the gutters and held in place with a fine-tip clamp while the gutter guide is removed. Gutter guides should allow for a predictable insertion of the hairpin, which results in an acceptable geometry and homogeneous dose distribution of the implant. The gutter guide technique is used primarily in smaller tumors of the oral cavity and in the anal region.

Removable Iodine 125 Plastic Tube Implants

Clarke and coworkers[20,21] at William Beaumont Hospital (WBH) described a temporary removable ^{125}I plastic tube implant technique. Iodine 125 seeds, 4.5 mm in length, were used with interseed spacing within the ribbons (from seed center to seed center) ranging from 4.5 (seeds back to back) to 12.5 mm (8-mm spacers). The operative technique using hollow stainless-steel 17-gauge trocars is identical to the ^{192}Ir implant procedure. Iodine 125 dosimetry is somewhat more complex because iodine seed dose distributions are more anisotropic, fall off more rapidly with distance, and are more sensitive to tissue heterogeneities than those of ^{192}Ir sources. However, the ^{125}I tubes must have a greater diameter to house the ^{125}I seed ribbons, which are larger than the ^{192}Ir ribbons. The seed ribbons are prepared by loading loose seeds into the hollow ribbons; the seeds are separated by spacers and held in position by a "pusher." The open end of the seed ribbon is heated for sealing. The seed separation varies depending on the activity, the geometry of the implant, and the desired dose rate, which is individualized for each patient and determined after the procedure in the operating room is completed. The most common clinical applications of temporary ^{125}I seeds are episcleral plaque therapy for ocular melanoma and volume implants in the breast, brain, sarcomas, and head and neck. Of particular relevance is its use in pediatric brachytherapy to decrease the dose to growing neighboring organs.

Compared with the ^{192}Ir implants, use of the ^{125}I seed ribbons requires additional physicist or dosimetrist time to assemble and disassemble the ribbons. This is offset by a compensatory decrease in other tasks that are required for the preparation of the ^{192}Ir seeds or wires.

Because of the lower energy of ^{125}I, shielding is easily accomplished, and doses to neighboring organs are lower. For example, when breast cancer is treated with ^{125}I seeds, the dose to the thyroid gland and opposite breast is much diminished when compared with ^{192}Ir. Similarly, for pelvic and lower extremity brachytherapy, ovarian, vaginal, and uterine dosages are significantly decreased with ^{125}I seeds. The lower energy of ^{125}I seeds also results in increased safety during the operation and decreased exposure to the nurses and paramedical personnel caring for the patient.

Permanent Interstitial Iodine 125 Implants

A system with 10 ^{125}I seeds contained within a braided synthetic absorbable carrier has been developed for implants in a shallow plane of tissue or for a tumor site that is inaccessible to standard implant devices.[22,23] The ^{125}I seeds are spaced at 1.0-cm intervals, center to center. The carrier retains a half-circle, taper-point surgical needle. Each strand of 10 seeds is contained within a stainless-steel tubular ring, which effectively shields radiation. The unopened package has a surface dose rate of less than .2 mR/h for a loading of ten .5-mCi seeds. Consequently, it can be handled and stored without additional shielding.

In circumstances in which the supplied surgical needle is unsuitable, it can be replaced by a tie-on needle (e.g., a French spring-eye needle). The placement of the strands and spacing of the seeds should follow appropriate dosimetric considerations. Martinez and associates described a methodology to insert seeds into an absorbable suture[24] and to sterilize them for intraoperative use.[25] The absorbable carrier material and ^{125}I seeds are implanted in the tumor tissues by successive advancing of the needle and gentle pulling of the carrier. The carrier material is absorbed by body tissue; the rate depends on the nature of the implanted tissue. Intramuscular implantation studies in rats showed that the absorption of the carrier is minimal until the 40th postoperative day. Absorption is essentially complete after 60 to 90 days.

Goffinet and coworkers[26] at Stanford University reported on 64 intraoperative ^{125}I implants with absorbable Vicryl suture carriers performed in 53 patients with head and neck cancers, many of them recurrent after initial definitive radiation therapy. Among 14 patients who had received no prior therapy, local control was achieved in 10 (71%), and 5 (40%) were alive 2 to 45 months after therapy. Among 34 patients who had received prior therapy, local control was achieved in 20 (59%), and no recurrences developed in any head and neck site in 13 (38%). Complications were noted in 7 (50%) of 14 patients treated definitively, including skin ulceration and intraoral and intrapharyngeal ulceration, which usually healed. In 34 patients who had ^{125}I suture implants after prior therapy, 7 (20%) had complications after the procedure. In a variation of this technique, the ^{125}I suture material is sewed through Gelfoam, which in turn is secured to the tumor bed with special clips.

TEMPLATES

A variety of templates have been designed in an attempt to more easily place interstitial sources and to obtain more homogeneous doses with implants.

Syed-Neblett Templates

Several Syed-Neblett templates are commercially available. These have been individualized by disease site.

Gynecologic

A template primarily used for gynecologic tumors consists of two Lucite plates joined by six screws that tighten to grasp as many as 38 afterloading, hollow, stainless-steel needles. An additional six needles fit into grooves of a 2-cm-diameter plastic vaginal cylinder that is placed inside an opening in the middle of the template. These needles are arranged in concentric circles or arcs with a spacing of 1 cm between adjacent needles. A 4 × 10-cm area can be implanted in a butterfly distribution. The 17-gauge needles supplied with the templates are 20 cm long, but they can be shortened to treat more shallow areas. The vaginal cylinder has a central opening for placement of a tandem if desired.

Rectal

A rectal template is similar to the one just described, but the two plates contain three concentric circular rings with a total of 36 needles with 1-cm spacing. Cylindrical volumes with diameters of 2, 4, or 6 cm can be implanted. A rectal tube can be placed in the central hole if necessary, but this hole can be left open if the template is placed in an area not covering the anus, such as the vulva.

Prostatic

Puthawala and associates[27] described a prostate template used to guide the insertion of metallic source guides transperineally. The template consists of two concentric rings with radii of 1 and 2 cm, containing 6 and 12 guide holes, respectively. Up to 18 metallic source guides (17-gauge, 20-cm-long needles) are inserted transperineally through the prostate and seminal vesicles as indicated. The tips of the guides are usually 1 cm above the level of the bladder neck. The template is fixed to the perineum by 00 silk sutures, and the space between the perineum and the template is filled with gauze soaked in antibiotic cream.

Urethral

The urethral template has two concentric rings with 17 needles with the same 1-cm spacing as the rectal template. A cylindrical volume with either a 2- or 4-cm diameter is implanted with this template. This is a single plate with no machine screws to other plates. A Foley urethral catheter is inserted through the central opening to drain the urinary bladder.

Modified Perineal Template

Hockel and Muller[28] described a modified Syed-Neblett type perineal template for HDR interstitial brachytherapy of gynecologic malignancies. The template can easily be disassembled after insertion of the central needles into the pelvis, allowing cystoscopic and rectoscopic control of the needle position. Needles penetrating the bladder or the rectum can be repositioned before reassembling the template, eliminating a high-irradiation zone in tumor-free bladder and rectum walls.

Martinez Universal Perineal Interstitial Template

The Martinez Universal Perineal Interstitial Template (MUPIT) was designed to treat locally advanced or recurrent tumors in the prostate, anorectal, perineal, or gynecologic areas. The device consists of two acrylic cylinders, one that can be placed in the vagina and the other in the rectum, an acrylic template with an array of holes that allows placement of the metallic guides in the tissues to be implanted, and a cover plate.[29] The cylinders are placed in the vagina, rectum, or both and fastened to the templates so that a fixed geometric relationship among the tumor volume, normal structures, and source placement is preserved throughout the course of the implantation. When the MUPIT interstitial template is used, no central intracavitary sources are inserted, except in some patients requiring an intrauterine tandem (beyond the volume treated with the interstitial sources). Differential loading (using ^{192}Ir seeds of different activity) has always been used for the MUPIT implants to optimize LDR dose distribution.

Template Versus Intracavitary Brachytherapy in Locally Advanced Gynecologic Tumors

Patients with locally advanced or recurrent gynecologic malignancies have relatively few treatment options. Radical surgery and traditional irradiation have been associated with high rates of local failure and can produce significant morbidity. Local recurrence rates range from 24% to 45% following radical hysterectomy for patients with large lesions.

Results with definitive radiation using intracavitary treatment as a boost have served as a benchmark for comparison. In advanced stage or bulky disease, however, local control rates drop to 25% to 60%. In the patterns of care study, local control in stage III disease was only 49%. Local control rates of 60% have been reported in stage II disease with lesions greater than 6 cm. Despite these aggressive therapies, local failure has been thought to be secondary to inadequate tumor clearance by surgery or inadequate coverage and/or dose inhomogeneities by radiotherapy.

In an effort to improve on these results, LDR transperineal interstitial brachytherapy techniques were developed as a supplement to external beam radiation therapy (EBRT). Prempree[30] used radium needle implants in conjunction with a tandem in 49 patients with stage IIIB cervical carcinoma. All patients were followed for a minimum of 5 years. The control rate in the cervix, vagina, and parametrium was 84% and the major complication rate was 8%. Gaddis and colleagues[31] have reported the results of treating 75 patients with primary cervical carcinoma using the Syed-Neblett template. With a median follow-up of 17 months, the overall pelvic control rate was 71% (77% in stage IE/IIA, 80% in stage IIB, 54% in stage III, and 0% in stage IV). It is difficult to compare interstitial brachytherapy with traditional intracavitary treatment owing to differences in patient populations, length of follow-up, and methods of reporting results.

Monk and coworkers[32] have reported results in 70 patients with stage II, III, or IVA cervical cancer treated with interstitial therapy using the Syed-Neblett template retrospectively compared with 61 patients with similar disease treated with intracavitary treatment. They reported similar results in stage III and IVA patients; however, patients with stage II disease had a significantly improved 5-year disease-free survival (50% versus 21%) and 5-year local control (61% versus 32%) with intracavitary treatment. A greater percentage of the patients in the interstitial group had unknown tumor size (27% versus 7%), and the stage distribution was slightly in favor of the intracavitary group.

Gupta and associates[33] reviewed the outcomes of patients with locally advanced or recurrent gynecologic malignancies who were treated with LDR brachytherapy using the MUPIT. The 3-year actuarial local control rate, disease-free survival, and overall survival for all patients were 60%, 55%, and 41%, respectively. For patients with primary cervical cancer, the 3-year actuarial local control rate was 44%. However, 12 of the 30 patients with primary cervical cancer had disease volume of 100 cm^3 or greater. In patients with recurrent disease, the control rates were 68%. The overall complication rate was 13%. These results suggest that in patients with locally advanced or recurrent disease, interstitial implants using the MUPIT applicator can produce acceptable results with acceptable rates of toxicity.

Some concern exists regarding operator variability for interstitial implants. Although patient numbers are small, Gupta and associates[33] retrospectively analyzed local control with respect to physician performing the implant. No difference in outcome was found for those patients undergoing this procedure by the senior author versus the other four operators.[33]

In Gupta and associates' report,[33] 41% of the patients had recurrent disease, 22% of the patients had received prior irradiation, and 26% had disease greater than 100 cm^3 in volume. The 3-year local control rate with a disease volume of 100 cm^3 or less was 89%. The 3-year actuarial local control rate in the 15 patients who had received prior irradiation was 49%. The major complication rate using interstitial treatment in this group of patients was only 13%.

Russell and colleagues[34] have reported their results with reirradiation of recurrent gynecologic malignancies using intracavitary treatment in 25 patients. They report crude local control rates of 56% and major complication rates of 50%. Similar results have been reported by Puthawala and coworkers[35] using interstitial implants for recurrent pelvic malignancies. After a minimum follow-up of 2 years in 40 patients, they reported a pelvic control rate of 67% and a grade 4 complication rate of 15%.

DOSE-RATE DELIVERY ISSUES

Low-Dose Rate: Manual Versus Remote Afterloading

Few studies compare results of intracavitary therapy with LDR remote afterloading implants with those for manual afterloading systems because there are no significant changes in isotopes or dose rates. Battermann and Szabol[36] reported their experience with the LDR Selectron afterloading machine for patients with cancer of the cervix using the same treatment policy as previously used for manual afterloading. Local tumor control and complications were the same for both groups.

High-Dose Rate Remote Afterloading: Potential Advantages Over Low-Dose Rate

Some of the advantages of HDR remote afterloading techniques relative to LDR manual or remote afterloading are as follows:

1. Patient treatment and immobilization times are short; therefore, complications resulting from prolonged bed rest, such as pulmonary emboli, are eliminated; general anesthesia is avoided, and patient discomfort is decreased.
2. Use of external applicator fixation devices during the short treatment time allows more constant and reproducible geometry of source positioning. Dose inaccuracy is minimized since internal organ and patient motion are overcome.
3. Treatment planning and dosimetry are more exact, and optimization is possible using varying source dwelling times. Dose prescribed and dose delivered is the same.
4. Treatment can be performed on an outpatient basis without the need for an operating room and hospitalization; thus, health care costs are reduced.

Fractionation and adjustment of total dose are crucial factors in lowering the frequency of complications without compromising the results of therapy with HDR systems.[37] Scalliet and coworkers[38] compared HDR and LDR in gynecologic brachytherapy, especially regarding the conversion of LDR total dose into equivalent HDR dose per fraction and total dose. Calculation of biologically equivalent schedules requires knowledge of repair capacity and repair kinetics of tumors and normal tissues, both of which influence the biologic effect of any radiation dose. The emerging clinical experience with HDR is equivalent to that of classic LDR. However, although treatment with LDR has proven to be quite tolerant to a lack of absolute precision, that would be disastrous with HDR techniques due to large dosages per fraction.

Pulsed-Dose Rate Brachytherapy

Pulsed-dose rate (PDR) was proposed[39] to exploit the advantages of HDR computer-controlled remote afterloading technology. It was noted that by varying the dwell times of the stepping source, dose optimization could be achieved, maintaining the potential benefits of LDR, including improved radiation protection. The inactive source times, when the sources are in the safe between pulses, should allow for improved nursing care and patient visiting. The pulse delivers about .5 Gy per 10-minute exposure every hour. As the dose rate gradually decreases because of radioactive decay of the source, somewhat longer periods of pulsed times are required.

Pulsed LDR brachytherapy has been made possible with the development of commercial devices modified from HDR intracavitary brachytherapy applications. A single high-activity source that can be programmed for a dwell time in each position at appropriate periods, to reflect the required differential loading of activity, and with a dose rate of .5 Gy/h, has been used at a few institutions. Using the linear-quadratic formula, Brenner and Hall[39] determined the pulse lengths and frequencies based on radiobiologic data that were equivalent to conventional continuous LDR irradiation. They determined that for a regimen of 30 Gy in 60 hours, a 1-hour period between 10-minute pulses might produce up to a 2% increase in late effects probability.

Visser and associates[40] described a radiobiologic model and equations to determine the PDR or HDR schedules equivalent to certain LDR schedules, similar to that proposed by Brenner and Hall,[39] by applying probable ranges for the values for alpha/beta ratio and repair time. They concluded that eight fractions of 1 to 1.5 Gy per 24 hours, up to 3 hours apart, would be equivalent to commonly used LDR treatment schedules. Hall pointed out that Visser and associates[40] showed that the more different the proposed regimen is from continuous LDR, the longer the overall treatment time needs to be extended to preserve the therapeutic ratio.

Erickson and Shadley,[41] using in vitro irradiation experiments on rodent tumor cell lines, showed that there was a slight increase in cell killing with PDR relative to continuous LDR irradiation of hourly 5-, 10-, or 20-minute pulses, or a 20-minute pulse every 2 hours. In no case was the increased killing statistically significant, and the cells did appear to be clinically indistinguishable as determined by the Brenner and Hall criteria.

In an editorial, Hall and Brenner[42] noted that although the linear-quadratic model has been widely used and accepted, it has not been tested in extreme cases and that the biologic data needed for the model calculations are not well known. Armour, White, and colleagues[43,44] at WBH developed a reproducible rat model for comparing late rectal toxicity from different brachytherapy techniques, that is, LDR, HDR, and PDR. Later, Armour and coworkers using the same rat model reported PDR results with a very strong dependence of late rat rectal injury on radiation pulse size.[45]

Although PDR has prospered in Europe and Asia, unfortunately, in the United States it has floundered, because the Nuclear Regulatory Committee (NRC) requires that a physicist and/or radiation oncologist (or other suitably qualified person) be present throughout the treatment, which is almost impossible to accomplish in a long treatment schedule in a hospital setting.

QUALITY ASSURANCE, RADIATION SAFETY, AND IMPLANT REMOVAL

Dosimetry

In the United States and most other countries, the brachytherapy dosimetric calculations are performed with the aid of computers. Orthogonal radiographs, stereo-shift, and/or computed tomography (CT)-based reconstruction are used. The greatest advantage of CT, magnetic resonance imaging (MRI), or ultrasound-based reconstruction is the ability to see the relationship of the tumor boundaries, surrounding normal tissues, and catheters and applicators. This allows the most critical assessment of implant quality parameters such as target volume coverage, dose homogeneity through the implant volume, dose to neighboring critical structures, and three-dimensional (3D) graphics for documentation of isodose distributions. For interstitial brachytherapy the use of image-guided dosimetric analysis with CT, MRI, or ultrasound is strongly recommended.

It is extremely important in the use of brachytherapy to formulate and strictly observe radiation safety procedures at each institution in compliance with U.S. NRC regulations. The safety of personnel, patients, and visitors is based on three factors: (1) time of radiation exposure as short as possible, (2) distance as great as practically allowed between the radioactive sources and the operator, and (3) shielding to diminish radiation exposure to all concerned.

Careful quality control procedures should be followed in the prescription and calculation of doses; preparation, calibration, and handling of radioactive sources; and verification of treatment parameters. If promptly discovered, an error in brachytherapy can be corrected, but this is more difficult to do than in fractionated EBRT. The prescription is written on a form that is given to the brachytherapy medical physicist specifying the configuration of source strengths for intracavitary treatment or the array of active lengths and linear activity. Treatment duration is generally determined after conjointly reviewing the computer isodose rate distributions and is double-checked with hand calculations. The physicist documents the preparation of sources in a treatment logbook, on a source inventory sheet that is posted on the patient's door, and on a magnetic source inventory in the radioactive source room. A well-type ion chamber is used to verify the source activity in accord with American Association of Physicists in Medicine (AAPM) recommendations.

When manual intracavitary afterloading is used, for the sake of prompt patient loading, the various cesium tubes are color-coded. The attending physician or resident (after verifying the source loading) and the dosimetrist/physicist load the applicator in the patient. The loading time is documented by the physician, and the physicist measures the radiation exposure levels around the patient and arranges lead shields appropriately. The nursing division is also actively involved in checking every 3 to 4 hours that applicators or sources do not become dislodged over the course of treatment. For further discussion of LDR brachytherapy quality assurance techniques and programs, the reader is referred to a review by Williamson[46] and published AAPM recommendations.

The physician's order sheets contain the home telephone number and the beeper number of at least two physicians who can be contacted in case of an emergency if source removal is required. The attending physician or resident is responsible for the unloading of an implant. Afterward, the physician counts the sources removed and places them in a lead carrier. After removal of the sources, the patient is surveyed to ensure that no radioactivity remains in the patient or in the patient's room. The time of unloading is documented, and all radiation warning signs are removed from the patient's door. The source curator checks that all sources have been recovered and returns the sources to their designated storage area. The magnetic inventory board is revised to show that the sources have been returned to their storage area. Additionally, source recovery is documented in the source logbook.

Safety Regulations in the United States

The U.S. NRC and states that have negotiated agreements with NRC regulate the use and safety of all reactor by-product materials (excluding naturally occurring radionuclides such as ^{226}Ra and electronically generated radiation). Specific regulations for medical use of by-product materials are outlined in Title 10 Code of Federal Regulations, Part 35.

At the institutional level, a radiation safety committee and radiation safety officer are responsible for supervising the use of by-product materials and seeing that all NRC license requirements are in compliance. The NRC mandates an institutional quality management program (QMP) philosophy aimed to zero incidence of misadministration or recordable events. When misadministration occurs, the licensee is required to report to the NRC by telephone within 24 hours and in writing within 15 days; the patient and referring physician should be informed verbally within 24 hours and by written report within 15 days. If informing the patient would be medically harmful, a relative or friend of the patient must be selected to receive this information. A QMP review must be conducted at least annually to determine compliance and whether modifications are required. For HDR or PDR procedures, the NRC requires the presence of an authorized radiation oncologist and physicist at all times when a procedure is being performed. Imaging or techniques must be in place to verify source position and accuracy before a procedure is performed. A physicist must verify the accuracy of plan input date, dose calculation, and information transfer. Before treatment, the technologist verifies treatment site, isotope, total dose, dose per fraction and treatment modality, program sequence of source position, and dwell times, which must agree with the treatment plan calculation; the technologist also must verify that the HDR treatment channels are correctly connected to corresponding applicators. Before treatment, the attending physician must review the record and sign forms as required.

Radiation Safety in the Operating Room

If radioactive sources are prepared in the operating room (preloaded needles for prostatic implants), a workbench with shielding should be placed in one comer of the room so no one except the brachytherapy technician preparing them is exposed to radiation. The workbench is designed with a frontal working area with an L-shaped lead screen to protect the trunk, lower extremities, and medial aspect of the arms. In addition, a leaded-glass screen reduces exposure to the eyes. Behind the barrier there should be a lead well to store the remaining radioactive material while the individual needles or seeds are being prepared for insertion into the patient. The bench is covered with sterile drapes.

Exposure to the eyes and hands can be reduced only by distance and by dexterity gained through experience. All radioactive sources should be handled with long instruments. After insertion of the sources and removal of the patient, the remaining sources should be carefully inventoried and the operating room surveyed using a Geiger-Muller detector.

Removal of Implants

The carrier housing the interstitial implants (nylon catheter) can generally be removed in the brachytherapy suite and/or in the patient's room. For patients with standard implants of the oropharynx or for less-than-cooperative patients, it is preferable, and sometimes essential, to remove the implant in the operating room, at times with the patient under general anesthesia; thus, adequate lighting, suction, and assistants are available. Bleeding at the time of catheter removal is infrequent, but when it occurs, it may cause the patient or the assisting staff to panic. Firm and steady pressure with a finger on a compress over the bleeding point for several minutes usually is adequate treatment; occasionally a surgeon's assistance is required for bleeding control.

For the sake of radiation protection, it is advisable, initially, to uncrimp the metallic buttons and carefully remove the radioactive sources, which are accounted for and immediately placed in a portable safe or shielded cart. After this is done, each individual tube is removed by freeing one end. For oral cavity or oropharynx implants, we prefer to cut the two ends of the tubing at the skin and pull it out through the oral cavity. A previously tied silk thread inside the cavity on the nylon tube loop is helpful in this maneuver.

BRACHYTHERAPY TECHNIQUES FOR SPECIFIC SITES

Brain Implants

Brachytherapy may allow delivery of interstitial irradiation boosts to primary brain tumors after conventional EBRT or may be used to treat recurrent brain tumors. Patients with primary malignant brain tumors who received initial doses of more than 50 Gy of EBRT to the whole brain survived 20.5 weeks longer than did patients treated by surgery only. Walker and colleagues,[47] analyzing the Brain Tumor Study Group data, showed stepwise increments in survival in patients receiving 50, 55, or 60 Gy. At the same time, it is well known that higher irradiation doses may significantly increase risk of brain necrosis.

At some institutions, permanent implants have been used; however, removal implants are more popular. The advantages of removable implants include (1) greater control of the irradiation dose because the source placement can be rearranged and differential activity can be used to improve dose distribution; (2) no possibility of migration of the radioactive sources; (3) easy removal of the sources if emergency decompressive surgery is required; and (4) provision of dose rates greater than .3 Gy/h, which may be necessary to treat fast-growing malignant brain tumors as suggested by some data.

Several techniques have been used for interstitial irradiation of the brain, some using multiple planar implants (with or without templates) and ^{192}Ir wires or seeds and others with a few higher intensity ^{125}I sources. The same concept has been used in the treatment of patients with tumors of the base of the skull or spine, placing .5-mCi ^{125}I sources intraoperatively at the time of neurosurgical tumor resection. Doses of 50 to 200 Gy were delivered with permanently implanted sources.

Prados and coworkers[48] reported results in 56 patients with glioblastoma multiforme and 32 patients with anaplastic glioma treated with temporary ^{125}I interstitial implants. Patients received external irradiation (median, 59.4 Gy), most with concomitant hydroxyurea, followed by interstitial implant. Eight patients (14%) survived 3 years or longer, and 16 (29%) survived 2 years or longer. A second operation was necessary in 50% of patients to remove symptomatic necrosis produced by the implant. Prolonged steroid use was necessary in many patients.

Another technique described was developed at Washington University using radioactive sources placed in Teflon catheters inserted into the brain under direct CT monitoring. Multiple burr holes are made in the brain at I-cm intervals (patient under local anesthesia). The locations of the burr holes are determined using a template, which is attached to a stereotactic frame and to the patient's head. The template used is a thick acrylic block containing a 7 × 7-cm array of 49 holes spaced at 1-cm intervals. The holes along the diagonal axis of the template have slightly larger diameters to provide a method of orientation for each CT slice. The tumor is outlined on the CT screen with the aid of intravenously administered contrast material. The template is placed against the scalp at the site allowing best access to the tumor, usually a lateral surface. Intravenous contrast material is administered and scanning is performed with the scan plane parallel to the rows of the template. The target volume for the implant is the contrast-enhancing ring seen on CT scans, with a 1.0-cm margin. The number of catheters required to encompass the target at each level is determined at the CT console. Seventeen-gauge catheters, 15 cm long spaced at 1-cm intervals, are then placed through the template into the brain to the desired depths with CT monitoring. Following the grid pattern, under CT observation, the Teflon angiocatheters with a metallic stylet are inserted through the burr holes into the brain substance to ensure straight and parallel insertion. After the tumor volume is implanted, the length of the radioactive sources is determined, and films, with the distribution of the catheters, are obtained for dosimetry calculations. Dummy seeds and ribbons are loaded in each of the catheters. Once the catheters are secured, the patient is transferred to the intensive care unit, where the dummy sources are replaced by ribbons of active ^{192}Ir seed with a specific activity of about .6 mCi per seed. Metal buttons are attached to the catheters to fasten them to the scalp.

Careful records are maintained of the position and length of all the catheters. Computer-generated isodose calculations are used to determine the dose and distribution in the implant volume. The dose rate ranges from .5 to .8 Gy/h at .5 to 1 cm. In general, the implant duration is 70 to 100 hours to deliver 60 to 70 Gy total dose to the entire tumor. Verification dosimetry with thermoluminescent dosimeters placed in catheters disclosed an agreement of ± 5% to 10% between the computer calculations and the actual doses at any point within the irradiated volume. This method has been used in more than 70 patients at Washington University, most of them with glioblastoma multiforme, sometimes recurrent after external irradiation, and in a few patients with solitary brain metastasis. Fatal intracranial bleeding has been rare (<5%), and edema is not severe enough to represent a significant management problem. Brain necrosis has been observed in about 25% of patients.

Eye

Episcleral Plaque

Episcleral plaque therapy is a cost-effective approach to treat localized intraocular malignancies such as retinoblastoma and choroidal melanoma. Intraorbital tumors (extraocular) such as rhabdomyosarcomas can also be treated. The technique consists of fabricating a small, spherically curved plaque containing radioactive sources, immobilizing the patient's eye, and suturing the plaque onto the sclera opposite the tumor, where it remains for 3 to 10 days. Because of the close proximity of the radioactive sources to the tumor, a highly localized and intense dose of irradiation is delivered to the tumor, which spares more normal tissue than is possible by conventional EBRT techniques and is competitive with the precision of heavy particle therapy.

The Collaborative Ocular Melanoma Study (COMS) was conducted as a multicenter randomized phase III clinical trial comparing eye plaque therapy to enucleation with survival and preservation of vision as end points. The study enrolled 1317 patients and demonstrated equivalent 5-year overall survival of 81% in both arms (see Chapter 28). In the brachytherapy arm, visual acuity decreased over time, with vision 20/200 or worse in 43% of treated eyes. At the interval of 5 years following plaque therapy, enucleation was needed in 10% of patients because of tumor relapse and in 3% due to treatment related complications (see Chapter 28).

Historically, plaque therapy has been delivered using the ^{60}Co plaque system originally developed by Stallard[49] for treatment of retinoblastoma. These plaques are available in a limited range of sizes (8- to 12-mm diameters). Both circular and semicircular-notched plaques are available for treatment of posterior lesions abutting the optic nerve. Although easy to prepare and use, ^{60}Co plaques do not allow customization of the dose distribution, shielding of critical structures, or treatment of eye tumors on an outpatient basis.

Within the COMS clinical trial, ^{125}I seeds were used in conjunction with standardized gold alloy plaques ranging from 12 to 20 mm in diameter.[40] A COMS plaque can be assembled within 30 minutes, almost entirely eliminates the possibility of seed loss during treatment, fixes the seeds in a rigid geometry, and retains a high degree of individualization.

Iodine 125 plaques offer several dosimetric advantages over ^{60}Co plaques. The .5-mm-thick gold plaque almost completely attenuates ^{125}I primary x-rays, providing a high degree of protection (95%) to tissue posterior to the eye. The 2.5- to 3.3-mm-high lip of the COMS plaque produces limited collimation of the ^{125}I x-rays, which reduces the area of the retina treated to a high dose. Moreover, a thick lead foil (.2 mm thick) placed over the patient's eye affords substantial radiation protection, making it possible to treat with plaques on an outpatient basis.

Before plaque fabrication, all relevant imaging studies should be examined to define the basal dimensions and location of the tumor. A good collaboration between ophthalmologists and radiation oncologists is required. A-mode ultrasound study is used to define the maximum height of the tumor. If the tumor height is less than 5 mm, the prescription point is defined at 5 mm. Otherwise, the actual height is used. Fluorescein angiograms are often helpful in determining the posterior boundary of the tumor. When the anterior margin of the tumor is anterior to the equator, every attempt should be made to localize the margin relative to the ora serrata using transillumination. After the basal diameters, height, and location of the tumor are defined, a plaque is fabricated such that its diameter is 2 to 6 mm larger than the assumed diameter of the tumor. A dummy plaque of identical size is used to define the plaque position in the operating room using transillumination as the definitive guide to tumor localization and size. A small caliper should be available for measuring the orthogonal dimensions and location of the tumor relative to the ora serrata. These data should be used as the basis for the final treatment plan. Both fundus view isodose curves, which give the dose distribution on the retinal surface, and the conventional transverse views are useful.

Pterygium

It is common practice to administer radiation therapy after surgical resection of the pterygium, because of the high local recurrence rate (20% to 69%).[50,51] In most institutions a ^{90}Sr β-ray applicator is used for treatment of these patients. The overall diameter of the applicator is 12.7 mm; the center is a circular radioactive disk 5 mm in diameter containing the isotope. The dose rate is generally about 5 Gy/min. Irradiation is begun within 24 hours after resection because local relapse increases with greater time delays.[51]

A lid retractor is inserted to hold the eye open. The cornea and conjunctiva are anesthetized with a few drops of .5% to 1% lidocaine. The applicator is carefully applied on the surface of the resected sclera. Doses of about 10 Gy are delivered. The application is repeated in three consecutive weekly fractions for a total of 30 Gy. If a larger area of resection is to be irradiated, it may require application to two contiguous areas, each receiving the same dose. The lens, which is located at the depth of 3.5 to 5 mm from the surface, receives less than 5% of the dose.[52]

Maxillary Sinus

Rosenblatt and colleagues[53] described the use of a surgical obturator made of vinyl polysiloxane as a carrier for afterloading ^{192}Ir seed ribbons to treat patients with maxillary antrum tumors after partial or total maxillectomy. Two weeks after the surgical procedure, an impression was made of the maxillary cavity, and the obturator mold was built. Multiple nylon catheters were inserted, depending on the geometry and dosimetry of the implant. Prescribed doses were 45 to 70 Gy at .5 cm from the outermost source plane. The obturator mold previously loaded with ^{192}Ir was carefully coated with acylmethacrylate resin to secure it in place and prevent disturbance of the dosimetry once inserted in the surgical cavity.

Nasal Vestibule

Small lesions of the nasal vestibule can be adequately treated with either external or interstitial irradiation, whereas more advanced lesions require a combination of both modalities. Irradiation is an excellent alternative to surgery in the treatment of these tumors because tumor control can be very good and cosmetic results are better than with surgery.[54,55]

These tumors are implanted with single- or double-plane techniques using rigid radium or cesium needles or ^{192}Ir nylon tubing techniques. According to Mendenhall and associates,[54,55] the distal vertical needles (perpendicular to the dorsum of the nose) in each plane may be mounted in a nylon bar to stabilize the distal needles.

For small or large primaries, at WBH we always recommend the use of a cast and/or template to improve the geometric coverage of the implant. Both afterloading, LDR, and HDR treatment techniques can be used. It is important to pack all empty spaces to minimize the cavities. Figure 13-1 illustrates a patient treatment with the cast technique.

Skin and Lip

Interstitial single- or double-plane implants could be performed to encompass the tumor with a safe margin. Doses of 50 to 70 Gy are delivered in 5 to 7 days. Carcinoma of the skin has been treated with surface molds or interstitial brachytherapy.[56] Jorgensen and coworkers[57] reported on 869 patients with squamous cell carcinoma of the lip for whom irradiation was the initial form of treatment in all but 25. Radium implants were used in 766 patients, with local tumor control rates of 93% in T1, 87% in T2, and 75% in T3 tumors. Brachytherapy is recommended over surgery in lesions at or close to the commissure. Functional results are superior to surgery without the postsurgical drooling of saliva.

Nasopharynx

Some investigators have used interstitial techniques, which are more difficult to perform because of difficulty in positioning the needles/seeds in the tumor area and limitation of effective depth dose. Palatal fenestration may be required in patients with lesions in the superior and high posterior nasopharyngeal walls, which are more difficult to reach through the nasal or oral cavities.[58,59] The use of ^{103}Pd seeds for permanent implant of nasopharyngeal tumors has been described by Porrazzo and associates.[60]

Wang[61] described the use of intracavitary brachytherapy alone or combined with external irradiation to boost the dose to the nasopharynx. Two pediatric endotracheal tubes with inner and outer diameters of 5 mm and 6.9 mm, respectively,

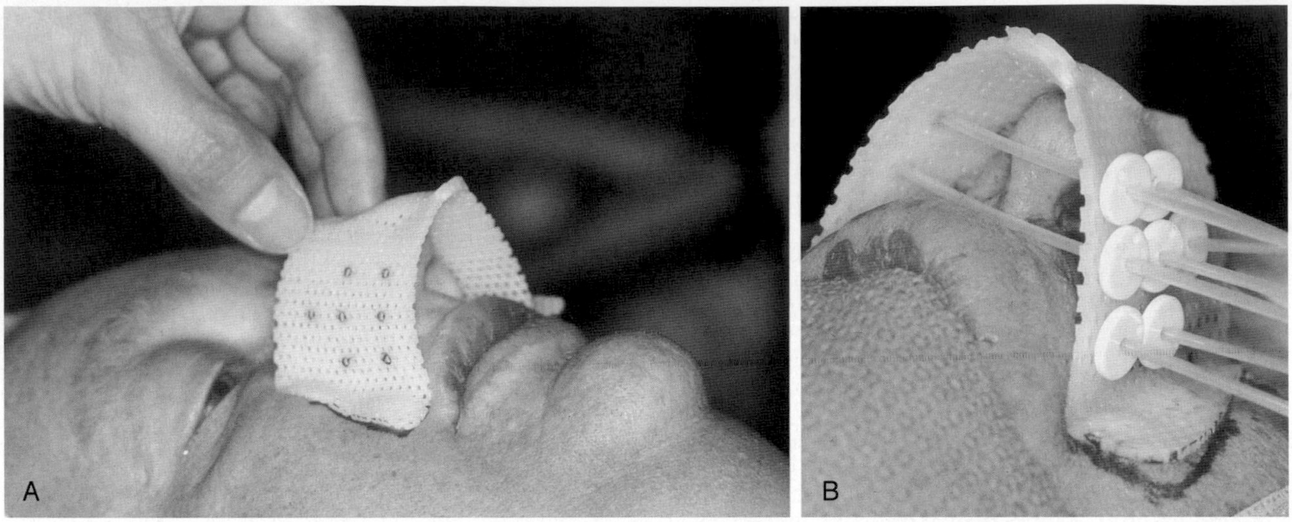

Figure 13-1 Application of a thermoplastic cast. **A,** Standard nasal splint is measured and marked for catheter placement. **B,** The cast in place. The volume below the nares will be packed with wet gauze to provide full scatter (not shown for clarity).

each loaded with two 20-mg RaEq ^{137}Cs sources are used. Local anesthesia of the nasal cavity is achieved using cocaine. The endotracheal tubes are introduced through the nares into the nasopharynx with the head hyperextended. Under fluoroscopic control on the simulator, the tips of the cesium sources are placed at the free edge of the soft palate posteriorly and behind the posterior wall of the maxillary sinus anteriorly. A 5-mL balloon attached to the distal end of the endotracheal tube is inflated for anchoring purposes. The dose reference point is .5 cm below the mucosa of the nasopharyngeal vault; the dose rate is approximately 1.2 Gy/h.

For all interstitial implants in the head and neck area, CT or MRI reconstruction is strongly recommended. Standard orthogonal films and/or stereo-shift techniques are suboptimal.

Oral Cavity

For implants of the oral cavity, it is desirable to outline the tumor with gentian violet, Castellani's paint, or a surgical marker before starting the implantation of sources. For small lesions, the intraoral approach is preferable. For larger lesions, usually the submental approach is recommended.

The anterolateral needles of an implant of the oral cavity should be kept away from the thin mucous membrane that covers the bone in the upper and lower gum, as well as from the periosteum, teeth, and bone. To increase and maintain the distance, a regular fluoride carrier is thickened on the inside by one to four layers (one layer = 2 mm) of lead to increase the distance and shield part of the dose to the mandible.

Floor of Mouth and Tongue

Lesions beneath the tongue, or in the floor of the mouth, usually are implanted through the dorsum of the tongue. The anterolateral needles emerge from the undersurface of the tongue and are reinserted into the floor of the mouth. The implants should extend beyond the visible or palpable tumor by at least 2 cm in all directions. A popular technique of interstitial implants with nylon tubing and ^{192}Ir sources for lesions of the oral tongue or floor of the mouth uses a submental or submaxillary approach for the insertion of metallic guides into the oral cavity. The exit points of the guides in the oral cavity are carefully verified with the index finger of the other hand (through-and-through technique).

The nylon tubing is threaded through the metallic guides and looped around the dorsum of the tongue and exits through a parallel metallic guide. The metallic guides are pulled out externally, and the nylon thread is secured by crimping with a metallic button at one end. The procedure continues as described previously, leaving the other end open momentarily for insertion of the radioactive sources. For the nonloop technique several buttons are placed over the surface of the tongue with the last button being of gold to shield and decrease the dose to the palate and ensure an adequate surface dose. To facilitate removal, it is preferred that a silk thread be tied on the end loop of each nylon tube inside the oral cavity.

After position of the sources is verified on x-ray films using radiopaque inactive dummy sources, the appropriate ^{192}Ir wires (or seeds in nylon tubing) are inserted, and the other end of the larger nylon tube is crimped. For implant reconstruction and assessment of implant quality, CT- or MRI-based dosimetry is recommended.

Marcus and associates[62] described a template for floor-of-mouth implants made of aluminum, stainless steel, or nylon that is individually customized to fit the lesion of each patient. The device is inserted into the floor of the mouth under general anesthesia and is secured by one suture through the submental area, which is tied to a cotton cigarette roll. The active ends of the radium needles may be positioned above the level of the mucosa to ensure an adequate surface dose. Crossing is accomplished by placing a needle parallel to the mucosal surface on the implant device. The system is not afterloaded, but the procedure can be performed rapidly with predictable geometry so irradiation exposure to the operating staff is lower than with the hairpin technique. According to the investigators, the advantage of this technique over use of iridium hairpins is that all needles with the template are rigidly fixed in relationship to one another, and the isodose distributions can be calculated before the procedure or can be modified if necessary by adjusting the arrangement of the needles.

Implantation with rigid needles of the posterolateral border of the tongue via the oral cavity requires pulling the tongue forward to start the implant at the base of the tongue.

The first needle is inserted pointing posteriorly and inferiorly at about 45 degrees; a lesser angle is used for successive needles. At the end of the implant, when the tongue returns to its normal position, the implant needles adopt a vertical position.

The advantage of the iridium hairpin technique over the radium or cesium rigid needles is that the overall source length is shorter for the same active length because of the 6-mm inactive tips at either end of the rigid needles. Furthermore, there are only two vertical sources per hairpin as opposed to three or four radium or cesium needles on each bar so that it is easier to position the hairpins in the tongue. This is particularly helpful in patients with small mouths, trismus, or full dentition, where it is difficult to adequately position the rigid needles.

For early lesions (T1), brachytherapy alone gives excellent local control with minimal impact on salivary gland function. For T2, T3, or T4 lesions, a combination of EBRT followed by brachytherapy is most commonly used.

Base of Tongue

Because of the possibility of airway obstruction, it is imperative to perform an elective temporary tracheostomy before the implant procedure is initiated. Implantation of the base of the tongue (and sometimes the posterolateral border of the oral tongue) is best accomplished by using long metallic needles inserted through the submaxillary/subdigastric region, with the index finger of the other hand in the oropharynx to verify the position of the guide at the exit point, the base of the tongue. As described earlier, the nylon thread is inserted through the tubing into the oropharynx, looped around, and brought out through the opposite guide, thus providing the equivalent of a crossing needle in the cephalad end of the implant. The metallic guides are withdrawn from the submental region and the nylon tubes are secured externally with metallic buttons as described earlier. As in lesions of the oral tongue, a single row of needles with a gold button without a loop could be used. Double-plane or volume implants can be easily performed. After implant localization x-ray films (CT or MRI based) are taken, afterloading ^{192}Ir wire or seeds or ^{125}I seeds in nylon threads are inserted into the nylon tubing or metallic guides, and isodose distributions are obtained. Most patients are treated with EBRT followed by a brachytherapy boost (LDR or HDR) to increase local control and decrease complications related to the temporomandibular joint and middle ear.

Tonsillar Region Including Faucial Arch

Iridium 192 hairpin or plastic tube techniques have been used by Mazeron and coworkers.[63] The nylon tube technique also may be used to implant the soft palate.[64] The iridium hairpin technique is used with one gutter guide placed in the soft palate in the transverse plane and additional gutter guides placed vertically into the anterior tonsillar pillars, depending on the extent of the lesion. Iridium hairpins are afterloaded into the gutter guides, which are removed as described earlier.

Mendenhall and associates[65] reviewed the techniques for implantation of the anterior tonsillar pillars, soft palate, or tonsillar region using two nylon bars, each containing three full-intensity, 2- to 3-cm active-length radium or cesium needles implanted into the anterior tonsillar pillar and the other 1 cm medial to the tonsillar pillar bar, in the base of the tongue. A crossing needle is sometimes included in the anterior pillar bar to ensure adequate mucosal dose. Goffinet and associates[66] developed a method for intraoral tonsillopallatine implants.

Breast Implants as a Boost

Interstitial irradiation of the breast has been used as a boost in conjunction with conservation surgery after the whole organ is given external irradiation (45 to 50 Gy). Bartelink and Borger in Europe[67] and Martinez and Goffinet in the United States[68] pioneered this technique. Selection of patients for this technique is limited to those with an adequate breast volume and lesions less than 5 cm in diameter.

The procedure can be performed with the patient under general anesthesia, although at some institutions it is performed with local anesthetic. Implantation is also performed in conjunction with resection of the primary tumor (and when indicated, the axillary dissection) or as a separate operating room procedure. The former approach has the advantages of eliminating one anesthesia, reducing the cost of treatment, and allowing the surgeon and radiation oncologist to interact closely in determining the extent and location of the tumor bed and to better plan the placement of the needles.

After the volume to be implanted is determined and for free hand implants, lines are drawn on the surface of the breast to determine the position of the planes of the implant. The implant planes are drawn with 1.5-cm separation, and the placement of the metallic or plastic guides is set at 1.2 to 1.5 cm from each other. Depending on the configuration of the breast and the location of the tumor, the needles may be inserted on a coronal or a transverse plane. For template-guided implants, which we strongly recommend, the comers of the template are drawn on the patient's skin. The needles are then placed based on the predrilled hole pattern of the template.

Rigid metallic guides or Teflon catheters with metallic guides are inserted into the breast, passing through the tumor excision site until the end of the guide reaches the opposite portion of the breast. In general, for multiple plane implants the guides for the deep plane are inserted first, followed by those for the superficial planes. For closed cavity implants, percutaneous ultrasound is recommended for needle guidance and good deep plane coverage. Next, the nylon tubing for afterloading insertion of the ^{192}Ir seed nylon thread is inserted through the metallic guides, which are withdrawn progressively. The distal end of the nylon tubing is secured by crimping metallic buttons at the level of the skin surface. The length of the ^{192}Ir seed nylon thread is determined by inserting dummy sources and measuring the bed cavity, which should be .5 to 1.5 cm from the skin surface at both ends to prevent excessive skin dose. Radiopaque dummy sources are inserted into the nylon tubing with appropriate identification (colored) tags. The proximal end of the tubing is left open for future removal of the dummy sources and insertion of the radioactive seeds. Radiographic films (anteroposterior and lateral) of the breast are obtained after the patient is recovered from the anesthesia. However, CT-based reconstruction for dosimetric analysis and implant quality is recommended.

The patient is then taken to her hospital room, and the radioactive sources of appropriate length and strength are inserted into the plastic tubing, which is cut about 2 cm from the skin surface. Metallic buttons are crimped at the level of the skin to secure the plastic tubes in place.

The minimal desired dose rate is .5 to .6 Gy/h. In general, doses of 10 to 20 Gy are delivered to the volume of interest. Optimally, the maximum dose distribution throughout the implant volume should be within 10% to 15% of the minimum tumor dose.

Mansfield and associates[69] described an intraoperative technique at the time of the breast tumor excision. The plastic tubes were loaded with the active sources within 6 hours of surgery. The dose rate was .3 to .5 Gy/h; usual dose was 20 Gy delivered in 50 to 60 hours. Ten days later breast irradiation was begun with tangential fields, 6-MV photons, to deliver 45 Gy at 1.8 Gy per day. The 10-year local tumor control rates for stage T1 and T2 were 93% and 87%, respectively, and the 10-year disease-free survival rates were 82% and 75%, respectively.

Mazeron and associates[70] used a technique for interstitial brachytherapy of the breast with rigid metallic needles inserted through a template in single or double planes. After external breast irradiation (45 Gy in 25 fractions), a boost of 37 Gy to the primary tumor was prescribed at the 85% basal dose rate (Paris system). Implanted volume was adapted to tumor extent by varying the number of sources and active length according to the Paris system rules. Fifty-eight patients were treated with single-plane and 340 with two-plane implants. Local recurrence rates were 10% for T1 (2 of 20), 15% for T2a (21 of 138), 23% for T2b (30 of 129), and 25% for T3 (13 of 53). The local tumor control rates at 15 years were 76% for T1 and T2a and 70% for T2b and T3 lesions. Mean dose rates were .53 Gy/h for patients with local recurrence and .56 Gy/h for recurrence-free patients ($p < .01$). Local tumor control correlations with dose rate and tumor size were shown.

Accelerated Partial Breast Irradiation

Accelerated partial breast irradiation (APBI) is the delivery of a shortened course of adjuvant radiation to the planning target volume (PTV) (lumpectomy cavity plus 1- to 2-cm margin) after breast-conserving surgery. The treatment is completed in 4 to 5 days, thus the term "accelerated treatment."

In an effort to improve the accessibility, convenience, and logistics of breast-conserving therapy (BCT) at WBH, we initiated pilot trials to test the technical feasibility and acute toxicity of interstitial brachytherapy directed only to the tumor bed after lumpectomy in selected patients with early-stage breast cancer treated with BCT.[71] An LDR APBI trial was initiated in 1991; in 1995 we switched to HDR interstitial breast brachytherapy and started an HDR APBI trial. Figure 13-2 demonstrates the application and use of one particular template system.

The interim findings of our in-house protocol treating the tumor bed alone after lumpectomy with LDR interstitial brachytherapy in selected patients with early-stage breast cancer treated with BCT were published by Vicini and associates.[72] From March 1, 1993, through January 1, 1995, 50 women with early-stage breast cancer were entered into a protocol of tumor bed irradiation alone using an interstitial LDR implant. Patients were eligible if their tumor was an infiltrating ductal carcinoma 3 cm or smaller in diameter, surgical margins were clear by at least 2 mm, the tumor did not contain an extensive intraductal component, the axilla was surgically staged with three or fewer nodes involved with cancer, and a postoperative mammogram was performed. Implants were positioned using a template guide delivering 50 Gy over 96 hours to the lumpectomy bed plus a 1- to 2-cm margin. With relative short follow-up, local control, cosmetic outcome, and complications were encouraging.[72] Patients ranged in age 40 to 84 years (median, 65 years). The median tumor size was 10 mm (range, 1 to 25 mm). Seventeen (34%) of 50 patients had well-differentiated tumors, 22 (44%) had moderately differentiated tumors, and in 11 (22%) the tumor was poorly differentiated. Forty-five patients (90%) were node negative, whereas five (10%) had one to three positive nodes. A total of 23 (46%) patients were placed on tamoxifen and 3 (6%) received adjuvant systemic chemotherapy. No patient was lost to follow-up. The median follow-up for surviving patients is 47 months (range, 37 to 59 months). No patient has experienced a local, regional, or distant failure. Three patients have died at 19, 33, and 39 months after treatment. All were without clinical evidence of recurrent disease and all deaths were unrelated to treatment. Good-to-excellent cosmetic results have been observed in 49 (98%) of 50 patients (median cosmetic follow-up was 44 months with a range of 19 to 59 months). No patient has experienced significant sequelae related to the implant.

Vicini and associates[73] published results in 199 breast cancer patients treated with APBI interstitial brachytherapy at WBH using either LDR or HDR treatment. At 5 years, the results (local control, cosmesis) are as good as those obtained with the more standard 6 weeks of whole-breast external beam treatment. Chen and colleagues updated the toxicity analysis in these 199 patients with a mean follow-up of 5.4 years.[74] The long-term toxicity was as low as conventional 6-week treatment. Benitez and colleagues[75] reported on the acute and long-term surgical complications of APBI with interstitial brachytherapy. She reported no increase in either intraoperative, perioperative, or postoperative complications.

Results in various series using APBI with either HDR or LDR techniques are shown in Tables 13-1 and 13-2. Table 13-1 summarizes the phase I/II APBI using interstitial HDR breast

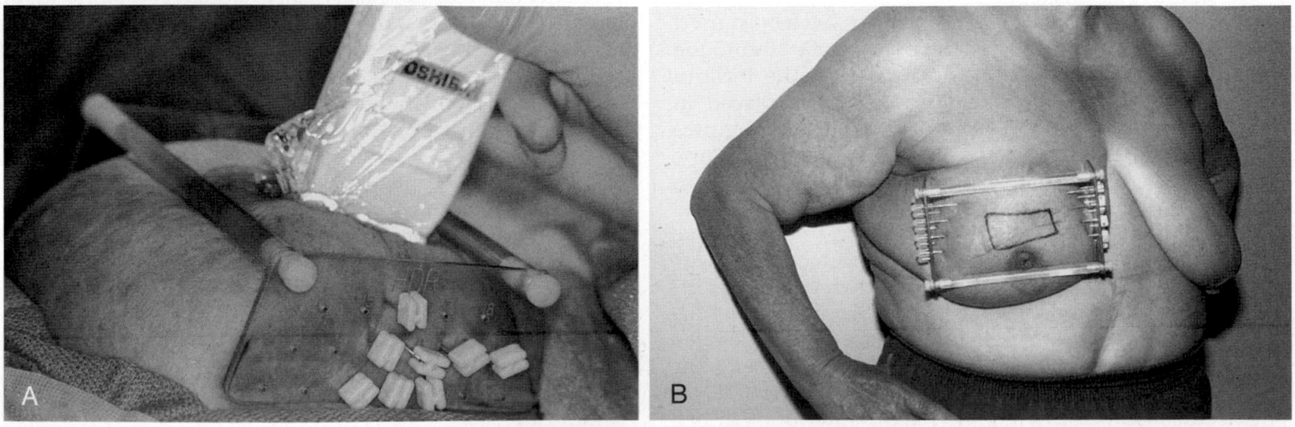

Figure 13-2 Breast template technique. **A,** Accurate application is often aided with intraoperative ultrasonography. **B,** Template in place for fractionated outpatient treatment. Sterile dressings and a support bra will complete the application.

Table 13-1 Partial Breast Irradiation Phase I/II Trials Using High-Dose Rate Brachytherapy

Institution	Patients	F/U (mo)	cGy/fx	Total Dose	% LR	Good Cosmesis (%)
Ochsner Clinic	26	75	400 × 8	3200	<2	75
Exeter, England	45	18	1000 × 2	2000	8.8	95
			700 × 4	2800		
			600 × 6	3600		
Hungary	72	21	520 × 7	3640	2.8	98
			433 × 7	3030		
London, Ontario	39	20	372 × 10	3720	2.6	NS
William Beaumont Hospital	54	>36	400 × 8	3200	0	>90
			340 × 10	3400		
RTOG 95-17	68	NS	340 × 10	3400	NS	NS
Mammosit Device (Proxima Corp)	42	<12 (mo)	340 × 10	3400	NS	NS
Tufts	30	24	340 × 10	3400	NS	NS

Total patients, 376. LR, local relapse; F/U, follow-up; Mo, maths; fx, fraction.

Table 13-2 Partial Breast Irradiation Phase I/II Trials Using Low-Dose Rate Brachytherapy

Institution	Patients	F/U (mo)	cGy	Total Dose	% LR	Good Cosmesis (%)
Ochsner Clinic	25	75	—	4500	<2	75
Guy's Hospital	27	72	40 cGy/hr	5500	37	83
Cionini	90	27	—	50-60 Gy	4.4	NS
William Beaumont Hospital	120	>36	52 cGy/hr	4992	0	>90
RTOG 95-17	31	NS	42 cGy/hr	4500	NS	NS
University Kansas	25	47	—	20-25 Gy	0	100

Total patients, 318.

brachytherapy, and Table 13-2 describes the phase I/II APBI using interstitial LDR breast brachytherapy.

A new applicator, the mammosite balloon, was introduced as an alternative to the multiple catheter brachytherapy technique. Edmundson and associates[76] reported the dosimetry and excellent conformality in dose distribution. Keish and colleagues[77] published the preliminary results using the mammosite balloon technique.

In the summer of 2005, the National Surgical Adjuvant Breast and Bowel Project (NSABP) and Radiation Therapy Oncology Group (RTOG) opened a randomized clinical trial testing the long-term effectiveness of APBI compared with the more standard 6 weeks of whole-breast irradiation. The accrual objective is 3000 women. Alternate acceptable methods of APBI include multiple catheter interstitial brachytherapy techniques (LDR or HDR), mammosite balloon technique, or EBRT.

Lung and Mediastinum

Lung

The group at MSKCC has published several reports[78] on the use of ^{125}I seeds and ^{198}Au grains for permanent perioperative brachytherapy in patients with persistent or recurrent bronchogenic carcinoma after EBRT or for residual disease after surgical resection. The radioactive seeds or grains are directly implanted in the tumor at the time of thoracotomy under general anesthesia.

Temporary removable implants of the mediastinum with or without resection followed by a moderate dose of postoperative EBRT (35 to 40 Gy) have been used alone or combined with ^{125}I implantation of the known primary tumor. The MSKCC report described local tumor control in 78% of patients with stage I and II tumors and 67% of those with stage III lesions.[78] Furthermore, patients with microscopic residual tumor have significantly better tumor control and survival than those with gross residual disease.

Intrabronchial Site

Intrabronchial insertion of LDR or HDR radioactive sources has gained popularity for treatment of patients with symptoms related to malignant airway obstruction. Figure 13-3 illustrates the use of a bronchoscopically placed endobronchial catheter.

Lo and colleagues[79] described results in 110 patients (group 1) treated with LDR brachytherapy (133 procedures) and 59 patients (group 2) treated with HDR brachytherapy (161 procedures). In group 1, patients were treated with one or two sessions of 30 to 60 Gy each, calculated at a 1-cm radius. In patients in group 2, three weekly sessions of 7 Gy each, calculated at a 1-cm radius, were used. EBRT had previously been given to 88% of patients in group 1 and to 85% of patients in group 2. Laser bronchoscopy was performed in 36% of patients in group 1 and in 24% of patients in group 2 before brachytherapy. Clinical or bronchoscopic improvement was noted in 72% of patients in group 1 and in 85% of patients in group 2 ($p > .05$). Complication rates were low and equivalent in both groups. Survival was similar in both groups (median, <6 months).

Esophagus

Irradiation, both external beam and intracavitary, has been used in the curative and palliative treatment of patients with esophageal cancer, either alone or combined with surgery. LDR intracavitary insertions have been performed using ^{226}Ra, ^{60}Co, ^{137}Cs, or ^{192}Ir sources.

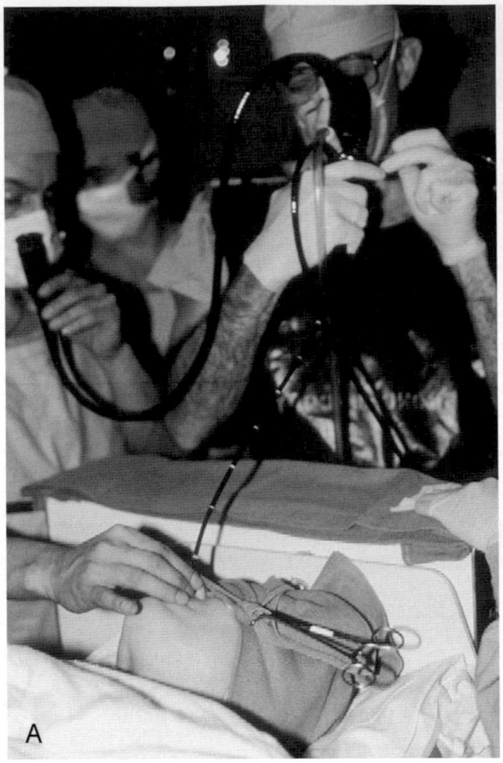

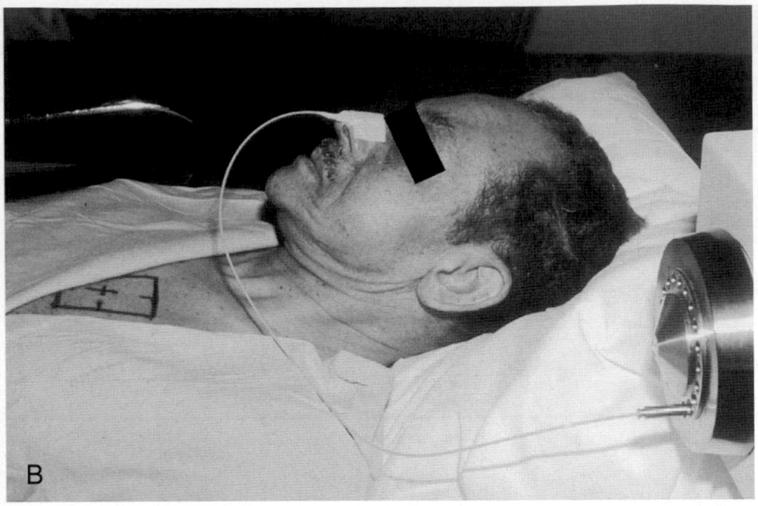

Figure 13-3 Bronchoscope-guided brachytherapy. **A**, Treatment catheter is passed through the biopsy channel of the bronchoscope under direct visualization. **B,** Catheter is taped in position at the nares for treatment.

Flores and coworkers[80] outlined the advantages of intracavitary brachytherapy. Radiation sources can be easily placed at the desired tumor site and subsequently removed. Normal anatomy is preserved. Radiation dose to the tumor is higher than to the adjacent tissues. With remote afterloading, radiation exposure to the staff can be eliminated. The insertion technique can be performed as an outpatient procedure under mild sedation. A soft rubber bougie or French catheter (No. 24 to 26) is inserted, preferably through the nose. The cut-end feeding tube is removed, and the esophageal stricture is dilated to 32-French by a balloon dilator (2 minutes required). The esophageal bougie containing dummy markers for intracavitary treatment is placed and secured in the desired position using fluoroscopy. After the position of the dummy sources is verified on radiograph, the patient is taken to the treatment room where the remote-controlled afterloading device is connected for treatment. If LDR sources are used, the usual dose rate is .4 Gy/h at .5 to 1 cm. Depending on the EBRT dose given, the total intracavitary dose is prescribed to complete 65 to 70 Gy to the tumor volume. With higher dose rates, corresponding lower treatment times and total doses are used.

Syed and colleagues[81] described a comparable technique used in 47 patients with carcinoma of the esophagus (37 with primary and 10 with recurrent lesions). After completion of EBRT, patients received intraluminal brachytherapy to deliver 30 to 40 Gy at .5 cm from the surface of the applicator in two applications, 2 weeks apart. In patients with minimum residual tumor, only one application was used to deliver 20 to 25 Gy minimal tumor dose. Most patients also received concomitant 5-fluorouracil infusion. Intraluminal application was performed with a Syed-Puthawala-Hedger esophageal applicator. The total length of the applicator is 65 cm. Marked rings are present at 10-cm intervals from the tip of the applicator for identification on localization films. The central nasogastric tube can be used for both feeding and suction. The procedure is performed under either general anesthesia or deep sedation and local anesthesia. Extent of the tumor, stricture, ulceration, and impending tracheoesophageal fistula are evaluated by endoscopy. Determination is made of the proximal and distal end of the tumor from the level of the incisor teeth, on endoscopy, and on review of the initial barium swallow x-ray films. Orthogonal anteroposterior and lateral x-ray films of the chest are obtained after inactive dummy sources have been inserted into the afterloading catheters in the applicator. The location of the tumor is marked on the x-ray films, and appropriate margins are determined to perform the dose calculations. Radioactive sources are spaced .5 to 1 cm apart, and margins of 3 cm above and below the tumor are allowed.

Pancreas

Interstitial irradiation, most frequently using ^{125}I permanent implants, has been used in patients with locally advanced unresectable carcinoma of the pancreas. With the patient under general anesthesia, after the tumor is exposed by the surgeon, tumor volume is evaluated and biliary and/or gastric bypasses are performed as required. Multiple seeds are implanted in the pancreas with ^{125}I implantation techniques (with a device such as the Mick applicator). The posterior wall of the stomach can be displaced away from the implant with an omental pedicle flap. After localization x-ray films are obtained by the stereo-shift or orthogonal technique, computer dose calculations to determine the minimal peripheral dose are obtained.

In 98 patients described by Peretz and associates[82] the mean matched peripheral dose was 136.6 Gy. The mean activity of the implant was 35 mCi, and the mean volume was 53 cm^3. Ten patients (10%) survived more than 18 months, and three patients are long-term survivors. Twenty-eight of 68 patients (45%) who had one or more follow-up radiographic studies to assess tumor response showed 30% or more reduction in tumor size. Significant pain relief was observed in 37 (65%) of 57 patients. Nineteen patients (20%) experienced postoperative complications; one patient died with a pancreatic fistula and generalized sepsis, and eight patients (8%) experienced major complications that included fistula formation, gastrointestinal bleeding, gastrointestinal obstruction, and intra-abdominal abscess. Similar survival results have been reported from other institutions. Because of potential biologic disadvantages of ^{125}I (long half-life and LDR), Peretz and associates[82] introduced ^{103}Pd (half-life of 17 days and 20 to 23 KeV) as a new isotope for pancreatic implants.

Biliary Tree

An increasingly popular technique is the insertion of radioactive sources via Teflon catheters in the biliary tree under fluoroscopic conditions. The main objective is to drain bile and palliate obstructive jaundice. Intracatheter irradiation is best delivered as a boost supplement to EBRT, which is delivered to a larger target volume, including nodal drainage.[83]

A transhepatic cholangiogram is initially performed, usually percutaneously. After the site of obstruction is identified, flexible catheters are inserted into the biliary tree to appropriate lengths, under fluoroscopic control. A dual-lumen catheter or two separate catheters should be inserted, one for lodging the radioactive sources and the other for bile drainage. The patency of the biliary tree is monitored with injection of radiopaque material under fluoroscopic control. Special care must be taken to maintain biliary drainage. The catheter is sutured to the skin. Radiographs are obtained to determine the length of active radioactive sources to be inserted and the exact position of the catheter for dosimetric purposes.

An alternative method of insertion for the radioactive sources is via an endoscopic approach under fluoroscopic control. This has become the preferred technique in institutions who consider liver transplant after planned preoperative chemoradiation, since it prevents potential tumor implantation in the catheter tract that transgresses the chest or abdominal wall.

Doses of 20 to 30 Gy are delivered at a 1-cm radius (2-cm diameter) from the catheter when combined with EBRT (45 to 50 Gy in 1.8- to 2.0-Gy fractions preferably) plus concomitant 5-fluorouracil. If only intracavitary irradiation is prescribed, the doses with this modality are 60 to 65 Gy at a 1-cm radius. HDR brachytherapy with 4 Gy × 10 in a twice-per-day fractionation is also an alternative.

Meerwaldt and associates[84] reported on 42 patients with bile duct tumors treated with one or two brachytherapy sessions plus EBRT, alone or combined with palliative resection. A dose of 15 Gy was delivered at each of two sessions or 25 Gy in one session, calculated at 2 cm from the wire, combined with EBRT (40 Gy in 16 fractions). Fourteen percent of the 42 patients survived for 2 years or more. Median and long-term survival was best in the 11 patients who had a noncurative resection in addition to irradiation (median survival of 15 versus 8 months; 3-year survival of 36% versus 6%; $p = .06$). Fever occurred shortly after insertion of the ^{192}Ir wire in 6 of 38 brachytherapy sessions; it was usually controlled with antibiotics.

Fritz and colleagues[85] reported on 18 patients with carcinoma of the hepatic duct bifurcation and 12 patients with carcinoma of the common duct or the common hepatic duct treated with EBRT and intraluminal HDR brachytherapy alone or combined with noncurative resection. Nine patients received radiation therapy after palliative tumor resection, and 21 patients were primarily irradiated. Twenty-five patients completed the full course of radiation therapy. EBRT dose varied from 30 to 45 Gy and brachytherapy doses from 20 to 45 Gy. Biliary drainage after irradiation was achieved using percutaneous catheters, endoprostheses, or stents. The median survival for the entire group was 10 months. The actuarial survival rate was 34% after I year, 18% after 2 and 3 years, and 8% after 5 years. Three patients were still living without evidence of disease at 35 to 69 months. Major complications such as bacterial cholangitis could be lowered from 37% to 28% through exchange of percutaneous transhepatic catheters to endoprosthesis or stents. The longest lasting drainage was achieved using stents. The incidence of radiogenic ulcers was lowered from 23% to 7.6% after the total dose of HDR afterloading boost was reduced to 20 Gy.

Mayo Clinic investigators published results in a series of 24 patients with unresectable bile duct cancers treated with EBRT plus ^{192}Ir alone or with concomitant 5-fluorouracil during EBRT. EBRT was delivered at a dose of 45 to 54 Gy in 25 to 30 fractions over 5.5 to 6 weeks, and the brachytherapy dose was 20 to 30 Gy at a 1-cm radius. Three of the 24 patients were 5-year survivors and results appeared best in the nine patients who received concomitant 5-fluorouracil during EBRT (5-year survival of 22% versus 8%).

Soft Tissue Sarcomas

In treatment of soft tissue sarcomas, EBRT combined with limb-preservation surgery has been successful in achieving the same results as obtained with radical surgical resection. Interstitial brachytherapy can be successfully combined with EBRT in patients who have a marginal gross total resection with narrow margins or microscopic residual disease. The theoretical advantages of such a combination include (1) less extensive surgery; (2) synchronous brachytherapy, which allows aggressive treatment of microscopic residual malignant cells at a time when these cells are still oxygenated and before they are embedded in scar tissue; (3) placing of the implant plane(s) on the tumor bed, which ensures that this site will receive the highest irradiation dose; and (4) short treatment (4 to 5 days as primary treatment; 2 days if combined with EBRT) completed before discharge of the patient from the hospital, which presents considerable medical, psychological, and economic advantages. Brachytherapy alone (no EBRT) can be either combined with surgery in the primary treatment of high-grade sarcomas or used as a potentially curative salvage procedure for locally recurrent sarcomas when surgery and EBRT have failed to prevent relapse.

Usually a single-plane implant is satisfactory. A margin of 2 to 5 cm beyond the boundaries of gross or suspected tumor must be added; the extent of the margin is normally larger along muscles, nerves, and vessels that transverse to those structures. The dimensions of the area to be implanted are measured and recorded. The number of afterloading tubes to be placed at intervals of 1 to 1.5 cm in the target area to deliver 10 Gy/day is determined using the planar implant nomogram of the MSKCC or comparable dosimetry system. To ensure a proper implant, the points of needle insertion are marked on the skin with a sterile pen. The tubes are inserted through normal skin after surgical resection but before completion of any reconstruction and wound closure. At MSKCC, the tubes are placed parallel to the surgical incision, but at Mayo Clinic and other institutions, physicians usually prefer placement of the tubes vertical or perpendicular to the incision plane.

With the perpendicular or vertical placement, parallel stainless-steel needles are spaced uniformly and embedded in the depth of the operative field. The closed end of each afterloading nylon tube (in the sealed-end technique) is threaded through the needle until it emerges from the opposite end of the needle. The needle is withdrawn while the plastic tube is held in place until the needle is out of the skin. This process is repeated for the total planned number of afterloading tubes. Each tube is secured in proper position in the tumor bed either by anchoring the needle (and subsequently the tube) in the fascia or muscle, or by securing the nylon tube with No. 2 or 3 absorbable suture material. Metallic clips are placed near each blind end of the nylon tube for later identification of this end on the localization radiographs. The afterloading tubes are individually secured to the skin by means of a stainless-steel button that is threaded over the tube, fixed to it by crimping, and anchored to the underlying skin by silk sutures. A plastic hemispheric bead cushions the button on the skin, protecting it from undue pressure.

Because of the use of irradiation, wound closure requires extra planning and care to avoid undue tension predisposing to wound breakdown. To further diminish wound complications, the loading of the ^{192}Ir ribbon or ^{125}I seeds is delayed until 3 or 5 days after surgery (3 days is adequate if there is no wound tension).[86] Before loading, anteroposterior and lateral radiographs with radiopaque dummy sources in the plastic tubes provide the information necessary for computerized dosimetry calculations and dose-rate determination. CT planned dosimetry is recommended.

The LDR dose for tumor bed implants is 45 to 50 Gy in 4 to 5 days if used as the sole therapy for high-grade sarcomas. For HDR implants the dose is 4 Gy × 10 (40 Gy) in a bid schedule or 15 to 20 Gy if used as a supplement to EBRT doses of 45 to 50 Gy and a marginal gross total resection. At MSKCC, EBRT is now combined with brachytherapy for high-grade sarcomas with positive margins of resection and for all low-grade lesions. In such cases the implant boost dose is 15 to 30 Gy, supplemented by 45 to 50 Gy of EBRT (15 to 20 Gy for narrow or microscopic positive margins, 30 Gy for grossly positive margins). For additional technical details, the reader is referred to the textbook by Hilaris and colleagues.[87]

Pisters and coworkers[88] reported on 164 patients with soft tissue sarcomas randomized to receive or not receive brachytherapy as the sole method of irradiation after complete wide local tumor resection at MSKCC (78 and 86 patients in either group, respectively). A target region in the tumor bed was identified by adding 2 cm to the superior and inferior dimensions and 1.5 to 2 cm in the medial and lateral directions. Afterloading catheters were placed approximately 1 cm apart and were fixed in treatment position with absorbable sutures, secured to the skin at the catheter exit site with buttons and nonabsorbable sutures. Implant dose was 42 to 5 Gy over 4 to 6 days using ^{192}Ir. Sources were loaded on the fifth or sixth postoperative day to decrease interference with wound healing. There were 13 local recurrences in 78 patients (16%) who received brachytherapy and 25 (29%) in 86 patients treated with surgery only. Actuarial estimates of local recurrence at 60 months were 18% in the brachytherapy and 31% in the no-irradiation group. It is highly likely that the prescribed dose of irradiation was not adequate to eliminate microscopic disease, and higher doses (55 to 60 Gy) would have been more effective. Subsequent evaluations of the MSKCC data show inadequate local control with low-grade sarcomas using brachytherapy alone and for high-grade lesions with positive margins of resection. Such patients are now treated with combined EBRT and brachytherapy.

Potter and colleagues[89] reported on 12 patients with soft tissue sarcomas treated with HDR or PDR brachytherapy. Brachytherapy was part of the recurrence treatment regimen in eight patients and part of the primary treatment alone or combined with EBRT in four patients. In HDR treatment a dose of 15 to 43 Gy was delivered in 3 to 16 fractions, and in PDR treatment 13 to 36 Gy in fractions of 1 Gy/h were used. With median follow-up of 14 months, 7 of the patients showed no evidence of disease, 9 of 12 patients had local control, and 3 patients progressed locoregionally. In 6 patients with Ewing's sarcoma, brachytherapy was performed intraoperatively as a boost treatment after EBRT (50 to 55 Gy), if no wide resection could be achieved. A dose of 10 to 12 Gy was applied in one fraction to a limited volume (20 to 50 cm^3) at the time of surgery. Follow-up is 13 to 26 months (median, 21 months). All patients are disease free, and perioperative and subacute morbidity were not increased.

Brachytherapy (15 to 20 Gy with LDR) was combined with EBRT (45 to 50 Gy) either preoperatively or postoperatively by Schray and associates at Mayo Clinic.[90] Three-dimensional reconstruction of the tumor or tumor bed was accomplished by CT scan or MRI. Margins beyond the tumor were 5 to 10 cm axially or along tissue planes and 2 to 4 cm radially or perpendicular to tissue planes for the EBRT component of treatment. Brachytherapy was performed with standard nylon afterloading tubes positioned to encompass the boost volume with a 2- to 4-cm margin (Fig. 13-4). The boost volume was considered to be the tumor bed after preoperative irradiation and the surgical bed and incision if no previous irradiation had been given. With rare exceptions (distal extremities, groin), needles were placed transversely to the incision (and axis of the extremity) under direct visualization of the tumor bed and with entry and exit points outside the tumor and surgical bed. Nylon tubes were commonly placed in contact with bone and neurovascular structures and were maintained in place by skin fascia and muscle, sutures being rarely used. After the implant was in place, the skin was closed with sutures. Implants were loaded 72 to 96 hours postoperatively with ^{192}Ir; the sources were placed 1 cm deep to the skin surface along the tube axis. Average implant activity was 107 mCi, and a portion of the implants used two or more planes. The average dose rate was 48.6 Gy/h, average time was 44.2 hours, and average dose was 20.52 Gy. In 63 patients, 65 brachytherapy procedures were performed. With median follow-up of 20 months, there were two local failures in 56 patients (4%) treated initially and in three of nine patients treated for recurrent tumors. Only one of the five local recurrences was within the implanted volume. Two of 40 implants (5%) performed at initial resection followed by postoperative irradiation led to wound complications, in contrast to 4 of 16 implants (25%) performed at resection after preoperative EBRT.

Uterine Cervix

Intracavitary insertions in carcinoma of the cervix are performed under general, spinal, or local (block) anesthesia. The patient is placed in the lithotomy position, and a complete bimanual pelvic and rectal examination is performed. After adequate preparation, the cervix is grasped with a tenaculum, and the uterus is sounded carefully to prevent a perforation. If the cervical os/canal is not identified, a small metallic probe may be used. Bimanual pelvic examination may be extremely helpful in determining the position of the uterus and the probe or sound. In most patients, dilation and curettage is performed at the time of the first intracavitary insertion (if not performed at initial work-up). Radiopaque markers (lead shots or metallic clips) are placed in the anterior and posterior lips of the cervix. The tandem is inserted in the uterus to the appropriate depth (as determined by a stopper), and subsequently each

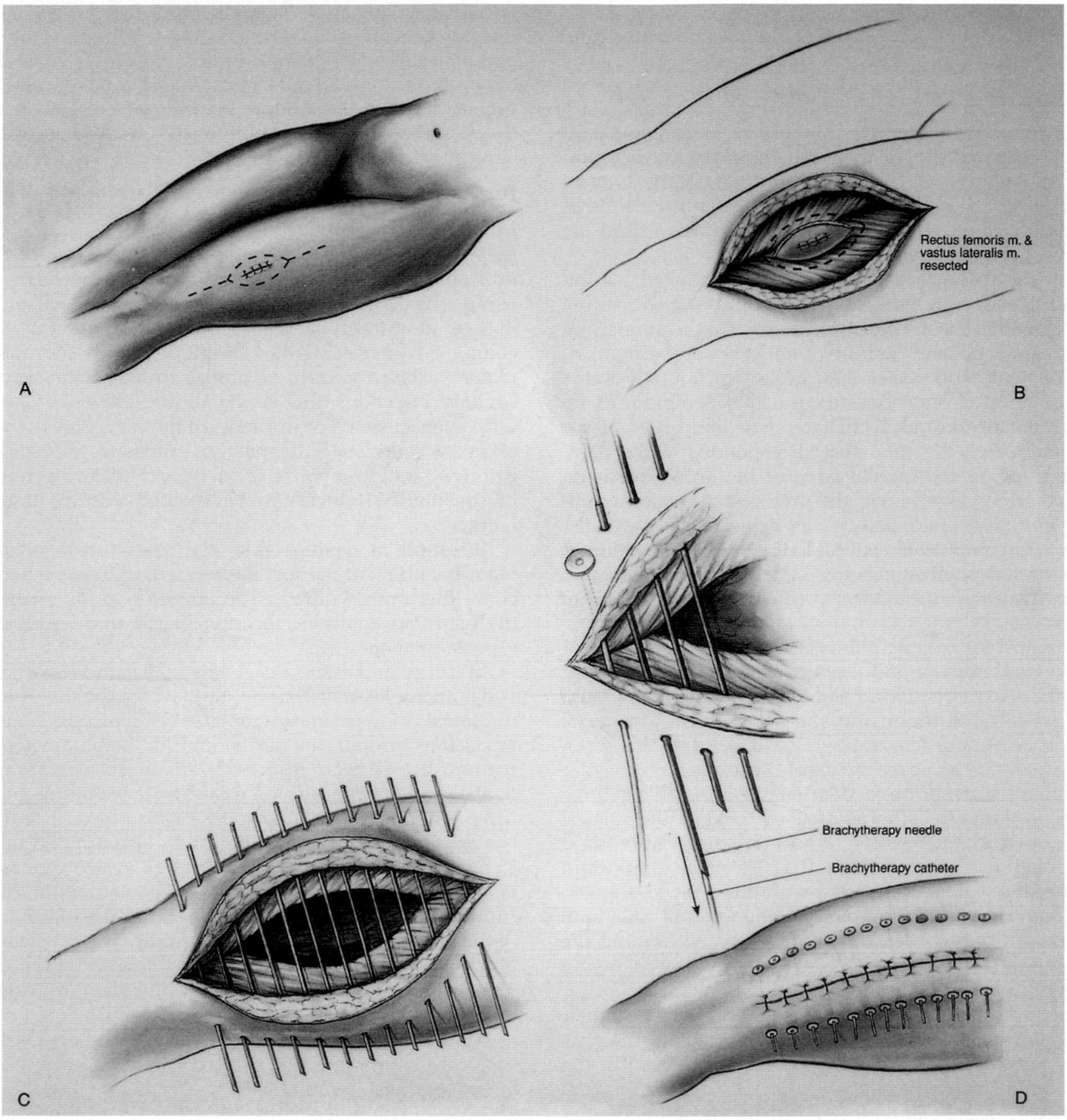

Figure 13-4 Artist's idealized depiction of surgical technique of wide excision of extremity sarcoma with placement of afterloading tubes for brachytherapy (LDR or HDR). **A,** Elliptical incision of biopsy site for wide excision of soft tissue sarcoma involving the vastus lateralis. **B,** Anterior and posterior flaps are raised. Dissection is carried down through the muscle, with care taken to maintain a 1- to 2-cm margin of soft tissue around the tumor. **C,** Hollow needles are placed to cover the surgical bed at 1- to 1.5-cm intervals. **D,** Plastic hollow catheters are threaded through the needles and anchored with barium buttons for afterloading with Ir^{192} (LDR brachytherapy) or HDR source. (Copyright © Mayo Clinic, 2006.)

ovoid is gently inserted to prevent injury to the vaginal mucosa.

If ideally inserted in the patient, the tandem should be in the midline or as nearly as possible equidistant from the lateral pelvic wall, and the vaginal colpostats should be symmetrically positioned against the cervix in relation to the tandem. The tandem should be kept along the sagittal axis of the pelvis, equidistant from the pubis, sacral promontory, and lateral pelvic wall as allowed by the geometry of the patient and the tumor to avoid overdosage to the bladder, rectosigmoid, or either ureter. Corn and colleagues,[91] in a retrospective evaluation of the technical quality of brachytherapy procedures with respect to ovoid and tandem placement, demonstrated a significantly worse outcome for patients whose implants were judged to be unacceptable.

After the tandem and colpostat positions are judged to be correct, careful packing of the vagina should be performed. A small amount of packing in front of and behind the colpostats (making sure overpacking does not separate the cervix from the colpostats) decreases the dose to the bladder base and the anterior rectal wall.

An indwelling Foley catheter should be inserted in the bladder; 7 mL of radiopaque contrast material in the Foley balloon will aid in determining a point dose to the bladder neck. For difficult insertions, intraoperative x-rays with C-ARM are recommended. After the patient recovers from anesthesia, anteroposterior and lateral x-ray films of the pelvis are obtained to document the position of the applicator, and isodose curves are generated.

Brachytherapy Systems for Carcinoma of the Cervix

Initially, three systems for brachytherapy in carcinoma of the uterine cervix were developed: the Paris, the Swedish, and the Manchester systems. The systems differ in the type of applicator used, the strength of the source, and the time of administration. In the United States, most systems used are derivations of the Manchester technique.

The Manchester intracavitary system, introduced by Tod and Meredith[92] in 1938, was the first applicator and loading system designed to meet certain dosimetric specifications, and it used a dosimetric field quantity, total exposure at point A, to prescribe treatment, rather than milligram hours. Point A was defined as being 2 cm above the mucous membrane of the lateral vaginal fornix and 2 cm lateral to the center of the uterine canal. Allegedly this area corresponded to the paracervical triangle, in the medial edge of the broad ligament, where the uterine vessels cross the ureter. A subsequent arbitrary convention defined point A as being 2 cm above the external cervical os and 2 cm lateral to the midline. Yet another definition located point A as being 2 cm above the distal end of the lowest source in the cervical canal and 2 cm lateral to the tandem.

The two most vulnerable points in the pelvis were thought to be the vaginal mucosa and the rectovaginal septum, opposite the cervix. No more than 40% of total dose at point A could be delivered safely through the vaginal mucosa. The rectal dose should be 80% or less of the dose at point A; this rectal dose can usually be achieved by careful packing.

The tandems, about 6 mm in diameter, are available in three curvatures. A flange or stopper is used to keep the uterine tandem in the selected position; a keeled flange can be used to avoid rotation of the tandem. It is extremely important when applicators are purchased to examine the design, to obtain radiographs to identify the position of the shielding, and to take dosimetric measurements after determining the diameter and thickness of the walls of the applicator to exactly determine the dose distribution around the applicators.

Mini-colpostats have a diameter of 1.6 cm and a flat inner surface to allow their insertion in patients in whom the only alternative would be protruding vaginal sources in the tandem.[93] Some mini-ovoids have no shielding; thus, the surface dose is significantly higher than with the regular ovoids (with 3M cesium sources, the surface dose is 9.8 cGy/mg/h with the mini-ovoids, in contrast to 6.3 cGy with the 2-cm-diameter ovoids), and they are usually loaded with 10-mg sources. The 3M mini-ovoids have internal shielding. However, phantom measurements did not demonstrate a significant decrease in dose for the newer mini-colpostats with rectal shielding for a source separation of 3 cm, which potentially could allow undue user confidence in the doses delivered.

Henschke Applicator

The Henschke[94] and other applicators are commercially available. The basic configuration of the ovoids is hemispheres that are inserted parallel to the lateral wall of the vaginal vault and the intrauterine tandem. Three ovoid diameters and various tandems are available. Although this applicator's configuration conforms better to a narrow vaginal vault, the radioactive sources are placed parallel to the long axis of the bladder and the rectum and do not have any shielding, thus, potentially delivering a higher dose to these organs. Users should familiarize themselves with the dosimetric aspects of these devices. Delclos and colleagues[93] emphasized that the dosimetry with the Fletcher colpostats is unique and that treatment techniques and tables derived for this applicator should not be used with other applicators because this might result in significantly higher doses to the vagina, bladder, or rectum. Appropriate source loading and dose prescription produce satisfactory clinical results.

Interstitial Implants for Cervical Carcinoma

Metallic needles containing ^{226}Ra, ^{60}Co, or ^{137}Cs or afterloading metallic guides or Teflon catheters for insertion of ^{192}Ir wires or seeds have been implanted in the parametrium or cervix, using a transvaginal or transperineal approach (sometimes in lieu of intracavitary insertions when the cervical canal cannot be identified) and frequently with the aid of templates.[95] The procedure is similar to that followed for intracavitary insertions. The cervix should always be held firmly with a tenaculum. For implants in the cervix itself, the needles or nylon catheters with metallic guides (5 to 6 cm long) are inserted straight, about 1.2 cm apart, following the position of the uterus (which can be verified with a finger in the rectum).

Insertion of needles into vital structures, including the bladder and rectum, must be avoided, unless it is necessary to cover the tumor volume. The operator should keep in mind the expected anatomic location of the major pelvic vessels, especially veins.

Martinez and associates,[95] Aristizabal and coworkers,[96] and Feder and colleagues[97] have popularized the use of interstitial implants, using perineal templates with introduction of metallic needles through the perineum into the parametrial tissues. Iridium 192 seeds are inserted in an afterloading fashion. Aristizabal and colleagues[96] modified their technique by deleting three anteriorly and three posteriorly placed needles in the central row; the central tandem was also omitted in an effort to decrease an initial high incidence of vesicovaginal or rectovaginal fistula. The investigators reported about 75% pelvic tumor control in 118 patients with stages IIB and III carcinoma of the uterine cervix. The major complication rate was 6% with less than 4500 mg/h, 16% with 4500 to 4999 mg/h, 28% with 5500 mg/h, and 87% with higher intracavitary doses (combined with 45 to 50 Gy to the whole pelvis).

Martinez and coworkers[29] described results in 104 patients with locally advanced or recurrent pelvic tumor using a universal perineal template (32 to 35 Gy at dose rates of 2: 75 cGy/h) combined with EBRT (36 Gy to the whole pelvis and 14 Gy to the pelvic side wall with midline block using four-field techniques, 4- or 10-MV photons). Local tumor control was obtained in 82% of 63 patients with gynecologic lesions. The major complication rate requiring surgical intervention was 3.2%.

Leborgne and colleagues[98] reported their experience with MDR brachytherapy (1 to 12 Gy/h). In carcinoma of the cervix, EBRT with a central block was given to the pelvis (40 Gy at 2 Gy/fraction), and patients with stage IIB disease received an additional 20 Gy to the whole pelvis without central shielding. A control group of 102 patients was treated with LDR brachytherapy (average dose rate was .44 Gy/h, two 32.5-Gy fractions to point A in 74 hours each, 2 weeks apart). The MDR group was treated at 1.6 to 1.7 Gy/h to point A. Dose fractionation schedules for MDR were derived using the linear-quadratic equation to arrive at a biologically equivalent dose. Grade 2 and 3 sequelae were noted in 1 of 102 patients treated with LDR brachytherapy, in 25 (83%) of 30 patients treated with MDR with a 5% dose reduction compared with LDR therapy (61.75 Gy), and in 4 (40%) of 10 and 0 of 38 patients treated with 3 or 6 MDR fractions for a total of 58 or 55.5 Gy to point A, respectively. The average nominal biologically effective dose (BED) for the various groups ranged from 78 to 124 Gy. The incidence of the late rectal complications was zero for patients receiving rectal BED of less than 50 Gy, 24% to 36% for 50 Gy to 199 Gy, and 67% for doses of 200 Gy BED or greater. The investigators concluded that the safest schedule was to deliver 18 Gy to the whole pelvis with EBRT, plus brachytherapy delivering a dose rate to point A of 1.6 Gy/h, in 6 fractions of 8 Gy, 2 in each treatment day, 10 days apart. Two fractions are given on a single day, 6 hours apart, to reduce the number of insertions to three. This study emphasizes the importance of conducting prospective dose fractionation studies based on sound biologic data.

Endometrium

Carcinoma of the endometrium may grow irregularly into the uterine cavity and produce deformity of the lumen. It is important to determine the size and shape of the uterine cavity as well as the thickness of the uterine wall. This is accomplished by rotating the uterine sound and measuring the width and depth of the uterine cavity as well as by bimanual palpation or hysterogram. Special care should be taken to avoid a perforation; if this occurs, packing with Heyman capsules should not be performed at that time. However, a carefully inserted tandem may be used, avoiding the site of perforation. Ultrasound may help in ascertaining the exact position of the tandem. Rupture (splitting) of the cervix, which may be caused by excessive careless dilation, should be avoided. Assessment of uterine wall thickness is done by MRI, CT, or ultrasound. This is important to determine dose prescription point.

Uterine packing with capsules was originally described by Heyman in 1934. The practice of introducing as many capsules as possible to stretch the wall of the uterus has several advantages: a bulky tumor can be flattened out, allowing the base of the lesion to be more effectively irradiated; stretching of the uterine wall to make it thinner permits higher doses to be delivered to the serosa of the organ; and a more uniform distribution of the radiation is delivered to the entire myometrium. Afterloading Heyman-Simon capsules are available in 6-, 8-, and 10-mm diameters and 2- to 3-cm lengths.

When capsules are used, it is convenient to insert an afterloading tandem to cover the lower uterine segment because this permits more flexibility in the loading, to obtain improved coverage of this portion of the uterus and the cervical canal. Afterloading colpostats should be routinely used to irradiate the vaginal cuff. A technical problem with the afterloading Heyman-Simon capsules is the relatively large thickness of the sterns, which requires continued dilation of the cervical canal (Hegar dilators) after a few capsules have been inserted. It is critical to record the order of insertion of the capsules (by numbers that are printed on each capsule), so that removal is performed in the reverse order of insertion. Otherwise, the capsules may become jammed, making removal more difficult. Ideally, a minimum of four capsules should be inserted. If fewer are allowed by the size of the endometrial cavity, it may be better to insert an afterloading tandem.

The dose of irradiation delivered with this system is somewhat empirically derived. In general, in preoperative insertions we use 3500 mg/h in the uterine cavity; however, cavities larger than 8 cm receive doses of approximately 4000 mg/h. Doses of about 65 Gy to the mucosal surface of the vagina are delivered (1900 to 2000 mg/h) with 2-cm-diameter vaginal ovoids. Grigsby and colleagues[99] reported higher survival and fewer pelvic recurrences and distant metastases in patients with stage I poorly differentiated endometrial carcinoma when doses higher than 3500 mg/h were delivered in the uterus. A lesser beneficial impact was noted in moderately differentiated tumors.

In patients treated with radiation therapy alone, higher intracavitary doses (in the range of 8000 mg/h) are given in two or three insertions. This is combined with EBRT 20 Gy whole pelvis and an additional 30 Gy to the parametria with midline shielding.

For postoperative irradiation in endometrial carcinoma, if no preoperative irradiation was delivered, we use afterloading colpostats to deliver 55 to 65 Gy to the vaginal mucosa with LDR brachytherapy in patients with poorly differentiated tumors even in the absence of deep myometrial invasion. When there is deep myometrial invasion (>50%), regardless of the histologic features, the intracavitary therapy is combined with EBRT (20 Gy whole pelvis and additional 30 Gy to parametria with midline shielding).

Chao and colleagues[100] described the medical complications associated with 150 intracavitary implants performed in 96 patients treated with irradiation alone for inoperable carcinoma of the endometrium. General anesthesia was used in 98 implants, spinal in 26, local in 25, and epidural in 1. Preventive measures included low-dose cutaneous doses of heparin in 55 patients and intermittent pneumatic compression boots in 29. Four patients (4.2%) developed life-threatening complications (myocardial infarction in two, congestive heart failure in one, and pulmonary embolism in one patient). Two patients died (of myocardial infarction and pulmonary embolism).

Rotte[101] reported an incidence of 7.5% thromboembolic complications in 106 patients with carcinoma of the endometrium undergoing LDR implants. In contrast, none of the patients treated at the institution with HDR devices had thromboembolic phenomena. It is important to identify patients at high risk for thromboembolic complications, such as those with trauma to the lower extremities or pelvis, obesity, advanced age, and a history of prior thromboembolism. For these patients, outpatient HDR brachytherapy is the recommended intracavitary treatment.

Vagina, Vulva, and Female Urethra

Indications for and techniques of interstitial therapy for carcinoma of the vagina, vulva, and urethra have been described.[32,95,102] These areas are potentially vulnerable to severe complications because of the reported lower tolerance of the surrounding tissues to irradiation and because they are exposed to the constant irritation of perspiration, urine, and occasionally feces; therefore, it is important to minimize irradiation to the surrounding normal areas.

Use of interstitial implants ideally should be limited to a volume encompassing 75% or less of the circumference of the vagina, particularly when the lesion involves the posterior wall and rectovaginal septum. The remaining normal tissues should be kept away from the implanted area as much as possible, with the judicious use of gauze packing, cylinders, or templates. The use of abductor pillows helps by separating the inner thighs from the sources in or at the perineum.

Afterloading vaginal cylinders have a central, hollow tandem cylinder, in which the sources are placed, and plastic rings 2.5 cm in length and of varying diameters are inserted over the tandem. Domed cylinders are used to irradiate the vaginal cuff homogeneously, when indicated.

An intracavitary application with a vaginal cylinder or similar applicator (e.g., Bloedorn, Burnett, Delclos, MIRAv) delivering about 65 to 75 Gy to the mucosa is adequate to control carcinoma in situ. Because of the multicentric nature of this tumor, the entire vaginal mucosa must be treated. When HDR vaginal cylinders are used, 3.6 to 4.0 Gy × 8 to 10 fractions delivered to the mucosal surface is recommended.

The most superficial tumors are treated with an intracavitary insertion alone, with the largest cylinder covering the entire vagina. If the lesion is thicker, a single-plane needle implant is used in addition to the intracavitary cylinder. This has the advantage of increasing the tumor depth dose without delivering excessive irradiation to the uninvolved vaginal mucosa, which receives 60 to 65 Gy. The gross tumor is treated with 65 to 75 Gy calculated to .5 cm beyond the plane of the implant; the vaginal mucosa in this area receives an estimated 80 to 100 Gy, depending on the size of the lesion and tumor dose prescribed. More extensive tumors are treated with intracavitary and interstitial therapy supplemented with EBRT. When EBRT is used, the brachytherapy dose is adjusted downward, adding it to the whole pelvis to achieve the prescribed total vaginal tumor dose.

Patients with more advanced paravaginal tumors without extensive parametrial infiltration (stage II lesions) are always treated with a greater external irradiation dose of 40 Gy to the whole pelvis and an additional parametrial dose with midline block, to deliver a total of 50 to 60 Gy to the lateral pelvic wall. In these patients interstitial therapy should also be used delivering 30 Gy to the tumor to administer about 70 Gy to a volume .5 to 1 cm around the palpable tumor (dose includes whole pelvis external beam contribution). Because of the more extensive tumor, double-plane or volume implants are necessary.

Tumors of the Vulva or Distal Urethra

Vulvar or distal urethral tumors can be treated with similar brachytherapy techniques. Erickson[103] published a historical review of interstitial implants for vulvar carcinoma.

The patient is placed in a lithotomy position, and ring, double-plane, or volume implants can be designed around the urethra or in the vulvar labia. When the procedure is completed, cystoscopy is performed to ascertain the position of the catheters in the bladder and an indwelling three-way catheter is inserted. If there is intravesical bleeding, periodic irrigation of the bladder is necessary while the implant is in place, and it is preferable to leave a three-way catheter in place for a few days (up to 1 week) to facilitate bladder irrigation and avoid clot formation with bladder neck obstruction. When the vulva is involved, the sources must protrude into the perineum. If the tumor extends into the vagina, an intravaginal cylinder with some sources may be necessary to increase the dose to the vaginal mucosa. Gupta and associates[33] reported excellent local controls with minimal urinary incontinence. The design of the implant, placement of the radioactive sources, and tumor doses are similar to those for comparable lesions in the vagina.

Anal Canal and Rectum

Interstitial and intracavitary techniques have been used for many years for the treatment of anorectal carcinoma. Ideally, implants should be restricted to lesions that require implantation of no more than half the circumference of the anal canal for preservation of sphincter function. Single-plane, double-plane, or volume implants may be necessary, depending on the extent of the tumor. Because of the excellent response to chemoradiation in anal canal carcinoma, brachytherapy is now seldom used.

The catheters are inserted through the perianal area in the central plane .5 cm from the anal or rectal mucosa with one finger (double gloved) in the rectum to verify appropriate placement. Peripheral planes are placed at 1- to 1.5-cm spacing. The anal canal is kept distended with a custom-designed rectal plug, which reduces the dose to the opposite side of the canal to less than 15% of the minimum tumor dose at the implanted area. Perineal templates are strongly recommended.

Papillon and coworkers[104] reported on 221 patients with epidermoid carcinoma of the anal canal treated with EBRT (35 Gy) combined with 5-fluorouracil and mitomycin C, followed by an ^{192}Ir implant 2 months later. The implants were performed with either a plastic template or a steel fork, using four to eight wires, 5 to 7 cm long, adapted to the tumor extent covering the quadrants of the anal circumference involved by the tumor. A minimum dose of 15 to 20 Gy was delivered in 15 to 28 hours. Of 179 patients followed for 5 years, 118 (65.9%) were alive and well, and 110 (61.4%) had anal preservation. Thirty-three patients (18.4%) died of cancer. Of patients with tumors measuring less than 4 cm, 50 (75.7%) of 66 were alive with anal preservation at the time of the report, and only 5 (7.5%) died of cancer.

Papillon and colleagues[104] also reported on 90 patients with T1 or T2 rectal carcinoma treated with contact x-ray endocavitary therapy followed by ^{192}Ir implant with an iridium fork. Doses were similar to those administered to the patients with anal carcinoma. The 5-year survival rate was 77.8%; 67 (74%) were alive with anal preservation, and only 10 (11.1%) died of cancer. They also reported on a third group of patients with more advanced, moderately infiltrating low lying T2 or T3 tumors, who would have been treated by abdominoperineal resection but because of age or poor operative risk were treated with radiation therapy including interstitial implants. At 4 years, 37 (59.6%) of 62 patients were alive, and 36 (58%) had anal preservation. Only nine patients (14.5%) died of cancer; three had unresectable lesions and one died after major surgery.

Puthawala and colleagues[105] reported on 40 patients with anorectal cancer who were treated with EBRT (40 to 50 Gy in 25 to 30 fractions) followed by two ^{192}Ir implants using the Syed template to deliver a total tumor dose of 65 to 75 Gy. Local tumor control was achieved in 70% of tumors with 20% major morbidity.

Interstitial implants with 10- to 15-cm nylon catheters for ^{192}Ir ribbons are used to treat patients with recurrent carcinoma of the rectum in the perineal and presacral fossa after abdominoperineal resection. Care should be exercised to direct the metallic guides initially inserted or catheters with a posterior orientation (5 to 10 degrees from the horizontal plane). In many instances, the needles find resistance from the sacrum; occasionally the sources are inadvertently placed in the bladder. Occasionally we have performed intraoperative implants at the time of resection of the recurrent tumor, which allows for better identification of the volume to be treated and placement of the catheters.

Bladder

Van der Werf-Messing[106] popularized bladder implants with radium or cesium needles. Apart from surgery and general anesthesia, disadvantages of this technique were radiation safety, impaired wound healing because of acute side effects, and sometimes difficulties in removing the radioactive sources. In a series of 160 patients, the mean hospitalization was 36 days after the operation. In 10% of the patients, the abdomen had to be reopened to remove one or more needles. Van der Werf-Messing and associates used radium implants in 328 patients with T2 and 63 patients with T3 tumors after a small dose of preoperative irradiation (3.5 Gy for 3 fractions).

The recurrence rates were 16% for the T2 and 28% for the T3 tumors. Disease-free survival rates were 75% and 62%, respectively. Battermann and Tierie,[107] using a similar technique, obtained local tumor control in 69 (81%) of 85 patients with T2 tumors, and a 10-year disease-free survival rate of 56%. Subsequently, van der Werf-Messing and van Putten[108] used 40-Gy external irradiation followed by ^{137}Cs implants in 48 patients with T2 and in 42 patients with T3 bladder cancer. The 5-year disease-free survival rate was 70%.

A different method using iridium wires was designed in France; it was modified by Battermann and Boon[109] to overcome most of the disadvantages of the rigid needle technique. After a lower abdominal incision, the bladder is opened to visualize the tumor area. Plastic carriers consisting of a hollow part and a thinner leading end are inserted 1.5 cm apart. The tubes penetrate the abdominal wall, are tunneled in the bladder muscle through the tumor and out of the bladder, and penetrate the abdominal wall again. The catheters should be placed in such a way that removal is feasible without a second laparotomy, although in more complex cases this may be necessary. Dummy sources are introduced in the carriers to visualize the length of the source to be used while the bladder is still open. After the position of the sources is checked, the bladder is closed, and subsequently the abdomen is closed. A Foley catheter is placed for drainage. After film localization, the dose distribution is determined. The carriers are connected to the MicroSelectron (LDR or HDR), and the radioactive phase of the procedure is started. The tubes are well tolerated and, after completion of irradiation, can be removed easily. All patients receive preoperative EBRT to prevent tumor seeding during operation (30 Gy). A dose of 40 Gy is given by brachytherapy at a dose rate of .3 to .5 Gy/h.

Prostate

Permanent Iodine 125 Implants

Hilaris and colleagues[110] popularized the use of ^{125}I seeds for treatment of stage A (T1), B (T2), or occasionally early C (T3) prostate carcinoma. The ^{125}I seeds were implanted permanently in the prostate through open retropubic laparotomy incision with the patient in a modified lithotomy position.

Critz and associates,[111] in a report of 239 patients with clinical T1 or T2 surgically negative-node carcinoma of the prostate treated with ^{125}I prostate implants (80 Gy MPD [minimal peripheral dose]) after pelvic EBRT (10 × 8-cm portals, bilateral 120-degree arcs, 45 Gy in 5 weeks), described a good correlation between the prostate volume and amount of ^{125}I required for implant (15 to 20 mCi for a 30-mL prostate volume versus 25 mCi for a 60-mL prostate volume). Five patients developed rectal ulcers that were treated conservatively, and one patient required a colostomy. One patient had superficial urethral necrosis and two urethral strictures (history of previous transurethral resection). Sexual potency was maintained at 5 years in 75% of patients.

The treatment of organ-confined carcinoma of the prostate with permanent radioisotopes by the retropubic method has generated variable and controversial results. Advances in radioisotope development, computer-based dosimetry, and transrectal ultrasound and CT imaging have fostered techniques of closed transperineal implantation that produce more homogeneous, reproducible, and larger-volume implants with a higher peripheral dose than was possible in the past.[112] With a median follow-up of 37 months (range, 12 to 78 months), 93% of 291 early-stage A-B patients treated with ^{125}I or ^{103}Pd alone had a normal posttreatment prostate-specific antigen (PSA) level (median value, .4). Of 160 more advanced stages A to C patients treated with EBRT and implant boost, 85% had a normal PSA level (median value, .3). The elimination of surgery with these techniques permits outpatient treatment, resulting in high patient acceptance. If longer follow-up substantiates the favorable early results, these methods may offer the least morbid and least expensive method of treatment for early-stage carcinoma of the prostate.[113]

Palladium 103 Implants

Palladium 103 is currently available in seed form for use in permanent implants. The ^{103}Pd seed is physically similar to ^{125}I; therefore, techniques of ^{125}I implantation are applicable to ^{103}Pd. However, ^{103}Pd differs from ^{125}I in possessing a slightly lower energy (21 KeV versus 27 KeV) and a significantly shorter half-life (17 days compared with 60 days). These differences in energy and half-life require a change in dose prescription. Both radioisotopes are available for permanent implantation of single seeds or as a strand in an absorbable suture material to decrease seed migration.

The lower energy of ^{103}Pd results in a minor reduction of tissue penetration when compared with ^{125}I. The dose distribution effect of this difference is insignificant for seed-to-seed distances of 1.7 cm or less, and linear, planar, biplanar, and cubic configurations are similar for both sources, provided proper spacing requirements are met.

Transperineal Implants: Ultrasound Guided

Implants are performed on an outpatient basis under spinal anesthesia. With the patient in an exaggerated pelvic tilt lithotomy position, the 7.5-MHz biplanar ultrasound probe is inserted in the rectum to guide the physician in the positioning of the needle insertion. Transverse images are recorded at 5-mm increments from the base of the prostatic apex. The optimal seed distribution is determined by superimposing the computer-generated isodose distribution over the target volume. Disposable guides preloaded with sources and absorbable spacers and/or seeds in a strand of absorbable suture are introduced through the appropriate template holes as indicated in the plan. Alternatively, the Mick applicator (Mick Radionuclear Instruments, Bronx, NY) may be used. Each needle is guided to its predetermined position within the prostate under direct ultrasound visualization. Figure 13-5 demonstrates the use of ultrasound volume studies in treatment planning for prostate implants. The on-screen template coordinates of the ultrasound unit allow accurate visualization of the needle position in the prostate. Some institutions have used CT-based fluoroscopic methods for monitoring needle insertion. CT-based dosimetry is performed on every patient.

The recommendation for use of permanent implants is based on both patient and disease factors. These include prostate volume less than 60 cm^3, no severe pubic arch interference, no severe urinary obstructive symptoms, and clinically intracapsular disease; prior transurethral resection of the prostate is discouraged. The Gleason score should be 6 or less and the PSA level 10 or less; the patient should be stage T1 or T2a. In addition one can use either ^{125}I or ^{103}Pd, alone or as a boost after EBRT (for patients with larger tumor volume or those at higher risk for extraprostatic extension such as larger T2B, T3, or higher-grade or -stage patients). Use of ^{125}I and/or Pd^{103} seeds embedded in a stiffened Vicryl carrier has decreased the possibility of seeds migrating and causing lung embolization.

Because tissue tolerance is a function of total dose as well as dose rate, some adjustment of target dose must be made when considering ^{103}Pd rather than ^{125}I for implantation. Clinical observations of the normal tissue effects of permanent

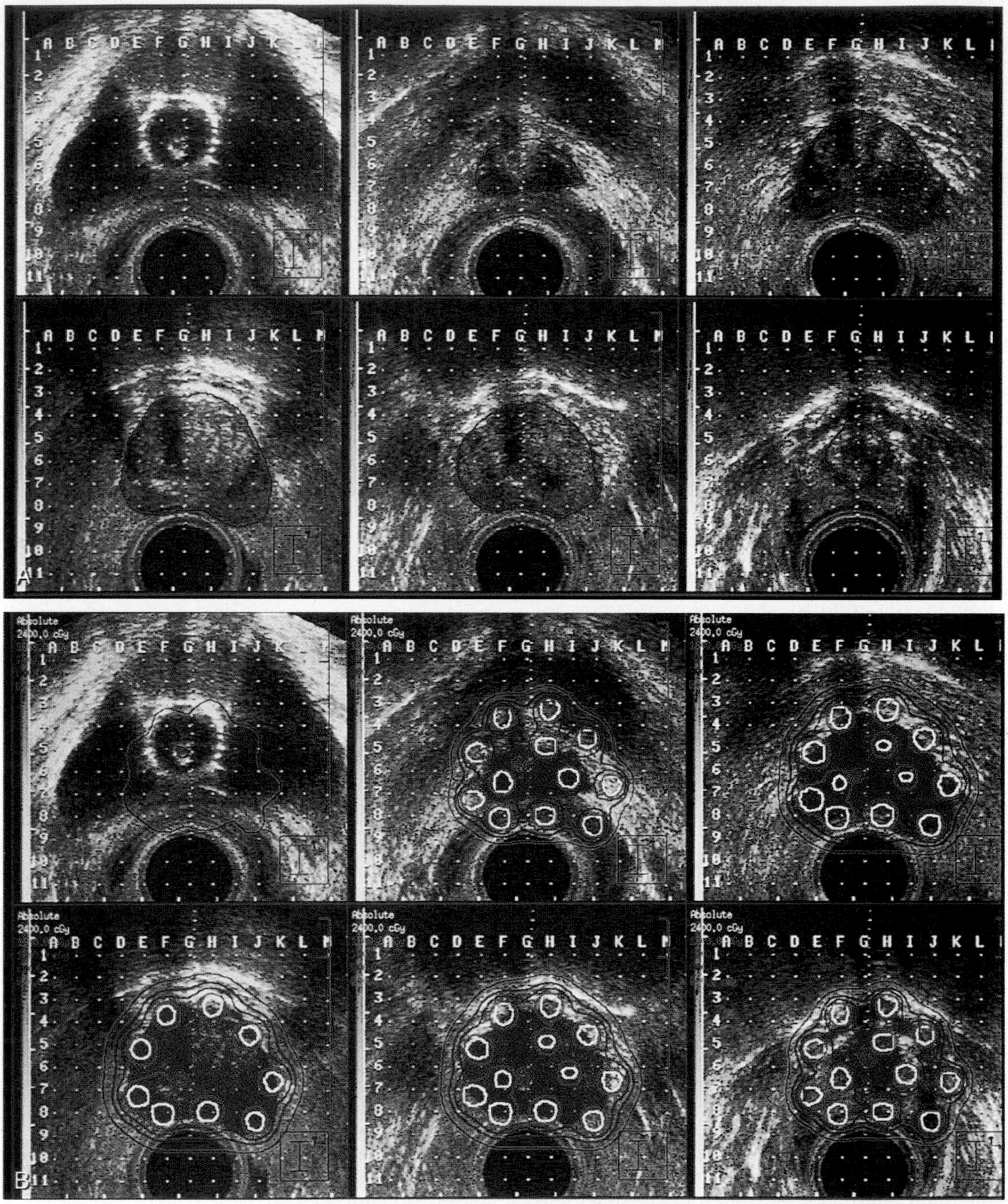

Figure 13-5 Ultrasound-guided permanent implant planning. **A,** Volume study with prostate and urethra identified. Note the eccentric positioning of the urethra. **B,** Isodose distribution of the same patient. Red color wash is 100%; blue line indicates 75%.

implants have been mathematically quantified into biologic dosimetry in terms of time-dose factors.

A typical ^{125}I prostate implant (MPD of 160 Gy) yields an initial dose rate of .08 to .1 Gy/h. The substantially larger amounts of total activity implant with ^{103}Pd (typically 110 to 130 mCi versus 30 to 35 mCi for ^{125}I) result in an initial dose rate two or three times greater (.18 to .2 Gy/h) than ^{125}I. However, because of the half-life difference, the dose rate of ^{103}Pd decreases more rapidly with time than that of ^{125}I. At 5 weeks after implantation, the dose rates of the two radionuclides will be approximately equal, but thereafter ^{125}I will deliver a somewhat higher dose rate to full decay. At 5 weeks, the ^{103}Pd will have delivered approximately 76% of a 115-Gy dose, and the ^{125}I implant will have delivered only 33% of the 160-Gy dose.

Wallner and associates,[114] in a review of 65 patients treated with a transperineal ^{125}I implant for T1 and T2 prostatic carcinoma, noted that a greater incidence of urinary grades 2 and 3 morbidity was associated with maximum central urethral dose, length of urethra that received more than 300 Gy, and large prostate volume. Rectal ulceration was associated with irradiation of the rectal wall to doses greater than 100 Gy.

Efforts should be made to keep the central urethral dose below 400 Gy and rectal surface dose below 100 Gy to decrease toxicity.

Removable Interstitial Implants with Iridium 192

Syed[115] and Martinez[116] and their colleagues developed an interstitial implant LDR technique using removable ^{192}Ir sources with a transperineal template for treatment of carcinoma of the prostate. After the patient has recovered from anesthesia, anteroposterior and lateral x-ray films of the pelvis are obtained for dose computations. Later, ^{192}Ir seeds, about eight per ribbon with .3-mCi RaEq, are inserted in the guides (dose rate, .7 to .8 Gy/h to periphery of gland). Minimum tumor doses of 30 to 35 Gy are delivered. This is combined with 40 Gy (2 Gy/fraction) to the prostate or the whole pelvis as required.

In an update of the initial publication, Stromberg and associates[117] described implantation of the prostate with a transperineal template (MUPIT). A bilateral staging pelvic lymphadenopathy is performed; the length of metallic guides is determined by palpation, and palpable tumor margins are identified with inactive gold seeds. In a modification of the technique, the first needle is placed with the guidance of a finger in the rectum to prevent piercing of that organ. A rectal tube is inserted to help position the template to allow for proper spacing of the rest of the needles. The template is carefully aligned parallel to the floor of the pelvis, not conforming to the perineal slope, to avoid posterior angling of the needles. The needles are differentially loaded with ^{192}Ir seeds on nylon ribbons of varying activity, number of seeds, and the use of ribbon spacers. The posterior needles, in particular, which are primarily directed to the seminal vesicles, are loaded only in the superior half. The implant dose is 33 Gy, which is combined with EBRT (5 Gy in one dose before implant and 30 Gy in 17 fractions after implant). Local control rates of 100% by clinical examination and 84.5% by biopsy and 89% actuarial disease-free survival have been reported.

Image-Guided Intensity-Modulated High-Dose Rate Prostate Brachytherapy

Image-guided intensity-modulated prostate brachytherapy began in 1988 at Kiel University in Germany and soon after in 1991 at WBH in Royal Oak, Michigan, and Seattle Tumor Institute.[118] This section will be subdivided between intensity-modulated HDR prostate brachytherapy (IMBT) as a boost and as monotherapy.

INTENSITY-MODULATED HIGH-DOSE RATE PROSTATE BRACHYTHERAPY TO THE PROSTATE AS A BOOST

To improve treatment results in prostatic adenocarcinoma, studies were designed to optimize treatment planning toward more conformal radiation therapy (CRT) delivery. Three major drawbacks of external beam CRT are variations in internal organ motion/deformation, daily setup inaccuracies, and exclusion of several patients for CRT based on poor geometric relationships as identified by 3D treatment planning. To overcome these problems, we began the first prospective phase I/II dose-escalating clinical trial of conformal IMBT combined with fractionated EBRT. As stated before, the modulation on energy deposition from HDR is related to the computer-controlled spatial distribution of dwell positions and dwell times.

With ultrasound guidance and the interactive online dosimetry system, organ motion and setup inaccuracies (as compared with EBRT) are insignificant because they can be corrected during the procedure without increasing target volume margins. Common pitfalls of brachytherapy, including operator dependence and difficulty with reproducibility, have been eliminated with the intraoperative online planning system[119,120] (Fig. 13-6).

PSA levels have been used as a surrogate to judge disease control of prostate cancer. Several published data sets now attest to the greater ability of IMBT using HDR to control disease compared with conventional radiation.

From November 1991 through November 1995, 58 patients received 45.6-Gy pelvic EBRT and three HDR ^{192}Ir boost implants of 5.5 to 6.5 Gy each.[121] They were compared with 278 similarly staged patients treated from January 1987 through December 1991 with EBRT to prostate-only fields (median dose, 66.6 Gy).[122] No patient received androgen deprivation. Patient outcome was analyzed for biochemical control. Biochemical failure was defined as a PSA level higher than 1.5 ng/mL and rising on two consecutive values. If serial posttreatment PSA levels were showing a continuous downward trend, failure was not scored. Median follow-up was 43 months for the conventionally treated group and 26 months for the IMBT boost group. The median pretreatment PSA level was 14.3 ng/mL for the EBRT-alone group and 14.0 ng/mL for the IMBT boost group. The median Gleason scores were 6 and 7, respectively, for the two groups. The biochemical control rate was significantly higher in the IMBT boost treatment group. Three-year actuarial biochemical control rates were

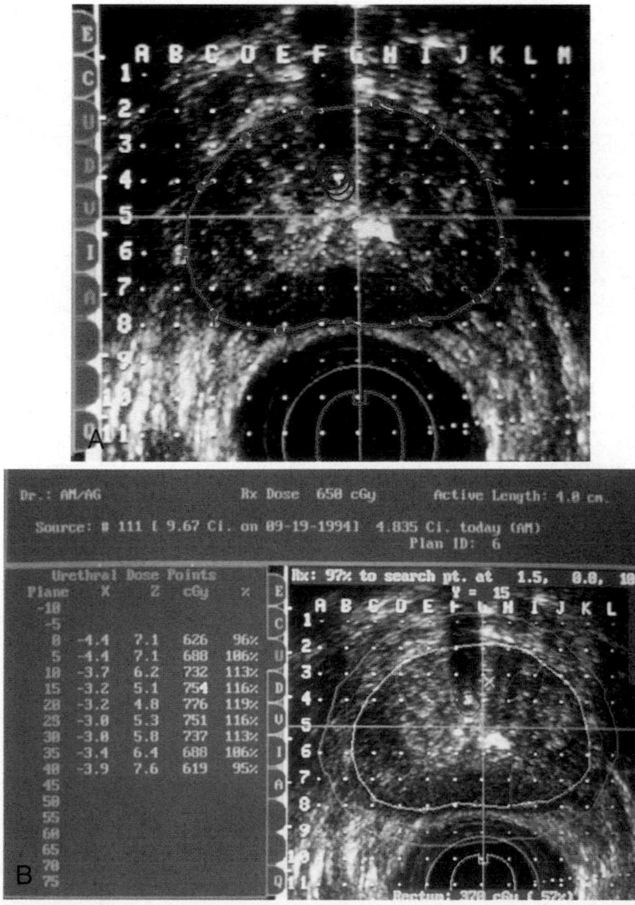

Figure 13-6 HDR planning for prostate. **A,** Prostate is contoured at its maximum extent. Blue arrows denote needle positions proposed by the computer. **B,** Same plan, showing isodose distribution and urethral and rectal doses.

85% and 52% for the conformal IMBT boost and conventionally treated patients, respectively. In a multivariate analysis, the use of IMBT boost and pretreatment PSA level were significant prognostic determinants of biochemical control. The 3-year actuarial rates of biochemical control for conformal IMBT boost versus conventionally treated patients, respectively, were 83% versus 72% for a pretreatment PSA level of 4.1 to 10.0 ng/mL, 85% versus 47% for a PSA level of 10.1 to 20.0 ng/mL, and 89% versus 29% for a PSA level higher than 10 ng/mL. When the analysis was limited to patients in both groups with a minimum 12-month follow-up, the IMBT boost group continued to show a higher biochemical control rate than the conventional radiation group (3-year actuarial rates of 86% versus 53%).[122]

Martinez and associates[123] updated the series with an analysis of 207 patients treated on the dose-escalation IMBT-HDR prostate brachytherapy trial. It demonstrated to be a precise and accurate dose delivery system and a very effective treatment for patients with unfavorable prostate cancer. The improved outcomes coupled with the low risk of complications and the advantage over permanent seed of not being radioactive after implantation, define a new standard for treatment. Using the same database, Brenner, Martinez, and associates[124] reported a low α/β ratio of 1.2 showing high sensitivity to fractionation similar to the late responding tissues.

With longer follow-up and a larger number of patients, Martinez and associates[125] published the long-term results of the WBH prostate HDR dose-escalation trial. Data demonstrated that a conformal IMBT HDR brachytherapy boost improves biochemical control and cause-specific survival in patients with prostate cancer and poor prognostic factors. At the 2005 ASTRO annual meeting, Vargas and colleagues[126] from WBH reported the final analysis of the HDR boost dose-escalation trial. For the first time, an improvement on biochemical control led to a decrease in metastatic rate and improved overall survival.

Galalee and colleagues[118] reported on the collaborative trial between Kiel University in Germany, Seattle Tumor Institute, and WBH on long-term outcomes by risk factor using a conformal HDR brachytherapy boost for patients with localized prostate cancer during the PSA era. Similar results were found at the three institutions in 611 patients with prostate cancer harboring intermediate and high risk factors. With a mean follow-up of 5 years, the 5- and 10-year biochemical control was 77% and 73%, the disease free-survival was 67% and 49%, and the cause-specific survival was 96% and 92%, respectively. The similarity in results at the three institutions gives credence to the reproducibility of the brachytherapy boost treatment. Dose escalation greater than 95 Gy resulted in better 5-year biochemical control for conformal HDR boost (59% versus 85%; $p < .001$) for the entire cohort of hormonal-naïve men. Discriminating by risk factors, a striking dose-escalation effect was seen in the group of patients with two or three poor prognostic factors ($p = .02$ and $p < .001$). This unfavorable group has a remarkable 5-year biochemical control of 85%.

Martinez and associates[127] looked at the question of long-term survival impact with a short course (≤6 months) of adjuvant androgen deprivation when a very high radiation dose was delivered to 934 patients treated with an IMBT-HDR brachytherapy boost in a hypofractionated regime. At 8 years, the addition of a course of 6 months or less of ADT to a very high hypofractionated radiation dose had not conferred a therapeutic advantage but added side effects and cost. Furthermore, for the most unfavorable group of patients harboring all three poor risk factors, there was a higher rate of distant metastasis and more prostate cancer–related deaths. This result questions the value of a short course of ADT and the impact on delaying curative treatment.

Intensity-Modulated High-Dose Rate Brachytherapy to the Prostate as Monotherapy

The twice-per-day accelerated hypofractionated regime was selected based on HDR favorable radiobiological considerations and physical dose delivery advantages of TRUS guidance,[128] with conformal intensity modulated real-time dosimetry of prostate HDR brachytherapy. The Beaumont HDR dose schedule is 9.5 Gy × 4 in a twice-per-day (bid) fractionation in a single implant. This is biologically equivalent to 74 Gy in daily fractions of 2 Gy of external beam radiation (EBRT). For California Endocuritherapy (CET) Cancer Center, the HDR dose schedule is 42 Gy in 6 fractions (bid) in two separate implants 1 week apart. The biologic equivalence is 76 Gy in 2-Gy daily fractions of EBRT.

Patients with clinical stage II (T1c-T2a) disease, Gleason score less than 7 (unilobar, 3 + 4, no perineural invasion), and pretreatment PSA less than 12 ng/mL were treated with monotherapy. The majority of patients presented with what would be considered low-risk or favorable prostate cancer. Patients were offered either HDR or LDR brachytherapy as treatment options, and then the patient selected the brachytherapy modality. A short course of neoadjuvant androgen deprivation (<6 months) was used for downsizing the gland volume in 31% of WBH patients, in equal proportions between permanent seeds and HDR and in 30% of the CET Cancer Center patients.[129] All procedures were done under spinal anesthesia. Figure 13-7 depicts an HDR intraoperative implant using the Nucletron Swift guidance system.

Between January 1996 and December 2002, 378 consecutive patients with clinically localized prostate cancer were treated with accelerated hypofractionated brachytherapy as the sole treatment modality. Of the patients, 172 were treated with HDR brachytherapy alone using ^{192}Ir, and 206 patients were treated with LDR brachytherapy alone using ^{103}Pd.

For the implant procedure and for pain control during the entire treatment time, spinal anesthesia was administered following placement of an epidural catheter for analgesia. Dosimetry was continuously updated in real-time based on the actual location of needles to compensate for organ distortion and motion and to ensure conformal coverage of the gland.[119,120] Gold seed markers were then placed under TRUS guidance at the base and at the apex of the prostate to assess and measure possible interfraction needle displacement. Before delivery of the radiation, the entire prostate was imaged again, with final needle and urethral positions captured by TRUS, and a final treatment plan was created.

At CET, after recovery the patient underwent a dual method of simulation radiography consisting of plain film localization for applicator adjustment and quality control, and a CT scan was performed. The images were downloaded to the "treatment-planning" computer and a 3D reconstruction was carried out. A dose-volume histogram (DVH) and virtual images of the anatomy, clinical target volume (CTV), and PTV were obtained.

The toxicity profile of IMBT-HDR monotherapy was first described by Grills and colleagues[130] from WBH, demonstrating less acute and chronic toxicity with HDR when compared with permanent seeds with ^{103}Pd. Also, the impotency rate was decreased in the HDR group of treated patients by half compared with permanent seeds. The following toxicity analysis is an updated report from the combined experience from WBH

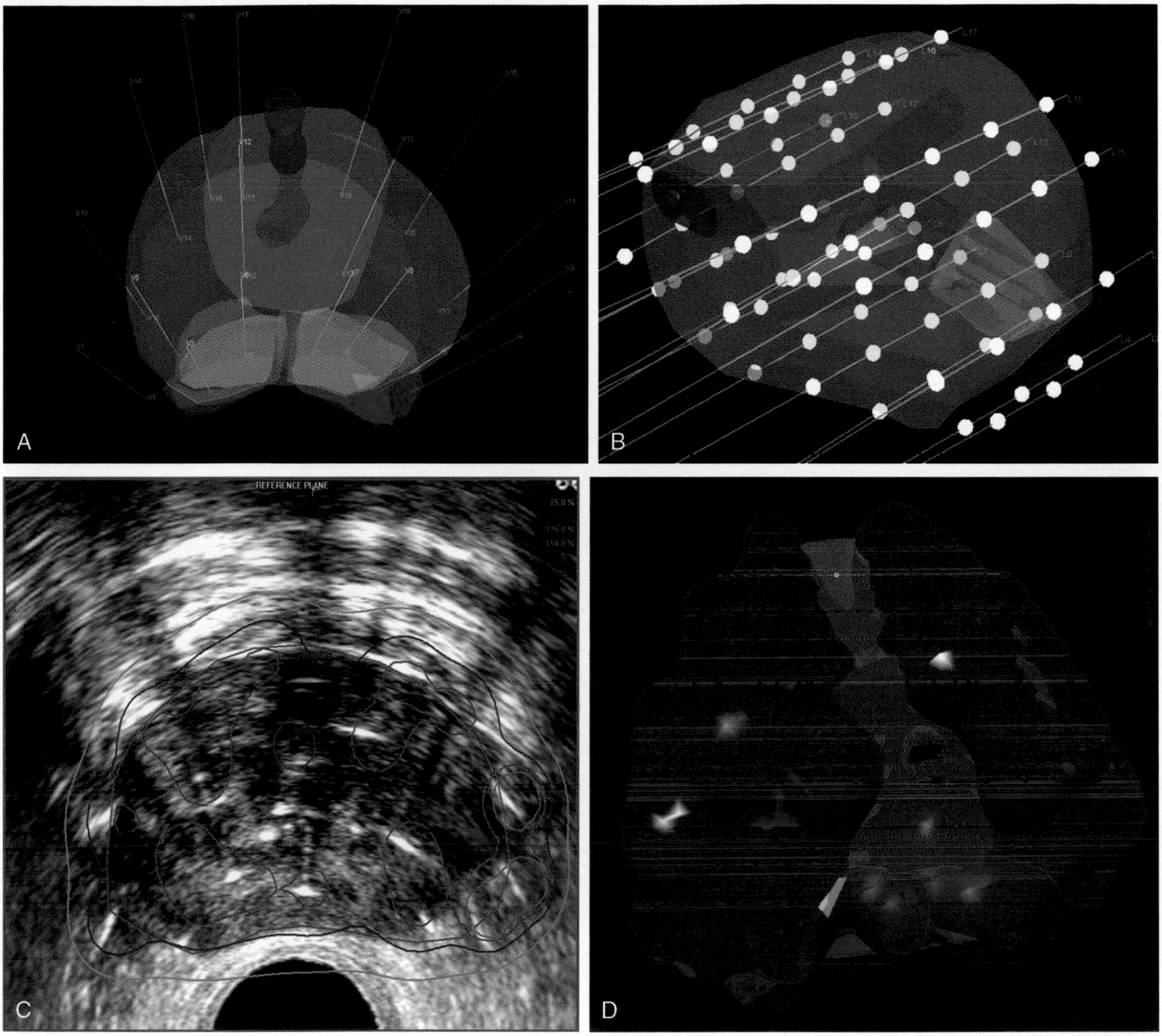

Figure 13-7 HDR intraoperative implant using the Nucletron Swift guidance system. **A,** The 3D reconstruction of the prostate gland, urethral trajectory, and needle orientation. **B,** Anatomical relationship of the prostate, urethra, and the needles with the selected dwell positions on each needle. **C,** Final TRUS-based intraoperative dosimetry and coverage of the PTV. **D,** Dosimetric rendition of the prostate coverage by the 100% isodose cloud in red with urethral sparing from modulating the dwell times and dwell positions.

and CET.[131] The median follow-up for all patients was 4.1 years (range, .8 to 12.3 years).

Acute Toxicity

HDR brachytherapy alone was associated with statistically significant reductions in the acute rates of dysuria (65% with ^{103}Pd seeds versus 38% with HDR monotherapy; $P < .001$), as well as urinary frequency and/or urgency (^{103}Pd: 94% versus 53%, HDR; $P < .001$) and urinary retention (^{103}Pd: 43% versus 29%, HDR; $P = .012$). In addition to reduced acute genitourinary symptoms, HDR was also associated with lower rates of rectal pain (18% with LDR versus 7%, HDR; $P = .025$). The majority of acute toxicities in both groups were grade 1. Hormonal androgen ablation for gland downsizing was given to 31% of patients in both groups.

Chronic Toxicity

HDR brachytherapy alone was again associated with reduced urinary frequency and urgency (^{103}Pd: 54% versus 32%, HDR; $P < .001$). The majority of toxicities were grade 1. There were no differences in the remaining chronic toxicity rates of urinary incontinence or retention, hematuria, diarrhea, rectal pain, or rectal bleeding between the two treatment groups. The rate of urethral stricture requiring dilatation was 3% with HDR compared with 1% with ^{103}Pd ($P = .3$). The median time to development of urethral stricture was 17 months, with a

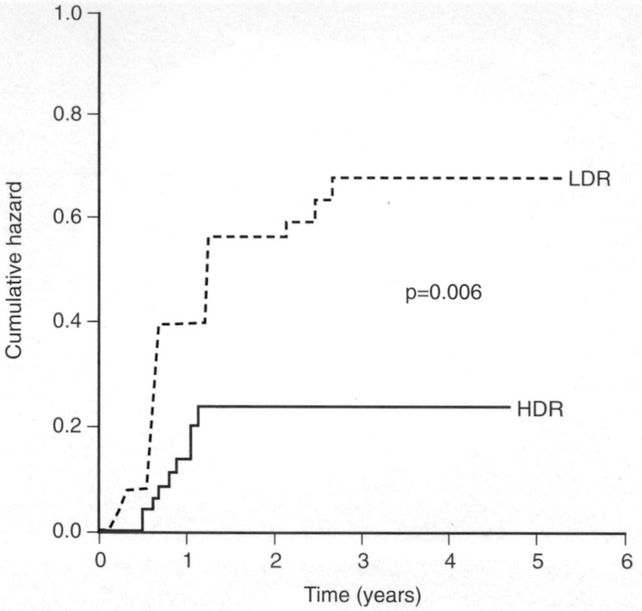

Figure 13-8 Probability of sexual impotence by treatment method.

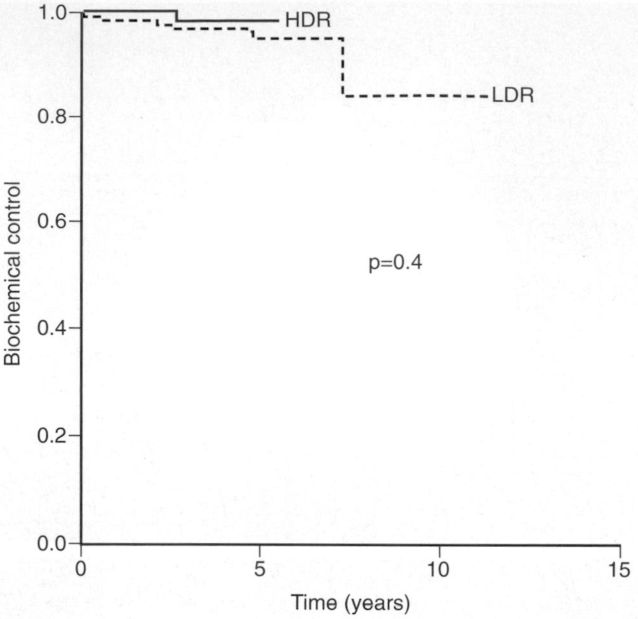

Figure 13-9 Actuarial analysis of biochemical control, ASTRO definition.

range of 4 to 37 months. The cumulative proportion of chronic grade 3 toxicity by treatment modality did not differ between the two treatment types.

POTENCY

Regardless of the use of adjuvant hormonal therapy, all cases were included for which complete pretreatment and post-treatment information was available. This included 61 patients treated with HDR brachytherapy alone and 81 patients treated with permanent ^{103}Pd. The 5-year probability of impotency was 38% for all patients with available data. As shown in Figure 13-8, the probability was 49% for LDR patients and 21% for HDR patients ($P = .006$). The mean times to impotency for the HDR and LDR treatments were 3.9 and 3.2 years, respectively.

SURVIVAL OUTCOMES

The 5-year actuarial outcomes for monotherapy showed no difference in terms of ASTRO definition for biochemical failure, cancer mortality, or overall survival between HDR alone versus permanent seeds. In Figure 13-9, the actuarial 5-year biochemical control curves for HDR and LDR are depicted. No difference in biochemical control ASTRO definition can be seen by treatment modality.

ENDOVASCULAR BRACHYTHERAPY

A new application of brachytherapy was intended to prevent restenosis after coronary angioplasty, stenting, peripheral vascular bypass surgery, or access procedures for renal dialysis, since restenosis after coronary angioplasty and stenting was reported in about 30% to 60% of patients. Most restenosis occurs 3 to 9 months after the angioplasty procedure; also, restenosis of aortofemoral bypasses has been reported in 15% to 30% of patients with arterial and vein bypass and in 40% to 50% with prosthetic bypasses. The results of treatment for coronary restenosis and peripheral vascular restenosis were traditionally poor until endovascular brachytherapy began to be tested in multi-institutional clinical trials. Phase III trials subsequently demonstrated an advantage in patients who were treated versus not treated with endovascular brachytherapy (see Human Studies). Coronary brachytherapy is now used infrequently, as the recently approved drug-eluting stents (DESs) virtually eliminated in-stent restenosis, thereby significantly decreasing the need for endovascular brachytherapy (see Current Indications).

Stenosis of coronary vessels after angioplasty is due to thrombosis, plaque dissection, arterial remodeling (enlargement of the lumen), and cellular proliferation that takes place in the intima of the coronary vessel (endothelial cells), media (smooth muscle), or external elastic lamina and adventitia (myofibroblasts). Causes of peripheral vascular bypass failure are operative techniques (skill of surgeon), low flow/poor runoff of blood (<100 mL/min), graft surface thrombogenesis, obstructive venous disease (outer flow), neointimal hyperplasia, graft structural abnormalities in both venous or prosthetic grafts, progressive arteriosclerotic plaques, and other factors such as smoking and hyperlipidemia.

Animal Studies

Animal experiments in pigs[132,133] using coronary endovascular brachytherapy with ^{192}Ir at doses ranging from 7 to 25 Gy have shown a significant reduction in the incidence and degree of restenosis after injury of the swine coronary vessels with a stretching balloon. Most of the studies have been done at 1 month after the procedure and irradiation. Wiedermann and colleagues,[133] with 20 Gy at 1.5 mm, observed a 70% reduction in restenosis. Waksman and coworkers,[134] with doses of 7 or 14 Gy at 2 mm, noted a reduction of 30% and 67%, respectively, in restenosis at 6 months, and Raizner[132] observed not only a dose effect but a dose-rate effect as well with regard to restenosis.

Biologic and pathophysiologic observations from in vitro and in vivo experiments on radiation effects have shown that, in addition to clonogenic cell death (postmitotic), a significant portion of irradiated endothelial cells succumbs to apoptosis. Studies have also demonstrated that basic fibroblast growth factor, a known mitogen for endothelial cells, protected them against radiation-induced apoptosis but not against clonogenic cell kill. Immunohistochemical studies showed that basic fibroblast growth factor is present in large arteries and veins, whereas there are very small amounts in vasa vasorum and small capillaries. Thus, small capillaries undergo apoptosis because of this fibroblast growth factor deficiency, whereas larger vessels are immune to apoptosis.

In addition to endothelial proliferation, there is smooth muscle degeneration and hyperplasia, which contribute to restenosis after angioplasty and stenting. Waksman and colleagues[134,135] have shown experimentally that intravascular irradiation modifies this response, inhibiting early adventitial cell proliferation and modifying the production of α-actinin by the adventitia myofibroblasts at later times after injury. Intravascular irradiation may be expected to reduce the growth of the restenosis lesion and has the potential to positively affect vascular remodeling.

Human Studies

Schopohl and colleagues[136] used a Nucletron MicroSelectron HDR device, a 5-French catheter, and a 9-French ReKa catheter to deliver 12 Gy at 3 mm from the ^{192}Ir source. With a follow-up of 8 to 69 months, of 29 patients treated after repair (stent) of femoral restenosis, 21 remained without restenosis, 4 had reocclusion, 1 died at 36 months of ovarian cancer, and 2 had no follow-up because they moved and had no forwarding address.

Condado and coworkers[137] treated 21 patients using HDR ^{192}Ir to deliver 20 to 25 Gy. Three of 11 patients treated with 20 Gy developed restenosis in contrast with no restenoses in 10 patients treated with 25 Gy. One patient developed a coronary aneurysm. Initially, the dose was prescribed at 25 Gy, but review of the dosimetry showed that the actual dose delivered was 54 Gy.

Scripps Clinic investigators conducted a randomized study comparing sham radiation to coronary intravascular irradiation with LDR.[138-140] Eligibility for the study included patients with stenosed vessels who had previous successful stenting or angioplasty in lesions in coronary vessels larger than 3 mm. The iridium source was 100 mCi strength, and mean treatment time was approximately 35 minutes. Maximum vessel and the minimum dose in the adventitia was 80 Gy (average). One patient died, and one required restenting. Results were reported in 26 patients assigned to ^{192}Ir and 29 assigned to a placebo. Angiographically identified restenosis (>50% of luminal diameter) was noted in 17% of the ^{192}Ir group and 54% of patients not irradiated ($p = .01$). The mean luminal diameter was larger with irradiation (2.43 mm) than with placebo (1.85 mm). Updated 3-year angiographic restenosis rates favored radiated patients (64% with placebo versus 33% with radiation, $P < .05$), and the target lesion revascularization (TLR) rate at 5-year follow-up was significantly lower in irradiated patients (48% versus 23%, $P = .05$).

Subsequently, three multi-institution phase III trials were performed that demonstrated the advantage of endovascular radiation versus placebo (GAMMA I, START, and INHIBIT).[141-144] The GAMMA I trial[141] was a multi-institutional phase III trial of 252 patients (12 institutions) testing the value of ^{192}Ir (gamma radiation) in preventing coronary in-stent restenosis. At 6-month follow-up, the rate of angiographic restenosis was reduced from 50.5% to 21.5% in favor of irradiated patients, and the TLR rate at 9 months was reduced from 45% to 24% (p = .03) . The START trial[142] was a multi-institution phase III trial, involving 476 patients (50 centers) with in-stent restenosis, which tested ^{90}Sr/Y (beta radiation). At 8-month follow-up, the angiographic in-stent restenosis rate was significantly decreased from 41% with placebo to 14% with radiation, and the TLR rate was decreased from 22% to 13% ($P < .008$). The INHIBIT trial[143,144] randomized 332 patients (27 institutions) with in-stent restenosis to placebo versus irradiation with ^{32}P (beta radiation). The in-stent angiographic restenosis rate at 9 months was decreased from 49% with placebo to 16% with radiation ($P < .0001$), and the rate of major adverse cardiac events was decreased from 31% to 15% ($P = .0006$).

While the above reported trials demonstrated a favorable response to endovascular irradiation, the complex interactions of two specialties (cardiology, radiation oncology) coupled with a difficult delivery system led the cardiologist to seek other treatment alternatives. DESs were developed and tested. The results of the DES trials demonstrated equal effectiveness in preventing restenosis with a much simpler cardiology approach.[145]

Current Indications

Both the indications for and utilization of endovascular coronary brachytherapy have markedly changed. This is primarily due to the availability and success of DES that dramatically decreased, or in some instances virtually eliminated, in-stent restenosis, thereby eliminating the need for routine endovascular brachytherapy. Most U.S. institutions are no longer using coronary brachytherapy in view of the DES success.

In those institutions that still use coronary brachytherapy, both indication and system availability have changed dramatically. The main indication for endovascular brachytherapy is "drug-resistant in-stent restenosis" after the deployment of a DES, either rapamycin- or Taxol-coated stents. The only endovascular brachytherapy system available is the Betacath system (Novoste Corporation, Norcross, GA) using ^{90}Sr.

REFERENCES

1. Henschke UK: Afterloading applicator for radiation therapy of carcinoma of the uterus. Radiology 74:834, 1960.
2. Fletcher GH: Cervical radium applicators with screening in the direction of bladder and rectum. Radiology 60:77-84, 1953.
3. Henschke UK: Interstitial implantation with radioisotopes. *In* Hahan PF (ed): Therapeutic Use of Artificial Radioisotopes. New York, Wiley, 1956.
4. Batley F, Constable WE: The use of the "Manchester System" for treatment of cancer of the uterine cervix with modern afterloading radium applicators. J Can Assoc Radiol 18:396, 1967.
5. Henschke UK: Afterloading applicator for radiation therapy of carcinoma of the uterus. Radiology 74:834, 1960.
6. Henschke UK, Hilaris BS, Mahan GD: Afterloading in interstitial and intracavitary radiation therapy. AJR Am J Roentgenol 90:386-395, 1963.
7. International Commission on Radiation Units (ICRU): ICRU Report No. 38: Dose and Volume Specification for Reporting Intracavitary Therapy in Gynecology. Bethesda, MD, ICRU, 1985, pp 1-16.
8. Hames F: A new method in the use of radon gold seeds. Am J Surg 38:235, 1937.
9. Morton JL, Callendine GW Jr, Myers WG: Radioactive cobalt 60 in plastic tubing for interstitial radiation therapy. Radiology 56:553, 1951.
10. Pierquin B, Chassagne D, Bailiet F, et al: The place of implantation in tongue and floor of mouth cancer. JAMA 215:961, 1971.
11. Alden ME, Mohiuddin M: The impact of radiation dose in combined external beam and intraluminal ^{192}Ir brachytherapy for bile duct cancer. Int J Radiat Oncol Biol Phys 28:945-951, 1994.
12. Bier R, Small RC, Leake DL, et al: An afterloading technique for radium needles in the treatment of carcinoma of the oral cavity. Radiology 108:711, 1973.

13. Delclos L: Are interstitial radium applications passé? Front Radiat Ther Oncol 12:42, 1978.
14. Hilaris BS, Henschke UK, Holt JG: Clinical experience with long half-life and low-energy encapsulated radioactive sources in cancer radiation therapy. Radiology 91:1163, 1968.
15. Henschke UK: Artificial radioisotopes in nylon ribbons for implantation in neoplasms. *In* International Conferences on the Peaceful Uses of Atomic Energy. New York, United Nations, 1956.
16. Hilaris BS: Handbook of Interstitial Brachytherapy. Acton, MS, Acton Publishing, 1975.
17. Morphis OL: Teflon tube method of radium implantation. AJR Am J Roentgenol 83:455, 1960.
18. Mowatt KS, Stevens KA: Afterloading: a contribution to the protection problem. J Fac Radiol 8:28, 1956.
19. Paine CH: Modem afterloading methods for interstitial radiotherapy. Clin Radiol 23:263, 1972.
20. Clarke DH, Edmundson GK, Martinez A, et al: The utilization of I-125 seeds as a substitute for Ir-192 seeds in temporary interstitial implants: an overview and a description of the William Beaumont Hospital technique. Int J Radiat Oncol Biol Phys 15:1027-1033, 1988.
21. Clarke DH, Edmundson GK, Martinez A, et al: The clinical advantages of I-125 seeds as a substitute for Ir-192 seeds in temporary plastic tube implants. Int J Radiat Oncol Biol Phys 17:859-863, 1989.
22. Harter DJ, Delclos L: Sealed sources in synthetic absorbable suture. Radiology 116:727, 1975.
23. Scott WP: Simplified interstitial therapy technique (Vicryl) for unresectable lung cancer. Radiology 117:734, 1975.
24. Palos B, Pooler D, Goffinet DR, Martinez A: A method for inserting I-125 seeds into the absorbable sutures for permanent implantation in tissue. Int J Radiat Oncol Biol Phys 6:381-385, 1980.
25. Martinez A, Goffinet DR, Palos B, et al: Sterilization of 125-iodine seeds encased in Ethicon Vicryl sutures for permanent interstitial implantation. Int J Radiat Oncol Bio Phys 5:411-413, 1979.
26. Goffinet DR, Martinez A, Fee WE Jr: ^{125}I Vicryl suture implants as a surgical adjuvant in cancer of the head and neck. Int J Radiat Oncol Biol Phys 11:399, 1985.
27. Puthawala AA, Syed AM, Tansey LA, et al: Temporary iridium 192 implant in the management of carcinoma of the prostate. Endocurie Hypertherm Oncol 1:25, 1985.
28. Hockel M, Muller T: A new perineal template assembly for high-dose rate interstitial brachytherapy of gynecologic malignancies. Radiother Oncol 31:262-264, 1994.
29. Martinez AM, Edmundson GK, Cox RS, et al: Combination of external beam irradiation and multiple-site perineal applicator (MUPIT) for treatment of locally advanced or recurrent prostatic, anorectal, and gynecologic malignancies. Int J Radiat Oncol Biol Phys 11:391-398, 1985.
30. Prempree T: Parametrial implant in stage IIIB cancer of the cervix: III. A five-year study. Cancer 52:748, 1983.
31. Gaddis O Jr, Morrow CP, Klement V, et al: Treatment of cervical carcinoma employing a template for transperineal interstitial ^{192}Ir brachytherapy. Int J Radiat Oncol Biol Phys 9:819-827, 1983.
32. Monk BJ, Tewari K, Burger RA, et al: A comparison of intracavitary versus interstitial irradiation in the treatment of cervical cancer. Gynecol Oncol 67:241-247, 1997.
33. Gupta AK, Vicini FA, Frazier AI, et al: Iridium 192 transperineal interstitial brachytherapy for locally advanced or recurrent gynecological malignancies. Int J Radiat Oncol Biol Phys 43:1055-1060, 1999.
34. Russell AH, Koh WJ, Markette K, et al: Radical reirradiation for recurrent or second primary carcinoma of the female reproductive tract. Gynecol Oncol 27:226-232, 1987.
35. Puthawala AA, Syed AM, Fleming PA, et al: Re-irradiation with interstitial implant for recurrent pelvic malignancies. Cancer 50:2810-2814, 1982.
36. Battermann JJ, Szabol B: Preliminary results of radiation therapy for carcinoma of the uterine cervix, using the Selectron afterloading machine. *In* Mould RF (ed): Brachytherapy 2. Leersum, The Netherlands, Nucletron International BV, 1989, pp 229-234.
37. Gupta BD, Ayyagari S, Sharma SC, et al: Carcinoma of the cervix: Optimal time-dose fractionation of HDR brachytherapy and comparison with conventional dose-rate brachytherapy. *In* Mould RF (ed): Brachytherapy 2. Leerum, The Netherlands, Nucletron International BV, 1989, pp 307-308.
38. Scalliet P, Gerbaulet A, Dubray B: HDR versus LDR in gynecological brachytherapy revisited. Radiother Oncol 28:118-126, 1993.
39. Brenner DJ, Hall EJ: Conditions for the equivalence of continuous to pulsed low-dose-rate brachytherapy. Int J Radiat Oncol Biol Phys 20:181-190, 1991.
40. Visser AG, van den Aardweg GJMJ, Levenday PC: Pulsed-dose-rate and fractionated high-dose-rate brachytherapy: choice of brachytherapy schedules to replace low-dose-rate treatments. Int J Radiat Oncol Biol Phys 34:497-505, 1996.
41. Erickson BA, Shadley JD: In vitro test of the cytotoxic equivalence between pulsed dose rate and continuous low dose rate. Radiat Oncol Invest 3:217-244, 1996.
42. Hall EJ, Brenner DJ: Pulsed dose rate brachytherapy: can we take advantage of new technology? [Editorial] Int J Radiat Oncol Biol Phys 34:511-512, 1996.
43. Armour E, White J, DeWitt C, et al: Effects of continuous low-dose-rate brachytherapy on the rectum of the rat. Radiat Res 145:474-480, 1996.
44. White JR, Armour EP, Armin AR, et al: Reproducible rat model for comparing late rectal toxicity from different brachytherapy techniques. Int J Radiat Oncol Biol Phys 37:1155-1161, 1997.
45. Armour EP, White JR, Armin AR, et al: Pulsed low-dose-rate brachytherapy in a rat model: dependence of late rectal injury on radiation pulse size. Int J Radiat Oncol Biol Phys 38:825-834, 1997.
46. Williamson JF: Practical quality assurance in low-dose-rate brachytherapy. *In* Proceedings of American College of Medical Physics-Sponsored Symposium on Quality Assurance in Radiotherapy Physics. Madison, WI, Medical Physics Publishing, 1991, pp 139-182.
47. Walker MD, Strike TA, Sheline GE: An analysis of dose-effect relationship in the radiotherapy of malignant gliomas. Int J Radiat Oncol Biol Phys 5:1733, 1979.
48. Prados MD, Gutin PH, Philips TL, et al: Interstitial brachytherapy for newly diagnosed patients with malignant gliomas: the UCSF experience. Int J Radiat Oncol Biol Phys 24:593-597, 1992.
49. Stallard HB: Malignant melanoma of the choroid treated with radioactive applicators. Trans Ophthalmol Soc UK 79:373-392, 1959.
50. Cameron ME: Pterygium Throughout the World. Springfield, IL, Charles C Thomas, 1965.
51. van den Brenk HAS: Results of prophylactic postoperative irradiation in 1300 cases of pterygium. AJR Am J Roentgenol 103:723-733, 1968.
52. Greenberg M: Eye: Choroidal melanomas and pterygium. *In* Pierquin B, Wilson J-F, Chassagne D (eds): Modern Brachytherapy. New York, Masson, 1987, pp 301-314.
53. Rosenblatt E, Rachmiel A, Blumenfeld I, et al: Intracavitary mould brachytherapy in malignant tumors of the maxilla. Endocurie Hypertherm Oncol 12:25-34, 1996.
54. Mendenhall NP, Parsons JT, Cassisi NJ, et al: Carcinoma of the nasal vestibule. Int J Radiat Oncol Biol Phys 10:627-637, 1984.
55. Mendenhall NP, Parsons JT, Cassisi NJ, et al: Carcinoma of the nasal vestibule treated with radiation therapy. Laryngoscope 97:626-632, 1987.
56. Marchese MI, Nori D, Anderson LL, et al: A versatile permanent planar implant technique utilizing iodine 125 seeds imbedded in Gel-foam. Int J Radiat Oncol Biol Phys 10:747, 1984.
57. Jorgensen K, Elbrond O, Andersen AP: Carcinoma of the lip: a series of 869 cases. Acta Radiol Ther Phys Biol 12:177-190, 1973.
58. Erickson BA, Wilson JF: Nasopharyngeal brachytherapy. Am J Clin Oncol 16:424-443, 1993.
59. Wang CC, Busse J, Gitterman M: A simple afterloading applicator for intracavitary irradiation of carcinoma of the nasopharynx. Radiology 115:737-738, 1975.
60. Porrazzo MS, Hilaris BS, Moorthy CR, et al: Permanent interstitial implantation using palladium 103: the New York Medical College preliminary experience. Int J Radiat Oncol Biol Phys 23:1033-1036, 1992.
61. Wang CC: Re-irradiation of recurrent nasopharyngeal carcinoma: treatment techniques and results. Int J Radiat Oncol Biol Phys 13:953-956, 1987.

62. Marcus RB Jr, Million RR, Mitchell TP: A preloaded, custom-designed implantation device for stage Tl-T2 carcinoma of the floor of mouth. Int J Radiat Oncol Biol Phys 6:111-113, 1980.
63. Mazeron N, Lusichini A, Marinello G, et al: Interstitial radiation therapy for squamous cell carcinoma of the tonsillar region: the Creteil experience (1971-1981). Int J Radiat Oncol Biol Phys 12:895-900, 1986.
64. Esche BA, Haie CM, Gerbaulet AP, et al: Interstitial and external radiotherapy in carcinoma of the soft palate and uvula. Int J Radiat Oncol Biol Phys 15:619-625, 1988.
65. Mendenhall WM, Parsons IT, Mendenhall JP, et al: Brachytherapy in head and neck cancer. Oncology 5:44-54, 1991.
66. Goffinet DR, Martinez A, Palos B, et al: A method of interstitial tonsillopallatine implants. Int J Radiat Oncol Biol Phys 22:155-162, 1977.
67. Bartelink H, Borger JH: Breast conservation therapy: current and future role of interstitial boost irradiation. *In* Mould RF (ed): Brachytherapy 2. Leersum, The Netherlands, Nucletron International BV, 1989, pp 497-502.
68. Martinez A, Goffinet DR: Irradiation with external beam and interstitial radioactive implant as primary treatment for early breast cancer. Surg Gynecol Obstet 152:285-290, 1981.
69. Mansfield CM, Domamicky LT, Schwartz GF, et al: Perioperative implantation of iridium 192 as the boost technique for stage I and II breast cancer: results of a 10-year study of 655 patients. Radiology 192:33-36, 1994.
70. Mazeron JJ, Simon JM, Crook J, et al: Influence of dose rate on local control of breast carcinoma treated by external beam irradiation plus iridium 192 implant. Int J Radiat Oncol Biol Phys 21:1173-1177, 1991.
71. Martinez AA, Chen PY, Gustafson G, et al: Irradiation of the tumor bed alone after lumpectomy with high-dose-rate brachytherapy. *In* Proceedings of the 19th Annual Meeting of the American Brachytherapy Society, Palm Beach, FL, 1997.
72. Vicini FA, Baglan KL, Kestin LL, et al: Accelerated treatment of breast cancer. J Clin Oncol 19:1993-2001, 2001.
73. Vicini FA, Kestin L, Chen P, et al: Limited-field radiation therapy in the management of early-stage breast cancer. JNCI 95:1205-1211, 2003.
74. Chen P, Vicini FA, Benitez P, et al: Long-term cosmetic results and toxicity after acclerated partial-breast irradiation: a method of radiation delivery by interstelial brachy therapy for the treatment of early-stage breast carcinoma. Cancer 166: 991-999, 2006.
75. Benitez PR, Chen PY, Vicini FA, et al: Surgical considerations in the treatment of early-stage breast cancer with accelerated partial breast irradiation (APBI) in breast conserving therapy via interstitial brachytherapy. Am J Surg 188:355-364, 2004.
76. Edmundson GK, Vicini FA, Chen P, et al: Dosimetric characteristics of the MammoSite RTS, a new breast brachytherapy applicator. Int J Radiat Oncol Biol Phys 52:1132-1139, 2002.
77. Keish M, Vicini F: Applying innovations in surgical and radiation oncology to breast conservation. Breast J 11(Suppl 1):S24-S29, 2005.
78. Hilaris BS, Gomez J, Nori D, et al: Combined surgery, intraoperative brachytherapy, and postoperative external radiation in stage III non-small cell lung cancer. Cancer 55:1226-1231, 1985.
79. Lo TC, Girshovich L, Healey GA, et al: Low-dose-rate versus high-dose-rate intraluminal brachytherapy for malignant endobronchial tumors. Radiother Oncol 35:193-197, 1995.
80. Flores AD, Nelems B, Evans K, et al: Impact of new radiotherapy modalities on the surgical management of cancer of the esophagus and cardia. Int J Radiat Oncol Biol Phys 17:937-944, 1989.
81. Syed AMN, Puthawala AA, Severance SR, et al: Intraluminal irradiation in the treatment of esophageal cancer. Endocurie Hypertherm Oncol 3:105-113, 1987.
82. Peretz T, Nori D, Hilaris B, et al: Treatment of primary unresectable carcinoma of the pancreas with I-125 implantation. Int J Radiat Biol Phys 17:931-935, 1989.
83. Fields JN, Emami B: Carcinoma of the extrahepatic biliary system: results of primary and adjuvant radiotherapy. Int J Radiat Oncol Biol Phys 13:331-338, 1987.
84. Meerwaldt JH, Veeze-Kuijpers B, Visser AG, et al: Combined modality radiotherapy in the treatment of bile duct carcinoma. *In* Mould RF (ed): Brachytherapy 2. Leersum, The Netherlands, Nucletron International BV, 1989, pp 577-583.
85. Fritz P, Brambs HJ, Schraube P, et al: Combined external beam radiotherapy and intraluminal high-dose-rate brachytherapy on bile duct carcinomas. Int J Radiat Oncol Biol Phys 29:855-861, 1994.
86. Lacerna M, Irwin R, Vicini F, et al: Iodine 125 temporary interstitial Implants and limb conserving surgery in the management of extremity soft tissue sarcomas. Endocurie Hypertherm Oncol 12:191-198, 1996.
87. Hilaris BS, Nori D, Anderson LL: Brachytherapy for soft tissue sarcomas. *In* Hilaris BS, Nori D, Anderson LL (eds): Atlas of Brachytherapy. New York, Macmillan, 1988, pp 170-182.
88. Pisters PWT, Harrison LB, Leung DHY, et al: Long-term results of a prospective randomized trial of adjuvant brachytherapy in soft tissue sarcoma. J Clin Oncol 14:859-868, 1996.
89. Potter R, Knocke TH, Kovacs G, et al: Brachytherapy in the combined modality treatment of pediatric malignancies: principles and preliminary experience with treatment of soft tissue sarcoma (recurrence) and Ewing's sarcoma. Klin Paediatr 207:164-173, 1995.
90. Schray MF, Gunderson LL, Sim FH, et al: Soft tissue sarcoma: integration of brachytherapy, resection, and external irradiation. Cancer 66:451-456, 1990.
91. Corn BW, Hanlon AL, Pajak TF, et al: Technically accurate intracavitary insertions improve pelvic control and survival among patients with locally advanced carcinoma of the uterine cervix. Gynecol Oncol 53:294-300, 1994.
92. Tod MC, Meredith WJ: A dosage system for use in the treatment of cancer of the uterine cervix. Br J Radiol 11:809, 1938.
93. Delclos L, Fletcher GH, Sampiere V, et al: Can the Fletcher gamma ray colpostat system be extrapolated to other systems? Cancer 41:970, 1978.
94. Henschke UK: Afterloading applicator for radiation therapy of carcinoma of the uterus. Radiology 74:834, 1960.
95. Martinez A, Cox RS, Edmundson GK: A multiple-site perineal applicator, MUPIT, for the treatment of prostatic, anorectal, and gynecological malignancies. Int J Radiat Oncol Biol Phys 10:297-305, 1984.
96. Aristizabal SA, Valencia A, Ocampo G, et al: Interstitial parametrial irradiation in cancer of the cervix stage IIB-IIIB. Endocurie Hypertherm Oncol 1:41, 1985.
97. Feder BH, Syed AM, Neblett D: Treatment of extensive carcinoma of the cervix with the transperineal parametrial butterfly: a preliminary report. Int J Radiat Oncol Biol Phys 4:735-742, 1978.
98. Leborgue F, Fowler JF, Leborgue JH, et al: Fractionation in medium-dose-rate brachytherapy of cancer of the cervix. Int J Radiat Oncol Biol Phys 35:907-914, 1996.
99. Grigsby PW, Perez CA, Kuten A, et al: Clinical stage I endometrial cancer: results of adjuvant irradiation and patterns of failure. Int J Radiat Oncol Biol Phys 21:379-385, 1991.
100. Chao CKS, Grigsby PW, Perez CA, et al: Brachytherapy-related complications for medically inoperable stage I endometrial carcinoma. Int J Radiat Oncol Biol Phys 31:37-42, 1995.
101. Rotte K: Technique and results of HDR afterloading in cancer of the endometrium. *In* Martinez AA, Orton CG, Mould RF (eds): Brachytherapy: HDR and LDR. Columbia, MD, Nucletron Corporation, 1990, pp 68-79.
102. Perez CA, Kuske R, Glasgow GP: Review of brachytherapy for gynecologic tumors. Endocurie Hypertherm Oncol 1:153, 1985.
103. Erickson BA: Interstitial implantation of vulvar malignancies: an historical perspective. Endocurie Hypertherm Oncol 12:101-112, 1996.
104. Papillon J, Montbarbon JR, Gerard JP, et al: Interstitial curietherapy in the conservative treatment of anal and rectal cancers. Int J Radiat Oncol Biol Phys 17:1161-1169, 1989.
105. Puthawala AA, Syed AMN, Gates TC, et al: Definitive treatment of extensive anorectal cancer by external and interstitial irradiation. Cancer 50:1746-1750, 1982.
106. van der Werf-Messing B: Interstitial radium therapy of superficial bladder cancer (category T1NxM9 and T2NxM0). *In* Smith PH, Prout GB Jr (eds): Bladder Cancer. London, Butterworth, 1984, pp 191-202.
107. Batterman JJ, Tierie AH: Results of implantation for T1 and T2 bladder tumors. Radiother Oncol 5:85-90, 1986.

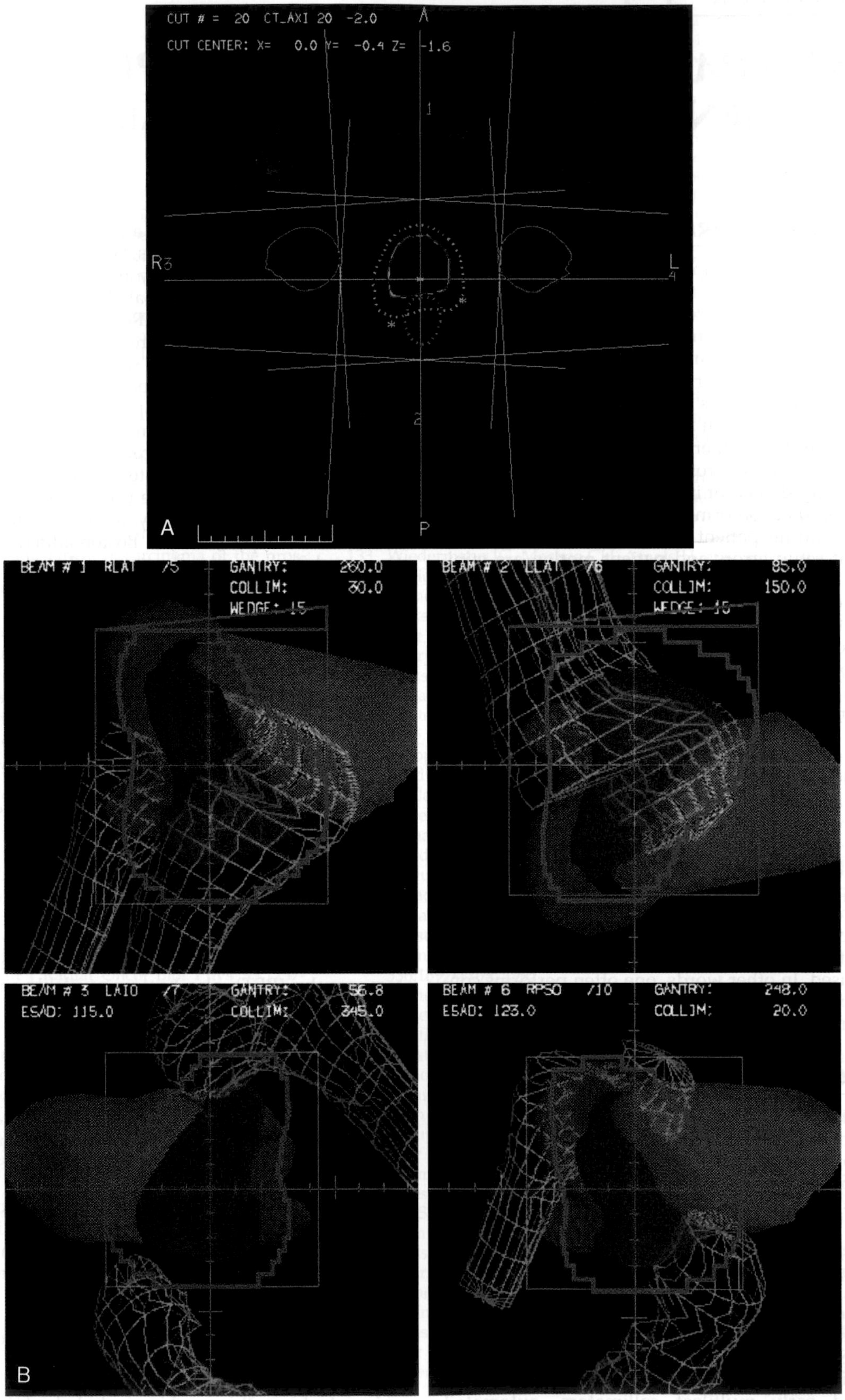

Figure 14-1 **A,** Four-field box treatment of the prostate. **B,** Beam's eye view of four fields from a conformal plan for prostate treatment.

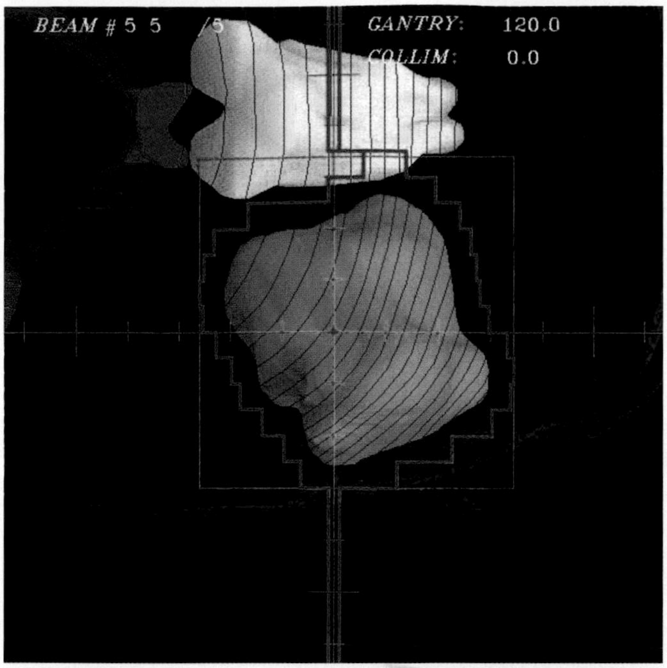

Figure 14-2 Beam's eye view of a brain tumor showing a multileaf collimator shaped to the *violet* target volume. Normal tissues include brainstem *(white)*, chiasm *(green)*, and optic nerves *(red)*.

machines have since that time also implemented computer control systems and MLC systems.[36-38]

The capabilities of computer control and multileaf collimator systems have made possible the delivery of very complicated plans, including those that make use of intensity modulation (changing the intensity in different parts of a single radiation beam). The most recent technological improvement in conformal radiotherapy makes use of intensity modulation (using multiple segments[39-44] or dynamic MLC motions[32,45,46] and computer plan optimization ("inverse planning"),[47-51] integrating them into a process called IMRT.[52] The basic concepts of IMRT were described by Brahme in 1987[32,47,53] and by Bortfeld,[54] while the first commercial IMRT system was introduced in 1992.[55] The combination of the flexibility of computer-controlled IMRT delivery with sophisticated plan optimization techniques has made IMRT an extremely powerful tool that can be used to perform conformal therapy.

ISSUES FOR CLINICAL USE

A number of important clinical features are crucial for planning and delivery of high-quality conformal therapy, and these issues should be carefully considered throughout the conformal therapy planning/delivery process:

- Conformal therapy attempts to carefully conform the dose to the target, so target delineation and the desired dose distribution should be carefully and accurately defined.
- Patient immobilization and localization (setup accuracy and motion) must be considered throughout the process to minimize normal tissue that will be irradiated.
- Improvement of the clinical results achieved by conformal therapy, compared with standard techniques, depends on choosing the correct tradeoffs between target coverage and normal tissue sparing, so these choices must be made appropriately.

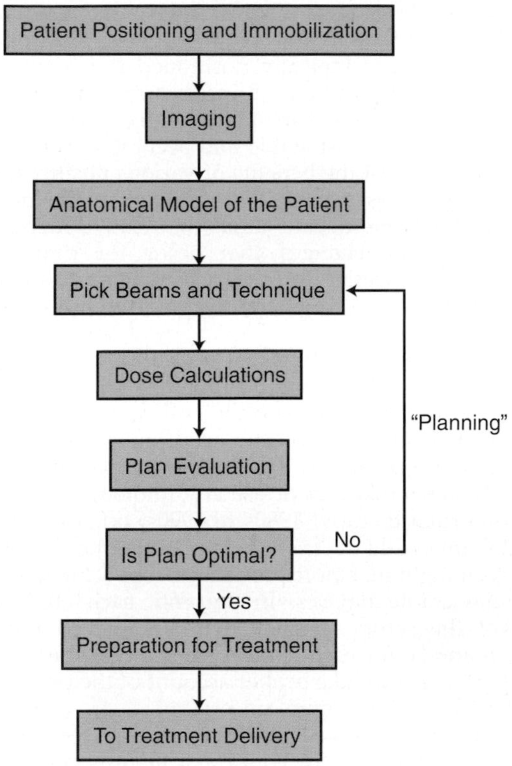

Figure 14-3 Schematic chart of the basic components of the planning process.

- The dose distribution that is achieved (or desired) is the crucial thing—the techniques used for planning and delivery are simply the means to achieve the desired dose distribution.

PLANNING FOR CONFORMAL THERAPY

Treatment planning is one of the most critical parts of the conformal therapy process. In this description, we include all preparatory aspects of the planning process, including many activities that occur outside the RTP system. Many treatment delivery issues (e.g., setup accuracy, patient motion, portal and localization imaging) are mentioned here, although they are more completely described later. A schematic of the basic components of the planning process is given in Figure 14-3.

Positioning and Immobilization

One of the basic ideas of conformal therapy is to minimize the dose to normal tissues while conforming the dose to the target, so it is of course crucial to accurately position and immobilize the patient for each procedure in the planning/delivery process. One of the first clinical decisions to be made for each patient includes what position to use for the patient's treatment and whether any positioning and immobilization devices or aids will be used.

Basic patient positioning, including location of the arms and legs, and whether the patient is to be treated supine, prone, or in some other more unusual position, depends mainly two issues: (1) patient comfort and stability and (2) the beam directions that will be used. In most cases, conformal therapy plans make use of three or more beams that crossfire on the target from a number of different positions arranged around the patient, so the patient is typically positioned with both arms up (if the target is somewhere in the torso) or arms down (head and neck and brain targets). For superficial targets, the target is typically positioned facing up, but for most deep tumors, the crossfiring beam directions can be achieved with the patient in standard supine or prone positions, whichever is most stable and accurately set up. There have been studies of the benefits of various positioning decisions (prone versus supine, for example) in the prostate,[56] where there is some debate about the relative merits of the possible anatomic changes that occur for prone versus supine position, relative to other advantages/disadvantages for planning, daily setup, and respiratory motion–related stability.

The use of various types of so-called "immobilization devices" to help with patient positioning and immobilization for conformal therapy has run the entire gamut of possibilities, from the use of stereotactic headframes and other such devices that are physically attached to the patient's skull, to other techniques that do not use any immobilization device. Early conformal therapy (1980s to 1990s) often incorporated use of a foam cradle device to help position the patient[57]; it is currently thought that more precision can be achieved without use of the cradle devices. In the end, each clinic should document the setup accuracy that is achieved with their chosen methods, for each clinical site, so that the planning/delivery process can take proper account of the expected systematic and random setup uncertainties. As new in-room imaging systems (diagnostic and megavoltage cone-beam CT) establish their place in the conformal therapy process, there will be a new opportunity to further improve the accuracy with which the patient is positioned and localized for each fraction's treatment.

Table 14-1 Treatment Planning CT Scan Features

Use flat table top to mimic treatment machine couch.
Use patient immobilization devices to position patient same as for treatment.
Scan patient from the top of any critical structure to the bottom of any other important structure, since planning typically requires delineation of entire organs to make use of biological effect data. For example, treatment anywhere in the thorax would typically require scanning from the apex of the lung to below the diaphragm, so that the entire lung can be delineated.
Modern CT scanners are efficient enough that 1- to 3-mm-thick slices are obtained through the target region, while 3- to 5-mm-thick slices can be used in other regions. This can amount to several hundred CT slices per study.
Careful consideration must be given to the advantages and disadvantages of using contrast during the scans. Contrast can help identify organs but can also make accurate dose calculations difficult (since it distorts the apparent electron density of the tissue, affecting dose calculations).
The treatment planning CT scan study is used for (1) target definition and delineation, (2) normal tissue delineation, (3) the overall anatomic model of the patient, (4) planning, (5) dose calculations based on electron density obtained from CT numbers, and (6) creation of digital reconstructed radiographs (DRRs) used to set up and verify patient position. Each of these uses may require some individualization of the CT scan protocol or use.
The CT scan protocol should be defined for each clinical site, including slice thicknesses, scan extent (top and bottom), reconstruction window size, use of contrast, patient positioning and immobilization, patient breathing control or instructions, etc.

Imaging (Computed Tomography, Magnetic Resonance Imaging, and Others)

The development of x-ray CT in the 1970s and its application to radiotherapy planning[18] were absolutely crucial milestones in the development of conformal therapy techniques. Without the cross-sectional anatomic imaging provided by CT (and MRI), there was not enough anatomic knowledge about the tumor or normal anatomy to consider the use of highly conformal dose distributions. Certainly, once the detailed anatomic information provided by CT became available, it was clear that radiotherapy planning and treatment should make use of this new and detailed description of the patient to better spare normal tissues and more accurately deliver dose to the tumor. Conformal therapy is a logical response to the new information provided by CT.

Modern conformal therapy is always based on a 3D anatomic model of the patient that is based on a CT scan of the involved region. Typically, a treatment planning CT scan of the patient is obtained to use as the basis for treatment planning. Features of the treatment planning scan are listed in Table 14-1.

Developments in CT and treatment delivery technology have made the consideration of motion during CT scanning (and radiotherapy treatment) an important research topic. "4D CT" describes various different techniques for obtaining CT data correlated with patient respiratory phase information so that the changes associated with respiration (or other motion) are displayed. For certain clinical sites (lung, breast, etc.), it is clear that consideration of respiratory (and maybe cardiac) motion will be an important aspect of the initial imaging of the patient, so that an appropriate model (maybe a time-varying or 4D model) of the patient can be used for further planning and analysis. Whether 4D CT,[58] respiratory gating,[59] active breathing control (ABC),[60,61] or other methods will eventually be shown to be necessary for each site will be determined during the next several years.

CT provides anatomic and electron density information that is critical for most treatment planning and provides a geometrically accurate base for planning. However, it provides only anatomic information, not the physiologic and functional information that would also be helpful for planning, and it provides only a limited amount of soft tissue contrast. MRI can provide complementary kinds of data, including excellent soft tissue contrast and different kinds of physiologic information. In addition, functional MR studies can provide some of the functional information that to this point has been unavailable. Other kinds of imaging also contain complementary or new information. PET and single-photon emission computed tomography (SPECT) provide different types of functional and physiologic information and can be quite important in helping define target volumes and regions that should be included or excluded from the radiation fields. Which modalities, scans, tracers, and analysis methods should be used for specific features is well beyond the scope of this work. To make quantitative use of any additional imaging modality for treatment planning, one should incorporate a number of important procedures into the imaging process, as listed in Table 14-2.

The main difference between the original CT dataset and these new imaging modality image sets is the fact that for any quantitative use of the new imaging study, it will have to be registered geometrically to the base CT dataset, so that one can relate information found on the new dataset to the relevant part of the original CT scan. This geometric registration watch process, called "dataset registration" or "image fusion," is typically performed within the treatment planning system as one is creating the anatomic model of the patient. It is important during the imaging process to (1) position and align the patient similarly for each of the imaging studies, as this makes the registration process more straightforward, and (2) ensure that you obtain all the information necessary so that the dataset registration/fusion process can be performed quickly and accurately. Registration/fusion is discussed in more detail in the Normal Tissues section.

Anatomy for Treatment Planning

RTP is a computer simulation of the process of radiotherapy treatment, and it is based on creating a model of the patient inside the RTP software and simulating radiation beams and the dose that those beams deliver to the patient. The definition of the virtual model of the patient, based on CT, MR, and other types of imaging data, and how that anatomic model is used are crucial parts of the RTP process.

Three-Dimensional Anatomic Model

To allow conformal therapy planning, the representation of the patient that is used for treatment planning must be fairly realistic and 3D. In general, the basic data used to define the anatomy come from a CT study, typically consisting of 50 to 200 CT scan slices. The anatomic model of the patient is based on this CT data and consists of a number of objects (structures) that delineate organs or other objects (e.g., target volumes) in 3D (or 4D, see Motion, Setup, and Four-Dimensional Anatomy). These structures can be defined by (1) a series of contours, (2) a 3D surface description, (3) a voxel-based description, or (4) a set of points distributed either randomly or on a grid. Methods used to delineate these structures are described in Structure Delineation and Contouring.

The 3D anatomic structures are crucial to the planning process. The various target and normal tissue structures describe the areas to be irradiated or to be spared (respectively) so that beams can be oriented and shaped. Graphical display of the 3D structures can also be used for geometrical registration of the treatment planning anatomy to localization images obtained during simulation or treatment procedures. The external surface (and any inhomogeneities) are used for the dose calculation process. Most plan evaluation tools (e.g., dose-volume histograms [DVHs]) make use of these 3D structures for plan evaluation of the planned dose distribution.

Table 14-2 Imaging for Treatment Planning (non-CT)

- Use flat table top to mimic radiotherapy Linac couch.
- Use patient immobilization devices to position patient same as for treatment.
- Ensure the imaging protocol provides enough anatomic information to allow geometric registration of the new scan study with the base CT information.
- Imaging protocol parameters should be optimized to provide the anatomic, physiologic, or function data that are desired.
- The scan protocol should be defined for each clinical site and protocol, including slice thicknesses, scan extent (top and bottom), scan orientation (nonaxial slices are possible in most non-CT methods), reconstruction window size, use of contrast, patient positioning and immobilization, patient breathing control or instructions, etc. For MRI, many additional scan technique parameters must be defined.
- Consideration of the time behavior, compared with the base CT. For example, most PET scans occur in a respiration-averaged technique, because the scan times are tens of minutes.

Structure Delineation and Contouring

One of the most important and time-consuming aspects of the entire conformal therapy process is the delineation of the 3D anatomic objects (structures) used for planning and plan evaluation. It would be nice if all the anatomic structures could be automatically delineated once the CT (and other imaging data) were obtained, but in general this technology does not yet exist. Most anatomic structures are delineated by drawing contours on top of each of the CT (or other) images that are available. Because more than 100 CT slices are often used, and there are many organs of interest that appear on each CT slice, there are many contours to be defined. Clever computer graphics drawing tools and techniques can make this easier, but defining the contours still requires much effort.

Accurately defining the structure contours is a critically important aspect of the conformal therapy process; because it defines the target and normal structure extents for the entire process, any error or inaccuracy becomes a systematic error throughout the entire conformal process. Errors in the process may come from sloppiness, from not knowing what is being visualized on the image on which contours are drawn, from limitations in the accuracy of the scan information (e.g., motion during the scan acquisition), and from many other problems. It is important that the 3D character of the objects being outlined is handled correctly: for example, sharp corners or spikes in a contour on just one slice are usually incorrect, because such a structure will usually show related features on a number of images. To avoid this type of drawing problem, it is important to review all the contours serially or to visualize the 3D shape of the object, so that any unphysical "spikes" can be identified and edited.

Target Volume Definition and Margins

To plan and deliver conformal therapy, it is essential to accurately define the volumes that must receive high radiation doses, the "target volumes." As described in detail by ICRU-50,[62] three kinds of target volumes are typically defined, as summarized in Table 14-3. For an individual patient, there can

Table 14-3 ICRU-50 Target Volume Definitions

Abbreviation	Name	Description
GTV	Gross tumor volume	Volume of macroscopic tumor that is visualized on imaging studies
CTV	Clinical target volume	Volume that should be treated to high dose, typically incorporating both the GTV and volumes that are assumed to be at risk due to microscopic spread of the disease
PTV	Planning target volume	Volume that should be treated in order to ensure that the CTV is always treated, including considerations of systematic and random daily setup errors and intertreatment and intratreatment motion

be multiple sets of gross tumor volume (GTV)–clinical target volume (CTV)–planning target volume (PTV), one for each area of disease. For example, in the head and neck, there are often CTV-PTV combinations for each potentially involved nodal group, and the GTV-CTV-PTV defined for the gross disease.

The GTV is typically delineated by drawing the imaged tumor on each of the imaging studies that are available. CT is used often, but for many sites, MR and PET can be very useful. When multiple imaging studies are available, the GTV can be drawn on each study, and then using dataset registration to geometrically align the different datasets (see Multiple Imaging Modalities: Dataset Registration and Fusion), one can transfer the different GTV contours onto a single dataset. How to combine the various GTVs thus defined is the subject of ongoing research; however, typically one will combine or take the union of all the defined GTVs in order to make sure that no gross tumor is missed within the defined GTV.

The definition of the CTV is probably the most important thing that the physician does in the conformal therapy process, as the CTV defines the region that is supposed to be treated with the prescribed dose. The CTV typically combines the GTVs plus any volumes that may contain microscopic disease that has not been imaged. The CTV depends on knowledge of the patterns of disease spread and incorporates any other clinical knowledge of the disease or the specific risks for spread that apply to the individual patient. The CTV is usually created by combining two kinds of information: (1) often, an expansion of the GTV by some margin (0.5-1 cm, typically) is used to account for microscopic invasion, and (2) additional anatomic areas may be included in the CTV based on standard directions of spread for the particular tumor type. In the end, the goal is to outline all the areas that should receive the intended dose.

While GTV and CTV definition are the job of the physician, definition of the PTV is the responsibility of the physicist and treatment planner, as the goal of the PTV is to make sure that the CTV is adequately treated in the face of setup error, intertreatment and intratreatment motion, delineation errors, and other errors in the planning and delivery process. The definition of the PTV should be done with as much information as possible, because the region between the CTV and PTV contours is all "normal tissue" and increasing the PTV margin will just cause more normal tissue to be irradiated.

Often, the PTV is designed by simply defining an isotropic margin (e.g., 1 cm), and the CTV is expanded by this margin (hopefully in 3D) to create the PTV (Fig. 14-4). This expansion should be performed in 3D, because expansion of contours only in the axial plane will lead to PTVs that are not correct in the third dimension. If the uncertainties are not isotropic, but are larger in one direction than in the others (e.g., due to respiration), then the margin to be applied should be anisotropic.

There has been a great deal of work studying patient positioning, motion, and target volume delineation errors, and analysis of these issues has led to specific recommendations for the size of the margin (between the CTV and the PTV) that should be used for the PTV. As described in Consideration of Setup Error and Patient Motion, one reasonable method for deciding the PTV-CTV margin has been determined to be $2.5 \times \Sigma + 0.7 \times \sigma$, where Σ is the standard deviation of the systematic error and σ is the standard deviation of the random errors for the population of patients treated in that particular site.[63] To apply this formula, it is important to have measured, for the institution and clinical site, the two standard deviations. Note that the systematic errors in the process, such as incorrect contouring or use of a nonrepresentative CT scan for target delineation, are much more important issues than random day-to-day setup errors.

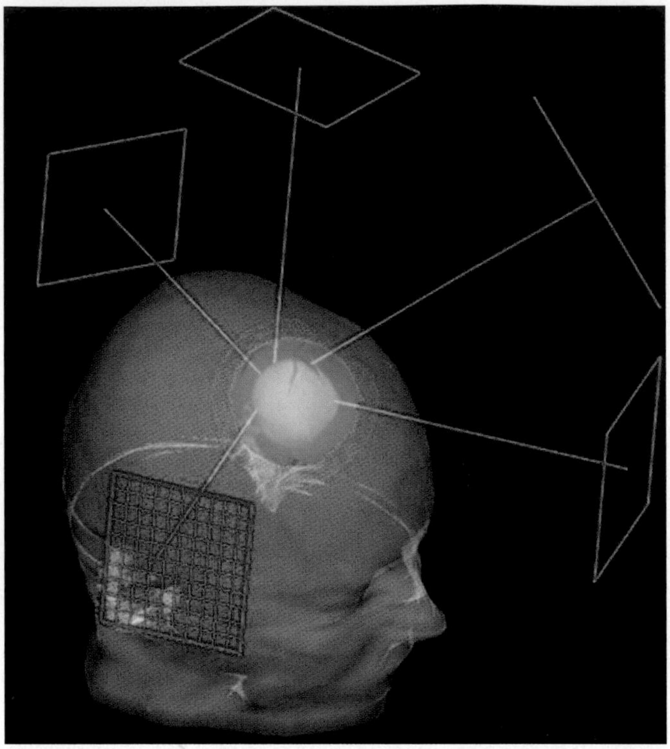

Figure 14-4 Plan for treating a brain tumor shows non-coplanar IMRT ICRU-50 target volumes: gross tumor volume *(white)*, clinical target volume *(pink)*, and planning target volume *(yellow)*.

Normal Tissues

Definition of *normal tissues* is also a critical task for conformal therapy, because identifying the critical tissues will allow the treatment planner to avoid or at least minimize dose delivery to those normal tissues. The planning tools used to avoid these structures can be simple graphic tools like the BEV display, which allows the planner to shape the radiation fields to avoid important structures, or it may involve detailed dosimetric and DVH analysis, as is often the case for IMRT planning.

In the case of DVH or other dosimetric analysis, it is important that each organ to be analyzed is contoured completely, because most current DVH data are characterized with respect to the whole organ's volume (either absolute volume or as a percentage of the whole organ). This has several implications:

1. The CT scans or other studies for a given site must image all the relevant normal tissues completely and the tumor. For example, a lung tumor CT scan should always include images from the neck down to below the bottom of the diaphragm, so that the complete volume of the normal tissues can be identified (e.g., lung, heart, esophagus, spinal cord, etc.).
2. Contouring of normal structures must be done consistently if the DVH information is to be useful. Whole organs should always be contoured. For tube-like structures (spinal cord, rectum, esophagus, etc.) that can often extend out of the region of the tumor, it is important to have a

defined protocol for how the structure will be defined, and how far superiorly and inferiorly contours for a given structure (e.g., the rectum during prostate planning) should be drawn.

Multiple Imaging Modalities: Dataset Registration and Fusion

Although CT scans are the primary imaging modality used for radiotherapy planning, information from other types of imaging, particularly including MRI and PET, can be very useful for identifying disease or better identifying functional or anatomic areas that should be spared. Target volumes and normal structures can be identified on these additional imaging datasets, and that information can be incorporated into the treatment plan along with the contours and data from the CT scans. Typically, a CT scan set is taken to be the geometric basis for the treatment planning, because the CT data are high resolution, geometrically accurate, and quickly obtained.

Several issues need to be solved to make quantitative use of the additional imaging information.

- For each imaging procedure, the patient should be positioned within the imaging device using the same position and immobilization/localization devices as for treatment. However, there are usually positioning differences that must be accounted for.
- Even if the patient positioning is perfect, the coordinate system used in the new imaging device is usually different than the coordinates used by the base CT scan. Therefore, a geometric registration of the new imaging information must be performed, to align the new images with the base imaging information. Otherwise, with different coordinates, one does not know how to map pixels in the new image dataset to the coordinates of the original image set.
- For many imaging modalities, for example MRI, various kinds of distortion are possible. If the new image dataset has geometric distortions, then these must be corrected before the imaging information can be transferred into the base coordinate system for use in planning.
- The resolution, slice thickness, and slice orientations of different imaging modalities can often be different than those of the original CT dataset, so any quantitative use of the new imaging data must also handle these kinds of differences.

To address these issues, the process of dataset (or image) registration is used to align the coordinates for the various imaging datasets so that information can be passed from one image set into a coordinate system to be used for treatment planning. The registration process finds the geometrical transform between the new dataset's coordinate system and the base coordinate system (typically the CT scan). If one considers only rigid body registration, the transform can consist of x, y, and z translations, or both translations and rotations, and it can include scaling as well (although typically, the scale of each dataset is known accurately and should not be modified). Research is developing methods for mapping distortions from one system to another, so distortions due to imaging or to patient motion (e.g., respiration) can be taken into account.

To determine the best transform, an optimization algorithm is applied to the problem. The optimization process consists of choosing the metric to be optimized (some metric that describes the quality of the registration), and choosing an optimization search algorithm that will perform the search over possible transforms so that the optimal one can be found. The metric can be something as simple as the sum of the squares of the distances between predicted and actual point locations, if it were possible to define point-based landmarks on both imaging studies, or it can be image-based metrics like the correlation between gray scale values of two CT scans, or mutual information, that can be used to register different image studies (e.g., CT and MRI or PET). This is a rapidly developing area of research.

No matter what kind of registration algorithm is used, it is necessary to verify the registration, and then to use the data from the various imaging studies. Verification typically consists of image or structure-based comparisons between the two datasets, with the goal of confirming that known structures from the two imaging studies accurately line up (Fig. 14-5). The quality of the registration depends on what parts of the images are most important clinically and must be reviewed by the planner/physician, because at this point, no quantitative measure accurately takes into account all the clinical knowledge of the case. Once the registration is verified, then contours or 3D structure definitions from one dataset can be transferred into the base coordinate system for planning. This combination of data from multiple imaging sources is sometimes called image fusion.

Motion, Setup, and Four-Dimensional Anatomy

So far, there has been little consideration of the facts that real patients breathe, move, are different from day to day, and

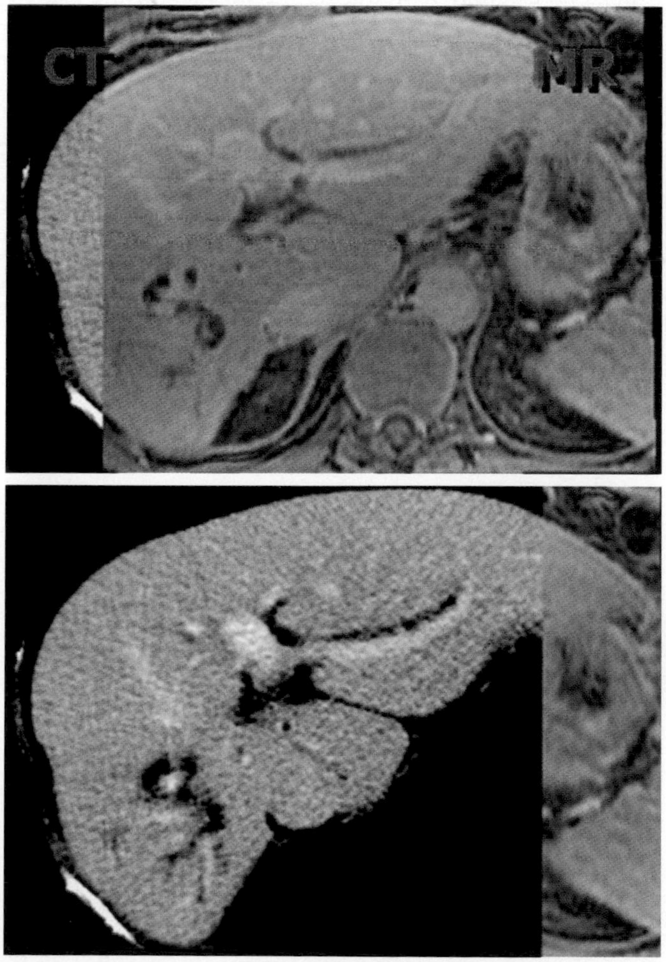

Figure 14-5 Split-screen comparisons of CT *(left)* and MR *(right)* image data to confirm the accuracy of the geometric registration of CT and MR scans of the liver.

change over time. Until recently, it was difficult to take such motions and localization differences into account within treatment planning, with the exception of defining appropriate PTV margins for the tumor. Fast helical CT scans, fast MRI, 4D CT, and 4D cone-beam CT imaging using the treatment machine have begun to provide detailed anatomic data as a function of time. These data have clearly demonstrated that a static anatomic description of the patient is not always appropriate and that treatment delivery schemes must also consider setup and motion effects if we are to achieve the optimal delivery of dose to the patient.

Several methods to handle motion and setup effects are in use or being investigated:

- As described in Target Volume Definition and Margins, the standard way to handle motion and setup error is to determine the appropriate margin, and then to expand the CTV by that margin to make a PTV that is the target for planning. If done correctly, the PTV makes sure that the high dose region always encompasses the CTV, even as the CTV moves around due to motion or setup error. The price, however, is that the larger the margin is, the more normal tissue is irradiated. Therefore, if the motion and setup error are taken more directly into account, this margin may be decreased, reducing the amount of normal tissue irradiated.
- Stereotactic treatments and treatments using daily setup correction try to significantly reduce the daily setup variations by carefully reproducing the position of the patient each day.
- With use of 4D CT, respiratory-correlated cone-beam CT, and other such "4D" imaging, it is now possible to visualize the motions of the tumor (and normal tissue) with the CT data, and to create structure outlines that better approximate the clinical targets and structures to be avoided. However, this technology is currently undergoing very rapid developments.
- With use of ABC, it is possible to control the breathing of the patient with the goal of turning on the treatment beam only when the patient is in the correct breathing state.
- It is also possible to gate the radiation beam, turning it on only when the target structure is in the correct location, based either on external markers or, potentially, on internal markers.

Over the next several years, a great deal of technical progress can be expected in this area.

Plan and Beam Definition

After the anatomic model of the patient has been established, the next major step in the planning process is to use the RTP system to create a set of beams to be used for planning. This collection of beams, usually known as a "plan," can be created using standard protocols ("treat all prostates with a four-field box of conformal fields") or designed based on the specific anatomy of the case. Basic decisions on beam technique are typically made very early in the planning process, based on experience and site-specific protocols. Typically, these decisions include picking the energy and number of beams, the basic orientations for the beams, and the type of beam shaping or intensity modulation to be used.

Beam Technique (Energy, Direction, Type)

The first things to be decided as a treatment plan is generated are the number of beams to be used, their energy (and modality), and their direction. These choices are all interrelated, so typically this decision is based on standard experience or protocols. Although it is hard to summarize all of the useful ways to make this decision, there are a few standard rules that apply to most conformal planning.

- Avoid opposed beams. Simple nonconformal planning often used opposed beams (AP-PA and opposed laterals or obliques) to create a relatively uniform region of high dose extending throughout the patient. For conformal planning, one typically wants to avoid pairs of opposed beams, because we want to conform the dose to the target. For IMRT plans, this is even more important, because opposed beams can cause degenerate solutions for the optimization search, leading to the optimization bouncing between two fairly equivalent solutions for opposing beamlets.
- Typically, lower energies are used for relatively superficial targets, or for beams that traverse less normal tissue on the way to the target, while beams that must penetrate lots of tissue are typically higher energy. Changing energies for individual beams often makes a relatively small difference in the dose distribution achieved, and this possible improvement should be balanced against the additional complexity of the plan if multiple photon energies are used.
- For sites in which one is attempting to make sure the dose in the buildup region is relatively high, lower energies are usually used, because there is less skin sparing for these beams.
- The most conformal plans can be achieved by ensuring that there are beams arranged around the target in all three dimensions, so that the plan includes some nonaxial beams.
- There is a great deal of debate (still) over the best energy beams to use for plans that involve large inhomogeneities like the lung.
- As one creates more complex IMRT plans that have many degrees of freedom available to be optimized, it is possible to achieve very conformal plans. Typically, these plans include an odd number of fields, although the goal is just to make sure there are no opposing fields. There has been much discussion saying that IMRT plans can all be accomplished with 6-MV photons and that higher energies are not necessary, but there is little hard evidence to really demonstrate that conclusion in general. In addition, it is often said that IMRT plans can be achieved with only axial beams, but the use of non-coplanar beam arrangements will still result in at least slightly better plans (typically reducing somewhat the normal tissue dose for the same target conformality).

Shaping with Blocks and Multileaf Collimator

While beam directions are important, shaping the radiation field to conform to the shape of the target volume is one of the crucial and defining concepts for "conformal therapy." The shaping can be accomplished equally well by focused blocks or with an MLC, as illustrated in Figure 14-6. The conformal shaping of focused blocks is in fact "more conformal" than the jagged shape created by an MLC, although the MLC has a number of other advantages that have led to its popularity.

The routine use of conformally shaped fields designed during treatment planning depends in large part on the availability of the BEV display in the planning system, as this view of the target shows the projection of the shape of the targets from the point of view of the radiation beam, so it is exactly the right view to use to design the field shaping. The simplest method used to conformally shape the fields (with either blocks or MLC) is to create a uniform geometric margin around the projection of the targets in the BEV and to set the

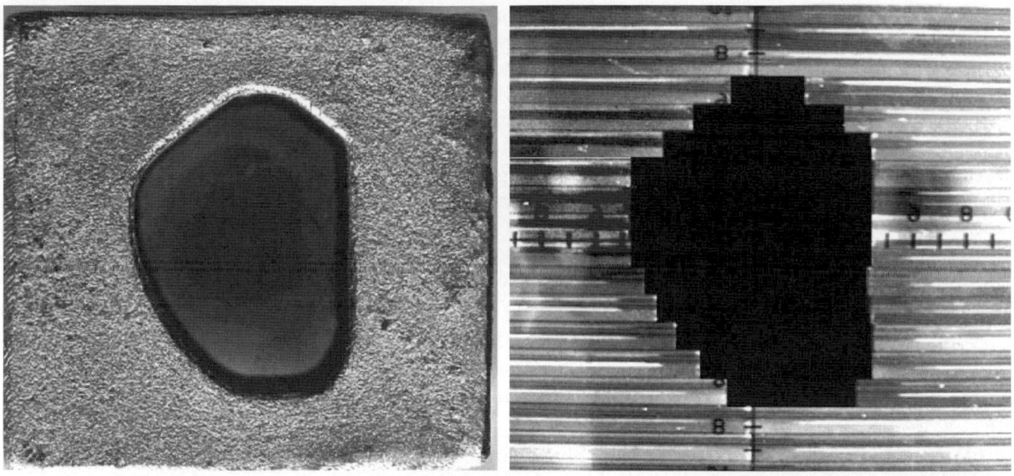

Figure 14-6 Shaped blocks and multileaf collimators can be used to shape the beam conformally.

shape to that margin, as shown in Figure 14-7. This method, the basis of the most simple type of conformal therapy, is sometimes called geometrical conformation, or beam's eye view targeting. Shaping a block to a given contour is easy, but there are several methods used to define where each leaf of an MLC goes when conforming to a BEV contour[38]: the most commonly used method is the so-called equal area method (Fig. 14-7).

Using a uniform geometric margin for the field shaping does not lead to the most conformal dose distribution, because there are a limited number of beams. To truly conform the dose distribution to the target, one must optimize the shaping of each of the beams so that the dose distribution is conformal. Figure 14-8 demonstrates the type of differences that occur when beam shapes are designed with a uniform margin and when the shapes are optimized to conform the dose to the target. Beam directions, penumbra, and how the beams cross-fire on the target affect the margins required for individual beam shapes.

Collimator angle is one more thing that can directly affect the conformality of a plan, mainly when an MLC is used. The

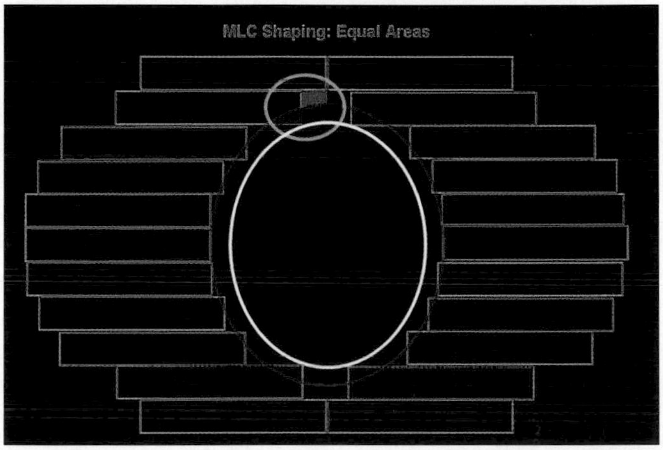

Figure 14-7 When using geometric conformal shaping for an MLC, the most common method is to create a contour at the desired margin *(red contour)* and then push the MLC leaves up to that contour so the areas overlapped and underlapped by each leaf are equal.

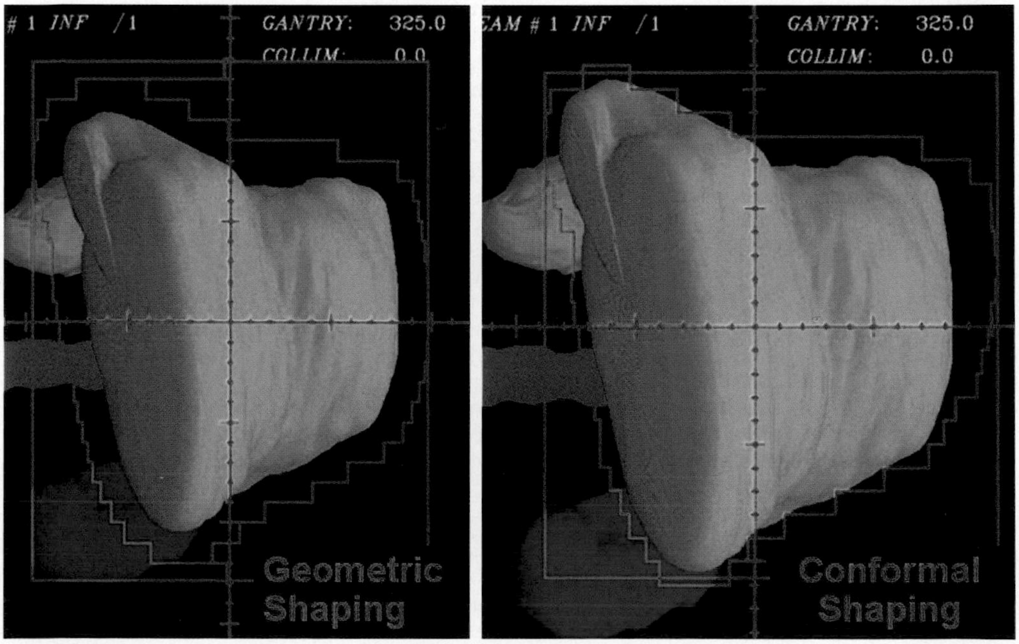

Figure 14-8 Beam's eye view of conformal fields: uniform geometric margin *(left)* and conformal dose distribution *(right)*. Using a uniform geometric margin typically does not achieve a dose distribution that is as conformal as possible. For this three-field pancreas treatment plan, the beam on the right had its shape optimized to make the dose distribution more conformal to the target.

leaves from an MLC move in only one direction, so to minimize the "stairstep" or jagged edges caused by MLC leaves when shaped to an angled contour, one may use collimator rotation to cause the MLC leaves to best fit the shape of the target or normal tissue. By minimizing the jaggedness of the MLC edges, one can decrease the amount of penumbra in that particular region of the beam, thereby allowing the beam to do a better job making a sharp penumbra between a target and normal tissue. For example, for beams trying to make a sharp dose gradient between the prostate and the rectum, rotating the collimator to parallel the edge of the rectum can help make the edge sharper.

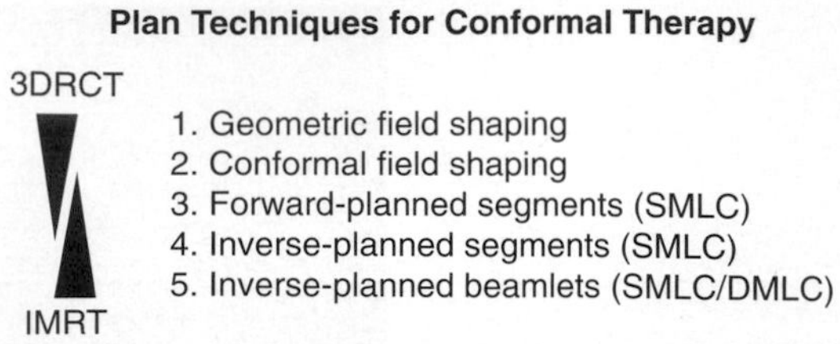

Figure 14-9 The terms *three-dimensional conformal radiation therapy* (3DCRT) and *intensity-modulated radiation therapy* (IMRT) can be applied to a range of different treatment techniques.

Other Beam Technique Decisions

There are numerous other decisions to be made while creating the plan.

- One must choose the intensity of each beam, typically called the beam weight. How this decision is made depends on the specific beam normalization methods used within the planning system. Because the beam weight or intensity is directly related to the number of monitor units (MU) that will be delivered from each beam, it is essential that translation of beam weights into MU be understood and carefully handled, because errors in this step deliver the wrong dose to the entire field.
- For certain beam combinations, use of wedges in the field can help achieve a more uniform dose in the target volume. Standard two-dimensional planning makes routine use of pairs of fields known as "wedged pairs," where the wedges help compensate for the fields entering the patient at 90 degrees (or some other angle) to each other. For conformal planning in 3D, there is a broader range of combinations of fields for which wedges are useful. For example, a 3D cone has some number of fields placed around a cone, and each of the fields usually requires a wedge to keep the target dose uniformity. This beam distribution is the 3D analog of the wedged pair.
- When the target is near the surface of the patient, it is often difficult to achieve the desired dose coverage of the target due to the low doses in the entrance region of megavoltage photon beams. In this case, some amount of bolus can be added to the skin of the patient, for one or more beams, so that the photon beams can transit more material, thus decreasing the skin sparing. This bolus description can be designed using the planning system, as long as care is taken in creating the physical bolus so that it actually matches the description that was put into the planning system.
- Most conformal treatment plans are isocentric, with the isocenter of the machine placed within the center of the target, and the beams rotating around the isocenter in the target. Other arrangements are possible, depending on the geometry of the normal anatomy and targets. For some situations, it is also possible to create pseudo-isocentric beams, which use 3D table motions to move the patient away from the head of the machine along the beam central axis, so that the plan is apparently isocentric but with a larger source-to-isocenter distance than the machine has. This technique can be used to create a larger range of table and gantry angles that can be used for treatment without the machine's head getting too close to the patient.[64]

Intensity-Modulated Radiation Therapy

Soon after conformal therapy began to be used clinically in the late 1980s, Brahme,[53] Bortfeld,[54] and others introduced the idea of modulating the intensity across each radiation beam, assisted by computer-based optimization algorithms to help determine the intensities required of the different parts of the beam. IMRT is now commonly used to create highly conformal treatment plans.

Intensity-modulated fields can be achieved in a number of different ways, and whether all plans that include any nonflat beams (including wedged fields?) are IMRT has been a semantic debate over the years. A more realistic way to consider this issue is shown in Figure 14-9, which illustrates the continuum of different types of planning, ranging from simple geometrically conformed flat fields (top) to inverse-planned beamlet IMRT created with dynamic MLC (DMLC) or multiple segment (SMLC) delivery of the intensity-modulated fields, all of which are conformal techniques. In Figure 14-9, the first three types of planning make use of standard forward planning, where iterative plan modifications by the planner are used to achieve the final plan (see Forward Planning), while the last two types make use of inverse planning (see Inverse Planning) involving use of computerized optimization algorithms to help with the plan optimization. IMRT typically combines inverse planning with the use of highly modulated beam intensities, although inverse planning with few segments and even simple flat fields is also possible.[65]

Beam design for IMRT depends on the type of planning to be used (forward or inverse) and the photon energies and beam arrangement expected and should consider the tradeoff between the planning goals chosen and the complexity of the plan that will be allowed. If simple multiple segments are planned, then the individual segments may be created by the planner, while for more complex IMRT planned with "beamlets," the beamlet size (1 × 1 cm, 0.5 × 0.5 cm, etc.) to be used for planning will be chosen by the planner.

Dose Calculations

Once the initial treatment plan is designed, the next step is typically to perform a dose calculation, so that the planner and physician can evaluate the dose distribution expected from the plan. Currently, because biological effects are not well documented and understood in general, the physical dose distribution is the main parameter that is used (1) to choose between plans, (2) to choose what dose to deliver to the patient, and (3) to evaluate the quality of various plans proposed by the planner.

Three-Dimensional Calculations

Treatment planning dose calculations have been performed on one (or more) two-dimensional slices (or contours) of the patient since the 1940s. Often, these calculations were performed by hand, from table or chart look-ups, using a single traced contour of the external shape of the patient on a single axial slice of the patient at the center of the treatment fields. Even if performed on a number of slices, these dose distributions were in principle two dimensional and did not give a complete description of the dose to be delivered to the patient.

Continuing increases in computer capabilities and improved treatment planning and dose calculation algorithm developments resulted in availability of so-called 3D dose calculations in the 3D planning systems that became available in the late 1980s. However, "3D" could mean (1) that the dose was calculated throughout a volume of points, (2) that the dose was calculated with an algorithm that took 3D scatter into account, (3) that the 3D effects of inhomogeneities were taken into account, (4) that a 3D description of the anatomy was used, (5) that full 3D beam divergence issues were considered, and so on. Because the calculation of dose with high resolution using an accurate and realistic dose calculation algorithm still takes a significant amount of time, even with the fastest computers available currently, every dose calculation algorithm and implementation makes tradeoff choices between accuracy, speed, computer resources needed, resolution, features and effects that are correctly modeled, and other factors. Determination of the appropriate mix of approximation, compromise, and robustness needed for particular kinds of clinical planning dose calculations is an important responsibility of the radiation oncology physicist.

To accurately perform planning for conformal therapy, 3D dose calculations must be performed. This is basically true for each of the different types of "3D" described earlier. A 3D anatomic model is required, the dose must be determined throughout the volume encompassing the targets and the critical normal tissues, the calculations should be done at high resolution if one wants to know how conformal the plan actually is, the calculation algorithm should model all the 3D dosimetric effects, and so on. It is critical that all limitations in the calculations be understood and the effects of those limitations should be considered in any clinical decisions that are based on the results of the calculations.

Algorithms

Many different types of calculation algorithms have been developed for photon and electron beams, and new improvements or implementations are continually becoming available. It is beyond the scope of this text to describe any algorithms in any detail. Algorithms ranging from simple table look-ups based on measured data to Monte Carlo simulations that require many hours of CPU time of the fastest computers all have their place and are the appropriate choice of algorithm for one particular situation or another.

It is possible to group most photon and electron beam dose calculation algorithms into a number of basic classes (Table 14-4). This table attempts to summarize, in a very general way, some of the advantages and disadvantages of each class. If there is a choice of algorithms for conformal planning, then the choice should be made with careful consideration of the potential limitations of the chosen algorithm, and the radiation oncology physicist should carefully commission

Table 14–4 Classes of Dose Calculation Algorithms for Photon

Algorithm Class	Description	Limitations	References
Matrix, data based	Based on measured data, often used for situations with specific field size capabilities (e.g., stereotactic applicator systems, very small field techniques). Very fast.	Only usable for specific measured situations—mainly radiosurgery applicators	66
Analytical beam models	Algebraic formulas model different aspects of the dose distribution. Very useful for fast 2D calculation models, limited in ability to model all the features in 3D dose distributions. Very fast.	Does not accurately model shaped beam scatter, patient contour changes, inhomogeneities	67-69
Scatter integration	The most used class of models from the 1970s until the last few years. Includes the well-known TAR-SAR (tissue-air ratio/scatter-air ratio) integration method developed by Cunningham.[70] 2D integration of scatter around the field handles most field-dependent scatter well but does not handle 3D inhomogeneities. Pencil beam models, often used for IMRT calculations, fall into this class. Fast.	OK for field shaping, 3DCRT except for inhomogeneities	70,71
3D integration	Convolution/superposition algorithms are the most popular of the 3D integration models. These algorithms calculate, for every point inside the 3D calculation grid, the scatter contribution from each voxel. To be done completely, this involves a seven-dimensional integration over all voxels, all primary dose deposition points, and energies, although many implementations compromise in order to speed up the calculations. Based on a dose-spread kernel typically calculated once by Monte Carlo and then used for all calculations.	In principle should get most photon-related effects correct, though inhomogeneities can still be a problem if energy spectrum and other issues are compromised	72,73
Monte Carlo	This method tracks dose deposition for millions of particle histories, using the basic physics interactions to determine what happens in each history. This algorithm has the best potential for accurate results but is costly in terms of calculation time and needs accurate simulation of the behavior and scattering, which occurs in the head of the machine. Slower, but easily parallelizable.	Most reliable if it includes good simulations of particle behavior in head of machine	74,75

the algorithm for clinical use by comparison to appropriately measured data for the local machines in order to demonstrate the adequacy and limitations of the algorithm for clinical use.[76]

Other Dose Calculation Issues: Grids, Resolution, Inhomogeneities, and Others

Aside from the inherent accuracy of the dose calculation algorithm that is used, many other user-controlled factors affect the final accuracy of the doses predicted by the calculations that are performed for a plan. Unfortunately, it is not possible to address all these issues with a few simple guidelines.

Every step of the treatment planning, dose calculation, and plan evaluation process involves decisions about how much time, effort, and precision to spend defining or reviewing each aspect of the planning, and the accuracy of the final product depends on all those individual decisions. If one chooses to calculate the dose on a grid of 0.5 ×. 0.5 × 0.5 cm spacing, then it will be hard to evaluate the dose 2 mm from the target with a significant degree of confidence, given that dose gradients at the edge of a beam can be approximately 10%/mm. Highly conformal therapy will require that dose calculations be performed with high-resolution grids (perhaps 2-3 mm), leading to very large numbers of points that need to be calculated and longer calculation times. Similarly, if truly conformal therapy is going to be performed in lung tumors, where inhomogeneities are significant, an advanced calculation algorithm that can accurately predict the dose in inhomogeneities should be used if one wants to understand the real dosimetric situation in the patient.

Plan Evaluation Tools

After the dose distribution from the plan has been calculated, the next step in the process is to evaluate the plan and the predicted dose distribution. Typically, the dose distribution is evaluated by looking at isodose curves on individual cuts through the plan, looking at isodose surfaces (3D displays of the isosurfaces) if available, and then using DVH analysis of the dose delivered to individual organs. If the capability and appropriate data are available, it is also possible to use biological modeling results like normal tissue complication probability (NTCP), tumor control probability (TCP), and the equivalent uniform dose (EUD) to help with the plan evaluation.

Dose Display

The most commonly used type of display of the dose distribution for a plan consists of displaying contour lines of constant dose, "isodose lines," on top of the anatomic information that was used for the plan. These kinds of displays have been used for many years—first with only the contours of the patient, obtained by hand measurement using solder wire or other techniques, and then later displaying the isodose lines on top of the CT scan. For conformal planning, not only axial cuts should be used for the isodose lines but also coronal and sagittal reformatted CT images, because display of isodose lines on multiple orthogonal cuts can give the planner a more 3D sense of the coverage of the target volume. The 3D graphics techniques can be used to put the images and dose lines in 3D perspective, as shown in Figure 14-10. A variation of the isodose line display is the colorwash display, in which the dose level calculated for each pixel of the image is used to assign a color value (Fig. 14-10C).

Any image that is part of the anatomic model of the patient can, in principle, be used for dose calculation and dose display. If MRI, PET, or other image datasets have been registered with the basic anatomy, then the PET or MR images can also be the backdrops for the dose display. By comparing the location of the isodose lines with the contours of the targets and critical normal tissues, the planner and physician can evaluate the quality of the dose distribution that is obtained for this particular beam arrangement and decide whether the plan is adequate or whether further modification of the plan is necessary.

In conformal therapy, the goal is to conform the shape of the high-dose region to the target in three dimensions, so display of the 3D dose distribution shape may be a help when evaluating the conformality of the plan. The 3D analog of an isodose line is called an isodose surface. Also sometimes called "dose clouds," isodose surfaces are typically displayed in a 3D perspective graphical image (see Fig. 14-10D).

The dose displayed in isodose curves or surfaces, or any other dose display, can be shown in a number of ways. The most common mode used for conformal therapy is the relative dose distribution, where all the dose display is normalized to the dose value at the isocenter or center of the target. With this kind of relative dose normalization, typical conformal therapy plans would have the 95% isodose surface surrounding the target, with the shape of the 95% surface (or isodose lines) conforming to the target. One could, however, equally well display the dose in absolute terms so that the high-dose region demonstrated the desired total dose for the plan (e.g., 60 Gy) or the desired dose/fraction (e.g., 2.0 Gy/fraction). It is of course essential that the output of the plan that is used for treatment preparation should be carefully understood and documented, so that there is no confusion between the different ways the dose can be displayed.

Dose-Volume Histograms

Review and evaluation of the dose throughout the patient in three dimensions can be complex and time-consuming processes, and it is also difficult to give specific guidelines for normal tissue or tumor responses with respect to that complex data. It has become standard to evaluate the dose received by the target volumes and normal tissues using DVHs. To form a DVH for any 3D object, one looks at the dose for each voxel in the object and forms a histogram, counting the number of voxels that receive each different dose level. Because the volume of each voxel is known, the volume of the organ receiving each dose level is known. See Kessler[77] for more detail.

Both the volume (vertical) and dose (horizontal) axes can be displayed in absolute terms (cc or Gy) or in relative terms (% volume or % dose), depending on how the planner wants to analyze the results. DVHs are displayed in three different forms: direct, cumulative, and differential.

- The direct histogram is the generic form of any histogram, displaying the volume of the organ that receives dose within each dose bin (1% or 0.5 to 1 Gy is a typical dose bin width). The direct DVH is most useful for display of the dose-to-target volumes, because one can easily visualize the minimum dose, maximum dose, and which dose is most representative of the dose to the entire target volume (Fig. 14-11B).
- The DVH display most commonly used in radiotherapy is the cumulative DVH, in that the volumes receiving at least a given dose value are plotted. The cumulative DVH integrates the direct histogram, so it always begins at 100% (100% of the organ receives at least 0 dose), and ends at the maximum dose (see Fig. 14-11A). Figure 14-11A illustrates a desirable cumulative DVH for a target (PTV, which has a uniform target dose with no underdosing or overdosing of the target). Figure 14-11A also shows two normal tissue

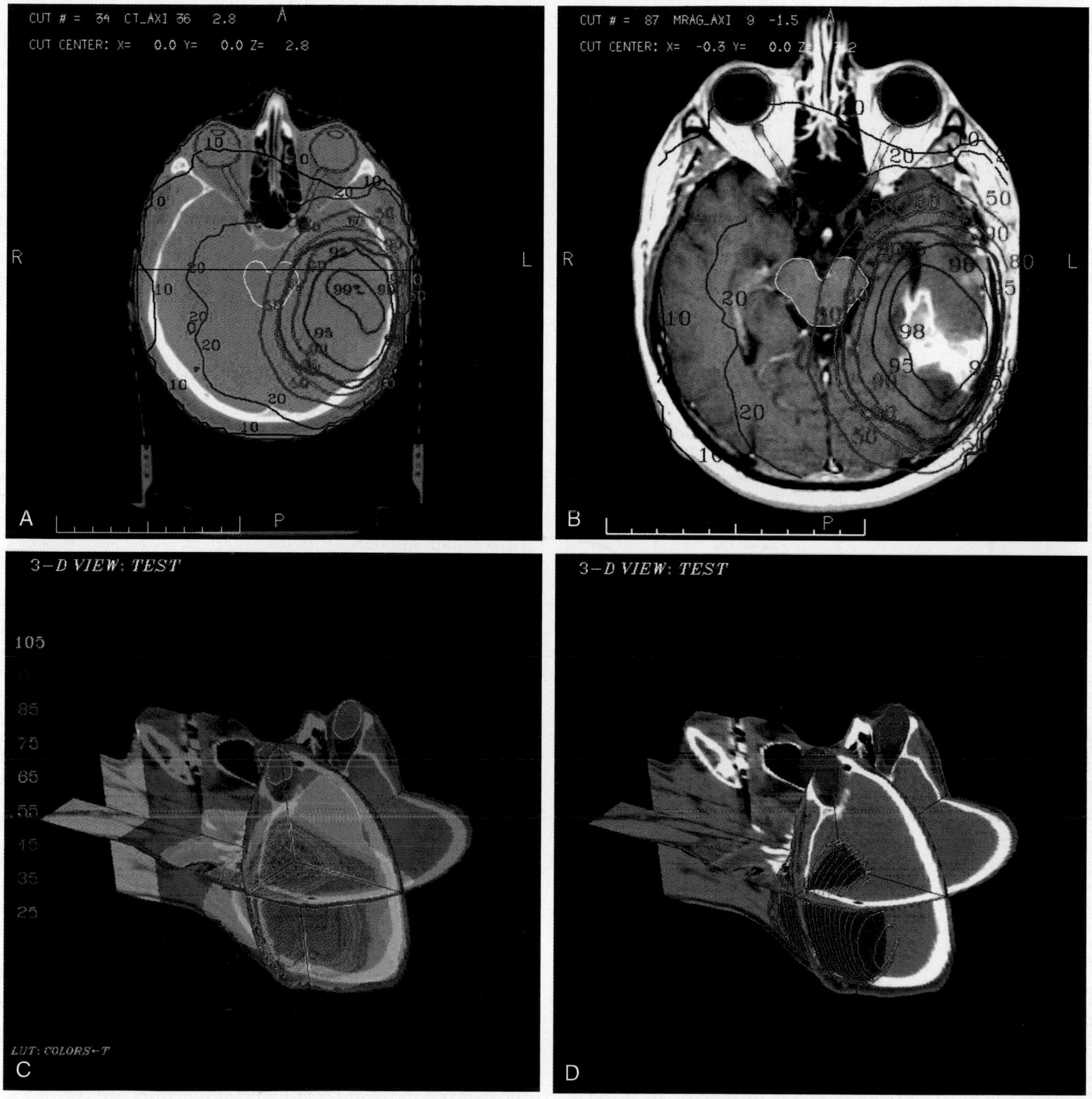

Figure 14-10 Dose display for a conformal brain plan. **A,** Axial CT with isodose lines. **B,** Axial MRI with isodose lines. **C,** Three-dimensional axonometric view with dose color wash. **D,** Target volume *(red contour)* and isodose surface *(yellow contour)*.

DVHs: Normal brain, which has some volume of the organ receiving a high dose, and chiasm, with a smaller volume of organ receiving high dose, even though the mean dose of the two DVHs is about the same. Whether a normal tissue DVH like normal brain is better than one like chiasm is only known once reliable clinical data are obtained for the two situations.

- The third type of DVH used for radiotherapy analysis is the differential DVH. This type is necessary in order to appropriately compare DVHs formed with different dose bin sizes, because the volume contained in any dose bin changes as the dose bin size changes. The differential DVH plots $(1/D_{bin})$*DV/DD and differential DVHs can be compared even if the dose bin size is different.

DVH analysis is a very important part of conformal therapy planning, but DVHs of target and normal structures do not tell the entire story. The DVH of an organ summarizes the dose to that organ, but it does not give any information about the geometric distribution of the different doses within the organ. If the DVH for a PTV shows cold and hot spots, it is not possible to tell if either the hot spots or the cold spots are in the center of the PTV or along the edges. Whenever the location of some dosimetric feature may make a difference, it is

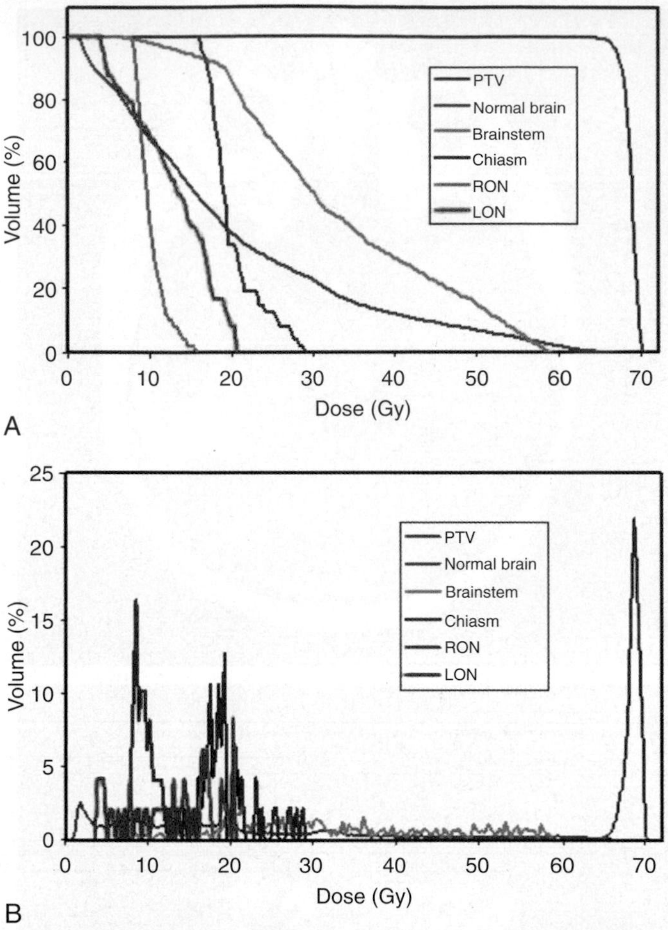

Figure 14-11 DVH displays for a brain treatment plan. **A,** Cumulative DVHs. **B,** Direct DVHs. LON, left optic nerve; RON, right optic nerve.

important to review the dose distribution using dose display tools.

Other Quantitative Metrics (Minimum, Maximum, and Others)

DVHs are only one kind of dosimetric analysis that can be used for conformal planning, and many other kinds of analysis are possible. For example, simple dosimetric metrics are often used to help make planning decisions. The maximum dose allowed within a target volume, or inside critical organs, is often specified in conformal therapy protocols. Particularly for IMRT conformal plans, the maximum dose may be a fairly difficult metric to use clinically, because it may depend strongly on the dose calculation grid spacing used and on details of the dose calculation algorithm implementation. A volume-based maximum dose criterion (e.g., the maximum dose to 1 cc of the object) may be less sensitive to algorithmic details. Similarly, the minimum dose to the PTV is subject to the same algorithm-related limitations and may be of limited value, particularly for IMRT planning. Another common dose metric is the mean dose to a structure, often used to describe target doses and for certain volume-effect organs like lung and liver, where the NTCP scales with the mean dose to the normal tissue.[78]

Use of "Biological Models"

To this point, all the treatment plan analysis has been based directly on the dose distribution. In reality, of course, it is the biological effects that are important, especially the probability of controlling the tumor and the probabilities of causing acute or late complications in the normal tissues. Analyzing the dose distribution is in many ways a surrogate for the analysis that is really needed, the biological effect analysis. It is expected that there will be major and continuing improvements in biological effect knowledge and modeling over the coming years, and as these improvements happen, they should be integrated into use for treatment planning. At the moment, however, the only biologically related parameters that are commonly used in treatment planning are the NTCP, the TCP, and the EUD. This section discusses each briefly.

The most commonly used "biologically related" parameter used in treatment planning is the NTCP. The term NTCP actually has several meanings: (1) the NTCP is a probability that can be determined clinically for an organ, (2) there are NTCP models that attempt to model how the probability of a particular complication changes as a function of dose, volume of the organ irradiated, and potentially other factors, and (3) the NTCP is used as the value of the complication probability that has been determined by an NTCP model for a particular situation. It is important to make sure it is clear how to differentiate between the real clinical NTCP, an NTCP model, or the particular expected value of the NTCP for a situation.

There are many kinds of models that have been developed for the NTCP, and these models have been applied to specific complications for many different organs. Discussion of these different models is beyond the scope of this work, and here we briefly describe only the most well known model, the Lyman NTCP model. John Lyman developed the three-parameter "Lyman" model early in the 1980s.[79,80] This power law model is a phenomenological model that characterizes complications using three parameters: TD_{50} for uniform irradiation, the slope of the dose sensitivity (n), and the volume parameter (m):

$$NTCP = \left(1/(2\pi)^{1/2}\right) \bullet \int_{-\infty}^{t} \exp(t^2/2)dt \qquad \text{(Eq. 1)}$$

where

$$t = [D - TD_{50}(v)]/[m \bullet TD_{50}(v)] \qquad \text{(Eq. 2)}$$

$$v = V/V_{ref} \qquad \text{(Eq. 3)}$$

$$TD_{50}(v) = TD_{50}(1) \bullet v^{-n} \qquad \text{(Eq. 4)}$$

To use this model for a real clinical DVH, one typically uses the Kutcher-Burman DVH reduction method[81] to convert the clinical DVH curve into a DVH with a single dose and volume, which are then used inside Equation 1. Together, these techniques are typically called the LKB (Lyman-Kutcher-Burman) model.

When developing this model, Lyman made no claim that it was a real biological model; he simply developed the simplest model that agreed with some of the most basic behavior of NTCPs, at least as characterized at that time. The model has been used extensively, either as a way to characterize complication data, or for plan evaluation and comparison. A very important starting point for study of NTCPs of various organs was published by Emami,[82] who summarized a tabulation of the current knowledge of clinical complication expectations (based on a physician working group), using Lyman NTCP model parameters. These parameterizations have sometimes been the starting points for clinical studies of complication probabilities; however, studies in many clinical sites have shown that the Emami parameters should be replaced by more modern results when possible. The Lyman model has proven to be a useful way to parameterize clinical NTCP data and has been used as part of dose escalation studies based on treating patients with a specific isocomplication level (for liver[83] and lung[84]).

One of the most important things that can be done to improve conformal therapy planning is to perform clinical studies that document, for each normal organ, the distribution of doses and volumes of various organs that are irradiated, include careful patient follow-up, and are analyzed to find the dose-volume-complication relationship for each organ. The dose-volume-complication relationship for each organ (and each complication) is unique and must be determined clinically. Once these kinds of results are known for all normal tissues, we will know better how to optimize treatment plans.

Just as the dose-volume-effect relationship is important to know for normal tissues, it is also very important to know it for the tumor. The TCP is the subject of clinical studies and modeling, and as a way of comparing expected tumor responses to planned dose distributions. A number of different models exist, including the Niemierko/Goitein[85] and Nahum[86] TCP models. Most of these models use various basic assumptions about tumor cell density and distribution, the statistical interactions between dose and tumor cell survival, and incorporation of population-based statistics for tumor heterogeneity, and may also consider effects that depend on tumor stage, hypoxia, and other issues. Tumor cell biology and predicting local tumor control are very complicated subjects that are well beyond the abilities of current models. TCP modeling is used in a reasonably limited way, because it is known that the predictions are of limited accuracy.

The last biologically related parameter used for treatment plan evaluation and optimization is the EUD. The EUD was originally described by Niemierko[87] by using a biologically and statistically influenced method to derive a dose parameter that was related to the effects one would expect on the tumor. The EUD has been generalized further[88,89] to be useful for normal tissues and targets. Because the EUD is in principle a generalized mean of the dose distribution according to a specific weighting method, one may use the parameters to represent the sensitivity of the tumor to underdosing in a small region, or the effect of hot spots in the tumor. Because the concept of the EUD is relatively new, numerous publications and analysis continue to explore and expand the characterization of tumor and normal tissue responses using various EUD representations.

Forward Planning

Since the 1950s, nearly all treatment planning has used the basic paradigm that is currently called "forward" planning. The treatment planner typically uses the following process:

1. Define the anatomy. The definition of the anatomic model to be used for the planning is the first step in planning, particularly involving delineation of the target volumes to be targeted for treatment.
2. Create the plan. Create a beam arrangement, choosing energy, beam location, direction and shape, beam weights, and addition of modifiers (wedges, compensators, etc.).
3. Calculate the dose. Calculate the dose distribution from that beam arrangement.
4. Evaluate. Evaluate the dose distribution, usually by looking at isodose line displays relative to the anatomy, and (in recent years) by calculating DVHs for the normal tissues and targets.
5. Iterative plan optimization. If plan is not adequate, or if the planner wishes to try to improve the plan, then the planner will iteratively modify the plan technique in an attempt to improve the plan result. Each iteration involves modifying the plan, performing a new dose calculation, and reevaluating the plan.
6. Plan completion. Once the plan is judged acceptable (or complete) by the planner and physician, the iterative optimization stops, and the plan is prepared for use. This involves calculation of MU for treatment, calculation of digital reconstructed radiographs (DRRs) to be used for patient localization, and transfer of the plan to the treatment delivery system.

Iterative forward planning is driven by the treatment planner and usually relies a great deal on the visual dosimetric evaluation performed by the planner or physician.

Setting Planning Goals

Creation of a high-quality conformal plan using forward planning depends crucially on the planning goals set by the physician. A typical set of conformal therapy planning goals may include the following:

- Typically the plan normalization point is chosen to be at the isocenter of the plan.
- The plan should make the 95% isodose line, for example, conform to the PTV (target volume) shape, so the minimum dose to the PTV is 95% of the plan reference point dose.
- The dose uniformity inside the PTV should be specified (e.g., ±5%), which will determine the maximum dose allowed in the PTV (in this example, 105%).
- Keep the maximum dose to the spinal cord less than some limit (typically 45-50 Gy).
- Minimize the dose to all normal tissues.
- Prescribe the target dose—either prescribe the dose to the plan normalization point and accept ±5% uniformity throughout the target, or prescribe the minimum dose to the target volume, and accept that the dose in the target may be as much as 10% (for example) higher.
- If normal tissue responses are known, specify reasonable normal tissue limits for the planner. For example, one can specify that the mean dose to the normal lung stay below some given value, because it is known that mean dose can be used to predict pneumonitis.

The physician should also specify any other constraints or evaluation expectations that will be used for final plan evaluation. One of the primary causes of additional iterations and frustrated planners is a physician who uses some plan evaluation criterion or rule that was not described to the planner as a goal or expectation.

Beam Arrangements

The basic beam arrangements useful for conformal therapy planning are site specific and depend on the geometry of the target volumes and normal tissues. Virtually all conformal plans have at least three different beams, and seven, nine, or many more beam directions are sometimes used (e.g., conformal stereotactic radiosurgery). Plans with more than seven beam directions are relatively uncommon when forward conformal planning is used, mainly due simply to the complexity involved in designing and determining the correct beam orientations, shapes, and weights interactively when there are so many different beams to consider. Nonopposing beam directions are very useful, as are beams that separate the target from the most critical normal tissues (increasing the distance between the target and normal tissues when viewed in BEV display). It is useful to have beams not in the axial plane, as they can help improve the conformality of the plan in all three dimensions.

Iterative Planning

Shaping beams is a very important part of the iterative planning process. Typically, a BEV margin of 6 to 7 mm is a good starting point for conformal beam shaping, but the shape of each field will then need to be modified to improve the conformality of the calculated dose distribution, as discussed earlier. This is the part of the iterative forward planning process that is most time-consuming, potentially, because in principle one needs to optimize the location of each leaf of the MLC for each beam, and there often are more than 100 involved MLC leaves in each field. The changes in shape that are needed are somewhat predictable, though, because larger MLC margins are needed in regions where there are no other beams (e.g., the superior and inferior aspects of the PTV for a plan with axial-only fields), while the margins can be much smaller if there are other beams that are transiting from an orthogonal direction. In the end, however, many iterations of the shapes may be necessary to get close to the optimal shaping. This is the part of forward planning that is often time-limited by clinical needs, and it could potentially be significantly improved by the application of computerized optimization methods to perform this shaping automatically.[65] Beam weights, use of wedges, and collimator angle rotation followed by revised beam shaping can also be part of the iterative planning process.

Plan Evaluation for Forward Planning

Evaluation of the plans resulting from forward planning is typically based on isodose line display and DVH plots for target (PTV) and normal tissues. Typically, the physician evaluates the plan using these tools and decides if the plan is adequate for clinical use, as well as whether the plan has the potential to be improved through plan technique changes, or by the physician modifying the dosimetric planning goals that were specified initially for the planning. Most clinical tradeoff decisions are made in a qualitative way, by inspection of the displayed dose distribution and the DVHs.

Inverse Planning

Rather than trying plans and seeing what kind of dose distribution can be achieved, as in forward planning, the basic concept of inverse planning is to decide up front what the dose distribution should look like and to then "invert" the problem to solve for the beams (and beam intensities) that will give the desired doses. This inverse problem, which is the inverse of the CT backprojection process, would be wonderful except for two small problems: (1) because there are no negative radiation intensities, it is not possible to invert the problem, and (2) we probably do not know what the best "achievable" dose distribution would be to use as our goal. We do know that the goal of full dose to the target and zero dose to the normal tissues is not possible.

To get around these problems, inverse planning makes use of computerized optimization techniques to search for the best plan among all possible candidate plans, using an objective or cost function to drive the optimization toward the plan that is "optimal." This kind of inverse planning or plan optimization process could be performed for any kind of radiotherapy plan. In practice, however, the plan needs to have many adjustable (optimizable) parameters that give enough flexibility to allow the optimization search to find a good solution to the planning problem. Therefore, until now, most inverse planning and optimization efforts have been applied to IMRT plans, particularly plans in which the individual beams are divided up into many separate beamlets or intensity "bixels." Plans created with beamlet IMRT may have hundreds or thousands of beamlet intensities to determine, and this large number of degrees of freedom makes it possible for the optimization process to work effectively.

The inverse planning process can be summarized as follows:

1. Define the anatomy. The definition of the anatomic model to be used for the planning is the first step in planning, particularly involving delineation of the target volumes to be targeted for treatment. Whereas in forward planning one is not "forced" to delineate all important structures, in inverse planning one must define all anatomic objects that are to be considered by the optimization. One must also define how calculation points are to be distributed throughout the involved objects.
2. Create the plan. Define the beam energies and directions, determine the largest extent of the beam shape, and divide the beams into beamlets (intensity bixels).
3. Calculate the dose per beamlet. For each relevant dose point, calculate the dose/unit fluence from each beamlet, the "D_{ij}" or "influence" matrix that tells how much dose each point receives as the intensity in an individual beamlet is changed.
4. Define the optimization method. One must define the cost function and optimization search algorithm to be used for the inverse plan. For an automated optimization algorithm to search the space of possible plans for the best one, one must define the cost (or objective) function that will be used to evaluate each plan iteration and drive the search algorithm toward the desired dose distribution. The cost function is defined individually, at least for each planning protocol, and perhaps for each patient, and is the most crucial decision involved in determining what kind of plan will result from the optimization process.
5. Iterative plan optimization. Inverse planning uses the optimization search algorithm, driven by the evaluation of the chosen cost function, to perform iterative plan optimization, with the search algorithm determining how the plans are modified, and the cost function serving as the judge of plan quality. In most current inverse planning, only the beamlet intensities are varied, so to recalculate the change in the plan dose distribution and cost function, one only needs to re-sum the dose contributions from the changed beamlets, a calculation that can be performed quickly. The optimization search will continue until predefined stopping criteria are achieved.
6. Plan evaluation and reoptimization. Once the optimization process is complete, the physician and planner must evaluate the plan, dose distribution, cost function results, and any other relevant information, to decide if the plan is acceptable. If it is not, then the plan optimization process must be rerun; however, it is necessary to make changes in the cost function to drive the plan toward a different result, because the running the optimization again using the same cost function should result in approximately the same plan as the first time.
7. Plan completion. Once the plan is judged acceptable (or complete) by the planner and physician, the iterative optimization stops, and the plan is prepared for use. For a beamlet-optimized IMRT plan, this includes leaf sequenc-

ing: the preparation of the MLC leaf trajectories (DMLC delivery) or MLC segment shapes (SMLC delivery) that will create the desired beamlet distribution. Other preparation steps include calculation of MU for treatment (usually included in leaf sequencing), calculation of DRRs to be used for patient localization, and transfer of the plan to the treatment delivery system.

Comparison of this process for inverse planning with the previously described forward planning process (see Forward Planning) shows that only a couple of steps are really different; most of the planning process is approximately the same.

Goals for Inverse Planning

As with forward planning, it is critical for the physician and planner to decide the overall goals for the inverse plan and to prioritize the various clinical issues. Goals for inverse planned IMRT may include the following:

- The dose to the target volumes should be specified: typically, this is the minimum dose, the mean dose, or the dose to a specific point inside the targets.
- Often, the dose distribution is defined in absolute terms (i.e., a plan will specify either the total dose [for the course of treatment, e.g., 60 Gy] or the dose/fraction [e.g., 2 Gy/fraction]). Relative dose can also be used, but given the use of IMRT, the dose to any defined reference point can be variable, so the relative dose mode of treatment planning is somewhat less useful than it is for flat field conformal therapy. In addition, if one wants to use biological model or other such evaluation or analysis tools, then the absolute dose mode of planning is much more useful than relative dose.
- The dose uniformity inside the PTVs should be specified (e.g., ±5%). Many current inverse planning systems may have a hard time achieving the ±5% uniformity in the target volume that is commonly used for conformal treatments, but this is not caused by using IMRT per se but rather by the kinds of cost functions used within those planning systems.[90]
- Keep the absolute maximum dose to the spinal cord less than 50 Gy. Note that for many (but not all, see earlier) cost functions, there are tails on the DVH of many structures that may allow higher doses to a small volume of the organ.
- Minimize the dose to all normal tissues.
- If normal tissue responses are known, specify reasonable normal tissue limits for the planner. For example, one can specify that the mean dose to the normal lung stay below some specified value, because it is known that mean dose can be used to predict pneumonitis.

The physician should also define and specify any other constraints or evaluation expectations that will be used for the cost function, because there is no other way to specify to the optimization method what it should do or should not do.

Beam Arrangements for Inverse Planned Intensity-Modulated Radiation Therapy

The rules usually applied to beam arrangements for forward planned conformal therapy also apply to inverse planned IMRT beams, in general. The beam arrangements that are most useful still depend on the site to be treated and on the geometry of the target volumes and normal tissues. Virtually all conformal plans have at least three different beams, and many beam directions are sometimes used. In much of the early IMRT literature, it was common to find plans with seven or nine axial beams, with beam directions evenly distributed about the patient. This number of beams allowed enough flexibility for the optimization to achieve a good plan, even if the beam directions were not tuned with respect to the anatomy. However, as IMRT planning has progressed, the use of nonaxial and geometrically optimized beam directions has become more popular. Contrary to some early IMRT literature, it is still useful to use beams from outside the axial plane, as they help improve conformality. However, with IMRT, it is often only obvious that the nonaxial beams are useful when considering low-priority normal tissues, because the IMRT optimization can typically achieve all of the higher priority goals without use of nonaxial beams. One feature of most IMRT plans still remains the same: typically, one avoids the use of opposed beams, because opposing beams tend to lead to degenerate solutions that can cause difficulties for some optimization search algorithms, preventing them from reaching the optimal solution.

Optimization Method

The most important issue affecting the quality of the final IMRT plan is typically the type of cost function used, and in particular how the different parts of the cost function are defined for each relevant organ or other anatomic object. In some systems, there is very limited flexibility in type of cost function used, as the cost function is limited to a simple method (often, a quadratic function of dose) in order to allow the gradient descent–based optimization search method to easily calculate the derivative of the cost function for each variable. However, other cost function methods can be quite general, allowing the use of dose, dose-volume, biological model, or other types of costlets that can be combined into an overall cost function.[91] In any event, it is the relationship of the different costlets (individual pieces of the cost function) that determine how important the various parts of the plan evaluation are, and so by changing one or more parameters in a costlet or costlets, one can drive the solution of the plan toward a different type of solution. Learning how to modify the cost function to modify the kind of solution achieved for the plan is one of the most important aspects of inverse planning and may take a significant amount of effort to master.

Regardless of the type of inverse planning system or cost functions used for inverse planning, one of the easiest ways to choose the appropriate cost function parameters for the plan is to first make sure that the clinical goals for the plan have been prioritized. Then, one constructs the cost function using the highest weights or power or importance for the high priority issues and decreasing weights (or whatever) for the lower priority issues. How this works in detail is specific for each type of inverse planning system, search method, and clinical site, but the general concept holds true for most inverse planning methods.

A number of different types of search algorithms are used for IMRT optimization, and these different methods can have some specific characteristics that are useful to know. Many current inverse planning systems, however, make use of only one search method, so many planners will not be able to choose different methods for specific patients or plans. Many inverse planning systems use gradient descent–based search methods, because they are fast, but this forces their cost functions to be limited to easily differentiable functions, typically quadratic dose penalties with a form like $w_i(D - D_i)^2$, where w_i is the weight of the penalty, and D_i is the dosimetric goal for the ith object. This type of cost function tends to lead to tails on the DVHs, because a small volume of the object can go higher than the desired dose without causing too much of a penalty. Another common concern about gradient descent algorithms is the possibility of local minima in the cost function. For simple cost functions this is not a problem, but use of many costlets or complex functions can lead to a local minimum that may trap the optimization search at a solution that is not the "global" minimum (the optimal solution). To avoid the possibility of being trapped in such local minima, stochastic search algorithms such as simulated annealing[51] and others can be used. These algorithms can perform a global search that is more certain to achieve the global minimum of the cost function, but they often are quite slow and can also be sensitive to the search parameters used (as in fact are all the search algorithms).

Plan Evaluation for Inverse Planning

If we knew exactly how to define the cost function so that it correctly summarized all of the physician's goals and desires for the treatment plan, then if the optimization method worked correctly and achieved the global minimum, we would know that the best plan had been found, and that would complete the plan evaluation. However, this is not the case at the current time. Most clinical inverse planning is still limited by many things, and so many IMRT plans still involve some "forward" iterative plan optimization, where an inverse plan is performed, the plan is evaluated by the physician or planner, and the cost function is modified and then the plan is reoptimized, as the planner or physician attempt to push the plan toward some goal that he or she believes is a better clinical result than what the inverse plan gave on the first attempt. As cost functions and search methods become more sophisticated, we can expect that this iterative forward planning use of inverse planning technology will become less necessary.

This problem demonstrates that there are some important issues for plan evaluation. The greatest problem to resolve is that the cost function determines what the search method will choose as the optimal plan, but the physician evaluation of the plan may not be consistent with what the cost function is telling the optimization to do. Whenever this happens, the physician will find the plan to be less good than desired and normally have to make modifications in the cost function and reoptimize the plan, perhaps many times, in order to achieve what was desired. A second complication is the fact that the metrics that physicians use to evaluate plans are many times not the same kinds of metrics used by the cost functions, causing another mismatch between physician and cost function. Methods that use clinically relevant metrics as part of the cost function may help decrease the severity of this problem somewhat. A third problem with IMRT plan evaluation is that most planners and physicians still have a difficult time knowing what is actually achievable with a given plan, beam arrangement, and anatomic situation, and thus even when an acceptable plan is achieved, they are not sure if they could achieve a "better" plan by changing something. New methods are needed to help give the planner and physician tools that can show them the kinds of changes that may be possible, so they can better know when the "optimal" plan is achieved.

One final plan evaluation issue involves the many compromises and approximations that are involved in current inverse planning and IMRT processes. Due to the huge number of calculations involved in a single iteration of the optimization method, and the large number of iterations that are necessary to optimize a given plan for some search methods, it is essential to make compromises in the dose calculation method, the evaluation of the cost function, and other parts of the process, and to limit the resolution of dose calculation points used within the calculation. In addition, as described in more detail in the next section, various compromises in the plan must be made when converting the ideal intensities of the beamlets into a deliverable set of MLC segments (SMLC) or trajectories (DMLC), and these compromises will generally degrade the quality of the plan that is delivered to the patient. As any plan is evaluated, one must also keep in mind the further degradation that will occur. The limited resolution used for dose calculations can often lead to changes in apparent conformality or target coverage if a new dose calculation (with different resolution or calculation grid placement) is used. More discussion about plan degradation caused by MLC sequencing is included in Conformal Therapy Delivery.

Plan Preparation

After a plan has been approved by the physician for clinical use, it must be prepared for treatment delivery and transfer to the delivery system. These preparations include the following:

- Documentation of plan approval. Documentation of the physician's approval of the plan for treatment should be clearly performed (e.g., signature on the treatment plan output, or electronic signature in the electronic chart). Other approvals (e.g., QA approval for IMRT treatments) may also be required.
- Preparation of treatment instructions. Creating a treatment plan for the patient usually involves determining the treatment beams to be used, but often does not consider other parts of the treatment delivery process, including patient setup and localization imaging, the treatment delivery methods to be used (e.g., automated delivery of all the beams, or manual delivery). For complex or automated treatments, creation of a complete treatment delivery script may be required. A graphical treatment delivery simulator can be quite useful.[92]
- Calculation of MUs may be required for non-IMRT fields, although some treatment planning systems also provide the MUs for the plan. In any event, an independent check of the MUs required for treatment should always be part of the process.
- Quality assurance (QA) checks for IMRT and other complex plans. Before delivery of a complex plan to the patient, it is often appropriate to perform various quality assurance checks on the treatment plan delivery, to assure that the treatment will work correctly and accurately. These kinds of QA checks are routine for IMRT treatments to confirm the correct dosimetric delivery of the complex beam intensity patterns that IMRT uses, and for stereotactic radiosurgery treatments to verify that the geometric accuracy of the treatment delivery is adequate, because large single doses are often delivered for these treatments.
- Hardcopy plan output. Once a plan is finalized, it is important to create a hard copy (or electronic) output describing the treatment plan, to be used in the patient's chart.
- Calculation of DRRs. The creation of DRRs is an important part of the plan preparation process, because these DRRs will be used for localization checks of the patient position while performing the setup of the patient.
- Plan transfer. Transfer of the plan information into the (paper or electronic) treatment chart and the treatment delivery system is a very important part of the process. For manual transfer methods, one of the biggest potential problems is the large probability of transcription errors as the various parameters for each field are transferred from the planning system to the delivery system or chart. For electronic transfers of the plan information to a computer-based delivery system, the errors that happen are typically not random transcription errors, but systematic errors are more

likely. The difference between the manual and electronic methods and their most likely errors means that the QA procedures for the two methods should be carefully defined to be appropriate for the method in use.

- If IMRT beams are used, then rather than calculation of MUs, "leaf sequencing" is performed for each beam to convert the planned IMRT intensity pattern into either multiple fixed MLC segments (SMLC) or dynamic trajectories of each leaf pair if the DMLC method is used.

Leaf Sequencing

To convert an IMRT intensity pattern into a delivery prescription that will create such a pattern of intensities, a leaf sequencing algorithm is used. Many different leaf sequencing algorithms exist, and all have advantages and disadvantages. Any leaf sequencing algorithm is really an optimization procedure that attempts to find the best way to create the desired intensity pattern while still adhering to all the constraints or limitations of the MLC and machine that are to deliver the IMRT intensity pattern. There are always compromises in the final result achieved by any of these algorithms, so one always knows that the plan has been changed (usually degraded) by those compromises. It is thus important to verify that the final "deliverable" plan is still acceptable. Many IMRT systems use a second dose calculation, based on the actual delivery sequence, to check that the plan is still within acceptable limits even after the compromises.

Two main methods of IMRT delivery are used with MLC systems (Fig. 14-12). SMLC, or segmental MLC, uses a set of fixed MLC segment shapes to deliver the intensity pattern, with the beam off as the MLC moves from one shape to the next. Many algorithms have been developed for this kind of MLC sequencing.[44,93] The other method is called DMLC, or dynamic MLC, in that the MLC leaves move on a trajectory that is defined so that the desired intensity pattern is created. Typically, a "sliding window" algorithm is used to derive the trajectories required.[46] Development of more efficient or effective algorithms or methods and characterization of the details of the differences between the various methods already in use are areas of active research. It appears that no one method or system is clearly better than the others, although there can be specific advantages or disadvantages for particular treatment types that are associated with a particular sequencing or delivery method.

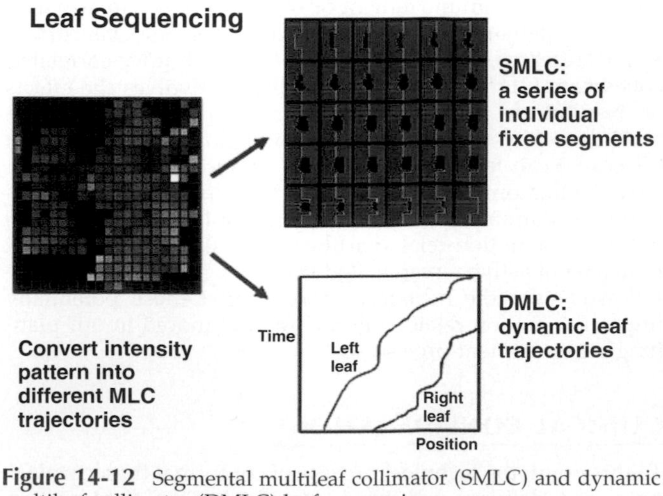

Figure 14-12 Segmental multileaf collimator (SMLC) and dynamic multileaf collimator (DMLC) leaf sequencing.

CONFORMAL THERAPY DELIVERY

Careful, efficient, and accurate treatment delivery is just as important as sophisticated treatment planning if the patient is to receive the benefits typically ascribed to conformal therapy.

Patient Setup and Localization

One of the most crucial aspects of patient treatment involves the setup and localization of the patient for each treatment fraction. For many years, this process has typically involved lining the patient up to laser lines using skin marks defining lateral and anteroposterior (AP) projections of the plan isocenter. To verify correct patient positioning, lateral and AP localization films were obtained (typically once per week) to confirm the correct placement of the isocenter inside the patient. The "orthogonal pair" films were compared by eye to the expected location (shown by DRR or BEV display from treatment planning) to document the accuracy of the setup. Use of a calibrated gradicule in the accelerator head when making the megavoltage images[94] was very helpful in making the comparison somewhat quantitative.

In the last several years, many new developments have begun to change the setup/localization process to allow much more quantitative and automated setup procedures. The development and implementation of electronic portal imaging devices (EPIDs)[95] for megavoltage imaging, diagnostic x-ray imagers,[96] and megavoltage or diagnostic cone-beam CT scanning[97] using accelerator-based systems are revolutionizing the setup and localization process. If the new digital imaging capabilities are integrated with the computer-control system of the treatment accelerator, it is possible to perform relatively automated patient setup with accuracy much improved over the old manual method.[98] Over the next years, it is clear that integration of cone-beam imaging into the treatment localization and setup process will lead to significantly improved accuracy for routine patient setup.

Manual and Computer-Controlled Treatment

The treatment delivery process used for modern conformal therapy has also changed. The usual method involved two or more therapists carrying the paper treatment chart into the treatment room, setting up the patient (as described above using lasers and skin marks), and then positioning the accelerator manually for each treatment field using the accelerator hand pendant controls. The therapists would exit the room in order to allow the treatment of each field, controlled using the treatment machine console in the control room. Although some machines were equipped with computer-based "record and verify" systems that would confirm the parameters to be used for each field, many of these systems were of limited sophistication. Most parameters used for patient treatment were set by hand and susceptible to various random errors.

Since the 1990s, integrated computer-controlled systems have entered widespread use for control of the treatment process, usually tied to a treatment plan or information system database that contains all the treatment plan information. To varying degrees, the progression through the setup process and treatment delivery is often automated, controlled via the machine's system. However, much remains to be done to optimize the efficiency, safety, and accuracy of the computer-controlled treatment delivery process. There has been some published work on the treatment delivery process,[92,99-101] but too often a treatment process taken directly from the old manual techniques is implemented with the computer-controlled system, without attention to changes needed for accuracy, safety, or efficiency. As the patient setup process, along with cone-beam CT or localization imaging using integrated electronic imaging systems, is integrated into the computer-controlled treatment process, additional effort to optimize the process will be required. Much work is needed in this area.

The use of IMRT treatment delivery has also caused a dramatic change in aspects of the delivery process. With simple nonconformal fields, it was common to outline the shape of each treatment field on the patient's skin and to confirm at treatment that the shape and placement of each radiation field agreed with the shape drawn on the skin. This limited very large errors but certainly was not a highly accurate positioning check. With modern IMRT treatment fields, understanding the fluence pattern that will be delivered requires computer-generated images, and there is no intuitive way to check the field shape, position, or intensity pattern directly on the patient, so more sophisticated QA checks or procedures are necessary. With modern EPID systems, so-called portal dose measurements (intensity or "dose" measured with the EPID) can be compared with that which is expected, and used as a quality assurance check that can potentially identify both geometric and dosimetric differences between the desired and delivered dose distributions.[102,103] It is also possible to reconstruct the delivered intensity distribution by analysis of MLC trajectory information.[104] The further development of quantitative online delivery quality assurance checks along with their integration into the treatment delivery process is an area of significant ongoing experience that is expected to lead to much more sophisticated delivery systems.

Patient Treatment Chart

As computer systems have increased the sophistication of planning, treatment delivery, and treatment verification and quality assurance, the need for more sophisticated treatment documentation has also grown. Computer-controlled treatment plans and IMRT require the use of electronic patient treatment charts, as there is just too much technical information to allow sole use of a paper treatment chart. The trend toward the use of electronic patient charts is certainly mirrored throughout the health care system, as all major medical systems convert their paper-based record system to an electronically based system.

It is incumbent on all users of such new electronic chart systems to carefully implement and use the new technology. It is not appropriate to just convert all the old paper-based documentation practices into electronic forms, as some standard paper-based methods just do not work well in the electronic world, such as writing notes in a chart in pencil to show what should happen in some number of future treatments. Some analysis of the needs for electronic treatment charts has been published,[101] but the ongoing transition from paper to electronic charts should be evaluated and performed with care. Complex IMRT-based prescriptions and plans probably require new methods that were not supportable in a paper-based chart, and users of highly sophisticated conformal therapy will have to develop their own migration from paper to electronic prescriptions and treatment charts.

Consideration of Setup Error and Patient Motion

As the field of radiation therapy has made the transition from four-field boxes and AP-PA fields to sophisticated conformal therapy based on 3D treatment planning and IMRT, it has become more obvious that considerations of daily setup uncertainties and errors and patient/organ motion during treatment are important considerations that should affect both treatment planning and treatment delivery methods. During multiple fraction treatment, all of the following effects should be considered:

- Daily setup variations
- Changes in patient anatomy and target shape over time
- Patient movement and organ motion during treatment

For many years, the ICRU-50 concept of the PTV[62] has been the sole response to these issues. However, the desire to perform precise conformal therapy has led many institutions to study these issues in more detail and to measure the uncertainties associated with these different issues. Daily setup uncertainty can be broken down into two parts: systematic and random errors. The systematic error (typically written as Σ) is more important for maintaining coverage of the target than the random error (σ), and Van Herk et al[63] have shown that one reasonable recipe for picking an appropriate margin between the CTV and PTV is to use a PTV margin given by

$$\text{PTV margin} = 2.5 \times \Sigma + 0.7 \times \sigma$$

This margin rule should cause a minimum dose of 95% to the CTV for 90% of the patients. In order to apply this rule, an institution must determine its systematic and random setup uncertainties by careful study of treatment accuracy (these values are often site dependent).

The importance of correcting the systematic setup uncertainty, if possible, has also led many institutions to convert their positioning verification procedure from the use of weekly port films, with position correction if a large-enough error is seen, to a more sophisticated offline or online repositioning scheme. Most accurate, although also requiring more effort, is to perform daily repositioning of the patient. Using EPID imaging and automated repositioning of the treatment table, it is possible to demonstrate large improvements in setup accuracy (e.g., improvement in Σ from >8 mm to 2.3 mm for liver patients).[105] It is also possible to apply "decision rule" protocols[106,107] in an offline manner: verification imaging is performed several days in a row, and only after the systematic error in the setup is determined is a correction made. However, it is expected that as the new online imaging with cone-beam CT and other accelerator-based imaging systems becomes better integrated with the treatment process, daily repositioning will eventually become a routinely used setup technique, thereby significantly decreasing the overall setup uncertainties that must be considered during treatment planning.

Changes in the patient anatomy from fraction to fraction, and intratreatment movement or organ motion, can also lead to both systematic and random geometric errors. One current area of research, now that 4D CT[58] and respiratory-correlated cone-beam CT[108] are becoming available, involves the effects of respiratory motion on treatments in the thorax and abdomen. Any non–time-resolved imaging (e.g., all normal CT scans) can lead to both systematic and random errors in how the anatomy is represented, so it is important to determine CT scanning protocols for planning (especially) that do not build in motion-related artifacts or systematic errors. This is an area of active research, and this work should be carefully followed over the next few years so that these potentially important motion-related effects are not ignored in our planning and treatment processes.

CLINICAL CONSIDERATIONS

To this point, the technical process of conformal therapy planning and delivery has been described. This final section describes some of the clinical considerations involved in the application of conformal therapy techniques and provides a very brief summary of some clinical results of IMRT treatments.

Immobilization, Setup Uncertainties, and Patient and Organ Motion

Patient positioning and immobilization should be comfortable but minimize motion and setup uncertainties. The clinically measured range of motion and setup uncertainties for each clinical site should be known, as they will determine the margins required for the PTVs (and PRVs, if used). Additional margin information can be obtained from the literature, as margins for a sample of patient populations using commercial, widely available immobilization systems have been determined and published; for example, the setup error standard deviation when using a commercial thermoplastic mask for head and neck immobilization has been determined to be 3 to 4 mm if patient-specific information is obtained and patient repositioning protocols using portal imaging are enacted.[109] While weekly verification is considered the standard method for conventional radiation therapy and 3DRT, daily imaging of the skeletal anatomy or implanted fiducial markers using an EPID has reduced systematic and random variations.

The systematic error can be established from imaging during the first three to five treatments[110] and can then be corrected, leaving only the random deviation to be accounted for by adequate PTV margins. Daily patient imaging and correction of setup deviations can reduce it even further, making it possible to reduce the PTV margin further, thereby increasing the sparing of adjacent noninvolved tissue. Individual measurements of motion and setup uncertainties, and their corrections, are especially important in sites where breathing or internal motion is significant. Techniques for dealing with this motion include active breath hold or gating for respiratory motion,[59,111] beam tracking of moving targets,[112] or fiducial markers for correction of prostate movement due to rectal filling-related changes in target position.[113]

Considerations of patient setup and immobilization approaches are complex. For example, in prostate cancer, prone patient position improves the separation between the prostate and the rectum compared with supine position,[114] thus potentially improving sparing of the rectum. However, prone positioning also increases breathing-related motion of the prostate.[115] In head and neck cancer, immobilization of the shoulders is essential if targets in the low neck are included in the conformal plan but is not required if the low neck is treated with an anterior field matched with the IMRT plan for the high neck.

Determining the Targets

The dosimetric advantages of IMRT need to be balanced with potential pitfalls related to the production of tight dose distributions around targets outlined on the CT scan. The most important issues are the reliability and reproducibility of outlining the targets that typically rely on a single planning scan performed prior to the start of treatment. The GTV is outlined on the treatment planning CT scan using clinical and radiologic information. In many cases, contrast-enhanced CT combined with clinical information derived from physical examination is the only modality required for the delineation of the targets. For some sites, CT is not the best imaging modality for the definition of the extent of the macroscopic tumor, and ancillary studies like MRI or fluorodeoxyglucose (FDG)-PET may add important information. MRI can be limited by its sensitivity to artifacts, difficulty in interpretation, long examination time, and cost. FDG-PET is often limited by a lack of specificity regarding tumor versus inflammation, and by uncertainties in interpretation, which may be subjective and differ depending on the observer's experience. PET-defined target volumes can also depend substantially on the standardized uptake value (SUV) chosen to contour the PET scan. The best added information from these studies is derived following their registration either with diagnostic CT or with the planning CT scans. Rigid body geometric registration of multiple scan types can now be performed in many cases using commercially available software, while registration of nonrigid structures like rectum, bladder, and others is the subject of ongoing research.[116]

Future improvements in the anatomic and metabolic imaging of tumors are expected to decrease the uncertainties in outlining the GTV to determine the volume to receive high radiation dose. However, the definition and outlining of the tissue volumes at risk of harboring subclinical disease (CTVs) depend on clinical judgment alone. It is not surprising that large interobserver differences have been noted in outlining these volumes.[117,118] The uncertainties in outlining the target volumes raise concerns about the potential of highly conformal radiotherapy to miss disease while striving to spare organs adjacent to the targets. Efforts to define the volumes at risk for subclinical disease for each tumor site have been made for head and neck cancer,[119,120] breast cancer,[121] and cancer at other sites.[122] They constitute the initial steps in this direction. Clinical validation, based on data regarding the sites of local/regional tumor recurrence and their relationships to the targets, is necessary. To date, relevant data are scant. It suggests that when target outlining is performed by experienced investigators, the large majority of the local/regional tumor recurrences are in-field, and only few marginal failures are observed.[123-125] Until more data are available, target outlining should be done in a conservative manner. Target volume definition requires thorough knowledge and understanding by the radiation oncologist of the anatomy and the local/regional tumor spread pattern.

An outline of imaging studies required for each tumor site, and other considerations for determining the targets, are described next.

Head and Neck Cancer

GTV

Most head and neck target volumes are defined using CT information. However, MRI is a necessary adjunct to CT for tumors close to the base of skull (i.e., nasopharyngeal and paranasal sinus cancer), where it provides better details of tumor extension and better details of the parapharyngeal and retropharyngeal spaces, compared with CT.[126] MRI is essential for delineating the targets in these cases. FDG-PET, in most cases, defines smaller primary targets compared with CT, and the volumes depicted by each modality do not completely overlap.[127] Relying on FDG-PET may result in changes in the outlining of the GTVs compared with outlining based on CT, at least in some patients.[127,128] Whether FDG-PET is more accurate than CT in delineating the primary tumor GTV has not yet been established, due to the paucity of data correlating the imaged extent of the gross tumor and its size in pathologic specimens following resection. Current data from series involving imaging followed with surgical validation suggest slightly more accurate definition of the gross tumor by FDG-PET compared with CT. In the delineation of neck lymph node metastases, FDG-PET has a higher sensitivity than CT.[127,129] Until more data are available, the most prudent practice seems to be outlining the GTV as the composite of the lesions observed on CT and PET. FDG-PET is a useful adjunct to CT in defining the GTV for head and neck cancer. It should be emphasized that FDG-PET has poor sensitivity for occult disease (25% in the clinically negative neck[130]) and cannot be relied on to determine the CTV. In cases of recurrent cancer, where extensive scars from previous surgeries confound the CT-based delineation of the tumor, FDG-PET has a clear advantage[131] and should be used for the delineation of the GTV.

CTV

The CTVs for head and neck cancer include subclinical disease in the vicinity of the primary tumor and lymph node groups at risk of subclinical disease. Outlining the CTVs requires knowledge of the natural history and pattern of failure of each tumor site. Suggestions for the selection and delineation of the targets have been published,[119,120,132-135] and atlases detail the recommended delineation of various lymph nodal groups. Studies detailing tumor failure patterns and how these patterns can affect modification of target outlining rules are emerging.[123,125]

Lung Cancer

GTV

In lung cancer, the primary lesion should be contoured on the CT scan using window/level settings for pulmonary visualization (i.e., a pulmonary window). FDG-PET adds significantly to the staging information gained from CT regarding the tumor extent and is an essential tool for the delineation of the GTV, with significantly better accuracy gained by fused PET-CT compared with each modality performed separately.[136] PET can differentiate atelectasis from tumor, preventing unnecessary inclusion of noninvolved lung tissue in the GTV.[137] In the free-breathing patient, FDG-PET depicts the tumor extent in both expiration and inspiration, providing information about breathing-related tumor motion and position changes that is not gained from the fast CT. FDG-PET is expected to improve significantly the outlining of the GTV for radiation therapy purposes.[138]

CTV

The CTV for the primary tumor requires 6- and 8-mm expansions for squamous cell and adenocarcinoma, respectively, according to a histopathologic study.[139] Outlining mediastinal lymph nodes at risk of harboring subclinical disease may be performed using the surgical definition of the mediastinal nodes and an atlas describing their positions for radiotherapy planning purposes.[140] Some centers (University of Michigan[141] and Memorial Sloan Kettering[142]) do not define mediastinal nodal CTVs and do not intend to irradiate lymph nodes at risk without evidence of involvement, due to the pattern of local-regional failures in these patients that is predominantly within the GTVs.

Lung target volumes often require use of an ITV-like margin (internal target volume from ICRU-62[143]) for respiratory motion of the target, depending on whether measures to reduce the motion are used (e.g., ABC or gating). In the absence of such measures, large variability in tumor motion is observed among patients, on average 1 cm in different directions. However, the variability among patient is large and requires individual measurements.[144]

Brain Cancer

GTV

The GTV is defined using MRI with and without contrast and then registered with the planning CT. MR T1-weighted images with contrast show contrast-enhancing tumors like meningioma and glioblastoma. T2-weighted images show edema that is likely to contain microscopic tumor in cases of high-grade glioma. T1-weighted fluid-attenuated inversion recovery (FLAIR) images can differentiate brain infiltrated by tumor from edema caused by a mass effect and may enhance the definition of nonenhancing tumors.[145]

CTV

Lacking well-defined anatomic compartments, the CTV for a brain tumor typically consists of a uniform expansion of the GTV by 1 to 2 cm depending on tumor grade. At the University of Michigan, dose-escalation studies are aimed at increasing the dose to the GTV alone, while the CTV dose remains constant in order to limit brain volume receiving a high dose.[146]

Gastrointestinal Cancer

Most clinical trials in conformal radiation therapy in gastrointestinal cancer have been performed in pancreatic cancer, in which tumor control rates are poor and 3DCRT and IMRT may reduce the volume of small bowel and duodenum irradiated, potentially allowing higher radiation doses.[147] Outlining the targets must take into account significant respiratory-related organ motion, ranging up to 25 mm in various directions.[148] Without methods to reduce respiratory movement, the large PTV margins required to accommodate this motion are expected to increase markedly the volumes of the small bowel and duodenum receiving target doses and limit the ability to escalate tumor dose.

Prostate Cancer

The gross disease within the prostate gland cannot accurately be defined using conventional imaging, and routine practice is to outline the CTVs. Research in magnetic resonance spectroscopy (MRS) suggests that it may be used to identify tumor cell foci within the prostate using the choline-to-citrate ratio, which is higher in tumor cells compared with prostatic cells.[149] If confirmed, MRS imaging may be used to define the GTV, or the boost volume, within the prostate.[150] The prostate's superior margins at the base of the bladder and its inferior margin (apex) are better defined on MRI compared with CT. MRI is also better at defining the rectal and bladder boundaries and the penile bulb. Prostatic motion is on average 5 mm in both anterior-posterior and superior-inferior directions. If adjustments for this motion are not made, 1-cm margins are required to take into account motion and setup uncertainties. The PTV is typically defined using these margins around the prostate alone in good-prognosis cancer; around the prostate and seminal vesicles in intermediate-risk and high-risk patients; and including the pelvic nodes in high-risk patients. Some centers limit the margin posteriorly at the interface with the rectum to 0.6 cm.[151]

Gynecologic Cancer

MRI defines gross abdominal disease better than CT, and it may be aided by FDG-PET.[152] Most clinical studies included patients receiving postoperative therapy in whom the CTVs include the pelvic lymph nodes, typically outlined along blood vessels with margins of 0.5 to 1.5 cm.[153] Organ motion may be significant in the lower pelvis, varying in different series,[154] and most likely is similar to prostatic motion. Whether IMRT can be useful in the treatment of intact cervix, replacing brachytherapy or, more likely, serving to augment GTV doses after brachytherapy, is not yet known.

Breast Cancer

Some work on breast cancer treatment has used targets obtained by outlining the whole breast or chest wall while trying to reproduce the tissue volume that would have been irradiated with standard tangential fields, although this target is not really based on anatomy but on the older type of treatment. In order to achieve such a reproduction, marking the borders of clinical tangential fields by radiopaque wires such that they are apparent on the planning CT ensures inclusion of all tissue irradiated traditionally. There have been some efforts to define anatomic target volumes.[155,156] For boost planning, the lumpectomy scar is outlined as the CTV and a 1-cm margin is assigned as PTV, for breathing motion and setup uncertainties. When regional lymph nodes require irradiation, treatment complexity is higher, and heart volumes in left-sided breast cancer therapy may be substantial. For the outlining of the lymphatic CTVs, particularly the supraclavicular lymphatics, some anatomic guidelines have been published.[121,157]

Noninvolved Normal Tissue

Forward planned 3DCRT allows intuitive decisions by the planner regarding beam apertures and directions, but such decisions cannot be made in inverse planned IMRT. This requires that all targets and organs at risk be determined and outlined in the planning CT for use in the inverse planning. In addition, inverse planning typically also requires the definition of "nonspecified tissue." This information is usually obtained by subtracting all targets and specified organs at risk from the external contour of the patient in the CT dataset. It allows constraints on the maximum doses delivered outside the targets and the organs at risk, which is necessary to reduce unexpected damage to soft tissue, nerves, blood vessels, and so on.

Treatment Goals and Rationale for Highly Conformal Radiotherapy

Head and Neck Cancer

Delivery of the prescribed dose to the targets in advanced head and neck cancer is often limited by the dose to the spinal cord and brainstem, especially in advanced nasopharyngeal cancer, posterior pharyngeal wall cancer, and thyroid cancer. Also, irradiation of gross disease in the posterior neck may be suboptimal due to dosimetric deficiencies due to the off-cord photon and posterior neck electron beams. By making possible concave dose distributions, IMRT can overcome these deficiencies and potentially improve tumor control rates. Dose escalation to the GTVs[158] or to hypoxic subvolumes within the GTV[159] using IMRT has been proposed.

Sparing of the parotid glands, in an effort to reduce xerostomia, has been a major goal of earlier 3DCRT[160] and subsequent IMRT studies.[90,161-163] However, IMRT cannot substantially preserve the function of submandibular glands. These glands lie anterior to the subdigastric nodes that are important targets in both sides of the neck, and the inability to reduce their doses meaningfully poses a limitation on reducing xerostomia by IMRT. Similarly, reducing the doses to the noninvolved oral cavity, striving to spare the minor salivary glands[164] and to reduce mucositis, is an important planning goal. Additional objectives include reduced doses to the optic pathways and inner ears in patients treated for advanced nasopharyngeal and paranasal sinus cancer,[163,165,166] to the skin,[167] and to the swallowing structures whose damage following intensive chemoirradiation may cause dysphagia and aspiration.[168]

Brain Cancer

Dose-escalation trials attempting to increase the currently poor local control of high-grade gliomas have been conducted at the University of Michigan.[146] These trials used 3DCRT or IMRT delivering a high dose to the GTV while keeping constant dose to the CTV and limiting the doses to the optic pathways and noninvolved brain. IMRT may be superior to 3DCRT in some cases in that tumors are close to the optic nerves or chiasm.

Lung Cancer

Facing low local/regional tumor control, the goals of conformal irradiation are to improve target irradiation while reducing lung volumes receiving a high dose. Using 3DCRT, trials of dose escalation have been conducted using various constraints on uninvolved lung doses, like the mean dose, the effective dose (V_{eff}), or the lung volume receiving greater than 20 Gy (V_{20}).[169] These constraints require that only grossly involved lymph nodes be included in the targets because inclusion of nodes at risk but without evidence of involvement increases significantly the lung volumes treated to high dose.[142] To this point, the clinical use of IMRT for lung cancer has been restricted by respiratory motion and by uncertainties about beamlet doses in lung tissue.[170]

Breast Cancer

IMRT can produce more homogeneous doses to the intact breast compared with lateral tangential beams, potentially improving cosmetic results. In addition, lung doses can be reduced and heart doses in the therapy of the left breast, especially in patients requiring comprehensive breast and nodal irradiation.[171] Accelerated hypofractionated irradiation to the lumpectomy site has been investigated, taking into account the pattern of breast relapse that predominates in the original tumor quadrant and the assumption that good cosmetic outcome may be achieved if high fraction doses are delivered to limited breast volumes using IMRT.

Prostate Cancer

Dose escalation to the prostate[114,172-174] and concomitant delivery of a high dose to the intraprostatic gross tumor defined by various imaging modalities described above, while limiting the doses to the rectum and bladder to reduce the main toxicities of therapy, have been the major goals of 3DCRT and IMRT. Efforts have been reported to reduce the doses to the penile bulb[175] or pudendal arteries[176] to reduce the rates of treatment-related erectile dysfunction.

Gynecologic Cancer

Most current studies of IMRT for gynecologic cancer aim at reducing the volume of small bowel irradiated during postoperative treatment.[177] Escalating the dose to the GTV using IMRT as a replacement for brachytherapy has been proposed,[178] but it is unlikely that escalated external beam doses can match the extremely high doses delivered safely by implants to tumor in the vicinity of the implant sources. An interesting concept of bone marrow sparing using IMRT in conjunction with bone marrow imaging has been proposed at the University of Chicago.[179]

Pediatric Tumors

The rationale for highly conformal radiotherapy in pediatric tumors is to limit the high-dose volumes in growing organs, especially bones. While IMRT may achieve this goal better than 3D radiation therapy in some cases, it increases the volumes receiving low-dose radiation and the potential for future radiation-related malignancies. This should be an important consideration. Only when an obvious benefit is expected should IMRT rather than simpler techniques be used in children. For example, in medulloblastoma, IMRT can reduce the dose delivered to the cochleae when posterior fossa boost is planned with IMRT compared with parallel-opposed beams,[180] but similar benefit may be gained by the use of 3DCRT.[181]

Target and Organ Prescription: Dose Constraints

Standard radiotherapy is typically delivered in two or three phases. For a typical head and neck example, in the first phase radiation is delivered to all targets, including nodal and high-risk volumes. After a dose that is likely to eradicate subclinical disease is delivered (typically 46-50 Gy), additional irradiation is delivered only to the high-risk targets, to a total of approximately 70 Gy. In this scheme, all of the targets receive the same daily dose of 1.8 to 2.0 Gy. In contrast, using IMRT, one may use a single treatment plan that improves dose conformity compared with sequentially optimized plans.[182] In this single integrated boost (SIB) technique, the high-risk targets receive both a higher total dose and a higher daily dose compared with the lower-risk targets, and compared with critical normal structures whose total maximal dose is constrained at total doses that are lower than the prescribed target doses. Smaller daily doses reduce the biological effect of the doses delivered to the critical organs (normalized total dose [NTD]), so the SIB technique creates the situation in which the maximum critical organ doses usually allowed in standard radiotherapy become much more conservative when used within the SIB IMRT technique. In addition, the maximum doses specified in IMRT or 3DCRT are delivered to smaller (or much smaller) organ volumes compared with conventional radiotherapy. IMRT or highly conformal 3DCRT treatments may be safer than corresponding standard radiotherapy treatments even if nominal maximum critical organ doses are similar. On the other hand, higher-than-standard total target doses, delivered inadvertently due to nonuniform dose distributions typical of many IMRT plans, or due to intentional GTV dose escalation in an effort to increase tumor control rates,[183] are associated with increased daily doses, causing a further increase of the NTD. This has the potential to increase toxicity related to tissue embedded within the target. Such toxicity may be apparent long after therapy and its prevalence is not yet known. Dose escalation relying on the ability of IMRT to restrict the high-dose volume to the GTVs should be conducted only within careful clinical trials.

When Should the Use of Highly Conformal Radiotherapy/Intensity-Modulated Radiation Therapy Be Considered?

Planning, delivery, and quality assurance of 3DCRT/IMRT is more complex, costly, and work-intensive compared with previous technologies. Its use is justified if it offers apparent clinical advantages. The advantage in the dose distributions achieved by IMRT compared with 3DRT is mainly in the ability to form concave, horseshoe-like dose distributions. Such distributions are desirable in cases where the target partly encircles a critical involved structure whose tolerance is less than the desired target dose. This includes cases like head and neck cancer, where the targets are arranged anterior and lateral to the spinal cord and are bounded laterally by the major salivary glands; in prostate cancer, where the rectum invaginates into the prostate target; cases of lung cancer, in which the target (usually mediastinal lymph nodes) may lay close to the esophagus; in cases of esophageal cancer, in which sparing the lungs from high doses is an objective; in gynecologic malignancies, in which the lymph node targets are arranged lateral to and posterior to the small bowel; in left-sided breast cancer, in which the target is concave anterior to part of the lung and heart; in brain tumors near the optic pathways; in medulloblastoma where the posterior fossa partly surrounds the inner ear; and in others. IMRT may also be indicated in cases in which minimizing the extent of the tissues receiving a high dose (at the expense of higher volumes receiving low doses) is likely to be beneficial, like re-treatment of recurrent cancer.[184] On the other hand, it is less likely that a dosimetric benefit will be gained from IMRT in cases in which tumors are remote from sensitive tissues or are adjacent to a sensitive tissue but do not (partly) surround it, compared with simpler conformal techniques. An example of a case where the dosimetric differences between 3DCRT and IMRT are small is prostate cancer, where the anterior wall of the rectum invaginates somewhat into the posterior prostatic target. Even these small differences may be translated into a clinically meaningful benefit in reducing rectal complications by IMRT compared with 3DCRT.[151]

Patient-related issues include the ability to tolerate treatment times that are longer than those required for less complex treatments. Poor immobilization and breathing-related motion increase uncertainties regarding the accurate positions of the targets and adjacent normal tissue in the chest and abdomen and, to a lesser degree, in the pelvis. Daily changes in the shapes of organs like the rectum and bladder may affect their spatial relationships with the prostate target. Due to the tight dose distributions produced by 3DCRT and IMRT, these uncertainties require the use of techniques that minimize, or take into account, target and organ at risk (OAR) internal motion in most sites apart from the brain and head and neck. An additional concern is tumor shrinkage during therapy, which may also change the shape and relative position of adjacent organs.[185] Whether these changes over the course of treatment require modifications of the treatment plans in most patients is the subject of current investigations.[186]

The high flexibility in creating desired dose distributions by IMRT provides the ability to deliver high doses to part of tumors judged to be at higher risk than other parts. Clinical accomplishment of this concept, termed "dose sculpting,"[187] depends on the verification of the utility of innovative imaging of tumor physiology and early tumor response prediction.[188]

IMRT treatment plans are often characterized by nonhomogeneous dose distributions in the targets that produce "hot spots," such as target volumes receiving substantially more than the prescribed dose. This characteristic has been credited with a high rate of tumor control in nasopharyngeal cancer.[163] The potential for increased local toxicity due to "hot spots" is not yet clear and may depend on the site irradiated: very high doses delivered to the nasopharynx may be well tolerated, as attested by the common use of intracavitary boost with radioactive sources for nasopharyngeal cancer, but may not be well tolerated by the mucosa in other sites in the head and neck. In any case, heterogeneous dose distributions by IMRT are not a necessity, because relatively homogeneous doses can be obtained. The decision of whether to deliver homogeneous dose belongs to the planner.[90]

Negative Aspects of Intensity-Modulated Radiation Therapy

Several potential negative aspects of IMRT exist, for which there is as yet no clinical validation. While IMRT reduces the tissue volumes receiving high doses, larger tissue volumes receive low doses compared with standard radiation therapy or 3DCRT. This is due primarily to use of many beams (often), many MUs, and leakage through the MLC leaves. This characteristic may increase the risk of radiation therapy–related malignancies, as the risk of radiation therapy–related mutations and carcinogenesis increases at intermediate rather than at high doses.[189] This risk is especially relevant for young patients. As the risk of radiation therapy–related malignancies increases over time, usually past 5 to 10 years after therapy, clinical data are not expected to be available at this time.

Another theoretical concern is the loss of biological effect of radiation therapy when treatment delivery time is prolonged.[190] Prolonged treatment delivery time is characteristic of some IMRT delivery techniques. There are differences in IMRT delivery modes that make a difference in this respect. For example, tomotherapy delivers sequential treatment throughout the target volumes, so that the exposure time of each tumor cell to daily radiation is short. In contrast, other systems irradiate all the targets simultaneously over a relatively prolonged daily treatment time. Whether the prolonged fraction delivery time translates into a clinical difference is not known.

Intensity-Modulated Radiation Therapy Clinical Results

Clinical results of the use of IMRT are still quite limited but have begun to emerge in recent years, mainly in head and neck and prostate cancer.

Head and Neck Cancer

The tumor control results of clinical series reported to date are very heterogeneous regarding tumor sites and stages, have relatively small patient numbers or patient selection factors, and are characterized by relatively short follow-up periods.[123-125,163] These factors prevent meaningful direct comparisons of tumor control rates with similar patient series treated with standard radiation therapy. The series cited earlier reported local/regional tumor control rates ranging between 81% and 97%. These rates seem to be better than those of most series of standard radiation therapy for similar tumors, suggesting that there may be no compromise in tumor control rates following IMRT. A randomized study comparing IMRT with standard radiation therapy for head and neck cancer has started in Europe (C. Nutting, MD, personal communication), and preliminary results of a small randomized study of nasopharyngeal cancer comparing IMRT with conventional radiation therapy have been presented by researchers from Hong Kong.[191] Long-term results of these and other studies are expected to accumulate rapidly in the near future, providing an opportunity to assess whether tumor control rates are indeed superior to those achieved following standard radiation therapy.

Most head and neck IMRT studies use fractionation schemes that strive to mimic those used in standard radiation therapy: total GTV doses of 70 to 73 Gy at 2.0 Gy/fraction and high-risk nodal volume (CTV) doses of 64 to 56 Gy at 1.8 to 1.6 Gy/fraction, all in 35 fractions.[161,163] For advanced tumors, these schemes should be delivered concurrent with chemotherapy. For early oropharyngeal cancer, the Radiation Therapy Oncology Group (RTOG) conducted a phase II study in which the GTV, high-risk CTV (subclinical disease surrounding the GTV and first echelon nodes), and low-risk CTV (other lymph nodes at risk) were prescribed 66, 60, and 54 Gy, respectively, in 30 fractions (2.2, 2.0, and 1.8 Gy, respectively). This scheme represents a moderately accelerated course (biologically equivalent GTV dose of 70 Gy at 2.0 Gy/fraction, delivered over 6 weeks). More aggressive schemes include the Simultaneous Modulated Accelerated Radiation Therapy (SMART) scheme developed at Baylor University, consisting of GTV dose of 60 Gy at 2.4 Gy/fraction and CTV dose of 50 Gy over 5 weeks for advanced cancer.[192] This group reported that delivering this scheme concurrent with chemotherapy resulted in intolerable acute toxicity.[193] Using a similar scheme (SIB), the Medical College of Virginia group performed a phase I dose-escalation study in which they determined that 70.8 Gy in 30 fractions at 2.36 Gy/fraction delivered to the GTV was the maximally tolerated dose.[194] It is likely that different sizes and locations of the GTVs affect potential toxicity, thus determining this regimen should not yet be done outside of a clinical study. Also, the inability to deliver concurrent chemotherapy safely is expected to limit the acceptance of similar regimens by other institutions.

Partial sparing of the parotid glands has been reported to result in partial preservation of salivary flows and in improved patient-reported[164] and observer-rated[195,196] xerostomia, which improves even further over time.[164,196] The improvement in xerostomia seems to be translated into improvements in broad aspects of quality of life (QOL).[197,198] It is possible, however, that the sparing of additional tissue may play a role in improving QOL. For example, IMRT may reduce the irradiated volumes of tissues whose damage or malfunction causes late dysphagia and aspiration after intensive chemoirradiation therapy.[168] Dose-response relationships in the parotid glands have been reported by several investigators. The mean dose has been established as the most important dosimetric factor predicting salivary output after irradiation, and the relationships between the mean dose and the salivary output have been characterized as threshold relationships,[199] exponential,[200] or linear.[201] The mean doses below which substantial sparing of the salivary output was achieved were reported to be in the range of 20 to 39 Gy.[202] The reasons for these discrepancies lie in different methods of determining salivary gland function, different models used to assess response relationships, and the neglect (in most studies) of clinical factors like certain medications and dehydration that have been found to contribute to the dose-related reduced salivary production.[199]

Excess toxicity associated with IMRT (compared with conventional radiation therapy) includes higher acute skin toxicity, which may be addressed by including the sparing of the skin in the optimization cost function,[167] by treating the low neck using an anterior beam matched to the upper neck IMRT fields (in cases of N0 neck), or by cutting the mask such that a bolus effect in the low lateral neck is avoided. Excess mucositis may be the result of inhomogeneous GTV doses in cases of oral cavity or oropharyngeal cancer or excess doses in the oral cavity outside the targets that can be reduced by sparing the noninvolved oral cavity.

Prostate Cancer

Several prospective and retrospective series suggest that prostate doses of greater than 75.6 Gy, delivered via conformal radiotherapy, increase freedom from biochemical failure rates compared with lower doses, especially in intermediate-risk patients.[172-174] A randomized dose-escalation study at M. D. Anderson compared 70 with 78 Gy using a four-field box boost technique in the low-dose patients and a conformal six-field boost in the high-dose patients. Biochemical freedom from relapse in intermediate to high-risk patients (PSA >10 ng/mL) was significantly higher in the high-dose compared with the low-dose group, while no significant difference was observed in low-risk patients (PSA <10 ng/mL).[174]

Reducing rectal toxicity, a major dose-limiting factor in the therapy of prostate cancer, may allow dose escalation and a potential for improved cure rates. Partial sparing of the rectal wall seems to be the major advantage of IMRT, which may be essential in securing low rates of rectal toxicity while higher-than-standard doses are delivered to the prostate. The largest experience in this regard has been accumulated at Memorial Sloan-Kettering Hospital in more than 700 patients.[114] This group reported that when doses of 81 Gy were delivered, IMRT resulted in significantly less acute[114] and late[172] rectal toxicity compared with previous techniques. They found that an average of 98% of the CTV could receive the prescribed dose of 81 Gy by IMRT compared with 95% with 3DCRT, and smaller volumes of the rectal wall (9% versus 13%, respectively) and bladder wall (29% versus 32%, respectively) receiving less than 75 Gy. While statistically significant, it is not usually expected that these relatively small differences would be apparent clinically. However, the authors reported that a nonrandomized comparison of toxicity between patients receiving CTV doses of 81 Gy using IMRT or 3DCRT showed significant reduction in acute rectal side effects and late rectal bleeding, suggesting that these high target doses should only be delivered with IMRT.[151]

The relationships between the rectal wall volumes, dose, and rectal toxicity have been explored by several groups. The results vary depending on whether the percentage of the rectum versus absolute volume is used.[203-205] The adoption of a certain set of volumes and doses, chosen from one of these publications, is necessary for the optimization of IMRT plans for prostate cancer. An example of one of the possibilities is provided by Zelefsky and colleagues[151] following their experience with dose escalation using IMRT. Another example can be derived from the M. D. Anderson randomized trial, in which an increase in rectal toxicity grade greater than 2 was observed when greater than 25% of the rectal volume received greater than 70 Gy.[174] To reduce rectal dose, several investigators reported partial blockage of the overlap region between the PTV and the rectum such that the maximal dose to the rectum is limited at 72 Gy, notwithstanding the blockage of part of the target in the posterior prostate.[151] A hypofractionated schedule delivering 70 Gy in 2.5 Gy/fraction using IMRT and resulting in a low rectal toxicity rate was reported from the Cleveland Clinic.[206] In addition to the rectum, constraints regarding bladder and femoral head doses are required for IMRT planning. However, dose/volume/complication data for these organs are scarce, or relationships are weak, and published constraints for these organs are quite arbitrary to date.

Lung Cancer

Efforts to increase local/regional control in lung include escalating radiation dose using conformal radiotherapy. The results of several studies suggest that increased dose using 3DCRT tends to increase local tumor control.[207-210] These studies aim to treat gross disease alone (primary tumor and FDG-PET avid lymph nodes) without adjuvant irradiation of subclinical mediastinal disease. At the same time that radiation dose-escalation studies have suggested that local control can be improved, randomized studies have demonstrated that sequential chemotherapy combined with standard-dose radiation is superior to standard-dose radiation alone and that concurrent chemoirradiation is superior to sequential therapy. The next logical step in improving both local and systemic control of unresectable non–small cell lung cancer would be to escalate radiation dose, using conformal therapy, with concurrent systemic chemotherapy. As the time periods required for dose-escalation regimens using daily 1.8- to 2.0-Gy fraction doses are exceedingly long, recent trials use a strategy of escalating the dose per fraction, keeping overall time constant. When combined with concurrent chemotherapy, such regimens may be associated with prohibitive esophageal and lung toxicity, so a strategy that allows safe delivery of higher-than-standard fraction doses and chemotherapy using highly conformal radiation therapy is currently being sought in several institutions.

Data about dose/volume/pneumonitis risk following 3DCRT of lung cancer have been accumulated in recent years and should aid in evaluating treatment plans and protocols. Partial lung volumes receiving specified maximal doses, like V_{20} (the partial volume receiving >20 Gy), and others, have been used as metrics related to significant prognostic factors for pneumonitis risk.[169] These partial volumes are highly correlated with measures that have been found to correlate with the risk of pneumonitis, like the mean lung dose[169] or the effective volume (V_{eff}), which denotes the lung volume receiving a homogeneous dose causing the same complication probability as the prescribed nonhomogeneous dose distribution.[209] It should be noted that clinical factors, in addition to dosimetric ones, are likely to play a role in the risk of pneumonitis, like the location of the tumor, preexisting lung function abnormalities, added chemotherapy, and others.[169]

Acute esophagitis is another common toxicity of high-dose irradiation of lung cancer. Data suggest that this toxicity has a relationship with dose and length of esophagus receiving a high dose.[211] The addition of concurrent chemotherapy markedly increases the risk of this complication.

While dosimetric studies show advantages of IMRT over 3DCRT in some lung tumors, especially large tumors and those close to the esophagus, no clinical data are yet available for such treatment, as issues regarding lung motion, dose calculation accuracy, and treatment dose need to be addressed before large-scale clinical trials are conducted.

Breast Cancer

Clinical experience with breast-only IMRT has been reported by several groups using simple dosimetric requirements as the IMRT technique goals.[212,213] Excellent cosmetic results, assumed to relate to the high degree of dose uniformity achieved with this technique, have been reported by Vicini.[212] Using IMRT for comprehensive treatment in patients requiring breast and regional nodal irradiation may have dosimetric benefits in reducing lung and heart dose,[155] compared with 3DCRT, but it is limited by respiratory motion. Clinical studies of therapy using various techniques to accommodate motion are ongoing.

Gynecologic Cancer

Tumor control rates following postoperative IMRT of endometrial cancer are high, suggesting that irradiation of carefully selected targets, rather than the whole pelvis, does not compromise tumor control rates.[214] These studies also suggest that acute gastrointestinal toxicity (and to a lesser extent, genitourinary toxicity) is reduced compared with historic control patients who had received standard four-field radiation therapy.[215] Late gastrointestinal toxicity was also found to be reduced following IMRT compared with standard radiation therapy in a retrospective analysis.[216] Another normal tissue that is relatively spared by IMRT compared with standard radiation therapy is the bone marrow, where sparing is especially relevant for patients receiving combined chemoirradiation therapy. Relative bone marrow sparing and improved blood counts were found following "standard" IMRT compared with conventional radiation therapy, and they may improve even further when the sparing of the bone marrow is included in the optimization cost function following bone marrow imaging.[217]

Future Efforts

In order to further improve the technical clinical contribution of IMRT to cancer therapy, further steps need to be taken. They include studies of IMRT delivery together with normal tissue protectors like amifostine, better understanding of tumor and organ motion and changes during each treatment fraction and during the total course of therapy, and an improved ability to image the anatomic extent and the metabolic activity of tumors. Detailed knowledge of the clinical dose-volume-response relationships for all tissues involved in irradiation, to be gained from careful clinical studies and analyses, will help lead to improved treatments using the tools provided by conformal therapy and IMRT planning and delivery.

CONCLUSION

Conformal therapy is a term that embodies a general strategy for conforming the high-dose region to the target volume while minimizing dose to all the normal tissues. Many different techniques can be applied, including multiple flat shaped fields and complex intensity-modulated (IMRT) plans. The key to conformal therapy is the accuracy and precision with which targets and tissues are defined, planning is performed, and treatments are delivered, so any technical improvement that can enhance any of those capabilities will potentially improve the outcome of the therapy. The most important remaining task is the clinical study of normal tissue complications and tumor control as a function of dose and volume (and other factors), so that we have the basic data that can be used to better optimize our conformal therapy treatments.

REFERENCES

1. Takahashi S: Conformation radiotherapy: rotation techniques as applied to radiography and radiotherapy of cancer. Acta Radiol Suppl 242:1-141, 1965.
2. Mantel J, Perry H, Weinham JJ: Automatic variation of field size and dose rate in rotation therapy. Int J Radiat Oncol Biol Phys 2:697-704, 1977.
3. Proimos BS: Beam-shapers oriented by gravity in rotational therapy. Radiology 87:928-932, 1966.
4. Proimos BS: Shaping the dose distribution through a tumor model. Radiology 92:130-135, 1969.
5. Proimos BS: Synchronous field shaping in rotational megavolt therapy. Radiology 74:753-757, 1960.
6. Trump JG, Wright KA, Smedal MI, et al: Synchronous field shaping and protection in 2-million-volt rotational therapy. Radiology 76:275, 1961.
7. Wright KA, Proimos BS, Trump JG, et al: Field shaping and selective protection in megavolt radiation therapy. Radiology 72:101, 1959.
8. Jennings WA: The Tracking Cobalt Project: From moving-beam therapy to three-dimensional programmed irradiation. *In* Orton C (ed): Progress in Medical Radiation Physics. New York, Plenum Press, 1985, pp 1-44.
9. Green A: Tracking Cobalt Project. Nature 207:1311, 1965.
10. Green A, Jennings WA, Christie HM: Radiotherapy by tracking the spread of disease. *In* Transactions of the Ninth International Congress of Radiology, Munchen 1959, Munchen, Verlag, 1960, pp 766-772.
11. Brace JA, Davy TJ, Skeggs DBL, Williams HL: Conformation therapy at the Royal Free Hospital: a progress report on the Tracking Cobalt Project. BJR 54:1068-1074, 1981.
12. Chin L, Kijewski PK, Svensson GK, et al: A computer-controlled radiation therapy machine for pelvic and paraaortic nodal areas. Int J Radiat Oncol Biol Phys 7:61-70, 1981.
13. Chin LM, Kijewski PK, Svensson GK, Bjarngard BE: Dose optimization with computer-controlled gantry rotation, collimator motion and dose-rate variation. Int J Radiat Oncol Biol Phys 9:723-729, 1983.
14. Kijewski PK, Chin LM, Bjarngard BE: Wedge-shaped dose distributions by computer-controlled collimator motion. Med Phys 5:426-429, 1978.
15. Levene MB, Kijewski PK, Chin LM, et al: Computer-controlled radiation therapy. Radiology 129:769-775, 1978.
16. Brizel HE, Livingston PA, Grayson EV: Radiotherapeutic applications of pelvic CT. J Comput Assist Tomogr 4:453-466, 1974.
17. Goitein M, Wittenberg J, Mendiondo M, et al: The value of CT scanning in radiation therapy treatment planning: a prospective study. Int J Radiat Oncol Biol Phys 5:1787-1793, 1979.
18. Munzenrider JE, Pilepich M, Rene-Ferrero J, et al: Use of body scanner in radiotherapy treatment planning. Cancer 40:170-179, 1977.
19. Ling CC, Rogers CC, Morton RJ (eds): Computed Tomography in Radiation Therapy. New York, Raven Press, 1983.
20. Cunningham JR: Current and future development of tissue inhomogeneity corrections for photon beam clinical dosimetry with use of CT. *In* Ling CC, Rogers CC, Morton RJ (eds): Computed Tomography in Radiation Therapy. New York, Raven Press, 1983, pp 209-218.
21. Goitein M, Abrams M: Multi-dimensional treatment planning: I. delineation of anatomy. Int J Radiat Oncol Biol Phys 8:777-787, 1983.
22. Goitein M, Abrams M, Rowell D, et al: Multi-dimensional treatment planning: II. beam's eye-view back projection, and projection through CT sections. Int J Radiat Oncol Biol Phys 9:780-797, 1983.
23. McShan DL, Reinstein LE, Land RE, Glicksman AS: Automatic contour recognition in three-dimensional treatment planning. *In* Ling CC, Rogers CC, Morton RJ (eds): Computed Tomography in Radiation Therapy. New York, Raven Press, 1983, pp 167-173.
24. McShan DL, Silverman A, Lanza D, et al: A computerized three-dimensional treatment planning system utilizing interactive color graphics. BJR 52:478-481, 1979.
25. Reinstein LE, McShan DL, Land RE, Glicksman AS: Three-dimensional reconstruction of CT images for treatment planning in carcinoma of the lung. *In* Ling CC, Rogers CC, Morton RJ (eds): Computed Tomography in Radiation Therapy. New York, Raven Press, 1983, pp 155-165.
26. McShan DL, Fraass BA, Lichter AS: Full integration of the beam's eye view concept into clinical treatment planning. Int J Radiat Oncol Biol Phys 18:1485-1494, 1990.
27. Fraass BA, McShan DL: 3D treatment planning: I. Overview of a clinical planning system. *In* Bruinvis IAD, van der Giessen FH, van Kleffens HJ, Wittkamper FW (eds): The Use of Computers in Radiation Therapy. North Holland, Elsevier Science Publishers BV, 1987, pp 273-276.
28. Bauer-Kirpes B, Schlegel W, Boesecke R, Lorenz WJ: Display of organs and isodoses as shaded 3D objects for 3D therapy planning. Int J Radiat Oncol Biol Phys 13:130-140, 1987.
29. Mohan R, Barest G, Brewster LJ, et al: A comprehensive three-dimensional radiation treatment planning system. Int J Radiat Oncol Biol Phys 15:481-495, 1988.
30. Rosenman J, Sherouse GW, Fuchs H, et al: Three-dimensional display techniques in radiation therapy treatment planning. Int J Radiat Oncol Biol Phys 16:263-269, 1989.
31. Sherouse GW, Mosher CE, Novine K, et al: Virtual simulation: concept and implementation. *In* Bruinvis IAD, van der Giessen FH, van Kleffens HJ, Wittkamper FW (eds): The Use of Computers in Radiation Therapy. North Holland, Elsevier Science Publishers BV, 1987, pp 423-436.
32. Brahme A: Design principles and clinical possibilities for a new generation of radiation therapy equipment. Acta Oncol 26:403-412, 1987.
33. Brahme A, Eenmaa J, Lindback S, et al: Neutron beam characteristics from 50 MeV photons on beryllium using a continuously variable multileaf collimator. Radiother Oncol 1:65-76, 1983.

34. Brahme A, Kraepelien T, Svensson H: Electron and photon beams from a 50 MeV racetrack microtron. Acta Radiol Oncol 19:305-319, 1980.
35. Brahme A, Reisstad D: Microtrons for electron and photon radiotherapy. IEEE Trans Nucl Sci NS-28:1880-1883, 1981.
36. Galvin JM, Smith AR, Lally B: Characterization of a multileaf collimator system. Int J Radiat Oncol Biol Phys 25:181-192, 1993.
37. Jordan TJ, Williams PC: The design and performance characteristics of a multileaf collimator. PMB 39:231-251, 1994.
38. Mohan R: Field shaping for three-dimensional conformal radiation therapy and multileaf collimation. Semin Radiat Oncol 5:86-99, 1995.
39. Fraass BA, Marsh L, Martel MK, et al: Multileaf collimator-based intensity modulation for conformal therapy (abstract). Med Phys 21:1008, 1994.
40. Galvin JM, Chen X-G, Smith RM: Combining multileaf fields to modulate fluence distributions. Int J Radiat Oncol Biol Phys 27:697-705, 1993.
41. Lane RG, Loyd MD, Chow CH, et al: Custom beam profiles in computer-controlled radiation therapy. Int J Radiat Oncol Biol Phys 22:167-174, 1991.
42. Zacarias AS, Lane RG, Rosen II: Assessment of a linear accelerator for segmented conformal radiation therapy. Med Phys 20:193-198, 1993.
43. De Neve W, De Gersem W, Derycke S, et al: Clinical delivery of intensity modulated conformal radiotherapy for relapsed or second-primary head and neck cancer using a multileaf collimator with dynamic control. Radiother Oncol 50:301-314, 1999.
44. Bortfeld TR, Kahler DL, Waldron TJ, Boyer AJ: X-ray field compensation with multileaf collimators. Int J Radiat Oncol Biol Phys 28:723-730, 1994.
45. Kallman P, Lind B, Eklof A, Brahme A: Shaping of arbitrary dose distributions by dynamic multileaf collimation. PMB 33:1291-1300, 1988.
46. Spirou SV, Chui CS: Generation of arbitrary intensity profiles by dynamic jaws or multileaf collimators. Med Phys 21:1031-1041, 1994.
47. Brahme A: Optimization of stationary and moving beam radiation therapy techniques. Radiother Oncol 12:129-140, 1988
48. Holmes T, Mackie TR: A filtered backprojection dose calculation method for inverse planning. Med Phys 21:303-313, 1994.
49. Mohan R, Mageras GS, Baldwin B, et al: Clinically relevant optimization of 3D conformal treatments. Med Phys 19:933-944, 1992.
50. Webb S: Optimisation of conformal radiation therapy dose distributions by simulated annealing. Phys Med Biol 34:1349-1370, 1989.
51. Webb S: Optimization by simulated annealing of three-dimensional treatment planning for radiation fields defined by a multileaf collimator. Phys Med Biol 36:1201-1226, 1991.
52. Boyer AL, Butler EB, DiPetrillo TA, et al: Intensity Modulated Radiation Therapy Collaborative Working Group. Intensity modulated radiotherapy: current status and issues of interest. Int J Radiat Oncol Biol Phys 51:880-914, 2001
53. Brahme A: Optimization of conformation and general moving beam radiation therapy techniques. Use Comput Radiat Ther (9th ICCR):227-234, 1987.
54. Bortfeld T, Burkelbach J, Boesecke R, Schlegel W: Methods of image reconstruction from projection applied to conformation radiotherapy. PMB 35:1423-1434, 1990
55. Carol M: Integrated 3D conformal multivane intensity modulation delivery system for radiotherapy. *In* Hounsell A, Wilkinson J, Williams P (eds): Proceedings of the XIth International Conference on the Use of Computers in Radiation Therapy. Manchester, UK, Medical Physics, 1994, p 172.
56. McLaughlin PW, Wygoda A, Sahijdak W, et al: The effect of patient position and treatment technique in conformal treatment of prostate cancer. Int J Radiat Oncol Biol Phys 45:407-413, 1999.
57. Bentel GC, Marks LB, Krishnamurthy R: Impact of cradle immobilization on setup reproducibility during external beam radiation therapy for lung cancer. Int J Radiat Oncol Biol Phys 38: 527-531, 1997.
58. Low DA, Nystrom M, Kalinin E, et al: A method for the reconstruction of four-dimensional synchronized CT scans acquired during free breathing. Med Phys 30:1254-1263, 2003.
59. Kubo HD, Hill BC: Respiration gated radiotherapy treatment: a technical study. Phys Med Biol 41:83-91, 1996.
60. Wong JW, Sharpe MB, Jaffray DA, et al: The use of active breathing control (ABC) to reduce margin for breathing motion. Int J Radiat Oncol Biol Phys 44:911-919, 1999.
61. Dawson LA, Brock KK, Kazanjian S, et al: The reproducibility of organ position using active breathing control (ABC) during liver radiotherapy. Int J Radiat Oncol Biol Phys 51:1410-1421, 2001.
62. ICRU Report 50, Prescribing, Recording, and Reporting Photon Beam Therapy. Bethesda, MD, International Commission on Radiation Units and Measurements, 1993.
63. van Herk M, Remeijer P, Rasch C, Lebesque JV: The probability of correct target dosage: dose-population histograms for deriving treatment margins in radiotherapy. Int J Radiat Oncol Biol Phys 47:1121-1135, 2000.
64. Fraass BA, Lash KL, Matrone GM, et al: The impact of treatment complexity and computer-control delivery technology on treatment delivery errors. Int J Radiat Oncol Biol Phys 42:651-659, 1998.
65. Fraass BA, McShan DL, Kessler ML: Dose-based conformal field shaping using automated optimization. *In* Bortfeld T, Schlegel W (eds): Proceedings of the XIIIth International Conference on the Use of Computers in Radiotherapy. Heidelberg, Germany, 2000, pp 32-35.
66. Milan J, Bentley RE: An interactive digital computer system for radiotherapy treatment planning. Br J Radiol 47:115-121, 1974.
67. Sterling TD, Perry H, Katz L: Automation of radiation treatment planning. Br J Radiol 37:544-550, 1964.
68. van de Geijn J: The computation of two and three dimensional dose distributions in cobalt-60 teletherapy. Br J Radiol 38:369-377, 1965.
69. van de Geijn J, Fraass BA: Net fractional depth dose: a basis for a unified analytical description of FDD, TAR, TMR and TPR. Med Phys 11:784-793, 1984.
70. Cunningham JR, Shrivastava PN, Wilkinson JM: Program IRREG: calculation of dose from irregularly shaped radiation beams. Comput Prog Biomed 2:192-199, 1972.
71. Fraass BA, McShan DL, Ten Haken RK, Hutchins KM: 3D treatment planning: V. a fast 3D photon calculation model. *In* Bruinvis IAD, van der Giessen FH, van Kleffens HJ, Wittkamper FW (eds): The Use of Computers in Radiation Therapy. North Holland, Elsevier Science Publishers BV, 1987, pp 521-525.
72. Mackie TR, Scrimger JW, Battista JJ: A convolution method of calculation dose for 15-MV X-rays. Med Phys 12:188-196, 1985.
73. Ahnesjo A: Collapsed cone convolution of radiant energy for photon dose calculation in heterogeneous media. Med Phys 16:577-592, 1989.
74. Rogers DWO, Bielajew AF: Monte Carlo techniques of electron and photon transport of radiation dosimetry. *In* Kase KR, Bjarngard BE, Attiz FH (eds): The Dosimetry of Ionizing Radiation, Vol III. New York, Academic Press, 1985.
75. Andreo P: Monte Carlo techniques in medical radiation physics. Phys Med Biol 26:861-920, 1991.
76. Fraass BA, Doppke KP, Hunt MA, et al: American Association of Physicists in Medicine Task Group 53: quality assurance for clinical radiotherapy treatment planning. Med Phys 25:1773-1829, 1998
77. Kessler ML, Ten Haken RK, Fraass BA, McShan DL: Expanding the use and effectiveness of dose-volume histograms for 3D treatment planning, I: integration of 3D dose-display. Int J Radiat Oncol Biol Phys 29:1125-1131, 1994.
78. Ten Haken RK, Martel MK, Kessler ML, et al: Use of Veff and iso-NTCP in the implementation of dose escalation protocols. Int J Radiat Oncol Biol Phys 27:689-695, 1993
79. Lyman JT: Complication probability as assessed from dose volume histograms. Radiat Res 104:5-13, 1985.
80. Lyman JT, Wolbarst AB: Optimization of radiation therapy, III: a method of assessing complication probabilities from dose volume histograms. Int J Radiat Oncol Biol Phys 13:103-109, 1987.
81. Kutcher GJ, Burman C, Brewster L, et al: Histogram reduction method for calculating complication probabilities for 3D treat-

ment planning evaluations. Int J Radiat Oncol Biol Phys 21:137-146, 1991.
82. Emami B, Lyman J, Brown A, et al: Tolerance of normal tissue to therapeutic irradiation. Int J Radiat Oncol Biol Phys 21:109-122, 1991.
83. Dawson LA, Normolle D, Balter JM, et al: Analysis of radiation induced liver disease using the Lyman NTCP model. Int J Radiat Oncol Biol Phys 53:810-821, 2002.
84. Hayman JA, Martel MK, Ten Haken RK, et al: Dose escalation in non-small-cell lung cancer using three-dimensional conformal radiation therapy: update of a phase I trial. J Clin Oncol 19:127-136, 2001.
85. Niemierko A, Goitein M: Implementation of a model for estimating tumor control probability for an inhomogeneously irradiated tumor. Radiother Oncol 29:140-147, 1993.
86. Webb S, Nahum AE: A model for calculating tumour control probability including the effects of inhomogeneous distributions of dose and clonogenic cell density. Phys Med Biol 38:653-666, 1993.
87. Niemierko A: Reporting and analyzing dose distributions: a concept of equivalent uniform dose. Med Phys 24:103-110, 1997.
88. Niemierko A: A generalized concept of equivalent uniform dose. Med Phys 26:1100, 1999.
89. Wu Q, Mohan R, Niemierko A: IMRT optimization based on the generalized equivalent uniform dose (EUD). Int J Radiat Oncol Biol Phys 52:224-235, 2002.
90. Vineberg KA, Eisbruch A, Kessler ML, et al: Is uniform target dose possible in IMRT plans for head and neck cancer? Int J Radiat Oncol Biol Phys 52:1159-1172, 2002.
91. Kessler ML, McShan DL, Epelman MA, et al: Costlets: a generalized approach to cost functions for automated optimization of IMRT treatment plans. Optim Eng 6:421-448, 2005.
92. Kessler ML, McShan DL, Fraass BA: A computer-controlled conformal radiotherapy system: III: graphical simulation and monitoring of treatment delivery. Int J Radiat Oncol Biol Phys 33:1173-1180, 1995.
93. Siochi RA: Minimizing static intensity modulation delivery time using an intensity solid paradigm. Int J Radiat Oncol Biol Phys 43:671-680, 1999.
94. van de Geijn J, Harrington FS, Fraass BA: A graticule for evaluation of megavolt X ray port films. Int J Radiat Oncol Biol Phys 8:1999-2000, 1982.
95. Boyer AL, Antonuk LE, Fenster A, et al: A review of electronic portal imaging devices (EPIDs). Med Phys 19:1-16, 1992.
96. Antonuk LE, Boudry J, Huang W, et al: Demonstration of megavoltage and diagnostic x-ray imaging with hydrogenated amorphous silicon arrays. Med Physics 19:1455-1466, 1992.
97. Jaffray DA, Siewerdsen JH, Wong JW, Martinez AA: Flat-panel cone-beam computed tomography for image-guided radiation therapy. Int J Radiat Oncol Biol Phys 53:1337-1349, 2002.
98. Balter JM, McShan DL, Lam KL, et al: Incorporation of patient setup measurement and adjustment within a computer controlled radiotherapy system. *In* Starkschall G, Leavitt DD (eds): Proceedings of the XIIth International Conference on the Use of Computers in Radiation Therapy-ICCRT, Madison, Advanced Medical Publishing, 1997.
99. Fraass BA, McShan DL, Kessler ML, et al: A computer-controlled conformal radiotherapy system: I. overview. Int J Radiat Oncol Biol Phys 33:1139-1157, 1995.
100. McShan DL, Fraass BA, Kessler ML, et al: A computer-controlled conformal radiotherapy system: II: sequence processor. Int J Radiat Oncol Biol Phys 33:1159-1172, 1995.
101. Fraass BA, McShan DL, Matrone GM, et al: A computer-controlled conformal radiotherapy system: IV. electronic chart. Int J Radiat Oncol Biol Phys 33:1181-1194, 1995.
102. de Boer JC, Heijmen BJ, Pasma KL, Visser AG: Characterization of a high-elbow, fluoroscopic electronic portal imaging device for portal dosimetry. Phys Med Biol 45:197-216, 2000.
103. Louwe RJW, McDermott LN, Sonke J-J, et al: The long-term stability of amorphous silicon flat panel imaging devices for dosimetry purposes. Med Physics 31:2989-2995, 2004.
104. Litzenberg DW, Moran JM, Fraass BA: A semi-automated analysis tool for evaluation of dynamic MLC delivery. J Appl Clin Med Phys 3:63-72, 2002.
105. Balter JM, Brock KK, Litzenberg DW, et al: Daily targeting of intrahepatic tumors for radiotherapy. Int J Radiat Oncol Biol Phys 52:266-271, 2002.
106. Bel A, Vos PH, Rodrigus PTR, et al: High-precision prostate cancer irradiation by clinical application of an offline patient setup verification procedure, using portal imaging. Int J Radiat Oncol Biol Phys 35:321-332, 1997.
107. de Boer HC, Heijmen BJ: A protocol for the reduction of systematic patient setup errors with minimal portal imaging workload. Int J Radiat Oncol Biol Phys 50:1350-1365, 2001.
108. Sonke JJ, Zijp L, Remeijer P, van Herk M: Respiratory correlated cone-beam CT. Med Phys 32:1176-1186, 2005.
109. van Lin EN, van der Vight L, Huizenga H, et al: Set up improvement in head and neck radiotherapy using a 3D off-line EPID-based correction protocol and a customized head and neck support. Radiother Oncol 68:137-148, 2003.
110. De Boer JC, Heijman BJ: A new approach to off-line setup corrections: combining safety with minimal workload. Med Phys 29:1998-2012, 2002.
111. Balter JM, Brock KK, Litzenberg DW, et al: Daily targeting of intrahepatic tumors for radiotherapy. Int J Radiat Oncol Biol Phys 52:266-271, 2002.
112. Keall PJ, Joshi S, Vedam SS, et al: Four-dimensional radiotherapy planning for DMLC-based respiratory motion tracking. Med Phys 32:942-951, 2005.
113. Shirato H, Oita M, Fujita K, et al: Three dimensional conformal setup of patients using the coordinate system provided by three internal fiducial markers and two orthogonal diagnostic x-ray systems in the room. Int J Radiat Oncol Biol Phys 60:607-612, 2004.
114. Zelefsky MJ, Fuks Z, Hunt M, et al: High-dose intensity modulated radiation therapy for prostate cancer: early toxicity and biochemical outcome in 772 patients. Int J Radiat Oncol Biol Phys 53:1111-1116, 2002.
115. Dawson LA, Litzenberg DW, Brock KK, et al: A comparison of ventilatory prostate movement in four treatment positions. Int J Radiat Oncol Biol Phys 48:319-323, 2000.
116. Kessler ML, Meyers C, Balter J, et al: A robust system for registration of 3D and 4D image data. *In* Yi BY, Ahn SD, Choi EJ, Ha SW (eds): Proceedings of the XIVth International Conference on Computers in Radiation Therapy. South Korea, Jeong Publishing, 2004, pp 383-385.
117. Logue JP, Sharrock CL, Cowan RA, et al: Clinical variability of target volume description in conformal radiotherapy planning. Int J Radiat Oncol Biol Phys 41:929-931, 1998.
118. Nowak P, van Dieren E, van Sornsen J, et al: Treatment portals for elective radiotherapy of the neck: an inventory in the Netherlands. Radiother Oncol 43:81-86, 1997.
119. Eisbruch A, Foote RL, O'Sullivan B, et al: IMRT for head and neck cancer: Emphasis on the selection and delineation of the targets. Semin Radiat Oncol 12:238-249, 2002.
120. Gregoire V, Coche E, Cosnard G, et al: Selection and delineation of lymph node target volumes in head and neck conformal radiotherapy. Proposal for standardizing terminology and procedure based on the surgical experience. Radiother Oncol 56:135-150, 2000.
121. Madu CN, Quint DJ, Normolle DP, et al: Definition of supraclavicular and infraclavicular nodes: implications for three-dimensional CT-based conformal radiation therapy. Radiology 221:333-339, 2001.
122. Gregoire V, Scalliet P, Ang KK (eds): Clinical Target Volumes in Conformal and Intensity Modulated Radiation Therapy. Berlin, Springer-Verlag, 2004.
123. Chao KS, Ozygit G, Tran BN, et al: Pattern of failure in patients receiving definitive and postoperative IMRT for head and neck cancer. Int J Radiat Oncol Biol Phys 56:312-321, 2003.
124. Lee N, Xia P, Fischbain NJ, et al: Intensity-modulated radiation therapy for head and neck cancer: the UCSF experience focusing on target volume delineation. Int J Radiat Oncol Biol Phys 57:49-60, 2003.
125. Eisbruch A, Marsh LH, Dawson LA, et al: Recurrences near the base of skull following IMRT of head and neck cancer: implications for target delineation in the high neck and for parotid gland sparing. Int J Radiat Oncol Biol Phys 59:28-42, 2004.

126. Som PM: The present controversy over the imaging method of choice for evaluating the soft tissue of the neck. AJNR Am J Neuroradiol 18:1869-1872, 1997.
127. Daisne JF, Duprez T, Weynand B, et al: Tumor volume in pharyngolaryngeal squamous cell carcinoma: comparison at CT, MR imaging, and FDG PET and validation with surgical specimen. Radiology 233:93-100, 2004.
128. Nishioka T, Shiga T, Shirato H, et al: Image fusion between 18FDG PET and MRI/CT for radiotherapy planning of oropharyngeal and nasopharyngeal carcinomas. Int J Radiat Oncol Biol Phys 53:1051-1057, 2002.
129. Schechter NR, Gillenwater AM, Byers RM, et al: Can positron emission tomography improve the quality of care for head and neck cancer patients? Int J Radiat Oncol Biol Phys 51:4-9, 2001.
130. Stoeckli SJ, Steinert H, Pfaltz M, Schmidt S: Is there a role for positron emission tomography with 18F-fluorodeoxyglucose in the initial staging of nodal negative oral and oropharyngeal squamous cell carcinoma. Head Neck 24:345-349, 2002.
131. Greven KM: Positron emission tomography for head and neck cancer. Semin Radiat Oncol 14:121-129, 2004.
132. Gregoire V, Levendag P, et al: CT-based delineation of lymph node levels in the node negative neck: consensus guidelines. Available at: www.rtog.org/hnatlas/main.htm.
133. Nowak PJCM, Wijers OB, Lagerwaard FJ, Levendag PC: A three-dimensional CT-based target definition for elective irradiation of the neck. Int J Radiat Oncol Biol Phys 45:33-39, 1999.
134. Wijers OB, Levendag PC, Tan T, et al: A simplified CT-based definition of the lymph node levels in the node negative neck. Radiother Oncol 52:35-42, 1999.
135. Chao KSC, Wippold FJ, Ozygit G, et al: Determination and delineation of nodal target volumes for head and neck cancer based on patterns of failure in patients receiving definitive and postoperative IMRT. Int J Radiat Oncol Biol Phys 53:1174-1184, 2002.
136. Lardinois D, Weder W, Hany TF, et al: Staging of non-small cell lung cancer with integrated positron-emission tomography and computed tomography. N Engl J Med 348:2500-2507, 2003.
137. Nestle U, Walter K, Schmidt S, et al: 18F-Deoxyglucose positron emission tomography for the planning of radiotherapy in lung cancer: high impact in patients with atelectasis. Int J Radiat Oncol Biol Phys 44:593-597, 1999.
138. Mah K, Caldwell CB, Ung YC, et al: The impact of 18FDG-PET on target and critical organs in CT-based treatment planning of patients with poorly defined non-small cell lung carcinoma: prospective study. Int J Radiat Oncol Biol Phys 52:339-350, 2002.
139. Giraud P, Antoine M, Larrouy A, et al: Evaluation of microscopic tumor extent in non-small cell lung cancer for three-dimensional conformal radiotherapy planning. Int J Radiat Oncol Biol Phys 48:1015-1024, 2000.
140. Chapet O, Kong FM, Quint L, et al: CT-based definition of thoracic lymph node station. An atlas from the University of Michigan. Int J Radiat Oncol Biol Phys 63:170-178, 2005.
141. Narayan S, Henning GT, Ten Haken RK, et al: Results following treatment to doses of 92.4 or 102.9 Gy on a phase I dose escalation study for non-small cell lung cancer. Lung Cancer 44:79-88, 2004.
142. Rosenzweig KE, Fox JL, Yorke E, Amols H, et al: Results of a phase I dose escalation study using three-dimensional conformal radiotherapy in the treatment of inoperable nonsmall cell lung carcinoma. Cancer 103:2118-2127, 2005.
143. ICRU Report 62, Prescribing, Recording and Reporting Photon Beam Therapy (Supplement to ICRU Report 50). Bethesda, MD, International Commission on Radiation Units and Measurements.
144. Stevens CW, Munden RE, Forster KM, et al: Respiratory driven lung tumor motion is independent of tumor size, tumor location and pulmonary function. Int J Radiat Oncol Biol Phys 51:62-68, 2001.
145. Husstedt HW, Sickert M, Kostler H, et al: Diagnostic value of fast-FLAIR sequence in MR imaging of intracranial tumors. Eur Radiol 10:745-752, 2000.
146. Chan JL, Lee SW, Fraass BA, et al: Survival and failure patterns of high grade gliomas after three-dimensional conformal radiotherapy. J Clin Oncol 20:1635-1642, 2002.
147. Ben Josef E, Shields AF, Vaishampayan U, et al: Intensity modulated radiotherapy and concurrent capecitabine for pancreatic cancer. Int J Radiat Oncol Biol Phys 59:454-459, 2004.
148. Bussels B, Goethals L, Feron M, et al: Respiration-induced movement of the upper abdominal organs: a pitfall for the three-dimensional conformal radiation treatment of pancreatic cancer. Radiother Oncol 68:69-74, 2003.
149. Kurhanewicz J, Vigneron DB, Hricak H, et al: Three-dimensional H-1 MR spectroscopic imaging of the in situ human prostate with high spatial resolution. Radiology 198:795-805, 1996.
150. Xia P, Pickett B, Vigneault E, et al: Forward or inversely planned segmental multileaf collimator IMRT and sequential tomotherapy to treat multiple dominant intraprostatic lesions of prostate cancer. Int J Radiat Oncol Biol Phys 51:244-254, 2001.
151. Zelefsky MJ, Fuks Z, Leibel SA: Intensity modulated radiation therapy for prostate cancer. Sem Radiat Oncol 12:229-237, 2002.
152. Kumar R, Alavi A: PET imaging in gynecologic malignancies. Radiol Clin North Am 42:1155-1167, 2004.
153. Chao KS, Lin M: Lymphangiogram-assisted lymph node target delineation for patients with gynecologic malignancies. Int J Radiat Oncol Biol Phys 54:1147-1152, 2002.
154. Schefter TE, Kavanagh BD, Wu Q, et al: Technical considerations in the application of intensity-modulated radiotherapy for locally advanced cervical cancer. Med Dosimetry 27:177-184, 2002.
155. Krueger EA, Fraass BA, McShan DL, et al: Potential gains for irradiation of chest wall and regional nodes with intensity modulated radiation therapy (IMRT). Int J Radiat Oncol Biol Phys 56:1023-1037, 2003.
156. Bentel G, Marks LB, Hardenbergh P, Prosnitz L: Variability of the location of internal mammary vessels and glandular breast tissue in breast cancer patients undergoing routine CT-based treatment planning. Int J Radiat Oncol Biol Phys 44:1017-1025, 1999.
157. Krueger EA, Fraass BA, Pierce LJ: Clinical aspects of intensity modulated radiotherapy in the treatment of breast cancer. Semin Radiat Oncol 12:250-259, 2002.
158. Wu Q, Manning M, Schmidt-Ullrich R, Mohan R: The potential for sparing of parotids and escalation of biologically equivalent dose with intensity modulated radiation treatments of head and neck cancers: a treatment design study. Int J Radiat Oncol Biol Phys 46:195-205, 2000.
159. Chao KSC, Bosch WR, Mutic S, et al: A novel approach to overcome hypoxic tumor resistance: Cu-ATSM guided intensity-modulated radiation therapy. Int J Radiat Oncol Biol Phys 49:1171-1182, 2001.
160. Eisbruch A, Ship JA, Martel MK, et al: Parotid gland sparing in patients undergoing bilateral head and neck irradiation: techniques and early results. Int J Radiat Oncol Biol Phys 36:469-480, 1996.
161. Eisbruch A, Marsh LH, Martel MK, et al: Comprehensive irradiation of head and neck cancer using conformal multisegmental fields: assessment of target coverage and noninvolved tissue sparing. Int J Radiat Oncol Biol Phys 41:559-568, 1998.
162. Chao KS, Low D, Perez CA, Purdy JA: Intensity-modulated radiation therapy in head and neck cancer: The Mallinckrodt experience. Int J Cancer 90:92-103, 2000.
163. Lee N, Xia P, Akazawa P, et al: Intensity modulated radiotherapy in the treatment of nasopharyngeal carcinoma: an update of the UCSF experience. Int J Radiat Oncol Biol 53:12-21, 2002.
164. Eisbruch A, Kim HM, Terrell JE, et al: Xerostomia and its predictors following parotid-sparing irradiation of head and neck cancer. Int J Radiat Oncol Biol Phys 50:695-704, 2001.
165. Tsien C, Eisbruch A, McShan D, et al: IMRT for locally advanced paranasal sinus tumors: incorporating clinical decisions in the automated optimization process. Int J Radiat Oncol Biol Phys 55:776-784, 2003.
166. Pan CC, Eisbruch A, Lee SJ, et al: Prospective study of dose and inner ear function relationships in irradiated head and neck cancer patients. Int J Radiat Oncol Biol Phys 61:1393-1402, 2005.
167. Lee N, Chuang C, Quivey IM, et al: Skin toxicity due to intensity modulated radiotherapy for head and neck cancer. Int J Radiat Oncol Biol Phys 53:630-637, 2002.
168. Eisbruch A, Schwartz M, Rasch C, et al: Dysphagia and aspiration following chemo-irradiation of head and neck cancer: which

anatomical structures are affected, and can they be spared by IMRT? Int J Radiat Oncol Biol Phys 60:1425-1439, 2004.
169. Kong FM, Ten Haken R, Eisbruch A, Lawrence T: Non-small cell lung cancer therapy-related pulmonary toxicity: an update on radiation pneumonitis and fibrosis. Semin Oncol 32(Suppl 3): S42-S54, 2005.
170. Wang I, Yorke E, Desobry G, et al: Dosimetric advantage of using 6 MV over 15 MV photons in conformal therapy of lung cancer: Monte Carlo studies in patient geometries. J Appl Clin Med Phys 3:51-59, 2002.
171. Kestin LL, Sharpe MB, Frazier RC, et al: Intensity modulation to improve dose uniformity with tangential breast radiotherapy: initial clinical experience. Int J Radiat Oncol Biol Phys 48:1559-1568, 2000.
172. Zelefsky MJ, Fuks Z, Hunt M, et al: High dose radiation delivered by IMRT improves the outcome of localized prostate cancer. J Urol 166:876-881, 2001.
173. Symon Z, Griffith KA, McLaughlin PW, et al: Dose escalation for localized prostate cancer: substantial benefit observed with 3D conformal therapy. Int J Radiat Oncol Biol Phys 57:384-390, 2003.
174. Pollack A, Hanlon AL, Horwitz EM, et al: Prostate cancer radiotherapy dose response: an update of the Fox Chase experience. J Urol 171:1132-1136, 2004.
175. Kao J, Turian J, Hamilton RJ, et al: Sparing of the penile bulb and proximal penile structures with intensity modulated radiation therapy for prostate cancer. Br J Radiol 77:129-136, 2004.
176. McLaughlin PW, Narayana V, Meirovitz A, et al: Vessel-sparing prostate radiotherapy: dose limitation to critical erectile vascular structures defined by MRI. Int J Radiat Oncol Biol Phys 61:20-31, 2005.
177. Roeske JC, Lujan A, Rotmensch J, et al: Intensity modulated whole pelvis radiation therapy in patients with gynecologic malignancies. Int J Radiat Oncol Biol Phys 48:1613-1621, 2000.
178. Mundt AJ, Roeske JC: Could intensity modulated radiation therapy replace brachytherapy in the treatment of cervical cancer? Brachyther J 1:195-196, 2002.
179. Lujan AE, Mundt AJ, Yamada SD, et al: Intensity modulated radiotherapy as a means to reducing dose to bone marrow in gynecologic patients receiving whole pelvic radiotherapy. Int J Radiat Oncol Biol Phys 57:516-521, 2003.
180. Huang E, Teh BS, Strother DR, et al: Intensity modulated radiotherapy for pediatric medulloblastoma: early report on the reduction of ototoxicity. Int J Radiat Oncol Biol Phys 52:599-605, 2003.
181. Fukunaga-Johnson N, Sandler HM, Marsh R, et al: The use of 3D conformal radiotherapy to spare the cochlea in patients with medulloblastoma. Int J Radiat Oncol Biol Phys 41:77-82, 1998.
182. Mohan R, Wu Q, Manning M, Schmidt-Ullrich R: Radiobiological considerations in the design of fractionation strategies for intensity modulated radiation therapy of the head and neck. Int J Radiat Oncol Biol Phys 46:619-630, 2000.
183. Wu Q, Manning M, Schmidt-Ullrich R, Mohan R: The potential for sparing of parotids and escalation of biologically equivalent dose with intensity modulated radiation treatments of head and neck cancers: a treatment design study. Int J Radiat Oncol Biol Phys 46:195-205, 2000.
184. Lu Tx, Mai WY, The BS, et al: Initial experience using intensity modulated radiotherapy for recurrent nasopharyngeal carcinoma. Int J Radiat Oncol Biol Phys 58:682-687, 2004.
185. Mohan R, Zhang X, Wang H, et al: Use of deformed intensity distributions for on-line modification of image-guided IMRT to account for interfractional anatomic changes. Int J Radiat Oncol Biol Phys 61:1258-1266, 2005.
186. Barker JL, Garden AS, Ang K, et al: Quantification of volumetric and geometric changes occurring during fractionated radiotherapy for head and neck cancer using an integrated CT/linear accelerator system. Int J Radiat Oncol Biol Phys 59:960-970, 2004.
187. Ling CC, Humm J, Larson S, et al: Toward multidimensional radiotherapy: biological imaging and biological conformality. Int J Radiat Oncol Biol Phys 47:551-560, 2000.
188. Hockel M, Schlenger K, Mitze M, et al: Hypoxia and radiation response in human tumors. Semin Radiat Oncol 6:3-9, 1996.
189. Lindsay KA, Wheldon EG, Deehan C, et al: Radiation carcinogenesis modeling for risk of treatment-related second tumors following radiotherapy. Br J Radiol 74:529-536, 2001.
190. Fowler JF, Welsh JS, Howard SP: Loss of biological effect in prolonged fraction delivery. Int J Radiat Oncol Biol Phys 59:242-249, 2004.
191. Kam MK, Leung SF, Zee B, et al: Impact of intensity modulated radiotherapy on salivary gland function in early stage nasopharyngeal carcinoma: a prospective randomized study. J Clin Oncol 23(Suppl 16):500s, 2005.
192. Butler EB, The BS, Grant WH, et al: SMART (simultaneous modulated accelerated radiation therapy) boost: a new accelerated fractionation schedule for the treatment of head and neck cancer with intensity modulated radiotherapy. Int J Radiat Oncol Biol Phys 45:21-32, 1999.
193. Amosson CM, Teh AK, Garg WY, et al: Accelerated fractionation for head and neck cancer using the SMART boost technique. Int J Radiat Oncol Biol Phys 57(2 Suppl):S306, 2003.
194. Lauve A, Morris M, Schmidt-Ullrich R, et al: Simultaneous integrated boost intensity modulated radiotherapy for locally advanced head and neck squamous cell carcinomas: II, clinical results. Int J Radiat Oncol Biol Phys 60:374-387, 2004.
195. Chao KSC, Deasy JO, Markman J, et al: A prospective study of salivary function sparing in patients with head and neck cancers receiving intensity-modulated or three-dimensional radiation therapy: initial results. Int J Radiat Oncol Biol Phys 49:907-916, 2001.
196. Sultanem K, Shu HK, Xia P, et al: Three-dimensional intensity-modulated radiotherapy in the treatment of nasopharyngeal carcinoma: the University of California-San Francisco experience. Int J Radiat Oncol Biol Phys 48:711-722, 2000.
197. Lin A, Kim HM, Terrell JE, et al: Quality of life following parotid-sparing IMRT of head and neck cancer: a prospective longitudinal study. Int J Radiat Oncol Biol Phys 57:61-70, 2003.
198. Parliament MB, Scrimger R, Anderson SG, et al: Preservation of oral health-related quality of life and salivary flow rates after inverse-planned intensity-modulated radiotherapy (IMRT) for head and neck cancer. Int J Radiat Oncol Biol Phys 58:663-673, 2004.
199. Eisbruch A, Kim HM, Ten Haken R, et al: Dose, volume and function relationships in parotid glands following conformal and intensity modulated irradiation of head and neck cancer. Int J Radiat Oncol Biol Phys 45:577-587, 1999.
200. Chao KSC, Deasy JO, Markman J, et al: A prospective study of salivary function sparing in patients with head and neck cancers receiving intensity-modulated or three-dimensional radiation therapy: initial results. Int J Radiat Oncol Biol Phys 51:938-946, 2001.
201. Roesink JM, Moerland MA, Battersmann JJ, et al: Quantitative dose-volume response analysis of changes in parotid gland function after radiotherapy in the head and neck region. Int J Radiat Oncol Biol Phys 51:938-946, 2001.
202. Eisbruch A, Rhodus N, Rosenthal D, et al: How should we measure and report xerostomia? Sem Radiat Oncol 13:226-234, 2003.
203. Kupelian PA, Reddy CA, Carlson TP, et al: Dose/volume relationships of late rectal bleeding after external beam radiotherapy for localized prostate cancer: absolute or relative rectal volume? Cancer J 8:62-66, 2002.
204. Huang EH, Pollack A, Levy L, et al: Late rectal toxicity: dose-volume effects of conformal radiotherapy for prostate cancer. Int J Radiat Oncol Biol Phys 54:1314-1321, 2002.
205. Skwarchuk MW, Jackson A, Zelefsky MJ, et al: Late rectal toxicity after conformal radiotherapy of prostate cancer: multivariate analysis of dose-response. Int J Radiat Oncol Biol Phys 47:103-113, 2000.
206. Kupelian PA, Reddy CA, et al: Short course intensity modulated radiotherapy (70 Gy at 2.5 Gy per fraction) for localized prostate cancer: preliminary results on late toxicity and quality of life. Int J Radiat Oncol Biol Phys 51:988-993, 2001.
207. Rosenzweig KE, Mychalczak B, Fuks Z, et al: Final report of the 70.2 Gy and 75.6 Gy dose levels of a phase I dose escalation study

using three-dimensional conformal radiotherapy in the treatment of inoperable non-small cell lung cancer. Cancer 6:82-87, 2000.
208. Wu KL, Liao Y, Qian H, et al: Three-dimensional conformal radiation therapy for non-small cell lung cancer: a phase I/II dose escalation clinical trial. Int J Radiat Oncol Biol Phys 57:1336-1344, 2003.
209. Hayman J, Martel MK, Ten Haken RK, et al: Dose escalation in non-small-cell lung cancer using three-dimensional conformal radiation therapy: update of a phase I trial. J Clin Oncol 19:127-136, 2001.
210. Belderbos JS, De Jaeger K, Heemsbergen WD, et al: First results of a phase I/II dose escalation trial in non-small cell lung cancer using three dimensional conformal radiotherapy. Radiother Oncol 66:119-126, 2003.
211. Singh AK, Lockett MA, Bradley JD: Predictors of radiation-induced esophageal toxicity in patients with non-small cell lung cancer treated with three-dimensional conformal radiotherapy. Int J Radiat Oncol Biol Phys 55:337-341, 2000.
212. Vicini FA, Sharpe M, Kestin L, et al: Optimizing breast cancer treatment efficacy with intensity modulated radiotherapy. Int J Radiat Oncol Biol Phys 54:1336-1344, 2002.
213. Hong L, Hunt M, Chui C, et al: Intensity-modulated tangential beam irradiation of the intact breast. Int J Radiat Oncol Biol Phys 44:1155-1164, 1999.
214. Knab B, Mehta N, Roeske JC, et al: Outcome of endometrial cancer patients treated with adjuvant intensity modulated pelvic radiation therapy. Paper presented at the 46th Annual Meeting of the American Society for Therapeutic Radiology and Oncology, October 6-7, 2004, Atlanta, GA.
215. Mundt AJ, Lujan AE, Rotmensch J, et al: Intensity-modulated whole pelvic radiotherapy in women with gynecologic malignancies. Int J Radiat Oncol Biol Phys 52:1330-1337, 2002.
216. Mundt AJ, Mell LK, Roeske JC, et al: Preliminary analysis of chronic gastrointestinal toxicity in gynecologic patients treated with intensity modulated whole pelvic radiation therapy. Int J Radiat Oncol Biol Phys 56:1354-1360, 2003.
217. Roeske JC, Lujan AE, Reba RC, et al: Incorporation of SPECT bone marrow imaging into intensity modulated whole-pelvic radiation therapy treatment planning for gynecologic malignancies. Radiother Oncol 77:11-17, 2005.

CHAPTER 15

INTRAOPERATIVE IRRADIATION

Brian G. Czito and Christopher G. Willett

Intraoperative radiation therapy (IORT) is the delivery of radiation at the time of surgery. The rationale is straightforward: increasing doses of radiation therapy enhance local tumor control. In many clinical situations, the dose delivered by external beam radiation techniques is limited by tolerance of surrounding normal tissues. To overcome this, intraoperative irradiation has been used as a technique facilitating tumor dose escalation.

This chapter reviews the rationale and treatment strategies of intraoperative electron radiation therapy (IOERT) and intraoperative high-dose-rate brachytherapy (HDR-IORT) with surgery. These strategies usually integrate external beam irradiation (EBRT) and chemotherapy.

HISTORY

Intraoperative radiation was first used almost 100 years ago.[1] The contemporary approach to intraoperative radiation was initiated in the 1960s by Abe and colleagues[2] in Japan. These investigators advocated resection (where possible) with large single-dose radiation (25 to 40 Gy using cobalt-60). In the mid-to-late 1970s, many institutions in the United States had adopted IORT as a treatment approach using linear accelerator–based electron treatment in the operating room, including Howard University, Massachusetts General Hospital (MGH), the Mayo Clinic, and the National Cancer Institute (NCI). There are about 90 centers in at least 16 countries worldwide with active IORT programs.

RATIONALE

IORT has the potential to improve local control and the therapeutic ratio in many tumor sites by (1) reducing the volume of the irradiation "boost" field by direct tumor/tumor bed visualization and conformal treatment, (2) excluding part or all of dose-limiting normal structures by operative mobilization, direct shielding, or varying electron beam energy, and (3) allowing the delivery of high-dose irradiation by the above methods.

Although early investigators studied this modality separately in the treatment of resected and unresectable malignancies, current approaches use this technique in combination with fractionated EBRT (with or without concomitant chemotherapy) and resection. The rationale is that EBRT fields encompass the primary tumor and surrounding tissues harboring potential microscopic disease. In contrast to a large single fraction of irradiation, fractionated radiation (EBRT) is radiobiologically advantageous in promoting tumor control while minimizing late normal tissue injury.

Shrinking field techniques permit dose escalation. This approach is used in many malignancies, including head and neck cancer, breast cancer, and cervical cancer, with excellent local control and acceptable morbidity to dose-limiting normal tissues. These boost fields can be delivered in a multitude of ways, including interstitial and intracavitary techniques, as well as superficial electrons. For selected intra-abdominal, pelvic, and thoracic malignancies, IORT is a technique for localized dose escalation.

BIOLOGY OF INTRAOPERATIVE RADIATION

When external beam irradiation is fractionated, there is a preferential therapeutic advantage for normal tissues relative to tumor as defined by the "4Rs" of classic radiobiology (repair, reoxygenation, redistribution, and repopulation). With a single large fraction of radiation therapy, these advantages are lost. In addition, large doses per fraction may result in increased risk of late effects. There is evidence that small vessel injury caused by large doses per fraction may contribute to late effects, and ischemic complications are dose dependent.[3] Furthermore, tumor response to single and fractionated radiation therapy depends on the percentage of hypoxic cells within a tumor. This differential sensitivity between hypoxic and well-oxygenated cells increases with increasing dose.

With alpha/beta calculations (α/β), biologically equivalent doses to a fractionated EBRT course using 2 Gy/fraction for varying IORT doses have been estimated (Table 15-1). As shown, there are disadvantages from a late effects standpoint with IORT; however, many of these disadvantages are mitigated by exclusion of nontarget tissues from the radiation field by direct inspection, mobilization, and shielding.[4] When combined with EBRT and resection, IORT doses of 10 to 20 Gy provide local control for most solid tumors, especially in the setting of microscopic residual. When combined with EBRT and surgery, there is little reason to exceed IORT doses of 10 to 20 Gy. Late normal tissue complications are often the limiting sequelae of IORT administration, and careful planning and administration with techniques designed to reduce dose to nontarget tissues are of paramount importance.

LOCAL CONTROL: AN IMPORTANT END POINT

For any treatment, a patient is incurable if local control of the tumor is not achieved. If conventional treatment methods of EBRT, chemotherapy, and surgery provided high local control rates, IORT as a component of treatment would be unnecessary. Although local control rates are satisfactory in many tumor sites using conventional techniques, local failure is problematic in other sites, including abdominal and pelvic malignancies. Treatment of these areas using standard external beam techniques is limited by normal tissue tolerance. Examples of such sites are discussed next.

Pancreatic Cancer

EBRT with 5-fluorouracil (5-FU)–based chemotherapy used in the treatment of unresectable pancreatic cancer results in a doubling of median survival compared with surgical bypass/stenting alone (3 to 6 months versus 9 to 13 months) and an increase in 2-year survival from 0% to 5% to 10% to 20%.[5] Unfortunately, these techniques result in poor local control rates. Series from the Mayo Clinic and Thomas Jefferson University report local failure rates exceeding 70% to 80%[6-10] (Table 15-2).

Retroperitoneal Sarcoma

When surgery is used as the primary treatment modality for retroperitoneal sarcomas, local failure has been reported to

Section Title

range from 40% to 90%. Despite the addition of EBRT to surgery, local failure rates are 40% to 80%. This is in contrast to extremity sarcomas, where local control rates approach 90%. Because of the limited tolerance of surrounding normal tissue (small intestine, stomach, liver, kidney, spinal cord), EBRT doses are limited. A randomized NCI trial evaluating IORT in retroperitoneal sarcomas demonstrated that patients receiving IORT plus EBRT experienced significantly improved local control and less small bowel toxicity versus patients treated with EBRT-alone (80% in-field relapse) techniques[11] (discussed later).

Colon and Rectal Cancer

In patients with locally advanced (T4) or locally recurrent colon and rectal cancer, local control is difficult to achieve, despite multimodality therapy. Studies from Princess Margaret Hospital and Mayo Clinic report local failure rates of 90% or greater in evaluable patients treated with EBRT with or without systemic therapy.[12,13] In radiation-naïve patients, the optimal approach in locally advanced patients is preoperative EBRT combined with 5-FU–based chemotherapy followed by resection. Despite this, local recurrence occurs in 30% to 70% of patients.[14]

Cervical Cancer

For patients with cervical cancer, para-aortic nodal metastases are common. Despite the presence of "distant" metastases, approximately 15% to 20% of patients are cured by radical radiotherapy techniques, using EBRT doses of 55 to 60 Gy. However, high complication rates have been reported with these doses and techniques.[15,16] As in rectal cancer, patients with recurrent cervical cancer in the pelvis or para-aortic region have a poor long-term prognosis, with 5-year survival rates ranging from 5% to 30%. These patients have often been previously irradiated, and retreatment with meaningful doses of EBRT is usually not feasible given normal tissue tolerance. When patients have para-aortic or locally recurrent disease, administration of IORT is a feasible technique to dose escalate and enhance local control.

Table 15-1 Estimated Biologically Equivalent External Beam Irradiation Doses (2 Gy/d) of Varying Intraoperative Irradiation Doses

IORT dose	10 Gy	15 Gy	20 Gy
Normal tissue (acute) ($\alpha/\beta = 7$)	20 Gy	37 Gy	60 Gy
Tumor ($\alpha/\beta = 10$)	17 Gy	31 Gy	50 Gy
Normal tissue (late) ($\alpha/\beta = 2$)	30 Gy	65 Gy	120 Gy

LOCAL CONTROL: RELATIONSHIP TO RADIATION DOSE, DOSE-RELATED COMPLICATIONS, SHRINKING FIELD TECHNIQUES, AND DISTANT METASTASES

Influence of Dose

In both animal and human models, the probability of local control of a tumor by radiation is proportional to the total dose administered. The dose of radiation to control a tumor locally depends on several factors, including tumor type, clonogen number, and tumor microenvironment. A given radiation dose may be able to control a small tumor with high probability and acceptable morbidity; however, that same dose may be insufficient against disease of larger volume. Clinical experience has generated a body of data correlating local control by tumor type and radiation dose. Figure 15-1 summarizes in vivo data for a variety of irradiated human tumors of varying sizes and types.

The studies of Fletcher examined local control probability as a function of radiation dose for patients undergoing treatment for breast carcinoma and squamous cell carcinoma (SCC) of the upper aerodigestive tract. For breast cancer patients, control of subclinical disease was approximately 60% to 70% with 30 to 35 Gy, 85% with 40 Gy, and 95% with 45 to 50 Gy. For larger/palpable tumors, EBRT doses of 46 Gy, 59 Gy, and 76 to 90 Gy result in a local control probability of 20%, 35% to 50%, and 70% to 80%, respectively.[17-20] Dose-response data are summarized for patients with SCC of the upper aerodigestive tract and breast cancer in Table 15-3. These data suggest that marked improvements in local control can be achieved by escalating radiation doses.

Table 15-2 Selected Series of Intraoperative Radiation Therapy in Unresectable Pancreatic Adenocarcinoma

Series[ref no.]	Survival No. Pts.	Median (mo)	2-Y (%)	5-Y (%)	Relapse (%) Local (2 Y)	Liver or Peritoneal
Massachusetts General Hospital[52,75-77]						
^{125}I + EBRT (40-45 Gy/5 wk) ± CT	12	11	20	—	25	—
EBRT (40-50 Gy/6 wk) + IOERT ± CT	29	16.5	28	—	36 (1 y)	—
EBRT (45-50 Gy) + IOERT ± CT	150	13	15	4‡	—	—
Mayo Clinic[6,7]						
EBRT (40-60 Gy) ± CT	122	12.6	16.5	0	80	56 (det)
IOERT + EBRT (45-55 Gy) ± CT	56	10.5	6	0	35	54 (det)
Preop EBRT/5FU (45-54 Gy) + IOERT	27	14.9	27	7	32	52 (det)
Thomas Jefferson University[8-10]						
EBRT 63-67 Gy/7-9 wks ± CT	46	12.4†	—	—	78 (det)	—
EBRT (5 Gy-Pre/50 Gy-Post implant/^{125}I/CT	54	12.5	18	—	12 (det)	—
IOERT + EBRT/5FU + Leucovorin (20)*	49	16	22	7 (4 y)	31 (det)	55 (det)

EBRT, external radiation therapy; IOERT, intraoperative electron radiation therapy; CT, chemotherapy; det, determinate.
*Concurrent and maintenance 5FU-leucovorin. †12.4 mo median SR with CT vs 7.3 mo without CT.
‡5 pts survived beyond 5 yr; 6th pt alive NED at 4-yr 8 mo.

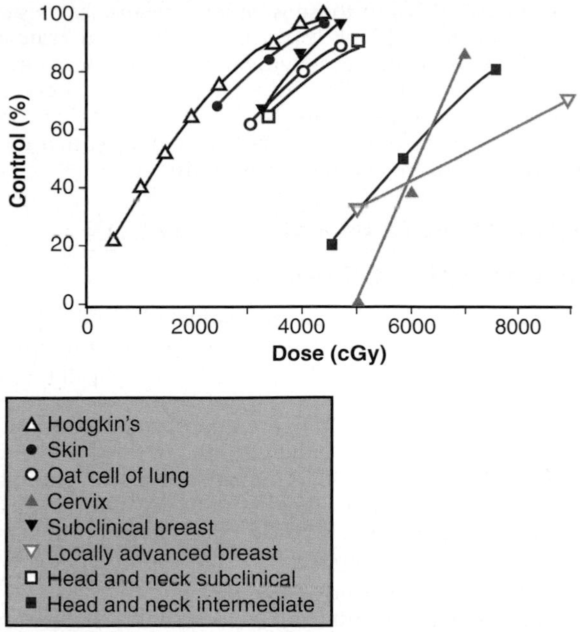

Figure 15-1 Local control versus dose of irradiation. (From Gunderson LL, Tepper JE, Biggs DJ, et al: Intraoperative +/− external beam irradiation. Curr Probl Cancer 7:8, 1983.)

Dose Versus Complications

The chief limitation of external radiation therapy to control macroscopic disease in the abdomen and pelvis is normal tissue tolerance. Normal organs such as stomach, small bowel, and kidney have tolerance levels well below the radiation doses required to eradicate most abdominal and pelvic malignancies. Exceeding these EBRT doses results in a prohibitive risk of late normal tissue damage (Table 15-4). Because of this, "conventional" tolerable doses of EBRT of 45 to 55 Gy using 1.8 to 2 Gy/fraction are not curative in most abdominal and pelvic malignancies, with resultant local persistence/local recurrence of disease common in patients treated with radiation therapy alone. This often results in tumor-related morbidity and mortality such as bowel obstruction and perforation, ureteral obstruction, and neuropathy.

Although local control is enhanced with increasing doses of radiation, tumor dose-response curves with EBRT closely resemble normal tissue complication curves. Efforts to improve local control through escalating EBRT doses may also result in treatment-related complications (Fig. 15-2). In an R1 (microscopic residual) resection, EBRT doses of 60 Gy or higher using conventional fractionation schemes are necessary to achieve a high probability of local control. In an R2 (gross residual) resection, even higher doses are usually required. Such doses exceed normal tissue tolerance (see Table 15-4).

Because of the risks associated with dose escalation beyond normal tissue tolerance, an attractive alternative in patients with locally advanced malignancies is to deliver moderate doses of EBRT (i.e., at or below accepted tolerance of surrounding normal tissue). A typical course would range from 45 to 50 Gy at 1.8 to 2 Gy/fraction, followed by surgical explo-

Table 15-3 Tumor Control Probability Correlated with Irradiation Dose and Volume of Cancer

Dose (Gy)	Tumor Control Probability
SQUAMOUS CELL CARCINOMA: UPPER AERODIGESTIVE TRACT	
50*	>90% subclinical
	60% T1 lesions of nasopharynx
	≈50% 1- to 3-cm neck nodes
60*	≈90% T1 lesions of pharynx and larynx
	≈50% T3 and T4 lesions of tonsillar fossa
	≈90% 1- to 3-cm neck nodes
	≈70% 3- to 5-cm neck nodes
70*	≈90% T2 lesions of tonsillar fossa and supraglottic larynx
	≈80% T3 and T4 lesions of tonsillar fossa
ADENOCARCINOMA OF THE BREAST	
50*	>90% subclinical
60*	90% clinically positive axillary nodes 2.5-3 cm
70*	65% 2- to 3-cm primary
70-80 (8-9 wk)	30% >5-cm primary
80-90 (8-10 wk)	56% >5-cm primary
80-100 (10-12 wk)	75% 5- to 15-cm primary

*10 Gy in five fractions each week.

Modified from Fletcher GH, Shukovsky LJ: The interplay of radiocurability and tolerance in the irradiation of human cancers. J Radiol Electrol 56:383-400, 1975.

Table 15-4 Gastrointestinal Radiation Tolerance

		Doses (in Gy)*		
Organ	**Injury at 5 y**	**1-5%$TD_{5/5}$**	**25-30%$TD_{50/5}$**	**Volume or Length**
Esophagus	Ulcer, stricture	60-65	75	75 cm^3
Stomach	Ulcer, perforation	45-50	55	100 cm^3
Intestine (small)	Ulcer, stricture	45-50	55	100 cm^3
Colon	Ulcer, stricture	55-60	75	100 cm^3
Rectum	Ulcer, stricture	55-60	75	100 cm^3
Anus	Ulcer, stricture	60-65	≥75	—
Pancreas	Secretory functions	—	—	—
Liver	Liver failure, ascites	35	45	Whole
Biliary ducts	Stricture, obstruction	50	70†	—

*Data based on supervoltage (6/18 MV), 9 Gy/wk (5 × 1.8).

†External beam radiation therapy to 50.4 Gy (28 × 1.8/5½ weeks) plus 20 Gy at 1-cm radius with iridium 192.

$TD_{5/5}$, 5% chance of severe intolerance within 5 y; $TD_{50/5}$, 50% chance of severe intolerance within 5 y.

Modified from Gunderson LL, Martenson JA: Gastrointestinal tract radiation tolerance. Front Radiat Ther Oncol 23:277-298, 1989.

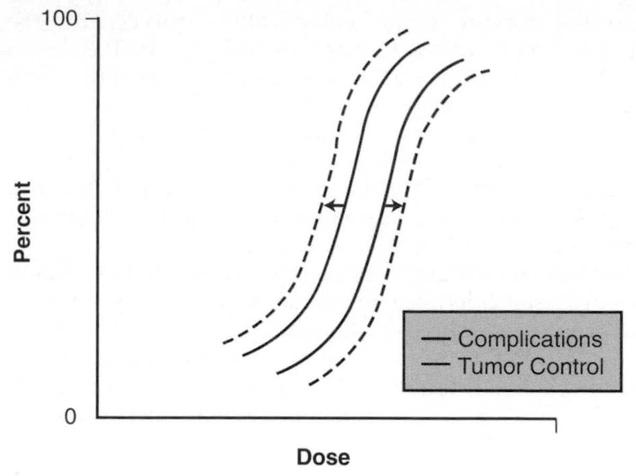

Figure 15-2 Radiation dose versus incidence of tumor control or complications. (From Gunderson LL, Tepper JE, Biggs DJ, et al: Intraoperative ± external beam irradiation. Curr Probl Cancer 7:8, 1983.)

ration. After resection, IORT would be performed, avoiding or minimizing irradiation of surrounding organs by shielding or mobilization. With this approach, an increase in local control with decreased risk of normal tissue complications (relative to an EBRT-only approach) can be achieved. In Figure 15-2, the local control curve shifts to the left with IORT, and the complication curve shifts to the right with increasing EBRT doses.

Shrinking-Field (Boost) Techniques

The concept of shrinking-field irradiation, otherwise known as administering "boost" treatments, has been used for decades by radiation oncologists. This strategy entails treating larger fields encompassing the primary/recurrent tumor along with local-regional lymph node basins and other tissues at risk for subclinical disease. These larger fields receive a dose sufficient to control microscopic disease yet respect normal organ tolerance (often 45 to 50 Gy using 1.8 to 2 Gy/fraction). Fields are then reduced to encompass gross disease with smaller margins, excluding dose-limiting normal tissues. An additional 20 to 35 Gy may then be administered to these fields using either EBRT or brachytherapy techniques, bringing the cumulative dose to 65 to 80 Gy. These approaches are used in many tumor sites, including gynecologic and head and neck cancers, with excellent long-term outcomes and local control with relatively low and acceptable morbidity levels. The concept of administering IORT in conjunction with EBRT is a logical application of this approach.

Local Control and Development of Distant Metastases

Preclinical data suggest that the incidence of distant metastases is related to both tumor size and the development of locally recurrent disease in multiple spontaneous tumor systems.[21-23] In fibrosarcoma and squamous cell carcinoma cell lines in rodent models, Ramsay and coworkers[21] reported increased rates of distant metastases in tumors measuring 6 mm versus 12 mm in size, as well as primary versus recurrent tumors. Additionally, Suit and colleagues[23] showed that in mouse mammary tumors treated with single-dose irradiation, increasing rates of local failure were associated with increasing rates of distant metastases. Specifically, the incidence of metastatic disease was 31% (16 of 52) in mice with local control, 50% (9 of 18) in those with local relapse salvaged by resection, and 80% (12 of 15) in mice with local relapse in which salvage was not attempted. Similar high rates of metastases associated with local failure have been observed in human malignancies, including cervix,[24] prostate,[25] and head and neck[26] cancers. These and other data suggest that metastases may arise from locally recurrent disease.

PATIENT SELECTION AND EVALUATION

Patient Selection Criteria

Candidates for IORT should be evaluated by the treating surgeon and radiation oncologist in the multidisciplinary setting. This allows for joint decisions regarding the appropriateness of IORT and whether further studies that may influence IORT and EBRT planning are appropriate. Additionally, joint decisions can be made defining the optimal sequencing of surgery/IORT and EBRT. Informed consent should be obtained from both specialties, specifically with regard to potential risks, benefits, and side effects of proposed treatments. Criteria for the appropriate selection of patients for IORT include the following:

1. Surgery alone will result in a high probability of incomplete resection (microscopic or gross residual disease) and resultant high probability of failure within the tumor bed. Potential candidates must be appropriate for surgical attempts at gross total resection. IORT administration should be performed at the time of a planned operation.
2. There is no evidence of distant metastases. Rare exceptions include resectable single-organ metastasis, slow progression of systemic disease, excellent chemotherapy options, and patients with oligometastatic disease with slow systemic progression and high probability of symptomatic local failure.
3. EBRT doses required for high probability of local control following subtotal or no resection exceed normal tissue tolerance (total doses required for eradication in this setting: 60 to 70 Gy for microscopic disease and 70 to 90 Gy for gross disease at 1.8 to 2 Gy/fraction).
4. Surgical displacement or shielding of dose-limiting structures or organs can be accomplished during IORT administration, allowing for acceptable risks of immediate and late effects. Theoretically, EBRT in conjunction with IORT should result in an improved therapeutic ratio between disease eradication and normal tissue complications.

Patient Evaluation

Pretreatment patient evaluation in patients eligible for IORT should include a thorough history and physical examination, with attention to palpable disease and its relationship to anatomically immobile normal structures. Examples include pelvic disease and its relationship to the pelvic sidewall, presacral space, prostate, or vagina. Computed tomography (CT), magnetic resonance imaging (MRI), and endoscopic ultrasound can aid in identifying adherence to structures (e.g., bony pelvis, large vessels) that may be surgically unresectable for cure. Examination under anesthesia may be helpful in some situations, including locally advanced gynecologic and rectal cancers. Routine blood counts, including complete blood cell count, liver function tests, renal function tests, and tumor-specific serum test (e.g., carcinoembryonic antigen, CA19-9), should be obtained where appropriate. Patients should be evaluated clinically and radiographically for evidence of distant spread. Positron emission tomography (PET), preferably in conjunction with CT, may facilitate defining local disease extent as well as unsuspected distant metastases.

Evaluation of distant metastases is particularly important in the recurrent setting where concurrent distant failure is common. Biopsy confirmation of disease should usually be obtained prior to proceeding with resection.

SEQUENCING AND DOSE OF EXTERNAL BEAM AND INTRAOPERATIVE RADIATION

Sequencing with Surgery

For patients with localized malignancy, the goal of curative oncologic surgery is an R0 (margin-negative) resection. Because of the locally advanced and infiltrative nature of many primary tumors (including colorectal, gynecologic, and upper gastrointestinal malignancies; sarcomas; etc.) and locally recurrent malignancies, surgery may be compromised with close margins or microscopic/gross residual. For patients with locally advanced tumors, preoperative EBRT to doses of 45 to 50 Gy using 1.8 to 2 Gy/fraction (with or without chemotherapy) followed by laparotomy, resection and IORT offers theoretical and clinical advantages over resection and IORT followed by EBRT. These are listed as follows:

1. By postponing surgical resection until after preoperative therapy is completed, patients with disease that is rapidly progressive may avoid an unnecessary surgical procedure with associated morbidity.
2. Preoperative therapy may allow for tumor downstaging and facilitate resection with curative intent.
3. Preoperative therapy may reduce the risk of tumor seeding/dissemination at resection.
4. Preoperative therapy allows delivery of treatment to disease with an intact vasculature, potentially improving the delivery of chemotherapy and improving oxygen delivery for EBRT.
5. The morbidity and delayed recovery time associated with extensive surgical procedures may prevent the timely delivery of postoperative therapy in a high percentage of patients.[27,28]

The role of preoperative versus postoperative therapy has been evaluated in rectal cancer. A large German randomized trial demonstrated that patients undergoing neoadjuvant radiation therapy and chemotherapy experienced significantly improved local control and less toxicity than did patients receiving postoperative radiation therapy and chemotherapy.[29]

Radiation Dose and Technique

Techniques combining EBRT and IORT have been fairly uniform in the United States and Europe. In previously untreated patients, EBRT doses of 45 to 54 Gy have been used delivering 1.8 to 2 Gy/fraction, 5 days per week, over a period of 5 to 6 weeks. Because of the anatomical location of pelvic and abdominal malignancies, high-energy (>10 MV) photons delivered via linear accelerators using multifield, shaped techniques are required. CT-, PET-, or MRI-based treatment planning permits accurate definition of the target volume. For extrapelvic, unresected, or residual disease following resection, radiation doses of 40 to 45 Gy delivered at 1.8 to 2 Gy/fraction with a 3- to 5-cm margin accounting for microscopic extension and target mobility are used. Treatments are generally delivered through multifield techniques aided by three-dimensional–based treatment planning. Reduced-field or boost techniques are often used to bring the total dose to 45 to 54 Gy as dictated by tolerance of surrounding normal tissue (see earlier). Chemotherapy administration varies by tumor site, although in gastrointestinal malignancies concurrent treatment with 5-FU–based regimens, cisplatin, or mitomycin C is frequently implemented. In carefully selected patients receiving prior irradiation, low-dose preoperative EBRT doses of 20 to 30 Gy at 1.5 to 1.8 Gy/fraction (often in conjunction with appropriate systemic agents) may be used.

Dosing of Intraoperative Radiation

IORT dose should be based on extent of residual disease at resection, the amount of EBRT delivered previously, and the type and volume of normal tissue irradiated. For patients who have received preoperative doses of 45 to 54 Gy (1.8 to 2 Gy/fraction, 5 days per week), IORT doses usually range from 10 to 20 Gy. For patients with microscopic residual or close margins, doses of 10 to 12.5 Gy are often administered. Patients with gross residual disease require higher doses and 15 to 20 Gy is usually administered. In previously irradiated patients, in whom additional EBRT is feasible (20 to 30 Gy), the dose of IORT generally ranges between 15 and 20 Gy. In patients in whom no or very limited EBRT is planned, IORT doses from 25 to 30 Gy have been administered; however, doses in this range should be judiciously used given the risk of normal tissue damage, specifically peripheral nerve injury.

The biological effectiveness of single-dose IORT in early responding tissues (tumor) relative to an equivalent total dose of fractionated EBRT has been estimated to be 1.5 to 2.5 times the IORT dose delivered[4,30,31] (see Table 15-1). The effective tumor dose (when "normalized" to fractionated EBRT doses) of IORT treatment added to 45 to 50 Gy given by EBRT are as follows: 10-Gy IORT dose, 60 to 80 Gy; 15-Gy IORT dose, 75 to 87.5 Gy; 20-Gy IORT dose, 85 to 100 Gy. These figures are not intended to be exact but represent educated estimates.

Technical Aspects

The technical aspects of IORT administration are beyond the scope of this chapter and have been discussed in other publications (see reference list). In brief, the implementation of IORT-based treatment is a multidisciplinary effort that includes one or multiple surgeons, radiation oncologist, anesthesiologist, operating room nurse, radiation physicist/dosimetrist, and therapist. In its broadest sense, IORT may be administered with either electrons (IOERT) or HDR photon afterloading techniques (HDR-IORT). Each method has potential advantages and disadvantages, which are summarized later (see Tables 15-12 and 15-13). In addition, differences in physical characteristics of electrons versus low-energy photon (HDR-IORT) therapies are illustrated in Figure 15-6.

INTRAOPERATIVE RADIATION DOSE-LIMITING STRUCTURES AND TOLERANCE

The development of normal tissue late effects increases with increasing radiation dose as well as dose delivered per fraction. The incidence of late normal tissue effects in patients receiving IORT plus EBRT would be higher than those receiving EBRT alone. However, the severe morbidity and mortality associated with locally recurrent tumor are often overlooked. As an example, when EBRT alone is used as the primary treatment modality for locally advanced rectal cancer, more than 90% of patients experience local persistence or local recurrence of disease with associated symptomatology. These symptoms include severe pelvic pain and neuropathy, which are difficult to manage clinically. The vast majority of patients experience disease-related death within 2 to 3 years. An argument can be made that the tumor-related morbidity/mortality approaches 100% in these patients.[32]

IORT tolerance for intact or surgically manipulated organs or structures in animals (primarily canines) is seen in Table 15-5. Much of this information has been derived from studies from the National Cancer Institute (NCI)[33-38] and Colorado State University (CSU).[39-41]

Several dose-sensitive structures have been studied in humans receiving IORT, including the ureter and peripheral nerve. These are discussed next.

Ureter

Clinical studies of the effect of IOERT on the ureters of human cancer patients have been undertaken at the Mayo Clinic. Doses of 10 Gy administered intraoperatively resulted in a 50% incidence of ureteral obstruction, increasing to 70% with doses from 15 to 25 Gy. This high complication rate relative to canine models may be due to age-related factors, surgical manipulation, EBRT, or tumor bed effects.[42] In an update of this experience, investigators from the Mayo Clinic reported on 146 patients with locally advanced malignancies receiving intraoperative radiotherapy to one or both ureters. They reported the risk of obstruction following IOERT is significant and increases with time. At 5 years, ureteral obstruction rates were 56%; this risk was relatively constant across the "normal" dose ranges of IOERT (10 to 20 Gy).[43]

Peripheral Nerve

Peripheral nerve is the principal dose-limiting normal tissue for IORT in the pelvis and retroperitoneum. Data regarding peripheral nerve tolerance and neuropathy come from canine models and from clinical analyses from patients treated intraoperatively.[37,39-42,44-48] Peripheral nerve is often situated adjacent to or directly involved by tumor in the abdomen and pelvis. Because of this, the relative surgical "immobility" of peripheral nerve, and inability to shield the nerve from the IORT field, nerve tissue often receives full-dose EBRT and IORT.

The mechanism of neuropathy following IORT is poorly understood. Peripheral nerve tolerance depends on the volume of nerve irradiated and total dose delivered. In animal models, histomorphologic findings following IORT have demonstrated decreased central nerve fiber density, particularly in large nerve fibers receiving more than 20 Gy. Electron microscopy analysis has demonstrated increased microtubule density and neurofilament accumulation within axons without associated myelin changes, suggesting possible hypoxic injury related to vascular changes.[48]

A Spanish study evaluated 45 patients with primary or locally recurrent extremity soft tissue sarcoma undergoing resection with IOERT (10 to 20 Gy). Nine patients received IOERT alone secondary to prior EBRT or patient refusal. Five patients developed neurotoxicity at a median of 13 months; four of five showed objective weakness and/or sensory loss. Most patients developing neuropathy received IOERT doses of greater than 15 Gy.[49]

An analysis from the Mayo Clinic evaluated peripheral nerve tolerance in 51 patients undergoing IOERT for primary or recurrent pelvic malignancies. Patients received EBRT (median dose, 50.4 Gy), maximal resection where possible, and IOERT boost from 10 to 25 Gy using 9- to 18-MeV electrons. Sixteen (32%) of patients experienced grade I to III peripheral neuropathy as manifested by pelvic/extremity pain, leg weakness, numbness, or tingling. Pain was severe (grade III) in 3 of 51 patients (6%)[42] (Table 15-6).

Table 15-5 Normal Tissue Tolerance to Intraoperative Electron Irradiation in Animals (Usually Dogs)

Tissue	Maximum Tolerated Dose (Gy)	Tissue Effect	Dose (Gy)
Intact Structure			
Aorta, vena cava	50	Fibrosis of wall (patency up to 50 Gy)	≥30
Peripheral nerve	15	Neuropathy, sensory-motor	≥20
Bladder	30	Contraction and ureterovesical narrowing	≥25
Ureter	30	Fibrosis and stenosis	≥30
Kidney	<15	Atrophy and fibrosis	≥20
Bile duct	20	Fibrosis and stenosis	≥30
Small intestine	<20	Ulceration, fibrosis, stenosis	≥20
Large bowel	15	Ulceration, fibrosis, stenosis	≥17.5
		Perforation	50
Esophagus			
Full thickness	≤20	Ulceration, stricture	≥30
Partial thickness	40	No sequelae at this dose	≥40
Muscle (psoas)	23	50% Decrement muscle fibers	38
Heart (right atrium)	20	Fibrosis	≥30
Lung	20	Fibrosis	≥20
Trachea	30	Submucosal fibrosis	≥30
Surgically Manipulated			
Aorta anastomosis (end to end)	20	Fibrosis and stenosis	≥20
		No anastomosis disruption	≤45
Aortic prosthetic graft	25	Graft occlusion	25
Portal vein anastomosis	40	Stenosis	>40
Biliary-enteric anastomosis	<20	Anastomotic breakdown	≥20
Small intestine (defunctionalized)	45	Fibrosis and stenosis	≤20
		No suture line breakdown	≤45
Bladder	30	Healing but contraction	≥30
Bronchial stump	>40	Absence of air leak	>40

Table 15-6 Clinical Peripheral Neuropathy Characteristics With Pelvic IOERT, Mayo Clinic

Characteristic	Incidence*	Severity: Mild/Moderate	Severity: Severe	Time Course (Mo From IORT): Onset†	Time Course (Mo From IORT): Resolution, Range
Pain	16/50 (32%)	13 (26%)	3 (6%)	½-18 (15)	6/14 (42%),‡ 5-32§
Motor	8/50 (16%)	6 (12%)	2 (4%)	3-22 (7)	1/8 (13%), 20
Sensory	11/50 (22%)	11 (22%)	0 (0%)	3-22 (7)	4/11 (36%), 1-20

*One patient excluded who died postoperatively.
†Values in parentheses represent median.
‡Two patients excluded who were lost to follow-up.
§Median, 15 mo.
IOERT, intraoperative electron irradiation; IORT, intraoperative irradiation.
Modified from Shaw E, Gunderson LL, Martin JK, et al: Peripheral nerve and ureteral tolerance of intraoperative radiation therapy: clinical and dose-response analysis. Radiother Oncol 18:247-255, 1990.

Table 15-7 Colorectal IOERT, Mayo Clinic IOERT Dose Versus Neuropathy

Disease Presentation	IOERT Dose Versus Grade 2 or 3 Neuropathy: ≤12.5 Gy	≥15 Gy	P
Primary[47]*	1/29 (3%)	6/28 (21%)	.03
Recurrent, no prior EBRT[46]†	2/29 (7%)	19/101 (19%)	.12
Primary + recurrent	3/58 (5%)	25/129 (19%)	.01

*57 IOERT fields in 55 evaluable patients. Incidence of grade 3 neuropathy by dose: ≤12.5 Gy, 0 of 9; 15 or 17.5 Gy, 1 of 19, or 5%; ≥20 Gy, 2 of 9, or 22%.
†130 IOERT fields in 123 patients.
EBRT, external beam irradiation; IOERT, intraoperative electron irradiation.

A follow-up study from the Mayo Clinic evaluated 178 patients with locally advanced colorectal cancer receiving IOERT. This study suggested a relationship between increasing doses of IOERT and the incidence of clinically significant neuropathy (Table 15-7). In primary and locally recurrent colorectal patients, the incidence of severe (grade III) neuropathy was approximately 5%, and the incidence of any neuropathy was approximately one third. This is consistent with canine studies suggesting increasing IOERT doses are related to the incidence of clinical and electrophysiologic neuropathy.[46,47]

Conclusion

All patients considered for IORT should undergo thorough pretreatment informed consent, including a discussion regarding neuropathy-related side effects. It should also be remembered that uncontrolled tumor frequently causes symptoms related to neural impingement, and in fact many potential IORT candidates present with neuropathic symptoms caused by primary or recurrent disease. Based on human and animal data evaluating IORT-induced neuropathy, IORT doses are generally limited to 10 to 20 Gy when a full course of EBRT is administered (45 to 54 Gy using 1.8 to 2 Gy/fraction). Doses exceeding 20 Gy in the intraoperative setting should be used with caution, and our general policy regarding such is to administer higher doses only in the setting of limited EBRT options (i.e., prior EBRT treatment).

INTRAOPERATIVE RADIATION RESULTS FOR SELECTED DISEASE SITES

A summary of IORT results and future possibilities in selected disease sites (pancreas, breast, colorectal, gynecologic cancers, and retroperitoneal/pelvic sarcomas) is now presented. For a more detailed discussion, the reader is referred to dedicated chapters on each site in an IORT text.[50]

Pancreas Cancer: External Beam and Intraoperative Radiation

Because of poor local control results achieved with conventional EBRT and chemotherapy, the use of IORT in the setting of pancreatic cancer is rational. The combination of EBRT plus IOERT in the setting of locally advanced/unresectable pancreatic adenocarcinoma has resulted in improvement in local control in separate series from MGH, Mayo Clinic and Thomas Jefferson Hospital (see Table 15-2). However, most patients ultimately develop liver metastases, peritoneal seeding, or both.

Mayo Clinic investigators reported on 27 patients with locally advanced pancreatic carcinoma who received IOERT following EBRT with chemotherapy. Local control was achieved in 78% of patients. Median and 2- and 5-year survivals were 14.9 months and 27% and 7%, respectively. This compared favorably to similarly matched patients treated with IOERT followed by EBRT (median survival, 10.5 months; 2-year survival, 6%; $P = .001$ in favor of preoperative therapy).[51]

In a report from the MGH, Willett and coworkers[52] described 150 patients with locally advanced pancreatic cancer who received IOERT, EBRT, and 5-FU–based chemotherapy. The 1-, 2-, and 5-year actuarial survival rates were 54%, 15%, and 4%, respectively. Median survival for the entire cohort was 13 months. Five patients survived beyond 5 years. Long-term survivors were treated by smaller applicator sizes, reflecting smaller tumor size.

Future Possibilities

Although slight gains in survival may be achieved by improving local control in pancreatic cancer patients, the high rate of distant metastases precludes significant improvements in long-term survival by IORT approaches. Because of the high incidence of failure in the peritoneal cavity as well as the liver, pilot studies are evaluating novel systemic agents in the treatment of this disease, including "targeted" agents such as epidermal growth factor receptor (EGFR) inhibitors, vascular endothelial growth factor (VEGF) inhibitors, and others.

Breast Cancer

Intraoperative Radiation Therapy Alone

Randomized trials have demonstrated equivalent disease-free and overall survival in selected breast cancer patients undergoing either mastectomy or breast-conserving surgery followed by EBRT.[53] Local recurrences frequently occur at or adjacent to the original tumor bed following breast-conserving surgery. There is increasing interest in the use of IORT as a supplement to or alternative to EBRT in selected cases.

Veronesi and colleagues[54] reported on 237 patients with primary tumors less than 2 cm undergoing wide excision with either sentinel lymph node biopsy and/or axillary lymph node dissection. Patients received IOERT using 3- to 9-MeV electrons with doses of 17 to 21 Gy (>90% received 21 Gy as the prescribed dose). At a median follow-up of 19 months, the rate of posttreatment complications was low with 1.7% developing breast fibrosis. Follow-up was too short to provide meaningful local recurrence data.

A systematic review of seven published IORT alone series in early breast cancer suggested that short-term local control and disease-free and overall survival results were similar to reported EBRT series. Local control rates ranged from 0% to 29% with IORT. However, many of these small, single-institution studies had short follow-up (median, 2 years).[55]

Intraoperative plus External Beam Radiation

In combined series from the Medical College of Ohio and Centre Regional de Lutte Contre le Cancer (France), 72 patients with early-stage breast cancer underwent lumpectomy with axillary lymph node dissection followed by 10- to 15-Gy IOERT using 6- to 20-MeV electrons. Patients later received EBRT doses of 45 to 50 Gy at 1.8 to 2 Gy/fraction. No significant complications were observed and cosmetic results were described as excellent. Eight of 72 patients developed minor palpable fibrosis at the lumpectomy site. At a minimum 2-year follow-up in all patients, no patients have experienced local relapse.[56]

The University of Salzburg used IOERT combined with EBRT in 351 consecutive patients from October 1998 to April 2002 and reported their results in the initial 170 patients treated through December 2000.[57] Local control results were compared with those of patients treated with EBRT alone. At the time of publication, 3-year local control was 100% with an IOERT boost versus about 97% with EBRT boost.

Future Possibilities

Multiple phase II or III trials evaluating adjuvant IORT are actively accruing patients in the United States (phase II), Europe, United Kingdom, and Australia. These trials use varying IORT techniques including 50-kV photons as well as low-energy electrons. Final results are likely years away, and identification of patients appropriate for breast IORT remains an ill-defined area. Long-term results from these and other trials will be necessary to demonstrate ultimate local recurrence, late effect, and survival data with these approaches.

Retroperitoneal and Pelvic Soft Tissue Sarcomas

National Cancer Institute Randomized Phase III Trial

The National Cancer Institute (NCI) conducted a randomized trial in patients undergoing surgical resection of primary retroperitoneal sarcoma. All patients underwent gross total resection, although most had microscopically involved margins. Patients were randomized to receive 20 Gy IOERT followed by 35 to 40 Gy of EBRT postoperatively versus postoperative EBRT alone to a dose of 50 to 55 Gy. Patients receiving IOERT were treated with concurrent misonidazole given 15 to 30 minutes pretreatment. EBRT treatments were delivered over 4 to 5 weeks at 1.5 to 1.8 Gy per fraction in both arms; however, patients receiving EBRT only received an additional 15 Gy using similar fractionation by reduced fields. The incidence of in-field local-regional recurrence was significantly lower among patients receiving IOERT compared with patients receiving EBRT only (3/15 vs. 16/20, $p < .001$). Patients receiving IOERT experienced fewer episodes of radiation enteritis than EBRT-alone patients (2/15 vs 10/20, $p < .05$); however, radiation-related peripheral neuropathy was more frequent in patients receiving IOERT (9/15 vs 1/20, $p < .01$).[11]

Mayo Clinic Experience

Investigators at the Mayo Clinic reported on 87 patients with primary or recurrent retroperitoneal/intrapelvic sarcomas receiving IOERT as a component of treatment. Seventy-seven patients received EBRT (53 preoperatively, 12 postoperatively, 12 both) to a median dose of 48 Gy, usually through a shrinking field technique. Fifteen patients (17%) had gross residual disease following resection, fifty-six (64%) microscopic residual, and sixteen (18%) either negative margins or no residual disease. Median IOERT dose was 15 Gy (range 9-30 Gy). Five-year actuarial survival was 47%. Patients with tumors >10 cm experienced a significantly worse survival compared with smaller lesions (five-year survival 28% versus 60%, $p = .01$) and patients with gross residual disease following resection experienced worse five-year survival versus gross totally resected patients (37% versus 52%, $p = .08$). Five-year local control rates in patients with gross residual, microscopic residual and no residual tumor were 41%, 60% and 100%, respectively. Factors influencing local control at five years are shown in Table 15-8. Patients with gross total resection experienced significantly improved local control. Table 15-9 shows factors influencing survival following treatment. Patients with tumors greater than 10 cm were significantly less likely to be long-term survivors.[58]

Massachusetts General Hospital Experience

Investigators from the Massachusetts General Hospital described 37 patients with primary or recurrent retroperitoneal sarcoma who underwent EBRT (median dose 45 Gy) and resection. Twenty patients received IOERT (10-20 Gy). In 16 patients receiving gross total resection and IOERT, five-year survival and local control rates were 74% and 83%, respectively. In comparison, 13 patients undergoing gross total resection without IOERT had five-year survival and local control rates of 30% and 61%, respectively. Four patients receiving IOERT experienced significant complications including neuropathy, hydronephrosis and fistula formation.[59]

Conclusions and Future Possibilities

IORT combined with EBRT and resection offers an effective means of improving local control in patients with primary and recurrent retroperitoneal sarcomas, as demonstrated in a randomized trial from the NCI as well as multiple American and European single-institution studies.[58-62] A randomized NCI trial showed an 80% tumor bed relapse rate with adjuvant EBRT alone, likely due to an inability to deliver effective EBRT doses given normal tissue constraints. Because these results are similar to reports of resection alone, the use of adjuvant EBRT without IORT following marginal resection could be questioned. A more practical approach would be to adminis-

Table 15-8 **Mayo Clinic Analysis: Factors Influencing Local Control in Resected Retroperitoneal Sarcomas With IOERT**

Factor	Primary Tumors n	Primary Tumors LC (%)	Primary Tumors *P*	Recurrent Tumors n	Recurrent Tumors LC (%)	Recurrent Tumors *P*	All n	All LC (%)	All *P*
Residual at IOERT									
None	11	100		5	100		16	100	
Microscopic	25	92		31	36		56	57	
Gross	7	60	<.01	8	67	.12	15	37	.04
Broders grade									
1-2	9	100		24	28		33	47	
3-4	34	84	.32	20	58	.52	54	75	.16
Tumor size (cm)									
≤10	23	83		30	50		17	64	
>10	19	92	.80	14	34	.69	69	62	.96

IOERT, intraoperative electron beam radiotherapy; LC, local control.

Table 15-9 **Mayo Clinic Analysis: Factors Influencing Survival in Resected Retroperitoneal Sarcomas With IOERT at 5 Years**

Factor	Primary Tumors n	Primary Tumors OS (%)	Primary Tumors *P*	Recurrent Tumors n	Recurrent Tumors OS (%)	Recurrent Tumors *P*	All n	All OS (%)	All *P*
Residual at IOERT									
None	11	62		5	80		16	68	
Microscopic	25	54		31	44		56	48	
Gross	7	29	.15	8	45	.60	15	37	.12
Broders grade									
1-2	9	42		24	53		33	50	
3-4	34	54	.70	20	35	.36	54	48	.32
Tumor size* (cm)									
≤10	23	66		30	54		53	60	
>10	19	33	.15	14	19	.04	33	28	.01

IOERT, intraoperative electron beam radiotherapy; OS, overall survival.
*One value missing.

ter preoperative EBRT following confirmation of diagnosis by thin-needle biopsy. This would be followed by resection at an institution with IORT capabilities. Even with improved local control rates, locoregional and distant failure remain common modes of failure, emphasizing the need for improved therapies. Pilot studies are evaluating the role of concomitant radiochemotherapy with preoperative EBRT, IORT and maintenance chemotherapy for resectable moderate- and high-grade retroperitoneal and pelvic sarcomas.[63]

Gynecologic Cancers

Patients with locally advanced or locally recurrent gynecologic cancers often have involvement of the pelvic sidewall, pelvic lymph nodes or paraaortic nodes. The use of radical resection and IORT with or without EBRT and/or chemotherapy may benefit patients when compared with EBRT alone.

Mayo Clinic Experience

A Mayo Clinic analysis described 121 patients with primary (16 patients) or recurrent (105 patients) gynecologic malignancies treated with IOERT-containing regimens.[64,65] Preoperative or postoperative EBRT was delivered in 90 patients; 71 (59%) had received prior EBRT. Multiple tumor types were analyzed including cervical, endometrial, ovary and vaginal carcinomas and uterine sarcomas. The five-year survival rate for all patients was 25%, and the 5-year local failure rate was 34%[65] (Table 15-10). On subset analysis, patients with gross total resection (N = 94) had improved 5-year survival rates compared with patients with gross residual (30% versus 10%, $P = .02$); patients with uterine or ovarian primary origin had better survival than patients with cervical or vaginal primaries (5-yr SR—43% versus 16%, $P = .001$) The rate of distant metastases at 5 years was 48% (75% gross residual vs 41% microscopic residual, $P = .02$). Fewer metastases were seen in patients treated with MVAC chemotherapy (methotrexate, vinblastine, doxorubicin, cisplatin) in a prior analysis.[65]

Pamplona Experience

Spanish investigators reported on 67 patients with primary (31) or recurrent (36) cervical cancer. Previously unirradiated patients were generally treated with preoperative EBRT to 45 Gy at 1.8 Gy per fraction with concurrent cisplatin and 5-FU. Previously irradiated patients underwent immediate resection or neoadjuvant chemotherapy if unresectable. A median IOERT dose of 12 Gy was delivered for primary disease and 15 Gy for recurrent disease following resection. Ten-year local control rate (within the IOERT field) was 69% for the entire group; local control rates for primary and recurrent disease were 93% and 46%, respectively. Factors adversely influencing local control included involved parametrial margins, gross residual disease and pelvic lymph node involvement. Patients with two or more risk factors had a ten-

Table 15-10 Mayo Clinic Analysis: Factors Influencing Local Control and Survival in Resected Gynecologic Malignancies with IOERT

Treatment Group	No. of Patients	SURVIVAL (%) Median (mo)	2-y	5-y	RELAPSE—5 Y (%) Local	Distant	Central[§]
All patients	121	20	41	25	34	48	27
Amount residual							
≤ Microscopic	94	21	43	30*	29	41*	37
Gross	27	12	35	10	18	75	18
Site of primary lesion							
Uterine, ovary	47	35	59	43‡	NA	NA	14‡
Cervix, vagina	74	16	32	16	NA	NA	34

*P = .02; †P = .001; ‡P = .017.
§Central, within IOERT field.

Table 15-11 Primary Rectal (MGH) or Colorectal (Mayo Clinic) IOERT Series: Disease Control and Survival by Degree of Resection and Amount of Residual Disease

Degree of Resection	MGH RESULTS 5-Y ACT (%)*† n	LF	DSS	MAYO CLINIC RESULTS 5-Y ACT (%) n	LF	DF	OS
No tumor	—	—	—	2	0	0	100
Complete resection	40	9	63	18	7	54†	69
Partial (subtotal) resection	24	37	35	—	—	—	—
Microscopic residual	17	35	47	19	14	50†	55
Gross residual	7	43	14	16	27	83†	21
No resection	—	—	—	1	—	—	0
Total series	64			56	16	59	46

*Data from Willett et al.[69]
†Three-year actuarial DF of 43%, 38%, and 66% for complete resection, microresidual, and gross residual, respectively.
Act, actuarial; DF, distant failure; DSS, disease-specific survival; LF, local failure; MGH, Massachusetts General Hospital; OS, overall survival.

year local control rate of 0%. Ten-year survival for the entire group was 35% (primary disease 58%, recurrent disease 14%). Patients with gross residual, microscopic residual, and no residual disease had ten-year survival rates of 0%, 9% and 45%, respectively. Eight of 67 (12%) patients experienced chronic pain; motor neuropathy was noted in one patient (3%). All failures within the IOERT field occurred concomitant with relapse in the pelvis and/or distant metastases.[66]

Future Possibilities

Because of the high incidence of distant metastases observed in patients with microscopic and gross residual disease following resection, evaluation of newer chemotherapeutic agents is indicated. The use of MVAC (methotrexate, vinblastine, doxorubicin [Adriamycin] and cisplatin) chemotherapy showed a trend toward fewer metastases in patients treated in the Mayo Clinic experience. Investigation of this regimen along with newer chemotherapeutic and targeted biologic agents may hold promise in improving distant metastases rates and ultimate survival in this disease.

Colorectal Cancer: Primary and Recurrent Disease

Primary Locally Advanced Cancers

Locally advanced colorectal cancers are tumors that cannot be resected without microscopic or gross residual secondary to tumor adherence to adjacent structures. In selected patients, the optimal approach is to administer preoperative chemoradiation in efforts to "downstage" disease and facilitate surgical resection. At the time of resection, if clinical suspicion for involved margins is high, the use of IORT may be appropriate.

In a report from the MGH, 64 patients with locally advanced primary rectal cancer underwent preoperative irradiation (with or without 5-FU) followed by resection and IOERT. Patients undergoing margin negative resection had a five-year actuarial local control and disease-specific survival of 91% and 63%, respectively. Patients with microscopically involved margins experienced five-year local control and disease-specific survivals of 65% and 47%, respectively, and patients with gross disease 57% and 14%, respectively[67] (Table 15-11).

A Mayo Clinic report described 56 patients with primary locally advanced colorectal cancer undergoing EBRT (45-55 Gy, usually with concurrent 5-FU administration) followed by resection and IOERT (10-20 Gy). Five-year survival for all patients was 46%. Patients with microscopic/no residual disease following resection had an improved survival relative to patients with gross residual (5-year survival of 59% versus 21%, P = .0005). Failure within the IOERT field occurred in 4 of 16 patients (25%) with gross residual following resection versus 2 of 39 (5%) with microscopic residual or less (P = .01) (see Table 15-11).[47]

Locally Recurrent Colorectal

Patients developing local recurrence following curative resection of primary colon or rectal cancer are treated with palliative intent at most institutions. Local recurrence from rectosigmoid cancer often causes pelvic pain due to nerve involvement in the presacral space or pelvic sidewall. The likelihood of margin negative resection is low. For patients undergoing surgery alone for pelvic recurrence from rectal cancer, reported five-year survival rates are 0%.[68] When IOERT is combined with EBRT ± chemotherapy and surgical salvage, five-year survival in the range of 20% has been achieved.[46,68-71] In an MGH analysis of 41 patients with locally recurrent rectosigmoid cancer undergoing IOERT, patients with gross residual disease experienced five-year local control and disease-free survival rates of 21% and 7%, respectively, versus 47% and 21% with clear or microscopically positive margins.[69]

Similarly, a Mayo Clinic report described the outcome of 106 patients undergoing palliative resection of locally recurrent, nonmetastatic rectal cancer. Forty-two patients received IOERT as a component of treatment (most 15-20 Gy) and 41 EBRT (most >45 Gy). Patients with gross residual disease experienced a significantly worse outcome versus microscopically involved margins (5-year survival 9% versus 33%, p = .03). Patients receiving IOERT had a five-year survival rate of 19% versus 7% without IOERT (p = .0006).[68]

An updated Mayo Clinic analysis described 175 patients with locally recurrent colorectal cancer (123 no prior EBRT, 52 prior EBRT) undergoing IOERT. Five-year survival in previously unirradiated patients was 20% versus 12% in previously irradiated patients. Three-year local control rate in previously unirradiated patients was 75% versus 51% in those previously irradiated. Three-year distant metastases rates were 64% and 71%, respectively.[72]

Future Possibilities

Based on the above and other data, it appears improved local control and survival may be achieved when IORT is combined with preoperative chemoradiation for locally advanced or locally recurrent colorectal cancer. Most patients will develop distant metastases, and relapse within the IORT and EBRT fields is common if gross total resection is not obtained. Based on the proven survival benefit of concurrent 5-FU with EBRT in colorectal and other gastrointestinal malignancies, 5-FU should be administered concurrent with EBRT. Although adjuvant 5-FU with leucovorin has previously been shown to improve survival in advanced stage colorectal cancer patients, the addition of newer therapies (oxaliplatin, capecitabine, irinotecan, bevacizumab) has recently demonstrated further survival benefit in stage IV patients. These agents are being evaluated as adjuvant therapy in Stage II and III patients. Given the high rate of subsequent distant metastases in locally advanced and recurrent colorectal cancer patients, significant improvement in long-term survival will likely be achieved through improvements in systemic agents.

CONCLUSIONS AND FUTURE POSSIBILITIES

IORT is the delivery of radiation at the time of operation. This can be accomplished using different techniques including IOERT and HDR-IORT. IORT is usually given in combination with EBRT +/− chemotherapy and surgical resection. IORT allows exclusion of part or all dose limiting sensitive structures, thereby increasing the effective dose to the tumor bed (and therefore local control) without significantly increasing normal tissue morbidity.

Intraoperative Radiation: Technical Considerations

Many limitations and perceived drawbacks of IORT in past decades were due to inefficiencies associated with non-dedicated facilities. Patients were often transported from the operating suite to the radiation oncology department where they were treated with non-dedicated linear accelerators. These inconveniences have been overcome with dedicated IOERT and/or HDR-IORT facilities. Presently, dedicated IORT suites within or adjacent to the operating room exist at many institutions in the United States and Europe. These facilities simplify treatment by avoiding transportation and sterility problems. A major limiting factor is the expense associated with outfitting a dedicated room (i.e., retrofitting an operating room with proper shielding, purchase of a linear accelerator dedicated for use in the operating room, construction of a separate IORT suite adjacent to the operating room, etc.). However, newer technologies have lowered these costs. Contemporary options include mobile IOERT units (Mobetron) as well as mobile HDR-IORT.[73] The Mobetron is a mobile, self-shielded compact linear accelerator with C-arm design that generates electron energies of 4 to 12 MeV (Intraop Medical, Inc., Santa Clara, CA) (Fig. 15-3). HDR-IORT units are remote afterloading devices that use an Ir-192 source (Figs. 15-4 and 15-5). In contrast to the Mobetron, HDR-IORT requires room shielding, which may be achieved by retrofitting an existing room or construction of a smaller shielded room adjacent to the operating suite. In either situation, patients are monitored by camera during radiation administration. After completion, the HDR-IORT unit can be transported to the radiation oncology department for outpatient HDR appropriate malignancies, including gynecologic and prostate malignancies. Another mobile IOERT device used in Europe is the NOVAC7, which consists of a miniature linear accelerator mounted on a robotic arm. The highest electron energies available with the NOVAC7 are 7 to 10 MeV.

A detailed description of the relative advantages/disadvantages of IOERT and HDR-IORT has been provided elsewhere and is beyond the scope of this chapter (Tables 15-12 and 15-13).[31] In summary, treatment/procedure times are generally shorter with IOERT compared with HDR-IORT. Additionally, IOERT allows variation of electron energies and therefore treatment of both superficial and deeper-seated targets, whereas HDR-IORT is appropriate for targets ≤.5 cm in thickness (Fig. 15-6). The flexible Harrison-Anderson-Mick (HAM) applicator used in HDR-IORT may allow more conformal treatment along curved body surfaces (e.g., large pelvic sidewall fields, lateral abdominal wall, and thoracic cage) which may prove difficult with rigid IOERT cone applicators (see Fig. 15-5). Separate, matching fields may be required to treat larger target areas with IOERT-based cone applicators. A comprehensive intraoperative program would ideally have IOERT, HDR-IORT as well as perioperative brachytherapy available to treat all disease sites and situations. These modalities should be viewed as complementary and not competitive.

Future Possibilities

Despite optimal therapy with non-IORT approaches, high rates of local relapse occur in patients with retroperitoneal sarcoma, pancreatic cancer, colorectal, gynecologic and other malignancies. The addition of IORT to conventional treatment methods has improved local control as well as survival in many disease sites in both the primary and recurrent disease settings. In view of newer, lower cost treatment devices, the use of IORT in clinical practice will likely grow, with increasing integration into the treatment of "non-conventional" malignancies.

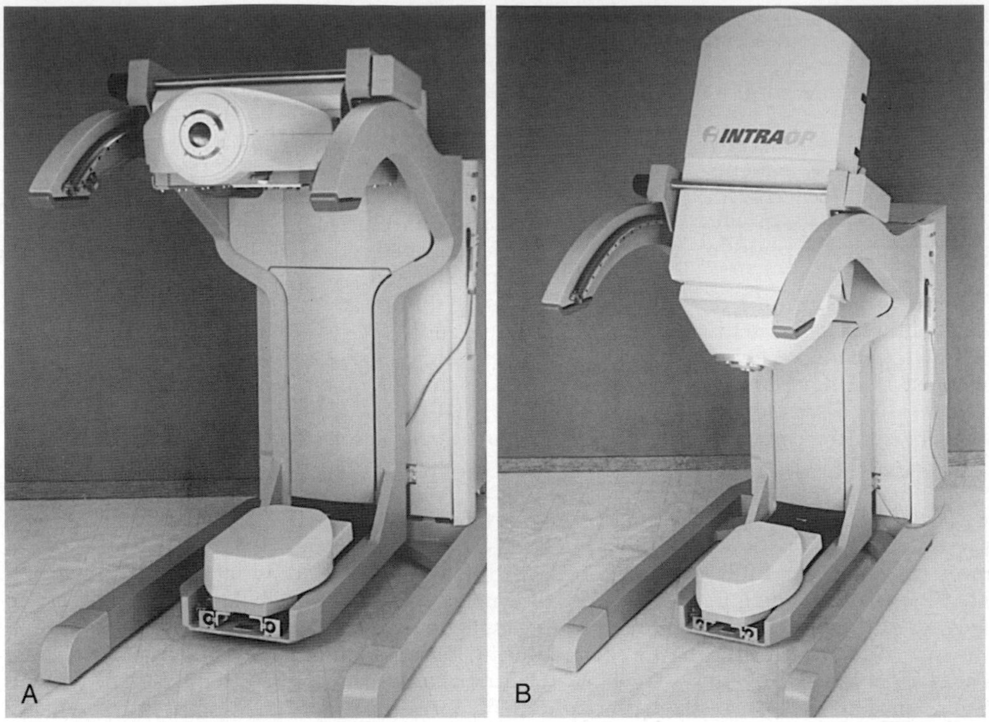

Figure 15-3 Mobile intraoperative electron irradiation system (Mobetron) with compact beam stopper allows use in existing operating rooms with little or no additional shielding required. **A,** Transport configuration. **B,** Treatment configuration. (From Gunderson LL, Willett CG, Harrison LB, et al: Intraoperative irradiation: current and future status. Semin Oncol 24:715-731, 1997.)

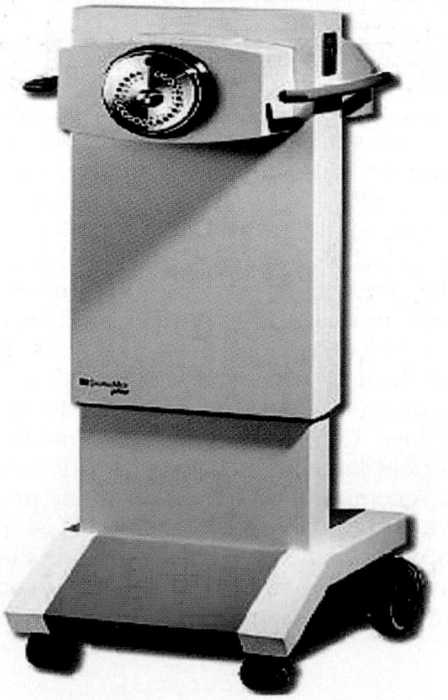

Figure 15-4 Source housing for an iridium-192 source. This device allows computer-assisted treatment delivery during intraoperative radiation therapy. (Courtesy of Varian Medical Systems, Palo Alto, CA.)

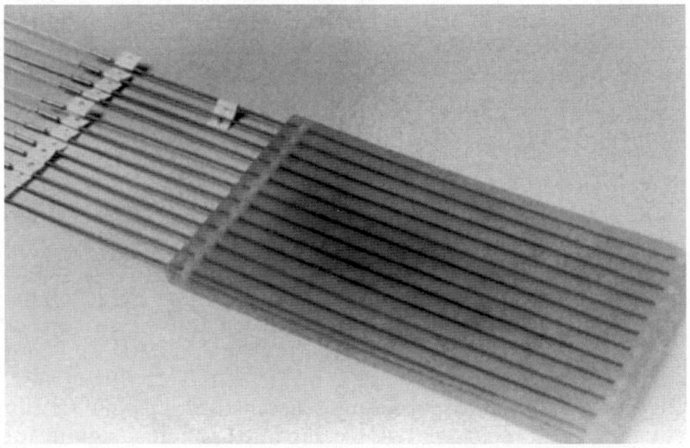

Figure 15-5 Harrison-Anderson-Mick (HAM) applicator is used to guide an iridium-192 source during high-dose-rate intraoperative radiation therapy.

Although there is a large body of data supporting the use of IORT in varying malignancies, there is a relative paucity of Phase III randomized trials. This is at least in part secondary to the limited number of IORT facilities in any given country as well as relative rarity of diseases commonly treated with IORT. Completion of Phase II/III trials will likely require cooperation among multiple institutions and countries. Future treatment approaches should include "standard" courses of EBRT +/− concurrent chemotherapy and surgical resection with the integration of novel radiation sensitizers, protectors, and targeted biologic agents with IORT.[74]

ACKNOWLEDGMENTS

The chapter authors would like to thank Wanda Lawrence for her assistance in the preparation of this work.

Table 15-12 Relative Advantages and Disadvantages of IOERT Versus HDR-IORT Brachytherapy After Gross Total or Near-Total Resection (Maximum Tumor Thickness ≤0.5 cm)

IOERT Potential Advantage If Technically Feasible	Potential Disadvantages of IOERT	Potential Solution to Disadvantage
Better dose homogeneity Faster treatment time Less shielding required in OR Can treat full thickness of organ or structure at risk with relative homogeneity (e.g., aorta or vena cava, bladder side wall)	Surface dose <90% with 6 ± 9 MeV	Add bolus over tumor bed to improve surface dose; use HDR-IORT
	Unable to include some areas at risk in single field within either abdomen or pelvis	Use abutting IOERT fields (difficult in pelvis); use HDR-IORT
	Area at risk is technically inaccessible because of location	Use HDR-IORT; surgically displace small bowel or stomach with vascularized flap (omentum, muscle) and give postoperative EBRT boost or perioperative brachytherapy

EBRT, external beam irradiation; HDR, high-dose rate; IOERT, intraoperative electron irradiation; IORT, intraoperative irradiation; OR, operating room.
From Nag S, Gunderson LL, Willett CG, et al: Intraoperative irradiation with electron beam or high-dose-rate brachytherapy: methodological comparisons. *In* Gunderson LL, Willett CG, Harrison LB, Calvo FA (eds): Intraoperative Irradiation: Techniques and Results. Totowa, NJ, Humana Press, 1999, pp 111-130.

Table 15-13 Potential Differences Between IOERT and HDR-IORT

	IOERT	HDR-IORT
Actual treatment time	2-4 min	5-30 min
Total procedure time	30-45 min	45-120 min
Treatment sites	Accessible locations	All areas where depth at risk is ≤0.5 cm from surface of applicator*
Surface dose	Lower (75%-93%)†	Higher (150%-200%)
Dose at depth (2 cm)	Higher (70%-100%)†	Lower (30%)
Dosimetric homogeneity (surface to depth)	≤10% variation	≥100% variation

From Nag S, et al: Intraoperative irradiation with electron-beam or high-dose-rate brachytherapy. *In* Gunderson L, Willett C, Harrison L, Calvo F (eds): Intraoperative Irradiation. Totowa, NJ, Humana Press, 1999, pp 111-130.
*Precludes aortocaval region, mediastinum, and any unresected disease >0.5 cm.
†Based on electron energy of 6 MeV and energies of 6-18 MeV with 7-cm flat-end Lucite applicator.

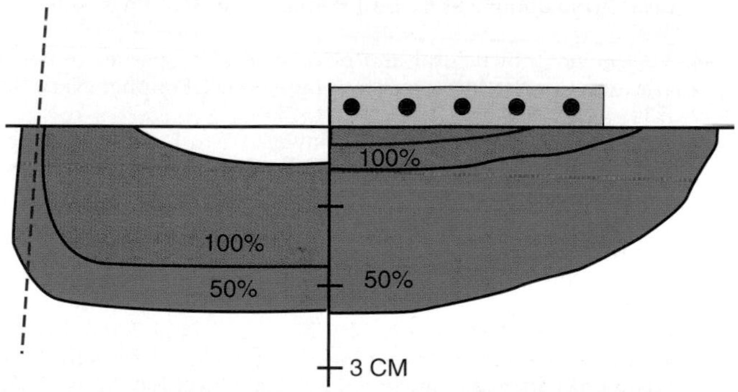

Figure 15-6 Dose distribution characteristics of intraoperative electron radiation therapy (IOERT) *(left)* in high-dose-rate intraoperative radiation therapy (HDR-IORT) *(right)*. IOERT uses 6-MeV electrons, and HDR-IORT uses a 1-cm surface applicator with a dose prescribed to a depth of 0.5 cm.

REFERENCES

1. Medina R, Casas F, Calvo F: Radiation oncology in Spain: historical notes for the radiology centennial. Int J Radiat Oncol Biol Phys 35:1075-1097, 1996.
2. Abe M, Fukada M, Yamano K, et al: Intraoperative radiation in abdominal and cerebral tumors. Acta Radiol 10:408-416, 1971.
3. Rubin P, Cassarett GW: Clinical Radiation and Pathology. Philadelphia, WB Saunders, 1968.
4. Okunieff P, Sundararaman S, Chen Y: Biology of large dose per fraction radiation therapy. *In* Gunderson LL, Willett CG, Harrison LB, Calvo FA (eds): Intraoperative Irradiation: Techniques and Results. Totowa, NJ, Humana Press, 1999, pp 25-46.
5. Gunderson LL, Nagorney DM, Martenson JA, et al: External beam plus intraoperative radiation for gastrointestinal cancers. World J Surg 19:191-197, 1995.
6. Roldan GE, Gunderson LL, Nagorney DM, et al: External beam versus intraoperative and external beam irradiation for locally advanced pancreatic cancer. Cancer 61:1110-1116, 1988.
7. Garton GR, Gunderson LL, Nagorney DM, et al: High dose preoperative external beam and intraoperative irradiation for locally advanced pancreatic cancer. Int J Radiat Oncol Biol Phys 27:1153-1157, 1993.
8. Whittington R, Solin L, Mohiuddin M, et al: Multimodality therapy of unresectable pancreatic adenocarcinoma. Cancer 54:1991-1998, 1984.
9. Mohiuddin M, Regine WF, Stevens J, et al: Combined intraoperative radiation in perioperative chemotherapy for unresectable cancers of the pancreas. J Clin Oncol 13:2764-2768, 1995.
10. Mohiuddin M, Cantor RJ, Bierman W, et al: Combined modality treatment of localized unresectable adenocarcinoma of the pancreas. Int J Radiat Oncol Biol Phys 14:79-84, 1988.
11. Sindelar WF, Kinsella TJ, Chen PW, et al: Intraoperative radiotherapy and retroperitoneal sarcomas: final results of a prospective, randomized, clinical trial. Arch Surg 128:402-410, 1993.
12. Brierly JD, Cummings BJ, Wong CS, et al: Adenocarcinoma of the rectum treated by radical external radiation therapy. Int J Radiat Oncol Biol Phys 31:255-259, 1995.
13. O'Connell MJ, Childs DS, Moertel CG, et al: A prospective controlled evaluation of combined pelvic radiotherapy and methanol extraction residue of BCG (MER) for locally unresectable or recurrent rectal carcinoma. Int J Radiat Oncol Biol Phys 8:1115-1119, 1982.
14. Gunderson LL, Cohen AC, Dosoretz DD, et al: Residual, unresectable or recurrent colorectal cancer: external beam irradiation and intraoperative electron beam boost + resection. Int J Radiat Oncol Biol Phys 9:1597-1606, 1983.

15. Tewfik HH, Bushsbuam HJ, Latourette HB, et al: Para-aortic lymph node irradiation in carcinoma of the cervix after exploratory laparotomy and biopsy-proven aortic nodes. Int J Radiat Oncol Biol Phys 8:13-18, 1982.
16. Piver MS, Barlow JJ: High dose irradiation to biopsy confirmed aortic node metastases from carcinoma of the uterine cervix. Cancer 39:1243-1246, 1977.
17. Fletcher GH: Clinical dose response curves of human malignant epithelial tumors. Br J Radiol 46:1-12, 1973.
18. Fletcher GH, Shukovsky LJ: The interplay of radiocurability and tolerance in the irradiation of human cancers. J Radiol Electrol 56:383-400, 1975.
19. Griscom NT, Wang CC: Radiation therapy in inoperable breast carcinoma. Radiol 79:18-23, 1962.
20. Tepper J: Clonogenic potential of human tumors: a hypothesis. Acta Radiol Oncol 20:283-288, 1981.
21. Ramsay J, Suit HD, Sedlacek R: Experimental studies on the incidence of metastases after failure of radiation treatment and the effect of salvage surgery. Int J Radiat Oncol Biol Phys 14:1165-1168, 1988.
22. Suit HD: Local control in patient survival. Int J Radiat Oncol Biol Phys 23:653-660, 1992.
23. Suit HD, Sedlacek RS, Gillette EL: Examination for a correlation between probabilities of development of distant metastasis and of local recurrence. Radiology 95:189-194, 1970.
24. Suit HD: Potential for improving survival rates for the cancer patient by increasing efficacy of treatment of the primary lesion. Cancer 50:1227-1234, 1982.
25. Fuks Z, Leibel SA, Wallner KE, et al: The effect of local control in metastatic dissemination in carcinoma of the prostate: Long-term results in patients treated with I-125 implantation. Int J Radiat Oncol Biol Phys 21:537-547, 1991.
26. Leibel SA, Scott CB, Mohiuddin M, et al: The effect of local-regional control on distant metastatic dissemination in carcinoma of the head and neck: the results of an analysis of the RTOG head and neck database. Int J Radiat Oncol Biol Phys 21:549-556, 1991.
27. Sohn TA, Yeo CF, Cameron JL, et al: Resected adenocarcinoma of the pancreas: 616 patients: results, outcomes, and prognostic indicators. J Gasterointest Surg 4:567-579, 2000.
28. Spitz FR, Abbruzzese JL, Lee JE, et al: Preoperative and postoperative chemoradiation strategies in patients treated with pancreaticoduodenectomy for adenocarcinoma of the pancreas. J Clin Oncol 15:928-937, 1997.
29. Sauer R, Becker H, Hoheberger W, et al: Preoperative versus post-operative chemoradiotherapy for rectal cancer. N Engl J Med 351:1731-1740, 2004.
30. Gunderson LL, Shipley WU, Suit HD, et al: Intraoperative irradiation: A pilot study combining external beam photons with "boost" dose intraoperative electrons. Cancer 49:2259-2266, 1982.
31. Nag S, Gunderson LL, Willett CG, et al: Intraoperative irradiation with electron beam or high dose rate brachytherapy: methodological comparisons. *In* Gunderson LL, Willett CG, Harrison LB, Calvo FA (eds): Intraoperative Irradiation—Techniques and Results. Totowa, NJ, Humana Press, 1999, pp 111-130.
32. Tepper JE, Gunderson LL, Orlow E, et al: Complications of intra-operative radiation therapy. Int J Radiat Oncol Biol Phys 10:1831-1839, 1984.
33. Johnstone PA, Sindelar WF, Kinsella TJ: Experimental and clinical studies of intraoperative radiation. Int J Radiat Oncol Biol Phys 12:1687-1695, 1986.
34. Kinsella TJ, DeLuca AM, Barnes M, et al: Threshold dose for peripheral neuropathy following intraoperative radiotherapy (IORT) in a large animal model. Int J Radiat Oncol Biol Phys 20:697-701, 1991.
35. Kinsella TJ, Sindelar WF, DeLuca AM, et al: Tolerance of the canine bladder to intraoperative radiation therapy: an experimental study. Int J Radiat Oncol Biol Phys 14:939-946, 1988.
36. Sindelar WF, Tepper JE, Travis EL: Tolerance of bile duct to intra-operative irradiation. Surgery 92:533-546, 1982.
37. Sindelar WF, Tepper JE, Kinsella TJ: Late effects of intraoperative radiation therapy on retroperitoneal structures, intestine, and bile duct in a large animal model. Int J Radiat Oncol Biol Phys 29:781-788, 1994.
38. Sindelar WF, Johnstone PA, Hoekstra H, et al: Normal tissue tolerance to IORT: The NCI experimental studies. *In* Gunderson LL, Willett CG, Harrison LB, Calvo FA (eds): Intraoperative Irradiation—Techniques and Results. Totowa, NJ, Humana Press, 1999, pp 131-146.
39. LeCouteur RA, Gillette EL, Powers EL, et al: Peripheral neuropathies following experimental intraoperative radiation therapy (IORT). Int J Radiat Oncol Biol Phys 17:583-590, 1989.
40. Gillette EL, Gillette SM, Vujaskovic Z, et al: Influence of volume on canine ureters and peripheral nerves irradiated intraoperatively. *In* Schildberg FW, Willich N, Krämling H (eds): Intraoperative Radiation Therapy. Proceedings of the 4th International IORT Symposium. Munich, 1992. Essen, Germany, Verlag Die Blaue Eule, 1993, pp 61-63.
41. Gillette EL, Gillette SM, Powers BE: Studies at Colorado State University of normal tissue tolerance of beagles to IOERT, EBRT or a combination. *In* Gunderson LL, Willett CG, Harrison LB, Calvo FA (eds): Intraoperative Irradiation—Techniques and Results. Totowa, NJ, Humana Press, 1999, pp 147-164.
42. Shaw EG, Gunderson LL, Martin JK, et al: Peripheral nerve and ureteral tolerance of intraoperative radiation therapy: clinical and dose response analysis. Radiother Oncol 18:247-255, 1990.
43. Miller RC, Haddock MG, Peterson IA, et al: Intraoperative electron beam radiotherapy in human ureteral obstruction. Proceedings of ASTRO 2004, Abstract 2136.
44. Johnstone PA, Sindelar WF, Kinsella TJ: Experimental and clinical studies of intraoperative radiation therapy. Curr Probl Cancer 18:249-292, 1994.
45. Kinsella TJ, DeLuca AM, Barnes M, et al: Threshold dose for peripheral neuropathy following intraoperative radiotherapy (IORT) in a large animal model. Int J Radiat Oncol Biol Phys 20:697-701, 1991.
46. Gunderson LL, Nelson H, Martenson JA, et al: Intraoperative electron and external beam irradiation with or without 5-fluorouracil and maximum surgical resection for previously unirradiated, locally recurrent colorectal cancer. Dis Colon Rectum 39:1379-1395, 1996.
47. Gunderson LL, Nelson H, Martenson JA, et al: Locally advanced primary colorectal cancer: intraoperative electron and external beam irradiation ± 5-FU. Int J Radiat Oncol Biol Phys 37:601-614, 1997.
48. Vujaskovic Z: Structural and physiological properties of peripheral nerves after intraoperative radiation. J Peripher Nerv Syst. 2:343-349, 1997.
49. Azinovic I, Martinez-Monge R, Javier-Aristu J, et al: Intraoperative radiotherapy electron boost followed by moderate doses of external beam radiotherapy in resected soft-tissue sarcoma of the extremities. Radiother Oncol 67:331-337, 2003.
50. Gunderson LL, Willett CG, Harrison LB, Calvo FA: Intraoperative Irradiation—Techniques and Results. Totowa, NJ, Humana Press, 1999.
51. Garton GR, Gunderson LL, Nagorney DM, et al: High-dose preoperative external beam and intraoperative irradiation for locally advanced pancreatic cancer. Int J Radiat Oncol Biol Phys 27:1153-1157, 1993.
52. Willett CG, Del Castillo CF, Shih HA, et al: Long-term results of intraoperative electron beam irradiation (IOERT) for patients with unresectable pancreatic cancer. Ann Surg 241:295-299, 2005.
53. Early Breast Cancer Trialist Collaborative Group: Favourable and unfavourable effect on long-term survival of radiotherapy for early breast cancer: an overview of the randomized trials. Lancet 355:1757-1770, 2000.
54. Veronesi U, Gatti G, Luini A, et al: Full-dose intraoperative radiotherapy with electrons during breast-conserving surgery. Arch Surg 138:1253-1256, 2003.
55. Cuncins-Harn A, Saunders C, Walsh D: A systematic review of intraoperative radiotherapy in early breast cancer. Breast Cancer Res Treat 85:271-280, 2004.
56. Battle JA, DuBois JB, Merrick HW, et al: IORT for breast cancer. *In* Gunderson LL, Willett CG, Harrison LB, Calvo FA (eds): Intraoperative Irradiation—Techniques and Results. Totowa, NJ, Humana Press, 1999, pp 521-526.
57. Reitsamer R, Peintinger F, Kopp M, et al: Local recurrence rated in breast cancer patients treated with intraoperative electron-boost

radiotherapy versus postoperative external beam electron boost irradiation. Strahlenther Onkol 1:38-44, 2004.
58. Petersen IA, Haddock MG, Donohue JH: Use of intraoperative electron beam radiotherapy in the management of retroperitoneal soft tissue sarcomas. Int J Radiat Oncol Biol Phys 52:469-475, 2002.
59. Gieschen HL, Spiro IJ, Suit HD, et al: Long-term results of intraoperative electron beam radiotherapy for primary and recurrent retroperitoneal soft tissue sarcoma. Int J Radiat Oncol Biol Phys 50:127-131, 2001.
60. Gunderson LL, Nagorney DM, McIlrath DC, et al: External beam and intraoperative electron irradiation for locally advanced soft tissue sarcomas. Int J Radiat Oncol Biol Phys 25:647-656, 1993.
61. Calvo FA, Azinovic I, Martinez R, et al: Intraoperative radiotherapy for the treatment of soft tissue sarcomas of central anatomic sites. IORT 94-5th International Symposium Abstracts. Hepatogastroenterology 41:4, 1994.
62. Dubois JB, Hay MH, Gely S, et al: Intraoperative radiation therapy (IORT) in soft tissue sarcomas. IORT 94-5th International Symposium Abstracts. Hepatogastroenterology 41:3, 1994.
63. Pisters PWT, Ballo MT, Fenstermacher MJ, et al: Phase I trial of preoperative concurrent doxorubicin and radiation therapy, surgical resection an intraoperative electron-beam radiation therapy for patients with localized retroperitoneal sarcoma. J Clin Oncol 21:3092-3097, 2003.
64. Haddock MG, Petersen IA, Webb MJ, et al: Intraoperative radiotherapy for locally advanced gynecologic malignancies. Front Radiat Ther Oncol 31:256-259, 1997.
65. Haddock MG, Petersen IA, Webb MJ, et al: Intraoperative radiation therapy for locally advanced gynecological (GYN) malignancies. 3rd International ISIORT Meeting, Aachen, Germany. ISIORT Abstract 5.555, 2002.
66. Martinez-Monge R, Jurado M, Arist J, et al: Intraoperative electron beam radiotherapy during radical surgery for locally advanced and recurrent cervical cancer. Gynecol Oncol 80:538-543, 2001.
67. Willett CG, Shellito PC, Tepper JE, et al: Intraoperative electron beam radiation therapy for primary locally advanced rectal and rectosigmoid carcinoma. J Clin Oncol 9:843-849, 1991.
68. Suzuki K, Gunderson L, Devine R, et al: Intraoperative radiation after palliative surgery for locally recurrent rectal cancer. Cancer 75:939-952, 1995.
69. Willett CG, Shellito PC, Tepper JE, et al: Intraoperative electron beam radiation therapy for recurrent locally advanced rectal and rectosigmoid carcinoma. Cancer 67:1504-1508, 1991.
70. Wallace HJ, Willett CG, Shellito PC, et al: Intraoperative radiation therapy for locally advanced recurrent rectal and rectosigmoid cancer. J Surg Oncol 60:122-127, 1995.
71. Abuchaibe O, Calvo FA, Tangeo E, et al: Intraoperative irradiation in locally advanced recurrent colorectal cancer. Int J Radiat Oncol Biol Phys 26:859-867, 1993.
72. Haddock MG, Gunderson LL, Nelson H, et al: Intraoperative irradiation for locally recurrent colorectal cancer in previously irradiated patients. Int J Radiat Oncol Biol Phys 49:1267-1274, 2001.
73. Meurk ML, Goer DA, Spalek G, et al: The Mobetron: a new concept for intraoperative radiotherapy. Front Radiat Ther Oncol 31:65-70, 1997.
74. Merrick HW, Gunderson LL, Calvo FA: Future directions in intraoperative radiation therapy in surgical oncology clinics. North Am Surg Oncol Clin 12:1099-1105, 2003.
75. Shipley WU, Nardi GL, Cohen AM, et al: Iodine-125 implant and external beam irradiation in patients with localized pancreatic carcinoma: a comparative study to surgical resection. Cancer 45:709-714, 1980.
76. Shipley WU, Wood WC, Tepper JE, et al: Intraoperative electron beam irradiation for patients with unresectable pancreatic carcinoma. Ann Surg 200:289-296, 1984.
77. Tepper JE, Shipley WU, Warshaw AL, et al: The role of misonidazole combined with intraoperative radiation therapy in the treatment of pancreatic carcinoma. J Clin Oncol 5:579-584, 1987.

CHAPTER 16

STEREOTACTIC IRRADIATION: LINEAR ACCELERATOR AND GAMMA KNIFE

Deepak Khuntia, John H. Suh, Wolfgang Tomé, and Minesh P. Mehta

Radiosurgery was first described in 1951 by Lars Leksell, a neurosurgeon at the Karolinska Institute in Stockholm, Sweden.[1] The term *radiosurgery* was selected because of the similarity of this technique to stereotactic neurosurgery. The initial work by Leksell first involved the treatment of patients with functional disorders and benign conditions such as chronic pain and arteriovenous malformations but later included benign and malignant tumors. The first patient was treated with Gamma Knife (GK) in 1968.[2] The limited availability, skepticism regarding this technology, and prohibitive costs initially limited the spread of this technology. By the 1980s, linear accelerator–based radiosurgery had evolved and further renewed the interest in stereotactic radiosurgery (SRS).

Because of hardware and software improvements, radiosurgery has proliferated and several hundreds of thousands of patients have been treated. In this chapter, we discuss the physics and radiobiologic principles of radiosurgery and the clinical application of this technology. Particle beam therapy is not the focus of this chapter.

BASIC PRINCIPLES OF RADIOSURGERY

Radiosurgery differs significantly from conventional fractionated radiotherapy. By definition, *radiosurgery* implies a single treatment. With conventional fractionation regimens, some normal brain tissue adjacent to the target receives a near full dose of radiation. Because normal brain parenchyma is relatively unforgiving in regard to late toxicity, the ability of radiosurgery to treat with high-dose gradients adjacent to a nonmobile target makes its use in the brain attractive. The use of a very large number of beams ensures that no single beam has substantial energy on its own, and this minimizes dose to normal tissues in its path. This geometry provides physical dose distribution advantages for relatively small targets, usually less than 4 cm in diameter. Targets larger than 4 cm result in an unacceptable increase in dose to adjacent normal brain tissue.

Radiosurgery can be performed using various devices, including the GK, particle beam devices, or modified linear accelerators. With technologic advances in software and hardware, clear superiority of one technology over the other has disappeared and mature clinical results demonstrate no outcome differences based on technology.[3] A comparison of some of the features of these two techniques is presented in Table 16-1. Because the linear accelerator–based units can be used to treat patients not receiving radiosurgery during its "down-time," cost and volume considerations are key features that determine equipment selection.[3]

Radiosurgery and neurosurgical approaches are often complementary, but there are key differences. Radiosurgery does not require a craniotomy, and hence general anesthesia is not required and patients are usually discharged the same day. In a cost-effectiveness/cost-utility analysis by Mehta and colleagues[4] in the 1990s, the authors showed that the average cost per week of survival for single brain metastasis was $310 for radiotherapy, $524 for resection plus radiation, and only $270 for radiosurgery plus whole brain radiation. With the advent of shorter hospital stays following neurosurgical procedures, these numbers have probably changed somewhat. Other advantages include lower postoperative risks for bleeding or infection and rapid recovery times. Patients who are working prior to treatment often can return to work within 1 to 2 days. More important, neurosurgically inaccessible lesions and patients who are deemed unfit for surgery or anesthesia can often be treated with radiosurgery.

The clinical applications of radiosurgery have grown substantially over the past decade. There are multiple disease processes where the use of SRS has been found to be clinically effective. Current indications, discussed later in greater detail, include arteriovenous malformations, benign brain tumors, malignant brain tumors, and functional disorders (Table 16-2). With the ability to localize targets outside of the brain, an interest in expanding radiosurgery outside the cranium is developing, with early reports of experience in treating some spinal and paraspinal tumors, as well as hepatic and pulmonary tumors. Some principles of the radiosurgery paradigm have been incorporated into a strategy employing fractionated treatments; this approach, referred to as fractionated stereotactic radiotherapy, as opposed to radiosurgery, is applied to both intracranial and extracranial lesions.

Radiosurgery is an important tool available to the neurosurgeon and radiation oncologist. Proper implementation of the treatment requires the coordination of care by the neurosurgeon, radiation oncologist, and physicist. This allows for appropriate coordination of care, improved quality of care, reduction in practice variation, a strategic marketing advantage, and improved patient satisfaction. Each specialty brings unique skills that are required for a successful radiosurgery program.[5]

PHYSICS OF RADIOSURGERY

SRS involves the use of numerous beamlets of radiation aimed precisely at an immobilized target to deliver a single session of high-dose radiation. Although no single beamlet carries significant energy, a large dose is deposited at the intersection of these beamlets with a steep dose fall-off outside the target. As tumor size increases, this fall-off becomes shallower,[6] and typically radiosurgery becomes prohibitive at sizes in excess of 4 to 5 cm.

Physics Fundamentals

Therapeutic radiation can either be delivered via photons or charged or neutral particles. Photons (x-rays and gamma rays) have no mass but have significant energy (usually in the range of 4 to 6 MV for linac [linear accelerator]-based and 1.25 MV for GK). Charged particles, including electrons, protons, and ions, have both mass and an electrical charge, whereas neutrons have significant mass but no charge. Multicobalt units containing cobalt 60 sources include devices such as the Gamma Knife and the Rotating Gamma System (American Radiosurgery Inc., San Diego, CA) (Figs. 16-1 and 16-2). Cobalt

Table 16-1 Comparing Gamma Knife and Linear Accelerator Radiosurgery Characteristics

	Gamma Knife	Linac Radiosurgery
Clinical experience	Over 3 decades	Over 2 decades
Accuracy	Submillimeter	Submillimeter
QA	Fewer QA checks	More QA checks
Machine use	Dedicated machine	Usually not a dedicated machine
Functional disorders	Longer experience	Shorter experience
Extracranial radiosurgery capable	No	Yes
Price	High. Must replace source every 5-7 y	Less expensive, no source replacement
Tumor location	Difficult to radiate peripheral lesions	Can treat peripheral lesions
Fractionated treatments	Not practical	Can treat with fractionated regimens
Treatment time	About equal	About equal

Table 16-2 Clinical Applications of Radiosurgery

Vascular (≈15%)	Benign Tumors (≈30%)	Malignant (≈45%)	Functional Disorders (≈10%)
Arteriovenous malformations (95%)	Meningiomas (45%)	Metastasis (65%)	Trigeminal neuralgia (90%)
Cavernous angiomas and other vascular lesions (5%)	Vestibular schwannomas (30%)	Glioblastoma multiforme, low-grade astrocytomas, and recurrent gliomas (30%)	Cluster headaches, obsessive-compulsive disorder, Parkinson's, and epilepsy (10%)
	Pituitary adenomas (15%)	Choroidal melanomas and other malignant tumors (5%)	
	Craniopharyngiomas, chemodectomas (10%)		

60 decays with a half-life of 5.26 years by the release of gamma rays with an average energy of approximately 1.25 MeV. A gamma ray and an x-ray cannot be discriminated and differ only in terms of source. Gamma rays result from radioactive decay, whereas x-rays are generated by accelerating electrons (in a linear accelerator) and colliding them into a tungsten target. Protons are charged particles that have been adopted in a few centers for use in radiosurgery. One of the advantages of protons is that they deposit most of their energy over a finite distance, with very little release of energy beyond this. This narrow region of energy deposition is known as the Bragg peak, and it may allow for reducing the integral dose (total dose to the patient) because of the reduced exit dose.

Components of a Radiosurgery Unit

Both multicobalt and linear accelerator units have at their heart a source of radiation (cobalt for GK and linear accelerator for linac), a couch, a stereotactic helmet or frame system to ensure precise localization and immobilization, and sophisticated treatment planning software. When properly calibrated, an isocenter alignment to better than 1 mm can be achieved with either GK or a linac radiosurgery system, although it is important to recognize that image resolution, which depends on the slice thickness, is usually of a cruder magnitude than this.[7]

The use of the stereotactic frame that is invasively attached to the patient's skull ensures that the position of the patient at the time of treatment is the same as it was at the time when the treatment planning imaging study was acquired, because the frame serves as the platform to which various coordinate localization devices can be attached. Generally, the frames are applied with the patient under a local anesthetic and sedation with multiple pins that penetrate the skin and abut the skull without penetrating the bone. Coordinate systems used for radiosurgery are based on Cartesian coordinates and allow for the precise definition of the target relative to the origin of the stereotactic localization system one is using. This permits precise geometric definition for the placement of various isocenters (or "shots") and the correct beam geometry. The coordinate system is established in the treatment planning system and is used during treatment planning to define each of the shots or groups of arcs used to deliver focused radiation to the target.

Pretreatment Quality Assurance

Because GK radiosurgery uses live sources, radiation exposure and safety are important issues. Exposure maps of the entire room and surrounding environment are necessary. The central dogmas of radiation safety, namely time, distance, and shielding are paramount, especially when live sources are used. Principles of ALARA (as low as reasonably achievable) need to be implemented. Typical "action levels" include level I with 10% exposure (125 mR/quarter) and level II of 30% (375 mR/quarter) of the maximum allowable. Obtaining these action levels will result in consequences that vary, depending on the rules set by the specific institution's radiation safety department.

In regard to actual operation, only trained oncologists or therapists can operate radiosurgery units. All operators must be in the vicinity of the control area during the treatment. The operator ensures that all required safety checks have been performed and that the written directive has been completed. With GK, a "dummy run" with a helmet must be performed prior to each patient treatment to ensure procedural safety. In addition to the calibration and treatment planning, the physicist plays a major role in ensuring that radiation safety measures are in concordance with regulatory guidelines.

An in-depth description of the various linac radiosurgery systems is beyond the scope of this chapter, and the interested reader is referred to the Task Group Report 54 of the

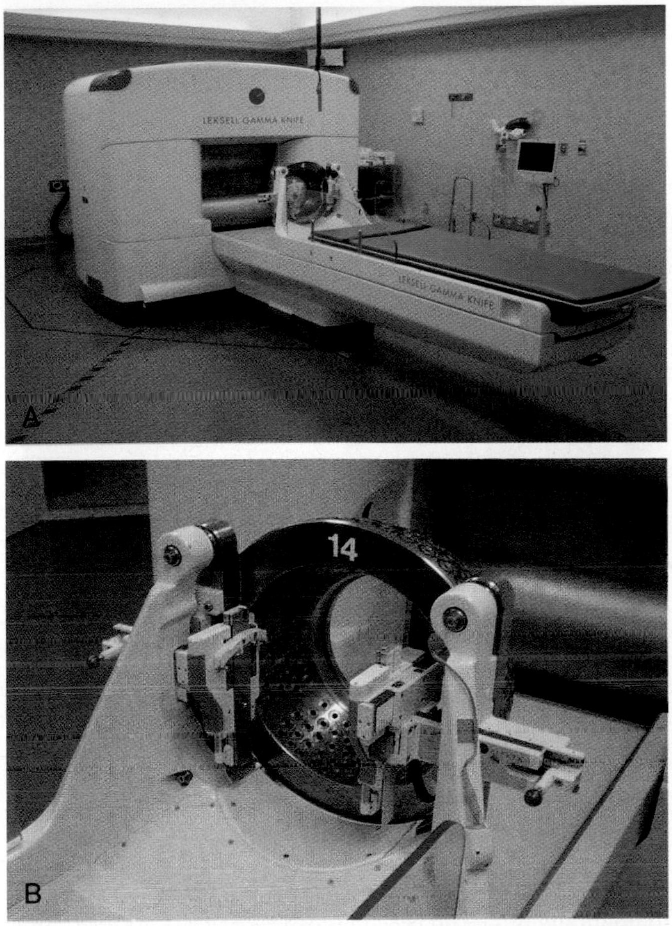

Figure 16-1 **A,** The Gamma Knife Model C unit is the most common gamma ray–based radiosurgery unit used in the world. **B,** The Model C unit is equipped with an automatic positioning system that reduces the need for manual position adjustments during the treatment. The 14-mm collimator helmet is shown.

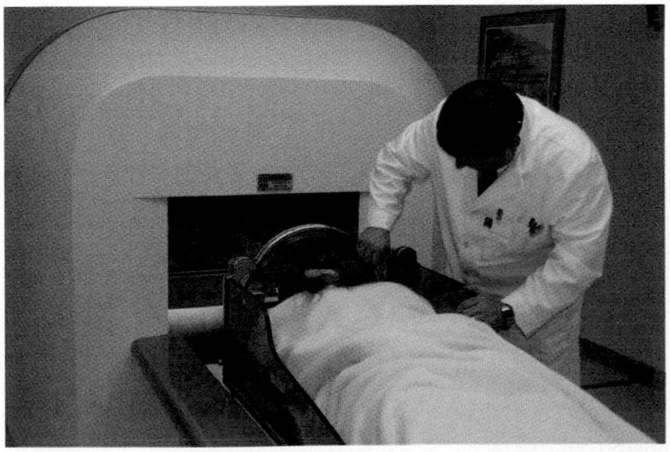

Figure 16-2 The Rotating Gamma System was originally developed in China, but the device is commercially used in a few centers in the United States. Model Gamma ART-6000 is shown. (Courtesy of Tomasz Helenowski, MD, Rotating Gamma System Institute, Gurnee, IL.)

American Association of Physicists in Medicine.[7] In general, linac radiosurgery systems can be classified into three groups. First, there are couch-mounted systems that use the treatment lasers or implanted fiducial markers as their target verification system; these systems are probably the least accurate because they have an isocenter stability of at best ±2 mm for any couch and gantry angle. Next, there are so-called floor stand–mounted systems that connect to the treatment couch and allow the user to correct for inaccuracies in the rotation of the treatment couch during treatment. However, these systems do not allow for corrections of inaccuracies in gantry rotation, and therefore such systems have at best an isocenter stability of ±1 mm for any couch and gantry angle. The most accurate linac radiosurgery system uses a floor stand with a high-precision bearing that is indexed to the linac machine but does not connect to the treatment couch. In this system, the floor stand is decoupled from the linac treatment couch, which allows for a high couch rotational accuracy in the order of a few hundredths of a millimeter to be achieved. This system has a separate arm rotating around a high-precision bearing that holds the collimator, which is coupled to the linac gantry using a gimble bearing. Because all translational and rotational degrees of freedom are decoupled from the linac, this system can be calibrated to have an isocenter stability that is equal to that of a GK of ±0.25 mm for any gantry and couch angle.[8]

Regardless of which radiosurgery system one is using, a comprehensive pretreatment quality assurance program should be implemented. At the University of Wisconsin, this program consists of three parts. First, one verifies that the frame has not slipped, using a depth helmet that allows one to measure the distance of the patient's skull to the helmet using various predefined access points. A measurement is taken before the patient is imaged, after the patient is imaged, and before the patient is set up on the floor stand. Only if all measurements are within 1 mm does one proceed with the treatment. Second, a pretreatment isocenter verification film is obtained. In this test, the coordinates of the first isocenter are set up on the floor stand and a quality assurance (QA) phantom independently. This test film serves two purposes: (1) it checks that the isocenter has been correctly set up on the floor stand and (2) it allows one to verify the integrity of the radiosurgery system. Last, an independent thorough pretreatment check is carried out by the attending physician that includes verification of the isocenter coordinates, the collimator setting, the collimator angle, the cone size, the system interlocks, and a final check verifying patient positioning.

RADIOBIOLOGIC CONSIDERATIONS

Radiosurgery differs from conventional fractionated external beam radiation treatments in the use of single fractions that treat small volumes. This poses unique radiobiologic challenges in that the increased biological effect on normal tissues is higher than that for tumors[9] (Fig. 16-3). The most important factor influencing the risk of developing late side effects is fraction dose. Single-fraction radiosurgery needs to be exquisitely accurate and must minimize dose to normal tissue.

Another potential disadvantage of using single-fraction treatment is the inability to exploit the temporal effects of cell cycle distribution. Because cells are thought to be most sensitive in the G2 and M phases of the cell cycle, fractionating radiation treatment allows redistribution of cells into the radiosensitive phases, which may improve cell kill. This opportunity is lost with radiosurgery. Hypoxia is another important variable to recognize. Malignant tumors are usually partially hypoxic, and fractionated treatments take advantage

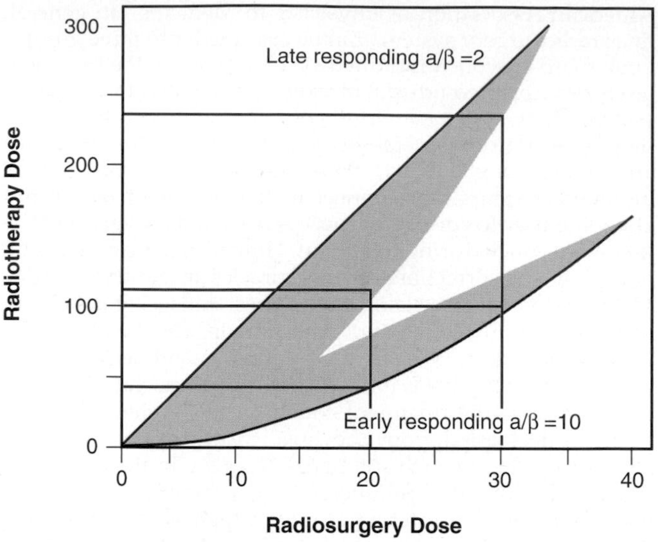

Figure 16-3 Representation of radiosurgery versus radiotherapy dose for both early and late responding tissues.[9]

of reoxygenation of the tumor, which occurs between fractions. This benefit is not realized with single-fraction SRS.

Despite these disadvantages of single-fraction radiation, efficacy with minimal toxicity has been shown in clinical trials in a multitude of disease sites. Potential explanations for this include the fact that by treating with a high single-fraction regimen, the effect of repopulation (tumor regrowth between fractions) is minimized. Uncertainties in day-to-day variations are minimized with radiosurgery. Accumulation of uncertainties ("geographic miss") during the entire course of fractionated treatment may hinder optimal therapeutic gain. Further, as the volume of normal tissue in the field is minimized, toxicity can be significantly reduced and very high radiation doses can be delivered; these high total doses might overcome some of the disadvantages of single-fraction delivery.

TREATMENT PLANNING

Treatment planning methods vary based on the software, but the ultimate obtained plans are similar. With the GK system, multiple circular collimators are used to generate "shots" to fill a particular volume. There are four helmets with varying collimator sizes used in GK systems: 4, 8, 14, and 18 mm. For linac-based radiosurgery, a variety of collimators ranging in size from 4 to 50 mm are available for different systems. Whenever multiple isocenters are used, homogeneity is sacrificed for conformality. Ideally, a desirable conformality index (prescribed isodose volume [PIV] divided by target volume [TV]) should be 2 and the heterogeneity index (maximum dose [MD] divided by prescribed dose [PD]) should be ≤2.

With some Linac-based radiosurgery, optimal distributions can be obtained by using a micromultileaf collimator (such as the Novalis system by Brain Lab), circular collimators such as with the Gamma Knife or circular collimator with jaw leaves that "shape" the beam. These devices allow for fractionation, more flexibility with beam shaping, and modulation of beam intensity. Linac-based devices are more readily adaptable for extracranial radiosurgery or fractionated delivery.

Almost every SRS treatment–planning procedure begins with the placement of the stereotactic head ring on the patient. The head ring is used for localization and to guarantee that

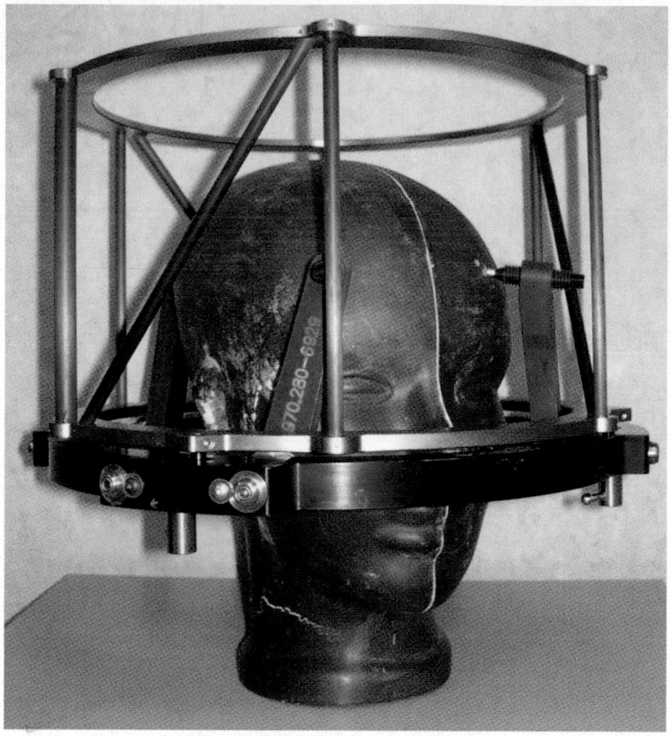

Figure 16-4 Phantom with head ring and the Brown-Roberts-Wells coordinate system in place.

the patient's position from the time of imaging to the time of treatment does not change. Before the stereotactic computed tomography (CT) scan is acquired, a stereotactic localizer ring is attached to the head ring. For linac radiosurgery, the most commonly used independent stereotactic localization system is the Brown-Roberts-Wells (BRW) system (Fig. 16-4). The BRW localizer has an inner diameter of 29 cm and a height of 16 cm and consists of nine carbon fiber rods that are arranged into three N-shaped structures between two aluminum rings, which are placed at 120-degree angles around the ring. Because three N-shaped fiducials are used, one obtains a system of linear equations that allow for definition of an independent, absolute coordinate system. Therefore, one does not have to QA the table indexing of the CT scanner because the slice position of each scan can be uniquely determined.

The origin of the BRW system lies within the localizer and divides the brain into eight distinct quadrants. Any point within this geometric configuration can be uniquely defined by specifying anteroposterior, lateral, and axial coordinates. During the stereotactic CT scan, portions of these N-shaped structures are included in each image, which allows for their identification during treatment planning. In order to reduce the error in localization, the slice thickness of the CT scan should be the smallest attainable on the scanner. Once the stereotactic CT scan has been acquired, it is transferred to the treatment planning system and the BRW coordinate system is defined by localizing each of the nine rods in each of the CT slices (Fig. 16-5).

Next, the TV is outlined. Because magnetic resonance imaging (MRI) often provides better tumor visualization than CT scanning, the TV is often delineated directly from MRI studies. MRI alone does not provide a sufficient database for stereotactic treatment planning, because magnetic field nonuniformity, gradient field nonlinearity, eddy current effects, and susceptibility artifacts at air-tissue interfaces can

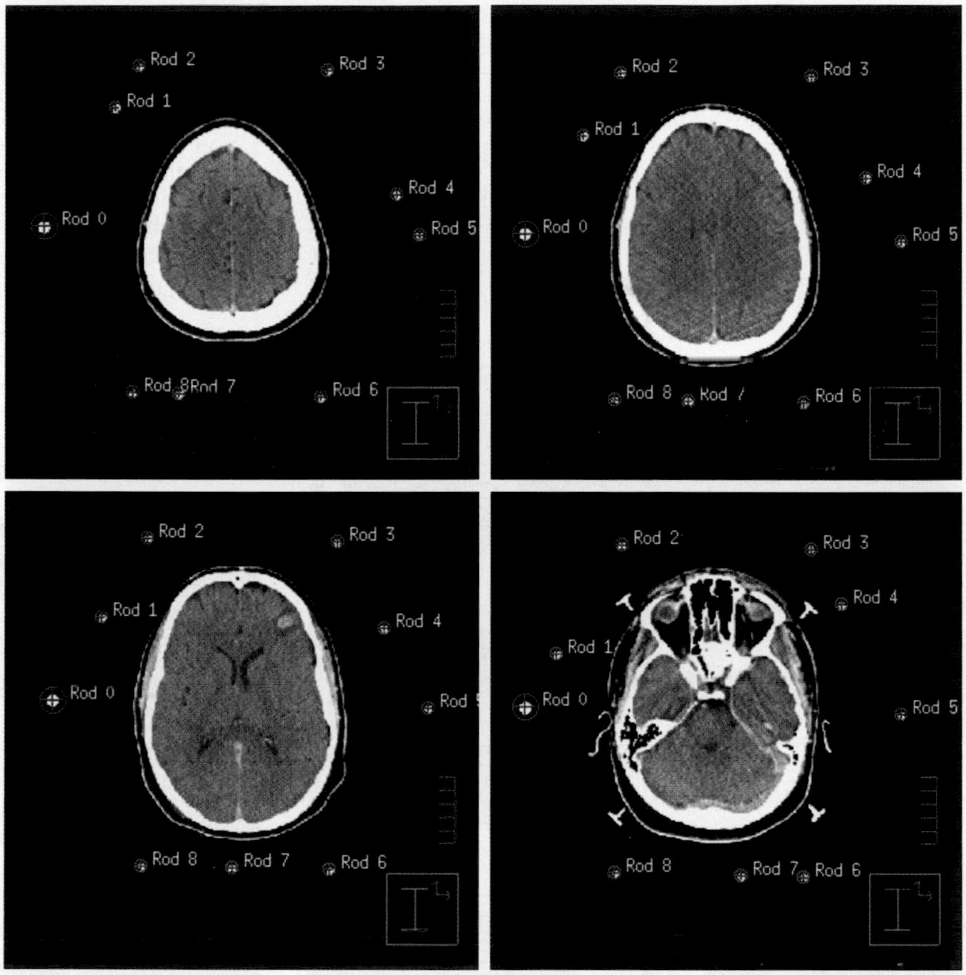

Figure 16-5 Four-panel view of acquired stereotactic CT shows how the Brown-Roberts-Wells localizer rods are imbedded into the CT images.

introduce significant geometric image distortions that affect the accuracy of treatment plans generated using MRI alone. Three-dimensional volumetric MRI is acquired either before or after head ring placement. After acquiring the stereotactic CT scan, the MRI dataset (which may or may not be stereotactically generated) is mapped onto the CT image space through correlation of anatomic landmarks in both image sets. During treatment planning, the regions of interest and dose distribution may be displayed on either the CT or fused MRI images, but dosimetric calculations are ideally performed on the underlying CT database (Fig. 16-6). If MRI is to be obtained after head ring placement, MR-compatible head rings need to be used. Some investigators use a "noninvasive" fiducial system where several fiducials are either implanted subcutaneously or taped on the patient, and the fiducials provide the frame of reference for obtaining stereotactic coordinates. This approach has not become very popular because of the perceived problems with patient immobilization during treatment.

Conventional linac radiosurgery uses a multiple-noncoplanar arc set to treat the TV (Fig. 16-7). For irregularly shaped lesions such as vestibular schwannomas and arteriovenous malformations (AVMs), arcs delivered through a single circular collimator would lead to the inclusion of a large amount of normal brain tissue, which yields inferior conformality. In these cases, it is advantageous to use multiple isocenters to conform the prescription isodose shell to the TV (Fig. 16-8).

CLINICAL APPLICATION

Both GK radiosurgery and linac-based radiosurgery have been used in a variety of benign and malignant diseases. Table 16-2 summarizes the most common clinical applications for radiosurgery. In this section, we outline some of the basic applications of radiosurgery and results of therapy. Specifics pertaining to each disease are discussed in greater detail in their respective chapters.

Benign Tumors

Meningiomas

Benign diseases make up a considerable proportion of the applications for radiosurgery, with meningiomas being one of the most common applications in this setting.

Although meningiomas are often resected, radiosurgery plays an important role when either the lesion is small and surgically inaccessible or there is residual disease postoperatively. The two largest series that have examined the results of radiosurgery are from the Mayo Clinic and University of Pittsburgh.[10-12] The University of Pittsburgh series analyzed the results of 159 cavernous sinus meningiomas treated to 13 to 14 Gy, while the Mayo Clinic series reports the results of 206 patients treated with a median marginal dose of 16 Gy in a single fraction. Both series have shown local control in excess of 90% for benign meningiomas. The Mayo Clinic series had a significant complication rate of 13% versus 7% for

University of Pittsburgh. However, in the former, a small portion of the optic chiasm was allowed to receive up to 12 Gy while the University of Pittsburgh kept the chiasmal dose at 8 Gy.

Table 16-3 summarizes the various series reported in the literature. Based on these results, it is reasonable to conclude that small meningiomas can be controlled in the majority of patients with radiosurgery. It must, however, be borne in mind that the majority of the experience with this approach has relatively short follow-up and long-term results (>10-year follow-up in each patient) are indeed very sparse. Because these data are for the most part not obtained in the setting of controlled clinical trials, absolute statements about the value of radiosurgery in managing meningiomas must be approached with caution (Fig. 16-9). To determine, with scientific merit, the value of radiosurgery, the European Organization for Research and Treatment of Cancer (EORTC) is conducting a phase III prospective randomized trial, EORTC 26021, randomizing patients with benign meningiomas to either radiation or observation after nonradical surgery for benign meningiomas.

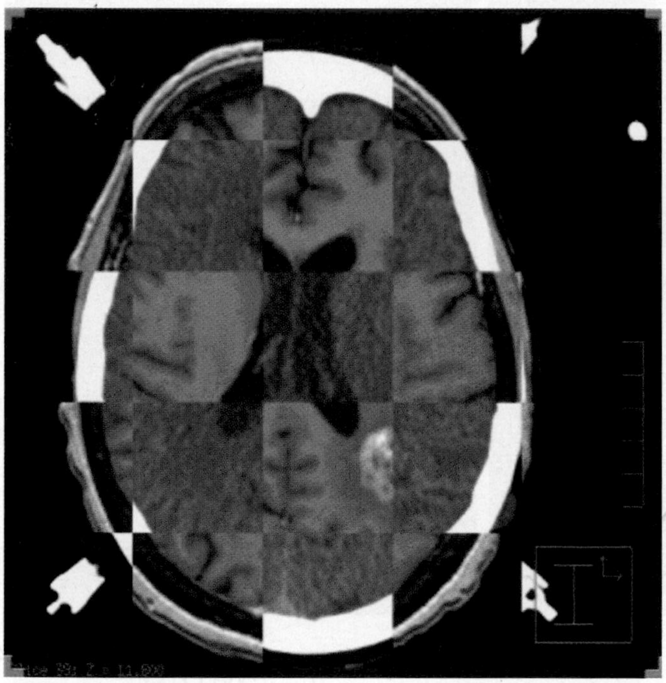

Figure 16-6 Image fusion of stereotactic CT with a T1-weighted, three-dimensional, spoiled gradient echo MRI image set. The MRI scan has been pixilated to show the underlying CT. The difference in tumor visualization between the two imaging modalities is demonstrated.

Vestibular Schwannomas

Vestibular schwannomas make up between 6% and 8% of all primary intracranial tumors. There are approximately 1200 cases per year. They are thought to arise at the point where nerve sheaths are replaced by fibroblasts. This transition is referred to as the Obersteiner-Redlich zone and is usually

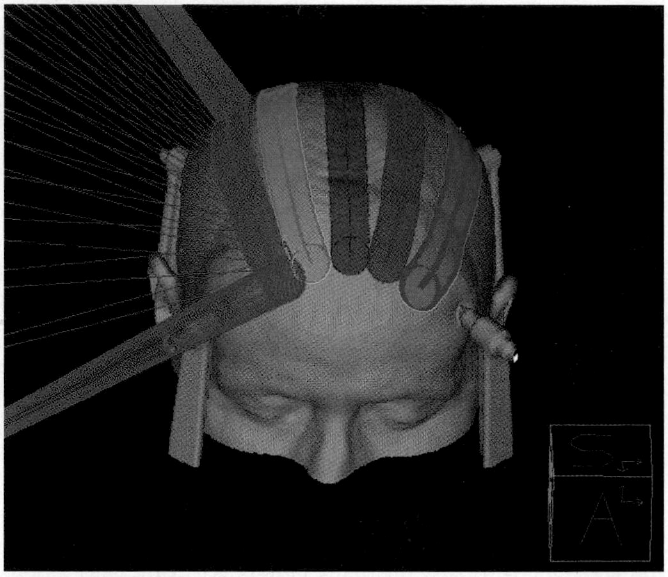

Figure 16-7 Typical nonopposing five arrangements used in multi-isocenter treatment planning for linear accelerator (linac)-based radiosurgery.

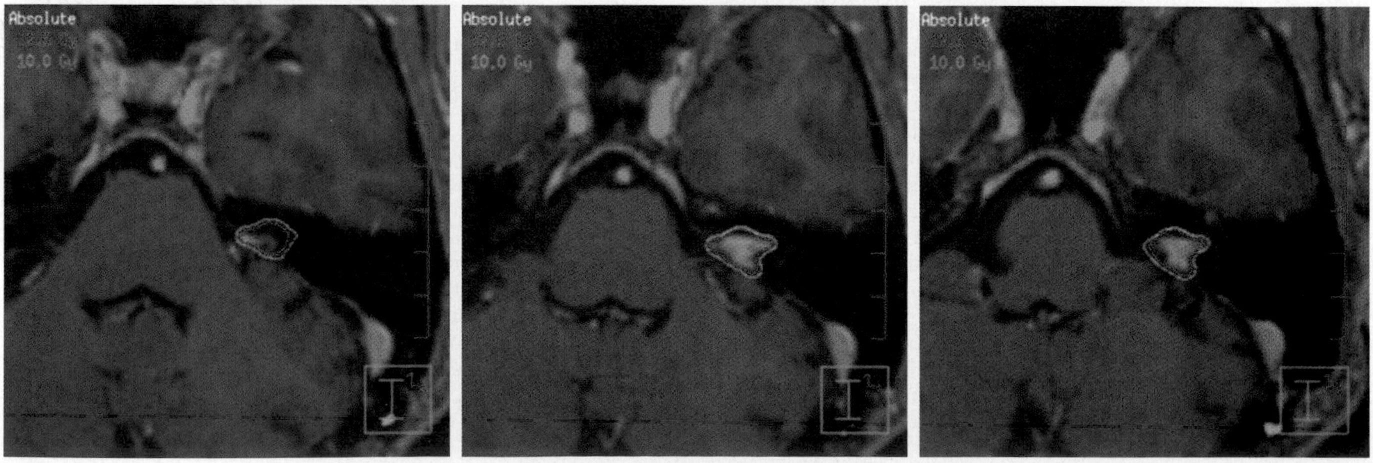

Figure 16-8 Three selected axial cuts through a vestibular schwannoma demonstrate the resulting conformal treatment plan using four different isocenters. The gadolinium contrast-enhanced, thin-slice, T1-weighted, three-dimensional, spoiled gradient echo MRI data set has been fused to the underlying stereotactic CT to visualize the vestibular schwannoma. The 12.5-Gy treatment isodose line and the 10-Gy isodose line are shown.

Table 16-3 Radiosurgery Results with Meningiomas[45]

Author (y)	n	No Histology	Margin Dose (Gy) (range)	Progression-free 5-y Survival
Hakim (1998)	106	54%	15 (9-20)	91%
Kondziolka (1999)	99	43%	16 (9-25)	93%
Roche (2000)	80	63%	14 (6-25)	93%
Stafford (2001)	168	41%	16 (12-36)	93%
Shin (2001)*	15	30%	>10-12	75% (10 y)†
	22	30%	14-18	100% (10 y)†
	3	30%	No SRS	0% at 3 y
Nicolato (2002)	111	50%	15 (11-23)	96%
Range:		30-63%	9-36 Gy	75-100% (≥14 Gy had 5-y PFS between 91% and 100%)

*Cavernous sinus.
†Overall 86.4% at 3 y, 82.3% at 10 y.

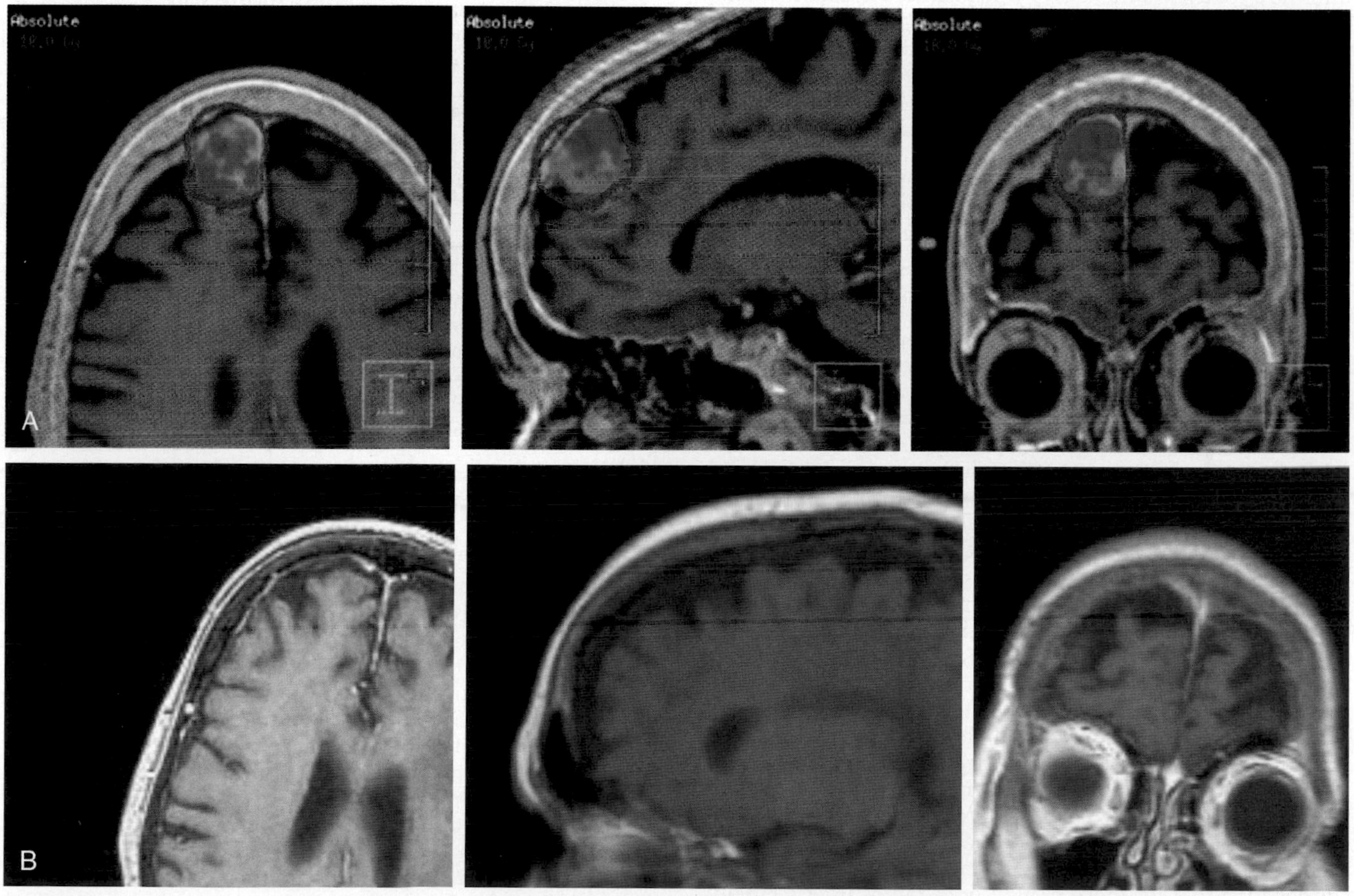

Figure 16-9 **A,** Radiosurgery plan showing the tumor volume and 18-Gy isodose line covering the entire tumor. **B,** Posttreatment MRI with complete resolution of the lesion.

located with the internal auditory canal. Although benign, they can cause severe local symptoms. Typical growth rates are less than 2 mm per year. Common symptoms include unilateral sensorineural hearing loss (>90%), unsteady gait (77%), tinnitus (70%), otalgia or mastoid pain (30%), and headaches (30%). Typical appearance on a CT scan shows an isodense or hypodense lesion centered upon the internal auditory meatus, resembling an "ice cream cone" on its side.

Traditionally, microsurgery has been the treatment of choice. Mortality from this procedure is generally less than 1% in modern times. However, if patients are not good surgical candidates and, more frequently, on the basis of patient choice, radiosurgery is used. The typical radiation dose is 12 to 13 Gy in a single fraction.[13] Pollock and colleagues[14] reviewed 87 patients with unilateral vestibular schwannomas of less than 3 cm. Using similarly matched treatment groups (treated with microsurgery), patients undergoing SRS were found to have improved facial nerve and hearing preservation with decreased morbidity. Tumor control in this series was 98% for surgery versus 94% for radiosurgery. Hearing was preserved in 14% of the surgery patients and 75% of the radiosurgery patients. Facial nerve preservation was observed in 83% of the radiosurgery group and only 63% in the surgery group. There also was a trend favoring radiosurgery in regard to patient satisfaction and functional outcomes. Similar results have been found by the Marseilles group.[15] In properly selected patients, radiosurgery may be the preferred treatment.

Single-institution patient series have shown excellent tolerability and efficacy in using radiosurgery with local control rates in excess of 90%. However, radiosurgery is not free of complications. In the early experience using 16 to 18 Gy, high rates of cranial neuropathies were observed and the variables predicting these included total dose, length of nerve irradiated, and tumor dose. Two distinct approaches were pursued to reduce these complications: one approach was to reduce the total dose to 12 to 13 Gy, and the experience with this was reported by Flickinger and colleagues.[13] Local control was achieved in nearly 99% of patients. A second approach to minimize toxicity is the use of fractionation, because smaller fractions produce lesser long-term damage. In this context, Williams[16] reported a series of 80 consecutive patients treated with fractionated radiosurgery. Patients with tumors of 3 cm or less received 25 Gy in five fractions, and patients with tumors greater than 3 cm received 30 Gy in 10 fractions. All received radiation prescribed to the 80% isodose line using 10-MV photons. There was no facial weakness or hearing loss in the 80 patients in this study. Others have found similar hearing rates in the range of 80% to 85% using more conventional fractionation regimens (50 Gy/25 fractions–57 Gy/23 fractions).[17,18]

The best series to date is a trial done by Meijer and colleagues in the Netherlands.[19] Their group prospectively evaluated 129 patients with vestibular schwannomas. Patients were assigned to receive either 20 to 25 Gy in four or five fractions if they were dentate (80 patients) versus 10 to 12.5 Gy in a single fraction if they were edentate (49 patients). Local control rates, hearing preservation, and cranial nerve VII complications were not statistically different. However, there was a fourfold increase in cranial nerve V complications with single-fraction radiosurgery compared with fractionated radiation (8% versus 2%).

Based on the data just presented, most investigators regard radiosurgery and fractionated radiotherapy as having comparable efficacy. If patients are at higher risk of developing complications, one may consider fractionated treatment. With single-fraction radiosurgery, doses should be kept below 13 Gy to reduce toxicity. Further, MRI-based planning has been shown to reduce the risk of toxicity in comparison to CT-based planning.[20] Patients with tumors greater than 2 cm or with previous surgeries may also be at higher risk of developing complications. It must, however, be borne in mind that the follow-up of patients treated with fractionated approaches is shorter than that for those treated with radiosurgery. Finally, neither radiosurgery nor fractionated approaches have been tested in prospective, controlled clinical trials for this disease.

Pituitary Adenomas

Ten percent of intracranial neoplasms arise in the pituitary region. Radiation is generally reserved for patients who have incompletely resected tumors or recurrent tumors. Based on the size and location, one may consider either SRS or conformal external beam radiation. Typical radiosurgery doses to the pituitary have ranged from 10 to 30 Gy, but doses in the 13- to 14-Gy range have been found to be equivalent to higher doses.[21] Local control using radiosurgery is generally in excess of 90% for nonsecretory tumors. When patients are on hormone suppressing therapies, markedly inferior control rates have been seen in several series and could be explained by possible underestimation of tumor size.[22,23]

Malignant Tumors

Brain Metastasis

Brain metastases affect over 100,000 patients in the United States annually. Radiosurgery is used more for brain metastasis than for any other malignant tumor. Here, we briefly describe the rationale for radiosurgery for brain metastasis.

Dose selection parameters for treating brain metastases were defined in part by a phase I Radiation Therapy Oncology Group (RTOG) trial.[24] As a result of this trial, typical recommended doses for brain metastasis are based on maximal diameter: 21 to 24 Gy for lesions of 2 cm, 18 Gy for lesions 2 to 3 cm, and 15 Gy for lesions 3 to 4 cm.

The RTOG reported results from a randomized trial of whole brain radiation therapy (WBRT) (37.5 Gy/15 fractions) with or without radiosurgery. The results of this trial suggest a survival benefit for patients with single brain metastases. Additionally, post-hoc subgroup analysis suggests the potential for benefiting some patients with up to three brain metastases.[25]

Eliminating whole brain radiation in SRS patients is controversial. Several retrospective series have been conducted that suggest that eliminating whole brain radiation will increase the likelihood of relapse but not necessarily affect survival.[26-28] The impact on neurologic function is a fine balance between the toxicity of brain irradiation and the negative consequences of tumor relapse,[29] and it must be borne in mind that exclusion of whole brain radiotherapy results in high intracranial relapse rates.[30] The American College of Surgical Oncologists (ACOSOG) initiated a phase III trial comparing SRS versus SRS followed by WBRT which is currently on hold.

Gliomas

Because at least 80% of gliomas fall within 2 cm of the primary, high-dose local radiation has been hypothesized as a means of improving tumor control rates. However, many patients with malignant gliomas have large tumors, or at least a significant amount of edema that harbors microscopic disease, reducing the likelihood of success of radiosurgery. In an effort to delineate the role of SRS, the RTOG conducted a randomized trial of 203 patients with glioblastoma multiforme who received either 60 Gy external beam radiation at 2 Gy/fraction with BCNU versus SRS prior to external beam and BCNU.[31] Radiosurgery did not add to overall survival, quality of life, or neurologic function as performed in this trial.

SRS for recurrent malignant gliomas has been reported from small institutional series and is succinctly summarized by Sanghavi and colleagues.[32] No prospective studies have defined its role adequately. The role of radiosurgery for malignant gliomas is limited. Patients with small-volume recurrent disease may be candidates for this modality. In the adjuvant or definitive setting, SRS has not been shown to be beneficial.

Vascular Lesions

Arteriovenous Malformations

AVMs represent abnormal clusters of arteries and veins that shunt blood from the arterial system to the venous system without an intervening capillary network. If left untreated, there is a risk of hemorrhage of about 1% to 4% per year. Treatment is often considered in an asymptomatic patient. Surgery is the treatment of choice, whenever feasible, as it immediately removes the risk of hemorrhage. If the volume of the nidus is small and it is inoperable, radiosurgery is a safe and effective alternative.

The high dose of radiation presumably unleashes a cytokine cascade that induces endothelial proliferation and eventual obliteration of the AVM nidus, over 1 to 3 years. Typical doses used are in the 15- to 30-Gy range.

Complete obliteration of the nidus leading to control of the AVM has been reported at levels at or above 90%.[33] Rates are on the higher end for lesions of less than 4 cm^3. However, it may take up to 2 years for complete obliteration. Patients are still at risk of developing a hemorrhage during this time period.

Functional Disorders

Trigeminal Neuralgia

Trigeminal neuralgia (also known as tic douloureux) is a syndrome characterized by paroxysmal facial pain and affects about 150,000 people worldwide each year. This disorder is characterized by brief attacks of severe pain in the face, mouth, and teeth that tend to radiate into the face on the affected side. It is not known what causes trigeminal neuralgia, although most people believe that pressure against the trigeminal nerve near the pons by adjacent vessels causes most cases of the condition. It is this region of the brain where local treatments are directed.

Typically, medications such as carbamazepine are the treatment of choice. If patients are refractory to medications, microvascular decompression, balloon compression, glycerol rhizotomy, and radiofrequency rhizotomy have been used, all with pain relief in the majority of the patients.

For patients refractory to medications, radiosurgery is the next least invasive procedure. Typical doses are 70 to 90 Gy in a single fraction directed at the root entry zone of cranial nerve V into the pons (Fig. 16-10). It is thought that delivering high doses of radiation to this region induces a block of the emphatic transmission through the pain fibers only. Sensorimotor function, however, is spared.

Results from the University of Pittsburgh suggest that approximately 70% of patients have some pain relief, with about 40% experiencing complete pain relief and coming off all medications.[34] Patients with typical symptoms (i.e., sharp, electric shock–like pains as opposed to dull aching or burning pain) have superior results compared with those with atypical symptoms. Patients with no previous surgical manipulations have a higher likelihood of complete pain relief.

It has been postulated that using an elliptical target as opposed to a spherical target would also add to improving the efficacy of radiosurgery. Flickinger and colleagues[35] randomized 87 patients with trigeminal neuralgia to receive either a single isocenter (spherical) or a two-isocenter (elliptical treatment volume) setup using GK. A maximal dose of 75 Gy was delivered with 4-mm-diameter collimators. Fifty-seven patients realized complete pain relief (45 without medication and 12 with low-dose medication), relief was partial in 15, and relief was minimal in another 15 patients. The actuarial rate of obtaining complete pain relief was 67.7 ± 5.1%. The pain relief was identical for one- and two-isocenter radiosurgery. Pain relapsed in 30 of 72 responding patients. Numbness and paresthesias correlated with the length of nerve irradiated. The authors concluded that treatment volume to include a longer nerve length for trigeminal neuralgia radiosurgery does not significantly improve pain relief but may increase complications.

Similar results using linac-based radiosurgery have been reported by Bradley and colleagues[36] from the University of Wisconsin. In their series, the actuarial 6-month complete/major response rate was 77.5% with an actuarial 6-month relapse rate of 21.3%.

Attempts for retreatment with radiosurgery have been reported. The University of Pittsburgh reports approximately 50% complete pain relief after retreatment, whereas the Mayo series reports 90% pain relief with retreatment. The University of Pittsburgh reported a modest rate of numbness at 13%, while all of the Mayo series patients developed minor numbness.[37,38] Similar results have been reported by others.[39]

Other Functional Disorders

Other functional disorders treated with radiosurgery include cluster headaches, obsessive-compulsive disorder (OCD),

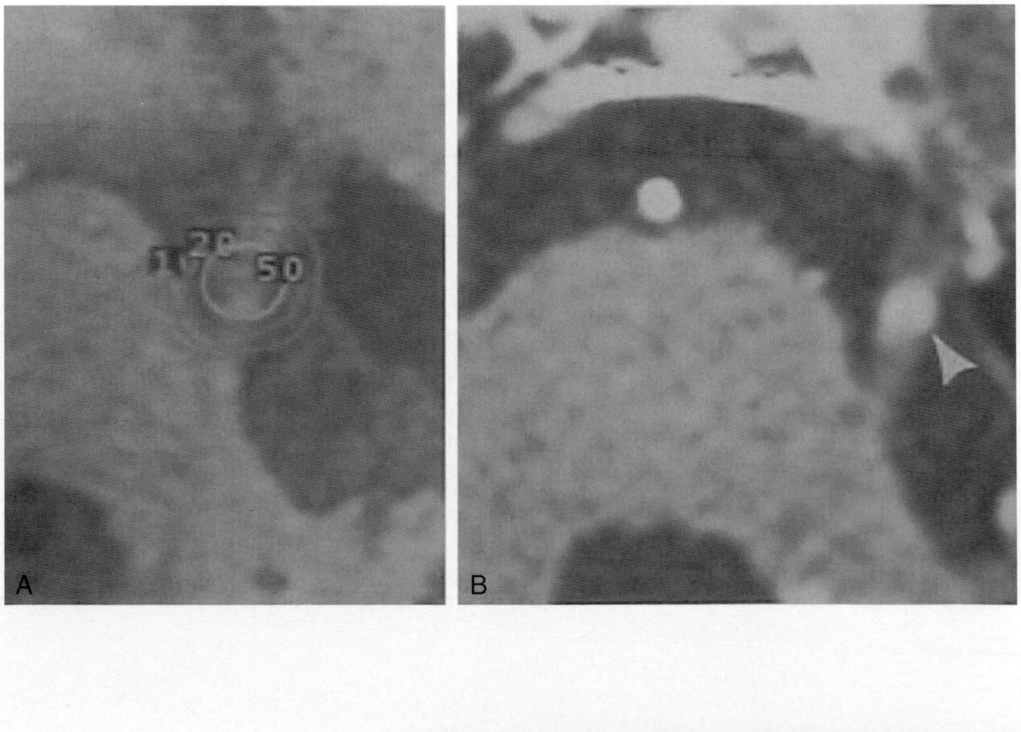

Figure 16-10 **A,** Typical Gamma Knife radiosurgery dose distribution targeted at the root entry zone of cranial nerve V. The prescription dose is typically 70 to 90 Gy, prescribed to the 100% isodose line. **B,** MRI 6 months after radiosurgery demonstrates the radiographic changes for cranial nerve V.

Parkinson's disease, and epilepsy. Standard radiation recommendations for these disorders have not been developed, and conclusive evidence of efficacy has not been established. In regard to cluster headaches, medical management is generally the first line. If patients are refractory to medical or surgical techniques, radiosurgery can be considered. The target, like trigeminal neuralgia, is the root entry zone of cranial nerve V. Typical doses are 70 to 80 Gy to the 100% isodose line.

For Parkinson's disease, medical, surgical, and electrotherapy are first considered. If the patient is refractory to this management, radiosurgery can be considered. The target for this disease is the globus pallidus (posteroventral region) for patients experiencing dyskinesia or akinesisa. If patients are experiencing tremors, the ventrolateral thalamus region is targeted. Typical doses are in the range of 130 to 140 Gy prescribed to the 100% isodose line.

Patients with OCD who are refractory to medications, surgery, or radiofrequency capsulotomy may be considered for radiosurgery. The target is the anterior capsule, bilaterally. Typical doses are 120 Gy to the 100% isodose line. Patients with epilepsy can also be treated with radiosurgery if they are refractory to other modalities. Doses are typically 18 Gy to the 50% isodose line centered on the hippocampus.

Extracranial Radiosurgery

With improvements in hardware, image guidance, and immobilization, radiosurgery is now possible outside of the brain. Extracranial stereotactic body radiosurgery (SBRT) is being investigated in a variety of tumors, including early stage non–small cell lung cancer (NSCLC), spinal cord tumors, liver metastases, and other abdominal tumors. We briefly introduce some of the concepts that have allowed extracranial radiosurgery to flourish.

Because of the high doses delivered, SBRT requires very high confidence in targeting. However, because of issues of target motion, this becomes a difficult task to accomplish outside of the brain. The prescription isodose must be shaped with a high degree of conformality to keep high doses off normal tissue. During the CT-simulation process, immobilization, such as with a whole-body vacuum mold, is necessary (Fig. 16-11A). At the University of Wisconsin, chest wall motion can be reduced to 2 mm by using a vacuum system with an abdominal pressure pillow (see Fig. 16-11B). Four-dimensional CT scans or fluoroscopic motion studies are then conducted to assist with planning target volume (PTV) measurements. For tumors that are positron emission tomography (PET) avid, often times ^{18}F-fluorodeoxyglucose (FDG)-PET imaging is conducted while the patient is in the body mold to improve the accuracy of delineating the tumor. Because the PET is a slow scan, motion is already accounted for in the fusion of the PET to the four-dimensional CT.

Treatment planning usually involves a multiple beam arrangement, very often non-coplanar, to produce distributions with very rapid fall-off (Fig. 16-12). Typically, dosimetric margins around the PTV are selected so that the 80% isodose line encompasses 100% of the PTV. Localization with orthogonal x-rays, kilovoltage or megavoltage CT guidance, or optical guidance with three-dimensional ultrasound, x-rays, or CT is usually necessary to ensure that there is not a geographic miss for each fraction. Once this is accomplished, radiation treatment is delivered. A variety of systems are in use for SBRT. These include using standard linac machines, the Novalis Brain Lab system, and the Accuray Cyberknife system (among many others.)

Long-term clinic results are still pending. Stage I lung cancers represent the majority of the recent experience using SBRT. Typically, patients with NSCLC have survivals of about 70% with resection. With standard "postage stamp" radiation (typically between 60 and 70 Gy), results are about half that of surgery.[40] However, with modern techniques, dose escalation is possible, and improved results with single-institution experiences have been reported.[41,42] Timmerman and colleagues[43] completed a phase I dose-escalation protocol for medically inoperable patients with stage I lung cancer. Initial doses started at 8 Gy × 3 fractions over 2 weeks. Dose per fraction was increased by 2 Gy per fraction in the three cohorts. The maximum tolerated dose in this trial has not been reached, and this has led to the ongoing RTOG 0236 phase II trial delivering 20 Gy per fraction for 3 fractions.

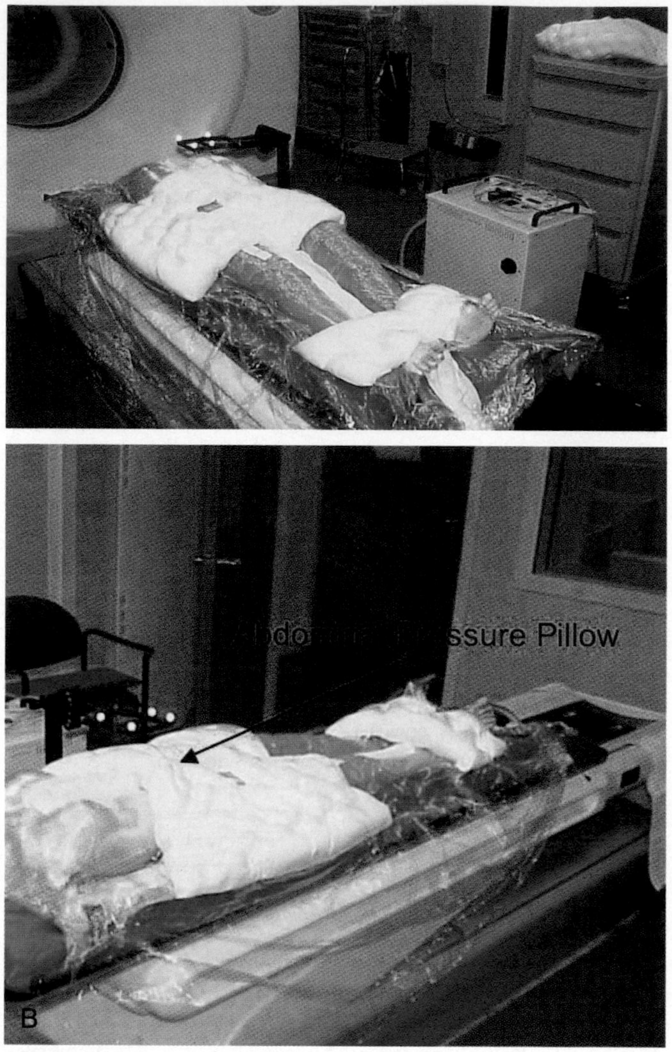

Figure 16-11 **A,** CT simulation is conducted with the patient in an immobilization device. The VacLoc bag is immobilized using –80 mbar of pressure in the vacuum. **B,** Abdominal pressure pillow.

In addition to primary lung tumors, SBRT has been used for lung and liver metastasis. Excellent local control of 66% to 100% has been reported.[44]

Other areas where SBRT has been used includes the abdomen, spine, and liver. Data have been restricted to single-institution series, and follow-up is short in these regards.

The initial experience with SBRT is very promising. A high degree of local control should be expected, at least in the short run. However, toxicity will remain the rate-limiting factor as

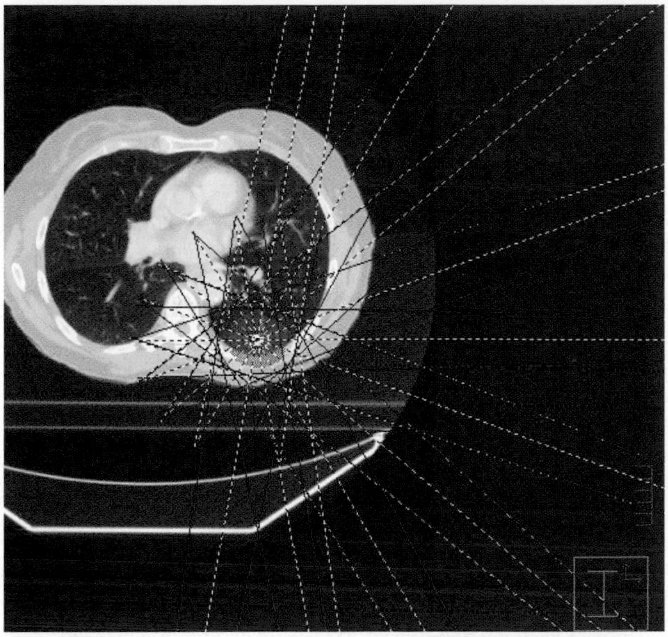

Figure 16-12 Beam arrangements are shown for a T1 non–small cell lung cancer. Ideally, all beams are selected to minimize exit to the contralateral lung. Dosimetric margins are selected to ensure that the planning target volume is enclosed by the 80% of maximum isodose shell.

to the success of this treatment. Because tumors are often close to critical structures (e.g., brain, lung, kidneys), special care and expertise are necessary to deliver SBRT accurately and safely, and treatment should be restricted to those with expertise and experience with the procedure.

CONCLUSION

In this chapter, basic concepts of radiosurgery have been introduced. Radiosurgery is an effective treatment modality for arteriovenous malformations, benign and malignant tumors, and functional disorders. Future directions using this technology may incorporate the use of biologic imaging to better define targets. This may allow potential escalation of doses to improve tumor control. The improved conformality may also allow a decrease in complication rates. The role of radiosurgery for functional disorders beyond trigeminal neuralgia needs to be defined. Initial experience with extracranial radiosurgery looks promising, and further trials will be needed to evaluate the efficacy and toxicity of the treatment.

REFERENCES

1. Leksell L: The stereotaxic method and radiosurgery of the brain. Acta Chir Scand 102:316-319, 1951.
2. Leksell L. [Trigeminal neuralgia. Some neurophysiologic aspects and a new method of therapy]. Lakartidningen 68:5145-5148, 1971.
3. Stieber VW, Bourland JD, Tome WA, et al: Gentlemen (and ladies), choose your weapons: gamma knife vs. linear accelerator radiosurgery. Technol Cancer Res Treat 2:79-86, 2003.
4. Mehta M, Noyes W, Craig B, et al: A cost-effectiveness and cost-utility analysis of radiosurgery vs. resection for single-brain metastases. Int J Radiat Oncol Biol Phys 39:445-454, 1997.
5. Larson DA, Bova F, Eisert D, et al: Current radiosurgery practice: results of an ASTRO survey. Task Force on Stereotactic Radiosurgery, American Society for Therapeutic Radiology and Oncology. Int J Radiat Oncol Biol Phys 28:523-526, 1994.
6. Kubsad SS, Mackie TR, Gehring MA, et al: Monte Carlo and convolution dosimetry for stereotactic radiosurgery. Int J Radiat Oncol Biol Phys 19:1027-1035, 1990.
7. Schell M, Bova F, Larson V: AAPM Report 54: Stereotactic radiosurgery. Am Assoc Physicist Med 1995.
8. Friedman WA, Bova FJ: The University of Florida radiosurgery system. Surg Neurol 32:334-342, 1989.
9. Mehta MP: The physical, biologic, and clinical basis of radiosurgery. Curr Probl Cancer 19:265-329, 1995.
10. Stafford SL, Pollock BE, Foote RL, et al: Meningioma radiosurgery: tumor control, outcomes, and complications among 190 consecutive patients. Neurosurgery 49:1029-1037; discussion 1037-1038, 2001.
11. Kondziolka D, Niranjan A, Lunsford LD, et al: Stereotactic radiosurgery for meningiomas. Neurosurg Clin N Am 10:317-325, 1999.
12. Lee JY, Niranjan A, McInerney J, et al: Stereotactic radiosurgery providing long-term tumor control of cavernous sinus meningiomas. J Neurosurg 97:65-72, 2002.
13. Flickinger JC, Kondziolka D, Niranjan A, et al: Acoustic neuroma radiosurgery with marginal tumor doses of 12 to 13 Gy. Int J Radiat Oncol Biol Phys 60:225-230, 2004.
14. Pollock BE, Lunsford LD, Kondziolka D, et al: Outcome analysis of acoustic neuroma management: a comparison of microsurgery and stereotactic radiosurgery. Neurosurgery 36:215-224; discussion 224-229, 1995.
15. Regis J: [New developments in the management of vestibular schwannomas in the modern era of radiosurgery]. Neurochirurgie 50(2-3 Pt 2):156-158, 2004.
16. Williams JA: Fractionated stereotactic radiotherapy for acoustic neuromas: preservation of function versus size. J Clin Neurosci 10:48-52, 2003.
17. Andrews DW, Suarez O, Goldman HW, et al: Stereotactic radiosurgery and fractionated stereotactic radiotherapy for the treatment of acoustic schwannomas: comparative observations of 125 patients treated at one institution. Int J Radiat Oncol Biol Phys 50:1265-1278, 2001.
18. Fuss M, Debus J, Lohr F, et al: Conventionally fractionated stereotactic radiotherapy (FSRT) for acoustic neuromas. Int J Radiat Oncol Biol Phys 48:1381-1387, 2000.
19. Meijer OW, Vandertop WP, Baayen JC, et al: Single-fraction vs. fractionated Linac-based stereotactic radiosurgery for vestibular schwannoma: a single-institution study. Int J Radiat Oncol Biol Phys 56:1390-1396, 2003.
20. Suh JH, Barnett GH, Sohn JW, et al: Results of linear accelerator-based stereotactic radiosurgery for recurrent and newly diagnosed acoustic neuromas. Int J Cancer 90:145-151, 2000.
21. Sheehan JP, Kondziolka D, Flickinger J, et al: Radiosurgery for residual or recurrent nonfunctioning pituitary adenoma. J Neurosurg 97(Suppl 5):408-414, 2002.
22. Landolt AM, Lomax N: Gamma knife radiosurgery for prolactinomas. J Neurosurg 93(Suppl 3):14-18, 2000.
23. Pollock BE, Nippoldt TB, Stafford SL, et al: Results of stereotactic radiosurgery in patients with hormone-producing pituitary adenomas: factors associated with endocrine normalization. J Neurosurg 97:525-530, 2002.
24. Shaw E, Scott C, Souhami L, et al: Single dose radiosurgical treatment of recurrent previously irradiated primary brain tumors and brain metastases: final report of RTOG protocol 90-05. Int J Radiat Oncol Biol Phys 47:291-298, 2000.
25. Andrews DW, Scott CB, Sperduto PW, et al: Whole brain radiation therapy with or without stereotactic radiosurgery boost for patients with one to three brain metastases: phase III results of the RTOG 9508 randomised trial. Lancet 363:1665-1672, 2004.
26. Sneed PK, Suh JH, Goetsch SJ, et al: A multi-institutional review of radiosurgery alone vs. radiosurgery with whole brain radiotherapy as the initial management of brain metastases. Int J Radiat Oncol Biol Phys 53:519-526, 2002.
27. Chidel MA, Suh JH, Reddy CA, et al: Application of recursive partitioning analysis and evaluation of the use of whole brain radiation among patients treated with stereotactic radiosurgery for newly diagnosed brain metastases. Int J Radiat Oncol Biol Phys 47:993-999, 2000.

28. Sneed PK, Lamborn KR, Forstner JM, et al: Radiosurgery for brain metastases: is whole brain radiotherapy necessary? Int J Radiat Oncol Biol Phys 43:549-558, 1999.
29. Regine WF, Huhn JL, Patchell RA, et al: Risk of symptomatic brain tumor recurrence and neurologic deficit after radiosurgery alone in patients with newly diagnosed brain metastases: results and implications. Int J Radiat Oncol Biol Phys 52:333-338, 2002.
30. Patchell RA, Tibbs PA, Regine WF, et al: Postoperative radiotherapy in the treatment of single metastases to the brain: a randomized trial. JAMA 280:1485-1489, 1998.
31. Souhami L, Seiferheld W, Brachman D, et al: Randomized comparison of stereotactic radiosurgery followed by conventional radiotherapy with carmustine to conventional radiotherapy with carmustine for patients with glioblastoma multiforme: report of Radiation Therapy Oncology Group 93-05 protocol. Int J Radiat Oncol Biol Phys 60:853-860, 2004.
32. Sanghavi SN, Miranpuri SS, Chappell R, et al: Radiosurgery for patients with brain metastases: a multi-institutional analysis, stratified by the RTOG recursive partitioning analysis method. Int J Radiat Oncol Biol Phys 51:426-434, 2001.
33. Friedman WA: Radiosurgery versus surgery for arteriovenous malformations: the case for radiosurgery. Clin Neurosurg 45:18-20, 1999.
34. Maesawa S, Salame C, Flickinger JC, et al: Clinical outcomes after stereotactic radiosurgery for idiopathic trigeminal neuralgia. J Neurosurg 94:14-20, 2001.
35. Flickinger JC, Pollock BE, Kondziolka D, et al: Does increased nerve length within the treatment volume improve trigeminal neuralgia radiosurgery? A prospective double-blind, randomized study. Int J Radiat Oncol Biol Phys 51:449-454, 2001.
36. Bradley K, Tome W, Resnick D, et al: Treatment of Trigeminal Neuralgia Using Linear Accelerator-Based Radiosurgery. Basel, Karger, 2004.
37. Hasegawa T, Kondziolka D, Spiro R, et al: Repeat radiosurgery for refractory trigeminal neuralgia. Neurosurgery 50:494-500; discussion 500-502, 2002.
38. Pollock BE, Foote RL, Stafford SL, et al: Results of repeated gamma knife radiosurgery for medically unresponsive trigeminal neuralgia. J Neurosurg 93(Suppl 3):162-164, 2000.
39. Cheuk AV, Chin LS, Petit JH, et al: Gamma knife surgery for trigeminal neuralgia: outcome, imaging, and brainstem correlates. Int J Radiat Oncol Biol Phys 60:537-541, 2004.
40. Haffty BG, Goldberg NB, Gerstley J, et al: Results of radical radiation therapy in clinical stage I, technically operable non-small cell lung cancer. Int J Radiat Oncol Biol Phys 15:69-73, 1988.
41. Sibley GS, Jamieson TA, Marks LB, et al: Radiotherapy alone for medically inoperable stage I non-small-cell lung cancer: the Duke experience. Int J Radiat Oncol Biol Phys 40:149-154, 1998.
42. Slotman BJ, Njo KH, Karim AB: Curative radiotherapy for technically operable stage I nonsmall cell lung cancer. Int J Radiat Oncol Biol Phys 29:33-37, 1994.
43. Timmerman R, Papiez L, McGarry R, et al: Extracranial stereotactic radioablation: results of a phase I study in medically inoperable stage I non-small cell lung cancer. Chest 124:1946-1955, 2003.
44. Song DY, Kavanagh BD, Benedict SH, et al: Stereotactic body radiation therapy. Rationale, techniques, applications, and optimization. Oncology (Huntingt) 18:1419-1430; discussion 1430-1436, 2004.
45. Rogers L: Adult brain tumors: Educational Session 401. Paper presented at the 46th Annual Meeting of the American Society for Therapeutic Radiology and Oncology, 2004, Atlanta, Georgia.

CHAPTER 17

TOTAL BODY IRRADIATION

Brenda Shank

PURPOSES OF TOTAL BODY IRRADIATION

Total body irradiation (TBI) and other large-field variations, such as total lymphoid irradiation (TLI) and total abdominal irradiation (TAI), have played an important role in preparative cytoreductive regimens for hematopoietic cell transplantation (HCT), defined as the intravenous infusion of hematopoietic progenitor cells, in order to restore marrow function in patients with damaged or ablated bone marrow. There are three main purposes of TBI: immunosuppression (lymphocyte cell kill) to allow engraftment of donor stem cells (aplastic anemia); eradication of malignant cells (leukemias, lymphomas, and some solid tumors); and eradication of cell populations with genetic disorders (e.g., Fanconi's anemia, thalassemia major).

ADVANTAGES OF TOTAL BODY IRRADIATION

Theoretical advantages of TBI as a systemic agent compared with chemotherapy are that (1) there is no sparing of "sanctuary" sites such as the testes; (2) the dose delivered is relatively homogeneous and independent of blood supply; (3) there is no cross-resistance with other agents; (4) because no detoxification or excretion of a chemical agent is necessary, there is no alteration of dose distribution if these mechanisms are impaired; and (5) the dose distribution within the body may be tailored by either blocking more sensitive normal tissues or "boosting" sites at greater risk of recurrence.

TBI can have deleterious effects on normal tissues, most notably on the gastrointestinal tract acutely and on lung and lens for late complications, when given in high doses. Because of the toxicity of the high TBI doses, if used alone, that would be required to immunosuppress adequately for consistent donor marrow engraftment and for sufficient eradication of malignancies to obtain cures, TBI has been used at somewhat lower doses, but combined with chemotherapeutic agents. Most commonly in leukemias, cyclophosphamide (Cy) has been used, with the most frequently used schedule being 60 mg/kg/d for 2 days, either before or after TBI. Etoposide (VP-16) has also been frequently used, either instead of Cy or in addition to Cy.

Investigators have attempted to replace TBI with busulfan (Bu) in order to avoid toxicities associated with TBI, but new toxicities attributable to Bu have occurred. It should be noted that one long-term quality-of-life (QOL) study in 22 young adults, who had received a bone marrow transplant 14 years prior on average, demonstrated a generally normal range of functioning, with no influence on QOL based on whether or not they had received TBI as part of their conditioning regimen.[1]

TBI has also been used in considerably lower or "nonmyeloablative" doses (1 to 2 Gy) along with immunotherapy (donor lymphocyte infusions [DLIs]) to achieve marrow chimeras and even sustained remissions in some leukemia patients after autologous grafting.

CYTOREDUCTIVE THERAPY REGIMENS

The International Bone Marrow Transplant Registry (IBMTR), indicated that the majority of allogeneic hematopoietic stem cell transplants (74%) are performed for leukemia.[2] Other malignancies make up 10%, aplastic anemia, 7%, with the remainder being for genetic disorders and immune deficiencies. Because of the continued widespread use of TBI for the leukemias, the use of this modality for the leukemias will be emphasized in this chapter, but important results in other diseases are also included.

In addition, the indications for the use of TAI and TLI are covered briefly. These irradiation fields are often adequate when only immunosuppression is needed, as for aplastic anemia, or when only nodal areas need to be treated, as in refractory Hodgkin's disease without marrow involvement.

Many investigators have been looking at alternative regimens to the standard TBI/Cy regimen, containing only chemotherapy for cytoreduction, to avoid the toxicities attributed to TBI.[3] Although a variety of regimens have been tried, the most common alternative in patients with leukemia has been the use of Bu, in various doses, to replace TBI.[4] However, other toxicities are associated with such regimens, such as seizures,[5,6] a high incidence of veno-occlusive disease (VOD) compared with TBI/Cy,[7-10] and a high incidence of hemorrhagic cystitis compared with TBI/Cy.[7] The incidence of fatal interstitial pneumonitis (IP), however, appears to be low compared with that from TBI/Cy (5% versus 32%), in patients who had received prior thoracic irradiation to doses greater than 20 Gy.[11] Without prior thoracic irradiation, IP incidence and fatalities have been similar in both groups.[7,9,12] A long-term study showed greater long-term lung toxicity with Bu than with TBI on pulmonary function tests in a study of 80 children who had undergone allogeneic BMT.[13] Growth in children given Bu/Cy was found to be no better than that in children who received TBI/Cy in a study from Johns Hopkins University.[14]

An analysis of 123 patients in the Japanese Bone Marrow Transplant Registry indicated a decreased relapse rate (16% versus 37%) and improved overall survival (OS) (77% versus 51%) with TBI-containing regimens (mostly TBI/Cy) compared with chemotherapy-only regimens (mostly Bu/Cy).[12] The importance of Cy dose in the Bu/Cy combination was noted in a retrospective study of children 16 years or younger with acute myeloid leukemia (AML) in first complete remission (CR).[15] The combination of Bu/Cy with 200 mg/kg Cy was equivalent to TBI/Cy for relapse (13% and 10%, respectively) and event-free survival (EFS) (82% and 80%), but inferior to TBI/Cy at a lower dose of Cy (120 mg/kg) in the Bu/Cy regimen, with a 54% relapse rate and only 46% EFS.

Several randomized studies compared Bu/Cy with TBI-containing regimens[16-25] (Table 17-1). In a French multi-institutional study (Groupe d'Etudes de la Greffe de Moelle Osseuse [GEGMO]),[16] there was an advantage to the TBI/Cy regimen over Bu/Cy in AML patients in first remission, in terms of relapse rate, OS and disease-free survival (DFS), and mortality. A long-term follow-up of four randomized studies for myeloid leukemia, which included this GEGMO study, still demonstrated a 10% lower survival rate after Bu/Cy compared with TBI/Cy, but this was not statistically significant.[26] A randomized study of TBI/Cy versus Bu/Cy for autologous purged marrow transplants in AML patients demonstrated that for all end points (relapse, relapse-free survival [RFS], OS,

Table 17-1 **Randomized Studies Comparing Total Body Irradiation–Containing Regimens with Busulfan-Cyclophosphamide for Conventional Allogeneic Bone Marrow Transplantation**

Disease/Stage	ACTUARIAL Regimen/No.	Patients, n	Time of Analysis, y	Disease-Free Survival, %	Actuarial Overall Survival, %	Actuarial Relapse, %	References
AML-1st (GEGMO)	TBI/Cy	50	2	72 (P < .01)	75 (P < .02)	14 (P < .04)	Blaise et al.[16]
	Bu/Cy	51	2	47	51	34	
CML-CP (Seattle)	TBI/Cy	66	3	—	80 (NS)	13 (NS)	Clift et al.[17-19]
	Bu/Cy	68	3	—	78	11	
Acute leukemia >1st and CML >1st CP (SWOG)	TBI/VP16	61	3	25	52*/11† (NS)*/(NS)†	—	Blume et al.[20]
	BU/Cy	61	3	28	37*/24†	—	
CML-CP (GEGMO)	TBI/Cy	56	2	— (NS)	— (NS)	11‡,31§ (P = .04)	Devergie et al.[21]
	Bu/Cy	66	2	—	—	4	
CML-CP (Berlin)	TBI/Cy	16	2	—	63 (P = .24)	—	Schwerdtfeger et al.[22]
	Bu/Cy	16	2	—	81	—	
CML-CP (Baltimore)	TBI/Cy	18	1.7	56	56 (NS)	0 (NS)	Miller et al.[23]
	Bu/Cy	19	1.7	52	52	0	
Acute leukemia/ CML, Early disease	TBI/Cy	61	7	66 (NS)	67 (NS)	27 (NS)	Ringden et al.[24,25]
	Bu/Cy	59	7	68	72	21	
Late disease (Nordic BMTG)	TBI/Cy	18	7	49 (P = .09)	49 (P = .05)	36 (NS)	
	Bu/Cy	29	7	17	17	50	

*"Good-risk" patients.
†"Bad-risk" patients.
‡Single-dose TBI (11%).
§Fractionated TBI (31%).
AML, acute myeloid leukemia; BMTG, Bone Marrow Transplant Group; Bu, busulfan; CML, chronic myeloid leukemia; CP, chronic phase; Cy, cyclophosphamide; GEGMO, Groupe d'Etudes de la Greffe de Moelle Osseuse; NS, not statistically significant; SWOG, Southwest Oncology Group; TBI, total body irradiation; VP-16, etoposide; 1st, first remission.

and incidence of VOD), TBI/Cy was equivalent to or better than Bu/Cy, although with only 35 patients randomized, none of these reached statistical significance.[27] When these randomized patients were analyzed in combination with 40 nonrandomized AML patients, there was a statistically significant improvement in DFS at 2 years (P = .04) in the TBI/Cy subset of patients who were in second or later remission (38% versus 7%).[28]

In chronic myeloid leukemia (CML), TBI-containing regimens appear to be equivalent to Bu/Cy in five randomized studies[17-23] in terms of DFS and OS; however, in the French study,[21] the relapse rate was higher (P = .04) in the TBI/Cy arms (11% for single-dose TBI and 31% for fractionated TBI) compared with the Bu/Cy arm (4%), but there were no differences in either DFS or OS rates. It should be noted that the SWOG study[20] also included acute leukemia patients in greater than first remission as well as CML patients in greater than first chronic phase. The Nordic study,[24,25] however, favored TBI/Cy over Bu/Cy in advanced disease patients, with highly significant differences out to 7 years in both OS and DFS rates.

A randomized trial (allogeneic HCT conditioned with Cy/VP16 with either Bu or TBI) in 43 children younger than 21 years with acute lymphoblastic leukemia (ALL) in first or second remission in 86% found that EFS at 3 years was 58% in the TBI arm and 29% in the Bu arm (P = .03).[29] There was a significant difference for the patients who had received their stem cells from unrelated donors, when subsets were analyzed.

A meta-analysis of randomized studies showed that although DFS and OS were better in the allogeneic transplant groups who had received the TBI-based regimens compared with Bu/Cy, the difference was not significant.[9]

Many other chemotherapeutic agents have been used with or without TBI for cytoreduction prior to transplant. Most frequently used have been VP-16[31] or cytosine arabinoside (AraC).[24] Further discussion of these agents will follow in the section regarding the interaction with chemotherapy under Biological Principles; these agents and others have been reviewed in detail elsewhere.[3,32] Nonmyeloablative TBI regimens are discussed in Engraftment under Results of Clinical Studies.

BIOLOGICAL PRINCIPLES

In Vitro Data

Normal Lymphocytes

Immunosuppression, the clinical manifestation of reduced lymphocyte numbers or activity, is one important function of TBI. Cell culture studies, supported by studies of lymphocyte survival in vivo, demonstrate either no or a very small shoulder to the cell survival curve, indicating minimal repair.[33,34]

Lymphocyte survival in patients undergoing TBI appears similar to the in vitro data; one study of the decrease in absolute lymphocyte concentration during the course of a hyperfractionated TBI regimen showed no shoulder to the survival curve and an *effective* D_0 of about 3.8 Gy, where *effective* D_0 was defined as the fractionated dose required by a given regimen to reduce the cell population to 37% in the straight line portion of the survival curve.[35]

Leukemic Cells

Leukemic cells have also been considered to have either no shoulder or a minimal shoulder to the cell survival curve. Because many investigators have studied survival in a variety of leukemic cells, there are sufficient data to indicate the following: (1) the shoulder and slope of survival curves vary widely for different cell types and for different cell lines from the same type of leukemia[36,37]; (2) some cell lines have no repair at all, whereas others exhibit definite repair[37-39]; and (3) most human hematopoietic cell lines studied have survival curves that fit the linear quadratic (LQ) model of cell survival.[37,39]

In a human acute lymphoblastic leukemia (ALL) cell line (Reh), using a common TBI hyperfractionation regimen (1.25 Gy/fraction, 3 fractions per day), the resulting survival curve could be readily explained by complete repair between fractions and minimal regrowth between fractions.[39] The single-dose survival curve fit the LQ model, with a continuously downward curving appearance.

Animal Data

Immunosuppression

In stem cell transplantation, the degree of immunosuppression is reflected clinically in the success of engraftment of donor stem cells. It was shown in dogs that the rate of bone marrow engraftment increases with increasing doses of irradiation.[40,41] Furthermore, single-dose irradiation was more immunosuppressive in dogs than fractionated irradiation, for the same total dose.[41] This was also demonstrated in mice as measured by splenic lymphocyte cell kill, but in contrast, there was greater bone marrow myeloid eradication with hyperfractionation (total dose of 14.4 Gy) compared with single-dose TBI.[42] Other studies in mice, rats, and monkeys have shown that, with fractionated irradiation, higher total doses are necessary for engraftment with single-dose irradiation.[43,44]

In one murine study,[45] both low-dose-rate, single-dose TBI (0.05 Gy/min) and fractionated TBI required higher total doses for engraftment compared with high-dose-rate, single-dose TBI (1 Gy/min); increasing the interval between fractions from 6 to 24 hours required an additional dose increase. In another murine study, low-dose-rate, single-dose TBI (0.04 Gy/min) to 7.5 Gy total dose was equivalent to a hyperfractionated TBI schedule of 1.25 Gy three times a day to the same total dose, in terms of the effect on the hematopoietic system.[46] No significant repopulation between fractions was seen with the fractionated course.

Using a variety of mouse strains, one group attempted to come up with an optimum TBI protocol, as measured by complete reconstitution with donor cells in hematolymphoid tissues and a high survival rate.[47] They found the optimum regimens to be either 6 Gy or 6.5 Gy twice a day with a 4-hour interval between fractions.

A murine study across various degrees of genetic disparity between donor and host demonstrated that engraftment depended critically on the TBI dose; the required TBI dose increased with greater genetic disparity.[48] Although one might expect that donor T cells would suppress host marrow and therefore enhance engraftment, another murine study showed that the addition of an increasing number of donor T cells did not affect the TBI dose required to achieve equivalent erythroid engraftment.[49]

Leukemia

One important issue has been the sequencing of TBI with Cy; in early marrow transplantation regimens, Cy was given before TBI, but now many centers deliver TBI first, with the advantage of better tolerance of the many fractions of TBI in fractionated regimens, especially when the patient is in the standing position. The results of a murine study suggested that there is a greater antileukemic effect of Cy followed by TBI, compared with the reverse order.[50] This study was done by transferring the spleens from leukemic mice treated with either regimen to nonleukemic mice and monitoring the development of leukemia and survival in the recipient mice.

Lung Toxicity

Radiobiological studies in animals and humans have shown that increasing the number of fractions, for a given total dose, contributes greatly to decreasing the incidence of IP.[51,52] As a corollary, increasing the number of fractions allows one to increase the total dose for the same biological effect. In a murine study, the $LD_{50/30}$ (lethal dose for 50% of the animals in 30 days) due to IP was increased by 21% with an increase from one to six fractions, with a dose rate of 0.25 Gy/min.[51] With a lower dose rate (0.08 Gy/min), the increase in $LD_{50/30}$ with the increased number of fractions was less (14%), but still evident.

Graft-versus-host disease (GVHD) also plays a significant role in the development of IP. In the murine study cited previously that looked at the issue of engraftment as a function of the addition of varying amounts of donor T lymphocytes, it was found that the increasing numbers of T cells significantly increased the risk of pulmonary toxicity.[49]

Sequencing studies in mice have shown that there is less lung damage when Cy is given 12 to 24 hours after TBI compared with 24 to 48 hours before TBI.[53,54] In contrast, a different murine study showed a high incidence of early deaths when the majority of irradiation was given before chemotherapy.[55]

Schedule Optimization (Theoretical)

In 1979 and 1980, Peters and his associates[56,57] suggested that the use of fractionated TBI would be better than single-dose TBI; this suggestion was based on basic radiobiological knowledge of hematopoietic and normal tissue effects. Many clinical studies have shown that a fractionated regimen, either daily fractionation or multiple fractions per day, decreased toxicity in a number of organs. Since then, many investigators have attempted to model the effects of TBI and to optimize its schedule.

Vriesendorp[43,58] took the approach of calculating the surviving fraction of cells, which determines tissue damage and organ function, for various fractionation schemes of TBI, using the multihit multitarget model of cell survival. His calculated results show the impressive sparing of lung and intestines that could be expected with increasingly fractionated TBI regimens. Immune system survival results in this study suggested that immunosuppression with these highly fractionated regimens would be poor; however, when corrected and expanded to include some of the high total dose regimens (15 Gy) in use, immunosuppression was predicted to be excellent with these high total doses, and normal tissues continue to be spared.[59]

Vitale and his colleagues[60] performed calculations on the effectiveness of various dose rates and fractionation schemes for lung and leukemia relative to their own regimen of 9.9 Gy in three fractions at a dose rate of 0.05 Gy/min. They found a greater dose rate effect in lung than in leukemic cells, but this became insignificant in the more highly fractionated schemes such as 15 Gy in 12 fractions. At any dose rate, the antileukemic effect relative to lung was greatest with this highly fractionated regimen which allowed the greatest total dose to be given.

When O'Donoghue and colleagues[61] compared schedules that were isoeffective for lung damage, using a mathematical model for leukemic cell kill that considered leukemic cell doubling time, they concluded that "accelerated hyperfractionation" schedules were optimal. With a minimum of 6 hours between fractions for maximal repair, two fractions per day was considered to be most practical. With no treatments on weekends, they concluded that the optimal schedule for rapidly dividing cells (doubling time of 2 to 4 days) would be 10 fractions of 1.37 Gy per fraction in 5 days. For longer doubling times, a smaller dose per fraction would be optimal. Their recommendation for a practical schedule is 1.3 to 1.5 Gy per fraction for 10 fractions in 5 days. Data at Mount Sinai Medical Center suggested that immunosuppression at 1.5 Gy per fraction as suggested is equivalent to that for the three fractions per day regimen (1.25 Gy/fraction) used extensively at Memorial Sloan-Kettering Cancer Center (MSKCC) to the same total dose (15 Gy); in CML patients, excellent clinical results were achieved with no untoward toxicity.[62,63]

In another publication, O'Donoghue[64] suggested that single-dose, low-dose-rate TBI could potentially be radiobiologically equivalent to fractionated TBI, but this would require unduly long treatment times (about 24 hours), which would be very impractical for most centers.

Calculation of biologically effective doses (BEDs) of multiple regimens in the literature was compared with literature results for relapse incidence, transplant-related mortality, DFS, and OS.[65] It was concluded that "more BED is better," that high-dose TBI regimens were preferable, provided that the dose to lung and kidneys would not cause late normal tissue damage. Highly fractionated regimens, with minimal shielding of lungs only, were thought to be maximally effective, such as 1.65 Gy × 8, 1.5 Gy × 9, or 1.4 Gy × 10 fractions.

Interaction with Chemotherapy

The principal chemotherapeutic agents that have been used with TBI are Cy, VP-16, and AraC. With Cy, toxicities of greatest concern have been IP and hemorrhagic cystitis. In the literature, either Cy alone[66,67] or AraC alone[31,68] can cause IP; it has been difficult to separate the contribution of Cy or AraC to IP when used in combination with TBI, especially when so many other factors are involved. IP is considered further in the section on Toxicity under Results of Clinical Studies.

The agent VP-16 has been increasingly used in regimens for ALL. Major toxicities in combination with TBI have not appeared to be a problem. AraC, on the other hand, has been implicated in an increased risk of renal toxicity, which had been seen rarely in transplant patients when Cy was the only chemotherapeutic agent used.

An aggressive regimen using Cy, VP-16, and carboplatin with TBI (10 to 12.95 Gy in 3 days) was used as a preparative regimen in 60 patients with hematologic malignancies who received autologous marrow, peripheral blood stem cells, or both.[69] Encouraging outcomes were noted in 12 patients with high-risk or advanced AML, with 7 alive and free of disease beyond 5 years.

Optimum sequencing of Cy with TBI has been a major question. In early transplant studies, TBI was given after Cy; when institutions began fractionating irradiation, it was found to be more advantageous for the patient and the department to give TBI before Cy, so that the patient experienced less nausea and vomiting during TBI, especially when the patient was in the standing position as in the treatment protocol developed at MSKCC. There was improved acute tolerance of TBI when this was done, although no randomized studies have addressed this issue. Animal studies (see the previous section on leukemia) have suggested potential advantages for either alternative[50,70]; clinical results have not suggested any advantage for either in terms of relapse or survival, but no randomized studies have been done.

Physiologic Considerations

Orthostatic Hypotension

Occasionally, patients have experienced syncope during the course of TBI in the standing position; most often, this has been attributable to the administration of a phenothiazine, which can cause orthostatic hypotension. Use of nonphenothiazine antiemetics usually ameliorates this problem. Occasionally, especially in patients with aplastic anemia, syncope may be caused by brain hypoxia resulting from a combination of anemia and hypotension in the standing position. Transfusion with packed red cells usually eliminates this problem.

Nausea and Vomiting

The most common acute side effects, regardless of regimen used, have been nausea and vomiting. These have been noted to be less intense with fractionated regimens compared with single dose regimens,[71] but they have persisted. One report indicated that emesis was universal after one fraction of 1.2 Gy in a hyperfractionated regimen and showed that there was a statistically significant diminution over the 4 days of that regimen.[72]

Many agents other than phenothiazines, such as metoclopramide and dexamethasone, have been used in attempts to control emesis. Several studies have attested to the antiemetic efficacy of ondansetron and granisetron, 5-hydroxytryptamine subtype 3 (5-HT_3) antagonists, for TBI.[73,74]

A randomized double-blind, placebo-controlled trial of ondansetron during fractionated TBI showed that ondansetron was superior to placebo for both number of emetic episodes ($P = .005$) and the time to the onset of emesis ($P = .003$) when given prophylactically 1.5 hours before each fraction of TBI.[75] Another double-blind, placebo-controlled trial during single-dose TBI also showed a statistically significant reduction in emetic events with a single 8-mg dose of ondansetron at the initiation of TBI.[76] In a study from Japan of 50 patients conditioned for HCT with high-dose chemotherapy with or without TBI, dexamethasone added to granisetron resulted in better emetic control than granisetron alone, although other nonserious side effects were more frequent, such as insomnia, headache, flushing, and hyperglycemia.[77]

PHYSICAL PRINCIPLES

Reproducibility

To ensure reproducibility from one fraction to another and consistency throughout the course of one fraction, patient position and immobilization must be considered and controlled. Various patient positions were described by Shank.[78] In brief, patients are either treated standing up with anterior and posterior fields, or lying supine and/or prone with anterior and posterior fields, lateral fields, or a combination of both. When the patient is lying down, the patient is comfortable and motion during relatively short fractions (10 to 15 minutes) is minimal. When the patient is standing for that long, however, some form of immobilization is necessary.

Many centers have developed some form of TBI stand to help support and immobilize the patient.[79-82] An example of such a stand developed at MSKCC is shown in Figure 17-1.[59,80] It incorporates a bicycle seat and hand grips for greater patient security, as well as devices to control movement of the thorax region and to support lung shields and port film holders. This stand increased the accuracy and reproducibility of lung shield placement. Another device described in the literature is a plaster vest that also supports lung shields.[83]

Homogeneity

Leukemic cells may be distributed anywhere in the body, including within the skin. Most centers in the United States have used energies that range from that of ^{60}Co (1.25 MV) to 10 MV with a linear accelerator; these energies result in a dose buildup region upon entering tissue, which could potentially result in underdosing the skin. Even higher energies, up to 25 MV, have also been used, especially in Europe, but these would appear to have little advantage.

When energies greater than that of ^{60}Co are used for TBI, it is necessary to introduce a screen made of a tissue-equivalent material between the beam and the patient to maintain dose homogeneity.[78] This screen allows adequate buildup of dose in the skin to prevent underdosage; for example, with 6 MV photons, a screen made of 1 cm Lexan results in a surface dose (at 1 mm) of about 95% relative to the prescribed dose at the midline from that single beam. Of course, the final dose to the surface depends on the exit dose from the opposing beam as well.

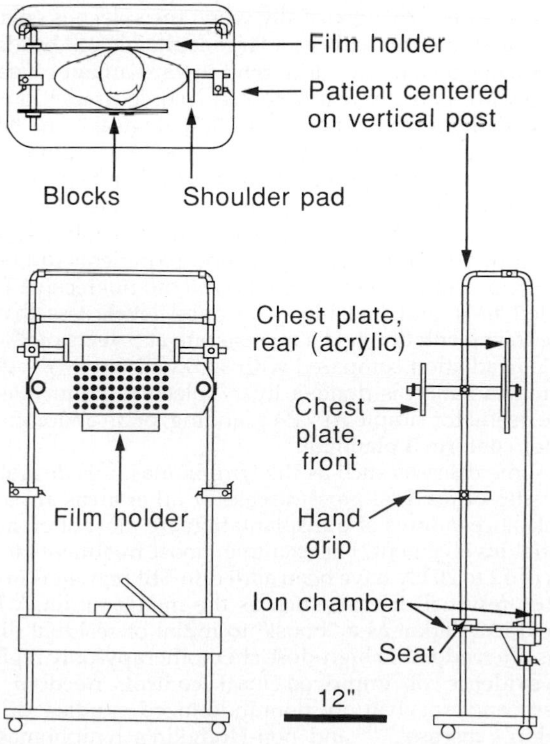

FIGURE 17-1 Total body irradiation support stand designed at the Memorial Sloan-Kettering Cancer Center.

At some institutions, compensators have also been used at the neck, feet, and other areas to increase homogeneity, especially when beams of 10 MV or greater have been used.[78] TBI dose variability within the patient of +5% is considered excellent, but +10% is considered acceptable.

Dose Rate and Dose

When TBI is given in a single dose to a total dose of 10 Gy, it is necessary to use a low dose rate (≤0.05 Gy/min) to decrease the probability of IP.[84,85] When higher dose rates are used, it is necessary to decrease the total dose given,[86,87] although this may contribute to a higher relapse rate as noted in one study when 5 Gy total dose was used at a dose rate of 0.4 to 0.9 Gy/min.[87] For fractionated TBI schedules, the dose rate becomes less important, although in a mouse study, there was still a dose-rate effect for fraction sizes of 2 Gy/fraction or more.[88] When fraction sizes of 1.5 Gy or less are used, dose rates usually range from 0.05 to 0.18 Gy/min.

One group has been studying a TBI regimen at a high dose rate (0.3 Gy/min) to a total dose of 5.5 Gy with Cy for conditioning, and cyclosporine as GVHD prophylaxis.[89-91] When related donor HCT was done, there were no graft failures in 27 good-risk patients (acute leukemia in first remission and CML in chronic phase) and 53 poor-risk patients (all others).[89] In the good-risk group, transplant-related mortality (TRM) through 2 years or more was 7%, relapse was 15%, and 3-year DFS and OS were 77% and 85%, respectively. In the poor-risk group, TRM was 19%, relapse was 45%, and DFS and OS were 34% and 36%, respectively.

The same group looked at chimerism and outcomes using this 5.5-Gy TBI regimen with HCT from HLA-matched unrelated donors (26 good-risk patients as defined in their matched donor study earlier and 84 poor-risk patients).[90] Donor chimerism was 100% in 86% (78 of 91) evaluable patients. DFS and OS were 40% and 47%, respectively, in the good-risk group, and 21% and 25%, respectively, in the poor-risk group.

In another publication from this group,[91] they looked only at 32 consecutive adults with AML who underwent this 5.5-Gy TBI regimen (15 in first remission [CR1] and 17 in second or greater remission [CR ≥2]). There was no graft failure. TRM was 13% in CR1 patients and 41% in CR ≥2 patients. Relapse occurred in 22%. At median follow-up of 2.2 years, DFS and OS Kaplan-Meier estimates were 57% and 55% for the CR1 patients and 39% for both in the CR ≥2 patients.

At the large distances used to ensure that the entire unflexed body is in the beam with some margin around the patient, the dose rate is usually in the desired range. For infants, who may be treated supine and prone on a mat on the floor (closer to the head of the machine compared with adults), it may be desirable to reduce the dose rate by means of Pb (lead) beam attenuators.

Blocking

Many centers use lung shields during TBI. Most use partially attenuating shields (one half-value layer [HVL]) throughout the course of treatment,[92] but at least one institution has used thick blocks (seven HVLs) for one treatment of the TBI course with none the remainder of the time.[93] Some institutions have attempted to shield the lungs with the patient's arms, by treating the patient laterally. However, the position is difficult to reproduce and it is difficult to assess the dosimetry; this method is not recommended.

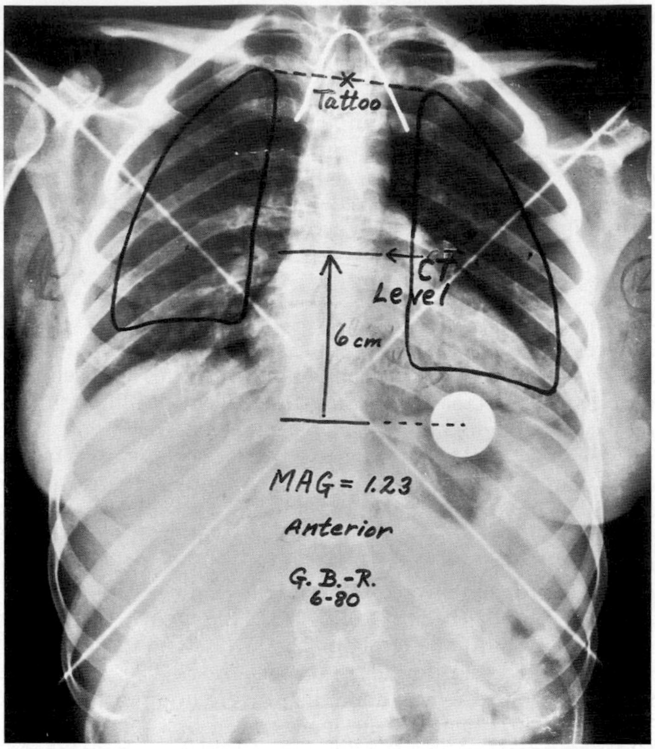

FIGURE 17-2 Example of a simulation for lung blocks. The patient is in the standing position with a wire marker on the skin as a reference point and a quarter on the skin to aid in the calculation of magnification.

It is relatively easy to simulate treatment with the patient in the standing position (Fig. 17-2). Films are taken in both the anterior and the posterior position with a wire marker on the skin as a reference point. After the blocks are designed on the anterior film, a final reference point may be determined both anteriorly and posteriorly for a tattoo to guide block placement during the course of treatment: midway between the blocks at a level corresponding to the superior edge of the blocks. The same blocks, carefully labeled as to *right* and *left*, may be used both anteriorly and, when reversed, posteriorly for treatment.

One institution has used partial-transmission liver shielding to decrease the incidence of VOD and has also used renal shielding (70% transmission) to minimize renal dysfunction in the setting of cytoreduction that includes both AraC and Cy.[94] Late renal dysfunction (at 18 months) was significantly less with the use of these blocks.[95] Long-term results with respect to relapse and survival are not available.

With leukemias, it has been thought that the lenses should not be shielded because of possible eye or orbital involvement with disease. In practice, this may not be an issue (see discussion on cataracts in Toxicity under Results of Clinical Studies). With some diseases, it is useful to use eye shielding. For example, in aplastic anemia, when the donor is unrelated, intensive cytoreduction is necessary for engraftment, but there are no malignant cells to be concerned about. When TBI is part of such a cytoreductive regimen, adjustable eye shields can be used, as was done at MSKCC in a protocol for aplastic anemia patients.[96] Of course, if intensive cytoreduction is not necessary, TLI or TAI may be used with the eyes outside of the fields.

"Boosting"

When lung blocks were instituted during TBI, it was thought necessary to supplement the dose to marrow-containing ribs in the area of the lung blocks to ensure that an adequate dose was given to all potential sites of leukemia.[92] When this was done, careful CT treatment planning through the area beneath the lung blocks was necessary so that the appropriate energy of electrons and thickness of bolus were used.

Such "boosting" is probably not necessary. Dutreix and colleagues[97] calculated that blocking lungs was theoretically equivalent to merely lowering the total body dose by a small percentage. On that basis, the Institut Gustave-Roussy did not add an electron boost to lungs. They reported no difference in relapse rate in their patients compared with other centers where lung boosts were given.[98] As a result, many centers have eliminated this step.

In the Seattle experience, 25% of the boys who survived more than 5 months after transplantation developed primary testicular relapse.[99] After noting a high relapse rate in the testes in the MSKCC patients with leukemia (4 of 28 males), Shank and colleagues[100] added a 4-Gy testes boost with electrons to all their leukemia TBI protocols. This was usually given in one fraction unless prior testicular irradiation had been given. With prior testicular treatment, this dose was split into two fractions in 2 days, or not given at all if that treatment was within 1 to 2 months of the transplantation. No further relapses occurred in greater than 300 male patients after this added boost. In 94 boys with acute leukemia treated with a testicular boost added to TBI at Duke University Medical Center, two boys had relapse in the testes, for a failure rate of 4.2% in those who survived for at least 1 year.[101] In 36 boys who received chemotherapy alone, none had primary testicular failure. The authors concluded that there was a low incidence of primary testicular failure in either group.

Splenic irradiation before TBI is a logical boost treatment in patients with CML, especially when the spleen is enlarged, because it frequently harbors a large leukemic cell burden. In a European study, there was a trend toward an improved survival in CML patients who received splenic irradiation compared with those who did not.[102] Radiobiological[103] and clinical studies[104] support this concept. In a prospective randomized study, however, no significant survival advantage was seen when splenic irradiation was given up to 14 days before BMT in 239 patients with chronic-phase CML, but follow-up was quite short.[105] In an update, one subset of patients did benefit with splenic irradiation.[106] Patients who did not receive T cell–depleted BMT and had blood basophil levels less than 3% before transplantation had a relapse rate at 8 years of 8% with splenic irradiation compared with 30% without it ($P < .05$). If splenic irradiation is done, a liver/spleen radionuclide scan can be useful for simple AP/PA planning, or an abdominal CT scan for conformal planning.

In some diseases such as the lymphomas, it is desirable to boost sites of residual gross disease or other areas at particular risk since failures of transplantation are most often in sites of initial involvement. For example, boost treatments to total doses of 12 to 20 Gy have been added to TBI regimens in areas of gross residual disease, such as the mediastinum.[107] Locoregional irradiation as a "boost" to initial or residual disease sites is often added to high-dose chemotherapy-only regimens with evidence of improved local control, freedom from relapse, and survival in nonrandomized studies of both Hodgkin's disease[108-111] and non-Hodgkin's lymphomas.[112-114] The treatment volume and optimal timing of such a boost (pre- or post-TBI and transplant) is not established. One group is doing a clinical trial to investigate prospectively this timing.[115]

A novel type of supplemental treatment that may be thought of as a hematopoietic boost is the use of antibody radionuclide conjugates, with or without TBI and/or chemotherapy; various radionuclide and antibody combinations are under active investigation.[116-121]

Special Dosimetry

Special considerations contribute to the dose distribution in the patient when TBI is used. For example, with a patient in the standing position at one end of a room at a large distance from the source, the gantry may be angled in a way that increases the distance from the source to the feet compared with the distance from the source to the vertex, resulting in a lesser dose to the feet than to the vertex. There is a large amount of internal scatter from within the patient, and scatter from the wall behind the patient and even from the TBI stand itself. With any given setup at an institution, it is important to make careful measurements on many patients of the dose at various sites, including behind lung blocks, to understand the dose distribution for that system. At the low dose rates encountered, ion chambers are usually the best means of measuring the doses. For extensive discussions of dosimetry and dose calibration, see the publications of Briot and colleagues[122] and Van Dyk and colleagues.[123,124]

RESULTS OF CLINICAL STUDIES

Immunosuppression

Engraftment

With conventional matched sibling allografts, nonengraftment is rare (1% to 2%);[125,126] engraftment, as measured by a white blood cell greater than 500/mm^3, is noted from 1.5 to 3 weeks from the day of BMT (median, 17 days).[35] In human leukocyte antigen (HLA)-nonidentical transplants from related nonsibling donors, graft failure was found to be a function of the degree of donor incompatibility.[126]

When donor marrow has been T cell–depleted as a means of preventing GVHD, graft failures have been more frequent. Single-dose TBI (7.5 to 10 Gy) has been shown to be more effective in preventing rejection than fractionated TBI to a relatively low total dose of 10 to 12 Gy.[127-130] Many reports have indicated that either higher total doses of fractionated TBI[131-134] or the addition of TLI to TBI[127,135-139] may prevent graft rejection in a large proportion of patients receiving T cell–depleted marrow, although this improvement has not always been found with either increased TBI dose[140,141] or the addition of TLI.[142] In the analysis of T cell–depleted transplants performed by the IBMTR,[130] higher total doses (≥11 Gy) and higher dose rates (≥0.14 Gy/min) were associated with significantly fewer rejections.

Single fraction low-dose "nonmyeloablative" TBI (1 to 2 Gy) has been used as immunosuppressive therapy prior to HCT and allogeneic DLI.[143,144] Donor chimerism, often unstable, has been achieved, as have sustained complete remissions in some patients, but GVHD has been a problem. In a multicenter study, 45 patients with HLA-identical sibling donors, who were ineligible for conventional preparation for HCT due to age or medical contraindications, were treated with 2-Gy single-fraction TBI prior to HCT, with cyclosporine and mycophenolate mofetil (MMF) given concurrently and after HCT for additional immunosuppression and GVHD prevention.[143] DLI was given based on the presence of stable mixed chimerism and absence of GVHD, or for persistent or progressive disease. Approximately 80% achieved an early mixed chimerism, but it was usually unstable. Acute and chronic GVHD were appreciable. Of those with sustained engraftment, 53% were in CR. In a study of 11 patients with refractory hematologic malignancies treated with 1-Gy single-fraction TBI and sibling donor cells, 9 achieved donor chimerism and 4 had sustained CR.[144] Such studies have shown the feasibility and potential of such an approach.

Comparisons between nonmyeloablative and myeloablative conditioning regimens have been published for HCT from HLA-matched related donors[145] and from HLA-matched unrelated donors,[146] as well as a comparison between a nonmyeloablative regimen and a "reduced-intensity" conditioning (RIC) regimen for HCT in a mix of leukocyte antigen-identical sibs and unrelated donors.[147] The nonmyeloablative regimen was, in all of these reports, 2-Gy single-fraction TBI combined with fludarabine, or, in the HLA-matched related donor study,[145] the same TBI alone in 40 of the 73 patients studied. In all studies, post-HCT immunosuppression was done in these groups with cyclosporine and MMF. Myeloablative conditioning regimens were TBI/Cy or Bu/Cy primarily, with post-HCT immunosuppression with methotrexate and cyclosporine. RIC consisted of fludarabine combined with Bu or Cy, ATG, and post-HCT methotrexate and cyclosporine. In general, there was less regimen-related toxicity (RRT)[145] and fewer grade III-IV toxicities[146] in the nonmyeloablative groups than in the myeloablative group. In the unrelated donor study, there was also a lesser incidence of Grade III-IV acute GVHD in the nonmyeloablative group. These results were obtained in spite of greater age and comorbidities in the nonmyeloablative groups. In contrast, in the study where the comparison group was RIC, the nonmyeloablative group had more acute GVHD and transplant-related mortality, as well as more graft failures than the RIC group.[147]

Aplastic Anemia and Fanconi's Anemia

In severe aplastic anemia, large-field irradiation is useful only to prevent rejection since there are no malignant cells to eradicate. To prevent rejection, Cy alone is insufficient, so cytoreductive regimens have usually included either TBI or TLI to enhance engraftment, either as a single dose[148,149] or fractionated.[96] The advantage of using TLI for immunosuppression is that normal tissues outside of the field can be spared, namely brain and eye, kidneys, lungs, and much of the small bowel. Shank and colleagues[96] have determined that, for a one-log peripheral blood lymphocyte decrease, TBI to 6 Gy is equivalent to TLI to 10 Gy, when fractionated as done at MSKCC: TBI in 2-Gy daily fractions and TLI given in 1-Gy fractions, three fractions per day.

In patients with aplastic anemia who receive T cell–depleted marrow transplants, no rejection and no GVHD was seen when the TLI dose was increased to 18 Gy with twice-daily fractions, although follow-up was short.[137,138] TAI has also been used for severe aplastic anemia and, more commonly, for Fanconi's anemia.[150,151] These fields do not spare small bowel and kidneys, but they spare brain, eyes, and lung and are easy to administer in small children, because the block arrangement is less complicated. The Seattle group has reported on one patient with Fanconi's anemia who had reduced toxicity and prompt sustained engraftment (>10-month follow-up) with a minimal conditioning regimen of TBI to 2 Gy and 90 mg/m^2 fludarabine, and postgrafting immunosuppression with cyclosporine and mycophenolate for HCT from an HLA-matched unrelated donor.[152] Some regimens do not use any irradiation, such as one reported by the Seattle group, which consists of only Cy and antithymocyte globulin.[153]

Long-term survival in severe aplastic anemia is generally in the range of 65% to 75%, but GVHD has remained a problem.[154] Survival at 5 years for Fanconi's anemia patients who have been transplanted is similar.[155] The most serious long-term complication encountered with the anemias has been second malignancies; this is discussed in the section on Toxicity.

Eradication of Malignancy

Dose, Dose Rate, Fractionation Studies

Leukemic relapse is a reflection of the efficacy of leukemic cell kill, which is dependent on many factors in addition to the cytoreductive transplant regimen; these factors include the leukemic cell burden, pretransplant chemotherapy, drug resistance, and graft-versus-leukemia effect.

Several studies have examined the influence of total TBI dose, dose rate, and fractionation on leukemic relapse. Three randomized studies in Seattle compared schedules.[156-161] These studies showed that the higher doses, which can be achieved with fractionation, decrease the relapse rate as might be expected radiobiologically. In the CML study, survival was initially lower in the high-dose group because of an increased early mortality, but at 5 years, there was no statistically significant difference in survival.[156,159] In the first AML study comparing single-dose TBI with fractionated daily TBI, survival was significantly better with fractionated TBI.[157,160] In the second study, which compared two daily fractionation schemes, no difference in survival was seen.[158,161]

Dose escalation has been attempted to levels above 15 Gy for TBI.[162,163] One study achieved a maximum tolerated dose of 16 Gy in 2-Gy fractions given twice a day 6 hours apart.[162] Another study used 50% lung transmission blocks with electron chest wall boosts in those areas, and kidney shielding to a maximum dose of 16 Gy.[163] In nine patients receiving autologous peripheral blood stem cells, with three patients each at 16 Gy, 18 Gy, and 20 Gy (2 Gy/fraction twice daily), toxicity was moderate with four patients achieving complete remissions, and one remaining disease free at 5 years posttransplant.

Results from nonrandomized studies with regard to relapse rate are quite variable, with only a study from Genoa showing a significant difference in relapse rate.[164-165] In that study, patients with CML and AML were treated with a nominal dose of 9.9 Gy given in three fractions of 3.3 Gy each. Actual doses calculated retrospectively, however, were found to differ considerably. The difference in relapse between patients who received greater than 9.9 Gy compared with patients who received less than 9.9 Gy translated into a highly significant difference in survival (74% at 8 years compared with only 38%, respectively). The total dose was the most significant factor influencing relapse; dose rate was of only borderline significance.

In a more recent study from Genoa of leukemia patients who received HCT from HLA-matched unrelated donors, low-dose TBI (9.9 Gy in 3 daily fractions) with Cy was inferior to 12 Gy TBI (2-Gy fractions twice a day for 3 days) with Cy.[166] The relapse rate at 5 years was 13% for the 12-Gy regimen compared with 31% for the 9.9-Gy regimen. Multivariate analysis demonstrated that the 9.9-Gy daily regimen was an adverse predictor for 5-year OS (51% versus 68% for the 12-Gy regimen) and for relapse rate.

Acute Lymphoblastic Leukemia

Comparative studies between allogeneic BMT and maintenance chemotherapy for ALL have shown decreased relapse rates and improved DFS in the BMT arm of the studies,[167-171] but this was not statistically significant in all. The success of transplant depends upon remission status. In children with ALL in second remission, the relapse rate at 5 years is only 13% and DFS is 64%.[172]

The Seattle group compared two fractionated dose schedules in a nonrandomized study: 2.25 Gy daily for 7 days to 15.75 Gy total dose (26 patients), and 1.2 Gy three times daily for 4 days to 14.4 Gy total dose (23 patients).[173] The group receiving the 15.75 Gy total dose had a lower relapse rate and better DFS at 3 years, but these differences were not statistically significant.

Allogeneic transplant, when a matched donor is available, has the advantage over autologous transplant, based on the available data (Table 17-2). A study from Rome has demonstrated a significantly better DFS and lower relapse rate for allogeneic BMT compared with autologous BMT,[174] whereas others show a significantly lower relapse rate but no difference in disease-free survival[169] or a trend toward a higher DFS rate with allogeneic transplants.[175-177] For patients who do not have matched donors for an allogeneic transplant, however, an autologous BMT is possible using marrow that was obtained in remission and then purged of leukemic cells by chemotherapeutic or immunologic methods.[169,174-177] An advantage of autologous BMT over chemotherapy alone has not been conclusively demonstrated, but data suggest an improved DFS with autologous BMT[169]; the major disadvantage is a high relapse rate, which suggests either that the graft-versus-leukemia effect is important or that purging is insufficient. Long-term DFS is in the range of 25% to 30%, with the best results in patients in first remission.

Acute Myeloid Leukemia

In AML, a large number of studies have shown an improved DFS rate with BMT compared with continued chemotherapy (Table 17-3) in adults[178-184] and children.[181,185-187] OS or crude OS was better with BMT than with continued chemotherapy in two studies in adults.[188,189] Not much difference has been observed between allogeneic and autologous BMT (see Table

Table 17-2 Percentage Disease-Free Survival of Acute Lymphoblastic Leukemia Patients According to Type of Transplant

Study/Reference No.	Population	Disease-Free Survival, % *Allo BMT*	*Auto BMT*	Time of Analysis (y)
Rome[174]	C+A, CR1	52	29	3
Italy[177]	C, CR1	57	50	2.5
Newcastle[169]	A, CR1	30	30	3
France[175]	C+A, CRl	71	40	4
Minneapolis[176]	C, CR2	27	20	4

A, adults; Allo, allogeneic; Auto, autologous; BMT, bone marrow transplantation; C, children; CR1, first remission; CR2, second remission.

Table 17-3 **Percentage Disease-Free Survival of Acute Myeloid Leukemia Patients According to Postinduction Treatment**

Study/Reference	Population	Disease-Free Survival, % Allo BMT	Auto BMT	Chemo	Time of Analysis, y
UCLA[188]	Adults	40*	—	27*	4
Seattle/SWOG[180]	Adults	48	—	26	4
Royal Marsden[181]	Children + adults	61	—	29	3
CCG[185]	Children	47	—	34	8
CCG†[192]	Children	55	51	—	3
IBMTR-German AML Coop. Group[178]	Adults	54	—	40	3
Paris (SHIP)[186]	Children	83	—	52	3
	Adults	54	49	30	4
EORTC[179]	Adults	42	54	—	3
ECOG[190]	Adults	36‡	—	19‡	3
M. D. Anderson[189]	Children	43	—	31	6
AML-80[187]	Adults	51	35	—	3
Netherlands[191]	Adults	66	41	16	2.5
Bordeaux (BGMT)[182]	Adults	41	—	27	7
Lyon[183]					
Spain[184]	Adults	70	—	10	3
	Adults <45 y	70	—	17	3

*Overall survival.
†Included patients with myelodysplastic syndrome.
‡Crude overall survival.
Allo, allogeneic; AML, acute myeloid leukemia; Auto, autologous; BMT, bone marrow transplantation; Chemo, chemotherapy; IBMTR, International Bone Marrow Transplant Registry.

17-3),[179,182,190-192] with DFS for either being about 50%. Long-term leukemia-free survival from IBMTR data is 51% for patients in first remission, 31% in second or greater remission, and 21% in relapse.[130] In an analysis from MSKCC, children with AML had a 0% relapse rate when transplanted in first remission and 13% in second remission, and DFS was about 70% for either first or second remission.[172] These low relapse rates were attributed to the high total TBI dose (13.2 to 14.4 Gy) used with their hyperfractionated regimen, the addition of a 4-Gy testes boost, and the sequencing of Cy after TBI.

Two randomized scheduling trials for AML in first remission have been done in Seattle.[157,158,160,161] First, single-dose TBI was compared with daily fractionation[157,160] (six fractions of 2 Gy each for a total dose of 12 Gy). EFS was significantly better with the daily fractionation scheme, primarily due to decreased early mortality. When this same fractionation scheme was compared with another daily fractionation scheme (seven fractions of 2.25 Gy each for a total dose of 15.75 Gy) in a second trial, there was no difference in RFS (both about 55% at 6 years).[158,161] Although the relapse rate was less with the regimen with the higher total dose of 15.75 Gy, mortality was also greater.

Chronic Myeloid Leukemia

Many studies have shown that CML patients have a better survival rate when transplanted in the first chronic phase. Long-term DFS for patients in first chronic phase who have been transplanted with nonmanipulated marrow from a matched sibling donor is about 60% to 70%.[159,193,194] With T cell depletion of donor marrow, there is an increased risk of relapse, resulting in a lower DFS rate.[195] In either group, with or without T cell depletion, patients who develop chronic GVHD have less risk of relapse, demonstrating a graft-versus-leukemia effect as well.

In the same patients in the Genoa study described at the beginning of this section on the eradication of malignancy, a later analysis was done that looked at the presence of mixed chimerism, that is, the presence of host marrow cells as well as donor cells.[196] It was found that the patients who did not have mixed chimerism were the patients who had received the higher mean TBI dose (>9.9 Gy); these patients were more likely to remain in remission.

In elderly CML patients with matched sibling or unrelated donors, a reduced-intensity conditioning regimen using TBI to 8 Gy, combined with lower-dose Cy, with fludarabine, ATG, cyclosporine, and methotrexate for immunosuppression, good early results have been obtained, especially when performed within the first year of diagnosis (OS = 79%).[197] Transplant-related mortality was only 11% at day 100+.

Lymphomas

Non-Hodgkin's Lymphomas

The first marrow transplants in patients with non-Hodgkin's lymphoma were done on patients in relapse; the surprising success in some of these otherwise hopeless patients encouraged others to perform BMT earlier in the course of intermediate or high-grade non-Hodgkin's lymphoma. It was shown that aggressive cytoreduction (TBI/Cy) followed by autologous BMT as early treatment was highly successful in patients with the poor prognostic features of high serum lactic dehydrogenase or bulky mediastinal or abdominal disease.[107,198,199] At 5 years, 79% of patients were alive and free of disease in the group who underwent autologous BMT after induction chemotherapy, compared with only 31% in the group of patients who elected to wait and undergo BMT only at failure of chemotherapy.

From data gathered by the European Bone Marrow Transplant Group (EBMTG), patients who have relapsed but responded to chemotherapy, achieving a complete or partial response, may achieve a 40% progression-free survival at 5 years after an autologous BMT.[200] With a more aggressive cytoreductive regimen (TBI/VP-16/Cy), even patients with relapsed and resistant disease may be successfully treated (57% DFS at a median follow-up of >42 months).[201-203]

Some patients may not be considered good candidates for an autologous BMT, because of severe marrow dysfunction or the presence of lymphoma in the marrow, but may have a matched donor for an allogeneic BMT. Although GVHD and regimen-related toxicity are higher than with an autologous BMT, the relapse rate is low, perhaps as a result of a "graft-versus-lymphoma" effect. A case-control study by the EBMTG demonstrated that there was no difference in progression-free survival, even though there was a statistically significant greater relapse rate in the autologous group (48% versus 24%).[204]

When locoregional "boost" irradiation to areas of gross or residual disease has been added to cytoreductive regimens for SCT in non-Hodgkin's lymphoma patients, relapse has been less and EFS is greater than when no irradiation is done.[112-114]

The role of BMT in low-grade non-Hodgkin's lymphoma is as yet undefined.[205] The indolent course of most of these patients makes it difficult to justify the risks of early mortality from BMT, and makes investigational studies difficult to assess, because results will be meaningful only after a decade or more.

Nonmyeloablative conditioning regimens may prove to be particularly advantageous in low-grade lymphoproliferative disorders in preparation for allogeneic HCT.[206] The addition of involved field irradiation prior to TBI did not increase short-term toxicity in 11 patients undergoing autologous HCT for advanced-stage low-grade non-Hodgkin's lymphoma after induction chemotherapy, compared with patients who received TBI alone.[207]

There is a long history (since 1923) of reports documenting excellent symptomatic and objective responses in patients with highly radiosensitive tumors (lymphomas and leukemias) treated with low-dose TBI without BMT. The most rewarding responses were in the indolent non-Hodgkin's lymphomas and in chronic lymphocytic leukemia. Typical regimens, from 1975 on, consisted of 10 to 15 cGy per fraction, two or three fractions per week, to a total dose of 150 to 200 cGy. Although as many as 80% to 85% of lymphoma patients achieved a complete response,[208,209] few studies had long-term follow-up, and hematopoietic toxicity has been severe in some studies. Results of randomized comparisons of TBI versus chemotherapy for chronic lymphocytic leukemia have been mixed, with two studies favoring TBI[210,211] and one favoring chemotherapy (chlorambucil and prednisone),[212] but in all of these studies, follow-up was short. In another study with both chronic lymphocytic leukemia and indolent lymphoma patients, TBI and chemotherapy with the same agents as above were equivalent.[213] One long-term study demonstrated a recurrence-free survival of 19% at 10 years after TBI for advanced-stage low-grade non-Hodgkin's lymphoma. This excellent survival without any maintenance therapy suggested that low-dose TBI should be first-line therapy in this group of patients.[214]

Hodgkin's Disease

Patients with refractory or relapsed Hodgkin's disease also may be salvaged by BMT. In patients who had not had prior irradiation, a group at MSKCC found DFS to be 65% at 20+ month follow-up using a regimen involving boost irradiation to any areas of gross disease, followed by TLI/VP-16/Cy and autologous BMT.[215,216] A later analysis in 56 patients who underwent transplantation yielded a 68% EFS and 81% OS.[217]

In Seattle, various regimens were used over a period of 21 years for such patients; more than half of the regimens did not use irradiation, and the rest incorporated TBI.[218] These investigators concluded that (1) BMT should be performed early after relapse and (2) HLA-matched sibling marrow resulted in a lower relapse rate compared with autologous marrow.

Patients who have received prior irradiation usually are not eligible for either a TLI- or TBI-containing preparative regimen. At Stanford, a nonrandomized comparison of patients receiving an autologous BMT after either chemotherapy (bis-chloroethyl-nitrosourea [BCNU]) or TBI/VP-16/Cy demonstrated no difference at 4 years in relapse, OS, or EFS between the two regimens, but the populations differed with respect to prior therapy.[219] In a later study, Stanford patients with relapsed Hodgkin's disease who had locoregional irradiation added to their high-dose therapy regimens did better than those who did not, based on 3-year freedom-from-relapse survival and EFS.[220] Other studies have shown similar improved results with the addition of involved field irradiation.[221,222]

A SWOG Phase II trial studied augmented preparative regimens prior to autologous BMT in 81 relapsed or refractory Hodgkin's disease patients.[223] Conditioning was done with VP-16/Cy/TBI or, if previously irradiated, with VP-16/Cy/carmustine. Results were promising with a 5-year progression-free survival and OS of 41% and 54%, respectively, without an increase in regimen-related mortality.

Toxicity

Acute Side Effects

The most obvious acute side effects are nausea and vomiting, which usually occur a few hours after the first fraction of fractionated irradiation and have been noted to decrease with time over a course of hyperfractionated irradiation. The successful use of ondansetron or granisetron to control this has been described in the section on physiologic considerations.

Other acute side effects frequently encountered include oral mucositis, diarrhea, and parotiditis. These, along with nausea and vomiting, have been shown to be less with hyperfractionated (twice-daily) irradiation compared with single-dose irradiation in a French study that randomized dose rates but not fractionation.[224,225] The dose rate per se had no obvious effect on acute side effects for either fractionation. Another study showed that no parotiditis occurred with fractionated TBI (12 Gy in six fractions) compared with a 40% incidence with single-dose TBI (10 Gy).[226]

The major factor responsible for the transient xerostomia associated with BMT is probably TBI.[227] Some patients develop severe dental caries without fluoride prophylaxis; dental assessment and fluoride prophylaxis are recommended for all TBI patients. Prophylactic acyclovir, effective against herpes simplex virus, was found to be very effective in decreasing the severity of mucositis.[228] Pentoxyfylline was thought initially in clinical observations to decrease mucositis and other later toxicities of acute GVHD, VOD, and renal insufficiency; however, in a randomized controlled trial, it was found to be of no benefit.[229] In an analysis from Seattle of CML patients who underwent allogeneic HCT, predictors of oral mucositis were TBI in the conditioning regimen rather than Bu, elevated body mass index ($\geq$25), or having the methylenetetrahydrofolate reductase *677TT* genotype.[230] Pretransplant multivitamin use resulted in lower mucositis scores compared with patients who did not use vitamin supplements.

Fatigue occurs over the course of TBI with any fractionation scheme. Some patients will develop skin erythema and, later, even hyperpigmentation.

Late Toxicities

Regimen-Related Toxicity

The term *regimen-related toxicity* refers to all toxicities related to the preparative (cytoreductive) regimen[231] and should be distinguished from transplant-related morbidity, which can refer to other toxicities related to transplantation, such as from prophylactic medications, pancytopenia, or GVHD. An empirical grading system for eight individual organs was devised by the Seattle group.[232] When all regimen-related toxicities were grouped together, one study showed that the only major factor that increased the risk in allogeneic transplant patients was higher TBI dose, in a comparison of two regimens with daily fractionation (12 Gy in six fractions of 2 Gy, versus 15.75 Gy in seven fractions of 2.25 Gy).[231] Although the higher dose was administered more commonly to relapsed patients and patients who received mismatched grafts, the TBI dose was still the only high-risk factor for allogeneic transplant patients that emerged in a multivariate analysis. An allogeneic BMT per se increased the risk for regimen-related toxicity compared with an autologous transplant.

Graft-Versus-Host Disease

The immune response of donor T lymphocytes against host normal tissues despite apparent histocompatibility between donor and host, that is, GVHD, can be a significant contributor to organ toxicity. Acute GVHD is a distinctive syndrome consisting, to variable degrees, of dermatitis, hepatitis, and enteritis, appearing within 100 days of allogeneic transplant.

Acute GVHD may be staged (+1 to +4) at each organ site by severity, based on (1) the intensity of the skin rash and percentage of body surface area involved, (2) the extent of bilirubin elevation for liver involvement, and (3) the severity of diarrhea for the gastrointestinal tract.[233] An overall grade of GVHD from 0 (none) to IV (life-threatening), which predicts the clinical course, is then assigned based on the staging at each organ site. IP, as discussed later, is related to the severity of acute GVHD. The histopathology has been well described in the literature.[234]

Chronic GVHD, which is considered to develop more than 100 days after allogeneic transplantation, tends to result in more widespread organ involvement (skin, liver, lung, eye, and gastrointestinal tract) and behaves more like an autoimmune process.

Many agents have been used for the prevention of acute GVHD, such as methotrexate alone, cyclosporine alone, combined methotrexate and cyclosporine, or a regimen of methotrexate, antithymocyte globulin, and prednisone. The latter regimen decreased the incidence of GVHD when compared in a randomized study to methotrexate alone.[235] Methotrexate combined with cyclosporine was superior to cyclosporine alone in another randomized study, demonstrating an advantage in survival as well as in GVHD reduction.[236]

Other approaches to reducing GVHD include the use of polyvalent intravenous immunoglobulin,[237] thalidomide,[238] and donor marrow T lymphocyte depletion.[239,240] Although the latter technique can be highly successful in eliminating GVHD, problems encountered include graft failure and, in patients with CML, a higher incidence of relapse, presumably due to the loss of a graft-versus-leukemia capability during the T lymphocyte–depletion process.

Interstitial Pneumonitis

One of the major contributors to mortality after BMT has been IP, with a minimum incidence of about 20% even in patients who have not received TBI as part of their cytoreductive regimen.[93] IP had been fatal in approximately two thirds of patients who developed it,[92,93] but there are fewer fatalities with the advent of treatment with combined ganciclovir and immunoglobulin,[241,242] for IP caused by one of the organisms most frequently responsible, cytomegalovirus.

Complicating any analysis of IP and its risk factors is the use of varying definitions of IP in the literature. Some investigators consider only idiopathic IP, while others consider all IP, including that of known infectious cause. The time frame also varies, with some considering only IP which develops in 100 days or less, while others may consider any IP, even as remote as 1 to 2 years after BMT. It is advisable to consider all IP, but to define the causes, since the cytoreductive regimen could potentially play a role in IP of any cause, even infectious.

Despite the difficulties cited, some factors that put patients at risk for developing IP have been identified. Factors that may increase the risk can be divided into patient-related factors over which we have no or little control, such as older patient age, increased body weight,[243] 1.5 m^2 or greater body surface area,[244] male sex,[245] and a diagnosis of CML compared with other leukemias.[232,246] GVHD, over which we only have partial control, has been shown in many studies to increase the risk of IP.[244-250] The use of T cell–depleted transplants, which minimizes the incidence and severity of GVHD, results in a very low incidence of IP.[71,140,251-253]

The immediate cause of IP can often be diagnosed as an infectious agent, such as cytomegalovirus or *Pneumocystis carinii*. Patients who are seropositive for cytomegalovirus, or who develop cytomegalovirus viruria or viremia, are at increased risk for cytomegalovirus IP.[242]

Factors related to the transplant procedures that influence IP are the cytoreductive regimen, including Cy[65,66] and TBI, and agents used after BMT for GVHD prophylaxis, such as methotrexate.[254] In a nonrandomized retrospective comparison of TBI/Cy and Bu/Cy, patients who had the TBI/Cy preparation for BMT had a greater decrease in carbon monoxide diffusion than did patients who had Bu/Cy.[245]

TBI techniques may be altered in various ways to minimize IP. Fractionation has been found to be extremely important. There is a lower incidence of IP and fewer fatalities from IP when TBI is fractionated than when single-dose TBI is used, even though the total dose with the fractionated regimen is higher. This was found in a large number of nonrandomized studies[93,98,100,250,255-260] and in the randomized study from Seattle.[157] The only exception was in the low-dose-rate arm of a study that randomized patients to high and low dose rates; in that low-dose-rate arm, there was no significant difference between single-dose and hyperfractionated TBI.[224]

Lung shields can reduce the dose to a large percentage of the lung and, theoretically, reduce IP as a result. Some of the decrease in IP in fractionation studies may be attributable to the concomitant use of lung blocks as in the study from MSKCC.[100] In the study from the Institut Gustave-Roussy, however, lung shields were used in both single-dose and fractionated TBI, and the beneficial effect of fractionation in reducing IP was still observed.[98] In a study from Croatia, using the same TBI regimen with and without lung blocks, IP was 8% with lung shielding compared with 27% without such shields.[261]

Idiopathic pneumonia syndrome was significantly lower with nonmyeloablative regimens (2.2%) than with conventional conditioning regimens (8.4%) in a study with allogeneic transplantation from Seattle.[262]

Investigators from Glasgow studied the effects of different TBI regimens, which incorporated lung shielding, on pulmonary function at various times after BMT.[263] The regimens were single-dose TBI to 9.5 Gy with a lung dose of 8 Gy, and fractionated regimens, which varied from 12 to 14.4 Gy in six to eight fractions with lung doses between 11 and 13.5 Gy. Impairment of lung function was seen in all instances after BMT, especially with respect to gas exchange; these gradually improved to normal, as is also seen in a Milan study of pulmonary function tests.[264] There was a significantly less marked impairment in patients who had undergone the fractionated regimens compared with single-dose TBI, despite the lesser total lung dose received with single-dose TBI. In addition, patients who had the single-dose regimen had a slower and less complete recovery of gas exchange.

Reducing the total lung dose by shielding, in a single-dose (10 Gy) regimen, does not appear to be the answer to reducing IP. When this was attempted in a study that randomized patients between total lung doses of 6 and 8 Gy, IP was essentially the same (23% versus 28%, respectively), and relapse was significantly higher in the 6-Gy group.[265]

Dose rate is important with single-dose TBI, with very low dose rates (0.025 Gy/min) resulting in a low incidence of IP (10%) and fatal IP (5%), but treatment times are extremely lengthy to achieve this, as long as 7 hours.[266] One study using a high instantaneous dose rate (0.21 to 0.235 Gy/min) reported a very high IP incidence (8 of 11 patients), which was fatal in half of the patients.[259] Two studies suggest that with fractionated TBI, dose rate is of little importance, which is the result expected if the dose per fraction is within the shoulder of the cell survival curve for the tissue of interest.[224,247] Two studies suggest that, with a regimen of 12 Gy in 6 fractions, dose rate may still be important, with higher dose rates increasing the risk of pneumonitis.[267,268]

Prior pulmonary irradiation is also a consideration in the development of lung toxicity. The carbon monoxide transfer coefficient dropped to a significantly greater extent after BMT in patients who had received prior pulmonary irradiation.[248] In a study in which lymphoma patients were treated with high-dose therapy and autologous BMT, an acute respiratory failure thought to be secondary to pulmonary alveolar hemorrhage occurred in 26% of patients and was associated with the use of thoracic radiation for malignant disease just before BMT.[269] Prior bleomycin treatment was found to significantly enhance lung toxicity in patients who received TBI.[245]

Cataracts

With single-dose TBI, it has been found that the incidence of cataract development is very high, 80% to 100%, when patients are followed 8 to 10 years.[270-276] As many as 59% of these patients required surgery for this condition.[271]

The incidence of cataract development is considerably less (5% to 30%) when TBI is fractionated,[256,270-272,274,276-281] with only about 20% requiring surgery.[270,271,275] One exception is a study with rapid fractionation (10.5 to 12 Gy in only 1.5 to 3 days), in which 63% of patients developed cataracts.[282] Other factors that contribute to the development and severity of cataracts include the use of steroids,[270,278,283] high-dose-rate TBI,[277,284] the use of non–T cell–depleted grafts,[275,281] prior cranial irradiation,[285,286] the development of GVHD,[270] and the use of Bu.[287]

Eye shielding has been studied in a retrospective analysis in 188 children who underwent TBI in only 1 to 2 fractions prior to BMT for hematologic disorders.[288] Shielding in 139 children decreased the incidence of cataracts to 31% compared with 90% in 49 children without shielding; severe cataracts decreased to 3% with shielding compared with 38% without shielding. The incidence of relapse in the eyes was zero and in the CNS (partially shielded behind the eyes) was 2 of 139 (1.4%) with shielding; there were no eye or CNS relapses in the nonshielded group (not significantly different). This same group has studied the parameters for the LQ formula for the lens based on results in patients with ALL treated with single-dose TBI and BMT and determined the BEDs.[289] Patients were excluded if they received heparin or posttransplant steroid treatment. The values of the parameters obtained for lens are characteristic of late-responding tissues and allow prediction of cataract formation, based on TBI dose and dose rate.

Hepatic Dysfunction

Many hepatic disorders may occur after BMT: GVHD, chronic hepatitis, infections (viral, fungal, bacterial), drug reactions, leukemic infiltrates, and a potentially fatal complication, VOD of the liver, which rose in incidence as cytoreductive regimens became more intense. Clinically, the disease is defined by the triad of hepatomegaly, weight gain, and jaundice.[290]

Chemotherapy and TBI are the principal causes of VOD, but the etiology of the disease is undoubtedly multifactorial. With respect to TBI, a higher total dose (>12 Gy compared with 12 Gy) played a role in one study.[291] Fractionation has usually resulted in a lower incidence of VOD when results of single-dose (10 Gy) TBI have been compared with those of fractionated TBI (12 to 14 Gy),[98,160,256,292-294] but a few exceptions have been noted.[224,226,295] In single-dose regimens, the dose rate has been important, with minimal VOD with dose rates of 0.07 Gy/min or less compared with an incidence as high as 50% with dose rates of 0.18 to 1.20 Gy/min.[296] A randomized study of dose rate, in both single-dose and fractionated TBI, did not show a difference in VOD.[224] There was a significantly higher incidence of chronic hepatitis in one study in patients who had an abnormal alanine aminotransferase level prior to BMT, but survival was unaffected.[297]

Renal Dysfunction

Renal changes have been noted in some studies after BMT.[298-303] Characteristics include (1) increased serum creatinine and decreased creatinine clearance, (2) increased blood urea nitrogen, (3) a decreased glomerular filtration rate, (4) anemia, (5) hypertension without obvious cause, (6) peripheral edema, and (7) elevated lactic dehydrogenase.[298,299]

Analyses have suggested various risk factors that contribute to this morbidity. The combination of AraC plus Cy was suggested in one study.[298] In another, a stepwise regression analysis suggested contributions from TBI, the use of cyclosporine for GVHD prophylaxis, and the use of the antifungal agent amphotericin B.[300] Renal dysfunction was strongly correlated with total TBI dose and dose per fraction in two studies.[302,303] In contrast, one study demonstrated only one radiation nephritis case in 59 adult patients with no renal abnormalities prior to TBI, studied at 24 months post-BMT.[304] Another study in 66 children indicated that TBI was not a risk factor for chronic renal insufficiency.[305] Acute renal insufficiency was the sole risk factor for chronic renal insufficiency, while VOD, high cyclosporine serum levels, and foscarnet therapy were the only risk factors for acute renal insufficiency.

A prospective study from Switzerland in 71 patients with normal renal function who underwent BMT for various hematologic malignancies used either 12 Gy fractionated TBI (45 patients) or 13.5 Gy (26 patients).[306] In 21 patients who received 12 Gy, kidney dose was limited to 10 Gy using partial transmission blocks planned with renal opacification for shaping the blocks by means of nonionic, hypo-osmolar contrast medium. Surprisingly, an inverse correlation with TBI dose was noted, with the patients whose kidneys were shielded to 10 Gy having significantly greater renal dysfunction (GFR reduction) at 4 months. The authors suggested that the potentially nephrotoxic contrast agents used for planning may have been the reason. Another contributing factor was the number of days of aminoglycoside/vancomycin use.

Endocrine Dysfunction

Many abnormalities in endocrine function have been noted after BMT, manifested as hypothyroidism, growth deficits, impaired sexual development, and infertility. Decreased morbidity has generally been noted with fractionated TBI compared with single-dose TBI. Excellent reviews of this subject by Sanders and her colleagues from Seattle have been published.[307,308]

Thyroid function has been shown to be altered more frequently with transplant regimens containing TBI.[309] In several studies, a much higher incidence of compensated hypothyroidism and overt hypothyroidism was found in children who had received single-dose TBI (10 Gy) compared with fractionated TBI (12 to 15.75 Gy over 4 to 7 days).[274,307,310,311] Even in regimens without TBI, however, thyroid dysfunction may occur, as noted in two studies of BMT using Bu/Cy for conditioning, one in children[312] and one in adults.[313]

Gonadal function is depressed in the majority of patients who receive single-dose TBI but is less frequently affected in patients who receive fractionated TBI,[309] as measured by basal and stimulated luteinizing hormone levels and follicle-stimulating hormone levels. With single-dose TBI, menarche and the development of secondary sexual characteristics are significantly delayed, but with fractionated TBI, about 50% of the patients experience normal pubertal development.[276]

Although most women develop primary gonadal failure, a few have recovered, and pregnancies have been reported from several institutions.[276,307,310,314,315] The first report of a successful full-term pregnancy with an embryo from donated oocytes in a woman who had undergone an allogeneic BMT appeared in 1994.[316] There has been a report of successful paternity with micro-assisted fertilization 14 years after TBI-based conditioning for autologous BMT in a 20-year-old man with ALL.[317]

Growth Retardation

Two factors can contribute to growth retardation of children who receive TBI: depressed growth hormone and a direct radiation effect on bone growth. Growth hormone deficiency is found in about 40% to 55% of children who have received TBI, but if they have had prior cranial irradiation, this incidence climbs to as high as 90%.[276] Less growth retardation occurs with fractionated TBI compared with single-dose TBI.[318-320] Two recent studies support the use of growth hormone therapy in young children who receive TBI prior to transplantation.[321,322]

Cognitive Dysfunction

Few studies have looked at cognitive function after marrow transplantation. A case report described somnolence syndrome 8 weeks after irradiation in an adult with AML who underwent cytoreduction with Cy and a rapid TBI course (2.2 Gy twice daily for 3 days to a total dose of 13.2 Gy).[323] A study in children showed no significant changes in IQ or in an adaptive behavior scale.[324] Hyperfractionated TBI resulted in no alterations in cognitive testing in a study of 58 patients.[325]

One study demonstrated an increasing cognitive dysfunction with increasing TBI dose, by both univariate and multivariate analyses.[326] Another study by the same group showed that 75% of adults with malignant disease (primarily leukemia) who are candidates for marrow transplantation had a cognitive impairment prior to the transplant procedure, when tested for 11 functional indices.[327] Most common was a memory impairment. Prior history of cranial irradiation was the variable most strongly associated with impaired function, but there were also trends associating impairment with high-dose AraC, as well as central nervous system disease treated with intrathecal chemotherapy. Children with ALL who have more than one course of cranial irradiation also have increasing toxicity, with greater decrements in IQ and achievement.[328]

TBI was a risk factor (among many others including metabolic factors) for higher delirium severity, but not for the incidence of delirium in a study in adults who underwent HCT.[329] In a study in children who had undergone HCT, TBI was a risk factor for severe neurologic events; other risk factors were transplant from an allogeneic donor, especially if unrelated, and development of severe acute GVHD greater than grade 2.[330]

Secondary Malignancies

An association between irradiation for BMT and the development of secondary malignancies (SMs) is controversial. A report from Paris implicated TAI, which was used in preparation for BMT for severe aplastic anemia and Fanconi's anemia, in an unusually high incidence of SM at 8 years (22% ± 11% SE).[331] In contrast, there was only a 1.4% incidence at 10 years when aplastic anemia patients in Seattle were prepared with chemotherapy only.[153] It should be noted that there is an association of squamous cell carcinoma with Fanconi's anemia, even without irradiation.[332] Another analysis from Seattle with 2246 patients (320 with aplastic anemia and 1926 with hematologic malignancies) cited a 1.4% incidence of SM and implicated TBI as well as antithymocyte globulin for GVHD as risk factors.[333] An analysis of European BMT data that compared immunosuppression with BMT for aplastic anemia showed that patients who were immunosuppressed had a similar incidence of SM (0.9%) compared with those who had a BMT (0.8%).[334] In the patients who developed solid tumors in the BMT group, there was a relative risk of 20.7 for irradiation. Surprisingly, all 15 patients who developed solid tumors were male.

An analysis of 493 non-Hodgkin's lymphoma patients who had undergone autologous HCT found 22 patients who had developed persistent cytopenia in at least one cell line and with morphologic or cytogenetic evidence of therapy-related myelodysplastic syndrome or AML.[335] TBI was independently associated with an increased risk of developing myelodysplastic syndrome or AML. When combined with Cy/VP-16, the risk was greater.

In contrast to the above studies, other investigators suggest no association with irradiation.[336,337] In a registry study of 9880 patients, the distribution of the 127 SMs seen was similar to that in other organ transplant patients not given irradiation, only immunosuppression.[336]

STATUS OF TOTAL BODY IRRADIATION USE AND FUTURE DIRECTIONS IN SELECTED DISEASES

Leukemias and Lymphomas

In these diseases, the major challenges continue to be the reduction of early morbidity and GVHD without compromising malignant cell kill. Innovative techniques of radiolabeled antibodies appear promising, and newer supportive care measures are continually being developed. Low-dose nonmyeloblative TBI with DLI holds promise, providing that the high rate of severe GVHD can be reduced. Outpatient TBI as a component of a comprehensive outpatient transplant program appears safe, with no difference in 100-day mortality for TBI as an outpatient compared with inpatient TBI (9% versus 16%, respectively).[338]

Multiple Myeloma

Several promising regimens have appeared in reports in the literature for autologous BMT in multiple myeloma patients who have a large tumor burden; many contain melphalan plus TBI, and others have multiple chemotherapeutic agents and TBI. The value of purging in this disease is unclear. In a study from France, which used multiagent chemotherapy and TBI, a 40% event-free survival rate was reported.[339] This was a relatively young group of patients with a median age of 44 years. A group from Milan achieved a survival benefit in a high-risk group defined by a high labeling index of the tumor.[340]

Most regimens for cytoreduction have consisted of high-dose chemotherapy without TBI prior to BMT. A European Bone Marrow Transplant Group study indicated that non-TBI conditioning, among other factors, was independently predictive of longer survival in a multivariate analysis.[341] Some investigators have described improved response rates with double or tandem transplants,[342] but a French randomized study, comparing single to double high-dose therapy, did not show a significant difference at 2-year median follow-up.[343] A prospective study from Bologna demonstrated a significantly improved EFS by 12 months and projected 6-year OS for double transplant versus single transplant (63% versus 44%, respectively).[344] Because toxicity is still a major problem and long-term survival is poor, efforts at more-effective, less-toxic regimens are needed.

Anemias

Severe aplastic anemia was considered in some detail in Results of Clinical Studies. Patients who have been heavily transfused require sufficiently aggressive treatment to allow engraftment because they have been sensitized to allografts by their transfusions. TLI, which spares many sensitive structures, along with Cy, is theoretically ideal for this purpose, providing that a sufficiently high dose is given. Although the optimal dose is not defined, our prior studies suggest that somewhere in the range of 900 cGy may be recommended.[96]

Genetic Disorders

Many patients with genetic disorders have successfully received allogeneic transplants after preparation with regimens containing TBI. Examples of diseases treated include Wiskott-Aldrich syndrome,[345] thalassemia major,[346] and infantile malignant osteopetrosis.[347] Total TBI doses may be kept low (4 to 7 Gy), minimizing any effects on bone growth and endocrine function in these children.

REFERENCES

1. Helder DI, Bakker B, de Heer P, et al: Quality of life in adults following bone marrow transplantation during childhood. Bone Marrow Transplant 33:329, 2004.
2. Horowitz NM, Rowlings PA: An update from the International Bone Marrow Transplant Registry and the Autologous Blood and Marrow Transplant Registry on current activity in hematopoietic stem cell transplantation. Curr Opin Hematol 4:395, 1997.
3. Copelan EA, Deeg HJ: Conditioning for allogeneic marrow transplantation in patients with lymphohematopoietic malignancies without the use of total body irradiation [review]. Blood 80:1648, 1992.
4. Tutschka PJ, Copelan EA, Kapoor N: Replacing total body irradiation with busulfan as conditioning of patients with leukemia for allogeneic marrow transplantation. Transplant Proc 21:2952, 1989.
5. DeLaCamara R, Tomas JF, Figuera A, et al: High dose busulfan and seizures. Bone Marrow Transplant 7:363, 1991.
6. Lanteenmaki PM, Chakrabarti S, Cornish JM, et al: Outcome of single fraction total body irradiation-conditioned stem cell transplantation in younger children with malignant disease-comparison with a busulphan-cyclophosphamide regimen. Acta Oncol 43:196, 2004.
7. Morgan M, Dodds A, Atkinson K, et al: The toxicity of busulphan and cyclophosphamide as the preparative regimen for bone marrow transplantation. Br J Haematol 77:529, 1991.
8. Rozman C, Carreras E, Qian C, et al: Risk factors for hepatic veno-occlusive disease following HLA-identical sibling bone marrow transplants for leukemia. Bone Marrow Transplant 17:75, 1996.
9. Hartman AR, Williams SF, Dillon JJ: Survival, disease-free survival and adverse effects of conditioning for allogeneic bone marrow transplantation with busulfan/cyclophosphamide versus total body irradiation: a meta-analysis. Bone Marrow Transplant 22:439, 1998.
10. Litzow MR, Perez WS, Klein JP, et al: Comparison of outcome following allogeneic bone marrow transplantation with cyclophosphamide-total body irradiation versus busulphan-cyclophosphamide conditioning regimens for acute myelogenous leukaemia in first remission. Br J Haematol 119:1115, 2002.
11. Van der Jagt RHC, Appelbaum FR, Petersen FB, et al: Busulfan and cyclophosphamide as a preparative regimen for bone marrow transplantation in patients with prior chest radiotherapy. Bone Marrow Transplant 8:211, 1991.
12. Inoue T, Ikeda H, Yamazaki H, et al: Role of total body irradiation as based on the comparison of preparation regimens for allogeneic bone marrow transplantation for acute leukemia in first complete remission. Strahlenther Onkol 169:250, 1993.
13. Bruno B, Souillet G, Bertrand Y, et al: Effects of allogeneic bone marrow transplantation on pulmonary function in 80 children in a single paediatric centre. Bone Marrow Transplant 34:143, 2004.
14. Wingard JR, Plotnick LP, Freemer CS, et al: Growth in children after bone marrow transplantation: busulfan plus cyclophosphamide versus cyclophosphamide plus total body irradiation. Blood 79:1068, 1992.
15. Michel G, Gluckman E, Esperou-Bourdeau H, et al: Allogeneic bone marrow transplantation for children with acute myeloblastic leukemia in first complete remission: impact of conditioning regimen without total body irradiation: a report from the Société Française de Greffe de Moelle. J Clin Oncol 12:1217, 1994.
16. Blaise D, Maraninchi D, Archimbaud E, et al: Allogeneic bone marrow transplantation for acute myeloid leukemia in first remission: a randomized trial of a busulfan-Cytoxan versus Cytoxan-total body irradiation as preparative regimen: a report from the Groupe d'Etudes de la Greffe de Moelle Osseuse. Blood 79:2578, 1993.
17. Clift RA, Buckner CD, Thomas ED, et al: Marrow transplantation for chronic myeloid leukemia: a randomized study comparing cyclophosphamide and total body irradiation with busulfan and cyclophosphamide. Blood 84:2036, 1994.
18. Clift RA, Storb R: Marrow transplantation for CML: the Seattle experience. Bone Marrow Transplant 17(Suppl 3):S1, 1996.
19. Clift RT, Radich J, Appelbaum FR, et al: Long-term follow-up of a randomized study comparing cyclophosphamide and total body irradiation with busulfan and cyclophosphamide for patients receiving allogeneic marrow transplants during chronic phase of chronic myeloid leukemia. Blood 94:3960, 1999.
20. Blume KG, Kopecky KJ, Henslee-Downey JP, et al: A prospective randomized comparison of total body irradiation-etoposide versus busulfan-cyclophosphamide as preparatory regimens for bone marrow transplantation in patients with leukemia who were not in first remission. Blood 81:2187, 1993.
21. Devergie A, Blaise D, Attal M, et al: Allogeneic bone marrow transplantation for chronic myeloid leukemia in first chronic phase: a randomized trial of busulfan-Cytoxan versus Cytoxan-total body irradiation as preparative regimen: a report from the French Society of Bone Marrow Graft (SFGM). Blood 85:2263, 1995.
22. Schwerdtfeger R, Kirsch A, Sonntag S, et al: Allogeneic bone marrow transplantation in chronic myeloid leukemia: what is the best conditioning regime? Bone Marrow Transplant 12(Suppl 2): 13, 1993.

23. Miller G, Wagner JE, Vogelsang GB, et al: A randomized trial of busulfan-cyclophosphamide (Bu-Cy) versus cyclophosphamide-total body irradiation (Cy-TBI) as preparative regimen for patients with chronic myelogenous leukemia (CML) [abstract]. Blood 78(Suppl 1):291a, 1991.
24. Ringden O, Ruutu T, Remberger M, et al: A randomized trial comparing busulfan with total body irradiation as conditioning in allogeneic marrow transplant recipients with leukemia: a report from the Nordic Bone Marrow Transplant Group. Blood 83:2723, 1994.
25. Ringden O, Remberger M, Ruutu T, et al: Increased risk of chronic graft-versus-host disease, obstructive bronchiolitis, and alopecia with busulfan versus total body irradiation: long-term results of a randomized trial in allogeneic marrow recipients with leukemia. Blood 93:2196, 1999.
26. Socie G, Clift RA, Blaise D, et al: Busulfan plus cyclophosphamide compared with total body irradiation plus cyclophosphamide before marrow transplantation for myeloid leukemia: long-term follow-up of 4 randomized studies. Blood 98:3569, 2001.
27. Dusenbery KE, Daniels KA, McClure JS, et al: Randomized comparison of cyclophosphamide-total body irradiation versus busulfan-cyclophosphamide conditioning in autologous bone marrow transplantation for acute myeloid leukemia. Int J Radiat Oncol Biol Phys 31:119, 1995.
28. Dusenbery KE, Steinbuch M, McGlave PB, et al: Autologous bone marrow transplantation in acute myeloid leukemia: the University of Minnesota experience. Int J Radiat Oncol Biol Phys 36:335, 1996.
29. Bunin N, Aplenc R, Kamani N, et al: Randomized trial of busulfan versus total body irradiation containing conditioning regimens for children with acute lymphoblastic leukemia: a Pediatric Blood and Marrow Transplant Consortium study. Bone Marrow Transplant 32:543, 2003.
30. Blume KG, Forman SJ: High-dose etoposide (VP-16)-containing preparatory regimens in allogeneic and autologous bone marrow transplantation for hematologic malignancies. Semin Oncol 19:63, 1992.
31. Weyman C, Graham-Pole J, Emerson S, et al: Use of cytosine arabinoside and total body irradiation as conditioning for allogeneic marrow transplantation in patients with acute lymphoblastic leukemia: a multicenter survey. Bone Marrow Transplant 11:43, 1993.
32. Copelan EA: Conditioning regimens for allogeneic bone marrow transplantation. Blood Rev 6:234, 1992.
33. Kwan DK, Norman A: Radiosensitivity of human lymphocytes and thymocytes. Radiat Res 69:143, 1977.
34. Szcylik C, Wiktor-Jedrzejczak W: The effects of X-irradiation in vitro on subpopulations of human lymphocytes. Int J Radiat Biol 39:253, 1981.
35. Shank B, Andreeff M, Li D: Cell survival kinetics in peripheral blood and bone marrow during total body irradiation for marrow transplantation. Int J Radiat Oncol Biol Phys 9:1613, 1983.
36. Weichselbaum RR, Greenberger JS, Schmidt A, et al: In vitro radiosensitivity of human leukemia cell lines. Radiology 139:485, 1981.
37. Lehnert S, Rybka WB, Suissa S, et al: Radiation response of haematopoietic cell lines of human origin. Int J Radiat Biol 49:423, 1986.
38. Rhee JG, Song CW, Kim TH, et al: Effect of fractionation and rate of radiation dose on human leukemic cells, HL-60. Radiat Res 101:519, 1985.
39. Shank B: Hyperfractionation (T.I.D.) versus single dose irradiation in human acute lymphocytic leukemia cells: application to TBI for marrow transplantation. Radiother Oncol 27:30, 1993.
40. Vriesendorp HM, Johnson PM, Fey TA, et al: Optimal dose of total body irradiation for allogeneic bone marrow transplantation. Transplant Proc 1985;17:517, 1985.
41. Storb R, Raff RF, Appelbaum FR, et al: Comparison of fractionated to single-dose total body irradiation in conditioning canine littermates for DLA-identical marrow grafts. Blood 74:1139, 1989.
42. Terenzi A, Aristei C, Aversa F, et al: Comparison of immunosuppressive effects of single-dose and hyperfractionated total body irradiation. Transplant Proc 26:3217, 1994.
43. Vriesendorp HM: Radiobiological speculations on therapeutic total body irradiation. Crit Rev Oncol Hematol 10:211, 1990.
44. Down JD, Tarbell NJ, Thames HD, et al: Syngeneic and allogeneic bone marrow engraftment after total body irradiation: dependence on dose, dose rate, and fractionation. Blood 77:661, 1991.
45. Van Os R, Thames HD, Konings AWT, et al: Radiation dose-fractionation and dose-rate relationships for long-term repopulating hemopoietic stem cells in a murine bone marrow transplant model. Radiat Res 136:118, 1993.
46. Girinski T, Socie G, Cosset JM, et al: Similar effects on murine haemopoietic compartment of low dose rate single dose and high dose rate fractionated total body irradiation. Preliminary results after a unique dose of 750 cGy. Br J Radiol 61:797, 1990.
47. Cui YZ, Hisha H, Yang GX, et al: Optimal protocol for total body irradiation for allogeneic bone marrow transplantation in mice. Bone Marrow Transplant 30:843, 2002.
48. Van Os R, Konings AWT, Down JD: Radiation dose as a factor in host preparation for bone marrow transplantation across different genetic barriers. Int J Radiat Biol 61:501, 1992.
49. Down JD, Mauch P, Warhol M, et al: The effect of donor T lymphocytes and total body irradiation on hemopoietic engraftment and pulmonary toxicity following experimental allogeneic bone marrow transplantation. Transplant 54:802, 1992.
50. Loewenthal E, Weiss L, Samuel S, et al: Optimization of conditioning therapy for leukemia prior to BMT. I. Optimal synergism between cyclophosphamide and total body irradiation for eradication of murine B cell leukemia (BCL1). Bone Marrow Transplant 12:109, 1993.
51. Evans RG: Radiobiological considerations in magna-field irradiation. Int J Radiat Oncol Biol Phys 9:1907, 1983.
52. Wara WM, Phillips TL, Margolis LW, et al: Radiation pneumonitis: a new approach to the derivation of time-dose factors. Cancer 32:547, 1973.
53. Yan R, Peters LJ, Travis EL: Cyclophosphamide 24 hours before or after total body irradiation: effects on lung and bone marrow. Radiother Oncol 21:149, 1991.
54. Collis CH, Steel GG: Lung damage in mice from cyclophosphamide and thoracic irradiation: the effect of timing. Int J Radiat Oncol Biol Phys 9:685, 1983.
55. Okunewick JP, Kociban DL, Young CK, et al: Effect of radiation and drug order in preparatory regimens for bone marrow transplantation [abstract]. *In* Proceedings of the 36th Annual Meeting of the Radiation Research Society, Philadelphia, 1988, p 157.
56. Peters LJ, Withers HR, Cundiff JH, et al: Radiobiological considerations in the use of total body irradiation for bone-marrow transplantation. Radiology 131:243, 1979.
57. Peters L: Discussion: the radiobiological bases of TBI. Int J Radiat Oncol Biol Phys 6:785, 1980.
58. Vriesendorp HM: Prediction of effects of therapeutic total body irradiation in man. Radiother Oncol 1(Suppl):37, 1990.
59. Shank B, Hoppe RT: Radiotherapeutic principles of hematopoietic cell transplantation. *In* Blume KG, Forman SJ, Appelbaum FR (eds): Thomas' Hematopoietic Cell Transplantation, 3rd ed. Boston, Blackwell Scientific, 2004, pp 178-197.
60. Vitale V, Scarpati D, Frassoni F, et al: Total body irradiation: single dose, fractions, dose rate. Bone Marrow Transplant 4(Suppl 1):233, 1989.
61. O'Donoghue JA, Wheldon TE, Gregor A: The implications of *in-vitro* radiation-survival curves for the optimal scheduling of total body irradiation with bone marrow rescue in the treatment of leukaemia. Br J Radiol 60:279, 1987.
62. Fruchtman S, Scigliano E, Isola L, et al: Hyperfractionated total body irradiation (HF-TBI) and whole allogeneic marrow grafts: An intensive, safe, and highly efficacious approach to the cure of leukemia [abstract]. Blood 86(Suppl 1):945a, 1995.
63. Singh H, Isola L, Richards S, Scigliano E, Fruchtman SM: Higher dose total body irradiation with allogeneic BMT for CML-CP results in fewer relapses [abstract]. Blood 96:358b, 2000.
64. O'Donoghue JA: Fractionated versus low dose-rate total body irradiation. Radiobiological considerations in the selection of regimes. Radiother Oncol 7:241, 1986.

65. Kal HB, Van Kempen-Harteveld ML, Heijenbrok-Kal MH, et al: Biologically effective dose in total body irradiation and bone marrow transplantation. More dose is better [abstract]. Radiother Oncol 73(Suppl 1):S206, 2004.
66. Mark GJ, Lehimgar-Zadeh A, Ragsdale BD: Cyclophosphamide pneumonitis. Thorax 33:89, 1978.
67. Spector JI, Zimbler H, Ross JS: Early-onset cyclophosphamide-induced interstitial pneumonitis. JAMA 242:2852, 1979.
68. Andersson BS, Luna MA, Yee C, et al: Fatal pulmonary failure complicating high-dose cytosine arabinoside therapy in acute leukemia. Cancer 65:1079, 1990.
69. Shea TC, Bruner R, Wiley JM, et al: An expanded phase I/II trial of cyclophosphamide, etoposide, and carboplatin plus total body irradiation with autologous marrow or stem cell support for patients with hematologic malignancies. Biol Blood Marrow Transplant 9:443, 2003.
70. Blackett NM, Aguado M: The enhancement of haemopoietic stem cell recovery in irradiated mice by prior treatment with cyclophosphamide. Cell Tissue Kinet 12:291, 1979.
71. Shank B, O'Reilly RJ, Cunningham I, et al: Total body irradiation for bone marrow transplantation: the Memorial Sloan-Kettering Cancer Center experience. Radiother Oncol 1(Suppl):68, 1990.
72. Spitzer TR, Deeg HJ, Torrisi J, et al: Total body irradiation (TBI) induced emesis is universal after small dose fractions (120 cGy) and is not cumulative dose related [abstract]. Proc Am Soc Clin Oncol 9:14, 1990.
73. Hewitt M, Cornish J, Pamphilou D, et al: Effective emetic control during conditioning of children for bone marrow transplantation using ondansetron, a 5-HT3 antagonist. Bone Marrow Transplant 7:431, 1991.
74. Spitzer TR, Friedman CJ, Bushnell W, et al: Double-blind, randomized, parallel-group study on the efficacy and safety of oral granisetron and oral ondansetron in the prophylaxis of nausea and vomiting in patients receiving hyperfractionated total body irradiation. Bone Marrow Transplant 26:203, 2000.
75. Spitzer TR, Bryson JC, Cirenza E, et al: Randomized double-blind, placebo-controlled evaluation of oral ondansetron in the prevention of nausea and vomiting associated with fractionated total body irradiation. J Clin Oncol 12:2432, 1994.
76. Tiley C, Powles R, Catalano J, et al: Results of a double blind placebo controlled study of ondansetron as an antiemetic during total body irradiation in patients undergoing bone marrow transplantation. Leuk Lymphoma 7:317, 1992.
77. Matsuoka S, Okamoto S, Watanabe R, et al: Granisetron plus dexamethasone versus granisetron alone in the prevention of vomiting induced by conditioning for stem cell transplantation: a prospective randomized study. Int J Hematol 77:86, 2003.
78. Shank B: Techniques of magna-field irradiation. Int J Radiat Oncol Biol Phys 9:1925, 1983.
79. Glasgow GP, Wang S, Stanton J: A total body irradiation stand for bone marrow transplant patients. Int J Radiat Oncol Biol Phys 16:875, 1989.
80. Kutcher GJ, Bonfiglio P, Shank B, et al: Combined photon and electron technique for total body irradiation [abstract]. European Society for Therapeutic Radiology and Oncology, p 31, 1988.
81. Miralbell R, Rouzaud M, Grob E, et al: Can a total body irradiation technique be fast and reproducible? Int J Radiat Oncol Biol Phys 29:1167, 1994.
82. Gerbi BJ, Dusenbery KE: Design specifications for a treatment stand used for total body photon irradiation [abstract]. European Society for Therapeutic Radiology and Oncology, p 31, 1988.
83. Breneman JC, Elson HR, Little R, et al: A technique for delivery of total body irradiation for bone marrow transplantation in adults and adolescents. Int J Radiat Oncol Biol Phys 18:1233, 1990.
84. Bortin MM: Pathogenesis of interstitial pneumonitis following allogeneic bone marrow transplantation for acute leukemia. *In* Gale RP (ed): Recent Advances in Bone Marrow Transplantation. New York, Alan R Liss, 1983, p 445.
85. Fryer CJH, Fitzpatrick PJ, Rider WD, et al: Radiation pneumonitis: experience following a large single dose of radiation. Int J Radiat Oncol Biol Phys 4:931, 1978.
86. Kim TH, Kersey JH, Sewchand W, et al: Total body irradiation with a high-dose-rate linear accelerator for bone-marrow transplantation in aplastic anemia and neoplastic disease. Radiol 122:523, 1977.
87. Fyles GM, Messner HA, Lockwood G, et al: Long-term results of bone marrow transplantation for patients with AML, ALL, and CML prepared with single dose total body irradiation of 500 cGy delivered with a high dose rate. Bone Marrow Transplant 8:453, 1991.
88. Tarbell NJ, Amato DA, Down JD, et al: Fractionation and dose rate effects in mice: a model for bone marrow transplantation in man. Int J Radiat Oncol Biol Phys 13:1065, 1987.
89. Blum W, Brown R, Lin HS, et al: Low-dose (550 cGy), single-exposure total body irradiation and cyclophosphamide: consistent, durable engraftment of related-donor peripheral blood stem cells with low treatment-related mortality and fatal organ toxicity. Biol Blood Marrow Transplant 8:608, 2002.
90. Girgis M, Hallemeier C, Blum W, et al: Chimerism and clinical outcomes of 110 recipients of unrelated donor bone marrow transplants who underwent conditioning with low-dose, single-exposure total body irradiation and cyclophosphamide. Blood 105:3035, 2005.
91. Hallemeier C, Girgis M, Blum W, et al: Outcomes of adults with acute myelogenous leukemia in remission given 550 cGy of single-exposure total body irradiation, cyclophosphamide, and unrelated donor bone marrow transplants. Biol Blood Marrow Transplant 10:310, 2004.
92. Shank B, Hopfan S, Kim JH, et al: Hyperfractionated total body irradiation for bone marrow transplantation: I. Early results in leukemia patients. Int J Radiat Oncol Biol Phys 7:1109, 1981.
93. Pino y Torres JL, Bross DS, Lam W-C, et al: Risk factors in interstitial pneumonitis following allogeneic bone marrow transplantation. Int J Radiat Oncol Biol Phys 8:1301, 1982.
94. Lawton CA, Barber-Derus S, Murray KJ, et al: Technical modifications in hyperfractionated total body irradiation for T-lymphocyte deplete bone marrow transplant. Int J Radiat Oncol Biol Phys 17:319, 1989.
95. Lawton CA, Barber-Derus SW, Murray KJ, et al: Influence of renal shielding on the incidence of late renal dysfunction associated with T-lymphocyte deplete bone marrow transplantation in adult patients. Int J Radiat Oncol Biol Phys 23:681, 1992.
96. Shank B, Brochstein JA, Castro-Malaspina H, et al: Immunosuppression prior to marrow transplantation for sensitized aplastic anemia patients: comparison of TLI with TBI. Int J Radiat Oncol Biol Phys 14:1133, 1988.
97. Dutreix J, Janoray P, Bridier A, et al: Biologic and anatomic problems of lung shielding in whole-body irradiation. JNCI 76:1333, 1986.
98. Cosset JM, Baume D, Pico JL, et al: Single dose versus hyperfractionated total body irradiation before allogeneic bone marrow transplantation: a non-randomized comparative study of 54 patients at the Institut Gustave-Roussy. Radiother Oncol 15:151, 1989.
99. Sanders JE, Flournoy N, Thomas ED, et al: Marrow transplant experience in children with acute lymphoblastic leukemia: an analysis of factors associated with survival, relapse, and graft-versus-host disease. Med Pediatr Oncol 13:165, 1985.
100. Shank B, Chu FCH, Dinsmore R, et al: Hyperfractionated total body irradiation for bone marrow transplantation. Results in seventy leukemia patients with allogeneic transplants. Int J Radiat Oncol Biol Phys 9:1607, 1983.
101. Quaranta BP, Halperin EC, Kurtzberg J, et al: The incidence of testicular recurrence in boys with acute leukemia treated with total body and testicular irradiation and stem cell transplantation. Cancer 101:845, 2004.
102. Gratwohl A, Gluckman E, Goldman J, et al: Effect of splenectomy before bone marrow transplantation on survival in chronic granulocytic leukemia. Lancet 2:1290, 1985.
103. Barrett AJ, Longhurst P, Humble JG, et al: Effect of splenic irradiation on circulating colony-forming cells in chronic granulocytic leukemia. Br Med J 1:1259, 1977.
104. Ravalese J, III, Madoc-Jones H, Ling M, et al: Splenic irradiation prior to high dose chemotherapy and allogeneic bone marrow

transplantation for chronic myelogenous leukemia [abstract]. Int J Radiat Oncol Biol Phys 27:312, 1993.
105. Gratwohl A, Hermans J, Biezen AV, et al: No advantage for patients who receive splenic irradiation before bone marrow transplantation for chronic myeloid leukaemia. Bone Marrow Transplant 10:147, 1992.
106. Gratwohl A, Hermans J, Biezen AV, et al: Splenic irradiation before bone marrow transplantation for chronic myeloid leukaemia. Br J Haematol 95:494, 1996.
107. Chadha M, Shank B, Fuks Z, et al: Improved survival of poor prognosis diffuse histiocytic (large cell) lymphoma managed with sequential induction chemotherapy, "boost" radiation therapy, and autologous bone marrow transplantation. Int J Radiat Oncol Biol Phys 14:407, 1988.
108. Mundt AJ, Sibley G, Williams S, et al: Patterns of failure following high-dose chemotherapy and autologous bone marrow transplantation with involved field radiotherapy for relapsed/refractory Hodgkin's disease. Int J Radiat Oncol Biol Phys 33:261, 1995.
109. Poen JP, Hoppe RT, Horning SJ: High-dose therapy and autologous bone marrow transplantation for relapsed/refractory Hodgkin's disease: The impact of involved field radiotherapy on patterns of failure and survival. Int J Radiat Oncol Biol Phys 36:3, 1996.
110. Moskowitz CH, Nimer SD, Zelenetz AD, et al: A 2-step comprehensive high-dose chemoradiotherapy second-line program for relapsed and refractory Hodgkin disease: Analysis by intent to treat and development of a prognostic model. Blood 97:616, 2001.
111. Lancet JE, Rapoport AP, Brasacchio R, et al: Autotransplantation for relapsed or refractory Hodgkin's disease: long-term follow-up and analysis of prognostic factors. Bone Marrow Transplant 22:265, 1998.
112. Mundt AJ, Williams SF, Hallahan D: High dose chemotherapy and stem cell rescue for aggressive non-Hodgkin's lymphoma: Pattern of failure and implications for involved-field radiotherapy. Int J Radiat Oncol Biol Phys 39:617, 1997.
113. Fouillard L, Laporte JP, Labopin M, et al: Autologous stem-cell transplantation for non-Hodgkin's lymphomas: The role of graft purging and radiotherapy posttransplantation. Results of a retrospective analysis on 120 patients autografted in a single institution. J Clin Oncol 16:2803, 1998.
114. Philip T, Guglielmi C, Hagenbeek A, et al: Autologous bone marrow transplantation as compared with salvage chemotherapy in relapses of chemotherapy-sensitive non-Hodgkin's lymphoma. N Engl J Med 333:1540, 1995.
115. Wirth A, Prince HM, Wolf M, et al: Optimal timing to reduce morbidity of involved-field radiotherapy (IFRT) with transplantation for lymphomas: a prospective Australasian Leukemia and Lymphoma Group study [abstract]. Ann Oncol 13(Suppl 2):75, 2002.
116. Matthews DC, Appelbaum FR, Eary JE, et al: Phase I study of (131)I-anti-CD45 antibody + cyclophosphamide and total body irradiation for advanced leukemia and myelodysplastic syndrome. Blood 94:1237, 1999.
117. Matthews DC, Appelbaum FR, Eary JF, et al: Development of a marrow transplant regimen for acute leukemia using targeted hematopoietic irradiation delivered by 131I-labeled anti-CD45 antibody, combined with cyclophosphamide and total body irradiation. Blood 85:1122, 1995.
118. Bunjes D, Buchmann I, Duncker C, et al: Rhenium 188-labeled anti-CD66 (a,b,c,e) monoclonal antibody to intensify the conditioning regimen prior to stem cell transplantation for patients with high-risk acute myeloid leukemia or myelodysplastic syndrome: results of a phase I-II study. Blood 98:565, 2001.
119. Press OW, Eary JE, Appelbaum FR, et al: Phase II trial of 131I-B1 (anti-CD20) antibody therapy with autologous stem cell transplantation for relapsed B cell lymphomas. Lancet 346:336, 1995.
120. Knox SJ, Goris ML, Trisler KD, et al: 90Y-antiCD20 monoclonal antibody therapy of recurrent B-cell lymphoma. Clin Cancer Res 2:457, 1996.
121. Alyea E, Neuberg D, Mauch P, et al: Effect of total body irradiation dose escalation on outcome following T-cell-depleted allogeneic bone marrow transplantation. Biol Blood Marrow Transplant 8:139, 2002.
122. Briot E, Dutreix A, Bridier A: Dosimetry for total body irradiation. Radiother Oncol Suppl 1:16, 1990.
123. Van Dyk J: Dosimetry for total body irradiation. Radiother Oncol 9:107, 1987.
124. Van Dyk J, Galvin JM, Glasgow GP, Podgorsak EB: The physical aspects of total and half body photon irradiation. AAPM Report No 17. New York, American Institute of Physics, 1986.
125. Storb R, Appelbaum F, Schuening F, et al: Bone marrow transplantation and massive total body irradiation. *In* Ricks RC, Fry SA (eds): The Basis for Radiation Accident Preparedness: II. Clinical Experience and Follow-up Since 1979. New York, Elsevier, 1990, p 109.
126. Anasetti C, Amos D, Beatty PG, et al: Effect of HLA compatibility on engraftment of bone marrow transplants in patients with leukemia or lymphoma. N Engl J Med 320:197, 1989.
127. Champlin R, Ho WG, Mitsuyasu R, et al: Graft failure and leukemia relapse following T-lymphocyte depleted bone marrow transplantation; effect of intensification of immunosuppressive conditioning. Transplant Proc 19:2616, 1987.
128. Guyotat D, Dutou L, Ehrsam A, et al: Graft rejection after T-cell depleted marrow transplantation: Role of fractionated irradiation. Br J Haematol 65:499, 1987.
129. Patterson J, Prentice HG, Brenner MK, et al: Graft rejection following HLA matched T-lymphocyte depleted bone marrow transplantation. Br J Haematol 63:221, 1986.
130. Bortin MM, Horowitz MM, Rimm AA: Progress report from the international bone marrow transplant registry. Bone Marrow Transplant 10:113, 1992.
131. Burnett AK, Robertson AG, Hann IM, et al: In vitro T-depletion of allogeneic bone marrow: prevention of rejection in HLA-matched transplants by increased TBI. Bone Marrow Transplant 1(Suppl 1):121, 1986.
132. Racadot E, Herve P, Beaujean F, et al: Prevention of graft-versus-host disease in HLA-matched bone marrow transplantation for malignant diseases: multicentric study of 62 patients using 3-pan-T monoclonal antibodies and rabbit complement. J Clin Oncol 5:426, 1987.
133. Iriondo A, Hermosa V, Richard C, et al: Graft rejection following T lymphocyte depleted bone marrow transplantation with two different TBI regimens. Br J Haematol 65:246, 1987.
134. Martin PH, Hansen JA, Torok-Storb B, et al: Graft failure in patients receiving T cell-depleted HLA-identical allogeneic marrow transplants. Bone Marrow Transplant 3:445, 1988.
135. Soiffer RJ, Mauch P, Tarbell NJ, et al: Total lymphoid irradiation to prevent graft rejection in recipients of HLA non-identical T cell-depleted allogeneic marrow. Bone Marrow Transplant 7:23, 1991.
136. James ND, Apperley JF, Kam KC, et al: Total lymphoid irradiation preceding bone marrow transplantation for chronic myeloid leukaemia. Clin Radiol 40:195, 1989.
137. Slavin S, Or R, Naparstek E, et al: New approaches for the prevention of rejection and graft-versus-host disease in clinical bone marrow transplantation. Israel J Med Sci 22:264, 1986.
138. Slavin S, Or R, Weshler Z, et al: The use of total lymphoid irradiation for abrogation of host resistance to T-cell depleted marrow allografts. Bone Marrow Transplant 1(Suppl 1):98, 1986.
139. Pipard G, Stepanian E, Chapuis B, et al: Total lymphoid irradiation (TLI), chemotherapy (CT) and total body irradiation (TBI) before T-cell depleted bone marrow allografts [abstract]. ESTRO, 7th annual meeting, Ben Haag, The Netherlands, 1988, p 36.
140. Kernan NA, Bordignon C, Heller G, et al: Graft failure after T-cell-depleted human leukocyte antigen identical marrow transplants for leukemia: I. Analysis of risk factors and results of secondary transplants. Blood 74:2227, 1989.
141. Poynton CH, MacDonald D, Byrom NA, et al: Rejection after T cell depletion of donor bone marrow. Bone Marrow Transplant 2(Suppl 1):153, 1987.
142. Ganem G, Kuentz M, Beaujean F, et al: Additional total lymphoid irradiation (TLI) in preventing graft failure of T cell depleted bone marrow transplantation (BMT) from HLA identical siblings: results of a prospective randomized study. Bone Marrow Transplant 2(Suppl 1):156, 1987.
143. McSweeney PA, Niederwieser D, Shizuru JA, et al: Hematopoietic cell transpantation in older patients with hematologic malig-

nancies: replacing high-dose cytotoxic therapy with graft-versus-tumor effects. Blood 97:3390, 2001.
144. Ballen KK, Becker PS, Emmons RV, et al: Low-dose total body irradiation followed by allogeneic lymphocyte infusion may induce remission in patients with refractory hematologic malignancy. Blood 100:442, 2002.
145. Diaconescu R, Flowers CR, Storer B, et al: Morbidity and mortality with nonmyeloablative compared with myeloablative conditioning before hematopoietic cell transplantation from HLA-matched related donors. Blood 104:1550, 2004.
146. Sorror ML, Maris MB, Storer B, et al: Comparing morbidity and mortality of HLA-matched unrelated donor hematopoietic cell transplantation after nonmyeloablative and myeloablative conditioning: influence of pretransplantation comorbidities. Blood 104:961, 2004.
147. Le Blanc K, Remberger M, Uzunel M, et al: A comparison of nonmyeloablative and reduced-intensity conditioning for allogeneic stem-cell transplantation. Transplantation 78:1014, 2004.
148. Ramsay NKC, Kim TH, McGlave P, et al: Bone marrow transplantation for severe aplastic anemia following preparation with cyclophosphamide and total lymphoid irradiation. *In* Young NS, Levine AS, Humphries RK (eds): Aplastic Anemia: Stem Cell Biology and Advances in Treatment. New York, Alan R Liss, 1984, p 315.
149. Kim TH, Kersey JH, Khan FM, et al: Single dose total lymphoid irradiation combined with cyclophosphamide as immunosuppression for human marrow transplantation in aplastic anemia. Int J Radiat Oncol Biol Phys 5:993, 1979.
150. Vitale V, Barra S, Corvo R, et al: The role of thoraco-abdominal irradiation before marrow transplantation. Bone Marrow Transplant 7(Suppl 3):35, 1991.
151. Gluckman E: Radiosensitivity in Fanconi anemia: application to the conditioning for bone marrow transplantation. Radiother Oncol 18(Suppl 1):88, 1990.
152. Kurre P, Pulsipher M, Woolfrey A, et al: Reduced toxicity and prompt engraftment after minimal conditioning of a patient with Fanconi anemia undergoing hematopoietic stem cell transplantation from an HLA-matched unrelated donor. J Pediatr Hematol Oncol 25:581, 2003.
153. Witherspoon RP, Storb R, Pepe M, et al: Cumulative incidence of secondary solid malignant tumors in aplastic anemia. Blood 79:289, 1992.
154. Storb R: Allogeneic marrow transplantation in patients with severe aplastic anemia. Transplant Rev 3:33, 1993.
155. Flowers MED, Doney KC, Storb R, et al: Marrow transplantation for Fanconi anemia with or without leukemic transformation: an update of the Seattle experience. Bone Marrow Transplant 9:167, 1992.
156. Thomas ED: Total body irradiation regimens for marrow grafting. Int J Radiat Oncol Biol Phys 19:1285, 1990.
157. Thomas ED, Clift RA, Hersman J, et al: Marrow transplantation for acute nonlymphoblastic leukemia in first remission using fractionated or single-dose irradiation. Int J Radiat Oncol Biol Phys 8:817, 1982.
158. Clift RA, Buckner CD, Appelbaum FR, et al: Allogeneic marrow transplantation in patients with acute myeloid leukemia in first remission: a randomized trial of two irradiation regimens. Blood 76:1867, 1990.
159. Clift RA, Buckner CD, Appelbaum FR, et al: Allogeneic marrow transplantation in patients with chronic myeloid leukemia in the chronic phase: a randomized trial of two irradiation regimens. Blood 77:1660, 1991.
160. Deeg HJ, Sullivan KM, Buckner CD, et al: Marrow transplantation for acute non lymphoblastic leukemia in first remission: toxicity and long-term follow-up of patients conditioned with single dose or fractionated total body irradiation. Bone Marrow Transplant 1:151, 1986.
161. Clift R, Buckner CD, Bianco J, et al: Marrow transplantation in patients with acute myeloid leukemia. Leukemia 6(Suppl 2):104, 1992.
162. Peterson FB, Deeg HJ, Buckner CD, et al: Marrow transplantation following escalating doses of fractionated total body irradiation and cyclophosphamide. A phase I trial. Int J Radiat Oncol Biol Phys 23:1027, 1992.
163. McAfee SL, Powell SN, Colby C, Spitzer TR: Dose-escalated total body irradiation and autologous stem cell transplantation for refractory hematologic malignancy. Int J Radiat Oncol Biol Phys 53:151, 2002.
164. Scarpati D, Frassoni F, Vitale V, et al: Total body irradiation in acute myeloid leukemia and chronic myelogenous leukemia: influence of dose and dose-rate on leukemia relapse. Int J Radiat Oncol Biol Phys 17:547, 1989.
165. Frassoni F: Eradication of leukaemic marrow and prevention of leukaemia relapse with total body irradiation and bone marrow transplantation. Med Oncol Tumor Pharmacother 8:189, 1991.
166. Corvo R, Lamparelli T, Bruno B, et al: Low-dose fractionated total body irradiation (TBI) adversely affects prognosis of patients with leukemia receiving an HLA-matched allogeneic bone marrow transplant from an unrelated donor (UD-BMT). Bone Marrow Transplant 30:717, 2002.
167. Chessells JM, Rogers DW, Leiper AD, et al: Bone-marrow transplantation has a limited role in prolonging second marrow remission in childhood lymphoblastic leukaemia. Lancet 1:1239, 1986.
168. Harris R, Feig S, Coccia P, et al: ALL in second remission: a CCSG study comparing intensive maintenance chemotherapy to bone marrow transplantation [abstract]. Proc Am Soc Clin Oncol 6:163, 1987.
169. Proctor SJ, Hamilton PJ, Taylor P, et al: A comparative study of combination chemotherapy versus marrow transplant in first remission in adult acute lymphoblastic leukaemia. Br J Haematol 69:35, 1988.
170. Mrsic M, Nemet D, Labar B, et al: Chemotherapy versus allogeneic bone marrow transplantation in adults with acute lymphoblastic leukemia. Transplant Proc 25:1268, 1993.
171. Johnson FL, Thomas ED: Treatment of relapsed acute lymphoblastic leukemia in childhood [letter]. N Engl J Med 310:263, 1984.
172. Brochstein JA, Kernan NA, Groshen S, et al: Allogeneic bone marrow transplantation after hyperfractionated total body irradiation and cyclophosphamide in children with acute leukemia. N Engl J Med 317:1618, 1987.
173. Buckner CD, Doney K, Sanders J, et al: Marrow transplantation for patients with acute lymphoblastic leukemia: the Seattle experience. Leukemia 6(Suppl 2):193, 1992.
174. Arcese W, Meloni G, Giona F, et al: Idarubicin plus ARA-C followed by allogeneic or autologous bone marrow transplantation in advanced acute lymphoblastic leukemia. Bone Marrow Transplant 7(Suppl 2):38, 1991.
175. Blaise D, Gaspard MH, Stoppa MA, et al: Allogeneic or autologous bone marrow transplantation for acute lymphoblastic leukemia in first complete remission. Bone Marrow Transplant 5:7, 1990.
176. Kersey JH, Weisdorf D, Nesbit ME, et al: Comparison of autologous and allogeneic bone marrow transplantation for treatment of high-risk refractory acute lymphoblastic leukemia. N Engl J Med 317:461, 1987.
177. Uderzo C, Coleselli P, Messina C, et al: Allogeneic BMT versus autologous BMT in childhood acute lymphoblastic leukemia (ALL): an Italian cooperative study of vincristine (VCR), R-TBI and cyclophosphamide. Bone Marrow Transplant 7(Suppl 2):132, 1991.
178. Gale RP, Buchner T, Horowitz MM, et al: Chemotherapy versus bone marrow transplants for adults with acute myelogenous leukemia (AML) in first remission [abstract]. Blood 82:168a, 1993.
179. Zittoun R, Mandelli F, Willemze R, et al: Prospective phase III study of autologous bone marrow transplantation (ABMT) v short intensive chemotherapy (IC) v allogeneic bone marrow transplantation (allo-BMT) during first complete remission (CR) of acute myelogenous leukemia (AML) [abstract]. Blood 82:85a, 1993.
180. Appelbaum FR, Fisher LD, Thomas ED: Chemotherapy v. marrow transplantation for adults with acute nonlymphocytic leukemia: a 5-year follow-up. Blood 72:179, 1988.
181. Powles RL, Morgenstern G, Clink HM, et al: The place of bone-marrow transplantation in acute myelogenous leukemia. Lancet 1:1047, 1980.

182. Reiffers J, Gaspard MH, Maraninchi D, et al: Allogeneic bone marrow transplantation versus chemotherapy in first-remission acute myeloid leukemia [letter]. J Clin Oncol 7:979, 1989.
183. Archimbaud E, Thomas X, Michallet M, et al: Prospective genetically randomized comparison between intensive postinduction chemotherapy and bone marrow transplantation in adults with newly diagnosed acute myeloid leukemia. J Clin Oncol 12:262, 1994.
184. Conde E, Iriondo A, Rayon C, et al: Allogeneic bone marrow transplantation versus intensification chemotherapy for acute myelogenous leukaemia in first remission: a prospective controlled trial. Br J Haematol 68:219, 1988.
185. Nesbit ME, Jr., Buckley JD, Feig SA, et al: Chemotherapy for induction of remission of childhood acute myeloid leukemia followed by marrow transplantation or multiagent chemotherapy: a report from the Childrens Cancer Group. J Clin Oncol 12:127, 1994.
186. Schalson G, Michel G, Landman-Parker J, et al: Allogeneic bone marrow transplantation (BMT) is the most effective treatment for acute myeloblastic leukemia in childhood [abstract]. Blood 82:169a, 1993.
187. Dahl GV, Kalwinsky DK, Mirro J, Jr., et al: Allogeneic bone marrow transplantation in a program of intensive sequential chemotherapy for children and young adults with acute nonlymphoblastic leukemia in first remission. J Clin Oncol 8:295, 1990.
188. Champlin RE, Ho WG, Gale RP, et al: Treatment of acute myelogenous leukemia. A prospective controlled trial of bone marrow transplantation versus consolidation chemotherapy. Ann Intern Med 102:285, 1985.
189. Zander AR, Keating M, Dicke K, et al: A comparison of marrow transplantation with chemotherapy for adults with acute leukemia of poor prognosis in first complete remission. J Clin Oncol 6:1548, 1988.
190. Cassileth PA, Andersen J, Lazarus HM, et al: Autologous bone marrow transplant in acute myeloid leukemia in first remission. J Clin Oncol 11:314, 1993.
191. Lowenberg B, Verdonck LJ, Dekker AW, et al: Autologous bone marrow transplantation in acute myeloid leukemia in first remission: results of a Dutch prospective study. J Clin Oncol 8:287, 1990.
192. Woods WG, Kobrinsky N, Buckley J, et al: Intensively timed induction therapy followed by autologous or allogeneic bone marrow transplantation for children with acute myeloid leukemia or myelodysplastic syndrome: a Childrens Cancer Group pilot study. J Clin Oncol 11:1448, 1993.
193. Gratwohl A, Hermans J, Niederwieser D, et al: Bone marrow transplantation for chronic myeloid leukemia: long-term results. Bone Marrow Transplant 12:509, 1993.
194. Clift RA, Appelbaum FR, Thomas ED: Treatment of chronic myeloid leukemia by marrow transplantation. Blood 82:1954, 1993.
195. Goldman JM, Gale RP, Horowitz MM, et al: Bone marrow transplantation for chronic myelogenous leukemia in chronic phase. Ann Intern Med 108:806, 1988.
196. Frassoni F, Strada P, Sessarego M, et al: Mixed chimerism after allogeneic marrow transplantation for leukaemia: correlation with dose of total body irradiation and graft-versus-host disease. Bone Marrow Transplant 5:235, 1990.
197. Weisser M, Schleuning M, Ledderose G, et al: Reduced-intensity conditioning using TBI (8 Gy), fludarabine, cyclophosphamide and ATG in elderly CML patients provides excellent results especially when performed in the early course of disease [Epub]. Bone Marrow Transplant, 2004.
198. Gulati SC, Shank B, Black P, et al: Autologous bone marrow transplantation for patients with poor-prognosis lymphoma. J Clin Oncol 6:1303, 1988.
199. Freedman AS, Takvorian T, Neuberg D, et al: Autologous bone marrow transplantation in poor-prognosis intermediate-grade and high-grade B-cell non-Hodgkin's lymphoma in first remission: a pilot study. J Clin Oncol 11:931, 1993.
200. Goldstone AH: High-dose therapy for the treatment of non-Hodgkin's lymphoma. *In* Armitage JO, Antman KH (eds): High-Dose Cancer Therapy: Pharmacology, Hematopoietins, Stem Cells. Baltimore, Williams & Wilkins, 1992, p 662.
201. Gulati S, Acaba L, Yahalom J, et al: Autologous bone marrow transplantation for acute myelogenous leukemia using 4-hydroperoxycyclophosphamide and VP-16 purged bone marrow. Bone Marrow Transplant 10:129, 1992.
202. Shepherd JD, Barnett MJ, Connors JM, et al: Allogeneic bone marrow transplantation for poor-prognosis non-Hodgkin's lymphoma. Bone Marrow Transplant 12:591, 1993.
203. Gulati S, Yahalom J, Acaba L, et al: Treatment of patients with relapsed and resistant non-Hodgkin's lymphoma using total body irradiation, etoposide, and cyclophosphamide and autologous bone marrow transplantation. J Clin Oncol 10:936, 1992.
204. Chopra R, Goldstone AH, Pearce R, et al: Autologous versus allogeneic bone marrow transplantation for non-Hodgkin's lymphoma: a case-controlled analysis of the European Bone Marrow Transplant Group Registry data. J Clin Oncol 10:1690, 1992.
205. Stewart FM: Indications and relative indications for stem cell transplantation in non-Hodgkin's lymphoma. Leukemia 7:1091, 1993.
206. Mahoney DG: Graft-versus-lymphoma effect in various histologies of non-Hodgkin's lymphoma. Leuk Lymphoma 44(Suppl 3): S99, 2003.
207. Ott M, Schmidberger H, Wormann B, et al: Involved-field irradiation in combination with total body irradiation (TBI) does not increase short-term toxicity compared with TBI alone in patients with advanced-stage low-grade non-Hodgkin lymphoma. Strahlenther Onkol 178:245, 2002.
208. Chaffey JT, Hellman S, Rosenthal DS, et al: Total body irradiation in the treatment of lymphocytic lymphoma. Cancer Treat Rep 61:1149, 1977.
209. Qasim MM: Total body irradiation as a primary therapy in non-Hodgkin lymphoma. Clin Radiol 30:287, 1979.
210. Johnson RE, Ruhl U: Treatment of chronic lymphocytic leukemia with emphasis on total body irradiation. Int J Radiat Oncol Biol Phys 1:387, 1976.
211. Kempin S, Shank B: Radiation in chronic lymphocytic leukemia. *In* Gale RP, Rai KR (eds): Chronic Lymphocytic Leukemia: Recent Progress and Future Direction. New York, Alan R Liss, 1987, p 337.
212. Rubin P, Bennett JM, Begg C, et al: The comparison of total body irradiation versus chlorambucil and prednisone for remission induction of active chronic lymphocytic leukemia: An ECOG study: Part I: Total body irradiation-response and toxicity. Int J Radiat Oncol Biol Phys 7:1623, 1981.
213. Jacobs P, King HS: A randomized prospective comparison of chemotherapy to total body irradiation as initial treatment for the indolent lymphoproliferative diseases. Blood 69:1642, 1987.
214. Lybeert MLM, Meerwaldt JH, Deneve W: Long-term results of low dose total body irradiation for advanced non-Hodgkin's lymphoma. Int J Radiat Oncol Biol Phys 13:1167, 1987.
215. Yahalom J, Gulati S, Shank B, et al: Total lymphoid irradiation, high-dose chemotherapy and autologous bone marrow transplantation for chemotherapy-resistant Hodgkin's disease. Int J Radiat Oncol Biol Phys 17:915, 1989.
216. Yahalom J, Gulati SC, Toia M, et al: Accelerated hyperfractionated total-lymphoid irradiation, high-dose chemotherapy, and autologous bone marrow transplantation for refractory and relapsing patients with Hodgkin's disease. J Clin Oncol 11:1062, 1993.
217. Moskowitz CH, Nimer SD, Zelenetz AD, et al: A two-step comprehensive high-dose chemoradiotherapy second-line program for relapsed and refractory Hodgkin disease: analysis by intent to treat and development of a prognostic model. Blood 97:616, 2001.
218. Anderson JE, Litzow MR, Appelbaum FR, et al: Allogeneic, syngeneic, and autologous marrow transplantation for Hodgkin's disease: the 21-year Seattle experience. J Clin Oncol 11:2342, 1993.
219. Horning SJ, Negrin RS, Chao NJ, et al: Autologous stem cell transplant for recurrent or refractory Hodgkin's disease: comparative results of total body irradiation (TBI) and chemotherapy-only high dose regimens [abstract]. Blood 82:445a, 1993.
220. Poen JP, Hoppe RT, Horning SJ: High-dose therapy and autologous bone marrow transplantation for relapsed/refractory

Hodgkin's disease: the impact of involved field radiotherapy on patterns of failure and survival. Int J Radiat Oncol Biol Phys 36:3, 1996.
221. Mundt AJ, Sibley G, Williams S, et al: Patterns of failure following high-dose chemotherapy and autologous bone marrow transplantation with involved field radiotherapy for relapsed/refractory Hodgkin's disease. Int J Radiat Oncol Biol Phys 33:261, 1995.
222. Lancet JE, Rapoport AP, Brasacchio R, et al: Autotransplantation for relapsed or refractory Hodgkin's disease: long-term follow-up and analysis of prognostic factors. Bone Marrow Transplant 22:265, 1998.
223. Stiff PJ, Unger JM, Forman SJ, et al: The value of augmented preparative regimens combined with an autologous bone marrow transplant for the management of relapsed or refractory Hodgkin disease: a Southwest Oncology Group phase II trial. Biol Blood Marrow Transplant 9:529, 2003.
224. Ozsahin M, Pene F, Touboul E, et al: Total body irradiation before bone marrow transplantation; results of two randomized instantaneous dose rates in 157 patients. Cancer 69:2853, 1992.
225. Belkacemi Y, Pene F, Touboul E, et al: Total body irradiation before bone marrow transplantation for acute leukemia in first or second complete remission. Results and prognostic factors in 326 consecutive patients. Strahlenther Onkol 174:92, 1998.
226. Valls A, Granena A, Carreras E, et al: Total body irradiation in bone marrow transplantation: fractionated versus single dose. Acute toxicity and preliminary results. Bull Cancer 76:797, 1989.
227. Jones LR, Toth BB, Keene HJ: Effects of total body irradiation on salivary gland function and caries-associated oral microflora in bone marrow transplant patients. Oral Surg Oral Med Oral Pathol 73:670, 1992.
228. Shepp DH, Dandliker PS, Flournoy N, et al: Sequential intravenous and twice-daily oral acyclovir for extended prophylaxis of Herpes simplex virus infection in marrow transplant patients. Transplant 43:654, 1987.
229. Clift RA, Bianco JA, Appelbaum FR, et al: A randomized controlled trial of pentoxifylline for the prevention of regimen-related toxicities in patients undergoing allogeneic marrow transplantation. Blood 82:2025, 1993.
230. Robien K, Schubert MM, Bruemmer B, et al: Predictors of oral mucositis in patients receiving hematopoietic cell transplants for chronic myelogenous leukemia. J Clin Oncol 22:1268, 2004.
231. Bearman SI, Appelbaum FR, Buckner CD, et al: Regimen-related toxicity in patients undergoing bone marrow transplantation. J Clin Oncol 6:1562, 1988.
232. Petersen FB, Bearman SI: Preparative regimens and their toxicity. *In* Forman SJ, Blume KG, Thomas ED (eds): Bone Marrow Transplantation. Boston, Blackwell Scientific, 1994, p 79.
233. Glucksberg H, Storb R, Fefer A, et al: Clinical manifestations of graft-versus-host disease in human recipients of marrow from HL-A-matched sibling donors. Transplant 18:295, 1974.
234. Slavin RE, Santos GW: The graft versus host reaction in man after bone marrow transplantation: pathology, pathogenesis, clinical features, and implication. Clin Immunol Immunobiol 1:472, 1973.
235. Ramsay NKC, Kersey JH, Robison LL, et al: A randomized study of the prevention of acute graft-versus-host disease. N Engl J Med 306:392, 1982.
236. Storb R, Deeg HJ, Whitehead J, et al: Methotrexate and cyclosporine compared with cyclosporine alone for prophylaxis of acute graft versus host disease after marrow transplantation for leukemia. N Engl J Med 314:729, 1986.
237. Sullivan KM, Kopecky KJ, Buckner CD, et al: Intravenous IgG to prevent graft-versus-host disease after bone marrow transplantation [letter]. N Engl J Med 323:705, 1990.
238. Vogelsang G, Farmer E, Hess A, et al: Thalidomide for the treatment of chronic graft-versus-host disease. N Engl J Med 326:1055, 1988.
239. Reisner Y, Kapoor N, Kirkpatrick D, et al: Transplantation for acute leukaemia with HLA-A and B non-identical parental marrow cells fractionated with soybean agglutinin and sheep red blood cells. Lancet 2:327, 1981.
240. Kernan NA: T-cell depletion for prevention of graft-versus-host disease. *In* Forman SJ, Blume KG, Thomas ED (eds): Bone Marrow Transplantation. Boston, Blackwell Scientific, 1994, p 124.
241. Emanuel D, Cunningham I, Jules-Elysee K, et al: Cytomegalovirus pneumonia after bone marrow transplantation successfully treated with the combination of ganciclovir and high-dose intravenous immune globulin. Ann Intern Med 109:777, 1988.
242. Enright H, Haake R, Weisdorf D, et al: Cytomegalovirus pneumonia after bone marrow transplantation: risk factors and response to therapy. Transplant 55:1339, 1993.
243. Ozsahin M, Schwartz LH, Pene F, et al: Is body weight a risk factor of interstitial pneumonitis after bone marrow transplantation? [correspondence]. Bone Marrow Transplant 10:97, 1992.
244. Ozsahin M, Belkacemi Y, Touboul E, et al: The influence of body surface on interstitial pneumonitis following bone marrow transplantation [abstract]. Int Congress Radiat Oncol 546, 1993.
245. Hartsell WF, Ghalie R, Rubin D, et al: Pulmonary complications of bone marrow transplantation (BMT): A comparison of total body irradiation and cyclophosphamide (TBI-Cy) to busulfan and cyclophosphamide (Bu-Cy) [abstract]. Int J Radiat Oncol Biol Phys 27(Suppl 1):186, 1993.
246. Granena A, Carreras E, Rozman C, et al: Interstitial pneumonitis after BMT: 15 years experience in a single institution. Bone Marrow Transplant 11:453, 1993.
247. Gogna NK, Morgan G, Downs K, et al: Lung dose rate and interstitial pneumonitis in total body irradiation for bone marrow transplantation. Australas Radiol 36:317, 1992.
248. Badier M, Guillot C, Delpierre S, et al: Pulmonary function changes 100 days and one year after bone marrow transplantation. Bone Marrow Transplant 12:457, 1993.
249. Wingard JR, Mellits ED, Sostrin MB, et al: Interstitial pneumonitis after allogeneic bone marrow transplantation: nine-year experience at a single institution. Medicine 67:175, 1988.
250. Sutton L, Kuentz M, Cordonnier C, et al: Allogeneic bone marrow transplantation for adult acute lymphoblastic leukemia in first complete remission: factors predictive of transplant-related mortality and influence of total body irradiation modalities. Bone Marrow Transplant 12:583, 1993.
251. Latini P, Aristei C, Aversa F, et al: Lung damage following bone marrow transplantation after hyperfractionated total body irradiation. Radiother Oncol 22:127, 1991.
252. Latini P, Aristei C, Aversa F, et al: Interstitial pneumonitis after hyperfractionated total body irradiation in HLA-matched T-depleted bone marrow transplantation. Int J Radiat Oncol Biol Phys 23:401, 1992.
253. Ho VT, Weller E, Lee SJ, et al: Prognostic factors for early severe pulmonary complications after hematopoietic stem cell transplantation. Biol Blood Marrow Transplant 7:223, 2001.
254. Ginsberg SJ, Comis RL: The pulmonary toxicity of antineoplastic agents. Semin Oncol 9:34, 1982.
255. Socie G, Devergie A, Girinsky T, et al: Influence of the fractionation of total body irradiation on complications and relapse rate for chronic myelogenous leukemia. Int J Radiat Oncol Biol Phys 20:397, 1991.
256. Kim TH, McGlave PB, Ramsay N, et al: Comparison of two total body irradiation regimens in allogeneic bone marrow transplantation for acute non-lymphoblastic leukemia in first remission. Int J Radiat Oncol Biol Phys 19:889, 1990.
257. Blume KG, Forman SJ, Snyder DS, et al: Allogeneic bone marrow transplantation for acute lymphoblastic leukemia during first complete remission. Transplant 43:389, 1987.
258. Devergie A, Reiffers J, Vernant JP, et al: Long-term follow-up after bone marrow transplantation for chronic myelogenous leukemia: factors associated with relapse. Bone Marrow Transplant 5:379, 1990.
259. Kim TH, Rybka WB, Lehnert S, et al: Interstitial pneumonitis following total body irradiation for bone marrow transplantation using two different dose rates. Int J Radiat Oncol Biol Phys 11:1285, 1985.
260. Bacigalupo A, van Lint MT, Frassoni F, et al: Late complications of allogeneic bone marrow transplantation. Med Oncol Tumor Pharmacother 8:261, 1991.

261. Labar B, Bogdanic V, Nemet D, et al: Total body irradiation with or without lung shielding for allogeneic bone marrow transplantation. Bone Marrow Transplant 9:343, 1992.
262. Fukuda T, Hackman RC, Guthrie KA, et al: Risks and outcomes of idiopathic pneumonia syndrome after nonmyeloablative and conventional conditioning regimens for allogeneic hematopoietic stem cell transplantation. Blood 102:2777, 2003.
263. Tait RC, Burnett AK, Robertson AG, et al: Subclinical pulmonary function defects following autologous and allogeneic bone marrow transplantation: relationship to total body irradiation and graft-versus-host disease. Int J Radiat Oncol Biol Phys 20: 1219, 1991.
264. Gandola L, Siena S, Bregni M, et al: Prospective evaluation of pulmonary function in cancer patients treated with total body irradiation, high-dose melphalan, and autologous hematopoietic stem cell transplantation. Int J Radiat Oncol Biol Phys 19:743, 1990.
265. Girinsky T, Socie G, Ammarguellat H, et al: Consequences of two different doses to the lungs during a single dose of total body irradiation: Results of a randomized study on 85 patients. Int J Radiat Oncol Biol Phys 30:821, 1994.
266. Barrett A, Depledge MH, Powles RL: Interstitial pneumonitis following bone marrow transplantation after low dose rate total body irradiation. Int J Radiat Oncol Biol Phys 9:1029, 1983.
267. Beyzadeoglu M, Oysul K, Dirican B, et al: Effect of dose-rate and lung dose in total body irradiation on interstitial pneumonitis after bone marrow transplantation. Tohoku J Exp Med 202:255, 2004.
268. Carruthers SA, Wallington MM: Total body irradiation and pneumonitis risk: a review of outcomes. Br J Cancer 90:2080, 2004.
269. Jules-Elysee K, Stover DE, Yahalom J, et al: Pulmonary complications in lymphoma patients treated with high-dose therapy and autologous bone marrow transplantation. Am Rev Resp Dis 146:485, 1992.
270. Deeg HJ, Flournoy N, Sullivan KM, et al: Cataracts after total body irradiation and marrow transplantation: a sparing effect of dose fractionation. Int J Radiat Oncol Biol Phys 10:957, 1984.
271. Benyunes MC, Sullivan KM, Deeg HJ, et al: Cataracts after bone marrow transplantation: Long-term follow-up of adults treated with fractionated total body irradiation. Int J Radiat Oncol Biol Phys 32:661, 1995.
272. Livesey SJ, Holmes JA, Whittaker JA: Ocular complications of bone marrow transplantation. Eye 3:271, 1989.
273. Calissendorff B, Bolme P, el Azazi M: The development of cataract in children as a late side-effect of bone marrow transplantation. Bone Marrow Transplant 7:427, 1991.
274. Sanders JE: Late effects in children receiving total body irradiation for bone marrow transplantation. Radiother Oncol Suppl 1:82, 1990.
275. Hamon MD, Gale RP, MacDonald ID, et al: Incidence of cataracts after single fraction total body irradiation: the role of steroids and graft versus host disease. Bone Marrow Transplant 12:233, 1993.
276. Deeg HJ: Delayed complications of marrow transplantation. Marrow Transplant Rev 2:10, 1992.
277. Ozsahin M, Belkacemi Y, Pene F, et al: Total body irradiation and cataract incidence: a randomized comparison of two instantaneous dose rates. Int J Radiat Oncol Biol Phys 28:343, 1993.
278. Dunn JP, Jabs DA, Wingard J, et al: Bone marrow transplantation and cataract development. Arch Ophthalmol 111:1367, 1993.
279. Lappi M, Rajantie J, Uusitalo RJ: Irradiation cataract in children after bone marrow transplantation. Graefe's Arch Clin Exp Ophthalmol 228:218, 1990.
280. Belkacemi Y, Labopin M, Vernant JP, et al: Cataracts after total body irradiation and bone marrow transplantation in patients with acute leukemia in complete remission: A study of the European Group for Blood and Bone Marrow Transplantation. Int J Radiat Oncol Biol Phys 41:659, 1998.
281. Aristei C, Alessandro M, Santucci A, et al: Cataracts in patients receiving stem cell transplantation after conditioning with total body irradiation. Bone Marrow Transplant 29:503, 2002.
282. Bray LC, Carey PJ, Proctor SJ, et al: Ocular complications of bone marrow transplantation. Br J Ophthalmol 75:611, 1991.
283. Van Kempen-Harteveld ML, Struikmans H, Kal HB, et al: Cataract after total body irradiation and bone marrow transplantation: degree of visual impairment. Int J Radiat Oncol Biol Phys 52:1375, 2002.
284. Beyzadeoglu M, Dirican B, Oysul K, et al: Evaluation of fractionated total body irradiation and dose rate on cataractogenesis in bone marrow transplantation. Haematologia (Budap) 32:25, 2002.
285. Fife K, Milan S, Westbrook K, et al: Risk factors for requiring cataract surgery following total body irradiation. Radiother Oncol 33:93, 1994.
286. Zierhut D, Lohr F, Schraube P, et al: Cataract incidence after total body irradiation. Int J Radiat Oncol Biol Phys 46:131, 2000.
287. Holmstrom G, Borgstrom B, Calissendorff B: Cataract in children after bone marrow transplantation: relation to conditioning regimen. Acta Ophthalmol Scand 80:211, 2002.
288. Van Kempen-Harteveld ML, van Weel-Sipman MH, Emmens C, et al: Eye shielding during total body irradiation for bone marrow transplantation in children transplanted for a hematological disorder: risks and benefits. Bone Marrow Transplant 31:1151, 2003.
289. Van Kempen-Harteveld ML, Belkacemi Y, Kal HB, et al: Dose-effect relationship for cataract induction after single-dose total body irradiation and bone marrow transplantation for acute leukemia. Int J Radiat Oncol Biol Phys 52:1367, 2002.
290. McDonald GB: Venoocclusive disease of the liver following marrow transplantation. Marrow Transplant Rev 3:50, 1993.
291. McDonald GB, Hinds MS, Fisher LD, et al: Veno-occlusive disease of the liver and multiorgan failure after bone marrow transplantation: a cohort study of 355 patients. Ann Intern Med 118:255, 1993.
292. McDonald GB, Sharma P, Matthews DE, et al: Veno-occlusive disease of the liver after bone marrow transplantation: diagnosis, incidence, and predisposing factors. Hepatology 4:116, 1984.
293. Resbeut M, Cowen D, Blaise D, et al: Fractionated or single-dose total body irradiation in 171 acute myeloblastic leukemias in first complete remission: Is there a best choice? Int J Radiat Oncol Biol Phys 31:509, 1995.
294. Girinsky T, Benhamou E, Bourhis J-H, et al: Prospective randomized comparison of single-dose versus hyperfractionated total body irradiation in patients with hematologic malignancies. J Clin Oncol 18:981, 2000.
295. Belkacemi Y, Ozsahin M, Rio B, et al: Is veno-occlusive disease incidence influenced by the total body irradiation technique? Semin Oncol 171:694, 1995.
296. Shulman HM, Hinterberger W: Hepatic veno-occlusive disease-liver toxicity syndrome after bone marrow transplantation. Bone Marrow Transplant 10:197, 1992.
297. Locasciulli A, Bacigalupo A, Alberti A, et al: Predictability before transplant of hepatic complications following allogeneic bone marrow transplantation. Transplant 48:68, 1989.
298. Lawton CA, Cohen EP, Barber-Derus SW, et al: Late renal dysfunction in adult survivors of bone marrow transplantation. Cancer 67:2795, 1991.
299. Bergstein J, Andreoli SP, Provisor AJ, et al: Radiation nephritis following total body irradiation and cyclophosphamide in preparation for bone marrow transplantation. Transplant 41:63, 1986.
300. Van Why SK, Friedman AL, Wei LJ, et al: Renal insufficiency after bone marrow transplantation in children. Bone Marrow Transplant 7:383, 1991.
301. Tarbell NJ, Guinan EC, Niemeyer C, et al: Late onset of renal dysfunction in survivors of bone marrow transplantation. Int J Radiat Oncol Biol Phys 15:99, 1988.
302. Rhoades JL, Lawson CA, Cohen EP, et al: Incidence of bone marrow transplant nephropathy (BMT-Np) after twice-daily hyperfractionated total body irradiation [abstract]. Cancer J Sci Am 3:116, 1997.
303. Miralbell R, Bieri S, Mermillod B, et al: Renal toxicity after allogeneic bone marrow transplantation: The combined effects of total body irradiation and graft-versus-host disease. J Clin Oncol 14:579, 1996.
304. Borg M, Hughes T, Horvath N, et al: Renal toxicity after total body irradiation. Int J Radiat Oncol Biol Phys 54:1165, 2002.

305. Kist-van Holthe JE, Goedvolk CA, Brand R, et al: Prospective study of renal insufficiency after bone marrow transplantation. Pediatr Nephrol 17:1032, 2002.
306. Miralbell R, Sancho G, Bieri S, et al: Renal insufficiency in patients with hematologic malignancies undergoing total body irradiation and bone marrow transplantation: a prospective assessment. Int J Radiat Oncol Biol Phys 58:809, 2004.
307. Sanders JE, Long-term Follow-up Team: Endocrine problems in children after bone marrow transplant for hematologic malignancies. Bone Marrow Transplant 8(Suppl 1):2, 1991.
308. Sanders JE: Endocrine complications of high-dose therapy with stem cell transplantation. Pediatr Transplant 8(Suppl 5):39, 2004.
309. Carlson K, Lonnerholm G, Smedmyr B, et al: Thyroid function after autologous bone marrow transplantation. Bone Marrow Transplant 10:123, 1992.
310. Sanders JE, Seattle Marrow Transplant Team: The impact of marrow transplant preparative regimens on subsequent growth and development. Semin Hematol 28:244, 1991.
311. Thomas BC, Stanhope R, Plowman PN, et al: Endocrine function following single fraction and fractionated total body irradiation for bone marrow transplantation in childhood. Acta Endocrinol 128:508, 1993.
312. Slatter MA, Gennery AR, Cheetham TD, et al: Thyroid dysfunction after bone marrow transplantation for primary immunodeficiency without the use of total body irradiation in conditioning. Bone Marrow Transplant 33:949, 2004.
313. Tauchmanova L, Selleri C, Rosa GD, et al: High prevalence of endocrine dysfunction in long-term survivors after allogeneic bone marrow transplantation for hematologic diseases. Cancer 95:1076, 2002.
314. Samuelsson A, Fuchs T, Simonsson B, et al: Successful pregnancy in a 28-year-old patient autografted for acute lymphoblastic leukemia following myeloablative treatment including total body irradiation. Bone Marrow Transplant 12:659, 1993.
315. Giri N, Vowels MR, Barr AL, et al: Successful pregnancy after total body irradiation and bone marrow transplantation for acute leukaemia. Bone Marrow Transplant 10:93, 1992.
316. Rio B, Letur-Konirsch H, Ajchenbaum-Cymbalista F, et al: Full-term pregnancy with embryos from donated oocytes in a 36-year-old woman allografted for chronic myeloid leukemia. Bone Marrow Transplant 13:487, 1994.
317. Petti N, Anghel G, Schimberni M, et al: Successful paternity with microassisted fertilization after total body irradiation-based conditioning for autologous bone marrow transplantation. Hematol J 4:285, 2003.
318. Hovi L, Saarinen UM, Siimes MA: Growth failure in children after total body irradiation preparative for bone marrow transplantation. Bone Marrow Transplant 8(Suppl 1):10, 1991.
319. Brauner R, Fontoura M, Zucker JM, et al: Growth and growth hormone secretion after bone marrow transplantation. Arch Dis Childhood 68:458, 1993.
320. Cohen A, Rovelli A, Bakker B, et al: Final height of patients who underwent bone marrow transplantation for hematological disorders during childhood: A study by the Working Party for Late Effects-EBMT. Blood 93:4109, 1999.
321. Frisk P, Arvidson J, Gustafsson J, et al: Pubertal development and final height after autologous bone marrow transplantation for acute lymphoblastic leukemia. Bone Marrow Transplant 33:205, 2004.
322. Sanders JE, Guthrie KA, Hoffmeister PA, et al: Final adult height of patients who received a childhood hematopoietic cell transplant [Epub]. Blood, 2004.
323. Goldberg SL, Tefferi A, Rummans TA, et al: Post-irradiation somnolence syndrome in an adult patient following allogeneic bone marrow transplantation. Bone Marrow Transplant 9:499, 1992.
324. Kramer JH, Crittenden MR, Halberg FE, et al: A prospective study of cognitive functioning following low-dose cranial radiation for bone marrow transplantation. Pediatrics 90:447, 1992.
325. Wenz F, Steinvorth S, Lohr F, et al: Prospective evaluation of delayed central nervous system (CNS) toxicity of hyperfractionated total body irradiation (TBI). Int J Radiat Oncol Biol Phys 48:1497, 2000.
326. Andrykowski MA, Altmaier EM, Barnett RL, et al: Cognitive dysfunction in adult survivors of allogeneic marrow transplantation: relationship to dose of total body irradiation. Bone Marrow Transplant 6:269, 1990.
327. Andrykowski MA, Schmitt FA, Gregg ME, et al: Neuropsychologic impairment in adult bone marrow transplant candidates. Cancer 70:2288, 1992.
328. Mulhern RK, Ochs J, Fairclough D, et al: Intellectual and academic achievement status after CNS relapse; a retrospective analysis of 40 children treated for acute lymphoblastic leukemia. J Clin Oncol 5:933, 1987.
329. Fann JR, Roth-Roemer, S, Burington BE, et al: Delirium in patients undergoing hematopoietic stem cell transplantation. Cancer 95:1971, 2002.
330. Faraci M, Lanino E, Dini G, et al: Severe neurologic complications after hematopoietic stem cell transplantation in children. Neurology 59:1895, 2002.
331. Socie G, Henry-Amar M, Cosset JM, et al: Increased incidence of solid malignant tumors after bone marrow transplantation for severe aplastic anemia. Blood 78:277, 1991.
332. Reed K, Ravikumar TS, Gifford RRM, et al: The association of Fanconi's anemia and squamous cell carcinoma. Cancer 52:926, 1983.
333. Sullivan KM, Mori M, Sanders J, et al: Late complications of allogeneic and autologous marrow transplantation. Bone Marrow Transplant 10:127, 1992.
334. Socie G, Henry-Amar M, Bacigalupo A, et al: Malignancies occurring after the treatment for aplastic anemia: A survey on 1680 patients conducted by the European Group for Bone Marrow Transplantation (EBMT)—Severe Aplastic Anemia Working Party [abstract]. Blood 80:169a, 1992.
335. Hosing C, Munsell M, Yazji S, et al: Risk of therapy-related myelodysplastic syndrome/acute leukemia following high-dose therapy and autologous bone marrow transplantation for non-Hodgkin's lymphoma. Ann Oncol 13:450, 2002.
336. Kolb HJ, Guenther W, Duell T, et al: Cancer after bone marrow transplantation. Bone Marrow Transplant 10:135, 1992.
337. Neglia J, Shapiro R, Haake R, et al: Second neoplasms following bone marrow transplantation (BMT) [abstract]. Blood 80:169a, 1992.
338. Bredeson C, Perry G, Martens C, et al: Outpatient total body irradiation as a component of a comprehensive outpatient transplant program. Bone Marrow Transplant 29:667, 2002.
339. Fermand J-P, Chevret S, Ravaud P, et al: High-dose chemoradiotherapy and autologous blood stem cell transplantation in multiple myeloma: results of a phase II trial involving 63 patients. Blood 82:2005, 1993.
340. Gandola L, Caracciolo D, Stern A, et al: High-dose sequential chemoradiotherapy, a widely applicable regimen, confers survival benefit to patients with high-risk multiple myeloma. J Clin Oncol 12:503, 1994.
341. Bjorkstrand B, Ljungman P, Bird JM, et al: Autologous stem cell transplantation in multiple myeloma: results of the European Group for Bone Marrow Transplantation. Stem Cells 13:140, 1995.
342. Barlogie B, Jagannath S, Desikan KR, et al: Total therapy with tandem transplants for newly diagnosed multiple myeloma. Blood 93:55, 1999.
343. Attal M, Harousseau JL, Facon T, et al: Single versus double autologous stem cell transplantation for multiple myeloma. N Engl J Med 349:2495, 2003.
344. Cavo M, Cellini C, Zamagni E, et al: Superiority of double over single autologous stem cell transplantation as first-line therapy for multiple myeloma [abstract]. Blood 104:155a, 2004.
345. Rimm IJ, Rappeport JM: Bone marrow transplantation for the Wiskott-Aldrich syndrome: long-term follow-up. Transplant 50:617, 1990.
346. Brochstein JA, Kirkpatrick D, Giardina PJ, et al: Bone marrow transplantation in two multiply transfused patients with thalassemia major. Br J Haematol 63:445, 1986.
347. Coccia PF, Krivit W, Cervenka J, et al: Successful bone-marrow transplantation for infantile malignant osteoporosis. N Engl J Med 302:701, 1980.

CHAPTER 18

CHARGED PARTICLE RADIOTHERAPY

William P. Levin and Thomas F. DeLaney

Interest in the use of charged particle radiotherapy has been primarily stimulated by the superior dose distributions that can be achieved with these particles compared with those produced by standard photon therapy techniques. Charged particles deposit energy in tissue through multiple interactions with electrons in the atoms of cells, although a small fraction of energy is also transferred to tissue through collisions with the nuclei of atoms. The energy loss per unit path length is relatively small and constant until near the end of the range, where the residual energy is lost over a short distance, resulting in a steep rise in the absorbed dose (i.e., energy absorbed per unit mass). This portion of the particle track, where energy is rapidly lost over a short distance, is known as the *Bragg peak* (Fig. 18-1).

The initial low-dose region in the depth-dose curve before the Bragg peak is referred to as the plateau of the dose distribution, and it is about 30% of the Bragg peak maximum dose. The Bragg peak is too narrow for practical clinical applications. For the irradiation of most tumors, the beam energy is modulated to achieve a uniform dose over a significant volume. This is accomplished by superimposing several Bragg peaks of descending energies (ranges) and weights to create a region of uniform dose over the depth of the target; these extended regions of uniform dose are called *spread-out Bragg peaks* (see Fig. 18-1). Although the beam modulation to spread out the Bragg peaks does increase the entrance dose, the proton dose distribution is still characterized by a lower dose region in normal tissue proximal to the tumor, a uniform high-dose region in the tumor, and zero dose beyond the tumor.

Charged particles are generally characterized as having high or low linear energy transfer (LET), the rate of energy loss by the particle in tissue. The LET influences the biologic impact of the energy deposited in tissue. X and gamma photons, protons, and helium ions are considered low-LET radiation. Heavier charged particles, such as neon and carbon, are considered high-LET radiation. There is an initial increase in the relative biologic effectiveness (RBE) with an increase in LET.[1] Carbon ions have a RBE of about 3, whereas the RBE of protons is estimated to be 1.1.[2] Higher LET radiation is less influenced by tissue oxygenation and less sensitive to variations in the cell cycle and DNA repair. For particle radiation, the gray equivalent (GyE) dose is calculated by multiplying the physical dose administered by the RBE for that particle.

PROTON BEAM RADIATION THERAPY

Most patients receiving charged particle therapy have been treated with protons. As of July 2004, more than 39,000 patients have received part or all of their radiation therapy by proton beams.[3] Table 18-1 lists operational proton beam treatment facilities worldwide. Several more sites are scheduled to come online over the next several years.

In 1946, Robert Wilson proposed the idea that proton beams could provide superior dose distributions over photons and should be considered for clinical radiation therapy.[4] Initially, patients were being treated at facilities designed and constructed for basic high-energy physics research, often resulting in very cumbersome treatments. The proton beams were limited to a fixed horizontal position, which meant that the patient had to be moved to align the tumor on the trajectory of the beam. This technique contrasts with the isocentric capabilities of the modern linear accelerator, which rotates around a point in space and can effectively target any site in the body. For many of the proton machines, the energy of the beam (which defined the depth of the Bragg peak) was sufficient to treat only superficial lesions (e.g., those of the eye) or intermediate-depth lesions (e.g., base of the skull). Because of these technical factors and the interests of the involved physicians, the clinical sites that had initially received the most attention were uveal melanomas in the eye and base of skull sarcomas. The major emphasis for proton therapy clinical research initially was dose escalation for tumors, for which local control with conventional radiotherapy was poor.

The development of hospital-based cyclotrons with higher energy beams capable of reaching deep-seated tumors (up to about 30 cm with a 235-MeV beam), field sizes comparable to linear accelerators, and rotational gantries has greatly facilitated proton radiation therapy. Increasingly, there is interest in protocols aimed at morbidity reduction in those tumor sites in which tumor control with photons is good. The competing technology for many patients is intensity-modulated radiation therapy (IMRT). Passively scattered proton fields and intensity-modulated proton therapy (IMPT) produce similar target dose distributions in the tumor, but IMPT delivers substantially higher integral dose to nontarget normal tissues.[5] This is thought to be most problematic for the pediatric population, and young patients are increasingly being referred for proton radiation therapy whenever possible. IMPT has also been developed using magnetically scanned proton pencil beams and permits even more conformal dose delivery than achievable with IMRT or passively scattered proton fields.[6,7]

Uveal Melanoma

Uveal melanoma is the most common primary ocular tumor. Historically, the primary treatment has been enucleation. Radiotherapy is an alternative to surgery, but it does not ensure preservation of sight due to the proximity of nearby structures, such as the cornea, lens, retina, fovea, and optic nerve. Because preservation of vision is of utmost importance (secondary only to tumor control), particle beam therapy, with its favorable dose distribution characteristics, has increasingly been employed in the treatment of these tumors.

At The Massachusetts General Hospital (MGH) in cooperation with The Massachusetts Eye and Ear Infirmary, a technique was developed in which patients undergo pretreatment placement of tantalum clips to demarcate the location of the tumor. When the patient is under treatment, these clips can be identified radiographically to allow for accurate daily set-up. Most institutions employ a fixed beam for treatment of these lesions, allowing the patient to sit upright. Immobilization is achieved with a mask and a bite block. Patients are asked to stare at a small light to help set eye position and are monitored with a video camera during treatment Typically, a total dose of 70 CGE (cobalt gray equivalent) is administered over 5 fractions.

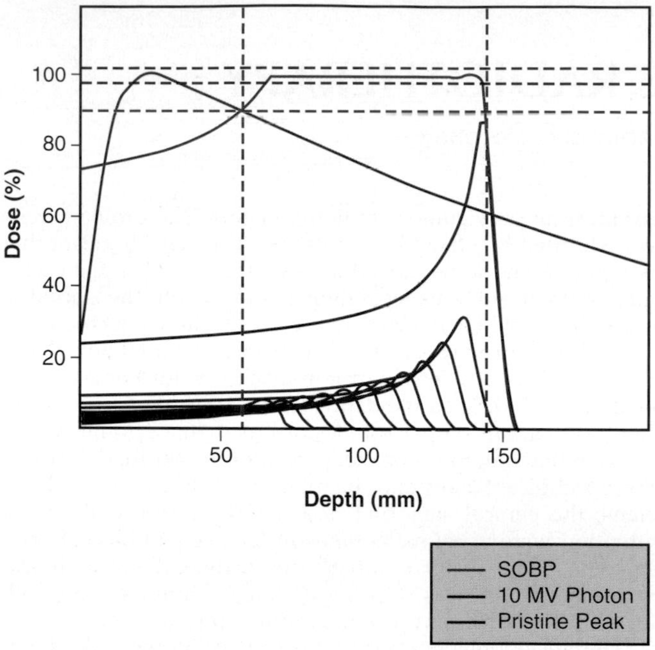

Figure 18-1 Depth-dose distributions for a spread-out Bragg peak (SOBP), its constituent pristine peaks, and a 10-MV photon beam. The SOBP dose distribution is created by adding the contributions of individually modulated pristine Bragg peaks. The penetration depth, or range (measured as the depth of the distal 90% of plateau dose) of the SOBP dose distribution, is determined by the range of the most distal pristine peak *(green line)*. The *black dashed lines* indicate the clinically acceptable variation in the plateau dose of ±2%. The *red dashed lines* indicate the 90% dose and spatial range and the modulation-width intervals. The SOBP dose distribution of even a single field can provide complete target volume coverage in depth and lateral dimensions, in sharp contrast to a single-photon field dose distribution; only a composite set of photon fields can deliver an appropriate clinical target dose distribution. Notice the absence of dose beyond the distal fall-off edge of the SOBP. (From Levin WP, Kooy H, Loeffler JS, DeLaney TF: Proton beam therapy. Br J Cancer 93:849-854, 2005.)

As of December 2002, more than 3000 patients with uveal melanoma have been treated with protons at the MGH in collaboration with The Massachusetts Eye and Ear Infirmary.[8] The 5-year actuarial local control rate is 96% for all sites within the globe, with an 80% survival rate. The probability of eye retention at 5 years was estimated to be 90% for the entire group and to be 97%, 93%, and 78% for patients with small, intermediate, and large tumors, respectively. Independent risk factors for enucleation were involvement of the ciliary body, tumor height greater than 8 mm, and distance between the posterior tumor edge and the fovea. These results compare favorably with local control rates of 89% reported with protons in Nice, France,[9] and similar results from the Paul Scherrer Institute in Villigen, Switzerland.[10]

Because some patients have experienced deteriorating vision after doses of 70 CGE, a randomized trial of 50 versus 70 CGE for small- and intermediate-sized lesions located within 6 mm of the optic disc or macula was conducted. Interim analysis of 188 patients, with a median follow-up of 60 months suggested no reduction in local control or survival. No significant improvement in visual outcome or complications has been observed. However, visual field analysis does show a smaller mean defect in the patients randomized to 50 CGE.[11]

Egger and colleagues reported long-term results of eye retention after treatment of uveal melanoma with proton beam therapy.[12] A total of 2645 patients (2648 eyes) was treated at Paul Scherrer Institute in Switzerland between 1984 and 1999. The overall eye retention rates at 5, 10, and 15 years after treatment were 89%, 86%, and 83%, respectively. Enucleation was related to large tumor size, mainly tumor height; male gender; high intraocular pressure; and a large degree of retinal detachment at treatment time.

Sarcomas of the Skull Base and Spine

Treatment of patients with sarcoma of the skull base is very challenging because of the proximity of critical structures, particularly the brain, brainstem, cervical cord, optic nerves, and chiasm. Surgery and conventional photon therapy have not been very successful at controlling these tumors. Because of the necessity to deliver dose in a precise manner, the use of proton therapy is becoming the treatment of choice for these tumors.

At the Harvard Cyclotron Laboratory (HCL), MGH physicians used a combination of protons and photons to treat patients with tumors of the skull base and cervical spine.[13] A total of 169 patients with chordoma and 165 patients with chondrosarcoma were treated. Ten-year local control was highest for chondrosarcomas, intermediate for male chordomas, and lowest for female chordomas (94%, 65%, and 42%, respectively). For cervical spine tumors, 10-year local control rates were not significantly different for chordomas and chondrosarcomas (54% and 48%, respectively), nor were there any significant differences in local control between male and female patients. In a Cox multivariate analysis, predictors of local control for base of skull chordomas included gender and equivalent uniform dose, gender and the target volume, or gender and the minimum target dose.[14] Five-year actuarial rates of endocrinopathy were as follows: 72% for hyperprolactinemia, 30% for hypothyroidism, 29% for hypogonadism, and 19% for hypoadrenalism. Minimum target dose (D_{min}) to the pituitary gland was found to be predictive of endocrinopathy; patients receiving 50 CGE or greater at D_{min} to the pituitary gland had a higher incidence and severity of endocrine dysfunction. Posterior pituitary dysfunction, represented by vasopressin activity with diabetes insipidus, was not observed.[15]

The French group at Orsay reported on the treatment of patients with skull base tumors, 34 with chordoma and 11 with chondrosarcoma.[16] Irradiation was done with a combination of photons and protons, with protons representing one third of the treatment. The median total dose delivered was 67 CGE (range, 60 to 70 CGE). With a mean follow-up of 30.5 months (range, 2 to 56 months), the 3-year local control rate was 83.1% for chordomas and 90% for chondrosarcomas. Three-year overall survival rates were 91% and 90%, respectively.

Like skull base tumors, treatment of spinal and paraspinal tumors is complicated by the proximity of the spinal cord. Radiation tolerance of the spinal cord is generally quoted at 45 to 50 Gy, well below that necessary to reliably control most sarcomas, which require doses of approximately 60 Gy for subclinical microscopic disease, 66 Gy for microscopically positive margins, and in excess of 70 Gy for gross residual disease. Proton radiotherapy, with its ability to spare adjacent tissues, offers advantages for treatment of tumors in this location.

Isacsson and colleagues compared conformal radiotherapy treatment plans with combination photon and proton plans for a patient with a cervical Ewing sarcoma.[17] The comparison showed small but clear advantages of protons for the boost.

Table 18-1 **Operational Proton Therapy Centers**

Facility	Location	Date of First Treatment	Patient Total	Date of Total
Institute of Theoretical and Experimental Physics (ITEP), Moscow	Russia	1969	3748	June 2004
St. Petersburg	Russia	1975	1145	April 2004
Chiba	Japan	1979	145	April 2002
Paul Scherrer Institute (PSI)	Switzerland	1984	4066	June 2004
Dubna	Russia	1999	191	Nov 2003
Uppsala	Sweden	1989	418	Jan 2004
Clatterbridge	England	1989	1287	Dec 2003
Loma Linda	California, USA	1990	9282	July 2004
Nice	France	1991	2555	April 2004
Orsay	France	1991	2805	Dec 2003
iThemba LABS	South Africa	1993	446	Dec 2003
University of California, San Francisco–Crocker Nuclear Laboratory (UCSF-CNL)	California, USA	1994	632	June 2004
Tri-University Meson Facility (TRIUMF), Vancouver	Canada	1995	89	Dec 2003
Paul Scherrer Institute (PSI)	Switzerland	1996	166	Dec 2003
Hahn-Meitner Institute (HMI), Berlin	Germany	1998	437	Dec 2003
National Cancer Center (NCC), Kashiwa	Japan	1998	270	June 2004
Hyogo Ion Beam Medical Center (HIBMC), Hyogo	Japan	2001	359	June 2004
Proton Medical Research Center (PMRC), Tsukuba	Japan	2001	492	July 2004
Northeast Proton Therapy Center (NPTC), Massachusetts General Hospital	Massachusetts, USA	2001	800	July 2004
Instituto Nazionale di Fisica Nucleare–Laboratori Nazionali del Sud (INFN-LNS), Catania	Italy	2002	77	June 2004
Wakasa Wan Energy Research Center (WERC)	Japan	2002	14	Dec 2003
Shizuoka	Japan	2003	69	July 2004
Midwest Proton Radiotherapy Institute (MPRI)	Indiana, USA	2004	21	July 2004

At 1% normal tissue complication probability in the spinal cord, the calculated tumor control probability was on average 5% higher for the photon plus proton boost combination.

Hug and coworkers presented results on combined photon and proton treatment of 47 patients with osteogenic and chondrogenic tumors of the axial skeleton.[18] Radiation was delivered postoperatively in 23 patients, preoperatively and postoperatively in 17, and as sole treatment in 7 patients. Mean radiation doses of 73.9 CGE, 69.8 CGE, and 61.8 CGE were delivered to group 1 (20 patients with recurrent or primary chordoma or chondrosarcoma), group 2 (15 patients with osteogenic sarcoma), and group 3 (12 patients with giant cell tumors, osteoblastomas, or chondroblastomas), respectively. Five-year actuarial local control and survival rates for patients with chondrosarcoma were 100% and 100%, and the rates for those with chordoma were 53% and 50%, respectively. The actuarial 5-year local control rate for patients with osteosarcoma was 59%. The 5-year actuarial local control and survival rates for the group 3 patients were 76% and 87%. Overall, improved local control occurred for primary versus recurrent tumors, gross total resection, and target doses of more than 77 Gy.

Weber and colleagues carried out a treatment planning comparison of intensity-modulated radiation therapy (IMRT) and intensity-modulated proton therapy (IMPT) for paraspinal sarcomas.[6] Plans for 5 patients were computed for IM photons (seven coplanar fields) and protons (three coplanar beams). Prescribed dose was 77.4 CGE for protons to the gross tumor volume. Surface and center spinal cord dose constraint for all techniques was 64 and 53 Gy/CGE, respectively. Gross tumor volume (GTV) coverage was optimal and equally homogeneous with IM photon and IM proton plans. Median heart, lung, kidney, stomach, and liver mean doses and doses at the 50% volume level were consistently reduced by a factor of 1.3 to 25. Although tumor target coverage and dose homogeneity were similar with IMPT and IMRT plans, integral doses were much lower with the IMPT plans. IMPT dose escalation (to 92.9 CGE to the GTV) was possible in all patients without exceeding the normal tissue dose limits.

At the Northeast Proton Therapy Center (MGH), a phase II study was completed in March 2005 of combined photon and proton beam radiation therapy in conjunction with maximal surgical resection (and dural plaque therapy when possible) for patients with spinal and paraspinal sarcomas. Doses of 77.4 CGE at 1.8 CGE per day to patients with gross residual disease and 70.2 CGE for patients with microscopic residual disease were employed.

Optic Pathway Glioma

At Loma Linda University (LLU), seven children with optic pathway gliomas were treated with proton radiation therapy.[19] At a median follow-up of 37 months, the tumors of all patients were locally controlled. A reduction in tumor volume was seen in three patients and was stable in the other four. Visual acuity was stable in those who presented with useful vision. Proton plans were compared with photon plans for individual patients. With proton radiation therapy, there was a 47% reduction in the dose to the contralateral optic nerve. There was an 11% reduction to the chiasm and a 13% reduction in dose to the pituitary gland. There was also a reduction in the dose to the temporal lobes and frontal lobes.

Astrocytoma

Between 1993 and 1998, 48 patients were treated for nonresectable grade II and III intracranial tumors at the Center for Proton Therapy in Orsay, France.[20] Mean tumor doses ranged from 63 to 67 Gy at 1.8 Gy per fraction. With a median follow-up of 18 months, local control was 97% (33 of 34) and 43% (6 of 14) for nonparenchymal and parenchymal lesions, respectively.

At the HCL/MGH, a phase II study was undertaken by MGH researchers to assess whether dose escalation to 90 CGE with conformal protons and photons in accelerated fractionation (twice daily) would improve local tumor control and survival.[21] A total of 23 patients were enrolled; they were between 18 and 70 years old. Actuarial survival rates at 2 and 3 years were 34% and 18%, respectively. The median survival time was 20 months, with 4 patients alive 22 to 60 months after diagnosis. All patients developed new areas of gadolinium enhancement during the follow-up period. Histologic examination of tissues obtained at biopsy, resection, or autopsy was conducted for 15 patients. Radiation necrosis only was demonstrated in seven patients, and their survival was significantly longer than that of patients with recurrent tumor. Tumor regrowth occurred most commonly in areas that received doses of 60 to 70 CGE or less; recurrent tumor was found in only one case in the 90-CGE volume. The investigators concluded that attempts to extend local control by enlarging the volume would likely be complicated by a high incidence of radionecrosis.

Benign Meningioma

Surgical resection of meningiomas is often limited by their location, such as the sphenoid ridge, parasellar area, and posterior fossa. Likewise, radiation therapy for these intracranial tumors is complicated by the proximity of critical structures, especially the visual system. Proton beam radiation, with its high degree of conformality, therefore would seem to be an attractive treatment modality.

Between 1981 and 1996, 46 patients with partially resected, biopsied, or recurrent benign meningiomas were treated with combined proton and photon radiation at the HCL/MGH.[22] The median dose to the tumor was 59 CGE. Overall survival rates at 5 and 10 years were 93% and 77%, respectively, and the recurrence-free rates at 5 and 10 years were 100% and 88%, respectively. Three patients presented with local tumor recurrence at 61, 95, and 125 months. One patient died of focal brain necrosis at 22 months. Neurologic complications, including memory deficits and hearing loss, were also seen. Four patients developed ophthalmologic toxicity. In all of these cases, maximum dose to the optic structures was greater than 58 CGE. Endocrine abnormalities after treatment were also seen.

Investigators from Paul Scherrer Institute in Switzerland reported the treatment of 16 patients with recurrent, residual, or untreated intracranial meningiomas.[7] The median prescribed dose was 56 CGE (range, 52 to 64 CGE) at 1.8 to 2 CGE per fraction. Cumulative 3-year local control, progression-free survival, and overall survival rates were 91%, 91%, and 92%, respectively. No patient died of recurrent meningioma. Radiographic follow-up (median, 34 months) revealed an objective response in three patients and stable disease in 12 patients. The cumulative 3-year, toxicity-free survival rate was 76%. One patient with an optic nerve sheath meningioma presented with sudden visual field deterioration of the ipsilateral eye 30 months after irradiation (56 Gy). Another patient, with optic nerve encasement by disease, developed visual deterioration at 9 months. A third patient developed symptomatic brain necrosis 7 months after treatment. No radiation-induced hypothalamic or pituitary dysfunction was observed.

Paranasal Sinus, Nasal, and Nasopharyngeal Tumors

Mock and associates performed a planning comparison study of various photon and proton techniques for the treatment of paranasal sinus carcinoma.[5] In five patients, proton plans were compared with conventional, conformal, and IMRT photon plans. The evaluations analyzed dose-volume histogram findings of the target volumes and organs at risk (OARs) (i.e., pituitary gland, optic pathway structures, and brain).

The mean and maximal doses, dose inhomogeneities, and conformity indices for the planning target volumes were comparable for all techniques. Photon plans resulted in greater volumes of irradiated nontarget tissues at the 10% to 70% dose level compared with the corresponding proton plans. Compared with conventional techniques, conformal and IMRT photon treatment planning options similarly reduced the mean dose to the OARs. The use of protons further reduced the mean dose to the OARs by up to 65% and 62% compared with conformal and IMRT technique, respectively.

Between 1991 and 1996, 32 patients with carcinomas of the paranasal sinuses were treated on an accelerated photon plus proton protocol.[23] The stage distribution was T3 in two cases and T4 in 30 cases, and all were N0 and M0. Four patients had undergone a gross total resection, and the others had undergone only biopsy or subtotal resection. The median follow-up was 2.7 years. Actuarial disease-specific survival at 3 years was 62%. There have been 10 deaths, 3 with intercurrent disease and 7 with metastatic disease. The 3-year actuarial local control rate was 89%. Late toxicity has included temporal lobe necrosis in three patients. Three patients have required surgical soft tissue repair.

Investigators at MGH performed a prospective study incorporating chemotherapy, surgery, and combined proton-photon therapy in the treatment of patients with neuroendocrine tumors of the sinonasal tract.[24] Nineteen patients with olfactory neuroblastoma or neuroendocrine carcinoma were treated between 1992 and 1998. Patients received chemotherapy with two courses of cisplatin and etoposide, followed by high-dose proton-photon radiotherapy to 69.2 CGE using 1.6 to 1.8 CGE per fraction twice daily in a concomitant boost schedule. Two additional courses of chemotherapy were given to responders.

With a median follow-up of 45 months (range, 20 to 92 months), 15 of the 19 patients were still alive. Four patients died of disseminated disease 8 to 47 months after their original diagnosis. The 5-year survival rate was 74%, and local control was 88%. Acute toxicity of chemotherapy was tolerable, with no patient sustaining more than grade 3 hematologic toxicity. One patient developed unilateral vision loss after the first course of chemotherapy; otherwise, visual preservation was achieved in all patients. Four patients who were clinically intact developed radiation-induced damage to the frontal or temporal lobe by magnetic resonance imaging criteria. Two patients showed soft tissue or bone necrosis, and one of these patients required surgical repair of a cerebrospinal fluid leak.

The investigators concluded that neoadjuvant chemotherapy and high-dose proton-photon therapy was a successful treatment for these patients. They also suggested that radiation-induced visual loss was avoided by the use of stereotactic setup and protons.

At LLU, 16 patients with recurrent nasopharyngeal carcinoma were treated with conformal proton radiation.[25] Patients had initially been treated with photon therapy using doses of 50 to 70 Gy. An additional 59 to 70 CGE was administered using conformal proton radiation. With a mean follow-up of 23 months, 24-month actuarial overall and locoregional progression-free survival rates were both 50%. No central nervous system complications were observed.

Acoustic Neuroma

Between 1991 and 1999, 30 patients with acoustic neuroma were treated with proton therapy at LLU.[26] Patients with useful hearing before treatment received 54 CGE in 30 fractions, and patients without useful hearing received 60 CGE. Follow-up ranged from 7 to 98 months (median, 34 months), during which no patients demonstrated disease progression on magnetic resonance imaging scans. Eleven patients demonstrated radiographic regression. Of the 13 patients with useful hearing before treatment, 4 (31%) maintained hearing. No transient or permanent treatment-related trigeminal or facial nerve dysfunction was observed. Investigators have become interested in evaluating reduction in tumor dose in an attempt to increase hearing preservation rates.

The group at MGH treated 88 patients with vestibular schwannoma using proton beam stereotactic radiosurgery. Two to four convergent fixed beams of 160-MeV protons were applied. Surgical resection had been performed previously in 15 patients (17%). Facial nerve function and trigeminal nerve function were normal in 90% of patients. Eight patients had good or excellent hearing, and 13 patients had serviceable hearing. A median dose of 12 CGE was prescribed to the 70% to 108% isodose lines (median, 70%). The median follow-up was 38 months (range, 12 to 102 months). The actuarial 2- and 5-year tumor control rates were 95% and 93%, respectively. Salvage radiosurgery was performed in one patient 32.5 months after treatment, and a craniotomy was required 19 months after treatment in another patient with hemorrhage in the vicinity of stable tumor. Three patients underwent shunting for hydrocephalus. The actuarial 5-year cumulative radiologic reduction rate was 94%. Of the 21 patients with functional hearing, 7 (33%) retained serviceable hearing ability. Actuarial 5-year normal facial and trigeminal nerve function was about 90%. Univariate analysis revealed that prescribed dose, maximum dose, and inhomogeneity coefficient were associated with a significant risk of long-term facial neuropathy. No other cranial nerve deficits were observed.

Carcinoma of the Prostate

Investigators at MGH completed a phase III trial comparing 67.2 Gy of photons with 75.6 CGE using a perineal proton boost to the prostate following whole pelvic photons.[27] From 1982 to 1992, 202 patients with T3 or T4 prostate cancer received 50.4 Gy by four-field photons. Patients then received 25.2 CGE with conformal protons or a 16.8-Gy photon boost. No differences between the two groups were found in overall survival, total recurrence-free survival, or local recurrence-free survival. The local recurrence-free survival at 7 years for patients with poorly differentiated tumors (Gleason 9 or 10) was 85% on the proton arm and 37% on the photon arm. Grade 1 and 2 rectal bleeding was higher in the proton arm (32% versus 12%), as was urethral stricture (19% versus 8%). Dose escalation to 75.6 CGE by conformal proton boost led to increased late radiation sequelae but not to increased total survival in any subgroup. However, there was improved local recurrence-free survival in patients with poorly differentiated tumors.

The Loma Linda University experience of proton therapy for prostate cancer was reported.[28] Between 1991 and 1997, 1255 patients with prostate cancer were treated using conformal proton therapy. The overall biochemical disease-free survival rate was 73%, and it was 90% for patients with an initial prostate-specific antigen (PSA) value less than 4.0; it was 87% in patients with PSA nadirs less than .50 after treatment. Rates dropped with rises in initial and nadir PSA values.

In general, conformal proton beam radiation therapy was well tolerated; the rate of Radiation Therapy Oncology Group (RTOG) grade 3 or higher acute gastrointestinal or genitourinary morbidity was less than 1%. RTOG grade 3 late morbidity was seen in 16 patients (1%) and grade 4 in 2 patients (0.2%). Late gastrointestinal toxicity included grade 3 bleeding and pain in two patients and a bowel obstruction requiring diverting colostomy in one patient. All severe gastrointestinal toxicity initially manifested within the first 2.5 years after treatment. The actuarial 5-year and 10-year rates for freedom from grade 3 and 4 gastrointestinal morbidity were both 99%.

Late genitourinary morbidity was seen more frequently than gastrointestinal morbidity. Fourteen patients developed grade 3 late toxicity; 8 patients had urethral strictures, 4 had hematuria, and 2 had dysuria. The actuarial 5- and 10-year rates for freedom from grade 3 and 4 genitourinary toxicity were both 99%. One patient developed necrosis of the symphysis, which was partially included in the treatment field. Because of the very small incidence of grade 3 and 4 side effects, no statistically significant prognostic variables for toxicity could be found. These results, when accounting for length of follow-up, compare favorably with conformal photon therapy and intensity-modulated photon therapy.

MGH and Loma Linda conducted a phase III randomized trial of dose in patients with early-stage prostate cancer.[29] Between 1996 and 1999, 393 patients with early-stage prostate cancer received a conformal proton radiation boost of 19.8 or 28.8 GyE. After the boost, all patients received 50.4 Gy using three-dimensional conformal photons to the prostate, seminal vesicles, and periprostatic tissues. No patient received adjunctive androgen-suppression therapy with irradiation. Median follow-up was 4 years.

The distribution of PSA nadirs of less than 0.5 or less than 1.0 ng/mL was 36.7% and 73% after 70.2 GyE and 50% and 79.9% after 79.2 GyE, respectively. The cumulative incidence estimates of the 5-year local failure rate using the surrogate of a PSA value more than 1 ng/mL 2 or more years after irradiation were 63.6% for the 70.2 GyE group and 36.3% for the 79.2 GyE group ($P < .0001$). The 5-year biochemical failure rates were 37.3% for the conventional-dose group and 19.1% for the high-dose group ($P = .00001$). This difference also held true when only those with low-risk disease were examined (T1B-2A, PSA < 10, Gleason ≤ 6). The 5-year biochemical failure rate was 34.9% in the conventional-dose arm and only 17.2% in the high-dose arm ($P = .002$). It was also significant for intermediate-risk patients (39.5% versus 21.3%, $P = .01$). There was no difference in the overall survival rates between the treatment arms. Only 2% of patients receiving conventional-dose and 1.5% receiving high-dose irradiation experienced acute urinary or rectal morbidity of RTOG grade 3 or higher. The respective proportions for those experiencing any grade 2 acute morbidity were 62% and 69%. Only 1.5% and 0.5%, respectively, have experienced late morbidities of RTOG grade 3 or higher.

The investigators concluded that there was an advantage in terms of freedom from biochemical failure for men with low- and intermediate-risk prostate cancer receiving high-dose versus conventional-dose conformal irradiation. They also indicated that this advantage was achieved without any associated increase in acute or late urinary or rectal morbidity.

Gastrointestinal Tumors

Investigators at Tsukuba University in Japan have reported impressive long-term control and survival results for 122 patients with primary hepatocellular carcinoma treated with proton radiotherapy.[30] The dose per fraction was 4 CGE, with a mean total dose of 72 CGE. The 7-year local control and survival rates were 94% and 27%, respectively. Irradiation with protons did not cause clinically symptomatic changes in liver function. The only notable change observed was a transient increase in the levels of liver transaminases.

Because of the presence of nearby critical structures, dose limitations are frequently an issue in the treatment of pancreatic cancer. Stripp and coworkers conducted a study comparing proton plans to conventional photon plans for patients with unresectable pancreatic cancer.[31] Dose-volume histograms were generated for the GTV, clinical target volume (CTV), spinal cord, liver, and right and left kidneys. Proton plans used a two- or three-field technique. With the CTV and GTV receiving the same dose from proton and photon plans, all individual proton plans were superior to the photon plans in reduction of normal tissue doses. For the four patients evaluated, the average dose reduction to 50% of the organ at risk was 78% to the spinal cord, 73% to the left kidney, 43% to the right kidney, and 55% to the liver.

Lung Cancer

At LLU, a prospective study was undertaken to assess the efficacy and toxicity of conformal proton beam radiotherapy for 37 patients with medically inoperable non–small cell lung cancer.[32] Eligible patients had clinical stage I to IIIa non–small cell lung cancer and were not candidates for surgical resection for medical reasons or because they refused surgery. Patients with adequate cardiopulmonary function received 45 Gy to the mediastinum and gross tumor volume with photons with a concurrent proton boost to the GTV of an additional 28.8 CGE. Total tumor dose was 73.8 CGE given over 5 weeks. Patients with poor cardiopulmonary function received proton beam radiotherapy to the GTV only, with 51 CGE given in 10 fractions over a 2-week period. Follow-up of evaluable patients ranged from 3 to 45 months, with a median of 14 months. Two patients in the proton and photon arm developed pneumonitis that resolved with oral steroids; otherwise, no significant toxicities were encountered. The 2-year actuarial disease-free survival for the entire group was 63%; for patients with stage I tumors, the 2-year disease-free survival rate was 86%, and the local control rate was 87%.

Between 1983 and 2000, patients with non–small cell lung cancer were treated with proton therapy at the University of Tsukuba.[33] There were 28 patients with stage I disease, 9 with stage II, 8 with stage III, 1 with stage IV, and 5 with recurrent disease. Thirty-three patients had squamous cell carcinoma, 17 had adenocarcinoma, and 1 had large cell carcinoma. Median fraction size was 3.0 Gy (range, 2.0 to 6.0 Gy). Median total dose delivered was 76 Gy (range, 49.0 to 93.0 Gy). The 5-year overall survival rate was 29% for all patients, 70% for stage IA patients, and 16% for stage IB patients. The 5-year in field local control rate was higher for patients with stage IA (89%) disease than those with IB (39%) disease. Forty-seven patients (92%) experienced acute lung toxicity of grade 1 or less; three had grade 2, one had grade 3, and no patient experienced grade 4 toxicity.

Pediatric Malignancies

Investigators in Switzerland looked at the potential influence of improved dose distribution with proton beams compared with conventional or intensity-modulated (IM) x-ray beams on the incidence of treatment-induced secondary cancers in children.[34] Two children, one with parameningeal rhabdomyosarcoma and a second with medulloblastoma, were used as models for this study. After defining the target and critical structures, treatment plans were calculated and optimized, four for the rhabdomyosarcoma case (i.e., conventional x-ray, IM x-rays, protons, and IM protons) and three for the irradiation of the spinal axis in medulloblastoma (i.e., conventional x-ray, IM x-rays, and protons). The secondary cancer incidence was estimated using a model by the International Commission on Radiologic Protection. This model allowed estimation of absolute risks of secondary cancer for each treatment plan based on dose-volume distributions for nontarget organs. Proton beams reduced the expected incidence of radiation-induced secondary cancers for the rhabdomyosarcoma patient by a factor equal to or greater than 2, and for the medulloblastoma cases, it was reduced by a factor of 8 to 15 compared with IM or conventional x-ray plans. This study underscores the concern with using radiation therapy in the treatment of pediatric malignancies. It is the goal of clinicians to eradicate the primary tumor and to minimize the risk of radiation-induced malignancies over the lifetime of these patients.

In a study done at MGH, treatment plans were compared from standard photon therapy or IMRT and protons for craniospinal axis irradiation and posterior fossa boost in a patient with medulloblastoma.[35] Substantial normal tissue sparing was realized with IMRT and proton irradiation of the posterior fossa and spinal axis (Figs. 18-2 and 18-3). The dose to 90% of the cochlea was reduced from 101% of the prescribed posterior fossa boost dose from conventional x-rays to 33% and 2% from IMRT and protons, respectively. The dose to 50% of the heart volume was reduced from 72% for photons to 30% for IMRT and 0.5% for protons.

The LLU group also compared photon and proton plans for pediatric patients receiving posterior fossa irradiation.[36] Using original planning CT scans, the posterior fossa, inner and middle ear, and temporal lobes were delineated. The 95% isodose encompassed the posterior fossa in all plans. Normal structures received markedly less radiation from proton plans than from photon plans. The cochlea received an average mean of 25% of the prescribed dose from the proton plan, and 75% from the photons. Forty percent of temporal lobe volume was completely excluded using protons; with photons, 90% of the temporal lobe received 31% of the dose.

LLU investigators evaluated the safety and efficacy of proton beam irradiation in the treatment of pediatric patients with intracranial low-grade astrocytoma.[37] Between 1991 and 1997, 27 patients underwent fractionated proton radiation therapy for progression of recurrent low-grade astrocytoma. Patients were between 2 and 18 years old. Twenty-five (92%) of the 27 patients were treated for progressive, unresectable, or residual disease after subtotal resection. The mean target dose was 55.2 CGE (range, 50.4 to 63.0 CGE), and the fraction size was 1.8 CGE. At a mean follow-up period of 3.3 years (range, 0 to 6.8 years), 6 of 27 patients experienced local failure within the irradiated field, and 4 of 27 had died. Local control and survival rates were 87% and 93%, respectively, for centrally located tumors; 71% and 86% for hemispheric tumors;

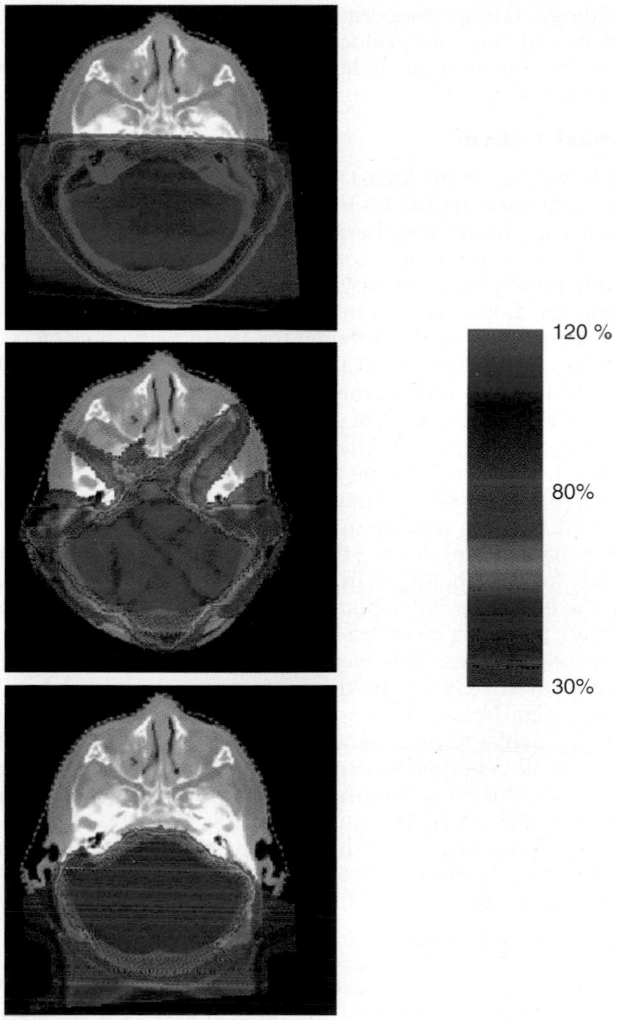

Figure 18-2 Three-dimensional, conformal photon *(upper panel)*, intensity-modulated radiation therapy (IMRT, *middle panel*), and passively scattered proton *(lower panel)* dose distributions for delivery of the posterior fossa boost in a patient with medulloblastoma. Notice the absence of dose to the temporal lobes, pituitary, orbits, and cochlea that can be achieved with protons that is not possible with three-dimensional, conformal photon therapy or IMRT. This additional dose to nontarget normal tissues offers only potential morbidity to these young patients. (From St Clair WH, Adams JA, Bues M, et al: Advantage of protons compared to conventional x-ray or IMRT in the treatment of a pediatric patient with medulloblastoma. Int J Radiat Oncol Biol Phys 58:727-734, 2004.)

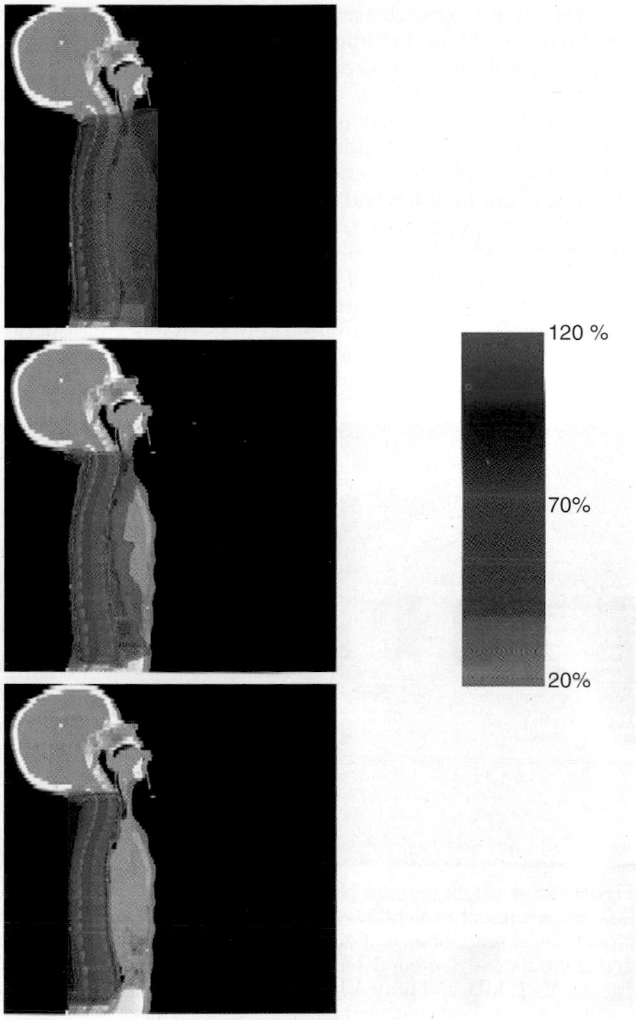

Figure 18-3 Sagittal dose displays for the spinal irradiation field in a child with medulloblastoma undergoing craniospinal irradiation with three-dimensional, conformal photons *(upper panel)*, intensity-modulated radiation therapy (IMRT, *middle panel*), or passively scattered proton *(lower panel)* fields. Notice the absence of a significant exit dose beyond the anterior border of the vertebral bodies with protons, sparing bowel, heart, and mediastinum from potential side effects of radiotherapy. (From St Clair WH, Adams JA, Bues M, et al: Advantage of protons compared to conventional x-ray or IMRT in the treatment of a pediatric patient with medulloblastoma. Int J Radiat Oncol Biol Phys 58:727-734, 2004.)

and 60% and 60% for tumors of the brainstem. All children with local control maintained their performance status, except one, who developed moyamoya disease. All six patients with optic pathway tumors and useful vision maintained or improved their visual status.

Four pediatric patients presenting with aggressive giant cell tumors of the skull base were treated with a combination of proton and photon beam radiation at MGH.[38] Three female patients and one male patient (10 to 15 years old) had undergone prior, extensive surgical resections and were treated for primary or recurrent disease. Gross residual tumor was evident in three patients, and microscopic disease was suspected in one patient. Combined proton and photon radiation therapy was based on three-dimensional planning. Target doses of 57.6 to 61.2 CGE were given in daily fractions of 1.8 CGE. With observation times between 3.1 and 5.8 years, all four patients were alive and well, disease remained locally controlled, and they had no evidence of recurrent disease. Except for one patient with partial pituitary insufficiency after radiotherapy for recurrent sellar disease, no late effects attributable to radiation therapy have been observed.

Retroperitoneal tumors, such as neuroblastoma, can be quite difficult to treat, given the proximity of the spinal cord, liver, and kidneys. In a comparison of proton and photon plans for a patient treated for neuroblastoma, a significant reduction in normal tissue exposure was achieved using protons.[39] Likewise, protons offered a preferable dose distribution to photons in two patients treated for orbital rhabdomyosarcoma.[40] Dose-volume histograms were obtained for target and nontarget regions, including the lens, bony orbit, pituitary gland, optic chiasm, optic nerves, lacrimal gland, and ipsilateral frontal and temporal lobes. Doses to 90%, 50%, and 5% of lens volume were kept at less than 1%, less than 2%, and less than 8%, respectively. At a mean follow-up of 3 years, visual acuity for both patients was excellent, and there was no evidence of cataract formation. Pituitary function was normal; cosmetically, only mild enophthalmos was noticeable. The steep dose gradient beyond the orbit minimized irradiation of normal brain parenchyma, with almost complete sparing of the pituitary gland (Fig. 18-4).

Ongoing clinical trials of proton beam radiation therapy are in progress at the Northeast Proton Therapy Center for pediatric patients with medulloblastoma, rhabdomyosarcoma, and retinoblastoma. Children being treated on the Children's Oncology Group cooperative studies who are to receive radiation therapy on protocol can be irradiated with protons, with the anticipation of less normal tissue irradiation and morbidity (Fig. 18-5).

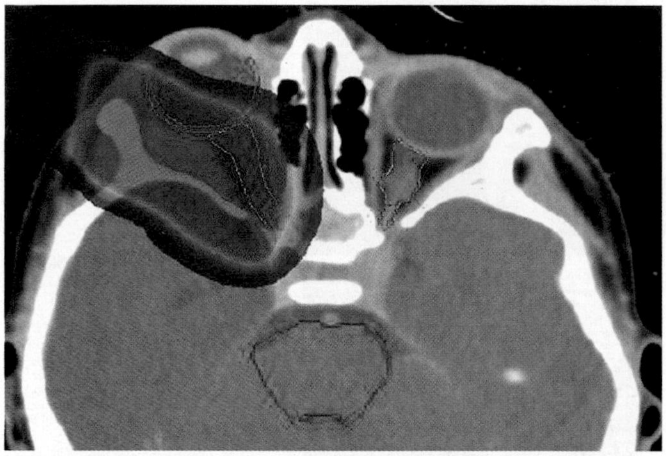

Figure 18-4 Right anterior oblique proton beam radiation therapy field for treatment of a child with a right orbital rhabdomyosarcoma. Notice the absence of an exit dose to the pituitary, contralateral orbit, and contralateral temporal lobe. (Courtesy of Nancy Tarbell, MD, Torunn Yock, MD, and Judy Adams, CMD, Northeast Proton Therapy Center, Massachusetts General Hospital, Boston, MA.)

Breast Cancer

Some patients with breast cancer have anatomic configurations that make it difficult to adequately treat the breast while sparing the underlying lung and heart. A treatment planning exercise was undertaken comparing standard photon therapy to IMRT and proton therapy in the treatment of breast cancer.[41] Using CT data from a breast cancer patient, treatment plans were computed for the different treatment techniques. A dose of 50 Gy was prescribed to the target volume consisting of the involved breast, internal mammary, supraclavicular, and axillary nodes. Comparison of plans revealed worse dose heterogeneity for the photon plan compared with the other two plans. Lung dose-volume histograms for the photon and IMRT plans were comparable, whereas the proton plan showed the best sparing over all dose levels. Mean doses to the ipsilateral lung for the three plans were 17 Gy, 15 Gy, and 13 Gy, for the photon, IMRT, and proton plans, respectively. For the heart, the IMRT plan delivered the highest mean dose (16 Gy), reflecting the extra dose delivered through this organ to spare the lungs. This was reduced somewhat by the standard plan (15 Gy), with the best sparing provided by the proton plan (6 Gy). When the IMRT plan was re-optimized with an increased precedence to the normal tissues, the mean doses to all neighboring organs at risk could be reduced, but only at the cost of substantial target dose heterogeneity. Only the two-field, energy-modulated proton plan had the potential to preserve target dose homogeneity while simultaneously minimizing the dose delivered to lungs, heart, and the contralateral breast.

Cost Comparisons

All of the clinical and treatment planning results that have been reported indicate that proton beams offer a significant

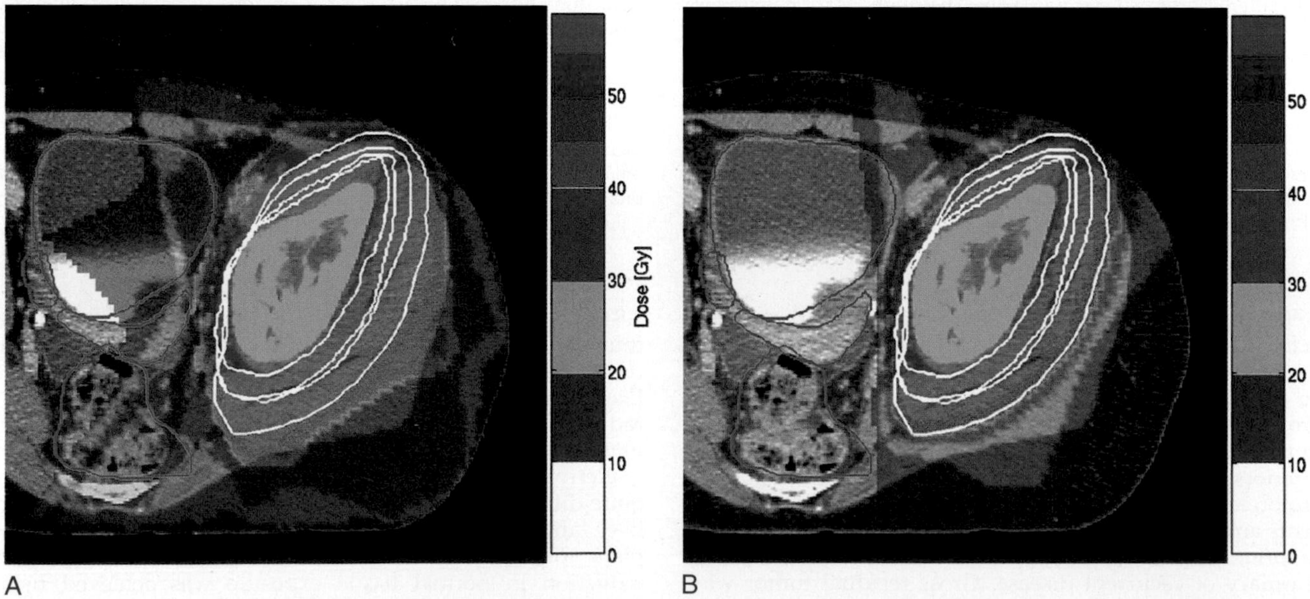

Figure 18-5 Intensity-modulated radiation therapy (IMRT) (**A**) and passively scattered proton dose distributions (**B**) for delivery of radiation therapy to a young patient with a Ewing's sarcoma of the left acetabulum after 12 weeks of chemotherapy. Protons deliver substantially less dose to the bladder, rectum, and other pelvic tissues, reducing the acute and late effects of treatment. (Courtesy of Torunn Yock, MD, and Judy Adams, CMD, Northeast Proton Therapy Center, Massachusetts General Hospital, Boston, MA.)

potential for improvements in clinical outcomes for cancer patients over a broad range of disease sites. It is hoped that the prospective clinical trials that have begun in hospital-based proton therapy facilities will establish the magnitude of these improvements. It will be important for society, physicians, and patients to have some sense of the cost for these benefits to place them in an appropriate context and allow comparison with other medical interventions. Goitein and Jermann performed cost comparisons between proton radiation therapy and technically sophisticated photon radiation therapy in an effort to define the relative costs of the technologies. The expense of proton therapy per patient will decrease as more facilities are built and greater numbers of patients are treated. When neither costs nor benefits are adequately determined, it is not possible to carry out a reliable cost-benefit analysis. Goitein and Jermann were able to estimate that the relative cost of proton beam radiation therapy compared with intensity-modulated photon beam radiation therapy was in the range of 2.4, but it may come down to 1.7 to 2.1 over the next 5 years.[42]

CARBON ION RADIATION THERAPY

The Heavy Ion Medical Accelerator (HIMAC) in Chiba, Japan, began clinical studies in 1994. Kamada and colleagues reported the results of a phase I/II study evaluating the tolerance for and effectiveness of carbon ion radiotherapy in patients with unresectable bone and soft tissue sarcomas.[43] Fifty-seven patients with 64 sites of bone and soft tissue sarcomas not suited for resection received carbon ion therapy. Tumors involved the spine or paraspinous soft tissues in 19 patients, pelvis in 32 patients, and extremities in 6 patients. The total dose ranged from 52.8 to 73.6 carbon GyE and was administered in 16 fractions over 4 weeks (3.3 to 4.6 GyE/fraction). Seven of seventeen patients treated with the highest total dose of 73.6 GyE experienced RTOG grade 3 acute skin reactions. Dose escalation was then halted at this level. No other severe acute reactions (grade > 3) were observed in this series. The overall local control rates were 88% and 73% at 1 and 3 years of follow-up, respectively. The 1- and 3-year overall survival rates were 82% and 46%, respectively. It is important to continue close follow-up of these patients to ensure that the large dose fractions are not associated with late injury of normal tissue.

Raster-scanned carbon ion radiation therapy at the Gesellschaft Schwerionenforschung Institut (GSI), Darmstadt, Germany, has been used to treat patients since 1997. Eighty-seven patients with chordomas and low-grade chondrosarcomas of the skull base received carbon ion radiation therapy alone (median dose, 60 GyE); 17 patients with spinal (n = 9) and sacrococcygeal (n = 8) chordomas and chondrosarcomas were treated with combined photon and carbon ion radiation therapy.[44] Actuarial 3-year local control was 81% for chordomas and 100% for chondrosarcomas. Local control was obtained in 15 of 17 patients with spinal (8 of 9) and sacral (7 of 8) chordomas or chondrosarcomas. Common toxicity criteria grade 4 or grade 5 was not observed. The investigators felt that carbon ion therapy was safe with respect to toxicity and offers high local control rates for skull base tumors such as chordomas and low-grade chondrosarcomas.

Kato and associates from Chiba, Japan, reported the results of a carbon ion dose escalation study for 24 patients with hepatocellular carcinoma.[45] Fifteen fractions were delivered over 5 weeks, and total doses ranged from 49.5 to 79.5 GyE. During a median follow-up of 71 months (range, 63 to 83 months), no severe adverse effects or treatment-related deaths occurred. The overall tumor response rate was 71%. The local control and overall survival rates were 92% and 92%, 81% and 50%, and 81% and 25% at 1, 3, and 5 years, respectively.

NEON ION RADIATION THERAPY

High-LET charged particle therapy with neon ions has been of interest in the treatment of malignant glioblastoma of the brain because of its increased biologic potential for destruction of radioresistant tumors. At the University of California, San Francisco (UCSF), and the Lawrence Berkeley Laboratories (LBL), 15 patients with glioblastoma multiforme were entered into a randomized protocol comparing two dose levels of neon ion irradiation.[46] Patients received 20 or 25 Gy in 4 weeks. However, there was no significant difference in overall survival (13 to 14 months). An optimal dose level was not identified.

π-MESON RADIATION THERAPY

Subatomic particles called π-mesons provide the nuclear binding force between nuclei. These particles are produced when protons (600+ MeV) impact a target. Three types of mesons are produced: a neutral form, a positive form, and a negative form. The negative form, π^-, is used for radiotherapy. When the π^- slows down, it is captured by a nucleus, causing it to "explode" in a starlike event, producing neutrons and charged nuclear fragments having high-LET properties (Fig. 18-6).

Negative π-mesons (i.e., pions) were used to treat 228 patients at Los Alamos Meson Physics Facility (LAMPF) between 1974 and 1981. One hundred twenty-nine patients received pion therapy only. All patients had locally advanced disease, and a number of different sites were treated. Local control was achieved in 86% of patients with prostate cancer, in 26% with head and neck cancers, and none with pancreatic cancer. A steep rise in the complication rate was seen beyond a dose level of 3750 cGy.[47]

At the Tri-University Meson Facility (TRIUMF), in Vancouver, British Columbia, 81 patients with high-grade gliomas

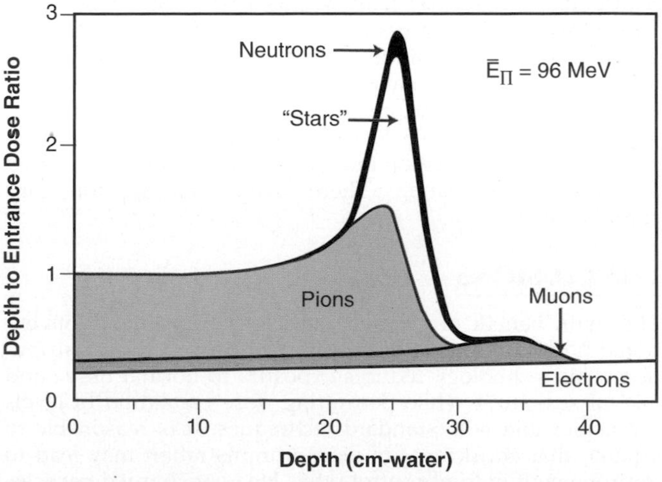

Figure 18-6 Negative π^- meson capture. When the π^- slows down, it is captured by a nucleus, causing it to "explode" in a starlike event, producing neutrons and charged nuclear fragments that have high linear energy transfer (LET) properties. (Adapted from Vecsey G: The PIOTRON. *In* Skarsguard LD [ed]: Pion and Heavy Ion Radiotherapy: Preclinical and Clinical Studies. New York, Elsevier Biomedical, 1981, p 23.)

were randomized to a 33- to 34.5-Gy pion dose given over 3 weeks or to a 60-Gy photon dose given over 6 weeks. Median survival was 10 months for both arms, and there was no significant difference in time to progression, radiation toxicity, performance status, or quality of life assessments.[48] TRIUMF was also the site for a phase III trial comparing pion therapy to photon therapy in the treatment of locally advanced prostate cancer. At a follow-up evaluation of 3.75 years, there was no difference in local control or survival. There was significantly more acute grade 3 or 4 bladder toxicity for the pion group, but there was no difference in late effects.[49]

HELIUM RADIATION THERAPY

A retrospective study done at UCSF and LBL evaluated the use of helium ions in the treatment of uveal melanomas.[50] Ten years after helium ion radiation, 208 (95.4%) of the 218 eyes irradiated had local tumor control. At 10 years, 46 eyes (22%) had been enucleated, with most resulting from anterior ocular segment complications. At 10 years, 51 patients (23%) had died of metastatic melanoma. Best corrected visual acuity after radiation was greater than 20/40 in 21 (23%) of 93 eyes of patients who were alive and who had retained their eyes 10 or more years after treatment. Visual acuity was related to height of the tumor and location near the nerve or fovea.

A study was recently completed comparing ^{125}I plaques with helium ions by the group at UCSF and LBL.[51] Patients with melanomas less than 10 mm high and less than 15 mm in diameter were randomized by the UCSF/LBL group to receive 70 CGE in five treatments with helium ions or 70 Gy to the tumor apex with ^{125}I plaque brachytherapy. Local control was 100% in patients treated with helium ions and 87% in patients treated with ^{125}I plaques.

Schoenthaler and colleagues reported the use of charged particle irradiation for sacral chordomas.[52] At LBL, 14 patients with sacral chordomas were treated with charged particles helium and neon. All patients were treated postoperatively; 10 had gross disease. The median dose was 7565 cGy and the median follow-up was 5 years. Kaplan-Meier survival at 5 years was 85%, and overall 5-year local control was 55%. A trend to improved local control at 5 years was seen in patients treated with neon when compared with patients treated with helium (62% versus 34%), in patients after complete resection versus patients with gross residual tumor (75% versus 40%), and in patients who had treatment courses less than 73 days (61% versus 21%). No patient developed neurologic sequelae or pain syndromes. One previously irradiated patient required colostomy, one patient had delayed wound healing after a negative postirradiation biopsy, and one patient developed a second malignancy. There were no genitourinary complications.

CONCLUSIONS

The main benefit of charged particle therapy over conventional photon beam radiotherapy is improved dose distribution. This technology reduces exposure to normal tissue and critical structures while permitting dose escalation to levels not achievable with standard techniques. It is reasonable to assume that an increase in dose administration may lead to improvement in local control rates. Heavier charged particles may also confer a biologic advantage against tumor because of the higher RBE, although additional follow-up is necessary to see if sensitive normal tissues in the high-dose region are subject to late toxicity. By reducing the volume of irradiated normal tissue, charged particles also offer the potential for a decrease in the appearance of radiation-induced malignancies. The importance of this issue cannot be overemphasized when considering the irradiation of pediatric patients. With minimization of normal tissue morbidity, charged particle therapy should also allow for better tolerance of combined chemotherapy and radiation therapy regimens.

In the United States, at LLU, the Northeast Proton Therapy Center (MGH), and the Midwest Proton Radiotherapy Clinic in Bloomington, Indiana, patients are being treated with proton radiotherapy for a number of the diseases and sites described previously, for which proton radiotherapy has been shown to confer a treatment advantage. Investigational proton radiation treatment protocols for newer indications, such as craniospinal irradiation for medulloblastoma, chemoradiation for pediatric rhabdomyosarcoma, and concurrent chemoradiation for locally advanced nasopharyngeal and medically inoperable lung cancer, are open for enrollment. Additional proton centers are under construction at M. D. Anderson Cancer Center in Houston and at the University of Florida facility in Jacksonville, Florida; both plan to begin patient treatments in 2006. Pediatric patients should be considered for referral, as should all patients for whom the proximity of tumor to critical structures prohibits the administration of adequate radiation doses using conventional techniques. Active research programs into carbon ion particle radiotherapy continue in Europe and Japan.

REFERENCES

1. Demizu Y, Kagawa K, Ejima Y: Cell biological basis for combination radiotherapy using heavy-ion beams and high energy x-rays. Radiother Oncol 74:207, 2004.
2. Koike S, Ando K, Oohira C, et al: Relative biological effectiveness of 290 MeV/u carbon ions for the growth delay of a radioresistant murine fibrosarcoma. J Radiat Res (Tokyo) 43:247-255, 2002.
3. Sisterson J: World wide charged particle patient totals. Particles 34:1-12, 2004.
4. Wilson RR: Radiological uses of fast protons. Radiology 47:487, 1946.
5. Mock U, Georg D, Bogner J, et al: Treatment planning comparison of conventional, 3D conformal, and intensity-modulated photon (IMRT) and proton therapy for paranasal sinus carcinoma. Int J Radiat Oncol Biol Phys 58:147-154, 2004.
6. Weber DC, Trofimov AV, Delaney TF, Bortfeld T: A treatment planning comparison of intensity modulated photon and proton therapy for paraspinal sarcomas. Int J Radiat Oncol Biol Phys 58:1596-1606, 2004.
7. Weber DC, Lomax AJ, Rutz HP: Spot-scanning proton radiation therapy for recurrent, residual or untreated intracranial meningiomas. Radiother Oncol 71:251-258, 2004.
8. Munzenrider JE: Proton therapy for uveal melanomas and other eye lesions. Strahlenther Onkol 175(Suppl 2):68, 1999.
9. Courdi A, Caujolle JP, Grange JD, et al: Results of proton therapy of uveal melanomas treated in Nice. Int J Radiat Oncol Biol Phys 45:5-11, 1999.
10. Egger E, Schalenbourg A, Zografos L, et al: Maximizing local tumor control and survival after proton beam radiotherapy of uveal melanoma. Int J Radiat Oncol Biol Phys 51:138-147, 2001.
11. Gragoudas ES, Lane AM, Regan S, et al: A randomized controlled trial of varying radiation doses in the treatment of choroidal melanoma. Arch Ophthalmol 118:773-778, 2000.
12. Egger E, Zografos L, Schalenbourg A, et al: Eye retention after proton beam radiotherapy for uveal melanoma. Int J Radiat Oncol Biol Phys 55:867-880, 2003.
13. Munzenrider JE, Liebsch NJ: Proton therapy for tumors of the skull base. Strahlenther Onkol 175(Suppl 2):57-63, 1999.
14. Terahara A, Niemierko A, Goitein M, et al: Analysis of the relationship between tumor dose inhomogeneity and local control in patients with skull base chordoma. Int J Radiat Oncol Biol Phys 45:351-358, 1999.
15. Pai HH, Thornton A, Katznelson L, et al: Hypothalamic/pituitary function following high-dose conformal radiotherapy to the base

of skull: demonstration of a dose-effect relationship using dose-volume histogram analysis. Int J Radiat Oncol Biol Phys 49:1079-1092, 2001.
16. Noel G, Habrand JL, Mammar H, et al: Combination of photon and proton radiation therapy for chordomas and chondrosarcomas of the skull base: the Centre de Protontherapie D'Orsay experience. Int J Radiat Oncol Biol Phys 51:392-398, 2001.
17. Isacsson U, Hagberg H, Johansson KA, et al: Potential advantages of protons over conventional radiation beams for paraspinal tumours. Radiother Oncol 45:63-70, 1997.
18. Hug EB, Fitzek MM, Liebsch NJ: Locally challenging osteo- and chondrogenic tumors of the axial skeleton: results of combined proton and photon radiation therapy using three-dimensional treatment planning. Int J Radiat Oncol Biol Phys 31:467-476, 1995.
19. Fuss M, Hug EB, Schaefer RA, et al: Proton radiation therapy (PRT) for pediatric optic pathway gliomas: comparison with 3D planned conventional photons and a standard photon technique. Int J Radiat Oncol Biol Phys 45:1117-1126, 1999.
20. Habrand JL, Haie-Meder C, Rey A, et al: Radiotherapy using a combination of photons and protons for locally aggressive intracranial tumors. Preliminary results of protocol CPO 94-C1 [in French]. Cancer Radiother 3:480-488, 1999.
21. Fitzek MM, Thornton AF, Rabinov JD, et al: Accelerated fractionated proton/photon irradiation to 90 cobalt gray equivalent for glioblastoma multiforme: results of a phase II prospective trial. J Neurosurg 91:251-260, 1999.
22. Wenkel E, Thornton AF, Finkelstein D, et al: Benign meningioma: partially resected, biopsied, and recurrent intracranial tumors treated with combined proton and photon radiotherapy. Int J Radiat Oncol Biol Phys 48:1363-1370, 2000.
23. Thornton AF, Fitzek MM, Varvares M, et al: Accelerated, hyperfractionated photon/proton irradiation for advanced paranasal sinus cancer: results of a prospective phase I-II study (abstract). Int J Radiat Oncol Biol Phys 42:S222, 1998.
24. Fitzek MM, Thornton AF, Varvares M, et al: Neuroendocrine tumors of the sinonasal tract. Results of a prospective study incorporating chemotherapy, surgery, and combined proton-photon radiotherapy. Cancer 94:2623-2634, 2002.
25. Lin R, Slater JD, Yonemoto LT, et al: Nasopharyngeal carcinoma: repeat treatment with conformal proton therapy—dose-volume histogram analysis. Radiology 213:489-494, 1999.
26. Bush DA, McAllister CJ, Loredo LN, et al: Fractionated proton beam radiotherapy for acoustic neuroma. Neurosurgery 50:270-273, 2002.
27. Shipley WU, Verhey LJ, Muzenrider JE, et al: Advanced prostate cancer: results of a randomized comparative trial of high dose irradiation boosting with conformal protons compared with conventional dose irradiation using protons alone. Int J Radiat Oncol Biol Phys 32:3-12, 1995.
28. Slater JD, Rossi CJ Jr, Yonemoto LT, et al: Proton therapy for prostate cancer: the initial Loma Linda University experience. Int J Radiat Oncol Biol Phys 59:348-352, 2004.
29. Zietman AL, DeSilvio M, Slater JD, et al: A randomized trial comparing conventional dose (70.2 GyE) and high-dose (79.2 GyE) conformal radiation in early stage adenocarcinoma of the prostate: results of an interim analysis of PROG 95-09. Int J Radiat Oncol Biol Phys 60(Suppl):S131, 2004.
30. Matsuzaki Y, Osuga T, Chiba T, et al: New, effective treatment using proton irradiation for unresectable hepatocellular carcinoma. Intern Med 34:302-307, 1995.
31. Hsiung-Stripp DC, McDonough J, Masters HM, et al: Comparative treatment planning between proton and x-ray therapy in pancreatic cancer. Med Dosim 26:255-259, 2001.
32. Bush DA, Slater JD, Bonnet R, et al: Proton-beam radiotherapy for early-stage lung cancer. Chest 116:1313-1319, 1999.
33. Shioyama Y, Tokuuye K, Okumura T, et al: Clinical evaluation of proton radiotherapy for non-small-cell lung cancer. Int J Radiat Oncol Biol Phys 56:7-13, 2003.
34. Miralbell R, Lomax A, Cella L, Schneider U: Potential reduction of the incidence of radiation-induced second cancers by using proton beams in the treatment of pediatric tumors. Int J Radiat Oncol Biol Phys 54:824-829, 2002.
35. St Clair WH, Adams JA, Bues M, et al: Advantage of protons compared to conventional x-ray or IMRT in the treatment of a pediatric patient with medulloblastoma. Int J Radiat Oncol Biol Phys 58:727-734, 2004.
36. Lin R, Hug EB, Schaefer RA, et al: Conformal proton radiation therapy of the posterior fossa: a study comparing protons with three-dimensional planned photons in limiting dose to auditory structures. Int J Radiat Oncol Biol Phys 48:1219-1226, 2000.
37. Hug EB, Muenter MW, Archambeau JO, et al: Conformal proton radiation therapy for pediatric low-grade astrocytomas. Strahlenther Onkol 178:10-17, 2002.
38. Hug EB, Muenter MW, Adams JA, et al: 3-D conformal radiation therapy for pediatric giant cell tumors of the skull base. Strahlenther Onkol 178:239-244, 2002.
39. Hug EB, Nevinny-Stickel M, Fuss M, et al: Conformal proton radiation treatment for retroperitoneal neuroblastoma: introduction of a novel technique. Med Pediatr Oncol 37:36-41, 2001.
40. Hug EB, Adams J, Fitzek M, et al: Fractionated, three-dimensional, planning-assisted proton-radiation therapy for orbital rhabdomyosarcoma: a novel technique. Int J Radiat Oncol Biol Phys 47: 979-984, 2000.
41. Fogliata A, Bolsi A, Cozzi L: Critical appraisal of treatment techniques based on conventional photon beams, intensity modulated photon beams and proton beams for therapy of intact breast. Radiother Oncol 62:137-145, 2002.
42. Goitein M, Jermann M: The relative costs of proton and x-ray radiation therapy. Clin Oncol (R Coll Radiol) 15:S37-S50, 2003.
43. Kamada T, Tsujii H, Tsuji H, et al: Efficacy and safety of carbon ion radiotherapy in bone and soft tissue sarcomas. J Clin Oncol 20:4466-4471, 2002.
44. Schulz-Ertner D, Nikoghosyan A, Thilmann C, et al: Results of carbon ion radiotherapy in 152 patients. Int J Radiat Oncol Biol Phys 58:631-640, 2004.
45. Kato H, Tsujii H, Miyamoto T: Results of the first prospective study of carbon ion radiotherapy for hepatocellular carcinoma with liver cirrhosis. Int J Radiat Oncol Biol Phys 59:1468-1476, 2004.
46. Castro JR, Phillips TL, Prados M, et al: Neon heavy charged particle radiotherapy of glioblastoma of the brain. Int J Radiat Oncol Biol Phys 38:257-261, 1997.
47. von Essen CF, Bagshaw MA, Bush SE, et al: Long-term results of pion therapy at Los Alamos. Int J Radiat Oncol Biol Phys 3:1389-1398, 1987.
48. Pickles T, Goodman GB, Rheaume DE, et al: Pion radiation for high grade astrocytoma: results of a randomized study. Int J Radiat Oncol Biol Phys 37:491-497, 1997.
49. Thornton AF, Laramore GE: Particle radiation therapy. *In* Gunderson LL, Tepper JE (eds): Clinical Radiation Oncology. Philadelphia, Churchill Livingstone, 2000, pp 225-234.
50. Char DH, Kroll SM, Castro J: Ten-year follow-up of helium ion therapy for uveal melanoma. Am J Ophthalmol 125:81-89, 1998.
51. Char DH, Quivey JM, Castro JR, et al: Helium ions versus iodine 125 brachytherapy in the management of uveal melanoma. A prospective, randomized, dynamically balanced trial. Ophthalmol 100:1547-1554, 1993.
52. Schoenthalar R, Castro JR, Petti PL: Charged particle irradiation of sacral chordomas. Int J Radiat Oncol Biol Phys 26:291-298, 1993.

CHAPTER 19

NEUTRON RADIOTHERAPY

Jason K. Rockhill and George E. Laramore

The neutron was discovered by Sir James Chadwick in 1932 during an analysis of certain nuclear reactions. Shortly thereafter, investigators proposed using it to treat various human malignancies. There have been two main areas of clinical investigation: fast neutron radiotherapy and boron neutron capture therapy (BNCT). We briefly describe the underlying physics of each type of therapy, summarize their historical development, and discuss their current clinical usage. Space does not permit us to discuss neutron brachytherapy using ^{252}Cf sources, which is in very limited clinical use today.

FAST NEUTRON RADIOTHERAPY

Overview

Fast neutron radiotherapy refers to using neutrons having an energy of several tens of MeV that are generated by accelerating either protons or deuterons with cyclotrons or particle accelerators and then impacting them onto an appropriate target, most generally beryllium. The resulting distribution of neutrons is approximately spherically symmetric and the beams used in therapy are collimated out in much the same manner as the photon therapy beams generated by electron linear accelerators. These fast neutrons are neutral particles and interact directly with the atomic nuclei in tissue producing recoil protons and nuclear fragments, which in turn create a dense chain of ionization events. For therapy neutrons about 85% of the deposited energy is via a "knock on" reaction involving the ^{1}H nucleus, meaning that the KERMA (kinetic energy release in matter) is larger in high-hydrogen-content tissue such as fat or myelin.

The resulting energy transfer is in the range of 20 to 100 keV/μ compared with 0.2 to 2.0 keV/μ for the megavoltage photons and electrons used in conventional radiotherapy. It is this higher energy transfer that gives rise to the different radiobiological properties of fast neutrons, which are advantageous in certain clinical situations. The higher relative biological effectiveness (RBE) accounts for the different clinical response observed with neutrons as opposed to conventional photon irradiation. Fast neutrons have RBEs in the range of 3.0 to 3.5 in terms of most normal tissue late effects, RBEs in the range of 4.0 to 4.5 in terms of damage to the central nervous system (CNS), and RBEs in the range of 8.0 for salivary gland malignancies.[1,2,3] High LET radiation causes a dense chain of ionizing events to both strands of the DNA and thus makes the DNA repair more difficult. Furthermore, high LET radiation from fast neutrons is less sensitive to the effects of hypoxia in terms of causing a reduced cell killing.

Historical Perspective

Patients were first treated with fast neutron radiotherapy in 1938 by Robert Stone and coworkers[4] at the Crocker Radiation Laboratory (later to become Lawrence Berkeley Laboratory). Two hundred forty patients were treated between 1938 and 1942. Many of these patients had received prior photon irradiation. There were significant radiation sequelae in the few long-term survivors such that clinical interest in fast neutron radiotherapy dropped off significantly for the next 20 years. Brennan and Phillips[5] subsequently reviewed the initial work by Stone and colleagues and showed that an inappropriate value for the neutron RBE had been used in the dose calculations. Hence, many of those initial patients had been inadvertently overdosed. With a better understanding of the RBE of fast neutron radiotherapy in different tissue types, in the 1970s Catterall and coworkers resumed neutron clinical trials at Hammersmith Hospital in London, England.[6-8] Their results indicated that many advanced head and neck cancers exhibited a good response with acceptable side effects. The interest in fast neutron radiotherapy grew so that at one point there were 39 different centers in North America, Europe, Asia, and Africa treating patients with fast neutrons. Clinical utility has been further elucidated through clinical trials and single institution experience and now neutron radiotherapy has fairly well-defined and limited indications. There are currently only seven operating fast neutron radiotherapy centers throughout the world. These are listed in Table 19-1 along with some of their more important characteristics.

Below is a summary of tumor histologies where neutrons have been shown to be advantageous compared with standard photon irradiation.

Salivary Gland Tumors

The major therapeutic advantage of fast neutron radiotherapy over conventional radiotherapy is best established in salivary gland tumors. The RBE for salivary gland tumors is 8 while for the surrounding normal tissues the RBE is 3 to 3.5.[1] A typical neutron dose for a salivary gland cancer is approximately 20 nGy (neutron gray). The approximate equivalent photon dose is 60-70 Gy-equivalent as far as normal tissues are concerned but in the range of 160 Gy-equivalent as far as the tumor is concerned. The therapeutic gain factor for salivary gland tumors is thus in the range of 2.3 to 2.6.

Early, single institutions showed neutrons to be beneficial in the treatment of salivary gland tumors. These results led to a prospective randomized trial sponsored by the Radiation Therapy Oncology Group (RTOG) and the Medical Research Council (MRC) of Great Britain.[9] Local control at 10 years was improved in the neutron arm (56% versus 17%, $P = .009$). The final report showed a trend toward increased median survival of about 8 months in the neutron arm, but this was not statistically significant. However, the cause of death differed between the two subgroups. Metastatic disease was the main cause of death for the neutron patients, while local/regional tumor failure was the main cause of death for the photon patients. Of note, the study was stopped early for ethical reasons when 2-year survival data showed a strong trend in favor of the neutron patients. Local tumor control curves for this study are shown in Figure 19-1.

The University of Washington experience was reviewed by Douglas and colleagues.[10] Two hundred seventy nine patients treated with curative intent were included in the analysis. A majority (263 patients) had evidence of gross disease, with 141 having major salivary gland neoplasms and 138 having minor salivary gland neoplasms. The 6-year actuarial cause-specific survival rate was 67%. On multivariate analysis, stage I/II disease, minor salivary gland primaries, lack of base-of-skull involvement, and primary (rather than recurrent) disease were associated with improved survival. Local-regional control was improved for tumors less than 4 cm in greatest diameter, with

Table 19-1 Location of Operating Fast Neutron Radiotherapy Centers—2004

Location	Beam Reaction	Comments
UNITED STATES		
University of Washington Medical Center—Seattle, WA	50 MeV p→Be	Isocentric gantry and multileaf collimator
Harper-Grace Hospital—Detroit, MI	48 MeV d→Be	Isocentric gantry and multirod collimator
Fermi Laboratories—Batavia, IL	66 MeV p→Be	Horizontal beam, fixed collimators with blocking inserts
EUROPE		
Centre Hospitalier Regional—Orleans, France	34 MeV p→Be	Vertical beam, fixed collimators with blocking inserts
University of Essen—Essen, Germany	14 MeV d→Be	Isocentric gantry with collimator inserts and wedge capability
ASIA		
National Institute of Radiological Sciences—Chiba, Japan	30 MeV d→Be	Vertical beam, multileaf collimator
AFRICA		
National Accelerator Centre—Faure, South Africa	66 MeV p→Be	Isocentric gantry and jaw collimator

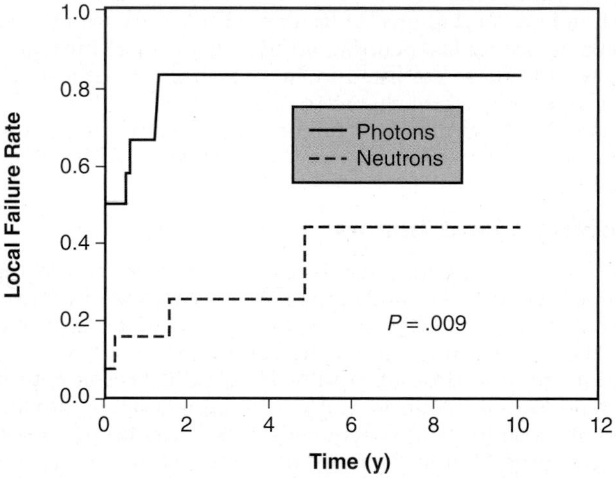

Figure 19-1 Actuarial local-regional control curves for patients with unresectable salivary gland tumors from the Radiation Therapy Oncology Group/Medical Research Council (RTOG/MRC) randomized study (80-01). The difference between the neutron curve (*red dashed line*) and the photon curve (*blue solid line*) is statistically significant at the $P = .009$ level. (Adapted from Laramore GE, Krall JM, Griffin TW, et al: Neutron versus photon irradiation for unresectable salivary gland tumors: final report of an RTOG-MRC randomized clinical trial. Int J Radiat Oncol Biol Phys 27:235, 1993.)

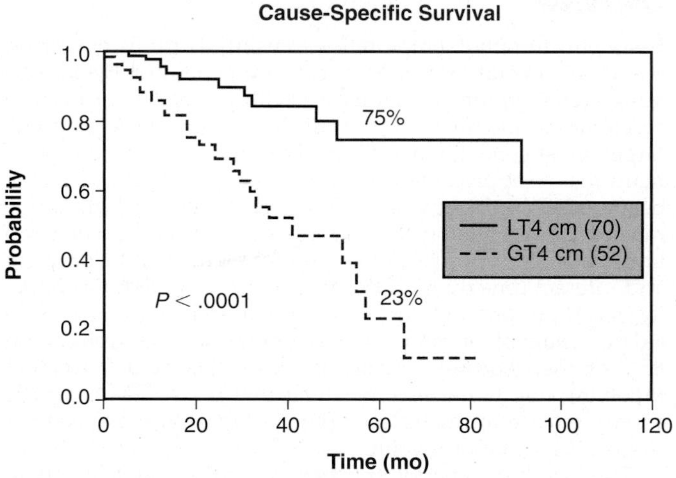

Figure 19-2 Actuarial cause-specific survival curves as a function of tumor size for patients with major salivary gland tumors treated with curative intent at the University of Washington neutron treatment facility. The *blue solid curve* depicts the results for patients with tumors smaller than 4 cm in the greatest diameter, and the *dashed red curve* depicts the results for patients with tumors larger than 4 cm in the greatest diameter. The difference between the two curves is statistically significant at the $P < .0001$ level. (Adapted from Douglas JG, Lee S, Laramore GE, et al: Neutron radiotherapy for the treatment of locally advanced major salivary gland tumors. Head Neck 21:255, 1999.)

lack of base-of-skull invasion, with prior surgical resection, and with no previous radiation therapy. The 6-year actuarial freedom from the development of metastases was 64% for patients without lymph node involvement or base-of-skull involvement. There was a 6-year actuarial rate of 10% for developing RTOG grade 3 or 4 toxicity. Cause-specific survival curves for the major salivary gland patients as a function of tumor size are shown in Figure 19-2.[11]

The poorer outcome of salivary tumors with base-of-skull involvement is likely due to the need to reduce the dose to portions of tumors that are adjacent to critical CNS structures (recall that the RBE for fast neutrons for CNS tissue is 4 to 4.5). With a standard 20-nGy dose to the involved site, the dose to the temporal tips could be approximately 80 photon Gy-equivalent. Reducing the temporal lobe dose to a safe level sometimes necessitated blocking portions of tumor. In an attempt to try to compensate for the reduced neutron dose, a stereotatic radiosurgery boost with photon radiation has been instituted at the University of Washington. Initial results suggest that this is both feasible and well tolerated.[12]

The use of both neutrons and photons as a composite "mixed beam" treatment has been explored by Huber and coworkers[13] in a series of patients with advanced adenoid cystic carcinomas treated at the Heidelberg neutron facility. They found a 5-year local control rate of 75% for patients treated with neutrons alone compared with 32% for groups of patients treated with "mixed beam" or with photons alone. It appears that patients having a greater portion of their treatment with neutrons fared better. Distant metastatic disease once again prevented improved local control from translating into an increase in overall survival.

The neutron facility in Orleans has reported similar results for 59 patients treated with fast neutron radiotherapy.[14] The

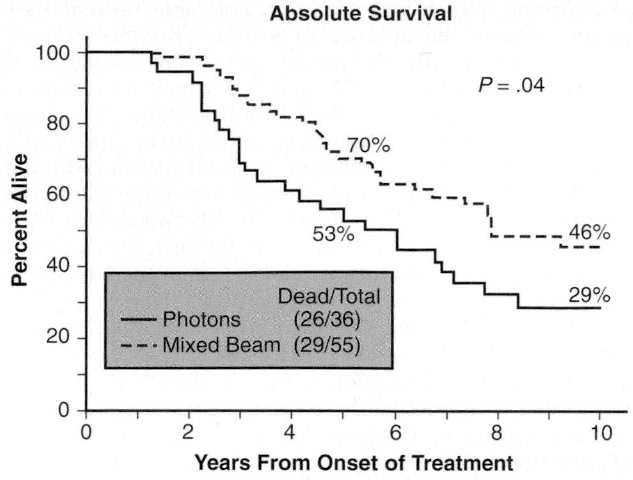

Figure 19-3 Actuarial survival curves for patients with locally advanced prostate cancer treated on Radiation Therapy Oncology Group (RTOG) protocol 77-04. The mixed (neutron and photon) beam group is shown by the *dashed red curve*, and the photon control arm is shown as the *solid blue curve*. The difference between the curves is statistically significant at the $P = .04$ level. (Adapted from Laramore GE, Krall JM, Griffin TW, et al: Fast neutron radiotherapy for locally advanced prostate cancer. Am J Clin Oncol 16:164, 1993.)

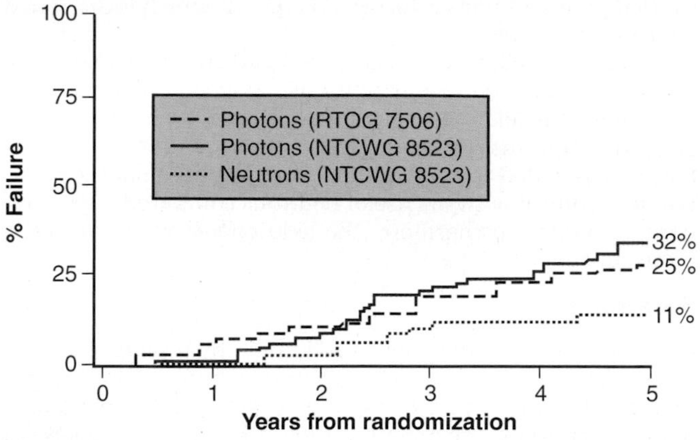

Figure 19-4 Actuarial percent local failure curves for patients with locally advanced prostate cancer treated on Neutron Therapy Collaborative Working Group (NTCWG) protocol 85-23. The group treated with neutrons is shown as the *dotted green curve*, and the group treated with photons is shown as the *dashed blue curve*. The difference between these two curves is statistically significant at the $P < .01$ level. A local control curve (*solid red line*) for photon-treated patients from another Radiation Therapy Oncology Group study (RTOG 75-06) is shown for comparison. There is no statistical difference between the latter curve and the photon control arm of the neutron study. (Adapted from Russell KJ, Caplan RJ, Laramore GE, et al: Photon versus fast neutron external beam radiotherapy in the treatment of locally advanced prostate cancer: results of a randomized prospective trial. Int J Radiat Oncol Biol Phys 28:47, 1993.)

5-year local control was 69.5%, with a crude 5-year survival of 66% and a 5-year tumor-free survival of 64.5%.

Prostate Cancer

Prostate cancer is another tumor for which there has been significant clinical work using fast neutron radiotherapy. The National Cancer Institute (through RTOG 77-04) conducted a randomized trial for patients with T3 N0/N1 disease.[15] One arm received a mixed beam (neutron/photon) dose to 70 Gy-equivalent versus a second arm that received standard photons to 70 Gy. At the 10-year end point, survival (46% versus 29%, $P = .04$) was improved in the mixed beam arm. There was also improved local/regional control (70% versus 58%, $P = .03$) for the mixed beam subgroup. There was no difference in the rate of significant complications between the two arms. Survival curves for the patients in this study are shown in Figure 19-3.

A follow-up randomized trial was conducted that compared 70-Gy standard photon irradiation versus 20.4 nGy with fast neutrons. This was carried out by the National Cancer Institute (NCI)-sponsored Neutron Therapy Collaborative Working Group (NTCWG) and included patients with high grade T2 or any grade T3-T4, N0-N1, M0 tumors.[16] With a median follow-up of 68 months, the 5-year actuarial local-region failure rate was 11% for neutrons versus 32% for photons ($P < .01$). Actuarial overall survival and cause-specific survival were statistically equivalent. The incidence of severe complications was higher in the neutron group than in the photon group (11% versus 3%). Complications were less severe and fewer in the centers that had more sophisticated beam-shaping abilities. Local failure curves for the patients on this study are shown in Figure 19-4.

Work on fast neutron radiotherapy and prostate cancer continues at many centers in the United States,[17-21] Europe,[22,23] and Asia.[24,25] These single-institution results show good local and regional control and appear to corroborate the results of the randomized trials described earlier.

Sarcomas

Sarcomas are generally considered to be among the more "radioresistant" tumor histologies and so would fall into the category of tumors thought to be more responsive to high LET radiation.[26] In a retrospective review by Schwarz and coworkers,[27] 1171 soft tissue sarcoma patients from 11 European centers were treated with fast neutron radiotherapy. In those patients with either inoperable tumors or gross disease after surgery, the local control was approximately 50%. Toxicity was higher than what was generally seen with photon radiation. The local control rates were thought by the authors to be better that what would have been expected with standard radiotherapy. This conclusion is supported by other single-institution studies.[28]

Other Tumor Types

Fast neutron radiation has been tested on a variety of other tumor types. Generally, the rationale for the use of fast neutrons came from trying to overcome a perceived limitation of standard photon irradiation. A good example of this is for malignant gliomas of the brain. Dose-escalation studies with photons have failed to increase overall survival.[29] By definition, *glioblastoma multiforme* have areas of necrosis associated with the tumor. These areas of necrosis are likely surrounded by regions of hypoxia, which might make the tumors more radioresistant. Studies for malignant gliomas in the 1970s and 1980s used neutrons either alone or combination with photons.[30] None of these initial trials showed an improvement in overall survival with the addition of neutrons. However, with relatively high doses of fast neutrons alone, autopsy and second-look surgical data indicated that tumor cells were sterilized in the treated region.[31] Unfortunately, there was also significant coagulative necrosis caused by the neutron irradiation, which indicated too much damage to normal brain tissue. Much of the current interest in neutron radiotherapy for malignant gliomas is focused on BNCT, which is discussed later in this chapter.

Squamous cell carcinomas of the head and neck region are another tumor type where neutrons have been used to try to overcome the relative radiation resistance of hypoxic cells. Several single institutional trials in Europe and the United States have failed to show a significant improvement in local-regional control with the use of neutrons compared with standard photons. Furthermore, the side effects were generally more severe.

Summary

Neutron radiotherapy is best used in the treatment of certain tumors that exhibit a "resistance" to standard low LET radiotherapy. The niche that it occupies is small but it remains a highly important treatment option for small numbers of patients for whom it appears to be better than more traditional forms of treatment. Examples are patients with inoperable or recurrent salivary gland malignancies or in high-risk situations where there has been an incomplete surgical extirpation, inoperable or incompletely resected sarcomas of bone, cartilage, and soft tissue, or locally advanced prostate cancers—particularly those that are not hormonally responsive. In highly selected circumstances, it may also be beneficial in the treatment of metastases from melanoma and renal cell cancer. Future research may extend these indications.

BORON NEUTRON CAPTURE THERAPY

Overview

Conceptually, BNCT is a "magic bullet" approach to treating tumors. Pure beams of very low energy neutrons do not directly deposit much energy in tissue via collisions but rather interact via nuclear transmutation reactions. The basic idea is to selectively attach to the cancer cells a nuclide having a large cross section for capturing a thermal neutron. The nuclide then undergoes a nuclear reaction with the localized release of a substantial amount of energy. In principle, this kills the "tagged" cell but does not damage the surrounding "untagged" normal cells. While there is ongoing work in developing high current particle accelerators to produce low energy thermal or epithermal beams for BNCT, at the present time, all clinical work is being done using moderated neutron beams from nuclear reactors. There are other nuclides besides ^{10}B that have a high neutron capture therapy cross section, and some of these (e.g., ^{157}Gd) are of interest in neutron capture therapy for cancer. However, we confine our discussion to BNCT. We also confine ourselves to the clinical perspective and not attempt to describe the ongoing research in radiobiology, compound development, and the physics research into nonreactor sources of appropriate beams.

Historical Perspective

The basic idea of BNCT dates to 1936, when Locher[32] proposed treating malignant tumors with low energy thermal neutrons mediated via a capture cross section with ^{10}B. A few years later, Kruger[33] and Zahl and colleagues[34] experimentally verified some of the basic tenets of this concept and demonstrated the high RBE of the ^{4}He and ^{7}Li fission fragments. The theoretical advantage of "tagging" the tumor-specific carrier with an innocuous substance such as ^{10}B and then activating it, rather than "tagging" it with a toxic compound such as ricin, is that the "binary approach" is more forgiving of other body tissues that might also display some avidity for the carrier agent. In the real world, the thermal and epithermal beams produced by nuclear reactors are contaminated with gamma rays and fast neutrons, which can cause considerable normal tissue damage even in the absence of a high ^{10}B concentration.[35] Moreover, even in the absence of such beam contaminants, nuclear species such as ^{1}H, ^{14}N, and ^{35}Cl, which are commonly found in tissue, interact with thermal neutrons via capture events of their own and their reaction products cause biological damage to non–^{10}B-containing normal tissues. Although the respective capture cross sections for these commonly found nuclei are much lower than for ^{10}B and other nuclear species of interest for neutron capture therapy, the concentrations of these commonly found nuclei are many orders of magnitude greater than the ^{10}B concentration. Hence, reactions involving these nuclides can result in an appreciable tissue dose, even in the absence of ^{10}B. The key to BNCT as a practical therapy is the development of compounds that localize specifically in tumors and deliver sufficient ^{10}B concentrations to yield a significant therapeutic advantage compared with the radiation doses delivered to normal tissues.

Early Clinical Studies

The first set of human clinical trials was carried out in the 1950s at Brookhaven National Laboratory (BNL) using ^{10}B-enriched, boric acid derivatives.[36,37] These compounds yielded high concentrations of ^{10}B in the blood at the time of irradiation and unfortunately produced relatively low ^{10}B levels in the tumors. This resulted in considerable blood vessel endothelial damage and no therapeutic benefit from treatment either in these trials or in subsequent trials that were carried out in the 1960s.[38-40] Interest in the technique waned until Hatanaka and others in Japan[41] reinstituted BNCT for malignant gliomas using a different ^{10}B-carrier, ^{10}B-sodium-mercaptoundecahydrododecaborate (BSH). This compound produced better tumor-to-blood boron ratios than the compounds used in the prior BNL studies and the treatments caused less damage to normal brain tissue. Favorable reports regarding its efficacy[41-43] led to renewed worldwide interest in the technique. Many patients have received BNCT treatments using thermal neutron beams from various reactors in Japan but to date, no randomized, clinical trials have been carried out. An analysis of the RTOG database by Curran and colleagues[44] has demonstrated that there are some subsets of patients with high-grade gliomas who will do well with conventional photon irradiation. A few years ago, an analysis of a subset of patients from the United States who were treated with BNCT in Japan showed no improvement over that which would have been expected with conventional therapy after correcting for the appropriate prognostic factors.[45] A comparison of the survival of these patients with that expected for a pseudo-matched set of conventionally treated patients generated using the prognostic factors identified by Curran and colleaguesl[44] from the RTOG data base is shown in Figure 19-5. There is no statistical difference between the two curves. Moreover, review of the data for the entire group of evaluable patients showed that in all except one patient there was a documented tumor recurrence within the primary radiation field.[45] The only long-term survivor in this group of American patients had an anaplastic astrocytoma and fell into the most favorable category I of Curran and coworkers.[44]

There is no doubt that many aspects of the early Japanese BNCT clinical research program were suboptimal. The use of a poorly penetrating beam of thermal neutrons meant that an open craniotomy was required in order to expose the tumor bed. Due to the low neutron fluxes, treatment times of 4 to 8 hours were required to deliver a surface fluence of approximately 10^{13} neutrons/cm^{2}, and during treatment the patient had to be under general anesthesia with the brain exposed in

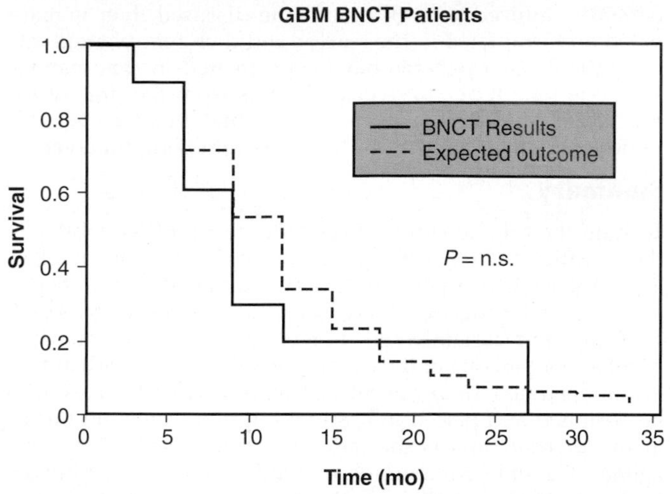

Figure 19-5 Actuarial survival curves for a group of 10 patients from the United States with glioblastoma multiforme (GBM) histology who were treated with boron neutron capture therapy (BNCT) *(solid blue curve)* and the expected survival curve for a matched cohort who received conventional treatment according to various Radiation Therapy Oncology Group study (RTOG) protocols *(dashed red curve)*. There is no statistically significant difference between the two curves. (Adapted from Laramore GE, Spence AM: Boron neutron capture therapy [BNCT] for high grade gliomas of the brain: a cautionary note. Int J Radiat Oncol Biol Phys 36:241, 1996.)

a converted operating room adjacent to the nuclear reactor. While BSH is conceptually attractive as a ^{10}B-carrier agent in that it is excluded from normal brain by the blood-brain barrier, typical tumor boron concentrations for glioblastoma multiforme were in the range of only 15 to 25 µg/g. It is now possible to improve on many of these shortcomings.

Modern Clinical Trials

There is ongoing clinical work in Japan, Europe, Argentina, and the United States in the treatment of malignant brain tumors.

In Japan there are three reactor facilities currently involved in patient treatments: (1) KUR in Kyoto, (2) MITR in Musashi, and (3) JRR-4 at the Japan Atomic Energy Research Institute in Tokai.[46] While most patients have been treated using thermal neutron beams, the KUR facility has been modified to produce a higher energy epithermal beam allowing treatment through the intact skull. The majority of the treated patients have been treated for various types of brain tumors using BSH as the ^{10}B-carrier agent and with a single fraction of neutron radiation. A report by Nakagawa and colleagues[47] shows that in the subset of GBM patients, 12% of treated patients lived longer than 2 years. Depending on other prognostic factors, this may or may not be better than expected with more conventional forms of treatment.

There are several reactor facilities in Europe with BNCT clinical programs for malignant brain tumors, all using epithermal neutron beams. The program that has treated the most patients is based at the HFR reactor in Petten (the Netherlands) and is being directed by the European Collaboration on Boron Neutron Capture Therapy. BSH at 100 mg/kg is used as the ^{10}B-carrier and there is an ongoing Phase I dose-searching study. This study is restricted to the subsets of glioblastoma multiforme patients whose expected median survival with conventional radiotherapy is less than 10 months. Unlike the other ongoing treatment regimens, which use a single BNCT treatment, the Petten program uses four fractions requiring multiple administrations of the boron carrier compound. BNCT dose reporting is complex, and the Petten group has chosen to specify each component of the radiation field separately rather than stating a Gy-equivalent dose.[48] The starting dose from the ^{10}B component was set at 80% of the dose that produced neurological changes in a dog brain study, $D_B = 8.6$ Gy. The other components of the radiation dose were limited to $D_n < 0.9$ Gy, $D_N < 1.1$ Gy, and $D_g < 5.8$ Gy where D_n is the neutron absorbed dose delivered by the thermal, epithermal, and fast neutrons and the charged particles produced by their reactions, D_g is the gamma ray absorbed dose, and D_N is the absorbed dose from the protons produced by the ^{14}N capture reaction. Twenty-five patients were entered into the initial dose arm of the study with 21 actually receiving BNCT treatment.[49] The median survival of the BNCT treated patients was 31 weeks with 6 patients alive at the time of a preliminary report. All 21 patients exhibited tumor recurrence. A second BNCT program is based at the FiR No. 1 reactor in Helsinki, Finland. The initial protocol was a phase I dose searching study that used L-*para*-boronophenylalanine (BPA) in a fructose solution at 290 mg BPA/kg as the ^{10}B-carrier. Only a single treatment was given using two radiation fields. Thus far 10 patients have been treated with tumor doses between 35.1 and 66.7 Gy-equivalent. This effective dose has been determined using weighting factors for each of the radiation components (see Kankaanranta and colleagues[50] for specific details). With a median follow-up of 9 months, 7 of 10 patients have recurrent or persistent tumor with the median time to tumor progression being 8 months.[50] The toxicity in both of the European trials has been thought to be acceptable, making future escalations of the radiation dose possible. Small numbers of patients also have been treated at Studsvik Medical AB in Uppsala University[51] and at the Nuclear Research Institute in the Czech Republic.[52]

After approximately a 30-year hiatus, the first "modern era" BNCT clinical program in the United States was begun at the MIT research reactor in collaboration with Tufts Medical Center. The first patient was treated in September 1994. This project is now under the clinical direction of the New England Deaconess Hospital. Treatments are delivered using an epithermal beam with BPA as the ^{10}B-carrier agent. Between 1996 and 1999, a total of 22 patients with intracranial lesions, either GBM or metastatic melanoma, were treated.[20] The initial clinical trial was a dose-searching, toxicity study with the target dose ranging between 8.8 and 14.2 Gy-equivalent. At the higher radiation doses, the time required to deliver the dose ranged up to 3 hours. At the higher dose levels, significant skin and mucosal reactions were observed. No adverse effects were noted due to the BPA administration and no long-term complications relating to the BNCT treatment were noted. Some tumor responses were noted in the patients with metastatic melanoma, but there was no obvious prolongation of survival in either group of the treated patients. This is now the only operating BNCT treatment facility in the United States.

A second clinical BNCT program focusing on high-grade gliomas of the brain was initiated at BNL. This program differed from the Japanese glioma program in two main respects: (1) a higher energy epithermal neutron beam was used rather than a thermal neutron beam, and (2) a different ^{10}B-carrier agent (BPA) was used rather than BSH. The epithermal beam meant that patients could be treated without recourse to a craniotomy and intraoperative irradiation and that more deeply located tumors could be given adequate doses. It was expected that BPA would produce higher tumor ^{10}B concentrations than could be achieved with BSH. Based on ^{10}B blood levels, it appeared that tumor ^{10}B concentrations of approximately 35 to 50 μg/g were achieved. However, unlike the case of BSH, BPA is not excluded from the normal brain by the blood-brain barrier, and tumor enrichment depends on other mechanisms of selective uptake (perhaps relating to an enhanced amino acid transport system). A dose-escalation approach was used. Prior to June 1996, all patients were treated using a simple appositional field with a single treatment fraction being given. A critique of this early BNL treatment technique indicated significant deficiencies in the basic approach relating to the inability to achieve a tumor dose adequate to sterilize GBMs using a single appositional field.[54]

Between September 1994 and May 1999, 53 patients with primary GBM received BPA-fructose–mediated BNCT at BNL using one, two, or three irradiation fields on a sequential, dose-searching protocol. The median age for the subjects treated with one field was 56.5 years, with a median tumor volume of 20.5 cm^3 (2 to 70 cm^3) and a median KPS of 80. The volume-weighted average radiation dose to normal brain (ABD) varied from 1.9 to 4.1 Gy-equivalent for one field, from 4.1 to 6.6 Gy-equivalent for two fields, and from 6.7 to 9.5 Gy-equivalent for the three-field group.

Fifty of the 53 subjects have exhibited tumor persistence/recurrence within the treatment volume.[55] The median time to progression was independent of dose. In fact, there was a significant trend toward worse local control in subjects treated using three fields. Survival as an end point was found to be more dependent on the aggressiveness of the postrecurrence treatment than the BNCT dose given and, as such, was not a useful indicator of treatment-dependent tumor control.[23] The functional brain tolerance was reached in the three-field group. All except one patient treated with three fields exhibited significant acute or subacute functional neurologic toxicity at average brain doses as low as 6.7 Gy-equivalent. This may indicate a "volume effect" in that multiple fields generally treat a larger volume of normal brain to a lower dose compared with when a single field is used. The early stopping criterion of more than 20% incidence of grade 3 or 4 toxicity (RTOG/EORTC criteria) was reached during this study. However, no significant tumor response was observed in the patients in this protocol treated to minimum tumor doses above those predicted by Laramore and coworkers[54] to be therapeutic. We also note that preclinical studies using 9-L rat gliosarcoma model showed significant tumor response of the tumor to BPA-F–mediated BNCT at comparable doses.[56] Hence, neither the preclinical radiobiological studies nor the mathematical modeling based on fast neutron data provided an accurate guide to the necessary therapeutic dose. The BNL clinical program is no longer in operation.

In parallel with the BNCT program for malignant gliomas, a second area of major interest is the treatment of malignant melanoma metastatic to the brain. This work was instigated by Mishima and coworkers[57,58] in Japan. They used BPA as the ^{10}B-carrier agent with a single fraction of thermal neutrons used. BPA acts as a dopamine analogue in the melanin synthetic pathway and concentrates well in pigmented tumors. Initial reports describe good clinical results with this treatment,[59,60] but no randomized trials have been performed. Reports from the MIT/MGH program indicate that responses are better in this setting than in the treatment of GBMs, which is consistent with BPA being better suited to the treatment of pigmented tumors. Under the auspices of the Atomic Energy Commission of Argentina, a program for the treatment of metastatic melanoma has been instituted at the RA-6 research reactor in San Carlos de Bariloche.[61]

A very interesting approach to the treatment of liver metastases has been instituted at the University of Pavia in Italy. The patient is infused with BPA, and the diseased liver is extirpated and irradiated in the reactor and then reimplanted into the patient. Two patients have been treated in this manner, with one long-term survivor at 3 years from the time of the procedure. Model calculations indicate that it may be possible to perform this treatment without first removing the liver.[62]

Summary

To date there is no convincing evidence that BNCT offers a therapeutic advantage over conventional treatments for GBM. Reactor-based treatment centers are sufficient in number to conduct well-designed clinical trials to provide a "proof-of-concept," but certainly will not be adequate to treat large numbers of patients in the event that a therapeutic advantage is demonstrated. In this event, accelerator-based sources must be designed and placed in hospital settings. The main hurdle at the present time is the lack of tumor-specific ^{10}B carrier agents. The only compounds currently approved for human trials are BSH and BPA—both of which are suboptimal in many ways. Support of research in compound development will be key to further development of the field.[63]

REFERENCES

1. Batterman JJ, Breur K, Hare GAM, et al: Observations on pulmonary metastases in patients after single doses and multiple fractions of fast neutrons and cobalt-60 gamma rays. Eur J Cancer 17:539, 1981.
2. Hall EJ: Radiobiology for the Radiologist. 4th ed. Philadelphia: Lippincott, 1992, Chapters 9 and 14.
3. Laramore GE, Austin-Seymour MM: Fast neutron radiotherapy in relation to the radiation sensitivity of human organ systems. Adv Radiat Biol 15:153, 1992.
4. Stone RS: Neutron therapy and specific ionization. AJR Am J Roentgenol 59:771, 1948.
5. Brennan JT, Phillips TL: Evaluation of past experience with fast neutron teletherapy and its implications for future applications. Eur J Cancer Clin Oncol 7:219, 1971.
6. Catterall M: The treatment of advanced cancer by fast neutrons from the Medical Research Council's cyclotron at Hammersmith Hospital, London. Eur J Cancer Clin Oncol 10:343, 1974.
7. Catterall M, Bewley DK, Sutherland I: Second report on results of a randomized clinical trial of fast neutrons compared with x or gamma rays in treatment of advanced tumor of head and neck. Br Med J 1:1642, 1977.
8. Catterall M, Sutherland I, Bewley DK: First results of a randomized clinical trial of fast neutrons compared with X or gamma rays in treatment of advanced tumors of the head and neck. Br Med J 2:653, 1975.
9. Laramore GE, Krall JM, Griffin TW, et al: Neutron versus photon irradiation for unresectable salivary gland tumors: final report of an RTOG-MRC randomized clinical trial. Int J Radiat Oncol Biol Phys 27:235, 1993.
10. Douglas JG, Koh W, Austin-Seymour M, Laramore GE: Treatment of salivary gland neoplasms with fast neutron radiotherapy. Arch Otolaryngol Head Neck Surg 129:944, 2003.
11. Douglas JG, Lee S, Laramore GE, et al: Neutron radiotherapy for the treatment of locally-advanced major salivary gland tumors. Head Neck 21:255, 1999
12. Douglas JG, Silbergeld DL, Laramore GE: Gamma knife stereotactic radiosurgical boost for patients treated primarily with neutron radiotherapy for salivary gland neoplasms Stereotact Funct Neurosurg 82:84, 2004.
13. Huber PE, Debus J, Latz D, et al: Radiotherapy for advanced adenoid cystic carcinoma: neutrons, photons, or mixed beam? Radiother Oncol 59:161, 2001.
14. Breteau N, Wachter T, Kerdraon R, et al: Use of fast neutrons in the treatment of tumors of the salivary glands: rationale, review of the literature and experience in Orleans. Cancer Radiother 4:181, 2000.

15. Laramore GE, Krall JM, Griffin TW, et al: Fast neutron radiotherapy for locally-advanced prostate cancer. Am J Clin Oncol (CCT) 16:164, 1993.
16. Russell KJ, Caplan RJ, Laramore GE, et al: Photon versus fast neutron external beam radiotherapy in the treatment of locally advanced prostate cancer: results of a randomized prospective trial. Int J Radiat Oncol Biol Phys 28:47, 1993.
17. Chuba PJ, Maughan R, Forman JD: Three dimensional conformal neutron radiotherapy for prostate cancer. Strahlenther Onkol 175:79, 1999.
18. Forman JD, Duclos M, Sharma R, et al: Conformal mixed neutron and photon irradiation in localized and locally advanced prostate cancer: preliminary estimates of the therapeutic ratio. Int J Radiat Oncol Biol Phys 35:259, 1996.
19. Forman JD, Porter AT: The experience with neutron irradiation in locally advanced adenocarcinoma of the prostate. Semin Urol Oncol 15:239, 1997.
20. Haraf DJ, Rubin SJ, Sweeney P, et al: Photon neutron mixed-beam radiotherapy of locally advanced prostate cancer. Int J Radiat Oncol Biol Phys 33:3, 1995.
21. Maughan RL, Brambs B, Porter AT, et al: The cost-effectiveness of mixed beam neutron-photon radiation therapy in the treatment of adenocarcinoma of the prostate. Strahlenther Onkol 175:104, 1999.
22. Scalliet PG, Remouchamps V, Lhoas F, et al: A retrospective analysis of the results of p(65) + Be neutron therapy for the treatment of prostate adenocarcinoma at the cyclotron of Louvain-la-Neuve. Part I: survival and progression-free survival. Cancer Radiother 5:262, 2001.
23. Schwarz R, Krull A, Heyer D, et al: Present results of neutron therapy. The German experience. Acta Oncol 33:281, 1994.
24. Fuse H, Katayama T, Akimoto S, et al: Radiotherapy of prostatic carcinoma. Hinyokika Kiyo 37:801, 1991 [in Japanese].
25. Tsunemoto H, Morita S, Shimazaki J: Fast neutron therapy for carcinoma of the prostate. *In* Karr JP, Yamanaka H (eds): Prostate Cancer: The Second Tokyo Symposium. New York, Elsevier Science Publishing Co., 1989, pp 383-391.
26. Batterman JJ, Breur K, Hare GAM, et al: Observations on pulmonary metastases in patients after single doses and multiple fractions of fast neutrons and cobalt-60 gamma rays. Eur J Cancer 17:539, 1981.
27. Schwarz R, Krull A, Heyer D, et al. Neutron therapy in soft tissue sarcomas: a review of European results. Bull Cancer/Radiother 83(Suppl):110, 1996.
28. Schwartz DL, Einck J, Bellon J, Laramore GE: Fast neutron radiotherapy for soft tissue and cartilaginous sarcomas at high risk for local recurrence. Int J Radiat Oncol Biol Phys 50:449, 2001.
29. Fitzek MM, Thornton AF, Rabinov JD, et al: Accelerated fractionated proton/photon irradiation to 90 cobalt gray equivalent for glioblastoma multiforme: results of a phase II prospective trial. Accelerated fractionated proton/photon irradiation to 90 cobalt gray equivalent for glioblastoma multiforme: results of a phase II prospective trial. J Neurosurg 91:251, 1999.
30. Griffin BR, Berger MS, Laramore GE, et al: Neutron radiotherapy for malignant gliomas. Am J Clin Oncol 12:311, 1989.
31. Silbergeld DL, Rostomily RC, Alvord EC Jr: The cause of death in patients with glioblastoma is multifactorial: clinical factors and autopsy findings in 117 cases of supratentorial glioblastoma in adults. J Neurooncol 10:179, 1991.
32. Locher GL: Biological effects and therapeutic possibilities of neutrons. Am J Roentgenol Radium Ther 36:1, 1936.
33. Kruger PG: Some biological effects of biological disintegration products on neoplastic tissue. Proc Natl Acad Sci U S A 26:181, 1940.
34. Zahl PA, Cooper FS, Dunning JR: Some in vivo effects of localized nuclear disintegration products on a tranplantable mouse sarcoma. Proc Natl Acad Sci U S A 26:589, 1940.
35. Moss RL: Review of reactor-based neutron beam development of BNCT applications. *In* Soloway AH, Barth RE, Carpenter DE (eds): Advances in Neutron Capture Therapy. New York, Plenum Press, 1993, pp 1-7.
36. Farr LE, Sweet WH, Robertson JS, et al: Neutron capture therapy with boron in the treatment of glioblastoma multiforme. AJR Am J Roentgenol 71:279, 1954.
37. Godwin JT, Farr LE, Sweet WH, et al: Pathological study of eight patients with glioblastoma multiforme treated by neutron capture therapy using boron 10. Cancer 8:601, 1956.
38. Asbury AK, Ojemann R, Nielsen SL, et al: Neuropathologic study of fourteen cases of malignant brain tumors treated by boron-10 slow neutron capture therapy. J Neuropathol Exp Neurol 31:278, 1972.
39. Brownell GL, Murray BW, Sweet WH, et al: A reassessment of neutron capture therapy in the treatment of cerebral gliomas. *In* Seventh National Cancer Conference Proceedings, Philadelphia, Lippincott; 1973, pp 827-837.
40. Slatkin DN: A history of boron neutron capture therapy of brain tumors. Postulation of a brain radiation dose tolerance limit. Brain 114:1609, 1991.
41. Hatanaka H: Boron Neutron Capture Therapy for Tumors. Niigata, Japan, Nishimura Press, 1986.
42. Hatanaka H, Nakagawa N: Clinical results of long-surviving brain tumor patients who underwent boron neutron capture therapy. Int J Radiat Oncol Biol Phys 28:1061, 1994.
43. Nakagawa N: Recent study of boron neutron capture therapy for brain tumors. *In* Nigg DW, Wiersema RJ (eds): Proceedings of the First International Workshop on Accelerator-Based Neutron Sources for Boron Neutron Capture Therapy, Vol I, United States Department of Energy Report CONF-940976, 1994, pp 11-23.
44. Curran WJ, Scott CB, Horton J, et al: Recursive partitioning analysis of prognostic factors in three Radiation Therapy Group malignant glioma trials. J Natl Cancer Inst 85:704, 1993.
45. Laramore GE, Spence AM: Boron neutron capture therapy (BNCT) for high-grade gliomas of the brain: a cautionary note. Int J Radiat Oncol Biol Phys 36:241, 1996.
46. Kanda K: Experience of boron neutron capture therapy in Japan. *In* Larsson B, Crawford JF, Higgs CE, et al (eds): Proceedings of the Seventh International Symposium on Neutron Capture Therapy for Cancer, Vol I, Medicine and Physics, Amsterdam, Elsevier Scientific, 1997, pp 71-76.
47. Nakagawa Y, Kyonghon P, Kitamura K, et al: What were important factors in patients treated by BNCT in Japan? *In* Larsson B, Crawford JF, Higgs CE, et al (eds): Proceedings of the Seventh International Symposium on Neutron Capture Therapy for Cancer, Vol I, Medicine and Physics, Amsterdam, Elsevier Scientific, 1997, pp 65-70.
48. Sauerwein W, Rassow J, Mijnheer B. Considerations about specification and reporting of dose in BNCT. *In* Larsson B, Crawford JF, Higgs CE, et al (eds): Proceedings of the Seventh International Symposium on Neutron Capture Therapy for Cancer, Vol II, Chemistry and Biology, Amsterdam, Elsevier Scientific, 1997, pp 531-534.
49. Sauerwein W, Hideghety K, de Vries MJ, et al: Preliminary clinical results from the EORTC 11961 trial at the Petten irradiation facility. *In* Program and Abstracts, Ninth International Symposium on Neutron Capture Therapy for Cancer, Osaka, Japan, 2000, pp 15-16.
50. Kankaanranta L, Seppala T, Kallie M, et al: First clinical results on the Finnish study on a BPA-medicated BNCT in glioblastoma. *In* Program and Abstracts, Ninth International Symposium on Neutron Capture Therapy for Cancer, Osaka, Japan, 2000, pp 31-32.
51. Capala J, Stenstam BH, Skold K, et al: Boron neutron capture therapy for glioblastoma multiforme: clinical studies in Sweden. J Neurooncol 62:1354, 2003.
52. Honova H, Safanda M, Petruzelka L, et al: Neutron capture therapy in the treatment of glioblastoma multiforme. Initial experience in the Czech Republic. Cas Lek Cesk 143:44, 2004.
53. Busse PM, Harling OK, Palmer MR, et al: A phase-I clinical trial for cranial BNCT at Harvard-MIT. *In* Program and Abstracts, Ninth International Symposium on Neutron Capture Therapy for Cancer, Osaka, Japan, 2000, pp 27-28.
54. Laramore GE, Wheeler FJ, Wessol DE, et al: A tumor control curve for malignant gliomas derived from fast neutron radiotherapy data: implications for treatment delivery and compound selection. *In* Larsson B, Crawford JF, Higgs CE, et al (eds): Proceedings of the Seventh International Symposium on Neutron Capture Therapy for Cancer, Vol I, Medicine and Physics, Amsterdam, Elsevier Scientific, 1997, pp 580-587.

55. Diaz AZ: Assessment of the results from the phase I/II boron neutron capture therapy trials at the Brookhaven National Laboratory from a clinician's point of view. J Neuro-Oncol 62:101, 2003.
56. Coderre JA, Button TM, Micca PL, et al: Neutron capture therapy of the 9L rat gliosarcoma using the p-boronophenylalanine-fructose complex. Int J Radiat Oncol Biol Phys 30:643, 1994.
57. Mishima Y, Honda C, Ichihashi M, et al: Treatment of malignant melanoma by single neutron capture treatment with melanoma-seeking +10B-compound. Lancet 11:388, 1989.
58. Mishima Y, Honda C, Ichihashi M, et al: Selective melanoma thermal neutron capture therapy for lymph node metastases. *In* Soloway AH, Barth RF, Carpenter DE (eds): Advances in Neutron Capture Therapy, New York, Plenum Press, 1993, pp 705-710.
59. Mishima Y: Melanoma and non-melanoma neutron capture therapy using gene therapy: overview. *In* Larsson B, Crawford JF, Higgs CE, et al (eds): Proceedings of the Seventh International Symposium on Neutron Capture Therapy for Cancer, Vol I, Medicine and Physics, Amsterdam, Elsevier Scientific, 1997, pp 10-25.
60. Ichihasi I: Boron neutron capture therapy for malignant melanoma—retrospective and perspective of clinical trials. *In* Program and Abstracts, Ninth International Symposium on Neutron Capture Therapy for Cancer, Osaka, Japan, 2000, pp 3-4.
61. Gonzalez SJ, Bonomi MR, Santa Cruz GA, et al: First BNCT treatment of a skin melanoma in Argentina: dosimetric analysis and clinical outcome. Appl Radiat Isotop 61:1101, 2004.
62. Koivunoro H, Bleul DL, Nastasi U, et al: BNCT dose distribution in liver with epithermal D-D and D-T fusion based neutron beams. Appl Radiat Isot 61:853, 2004.
63. Chamberlin RL: Clinical research in neutron capture therapy. NCI Radiation Research Program meeting report. Int J Radiat Oncol Biol Phys 54:992, 2002.

CHAPTER 20

HYPERTHERMIA

Mark Dewhirst, Ellen L. Jones, Thaddeus Samulski, Shiva Das, Oana Craciunescu, Zeljko Vujaskovic, Chuan Li, and Leonard Prosnitz

The biological rationale for hyperthermia (HT) as a cancer treatment is based on several mechanisms, particularly relating to its combination with other therapies: HT is directly cytotoxic. When used with radiation therapy (RT), HT inhibits potentially lethal and sublethal damage repair and has complementary cytotoxicity with reference to the cell cycle. Hyperthermic killing is not influenced by hypoxia, whereas hypoxia has a significant effect on radiosensitivity. HT causes reoxygenation, which can increase RT sensitivity. HT increases drug uptake into cells, enhances DNA damage, and at least partially reverses drug resistance. HT improves delivery of nanoparticle drug carriers and macromolecular drugs, such as antibodies and drug-carrying polymers. The process of thermal adaptation (thermotolerance) may enhance exposure of tumor cell antigens to immune cells and increase innate immunity, thereby augmenting host immune responses against tumor cells. Developments in the field of gene therapy show that the heat shock promoter can be used with HT to trigger targeted, localized induction of therapeutic genes.

Despite the strong biological rationale, delivery of HT presents significant challenges. The goal is to be able to heat tumor tissue volumes precisely and reproducibly and to do so using methods that are clinically practical. A significant impediment to this goal is that current thermometry is invasive. Consequently, definition and calculation of thermal dose are not well defined. Priorities in the area of engineering and physics center on improvements in technologies to deliver HT and measure thermal dose.

Despite the technical difficulties in delivering HT, however, nine positive randomized trials of HT in human cancer patients have been published in addition to three positive canine randomized trials. The majority have demonstrated local control or survival advantages with the addition of HT to RT. Thus, even with the limitations of current technology, the promise of HT is emerging from clinical trials. As the technology improves, the benefits of this form of therapy will only become more visible. In this chapter, the biological rationale for using HT will be examined in more detail, a survey of methods used to heat tissues will be provided, and a comprehensive overview of key phase III studies will be presented.

BIOLOGY OF HYPERTHERMIA

Definition of Hyperthermia

Hyperthermia means elevation of temperature to a supraphysiologic level, between 40° and 45°C. Higher temperatures are used for thermal ablation but are not discussed in this chapter.

Arrhenius Relationship and Thermal Isoeffect Dose

Arrhenius found a temperature dependence of sucrose hydrolysis in the presence of various acids that was a logarithmic function of the absolute temperatures at which the reactions were conducted.[1] These observations were physiologically relevant in that the rate of cellular metabolism increases as temperature rises in cells or tissues, up to a point where thermal damage is created. The principles discovered by Arrhenius extend to cell killing by HT as well. The temperature dependence of the rate of cell killing is referred to as the "Arrhenius relationship."

The temperature dependence of the rate of cell killing has been used as a method for thermal dosimetry. This is done by plotting temperature versus log of the slope of the survival curve (1/Do). Do is analogous to a Do in a radiation survival curve (the dose to reduce survival to 37% of a starting value on the exponential portion of the survival curve). In the case of HT, "dose" is the number of minutes at a specified temperature (Fig. 20-1). Typically, Arrhenius plots have a biphasic curve and the point at which the slope changes is referred to as a "breakpoint." Above the breakpoint for nearly all cell types, a change in temperature of 1.0°C will double the rate of cell killing. Acquired resistance to HT killing (thermotolerance) that occurs during HT is responsible for the change in slope below the breakpoint. Arrhenius plots for human cell and rodent lines are well described. The breakpoint for human cells is near 43.5°C, and the slope below the breakpoint is between 2 and 4. The breakpoint for rodent cell lines is lower than that of humans, at about 43°C. The slopes of Arrhenius plots derived from in vivo studies are virtually identical to those that are derived from in vitro studies.

Sapareto and Dewey[2] proposed using the Arrhenius relationship to normalize thermal data from HT treatments. The rationale came from the observations that time-temperature histories are not stable, that they vary from patient to patient, and that temperatures within tumors were almost always nonuniform. Using the Arrhenius relationship, it would be possible to convert all time-temperature data to an equivalent number of minutes at a standard temperature. The formulation takes the following form.

$$\text{CEM } 43°\text{C} = tR^{(43-T)} \qquad \text{(Eq. 1)}$$

where CEM 43°C is cumulative equivalent minutes at 43°C (the temperature most commonly used for normalization), t is time of treatment, T is average temperature during desired interval of heating, and R is a constant. When above the breakpoint, which is usually assumed to be 43°C, R = 0.5. When below the breakpoint, R = 0.25.

For a complex time-temperature history, the heating profile is broken into intervals of time "t" length, where the temperature remains relatively constant. CEM 43°C is calculated using the average T (T_{avg}) for each interval, and the resultant data are summed to give a final CEM 43°C for the entire heating regimen.

$$\text{CEM } 43°\text{C} = \sum tR^{(43-T_{avg})} \qquad \text{(Eq. 2)}$$

The CEM 43°C (thermal isoeffect dose) formulation has been used extensively and successfully in clinical trials to assess the efficacy of heating. This is despite the fact that the R values and breakpoints have historically been derived from studies done in rodents, which are not exactly equivalent to human cells.[3]

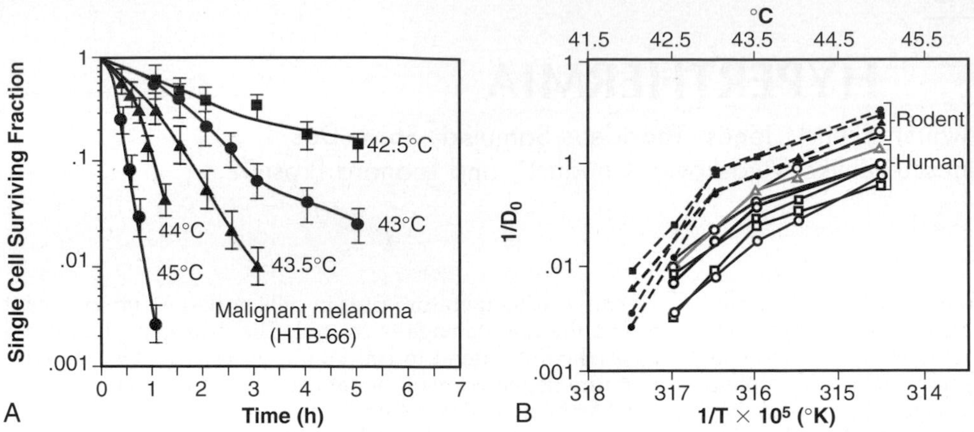

Figure 20-1 **A,** Cell survival curves for human melanoma cells are plotted as the log of the surviving fraction as a function of time of heating at a defined temperature. **B,** Arrhenius plots derived from survival curve data of several human and rodent tumor lines. Notice the change in slope (i.e., breakpoint) of the Arrhenius plots for both types of cells. For human cell lines, this appears to occur at about 43.5°C, whereas for rodent lines, it is approximately 43°C. (Data from Roizin-Towle L, Pirro JP: The response of human and rodent cells to hyperthermia. Int J Radiat Oncol Biol Phys 20:751-756, 1991.)

Modifiers of Thermal Cytotoxicity

Thermotolerance

Thermotolerance is defined as a transient adaptation to thermal stress that renders surviving heated cells more resistant to additional heat stress. Historically, thermotolerance has been avoided by using 2- to 3-day intervals between HT fractions to allow for decay of thermotolerance. Accordingly, clinical trials have not been designed to maximize the interactions between HT and conventionally fractionated radiation, as might be achieved by using HT every day with RT. It has been argued that daily HT with RT should be attempted, because heat radiosensitization is not affected by thermotolerance.

Acute Acidification

Acute acidification sensitizes cells to killing in two ways. It inhibits thermotolerance induction, and it increases cellular sensitivity to HT. Methods for achieving acute acidification in tumors have been studied extensively in preclinical models and in humans and are reviewed briefly in Physiologic Response to Hyperthermia.

Step-Down Heating

Step-down heating occurs when temperatures rise above the breakpoint and then drop below the breakpoint for the remainder of a treatment.[4] This occurs clinically in two circumstances: when power is turned down after heating has started in response to pain or excessively high normal tissue temperatures or when perfusion is increased in response to increased temperatures. When step-down heating occurs, thermotolerance induction is prevented during that heating session, and this effectively sensitizes cells to the cytotoxic effects of the treatment as delivered at the lower temperature.

Mechanisms of Hyperthermic Cytotoxicity

Cellular and Tissue Responses to Hyperthermia

Protein Is the Primary Target for Hyperthermic Cytotoxicity

When cells are exposed to elevated temperatures (≥41.0°C), damage is inflicted in multiple sites, but the predominant molecular target appears to be protein. The heat of inactivation for cell killing and thermal damage to tissues is in the range of that necessary for protein denaturation (130 to 170 kcal/mol). Additional evidence for proteins as being the primary target for cell killing is the importance of heat shock proteins in protecting thermotolerant cells from thermal damage. One of the primary functions of heat shock proteins is to refold other proteins that have been denatured or damaged.[5]

Some organelles are especially important in controlling thermal response. For example, modification of membrane lipid content or use of membrane active agents, such as alcohols, can sensitize cells to heat killing, but the sensitization is probably related to destabilization of the membrane as it relates to lipid-protein interactions.[6] The cytoskeleton of cells is particularly heat sensitive.[7] When it is collapsed by heat, there is disruption of cytoskeletal-dependent signal transduction pathways as well as inhibition of cell motility.[8,9] Enzymes in the respiratory chain are more heat sensitive than enzymes in the glycolytic pathway.[10] The heat sensitivity of the centriole leads to chromosomal aberrations following thermal injury.[11] Finally, the DNA repair process is heat sensitive, and this may be one of the mechanisms that leads to heat-induced radiosensitization and chemosensitization.[12]

Physiologic Response to Hyperthermia

Tumor blood flow and metabolism have important influences on the efficacy of HT and, conversely, the physiologic consequences of HT can influence the efficacy of other treatments.

As temperatures are increased, there is an increase in blood flow. The temperature threshold for this change is 41° to 41.5°C in skin.[13] Changes in vascular permeability also occur, leading to edema formation in the heated volume. At higher thermal doses, vascular stasis and hemorrhage develop. The change in normal tissue perfusion upon heating is much greater (10-fold) than one sees in tumors (1.5- to 2-fold).[14] Mechanisms underlying vascular stasis may include arteriovenous shunting, thrombus formation, and leukocyte plugging.[15] However, it is rare to achieve temperatures clinically that are sufficient to cause vascular damage. Importantly, physiologic changes occur in tumors at lower temperatures that are potentially beneficial (Fig. 20-2).

Taking Advantage of Physiologic Response to Hyperthermia

Improvement in Macromolecular and Liposomal Drug Delivery. A liposome is a small lipid vesicle (≈100-nm diameter) that contains water or saline in the center. Drugs can be loaded into liposomes at high concentration. It has been shown that HT increases microvascular pore sizes preferentially in tumor microvessels, which leads to enhanced liposomal accumulation in tumor.[16] The threshold for increased liposomal extravasation is 40°C and increases by a factor of two for every degree temperature rise until vascular damage occurs.[17] The effects of HT on liposomal extravasation have been studied extensively in preclinical models, but 2- to 13-fold enhancement in accumulation occurs in spontaneous soft tissue sarcomas of pet cats, an encouraging result that may translate to human tumors[18] (Fig. 20-3). HT also increases the available volume fraction (fraction of tissue not occupied by cells or stromal fibers), which may develop as cells undergo either necrosis or apoptosis following heat treatment.[19] This increases the tissue space available for liposomes to be deposited. The increase in liposomal drug delivery has been shown to result in increased anti-tumor effect in many preclinical studies.[20] HT has been used in conjunction with liposomal doxorubicin and radiation in one small clinical series of patients with chest wall recurrences of breast cancer and encouraging results were obtained, although drug concentrations were not measured in this series.[21]

For relatively small agents, such as most chemotherapeutic drugs, there is no advantage gained via increased vascular permeability to macromolecules or nanoparticles, unless the drugs are protein bound.[22] For drugs with molecular weight less than 1000 MW, the primary mechanism that governs drug transport is diffusion,[23] which is not highly temperature dependent. However, for molecules greater than 1000 MW, the primary driving force for transport is convection, which is controlled by the pressure gradient across the vessel wall. Accordingly, HT can augment the transvascular delivery of agents such as monoclonal antibodies[24] and polymeric peptides that carry drugs or radioisotopes.[25]

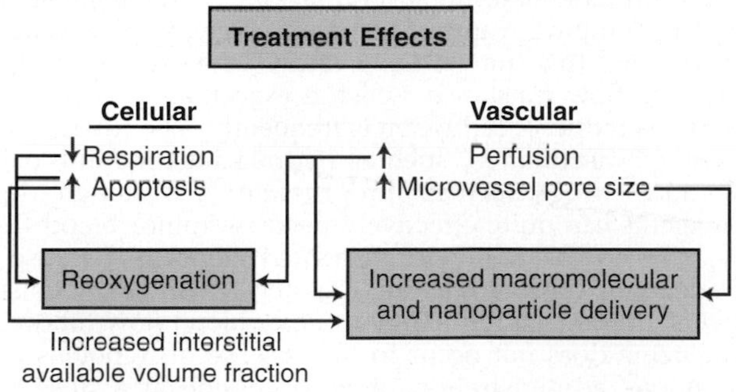

Figure 20-2 Overview of the beneficial physiologic and metabolic effects of hyperthermia.

Effects of Hyperthermia on Tumor Metabolism and Oxygenation. Enzymes for aerobic metabolism are more heat sensitive than those involved in anaerobic metabolism.[10] Decreases in ATP and increases in lactate concentration have been reported to occur following tumor blood flow reduction after HT.[26] In human patients with soft tissue sarcomas who were treated preoperatively with HT and RT, reduction in ATP/P_i ratio (measured using ^{31}P magnetic resonance spectroscopy; P_i = inorganic phosphate) was significantly correlated with a higher probability for pathologic complete response (pCR).[27] These results are consistent with the theory that tumor respiration can decrease after HT treatment.

A shift toward anaerobic metabolism would decrease oxygen consumption rates, which could lead to improvement in tumor oxygenation. Some of the benefits of HT may therefore result from improvements in oxygenation.[28] Several preclinical studies have shown that mild temperature heating (between 40° and 42°C for 1 hour) can lead to improvements in tumor Po_2 up to 24 hours after heating.[29] It has been reported that HT improves tumor oxygenation in canine and human soft tissue sarcomas, with reoxygenation being associated with greater probability for pCR in the human series.[30,31] In the canine study, median temperatures less than 44°C improved oxygenation, whereas median temperatures greater than 44°C for 60 minutes led to decreased oxygenation.[30] In a recent report of patients with locally advanced breast cancer who were treated in a phase II study with preoperative HT plus RT and Taxol, there was a significantly increased

Techniques and Modalities

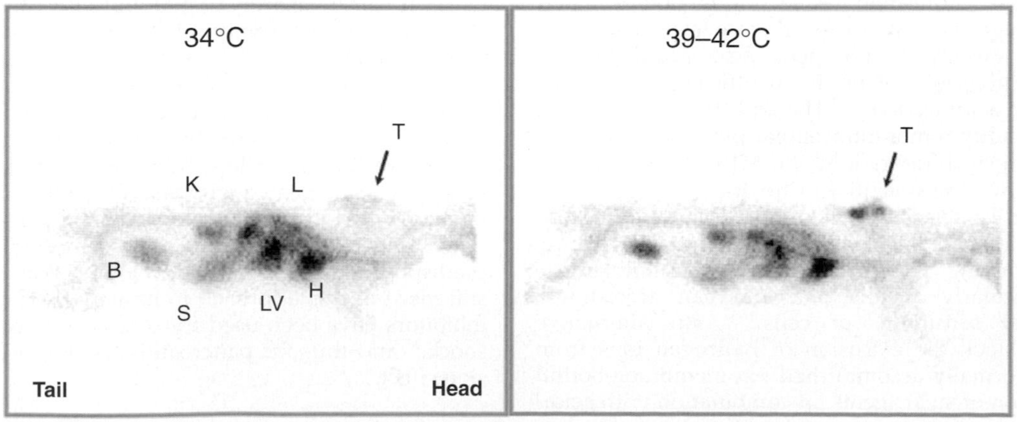

Figure 20-3 Gamma camera images of the effect of hyperthermia on radiolabeled pegylated liposomal accumulation in a spontaneous soft tissue sarcoma in a pet cat. The animal is lying in left lateral recumbency with the head to the right, and the tumor is located on the dorsal surface of the upper thorax (T, *arrow*). Other organs are indicated: lung (L), heart (H), liver (LV), spleen (S), kidney (K), and bladder (B). These liposomes also tend to accumulate in the reticuloendothelial system, as exhibited by the localization of relatively enhanced signal in the liver and spleen. Notice that there is greatly enhanced accumulation of liposomes when the tumor is heated compared with the control. Images were obtained serially on the same animal, allowing time for decay of the signal between the two sessions. The relative improvement in accumulation created by hyperthermia in this series of tumor-bearing cats ranged between 2- and 13-fold, with an average of a 4-fold improvement. (From Matteucci ML, Anyarambhatla G, Rosner G, et al: Hyperthermia increases accumulation of technetium-99m-labeled liposomes in feline sarcomas. Clin Cancer Res 6:3748-3755, 2000.)

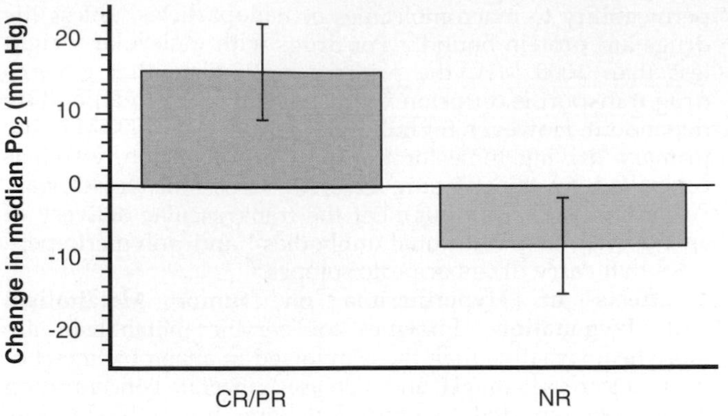

Figure 20-4 Change in Po_2 after the first hyperthermia treatment in series of patients with locally advanced breast cancer who were treated with neoadjuvant taxol, radiation, and hyperthermia. Notice that oxygenation improved in the subgroup of patients who achieved a response compared with those who did not respond favorably to treatment. These results strongly suggest that reoxygenation created by hyperthermia is beneficial for radiation therapy (and perhaps taxol treatment). Oxygen tension profile data were obtained using the Eppendorf oxygen sensor device. NR, no response; PR, partial response. (Data from Jones EL, Prosnitz LR, Dewhirst MW, et al: Thermochemoradiotherapy improves oxygenation in locally advanced breast cancer. Clin Cancer Res 10:4287-4293, 2004.)

likelihood for achieving pCR if the tumors showed reoxygenation after the first HT treatment. The probability for achieving a pCR was greater when the median temperatures during treatment were below 41.5°C[32] (Fig. 20-4). The benefit was restricted to those tumors that were hypoxic prior to treatment. These results confirm the preclinical studies, showing that mild temperature elevations during HT are more likely to be beneficial when they are combined with RT because such temperatures often lead to reoxygenation.[29]

Physiologic Approaches to Enhance Thermal Cytotoxicity

pH Modification

It is well established that acidification can enhance sensitivity to HT. Changes in intracellular pH are responsible for increased thermal sensitivity.[33,34] The most widely studied method to achieve acidification has been induction of hyperglycemia. The logic is that excess glucose load will push tumors toward glycolysis and lactic acid production.[35,36] However, hyperglycemia alone is insufficient to reliably achieve adequate acidification.[37,38] The addition of agents that can selectively acidify tumor intracellular pH, such as glucose combined with the respiratory inhibitor MIBG (metaiodobenzylguanidine), have the potential to further enhance hyperthermic cytotoxicity selectively in tumor tissues[39,40] because the acidification appears to be selective for tumors. Quercetin, a naturally occurring flavonoid, inhibits thermotolerance induction, particularly at low pH, and can accordingly increase thermal sensitivity of cells.[41-43] An alternative approach is to block the extrusion of hydrogen ions from cells, which is normally accomplished via membrane-bound pumps. Utilization of such agents, in combination with acidification of the extracellular space, can lead to enhanced hyperthermic cell killing both in vitro and in vivo.[44]

Blood Flow Manipulation

Blood perfusion is a major impediment to effective heating. Thus, selective reduction in tumor perfusion could prove beneficial. A number of vasoactive agents have been shown to reduce tumor blood flow, including those that are normally considered to be vasodilators. The reason for this paradoxical effect in tumors relates to several factors: (1) the relative lack of arteriolar input to tumors, (2) preexisting vasodilation in the few arterioles that tumors have, and (3) the presence of relatively high flow resistance, which is exacerbated when blood pressure is reduced; reduction is frequently encountered with the use of vasodilators, such as hydralazine, or nitric oxide (NO) donor drugs, such as nitroprusside.[45-47] Although use of such agents can quite effectively decrease tumor blood flow, they may not be easily implemented clinically because of the attendant risks of creating hypotension in normotensive patients. In humans reduction in tumor blood flow following hydralazine does not occur in the absence of hypotension.[48] Continuous administration of nitroprusside at a dose that decreases mean arterial pressure by 40% improves temperatures in spontaneous canine tumors. However, a safer dose for human use that reduced arterial pressure by 20% did not yield adequate improvement in temperature to create significant enhancement in cytoxicity.[49] Agents such as angiotensin II cause vasoconstriction but also cause hypertension. The net effect on tumor blood flow is unpredictable and heterogeneous.[50,51]

Another approach would be to use agents that cause peripheral vasoconstriction, such as NO synthase inhibitors. Such approaches effectively reduce tumor perfusion[52,53] and Po_2 in preclinical models.[54] Pet dogs with spontaneous soft tissue sarcomas treated with an NO synthase inhibitor in combination with local HT developed pancreatitis posttreatment.[55] These effects were attributed to comorbid conditions that predisposed them toward developing pancreatitis. There is still merit in this approach in humans, because NO synthase inhibitors have been used for other conditions such as septic shock,[56] and thus far pancreatitis has not been reported as a side effect.

Hyperthermia and Metastases

HT causes abrupt changes in tumor microvascular function, as described above, which could enhance tumor cell shedding from the heated site. Preclinical studies are mixed on this issue. One report showed that local HT enhanced the metastatic rate of B16 melanoma.[57,58] However, two other preclinical studies with different tumor models showed either a reduction in metastases following local HT[59] or no effect on the incidence of metastases, relative to controls.[60]

The question of whether local HT increases the risk for metastasis is difficult to answer in clinical trials unless the primary therapy has a high probability for local control. This is because of the problem of competing risks. In a phase III trial of canine patients with primary malignant melanomas treated with the combination of HT and radiation or radiation alone, no difference in the likelihood for metastasis between the two groups was seen.[61] However, local recurrence was a common event, and its onset was frequently followed by appearance of distant metastases. In a recently completed phase III randomized trial of human melanomas treated in a similarly designed trial, there was significant improvement in the likelihood for survival when the local tumor was controlled. Because the use of HT in that trial resulted in improved local control, the implication is that the combination therapy reduced the probability for metastases.[62,63] In a study comparing graded doses of radiation with or without HT for treatment of canine soft tissue sarcomas, higher normal tissue temperatures in the region of the tumor were correlated with lower likelihood for distant metastases.[64] A large series of patients (N = 95) with previously untreated high-grade soft tissue sarcomas who were treated preoperatively with HT and radiation achieved a local control rate near 90%, but 50% developed distant metastases.[65] This rate of metastasis is essentially identical to that seen with preoperative RT alone, however, suggesting that HT had an undetectable influence on metastases.[66]

The data are somewhat clearer when the effects of whole body hyperthermia (WBH) are considered. Urano and colleagues[67] reported that WBH increased the frequency of metastases in one of two preclinical fibrosarcoma models. Studies with the Lewis lung tumor model demonstrated that WBH could increase the rate of metastasis in tumor-bearing mice and, interestingly, even when tumor cells were given to animals after WBH exposure.[68] Whole body temperatures achieved during these relatively old studies were high, in the range of 41.8° to 42°C. There has been a trend toward reducing temperature of WBH to 40°C with longer-duration heating. In one preclinical study using this type of regimen, WBH had no discernible effect on metastases in a highly metastatic rat fibrosarcoma line.[69]

Published clinical studies have involved the higher temperature types of regimens. In a small pilot study, numbers of circulating tumor cells in peripheral blood were determined for 20 patients who received platinum-based chemotherapy plus HT (41.8°C, 60 minutes). Numbers of circulating tumor cells increased during WBH, but the impact of this observation on metastases was not reported.[70] In a randomized phase II study, dogs with soft tissue sarcomas received RT in combination with local HT alone or local HT plus whole body HT.[71] The addition of whole body HT increased the likelihood of distant metastases. In a separate study, aberrant metastasis locations were observed in dogs with primary osteosarcomas following treatment with whole body HT.[72] It has also been reported that patients who had a fever during or shortly after receiving brachytherapy for carcinoma of the cervix had an increased risk for developing distant metastases.[73]

The conclusion is that with the exception of one study with the B16 melanoma murine model, there is no evidence from preclinical models or human trials that local-regional HT causes an increase in metastases. When whole body HT is used, the issue is unresolved.

Normal Tissue Damage From Hyperthermia

Thresholds for thermal damage depend on the tissue type being heated and the severity of the injury. Mild damage can merely lead to edema, whereas more severe injury can lead to massive necrosis and organ failure. This subject has been reviewed in detail recently.[3] The ranking of tissue thermal sensitivities does not follow classic principles derived from other cytotoxic agents, such as radiation or chemotherapy. With such agents, the most sensitive tissues are those with the highest proliferative potential or activity. For HT, the most sensitive tissue classification includes brain, which is composed of cells with almost no proliferative potential, as well as testis, which has high proliferative potential. There has been speculation as to whether tumor tissues might be more sensitive to thermal damage than normal tissues. Many studies have compared tumor with normal cells, in vitro. There is no inherent difference in the thermal sensitivity. However, the microenvironment of tumors, which is often acidotic and nutritionally deprived, leads to an increase in thermal sensitivity that has been reported in a clinical series.[74]

Radiation and Hyperthermia

Rationale for Combining Hyperthermia With Radiation Therapy

When radiation is combined with HT, complementary effects occur. Cells in S-phase are radioresistant but sensitive to HT. Hypoxic cells are threefold more resistant to radiation, compared with aerobic cells, but there is no difference in thermal sensitivity between aerobic and hypoxic cells. As discussed earlier, HT can lead to reoxygenation, which will further improve RT response.[29-31] Finally, HT inhibits the repair of both sublethal and potentially lethal damage by inactivating crucial DNA repair pathways.[75-77]

Factors to Consider When Combining Hyperthermia With Radiation Therapy

The interaction between radiation and HT is described by the "thermal enhancement ratio" (TER), which is defined as the ratio of doses of radiation to achieve an isoeffect for RT/RT + HT. TERs for local control have been estimated for a number of human tumors using historical control data for radiation alone.[78] In most tumor types examined, these ratios were greater than 1. Assessment of normal tissue TER has not been attempted except in a few cases. For those examples, TER values for normal tissue damage have been less than those for tumor in the same patient population, suggesting potential for therapeutic gain for RT + HT compared with RT alone.[78] Prospective randomized trials in dogs with spontaneous tumors have also shown evidence for improved local tumor control with RT + HT compared with RT alone,[64,79-81] with no clinically observable increase in the frequency of clinically relevant late normal tissue complications. In one canine trial, enhancement of late radiation damage (as assessed histologically) was reported and the duration of acute radiation complications was prolonged.[81] There is clinical evidence, however, that excessively high intratumoral temperatures (i.e., >45°C for 60 minutes) can lead to damage to surrounding normal tissues, an effect that is often caused by rapid tumor regression.[79,82] Such damage is not easily repaired and can lead to chronic tissue consequences, such as fibrosis, fistula formation, and bone necrosis.

In summary, most available data from preclinical and clinical studies indicate that therapeutic gain is achievable for the combination of HT with RT. There is very little evidence to suggest that HT enhances the incidence or severity of late normal tissue complications from RT, particularly when excessively high intratumoral temperatures are avoided.

Hyperthermia and Chemotherapy

Rationale for Using Hypertherma With Chemotherapy

Many chemotherapeutic agents have been shown to exhibit synergism with HT, including cisplatin and related compounds, melphalan, cyclophosphamide, nitrogen mustards, anthracyclines, nitrosoureas, bleomycin, mitomycin C, and hypoxic cell sensitizers.[22] The mechanisms that underlie the synergy may include (1) increased cellular uptake of drug, (2) increased oxygen radical production, (3) increased DNA damage and inhibition of repair, and (4) reversal of drug resistance mechanisms.[83-86] Hypoxia and pH are also important in the thermochemotherapeutic response.[87-91] There are some classes of drugs, such as etoposide and vinca alkaloids, that do not synergistically interact with HT.[22]

Factors to Consider When Combining Hyperthermia With Chemotherapy

Temperature Dependence

The degree of enhancement of cytotoxicity has been shown to be temperature dependent for many drugs.[92] Combinations of camptothecins with HT have not shown consistent results in vitro. The interaction between these agents and HT is schedule and temperature dependent.[93,94] In one report, temperatures up to 41.8°C increased the activity of topoisomerase II, which may be the explanation for the increased activity of these drugs at elevated temperatures.[93] Enhancement of drug activity has been seen in vivo.[95]

In Vitro Results May Not Predict In Vivo Activity

Tubulin binding agents, such as Taxol, show no evidence for interaction in vitro,[96] but studies in combination with RT in vivo are more encouraging.[97] There may be physiologic consequences of the combination of Taxol and HT that make the combination work better than predicted from in vitro studies.

Sequencing

For most drugs (excluding 5-FU and perhaps other antimetabolites), the optimal sequence between heat and drug is to administer them simultaneously or to give the drug immediately before the onset of heating. For platinum-containing drugs, the tissue extraction rate of drug may be increased with HT, further substantiating the rationale for use of this sequence.[98] Most antimetabolites do not interact with HT when given concomitantly.[22] However, 5-FU has been shown to interact supra-additively with HT by maintaining temperatures between 39° and 41°C. Temperatures in this range lead to enhanced conversion to active metabolites, thereby increasing drug cytotoxicity. In addition, continuous infusion protocols with this drug may lead to cell cycle block in S phase, a relatively sensitive part of the cell cycle to HT.[99]

Hyperthermia and Gene Therapy

Several investigators have exploited the heat shock response as a means to perform gene therapy.[100-109] The heat shock promoter is highly inducible and relatively quiescent under normothermic conditions. For example, 42°C for 30 minutes yielded several hundredfold induction of reporter protein expression under control of the HSP70 promoter.[106] Similar results have been reported for other cell lines.[109-111] In one series of studies, tumor growth delay was improved in the B16 melanoma model treated with HT and gene therapy involving the immune modulator interleukin-12 under control of the HSP70 promoter.[106] When RT was added, superior results were obtained, relative to all controls.[107] An additional advantage to this approach is that HT allows for control of gene expression to the tissue of interest.[108] Further improvements in HT-mediated gene therapy may be obtained by combining the HSP70 promoter with a constitutive promoter[112] (Fig. 20-5). The same basic approach could be used to drive suicide gene therapy, induce wild-type *TP53* to induce apoptosis, or control production of other cytokines such as tumor necrosis factor α.[111,113-115]

Immunologic Effects of Hyperthermia

Heat shock proteins have been recently recognized for their potential role in regulating immune responses. There are several recognized functions of these proteins: (1) They are known to bind, in a noncovalent fashion, to immunogenic peptides. (2) When tumor cells are exposed to HT, heat shock protein–peptide complexes are presented on the cell surface.

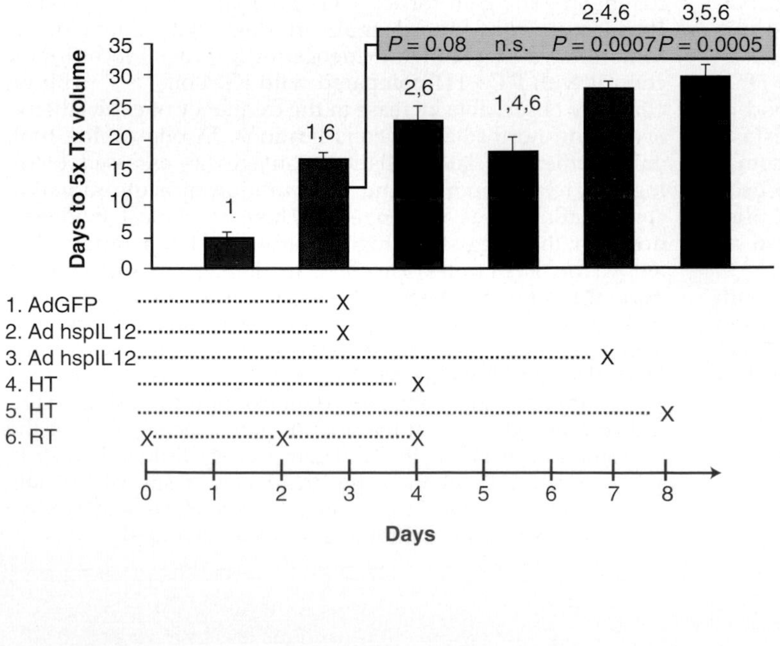

Figure 20-5 Days to reach five times treatment volume for adenovirus-mediated (Ad), heat-regulated gene therapy in combination with fractionated radiotherapy (RT) in the B16 mouse melanoma model. The heat shock protein 70 (HSP70) promoter was used to drive gene expression of interleukin-12 (hspIL12). An adenoviral vector containing the gene for green fluorescence protein (GFP), under control of a constitutive promoter, was used as a control. The timing of treatments is shown in the time line below the plot. The particular treatment and sequence used are indicated by the numbers listed above each bar in the graph. There were significant increases in growth time for combinations involving the interleukin-12 genes, hyperthermia (HT), and RT, compared with the use of hyperthermia plus the GFP-containing virus, when combined with radiotherapy. Equivalent results were obtained when the gene therapy was administered before the last radiation fraction or 3 days later. (Data from Lohr F, Huang Q, Hu K, et al: Systemic vector leakage and transgene expression by intratumorally injected recombinant adenovirus vectors. Clin Cancer Res 7:3625-3628, 2001.)

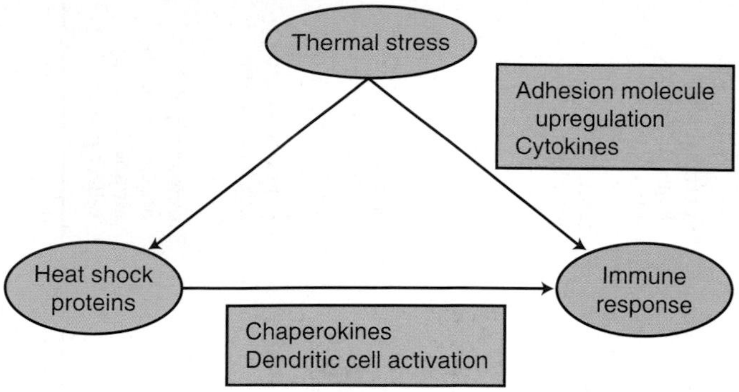

Figure 20-6 Summary of known beneficial immunologic effects of mild temperature hyperthermia. In this context, mild heating refers to temperatures between 39°C and 41°C. (Adapted from Repasky E, Issels R: Physiological consequences of hyperthermia: heat, heat shock proteins and the immune response. Int J Hyperthermia 18:486-489, 2002.)

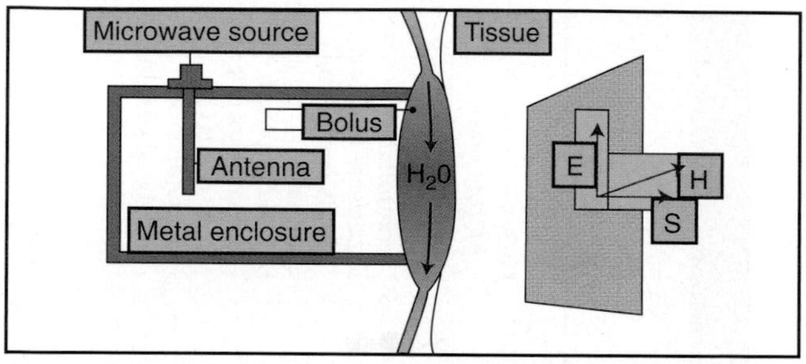

Figure 20-7 Diagram of a simple microwave waveguide applicator. Energy is often coupled to the tissue using a water bolus, which can also be temperature controlled to regulate skin temperature. This type of device usually operates at frequencies between 400 and 2500 MHz. The depth of penetration is better with lower frequency, but it is still limited to no more than 4 cm at 400 MHz. At 915 MHz, the penetration depth is about 2 cm. There is no control of power in the x-y plane, other than what can be achieved by physically moving the applicator.

These complexes can be recognized by antigen-presenting cells (dendritic cells) via MHC class I molecules. Once dendritic cells have received this type of stimulus, they migrate to lymph nodes, where they prime T cell lymphocytes to be cytotoxic toward cells that express the peptide–heat shock protein complex. HT has been shown to enhance the rate of dendritic cell migration.[116] (3) Heat shock proteins also induce dendritic cell maturation and proinflammatory cytokine release.[117,118] (4) Cell membrane localization of heat shock proteins also activates the innate immune system by activating natural killer (NK) cells.[119] Other sources of cellular stress, such as viral infection, fever, hypoxia, and radiation exposure, have been shown to upregulate heat shock proteins as well. Because this process appears to occur naturally, there have been efforts to exploit the use of HT to produce tumor-derived vaccines and to augment the in vivo response to such vaccines.[118] HT has also been reported to upregulate a number of proinflammatory cytokines and adhesion molecules that facilitate immune cell trafficking across endothelial cells to gain access to tumor interstitium.[120] Additionally, shed heat shock proteins, with or without associated peptides, may act as chemokines to attract immune cells (particularly macrophages) toward a region tissue that has undergone heat stress.[121] A summary of some key immunologic effects of HT is shown in Figure 20-6.

HYPERTHERMIA PHYSICS

Clinical HT is usually achieved by exposing tissues to conductive heat sources, or nonionizing radiation (e.g., electromagnetic [EM] or ultrasonic [US] fields). Although these modalities deposit energy in tissue by different physical mechanisms, they have general similarities. They are sensitive to the heterogeneity of tissue properties, geometry of blood flow, and the practical problems of coupling the energy source into tissue. HT can be administered using either invasive sources or noninvasively using externally applied power. A brief discussion of the noninvasive methods is provided later and is summarized in Table 20-1. Invasive methods have been developed extensively and include radiofrequency (RF) antennas, RF electrodes, hot water tubes, ferromagnetic metals, and ultrasound transducers. These types of devices have been designed for direct implantation into tissue or for intracavitary use. Further details on all methods are available elsewhere.[122,123]

Electromagnetic Heating

When an electric field (E-field) propagates through materials of finite electrical conductivity, resistant heating occurs. Improved penetration is seen for low-frequency or long wavelengths, but the ability to localize EM energy deposition is dependent on the wavelength. The longer the wavelength, the broader is the focus of heating. Accordingly, there is a tradeoff between depth of penetration and ability to focus energy. There is a fundamental constraint on noninvasive heating by EM techniques that does not allow *localized* heating at depths greater than 2 to 5 cm from a single applicator. Utilization of EM techniques with multiple applicators results in regional energy deposition that can then involve substantial volumes of normal tissue around the tumor.

Electromagnetic Heating Devices

These devices can be separated into two categories: superficial applicators with effective penetration into tissue in the range of 2 to 5 cm and deep heating devices that have effective penetration greater than 5 cm. Superficial devices include waveguides and microstrip or patch antennas operating at RF and microwave frequencies of 433, 915, or 2450 MHz.[124] Energy is usually coupled into tissue through a temperature-controlled deionized water bolus to maintain skin temperature below 43°C (Figs. 20-7 and 20-8).

To heat at depths greater than 5 cm, RFs between 5 and 200 MHz are used. There are three basic techniques for EM deep heating: magnetic induction, capacitive coupling, and phased arrays. *Magnetic induction* heating uses a time-varying magnetic field to induce eddy currents in conductive tissue. The magnetic field distribution is not sensitive to tissue type and is consistently predictable. However, the eddy current distribution is governed by paths of least resistance and is affected by tissue conductivity. Deep heating using the *capacitive technique* uses RF fields between 5 and 30 MHz with ion currents being driven between two or more conductive electrodes. Heating tends to be concentrated at the electrodes, but saline bolus can be temperature controlled to prevent hot spots on the skin surface and help to cool superficial fat.[125] Varying electrode size can shift current distribution toward the smallest of the electrodes. For example, this can be done with a balloon electrode for intracavitary applications (e.g., esophagus).[126] The thickness of the superficial fat layer is a significant limitation to this method because of resistive heating.

Table 20-1 Summary of Methods Used to Heat Tissues

Class	Method	Power Directed to Tumor Site?	Frequency	Coupling Medium	Invasive Thermometry Requirements	Advantages	Disadvantages
Electromagnetic	**SUPERFICIAL**						
	Magnetic induction	No		Air	Fiberoptic or high-resistance lead thermistors	Simple to operate	Eddy currents follow path of least resistance; heating pattern is not controllable
	Capacitive radiofrequency	Sometimes—use different sized applicators	5-30 MHz	Saline	Same as above	Simple to operate	Superficial fat heats; limits use to thin patients
	Microwave wave guide	Yes, by physical placement of waveguides over tumor	433, 915, 2450 MHz	Water	Same as above	Simple to operate	Limited depth of heating; heating pattern highly dependent on power deposition pattern
Electromagnetic	**DEEP**						
	Magnetic induction	No		Air	Same as above	Simple to operate	Eddy currents follow path of least resistance; heating pattern is not controllable
	Capacitive radiofrequency	Partially—by physical location of applicators	5-30 MHz	Saline	Same as above	Simple to operate	Superficial fat heats; limits use to thin patients
	Phased radiofrequency or microwave arrays	Partially—by altering phase and amplitude of power from different antennas	100-200 MHz	Water	Same as above	Better focus capability than other EM methods	Technically challenging
Ultrasound	**SUPERFICIAL**						
	Planar ultrasound transducers—single or multiple	Yes, mainly by physical placement of transducers over region of tumor	1-3 MHz	Degassed water	Metal device preferable (i.e., thermocouple or thermistor); Avoid plastic	Similar to waveguides	Good coupling to body required—air and bone prohibit penetration and can lead to pain
Ultrasound	**DEEP**						
	Focused transducer arrays	Yes	0.5-2 MHz	Degassed water	Same as above	The most focusable method	Limited size of acoustic windows, air and bone reflect power

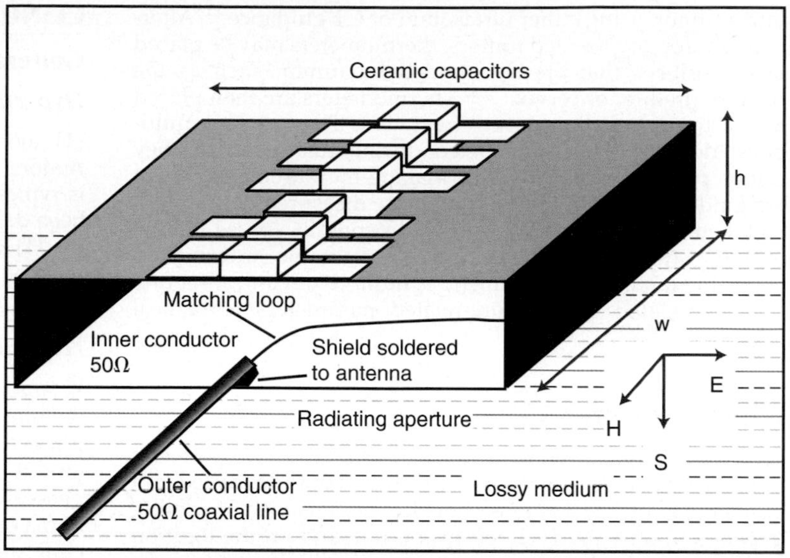

Figure 20-8 Diagram of a radiofrequency current sheet applicator. This type of applicator is composed of multiple elements that facilitate power control in the x-y plane, and it is particularly useful for superficial tumors, such as chest wall recurrences of breast cancer. This applicator was designed to operate at 125 MHz, and it demonstrated a penetration depth of 4 cm. (From Hoffmann W, Rhein KH, Wojcik F, et al: Performance and use of current sheet antennae for RF-hyperthermia of a phantom monitored by 3 tesla MR-thermography. Int J Hyperthermia 18:454-471, 2002. With permission from Taylor & Francis Ltd. http://www.tandf.co.uk/journals).

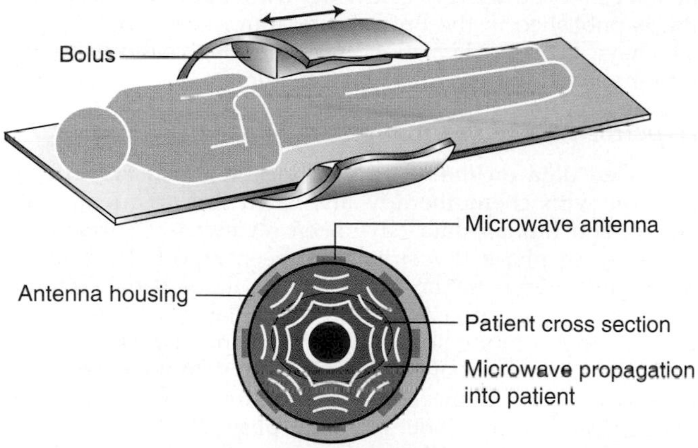

Figure 20-9 Diagram of a radiofrequency phased-array system. This type of device operates in the range of 100 MHz. Heating the body center can be achieved with this type of device when the antennas are driven in phase, leading to phase addition from each of the contributing antennas in the center of the target volume. Additional spatial control of temperatures is achieved by varying the amount of power delivered to each antenna. Coupling of energy to the body is achieved using a water-filled bolus.

Therefore, RF capacitive heating is used almost exclusively in Asia, where patients tend to be thinner. The third option is the *RF phased array*.[127] These devices consist of an array of RF antennas arranged in a geometric pattern surrounding the target body region.[124] Antennas are driven from a common RF source, allowing the RF fields from the antennas to add together to form a null (phase subtraction; the EM waves cancel each other out) or a focus (phase addition; the EM waves from the sources add together). In the latter case, one can achieve better and deeper power deposition into tissue than what one would achieve by operating the antennas independently (i.e., driving the antennas without phase addition). In general, the phased array technique has more flexibility for controlling power deposition than magnetic induction and capacitive techniques (Fig. 20-9).

Ultrasound Heating

Energy transfer from ultrasound is associated with viscous friction. Penetration of US field decreases with frequency. Because the wavelength of an US field is several orders of magnitude smaller than that of EM fields, the problems of applicator size and focusing of US field energy in deeper tissues are greatly reduced. Anatomic geometry and tissue heterogeneity (air reflects, bone preferentially absorbs) severely limit the utility of US. The availability of an adequate "acoustic window" (a path unobstructed by bone or air proximal and distal to the target) is often a problem in clinical applications. The entry window size determines the size and depth of the target volume.

There are several types of ultrasound applicators. Energy is coupled into tissue using temperature-controlled degassed water. Single and multiple transducer plane wave devices have been designed for superficial tumor (2 to 5 cm) heating,[124] and they typically operate in the 1- to 3-MHz range.[128-130] Deep heating with ultrasound is accomplished by using scanned focused transducers, phased arrays, or multiple scanned focused transducers.[124] Ultrasound frequencies for deep heating are in the 0.5- to 2-MHz range.

Measurement of Temperatures During Hyperthermia

Invasive thermometry is the current standard, which involves physically placing thermometers into the tumor. Alternatively, for superficial tumors (<0.5-cm depth), probes can be attached in fixed positions on the skin surface or mapped through catheters lying on the skin. Although the accuracy of invasive thermometers is sufficiently precise (typically ±0.2°C) to resolve important differences in thermal dose (as described earlier), this type of thermometry has many disadvantages. Disadvantages include discomfort to the patient and risk of hemorrhage and/or infection, the expense of physician time required for catheter placement, and necessity for imaging to verify placement of thermometers. In addition, the sparse nature of the data obtained makes it difficult to spatially control power deposition or alter treatment to improve temperature distibutions.[131,132] The most common method for doing invasive thermometry is to insert blind ended catheters into a tumor, using either ultrasound or CT guidance.[133] Alternatively, for deep-seated tumors, thermometers may be placed inside orifices that are surrounded by tumor, such as the rectum, urethra, or cervix.[134,135] Thermometers are then placed inside these catheters during treatment. They can be multipoint devices that remain fixed during treatment, or they can be physically moved while making measurements. There are guidelines published for how these measurements should be taken for all HT devices.[133,136-138] Despite its sparse nature, invasive thermometry can provide valuable information about the quality of a treatment. A number of clinical reports have correlated temperature-related parameters to clinical response.[79,139-143]

Bioheat Transfer

Temperatures achieved with any heating method are the result of the net balance between how much power is deposited and how efficiently the tissue is cooled. The efficiency of cooling depends upon bulk tissue perfusion rate and on the location and density of relatively large, thermally significant vessels, such as small arteries. Considerable effort has gone into the development of methods to predict or calculate the efficiency of heat transfer.[144-147] Such information could prove valuable for treatment planning and treatment optimization.[134,148] Advances in this methodology have included use of MR contrast enhancement and flow-sensitive pulse sequences to identify the perfusion distribution pattern and location of thermally significant vessels, respectively.[145,149]

Noninvasive Thermometry

MRI is currently the preferred technology. Several basic MR parameters are sensitive to changes in temperature, including the relaxation times T1 and T2, the bulk magnetization, the diffusion coefficient of water, and the resonance frequency of the water atoms. Currently, temperature changes are monitored with MR by measuring the water proton resonance frequency shift (PRFS), although improvements in MR hardware may revive the use of the diffusion coefficient–based methods. The latter has shown to provide the best temperature sensitivity and is most commonly used.[150-152] MRI thermometry has been used for measuring power deposition distributions in phantoms with resolution of 0.3° to 0.5°C.[146] Clinical studies in patients with soft tissue sarcomas have reported resolution of 0.5° to 1°C.[153] MRI thermometry has also been used to monitor changes in temperature for thermal ablation.[154,155] There are important technical issues that need to be solved for application of HT in more important tumor sites, such as the abdomen and pelvis. Drift in MR magnet coils and motion of the patient or parts of the patient, created by factors such as peristalsis or respiration, are not easily corrected and create artifacts in the thermal data. If methods can be developed that correct artifact MR, then MR thermometry could be used for modulation of power during treatment to achieve more controlled delivery of heat.

Other methods that have been investigated for imaging temperatures have included ultrasound[156,157] and microwave thermography.[158-160] The temperature resolution of ultrasound is marginal for HT temperature ranges, although it has proved useful for monitoring thermal ablation. Microwave thermography is fairly well developed, but it is only useful for relatively superficial tumors. Electron paramagnetic resonance (EPR) has been investigated for its potential usefulness in thermometry.[161] EPR is a much cheaper technology than MR, but EPR imaging is still in its infancy.

CLINICAL HYPERTHERMIA

General Considerations

Hyperthermia Alone

HT alone has been studied in the treatment of superficial tumors. While an occasional response is noted, the duration is typically quite short.[162,163] No long-term tumor control has been described with the use of HT as a sole treatment modality. HT alone remains widely practiced in certain alternative and complementary medicine clinics. Its use, however, is not supported by any peer-reviewed published scientific data.

Hyperthermia With Radiation Therapy

A large number of reports attest to the efficacy of HT in combination with RT. The majority of publications have been from phase II trials involving patients with superficial malignancies (and thus more amenable to heating) as a component of more generalized disease, such as local recurrence of breast carcinoma on the chest wall. With the addition of HT to radiation, clinical response rates have approximately doubled from 25% to 35% with radiation alone to 50% to 70% with RT + HT.[164] In addition to phase II studies, several phase III trials have now been conducted worldwide with approximately two thirds published in the English literature. These trials generally have been positive, lending additional validity to the information obtained from phase II studies.

Hyperthermia With Chemotherapy

Published data on the efficacy of local-regional HT in conjunction with chemotherapy are much less frequent. Both animal and human data have been reviewed.[164] Particularly encouraging phase II results have been reported for sarcomas[165] and breast carcinoma (J. Park et al., personal communication). A small phase III study from Japan compared the preoperative combination of bleomycin and cisplatin with or without HT for esophageal cancer.[166] The pathologic response rate was higher in the combined treatment arm compared with chemotherapy alone. No other phase III data are as yet reported, but a phase III trial, being conducted by EORTC, is nearly completed for locally advanced soft tissue sarcomas.

Trimodality Therapies With Hyperthermia, Chemotherapy, and Radiation Therapy

The combination of HT, chemotherapy, and radiation has been evaluated preclinically and has been shown to yield superior antitumor effects.[167] Clinical studies have reported encouraging results with this approach as well. For example, pilot clinical studies have evaluated the combination of the hypoxic cell sensitizer etanidazole, radiation, and HT for superficial tumors.[168] A small randomized phase III trial involving patients with esophageal cancer showed a higher pCR rate when HT was added to chemoradiotherapy compared with chemoradiotherapy alone.[169] More recently, the combination of HT plus cisplatin plus RT has been evaluated in patients with locally advanced cervix cancer. Twelve patients were treated in this series, with local control being achieved in 10. The two patients with local failure presented with local recurrence following hysterectomy.[170] These trials formed the basis for a recently initiated multi-institutional phase III trial comparing the trimodality approach to chemoradiotherapy alone that is being conducted by investigators in the United States and Europe, with Duke University serving as the trial center. The combination of 5-FU, HT, and RT yielded favorable responses in patients with locally advanced colorectal cancer in a phase II study,[171] which formed the basis for a randomized phase III trial of 5-FU plus radiation with or without HT by investigators in Germany.

Normal Tissue Damage from Hyperthermia

HT does not significantly increase early or late toxicity of radiation.[64,78-81] The most common toxicities of HT are superficial or subcutaneous tissue burns. They are usually first or second degree and small in volume. Such burns occur in approximately 5% of patients treated in the Duke experience; characteristically they do not exceed 3 to 4 cm in maximum diameter. Third-degree burns are infrequently observed (<1% incidence). Complications from thermometry catheters are infrequent if the catheters are removed following each HT treatment.[172] When catheters are left in place throughout the course of HT (e.g., for several weeks), the frequency of complications rises significantly, particularly secondary infections.[173] There are potential medical contraindications to deep-regional HT related to the physiologic stress. Guidelines for patient selection for deep HT have been developed by the Radiation Therapy Oncology Group (RTOG).[138]

Relationship between Thermal Dose and Outcome

Quality assurance for delivery and measurement of temperatures during HT is essential to identify quantifiable thermal dose parameters. Negative early phase III clinical trials conducted by the RTOG were attributed to this issue.[174-177] Quality assurance standards and data acquisition procedures were subsequently established by both the RTOG[133,138] and European Society of Hyperthermic Oncology (ESHO).[178,179] The biological underpinning for thermal dosimetry was discussed previously in the biology section of this chapter.

Dosimetry for HT is distinctly different from that for RT in that the amount of energy deposited does not correlate with the degree of damage. This is because damage is related to the amount of temperature rise and the time of exposure, both of which are governed by the net balance between how much energy is deposited versus how much is carried away by thermal conduction and perfusion. In the case of HT, the dosimetric unit used most often has been one that was derived empirically from evaluation of the Arrhenius relationship for cell killing in vitro as well as from numerous studies of degree of tissue damage as a function of temperature and time of exposure.[3] As was described in detail above, the unit most often used has been equivalent minutes at 43°C (CEM43°C). Application of this concept to the clinic, however, requires integration of nonuniform temperature history data with CEM43°C.

Because temperatures during HT treatment are nonuniform, it is necessary to derive descriptive parameters from the temperature distribution to which the CEM43°C parameter can be applied. A number of clinical parameters have been described based on simple descriptions of the multipoint thermometry, such as minimum temperature, average temperature, etc. Parameters that have proved useful for describing temperature distributions are the 10th percentile of the temperature distribution, which is commonly referred to as the T_{90} (90% of measured points exceed this value) or the T_{50}, which is the median temperature. Use of these types of parameters leads to dosimetry that is comparable across patients and studies, as long as quality assurance guidelines are followed with respect to the placement and number of thermometers used. The resultant units are referred to as CEM43°CT_{90} or CEM43°CT_{50}.

Retrospective evaluation of many phase II and phase III trial results has shown positive relationships between measures of thermal dose and treatment outcome, suggesting that higher thermal doses yield better responses when HT is combined with RT.[139-143] In all positive studies reported to date, thermal analysis was performed retrospectively. It has been more difficult to correlate variations in thermal dose administered a priori and clinical outcome. Two studies compared various numbers of heat treatments given in combination with fractionated RT,[180,181] using the assumption that more treatments would yield greater cumulative thermal dose. Neither study showed any benefit with higher numbers of HT fractions, which could in part be due to the fact that there was considerable overlap in thermal doses between the treatment arms. This is because temperature is a stronger determinant of thermal dose than time at temperature (see earlier section on biology). A canine study compared RT combined with whole body HT plus local HT compared with local HT alone. The CEM43°CT_{90} was higher in the group that received whole body HT, but there was no difference in duration of local control between the two treatment arms.[71] One potential explanation for the lack of improvement in local control might have been the induction of thermotolerance during the whole body HT, which was administered prior to application of local heating.

The first attempt to prospectively control thermal dose, as prescribed by the CEM43°CT_{90}, was a study of preoperative RT plus HT for soft tissue sarcomas. The outcome variable was pCR assessed at the time of surgery, and the percentage of patients predicted to achieve a pCR as a result of achieving CEM43T_{90} greater than 10 minutes was predicted to be 75%, based on prior phase II studies.[140] The pCR rate in this study was 54%, which was below the 95% confidence level for the projected rate.[65] A number of explanations are possible for failing to achieve the projected pCR rate, including the sparseness of the temperature information gained. Recently, it was reported that other mitigating physiologic factors may have confounded the results of this study.[182] Two additional phase III trials have been completed by the same group—one in patients with superficial tumors and the other in pet dogs with soft tissue sarcomas. In both of these trials, there was clear separation in thermal doses between the two treatment arms.[183,184] Most important, improved response and duration of local control were observed in the groups that prospectively received the higher thermal dose.[184,185] These are the first two trials conducted in which prospective control of thermal dose has yielded demonstrated improvement in local tumor response or control or both. They clearly indicate that better prospective control of thermal dose may ultimately lead to methods to truly optimize HT treatment.

Phase III Clinical Trials Overview

Phase III trials have involved a wide variety of diseases, including superficial malignancies and tumors deep within the body. Trials have been conducted with either palliative or curative intent. A summary of the most important of these trials is presented in Table 20-2.

Breast Cancer

Chest wall recurrences of breast cancer are difficult to control with conventional approaches, and many patients develop such recurrences despite prior adjuvant RT or systemic therapy. Because they are superficial tumors, they have been amenable to HT trials. Five separate phase III trials were combined for analysis in an international collaborative study.[186] Patients were randomized to either RT alone or RT with HT. Treatment was prescribed according to ESHO and RTOG guidelines. HT techniques differed somewhat between

Table 20-2 Summary of Key Phase III Trial Results

Author	Tumor Type/ Location	Type of Trial	No.	Rx Arm: RT	Rx Arm: RT + HT	Total RT Dose (Gy)	Dose/Fx and/or Dose Rate	# Fx	Mean Tx Time	Hyperthermia: # Fx	Hyperthermia: Thermal dose goals or reported data	End Points: Control arm (RT)	End Points: Treatment arm (RT + HT)	Significance ($P < .05$)	Effect of Heating Quality
Van der Zee[207]	Pelvic	Multicenter	358	176	182					1/wk up to 5 treatments	Target = 60 min after any point in tumor is 42°C	CR 39% at 3 mo	CR 55% at 3 mo	Yes	41% of patients received fewer than 5 HT treatments because of refusal
										1-4 h post-RT	Average total HT duration = 90 min	OS 24% at 3 y	OS 30% at 3 y	Yes	
	Rectal		143	71	72	46-50	1.8-2.3 Gy + 10-24 Gy boost		42 d (29-81)			LC 26% at 3 y CR 15% at 3 mo OS 22% at 3 y LC 8% at 3 y	LC 38% at 3 y CR 21% at 3 mo OS 13% at 3 y LC 16% at 3 y	Yes No No NR	
	Bladder		101	49	52	66-70	2 Gy		48 d (21-127)			CR 51% at 3 mo OS 22% at 3 y LC 33% at 3 y	CR 73% at 3 mo OS 28% at 3 y LC 42% at 3 y	Yes No No	
	Cervical		114	56	58	46-50	1.8-2.0 Gy + brachytherapy boost	23-28	48 d (35-121)			CR 57% at 3 mo OS 27% at 3 y LC 41% at 3 y	CR 83% at 3 mo OS 51% at 3 y LC 61% at 3 y	Yes Yes Yes	
Sneed[190]	Glioblastoma (after RT)	Single institution	68	33	35	59.4	1.8 Gy	33	32 d	2 Fx (pre/ post-BT)	Median (range) CEM43°$_{90}$: 14.1 (0-771)	TTP median 33 wk	TTP median 49 wk	Yes	8 Patients had only 1 HT treatment
						60	0.4-0.6 Gy/h ^{125}I		100 h		Median (range) CEM43° T_{50}: 74.6 (0.1-4652)	TTLTP 35 wk	TTLTP 57 wk	Yes	
												OS 15% at 2 y Median survival 76 wk	OS 31% at 2 y Median survival 85 wk	Yes	No thermal-dose relationship found
Emami[175]	Various	Multicenter	173	87	86	Prior dose + study dose <100 Gy	10 Gy ± 10%/d (0.4-0.5 Gy/h)		1 d	1 or 2 (pre- ± post-RT)	Goal: T_{min} 43°C for 60 min	CR 54%	CR 57%	No	Only 1 patient met criteria for "adequate HT treatment"
												PR 24%	PR 14%	No	T_{90} <40.5°C versus T_{90} >40.5°C; CR 53% versus 68%, respectively
	Head and neck		75	35	40							LC 37% at 2 y OS 29% at 2 y CR 52% PR 37%	LC 43% at 2 y OS 36% at 2 y CR 62% PR 10%	No NR No No	
	Pelvis		75	37	38							CR 57% PR 8%	CR 60% PR 10%	No No	
Vernon[186]	Breast	Multicenter	306	135	171	29-50 Gy ± boost	1.8-4 Gy	Varied	2-5 wk	1 to 8	Goal: T >42.5°C every 30 min	CR 41% Actuarial survival 40% at 2 y	CR 59% Actuarial survival 40% at 2 y	Yes No	

Overgaard[63]	Melanoma	Multicenter	68	65	63	24-27	8 or 9 Gy	3	8 d	3	Goal: 43°C for 60 min	CR 35% at 3 mo	CR 62% at 3 mo	Yes	62% Had T_{max} >60 CEM43°C
				Patients had more than one tumor								LC 28% at 5 y	LC 46% at 5 y	Yes	9% Reached T_{min} target >60 CEM43°C
												RR (RT + HT versus RT alone): CR = 4.01; 2-y local control = 1.73			Local control at 5 y:
															When average T_{max} >76 CEM 43°C (n = 27) 54% When average T_{max} >1-76 CEM 43°C (n = 27) 36%
Sugimachi[166]	Esophagus	Single institution	66	34*	32*	30	2 Gy	13	3 wk	6	42.5°-44.0°C every 30 min	Downstaging effect of neoadjuvant therapy			
						*Patients also received chemotherapy								NR NR	
												Effective in 44%	Effective in 69%	Yes	
												OS 24% at 3 y	OS 50% at 3 y	NR	
Valdagni[188]	Head and neck	Single institution	41	23	21	64-70	2.0-2.5 Gy	NR	30 d	2 versus 6 Fx	Goal: T_{min} + 42.5°C every 30 min	CR 37% at 3 mo	CR 82% at 3 mo	Yes	CR 86% versus 80% for 2 versus 6 HT doses; no correlation for CR versus thermal parameters
				Multiple nodes in some											
Valdagni[189]	5-y follow-up on above patients			21/22 nodes	16/18 nodes	" "	" "	" "	" "	" "	" "	Actuarial probability of control 24% at 5 y	Actuarial probability of control 69% at 5 y	Yes	
												OS 0% at 5 y	OS 53% at 5 y	Yes	
Perez[176]	Head and neck	Multicenter	218	107	111	32 Gy	4 Gy	8	4 wk	8	Goal: 42.5°C for 60 min 2×/wk; "Good" HT = 45 min at 42.5°C × 4 Fx	CR 28%	CR 32%	No group	52% Patients in RT + HT received full Rx; few received "good HT"
Perez[177]	Final report on trial		236	117	119	" "	" "	" "	" "	" "	" "	Overall CR 30%; CR for lesions <3 cm, 25%	Overall CR 32%; CR for lesions <3 cm, 52%	No overall and in subgroup	" "
Datta[187]	Head and neck	Single institution	65	32	33	50 Gy + boost	2.0 Gy/d	25	5 wk	BIW	Goal: 20 min at 42.5°C	CR 31% at 8 wk	CR 55% at 8 wk	Yes	NR
												DFS difference		No overall Yes, in stage III/IV	

RT, radiation therapy; HT, hyperthermia; Rx, treatment; Fx, fraction; BT, brachytherapy; CR, complete response; DFS, disease-free survival; PR, partial response; OS, overall survival; LC, local control; TTP, time to progression; TTLTP, time to local tumor progression.

institutions but are well documented, as is information concerning temperature distributions and thermal dosimetry.[143] Overall, the five trials demonstrated a significant improvement in the CR rate for patients receiving HT plus RT (59%) compared with RT alone (41%), with an odds ratio of 2.3 (95% confidence interval, 1.4 to 3.8). The greatest effect was observed in patients with recurrent lesions in previously irradiated areas where further irradiation was of necessity limited to low doses. No survival advantage was seen.

Other Superficial Malignancies

A study was conducted by the RTOG in the 1980s comparing RT alone with RT plus HT in superficial measurable tumors (RTOG 8104).[176,177] Three hundred seven patients were included in the study; approximately half of the patients had head and neck tumors, one third had breast carcinoma (chest wall recurrences), and the remaining had a variety of superficial malignancies. Patients treated with RT plus HT had a CR rate of 32% compared with 30% for those receiving RT alone. Subgroup analysis revealed significant improvements in duration of local control only in patients with tumors less than 3 cm and in those with breast or chest wall recurrences. It was postulated that the better outcome in smaller tumors was a consequence of better heating. This trial was plagued by highly variable heating techniques and crude thermal dosimetry. These problems led to the development of subsequent RTOG guidelines for performing HT.[133]

Head and Neck Cancer

There are two randomized series demonstrating an advantage to HT combined with RT. The first study randomized 65 patients to radiation alone versus RT and HT.[187] RT doses consisted of 50 Gy in 5 weeks to the primary site and regional lymphatics followed by 10 to 15 Gy given to sites of gross disease in daily fractions of 2 Gy. HT was given twice a week with 72 hours between each session. The HT-plus-RT arm showed significant improvement in response in patients with stage III or IV disease. For example, patients with stage III disease receiving combined treatment had a 58% CR compared with 20% in the RT-alone group. There was no benefit for patients with stage I or II disease, with greater than 90% of these patients achieving a CR with either treatment. This trial from India evaluated both the primary site and neck nodes, despite the recognized difficulties of effectively delivering heat to most primary head and neck tumors.

A second trial from Italy restricted treatment and evaluation to metastatic cervical lymph nodes. This study randomized 41 patients with advanced local regional squamous cell carcinoma of the head and neck to treatment with either RT alone or RT combined with HT.[188,189] Long-term follow-up allowed for analysis of response, duration of local control, and survival. The 5-year actuarial probability of local control in the neck was 24% in the RT-alone group versus 69% in the combined arm. Five-year survival was 0% in the RT-alone patients versus 53% in the RT-plus-HT group. All of these differences were statistically significant. There was no clear enhancement of toxicity or any clear relationship between thermal dose received and outcome. Nonetheless, this well-executed and described phase III trial, despite the relatively small number of patients, is an important component of the evidence suggesting the value of HT.

A trial of interstitial HT was carried out primarily in head and neck patients by the RTOG.[175] This trial entered 173 patients with persistent or recurrent tumors after prior RT and/or surgery that were amenable to interstitial RT. The lesion site was the head and neck in approximately 45% of patients, the pelvis in approximately 40%, and miscellaneous sites accounting for the rest. The patients were randomized to receive interstitial RT alone with or without interstitial HT. Overall, there was no difference in CR rates or 2-year survival. There were major quality assurance issues with this trial. Only one patient in the entire group was considered to have had adequate HT. This trial, as well as the previously mentioned RTOG trial, provided impetus for the subsequent development of HT guidelines by the RTOG.[137]

Esophagus Cancer

Two randomized studies demonstrated an advantage to the addition of HT to chemoradiotherapy or chemotherapy alone in the neoadjuvant treatment of esophagus cancer. In the first study, 53 patients with squamous cell carcinoma of the thoracic esophagus were randomized to preoperative HT, RT, and CT, compared with chemoradiotherapy alone.[169] The chemotherapy (bleomycin) and HT were given concurrently 1 hour prior to the radiation in a 3-week regimen with a total RT dose of approximately 32 Gy. Clinical CRs and pathologic responses were significantly improved in the trimodality arm, with a pCR of 26% combined in the trimodality group versus 8% in the chemoradiotherapy group.

In a follow-up study, an additional 40 patients were treated with chemotherapy alone (bleomycin and cisplatin) or combined with HT.[166] No RT was given in this trial. Again, an improvement in histopathologic response was noted favoring the HT group (19% versus 41%).

Malignant Melanoma

A major multicenter trial was conducted in patients with metastatic melanoma. Seventy patients with 134 metastatic or recurrent malignant melanoma lesions were randomized to receive RT with or without HT. Overall, there was a significant benefit for the addition of HT with a 2-year local control of 46% in the combined group compared with 28% for those receiving RT alone. Quality assurance issues were problematic in this trial, with only 14% of treatments achieving the protocol objective of 43°C for 60 minutes. Despite this, positive benefits were seen.[63]

Glioblastoma Multiforme

A University of California in San Francisco study evaluated interstitial HT combined with a brachytherapy boost for selected patients with glioblastoma multiforme. One hundred twelve patients were entered into this trial, which randomized patients whose tumor was implantable following external beam RT and chemotherapy to receive brachytherapy with or without HT. Seventy-nine were randomized; 33 patients were dropped from the protocol due to disease progression. Both time to tumor progression and survival were significantly improved for the HT patients compared with those treated with brachytherapy alone. Two-year survival in the two groups was 31% and 15%, respectively. Toxicity appeared to be slightly greater in the HT patients, with seven grade 3 toxicities reported compared with one in the brachytherapy alone group. Thermal dose data showed that good heating was achieved in most patients. No good correlation was seen between thermal dose and response.[190]

Pelvic Tumors (Cervix, Bladder, Colorectum)

A Dutch study randomized 361 patients with previously untreated locally advanced pelvic tumors to receive RT alone or RT plus HT. HT treatments were given once weekly for a total of five treatments.[207] Generally, thermal goals were not achieved. Detailed thermal dose analyses have not been published.

There were approximately equal numbers of patients with bladder, colorectal, and cervical carcinomas. CR rates were 39% and 55% after RT alone and RT plus HT, respectively ($P \leq .001$). Duration of local control was also significantly improved with RT plus HT. Patients with cervical carcinoma benefited the most. Three-year survivals were 27% and 51% in the RT and RT-plus-HT groups, respectively ($P = .003$).

This study has been criticized for suboptimal therapy in the control arm, namely RT alone as opposed to the combination of RT plus CT. At the time the trial was initiated in 1990, the role of chemotherapy in cervix carcinoma was not established. Subsequently, a number of studies published in 1999/2000 have demonstrated a survival advantage for concurrent cisplatin-based chemotherapy in cervical carcinoma.[191-195] Two follow-up phase III trials are now being conducted. The United States–led trial tests best conventional therapy with and without HT. The Dutch trial considers RT plus HT to be best conventional therapy and therefore is testing RT plus HT with or without chemotherapy.

Summary of Clinical Trials

Results of the published phase III trials above are intriguing. Apart from the RTOG trials, they all appear to demonstrate substantial benefits with the addition of HT to RT. All of the trials were associated with significant design and implementation problems, including relatively small numbers of patients, thermal dosimetry information that was highly variable in nature, thermal goals that were often not achieved, and control arms that may not have represented optimal standard therapy. Despite these difficulties, the positive clinical outcome of these trials and the sound scientific rationale for adjuvant HT justify continued efforts in technologic refinements and the conduct of well-designed clinical trials.

CHALLENGES, CONTROVERSIES, AND FUTURE POSSIBILITIES

There are significant challenges to the continued development of HT. These can be roughly categorized into three types: (1) technology developments in application of RT, (2) widespread establishment of chemoradiation for many locally advanced cancers and (3) emphasis for development of targeted therapies, such as tyrosine kinase inhibitors and antiangiogenic drugs, which show promise for selective targeting of tumors while greatly minimizing normal tissue toxicities. It is important to consider how HT can fit into this rapidly changing landscape of oncology research and practice, and this is discussed next.

Technical Challenges

The use of HT for deep-seated tumors is still experimental. As such, a dedicated team involving highly skilled physicists, engineers, physicians, and nurses is needed to perform it safely and accurately. Invasive thermometry requires dedicated physician time to place thermometry catheters, and imaging is needed to document thermometry placement. Control of applied power requires significant technical skill and experience. These issues place important constraints on the promulgation of HT to the broader medical community and will continue to impede progress until the technology is made more user-friendly.

Noninvasive Thermometry

The development of noninvasive thermometry is of paramount importance in breaking this cycle. If noninvasive thermometry can be proved to be safe and accurate, then sophisticated power control algorithms can be developed to control temperatures in real time and in full three-dimensional space (Fig. 20-10). This will reduce the size of the team needed

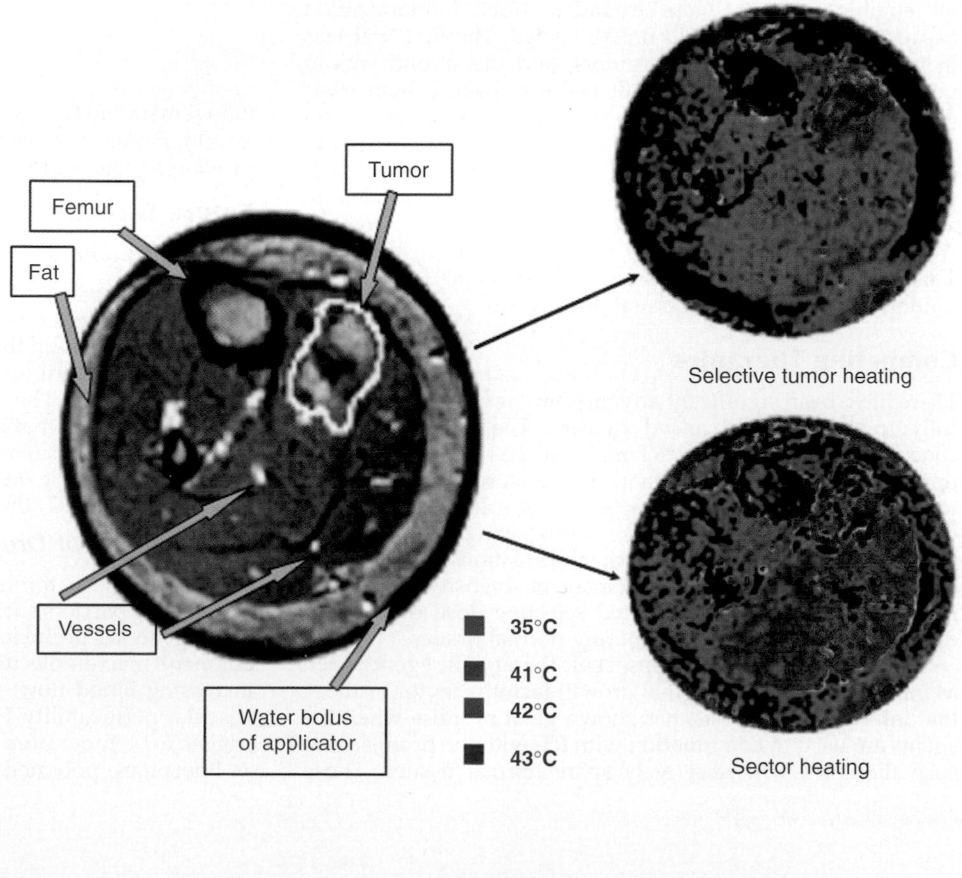

Figure 20-10 Example of noninvasive thermometry data acquired from a patient with a lower extremity soft tissue sarcoma. The patient was placed inside a 1.5-T magnetic resonance (MR) imager, and hyperthermia was administered using an MRI-compatible radiofrequency phased array designed for the lower extremity. MR thermal data were obtained during the heating procedure. The measurement was made using phase-difference (i.e., chemical shift) magnetic resonance imaging. The temperature coefficient of this measurement is approximately 0.01 ppm/1°C. The method in human patients has yielded a temperature resolution of 1.0°C, as calibrated against invasive measurements. *Left panel,* T2-weighted image acquired before treatment started. The tumor location is outlined *(white). Upper right panel,* Antenna settings provided selective heating of the tumor region. *Lower right panel,* Antenna settings heated the entire right side of the calf region. (Data from Carter DL, MacFall JR, Clegg ST, et al: Magnetic resonance thermometry during hyperthermia for human high-grade sarcoma. Int J Radiat Oncol Biol Phys 40:815-822, 1998.)

to safely operate the equipment and eliminate the need for extensive invasive thermometry. While still in its infancy, progress is being made toward the realization of accurate noninvasive thermometry. The lead technology is MRI. MRI methods have been used rather extensively to monitor temperature and tissue changes during thermal ablation,[196,197] and two centers are now testing this technology with MR compatible RF phased arrays for HT treatment (Duke University Medical Center and Charité Hospital in Berlin, Germany).[198,153] Importantly, the German group has established the feasibility of using data derived from noninvasive thermometry to predict treatment outcome from thermochemoradiotherapy treatment.[198]

Thermal Dose Prescription

Even if noninvasive thermometry were available, until recently there has been no information on what target temperature ranges are needed to optimize this therapy. Such information is the second key for providing a quantitative assessment of HT treatment adequacy (i.e., establishes a method for writing a HT prescription). Despite extensive phase II data suggesting that higher temperatures yield improved likelihood for effective therapy, there have not been any successful prospective trials showing that escalation of thermal dose yields improved antitumor effect. This has proved to be a significant roadblock to development of a thermal prescription. However, two clinical trials have been reported where thermal dose was controlled during application of HT. These trials have set the stage for establishing realistic goals for how to administer this treatment.

These two trials were designed to perform a "test" HT treatment first, to determine whether the tumor was heatable, as defined by preestablished criteria. If the tumor was "heatable," then the patient was randomized to receive either a low cumulative thermal dose or a high thermal dose that was at least 10-fold higher than the low-dose group. The inclusion of the "test" treatment was key in both studies, as about 12% of all eligible patients were excluded from randomization because their tumors could not be heated. The first trial was in patients with superficial tumors, and the second was in pet dogs with spontaneous soft tissue sarcomas. Both trials demonstrated that cumulative thermal doses greater than 10CEM 43°CT$_{90}$ yielded improved tumor responses and durations of local control[184,185] (Fig. 20-11). To put this into perspective, this cumulative thermal dose is equivalent to achieving a temperature of 40°C for 1 hour, once or twice a week, at the 10th percentile of the temperature distribution. This thermal goal was reached in more than 90% of patients randomized to the high thermal dose group.

Competing Therapies

There have been significant advances in the ability to successfully treat locally advanced cancers. The development of concurrent chemotherapy/RT regimens has made significant improvements in diseases that were historically considered to be refractory to RT. Examples include locally advanced cancers of the head and neck, cervix, and colon.[191,192,199,200] Coupled with the advent of chemoradiation has been the rapid development and deployment of intensity-modulated RT, which has greatly facilitated selective dose delivery to desired target tissues, while sparing normal tissues.

The development of target-specific therapeutic agents, such as inhibitors of the epidermal growth factor receptor or those that inhibit angiogenesis, has shown great promise when the agents are used in combination with RT, with the promise that such therapies will selectively spare normal tissues. Those who remain in HT research need to remain cognizant of these developments and determine where this technology can provide added value.

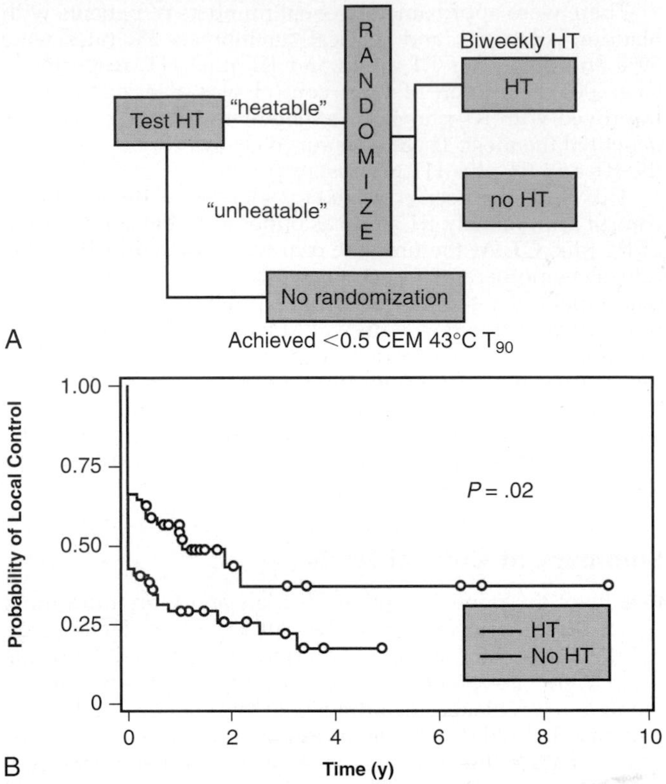

Figure 20-11 **A,** Clinical trial design. **B,** Duration of local control in patients with superficial tumors treated with a low or high cumulative thermal dose combined with radiation therapy. The difference in the complete response rate was significant, as was the duration of local control after administration of a higher cumulative thermal dose. CEM 43°C, cumulative equivalent minutes at 43°C; HT, hyperthermia; T$_{90}$, interval of heating. (From Jones E, Oleson JR, Dewhirst MW, et al: A randomized trial of hyperthermia and radiation for superficial tumors. J Clin Oncol 23:3079-3085, 2005.)

Future Directions

Trimodality Therapies

There are important observations that have been made about HT that provide strong rationale for its continued development. First, although the addition of chemotherapy to RT has improved treatment outcome for many diseases, there is still a long way to go. The addition of HT to chemoradiotherapy protocols may be what is needed to push the therapies further toward the goal of reaching 100% local control. Because HT provides synergistic interaction with many chemotherapeutic drugs as well as RT, this general approach is compelling.

Augmentation of Drug Delivery

Drug delivery to tumors remains a major challenge due to physiologic barriers such as high interstitial fluid pressure and heterogeneous perfusion. As noted, HT has been shown to augment macromolecule and nanoparticle drug delivery by increasing blood flow, available volume fraction, and tumor vascular permeability. Furthermore, local HT can be used as a trigger for temperature-sensitive drug delivery systems such as liposomes, polymers, and hydrogels.[201-206] In this manner, site-specific bioavailability can be achieved. For example, a temperature-sensitive liposome containing doxorubicin (ThermoDox) has been developed to release rapidly at clinically achievable temperatures of 40° to 42°C. This formulation has shown dramatic improvement in tumor drug concentration and antitumor efficacy in preclinical studies and is being investigated in phase I clinical trials for advanced prostate cancer and RF ablation of liver metastases.[205,206] As thermal technology and liposomal formulations advance, this method has the potential for precise control of drug delivery independent of tumor phenotype and drug composition.

ACKNOWLEDGMENTS

This work supported by grant CA42745 from the National Institutes of Health/National Cancer Institute.

REFERENCES

1. Arrhenius S: Uber die reaktionsgeschwindigkeit bei der inversion von rohrzucker durch Sauren. Zeitschr Physik Chem 4:226, 1889.
2. Sapareto SA, Dewey WC: Thermal dose determination in cancer therapy. Int J Radiat Oncol Biol Phys 10:787, 1984.
3. Dewhirst MW, Viglianti BL, Lora-Michiels M, et al: Basic principles of thermal dosimetry and thermal thresholds for tissue damage from hyperthermia. Int J Hyperthermia 19:267, 2003.
4. Dewhirst MW: Thermal dosimetry. *In* Seegenschmiedt M, Fessenden P, Vernon CC (eds): Thermoradiotherapy and Thermochemotherapy. Berlin, Springer Verlag, 1995, p 123.
5. Morimoto RI, Kroeger PE, Cotto JJ: The transcriptional regulation of heat shock genes: a plethora of heat shock factors and regulatory conditions. EXS 77:139, 1996.
6. Raaphorst G: Fundamental aspects of hyperthermic biology. *In* Field S, Hand J (eds): An Introduction to the Practical Aspects of Clinical Hyperthermia. London, Taylor and Francis, 1990, p 10.
7. Coss RA, Linnemans WA: The effects of hyperthermia on the cytoskeleton: a review. Int J Hyperthermia 12:173, 1996.
8. Pratt WB, Silverstein AM, Galigniana MD: A model for the cytoplasmic trafficking of signalling proteins involving the hsp90-binding immunophilins and p50cdc37. Cell Signal 11:839, 1999.
9. Liang P, MacRae TH: Molecular chaperones and the cytoskeleton. J Cell Sci 110:1431, 1997.
10. Streffer C: Metabolic changes during and after hyperthermia. Int J Hyperthermia 1:305, 1985.
11. Vidair CA, Doxsey SJ, Dewey WC: Heat shock alters centrosome organization leading to mitotic dysfunction and cell death. J Cell Physiol 154:443, 1993.
12. Kampinga HH, Dikomey E: Hyperthermic radiosensitization: mode of action and clinical relevance. Int J Radiat Biol 77:399, 2001.
13. Dewhirst MW, Sim D, Gross J, et al: Effects of heating rate on normal and tumor microcirculatory function. *In* Heat and Mass Transfer in the Microcirculation of Thermally Significant Vessels. Anaheim, CA, 1986, ASME.
14. Song CW: Effect of local hyperthermia on blood flow and microenvironment: a review. Cancer Res 44:4721s, 1984.
15. Reinhold HS: Physiological effects of hyperthermia. Rec Results Cancer Res 107:32, 1988.
16. Kong G, Braun RD, Dewhirst MW: Hyperthermia enables tumor-specific nanoparticle delivery: effect of particle size. Cancer Res 60:4440, 2000.
17. Kong G, Braun RD, Dewhirst MW: Characterization of the effect of hyperthermia on nanoparticle extravasation from tumor vasculature. Cancer Res 61:3027, 2001.
18. Matteucci ML, Anyarambhatla G, Rosner G, et al: Hyperthermia increases accumulation of technetium-99m-labeled liposomes in feline sarcomas. Clin Cancer Res 6:3748, 2000.
19. Krol A, Dewhirst MW, Yuan F: Effects of cell damage and glycosaminoglycan degradation on available extravascular space of different dextrans in a rat fibrosarcoma. Int J Hyperthermia 19:154, 2003.
20. Kong G, Dewhirst MW: Hyperthermia and liposomes. Int J Hyperthermia 15:345, 1999.
21. Kouloulias VE, Dardoufas CE, Kouvaris JR, et al: Liposomal doxorubicin in conjunction with reirradiation and local hyperthermia treatment in recurrent breast cancer: a phase I/II trial. Clin Cancer Res 8:374, 2002.
22. Dahl O: Interaction of heat and drugs in vitro and in vivo. *In* Seegenschmiedt M, Fessenden P, Vernon C (eds): Thermoradiotherapy and Thermochemotherapy. Berlin, Springer Verlag, 1995, p 103.
23. Curry FE: Determinants of capillary permeability: a review of mechanisms based on single capillary studies in the frog. Circ Res 59:367, 1986.
24. Hauck M, Zalutsky M, Dewhirst MW: Enhancement of radiolabeled monoclonal antibody uptake in tumors with local hyperthermia. *In* Torchilin V (ed): Targeted Delivery of Imaging Agents. Boca Raton, CRC Press, 1995, p 335.
25. Meyer DE, Kong GA, Dewhirst MW, et al: Targeting a genetically engineered elastin-like polypeptide to solid tumors by local hyperthermia. Cancer Res 61:1548, 2001.
26. Kelleher DK, Engel T, Vaupel PW: Changes in microregional perfusion, oxygenation, ATP and lactate distribution in subcutaneous rat tumours upon water-filtered IR-A hyperthermia. Int J Hyperthermia 11:241, 1995.
27. Prescott DM, Charles HC, Sostman HD, et al: Therapy monitoring in human and canine soft tissue sarcomas using magnetic resonance imaging and spectroscopy. Int J Radiat Oncol Biol Phys 28:415, 1994.
28. Oleson JR: Eugene Robertson Special Lecture. Hyperthermia from the clinic to the laboratory: a hypothesis. Int J Hyperthermia 11:315, 1995.
29. Song CW, Park H, Griffin RJ: Improvement of tumor oxygenation by mild hyperthermia. Radiat Res 155:515, 2001.
30. Vujaskovic Z, Poulson J, Gaskin A, et al: Temperature dependent changes in physiologic parameters of spontaneous canine soft tissue sarcomas after combined radiotherapy and hyperthermia. Int J Radiat Oncol Biol Phys 46:179, 2000.
31. Brizel DM, Scully SP, Harrelson JM, et al: Radiation therapy and hyperthermia improve the oxygenation of human soft tissue sarcomas. Cancer Res 56:5347, 1996.
32. Jones EL, Prosnitz LR, Dewhirst MW, et al: Thermochemoradiotherapy improves oxygenation in locally advanced breast cancer. Clin Cancer Res 10:4287, 2004.
33. Wahl ML, Bobyock SB, Leeper DB, et al: Effects of 42 degrees C hyperthermia on intracellular pH in ovarian carcinoma cells during acute or chronic exposure to low extracellular pH. Int J Radiat Oncol Biol Phys 39:205, 1997.
34. Coss RA, Storck CW, Wachsberger PR, et al: Acute extracellular acidification reduces intracellular pH, 42 degrees C-induction of heat shock proteins and clonal survival of human melanoma cells grown at pH 6.7. Int J Hyperthermia 20:93, 2004.
35. Crabtree H: Observations on the carbohydrate metabolism of tumours. Biochem J 23:536, 1929.
36. Newsholme E, Crabtree B, Ardawi M: The role of high rates of glycolysis and glutamine utilization in rapidly dividing cells. Biosci Rep 5:393, 1985.
37. Leeper DB, Engin K, Thistlethwaite AJ, et al: Human tumor extracellular pH as a function of blood glucose concentration. Int J Radiat Oncol Biol Phys 28:935, 1994.
38. Prescott DM, Charles HC, Sostman HD, et al: Manipulation of intra- and extracellular pH in spontaneous canine tumours by use of hyperglycaemia. Int J Hyperthermia 9:745, 1993.
39. Biaglow JE, Manevich Y, Leeper D, et al: MIBG inhibits respiration: potential for radio- and hyperthermic sensitization. Int J Radiat Oncol Biol Phys 42:871, 1998.
40. Zhou R, Bansal N, Leeper DB, et al: Intracellular acidification of human melanoma xenografts by the respiratory inhibitor m-iodobenzylguanidine plus hyperglycemia: a 31P magnetic resonance spectroscopy study. Cancer Res 60:3532, 2000.

41. Wachsberger PR, Burd R, Bhala A, et al: Quercetin sensitizes cells in a tumour-like low pH environment to hyperthermia. Int J Hyperthermia 19:507, 2003.
42. Asea A, Ara G, Teicher BA, et al: Effects of the flavonoid drug quercetin on the response of human prostate tumours to hyperthermia in vitro and in vivo. Int J Hyperthermia 17:347, 2001.
43. Jones EA, Zhao M, Stevenson MA, et al: The 70 kilodalton heat shock protein is an inhibitor of apoptosis in prostate cancer. Int J Hyperthermia 2005.
44. Song CW, Kim GE, Lyons JC, et al: Thermosensitization by increasing intracellular acidity with amiloride and its analogs. Int J Radiat Oncol Biol Phys 30:1161, 1994.
45. Sevick EM, Jain RK: Geometric resistance to blood flow in solid tumors perfused ex vivo: effects of tumor size and perfusion pressure. Cancer Res 49:3506, 1989.
46. Sevick EM, Jain RK: Viscous resistance to blood flow in solid tumors: effect of hematocrit on intratumor blood viscosity. Cancer Res 49:3513, 1989.
47. Jirtle RL: Chemical modification of tumour blood flow. Int J Hyperthermia 4:355, 1988.
48. Dewhirst MW, Prescott DM, Clegg S, et al: The use of hydralazine to manipulate tumour temperatures during hyperthermia. Int J Hyperthermia 6:971, 1990.
49. Poulson J, Vujaskovic Z, Gaskin A, et al: Effect of calcitonin gene related peptide to increase tissue temperature in spontaneous canine tumors during local hyperthermia. Int J Hyperthermia 20:477, 2004.
50. Tozer GM, Shaffi KM, Prise VE, et al: Spatial heterogeneity of tumour blood flow modification induced by angiotensin II: relationship to receptor distribution. Int J Cancer 65:658, 1996.
51. Bell KM, Prise VE, Shaffi KM, et al: A comparative study of tumour blood flow modification in two rat tumour systems using endothelin-1 and angiotensin II: influence of tumour size on angiotensin II response. Int J Cancer 67:730, 1996.
52. Meyer RE, Shan S, DeAngelo J, et al: Nitric oxide synthase inhibition irreversibly decreases perfusion in the R3230Ac rat mammary adenocarcinoma. Br J Cancer 71:1169, 1995.
53. Fukumura D, Yuan F, Endo M, et al: Role of nitric oxide in tumor microcirculation. Blood flow, vascular permeability, and leukocyte-endothelial interactions. Am J Pathol 150:713, 1997.
54. Hahn JS, Braun RD, Dewhirst MW, et al: Stroma-free human hemoglobin A decreases R3230Ac rat mammary adenocarcinoma blood flow and oxygen partial pressure. Radiat Res 147:185, 1997.
55. Poulson JM, Dewhirst MW, Gaskin AA, et al: Acute pancreatitis associated with administration of a nitric oxide synthase inhibitor in tumor-bearing dogs. In Vivo 14:709, 2000.
56. Schoonover LL, Stewart AS, Clifton GD: Hemodynamic and cardiovascular effects of nitric oxide modulation in the therapy of septic shock. Pharmacotherapy 20:1184, 2000.
57. Nathanson SD, Cerra RF, Hetzel FW, et al: Changes associated with metastasis in B16-F1 melanoma cells surviving heat. Arch Surg 125:216, 1990.
58. Nathanson SD, Nelson L, Anaya P, et al: Development of lymph node and pulmonary metastases after local irradiation and hyperthermia of footpad melanomas. Clin Exp Metastasis 9:377, 1991.
59. Ando K, Urano M, Kenton L, et al: Effect of thermochemotherapy on the development of spontaneous lung metastases. Int J Hyperthermia 3:453, 1987.
60. Bataille N, Vallancien G, Chopin D: Antitumoral local effect and metastatic risk of focused extracorporeal pyrotherapy on Dunning R-3327 tumors. Eur Urol 29:72, 1996.
61. Dewhirst MW, Sim DA, Forsyth K, et al: Local control and distant metastases in primary canine malignant melanomas treated with hyperthermia and/or radiotherapy. Int J Hyperthermia 1:219, 1985.
62. Overgaard J, Gonzalez D, Hulshof MC, et al: Hyperthermia as an adjuvant to radiation therapy of recurrent or metastatic malignant melanoma. A multicentre randomized trial by the European Society for Hyperthermic Oncology. Int J Hyperthermia 12:3, 1996.
63. Overgaard J, Gonzalez D, Hulshof MC, et al: Randomised trial of hyperthermia as adjuvant to radiotherapy for recurrent or metastatic malignant melanoma. European Society for Hyperthermic Oncology. Lancet 345:540, 1995.
64. Gillette SM, Dewhirst MW, Gillette EL, et al: Response of canine soft tissue sarcomas to radiation or radiation plus hyperthermia: a randomized phase II study. Int J Hyperthermia 8:309, 1992.
65. Maguire PD, Samulski TV, Prosnitz LR, et al: A phase II trial testing the thermal dose parameter CEM43 degrees T90 as a predictor of response in soft tissue sarcomas treated with preoperative thermoradiotherapy. Int J Hyperthermia 17:283, 2001.
66. Pisters WT, O'Sullivan BO, Demetri GD: Sarcomas of nonosseous tissues. *In* Bast RC, et al (eds): Cancer Medicine. Hamilton, Ontario, Canada, BC Decker, 2000, p 1906.
67. Urano M, Rice L, Epstein R, et al: Effect of whole-body hyperthermia on cell survival, metastasis frequency, and host immunity in moderately and weakly immunogenic murine tumors. Cancer Res 43:1039, 1983.
68. Oda M, Koga S, Maeta M: Mechanism of metastatic spread by 42 degrees C total-body hyperthermia in Lewis lung carcinoma. Cancer Res 46:1102, 1986.
69. Matsuda H, Strebel FR, Kaneko T, et al: Long duration-mild whole body hyperthermia of up to 12 hours in rats: feasibility, and efficacy on primary tumour and axillary lymph node metastases of a mammary adenocarcinoma: implications for adjuvant therapy. Int J Hyperthermia 13:89, 1997.
70. Hegewisch-Becker S, Braun K, Otte M, et al: Effects of whole body hyperthermia (41.8 degrees C) on the frequency of tumor cells in the peripheral blood of patients with advanced malignancies. Clin Cancer Res 9:2079, 2003.
71. Thrall DE, Prescott DM, Samulski TV, et al: Radiation plus local hyperthermia versus radiation plus the combination of local and whole-body hyperthermia in canine sarcomas. Int J Radiat Oncol Biol Phys 34:1087, 1996.
72. Lord PF, Kapp DS, Morrow D: Increased skeletal metastases of spontaneous canine osteosarcoma after fractionated systemic hyperthermia and local X-irradiation. Cancer Res 41:4331, 1981.
73. Kapp DS, Lawrence R: Temperature elevation during brachytherapy for carcinoma of the uterine cervix: adverse effect on survival and enhancement of distant metastasis. Int J Radiat Oncol Biol Phys 10:2281, 1984.
74. Engin K, Leeper D, Thistlethwaite A, et al: Tumor extracellular pH as a prognostic factor in thermoradiotherapy. Int J Radiat Oncol Biol Phys 29:125, 1994.
75. Mivechi NF, Dewey WC: DNA polymerase alpha and beta activities during the cell cycle and their role in heat radiosensitization in Chinese hamster ovary cells. Radiat Res 103:337, 1985.
76. Raaphorst GP, Ng CE, Yang DP: Thermal radiosensitization and repair inhibition in human melanoma cells: a comparison of survival and DNA double strand breaks. Int J Hyperthermia 15:17, 1999.
77. Raaphorst GP, Yang DP, Ng CE: Effect of protracted mild hyperthermia on polymerase activity in a human melanoma cell line. Int J Hyperthermia 10:827, 1994.
78. Overgaard J: The current and potential role of hyperthermia in radiotherapy. Int J Radiat Oncol Biol Phys 16:535, 1989.
79. Dewhirst MW, Sim DA: The utility of thermal dose as a predictor of tumor and normal tissue responses to combined radiation and hyperthermia. Cancer Res 44:4772s, 1984.
80. Gillette EL, McChesney SL, Dewhirst MW, et al: Response of canine oral carcinomas to heat and radiation. Int J Radiat Oncol Biol Phys 13:1861, 1987.
81. Denman DL, Legorreta RA, Kier AB, et al: Therapeutic responses of spontaneous canine malignancies to combinations of radiotherapy and hyperthermia. Int J Radiat Oncol Biol Phys 21:415, 1991.
82. Kapp DS, Cox RS, Fessenden P, et al: Parameters predictive for complications of treatment with combined hyperthermia and radiation therapy. Int J Radiat Oncol Biol Phys 22:999, 1992.
83. Hettinga JV, Konings AW, Kampinga HH: Reduction of cellular cisplatin resistance by hyperthermia—a review. Int J Hyperthermia 13:439, 1997.
84. Laskowitz DT, Elion GB, Dewhirst MW, et al: Hyperthermia-induced enhancement of melphalan activity against a melphalan-resistant human rhabdomyosarcoma xenograft. Radiat Res 129:218, 1992.

85. Da Silva VF, Feeley M, Raaphorst GP: Hyperthermic potentiation of BCNU toxicity in BCNU-resistant human glioma cells. J Neurooncol 11:37, 1991.
86. Averill DA, Su C: Sensitization to the cytotoxicity of adriamycin by verapamil and heat in multidrug-resistant Chinese hamster ovary cells. Radiat Res 151:694, 1999.
87. Herman TS, Teicher BA, Varshney A, et al: Effect of hypoxia and acidosis on the cytotoxicity of mitoxantrone, bisantrene and amsacrine and their platinum complexes at normal and hyperthermic temperatures. Anticancer Res 12:827, 1992.
88. Teicher BA, Holden SA, Rudolph MB, et al: Effect of environmental conditions (pH, oxygenation and temperature) on the cytotoxicity of flavone acetic acid and its dimethylaminoethyl ester. Int J Hyperthermia 7:905, 1991.
89. Teicher BA, Herman TS, Holden SA, et al: Effect of oxygenation, pH and hyperthermia on RSU-1069 in vitro and in vivo with radiation in the FSaIIC murine fibrosarcoma. Cancer Lett 59:109, 1991.
90. Holden SA, Teicher BA, Herman TS: Effect of environmental conditions (pH, oxygenation, and temperature) on misonidazole cytotoxicity and radiosensitization in vitro and in vivo in FSaIIC fibrosarcoma. Int J Radiat Oncol Biol Phys 20:1031, 1991.
91. Teicher BA, Herman TS, Holden SA: Effect of pH, oxygenation, and temperature on the cytotoxicity and radiosensitization by etanidazole. Int J Radiat Oncol Biol Phys 20:723, 1991.
92. Urano M, Kuroda M, Nishimura Y: For the clinical application of thermochemotherapy given at mild temperatures. Int J Hyperthermia 15:79, 1999.
93. Katschinski DM, Robins HI: Hyperthermic modulation of SN-38-induced topoisomerase I DNA cross- linking and SN-38 cytotoxicity through altered topoisomerase I activity. Int J Cancer 80:104, 1999.
94. Ng CE, Bussey AM, Raaphorst GP: Sequence of treatment is important in the modification of camptothecin induced cell killing by hyperthermia. Int J Hyperthermia 12:663, 1996; discussion, 679.
95. Teicher BA, Holden SA, Khandakar V, et al: Addition of a topoisomerase I inhibitor to trimodality therapy [cis-diamminedichloroplatinum (II)/heat/radiation] in a murine tumor. J Cancer Res Clin Oncol 119:645, 1993.
96. Leal BZ, Meltz ML, Mohan N, et al: Interaction of hyperthermia with Taxol in human MCF-7 breast adenocarcinoma cells. Int J Hyperthermia 15:225, 1999.
97. Cividalli A, Cruciani G, Livdi E, et al: Hyperthermia enhances the response of paclitaxel and radiation in a mouse adenocarcinoma. Int J Radiat Oncol Biol Phys 44:407, 1999.
98. Vaden SL, Page RL, Williams PL, et al: Effect of hyperthermia on cisplatin and carboplastin disposition in the isolated, perfused tumour and skin flap. Int J Hyperthermia 10:563, 1994.
99. Kido Y, Kuwano H, Maehara Y, et al: Increased cytotoxicity of low-dose, long-duration exposure to 5-fluorouracil of V-79 cells with hyperthermia. Cancer Chemother Pharmacol 28:251, 1991.
100. Ito A, Matsuoka F, Honda H, et al: Heat shock protein 70 gene therapy combined with hyperthermia using magnetic nanoparticles. Cancer Gene Ther 10:918, 2003.
101. Guilhon E, Quesson B, Moraud-Gaudry F, et al: Image-guided control of transgene expression based on local hyperthermia. Mol Imaging 2:11, 2003.
102. Higuchi Y, Asaumi J, Murakami J, et al: Effects of p53 gene therapy in radiotherapy or thermotherapy of human head and neck squamous cell carcinoma cell lines. Oncol Rep 10:671, 2003.
103. Brade AM, Szmitko P, Ngo D, et al: Heat-directed suicide gene therapy for breast cancer. Cancer Gene Ther 10:294, 2003.
104. Xu M, Myerson RJ, Hunt C, et al: Transfection of human tumour cells with Mre11 siRNA and the increase in radiation sensitivity and the reduction in heat-induced radiosensitization. Int J Hyperthermia 20:157, 2004.
105. Xu L, Zhao Y, Zhang Q, et al: Regulation of transgene expression in muscles by ultrasound-mediated hyperthermia. Gene Ther 11:894, 2004.
106. Huang Q, Hu JK, Lohr F, et al: Heat-induced gene expression as a novel targeted cancer gene therapy strategy. Cancer Res 60:3435, 2000.
107. Lohr F, Hu K, Huang Q, et al: Enhancement of radiotherapy by hyperthermia-regulated gene therapy. Int J Radiat Oncol Biol Phys 48:1513, 2000.
108. Lohr F, Huang Q, Hu K, et al: Systemic vector leakage and transgene expression by intratumorally injected recombinant adenovirus vectors. Clin Cancer Res 7:3625, 2001.
109. Borrelli M, Schoenherr D, Wong A, et al: Heat-activated transgene expression from adenovirus vectors infected into human prostate cancer cells. Cancer Res 61:1113, 2001.
110. Brade AM, Ngo D, Szmitko P, et al: Heat-directed gene targeting of adenoviral vectors to tumor cells. Cancer Gene Ther 7:1566, 2000.
111. Braiden V, Ohtsuru A, Kawashita Y, et al: Eradication of breast cancer xenografts by hyperthermic suicide gene therapy under the control of the heat shock protein promoter. Hum Gene Ther 11:2453, 2000.
112. Gerner EW, Hersh EM, Pennington M, et al: Heat-inducible vectors for use in gene therapy. Int J Hyperthermia 16:171, 2000.
113. Blackburn RV, Galoforo SS, Corry PM, et al: Adenoviral-mediated transfer of a heat-inducible double suicide gene into prostate carcinoma cells. Cancer Res 58:1358, 1998.
114. Okamoto K, Shinoura N, Egawa N, et al: Adenovirus-mediated transfer of p53 augments hyperthermia-induced apoptosis in U251 glioma cells. Int J Radiat Oncol Biol Phys 50:525, 2001.
115. Qi V, Weinrib L, Ma N, et al: Adenoviral p53 gene therapy promotes heat-induced apoptosis in a nasopharyngeal carcinoma cell line. Int J Hyperthermia 17:38, 2001.
116. Ostberg JR, Kabingu E, Repasky EA: Thermal regulation of dendritic cell activation and migration from skin explants. Int J Hyperthermia 19:520, 2003.
117. Menoret A, Chaillot D, Callahan M, et al: Hsp70, an immunological actor playing with the intracellular self under oxidative stress. Int J Hyperthermia 18:490, 2002.
118. Manjili MH, Wang XY, Park J, et al: Cancer immunotherapy: stress proteins and hyperthermia. Int J Hyperthermia 18:506, 2002.
119. Multhoff G: Activation of natural killer cells by heat shock protein 70. Int J Hyperthermia 18:576, 2002.
120. Shah A, Unger E, Bain MD, et al: Cytokine and adhesion molecule expression in primary human endothelial cells stimulated with fever-range hyperthermia. Int J Hyperthermia 18:534, 2002.
121. Asea A, Kabingu E, Stevenson MA, et al: HSP70 peptide-bearing and peptide-negative preparations act as chaperokines. Cell Stress Chaperones 5:425, 2000.
122. Hand JW, James JR: Physical Techniques in Clinical Hyperthermia. New York, John Wiley and Sons, 1986.
123. Cossett JM: Interstitial, Endocavitary, and Perfusional Hyperthermia. Clinical Thermology. Berlin, Springer Verlag, 1990.
124. Dewhirst MW, Samulski TV: Hyperthermia in the Treatment of Cancer. Current Concepts. Kalamazoo, Upjohn, 1988, pp 3-49.
125. Rhee JG, Lee CK, Osborn J, et al: Precooling prevents overheating of subcutaneous fat in the use of RF capacitive heating. Int J Radiat Oncol Biol Phys 20:1009, 1991.
126. Maehara Y, Kuwano H, Kitamura K, et al: Hyperthermochemoradiotherapy for esophageal cancer (review). Anticancer Res 12:805, 1992.
127. Turner PF: Regional hyperthermia with an annular phased array. IEEE Trans Biomed Eng 31:106, 1984.
128. Moros EG, Straube WL, Klein EE, et al: Simultaneous delivery of electron beam therapy and ultrasound hyperthermia using scanning reflectors: a feasibility study. Int J Radiat Oncol Biol Phys 31:893, 1995.
129. Moros EG, Straube WL, Myerson RJ: Potential for power deposition conformability using reflected-scanned planar ultrasound. Int J Hyperthermia 12:723, 1996.
130. Underwood HR, Burdette EC, Ocheltree KB, et al: A multi-element ultrasonic hyperthermia applicator with independent element control. Int J Hyperthermia 3:257, 1987.
131. Edelstein-Keshet L, Dewhirst MW, Oleson JR, et al: Characterization of tumour temperature distributions in hyperthermia based on assumed mathematical forms. Int J Hyperthermia 5:757, 1989.

132. Dewhirst MW, Winget JM, Edelstein-Keshet L, et al: Clinical application of thermal isoeffect dose. Int J Hyperthermia 3:307, 1987.
133. Dewhirst MW, Phillips TL, Samulski TV, et al: RTOG quality assurance guidelines for clinical trials using hyperthermia. Int J Radiat Oncol Biol Phys 18:1249, 1990.
134. Tilly W, Wust P, Rau B, et al: Temperature data and specific absorption rates in pelvic tumours: predictive factors and correlations. Int J Hyperthermia 17:172, 2001.
135. Wust P, Gellermann J, Harder C, et al: Rationale for using invasive thermometry for regional hyperthermia of pelvic tumors. Int J Radiat Oncol Biol Phys 41:1129, 1998.
136. Waterman FM, Dewhirst MW, Fessenden P, et al: RTOG quality assurance guidelines for clinical trials using hyperthermia administered by ultrasound. Int J Radiat Oncol Biol Phys 20:1099, 1991.
137. Emami B, Stauffer P, Dewhirst MW, et al: RTOG quality assurance guidelines for interstitial hyperthermia. Int J Radiat Oncol Biol Phys 20:1117, 1991.
138. Sapozink MD, Corry PM, Kapp DS, et al: RTOG quality assurance guidelines for clinical trials using hyperthermia for deep-seated malignancy. Int J Radiat Oncol Biol Phys 20:1109, 1991.
139. Seegenschmiedt MH, Martus P, Fietkau R, et al: Multivariate analysis of prognostic parameters using interstitial thermoradiotherapy (IHT-IRT): tumor and treatment variables predict outcome. Int J Radiat Oncol Biol Phys 29:1049, 1994.
140. Oleson JR, Samulski TV, Leopold KA, et al: Sensitivity of hyperthermia trial outcomes to temperature and time: implications for thermal goals of treatment. Int J Radiat Oncol Biol Phys 25:289, 1993.
141. Kapp DS, Cox RS: Thermal treatment parameters are most predictive of outcome in patients with single tumor nodules per treatment field in recurrent adenocarcinoma of the breast. Int J Radiat Oncol Biol Phys 33:887, 1995.
142. Hand JW, Machin D, Vernon CC, et al: Analysis of thermal parameters obtained during phase III trials of hyperthermia as an adjunct to radiotherapy in the treatment of breast carcinoma. Int J Hyperthermia 13:343, 1997.
143. Sherar M, Liu FF, Pintilie M, et al: Relationship between thermal dose and outcome in thermoradiotherapy treatments for superficial recurrences of breast cancer: data from a phase III trial. Int J Radiat Oncol Biol Phys 39:371, 1997.
144. Clegg ST, Samulski TV, Murphy KA, et al: Inverse techniques in hyperthermia: a sensitivity study. IEEE Trans Biomed Eng 41:373, 1994.
145. Craciunescu OI, Raaymakers BW, Kotte AN, et al: Discretizing large traceable vessels and using DE-MRI perfusion maps yields numerical temperature contours that match the MR noninvasive measurements. Med Phys 28:2289, 2001.
146. Das SK, Jones EA, Samulski TV: A method of MRI-based thermal modelling for a RF phased array. Int J Hyperthermia 17:465, 2001.
147. DeFord JA, Babbs CF, Patel UH, et al: Accuracy and precision of computer-simulated tissue temperatures in individual human intracranial tumours treated with interstitial hyperthermia. Int J Hyperthermia 6:755, 1990.
148. Das SK, Clegg ST, Anscher MS, et al: Simulation of electromagnetically induced hyperthermia: a finite element gridding method. Int J Hyperthermia 11:797, 1995.
149. van der Koijk JF, Lagendijk JJ, Crezee J, et al: The influence of vasculature on temperature distributions in MECS interstitial hyperthermia: importance of longitudinal control. Int J Hyperthermia 13:365, 1997.
150. Wlodarczyk W, Hentschel M, Wust P, et al: Comparison of four magnetic resonance methods for mapping small temperature changes. Phys Med Biol 44:607, 1999.
151. MacFall J, Prescott DM, Fullar E, et al: Temperature dependence of canine brain tissue diffusion coefficient measured in vivo with magnetic resonance echo-planar imaging. Int J Hyperthermia 11:73, 1995.
152. Wust P, Nadobny J, Felix R, et al: Strategies for optimized application of annular-phased-array systems in clinical hyperthermia. Int J Hyperthermia 7:157, 1991.
153. Carter DL, MacFall JR, Clegg ST, et al: Magnetic resonance thermometry during hyperthermia for human high-grade sarcoma. Int J Radiat Oncol Biol Phys 40:815, 1998.
154. Sokka SD, Hynynen KH: The feasibility of MRI-guided whole prostate ablation with a linear aperiodic intracavitary ultrasound phased array. Phys Med Biol 45:3373, 2000.
155. Hynynen K, Freund WR, Cline HE, et al: A clinical, noninvasive, MR imaging-monitored ultrasound surgery method. Radiographics 16:185, 1996.
156. Sun Z, Ying H: A multi-gate time-of-flight technique for estimation of temperature distribution in heated tissue: theory and computer simulation. Ultrasonics 37:107, 1999.
157. Hynynen K, Darkazanli A, Damianou CA, et al: Tissue thermometry during ultrasound exposure. Eur Urol 23(Suppl 1):12, 1993.
158. Meaney PM, Fanning MW, Paulsen KD, et al: Microwave thermal imaging: initial in vivo experience with a single heating zone. Int J Hyperthermia 19:617, 2003.
159. Meaney PM, Paulsen KD, Fanning MW, et al: Image accuracy improvements in microwave tomographic thermometry: phantom experience. Int J Hyperthermia 19:534, 2003.
160. Jacobsen S, Stauffer P: Non-invasive temperature profile estimation in a lossy medium based on multi-band radiometric signals sensed by a microwave dual-purpose body-contacting antenna. Int J Hyperthermia 18:86, 2002.
161. Dreher MR, Elas M, Ichikawa K, et al: Nitroxide conjugate of a thermally responsive elastin-like polypeptide for non-invasive thermometry. Med Phys 31:2755, 2004.
162. Meyer JL: The clinical efficacy of localized hyperthermia. Cancer Res 44:4745s, 1984.
163. Dewhirst MW, Connor WG, Sim DA: Preliminary results of a phase III trial of spontaneous animal tumors to heat and/or radiation: early normal tissue response and tumor volume influence on initial response. Int J Radiat Oncol Biol Phys 8:1951, 1982.
164. Falk MH, Issels RD: Hyperthermia in oncology. Int J Hyperthermia 17:1, 2001.
165. Issels RD, Abdel-Rahman S, Wendtner C, et al: Neoadjuvant chemotherapy combined with regional hyperthermia (RHT) for locally advanced primary or recurrent high-risk adult soft-tissue sarcomas (STS) of adults: long-term results of a phase II study. Eur J Cancer 37:1599, 2001.
166. Sugimachi K, Kuwano H, Ide H, et al: Chemotherapy combined with or without hyperthermia for patients with oesophageal carcinoma: a prospective randomized trial. Int J Hyperthermia 10:485, 1994.
167. Herman TS, Teicher BA: Sequencing of trimodality therapy [cis-diamminedichloroplatinum (II)/hyperthermia/radiation] as determined by tumor growth delay and tumor cell survival in the FSaIIC fibrosarcoma. Cancer Res 48:2693, 1988.
168. Bornstein BA, Herman TS, Hansen JL, et al: Pilot study of local hyperthermia, radiation therapy, etanidazole, and cisplatin for advanced superficial tumours. Int J Hyperthermia 11:489, 1995.
169. Sugimachi K, Kitamura K, Baba K, et al: Hyperthermia combined with chemotherapy and irradiation for patients with carcinoma of the oesophagus—a prospective randomized trial. Int J Hyperthermia 8:289, 1992.
170. Jones EL, Samulski TV, Dewhirst MW, et al: A pilot phase II trial of concurrent radiotherapy, chemotherapy, and hyperthermia for locally advanced cervical carcinoma. Cancer 98:277, 2003.
171. Rau B, Wust P, Gellermann J, et al: [Phase II study on preoperative radio-chemo-thermotherapy in locally advanced rectal carcinoma]. Strahlenther Onkol 174:556, 1998.
172. Sneed PK, Dewhirst MW, Samulski T, et al: Should interstitial thermometry be used for deep hyperthermia? [editorial. comment] Int J Radiat Oncol Biol Phys 40:1015, 1998.
173. van der Zee J, Peer-Valstar JN, Rietveld PJ, et al: Practical limitations of interstitial thermometry during deep hyperthermia. Int J Radiat Oncol Biol Phys 40:1205, 1998.
174. Dewhirst MW, Griffin TW, Smith AR, et al: Intersociety Council on Radiation Oncology essay on the introduction of new medical treatments into practice. J Natl Cancer Inst 85:951, 1993.
175. Emami B, Scott C, Perez CA, et al: Phase III study of interstitial thermoradiotherapy compared with interstitial radiotherapy alone in the treatment of recurrent or persistent human tumors.

A prospectively controlled randomized study by the Radiation Therapy Group. Int J Radiat Oncol Biol Phys 34:1097, 1996.
176. Perez CA, Gillespie B, Pajak T, et al: Quality assurance problems in clinical hyperthermia and their impact on therapeutic outcome: a report by the Radiation Therapy Oncology Group. Int J Radiat Oncol Biol Phys 16:551, 1989.
177. Perez CA, Pajak T, Emami B, et al: Randomized phase III study comparing irradiation and hyperthermia with irradiation alone in superficial measurable tumors. Final report by the Radiation Therapy Oncology Group. Am J Clin Oncol 14:133, 1991.
178. Hand JW, Lagendijk JJ, Bach Andersen J, et al: Quality assurance guidelines for ESHO protocols. Int J Hyperthermia 5:421, 1989.
179. Lagendijk JJ, Van Rhoon GC, Hornsleth SN, et al: ESHO quality assurance guidelines for regional hyperthermia. Int J Hyperthermia 14:125, 1998.
180. Engin K, Tupchong L, Moylan DJ, et al: Randomized trial of one versus two adjuvant hyperthermia treatments per week in patients with superficial tumours. Int J Hyperthermia 9:327, 1993.
181. Kapp DS, Petersen IA, Cox RS, et al: Two or six hyperthermia treatments as an adjunct to radiation therapy yield similar tumor responses: results of a randomized trial. Int J Radiat Oncol Biol Phys 19:1481, 1990.
182. Dewhirst MW, Poulson JM, Yu D, et al: Relation between pO2, 31-P MRS parameters and treatment outcome in patients with high grade soft tissue sarcomas (STS) treated with thermoradiotherapy. Int J Radiat Oncol Biol Phys 2004.
183. Thrall DE, Rosner GL, Azuma C, et al: Using units of CEM 43 degrees C T90, local hyperthermia thermal dose can be delivered as prescribed. Int J Hyperthermia 16:415, 2000.
184. Jones EA, Oleson JR, Prosnitz LR, et al: Randomized trial of hyperthermia and radiation for superficial tumors. J Clin Oncol 23:3079, 2005.
185. Thrall DE, Dewhirst MW, Jones EL, et al: A clinically proven, prospective thermal dose descriptor exists. Clin Cancer Res 12:1944, 2006.
186. Vernon CC, Hand JW, Field SB, et al: Radiotherapy with or without hyperthermia in the treatment of superficial localized breast cancer: results from five randomized controlled trials. International Collaborative Hyperthermia Group. Int J Radiat Oncol Biol Phys 35:731, 1996.
187. Datta NR, Bose AK, Kapoor HK, et al: Head and neck cancers: results of thermoradiotherapy versus radiotherapy. Int J Hyperthermia 6:479, 1990.
188. Valdagni R, Amichetti M, Pani G: Radical radiation alone versus radical radiation plus microwave hyperthermia for N3 (TNM-UICC) neck nodes: a prospective randomized clinical trial. Int J Radiat Oncol Biol Phys 15:13, 1988.
189. Valdagni R, Amichetti M: Report of long-term follow-up in a randomized trial comparing radiation therapy and radiation therapy plus hyperthermia to metastatic lymph nodes in stage IV head and neck patients. Int J Radiat Oncol Biol Phys 28:163, 1994.
190. Sneed PK, Stauffer PR, McDermott MW, et al: Survival benefit of hyperthermia in a prospective randomized trial of brachytherapy boost +/− hyperthermia for glioblastoma multiforme. Int J Radiat Oncol Biol Phys 40:287, 1998.
191. Keys HM, Bundy BN, Stehman FB, et al: Cisplatin, radiation, and adjuvant hysterectomy compared with radiation and adjuvant hysterectomy for bulky stage IB cervical carcinoma. N Engl J Med 340:1154, 1999.
192. Morris M, Eifel PJ, Lu J, et al: Pelvic radiation with concurrent chemotherapy compared with pelvic and para-aortic radiation for high-risk cervical cancer. N Engl J Med 340:1137, 1999.
193. Peters WA 3rd, Liu PY, Barrett RJ 2nd, et al: Concurrent chemotherapy and pelvic radiation therapy compared with pelvic radiation therapy alone as adjuvant therapy after radical surgery in high-risk early-stage cancer of the cervix. J Clin Oncol 18:1606, 2000.
194. Rose PG, Bundy BN, Watkins EB, et al: Concurrent cisplatin-based radiotherapy and chemotherapy for locally advanced cervical cancer. N Engl J Med 340:1144, 1999.
195. Whitney CW, Sause W, Bundy BN, et al: Randomized comparison of fluorouracil plus cisplatin versus hydroxyurea as an adjunct to radiation therapy in stage IIB-IVA carcinoma of the cervix with negative para-aortic lymph nodes: a Gynecologic Oncology Group and Southwest Oncology Group study. J Clin Oncol 17:1339, 1999.
196. Hynynen K, McDannold N: MRI guided and monitored focused ultrasound thermal ablation methods: a review of progress. Int J Hyperthermia 20:725, 2004.
197. McDannold N, Hynynen K, Jolesz F: MRI monitoring of the thermal ablation of tissue: effects of long exposure times. J Magn Reson Imaging 13:421, 2001.
198. Gellerman J, Wlodarczyk W, Hildebrandt B, et al: Non-invasive magnetic resonance thermography of recurrent rectal carcinoma in a 1.5 Tesla hybrid system. Cancer Res 65:5872, 2005.
199. Brizel DM, Albers ME, Fisher SR, et al: Hyperfractionated irradiation with or without concurrent chemotherapy for locally advanced head and neck cancer. N Engl J Med 338:1798, 1998.
200. Wolmark N, Wieand HS, Hyams DM, et al: Randomized trial of postoperative adjuvant chemotherapy with or without radiotherapy for carcinoma of the rectum: National Surgical Adjuvant Breast and Bowel Project Protocol R. J Natl Cancer Inst 92:388, 2000.
201. Allen TM, Cullis PR: Drug delivery systems: entering the mainstream. Science 303:1818, 2004.
202. Mills JK, Needham D: The materials engineering of temperature-sensitive liposomes. Methods Enzymol 387:82, 2004.
203. Chilkoti A, Dreher MR, Meyer DE: Design of thermally responsive, recombinant polypeptide carriers for targeted drug delivery. Adv Drug Deliv Rev 54:1093, 2002.
204. Liu XY, Ding XB, Guan Y, et al: Fabrication of temperature-sensitive imprinted polymer hydrogel. Macromolecular Biosci 4:412, 2004.
205. Kong G, Anyarambhatla G, Petros WP, et al: Efficacy of liposomes and hyperthermia in a human tumor xenograft model: importance of triggered drug release. Cancer Res 60:6950, 2000.
206. Needham D, Anyarambhatla G, Kong G, et al: A new temperature-sensitive liposome for use with mild hyperthermia: characterization and testing in a human tumor xenograft model. Cancer Res 60:1197, 2000.
207. Van der Zee J, Gonzalez G, van Rhoon GC, et al: Comparison of radiotherapy along with radiotherapy plus hyperthermia in locally advanced pelvic tumors: A prospective randomized multi-center Dutch Deep Hyperthermia Group. Lancet 355:1119, 2000.

CHAPTER 21

TARGETED RADIONUCLIDE THERAPY

Ruby F. Meredith, Jeffrey Y. C. Wong, and Susan J. Knox

Selective delivery of radionuclides to cancer cells using an antibody or other conjugate has been under investigation for longer than 20 years. In 2002, the first Food and Drug Administration (FDA) approval was issued for a radiolabeled antibody. This form of radionuclide therapy has mainly involved the use of antibodies, or antibody-derived constructs as carriers of radionuclides, and is called radioimmunotherapy (RIT). Because the concept also includes binding to nonantigen receptors, targeted radionuclide therapy (TaRT) is a more comprehensive term. The development of TaRT has required the cooperation of basic scientists in the areas of radiation biology, chemistry, physics, and immunology with multiple clinical specialists. With the exception of some gene therapy approaches, TaRT differs from external beam radiation therapy in that selective targeting can be at the cellular rather than at the target volume level. Among its potential applications, TaRT provides a means of irradiating multiple tumor sites throughout the body with relative sparing of normal tissues. A number of challenges hampering use of TaRT have been met, while others remain under active investigation. Many of these are covered in more detail in other reviews.[1-7]

TUMOR TARGETING

Antibody Targeting

The efficacy of RIT is dependent on a number of factors, including properties of the targeted antigen, tumor, and antibody. Antigen variables include density, availability, shedding, and heterogeneity of expression. Tumor factors include vascularity, blood flow, and permeability. Antibody features to consider are specificity of the binding site, which affects selective tumor uptake; immunoreactivity, which can affect localization; stability in vivo; and both avidity and affinity.[8,9] Affinity can be described by an intrinsic association constant *K* that characterizes binding of a univalent ligand (formation of a stable antibody-antigen complex) and can be calculated from the ratio of the rate constants for association and dissociation. Because intact antibodies and most antigens are multivalent, the tendency to bind depends on the affinity, number of binding sites, and other nonspecific factors involved in aggregation. The term *avidity* is used to describe the overall tendency of antibody to bind to antigen.

The optimal level of binding affinity for maximal in vivo effectiveness is controversial, and binding affinity does not always correlate with activity in vivo.[8,10] One might expect that high, compared with low, affinity antibodies would result in increased tumor uptake, retention, and improved efficacy, as shown in some studies.[11-13] However, high-affinity antibodies may preferentially bind to perivascular regions in the periphery of tumors, while antibodies of lower affinity are able to penetrate deeper into tumors.[14-16]

A wide variety of antibodies have been made against a number of tumor-specific and tumor-associated antigens that, although present on some normal cells, are usually expressed at lower levels on normal cells than on the targeted tumor cells. Most RIT trials have used monoclonal antibodies, and many have used intact murine IgG antibodies. Early on, the immunogenicity of the nonhuman antibodies was recognized as a serious limitation of RIT.[17] With the exception of patients with lymphoma, who are less prone to develop an immune response to murine antibodies (human anti-mouse antibody [HAMA] response), more than 80% of patients usually develop an immune response against a therapeutically administered murine or other species antibody after a single injection of antibody.[17] Such an immune response can occur even after doses as small as 1 mg used for imaging studies or following administration of antibody fragments or smaller constructs (but with less frequency than found following administration of intact IgG). Administration of antibody in a patient with an HAMA response can result in a severe immune reaction and rapid blood clearance, limiting tumor uptake of radiolabeled antibody.[18] Several approaches have been used in an effort to ameliorate the problem of antibody immunogenicity, such as (1) the development of less immunogenic (chimeric and humanized) antibodies, (2) the use of immunosuppression by cyclosporine or deoxyspergualin to prevent an immune response, (3) the removal of HAMA directed to the therapeutic antibody by administration of an excess of unlabeled antibody prior to the administration of the radioimmunoconjugate, and (4) posttreatment removal of immune complexes by passing the patient's blood through an extracorporeal immunoadsorption column.[19]

Genetic engineering has been successful in providing numerous targeting agents with reduced immunogenicity and has allowed for optimization of other aspects of the therapy.[20,21] Genetic constructs have been produced that vary in and can be altered by conjugating them to other agents (e.g., cytokines, toxins, or radiosensitizers) to form fusion proteins.[22]

Technologic advances have provided a wide variety of antibodies and constructs varying in specificity, size and number of antigen-combining sites, rapidity of distribution, immunogenicity, and immunologic function. Use of small antibody constructs such as single-chain antigen binding proteins may be most useful for diagnostic studies or for multistep targeting strategies. The decreased immunogenicity of fragments/constructs and human and humanized antibodies now allows for administration of repeat courses or fractionated RIT dosing.[23]

As immunogenicity of antibodies has been ameliorated, some investigators have had concern about the potential immunogenicity of other components of therapy. For example, as more macrocyclic chelators have been developed to improve stability of conjugates, some data suggest that these molecules may be immunogenic. Furthermore, the immunogenicity of streptavidin used in some pretargeting schemes has generally limited it to single-dose therapy.[24-26] Work continues to diminish the immunogenicity of these other components of RIT.

Nonantibody Targeting

Several of the factors affecting antibody development/efficacy for TaRT are also pertinent to nonantigen targeting such as receptor density, availability, affinity, shedding, and heterogeneity of receptor expression, as well as features of the tumor, including vascularity, blood flow, and permeability. The discovery more than a decade ago that many tumors overexpress receptors for peptide hormones opened the field for TaRT and other forms of targeted therapy. Radiolabeled peptide analogs such as those for somatostatin, bombesin, calcitonin, oxytocin, and epidermal growth factor have been studied. Analogs of somatostatin are the most studied to date, with radiolabeled peptides being used for detection and treatment of a variety of neuroendocrine tumors.[27] Initial treatment of tumors expressing somatostatin receptor subtype 2 was with higher doses of the diagnostic agent [^{111}In-DTPA]octreotide.[28] Subsequently, the higher-affinity [DOTA,Tyr^3]octreotide and [DOTA,Tyr^3]octreotate were introduced and used with ^{90}Y and ^{177}Lu labeling as the therapeutic beta emitter. [Tyr^3]Octreotate differs from octreotide by substitution of tyrosine as the third residue and the replacement of threoninol by threonine. Early studies showed impressive response rates and that fractionation of administered dose as well as infusion of amino acids ameliorated the dose-limiting renal toxicity.[4,29,30] Various multicenter studies are ongoing for optimization of ^{90}Y-[DOTA,Tyr^3]octreotide, ^{177}Lu-[DOTA,Tyr^3]octreotate, and ^{90}Y-[DOTA]lanreotide, another somatostatin analog.[31] In addition to objective clinical response rates often higher than 25% and improved survival, clinical benefit in terms of decreased symptoms has usually been observed in the majority of patients with progressive neuroendocrine tumors.[30,32] Radiolabeled peptides targeting tumor neovasculature are also under investigation and may provide therapy to nonendocrine malignancies.[33] Another targeting entity under investigation is the use of liposomes or nanoparticles as carriers of radionuclides.[34-36]

SELECTION OF RADIONUCLIDES

Other reviews provide detail on the importance of radionuclide selection, primarily with regard to the radiolabeling of whole immunoglobulins.[37-39] Some studies have focused on the selection of radionuclides for use with smaller, engineered antibody-derived constructs.[40] The emission profile of radionuclides determines their suitability for therapy and imaging. Particle energy and mean path length in tissue are important determinants of therapeutic efficacy, whereas the presence of gamma emissions at an appropriate energy is best for imaging. Some radionuclides such as ^{131}I have beta and gamma emissions that allow for both therapy and imaging. The therapeutic effect from such radionuclides is primarily due to the beta radiation, while the gamma component allows for imaging but contributes substantially more to normal tissue toxicity than efficacy. Important considerations for selection of radionuclides for TaRT include the size and biological features of the tumor and antibody (or other targeting agent). In a one-step RIT administration using directly labeled antibodies, matching of the physical half-life of the radionuclide with the initial peak of tumor/nontumor antibody concentration was reported to be the most important factor for optimal radionuclide selection.[37] For example, a good therapeutic ratio would not be obtained if one used a radionuclide that decays within several hours linked to an antibody that has a circulation time of several days, because most of the radiation exposure would have occurred before the radiolabeled antibody localized in the tumor. In this case, the resulting radiation dose to normal tissues would be nearly as great as that to the targeted tumor. Pretargeting strategies, discussed in more detail in the Optimization section, allow for use of radionuclides with shorter half-lives, because unlabeled antibody-tumor targeting precedes administration of the radionuclide.

With direct targeting by radioimmunoconjugates, the size and composition of the carrier molecule determine, in part, the biological half-life and effector function of the molecule. Tumor characteristics such as size (e.g., micrometastases versus bulky masses) and the level and heterogeneity of antigen expression affect antibody distribution. Beta emitting radionuclides will be suitable for sizable tumors with heterogeneous antigen expression because crossfire of the associated penetrating radiation allows for killing of cells some distance (along the path length of the beta particles) from bound antibody. Auger electron emitters, such as ^{125}I, may be suitable for treatment of micrometastases that abundantly express internalizing antigen on every cell, because targeting of the nucleus is necessary for effective cell killing with this very short range emitter. Alpha emitters may be most useful for the treatment of micrometastatic disease, such as leukemia in bone marrow, minimal intraperitoneal (IP) disease, and intratumoral delivery. High levels of antigen/receptor expression are not necessary for effective killing by alpha emitters because of the associated high linear energy transfer (LET) radiation and path length of several cell diameters.

The development of labeling and chelation chemistry for the production of stable radioconjugates has greatly facilitated TaRT. ^{131}I can be directly attached to antibody without a chelator. However, if a targeted antigen/receptor undergoes modulation (internalization), the tumor cells can dehalogenate the conjugate and release free iodine. ^{131}I can also be attached by a secondary molecule conjugated through an iodinatable linker rather than directly linked to antibodies. These radioimmunoconjugates appear to be more resistant to dehalogenation.[41]

A variety of increasingly stable chelators have been developed for ^{90}Y and other metal radionuclides, but some have been found to be immunogenic (probably due in part to aggregation).[24,26] The chemistry, stability, and in vivo processing of radioimmunoconjugates also have implications for toxicity. The filtration of small radioconjugates or their metabolites through the kidneys may result in considerable radiation to the kidneys. Renal toxicity has been reported to be the dose-limiting toxicity for some small-molecular-weight peptide conjugates.[42] Hepatic uptake, metabolism of radioimmunoconjugates, and retention of ^{90}Y complexes in the liver is potentially dose limiting in myeloablative TaRT. With some antibodies, comparison of radionuclides for optimization purposes has been studied, using human tumors in xenograft models or theoretical modeling based on prior patient pharmacokinetics data.[43-45]

In summary, there are a variety of radionuclides that are suitable for TaRT. These include alpha emitters; low-, medium-, and high-energy beta emitters; and those that work through electron capture and/or internal conversion (Auger electrons). Beta emitters (e.g., ^{131}I and ^{90}Y) have been the most popular radionuclides for clinical TaRT trials to date. These radionuclides have the advantage of not needing to target every individual tumor cell since the mean radiation range is approximately 0.4 and 2.5 mm, respectively. Features of some of these radionuclides are compared in Table 21-1. Alpha emitters offer promise for the future, especially when used to treat microscopic disease or administered intratumorally. Their suitability includes relatively short half-lives of most alpha emitters (e.g., $t_{1/2}$ = 45.6 minutes for ^{213}Bi and 7 hours for ^{211}At) and short range of the high LET alpha particles (e.g., limited to 40 to 80 μm). These radionuclides may prove to be advantageous for the treatment of small-volume disease.[46] Designing chelators with special characteristics can also affect radionuclide "matching" with the targeting agent. For example, selective degradation of a cathepsin-sensitive chelate

Table 21-1 Radionuclides Used for Therapy

Isotope	$T_{1/2}$ (d)	γ Energy (kev)	Percent γ Intensity	β Range in Tissue (mm) Maximum	Mean	Advantages	Disadvantages
^{90}Y	2.7			11.9	2.5	Long β range	Chelator, bone seeker
^{131}I	8.0	364	81	2.4	0.3	No chelator needed	Dehalogenation, toxicity from γ
^{186}Re	3.7	137	9	5.0	0.9	Less γ than ^{131}I	Chelator, scarce
^{67}Cu	2.5	184	48	2.2	0.4	Less γ than ^{131}I	Chelator, scarce
^{177}Lu	6.7	208/113	11 and 7	2.2	0.3	Less γ than ^{131}I	Chelator, scarce
^{125}I	60.4	35	7	0.02	—	Low-normal tissue toxicity	Does not image well
^{188}Re	0.8	155	15	11.0	2.4	Long β range	Chelator, scarce

reduced liver uptake of radiometal.[47] The use of such chelators may allow for dose escalation of radiometal conjugates such as ^{67}Cu that otherwise would be limited by hepatic toxicity. Other conditionally cleavable chelators are also under study.[48]

RADIOBIOLOGY

Biological effects of TaRT may be associated with both the radionuclides and their carriers, either alone or in combination.[49,50] This is particularly true for certain antibody carriers that may have antitumor efficacy alone (e.g., anti-CD20 antibodies). Antibody-induced responses can include apoptosis, complement-dependent cytotoxicity, and antibody-dependent cell-mediated cytotoxicity. Radiation effects can result in cell death during mitosis or by apoptosis, necrosis, and/or a metabolic cell death. The relative importance of these types of cell death depends on factors such as inherent genetic makeup of the cells. For lymphomas, apoptosis is an important mechanism of cell death, whereas apoptosis usually plays less of a role in killing solid tumor cells.

Lymphomas are especially sensitive to apoptosis induced not only by radiation but also by a variety of cytotoxic agents including antibody therapy alone.[51-54] Several signal transduction pathways have been found to be associated with radiation-induced apoptosis; these were reviewed by Hernandez and Knox.[50]

Several studies have shown that cells exposed to either continuous or exponentially decreasing low-dose-rate radiation arrest in the radiosensitive G_2/M phase of the cell cycle and undergo apoptosis.[55-58] This G_2/M block from low-dose-rate radiation as delivered via TaRT may also sensitize tumor cells to killing by other therapies such as external beam radiation.[59] Data from some experiments showing this effect suggest that therapy may be optimized by using TaRT prior to external beam radiation[59] (external beam[60] has also been given before radiation to increase tumor uptake of radionuclide conjugates, as discussed later). In addition, regulating cell-cycle distribution or altering the underlying apoptotic potential by drugs or biological response modifiers in tumor cells can affect the susceptibility of such cells to radiation-induced apoptosis.[61,62]

Although there is usually a positive correlation between the level of radiation-induced cell killing and dose rate, an inverse dose-rate effect has been reported with low-dose-rate irradiation in the range of about 0.3 Gy/h, with some cell types being more sensitive to this inverse dose-rate effect than others.[63] Knox and colleagues[64] showed lymphoma cells to be very sensitive to ^{131}I-labeled antibody low-dose-rate radiation in a direct comparison to high-dose-rate external beam irradiation. At least one mechanism for this observation appears to be greater arrest in the G_2/M phase of the cell cycle. Another mechanism of lymphoma radiation sensitivity may be less efficient DNA repair among lymphomas compared with some other cell types.[49,50] Ongoing studies will help elucidate the radiobiology of TaRT, which will facilitate optimization of TaRT therapy in the future and provide the prerequisite understanding of underlying biological mechanisms to determine how best to use TaRT in combination with other treatment modalities.

CLINICAL RESULTS

A wide variety of human malignancies have been treated with RIT in the setting of clinical trials. Antibodies carrying radionuclides have targeted tumor-associated antigens, growth factor receptors, and other cell surface markers, usually expressed at a high level on malignant cells and to a lesser extent on subsets of normal cells. Nonantibody targeting has primarily been against neuroendocrine receptors. Several routes of administration have been used, including intravenous (IV), intra-arterial, intrathecal, IP, intratumoral, and, rarely, intrapleural administration. The most prevalent route of administration has been IV for systemic therapy. However, for localized disease, regional or intracavitary administration may be advantageous. IP RIT has generally been more efficacious than IV RIT for the treatment of small-volume disease confined to the peritoneal cavity, but there are conflicting reports concerning the relative merits of arterial and venous routes of administration of radiolabeled antibodies for other sites.[65-69]

RADIOIMMUNOTHERAPY OF SOLID NONHEMATOLOGIC TUMORS

RIT of solid tumors has been actively investigated for decades and continues to hold promise as a form of systemic targeted radiation therapy in the appropriate clinical settings. Initial efforts date back to 1951 when Beierwaltes and colleagues[70] administered ^{131}I-labeled polyclonal antibodies produced from rabbits immunized with tumor extracts from patients with metastatic melanoma and noted a pathologic complete response (CR) in 1 of 14 patients. Phase I/II clinical trials conducted by Order and colleagues[71] followed, evaluating ^{131}I-polyclonal anti-ferritin in patients with hepatoma and Hodgkin's lymphoma. Beginning in the 1970s, with the development of hybridoma technology,[72] large-scale production of clinical-grade monoclonal antibodies (mAbs) selected against specific tumor-associated antigens became possible and greatly expanded the number of clinical trials evaluating radiolabeled mAbs as agents for tumor detection and therapy. The application of molecular engineering techniques permits the customized design and production of antibody constructs with reduced immunogenicity and pharmacokinetic properties optimized for therapy.

The mAbs conjugated to radionuclides demonstrated significant promise in animal models as a form of systemic targeted therapy. Dozens of studies in tumor-bearing animal models documented significant tumor growth delay and cures after RIT in a wide variety of solid tumor types,[73-77] with tumor doses often exceeding 10 to 15 Gy after a single infusion.[77,78] In some studies, RIT achieved comparable tumor growth delays to equivalent doses of single-fraction or conventionally fractionated external beam radiation therapy.[77,79-86] Initial clinical trials evaluating biodistribution and pharmacokinetics confirmed tumor targeting and demonstrated that therapeutic doses of radiation to tumor were achievable.[87-92]

The promise of RIT is being realized in the clinic for the more radiosensitive hematologic malignancies, with overall response rates ranging from 30% to 85%.[93-99] The FDA approved two radiolabeled anti-CD20 monoclonal antibodies for clinical use in patients with low-grade non-Hodgkin's lymphoma (NHL).[97,100] For solid tumors, results have been less impressive but remain encouraging. Results from solid tumor therapy trials using nonmyeloablative systemic RIT as single-modality therapy are summarized in Table 21-2. Early trials used ^{131}I as the radionuclide because it was readily available and easy to link to antibody molecules, with subsequent trials using radiometals such as ^{90}Y, ^{186}Re, and ^{177}Lu. Although different mAbs, tumor types, and radionuclides have been evaluated, comparable results have been observed in most trials. The majority have been phase I trials reporting on a relatively limited number of patients. Almost all of the antibodies studied have been administered at low protein doses (about 5 to 50 mg), have had no demonstrated clinical immunomodulatory or antitumor properties, and have therefore served primarily as a delivery vehicle for radiation. Most patients have received a single therapy infusion, with only a small subset receiving a limited number of additional infusion cycles. Dose-limiting toxicity has been hematologic, primarily thrombocytopenia and leukopenia. As is typical of phase I trials, patients who were entered often had advanced, bulky, chemotherapy refractory disease, with progressive disease at the time of therapy. In this patient population, studies have reported primarily stable disease and serologic, mixed, or minor responses (MRs) of 25% to 49% decrease from baseline in overall tumor size for ≥1 month,[91,101-123] with infrequent partial responses (PRs) of ≥50% decrease from baseline in overall tumor size for ≥1 month[124-130] and rare CRs where there is no evidence of disease for ≥1 month.[101,131,132] Based on the clinical experience thus far, there appears to be no clear advantage to any particular radionuclide-antibody combination.

Tumor radiation doses and objective response rates from selected solid tumor RIT trials are shown in Table 21-3. Regardless of the antibody, antigen target, radionuclide, or tumor type studied, radiation doses to tumors have been comparable for most antibodies, with median or mean doses in the range of 1000 to 2000 cGy, and subsets of tumors receiving approximately 2000 to 7000 cGy after single infusion. Also shown for comparison are tumor doses from lymphoma RIT trials. The range and reported median and mean tumor doses are comparable for solid tumor and lymphoma antibody delivery systems, yet objective responses are more frequent for lymphomas, in large part due to their greater radiosensitivity.[50]

Although tumor doses from RIT are usually a fraction of what can be delivered by teletherapy or brachytherapy systems, doses currently achievable are at levels that can potentially result in clinically important antitumor effects in solid tumors. This is particularly pertinent in subclinical or microscopic disease, with TaRT alone or when combined with radiation-enhancing chemotherapeutic or biological response agents. With conventionally fractionated external beam radiotherapy of solid tumors, an inverse linear relationship has been reported between radiation dose and tumor recurrence rate with doses ranging from 2000 to 5000 cGy.[133] More important, there was no threshold effect and doses in the range of 2000 cGy had measurable effects in the adjuvant setting. Other clinical trials have demonstrated clinically important antitumor effects in rectal cancer with doses in the range of 3000 cGy.[134,135] Finally, doses as low as 3000 cGy conventionally fractionated have been effectively combined with chemotherapy in esophageal and anal cancer, resulting in pathologic CRs, again suggesting that doses achievable from RIT, either alone or in combination with chemotherapy, may be clinically meaningful.[136-138]

Strategies that have proved successful in optimizing external beam radiotherapy should also prove successful with RIT. These strategies have followed three general approaches: (1) increasing antibody targeting and delivery of radiation dose to the tumor, (2) decreasing radiation dose to normal organs and dose-limiting side effects, thereby permitting escalation of administered activity, and (3) enhancing the tumoricidal effects of the targeted tumor dose through combined-modality approaches. Multiple optimization strategies have been explored in preclinical models and are described elsewhere in this chapter. Those that have been promising and translatable to the clinic are being actively investigated. These include overcoming the dose-limiting hematologic toxicity of RIT through stem cell transplantation (SCT) or bone marrow transplantation (BMT), the use of agents to upregulate antigen expression, novel engineered immunoconstructs, regional administration, combined-modality approaches, and therapy in the minimal tumor burden or adjuvant setting. Pretargeting delivery strategies that seek to amplify the differences between tumor and normal organ uptake are also promising and are described in detail later in this chapter.

Because hematologic toxicity is dose limiting, groups have explored dose intensification strategies using stem cell or bone marrow reinfusion after myeloablative doses of radiolabeled mAbs. Most have been phase I studies treating a limited number of patients. Schrier and coworkers[139] observed PRs in four of eight patients with measurable disease and decreased bone pain in another patient after a myeloablative dose of ^{90}Y-BrE3. The same group evaluated the humanized version of BrE-3 in a similarly designed trial and noted 2 of 12 patients with a PR and 7 of 12 with stable disease.[140] Richman and colleagues[141,142] reported a progression-free survival (PFS) and stable disease in three patients with breast cancer treated with ^{131}I-170H.82, and stable disease in one of three receiving ^{131}I-chL6. Other myeloablative RIT studies have reported fewer or no objective responses.[126,143-146] Stem cell and bone marrow reinfusion has permitted higher myeloablative doses to be administered, but it appears that dose-intensification alone will not result in the level of objective response rates initially hoped for and may need to be combined with other optimization strategies and/or other therapeutic approaches.

Delivering multicycle therapy to increase antibody targeted radiation dose to tumor has been hampered by antibody immunogenicity. Table 21-4 compares the immunogenicity of murine, chimeric, and humanized radiolabeled mAbs that have been evaluated in clinical trials. Chimerization and humanization have decreased the immunogenicity of most antibody constructs.[23,147-150] For example, humanization of anti-CD44v66 BIWA 4 resulted in an immune response in 10% of patients, compared with 40% with the chimeric version U36 and 90% with the parental murine mAb BIWA 1.[117,118,151] Not all humanized mAbs have low immunogenicity. A 47%

Table 21-2 Selected Systemic Monoclonal Antibody Radioimmunotherapy Clinical Trials in Solid Tumors

Study (First Author)	Year	Radiolabeled Antibody	Study Type	No. of Patients	Tumor Type	Activity per Cycle	Objective Responses (%)	Minor/Mixed Response or Stable Disease (%)
Carasquillo[160]	1984	^{131}I-anti-p97	Pilot	10	Melanoma	30-342 mCi	1/3 (33)	1/3 (33)
Lashford[101]	1987	^{131}I-UJ13A	Pilot	5	Neuroblastoma	33-55 mCi	1/5 (20)	1/5 (20)
Meredith[102]	1992	^{131}I-cB72.3	I	12	Colorectal	12-18 mCi/m^2 weekly ×2-3		4/12 (33)
Lane[132]	1994	^{131}I-A5B7 intact/F(ab′)$_2$	Pilot	19	CEA+		2/19 (11)	
Meredith[103]	1994	^{131}I-CC49	II	15	Prostate	75 mCi/m^2		10/15 (67) 5/15 >50% ↓PSA (33) 6/10 ↓Bone pain (60)
Welt[104]	1994	^{131}I-A33	I/II	23	Colorectal	30-90 mCi/m^2		3/20 (15)
Murray[105]	1994	^{131}I-CC49	II	15	Colorectal	75 mCi/m^2		3/14 (21)
Juweid[159]	1996	^{131}I-NP4 F(ab′)$_2$	I	13	CEA+	70-296 mCi		4/13 (31)
Yu[107]	1996	^{131}I-COL-1	I	18	Gastrointestinal	10-75 mCi/m^2		4/18 (22)
Behr[124]	1997	^{131}I-NP-4	I/II	57	CEA+	44-268 mCi	1/57 (2)	4/57 (7)
DeNardo[125]	1997	^{131}I-chL6	I	10	Breast	20-70 mCi/m^2	4/10 (40)	2/10 (20)
Juweid[131]	1997	^{131}I-MN-14	I	14	Ovary	30-50 mCi/m^2	1/14 (7)	2/14 (14)
Divgi[103]	1998	^{131}I-G250	I/II	33	Renal	30-90 mCi/m^2		17/33 (52)
Ychou[126]	1998	^{131}I-F6 F(ab′)$_2$	I/II	10	Colon	100-300 mCi	1/9 (11)	3/9 (33)
Behr[127]	1999	^{131}I-hMN-14	I	12	Colorectal	50-70 mCi/m^2	2/11 (16)	5/11 (45)
Juweid[128]	1999	^{131}I-MN-14 F(ab′)$_2$	I/II	15	Thyroid	110-267 mCi	1/12 (8)	11/12 (92)
Steffens[129]	1999	^{131}I-cG250	I	8	Renal	45-75 mCi/m^2	1/8 (13)	1/8 (13)
Van Zanten-Przybysz[109]	1999	^{131}I-cMOv18	Pilot	3	Ovary	74.5-81.4 mCi/m^2		3/3 (100)
Meredith[110]	1995	^{125}I-chimeric 17-1A	I	28	Colorectal	20-250 mCi		10/28 (36)
Deb[111]	1996	^{90}Y-CYT-356	I	12	Prostate	1.83-12.0 mCi/m^2		2/12 ↓Pain (17)
DeNardo[112]	1997	^{90}Y-BrE-3	I	6	Breast	6.25-9.25 mCi/m^2		3/6 (50)
Kahn[113]	1999	^{90}Y-CYT-356	II	8	Prostate (rising postoperative PSA)	9 mCi/m^2		4/8 Stable PSA (50)
Wong[114]	2000	^{90}Y-cT84.66	I	22	CEA+	5-22 mCi/m^2		12/22 (54) 7/22 >50% ↓CEA (33)
O'Donnell[115]	2001	^{90}Y-m170	I	17	Prostate	5-20 mCi/m^2		8/13 ↓Pain (62) 7/17 State PSA (41)
Milowsky[123]	2002	^{90}Y-huJ591	I	19	Prostate	5-20 mCi/m^2		6/19 Stable/↓PSA (32)
Breitz[130]	1992	^{186}Re-NR-LU-10	I	15	Colorectal, lung, breast	25-120 mCi/m^2		
Breitz[130]	1992	^{186}Re-NR-CO-2 F(ab′)$_2$	I	26	Colorectal, lung, breast	25-200 mCi/m^2	1/26 (4)	11/26 (42)
Weiden[116]	1993	^{186}Re-NR-LU-13	I	9	Gastrointestinal, lung, breast	25-60 mCi/m^2		2/9 (22)
Colnot[117]	2000	^{186}Re-chimeric U36	I	13	Head and neck	10.8-40.5 mCi/m^2		1/13 (8)
Borjesson[118]	2003	^{186}Re-hu BIWA 4	I	17	Head and neck	20-60 mCi/m^2		4/17 (24)
Juweid[119]	1997	^{186}Re-MN-14	I	11	Colon, pancreas	30-80 mCi/m^2		
Mulligan[120]	1995	^{177}Lu-CC49	I	9	Colorectal, breast, lung	10-25 mCi/m^2		2/9 (22)
Vallabahajosula[122]	2002	^{177}Lu-huJ591	I	9	Prostate	10-60 mCi/m^2		6/9 (67)

CEA, carcinoembryonic antigen; PSA, prostate-specific antigen.

immune response rate was seen with hMN-14 and a 63% immune response rate was seen with humanized mAb A33.[152,153] However, this is still substantially lower than the 100% rate of immunization observed with their murine counterparts.[104,131]

Genetically engineered modifications to the antibody molecule to optimize its biodistribution and pharmacokinetic properties for therapy are also being explored. A limiting factor of intact antibodies is their relatively slow blood clearance with serum half-lives of several days, resulting in

Table 21-3 Tumor Doses and Objective Response Rates From Selected Solid Tumor and Lymphoma Radioimmunotherapy Trials

Study (First Author)	Radionuclide-Antibody	Tumor Type	No. of Tumors Analyzed	Tumor Dose (cGy/cycle)	Objective Response Rate (%)
Meredith[103]	^{131}I-CC49	Prostate	4	208-1083	0
Juweid[159]	^{131}I-NP4 F(ab′)$_2$	Colorectal, lung, pancreas, thyroid	4	511-6476	0
DeNardo[125]	^{131}I-chL6	Breast	7	120-3700 (~1300 mean)	40
Van Zanten-Przybysz[109]	^{131}I-cMOv18	Ovary	3	600-3800	0
Breitz[130]	^{186}Re-NR-CO-2 F(ab′)$_2$	Lung, colorectal, breast, ovary, renal	5	500-2100	4
Postema[118,438]	^{186}Re-hu BIWA 4	Head and neck	16	380-7610 (1240 median)	0
DeNardo[112]	^{90}Y-BrE-3	Breast	16	442-1887	0
Wong[257]	^{90}Y-cT84.66	Colorectal	31	46-6400 (1320 mean)	0
Wiseman[439]	^{90}Y-2B8	Non-Hodgkin's lymphoma	18	580-6700 (1700 median)	67
Kaminski[435]	^{131}I-anti-B1	Non-Hodgkin's lymphoma	NS	141-2584 (925 mean)	79
Lamborn[436]	^{131}I-Lym-1	Non-Hodgkin's lymphoma	45	16-1485 (241 median)	54
Vose[437]	^{131}I-LL2	Non-Hodgkin's lymphoma	NS	166-861	33

Table 21-4 Antibody Immunogenicity after Single Administration (Selected Solid Tumor Radioimmunotherapy [RIT] Trials)

Study (First Author)	Year	Antibody	Type	No. of Patients	Percent Antiantibody Response
Breitz[130]	1992	^{186}Re-NR-LU-10	Murine	15	100
Meredith[103]	1994	^{131}I-CC49	Murine	15	100
Welt[104]	1994	^{131}I-mAb A33	Murine	23	100
Mulligan[120]	1995	^{177}Lu-CC49	Murine	9	100
Yu[107]	1996	^{131}I-COL-1	Murine	18	83, prevented additional RIT in 2
DeNardo[112]	1997	^{90}Y-BreE-3	Murine	6	80, prevented additional RIT in 3
Behr[124]	1997	^{131}I-NP-4	Murine	32	94
Juweid[131]	1997	^{131}I-MN-14	Murine	14	100
Divgi[108]	1998	^{131}I-mG250	Murine	33	100
Meredith[102]	1992	^{131}I-cB72.3	Chimeric	12	58
Weiden[116]	1993	^{186}Re-NR-LU-13	Chimeric	8	75
Meredith[110]	1995	^{125}I-17-1A	Chimeric	15	13
DeNardo[125]	1997	^{131}I-chL6	Chimeric	10	80, prevented additional RIT in 4
Steffens[129]	1999	^{131}I-cG250	Chimeric	12	8
van Zanten-Przybysz[109]	2000	^{131}I-cMOv18	Chimeric	3	0
Colnot[117]	2000	^{186}Re-U36	Chimeric	12	42
Wong[114]	2002	^{90}Y-cT84.66	Chimeric	21	52, prevented additional RIT in 8
Hajjar[152]	2002	^{131}I-hMN-14	Humanized	15	47
Goldsmith[121]	2002	^{90}Y-huJ591	Humanized	19	0
Borjesson[118]	2003	^{186}Re-BIWA 4	Humanized	20	10

higher doses to marrow and hematologic toxicity. Antibody fragments and other smaller, lower-molecular-weight engineered immunoconstructs may ultimately prove superior for therapy due to potentially greater tumor penetration, more uniform distribution in tumor, higher initial dose rate in tumor, decreased immunogenicity, faster blood clearance, and higher tumor-to-background ratios, which allow for higher administered activities and higher tumor doses for the same level of toxicity.[14,154-156] Initial efforts evaluated F(ab′)$_2$ and Fab′ fragments produced after enzymatic digestion of the parental intact mAb, with in vivo studies demonstrating a superior ratio of tumor to blood dose for fragments compared with the intact antibody.[76,157,158] Radiolabeled F(ab′)$_2$ and Fab′ fragments have also been evaluated as radioimmunotherapeutics in the clinic with reported success[126,128,130,132,155,159,160] (see Table 21-2).

Efforts have used recombinant DNA technology to genetically engineer antibody constructs with properties to improve tumor to normal organ biodistribution, enhance in vivo stability, reduce immunogenicity, aid in conjugation and radiolabeling, and increase clearance kinetics. Constructs have ranged from approximately 25 to 160 kd in size.[161-168] Single-chain monovalent constructs (scFv) of approximately 28 kd MW are composed of the variable heavy (V_H) and variable light (V_L) regions linked by a contiguously encoded peptide. These low-molecular-weight constructs clear rapidly compared with intact antibodies. This results in increased tumor/blood ratios and reduced background activity, which make them attractive as potential imaging agents.[169,170] However, peak uptake and retention time in tumor are often reduced, limiting their use as therapy agents.[161,169-171]

A more suitable therapy construct may be of intermediate molecular weight, with antibody uptake and retention in tumor comparable to intact antibodies but with faster clearance times, resulting in an improved therapeutic ratio. Multivalent, intermediate-molecular-weight constructs have been produced through covalent linking of monovalent fragments.[162,165,172-174] Alternatively, single-chain monomers can be engineered with properties that promote spontaneous formation of dimeric and trimeric species. For example, Wu and coworkers[175] engineered a series of recombinant fragments derived from the intact anti-CEA mAb, chimeric T84.66, and have compared each radioiodinated construct in animal models. The scFv monomer (28 kd) gave low peak tumor uptake of 2% to 3% injected dose/gram (% ID/g). The diabody (55 kd), which is formed by the cross-pair dimerization of two scFv monomers, gave improved peak tumor uptake of 10% to 15% ID/g with longer retention time in tumor than the scFv monomer. The minibody (80 kd MW), formed by the self-association of two scFv-C_H3 single-chain monomers, gave peak tumor uptake of over 20% to 30% injected dose per gram, which exceeded that of the diabody and $F(ab')_2$ and approached that of the intact antibody. In addition, the minibody demonstrated faster clearance compared with the intact antibody, predicting for a 60% increase in radiation dose to tumor for equitoxic administered activities of the minibody compared with the intact mAb.[40] Other groups have investigated similar strategies with encouraging results.[171,176-180]

Constructs that were promising in preclinical studies are now being evaluated in pilot biodistribution trials to assess their potential as radioimmunotherapy delivery agents.[173,174,181-183] Forero and coworkers[181] confirmed faster blood clearance rates and decreased immunogenicity of ^{131}I-HuCC49$\Delta$$CH_2$ (153 kd), which resulted in a greater than threefold increase in predicted radiation dose to tumor versus blood compared with the parental intact murine CC49. A phase I dose escalation therapy trial was initiated and preliminary results indicate reduced hematologic toxicity of the construct compared with the murine CC49 antibody. Wong and colleagues[183] completed a pilot biodistribution trial of ^{123}I-cT84.66 minibody and confirmed reduced immunogenicity, faster blood clearance, and blood residence times than intact cT84.66. A pretherapy biodistribution trial with ^{111}In-cT84.66 minibody is ongoing to further evaluate its potential as a therapy agent.

Upregulation of tumor antigen expression has been explored as a means of increasing antibody targeting and radiation dose to tumor. Alpha and gamma interferon have been shown to increase tumor-associated antigen expression, including CEA and TAG-72, in vitro and in vivo in preclinical studies and in patients, resulting in increased tumor antibody uptake and enhanced efficacy of radioimmunotherapy in animal models.[184-193] Macey[194] and Slovin[195] and their colleagues documented a significant increase in TAG-72 expression and antibody uptake in tumor with interferon administered prior to ^{131}I-CC49 radioimmunotherapy in breast cancer and prostate cancer patients, respectively. Meredith and coworkers[196,197] noted an increase in estimated radiation dose to tumors in patients with colorectal cancer and prostate cancer receiving interferon prior to RIT. The impact of this strategy on the efficacy of RIT continues to be actively investigated in the clinic.

Tumor size plays a dominant role in influencing antibody uptake and, as a result, clinically important outcomes are predicted if systemic RIT is used to treat subclinical or microscopic disease. Jain and colleagues[14,198] identified key physiologic factors in tumors that limit uptake of macromolecules. These factors include spatial heterogeneity of tumor vascularity, increased interstitial pressure in poorly vascularized areas, and limited diffusion distances of macromolecules, which work to significantly limit the ability of the antibody to reach all sites within the tumor, particularly the most poorly vascularized and central necrotic regions. As a consequence, a physiologic barrier is created that impedes the delivery of radiation to tumor through antibody-targeted approaches. These factors are amplified as the tumor grows, resulting in an exponential decrease in tumor antibody uptake. Investigators have documented an inverse log relationship between tumor antibody uptake and tumor size in a variety of experimental systems and clinical trials.[199-205] These data indicate that exponential increases in cGy dose to tumor result as RIT moves from treating macroscopic to microscopic tumors and predict that RIT will have its greatest impact in the adjuvant setting. For example, Behr and colleagues[127,206] demonstrated improved survival and prevention of liver metastases in animal models, leading to a clinical trial evaluating adjuvant ^{131}I-hMN14 anti-CEA in patients after resection of limited hepatic metastases from colon cancer. Of nine patients receiving adjuvant RIT, eight remain disease free at 24+ months, which compares favorably to historical control patients treated with other therapies post hepatic resection.

Regional administration to optimize uptake at the tumor site relative to dose-limiting normal organs has been extensively explored with the most encouraging results in the adjuvant setting. Preclinical and clinical studies indicate that IP administration has pharmacologic advantages over IV administration for cancers confined to the peritoneal cavity, due to reduced circulating activity and lower hematologic toxicity secondary to increased antibody uptake in tumor, particularly for small-volume disease.[207-209] For example, Ward and coworkers[210] administered radioiodinated HMFG2 to patients with ovarian cancer prior to exploratory laparotomy and noted a 3.8- to greater than 70-fold increase in antibody uptake in malignant ascites cells when delivered via IP versus IV route. In a similar study, Chatal and coworkers[211] noted an advantage to IP administered antibody primarily in patients with small tumor nodules. At 72 hours, uptake of ^{111}In-OC125 was 128% injected dose per kilogram (ID/kg) for malignant ascites cells compared with 3.4% ID/kg for tumors larger than 10 cm.

Table 21-5 summarizes RIT trials that have administered therapy through the IP route. The antibody furthest along in development as a therapy agent is HMFG1. Epenetos and colleagues[212] first evaluated HMFG1, along with a panel of other anti–ovarian cancer antibodies, radiolabeled with ^{131}I in patients with ovarian cancer after debulking surgery, first-line chemotherapy, and second-look laparoscopy. Objective responses were more frequent in patients with smaller tumors or lower tumor burden. On follow-up laparoscopy, no responses were observed in patients with residual tumors larger than 2 cm, but CRs were seen in three of six patients with positive cytology only. Of particular interest were four patients with a negative second-look laparoscopy who

Table 21-5 Selected Intraperitoneal Solid Tumor Radioimmunotherapy Trials

Study (First Author)	Year	Antibody	Phase	Tumor Type	No. of Patients	Administered Activity/ Cycles	Objective Responses	Other Antitumor Effects
Stewart[212]	1989	^{131}I-HMFG1, AUA1, HMFG2, HE17E2	I/II	Ovary (after surgery, chemotherapy and second-look laparoscopy)	36	20-158 mCi	0/10 if >2-cm tumors 2/15 PR if <2-cm tumors 3/6 CR if positive cytology 4/4 NED at 6-12 mo if negative cytology	
Stewart[240]	1990	^{90}Y-HMFG1, AUA1	I/II	Ovary (after surgery, chemotherapy, and second-look laparoscopy)	25	5-25.2 mCi	0/3 if >2-cm tumors 1/10 PR if <2-cm tumors 0/1 if positive cytology 10/11 NED at 6-15 mo if negative cytology	
Nicholson[213]	1998	^{90}Y-HMFG1	II	Ovary (after surgery, chemotherapy, and negative second-look laparoscopy)	25	18 mCi/m^2	5-y actuarial survival 80% versus 55% matched historical controls ($P = .0035$); median follow-up 59 mo	
Rosenblum[441]	1999	^{90}Y-B72.3	I	Ovary, fallopian tube, papillary serous	58	1-40 mCi	2/57 CR 9-12 mo (both <3 cm)	2/57 Minor 30/57 Stable median 6 mo
Jacobs[443]	1993	^{186}Re-NR-LU-10	I	Ovary (recurrent or persistent)	17	25-180 mCi/m^2	4/7 PR if ≤1 cm 0/10 if >1 cm ($P < .05$)	4/13 ↓ CA-125
Meredith[217]	1998	^{177}Lu-CC49	I	Ovary (residual disease at second-look laparoscopy)	27	10-45 mCi/m^2	1/12 PR if >1 cm 3/15 NED for 3-5 y if <1 cm or positive cytology	
Crippa[216]	1995	^{131}I-Mov18	I	Ovary (<.5 cm residual after second-look laparoscopy)	16	100 mCi	5/16 CR	6/16 Stable
Mahe[442]	1999	^{131}I-OC125 F(ab′)$_2$	II	Ovary (<.5 cm residual after second-look laparoscopy)	6	120 mCi		3/6 Stable
Riva[444]	1991	^{131}I-FO23C5, BW494/32, B72.3, AUA1	II	Colorectal	16	21-150 mCi	2/15 CR (6-12 mo) 2/15 PR (3-16 mo)	3/15 Stable 6/10 ↓ CEA
Muto[445]	1992	^{131}I-OC125 F(ab′)$_2$	I	Ovary (refractory)	29	20-140 mCi		1/28 NED at 41 mo
Buckman[446]	1992	^{131}I-mab 2G3	I/II	Malignant ascites—ovary, breast	9	15-150 mCi		3/4 Temporary, ↓ ascites if >50 mCi administered
Wong (unpublished)		^{90}Y-cT84.66	I	Gastrointestinal, pseudomyxoma	13	5-19 mCi/m^2		5/13 Stable 2/13 Resolution of ascites

received RIT as adjuvant therapy. At the time of the analysis, all four were without evidence of disease 6 to 12 months posttherapy. This led to a phase II trial evaluating adjuvant IP ^{90}Y-HMFG1 at 18 mCi/m^2 in patients with initial stage Ic-IV after surgery, first-line chemotherapy, and negative second-look laparoscopy.[213] With a median follow-up of 59 months, a 5-year actuarial survival of 80% was reported, which was significantly better than the 55% observed for a matched historical control group ($P = .0035$). These results were recently updated with an actuarial 10-year survival of 73% reported.[214] ^{90}Y-HMFG1 is being evaluated in a multi-institutional randomized phase III trial for ovarian cancer patients with negative second-look laparoscopy after surgery and platinum-based chemotherapy.

Others have also seen encouraging results with IP RIT in patients with ovarian cancer in the minimal tumor burden setting. Jacobs and coworkers[215] observed PR in four of seven ovarian cancer patients with tumors less than 1 cm, but no responses in the 10 patients with larger tumors after treatment with IP ^{186}Re-NR-LU-10. Crippa and coworkers[216] noted CRs in 5 of 16 patients with residual disease less than 0.5 cm after IP ^{131}I-Mov18. In a phase I trial conducted by Meredith and colleagues, 3 of 15 ovarian cancer patients with microscopic or tumor less than 1 cm burden were without evidence of disease (NED) 3 to 5 years after ^{177}Lu-CC49 IP RIT.[217]

Regional delivery of RIT has also been evaluated in central nervous system malignancies, primarily high-grade gliomas (Table 21-6). Studies have investigated intracavitary administration after surgical resection, intralesional, intra-arterial, or intrathecal administration. Early efforts in patients with recurrent disease were encouraging, leading to trials evaluating this approach as adjuvant therapy in combination with standard surgical resection, external beam radiotherapy, and chemotherapy in patients with newly diagnosed high-grade gliomas. In general, therapy has been well tolerated. Reported toxicities have been neurologic and hematologic and have included temporary headache, seizure, and worsening of neurologic symptoms, with a few studies reporting irreversible neurologic symptoms in a small subset of patients at maximum tolerated doses.[218,219]

Intracavitary and intralesional delivery of radioiodinated antibodies against tenascin, an extracellular matrix protein expressed by gliomas but not by normal brain tissue, has been evaluated as single-cycle therapy in multi-institutional trials coordinated by investigators at Duke University and as multicycle therapy in Italy. Bigner and colleagues[218,220] have evaluated single administration of intracavitary ^{131}I-81C6 in recurrent and newly diagnosed high-grade gliomas (see Table 21-6). Phase II adjuvant RIT trial results were recently reported by Reardon and coworkers.[219] Thirty-three patients with previously untreated high-grade gliomas received a single treatment with 120 mCi of ^{131}I-81C6 directly into the surgical resection cavity, followed by conventional radiation therapy and 1 year of alkylator-based chemotherapy. The average radiation dose from RIT to the 2-cm rim around the resection cavity was 48 Gy. A median survival of 86.7 weeks for all patients and 79.4 weeks for glioblastoma patients was observed. A chimeric version of 81C6, radiolabeled with the alpha-emitter ^{211}At, is currently being evaluated.[221,222] Riva and colleagues in Italy have also investigated intracavitary and intralesional radiolabeled anti-tenascin RIT in resected high-grade glioma patients.[223-227] Goetz and coworkers[226] reported results of a multi-institutional trial in 37 patients with newly diagnosed disease receiving intracavitary ^{131}I- or ^{90}Y-labeled BC-4 after surgical resection and conventional radiotherapy. A mean of 2.96 cycles were administered. Median survival for patients with glioblastoma was 17 months. For grade III astrocytoma, the median survival has not yet been reached and an 85% 5-year probability of survival was predicted. Other antibodies have also been evaluated in a similar approach, with mean doses to the cavity rim of 5120 and 5500 cGy.[228-230] In addition, regional intrathecal administration has been evaluated in meningeal carcinomatosis and medulloblastoma with objective responses observed.[231-233]

Central nervous system malignancies have also been treated through intra-arterial and IV infusion of RIT using antibodies directed against EGFR.[234-236] Brady and colleagues[69,235-238] have administered ^{125}I-mAb 425, an internalizing murine IgG_{2a} directed against epidermal growth factor receptor (EGFR), in patients with high-grade gliomas. Emrich and coworkers[235,237,238] recently reported results of 180 patients treated on a Phase II trial delivering ^{125}I-mAb 425 as adjuvant therapy in patients with previously untreated disease. Most underwent prior surgical debulking and conventional radiotherapy, with approximately one third also receiving chemotherapy. RIT consisted of weekly intra-arterial or IV administrations of approximately 50 mCi for a mean of three cycles. For glioblastoma patients, which comprised the majority of the patients in the study population, median survival was 13.4 months, and 25.4 months for patients younger than 40 years with a Karnofsky Performance Status (KPS) greater than 70, with 10 patients still alive more than 5 years after therapy.

Hepatic arterial regional delivery of RIT in hepatocellular carcinoma has been investigated. Zeng and coworkers[239,240] reported their single-institution experience and observed a significantly higher rate of conversion to resectability for the group receiving hepatic arterial ^{131}I–Hepama-1 RIT compared with patients receiving hepatic arterial 5-fluorouracil (5-FU), cisplatin, and Adriamycin or chemoembolization and 46 Gy external beam radiotherapy. A 5-year survival rate of 28.1% for the RIT group was reported, which compared favorably to 9.1% for the chemotherapy group.

In summary, regional delivery of RIT to increase antibody uptake at the tumor site has shown promise in ovarian and central nervous system malignancies, particularly in the adjuvant setting. Randomized phase III trials evaluating the addition of adjuvant RIT to conventional multimodality therapy are under way for ovarian cancer and are needed to confirm the encouraging results in high-grade gliomas.

Multiple preclinical studies have documented additive or supra-additive antitumor effects with RIT and concurrent radiation-enhancing chemotherapy agents, such as gemcitabine, taxanes, cisplatin, 5-FU, halogenated pyrimidines, and topoisomerase inhibitors.[241-253] A growing number of clinical trials are evaluating the feasibility and potentially improved efficacy of concomitant chemotherapy and RIT, either adding chemotherapy to maximum tolerated doses of RIT or adding RIT as additional therapy to established chemotherapy regimens. In some studies, chemotherapy and RIT has been combined with other strategies to increase antibody delivery to tumor. For example, Meredith and coworkers[254] evaluated a regional combined-modality approach administering a single cycle of IP ^{177}Lu-CC49 RIT, IP paclitaxel, and subcutaneous α-interferon to enhance antigen expression and antibody targeting to tumor in patients with recurrent or refractory ovarian cancer. A maximum tolerated dose of 40 mg/m^2 of ^{177}Lu-CC49 and of 100 mg/m^2 of paclitaxel was achieved, demonstrating the feasibility of this approach. Four of 17 patients with computed tomography–measurable disease had a PR, and 4 of 27 patients with nonmeasurable disease remained progression free at 18+ to 37+ months. A subsequent phase I study of the same design evaluated IP ^{90}Y-CC49 in combination with IP paclitaxel and α-interferon.[255] With paclitaxel doses of 100 mg/m^2, a maximum tolerated dose of 24.2 mCi/m^2 of ^{90}Y-CC49 was achieved, which is comparable to administered activities achievable with IP RIT alone. Two of nine patients with measurable disease demonstrated a PR and 4 of 11 with nonmeasurable disease remained progression free at 15+ to 23+ months. Richman and coworkers[256] are also evaluating the combination of systemic paclitaxel and ^{90}Y-m170 anti–MUC-1 RIT in patients with metastatic breast and prostate cancer. Wong and coworkers reported the results of a phase I trial combining systemic ^{90}Y-cT84.66 anti-CEA RIT and 5-day continuous infusion 5-FU in patients with metastatic colorectal cancer. The maximum tolerated dose was 16.6 mCi/m^2 of ^{90}Y-cT84.66 and 1000 mg/m^2/day 5-FU, comparable to that expected for each agent alone, demonstrating the feasibility of

Table 21-5 **Selected Central Nervous System Radioimmunotherapy Trials**

Study (First Author), Year	Phase	Antibody	Route	Tumor Type	No. of Patients	Administered Activity/ Cycle	Other Therapies	Antitumor Effects	Survival
Brady,[236] 1990	I	^{125}I-425	IA	Glioma, grade II-IV recurrent	15	7-50 mCi		1/12 CR 11/12 Stable	8 mo median
Emrich,[238] 2002	II	^{125}I-425	IV or IA	Glioma, grade III/IV newly diagnosed	180	50 mCi	S, RT, C (56 patients)		13.4 mo median grade IV 25.4 mo age <40, KPS ≥70 50.9 mo grade III 62.3 mo age <40, KPS ≥70
Bigner,[220] 1998	I	^{131}I-81C6	IC	Recurrent glioma or metastases amenable to surgery	34	20-120 mCi	S	14/33 Stable	10 patients alive >5 y 60 wk median 56 wk for grade IV
Cokgor,[218] 2000	I	^{131}I-81C6	IC	Glioma, grade III/IV newly diagnosed	42	20-180 mCi	S, RT, C		79 wk median all patients, 69 wk for grade IV
Reardon,[219] 2002	II	^{131}I-81C6	IC	Glioma, grade III/IV newly diagnosed	32	120 mCi	S, RT, C		86.7 wk median 79.4 wk for grade IV
Riva,[223] 1995	I	^{131}I-BC-2 and BC-4	IC and intralesional	Glioma, grade III/IV recurrent and newly diagnosed	50	5-65 mCi	S, RT	3/50 CR 6/50 PR 11/50 Stable 11/50 NED mean 13 mo	20 mo median 18 mo recurrent 23 mo newly diagnosed
Goetz,[226] 2003	Pilot	^{131}I or ^{90}Y-BC-4	IC	Glioma, grade III/IV newly diagnosed	37	29.7 mCi mean	S, RT		17 mo median for grade IV For grade III, median not reached, estimate 85% 5-y survival
Kalofaonos,[234] 1989	I	^{131}I-EGFR1 or H17E2	IV or IA	Glioma, grade III/IV recurrent	10	40-140 mCi			1/10 NED for 3+ y
Papanastassiou,[229] 1993	Pilot	^{131}I-ERIC-1	IC	Glioma, grade III/IV recurrent	7	36-59 mCi		3/7 Stable	
Hopkins,[228] 1995	Pilot	^{90}Y-ERIC-1	IC	Glioma, grade III/IV recurrent	15	11-25 mCi			6 mo median 3 Alive at 4, 6, and 26 mo
Casaco,[230] 2004	I	^{188}Re-h-R3	IC	Glioma, grade III/IV newly diagnosed	5	10-15 mCi	S	2/4 Stable	2/4 (Grade IV glioma) alive at 1 y
Kemshead,[231] 1996	Pilot	^{131}I-HMFG1, Mel-14, M340	IT	Meningeal disease from carcinoma, melanoma and PNET	27	17-196 mCi		3/7 CR Carcinoma patients 7/18 PR in PNET	
Pizer,[232] 1991	Pilot	^{131}I-UJ181.4, M340, UJ13A, Mel-14	IT or intraventricular	Relapsed medulloblastoma	14	17-62 mCi		2/11 CR 2/11 PR 1/11 Stable	
Brown,[233] 1996	I	^{131}I-81C6	IT or IC with subarachnoid communication	High-grade glioma, ependymoma, medulloblastoma	31	40-100 mCi		1/31 PR 13/31 Stable	

C, chemotherapy; IA, intra-arterial; IC, intracavitary; IT, intrathecal; IV, intravenous; RT, external beam radiotherapy; S, surgery.

this combination.[257] Of 21 patients treated, there was 1 patient with a mixed response and 11 patients with stable disease of 3 to 8 months' duration. Phase I studies evaluating concomitant ^{90}Y-cT84.66 and gemcitabine systemically or intraperitoneally are ongoing at the same institution.

A few studies have combined external beam radiation therapy with RIT. Buchegger and coworkers[258] combined external beam radiotherapy to the liver with ^{131}I–anti-CEA mAb with acceptable toxicity. There has also been interest in combining various forms of systemic radiotherapy. For example, a pilot trial of 1320 cGy of total body irradiation (TBI) and ^{131}I-CC49, followed by stem cell reinfusion, in breast and prostate cancer patients resulted in four objective responses in 12 patients.[259] Similar studies are ongoing in lymphohematopoietic malignancies and are discussed later in this chapter. With the next generation of tomotherapy intensity-modulated radiation therapy technology, standard total body irradiation (TBI) may be replaced with conformal radiation therapy to large target regions, such as the marrow cavity, resulting in conformal avoidance of normal organs, such as the kidneys, heart, lungs, and liver.[260,261] The combination of antibody-guided radiation therapy and image-guided total marrow conformal radiation therapy should be associated with reduced nonhematologic toxicity in patients undergoing BMT. These strategies under study in lymphohematopoietic malignancies may eventually have applicability to patients with solid tumors.

As one of the first forms of targeted therapy, the introduction of radiolabeled antibodies into the clinic was understandably accompanied by high expectations and initially viewed by many as the "magic bullet" that would replace other established forms of therapy. In hindsight and in comparison with the results of other emerging biological and targeted therapies, these initial expectations were unrealistic. What has been gained through preclinical and clinical studies is a better understanding of the limitations and the challenges associated with RIT, many of which apply to both solid tumors and hematologic malignancies. As with other emerging therapies, RIT will find its role not as a monotherapy in most cases but rather as a therapy used rationally in combination with other modalities. Although a number of strategies to increase tumor uptake and antitumor effects of these agents have been encouraging, it is likely that no one strategy will be sufficient and that multiple strategies will be needed to achieve clinically important results in the solid tumor setting. Most important, RIT will probably be most effective for the treatment of solid tumors in patients with minimal tumor burden or when used in an adjuvant setting.

RADIOIMMUNOTHERAPY OF LYMPHOMA AND LEUKEMIA

RIT has been most successful for the treatment of lymphoma and leukemia. Representative clinical trials using RIT for B-cell NHL and T-cell lymphoma and leukemia have been summarized in Tables 21-7[94,262-293] and 21-8[294-297] in terms of general study design (nonmyeloablative versus myeloablative), radionuclide and antibody used, number of treatments, number of treated evaluable patients, and responses to date. Myeloablative studies have included bone marrow and/or peripheral stem cell collection and reinfusion. These trials differ in terms of eligibility criteria, antibody and radionuclides used, dose, number of treatments, doses of unlabeled antibody preinfused or coinfused, and the biodistribution or dosimetry estimations required for administration of a therapeutic dose of radiolabeled antibody. The results summarized in Table 21-7 are particularly promising and show a relatively high response rate with a number of durable PRs and CRs, with a subset of these responses ongoing at 5 years, and many patients experiencing remissions of longer duration than had been achieved with previous chemotherapy. The highest overall response and CR rates, and the longest remission durations, have been reported in patients treated with very high doses of radiolabeled antibody in single doses in conjunction with autologous BMT or SCT.[289-293] Although higher doses of RIT have tended to be more efficacious, there has not been a direct correlation between dose and response in most reported studies. These results are particularly encouraging because all of the patients treated in these trials have had recurrent disease following at least one form of conventional therapy. Many of the patients have had failed multiple courses of therapy, and some were unable to tolerate additional chemotherapy for a variety of reasons.

Two anti-CD20 mAbs conjugated to either ^{131}I (^{131}I-Tositumomab or Bexxar) or ^{90}Y (^{90}Y-ibritumomab tiuxetan or Zevalin) have been approved by the FDA for patients with relapsed or refractory low-grade or transformed B-cell NHL[281,282,286] and have demonstrated efficacy in patients even after the use of rituximab (Rituxan).[284,288] The Bexxar (Tositumomab and ^{131}I-Tositumomab) regimen consists of the sequential administration of a dose of unlabeled murine mAb, Tositumomab, to optimize biodistribution and increase tumor localization[298,299] of the ^{131}I-Tositumomab that is administered thereafter. An initial biodistribution study uses a dosimetric dose to allow for the calculation of a patient-specific therapeutic dose to deliver an absorbed whole-body dose of 75 cGy in patients with a platelet count of ≥150,000/μL. FDA approval was based on a study in 40 patients with relapsed/refractory disease after rituximab therapy and was further supported by the demonstration of durable responses in four other studies enrolling 190 patients with relapsed/refractory disease following chemotherapy. Objective tumor responses occurred in approximately 60% of patients, with CRs in approximately 30%. Median response durations have been in excess of 12 months, with occasional durable CRs[281,282,300,301] lasting for years.

The ^{90}Y-ibritumomab tiuxetan or Zevalin regimen uses the chimeric anti-CD20 antibody rituximab for predosing. The pivotal study that supported FDA approval of Zevalin randomized 143 patients to receive either rituximab alone (four weekly doses of 375 mg/m^2, as it is used as a therapeutic agent) or RIT with a lower dose (250 mg/m^2) of rituximab for purposes of optimizing the biodistribution of ^{111}In-labeled ibritumomab tiuxetan for an imaging/dosimetry study. Seven days later, patients received 250 mg/m^2 rituximab followed by 0.4 mCi/kg ^{90}Y-labeled ibritumomab tiuxetan. Based on the International Workshop NHL Response Criteria, the overall response rate was 80% for Zevalin versus 56% in the rituximab arm (P = .002). CRs were achieved in 30% of patients with Zevalin versus 16% for rituximab (P = .04).[286] Of those patients who have since progressed, the time to next therapy was 11.5 months after Zevalin and 7.8 months after rituximab.

Two randomized studies of either ^{90}Y–anti-CD20 mAb[286] or ^{131}I–anti-CD20 mAb[283] versus unlabeled anti-CD20 mAb have demonstrated the importance of the radiation associated with RIT as a determinant of both the efficacy and toxicity of the RIT treatment. The radiobiology of RIT targeting the CD20 antigen is critical to tumor and normal tissue effects associated with this therapy and was reviewed.[50] Retreatment with radiolabeled anti-CD20 mAb has also been reported to be well tolerated and efficacious in a subset of patients.[274,279,302]

The optimal time to use RIT in the course of NHL has not been defined. A trial using ^{131}I-Tositumomab as primary therapy for low-grade disease has shown impressive results,

Table 21-7 Radioimmunotherapy Trials for B-Cell Lymphoma

Antibody (Cumulative mg)	Radionuclide (Cumulative mCi)	Treatments	No. of Evaluable Patients	Responses	References
NONMYELOABLATIVE					
LYM-1 (8-676)	^{131}I (26-1044)	1-16	57	11 CR, 20 PR	DeNardo, 1994[262]; Lewis, 1995[263]; DeNardo, 1998[264]
	^{131}I-(40-100/m^2/ treatment)	1-4	21	7 CR, 4 PR	DeNardo, 1998[265]
LYM-1 (30-67)	^{131}I (50-267)	1-2	13	4 PR	Kuzel, 1993[266]; Meredith, 1993[267]
LYM-1 (17-290)	^{67}Cu (40-438)	1-4	12	1 CR, 4 PR, 2 MR	O'Donnell, 1999[268,269]
	^{90}Y (.185-0.370 GBq/ m^2)	1	8	5 PR or SD	O'Donnell, 2000[270]
LL2- (epratuzumab) [1.1 mg IgG-157 mgF/(ab')$_2$]	^{131}I (15-343)	1-7	17	2 CR, 2 PR, 2 MR	Juweid, 1995[94]
LL2 (N/A)	^{186}Re (.5-2.0 GBq/m^2)	1	15	1 CR, 4 PR	Postema, 2003[271]
Humanized LL-2 (41-139)	^{131}I (15-59)	1	13	1 CR, 1 PR	Juweid, 1999[272]
	^{90}Y (15-22.5 mCi/m^2)	1	13	8 Objective responses	Chatal, 2004[273]
LL2 (0-160)	^{131}I (30-120 mCi/m^2)	2-8	21	5 CR, 2 PR	Vose, 1997[274]
MB-1 (40)	^{131}I (25-161)	1	10	1 CR, 2 PR, 1 MR	Kaminski, 1992[275]
OKB7 (25)	^{131}I (90-200)	3-4	18	1 PR, 12 MR	Czuczman, 1993[276]
Anti-idiotype (1000-4050)	^{90}Y (10-54)	1-4	9	2 CR, 1 PR, 1 MR	Parker, 1990[277]; White, 1996[278]
Tositumomab (2-110)	^{90}Y (14-22)	1	4	1 CR, 1 PR	Knox, 1996[279]
Tositumomab (10-518)	^{131}I (33-161)	1	59	20 CR, 22 PR	Kaminski, 2000[280]
Tositumomab (484-487)	^{131}I (45-177)	1	47	15 CR, 12 PR	Vose, 2000[281]
Tositumomab (450-506)	^{131}I ($0 \leq 198$)	1	60	10 CR, 29 PR	Kaminski, 2001[282]
Tositumomab (485)	^{131}I (NA)	1	42	14 CR, 9 PR	Davis, 2003[283]
Tositumomab (485)	^{131}I (NA)	1	38	8 CR, 14 PR	Horning, 2002[284]
Chimeric C2B8 (Rituximab; cumulative mg N/A)	^{90}Y (51-109)	1	7	3 CR, 1 PR, 2 MR	Weiden, 2000[285]
Ibritumomab Tiuxetan 2B8 (55-294)	^{90}Y (20-53)	1-2	14	5 CR, 6 PR	Knox, 1996[279*]
Ibritumomab Tiuxetan 2B8 (Rituximab; 100-250 mg/m^2 × 2)	^{90}Y (12-32)	1	50	13 CR, 21 PR	Witzig, 1999[287]
Ibritumomab Tiuxetan 2B8 (Rituximab; 250 mg/m^2 × 2)	^{90}Y (≤32)	1	73	25 CR, 33 PR	Witzig, 2002[286]
Ibritumomab Tiuxetan 2B8 (Rituximab; 250 mg/m^2 × 2)	^{90}Y (NA)	1	54	8 CR, 32 PR	Witzig, 2002[288]
MYELOABLATIVE					
^{131}I (280-785)	Tositumomab (58-1168)	1	29	23 CR, 2 PR	Press, 1993[289]; Liu, 1998[290]; Press, 1995[291]
^{131}I (608)	1F5 (274)	1	1	1 PR	Press, 1993[289]
^{131}I (234-628)	MB1 (275-970)	1	6	6 CR	Press, 1993[289]; Press, 1989[292]
^{131}I (232)	Anti-idiotype (1000)	1	1	1 CR	Badger, 1987[293]
^{131}I (145-323)	LL2 (epratuzumab) (97-111)	1	7	2 PR, 3 MR	Unpublished data[†]; Juweid, 1995[94]
^{90}Y (5-10 mCi/m^2)	LL2 (NA)	1	9	5 Objective responses	Chatal, 2004[273]
^{90}Y (20)	Tositumomab (NA)[§]	1	3	1 PR, 1 MR	Unpublished data[‡]

*A Phase I dose escalation trial; two patients required stem cell reinfusion, of four patients treated at the highest dose (50 mCi)
[†]Personal communication from Dr. D. M. Goldenberg, 1997.
[‡]Personal communication from Drs. S. O'Day and L. M. Nadler, 1994.
[§]NA, not available.
Adapted from Knox SJ: Radioimmunotherapy of the non-Hodgkin's lymphomas. Semin Radiat Oncol 5:331-341, 1995.

Table 21-8 Radioimmunotherapy Trials for T-Cell Lymphoma and Leukemia

Radionuclide (Cumulative mCi)	Antibody (Cumulative mg)	Treatment	No. of Evaluable Patients	Responses	References
NONMYELOABLATIVE					
^{131}I (25-50)	T101 (10)	1	4	0*	Zimmer, 1988[294†]
^{131}I (100-150)	T101 (10-16)	1‡	6	2 PR, 4 MR	Rosen, 1989[295]
^{90}Y (NA)	T101 (NA)§	1	6	3 CR	Raubitschek, 1990[296‖]
^{90}Y (5-15)	Anti-Tac (2-10)	1-9	16	2 CR, 9 PR	Waldmann, 1995[297¶]

*No objective clinical responses were observed; however, a transient decrease in peripheral blood lymphocytes was observed in one patient.
†CLL, chronic lymphocytic leukemia.
‡Three patients were subsequently re-treated, but responses shown are for the first treatment with a single dose of ^{131}I-T101.
§NA, not available.
‖CLL, chronic lymphocytic leukemia; CTCL, cutaneous T-cell lymphoma.
¶Adult T-cell leukemia.
Adapted from Knox SJ: Radioimmunotherapy of the non-Hodgkin's lymphomas. Semin Radiat Oncol 5:331-341, 1995.

with a response rate of 95% and evidence of conversion to molecular negativity by polymerase chain reaction (PCR) testing for Bcl-2 rearrangements in 84% of patients.[303] Response durations have not yet been defined. Patients for whom BMT failed have experienced excellent tumor responses to RIT as well.[273,304] RIT has also been useful as a preparatory regimen for transplantation.[289-293] In a clinical trial comparing high-dose RIT with conventional high-dose chemotherapy with hematopoietic SCT, the RIT group had higher overall survival (OS) and progression-free survival (PFS) than the group of patients who received the conventional preparatory regimen for transplantation.[305] Other trials of ^{131}I-Tositumomab combined with etoposide, cyclophosphamide, and autologous stem cell transplantation (ASCT) compared with TBI combined with etoposide, cyclophosphamide, and ASCT also demonstrated improved OS and PFS in the group receiving RIT.[306] The same regimen has yielded very encouraging results in patients with mantle cell lymphoma, with 3-year PFS of 61%.[307] ^{131}I-Tositumomab has also been studied in combination with BEAM (BCNU, etoposide, Ara-C, and melphalan) followed by ASCT. Toxicity was similar to BEAM alone. The CR rate was 59% and overall response rate was 68%, with 3-year event-free survival of 39% and overall survival of 55%.[308]

Other approaches to increase the efficacy of RIT in B-cell NHL include the use of a pretargeting regimen using an anti–CD20-fusion peptide.[309] This approach is based on the dissociation of the delivery of antibody from the delivery of radionuclide, with a clearing agent used in between to eliminate unbound circulating antibody, which, if radiolabeled, would be a source of nonspecific radiation and therefore toxicity. Proof of principle for this platform technology has been demonstrated in a clinical trial[309] with significantly increased tumor/whole-body, tumor/blood, and tumor/normal organ ratios than achievable with directly labeled mAb.

Another area of active investigation is the study of RIT as part of a combined-modality approach with either chemotherapy or conventional radiation therapy. A variety of clinical trials are under way to study the safety and efficacy of radiolabeled anti-CD20 mAb as a component of combined-modality therapy. For example, a phase II trial (SWOG 9911) of CHOP chemotherapy combined with ^{131}I–anti-CD20 mAb in 90 newly diagnosed follicular NHL patients resulted in a CR and PR rate of 67% and 23%, respectively. Two-year PFS was 81%, and OS was 97%.[310] These results provided the rationale for an ongoing phase III trial (SWOG 0016) of CHOP plus rituximab and CHOP combined with ^{131}I–anti-CD20 mAb. It is noteworthy that patients with NHL who undergo RIT therapy can well tolerate subsequent chemotherapy regimens or ASCT,[311] with toxicity from subsequent therapy being similar to that observed in patients not previously treated with RIT.

Results from clinical studies of RIT for the treatment of patients with recurrent Hodgkin's disease have been encouraging. These studies have used ^{131}I labeled anti-ferritin antibody[312] or ^{90}Y labeled anti-ferritin antibody.[93,313-315] Overall, 134 patients with recurrent Hodgkin's disease have been treated in five different studies with radiolabeled antiferritin antibody.[316] Results obtained with ^{90}Y-antiferritin antibody were better than those obtained with ^{131}I-antiferritin antibody. ^{90}Y-antiferritin antibody therapy resulted in a response rate of 60%, with a CR rate of 30%. The extent of response was associated with survival, with 50% of patients with CR, PR, and progressive disease alive at 2 years, 1 year, and 4 months, respectively.[316] Responses in these studies were more common in patients with disease histories longer than 3 years, tumor volumes less than 30 cm^3, and patients receiving at least 0.4 mCi/kg of ^{90}Y-labeled antiferritin antibody.[316]

A variety of radiolabeled antibodies have been safely administered to patients with advanced acute leukemia and have been shown to have significant antileukemic activity and to enhance the antileukemic effects of SCT-conditioning regimens (e.g., beta-emitting ^{131}I–anti-CD33, ^{90}Y–anti-CD33, ^{131}I–anti-CD45, and ^{188}Re–anti-CD66c). Radioimmunoconjugates that emit alpha particles with a very short range (e.g., ^{213}Bi) may be most useful for low-volume and/or microscopic residual leukemic disease.[317] Studies using RIT targeting the CD33 antigen, which is expressed on early myeloid progenitor cells and myeloid leukemia cells, have yielded promising results that may improve the efficacy of marrow transplantation. In a dose-escalation trial of ^{131}I-murine anti-CD33 (M195) in patients with relapsed or refractory myeloid leukemia,[83] 8 of 24 patients treated with 50 to 210 mCi/m^2 in divided doses had sufficient marrow cytoreduction to proceed to BMT, and 3 of these patients achieved marrow remission, but 37% of assessable patients developed HAMA. ^{131}I-M195 (120 to 230 mCi/m^2) was then combined with busulfan (BU) and cyclophosphamide (CY) in an effort to intensify therapy prior to first or second BMT.[95] All patients engrafted, and 18 achieved CRs, with 3 patients following first BMT remaining in nonmaintained remission for 18+ and 29+ months. Six patients relapsed, and 10 patients died in CR of transplant-related complications.[95] HAMA occurred in 37.5% of evaluable patients. Nevertheless, these studies provided data that suggest leukemic cytoreduction could be safely achieved with ^{131}I–anti-CD33, even in multiply relapsed or chemotherapy-refractory leukemia, and that RIT may be useful as part of a preparatory regimen for BMT in myeloid leukemia.

Next, a study was performed with ^{131}I-M195 (50 or 70 mCi/m^2) in seven patients with relapsed acute promyelocytic leukemia (APL) in second remission following treatment with all-*trans* retinoic acid.[318] Two of six patients with detectable promyelocytic leukemia/retinoic acid receptor-α gene translocation (PML/RAR-α) messenger RNA after all-*trans* retinoic acid therapy had negative reverse transcriptase-PCR determinations following ^{131}I-MI95. Median disease-free survival was 8 months, and median overall survival was longer than 21+ months, demonstrating that this regimen compared favorably with other approaches for the treatment of relapsed APL,[318] but HAMA developed in five of the seven patients. Because of the immunogenicity of the murine M195 antibody, a humanized M195 antibody was developed that had an avidity 4 to 8.6 times higher than the murine antibody.[319] A homodimeric humanized IgG1 antibody was also developed that had improved effector function, as well as the ability to internalize and retain radioisotope in targeted leukemia cells.[319] This humanized M195 (Hu-M195) was subsequently used in a phase 1B trial,[320] in which patients with relapsed or refractory myeloid leukemia were treated at dose levels of 0.5 to 10.0 mg/m^2 and patients received six doses over 8 days. Optimal biodistribution occurred at 3 mg/m^2, and HAMA responses were not observed.[320]

^{131}I-M195 and HuM195 have also been studied in combination with chemotherapy as a conditioning regimen for allogeneic transplant. Absorbed doses to the bone marrow ranged between 272 and 1470 cGy. Median survival was 4.9 months (range, 0.3 to 90+), and three patients with relapsed AML have ongoing CRs at 59+ to 90+ months following BMT. These results demonstrate the feasibility of using radiolabeled anti-CD33 in combination with a standard BMT preparatory regimen, but randomized trials will be needed to determine whether there is a statistically significant benefit to intensified conditioning with RIT.[321]

The alpha emitter ^{213}Bi has been conjugated to Hu-M195 in an effort to increase the efficacy of RIT with this antibody without the nonspecific effects of beta-emitting radionuclides. ^{213}Bi has a $t_{1/2}$ of 45.6 minutes and emits high LET alpha particles (8 MeV) with a path length of approximately 60 to 90 μm in tissue. Therefore, ^{213}Bi-labeled mAb can theoretically kill leukemia cells with one or two alpha particles with minimal bystander effect. A phase I dose-escalation study at Memorial Sloan-Kettering Cancer Center using ^{213}Bi-Hu-M195 in patients with refractory and relapsed myeloid leukemias demonstrated rapid targeting of disease sites within minutes, with evidence of antileukemic effects even at low-dose levels.[322] In a study of 18 patients with relapsed and refractory AML or chronic myelomonocytic leukemia treated with 37.0 MBq/kg ^{213}Bi-HuM195, there was no significant extramedullary toxicity. The median time to hematologic recovery was 22 days. Target/background and target/whole-body ratios were greatly enhanced compared with those seen with immunoconjugates using beta emitters in this patient population. With this therapy, 78% of patients had a decrease in the percentage of bone marrow blasts.[323]

Other very encouraging results have been achieved using RIT targeting the CD45 antigen with ^{131}I–anti-CD45 (BC8 antibody) combined with CY and TBI as a marrow transplant regimen for acute leukemia and myelodysplastic syndrome (MDS).[324] Forty-four patients received a biodistribution dose of 0.5 mg/kg ^{131}I–anti-CD45, which delivered 6.5 ± 0.5 cGy/mCi to the marrow, with a mean dose to the spleen of 13.5 ± 1.3 cGy/mCi. Doses to liver, lung, kidney, and total body were significantly less, and 84% of patients had a favorable biodistribution of antibody, with higher estimated radiation absorbed doses to the marrow and spleen than to normal organs. Thirty-four patients received a therapeutic dose of ^{131}I–anti-CD45 labeled with 76 to 612 mCi of ^{131}I in addition to CY and TBI. The maximum tolerated dose delivered 10.5 Gy to the liver. Seven of 25 treated patients with AML/MDS survived disease free 15 to 89 months (median, 65 months) post-transplant, and three of nine patients with ALL were disease free 19, 54, and 66 months posttransplant. This study demonstrates that RIT with ^{131}I–anti-CD45 can be used safely to deliver additional targeted radiation to bone marrow (approximately 24 Gy) and spleen (approximately 50 Gy) when combined with CY/TBI.[324]

TOXICITY ASSOCIATED WITH TARGETED RADIONUCLIDE THERAPY

Bone marrow suppression has been the primary dose-limiting toxicity of most conventional TaRT. Among multiple factors that may influence the extent and duration of myelosuppression, marrow reserve, recovery from prior therapy, and radioconjugate stability appear to be predominant determinants of this effect.[325,326] Hematologic support with transfusions and growth factors has been helpful, and bone marrow or peripheral stem cell reinfusion has allowed dose escalation of radioconjugates to at least threefold over the dose that results in dose-limiting hematopoietic toxicity.[305] Interleukin-1 and GM-CSF have been reported to have radioprotective effects on the hematopoietic system.[327,328] The adjuvant use of these cytokines with TaRT has resulted in modest protection. Additionally, the radioprotector Amifostine has been helpful in preclinical radionuclide studies and for the therapy of thyroid disease with ^{131}I.[329,330] Similar effects with radioconjugates are expected, but this potential effect has not been well studied. Adjuvant use of chelating agents in combination with unstable metal radioconjugates can help to minimize toxicity but has had only a minor protective effect when used with stable chelators.[331,332] In addition to chelators that remove unbound radioactivity from the blood, "chasing" the radiolabeled antibody with a second unlabeled antibody directed against the radiolabeled antibody has been reported to modestly decrease toxicity.[333] Pretargeting approaches, which dissociate and delay the delivery of the radionuclide from that of the targeting agent, can decrease toxicity and are discussed in more detail in the Optimization section. Although second dose-limiting organ toxicity for myeloablative TaRT may vary with radionuclide, cardiopulmonary and liver toxicity has been reported for ^{131}I and ^{90}Y immunoconjugates, respectively.[146,291,334]

Acute symptoms from RIT are usually related to administration of antibody products. The symptoms have generally been mild and have included rash, fever, chills, myalgia, diaphoresis, pruritus, nausea, vomiting, diarrhea, nasal congestion, and hypotension.[335] These side effects are very transient and usually respond to antihistamines, acetaminophen, and nonsteroidal anti-inflammatory drugs. Rarely, more severe symptoms, including rigors, bronchospasm, or laryngeal edema, have been noted. These often respond quickly to steroids, antihistamines, oxygen, and meperidine. With central nervous system administration, various transient symptoms have been described, which are usually mild but can include cerebral edema, nuchal rigidity, aseptic meningitis, increased intracranial pressure, and seizure. Steroids have usually ameliorated these symptoms.

A serum sickness–like phenomenon has been commonly observed with IP administration of murine antibody conjugates (affecting about one third of patients), but it is rare among patients receiving IV RIT, even with the same radioimmunoconjugate. Serum sickness–like symptoms occur about 2 weeks after treatment and may persist for longer than 1 week. Variation in the manifestation of symptoms may depend in part on the particular radioimmunoconjugate used, because skin rash has been noted by the Hammersmith group, whereas fever with joint and/or muscle aches, but no rash, has been common among patients treated at the University of Alabama at Birmingham with a different radiolabeled monoclonal antibody.[212,336]

Late bowel toxicity after IP RIT has been infrequent, which is an advantage compared with nonspecific radionuclide therapy (e.g., ^{32}P). Thus far, late toxicity following RIT with ^{131}I-labeled antibodies has been uncommon except for abnormal thyroid function.[290] Elevated thyroid-stimulating hormone levels occurred in 59% of patients treated with myeloablative doses of ^{131}I–anti-CD20 antibodies, at a median of 6 months after treatment. Some patients who received nonmyeloablative doses of ^{131}I have also had elevated thyroid-stimulating hormone levels at later times. Salivary gland inflammation and damage can be an acute and/or late toxicity. Parotiditis, which may result in xerostomia, has been more common with treatment of thyroid cancer than high-dose radioconjugate therapy. However, this remains a potential toxicity of ^{131}I-antibody therapy.[337] A small percentage of patients have developed second malignancies. Of most concern for TaRT treatment–related effects is myelodysplasia. It is difficult to quantify any increased risk for myelodysplasia due to TaRT because patients have often received alkylating agents with or without conventional external beam radiation (also a risk factor in combination with alkylating agents), and some patients have shown evidence of dysplasia prior to radionuclide therapy.[282]

In TaRT using small molecules, such as peptides or radionuclide conjugates used in pretargeting approaches, the kidney and bladder usually receive much higher doses than other normal organs. For these therapies, renal, rather than bone marrow, toxicity can be dose limiting.[29,26] Fractionated radionuclide delivery may reduce toxicity and increase efficacy.[338] Limited clinical studies and radiobiological considerations of fractionated TaRT have been reviewed elsewhere.[339] Fractionation of dosing has been helpful for decreasing toxicity associated with peptide-radionuclide therapy and has been investigated in other TaRTs.[339]

DOSIMETRY

Dosimetry is the process of relating the administered amount of radioactivity to the absorbed radiation dose in tumors, organs, or the whole body. Dosimetry is important for dose correlation with clinical results, and in some instances, for treatment planning to avoid excess toxicity. The doses calculated for TaRT are less accurate than for external beam radiation therapy for a variety of reasons. These include limited radiation dose input data (e.g., few sample points for a therapy utilizing continuous exponentially decreasing irradiation), inhomogeneous dose distributions, and the assumptions/calculation methodology used to estimate TaRT absorbed doses. Dose calculation is also more complicated for internally distributed radionuclides than for external beam irradiation.

Data required for TaRT dose estimate calculations include the mass of tumors and normal organs, the cumulative radioactivity taken up by organs and tumors, and the pharmacokinetics of the administered radioactivity.[340] Data are usually acquired by serial gamma camera imaging. Bone marrow dose estimates are based on imaging studies of bony regions of active marrow such as the spine or blood pharmacokinetics.[341,342] Although there have been attempts to provide dosimetry based on Bremsstrahlung images from radionuclides that do not have gamma emissions, this is not commonly done. The images are of suboptimal quality, making accurate quantitation difficult. Instead, estimates are made for nongamma emitters from tracer studies using a gamma emitter that has a similar chemistry to that of the therapeutic radionuclide. Because animal studies have shown that the biodistribution is similar, although not usually identical, for ^{111}In and ^{90}Y, tracer/dosimetry studies with ^{111}In-labeled antibody have frequently been performed in conjunction with ^{90}Y-labeled antibody therapy to estimate the subsequent biodistribution/dosimetry of the ^{90}Y-immunoconjugate.[146,343] Quantitative immuno-PET with ^{89}Zr-labeled antibody has shown good correlation with ^{111}In-labeled antibody biodistribution and may be useful as a positron-emitting surrogate for ^{90}Y-labeled antibody therapy.[344] Other examples include use of ^{99m}Tc-antibody for imaging/dosimetry studies in conjunction with ^{186}Re-antibody therapy.[89] Another variable in estimating the expected dose from therapeutic RIT using preliminary biodistribution/dosimetry is that even when a small amount of a therapeutic agent (trace labeled study using the same antibody and radionuclide that will be used for therapy) is used, there can be either extremely good correlation between doses predicted and later delivered, or a significant discrepancy in the range of approximately 30% between estimated absorbed doses for the two procedures in the same patient.[267,345,346]

To estimate dose, conjugate views of the whole body and regions of interest (ROIs) (e.g., tumors and normal organs such as liver) are obtained. The activity for each ROI is measured from the counts in that region at multiple time points. The counts in each ROI are corrected for background. Attenuation correction factors are calculated for each patient, and a sample of the administered radionuclide is used for calibration so that counts per minute can be converted to units of radioactivity (mCi or MBq). SPECT (single-photon emission computed tomography) of an ROI may provide superior definition and quantitation, but this has not yet become the standard for quantitation and is more time consuming than planar conjugate view methodology.[347] Absorbed radiation doses can be calculated from radioactivity quantitation and the specific absorbed fraction for the target. The specific absorbed fraction takes into account the type and energy of radiation emissions, the fraction of energy from the source absorbed by the target, and mass of the target.[348] The mass of each ROI is usually determined by estimating volumes from CT, MRI, or other methods such as ^{99m}Tc-sulphur colloid liver scans, and converting volume to mass by assuming a unit density of 1 g/mm^3. Accounting for excretory routes is needed in quantitating changes in radioactivity distribution over time. For radionuclides such as ^{131}I where the major route of excretion is renal, urinary activity measurements can provide an estimate of total body clearance if it is not feasible to obtain whole-body counts.

The Medical Internal Radiation Dose (MIRD) committee of the Society of Nuclear Medicine provides guidance for methods to calculate radiation absorbed dose estimates for the whole body and organs.[349] This methodology has been adapted for TaRT, with continuing effort by this committee and others to further improve the models and methods available.[348-353] MIRD 16, other informational publications, Web sites, and computer programs have been developed to assist with these calculations.[354,355] Among available Web sites, www.doseinfo-radar.com was developed to provide information in a number of areas including standardized dose estimates, decay data, and absorbed fractions. With fusion of anatomic and physiologic images, dose estimates can be calculated in three dimensions at the voxel level, taking into account heterogeneity of radioactivity distribution within an organ.[356,357]

Biopsy results are infrequently used for dosimetry. Although biopsy provides a direct measurement and can be used for autoradiography, it is invasive and not practical for most tumor and organ dosimetry. Although biopsy data are of interest to correlate with other methods of dosimetry, they are of limited value alone because of the small sample size, which may not be representative, and are usually only done once. Thus, biopsy dosimetry does not allow a time-activity curve to be generated. Implanted dosimeters have also been used for quantitation in experimental preclinical studies and in limited clinical trials.[358] When used in patients with ovarian cancer treated with IP RIT, TLD-obtained dose measurements were in the range of those estimated with other methods.[89] As with biopsy, TLDs provide a direct measurement of absorbed dose, but also usually require an invasive procedure for placement that has the disadvantage of potentially introducing a sampling error. Like most other dosimetry methods, TLDs do not account for dose rate, which may be an important determinant of dose-response relationships. As stated earlier, PET scanning with ^{124}I-labeled antibody or other agents is an interesting new approach to RIT dosimetry and may prove to be useful in the future.[359] Thus far PET images from ^{89}Zr-cG250 antibody have been superior to those of ^{111}In-cG250 antibody in an animal model.[360]

The relationship between outcome and radiation dose–related factors is variable, with some studies showing a strong correlation while others show no correlation.[100,361,362] Some of the factors making it more difficult to establish a dose-response relationship for TaRT, compared with external beam radiation therapy, may include relative uncertainty associated with TaRT dose calculations, the heterogeneity of dose deposition that occurs with TaRT, dose-rate effects, and agent/patient variation in excretion/clearance. Whereas most normal organ tolerance levels for external beam radiation have been established using high-dose-rate radiation and vary as a function of fraction size, the dose rate is often low and variable with TaRT, limiting the validity of extrapolating from high-dose-rate tolerance levels to those expected with TaRT. Fractionation of TaRT, as with external beam, increases the total radionuclide dose tolerated.[29,339] Several studies have demonstrated how biological factors affect tolerance but are not accounted for in standard dose/toxicity reporting. To date, one of the strongest dose/toxicity correlations has been with adjustment of calculated absorbed marrow dose for levels of a biomarker involved in hematopoiesis.[326] Although data suggest the presence of a relationship between TaRT radiation dose and tumor response, analyses to date with relatively small numbers of patients fail to show strong correlation between these two factors.[362,363]

OPTIMIZATION OF TARGETED RADIONUCLIDE THERAPY

Encouraging results have been obtained in TaRT studies using a variety of targeting agents, radionuclides, and study designs. The success with lymphomas has spurred much investigation to further optimize this form of therapy in NHL and other malignancies.[2,7,74,96] Multiple presentations from recent meetings, including ASTRO, ASCO, ASH, and SNM, have reported encouraging results from attempts to further optimize TaRT. Although much progress has been made, especially in reducing immunogenicity of antibody-derived targeting agents and improving radionuclide conjugate chemistry, many challenges remain.

One of the main limitations of systemic TaRT has been the low uptake of radioactivity (generally <0.001% ID/g) in tumors. This low uptake is affected by such factors as tumor vascularity, size, charge, affinity and avidity of the targeting agent, and the interstitial pressure in tumors.[365] The use of small targeting agents may improve tumor penetration with more rapid tumor uptake, but they are generally limited by a relatively short retention time/half-life.[366,367] Other approaches for increasing tumor uptake of radiolabeled antibody include the use of external beam therapy. In early studies, external beam radiation therapy was used to increase vascular permeability.[368] More recent studies show it may also increase the expression of some targeted antigens that could potentially enhance efficacy.[369] In patients, the combination of external beam therapy with TaRT increased the objective response rate of liver tumors to RIT. This combined approach has used both local and TBI in stem cell rescue studies during which radiolabeled antibody was still circulating.[259,370] In colon cancer, RIT has been combined with proton therapy in preclinical studies.[371] The use of hyperthermia and vasoactive cytokines such as interleukin-2 and tumor necrosis factor have also resulted in higher tumor uptake of radiolabeled antibody in early studies.[372-374] Many studies have been preclinical; however, hyperthermia and interleukin-2 have been used clinically in conjunction with RIT with some success.[375] Of note, hyperthermia can have multiple effects including increased antigen expression, direct cytotoxic activity, and reduced interstitial fluid pressure.[376-378] Hyperthermia enhances both antibody uptake in tumor via vascular mechanisms and low-dose-rate radiation effects.[378,379] Neovascular targeting is also a promising approach to use in combination with TaRT, such as targeting upregulated receptors on new tumor vessels.[33,379] Antiangiogenic agents can also be combined with TaRT.[36,381] For example, a selective peptide agonist of human C5a, given before and after radiolabeled antibody therapy to increase vascular permeability of tumor capillaries, improved the therapeutic outcome of TaRT in xenograft tumors.[382] Fractionation of TaRT dosing has generally been favorable in many preclinical investigations and in limited clinical experience.[339] However, more study is needed, as some preclinical studies have shown decreased vascular permeability with fractionation, which could have a deleterious effect.[383] As previously discussed, high-affinity antibodies have been reported to improve antibody uptake but not necessarily intratumor distribution, and in some cases high-affinity antibodies have produced a more favorable therapeutic ratio. Clinical trials using high-affinity antibodies have been performed for cancer of the colon, breast, prostate, lung, and ovary.[103,105,332,384,385] Targeting may also be enhanced by increasing antigen expression on target cells.[386] Several studies show that interferon can increase the expression of some common tumor-associated antigens, including CEA, TAG-72, and an antigen expressed on melanomas.[190,387] Applications of this approach in vivo using human tumor xenografts in mice have shown greater tumor growth inhibition with interferon administration before RIT compared with similarly treated mice without interferon.[192] Human tumor biopsy material has also confirmed increased antigen expression following interferon administration. However, benefit from adjuvant interferon in clinical trials has been difficult to demonstrate. Potential benefit may be inferred because increased tumor antigen expression was demonstrated by biopsy, and imaging of antibody localization in known sites of disease was improved by interferon compared with results obtained in other trials with similar radiolabeled antibodies that did not use interferon.[197,388]

Several pretargeting methods have been proposed to overcome some of the limitations of conventional one-step TaRT, where prolonged radiation exposure of the bone marrow results in dose-limiting marrow suppression. As previously mentioned, pretargeting approaches dissociate the delivery of unlabeled antibody, or other targeting entity, from the delivery of the radionuclide. Ideally, this approach delays the delivery of the radioactivity until the ratio of tumor-bound to non–tumor-bound targeting agent has reached its maximum. Because the radionuclide is usually given conjugated to a small hapten that interacts with the targeting entity, any nonbound radioactivity will clear quickly because of the small molecular weight of the radionuclide conjugate. Thus, the pretargeting approach has the potential to improve tumor/normal tissue ratios severalfold over that achieved with directly labeled antibodies by minimizing circulation time of unbound radionuclide. Proof of principle of the pretargeting approach has been established in multiple preclinical and early phase clinical trials while studies continue for further optimization.[26,309,389]

Several pretargeting designs have been devised and others are in development. To date, the most popular are based on the use of bifunctional antibodies or biotin-streptavidin interactions, with these components complexed to a targeting agent and radionuclide. Less common pretargeting approaches include the use of antibody-oligonucleotide conjugates, a prodrug/enzyme strategy, and DNA/DNA systems.[390,391] Other mechanisms that allow for amplification/enhancement of targeting are under study.[392] Common to all methods is the desire for (1) high specificity and retention of the targeting agent, without shedding or internalization, (2) high specificity of the radionuclide conjugate for the bound targeting agent, and (3) rapid clearance of radionuclide that does not localize to target.

Some bifunctional antibodies have been constructed by cross-linking Fab′ fragments from two antibodies that have different specificities.[393-395] For RIT, one end of a bifunctional antibody contains an unlabeled fragment directed toward a tumor-associated antigen, while the other binding site reacts with a hapten linked to a radionuclide. Sharkey and colleagues[394] designed a "universal" system by making one Fab′ fragment specific for the chelating agent that is conjugated to the radionuclide. Thus, different radionuclides can be used as long as they are complexed to that chelating agent. Bivalent nonantibody peptides have also been developed.[393,396]

Advantages of the biotin-streptavidin system include not only the small molecular weight of biotin, which can quickly circulate throughout the body, but also the high binding affinity between biotin and avidin or streptavidin (10^{15}/mol/L). Streptavidin is tetravalent (has four biotin binding sites) and can thereby increase the amount of radionuclide localization in tumor. On the other hand, a disadvantage of the biotin/streptavidin system is the immunogenicity of streptavidin or avidin. Polyethylene glycol (PEG) modification can reduce this immunogenicity, but may also decrease the binding capacity of biotin.[393,397]

Although the concept of pretargeting does not require a clearing step between administration of the targeting agent and radionuclide, use of a clearing agent can further enhance the tumor/normal tissue ratio. Theoretical and experimental pharmacokinetic modeling studies suggest that pretargeting approaches using a two-step method will result in a twofold to threefold enhancement of efficacy compared with conventional one-step RIT.[393,398] Use of a clearing agent can further improve tumor/normal tissue ratios severalfold. A variety of clearing mechanisms have been studied to date, including use of an antibody that reacts with the targeting agent, plasmapheresis/extracorporeal immunoadsorption, and large-molecular-weight agents that react with the targeting agent in the circulation or other agents that are primarily confined to vasculature.[399-402] The primary objective of clearing strategies is to remove unbound targeting agent from the circulation without affecting that bound to tumor.

Clearing designs for biotin-streptavidin systems have included use of three to five steps to promote clearance of unbound targeting agent to which the radionuclide complex would otherwise bind.[403] By using a three-step approach, a mean tumor/marrow ratio of 19 was achieved in glioma patients. Using this three-step pretargeting approach, 12 of 48 glioma patients with residual or recurrent disease after conventional therapy achieved a greater than 25% reduction in tumor, with 8 of 48 patients in remission at 12 months.[404,405] Efficacy has been reported by Paganelli and his European Institute of Oncology colleagues using this biotinylated antibody in a three-step approach for therapy in patients with other solid tumors as well.[404,406]

One of the most efficient clearing agents is a complex of galactosamine-biotin molecules that bind streptavidin-antibody and are extracted via the liver. After optimal tumor targeting, antibody complexes were efficiently removed such that blood concentrations of streptavidin were reduced by greater than 95% within 6 hours of administration of a synthetic monobiotin poly-*N*-acetyl-galactosamine compound developed by NeoRx Corp. investigators.[309,407] Extraction of clearing agent from blood occurs via interaction with Ashwell receptors in the liver. Use of clearing agents that complex with the targeting agent and are trapped in the liver has allowed dose escalation as high as 140 mCi/m^2 ^{90}Y, whereas the MTD for conventional RIT of ^{90}Y-antibody conjugates is usually less than 30 mCi/m^2 due to myelosuppression.[26,332,408] This synthetic monobiotin poly-*N*-acetyl-galactosamine compound has been used with antibodies conjugated chemically with streptavidin and more recently with Fusion proteins.[309,409] The genetically engineered Fusion proteins have been produced by fusing single-chain antibody fragments with streptavidin. This has provided tetrameric products with four binding sites for the bivalent antibody and four binding sites for biotin.[410] Early study of an anti-CD20/streptavidin fusion protein in a pretarget approach with the synthetic biotin-poly-*N*-acetyl-galactosamine compound resulted in an average tumor–to–whole-body radiation dose ratio of 49, with most patients having no significant hematologic toxicity at 15 mCi/m^2 of ^{90}Y.[309]

The pretargeting approach is very promising for treating solid tumors where efficacy has been limited primarily by the inability to deliver sufficient tumor doses with acceptable toxicity. Meaningful responses in a variety of nonmyelogenous solid tumors and lymphomas have been achieved with pretargeting.[26,402,411,412] Several reviews provide additional details of pretargeting development.[6,389,393]

Use of regional or direct injection of TaRT into tumors or tumor cavities has allowed dose escalation for treatment of relatively radioresistant tumors, with encouraging results as discussed in the Solid Tumor section.[68,215,216,232,233,254,331,413-417] Other approaches that may improve uptake of radiolabeled antibody in tumors include the use of unlabeled antibody to bind circulating antigen and nonspecific binding sites and the use of cocktails or mixtures of antibodies reactive with different tumor-associated antigens.[418-420] An advantage of antibody mixtures has been confirmed in animal studies that showed superior detection and localization to smaller tumors and greater tumor growth inhibition with the combination of two ^{131}I-labeled antibodies than either antibody alone using the same total amount of radionuclide.[421,422] Several human trials have used two or more antibodies simultaneously. However, it has not been possible to make a direct comparison of one versus two or more antibodies in patients, because most trials did not test one antibody alone compared with a combination of antibodies in the same study.[196] When optimized, antibody cocktails may include the combination of whole antibodies with smaller constructs, the use of different radionuclides, or both. Radionuclides are chosen on the basis of their physical half-life, radiation emission characteristics, and pharmacokinetics in a manner that would complement one another and be matched with the half-life of the antibody or antibody constructs. In addition, the use of antibodies with different affinities and/or the use of genetically engineered antibodies with greater avidity may also increase the targeting and retention of radioimmunoconjugates in tumors.

In an effort to increase the efficacy of TaRT in relatively radioresistant malignancies, TaRT is being studied in conjunction with other agents or therapies (e.g., external beam radiation, which may increase targeting by affecting tumor vasculature while causing G_2/M arrest in a radiosensitive phase of the cell cycle). During the radiosensitive phase of the cell cycle, tumors receive prolonged low-dose-rate radiation from radionuclide emissions associated with TaRT. Other approaches for improving the therapeutic ratio and efficacy of TaRT include the use of radiosensitizers and radioprotectors.[423] TaRT is now being studied in combination with chemotherapy and a variety of other therapeutic agents as previously described, but these combined-modality approaches have generally not been optimized (e.g., in terms of dose sequence and timing).[424] Optimization of these regimens may vary with tumor/radionuclide systems.[425-427] PEG modification of targeting agents is an example of an optimization strategy under study that provides multiple carrying sites for molecules such as radiosensitizers.[428,429] TaRT has been studied in combination with a variety of agents including the radiosensitizer SR2508, intercalating agents, and the hypoxic cytotoxin, SR 4233 (Tirapazamine).[378] A variety of chemotherapy agents have also been studied as radiosensitizing agents in conjunction with TaRT.[245,257,430] The taxanes radiosensitize tumors by arresting cells in the G_2/M cell cycle phase and have demonstrated synergistic effects in preclinical TaRT studies. They are now being studied in clinical trials in combination with RIT.[254,424] Cisplatin has also been shown to have a supra-additive effect in combination with low-dose-rate radiation.[431] Buchsbaum and coworkers[248] have reported increased growth inhibition in human tumor xenografts in nude mice when bromodeoxyuridine, which is incorporated into the DNA in place of thymidine, was given for 4 days before RIT with a 1-day washout. Tirapazamine potentiated cytotoxicity by RIT in mice bearing human tumor xenografts.[378,432] Caffeine has also been shown to modulate sensitivity to RIT in lymphoma cells.[53] Although sensitization may be achieved with low doses of adjuvant agents, it has been feasible to use nearly full doses of each agent with acceptable toxicity in some trials.[254,332]

At the preclinical level, it was recognized that gene therapy may enhance the efficacy of TaRT. Gene transfer methods have been used to genetically induce tumor cells to express enhanced levels of cell surface tumor-associated antigens or receptors that have resulted in increased tumor uptake of radiolabeled antibody or peptide in animal models.[433] This approach could potentially result in enhanced therapeutic efficacy. There is also the potential to use gene transfer techniques to radiosensitize tumors by knocking out genes involved in DNA repair, signal transduction, and control of the cell cycle, which would result in sensitization of tumors to TaRT. Alternatively, gene therapy may be used to provide radioprotection of bone marrow. Furthermore, specific genes can be targeted with short range radionuclides such as Auger emitters as demonstrated by ^{125}I-labeled triplex-forming oligonucleotides.[434] The combination of toxin-gene delivery and TaRT also offers the potential for improved therapeutic efficacy.[433]

FUTURE CONSIDERATIONS

TaRT is a promising therapeutic modality, and ongoing work in this area will result in expansion of indications and improved efficacy. In addition to acceptance of TaRT as a component of the standard armamentarium for lymphohematopoietic malignancies, its efficacy for selected nonhematologic entities is continually being improved. It is expected that for many diseases TaRT will be most useful as a component of multimodality therapy.[257] Future studies should define how to optimally combine TaRT with other therapeutic modalities. More investigation is needed to determine agents/schedules that result in synergistic antitumor activity without significantly greater toxicity. TaRT has been useful both as a component of early therapy and as a salvage therapy (e.g., improved survival of glioma patients). It is also being studied in lymphoma in combination with other agents by national cooperative groups in an effort to further improve therapeutic outcome. Active areas of investigation include studies of TaRT using alpha particles, nonantibody targeting agents, gene therapy, and other approaches for increasing tumor uptake of radionuclide and enhancing efficacy.[382]

ACKNOWLEDGMENTS

The authors thank Chuck DiBari and Tracey Cotton for preparation of the manuscript. Work was supported by National Institutes of Health grants P50 CA83591, NIH 1 R01 CA82617, and P50 CA89019. The authors would also like to thank the American Association for Cancer Research, Inc. for granting permission to use material presented in a paper published in Cancer Research (Suppl)55:5832s, 1995.

REFERENCES

1. Press OW, Rasey J: Principles of radioimmunotherapy for hematologists and oncologists, Semin Oncol 27:62, 2000.
2. Goldenberg DM: Advancing role of radiolabeled antibodies in the therapy of cancer. Cancer Immunol Immunother 52:281, 2003.
3. Juweid M, DeNardo GL, Graham M, et al: Radioimmunotherapy: a novel treatment modality for B-cell non-Hodgkin's lymphoma. Cancer Biother Radiopharm 18:673, 2003.
4. Bodei L, Cremonesi M, Grana C, et al: Receptor radionuclide therapy with [(90)Y-DOTA](0)-Tyr(3)-octreotide ((90)Y-DOTATOC) in neuroendocrine tumours. Eur J Nucl Med Mol Imaging 31:1038, 2004.
5. Hagenbeek A: Radioimmunotherapy for NHL: experience of 90Y-ibritumomab tiuxetan in clinical practice. Leuk Lymphoma 44(Suppl 4):S37, 2003.
6. Abrams PG, Fritzberg AR: Radioimmunotherapy of Cancer. New York, Marcel Dekker, 2000.
7. Buchsbaum DJ: Experimental radioimmunotherapy. Semin Radiat Oncol 10:156, 2000.
8. Buchsbaum DJ, Langmuir VK, Wessels BW: Experimental radioimmunotherapy. Med Phys 20:551, 1993.
9. Zola H: Monoclonal Antibodies, the Second Generation. Oxford, BIOS, 1995.

10. Tempest PR, Bremner P, Lambert M, et al: Reshaping a human monoclonal antibody to inhibit human respiratory syncytial virus infection in vivo. Biotechnology (N Y) 9:266, 1991.
11. Muraro R, Kuroki M, Wunderlich D, et al: Generation and characterization of B72.3 second generation monoclonal antibodies reactive with the tumor-associated glycoprotein 72 antigen. Cancer Res 48:4588, 1988.
12. Colcher D, Minelli MF, Roselli M, et al: Radioimmunolocalization of human carcinoma xenografts with B72.3 second generation monoclonal antibodies. Cancer Res 48:4597, 1988.
13. Andrew SM, Johnstone RW, Russell SM, et al: Comparison of in vitro cell binding characteristics of four monoclonal antibodies and their individual tumor localization properties in mice. Cancer Res 50:4423, 1990.
14. Jain RK: Physiological barriers to delivery of monoclonal antibodies and other macromolecules in tumors. Cancer Res 50:814s, 1990.
15. Langmuir VK, Mendonca HL, Woo DV: Comparisons between two monoclonal antibodies that bind to the same antigen but have differing affinities: uptake kinetics and 125I-antibody therapy efficacy in multicell spheroids. Cancer Res 52:4728, 1992.
16. Yokota T, Milenic DE, Whitlow M, et al: Rapid tumor penetration of a single-chain Fv and comparison with other immunoglobulin forms. Cancer Res 52:3402, 1992.
17. Khazaeli MB, Conry RM, LoBuglio AF: Human immune response to monoclonal antibodies. J Immunother 15:42, 1994.
18. Meredith RF, Khazaeli MB, Plott WE, et al: Effect of human immune response on repeat courses of 131I-chimeric B72.3 antibody therapy. Antibody Immunoconj Radiopharm 6:39, 1993.
19. Weiden PL, Wolf SB, Breitz HB, et al: Human anti-mouse antibody suppression with cyclosporin A. Cancer 73:1093, 1994.
20. Reichmann L, Clark MR, Waldmann H, et al: Reshaping antibodies for therapy. Nature 332:323, 1988.
21. Mark GE: Reengineered monoclonal antibodies. Antibody Immunoconj Radiopharm 5:347, 1992.
22. Schrama D, Straten P, Brocker EB, et al: Cytokine fusion protein treatment. Recent Results Cancer Res 160:185, 2002.
23. Khazaeli MB, Wheeler R, Rogers K, et al: Initial evaluation of a human immunoglobulin M monoclonal antibody (HA-1A) in humans. J Biol Response Mod 9:178, 1990.
24. Gansow OA: Newer approaches to the radiolabeling of monoclonal antibodies by use of metal chelates. Int J Rad Appl Instrum B 18:369, 1991.
25. Meyer DL, Schultz J, Lin Y, et al: Reduced antibody response to streptavidin through site-directed mutagenesis. Prot Sci 10:491, 2001.
26. Knox SJ, Goris ML, Tempero M, et al: Phase II trial of yttrium-90-DOTA-biotin pretargeted by NR-LU-10 antibody/streptavidin in patients with metastatic colon cancer. Clin Cancer Res 6:406, 2000.
27. Reubi JC, Schaer JC, Waser B, et al: Expression and localization of somatostatin receptor SSTR1, SSTR2, and SSTR3 messenger RNAs in primary human tumors using in situ hybridization. Cancer Res 54:3455, 1994.
28. Anthony LB, Woltering EA, Espenan GD, et al: Indium-111-pentetreotide prolongs survival in gastroenteropancreatic malignancies. Semin Nucl Med 32:123, 2002.
29. Rolleman EJ, Valkema R, de Jong M, et al: Safe and effective inhibition of renal uptake of radiolabelled octreotide by a combination of lysine and arginine. Eur J Nucl Med Mol Imaging 30:9, 2003.
30. de Jong M, Valkema R, Jamar F, et al: Somatostatin receptor-targeted radionuclide therapy of tumors: preclinical and clinical findings. Semin Nucl Med 32:133, 2002.
31. Virgolini I, Traub T, Leimer M, et al: New radiopharmaceuticals for receptor scintigraphy and radionuclide therapy. Q J Nucl Med 44:50, 2000.
32. Waldherr C, Pless M, Maecke HR, et al: Tumor response and clinical benefit in neuroendocrine tumors after 7.4 GBq (90)Y-DOTATOC. J Nucl Med 43:610, 2002.
33. Harris TD, Kalogeropoulos S, Nguyen T, et al: Design, synthesis, and evaluation of radiolabeled integrin alpha v beta 3 receptor antagonists for tumor imaging and radiotherapy. Cancer Biother Radiopharm 18:627, 2003.
34. Sofou S, Thomas JL, Lin HY, et al: Engineered liposomes for potential alpha-particle therapy of metastatic cancer. J Nucl Med 45:253, 2004.
35. Harrington KJ, Mohammadtaghi S, Uster PS, et al: Effective targeting of solid tumors in patients with locally advanced cancers by radiolabeled pegylated liposomes. Clin Cancer Res 7:243, 2001.
36. Li L, Wartchow CA, Danthi SN, et al: A novel antiangiogenesis therapy using an integrin antagonist or anti-Flk-1 antibody coated 90Y-labeled nanoparticles. Int J Radiat Oncol Biol Phys 58:1215, 2004.
37. Wessels BW, Rogus RD: Radionuclide selection and model absorbed dose calculations for radiolabeled tumor associated antibodies. Med Phys 11:638, 1984.
38. Yorke ED, Beaumier PL, Wessels BW, et al: Optimal antibody-radionuclide combinations for clinical radioimmunotherapy: a predictive model based on mouse pharmacokinetics. Int J Rad Appl Instrum B 18:827, 1991.
39. Wessels BW, Meares CF: Physical and chemical properties of radionuclide therapy. Semin Radiat Oncol 10:115, 2000.
40. Williams LE, Wu AM, Yazaki PJ, et al: Numerical selection of optimal tumor imaging agents with application to engineered antibodies. Cancer Biother Radiopharm 16:25, 2001.
41. Shankar S, Vaidyanathan G, Affleck D, et al: N-Succinimidyl 3-[(131)I]iodo-4-phosphonomethylbenzoate ([(131)I]SIPMB), a negatively charged substituent-bearing acylation agent for the radioiodination of peptides and mAbs. Bioconjug Chem 14:331, 2003.
42. Jamar F, Barone R, Mathieu I, et al: 86Y-DOTA(0)-D-Phe1-Tyr3-octreotide (SMT487)—a phase 1 clinical study: pharmacokinetics, biodistribution and renal protective effect of different regimens of amino acid co-infusion. Eur J Nucl Med Mol Imaging 30:510, 2003.
43. Brouwers AH, van Eerd JE, Frielink C, et al: Optimization of radioimmunotherapy of renal cell carcinoma: labeling of monoclonal antibody cG250 with 131I:90Y:177Lu, or 186Re. J Nucl Med 45:327, 2004.
44. Macey DJ, Meredith RF: A strategy to reduce red marrow dose for intraperitoneal radioimmunotherapy. Clin Cancer Res 5:3044s, 1999.
45. Buchsbaum DJ, Lawrence TS, Roberson PL, et al: Comparison of 131I- and 90Y-labeled monoclonal antibody 17 A for treatment of human colon cancer xenografts. Int J Radiat Oncol Biol Phys 25:629, 1993.
46. Borchardt PE, Yuan RR, Miederer M, et al: Targeted actinium-125 in vivo generators for therapy of ovarian cancer. Cancer Res 63:5084, 2003.
47. DeNardo GL: Evaluation of a cathepsin-cleavable peptide linked radioimmunoconjugate of a panadenocarcinoma MAb, m170, in mice and patients. Cancer Biother Radiopharm 19:85, 2004.
48. Beeson C, Butrynski JE, Hart MJ, et al: Conditionally cleavable radioimmunoconjugates: a novel approach for the release of radioisotopes from radioimmunoconjugates. Bioconjug Chem 14:927, 2003.
49. Hernandez MC, Knox SJ: Radiobiology of radioimmunotherapy with 90Y ibritumomab tiuxetan (Zevalin). Semin Oncol 30:6, 2003.
50. Hernandez MC, Knox SJ: Radiobiology of radioimmunotherapy: targeting CD20 B-cell antigen in non-Hodgkin's lymphoma. Int J Radiat Oncol Biol Phys 59:1274, 2004.
51. Riccobene TA, Miceli RC, Lincoln C, et al: Rapid and specific targeting of 125I-labeled B lymphocyte stimulator to lymphoid tissues and B cell tumors in mice. J Nucl Med 44:422, 2003.
52. Kroger LA, DeNardo GL, Gumerlock PH, et al: Apoptosis-related gene and protein expression in human lymphoma xenografts (Raji) after low dose rate radiation using 67Cu-2IT-BAT-Lym-1 radioimmunotherapy. Cancer Biother Radiopharm 16:213, 2001.
53. Macklis RM, Beresford BA, Humm JL: Radiobiologic studies of low-dose-rate 90Y-lymphoma therapy. Cancer 73:966, 1994.
54. Rupnow BA, Murtha AD, Alarcon RM, et al: Direct evidence that apoptosis enhances tumor responses to fractionated radiotherapy. Cancer Res 58:1779, 1998.

55. Ning S, Knox SJ: G2/M-phase arrest and death by apoptosis of HL60 cells irradiated with exponentially decreasing low-dose-rate gamma radiation. Radiat Res 151:659, 1999.
56. Knox SJ, Sutherland W, Goris ML: Correlation of tumor sensitivity to low-dose-rate irradiation with G2/M-phase block and other radiobiological parameters. Radiat Res 135:24, 1993.
57. Palayoor ST, Macklis RM, Bump EA, et al: Modulation of radiation-induced apoptosis and G2/M block in murine T-lymphoma cells. Radiat Res 141:235, 1995.
58. Macklis RM, Beresford BA, Palayoor S, et al: Cell cycle alterations, apoptosis, and response to low-dose-rate radioimmunotherapy in lymphoma cells. Int J Radiat Oncol Biol Phys 27:643, 1993.
59. Williams JR, Zhang YG, Dillehay LE: Sensitization processes in human tumor cells during protracted irradiation: possible exploitation in the clinic. Int J Radiat Oncol Biol Phys 24:699, 1992.
60. Ruan S, O'Donoghue JA, Larson SM, et al: Optimizing the sequence of combination therapy with radiolabeled antibodies and fractionated external beam. J Nucl Med 41:1905, 2000.
61. Pawlik TM, Keyomarsi K: Role of cell cycle in mediating sensitivity to radiotherapy. Int J Radiat Oncol Biol Phys 59:928, 2004.
62. Rupnow BA, Alarcon RM, Giaccia AJ, et al: p53 mediates apoptosis induced by c-Myc activation in hypoxic or gamma irradiated fibroblasts. Cell Death Differ 5:141, 1998.
63. Hall EJ: Radiobiology for the Radiologist, 5th ed. Philadelphia, Lippincott Williams & Wilkins, 2000.
64. Knox SJ, Levy R, Miller RA, et al: Determinants of the antitumor effect of radiolabeled monoclonal antibodies. Cancer Res 50:4935, 1990.
65. Zalutsky MR, Moseley RP, Benjamin JC, et al: Monoclonal antibody and F(ab')2 fragment delivery to tumor in patients with glioma: comparison of intracarotid and intravenous administration. Cancer Res 50:4105, 1990.
66. Breitz HB, Durham JC, Fisher DR, et al: Radiation-absorbed dose estimates to normal organs following intraperitoneal 186Re-labeled monoclonal antibody: methods and results. Cancer Res 55:5817s, 1995.
67. Hnatowich DJ, Chinol M, Siebecker DA, et al: Patient biodistribution of intraperitoneally administered yttrium-90-labeled antibody. J Nucl Med 29:1428, 1988.
68. Epenetos AA, Munro AJ, Stewart S, et al: Antibody-guided irradiation of advanced ovarian cancer with intraperitoneally administered radiolabeled monoclonal antibodies. J Clin Oncol 5:1890, 1987.
69. Miyamoto C, Brady LW, Rackover M, et al: Utilization of 125I monoclonal antibody in the management of primary glioblastoma multiforme. Radiation Oncology Investigations 3:126, 1995.
70. Beierwaltes WH, Sturman MF, Ryo U, et al: Imaging functional nodules of the adrenal glands with 131-I-19-iodocholesterol. J Nucl Med 15:246, 1974.
71. Order SE, Klein JL, Ettinger D, et al: Phase I-II study of radiolabeled antibody integrated in the treatment of primary hepatic malignancies. Int J Radiat Oncol Biol Phys 6:703, 1980.
72. Kohler G, Milstein C: Continuous cultures of fused cells secreting antibody of predefined specificity. Nature 256:495, 1975.
73. Buchsbaum D: Experimental Radioimmunotherapy and Methods to Increase Therapeutic Efficacy. Boca Raton, CRC Press, 1995, chapter 10.
74. Knox SJ: Overview of studies on experimental radioimmunotherapy. Cancer Res 55:5832s, 1995.
75. Buras RR, Beatty BG, Williams LE, et al: Radioimmunotherapy of human colon cancer in nude mice. Arch Surg 125:660, 1990.
76. Pedley RB, Boden JA, Boden R, et al: Comparative radioimmunotherapy using intact or F(ab')2 fragments of 131I anti-CEA antibody in a colonic xenograft model. Br J Cancer 68:69, 1993.
77. Buras RR, Wong JY, Kuhn JA, et al: Comparison of radioimmunotherapy and external beam radiotherapy in colon cancer xenografts. Int J Radiat Oncol Biol Phys 25:473, 1993.
78. Buchsbaum DJ, ten Haken RK, Heidorn DB, et al: A comparison of 131I-labeled monoclonal antibody 17-1. A treatment to external beam irradiation on the growth of LS174T human colon carcinoma xenografts. Int J Radiat Oncol Biol Phys 18:1033, 1990.
79. Neacy WP, Wessels BW, Bradley EW, et al: Comparison of radioimmunotherapy (RIT) and 4MV external beam radiotherapy of human tumor xenografts in athymic mice (abstract). J Nucl Med 27:902, 1986.
80. Wessels BW, Vessella RL, Palme DF 2nd, et al: Radiobiological comparison of external beam irradiation and radioimmunotherapy in renal cell carcinoma xenografts. Int J Radiat Oncol Biol Phys 17:1257, 1989.
81. Knox SJ, Goris ML, Wessels BW: Overview of animal studies comparing radioimmunotherapy with dose equivalent external beam irradiation. Radiother Oncol 23:111, 1992.
82. Langmuir VK, Fowler JF, Knox SJ, et al: Radiobiology of radiolabeled antibody therapy as applied to tumor dosimetry, Med Phys 20:601, 1993.
83. Schwartz MA, Lovett DR, Redner A, et al: Dose-escalation trial of M195 labeled with iodine 131 for cytoreduction and marrow ablation in relapsed or refractory myeloid leukemias. J Clin Oncol 11:294, 1993.
84. Fowler JF: Radiobiological aspects of low dose rates in radioimmunotherapy. Int J Radiat Oncol Biol Phys 18:1261, 1990.
85. Wong JY, Buras R, Kuhn JA, et al: Strategies to Improve the Efficacy of Radioimmunotherapy: Radiobiologic and Dosimetric Considerations II. New York, Academic Press, 1992.
86. Buras R, Wong JY, Beatty B, et al: Comparison of Y 90-labeled anti-CEA monoclonal antibody therapy with external beam radiotherapy in colon cancer. Presented at 38th Annual Meeting of the Radiation Research Society and 10th Annual Meeting of the North American Hyperthermia Group, 1990.
87. Wong JY, Thomas GE, Yamauchi D, et al: Clinical evaluation of indium-111-labeled chimeric anti-CEA monoclonal antibody. J Nucl Med 38:1951, 1997.
88. de Bree R, Roos JC, Plaizier MA, et al: Selection of monoclonal antibody E48 IgG or U36 IgG for adjuvant radioimmunotherapy in head and neck cancer patients. Br J Cancer 75:1049, 1997.
89. Breitz HB, Fisher DR, Weiden PL, et al: Dosimetry of rhenium-labeled monoclonal antibodies: methods, prediction from technetium-99m-labeled antibodies and results of phase I trials. J Nucl Med 34:908, 1993.
90. Colnot DR, Roos JC, de Bree R, et al: Safety, biodistribution, pharmacokinetics, and immunogenicity of 99mTc-labeled humanized monoclonal antibody BIWA 4 (bivatuzumab) in patients with squamous cell carcinoma of the head and neck. Cancer Immunol Immunother 52:576, 2003.
91. Nanus DM, Milowsky MI, Kostakoglu L, et al: Clinical use of monoclonal antibody HuJ591 therapy: targeting prostate specific membrane antigen. J Urol 170:S84; discussion S88, 2003.
92. Larson SM, Carrasquillo JA, Krohn KA, et al: Localization of 131I-labeled p97-specific Fab fragments in human melanoma as a basis for radiotherapy. J Clin Invest 72:2101, 1983.
93. Vriesendorp HM, Herpst JM, Germack MA, et al: Phase I-II studies of yttrium-90-labeled antiferritin treatment for end-stage Hodgkin's disease, including Radiation Therapy Oncology Group 87. J Clin Oncol 9:918, 1991.
94. Juweid M, Sharkey RM, Markowitz A, et al: Treatment of non-Hodgkin's lymphoma with radiolabeled murine, chimeric, or humanized LL2, an anti-CD22 monoclonal antibody. Cancer Res 55:5899s, 1995.
95. Jurcic JC, Caron PC, Nikula TK, et al: Radiolabeled anti-CD33 monoclonal antibody M195 for myeloid leukemias. Cancer Res 55:5908s, 1995.
96. Knox SJ, Meredith RF: Clinical radioimmunotherapy. Semin Radiat Oncol 10:73, 2000.
97. Gordon LI, Witzig TE, Wiseman GA, et al: Yttrium 90 ibritumomab tiuxetan radioimmunotherapy for relapsed or refractory low-grade non-Hodgkin's lymphoma. Semin Oncol 29:87, 2002.
98. Press OW: Radiolabeled antibody therapy of B-cell lymphomas. Semin Oncol 26:58, 1999.
99. Kaminski MS, Leonard J, Zelenetz AD, et al: Bexar therapy (tositumomab and iodine I-131 tositumomab) has high response rates in the treatment of bulky low grade (LG) relapsed or refractory non-Hodgkin's lymphoma (NHL). Am Soc Clin Oncol 21(1):5, 2002.
100. Zelenetz AD: A clinical and scientific overview of tositumomab and iodine I-131 tositumomab. Semin Oncol 30:22, 2003.

101. Lashford L, Jones D, Pritchard J, et al: Therapeutic application of radiolabeled monoclonal antibody UJ13A in children with disseminated neuroblastoma. NCI Monogr 53, 1987.
102. Meredith RF, Khazaeli MB, Liu T, et al: Dose fractionation of radiolabeled antibodies in patients with metastatic colon cancer. J Nucl Med 33:1648, 1992.
103. Meredith RF, Bueschen AJ, Khazaeli MB, et al: Treatment of metastatic prostate carcinoma with radiolabeled antibody CC49. J Nucl Med 35:1017, 1994.
104. Welt S, Divgi CR, Kemeny N, et al: Phase I/II study of iodine 131-labeled monoclonal antibody A33 in patients with advanced colon cancer. J Clin Oncol 12:1561, 1994.
105. Murray JL, Macey DJ, Kasi LP, et al: Phase II radioimmunotherapy trial with 131I-CC49 in colorectal cancer. Cancer 73:1057, 1994.
106. Wheeler R, Meredith RF, Saleh MN, et al: A phase II trial of IL + radioimmunotherapy (RIT) in patients (pts) with metastatic colon cancer. Proc Am Soc Clin Oncol 13:295, 1994.
107. Yu B, Carrasquillo J, Milenic D, et al: Phase I trial of iodine-131-labeled COL in patients with gastrointestinal malignancies: influence of serum carcinoembryonic antigen and tumor bulk on pharmacokinetics. J Clin Oncol 14:1798, 1996.
108. Divgi CR, Bander NH, Scott AM, et al: Phase I/II radioimmunotherapy trial with iodine-labeled monoclonal antibody G250 in metastatic renal cell carcinoma. Clin Cancer Res 4:2729, 1998.
109. van Zanten-Przybysz I, Molthoff CF, Roos JC, et al: Radioimmunotherapy with intravenously administered 131I-labeled chimeric monoclonal antibody MOv18 in patients with ovarian cancer. J Nucl Med 41:1168, 2000.
110. Meredith RF, Khazaeli MB, Plott WE, et al: Initial clinical evaluation of iodine-125-labeled chimeric 17-1A for metastatic colon cancer. J Nucl Med 36:2229, 1995.
111. Deb N, Goris M, Trisler K, et al: Treatment of hormone-refractory prostate cancer with 90Y-CYT-356 monoclonal antibody. Clin Cancer Res 2:1289, 1996.
112. DeNardo SJ, Kramer EL, O'Donnell RT, et al: Radioimmunotherapy for breast cancer using indium-111/yttrium-90 BrE-3: results of a phase I clinical trial. J Nucl Med 38:1180, 1997.
113. Kahn D, Austin JC, Maguire RT, et al: A phase II study of [90Y] yttrium-capromab pendetide in the treatment of men with prostate cancer recurrence following radical prostatectomy. Cancer Biother Radiopharm 14:99, 1999.
114. Wong YC, Chu DZ, Yamauchi DM, et al: A phase I radioimmunotherapy trial evaluating 90yttrium-labeled anti-carcinoembryonic antigen (CEA) chimeric T84.66 in patients with metastatic CEA-producing malignancies. Clin Cancer Res 6:3855, 2000.
115. O'Donnell RT, DeNardo SJ, Yuan A, et al: Radioimmunotherapy with (111)In/(90)Y-2IT-BAD-m170 for metastatic prostate cancer. Clin Cancer Res 7:1561, 2001.
116. Weiden PL, Breitz HB, Seiler CA, et al: Rhenium-labeled chimeric antibody NR-LU-13: pharmacokinetics, biodistribution and immunogenicity relative to murine analog NR-LU-10. J Nucl Med 34:2111, 1993.
117. Colnot DR, Quak JJ, Roos JC, et al: Phase I therapy study of 186Re-labeled chimeric monoclonal antibody U36 in patients with squamous cell carcinoma of the head and neck. J Nucl Med 41:1999, 2000.
118. Borjesson PK, Postema EJ, Roos JC, et al: Phase I therapy study with (186)Re-labeled humanized monoclonal antibody BIWA 4 (bivatuzumab) in patients with head and neck squamous cell carcinoma. Clin Cancer Res 9:3961S, 2003.
119. Juweid M, Sharkey RM, Swayne LC, et al: Pharmacokinetics, dosimetry and toxicity of rhenium-188-labeled anti-carcinoembryonic antigen monoclonal antibody, MN, in gastrointestinal cancer. J Nucl Med 39:34, 1998.
120. Mulligan T, Carrasquillo JA, Chung Y, et al: Phase I study of intravenous Lu-labeled CC49 murine monoclonal antibody in patients with advanced adenocarcinoma. Clin Cancer Res 1:1447, 1995.
121. Goldsmith SJ, Vallabahajosula S, Kostakoglu L, et al: 90Y-DOTA-huJ591: radiolabeled anti-PSMA humanized monoclonal antibody for the treatment of prostate cancer: phase I dose escalation studies. J Nucl Med 43:158p, 2002.
122. Vallabahajosula S, Kostakoglu L, Goldsmith SJ, et al: Phase I dose escalation clinical studies with 177 Lu-DOTA-Hu-J591: a new radiolabeled antibody for the treatment of prostate cancer. J Nucl Med 43:159p, 2002.
123. Milowsky MI, Nanus DM, Kostakoglu L, et al: Phase I trial of yttrium-90-labeled anti-prostate-specific membrane antigen monoclonal antibody J591 for androgen-independent prostate cancer. J Clin Oncol 22:2522, 2004.
124. Behr TM, Sharkey RM, Juweid ME, et al: Phase I/II clinical radioimmunotherapy with an iodine-131-labeled anti-carcinoembryonic antigen murine monoclonal antibody IgG. J Nucl Med 38:858, 1997.
125. DeNardo SJ, O'Grady LF, Richman CM, et al: Radioimmunotherapy for advanced breast cancer using I-131-ChL6 antibody. Anticancer Res 17:1745, 1997.
126. Ychou M, Pelegrin A, Faurous P, et al: Phase-I/II radioimmunotherapy study with iodine-131-labeled anti-CEA monoclonal antibody F6 F(ab')2 in patients with non-resectable liver metastases from colorectal cancer. Int J Cancer 75:615, 1998.
127. Behr TM, Salib AL, Liersch T, et al: Radioimmunotherapy of small volume disease of colorectal cancer metastatic to the liver: preclinical evaluation in comparison to standard chemotherapy and initial results of a phase I clinical study. Clin Cancer Res 5:3232s, 1999.
128. Juweid ME, Hajjar G, Swayne LC, et al: Phase I/II trial of (131)I-MN F(ab)2 anti-carcinoembryonic antigen monoclonal antibody in the treatment of patients with metastatic medullary thyroid carcinoma. Cancer 85:1828, 1999.
129. Steffens MG, Boerman OC, de Mulder PH, et al: Phase I radioimmunotherapy of metastatic renal cell carcinoma with 131I-labeled chimeric monoclonal antibody G250. Clin Cancer Res 5:3268s, 1999.
130. Breitz HB, Weiden PL, Vanderheyden JL, et al: Clinical experience with rhenium-186-labeled monoclonal antibodies for radioimmunotherapy: results of phase I trials. J Nucl Med 33:1099, 1992.
131. Juweid M, Swayne LC, Sharkey RM, et al: Prospects of radioimmunotherapy in epithelial ovarian cancer: results with iodine 131-labeled murine and humanized MN-14 anti-carcinoembryonic antigen monoclonal antibodies. Gynecol Oncol 67:259, 1997.
132. Lane DM, Eagle KF, Begent RH, et al: Radioimmunotherapy of metastatic colorectal tumours with iodine 131-labelled antibody to carcinoembryonic antigen: phase I/II study with comparative biodistribution of intact and F(ab')2 antibodies. Br J Cancer 70:521, 1994.
133. Withers HR, Peters LJ, Taylor JM: Dose-response relationship for radiation therapy of subclinical disease. Int J Radiat Oncol Biol Phys 31:353, 1995.
134. Dahl O, Horn A, Morild I, et al: Low-dose preoperative radiation postpones recurrences in operable rectal cancer. Results of a randomized multicenter trial in western Norway. Cancer 66:2286, 1990.
135. Gerard A, Buyse M, Nordlinger B, et al: Preoperative radiotherapy as adjuvant treatment in rectal cancer. Final results of a randomized study of the European Organization for Research and Treatment of Cancer (EORTC). Ann Surg 208:606, 1988.
136. Franklin R, Steiger Z, Vaishampayan G, et al: Combined modality therapy for esophageal squamous cell carcinoma. Cancer 51:1062, 1983.
137. Nigro ND, Seydel HG, Considine B, et al: Combined preoperative radiation and chemotherapy for squamous cell carcinoma of the anal canal. Cancer 51:1826, 1983.
138. Roth JA, Putnam JB, Lichter AS, et al: Cancer of the Esophagus. Philadelphia, JB Lippincott, 1993.
139. Schrier DM, Stemmer SM, Johnson T, et al: High-dose 90Y Mx-diethylenetriaminepentaacetic acid (DTPA)-BrE-3 and autologous hematopoietic stem cell support (AHSCS) for the treatment of advanced breast cancer: a phase I trial. Cancer Res 55:5921s, 1995.
140. Cagnoni PJ, Ceriani R, Cole WC, et al: High-dose radioimmunothrapy with 90 Y-hu-BrE followed by autologous

hematopoietic stem cell support (AHSCS) in patients with metastatic breast cancer. Cancer Biother Radiopharmaceut 14:318, 1999.
141. Richman CM, DeNardo SJ, O'Grady LF, et al: Radioimmunotherapy for breast cancer using escalating fractionated doses of 131I-labeled chimeric L6 antibody with peripheral blood progenitor cell transfusions. Cancer Res 55:5916s, 1995.
142. Richman CM, DeNardo SJ, O'Donnell RT, et al: Dosimetry-based therapy in metastatic breast cancer patients using 90Y monoclonal antibody 170H.82 with autologous stem cell support and cyclosporin A. Clin Cancer Res 5:3243s, 1999.
143. Wong JY, Somlo G, Odom-Maryon T, et al: Initial clinical experience evaluating yttrium-90-chimeric T84.66 anticarcinoembryonic antigen antibody and autologous hematopoietic stem cell support in patients with carcinoembryonic antigen-producing metastatic breast cancer. Clin Cancer Res 5:3224s, 1999.
144. Juweid MR, Hajjar G, Stein R, et al: Initial experience with high-dose radioimmunotherapy of metastatic medullary thyroid cancer using 131I-MN-14 F(ab)2 anti-carcinoembryonic antigen MAb and AHSCR. J Nucl Med 41:93, 2000.
145. Tempero M, Leichner P, Dalrymple G, et al: High-dose therapy with iodine 131-labeled monoclonal antibody CC49 in patients with gastrointestinal cancers: a phase I trial. J Clin Oncol 15:1518, 1997.
146. Tempero M, Leichner P, Baranowska-Kortylewicz J, et al: High-dose therapy with 90yttrium-labeled monoclonal antibody CC49: a phase I trial. Clin Cancer Res 6:3095, 2000.
147. Khazaeli MR, Saleh MN, Liu TP, et al: Pharmacokinetics and immune response of 131I-chimeric mouse/human B72.3 (human gamma 4) monoclonal antibody in humans. Cancer Res 51:5461, 1991.
148. LoBuglio AF, Wheeler RH, Trang J, et al: Mouse/human chimeric monoclonal antibody in man: kinetics and immune response. Proc Natl Acad Sci U S A 86:4220, 1989.
149. Goodman GE, Hellstrom I, Yelton DE, et al: Phase I trial of chimeric (human-mouse) monoclonal antibody L6 in patients with non-small-cell lung, colon, and breast cancer. Cancer Immunol Immunother 36:267, 1993.
150. LoBuglio AF, Khazaeli MR, Meredith R, et al: Chimeric monoclonal antibodies in cancer therapy. Ann Oncol 3:196, 1992.
151. Stroomer JW, Roos JC, Sproll M, et al: Safety and biodistribution of 99mTechnetium-labeled anti-CD44v6 monoclonal antibody BIWA 1 in head and neck cancer patients. Clin Cancer Res 6:3046, 2000.
152. Hajjar G, Sharkey RM, Burton J, et al: Phase I radioimmunotherapy trial with iodine–labeled humanized MN-14 anti-carcinoembryonic antigen monoclonal antibody in patients with metastatic gastrointestinal and colorectal cancer. Clin Colorectal Cancer 2:31, 2002.
153. Ritter G, Cohen LS, Williams C Jr, et al: Serological analysis of human anti-human antibody responses in colon cancer patients treated with repeated doses of humanized monoclonal antibody A33. Cancer Res 61:6851, 2001.
154. Dale RG: Radiobiological assessment of permanent implants using tumour repopulation factors in the linear-quadratic model. Br J Radiol 62:241, 1989.
155. Juweid M, Sharkey RM, Behr T, et al: Targeting and initial radioimmunotherapy of medullary thyroid carcinoma with 131I-labeled monoclonal antibodies to carcinoembryonic antigen. Cancer Res 55:5946s, 1995.
156. Kaminski MS, Zasadny KR, Francis IR, et al: Iodine-131 anti-BI radioimmunotherapy for B-cell lymphoma. J Clin Oncol 14:1974, 1996.
157. Buchegger F, Mach JP, Folli S, et al: Higher efficiency of 131I-labeled anti-carcinoembryonic antigen-monoclonal antibody F(ab')2 as compared with intact antibodies in radioimmunotherapy of established human colon carcinoma grafted in nude mice. Recent Results Cancer Res 141:19, 1996.
158. Buchegger F, Pelegrin A, Delaloye B, et al: Iodine 131-labeled MAb F(ab')2 fragments are more efficient and less toxic than intact anti-CEA antibodies in radioimmunotherapy of large human colon carcinoma grafted in nude mice. J Nucl Med 31:1035, 1990.
159. Juweid MR, Sharkey RM, Behr T, et al: Radioimmunotherapy of patients with small-volume tumors using iodine 131-labeled anti-CEA monoclonal antibody NP F(ab')2. J Nucl Med 37:1504, 1996.
160. Carrasquillo JA, Krohn KA, Beaumier P, et al: Diagnosis of and therapy for solid tumors with radiolabeled antibodies and immune fragments. Cancer Treat Rep 68:317, 1984.
161. Milenic DE, Yokota T, Filpula DR, et al: Construction, binding properties, metabolism, and tumor targeting of a single-chain Fv derived from the pancarcinoma monoclonal antibody CC49. Cancer Res 51:6363, 1991.
162. Beresford GW, Pavlinkova G, Booth BJ, et al: Binding characteristics and tumor targeting of a covalently linked divalent CC49 single-chain antibody. Int J Cancer 81:911, 1999.
163. Yazaki PJ, Wu AM, Tsai SW, et al: Tumor targeting of radiometal labeled anti-CEA recombinant T84.66 diabody and t84.66 minibody: comparison to radioiodinated fragments. Bioconjug Chem 12:220, 2001.
164. Iliades P, Kortt AA, Hudson PJ: Triabodies: single chain Fv fragments without a linker form trivalent trimers. FEBS Lett 409:437, 1997.
165. King DJ, Turner A, Farnsworth AP, et al: Improved tumor targeting with chemically cross-linked recombinant antibody fragments. Cancer Res 54:6176, 1994.
166. Slavin-Chiorini DC, Horan Hand PH, Kashmiri SV, et al: Biologic properties of a CH2 domain-deleted recombinant immunoglobulin. Int J Cancer 53:97, 1993.
167. Santos AD, Kashmiri SV, Hand PH, et al: Generation and characterization of a single gene-encoded single-chain-tetravalent antitumor antibody. Clin Cancer Res 5:3118s, 1999.
168. Wu AM, Williams LE, Zieran L, et al: Anti-carcinoembryonic antigen (CEA) diabody for rapid tumor targeting and imaging. Tumor Targeting 4:47, 1999.
169. Begent RH, Verhaar MJ, Chester KA, et al: Clinical evidence of efficient tumor targeting based on single-chain Fv antibody selected from a combinatorial library. Nat Med 2:979, 1996.
170. Larson SM, El-Shirbiny AM, Divgi CR, et al: Single chain antigen binding protein (sFv CC49): first human studies in colorectal carcinoma metastatic to liver. Cancer 80:2458, 1997.
171. Adams GP, McCartney JE, Tai MS, et al: Highly specific in vivo tumor targeting by monovalent and divalent forms of 741F8 anti-c-erbB-2 single-chain Fv. Cancer Res 53:4026, 1993.
172. Goel A, Augustine S, Baranowska-Kortylewicz J, et al: Single-dose versus fractionated radioimmunotherapy of human colon carcinoma xenografts using 131I-labeled multivalent CC49 single-chain fvs. Clin Cancer Res 7:175, 2001.
173. Storto G, Buchegger F, Waibel R, et al: Biokinetics of a F(ab')3 iodine-131-labeled antigen binding construct (mAb 35) directed against CEA in patients with colorectal carcinoma. Cancer Biother Radiopharm 16:371, 2001.
174. Casey JL, Napier MP, King DJ, et al: Tumour targeting of humanised cross-linked divalent-Fab' antibody fragments: a clinical phase I/II study. Br J Cancer 86:1401, 2002.
175. Wu AM, Williams LE, Bebb GG, et al: Selection of engineered antibody fragments for targeting and imaging applications: Southborough, MA, IBC BioMedical Library, 1997.
176. Whitlow M, Bell BA, Feng SL, et al: An improved linker for single-chain Fv with reduced aggregation and enhanced proteolytic stability. Prot Eng 6:989, 1993.
177. Cumber AJ, Ward ES, Winter G, et al: Comparative stabilities in vitro and in vivo of a recombinant mouse antibody FvCys fragment and a bisFvCys conjugate. J Immunol 149:120, 1992.
178. Pack P, Pluckthun A: Miniantibodies: use of amphipathic helices to produce functional, flexibly linked dimeric FV fragments with high avidity in *Escherichia coli*. Biochemistry 31:1579, 1992.
179. Holliger P, Prospero T, Winter G: Diabodies: small bivalent and bispecific antibody fragments. Proc Natl Acad Sci U S A 90:6444, 1993.
180. Kostelny SA, Cole MS, Tso JY: Formation of a bispecific antibody by the use of leucine zippers. J Immunol 148:1547, 1992.
181. Forero A, Meredith RF, Khazaeli MR, et al: A novel monoclonal antibody design for radioimmunotherapy. Cancer Biother Radiopharm 18:751, 2003.

182. Khazaeli MR, Forero A, Meredith R, et al: An improved monoclonal antibody design for radioimmunotherapy (RIT). Presented at American Association for Cancer Research, meeting, San Francisco, March 2002.
183. Wong JY, Chu DZ, Williams LE, et al: A pilot trial evaluating a I-123-labeled 80 kd engineered anti-CEA antibody fragment (cT84.66 minibody) in patients with colorectal cancer. Clin Cancer Res 10:5014, 2004.
184. Greiner JW, Hand PH, Noguchi P, et al: Enhanced expression of surface tumor-associated antigens on human breast and colon tumor cells after recombinant human leukocyte alpha-interferon treatment. Cancer Res 44:3208, 1984.
185. Greiner JW, Guadagni F, Hand PH, et al: Augmentation of tumor antigen expression by recombinant human interferons: enhanced targeting of monoclonal antibodies to carcinomas. Cancer Treat Res 51:413, 1990.
186. Kantor J, Tran R, Greiner J, et al: Modulation of carcinoembryonic antigen messenger RNA levels in human colon carcinoma cells by recombinant human gamma-interferon. Cancer Res 49:2651, 1989.
187. Yan XW, Wong JY, Esteban JM, et al: Effects of recombinant human gamma-interferon on carcinoembryonic antigen expression of human colon cancer cells. J Immunother 11:77, 1992.
188. Greiner JW, Guadagni F, Noguchi P, et al: Recombinant interferon enhances monoclonal antibody-targeting of carcinoma lesions in vivo. Science 235:895, 1987.
189. Guadagni F, Roselli M, Schlom J, et al: In vitro and in vivo regulation of human tumor antigen expression by human recombinant interferons: a review. Int J Biol Markers 9:53, 1994.
190. Greiner JW, Guadagni F, Goldstein D, et al: Evidence for the elevation of serum carcinoembryonic antigen and tumor-associated glycoprotein-72 levels in patients administered interferons. Cancer Res 51:4155, 1991.
191. Greiner JW, Guadagni F, Goldstein D, et al: Intraperitoneal administration of interferon-gamma to carcinoma patients enhances expression of tumor-associated glycoprotein-72 and carcinoembryonic antigen on malignant ascites cells. J Clin Oncol 10:735, 1992.
192. Greiner JW, Guadagni F, Roselli M, et al: Improved experimental radioimmunotherapy of colon xenografts by combining 131I-CC49 and interferon-gamma. Dis Colon Rectum 37:S100, 1994.
193. Kuhn JA, Beatty BG, Wong JY, et al: Interferon enhancement of radioimmunotherapy for colon carcinoma. Cancer Res 51:2335, 1991.
194. Macey DJ, Grant EJ, Kasi L, et al: Effect of recombinant alpha-interferon on pharmacokinetics, biodistribution, toxicity, and efficacy of 131I-labeled monoclonal antibody CC49 in breast cancer: a phase II trial. Clin Cancer Res 3:1547, 1997.
195. Slovin SF, Scher HI, Divgi CR, et al: Interferon-gamma and monoclonal antibody 131I-labeled CC49: outcomes in patients with androgen-independent prostate cancer. Clin Cancer Res 4:643, 1998.
196. Meredith RF, Khazaeli MR, Plott WE, et al: Phase II study of dual 131I-labeled monoclonal antibody therapy with interferon in patients with metastatic colorectal cancer. Clin Cancer Res 2:1811, 1996.
197. Meredith RF, Khazaeli MR, Macey DJ, et al: Phase II study of interferon-enhanced 131I-labeled high affinity CC49 monoclonal antibody therapy in patients with metastatic prostate cancer. Clin Cancer Res 5:3254s, 1999.
198. Jain RK: Haemodynamic and transport barriers to the treatment of solid tumours. Int J Radiat Biol 60:85, 1991.
199. Buras R, Williams LE, Beatty BG, et al: A method including edge effects for the estimation of radioimmunotherapy absorbed doses in the tumor xenograft model. Med Phys 21:287, 1994.
200. Wong JY, Williams LE, Demidecki AJ, et al: Radiobiologic studies comparing yttrium irradiation and external beam irradiation in vitro. Int J Radiat Oncol Biol Phys 20:715, 1991.
201. Tempero M, Colcher D, Dalrymple G, et al: High-dose therapy with 131I-conjugated monoclonal antibody CC49: a phase I trial. Antibody Immunoconj Radiopharm 6:90, 1993.
202. Philben VJ, Jakowatz JG, Beatty BG, et al: The effect of tumor CEA content and tumor size on tissue uptake of indium 111-labeled anti-CEA monoclonal antibody. Cancer 57:571, 1986.
203. O'Donoghue JA, Bardies M, Wheldon TE: Relationships between tumor size and curability for uniformly targeted therapy with beta-emitting radionuclides. J Nucl Med 36:1902, 1995.
204. Behr TM, Sharkey RM, Juweid ME, et al: Variables influencing tumor dosimetry in radioimmunotherapy of CEA-expressing cancers with anti-CEA and antimucin monoclonal antibodies. J Nucl Med 38:409, 1997.
205. de Bree R, Kuik DJ, Quak JJ, et al: The impact of tumour volume and other characteristics on uptake of radiolabelled monoclonal antibodies in tumour tissue of head and neck cancer patients. Eur J Nucl Med 25:1562, 1998.
206. Behr T, Liersch T, Griesinger F, et al: Radioimmunotherapy of small volume disease of metastatic colorectal cancer. Results of an ongoing Phase II trial with the 131I-labeled humanized anti-CEA antibody, hMN. Cancer Biother Radiopharm 15:413, 2000.
207. Rowlinson G, Snook D, Busza A, et al: Antibody-guided localization of intraperitoneal tumors following intraperitoneal or intravenous antibody administration. Cancer Res 47:6528, 1987.
208. Braakhuis BJ, Ruiz van Haperen VW, Boven E, et al: Schedule-dependent antitumor effect of gemcitabine in vivo model system. Semin Oncol 22:42, 1995.
209. Colcher D, Esteban J, Carrasquillo JA, et al: Complementation of intracavitary and intravenous administration of a monoclonal antibody (B72.3) in patients with carcinoma. Cancer Res 47:4218, 1987.
210. Ward BG, Mather SJ, Hawkins LR, et al: Localization of radioiodine conjugated to the monoclonal antibody HMFG2 in human ovarian carcinoma: assessment of intravenous and intraperitoneal routes of administration. Cancer Res 47:4719, 1987.
211. Chatal JF, Saccavini JC, Gestin JF, et al: Biodistribution of indium-111-labeled OC 125 monoclonal antibody intraperitoneally injected into patients operated on for ovarian carcinomas. Cancer Res 49:3087, 1989.
212. Stewart JS, Hird V, Snook D, et al: Intraperitoneal radioimmunotherapy for ovarian cancer: pharmacokinetics, toxicity, and efficacy of I-131 labeled monoclonal antibodies. Int J Radiat Oncol Biol Phys 16:405, 1989.
213. Nicholson S, Gooden CS, Hird V, et al: Radioimmunotherapy after chemotherapy compared with chemotherapy alone in the treatment of advanced ovarian cancer: a matched analysis. Oncol Rep 5:223, 1998.
214. Epenetos AA, Hird V, Lambert H, et al: Long term survival of patients with advanced ovarian cancer treated with intraperitoneal radioimmunotherapy. Int J Gynecol Cancer 10:44, 2000.
215. Jacobs AJ, Fer M, Su FM, et al: A phase I trial of a rhenium 186-labeled monoclonal antibody administered intraperitoneally in ovarian carcinoma: toxicity and clinical response. Obstet Gynecol 82:586, 1993.
216. Crippa F, Bolis G, Seregni E, et al: Single-dose intraperitoneal radioimmunotherapy with the murine monoclonal antibody I-131 MOv18: clinical results in patients with minimal residual disease of ovarian cancer. Eur J Cancer 31A:686, 1995.
217. Meredith R, Alvarez RD, Khazaeli MR, et al: Intraperitoneal radioimmunotherapy for refractory epithelial ovarian cancer with 177 Lu-CC49. Minerva Biotecnol 10:100, 1998.
218. Cokgor I, Akabani G, Kuan CT, et al: Phase I trial results of iodine 131-labeled antitenascin monoclonal antibody 81C6 treatment of patients with newly diagnosed malignant gliomas. J Clin Oncol 18:3862, 2000.
219. Reardon DA, Akabani G, Coleman RE, et al: Phase II trial of murine (131)I-labeled antitenascin monoclonal antibody 81C6 administered into surgically created resection cavities of patients with newly diagnosed malignant gliomas. J Clin Oncol 20:1389, 2002.
220. Bigner DD, Brown MT, Friedman AH, et al: Iodine 131-labeled antitenascin monoclonal antibody 81C6 treatment of patients with recurrent malignant gliomas: phase I trial results. J Clin Oncol 16:2202, 1998.
221. Zalutsky MR, Vaidyanathan G: Astatine-211-labeled radiotherapeutics: an emerging approach to targeted alpha-particle radiotherapy. Curr Pharm Des 6:1433, 2000.
222. Zalutsky MR: Targeted radiotherapy of brain tumours. Br J Cancer 90:1469, 2004.

223. Riva P, Arista A, Franceschi G, et al: Local treatment of malignant gliomas by direct infusion of specific monoclonal antibodies labeled with 131I: comparison of the results obtained in recurrent and newly diagnosed tumors. Cancer Res 55:5952s, 1995.
224. Riva P, Franceschi G, Arista A, et al: Local application of radiolabeled monoclonal antibodies in the treatment of high grade malignant gliomas: a six-year clinical experience. Cancer 80:2733, 1997.
225. Riva P, Franceschi G, Frattarelli M, et al: Loco-regional radioimmunotherapy of high-grade malignant gliomas using specific monoclonal antibodies labeled with 90Y: a phase I study. Clin Cancer Res 5:3275s, 1999.
226. Goetz C, Riva P, Poepperl G, et al: Locoregional radioimmunotherapy in selected patients with malignant glioma: experiences, side effects and survival times. J Neurooncol 62:321, 2003.
227. Goetz C, Rachinger W, Poepperl G, et al: Intralesional radioimmunotherapy in the treatment of malignant glioma: clinical and experimental findings. Acta Neurochir Suppl 88:69, 2003.
228. Hopkins K, Chandler C, Bullimore J, et al: A pilot study of the treatment of patients with recurrent malignant gliomas with intratumoral yttrium-90 radioimmunoconjugates. Radiother Oncol 34:121, 1995.
229. Papanastassiou V, Pizer BL, Coakham HB, et al: Treatment of recurrent and cystic malignant gliomas by a single intracavity injection of 131I monoclonal antibody: feasibility, pharmacokinetics and dosimetry. Br J Cancer 67:144, 1993.
230. Casaco A, Lopez G, Fernandez R, et al: Loco-regional radioimmunotherapy of high grade malignant gliomas using the humanized monoclonal antibody, h-R3, labeled with 188-Re. J Clin Oncol 23:170, 2004.
231. Kemshead JT, Hopkins KI, Chandler CL: Treatment of diffuse leptomeningeal malignancy by intrathecal injection of 131I radioimmunoconjugates. Recent Results Cancer Res 141:145, 1996.
232. Pizer BL, Papanastassiou V, Moseley R, et al: Meningeal leukemia and medulloblastoma: Preliminary experience with intrathecal radioimmunotherapy. Antibody Immunoconj Radiopharm 4:753, 1991.
233. Brown MT, Coleman RE, Friedman AH, et al: Intrathecal 131I-labeled antitenascin monoclonal antibody 81C6 treatment of patients with leptomeningeal neoplasms or primary brain tumor resection cavities with subarachnoid communication: phase I trial results. Clin Cancer Res 2:963, 1996.
234. Kalofonos HP, Pawlikowska TR, Hemingway A, et al: Antibody guided diagnosis and therapy of brain gliomas using radiolabeled monoclonal antibodies against epidermal growth factor receptor and placental alkaline phosphatase. J Nucl Med 30:1636, 1989.
235. Brady LW, Markoe AM, Woo DV, et al: Iodine 131-labeled anti-epidermal growth factor receptor in the treatment of glioblastoma multiforme. A pilot study. Front Radiat Ther Oncol 24:151; discussion 161, 1990.
236. Brady LW, Woo DV, Markoe AM, et al: Treatment of malignant gliomas with 125I-labeled monoclonal antibody against epidermal growth factor receptor. Antibody Immunoconj Radiopharm 3:169, 1990.
237. Brady LW, Miyamoto C, Woo DV, et al: Malignant astrocytomas treated with iodine labeled monoclonal antibody 425 against epidermal growth factor receptor: a phase II trial. Int J Radiat Oncol Biol Phys 22:225, 1992.
238. Emrich JG, Brady LW, Quang TS, et al: Radioiodinated (I) monoclonal antibody 425 in the treatment of high grade glioma patients: ten-year synopsis of a novel treatment. Am J Clin Oncol 25:541, 2002.
239. Zeng ZC, Tang ZY, Liu KD, et al: Improved long-term survival for unresectable hepatocellular carcinoma (HCC) with a combination of surgery and intrahepatic arterial infusion of 131I-anti-HCC mAb. Phase I/II clinical trials. J Cancer Res Clin Oncol 124:275, 1998.
240. Zeng ZC, Tang ZY, Yang BH, et al: Comparison between radioimmunotherapy and external beam radiation therapy for patients with hepatocellular carcinoma. Eur J Nucl Med Mol Imaging 29:1657, 2002.
241. Gold DV, Schutsky K, Modrak D, et al: Low-dose radioimmunotherapy ((90)Y-PAM4) combined with gemcitabine for the treatment of experimental pancreatic cancer. Clin Cancer Res 9:3929S, 2003.
242. Scott AM, Wiseman G, Welt S, et al: A Phase I dose-escalation study of sibrotuzumab in patients with advanced or metastatic fibroblast activation protein-positive cancer. Clin Cancer Res 9:1639, 2003.
243. DeNardo SJ, Kukis SL, Kroger LA, et al: Synergy of Taxol and radioimmunotherapy with yttrium-90-labeled chimeric L6 antibody: efficacy and toxicity in breast cancer xenografts. Proc Natl Acad Sci U S A 94:4000, 1997.
244. O'Donnell RT, DeNardo SJ, Miers LA, et al: Combined modality radioimmunotherapy with Taxol and 90Y-Lym-1 for Raji lymphoma xenografts. Cancer Biother Radiopharm 13:351, 1998.
245. Kievit E, Pinedo HM, Schluper H, et al: Addition of cisplatin improves efficacy of 131I-labeled monoclonal antibody 323/A3 in experimental human ovarian cancer. Int J Radiat Oncol Biol Phys 38:419, 1997.
246. Kinuya S, Yokoyama K, Tega H, et al: Efficacy, toxicity and mode of interaction of combination radioimmunotherapy with 5-fluorouracil in colon cancer xenografts. J Cancer Res Clin Oncol 125:630, 1999.
247. Remmenga SW, Colcher D, Gansow O, et al: Continuous infusion chemotherapy as a radiation-enhancing agent for yttrium 90-radiolabeled monoclonal antibody therapy of a human tumor xenograft. Gynecol Oncol 55:115, 1994.
248. Buchsbaum DJ, Khazaeli MR, Davis MA, et al: Sensitization of radiolabeled monoclonal antibody therapy using bromodeoxyuridine. Cancer 73:999, 1994.
249. Roffler SR, Chan J, Yeh MY: Potentiation of radioimmunotherapy by inhibition of topoisomerase I. Cancer Res 54:1276, 1994.
250. Graves S, Dearstyne E, Hylarides M, et al: Gemicitabine improves the efficacy of 90yttrium-based pretarget radioimmunotherapy against LS174T tumor xenografts. Presented at American Association for Cancer Research meeting, San Francisco, March 2002.
251. Okazaki S, Tempero M, Colcher D: Combination radioimmunotherapy and chemotherapy using 131I-B72.3 and gemcitabine. Presented at American Association for Cancer Research meeting, New Orleans, March 1998.
252. Blumenthal RD, Osorio L, Leon E, et al: Multimodal preclinical radioimmunotherapy (RAIT) in combination with chemotherapy of human colonic tumors: Selection between 5-fluorouracil (%-FU) and irinotecan (CPT). Presented at American Association for Cancer Research meeting, San Francisco, March 2002.
253. Ng B, Liebes L, Kramer E, et al: Synergistic activity of radioimmunotherapy with prolonged toptecan infusion in human breast cancer xenograft. Presented at American Association for Cancer Research 38, 1997.
254. Meredith RF, Alvarez RD, Partridge EE, et al: Intraperitoneal radioimmunochemotherapy of ovarian cancer: a phase I study. Cancer Biother Radiopharm 16:305, 2001.
255. Alvarez RD, Huh WK, Khazaeli MR, et al: A phase I study of combined modality (90)yttrium-CC49 intraperitoneal radioimmunotherapy for ovarian cancer. Clin Cancer Res 8:2806, 2002.
256. Richman CM, DeNardo SJ, O'Donnell RT, et al: Combined modality radioimmunotherapy (RIT) in metastatic prostate (PC) and breast cancer (BC) using paclitaxel (PT) and a MUC monoclonal antibody m170, linked to yttrium (Y). J Clin Oncol 23:176, 2004.
257. Wong JY, Shibata S, Williams LE, et al: A phase I trial of 90Y-anti-carcinoembryonic antigen chimeric T84.66 radioimmunotherapy with 5-fluorouracil in patients with metastatic colorectal cancer. Clin Cancer Res 9:5842, 2003.
258. Buchegger F, Allal AS, Roth A, et al: Combined radioimmunotherapy and radiotherapy of liver metastases from colorectal cancer: a feasibility study. Anticancer Res 20:1889, 2000.
259. Carabasi M, Khazaeli MR, Tilden AB, et al: Autologous stem cell transplantation for breast and prostate cancer after combined modality therapy with radioimmunotherapy plus external beam radiation. Blood 94:333a, 1999.
260. Schultheiss T, Liu A, Wong JY, et al: Total marrow and total lymphatic irradiation with helical tomotherapy. Med Phys 31:1845, 2004.

261. Schultheiss T, Wong JY, Olivera G, et al: Normal tissue sparing in total marrow and total lymphatic irradiation with helical tomotherapy. Presented at American Society for Therapeutic Radiology and Oncology, 2004.
262. DeNardo GL, DeNardo SJ: Treatment of B-lymphocyte malignancies with 131I-Lym-1 and 67Cu IT-BAT-Lym-1 and opportunities for improvement. Boca Raton: CRC Press, 1994.
263. Lewis JP, DeNardo GL, DeNardo SJ: Radioimmunotherapy of lymphoma: a UC Davis experience. Hybridoma 14:115, 1995.
264. DeNardo GL, DeNardo SJ, Lamborn KR, et al: Low-dose, fractionated radioimmunotherapy for B-cell malignancies using 131I-Lym-1 antibody. Cancer Biother Radiopharm 13:239, 1998.
265. DeNardo GL, DeNardo SJ, Goldstein DS, et al: Maximum-tolerated dose, toxicity, and efficacy of (131)I-Lym-1 antibody for fractionated radioimmunotherapy of non-Hodgkin's lymphoma. J Clin Oncol 16:3246, 1998.
266. Kuzel T, Rosen ST, Zimmer AM, et al: A phase I escalating-dose safety, dosimetry and efficacy study of radiolabeled monoclonal antibody LYM. Cancer Biother 8:3, 1993.
267. Meredith RF, Khazaeli MR, Plott G, et al: Comparison of diagnostic and therapeutic doses of I-131-Lym-1 in patients with non-Hodgkin's lymphoma. Antibody Immunoconj Radiopharm 6:1, 1993.
268. O'Donnell RT, DeNardo GL, Kukis DL, et al: A clinical trial of radioimmunotherapy with 67Cu-2IT-BAT-Lym-1 for non-Hodgkin's lymphoma. J Nucl Med 40:2014, 1999.
269. O'Donnell RT, DeNardo GL, Kukis DL, et al: 67Copper-2-iminothiolane-6-p-(bromoacetamido)benzyl-TETA-Lym-1 for radioimmunotherapy of non-Hodgkin's lymphoma. Clin Cancer Res 5:3330s, 1999.
270. O'Donnell RT, Shen S, DeNardo SJ, et al: A phase I study of 90Y IT-BAD-Lym-1 in patients with non-Hodgkin's lymphoma. Anticancer Res 20:3647, 2000.
271. Postema EJ, Raemaekers JM, Oyen WJ, et al: Final results of a phase I radioimmunotherapy trial using (186)Re-epratuzumab for the treatment of patients with non-Hodgkin's lymphoma. Clin Cancer Res 9:3995S, 2003.
272. Juweid ME, Stadtmauer E, Hajjar G, et al: Pharmacokinetics, dosimetry, and initial therapeutic results with 131I- and (111)In-/90Y-labeled humanized LL2 anti-CD22 monoclonal antibody in patients with relapsed, refractory non-Hodgkin's lymphoma. Clin Cancer Res 5:3292s, 1999.
273. Chatal JR, Harousseau JL, Griesinger F, et al: Radioimmunotherapy in non-Hodgkin's lymphoma (NHL) using a fractionated schedule of DOTA-conjugated:90Y-radiolabeled, humanized anti-CD22 monoclonal antibody. Epratuzumab. J Clin Oncol 23:174, 2004.
274. Vose JM, Colcher D, Bierman PJ, et al: I-131-LL2 (anti-CD20) radioimmunotherapy (RIT) of refractory non-Hodgkin's lymphoma (NHL): results of a repetitive dosing trial. J Clin Oncol 10:1696, 1997.
275. Kaminski MS, Fig LM, Zasadny KR, et al: Imaging, dosimetry, and radioimmunotherapy with iodine 131-labeled anti-CD37 antibody in B-cell lymphoma. J Clin Oncol 10:1696, 1992.
276. Czuczman MS, Straus DJ, Divgi CR, et al: Phase I dose-escalation trial of iodine 131-labeled monoclonal antibody OKB7 in patients with non-Hodgkin's lymphoma. J Clin Oncol 11:2021, 1993.
277. Parker BA, Vassos AB, Halpern SE, et al: Radioimmunotherapy of human B-cell lymphoma with 90Y-conjugated antiidiotype monoclonal antibody. Cancer Res 50:1022s, 1990.
278. White CA, Halpern SE, Parker BA, et al: Radioimmunotherapy of relapsed B-cell lymphoma with yttrium 90 anti-idiotype monoclonal antibodies. Blood 87:3640, 1996.
279. Knox SJ, Goris ML, Trisler K, et al: Yttrium-90-labeled anti-CD20 monoclonal antibody therapy of recurrent B-cell lymphoma. Clin Cancer Res 2:457, 1996.
280. Kaminski MS, Estes J, Zasadny KR, et al: Radioimmunotherapy with iodine (131)I tositumomab for relapsed or refractory B-cell non-Hodgkin lymphoma: updated results and long-term follow-up of the University of Michigan experience. Blood 96:1259, 2000.
281. Vose JM, Wahl RL, Saleh M, et al: Multicenter phase II study of iodine tositumomab for chemotherapy-relapsed/refractory low-grade and transformed low-grade B-cell non-Hodgkin's lymphomas. J Clin Oncol 18:1316, 2000.
282. Kaminski MS, Zelenetz AD, Press OW, et al: Pivotal study of iodine I-131 tositumomab for chemotherapy-refractory low-grade or transformed low-grade B-cell non-Hodgkin's lymphomas. J Clin Oncol 19:3918, 2001.
283. Davis T, Kaminski MS, Leonard J, et al: Long-term results of a randomized trial comparing Tositumomab alone in patients with relapsed or refractory low-grade (LG) or transformed low grade (T-LG) non-Hodgkin's lymphoma (NHL). Blood 102:405a, 2003.
284. Horning SJ, Younes A, Lucas JB, et al: Rituximab treatment failures: tositumomab and iodine I-131 tositumomab (Bexxar) can produce meaningful dupable responses. Blood 100:1385, 2002.
285. Weiden PL, Breitz HB, Press O, et al: Pretargeted radioimmunotherapy (PRIT) for treatment of non-Hodgkin's lymphoma (NHL): initial phase I/II study results. Cancer Biother Radiopharm 15:15, 2000.
286. Witzig TW, Gordon LI, Cabanillas F, et al: Randomized controlled trial of yttrium-90-labeled ibritumomab tiuxetan radioimmunotherapy versus rituximab immunotherapy for patients with relapsed or refractory low-grade, follicular, or transformed B-cell non-Hodgkin's lymphoma. J Clin Oncol 20:2453, 2002.
287. Witzig TW, White CA, Wiseman GA, et al: Phase I/II trial of IDEC-Y2B8 radioimmunotherapy for treatment of relapsed or refractory CD20(+) B-cell non-Hodgkin's lymphoma. J Clin Oncol 17:3793, 1999.
288. Witzig TE, Flinn IW, Gordon LI, et al: Treatment with ibritumomab tiuxetan radioimmunotherapy in patients with rituximab-refractory follicular non-Hodgkin's lymphoma. J Clin Oncol 20:3262, 2002.
289. Press OW, Eary JW, Appelbaum FR, et al: Radiolabeled-antibody therapy of B-cell lymphoma with autologous bone marrow support. N Engl J Med 329:1219, 1993.
290. Liu SY, Eary JF, Petersdorf SH, et al: Follow-up of relapsed B-cell lymphoma patients treated with iodine 131-labeled anti-CD20 antibody and autologous stem-cell rescue. J Clin Oncol 16:3270, 1998.
291. Press OW, Eary JR, Appelbaum FR, et al: Phase II trial of 131I-B1 (anti-CD20) antibody therapy with autologous stem cell transplantation for relapsed B cell lymphomas. Lancet 346:336, 1995.
292. Press OW, Eary JR, Badger CC, et al: Treatment of refractory non-Hodgkin's lymphoma with radiolabeled MB (anti-CD37) antibody. J Clin Oncol 7:1027, 1989.
293. Badger CC, Eary JF, Brown BA: Therapy of lymphoma with I-131-labeled anti-idiotype antibodies. Presented at AACR, 1987.
294. Zimmer AM, Kaplan EH, Kazikiewicz JM, et al: Pharmacokinetics of I-131 T101 monoclonal antibody in patients with chronic lymphocytic leukemia. Antibody Immunoconj Radiopharm 1:291, 1988.
295. Rosen ST, Zimmer AM, Goldman-Leikin R, et al: Progress in the treatment of cutaneous T cell lymphomas with radiolabeled monoclonal antibodies. Int J Rad Appl Instrum B 16:667, 1989.
296. Raubitschek A: Yttrium 90-labeled T101 in the treatment of hematologic malignancies. Presented at Fifth International Conference of Monoclonal Antibody Conjugates for Cancer, San Diego, CA, March 1990.
297. Waldmann TA, White JD, Carrasquillo JA, et al: Radioimmunotherapy of interleukin R alpha-expressing adult T-cell leukemia with yttrium-90-labeled anti-Tac. Blood 86:4063, 1995.
298. Wahl RL, Kroll S, Zasadny KR: Patient-specific whole-body dosimetry: principles and a simplified method for clinical implementation. J Nucl Med 39:14S, 1998.
299. Kaminski MS, Zasadny KR, Francis IR, et al: Radioimmunotherapy of B-cell lymphoma with [131I]anti-B1 (anti-CD20) antibody. N Engl J Med 329:459, 1993.
300. Zelenetz AD, Leonard J, Bennett J, et al: Long-term follow-up of patients with low-grade and transformed low-grade NHL treated with Bexxar therapy. J Clin Oncol 21:283a, 2002.
301. Kaminski MS, Zasadny KR, Francis IR, et al: Iodine 131-anti-B1 radioimmunotherapy for B-cell lymphoma. J Clin Oncol 14, 1974, 1996.
302. Kaminski MS, Knox S, Radford JA, et al: Re-treatment with tositumomab and iodine I-131 tositumomab (the Bexxar Therapeu-

tic Regimen) in patients with non-Hodgkin's lymphoma (NHL) with a previous response to the Bexxar Therapeutic Regimen. Blood 102:30a, 2003.
303. Kaminski MS, Tuck M, Regan D, et al: High response rates and durable remissions in patients with previously untreated, advanced stage, follicular lymphoma treated with tositumomab and iodine I-131 tositumomab (Bexxar). Blood 100:356a, 2002.
304. Vose JM, Bierman PJ, Lynch J, et al: Phase I clinical trial of Zevalin (90Y-ibritumomab) in patients with B-cell non-Hodgkin's lymphoma (NHL) with relapsed disease following high-dose chemotherapy and autologous stem cell transplantation (ASCT). Blood 102:304a, 2003.
305. Gopal AK, Gooley TA, Maloney DG, et al: High-dose radioimmunotherapy versus conventional high-dose therapy and autologous hematopoietic stem cell transplantation for relapsed follicular non-Hodgkin lymphoma: a multivariable cohort analysis. Blood 102:2351, 2003.
306. Press OW, Eary JF, Gooley T, et al: A phase I/II trial of iodine 131-tositumomab (anti-CD20), etoposide, cyclophosphamide, and autologous stem cell transplantation for relapsed B-cell lymphomas. Blood 96:2934, 2000.
307. Gopal AK, Rajendran JG, Petersdorf S, et al: High-dose chemoradioimmunnotherapy with autologous stem cell support for relapsed mantle cell lymphoma. Blood 99:3158, 2002.
308. Vose JM, Bierman PJ, Lynch J, et al: Long term results of radioimmunotherapy with Bexxar/BEAM and autologous stem cell transplantation (ASCT) for chemotherapy resistant aggressive non-Hodgkin's lymphoma (NHL). Blood 102:248a, 2003.
309. Forero A, Weiden PL, Vose JM, et al: Phase I-131 trial of a novel anti-CD20 fusion protein in pretargeted radioimmunotherapy for B-cell non-Hodgkin's lymphoma. Blood 104:227, 2004.
310. Press OW, Unger JM, Braziel RM, et al: A phase 2 trial of CHOP chemotherapy followed by tositumomab/iodine I-131 tositumomab for previously untreated follicular non-Hodgkin lymphoma: Southwest Oncology Group Protocol S9911. Blood 102:1606, 2003.
311. Ansell SM, Ristow KM, Habermann TM, et al: Subsequent chemotherapy regimens are well tolerated after radioimmunotherapy with yttrium ibritumomab tiuxetan for non-Hodgkin's lymphoma. J Clin Oncol 20:3885, 2002.
312. Lenhard RE Jr, Order SE, Spunberg JJ, et al: Isotopic immunoglobulin: a new systemic therapy for advanced Hodgkin's disease. J Clin Oncol 3:1296, 1985.
313. Bierman PJ, Vose JM, Leichner PK, et al: Yttrium 90-labeled antiferritin followed by high-dose chemotherapy and autologous bone marrow transplantation for poor-prognosis Hodgkin's disease. J Clin Oncol 11:698, 1993.
314. Herpst JM, Klein JL, Leichner PK, et al: Survival of patients with resistant Hodgkin's disease after polyclonal yttrium 90-labeled antiferritin treatment. J Clin Oncol 13:2394, 1995.
315. Morton JD, Quadri SM, Tang XZ, et al: Yttrium 90 polyclonal antiferrtin therapy in patients with refractory end-stage Hodgkin's disease. Int J Radiat Onc Biol Phys 30:181, 1994.
316. Vriesendorp HM, Morton JD, Quadri SM: Review of five consecutive studies of radiolabeled immunoglobulin therapy in Hodgkin's disease. Cancer Res 55:5888s, 1995.
317. Burke JM, Jurcic JG, Scheinberg DA: Radioimmunotherapy for acute leukemia. Cancer Control 9:106, 2002.
318. Jurcic JG, Caron PC, Miller WH Jr, et al: Sequential targeted therapy for relapsed acute promyelocytic leukemia with all-trans retinoic acid and anti-CD33 monoclonal antibody M195. Leukemia 9:244, 1995.
319. Caron MA, Schwartz MS, Co, et al: Murine and humanized constructs of monoclonal antibody M195 (anti-CD33) for the therapy of acute myelogenous leukemia. Cancer 73:1049, 1994.
320. Caron PC, Jurcic JG, Scott AM, et al: A phase 1B trial of humanized monoclonal antibody M195 (anti-CD33) in myeloid leukemia: specific targeting without immunogenicity. Blood 83:1760, 1994.
321. Burke JM, Caron PC, Papadopoulos EB, et al: Cytoreduction with iodine-anti-CD33 antibodies before bone marrow transplantation for advanced myeloid leukemias. Bone Marrow Transplant 32:549, 2003.
322. Sgouros G, Ballangrud AM, Jurcic JG, et al: Pharmacokinetics and dosimetry of an alpha-particle emitter labeled antibody: 213Bi-HuM195 (anti-CD33) in patients with leukemia. J Nucl Med 40:1935, 1999.
323. Jurcic JG, Larson SM, Sgouros G, et al: Targeted alpha particle immunotherapy for myeloid leukemia. Blood 100:1233, 2002.
324. Matthews DC, Appelbaum FR, Eary JF, et al: Phase I study of (131)I-anti-CD45 antibody plus cyclophosphamide and total body irradiation for advanced acute leukemia and myelodysplastic syndrome. Blood 94:1237, 1999.
325. Juweid ME, Zhang CH, Blumenthal RD, et al: Prediction of hematologic toxicity after radioimmunotherapy with (131)I-labeled anticarcinoembryonic antigen monoclonal antibodies. J Nucl Med 40:1609, 1999.
326. Siegel JA, Yeldell D, Goldenberg DM, et al: Red marrow radiation dose adjustment using plasma FLT3-L cytokine levels: improved correlations between hematologic toxicity and bone marrow dose for radioimmunotherapy patients. J Nucl Med 44:67, 2003.
327. Blumenthal RD, Sharkey RM, Goldenberg DM: Dose escalation of radioantibody in a mouse model with the use of recombinant human interleukin and granulocyte-macrophage colony-stimulating factor intervention to reduce myelosuppression. J Natl Cancer Inst 84:399, 1992.
328. Neta R, Douches S, Oppenheim JJ: Interleukin 1 is a radioprotector. J Immunol 136:2483, 1986.
329. Brenner W, Kampen WU, Brummer C, et al: Myeloprotective effects of different amifostine regimens in rabbits undergoing high-dose treatment with 186rhenium-(tin)1,1-hydroxyethylidene diphosphonate (186Re-HEDP). Cancer Biother Radiopharm 18:887, 2003.
330. Bohuslavizki KH, Klutmann S, Brenner W, et al: Radioprotection of salivary glands by amifostine in high-dose radioiodine treatment. Results of a double-blinded, placebo-controlled study in patients with differentiated thyroid cancer. Strahlenther Onkol 175(Suppl 4):6, 1999.
331. Hird V, Stewart JS, Snook D, et al: Intraperitoneally administered 90Y-labelled monoclonal antibodies as a third line of treatment in ovarian cancer. A phase 1 trial: problems encountered and possible solutions. Br J Cancer Suppl 10:48, 1990.
332. Forero A, Meredith RF, Khazaeli MB, et al: Phase I study of ^{90}Y-CC49 monoclonal antibody therapy in patients with advanced non–small cell lung cancer: effect of chelating agents and paclitaxel co-administration. Cancer Biother Radiopharm 20:467, 2005.
333. Blumenthal RD, Sharkey RM, Snyder D, et al: Reduction by anti-antibody administration of the radiotoxicity associated with 131I-labeled antibody to carcinoembryonic antigen in cancer radioimmunotherapy. J Natl Cancer Inst 81:194, 1989.
334. Press OW, Appelbaum FR, Eary JF, et al: Radiolabeled antibody therapy of lymphomas. Important Adv Oncol:157, 1995.
335. Dillman RO: Monoclonal antibodies for treating cancer. Ann Intern Med 111:592, 1989.
336. Alvarez RD, Partridge EE, Khazaeli MR, et al: Intraperitoneal radioimmunotherapy of ovarian cancer with 177Lu-CC49: a phase I/II study. Gynecol Oncol 65:94, 1997.
337. Mandel SJ, Mandel L: Radioactive iodine and the salivary glands, Thyroid 13:265, 2003.
338. Schlom J, Molinolo A, Simpson JF, et al: Advantage of dose fractionation in monoclonal antibody-targeted radioimmunotherapy. J Natl Cancer Inst 82:763, 1990.
339. DeNardo GL, Schlom J, Buchsbaum DJ, et al: Rationales, evidence, and design considerations for fractionated radioimmunotherapy. Cancer 94:1332, 2002.
340. Stabin MG: Radiotherapy with internal emitters: what can dosimetrists offer? Cancer Biother Radiopharm 18:611, 2003.
341. Siegel JA, Lee RE, Pawlyk DA, et al: Sacral scintigraphy for bone marrow dosimetry in radioimmunotherapy. Int J Rad Appl Instrum B 16:553, 1989.
342. Sgouros G: Bone marrow dosimetry for radioimmunotherapy: theoretical considerations. J Nucl Med 34:689, 1993.
343. Wiseman GA, Leigh BR, Erwin WD, et al: Radiation dosimetry results from a Phase II trial of ibritumomab tiuxetan (Zevalin)

radioimmunotherapy for patients with non-Hodgkin's lymphoma and mild thrombocytopenia. Cancer Biother Radiopharm 18:165, 2003.

344. Verel I, Visser GW, Boellaard R, et al: Quantitative 89Zr immuno-PET for in vivo scouting of 90Y-labeled monoclonal antibodies in xenograft-bearing nude mice. J Nucl Med 44:1663, 2003.
345. Eary JF, Press OW, Badger CC, et al: Imaging and treatment of B-cell lymphoma. J Nucl Med 31:1257, 1990.
346. Clarke KG, Odom-Maryon TL, Williams LE, and coworkers Intrapatient consistency of imaging biodistributions and their application to predicting therapeutic doses in a phase I-131 clinical study of 90Y-based radioimmunotherapy. Med Phys 26:799, 1999.
347. Tsui BMW: Quantitative SPECT. St. Louis, Mosby-Year Book, 1996.
348. Stabin MG: Developments in the internal dosimetry of radiopharmaceuticals. Radiat Prot Dosimetry 105:575, 2003.
349. Howell RW, Wessels BW, Loevinger R, et al: The MIRD perspective 1999. Medical Internal Radiation Dose Committee. J Nucl Med 40:3S, 1999.
350. Stabin MG, Siegel JA: Physical models and dose factors for use in internal dose assessment. Health Phys 85:294, 2003.
351. Bolch WE, Bouchet LG, Robertson JS, et al: MIRD pamphlet No. 17: the dosimetry of nonuniform activity distributions—radionuclide S values at the voxel level. Medical Internal Radiation Dose Committee. J Nucl Med 40:11S, 1999.
352. Bouchet LG, Bolch WE, Blanco HP, et al: MIRD Pamphlet No 19: absorbed fractions and radionuclide S values for six age-dependent multiregion models of the kidney. J Nucl Med 44:1113, 2003.
353. Meredith RF, Johnson TK, Plott G, et al: Dosimetry of solid tumors. Med Phys 20:583, 1993.
354. Johnson TK, McClure D, McCourt S: MABDOSE. II: Validation of a general purpose dose estimation code. Med Phys 26:1396, 1999.
355. Seigel JA, Thomas SR, Stubbs JB, et al: MIRD Pamphlet No. 16: techniques for quantitative radiopharmaceutical biodistribution data acquisition and analysis for use in human radiation dose estimates. J Nucl Med 37, 1999.
356. Ljungberg M, Frey E, Sjogreen K, et al: 3D absorbed dose calculations based on SPECT: evaluation for 111-In/90-Y therapy using Monte Carlo simulations. Cancer Biother Radiopharm 18:99, 2003.
357. Yoriyaz H, Stabin MG, dos Santos A: Monte Carlo MCNP B-based absorbed dose distribution estimates for patient-specific dosimetry. J Nucl Med 42:662, 2001.
358. Griffith MH, Yorke ED, Wessels BW, et al: Direct dose confirmation of quantitative autoradiography with micro-TLD measurements for radioimmunotherapy. J Nucl Med 29:1795, 1988.
359. Larson SM, Pentlow KS, Volkow ND, et al: PET scanning of iodine F9 as an approach to tumor dosimetry during treatment planning for radioimmunotherapy in a child with neuroblastoma. J Nucl Med 33:2020, 1992.
360. Brouwers A, Verel I, Van Eerd J, et al: PET radioimmunoscintigraphy of renal cell cancer using 89Zr-labeled cG250 monoclonal antibody in nude rats. Cancer Biother Radiopharm 19:155, 2004.
361. Wiseman GA, Kornmehl E, Leigh B, et al: Radiation dosimetry results and safety correlations from 90Y-ibritumomab tiuxetan radioimmunotherapy for relapsed or refractory non-Hodgkin's lymphoma: combined data from 4 clinical trials. J Nucl Med 44:465, 2003.
362. Helisch A, Forster GJ, Reber H, et al: Pre-therapeutic dosimetry and biodistribution of (86) Y-DOTA-Phe(1)-Tyr(3)-octreotide versus (111)In-pentetreotide in patient with advanced neuroendocrine tumours. Eur J Nucl Med 31:1386, 2004.
363. Sgouros G, Squeri S, Ballangrud AM, et al: Patient-specific: 3-dimensional dosimetry in non-Hodgkin's lymphoma patients treated with 131I-anti-B1 antibody: assessment of tumor dose-response. J Nucl Med 44:260, 2003.
364. Koral KF, Kaminski MS, Wahl RL: Correlation of tumor radiation-absorbed dose with response is easier to find in previously untreated patients. J Nucl Med 44:1541; author reply 1543, 2003.
365. van Osdol W, Fujimori K, Weinstein JN: An analysis of monoclonal antibody distribution in microscopic tumor nodules: consequences of a binding site barrier. Cancer Res 51:4776, 1991.
366. Chatal JF, Saccavini JC, Fumoleau P, et al: Immunoscintigraphy of colon carcinoma. J Nucl Med 25:307, 1984.
367. Quadri SM, Lai J, Mohammadpour H, et al: Assessment of radiolabeled stabilized F(ab')2 fragments of monoclonal antiferritin in nude mouse model. J Nucl Med 34:2152, 1993.
368. Msirikale JS, Klein JL, Schroeder J, et al: Radiation enhancement of radiolabelled antibody deposition in tumors. Int J Radiat Oncol Biol Phys 13:1839, 1987.
369. Raben D, Buchsbaum D: Combined External Beam Radiotherapy and Radioimmunotherapy. Oxford. England, Oxford University Press, 2003.
370. Order SE, Stillwagon GB, Klein JL, et al: Iodine 131 antiferritin, a new treatment modality in hepatoma: a Radiation Therapy Oncology Group study. J Clin Oncol 3:1573, 1985.
371. Gridley DS, Mackensen DG, Slater JB, et al: Effects of proton irradiation on radiolabeled monoclonal antibody uptake in human colon tumor xenografts. J Immunother Emphasis Tumor Immunol 17:229, 1995.
372. Folli S, Pelegrin A, Chalandon Y, et al: Tumor-necrosis factor can enhance radio-antibody uptake in human colon carcinoma xenografts by increasing vascular permeability. Int J Cancer 53:829, 1993.
373. Schuster JM, Zalutsky MR, Noska MA, et al: Hyperthermic modulation of radiolabelled antibody uptake in a human glioma xenograft and normal tissues. Int J Hyperthermia 11:59, 1995.
374. DeNardo GL, DeNardo SJ, Lamborn KR: Enhancement of tumor uptake of monoclonal antibody in nude mice with PEG-IL. Antibody Immunoconj Radiopharm 4:859, 1991.
375. DeNardo SJ, Mirick GR, Kroger LA, et al: The biologic window for chimeric L6 radioimmunotherapy. Cancer 73:1023, 1994.
376. Leunig M, Goetz AE, Dellian M, et al: Interstitial fluid pressure in solid tumors following hyperthermia: possible correlation with therapeutic response. Cancer Res 52:487, 1992.
377. Leunig M, Goetz AE, Gamarra F, et al: Photodynamic therapy-induced alterations in interstitial fluid pressure, volume and water content of an amelanotic melanoma in the hamster. Br J Cancer 69:101, 1994.
378. Wilder RB, Langmuir VK, Mendonca HL, et al: Local hyperthermia and SR 4233 enhance the antitumor effects of radioimmunotherapy in nude mice with human colonic adenocarcinoma xenografts. Cancer Res 53:3022, 1993.
379. Schuster JM, Bigner DD: Immunotherapy and monoclonal antibody therapies. Curr Opin Oncol 4:547, 1992.
380. DeNardo SJ, Burke PA, Leigh BR, et al: Neovascular targeting with cyclic RGD peptide (cRGDf-ACHA) to enhance delivery of radioimmunotherapy. Cancer Biother Radiopharm 15:71, 2000.
381. Kinuya A, Yokoyama K, Koshida K, et al: Improved survival of mice bearing liver metastases of colon cancer cells treated with a combination of radioimmunotherapy and antiangiogenic therapy. Eur J Nucl Med Mol Imaging 31:986, 2004.
382. Kurizaki T, Okazaki S, Sanderson SD, et al: Potentiation of radioimmunotherapy with response-selective peptide agonist of human C5a. J Nucl Med 43:957, 2002.
383. Blumenthal RD, Sharkey RM, Kashi R, et al: Changes in tumor vascular permeability in response to experimental radioimmunotherapy: a comparative study of 11 xenografts, Tumour Biol 18:367, 1997.
384. Schlom J, Eggensperger D, Colcher D, et al: Therapeutic advantage of high-affinity anticarcinoma radioimmunoconjugates. Cancer Res 52:1067, 1992.
385. Meredith RF, Plott WE, Brezovich IA, et al: Radiation dose estimates from intraperitoneal radioimmunotherapy with 177Lu-CC49. Proc Int Radiopharmaceut Dosimetry Symp 1:158, 1999.
386. Murray JL, Macey DJ, Grant EJ, et al: Enhanced TAG expression and tumor uptake of radiolabeled monoclonal antibody CC49 in metastatic breast cancer patients following alpha-interferon treatment. Cancer Res 55:5925s, 1995.

387. Rosenblum MG, Lamki LM, Murray JL, et al: Interferon-induced changes in pharmacokinetics and tumor uptake of 111In-labeled antimelanoma antibody 96.5 in melanoma patients. J Natl Cancer Inst 80:160, 1988.
388. Murray JL, Grant EJ, Rosenblum MG, et al: Enhanced RAG expression and tumor uptake of radiolabeled monoclonal antibody CC49 in metastatic breast cancer patients following α-interferon treatment. Cancer Res Suppl 55:5925s, 1995.
389. Boerman OC, van Schaijk FG, Oyen WJ, et al: Pretargeted radioimmunotherapy of cancer: progress step by step. J Nucl Med 44:400, 2003.
390. Bos ES, Kuijpers WH, Meesters-Winters M, et al: In vitro evaluation of DNA-DNA hybridization as a two-step approach in radioimmunotherapy of cancer. Cancer Res 54:3479, 1994.
391. Pedley RB, Sharma SK, Boxer GM, et al: Enhancement of antibody-directed enzyme prodrug therapy in colorectal xenografts by an antivascular agent. Cancer Res 59:3998, 1999.
392. Liu G, He J, Dou D, et al: Pretargeting in tumored mice with radiolabeled morpholino oligomer showing low kidney uptake. Eur J Nucl Med Mol Imaging 31:417, 2004.
393. Marshall D, Pedley RB, Boden JA, et al: Polyethylene glycol modification of a galactosylated streptavidin clearing agent: effects on immunogenicity and clearance of a biotinylated anti-tumour antibody. Br J Cancer 73:565, 1996.
394. Sharkey RM, McBride WJ, Karacay H, et al: A universal pretargeting system for cancer detection and therapy using bispecific antibody. Cancer Res 63:354, 2003.
395. Stickney DR, Anderson LD, Slater JB, et al: Bifunctional antibody: a binary radiopharmaceutical delivery system for imaging colorectal carcinoma. Cancer Res 51:6650, 1991.
396. van Schaijk FG, Oosterwijk E, Soede AC, et al: Pretargeting with labeled bivalent peptides allowing the use of four radionuclides: (111)In, (131)I, (99m)Tc, and (188)Re. Clin Cancer Res 9:3880S, 2003.
397. Chinol M, Casalini P, Maggiolo M, et al: Biochemical modifications of avidin improve pharmacokinetics and biodistribution, and reduce immunogenicity. Br J Cancer 78:189, 1998.
398. Sung C, van Osdol WW: Pharmacokinetic comparison of direct antibody targeting with pretargeting protocols based on streptavidin-biotin binding. J Nucl Med 36:867, 1995.
399. Sharkey RM, Karacay H, Griffiths GL, et al: Development of a streptavidin-anti-carcinoembryonic antigen antibody, radiolabeled biotin pretargeting method for radioimmunotherapy of colorectal cancer. Studies in a human colon cancer xenograft model. Bioconjug Chem 8:595, 1997.
400. Zhu H, Jain RK, Baxter LT: Tumor pretargeting for radioimmunodetection and radioimmunotherapy. J Nucl Med 39:65, 1998.
401. Chen JQ, Strand SE, Tennvall J, et al: Extracorporeal immunoadsorption compared with avidin chase: enhancement of tumor-to-normal tissue ratio for biotinylated rhenium-chimeric BR96. J Nucl Med 38:1934, 1997.
402. Goodwin DA, Meares CF, McCall MJ, et al: Pre-targeted immunoscintigraphy of murine tumors with indium 111-labeled bifunctional haptens. J Nucl Med 29:226, 1988.
403. Grana C, Chinol M, Robertson C, et al: Pretargeted adjuvant radioimmunotherapy with yttrium 90-biotin in malignant glioma patients: a pilot study. Br J Cancer 86:207, 2002.
404. Paganelli G, Orecchia R, Jereczek-Fossa B, et al: Combined treatment of advanced oropharyngeal cancer with external radiotherapy and three-step radioimmunotherapy. Eur J Nucl Med 25:1336, 1998.
405. Paganelli G, Grana C, Chinol M, et al: Antibody-guided three-step therapy for high grade glioma with yttrium-90 biotin. Eur J Nucl Med 26:348, 1999.
406. Paganelli G, Magnani P, Fazio F: Pretargeting of carcinomas with the avidin-biotin system. Int J Biol Markers 8:155, 1993.
407. Theodore LJ, Axworthy D: Cluster Clearing Agents. Wichtig Editore, Milan, Italy, 1997.
408. Wiseman GA, White CA, Witzig TE, et al: Radioimmunotherapy of relapsed non-Hodgkin's lymphoma with zevalin, a 90Y-labeled anti-CD20 monoclonal antibody. Clin Cancer Res 5:3281s, 1999.
409. Weiden PL: Pretargeted radioimmunotherapy (PRIT) using an antibody-streptavidin fusion protein in non-Hodgkin's lymphoma. Leuk Lymphoma 43:1971, 2002.
410. Schultz J, Lin Y, Sanderson J, et al: A tetravalent single-chain antibody-streptavidin fusion protein for pretargeted lymphoma therapy. Cancer Res 60:6663, 2000.
411. Vuillez JP, Kraeber-Bodere F, Moro D, et al: Radioimmunotherapy of small cell lung carcinoma with the two-step method using a bispecific anti-carcinoembryonic antigen/anti-diethylenetriaminepentaacetic acid (DTPA) antibody and iodine Di-DTPA hapten: results of a phase I/II trial. Clin Cancer Res 5:3259s, 1999.
412. Kraeber-Bodere F, Bardet S, Hoefnagel CA, et al: Radioimmunotherapy in medullary thyroid cancer using bispecific antibody and iodine 131-labeled bivalent hapten: preliminary results of a phase I/II clinical trial. Clin Cancer Res 5:3190s, 1999.
413. Hird V, Maraveyas A, Snook D, et al: Adjuvant therapy of ovarian cancer with radioactive monoclonal antibody. Br J Cancer 68:403, 1993.
414. Stewart JS, Hird V, Sullivan M, et al: Intraperitoneal radioimmunotherapy for ovarian cancer. Br J Obstet Gynaecol 96:529, 1989.
415. Paganelli G, Pervez S, Siccardi AG, et al: Intraperitoneal radiolocalization of tumors pre-targeted by biotinylated monoclonal antibodies. Int J Cancer 45:1184, 1990.
416. Riva P, Arista A, Sturiale C, et al: Treatment of intracranial human glioblastoma by direct intratumoral administration of 131I-labelled anti-tenascin monoclonal antibody BC. Int J Cancer 51:7, 1992.
417. Riva P, Arista A, Tison V, et al: Intralesional radioimmunotherapy of malignant gliomas. An effective treatment in recurrent tumors. Cancer 73:1076, 1994.
418. Buchsbaum DJ, Sinkule JA, Stites MA, et al: Localization and imaging with radioiodine-labeled monoclonal antibodies in a xenogeneic tumor model for human B-cell lymphoma. Cancer Res 48:2475, 1988.
419. Mattes MJ, Major PP, Goldenberg DM, et al: Patterns of antigen distribution in human carcinomas. Cancer Res 50:880s, 1990.
420. Munz SL, Alavi A, Koprowski H, et al: Improved radioimmunoimaging of human tumor xenografts by a mixture of monoclonal antibody F(ab')2 fragments. J Nucl Med 27:1739, 1986.
421. Fleshman JW, Connett JM, Neufeld DM, et al: Tumor localization and radioimaging with mixtures of radioiodinated monoclonal antibodies directed to different colon cancer associated antigens. Int J Rad Appl Instrum B 19:659, 1992.
422. Blumenthal RD, Kashi R, Stephens R, et al: Improved radioimmunotherapy of colorectal cancer xenografts using antibody mixtures against carcinoembryonic antigen and colon-specific antigen-P. Cancer Immunol Immunother 32:303, 1991.
423. Wilder RB, DeNardo GL, DeNardo SJ: Radioimmunotherapy: recent results and future directions. J Clin Oncol 14:1383, 1996.
424. O'Donnell RT, DeNardo SJ, Miers LA, et al: Combined modality radioimmunotherapy for human prostate cancer xenografts with taxanes and 90yttrium-DOTA-peptide-ChL6. Prostate 50:27, 2002.
425. Blumenthal RD, Leone E, Goldenberg DM: Tumor-specific dose scheduling of bimodal radioimmunotherapy and chemotherapy. Anticancer Res 23:4613, 2003.
426. Blumenthal RD, Leone E, Goldenberg DM, et al: An in vitro model to optimize dose scheduling of multimodal radioimmunotherapy and chemotherapy: effects of p53 expression. Int J Cancer 108:293, 2004.
427. DeNardo SJ, Kroger LA, Lamborn KR, et al: Importance of temporal relationships in combined modality radioimmunotherapy of breast carcinoma. Cancer 80:2583, 1997.
428. DeNardo DG, Xiong CY, Shi XB, et al: Anti-HLA-DR/anti-DOTA diabody construction in a modular gene design platform: bispecific antibodies for pretargeted radioimmunotherapy. Cancer Biother Radiopharm 16:525, 2001.
429. Goodwin DA, Meares CF: Advances in pretargeting biotechnology. Biotechnol Adv 19:435, 2001.

430. Ng B, Kramer E, Liebes L, et al: Radiosensitization of tumor-targeted radioimmunotherapy with prolonged topotecan infusion in human breast cancer xenografts. Cancer Res 61:2996, 2001.
431. Fu KK, Lam KN, Rayner PA: The influence of time sequence of cisplatin administration and continuous low dose rate irradiation (CLDRI) on their combined effects on a murine squamous cell carcinoma. Int J Radiat Oncol Biol Phys 11:2119, 1985.
432. Langmuir VK, Mendonca HL: The combined use of 131I-labeled antibody and the hypoxic cytotoxin SR 4233 in vitro and in vivo. Radiat Res 132:351, 1992.
433. Buchsbaum DJ, Rogers BE, Khazaeli MR, et al: Targeting strategies for cancer radiotherapy. Clin Cancer Res 5:3048s, 1999.
434. Panyutin IG, Sedelnikova OA, Karamychev VN, et al: Antigene radiotherapy: targeted radiodamage with 125I-labeled triplex-forming oligonucleotides. Ann N Y Acad Sci 1002:134, 2003.
435. Kaminski MS, Zasadny KR, Francis IR, et al: Iodine-131-anti-B1 radiommunotherapy for B-cell lymphoma. J Clin Oncol 14:1974, 1996.
436. Lamborn KR, DeNardo GL, DeNardo SJ, et al: Treatment-related parameters predicting efficacy of Lym-1 radioimmunotherapy in patients with B-lymphocytic malignancies. Clin Cancer Res 3:1253, 1997.
437. Vose JM, Colcher D, Gobar L, et al: Phase I/II trial of multiple dose ^{131}iodine-MAb LL2 (CD22) in patients with recurrent non-Hodgkin's lymphoma. Leuk Lymphoma 38:91, 2000.
438. Postema EJ, Borjesson PK, Buijs WC, et al: Dosimetric analysis of radioimmunotherapy with ^{186}Re-labeled bivatuzumab in patients with head and neck cancer. J Nucl Med 44:1690, 2003.
439. Wiseman GA, White CA, Stabin M, et al: Phase I/II ^{90}Y-Zevalin (yttrium-90 ibritumomab tiuxetan, IDEC-Y2B8) radioimmunotherapy dosimetry results in relapsed or refractory non-Hodgkin's lymphoma. Eur J Nucl Med 27:766, 2000.
440. Stewart JSW, Hird V, Snook D, et al: Intraperitoneal yttrium-90-labeled monoclonal antibody in ovarian cancer. J Clin Oncol 8:1941, 1990.
441. Rosenblum MG, Verschraegen CF, Murray JL, et al: Phase I study of ^{90}Y-labeled B72.3 intraperitoneal administration in patients with ovarian cancer: effect of dose and EDTA coadministration on pharmacokinetics and toxicity. Clin Cancer Res 5:953, 1999.
442. Mahe MA, Fumoleau P, Fabbro M, et al: A phase II study of intraperitoneal radioimmunotherapy with iodine-131-labeled monoclonal antibody OC-125 in patients with residual ovarian carcinoma. Clin Cancer Res 5:3249s, 1999.
443. Jacobs AJ, Fer M, Su FM, et al: A phase I trial of a rhenium 186-labeled monoclonal antibody administered intraperitoneally in ovarian carcinoma: toxicity and clinical response. Obstet Gynecol 82:586, 1993.
444. Riva P, Marangolo M, Tison V, et al: Treatment of metastatic colorectal cancer by means of specific monoclonal antibodies conjugated with iodine-131: a phase II study. Nucl Med Biol 18:109, 1991.
445. Muto MG, Finkler NJ, Kassis AI, et al: Intraperitoneal radioimmunotherapy of refractory ovarian carcinoma utilizing iodine-131-labeled monoclonal antibody OC125. Gynecol Oncol 45:265, 1992.
446. Buckman R, De Angelis C, Shaw P, et al: Intraperitoneal therapy of malignant ascites associated with carcinoma of ovary and breast using radioiodinated monoclonal antibody 2G3. Gynecol Oncol 47:102, 1992.

CHAPTER 22

PALLIATIVE CARE FOR BONE, SPINAL CORD, BRAIN, AND LIVER METASTASES

Arthur T. Porter and Marc David

Although palliative care comprises a large part of the clinical practice of oncology, studies show that cancer pain is often inadequately managed.[1,2] Osseous metastases[3] remain the most common cause of intractable pain in cancer patients. Bone is the third most common site of metastases after lung and liver.[4] Metastases usually become apparent after the diagnosis of the primary tumor, but in up to 23% of patients they are the presenting problem. Bone pain results in immobility, anxiety, and depression, and severely impacts on a patient's quality of life.

Table 22-1 shows the prevalence of skeletal metastases in several autopsy series.[5] The marked variation may be attributed to differences in the thoroughness of the pathologic examination of the skeleton. Bone scintigraphic surveys have, in general, reported higher rates of bone metastases. In a study by Tofe and colleagues,[6] bone scans of 1143 patients with a nonosseous primary tumor were examined; 61% of the patients had an abnormal bone scan finding, and 33% had breast, lung, or prostate primary cancer.

In a prospective series of hospital patients with bone metastases, the tumors carrying the highest risk of bone metastases were those originating in the prostate (32.4%), breast (21.9%), kidney (16.4%), thyroid (11.7%), lung (10.9%), and testes (10.2%).[2] The incidence of patients developing bone metastases by primary site is shown in Table 22-2.[6]

The distribution of skeletal metastases from breast cancer is shown in Table 22-3. Similar distributions have been noted from prostate, lung, and breast primary cancers.[7-10]

BONE METASTASES

Pathophysiology

Numerous tumor cells gain access to the systemic circulation, primarily through the capillary system, but some gain access through the lymphatics; only a few of these cells are able to establish a metastatic focus successfully.[11]

The metastatic process is described pathologically as a five-step process: (1) release of tumor cells from the primary, (2) invasion of efferent lymphatic or vascular channels, (3) dissemination through the vascular and lymphatic channels to distant sites, (4) endothelial attachment and invasion of the new host, and (5) growth of the original colony into a metastatic focus.

Cancer cells metastasize to bone *mostly* via hematogenous spread. Skeletal blood flow accounts for only 4% to 10% of the cardiac output,[12] and some authors believe that the incidence of skeletal metastases is higher than expected from the relatively low perfusion of bone. A mechanism explaining the high incidence has been described by Weiss.[13] The microstructure of the hematopoietic marrow renders it particularly vulnerable to tumor cell accumulation and ultimate invasion. Nutrient arteries to the bone tend to subdivide into capillaries as they near the endosteal margin of the bone. These capillaries become continuous with a rich venous sinusoidal system, with a capacity six to eight times that of the osseous arterial system. More important, the circulation comes to a near standstill at this point, allowing tumor cells more time to invade the matrix.

To sustain growth, a colony of tumor cells needs to obtain its own vascular supply once it has been established. A hypothesis is that a tumor angiogenesis factor attracts vessels to a small tumor colony that would otherwise be dependent on local tissue circulation and incapable of further invasion.[14] The production of such tumor angiogenesis factor may be partly blocked by the immune responses, presumably mediated through lymphocytes. Therefore, an established micrometastasis may attract vasculature required for growth several years later. This theory may explain the late appearance of metastases long after definitive treatment of the primary.

Some tumors, notably of breast, prostate, lung, renal, and thyroid cancer, produce and secrete humeral mediators that stimulate osteoclast activity. These include transforming growth factor, platelet-derived growth factor, tumor necrosis factor, prostaglandins, procathepsin D, interleukins, parathyroid hormone–related protein, and granulocyte-macrophage colony-stimulating factors.[15,16]

The distribution of metastases in the skeletal system is not uniform. Bone metastases tend to involve the axial skeleton more often than the appendicular skeleton. Considering the equally rich hematopoietic system in the appendicular skeleton, this higher predilection argues for specific circulatory factors outside the general arterial system.[12]

Diagnosis

Laboratory

The biochemical parameters available include alkaline phosphatase, urinary hydroxyproline, and the urinary hydroxyproline-creatinine ratio. These lack specificity and are of no value in the diagnosis of skeletal metastases.[17,18]

Imaging

Skeletal scintigraphy is usually the first-line imaging technique used for detecting skeletal metastases. A bone scan is more sensitive than plain radiographs and has the advantage of examining the entire skeleton. Most lesions evoke an osteoblastic response, which shows up as an increased tracer uptake.[19] Occasionally, metastases may show up as areas of decreased uptake. This may be observed in rapidly growing lesions, when bone destruction far exceeds new bone formation, or secondary to an infarction. Highly vascular metastases, such as those from a renal primary cancer, may be seen on the early vascular phase of the bone scan. Metastases not detected by a bone scan include tumors that do not evoke an osteoblastic response such as myeloma, some lymphomas, and very small deposits.[20]

Widespread metastatic disease may be misinterpreted as a normal scan with symmetric uptake. In these situations, a reduction in urinary excretion of isotope and faint or absent renal uptake with decreased bladder activity are clues of an abnormal scan.[21]

Table 22-1 **Prevalence of Skeletal Metastases at Autopsy**

Primary Site	Prevalence (%)
Breast	47-85
Prostate	54-85
Thyroid	28-60
Kidney	33-40
Bronchus	32-40
Esophagus	5-7
Other gastrointestinal	3-11
Rectum	8-13
Bladder	42
Cervix	0
Ovaries	9
Liver	16

Data from Galasko CSB: Incidence and distribution of skeletal metastases. Clin Orthop 210:14-22, 1986.

Table 22-2 **Incidence of Bone Metastases According to Primary Site**

Primary Site	No. of Patients	Patients With Bone Metastases (%)
Breast	6423	17
Prostate	144	16
Esophagus	451	6
Lung	589	5
Bladder	172	5
Rectum	274	4
Thyroid	107	4
Uterine cervix	1981	3
Uterine corpus	509	3
Head and neck	2860	2
Ovaries	586	1
Colon	153	1
Stomach	118	1

Data from Tubiana-Hulin M: Incidence, prevalence and distribution of bone mets. Bone 12:S9-S10, 1991.

Table 22-3 **Distribution of Skeletal Metastases in 212 Breast Cancer Patients**

Anatomic Site	At Presentation (%*)	At Any Time (%*)
Lumbar spine	52	59
Thoracic spine	35	57
Pelvis	31	49
Ribs	18	30
Femur	15	24
Skull	12	20
Cervical spine	11	17
Humerus	8	13
Other	3	3
Diffuse	1	12

*Of all patients.
Data from Tubiana-Hulin M: Incidence, prevalence and distribution of bone mets. Bone 12:S9-S10, 1991.

Most skeletal metastases develop in the medulla and involve the cortex late; therefore, radiographs are generally insensitive.[21] Within the spine, the vertebral body is affected first, although the radiologic findings of pedicle destruction are noted first.[22]

Although plain films cannot be relied on to diagnose skeletal metastases, they have an important role in patients with painful lesions and a positive bone scan. Radiographs of a painful lesion may uncover a pathologic fracture or an impending fracture. Two views are recommended to diagnose the latter. The lesions may be lytic, sclerotic, or mixed. Sclerotic metastases are commonly from prostate carcinoma but may be from breast, gastrointestinal, and bladder carcinoma. Lytic metastases are seen with all sites, and mixed metastases are commonly from a breast primary.

Computed tomography (CT) scanning has been found to differentiate between metastases and degenerative joint disease, even though the two coexist, and the latter is a common cause of increased uptake on a bone scan. Muindi and colleagues[23] reported that 50% of breast cancer patients with a positive bone scan and a normal radiograph had obvious skeletal metastases on a CT scan, 25% had a benign cause, and 25% had a negative CT. None of the patients with a CT scan that was negative for metastases subsequently experienced metastases. CT scan is also valuable in evaluating soft tissue involvement and can be combined with myelography for detecting extradural tumor spread in patients unable to undergo magnetic resonance imaging (MRI).

MRI has been described as the method of choice for examining the spine. It is more sensitive than a bone scan for detecting early metastases within the medulla, but both T1- and T2-weighted images are required.[24] It is the procedure of choice when neural compression is suspected,[24] because it is less invasive than CT myelography, and a small incidence of acute deterioration of neurologic function has been reported by CT myelography.[25] When cord impingement is suspected, imaging of the entire spine should be considered because approximately 10% of patients have multiple levels of cord impingement.[26] It is also used in discriminating between benign and malignant vertebral collapse. In the future, whole-body MRI could emerge for metastasis screening.[27] Disadvantages of MRI include the high cost, exclusion of patients with metal implants, patients with severe claustrophobia, and inferior visualization of the cortex compared with a CT scan.

PET (positron emission tomography) using ^{18}F-fluoride or 2-fluoro-2-deoxy-D-glucose (FDG) has emerged as a new imaging tool for initial staging of malignancy (lung and breast) and to diagnose bony metastasis. ^{18}F-fluoride is a bone-imaging agent, and it forms fluoroapatite in osteoblastic cells. Uptake is higher than that for ^{99m}Tc, used for bone scintigraphy.[28] FDG is a tumor-imaging agent that uses the higher glycolysis activity in the tumor cells.[29] FDG-PET scan compared to bone scintigraphy shows a similar high sensitivity (range from 74% to 95%) but a higher specificity (range of 90% to 97%).[30-34] Limitations include traumatic, infectious, and inflammatory processes. In 1998, Cook and coworkers[35] revealed a possible limitation linked to sclerotic bone lesion, but in a later, larger series it did not materialize. Better differentiated neoplasms, like prostate adenocarcinoma, uptake less FDG and the PET scan is not used as a screening modality.[36,37] A new modality combining PET and CT (PET/CT) offers a better spatial resolution to improve the sensibility of the test.[28,38,39]

Arteriography has a role when considering surgery for vascular lesions, such as renal cell carcinoma. Preoperative embolization may be required to decrease the risk of major hemorrhage.

Biopsy

Bone biopsy is not necessary routinely. It is helpful in patients with no history of malignancy, in patients with a solitary lesion (in whom a more aggressive treatment approach may be indicated), and in patients with more than one suspected primary. In the latter situation, it may make a difference in the systemic therapy.

Treatment

The primary goal of therapy is to improve quality of life. To achieve this goal, we need to decrease or eliminate pain and improve or maintain function for the duration or as a major component of the patient's remaining life. The complexity, duration, and cost of therapy should be low, and complications should be avoided.

Treatment recommendations must be individualized. A key consideration is the patient's overall prognosis. This assessment should be based on an understanding of the natural course of the specific disease. Although the survival of patients with bone metastases is generally poor, potential long-term survivors must be identified. Not only would they require a more durable relief, but they are also more at risk for a late, treatment-related complication. In the Radiation Therapy Oncology Group (RTOG) trial,[40] median survival (MS) in patients with solitary and multiple bone metastases was 36 and 24 weeks, respectively. Patients with breast and prostate primaries survived significantly longer (30 to 73 weeks), whereas patients with lung cancer died within a median of 12 to 14 weeks. Patients with renal cell carcinoma with solitary metastasis are also likely to be long-term survivors. Mogens[41] monitored 25 such patients for 10 to 14 years. The MS was 4.3 years, 5-year survival was 36%, and 10-year survival was 16%.

Pharmacologic Treatment

ENDOCRINE THERAPY

Endocrine therapy is widely used in breast and prostate cancer. Tamoxifen has been the first-line hormonal therapy in postmenopausal women with advanced breast cancer since the 1970s. It is most effective in patients with estrogen receptor–positive tumors, with response rates as high as 50% compared with only 10% response rates for patients with estrogen-negative tumors.[42] Median duration of response to first-line treatment is approximately 15 months, although a prolonged response lasting several years may be seen in patients with bone metastases.

The role of tamoxifen as first-line therapy has since been challenged by anastrozole and letrozole, two aromatase inhibitors.[43,44] Mouridsen and colleagues[43-45] reported statistical significant superiority of letrozole against tamoxifen in a randomized double-blind double-dummy trial with regard to 1- and 2-year survival, time to progression, tolerability, and clinical benefit. Nine hundred seven patients with advanced or metastatic breast cancer and positive or unknown (30%) receptors were randomized to letrozole 2.5 mg versus tamoxifen 20 mg. Objective response rates were 32% for letrozole versus 21% for tamoxifen ($P = .0002$). Median time to progression was 9.4 months against 6 months in favor of letrozole (Cox hazards ratio, 0.70; 95% confidence interval, 0.6 to 0.82; $P < .0001$).[43] Survival at 2 years is 64% for letrozole versus 58% for tamoxifen.[45]

Bonneterre and coworkers combined European and North American data in a randomized double-blind trial comparing anastrozole to tamoxifen in the same group of patients. All end points showed equivalence between the two drugs.[44] Survival at 2 years of 69.9% and 68% is superior to that of a previous trial, which "suggests a high level of benefit for adequately selected patients." Milla-Santos and coworkers[46] conducted a randomized controlled trial on 238 postmenopausal patients with advanced breast cancer. Patients received anastrozole 1 mg or tamoxifen 40 mg daily; this dose is higher than what is usually used in North America. All end points of clinical benefit, time to progression, and overall survival showed statistical significance in favor of the anastrozole group.[46] Median time to progression was 18 months for anastrozole and 7 months for tamoxifen (hazards ratio, 0.13; 95% confidence interval, 0.08 to 0.20; $P < .01$). It is now accepted that third-generation aromatase inhibitors can be used as first-line therapy for metastatic breast cancer in postmenopausal status.

Patients who relapse after initially responding to one type of endocrine therapy often respond to a second line of hormones. Available agents that have demonstrated efficacy are aminoglutethimide, megestrol acetate, and aromatase inhibitors. Patients who have failed first-line aromatase inhibitors therapy can receive tamoxifen as second-line therapy.[47] An advantage of aromatase inhibitors is selective peripheral blockage of the conversion of androgen to estrogen. Aminoglutethimide is a nonsteroidal agent that also blocks synthesis of glucocorticoids and mineralocorticoids, which requires administration of cortisone with concomitant side effects. Five randomized trials compared third-generation aromatase inhibitors with aminoglutethimide and megestrol acetate.[48-52] Overall response rates (ORs) vary from 12% to 24%. Overall survival ranges from 21 to 33 months (Table 22-4). Premenopausal women are usually treated with ovarian ablation (bilateral oophorectomy or radioablation) or with luteinizing hormone–releasing hormone (LHRH) agonists.[16]

Prostate cancer is very sensitive to hormones; as many as 80% of patients show some degree of response.[53] Similar response has been reported with orchiectomy or LHRH agonists. A flare response is noted in 8% to 30% of patients treated with an LHRH agonist. This can be easily avoided by the use of an antiandrogen during the first 2 to 4 weeks. The National Cancer Institute (NCI) trial[54] comparing total androgen blockade using leuprolide with and without flutamide showed a significant benefit to combined therapy. The 303 patients receiving the combined therapy had a longer progression-free survival (16.5 versus 13.9 months, $P = .039$), and a longer MS (35.6 versus 28.3 months, $P = .035$) compared with the 300 patients receiving leuprolide with a placebo.[54] Similar results were seen in a phase III European Organization for Research and Treatment of Cancer (EORTC) trial.[55] In both trials, the superiority of the total androgen blockade was demonstrated for patients with low-burden disease only. Antiandrogen monotherapy is also used for treatment of metastatic prostate cancer. Few randomized trials were realized, but Tyrrell and colleagues[56] compared bicalutamide (Casodex) 150 mg with castration and found statistically significant differences in terms of subjective response (70% versus 58%) and quality of life.

Other effective agents include cyproterone acetate, flutamide, and ketoconazole. Treatment of patients who relapse through first-line hormonal therapy is unsatisfactory; response rates rarely exceed 20% and usually last less than 6 months.[57]

BIOLOGIC THERAPY

Her-2/neu (also referred as c-erbB-2) represents the human epidermal growth factor and is overexpressed or amplified in 20% to 30% of cases of breast cancer.[58] Other tumors also

Techniques and Modalities

Table 22-4 Summary of Clinical Trials on Aromatase inhibitors

Trial (First Author)	Treatment	*n*	Overall Response (%)	Overall Median Survival (mo)
Gershanovich[48]	Letrozole 0.5 mg	192	16.7	21
	Letrozole 2.5 mg	185	9.5	28
	AG 250 mg	178	12.4	20
Dombernowsky[49]	Letrozole 0.5 mg	188	12.8	21.5
	Letrozole 2.5 mg	174	23.6	25.3
	MA 160 mg	189	16.4	21.5
Buzdar[50]	Letrozole 0.5 mg	202	21	33
	Letrozole 2.5 mg	199	16	29
	MA 160 mg	201	15	26
Buzdar[51]	Anastrozole 1 mg	263	12.5	26.7
	Anastrozole 1 mg	248	12.5	25.5
	MA 40 mg	253	12.2	22.5
Kaufmann[52]	Examestane 25 mg	366	15	NA
	MA 40 mg	403	12.4	28.8

AG, aminoglutethimide; MA, megestral acetate.

overexpress Her-2/neu, such as ovary, lung, and salivary gland. Amplification is associated with an increase in tumor growth rate and metastatic rate and shorter overall survival.[58]

Trastuzumab is a humanized antibody directed against the extracellular domain of the receptor. Higher tumor response to trastuzumab is correlated with high levels of overexpression measured by immunohistochemical assay (grade 3+) or positive fluorescent in situ hybridization (FISH) compared with immunohistochemical assay 2+ (34% versus 7%).[59] As a single agent, clinical benefit ranges from 13% to 20%.[60] Trastuzumab is used in combination with chemotherapeutic agents such as palliate, docetaxel, platinum salts, vinorelbine, and gemcitabine. OR and MS are significantly improved by the addition of trastuzumab (50% versus 34% for OR and 25 versus 20 months for MS, respectively).[61] Toxicity is mostly related to low-grade fever, chills, and fatigue and is seen primarily at the first infusion. Cardiac toxicity (congested heart failure) has been reported in 16% of patients when used with doxorubicin combination. Other chemotherapeutic agents exhibit an acceptable rate of cardiotoxicity of 1% to 2%.[61] Although clinical trials have not established optimal duration of treatment, it is usually the practice to stop the trastuzumab at the time of progression. Ongoing studies should clarify these issues, but the evidence is present to incorporate this new weapon in the treatment of advanced and metastatic breast cancer.[62]

Chemotherapy

Chemotherapy has an important role in palliation of pain in different tumor types. Response rates in bone are poor; varying between 0% and 30%.[63] Responses are nearly always partial, with a median duration of 9 to 12 months. Good responses can be expected in adenocarcinoma of the breast and in small cell lung carcinoma. The side effect of myelosuppression can be especially hazardous to patients with extensive bone disease involving the marrow and in those previously treated with bone irradiation.

Chemotherapy can be curative for bone metastases resulting from germ cell tumors and Hodgkin's and non-Hodgkin's lymphoma. In multiple myeloma, continuous or intermittent alkylating agents such as melphalan or cyclophosphamide (Cytoxan) with or without steroids is the mainstay of treatment. Approximately 50% of myeloma patients respond to chemotherapy, with a decrease in paraprotein levels and subjective improvement.[64]

Bisphosphonates

The discovery of compounds inhibiting calcium phosphate precipitation in plasma and urine led to an interest in the use of bisphosphonates as therapeutic agents. The inhibitory activity was attributed to inorganic pyrophosphate, but the use of this agent was limited because of its rapid hydrolysis when given parenterally. Subsequent research led to the development of pyrophosphate analogues resistant to endogenous phosphatases, now known as bisphosphonates.

The bisphosphonates have a phosphate-carbon-phosphate backbone that binds tightly to calcified bone matrix. They inhibit osteoclast-mediated bone resorption; potency depends on the structure of the molecule. The exact mechanism is unclear, but postulated mechanisms include direct biochemical effects on the osteoclast, prevention of osteoclast attachment to the bone matrix, and inhibition of differentiation of osteoclast precursors and recruitment.

Four phase II trials of intravenous pamidronate every 2 to 4 weeks as the sole treatment of osteolytic bone metastases in breast cancer reported similar results.[65-68] Relief of pain was noted in approximately 50% of patients, and approximately 25% showed radiographic evidence of bone healing. Similar results for bone pain have been reported in patients with prostate cancer.

One phase II trial[69] and one phase III trial[70] showed equivalence between zoledronic acid and pamidronate. Rosen conducted a three-arm study for patients with bone lytic or mixed disease from either breast cancer or multiple myeloma.[70] One thousand six hundred forty-eight patients received intravenous pamidronate 90 mg, zoledronate 4 mg or 8 mg every 3 weeks for 13 months. The primary end point was the incidence of skeletal events, and secondary end points were pain relief and performance status (ECOG). All treatment groups showed equivalence with a skeletal event at 12 months, and pain scores decreased by an average of .5 on a scale of 1 to 5. This randomized trial led to modification of the ASCO 2003 and the Cochrane Breast Cancer Review Group update recommendations on the use of bisphosphonates in breast cancer.[71,72] Both boards now recommend either pamidronate 90 mg IV over 2 hours or zoledronate acid 4 mg IV over 15 minutes for patients with an abnormal bone scan and abnormal imaging on plain radiography, CT, or MRI. There is no evidence to treat asymptomatic patients with an abnormal bone scan.

Zoledronic acid has also been used in prostate cancer to treat blastic metastasis. Saad and colleagues[73] randomized 643 patients to placebo or zometa 4 or 8 mg IV every 3 weeks for 15 months. Results show a reduction in skeletal related events from 44% to 33% with a significant *P* value of .021. Pathologic fractures were reduced from 22% to 13% (*P* = .015). Onset of the events occurred at a median time of greater than 420 days (median not reached) in the group receiving zometa and at 321 days in the placebo group. Time to disease progression or survival was similar in both groups. The need for local field radiation was not significantly different in the two groups.

Zometa has also been evaluated for the treatment of bone metastasis from other disease sites: 773 patients with lung, renal, head and neck, thyroid, and unknown primary received either placebo or zometa 4 or 8 mg.[74] Skeletal events including hypercalcemia were significantly reduced from 47% to 38% (*P* = .039), and median time to first event was slower in the zometa group (225 versus 155 days, *P* = .023).

Although zoledronic acid is well tolerated, the treating physician is advised to monitor serum creatinine before each administration. Caution is also advised for patients receiving concomitant aminoglycoside or loop diuretic due to an increased risk of hypocalcemia. Ruggiero and colleagues[75] published a retrospective review of 63 patients on bisphosphonates who sustained osteonecrosis of the jaw; 57% received pamidronate and 21% received zoledronic acid. Surgical treatment was required.

Oral agents, like clodronate, have low bioavailability (2%) and produce gastrointestinal side effects. Dearnaley and coworkers[76] randomized 311 men with bone metastasis from prostate cancer who were starting LHRH to receive daily placebo or 2080 mg of oral clodronate for 3 years. Although statistical significance was not reached this study showed a reduction in bone progression-free survival with a hazard ratio of .79 (95% confidence interval, .61 to 1.02; *P* = .066). Overall survival was not different. Another study randomized 302 women with breast cancer to receive clodronate or standard care for 2 years. Patients were all known to have cancer cells in their bone marrow and were therefore at high risk for symptomatic bone metastasis.[77] Results showed a significant reduction in the incidence of distant metastasis, as well as bone and visceral metastasis.

ANALGESICS

The optimal management of pain begins with careful assessment of the degree of pain, site, functional limitations, and concurrent neurologic symptoms.[78] The World Health Organization (WHO) analgesic ladder for cancer pain management provides a good guideline for analgesic use.[79]

Step I. Nonopioid with or without adjuvant therapy
Step II. Opioid for mild to moderate pain plus nonopioid with or without adjuvant therapy
Step III. Opioid for moderate to severe pain with or without nonopioid with or without adjuvant therapy

Step I nonopioid analgesics include acetaminophen, aspirin, and other nonsteroidal anti-inflammatory drugs (NSAIDs). The dose of acetaminophen should not exceed 4 g/day. Step II opioids include codeine, dihydrocodeine, hydrocodone, oxycodone, and propoxyphene. Step III opioids include morphine, oxycodone, hydromorphone, and fentanyl.

Attention should be paid to selection of the appropriate analgesic, dose, route, and schedule. Continuous, slow-release medications are generally preferred over short-acting medications. The latter can be effectively used for breakthrough pain. Allowing pain to recur between doses causes unnecessary suffering and may allow tolerance to develop. When prescribing oral opioids, the dose is about two times that of the subcutaneous dose and three times that of the intravenous dose. For

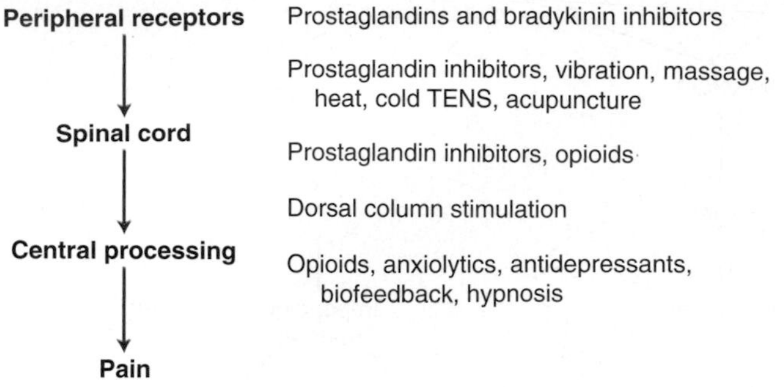

Figure 22-1 Pain pathway and analgesia interventions. TENS, transcutaneous electrical nerve stimulation.

patients unable to take oral medications, suppositories and transdermal patches are good options. When combining drugs, it is important to use drugs that act at different levels of the pain pathway (Fig. 22-1). The combined effect can be additive and at times synergistic.

The pain of bone metastases is generally only partially responsive to opioids.[80] Many osseous metastases produce prostaglandins that induce osteolysis. NSAIDs alleviate pain by inhibiting the synthesis of prostaglandins. Corticosteroids prevent the formation of arachidonic acid (the precursor of prostaglandins) from cell membrane phospholipids. The use of NSAIDs or corticosteroids in combination with morphine is usually effective.

Corticosteroids can be used when pain is caused by nerve compression. They decrease edema and reduce the pressure on the nerve. Pain relief can be achieved within 48 hours. Corticosteroids can be used as a temporary measure, before a more definitive decompression is achieved with radiotherapy or surgery.

Side effects associated with the use of opioids include nausea, vomiting, constipation, urinary retention, dysphoria, mental clouding, tolerance, and addiction. Nausea and vomiting are usually self-limiting and resolve during the first week. Side effects should be anticipated, prevented, and managed aggressively.

Surgery

Surgery should be considered for patients with pathologic fractures or impending fractures (Fig. 22-2). In the former situation, fixation can reduce pain and expedite healing. In the latter, prophylactic fixation may prevent a fracture, thereby eliminating the functional loss and reducing the risk of nonunion of a fracture.

To better understand the role of surgery, we need first to elaborate on the biomechanics of pathologic fractures. Cortical defects weaken bone, especially in the setting of torsional stress. The two general categories of cortical defects are (1) stress riser, a defect with dimensions less than the diameter of the bone, and (2) open-section defect, a discontinuity of dimensions greater than the diameter of the bone.[81] By creating a nonuniform distribution of stresses in bone, stress risers can decrease bone strength by 60% to 70%.[82] In a normal bone under torsional loading, the shear stresses are evenly distributed in the cross-section. An open-section defect has a greater impact on decreasing shear and torque-loading resistance. These defects lack a continuous outer surface; hence, only the shear stress developed at the periphery of the section can resist the applied torque.[83] The volume of bone able to resist the load is significantly decreased compared with a closed section. A 90% reduction in load to failure and energy storage to failure is noted in torsion testing of the human adult tibia with open

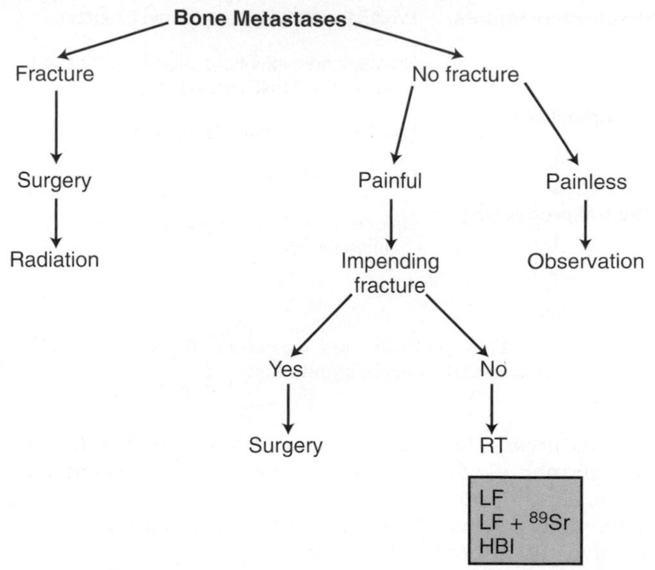

Figures 22-2 Treatment algorithm for bone metastases. LF, local field; LF + ^{89}Sr, local field plus strontium 89; HBI, hemibody irradiation; RT, radiation therapy.

Table 22-5 Distribution of Pathologic Fractures[58]

Location	No.	%
Femur	258	65.0
Femoral neck	69	17.0
Peritrochanteric	50	13.0
Subtrochanteric	84	21.0
Femoral shaft	38	10.0
Supracondylar	17	4.0
Acetabulum	34	8.5
Tibia	31	7.5
Humerus	68	17.0
Forearm	8	2.0
Total	399	100

From Mirels H: Metastatic disease in long bones: A proposed scoring system. Clin Orthop 249:256, 1989.

section.[83] Torsional or rotational forces occur in various daily movements such as getting out of a chair. Bone is weakest during torsion. A single quarter-inch hole made for a bone biopsy can decrease torsional strength by 50%.[84]

The nature of the metastatic lesion affects the overall bone strength. Both lytic and blastic lesions dramatically alter bone elasticity; lytic lesions reduce bone strength more than blastic lesions. Irregular lesions are not necessarily more detrimental to the bone than are smooth lesions, but elongated lesions drastically reduce bone strength.[85]

Fidler[85] described a technique for estimating the percentage of cortical bone involvement at any level of a long bone using anteroposterior (AP) and lateral films. This technique is thought to be as accurate a prognostic indicator as cross-sectional CT images, except when cortical destruction progresses in a patchy or spiral form.[81]

The distribution of pathologic fractures is shown in Table 22-5. Several series have examined various criteria predicting the risk of a pathologic fracture. Keene and associates[86] evaluated 2673 breast cancer patients in an attempt to predict pathologic fracture of the femur using clinical and radiologic criteria. Only 26 (13%) of 203 patients with evaluable proximal femur metastasis had pathologic fractures. They were unable to correlate lesion size and risk of pathologic fracture. No other risk factor was identified. The authors concluded that plain radiographs are insufficient diagnostic tools in the identification of high-risk lesions. Three reasons were cited. First, 57% of the lesions were permeative, did not have clear boundaries, and were, therefore, unmeasurable. Second, 14 (54%) of the 26 fractures observed occurred through unmeasurable lesions. Third, the 12 measurable lesions that fractured had defect sizes overlapping with those that did not fracture. Of note is that this study was limited to single AP films.

Table 22-6 Scoring System by Mirels

Variable	POINTS 1	2	3
Site	Upper extremity	Lower extremity	Peritrochanteric
Pain	Mild	Moderate	Mechanical
Radiograph	Blastic	Mixed	Lytic
Size (% of shaft)	0-3	34-67	68-100

From Mirels H: Metastatic disease in long bones: A proposed scoring system. Clin Orthop 249:256, 1989.

Table 22-7 Pathologic Fracture Rate

Score	No. of Patients	Fracture Rate (%)
0-6	11	0
7	19	5
8	12	33
9	7	57
10-12	18	100

From Mirels H: Metastatic disease in long bones: A proposed scoring system. Clin Orthop 249:256, 1989.

Mirels[87] designed a score system to predict the risk of a pathologic fracture (Tables 22-6 and 22-7). Of 78 patients, 51 experienced a fracture and 27 did not. The mean score for the nonfracture group was 7 versus 10 for the fracture group. This system provides a useful tool to evaluate patients for prophylactic fixation. Patients with a score of 10 to 12 should undergo surgery. Patients with scores of 7 or less are not likely to benefit from such therapy. In patients with a "gray zone" score, consideration should be given to the status of surrounding bone and lifestyle (old, osteoporotic woman versus young athlete).

The following guidelines may help make a decision regarding prophylactic fixation. Because each patient presents with unique circumstances, these guidelines cannot replace sound clinical judgment on the part of the attending physician.

1. Life expectancy is longer than 3 months.
2. Patient is medically fit to tolerate major surgery.
3. Procedure planned is expected to expedite mobilization.
4. Quality of bone both proximal and distal to the lesion is adequate to support any fixation device.
5. There is cortical bone destruction of 50% or more.
6. Lesion measuring 2.5 cm or larger is located in the proximal femur.
7. There is pathologic avulsion fracture of the lesser trochanter.
8. Stress pain persists after irradiation.

The following principles govern the surgery of impending fractures:

1. Maximum effort is made to avoid disruption of the surrounding soft tissue to preserve the periosteal blood supply. This is of particular importance in these patients because the endosteal circulation has usually been disrupted by the metastatic deposits.
2. Highly vascular lesions (metastasis from renal cell carcinoma, for instance) should be considered for arteriographic evaluation and possible embolization before open curettage.
3. Defects that include the entire circumference of the cortex should be plugged by acrylic cement at fixation to reduce the biomechanical risks associated with stress risers or open-section defects.
4. When large, thin-walled lesions exist, the intramedullary nailing techniques should be augmented by direct reinforcement of the lesion using methyl methacrylate. This will enhance fixation of the distal long bone, particularly with regard to the torsional stability, and will also prevent shortening of the bone.

Pathologic fractures of the humerus commonly occur in the diaphysis followed by the proximal humerus. Fractures of the diaphysis can be fixed using an intramedullary interlocking device, such as a Brooker-Wills nail, which provides excellent strength and effective resistance against varus, torque, and distraction forces.[88] Proximal humerus fractures commonly require a prosthesis. These patients usually achieve a limited flexion and abduction of about 90 to 100 degrees and enjoy good overall function, joint stability, and pain relief.[81]

Fixation of the femoral neck–intertrochanteric area can be achieved with the use of a compression hip screw and side plate. Fractures involving the femoral neck may be better treated with prosthetic replacement because they are rarely amenable to internal fixation.[89] Subtrochanteric, femoral shaft, and supracondylar femoral lesions are amenable to internal fixation, but large cortical lesions may benefit from an intramedullary acrylic cement filling.

The common problem encountered in acetabular lesions is the failure to appreciate the extent of bone lysis radiographically. Extensive destruction of bone may render efforts to reinforce such lesions with bone graft fruitless. Pathologic fractures of the acetabulum should be managed by total hip arthroplasty.

The spine is the most common site of skeletal metastases. The vertebral body is typically affected first, although pedicle destruction is noted first radiographically. In the absence of a blastic lesion, 30% to 50% of the vertebral body needs to be destroyed before any destruction can be noted on a radiograph. Vertebral metastases are often asymptomatic. Symptoms are usually a result of one of the following: (1) an enlarging mass within the vertebral body that breaks through the cortex and invades the paravertebral soft tissues, (2) a mass compressing or invading local nerve roots, (3) a pathologic fracture, (4) spinal instability secondary to a pathologic fracture (in particular when the posterior elements are involved), and (5) spinal cord compression.

An aggressive surgical approach to spine metastases is usually not warranted.[90] Spinal stabilization is a major surgery involving multiple risks and prolonged recovery. Most patients with spinal metastases do not have progressive spinal instability or neurologic involvement and can be treated with radiation, hormones, chemotherapy, or temporary bracing. Even patients with vertebral body compression fractures can be treated with temporary bed rest and soft bracing. Indications for surgical intervention include (1) progressive spinal canal impingement and cord compression by a radioresistant tumor or a recurrence after maximum tolerance dose to the intended area; (2) bone or soft tissue detritus extruded into the canal as a result of progressive spinal deformity, with or without spinal instability; (3) progressive spinal deformity; (4) progressive kyphotic deformity associated with posterior disruption and shear deformity; and (5) solitary metastases of a histology that is unlikely to be controlled long term with tolerable doses of radiation.

Vertebroplasty of bone metastasis was first described in 1987 and consists of direct injection of the affected vertebra with cement. Polymethylmethacrylate (PMMA) is active through several pathways and produces pain relief in 80% of patients.[91] The procedure is done under intravenous sedation or general anesthesia. Pain receptor destruction is achieved with exothermic reaction of the polymonomer and compressive effect on small nerves. Vertebroplasty effects are not modified by external beam radiation, and PMMA conserves its properties despite radiation.[91] Both could become complementary measures in the future.

Radiotherapy

LOCAL-FIELD RADIOTHERAPY

The vast majority of patients can be managed successfully with external beam radiotherapy. A large body of clinical evidence documents the effectiveness of such therapy.[92] The optimal dose and fractionation schedule is still not resolved. A summary of the major prospective clinical trials that addressed these issues is provided in Table 22-8. The results of these studies should be interpreted with caution because the inherent heterogeneity within the randomization groups may have precluded detection of significant differences, even when such differences could have existed. The use of different pain-scoring systems (physician based versus patient based) and different handling of concomitant use of analgesics, chemotherapy, or hormonal therapy preclude meaningful comparison of the results of these studies.

Between 1974 and 1980, the RTOG conducted a large national study to determine the effectiveness of five different dose fractionation schedules.[40] A total of 1016 patients were entered: 266 into a solitary metastasis stratum and 750 into a multiple metastasis stratum. The former were randomly assigned to treatment with 40.5 Gy in 15 fractions or 20 Gy in 5 fractions. The latter were assigned to 30 Gy in 10 fractions, 15 Gy in 5 fractions, 20 Gy in 5 fractions, or 25 Gy in 5 fractions. A quantitative measure of pain, based on severity and frequency of pain and the type and frequency of pain medications used, was devised to evaluate response. Overall, 89% of patients experienced minimal relief, whereas 83% achieved partial relief and 54% obtained complete relief. There were no significant differences between the treatment arms in both strata. The initial pain score was found to be a useful predictor; patients with high scores were less likely to respond and less likely to experience a complete response. Patients with breast and prostate cancer were significantly more likely to respond than were those with lung or other primary lesions. Patients completing their treatment as planned had a significantly higher rate of complete response than those who did not. Although some pain relief was experienced almost invariably within the first 4 weeks, complete relief was first reported later than 4 weeks after the start of treatment in about 50% of patients. The median duration of minimal and complete pain relief was 20 and 12 weeks, respectively. There were no significant differences in the duration of pain relief between the different arms. The authors concluded that all treatment dose schedules were equally effective.

Table 22-8 **Summary of Prospective Clinical Trials of Radiotherapy for Painful Osseous Metastases**

Study	No. of Patients	Total Dose (Gy)	No. of Fractions	BED (Gy)	Overall Response (%)	Complete Response (%)
Tong et al[40]	1016	40.5	15	51.4	85*	61*
		20.0	5	28.0	82*	53*
		30.0	10	39.0	87	57
		15.0	5	19.5	85	49
		20.0	5	28.0	83	56
		25.0	5	37.5	78	49
Price et al[95]	288	8.0	1	14.4	82	45
		30.0	10	39.0	71	28
Hoskin et al[96]	270	4.0	1	5.6	44	36
		8.0	1	14.4	69	39
Okawa et al[160]	92	30.0	15	36.0	76	—
		22.5	5	32.6	75	—
		20.0	10 (bid)	24.0	78	—
Madsen et al[161]	57	24.0	6	33.6	47	—
		20.0	2	40.0	48	—

*Patients with solitary metastases.
BED, biologically effective dose; bid.

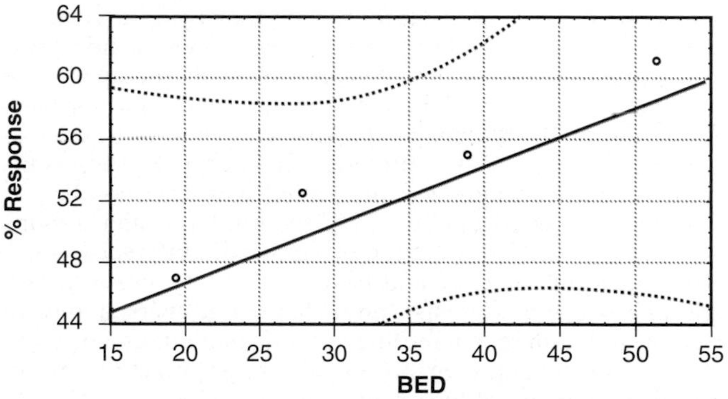

Figure 22-3 Pain response as a function of biologically effective dose (BED) by means of linear regression analysis. Response = 39.1 + .38 × BED; r = .74; P = .15. The *solid red line* indicates the regression function, and the *dotted blue lines* indicate the 95% confidence intervals.

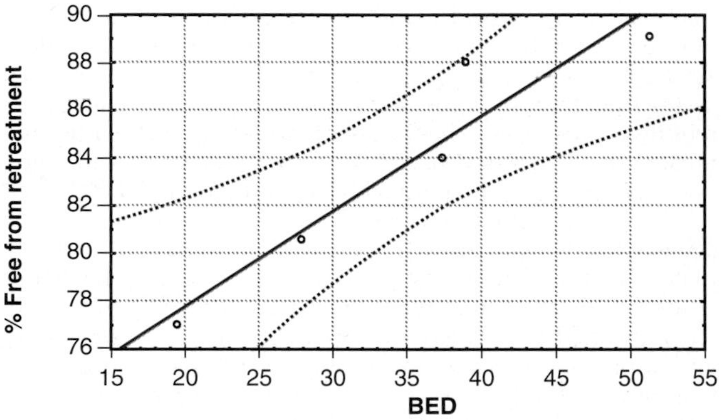

Figure 22-4 Freedom from retreatment as a function of biologically effective dose (BED) by means of linear regression analysis. Response = 69.7 + .4 × BED; r = 0.95; P = .05. The *solid red line* indicates the regression function, and the *dotted blue lines* indicate the 95% confidence intervals.

Blitzer[93] performed a reanalysis of the RTOG study. Using a stepwise logistic regression, he examined the effect of the number of fractions, the dose per fraction, and solitary versus multiple metastases on the probability of attaining complete pain relief and the need for retreatment. This multivariate technique allowed patients with solitary and multiple metastases to be analyzed together. By increasing the number of patients and events, the statistical power of the analysis was increased. The number of fractions was the only variable that was significantly associated with outcome. There was no correlation of the time-dose factor (TDF)[94] with outcome. It was concluded that the more protracted schedules resulted in improved pain relief.

The concept of TDF has long been replaced by the linear quadratic model. Using this model, and assuming an α/β of 10 for tumor, we calculated the biologically effective dose (BED) for the various schedules tested by the RTOG. Figures 22-3 and 22-4 depict pain response and freedom from retreatment as a function of BED, respectively. The solid lines are the regression functions, and the dotted lines represent the 95% confidence intervals. The results suggest that schedules with higher BED resulted in better pain relief and reduced the need for retreatment.

Price and others[95] randomized 288 patients to receive either 8 Gy in one fraction or 30 Gy in 10 daily fractions. Pain was assessed using a daily questionnaire completed by the patient at home. No differences were found in the probability of attaining pain relief, speed of onset, or duration of relief between the two arms.

Hoskin and colleagues[96] randomized 270 patients to receive either 4 Gy or 8 Gy in one fraction. Pain (assessed by the patient) and analgesic usage were recorded before treatment and at 2, 4, 8, and 12 weeks. At 4 weeks, the response rates were 69% for 8 Gy and 44% for 4 Gy (P < .001). The duration of the effect was independent of dose.

Additional studies have evaluated single versus multiple fraction regimens. A Danish randomized trial of 241 patients showed no significant difference with regard to pain relief or quality of life after receiving either 8 Gy in a single fraction or 20 Gy in 5 fractions.[97] Wu and colleagues[98] performed a meta-analysis of 16 trials including 5455 patients and proclaimed equivalence between single and multiple fractions.

Van der Linden and colleagues[99] recently published a reanalysis of a Dutch Bone Metastasis Study that included 1171 patients. This study randomized patients to either single 8 Gy versus 24 Gy in 6 fractions. This new publication focuses on retreatment need. Mean time to retreatment was shorter (13 versus 21 weeks) with single fraction. It was also more frequent: 24% after single fraction and 6% after 6 fractions (P = .001). Initial high pain score also influenced the need for retreatment.

Treatment Techniques

The target volumes for external beam radiotherapy should be defined after review of all appropriate diagnostic studies. Attention should be paid to soft tissue masses, which are often associated with bone metastases and at times responsible for the observed symptoms. Such lesions are best assessed by CT or MRI. The target volumes are treated with appropriate margins. Depending on the treatment site and volume, suppression of the bone marrow should be anticipated. In patients for whom chemotherapy is planned, treatment volumes should be kept to a minimum to preserve marrow reserves. Because many patients have repeated courses of therapy, all previous ports and radiation records must be reviewed. To minimize late radiation damage, overlap of radiation fields should be avoided. Depending on the clinical circumstances, overlapping retreatment may be appropriate in patients with short life expectancy. Figures 22-5 to 22-8 demonstrate typical field arrangements used to treat bone metastases.

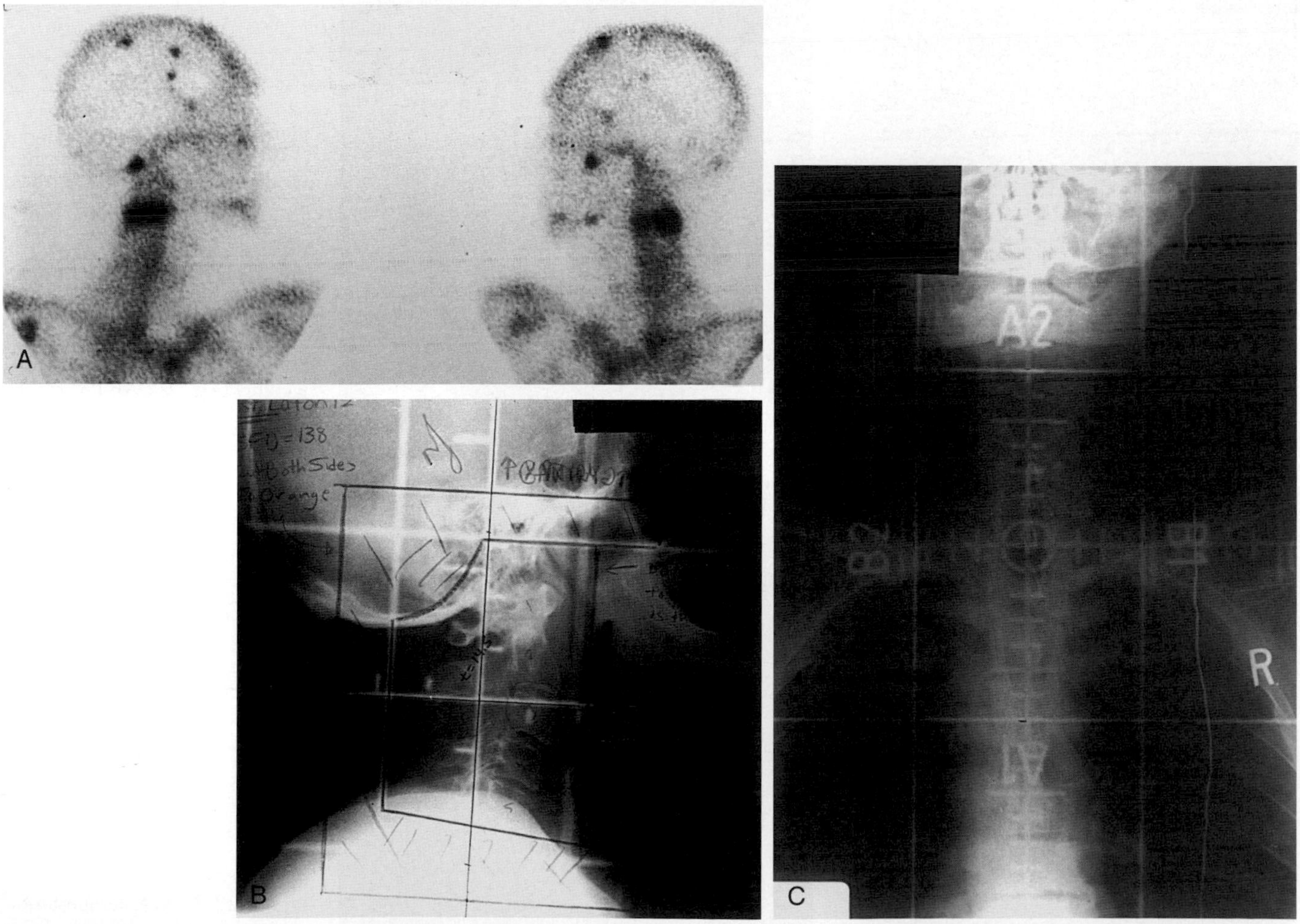

Figure 22-5 Treatment of the cervical spine. **A,** Radionuclide bone scan demonstrates increased tracer uptake in the skull and cervical spine. **B,** Therapy with two opposing lateral fields. The dose is prescribed at the middle depth. **C,** Therapy with a single posterior field. The dose is prescribed at 5 cm at the depth of the target volume.

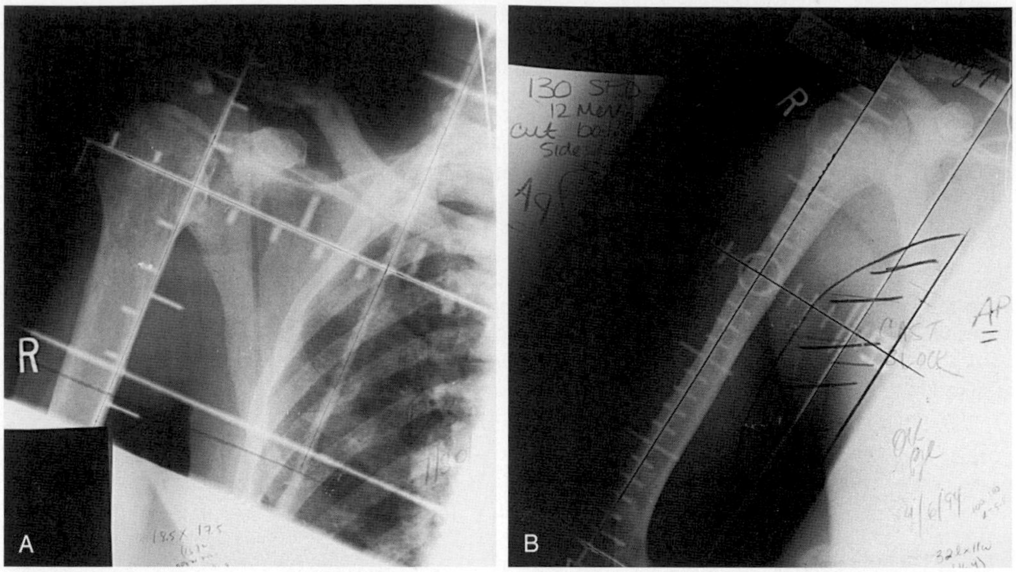

Figure 22-6 Treatment of the upper extremity. **A,** The shoulder girdle is treated with an antero-posterior-posteroanterior (AP-PA) pair of fields. **B,** AP-PA fields for treating the humerus.

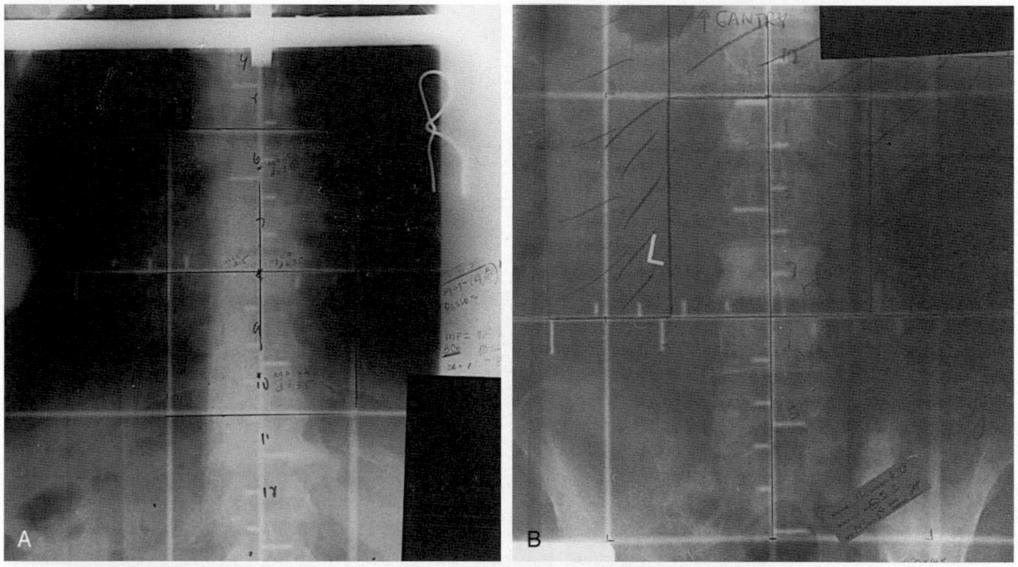

Figure 22-7 **A,** Posteroanterior (PA) field for treatment of the thoracic spine. The dose is prescribed at 5 cm or at the depth of the target volume. **B,** Anteroposterior-posteroanterior (AP-PA) inverted T-shaped fields for treatment of the lumbosacral spine. The dose distribution from a single PA field typically would not be adequate. Differential weights (e.g., 1:2 AP-PA) can be used.

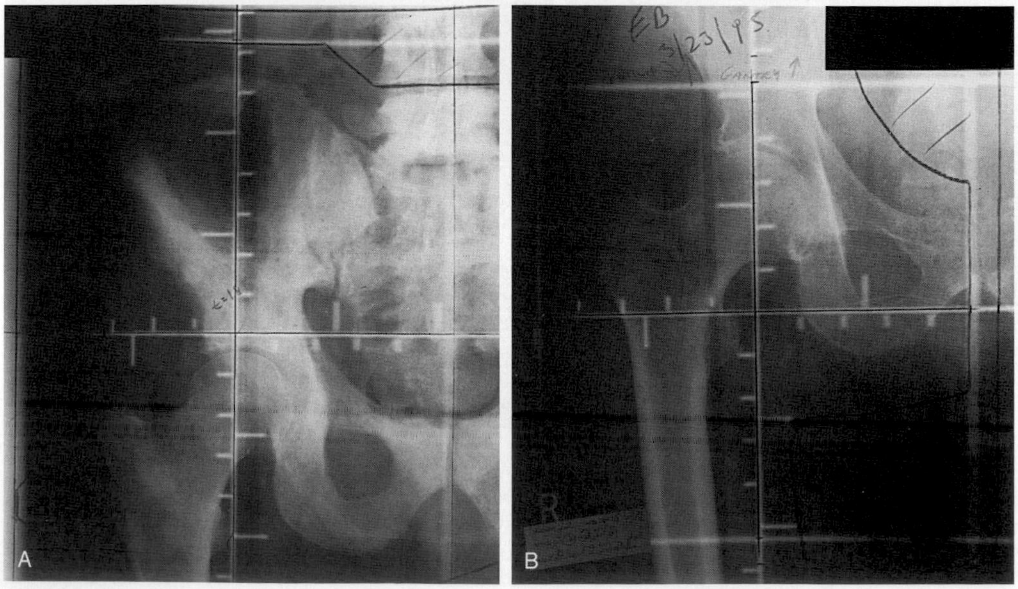

Figure 22-8 **A,** Anteroposterior-posteroanterior (AP-PA) fields used to treat the left hemipelvis and upper femur. **B,** AP-PA fields used to treat the upper femur acetabulum and pubic bone.

HEMIBODY IRRADIATION

Most patients with bone metastases have multiple sites of involvement. As many as 76% of patients receiving therapy to a local field require additional treatment for pain at other sites within 1 year.[100] Wide-field radiotherapy has been used to address this problem. A summary of results of this form of therapy is provided in Table 22-9. Response rates are similar to those observed with local-field radiotherapy, but the onset of relief is more rapid, occurring often within 24 hours of treatment. Hemibody irradiation (HBI) may require hospitalization for hydration and premedication with steroids and antiemetics and tends to be associated with substantial morbidity. Most patients experience acute gastrointestinal toxicity, with nausea, vomiting, and diarrhea persisting for 24 to 48 hours. Myelosuppression is commonly observed but is rarely of clinical significance. Radiation pneumonitis is rare at doses below 7 Gy to the lungs.

RTOG conducted a phase III study to evaluate the efficacy of HBI in addition to local-field irradiation.[100] A total of 499 patients were randomized to receive either HBI or no further therapy after completion of local-field irradiation to a symptomatic site. Entry was stratified by extent of metastatic disease (solitary or multiple) and the targeted hemibody area (upper, middle, or lower). Local-field irradiation consisted of 30 Gy in 10 fractions. HBI consisted of 8 Gy in 1 fraction given within 7 days of completion of the local field. Partial transmission blocks were used to reduce the dose to the lungs to 7 Gy. Time to disease progression, time to new disease, and time to new course of therapy were significantly longer in the HBI arm. Progression of disease was faster in patients with involvement of the upper and middle hemibody (compared with lower hemibody) and in patients with multiple metastases (compared with solitary tumor). As expected, toxicity was significantly higher in the HBI arm, but there were no fatalities and no occurrences of radiation pneumonitis. Although the impact of HBI on clinically occult metastatic disease was demonstrated unequivocally, the long-term benefit was relatively small. The ultimate progression rates were not significantly different between the arms, and at 1 year 60% of the HBI patients had to be retreated.

Table 22-9 Wide-Field Radiotherapy for Painful Osseous Metastases

Study	No. Fields Treated	Dose (Gy) Upper	Dose (Gy) Lower	Response (%)
Fitzpatrick[162]	570	3-6	10	55-72
Rowland et al[163]	96	7.5	10	80
Qasim[164]	129	7-8*	7-8*	76
Salazar et al[165]	168	6	8	73
Wilkins et al[166]	141	6	8	82
Poulter et al[100]	229	8	8	93

*3 to 4 Gy in multiple myeloma patients.

SYSTEMIC RADIONUCLIDE THERAPY

The first report on the use of systemic radionuclides for the treatment of bone metastases was published by Pecher in the 1940s.[101] Using this modality, all involved osseous sites can be addressed simultaneously with little toxicity. Selective absorption into bone metastases limits irradiation of normal tissues and increases the therapeutic ratio. Administration as a single intravenous injection in the outpatient clinic is a further advantage for many patients.

Systemic radionuclides should be considered in the following circumstances:

1. In patients with widely metastatic disease, as adjuvant to external beam radiotherapy
2. In patients without a predominantly painful site, as a first-line therapy
3. When external beam therapy options have been exhausted, and normal tissue tolerance has been reached
4. In patients with a life expectancy of at least 3 months
5. There is no evidence of imminent epidural cord compression, pathologic fracture, or mechanical instability
6. In patients with good marrow reserve with a white blood cell count of greater than 2400 and a platelet count of greater than 100,000

Historically, phosphorus 32 was the first radionuclide to be widely used in the treatment of bone metastases. It decays by beta emission to sulfur 32 with a half-life of 14.3 days. The maximum beta energy is 1.71 MeV. After parenteral administration, phosphorus 32 skeletal uptake exceeds that of muscle, fat, or skin by a factor of 6 to 10. Silberstein[102] reviewed the results of 28 reported human studies. Subjective decrease in pain occurs in 60% to 80% of patients. Pain relief is rapid, most often obtained within 14 days. The major toxicity reported is myelosuppression with pancytopenia. Nausea and vomiting are not uncommon. An increased incidence of acute leukemia has also been reported.[103] Phosphorus 32 has since been replaced by newer, less toxic radionuclides (Tables 22-10 and 22-11).

Strontium 89 Strontium 89 decays by beta emission to yttrium 89 with a half-life of 50.6 days. The average beta energy is 1.46 MeV. Chemically similar to calcium, strontium 89 is quickly taken up into the mineral matrix of bone. The fraction of strontium 89 retained is proportional to the metastatic tumor burden and varies between 20% and 80% of the administered dose.[104] Preferential accumulation in and around metastatic deposits, where active bone formation takes place, has been demonstrated by bone scans with the gamma emitter strontium 89[104,105] and by direct comparison of autoradiography and histologic sections of affected bone.[106] Once incorporated into the metastatic lesion, strontium 89 is not removed metabolically and remains deposited for as long as 100 days.[104] Normal bone takes up only a small fraction of the

Table 22-10 Physical Characteristics of Various Radionuclides

Radionuclide	Physical Half-Life	Beta Energy (MeV)	Gamma Energy (keV)	Chelate
Phosphorus 32	14.3 d	1.71	—	Orthophosphate
Strontium 89	50.6 d	1.46	—	Chloride
Rhenium 186	90.6 h	1.07	137	HEDP
Samarium 153	46.3 h	0.84	103	EDTMP

HEDP, hydroxyethylenediphosphonic acid; EDTMP, ethylenediaminetetramethylene phosphonate.

Table 22-11 Summary of Clinical Trials With Systemic Radionuclides

Radionuclide	Response Rate (%)	Complete Response (%)	Response Duration
Phosphorus 32[103]	60-80	—	~5 mo
Strontium 89			
Laing et al[111]	75	22	6 mo
Robinson et al[112]	80	11	NA
Quilty et al[117]	65-70	30*	NA
Rhenium 186			
Maxon[121-123]	77	21	5 wk
Samarium 153			
Collins et al[120]	76	NA	2.6
Ahonen et al[167]	80	54	2-17 wk

*Substantial or dramatic response, estimated from a graph.
NA, not applicable.

injected dose and retains it for a much shorter period of time.[71] Estimates of the total dose absorbed within the metastatic lesion vary between 0.9 and 231 cGy/MBq.[105-108] Elimination is through the kidneys, and careful disposal of urine is needed for 7 to 10 days after administration. Extra care is advised for incontinent patients. Because strontium 89 emits extremely little gamma radiation, the patient is not a radiation hazard to family members or hospital staff.

The efficacy of strontium 89 has been well documented.[104,108-114] Lewington and coworkers,[115] in a randomized, double-blind study, demonstrated the superiority of strontium 89 over stable elemental strontium. Thirty-two patients were randomized to receive a first injection, and response was assessed at 5 weeks. Nonresponders received a second injection at 6 weeks, and response was assessed again after 5 weeks. At 5 weeks, of 12 patients receiving strontium 89, dramatic and any relief of pain were noted in 4 and 8 patients, respectively; of 14 patients receiving elemental strontium, dramatic and any relief of pain were noted in 3 and 6 patients, respectively. Combined with the results of the second evaluation, dramatic and any relief of pain were noted in 4 and 10 patients, respectively, of 20 who received strontium 89 and in 4 and 0 patients, respectively, of 18 who received elemental strontium. These differences were statistically significant, confirming that the palliative effects of strontium 89 were due to its radioactive emission.

Laing and associates[111] reported on the results of a dose-escalation study. The optimal dose was found to be 1.5 MBq/kg with no appreciable increment in efficacy above this dose. Of 83 patients treated with at least 1.5 MBq/kg, 75% had partial relief of pain and 22% were rendered pain free. Pain relief began 10 to 20 days after treatment and peaked at 6 weeks. Response was maintained for a median of 6 months (range, 4 to 15 months). The RTOG conducted a dose-escalation study and concluded that the maximum tolerated dose of strontium 89 is 6.5 mCi (approximately 3.4 MBq/kg).

Toxicity of strontium 89 is mainly hematologic. Platelet depression is dose dependent. Most patients have a 20% to 30% drop in their counts after doses of 3 to 4 mCi (1.5 to 2 MBq/kg). Grade III toxicity is rare. Other adverse effects include a transient increase in bone pain in up to 10% of patients and, rarely, facial flushing. The pain flare occurs 1 to 2 weeks after treatment, may last a few days, and usually heralds a favorable response.

Porter and colleagues[116] reported the results of the Trans-Canada study. This trial evaluated the efficacy of strontium 89 adjuvant to local-field external beam radiotherapy in patients with hormone-refractory prostate cancer. A total of 126 patients were randomized to local-field radiotherapy (20 Gy in 5 fractions or 30 Gy in 10 fractions) followed by placebo or by strontium 89 (10.8 mCi). Overall and complete responses (relief of pain at the index site) were higher in the treatment arm, but the differences did not reach statistical significance. Objectively measured responses (greater than 50% reduction in serum prostate-specific antigen and alkaline phosphatase) were also significantly superior in the treatment arm. A significantly greater proportion of patients in the treatment arm had stopped taking analgesics and experienced an improvement in physical activity and quality of life. Strontium 89–treated patients had a significant delay in the appearance of new painful sites and prolongation in the time before further radiotherapy was required. At 3 months after treatment, 58.7% and 34% of patients in the treatment arm and control arm, respectively, were free of new painful metastases. The median time to further radiotherapy was 35.3 and 20.3 weeks in the treatment arm and control arm, respectively. Hematologic toxicity was, as expected, higher in strontium 89–treated patients.

The U.K. Metastron Investigators Group Study[117] was designed to compare pain relief after strontium 89 with that after external beam radiotherapy. Entry criteria were similar to those in the Trans-Canada study. Eligible patients were stratified as suitable for treatment with either local or hemibody radiotherapy. They were then randomized to treatment with that form of external beam irradiation or strontium 89. Local-field radiation schedules were usually 20 Gy in five fractions, but a single 8-Gy fraction was occasionally used. HBI was given as a single fraction of 6 Gy (upper half) or 8 Gy (lower half). Strontium 89 was given at a dose of 200 MBq (5.4 mCi). Pain at each site was graded according to severity (mild to intractable) and type (intermittent or constant). Additional end points scored included analgesic use, performance status, and mobility. Overall response was scored using a scale ranging from "deterioration" to "dramatic improvement." A total of 284 patients were treated according to protocol. Both overall pain relief and dramatic pain relief were similar with strontium 89 (61% and 44.1%, respectively), local radiotherapy (65.9% and 36.4%, respectively), or HBI (63.6% and 43.2%, respectively). Patients receiving strontium 89 were significantly less likely to experience new sites of pain or require additional therapy than were those treated with either form of external beam irradiation. The incidence of symptomatic side effects was markedly less after strontium 89 than after HBI.

Samarium 153 Samarium 153 is a man-made radionuclide that emits beta particles of 0.81 MeV (20%), 0.71 MeV (30%), and 0.64 MeV (50%) and gamma photons of 103 keV (28%). It has a relatively short half-life of 46.3 hours and, consequently, a relatively high-dose rate. Samarium 153 has been chelated to a phosphonate, ethylenediaminetetramethylene (EDTMP), to produce a bone-seeking complex. About 50% of an intravenously administered dose is retained in bone.[118,119] Absorbed dose in bone and red marrow has been estimated at 2.5 and 0.57 cGy/MBq, respectively.[119] Clinical experience with samarium 153 is still limited. In a phase I/II clinical trial,[120] the maximally tolerated dose was determined to be 2.5 mCi/kg. The principal toxicity observed was hematologic; maximum myelosuppression occurred at 3 to 4 weeks. A flare of bone pain occurred in 12% of patients. The overall pain relief rate was 74%, with a median duration of palliation of 2.6 months. In responders, relief was obtained promptly within 7 to 14 days of treatment. Response rates were significantly higher with 2.5 mCi/kg than with 1.0 mCi/kg.

Rhenium 186 Rhenium 186 emits beta particles of 1.07 MeV and a 137-keV gamma ray and has a short half-life of 3.8 days. Like samarium 153, it has been complexed to a bone-seeking phosphonate, hydroxyethylenediphosphonic acid (HEDP). Retention in bone is about 50% of the injected dose; the rest is excreted through the kidneys into the urine.[121] Rhenium 186 has been studied in a small number of patients with metastatic cancer of the prostate, breast, colon, and lung.[122] After administration of 33 to 35 mCi, 75% to 80% of patients experienced pain relief, most often within 2 weeks.[121-123] The therapeutic efficacy of rhenium 186 has been confirmed in a double-blind, crossover comparison with placebo.[123] Myelosuppression begins 2 weeks after treatment, peaks at 4 to 6 weeks, and resolves by 8 weeks.[122] A pain flare occurs in 10% of patients 2 to 3 days after treatment and resolves within 1 week.

American Society for Therapeutic Radiology and Oncology Survey

We surveyed the membership of the American Society for Therapeutic Radiology and Oncology (ASTRO) regarding the management of painful osseous metastases. The survey consisted of 30 multiple-choice questions regarding four hypothetical clinical scenarios likely to be encountered in daily practice. Questions related to the technique of choice (local-field versus hemibody radiotherapy), the use of systemic radionuclides, fractionation schemes, dose, integration of modalities, and follow-up of these patients. Eight hundred seventeen responses have been received and analyzed. The results indicated that systemic radionuclides have gained popularity in the management of metastatic prostate cancer, where they are used alone in up to 11% of patients or in combination with local-field irradiation in up to 79% of patients. Strontium 89 is the most common radionuclide in use (99% of users). The administered doses are 4 mCi (73%) and 10.8 mCi (26%). Systemic radionuclide therapy appears to have replaced HBI. The latter is seldom (0.9% to 4% of responders) considered in the management of patients with prostate cancer. In patients with breast cancer, local-field irradiation continues to be the preferred therapy. It is possible that concerns regarding bone marrow reserves sway physicians away from systemic radionuclides in this chemotherapy-responsive disease.

These results demonstrate a change in the management of painful osseous metastases with increased acceptance of a new paradigm: local-field external beam radiotherapy to the painful index site in combination with prophylactic administration of systemic radionuclides for clinically occult metastases.

SPINAL CORD COMPRESSION

Malignant spinal cord compression occurs in 5% of all patients with malignant disease and in approximately 20% of patients with metastases to the vertebral column.[124] More than 95% of spinal cord compressions are due to extramedullary malignancy, most commonly secondary to involvement of the vertebral column anterior to the spinal cord, less frequently by tumors posterior to the spinal cord, and occasionally by invasion of the epidural space.

Any tumor that metastasizes to the bone can eventually result in a cord compression. Most commonly seen primaries include lung, breast, prostate, kidney, lymphoma, myeloma, sarcoma, and unknown primaries.

Clinical Manifestations and Patient Evaluation

The majority of patients present with pain, motor loss, autonomic dysfunction, and sensory loss.[125] Pain is often radicular for weeks or months before onset of the neurologic symptoms. Autonomic dysfunction may occur early and manifest as hesitancy and urgency. Weakness usually precedes sensory loss; incontinence, paraplegia, and paralysis are late effects. Pain was the initial symptom in 96% of the patients but is a poor indicator of spinal-epidural involvement.[126] In contrast, 75% of patients with major neurologic involvement have involvement of the epidural space.

Diagnosis

Early diagnosis is essential because recovery of neurologic function is related to the degree of loss. A careful history and physical examination focusing on neurologic assessment with a high index of suspicion in patients with known malignancy is key to early diagnosis. Diagnostic investigations varying from plain spine radiographs to myelograms have been used in the past. MRI is now the diagnostic study of choice. The entire length of the spinal cord and its relationship with surrounding structures can be visualized without the use of intrathecal contrast.[127,128] Distortion of the theca by extradural lesions and soft tissue abnormalities can be easily identified.[126,129] In case of compression fracture, protrusion of the vertebral body or tumor into the spinal canal is seen clearly, as is the impingement of nerve roots and neural foramina.[127] Approximately 10% of patients have multiple sites of cord compression and perhaps benefit from imaging of the entire spine.

Treatment

A multidisciplinary approach is recommended to treat spinal cord compression. High-dose steroids should be administered after a clinical diagnosis. An initial dose of 20 mg of dexamethasone (Decadron) followed by 4 mg four times daily improves pain and neurologic symptoms in most patients. Steroids should be tapered gradually after completion of radiation. Patients receiving dexamethasone should be placed on H_2 blockers and monitored for hyperglycemia, hypertension, and electrolyte imbalances.

A randomized trial comparing laminectomy followed by radiation versus radiation alone in the treatment of spinal epidural metastasis showed no significant difference in the effectiveness of treatment in regard to pain relief, improved ambulation, and improved sphincter function.[130] Although most cases of spinal cord compression can be managed with steroids and radiotherapy, patients without a histologically proven cancer, radioresistant tumors, previously radiated sites, or mechanical instability should be seen by a neurosurgeon for a laminectomy (Fig. 22-9).

Treatment outcome is dependent on pretreatment function. In a study of 137 patients with malignant spinal cord compression, 81% of patients who were ambulatory pretreatment remained ambulant, whereas only 16.5% of those who were nonambulant before treatment became ambulant after treatment. Pain improved after treatment in 73% of the patients regardless of their ambulatory status.[124] This was confirmed by Zelefsky and colleagues[131] in a retrospective review of 42 patients. They also reported that the presence of a compression fracture of greater than 50% at the level of the spinal cord compression was associated with poor response on refluoromyelography (RFM). Sixty-seven percent with severe compression fractures had no response on RFM versus 11% without compression fracture ($P = .01$).

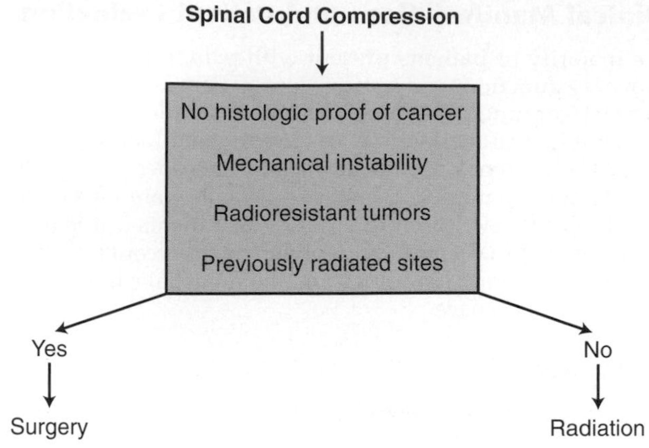

Figure 22-9 Treatment algorithm for spinal cord compression.

Irradiation Technique and Doses

The depth of the tumor mass can be determined by MRI. If MRI is unavailable at the time of simulation, a lateral film taken at simulation can help determine the prescription depth. The width of the field is dependent on the extent of the soft tissue mass as determined by MRI.

Treatment fields are dependent on the site of involved spinal cord. The cervical spine is usually treated using opposed laterals to avoid the oral cavity. For the thoracic spine, a posterior field alone can be used. When treating the lumbar spine or when the target appears to be more midline, a parallel opposed AP: PA beam arrangement may be preferred. For either the thoracic or lumbar spine, acceptable alternative techniques include paired posterior obliques or PA and paired laterals.

The dose of irradiation used for the treatment of spinal cord compression is dependent on both the histopathologic findings and the clinical situation (ambulatory versus nonambulatory, solitary versus multiple metastases, systemic therapy options and efficacy). The typical dose is 30 Gy in 10 fractions over 2 weeks or 20 Gy in 5 fractions. If life expectancy exceeds a few months, a more protracted regimen (35 to 40 Gy in 3 to 4 weeks) is reasonable with regard to the issue of spinal cord tolerance.

BRAIN METASTASES

Secondary brain tumors are a common complication of systemic cancer. The incidence ranges from 20% to 40% of all patients diagnosed with cancer.[132] Cancers known to generate systemic disease are the most common primary tumors involved: lung, breast, colon, and melanoma. Current improvements in systemic therapy have improved survival significantly for several cancers but may leave untreated tumor cells beyond the blood-brain barrier. More precise diagnostic tools, like MRI, also have an impact on the increasing discovery of brain metastases.

The prognosis of brain metastases is poor and the impact on the patient's quality of life is important due to the functional neurologic deficits associated. Symptom management is successful in most patients and efforts can be concentrated on improving the outcome of the patients.[132]

Arterial hematogenous spread results in tumor emboli growth at the gray-white junction[133]; the most common neuroanatomical sites are the cerebral hemispheres (80%), the cerebellum (15%), and the brainstem (5%).[134] Multiple metastases are more common than single metastasis and the contribution of MRI to this statistic has reached 80% to 90%.[132]

Presenting symptoms are various and require that any new neurologic symptom be investigated in a patient known to have cancer. Symptoms reflect increasing intracranial pressure and focal neurologic deficit—headache, nausea, lateralized weakness, seizures, modified higher neurologic function. In most patients, the cancer is already diagnosed, but in as many as 20%, it may be the first manifestation; histologic confirmation is then necessary.

Contrast-enhanced MRI is the diagnostic modality of choice. The radiologic differential diagnosis includes primary brain tumor, inflammatory lesion, abscess, and brain infarction or hemorrhage. CT may also be used, but it is less specific and warrants MRI confirmation in case of single metastasis. Patchell and colleagues[135] reported a false-positive rate of MRI of 11%, confirmed by histology.

Treatment

Palliative treatment of brain metastases requires rapid control of the symptoms, which are decreasing the patient's quality of life. Collaboration with colleagues in neurology is preferable. Pharmacologic treatment includes corticosteroids, antiepileptic drugs, and H_2 inhibitors. Rapid regression of cerebral edema is the first step and can be achieved with intravenous corticosteroids. Optimal dosage is unknown, but the general practice is to administer a loading dose of Decadron (8 to 32 mg) followed by oral medication (4 mg four times a day).[136] Side effects are numerous, and a tapering dose schedule should be planned as symptoms improve. As a single modality, corticosteroids achieve poor survival results of 1 to 3 months.

Treatment depends on several prognostic factors; Gaspar and coworkers[137] have evaluated results of RTOG trials to produce a recursive partitioning analysis. Pretreatment and treatment-related variables were analyzed. Class 1 (Karnofsky Performance Status [KPS] > 70, age < 65 years, and controlled primary tumor) patients have a better median prognostic of 7 months. Class 2 (KPS < 70, age > 65 years, or uncontrolled primary tumor) patients have a median prognostic of 4 months, and class 3 (KPS < 70, age > 65 years, and uncontrolled primary tumor) patients have a median of 2 months. Other factors, such as histology of the tumor and the number and size of metastases, are important in the initial evaluation. Treatment options are evolving and now include whole brain radiotherapy (WBRT), surgical resection, and radiosurgery (linear accelerator or gamma knife)

Patients with a single brain metastasis in RPA class 1 are treated aggressively with surgical resection and WBRT. Multiple metastases from any RPA class receive standard WBRT alone. Patients with two or three metastases in class 1 or 2 may be considered for single or multiple modalities.

Whole Brain Radiotherapy

WBRT is the treatment of choice for most patients because of the high incidence of multiple metastatic sites or uncontrolled primary tumor.[132,136,137] The goal of WBRT is to limit tumor progression and, in the middle term, to limit the use of corticosteroids. MS is expected to reach 4 to 6 months with WBRT.[138] The optimal dose of radiation is unknown, but in clinical practice, the range is 20 Gy in 5 fractions over 1 week to 40 Gy in 20 fractions over 4 weeks.[132]

Complications of treatment include alopecia, transient worsening of neurologic symptoms, and otitis. Continuing use of corticosteroids during WBRT may limit the incidence of most side effects. Long-term side effects such as memory loss, dementia, and decreased concentration are possible in survivors but are not expected to appear in the majority of patients with short survival.

Technique of Whole Brain Radiotherapy

The patient is undergoing simulation for palliative treatment and therefore should be conscious and cooperative. Agitated or unresponsive patients should be stabilized before this step to decrease the risk of injury. Simulation is done in a supine position with head rest, and immobilization is achieved with a custom mask or at least tape between the forehead and table. CT simulation requires the use of a mask.

Portal films with the gantry at 90 and 270 degrees will give parallel-opposed lateral fields. The collimator should be rotated to allow the inferior border to parallel the base of skull. The field borders should go beyond the skull anterior, superior, and posterior bony limits by 2 cm to allow dosimetric homogeneity. The inferior border can be set from the bony canthus to the C1-2 intervertebral space. This should cover the base of skull with a 1-cm margin. CT simulation is now commonly used with the same parameter but allows for custom block design to avoid irradiation of the lens and facial structures. All fields are treated daily. Megavoltage energy of 4-6 MV is used.

Surgical Resection

The role of surgery has evolved over the past decade and is now part of the aggressive management of brain metastases. Three randomized controlled trials comparing WBRT alone versus surgery plus WBRT have been published.[139-141] Although they were relatively small studies, two of them demonstrated a survival advantage of the combined modalities over WBRT alone (Table 22-12).

All three trials addressed the issue of single metastases, and one cannot extrapolate the results to multiple lesions. The negative results of Mintz contradict those of others, but this trial also contained a lower complete surgical resection rate and lower WBRT dose.

Radiosurgery

Stereotactic radiosurgery (SRS) is a competing modality to surgical resection for small brain lesions, without the disadvantage of craniotomy. Size is limited to metastases smaller than 3 to 4 cm in diameter. The RTOG published the results of RTOG 9805 in 2004.[142] One hundred sixty-four patients were assigned to receive WBRT alone versus 167 receiving WBRT followed by SRS boost. All histologies were welcomed, and patients were stratified according to the number of metastases. WBRT consisted of 37.5 Gy in 12 fractions in both groups, SRS was given to different doses according to size and varied from 24 Gy for smaller lesions to 15 Gy for larger lesions. Andrews reports significantly improved MS for single metastasis from 4.9 to 6.5 months ($P = .0393$). Thus, WBRT plus SRS is considered an alternative treatment for single metastasis. Nonsignificant results in term of survival were reported for all other patients. Technical aspects of SRS are beyond the scope of this chapter and can be found in other sections of this book (see Chapter 16, Stereotactic Irradiation: Linear Accelerator and Gamma Knife).

LIVER METASTASES

Colorectal cancer is one of the most common cancers with a yearly incidence of 145,000 new cases in the United States, and 56,000 will die annually of the disease[143]; many patients (50% to 60%)[144] with colorectal cancer will develop liver metastases in the course of their disease. Liver is also a frequent site of systemic spread for other solid tumors (breast, lung, melanoma). The burden of this clinical entity is important.

Colorectal Cancer

Systemic chemotherapy is administered to patients with the hope of prolonged survival, symptom control, and maintained quality of life. A meta-analysis by Simmonds[145] proved the value of this approach over best supportive care with an improvement of 16% in survival, which translated into an increase in MS from 8 to 11.7 months. Early administration of chemotherapy is favored over delayed treatment when symptoms arise.[146] The chemotherapy regimen is not yet standardized and is still the scope of many recent and ongoing trials. Combinations are preferred and include 5-fluorouracil (5-FU) and leucovorin plus either irinotecan (Saltz,[147] FOLFIRI[148] regimen) or oxaliplatin (FOLFOX[149] regimen).

A small proportion of patients can be selected for regional management of liver metastases with curative intent (surgical resection, radiofrequency ablation, cryosurgery). From 10% to 20% of the patients will present with liver-confined disease and may be addressed by metastasectomy.[150] Unresectable extrahepatic metastases are a contraindication to aggressive regional treatment of liver metastases.[144] Cure rates range from 20% to 45% at 5 years[151]; they are influenced by the number of metastases and the surgeon's experience. Laparotomy with surgical resection is the standard approach; radiofrequency ablation and cryosurgery are also used. Local recurrence in the liver occurs in about 30% of patients, and relapse outside the liver is frequent. Ways to improve outcomes have been developed.

The liver has dual blood supply, and it is possible to deliver chemotherapy directly into the hepatic artery (hepatic arterial chemotherapy [HAC]). HAC has been used to increase respectability (downstaging) and to consolidate treatments. Most regimens are fluoropyrimidine-based, and response rates vary greatly between trials (10% to 62%).[152] HAC has been compared with systemic chemotherapy without defini-

Table 22-12 WBRT Alone or Plus Surgical Resection in the Management of Brain Metastases

Trial	Treatment	Radiotherapy Schedule	*n*	Median Survival (mo)	*P* Value
Patchell[139]	Biopsy + WBRT	36 Gy/12	23	4.2	<.01
	S + WBRT	36 Gy/12	25	10	
Vecht[140]	WBRT	40 Gy/10 bid	31	6.5	NA
	S + WBRT	40 Gy/10 bid	32	10.8	
Mintz[141]	WBRT	30 Gy/10	43	6.3	.24
	S + WBRT	30 Gy/10	41	5.9	

S, surgery; WBRT, whole body radiotherapy.

Techniques and Modalities

tive conclusions.[153,154] The European Organization for the Research and Treatment of Cancer (EORTC)/Medical Research Council (MRC) and the CALGB have randomized patients to a comparable regimen of HAC versus systemic chemotherapy. The final publication of the CALGB trial is awaited, but Kerr and colleagues[153] reported similar overall survival of 14 months in both groups.

Liver Irradiation

Normal liver has poor tolerance to external beam radiotherapy if the entire liver is irradiated, and clinical liver failure can arise from low to moderate doses of whole liver radiation (25 to 35 Gy in 1.8- to 2-Gy fractions). Radiation has not had a significant role in the treatment of liver metastases in most institutions. It should be noted, however, that the risk for radiation-induced liver disease (RILD) is low if the whole liver dose is restricted to 30 Gy or less in fractions of 2 Gy or less. Liver radiation for metastatic disease can be of palliative benefit, as found in an RTOG phase II trial of 100 patients in whom palliation of pain was noted in 55%.[155]

Partial liver irradiation using three-dimensional conformal or intensity-modulated radiation therapy techniques with external beam radiation, high-dose rate brachytherapy implants, and selective hepatic artery delivery of radiation using different isotopes are under investigation. These techniques have stimulated greater interest, because higher radiation doses can be delivered with acceptable tolerance and have already produced interesting results that warrant further investigation.[156-158]

Tolerance issues using partial liver radiation with conformal techniques are discussed in detail in Chapter 46 and are not discussed in detail in this section. Lawrence and colleagues have done extensive investigations at the University of Michigan evaluating the relationship between dose and liver volumes irradiated and the probability of RILD. Ben-Josef and Lawrence note in their chapter in this textbook that, using three-dimensional treatment planning, it is possible to safely irradiate two thirds of the normal liver to 48 to 52.8 Gy and one third of the liver to 66 to 72.6 Gy (1.5 to 1.65 Gy twice a day with separation of 4 or more hours).

Other Solid Tumors

Other solid tumors also frequently result in liver metastases. Usually the metastasis is found late, at the end of metastatic progression, but in 5% to 10%, an isolated liver metastasis is found. For patients with liver metastases from sarcoma, breast, lung, and gynecologic malignancies, metastasectomy should be contemplated for cytoreduction. MS ranges from 20 to 35 months for liver metastases from breast cancer.[159]

REFERENCES

1. Von Roenn JH, Cleeland CS, Gonin R, et al: Physician attitudes and practice in cancer pain management: a survey from the Eastern Cooperative Oncology Group. Ann Intern Med 119:121-126, 1993.
2. Cleeland CS, Gonin R, Hatfield AK, et al: Pain and its treatment in outpatients with metastatic cancer. N Engl J Med 330:592-596, 1994.
3. Foley KM: The treatment of cancer pain. N Engl J Med 313:84-94, 1985.
4. Abrams HL, Spiro R, Goldstein A: Metastases in carcinomas. Analysis of 1000 autopsied cases. Cancer 23:74-85, 1950.
5. Galasko CSB: Incidence and distribution of skeletal metastases. Clin Orthop 210:14-22, 1986.
6. Tofe AJ, Francis MD, Harvey WJ: Correlation of neoplasms with incidence and localization of skeletal metastases: An analysis of 1,355 diphosphonate bone scans. J Nucl Med 16:986-989, 1975.
7. Clain A: Secondary malignant disease of bone. Br J Cancer 19:15-29, 1965.
8. Tubiana-Hulin M: Incidence, prevalence and distribution of bone metastases. Bone 12:S9-S10, 1991.
9. Morgan JWM, Adcock LA, Donohue RE: Distribution of skeletal metastases in prostatic and lung cancer. Urology 36:31-34, 1990.
10. Wilson MA, Calhoun FW: The distribution of skeletal metastases in breast and pulmonary cancer: concise communication. J Nucl Med 22:594-597, 1981.
11. Harrington KD: Mechanisms of metastases. *In* Harrington KD (ed): Orthopedic Management of Metastatic Bone Disease. St. Louis, CV Mosby, 1988, pp 19-30.
12. Cumming JD: A study of blood flow through bone marrow by a method of venous effluent collection. J Physiol 162:13, 1962.
13. Weiss L: Dynamic aspects of cancer cell populations in metastases. Am J Pathol 97:601, 1979.
14. Springfield DS: Mechanisms of metastases. Clin Orthop 169:15, 1982.
15. Garrett RI: Bone destruction in cancer. Semin Oncol 20:4-9, 1993.
16. Houston SJ, Rubens RD: The systemic treatment of bone metastases. Clin Orthop 312:95-104, 1995.
17. Galasko CSB: Skeletal metastases and mammary cancer. Ann R Coll Surg Engl 50:3-28, 1972.
18. Cuschieri A, Jarvie R, Taylor WH, et al: Three centre study on urinary hydroxyproline excretion in cancer of the breast. Br J Cancer 37:1002-1005, 1978.
19. Galasko CSB: The mechanism of uptake of bone-seeking isotopes by skeletal metastases. *In* Medical Radionuclide Imaging, Vol. 2. Vienna, International Atomic Energy Agency, 1977, pp 125-134.
20. Galasko CSB: The pathophysiological basis for skeletal scintigraphy. *In* Galasko CSB, Weber DA (eds): Radionuclide Scintigraphy in Orthopaedics. Edinburgh, Churchill Livingstone, 1984, pp 210-234.
21. Galasko CSB: Diagnosis of skeletal metastases and assessment of response to treatment. Clin Orthop 312:64-75, 1995.
22. Johnston AD: Pathology of metastatic tumors in bone. Clin Orthop 73:8, 1970.
23. Muindi J, Coombes RC, Golding S, et al: The role of computed tomography in the detection of bone metastases in breast cancer patients. Br J Radiol 56:233-236, 1983.
24. Daaffner RH, Lupetin AR, Dash N, et al: MRI in the detection of malignant infiltration of bone marrow. AJR Am J Roentgenol 146:353-358, 1986.
25. Hollis PH, Malis LI, Zappulla RA: Neurological deterioration after lumbar puncture below complete spinal subarachnoid block. J Neurosurg 64:253-256, 1986.
26. Bonner JA, Lichter AS: A caution about the use of MRI to diagnose spinal cord compression. N Engl J Med 322:556-557, 1990.
27. Lauenstein TC, Goehde SC, Herborn CU, et al: Whole-body MR imaging: evaluation of patients for metastases. Radiology 233:139-148, 2004.
28. Sapir EE, Metser UR, Flusser G, et al: Assessment of malignant skeletal disease: initial experience with ^{18}F-fluoride PET/CT and comparison between ^{18}F-fluoride PET/CT. J Nucl Med 45:272-278, 2004.
29. Yang SN, Liang JA, Lin FJ, et al: Comparing whole body (18)F-2-deoxyglucose positron emission tomography and technetium-99m methylene diphosphonate bone scan to detect bone metastases in patients with breast cancer. J Cancer Res Clin Oncol 128:325-328, 2002.
30. Duarte PS, Zhuang H, Castellucci P: The receiver operating characteristic curve for the standard uptake value in a group of patients with bone marrow metastasis. Mol Imaging Biol 4:157-160, 2002.
31. Gayed I, Vu T, Johnson M, et al: Comparison of bone and 2-deoxy-2[18F] fluoro-D-glucose positron emission tomography in the evaluation of bony metastases in lung cancer. Mol Imaging Biol 5:26-31, 2003.
32. Ohta M, Tokuda Y, Suzuki Y: Whole body PET for the evaluation of bony metastases in patients with breast cancer: comparison with 99 Tcm-MDP bone scintigraphy. Nucl Med Commun 22:875-879, 2001.

33. Hsia TC, Shen YY, Yen RF: Comparing whole body 18F-2-deoxyglucose positron emission tomography and technetium-99m methylene diophosphate bone scan to detect bone metastases in patients with non-small cell lung cancer. Neoplasma 49:267-271, 2002.
34. Hamaoka T, Madewell JE, Podoloff DA: Bone imaging in metastatic breast cancer. J Clin Oncol 22:2942-2953, 2004.
35. Cook GJ, Houston S, Rubens R, et al: Detection of bone metastases in breast cancer by 18FDG PET: differing metabolic activity in osteoblastic and osteolytic lesions. J Clin Oncol 16:3375-3379, 1998.
36. Hoh CK, Seltzer MA, Franklin J, et al: Positron emission tomography in urological oncology. J Urol 159:347-356, 1998.
37. Shreve PD, Grossman HB, Gross MD, et al: Metastatic prostate cancer: initial findings of PET with 2-deoxy-18-fluoro-D-glucose. Radiology 199:751-756, 1996.
38. Charron M, Beyer T, Bohnen N: Image analysis in patients with cancer studied with a combined PET and CT scanner. Clin Nucl Med 25:905-910, 2000.
39. Metser U, Lerman H, Blank A: Malignant involvement of the spine: assessment by 18F-FDG PET/CT. J Nucl Med 45:279-284, 2004.
40. Tong D, Gillick L, Hendrickson FR: The palliation of symptomatic osseous metastases: the results of the Radiation Therapy Oncology Group. Cancer 50:893, 1982.
41. Mogens K: The treatment and prognosis of patients with renal adenocarcinoma with solitary metastases: 10 year survival results. Int J Radiat Oncol Biol Phys 13:619-621, 1987.
42. Lote K, Walloe A, Bjersand A: Bone metastasis. Prognosis, diagnosis and treatment. Acta Radiol Oncol 25:227-232, 1986.
43. Mouridsen H, Gershanovich M, Sun Y, et al: Superior efficacy of letrozole versus Tamoxifen at first-line women with advanced breast cancer: results of phase III Letrozole Breast Cancer Group. J Clin Oncol 19:3302, 2001.
44. Nabholtz JM, Bonneterre J, Buzdar A et al: Anastrozole (Arimidex) versus Tamoxifen as first-line therapy for advanced breast cancer in postmenopausal women: survival analysis and updated safety results. Eur J Cancer 39:1684-1689, 2003.
45. Mouridsen H, Gershanovich M: The role of aromatase inhibitors in the treatment of metastatic breast cancer. Semin Oncol 30(Suppl 14):33-45, 2003 .
46. Milla-Santos A, Milla L, Portella J, et al: Anastrozole versus Tamoxifen as first-line therapy in postmenopausal patients with hormone-dependent advanced breast cancer: a prospective, randomized, phase III study. Am J Clin Oncol 26:317-322, 2003.
47. Goss PE, Strasser K: Tamoxifen resistant and refractory breast cancer: the value of aromatase inhibitors. Drugs 62:957-966, 2002.
48. Gershanovich M, Chaudri HA, Campos D, et al: Letrozole, a new oral aromatase inhibitor: randomized trial comparing 2.5 mg daily, 0.5 mg daily and aminoglutethimide in postmenopausal women with advanced breast cancer. Letrozole International Trial Group (AR/BC3). Ann Oncol 9:639-645, 1998.
49. Dombernowsky P, Smith I, Falkson G, et al: Letrozole, a new oral aromatase inhibitor for advanced breast cancer: double-blind randomized trial showing a dose effect and improved efficacy and tolerability compared with megestrol acetate. J Clin Oncol 16:453-461, 1998.
50. Buzdar A, Douma J, Davidson, et al: Phase III, multicenter, double-blind, randomized study of letrozole, an aromatase inhibitor, for advanced breast cancer versus megestrol acetate. J Clin Oncol 19:3357-3366, 2001.
51. Buzdar AU, Jonat W, Howell A, et al: Anastrozole versus megestrol acetate in the treatment of postmenopausal women with advanced breast carcinoma: results of a survival update based on a combined group analysis of data from two mature phase III trials. Arimidex Study Group. Cancer 83:1142-1152, 1998.
52. Kaufmann M, Bajetta E, Dirix LY, et al: Exemestane is superior to megestrol acetate after Tamoxifen failure in postmenopausal women with advanced breast cancer: results of a phase III randomized double-blind trial. The Exemestane Study Group. J Clin Oncol 18:1399-1411, 2000.
53. Soloway MS: Newer methods of hormonal therapy for prostate cancer. Urology 5(Suppl):30-38, 1984.
54. Crawford ED, Eisenberger MA, McLeod DG, et al: A controlled trial of leuprolide with and without flutamide in prostatic carcinoma. N Engl J Med 321:419-424, 1989.
55. Denis LJ, Whelan P, Carneiro de Moura JL, et al: Goserelin acetate and flutamide versus bilateral orchidectomy: a phase III EORTC trial (30853). Urology 42:119-130, 1993.
56. Tyrrell CJ, Kaisary AV, Iversen P. A randomized comparison of Casodes bicalutamide 150 mg monotherapy versus castration in the treatment of metastatic and locally advanced prostate cancer. Eur Urol 33:447-456, 1998.
57. Mahler C, Denis L: Management of relapsing disease in prostate cancer. Cancer 70S:329-334, 1992.
58. Press MF, Jones LA, Godolphin W, et al: HER-2/neu oncogene amplification and expression in breast and ovarian cancers. Prog Clin Biol Res 354A:209-221, 1990.
59. Vogel CL, Cobleigh MA, Tripathy D, et al: Efficacy and safety of trastuzumab as a single agent in first-line treatment of HER-2-overexpressing metastatic breast cancer. J Clin Oncol 20:719-726, 2002.
60. Tedesco KL, Thor AD, Johnson DH, et al: Docetaxel combined with trastuzumab is an active regimen in HER-2 3+ over expressing and fluorescent in situ hybridization-positive metastatic breast cancer: a multi-institutional phase II trial. J Clin Oncol 22:1071-1077, 2004.
61. Hortobagyi GN, Overview of treatment results with Trastuzumab (Hepceptin) in metastatic breast cancer. Semin 28(Suppl 18):43-47, 2001.
62. Cobleigh MA, Vogel CL, Tripathy D, et al: Efficacy and safety of Herceptin (humanized anti HER/2 antibody) as a single agent in 222 women with HER 2 overexpression who relapsed following chemotherapy for metastatic breast cancer [abstract]. Proc Am Soc Clin Oncol 17:97a, 1998.
63. Whitehouse JMA: Site-dependent response to chemotherapy for carcinoma of the breast. J R Soc Med 9(Suppl):18-22, 1985.
64. Medical Research Council: Report on the second myelomatosis trial after 5 years of follow up. Br J Cancer 42:823, 1980.
65. Burckhardt P, Thiebaud D, Perey L, et al: Treatment of tumor induced osteolysis by APD. Recent Results Cancer Res 116:54-66, 1989.
66. Coleman RE, Whitaker KD, Moss DW, et al: 3-Amino-1,1 hydroxypropylidene bisphosphonate (APD) for the treatment of bone metastases from breast cancer. Br J Cancer 58:621-625, 1988.
67. Lipton A, Glover D, Harvey H, et al: Pamidronate in the treatment of bone metastases: results of 2 dose-ranging trials in patients with breast or prostate cancer. Ann Oncol 5(Suppl 7):S31-S35, 1994.
68. Morton AR, Cantrill JA, Pillai GV, et al: Sclerosis of lytic bone metastases after disodium aminohydroxypropylidene bisphosphonate (APD) in patients with breast cancer. BMJ 297:772-773, 1988.
69. Berenson JR, Rosen LS, Howell A, et al: Zoledronic acid reduces skeletal-related events in patients. Cancer 91:1191-1200, 2001.
70. Rosen LS, Gordon D, Kaminski M: Zoledronic acid versus pamidronate in the treatment of skeletal metastases in patients with breast cancer or osteolytic lesions of multiple myeloma: a phase III, double-blind, comparative trial. Cancer J 7:3377-3387, 2001.
71. Hillner E, Rowan I, et al: American Society of Clinical Oncology 2003 update on the role of bisphosphonates and bone health issues in women with breast cancer. J Clin Oncol 21:4042-4057, 2003.
72. Pavlakis N, Stockler M: Bisphosphonates for breast cancer. Cochrane Database Syst Rev CD003474, 2002.
73. Saad F, Gleason DM, Murray R: A randomized, placebo-controlled trial of zoledronic acid in patients with hormone-refractory metastatic. J Natl Cancer Inst 96:879-882, 2004.
74. Zoledronic Acid Lung Cancer and Other Solid Tumors Study Group: Zoledronic acid versus placebo in the treatment of skeletal metastases in patients with lung cancer and other solid tumors: phase III, double-blind, randomized trial. J Clin Oncol 21:3150-3157, 2003.

75. Ruggiero SL, Mebrotra B, Tracey J, et al: Osteonecrosis of the jaws associated with the use of bisphosphonates: a review of 63 cases. J Oral Maxillofac Surg 62:527-534, 2004.
76. Dearnaley DP, Sydes MR, Mason MD, et al: A double-blind, placebo-controlled, randomized trial of oral sodium clodronate for metastatic prostate cancer (MRC PR05 Trial). J Natl Cancer Inst 95:1300-1311, 2003.
77. Diel IJ, Solomayer EF, Costa SD, et al: Reduction in new metastases in breast cancer with adjuvant clodronate treatment. N Engl J Med 339:357-363, 1998.
78. Bonica JJ: The Management of Pain, 2nd ed. Philadelphia, Lea & Febiger, 1990.
79. Levy MH: Pharmacologic treatment of cancer pain. N Engl J Med 335:1124-1132, 1996.
80. Twycross RG: Management of pain in skeletal metastases. Clin Orthop 312:187-196, 1995.
81. Harrington KD: Prophylactic management of impending fractures. *In* Harrington KD (ed): Orthopaedic Management of Metastatic Bone Disease. St Louis, CV Mosby, 1988, pp 283-307.
82. Pugh J, Sherry HS, Futterman B, et al: Biomechanics of pathological fractures. Clin Orthop 169:109, 1982.
83. Healey JH: Metastatic cancer to the bone. *In* DeVitta VT, Hellman S, Rosenberg SA (eds): Cancer: Principles and Practice of Oncology, 5th ed. Philadelphia, Lippincott-Raven, 1997, pp 2570-2583.
84. Hipp JA, Katz G, Hayes WC: Local demineralization as a model for bone strength reductions in lytic transcortical metastatic lesions. Invest Radiol 26:934, 1991.
85. Fidler M: Prophylactic internal fixation of secondary neoplastic deposits in long bones. BMJ 1:341, 1973.
86. Keene JS, Sellinger DS, McBeath AA, Engber WD: Metastatic breast cancer in the femur: a search for the lesion at risk of fracture. Clin Orthop 203:282, 1986.
87. Mirels H: Metastatic disease in long bones: a proposed scoring system. Clin Orthop 249:256, 1989.
88. Hipp JA, Springfield DS, Hayes WC: Predicting pathological fracture risk in the management of metastatic bone defects. Clin Orthop 312:120-135, 1995.
89. Harrington KD: Management of lower extremity metastases. *In* Harrington KD (ed): Orthopaedic Management of Metastatic Bone Disease. St Louis, CV Mosby, 1988, pp 141-214.
90. Harrington KD: Metastatic disease of the spine. *In* Harrington KD (ed): Orthopaedic Management of Metastatic Bone Disease. St Louis, CV Mosby, 1988, pp 309-383.
91. Wenger M: Vertebroplasty for metastasis. Med Oncol 20-29, 2003.
92. Hoskin PJ: Scientific and clinical aspects of radiotherapy in the relief of bone pain. Cancer Surv 7:69, 1988.
93. Blitzer PH: Reanalysis of the RTOG study of the palliation of symptomatic osseous metastasis. Cancer 55:1468-1472, 1985.
94. Orton CG, Ellis F: A simplification in the use of the NSD concept in practical radiotherapy. Br J Radiol 46:529-537, 1973.
95. Price P, Hoskin PJ, Easton D, et al: Prospective randomized trial of single and multifraction radiotherapy schedules in the treatment of painful bony metastases. Radiother Oncol 6:247-255, 1986.
96. Hoskin PJ, Price P, Easton D, et al: A prospective randomized trial of 4 Gy or 8 Gy single doses in the treatment of metastatic bone pain. Radiother Oncol 23:74-78, 1992.
97. Nielsen OS, Bentzen SM, Sandberg E, et al: Randomized trial of single dose versus fractionated palliative radiotherapy of bone metastases. Radiother Oncol 47:233-240, 1998.
98. Wu JSY, Wong R, Johnston M, et al: Meta-analysis of dose-fractionation radiotherapy trials for the palliation of painful metastases. Int J Radiat Oncol Biol Phys 55:594-605, 2003.
99. Van der Linden YM, Steenland E, Martijn H, et al: Single fraction radiotherapy is efficacious: a further analysis of the Dutch Bone Metastasis Study controlling for the influence of retreatment. Int J Radiat Oncol Biol Phys 59:528-537, 2004.
100. Poulter CA, Cosmatos D, Rubin P, et al: A report of RTOG 8206: a phase III study of whether the addition of single dose hemibody irradiation to standard fractionated local field irradiation is more effective than local field irradiation alone in the treatment of symptomatic osseous metastases. Int J Radiat Oncol Biol Phys 23:207-214, 1992.
101. Pecher C: Biological investigations with radioactive calcium and strontium: preliminary report on the use of radioactive strontium in treatment of metastatic bone cancer. Univ Calif Publ Pharmacol 11:117-149, 1942.
102. Silberstein EB: The treatment of painful osseous metastases with phosphorus-32 labeled phosphates. Semin Oncol 20(Suppl 2):10-21, 1993.
103. Landaw SA: Acute leukemia in polycythemia vera. Semin Hematol 23:156-165, 1986.
104. Blake GM, Zivanovic MA, McEwan AJ, et al: Sr 89 therapy: strontium kinetics in disseminated carcinoma of the prostate. Eur J Nucl Med 12:447-454, 1986.
105. Breen SL, Powe JE, Porter AT: Dose estimation in strontium 89 radiotherapy of metastatic prostatic carcinoma. J Nucl Med 33:1316-1323, 1992.
106. Ben-Josef E, Lucas RD, Vasan S, Porter AT: Selective accumulation of strontium 89 in metastatic deposits in bone: radio-histological correlation. Nucl Med Commun 16:457-463, 1995.
107. Blake GM, Zivanovic MA, Blaquiere RM, et al: Strontium 89 therapy: measurement of absorbed dose to skeletal metastases. J Nucl Med 29:549-557, 1988.
108. Ben-Josef E, Maughan RL, Vasan S, Porter AT: A direct measurement of ^{89}Sr activity in bone metastases. Nucl Med Commun 16:452-456, 1995.
109. Tennvall J, Darte L, Lindgren R, El Hassan AM: Palliation of multiple bony metastases from prostatic carcinoma with strontium 89. Acta Oncol 27:365-369, 1988.
110. Silberstein EB, Williams C: Strontium 89 therapy for the pain of osseous metastases. J Nucl Med 26:345-348, 1985.
111. Laing AH, Ackery DM, Bayly RJ, et al: Strontium 89 chloride for pain palliation in prostatic skeletal malignancy. Br J Radiol 64:816-822, 1981.
112. Robinson RG, Spicer JA, Preston DF, et al: Treatment of metastatic bone pain with strontium 89. Nucl Med Biol 14:219-222, 1987.
113. Correns HJ, Mebel M, Buchali K, et al: Strontium 89 therapy of bone metastases of carcinoma of the prostate gland. Eur J Nucl Med 4:33-35, 1979.
114. Firusian N, Mellin P, Schmidt CG: Results of strontium 89 therapy in patients with carcinoma of the prostate and incurable pain from bone metastases: a preliminary report. J Urol 116:764-798, 1976.
115. Lewington VJ, McEwan AJ, Ackery DM, et al: A prospective randomized double-blind crossover study to examine the efficacy of strontium 89 in pain palliation in patients with advanced prostate cancer metastatic to bone. Eur J Cancer 27:954-958, 1991.
116. Porter AT, McEwan AJB, Powe JE, et al: Results of a randomized phase-III trial to evaluate the efficacy of strontium 89 adjuvant to local field external beam irradiation in the management of endocrine resistant metastatic prostate cancer. Int J Radiat Oncol Biol Phys 25:805-813, 1993.
117. Quilty PM, Kirk D, Bolger JJ, et al: A comparison of the palliative effects of strontium 89 and external beam radiotherapy in metastatic prostate cancer. Radiother Oncol 31:33-40, 1994.
118. Bayouth JE, Macey DJ, Kasi LP, Fossella FV: Dosimetry and toxicity of samarium-153-EDTMP administered for bone pain due to skeletal metastases. J Nucl Med 35:63-69, 1994.
119. Eary JF, Collins C, Stabin M, et al: Samarium-153-EDTMP biodistribution and dosimetry estimation. J Nucl Med 34:1031-1036, 1993.
120. Collins C, Eary JF, Donaldson G, et al: Samarium-153-EDTMP in bone metastases of hormone refractory prostate carcinoma: a phase I/II trial. J Nucl Med 34:1839-1844, 1993.
121. Maxon HR, Schroder LE, Thomas SR, et al: Re-186(Sn) HEDP for treatment of painful osseous metastases: initial clinical experience in 20 patients with hormone-resistant prostate cancer. Radiology 176:155-159, 1990.
122. Maxon HR, Thomas SR, Hertzberg VA, et al: Rhenium 186 hydroxyethylidene diphosphonate for the treatment of painful osseous metastases. Semin Nucl Med 22:33-40, 1992.
123. Maxon HR, Schroder LE, Hertzberg VA, et al: Re-186(Sn) HEDP for treatment of painful osseous metastases: results of a double-blind crossover comparison with placebo. J Nucl Med 32:1877-1881, 1991.

124. Turner S, Marosszeky B, Timms I, Boyages J: Malignant spinal cord compression: a prospective evaluation. Int J Radiat Oncol Biol Phys 26:141-146, 1993.
125. Gilbert RN, Kim JH, Posner JB: Epidural spinal cord compression from metastatic tumors: diagnosis and treatment. Ann Neurol 3:40-51, 1978.
126. Graus F, Krol G, Foley K: Early diagnosis of spinal epidural metastases: correlation with clinical and radiological findings. Proc ASCO 4:269, 1985.
127. Han JS, Benson JE, Yoon YS: Magnetic resonance imaging in the spinal column and craniovertebral junction. Radiol Clin North Am 22:805-827, 1984.
128. Modic MT, Weinstein MA, Pavlicek W, et al: Nuclear magnetic resonance imaging of the spine. Radiology 148:757-762, 1983.
129. Paushter DM, Modic MT: Magnetic resonance imaging of the spine. Appl Radiol 13:61-68, 1984.
130. Young RF, Post EM, King GA: Treatment of spinal epidural metastases. Randomized prospective comparison of laminectomy and radiotherapy. J Neurosurg 53:741, 1980.
131. Zelefsky MJ, Scher HI, Knol G, et al: Spinal epidural tumor in patients with prostate cancer: clinical and radiologic predictors of response to radiation therapy. Cancer 70:2319-2325, 1992.
132. Patchell RA: The management of brain metastases. Cancer Treat Rev 29:533-540, 2003.
133. Hwang T, Close TP, Grego JM, et al: Predilection of brain metastasis in gray and white matter junction and vascular border zones. Cancer 77:1551-1555, 1996.
134. Delattre JY, Krol G, Thaler HT, et al: Distribution of brain metastases. Arch Neurol 45:741-744, 1988.
135. Patchell RA, Tibbs PA, Walsh JW, et al: A randomized trial of surgery in the treatment of single metastases to the brain. N Engl J Med 322:494-500, 1990.
136. El Kamar FG, Posner JB: Brain metastases. Semin Neurol 24:347-362, 2004.
137. Gaspar L, Scott C, Rotman M, Asbell S, et al. Recursive partitioning analysis (RPA) of prognostic factors in three Radiation Oncology Group (RTOG) brain metastases trials. Int J Radiat Oncol Biol Phys 37:745-751, 1997.
138. Borgelt B, Gelber R, Kramer S, et al: The palliation of brain metastases: final results of the first two studies by the Radiation Oncology Group. Int J Radiat Oncol Biol Phys 6:1-9, 1980.
139. Patchell RA, Tibbs PA, Walsh JW, et al: A randomized trial of surgery in the treatment of single metastases to the brain. N Engl J Med 322:494-500, 1990.
140. Vecht CJ, Haaxma-Reiche H, Noordijk EM, et al: Treatment of single brain metastasis: radiotherapy alone or combined with neurosurgery. Ann Neurol 33:583-590, 1993.
141. Mintz AH, Kestle J, Rathbone MP: A randomized trial to assess the efficacy of surgery in addition to radiotherapy in patients with a single cerebral metastasis. Cancer 78:1470-1476, 1996.
142. Andrews DW, Scott CB, Sperduto PW, et al: Whole brain radiation therapy with or without stereotactic radiosurgery boost for patients with one to three brain metastases: a phase III results of the RTOG 9805 randomised trial. Lancet 363:1665-1672, 2004.
143. Jemal A, Murray T, Ward E, et al: Cancer statistics, 2005. Cancer J Clin 55:10-30, 2005.
144. Adam R, Vinet E: Regional treatment of metastasis: surgery of colorectal liver metastases. Ann Oncol 15(Suppl 14):103-106, 2004.
145. Simmonds PC: Palliative chemotherapy for advanced colorectal cancer: systematic review and meta-analysis. Colorectal Cancer Collaborative Group. BMJ 321:531-535, 2000.
146. Nordic Gastrointestinal Tumor Adjuvant Therapy Group: Expectancy or primary chemotherapy in patients with advanced asymptomatic colorectal cancer: a randomized trial. J Clin Oncol 10:904-911, 1992.
147. Saltz LB, Cox JV, Blanke C, et al: Irinotecan plus fluorouracil and leucovorin for metastatic colorectal cancer. N Engl J Med 343:905-914, 2000.
148. Tournigand C, Andre T, Achille E, et al: FOLFIRI followed by FOLFOX6 or the reverse sequence in advanced colorectal cancer: a randomized GERCOR study. J Clin Oncol 22:229-237, 2004.
149. Goldbert RM, Sargent DJ, Morton RF, et al: A randomized controlled trial of fluorouracil plus leucovorin, irinotecan, and oxaliplatin combinations in patients with previously untreated metastatic colorectal cancer. J Clin Oncol 22:23-30, 2004.
150. Venook AP: Colorectal metastases confined to the liver: a unique opportunity? Semin Oncol 30(Suppl 15):34-39, 2003.
151. Fong Y, Cohen AM, Fortner JG, et al: Liver resection for colorectal metastases. J Clin Oncol 15:938-946, 1997.
152. Chan R, Kerr DJ: Hepatic arterial chemotherapy for colorectal cancer liver metastases: a review of advances in 2003. Curr Opin Oncol 16:378-384, 2004.
153. Kerr DJ, McArdle CS, Ledermann J, et al: Intravenous arterial versus intravenous fluorouracil and folinic acid for colorectal cancer liver metastases: a multicenter randomized trial. Lancet 361:368-373, 2003.
154. Kemeny NE, Niedzwiecki D, Hollis DR, et al: Hepatic arterial infusion versus systemic therapy for hepatic metastases from colorectal cancer: a CALGB randomized trial of efficacy, quality of life, cost effectiveness and molecular markers. Proc Am Soc Clin Oncol 22:252a, 2003.
155. Borgelt BB, Gelber R, Brady LW, et al: The palliation of hepatic metastases: results of the Radiation Therapy Oncology Group pilot study. Int J Radiat Oncol Biol Phys 7:587-591, 1981.
156. Robertson JM, McGinn CJ, Walker S, et al: A phase I trial of hepatic arterial bromodeoxyuridine and conformal radiation therapy for patients with primary hepatobiliary cancers or colorectal liver metastases. Int J Radiat Oncol Biol Phys 39:1087-1092, 1997.
157. Salem CL, Dritschilo A: Radiation ablation of liver metastases: HDR-IORT with or without EBRT. *In* Gunderson LL, et al (eds): Intraoperative Irradiation: Techniques and Results. Totowa, NJ, Humana, 1999, pp 315-328.
158. Gray B, Van Hazel G, Hope M, et al: Randomised trial of SIR-spheres plus chemotherapy versus chemotherapy alone for treating patients with liver metastases from primary large bowel cancer. Ann Oncol 12:1711-1720, 2001.
159. Bathe OF, Kaklamanos IG, Moffat FL, et al: Metastasectomy as a cytoreductive strategy for treatment of isolated pulmonary and hepatic metastases from breast cancer. Surg Oncol 8:35-42, 1999.
160. Okawa T, Kita M, Goto M, et al: Randomized prospective clinical study of small, large and twice-a-day fraction radiotherapy for painful bone metastases. Radiother Oncol 13:99-104, 1988.
161. Madsen EL: Painful bone metastases: Efficacy of radiotherapy assessed by the patients: A radomized trial comparing 4 Gy × 6 versus 10 Gy × 2. Int J Radiat Oncol Biol Phys 9:1775-1779, 1983.
162. Fitzpatrick PJ: Wide-field irradiation of bone metastases. In Weiss L, Gilbert HA (eds): Bone Metastases. Boston, GK Hall, 1981, pp 83-113.
163. Rowland CG, Bullimore JA, Smith PJB, Roberts JBM: Half body irradiation in the treatment of metastatic prostatic carcinoma. Br J Urol 53:628-629, 1981.
164. Qasim MM: Half body irradiation in the treatment of metastatic carcinomas. Clin Radiol 32:215-219, 1981.
165. Salazar OM, Rubin P, Hendrikson FR, et al: Single-dose half-body irradiation for palliation of multiple bone metastases from solid tumors: Final Radiation Therapy Oncology Group report. Cancer 58:29, 1986.
166. Wilkins MF, Keen CW: Hemibody radiotherapy in the management of metastatic carcinoma. Clin Radiol 38:267-268, 1987.
167. Ahonen A, Joensuu H, Hiltunen J, et al: Samarium-153-EDTMP in bone metastases. J Nucl Biol Med 38(4, Suppl 1):123-127, 1994.

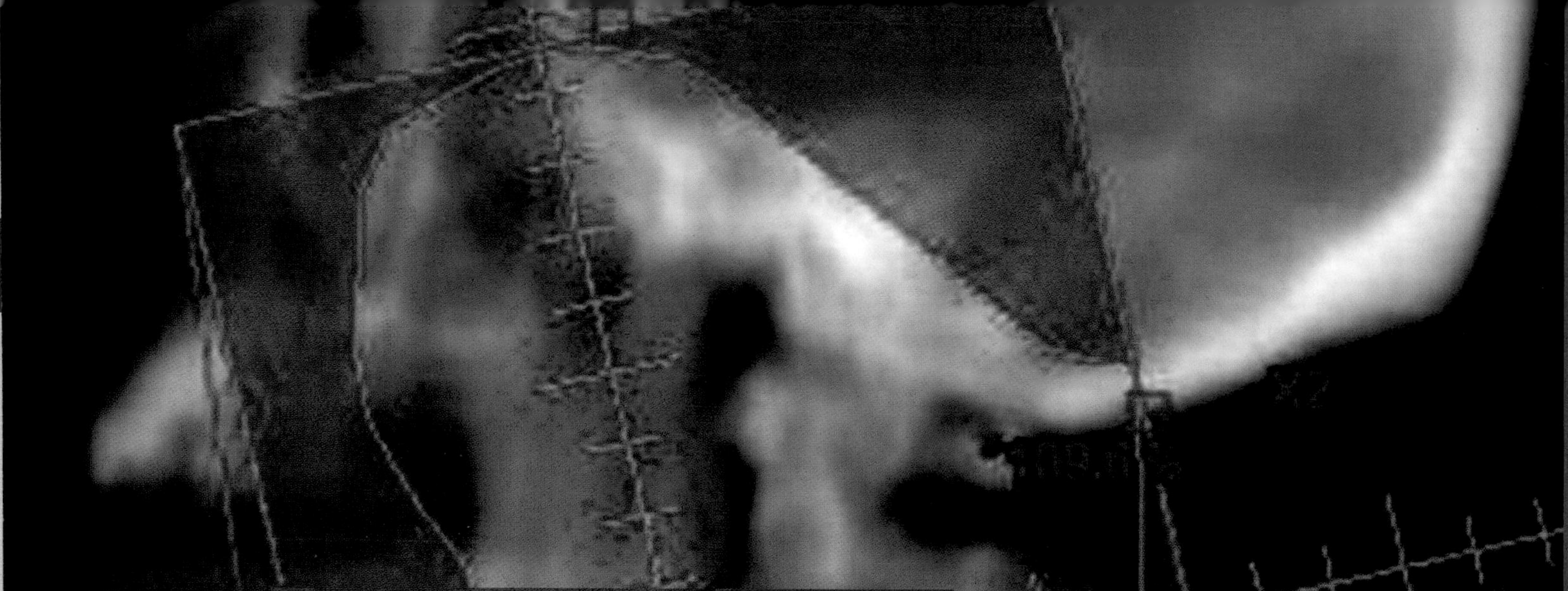

SECTION III

DISEASE SITES

This overview provides background information on the causes, incidence, heredity patterns, pathology, molecular genetics, clinical manifestations, patient evaluation, general principles of radiation therapy, and specific techniques of irradiation for primary central nervous system (CNS) tumors. Subsequent chapters focus on the multidisciplinary treatment of the more common primary CNS tumors, including low- and high-grade gliomas, ependymomas and meningiomas, ocular tumors, pituitary adenomas, and spinal cord tumors, as well as less common tumors (e.g., chemodectomas, chordomas, choroid plexus tumors, craniopharyngiomas, germ cell tumors, hemangioblastomas, hemangiopericytomas, pineal region tumors) and the radiotherapeutic modality of stereotactic radiosurgery for primary and metastatic CNS tumors.

ETIOLOGY, EPIDEMIOLOGY, AND HEREDITY

Etiology

The origin of primary CNS tumors is largely unknown. Numerous associations with brain tumors have been reported, including occupational and environmental exposures, lifestyle and dietary factors, medical conditions, and genetic factors, although cause-and-effect relationship has not been proved in most instances. Occupational and environmental exposures include chemicals (especially organic solvents), petrochemicals, synthetic rubber, formaldehyde, polyvinyl chloride, pesticides, herbicides, ionizing radiation, and electromagnetic fields. Lifestyle and dietary factors include cellular telephones, dietary *N*-nitroso compounds (nitrates and nitrosamines), cholesterol, higher social class, hair dyes and sprays, and smoking.

Medical conditions associated with brain tumors include drugs, viral and parasitic infections (e.g., toxoplasmosis), acquired immunodeficiency syndrome (AIDS) and immunosuppression, head injury, and other conditions. In general, the associations are strongest for gliomas, especially astrocytomas (i.e., polyvinyl chloride exposure), meningiomas (i.e., ionizing radiation), and lymphoma (i.e., AIDS or immunosuppression). In utero or postnatal exposure to environmental or dietary factors has been suggested as the cause of primary CNS tumors occurring in young children (i.e., birth to 9 years old).[1]

Some associations appear to protect from CNS tumors. These include vitamins A, C, and E and having allergies, asthma, and frequent colds.

Epidemiology

In 2006, an estimated 18,820 new cases of primary CNS tumors will be diagnosed in the United States, representing 1.4% of all new cancers.[2] The estimated number of related deaths was 12,820, or 2.2% of all cancer deaths. In children younger than 15 years, primary CNS tumors are the second most common cause of cancer death, with only leukemia being more common. The incidence and mortality rates from primary CNS tumors are higher for male than female patients by a ratio of 1.2:1.3. In male and female patients 15 to 34 years old, primary CNS tumors are the third and fourth most common causes of death, respectively. Racial differences in mortality have been observed.[3] Brain and other nervous system tumors are the ninth most common of cancer deaths among whites, but they are not among the 10 most common causes of cancer deaths in blacks.[4]

Heredity

Five percent or fewer of primary CNS tumors are hereditary, although a family history positive for cancer of any type is present in 20% to 30% of patients with brain tumors.[1] Certain hereditary syndromes have been associated with various common and uncommon primary CNS tumors. The best known of these is von Recklinghausen's disease, or neurofibromatosis type 1 (NF1), which is an autosomal dominant disorder. Patients with NF1 may have intracranial astrocytomas of all grades (World Health Organization [WHO] I to IV), particularly pilocytic astrocytomas (WHO I) of the optic pathways or cerebellum. Those with NF2, which is also an autosomal dominant disorder, may have schwannomas, particularly acoustic schwannomas, which are usually bilateral. Other primary CNS tumors in patients with NF2 include intracranial meningiomas and spinal cord astrocytomas or ependymomas, although intracranial astrocytomas (WHO I to IV) can occur. The *NF1* gene is located on chromosome 17, and the *NF2* gene is on chromosome 22. Both are tumor suppressor genes. Cerebellar, brainstem, and spinal cord hemangioblastomas occur in patients with the autosomal dominant disorder von Hippel–Lindau (VHL) disease, although hemangioblastomas may also arise sporadically. The tumor suppressor gene causing VHL syndrome is on chromosome 3. Subependymal giant cell astrocytomas occur only in patients with tuberous sclerosis (Bourneville's disease), an autosomal dominant trait with a high incidence of sporadic cases. The two genes responsible for tuberous sclerosis are located on chromosomes 9 and 16. Less common inherited syndromes in which primary CNS tumors occur include Li-Fraumeni, Cowden's, Turcot's, and nevoid basal cell carcinoma (Gorlin's) syndrome.[5]

PATHOLOGY

Tumors of the CNS, including those of the brain and spinal cord and their coverings, are a pathologically and biologically diverse group of neoplasms. Table A-1 shows the current WHO histologic classification of CNS tumors,[6] a classification that divides them by their putative embryonic tissue of origin. Table A-2 shows a breakdown of the incidence of the most common primary CNS tumors.[7] Although numerous types of CNS tumors occur, practically speaking, 82% are WHO grade II, III, and IV astrocytomas (i.e., astrocytomas, anaplastic astrocytomas, and glioblastomas) (Fig. A-1).[7,8] The next most common tumors, including pilocytic astrocytomas, oligodendrogliomas, mixed oligoastrocytomas, ependymomas, meningiomas, and medulloblastomas, together account for another 14% of primary CNS tumors (Fig. A-2),[7,8] leaving all the other pathologic types shown in Table A-1 to account for the remaining 4%.[7] Primary CNS tumors can also be classified based on their anatomic site of origin—supratentorial, infratentorial, sellar, parasellar, suprasellar, skull base, or spinal cord—and on their propensity to affect children or adults, or both, as shown in Table A-3.[6,8,9]

BIOLOGIC CHARACTERISTICS AND PROGNOSTIC FACTORS

The 5-year survival rates for patients with primary CNS tumors have increased over the past 3 decades, from 18% to 19% during 1960 to 1983 to 29% to 35% during 1986 to 1993. Survival in children younger than 15 years with primary CNS tumors has nearly doubled (from 35% to 61%) over a similar

Table A-1 **World Health Organization (WHO) Histologic Classification of Primary Central Nervous System Tumors**

Origin	Tumor Type	WHO Classification
Neuroepithelial	Astrocytic	Pilocytic astrocytoma (WHO I)
		Pleomorphic xanthoastrocytoma
		Subependymal giant cell astrocytoma (tuberous sclerosis)
		Astrocytoma (WHO II)
		Anaplastic (malignant) astrocytoma (WHO III)
		Glioblastoma (WHO IV)
	Oligodendroglial	Oligodendroglioma
		Anaplastic (malignant) oligodendroglioma
	Ependymal	Subependymoma
		Myxopapillary ependymoma
		Ependymoma
		Anaplastic (malignant) ependymoma
	Mixed glial	Oligoastrocytoma
		Anaplastic (malignant) oligoastrocytoma
	Choroid plexus	Choroid plexus papilloma
		Choroid plexus carcinoma
	Uncertain	Gliomatosis cerebri
	Neuronal/mixed neuronal-glial	Dysembryoplastic neuroepithelial tumor
		Ganglioglioma
		Anaplastic (malignant) ganglioglioma
		Central neurocytoma
		Olfactory neuroblastoma
	Pineal parenchymal	Pineocytoma
		Pineoblastoma
	Embryonal	Neuroblastoma
		Ependymoblastoma
		Primitive neuroectodermal tumor (PNET)
		Medulloblastoma
Cranial/spinal nerves		Schwannoma
		Neurofibroma
		Malignant schwannoma/anaplastic neurofibroma
Meninges	Meningothelial	Meningioma
		Atypical meningioma
		Papillary meningioma
		Anaplastic (malignant) meningioma
	Mesenchymal	Hemangioblastoma
Lymphoma		Malignant lymphoma
Germ cell		Germinoma
		Embryonal carcinoma
		Yolk sac (endodermal sinus) tumor
		Choriocarcinoma
		Teratoma
Sellar region		Pituitary adenoma
		Pituitary carcinoma
		Craniopharyngioma
Other		
Neuroendocrine		Paraganglioma (chemodectoma)
Notochord		Chordoma

Data from Kleihues P, Burger PC, Scheithauer BW: Histological Typing of Tumours of the Central Nervous System, 2nd ed. Berlin, Springer, 1993.

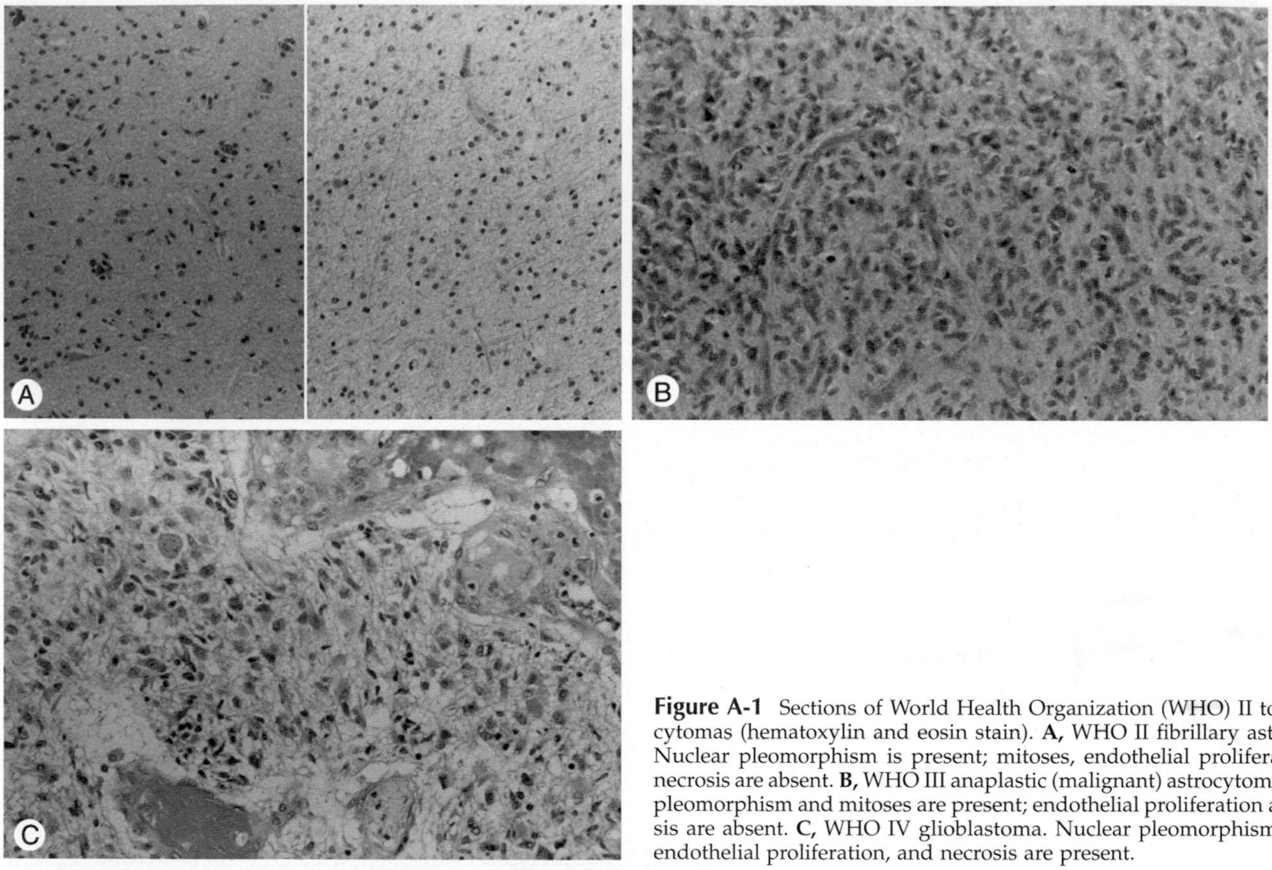

Figure A-1 Sections of World Health Organization (WHO) II to IV astrocytomas (hematoxylin and eosin stain). **A,** WHO II fibrillary astrocytoma. Nuclear pleomorphism is present; mitoses, endothelial proliferation, and necrosis are absent. **B,** WHO III anaplastic (malignant) astrocytoma. Nuclear pleomorphism and mitoses are present; endothelial proliferation and necrosis are absent. **C,** WHO IV glioblastoma. Nuclear pleomorphism, mitoses, endothelial proliferation, and necrosis are present.

Table A-2 **Incidence of Primary Central Nervous System Tumors Based on Survival, Epidemiology, and End Results (SEER) Data**

Pathologic Type	Frequency (%)
Pilocytic astrocytoma (WHO I)	1.4
Astrocytoma (WHO II)/ anaplastic astrocytoma (WHO III)*	41.9
Glioblastoma (WHO IV)	40.1
Oligodendroglioma	3.4
Oligoastrocytoma	1.6
Medulloblastoma	3.6
Ependymoma	3.0
Meningioma (malignant)	1.9

*Includes the fibrillary, protoplasmic, and gemistocytic astrocytoma subtypes, as well as glioma not otherwise specified.

WHO, World Health Organization.

Data from Polednak AP, Flannery JT: Brain, other central nervous system, and eye cancer. Cancer 75(Suppl 1):330-337, 1995.

period.[2] Tables A-4 and A-5 show overall survival data and survival as a function of age derived from the Survival, Epidemiology, and End Results (SEER) database for the more common types of primary CNS tumors. The SEER data exclude "benign" histologies such as meningiomas and pituitary adenomas, which have an approximate incidence of 18% and 3%, respectively.[10] Survival decreases with increasing patient age for all tumor types, except ependymoma, for which children and older adults have better survival than adults 21 to 64 years old.[11] The only other CNS tumors with which adults fare better than children are brainstem gliomas, which are universally fatal in children but not in adults.[12,13] The concept of conditional probability of survival (i.e., the probability of surviving to 5 years if a person has survived to 2 years after diagnosis) has been introduced. Table A-6 summarizes the 2-year and conditional survival probabilities for the more common types of primary CNS tumors.[14]

To assess the impact of various prognostic factors on survival in patients with malignant astrocytomas (i.e., anaplastic astrocytomas and glioblastomas), the Radiation Therapy Oncology Group (RTOG) performed recursive-partitioning analysis for a large group of patients. This effort resulted in six classes, each with a significantly different survival rate (Table A-7).[15] These data emphasize the importance of prognostic factors such as histology, patient age, and performance status on survival. Microarray analysis has revealed that the gene expression profile may be even a better prognostic factor than histologic classification.[16]

MOLECULAR GENETICS

An understanding of the molecular genetics of gliomas, such as those primary CNS tumors believed to arise from an astrocytic lineage, provides a framework for understanding how the accumulated genetic alterations lead to cellular transformation and result in the progression to a more malignant tumor (e.g., from astrocytoma to anaplastic astrocytoma or glioblastoma). However, the origin and the stimulus for further progression of primary brain tumors have been recently attributed to cancer stem cells.[17] The most common

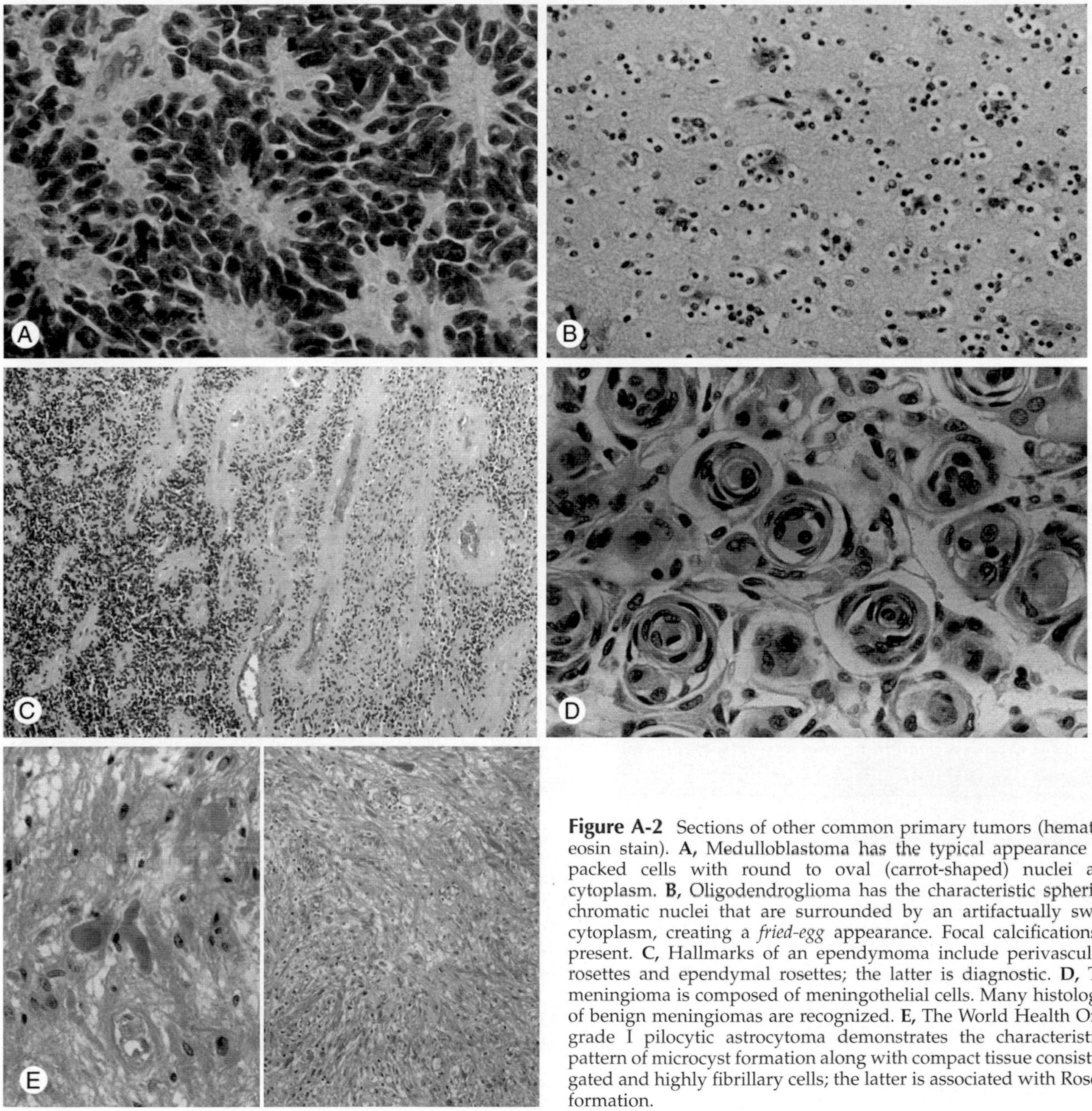

Figure A-2 Sections of other common primary tumors (hematoxylin and eosin stain). **A,** Medulloblastoma has the typical appearance of densely packed cells with round to oval (carrot-shaped) nuclei and scanty cytoplasm. **B,** Oligodendroglioma has the characteristic spherical, hyperchromatic nuclei that are surrounded by an artifactually swollen clear cytoplasm, creating a *fried-egg* appearance. Focal calcifications are often present. **C,** Hallmarks of an ependymoma include perivascular pseudorosettes and ependymal rosettes; the latter is diagnostic. **D,** The benign meningioma is composed of meningothelial cells. Many histologic variants of benign meningiomas are recognized. **E,** The World Health Organization grade I pilocytic astrocytoma demonstrates the characteristic biphasic pattern of microcyst formation along with compact tissue consisting of elongated and highly fibrillary cells; the latter is associated with Rosenthal fiber formation.

alteration is a chromosome 17 mutation, which is associated with the tumor suppressor gene *TP53,* and its gene product TP53, a multifunctional protein involved in the regulation of cell growth, cell death (i.e., apoptosis), and transcription.[18] Other chromosomes commonly involved include 10 (loss of heterozygosity [LOH]) and 19q (LOH), both of which are thought to contain tumor suppressor genes. Chromosome 10 is also thought to contain a gene that encodes for a protein tyrosine phosphatase called PTEN (formerly designated MMAC1), which is involved in tumor invasion and can be mutated in glioblastoma. The retinoblastoma gene *(RB1),* located on chromosome 13, and the *CDKN2A* gene (formerly designated *MTS1*), which encodes the CDKN2A protein (formerly designated p16), are thought to be important in the control of the cell cycle. Alterations to the *RB1* gene and CDKN2A protein occur in anaplastic astrocytoma and glioblastoma. The *MDM2* gene, located on chromosome 12, is amplified and its protein is overexpressed in glioblastoma, and it is thought to be involved in the malignant transformation process. Loss of expression of the so-called deleted in colorectal cancer gene *(DCC),* which is on chromosome 18, is also thought to be involved in malignant transformation. The involvement of epigenetic factors, such as DNA methylation, in the etiopathology of brain tumors and in their response to therapies has been documented.[19-21]

A more detailed analysis of the noncircumscribed or infiltrative tumors has uncovered different genetic profiles corresponding to different properties of cells residing in the solid tumor tissue core compared with the surrounding normal brain tissue infiltrated by isolated tumor cells.[22] The overexpression or amplification of certain growth factor genes, growth factors, and growth factor receptors has been observed

Table A-3 Common Anatomic Sites of Primary Central Nervous System Tumors

Anatomic Site	Pathologic Type: More Common Tumors	Less Common Tumors
Supratentorial (hemispheric)	Pilocytic astrocytoma (WHO I)* Astrocytoma (WHO II)† Anaplastic astrocytoma (WHO III)† Glioblastoma (WHO IV)‡ Oligodendroglioma† Oligoastrocytoma† Meningioma (meninges, tentorium)‡	Primitive neuroectodermal tumor* Pineocytoma/pineoblastoma (pineal region) Germ cell (pineal region)† Choroid plexus papilloma/carcinoma (third ventricle)*
Infratentorial	Astrocytoma (brainstem) (WHO II)† Pilocytic astrocytoma (cerebellum) (WHO I)* Medulloblastoma (cerebellum)* Ependymoma (fourth ventricle)†	Hemangioblastoma (cerebellum)‡
Sellar/parasellar/suprasellar	Pilocytic astrocytoma (optic pathway) (WHO I)* Astrocytoma (optic pathway) (WHO II)† Meningioma (cavernous sinus)‡	Pituitary adenoma† Germ cell tumors† Craniopharyngioma†
Skull base	Meningioma‡	Schwannoma (acoustic nerve)‡ Chordoma (clivus)‡
Spinal cord§	Pilocytic astrocytoma (WHO I)* Astrocytoma (WHO II)† Meningioma‡ Ependymoma†	Chordoma (sacrum)‡

*More common in children.
†Occur more commonly in both children and adults.
‡More common in adults.
§Together with schwannoma, the pathologic types shown account for more than 90% of primary spinal cord tumors.

Table A-4 Survival, Epidemiology, and End Results (SEER) Data from 1973 to 1991 for the More Common Types of Primary Central Nervous System Tumors

Pathologic Type	2-Year Survival (%)	5-Year Survival (%)
Glioblastoma	6	1
Astrocytoma*	46	34
Oligodendroglioma	81	65
Medulloblastoma	66	60
Ependymoma	83	60

*Includes astrocytoma (World Health Organization [WHO] II) and anaplastic astrocytoma (WHO III).

Data from Davis FG, Freels S, Grutsch J, et al: Survival rates in patients with primary malignant brain tumors stratified by patient age and tumor histological type: an analysis based on Surveillance, Epidemiology, and End Results (SEER) data, 1973-1991. J Neurosurg 88:1-10, 1998.

in WHO grade II to IV astrocytomas, including platelet-derived growth factor A (PDGFA), PDGFA receptor (PDGFRA), and the epidermal growth factor receptor *(EGFR)* gene, contributing to an unregulated cell growth.[23,24] The overexpression of plasma membrane receptors of unknown pathobiologic function, but suitable for molecular therapies, has been found in most patients with high-grade gliomas.[25] Figure A-3 summarizes the molecular genetic events occurring in the process of astrocytic malignant transformation. Table A-8 summarizes the chromosomal abnormalities observed in the other common types of primary CNS tumors.[5]

CLINICAL MANIFESTATIONS AND PATIENT EVALUATION

Signs and Symptoms

The signs and symptoms of primary CNS tumors are shown in Table A-9. They depend on their anatomic site of origin.[10]

Table A-5 Survival, Epidemiology, and End Results (SEER) Data as a Function of Age

	SEER Data, 1986-1991* 2-Year Survival (%)			5-Year Survival (%)		
Pathologic Type	*<20*	*21-64*	*>65*	*<20*	*21-64*	*>65*
Glioblastoma	31	13	6	21	4	2
Astrocytoma	78	39	7	72	26	2
Medulloblastoma	80	78	n/a	70	70	44
Oligodendroglioma	81	42	42	74	28	13
Ependymoma	64	82	54	43	70	42

*Or most recent period between 1973-1991 for which data is available.

Data from Davis FG, Freels S, Grutsch J, et al: Survival rates in patients with primary malignant brain tumors stratified by patient age and tumor histological type: an analysis based on Surveillance, Epidemiology, and End Results (SEER) data, 1973-1991. J Neurosurg 88:1-10, 1998.

Table A-6 Conditional Probability of Survival for the Common Types of Primary Central Nervous System Tumors Based on Survival, Epidemiology, and End Results (SEER) Data

	SEER DATA, 1979-1993	
Pathologic Type	*2-yr Survival (%)*	*Conditional Survival* (%)*
Pilocytic astrocytoma (WHO I)	90	96
Astrocytoma† (WHO II)	66	73
Anaplastic astrocytoma (WHO III)	45	68
Glioblastoma multiforme (WHO IV)	9	36
Medulloblastoma	70	80
Oligodendroglioma	79	79
Anaplastic oligodendroglioma	60	63
Ependymoma‡	80	83

*Given survival to 2 years, probability of surviving another 3 years.
†Also referred to as diffuse (fibrillary) astrocytoma
‡Includes anaplastic ependymoma.
WHO, World Health Organization.
Data from Davis FG, McCarthy BJ, Freels S, et al: The conditional probability of survival of patients with primary malignant brain tumors: surveillance, epidemiology and end results (SEER) data. Cancer 85:485-491, 1999.

Table A-7 The Six Radiation Therapy Oncology Group Recursive Partitioning Analysis Classes for Malignant Astrocytomas

		SURVIVAL	
RPA Class	Definition	*Median (mo)*	*2-Year (%)*
I	AA, age < 50, nl MS	58.6	76
II	AA, age ≥ 50, KPS ≥ 70, sx > 3 mo	37.4	68
III	GBM, age < 50, KPS 90-100	17.9	35
IV	GBM, age < 50, KPS < 90	11.1	15
V	GBM, age ≥ 50, KPS ≥ 70, mixed other PF	8.9	6
VI	GBM, age ≥ 50, KPS < 70, abnl MS	4.6	4

AA, anaplastic astrocytoma; abnl, abnormal; GBM, glioblastoma multiforme; KPS, Karnofsky performance status; MS, mental status; nl, normal; PF, prognostic factors; RPA, recursive partitioning analysis; sx, symptoms.
Data from Curran WJ, Scott CB, Horton J, et al: Recursive partitioning analysis of prognostic factors in three Radiation Therapy Oncology Group malignant glioma trials. J Natl Cancer Inst 85:704-710, 1993.

Table A-8 Molecular Genetic (Chromosomal) Abnormalities Observed in the Common Types of Central Nervous System Tumors

Pathologic Type	Chromosomal Abnormalities
Pilocytic astrocytoma (WHO I)	17q−
Oligodendroglioma	19q− and 1p−
Medulloblastoma	Isochromosome 17q, 17p−, *TP53* mutations
Ependymoma	22 abnormalities, 17p−
Meningioma	Allelic losses on 1p, 9q, 10q, 14q, 17p, and 22q (including the *NF2* gene)

Kleihues P, Burger PC, Scheithauer BW: Histological Typing of Tumours of the Central Nervous System, 2nd ed. Berlin, Springer, 1993.

Table A-9 Common Symptoms of Primary Central Nervous System Tumors

Aphasia (including dysphasia) (T)
Ataxia (including truncal and limb) (BS, CB)
Back pain (including neck pain) (SC)
Bowel/bladder continence problems (F, SC)
Deafness (BS, CPA, CN VIII)
Dementia (T)
Diplopia (BS, CS, CN III, IV, VI)
Dizziness (BS, CB, CPA, CN VIII)
Dysarthria (BS, CN IX/X)
Dysphagia (BS, CN IX/X)
Facial numbness (BS, CN VII, CPA)
Facial pain (BS, CS, CN VII)
Headache (G, 3/4V, HC)
Impotence (SC)
Memory impairment (T)
Nausea (G, CB, BS, 3/4V, HC)
Personality changes (including mood, mentation, concentration) (G, F, T)
Seizures (G)
Sensory changes (including numbness, tingling, paresthesias) (P, BS, SC)
Visual field deficits (including blindness) (T, P, S/PIT,* SS)
Vomiting (G, CB, BS, 3/4V, HC)
Weakness (F, BS, SC)

*Pituitary adenomas may also cause hormonal syndromes resulting from excess production of prolactin (amenorrhea, galactorrhea, impotence), growth hormone (acromegaly), ACTH (Cushing's syndrome), or thyroid-stimulating hormone (hyperthyroidism).
BS, brainstem; CB, cerebellum; CN, cranial nerve; CPA, cerebellopontine angle; CS, cavernous sinus; F, frontal lobe; G, general cerebral (including any intracranial location); HC, symptoms associated with hydrocephalus; P, parietal lobe; PIT, pituitary gland; S, sellar; SC, spinal cord; SS, suprasellar; T, temporal lobe; 3/4V, third or fourth ventricle.
Data from Levin VA, Gutin PH, Leibel S: Neoplasms of the central nervous system. *In* DeVita VT, Hellman S, Rosenberg SA (eds): Cancer: Principles and Practice of Oncology, 4th ed. Philadelphia, JB Lippincott, 1993, pp 1679-1737.

Patient Evaluation

Studies that image primary CNS tumors define the anatomic extent of these tumors and determine and guide surgery, radiation therapy, and chemotherapy. Computed tomography (CT), although less expensive than magnetic resonance imaging (MRI), gives less anatomic detail of the soft tissues, but it may be more useful in imaging bony structures, particularly the skull base (Fig. A-4). CT is also useful in planning radiation therapy, to facilitate image fusion with MRI scans, and to provide the bony anatomy necessary to generate digitally reconstructed radiographs that are used as simulator

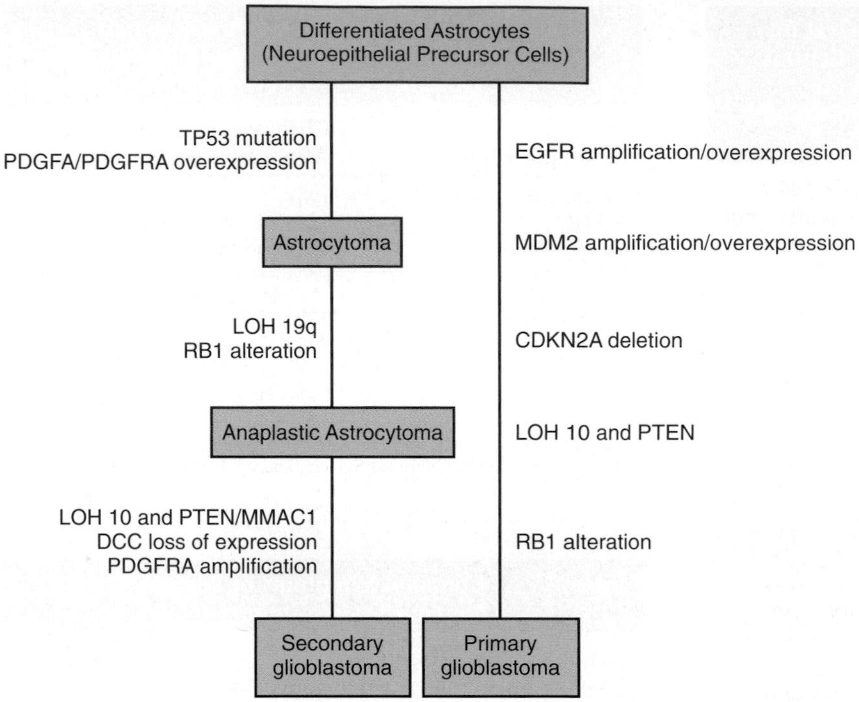

Figure A-3 Molecular genetic events occurring in the malignant transformation process of differentiated astrocytes (or neuroepithelial precursor cells) to astrocytoma, anaplastic astrocytoma, and glioblastoma or directly to glioblastoma. (Adapted from Kleihues P, Ohgaki H: Genetics of glioma progression and the definition of primary and secondary glioblastoma. Brain Pathol 7:1131-1136, 1997.)

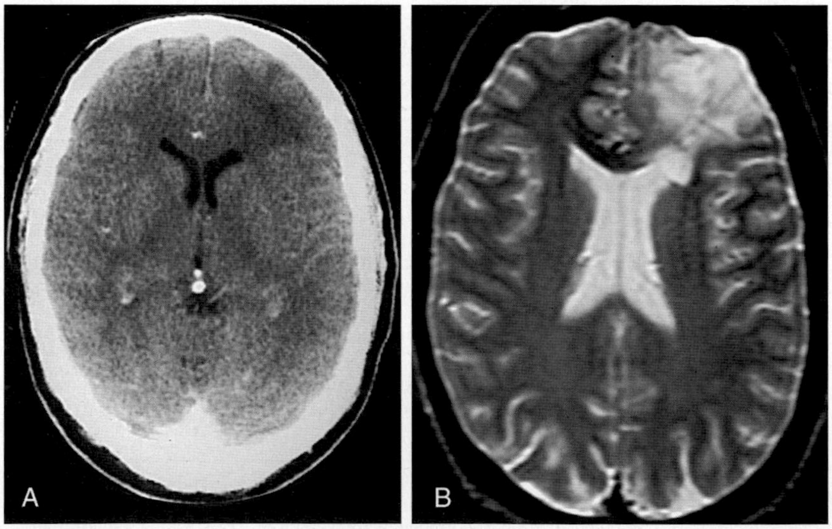

Figure A-4 Contrast-enhanced CT (**A**) and MRI (**B**) scans of a patient with a low-grade diffuse astrocytoma of the left frontal lobe.

films. As a baseline, almost without exception, patients with a brain or spinal cord tumor, or both, should undergo MRI with and without intravenous contrast (see Fig. A-4). CNS tumors rarely metastasize outside the CNS, but they may spread within it. For example, certain brain tumors, such as medulloblastomas, primitive neuroectodermal tumors, anaplastic ependymomas, choroid plexus carcinomas, pineoblastomas, germ cell tumors, and lymphomas, may involve the cerebrospinal fluid (CSF) and leptomeninges (i.e., the coverings) of the brain or spinal cord. Studies that stage or determine the anatomic extent of CNS involvement of these tumors include MRI of the brain and spine, CSF cytology, and myelography.

Other imaging studies, such as functional (diffusion/perfusion) MRI, MRI spectroscopy, positron emission tomography (PET), and single-photon emission tomography (SPECT), better reflect biologic or physiologic characteristics of primary CNS tumors, such as tumor metabolism, glucose use, and blood flow. These imaging techniques, useful for differentiating postirradiation tumor recurrence (Fig. A-5) from radiation necrosis (Fig. A-6), will play increasingly important roles in bioanatomic radiation therapy planning and delivery for patients with primary CNS tumors.[26]

CENTRAL NERVOUS SYSTEM TOLERANCE

Normal Tissue Tolerance

Radiation tolerance of any normal tissues, including those of the CNS, depends on a number of factors, including total dose, dose per fraction, total time, volume, host factors, radiation

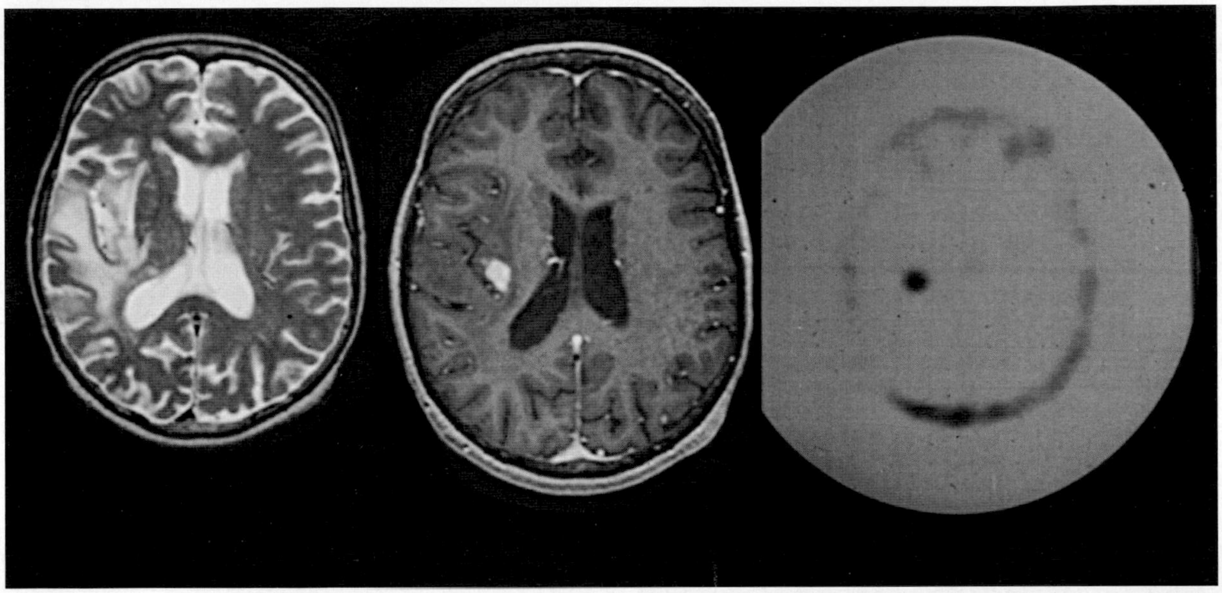

Figure A-5 MRI *(left, center)* and single photon emission CT *(right)* scans of a patient with a recurrent low-grade oligodendroglioma of the right temporal lobe.

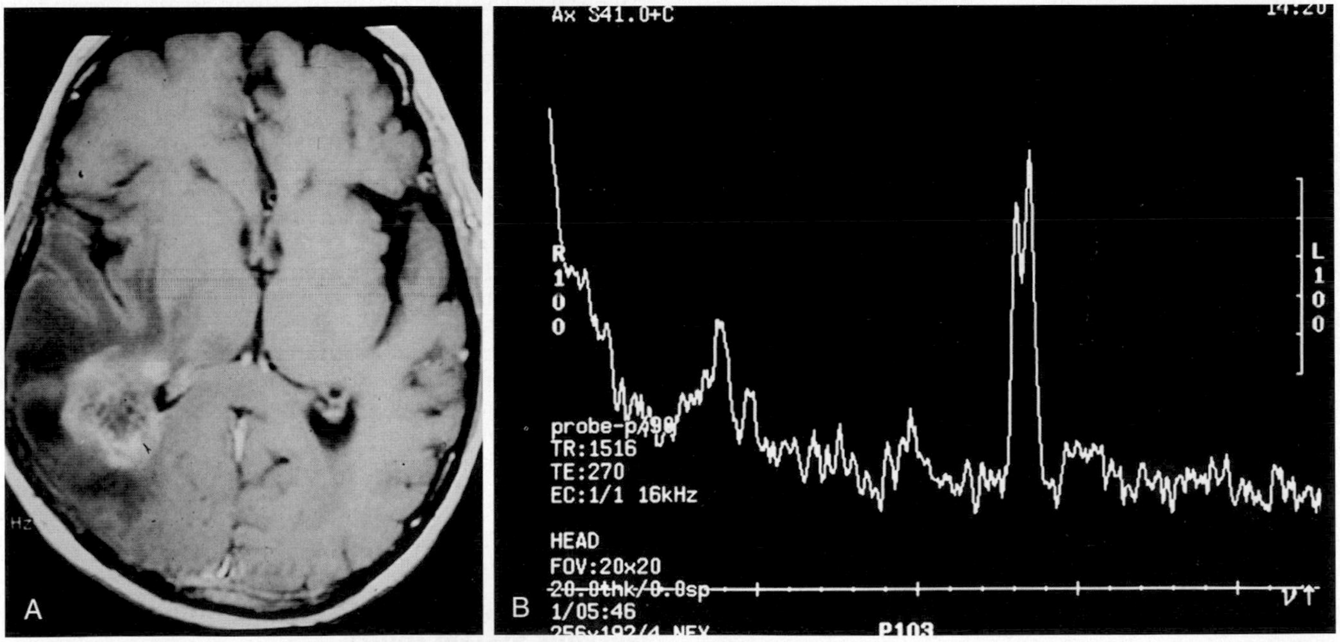

Figure A-6 **A,** MRI scan of a patient with radionecrosis of the right temporoparietal lobes. **B,** MRI spectroscopy shows a large lactate peak, with depressed choline, creatine, and *N*-acetyl-aspartate peaks.

quality (linear energy transfer), and adjunctive therapies. Table A-10 defines the role of these factors in radiation tolerance and injury to normal CNS tissues, as well as ways they may be modified to increase tolerance (i.e., reduce injury).[27,28]

Table A-11 shows partial- and whole-organ tolerance doses for the brain and spinal cord and includes doses predicted to result in a 5% and 50% probability of injury 5 years after treatment with irradiation ($TD_{5/5}$ and $TD_{50/5}$, respectively).[29,30] These values are derived from mathematical models of brain and spinal cord tolerance based on clinical data describing instances of radiation injury and the total doses and fraction sizes at which they occurred. None of the mathematical models accounts for the factors listed in Table A-10, nor do they adequately predict radiation tolerance or injury. The best of the models is that described by Sheline and associates,[27] which represents a modification of the Ellis nominal standard dose formula[31]:

$$\text{neuret} = (D)(N^{-0.41})(T^{-0.03})$$

In the equation, D is the total dose, N is the number of fractions, and T is time. Based on various models, the $TD_{5/5}$ for the whole brain is 50 ± 10 Gy; for part of the brain, it is 60 ± 10 Gy; and for a 10-cm segment of spinal cord, it is 45 to 50 Gy (see Table A-11). Although the $TD_{50/5}$ for spinal cord is

Table A-10 Factors Associated with Radiation Tolerance of the Normal Central Nervous System Tissues

Factor*	Factors for Increased Risk of Injury	Tolerance Increased by
Total dose	Higher total dose	Decreasing total dose, hyperfractionation,‡ radiosensitizers
Dose per fraction	Dose per fraction >180-200 cGy	Decreasing dose/fraction to ≤180-200 cGy
Volume	Increased volume (e.g., whole-organ radiation)	Decreasing volume (e.g., partial-organ radiation)
Host factors	Medical illness (e.g., hypertension, diabetes)	Unknown, possibly radioprotectors
Beam quality	High-LET radiation beams (e.g., neutrons)	Low-LET beams (e.g., photons)
Adjunctive therapy	Concomitant use of CNS toxic drugs (e.g., methotrexate)	Avoid concomitant use of CNS toxic drugs or use sequentially

*Total time is not a major determinant of normal CNS tissue tolerance.

‡Defined as multiple daily fractions, usually two with doses per fraction of ≤180 to 200 cGy, usually 100 to 120 cGy, separated by 4 to 8 hours, to total doses higher than those given with standard fractionation.

CNS, central nervous system; LET, linear energy transfer.

Some data from Schueltheiss TE, Kun LE, Ang KK, Stephens LC: Radiation response of the central nervous system. Int J Radiat Oncol Biol Phys 31:1093-1112, 1995.

Table A-11 Tolerance Doses for Normal Central Nervous System Tissues*

CNS Tissue	$TD_{5/5}$ (Gy)	$TD_{50/5}$ (Gy)	End Point
RUBIN[29]			
Brain			Infarction, necrosis
Whole	60	70	
Partial (25%)	70	80	
Spinal cord			Infarction, necrosis
Partial (10-cm length)	45	55	
EMAMI ET AL[30]			
Brain			Infarction, necrosis
One-third	60	75	
Two-thirds	50	65	
Whole	40	60	
Brainstem			Infarction, necrosis
One-third	60	—	
Two-thirds	53	—	
Whole	50	65	
Spinal cord			Myelitis, necrosis
5 cm	50	70	
10 cm	50	70	
20 cm	47	—	
Cauda equina	60	75	Clinically apparent nerve damage
Brachial plexus			Clinically apparent nerve damage
One-third	62	77	
Two-thirds	61	76	
Whole	60	75	

*Assumes 2 Gy per fraction, 5 days per week.

CNS, central nervous system; $TD_{5/5}$ and $TD_{50/5}$, doses predicted to result in a 5% and 50% probability of complications in 5 years, respectively.

Data from Rubin P: Radiation Biology and Radiation Pathology Syllabus. Chicago, American College of Radiology, 1975; Emami B, Lyman J, Brown A, et al: Tolerance of normal tissues to therapeutic irradiation. Int J Radiat Oncol Biol Phys 21:109-122, 1991.

reportedly lower than that for brain, no definitive data support this difference. Instead, the sequelae of spinal cord radiation injury are perceived as greater than those of brain injury; therefore, tolerance doses have been arbitrarily lowered. In clinical practice, $TD_{5/5}$ values of 60 Gy for partial brain and 50 Gy for a limited segment of spinal cord are commonly used.

As important as total dose is the dose per fraction. It is implied in the neuret model of brain tolerance that the fraction size, which is related to N (number of fractions), is far more important than T (time), given that the exponent for N is much larger than that for T. The $TD_{5/5}$ values given for brain and spinal cord tolerance assume a fraction size of 1.8 to 2.0 Gy per day. The only prospective study assessing brain tolerance for partial brain irradiation using conventional 1.8-Gy fractions was published by Shaw and associates.[32] This clinical trial enrolling approximately 200 adults with supratentorial low-grade glioma randomized patients to 50.4 Gy in 28 fractions or to 64.8 Gy in 36 fractions. The crude 5-year incidence of radiation necrosis at 50.4 Gy was 1% (actuarial incidence, 2%) compared with 5% at 64.8 Gy (actuarial incidence, 10%).[32] These data suggest that the $TD_{1/5}$ and $TD_{5/5}$ for partial-brain irradiation using conventional fraction size are 50 and 65 Gy, respectively. For patients with primary CNS tumors who are being treated with curative intent, fraction size should rarely exceed 2.0 Gy daily, and in most situations, it should be 1.8 to 2.0 Gy. Fraction sizes greater than 2.0 Gy daily (usually 2.5 to 3.0 Gy) are commonly used for palliation of brain metastases and spinal cord compression, but only because these patients are not expected to live long enough to manifest late normal tissue injury.

Table A-12 shows the tolerance doses for other normal tissues of the CNS, including the ear, eye, and optic chiasm or optic nerve. The clinical manifestations of severe injury to these structures are also listed.[28,33,34]

Pathogenesis of Late Radiation-Induced Central Nervous System Injury

Classic Model of Parenchymal or Vascular Target Cells

Vascular abnormalities and demyelination are the predominant histologic changes seen in radiation-induced CNS injury. Classically, late delayed injury was viewed as resulting solely from a reduction in the number of surviving clonogens of parenchymal (i.e., oligodendrocyte[35]) or vascular (i.e., endothelial[36]) target cell populations, leading to white matter necrosis. Later findings suggest that the classic model is simplistic. Pathophysiologic data from a variety of late-responding tissues, including the CNS, indicate that the expression of radiation-induced normal tissue injury involves complex and dynamic interactions between several cell types within a particular organ.[37-39] In the brain, these include oligodendrocytes, endothelial cells, astrocytes, microglia, and neurons. These cells are no longer viewed as passive bystanders, merely dying

Table A-12 Tolerance Doses for Miscellaneous Normal Tissues of the Cranium

Normal Tissue	$TD_{5/5}$ (Gy)	$TD_{50/5}$ (Gy)	Manifestations of Severe Injury
Ear (middle/external)	30-55	40-65	Acute or chronic serous otitis
Eye			
Retina	45	65	Blindness
Lens	10	18	Cataract formation
Optic nerve or chiasm	50	65	Blindness

$TD_{5/5}$ and $TD_{50/5}$, doses predicted to result in a 5% and 50% probability of complications in 5 years, respectively.
Data from references 30, 33, 34.

as they attempt to divide, but are seen as active participants in an orchestrated, yet limited, response to injury.[40] This new paradigm offers an exciting new approach to radiation-induced normal tissue morbidity—the possibility that radiation injury can be modulated by the application of therapies directed at altering steps in the cascade of events leading to the clinical expression of normal tissue injury. Because such a cascade of events does not occur in tumors, where direct clonogenic cell kill predominates, such treatments should not negatively impact antitumor efficacy.

Contemporary Model of Radiation-Induced Central Nervous System Injury

A contemporary model of radiation-induced injury to the CNS has been published by Tofilon and Fike.[40] In this model, radiation causes acute cell death and induces an intrinsic recovery and repair response in the form of specific cytokines, and it may initiate secondary reactive processes that result in the generation of a persistent oxidative stress or chronic inflammation.

Treatment of Radiation-Induced Central Nervous System Injury

Radiation-induced CNS injury has been well characterized in terms of histologic criteria and radiobiologic parameters. In contrast, details of the molecular, cellular, and biochemical processes responsible for the expression and progression of radiation-induced CNS injury are limited. The rational application of interventional procedures directed at reducing the severity of late radiation injury is problematic.

Several approaches have been used but remain clinically unproven. Intrathecal administration of the classic radioprotector WR-2721 (amifostine) before spinal cord irradiation resulted in a dose-modifying factor of 1.3 and a prolongation of median latency to myelopathy by 63% at the TD_{50}.[41] Fike and colleagues observed that the polyamine synthesis inhibitor α-difluoromethylornithine reduced the volume of radionecrosis and contrast enhancement in the irradiated dog brain[42]; a delayed increase in microglia was also seen.[43] Based on the vascular target cell hypothesis, Hornsey and coworkers hypothesized that treating rats with the iron-chelating agent desferrioxamine would reduce hydroxyl-mediated reperfusion-related injury in the irradiated spinal cord.[44] Rats were fed a low-iron diet from 85 days after local spinal cord irradiation and received desferrioxamine (30 mg in 0.3 mL, SC, three times per week) from day 120, the time at which changes in vascular permeability were observed. The onset of ataxia due to white matter necrosis was delayed, and the incidence of lesions was reduced after single doses of 25 and 27 Gy. Dexamethasone also delayed the development of radiation-induced ataxia, along with a reduction in regional capillary permeability. In contrast, indomethacin did not appear to affect any of these end points. In the pig, administration of the polyunsaturated fatty acids γ-linolenic acid (GLA; 18C: 3n-6) and eicosapentaenoic acid (EPA; 20C:5n-3) starting the day after spinal cord irradiation reduced the incidence of paralysis from 80% to 20%.[45] El-Agamawi and colleagues reported that GLA significantly reduced the onset of paralysis after spinal cord irradiation in 5-week-old rats.[46]

Attempts have been made to rectify the radiation-induced decrease in neurogenesis. Rezvani and associates[47] transplanted neural stem cells 90 days after irradiation of the rat spinal cord with a single dose of 22 Gy. Although 100% of irradiated rats treated with saline exhibited paralysis within 167 days of irradiation, the paralysis-free survival rate of rats treated with neural stem cells was approximately 34% at 183 days. These findings are somewhat controversial; nonirradiated stem cells transplanted into the irradiated rat hippocampus failed to generate neurons, although gliogenesis was spared.[48] Preliminary data suggest that insulin-like growth factor-1 (IGF-1) may show efficacy in preventing radiation myelopathy in adult rats[49] and in ameliorating the radiation-induced cognitive dysfunction observed in the rat after whole-brain irradiation.[50]

Toxicity Scoring Systems

Radiation injury is usually described in terms of its time course and severity. Acute injury occurs during the course of brain and spinal cord irradiation and is extremely uncommon, although acute side effects of radiation do occur, such as fatigue, hair loss, and erythema of the skin. More common are early delayed reactions, which occur several weeks to months after radiation has been completed, and late delayed reactions, which occur beyond several months (usually between 1 and 2 years) after treatment.

Toxicity values for CNS tumor radiation therapy are provided in Tables A-13 and A-14. Table A-13 shows the toxicity assessments for CNS tumor clinical research protocols used by the RTOG and its European counterpart, the European Organization for the Research and Treatment of Cancer (EORTC).[51] In Table A-14, the proposed late effects on normal tissues (LENT) subjective-objective management-analytical (SOMA) CNS toxicity tables, which are in the process of being validated by the RTOG, are shown.[52] They may eventually replace the RTOG/EORTC tables.

Early delayed reactions in the brain clinically manifest as somnolence, increased irritability, loss of appetite, and sometimes an exacerbation of tumor-associated symptoms or signs. When these symptoms occur in children, usually after whole-brain irradiation, it is called the *somnolence syndrome*. In the spinal cord, clinical findings include electric shock–like paresthesias that occur with flexion of the neck, or Lhermitte's syndrome. These early delayed reactions are usually transient

Table A-13 **Radiation Therapy Oncology Group and European Organization for Research and Treatment of Cancer Central Nervous System Toxicity Tables**

Toxicity, Organ	Toxicity Grade* 1	2	3	4
Acute toxicity, brain	Fully functional status (i.e., able to work) with minor neurologic findings; no medication needed	Neurologic findings sufficient to require home care; nursing assistance may be required; medications (e.g., steroids, antiseizure agents) may be required	Neurologic findings requiring hospitalization for initial management	Serious neurologic impairment that includes paralysis, coma, or seizures (>3 per week) despite medication and/or hospitalization required
Chronic toxicity, brain	Mild headache; slight lethargy	Moderate headache; significant lethargy	Severe headaches; severe central nervous system dysfunction (partial loss of strength)	Seizure or paralysis; coma
Chronic toxicity, spinal cord	Mild Lhermitte's syndrome	Severe Lhermitte's syndrome	Objective neurologic findings at or below cord level treated	Monoplegia, paraplegia, or quadriplegia

*Grade 0 toxicity, none; grade 1, mild; grade 2, moderate; grade 3, severe; grade 4, life threatening; grade 5, fatal.

Data from Cox JD, Stetz J, Pajak TF: Toxicity criteria of the Radiation Therapy Oncology Group and the European Organization for Research and Treatment of Cancer. Int J Radiat Oncol Biol Phys 31:1341-1346, 1995.

(lasting several weeks to months) and do not predict subsequent injury. Late delayed reactions are usually irreversible.

For early and late delayed reactions, the result is radiation necrosis, which is tissue damage to the substance or white matter of the brain or spinal cord. The clinical symptoms and signs are the direct result of the tissue damage or the indirect result of swelling of the adjacent normal tissues in response to the necrotic material. Brain necrosis may be asymptomatic if it occurs in a noncritical area, but it usually is associated with location-specific symptoms (e.g., necrosis in the right posterior frontal lobe [motor strip] results in left hemiparesis). Spinal cord necrosis is usually symptomatic and may include sensory and motor loss in the legs or arms and legs, depending on the level of the injury, as well as sphincter impairment of the bowel and bladder. Certain treatments of cerebral radiation necrosis, such as hyperbaric oxygen and warfarin, have been anecdotally described as being helpful to arrest or reverse the process, although such interventions have no proven value.[53,54] Some radiologists believe pentoxifylline may have therapeutic value based on the use of this platelet antagonist to treat soft tissue fibrosis,[55] although there are no data to support the efficacy of this drug in cerebral radionecrosis.

IRRADIATION TARGET AND DOSE

Target Volume Determinations

For the purposes of this overview, the nomenclature described in the physics publication Report 50 of the International Commission on Radiation Units and Measurements (ICRU-50)[56] is used, including gross tumor volume (GTV), clinical target volume (CTV), planning target volume (PTV), treated volume (TV), and irradiated volume, which are defined in Table A-15. The initial step in the treatment planning process is the identification of the GTV, which is an imaging-based process. Typically, the GTV is the enhancing gross tumor seen on MRI or CT with contrast. However, tumor does not always enhance. For example, the edematous brain tissue surrounding enhancing gross disease often contains microscopic tumor. The CTV extends 1 to 3 cm beyond the GTV and represents the volume of tissue at risk for harboring microscopic tumor. The PTV, which usually extends 0.5 to 1 cm beyond the margin of the GTV and CTV, accounts for factors such as internal organ motion, set-up variation, and patient movement.

Most primary gliomas of the brain can be classified as circumscribed and noninfiltrative tumors, noncircumscribed and infiltrative (into surrounding normal brain tissue) tumors, or a combination of both.[57] Figure A-7A shows the MRI scan of a patient with a cerebral pilocytic astrocytoma, which is a circumscribed, noninfiltrative tumor. The scan shows a well-defined contrast-enhancing tumor without surrounding edema. Biopsy of the enhancement area would reveal pure tumor tissue, whereas biopsy beyond the enhancement area would reveal normal brain tissue. Tumors such as these are amenable to cure with complete surgical removal. Alternatively, radiosurgery, which delivers a highly focal dose of radiation to an intracranial lesion with minimal dose to the surrounding normal tissues (see Chapter 16), may also be a curative treatment. Other examples of circumscribed, noninfiltrative tumors include meningiomas, pituitary adenomas, and craniopharyngiomas. In cases such as pilocytic astrocytoma and other circumscribed, noninfiltrative tumors, the GTV is the enhancing tumor, and the CTV adds a 1- to 2-cm margin beyond the GTV (see Fig. A-7B).

Figure A-8 shows the MRI scan of a patient with a cerebral glioblastoma, which is a noncircumscribed, infiltrative tumor. The T1-weighted images with contrast (see Fig. A-8B) show a well-defined enhancing tumor with a necrotic center that is surrounded by edema, which is better seen on the T2-weighted images (see Fig. A-8A). Biopsy of the enhancement would show pure tumor tissue, whereas biopsy of the edema would reveal normal brain tissue infiltrated with microscopic tumor. Such tumors are not likely to be cured by complete surgical removal (or radiosurgery) alone, because tumor may be present several centimeters beyond the MRI-defined extent of the edema.[57] Surgical removal (or radiosurgery) of the edematous brain tissue, which contains normal brain and tumor tissue, may result in a neurologic deficit if the tumor is located in a functionally critical area of the brain. In this example of a glioblastoma, the initial GTV is the enhancing tumor plus surrounding edema. The initial CTV adds a 2-cm margin beyond

Table A-14 Modified Late Effects on Normal Tissues (LENT) Central Nervous System Toxicity Tables

	Grade 1*	Grade 2*	Grade 3*	Grade 4*
SPINAL CORD				
Subjective				
Paresthesia, including tingling pain, and Lhermitte's syndrome	Occasional	Intermittent	Persistent	Refractory
Sensory (numbness)	Minimal change	Mild unilateral sensory loss; works with some difficulties	Partial unilateral sensory loss; needs assistance for self-care	Total loss of sensation; danger of self-injury
Motor (weakness)	Minor loss of strength	Weakness interfering with normal activities	Persistent weakness preventing basic activities	Paralysis
Sphincter control	Occasional loss	Intermittent loss	Incomplete control	Complete incontinence
Objective				
Neurologic evaluation	Barely detectable unilateral decrease in sensation or motor strength; no effect on function	Easily detectable unilateral decrease in sensation or motor strength; disturbs but does not prevent function	Full Brown-Séquard syndrome, loss of sphincter function; prevents function	Complete transection, disabling; requiring continuous care
Management				
Pain	Occasional non-narcotic analgesics	Intermittent low-dose steroids	Intermittent high-dose steroids	Persistent high-dose steroids
Neurologic function	Minor adaptation to continue work	Regular physical therapy	Intensive physical therapy plus regular supervision	Intensive nursing or life support
Incontinence	Physical therapy	Occasional use of incontinence pads	Regular use of incontinence pads	Permanent incontinence pads
Analytic†				
MRI	Edema	Local demyelination	Extensive demyelination	Necrosis
BRAIN				
Subjective				
Headache	Occasional	Intermittent	Persistent	Refractory
Somnolence	Occasional; able to work or perform normal activity	Intermittent; interferes with work	Persistent; needs some assistance for self-care	Refractory; prevents daily activity; coma
Intellectual deficit	Minor loss of ability to reason and judge	Moderate loss of ability to reason and judge	Major loss of ability to reason and judge	Complete loss of reasoning and judgment
Functional competence	Perform complex tasks with minor inconvenience	Inability to perform complex tasks	Inability to perform simple tasks	Need for continuous care and supervision; coma
Memory loss	Minor short- or long-term	Moderate short- or long-term	Severe short- or long-term	Complete disorientation
Objective				
Neurologic deficit	Barely detectable neurologic abnormalities; interferes with normal activities	Easily detectable neurologic abnormalities; interferes with normal activities	Focal motor signs; disturbances in speech, vision; interferes with daily activities	Hemiplegla, hemisensory deficit, aphasia, or blindness; need for continuous care; coma
Cognitive functions	Minor loss of memory, reason, and judgment	Moderate loss of memory, reason, and judgment	Major intellectual impairment	Complete memory loss or incapacity for rational thought
Seizures	Focal, without impairment of consciousness	Focal, with impairment of consciousness	Generalized, tonic-clonic or absence attack	Uncontrolled, with loss of consciousness > 10 minutes
Management				
Headache, somnolence	Occasional non-narcotic analgesics	Persistent non-narcotic medication	High-dose steroids	Parenteral high-dose sterolds, mannitol, and/or surgery
Seizures	Behavioral modification	Behavioral modification and occasional oral medication	Permanent oral medication	Intravenous anticonvulsive medication

Continued

Table A-14 Modified Late Effects on Normal Tissues (LENT) Central Nervous System Toxicity Tables—cont'd

	Grade 1*	Grade 2*	Grade 3*	Grade 4*
Cognition, memory	Minor adaptation	Psychosocial plus educational intervention	Occupational and physical therapy	Custodial care
Analytic[†]				
Neuropsychologic	Minor deficits in memory, IQ, attention	10-19 point decrease in IQ	20-29 point decrease in IQ	More than 30-point decrease in IQ but can learn simple tasks
MRI	Focal white matter changes; dystrophic cerebral calcification	White matter changes affecting <1 cerebral lobe; limited perilesional necrosis	Focal necrosis with mass effect	Pronounced white matter changes: mass effect requiring surgical intervention

*Grade 1, mild toxicity; grade 2, moderate; grade 3, severe; grade 4, life-threatening; grade 5, fatal.
[†]Other analytic studies include CT, MRI, MRI spectroscopy, positron emission tomography, functional MR, serum studies, cerebrospinal fluid studies.
Data from Pavy JJ, Denekamp J, Letschert J, et al: Late effects toxicity scoring: the SOMA scale. Int J Radiat Oncol Biol Phys 32:1043-1047, 1995.

Table A-15 Definitions of Gross, Clinical, and Planning Tumor Volumes Related to Primary Central Nervous System Tumors

Abbreviation	Volume Represented	Definition
GTV	Gross tumor volume	Gross (often enhancing) tumor seen on MRI, CT, or other imaging study
CTV	Clinical target volume	Other central nervous system tissue with suspected microscopic tumor; contains and usually extends 1-3 cm beyond the GTV
PTV	Planning target volume	Margin beyond the GTV and CTV accounting for factors such as internal organ motion, set-up variation, and patient movement; contains and usually extends 0.5 to 1 cm beyond the GTV and CTV
TV	Treated volume	Volume enclosed by the desired prescription isodose line (usually ≥95%); contains the GTV, CTV, and PTV
IV	Irradiated volume	Tissue volume that receives a significant dose of radiation; contains the GTV, CTV, PTV, and TV

Data from International Commission on Radiation Units and Measurements (ICRU): Prescribing, Recording, and Reporting Photon Beam Therapy: Report 50. Washington, DC, ICRU, 1993.

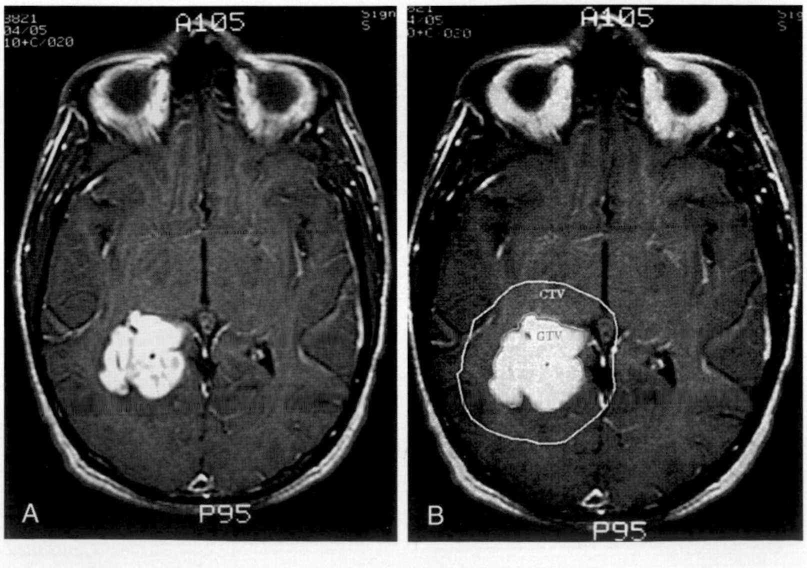

Figure A-7 **A,** MRI scan with contrast of a patient with a right temporoparietal pilocytic astrocytoma. **B,** The clinical target volume (CTV) is the gross tumor volume (GTV) plus a 1-cm margin.

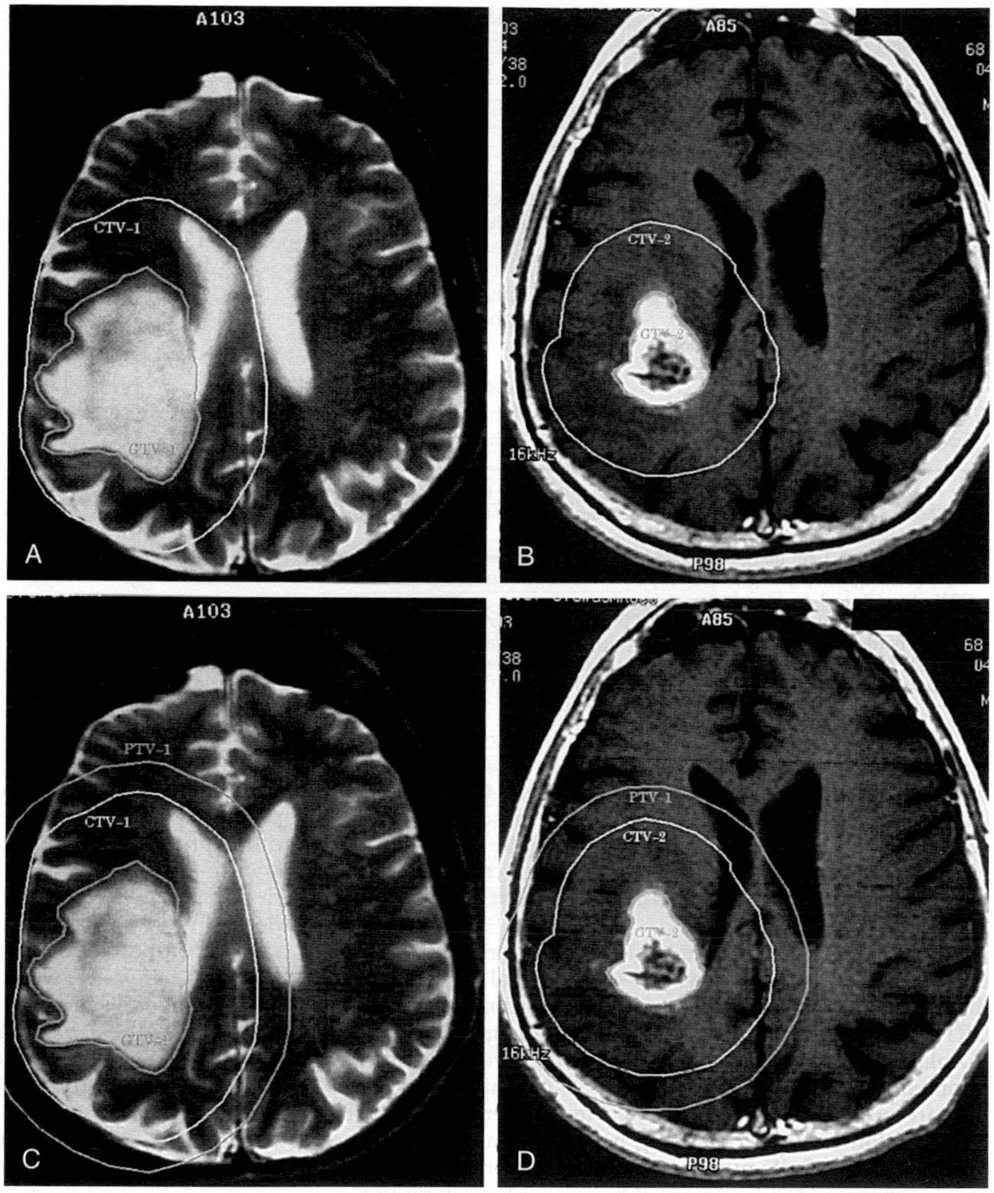

Figure A-8 MRI scan of a right parietal glioblastoma. The T2-weighted image (**A**) and the T1-weighted image with contrast (**B**) are shown. The initial clinical tumor volume (CTV-1) includes the enhancing tumor plus edema (i.e., the initial gross tumor volume [GTV-1]) with a 2-cm margin (**A**). The boost (CTV-2) includes only the enhancing tumor (i.e., the boost GTV) with a 2-cm margin (**B**). The planning target volume (PTV) adds another 1-cm margin to the initial and boost CTVs (**C** and **D**).

the GTV (see Fig. A-8C). Usually, an additional boost dose is given. The enhancing tumor is the boost GTV, and the boost CTV includes a 2-cm margin beyond the GTV (see Fig. A-8D).

Noncircumscribed, infiltrative tumors do not always have an enhancing component on CT or MRI scans with contrast, as in the case of cerebral low-grade gliomas (i.e., diffuse fibrillary astrocytoma, oligodendroglioma, or oligoastrocytoma). In this setting, the GTV is edematous brain tissue containing normal brain infiltrated with microscopic tumor. The initial CTV extends 2 to 3 cm beyond the GTV, and if there is a boost, the margin is reduced to 1 to 2 cm. In both examples of noncircumscribed, infiltrative tumors, the target of the initial GTVs was edematous brain tissue. CT (see Fig. A-4A) is inadequate to show this volume compared with T2-weighted MRI (see Fig. A-4B). MRI scans show greater detail in terms of the normal brain anatomy, specifically the critical normal structures that need to be dose-limited or avoided in the processes of treatment planning and delivery. Other than circumscribed, noninfiltrative tumors that enhance and appear comparable in anatomic extent on CT and MRI scans with contrast, MRI is the treatment planning study of choice for most patients with primary brain and spinal cord tumors.

Dose Recommendations

Table A-16 shows the GTVs and CTVs, as well as dose and fractionation guidelines, for the more common primary brain tumors.[10,58-60] In the context of the survival data presented in Tables A-1 and A-2, it is apparent that the radiation doses recommended do not cure many of the patients with primary CNS tumors, particularly adults. The reason is straightforward—the tolerance of the normal CNS tissues within and surrounding the tumor limits the amount of radiation that can be safely given.

TREATMENT PLANNING PRINCIPLES

Brain Tumors

Three general principles apply to the treatment of all brain tumors that do not require whole-brain irradiation. A single

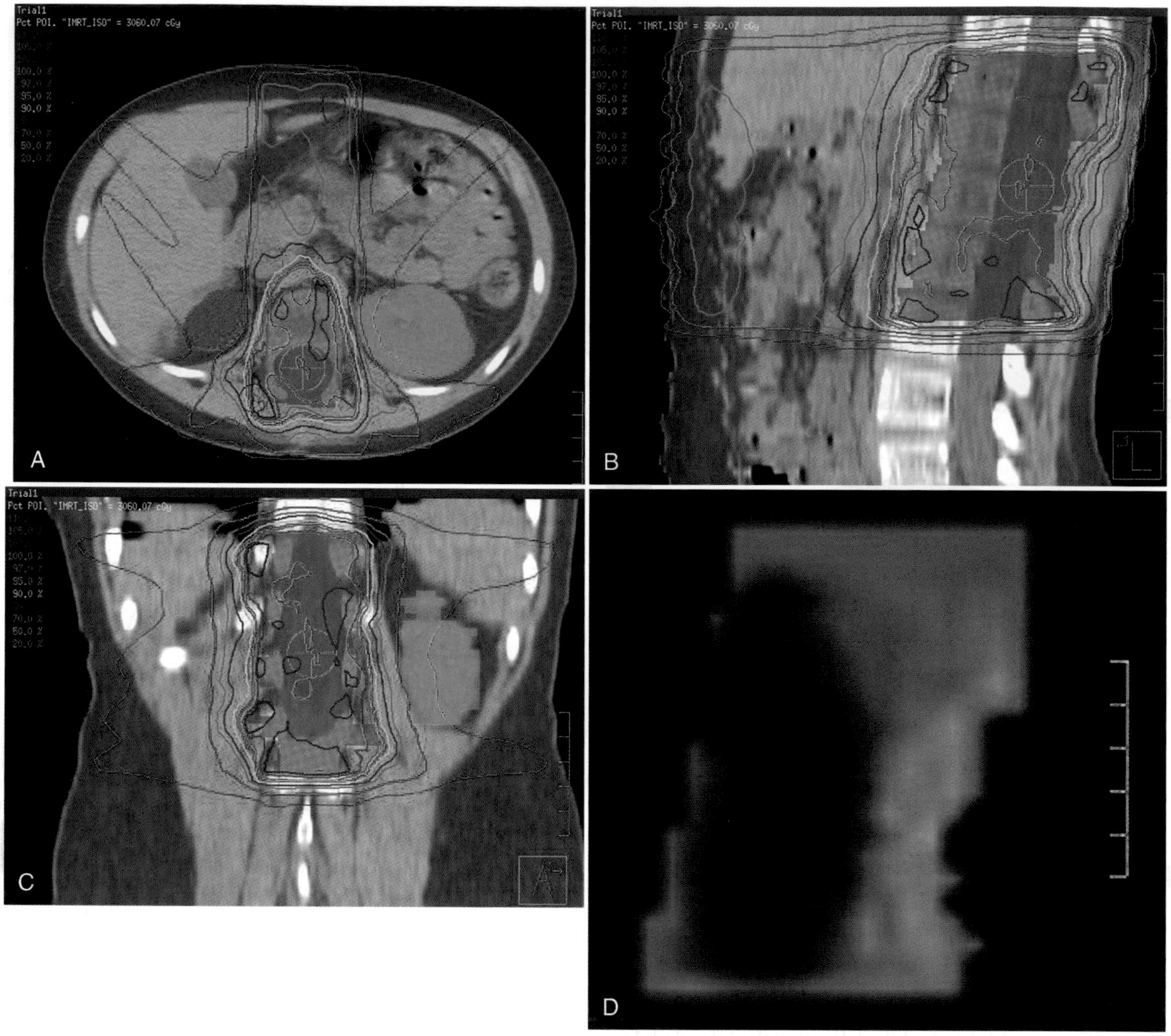

Figure A-14 Intensity-modulated radiation therapy (IMRT) treatment plan of a prepubertal child with a low-grade glioma involving the lumbar spinal cord. This approach allowed 50 Gy to be delivered to the tumor volume with a 1-cm dosimetric margin and a homogeneous low dose to be delivered to the adjacent vertebral bodies to prevent skeletal deformity, while limiting the kidneys to a dose well below the $TD_{5/5}$ level (i.e., 5% incidence of complications at 5 years). **A–C,** The axial, sagittal, and coronal isodose plots. **D,** Fluence map from a laterally directed beam, demonstrating the area of decreased fluence (i.e., reduced dose or intensity) corresponding to the patient's kidneys. (Courtesy of William H. Hinson, PhD, Wake Forest University School of Medicine, Winston-Salem, NC.)

selected institutions using 3D and IMRT radiation therapy planning approaches, only limited data exist about their clinical utility.

TECHNIQUES OF IRRADIATION

Patient Positioning and Immobilization

The first step in the treatment process is to decide how to position the patient for simulation and treatment. Two positioning issues are considered: whether to have the patient lie supine or prone and whether to have the patient's head and neck in a neutral, flexed, or extended position. In general, the supine position is the most stable and is used when treating most brain tumors. Exceptions include patients whose tumors are located posteriorly, such as those in the occipital lobes or posterior fossa, including the cerebellum and brainstem, and patients requiring craniospinal axis irradiation. In these situations, the prone position is preferred. With 3D irradiation and IMRT treatment planning of brain tumors, a neutral head and neck position is acceptable in most situations. Non-coplanar beam angles are accomplished by movements of the treatment couch and gantry. With 2D irradiation treatment planning, a neutral head and neck position may not be optimal for brain tumors in certain locations. For example, when treating a centrally located target such as a pituitary tumor, AP or PA beams enter and exit through the eyes. Flexion rotates the eyes inferiorly relative to the pituitary region, allowing for use of AP

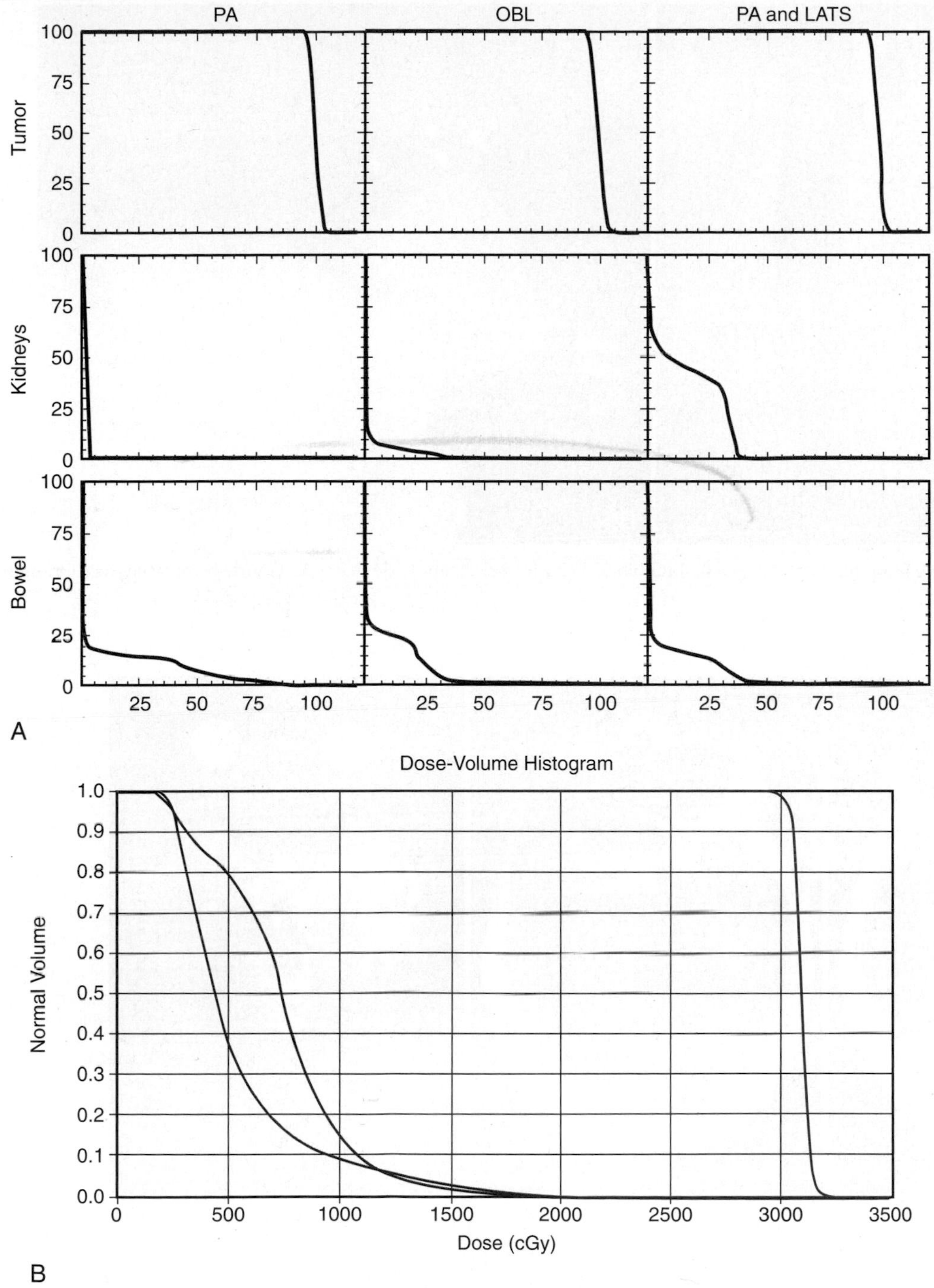

Figure A-15 Dose-volume histograms (DVH) for the isodose plans shown in Figures A-13 (**A**) and A-14 (**B**). Figure A-14B shows the DVH for the tumor (red) and both kidneys (blue, green).

and PA beams that avoid the eyes. When treating brain tumors located in the posterior fossa, such as a brainstem tumor, the supine position with neck extension allows a PA beam to be used because the eyes are rotated superiorly relative to the exit of the beam.

Once positioned, the patient must be immobilized. Various head immobilization devices are commercially available, most of which use a thermoplastic material that produces a custom fit and that is adequate for most 2D, 3D, and IMRT treatment plans (Fig. A-16A), or a more rigid bite-block (see Fig. A-16B), which is typically used for fractionated stereotactic radiotherapy. Once immobilized, the patient undergoes a treatment planning imaging study, which for most primary brain tumors should be an MRI scan for the reasons previously stated. However, most 3D irradiation or IMRT therapy planning systems have image fusion capability, allowing a diagnostic MRI scan not obtained in treatment position to be fused with a planning CT scan in treatment position (Fig. A-17). The remaining sections give examples of location-specific treatment approaches and plans for common types of primary brain tumors.

Centrally Located Tumors

A sellar or parasellar meningioma is one example of a centrally located primary brain tumor. Figure A-18A shows the treat-

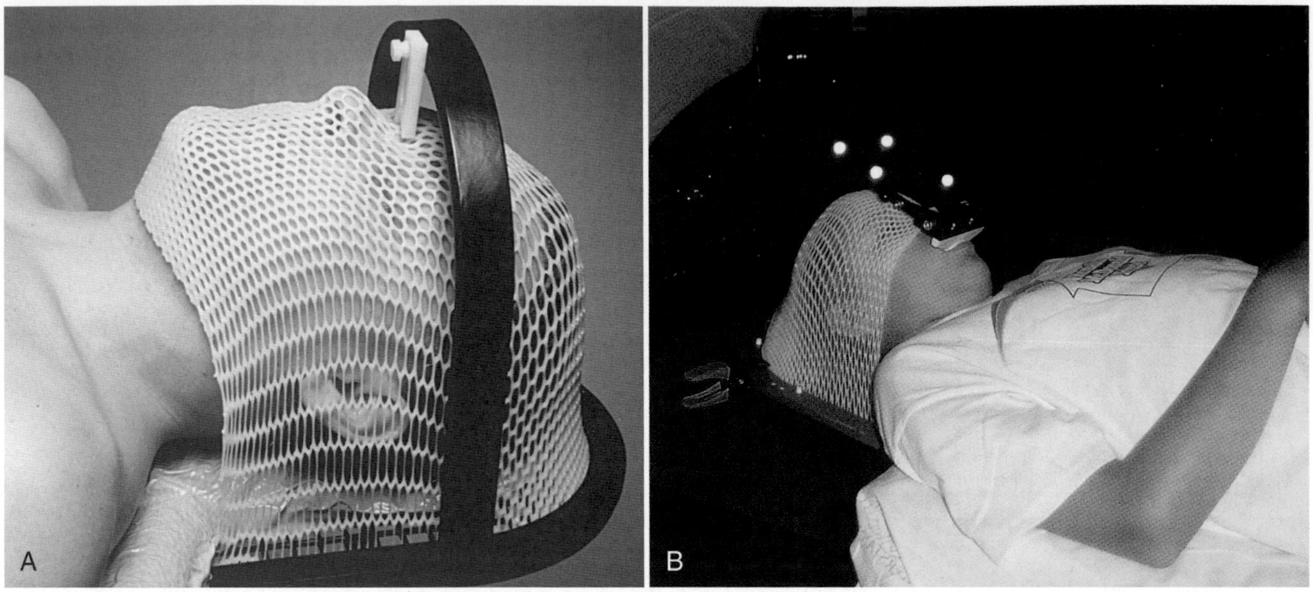

Figure A-16 **A,** Thermoplastic head-immobilization device. **B,** Bite-block head-immobilization device. (**A,** Courtesy of Med-Tec, Orange City, IA).

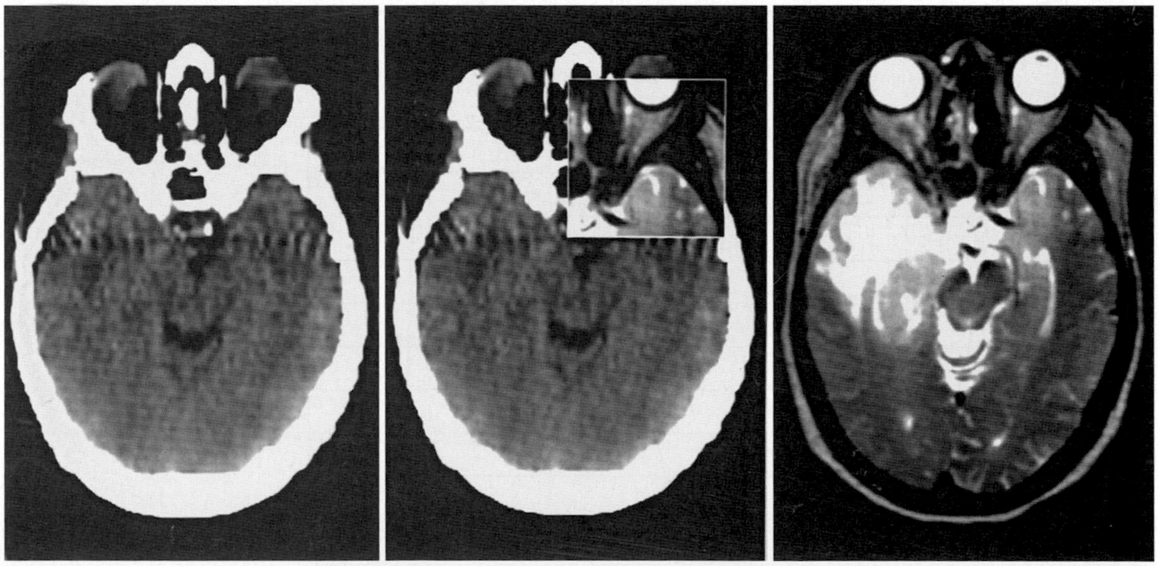

Figure A-17 Fusion of a CT scan *(left)* and MRI scan *(right)* results in a hybrid image *(center)*. (Courtesy of J. Rosenman, MD, PhD, University of North Carolina, Chapel Hill, NC.)

ment planning MRI scan of a patient who has undergone subtotal resection. The patient is supine, with a neutral head and neck position. The GTV is the residual enhancing tumor, and the CTV and PTV add a 1.5-cm margin. The prescription dose is 54 Gy in 30 fractions. Figure A-18B shows the isodose distribution from a 3D treatment plan that includes left lateral, superior, S35A, and P45S treatment fields. In Figure A-18C, these fields are shown as they project on the patient's skull. Another acceptable 3D approach would be a 3-field plan using a superior (or vertex) treatment field plus opposed lateral fields, or alternatively, an IMRT treatment plan could be used. The use of lateral treatment fields alone is discouraged because the temporal lobes, which lie lateral to the various target volumes, would receive the same dose as the PTV.

Laterally and Inferiorly Located Tumors

Posterior frontal or temporal lobe astrocytomas are examples of laterally and inferiorly placed primary brain tumors. Figure A-19A shows the postoperative treatment planning MRI scan of a patient after gross total resection of a right frontotemporal glioblastoma. The patient is supine, with a neutral head and neck position. The initial GTV is the resection cavity and surrounding edema; the initial CTV and PTV add a 2-cm margin. The boost GTV is the resection cavity alone; the boost CTV and PTV add a 2-cm margin. The prescription dose is 46 Gy in 23 fractions to the initial volume and 14 Gy in 7 fractions to the boost volume, for a total dose of 60 Gy in 30 fractions. Figure A-19B and C shows the isodose distribution from

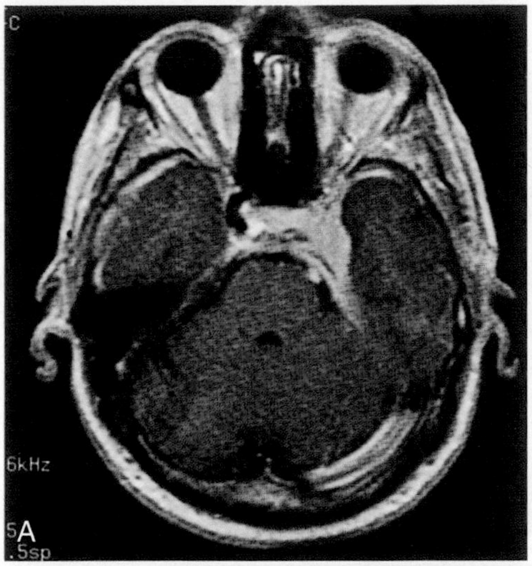

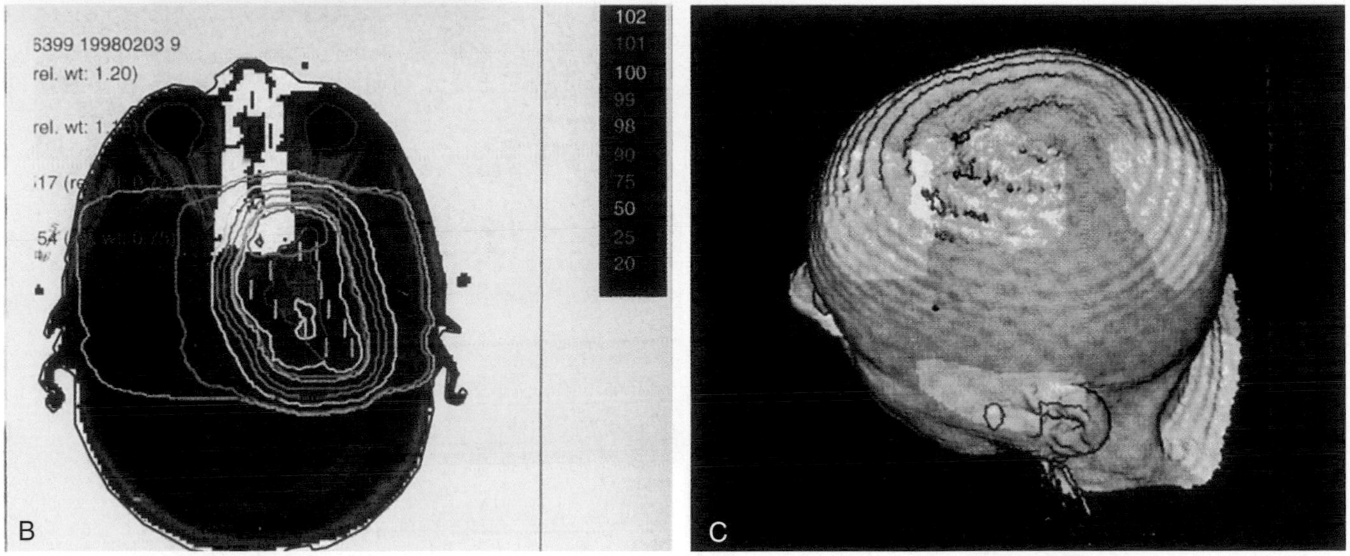

Figure A-18 Treatment planning process for a patient with a centrally located benign meningioma involving the sella and left cavernous sinus. The three-dimensional treatment plan used 10-MV photons with four treatment fields, including a left lateral field with a 45-degree wedge, heel out; a superior (vertex) field with a 60-degree wedge, heel left; and a P45S field (posterior field angled 45 degrees superiorly) with a 60-degee wedge, heel right. **A,** Axial slice of a treatment planning MRI scan. The T1-weighted, contrast-enhanced image is shown. **B,** The axial isodose distribution through the geometric center of the tumor corresponds to the image shown in **A**. **C,** Projection of the four treatment fields on the surface of the patient's skull.

a 3D treatment plan that initially includes A30S, right lateral, S15L, and PA treatment fields. For the boost, a P15L treatment field replaces the PA (other fields remain the same). In Figure A-19D, these fields are shown as they project on the patient's skull for the initial treatment fields. An alternative approach would be opposed lateral treatment fields off-weighted to the right side.[67] However, this treatment plan does a much poorer job of sparing the contralateral temporal lobe, as shown in Figure A-19E and F.

A better alternative would be the use of an IMRT treatment plan. Figure A-20 shows an IMRT approach for a patient with a non-enhancing left temporal anaplastic astrocytoma. The patient is supine, with the head in an Aquaplast mask and the head and neck in a neutral position. The initial GTV is based on the axial FLAIR MRI scan. The treatment planning system is given the following instructions: expand the GTV by 1.5 cm for dosimetric margin (CTV + PTV) and limit optic chiasm dose to less than 50 Gy and contralateral temporal lobe dose to less than 30 Gy. Figure A-20A shows the isodose distributions in the axial, coronal, and sagittal planes from an IMRT treatment plan that includes nine individually modulated beams, including an anterior, A30S, A45R, A45L, P30S, P55L, P60R, P85R, and P85L. A fluence map from the anterior beam shows an area of decreased fluence (i.e., dose) corresponding to the optic chiasm (see Fig. A-20B). The dose-volume histogram demonstrates that the treatment plan achieved the desired objectives of maximizing dose to the tumor while sparing the surrounding normal tissues (see Fig. A-20C).

Parasagittally Located Tumors

A thalamic astrocytoma is an example of a primary brain tumor that is parasagittally positioned; it is intermediately placed between the prior two examples of central and lateral-inferior lesions. Figure A-21A shows the MRI scan of a patient after biopsy of a pilocytic astrocytoma of the left thalamus. The patient is placed in a supine position, with maximum head and neck flexion. The GTV is the enhancing cystic tumor, and CTV and PTV add an additional 1.5 cm. The prescription dose is 55.8 Gy in 31 fractions. Figure A-21B shows the isodose distributions from a 2D treatment plan that uses a 360-degree arc rotation, an approach that minimizes dose to the surrounding normal tissues. Alternative plans include other 2D approaches such as three-field (opposed lateral fields plus a vertex field) or four-field (AP, PA, and opposed lateral fields) plans or a variety of 3D/IMRT approaches.

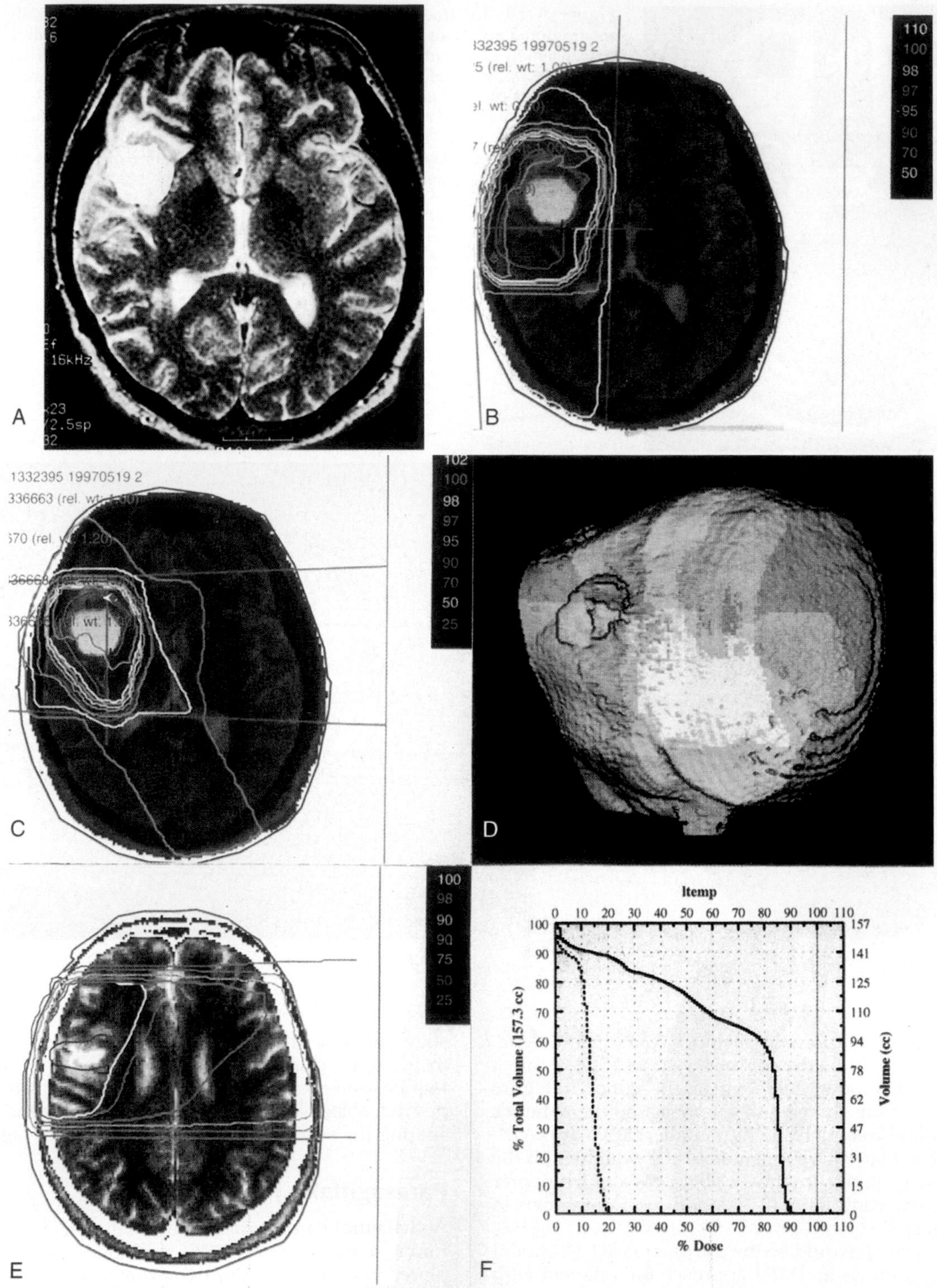

Figure A-19 Treatment planning process for a patient with a laterally and inferiorly located glioblastoma involving the right posterior frontal lobe and anterior temporal lobe. The three-dimensional treatment plan used 6-MV photons with four treatment fields, including a right lateral field with a 60-degree wedge, heel out; an A30S field (anterior field angled 30 degrees superiorly) with a 30-degree wedge, heel in; an S15L field (superior [vertex] angled 15 degrees left) with a 45 degree wedge, heel out; and a posteroanterior or P30L field (posterior field angled 30 degrees left) with a 30-degree wedge, heel right. **A,** Axial slice of a treatment planning MRI scan. The T2-weighted image is shown. **B,** Axial isodose distribution through the geometric center of the initial target volume, corresponding to the image shown in **A**, which includes the resection cavity plus the surrounding edema with a 2-cm margin (i.e., initial GTV + CTV + PTV). **C,** Axial isodose distribution through the geometric center of the boost target volume, corresponding to the image shown in **A**, which includes the resection cavity with a 2-cm margin (i.e., boost GTV + CTV + PTV). **D,** Projection of the four initial treatment fields on the surface of the patient's skull. **E,** Axial isodose distribution of the initial target volume, assuming opposed lateral treatment fields are used that include the resection cavity plus the surrounding edema with a 2-cm margin (i.e., initial GTV + CTV + PTV). The isodose distribution for the opposed lateral boost plan is not shown. **F,** Dose-volume histogram for the contralateral (left) temporal lobes using the three-dimensional, four-field treatment plan initially outlined *(dashed line)* and the treatment plan with opposed laterals *(solid line)*.

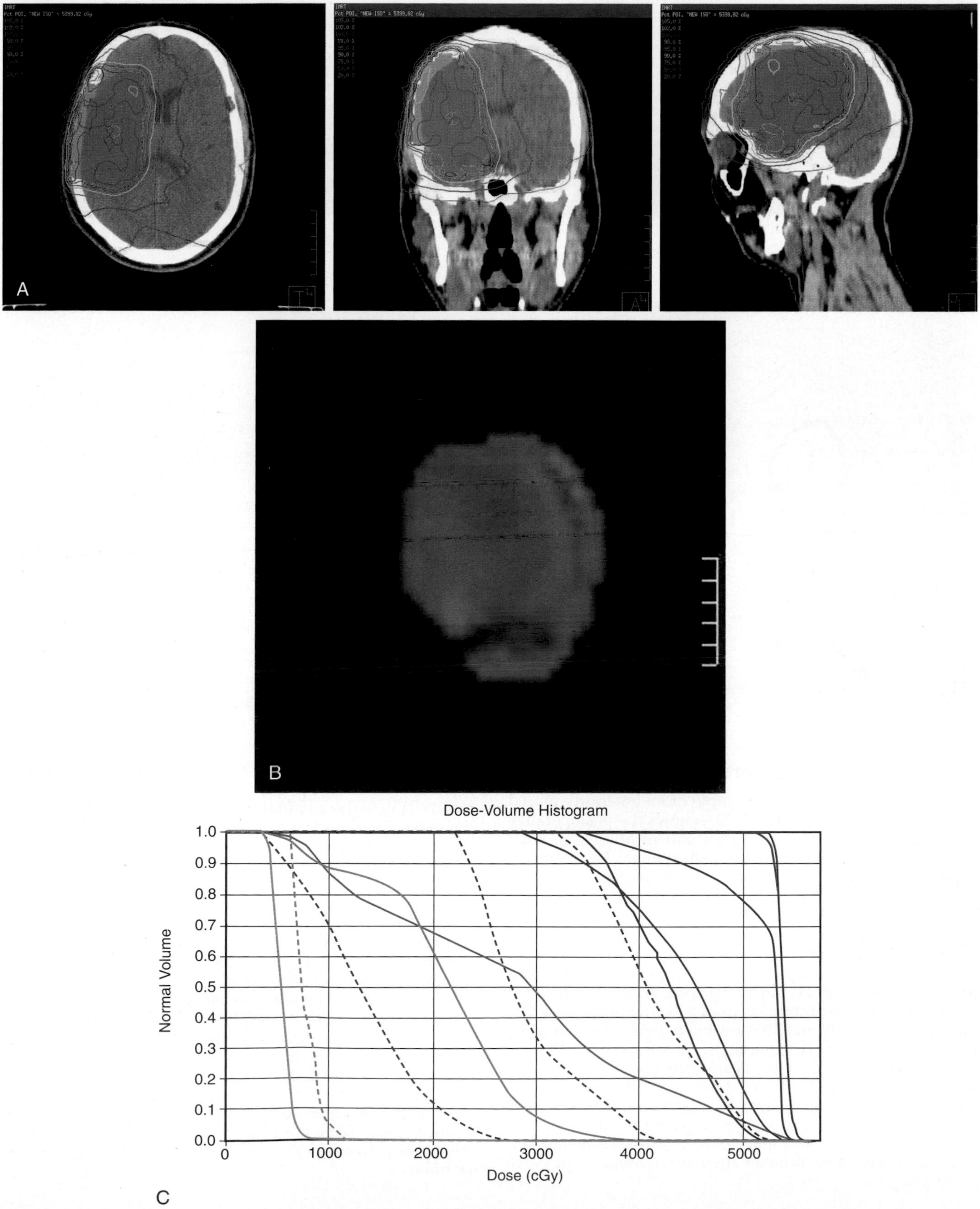

Figure A-20 Intensity-modulated radiation therapy (IMRT) approach for a patient with a left temporal anaplastic astrocytoma. **A,** Dose distributions in the three orthogonal planes (axial: *left*, coronal: *center*, sagittal: *right*) are shown for an IMRT treatment plan, which included P65L, A75L, A30L, A30R, A80R, P50R, and A40S beams. **B,** A fluence map from the anterior beam shows an area of decreased dose corresponding to the optic chiasm. **C,** The dose-volume histogram shows the dose-volume values for the planning target volume (PTV, *purple line*) and normal tissues *(other lines)*. (Courtesy of William H. Hinson, PhD, Wake Forest University School of Medicine, Winston-Salem, NC.)

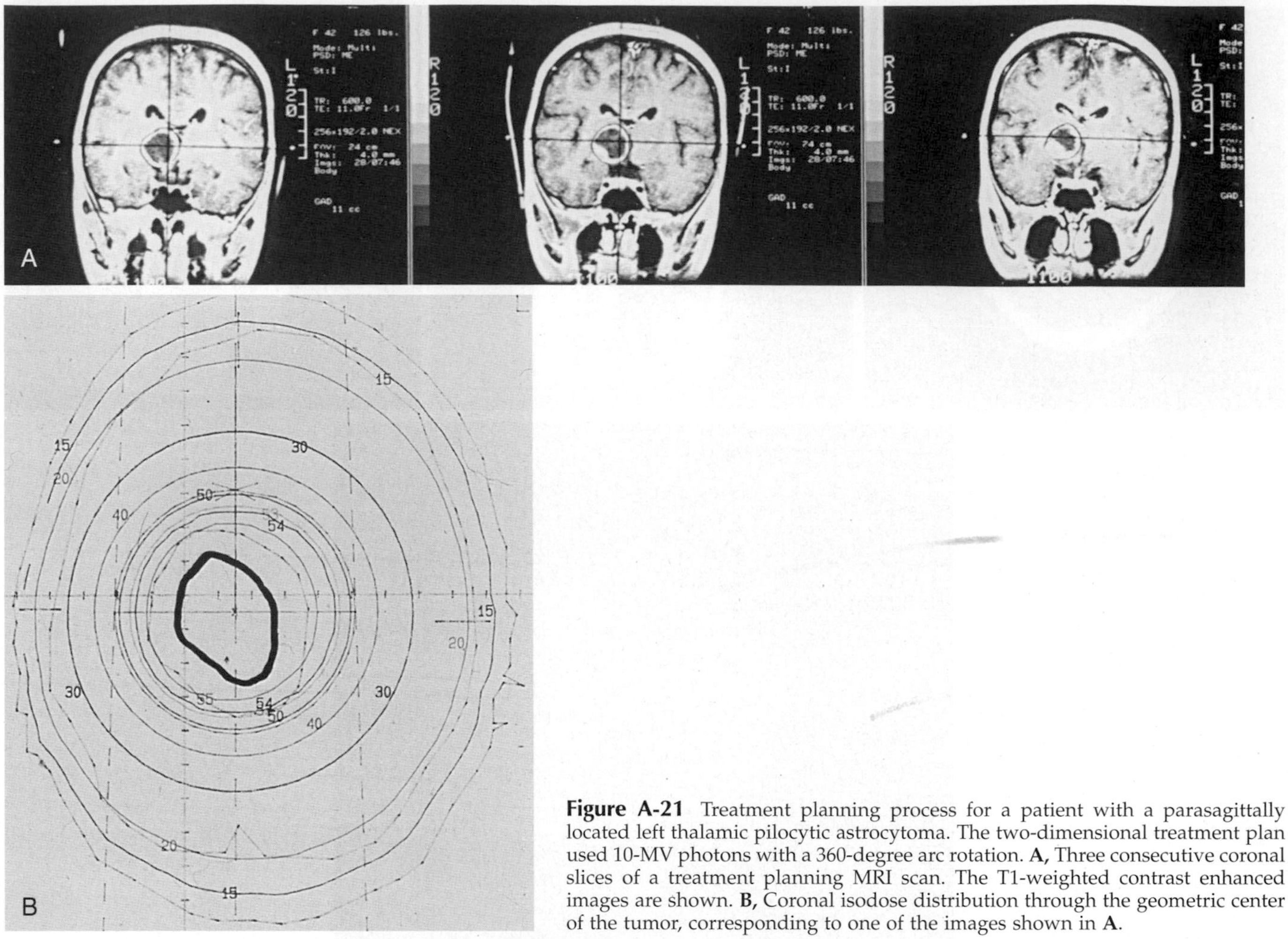

Figure A-21 Treatment planning process for a patient with a parasagittally located left thalamic pilocytic astrocytoma. The two-dimensional treatment plan used 10-MV photons with a 360-degree arc rotation. **A,** Three consecutive coronal slices of a treatment planning MRI scan. The T1-weighted contrast enhanced images are shown. **B,** Coronal isodose distribution through the geometric center of the tumor, corresponding to one of the images shown in **A**.

Anteriorly Located Tumors

A frontal astrocytoma is an example of an anteriorly placed primary brain tumor. Figure A-22A shows the postoperative treatment planning MRI scan of a patient after gross total resection of left frontal anaplastic astrocytoma. The patient is supine, with the head and neck in a neutral position. The initial GTV is the resection cavity and surrounding edema; the initial CTV and PTV add a 2-cm margin. The boost GTV is the resection cavity alone; the boost CTV and PTV add a 2-cm margin. The prescription dose is 45 Gy in 25 fractions to the initial volume and 14.4 Gy in 8 fractions to the boost volume, for a total dose of 59.4 Gy in 33 fractions. Figure A-22B and C show the isodose distributions from a 3D treatment plan that includes A10R, L10P, and S30A treatment fields. Because of the proximity of the left eye to the target volumes, eye blocks were required in each of the three beams (see Fig. A-22D to F). In Figure A-22G, these fields are shown as they project on the patient's skull. An alternative approach would be opposed lateral treatment fields off-weighted to the left side. However, this treatment plan does a much poorer job of sparing the contralateral frontal lobe. A better alternative would be an IMRT treatment plan.

Superiorly Located Tumors

A parietal astrocytoma is an example of a superiorly placed primary brain tumor. Figure A-23A shows the postoperative treatment planning MRI scan of a patient after subtotal resection of a small, right parietal glioblastoma. The patient is supine, with the head and neck in a neutral position. The initial GTV is the residual tumor and surrounding edema; the initial CTV and PTV add a 2-cm margin. The boost GTV is the residual tumor alone; the boost CTV and PTV add a 2-cm margin. The prescription dose is 46 Gy in 23 fractions to the initial volume and 14 Gy in 7 fractions to the boost volume, for a total dose of 60 Gy in 30 fractions. Figure A-23B shows the isodose distribution from a 3D treatment plan that includes a combination of AP-PA treatment fields plus a superior (vertex) field. In Figure A-23C, these fields are shown as they project on the patient's skull. An alternative 2D approach would use a right lateral treatment field (instead of the superior field) along with the AP-PA fields. This approach does result in some dose (exit from the right lateral) to the contralateral hemisphere, although less so than with the use of opposed lateral treatment fields.

For a superiorly located tumor, an IMRT approach is not likely to provide much benefit relative to 2D or 3D treatment plans, because there are really not any critical normal brain structures to avoid in the superior aspect of the supratentorial brain.

Posteriorly and Inferiorly Located Tumors

A brainstem glioma is an example of a posteriorly and inferiorly placed primary brain tumor. Cerebellar tumors also fit

Text continued on page 490

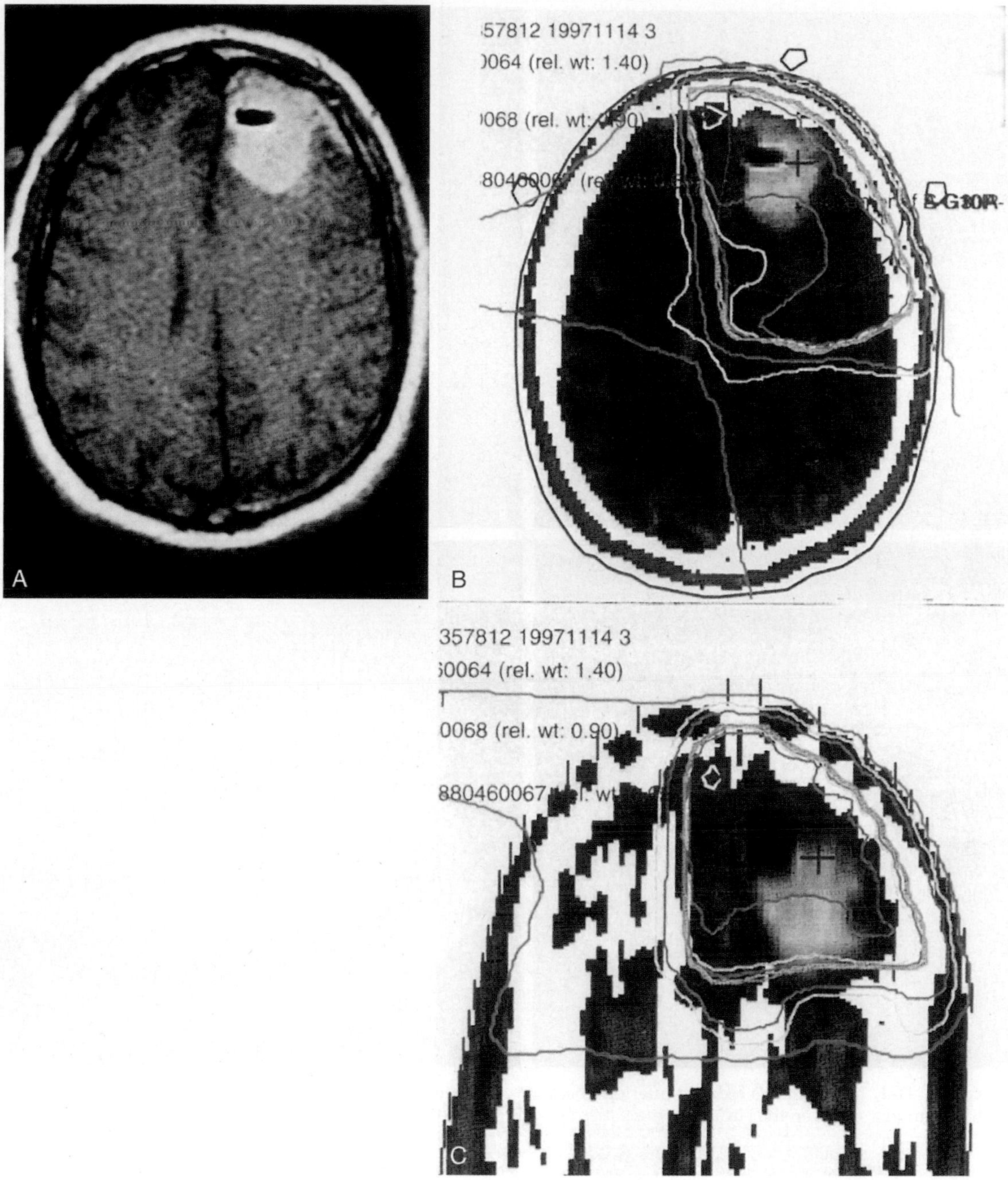

Figure A-22 Treatment planning process for a patient with an anteriorly located left frontal anaplastic astrocytoma. The three-dimensional treatment used 6-MV photons with three treatment fields, including an A10R field (anterior field angled 10 degrees to the right) with a 45-degree wedge, heel right; an L10P field (left lateral field angled 10 degrees posteriorly) with a 60-degree wedge, heel left; and an S30A field (superior [vertex] field angled 30 degrees anteriorly) with a 45-degree wedge, heel out. **A,** Axial slice of a treatment planning MRI scan. The T2-weighted image is shown. **B,** Axial isodose distribution through the geometric center of the initial target volume, corresponding to the image shown in **A,** which includes the resection cavity plus the surrounding edema with a 2-cm margin (i.e., initial GTV + CTV + PTV). **C,** Coronal isodose distribution through the geometric center of the initial target volume.

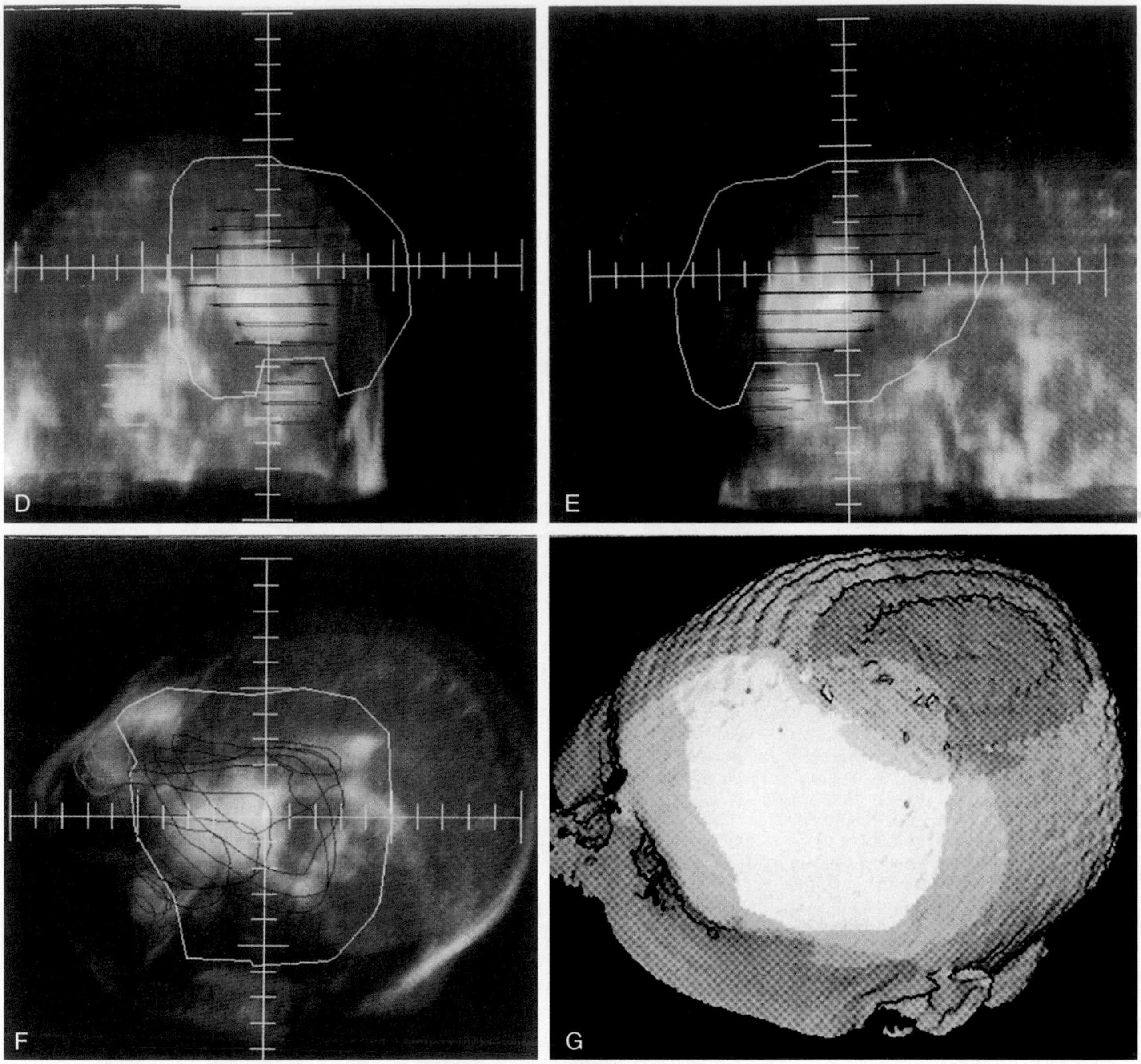

Figure A-22—cont'd **D–F,** The margin is reduced inferiorly because of an eye block placed in the A10R, L10P, and S30A beams. **G,** Projection of the three initial treatment fields on the surface of the patient's skull.

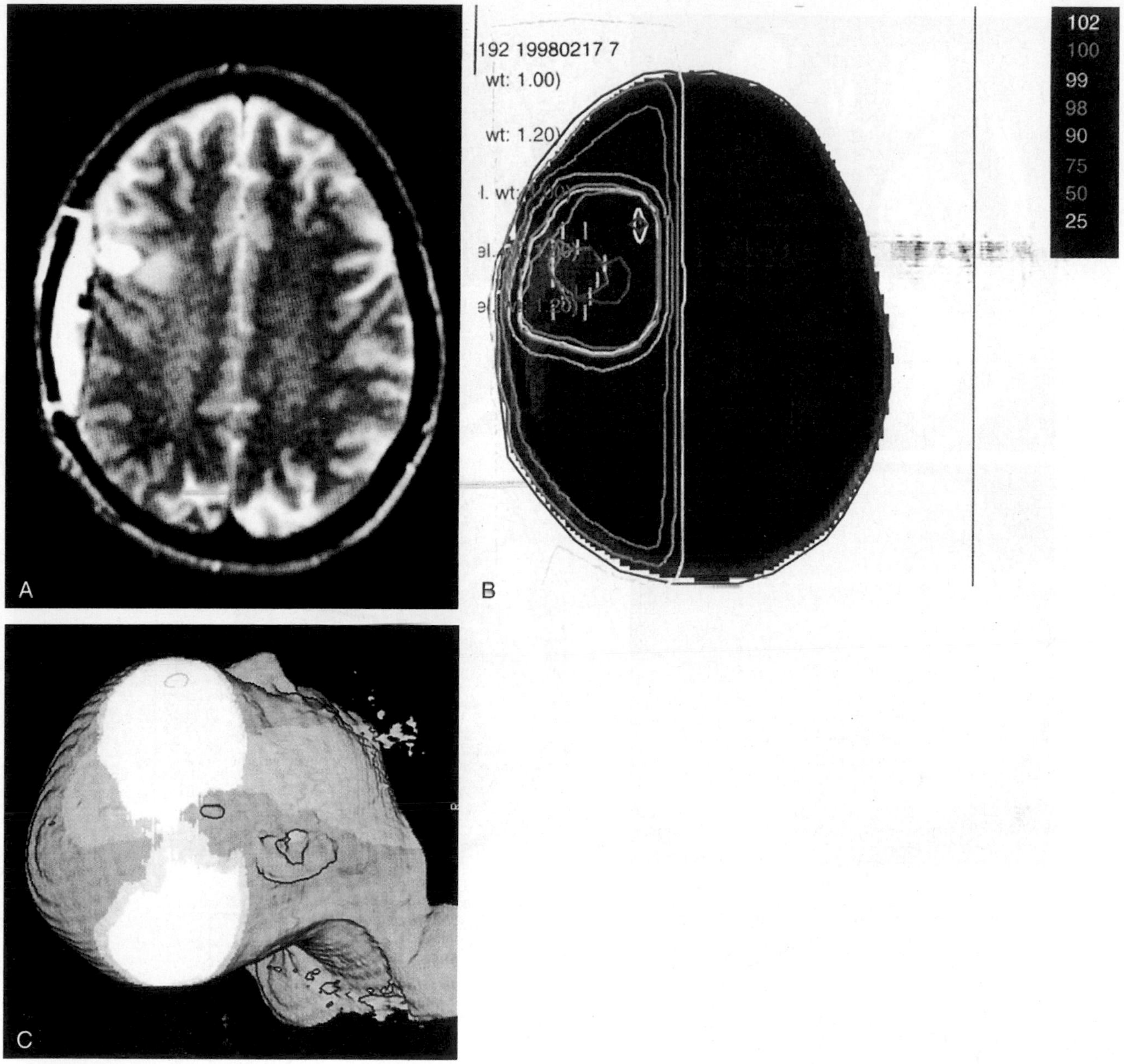

Figure A-23 Treatment planning process for a patient with a superiorly located right parietal glioblastoma. The 3-D treatment plan used 10-MV photons with three treatment fields, including an AP field with a 45-degree wedge, heel partially left and partially out; a PA field with a 45-degree wedge, heel partially right and partially out; and a superior (vertex) field with a 15-degree wedge, heel in. **A,** Axial slice of a treatment planning MRI scan. The T2-weighted image is shown. The resection cavity is lateral, and the residual tumor is medial. **B,** Axial isodose distribution through the geometric center of the initial target volume, corresponding to the image shown in **A**, which includes the resection cavity plus surrounding edema with a 2-cm margin (i.e., initial GTV + CTV + PTV). **C,** Projection of the three initial treatment fields on the surface of the patient's skull.

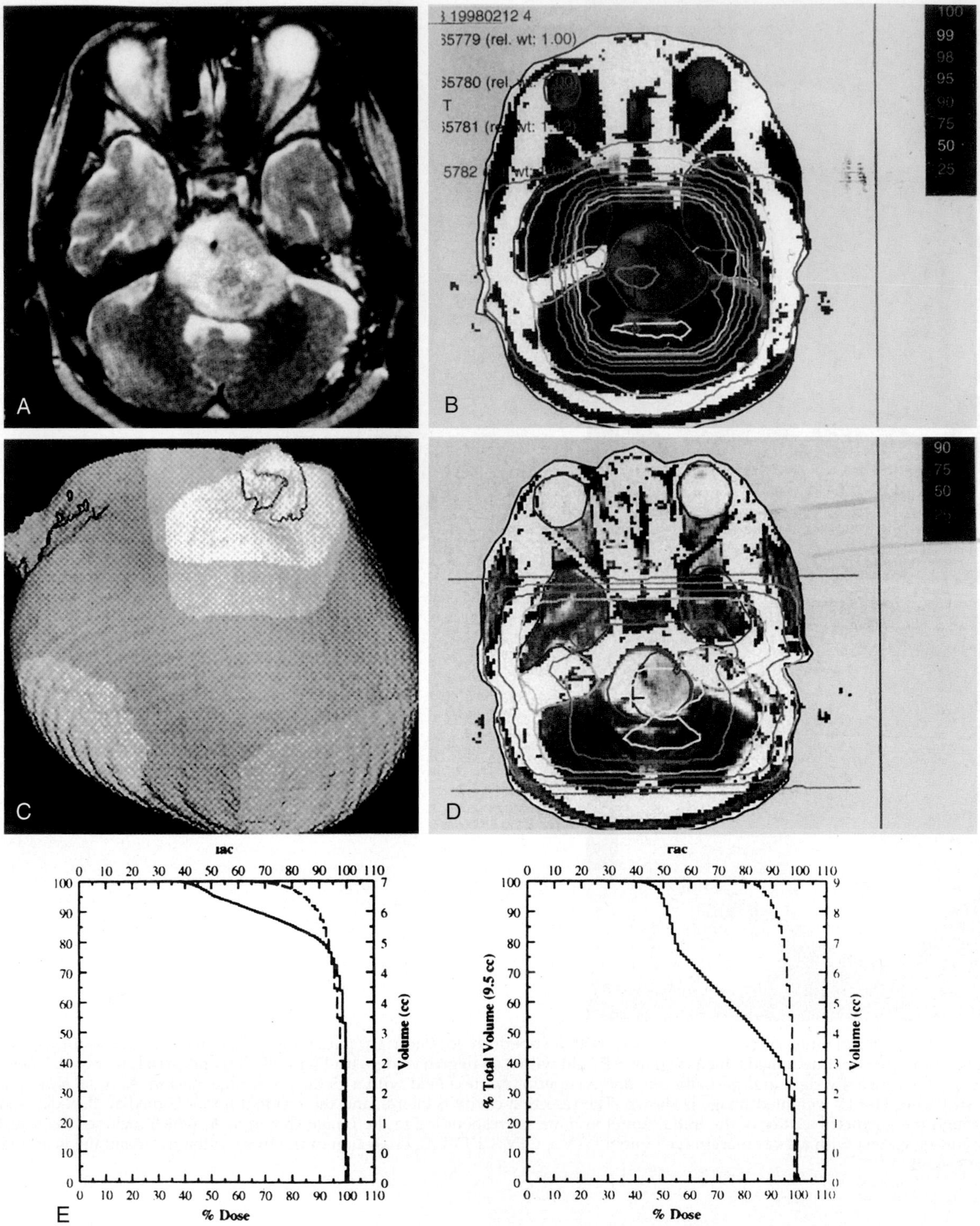

Figure A-24 Treatment planning process for a patient with a posteriorly and inferiorly located, low-grade, diffuse fibrillary astrocytoma involving the brainstem. The three-dimensional treatment plan used 18-MV photons with four treatment fields, including an A40S field (anterior field angled 40 degrees superiorly) with a 30-degree wedge, heel left; an S20P field (superior [vertex] field angled 20 degrees posteriorly) with a 30-degree wedge, heel right; an R15S field (right lateral field angled 15 degrees superiorly) with a 30-degree wedge, heel out; and an L15S field (left lateral with field angled 15 degrees superiorly) with a 30-degree wedge, heel out. **A,** Axial slice of a treatment planning MRI scan. The T2-weighted image is shown. **B,** Axial isodose distribution through the geometric center of the initial target volume, corresponding to the image shown in **A**, which includes the entire brainstem (normal plus abnormal) with a 2-cm margin (i.e., initial GTV + CTV + PTV). The axial isodose distribution through the geometric center of the target boost volume, which includes the area of increased signal with a 1-cm margin (i.e., boost GTV + CTV + PTV), is not shown. **C,** Projection of the four initial treatment fields on the surface of the patient's skull. **D,** Axial isodose distribution through the geometric center of the initial target volume, corresponding to the image shown in **A**, assuming opposed lateral treatment fields are used that include the entire brainstem (normal plus abnormal) with a 2-cm margin (i.e., initial GTV + CTV + PTV). The isodose distribution for the opposed lateral boost plan is not shown. **E,** Dose-volume histogram for the right (rac) and left (lac) external, middle, and internal auditory canals, using the 3-D treatment plan outlined previously *(solid line)* and the hypothetical plan with opposed laterals *(dashed line)*.

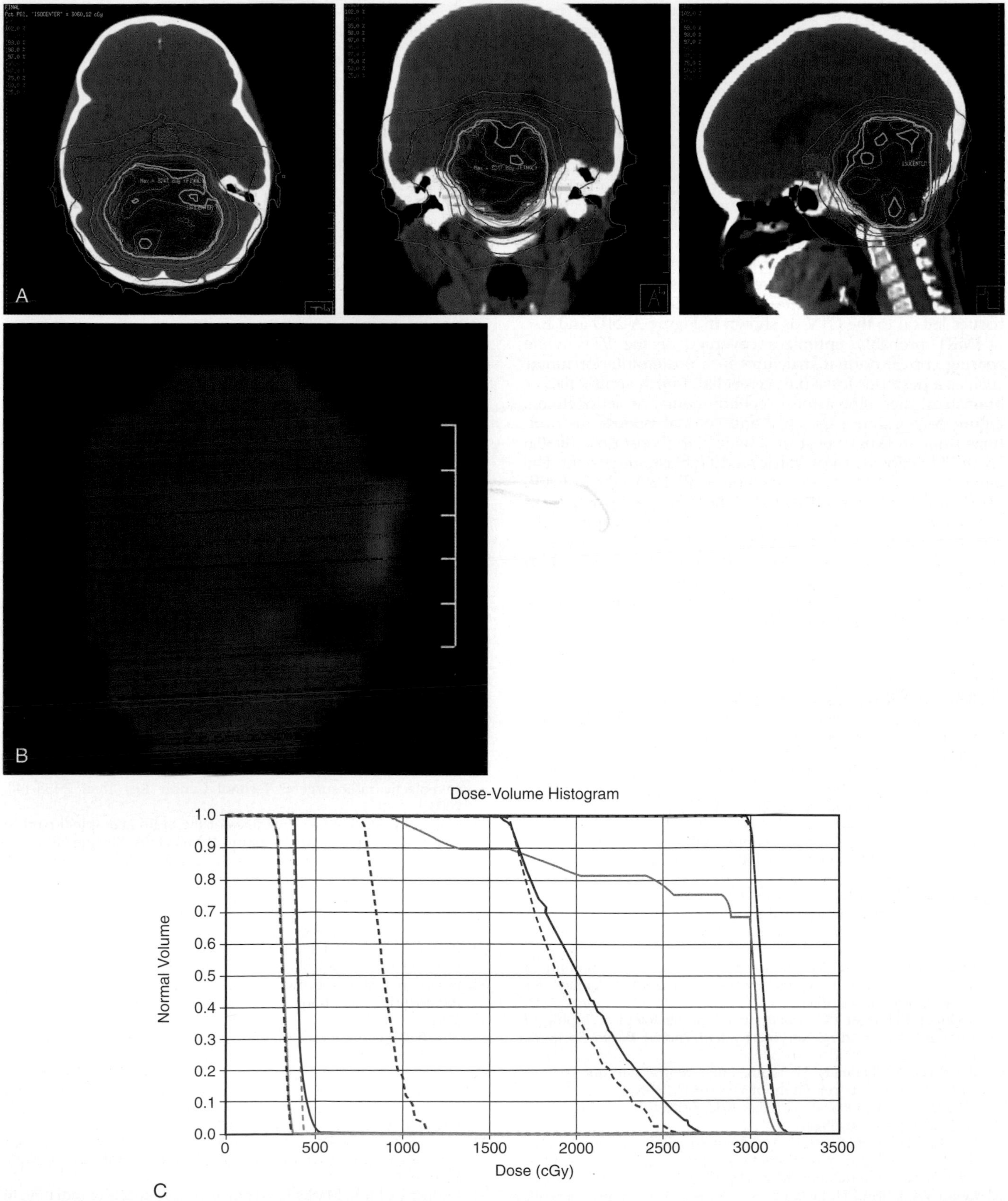

Figure A-25 **A,** Axial *(left)*, coronal *(center)*, and sagittal *(right)* isodose distributions from an intensity-modulated radiation therapy boost treatment plan for a pediatric patient with medulloblastoma. **B,** Fluence map from the left lateral beam shows a small volume of decreased fluence in the region of the cochlea. **C,** The dose-volume histogram shows the values for the PTV *(dashed purple line)* and normal tissues, including the right and left cochlea *(aquamarine and blue dashed lines)*. (Courtesy of William H. Hinson, PhD, Wake Forest University School of Medicine, Winston-Salem, NC.)

into this category. Figure A-24A shows the postbiopsy treatment planning MRI scan of a child with a pontine astrocytoma (WHO grade II). The patient is prone, with the head and neck in a neutral position. The initial GTV includes the midbrain, pons, and medulla; the initial CTV and PTV add a 2-cm margin. The boost GTV includes the areas of abnormal T2-weighted signal in the pons and medulla; the boost CTV and PTV add a 1-cm margin. The prescription dose is 45 Gy in 25 fractions to the initial volume and 10.8 Gy in 6 fractions to the boost volume, for a total dose of 55.8 Gy in 31 fractions. Figure A-24B shows the isodose distributions from a 3D treatment plan that includes A40S, S20P, R15S, and L15S treatment fields. In Figure A-24C, these fields are shown as they project on the patient's skull. An alternative approach would be opposed lateral treatment fields. However, this does a much poorer job of sparing the external auditory canals and normal brain tissues lateral to the GTV, as shown in Figure A-24D and E.

IMRT probably optimizes coverage of the PTV while sparing critical normal structures in a posteroinferior tumor such as a posterior fossa (i.e., cerebellar, fourth ventricular, or brainstem) medulloblastoma, ependymoma, or astrocytoma. Figure A-25A shows the axial and coronal isodose distributions from an IMRT boost treatment plan (boost dose of 30.6 Gy in 17 fractions) of a pediatric medulloblastoma patient. The intensity-modulated beams include S15P, P30L, P60L, P30R, P60R, and right and left laterals. There is a sharp fall-off of dose lateral to the midportion of the GTV in the location of the cochlea. The fluence map from the left lateral beam shows a small volume of decreased fluence in the region of the cochlea (see Fig. A-25B). The dose-volume histogram shows that despite their proximity to the GTV, 50% of the cochlear volume receives less than 20 Gy (see Fig. A-25C).

REFERENCES

1. Bohnen NI, Radhakrishnan K, O'Neill BP, Kurland LT: Descriptive and analytic epidemiology of brain tumors. *In* Black PM, Loeffler JS (eds): Cancer of the Nervous System. Oxford, Blackwell Scientific Publications, 1997, p 3.
2. Jemal A, Siegel R, Ward E, et al: Cancer statistics, 2006. CA Cancer J Clin 55:106-130, 2006.
3. Shaw EG, Seiferheld W, Scott C, et al: Ethnic differences in survival of glioblastoma (GBM): a secondary analysis of the Radiation Therapy Oncology Group (RTOG) recursive partitioning analysis (RPA) database [abstract]. Neurooncology 5:296, 2003.
4. Deorah S, Lynch CF, Sibenaller ZA, Ryken TC: Trends in brain cancer incidence and survival in the United States: surveillance, epidemiology and end results program, 1973 to 2001. Neurosurg Focus 20:E1, 2006.
5. Kleihues P, Cavenee WK: Pathology and Genetics of Tumours of the Nervous System. Lyon, France, International Agency for Research on Cancer, 1998.
6. Kleihues P, Burger PC, Scheithauer BW: Histological Typing of Tumours of the Central Nervous System, 2nd ed. Berlin, Springer, 1993.
7. Polednak AP, Flannery JT: Brain, other central nervous system, and eye cancer. Cancer 75(Suppl 1):330-337, 1995.
8. Scheithauer BW, Okazaki H (eds): Atlas of Neuropathology. New York, JB Lippincott, 1988.
9. Preston-Martin S: Descriptive epidemiology of primary tumors of the spinal cord and spinal meninges in Los Angeles County, 1972-1985. Neuroepidemiology 9:106-111, 1990.
10. Levin VA, Gutin PH, Leibel S: Neoplasms of the central nervous system. *In* DeVita VT, Hellman S, Rosenberg SA (eds): Cancer: Principles and Practice of Oncology, 4th ed. Philadelphia, JB Lippincott, 1993, pp 1679-1737.
11. Davis FG, Freels S, Grutsch J, et al: Survival rates in patients with primary malignant brain tumors stratified by patient age and tumor histological type: an analysis based on Surveillance, Epidemiology, and End Results (SEER) data, 1973-1991. J Neurosurg 88:1-10, 1998.
12. Freeman CR, Farmer JP: Pediatric brain stem gliomas: a review. Int J Radiat Oncol Biol Phys 40:265-271, 1998.
13. Guillamo JS, Monjour A, Taillandier L, et al: Brainstem gliomas in adults: prognostic factors and classification. Brain 124:2528-2539, 2001.
14. Davis FG, McCarthy BJ, Freels S, et al: The conditional probability of survival of patients with primary malignant brain tumors: surveillance, epidemiology and end results (SEER) data. Cancer 85:485-491, 1999.
15. Curran WJ, Scott CB, Horton J, et al: Recursive partitioning analysis of prognostic factors in three Radiation Therapy Oncology Group malignant glioma trials. J Natl Cancer Inst 85:704-710, 1993.
16. Nutt CL, Mani DR, Betensky RA, et al: Gene expression-based classification of malignant gliomas correlates better with survival than histological classification. Cancer Res 63:1602-1607, 2003.
17. Fomchenko EI, Holland EC: Stem cells and brain cancer. Exp Cell Res 306:323-329, 2005.
18. Ohgaki H, Kleihues P: Epidemiology and etiology of gliomas. Acta Neuropathol 109:93-108, 2005.
19. Baeza N, Weller M, Yonekawa Y, et al: *PTEN* methylation and expression in glioblastomas. Acta Neuropathol 106:479-485, 2003.
20. Esteller M, Garcia-Foncillas, Andion E, et al: Inactivation of the DNA-repair gene *MGMT* and the clinical response of gliomas to alkylating agents. N Engl J Med 343:1350-1354, 2000.
21. Debinski W, Gibo DM, Mintz A: Epigenetics in high-grade astrocytomas: opportunities for prevention and detection of brain tumors. Ann N Y Acad Sci 983:232-242, 2003.
22. Giese A, Bjerkvig R, Berens ME, Westphal M: Cost of migration: invasion of malignant gliomas and implications for treatment. J Clin Oncol 8:1624-1636, 2003.
23. Dudas SP, Rempel SA: Development, molecular genetics, and gene therapy of glial tumors. *In* Rock JP, Rosenblum ML, Shaw E, Cairncross G (eds): Practical Management of Low-Grade Primary Brain Tumors. Philadelphia, Lippincott-Raven, 1999.
24. Kleihues P, Ohgaki H: Genetics of glioma progression and the definition of primary and secondary glioblastoma. Brain Pathol 7:1131-1136, 1997.
25. Debinski W, Gibo DM, Hulet SW et al: Receptor for interleukin 13 is a marker and therapeutic target for human high-grade gliomas. Clin Cancer Res 5:985-990, 1999.
26. Bourland JD, Shaw EG: The evolving role of biological imaging in stereotactic radiosurgery. Technol Cancer Res Treat 2:135-140, 2003.
27. Leibel SA, Sheline GE: Tolerance of the brain and spinal cord to conventional irradiation. *In* Gutin P, Leibel SA, Sheline GE (eds): Radiation Injury to the Nervous System. New York, Raven Press, 1991, pp 211-238.
28. Schueltheiss TE, Kun LE, Ang KK, Stephens LC: Radiation response of the central nervous system. Int J Radiat Oncol Biol Phys 31:1093-1112, 1995.
29. Rubin P: Radiation Biology and Radiation Pathology Syllabus. Chicago, American College of Radiology, 1975.
30. Emami B, Lyman J, Brown A, et al: Tolerance of normal tissues to therapeutic irradiation. Int J Radiat Oncol Biol Phys 21:109-122, 1991.
31. Ellis F: Dose, time fractionation: a clinical hypothesis. Clin Radiol 20:1-7, 1969.
32. Shaw E, Arusell R, Scheithauer B, et al: A prospective randomized trial of low-versus high-dose radiation therapy in adults with supratentorial low-grade glioma: initial report of a NCCTG-RTOG-ECOG study. J Clin Oncol 20:2267-2276, 2002.
33. Gordon KB, Char DH, Sagerman RH: Late effects of radiation on the eye and ocular adnexa. Int J Radiat Oncol Biol Phys 32:1123-1140, 1995.
34. Cooper JS, Fu K, Marks J, Silverman S: Late effects of radiation in the head and neck region. Int J Radiat Oncol Biol Phys 31:1141-1164, 1995.
35. van den Maazen RWM, Kleiboer BJ, Berhagen I, van der Kogel AJ: Repair capacity of adult rat glial progenitor cells determined by an in vitro clonogenic assay after in vitro or in vivo fractionated irradiation. Int J Radiat Biol 63:661-666, 1993.

36. Calvo W, Hopewell JW, Reinhold HS, Yeung TK: Time-and dose-related changes in the white matter of the rat brain after single doses of x rays. Br J Radiol 61:1043-1052, 1988.
37. Schultheiss TE, Stephens LC: Permanent radiation myelopathy. Br J Radiol 65:737-753, 1992.
38. Jaenke RS, Robbins MEC, Bywaters T, et al: Capillary endothelium: target site of renal radiation injury. Lab Invest 57:551-565, 1993.
39. Moulder J, Robbins MEC, Cohen EP, et al: Pharmacologic modification of radiation-induced late normal tissue injury. *In* Mittal BB, Purdy JA, Ang KK (eds): Radiation Therapy. Norwell, MA, Kluwer, 1998, pp 129-151.
40. Tofilon PJ, Fike JR: The radioresponse of the central nervous system: a dynamic process. Radiat Res 153, 357-370. 2000.
41. Spence AM, Krohn KA, Edmonson SW, et al: Radioprotection in rat spinal cord with WR-2721 following cerebral lateral intraventricular injection. Int J Radiat Oncol Biol Phys 12:1479-1482, 1986.
42. Fike JR, Goebbel GT, Martob LJ, Seilhan TM: Radiation brain injury is reduced by the polyamine inhibitor alpha-difluoromethylornithine. Radiat Res 138:99-106. 1994.
43. Nakagawa M, Bellinzona M, Seilhan TM, et al: Microglial responses after focal radiation-induced injury are affected by alpha-difluoromethylornithine. Int J Radiat Oncol Biol Phys 36:113-123, 1996.
44. Hornsey S, Myers R, Jenkinson T: The reduction of radiation damage to the spinal cord by postirradiation administration of vasoactive drugs. Int J Radiat Oncol Biol Phys 18:1437-1442, 1990.
45. Hopewell JW, van den Aardweg GJMJ, Morris GM, et al: Unsaturated lipids as modulators of radiation damage in normal tissues. *In* Horrobin DF (ed): New Approaches to Cancer Treatment. London, Churchill Communications Europe, 1993, pp 88-106.
46. El-Agamawi AY, Hopewell JW, Plowman PN, et al: Modulation of normal tissue responses to radiation. Br J Radiol 69:374-375, 1996.
47. Rezvani M, Birds DA, Hodges H, et al: Modification of radiation myelopathy by the transplantation of neural stem cells in the rat. Radiat Res 156:408-412, 2002.
48. Monje ML, Mizumatsu S, Fike JR, Palmer T: Irradiation induced neural precursor-cell dysfunction. Nat Med 8:955-961, 2002.
49. Nieder C, Price RE, Rivera B, Ang KK: Both early and delayed treatment with growth factors can modulate the development of radiation myelopathy (RM) in rats. Radiother Oncol 56(Suppl 1):S15, 2000.
50. Lynch CD, Sonntag WE, Wheeler KT: Radiation-induced dementia in aged rats: effects of growth hormone and insulin-like growth factor 1. Neurooncology 4:354. 2002.
51. Cox JD, Stetz J, Pajak TF: Toxicity criteria of the Radiation Therapy Oncology Group and the European Organization for Research and Treatment of Cancer. Int J Radiat Oncol Biol Phys 31:1341-1346, 1995.
52. Pavy JJ, Denekamp J, Letschert J, et al: Late effects toxicity scoring: the SOMA scale. Int J Radiat Oncol Biol Phys 32:1043-1047, 1995.
53. Chuba PJ, Aronin P, Bhambhani K, et al: Hyperbaric oxygen therapy for radiation-induced brain injury in children. Cancer 30:2005-2012, 1997.
54. Liu CY, Yim BY, Wozniak AJ: Anticoagulation therapy for radiation-induced myelopathy. Ann Pharmacother 35:188-191, 2001.
55. Okunieff P, Augustine E, Hicks JE, et al: Pentoxifylline in the treatment of radiation-induced fibrosis. J Clin Oncol 22:2207-2213, 2004.
56. International Commission on Radiation Units and Measurements (ICRU): Prescribing, Recording, and Reporting Photon Beam Therapy: Report 50. Washington, DC, ICRU, 1993.
57. Kelly PJ, Daumas-Duport C, Scheithauer BW, et al: Stereotactic histologic correlations of CT and MRI defined abnormalities in patients with glial neoplasms. Mayo Clin Proc 62:450-459, 1987.
58. Karlsson UL, Leibel SA, Wallner K, et al: Brain. *In* Perez CA, Brady LW (eds): Principles and Practice of Radiation Oncology, 2nd ed. Philadelphia, JB Lippincott, 1992, pp 515-563.
59. Kun LE: Brain and spinal cord. *In* Cox JD (ed): Moss' Radiation Oncology: Rationale, Technique, Results, 7th ed. St. Louis, CV Mosby, 1994, pp 737-781.
60. Halperin EC, Constine LS, Tarbell NJ, Kun LE (eds): Pediatric Radiation Oncology, 2nd ed. New York, Raven Press, 1994.
61. Stieber VW, Munley MT: Central nervous system tumors. *In* Mundt AF, Roeske JC (eds): Intensity Modulated Radiation Therapy: A Clinical Perspective. Toronto, BC Decker, 2005, pp 231-241.
62. Suit H, Goldberg S, Niemierko A, et al: Proton beams to replace photon beams in radical dose treatments. Acta Oncol 42:800-808, 2003.
63. Bourland JD, McCollough KP: Static field conformal stereotactic radiosurgery: physical techniques. Int J Radiat Oncol Biol Phys 28:471-479, 1994.
64. Shrieve DC, Tarbell NJ, Alexander E, et al: Stereotactic radiotherapy: a technique for dose optimization and escalation for intracranial tumors. Acta Neurochir Suppl (Wien) 62:118-123, 1994.
65. Niemierko A: Treatment plan optimization. *In* Purdy JA, Emami B (eds): 3-D Radiation Treatment Planning and Conformal Therapy. Madison, WI, Medical Physics Publishing, 1995, pp 49-55.
66. Marks LB, Sherouse GW, Munley MT, et al: Incorporation of functional status into dose-volume analysis. Med Phys 26:196-199, 1999.
67. Cooley G, Gillin MT, Murray KJ, et al: Improved dose localization with dual energy photon irradiation in treatment of lateralized intracranial malignancies. Int J Radiat Oncol Biol Phys 20:815-821, 1991.

CHAPTER 23

LOW-GRADE GLIOMAS

Paul D. Brown and Edward G. Shaw

EPIDEMIOLOGY AND ETIOLOGY

The estimated annual incidence is 1800 cases. Etiologic factors are unknown. These tumors are seen with increased frequency in patients with types 1 and 2 neurofibromatosis.

PATHOLOGY

Most common pathologic types include pilocytic astrocytoma (World Health Organization [WHO] I), diffuse fibrillary astrocytoma, oligoastrocytoma, and oligodendroglioma (WHO II).

BIOLOGY

Increased proliferation, measured by Ki-67, or the presence of a mutant *p53* gene or protein, is associated with a worse outcome in some series. Both 1p and 19q deletions are associated with a superior outcome in anaplastic oligoastrocytoma and oligodendroglioma; similar evidence is accumulating for low-grade gliomas.

CLINICAL MANIFESTATIONS AND PATIENT EVALUATION

The mean age at presentation is 37 years.

The most common symptom is seizure.

Most patients do not have any signs of their disease (i.e., they are neurologically "intact").

Age is the most powerful clinical prognostic factor that affects survival. Children have a significantly better outcome than adults. Other prognostic factors associated with better overall and/or progression-free survival include oligodendroglioma histology and smaller tumor size.

The imaging features vary by pathologic type. Pilocytic astrocytomas are well circumscribed and contrast enhancing. Diffuse fibrillary astrocytomas are poorly circumscribed and nonenhancing, best seen on a T2-weighted or FLAIR (fluid-attenuated inversion recovery) magnetic resonance imaging scan.

PRIMARY THERAPY

Maximum surgical resection is associated with a more favorable outcome.

In pediatric low-grade glioma, after gross total resection, observation is recommended. After subtotal resection or biopsy, treatment (radiation therapy, chemotherapy) is usually deferred until the time of symptomatic imaging progression.

In adult low-grade glioma, after gross total resection of a pilocytic astrocytoma, observation is recommended. After gross total or subtotal resection (or biopsy) of a diffuse fibrillary astrocytoma, radiation may be given postoperatively or deferred until the time of imaging progression.

Recommended dose is 45-54 Gy in 25-30 fractions treating the MRI-defined tumor volume with a 2- to 3-cm margin.

Chemotherapy does not have a defined role in the management of adult low-grade glioma. The current European Organization for Research and Treatment of Cancer (EORTC) trial randomizes adult low-grade glioma patients with progressive disease, uncontrolled seizures despite anticonvulsants, or neurologic symptoms to standard radiotherapy or daily low-dose temozolomide. Patients will be stratified based on 1p status (intact versus deleted) as well as age, tumor size, and Karnofsky performance status. The primary end point is progression-free survival.

RECURRENT DISEASE

One cannot differentiate tumor recurrence from radionecrosis by clinical symptoms or signs or by conventional MRI or positron emission tomography.

Low-grade gliomas are a pathologically and clinically diverse group of uncommon central nervous system (CNS) tumors that occur primarily in children and young adults. Prognosis is principally affected by age and pathologic type. Studies assessing proliferation and molecular genetics may provide additional insight into prognostic groups that are at higher risk for developing tumor recurrence and therefore may benefit from adjunctive treatments such as radiation therapy (RT) and chemotherapy. In general, more extensive surgical resection is associated with better prognosis. The optimal timing of radiation, that is, "early" or postoperative versus "delayed" or at the time of tumor progression, remains to be determined, as does the role of chemotherapy.

In this chapter, a comprehensive overview of low-grade glioma is provided with an emphasis on adults. Topics covered include epidemiology, etiology, pathology, biology, clinical manifestations, patient evaluation, management (including surgery, RT, and chemotherapy), and radiation toxicity.

EPIDEMIOLOGY AND ETIOLOGY

In 2006 in the United States, it is estimated that 18,820 CNS tumors will be diagnosed,[1] of which approximately 16,400 will arise in the brain. Half of these will be gliomas, one fourth of which will be low grade, resulting in approximately 2000 new cases of low-grade gliomas per year.[2,3]

Etiologic factors for low-grade gliomas are largely unknown. Low-grade astrocytomas have been associated with von Recklinghausen's disease (type 1 neurofibromatosis) and type 2 neurofibromatosis.[4,5] In addition, a direct link has been made between subependymal giant cell astrocytoma, an uncommon pathologic type of low-grade astrocytoma, and tuberous sclerosis.[6-9]

PATHOLOGY

Pathologic Classification

Historically, low-grade gliomas have been thought of as a homogeneous group of neoplasms associated with a benign

Table 23-1 Low-Grade Gliomas* Included in World Health Organization (WHO) Classification of Gliomas

Type	WHO Grade
ASTROCYTIC TUMORS	
Astrocytomas	II
Fibrillary	
Gemistocytic	
Protoplasmic	
Pilocytic astrocytomas	I
Pleomorphic xanthoastrocytomas	II
Subependymal giant cell astrocytomas	I
Subependymomas	I
OLIGODENDROGLIAL TUMORS	
Oligodendrogliomas	I, II
MIXED GLIAL TUMORS	
Mixed oligoastrocytomas	I, II

*Exclusive of ependymal and glioneuronal neoplasms.

From Kleihues P, Burger PC, Scheithauer BW: Histologic Typing of Tumours of the Central Nervous System, 2nd ed. Berlin, Springer, 1993. Copyright 1993 Springer-Verlag.

or favorable natural history.[10,11] Actually, they are a diverse group of tumors found throughout the CNS whose outcome depends on a number of anatomic, pathologic, and treatment factors.

Table 23-1 summarizes the current WHO classification of primary CNS tumors as it applies to low-grade gliomas.[12,13] Astrocytic tumors can be classified broadly into three groups. The diffusely infiltrative low-grade astrocytomas are the most common and include the fibrillary, protoplasmic, and gemistocytic types (hereafter called the *diffuse astrocytomas*). They represent 70% of low-grade cerebral astrocytomas.[14] Diffuse astrocytomas are usually poorly circumscribed and are capable of undergoing anaplastic transformation with an incidence as high as 79%.[15] The pilocytic astrocytomas, which comprise nearly all the remainder of the cerebral astrocytomas, tend to be better circumscribed and rarely transform.[16] Although pilocytic astrocytomas occur more commonly in the cerebellum of children (juvenile pilocytic astrocytoma), several series have described the behavior of these tumors in the cerebral hemispheres.[17-19] Remaining are the uncommon low-grade glioma variants, including the pleomorphic xanthoastrocytomas,[20,21] subependymal giant cell astrocytomas,[6,8] subependymomas,[22] and others, which are discussed later in the chapter.

Grading Systems

The concept of dividing astrocytomas into discrete grades associated with a distinct clinical prognosis dates back to the mid-1920s and early 1930s and the work of Bailey and Cushing, who recognized a subset of astrocytomas that had a more favorable outcome than glioblastoma.[23,24] There have been many grading systems (e.g., Kernohan, St. Anne-Mayo, and Ringertz)[12,25-28] in the past, and most of these grading systems share an assessment of nuclear abnormalities, mitoses, endothelial proliferation, and necrosis, but the most widely used and accepted grading system today is the WHO[13] (Table 23-2). Although three-tier grading schemes such as that of the WHO[13] are the most widely used and accepted, all grading schemes are limited by their need to separate gliomas artificially into three or four groups, when, in fact, they exist along a biologic continuum. For the present, these proven but awkward methods retain their utility in both therapeutic decision making and prognostication. It is anticipated in future reiterations of the WHO grading system there will be incorporation of imaging and genetic testing.

BIOLOGIC CHARACTERISTICS

Since the 1990s, our understanding of the biology of low-grade astrocytomas has increased. This has included studies of DNA content, tumor proliferation, and both cytogenetic and molecular genetic studies.

Studies of Ploidy and Proliferation

In four separate series reporting the DNA content of 155 low-grade gliomas, the ratio of diploid to aneuploid tumors was approximately 2:1.[29-32] In the series by Danova and colleagues,[30] patients with all grades of astrocytoma had better survival if their tumors were DNA diploid versus aneuploid. However, Coons and associates[31] noted a weaker association between ploidy and survival, with aneuploid tumors having a similar or better survival than diploid tumors.

The assessment of tumor proliferation may offer greater insight into the malignant potential of the low-grade gliomas. Various methods are used to measure proliferation, including the use of Ki-67, a nuclear proliferation marker. Montine and colleagues,[33] using the Ki-67 proliferation index, observed a median value of 2.1% for 11 low-grade astrocytomas. All seven patients whose proliferation index was less than 3% were alive at the time of last follow-up, whereas only one of four patients whose index was more than 3% was alive. These authors also found that the proliferation index was more significantly related to survival than pathologic grade. McKeever and associates[34] found Ki-67 to be a superior predictor of survival compared with other markers of proliferation such as bromodeoxyuridine. However, Fisher and associates[35] found in their review of the Ki-67 index for 180 low-grade glioma patients that Ki-67 was not an independent prognostic factor and did not predict which patients would benefit from postoperative RT.

Genetic and Other Molecular Studies

The most common molecular genetic alteration, present in 30% to 45% of low-grade astrocytomas, occurs on the p arm of chromosome 17, which is where the tumor suppressor gene *TP53* resides. Its protein, p53, has multiple functions involved in the regulation of cell growth, apoptosis, transcription, and malignant transformation.[36]

Lang and colleagues[37] detected *TP53* mutations in 3 of 15 (20%) low-grade astrocytomas and mutant p53 protein accumulation in 5 of 8 (63%). Although these investigators could not explain the aberrant expression of p53 protein in the absence of a *TP53* gene mutation, they postulated that loss of p53 function in low-grade astrocytomas could be a predisposing factor for the accumulation of genetic damage leading to the progression of low-grade astrocytoma to glioblastoma.

Stander and colleagues[38] retrospectively assessed *TP53* mutation status and p53 expression/accumulation for 159 consecutive adult patients with heterogeneously treated low-grade astrocytoma or oligoastrocytoma. *TP53* mutations were present in 49% of all tumors, and p53 overexpression/accumulation was seen in 47% of patients. p53 overexpression/accumulation correlated with *TP53* status and was present in 93% of tumors with *TP53* mutations but was present in only 3% of tumors without *TP53* mutations. Positive *TP53*

Table 23-2 Comparison Grading for the Diffuse Astrocytomas

Grading Systems*	Grade 1	Grade 2	Grade 3	Grade 4
Kernohan[25]	Cells: no anaplasia Cellularity: mild Mitoses: none Vessels: minimal endothelial or adventitial proliferation Transition zone to normal brain: broad	Cells: most appear normal, anaplasia in small numbers Cellularity: mild Mitoses: none Vessels: as in grade 1 Transition zone: less broad	Cells: anaplasia in half of cells Cellularity: increased Mitoses: present Vessels: more frequent endothelial and adventitial proliferation Necrosis: frequent, regional Transition zone: narrowed	Cells: extensive anaplasia, few "normal" appearing Cellularity: marked Mitoses: numerous Vessels: marked proliferation Necrosis: extensive Transitional zone: may be sharply demarcated
WHO[13]	Pilocytic astrocytoma	Astrocytoma: tumor composed of astrocytes (fibrillary, protoplasmic, gemistocytic, giant cell, and combinations thereof); atypia evident, but no mitoses	Anaplastic astrocytoma: astrocytoma showing mitotic activity; such tumors are not difficult to distinguish from glioblastoma	Glioblastoma: anaplastic tumor, usually astrocytic, with high cellularity, endothelial proliferation, or necrosis with pseudopalisading
St. Anne-Mayo	None of the following four criteria: Nuclear abnormalities Mitoses Endothelial proliferation Necrosis	One criterion	Two criteria	Three or four criteria
Ringertz	Astrocytoma: tumor showing infiltrative growth pattern and mild to moderate hypercellularity; cytologic features resembling normal astrocytes with only mild nuclear abnormalities	Anaplastic astrocytoma: cellular infiltrative astrocytic tumor containing astrocytes with moderate pleomorphism; mitoses and moderate vascular proliferation may be seen but necrosis is absent		Glioblastoma multiforme: markedly pleomorphic astrocytic tumor with high cellularity, frequent mitoses, increased vascularity and necrosis; may show limited infiltration

Modified from Kleihues P, Burger PC, Scheithauer BW: Histologic Typing of Tumours of the Central Nervous System, 2nd ed. Berlin, Springer, 1993.

mutation status (but not p53 overexpression/accumulation) was found to be an independent unfavorable predictor of survival, progression-free survival, and time to malignant transformation. Chozick and colleagues[39] postulated that the accumulation of mutant p53 protein, or the inactivation of wild-type p53 protein, may predict poor survival in patients with astrocytomas. These workers observed accumulation of abnormal p53 protein in 29% of 81 patients with grade 2 astrocytomas; the 4-year survival of these patients was 25%, compared with 87% for those who did not accumulate abnormal p53 protein. Other than age, p53 status was the most significant prognostic factor predictive of survival in a multivariate analysis. In a review of 59 oligodendrogliomas (33 low-grade), p53 accumulation and mutations (along with grade) were found to be independent prognostic factors for poorer survival.[40]

Ritland and associates[41] observed allelic loss for chromosome 19 loci in 2 of 18 (11%) patients with grade 1, 2, and 3 astrocytomas compared with 21 of 54 (39%) patients with grade 4 astrocytomas. In most of these instances, the deletion was in the p arm of chromosome 19. These authors postulated that a tumor suppressor gene important in the malignant transformation of low-grade to high-grade astrocytomas may reside on chromosome 19p.

1p and 19q loss has become an established prognostic marker for anaplastic oligodendrogliomas,[42] and data also suggest a correlation between 1p and 19q loss and outcome for low-grade oligodendrogliomas. A prospective study of temozolomide in 60 patients with low-grade oligodendrogliomas and oligoastrocytomas found loss of 1p correlated with objective tumor response.[43] Buckner and colleagues[44] used FISH to analyze 1p19q status of 100 low-grade glioma patients enrolled on two North Central Cancer Treatment Group (NCCTG) protocols. 1p and 19q deletion was seen in 56%, 33%, and 5% of oligodendrogliomas, oligoastrocytomas, and astrocytomas, respectively. Both 1p and 19q loss was associated with superior 5-year progression free survival and overall survival in oligodendroglioma and oligoastrocytoma patients. Median survival with and without 1p and 19q deletion was 13 years versus 11 years for oligodendroglioma patients and was 11.7 years versus 7.3 years for patients with oligoastrocytomas.

O^6-Methylguanine-DNA methyltransferase (MGMT) is a DNA-repair enzyme that removes alkyl groups from the O^6 position of guanine in DNA and therefore repairs damage induced by alkylating agents (e.g., BCNU, temozolomide). Malignant gliomas that express high levels of *MGMT* are known to have worse outcomes.[45,46] Promoter methylation results in epigenetic silencing and thereby decreased *MGMT* expression, which is associated with longer survival in patients with glioblastoma who receive alkylating agents. Hegi and colleagues[47] determined the methylation status of the *MGMT* promoter by methylation-specific polymerase chain reaction (PCR) analysis in glioblastoma patients enrolled in a randomized trial comparing RT alone with RT combined with concomitant and adjuvant treatment with temozolomide. The *MGMT* promoter was methylated in 45% of 206 assessable cases. Irrespective of treatment, *MGMT* promoter methylation was an independent favorable prognostic factor. Among patients whose tumor contained a methylated *MGMT* promoter, a survival benefit was observed in the temozolomide and RT arm with a 2-year survival of 46% compared with 23% in the RT arm. In the absence of methylation of the *MGMT* promoter, there was a smaller and statistically insignificant difference in survival between the treatment groups.

Although little data pertaining to *MGMT* are available for patients with low-grade gliomas, it is expected in the future that there will be much research activity in this arena. One small study using PCR found *MGMT* promoter methylation in 21 of 49 low-grade gliomas.[48] A tight correlation existed between *MGMT* methylation and p53 protein accumulation, and the presence of *MGMT* methylation was significantly associated with a shorter progression-free survival. The authors noted that the presence of *MGMT* methylation predicted an increased sensitivity to alkylating chemotherapeutic agents, and therefore earlier chemotherapy could serve to improve an unfavorable natural history in low-grade gliomas with *MGMT* methylation.

Growth factor expression may be prognostic for survival in patients with low-grade astrocytomas. Abdulrauf and associates[49] found a significant correlation in both univariate and multivariate analyses between vascular endothelial growth factor (VEGF) expression and survival in a series of 74 adults with supratentorial cerebral low-grade diffuse astrocytomas. Median survival was 11.2 years in VEGF-positive patients compared with 5.3 years in those who were VEGF negative. Other growth factors, such as basic fibroblastic growth factor and epidermal growth factor, did not affect survival.

Immunohistochemical techniques also have been used to study the ontogeny of glial cells and have identified two lineages of astrocytes derived from distinct progenitor cells. Type II or fibrillary astrocytes are found in white matter and are derived from 02A cells, a bipotential precursor that can differentiate toward astrocytes or oligodendrocytes; type I or protoplasmic astrocytes reside in the cortex and are derived from a separate precursor cell. Type I and type II astrocytes express unique antigens that permit their characterization. Low-grade astrocytomas arising from the type I astrocyte lineage are associated with a more indolent clinical course, whereas those arising from the type II astrocyte lineage behave more aggressively.[50,51]

Clinically, the molecular and cellular biologic characterization of low-grade astrocytomas may help to predict which patients are more likely to require earlier and more aggressive therapy. Conversely, it may help determine which patients may be observed initially, withholding treatment until the time of disease progression. It is expected the knowledge in this field will continue to grow rapidly.

CLINICAL MANIFESTATIONS AND PATIENT EVALUATION

In this section, information is reviewed on the clinical presentation and imaging of supratentorial low-grade gliomas based on information from collected series in the literature reviewed by Shaw and associates.[52]

Clinical Presentation

Low-grade gliomas are generally a disease of patients in their 20s, 30s, or 40s with a mean age at presentation of 37 years. Cases have been reported in patients as young as 7 months and as old as 78 years. Low-grade astrocytomas are more common in men than in women by a ratio of 1.4:1.

The symptoms of low-grade astrocytomas are shown in Table 23-3. The most common symptom is seizure, occurring in two thirds of patients. Focal seizures are more common than generalized ones. Generalized tonic-clonic, simple partial, and complex partial seizures occur in 43%, 23%, and 34% of patients, respectively. Headache and weakness occur in approximately one third of patients. The remaining symptoms occur in 15% or fewer of patients with low-grade astrocytoma. The median duration from onset of symptoms to diagnosis is between 6 and 17 months, with a range of 1 day to 17 years.

The neurologic signs associated with low-grade astrocytomas have not been as rigorously reported in the literature as have neurologic symptoms. About one half of affected patients are reported to be neurologically intact—that is, have a normal neurologic examination. The frequency of other signs at presentation is as follows: sensory or motor deficit, 42%; altered mental status, 23%; papilledema, 22%; aphasia, dysphasia, or decreased memory, 20%; focal deficit, 15%; altered consciousness, 8%; and motor deficit, 8%. Overall, neurologic function is considered normal or mildly symptomatic or impaired in 63% of patients, moderately symptomatic or impaired in 25% of patients, and severely symptomatic or impaired in the remaining 12%.

Age, sex, symptoms, signs, and neurologic function have all been significantly associated with survival in univariate and multivariate analyses from a number of retrospective studies in the literature. Both preoperative and postoperative neurologic function and performance status are correlated with outcome.[15,53-58] Brown and colleagues[58] conducted an

Table 23-3 Symptoms of Low-Grade Astrocytomas

Symptom	Frequency (%) Mean	Range
Seizure	65	30-92
Headache	36	5-48
Weakness	30	6-53
Visual loss or change	15	4-16
Personality change	14	5-16
Focal symptom, NOS	13	6-20
Language dysfunction	13	4-17
Altered sensation	10	8-11
Nausea and vomiting	10	4-14
Altered mental status	9	7-12
Altered consciousness	8	4-20
Cranial neuropathy, NOS	7	—

NOS, not otherwise specified; —, data reported in only one series.

Data from Levin VA, Gutin PH, Leibel S: Neoplasms of the central nervous system. *In* DeVita V, Hellman J, Rosenberg S (eds): Cancer: Principles and Practice of Oncology, 4th ed. Philadelphia, JB Lippincott, 1993.

Table 23-4 Survival of Children with Low-Grade Astrocytoma

Series	*n*	Age (y)	5-y Survival (%)	10-y Survival (%)
North et al[59]	25	<20	79	NR‡
Dewit et al[60]	35*	8-14	94	82
Bloom et al[61]	72*	<15	80	75
Hoffman et al[62]	88*†	≤18	91	80
Pollack et al[63]	71	≤18	95	93

*Indicates that some posterior fossa tumors and pilocytic astrocytomas were included.
†Includes only midline tumors.
‡Data not reported.

Table 23-5 Imaging Characteristics of Supratentorial Low-Grade Astrocytoma

Characteristics	Frequency (%) Mean	Range
LOCATION		
Lobar	80	50-90
Deep/midline*	20	4-40
Right	50	42-55
Left	50	41-60
Bilateral	5	1-11
Hemispheric†	0.5	—
LOBAR SITES		
Single	84	—
Multiple	16	13-38
Frontal	44	38-65
Temporal	37	8-61
Parietal	18	5-40
Occipital	3	0-10
OTHER		
Enhancement	34	22-58
Size ≥5 cm	66	21-88
Calcification	10	3-18
Cyst	15	6-29
Mass effect‡	—	12-84

*Deep/midline sites include thalamus, basal ganglia, hypothalamus, third ventricle, and corpus callosum.
†Only one series presented data on hemispheric involvement.[56]
‡Only two series presented data on mass effect.[79,83]
From Shaw EG, Scheithauer BW, Dinapoli PR: Low-grade hemispheric astrocytomas. *In* Black PM, Loeffler JS (eds): Cancer of the Nervous System. Cambridge, Blackwell Scientific Publications, 1997.

analysis of baseline (before RT) Mini-Mental State Examination (MMSE) scores collected in patients with low-grade glioma on a prospective, intergroup clinical trial and found the presence of an abnormal baseline MMSE score (26 or less) was a strong predictor of worse outcome on univariate and multivariate analyses. Patients with an abnormal baseline MMSE score had a worse 5-year progression-free survival rate (27% versus 60%) and overall survival rate (31% versus 76%) compared with those with a normal score. Sex also appears to correlate with outcome, with female patients having a better survival than male patients.[55,57,59]

The most powerful predictor of survival in patients with low-grade glioma is age. Table 23-4 shows the survival of children with low-grade astrocytoma. The average 5- and 10-year survival rates from these series are 90% and 86%, respectively.[59-65] In one series, children younger than 5 years had a worse survival than those 5 years and older.[65] For adult patients with low-grade astrocytoma, there is also an association between age and survival. Those who are less than 40 years of age have a better survival than patients 40 years of age and older.[54,56,66-68] Piepmeier[66] reported a mean survival time of 8.5 years in his younger adult population (<40) versus 4.9 years for those 40 and older. In a more recent series, Leighton and associates[68] observed a median survival time of 10.7 years compared with 8.1 years for adults up to 40 years versus more than 40 years old, respectively.

Of all the neurologic symptoms associated with low-grade astrocytoma, seizures, particularly when preceding the diagnosis by 6 months or more and in the absence of other neurologic symptoms, are associated with a better prognosis.[53,54,59] In one series, the 5-year survival rate was 47% in patients presenting with seizures, 33% in those with headaches, 20% in those with altered mental status, and 0% when stupor was the presenting symptom.[69] In another series, the 5-year survival rate was 64% in patients with low-grade glioma who had seizures, compared with 14% in those without seizures.[70]

Patients who present with a history of chronic epilepsy resulting from an underlying cerebral neoplasm are frequently found to have a low-grade astrocytoma. These patients are usually children or young adults (30 years of age or younger) whose seizure disorder and underlying tumor are often cured by a complete resection.[71-73]

Imaging of Low-Grade Gliomas

Table 23-5 shows the imaging characteristics of supratentorial low-grade astrocytomas based on multiple series in the literature.[15,53,54,56,57,59,66,69,74-83] On computed tomography (CT), the typical low-grade astrocytoma is lobar in location, involves the frontal or temporal lobes, is larger than 5 cm in diameter, and is nonenhancing with the administration of intravenous contrast material. Because of the infiltrative nature of low-grade astrocytomas, the CT appearance of a typical nonenhancing tumor is a poorly defined area of low attenuation (Fig. 23-1A).

MRI (see Fig. 23-1B) has contributed to the diagnosis and treatment of low-grade astrocytomas. Both T2- and T1-weighted images (without and with contrast) provide anatomic detail that is useful in defining the extent of the tumor and for surgical and RT planning.

Daumas-Duport and Kelly and their colleagues performed imaging-histologic correlations of both CT and MRI scans in patients with astrocytic neoplasms of the brain who were undergoing stereotactic biopsies.[84,85] Three types of tumors can be identified, correlating with the three morphologic types of low-grade gliomas (Fig. 23-2). The CT (MRI) scan appearance of a type I tumor is that of a well-circumscribed area of contrast enhancement in the absence of surrounding low-attenuation change or edema (increased T2 signal). Pilocytic astrocytomas typically have this appearance (Fig. 23-3). The CT (MRI) scan appearance of a type II tumor is that of a poorly defined area of low attenuation (increased T2 signal) that contains a focal area of contrast enhancement (Fig. 23-4). The type II tumors are the 34% subset of low-grade astrocytomas that enhance (see Table 23-5). The CT (MRI) scan appearance of a type III tumor, which characterizes two thirds of low-grade gliomas, is that of a poorly defined area of low attenuation (increased T2 signal), as shown in Figure 23-1.

Stereotactic biopsy-histologic correlations have helped to define the underlying histopathologic features of type I, II, and

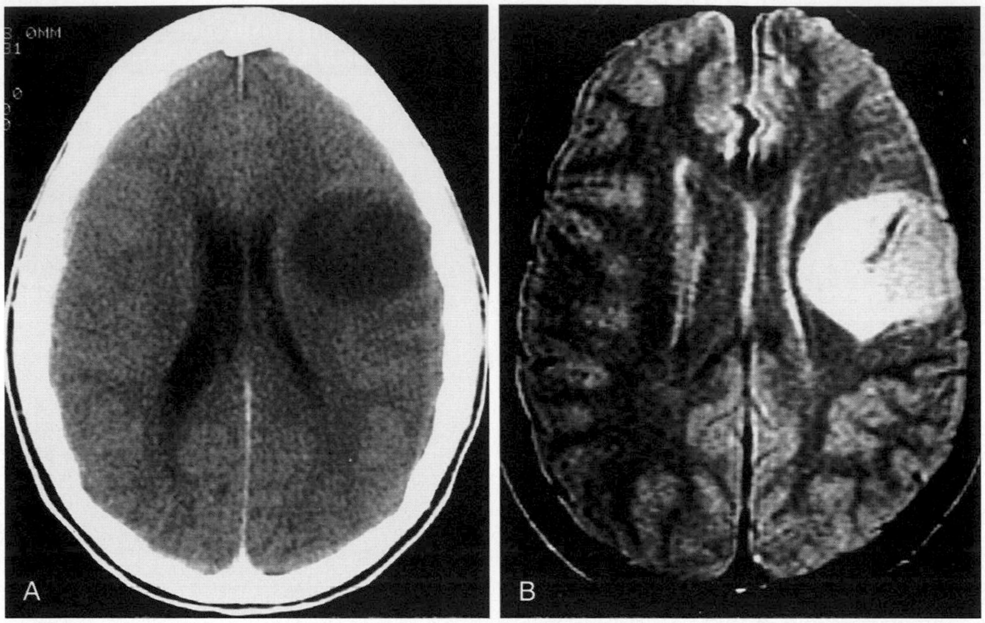

Figure 23-1 Postcontrast CT (**A**) and T1-weighted MRI (**B**) of an adult with a nonenhancing posterior left frontal WHO II astrocytoma.

Spatial configuration	Solid tumor tissue	Isolated tumor cells*
Type I ●	+	0
Type II	+	+
Type III	0	+

*Within intact parenchyma

Figure 23-2 Morphology of low-grade gliomas based on CT-histologic correlates, Adapted from Daumas-Duport C, Scheithauer BW, Kelly PJ: A histologic and cytologic method for spatial definition of gliomas. Mayo Clin Proc 62:435-449, 1987; Kelly PJ, Daumas-Duport C, Scheithauer BW, et al: Stereotactic histologic correlations of computed tomography and magnetic resonance imaging–defined abnormalities in patients with glial neoplasms. Mayo Clin Proc 62:450-459, 1987.

III tumors. Type I tumors comprise solid tumor tissue embedded in normal surrounding brain parenchyma. The contrast-enhanced portion of type II tumors also contains solid tumor tissue, whereas the surrounding low-attenuation area on a CT scan or the area of increased signal on a T2-weighted MR image contains intact brain parenchyma infiltrated by tumor cells. Type III tumors are characterized by intact parenchyma infiltrated by tumor cells in the absence of any focal areas of solid tumor tissue. Generally, the MRI scan defines a larger area of increased signal on T2-weighted images for both type II and III tumors in comparison with CT. In addition, microscopic tumor cells may extend several centimeters beyond the MRI-defined limits of the abnormalities seen in type II and III tumors.[85]

An understanding of these imaging-based anatomic-histopathologic relationships is important for both the neurosurgeon and the radiation oncologist. Removal of the CT nonenhancing portion of a type II or III tumor in a patient whose tumor is located in a functionally intact area of brain may lead to significant neurologic morbidity, whereas removal of the enhancing portion of a type I tumor should not, even in deep locations such as the thalamus or basal ganglia.[86] For the radiation oncologist treating a patient with a type II or III tumor, the initial treatment volume should include the MRI-based tumor extent, as defined by the T2-weighted MRI scan, with several centimeters of surrounding normal brain tissue as "margin," whereas a type I tumor could be irradiated with a minimal margin (1 cm or less) or conceivably by focal treatments such as stereotactic radiosurgery or brachytherapy.

The radiographic features of low-grade gliomas have been correlated with prognosis in a number of retrospective series. Single-lobe (versus multiple-lobe) involvement, a lobar site versus involvement of deep sites, and frontal or temporal location as opposed to parietal and occipital location have all been associated with a better prognosis.[59,83] Although the presence of contrast enhancement on a CT scan in nonpilocytic low-grade gliomas would seemingly be associated with worse prognosis because of presumed higher-grade elements or malignant transformation, the data from multiple series are mixed in that some associate contrast enhancement with a worse outcome,[54,57,66,69,87] whereas other series have found no difference in survival.[74,76,81,83] Other imaging findings, such as tumor size greater than 5 cm or the presence of mass effect, have been associated with worse outcome.[55,80,81] One series showed that the presence of a cyst predicted a more favorable outcome.[66]

Pignatti and colleagues[88] developed a prognostic scoring system using imaging, patient, and tumor characteristics derived from the databases of two large phase III adult low-grade glioma trials: European Organization for Research and Treatment of Cancer (EORTC) trial 22844 and EORTC trial 22845. By means of Cox regression, they identified and validated the following negative risk factors: age 40 years or more, astrocytoma histology subtype, largest diameter of the tumor of 6 cm or more, tumor crossing the midline, and presence of neurologic deficit before surgery. The total number of unfavorable factors present was found to be useful in predicting outcome. The presence of two of these factors or less identi-

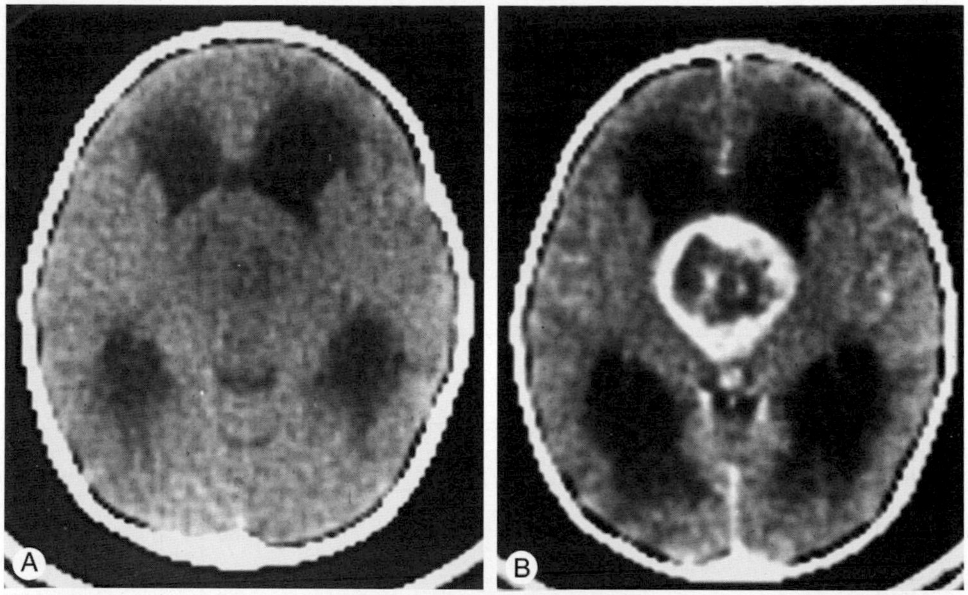

Figure 23-3 Precontrast (**A**) and postcontrast (**B**) CT scans of an 18-month-old child with a WHO I (pilocytic) astrocytoma of the third ventricle.

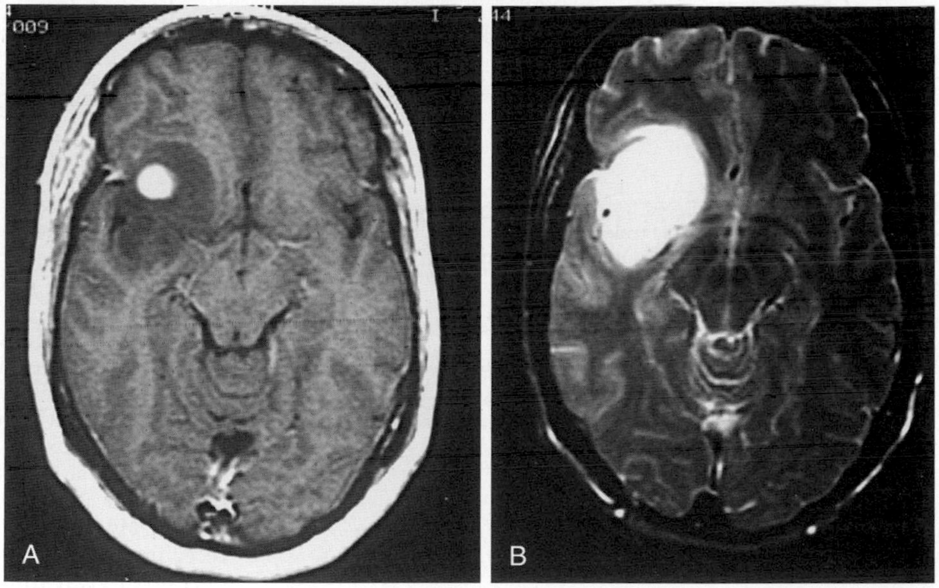

Figure 23-4 (**A**) Postgadolinium T1-weighted and T2-weighted (**B**) MRI scans of an adult with a WHO II astrocytoma of the right posterior frontal lobe.

fied a low-risk group (median survival, 7.7 years), whereas three risk factors or more identified a high-risk group (median survival, 3.2 years).

PRIMARY THERAPY OPTIONS

Observation

The decision to observe a low-grade glioma, either a presumed tumor based on clinical presentation and imaging findings or a histologically verified tumor, has been justified in the literature for several reasons. Reasons include the relatively favorable natural history of the disease, the lack of proven benefit for invasive interventions such as surgical resection or RT, and the potential morbidities of treatment.[80,89-92]

Despite the favorable survival observed in certain subsets of patients with low-grade glioma, the natural history of all pathologic types of supratentorial low-grade gliomas, including the pilocytic astrocytomas (WHO I), diffuse astrocytomas, oligoastrocytomas, and oligodendrogliomas (WHO II), is significantly worse than that of an age- and sex-matched control population, for which the expected survival is greater than 95%[10,91] (Table 23-6 and Fig. 23-5). Based on this observation, some have argued that all such patients should undergo maximally safe surgical resection followed by postoperative RT,[93] although a survival benefit for treatment, with either aggressive surgery or RT, even though suggested by the retrospective literature (see next two sections), has not been demonstrated in prospective clinical trials.

The Radiation Therapy Oncology Group (RTOG) phase II portion of protocol 9802 prospectively observed 111 low-risk (age younger than 40 years and gross total resection) low-grade glioma patients after gross total resection.[94] Histology and preoperative tumor diameter were found to be predictive of outcome. The 2- and 5-year progression-free survival rates were 93% and 78% for oligodendrogliomas (or oligo-dominant

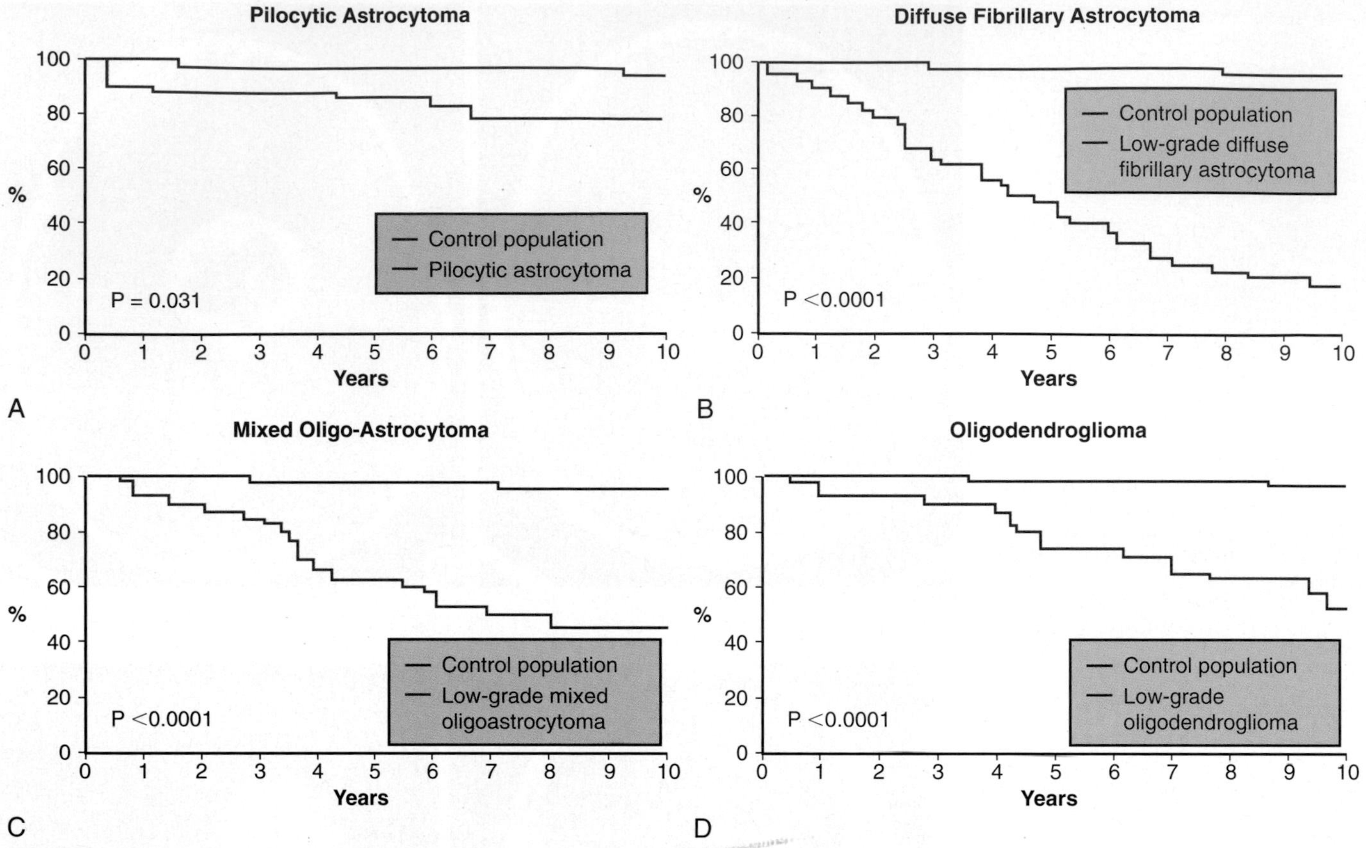

Figure 23-5 Survival curves for patients with the various subtypes of low-grade glioma compared with curves for an age- and sex-matched control population. **A,** WHO I (pilocytic) astrocytoma. **B,** WHO II (diffuse fibrillary) astrocytoma. **C,** WHO III (mixed) oligoastrocytoma, **D,** WHO II oligodendroglioma, **A–D,** Adapted from Shaw EG: The low-grade glioma debate: evidence defending the position of early radiation therapy. Clin Neurosurg 42:488-494, 1995.

Table 23-6 Survival of Supratentorial Low-Grade Gliomas, Mayo Experience

	Histologic Type			
Survival	**Pilo-A**	**Diff-A**	**OA**	**O**
Median (y)	—	4.7	7.1	9.8
2 y (%)	88	80	89	93
5 y (%)	85	46	63	73
10 y (%)	79	17	33	49
15 y (%)	79	7	17	49

A, astrocytoma: Diff, diffuse; O, oligodendroglioma; OA, oligoastrocytoma; Pilo, pilocytic.

Data from Shaw EG, Scheithauer BW, O'Fallon JR: Supratentorial gliomas: a comparative study by grade and histologic type. J Neurooncol 31:273-278, 1997; and Shaw E: The low-grade glioma debate: evidence defending the position of early radiation therapy. Clin Neurosurg 42:488-494, 1995.

mixed oligoastrocytomas) of less than 4 cm compared with 67% and 34% for diffuse astrocytomas (or astro-dominant mixed oligoastrocytomas) of 4 cm or greater. These data suggest observation is a reasonable strategy for some subsets of younger patients after a gross total resection of a low-grade glioma, but postoperative adjuvant treatment should be considered for higher-risk patients (i.e., large diffuse astrocytomas).

The EORTC has conducted a Phase III randomized trial (22845) in adults with supratentorial low-grade gliomas of all histologic types (excluding pilocytic astrocytomas) in which 311 patients were randomized to either observation with RT at progression (which should be considered a delayed RT arm since two thirds of the patients in the observation group received RT at the time of progression) or initial RT using 54 Gy to localized treatment fields.[95] The 5-year progression-free survival rate was significantly better for the patients receiving initial RT (55% versus 35%). However, median overall survival time was not affected (7.4 years versus 7.2 years). In patients still progression free at 2 years, there were no differences between the groups with respect to cognitive deficits, performance status, and headache. These data suggest that observation is a reasonable strategy in adults with asymptomatic supratentorial low-grade glioma.

Surgery

The key surgical issues in the management of supratentorial low-grade gliomas are twofold. The first issue is whether to perform a biopsy on a patient whose clinical presentation and imaging studies suggest a low-grade glioma. When a histologic diagnosis is established, the issue becomes whether to attempt gross total resection of the tumor.

Two series in the literature suggest that as many as half of patients with an imaging diagnosis of low-grade diffuse astrocytoma do not have pathologic confirmation of a low-grade tumor. Wilden and Kelly[96] reviewed their results in 35 patients who presented with a seizure disorder plus a nonenhancing tumor on CT scans. Stereotactic biopsy results revealed a low-grade glioma (astrocytoma, oligoastrocytoma, or oligodendroglioma) in 26 patients (73%), a high-grade glioma in 6 patients (18%), and a ganglioglioma in 2 patients (6%). Three patients had subsequent surgical resection confirming their stereotactic biopsy result. In another series with a similar outcome, Kondziolka and colleagues[97] reported the stereotactic biopsy results in 20 adults with CT evidence of a lobar, nonenhancing low-attenuation lesion. Seventeen of the 20 patients presented with a seizure. Only half the patients had a low-grade astrocytoma by stereotactic biopsy. Nine others (45%) had an anaplastic astrocytoma, and one patient (5%) had encephalitis.

Although one series in the literature suggests that the survival of patients irradiated for presumed low-grade glioma is comparable to that of patients irradiated for histologically verified low-grade astrocytoma,[98] the possibility of inappropriate management in 25% to 50% of cases underscores the need for histologic verification. For instance, patients with higher-grade astrocytomas typically receive high-dose external beam RT in addition to alkylating agents (e.g., temozolomide), whereas gross total resection without adjuvant RT constitutes curative treatment for a ganglioglioma.

In the largest neurosurgical series in the medical literature on the survival of patients with low-grade astrocytoma, Laws and associates[53] reported a significant increase in survival based on the calendar year the surgery was performed. Those patients operated on before 1950 had a 24% 5-year survival compared with those operated on between 1950 and 1975, in whom the 5-year survival was approximately 40% ($P < .0001$).

Extent of Resection

Table 23-7 summarizes the outcome by extent of surgery in "contemporary" (i.e., operated on in or later than 1950) supratentorial low-grade glioma series, with an emphasis on diffuse astrocytomas and oligoastrocytomas.[56,57,59,64,66,68,69,75,81,83,99-102] Collectively, the results show that 39% of patients with supratentorial low-grade gliomas underwent gross total or major subtotal resection, 23% underwent subtotal resection (not otherwise specified), and 38% had minor subtotal resection or a biopsy. Nine of the series demonstrated a significant survival advantage for gross total or major subtotal resection compared with minor subtotal resection or biopsy.[56,59,64,69,83,99-102] In the more aggressively operated patients in these series, the average 5-year survival rate was 87% (range, 82% to 100%), whereas the comparable survival rate was 60% in the less aggressively operated patients (range, 24% to 64%). Three other series did not find a significant difference in survival based on the extent of surgical resection.[66,75,81]

The surgical data are similar for the low-grade oligodendrogliomas (Table 23-8). In all three series, a significant survival benefit was seen in patients who underwent more aggressive surgery.[103-105] For both astrocytomas and oligodendrogliomas, it is important to recognize an inherent bias asso-

Table 23-7 Outcome by Extent of Surgical Resection in Contemporary Supratentorial Low-Grade Glioma Series (Mostly Diffuse Astrocytoma and Oligoastrocytoma)

Authors	Years of Study	Histologic Types Included	SURGICAL DATA Extent of Resection	*n*	SURVIVAL Median (y)	5-y (%)	10-y (%)	*P* Value
Westergaard et al[99]	1956-1991	A	Radical	218	5.9	—	—	.058
			Not radical		3.7	—	—	
Shaw et al[75]	1960-1982	A, OA	GTR; STR+	23	5.2	52	21	.82
			STR–; Bx	103	5.2	51	24	
Shibamoto et al[81]	1965-1989	A, OA	Extensive	15	—	64	56	.3
			Not extensive	86	—	59	39	
Reichenthal et al[69]	1970-1982	A	STR+	45	—	57	—	—
			STR–; Bx	11	—	38	—	
Janny et al[83]	1970-1989	A, OA	GTR; STR+	10	—	88	68	.03
			STR–; Bx	22	—	57	31	
North et al[59]	1975-1984	A, OA, PA	GTR	6	—	85	—	.002
			STR	62	—	64	—	
			Bx	9	—	43	—	
Piepmeier[66]	1975-1985	A, OA	GTR	19	8.5	—	—	.832
			STR	17	7.2	—	—	
			Bx	13	6.2	—	—	
Philippon et al[56]	1978-1987	A	GTR	45	—	80	—	<.001
			STR	95	—	—	—	
			Bx	39	—	45	—	
Nicolato et al[100]	1977-1989	A	GTR	17	—	87	—	.0001
			STR	59	—	26	—	
Piepmeier et al[102]	1982-1990	A	GTR	31	NR	—	—	.0013
			STR; Bx	24	12.0	—	—	
Bahary et al[101]	1974-1992	A, OA	GTR	14	NR	86	—	.002
			STR	34	10.8	74	—	
			Bx	15	4.2	38	—	
Scerrati et al[64]	1978-1989	A, OA, O	GTR	76	NR	100	76	<.001
			STR+	31	NR	94	71	
			STR–	24	8.0	92	21	
Leighton et al[68]	1979-1995	A, OA	GTR; STR+	128	10.7	82	59	.006
			STR–	101	8.4	64	41	

A, astrocytoma; Bx, biopsy; GTR, gross total resection; O, oligodendroglioma; OA, oligoastrocytoma; PA, pilocytic astrocytoma; STR+, more extensive subtotal resection; STR, extent of subtotal resection not reported; STR–, less extensive subtotal resection; —, data not reported; NR, not reached.

Table 23-8 Outcome by Extent of Surgical Resection in Contemporary Low-Grade Oligodendroglioma Series

Authors	Years of Study	Histologic Type Included	SURGICAL DATA Extent of Resection	*n*	SURVIVAL Median (y)	5-y (%)	10-y (%)	*P* Value
Celli et al[105]	1953-1986	LG > HG	GTR; STR+	29	9.3	66	—	<0.12
		O < OA	STR	71	4.8	48	—	
Mork et al[103]	1953-1977	LG > HG	GTR }	177	3.8	—	—	.051
			STR }		2.7	—	—	
Shaw et al[104]	1960-1982	LG < HG	GTR	19	12.6	74	59	.02
		O	STR	63	4.9	46	23	

A, astrocytoma; HG, high-grade, GTR, gross total resection; LG, low-grade; O, oligodendroglioma; OA, oligoastrocytoma; STR+, more extensive subtotal resection; STR, extent of subtotal resection not reported; —, data not reported.

ciated with extent of resection (i.e., more favorable "lobar" lesions resectable and unfavorable brainstem lesions unresectable) that makes any definitive conclusions about extent of resection dubious.[106]

External Beam Radiation Therapy

The key RT issues in the management of supratentorial low-grade gliomas are twofold. The issues include the timing of radiation with regard to when radiation is given (postoperative versus at recurrence), and the appropriate dose and treatment volume. Timing of RT has best been addressed by the phase III randomized trial EORTC 22845[95] and RTOG-Intergroup trial 98-02[94] as previously reviewed. However, radiation has several other effects besides the potential delay in tumor recurrence. In a small series of five patients with medically intractable epilepsy resulting from an underlying cerebral low-grade glioma, RT in doses of 54 to 61.2 Gy caused one patient to become seizure free, three had more than a 90% decrease in seizure frequency, and one patient had a more than 75% but less than 90% reduction in seizures.[107] In the EORTC phase III randomized trial 22845, there were no differences in seizure control at baseline, but at 1 year there were significantly more seizures in the observation group (41%) than in the irradiated group (25%).[95]

RT also may decrease the likelihood of malignant transformation or at least may delay its onset. Reichenthal and associates[69] observed a 9% incidence of malignant transformation in patients who received postoperative RT compared with 18% in those who had surgery alone. Vertosick and associates[79] reported a 56% likelihood of malignant transformation in their series and further observed that the median time to dedifferentiation was 5.4 years for patients who received RT compared with 3.7 years for those who had surgery alone. The series of Leighton and colleagues[68] reported an approximate 50% incidence of malignant transformation regardless of whether patients received postoperative RT. In the EORTC phase III randomized trial 22845, there were no differences in malignant transformation rate (observation group 66% versus 72% irradiated group) between the study arms at time of progression.[95] These data imply that radiation neither increases nor decreases the likelihood of malignant transformation, but rather dedifferentiation is a biologic phenomenon observed in low-grade gliomas independent of the treatment received.

External Beam Radiation Dose and Volume Considerations

For those patients who do receive RT, a decision must be made regarding the appropriate treatment field as well as the dose. Several series analyzing failure patterns in irradiated patients with low-grade hemispheric astrocytomas and oligodendrogliomas suggest that when tumor progression occurs, it almost always is at the site of the primary tumor within the treatment volume,[59,70,104,108] a finding implying that partial brain irradiation is appropriate. This was confirmed in NCCTG 86-72-51 (prospective dose-response trial) with 92% of failures occurring in field, 3% within 2 cm of the treatment field, and 5% more than 2 cm beyond the treatment field.[109] Furthermore, with the identification of tumor cells up to several centimeters beyond the margin of the tumor identified by T2-weighted MRI,[85] the appropriate radiation volume should include the MRI extent of tumor as defined by T2-weighted or FLAIR (fluid-attenuated inversion recovery) MR images with a 2- to 3-cm margin.

Regarding the potential benefit of higher doses of RT compared with lower doses, the retrospective data have been mixed[59,67,75]; however, two completed prospective randomized clinical trials have shown similar results. The issue of dose-response has been addressed in two separate phase III trials in adult patients with supratentorial low-grade gliomas (diffuse astrocytomas, oligoastrocytomas, and oligodendrogliomas), one from the EORTC and the other from the NCCTG. The EORTC randomized 379 patients to receive low-dose RT (45 Gy) or high-dose radiation (59.4 Gy) using multiple localized treatment fields. Initial analysis has failed to demonstrate a difference in survival between the two doses. The 5-year survival rate was 58% with 45 Gy and 59% with 59.4 Gy.[110] The NCCTG-led Intergroup trial compared 50.4 Gy with 64.8 Gy, also using multiple localized treatment fields. Initial analysis also failed to demonstrate a difference in survival between the two doses. The 5-year survival rate was 73% with 50.4 Gy and 68% with 64.8 Gy.[109] A single-institution prospective trial of 20 low-grade glioma patients treated with 68.2 cobalt Gray equivalents using a combination of protons and photons found no advantage with dose escalation compared with other published series.[111] Based on both retrospective and prospective dose-response data, the RTOG chose a total radiation dose of 54 Gy to localized treatment fields (tumor defined by the T2-weighted MRI scan plus a 2-cm margin) for its recently completed Intergroup study in adults with supratentorial low-grade glioma (Fig. 23-6).

Other Radiation Modalities

Several other radiation modalities have been used selectively in patients with low-grade gliomas, including stereotactic radiosurgery and stereotactic RT. In two series, radiosurgery for low-grade diffuse astrocytomas employing doses of 16 to 50 Gy in one or two fractions for tumors with maximum diameters of 30 to 40 mm resulted in radiographic responses in the majority of patients treated, without overt damage to normal tissue, although follow-up is short.[112,113] In another series of children with deep-seated pilocytic astrocytomas, single-dose radiosurgery (15 Gy) resulted in tumor shrinkage (five patients) or no further growth (four patients) without early or delayed morbidity.[114] In an effort to decrease neurocognitive complications and other possible toxicities, Marcus and colleagues[115] treated 50 pediatric low-grade astrocytoma patients with stereotactic RT (mean dose, 52.2 Gy in 1.8-Gy fractions) on a prospective single-institution protocol. The target volume generally included the preoperative tumor plus a 2-mm margin for the planning target volume. Six patients had local progression with no marginal failures. The progression-free survival rate was 83% at 5 years and 65% at 8 years.

Intraoperative radiation therapy (IORT) and brachytherapy, both interstitial and intracystic, have also been used selectively for patients with low-grade gliomas. Single-dose IORT (25 to 35 Gy, electrons) has been used in the setting of recurrent supratentorial low- to intermediate-grade gliomas with a reported 84% 2-year survival rate.[116] Interstitial implants, primarily with iodine-125, have been used for the treatment of some small, circumscribed, low-grade hemispheric astrocytomas. Five-year survival rates have ranged from 44% to 78%, similar to results achieved with external beam RT.[117,118] Chromic phosphate (^{32}P) also has been used for low-grade gliomas but primarily for cystic tumors, usually of the pilocytic type, as well as for recurrent astrocytomas with cyst formation.[119]

Chemotherapy

Chemotherapy has no proven role in the management of newly diagnosed low-grade gliomas in adults, although in the future, it is expected this may change. Eyre and associates[120] reported a randomized trial performed by the Southwest Oncology Group in which patients with subtotally resected supratentorial low-grade astrocytomas were randomized to 55 Gy with localized treatment fields, either alone or with oral CCNU chemotherapy (100 mg/m^2). Only 54 patients were entered on the study, which failed to identify any significant differences in survival between the two treatment arms. The most significant predictor of survival was age. Median survival time was not reached for patients younger than 30 years. It was 5.5 years for those 30 to 49 years old and 1.6 years for those 50 years of age and older. Shibamoto and colleagues[81] presented data from their retrospective series in which 19% of patients received chemotherapy, primarily with CCNU. Survival was not significantly affected.

The value of PCV (procarbazine, CCNU, vincristine) chemotherapy has also been tested. The NCCTG phase II study for adults with low-grade astrocytoma, oligoastrocytoma, or oligodendroglioma in which patients received six cycles of PCV every 8 weeks followed by localized external beam RT (54 or 59.4 Gy) revealed responses in 8 of 28 patients (29%), although 3 patients (11%) had tumor progression before their planned radiation.[121] Mason and colleagues[122] reported a 100% response rate in nine adult patients with cerebral low-grade oligodendrogliomas treated with initial PCV. Of the eight patients who were previously untreated, RT had to be given to only one patient who had stable disease after receiving six cycles of chemotherapy.

Figure 23-6 shows the schema of the recently completed RTOG-Intergroup low-grade glioma trial, designed for adults with supratentorial low-grade diffuse astrocytoma, oligoastrocytoma, and oligodendroglioma. Patients who are at low risk for recurrence (age younger than 40 years and gross total resection) are observed. Those at high risk for recurrence (age of 40 or older or subtotal resection/biopsy) are randomized between RT alone or radiation followed by six cycles of PCV. Figure 23-7 shows the prechemotherapy and postchemotherapy MRI of a patient with a newly diagnosed low-grade oligodendroglioma who received four cycles of PCV.

Temozolomide, an oral alkylating agent, has been tested initially in recurrent low-grade gliomas[123,124] and more recently in previously untreated (prior surgery only) diagnosed low-grade gliomas[43,125] (Table 23-9). Although the response rate is quite low in previously untreated low-grade gliomas (10% to 17%), the 1-year progression-free survival rates can be quite good at 73% or better.[43,125] It is important to emphasize these results should be considered preliminary, with median follow-up times ranging from less than 1 year to 3 years.[19]

An ongoing EORTC trial attempts to address the role of temozolomide in newly diagnosed low-grade glioma patients. This EORTC trial randomizes patients with progressive disease, uncontrolled seizures despite anticonvulsants, or neurologic symptoms to standard RT or daily low-dose

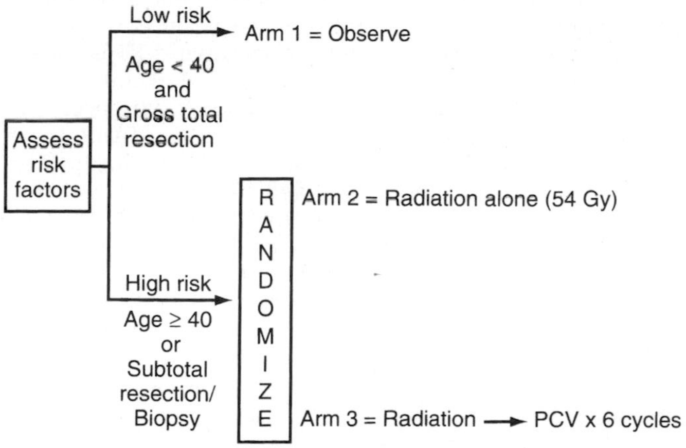

Figure 23-6 Schema of the Radiation Therapy Oncology Group–Intergroup Low-Grade Glioma Trial. PCV, procarbazine, CCNU, and vincristine.

Table 23-9 Temozolomide in Low-Grade Gliomas

Author	No. of Patients	Prior Radiotherapy (%)	Prior Chemotherapy (%)	Response, CR + PR (%)	1-y Progression-Free Survival (%)
Quinn, et al.[124]	46	15	20	61	76
Pace, et al.[123]	43	65	37	47	39
Brada, et al.[125]	30	None	None	10	93*
Hoang-Xuan, et al.[43]	60	None	None	17	73

*Derived from Figure 15-2.
CR, complete response; PR, partial response.

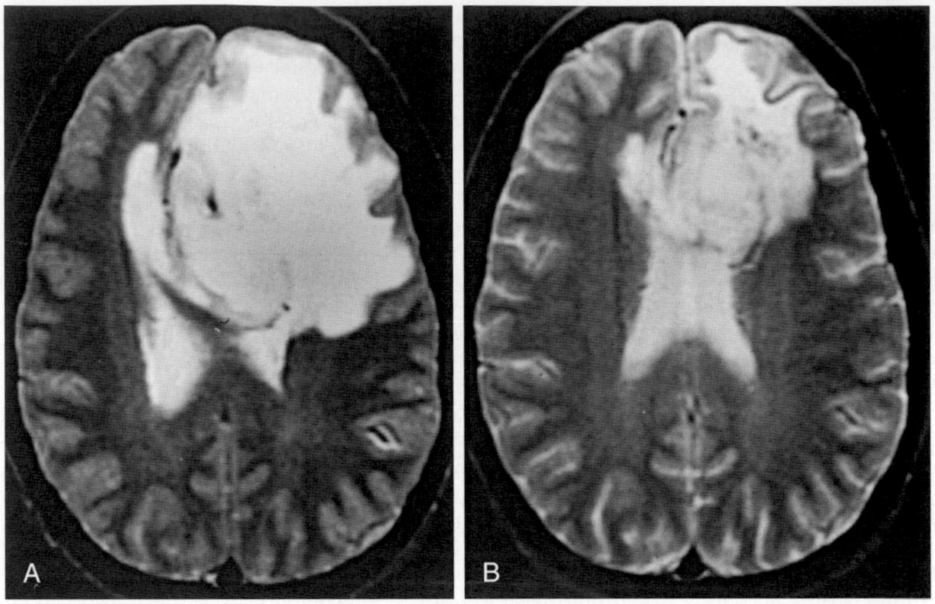

Figure 23-7 Prechemotherapy (**A**) and postchemotherapy (**B**) T2-weighted MRI of a young adult with a WHO II oligodendroglioma of the left frontal lobe.

temozolomide. Patients will be stratified based on 1p status (intact versus deleted), as well as age, tumor size, and Karnofsky performance status (KPS) with a primary end point of progression-free survival.

The response of recurrent, previously irradiated low-grade gliomas to chemotherapy has been variable. With astrocytomas or oligoastrocytomas, response rates range from 20% with MOP (nitrogen mustard, vincristine, and procarbazine)[127] to 33% to 40% with the combination of BCNU and interferon-α.[128] For recurrent low-grade oligodendrogliomas, response rates vary from 90% with PCV[42] to 47% for temozolomide.[123]

FAVORABLE LOW-GRADE GLIOMA VARIANTS

One group of primary CNS tumors has a distinctly more favorable prognosis than the low-grade diffuse astrocytomas, oligoastrocytomas, and oligodendrogliomas. This group includes the pilocytic astrocytomas (WHO I) and the other low-grade glioma variants, including the pleomorphic astrocytomas, subependymal giant cell astrocytomas, and subependymomas. Three other primary CNS tumors of neuronal or mixed neuronal-glial origin can also be grouped with the low-grade glioma variants because of their similar presentation and favorable prognosis, including the gangliogliomas, central neurocytomas, and dysembryoplastic neuroepithelial tumors. Other than the pilocytic astrocytomas, which make up approximately 20% of supratentorial low-grade gliomas and 80% of cerebellar gliomas,[14,129] the other six variants are uncommon, accounting for approximately 1% or less of primary CNS tumors. From an imaging standpoint, they are typically well circumscribed, enhancing, and sometimes cystic, calcified, or both.[130,131]

Pilocytic Astrocytomas

Pilocytic astrocytomas typically occur in children and young adults, with common locations being the cerebellum, optic pathways, hypothalamus/third ventricle, and cerebral hemispheres. They are the most common primary brain tumor occurring in patients with type 1 neurofibromatosis.[4,5] The overall 10-year survival rate is 80% or greater, independent of location in the brain,[17,18,56,129,132] although rarely, they behave more aggressively.[16] In patients undergoing gross total tumor resection, the 10-year disease-free and overall survival rates approach 100%.[17,18,129,132]

For those who have subtotal resection, particularly children, a reasonable strategy is observation with close follow-up because there is no apparent survival benefit to routine postoperative RT,[75,129] and a second surgical procedure accomplishing gross total resection appears curative.[132] RT is usually reserved for symptomatic subtotally resected or unresectable tumors, usually in the setting of tumor recurrence. This paradigm was tested and proved to be successful in an NCCTG prospective clinical trial of 20 adults with supratentorial pilocytic astrocytomas observed after gross (11 patients) or subtotal (6 patients) resection or treated with RT after biopsy (3 patients).[133] At the time of analysis (median follow-up, 10 years), 1 patient (5%) had died and 19 patients (95%) were alive. The 5-year progression-free and overall survival rates were 95%. When pilocytic astrocytomas require radiation, localized treatment fields (enhancing tumor with a 1-cm margin) to moderate doses (45 to 54 Gy) are recommended.[75]

Pleomorphic Xanthoastrocytomas

Pleomorphic xanthoastrocytomas also occur in children and young adults, usually presenting with seizures due to an underlying tumor in the cerebral cortex (temporal lobes), sometimes with adjacent meningeal and rarely with craniospinal leptomeningeal involvement. Despite their pleomorphism, they often behave in an indolent manner.[42,131] Treatment recommendations depend on the grade of the astrocytic component. When gross total resection has been achieved of a pleomorphic xanthoastrocytoma that contains a low-grade diffuse astrocytoma (WHO II), observation is appropriate, although local tumor recurrence, sometimes with malignant transformation, can occur. Indications for RT (doses, treatment fields similar to the more common forms of WHO II low-grade gliomas) include pleomorphic xanthoastrocytomas that contain an anaplastic astrocytoma or glioblastoma (WHO III/IV), symptomatic subtotally resected or unresectable tumors, or recurrent tumors, particularly if their astrocytic component dedifferentiates.[20,21,130]

Other Favorable Variants

Gangliogliomas consist of neoplastic ganglion (neuronal) cells and neoplastic glial (astrocytic) cells. They can occur in children and adults, although most are present in the first two to three decades of life. Gangliogliomas can develop anywhere in the CNS, but they tend to occur in the supratentorial brain, most often in a temporal location. Like pleomorphic xanthoastrocytomas, the glial component can be low grade (WHO II) or higher grade (WHO III/IV).[130,131] Treatment principles are similar to those of pleomorphic xanthoastrocytoma from both a surgical and radiotherapeutic standpoint.[134]

Dysembryoplastic neuroepithelial tumors, like gangliogliomas, also contain a mixture of neuronal and glial elements, although the neuronal component is mature, and the glial component is well differentiated and astrocytic or oligodendroglial. As such, they are classified as WHO I tumors. Typically, these tumors occur in a temporal location, are characteristically multinodular, and arise during the first two decades of life. Treatment principles are similar to those of pilocytic astrocytomas from both a surgical and radiotherapeutic standpoint, although radiation is rarely necessary.[130,131]

Central neurocytomas contain neuronal elements that are usually mature. They are classified as WHO II tumors. By definition, they arise in the ventricular system, usually as large tumors in the lateral ventricular system, and they rarely have been reported to disseminate craniospinally. The typical age at presentation is in the late 20s, although they can occur in children or adults.[130,131] Subtotally resected tumors have been reported to respond to RT.[135] Leenstra and colleagues[136] reviewed the Mayo Clinic experience of 45 patients with histologically confirmed central neurocytomas. Various combinations of surgery, RT (median dose, 55 Gy), and chemotherapy were used for treatment. The 5-year survival rate was 81% for the entire cohort. The 5-year local control rate was 100% for patients who received RT after subtotal resection compared with 48% for those who did not ($P = .013$); however, there was no difference in overall survival at 5 years, most likely due to the effectiveness of salvage RT. Therefore, patients with subtotally resected (especially "atypical neurocytomas"),[137] unresectable tumors, or recurrent tumors are usually offered RT postoperatively, whereas patients are usually observed after gross total resection.

Subependymal giant cell astrocytomas occur in patients with tuberous sclerosis, often during their first two decades of life but sometimes later. Characterized by large astrocyte-like cells, they are classified as WHO I tumors, like the pilocytic astrocytomas. Typically, they arise in an intraventricular or periventricular location (lateral ventricles, foramen of Monro).[5,6,132,138] Treatment recommendations parallel the pilocytic astrocytomas; that is, gross total resection is considered curative[8,9] and RT is reserved for sympathetic progression or relapse.

Subependymomas are also classified as WHO I/ II tumors. They contain both low-grade astrocytic and ependymal-like cells, and they usually arise in an intraventricular location (lateral or fourth ventricles, particularly in and around the foramen of Monro) in adults near the age of 50 years.[132,138] Treatment recommendations parallel those of pilocytic astrocytomas, both surgically and radiotherapeutically. Subtotally resected and recurrent tumors have been reported to respond to RT.[22]

RECURRENT LOW-GRADE GLIOMAS

As shown in Figure 23-5, patients with all histologic types of supratentorial low-grade gliomas have a significantly worse survival than expected for an age- and sex-matched control population. Essentially all patients who die do so because of tumor relapse and progression, because this young patient population (median age in the mid 30s) is unlikely to have other underlying diseases that would contribute to their mortality. As such, at some point in his or her illness, the typical patient with a low-grade glioma likely has the combination of progressive neurologic symptoms and signs in the face of neuroimaging evidence of tumor recurrence, usually the new development of contrast enhancement.[139]

The clinical and radiographic features of tumor recurrence are indistinguishable from radiation necrosis, even by positron emission tomography[140] or single-photon emission CT. MRI spectroscopy may prove to be more useful in this regard (Fig. 23-8). To differentiate between these diagnostic possibilities, tissue must be obtained. Data from pooled surgical series in which 100 patients with suspected recurrence of a cerebral low-grade astrocytoma underwent reoperation, pathologic examination revealed low-grade tumor in 33%, high-grade tumor in 64%, and radionecrosis in 3%.[14,41,54,55,59,83,141]

In general, survival after tumor recurrence is poor. In one series, patients whose disease progressed after treatment with surgery and postoperative RT had a median survival time of 9.7 months with a 2-year survival rate of 29%.[59] However, prognosis is significantly affected by the specific histologic findings at the time of biopsy or reoperation.

In the series of Forsyth and associates,[142] 51 previously irradiated patients (40 of whom had Kernohan grade 1 or 2 astrocytoma, oligoastrocytoma, or oligodendroglioma) underwent stereotactic biopsy for suspected tumor recurrence. Pathologic examination revealed the presence of tumor only in 30 biopsies (59%), tumor plus necrosis in 17 biopsies (33%), radionecrosis in 3 instances (6%), and 1 case of a radiation-induced sarcoma (3%). In patients in whom tumor was found, it was high grade in 63%. Median survival after biopsy was 10 months in patients with tumor only, a finding significantly worse than the 22-month median survival time in those with tumor plus necrosis. No deaths occurred among the two patients whose biopsies showed radionecrosis.

Postrecurrence survival is also influenced by pathologic type. In the series of Leighton and colleagues,[68] the median survival time after recurrence was 39 months for all patients, 16 months for those with recurrent low-grade diffuse astrocytomas, and 60 months for patients with recurrent low-grade oligodendrogliomas.

Several uncommon patterns of treatment failure can occur in patients with recurrent low-grade gliomas. Figure 23-9 demonstrates the MRI appearance of tumor infiltration across the deep, dense white matter tracts of the brain. The occurrence of leptomeningeal failure also has been reported. In one pediatric series of intracranial low-grade gliomas, its incidence was 4%.[143]

Treatment options for tumor recurrence include surgery, external beam radiation, brachytherapy, radiosurgery, intraoperative electron radiation, and chemotherapy. Each has been discussed in this chapter.

TECHNIQUES OF IRRADIATION

External Beam Radiation Dose and Volume Considerations

For patients who receive RT, a decision must be made regarding the appropriate treatment field as well as the dose. As

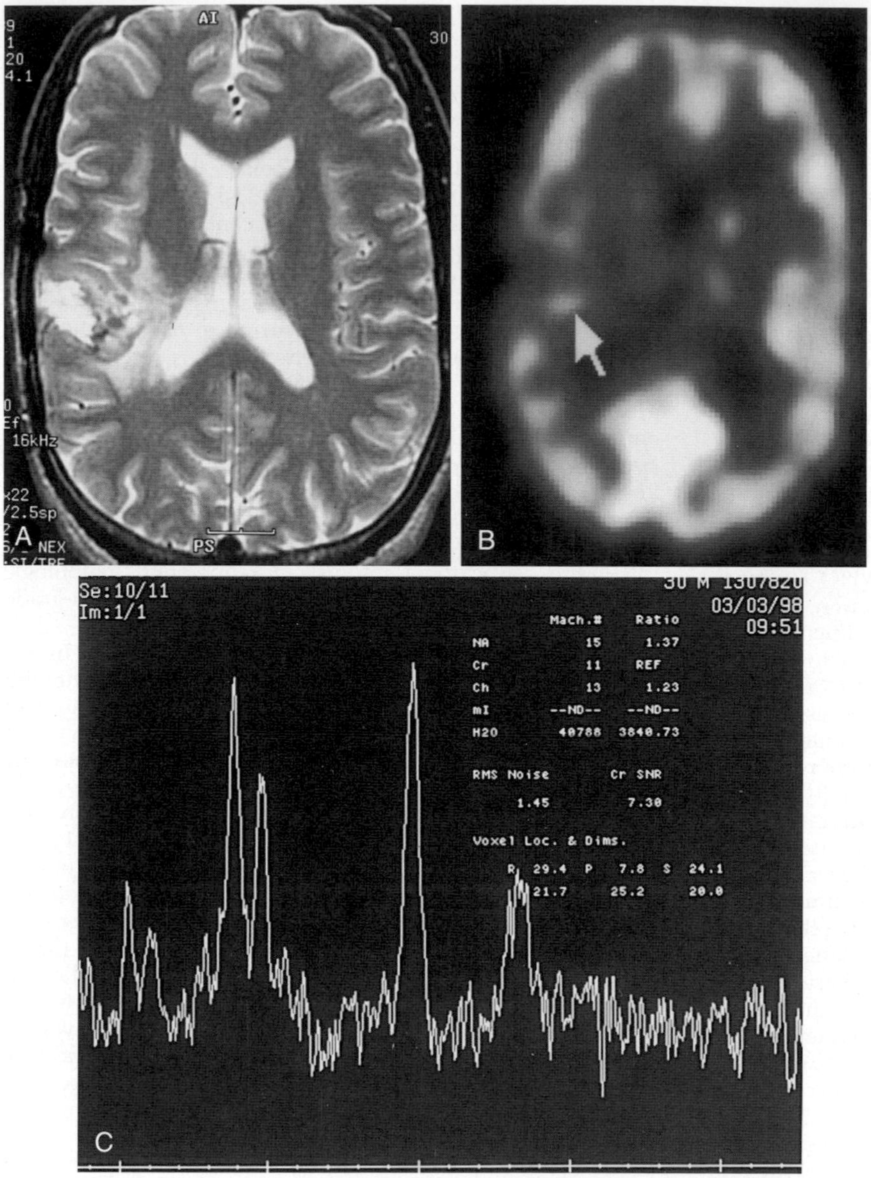

Figure 23-8 Postgadolinium T1-weighted MRI of a young adult with a WHO II oligoastrocytoma after subtotal resection, 50.4-Gy external beam radiation therapy, and 18 Gy given in 1 fraction in stereotactic radiosurgery for recurrent disease at the medial edge of the resection cavity. **A,** An area of increased contrast enhancement at the site of the stereotactic radiosurgery. **B,** Positron emission tomography using fluorodeoxyglucose showed increased uptake at the site of the contrast enhancement *(arrow)*. However, MRI spectroscopy (**C**) was more suggestive of radiation necrosis because the choline-to-creatine ratio was less than 2, and the lactate peak was elevated. Subsequent biopsy demonstrated radiation necrosis.

noted previously, in prior analyses of irradiated patients, tumor progression usually occurs at the site of the primary tumor within the treatment volume,[59,70,76,108] implying that partial brain irradiation is appropriate. In NCCTG 86-72-51 (prospective dose-response trial), 92% of failures occurred in field, 3% were within 2 cm of the treatment field, and 5% were more than 2 cm beyond the treatment field.[109] Furthermore, with the identification of tumor cells up to several centimeters beyond the margin of the tumor identified by T2-weighted MRI,[85] the appropriate radiation volume should include the MRI extent of tumor as defined by T2-weighted MRI or FLAIR with a 2- to 3-cm margin (see Central Nervous System Tumors Overview for an extensive discussion of radiation technique).

Toxicity of Radiation Therapy

A spectrum of radiation-induced toxicities can occur in patients receiving therapeutic brain irradiation. These range from neurocognitive sequelae, the pathogenesis of which is likely a white matter injury, to overt radiation necrosis, which is probably a consequence of vascular injury.[144,145]

Several studies have focused on the neurocognitive effects of RT in patients who are longer-term recurrence-free survivors, most of whom were irradiated for supratentorial low-grade gliomas. To assess the toxicity of RT, it is important to understand the neurologic and cognitive dysfunction that results from having a cerebral low-grade glioma.[146]

Prospective Neurocognitive and Quality-of-Life Analyses

In the series from Taphoorn and colleagues,[147] a subset of patients treated on the EORTC low-grade glioma trials[95,110] were assessed prospectively using the following: serial neurologic examinations; assessment of KPS; neuropsychological tests of attention, memory, language, visuospatial, and frontal lobe function; a quality-of-life questionnaire; and a profile of mood states.

Three groups of patients (about 20 patients per group) were studied. One group had histologically verified low-grade

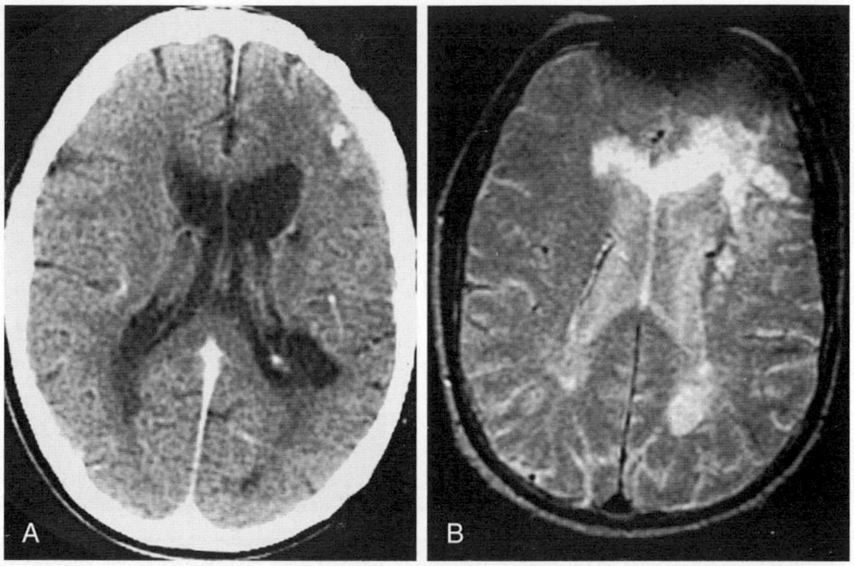

Figure 23-9 Postcontrast CT (**A**) and T2-weighted MRI (**B**) of an adult patient with a recurrent WHO II astrocytoma. MRI shows significant ipsilateral and contralateral white matter spread not seen on CT.

astrocytoma but did not receive postoperative RT. A second group received postoperative RT with 45 to 63 Gy, using multiple-shaped localized treatment fields. A third control group consisted of patients with hematologic malignant diseases in the absence of brain involvement. With an average follow-up of 3.5 years, neuropsychological test scores were similar for the patients with low-grade astrocytoma, whether they received RT or not, and were significantly worse than those of the control group, a finding implying that the disease, and not the RT, was the underlying cause of cognitive dysfunction. In addition, patients with left hemispheric tumors in the group who received postoperative RT scored significantly better on several neuropsychological tests than did patients with similarly located low-grade gliomas who did not receive RT.

Other observations made in the patients with low-grade glioma, independent of whether postoperative RT was given, included a higher frequency of the following: fatigue, memory, concentration, and speech difficulties; depression; tension; and impediment of the activities of daily living compared with the control group. The authors concluded that "RT had no negative impact on neurological, functional, cognitive, and affective status."[147]

An update of this study by Klein and associates[148] included 195 patients with low-grade glioma (of whom 104 had received RT 1 to 22 years earlier) compared with low-grade hematologic patients and healthy controls. Neurocognitive testing again found low-grade glioma patients, independent of whether postoperative RT was given, had lower ability in all cognitive domains than did low-grade hematological patients, and did even less well by comparison with healthy controls. However, there was poorer cognitive function associated with daily radiation fraction doses exceeding 2 Gy. Antiepileptic drug use was strongly associated with disability in attentional and executive function. The authors concluded that "the tumour itself has the most deleterious effect on cognitive function and that RT mainly results in additional long-term cognitive disability when high fraction doses are used."

A report from the EORTC compared the quality of life in patients with low-grade glioma who received either 45 Gy or 59.4 Gy on the dose-response trial.[110] Patients who received the higher dose reported significantly lower levels of functioning (especially emotional and in leisure time) and more symptom burden, especially fatigue, malaise, and insomnia.[149]

Along with radiation dose fraction and total dose, field size (i.e., volume irradiated) has a significant impact on neurocognitive function.[146] Kleinberg and associates[150] measured quality of life in 30 adult patients with hemispheric gliomas, 23 of whom had low- to intermediate-grade tumors. All patients were alive without evidence of tumor recurrence 1 year or more after surgery and postoperative RT. Quality of life was measured by KPS, employment history, and memory function comparing results 1 year after treatment with the last follow-up and comparing outcome in those patients who received localized brain irradiation versus whole brain treatment. KPS declined in none of 14 patients treated with localized fields versus 3 of 16 (19%) who received whole brain radiation. Although two thirds of patients were employed before their diagnosis, at 1 year or more after RT, 80% of those who received localized treatment fields were employed, compared with 38% to 46% who underwent whole brain irradiation. Moderate to severe memory deficits occurred in 43% of patients receiving whole brain irradiation as opposed to 6% with localized RT.

Because there is no convincing evidence that early RT improves overall survival, deferring irradiation until there is evidence of symptomatic tumor growth is an acceptable practice. The primary rationale for delaying radiation is to reduce the risk of radiation-induced neurocognitive damage. A number of retrospective studies have found increased neurocognitive difficulties after cranial RT. However, these studies have had many deficiencies,[146] besides the weaknesses inherent in retrospective studies, including outdated RT techniques (using whole brain RT for low-grade glioma patients),[92,150,151] unknown number of patients treated but not studied (unidentified denominator),[152] extremely heterogeneous groups,[153] and, most important, the lack of baseline neurocognitive testing because the brain tumor itself is often the primary cause of cognitive difficulties.[92,148,151,154,155]

In sharp contrast, a number of studies have prospectively performed extensive neuropsychological testing on adult patients with low-grade neoplasms before (baseline) and after RT (up to 6 years after RT) and have not found significant neurocognitive deficits when compared with either baseline[156-160] or a cohort of patients with low-grade brain neoplasms not

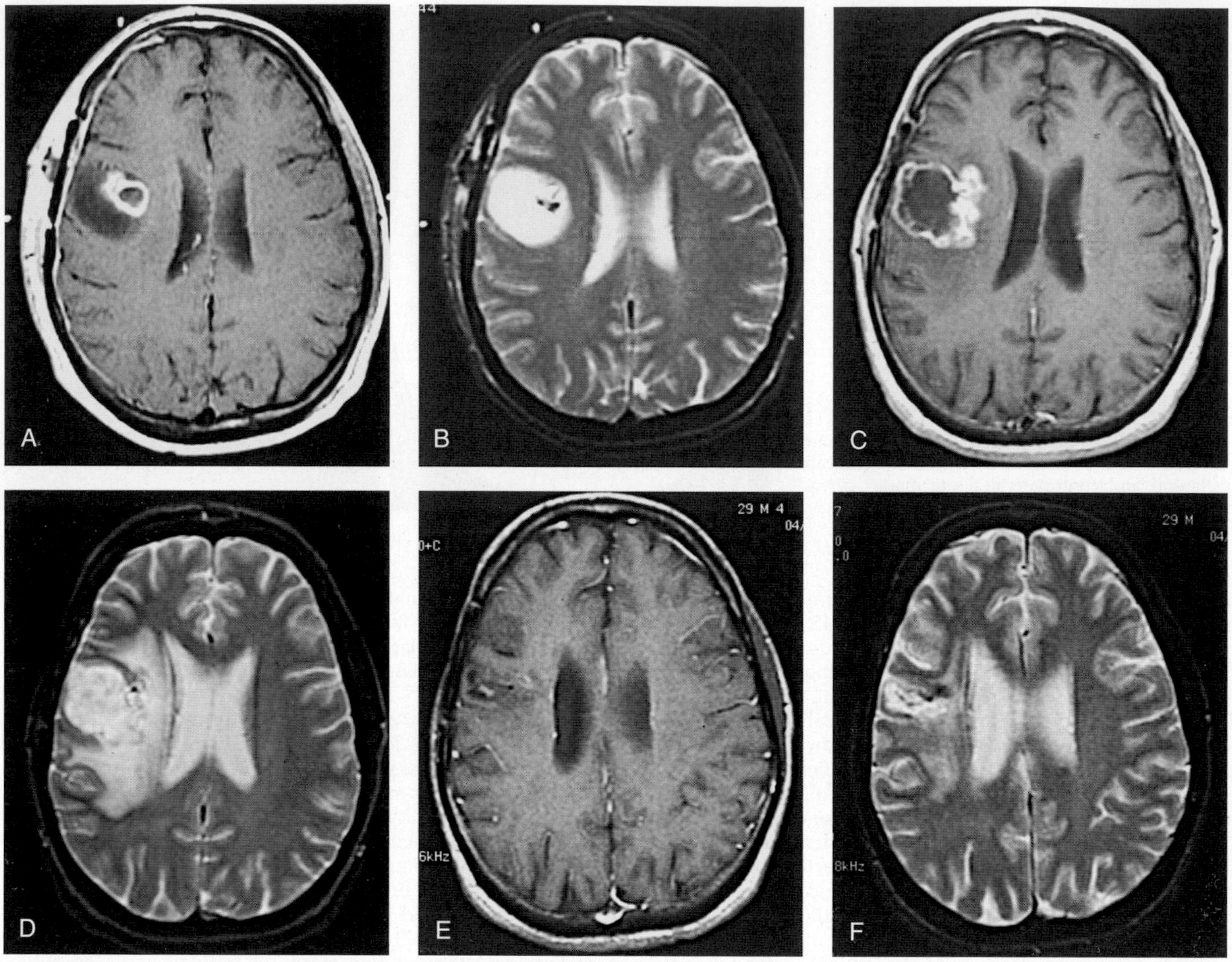

Figure 23-10 Preirradiation, postgadolinium T1-weighted (**A**) and T2-weighted (**B**) MR images of an adult with a WHO II oligodendroglioma of the right frontotemporal lobes. Seven months after 64.8-Gy external beam radiation therapy, the patient developed headaches. Postgadolinium T1-weighted (**C**) and T2-weighted (**D**) MR images are shown. The differential diagnosis considered recurrent tumor and radiation necrosis. After a brief course of oral corticosteroid medications, the imaging abnormalities resolved, a finding supporting the diagnosis of transient radiation necrosis. Postgadolinium T1-weighted (**E**) and T2-weighted (**F**) MR images are shown, Adapted from Daumas-Duport C, Scheithauer BW, Kelly PJ: A histologic and cytologic method for spatial definition of gliomas. Mayo Clin Proc 62:435-449, 1987; Kelly PJ, Daumas-Duport C, Scheithauer BW, et al: Stereotactic histologic correlations of computed tomography and magnetic resonance imaging-defined abnormalities in patients with glial neoplasms. Mayo Clin Proc 62:450-459, 1987.

treated with RT[161,162] (Table 23-10). For example in the NCCTG dose-response trial,[163] a subset of 20 of the 203 adult study patients who received either 50.4 or 64.8 Gy underwent psychometric testing before and up to 5 years after localized RT.[155] No significant losses in general intellectual function, new learning function, or memory function were seen, with the groups' mean test scores higher than their initial performances on all psychometric measures, although the improvement was not statistically significant. However, four patients, all in the 64.8-Gy arm, had a mild decline in one or more of the domains (immediate verbal memory, learning, and spatial problem solving) assessed. The weight of evidence indicates a low incidence of neurocognitive difficulties after focal, conventionally fractionated (1.8 to 2 Gy) RT using modern techniques to deliver moderate doses in adults.[146]

In contrast, a significant proportion of children who are long-term survivors after cranial RT do have significant sequelae of treatment. North and associates[59] reviewed a series of pediatric patients treated with cranial RT and found 54% of children were cognitively impaired (intelligence quotient [IQ] of 70, requiring special education) with major neurologic sequelae (e.g., requiring supervision, hospitalization, or nursing care). The comparable figure was 40% in children who had surgery but no postoperative RT. In several other pediatric low-grade astrocytoma series, a significant reduction in IQ was observed in 11% to 23% of patients, the majority of whom had surgery but not postoperative RT.[60,164] These studies highlight the underlying morbidity that occurs from the disease and its treatments, as well as the need for careful selection of patients with cerebral low-grade gliomas for surgery and postoperative RT.

The incidence of overt radiation necrosis after RT for a cerebral low-grade glioma is approximately 3% based on data from surgical series in which reoperation data were

Table 23-10 **Prospective Neurocognitive Trials (With Baseline Testing) of Low-Grade Neoplasms**

Author	Histology (No. Receiving RT)	Radiation Total Dose/Fraction Size (Gy)	Mean Follow-up (y)	Extensive Neurocognitive Assessment at Each Evaluation	Neurotoxicity After RT
Glosser, McManus et al., 1997	Chordoma, chondrosarcoma (17)	Proton RT median 68.4 CGE/1.8 CGE	4	Yes	No; mild decline in psychomotor speed with high doses
Vigliani, Sichez et al., 1996	LGG, AA (17)	Focal RT 54/1.8	4	Yes	No; transient decline in RcT
Armstrong, Hunter et al., 2002	LGG, pituitary, pineal, meningioma (26)	Focal RT mean 54.6/1.8–2.0	3	Yes	No; mild decline in visual memory after 5 y
Brown, Buckner et al., 2003	LGG (203)	Focal RT 50.4/1.8 or 64.8/1.8	7.4 (median)	No (MMSE and NFS)	5.3% with MMSE decline at 5 y
Torres, Mundt et al., 2003	Meningioma, LGG, GBM, ependymoma, adenoma (15)	Focal RT mean 54/1.8	2	Yes	No; decline in memory and attention only if tumor progression
Laack, Brown et al., 2003	LGG (20)	Focal RT 50.4/1.8 or 64.8/1.8	3	Yes	No; mild decline in 64.8-Gy arm in immediate verbal memory, learning, and spatial problem solving

AA, anaplastic astrocytoma; GBM, glioblastoma multiforme; LGG, low-grade glioma; MMSE, Folstein Mini-Mental State Examination; NFS, neurologic function scores; RcT, reaction time; RT, radiation therapy.

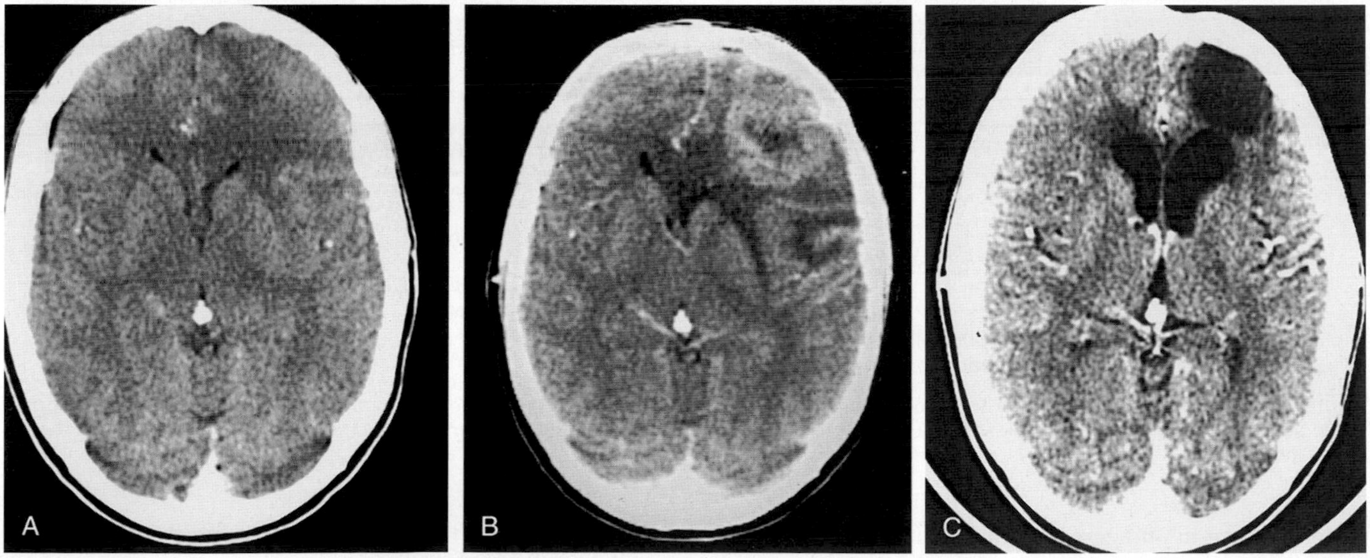

Figure 23-11 Contrast-enhanced CT demonstrates the progress of a left frontal WHO II astrocytoma in an adult patient. **A,** Before 64.8-Gy external beam radiation therapy. **B,** After irradiation, the patient had headaches. **C,** Eighteen months after gross total resection of what proved to be a combination of radiation necrosis and persistent low-grade astrocytoma, the patient had no evidence of further radiation necrosis or tumor.

reported.[11,55,59,66,69,76,83] This is consistent with findings from the NCCTG dose-response trial (50.4 versus 64.8 Gy) in which the 2-year actuarial incidence of severe, life-threatening, or fatal radionecrosis was 1% at 50.4 Gy and 5% at 64.8 Gy.[163] Examples of the clinical presentation, imaging changes, time course, management, and outcome of the spectrum of severe or worse radiation toxicities seen in patients with cerebral low-grade gliomas are shown in Figures 23-10 through 23-12.

CONCLUSIONS, TREATMENT ALGORITHM, AND FUTURE POSSIBILITIES

Low-grade gliomas are a heterogeneous group of CNS neoplasms, and their natural history depends primarily on pathologic type and patient age. Our preferred treatment algorithm for low-grade gliomas is given in Figure 23-13. Despite their having been considered "benign" historically, most of these

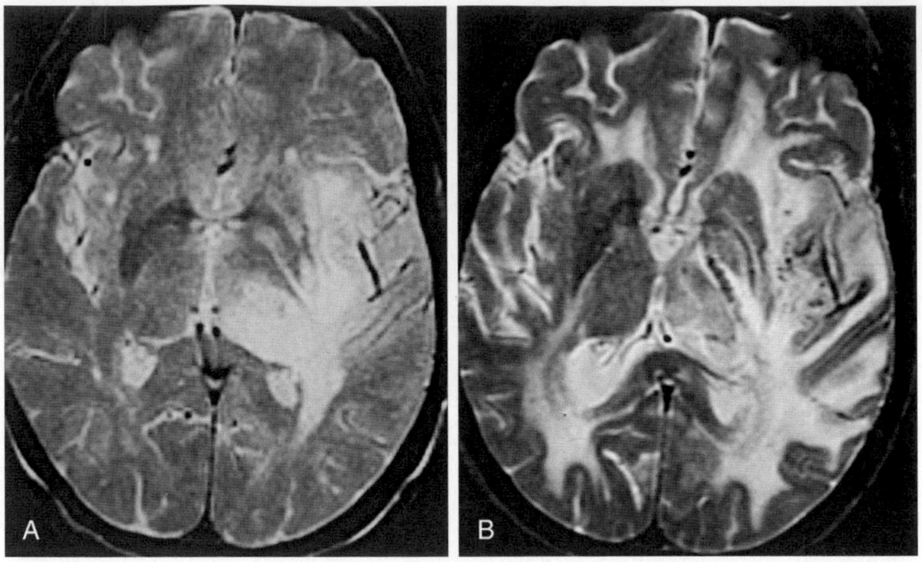

Figure 23-12 **A,** T2-weighted MRI scan of an older adult with an infiltrative, poorly defined WHO II astrocytoma whose epicenter was in the left temporal lobe. Six months after completing 64.8-Gy external beam radiation therapy, the patient developed a significant decline in cognitive function and overall performance status. **B,** Repeat MRI showed dramatic white matter changes. The patient subsequently died, and an autopsy showed radiation necrosis with a persistent low-grade astrocytoma.

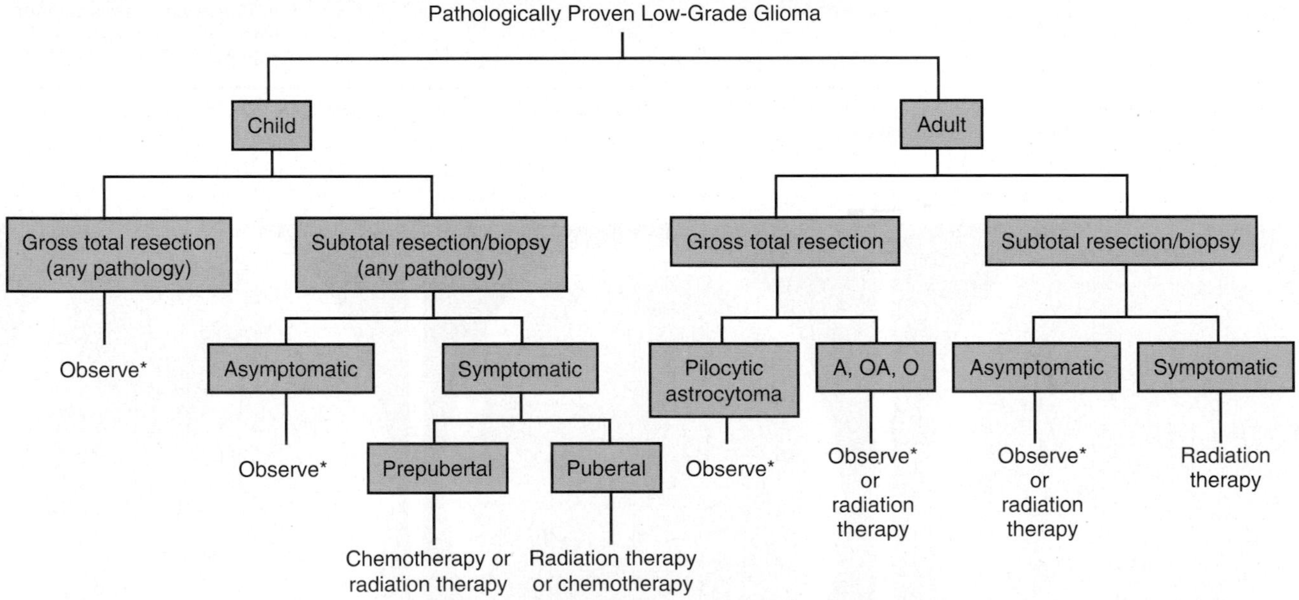

Figure 23-13 Treatment algorithm for low-grade glioma. *Treatment is deferred until the time of symptomatic or imaging progression. Appropriate treatment at the time of progression may include surgery, chemotherapy, or radiation therapy. A, astrocytoma; OA, oligoastrocytoma; O, oligodendroglioma.

tumors behave in an aggressive manner, even after surgery and RT. The role of chemotherapy remains to be determined. Translational research, including studies of proliferation, cytogenetics, and molecular genetics, will provide much needed insight for the next generation of biologically based therapies.

REFERENCES

1. Jemal A, Siegel R, Ward E, et al: Cancer statistics, 2006. Ca Cancer J Clin 56:106-130, 2006.
2. Okazaki H: Neoplastic and related lesions. *In* Okazaki H (ed): Fundamentals of Neuropathology. New York, Igaku-Shoin, 1983.
3. Levin VA, Gutin PH, et al: Neoplasms of the central nervous system. *In* DeVita V, Hellman J, Rosenberg S (eds): Cancer: Principles and Practice of Oncology. Philadelphia, JB Lippincott, 1993.
4. Blatt J, Jaffe R, et al: Neurofibromatosis and childhood tumors. Cancer 57:1225-1229, 1986.
5. Kleihues P, Ohgaki H: Genetics of glioma progression and the definition of primary and secondary glioblastoma. Brain Pathol 7:1131, 1997.
6. Kapp JR, Paulson GW, et al: Brain tumors with tuberous sclerosis. J Neurosurg 26:191-202, 1967.
7. Cooper JR: Brain tumors in hereditary multiple system hamartomatosis (tuberous sclerosis). J Neurosurg 34:194-202, 1971.
8. Chow CW, Klug GL, et al: Subependymal giant-cell astrocytoma in children. J Neurosurg 68:880-883, 1988.
9. Shepherd CW, Scheithauer BW, et al: Subependymal giant-cell astrocytomas: a clinical pathologic and flow cytometric study. Neurosurgery 28:864-868, 1991.
10. Horrax G: Benign (favorable) types of brain tumor: the end results (up to twenty years), with statistics of mortality and useful survival. N Engl J Med 250:981-984, 1954.

11. Gol A: The relatively benign astrocytomas of the cerebrum: a clinical study of 194 verified cases. J Neurosurg 18:501-506, 1961.
12. Kleihues P, Burger PC, et al: Histologic Typing of Tumours of the Central Nervous System. Berlin, Springer, 1993.
13. Kleihues P, Cavenee WK: Pathology and Genetics of Tumors of the Nervous System—WHO Classification of Tumours. Lyon, France, International Agency for Research on Cancer Press, 2000.
14. Shaw EG, Scheithauer BW, et al: Low-grade hemispheric astrocytomas. Cambridge, Blackwell Scientific Publications, 1997.
15. Sofietti R, Chio A, et al: Prognostic factors in well-differentiated cerebral astrocytomas in the adult. Neurosurgery 24:686-692, 1989.
16. Tomlinson F, Scheithauer B, et al: The significance of atypia and histologic malignancy in pilocytic astrocytoma of the cerebellum. J Child Neurol 9:301-310, 1993.
17. Garcia DM, Fulling DH: Juvenile pilocytic astrocytoma of the cerebrum in adults: a distinctive neoplasm with favorable prognosis. J Neurosurg 63:382-386, 1985.
18. Forsyth PA, Shaw EG, et al: Supratentorial pilocytic astrocytomas: a clinicopathologic, prognostic, flow cytometric study of 51 patients. Cancer 72:1335-1342, 1993.
19. Brown P, Buckner J: Temozolomide: too early for definitive conclusions. J Clin Oncol 21:3710, 2003.
20. Strom EH, Skullerud K: Pleomorphic xanthoastrocytoma: Report of 5 cases. Clin Neuropathol 2:188-191, 1982.
21. Whittle IR, Gordon A, et al: Pleomorphic xanthoastrocytoma: Report of four cases. J Neurosurg 70:463-468, 1989.
22. Lombardi D, Scheithauer BW, et al: Symptomatic subependymoma: a clinicopathologic and flow cytometric study. J Neurosurg 75:583-588, 1991.
23. Bailey P, Cushing H: A Classification of the Tumors of the Glioma Group on a Histogenetic Basis With a Correlated Study of Prognosis. Philadelphia, JB Lippincott, 1926.
24. Cushing H: Intracranial Tumors: Notes Upon a Series of 2000 Verified Cases with Surgical Mortality Percentages Pertaining Thereto. Springfield, IL, Charles C Thomas, 1932.
25. Kernohan JW, Mabon RF, et al: Symposium on new and simplified concept of gliomas: a classification of the gliomas. Proc Staff Meet Mayo Clin 24:71-75, 1949.
26. Daumas-Duport C, Scheithauer B, et al: Grading of astrocytomas. A simple and reproducible method. Cancer 62:2152-2165, 1988.
27. Burger PC, Scheithauer BW, et al: Brain tumors. *In* Burger PC, Scheithauer BW, Vogel FS (eds): Surgical Pathology of the Nervous System and Its Coverings. New York, Churchill Livingstone, 1991, pp 193-437.
28. Kim TS, Halliday AL, et al: Correlates of survival and the Daumas-Duport grading system for astrocytomas. J Neurosurg 74:27-37, 1991.
29. Zaprianov Z, Christov K: Histological grading, DNA content, cell survival. Cytometry 9:380-386, 1988.
30. Danova M, Giaretti W, et al: Prognostic significance of nuclear DNA content in human neuroepithelial tumors. Int J Cancer 48:663-667, 1991.
31. Coons SW, Johnson PC, et al: Prognostic significance of flow cytometry deoxyribonucleic acid analysis of human astrocytomas. Neurosurgery 35:119-126, 1994.
32. Struikmans H, Rutgers DH, et al: S-phase fraction, 5-bromo-2′-deoxyuridine labelling index, duration of S-phase, potential doubling time, and DNA index in benign and malignant brain tumors. Radiat Oncol Invest 5:170-179, 1997.
33. Montine TI, Vandersteenhoven JJ, et al: Prognostic significance of Ki-67 proliferation index in supratentorial fibrillary astrocytic neoplasms. Neurosurgery 34:674-679, 1994.
34. McKeever PE, Ross DA, et al: A comparison of the predictive power for survival in gliomas provided by MIB-1, bromodeoxyuridine and proliferating cell nuclear antigen with histopathologic and clinical parameters. J Neuropathol Exp Neurol 56:798-805, 1997.
35. Fisher BJ, Naumova E, et al: Ki-67: a prognostic factor for low-grade glioma? Int J Radiat Oncol Biol Phys 52:996-1001, 2002.
36. Dudas SP, Rempel SA: Development, Molecular Genetics, and Gene Therapy of Glial Tumors. Philadelphia, Lippincott-Raven, 1999.
37. Lang FF, Miller DC, et al: High frequency of p53 protein accumulation without p53 gene mutation in human juvenile pilocytic, low-grade and anaplastic astrocytomas. Oncogene 9:949-954, 1994.
38. Stander M, Peraud A, et al: Prognostic impact of TP53 mutation status for adult patients with supratentorial World Health Organization grade II astrocytoma or oligoastrocytoma: a long-term analysis. Cancer 101:1028-1035, 2004.
39. Chozick BS, Pezzulo JC, et al: Prognostic implications of p53 overexpression in supratentorial astrocytic tumors. Neurosurgery 35:351, 1994.
40. Hagel C, Krog B, et al: Prognostic relevance of TP53 mutations, p53 protein, Ki-67 index and conventional histological grading in oligodendrogliomas. J Exp Clin Cancer Res 18:305-309, 1999.
41. Ritland SR, Ganju V, et al: Region specific loss of heterozygosity on chromosome 19 is related to the morphologic type of human glioma. Genes Chromosomes Cancer 12:277-282, 1995.
42. Cairncross G, MacDonald D, et al: Chemotherapy for anaplastic oligodendroglioma. J Clin Oncol 12:2013-2021, 1994.
43. Hoang-Xuan K, Capelle L, et al: Temozolomide as initial treatment for adults with low-grade oligodendrogliomas or oligoastrocytomas and correlation with chromosome 1p deletions. J Clin Oncol 22:3133-3138, 2004.
44. Buckner JC, Ballman KV, et al: Diagnostic and prognostic significance of 1p and 19q deletions in patients (pts) with low-grade oligodendroglioma and astrocytoma. J Clin Oncol 23:1145, 2005.
45. Jaeckle KA, Eyre HJ, et al: Correlation of tumor O6 methylguanine-DNA methyltransferase levels with survival of malignant astrocytoma patients treated with bis-chloroethylnitrosourea: a Southwest Oncology Group study. J Clin Oncol 16:3310-3315, 1998.
46. Esteller M, Garcia-Foncillas, et al: Inactivation of the DNA-repair gene MGMT and the clinical response of gliomas to alkylating agents [erratum appears in N Engl J Med 343:1740, 2000]. N Engl J Med 343:1350-1354, 2000.
47. Hegi ME, Diserens AC, et al: MGMT gene silencing and benefit from temozolomide in glioblastoma. N Engl J Med 352:997-1003, 2005.
48. Komine C, Watanabe T, et al: Promoter hypermethylation of the DNA repair gene O6-methylguanine-DNA methyltransferase is an independent predictor of shortened progression free survival in patients with low-grade diffuse astrocytomas. Brain Pathol 13:176-184, 2003.
49. Abdulrauf SI, Edvardsen K, et al: Vascular endothelial growth factor expression and vascular density as prognostic markers of survival in patients with low-grade astrocytoma. J Neurosurg 88:513-520, 1998.
50. Piepmeier JM: Research strategies for evaluating the biological diversity of low-grade astrocytomas. Perspect Neurol Surg 4:1-20, 1993.
51. Piepmeier JM, Fried L, et al: Low-grade astrocytomas may arise from different astrocyte lineages. Neurosurgery 33:627-632, 1993.
52. Shaw EG, Scheithauer BW, et al: Supratentorial gliomas: a comparative study by grade and histologic type. J Neurooncol 31:273-278, 1997.
53. Laws ER Jr, Taylor WF, et al: Neurosurgical management of low-grade astrocytoma of the cerebral hemispheres. J Neurosurg 61:665-673, 1984.
54. McCormack BM, Miller DC, et al: Treatment and survival of low-grade astrocytoma in adults—1977-1988. Neurosurgery 31:636-642; discussion 642, 1992.
55. Miralbell R, Balart J, et al: Radiotherapy for supratentorial low-grade gliomas: results and prognostic factors with special focus on tumor volume parameters. Radiother Oncol 27:112-116, 1993.
56. Philippon JH, Clemenceau SH, et al: Supratentorial low-grade astrocytomas in adults. Neurosurgery 32:554-559, 1993.
57. Lote K, Egeland T, et al: Survival, prognostic factors, and therapeutic efficacy in low-grade glioma: a retrospective study in 379 patients. J Clin Oncol 15:3129-3140, 1997.
58. Brown PD, Buckner JC, et al: Importance of baseline Mini-Mental State Examination as a prognostic factor for patients with low-grade glioma. Int J Radiat Oncol Biol Phys 59:117-125, 2004.

59. North CA, North RB, et al: Low-grade cerebral astrocytomas. Survival and quality of life after radiation therapy. Cancer 66:6-14, 1990.
60. Dewit L, Van Der Schueren E, et al: Low-grade astrocytoma in children treated by surgery and radiation therapy. Acta Radiol 23:1-8, 1984.
61. Bloom HJ, Glees J, et al: The treatment and long-term prognosis of children with intracranial tumors: a study of 610 cases, 1950-1981 [erratum appears in Int J Radiat Oncol Biol Phys 19:829, 1990]. Int J Radiat Oncol Biol Phys 18:723-745, 1990.
62. Hoffman HJ, Soloniuk DS, et al: Management and outcome of low-grade astrocytomas of the midline in children: a retrospective review. Neurosurgery 33:964-971, 1993.
63. Pollack IF, Claassen D, et al: Low-grade gliomas of the cerebral hemispheres in children: An analysis of 71 cases. J Neurosurg 82:536-547, 1995.
64. Scerrati M, Roselli R, et al: Prognostic factors in low-grade (WHO grade II) gliomas of the cerebral hemispheres: the role of surgery. J Neurosurg Psychiatry 61:291-296, 1996.
65. Gajjar A, Sanford RA, et al: Low-grade astrocytoma: a decade of experience at St. Jude Children's Research Hospital. J Clin Oncol 15:2792-2799, 1997.
66. Piepmeier JM: Observations on the current treatment of low-grade astrocytic tumors of the cerebral hemispheres. J Neurosurg 67:177-181, 1987.
67. Medbery CA 3rd, Straus KL, et al: Low-grade astrocytomas: treatment results and prognostic variables. Int J Radiat Oncol Biol Phys 15:837-841, 1988.
68. Leighton C, Fisher B, et al: Supratentorial low-grade glioma in adults: an analysis of prognostic factors and timing of radiation. J Clin Oncol 15:1294-1301, 1997.
69. Reichenthal E, Feldman Z, et al: Hemispheric supratentorial low-grade astrocytomas. Neurochirurgia 35:18-22, 1992.
70. Rudoler S, Corn BW, et al: Patterns of tumor progression after radiotherapy for low-grade gliomas. Am J Clin Oncol 21:23-27, 1998.
71. Berger MS, Ghatan S, et al: Low-grade gliomas associated with intractable epilepsy: seizure outcome utilizing electrocorticography during tumor resection. J Neurosurg 79:62-69, 1993.
72. Kirkpatrick PJ, Honavar M, et al: Control of temporal lobe epilepsy following en bloc resection of low-grade tumors. J Neurosurg 78:19-52, 1993.
73. Fried I, Kim JH, et al: Limbic and neocortical gliomas associated with intractable seizures: a distinct clinicopathological group. Neurosurgery 34:815-824, 1994.
74. Silverman C, Marks J: Prognostic significance of contrast enhancement in low-grade astrocytomas of the adult cerebrum. Radiology 139:211-213, 1981.
75. Shaw EG, Daumas-Duport C, et al: Radiation therapy in the management of low-grade supratentorial astrocytomas. J Neurosurg 70:853-861, 1989.
76. Shaw EG, Scheithauer BW, et al: Postoperative radiotherapy of supratentorial low-grade gliomas. Int J Radiat Oncol Biol Phys 16:663-668, 1989.
77. Steiger JH, Markwalder RV, et al: Early prognosis of supratentorial grade 2 astrocytomas in adult patients after resection of stereotactic biopsy. Acta Neurochir (Wien) 106:99-105, 1990.
78. Whitton AC, Bloom HJC: Low-grade glioma of the cerebral hemispheres in adults: a retrospective analysis of 88 cases. Int J Radiat Oncol Biol Phys 18:783-786, 1990.
79. Vertosick FT, Selker RG, et al: Survival of patients with well-differentiated astrocytomas diagnosed in the era of computed tomography. Neurosurgery 28:496-450, 1991.
80. Recht LD, Lew R, et al: Suspected low-grade glioma: is deferring treatment safe? Ann Neurol 31:431-436, 1992.
81. Shibamoto Y, Kitakabu Y, et al: Supratentorial low-grade astrocytoma. Correlation of computed tomography findings with effect of radiation therapy and prognostic variables. Cancer 72:190-195, 1993.
82. Berger MS, Deliganis AV, et al: The effect of extent of resection on recurrence in patients with low grade cerebral hemisphere gliomas. Cancer 74:1784-1791, 1994.
83. Janny P, Cure H, et al: Low grade supratentorial astrocytomas. Management and prognostic factors. Cancer 73:1937-1945, 1994.
84. Daumas-Duport C, Scheithauer BW, et al: A histological and cytologic method for spatial definition of gliomas. Mayo Clin Proc 62:435-449, 1987.
85. Kelly PJ, Daumas-Duport C, et al: Stereotactic histologic correlations of computed tomography and magnetic resonance imaging-defined abnormalities in patients with glial neoplasms. Mayo Clin Proc 62:450-459, 1987.
86. McGirr SJ, Kelly PJ, et al: Stereotactic resection of juvenile pilocytic astrocytomas of the thalamus and basal ganglia. Neurosurgery 20:447-452, 1987.
87. Schuurman PR, Troost D, et al: 5-Year survival and clinical prognostic factors in progressive supratentorial diffuse low-grade astrocytoma: a retrospective analysis of 46 cases. Acta Neurochir (Wien) 139:2-7, 1997.
88. Pignatti F, van den Bent M, et al: Prognostic factors for survival in adult patients with cerebral low-grade glioma. J Clin Oncol 20:2076-2084, 2002.
89. Morantz RA: Radiation therapy in the treatment of cerebral astrocytoma. Neurosurgery 20:975-982, 1987.
90. Cairncross JG, Laperriere NJ: Low-grade glioma. To treat or not to treat? Arch Neurol 46:1238-1239, 1989.
91. Shaw E: The low-grade glioma debate: evidence defending the position of early radiation therapy. Clin Neurosurg 42:488-494, 1995.
92. Surma-aho O, Niemela M, Vilkki J, et al: Adverse long-term effects of brain radiotherapy in adult low-grade glioma patients. Neurology 56:1285-1290, 2001.
93. Shaw EG: Low-grade gliomas: to treat or not to treat? A radiation oncologist's viewpoint [editorial]. Arch Neurol 47:1138-1139, 1990.
94. Shaw EG, Won M, et al: Preliminary Results of RTOG Protocol 9802: A Phase II Study of Observation in Completely Resected Adult Low-Grade Glioma. Edinburgh, WFNO-II/EANO-VI, 2005.
95. van den Bent M, Afra D, et al: Long term results of EORTC study 22845: a randomized trial on the efficacy of radiation therapy of low-grade astrocytoma and oligodendroglioma in the adult. Lancet 366:985, 2005.
96. Wilden JN, Kelly PJ: CT computerized stereotactic biopsy for low density CT lesions presenting with epilepsy. J Neurol Neurosurg Psychiatry 50:1302-1305, 1987.
97. Kondziolka D, Lunsford D, et al: Unreliability of contemporary neurodiagnostic imaging in evaluating suspected adult supratentorial (low-grade) astrocytoma. J Neurosurg 79:533-536, 1993.
98. Rajan B, Pickuth D, et al: The management of histologically unverified presumed cerebral gliomas with radiotherapy. Int J Radiat Oncol Biol Phys 28:405-413, 1993.
99. Westergaard L, Gjerris F, et al: 3. Prognostic parameters in benign astrocytomas. Acta Neurochirurgica 123:1-7, 199.
100. Nicolato A, Gerosa MA, et al: Prognostic factors in low-grade supratentorial astrocytomas: a uni-multivariate statistical analysis in 76 surgically treated adult patients. Surg Neurol 44:208-221; discussion 221-223, 1995.
101. Bahary JP, Villemure JG, et al: Low-grade pure and mixed cerebral astrocytomas treated in the CT scan era. J Neurooncol 27:173-177, 1996.
102. Piepmeier J, Christopher S, et al: Variations in the natural history and survival of patients with supratentorial low-grade astrocytomas. Neurosurgery 38:872-878; discussion 878-879, 1996.
103. Mork SJ, Lindegaard K-F, et al: Oligodendroglioma: incidence and biologic behavior in a defined population. J Neurosurg 63:881-889, 1985.
104. Shaw EG, Scheithauer BW, et al: Oligodendrogliomas: the Mayo Clinic experience. J Neurosurg 76:428-434, 1992.
105. Celli P, Nofrone I, et al: Cerebral oligodendroglioma: prognostic factors and life history. Neurosurgery 35:1018-1035, 1994.
106. Florell RC, MacDonald DR, et al: Selection bias, survival, and brachytherapy for glioma [erratum appears in J Neurosurg 77:489, 1992]. J Neurosurg 76:179-183, 1992.
107. Rogers LR, Morris HH, et al: Effect of cranial irradiation on seizure frequency in adults with low grade astrocytoma and medically intractable epilepsy. Neurology 43:1599-1601, 1993.

108. Sunyach MP, Pommier P, et al: Conformal irradiation for pure and mixed oligodendroglioma: the experience of Centre Leon Berard Lyon. Int J Radiat Oncol Biol Phys 56:296-303, 2003.
109. Shaw E, Arusell R, et al: Prospective randomized trial of low- versus high-dose radiation therapy in adults with supratentorial low-grade glioma: initial report of a North Central Cancer Treatment Group/Radiation Therapy Oncology Group/Eastern Cooperative Oncology Group study. J Clin Oncol 20:2267-2276, 2002.
110. Karim AB, Maat B, et al: A randomized trial on dose-response in radiation therapy of low-grade cerebral glioma: European Organization for Research and Treatment of Cancer (EORTC) Study 22844. Int J Radiat Oncol Biol Phys 36:549-556, 1996.
111. Fitzek MM, Thornton AF, et al: Dose-escalation with proton/photon irradiation for Daumas-Duport lower-grade glioma: results of an institutional phase I/II trial. Int J Radiat Oncol Biol Phys 51:131-137, 2001.
112. Pozza F, Colombo F, et al: Low-grade astrocytomas: treatment with unconventionally fractionated external beam stereotactic radiation therapy. Radiology 171:565-569, 1989.
113. Souhami L, Olivier A, et al: Fractionated stereotactic radiation therapy for intracranial tumors. Cancer 68:2101-2108, 1991.
114. Somaza SC, Kondziolka D, et al: Early outcomes after stereotactic radiosurgery for growing pilocytic astrocytomas in children. Pediatr Neurosurg 25:109-115, 1996.
115. Marcus KJ, Goumnerova L, et al: Stereotactic radiotherapy for localized low-grade gliomas in children: final results of a prospective trial. Int J Radiat Oncol Biol Phys 61:374-379, 2005.
116. Hara A, Nishimura Y, et al: Effectiveness of intraoperative radiation therapy for recurrent supratentorial low grade glioma. J Neurooncol 25:239-243, 1995.
117. Mundinger F, Ostertag CB, et al: Stereotactic treatments of brain lesions. Appl Neurophysiol 43:198-204, 1980.
118. Szikla G, Schhenger M, et al: Interstitial and combined interstitial and external irradiation of supratentorial gliomas: results of 61 cases treated 1973-1981. Acta Neurochir (Wien) 33:355-362, 1984.
119. Schomberg PJ, Kelly P, et al: Phosphorus-32 therapy of cystic brain tumors [abstract]. Int J Radiat Oncol Biol Phys 15(Suppl 1):157, 1988.
120. Eyre HJ, Crowley JJ, et al: A randomized trial of radiotherapy versus radiotherapy plus CCNU for incompletely resected low-grade gliomas: a Southwest Oncology Group study. J Neurosurg 78:909-914, 1993.
121. Buckner JC, Gesme D, et al: Phase II trial of procarbazine, lomustine, and vincristine as initial therapy for patients with low-grade oligodendroglioma or oligoastrocytoma: efficacy and associations with chromosomal abnormalities. J Clin Oncol 21:251-255, 2003.
122. Mason WP, Krol GS, et al: Low-grade oligodendroglioma responds to chemotherapy. Neurology 46:203-207, 1996.
123. Pace A, Vidiri A, et al: Temozolomide chemotherapy for progressive low-grade glioma: clinical benefits and radiological response. Ann Oncol 14:1722-1726, 2003.
124. Quinn JA, Reardon DA, et al: Phase II trial of temozolomide in patients with progressive low-grade glioma. J Clin Oncol 21:646-651, 2003.
125. Brada M, Viviers L, et al: Phase II study of primary temozolomide chemotherapy in patients with WHO grade II gliomas. Ann Oncol 14:1715-1721, 2003.
126. Brown PD, Buckner JC, et al: Effects of radiotherapy on cognitive function in patients with low-grade glioma measured by the Folstein Mini-Mental State Examination. J Clin Oncol 21:2519-2524, 2003.
127. Buckner JC, Burch PA, et al: Phase II trial of nitrogen mustard, vincristine, and procarbazine (MOP) in patients with recurrent glioma: NCCTG results [abstract]. Proc ASCO 15:155, 1996.
128. Buckner JC, Brown LD, et al: Phase II evaluation of recombinant interferon alpha and BCNU in recurrent glioma. J Neurosurg 82:52-57, 1995.
129. Hayostek CJ, Shaw EG, et al: Astrocytomas of the cerebellum. A comparative clinicopathologic study of pilocytic and diffuse astrocytomas. Cancer 72:856-869, 1993.
130. Burger PC, Scheithauer BW: Tumors of the central nervous system. *In* Burger PC, Scheithauer BW (eds): Atlas of Tumor Pathology. Washington, DC, Armed Forces Institute of Pathology, 3rd series, fascicle 10, pp 96-105, 133-136, 163-172, 178-187, 1994.
131. Kleihues P, Cavanee WK: Pathology and Genetics of Tumours of the Nervous System. Lyon, France, International Agency for Research on Cancer Press, 1998, pp 34-36, 53, 182-184.
132. Morreale VM, Ebersold MJ, et al: Cerebellar astrocytoma: experience with 54 cases surgically treated at the Mayo Clinic, Rochester, Minnesota, from 1978 to 1990. J Neurosurg 87:257-261, 1997.
133. Brown PD, Buckner JC, et al: Adult patients with supratentorial pilocytic astrocytomas: a prospective multicenter clinical trial. Int J Radiat Oncol Biol Phys 58:1153-1160, 2004.
134. Krouwer HGJ, Davis RL, et al: Gangliogliomas: a clinicopathological study of 25 cases and review of the literature. J Neurooncol 17:139, 1993.
135. Kim DG, Paek SH, et al: Central neurocytoma: the role of radiation therapy and long term outcome. Cancer 79:1995, 1997.
136. Leenstra JL, Brown PD, et al: Central neurocytomas, the Mayo Clinic experience [abstract 2123]. 60S(Suppl):407-408, 2004.
137. Rades D, Fehlauer F, et al: Treatment of atypical neurocytomas. Cancer 100:814-817, 2004.
138. Sutton LN, Cnaan A, et al: Postoperative surveillance imaging in children with cerebellar astrocytomas. J Neurosurg 84:721-725, 1996.
139. Afra D, Muller W: Recurrent low-grade gliomas: dedifferentiation and prospects of reoperation. *In* Karim ABMF, Laws ERJ (eds): Glioma. Berlin, Springer, 1991, p 189.
140. Francavilla TL, Miletich RS, et al: Positron emission tomography in the detection of malignant degeneration of low-grade gliomas. Neurosurgery 24:1-5, 1989.
141. Bauman GS, Gaspar LE, et al: A prospective study of short-course radiotherapy in poor prognosis glioblastoma multiforme. Int J Radiat Oncol Biol Phys 29:835-839, 1994.
142. Forsyth PA, Kelly PJ, et al: Radiation necrosis or glioma recurrence: is computer assisted stereotactic biopsy useful? J Neurosurg 82:436-444, 1995.
143. Civetello LA, Packer RJ, et al: Leptomeningeal dissemination of low-grade gliomas in childhood. Neurology 38:562-566, 1988.
144. Sheline GE, Wara WM, et al: Therapeutic irradiation in brain injury. Int J Radiat Oncol Biol Phys 6:1215-1228, 1980.
145. Crossen JR, Garwood D, et al: Neurobehavioral sequelae of cranial irradiation in adults: a review of radiation-induced encephalopathy. J Clin Oncol 12:627-642, 1994.
146. Brown PD, Buckner JC, et al: The neurocognitive effects of radiation in adult low-grade glioma patients. Neuro-Oncology 5:161-167, 2003.
147. Taphoorn MJ, Schiphorst AK, et al: Cognitive functions and quality of life in patients with low-grade gliomas: the impact of radiotherapy [see comments]. Annals of Neurology 36:48-54, 1994.
148. Klein M, Heimans JJ, et al: Effect of radiotherapy and other treatment-related factors on mid-term to long-term cognitive sequelae in low-grade gliomas: a comparative study. Lancet 360:1361-1368, 2002.
149. Kiebert GM, Curran D, et al: Quality of life after radiation therapy of cerebral low-grade gliomas of the adult: results of a randomised phase III trial on dose response (EORTC trial 22844). EORTC Radiotherapy Co-operative Group. Eur J Cancer 34:1902-1909, 1998.
150. Kleinberg L, Wallner K, et al: Good performance status of long-term disease-free survivors of intracranial gliomas [published erratum appears in Int J Radiat Oncol Biol Phys 26:563, 1993]. Int J Radiat Oncol Biol Phys 26:129-133, 1993.
151. Gregor A, Cull A, et al: Neuropsychometric evaluation of long-term survivors of adult brain tumours: relationship with tumour and treatment parameters. Radiother Oncol 41:55-59, 1996.
152. Curnes JT, Laster DW, et al: MRI of radiation injury to the brain. AJR Am J Roentgenol 147:119-124, 1986.
153. Scheibel RS, Meyers CA, et al: Cognitive dysfunction following surgery for intracerebral glioma: influence of histopathology, lesion location, and treatment. J Neurooncol 30:61-69, 1996.

154. Imperato JP, Paleologos NA, et al: Effects of treatment on long-term survivors with malignant astrocytomas. Ann Neurol 28:818-822, 1990.
155. Laack NN, Brown PD: Cognitive sequelae of brain radiation in adults. Semin Oncol 31:702-713, 2004.
156. Armstrong C, Mollman J, et al: Effects of radiation therapy on adult brain behavior: evidence for a rebound phenomenon in a phase 1 trial. Neurology 43:1961-1965, 1993.
157. Armstrong, C, Ruffer J, et al: Biphasic patterns of memory deficits following moderate-dose partial-brain irradiation: neuropsychologic outcome and proposed mechanisms. J Clin Oncol 13:2263-2271, 1995.
158. Armstrong CL, Corn BW, et al: Radiotherapeutic effects on brain function: double dissociation of memory systems. Neuropsychiatry Neuropsychol Behav Neurol 13:101-111, 2000.
159. Armstrong CL, Hunter JV, et al: Late cognitive and radiographic changes related to radiotherapy: initial prospective findings. Neurology 59:40-48, 2002.
160. Laack N, Brown P, et al: Neurocognitive function after radiotherapy (RT) for supratentorial low-grade gliomas (LGG): results of a North Central Cancer Treatment Group (NCCTG) prospective study [abstract]. Int J Radiat Oncol Biol Phys 57(Suppl 1):34, 2003.
161. Vigliani MC, Sichez N, et al: A prospective study of cognitive functions following conventional radiotherapy for supratentorial gliomas in young adults: 4-year results. Int J Radiat Oncol Biol Phys 35:527-533, 1996.
162. Torres IJ, Mundt AJ, et al: A longitudinal neuropsychological study of partial brain radiation in adults with brain tumors. Neurology 60:1113-1118, 2003.
163. Shaw E, Arusell R, Scheithauer B, et al: A prospective randomized trial of low- versus high-dose radiation therapy in adults with supratentorial low-grade glioma: initial report of a NCCTG-RTOG-ECOG study [abstract]. Proc Am Soc Clin Oncol 17:401a, 1998.
164. Hirsch J-F, Sainte Rose C, et al: Benign astrocytic and oligodendrocytic tumors of the cerebral hemispheres in children. J Neurosurg 70:568-572, 1989.

CHAPTER 24

HIGH-GRADE GLIOMAS

John B. Fiveash, Robert A. Nordal, James M. Markert, Raef S. Ahmed, and Louis B. Nabors

INCIDENCE

There were 18,400 new cases of brain tumors in the United States in 2004. Glioblastoma multiforme (GBM) is the most common brain tumor. Gliomas account for 77% of malignant brain tumors.

BIOLOGICAL CHARACTERISTICS

World Health Organization grade III tumors, including anaplastic astrocytomas and anaplastic oligodendrogliomas, have a better prognosis than does GBM.

Better survival and response to therapy are associated with 1p/19q deletions commonly found in anaplastic oligodendrogliomas.

O^6-Methylguanine-DNA methyltransferase predicts for temozolomide sensitivity and is predictive of overall survival for GBM.

STAGING EVALUATION

Magnetic resonance imaging has generally replaced computed tomography for treatment planning in malignant gliomas. T2 or flair sequences demonstrate edema, which may or may not be infiltrated by neoplasm.

Magnetic resonance spectroscopy may be helpful in determining the extent of tumor within volume of T2 signal change. Postoperative day 1 imaging should be obtained to assess the extent of resection and for treatment planning.

PRIMARY THERAPY AND RESULTS

All patients with WHO grade III or IV neoplasms should have radiation therapy (RT) partial brain to approximately 60 Gy.

The only potential exception may be a select subset of patients with anaplastic oligodendrogliomas who have a complete response to chemotherapy.

ADJUVANT THERAPY

The routine use of RT plus concurrent and adjuvant temozolomide chemotherapy in patients with GBM is now supported by an EORTC randomized trial demonstrating an overall survival improvement.

Pure and mixed anaplastic oligodendrogliomas have at least a disease-free survival advantage to adjuvant PCV (procarbazine, CCNU, vincristine) chemotherapy in addition to adjuvant RT. Temozolomide has less toxicity than PCV and is preferred at many centers.

Interstitial BCNU wafers have a modest survival advantage in newly diagnosed patients with resected GBM.

Randomized trials do not show a survival advantage for either adjuvant radiosurgery or adjuvant brachytherapy when combined with fractionated partial brain radiation therapy.

LOCALLY ADVANCED DISEASE AND RETREATMENT

Older patients (more than 65 years of age) and those with a poor performance status that does not improve with steroids should be considered for hypofractionated regimens of radiation therapy or no therapy.

Additional radiation therapy utilizing stereotactic radiosurgery, brachytherapy, or retreatment with fractionated radiation using 3D conformal or intensity-modulated radiation therapy (IMRT) techniques may be considered for patients with selected focally recurrent malignant gliomas.

Malignant gliomas include a spectrum of primary brain tumors that represent some of the most lethal and debilitating neoplasms known. Long-term survival for glioblastoma multiforme (GBM), estimated at 2% to 5% at 5 years, has been the subject of case reports in young patients, genomic inquisition, and questioned diagnoses.[1-3] In contrast with other high-grade malignancies, recurrence of high-grade gliomas is predominantly a local problem. Proximity of tumor to eloquent brain often prevents wide margins of resection, and even when wide resection is possible, failure occurs most commonly at the resection margin.

Despite more than 30 years of extensive clinical trials, only recently has progress been made in the treatment of these neoplasms. Both surgery and radiation therapy (RT) have benefited from improvements in tumor imaging, allowing more accurate RT and more complete, safer tumor resections. The introduction of temozolomide chemotherapy has demonstrated a positive survival impact in patients with newly diagnosed GBM. Genomic analysis of anaplastic oligodendroglioma and the recognition of specific molecular markers enable physicians to identify a subset of patients with chemotherapy-sensitive tumors. Future studies will elucidate the underlying cancer biology of these resistant neoplasms and allow for molecularly targeted therapy, likely in combination with conventional therapies such as RT and chemotherapy.

ETIOLOGY AND EPIDEMIOLOGY

High-grade gliomas constitute 77% of malignant brain tumors.[4] Eighty-two percent of cases are GBM.[4] Incidence is greatest in the 65- to 75-year age group, and men are affected more commonly than women. Median survival decreases with increasing age.

There is little consensus on environmental influences that may contribute to gliomagenesis. Exposures suggested to play a role in brain tumor development include electromagnetic fields, cellular telephone use, and certain occupational exposures. As for studies on dietary factors such as nitrosamines, the results of epidemiologic studies assessing risk impact for these exposures have been inconclusive.[5,6] Therapeutic ionizing radiation is known to be associated with subsequent development of brain tumors.[7] While prior RT may increase relative risks by several-fold or higher, the vast majority of patients presenting with malignant glioma do not have a history of therapeutic radiation exposure.

Inherited genetic factors play a role in some cases of high-grade glioma. Genes involved in heritable tumor syndromes may have a role in sporadic gliomagenesis. Families with germline mutation of the *TP3* tumor suppressor gene exhibit an increased frequency of gliomas when other Li Fraumeni syndrome manifestations are present.[8] In addition to the more common optic gliomas, high-grade gliomas also occur in patients with neurofibromatosis type I, although mutations at the NF1 site are not frequently present in sporadic tumors.[9] Malignant gliomas also occur in Turcot's syndrome, where mutations in DNA mismatch repair enzymes appear to underlie colorectal and astroglial brain tumors. Genetic polymorphisms in detoxification enzyme or DJS repair loci may play a role in development of astrocytic tumors, although to date the data are inconclusive.[10,11]

PREVENTION AND EARLY DETECTION

There are no environmental factors with sufficient generality or importance to constitute a basis for preventive strategies aimed at decreasing glioma incidence. Further, evidence of curability with earlier detection, such as would support screening programs, is lacking. Screening approaches may have a role in familial brain tumor cohorts, although the rarity of these conditions hinders standardization of such assessment.

BIOLOGICAL CHARACTERISTICS AND MOLECULAR BIOLOGY

High-grade gliomas display a diversity of gene expression changes that may alter signal transduction pathways, cell growth control, cell cycle, apoptosis, and differentiation. Abnormal growth factor receptor expression and cell cycle arrest control are among the most common changes seen. Activating mutations or amplification of platelet-derived growth factor (PDGF), epidermal growth factor (EGF), or their receptors (PDGFR and EGFR) are often observed. Another growth-stimulatory change that may contribute to tumor development and progression is focal adhesion kinase (FAK) overexpression and associated signaling. FAK is overexpressed in astrocytomas and glioblastomas, and overexpression contributes to proliferation in vitro and in vivo and may also be important in malignant cell migration and tumor angiogenesis.[12-14]

Mutations of *CDKN2A* (previously designated *p16*) and the *RB1* gene are often present.[15,16] These tumor suppressor genes have key roles in the CDKN2A-CDK4/cyclin D1-RB1 cell cycle regulatory pathway. Other tumor suppressor genes, including *TP53* and *PTEN* (formerly designated *MMAC1*), and *MDM2* and other genes important in cell cycle regulation commonly bear mutations.[17,18]

High-grade gliomas commonly demonstrate deletion of *PTEN*, which results in cell growth–promoting de-repression of AKT phosphorylation.[19] This is believed to be a basis for the increased proliferation observed in *PTEN*-deleted astrocytes.[20]

The fact that the commonly affected growth factors are of key importance in differentiation of astrocytes has been hypothesized to indicate a link between astrocyte differentiation pathways and glioma formation, as suggested by Dai and Holland.[21] EGF and PDGF stimulation and disruption of cell cycle arrest pathways may maintain cells in an undifferentiated, progenitor-like state that allows continued proliferation.

Major Pathways

Molecular characterization of high-grade gliomas has revealed distinctive pathways of progression from cells of astrocytic lineage to glioblastoma (Fig. 24-1). De novo glioblastomas are more common in elderly patients and often involve nonsequential overexpression of EGFR and *MDM2* and mutation or loss of *PTEN, RB1*, or *CDKN2A. CDKN2A* deletion has been observed in tumors with EGFR amplification and is associated with higher proliferation rates.[22] Association of *p16/CDKN2* deletion and amplification of EGFR has been suggested to underlie the worse prognosis seen in elderly patients.[23] *PTEN* inactivation is most commonly seen in the de novo glioblastoma pathway.[24]

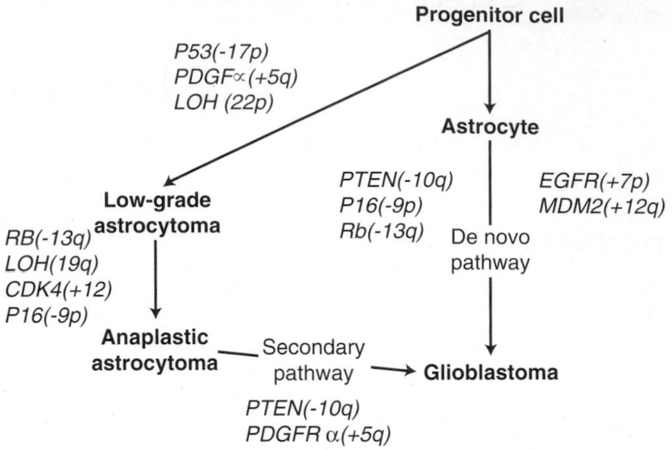

Figure 24-1 Secondary and de novo glioblastomas develop from specific molecular pathways. Epidermal growth factor receptor (EGFR) amplification is more frequent in de novo glioblastoma. Deletion of P16 (now designated CDKN2A) or amplification of CDK4 or cyclin D is believed to have a role in antagonizing RB protein function in these tumors. In combination with growth-stimulatory amplification of PDGFα, loss of wild-type P53 (TP53) function seems to be a foundation for development of low-grade astrocytic tumors. The TP53 mutation is less common in de novo glioblastoma. Loss of RB protein function (i.e., P16-CDK4-RB G_1/S checkpoint control) accompanies progression from low-grade to high-grade astrocytomas. PTEN deletion is seen frequently in glioblastomas that arise through either pathway.

In the secondary pathway, histologic progression occurs from a previously known low-grade astrocytoma. These patients are often younger, and their tumors display a sequence of genetic changes that parallel malignant progression. *TP53* mutation and overexpression of PDGFRs and ligands represent key steps in this pathway.

While these molecular changes exert effects in relevant pathways, the prognostic importance for specific genetic characteristics has not been firmly established. Enhanced expression and amplification of the EGFR gene are well established in glial tumors.[25] There is evidence that abnormal EGFR amplification/overexpression or internal gene rearrangement may portend poorer outcome in anaplastic astrocytoma (AA) and GBM, although this was not confirmed in all studies.[26-30] Newer cDNA or protein array technologies may provide insights into the interrelationships of important genetic alterations and their downstream effectors.

PATHOLOGY AND PATHWAYS OF SPREAD

High-grade astrocytic neoplasms demonstrate a diffuse infiltration of cells with an appearance similar to normal astrocytes. Astrocytes have small, round nuclei and numerous filaments composed of glial fibrillary acidic protein (GFAP). Tumor sections often contain reactive astrocytes, or gemistocytes, which display thickened and elongated cytoplasmic processes and enlarged cell bodies. Specific findings that support a diagnosis of malignancy are increased cellularity, nuclear and cytoplasmic pleomorphism, mitoses, small vessel or endothelial cell proliferation, and necrosis. These features are used for both diagnosis and grading. The World Health Organization (WHO) classification system uses criteria generally concordant with the Ste. Anne-Mayo system, with scoring based on the number of malignant features (cellular pleomorphism, mitotic activity, vascular endothelial proliferation, and necrosis) that are present.[31] AA (grade III) and GBM (grade IV) are characterized by the presence of three or four malignant features, respectively.[31]

High-grade gliomas spread by direct infiltration of surrounding brain. Tumors that originate near the corpus callosum may extend across the midline and involve the opposite cerebral hemisphere in a so-called butterfly pattern. While the extent of resection is generally believed to correlate with improved outcome, wide resection is not curative because of the diffuse and extensive infiltration of grossly normal brain. The diffuse character of the disease is most pronounced in multifocal presentations of AA or GBM. Tumor spread through the ventricular system and subarachnoid space can occur, and a small minority of patients develop spinal or spinal subarachnoid metastases, often as a late event. The absence of lymphatics eliminates that compartment as a pathway of spread. Hematogenous metastases, while possible, are very infrequent.

CLINICAL MANIFESTATIONS, PATIENT EVALUATION, AND STAGING

Most patients with malignant gliomas experience headache, nausea, or neurologic complaints including seizure as an initial presenting symptom. History and physical examination plus careful review of imaging studies may suggest a specific diagnosis, which will be confirmed by pathologic examination. Depending on the location, symptoms, and extent of tumor, pathologic confirmation of the diagnosis can be obtained through stereotactic needle biopsy, open biopsy, or attempted gross resection. An algorithm for the evaluation and management of patients with GBM is shown in Figure 24-3.

Most commonly, computed tomography (CT) without contrast performed in an emergency department reveals an intra-axial abnormality requiring further evaluation, including magnetic resonance imaging (MRI). An isolated ring enhancing or heterogeneously enhancing lesion in the brain in the absence of a history of cancer should be considered a possible malignant glioma. Differential diagnosis includes stroke, infectious etiologies, brain metastasis, and central nervous system (CNS) lymphoma. CNS lymphoma is more often multifocal and periventricular. If CNS lymphoma is strongly considered on the list of differential diagnoses, consideration should be given to withholding steroids in patients with limited symptoms, as this may interfere with biopsy. Chest radiography or body CT may demonstrate another primary neoplasm that is easier to biopsy than the brain.

Examples of imaging for GBM are shown in Figure 24-2. Approximately 5% to 10% of AAs will not enhance. Nonenhancement on MRI is more often suggestive of grade II astrocytic neoplasms. Pilocytic astrocytomas may enhance homogeneously even though they are lower grade. Malignant gliomas usually show nonspecific increased uptake on FDG positron emission tomography (PET), but background brain uptake has limited the applicability of PET in the diagnosis and follow-up of primary brain tumors. ^{1}H magnetic resonance spectroscopy (MRS) may help to distinguish the extent of the tumor within the T2-weighted or fluid-attenuated inversion recovery (FLAIR) abnormality and may augment conventional MRI to determine the extent of tumor after surgical resection.[32]

Prognostic Factors

Several prognostic factors have emerged from retrospective and prospective clinical trials. Until very recently, most clinical trials of malignant gliomas have included a variety of histologic subtypes rather than just glioblastoma, AA, or anaplastic oligodendroglioma. From these historical studies have emerged several prognostic factors. These studies have served as the background for clinical trial planning and patient stratification for modern clinical trials.

The RTOG database has served as a primary source of prognostic factors for malignant gliomas. In a review of patient outcomes from three large randomized trials with 1578 patients with malignant glioma treated in 1974 through 1989,

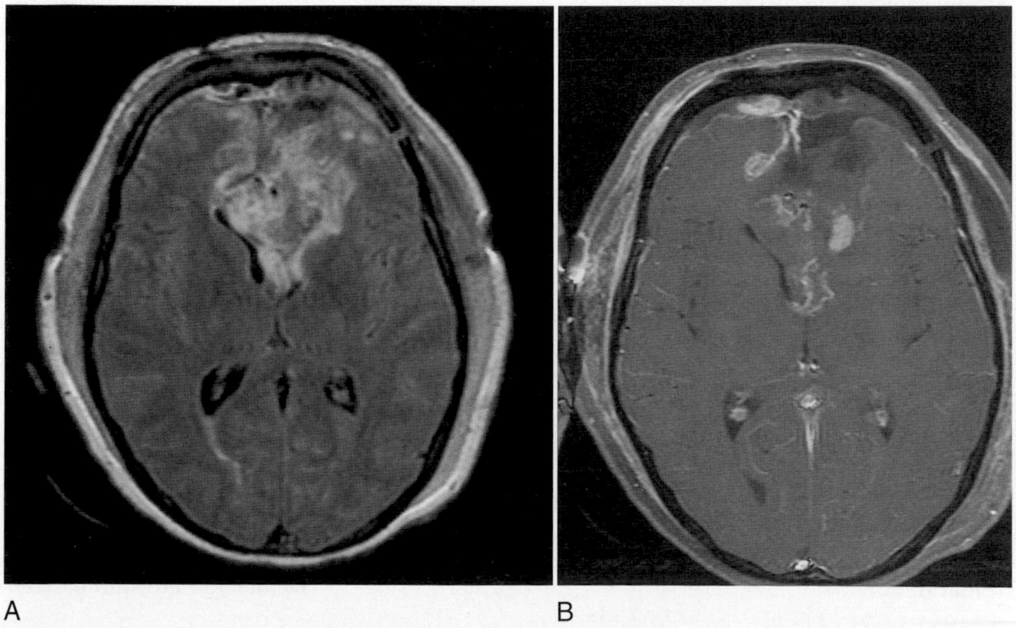

Figure 24-2 **A,** FLAIR MRI of radiographically typical glioblastoma multiforme shows extensive surrounding edema. **B,** Postcontrast MRI demonstrated typical bifrontal involvement. This tumor has been subtotally resected.

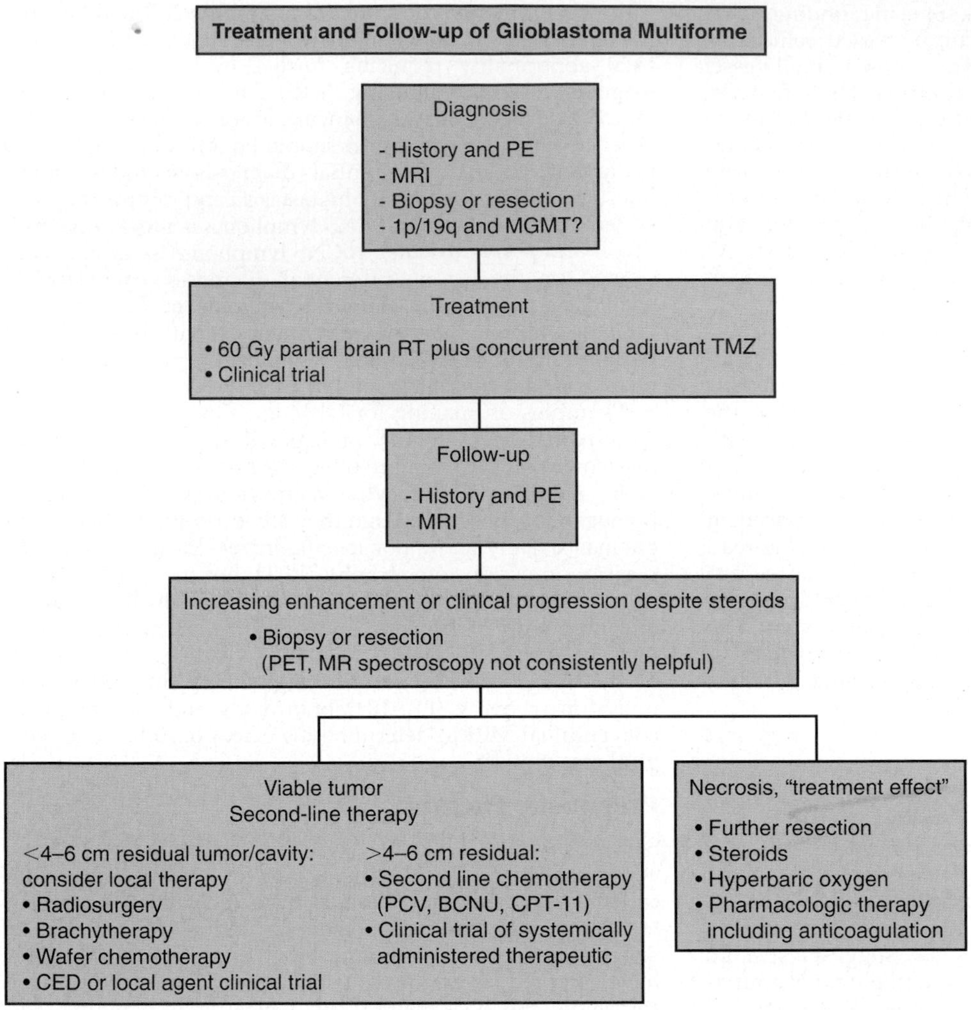

Figure 24-3 Algorithm for the diagnosis and treatment of glioblastoma multiforme.

Curran and colleagues used a recursive partitioning analysis (RPA) to group patients into six prognostic groups. Median survival among the six groups varied from 4.3 to 58.6 months. The important prognostic factors were age older than 50 years, histology (GBM versus AA), mental status, Karnofsky performance status (90 to 100 versus less than 90), length of symptoms prior to surgery (less than 3 months versus more than 3 months), extent of resection, neurologic function, and RT dose (less than 54.4 Gy versus more than 54 Gy). Table 24-1 shows the RPA tree and the survival curves for the resulting six prognostic classes demonstrating the heterogeneity of patients with malignant glioma. The RTOG RPA classification has been used to partially adjust for selection bias in phase I/II studies of promising new agents. It may also be helpful in counseling patients regarding their individual prognosis.

Newer clinical trials now recognize variations in prognosis among the histologic subtypes and do not include all subtypes of malignant glioma. Investigators from the University of California San Francisco have performed an RPA of patients with GBM, excluding other histologic subtypes of malignant glioma.[33] The most important prognostic factors in this analysis are similar to other studies: age, performance status, and extent of resection. The best prognostic subset in this analysis included patients less than 40 years of age with frontal tumors.

The extent of resection performed for malignant glioma remains variable within standard neurosurgical practices in the United States. Retrospective studies strongly suggest that patients with a subtotal resection do not live as long as those with gross total resections. It is unknown if this represents a therapeutic benefit or selection bias for those patients with less extensive tumors. For patients with controlled symptoms on steroids who are at risk for permanent serious neurologic injury with very aggressive resection, subtotal resection or biopsy only should be considered. No phase III data exist to verify the potential survival impact of very aggressive resections. In a large retrospective study of 416 patients treated at M. D. Anderson hospital with GBM, a volumetric analysis of the extent of resection on postoperative MRI suggested that at least 98% tumor removal was associated with a survival advantage compared with less complete resections (13.0 months versus 8.8 months, $P < .0001$).[34]

Building upon the clinical prognostic factors, several studies have searched for molecular markers that may predict for prognosis or response to therapy. In anaplastic oligodendroglioma and other histologies of malignant gliomas to a lesser extent, the predictive value of lesions with 1p19q loss of heterozygosity (LOH) is now well recognized.[35-37] A variety of other molecular markers have been studied as prognostic factors and are summarized in Table 24-2. This table includes

Table 24-1 RTOG Recursive Partitioning Analysis (RPA) Classification Showing Prognostic Groups of Malignant Glioma and Overall Survival by RPA Class

Class	Definition	Median Survival (mo)
I	Age <50, anaplastic astrocytoma, and normal mental status	58.6
II	Age ≥50, KPS 70 to 100, anaplastic astrocytoma, and at least 3 mo from time of first symptoms to initiation treatment	37.4
III	Age <50, anaplastic astrocytoma and abnormal mental status Age <50, glioblastoma multiforme and KPS 90-100	17.9
IV	Age <50, glioblastoma multiforme, KPS <90 Age ≥50, KPS 70 to 100, anaplastic astrocytoma and ≤3 mo from time of first symptoms to start of treatment Age >50, glioblastoma multiforme, surgical resection, and good neurologic function	11.1
V	Age ≥50, KPS 70 to 100, glioblastoma multiforme, either surgical resection and neurologic function that inhibits the ability to work or biopsy only followed by at least 54.4 Gy of radiation therapy Age ≥50, KPS <70, normal mental status	8.9
VI	Age ≥50, KPS <70, abnormal mental status Age ≥50, KPS 70 to 100, glioblastoma multiforme, biopsy only, receiving <54.4 Gy of radiation therapy	4.6

Table 24-2 Selected Molecular Markers of Prognostic Significance in Malignant Glioma

Marker	Function and Significance
1p/19q LOH	Loss of heterozygosity is associated with oligodendroglial phenotype, response to chemotherapy and RT, and better overall survival
PTEN	Tumor suppressor gene, regulator of PI3 kinase, correlated with activation of akt and mTOR
Survivin	Antiapoptotic protein associated with worse survival
EGFR including vIII mutant	Prognostic significance of overexpression is debated but may be associated with worse survival
p53	Tumor suppression gene, associated with age, mutation associated with better survival
Her-2/neu	Overexpression associated with worse survival
PI3 kinase	Regulator of survival pathways including akt and p70
P70	Inversely associated with caspase-3 activation, regulator of apoptosis
akt	Suppresser of apoptosis
MAP kinase	Mitogen-activated kinase is associated with MIB-1 labeling index and overall survival
O^6-Methylguanine-DNA methyltransferase (MGMT)	Inactivation of MGMT promoter by methylation is associated with longer survival for patients receiving temozolomide
VEGF/Flk-1	Regulator of angiogenesis and vascular permeability

only those markers that have been studied clinically. O^6-Methylguanine-DNA methyltransferase (MGMT) is of particular significance in patients receiving temozolomide. Methylation of the MGMT promoter has been associated with sensitivity to alkylating agents including temozolomide and BCNU preclinically. If methylation is not present, then MGMT can more effectively repair the DNA damage from temozolomide. Hegi and colleagues[38] reviewed the methylation status of MGMT in patients enrolled in a phase II trial of RT plus temozolomide. Twenty-six of the 38 patients (68%) had tumors with promoter methylation. These patients had superior survival of 62% at 18 months versus only 8% in patients without promoter methylation ($P = .0051$). This initial observation was later validated in a phase III trial of adjuvant temozolomide where 45% of' tumors had the methylated promoter.[39] Among patients receiving temozolomide and RT, 2-year survival was 46% with methylation of MGMT versus 13.8% without methylation ($P < .05$). There was only a borderline difference in survival by treatment arm for patients with a nonmethylated promoter ($P = .06$), suggesting that these patients should be considered for clinical trials of novel agents.

Because gliomas are genetically heterogeneous, more sophisticated prognostic analysis may be possible through gene expression profiling. Investigators from University of California Los Angeles defined and validated a limited set of genes that predict for prognosis independent of histology.[40] A large tissue study is under way by investigators at the National Cancer Institute that could eventually lead to a brain tumor–specific chip and a new standardized, objective staging system based upon gene expression profiling.

PRIMARY THERAPY

In discussing therapies for malignant gliomas, a comprehensive examination of failed therapies could fill an entire textbook. For review, a listing of selected promising approaches tested in negative phase III trials is shown in Table 24-3. This section focuses on the evolution of the standard of care over time and ongoing investigations with a look toward the future.

Surgery

General Considerations

Surgery is generally the first intervention for patients with suspected glioma. Surgery may consist of a simple biopsy to establish a diagnosis. More often, patients undergo a craniotomy aimed at removing as large a fraction of the tumor as is safely possible, with the goal of establishing a diagnosis and reducing the residual tumor burden. Surgical cure of gliomas is possible in only a few histologic subtypes (e.g., juvenile pilocytic astrocytoma, pleomorphic xanthoastrocytoma, etc.);

Table 24-3 **Selected Negative Phase III Randomized Trials in Malignant Glioma**

Modality or Agent	Initial Rationale and Comments
Hyperfractionated[148] and accelerated hyperfractionated RT[68]	Dose escalation, phase I/II studies suggested a benefit
Radiosurgery[84]	Retrospective studies suggested a benefit
Brachytherapy[88,149]	Retrospective studies suggested a benefit
Pions[150]	Intermediate LET
Fast neutrons[151,152]	High LET
DFMO[68]	Radiation sensitization
Misonidazole[148]	Hypoxic cell sensitization should be helpful in a necrotic tumor
Halogenated pyrimidines[153]	BUDR radiosensitization, promising phase II results in AA
Neoadjuvant BCNU and cisplatin[154]	Early chemotherapy may be more efficacious
Concurrent mitomycin C[155]	Malignant gliomas are hypoxic
Intra-arterial cisplatin[156]	Higher chemotherapy dose
Intra-arterial BCNU[157]	Higher chemotherapy dose
Cereport (RMP-7)[158]	Increase vascular permeability to deliver more chemotherapy
HSV/tk gene therapy with ganciclovir[159]	Suicide gene therapy

tk, thymidine kinase.

the vast majority of gliomas, including WHO grade II, III, and IV astrocytomas, oligodendrogliomas, ependymomas, and tumors with mixed histology, invade normal adjacent brain, and thus complete surgical removal is not possible. For high-grade gliomas, maximal tumor cytoreduction with minimal risk to the patient becomes the surgical objective. Surgery can rapidly reduce tumor bulk with potential benefits on secondary tumor mass effects, such as edema and hydrocephalus. While the benefits of cytoreductive surgery may be disputed by some, patients with symptoms clearly related to mass effect, impending herniation, or obstruction of cerebrospinal fluid outflow are universally accepted as candidates for surgical debulking.

Diagnosis of the histologic subtype of the lesion remains an undisputed goal of surgery. Certain lesions may have almost a classic MRI appearance (e.g., the butterfly glioma involving both hemispheres and the corpus callosum). Technological advancements in the area of MRS and perfusion can give further information about a tumor, including increasingly accurate preoperative appraisals of tumor grade.[41,42] However, important information about (1) histologic subtype, such as whether a particular tumor is an astrocytoma, oligodendroglioma, or a mixed tumor, and (2) increasingly relevant genetic information, such as the 1p and 19q chromosomal status of tumors, has become important in determining both patient prognosis and optimal treatment approaches. To date, such details have not been uniformly predictable based on preoperative testing alone.

Advances in surgical approaches, techniques and instrumentation, and the use of surgical navigation devices have rendered the majority of tumors amenable to resection and/or debulking; however, in some anatomic locations, the relative risk of open operation supports the choice of biopsy for obtaining tissue for diagnosis. Biopsy techniques include stereotactic biopsy using either CT or MRI to choose the target. Simple ultrasonic guidance can also be considered for obtaining diagnostic tissue. Metabolic imaging such as MRS or perfusion can be superimposed onto anatomic images (usually standard MRI) to choose biopsy sites that are likely to represent the most aggressive portions of the tumor. It is critical to obtain tissue from these regions of the tumor, as the overall behavior of a tumor is defined by its most aggressive portion. Otherwise, patients may be assigned a diagnosis that does not represent the most aggressive histology of the tumor based on sampling error. Such sampling error can result in both inaccurate prognostication and inappropriate therapeutic decision-making.

Either general endotracheal anesthesia or local anesthesia with sedation can be used for craniotomies. Patients undergoing "awake" craniotomy, that is, craniotomy with sedation and local anesthetic, for the resection of supratentorial tumors should be placed on anticonvulsants preoperatively, to minimize the possibility of a seizure occurring intraoperatively. The routine use of postoperative anticonvulsants for perioperative treatment of patients with supratentorial gliomas remains controversial, although a survey suggests that the majority of neurosurgeons do prescribe anticonvulsants, at least in the perioperative period.[43] Anticonvulsants are not generally prescribed for posterior fossa tumors due to the relative rarity of seizures associated with these lesions. Patients are generally given corticosteroids, usually dexamethasone, preoperatively and often for several days before glioma surgery to reduce cerebral edema and thus minimize secondary brain injury from cerebral retraction. Steroids are then continued in the immediate postoperative period and tapered as quickly as possible. Antibiotics are given shortly before incision to decrease the risk of wound infection.

Ordinarily, cranial fixation is used to minimize inadvertent patient movement during dissection. Steps are taken to minimize intracranial pressure (ICP), which may be high due to tumor bulk, edema, and blockage of cerebrospinal fluid outflow. The patient's head is placed slightly above the level of the heart to increase venous drainage and to avoid jugular venous compression. Mild hyperventilation is used. Mannitol is administered, often with furosemide, to decrease brain swelling. Minimizing ICP decreases the amount of brain retraction necessary during tumor resection; such retraction can result in neurologic injury. In extreme cases, high ICP can result in brain herniation when the dura is opened.

Craniotomy for Tumor Resection

The scalp incision or flap is designed to allow a complete exposure of the region of the proposed bony flap; the scalp's vascular supply is given careful consideration. The bony opening is designed to be large enough to facilitate surgery, without unduly exposing adjacent brain to the risk of inadvertent injury. An image-guided surgical navigation device can be used to minimize the size of the bone flap and scalp incision, by precisely locating the desired entry point for the procedure. After the scalp opening is made, burr holes are placed and connected with an air-powered device, the craniotome. The bone flap can then be removed, and the dura opened. Generally, the bone flap is reattached at the end of the resection, although many surgeons perform craniectomies for posterior fossa and temporal lobe lesions.

Tumors on the brain surface may be immediately visible. However, when the lesion is subcortical, the exposed field may appear normal. If the tumor is located near eloquent cortex, motor and speech function can be mapped intraoperatively using electrical cortical stimulation to allow for a safe approach for tumor resection.[44] Preoperative functional MRI or magnetoencephalography can also guide the surgeon. Motor mapping can be done under general anesthesia if muscle relaxants are avoided. Glioma resections in the dominant hemisphere are often done using local anesthesia with supplementary sedation to allow speech mapping.[44]

Frameless image-guided neuronavigation systems are widely used for localization of subcortical tumors along with intraoperative ultrasound and MRI.[45-47] During surgery, a neuronavigation system can display the location of a probe or surgical instrument superimposed on preoperative MR or CT images in real time. Neuronavigation can be used to determine the site of the scalp opening and the craniotomy flap, to localize subcortical tumors, and to estimate progress during tumor resection. There can be differences between the preoperative images and the actual position of the brain after portions of the tumor have been removed, resulting in "brain shift" and a loss of accuracy of these systems.[48] Intraoperative imaging using ultrasound, CT, and MRI can be used to provide an immediate estimate of the progress of the resection and to update the navigation system. While these systems do increase the degree of resection achieved, the impact on patient outcome has not yet been clarified. In one retrospective series, resection of more than 97% of enhancing tumor volume by MRI resulted in greater median survivals.[34]

Tumor removal is usually done with grasping and dissecting instruments, bipolar coagulation, and suction, but removal of firm, adherent, or calcified tumor tissue can require the use of a cavitational ultrasonic aspirator (CUSA), which uses ultrasound to disrupt the tissue at its tip and then aspirates it out of the field. Some surgeons prefer using the CO_2 laser, which can vaporize tumor tissue in situ. Tumor removal with a laser is slow, however, and is usually reserved for special circumstances. Tumors may be removed en bloc by circumferential dissection, or piecemeal, by entering the tumor directly. Piecemeal resection is favored by some surgeons, particularly when the tumor invades an adjacent region of eloquent brain; this is usually associated with more blood loss due to the tumor vasculature, which can make the resection more difficult; en bloc resection is usually faster with less associated blood loss but can be difficult if the tumor is deep, is recurrent, or lacks the pseudocapsule often seen in malignant gliomas.

In the rare situations in which brain swelling and elevations in ICP remain worrisome at the time of closure, a catheter can be left in the ventricle to measure the ICP and drain cerebrospinal fluid. Patients are routinely monitored in the intensive care unit overnight after surgery, and MRI is performed within 24 to 48 hours to evaluate the extent of any remaining tumor. MRI done after this time may result in an inaccurate assessment of residual tumor, as postoperative changes in the blood-brain barrier can result in enhancement occurring in regions outside the residual tumor.

Stereotactic Tumor Biopsy

For deeply situated intrinsic tumors or diffuse nonfocal tumors, resection is not practical. In these situations, needle biopsy is used for diagnosis. Open biopsy is reserved for unusual situations, such as a small lesion abutting a large blood vessel; these lesions are often simply resected. While tissue can be obtained through a needle directed by hand through a burr hole under ultrasound, CT, or MRI guidance, the simplicity and accuracy of CT- or MRI-directed stereotactic biopsy remains the gold standard for glioma biopsy.

For a typical stereotactic biopsy, the patient undergoes CT or MRI with a rigid frame including fiducial bars fixed to the skull to eliminate movement. A variety of systems are available.[49] For most adults, local anesthesia and intravenous sedation are used; children usually require general anesthesia. The MRI or CT shows the fiducials on each image. The desired biopsy target is selected, and an algorithm is used to generate the appropriate coordinates to pass a needle through a small burr hole in the skull to the target. Stereotactic biopsy can be done without a frame using a neuronavigation system. Fiducial markers are placed on the scalp and imaging is obtained. The target is chosen and an approach to the target is planned. The patient is placed in a rigid head holder, and the system guides the needle using the known location of the fiducials relative to the target. Whether or not a frame is used, a small tissue core is obtained from the target using a side-biting needle. Frozen section pathology confirms the acquisition of diagnostic tissue. Experienced surgeons obtain diagnostic tissue in more than 95% of patients.[50] An overnight stay or day surgery is the rule. Hemorrhage at the biopsy site, the principal risk of the surgery, occurs in few patients. Occasionally, cerebral edema is exacerbated by a biopsy. This usually responds to increased doses of corticosteroids.

External Beam Radiation Therapy

Radiation therapy has been used in the treatment of malignant gliomas for over six decades.[51] The first randomized trial demonstrating a survival advantage to RT over supportive care was performed by the Brain Tumor Study Group (BTSG).[52,53] The BTSG trial established a benefit for postoperative RT after demonstrating a 37.5-week median survival in RT alone versus 17 and 25 weeks for patients treated with conventional care and BCNU, respectively. BCNU and RT produced a 40.5-week median survival. Ninety percent of the patients enrolled in this trial had GBM.

Rationale for Current Radiation Volumes

Early clinical trials evaluating the role of RT in patients with malignant glioma used 50 to 60 Gy to the entire cranial contents, whole brain radiation therapy (WBRT).[52] This treatment was administered via large parallel-opposed lateral fields. With the advent of CT and MRI, tumor volumes can be more accurately defined. Although no large-scale randomized trials have been reported that directly compare WBRT versus partial brain RT, an intergroup trial changed design to include randomization to partial brain RT versus WBRT after initially accruing patients to WBRT alone.[54] In this large dataset, no overall survival difference was seen with smaller RT volumes. One additional small randomized trial of 50 patients with high-grade glioma found equivalent survival, similar patterns of recurrence, and possibly better KPS scores in patients receiving limited fields.[55] Furthermore, pathologic correlates with imaging and retrospective clinical studies support partial brain RT as an equivalent therapy.[56-58] The few long-term survivors may benefit from less toxicity with this approach. In addition, the patterns of failure of partial brain RT can now be assessed and suggest that progression is most likely to occur at the site or in close proximity to the previous enhancing abnormality. Hochberg and Pruitt[56] asserted in 1980 that partial brain RT could be administered rather than WBRT after finding that 90% of GBMs recurred on CT within 2 cm of the primary tumor site. Wallner and colleagues[59] studied the patterns of progression in 32 patients with unifocal malignant glioma treated with surgical resection and postoperative RT. Seventy-eight percent of patients progressed within 2 cm of the original tumor on CT scan. In a second follow-up study of the patterns of failure of 12 patients at second recurrence, 8 of 12 patients also progressed within 2 cm of the original tumor.[60] In a quantitative volumetric assessment of the patterns of failure after high-dose RT, Lee and colleagues[61] found that the vast majority of patients still progressed at the site of the primary tumor despite high-dose three-dimensional conformal therapy.

The conventional approach to MRI-based treatment planning for malignant gliomas assumes that the edema as represented by the T2 or FLAIR abnormality is at risk for microscopic tumor extension. This volume is generally targeted for 45 to 50 Gy followed by a boost to the gross tumor as represented by the T1-enhancing abnormality on MRI to a total dose of 60 Gy. One problem with this approach is that the T2 abnormality is not specific for microscopic tumor infiltration. Investigators at the University of California San Francisco have evaluated ^{1}H MRS as adjunctive imaging to better define the extent of tumor within the T2 abnormality.[32,62] Using a multivoxel technique, the relative signals from choline and *N*-acetylaspartate were combined to an index score that was correlated with histopathology obtained from surgical resection or biopsy. The specificity to distinguish tumor from a mixture of gliosis, necrosis, edema, and normal tissue was 86%. Sensitivity was 90%. Pirkall and colleagues[32] studied the impact this technique would have on RT treatment planning for malignant gliomas. The T2 abnormality both overestimated and underestimated the extent of tumor as defined by MRS. Although MRS has great potential to improve tumor targeting for RT and surgery, larger studies are needed to confirm its utility. In addition, many third party payors do not reimburse for this test and software tools in commercial radiation treatment planning systems are often inadequate to fully integrate MRS into the target volume definitions accurately.

Rationale for Current Radiation

Two papers published in the same journal issue in 1979 suggested that radiation dose beyond 50 Gy may be beneficial.[63,64] The larger study pooled data from three successive randomized trials performed by the Brain Tumor Study Group (BTSG 66-01, BTSG 69-01, BTSG 72-01).[64] A stepwise improvement in survival was seen with RT dose ranging from less than 45 Gy to 60 Gy strongly suggesting a dose response. A combined ECOG/RTOG trial of patients with malignant glioma was reported in 1983 by Chang and colleagues.[65] This four-arm study compared the standard arm of 60-Gy WBRT to three experimental arms: (1) 10-Gy partial brain RT boost (total 70 Gy), (2) 60 Gy plus BCNU, and (3) 60 Gy plus lomustine CCNU plus dacarbazine (DTIC). A 10-Gy boost did not improve survival over 60-Gy WBRT alone. In the United States, 60 Gy became the standard dose for all future studies. The standard dose of 60 Gy was further confirmed in a large randomized trial of patients with malignant glioma randomized to 45 Gy in 20 fractions versus 60 Gy in 30 fractions by the Medical Research Council.[66] Median survival was 9 months with the hypofractionated lower dose regimen versus 12 months with the conventional fractionation to 60 Gy. This modest difference has been interpreted by some as support for use of the lower dose in patients with limited life expectancy. Although 20 years of clinical trials have demonstrated that further dose escalation is safe beyond 60 to 70 Gy, no clinical benefit has been observed in randomized trials.

Three-dimensional Conformal Radiation for Dose Escalation

With the advent of improved computer hardware and software, the entire three-dimensional distribution of radiation to the tumor and normal tissue can be calculated. These same computer tools allow treatment plans to be designed that limit dose to normal tissue. Because the patterns of failure suggest a predominance of local tumor progression despite use of 60 Gy, a strategy of tumor dose escalation is appealing.

In the early years of conformal therapy development, several trials were conducted to determine if moderately higher doses of RT were beneficial. As technology has improved, additional dose escalation has been feasible but has not clearly improved survival. Lee and colleagues[61] reported the results of a dose-escalation study from the University of Michigan. Dose escalation was targeted against the enhancing central tumor while dose to the surrounding edema was held relatively constant. Escalation proceeded from 70 to 90 Gy. Dose-limiting toxicity was not seen at 90 Gy. No trend toward improvement in overall survival was seen with higher tumor dose. Follow-up scans were fused with the treatment plans to quantify the dose to the progressing tumor. Even after doses as high as 90 Gy, 91% of tumors progressed centrally or "in-field." No patient had isolated distant progression.

Altered Fractionation

In standard fractionated RT, treatment is administered 5 days per week once per day, generally at 1.8 to 2.0 Gy per fraction. Randomized trials of other tumor types suggest that altered fractionation may be more efficacious than conventional RT in selected tumor types.[67] Altered fractionation schedules may shorten treatment time, limiting accelerated repopulation of tumor cells, or may alter the dose per fraction, having enhanced biological effects with higher total doses without harming normal tissue. Many of these studies have incorporated dose escalation as well. In one study, an accelerated hyperfractionation schedule of 70.4 Gy delivery at 1.6 Gy twice daily for 44 fractions (about 4.5 weeks) was compared with a conventional regimen of 59.4 Gy at 1.8 Gy per fraction (about 6.5 weeks).[68] This four-arm trial had a second randomization to difluoromethylornithine (DFMO) or no DFMO. DFMO is an inhibitor of polyamine synthesis that inhibits sublethal and potentially lethal damage repair, but it did not prove beneficial for patients with GBM in this trial. Despite the higher radiation dose given in a shorter time, the accelerated hyperfractionation patients had the same survival as the conventional-dose patients. Investigators from Massachusetts General Hospital treated 23 patients with 90 cobalt gray equivalent (CGE) in 5 weeks with twice-daily proton-beam RT.[69] The median survival was 20 months, and patients were more likely to fail outside the 90 CGE volume, unlike other trials of radiation dose escalation.

The RTOG has extensively studied hyperfractionation for malignant gliomas. RTOG 83-02 was a dose escalation study assessing 1.2 Gy twice daily.[70] Patients were initially randomized to one of three arms (64.8 Gy, 72 Gy, or 76.8 Gy). Later patients also received 81.6 Gy. Late toxicity mildly increased with higher radiation dose. Because the best survival was observed in patients who received 72 Gy, this dose was selected for further study in a phase III trial, RTOG 90-06. Unfortunately, 72 Gy delivered at 1.2 Gy twice daily was not superior to 60-Gy delivery with conventional fractionation.[71] The RTOG and single institutions are actively investigating other approaches to altered fractionation. These include concomitant boost with intensity-modulated radiation therapy

(IMRT) and fractionated stereotactic radiosurgery where the dose to the enhancing tumor is escalated.

Intensity Modulated Radiation Therapy

Another approach to external beam dose escalation is to give differential dosing to the gross tumor (T1) and potential microscopic extension (T2 or FLAIR). Investigators from Wake Forest University have escalated the gross tumor to 80 Gy at 2.5 Gy per fraction using a forward planned field within a field IMRT approach.[79] This phase I study continues to dose escalate, but local tumor progression remains a problem.

Radiosurgery

Radiosurgery has been used for focal radiation delivery in patients with both newly diagnosed and recurrent malignant gliomas. With a predominant pattern of progression that is local, malignant gliomas are a rational target for radiation dose escalation with a variety of modalities including radiosurgery. Two early retrospective studies suggested a survival advantage for radiosurgery in newly diagnosed patients with malignant glioma; these results heavily influenced clinical practice and further prompted prospective studies in malignant gliomas.[80,81] Loeffler and colleagues[80] reported the results of 37 evaluable patients treated with 59.4 Gy followed by radiosurgery to a median dose of 12 Gy. After 19-month median follow-up, only 24% of patients had died. Sarkaria and colleagues[81] from the University of Wisconsin and University of Florida Joint Center retrospectively reviewed the results of stereotactic radiosurgery as a boost after external beam RT in 115 patients. In an attempt to adjust for potential confounding prognostic factors including histology, patient survival was compared with the RTOG RPA database. Median survival for the entire group treated with radiosurgery was 96 weeks, better than that for the historical controls.

To plan for prospective trials in GBM and brain metastases, the RTOG performed a radiosurgery dose-finding study, RTOG 9005.[82,83] In this trial, patients with recurrent malignant brain tumors, including gliomas and brain metastases, were stratified according to the maximum diameter of the enhancing volume. Dose-limiting toxicity in this study was irreversible grade 3 neurotoxicity, or any grade 4/5 neurologic toxicity within 3 months of therapy. The maximum tolerated dose was not reached in patients with tumors less than 2 cm in diameter, but dose was not escalated beyond 24 Gy (50% to 90% isodose line). The defined tolerable dose was 18 Gy for tumors 21 to 30 mm and 15 Gy for tumors 31 to 40 mm. On multivariate analysis, tumor diameter was an important predictor of toxicity. Forty-eight percent of patients failed locally; patients with gliomas were more likely to fail locally than those with metastases despite the high radiation doses.

Building on this phase I/II study, RTOG 9305 was conducted to determine the role of radiosurgery in newly diagnosed patients with malignant gliomas.[84] Two hundred three patients with newly diagnosed GBM less than 4 cm were randomized to postoperative radiosurgery, followed by standard 60-Gy partial brain RT plus BCNU versus standard chemoradiation alone. Radiosurgical dose was dependent upon tumor size and ranged from 15 to 24 Gy as defined in RTOG 9005. No difference was seen in overall survival or quality of life for patients who received a radiosurgery boost. Median survival was 13 months for both groups, and 92.5% of patients developed local progression. Crossover to radiosurgery at the time of local progression did occur in 19% of patients who were not randomized to radiosurgery at the time of initial diagnosis.

Although RTOG 9305 refutes the single arm and retrospective studies of radiosurgery that suggested a survival advantage for newly diagnosed patients with malignant glioma, there may be some efficacy for radiosurgery in recurrent patients. In all of these studies, the target volume for radiosurgery was the T1-enhancing tumor. It is conceivable that targeting by MRS or some other future modality may prove beneficial, especially if combined with a biological response modifier. Future studies will need to combine radiosurgery with other agents such as radiation sensitizers or biological therapies.

Brachytherapy

Brachytherapy has been performed in the brain with a variety of techniques. Traditionally, the more common techniques have included permanent or temporary ^{125}I or temporary ^{192}Ir. Sources can be after-loaded into stereotactically placed catheters or placed at the time of craniotomy. Loeffler and colleagues[85] reported on the patterns of failure after brachytherapy either for salvage or in combination with external beam radiation in the initial treatment of patients with malignant glioma. In an analysis based on CT scan results in 22 patients developing treatment failure, progression was either marginal or distant to the implant in 88% of patients.

In a prospective phase II clinical trial, Gutin and colleagues[86] from the University of California San Francisco treated malignant glioma patients with 60-Gy external beam RT, six cycles of adjuvant PCV chemotherapy, and a high activity ^{125}I temporary implant (50 to 60 Gy). Of 107 enrolled patients, 101 were evaluable, but only 63 received the implant, usually because the tumor was not an appropriate volume after external beam RT. Among evaluable non-GBM patients, median survival was similar whether brachytherapy was given (157 weeks) or not (165 weeks). However, median survival was longer in GBM patients who did receive brachytherapy at 88 weeks than in those patients who did not receive brachytherapy. One problem with this particular method of radiation dose escalation is highlighted in this series where nearly one half of the patients required reoperation due to mass effect, swelling, and steroid dependency.

Despite several reports that brachytherapy may be beneficial for patients with newly diagnosed malignant gliomas, concerns remain that the observed survival benefit was secondary to selection bias rather than treatment efficacy, as has been seen with radiosurgery. Most brachytherapy trials were limited to supratentorial tumors that were less than 6 cm in diameter that did not involve the corpus callosum. Florell and colleagues[87] reported that only 31% of their patients were eligible for brachytherapy based upon tumor size and patient performance status. In their cohort of patients who did not receive brachytherapy, patients theoretically eligible for brachytherapy had a longer median survival than did patients who were not eligible for brachytherapy (16.6 months versus 9.3 months). To answer the criticism that selection bias accounts for the survival benefit of brachytherapy, Videtic and colleagues performed a retrospective analysis of 75 patients with newly diagnosed malignant glioma that received brachytherapy in the initial management of their disease. Patients were stratified according to the RTOG RPA. Median survival was improved with brachytherapy, particularly in the worst prognosis classes, suggesting that selection biases alone do not account for the differences seen in retrospective studies.

Two randomized clinical trials of brachytherapy have been completed for patients with newly diagnosed malignant glioma. Investigators from Princess Margaret Hospital randomized 140 patients to external RT alone or external RT followed by implant. Eighty-nine percent of the patients in the study had GBM. High-activity ^{125}I was implanted intraoperatively. External beam RT consisting of 50 Gy in 25 fractions was given. An additional peripheral dose of 60 Gy was delivered via brachytherapy to all enhancing tumor. The median survivals were 13.2 and 13.8 months for the external beam and implant plus external beam groups, respectively. Selker and colleagues[88] from the Brain Tumor Cooperative Group performed a second randomized trial. Study 8701 included 270 valid enrollees with malignant glioma randomized after surgical resection to temporary ^{125}I brachytherapy followed by external beam RT plus BCNU or external beam RT plus BCNU. The brachytherapy patients received 6000 cGy prescribed to the 40 cGy/h isodose line, which was to include the residual enhancing tumor but not more than 1 cm beyond the enhancement. Figure 24-4 shows the survival curves for this trial. Median survival was 68.1 weeks in the brachytherapy group versus 58.9 weeks without brachytherapy. The difference in overall survival approached but did not reach statistical significance ($P = .101$). The lack of survival benefit for large boost doses of brachytherapy suggests a lack of dose response beyond 60 Gy. These two trials further weaken the rationale for other methods of radiation dose escalation, although the biology of alternative fractionation or radiosurgery schedules may be different.

A new brachytherapy device, the GliaSite RT system (GliaSite RTS, Proxima Therapeutics, Alpharetta, GA), was approved by the Food and Drug Administration (FDA) in 2002. This intracavitary device is implanted after resection of the tumor. A solution of ^{125}I is injected into the closed catheter balloon, which inflates to fill the resection cavity. Brachytherapy is delivery in doses of 40 to 60 Gy at 5 to 10 mm from the balloon surface over 4 to 6 days. Although the catheter is designed to be removed, many patients defer or refuse removal of the device. This design has allowed outpatient brachytherapy in many states. This Gliasite device is manufactured in three sizes: nominally 2 cm, 3 cm, and 4 cm.

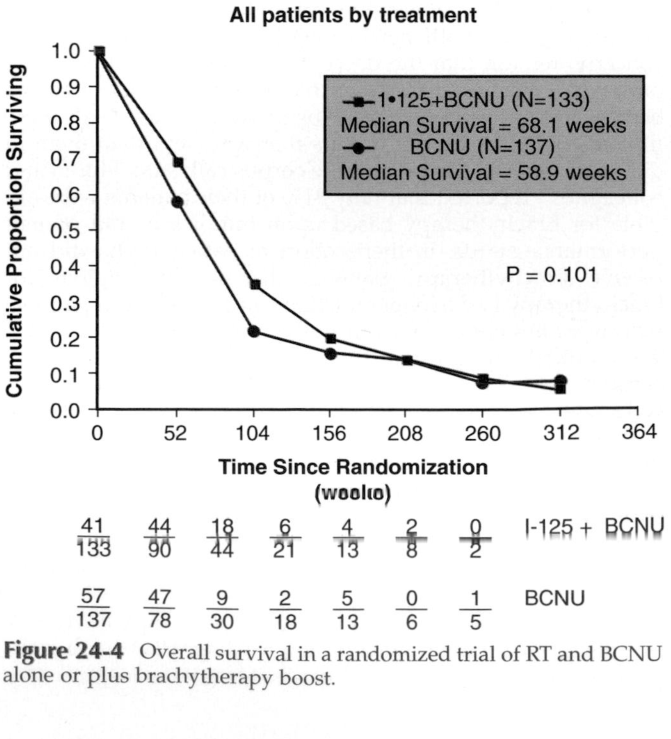

Figure 24-4 Overall survival in a randomized trial of RT and BCNU alone or plus brachytherapy boost.

Caution should be observed with high prescription doses using the 2-cm balloon for smaller resection cavities, as the ratio of surface dose to the prescription dose is much higher for smaller fill volumes. This may have resulted in a higher necrosis rate in a phase II trial of metastases than in prior studies of recurrent malignant glioma where a larger balloon was often used. The balloon, shown in Figure 24-5, is not a true point source and may have a theoretical advantage of avoiding hot spots around individual seeds or sources as is common with other methods of brain brachytherapy. With this device, brachytherapy prescription at 1 cm results in very high doses at the surface of the balloon compared with large balloon fill volumes. Studies of this brachytherapy device in combination with temozolomide and fractionated RT are planned within the New Approaches to Brain Tumor Therapy (NABTT) CNS consortium.

Toxicity of Radiation Therapy

The toxicity profile of cranial RT for GBM has changed modestly as improvements in imaging, localization, beam energy, and treatment planning have accompanied reductions in RT volumes. Acute radiation toxicity includes scalp irritation or erythema, alopecia, headache, nausea, and fatigue. Many of these symptoms are medically manageable with an adjustment in steroids. Patients receiving RT while on antiepileptics such as phenytoin may be at increased risk of a severe, but uncommon skin disorder, Stevens-Johnson syndrome.[72] There are case reports of this syndrome occurring with other antiepileptics as well.[73]

Late toxicity of RT can include somnolence and impaired cognitive function.[74] The extent of causation of RT in intellectual deterioration has been debated in patients receiving partial brain RT, as tumor progression may be a more common cause of impaired cognition than treatment effects.[75] In patients with left hemispheric malignant brain tumors, a considerable proportion of patients have preexisting dysfunction before RT is given.[76] In patients receiving partial brain RT for low-grade gliomas, where tumor progression occurs at a later date than high-grade gliomas, cognition may improve between 6 and 12 months after the completion of RT.[77] Use of conventional fractionation schedules rather than hypofractionated RT may play an important role in limiting neurocognitive sequelae.[74]

New enhancement of tumor or adjacent tissue is often seen after RT. In this situation, the differential diagnosis includes necrosis versus tumor progression. Modest asymptomatic changes in enhancement can often be observed and treated with steroids when symptoms develop. Some patients who have not had prior resection develop mass effect associated with enhancement and require surgical resection for symptom relief and diagnosis. The incidence of necrosis varies depending on how it was defined in the various trials, but it is clearly dose related for patients receiving partial brain RT.[78] In RTOG 83-02 with dose escalation from 64.8 to 81.6 Gy, late radiation toxicity was related to RT dose and occurred in 1.3% to 6.8% of patients.[70] One might expect that as survival improves for patients with malignant gliomas, subsets of patients will be at risk for late toxicity at greater rates than is reported in historical clinical trials.

Systemic Therapies

Steroids

Oral steroids were probably the first systemic therapy for glioma. The primary role of steroids is to reduce symptoms

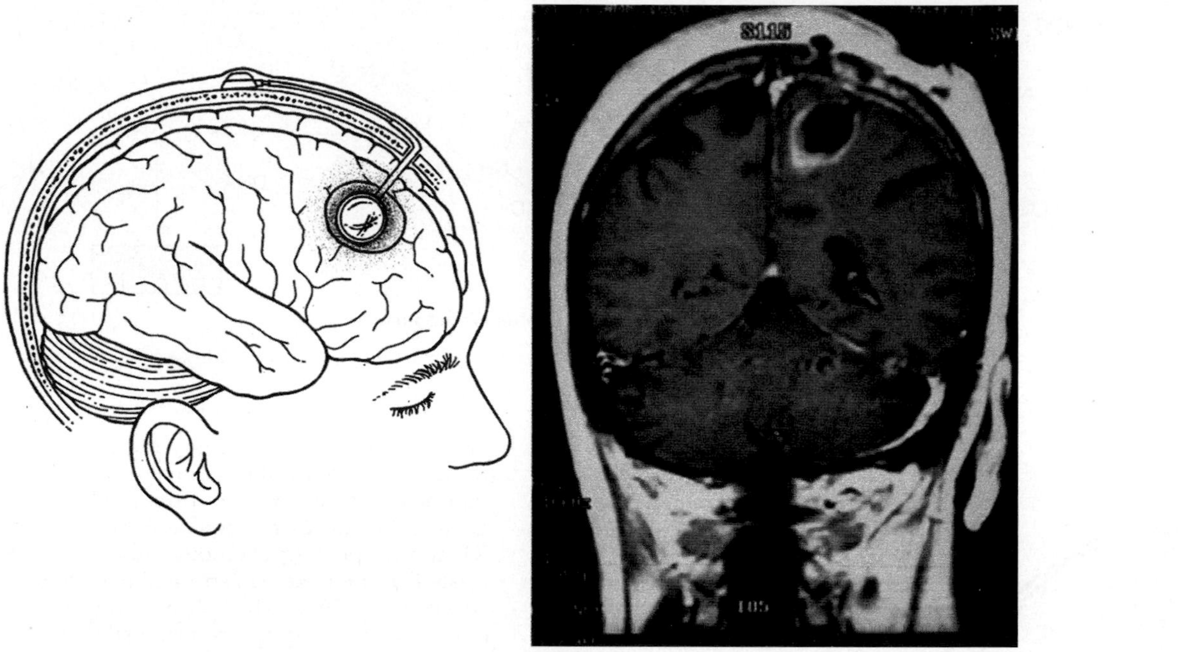

A B

Figure 24-5 **A,** The GliaSite RTS brachytherapy system consists of an inflatable balloon at the end of a closed catheter. Iotrex (^{125}I solution) is infused into the balloon through an access port beneath the scalp. **B,** Coronal MRI demonstrates an inflated balloon with a rim of enhancement at the edge of the resection cavity.

from cerebral edema. High-dose steroids with RT have not improved survival in a randomized trial, so patients should be maintained on the lowest dose of steroids that relieves symptoms.[89] Chronic steroid use is associated with significant toxicity including dyspepsia, oral and esophageal candidiasis, myopathy, and immunosuppression. The extent of immunosuppression from patients receiving oral steroids and cranial irradiation was studied by Klineberg and investigators from Johns Hopkins University.[90] Approximately one fourth of all patients developed a CD4 count below 200, a range diagnostic of AIDS in patients with HIV infection. This lymphopenia predisposes patients to opportunistic infections including pneumocystic pneumonia and is associated with hospitalization. There may be a role of prophylactic antibiotics in patients with low CD4 counts.

Chemotherapy

NITROSOUREA

Nitrosourea-based chemotherapy has been used extensively since the 1960s in the treatment of malignant gliomas. Brain Tumor Study Group trial 6901 was a four-arm trial comparing best supportive care with chemotherapy, RT, or chemoradiation.[52] In this trial, the chemotherapy was 1,3-bis-(chloroethyl)-1-nitrosourea (BCNU) given 80 mg/m^2/d for 3 days every 6 to 8 weeks. BCNU produced only marginally better overall survival than best supportive care with a median survival 14 versus 18 weeks (P = .11). No survival difference was seen in patients who received BCNU plus RT versus RT alone.

In a large Intergroup cooperative study of patients with malignant glioma, Chang and colleagues[65] compared two different radiation schedules without chemotherapy with two different chemoradiation regimens. The chemoradiation regimens included BCNU in one arm and methyl-CCNU plus DTIC in another. An exploratory subset analysis revealed that 40- to 60-year-olds administered BCNU had improved survival over the two RT-alone arms.[91] The methyl-CCNU–plus–DTIC arm was a borderline statistical significance (P = .08) but was more myelotoxic than BCNU.

Because of the perceived limited impact of nitrosourea chemotherapy in most randomized trials, Fine and colleagues[92] performed a meta-analysis of 16 randomized trials including more than 3000 patients. The absolute increase in overall survival was 10.1% at 1 year and 8.6% at 2 years with adjuvant chemotherapy.

TEMOZOLOMIDE

Temozolomide (Temodar) is a lipophilic second-generation alkylating agent developed especially for the treatment of malignant gliomas. At physiologic pH, this oral agent is spontaneously converted to MTIC [5-(3-methyltriazene-1-yl) imidazole-4-carboxamide]. The structure and mechanism of action of temozolomide are summarized in Figure 24-6. MTIC has a very short half-life (minutes) but leads to methylation of the O-6 position of guanine. If not repaired, this DNA methylation leads to double strand breaks. O^6-Benyl-guanine (O6-BG), another agent in clinical trials, inhibits repair of this process. An important enzyme responsible for repair of temozolomide-induced methylation is MGMT. Hypermethylation of the MGMT promoter leads to inactivation of this repair enzyme and increased sensitivity to temozolomide.[38,93]

Temolozomide was studied as a single agent in recurrent-glioma patients, where it first gained FDA approval. Yung and colleagues[94] performed a prospective randomized phase II study of patients with GBM at first relapse. Patients received either procarbazine (125 to 150 mg/m^2/d for 28 days repeated in 56-day cycles) or temozolomide (150 to 200 mg/m^2/d for 5 days repeated in 28-day cycles). The temozolomide-treated patients were more likely to objectively respond (21% versus 8%) and had a superior 6-month progression-free survival. The clinical benefit with the lower toxicity profile of temozolomide resulted in FDA approval of the drug.

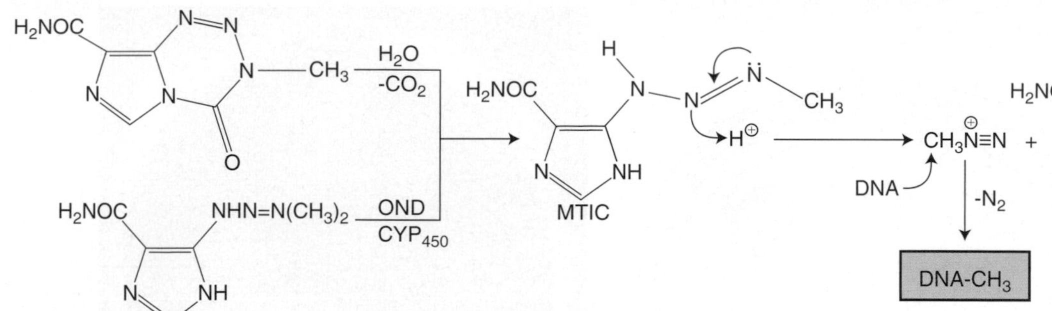

Temozolomide (Temodar)

Figure 24-6 Structure and mechanism of action of temozolomide.

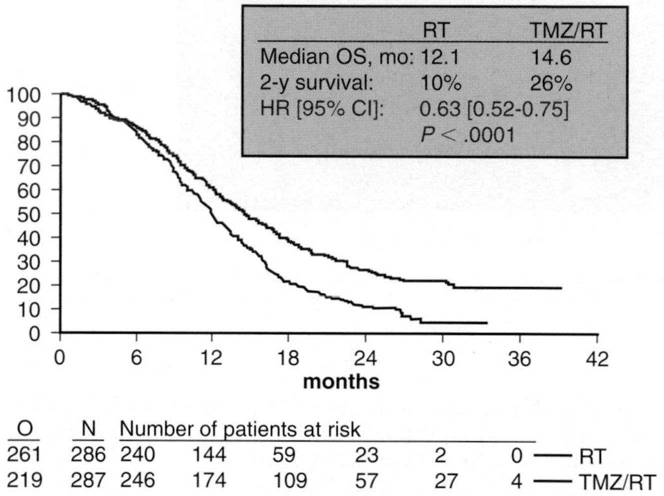

Figure 24-7 Survival is improved with RT plus concurrent and adjuvant temozolomide in a randomized trial in patients with newly diagnosed glioblastoma multiforme. CI, confidence interval; HR, hazard ratio; OS, overall survival; RT, radiation therapy; TMZ, temozolomide.

Preclinical studies suggested that temozolomide is a radiation sensitizer for some glioma cells in culture or is at least additive.[95,96] Building on positive results in recurrent patients and preclinical studies suggesting additive or possibly synergistic interactions with RT, Stupp and colleagues[97] performed a phase II study with 64 patients with newly diagnosed GBM. Treatment included daily temozolomide (75 mg/m^2) and concurrent conventional partial brain RT (60 Gy) followed by adjuvant temozolomide (200 mg/m^2/d for 5 days) given in 28 cycles. The median survival was promising at 16 months and 2-year survival was 31%.

A definitive phase III randomized trial of RT with or without temozolomide using the same schedule was subsequently performed by investigators from EORTC and NCI-Canada (NCI-C). Patients randomized to RT alone could crossover to receive temozolomide at the time of recurrence. Median survival was 12.1 months with RT alone and 14.6 months with temozolomide plus RT. At 2 years, the survival advantage was more pronounced (26% versus 10%, $P < .0001$) (Fig. 24-7). Toxicity of temozolomide included nausea and myelosuppression, but this was less cumulative than other regimens such as PCV. Based on this large randomized trial, RT plus temozolomide is now considered the standard of care for patients with newly diagnosed GBM.

Several questions remain regarding the ideal combination of temozolomide and RT. It is unknown whether concurrent or adjuvant use is more important. If the benefit was from radiosensitization, the adjuvant component may not be required. A phase II study from the University of Heidelberg gave only concurrent temozolomide 50 mg/m^2/d during RT and no post-RT chemotherapy.[98] Fifty-four patients were treated, and the median survival was 19 months with a 2-year survival of 29%. This study suggests that the post-RT chemotherapy may not be responsible for the majority of the benefit. The optimal number of cycles of adjuvant therapy is also unknown. In the EORTC study, 6 months of temozolomide therapy was administered for patients who did not progress. It is conceivable that a longer course of therapy in responders such as 1 to 2 years might be even more efficacious for selected patients.

The potential benefit of temozolomide is also being assessed in patients with anaplastic astrocytoma. The current NCI-sponsored clinical trial, RTOG 9813, for AAs excludes tumors with a dominant oligodendroglial component. This study includes RT for all patients and is comparing adjuvant BCNU with adjuvant temozolomide. This was originally designed as a three-arm study with the third arm to contain both agents. Unfortunately, the pilot portion of the trial found that combination therapy was too toxic. Most patients in the United States with AAs who are not enrolled in clinical trials receive adjuvant temozolomide chemotherapy based on its favorable toxicity profile and extrapolations from the EORTC/NCI-C randomized trial in GBM.

PCV Chemotherapy

Early clinical trials of malignant gliomas have suggested a survival advantage to adjuvant PCV chemotherapy. Levin and colleagues[99,100] reported a randomized trial for patients with malignant gliomas comparing adjuvant BCNU with PCV chemotherapy. All patients received 60 Gy RT plus hydroxyurea. For the subset of patients with anaplastic gliomas, there appeared to be a significant survival advantage to PCV chemotherapy over BCNU, with a doubling of median survival. During the time of these studies, there may have been a pathologic bias against classification of these tumors as having an oligodendroglial component. During the 1990s, the importance of oligodendroglial histology became apparent as a predictor of prognosis and response to chemotherapy.[36,101] More modern studies have treated tumors with an oligodendroglial component as distinct neoplasms.

For patients with pure or mixed anaplastic oligodendroglioma, there is better evidence of chemotherapy responses and a subsequent benefit. Cairncross[36] was one of the first investigators to demonstrate chemosensitivity of this subtype of malignant gliomas. In an initial report of 24 patients, 18 patients had objective responses to PCV chemotherapy. RTOG 9412 randomized patients with pure or mixed anaplastic oligodendroglioma to induction PCV chemotherapy for four cycles prior to RT versus RT alone with chemotherapy at the time of relapse. The early follow-up of this trial suggests similar overall survival but a better progression-free survival to upfront PCV (2.6 years versus 1.9 years, $P = .053$). It is conceivable that much of the perceived benefit to PCV in prior studies is actually attributable to unrecognized anaplastic oligodendrogliomas responding.[102]

Because of the observation that patients with anaplastic oligodendrogliomas that respond to PCV chemotherapy are likely to be long-term survivors, two clinical trials have explored dose-intensive chemotherapy for consolidation with deferred RT in patients with a complete response. Abrey and colleagues[103] reported the results of a transplant regimen in patients demonstrating chemosensitivity to induction therapy. Of 69 patients with anaplastic oligodendroglioma enrolled, 39 completed the transplant regimen. Of these 39 patients, median progression-free survival was 69 months and median overall survival had not been reached. A similar phase II study by the NABTT CNS consortium has completed accrual and follow-up is ongoing. Temozolomide has been proposed as primary treatment of anaplastic oligodendroglioma due to the toxicity of PCV and demonstrated efficacy of temozolomide in GBM. The omission of RT for patients with malignant gliomas has not been tested in a phase III trial and remains investigational.

The chemotherapy (and radiation) sensitivity of anaplastic oligodendrogliomas is very dependent upon 1p19q LOH. In RTOG 94-02, 46% of patients had this molecular marker. Survival was not reached in patients with the marker versus only 2.8 years for patients without the marker. This survival benefit for patients with 1p19q existed regardless of treatment arm, suggesting a better prognosis for these patients after RT as well. If future clinical trials are to select patient subsets to study the omission of RT, patient selection with molecular markers may be a better strategy than histology alone.

Intratumoral (Local) Chemotherapy

The local delivery of chemotherapy is one method of achieving greater concentrations of drug within the tumor. The most studied intratumoral chemotherapy is BCNU embedded in a polymer (Gliadel; Guilford Pharmaceuticals) shown in Figure 24-8. Brem and colleagues[104] randomized 222 patients with recurrent malignant glioma requiring operation to 3.8% BCNU wafer or placebo wafer. Patients receiving BCNU wafer had a modest median survival advantage of 31 versus 23 weeks. This trial has been criticized for not including an arm with BCNU delivered systemically as a control. Subsequently, BCNU wafers were studied in the upfront setting in a trial by Westphal and colleagues.[105] Two hundred forty patients with newly diagnosed malignant glioma were randomized to BCNU wafer or placebo after resection. All patients received postoperative RT but not adjuvant systemic chemotherapy. There was a modest overall survival advantage in the group of patients who received local BCNU wafer (median survival 13.9 versus 11.6 months). The survival curve is shown in Figure 24-9. The NABTT CNS consortium has performed additional dose-escalation studies of the BCNU wafer suggesting that 3.8% is not the maximum tolerated dose. Future studies will define the optimal dose of local BCNU delivered by polymer. Other polymer-delivered drugs are likely to be developed.

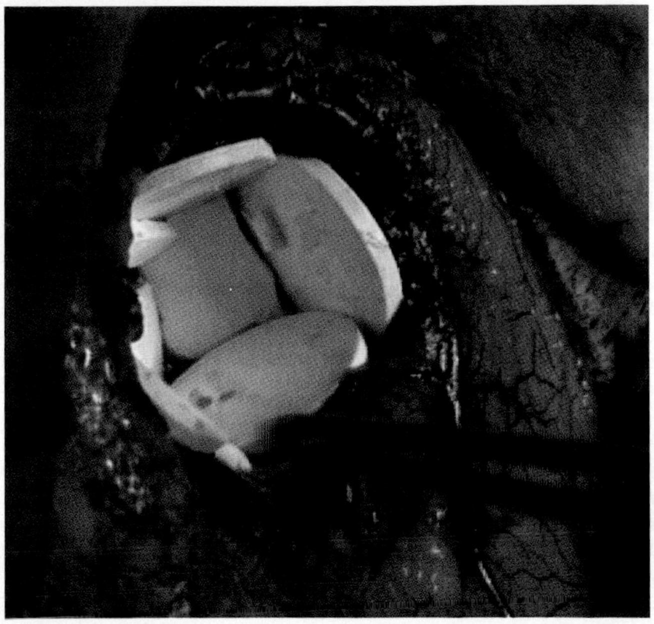

Figure 24-8 Gliadel wafer placement in tumor resection cavity.

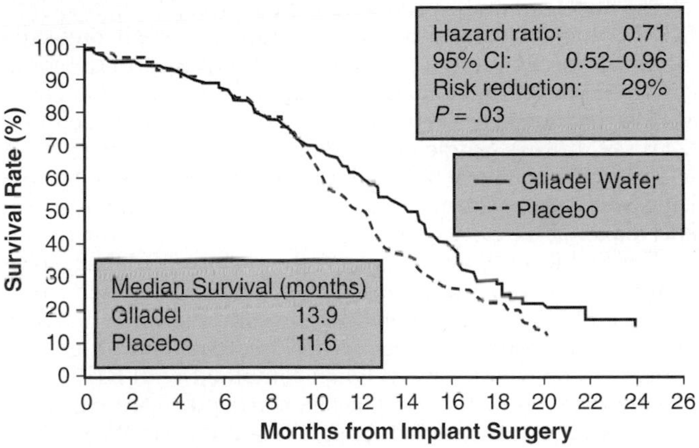

Figure 24-9 Overall survival in a randomized trial of RT alone or plus BCNU wafer (Gliadel Wafer; Guilford Pharmaceuticals) in patients with newly diagnosed malignant glioma. CI, confidence interval.

Targeted Therapies

The understanding of the molecular events important in the initiation and progression of malignant glioma is increasingly being explained. Several different pathways important in cellular processes may be aberrantly activated or deactivated in malignant glioma. These pathways support the cellular process of proliferation/survival, invasion/migration, and angiogenesis. This section describes these cellular pathways and the emerging inhibitors undergoing clinical evaluation for each.

Unregulated cell growth and proliferation are defining features of cancer. This may occur because of upregulation, overexpression, or constitutive activation of the components of signaling pathways or by loss of the mechanisms that trigger programmed cell death (apoptosis).

An increasing number of cell surface growth factor receptors appear to influence cellular behavior by the activation of gene transcription. A multistep process of intracellular signaling molecules effects this activation, offering a number of opportunities for amplification, divergent effects, and duplication. The mitogenic ras/raf/MAPKinase pathway is one of the best-described pathways in gliomas. Oncogenic mutations of ras leading to constitutive activation are present in approximately 30% of all cancers.[106] Malignant gliomas do not show oncogenic mutations of ras but have levels of activated ras similar to that seen in cancers with mutations of ras.[107] The implication has been that the upstream cell surface receptors are thus overly activated. The growth factor receptors for PDGF and EGF are the best understood.

The PDGF/PDGFR pathway is important in the normal development of glial cells in the nervous system and is present in all stages of glioma.[108,109] At the present, there are no descriptions of activating mutations in the PDGFR. Overexpression of the receptor in low-grade astrocytomas occurs in association with *p53* alterations, suggesting this pathway may play a role in early glioma initiation.[110] Inhibitors of the PDGF/PDGFR pathway that have undergone evaluation in glioma include SU101 and imatinib mesylate (Gleevec; STI571). In single-agent trials in recurrent malignant glioma, imatinib mesylate (STI571) appears to be well tolerated, however, with minimal activity.[111] In combination trials with cytotoxic agents for a recurrent disease population, a suggestion of enhanced activity has been reported.[112]

The EGF/EGFR pathway appears to play an important role in glioma progression. Overexpression of EGFR has been reported in 50% of GBMs and appears absent in lower-grade astrocytomas.[113] This suggests a role in the initiation of primary or de novo GBM. In addition, alternative-splicing events may lead to the production of a mutated form of EGFR, EGFRvIII, that is constitutively activated.[114] Small molecule inhibitors of EGFR tyrosine kinase activity are undergoing clinical investigation in patients with malignant glioma. These agents include erlotinib (Tarceva, OSI-774) and gefitinib (ZD1839, Iressa). Single-agent phase I trials in patients with recurrent glioma have been completed and demonstrated toxicities similar to systemic cancer trials.[115,116] These include rash and diarrhea.

The EGFR inhibitors are currently in clinical trials in combination with radiation and chemotherapy. The RTOG trial 0211 is a phase I/II trial of gefitinib in combination with RT in newly diagnosed patients with glioblastoma. Gefitinib appears to be well tolerated when combined with RT.[117]

Downstream of the growth factor receptors are signaling molecules that transmit the activation sequence to the nucleus for alterations in gene transcription. One of the major molecules important in this process is ras, which is a G protein that cycles between a GDP-bound inactive state and a GTP-bound active state.[118] The ras must be located in the plasma membrane for its activation but also for activation of the downstream elements. The process of membrane localization requires the protein to undergo prenylation by an enzyme, farnesyl transferase (FT).[119] Although direct inhibitors of ras are not in clinical evaluation, farnesyl transferase inhibitors (FTIs) have undergone clinical evaluation. The FTI tipifarnib (R115777, Zarnestra) has been evaluated in phase I and II trials of recurrent malignant glioma. The phase I findings demonstrated a difference in the maximum tolerated dose (MTD) depending on the use of enzyme-inducing anticonvulsants. Phase II evaluations in the same patient populations using the defined MTDs showed encouraging activity, with 23% of patients progression-free at 6 months.[120] Current studies are under way in newly diagnosed GBM in combination with RT. The possibility to interrupt this signaling pathway downstream of ras at the sequential steps of raf, MAPK kinase (MEK1), and MAP kinase (ERK1/2) does exist. The raf inhibitor, BAY 43-9006, has entered phase I evaluation in patients with recurrent malignant glioma. Inhibitors of MEK1 such as PD184322 have demonstrated potent and selective inhibition but are not currently under evaluation for gliomas.[121]

As opposed to the ras/raf/MAPK pathway's influence on growth and proliferation, the phosphoinositide 3-kinase (PI3K)/Akt pathway appears to influence cell survival. The tumor suppressor PTEN regulates the activity of this pathway. The activation of PTEN in glioma promotes cell cycle arrest and apoptosis.[122] PTEN is located on chromosome 10q and is mutated in a significant proportion of glioblastomas, resulting in a loss of this important growth control pathway.[123] The molecule mTOR (mammalian target of rapamycin) is downstream of Akt and a target for therapeutic intervention. Following activation by PI3K, Akt phosphorylates mTOR, promoting protein translation from mRNA. Inhibition of this pathway results in G_1 arrest. The analog of rapamycin, CCI-779, functions as an inhibitor of mTOR and is currently undergoing clinical evaluation in malignant glioma.

Angiogenesis is a significant component of malignant glioma. Angiogenesis in the setting of malignancy is a process required for tumor growth and spread. Without angiogenesis, solid tumors grow to only a few millimeters and do not metastasize or invade.[124] Pathologically, malignant gliomas are characterized by endothelial proliferation and neovascularization. An early step in glioma-associated angiogenesis is the secretion of angiogenic growth factors that activate the normally quiescent endothelial cells of the central nervous system. The best described and, in the case of malignant glioma, probably the most influential is VEGF (vascular endothelial growth factor). VEGF may bind to a number of VEGF receptors that include VEGFR-1 (Flt-1), VEGFR-2 (Flk-1/KDR), and VEGFR-3 (Flt-4). The dominant signaling pathway in malignant glioma appears to be dependent upon Flk-1/KDR.[125] Similar to EGFR, promising clinical activity has been seen in systemic solid cancer using anti-VEGF monoclonal antibodies. Bevacizumab (Avastin) is a humanized anti-VEGF monoclonal antibody derived from a murine antibody that has been approved for use in colon cancer. At this point, anti-VEGF antibody therapy has not been evaluated in glioma. The more promising line of clinical investigation in malignant glioma has involved the use of small molecule inhibitors of the major VEGF receptors, particularly Flt-1 and Flk-1/KDR. SU5416 (semaxanib) and PTK787 are undergoing phase I and II studies in recurrent malignant glioma as single agents and in combination with RT or temozolomide.[126]

The significant progress in defining the molecular events that promote glioma initiation and progression is leading to the development of agents specifically targeted to these biological processes. This class of biologically targeted therapy is completing the first phases of clinical investigation and appears to be largely safe and well tolerated in the malignant glioma population. Efforts to extend clinical research into combination therapy with conventional chemotherapy and RT are under way. It is in this setting that these agents hold the most promise for improvements in patient outcomes.

LOCALLY ADVANCED DISEASE AND RETREATMENT

Patients who are elderly or have a particularly poor performance status may be candidates for a hypofractionated course of RT or no therapy at all. This is particularly true for patients who do not improve with steroid administration and are not candidates for surgical resection. A variety of dose schedules have been proposed for this patient population including 30 Gy in 10 fractions to 50 Gy in 20 fractions. The treatment volume can be partial brain RT or WBRT depending on the extent of disease and dose schedule. Slotman and colleagues[127] performed a prospective study of 30 patients with poor-risk GBM, delivering 42 Gy in 14 fractions with overall survival similar to historical controls. No severe acute or late toxicity was observed in this series of 30 poor prognosis patients.

Two randomized trials have evaluated hypofractionated regimens in poor prognosis malignant glioma patients. Roa and colleagues[128] completed a randomized trial of newly diagnosed GBM patients who were 60 years old or older. One hundred patients were randomized to standard RT (60 Gy in 30 fractions) or hypofractionated RT (40 Gy in 15 fractions). No survival difference was observed with median survival of approximately 5 months in each arm. Patients receiving standard RT were more likely to require a post-treatment increase in steroid administration. This randomized trial suggests that a 3-week treatment schedule may be preferred in this patient population due to shorter overall treatment time, similar efficacy, and lower steroid requirements. Another randomized trial enrolled 69 patients and randomized to 60 Gy at 2 Gy per fraction versus 35 Gy in 10 fractions.[129] This trial was closed early due to poor accrual. Survival was not statistically different between the two arms but did slightly favor the conventional regimen.

For patients with local recurrence after prior RT, retreatment with a radiation modality may be an option, particularly in patients who have exhausted other therapeutic options including clinical trials. The best-studied modalities are radiosurgery and brachytherapy. The NABTT CNS consortium has performed a device-safety study of the Gliasite RTS device in patients with recurrent malignant glioma delivering 40 to 60 Gy over several days.[130] The device performed as designed and there was an observed low risk of toxicity. In a larger retrospective analysis of 80 patients with recurrent malignant glioma treated at nine institutions with the Gliasite device, the median survival was 38 weeks. The subset of patients with recurrent GBM had a median survival of 35 weeks. In this series, the mean brachytherapy dose was 60 Gy (range, 50 to 63 Gy) 5 to 10 mm from the balloon surface and the dose rate was 53 cGy/h. Only 3/80 patients developed symptomatic radionecrosis. Imaging changes including temporary increasing postcontrast enhancement commonly occur after brachytherapy with this device. This new enhancement should not be automatically interpreted as recurrent tumor with tissue confirmation.

Radiosurgery may be considered for small recurrences (less than 4 cm), particularly if the tumor cannot be resected. From 15 to 24 Gy may be administered to the T1-enhancing abnormality depending on tumor volume and location.[83] Retrospective studies suggest a range of survival depending on a variety of prognostic factors.[131]

Fractionated external beam retreatment is another modality that may be possible for patients whose tumors are too large for radiosurgery (more than 4 cm) or brachytherapy (more than 6 cm).[132-134] Animal studies suggest that neural tissue will "forgive" previous radiation to a great extent after 1 to 3 years.[135] Methods of improving dose to normal tissue including intensity-modulated radiation therapy (IMRT) and image guidance may minimize the risk of toxicity. Hudes and colleagues[134] found a dose response for radiographic tumor response with higher doses of hypofractionation stereotactic RT for retreatment. No dose-limiting toxicity was observed at 35 Gy in 10 fractions despite previous treatment to 60 Gy. A small study using IMRT for retreatment reported good tolerance with 6 × 5 Gy.[136] Although the efficacy of retreatment has not been clearly established, it is not unreasonable to consider additional radiation for patients who responded to therapy initially and who completed the initial course of treatment 2 years previously. Ideal candidates have exhausted other therapeutic options and have tumors that are limited in volume and are located away from the brainstem and optic structures.

Hyperthermia is another potential treatment modality for patients with recurrent malignant glioma. The best evidence of the efficacy of this modality is in a randomized trial performed by Sneed and colleagues[137] from University of California San Francisco. In a study of patients with newly diagnosed GBM 5 cm or less in greatest dimension, 112 patients received hydroxyurea plus conventional RT. Seventy-nine patients with focal tumors after fractionated RT were randomized to brachytherapy with or without hyperthermia. Survival was improved in the group of patients who received hypothermia (31% versus 15% in those who did not at 2 years, $P = .02$).

TECHNIQUES OF IRRADIATION

Partial brain RT has replaced WBRT techniques that were used in early clinical trials of malignant glioma. With improved imaging, more limited radiation volumes may limit later toxicity for those patients who are long-term survivors. Although malignant gliomas should be considered a whole CNS or whole brain disease, the patterns of failure suggest that local tumor control of the enhancing abnormalities is the predominant pattern of failure.[56,59,61]

Image registration with postoperative day 0-1 MRI has replaced CT-only treatment planning. The patient should be imaged in the similar position as the treatment planning CT scan to facilitate image registration. Postoperative CT scans are not adequate to evaluate the extent of resection. Patients are generally simulated approximately 10 to 14 days postoperatively after staples have been removed. The supine position with neutral neck position is comfortable for most patients. A custom aquaplast mask or similar system is required to minimize intrafraction and interfraction motion. Thin-slice (less than 3 mm) CT scans with or without contrast should be acquired of the head and neck region to allow enough anatomy for image fusion, assessment of exit dose dosimetry, and generation of high-quality digital reconstructed radiographs. Using the postoperative MRI, two datasets are fused with the treatment planning CT scan for target volume definition. The postcontrast T1 images are used to define the gross tumor volume (GTV). In cases of gross complete resection, the GTV is defined as the resection cavity. The T2 or FLAIR abnormality is contoured as the clinical target volume (CTV). The postoperative MRI should be compared with the preoperative study to confirm that postoperative changes have not been confused with tumor. If postoperative MRI is not obtained within 24 hours of surgery, postsurgical changes including hemorrhage can be confused with residual tumor on T1 postcontrast imaging. In this case, review of noncontrast T1 images will be helpful to distinguish tumor from hemorrhage. Preoperative T2 or FLAIR images should be reviewed to assess if signal has changed significantly due to surgery. In patients with significant gross residual disease, the defined CTV by T2/FLAIR MRI should be compared with the hypodensity on the treatment planning CT to further assess for possible progression since the postoperative MRI. Using this dataset, the GTV and CTV are defined as in Table 24-4. Example target volumes are shown in Figure 24-10 for GBM, and a less common case of partially enhancing or nonenhancing grade III tumor is shown in Figure 24-11.

To define the planning target volume (PTV) for three-dimensional planning, a margin is traditionally added to account for organ motion and setup error. In the brain, registration or fusion error may also exist. Organ motion of the brain is very small during therapy and approaches less than

Table 24-4 Target Volume Definition for Malignant Glioma

Target	Definition	Comments
GTV	T1 abnormality plus resection cavity	Subsets of tumors will be heterogeneously enhancing or grade III without enhancement. In these cases, CTV = GTV.
CTV	T2 or FLAIR abnormality including all of GTV	Extensions along pathways of spread such as corpus callosum may be considered
PTV1	CTV plus 1 cm	May be edited in areas where tumor progression is not likely to occur (bone, sinus, etc). Must still account for setup error (e.g., 3 to 5 mm).
PTV2	GTV plus 1 cm	May be compromised slightly where tumor is 5 to 10 mm from sensitive structures such as optic apparatus

CTV, clinical target volume; GTV, gross tumor volume; PTV, planning target volume.

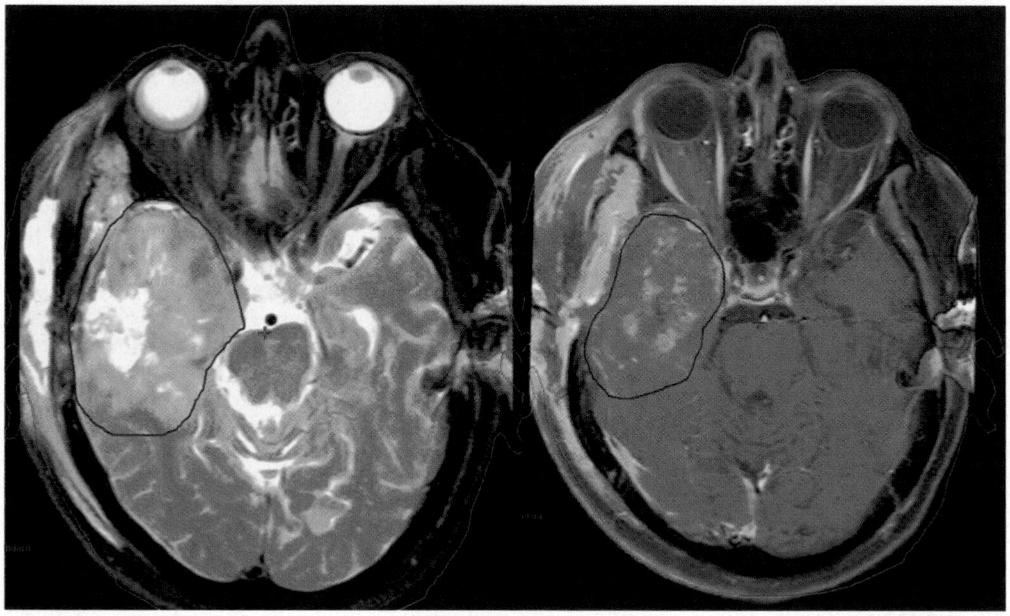

Figure 24-10 Example of gross tumor volume (*red outline*; T1-weighted, postcontrast scan) and clinical target volume (*blue outline*; T2-weighted or FLAIR scan) for a glioblastoma multiforme.

1 mm. Setup and localization error depend on the immobilization device and extent of image guidance used. An aquaplast mask has an error of 3 to 5 mm. Depending on the quality of MRI registration/fusion and immobilization, a margin of 1 to 2 cm on the CTV and GTV may be selected to define the PTV1 and PTV2. This includes additional margin for possible microscopic extension beyond radiographically detectable tumor. The PTVs may be further edited to exclude normal tissue volumes in areas where tumor is very unlikely to spread such as bone, but setup error must still be respected. If MRS is available with appropriate software tools, the target volumes may be altered further.[62]

Table 24-5 shows the partial brain RT volumes or margins used by several cooperative groups in current clinical trials investigating novel drugs in combination with radiation. The radiation volumes in studies implementing radiation dose escalation may differ slightly. The block edge margin or geometric margin has historically been utilized in treatment planning for GBM. The block edge typically represents approximately 50% of the radiation dose at the center of a single field. With the advent of three-dimensional conformal RT, the dose distribution to the entire target volume and normal tissue can now be assessed quantitatively in three dimensions. Some cooperative groups now specify RT dose and volume based on the ICRU 50 and ICRU 62 specifications, which define a PTV.[138] Three-dimensional volume definitions are preferred since different beam arrangements will produce different dose distributions with the same block edge or geometric margin. For example, an axial beam arrangement will have less dosimetric margin superiorly and inferiorly than in the axial directions. In addition, simple uniform block edge margins on gross tumor do not allow for differential margins in areas where tumor is more likely to spread (corpus callosum) or unlikely to spread (into bone).

Beam number and arrangement may vary from two parallel-opposed beams in selected cases of very extensive tumors to seven or more beams. Beam energy should be customized for the plan but is most commonly 6 MV. A larger number of beams will deliver lower doses of RT to a larger volume.

Because the dose, volume, and structural factors predictive of radiation toxicity are poorly understood, it is difficult to make generalizations regarding the relative merits of different RT plans. In a phase III study of RT dosage for low-grade gliomas, Shaw and colleagues found a greater risk of symptomatic necrosis in patients who received 64.8 Gy compared with 50.4 Gy. This study provides some rationale to limit the high dose volume receiving greater than 50 Gy. Alternatively, there is a greater theoretical potential for neurocognitive com-

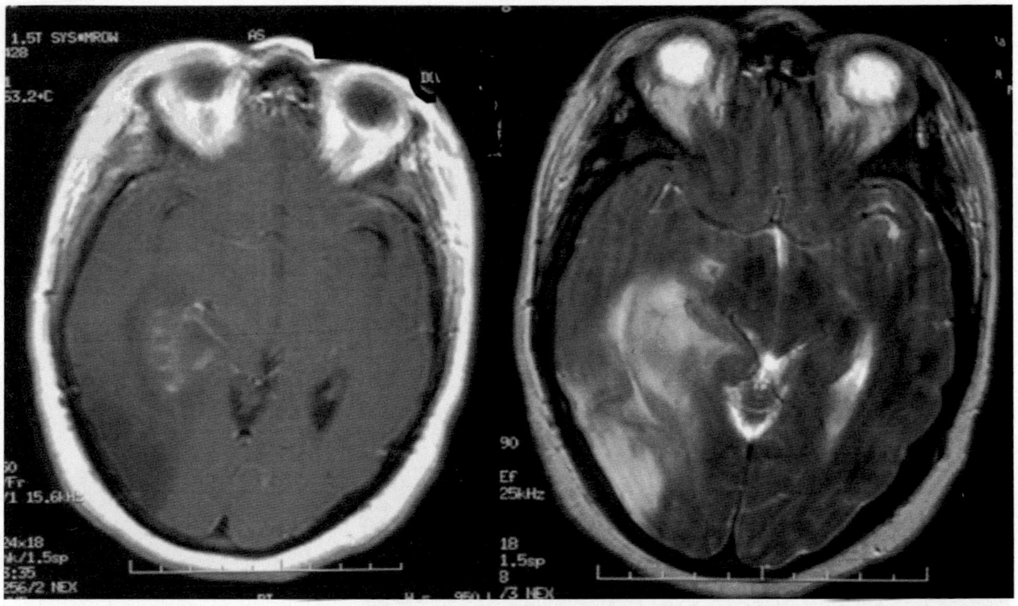

Figure 24-11 Heterogeneously enhancing grade III astrocytoma. In this case, the volume of enhancement is minimal and is probably not representative of the extent of the tumor. The suggested target volume in this case is the T2 or FLAIR abnormality unless additional data are available from a biopsy or possibly from magnetic resonance spectroscopy. The planning target volume is the T2 volume plus a 1-cm dosimetric margin prescribed to 60 Gy.

Table 24-5 Radiotherapy Volumes Used in Current Clinical Trials

	Block Edge (Geometric) Margin	Dosimetry (3D) Margin	RT Dose
RTOG	T2 plus 2 cm T1 plus 2.5 cm	—	46 Gy 14 Gy (60 Gy total)
North Central	—	T2 plus 2 cm T1 plus 2 cm	50 Gy 10 Gy (60 Gy total)
NABTT	—	T2 plus 1-2 cm T1 plus 1-2 cm	46 Gy 14 Gy (60 Gy total)

Table 24-6 Organs at Risk for Treatment Planning of Malignant Glioma

Organ	Dose Limit	Potential Complication and Comments
Optic apparatus	55-60 Gy	Optic neuritis is uncommon for dose <60 Gy. Gross tumor should not be underdosed.
Normal brain parenchyma away from tumor	>50 Gy	Radiation necrosis increases beyond 50 Gy.
Pons and medulla	>54 Gy	Radiation necrosis. Small volumes may tolerate slightly more.[160]
Cochlea, middle ear	>30 Gy?	Hearing loss, otitis media
Lens	>5-10 Gy	Cataracts
Hypothalamus/pituitary	>40 Gy?	Endocrine dysfunction
Parotid	26 Gy mean	Xerostomia

plications for large brain volumes receiving a moderate dose of RT. This may be of less importance in patients with GBM compared with those with anaplastic oligodendroglioma harboring 1p/19q LOH.

The most important organs at risk are shown in Table 24-6. Since there is a dose response for overall survival up to 60 Gy, the defined benefit of RT to gross tumor should not be overlooked because of a very low chance of optic nerve complications. For medial temporal or other tumors in close proximity to the optic apparatus, some physicians may consider limiting the dose to less than 50 Gy. The actual risk of optic complication with doses of 50 to 60 Gy is less than 5% and should not limit the tumor dose with proper informed consent.[139,140] In general, the optic nerves and chiasm are serial organs, but there is probably some volume effect that has not been well studied.

In planning beam design, the potential for less severe toxicity should be considered. Avoidance of entrance/exit through the eye (cataracts, dry, conjunctivitis) or external ear canals (otitis externa and otitis media) may limit both acute and late toxicity of therapy. Hematologic toxicity including lymphopenia has been recognized as a complication of partial brain RT plus steroids, even without systemic chemotherapy.[141] The mechanism of lymphopenia may be due to irradiation of circulating blood within the brain including the cavernous sinuses. Vertex beams exiting down the axis of the

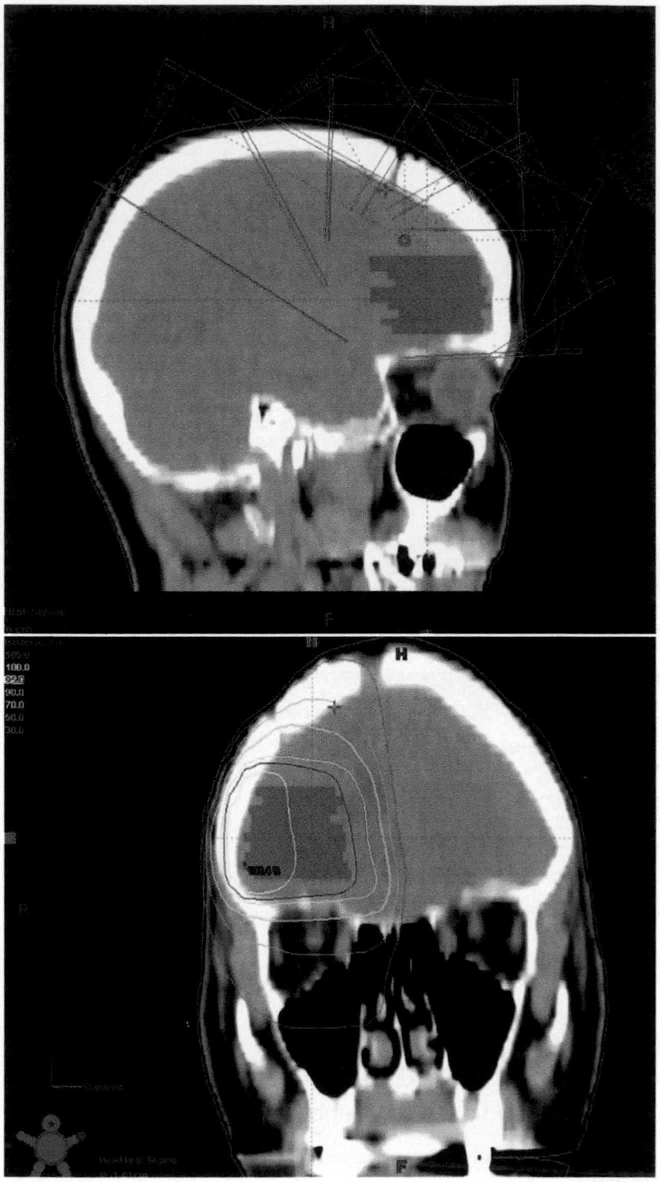

Figure 24-12 Preservation of the contralateral frontal lobe can be achieved by selection of beams that do not enter or exit the lobe. In this plan, all beams are in a sagittal plane.

spinal column could also contribute, but this has not been studied. Angulation of vertex beams to exit anterior or posterior to the vertebral column will prevent this. For anterior inferior temporal tumors, exit dose to the parotid should be considered. Bifrontal irradiation should be avoided for ipsilateral frontal tumors if alternative plans can be created. Multiple beams in the sagittal plane can be used to solve this treatment-planning problem as shown in Figure 24-12.

Treatment Planning Including Intensity-Modulated Radiation Therapy

Based on the prior studies, it is difficult to expect that computer optimization and IMRT will have a large impact on overall survival when standard fractionation is used, but altered fractionation studies may have a different biological effect. Treatment planning studies have demonstrated a physical dose advantage in the protection of normal tissue and that

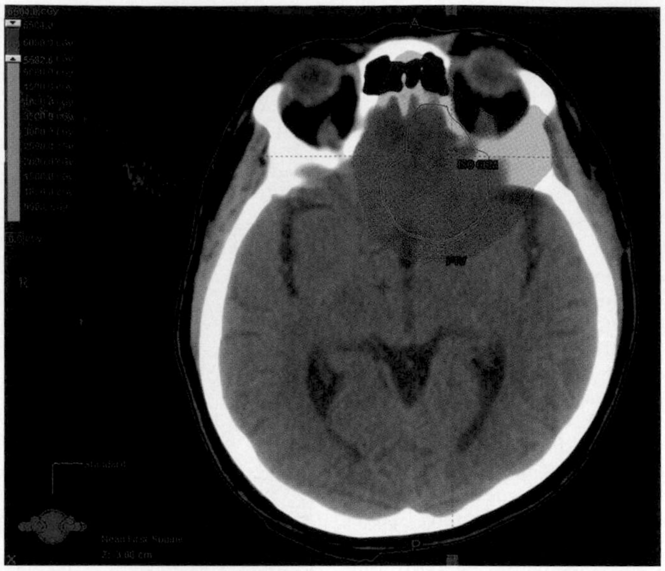

Figure 24-13 Computer-optimized, intensity-modulated radiation therapy was used to relatively protect the eye while treating a tumor with involvement of the frontal lobe near the cribriform plate. The gross tumor volume is outlined in *blue*.

dose escalation would likely be feasible, but it is doubtful that IMRT by itself will improve local tumor control.[142] There could still be some therapeutic benefit to IMRT with conventional dose of RT in selected cases with GBM. If 60 Gy is prescribed and there is a nearby sensitive normal structure such as the eye, optic apparatus, or brainstem, computer optimization may have a favorable therapeutic ratio. An example frontal tumor with extension of gross disease between the eyes is shown in Figure 24-13. Computer optimization was used to relatively protect the left eye. Improved image guidance through CT-based localization and setup may have a similar advantage to safely reduce margins as tumors approach certain critical structures.

After induction chemotherapy, it is intriguing to consider reducing treatment margins in patients who have responded to therapy. For anaplastic oligodendroglioma patients receiving induction PCV chemotherapy in RTOG 94-02, the boost volume was defined as the T1 enhancing tumor plus a 1-cm margin based upon the pretreatment MRI. In a pattern of failure analysis of a subset of patients, 10 of 40 (25%) failed outside the boost volume, suggesting that postchemotherapy volumes should not be used for treatment planning.[143]

TREATMENT ALGORITHMS, PROBLEMS, AND FUTURE POSSIBILITIES

Based on the treatment algorithm previously presented in Figure 24-3, future strategies in patients with malignant glioma will attempt to build on the modest benefit in overall survival that has been demonstrated in a randomized trial of concurrent/adjuvant temozolomide in patients with newly diagnosed GBM. Some of the problems and future strategies under consideration are described herein.

Problems

Local tumor control remains a problem in patients with malignant glioma. As new therapies are developed, especially in combination with RT, it is imperative to continue to examine the patterns of failure, as this is likely a whole brain or whole CNS disease. Local failure remains predominant, with isolated

CNS progression rare. Partial brain RT remains the standard, but this could change in the future.

One of the most difficult problems in managing patients with malignant glioma is the interpretation of imaging studies after treatment. New enhancement can be tumor progression or treatment effect including necrosis. Postsurgical changes, radiosurgery, and wafer chemotherapy can also mimic tumor recurrence. Clinical trials of gene therapy, liquid brachytherapy, radioimmunotherapy, and local cytotoxins are under way and will further complicate the interpretation of standard imaging. FDG PET and MRS have been proposed as potential solutions to this problem, but these evaluations have not been able to accurately distinguish mixtures of tumor and necrotic tissue. Furthermore, the prognostic significance and management of low-volume residual tumor within a background of necrosis are unknown. Future imaging improvements including novel PET tracers such as ^{18}F-fluoro-3′deoxy-3′-L-fluorothymidine (FLT) may hold some promise in this area.

Future Possibilities

The local administration of macromolecules or conventional chemotherapy is one method of overcoming the blood-brain barrier to deliver novel agents to brain tumors in greater concentrations than could be achieved systemically. In contrast to a simple intracavitary or intratumoral injection, convective enhanced delivery (CED) distributes an agent under pressure and is able to perfuse larger volumes of brain. One or more catheters are placed stereotactically or after surgical resection into the tumor or the parenchyma surrounding the tumor. The agent is then infused under pressure over many hours or a few days. One of the challenges of this method of treatment is predicting the distribution of the infused agent. Interleukin 13-PE38QQR (NeoPharm, Lake Forrest, IL) is one such agent undergoing clinical trials in patients with recurrent malignant glioma. Interleukin-13 receptors are present on most gliomas but not normal tissue. Combining interleukin-13 with *Pseudomonas* exotoxin leads to internalization of the toxin and cell death. Early clinical studies have demonstrated objective responses, with the main serious toxicity being local tissue reaction and mass effect. Another agent administered with CED techniques is paclitaxel. A small prospective study of 15 patients with recurrent malignant glioma has shown five clinical complete responses, some of which were confirmed histologically.[144] Systemic therapies of this agent in recurrent malignant gliomas have not demonstrated activity.

Many targeted therapies, as discussed, may have applications as radiation sensitizers. Other local novel therapeutics undergoing clinical evaluation may be of particular interest to radiation oncologists. Investigators from Duke University have evaluated intracavitary ^{131}I-radiolabeled monoclonal antibody in patients with malignant glioma. mAb 81C6 is a murine antibody directed against tenascin, an extracellular glycoprotein expressed on high-grade gliomas and some carcinomas. In a phase II study of surgical resection with instillation of ^{131}I-mAb 81C6 into the surgical cavity with conventional RT and chemotherapy, median survival was 79.4 weeks in the subset of patients with GBM.[145] Another locally administered radiolabeled macromolecule is ^{131}I-chlorotoxin (TM-601; TransMolecular Inc, Birmingham, AL). This 36–amino acid peptide derivative of a naturally occurring peptide specifically binds to many tumors including malignant gliomas. The peptide itself has antitumor activity by binding to lamellipoda and inducing cell cycle changes, but it also enhances radiation and chemotherapy response in preclinical studies. In the initial phase I/II imaging study of this agent directly injected once into tumor cavities with 10 mCi ^{131}I, there was no significant toxicity. Despite only a single low-dose injection, 5 of the 18 patients enrolled in this study were still alive at 1 year. Additional clinical trials are planned with multiple dosing and higher activity. One advantage of this agent is that it is not purely relying on radiation dose escalation for a therapeutic effect. ^{131}I-chTNT-1b (Cotara, Peregrine Pharmaceuticals), another local RT targeting agent, is a monoclonal antibody against DNA histone complex that preferentially binds to necrotic tissue. The NABTT CNS consortium has started a clinical trial evaluating this agent in recurrent malignant gliomas. Finally, although a subject of investigation for many years, boron neutron capture therapy (BNCT) represents another method of tumor specific targeting of RT. This treatment requires preferential boron tumor targeting. Upon treatment with neutrons, ^{10}B captures neutrons and leads to the production of high LET lithium and helium ions producing tumor cell–specific high relative biologic effectiveness (RBE) RT. The future of this therapy rests entirely on the development of tumor-specific boron-targeting agents.[146,147]

Another strategy to improve survival in a malignant glioma is gene therapy. Viral vectors can be directly oncolytic, deliver a suicide gene to the tumor cell, or cause the tumor cell to secrete a therapeutic agent locally. One of the current problems with current gene therapy vectors is efficient delivery to tumor cells and transfection. In preclinical models at the University of Alabama-Birmingham and the University of Chicago, modest doses of RT have increased transfection of G207, a modified oncolytic herpes virus, and act synergistically to kill tumor xenografts. A clinical trial of this approach in patients with recurrent malignant brain tumors is planned.

The molecular subset of patients most likely to benefit from chemotherapy can now be defined. Both genomics and proteomics should yield refinements in molecular diagnosis that will aid in a more biologically appropriate, patient-specific treatment approach. Both systemic small molecule–targeted therapies and local macromolecule therapies hold promise for the future, likely in combination with convention treatments such as RT and chemotherapy. Future genomic efforts will define patient prognosis and the ideal therapies for patients.

REFERENCES

1. Chandler KL, Prados MD, Malec M, Wilson CB: Long-term survival in patients with glioblastoma multiforme. Neurosurgery 32:716-720; discussion 720, 1993.
2. McLendon RE, Halperin EC: Is the long-term survival of patients with intracranial glioblastoma multiforme overstated? Cancer 98:1745-1748, 2003.
3. Senger D, Cairncross JG, Forsyth PA: Long-term survivors of glioblastoma: statistical aberration or important unrecognized molecular subtype? Cancer J 9:214-221, 2003.
4. CBTRUS: Central Brain Tumor Registry of the United States Statistical Report: Primary Brain Tumors in the United States, 1997-2001. Hinsdale, IL, CBTRUS, 2004.
5. Thomas TL, Stewart PA, Stemhagen A, et al: Risk of astrocytic brain tumors associated with occupational chemical exposures. A case-referent study. Scand J Work Environ Health 13:417-423, 1987.
6. Wrensch M, Minn Y, Chew T, et al: Epidemiology of primary brain tumors: current concepts and review of the literature. Neuro-oncology 4:278-299, 2002.
7. Wrensch M, Bondy ML, Wiencke J, Yost M: Environmental risk factors for primary malignant brain tumors: a review. J Neurooncol 17:47-64, 1993.
8. Tachibana I, Smith JS, Sato K, et al: Investigation of germline PTEN, p53, p16(INK4A)/p14(ARF), and CDK4 alterations in familial glioma. Am J Med Genet 92:136-141, 2000.

9. Jensen S, Paderanga DC, Chen P, et al: Molecular analysis at the NF1 locus in astrocytic brain tumors. Cancer 76:674-677, 1995.
10. Wiencke JK, Wrensch MR, Miike R, et al: Population-based study of glutathione S-transferase mu gene deletion in adult glioma cases and controls. Carcinogenesis 18:1431-1433, 1997.
11. Trizna Z, de Andrade M, Kyritsis AP, et al: Genetic polymorphisms in glutathione S-transferase mu and theta, N-acetyltransferase, and CYP1A1 and risk of gliomas. Cancer Epidemiol Biomarkers Prev 7:553-555, 1998.
12. Wang D, Grammer JR, Cobbs CS, et al: p125 focal adhesion kinase promotes malignant astrocytoma cell proliferation in vivo. J Cell Sci 113:4221-4230, 2000.
13. Zagzag D, Friedlander DR, Margolis B, et al: Molecular events implicated in brain tumor angiogenesis and invasion. Pediatr Neurosurg 33:49-55, 2000.
14. Haskell H, Natarajan M, Hecker TP, et al: Focal adhesion kinase is expressed in the angiogenic blood vessels of malignant astrocytic tumors in vivo and promotes capillary tube formation of brain microvascular endothelial cells. Clin Cancer Res 9:2157-2165, 2003.
15. Moulton T, Samara G, Chung WY, et al: MTS1/p16/CDKN2 lesions in primary glioblastoma multiforme. Am J Pathol 146:613-619, 1995.
16. Ueki K, Ono Y, Henson JW, et al: CDKN2/p16 or RB alterations occur in the majority of glioblastomas and are inversely correlated. Cancer Res 56:150-153, 1996.
17. Fulci G, Labuhn M, Maier D, et al: p53 gene mutation and ink4a-arf deletion appear to be two mutually exclusive events in human glioblastoma. Oncogene 19:3816-3822, 2000.
18. Henson JW, Schnitker BL, Correa KM, et al: The retinoblastoma gene is involved in malignant progression of astrocytomas. Ann Neurol 36:714-721, 1994.
19. Stambolic V, Suzuki A, de la Pompa JL, et al: Negative regulation of PKB/Akt-dependent cell survival by the tumor suppressor PTEN. Cell 95:29-39, 1998.
20. Fraser MM, Zhu X, Kwon CH, et al: PTEN loss causes hypertrophy and increased proliferation of astrocytes in vivo. Cancer Res 64:7773-7779, 2004.
21. Dai C, Holland EC: Astrocyte differentiation states and glioma formation. Cancer J 9:72-81, 2003.
22. Ono Y, Tamiya T, Ichikawa T, et al: Malignant astrocytomas with homozygous CDKN2/p16 gene deletions have higher Ki-67 proliferation indices. J Neuropathol Exp Neurol 55:1026-1031 1996.
23. Hayashi Y, Ueki K, Waha A, et al: Association of EGFR gene amplification and CDKN2 (p16/MTS1) gene deletion in glioblastoma multiforme. Brain Pathol 7:871-875, 1997.
24. Tohma Y, Gratas C, Biernat W, et al: PTEN (MMAC1) mutations are frequent in primary glioblastomas (de novo) but not in secondary glioblastomas. J Neuropathol Exp Neurol 57:684-689, 1998.
25. Libermann TA, Nusbaum HR, Razon N, et al: Amplification, enhanced expression and possible rearrangement of EGF receptor gene in primary human brain tumours of glial origin. Nature 313:144-147, 1985.
26. Zhu A, Shaeffer J, Leslie S, et al: Epidermal growth factor receptor: an independent predictor of survival in astrocytic tumors given definitive irradiation. Int J Radiat Oncol Biol Phys 34:809-815, 1996.
27. Etienne MC, Formento JL, Lebrun-Frenay C, et al: Epidermal growth factor receptor and labeling index are independent prognostic factors in glial tumor outcome. Clin Cancer Res 4:2383-2390, 1998.
28. Smith JS, Tachibana I, Passe SM, et al: PTEN mutation, EGFR amplification, and outcome in patients with anaplastic astrocytoma and glioblastoma multiforme. J Natl Cancer Inst 93:1246-1256, 2001.
29. Newcomb EW, Cohen H, Lee SR, et al: Survival of patients with glioblastoma multiforme is not influenced by altered expression of p16, p53, EGFR, MDM2 or Bcl-2 genes. Brain Pathol 8:655-667, 1998.
30. Waha A, Baumann A, Wolf HK, et al: Lack of prognostic relevance of alterations in the epidermal growth factor receptor-transforming growth factor-alpha pathway in human astrocytic gliomas. J Neurosurg 85:634-641, 1996.
31. Kleihues P, Louis DN, Scheithauer BW, et al: The WHO classification of tumors of the nervous system. J Neuropathol Exp Neurol 61:215-225; discussion 226-219, 2002.
32. Pirkall A, Li X, Oh J, et al: 3D MRSI for resected high-grade gliomas before RT: tumor extent according to metabolic activity in relation to MRI. Int J Radiat Oncol Biol Phys 59:126-137, 2004.
33. Lamborn KR, Chang SM, Prados MD: Prognostic factors for survival of patients with glioblastoma: recursive partitioning analysis. Neuro-oncology 6:227-235, 2004.
34. Lacroix M, Abi-Said D, Fourney DR, et al: A multivariate analysis of 416 patients with glioblastoma multiforme: prognosis, extent of resection, and survival. J Neurosurg 95:190-198, 2001.
35. Bello MJ, Vaquero J, de Campos JM, et al: Molecular analysis of chromosome 1 abnormalities in human gliomas reveals frequent loss of 1p in oligodendroglial tumors. Int J Cancer 57:172-175, 1994.
36. Cairncross G, Macdonald D, Ludwin S, et al: Chemotherapy for anaplastic oligodendroglioma. National Cancer Institute of Canada Clinical Trials Group. J Clin Oncol 12:2013-2021, 1994.
37. van den Bent M, Chinot OL, Cairncross JG: Recent developments in the molecular characterization and treatment of oligodendroglial tumors. Neuro-oncology 5:128-138, 2003.
38. Hegi ME, Diserens AC, Godard S, et al: Clinical trial substantiates the predictive value of O-6-methylguanine-DNA methyltransferase promoter methylation in glioblastoma patients treated with temozolomide. Clin Cancer Res 10:1871-1874, 2004.
39. Hegi ME, Diserens AC, Harnou M: Temozolomide (TMZ) targets only glioblastoma with a silenced MGMT gene. Results of a translational companion study to EORTC26981/NCIC CE.3 of radiotherapy +/− TMZ. Paper presented at 16th EORTC-NCI-AACR Symposium on Molecular Targets and Cancer Therapeutics, September 28-October 1, 2004, Geneva.
40. Freije WA, Castro-Vargas FE, Fang Z, et al: Gene expression profiling of gliomas strongly predicts survival. Cancer Res 64:6503-6510, 2004.
41. Law M, Yang S, Wang H, et al: Glioma grading: sensitivity, specificity, and predictive values of perfusion MR imaging and proton MR spectroscopic imaging compared with conventional MR imaging. AJNR Am J Neuroradiol 24:1989-1998, 2003.
42. Fountas KN, Kapsalaki EZ, Vogel RL, et al: Noninvasive histologic grading of solid astrocytomas using proton magnetic resonance spectroscopy. Stereotact Funct Neurosurg 82:90-97, 2004.
43. Vogelbaum MA, Angelov L, Siomin V, et al: Results of a survey of neurosurgical practice patterns regarding the prophylactic use of anti-epilepsy drugs in patients, with brain tumors. Paper presented at: Sixth Biennial Satellite Symposium, AANS/CNS Section on Tumors, 2004.
44. Matz PG, Cobbs C, Berger MS: Intraoperative cortical mapping as a guide to the surgical resection of gliomas. J Neurooncol 42:233-245, 1999.
45. Wadley J, Dorward N, Kitchen N, Thomas D: Pre-operative planning and intra-operative guidance in modern neurosurgery: a review of 300 cases. Ann R Coll Surg Engl 81:217-225, 1999.
46. Nimsky C, Ganslandt O, von Keller B, Fahlbusch R: Preliminary experience in glioma surgery with intraoperative high-field MRI. Acta Neurochir Suppl 88:21-29, 2003.
47. Metzger AK, Lewin JS: Optimizing brain tumor resection. Low-field interventional MR imaging. Neuroimaging Clin N Am 11:651-657, ix, 2001.
48. Nabavi A, Black PM, Gering DT, et al: Serial intraoperative magnetic resonance imaging of brain shift. Neurosurgery 48:787-797; discussion 797, 2001.
49. Heilbrun MP: Computed tomography-guided stereotactic systems. Clin Neurosurg 31:564-581, 1983.
50. Krieger MD, Chandrasoma PT, Zee CS, Apuzzo ML: Role of stereotactic biopsy in the diagnosis and management of brain tumors. Semin Surg Oncol 14:13-25, 1998.
51. Klar E, Becker J, Scheer KE: [Combined surgical and radiological therapy of glioblastoma multiforme with radiocobalt.]. Langenbecks Arch Klin Chir Ver Dtsch Z Chir 280:55-65, 1954.
52. Walker MD, Alexander E Jr, Hunt WE, et al: Evaluation of BCNU and/or radiotherapy in the treatment of anaplastic gliomas. A cooperative clinical trial. J. Neurosurg 49:333-343, 1978.

53. Walker MD, Strike TA: An evaluation of methyl-CCNU, BCNU and radiotherapy in the treatment of malignant glioma [abstract]. Proc Am Assoc Cancer Res 17:163, 1976.
54. Shapiro WR, Green SB, Burger PC, et al: Randomized trial of three chemotherapy regimens and two radiotherapy regimens and two radiotherapy regimens in postoperative treatment of malignant glioma. Brain Tumor Cooperative Group Trial 8001. J Neurosurg 71:1-9, 1989
55. Sharma RR, Singh DP, Pathak A, et al: Local control of high-grade gliomas with limited volume irradiation versus whole brain irradiation. Neurol India 51:512-517, 2003.
56. Hochberg FH, Pruitt A: Assumptions in the radiotherapy of glioblastoma. Neurology 30:907-911, 1980.
57. Garden AS, Maor MH, Yung WK, et al: Outcome and patterns of failure following limited-volume irradiation for malignant astrocytomas. Radiother Oncol 20:99-110, 1991.
58. Liang BC, Thornton AF Jr, Sandler HM, Greenberg HS: Malignant astrocytomas: focal tumor recurrence after focal external beam radiation therapy. J Neurosurg 75:559-563, 1991.
59. Wallner KE, Galicich JH, Krol G, et al: Patterns of failure following treatment for glioblastoma multiforme and anaplastic astrocytoma. Int J Radiat Oncol Biol Phys 16:1405-1409, 1989.
60. Massey V, Wallner KE: Patterns of second recurrence of malignant astrocytomas. Int J Radiat Oncol Biol Phys 18:395-398, 1990.
61. Lee SW, Fraass BA, Marsh LH, et al: Patterns of failure following high-dose 3-D conformal radiotherapy for high-grade astrocytomas: a quantitative dosimetric study. Int J Radiat Oncol Biol Phys 43:79-88, 1999.
62. Pirzkall A, McKnight TR, Graves EE, et al: MR-spectroscopy guided target delineation for high-grade gliomas. Int J Radiat Oncol Biol Phys 50:915-928, 2001.
63. Salazar OM, Rubin P, Feldstein ML, Pizzutiello R: High dose radiation therapy in the treatment of malignant gliomas: final report. Int J Radiat Oncol Biol Phys 5:1733-1740, 1979.
64. Walker MD, Strike TA, Sheline GE: An analysis of dose-effect relationship in the radiotherapy of malignant gliomas. Int J Radiat Oncol Biol Phys 5:1725-1731, 1979.
65. Chang CH, Horton J, Schoenfeld D, et al: Comparison of postoperative radiotherapy and combined postoperative radiotherapy and chemotherapy in the multidisciplinary management of malignant gliomas. A joint Radiation Therapy Oncology Group and Eastern Cooperative Oncology Group study. Cancer 52:997-1007, 1983.
66. Bleehen NM, Stenning SP: A Medical Research Council trial of two radiotherapy doses in the treatment of grades 3 and 4 astrocytoma. The Medical Research Council Brain Tumour Working Party. Br J Cancer 64:769-774, 1991.
67. Fu KK, Pajak TF, Trotti A, et al: A Radiation Therapy Oncology Group (RTOG) phase III randomized study to compare hyperfractionation and two variants of accelerated fractionation to standard fractionation radiotherapy for head and neck squamous cell carcinomas: first report of RTOG 9003. Int J Radiat Oncol Biol Phys 48:7-16, 2000.
68. Prados MD, Wara WM, Sneed PK, et al: Phase III trial of accelerated hyperfractionation with or without difluoromethylornithine (DFMO) versus standard fractionated radiotherapy with or without DFMO for newly diagnosed patients with glioblastoma multiforme. Int J Radiat Oncol Biol Phys 49:71-77, 2001.
69. Fitzek MM, Thornton AF, Rabinov JD, et al: Accelerated fractionated proton/photon irradiation to 90 cobalt gray equivalent for glioblastoma multiforme: results of a phase II prospective trial. J Neurosurg 91:251-260, 1999.
70. Nelson DF, Curran WJ Jr, Scott C, et al: Hyperfractionated radiation therapy and bis-chlorethyl nitrosourea in the treatment of malignant glioma—possible advantage observed at 72.0 Gy in 1.2 Gy B.I.D. fractions: report of the Radiation Therapy Oncology Group Protocol 8302. Int J Radiat Oncol Biol Phys 25:193-207, 1993.
71. Scott CB, Curran WJ, Yung WKA, et al: Long-term results of RTOG 90-06. A randomized trial of hyperfractionated radiotherapy to 72Gy and carmustine vs. standard RT and carmustine for malignant glioma patients with emphasis on anaplastic astrocytoma patients. J Clin Oncol 17:401, 1998.
72. Khafaga YM, Jamshed A, Allam AA, et al: Stevens-Johnson syndrome in patients on phenytoin and cranial radiotherapy. Acta Oncol 38:111-116, 1999.
73. Micali G, Linthicum K, Han N, West DP: Increased risk of erythema multiforme major with combination anticonvulsant and radiation therapies. Pharmacotherapy 19:223-227, 1999.
74. Klein M, Heimans JJ, Aaronson NK, et al: Effect of radiotherapy and other treatment-related factors on mid-term to long-term cognitive sequelae in low-grade gliomas: a comparative study. Lancet 360:1361-1368, 2002.
75. Torres IJ, Mundt AJ, Sweeney PJ, et al: A longitudinal neuropsychological study of partial brain radiation in adults with brain tumors. Neurology 60:1113-1118, 2003.
76. Hahn CA, Dunn RH, Logue PE, et al: Prospective study of neuropsychologic testing and quality-of-life assessment of adults with primary malignant brain tumors. Int J Radiat Oncol Biol Phys 55:992-999, 2003.
77. Vigliani MC, Sichez N, Poisson M, Delattre JY: A prospective study of cognitive functions following conventional radiotherapy for supratentorial gliomas in young adults: 4-year results. Int J Radiat Oncol Biol Phys 35:527-533, 1996.
78. Shaw E, Arusell R, Scheithauer B, et al: Prospective randomized trial of low- versus high-dose radiation therapy in adults with supratentorial low-grade glioma: initial report of a North Central Cancer Treatment Group/Radiation Therapy Oncology Group/Eastern Cooperative Oncology Group study. J Clin Oncol 20:2267-2276, 2002.
79. Steiber VW, Tatter SB, Lovato J, et al: A phase I dose escalating study of intensity modulated radiation therapy for the treatment of glioblastoma. Int J Radiat Oncol Biol Phys 2004, 2004.
80. Loeffler JS, Alexander E 3rd, Shea WM, et al: Radiosurgery as part of the initial management of patients with malignant gliomas. J Clin Oncol 10:1379-1385, 1992.
81. Sarkaria JN, Mehta MP, Loeffler JS, et al: Radiosurgery in the initial management of malignant gliomas: survival comparison with the RTOG recursive partitioning analysis. Radiation Therapy Oncology Group. Int J Radiat Oncol Biol Phys 2:931-941, 1995.
82. Shaw E, Scott C, Souhami L, et al: Radiosurgery for the treatment of previously irradiated recurrent primary brain tumors and brain metastases: initial report of Radiation Therapy Oncology Group Protocol (90-05). Int J Radiat Oncol Biol Phys 34:647-654, 1996.
83. Shaw E, Scott C, Souhami L, et al: Single dose radiosurgical treatment of recurrent previously irradiated primary brain tumors and brain metastases: final report of RTOG protocol 90-05. Int J Radiat Oncol Biol Phys 47:291-298, 2000.
84. Souhami L, Seiferheld W, Brachman D, et al: Randomized comparison of stereotactic radiosurgery followed by conventional radiotherapy with carmustine to conventional radiotherapy with carmustine for patients with glioblastoma multiforme: report of Radiation Therapy Oncology Group 93-05 protocol. Int J Radiat Oncol Biol Phys 60:853-860, 2004.
85. Loeffler JS, Alexander E 3rd, Hochberg FH, et al: Clinical patterns of failure following stereotactic interstitial irradiation for malignant gliomas. Int J Radiat Oncol Biol Phys 19:1455-1462, 1990.
86. Gutin PH, Prados MD, Phillips TL, et al: External irradiation followed by an interstitial high activity iodine-125 implant "boost" in the initial treatment of malignant gliomas: NCOG study 6G-82-2. Int J Radiat Oncol Biol Phys 21:601-606, 1991.
87. Florell RC, Macdonald DR, Irish WD, et al: Selection bias, survival, and brachytherapy for glioma. J Neurosurg 76:179-183, 1992.
88. Selker RG, Shapiro WR, Burger P, et al: The Brain Tumor Cooperative Group NIH Trial 87-01: a randomized comparison of surgery, external radiotherapy, and carmustine versus surgery, interstitial radiotherapy boost, external radiation therapy, and carmustine. Neurosurgery 51:343-355; discussion 355-347, 2002.
89. Green SB, Byar DP, Walker MD, et al: Comparisons of carmustine, procarbazine, and high-dose methylprednisolone as additions to surgery and radiotherapy for the treatment of malignant glioma. Cancer Treat Rep 67:121-132, 1983.
90. Kleinberg L, Grossman SA, Piantadosi S, et al: The effects of sequential versus concurrent chemotherapy and radiotherapy on

survival and toxicity in patients with newly diagnosed high-grade astrocytoma. Int J Radiat Oncol Biol Phys 44:535-543, 1999.
91. Nelson DF, Diener-West M, Horton J, et al: Combined modality approach to treatment of malignant gliomas—re-evaluation of RTOG 7401/ECOG 1374 with long-term follow-up: a joint study of the Radiation Therapy Oncology Group and the Eastern Cooperative Oncology Group. NCI Monogr 6:279-284, 1988.
92. Fine HA, Dear KB, Loeffler JS, et al: Meta-analysis of radiation therapy with and without adjuvant chemotherapy for malignant gliomas in adults. Cancer 71:2585-2597, 1993.
93. Friedman HS, McLendon RE, Kerby T, et al: DNA mismatch repair and O6-alkylguanine-DNA alkyltransferase analysis and response to Temodal in newly diagnosed malignant glioma. J Clin Oncol 16:3851-3857, 1998.
94. Yung WK, Albright RE, Olson J, et al: A phase II study of temozolomide vs. procarbazine in patients with glioblastoma multiforme at first relapse. Br J Cancer 83:588-593, 2000.
95. Wedge SR, Porteous JK, Glaser MG, et al: In vitro evaluation of temozolomide combined with X-irradiation. Anticancer Drugs 8:92-97, 1997.
96. van Rijn J, Heimans JJ, van den Berg J, et al: Survival of human glioma cells treated with various combination of temozolomide and X-rays. Int J Radiat Oncol Biol Phys 47:779-784, 2000.
97. Stupp R, Dietrich PY, Ostermann Kraljevic S, et al: Promising survival for patients with newly diagnosed glioblastoma multiforme treated with concomitant radiation plus temozolomide followed by adjuvant temozolomide. J Clin Oncol 20:1375-1382, 2002.
98. Combs SE, Gutwein S, Schultz-Ertner D, et al: Temozolomide combined with radiation as first-line treatment in primary glioblastoma multiforme: phase I/II-study. J Clin Oncol 22:1531, 2004.
99. Levin VA, Wara WM, Davis RL, et al: Phase III comparison of BCNU and the combination of procarbazine, CCNU, and vincristine administered after radiotherapy with hydroxyurea for malignant gliomas. J Neurosurg 3:218-223, 1985.
100. Levin VA, Wara WM, Davis RL, et al: Northern California Oncology Group protocol 6G91: response to treatment with radiation therapy and seven-drug chemotherapy in patients with glioblastoma multiforme. Cancer Treat Rep 70:739-743, 1986.
101. Donahue B, Scott CB, Nelson JS, et al: Influence of an oligodendroglial component on the survival of patients with anaplastic astrocytomas: a report of Radiation Therapy Oncology Group 83-02. Int J Radiat Oncol Biol Phys 38:911-914, 1997.
102. Levin VA, Silver P, Hannigan J, et al: Superiority of post-radiotherapy adjuvant chemotherapy with CCNU, procarbazine, and vincristine (PCV) over BCNU for anaplastic gliomas: NCOG 6G61 final report. Int J Radiat Oncol Biol Phys 18:321-324, 1990.
103. Abrey LE, Childs BH, Paleologos N, et al: High-dose chemotherapy with stem cell rescue as initial therapy for anaplastic oligodendroglioma. J Neurooncol 65:127-134, 2003.
104. Brem H, Piantadosi S, Burger PC, et al: Placebo-controlled trial of safety and efficacy of intraoperative controlled delivery by biodegradable polymers of chemotherapy for recurrent gliomas. The Polymer-brain Tumor Treatment Group. Lancet. 345:1008-1012, 1995.
105. Westphal M, Hilt DC, Bortey E, et al: A phase 3 trial of local chemotherapy with biodegradable carmustine (BCNU) wafers (Gliadel wafers) in patients with primary malignant glioma. Neuro-oncology 5:79-88, 2003.
106. Adjei AA: Blocking oncogenic Ras signaling for cancer therapy. J Natl Cancer Inst 93:1062-1074, 2001
107. Guha A, Feldkamp MM, Lau N, et al: Proliferation of human malignant astrocytomas is dependent on Ras activation. Oncogene 15:2755-2765, 1997.
108. Westermark B, Heldin CH, Nister M: Platelet-derived growth factor in human glioma. Glia 15:257-263, 1995.
109. Yeh HJ, Ruit KG, Wang YX, et al: PDGF A-chain gene is expressed by mammalian neurons during development and in maturity. Cell 64:209-216, 1991.
110. von Deimling A, Eibl RH, Ohgaki H, et al: p53 mutations are associated with 17p allelic loss in grade II and grade III astrocytoma. Cancer Res 52:2987-2990, 1992.
111. Wen P, Yung WK, Lamborn K, et al: Phase I/II study of Imatinib mesylate (STI571) for patients with recurrent malignant glioma (NABTC 99-08) [abstract]. Neuro-oncology 6:385, 2004.
112. Reardon D, Friedman A, Herndon J, et al: Phase II trial of imatinib mesylate plus hydroxyurea in the treatment of patients with malignant glioma [abstract]. Neuro-oncology 6:381, 2004.
113. Wong AJ, Bigner SH, Bigner DD, et al: Increased expression of the epidermal growth factor receptor gene in malignant gliomas is invariably associated with gene amplification. Proc Natl Acad Sci U S A 84:6899-6903, 1987.
114. Ekstrand AJ, Longo N, Hamid ML, et al: Functional characterization of an EGF receptor with a truncated extracellular domain expressed in glioblastomas with EGFR gene amplification. Oncogene 9:2313-2320, 1994.
115. Rich JN, Reardon DA, Peery T, et al: Phase II trial of gefitinib in recurrent glioblastoma. J Clin Oncol 22:133-142, 2004.
116. Volgelbaum M, Peereboom D, Stevens GH, et al: Initial experience with the EGFR tyrosine Tarceva (OSI-774) for single-agent therapy of recurrent/progressive glioblastoma multiforme [abstract]. Neuro-oncology 5:356, 2003.
117. Chakravarti A, Seiferheld W, Robins HI, et al: An update of phase I data from RTOG 0211: a phase I/II clinical study of ZD 1839 (Gefitinib) + radiation for newly diagnosed glioblastoma patients [abstract]. Neuro-oncology 6:372, 2004.
118. Buday L, Downward J: Epidermal growth factor regulates p21ras through the formation of a complex of receptor, Grb2 adapter protein, and Sos nucleotide exchange factor. Cell 73:611-620, 1993.
119. Goldstein JL, Brown MS: Regulation of the mevalonate pathway. Nature 343:425-430, 1990.
120. Cloughsey TF, Kuhn J, Wen P, et al: Two phase II trials of R115777 (zanestra) in patients with recurrent glioblastoma multiforme (GBM): a comparison of patients on enzyme-inducing anti-epileptic drugs (EIAED) and not on EIAED at maximum tolerated dose respectively: a North American Brain Tumor Consortium (NABTC) report [abstract]. Neuro-oncology 5:349, 2004.
121. Sebolt-Leopold JS, Dudley DT, Herrera R, et al: Blockade of the MAP kinase pathway suppresses growth of colon tumors in vivo. Nat Med 5:810-816, 1999.
122. Furnari FB, Lin H, Huang HS, Cavenee WK: Growth suppression of glioma cells by PTEN requires a functional phosphatase catalytic domain. Proc Natl Acad Sci U S A 94:12479-12484, 1997.
123. Wang SI, Puc J, Li J, et al: Somatic mutations of PTEN in glioblastoma multiforme. Cancer Res 57:4183-4186, 1997.
124. Hanahan D, Folkman J: Patterns and emerging mechanisms of the angiogenic switch during tumorigenesis. Cell 86:353-364, 1996.
125. Ellis LM, Takahashi Y, Liu W, Shaheen RM: Vascular endothelial growth factor in human colon cancer: biology and therapeutic implications. Oncologist 5(Suppl 1):11-15, 2000.
126. Reardon D, Friedman H, Yung W, et al: Preliminary phase I trial result: PTK787/ZK222584 (PTK/ZK), an oral VEGF tyrosine kinase inhibitor, in combination with either temozolomide or lomustine for patients with recurrent glioblastoma multiforme (GBM) [abstract]. Neuro-oncology 5:355, 2003.
127. Slotman BJ, Kralendonk JH, van Alphen HA, et al: Hypofractionated radiation therapy in patients with glioblastoma multiforme: results of treatment and impact of prognostic factors. Int J Radiat Oncol Biol Phys 34:895-898, 1996.
128. Roa W, Brasher PM, Bauman G, et al: Abbreviated course of radiation therapy in older patients with glioblastoma multiforme: a prospective randomized clinical trial. J Clin Oncol 22:1583-1588, 2004.
129. Phillips C, Guiney M, Smith J, et al: A randomized trial comparing 35Gy in ten fractions with 60Gy in 30 fractions of cerebral irradiation for glioblastoma multiforme and older patients with anaplastic astrocytoma. Radiother Oncol 68:23-26, 2003.
130. Tatter SB, Shaw EG, Rosenblum ML, et al: An inflatable balloon catheter and liquid 125I radiation source (GliaSite Radiation Therapy System) for treatment of recurrent malignant glioma: multicenter safety and feasibility trial. J Neurosurg 99:297-303, 2003.

131. Larson DA, Gutin PH, McDermott M, et al: Gamma knife for glioma: selection factors and survival. Int J Radiat Oncol Biol Phys 36:1045-1053, 1996.
132. Rostom AY, Sunderland K: Re-irradiation of astrocytoma of the brain. Br J Radiol 62:173-174, 1989.
133. Kim HK, Thornton AF, Greenberg HS, et al: Results of re-irradiation of primary intracranial neoplasms with three-dimensional conformal therapy. Am J Clin Oncol 20:358-363, 1997.
134. Hudes RS, Corn BW, Werner-Wasik M, et al: A phase I dose escalation study of hypofractionated stereotactic radiotherapy as salvage therapy for persistent or recurrent malignant glioma. Int J Radiat Oncol Biol Phys 43:293-298, 1999.
135. Ang KK, Jiang GL, Feng Y, et al: Extent and kinetics of recovery of occult spinal cord injury. Int J Radiat Oncol Biol Phys 50:1013-1020, 2001.
136. Voynov G, Kaufman S, Hong T, et al: Treatment of recurrent malignant gliomas with stereotactic intensity modulated radiation therapy. Am J Clin Oncol 25:606-611, 2002.
137. Sneed PK, Stauffer PR, McDermott MW, et al: Survival benefit of hyperthermia in a prospective randomized trial of brachytherapy boost +/− hyperthermia for glioblastoma multiforme. Int J Radiat Oncol Biol Phys 40:287-295, 1998.
138. Purdy JA: Dose-volume specification: new challenges with intensity-modulated radiation therapy. Semin Radiat Oncol 12:199-209, 2002.
139. Parsons JT, Bova FJ, Mendenhall WM, et al: Response of the normal eye to high dose radiotherapy. Oncology (Huntingt) 10:837-847; discussion 847-838, 851-832, 1996.
140. Parsons JT, Bova FJ, Fitzgerald CR, et al: Radiation optic neuropathy after megavoltage external-beam irradiation: analysis of time-dose factors. Int J Radiat Oncol Biol Phys 30:755-763, 1994.
141. Hughes MA, Parisi M, Kleinberg L, et al: Low CD4 counts and PCP prophylaxis in patients with primary brain tumors treated with steroids and radiation [abstract]. Proc Am Soc Clin Oncol 22:741, 2003.
142. Chan MF, Schupak K, Burman C, et al: Comparison of intensity-modulated radiotherapy with three-dimensional conformal radiation therapy planning for glioblastoma multiforme. Med Dosim 28:261-26, 2003.
143. Shaw EG, Seiferheld W, Cairncross G, et al: Radiation therapy (RT) alone vs intensive procarbazine-CCNU-vincristine (I-PCV) chemotherapy followed by radiation therapy for anaplastic oligodendroglioma (AO) and mixed oligoastrocytoma: results of Radiation Therapy Oncology Group—Intergroup Protocol 94-02. Int J Radiat Oncol Biol Phys 60:5163, 2004.
144. Lidar Z, Mardor Y, Jonas T, et al: Convection-enhanced delivery of paclitaxel for the treatment of recurrent malignant glioma: a phase I/II clinical study. J Neurosurg 100:472-479, 2004.
145. Reardon DA, Akabani G, Coleman RE, et al: Phase II trial of murine I-labeled antitenascin monoclonal antibody 81C6 administered into surgically created resection cavities of patients with newly diagnosed malignant gliomas. J Clin Oncol 1;20:1389-1397, 2002.
146. Hawthorne MF, Lee MW: A critical assessment of boron target compounds for boron neutron capture therapy. J Neurooncol 62:33-45, 2003.
147. Sauerwein W, Zurlo A, Group EBNCT: The EORTC Boron Neutron Capture Therapy (BNCT) Group: achievements and future projects. Eur J Cancer 38(Suppl 4):S31-S34, 2002.
148. Deutsch M, Green SB, Strike TA, et al: Results of a randomized trial comparing BCNU plus radiotherapy, streptozotocin plus radiotherapy, BCNU plus hyperfractionated radiotherapy, and BCNU following misonidazole plus radiotherapy in the postoperative treatment of malignant glioma. Int J Radiat Oncol Biol Phys 16:1389-1396, 1989.
149. Laperriere NJ, Leung PM, McKenzie S, et al: Randomized study of brachytherapy in the initial management of patients with malignant astrocytoma. Int J Radiat Oncol Biol Phys 41:1005-1011, 1998.
150. Pickles T, Goodman GB, Rheaume DE, et al: Pion radiation for high-grade astrocytoma: results of a randomized study. Int J Radiat Oncol Biol Phys 37:491-497, 1997.
151. Griffin TW, Davis R, Laramore G, et al: Fast neutron radiation therapy for glioblastoma multiforme. Results of an RTOG study. Am J Clin Oncol 6:661-667, 1983.
152. Laramore GE, Diener-West M, Griffin TW, et al: Randomized neutron dose searching study for malignant gliomas of the brain: results of an RTOG study. Radiation Therapy Oncology Group. Int J Radiat Oncol Biol Phys 14:1093-1102, 1988.
153. Prados MD, Seiferheld W, Sandler HM, et al: Phase III randomized study of radiotherapy plus procarbazine, lomustine, and vincristine with or without BUdR for treatment of anaplastic astrocytoma: final report of RTOG 9404. Int J Radiat Oncol Biol Phys 15;58:1147-1152, 2004.
154. Grossman SA, O'Neill A, Grunnet M, et al: Phase III study comparing three cycles of infusional carmustine and cisplatin followed by radiation therapy with radiation therapy and concurrent carmustine in patients with newly diagnosed supratentorial glioblastoma multiforme: Eastern Cooperative Oncology Group Trial 2394. J Clin Oncol 21:1485-1491, 2003.
155. Halperin EC, Herndon J, Schold SC, et al: A phase III randomized prospective trial of external beam radiotherapy, mitomycin C, carmustine, and 6-mercaptopurine for the treatment of adults with anaplastic glioma of the brain. CNS Cancer Consortium. Int J Radiat Oncol Biol Phys 34:793-802, 1996.
156. Hiesiger EM, Green SB, Shapiro WR, et al: Results of a randomized trial comparing intra-arterial cisplatin and intravenous PCNU for the treatment of primary brain tumors in adults: Brain Tumor Cooperative Group trial 8420A. J Neurooncol 25:143-154, 1995.
157. Shapiro WR, Green SB, Burger PC, et al: A randomized comparison of intra-arterial versus intravenous BCNU, with or without intravenous 5-fluorouracil, for newly diagnosed patients with malignant glioma. J Neurosurg 76:772-781, 1992.
158. Prados MD, Schold SJS, Fine HA, et al: A randomized, double-blind, placebo-controlled, phase 2 study of RMP-7 in combination with carboplatin administered intravenously for the treatment of recurrent malignant glioma. Neuro-oncology 5:96-103, 2003.
159. Rainov NG: A phase III clinical evaluation of herpes simplex virus type 1 thymidine kinase and ganciclovir gene therapy as an adjuvant to surgical resection and radiation in adults with previously untreated glioblastoma multiforme. Hum Gene Ther 11:2389-2401, 2000.
160. Debus J, Hug EB, Liebsch NJ, et al: Brainstem tolerance to conformal radiotherapy of skull base tumors. Int J Radiat Oncol Biol Phys 39:967-975, 1997.

CHAPTER 25

MENINGIOMA, EPENDYMOMA, AND OTHER ADULT BRAIN TUMORS

Glenn Bauman, Barbara Fisher, Steven Schild, and Edward G. Shaw

INCIDENCE AND PATHOLOGY

The tumors represented in this chapter represent a diverse collection of primary central nervous system (CNS) neoplasms that range from the relatively common (meningioma) to the relatively uncommon (base of skull chordoma and chondrosarcoma).

Overall, the incidence of these tumors ranges from 4/100,000 person-years (meningioma) to 0.2/100,000 person-years (chordoma/chondrosarcoma).

BIOLOGIC CHARACTERISTICS

These neoplasms present with varying pathologic features and patterns of spread that reflect their diverse origins. Some of these tumors present an almost solely locally aggressive entity (meningioma, craniopharyngioma, chordoma/chondrosarcoma, hemangioma/hemangioblastoma), while some present a risk of more widespread CNS dissemination (primary pineal tumors and CNS germ cell tumors, ependymoma, and choroid plexus tumors).

The natural history of these tumors may range from the very indolent (certain meningiomas and chondrosarcomas) to very aggressive (ependymoblastoma and choroid plexus carcinoma).

In all cases, the local extent of disease, presence of CNS spread, histology, and patient performance are important prognostic factors.

STAGING EVALUATION

As for all primary CNS tumors, a careful neurologic examination and assessment of the performance status of the patient are essential.

All these tumors are optimally staged using magnetic resonance imaging complemented by thin-slice computed tomography for tumors around the base of skull.

Magnetic resonance angiography or angiography may be useful for staging tumors with a tendency to vascularity (hemangioma, glomus tumors, meningiomas).

Craniospinal staging with spinal magnetic resonance imaging and cytology is recommended for those tumors with a potential for CNS spread (particularly ependymoma, pineal tumors, germ cell tumors, and choroid plexus tumors).

PRIMARY TREATMENT

In all cases, save primary CNS germinoma, maximum surgical resection while preserving function is the initial treatment (Table 25-1). Surgery in these instances will help relieve symptoms due to local compression or invasion and confirm histology and may facilitate subsequent therapy by debulking tumor around critical structures.

Many of these tumors occur in and around the skull base and arise in close proximity to critical structures like the brainstem, optic nerve and chiasm, cranial nerves, and eyes. In these instances, complete surgical resection without considerable morbidity may not be possible and adjuvant radiation therapy following a subtotal resection may be recommended.

In selected cases of small, noninvasive tumors such as small meningiomas, radiosurgery may be an acceptable alternative to surgical resection.

ADJUVANT TREATMENT

In instances of subtotal resection or high-grade/malignant variants, adjuvant radiation therapy may decrease the risk of local progression/recurrence following surgery. Adjuvant radiation therapy fields may need to include the ventricular system or whole cerebrospinal fluid (CSF) space for tumors at high risk of CSF dissemination or with established CSF dissemination.

Many of the tumors described in this chapter are localized neoplasms, and advanced radiation therapy delivery techniques (three-dimensional conformal or intensity-modulated radiation therapy, proton beam therapy) may help reduce the morbidity of treating these neoplasms where they occur around critical structures.

Some of these variants (chondrosarcoma and chordoma particularly) require adjuvant radiation therapy doses in excess of 70 Gy for optimal control; advanced delivery is necessary in these cases.

RECURRENT DISEASE AND PALLIATION

Radiosurgery may have a role for the treatment of small recurrences of these neoplasms.

Response to chemotherapy is variable and depends on the histology and ranges from highly sensitive (primary germ cell tumors) to totally insensitive (chordoma).

Palliative surgical debulking may play a role for selected, locally aggressive tumors such as chordomas and meningiomas, and in some instances, indolent biologic behavior argues for a conservative approach with minimal intervention for recurrent disease.

MENINGIOMA

Meningiomas arise from the arachnoid meninges of the brain and can cause symptoms by extra axial compression of adjacent structures. Typical locations for meningioma include the cerebral convexities, falx cerebri, tentorium cerebelli, cerebellopontine angle, and sphenoid ridge. Meningiomas can also occur within the spinal canal. Most meningiomas are of the "benign" or low-grade variety and are amenable to cure with surgical resection. Atypical or malignant meningiomas can be invasive, with aggressive behavior, and often require surgery and postoperative radiation therapy (RT).

Table 25-1 **Overview of Management of Tumors**

Histology	Incidence	Staging	Surgery	Radiation*	CTX	Outcome
Meningioma	25%	Not required	MSR	50-60 Gy CRT (1) (2)	No	LC >80%
Ependymoma	5%	Negative	MSR	50-60 Gy CRT (1) (3)	No	DFS 50-75%
		Positive	MSR	CSI (36 Gy) + CRT (to 50-60 Gy)	No	
Chordoma	<1%	Not required	MSR	70-80 Gy (1) (4)	No	LC >50%
Chondrosarcoma	<1%	Not required	MSR	65-70 Gy (1) (4)	No	LC >75%
Pineocytoma	<1%	Not required	Bx ± shunt	50-54 Gy CRT (5)	No	LC 50-75%
GGCT	<1%	Negative	Bx	WB (30 Gy) + CRT (to 50 Gy) (5)	± (6)	DFS >80%
		Positive	Bx	CSI (36 Gy) + CRT (to 50 Gy)	± (6)	DFS >80%
NGGCT	<1%	Negative	MSR	WB (30 Gy) + CRT (to 50 Gy) (5)	± (6)	DFS 50-75%
		Positive	MSR	CSI (36 Gy) + CRT (to 50 Gy)	± (6)	DFS 25-50%
Chemodectoma	<1%	Not required	MSR	45-50 Gy CRT (1) (2)	No	LC >80%
Hemangioblastoma	<1%	Suggested (7)	MSR	50-60 Gy CRT (1) (2)	No	LC >80%
Hemangiopericytoma	<1%	Suggested (8)	MSR	50-60 Gy CRT (1) (2)	No	LC >80%
Craniopharyngioma	5%	Not required	MSR	50-54 Gy CRT (1)	No	LC >80%
CPC	<1%	Negative	MSR	45-50 Gy CRT (1) (5)	± (6)	DFS 30-50%
		Positive	MSR	CSI (36 Gy) + CRT (to 50-60 Gy)		

Incidence, as a percentage of primary CNS tumors in adults; Staging, craniospinal axis staging (CSF cytology + spinal MRI); MSR, maximum safe resection; Bx, biopsy; CRT, conformal partial brain irradiation; CSI, craniospinal axis irradiation, typically 30-36 Gy; WB, whole brain irradiation; GGCT/NGGCT, germinomatous germ cell tumor/nongerminomatous germ cell tumor; CPC, choroid plexus carcinoma.

*Numbers in parentheses refer to following notes.

(1) Adjuvant radiation usually recommended for subtotally excised tumors; primary radiotherapy if MSR not feasible.

(2) Radiosurgery may be alternative to surgery for small (<3 cm) tumors (see text).

(3) Craniospinal radiation may be indicated for selected "high-risk tumors" even if CSAS negative (see text).

(4) Requires advanced radiation delivery to minimize morbidity and/or escalate dose (see text).

(5) Controversy exists as to optimum radiation volume (focal versus whole ventricular versus whole brain versus CSI).

(6) Chemotherapy may allow reduced radiation dose or volume (in GGCT) or improved outcome (in NGGCT or CPC).

(7) CSAS recommended for patients with von Hippel-Lindau.

(8) Systemic staging as well (bone scan, CT chest) if high grade/malignant hemangiopericytoma.

Etiology and Epidemiology

Prior exposure to ionizing radiation may be associated with the later development of meningioma.[1,2] Familial brain tumor syndromes such as neurofibromatosis type 2 may be associated with the development of meningioma or other primary brain tumors.[3] Meningiomas are more common among females and can express hormone receptors, suggesting hormonal factors may be important in their etiology. The exact role of hormones in the development and progression of meningioma remains to be determined. Other factors such as prior head trauma and exposure to cured foods have been postulated to play a role in the development of meningioma, but contradictory findings exist in the literature.[4]

Meningiomas comprise approximately a quarter of all adult brain tumors, making them the most common primary brain tumor. They are found twice as commonly among females versus males, and there is no difference in incidence noted according to race. The median age at diagnosis is 65 and the overall age-adjusted rate for the United States is estimated at approximately 4/100,000 person-years. An approximate 4-fold increase in incidence is noted from the fourth to eighth decades of age. In large multicenter clinical databases, overall survival at 5 years is estimated at approximately 60% with decreasing overall survival associated with older age (due to competing mortality) as well as atypical/malignant versus benign histology.[5,6]

Prevention and Early Detection

Exposure to ionizing radiation may increase the relative risk of meningioma by 10-fold versus unexposed populations. Among patients exposed to low-dose ionizing radiation (i.e., epilation for ringworm treatment), the latency period for development of meningioma is long, on the order of 40 years.[2] Among patients receiving therapeutic doses of radiation, latency periods may be shorter, on the order of 20 years.[7] Recognition of the carcinogenic effects of radiation has led to a sharp reduction in the use of radiation for nonmalignant conditions in children and the recommendation for regular imaging surveillance for children who have received therapeutic radiation to the CNS.[8]

Molecular Biology and Biologic Characteristics

Neurofibromatosis 2 (NF2) is an inherited autosomal dominant disorder in which affected individuals develop schwannomas, meningiomas, and ependymomas. The *NF2* gene is located on chromosome 22q and encodes a protein (merlin) from the 4.1 family of tumor suppressor proteins.[3] Loss of this tumor suppressor protein leads to loss of contact inhibition and increased invasiveness and motility among meningothelial cells. A second protein within this tumor suppressor family, 4.1b, is encoded at the 18p site, and alteration in either 22q or 18p affecting merlin or protein 4.1b is seen in over 90% of sporadic meningiomas.[9] Progression to higher tumor grades is associated with the accumulation of additional genetic changes, including loss of additional tumor suppresser genes on chromosomes 1p, 3p, 6q, 10, and 14q and gains of oncogenes on chromosomes 12q, 15q, 17q, and 20q.[3,10] Using high-density, oligonucleotide microarrays, Watson and colleagues[10] were able to identify gene expression profiles using a subset of 133 genes that distinguished between normal and neoplastic meningothelial tissue and between tumor grades.

Growth rates have been shown to be variable. Jaaskelainen and associates[11] correlated growth rate as measured on serial imaging with histologic grade in 43 patients with meningioma. For grade I tumors, a mean tumor volume doubling time of 415 days was noted with doubling times of 178 to 205 days in grades II (atypical) and III (anaplastic) meningiomas. In addition to grade, growth rate was correlated with mitotic index and absence of calcification on computed tomography (CT) scan. In contrast, Nakamura and colleagues[12] noted doubling times ranging from 1.27 to 143 years with a mean of 21 years in a group of 47 asymptomatic patients with meningiomas. Shorter doubling times were noted among younger patients and longer growth rates among patients with hypointense or isointense lesions on T2 MRI or calcified lesions on CT. Ultimately, 6 of the 41 patients required surgical treatment. Over a median follow-up of 85 months, Van Havenbergh and associates[13] noted tumor growth in three-quarters of a group of 21 patients with petroclival meningiomas. Functional deterioration was seen in approximately two thirds of patients and was associated with higher rates of tumor growth and infratentorial extension. Bindal and coworkers,[14] in reviewing 40 patients with skull base meningiomas, observed indolent growth and long periods of good function with observation alone. Thus, while indolent behavior of meningiomas is possible, unpredictability in biologic behavior requires careful clinical and imaging surveillance if observation is elected.

Pathology and Pathways of Spread

Grossly, meningiomas are well-circumscribed, firm, tan or grayish lesions arising from the meninges, usually with a broad dural attachment. Microscopically, benign meningiomas usually present a bland whorled appearance with little anaplasia or mitotic activity. Psammoma bodies may be present. A number of low-grade (World Health Organization [WHO] grade I) variants have been described but are of little prognostic consequence.

Malignant varieties are recognized and may be identified on the basis of clinical behavior (rapid growth or recurrence, invasiveness), microscopic features of malignancy (cellular or nuclear anaplasia, mitotic figures), or certain histologic variants.[3] Perry and colleagues[15] examined pathologic factors predicting recurrence after surgical resection and described atypical meningioma as those with brain invasion or mitotic index greater than 4 per 10 high-power field and the presence of features of sheeting, small cell formation, hypercellularity, and necrosis. Anaplastic meningomas were described as those with mitotic index greater than 20 per 10 high-power field and sarcoma-, carcinoma-, or melanoma-like histology.[15] Certain histologic variants predict more aggressive behavior, and the WHO grading system groups clear cell and chondroid histologic variants with atypical meningiomas as WHO grade II. Rhabdoid and papillary variants and anaplastic meningioma are grouped as WHO grade III.[3] An alternate grading system proposed by Jaaskelainen[11] grades meningiomas from I to IV according to a scoring system based on the number of adverse histologic features present, but the WHO system is most commonly used.

Meningiomas grow slowly in a localized fashion from the dura, eventually compressing and encasing surrounding vascular or neural structures. They are often quite vascular. Growth along the base of skull may be associated with invasion of the cavernous sinus, extension into the infratemporal space through cranial nerve foramen, or extension into the orbit. Sheet-like (en plaque) growth of meningiomas along meningeal surfaces may be seen. Invasion of dural sinus, particularly the superior sagittal sinus, may occur and may limit the ability to resect these tumors. Invasion of adjacent bone may occur and stimulate hyperostosis (Fig. 25-1). As meningiomas enlarge, compression of the overlying brain and associated edema is common but invasion of the brain is relatively rare. Atypical or malignant meningiomas may metastasize outside of the central nervous system, but this tends to be a feature of advanced/recurrent disease and does not occur with low-grade (WHO I) tumors.

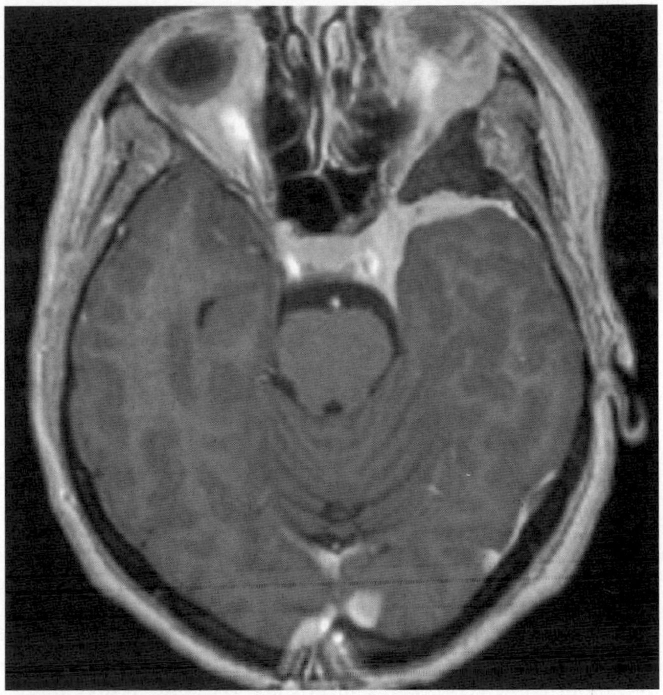

Figure 25-1 Axial-view, contrast-enhanced MRI demonstrates an enhancing en plaque meningioma involving the tip of the left temporal lobe with extension into the left cavernous sinus. Invasion of bone was associated with hyperostosis of the lateral orbital wall, with resulting proptosis.

Clinical Manifestations, Patient Evaluation, and Staging

In some cases, a meningioma may be discovered incidentally during investigation for an unrelated problem, in which case symptoms may not be present; otherwise, the presenting symptoms of meningioma are dependent on the site of origin of the tumor and tumor size. Meningiomas occurring over the cerebral convexity or falx may present with headache, seizures, or focal deficits due to compression of the surrounding brain by tumor or tumor-related edema. Tumors of the sphenoid wing and cerebellopontine angle may extend into the cavernous sinus and produce oculomotor deficits. Tumors of the suprasellar area may involve the optic nerve and chiasm and produce visual field defects. Proptosis may result from displacement of the orbital contents by hyperostotic bone or tumor. Additional cranial nerve deficits may result from extension along the base of skull and extension through cranial nerve fossae into the infratemporal space. Extension of the tumor through the bone table may result in a palpable soft tissue mass within the skull.

The patient history should include an assessment of risk factors including heritable tumor syndromes such as NF2 and prior exposure to ionizing radiation. Physical examination should include a careful neurologic examination to quantify existing deficits.

Magnetic resonance imaging (MRI) is the imaging modality of choice for meningiomas. The tumors typically appear as hypointense or isointense lesions on T1 with hyperintensity on T2-weighted images and enhance intensely and uniformly with gadolinium contrast. Thin-slice (<3 mm) CT may be useful for lesions around the base of skull to delineate bone involvement. Angiography may be useful for delineating the vascular supply of the tumor preoperatively, and embolization for large, vascular tumors may facilitate subsequent resection.

Occasionally, infiltrative meningiomas may be mistaken for primary or metastatic CNS parenchymal tumors. Bone metastasis or primary bone tumors (chondrosarcoma, chordoma, osteosarcoma) may present similarly to meningioma, particularly in the spine or base of skull. Within the cerebellopontine angle, acoustic neuromas may resemble meningiomas in location and in their densely enhancing CT/MRI appearance.

Primary Therapy

Treatment of meningioma may include observation alone, surgical resection, primary or postoperative radiation, or combinations of these treatments. Optimal management of these tumors is based largely on institutional reports of case series, and there are no large randomized trials comparing treatment options in these patients. A suggested algorithm for patient management is illustrated in Figure 25-2.

Observation

Patients with small, asymptomatic tumors may be suitable for imaging surveillance without immediate treatment. This may be especially appropriate for older (>age 65) patients, where competing morbidities and indolent tumor growth may allow deferral of any treatment. Regular surveillance MRI (every 4 to 6 months) in years 1 to 2 after diagnosis and yearly thereafter is recommended to rule out early, rapid tumor progression. Care should be taken to compare baseline images with subsequent images, as year-to-year progression may be subtle if comparisons are restricted to only the most recent and previous scan. Surveillance should also include regular neurologic examinations (including visual acuities and fields for tumors involving or near the optic apparatus) to detect subtle progression of deficits that may not be reflected with imaging alone.

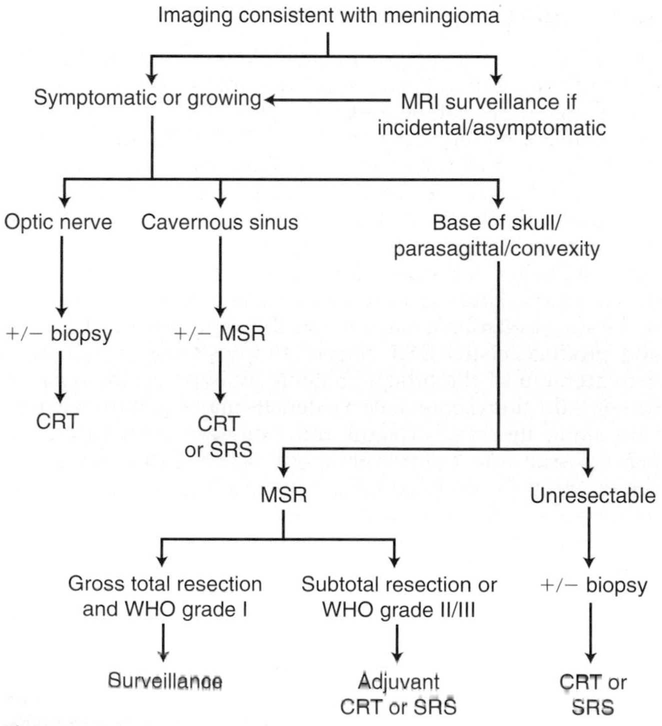

Figure 25-2 Treatment algorithm for meningioma. CRT, fractionated conformal radiotherapy (three-dimensional conformal radiotherapy or intensity-modulated radiotherapy); MSR, maximum surgical resection without anticipated neurologic deficits or morbidity; SRS, stereotactic radiosurgery (<3 cm tumor, minimal mass effect, no involvement of optic apparatus).

Surgical Resection

The current treatment of choice for benign meningiomas is complete surgical resection if this can be accomplished with low morbidity. Extent of resection is an important predictor of tumor recurrence. The Simpson[16] classification describes a grade I tumor as that which has been removed completely along with any dural attachment and involved bone or venous sinuses. Grade II tumors are those resected with coagulation of the dural attachment, grade III and IV tumors are those with incomplete resections of tumor or involved structures, and grade V tumors are those that only undergo biopsy. Even when complete resection is not possible, subtotal resections can relieve symptoms due to compression of normal structures, and a biopsy to establish a tissue diagnosis is usually possible even if an attempted resection is not.

Surgical issues in meningioma resection include hemostasis in these vascular tumors, resection of an adequate dural margin, and dissection of the brain tumor interface. Preoperative angiography and embolization may assist in resection of large or vascular tumors.[17,18] Image-guided surgical techniques may also facilitate resection with shorter hospital admissions and fewer complications.[19] For tumors of the parafalcine region, dural invasion may preclude complete resection, especially with involvement of the posterior two thirds of the sagittal sinus where the sinus is still patent (functioning). In these cases, maximum resection without sacrificing the sinus is recommended to avoid the risk of venous infarction in the immediate postoperative period.[20] Complete resection may also be difficult around the base of the skull and cerebellopontine angle due to location and involvement of contiguous structures. Advances in lateral skull base surgical approaches have provided extended exposures for more complete resections and decreased surgical morbidity in these areas.[21,22] Meningiomas originating within or invading into the cavernous sinus represent a unique surgical challenge. Successive aggressive surgical resections within these sites have been reported; however, there exists the potential for significant morbidity.[23,24]

Conservative subtotal resection followed by postoperative fractionated external beam radiation therapy (ERBT) or single-fraction stereotactic radiosurgery (SRS) is an alternative to aggressive base of skull resection. This approach may give good local control with decreased morbidity for patients with large or complex skull base or cavernous sinus tumors.[25]

For tumors of the optic nerve, conservative approaches with radiation alone or biopsy only followed by radiation has been associated with higher rates of preservation of visual function.[26] For patients with optic nerve meningioma and no useful vision, gross total surgical excision alone may be reasonable.

External Beam Radiotherapy

Fractionated EBRT may be used as primary therapy for unresectable or inoperable meningioma as adjuvant therapy following incomplete surgical resection or as salvage therapy for recurrence after surgery (Figs. 25-3 and 25-4). The clinical benefit of radiation is the arrest of tumor growth and stabilization of function; less often is significant tumor regression or recovery of deficits seen with radiation[27] (Fig. 25-5). For patients with symptoms due to compression of normal neural structures or significant mass effect from peritumoral edema, conservative decompressive surgery combined with adjuvant RT is a useful therapeutic strategy,[25,28] and tumor control rates

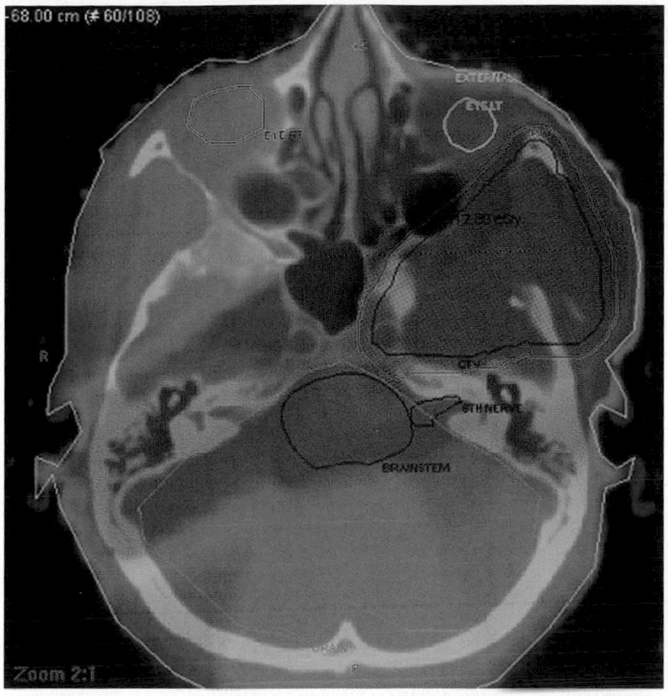

Figure 25-3 Intensity-modulated radiotherapy (IMRT) treatment plan for the adjuvant treatment of the large meningioma illustrated in Figure 25-1.

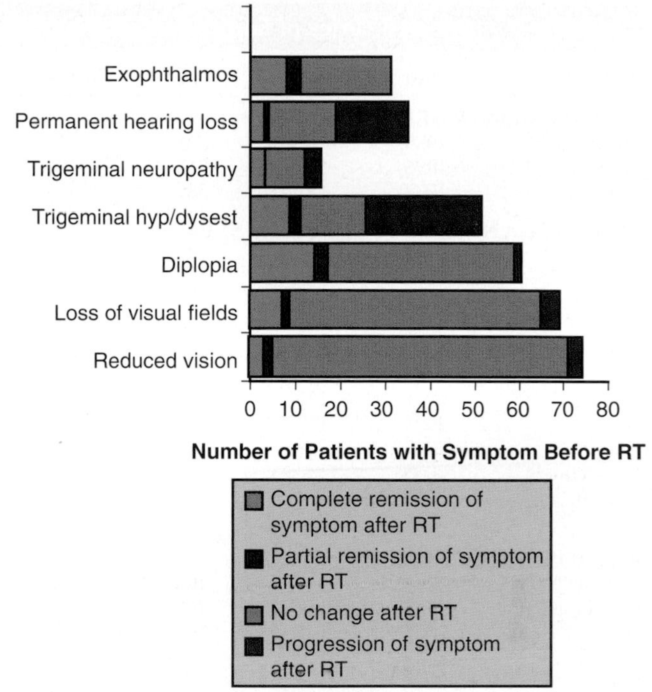

Figure 25-5 Response of symptoms to conventionally fractionated radiotherapy (RT). (From Debus J, Wuendrich M, Pirzkall A, et al: High efficacy of fractionated stereotactic radiotherapy of large base-of-skull meningiomas: long-term results. J Clin Oncol 19:3547-3553, 2001.)

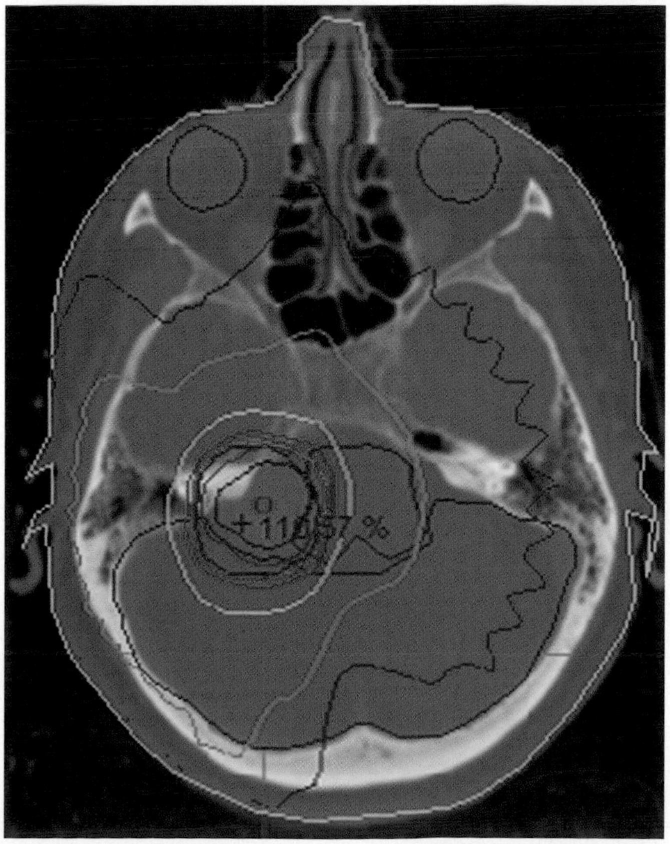

Figure 25-4 Fractionated stereotactic radiotherapy plan to treat a small cerebellopontine angle meningioma.

comparable to gross total resection are achieved (Table 25-2). For meningiomas in sites such as the cavernous sinus or optic nerve or for elderly patients with comorbidities, even limited decompressive surgery might be associated with significant complications. In these cases, primary radiation following a biopsy only (or empiric radiation based on an imaging diagnosis of meningioma) may be delivered. In cases of optic nerve sheath and cavernous sinus meningiomas, primary RT is associated with stabilization of cranial neuropathy symptoms in the majority of patients with improvement in function in up to one third of patients (see Table 25-2). For patients with atypical or malignant meningioma, high rates of tumor recurrence are noted even with gross total excision. In these cases, adjuvant RT is usually recommended even if a gross total excision is obtained (Table 25-3).

Stereotactic Radiosurgery

The well-circumscribed growth pattern and distinct enhancement on imaging render meningiomas an attractive target for SRS either as primary treatment or for adjuvant treatment of tumor residual following subtotal resection. The utility of SRS for neoplastic lesions has been questioned by some authors.[29] However, estimates of the alpha/beta ratio of meningioma suggest a value similar to that of late reacting tissue and a greater sensitivity to large dose per fraction radiation.[30] Good clinical results with single fraction linear accelerator or Gamma Knife–based radiosurgery confirm the efficacy of radiosurgery for tumor control with control rates in the 80% to 90% range (see Table 25-2). In a nonrandomized comparison of surgery and radiosurgery,[31] equivalent local control was noted for patients with a Simpson grade I tumor (complete resection) and those treated with radiosurgery. Radiosurgery may be considered for smaller tumors (<3 to 4 cm) without

Table 25-2 Selected Series of Surgery and Radiotherapy for Meningioma

Author	Year	Grade	No.	Follow-up	Outcome	GTR	STR	STR + XRT	XRT
SURGERY-ONLY SERIES									
Mirimanoff[197]	1985	I	225	—	10 y PFS	80%	45%		
Mathiesen[198]	1996	I	315	18 y	5 y PFS	96%	55%		
Stafford[199]	1998	I-III	581	—	10 y PFS	75%	39%		
SURGERY AND RADIOTHERAPY SERIES									
Taylor[200]	1988	I	132	2 y	10 y CSS	77%	18%	82%	
Glaholm[201]	1990	I-III	186	7 y	10 y CSS			77%	46%
Goldsmith[43]	1994	I	117	3 y	5 y PFS			85%	
Maire[202]	1995	I-III	91	3 y	5 y CSS			91%	
Condra[203]	1997	I-III	262	8 y	15 y CSS	88%	51%	86%	
Nutting[204]	1999	I	82		10 y PFS			83%	
Debus[27]	2001	I,II	180	3 y	5 y PFS			94%	
Uy[205]	2002	I	40	3 y	5 y PFS			88%	
Jalali[206]	2002	I	41	2 y	3 y PFS			100%	
Mendenhall[207]	2003	I	101	5 y	10 y CSS			92%	
Pirzkall[40]	2003	I	20	3 y	3 y PFS			100%	
Soyuer[208]	2004	I	92	8 y	5 y OS	72%	38%	91%	
RADIOSURGERY SERIES									
Hakim[209]	1998	I	106	3 y	3 y PFS				89%
Vermeulen[32]	1999	R	107	2 y	2 y PFS				80%
Stafford[199]	2001	I-III	190	4 y	5 y PFS			89%	
Lo[210]	2002	R	53	3 y	3 y PFS				97%
Eustaccchio[211]	2002	I	121	5 y	5 y PFS				98%
Lee[46]	2002		83	—	5 y PFS				97%
Pollock[31]	2003	I	198	—	7 y PFS	100%	34%		100%
Chuang[212]	2004	I	45	6 y	7 y LC			90%	
PROTON BEAM									
Wenkel[41]	2000	I	46	5 y	5 y PFS			100%	
Vernimmen[30]	2001	I	27	3 y	5 y PFS			88%	
Noel[213]	2002	I-III	17	3 y	4 y PFS			89%	
Weber[214]	2004	I	16	3 y	3 y PFS			92%	
CAVERNOUS SINUS MENINGIOMA									
Maguire[215]	1999	R	32	—	8 y PFS			81%	
Roche[47]	2000	R	80	3 y	5 y PFS			93%	
Dufour[216]	2001	R	31	6 y	10 y PFS			93%	
Nicolato[217]	2002	R	122	4 y	5 y PFS				97%
Lee[46]	2002	R	83	—	5 y PFS			97%	
Selch[218]	2004	R	45	3 y	3 y PFS			97%	
OPTIC NERVE SHEATH MENINGIOMA									
Andrews[57]	2002	R	30	2 y					30/30
Becker[56]	2002	R	39	3 y	3 y PFS				39/39
Naryana	2003	R	23	5 y	5 y PFS				23/23

CSS, cause-specific survival; Follow-up, median follow-up of patients in series; Grade, WHO tumor grade; GTR, gross total resection; Med PFS, median progression-free survival; OS, overall survival; Outcome, primary outcome reported in series; PFS, progression-free survival; R, radiologic diagnosis; STR, subtotal resection; STR + XRT, subtotal resection plus adjuvant radiotherapy; XRT, primary radiotherapy without surgery.

Table 25-3 Selected Series of Patients With Malignant or Atypical Meningioma

Author	Year	Grade	No.	Follow-up	Outcome	Sx	Sx + XRT	II	III
Goldsmith[43]	1994	II, III	23	3 y	5 y PFS			48%	
Milosevic[42]	1996	II, III	59		5 y CSS			28%	
Palma[219]	1997	II, III	71		10 y OS			79%	34%
Dziuk[220]	1998	II, III	38		5 y DFS	15%	80%		
Hakim[209]	1998	II, III	44	3 y	3 y OS			43%	
Ojemann[221]	2000	II, III	22		5 y PFS			26%	
Hug[222]	2000	II, III	31	5 y	5 y PFS			38%	52%
Goyal[223]	2000	II	22	5 y	5 y PFS	87%			
Harris[224]	2003	III	30	4 y	5 y PFS			83%	72%

CSS, cause-specific survival; Follow-up, median follow-up of patients in series; Grade, WHO tumor grade; OS, overall survival; Outcome, primary outcome reported in series; PFS, progression-free survival; Sx + XRT, surgical resection plus adjuvant radiotherapy; XRT, primary radiotherapy without surgery.

significant peritumoral edema or mass effect, located away from the optic apparatus. Treatment of larger tumors or tumors with significant mass effect from edema may be associated with a higher risk of symptomatic postradiosurgery edema.[32] Fractionated stereotactic RT may be an alternative to single-fraction radiosurgery for some patients with larger tumors or tumors involving the optic apparatus (see Figs. 25-2 and 25-4).

Proton Beam Radiotherapy

Proton beam RT has been used for the treatment of meningioma and exploits the range-limited nature of protons to produce highly conformal treatments. Fewer patients treated with proton beam have been reported in the literature compared with photon techniques and clinical results seem similar at least when moderate dose (50 to 54 Gy) radiation was used. SRS and hypofractionated stereotactic RT techniques with protons have also been reported (see Table 25-2).

Locally Advanced Disease and Palliation

While the majority of patients treated with complete resection or subtotal resection followed by RT have excellent long-term tumor control, some patients will experience disease recurrence. Patients with atypical or malignant tumors and those treated with subtotal resection alone are at higher risks of recurrence. For those patients treated with surgery alone, repeat resection or decompression followed by salvage radiation can be effective salvage therapy. For patients treated with prior RT, repeat surgery, radiosurgery, or interstitial brachytherapy may be options, albeit with a higher risk of late complications.[33] The use of hydroxyurea has been reported to stabilize disease progression for patients with recurrent meningioma.[34]

Techniques of Irradiation

The circumscribed nature of meningiomas combined with their propensity to occur in close proximity to critical structures makes them ideal targets for advanced radiation delivery techniques such as three-dimensional (3D) conformal radiotherapy (CRT), intensity-modulated radiotherapy (IMRT), and SRS. Meticulous treatment planning and delivery are essential given the overall favorable prognosis and possibility of late radiation toxicity in long-term survivors. Fabrication of a custom immobilization device and acquisition of a 3D CT data set for treatment planning are essential.

Fusion of the planning CT and the T1-weighted contrast-enhanced diagnostic MRI facilitates target volume delineation as each modality provides complementary information.[35] Typically, the composite volume of the enhanced tumor on CT and MRI is outlined as the gross tumor volume (GTV), with care to outline the tumor along its dural margins and in the orbital and cavernous sinus regions. The GTV may be expanded to include regions at risk (tumor bed, areas of hyperostotic bone, or soft tissue extension) to form the clinical target volume (CTV). For en plaque benign meningiomas, malignant meningiomas, and meningeal hemangiopericytomas, the CTV should also include a 2-cm margin on the GTV. The CTV is expanded by 3 to 5 mm (for conventional mask-based immobilization) or 1 to 2 mm (for stereotactic immobilization) to yield a planning target volume (PTV) to account for random set-up uncertainty.

Three-dimensional treatment planning using multiple (typically three to five) fields or IMRT (see Fig. 25-3) is recommended to conformally radiate the tumor with sparing of adjacent normal structures. For smaller tumors stereotactic techniques with non–coplanar-fixed circular collimator, multiple static fields shaped with 3- to 5-mm leaf multileaf collimation or dynamic arc techniques can provide highly conformal treatments (see Fig. 25-4). Comparisons of various planning and delivery options for patients with smaller meningioma have suggested improved conformality at higher isodoses, and improved dose homogeneity with IMRT or 3D CRT techniques compared with fixed circular collimator radiosurgery techniques, particularly for irregularly shaped lesions.[36-38] For lesions in close proximity to critical structures, proton beam RT may carry an advantage in terms of minimizing the irradiation dose received outside of the prescription dose volume.[36] The clinical significance of increased sparing of contiguous structures in the low-dose regions remains to be clarified, and even proton beam therapy may not spare critical structures embedded within a tumor volume.[39]

In a small series of 20 patients with recurrent or residual meningioma treated with IMRT, Pirzkall and associates[40] noted higher rates of symptom improvement and radiographic regression than noted with standard CRT. Using IMRT they were able to deliver a dose of 52 Gy to a mean prescription dose surface of 87% resulting in mean dose to the PTV of 55 to 58 Gy and a maximum dose of 60 to 65 Gy while respecting organ at risk tolerances. They hypothesized that the high-dose region within the tumor produced by the inhomogeneous IMRT distribution may have accounted for the somewhat higher rates of clinical and radiographic responses noted. They cautioned that follow-up was relatively short at a median of 36 months, and long-term results (control and toxicity) are not yet available.

Given the fact that many meningiomas may have critical normal tissue embedded within the target volume, heterogeneous dose delivery to the target with techniques like IMRT or multi-isocenter SRS may result in "hot spots" in critical structures with the possibility for higher rates of late toxicity. Careful evaluation of cumulative and differential dose-volume histograms and inspection of the 3D dose distributions in multiple planes is necessary to detect high dose regions associated with these techniques. Prescribing to the maximum target isodose and reducing target dose inhomogeneity will help minimize potential toxicity due to unrecognized hot spots within the treatment volume.

While a radiation dose response for meningioma has not clearly been established, most series reporting good clinical control and low toxicity have used doses of between 50 and 54 Gy (1.8 and 2.0 Gy/fraction) for benign meningioma. Dose escalation beyond 54 Gy was associated with increased toxicity in one series of meningioma patients treated with combined proton and photon beam, suggesting dose escalation should be cautiously applied.[41] Higher doses in the 55- to 60-Gy range (1.8 to 2.0 Gy/fraction) for atypical or malignant meningioma may be recommended given the propensity for recurrence even with aggressive surgical resection and moderate dose radiation.[42,43]

Using moderate-dose fractionated RT, rates of late toxicity (new focal deficits, neurocognitive impairment, necrosis) should be low. In a prospective study of meningioma patients treated with 3D conformal techniques no adverse effects on neurocognitive function at one year post treatment were noted.[44] In a large series of patients treated with fractionated 3D CRT, Debus and colleagues[27] noted a low incidence (3%) of worsening of preexisting deficits (see Fig. 25-5) and a low rate (3%) of other late toxicity. Similarly radiosurgical series report late toxicity rates of 10% or less (see Table 25-2). SRS within the cavernous sinus appears to be safe with similar low incidence of new cranial nerve deficits from treatment and stability or improvement of symptoms in the majority of patients.[45-47]

Critical structures to consider when treating meningiomas in the base of skull region include brainstem, optic apparatus, cranial nerves, hypothalamus/pituitary gland, and medial temporal lobes.

Radiation injury to the brainstem may be manifest as focal cranial nerve injury or long tract findings (hemisensory loss or hemiplegia) due to focal necrosis within the brainstem. Debus and colleagues[48] reported on 348 patients treated with combined photon/proton irradiation to the skull base. They found a crude incidence of 5.5% (19/348) for brainstem injury resulting in the death of three patients (0.9%). Within the 348 patients, the maximum dose to the brainstem ranged from 4 to 70 CGE (cobalt gray equivalent) and the median dose ranged from 3 to 55 CGE. Volume of brainstem receiving greater than 60 CGE was highly significant for predicting toxicity with a relative risk (RR) of 11.4 for brainstem injury in those patients receiving greater than 60 CGE to more than 0.9 cm^3 of brainstem. Castro and associates reported on 126 patients with base of skull tumors treated with charged particles. An overall severe (grade 4 or 5) complication rate (including brainstem injury) of 8% was noted. Higher prescribed dose and retreatment of recurrent tumors were associated with severe toxicity.[49] For photon irradiation, TD 5/5 levels of 60 Gy, 53 Gy, and 50 Gy to one third, two thirds, and three thirds of the brainstem have been suggested based on a review of the available literature.[50]

Radiation injury to the optic apparatus may be manifest as decreased visual acuity or visual field defects. These visual side effects may result from irradiation of the retina, optic nerve, or chiasm. In addition, irradiation of the lens or lacrimal gland of the eye may result in cataract formation or severe dry eye. Parsons and colleagues[51] found a threshold for radiation retinopathy of 45 Gy with the incidence increasing rapidly for doses between 45 and 55 Gy, especially for fraction sizes greater than 1.9 Gy. A similar threshold was found for irradiation of the optic nerves where no patients receiving less than 60 Gy to the optic nerves experienced optic neuropathy, while those patients receiving greater than 60 Gy had an incidence of optic neuropathy of 11% (for fraction size less than 1.9 Gy) and 47% (for fraction size greater than 1.9 Gy).[52] Threshold tolerance for severe dry eye (i.e., lacrimal gland tolerance) and cataracts (lens tolerance) has been estimated at 30 Gy and 10 Gy, respectively.[53] Kim and associates[54] noted a 4.4% incidence of optic nerve injury for base of skull tumors irradiated by proton beam with a median delivered dose to the optic apparatus of 59.4 CGE. In a review of the literature, Goldsmith found a low incidence of radiation-induced optic neuropathy with conventional-dose (50 to 54 Gy, 1.8 to 2.0 Gy/fraction) photon radiation and proposed radiobiologic models to predict optic nerve tolerance.[55]

For the treatment of primary optic nerve sheath meningioma with conventionally fractionated RT, high rates of visual function preservation and a low incidence of visual deterioration due to radiation have been reported.[26,56,57] With SRS, doses to the optic apparatus greater than 8 Gy are typically avoided because of concerns regarding radiation-induced optic neuropathy.[58] Stafford and associates,[59] however, reported a low risk of optic neuropathy in 215 patients treated for benign tumors with higher doses (median, 10 Gy; range, 0.4 to 16 Gy), suggesting the tolerance may be higher.

Focal brain injury has been noted following photon beam RT of brain lesions as well as proton/photon irradiation of base of skull lesions. In the treatment of brain tumors, CNS tolerance doses of 45 Gy, 50 Gy, and 60 Gy for treatment to whole brain, one-half brain, and one-third brain radiation have been quoted.[50] Santoni and colleagues[60] noted an incidence of temporal lobe injury of 10% among patients receiving between 66 and 72 Gy with combined proton/photon irradiation for patients with skull base tumors.

Conclusions and Future Possibilities

The lack of prospective and randomized trials in meningioma means that management for these tumors is based primarily on reports of single-institution experience. Controversies in treatment for meningioma exist in several areas: choice of surveillance versus treatment; role of aggressive surgery, especially for base of skull tumors; timing and dose of adjuvant RT; role of SRS as an alternative to surgery; and relative toxicity of treatment alternatives. Participation of physicians and their patients in randomized trials addressing these questions will be important in determining the optimal management of meningioma.

EPENDYMOMA

Etiology and Epidemiology

Ependymomas are glial neoplasms that account for 5% of intracranial tumors in adults and approximately 10% of intracranial tumors in children. The mean age at presentation is 5 years for children and in the third and fourth decades for adults.[6,61] Male and female incidence is equal. In children, 90% of ependymomas are intracranial and infratentorial, while in adults, tumors are more commonly supratentorial or spinal in location. While the overall incidence of spinal cord ependymomas is low, ependymomas make up the majority (60%) of primary spinal cord tumors.

Molecular Biology

Several chromosome abnormalities have been noted in ependymomas, including 22q11,[62] 6q, and 9.[63,64] Taylor and associates[65] performed whole genome analysis of 40 pediatric ependymoma patients. Using comparative genomic hybridization and RNA expression array analysis, they noted distinct chromosomal alteration and gene expression patterns according to the anatomic origin (spinal versus posterior fossa versus supratentorial) of the tumor. They hypothesized that different cell precursor and anatomic site–specific factors may account for the variable genetic patterns, and the differing genetic profiles may account for the heterogenous clinical behavior of these tumors.

Pathology and Pathways of Spread

Ependymal cells line the surface of the ventricular system of the brain and the central canal of the spinal cord. Migration of ependymal cells into the cerebral cortex from subependymal areas may occur. Ependymal tumors may arise anywhere within the brain or spinal cord and may be in close proximity to or distant from the ventricular system.

Two characteristic histologic features of ependymoma are "perivascular pseudo-rosettes" (anuclear perivascular collars radiating cellular processes around blood vessels) and true rosettes (characterized by organization of ependymal cells around a central lumen). Immunohistochemistry staining reveals diffuse S-100 positivity and focal GFAP positivity, especially around blood vessels composing the pseudorosettes. The presence of rosettes and pseudorosettes permits the diagnosis of ependymoma and can often allow the identification of even poorly differentiated ependymomas.

Ependymomas span a range of histologic appearance and biology from well-differentiated myxopapillary forms (WHO grade I) to anaplastic (WHO grade III).[66] The grade III or malignant variant of ependymoma (also termed anaplastic ependymoma) is characterized by the presence of angioproliferation, foci of necrosis, or evidence of anaplasia (increased cellularity, mitotic figures, multinucleation, giant cell formation). One third of ependymomas in children are histologically malignant. A solid squamous papillary subtype is identified in adults and may have a particularly good prognosis. Other subtypes include cellular and clear cell variants. Subependymomas are uncommon low-grade lesions that occur most often in the fourth and lateral ventricles of adults, and are often found incidentally at autopsy or during investigation of other intracranial pathology.[66] Ependymoblastomas, now considered a type of primitive neuroectodermal tumor, are highly malignant and most common in infants. Differentiation from medulloblastoma can occasionally be problematic, but the Homer-Wright rosettes seen in medulloblastoma lack the central lumen of ependymal rosettes and usually the cells surround a core of fibrillary material.

Ependymomas arise in variable locations within the brain or spinal cord. In children, two thirds of these tumors arise infratentorially from the floor of the fourth ventricle.[67] Infratentorial tumors may extend through the foramen magnum or protrude into the cervical subarachnoid space as low as the fifth or sixth cervical vertebra. Ependymomas also may arise from the brainstem and extend through the foramen of Luschka to the cerebellopontine angle. Spinal ependymomas (particularly WHO grade I myxopapillary ependymomas) commonly occur in the cauda equina region but may involve long segments of the spinal cord. Due to the proximity to ventricular spaces, ependymomas originating in the brain or spine can spread via the cerebrospinal fluid (CSF), most often at the time of relapse after initial treatment and less commonly at presentation.[68]

Clinical Manifestations, Patient Evaluation, and Staging

Presenting symptoms relate to site of origin or presence of metastasis. Infratentorial ependymoma may be suspected on the basis of posterior fossa symptomatology, that is, headache, vomiting, ataxia, neck stiffness or head tilt, cranial neuropathies (particularly cranial nerves VI, VII, and VIII), hydrocephalus, and long tract signs.[67,69,70] Supratentorial ependymomas present with focal neurologic deficits or mass effect. Spinal ependymoma, or intracranial ependymoma with spinal leptomeningeal metastases, presents with back pain, lower extremity weakness or sensory symptoms, or bowel/bladder dysfunction. Cranial leptomeningeal involvement usually presents with cranial nerve involvement without evidence of brainstem invasion.

These tumors appear heterogeneous on CT/MRI scan and enhance with CT contrast or gadolinium. Leptomeningeal deposits appear well circumscribed in the subarachnoid space on MRI and enhance with gadolinium. Careful neuraxis staging and pathology review (to differentiate ependymoblastomas and medulloblastomas) are important.[68,71]

Primary Therapy

Initial management may require corticosteroids and/or CSF diversion before primary therapy is initiated. A survival benefit and lower risk of CSF seeding are seen in patients who are able to undergo total excision of their tumors (Table 25-4). Surgery alone may be sufficient for selected patients with WHO grade I noninvasive tumors who undergo complete resections with negative CSF cytology and spinal MRI, although there is controversy on this point[67,72] (Fig. 25-6).

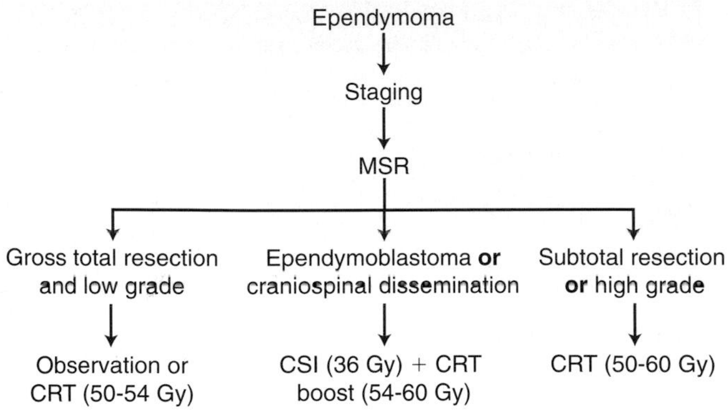

Figure 25-6 Treatment algorithm for ependymoma. Staging should include contrast-enhanced MRI spine and cerebrospinal cytology, especially for high-grade or infratentorial tumors. Controversy exists about whether high-grade, infratentorial ependymomas should routinely receive prophylactic craniospinal irradiation (CSI). CRT, conformal partial brain irradiation; MSR, maximum safe resection.

Age of patient at diagnosis, tumor location, invasiveness, neurologic symptoms, histologic grade, extent of surgical resection, and radiation dose and volume are proposed prognostic variables. Patients with high-grade tumors and patients with postoperative residual tumor are reported to have a worsened survival. Postoperative RT is often recommended for these patients.

The need for routine craniospinal radiation for patients with these tumors remains an area of controversy. Estimates of the frequency of the overall risk of CSF involvement range from 5% to 16%,[61,68,71,73] depending on tumor grade, location, and local control of the primary tumor. Supratentorial and low-grade tumors generally are associated with low rates of CSF dissemination, whereas infratentorial high-grade tumors are associated with higher rates of CSF relapse. Local relapse triples the rate of CSF failure (from 3% to 9% on average) and the higher incidence of CSF failure in high-grade infratentorial tumors is associated with poorer rates of local control rather than isolated CSF relapses. A review of the literature[68,71] suggests a very modest reduction in the incidence of spinal recurrence from 10% to 7% in high-grade tumors treated with routine prophylactic spinal irradiation.

Institutional reviews of treatment of ependymomas provide some general survival rates.[61,74-78] Patients with gross total resections have 5-year survivals on the order of 60% to 90%, and those with subtotal resections and radiation, 0% to 53%. Overall 5-year survival rates for patients treated with subtotal resection and radiation are in the range of 40% to 60%. A phase II prospective trial of conformal radiation for subtotally resected ependymoma reported an encouraging 75% progression-free survival and low neurocognitive toxicity at 3 years postradiation.[79] Among anaplastic tumors treated with surgery and radiation, 5-year survival rates in the range of 10% to 40% are reported. A prospective trial of combined surgery, RT, and chemotherapy reported a 3-year overall survival of 75%. Improved progression-free survival was noted among patients with completely resected versus subtotally resected tumors (3-year progression-free survival 83% versus 38%), confirming that complete surgical resection is an important therapeutic maneuver in these tumors.[80] Most series report local failure as the primary mode of tumor recurrence, and late failures at 5 to 10 years are not uncommon. Spinal cord ependymomas have an outlook comparable to intracranial tumors. High-grade/anaplastic lesions of the spinal

Table 25-4 Results of Selected Series of Patients Treated for Intracranial Ependymoma

Year	Author	No. of Patients	Patient Age	Treatment	5-y OS	5-y PFS
2005	Mansur[225]	60	Both	S + RT	71.2%	54.8%
2004	Massimino[226]	63	Pediatric	S + RT ± CT-GTR	82%	65%
				-STR	61%	35%
2004	Ben-Ammar[227]	31	Both	S + RT-all	63%	
				-CSI	86%	
				-WB	37.5%	
2004	Jaing[228]	43	Pediatric	RT	53.9%	45.9%
2004	Reni[229]	70	Adult	S ± RT	67%	43%
2002	Merchant[230]	88	Pediatric	S ± RT-anaplastic		3 y = 75%
				-diff		3 y = 84%
2002	Guyotat[231]	34	Adults	S	62%	47%
2002	van Veelen-Vincent[232]	83	Pediatric	S ± RT ± CT	73%	48%
2002	Merchant[233]	50	Pediatric	S ± RT-anaplastic		3 y = 28%
				-diff		3 y = 84%
2002	Paulino[234]	49	Both	S ± RT ± CT-CSRT	71.4%	
				-WB	60%	
				-CRT	80.8%	
2002	Oya[235]	48	Both	S + RT	10 y = 47%	10 y = 42%
2001	Grill[236]	73	Pediatric	S + CT-anaplastic	4 y = 59%	4 y = 22%
				-GTR	4 y = 74%	
				-STR	4 y = 35%	
2000	Akuyz[237]	62	Pediatric	S ± RT ± CT	10 y = 55%	10 y = 34%
2000	Timmerman[238]	55	Pediatric	S ± RT		3 y = 75.6%
2000	Figarella-Branger[239]	37	Pediatric	S ± RT ± CT	45%	25%
2000	Paulino[240]	34	Both	S ± RT	71.5%	61.8%
1999	Horn[241]	83	Pediatric	S ± RT ± CT	57%	42%
1998	McLaughlin[242]	41	Both	S ± RT	10 y = 51%	10 y = 46%
1998	Sala[243]	35	Pediatric	S ± RT	51%	
1998	Robertson[244]	32	Pediatric	S ± CSRT ± CT	69%	50%
1998	Schild[245]	70	Adult	S ± RT	67%	43%
1997	Merchant[246]	28	Pediatric	S ± RT	56%	
1997	Perilongo[247]	92	Pediatric	S ± RT ± CT	10 y = 55%	10 y = 35%
1997	Stuben[248]	56	Both	S ± RT	60%	51%
1996	Foreman[249]	31	Pediatric	S ± RT-GTR	69%	
				-STR	47%	
1995	Pollack[250]	40	Pediatric	S ± RT-GTR	80%	65%
				-STR	22%	8.9%

CRT, conformal radiotherapy; CSI, craniospinal radiotherapy; CT, chemotherapy; diff, differentiated; GTR, gross total resection; OS, overall survival; PFS, progression-free survival; RT, radiotherapy; S, surgery; STR, subtotal resection; WB, whole brain.

cord have a uniformly dismal prognosis and are frequently associated with leptomeningeal spread.

Chemotherapy is not routinely recommended for patients with ependymoma. Previous randomized trials of adjuvant chemotherapy in ependymoma have not demonstrated a survival benefit.[81] Neoadjuvant chemotherapy may be considered in order to defer RT in younger patients to allow time for more complete CNS maturation.[82] Chemotherapy for recurrent ependymoma may be useful for palliation with cisplatin among the more active agents for recurrent disease.[74]

Patients require regular imaging (CT/MRI every 3 to 6 months) and clinical follow-up posttreatment. Those patients who are treated with craniospinal irradiation need regular endocrinologic assessment as pituitary function and spinal growth may be impaired, particularly in prepubertal patients. Those patients treated with local fields only may benefit from routine spinal imaging. Most failures occur within the first 2 to 3 years posttreatment.

Long-term follow-up of patients is essential as late relapses (beyond 5 to 10 years) may occur. Surveillance spinal imaging may detect recurrences while they are still resectable. Repeat surgery, radiosurgery, or repeat fractionated EBRT can be considered for focal recurrences.[83] Salvage chemotherapy may be a palliative option for more extensive relapse.[74]

Techniques of Irradiation

In the era before routine spinal staging with CSF cytology and spinal MRI, routine craniospinal axis radiation was recommended in all ependymoma patients.[84] At present, regardless of the tumor site (supratentorial or infratentorial, intracranial and spinal) or grade, all patients with ependymoma should undergo MRI of the brain and entire spine as well as CSF cytology to stage the neuraxis. In those with low-grade intracranial or intraspinal tumors in whom the neuraxis is negative, localized radiation is adequate. In brain ependymomas, patterns of failure analysis with contemporary staging have suggested a low risk of isolated spine relapse in the absence of local intracranial failure, implying only minimal benefits to routine prophylactic spinal radiation.[68,71] Given the morbidity of large field radiation, particularly in younger patients, the use of craniospinal radiation should be restricted to patients with established positive CSF metastases or spinal MRI scan, or those with ependymoblastoma histology. Controversy remains in patients with anaplastic ependymoma (brain or spine) regarding the routine use of craniospinal axis radiation.

Patients with intracranial ependymoma who need localized radiation should be treated with multiple conformal fields with a 1- to 2-cm margin on the preoperative tumor volume to a total dose of 50.4 to 54 Gy (1.8 to 2.0 Gy/fraction). The use of conformal techniques to deliver higher doses (up to 59.4 Gy) to smaller volumes has been reported with good local control and low toxicity.[79] Doses of 30 to 36 Gy to the craniospinal axis with a boost to 50.4 to 59.4 Gy to the primary tumor are recommended when craniospinal radiation is indicated. The radiation technique is similar to that for medulloblastoma. Those with spinal ependymoma should either be treated with a single posteroanterior treatment field or multiple field techniques to the preoperative tumor volume with a 2-cm margin to 50 to 54 Gy.

Conclusions and Future Possibilities

The ability to achieve a gross total resection is the most important prognostic factor for patients with intracranial or spinal ependymoma. Conformal local field RT should be used for nondisseminated ependymomas of the brain or spine. Craniospinal RT should be restricted to patients who have CSF or MRI evidence of leptomeningeal spread or those with ependymoblastoma. The role of chemotherapy remains to be determined, although multimodality therapy (surgery, radiation, and chemotherapy) has resulted in encouraging survival rates in anaplastic/high-grade ependymoma.

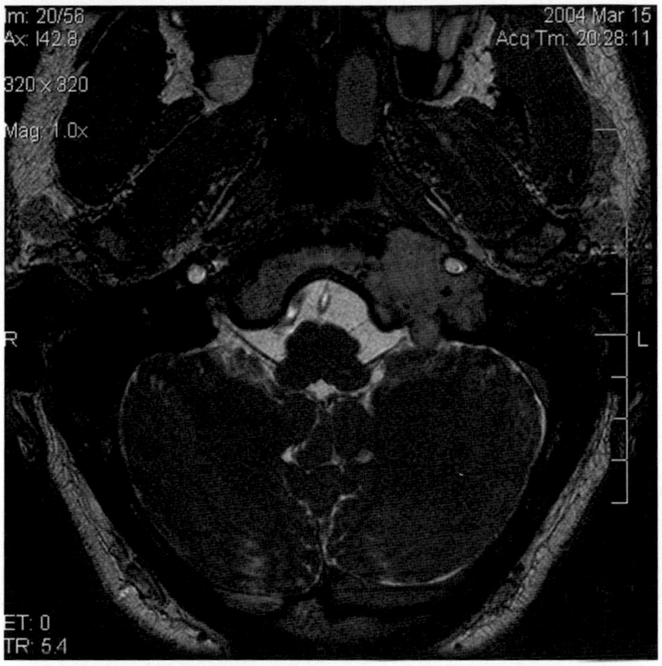

Figure 25-7 T2-weighted MRI demonstrates a low-grade chondrosarcoma arising from the clivus at the base of the skull.

CHORDOMA AND CHONDROSARCOMAS

Chordomas are rare tumors that are thought to originate from notochord remnants within the axial skeleton. Approximately one third of the tumors arise within the clivus/craniocervical junction, one third in the thoracic or lumbar spine, and one third in the sacrum. Chondrosarcomas arise from cartilaginous elements in bone and can occur in the base of skull or elsewhere in the axial skeleton. Taken together, chordomas and chondrosarcomas account for approximately 0.2% of primary brain tumors, with a median age at presentation of 47 and an age-adjusted incident rate of 0.03/100,000 person-years.[6]

Pathology and Patterns of Spread

Three varieties of chordoma are recognized: conventional (classic), chondroid, and dedifferentiated (atypical). Classic chordoma demonstrates no mesenchymal or cartilaginous differentiation and is characterized by physaliphorous cells (large, vacuolated mucus-containing cells) residing in a mucoid matrix. Chondroid chordomas possess a cartilaginous matrix and may be difficult to distinguish from chondrosarcoma. Immunohistochemistry positivity for keratin and epithelial membrane antigen can distinguish the two entities.[85] Dedifferentiated chordomas demonstrate features of malignancy such as cellular pleomorphism and mitotic figures. Chordomas arise within the cortex of bone and typically grow slowly, expanding and destroying bone and displacing and compressing adjacent neurologic structures. Within the base of skull, chordomas originate within the clivus and can expand to compress the brainstem and optic apparatus.[86]

Chondrosarcomas may have a clinical and histopathologic appearance similar to that of chordoma. Hyaline, mixoid, and mixed varieties are recognized as well as high-grade (grade 2) and low-grade (grade 1) lesions. Chondrosarcomas of the skull base may arise from the clivus but most arise laterally, from the sphenoid occipital junction and less commonly from the spheno-ethmoid complex. Like chordoma, chondrosarcomas exhibit locally aggressive growth and may expand and destroy bone and extend to compress or encase adjacent structures (Fig. 25-7). Intraparenchymal intracranial chondrosarcomas have also been reported.[87]

Histologically, chondroid chordomas and chondrosarcomas may appear similar. Rosenberg noted that of 200 chondrosarcomas referred for treatment at their institution, approximately one third had an original diagnosis of chordoma from the referring institution. S-100 protein positivity and keratin and epithelial membrane antigen negativity on immunohistochemistry distinguished chondrosarcoma from chordoma.[88]

Clinical Manifestations, Patient Evaluation, and Staging

The clinical presentation of chondrosarcoma and chordoma is similar to that of other base of skull lesions and is characterized by inexorable local growth and extension.[86] Tumors can be large at presentation and produce symptoms due to involvement/compression of adjacent critical structures. Compression of cranial nerves within the cavernous sinus or at the level of base of skull foramen may lead to multiple cranial neuropathies. Involvement or compression of the brainstem may lead to long tract findings, cranial nerve palsies, or symptoms due to obstructive hydrocephalus. Involvement of the optic nerves or chiasm may lead to loss of visual fields or acuity. Expansion of the periosteum and dura by the tumor may produce headache or neck pain. Involvement of the pituitary gland due to sellar/parasellar extension may produce endocrinopathies. Chordoma or chondrosarcoma of the spine may produce pain due to periosteal expansion or pathologic fracture as well as radiculopathies or myelopathy. Rarely, chordoma or chondrosarcoma may metastasize to viscera or bone.

A thorough history and physical examination are required to document any existing neurologic and endocrinologic deficits. Baseline neuro-ophthalmologic and endocrinologic work-up is recommended for base of skull tumors, given the propensity for these tumors to affect visual and pituitary function.

The value of different imaging techniques is dependent on location of the primary lesion. Contrast-enhanced thin-section CT with coronal reconstruction can provide valuable information regarding extend of bone involvement at the base of skull. Multiplanar contrast-enhanced MRI will provide the best assessment of local extension both intracranially and extracranially and the involvement of critical structures like the optic apparatus, brainstem, and cavernous sinus (see Fig. 25-7). Preoperative angiography can be useful for delineating vascular anatomy, particularly where the tumor is involving the internal carotid artery.[89] Unless the patient presents with symptoms suspicious for metastatic disease, routine systemic staging (bone scan, CT chest abdomen and pelvis) is usually not performed.

Primary Therapy

Surgery

The initial treatment for most patients with chordomas and chondrosarcomas is surgical resection to confirm the histologic diagnosis, relieve symptoms due to mass effect, and maximally debulk the tumor (Fig. 25-8). Gay and associates[90] reported on the results of surgery for patients with chondrosarcoma and chordoma in 60 patients (46 chordomas, 16 chondrosarcomas). A variety of surgical approaches were used, and staged surgical resections were performed in over half of the cases to obtain maximum tumor debulking. Total or near-total resection was achieved in two thirds of the patients and 20% of patients received postoperative RT. The 5-year relapse-free survival was 90% for chondrosarcoma and 65% for chordoma. Surgery for primary versus recurrent disease and total/near total resection was associated with improved survival. Tai and colleagues,[91] in a review of the literature, noted a 5-year survival of 20% among patients treated for chordoma with surgery alone and improved results among patients treated with surgery plus adjuvant radiation. Improvements in imaging, image-guided surgery, lateral and anterior skull base approaches, reconstructive surgery, and postoperative care have improved the ability to resect these tumors more completely. Gross total surgical resection alone may be sufficient treatment for patients where this can be achieved.[21,22,89]

Despite these innovations, the majority of patients with base of skull tumors have piecemeal or subtotal resections, and postoperative RT is usually recommended.[92,93] Gross total resection for patients with chordoma of the sacrum may often be more easily achieved. Improved results with surgery alone for sacral chordoma compared with clival chordoma have been reported.[94,95]

Photon Radiotherapy

As noted, achieving a gross total resection of tumors at the base of skull with acceptable morbidity is frequently not possible; for this reason, postoperative RT is often considered for subtotally excised chordomas and chondrosarcomas. Even for gross totally excised tumors, concerns about contamination of the operative field during a piecemeal excision or adherence to adjacent critical structures may increase the risk of microscopic residual disease and lead to a recommendation for postoperative RT.

The available literature suggests improved outcome with combinations of surgery and RT[86,91,94] (Table 25-5). Optimal treatment of residual chordoma and chondrosarcoma with radiation appears to require high radiation doses (>65 Gy), and this can be challenging to achieve in the base of skull. Results from series of patients with chordoma and chondrosarcoma treated with adjuvant RT have demonstrated inferior outcomes for patients with large tumor residuum or brainstem involvement.[86,96] Thus, even if adjuvant RT is being considered, maximum tumor debulkng to minimize the residual tumor volume and to remove tumor from adjacent, dose limiting structures like the brainstem will facilitate subsequent RT. Using conventional RT doses (50 to 60 Gy) and techniques, 10-year overall survival rates in the range of 50% to 60% are reported.[91] Debus and colleagues[97] reported on the use of fractionated stereotactic RT for the treatment of 45 patients with chordomas and chondrosarcomas. A median dose of 66.6 Gy for chordoma and 64.9 Gy for chondrosarcoma was used. Five-year local control rate was 100% for chondrosarcoma and 50% for chordoma.

Muthukumar and colleagues[98] reported on 15 patients treated with SRS (15 to 20 Gy) for small residual (4.6 mL) chordoma or chondrosarcoma at the base of skull. Twelve of the

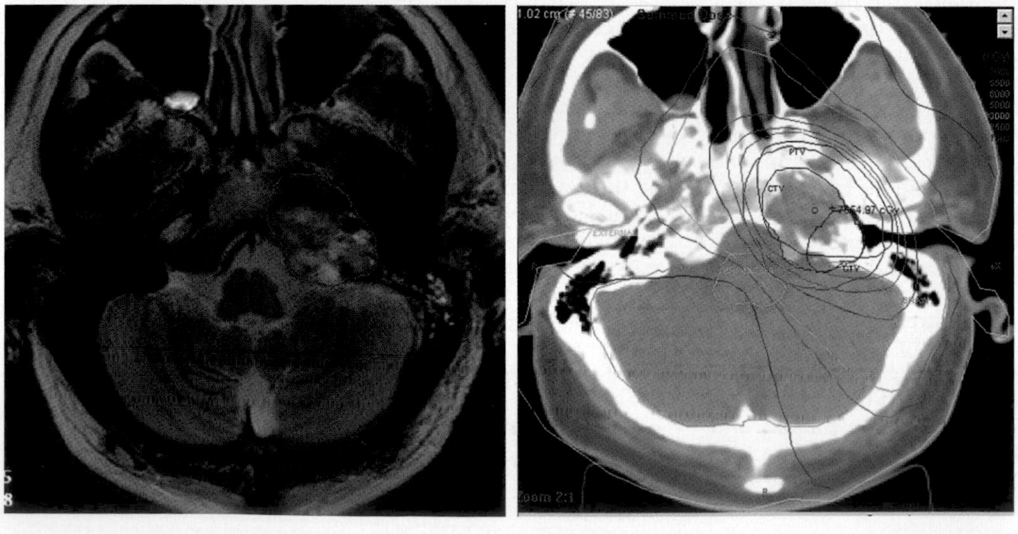

Figure 25-8 Postoperative T2-weighted MRI reveals a residual tumor at the base of the skull *(left)*. Non-coplanar dynamic arc radiotherapy plan to treat residual disease to a dose of 70 Gy in 35 fractions *(right)*.

Table 25-5 **Selected Series: Chordoma and Chondrosarcoma**

Author	Year	No.	Histology	End Point	Sx	Sx + XRT	Comments
Rich[94]	1985	48	Ch	5-y OS	75%	50%	
Gay[90]	1995	60	Ch	5-y RFS	90%		20% of patients received adjuvant photon radiation
			Cs	5-y RFS	65%		
Tai[91]	1995	159	Ch	5-y OS	20%	65%	Review included photon treatment only, 50-60 Gy
				10-y OS	20%	50%	
Castro[100]	1989	45	Ch, Cs	5-y LC		52%	Helium or neon ions to 36-80 GyE; variety of skull base tumors
Hug[86] (LLUMC)	1999	58	Ch	5-y LC		79%	Local control worse if brainstem involvement or >25 cm³ volume
			Cs	5-y LC		100%	
Hug[86] (MGH)	2000	290	Ch	10-y LC		40%	Late failures among Ch seen between 5-10 y after proton treatment
		229	Cs	10-y LC		95%	
Debus[97]	2000	45	Ch	5-y LC		50%	3D CRT XRT to 65-67 Gy
			Cs	5-y LC		100%	
Noel[96]	2003	67	Ch	3-y LC		71%	Mixed photon/proton treatment to median of 67 GyE
			Cs	3-y LC		85%	
Schultz[99]	2004		Ch	3-y LC		81%	Carbon ion; 60 GyE (RBE = 3)
			Cs	3-y LC		100%	

Ch, chordoma; Cs, chondrosarcoma; Sx, surgery; XRT, radiotherapy.

15 patients remained clinically controlled over an average follow-up period of 48 months. It remains to be seen whether the availability of advanced photon delivery with IMRT and stereotactic techniques is sufficiently conformal to allow dose escalation similar to that achieved with charged particles, particularly for chordoma where high doses (>70 Gy) are required for optimal results.[97]

Charged Particle Radiotherapy

Given the historically suboptimal results with conventional-dose RT for patients with chordomas, dose escalation has been attempted for these tumors. Prior to the introduction of 3D conformal photon and SRS techniques, charged particle therapy for chordomas and chondrosarcomas was introduced for dose escalation. The majority of patients treated with high-dose radiation have been treated with protons,[86] with a smaller number of patients treated with other charged particles (carbon, neon, helium).[49,99,100] For protons, the radiobiologic effectiveness (RBE) is close to that of photons (RBE of 1.1) and the major benefit is through the dose gradient advantages conferred by the Bragg peak deposition of energy, as sharp dose gradients at interfaces with critical structures can be established.[101] Charged particles such as carbon ions have a radiobiologic effect considerably higher than photons or protons due to a greater linear energy transfer (LET).

It is important to recognize that over the period of time charged particle therapy has been evaluated for treatment, advances in imaging and surgical resection have also contributed to the improved clinical results noted. For instance, detection and targeting of residual tumor following surgery has been facilitated by the availability of MRI. In addition, particularly for chordoma, late recurrences are common and long-term follow-up of patients treated with charged particles is necessary to best gauge efficacy.[86]

Using charged particles and moderately high doses (65 to 70 Gy), excellent results have been obtained for chondrosarcoma with 5- to 10-year local control rates in the 80% to 100% range. The results with chordoma are less optimal, with late failures up to 10 years noted and actuarial local control rates in the 80% range at 5 years and the 40% range at 10 years. Larger tumor residual (>25 mL); brainstem involvement and chordoma-versus-chondrosarcoma histology have been associated with inferior outcomes.[86] Among patients with chordoma, female gender and lower equivalent uniform dose have been associated with worse outcome.[102]

Locally Advanced Disease and Palliation

Recurrent chordoma and chondrosarcoma may be treated with repeat surgery for palliation of symptoms and may still be associated with prolonged survival.[94] Treatment of recurrences following surgery alone may be managed with repeat resection followed by postoperative fractionated EBRT, SRS, or a combination. Results are generally not as good in the treatment of recurrent disease compared with primary treatment.[86] Chemotherapy has not been found to be predictably effective for the treatment of recurrent chordoma or chondrosarcoma, emphasizing the need to optimize local control in the initial approach to these tumors.

Techniques of Irradiation

As previously noted, optimal treatment of chordoma and chondrosarcoma with radiation following surgery requires high-dose (>65 Gy) treatment. Given the proximity to adjacent critical structures, high-precision, conformal techniques are required with either SRS, fractionated stereotactic photon RT, or charged particle therapy. Typically, patients are treated with protons using a multifield technique using conformally shaped fields to treat the clinical target volume (surgical bed and areas of suspected tumor extension) with higher doses delivered to gross residual tumor. Tumor adherence to critical structures may limit the uniformity of dose that can be delivered and has been found to adversely affect outcome.[102] Similar 3D conformal or IMRT approaches are used (see Fig. 25-8) for patients treated with photons.[97,36] For tumors of the sacrum region (Fig. 25-9A), more complete surgical resections are usually possible, and RT may be more easily delivered with conformal techniques in the adjuvant setting (see Fig. 25-9B).

Dose-volume correlation with toxicity has been reported for patients with base of skull tumors treated with protons.[48,103-106] Tolerance may be influenced by other factors such as presence of comorbidity (diabetes) and the number of prior surgeries.

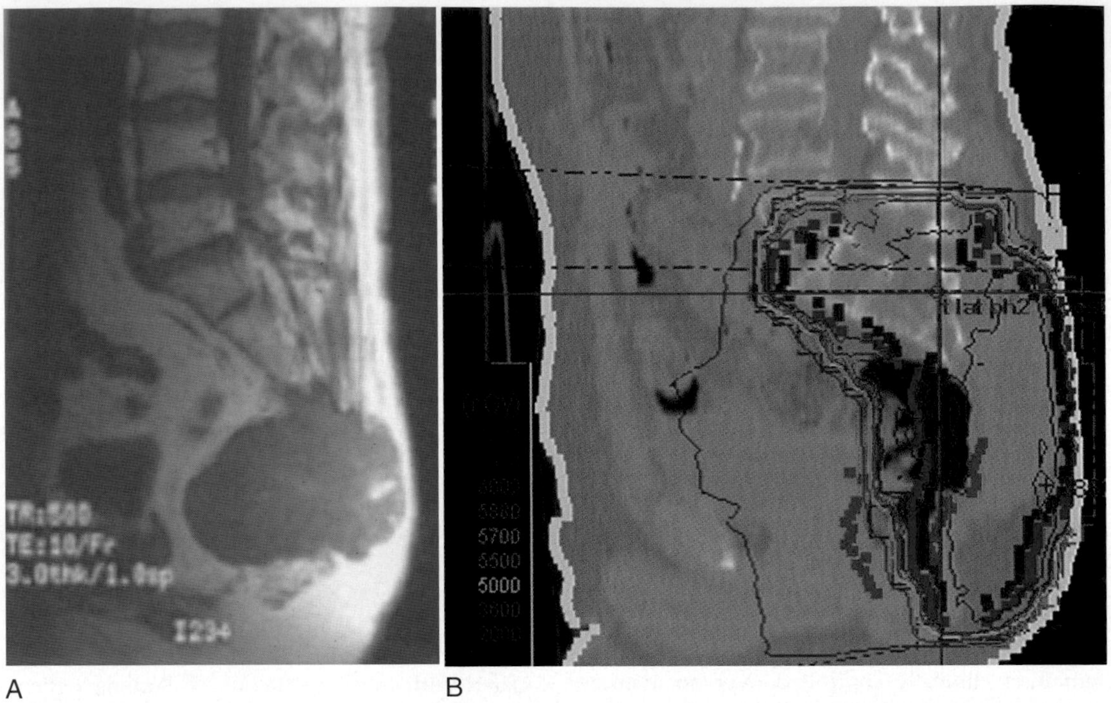

Figure 25-9 **A,** Large chordoma of the sacrum is demonstrated on preoperative, T1-weighted MRI. **B,** Sagittal distribution of postoperative treatment to the tumor bed (66 Gy in 33 fractions) after gross total resection.

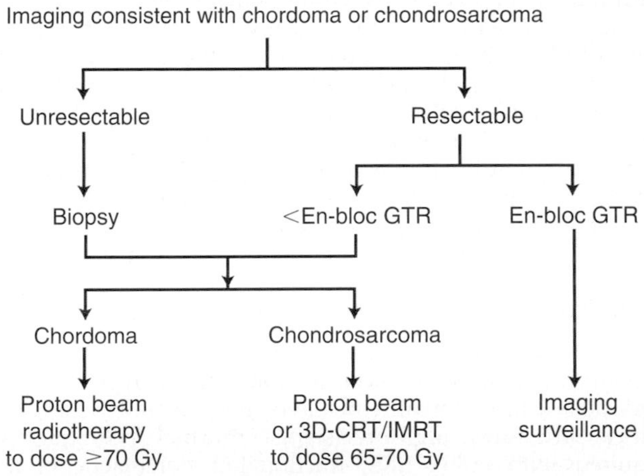

Figure 25-10 Treatment algorithm for chordoma and chondrosarcoma. GTR, gross total resection; 3D-CRT/IMRT, three-dimensional conformal or intensity-modulated radiotherapy.

Conclusions and Future Possibilities

Good results with optimal surgical resection and adjuvant photon or charged particle therapy to moderately high doses (60 to 70 Gy) have been achieved for chondrosarcoma (Fig. 25-10). Local control for chordoma still remains elusive and attempts at further dose escalation (beyond 70 Gy) and the use of novel charged particles (i.e., carbon ion) to improve results are underway. Treatment of skull base tumors requires the careful integration of neurosurgical, neurotologic, neuroradiologic, and radiation oncology expertise and radiation treatments (be it photons or protons) should be delivered by an experienced comprehensive multidisciplinary skull base team.

PINEAL REGION TUMORS

Pineal tumors are uncommon tumors and make up only 0.4% to 1% of all brain tumors.[6,107] Pineal region tumors are rare and include a large variety of lesions. Many studies have included patients whose tumor types were not histologically verified because of the risks associated with operative intervention.[108-112] As a result, these series may have included patients with benign processes such as cysts and vascular lesions.

The pineal gland is composed of pineal parenchymal cells or pineocytes. The pineocyte is a specialized neuron surrounded by blood vessels and astrocytes. The pineocytes produce the hormone melatonin, which affects circadian rhythms, inhibiting the release of both luteinizing and follicle-stimulating hormones. Serum concentrations of melatonin are low during exposure to light and increase in the dark.

Prognosis is dependent upon tumor histology. This finding has been reported by many investigators.[113-126] Patients with pineocytomas, germinomas, and mature teratomas have the most favorable survival rates.

Pathology

The pineal gland region is unusual in that a wide variety of primary tumors arise from this site.[127-131] Benign cysts can also occur in this site, as do ordinary brain tumors such as astrocytomas or meningiomas. However, these are not as common as the germ cell tumors, which make up about two thirds of the malignancies of the pineal region.

The most common site for a primary CNS germ cell tumor is the pineal gland, followed by the suprasellar region. It is assumed that germ cells migrate during embryogenesis and can lodge at this ectopic site, becoming malignant germ cell tumors later in life. The most common tumors are the germinomas, which are histologically indistinguishable from testicular seminomas and ovarian dysgerminomas.

Nongerminomatous germ cell tumors (NGGCTs) in the pineal region also occur in pure and mixed forms. Histologic varieties of NGGCTs include the teratoma, embryonal carcinoma, yolk sac tumor (endodermal sinus tumor), choriocarcinoma, or combinations referred to as mixed germ cell tumors. Teratomas typically include cell types derived from all three germ cell layers: endoderm, mesoderm, and ectoderm. Mature teratomas contain fully differentiated cells. Immature teratomas consist of cells and tissues resembling those of the developing fetus. By convention, tumors in which mature and immature components coexist are classified as immature. Other teratomas with malignant epithelial or mesenchymal elements are considered to be teratomas with malignant transformation. Embryonal carcinomas contain large, primitive-appearing epithelial cells. In rare instances they contain platelike miniature embryos or embryoid bodies. Yolk sac tumors are epithelial tumors that contain compact sheets, ribbons, cords, or papillae. Schiller-Duval bodies are diagnostic of yolk sac tumors. They contain tufted epithelium covered vessels projecting into clear spaces. In addition to Schiller-Duval bodies, yolk sac tumors often have a loose-knit vitelline pattern. Choriocarcinomas contain a bilaminar arrangement of both syncytiotrophoblasts and cytotrophoblasts. Combinations of any of these tumor types are referred to as mixed germ cell tumors. One specific mixed germ cell tumor, the teratocarcinoma, contains elements of both embryonal carcinoma and teratoma.[127-131]

Some of these tumors produce markers such as AFP (α-fetoprotein) or β-HCG (β-human chorionic gonadotropin). Yolk sac tumors (endodermal sinus tumors) can produce AFP, choriocarcinomas can produce β-HCG, and embryonal tumors can produce both markers. Pure germinomas can produce β-HCG but usually not in very high levels. These markers are generally found in higher concentration in the CSF than the serum and can aid in identifying the tumor type and monitoring the effects of therapy.

Tumors may also arise in the pineocytes, forming a group of tumors called pineal parenchymal tumors (PPTs), which compose 15% to 30% of all pineal tumors. These can be classified into four groups: pineocytomas, mixed PPTs, PPTs with intermediate differentiation, and pineoblastomas.[127-131] Pineocytomas are well-circumscribed masses that compress surrounding structures. They are composed of mature-appearing cells arranged in sheets or ill-defined irregular lobules. Fibrillary processes with clublike endings project from these cells, which take up silver stains. Pineocytomatous rosettes are formed around collections of these fibrillary processes. Pineoblastomas are grossly invasive and microscopically highly cellular with small mitotically active poorly differentiated cells with scant cytoplasm arranged in pattern-less sheets similar to other primitive neuroectodermal tumors (PNETs) and small blue cell tumors. They resemble retinoblastomas and medulloblastomas. Flexner-Wintersteiner rosette formation is a prominent feature of pineoblastomas. These are rosettes of cells forming around small lumens. Pineoblastomas occurring in patients with bilateral retinoblastomas are called trilateral retinoblastomas.

Clinical Manifestations, Pathways of Spread, and Patient Staging

Symptoms from pineal masses are related to the anatomy of the region. Pineal masses often obstruct the aqueduct of Sylvius, causing hydrocephalus, with the resulting increased intracranial pressure leading to headache, nausea, vomiting, cognitive dysfunction, and incontinence. Additionally, they can cause pressure on the superior colliculus (midbrain), causing Parinaud's syndrome or dorsal midbrain syndrome with a triad of signs consisting of vertical gaze palsy, light-near dissociation of the pupils, and convergence retraction nystagmus. Germ cell tumors and pineoblastoma have the potential to seed through the craniospinal axis, and symptoms due to craniospinal spread may be evident (symptoms from obstructive hydrocephalus, cranial neuropathy, radiculopathy, and cauda equina syndrome).

Jennings and colleagues[119] found that survival was dependent upon the extent of tumor, which emphasizes the importance of careful staging. The staging workup should include a careful history and physical examination, MRI of the entire brain (including eyes) and spine, spinal fluid cytology, complete blood cell count, chemistry panel, and tumor marker studies (AFP and β-HCG from both the CSF and serum). Caution should be exercised when obtaining CSF from patients with increased intracranial pressure as herniation of the brain may occur if pressure is rapidly reduced.

Primary Therapy

Diagnosis and treatment have changed markedly with advances in technology. The CT scanner, first introduced in 1973, made the diagnosis and localization of the pineal tumors easier, leading to a resurgence of surgical intervention with greater safety. Further improvements took place with the introduction of MRI, which aided in localization and the staging of the entire CNS. Prior to 1973, the operative risks of biopsy or resection were substantial, with mortality rates as high as 50%.[108,109,132] At that time, many experts recommended operative intervention be reserved for CSF shunting in patients with hydrocephalus and for the treatment of tumors that progressed after RT. Conservative therapy, including CSF shunting and RT, resulted in a generally favorable 5-year survival rate of approximately 70%.[108,109,132] However, therapy can only be customized to the specific tumor type if the exact tumor histology is known. Additionally, obtaining histologic confirmation, prior to therapy, allows one to avoid irradiating benign lesions such as cysts.[133,134] Computers are used to integrate data obtained from CT and MRI for surgical and RT treatment planning. Stereotactic techniques and operating microscopes have increased surgical and RT precision, reducing the risks of operative intervention. Cerebrospinal fluid diversion procedures are used to manage hydrocephalus. Corticosteroids are used to decrease edema caused by the tumor or intervention. Collectively, these technological advances have dramatically decreased the morbidity and mortality previously associated with biopsy or resection of pineal region tumors.[135]

The extent of surgery recommended is dependent on histologic type. Obtaining tissue for diagnosis is recommended in all patients with pineal region tumors whenever possible to guide therapies. Extent of resection appears to be important in patients with NGGCTs where survival appears dependent upon the extent of resection. In addition, immature and mature teratomas should be resected, if this can be safely achieved. Likewise, attempted gross total resection of primary parenchymal pineal tumors is usually recommended if this can be accomplished without excess morbidity.

With the ability to confirm histology safely in most patients through stereotactic techniques, the treatment of pineal and other primary CNS germ cell tumors should be guided by a precise knowledge of tumor histology. Obtaining histologic diagnosis is important because optimal therapy for the various tumor types differs significantly (Fig. 25-11).

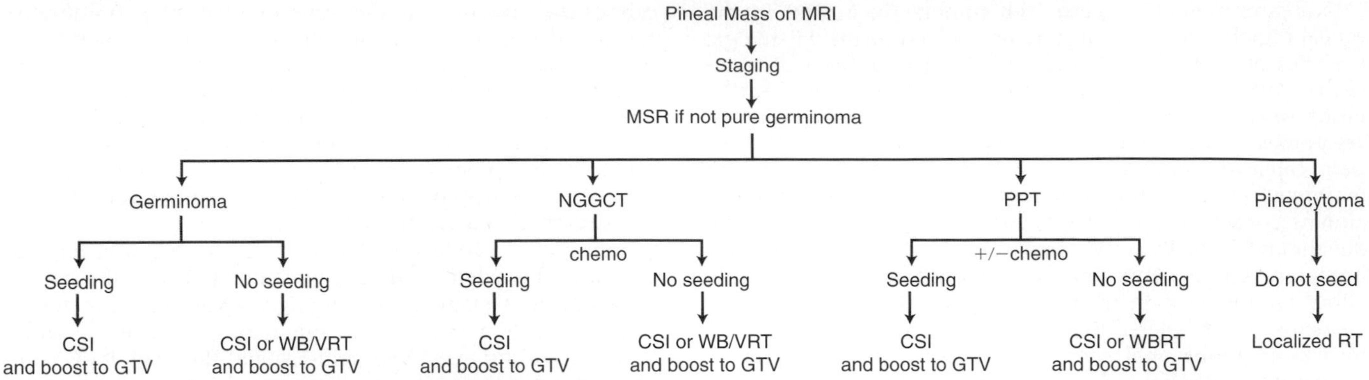

Figure 25-11 Treatment algorithm for pineal tumors. Staging is based on contrast-enhanced MRI of the whole brain and spine and on serum and cerebrospinal fluid (CSF) levels of alpha-fetoprotein and β-human chorionic gonadotropin. Maximal safe resection (MSR) appears most important for nongerminomatous germ cell tumors (NGGCTs) and some pineal parenchymal tumors (PPTs). CSF shunting should be performed when clinically indicated. Treatment volumes (craniospinal irradiation [CSI]. GVT, gross tumor volume; WBRT, whole-brain radiotherapy; WB/VRT, whole-brain or whole-ventricular radiotherapy.

Adjuvant Therapy and Techniques of Irradiation

Radiotherapy should be administered to most patients with pineal region tumors. The extent and dose of radiation should be tailored to the particular tumor type as outlined later.

Patients with pineocytomas can be irradiated to the local tumor alone, providing they have a negative CSF and MRI of the spine. It appears that the radiation dose (>50 Gy versus <50 Gy) delivered to the primary tumor is the most significant factor affecting survival in patients with pineal parenchymal tumors.[128,129] Radiation dose greater than 50 Gy (50.4 to 55.8 Gy in 1.8-Gy fractions) is recommended.

Patients with pineal parenchymal tumors other than pineocytomas have a higher risk of spinal failure, and craniospinal axis RT would appear reasonable (see Table 25-5). The primary tumor should receive 50.4 to 54.8 Gy and spinal metastases should receive 45 to 50.4 Gy in 1.8-Gy fractions. Prophylactic therapy can include the delivery of 30 to 36 Gy (1.5- to 1.8-Gy fractions) to uninvolved high-risk areas.

Patients with germinomas but no spinal seeding can be treated with either whole brain or ventricular radiation with a local boost or craniospinal radiation. In the Mayo Clinic series reported by Schild and associates, no patient who received craniospinal irradiation had a spine failure and only 1 of 11 (9%) patients treated with whole brain irradiation failed (Table 25-6). There appeared to be a substantially greater risk (28%) of spinal failure in those patients who received only local (tumor plus margin) radiation, although most experts in the field believe ventricular rather than whole brain radiation is adequate (personal communication, E. G. Shaw, First International Symposium on CNS Germ Cell Tumors, Kyoto, Japan, September 2003). The recommended dose for areas of gross disease is 40 to 50.4 Gy (1.8-Gy fractions). Prophylactic therapy can include the delivery of 20 to 30 Gy to high-risk areas (e.g., ventricular/whole brain field or craniospinal axis, depending on choice of approach). If spinal seeding is present, craniospinal irradiation is recommended.[129,136] Other institutions have reported similarly good results with limited volume radiation in nondisseminated germinoma.[137]

In one of the larger institutional series, Schild and colleagues[129,136] evaluated a multi-institutional cohort of 135 patients with histologically verified pineal region tumors.

Table 25-6 Probability of Spinal Seeding at Diagnosis According to Tumor Type

Histologic Types	No. With Spine Seeding/Total No. of Patients (%)
Mature and immature teratoma	0/20 (0%)
Mixed NGGCT	1/26 (4%)*
Other NGGCT	0/11 (0%)
Germinoma	2/48 (4%)†
Pineocytoma	0/9 (0%)
Pineoblastoma, PPTID, mixed PPT	4/21 (19%)‡
Total	7/135 (5%)

*This patient had a mixed germ cell tumor, composed of immature teratoma and germinoma, and had positive CSF cytology.

†Of these two patients with evidence of seeding at diagnosis, one had a positive CSF cytology and the other had radiographic evidence of spinal metastases.

‡Of the four patients with evidence of seeding at diagnosis, two had pineoblastomas (one with clinical evidence of spinal cord compression and one with radiographic evidence of spinal seeding) and two had pineal parenchymal tumors with intermediate differentiation (one with positive CSF cytology and one with radiographic evidence of spinal seeding).

All patients with evidence of spinal seeding at diagnosis received craniospinal irradiation and of these only one (with a pineoblastoma) had a subsequent treatment failure at the primary site and the spine.

From Schild SE, Scheithauer BW, Haddock MG, et al: Histologically confirmed pineal tumors and other germ cell tumors of the brain. Cancer 78:2564-2571, 1996.

There were two groups of neoplasms included in this series: pineal parenchymal tumors and germ cell tumors. At the time of diagnosis, 7 of the 135 (5%) patients were found to have evidence of spinal seeding (see Table 25-6). Spinal seeding most commonly occurred with pineoblastomas. One hundred patients underwent RT (Table 25-7). Regions treated included the craniospinal axis in 35 patients, the whole brain in 26 patients, and the partial brain in the remaining 39 patients. Doses delivered to the primary tumor bed ranged from 45 to 64.8 Gy (median dose = 41.3 Gy) in 1.5- to 2-Gy fractions. Chemotherapy was administered to 35 patients as a component of initial therapy (see Table 25-7).

Table 25-7 Pineal Tumors Summary of Therapy*

Histologic Type	RT	No RT	CTX	No CTX	Biopsy	Subtotal Resection	Gross Total Resection
Mature teratoma	2	5	1	6	0	3	4
Immature teratoma	2	7	0	9	3	2	4
Mixed NGGCT	19	6	17	8	3	12	10
Other pure NGGCT	5	4	3	6	4	3	2
Germinoma	48	0	8	40	29	16	3
Pineocytoma	6	1	0	7	3	4	0
PB, PPTID, mixed PPT	18	0	6	12	9	6	3

*Excludes 12 of the 135 patients who died postoperatively during the early years of the study.

CTX, chemotherapy; NGGCT, nongerminomatous germ cell tumor; PB, pineoblastoma; PPTID, pineal parenchymal tumor with intermediate differentiation; mixed PPT, mixed pineal parenchymal tumor; RT, radiotherapy.

From Schild SE, Scheithauer BW, Haddock MG, et al: Histologically confirmed pineal tumors and other germ cell tumors of the brain. Cancer 78:2564-2571, 1996.

The survival (with a median follow-up of 5.3 years) for the entire group of patients was 62% at 5 years. Tumor histology was evaluated for its relationship to survival. The 5-year patient survival rate was 86% for those with mature teratomas, 86% for those with pineocytomas, 80% for those with germinomas, 67% for those with immature teratomas, 49% for those with pineal parenchymal tumors other than pineocytomas (PBs, PPTIDs, and mixed PPTs), 38% for those with mixed germ cell tumors, and 17% for those with the other pure NGGCTs ($p = .0001$). The extent of resection was evaluated for its effect on patient survival. NGGCTs were the only tumors for which survival was associated with extent of tumor resection. The 3-year survival rate was 0% for patients having a biopsy, 36% for patients having a subtotal resection, and 73% for patients having a gross total resection ($p = .0002$). A significant survival advantage (3-year survival, 56% versus 8%, $p = .0001$) was noted for the use of chemotherapy among the subset of patients with NGGCT. Significant radiation dose-response relationships were noted for patients with NGGCT other than teratoma and PPT where doses of greater than 50 Gy were associated with significantly improved survival. For patients with germinoma, radiation doses of greater than 44 Gy were associated with significantly improved survival. There was no association between patient survival and radiation field arrangement (partial brain irradiation, whole brain irradiation, or craniospinal axis irradiation). Outcomes for patients with spinal seeding at diagnosis or relapse are summarized in Tables 25-8 and 25-9.

Table 25-8 Probability of Spinal Failure in Patients Without Evidence of Spinal Seeding at Diagnosis

Histologic Types	No. With Spine Failure/Total No. of Patients (%)*
Mature and immature teratoma	0/16 (0%)
Mixed NGGCT†	1/24 (4%)
Other NGGCT†	3/9 (33%)
Germinoma	8/46 (17%)
Pineocytoma	0/7 (0%)
Pineoblastoma, PPTID, mixed PPT	8/14 (57%)
Total	20/116 (17%)

*Some of these patients received no RT.

†Of the NGGCT patients with spinal failure, three of these patients had teratomas with malignant transformation and one had a yolk sac tumor. Not all of the patients with nongerminomatous germ cell tumors received RT.

From Schild SE, Scheithauer BW, Haddock MG, et al: Histologically confirmed pineal tumors and other germ cell tumors of the brain. Cancer 78:2564-2571, 1996.

The availability of platinum-based multiagent chemotherapy has dramatically improved the outcome for patients with NGGCTs over treatment with RT alone.[108,129,136] Significant increase in survival was associated with the administration of chemotherapy to patients with NGGCTs other than mature and immature teratomas. Many other authors have recommended the use of platinum-based multiagent chemotherapy for the treatment of NGGCTs of the brain.[114,115,119,120,126,138-140]

Buckner and associates[141] reported on a phase II trial of primary chemotherapy followed by reduced-dose RT for patients with CNS germ cell tumors. In that trial, induction chemotherapy with etoposide plus cisplatin was followed by RT (limited to the prechemotherapy tumor volume in localized disease and including the craniospinal axis in patients with disseminated disease). The dose of radiation to the craniospinal axis and primary tumor was tailored to the response to RT and varied between 20 and 36 Gy to the craniospinal axis and 30 and 60 Gy to the local tumor depending on the response to induction chemotherapy. Of 17 patients treated on the protocol (9 pure germinoma, 8 mixed germ cell tumors), 11 had complete responses to induction chemotherapy and all were alive and disease free at a median of 51-month follow-up. Only one patient relapsed (localized germinoma treated with induction chemotherapy and low-dose local field irradiation as per protocol), and this patient was subsequently salvaged with spinal radiation. This approach carries the potential advantage of lower neurocognitive toxicity by virtue of the ability to reduce radiation doses and use reduced volume irradiation for patients with localized disease. Matutani and colleagues[142,143] noted similar favorable benefits to induction chemotherapy followed by reduced-dose RT for germ cell tumors.

In general, for germ cell tumors, a combined chemoirradiation approach should be used for patients with NGGCTs (other than immature and mature teratomas). Outside the setting of a clinical trial, standard radiation doses should be used. For NGGCTs with negative CSF cytology and MRI of the spine, the ventricles or whole brain should be treated to 30 to 36 Gy, followed by a localized tumor boost to 54 to 59.4 Gy. If the CSF and/or MRI of the spine is positive, the craniospinal axis should be treated to 30 to 36 Gy, boosting spinal disease to 45 to 50.4 Gy and the primary to 54 to 59.4 Gy.[125,127] Chemotherapy may also be indicated for patients with pineoblastomas. Drugs and radiation doses and techniques

Table 25-9 **Probability of Spinal Failure According to the Radiotherapy Fields in Patients without Evidence of Spinal Seeding at Diagnosis***

Histologic Type	PB	WB	CSI	Total
NGGCT†	2/4 (50%)	0/8 (0%)	1/11 (9%)	3/23 (13%)
Germinoma	7/25 (28%)	1/11 (9%)	0/10 (0%)	8/46 (17%)
PPT‡	2/3 (66%)	2/5 (40%)	4/6 (66%)	8/14 (57%)
Total:	11/32 (34%)	3/24 (13%)	5/27 (19%)	19/83 (23%)

*This included only patients with potentially seeding tumors (NGGCTs excluding mature and immature teratomas, pineal parenchymal tumors excluding pineocytomas, and germinomas) who received RT. One patient with an NGGCT received no RT and later had a spinal failure.

†NGGCTs excluding mature and immature teratomas.

‡Excluding pineocytomas.

CSI, craniospinal irradiation; PB, partial brain fields; PPT, pineal parenchymal tumor; RT, radiotherapy; WB, whole brain fields.

From Mack EE, Wilson CB: Meningiomas induced by high-dose cranial irradiation. J Neurosurg 79:28-31, 1993.

similar to those used for medulloblastoma are typically used.[144]

SRS has a potential role to play in the treatment of pineal tumors, generally as single-fraction treatment modality for nonseeding tumors (e.g., pineocytomas) or for treatment of focal recurrences after EBRT. Pineocytomas and teratomas (especially mature teratomas) represent tumors in which this approach would be most applicable as they do not generally seed the CSF. Regarding PPTs, the University of Pittsburgh experience with SRS would support these contentions. Hasegawa and associates[145] reported 5-year survival of 90% in a series of 10 patients with pineocytomas using this approach. In contrast, the results of SRS with pineoblastomas were poor, with death occurring in four of six patients. Complications including upward gaze paralysis occurred in 2 of 16 (13%) and was likely due to the dose delivered to the superior colliculus, which lies in direct contact with pineal tumors. Hasegawa and colleagues[146] also reported on a small series of four patients treated for NGGCTs of the brain. These patients received a SRS boost after other therapies; three of four were alive without disease at last follow-up. While this was a small series, it shows potential for the use of SRS in the management of pineal region tumors.

Conclusions and Future Possibilities

Given the high curability of germinomas, current investigations are directed at minimizing the side effects of therapy through the reduction of radiation doses and volumes in patients receiving initial chemotherapy.[137,141] Combined chemoirradiation is now a standard of care for NGGCTs. The uses of focal techniques like single-fraction SRS for localized tumors like pineocytomas and the integration of chemotherapy with radiation for pineoblastoma are additional areas of investigation.

CHEMODECTOMA

The paraganglia are specialized cells that function as chemoreceptors and are located in close proximity to blood vessels. The cells of the paraganglia include chief (epithelial) cells grouped in small nests surrounded by vascular connective tissue trabeculae.[147] The chief cells are specialized neuroendocrine cells, which serve to maintain blood pressure homeostasis and contain neurotransmitter granules. Tumors arising in these cells are rare and generally called chemodectomas. They are also called glomus tumors and can be subdivided further by the site of origin as glomus jugulare, glomus tympanicum, or carotid body tumors. The most common locations for chemodectomas are the carotid body and temporal bone.

Epidemiology

Chemodectomas rarely metastasize and may be multiple or bilateral, especially in familial cases.[148] These tumors can be associated with the following conditions: neurofibromatosis, multiple endocrine neoplasia (MEN) syndromes, and thyroid malignancies. Rarely, these tumors produce an overabundance of catecholamines in a manner analogous to pheochromocytomas and carcinoid tumors.

Clinical Manifestations and Patient Evaluation

These tumors are generally slow growing, and symptoms are caused by local invasion of the adjacent structures or by the presence of a mass lesion. Chemodectomas can be diagnosed clinically with CT, MRI, or angiography. Additionally, diagnosis may be made pathologically with biopsy or resection. However, biopsy of these lesions can lead to serious hemorrhage because of their high vascularity.

Primary Therapy

Various treatments have been used, which include resection, RT, or a combination of resection and RT. Springate and associates published a very detailed review of the literature regarding the results of therapy for temporal bone chemodectomas. The local control was 86% for resection alone, 90% for a combination of RT plus resection, and 93% for RT alone.[149] Schild and colleagues[150] reviewed the Mayo Clinic experience with RT from 1974 and 1988. This included 10 patients: 5 with tumors of jugular bulb, 3 with tumors of the middle ear, and 2 with tumors of carotid body. Treatment was delivered with megavoltage photons and electrons. Doses ranged from 16.2 to 52 Gy (median, 46 Gy) in 1.6- to 2.0-Gy daily fractions. With a median follow-up of 7.5 years, all nine evaluable patients had improvement in symptoms and objective control of disease (no evidence of progression). Included in this report was a summary of the available literature regarding the reported RT series with chemodectomas of the temporal bone and the carotid bodies. Local control was reported in 91% of patients with temporal bone tumors and 97% of those with carotid body tumors. Additionally, these groups were added together to determine the overall local control for patients with chemodectomas treated with RT, which was 92%.

Regarding the optimal dose-fractionation pattern to be used in the RT of chemodectomas, Kim and associates[151] reported that local failures occurred in 25% of patients who received less than 40 Gy and in 2% of those who received 40 to 45 Gy. The usual dose using conventional fraction size is 45 Gy in 25 fractions. For intracranial chemodectomas (glomus tympanicum and jugulare) SRS using doses in the 12- to 14-Gy range resulted in a local control rate of 100% in several small series.[152-154] Extension of chemodectomas inferior to the skull base precludes SRS for technical reasons.

Acute side effects of RT generally include localized generally reversible alopecia and skin irritation. Other side effects depend on the technique (dose-fractionation and volume) used as well as the adjacent tissues irradiated. In a very large series of irradiated patients, Hinerman and colleagues[155] reported that 8 of 71 (11%) patients had radiation-related toxicity. One patient had severe mucositis that resulted in dehydration and hospitalization. One patient developed lethargy as a manifestation of a delayed transient CNS syndrome. One patient developed a temporary cranial nerve VII deficit. Two patients with prior histories of resection had bone exposure after RT. One patient had trismus from temporomandibular joint fibrosis, one had radiation-induced caries, and another developed serous otitis requiring tympanostomy tubes. None were thought to be severe complications and no second malignancies occurred.

Conclusions and Future Possibilities

Given the rarity of these tumors, a randomized prospective study comparing the efficacy of RT versus resection will likely never be performed. As such, we will continue to depend on retrospective reports regarding therapy and outcomes. It appears that resection and RT or RT alone (conventionally fractionated EBRT or SRS) offer equally high chances of local control. However, when attempting to optimally treat an individual patient, one must evaluate these two treatment options with respect to the potential for control and complications. Larger tumors in less accessible sites may be difficult to resect completely especially without severe morbidity. In these situations, primary RT would be preferable. For patients with small accessible tumors, resection may be preferable. The combination of subtotal resection plus RT appears to offer little advantage to the patient in regards to disease control. A reasonable approach to RT would include the delivery of 45 Gy in 1.8-Gy daily fractions to the tumor plus a small margin or if technically feasible, SRS delivering 12 to 14 Gy to the tumor. Stereotactic radiation, 3D treatment planning, or IMRT allows one to optimally spare the adjacent normal structures and could potentially decrease the risk of complications.[156]

HEMANGIOBLASTOMA AND HEMANGIOPERICYTOMA

Etiology and Epidemiology

Hemangioblastoma and hemangiopericytoma are rare mesenchymal tumors of the central nervous system. Each account for less than 1% of primary brain tumors with a median age at diagnosis of 40 to 50 years.[6] Hemangioblastomas may occur sporadically or in association with von Hippel-Lindau (VHL) syndrome, a familial cancer syndrome involving the germline mutation of the *VHL* tumor suppressor gene. Patients with VHL may develop hemangioblastoma at a younger age (20 to 30 years), may have multiple lesions, and develop new lesions on an ongoing basis.[157] Hemangiopericytomas occur sporadically and do not have a familial cancer association. Initially, hemangioblastomas and hemangiopericytomas were thought to represent vascular variants of meningioma ("angioblastic meningioma"); however, they are now recognized as separate entities.[158]

Pathology and Patterns of Spread

Hemangioblastomas macroscopically are well-circumscribed red, nodular lesions, often located in the wall of a large cyst and occurring within the brain or spinal cord parenchyma. Microscopically, the tumors are comprised of large vacuolated stromal cells in association with a rich capillary network. The stromal cells represent the neoplastic component of the tumor with development of the capillary network stimulated by stromal angiogenic factors. CNS hemangioblastomas occur primarily in the cerebellum but also in the brainstem and spinal cord and rarely occur supratentorially.[159] Hemangiopericytomas arise from the meninges, more commonly in the occipital region in association with the venous sinuses. Like meningiomas, they may enhance intensely and can be quite vascular but typically lack calcification; they tend to destroy adjacent bone and do not stimulate hyperostosis. Hemangiopericytomas are highly cellular, monotonous tumors composed of plump cells with scant cytoplasm, numerous small vascular spaces, and a dense reticulin fiber network. While the tumor exhibits features of pericytic differentiation, the cell of origin is thought to be an undifferentiated mesenchymal cell precursor. The clinical behavior of these tumors is similar to that of malignant meningioma with a propensity for local recurrence (even with gross total resection), leptomeningeal spread, and distant metastases.[158]

Molecular Biology and Biologic Characteristics

Hemangioblastomas are characterized by mutations in the *VHL* tumor suppressor gene located on chromosome 3p. In VHL disease, this mutation is found as a germline change, whereas in sporadic hemangioblastoma, the mutation is acquired. The *VHL* tumor suppressor gene is thought to be active in angiogenesis and cell cycle progression, and mutation of the gene results in upregulation of angiogenic factors such as VEGF, HIF-1, and erythropoietin. Diagnostic criteria for VHL disease include presence of capillary hemangioblastoma in the CNS or retina along with a family history of VHL or one of several characteristic visceral tumors (renal cell cancer, pancreatic islet cell tumor, visceral adenoma). Testing for germline *VHL* mutations is recommended for patients with evidence of a CNS hemangioblastoma, and MRI surveillance for new CNS hemangioblastoma is recommended for patients and affected family members.[159] Hemangiopericytomas are not characterized by any specific patterns of genetic change and do not exhibit the allelic losses on chromosome 22 (*NF2* gene) characteristic of meningioma. There is some correlation between markers of proliferation (Ki-57/MIB-1, mitotic index) and aggressiveness, as tumors with high mitotic indices or Ki-67 labeling exhibit more rapid recurrence and early metastatic spread.[158]

Clinical Manifestations, Patient Evaluation, and Staging

Hemangioblastomas are characterized by slow, indolent growth. They produce symptoms due to local pressure effects from either the cystic or solid components of the tumor. Cranial nerve deficits, long tract findings, ataxia, or obstructive hydrocephalus may be due to impingement on posterior fossa structures such as the brainstem, cerebellum, or fourth ventricle. Nonspecific symptoms such as headache and cognitive dysfunction due to mass effect may also be found. Capillary hemangioblastomas occurring in the context of VHL disease tend to present with signs and symptoms at a younger age, frequently have multiple lesions, and may develop new lesions over time.[157] Death from progressive CNS disease is the most common cause of mortality in VLH disease, with mortality from associated tumors such as renal cell carcinoma the next most common cause of death.

Hemangiopericytoma likewise grows in a locally aggressive fashion and may produce symptoms due to mass effect and impingement on normal neurologic structures. Unlike hemangioblastoma, hemangiopericytoma exhibits a propensity for recurrence even following a complete surgical resection. Late local, leptomeningeal and metastatic (lung and bone) failure in over 80% of patients has been noted after complete surgical resection with long-term (10- to 15-year) follow-up.[158,160,161]

Contrast-enhanced MRI best defines the extent of hemangioblastoma and hemangiopericytoma and may be supplemented with contrast-enhanced CT. Angiography may be helpful in presurgical planning to outline the vascular supply to the tumor. For patients with hemangioblastoma and VHL, imaging of the spine is recommended to assess for additional lesions within the spinal cord. For patients with hemangiopericytoma, bone scan and chest radiograph or CT scan of the chest and abdomen may be considered to rule out metastatic spread, especially for histologically aggressive or locally advanced lesions. Spinal MRI may also be necessary in patients with symptoms or signs of spinal axis dissemination.

Primary Therapy

Primary therapy for both hemangioblastoma and hemangiopericytoma is surgical resection. For patients with completely excised hemangioblastoma, additional therapy is unnecessary. For subtotally excised or unresectable lesions, RT or SRS has been associated with good rates of local control in the 60% to 90% range.[162-165] For hemangiopericytoma, adjuvant RT is recommended even following gross total resection given the propensity for local recurrence. In the series reported by Guthrie and colleagues, adjuvant radiation lengthened the interval to first recurrence from 34 to 75 months, and others have noted improved disease-free survival with adjuvant RT as well.[160,161]

Locally Advanced Disease and Palliation

Recurrences of hemangioblastoma or hemangiopericytoma following initial surgical resection are usually managed with salvage surgery plus adjuvant RT. SRS has been reported as a successful salvage modality for these tumors following prior surgery or conventional RT.[162,166,167] Conventional fractionated RT is the main treatment for large recurrent or unresectable lesions. Unfortunately, the effectiveness of conventional chemotherapy agents against recurrent or metastatic hemangiopericytoma and hemangioblastoma is limited and effective systemic salvage regimens are lacking.[165]

Techniques of Irradiation

Conventional fractionated RT treatments for hemangioblastoma and hemangiopericytoma are similar to those used for meningioma. Three-dimensional conformal and IMRT techniques may be useful to minimize the potential for late radiation toxicity in these potentially indolent tumors. Typically, the contrast-enhancing tumor is identified as the gross tumor volume. The CTV may include a small (1-cm) margin for hemangioblastoma and a larger 2-cm margin for hemangiopericytoma and should include the operative bed. Radiation dose in the range of 50 to 60 Gy at 1.8 to 2.0 Gy/day has been associated with improved tumor control and is recommended.[161,164,168,169]

Reports of SRS for hemangioblastoma and hemangiopericytoma have typically identified the target as the contrast-enhancing tumor without margin, and doses in the range of 12 to 20 Gy have been used. Higher control rates have been reported for the higher doses in this range and smaller tumor volumes. For instance, in a multi-institutional series of SRS for hemangioblastomas, a lower median radiation dose (14 versus 16 Gy) and larger tumor volume (7.85 versus 0.67 cm^3) were noted among patients with recurrence vs. control following treatment. A confounding effect is the tendency to prescribe lower doses for larger lesions out of concern for radiation toxicity (edema or necrosis), and therefore a clear SRS dose response remains to be determined. SRS is potentially attractive for patients with VLH disease where multiple hemangioblastomas may develop either concurrently or sequentially and may be difficult to treat or retreat with repeat surgery and/or conventional radiation techniques without excess cumulative toxicity.[162]

Conclusions and Future Possibilities

Surgery will remain the mainstay of therapy for hemangioblastomas and hemangiopericytomas. The role of RT in the management of these tumors continues to evolve. Early reports of radiosurgery for the management of small residual or recurrent tumor appear promising. Multi-institutional pooling of patient data for these rare tumors will help delineate the role of newer treatments.[162]

CRANIOPHARYNGIOMA

Etiology and Epidemiology

Craniopharyngiomas are benign suprasellar neoplasms that derive from squamous cell remnants of Rathke's pouch within the parasellar area. Craniopharyngiomas occur primarily among children and account for approximately 5% to 10% of primary intracranial tumors with a peak age of presentation between 5 and 10 years.[8,6] Peak age of presentation in adults is between ages 55 and 65 years.[6] The growth characteristics of craniopharyngiomas vary considerably.

Pathology and Pathways of Spread

Typically, these tumors have a solid nodule with a cystic component filled with lipoid, cholesterol-laden ("crankcase oil") fluid. Histologically, the tumors are characterized by pallisading epithelial cells lining cystic spaces. Prominent keratinization and keratin pearl formation may be present. Desquamation of these cells contributes to the lipoid nature of the cystic fluid containing cholesterol crystals. Calcification is frequently seen, especially among childhood craniopharyngioma. While grossly appearing well encapsulated, craniopharyngiomas typically demonstrate invaginations into adjacent brain and may provoke a vigorous glial reaction.[170]

Clinical Manifestations, Patient Evaluation, and Staging

Given the site of origin of these tumors in the parasellar region, local growth can give rise to symptoms from compression of adjacent structures. Severe headaches are present in approximately 50% of patients. Lesions may compress the pituitary and hypothalamic region, producing hormonal abnormalities, especially antidiuretic and growth hormone insufficiency in children and amenorrhea/impotence/galactorrhea syndrome in adults. Prechiasmal lesions typically compress the optic apparatus, leading to visual field cuts and/or decreased central visual acuity in 40% to 70% of patients.[171-173] Retrochiasmal lesions may grow into the third ventricle and precipitate hydrocephalus with associated papilledema or compress the optic tract to produce an homonymous hemianopsia. Craniopharyngiomas can occasionally reach an enormous size and produce neurologic impairment by direct impingement on cerebral parenchyma. Acute changes in intracerebral pressure can be precipitated by rapid cyst expansion or intratumoral bleed.

Adults typically present with craniopharyngiomas early and with visual symptomatology. The elderly may present with cognitive changes, increased intracranial pressure, and visual abnormalities. Children often present with larger tumors with advanced visual field loss, headaches, and papilledema and symptoms of endocrine abnormalities such as polyuria and polydipsia (diabetes insipidus) or growth retardation (growth hormone insufficiency).

The cystic nature of craniopharyngiomas is usually evident on CT and MRI and helps distinguish these tumors from other base of skull lesions and pituitary adenomas. The typical imaging appearance is that of a mixed cystic and solid lesion. The solid portion is often calcified and enhancing, while the cystic portion typically demonstrates a thin rim of enhancement.[174] On MRI, the lipoid nature of the cystic fluid produces a hyperintense T1-weighted image and differentiates the tumor from Rathke cleft and arachnoid cysts, which are typically low intensity on T1 scans. The finding of multiple cysts with varying intensity of T1 and T2 scans is characteristic of craniopharyngioma (Fig. 25-12). With contrast, both the cystic and solid components typically enhance. Solid craniopharyngiomas, especially in adults, need to be distinguished from other primary tumors at the base of skull such as osteosarcoma, chondrosarcoma, meningioma, acoustic neuroma, pituitary adenoma, glioma, and chordoma.

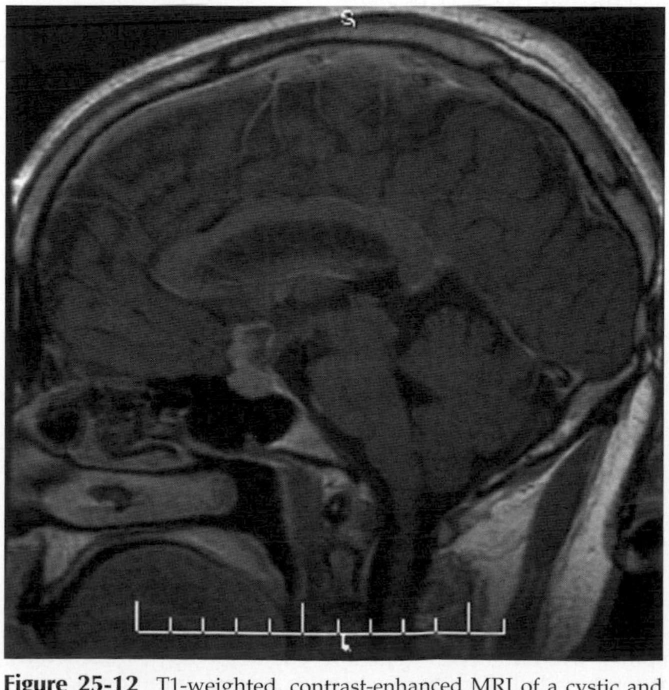

Figure 25-12 T1-weighted, contrast-enhanced MRI of a cystic and solid craniopharyngioma arising from the suprasellar area.

Primary Therapy

Complete surgical resection of craniopharyngiomas can result in long-term local control and cure[175,176] (Fig. 25-13). While surgical resection rapidly relieves compressive symptoms, most authors report significant rates of local recurrence,[177,178] even with gross complete resection. Aggressive resections of these parasellar tumors are also potentially associated with significant morbidity including optic nerve damage and hypothalamic damage with resulting visual and endocrinologic disturbances.[179,180] Partial resection or cyst aspiration and biopsy rapidly relieve local compressive symptoms and are associated with less operative morbidity but with eventual tumor progression in the majority of cases.

Complete surgical resection alone has been associated with local control and long-term survival in about 70% to 90% of patients,[175-177] but aggressive surgical resection has been associated with an estimated high incidence of perioperative mortality and morbidity. Partial resection alone is associated with fewer complications and rapid symptom relief, but long-term survival and local control are achieved in only about 30% of patients.[175] Van Effenterre and Boch[180] reported on 122 patients who underwent surgery. The operative mortality was 2.5%; 59% underwent gross total excision and 29% of those recurred postoperatively. Tsai and colleagues[183] reported on 90 patients with craniopharyngioma treated with surgery alone (gross total resection), limited surgery (subtotal resection) plus RT and RT alone. They noted a 10-year local control rate of 43% with surgery alone.

Radiotherapy combined with limited surgical procedures (partial resection or aspiration plus biopsy) has been used in an attempt to achieve good local control while limiting potential surgical morbidity.[179,181] The long-term local control following subtotal resection and RT has been reported as 75% to 90%.[182,183] In the report by Tsai and colleagues,[183] excellent long-term control with radiation alone was noted in a small (18 of 90) subset of patients. SRS may be useful in ablating small residual or recurrent tumors post surgery. The proximity of the optic chiasm and brainstem may prevent the use of SRS.[184]

The 20-year survival rate of children with craniopharyngioma has been noted to be 60%, but with recurrence this figure drops to 25%.[182,185,186] Favorable prognostic factors include lack of calcification (especially in adults), extent of surgical resection, age younger than 5 years, and hydrocephalus in children.

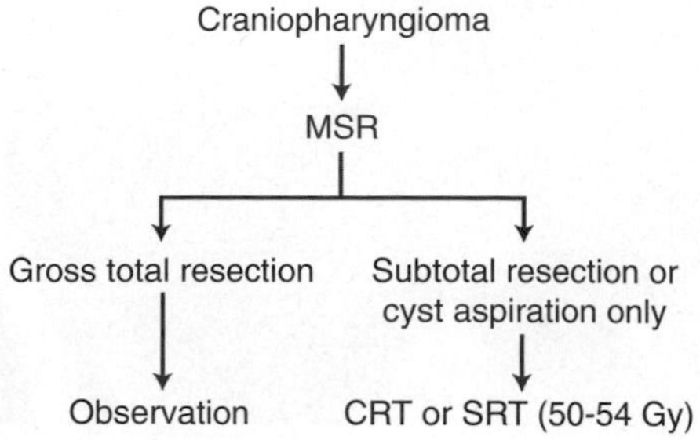

Figure 25-13 Treatment algorithm for craniopharyngioma. CRT, conformal partial-brain irradiation; MSR, maximum safe resection; SRT, stereotactic radiotherapy.

Recurrent symptoms are often due to reaccumulation of cyst fluid, which may be treated by intermittent aspiration, placement of an Ommaya reservoir, or sclerosis of the cyst wall by chemotherapeutic drugs such as bleomycin[187] or beta-emitting radioisotopes such as yttrium-90, rhenium-196, or phosphorus-32.[188] Preoperative intralesional bleomycin may be particularly effective at decreasing cyst size and fibrosing the cyst wall, thus facilitating more complete resection.

Techniques of Irradiation

In those patients with compressive symptoms, surgical decompression prior to RT is essential, the tumor typically responds slowly to RT and, in some patients, radiation-induced edema can worsen such symptoms. Typically, fractionated EBRT to doses of 50.4 to 54 Gy in 1.8-Gy fractions are delivered to the preoperative tumor volume (including cystic plus solid components) with a 1- to 2-cm margin. Given the well-circumscribed nature of the tumors and their location at the base of skull, multifield 3D-CRT or IMRT techniques are often necessary to provide maximum sparing of adjacent structures (Fig. 25-14). Radiotherapy combined with limited surgery (aspiration and biopsy or partial resection) achieves local control and survival nearly equivalent to that of complete resection, with lower morbidity.[175,182,185]

Close follow-up after treatment is essential and should include at least yearly ophthalmologic, endocrinologic, and imaging follow-up. The incidence of endocrinopathies after treatment is high, with more than 90% of patients manifesting insufficiency of at least one hormone. Low-dose radiation in prepubertal children can initially cause early or precocious puberty or pubertal delay due to gonadotropin deficiency. Decreased ADH leading to diabetes insipidus is particularly common as is growth hormone deficiency (40% to 90%). Cortisol and thyroid insufficiency are less common (20% to 40%).[189] Hypothalamic injury with associated weight, behavior, and sleep disturbances may occasionally occur. Visual acuity posttreatment is predicted primarily by pretreatment function. A subset of patients may improve posttreatment, but the majority demonstrate stable vision. The incidence of vascular injury or second malignancy in patients treated with radiation should be less than 1% to 2%.[175] The incidence of cognitive dysfunction appears to be similar following surgery alone or combined surgery and RT, with approximately 10% of patients severely disabled posttreatment.[175]

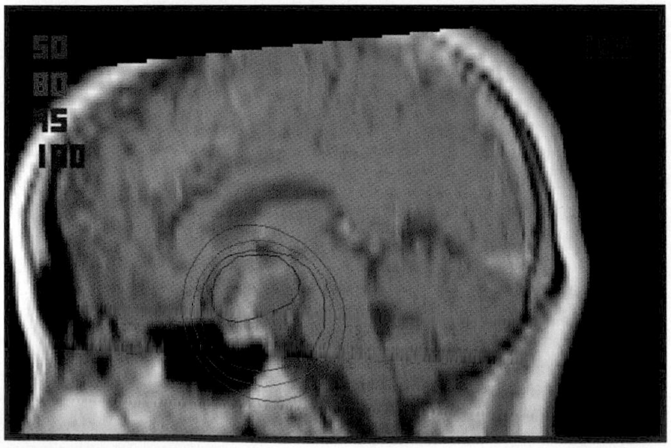

Figure 25-14 Sagittal dose distribution for stereotactic conformal radiotherapy of a craniopharyngioma using multiple circular collimator arcs.

Conclusions and Future Possibilities

Current knowledge would dictate a flexible approach to the treatment of craniopharyngioma. For those patients with small, resectable lesions, complete surgical resection has been associated with low morbidity and excellent local control. For those larger lesions less amenable to total resection, limited surgery (biopsy or subtotal resection) followed by RT may be the optimal approach. SRS is reserved for craniopharyngiomas that are at least 3 to 5 mm from critical structures such as the optic chiasm. In some patients (i.e., children younger than 3 years), limited surgery with careful follow-up and deferred radiation may be appropriate.

CHOROID PLEXUS TUMORS

Epidemiology

Choroid plexus tumors are rare (less than 2% of all glial tumors), intraventricular neoplasms. Most occur within the lateral ventricles of children. Tumors found in adult patients are more commonly fourth ventricular in location. Benign (choroid plexus papilloma [CPP]) and malignant (choroid plexus carcinoma [CPC]) varieties are identified. Cerebellopontine angle tumors are more frequently benign.

Pathology, Biology, and Patterns of Spread

Choroid plexus tumors produce symptoms of hydrocephalus due to obstruction of CSF flow and CSF overproduction. While both CPPs and CPCs may disseminate throughout the CSF, this is more common for the choroid plexus carcinomas.

Histologically, CPPs closely mimic the normal architecture of the choroid plexus (fibrovascular cores of connective tissue covered by modified ependymal cells).[190] Immunohistochemically, cytokeratin and vimentin are expressed by virtually all choroid plexus papillomas and most choroid plexus carcinomas, while transthretin and S-100 are present in 80% to 90% of cases, less frequently in CPCs. Glial fibrillary acidic protein can be found focally in about 25% to 55% of CPPs and 20% of CPCs. The mean Ki67 labeling index for CPPs is 2% compared with that of 13% for CPCs.[191]

The genetic changes associated with choroid plexus tumors are largely unknown; however, chromosome aberrations differ between choroid plexus papillomas and carcinomas as well as between pediatric and adult tumors. The gain of 9p and loss of 10q has been correlated with a more favorable prognosis in carcinomas.[192] Choroid plexus carcinomas have been reported in association with Li-Fraumeni syndrome with a p53 germline mutation and to occur in families with malignant rhabdoid tumor predispostion.[193,194]

Clinical Manifestations, Patient Evaluation, and Staging

Choroid plexus tumors present with signs and symptoms of increased intracranial pressure and hydrocephalus. CT/MRI demonstrates an intraventricular mass within the lateral or fourth ventricles with associated hydrocephalus usually noted. Neuraxis staging (CSF cytology and spinal MRI) is recommended for all patients.

Primary Therapy

Treatment is surgical resection. Completely excised choroid plexus papillomas that have no evidence of neuraxial dissemination are adequately treated with surgery alone. Craniospinal irradiation or adjuvant chemotherapy is generally recommended for those choroid plexus papillomas with CSF spread and for choroid plexus carcinomas. Systemic nitrosourea-based chemotherapy and/or intrathecal chemotherapy with methotrexate or AraC has been used in the adjuvant setting for these more aggressive tumors.[195]

The 5-year survival rate for gross totally excised choroid plexus papillomas is 80% to 95%.[194,196] Even after subtotal resection, only 50% of patients require a subsequent resection for recurrence/progression. SRS could be used following incomplete resection, depending on location of the tumor relative to critical normal structures.

Five-year survivals for patients with choroid plexus carcinomas are approximately 40%.[194,196] As in choroid plexus papillomas, complete surgical resection is prognostic. Adjuvant RT and chemotherapy are usually recommended for CPC given the high rates of recurrence and overall poor outlook.[195,196]

Conclusions and Future Possibilities

The prognosis of CPP tumors is related to the extent of surgical resection. Further improvements in the treatment of these tumors will be related to future improvements in neurosurgical technique to allow gross total resection. CPCs are rare tumors with a poor prognosis. Staging of the craniospinal axis with CSF cytology and spinal MRI is essential for selecting patients where craniospinal radiation is required. Continued efforts to develop and explore newer chemotherapeutic agents and combined modality treatment will be important to attempt to improve overall survival of patients and to reduce morbidity.

REFERENCES

1. Mack EE, Wilson CB: Meningiomas induced by high-dose cranial irradiation. J Neurosurg 79:28, 1993.
2. Sadetzki S, Flint-Richter P, Ben-Tal T, et al: Radiation-induced meningioma: a descriptive study of 253 cases. J Neurosurg 97:1078, 2002.
3. Louis DN, Scheithauer B, Budka H, et al: Meningiomas. *In* Kleihues P, Cavenee WK (eds): Pathology and Genetics: Tumors of the Nervous System. Lyon, IARC Press, 2000, p 176.
4. Minn Y, Wrensch M, Bondy M: Epidemiology of primary brain tumors. *In* Prados M (ed): American Cancer Society Atlas of Clinical Oncology: Brain Cancer. Hamilton, Ontario, BC Decker, 2002, p 1.
5. McCarthy BJ, Davis FG, Freels S, et al: Factors associated with survival in patients with meningioma. J Neurosurg 88:831, 1998.
6. CBTRUS (2002): Statistical Report: Primary Brain Tumors in the United States, 1995. Chicago, Central Brain Tumor Registry of the United States, 2003, p 2.
7. Wilson CB: Meningiomas: genetics, malignancy, and the role of radiation in induction and treatment. J Neurosurg 81:666, 1994.
8. Pollack IF: Brain tumors in children. N Engl J Med 331:1500, 1994.
9. Perry A, Cai DX, Scheithauer BW, et al: Merlin, DAL-1, and progesterone receptor expression in clinicopathologic subsets of meningioma: a correlative immunohistochemical study of 175 cases. J Neuropathol Exp Neurol 59:872, 2000.
10. Watson MA, Gutmann DH, Peterson K, et al: Molecular characterization of human meningiomas by gene expression profiling using high-density oligonucleotide microarrays. Am J Pathol 161:665, 2002.
11. Jaaskelainen J, Haltia M, Laasoen E, et al: The growth rate of intracranial meningiomas and its relation to histology. Surg Neurol 24:165, 1985.
12. Nakamura M, Roser F, Michel J, et al: The natural history of incidental meningiomas. Neurosurgery 53:62-70, 2003; discussion, 70.
13. Van Havenbergh T, Carvalho G, Tatagiba M, et al: Natural history of petroclival meningiomas. Neurosurgery 52:55-62, 2003; discussion, 62.
14. Bindal AK, Bindal RK, van Loveren H, et al: Management of intracranial plasmacytoma. J Neurosurg 83:218, 1995.
15. Perry A, Stafford SL, Scheithauer BW, et al: Meningioma grading: an analysis of histologic parameters. Am J Surg Pathol 21:1455, 1997.
16. Simpson D: The recurrence of intracranial meningiomas after surgical treatment. J Neurol Neurosurg Psychiatry 20:22, 1957.
17. Rosen CL, Ammerman JM, Sekhar LN, et al: Outcome analysis of preoperative embolization in cranial base surgery. Acta Neurochir (Wien) 144:1157, 2002.
18. Chun JY, McDermott MW, Lamborn KR, et al: Delayed surgical resection reduces intraoperative blood loss for embolized meningiomas. Neurosurgery 50:1231-1235, 2002; discussion, 1235.
19. Paleologos TS, Wadley JP, Kitchen ND, et al: Clinical utility and cost-effectiveness of interactive image-guided craniotomy: clinical comparison between conventional and image-guided meningioma surgery. Neurosurgery 47:40-47, 2000; discussion, 47.
20. Kondziolka D, Flickinger JC, Perez B: Judicious resection and/or radiosurgery for parasagittal meningiomas: outcomes from a multicenter review. Gamma Knife Meningioma Study Group. Neurosurgery 43:405-413, 1998; discussion, 413.
21. Ruckenstein MJ, Denys D: Lateral skull-base surgery—a review of recent advances in surgical approaches. J Otolaryngol 27:46, 1998.
22. Prabhu SS, Demonte F: Treatment of skull base tumors. Curr Opin Oncol 15:209, 2003.
23. DeMonte F, Smith HK, al-Mefty O: Outcome of aggressive removal of cavernous sinus meningiomas. J Neurosurg 81:245, 1994.
24. Cusimano MD, Sekhar LN, Sen CN, et al: The results of surgery for benign tumors of the cavernous sinus. Neurosurgery 37:1-9, 1995; discussion, 9.
25. Newman SA: Meningiomas: a quest for the optimum therapy. J Neurosurg 80:191, 1994.
26. Turbin RE, Thompson CR, Kennerdell JS, et al: A long-term visual outcome comparison in patients with optic nerve sheath meningioma managed with observation, surgery, radiotherapy, or surgery and radiotherapy. Ophthalmology 109:890-899, 2002; discussion, 899.
27. Debus J, Wuendrich M, Pirzkall A, et al: High efficacy of fractionated stereotactic radiotherapy of large base-of-skull meningiomas: long-term results. J Clin Oncol 19:3547, 2001.
28. Lunsford LD: Contemporary management of meningiomas: radiation therapy as an adjuvant and radiosurgery as an alternative to surgical removal. J Neurosurg 80:187, 1994.
29. Hall EJ, Brenner DJ: The radiobiology of radiosurgery: rationale for different treatment regimens for AVMs and malignancies. Int J Radiat Oncol Biol Phys 25:381, 1993.
30. Vernimmen FJ, Harris JK, Wilson JA, et al: Stereotactic proton beam therapy of skull base meningiomas. Int J Radiat Oncol Biol Phys 49:99, 2001.
31. Pollock BE, Stafford SL, Utter A, et al: Stereotactic radiosurgery provides equivalent tumor control to Simpson grade 1 resection for patients with small- to medium-size meningiomas. Int J Radiat Oncol Biol Phys 55:1000, 2003.
32. Vermeulen S, Young R, Li F, et al: A comparison of single fraction radiosurgery tumor control and toxicity in the treatment of basal and nonbasal meningiomas. Stereotact Funct Neurosurg 72(Suppl 1):60, 1999.
33. Larson DA, Suplica JM, Chang SM, et al: Permanent iodine 125 brachytherapy in patients with progressive or recurrent glioblastoma multiforme. Neuro-oncology 6:119, 2004.
34. Mason WP, Gentili F, Macdonald DR, et al: Stabilization of disease progression by hydroxyurea in patients with recurrent or unresectable meningioma. J Neurosurg 92:341, 2002.
35. Khoo VS, Adams EJ, Saran F, et al: A comparison of clinical target volumes determined by CT and MRI for the radiotherapy planning of base of skull meningiomas. Int J Radiat Oncol Biol Phys 46:1309, 2000.
36. Bolsi A, Fogliata A, Cozzi L: Radiotherapy of small intracranial tumours with different advanced techniques using photon and proton beams: a treatment planning study. Radiother Oncol 68:1, 2003.

37. Nakamura JL, Pirzkall A, Carol MP, et al: Comparison of intensity-modulated radiosurgery with gamma knife radiosurgery for challenging skull base lesions. Int J Radiat Oncol Biol Phys 55:99, 2003.
38. Baumert BG, Norton IA, Davis JB: Intensity-modulated stereotactic radiotherapy vs. stereotactic conformal radiotherapy for the treatment of meningioma located predominantly in the skull base. Int J Radiat Oncol Biol Phys 57:580, 2003.
39. Mirimanoff RO: New radiotherapy technologies for meningiomas: 3D conformal radiotherapy? radiosurgery? stereotactic radiotherapy? intensity-modulated radiotherapy? proton beam radiotherapy? spot scanning proton radiation therapy . . . or nothing at all? Radiother Oncol 71:247, 2004.
40. Pirzkall A, Debus J, Haering P, et al: Intensity modulated radiotherapy (IMRT) for recurrent, residual, or untreated skull-base meningiomas: preliminary clinical experience. Int J Radiat Oncol Biol Phys 55:362, 2003.
41. Wenkel E, Thornton AF, Finkelstein D, et al: Benign meningioma: partially resected, biopsied, and recurrent intracranial tumors treated with combined proton and photon radiotherapy. Int J Radiat Oncol Biol Phys 48:1363, 2000.
42. Milosevic MF, Frost PJ, Laperriere JN, et al: Radiotherapy for atypical or malignant intracranial meningioma. Int J Radiat Oncol Biol Phys 34:817, 1996.
43. Goldsmith BJ, Wara WM, Wilson CB, et al: Postoperative irradiation for subtotally resected meningiomas. A retrospective analysis of 140 patients treated from 1967 to 1990. J Neurosurg 80:195, 1994.
44. Steinvorth S, Welzel G, Fuss M, et al: Neuropsychological outcome after fractionated stereotactic radiotherapy (FSRT) for base of skull meningiomas: a prospective 1-year follow-up. Radiother Oncol 69:177, 2003.
45. Nicolato A, Foroni R, Alessandrini F, et al: The role of Gamma Knife radiosurgery in the management of cavernous sinus meningiomas. Int J Radiat Oncol Biol Phys 53:992, 2002.
46. Lee JY, Niranjan A, McInerney J, et al: Stereotactic radiosurgery providing long-term tumor control of cavernous sinus meningiomas. J Neurosurg 97:65, 2002.
47. Roche PH, Regis J, Dufour H, et al: Gamma knife radiosurgery in the management of cavernous sinus meningiomas. J Neurosurg 93(Suppl 3):68, 2000.
48. Debus J, Hug EB, Liebsch NJ, et al: Brainstem tolerance to conformal radiotherapy of skull base tumors. Int J Radiat Oncol Biol Phys 39:967, 1997.
49. Castro JR, Linstadt DE, Bahary J-P, et al: Experience in charged particle irradiation of tumors of the skull base: 1977. Int J Radiat Oncol Biol Phys 29:647, 1994.
50. Enami B, Lyman J, Brown A: Tolerance of normal tissue to therapeutic irradiation. Int J Radiat Oncol Biol Phys 21:109, 1991.
51. Parsons JT, Fitzgerald CR, Mendenhall WM, et al: Radiation retinopathy after external beam irradiation: analysis of time-dose factors. Int J Radiat Oncol Biol Phys 30:765, 1994.
52. Parsons JT, Fitzgerald CR, Mendenhall WM, et al: Radiation optic neuropathy after megavoltage external-beam irradiation: analysis of time-dose factors. Int J Radiat Oncol Biol Phys 30:755, 1994.
53. Parsons JT, Bova FJ, Fitzgerald CR, et al: Severe dry-eye syndrome following external beam irradiation. Int J Radiat Oncol Biol Phys 30:775, 1994.
54. Kim J, Munzenrider J, Maas A, et al: Optic neuropathy following combined proton and photon radiotherapy for base of skull tumors. Int J Radiat Oncol Biol Phys 39:272, 1997.
55. Goldsmith BJ, Rosenthal SA, Wara WM, et al: Optic neuropathy after irradiation of meningioma. Radiology 185:71, 1992.
56. Becker GE, Jeremic B, Pitz S, et al: Stereotactic fractionated radiotherapy in patients with optic nerve sheath meningioma. Int J Radiat Oncol Biol Phys 54:1422, 2002.
57. Andrews DW, Faroozan R, Yang BP, et al: Fractionated stereotactic radiotherapy for the treatment of optic nerve sheath meningiomas. Neurosurgery 51:890, 2002.
58. Shrieve DC, Hazard L, Boucher K, et al: Dose fractionation in stereotactic radiotherapy for parasellar meningiomas: radiobiological considerations of efficacy and optic nerve tolerance. J Neurosurg S3:390, 2004.
59. Stafford SL, Pollock BE, Leavitt JA, et al: A study on the radiation tolerance of the optic nerves and chiasm after stereotactic radiosurgery. Int J Radiat Oncol Biol Phys 55:1177, 2003.
60. Santoni R, Liebsch N, Finkelstein DM, et al: Temporal lobe (TL) damage following surgery and high-dose photon and proton irradiation in 96 patients affected by chordomas and chondrosarcomas of the base of the skull. Int J Radiat Oncol Biol Phys 41:59, 1998.
61. Shaw EG, Evans RG, Scheithauer BW, Ilstrup DM, et al: Postoperative radiotherapy of intracranial ependymoma in pediatric and adult patients. Int J Radiat Oncol Biol Phys 13:1457, 1987.
62. Debiec-Rychter M, Biernat W, Zakrzewski K, et al: Loss of chromosome 22 and proliferative potential in ependymomas. Folia Neuropathol 41:191, 2003.
63. Huang B, Starostik P, Schraut H, et al: Human ependymomas reveal frequent deletions on chromosomes 6 and 9. Acta Neuropathol (Berl) 106:357, 2003.
64. Goussia AC, Kyritsis AP, Mitlianga P, et al: Genetic abnormalities in oligodendroglial and ependymal tumours. J Neurol 248:1030, 2001.
65. Taylor M, Gajjar A, Hogg T, et al: Whole Genome Characterization of Pediatric CNS Ependymomas. Toronto, Society for Neuro-Oncology, 2004, p GE-14.
66. Kleihues P, Cavenee WK (eds): World Health Organization Classification of Tumors. Lyon, France, IARC Press, 2000.
67. Pollack IF: Pediatric brain tumors. Semin Surg Oncol 16:73, 1999.
68. Vanuytsel LJ: The role of prophylactic spinal irradiation in localized intracranial ependymoma. Int J Radiat Oncol Biol Phys 21:825, 1991.
69. Nazar GB, Becker LE, Jenkin D, et al: Infratentorial ependymomas in childhood: prognostic factors and treatment. J Neurosurg 72:408, 1990.
70. Rousseau P, Habrand JL, Sarrazin D, et al: Treatment of intracranial ependymomas of children: review of a 15-year experience. Int J Radiat Oncol Biol Phys 28:381, 1994.
71. Vanuytsel LJ, Bessell EM, Ashley SE, et al: Intracranial ependymoma: long-term results of a policy of surgery and radiotherapy. Int J Radiat Oncol Biol Phys 23:313, 1992.
72. Pollack IF: The role of surgery in pediatric gliomas. J Neuro-Oncol 42:271, 1999.
73. Goldwein JW, Packer RJ, Sutton LN, et al: Intracranial ependymomas in children. Int J Radiat Oncol Biol Phys 19:1497, 1990.
74. Grill J, Pascal C, Chantal K: Childhood ependymoma: a systematic review of treatment options and strategies. Paediatr Drugs 5:533, 2003.
75. Lyons MK: Posterior fossa ependymomas: report of 30 cases and review of the literature. Neurosurgery 28:659, 1991.
76. Healey EA, Kupsky WJ, Scott M, et al: The prognostic significance of postoperative residual tumor in ependymoma. Neurosurgery 28:666, 1991.
77. Chiu JK, Ater J, Connelly J, et al: Intracranial ependymoma in children: analysis of prognostic factors. J Neuro-oncol 13:283, 1992.
78. Kovalic JJ, Grigsby PW, Pirkowski M, et al: Intracranial ependymoma: long term outcome, patterns of failure. J Neuro-oncol 15:125, 1993.
79. Merchant TE, Mulhern RK, Krasin MJ, et al: Preliminary results from a phase II trial of conformal radiation therapy and evaluation of radiation-related CNS effects for pediatric patients with localized ependymoma. J Clin Oncol 22:3156, 2004.
80. Timmermann B, Kortmann RD, Kuhl J, et al: Combined postoperative irradiation and chemotherapy for anaplastic ependymomas in childhood: results of the German prospective trials HIT 88/89 and HIT 91. Int J Radiat Oncol Biol Phys 46:287, 2000.
81. Evans AE, Anderson JR, Lefkowitz-Boudreaux IB, et al: Adjuvant chemotherapy of childhood posterior fossa ependymoma: cranio-spinal irradiation with or without adjuvant CCNU, vincristine, and prednisone: a Children's Cancer Group study. Med Pediatr Oncol 27:8, 1996.
82. Duffner PK, Krischer JP, Fiedman HS, et al: Postoperative chemotherapy and delayed radiation in children less than three years of age with malignant brain tumor. N Engl J Med 328:1725, 1993.

83. Hodgson DC, Goumnerova LC, Loeffler JS, et al: Radiosurgery in the management of pediatric brain tumors. Int J Radiat Oncol Biol Phys 50:929, 2001.
84. Salazar OM: A better understanding of CNS seeding and a brighter outlook for postoperatively irradiated patients with ependymomas. Int J Radiat Oncol Biol Phys 9:1231, 1983.
85. Paulus W, Scheithauer BW: Mesenchymal, non-meningothelial tumors. *In* Kleihues P, Cavenee WK (eds): Pathology and Genetics of Tumors of the Nervous System. Lyon, IARC Press, 2000.
86. Hug EB, Slater JD: Proton radiation therapy for chordomas and chondrosarcomas of the skull base. Neurosurg Clin N Am 11:627, 2000.
87. Chandler JP, Yashar P, Laskin WB, et al: Intracranial chondrosarcoma: a case report and review of the literature. J Neuro-oncol 68:33, 2004.
88. Rosenberg AE, Nielsen GP, Keel SB, et al: Chondrosarcoma of the base of the skull: a clinicopathologic study of 200 cases with emphasis on its distinction from chordoma. Am J Surg Pathol 23:1370, 1999.
89. Boyle JO, Shah KC, Shah JP: Craniofacial resection for malignant neoplasms of the skull base: an overview. J Surg Oncol 69:275, 1998.
90. Gay E, Sekhar LN, Rubinstein E, et al: Chordomas and chondrosarcomas of the cranial base: results and follow-up of 60 patients. Neurosurgery 36:887, 1995.
91. Tai P, Craighead P, Bagdon F: Optimization of radiotherapy for patients with cranial chordoma. Cancer 75:749, 1995.
92. Al-mefty O, Borba LA: Skull base chordomas: a management challenge. J Neurosurg 86:182, 1997.
93. Raffel C, Wright DC, Gutin PH, et al: Cranial chordomas: clinical presentation and results of operative and radiation therapy in 26 patients. Neurosurgery 17:703, 1985.
94. Rich TA, Schiller A, Suit HD, et al: Clinical and pathologic review of 48 cases of chordoma. Cancer 56:182, 1985.
95. Cheng E, Ozerdemoglu RA, Transfeldt EE, et al: Lumbosacral chordoma: prognostic factors and treatment. Spine 24:1639, 1999.
96. Noel G, Habrand JL, Jauffret E, et al: Radiation therapy for chordoma and chondrosarcoma of the skull base and the cervical spine. Strahlenther Onkol 179:241, 2003.
97. Debus J, Schulsz-Erner D, Schad L, et al: Stereotactic fractionated radiotherapy for chordomas and chondrosarcomas of the skull base. Int J Radiat Oncol Biol Phys 47:591, 2000.
98. Muthumakar N, Kondziolka D, Lunsford LD, et al: Stereotactic radiosurgery for chordoma and chondrosarcoma: further experiences. Int J Radiat Oncol Biol Phys 41:387, 1998.
99. Schulz-Ertner D, Nikoghosyan A, Thilmann, et al: Results of carbon ion radiotherapy in 152 patients. Int J Radiat Oncol Biol Phys 58:631, 2004.
100. Castro JR, Collier M, Petti PL, et al: Charged particle radiotherapy for lesions encircling the brain stem or spinal cord. Int J Radiat Oncol Biol Phys 17:477, 1989.
101. Verhey LJ, Smith V, et al: Comparison of radiosurgery treatment modalities based on physical dose distributions. Int J Radiat Oncol Biol Phys 40:497, 1998.
102. Terahara A, Niemierko A, Goitein M, et al: Analysis of the relationship between tumor dose inhomogeneity and local control in patients with skull base chordoma. Int J Radiat Oncol Biol Phys 45:351, 1999.
103. Pai HH, Thornton A, Katznelson L, et al: Hypothalamic/pituitary function following high-dose conformal radiotherapy to the base of skull. Int J Radiat Oncol Biol Phys 2001.49:1079,
104. Marucci L, Niemierko A, Liebsch NJ, et al: Spinal cord tolerance to high-dose fractionated 3D conformal proton-photon irradiation as evaluated by equivalent uniform dose and dose volume histogram analysis. Int J Radiat Oncol Biol Phys 2004.59:551,
105. Hug EB, Munzenrider JE: Charged particle therapy for base of skull tumors: past accomplishments and future challenges. Int J Radiat Oncol Biol Phys 29:911, 1994.
106. Stelzer KJ: Acute and long-term complications of therapeutic radiation for skull base tumors. Neurosurg Clin N Am 11:597, 2000.
107. Zulch KJ: Biologie und Pathologie Der Hirgeschwulste. *In* Oliverona H, Tonnis J (eds): Handbuch der Neurochirurgie. Berlin, Springer Verlag, 1965, p 348.
108. Donat JF, Okazaki H, Gomez MR, et al: Pineal tumors. A 53-year experience. Arch Neurol 35:736, 1978.
109. Abay EO 2nd, Laws ER Jr, Grado GL, et al: Pineal tumors in children and adolescents. Treatment by CSF shunting and radiotherapy. J Neurosurg 55:889, 1981.
110. Linstadt DE, Wara WM, Edwards MSB, et al: Radiotherapy of primary intracranial germinomas: the case against routine craniospinal irradiation. Int J Radiat Oncol Biol Phys 15:291, 1988.
111. Rich TA, Cassady JR, Strand RD, et al: Radiation therapy for pineal and suprasellar germ cell tumors. Cancer 55:932, 1985.
112. Wara WM, Jenkin RD, Evans A, et al: Tumors of the pineal and suprasellar region: Children's Cancer Study Group treatment results 1960-1975: a report from Children's Cancer Study Group. Cancer 43:698, 1979.
113. Bjornsson J, Scheithauer BW, Okazaki H, et al: Intracranial germ cell tumors: pathobiological and immunohistochemical aspects of 70 cases. J Neuropathol Exp Neurol 44:32, 1985.
114. Bruce JN, Fetell MR, Stein BM: Incidence of spinal metastases in patients with malignant pineal regional tumors: avoidance of prophylactic spinal irradiation. J Neurosurg 75:354A, 1990.
115. Bruce J, Stein B, Balmaceda C, et al: Management of pineal region germ cell tumors: results and long-term follow-up. Proc Am Soc Clin Oncol 13:505A, 1994.
116. Dearnaley DP, Whittaker S, Bloom HJG: Pineal and CNS germ cell tumors: Royal Marsden Hospital Experience 1962. Int J Radiat Oncol Biol Phys 18:773, 1990.
117. Fuller BG, Kapp DS, Cox R: Radiation therapy of pineal region tumors: 25 new cases and a review of 208 previously reported cases. Int J Radiat Oncol Biol Phys 28:229, 1993.
118. Hoffman HJ, Otsubo H, Hendrick EB, et al: Intracranial germ-cell tumors in children. J Neurosurg 74:545, 1991.
119. Jennings MT, Gelman R, Hochberg F: Intracranial germ-cell tumors: natural history and pathogenesis. J Neurosurg 63:155, 1985.
120. Linggood RM, Chapman PH: Pineal tumors. J Neuro-oncol 12:85, 1992.
121. Mineura K, Sasajima T, Sakamoto T, et al: [Results of the treatment of intracranial germ cell tumors]. Gan No Rinsho 36:2399, 1990.
122. Sano K: Pineal region tumors: problems in pathology and treatment. Clin Neurosurg 30:59, 1983.
123. Sano K, Matsutani M, Seto T: So-called intracranial germ cell tumours: personal experiences and a theory of their pathogenesis. Neurol Res 11:118, 1989.
124. Takakura K: Intracranial germ cell tumors. Clin Neurosurg 32:429, 1985.
125. Wolden SL, Wara WM, Larson DA, et al: Radiation therapy for primary intracranial germ-cell tumors. Int J Radiat Oncol Biol Phys 32:943, 1995.
126. Yoshida J, Sugita K, Kobayashi T, et al: Prognosis of intracranial germ cell tumours: effectiveness of chemotherapy with cisplatin and etoposide (CDDP and VP-16). Acta Neurochir (Wien) 120:111, 1993.
127. Schild SE, Haddock MG, Scheithauer BW, et al: Nongerminomatous germ cell tumors of the brain. Int J Radiat Oncol Biol Phys 36:557, 1996.
128. Schild SE, Buskirk SJ, Frick LM, et al: Pineal parenchymal tumors: clinical, pathologic and therapeutic aspects. Cancer 72:870, 1993.
129. Schild SE, Schiethauer B, Haddock MG, et al: Histologically confirmed pineal tumors and other germ cell tumors of the brain: treatment and outcome. Cancer 78:2564, 1996.
130. Burger P, Scheithauer B: Pineal tumors. *In* Tumors of the Central Nervous System: Atlas of Tumor Pathology. Bethesda, MD, Armed Forces Institute of Pathology, 1994, p 227,
131. Mena H, Nakazato Y, Jouvet A, et al: Pineal parenchymal tumors. *In* Kleihues P, Cavenee WK (eds): World Health Organization Classification of Tumors, Pathology and Genetics. Tumors of the Nervous System. Lyon, IARC Press, 2000, p 115.
132. Marsh WR, Laws ER Jr: Shunting and irradiation of pineal tumors. Clin Neurosurg 32:384, 1985.
133. Fain JS, Tomlinson FH, Scheithauer BW, et al: Symptomatic glial cysts of the pineal gland. J Neurosurg 80:454, 1994.

134. Fleege MA, Miller GM, Fletcher GP, et al: Benign glial cysts of the pineal gland: unusual imaging characteristics with histologic correlation. AJNR Am J Neuroradiol 15:161, 1994.
135. Popovic EA, Kelly PJ: Stereotactic procedures for lesions of the pineal region. Mayo Clin Proc 68:965, 1993.
136. Schild SE, Scheithauer BW, Haddock MG, et al: Histologically confirmed pineal tumors and other germ cell tumors of the brain. Cancer 78:2564, 1996.
137. Haas-Kogan DA, Missett BT, Wara WM, et al: Radiation therapy for intracranial germ cell tumors. Int J Radiat Oncol Biol Phys 56:511, 2003.
138. Gobel U, Bamberg M, Calaminus G, et al: [Improved prognosis of intracranial germ cell tumors by intensified therapy: results of the MAKEI 89 therapy protocol]. Klin Padiatr 205:217, 1993.
139. Gobel U, Bamberg M, Engert J, et al: [Treatment of non-testicular germ cell tumors in children and adolescents with BEP and VIP: initial results of the MAKEI 89 therapy study]. Klin Padiatr 203:236, 1991.
140. Herrmann HD, Westphal M, Winkler K, et al: Treatment of nongerminomatous germ-cell tumors of the pineal region. Neurosurgery 34:524-529, 1994; discussion, 529.
141. Buckner JC, Peethambaram PP, Smithson WA, et al: Phase II trial of primary chemotherapy followed by reduced-dose radiation for CNS germ cell tumors. J Clin Oncol 17:933, 1999.
142. Matsutani M: Clinical management of primary central nervous system germ cell tumors. Semin Oncol 31:676, 2004.
143. Matsutani M: Combined chemotherapy and radiation therapy for CNS germ cell tumors—the Japanese experience. J Neurooncol 54:311, 2001.
144. Cohen BH, Zeltzer PM, Boyett JM, et al: Prognostic factors and treatment results for supratentorial primitive neuroectodermal tumors in children using radiation and chemotherapy: a Children's Cancer Group randomized trial. J Clin Oncol 13:1687, 1995.
145. Kondziolka D, Hadjipanayis CG, Flickinger JC, et al: The role of radiosurgery for the treatment of pineal parenchymal tumors. Neurosurgery 51:880, 2002.
146. Hasegawa T, Kondziolka D, Hadjipanayis CG, et al: Stereotactic radiosurgery for CNS nongerminomatous germ cell tumors. Report of four cases. Pediatr Neurosurg 38:329, 2003.
147. Delellis RA: The endocrine system: tumors of extra-adrenal paraganglia. *In* Cotra RS, Kumar V, Robbins SL (eds): Robbins Pathologic Basis of Disease. Philadelphia, WB Saunders, 1989.
148. Parry DM, Li FP, Strong LC, et al: Carotid body tumors in humans: genetics and epidemiology. J Natl Cancer Inst 68:573, 1982.
149. Springate SC, Haraf D, Weichselbaum RR: Temporal bone chemodectomas—comparing surgery and radiation therapy. Oncology (Huntingt) 5:131-137, 1991; discussion 140, 143.
150. Schild SE, Foote RL, Buskirk SJ, et al: Results of radiotherapy for chemodectomas. Mayo Clin Proc 67:537, 1992.
151. Kim JA, Elkon D, Lim ML, et al: Optimum dose of radiotherapy for chemodectomas of the middle ear. Int J Radiat Oncol Biol Phys 6:815, 1980.
152. Sheehan J, Kondziolka D, Flickinger J, et al: Gamma knife surgery for glomus jugulare tumors: an intermediate report on efficacy and safety. J Neurosurg 102(Suppl):241, 2005.
153. Pollock BE: Stereotactic radiosurgery in patients with glomus jugulare tumors. Neurosurg Focus 17:E10, 2004.
154. Lim M, Gibbs IC, Adler JR Jr, et al: Efficacy and safety of stereotactic radiosurgery for glomus jugulare tumors. Neurosurg Focus 17:E11, 2004.
155. Hinerman RW, Mendenhall WM, Amdur RJ, et al: Definitive radiotherapy in the management of chemodectomas arising in the temporal bone, carotid body, and glomus vagale. Head Neck 23:363, 2001.
156. Foote RL, Coffey RJ, Gorman DA, et al: Stereotactic radiosurgery for glomus jugulare tumors: a preliminary report. Int J Radiat Oncol Biol Phys 38:491, 1997.
157. Conway JE, Chou D, Clatterbuck RE, et al: Hemangioblastomas of the central nervous system in von Hippel-Lindau syndrome and sporadic disease. Neurosurgery 48:55, 2001.
158. Jaaskelainen J, Louis DN, Paulus W, et al: Hemangiopericytoma. *In* Kleihues P, Cavenee WK (eds): Pathology and Genetics: Tumors of the Central Nervous System. Lyon, IARC Press, 2000, p 190.
159. Bohling T, Plate KH, Haltia MJ, et al: von Hippel-Lindau disease and capillary hemangioblastoma. *In* Kleihues P, Cavenee WK (eds): Pathology and Genetics: Tumors of the Central Nervous System. Lyon, IARC Press, 2000, p 223.
160. Guthrie BL, Ebersold MJ, Scheithauer BW, et al: Meningeal hemangiopericytoma: histopathological features, treatment, and long-term follow-up of 44 cases. Neurosurgery 25:514, 1989.
161. Bastin KT, Mehta M: Meningeal hemangiopericytoma: defining the role for radiation therapy. J Neuro-Oncol 14:277, 1992.
162. Patrice JP, Sneed PK, Flickinger JC, et al: Radiosurgery for hemangioblastoma: results of a multiinstitutional experience. Int J Radiat Oncol Biol Phys 35:493, 1996.
163. Smalley SR, Schomberg PJ, Earle JD, et al: Radiotherapeutic considerations in the treatment of hemangioblastomas of the central nervous system. Int J Radiat Oncol Biol Phys 18:1165, 1990.
164. Sung DI, Chang CH, Harisiadis L: Cerebellar hemangioblastomas. Cancer 49:553, 1982.
165. Ecker RD, Marsh WR, Pollock BE, et al: Hemangiopericytoma in the central nervous system: treatment, pathological features and long-term follow-up in 38 patients. J Neurosurg 98:1182, 2003.
166. Galanis E, Buckner JC, Scheithauer BW, et al: Management of recurrent meningeal hemangiopericytoma. Cancer 82:1915, 1998.
167. Sheehan J, Kondziolka D, Flickinger J, et al: Radiosurgery for treatment of recurrent intracranial hemangiopericytomas. Neurosurgery 51:905, 2002.
168. Staples JJ, Wen BC, Hussey DH: Hemangiopericytoma: the role of radiotherapy. Int J Radiat Oncol Biol Phys 19:445, 1990.
169. Smalley S, Laws ER Jr, O'Fallon JR, et al. Resection for solitary brain metastasis. J Neurosurg 77:531, 1992.
170. Honegger J, Buchfelder M, Fahlbusch R: Surgical treatment of craniopharyngiomas: endocrinological results. J Neurosurg 90: 251, 1999.
171. Yasargil MG, Kis M, Siegenthaler G, et al: Total removal of craniopharyngiomas approaches and long-term results in 144 patients. J Neurosurg 73:3, 1990.
172. Carmel PW, Antunes JL, Chang CH: Craniopharyngiomas in children. Neurosurgery 11:382, 1982.
173. Sweet WH: Radical surgical treatment of craniopharyngioma. Clin Neurosurg 23:52, 1976.
174. Skarin AT: Atlas of Diagnostic Oncology. Philadelphia, JB Lippincott, 1991.
175. Zhang YQ, Wang CC, Ma ZY: Pediatric craniopharyngiomas: clinicomorphological study of 189 cases. Pediatr Neurosurg 36:80, 2002.
176. Fahlbusch R, Honegger J, Paulus W, et al: Surgical treatment of craniopharyngiomas: experience with 168 patients. J Neurosurg 90:237, 1999.
177. Stripp DC, Maity A, Janss AJ, et al: Surgery with or without radiation therapy in the management of craniopharyngiomas in children and young adults. Int J Radiat Oncol Biol Phys 58:714, 2004.
178. Hoffman HJ, Humphreys RP, Drake JM, et al: Aggressive surgical management of craniopharyngiomas in children. J Neurosurg 76:47, 1992.
179. Brada M: Craniopharyngioma Revisited. Int J Radiat Oncol Biol Phys 27:471, 1993.
180. Van Effenterre R, Boch AL: Craniopharyngioma in adults and children: a study of 122 surgical cases. J Neurosurg 97:3, 2002.
181. Wara WM, Larson DA: The role of radiation therapy in the treatment of craniopharyngioma. Pediatr Neurosurg 21:98, 1994.
182. Kahn EA, Gosch HH, Seeger JF, et al: Forty-five years experience with the craniopharyngiomas. Surg Neurol 1:5, 1973.
183. Tsai HK, Goumnerova LC, Pomery SL, et al: Long-term outcome after treatment of pediatric craniopharyngioma. Neurooncology. 6:RT-23, 2004.
184. Mokry M: Craniopharyngiomas: A six year experience with Gamma Knife radiosurgery. Stereotact Funct Neurosurg 72(Suppl 1):140, 1999.
185. Rajan B, Ashley S, Gorman C, et al: Craniopharyngioma—long-term results following limited surgery and radiotherapy. Radiother Oncol 26:1, 1993.

186. Rajan B, Ashley S, Thomas DG, et al: Craniopharyngioma: improving outcome by early recognition and treatment of acute complications. Int J Radiat Oncol Biol Phys 37:517, 1997.
187. Hader WJ, Steinbok P, Hukin J, et al: Intratumoral therapy with bleomycin for cystic craniopharyngiomas in children. Pediatr Neurosurg 33:211, 2000.
188. Pollack IF, Lunsford LD, Slamovits TL, et al: Stereotaxic intracavitary irradiation for cystic craniopharyngiomas. J Neurosurg 68:227, 1988.
189. Toogood AA: Endocrine consequences of brain irradiation. Growth Horm IGF Res 14(Suppl A):S118, 2004.
190. Kleihues P, Louis DN, Scheithauer BW, et al: The WHO classification of tumors of the nervous system. J Neuropathol Exp Neurol 61:215-225, 2002; discussion, 226.
191. Rickert CH, Paulus W: Tumors of the choroid plexus. Microsc Res Tech 52:104, 2001.
192. Wyatt-Ashmead J, Kleinschmidt-DeMasters B, Mierau GW, et al: Choroid plexus carcinomas and rhabdoid tumors: phenotypic and genotypic overlap. Pediatr Dev Pathol 4:545, 2001.
193. Gessi M, Giangaspero F, Pietsch T: Atypical teratoid/rhabdoid tumors and choroid plexus tumors: when genetics "surprise" pathology. Brain Pathol 13:409, 2003.
194. Krishnan S, Brown PD, Scheithauer BW, et al: Choroid plexus papillomas: a single institutional experience. J Neuro-oncol 68:49, 2004.
195. Gupta N: Choroid plexus tumors in children. Neurosurg Clin N Am 14:621, 2003.
196. Wolff JE, Sajedi M, Brant R, et al: Choroid plexus tumours. Br J Cancer 87:1086, 2002.
197. Mirimanoff RO, Dosoretz DE, Linggood RM, et al: Meningioma: analysis of recurrence and progression following neurosurgical resection. J Neurosurg 62:18, 1985.
198. Mathiesen T, Lindquist C, Kihlstrom L, et al: Recurrence of cranial base meningiomas. Neurosurgery 39:2-7, 1996; discussion, 8.
199. Stafford SL, Perry A, Suman VJ, et al: Primarily resected meningiomas: outcome and prognostic factors in 581 Mayo Clinic patients, 1978 through 1988. Mayo Clin Proc 73:936, 1998.
200. Taylor BW Jr, Marcus RB Jr, Friedman WA, et al: The meningioma controversy: postoperative radiation therapy. Int J Radiat Oncol Biol Phys 15:299, 1988.
201. Glaholm J, Bloom HJ, Crow JH: The role of radiotherapy in the management of intracranial meningiomas: the Royal Marsden Hospital experience with 186 patients. Int J Radiat Oncol Biol Phys 18:755, 1990.
202. Maire JP, Caudry M, Guerin J, et al: Fractionated radiation therapy in the treatment of intracranial meningiomas: local control, functional efficacy, and tolerance in 91 patients. Int J Radiat Oncol Biol Phys 33:315, 1995.
203. Condra KS, Buatti JM, Mendenhall WM, et al: Benign meningiomas: primary treatment selection affects survival. Int J Radiat Oncol Biol Phys 39:427, 1997.
204. Nutting C, Brada M, Brazil L, et al: Radiotherapy in the treatment of benign meningioma of the skull base. J Neurosurg 90:823, 1999.
205. Uy NW, Woo SY, Teh BS, et al: Intensity-modulated radiation therapy (IMRT) for meningioma. Int J Radiat Oncol Biol Phys 53:1265, 2002
206. Jalali R, Loughrey C, Baumert B, et al: High precision focused irradiation in the form of fractionated stereotactic conformal radiotherapy (SCRT) for benign meningiomas predominantly in the skull base location. Clin Oncol (R Coll Radiol) 14:103, 2002.
207. Mendenhall WM, Morris CG, Amdur RJ, et al: Radiotherapy alone or after subtotal resection for benign skull base meningiomas. Cancer 98:1473, 2003.
208. Soyuer S, Chang EL, Selek U, et al: Radiotherapy after surgery for benign cerebral meningioma. Radiother Oncol 71:85, 2004.
209. Hakim R, Alexander E 3rd, Loeffler JS, et al: Results of linear accelerator-based radiosurgery for intracranial meningiomas. Neurosurgery 42:446-453, 1998; discussion, 453.
210. Lo SS, Cho KH, Hall WA, et al: Single dose versus fractionated stereotactic radiotherapy for meningiomas. Can J Neurol Sci 29:240, 2002.
211. Eustacchio S, Trummer M, Fuchs I, et al: Preservation of cranial nerve function following Gamma Knife radiosurgery for benign skull base meningiomas: experience in 121 patients with follow-up of 5 to 9.8 years. Acta Neurochir Suppl 84:71, 2002
212. Chuang CC, Chang CN, Tsang NM, et al: Linear accelerator-based radiosurgery in the management of skull base meningiomas. J Neuro-oncol 66:241, 2004.
213. Noel G, Habrand JL, Mammar H, et al: Highly conformal therapy using proton component in the management of meningiomas. Preliminary experience of the Centre de Protontherapie d'Orsay. Strahlenther Onkol 178:480, 2002.
214. Weber DC, Lomax AJ, Peter Rutz H, et al: Spot-scanning proton radiation therapy for recurrent, residual or untreated intracranial meningiomas. Radiother Oncol 71:251, 2004.
215. Maguire PD, Clough R, Friedman AH, et al: Fractionated external-beam radiation therapy for meningiomas of the cavernous sinus. Int J Radiat Oncol Biol Phys 44:75, 1999.
216. Dufour H, Muracciole X, Metellus P, et al: Long-term tumor control and functional outcome in patients with cavernous sinus meningiomas treated by radiotherapy with or without previous surgery: is there an alternative to aggressive tumor removal? Neurosurgery 48:285-294, 2001; discussion, 294.
217. Nicolato A, Foroni R, Alessandrini F, et al: Radiosurgical treatment of cavernous sinus meningiomas: experience with 122 treated patients. Neurosurgery 51:1153-1159, 2002; discussion, 1159
218. Selch MT, Ahn E, Laskari A, et al: Stereotactic radiotherapy for treatment of cavernous sinus meningiomas. Int J Radiat Oncol Biol Phys 59:101, 2004.
219. Palma L, Celli P, Franco C, et al: Long-term prognosis for atypical and malignant meningiomas: a study of 71 surgical cases. Neurosurg Focus 2:e3, 1997.
220. Dziuk TW, Woo S, Butler EB, et al: Malignant meningioma: an indication for initial aggressive surgery and adjuvant radiotherapy. J Neuro-oncol 37:177, 1998.
221. Ojemann SG, Sneed PK, Larson DA, et al: Radiosurgery for malignant meningioma: results in 22 patients. J Neurosurg 93(Suppl 3):62, 2000.
222. Hug EB, Devries A, Thornton AF, et al: Management of atypical and malignant meningiomas: role of high-dose, 3D-conformal radiation therapy. J Neuro-oncol 48:151, 2000.
223. Goyal LK, Suh JH, Mohan DS, et al: Local control and overall survival in atypical meningioma: a retrospective study. Int J Radiat Oncol Biol Phys 46:57, 2000.
224. Harris AE, Lee JY, Omalu B, et al: The effect of radiosurgery during management of aggressive meningiomas. Surg Neurol 60:298-305, 2003; discussion, 305.
225. Mansur D, Perry A, Rajaram V, et al: Postoperative radiation therapy for grade II and III intracranial ependymoma. Int J Radiat Oncol Biol Phys 61:387, 2005.
226. Massimino M, Gandola M, Giangaspero F, et al: Hyperfractionated radiotherapy and chemotherapy for childhood ependymoma: final results of the first prospective AIEOP Study. Int J Radiat Oncol Biol Phys 58:1336, 2004.
227. Ben-Ammar C, Kochbati L, Frikha H, et al: Primitive intracranial ependymomas. Salah-Azaiz Institute experience. Cancer Radiother 8:75, 2004.
228. Jaing T, Wang H, Tsay P, et al: Multivariate analysis of clinical prognostic factors in children with intracranial ependymomas. J Neuro-oncol 68:255, 2004.
229. Reni M, Brandes A, Vavassori V, et al: A multicentre study of the prognosis and treatment of adult brain ependymal tumors. Cancer 100:1221, 2004.
230. Merchant T, Mlhern R, Krasin M, et al: Preliminary results from a phase ii trial of conformal radiation therapy and evaluation of radiation-related CNS effects for pediatric patients with localized ependymoma. J Clin Oncol 22:56, 2004.
231. Guyotat J, Signorelli F, Desme S, et al: Intracranial ependymomas in adult patients: analyses of prognostic factors. J Neuro-oncol 60:255, 2002.
232. van Veelen-Vincent M, Pierre-Kahn A, Kalifa C, et al: Ependymoma in childhood: prognostic factors, extent of surgery and adjuvant therapy. J Neurosurg 97:827, 2002.

233. Merchant T, Jenkins J, Burger P, et al: Influence of tumor grade on time to progression after irradiation for localized ependymoma in children. Int J Radiat Oncol Biol Phys 53:52, 2002.
234. Paulino AC, Wen B, Buatti, et al: Intracranial ependymomas: an analysis of prognostic factors and patterns of failure. Am J Clin Oncol 25:117, 2002.
235. Oya N, Shibamoto Y, Nagata Y, et al: Postoperative radiotherapy for intracranial ependymoma: analysis of prognostic factors and patterns of failure. J Neuro-oncol 56:87, 2002.
236. Grill J, Le Deley M, Gambarelli D, et al: Postoperative chemotherapy without irradiation for ependymoma in children under 5 years of age: a multicentre trial of the French Society of Pediatric Oncology. J Clin Oncol 19:1288, 2001.
237. Akuyz C, Emir S, Akalan N, et al: Intracranial ependymomas in childhood—a retrospective review of sixty-two children. Acta Oncol 39:97, 2000.
238. Timmerman B, Kortmann R, Kuhl J, et al: Combined postoperative irradiation and chemotherapy for anaplastic ependymomas in childhood: results of the German prospective trials HIT 88/89 and HIT 91. Int J Radiat Oncol Biol Phys 46:287, 2000.
239. Figarella-Branger D, Civatte M, Bouvier-Labit C, et al: Prognostic factors in intracranial ependymomas in children. J Neurosurg 93:605, 2000.
240. Paulino A, Wen B: The significance of radiotherapy treatment duration in intracranial ependymoma. Int J Radiat Oncol Biol Phys 47:585, 2000.
241. Horn B, Heideman R, Geyer R, et al: A multi-institutional retrospective study of intracranial ependymoma in children: identification of risk factors. J Pediatr Hematol Oncol 21:203, 1999.
242. McLaughlin M, Marcus RB Jr, Buatti JM, et al: Ependymoma: results, prognostic factors and treatment recommendations. Int J Radiat Oncol Biol Phys 40:845, 1998.
243. Sala F, Talacchi A, Mazz C, et al: Prognostic factors in childhood intracranial ependymomas: the role of age and tumor location. Pediatr Neurosurg 28:135, 1998.
244. Robertson P, Zeltzer P, Boyett J, et al: Survival and prognostic factors following radiation therapy and chemotherapy for ependymomas in children: a report of the Children's Cancer Group. J Neurosurg 88:695, 1998.
245. Schild S, Nisi R, Scheithauer B, et al: The results of radiotherapy for ependymomas: the Mayo Clinic experience. Int J Radiat Oncol Biol Phys 42:953, 1998.
246. Merchant T, Haida T, Wang M, et al: Anaplastic ependymoma: treatment of pediatric patients with or without craniospinal radiation therapy. J Neurosurg 86:943, 1998.
247. Perilongo G, Massimino M, Sotti G, et al: Analyses of prognostic factors in a retrospective review of 92 children with ependymoma: Italian Pediatric Neuro-oncology Group. Med Pediatr Oncol 29:79, 1997.
248. Stuben G, Sutschke M, Kroll M, et al: Postoperative radiotherapy of spinal and intracranial ependymomas: analysis of prognostic factors. Radiother Oncol 45:3, 1997.
249. Foreman N, Love S, Thorne R: Intracranial ependymomas: analysis of prognostic factors in a population-based series. Pediatr Neurosurg 24:119, 1996.
250. Pollack I, Gerszten P, Martinez A, et al: Intracranial ependymomas of childhood: long-term outcome and prognostic factors. Neurosurgery 37:655, 1995.

CHAPTER 26

PITUITARY TUMORS

Mahesh A. Varia, Matthew G. Ewend, Julie Sharpless, and David E. Morris

INCIDENCE

Each year, 70 new cases per million females and 28 new cases per million males are diagnosed. Pituitary tumors account for 10% to 15% of all intracranial tumors.

Ten percent of cases are identified by magnetic resonance imaging studies of otherwise normal adults, and 3% to 27% are identified in autopsy series.

BIOLOGIC CHARACTERISTICS

Most pituitary tumors are benign and monoclonal. Tumorigenesis involves an initiation event followed by clonal expansion.

Three nuclear transcriptional factors, AP-1, CREB, and Pit-1, appear to play critical roles in hormone secretion and neoplastic growth in hormone-secreting tumors.

STAGING EVALUATION

Evaluation of pituitary tumors requires the definition of the endocrine disorders and mass effects of the tumor with clinical and neuro-ophthalmic assessment, laboratory endocrine profile, and MRI to assess the size (microadenoma or macroadenoma) and anatomic extensions of the tumor.

Wilson's modification of the Hardy tumor classification system incorporates imaging and intraoperative criteria. Wilson's modifications are not routinely used for staging.

PRIMARY THERAPY AND RESULTS

Primary therapy is guided by the particular endocrine syndrome and the presence of mass effect.

Incidental findings of nonfunctioning pituitary adenomas may be followed with close surveillance.

Transsphenoidal and other surgical approaches, pharmacologic management of hormonal dysfunctions, medical treatment of the adenoma, and the selective use of radiation therapy in the form of fractionated therapy or stereotactic radiosurgery are effective treatment modalities.

The objectives of the treatments are to rectify the endocrine dysfunction, reverse the neuro-ophthalmic changes of the mass effect, and remove the pituitary adenoma or restrict its growth.

ADJUVANT THERAPY

Postoperative radiation therapy is indicated for extrasellar extensions and for residual tumor after repeat resections.

Medical therapy for endocrine management may be needed during and after surgery and radiation therapy.

LOCALLY ADVANCED DISEASE

Pituitary adenomas with suprasellar and parasellar extensions require management of the associated endocrine syndromes, surgical decompression for visual symptoms, and radiation therapy for the tumor.

PALLIATION

Metastases to the pituitary are infrequent. Breast and lung carcinomas are the common primary sites, and 70% of the metastases to the pituitary occur in the posterior lobe.

Palliative radiation therapy can be achieved with 30 Gy in 10 treatments.

The past century has witnessed dramatic advances in understanding the pituitary gland's endocrine functions and disorders. These remarkable advances have come about from the elucidation of the chemical structure of the hormones by biochemists and pharmacologists, progressive refinements in the laboratory techniques in the assessment of pituitary function, and noninvasive methods of imaging pituitary abnormalities. The skillful applications of these discoveries by neurosurgeons, endocrinologists, and radiation oncologists have brought major clinical advances in the management of pituitary diseases that now offer safer and sophisticated medical, surgical, and radiotherapeutic treatments of pituitary tumors.

Until a century ago, the pituitary gland (hypophysis cerebri) was considered a vestigial organ with no important functions. From its humble history, denoted by the origin of its name from Latin *pituitas,* meaning "mucus" (Galen believed that the pituitary secreted waste products from the brain as nasal mucus), it is now known that the pituitary has a preeminent position in the neuroendocrine hierarchy and that it influences the functions of multiple organs. It was not until 1886, a decade before the discovery of x-rays by Wilhelm Roentgen, that Pierre Marie[1] in Paris first described the abnormal pathologic findings of the pituitary in patients with acromegaly. Subsequent work by Harvey Cushing[2] and others led to an elucidation of the clinical syndromes associated with pituitary disorders and their treatments.

Pituitary tumors are generally benign and are associated with immense diversity in their endocrine manifestations secondary to hormone excess or deficiency, and neuro-ophthalmic manifestations from the mass effect of enlarging pituitary adenomas. Refinements in diagnostic evaluation of these clinical syndromes and advances in the surgical, medical, and radiation therapy of these tumors offer excellent prospects of successful therapeutic outcome by a multidisciplinary team. Application of molecular biology techniques is greatly advancing the understanding of the pathophysiology of pituitary tumors.

This chapter focuses on the current concepts and advances in the diagnosis, evaluation, and management of pituitary tumors. Oncologists are conversant with the importance of a multidisciplinary approach in the care of various malignancies. Although most pituitary tumors are benign, the paradigm of interdisciplinary approach is equally important in the management of patients with pituitary tumors. Such an approach, involving the endocrinologist, neurosurgeon, otorhinolaryngologist, radiation oncologist, neuroradiologist, ophthalmologist, and pathologist, greatly contributes to the optimal management of patients with pituitary tumors.

ETIOLOGY AND EPIDEMIOLOGY

Etiology

A major characteristic of pituitary adenoma is that tumor growth is under the control of an endocrinologic environment, and the improved knowledge of pituitary endocrine functions has served as a foundation for understanding pituitary oncogenesis. Faglia[3] and Tada and colleagues[4] provide excellent reviews of the concepts of tumor-initiating and tumor-promoting factors in the pathogenesis of pituitary adenomas. There has been considerable debate regarding the cause of pituitary tumors. Two rat pituitary models suggest two primary modes of pituitary oncogenesis.[4] The first model suggests a hormone-dependent pathway through hyperplasia to neoplasia, commonly referred to as the hyperplasia-adenoma sequence. The second model suggests a de novo occurrence without the development of hyperplasia, possibly because of a genetic alteration, and it is often the model for multiple endocrine neoplasia type 1 (MEN1) in humans. Investigative insights suggest merging of these two concepts, because neither is clearly identified in humans.

A unique cause of pituitary tumors has been elucidated in patients with MEN1, which is an autosomal dominant disease characterized by tumors in endocrine organs, typically the pancreas, parathyroid, thyroid, and pituitary. Less than 5% of pituitary tumors are associated with this syndrome. Pituitary tumors associated with the *MEN1* gene have demonstrated loss of heterozygosity of chromosome 11q13 (locale of the *MEN1* gene) and has been implicated in the malignant progression of pituitary adenomas.[5]

In the future, additional information may be learned from patients with Carney complex, McCune-Albright syndrome, and isolated familial somatotropinomas, because these patients also develop functioning pituitary tumors.

Epidemiology

Pituitary adenomas are the most common neoplasms near the sella. From the Central Brain Tumor Registry of the United States Annual Report for 2004 to 2005, 6% of central nervous system tumors, or just under 3500 cases of pituitary tumors, were reported between 1997 and 2001.[6] In neurosurgical series, these tumors comprise 10% to 15% of cases.[7] However, reports of the frequency of the pituitary neoplasms vary greatly by the type of epidemiologic survey methods used. Population studies such as that by Annegers and associates[8] report an increasing incidence of pituitary adenomas, from 8.2 to 14.7 per 100,000 women.

A high prevalence of pituitary adenomas is identified in radiologic[9] and autopsy[10] series. Ezzat and associates[11] performed a meta-analysis to determine the overall estimated prevalence of pituitary adenomas. There was an overall estimated prevalence of pituitary adenomas of 16.7%, with 14.4% observed in autopsy series and 22.5% in radiographic series.[11] Most are asymptomatic and remain undetected. Faglia[3] estimated that only 1 in 5000 pituitary adenomas becomes symptomatic.

Burrow and colleagues[10] reported a 25% prevalence of pituitary adenomas in unselected autopsy series. However, the incidence of pituitary tumors in autopsy series ranges widely between 3% and 27%.[12-14] This may be a result of the differences in criteria used for distinguishing hyperplasia from adenomas of the pituitary, the lack of immunohistochemical staining for pituitary hormones until recently, and the different slice thicknesses used in the magnetic resonance imaging (MRI) studies.

Radiologic series using recent neuroimaging studies permit detection of pituitary microadenomas that are 2 to 3 mm in diameter. Microadenomas are defined as pituitary adenomas smaller than 10 mm in diameter. In an MRI study of volunteers, Hall and coworkers[15] observed that 10% had pituitary adenomas. Teramoto and associates[16] found 178 incidental microadenomas in an imaging study of 1000 pituitary glands in unselected autopsy series, and they observed that a 6% false-positive rate might be expected when incidental pituitary lesions were found on imaging studies in the investigation of functioning pituitary tumors. Camaris and colleagues[17] found a 3% prevalence of microadenomas in unselected autopsy series of 434 pituitary glands. Using immunohistochemical testing of pituitary glands, they also observed prolactin (PRL) positivity (range, 30% to 60%) and absence of staining (range, 20% to 42%) as the two most frequent patterns in pituitary microadenomas. These data suggest that pituitary adenomas develop fairly commonly, but for the most part, they are asymptomatic and do not cause clinical, endocrine, or neurologic dysfunctions.

Age and Gender

Asymptomatic pituitary adenomas occur at all ages. In autopsy series, they are observed with equal frequency in males and females. This observation is in direct contrast with the female preponderance seen in clinical series. Seventy percent of pituitary tumors occur between the ages of 30 and 50 years.[18] Symptomatic presentations, however, are most common in women between the ages of 20 and 50 years.

The frequency of the various types of pituitary adenomas also differs widely according to age, gender, and type of hormone secretion (Table 26-1).[19,20] In these studies of more than 2300 patients treated surgically for pituitary adenomas, PRL adenomas were the most common, followed by nonfunctioning adenomas, growth hormone (GH)–releasing adenomas, and adrenocorticotropic hormone (ACTH)–releasing adenomas. Nelson's syndrome (i.e., growth of an ACTH-secreting pituitary adenoma after bilateral adrenalectomy) and thyroid-stimulating hormone (TSH)–releasing adenomas were rare.

Classification of Pituitary Tumors by Size and Growth Patterns

Pituitary tumors are referred to as *microadenomas* or *macroadenomas* depending on size (Jules Hardy classification).[21] Microadenoma is arbitrarily defined as smaller than 1 cm in diameter, and a macroadenoma has a diameter of 1 cm or larger. Incidental microadenomas have been observed with a frequency of 3% to 23% in large, unselected autopsy series. Macroadenomas are more common than microadenomas. Microadenomas are more frequently seen in females, whereas macroadenomas are about even in males and females. The term *picoadenoma* has been used to describe lesions less than 3 mm in diameter.[22]

Table 26-1 Frequency of Pituitary Adenomas by Age, Gender, and Type of Hormone

Variable	Type of Adenoma
AGE	
First decade	ACTH-releasing adenoma
Second to fourth decade	PRL
Fifth to ninth decade	Nonfunctioning adenomas
Fifth decade	Even distribution of adenomas
GENDER	
Males	Nonfunctioning and GH-releasing adenomas
Females	PRL-, ACTH-releasing adenoma TSH-releasing adenoma
TYPE OF HORMONE*	
PRL (28%)	
GH (23%)	
ACTH (8%)	
Gonadotropin (6%)	
TSH (1%)	
Nonfunctioning adenoma (33%)	

*Type of hormone was ascertained from the functional classification of 3000 surgically removed pituitary adenomas. Data from Thapar K, Kovacs K, Laws ER: Pituitary tumors. *In* Black P, Loeffler J (eds): Cancer of the Nervous System. Cambridge, Blackwell Scientific, 1997, p 363.

ACTH, adrenocorticotropic hormone; GH, growth hormone; PRL, prolactin; TSH, thyroid-stimulating hormone.

Table 26-2 Pituitary: Anatomic Data

ANATOMIC TERMS
Pituitary: hypophysis
Anterior lobe: adenohypophysis
Posterior lobe: neurohypophysis

AVERAGE DIMENSIONS
Vertical: 6 mm
Anteroposterior: 8 mm
Transverse: 12 mm

ANATOMIC RELATIONSHIPS
Inferiorly: floor of the sella, sphenoid sinus
Anteriorly: tuberculum sellae, anterior clinoids
Posteriorly: dorsum sellae, posterior clinoids
Superiorly: diaphragma sellae, optic chiasm, hypothalamus
Laterally: cavernous sinus, internal carotid artery, cranial nerves III, IV, V, and VI

ANATOMY, PATHOLOGY, AND PATHWAYS OF SPREAD

Anatomy

The pituitary gland is an ovoid, reddish gray, midline intracranial organ occupying the sella turcica at the base of the middle cranial fossa. Anatomic terms and data about the pituitary are provided in Table 26-2.

The structural relationships are shown in Figure 26-1. The sella, shaped like a Turkish saddle, which gives it its name, is part of the superior surface of the body of the sphenoid bone. The posterior aspect of the sella projects anterosuperiorly, forming the dorsum sellae, and the lateral aspects of the dorsum sellae are expanded to form the posterior clinoid processes. Lateral to the sella is the cavernous sinus, which is traversed by cranial nerves III, IV, V_1,V_2, and VI and the internal carotid artery. The pituitary is covered by the dura, which superiorly forms a circular fold, the diaphragm sella. The optic chiasm lies immediately anterior to the sella of the diaphragm. Parasellar tumor growth can affect cranial nerves III, IV, V, and VI, and the suprasellar tumor extension leads to compression of the optic chiasm, which explains the bitemporal visual field changes associated with pituitary tumors. The pituitary has two distinct developmental origins, giving rise to the anterior and the posterior lobes of the pituitary.

Anterior Pituitary

The anterior pituitary, or the adenohypophysis, is derived from Rathke's pouch. Rathke's pouch is an upward outgrowth from the primitive oral cavity and is ectodermal in origin. The anterior pituitary accounts for about 80% of the adult pituitary and produces at least six hormones[23]: PRL, ACTH (corticotropin), follicle-stimulating hormone (FSH), luteinizing hormone (LH), GH, and TSH.

A vascular network that forms the hypophyseal portal system surrounds the infundibulum and connects the anterior lobe of the pituitary with the hypothalamus and has an important role in the regulation of these anterior pituitary hormones through the mechanism of releasing hormones from the hypothalamus. The anterior pituitary hormones are also regulated by a feedback mechanism of circulating hormones from the target glands.

Fifty percent of the anterior pituitary cells produce GH. These are acidophil cells, occupying the lateral wings of the pituitary. PRL-producing cells (15%) are scattered throughout the pituitary. ACTH-secreting cells (15% to 20%) are found in the anterolateral aspect of the pituitary. Gonadotropin-producing cells (10%) are scattered in the acidophil lateral wings. TSH-secreting cell (<10%) distribution is in the anterolateral aspect of the pituitary.

Posterior Pituitary

The neurohypophysis develops as an outgrowth of the diencephalon to form the posterior lobe of the pituitary and the infundibulum, which connects the pituitary to the hypothalamus. The posterior pituitary stores and releases two hormones, vasopressin (antidiuretic hormone [ADH]) and oxytocin, which are produced by the hypothalamus.

Intermediate Lobe

The intermediate lobe produces the melanocyte-stimulating hormone (MSH) and is smallest of the three pituitary lobes.

Hypothalamus-Pituitary Axis

The hypothalamic nuclei secrete neuroendocrine factors that control the release of the pituitary hormones. The axons of these nuclei end in the median eminence region of the infundibulum, where the following neuroendocrine factors are released and are transported to the pituitary through the pituitary-hypothalamic portal circulation: corticotropin-releasing factor, gonadotropin-releasing factor, thyrotropin-releasing factor, GH-releasing inhibitor (i.e., somatostatin), PRL inhibitory factor, and others such as dynorphins, enkephalins, and β-endorphin.

Pathology

In the past, pituitary tumors were classified according to Mallory's trichrome histologic staining and their association with various endocrinopathies. For example, Cushing's disease was associated with basophil adenoma, acromegaly with eosinophil adenoma, and nonfunctioning adenomas with

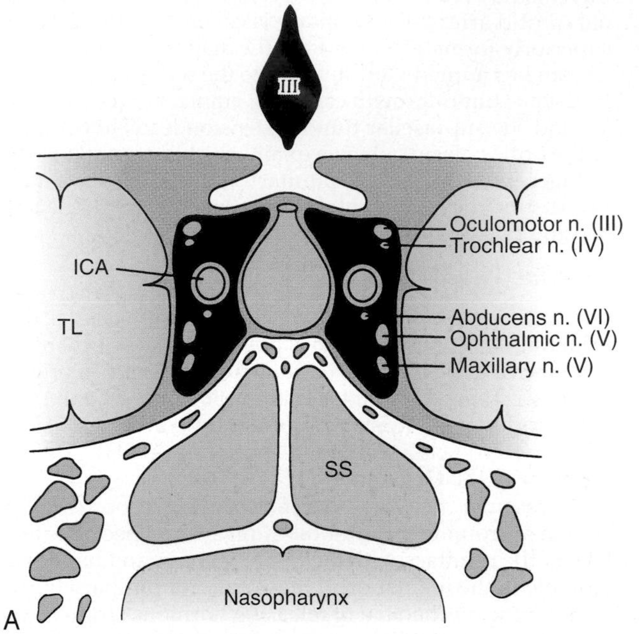

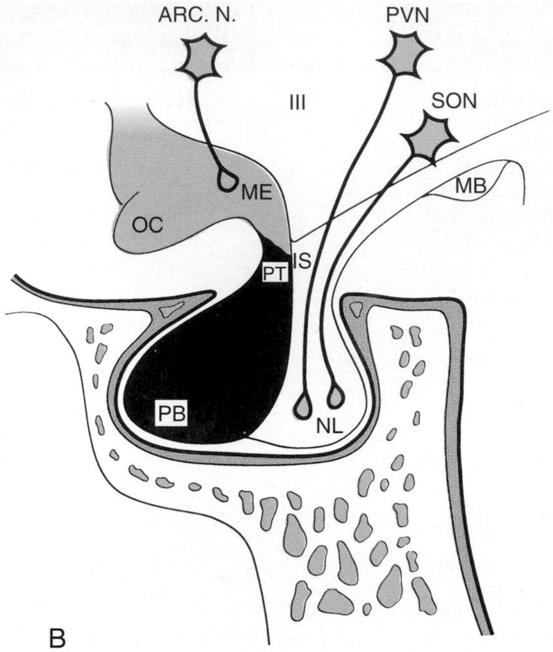

Figure 26-1 **A,** Anatomy of the sellar and parasellar regions. This coronal-view diagram illustrates the proximity of the pituitary gland to several important neural and vascular structures. The gland is laterally bordered by the cavernous sinuses *(black)*, which contain within their confines or their walls the carotid artery and the occulomotor, trochlear, maxillary, abducens, and first two divisions of the trigeminal nerves. The optic chiasm lies immediately superior to the gland. ICA, internal carotid artery; SS, sphenoid sinus; TL, temporal lobe; III, third ventricle. **B,** Anatomy of the pituitary gland. This sagittal-view diagram of the pituitary gland illustrates the hypothalamus, the pituitary stalk, and the pituitary gland located in the sella turcica. The anterior gland or adenohypophysis is composed of the pars distalis (PD), the rudimentary pars intermedia, and the pars tuberalis (PT). The posterior gland or neurohypophysis is composed of the median eminence (ME), located in the hypothalamus, the infundibular stem (IS), and the neural lobe (NL). The large neurons located in the supraoptic (SON) and paraventricular (PVN) nuclei project to the neural lobe where they store and release oxytocin and vasopressin into the systemic circulation under the appropriate stimulus. ARC N, arcuate nucleus; MB, mammillary bodies; OC, optic chiasm. (From Schwartz SI, et al [eds]: Principles of Surgery, 6th ed. New York, McGraw-Hill, 1994. Reproduced with permission of The McGraw-Hill Companies.)

chromophobe adenoma. With the advent of modern immunohistochemistry, electron microscopy, and studies of the distribution of the various secretory cells in the pituitary, a functional microscopic organizational view of the pituitary has emerged.[24] The pathologic hallmark of pituitary adenoma is described as the monotonous and monomorphous proliferation of neoplastic cells replacing the normal acinar pattern in the pituitary lobe. GH-producing cells are seen with greater frequency anteriorly in the lateral aspects of the pituitary. PRL-producing cells are distributed throughout the pituitary but have a greater density in the posterior aspects of the lateral aspect of the pituitary. ACTH-producing cells are present in the median wedge. TSH-producing cells are seen in the anterior aspect of the median wedge. Gonadotropin-producing cells are distributed throughout the anterior pituitary. There is overlap of the distribution of these functional hormonal secretory cells, and they do not reside in well-demarcated zones of the pituitary.

Burrow and associates[10] suggested the use of the following descriptions to distinguish hyperplasia from pituitary adenoma. *Pituitary adenomas* are characterized by uniformity of cells, a stromal pattern different from the gland, and evidence of compression of adjacent pituitary gland. *Pituitary hyperplasia* is characterized by diffuse or nodular accumulation of cells.

BIOLOGIC CHARACTERISTICS AND MOLECULAR BIOLOGY

Pituitary tumors occur sporadically or as part of hereditary endocrine syndromes. Hypothalamic, pituitary, and peripheral factors are involved in pituitary adenoma formation through complex genetic and hormonal signal disruptions.[25]

Pituitary tumors are monoclonal in origin, and tumorigenesis appears to be a multistep process through a sequence of initiation and tumor promotion steps. Several oncogenes and tumor suppressor genes appear to have a role in the initiation and progression of tumor growth. Initiation may occur with spontaneous or acquired mutations. This initial genetic event is associated with an allelic loss of an inhibitor gene or a hereditary or acquired genetic lesion. *MEN1* and *GSP1* (also designated *RAN*) genes have been implicated in the initiating events. Mutations have been shown in some GH-secreting adenomas[26] with up to 40% bearing the mutated *GSP1* gene. It may also play a role in nonfunctioning adenomas and ACTH-producing pituitary tumors. It has not been demonstrated to be of significance in prolactinomas or TSH-secreting tumors. *MEN1* gene mutations have been most commonly reported with familial pituitary tumors but have also been implicated with sporadic functioning and nonfunctioning tumors, including ACTH-secreting and prolactinomas.[27] Promotion, implying tumor expansion, is sustained by intrinsic or extrinsic promoting factors. The progression of tumors may be induced by the *TP53*, *RAS*, *RB1*, *NME1* (also designated *NM23*), and *MYC* genes.[27]

Tumor promotion and clonal expansion may involve hypothalamic hormones, paracrine growth factor, or peripheral hormone dysregulation of the pituitary.[25] Galectin-3 (Gal-3) is involved in cell growth, differentiation, and apoptosis. Immunohistochemical and Western blot analyses have demonstrated that only lactotroph (PRL) and corticotroph (ACTH) hormone-secreting cell lines and human tumor cells expressed Gal-3,[28] which may serve as a potential molecular target.

Increasing data support the hypothesis that intracellular signal transduction pathways important for hormonal regulation are also important in pituitary oncogenesis.[4] Three nuclear transcriptional factors that are targets of protein kinase C and A appear to play a role in hormone secretion and neoplastic growth for hormone-secreting tumors. These are activator protein-1 (AP-1), cAMP-responsive element binding protein (CREB), and pituitary-specific transcription factor (Pit-1). Most nonfunctioning adenomas do not appear to have a protein kinase C and A mediated mechanism. The cause of nonfunctioning pituitary adenomas remains unclear. However, epigenetic alterations such as hypermethylation of p16 have been associated with the formation of nonfunctioning pituitary adenomas.[28]

Seventy percent of the cases with tumor expansion and clinical presentations occur in 30- to 50-year-old patients, but tumors with the highest growth rate (PRL- and ACTH-secreting adenomas) are also seen in patients younger than 20 years. The doubling time for pituitary tumors ranges from 100 to 700 days, using Ki-67 antigen to assess the tumor growth fraction.[29,30]

A lack of inhibitory factors may also lead to tumor progression. For example, Nelson's syndrome results from ACTH-secreting pituitary adenomas after bilateral adrenalectomy for Cushing's disease and develops in 25% of such patients.[31] The resulting pituitary tumor, referred to as a corticotropinoma, can expand rapidly as a result of the negative feedback from the lack of adrenal glucocorticoids.

Prevalence of occult and clinically nonsignificant pituitary adenomas is not uncommon in unselected autopsy and imaging series.[3,9,10,12-15] This suggests that the initiating events are common. However, the prevalence of clinically overt tumors is quite low (0.02% to 0.025%),[18] suggesting that the influence of the tumor-promoting factors is uncommon. Non-cAMP–mediated activating oncogenes may play a role in the pathogenesis of aggressive adenomas.[32]

PREVENTION AND EARLY DETECTION

There is currently no prevention strategy to avoid the development of pituitary adenomas. When an endocrine abnormality is detected, referral to an endocrinologist is appropriate to correct and evaluate the cause of the abnormality, whether it is hypopituitarism, excess hormonal production, or management of diabetes insipidus. The routine use of endocrine or MRI screening of patients for detection of pituitary tumors is not recommended.

For patients with a familial disposition for the development of pituitary adenoma, as is the case with MEN1, mutational testing for the *MEN1* gene has been suggested for cases of classic MEN1, familial hyperparathyroidism, sporadic hyperparathyroidism with one other MEN1-related condition and for patients younger than 30 years with sporadic hyperparathyroidism and multigland hyperplasia. If MEN1 is detected or another familial syndrome associated with pituitary adenomas exists, consultation with an endocrinologist and a genetics specialist is appropriate, and diagnostic imaging should be used to detect suspected lesions based on clinical and laboratory findings. Obtaining a baseline MRI of the pituitary is reasonable; however, the routine imaging of the pituitary in the absence of clinical symptoms is not uniformly practiced.

CLINICAL MANIFESTATIONS, PATIENT EVALUATION, AND STAGING

Clinical Manifestations

The presence of a pituitary adenoma may come to attention as a result of the endocrine syndromes of pituitary dysfunction, neuro-ophthalmic manifestations from the pressure effects of an enlarging pituitary tumor, or the incidental discovery of pituitary adenoma during imaging studies of the brain for other reasons (Table 26-3). The usual cause of pituitary endocrine dysfunction in adults is a pituitary adenoma, whereas in children, it is craniopharyngioma. After a pituitary adenoma is suspected, evaluation and treatment of such patients benefit from a multidisciplinary management approach involving the endocrinologist, neurosurgeon, neuroradiologist, pathologist, ophthalmologist, radiation oncologist, and otorhinolaryngologist, depending on the nature of the abnormality detected.

Patient Evaluation

General Approach

As a first step, a detailed history and physical examination is obtained for the clinical assessment of the manifestations of the underlying endocrine disorder as well as neuro-ophthalmic changes from pressure effects of the tumor. Neurologic manifestations include headache from pressure effects on the dura, cranial nerve (III, IV, V, VI) abnormalities from extension into the cavernous sinus, and visual symptoms from suprasellar extension to the optic chiasm.

Ophthalmologic evaluation with formal visual field testing should be obtained in patients presenting with visual symptoms and those with extrasellar extensions of the tumor. Bi-temporal hemianopsia is classically associated with suprasellar extension of the pituitary tumor, causing compression of the anterior aspect of the optic chiasm. Other visual field defects can also occur. A baseline ophthalmologic assessment is appropriate for monitoring the results of therapy. This clinical assessment provides a useful guide for the subsequent laboratory and imaging evaluation of the patient by an endocrinologist, neuroradiologist, and ophthalmologist.

Laboratory Assessment

Initial tests of thyroid function and the PRL level are performed in addition to the individually tailored endocrine profile and specialized laboratory investigations determined by the clinical symptoms. The endocrine profile to be considered is influenced by the suspected clinical endocrine disorder and initial findings that would lead to a baseline measurement of ACTH, GH, FSH, LH, PRL, TSH (α subunit), thyroxine, cortisol, somatomedin C (i.e., insulin-like growth factor-1 [IGF-1]), testosterone, and estradiol as indicated (Table 26-4). There are physiologic variations in the blood and urine levels of these hormones, and the interpretation of results should be in the context of diurnal variations, age and gender of the patient, pregnancy, and menopausal status. The conditions under which the test samples are obtained (i.e., randomly, at specific times, or as part of a provocative test) also influence interpretations of the results that are obtained. In many circumstances, serum cortisol levels obtained during a hospitalization may not be reliable.

Imaging

MRI using gadolinium-diethylenetriaminepentaacetate (DTPA) enhancement is the imaging test of choice.[33,34] MRI has

Table 26-3 Clinical Manifestations of Pituitary Adenoma

Hormone or Type	Hypersecretion	Hyposecretion	Effect
ENDOCRINE SYNDROMES			
Prolactin	Galactorrhea-amenorrhea	As component of hypopituitarism	
Growth hormone	Gigantism Acromegaly	Short-stature disorders	
ACTH	Cushing's disease	Hypoadrenalism	
TSH	Hyperthyroidism	Hypothyroidism	
MSH	Nelson's syndrome		
FSH/LH		Hypogonadism	
TYPE OF MASS EFFECT			
General			Headache
Suprasellar			Headache, visual disturbances, bitemporal field loss
Parasellar			III, IV, V, VI cranial nerve palsy
Hypothalamus			Sleep, appetite, behavior disturbances
Third ventricle			Hydrocephalus
Temporal lobe			Seizures
Stalk compression			Hyperprolactinemia, usually <150 ng/mL
Intratumoral hemorrhage			Apoplexy; acute hypopituitarism/ visual field loss
INCIDENTAL DISCOVERY			
Asymptomatic disease			None; pituitary adenoma discovered on imaging study

ACTH, adrenocorticotropic hormone; FSH, follicle-stimulating hormone; LH, luteinizing hormone; MSH, melanocyte-stimulating hormone; TSH, thyroid-stimulating hormone.

Table 26-4 Normal Hormone Ranges

Hormone	Normal Level
Adrenocorticotropic hormone	10-52 pg/mL
Antidiuretic hormone	2-12 pg/mL
β-Human chorionic gonadotropin	Not detectable
Cortisol	
AM	3-20 μg/dL
PM	2.5-10 μg/dL
FSH	
Male	0.5-4.5 ng/mL
Premenopausal	1.1-5.3 ng/mL
Postmenopausal	11-66 ng/mL
Growth hormone	<5 ng/mL
Prolactin	
Adult female follicular	<20 ng/mL
Adult female luteal	<40 ng/mL
Adult male	<15 ng/mL
Somatostatin	
Fasting	<2.35 ng/mL
Postprandial	2.35-7.1 ng/mL
Thyroid-stimulating hormone	0.5-5.0 μU/mL

a high degree of sensitivity for microadenomas and macroadenomas of the pituitary, as well as other sellar and parasellar masses.[35] Thin slices, obtained before and after gadolinium sequences, and images in coronal, axial, and sagittal views provide detailed information for the initial diagnosis and are indispensable aids for surgical and radiotherapeutic treatment planning. The posterior lobe of the pituitary has high signal intensity on T1-weighted images ("posterior pituitary bright spot") that distinguishes it from the anterior lobe. The anterior lobe has a signal similar to the white matter. The diaphragma sellae has low signal intensity and aids the diagnosis of suprasellar extension. Microadenomas are usually hypointense, and macroadenomas are isodense on unenhanced T1-weighted image. Dynamic coronal imaging techniques after contrast medium administration enhance the normal pituitary earlier and more intensely and help delineate the presence of an adenoma.

In general, microadenomas have loss of signal intensity with gadolinium compared with the unaffected anterior pituitary gland. They often appear round or oval. High signal intensity, however, can be seen in the setting of internal hemorrhage, a finding frequently observed in prolactinomas.[22] On T2-weighted images, signal intensity of adenomas usually is hyperintense to that of the normal anterior lobe, but it may represent only a portion of the adenoma. Approximately 80% of microprolactinomas demonstrate high signal intensity, and approximately two thirds of those secreting GH are isointense or hypointense. Picoadenomas are often detected only on T2-weighted images.

Macroadenomas show compression of the adjacent pituitary and may distort the pituitary stalk, and the larger lesions demonstrate extrasellar extension (Fig. 26-2). When there is extrasellar extension, the diagnostic MRI helps delineate the relation to normal anatomic structures, particularly the cavernous sinus laterally and the optic chiasm superiorly. Compression and involvement of the cavernous sinus remain often difficult to distinguish, but more than 50% to complete encasement of the intracavernous carotid artery usually represents involvement. If a plane of normal pituitary tissue can be observed on coronal-view, T1-enhanced images, the likelihood of cavernous sinus involvement is extraordinarily low. When there is significant suprasellar extension, the optic chiasm can be difficult to identify and may be best seen on coronal-view, fast spin-echo T2-weighted images. Rarely, macroadenomas are so large that they cause obstruction of the

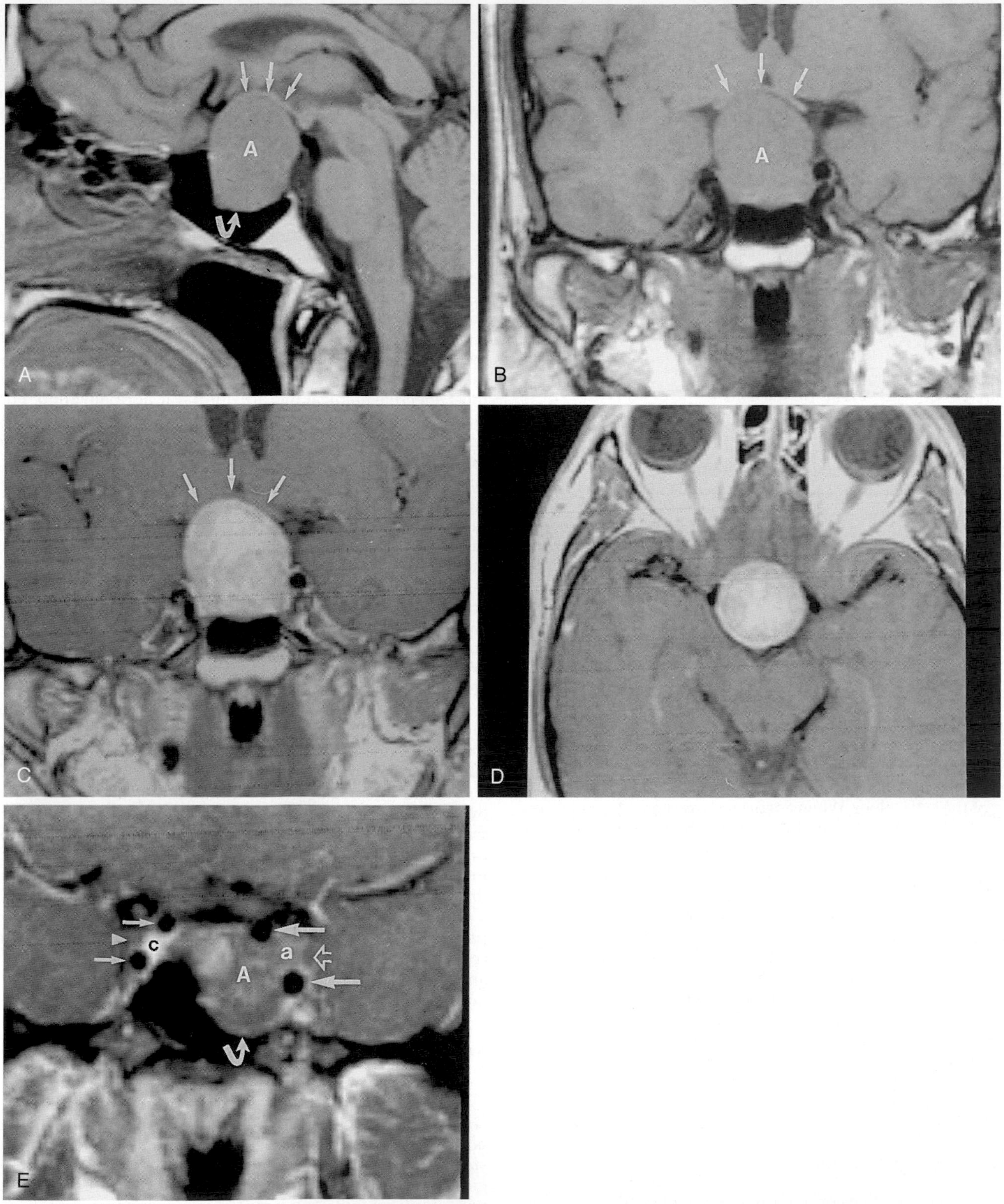

Figure 26-2 MRI of pituitary adenoma to demonstrate extrasellar extensions. **A,** Sagittal-view, non–contrast-enhanced, T1-weighted image demonstrates a large, homogeneous, intermediate-signal-intensity mass that is consistent with a pituitary macroadenoma (A). Inferiorly, the mass has enlarged the sella and extended into the superior aspect of the sphenoid sinus *(curved arrow)*. The mass extends into the suprasellar cistern and superiorly displaces the optic chiasm *(straight arrows)*. **B,** Coronal-view, non–contrast-enhanced, T1-weighted image of the same patient illustrated in **A** further demonstrates the suprasellar extension of the adenoma (A) and the superior displacement of the optic chiasm *(arrows)*. **C,** Coronal-view, contrast-enhanced T1-weighted image of the same patient illustrated in **A** shows dense, homogeneous enhancement of the mass. The *arrows* show the superiorly displaced optic nerve. **D,** Axial-view, contrast-enhanced, T1-weighted image of the same patient illustrated in **A** shows extension of the mass into the suprasellar cistern. **E,** Coronal-view, contrast-enhanced, T1-weighted image through the sella shows an enhancing pituitary adenoma in another patient. The mass extends inferiorly into the roof of the sphenoid sinus *(curved arrow)*. The mass extends laterally to invade the cavernous sinus (a). Notice the lateral displacement of the oculomotor nerve *(open arrow)* and the widening of the distance between the intracavernous segments of the internal carotid artery *(large straight arrows)*. Compare this with the normal appearance of the cavernous sinus on the uninvolved side. Other identified features are the normally enhancing cavernous sinus (c), oculomotor nerve *(arrowhead)*, and intracavernous segments of the internal carotid artery *(small straight arrows)*. (Courtesy of S. Mukherjee, MD, Department of Radiology, University of North Carolina at Chapel Hill, NC.)

Table 26-5 Classification of Pituitary Tumors*

GRADE: RELATIONSHIP OF ADENOMA TO SELLA AND SPHENOID SINUSES
Floor of sella intact
I: sella normal or focally expanded; tumor <10 mm
II: sella enlarged; tumor ≥10 mm
Sphenoid
III: localized perforation of sellar floor
IV: diffuse perforation of sellar floor
Distant spread
V: spread by cerebrospinal fluid or blood
STAGE: EXTRASELLAR EXTENSION
Suprasellar
O: none
A: occupies cistern
B: recesses of third ventricle obliterated
C: third ventricle grossly displaced
Parasellar extension
D: intracranial (intradural)
E: into or beneath cavernous sinus (extradural)

*Hardy classification[36] as modified by Wilson.[37]

Modified from Wilson CB: Neurosurgical management of large and invasive pituitary tumors. *In* Tinadall GT, Collins WF (eds): Clinical Management of Pituitary Disorders. New York, Raven Press, 1979, p 335.

third ventricle. Pituitary apoplexy is caused by intratumoral hemorrhage and can be seen on T1-weighted images as high signal intensity.

High-resolution computed tomography (CT) may be substituted when MRI is contraindicated or unavailable. CT scans are useful in neurosurgical planning for transsphenoidal surgery. Bone windows provide useful information about the pneumatization of the sphenoid sinus and about cortical thinning of the sellar floor. When aneurysms are considered within the radiographic differential diagnosis, the use of angiogram may be of assistance.

Staging

Most pituitary adenomas remain asymptomatic and undetected. Adenomas become clinically apparent with three growth patterns: intrasellar, extrasellar, or massive. Extrasellar growth includes tumor extension or invasion into suprasellar, parasellar, or infrasellar structures. Hardy's classification[36] is used in surgical assessment. Wilson's modification of Hardy's classification (Table 26-5) incorporates imaging and intraoperative findings of sellar destruction (grade) and extrasellar extension (stage).[37] Although stage and grade are defined, they are not routinely used in clinical radiation oncology practice.

PRIMARY THERAPY

The primary objectives of therapy are to rectify the endocrine dysfunction, reverse the neuro-ophthalmic changes of the mass effects, and remove the pituitary adenoma or restrict its growth. Modern pharmacologic management, neurosurgical procedures, and radiation therapy techniques increasingly accomplish these goals with a high degree of success.

Medical Therapy

Medical therapies are indicated to perform two activities: treat the hormonal dysfunction and reduce the size of the adenoma. Their role is primary therapy or as an adjunct to other interventions.

Dopamine agonists such as bromocriptine or cabergoline are the initial treatment of choice for prolactinomas, and they are highly efficacious in controlling hyperprolactinemia. Tumor regression of prolactinomas and improvement in the mass effect of enlarged adenomas are observed with medical treatment alone. Long-term maintenance treatment is necessary to control hyperprolactinemia and growth of prolactinoma.

For GH-secreting tumors, dopamine agonists are also used. However, somatostatin analogues such as octreotide or lanreotide are indicated for lowering the elevated GH levels before surgery and while awaiting radiation therapy control of GH-secreting adenoma. Pegvisomant, a GH receptor antagonist, has also been investigated and plays a role in management of acromegaly.[38] Early data suggest that IGF-1 normalization occurs in 97% of patients and appears to be the most effective medical therapy for IGF-1 normalization. Long-term follow-up studies are required, but its use in patients who have incomplete resection of tumors and who receive radiation is increasing.

Pharmacologic treatment can also restore hormone deficiencies resulting from the pressure effects of the pituitary tumor on adjacent normal pituitary and those resulting from the surgical and radiation therapy management of the pituitary adenomas. Hypopituitarism can have variable clinical manifestations, and management should be individualized and provided by an endocrinologist. The use of glucocorticoids, gonadal steroids, and thyroid hormones is often indicated. Commonly used glucocorticoid replacement therapies are hydrocortisone and cortisone acetate. Commonly used gonadal steroids are estrogen and progestin for women and testosterone for men. Thyroid replacement is typically done with L-thyroxine. GH deficiency as a component of hypopituitarism and the use of GH for treatment have been outlined in consensus guidelines.[39]

Medical management of hormonal dysfunction due to oversecretion or undersecretion can have significant effects on quality of life and longevity. Although it may not be an immediately life-threatening condition in a manner seen with many metastatic malignancies, its effects can be seen in activities of daily living, cognitive functioning, and life expectancy.

Central diabetes insipidus is an uncommon finding in patients presenting with a pituitary tumor, but it occurs more commonly after surgical intervention. Management with antidiuretic agents such as arginine vasopressin (pitressin) or desmopressin acetate (dDAVP) is typically indicated.

Surgery

Advances in transsphenoidal approaches with microsurgical techniques have made this procedure the initial treatment of choice for acromegaly, Cushing's disease, nonfunctioning adenomas, and in situations requiring immediate decompression, such as progressive visual loss or pituitary hemorrhage. Surgical therapy is used for patients with prolactinoma who are noncompliant with, intolerant to, or unresponsive to medical therapy. Surgery has also been useful in reducing the tumor bulk for combined management with radiation therapy and medical therapy.

In transsphenoidal surgery of the pituitary, the initial step involves one of the following four approaches to the sphenoid in conjunction with the otorhinologic surgeon: transnasal, sublabial/transseptal, transethmoidal, or transantral. The transsphenoidal approach has become less invasive with a newer approach of endoscopic, minimally invasive pituitary surgery (MIPS) (Fig. 26-3).[40] This approach avoids nasal or intraoral incisions, nasal speculums, or nasal packing. It

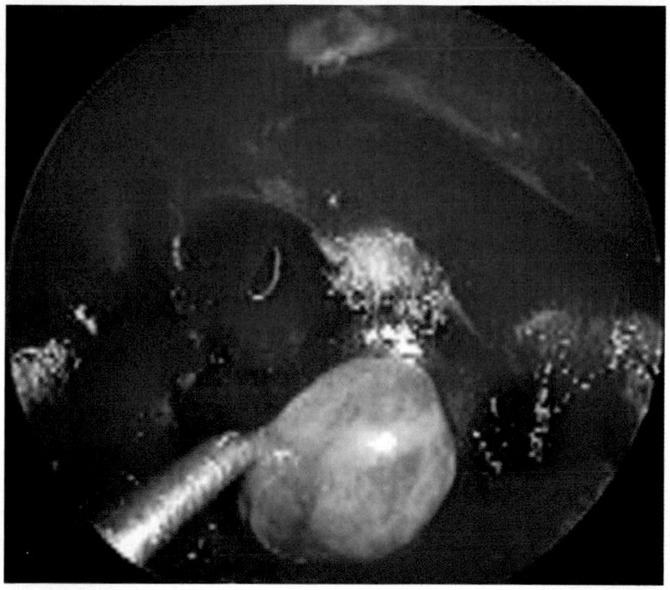

Figure 26-3 Transsphenoidal endoscopic removal of pituitary tumor.

appears to show a decreased complication rate compared with traditional sublabial transseptal approaches.

The transsphenoidal technique is the preferred approach for microadenoma and for pituitary tumors with extension toward the sphenoid sinus. Macroadenoma with suprasellar extension can also be approached transsphenoidally. Decompression of the optic chiasm is obtained, and removal of the intrasellar tumor permits removal of the suprasellar tumor. Transcranial surgery is reserved for large intracranial extensions and in cases in which transsphenoidal surgery has technical limitations, such as small sella and inadequate pneumatization of the sphenoid sinus.

Surgical series report a curative surgical resection rate of approximately 74% for microprolactinomas and 32% for macroprolactinomas, as characterized by a normalization of the prolactin level 1 to 12 weeks after completion of surgery.[41] Long-term surgical cure rates are 50% to 60% and 25% for microprolactinomas and macroprolactinomas, respectively. Surgical series for Cushing's disease suggest a curative surgical resection rate of greater than 75%, with no further requirement for treatment. Acromegaly is surgically cured in 50% or more of cases.

Radiation Therapy

Radiation therapy is selectively used as postoperative treatment after subtotal removal of the pituitary adenoma, in recurrent pituitary adenoma after surgical treatment, and as primary treatment when surgery is contraindicated. Options for the radiotherapeutic management of pituitary tumors include conventionally fractionated external beam radiation therapy or single-fraction stereotactic radiosurgery (SRS).

Radiation therapy equipment, techniques, and doses have evolved greatly since the first reports of radiation therapy for pituitary tumors in 1907 by Gramegna[42] and by Beclere.[43] Subsequent advances in radiation therapy have led to modern radiation techniques that include the use of megavoltage linear accelerators, sophisticated three-dimensional (3D) treatment planning systems, incorporation of CT and MRI radiologic studies, stereotactic guidance, and simulators for target localization.

Stereotactic Radiosurgery

SRS, the use of a highly focused, single, large fraction of ionizing radiation to a small, intracranial target volume, has been performed in the treatment of selected patients with pituitary adenomas.[44] Results of proton beam,[45] helium ions,[46] gamma knife,[47,48] and linear accelerator (Linac) SRS[49-51] techniques have been reported. In a review of the results of SRS and conventional radiation therapy of pituitary tumors, Alexander and Loeffler[51] stated that the radiographic and hormonal responses were more rapid with SRS for functioning tumors, but no data are available to demonstrate a long-term difference. Acute and subacute effects, such as edema and cranial neuropathies, are more likely with SRS for larger tumors, but late effects, such as cognitive dysfunction, encephalomalacia, and secondary tumors, are almost exclusively seen after conventional radiation therapy and not with SRS.[52]

Two systematic reviews were performed to evaluate the role of stereotactic radiosurgery. Jalali and Brada[53] concluded that there is little justification for the routine use of single-fraction stereotactic radiosurgery for most patients with benign pituitary adenomas because of the lack of convincing evidence for more rapid reduction of elevated hormones, minimal long-term control data, and higher toxicity than that seen with conventional radiation therapy techniques. On the contrary, Laws and coworkers[54] performed a review of the literature on SRS consisting of 34 published studies that included 1567 patients. In that review, the tumor growth control rate was approximately 90% (range, 68% to 100%), with various rates of hormonal normalization for functioning adenomas. The endocrine "cure" rate for functioning pituitary adenomas treated with SRS is approximately 50%, varying from 10% to 100% for Cushing's disease, 0% to 100% for acromegaly, 0% to 84% for prolactinomas, and 0% to 36% for Nelson's syndrome.

Results with SRS vary and are difficult to compare with other treatment modalities because of the wide range of peripheral doses used, different prescription isodose lines, variation in reporting response, and selection bias in its use. A wide range of doses to the periphery or margin of the tumor has been reported, ranging from 12 to 35 Gy at the 50% to 100% isodose line. No obvious dose-response relationship has been demonstrated, but it is believed that lower doses (12 to 18 Gy) are needed for nonfunctioning adenomas and higher doses (18 to 35 Gy) for functioning pituitary tumors. Efficacy of SRS for functioning pituitary adenomas may be compromised by the concomitant use of hormone suppressing medical therapies. These drugs are typically stopped several weeks before SRS and not restarted until several weeks afterward. The SRS dose given for pituitary adenomas is usually limited because of adjacent critical structures, particularly the optic nerves and chiasm.

The optic chiasm is a major dose-limiting critical structure in SRS treatment planning. Single-fraction dose to the optic chiasm in general should be limited to 8 Gy to minimize damage to the visual pathways, but the tolerance may be higher. Stafford and associates[55] performed a retrospective review to evaluate the risk of clinically significant radiation optic neuropathy (RON) for patients having undergone SRS of benign tumors adjacent to optic apparatus. With a median maximum radiation dose to the optic nerve of 10 Gy, 1.9% developed RON despite 73% of the patients receiving more than 8 Gy. The RON developed at a median of 48 months after radiosurgery. They suggested a clinically significant RON risk of 1.1% for those who receive 12 Gy or less to a small segment of the optic apparatus. Accurate localization of the target volume and the optic chiasm using MRI is essential.

Interstitial Therapy

Joplin[56] reviewed the technique and use of yttrium 90 (^{90}Y) for interstitial radiation therapy of pituitary adenomas. This technique was developed for pituitary ablation in the hormonal treatment of patients with advanced breast cancer using ^{198}Au, which was later replaced by ^{90}Y. ^{90}Y is a pure beta emitter with maximum energy of 2.2 MeV and half-life of 64 hours. In this permanent implant procedure, two 7-mm ^{90}Y seeds are implanted into the pituitary 3 mm apart through a transsphenoidal approach. A dose of 500 Gy is used for prolactinoma macroadenoma to suppress PRL, 1000 Gy for Cushing's disease, and up to 1500 Gy for acromegaly with highly active GH-producing adenoma. This approach is rarely used in clinical practice in the United States.

INDIVIDUAL SYNDROMES AND SPECIFIC TUMORS

Prolactinoma

Clinical Manifestations

Gonadal dysfunction (e.g., amenorrhea, oligomenorrhea, infertility, loss of libido) and galactorrhea are the more common symptoms related to hyperprolactinemia (Table 26-6). Headaches, visual field changes, and hypopituitarism resulting from pressure effects are more commonly seen with macroadenomas. In women with amenorrhea, 10% to 40% have hyperprolactinemia, and in women with amenorrhea and galactorrhea, 75% have PRL-secreting tumors. Prolactinomas are seen in 30% of women with amenorrhea after oral contraceptive use.

PRL excess in men causes impotence and infertility. Hyperprolactinemia leads to diminished FSH and LH levels and a decline in serum testosterone levels. Galactorrhea and gynecomastia are rarely seen in men with hyperprolactinemia.

Pathology

Prolactinomas are the most common functioning pituitary adenomas. Asymptomatic microadenomas are found in 5% to 20% of unselected autopsy series. PRL-secreting carcinomas are rare. Microprolactinomas are more common than macroprolactinomas and have earlier diagnosis in women because of symptoms of menstrual irregularities and galactorrhea. Ninety percent of microprolactinomas are found in women, whereas 60% of macroprolactinomas are found in men.

Prolactinomas may grow during pregnancy. With medical treatment of microprolactinomas, pregnancy outcome is uneventful in 95% of patients. Asymptomatic enlargement of prolactinomas occurs in 5% of microprolactinoma and symptomatic enlargement in 15% of macroprolactinoma patients during pregnancy.

Evaluation

A careful clinical and drug history, detection of elevated serum PRL level, and neuroradiologic examination of the pituitary region help establish a diagnosis of prolactinoma. Elevated PRL level can result from several different causes (Table 26-7) that should be carefully investigated. Elevated PRL level should be confirmed on at least two occasions because physiologic variations and elevations can occur from stress. Common conditions that have been associated with hyperprolactinemia besides prolactinomas include end-stage renal disease, renal insufficiency, depression, primary hypothyroidism, acquired immunodeficiency syndrome, sarcoidosis, and nonalcoholic cirrhosis.

Macroprolactinomas are associated with a serum PRL level higher than 200 ng/mL. Lower levels may indicate microprolactinoma or peripituitary tumor (i.e., pseudoprolactinoma), the result of tumor pressure on the infundibulum that interferes with the negative inhibitory control of PRL secretion by the hypothalamus. Pituitary stalk compression may cause elevated PRL levels in the range of 150 ng/mL or less. Determination of the source of the prolactin elevation is important because treatment of nonsecreting tumors typically is surgical, whereas others typically are managed medically with dopamine agonists.

Serum PRL should be assessed in all patients with galactorrhea or hypogonadism. A detailed drug history is necessary to evaluate drug-related causes of hyperprolactinemia. Common medications associated with elevated prolactin levels include antidepressants, protease inhibitors, verapamil, and phenothiazines. A pregnancy test is mandatory for women with amenorrhea or hyperprolactinemia. Elevated serum PRL levels result from a variety of causes; however, levels higher than 300 ng/mL are usually diagnostic of pituitary adenoma, and levels higher than 100 ng/mL in nonpregnant patients often are associated with a pituitary adenoma. Suckling-induced episodic elevation of PRL levels

Table 26-6 Prolactinoma: Key Points

- Most common functioning pituitary tumor, more common in females
- Microadenoma more common in females, macroadenoma in males
- Clinical presentation: amenorrhea, infertility, galactorrhea
- Diagnosis: hyperprolactinemia, MRI findings of adenoma
- Treatment
  - Use of a dopamine agonist (e.g., bromocriptine) is the primary approach.
  - Transsphenoidal surgery is used after failed medical therapy.
  - Radiation therapy has a limited role.
  - Asymptomatic adenomas require no treatment.
- Outcome: normal prolactin levels in 80% to 90% with dopamine agonists

Table 26-7 Prolactinoma: Causes of Hyperprolactinemia

Physiologic causes
- Pregnancy, breast-feeding, renal failure

Pharmacologic causes
- Tricyclic antidepressants, protease inhibitors, cocaine, verapamil, fluoxetine
- Dopamine-blocking drugs: phenothiazines, butyrophenones, metoclopramide
- Dopamine-depleting drugs: methyldopa, reserpine

Pathologic conditions
- Decreased clearance of prolactin in renal disease
- Dopamine inhibition overcome by estrogens and in hypothyroidism
- Decreased dopamine or dopamine inhibitory conditions
- Hypothalamic tumors: hyperprolactinemia in 20% to 50%
- Pituitary prolactin-secreting adenoma

Laboratory findings
- Normal prolactin levels
  - Women, nonpregnant: <20 ng/mL
  - Women, pregnant: 100-300 ng/mL
  - Men: <15 ng/mL
- Prolactinoma prolactin levels
  - Macroprolactinoma: >200 ng/mL

during breast-feeding declines after 6 months despite continued breast-feeding.

Imaging

MRI is the imaging modality of choice to detect abnormalities in the hypothalamic-pituitary region as a cause of hyperprolactinemia. Size and location of the tumor as well as extrasellar extent can be assessed. High-resolution CT and MRI can visualize microprolactinomas 2 to 3 mm and larger.

Treatment

INDICATIONS AND SELECTION OF TREATMENT

Treatment options include close surveillance, surgery, irradiation, and medical therapy (Fig. 26-4). Medical therapy is most often the treatment of choice when intervention is warranted. Treatment in patients with prolactinomas is indicated for the management of troublesome galactorrhea, menstrual irregularities, and infertility in women and for decreased libido, impotency, and infertility in men. Patients with macroprolactinomas require therapy for growth control of adenoma and hyperprolactinemia. Patients with asymptomatic microadenomas can be followed with periodic PRL assessments.[57] Most prolactin microadenomas do not progress to macroadenoma.[58] More than 90% fail to enlarge over a 4- to 6-year period of observation.[59] However, prolactin levels may change significantly without a significant change in tumor size. Most patients can be followed by serial prolactin levels, with repeat scanning indicated for significant rises in prolactin levels.

MEDICAL THERAPY

For patients with prolactinoma, medical management is the initial treatment of choice.[60] Dopamine agonists such as bromocriptine are successful in 80% to 90% of the patients. Bromocriptine is started at 1.25 mg, given orally once daily at night, with gradually increasing dose to reach a maintenance dose of 5 to 7.5 mg/day, adjusting for side effects of nausea and vomiting, fatigue, and postural hypotension. Menstrual and ovulatory irregularities and PRL levels are restored in more than 90% of the patients, despite the fact that prolactin levels returned to normal in 70% to 80% of patients. Tumor regression and relief of mass effects are observed with bromocriptine therapy in more than 80% of patients, with more than 40% having greater than 50% tumor size reduction. The time course for tumor reduction is variable with changes reported as late as 1 year of follow-up. Higher bromocriptine doses may be necessary in men with macroadenomas.

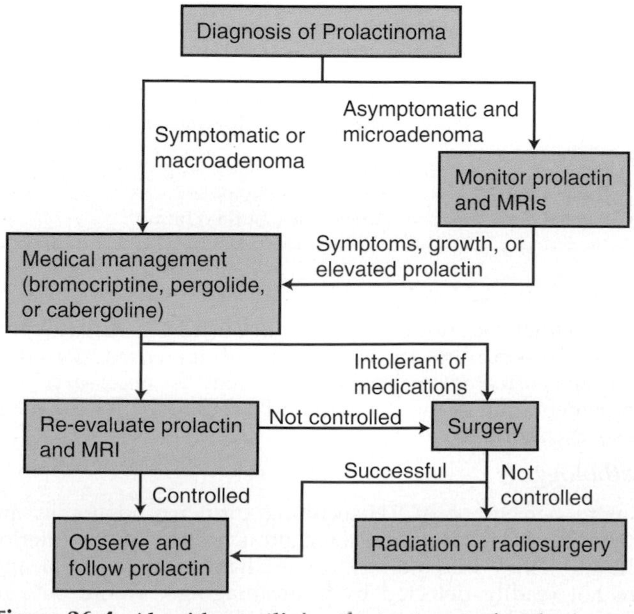

Figure 26-4 **Algorithm outlining the treatment of prolactinoma.**

Since the advent of bromocriptine, several other dopamine agonists have been developed, including pergolide, quinagolide, and cabergoline. Of the newer dopamine agonists, pergolide is not approved by the U.S. Food and Drug Administration (FDA) for hyperprolactinemia, but its use is well documented in the literature for microprolactinomas with single daily doses of 50 to 250 mg.

Quinagolide has fewer side effects and the convenience of once-daily dosage. It is a nonergot dopamine agonist, and approximately 50% of patients who are resistant to bromocriptine respond to quinagolide.[59]

Cabergoline has been demonstrated to be at least as effective as bromocriptine in lowering prolactin levels and reducing tumor size with fewer side effects. It needs to be taken only once or twice weekly because of its long half-life. In a double-blinded study of 459 women[61] comparing bromocriptine and cabergoline over 8 weeks, normoprolactinemia was achieved in 59% compared with 83%, respectively. Twelve percent stopped taking bromocriptine, and 3% discontinued cabergoline. A unique feature of cabergoline is that it can be administered intravaginally.

PRL level is monitored at 3-month intervals for the first year and then annually. PRL levels return to normal range in more than 80% of the patients by 6 months and in 90% by 1 year.[60] Tumor regression and visual field improvement also occur in 80% to 90% of the patients. Bromocriptine may be gradually withdrawn every 2 to 3 years to assess remission. Patients need to be assessed for surgery if they are noncompliant, cannot tolerate therapy, or do not respond to medical therapy.

SURGERY

Results of surgical therapy depend on the size of the prolactinoma and the baseline PRL level. In a review of several surgical series, Reilly[62] identified normal PRL levels in 60% to 90% of the patients with microadenomas, providing a prompt relief of hyperprolactinemia. However, long-term results show an appreciable relapse rate. From a review of 34 surgical series, the curative surgical resection rate for microprolactinomas is approximately 74%, and for macroprolactinomas, it is 32%, as characterized by a normalization of the prolactin level 1 to 12 weeks after completion of surgery.[41] Long-term surgical cure rates of 50% to 60% and 25% for microprolactinomas and macroprolactinomas, respectively, are reported.

Surgery is indicated in patients who are noncompliant with medications, do not tolerate long-term medical therapy, or who have an unsatisfactory response to medical management. Surgical therapy may be required for partial responders, those with macroadenomas, and patients who cannot tolerate medical management.

RADIATION THERAPY

With the successful results of dopamine agonists as primary therapy and transsphenoidal surgery as secondary therapy, radiation therapy is not required in the routine management of prolactinomas. The risk of hypopituitarism after radiation treatment makes radiation therapy a less favorable option in young women with prolactinoma. However, radiation therapy is valuable after unsuccessful medical and surgical therapy or when the patient's medical condition precludes surgical treatment. After radiation therapy, PRL levels decrease gradually

Table 26-8 Prolactinoma: Results of Radiation Therapy

Study	*N*	Treatment	Follow-Up (y)	Results
Grigsby et al[65] (1988)	17	RT	6.4 (minimum)	82% NED
Littley et al[63] (1991)	58	S + RT, RT	≤12.8	50% at 10 y, PRL <500 mU/L
Tsagarakis et al[64] (1991)	36	RT	8.5 (mean)	50%, normal PRL
Pan et al[66] (2000)	128	SRS	<3 (mean)	15% (<30 ng/mL)

NED, no evidence of disease; PRL, prolactin; RT, radiation therapy; S, surgery; SRS, stereotactic radiosurgery.

over several years and interval treatment with dopamine agonists is required.

Table 26-8 summarizes the results of radiation therapy reported in three studies.[63-65] and one SRS series.[66] In a series of 58 patients treated with external beam radiation therapy, Littley and associates[63] found a decrease in the serum PRL levels in all patients and 50% probability of PRL level reduction to 500 mU/L in 10 years. Patients with smaller tumors, pretreatment PRL levels higher than 6000 mU/L, and tumors with positive immunostaining for PRL were more likely to achieve normalization of serum PRL levels after radiation therapy. Tsagarakis and colleagues[64] reported normal serum PRL levels at a mean of 8.5 years after radiation treatment in 18 of 36 patients. Pituitary irradiation can lead to hypothalamic dysfunction and impairment of dopamine secretion that causes hyperprolactinemia and may explain the mildly elevated PRL levels (usually <50 mU/L) in some patients after radiation therapy of pituitary adenomas.

Twenty-three published studies of patients treated with SRS have been reported.[54] Median follow-up of greater than 12 months was reported in all except one study. Reported doses prescribed to the margin ranged between 13 and 33 Gy with a median dose of 20 Gy. The most commonly prescribed dose was 15 Gy to the tumor margin. Using a cure rate defined most frequently as a normal serum prolactin level, endocrine cure rates ranged between 0% and 84% (median 20%) with six reports having no endocrine cures and only three studies (all with less than 20 patients) having greater than 50% cure rates. Although a substantial reduction in prolactin levels has been seen, the use of SRS for prolactinomas should be selective.

CUSHING'S DISEASE

Clinical Manifestations

Cushing's syndrome results from manifestations of hypercortisolism from a variety of causes. These include excessive ACTH secretion (i.e., Cushing's disease), adrenal pathology, steroid therapy, or ectopic production from a variety of tumors (i.e., carcinoid, thymoma, small cell carcinoma, pheochromocytoma, islet cell tumor, and prostate cancer) (Table 26-9). Cushing's disease, first described by Harvey Cushing in 1912,[2] results from an ACTH-secreting adenoma of the corticotroph cells of the anterior pituitary, which is responsible for 80% of ACTH-dependent Cushing's syndrome cases. Non-ACTH–dependent causes include primary adrenocortical hyperplasia, adenoma or carcinoma, and prolonged glucocorticoid therapy, which is the most common cause of Cushing's syndrome.

Cushing's syndrome is more common in women and is recognized by a constellation of clinical and biochemical features that include truncal obesity, hirsutism, acne, easy bruisability, muscle weakness, moon facies, menstrual irregularities and gonadal dysfunction, hypertension, diabetes mellitus, and osteoporosis (Table 26-10).

Table 26-9 Cushing's Disease: Key Points

- Cushing's disease caused by an adrenocorticotropic hormone (ACTH)–secreting pituitary adenoma should be differentiated from causes of Cushing's syndrome
- Incidence: 0.4 to 2.4 cases per 1 million people; 10% of surgically resected pituitary tumors; 80% of endogenous Cushing's disease
- Age: 30 to 60 years
- Sex: 3-10:1 preponderance in females
- Onset: insidious, occurring over several years
- Clinical features: multiple-organ effects of hypercortisolism
- Laboratory tests: elevated ACTH and urinary cortisol levels, inferior petrosal sinus sampling
- Imaging: MRI; 90% of findings are microadenomas
- Other studies: neuro-ophthalmic, endocrine evaluation
- Treatment
  - Transsphenoidal surgery is the treatment of choice, with medical management of the complications of hypercortisolism.
  - Radiation therapy for patients not suitable for surgery, as adjunct to surgery, or for postsurgical recurrence.
  - Medical therapy uses inhibitors of steroidogenesis (e.g., mitotane, ketoconazole).

Table 26-10 Cushing's Syndrome: Clinical Features

- Cardiovascular disease: hypertension, atherosclerosis, congestive heart failure
- Gonadal and endocrine dysfunction: amenorrhea, infertility, diabetes mellitus
- Musculoskeletal disorders: osteoporosis, vertebral fractures, proximal muscle wasting, weakness
- Neuropsychiatric features: headache, visual symptoms less common; anxiety, irritability, steroid psychosis
- Skin changes: skin thinning, purple striae, plethora, hirsutism, acne
- Susceptibility to infections
- Tissue fragility: easy bruisability, ecchymoses
- Truncal fat deposition: moon facies, buffalo hump

It cannot be understated that Cushing's disease and Cushing's syndrome are associated with increased morbidity and age-corrected mortality. Treatment is necessary, and implementation of therapy should be initiated after the diagnosis is confirmed.

Pathology

Ninety percent of ACTH-secreting pituitary adenomas are microadenomas located in the central portion of the anterior pituitary; they infrequently cause changes in the sella and are not readily detected by neuroimaging.[67] About 50% of the macroadenomas are invasive. These adenomas have

Table 26-11 Cushing's Disease: Results of Surgery

Study	*N*	Remission (%)	Relapse (%)
Bochicchio et al[70] (1995)	668	76	13
Knappe and Luedecke[73] (1995)	287	92	11
Invitti et al[74] (1999)	288	69	17

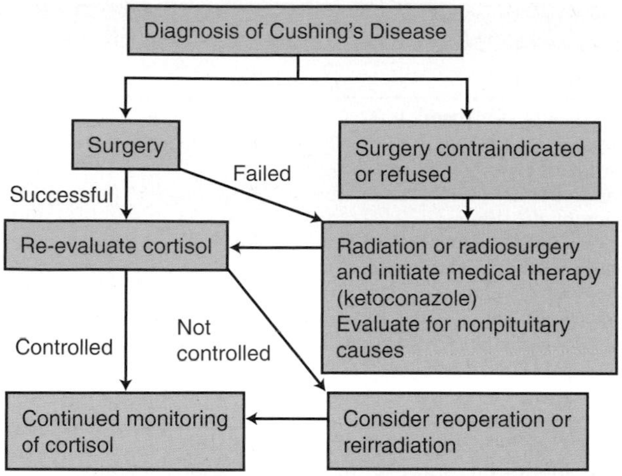

Figure 26-5 Algorithm outlining the treatment of Cushing's disease.

monomorphic basophil cells that are periodic acid–Schiff positive. Immunochemistry detects the presence of ACTH and its precursors in the adenoma.

Evaluation

It is critical to determine the precise cause of Cushing's syndrome, to establish the diagnosis of Cushing's disease, and to distinguish ACTH-secreting pituitary adenoma from other causes of the syndrome. This is accomplished by biochemical tests and pituitary MRI.

Laboratory Assessment

In Cushing's disease, serum ACTH level and urinary free cortisol excretion are elevated. Studies may have to be repeated on several occasions, because some tumors produce the hormones sporadically. An overnight 1-mg dose of dexamethasone fails to suppress the serum cortisol level in Cushing's disease. High-dose dexamethasone suppression test helps distinguish an ACTH-secreting pituitary adenoma from an ectopic ACTH-producing tumor. Serum cortisol levels are suppressed in ACTH-secreting pituitary adenoma but not in ectopic tumors. Bilateral venous blood sampling from the inferior petrosal sinus before and after corticotropin-releasing factor administration has a high sensitivity in detecting intrapituitary ACTH adenoma[68] and in differentiating this from an ectopic ACTH-secreting adenoma. This technique is helpful in lateralizing ACTH-secreting adenoma in the pituitary for consideration of hemihypophysectomy.

Imaging

Although MRI is the imaging modality of choice for Cushing's disease, microadenomas are not readily detectable by neuroimaging. T1-weighted images with and without gadolinium enhancement detect 70% of the pituitary macroadenomas in patients with Cushing's disease, and suprasellar and parasellar extensions can be assessed.[35,69] The presence of pituitary adenoma helps differentiate pituitary from ectopic tumor as a cause of Cushing's syndrome. Pituitary adenomas in Cushing's disease are mostly microadenomas and do not cause enlargement of the sella. Other significant radiologic findings may be related to osteoporosis and fractures of vertebrae and ribs.

Treatment

SURGERY

Transsphenoidal surgery is the established treatment of choice in the initial management of Cushing's disease (Table 26-11 and Fig. 26-5).[70-72] The advantages of surgical therapy are the rapid correction of the hypersecretion of ACTH and the removal of the adenoma that offers a potential cure. Surgery also provides rapid decompression of the pressure effects from an expanding adenoma. Normalization of cortisol and ACTH levels in the immediate postoperative period is to be expected with a curative resection. Hormonal control rate is 80% to 90% in microadenomas and up to 50% in macroadenomas.[70]

Bochicchio and coworkers[68] conducted a multicenter study of 668 consecutive patients with Cushing's disease treated with transsphenoidal surgery between 1975 and 1990 in several European centers. Operative mortality was 2%, and major complications were seen in 15%. The most frequent complications were cerebrospinal fluid rhinorrhea, diabetes insipidus, meningitis, vascular injury, and pulmonary embolism. Early treatment success, defined as clinical and biochemical remission without the need for further therapy within 6 months of surgery, was seen in 76% of the patients. Early failure was associated with the absence of response to corticotropin-releasing hormone in the initial evaluation. Recurrence of Cushing's disease at 6 to 104 months (median, 39 months) was observed in 13% of the patients who were in the early treatment success group. Disease-free survival is 83% at 5 years, but late recurrences continue to be identified.

After unsuccessful initial surgical therapy or relapse after surgical remission, treatment options to be considered are repeat pituitary surgery, medical therapy, radiation therapy, or bilateral adrenalectomy. Repeat surgery should not be routinely used with parasellar (cavernous sinus) tumor extension.

RADIATION THERAPY

Radiation therapy provides a treatment alternative for patients who are unable to undergo surgery for technical or medical reasons, for persistent postsurgical hormone secretion, and for postsurgical recurrences.[69] A dose of 45 to 50.4 Gy delivered in 25 to 28 fractions over 5 weeks is usually prescribed (Table 26-12).

Howlett and associates[75] reported the long-term results of clinical and biochemical assessment after megavoltage pituitary radiation therapy of 52 patients with Cushing's disease and Nelson's syndrome (i.e., growth of an ACTH-secreting pituitary adenoma and after bilateral adrenalectomy). A three-field technique was used to deliver 45 Gy in 25 fractions over 5 weeks. Median follow-up was 10 years (range, 6 to 16 years). Clinical remission with normal cortisol levels was achieved in 57% of patients without the need for medical therapy. Five patients required bilateral adrenalectomy, and four patients were placed on metyrapone or *ortho-para*-DDD (*op*′-DDD). No non-endocrine complications, such as optic nerve injury, brain necrosis, and cancer induction, were reported. The authors of the study concluded that pituitary irradiation has a valuable

Table 26-12 Cushing's Disease: Results of Radiation Therapy

Study	*N*	Treatment	Follow-Up (y)	Tumor Control (%)
Howlett et al[75] (1989)	52	RT	10	57
Hughes et al[76] (1993)	40	RT	10	59
Littley et al[77] (1990)	24	RT	8 (mean)	33
Sandler et al[78] (1987)	82	^{90}Y	11 (median)	77
Levy et al[79] (1991)	64	SRS	NR	86
Laws et al[80] (1999)	50	SRS	NR	58
Sheehan et al[81] (2000)	43	SRS	3.6	63
Devin et al[82] (2004)	35	SRS	3	49

NR, not recorded; RT, conventional fractionated megavoltage radiation therapy; SRS, stereotactic radiosurgery.

role as second-line therapy for Cushing's disease when transsphenoidal surgery has failed and for patients who cannot undergo the surgical procedure.[83]

Estrada and associates[84] reported the use of conventional radiation in the postoperative setting after unsuccessful transsphenoidal surgery, with a mean dose of 50 to 50.4 Gy in 1.8 to 2 Gy fractions. Eighty-three percent (25 of 30) adult patients achieved remission defined as the regression of signs and symptoms of Cushing's syndrome, normal urinary cortisol excretion, and a low morning plasma cortisol level after the administration of 1 mg of dexamethasone at midnight. Most remissions were achieved during the first year, but some occurred as late as 5 years after therapy.

Sandler and associates[78] reported long-term results of interstitial brachytherapy for Cushing's disease with yttrium and gold. Seventy-seven percent who were reassessed 1 year after treatment had a remission. Among 54 patients followed for a mean of 10.5 years since remission, there have been no recurrences and no complications, with the exception of hypopituitarism.

SRS has been used by numerous centers for the treatment of Cushing's disease, with 23 series reporting results for 349 patients. However, only four studies report findings involving more than 30 patients. The endocrine cure rates range between 49% and 86% in these four studies. Comparisons to conventional radiation therapy in the adult population have not been performed. There is a suggestion, however, that cortisol levels normalize at a faster rate with SRS compared with conventional radiation.

MEDICAL THERAPY

Although transsphenoidal surgery is the treatment of choice, medical management is an important aspect in the treatment of patients with Cushing's disease and its complications such as diabetes, hypertension, and osteoporosis. Medical therapy is required for the treatment of acute hypercortisolism and steroid-induced psychosis and in preoperative management. Similarly, for patients undergoing radiation therapy, medical therapy is required until radiation control of Cushing's disease is achieved. It is also used in patients unable to undergo surgical or radiation treatment.[84]

The mechanisms of action of medical therapy are categorized as steroidogenesis inhibitors, glucocorticoid antagonists, and compounds that modulate ACTH release from a pituitary tumor.[85] Glucocorticoid antagonists, such as mifepristone (RU486), have been used sparingly for Cushing's disease. Compounds that modulate ACTH, such as bromocriptine, cyproheptadine, octreotide acetate, and valproic acid, are of limited benefit.

For long-term medical therapy, steroidogenesis inhibitors are the medical treatment of choice and should be administered under the guidance of an endocrinologist. They include ketoconazole, aminoglutethimide, metyrapone, mitotane, and etomidate.[85] Etomidate is the only drug that can be given parenterally.

Ketoconazole is given as 400 to 1600 mg daily in divided doses and is frequently used for control of hypercortisolism. It is the best tolerated and is effective as monotherapy in 70% of patients. It is typically initiated at a daily dose of 400 to 600 mg and increased over 3 or more days to 1600 mg in four divided doses. Because gastric acidity is necessary for metabolism, proton pump inhibitors should be avoided in patients receiving this therapy.

Mitotane causes adrenal suppression of cortisol secretion and is cytotoxic to adrenocortical cells. It can be delivered in doses typically ranging in doses of 0.5 to 8.0 g daily, but with high doses, the entire adrenal cortex can be impaired permanently requiring replacement therapy with glucocorticoids and Florinef. Treatment is typically initiated at 0.5 to 1 g/day and increased gradually over weeks by 0.5 to 1 g at a time.

Metyrapone is begun at daily doses of 0.5 to 1 g and increased every few days to a maximum dose of 6 g maximum, but there is rarely an additional effect after 2 g. It is often used in conjunction with aminoglutethimide, which is started at doses of 500 mg given in divided doses, and it can be increased up to 2 g. However, neurologic complaints that include sedation, dizziness, and blurred vision are common.

ACROMEGALY

General

Acromegaly refers to a syndrome characterized by progressive enlargement of peripheral parts of the body, such as hands, feet, and head, resulting from the effects of the excessive secretion of human GH (Table 26-13). Acromegaly is associated with elevated levels of IGF-1 (i.e., somatomedin C).[86-88] Excessive amounts of these hormones lead to the growth and functional disturbances of multiple organs in the body. Acromegaly is an uncommon disease, and delay in diagnosis and treatment results in serious consequences of increased morbidity, decreased life expectancy, and high mortality. A mean interval of 8 years before diagnosis leads to insidious damage to multiple organ systems from the effects of chronic hypersecretion of GH. Excess GH secretion is primarily from pituitary adenomas.

The clinical findings, elevated serum IGF-1, and the neuroradiologic examination of the pituitary region readily establish the diagnosis of acromegaly. A careful assessment of multiple organ systems is required because elevated serum GH levels have such wide-ranging effects throughout the body.

Table 26-13 Acromegaly: Key Points

- Incidence: 3 cases per 1 million people
- Age: 30 to 60 years, but may occur at any age; gigantism in childhood
- Sex: equal preponderance in females and males
- Onset: insidious, occurring over 7 to 9 years before diagnosis
- Clinical features
  - Endocrine effects: coarsening facies, enlargement of hands and feet, multiple organ effects (e.g., skeletal, cardiovascular, skin, central nervous system, endocrine)
  - Mass effects: neuro-ophthalmic disorders
- Laboratory tests: elevated levels of GH, IGF-1; oral GTT, TRH-LHRH test, GHRH test
- Imaging: MRI; 50% are microadenoma
- Other studies: Neuro-ophthalmic, endocrine evaluation
- Treatment
  - Surgery is the primary treatment.
  - Radiation therapy is used for patients who are not suitable candidates for surgery, as an adjunct to surgery, or for treating postsurgical recurrence.
  - Medical therapy (e.g., somatostatin analogues such as octreotide for persistent elevation of GH after surgery) is used with radiation therapy.

GH, growth hormone; GHRH, growth hormone-releasing hormone; GTT, glucose tolerance test; IGF-1, insulin growth factor-1; LHRH, luteinizing hormone-releasing hormone; TRH, thyroid-releasing hormone.

Table 26-14 Acromegaly: Results of Surgical Therapy

Study	*N* (%)	GH < 5 μg/L (%)*	Recurrence (%)
Giovanelli et al[90] (1996)	277	55	4
Fahlbusch et al[91] (1997)	396	73	Rare
Abosch et al[92] (1998)	254	76	7

*An aim of surgery is to remove the growth hormone (GH)–secreting pituitary adenoma to normalize GH levels.

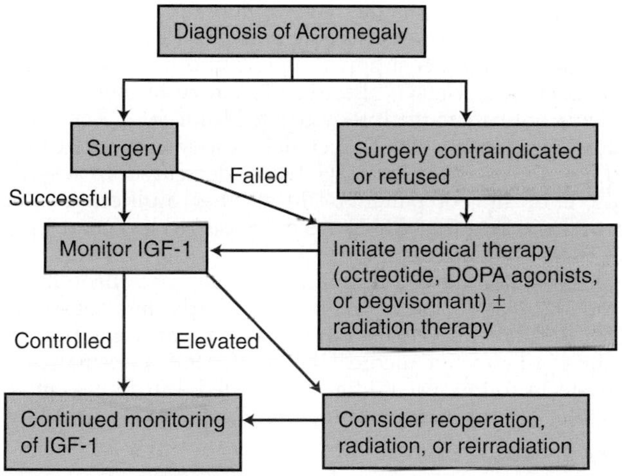

Figure 26-6 **Algorithm outlining the treatment of acromegaly.** IGF-1, insulin-like growth factor-1.

Clinical Manifestations

Excessive GH and IGF-1 levels cause myriad changes in skeletal and soft tissues that progress gradually and remain undetected for several years before increasing the size of the hands, feet, and mandible and causing frontal bossing; increasing body height; coarsening of facial features and skin; and enlarging the tongue, heart, and other organs, leading to the recognition of acromegaly.[88]

Manifestations of involvement of multiple organs include arthralgia, hyperhidrosis, skin tags, colon polyps, osteoporosis, apnea, dental malocclusion, diabetes mellitus, hypertension, respiratory symptoms, and cardiac failure.[88] Cardiovascular, respiratory, and other organ failures cause a twofold increase in mortality and a substantial decrease in longevity.[89]

Mass effects from the enlarging adenoma cause neuro-ophthalmic disturbances that include headache, visual field changes from suprasellar extension, and involvement of cranial nerves III, IV, V, and VI from the parasellar extension of the tumor into the cavernous sinus. Massive growth of the tumor leads to extensive involvement of the intracranial structures and sphenoid sinus, causing a wide variety of neurologic symptoms. Hypopituitarism may also result from the mass effect of the enlarging adenoma on the pituitary gland itself.

Laboratory Assessment

An elevated serum IGF-1 level (normal value <2.2 U/mL) readily leads to the diagnosis of acromegaly. Although serum GH levels in acromegaly are higher than 5 mU/L (normal basal serum GH level <1 mU/L), a single, random serum GH level measurement may not be elevated on account of the wide variations in GH secretion during the day. An oral glucose (75 g) tolerance test, which suppresses GH levels to less than 1 mU/L in normal individuals, reveals elevated GH levels in patients with acromegaly. Infusions of GH-releasing hormone and thyrotropin-releasing hormone also cause GH elevations in acromegaly patients.

Imaging

MRI of the pituitary is the imaging modality of choice. Giovanelli and colleagues[90] found microadenomas in 19%, intrasellar macroadenomas in 39%, and extrasellar macroadenomas in 42% of patients in a surgical series of 277 patients with acromegaly.

Treatment

SURGERY

Surgical management using transsphenoidal resection of the pituitary adenoma is the initial treatment of choice (Table 26-14 and Fig. 26-6).[91] Aims of the surgical treatment are to accomplish anatomic removal of the GH-secreting adenoma to normalize GH levels and to remove the mass effect from the suprasellar tumor extension, especially on the optic chiasm and nerves.

Giovanelli and coworkers[90] defined remission as GH level of less than 2 μg/L, normalization of the IGF-1 level, and no evidence of relapse within 6 months of surgery. Overall remission occurred in 55% of 277 patients in their series. Baseline GH level, tumor size, and invasiveness were important predictors of surgical outcome. Successful outcome was seen in 78% versus 37% of patients with baseline GH level less than 2 μg/L versus higher than 2 μg/L, respectively ($P < 0.01$). Success rates determined by tumor size revealed 81% for microadenoma, 59% for intrasellar macroadenoma, and 39% for extrasellar macroadenoma ($P < 0.01$). Remission occurred in 70% of patients without cavernous sinus invasion, compared with 18% of patients with cavernous sinus invasion ($P < 0.01$). The mortality rate was less than 1%.[90] Major morbidity such as cerebrospinal fluid leak, meningitis, and worsening of visual function occurs with low frequency (<5%). Diabetes insipidus and hypopituitarism are more common.

MEDICAL THERAPY

After surgical therapy, about one third of the patients have elevated GH levels and require additional therapy. In the past, radiation therapy was used, but the decline in GH levels is a gradual process occurring over several years. Eastman and coworkers[93] reported that GH falls about 50% from the baseline level by 2 years, about 75% by 5 years, and approaches 90% after 15 years. During this period, patients require medical therapy to control the excess GH levels.

Somatostatin analogues and bromocriptine are used for postsurgical therapy. Octreotide has 40-fold greater potency than somatostatin in suppressing GH and has been tested in several clinical trials.[88,89] Results of octreotide therapy in 189 patients entered in an International Multicenter Acromegaly Study Group trial show that clinical response in lowering the GH level was 88%, and GH levels decreased to less than 5 µg/L in 45% of patients.[94] In another multicenter study, Ezzat[81] reported that GH levels decreased to less than 5 µg/L in 45% of 182 patients.

Pegvisomant, a GH receptor antagonist, has been investigated and plays a role in acromegaly.[38] Early data suggest that IGF-1 normalization occurs in 97% of patients and appears to be the most effective medical therapy for IGF-1 normalization. Long-term follow-up studies are needed, but its use in conjunction with or in lieu of radiation treatment is increasing.

RADIATION THERAPY

Radiation therapy is effective in arresting the growth and causing regression of the pituitary adenoma. Earlier studies reported a higher than 80% control rate of tumor growth.[89] There are scarce data on long-term follow-up for a normal IGF-1 level or GH level criteria of less than 5 ng/mL in patients treated with radiation therapy. Some series report results of radiation therapy with GH level less than 10 ng/mL (Table 26-15).[95-97]

Radiation therapy should be considered after surgery for patients with extrasellar extensions, patients who fail or are intolerant to medical therapy, and patients who cannot undergo surgery. A dose of 45 to 50 Gy in 5 weeks is used. Pharmacologic therapy is required for several years until radiation therapy lowers the GH levels.

There have been 25 published reports of SRS for patients with acromegaly. Only three series had more than 30 patients. Endocrine criteria for cure varied in the studies. The endocrine cure rates ranged between 25% and 96%.

Thyroid-Stimulating Hormone–Secreting Pituitary Adenoma

TSH-secreting adenomas cause thyroid hyperfunction and are rare. Fewer than 300 cases have been reported and reviewed by Beck-Peccoz and associates.[101] Almost all arise in the anterior pituitary, and 72% secrete TSH alone. Hypersecretion of GH, PRL, and FSH/LH has been identified in the remainder. Most TSH-secreting adenomas are macroadenomas and are highly invasive. Unlike other pituitary adenomas, there is no gender or age predilection. Almost all patients have goiter, features of hyperthyroidism, and delayed diagnosis because they are initially treated for thyroid dysfunction. A high level of thyroid hormones in the presence of circulating TSH should lead to further evaluation for a TSH-secreting adenoma. The tumors have become more frequently diagnosed with the availability of more sensitive TSH and thyroid hormone immunoassays. Increased awareness leads to early diagnosis, with detection of small tumors by MRI.

Treatment

Surgical removal of the pituitary TSH-secreting adenoma is the initial treatment. Complete extirpation is difficult on account of extrasellar extensions into critical structures, invasiveness, and fibrosis. Pituitary irradiation has an important role when surgery is contraindicated or is incomplete.

Surgery and radiation therapy are successful in about two thirds of the patients. Patients who have persistent TSH level elevations after these treatments benefit from treatment with a somatostatin analogue or bromocriptine.

Nonfunctioning Adenomas

Clinical Manifestations

With the application of radioimmunoassays, the proportion of nonfunctioning pituitary adenomas has declined substantially. Most of the chromophobe adenomas are found to secrete PRL. Usually diagnosed late, chromophobe adenomas are larger than 10 mm (macroadenoma). These macroadenomas compress the adjacent pituitary, causing hypopituitarism; the optic chiasm, causing visual symptoms; and the cavernous sinus, causing cranial nerve deficits, and they can obstruct the third ventricle, causing hydrocephalus. Presenting symptoms include headache and visual symptoms, and further evaluation reveals endocrine deficiencies. Further evaluation includes visual field testing, endocrine hormone profile, and MRI of the pituitary region.

Treatment

Management of nonfunctioning adenomas depends on the size and endocrine disorders associated with these tumors.

Table 26-15 **Radiation Therapy of Growth Hormone–Secreting Pituitary Adenoma**

Study	*N*	Treatment	Control (%) of GH Secretion
Werner et al[95] (1985)	19	RT	84 (<10 ng/mL)
Ludecke et al[96] (1989)	30	RT	80 (<10 ng/mL)
Tran et al[97] (1991)	15	RT	60 (<10 ng/mL)
Laws et al[80] (1999)	56	SRS	25 (normal IGF-1)*
Zhang et al[98] (2000)	68	SRS	96 (<12 ng/mL)
Attanasio et al[99] (2003)	30	SRS	37 (<2.5 ng/mL)

*Reduction of insulin-like growth facter [IGF]-1 level to normal for age and sex is one of the measures to assess treatment success.[100]

GH, growth hormone; RT, conventional radiation therapy; SRS, stereotactic radiosurgery.

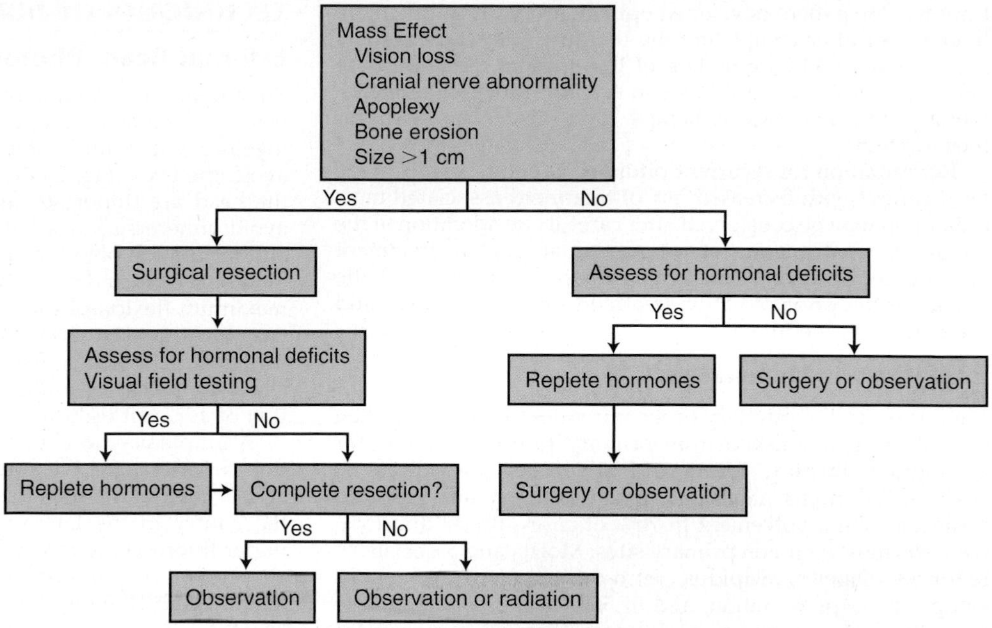

Figure 26-7 **Algorithm outlining the effect and treatment of nonfunctioning adenoma.**

Table 26-16 Radiation Therapy ± Surgery of Nonfunctional Pituitary Adenoma

Studies	*N*	Treatment	Tumor Control (%) at 10 Years
Brada et al[102] (1993)	199	S + RT	98
	31	RT only	98
Tsang et al[103] (1994)	160	S + RT	87
Breen et al[104] (1998)	120	S + RT	78
Feigl et al[105] (2002)	61	SRS	94
Petrovich et al[106] (2003)	56	SRS	100

RT, radiation therapy; S, surgery, SRS, stereotactic radiosurgery.

Observation or transsphenoidal surgery alone is an option for smaller tumors (Fig. 26-7).

When the tumors are incompletely resected, surgery followed by radiation therapy is used for macroadenomas. Excellent long-term control at 10 years has been documented in several large series (Table 26-16).[102-104]

Only two series with more than 50 patients treated with SRS have been published. Both studies had less than 5 years of follow-up, and they had local control rates of 94% and 100%.

Nelson's Syndrome

In 1958, Nelson and colleagues[31] reported the development of ACTH-secreting pituitary adenoma accompanied by hyperpigmentation that followed bilateral adrenalectomy in patients with Cushing's disease. Patients with a history of bilateral adrenalectomy later present with hyperpigmentation of the skin, ACTH-secreting pituitary adenoma, and an expanding intrasellar mass. About 30% of such patients develop Nelson's syndrome. These aggressive tumors are associated with extrasellar extension, causing compression of the chiasm and visual field changes, invasion to the cavernous sinus and associated cranial nerve palsies, and pituitary carcinoma.

Treatment

Surgical resection is made difficult by the rapid growth and infiltrative nature of the tumor. Postoperative radiation therapy or primary radiation therapy to a dose level of 45 to 50.4 Gy over 5 to 5.5 weeks is recommended. Howlett and coworkers[75] found improvement in 14 of 15 patients after radiation therapy.

REIRRADIATION AND PALLIATION OF METASTATIC DISEASE

Reirradiation of Pituitary Adenoma

Schoenthaler and coworkers[107] reirradiated 15 patients with a median dose of 42 Gy in 1.8- to 2.0-Gy fractions who had previously received a median dose of 40.84 Gy in standard fractions. Local control was achieved in 12 patients. All patients developed hypopituitarism from the initial or repeat course of radiation therapy. Two patients each later developed pituitary carcinoma and temporal lobe radionecrosis.

Flickinger and associates[108] reirradiated 10 patients with suprasellar or pituitary tumors with doses ranging from 35 Gy to 49.6 Gy in 1.8- to 2-Gy fractions. Six patients had pituitary tumors. One patient developed optic neuropathy a little more than 1 year after completing the therapy. The study authors suggest that a 40% estimation of the original radiation dose effect is a reasonable guideline to account for prior radiation therapy. SRS and brachytherapy have also been used for reirradiation.

Reirradiation for recurrent pituitary adenoma can provide local control with increased risk of treatment-associated morbidity and may be considered after careful consideration of the diagnostic confirmation of recurrence, alternative treatment options, the interval from prior radiation therapy, and the details of the prior radiation treatment technique, dose, and fractionation schedule.[107,108]

Palliation of Metastases

Metastases to the pituitary occur infrequently; however, they should be distinguished from primary pituitary tumors for appropriate therapy. Teears and Silverman[109] reviewed 88 cases of carcinoma metastatic to the pituitary and reported posterior lobe involvement in 70% of cases. Breast and lung were the most common primary sites. Morita and associates[110] reported diabetes insipidus, retro-orbital pain, and visual symptoms at presentation, and in 56% of the patients, these were the first manifestation of illness. Surgical management for diagnosis and decompression followed by radiation therapy was used for palliation. Median survival was 180 days. A dosage of 30 Gy in 10 fractions or any other comparable dose-fractionation scheme typically used for palliation of metastatic brain disease is appropriate.

TECHNIQUES OF IRRADIATION

External Beam Photons

The radiation technique that is widely used involves a three-field arrangement composed of two lateral opposing fields together with a third anterior field that is angled superiorly to avoid the eyes (Fig. 26-8). Positioning and immobilization of the head are important in the design of treatment fields to avoid unnecessary irradiation of the eyes from beam entrance and irradiation of the trunk from the exit beam of the anterior field. The head and neck are positioned on an incline to permit maximum flexion of the head toward the upper chest, and a custom Aquaplast facemask is prepared for reproducibility of the treatment setup. The fields are further shaped using shielding blocks or multileaf collimators to minimize irradiation of adjacent tissues.

A simple way to obtain the desired degrees of gantry rotation superiorly for the anterior field is to set up the isocenter at the center of the sella for the anterior and lateral fields. With the gantry in the lateral position, the collimator is rotated under fluoroscopic monitoring at the simulator console or on a treatment planning system so that the inferior border of the lateral beam is along the base of skull and avoids the orbital contents. The lateral view (see Fig. 26-4) also shows the exit path of the anterior beam through the upper cervical vertebrae and verifies that the beam has not been angled too superiorly such that the beam exits through the trunk. The number of degrees of the collimator rotation (usually 10 to 20) corresponds to the degrees the gantry is rotated superiorly from the

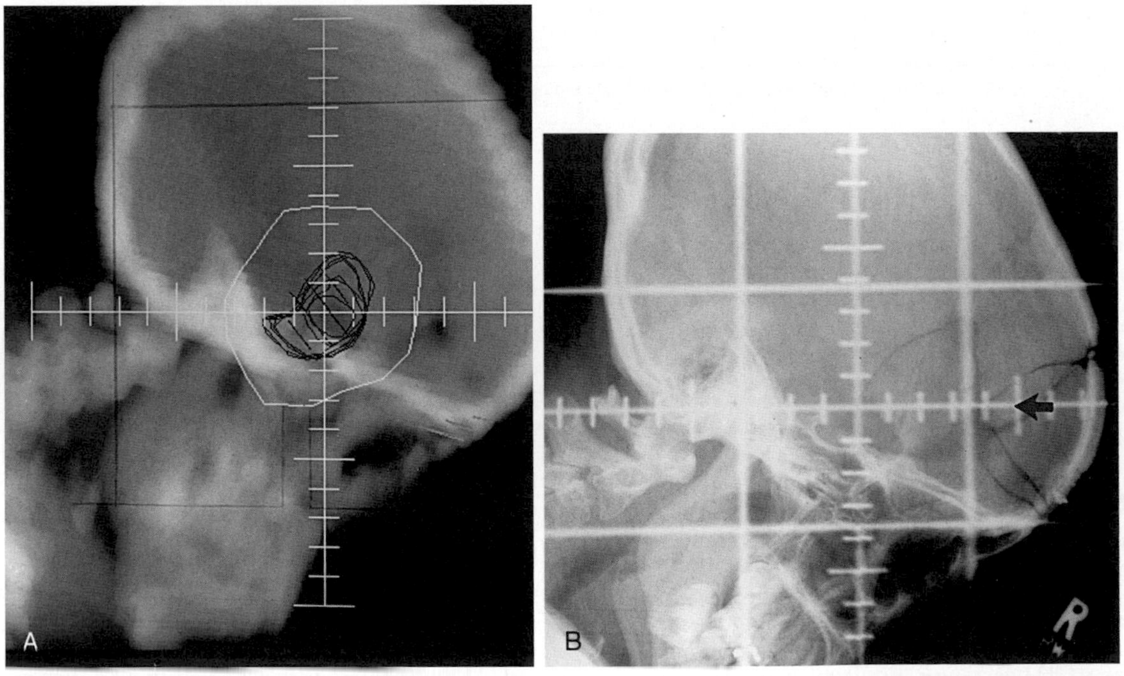

Figure 26-8 Three-field technique for pituitary irradiation. **A,** Digitally reconstructed radiograph from the treatment-planning CT, with the head in treatment position. The *dark lines* in the center represent the gross tumor volume obtained by image registration of the axial and sagittal MRI of a large pituitary adenoma with the treatment-planning CT. Isocentric arrangement of two opposed lateral fields and a third field, which is an anterior beam with gantry rotated 15 degrees superiorly (anterior 15 degrees superior), is planned using three-dimensional conformal treatment-planning software. **B,** A lateral simulation film is used to verify the treatment setup. The *arrow* shows the direction of the anterior 15-degree superior beam. Corresponding 15-degree collimator rotation to match the direction of the anterior 15-degree superior beam facilitates wedge alignment for dosimetry.

anterior field. This field is then set up by turning the couch to 90 degrees and rotating the gantry superiorly from the anterior position by the same number of degrees as the collimator rotation. The collimator for the lateral fields is rotated to match the anterior field. These lateral fields require wedges with heels anterosuperiorly to obtain a uniform dose distribution.

An alternative arrangement for small pituitary tumors involves bilateral 110-degree coronal arcs with a 30-degree wedge, which is reversed for the second arc.[111] Larger tumors are better treated with three or more stationary fields that permit the use of shaped shielding blocks and a conformal treatment plan.

Sohn and colleagues[112] evaluated five different techniques of pituitary irradiation using 3D treatment planning and dose-volume histograms. Two-field lateral opposed, three-field 110-degree bilateral arcs, 330-degree rotational arc, and four non-coplanar arc techniques were compared using 6-MV and 18-MV photons. The three-field technique delivered less dose to the temporal lobes than the two-field technique. The rotational techniques were superior to the stationary field techniques in sparing the temporal lobe but do not readily permit field blocking and also increase the total volume of the brain receiving low doses of radiation. Their four-field non-coplanar arc technique delivered less dose to the frontal lobe, but the dose to the lens was slightly higher.

Perks and associates[113] performed a similar study comparing 3 coplanar and 3, 4, 6, and 30 non-coplanar field arrangements to obtain 95% isodose coverage. Dose-volume histograms were calculated for the normal brain; a reduction was observed with a four-field non-coplanar arrangement when compared with the three-field coplanar arrangement of mean volume of normal brain receiving 80% or more and 60% or more by 22.3% and 47.6%, respectively. Near-equivalent tissue sparing was observed compared with the 30-field plan.

Dose

Selection of dose has emerged from retrospective data analysis using resolution of the presenting symptoms caused by hormone production or lack of tumor progression[114] as criteria for tumor control. Zierhut and coworkers[115] observed a recurrence frequency of 6 (11%) of 55 patients with doses lower than 45 Gy, compared with 1 (1%) of 83 patients receiving a dose of 45 Gy or more. A dose of 45 to 50.4 Gy over 5 to 5.5 weeks is recommended with daily fractions of 1.8 Gy to the target volume.[116]

In Cushing's disease, low-dose irradiation of 20 Gy in 8 fractions was attempted[117] with the intent of reducing the chance of hypopituitarism. Unfortunately, only 6 of 24 patients have remained in remission, with median follow-up of 93 months, suggesting that this regimen is suboptimal.

Doses used with SRS depend on whether the pituitary adenoma is a secreting or functioning tumor or a nonsecreting or nonfunctioning tumor. A wide range of doses to the periphery or margin of the tumor have been reported, ranging from 12 to 35 Gy at the 50% to 100% isodose line. No obvious dose response has been demonstrated, but it is thought that lower doses (12 to 18 Gy) are needed for nonfunctioning adenomas and higher doses (18 to 35 Gy) for functioning pituitary tumors. The dose-limiting structure has typically been the optic apparatus (i.e., optic chiasm and prechiasmal optic nerve), which has generally been limited to a dose of 8 Gy but is acceptably treated to a maximum of 12 Gy.

Treatment Outcome

Long-term tumor control rates of 90% are reported after radiation therapy of pituitary adenomas (Table 26-17). However, the data are limited on the restoration of hormone abnormalities as determined by current sensitive biochemical assays and dynamic testing of endocrine profiles.[118,120] Improvement in hormone abnormalities is gradual, occurring over 3 to 10 years. Long-term hormonal improvement rates are significantly lower than the high tumor control rates. Zierhut and associates[115] found improvement in 90% of patients with hormonally active tumors, but complete reduction of the excess hormone production was seen in only 38%, and partial reduction in 52% of the patients. Functioning pituitary adenomas appear to have lower control rates than nonfunctioning adenomas.[115,119] Results of treatment outcome are described further in the sections on individual pituitary adenomas. Improvement in visual impairment occurs in about 50% of patients.[102,119]

Treatment Morbidity

This outpatient treatment is well tolerated with no significant neurologic, endocrine, or systemic acute side effects during the course of radiation therapy. Temporary hair loss in the radiation treatment fields is usually followed by regrowth in 3 to 4 months.

Although radiation therapy of pituitary tumors has minimal acute morbidity, long-term radiation effects on the pituitary and the adjacent organs require meticulous attention to the selection of radiation modalities, techniques, and dose fractionations. Jones and colleagues[121] have drawn attention to increased anterior beam transmission through abnormally large frontal air sinuses in acromegalic patients, increasing the dose to the optic chiasm. A more superior beam and the use of 3D planning using air transmission corrections should be considered.

Hypopituitarism occurs commonly, requiring endocrine replacement of one or more hormones.[112,114] Pituitary insufficiency is multifactorial, resulting from the effects of the

Table 26-17 Pituitary Tumor Control with Radiation Therapy

Study	*N*	Treatment	Follow-Up (y)	Tumor Control (%) at 10 Years
Grigsby et al[118] (1989)	121	S + RT	13 (mean)	93
	70	RT only	13 (mean)	81
Hughes et al[76] (1993)	160	S + RT	13 (mean)	77
	108	RT only		60
Brada et al[102] (1993)	199	S + RT	10.5 (median)	98
Tsang et al[103] (1994)	128	S + RT	8.3 (median)	91
McCord et al[119] (1997)	98	S + RT	2 (minimum)	95

RT, radiation therapy; S, surgery.

adenoma on the normal pituitary-hypothalamic axis and from the results of surgical or radiation treatment of the pituitary adenoma. After 37.5 to 42.5 Gy in 15 or 16 fractions in the treatment of pituitary adenoma in 165 patients, Littley and coworkers[122] reported hormone deficiencies of 100%, 96%, 84%, and 49% at 8 years for GH, gonadotropins, corticotropin, and TSH, respectively. Radiation-induced hyperprolactinemia was seen in 45% of the patients.

Treatment complications such as temporal lobe radionecrosis,[123] damage to optic pathways,[124] and radiation-induced malignancies are rare with current techniques and dose-fractionation guidelines of 45 to 50 Gy in 1.8-Gy fractions.[125,126] Series of pituitary radiation therapy with long-term follow-up report absence of temporal lobe necrosis,[102,120] except as a rare complication of SRS. Previously reported cases of radiation optic neuropathy have been associated with a higher dose per fraction or higher total dose and is rare in contemporary series.[124] Secondary tumors reported include glioma, meningioma, and meningeal sarcoma, with a latent period of 8 to 15 years and cumulative risk of 1.3% over the first 10 years.[125] An area of concern that remains is the increased risk of cerebrovascular accidents in patients treated with conventional radiation techniques because the findings may not be seen for decades.

Table 26-18 Pituitary Tumors: Diagnostic and Treatment Algorithm

DIAGNOSIS AND EVALUATION

A. Clinical assessment of the endocrine and neuro-ophthalmic features
B. Laboratory assessment of endocrine abnormalities: PRL, GH, TSH, LH/FSH, plasma cortisol, ACTH
C. Imaging with MRI preferred over CT

TREATMENT DECISIONS

A. Prolactinoma
  - Bromocriptine is the primary treatment.
  - Surgery is chosen for bromocriptine intolerance, mass effects, apoplexy, or a desire to maintain fertility.
  - Radiation therapy has a limited role, usually for recurrences.

B. Cushing's disease
  - Transsphenoidal surgery is the primary treatment.
  - Radiation therapy is chosen for postoperative extrasellar residual or recurrent tumor or as primary treatment.
  - Medical therapy is used for postoperative management and while awaiting response from radiation therapy; it is primary therapy for patients who are unsuitable candidates for surgery or irradiation.

C. Acromegaly
  - Transsphenoidal surgery is the primary treatment.
  - Somatostatin analogues are used for persistent elevated GH.
  - Radiation therapy is used for residual or recurrent tumor.

D. Nelson's syndrome
  - Transsphenoidal surgery is the primary treatment.
  - Radiation therapy is used for postoperative residual or recurrent tumor.

E. Thyrotropin-secreting adenoma
  - Transsphenoidal surgery is the primary treatment.

F. Nonfunctioning adenoma
  - Observation is the approach for asymptomatic adenomas.
  - Transsphenoidal surgery is the primary treatment for symptomatic adenomas.
  - Radiation therapy for postoperative residual or recurrent tumor

ACTH, adrenocorticotropic hormone; FSH, follicle-stimulating hormone; GH, growth hormone; LH, luteinizing hormone; PRL, prolactin; TSH, thyroid-stimulating hormone.

TREATMENT ALGORITHMS, CONTROVERSIES, CHALLENGES, AND FUTURE POSSIBILITIES

Management of patients with pituitary neoplasms requires attention to the diversity of clinical syndromes of hyposecretion or hypersecretion of pituitary hormones, mass effects, imaging findings, and asymptomatic lesions. Surgery, medical management, and radiation therapy are effective, and, sometimes, competing therapy options add to the controversy and complexity of decision making for optimal treatment selection. The patient's age, medical condition, compliance, treatment tolerance, and preference also influence treatment decisions. Close collaboration among the various disciplines is necessary for comprehensive long-term care. Clinical findings, endocrine evaluation, and MRI findings can establish the diagnosis in most patients and define the initial treatment decisions. Table 26-18 outlines a diagnostic and treatment algorithm for all pituitary tumors.

Management of pituitary tumors requires a multidisciplinary approach. Initial diagnosis, evaluation, and medical management usually are under the direction of an endocrinologist. Laboratory investigations and pituitary imaging provide detailed information concerning endocrine dysfunctions and anatomic relationships of the pituitary adenoma. Sophisticated surgical approaches and refined radiation therapy techniques provide safe and successful management of patients with pituitary adenomas. Pathobiology of pituitary tumors is yielding new insights into the genetic and molecular biology of these tumors.

REFERENCES

1. Marie P: Sur deux cas d'acromegalie. Rec Med (Paris) 6:297-333, 1886.
2. Cushing H: The Pituitary Body and Its Disorders. Philadelphia, JB Lippincott, 1912.
3. Faglia G: Epidemiology and pathogenesis of pituitary adenomas. Acta Endocrinol 129(Suppl 1):1-5, 1993.
4. Tada M, Kobayashi H, Moriuchi T: Molecular basis of pituitary oncogenesis. Neuro-Oncol 45:83-96, 1999.
5. Bates AS, Farrell WE, Bicknell EJ, et al: Allelic deletion in pituitary adenomas reflects aggressive biologic activity and has potential value as a prognostic marker. J Clin Endocrinol Metab 82:818-24, 1997.
6. CBTRUS, Central Brain Tumor Registry of the United States: *Primary Brain Tumors in the United States, Statistical Report, 1997-2001, Years Data Collected.* Chicago: Central Brain Tumor Registry of the United States, 2005-2005.
7. Kernohan JW, Sayre GP: Tumors of the Pituitary Gland and Infundibulum, section X, fascicle 26. Washington DC, Armed Forces Institute of Pathology, 1956, p 7.
8. Annegers JF, Coulam CB, Abboud CF, et al: Pituitary adenoma in Olmsted County, Minnesota, 1935-1977. Mayo Clin Proc 53:641-643, 1978.
9. Hall WA, Luciano MG, Doppman JL, et al: Pituitary magnetic resonance imaging in normal human volunteers: Occult adenomas in the general population. Ann Intern Med 120:817-820, 1994.
10. Burrow GN, Wortzman G, Newcastle NB, et al: Microadenoma of the pituitary and abnormal sellar tomograms in unselected autopsy series. N Engl J Med 304:156-158, 1981.
11. Ezzat S, Asa SL, Couldwell WT, et al: The prevalence of pituitary adenomas: a systematic review. Cancer 101:613-619, 2004.
12. Parent AD, Beblin J: Incidental pituitary adenoma. J Neurosurg 54:228-231, 1981.
13. Chambers EF, Turski PA, LaMasters D, et al: Regions of low density in the contrast-enhanced pituitary and normal and pathological processes. Radiology 144:109-113, 1982.
14. Muhr C, Bergstrom K, Grimelius L, et al: A parallel study of the sella turcica and the histopathology of the pituitary gland in 205 autopsy specimens. Neuroradiology 21:55-65, 1981.

15. Hall WA, Luciano MG, Doppman JL, et al: Pituitary magnetic resonance imaging in normal human volunteers: occult adenomas in the general population. Ann Intern Med 120:817-820, 1994.
16. Teramoto A, Hirakawa K, Sanno N, et al: Incidental pituitary lesions in 1000 unselected autopsy specimens. Radiology 193:161-164, 1994.
17. Camaris C, Balleine R, Little D: Microadenomas of the human pituitary. Pathology 27:8-11, 1995.
18. Ambrosi B, Faglia G: Epidemiology of pituitary tumors. Excerpta Med Int Congr Ser 961:159-168, 1991.
19. Mindermann T, Wilson CB: Age-related and gender-related occurrence of pituitary adenomas. Clin Endocrinol 41:359-364, 1994.
20. Thapar K, Kovacs K, Laws ER: Pituitary tumors. *In* Black P, Loeffler J (eds): Cancer of the Nervous System. Cambridge, Blackwell Scientific, 1997, p 363.
21. Hardy J: Transsphenoidal surgery of hypersecreting pituitary tumors. *In* Kohler PO, Ross FT (eds): Diagnosis and Treatment of Pituitary Tumors. New York, Elsevier, 1973, p 179.
22. Bonneville J, Bonneville F, Cattin F: Magnetic resonance imaging of pituitary adenomas. Eur Radiol 15:543-548, 2005.
23. Asa SL, Kovacs K, Shlomad S: The hypothalamic-pituitary axis. *In* Melmed S (ed): The Pituitary. Cambridge, Blackwell Scientific, 1995, p 3.
24. Thapar K, Kovacs K, Laws ER: Classification and molecular biology of pituitary adenomas. Adv Tech Stand Neurosurg 22:3-53, 1995.
25. Melmed S: Pituitary neoplasia. Endocrinol Metab Clin North Am 23:81, 1994.
26. Vallar L, Spada A, Giannattasio G: Altered Gs and adenylate cyclase activity in human GH-secreting pituitary adenomas. Nature 330:566-568, 1987.
27. Suhardja AS, Kovacs KT, Rutka JT: Molecular pathogenesis of pituitary adenomas: a review. Acta Neurochir 141:729-736, 1999.
28. Kreutzer J, Fahlbusch R: Diagnosis and treatment of pituitary tumors. Curr Opin Neurol 17:693-703, 2004.
29. Landolt AM, Shibata T, Kleihues P, et al: Growth of human pituitary adenomas—facts and speculation: proliferation of human pituitary adenomas. Adv Biosci 69:53-62, 1988.
30. Knosp E, Kitz K, Perneczky A: Proliferation activity in pituitary adenomas: measurement by monoclonal antibody Ki-67. Neurosurgery 25:927-930, 1989.
31. Nelson DH, Meakin JW, Dealy JB, et al: ACTH-producing tumor of the pituitary gland. N Engl J Med 259:161-164, 1958.
32. Clayton RN, Boggild M, Bates AS, et al: Tumour suppressor genes in the pathogenesis of human pituitary tumours. Horm Res 47:185-193, 1997.
33. Hall-Craggs M, Kling Chong WK, Kendall B: Imaging of the pituitary. *In* Powell M, Lightman SL (eds): The Management of Pituitary Tumors. New York, Churchill Livingstone, 1996, p 77.
34. Schubiger O: Radiology of pituitary tumors. *In* Landolt AM, Vance ML, Reilly PL (eds): Pituitary Adenomas. New York, Churchill Livingstone, 1996, p 177.
35. Swallow CE, Osborn AG: Imaging of sella and parasellar disease. Semin Ultrasound CT MR 19:257-271, 1998.
36. Hardy J, Verzina JL: Transsphenoidal neurosurgery of intracranial neoplasm. *In* Thompson RA, Green JR (eds): Advances in Neurology. New York, Raven Press, 1976, p 261 (updated at the International Pituitary Conference, Zurich, 1987).
37. Wilson CB: Neurosurgical management of large and invasive pituitary tumors. *In* Tinadall GT, Collins WF (eds): Clinical Management of Pituitary Disorders. New York. Raven Press, 1979, p 335.
38. Stewart PM. Pegvisomant: an advance in clinical efficacy in acromegaly. Eur J Endocrinol 148:27-32, 2003.
39. Consensus guidelines for the diagnosis and treatment of adults with growth hormone deficiency: summary statement of the Growth Hormone Research Society on Adult Growth Hormone Deficiency. J Clin Endocrinol Metab 83:379-381, 1998.
40. White DR, Sonnenburg RE, Ewend MG, et al: Safety of minimally invasive pituitary surgery (MIPS) compared with a traditional approach. Laryngoscope 114:1945-1948, 2004.
41. Molitch ME: Prolactinoma. *In* Melmed S (ed): The Pituitary, 2nd ed., Malden MA: Blackwell Publishing, 2002, pp 455-495.
42. Gramegna A: Un cas d'acomegalie traite par la radiotherapie. Rev Nerul 17:15-17, 1909.
43. Beclere A: The radiotherapeutic treatment of tumors of the hypophysis, gigantism, and acromegaly. Arch Roentgen Ray 14:142-150, 1909.
44. Ganz JC, Backland E-O, Thorsen FA: The effects of gamma knife surgery of pituitary adenoma on tumor growth and endocrinopathies. Stereotact Funct Neurosurg 61(Suppl 1):30-37, 1993.
45. Kjellberg RN, Kliman B: Bragg peak proton treatment for pituitary-related conditions. Proc R Soc Med 67:32-33, 1974.
46. Levy RP, Fabrikant JI, Lyman JT, et al: Clinical results of stereotactic heavy-charged particle radiosurgery of the pituitary gland. *In* Steiner L (ed): Radiosurgery: Baselines and Trends. New York, Raven Press, 1992.
47. Ganz JC: Radiosurgery for pituitary tumors. *In* Gildenberg P, Tasker R (eds): Textbook of Stereotactic and Functional Neurosurgery. New York, McGraw-Hill, 1998, p 845.
48. Landolt AM, Haller D, Lomax N, et al: Stereotactic radiosurgery for recurrent surgically treated acromegaly: comparison with fractionated radiotherapy. J Neurosurg 88:1002-1008, 1998.
49. Yoon SC, Suh TS, Jang HS, et al: Clinical results of 24 pituitary macroadenomas with Linac-based stereotactic radiosurgery. Int J Radiat Oncol Biol Phys 41:849-853, 1998.
50. Mitsumori M, Shrieve DC, Alexander E III, et al: Initial clinical results of Linac-based stereotactic radiosurgery and stereotactic radiotherapy for pituitary adenomas. Int J Radiat Oncol Biol Phys 42:573, 1998.
51. Alexander E, Loeffler J: Clinical experience with Linac radiosurgery. *In* Gildenberg P, Tasker R (eds): Textbook of Stereotactic and Functional Neurosurgery. New York, McGraw-Hill, 1998, p 745.
52. Larson DA, Flickinger JC, Loeffler JS: Stereotactic radiosurgery: techniques and results. *In* DeVita VT, Hellman S, Rosenberg SA (eds): Cancer: Principles and Practice of Oncology Updates. Philadelphia, JB Lippincott, 1993, p 1.
53. Jalali R, Brada M. Radiosurgery for pituitary adenoma. Crit Rev Neurosurg 9:167-173, 1999.
54. Laws ER, Sheehan JP, Sheehan JM, et al: Stereotactic radiosurgery for pituitary adenomas: a review of the literature. J Neurooncol 69:257-272, 2004.
55. Stafford SL, Pollock BE, Leavitt JA, et al: A study on the radiation tolerance of the optic nerves and chiasm after stereotactic radiosurgery. Int J Radiat Oncol Biol Phys 55:1177-1181, 2003.
56. Joplin GF: The management of pituitary adenomas by yttrium 90 interstitial irradiation. *In* Lynn J, Bloom SR (eds): Surgical Endocrinology. London, Butterworth-Heineman, 1994, p 155.
57. Clayton RN, Wass JAH: Pituitary tumors: Recommendations for service provision and guidelines for management of patients. J R Coll Physicians Lond 31:628-636, 1997.
58. Schlete J, Dolan K, Sheraman B, et al: The natural history of untreated hyperprolactinemia: a prospective analysis. J Clin Endocrinol Metab 68:412-418, 1989.
59. Molitch ME: Medical management of prolactin-secreting pituitary adenomas. Pituitary 5:55-65, 2002.
60. Molitch ME, Elton RL, Blackwell RE, et al: Bromocriptine as primary therapy for prolactin-secreting macroadenomas: results of a prospective multicenter study. J Clin Endocrinol Metab 60:698-705, 1985.
61. Webster J, Piscitelli G, Polli A, et al: A comparison of cabergoline and bromocriptine in the treatment of hyperprolactinemic amenorrhea. Cabergoline Comparative Study Group. N Engl J Med 331:904-909, 1994.
62. Reilly PL: Prolactinomas: surgical results and prognosis. *In* Landoldt AM, Vance ML, Reilly PL (eds): Pituitary Adenomas. New York, Churchill Livingstone, 1996, p 363.
63. Littley MD, Shalet SM, Reid H, et al: The effect of external pituitary irradiation on elevated serum prolactin levels in patients with pituitary macroadenomas. Q J Med 81:985-998, 1991.
64. Tsagarakis S, Grossman A, Plowman PN, et al: Megavoltage pituitary irradiation in the management of prolactinomas: long-term follow-up. Clin Endocrinol 34:399-406, 1991.

65. Grigsby PW, Stokes S, Marks JE, et al: Prognostic factors and results of radiotherapy alone in the management of pituitary tumors. Int J Radiat Oncol Biol Phys 15:1103-1110, 1988.
66. Pan L, Zhang N, Wang EM, et al: Gamma knife radiosurgery as a primary treatment for prolactinomas. J Neurosurg. 93(Suppl 3):10-13, 2000.
67. Robert F, Hardy J: Cushing's disease: a correlation of radiological, surgical and pathological findings with therapeutic results. Pathol Res Pract 187:617-621, 1991.
68. Padayatty SJ, Orme SM, Nelson M, et al: Bilateral sequential inferior petrosal sinus sampling with corticotrophin-releasing hormone stimulation in the diagnosis of Cushing's disease. Eur J Endocrinol 139:161-166, 1998.
69. Escourolle H, Abecassis JP, Bertagna X, et al: Comparison of computerized tomography and magnetic resonance imaging for the examination of the pituitary gland in patients with Cushing's disease. Clin Endocrinol (Oxf) 39:307-313, 1993.
70. Bochicchio D, Losa M, Buchfelder M: Factors influencing the immediate and late outcome of Cushing's disease treated by transsphenoidal surgery: a retrospective study by the European Cushing's Disease Survey Group. J Clin Endocrinol Metab 80:3114-3120, 1995.
71. Melby JC: Therapy of Cushing disease: a consensus for pituitary microsurgery. Ann Intern Med 109:445-446, 1988.
72. Mampalam TJ, Tyrrell JB, Wilson CB: Transsphenoidal microsurgery for Cushing's disease: a report of 216 cases. Ann Intern Med 109:487-493, 1988.
73. Knappe UJ, Ludecke DK: Persistent and recurrent hypercortisolism after transsphenoidal surgery for Cushing's disease. Acta Neurochir Suppl (Wien) 65:31-34, 1996.
74. Invitti C, Giraldi FP, de Martin M, et al: Diagnosis and management of Cushing's syndrome: results of an Italian multicentre study. Study Group of the Italian Society of Endocrinology on the Pathophysiology of the Hypothalamic-Pituitary-Adrenal Axis. Clin Endocrinol Metab 84:440-448, 1999.
75. Howlett TA, Plowman PN, Wass JA, et al: Megavoltage pituitary irradiation in the management of Cushing's disease and Nelson's syndrome: long-term follow-up. Clin Endocrinol (Oxf) 31:309-323, 1989.
76. Hughes MN, Llamas KJ, Yelland ME, et al: Pituitary adenomas: long-term results for radiotherapy alone and postoperative radiotherapy. Int J Radiat Oncol Biol Phys 27:1035-1043, 1993.
77. Littley MD, Shalet SM, Beardwell CG, et al: Long-term follow-up of low-dose external pituitary irradiation for Cushing's disease. Clin Endocrinol (Oxf) 33:445-455, 1990.
78. Sandler LM, Richards NT, Carr DH, et al: Long-term follow-up of patients with Cushing's disease treated by interstitial irradiation. J Clin Endocrinol Metab 65:441-447, 1987.
79. Levy RP, Fabrikant JI, Frankel KA, et al: Heavy-charged-particle radiosurgery of the pituitary gland: clinical results of 840 patients, Stereotact Funct Neurosurg 57:22-35, 1991.
80. Laws ER Jr, Vance ML: Radiosurgery for pituitary tumors and craniopharyngiomas. Neurosurg Clin N Am 10:327-336, 1999.
81. Sheehan JM Vance ML, Sheehan JP, et al: Radiosurgery for Cushing's disease after failed transsphenoidal surgery. J Neurosurg 93:738-742, 2000.
82. Devin JK, Allen GS, Cmelak AJ, et al: The efficacy of linear accelerator radiosurgery in the management of Cushing's disease. Stereotact Funct Neurosurg 82:254-262, 2004.
83. Allolio B, Arlt W, Reincke M: Medical therapy of Cushing's syndrome. *In* Von Werder K, Fahlbusch KR (eds): Pituitary Adenomas: From Basic Research to Diagnosis and Therapy. Amsterdam, Elsevier, 1996, p 223.
84. Estrada J, Boronat M, Mielgo M, et al: The long-term outcome of pituitary irradiation after unsuccessful transsphenoidal surgery in Cushing's disease. N Engl J Med 336:172-177, 1997.
85. Nieman LK: Medical therapy of Cushing's disease. Pituitary 5:77-82, 2002.
86. Clemmons DR, Van Wyk JJ, Ridgway EC, et al: Evaluation of acromegaly by radioimmunoassay of somatomedin-C. N Engl J Med 301:1138-1142, 1979.
87. Ezzat S: Acromegaly. Endocrinol Metab Clin North Am 26:703-723, 1997.
88. Melmed S: Acromegaly. *In* Melmed S (ed): The Pituitary. Cambridge, Blackwell Scientific, 1995, p 413.
89. Bates AS, Van't Hoff W, Jones JM, et al: Does treatment of acromegaly affect life expectancy? Metabolism 44(Suppl 1):1-5, 1995.
90. Giovanelli M, Mortini P, Giugni E, et al: Surgical treatment of acromegaly. *In* Von Werder K, Fahlbusch KR (eds): Pituitary Adenomas: From Basic Research to Diagnosis and Therapy. Amsterdam, Elsevier, 1996, p 21.
91. Fahlbusch R, Honegger J, Buchfelder M: Evidence supporting surgery as treatment of choice for acromegaly. Endocrinology 155(Suppl 1):S53-S55, 1997.
92. Abosch A, Tyrrell JB, Lamborn KR, et al: Transsphenoidal microsurgery for growth hormone-secreting pituitary adenomas: initial outcome and long-term results. Clin Endocrinol Metab 83:3411-3418, 1998.
93. Eastman RC, Gorden P, Glatstein E, et al: Radiation therapy of acromegaly. Endocrinol Metab Clin North Am 21:693-712, 1992.
94. Vance ML, Harris AG: Long-term treatment of 189 acromegalic patients with the somatostatin analog octreotide. Results of the International Multicenter Acromegaly Study Group. Arch Intern Med 151:1573-1578, 1991.
95. Werner S, Trampe E, Palacios P, et al: Growth hormone-producing pituitary adenomas with concomitant hypersecretion of prolactin are particularly sensitive to photon irradiation. Int J Radiat Oncol Biol Phys 11:1713-1720, 1985.
96. Ludecke DK, Lutz BS, Niedworok G: The choice of treatment after incomplete adenomectomy in acromegaly: proton versus high-voltage radiation. Acta Neurochir (Wien) 96:32-38, 1989.
97. Tran LM, Blount L, Horton D, et al: Radiation therapy of pituitary tumors: results in 95 cases. Am J Clin Oncol 14:25-29, 1991.
98. Zhang N, Pan L, Wang EM, et al: Radiosurgery for growth hormone-producing pituitary adenomas. J Neurosurg 93(Suppl):3:6-9, 2000.
99. Attanasio R, Epaminonda P, Motti E, et al: Gamma-knife radiosurgery in acromegaly: a 4 year follow-up study. J Clin Endocrinol Metab 88:3105-3112, 2003.
100. Giustina S, Barkan A, Casanueva FF, et al: Criteria for cure of acromegaly: A censensus statement. J Clin Endocrinol Metab 85:3034-3040, 2000.
101. Beck-Peccoz P, Persani L, Asteris C, et al: TSH-secreting pituitary adenomas. *In* Von Werder K, Fahlbusch R (eds): Pituitary Adenomas. Amsterdam, Netherlands, Elsevier, 1996.
102. Brada M, Rajan B, Traish D, et al: The long-term efficacy of conservative surgery and radiotherapy in the control of pituitary adenomas. Clin Endocrinol 38:571-578, 1993.
103. Tsang RW, Brierley JD, Panzarella T, et al: Radiation therapy for pituitary adenoma: treatment outcome and prognostic factors. Int J Radiat Oncol Biol Phys 30:557-565, 1994.
104. Breen P, Flickinger JC, Kondziolka D, et al: Radiotherapy for nonfunctional pituitary adenoma: analysis of long-term tumor control. J Neurosurg 89:933-938, 1998.
105. Feigl GC, Bonelli CM, Berghold A, et al: Effects of gamma knife radiosurgery of pituitary adenomas on pituitary function. J Neurosurg 97(5Suppl):415-421, 2002.
106. Petrovich Z, Yu C, Giannotta SL, et al: Gamma knife radiosurgery for pituitary adenoma: early results. Neurosurgery 53:51-59, 2003.
107. Schoenthaler R, Albright NA, Wara WM, et al: Reirradiaton of pituitary adenoma. Int J Radiat Oncol Biol Phys 24:307-314, 1992.
108. Flickinger JC, Deutsch M, Lunsford LD: Repeat megavoltage irradiation of pituitary and suprasellar tumors. Int J Radiat Oncol Biol Phys 17:171-175, 1989.
109. Teears RJ, Silverman EM: Clinicopathologic review of 88 cases of carcinoma metastatic to the pituitary gland. Cancer 36:216-220, 1975.
110. Morita A, Meyer FB, Laws ER Jr: Symptomatic pituitary metastases. J Neurosurg 89:69-73, 1998.
111. Hallberg F: Pituitary tumors. *In* Liebel S, Phillips T (eds): Textbook of Radiation Oncology. Philadelphia, WB Saunders, 1998, p 357.
112. Sohn J, Dalzell JG, Suh JH, et al: Dose-volume histogram analysis of techniques for irradiating pituitary adenomas. Int J Radiat Oncol Biol Phys 32:831-877, 1995.

113. Perks JR, Jalali R, Cosgrove VP, et al: Optimization of stereotactically guided conformal treatment planning of sellar and parasellar tumors, based on normal brain dose volume histograms. Int J Radiat Oncol Biol Phys 45:507-513, 1999.
114. Chun M, Masko GB, Hetelekidis S: Radiotherapy in the treatment of pituitary adenomas. Int J Radiat Oncol Biol Phys 15:305-309, 1988.
115. Zierhut D, Flentje M, Adolph J, et al: External radiotherapy of pituitary adenomas. Int J Radiat Oncol Biol Phys 33:307-314, 1995.
116. McCollough WM, Marcus RB, Rhoton AL, et al: Long-term follow-up of radiotherapy for pituitary adenoma: the absence of late recurrence after ≥4500 cGy. Int J Radiat Oncol Biol Phys 21:607-614, 1991.
117. Littley J, Shalet SM, Beardwell CG, et al: Long-term follow-up of low dose external pituitary irradiation for Cushing's disease. Clin Endocrinol 33:445-455, 1990.
118. Grigsby PW, Simpson JR, Emami BN, et al: Prognostic factors and results of surgery and postoperative irradiation in the management of pituitary adenomas. Int J Radiat Oncol Biol Phys 16:1411-1417, 1989.
119. McCord M, Buatti JM, Fennell EM, et al: Radiotherapy for pituitary adenoma: long-term outcome and sequelae. Int J Radiat Oncol Biol Phys 39:437-444, 1997.
120. Tsang RW, Brierley JD, Panzarella T, et al: Role of radiation therapy in clinical hormonally active pituitary adenomas. Radiother Oncol 41:45-53, 1996.
121. Jones B, Samarasekara S, Tan LT: The influence of air cavities on the optic chiasm dose during pituitary radiotherapy for acromegaly. Br J Radiol 69:723-725, 1996.
122. Littley MD, Shalet SM, Beardwell CG, et al: Hypopituitarism following external radiotherapy for pituitary tumors in adults. Q J Med 70:145-160, 1989.
123. Griem ML: Clinical radiation tolerance of brain, spinal cord, and peripheral nerves: laboratory and patient data as clinical guides. Front Radiat Ther Oncol 23:367-389, 1989.
124. Goldsmith BJ, Shrieve DC, Loeffler JS: High efficacy without visual damage: the current status of pituitary radiotherapy. Int J Radiat Oncol Biol Phys 33:765-767, 1995.
125. Brada M, Ford D, Ashley S: Risk of brain tumor after conservative surgery and radiotherapy for pituitary adenoma. BMJ 304:1443, 1992.
126. Tsang RW, Laperriere NJ, Simpson WJ, et al: Glioma arising after radiation therapy for pituitary adenoma. Cancer 72:2227-2233, 1993.

CHAPTER 27

SPINAL CORD TUMORS

Volker W. Stieber and Edward G. Shaw

INCIDENCE AND PATHOLOGY

The incidence of spinal cord tumors in the United States is approximately 14 per 100,000.

Common histologies are tumors of glial origin (astrocytoma and ependymoma), meningioma, schwannoma, chordoma/chondrosarcoma, and vascular lesions.

Tumors are grouped according to extradural or intradural (extramedullary or intramedullary) origin.

BIOLOGIC CHARACTERISTICS

Histology is an important prognostic factor in spinal cord tumors.

Patients with ependymomas have a longer median survival than those with astrocytomas.

Additionally, low-grade (versus high-grade) and pilocytic (versus diffuse fibrillary) astrocytomas have a more favorable prognosis.

DIAGNOSTIC WORKUP

The workup should include a history and physical examination, with special attention given to a thorough neurologic assessment.

Radiographic imaging of the tumor should be magnetic resonance imaging (MRI).

Laboratory tests may include a cerebrospinal fluid (CSF) evaluation, which should be performed after the imaging study.

A tissue diagnosis should be obtained. For histologies with a high risk of seeding, spinal MRI should be performed to rule out an intracranial tumor presenting with drop metastasis.

There is no American Joint Committee on Cancer staging for spinal cord tumors.

PRIMARY THERAPY

If technically safe and achievable, complete surgical resection should be considered for all tumors, excluding spinal lymphomas. In general, if the tumor is completely resected, no postoperative adjuvant treatment is necessary.

If there is a subtotal resection, then postoperative radiation therapy should be given in adults for most histologic diagnoses.

In pediatric patients, observation with close imaging follow-up after subtotal resection is an alternative option.

Radiation treatment is also recommended for patients with spinal lymphomas, who typically undergo biopsy only, followed by both chemotherapy and radiation therapy.

Primary tumors of the spinal cord and canal are uncommon. Primary treatment for most spinal cord tumors involves surgical resection using advanced microsurgical techniques. Patients unable to undergo complete resection and those at high risk of recurrence are typically treated with radiation therapy. The role of chemotherapy in the management of most spinal cord tumors remains to be determined.

EPIDEMIOLOGY

United States tumor registry data demonstrate a combined incidence of all primary neural axis tumors of 14.0 in 100,000 person-years.[1,2] Table 27-1 shows the distribution by benign versus malignant, male versus female, and by racial group. Incidence rates for all primary neural axis tumors are lowest in the pediatric population under 20 years of age (3.9) and then rise notably after age 55 (17.2) and again after age 65 (39.7).[2]

The overall incidence of primary spinal cord tumors is approximately 10% to 19% that of all primary central nervous system (CNS) tumors[3] and increases with age. The incidence of primary spinal cord tumors is .7, 1.0, 2.8, and 3.6 per 100,000 person-years in the age groups of 0 to 24, 25 to 44, 45 to 64, and 65 and greater, respectively.[4] The incidence ratios of intracranial to intraspinal astrocytomas, ependymomas, and meningiomas are approximately 10:1, 3:1, and 18:1, respectively.[4] The incidence ratio of intracranial to intraspinal tumors is up to four times higher in pediatric patients than in adults. The age-adjusted incidence for spinal glioma is .11% to .14%; for meningioma, it is .08% to .28%, depending on sex (female higher than male subjects); and for nerve sheath tumors, it is .07% to .13%.[5] Schwannoma and meningioma account for approximately 60% of primary spinal tumors, with schwannoma being slightly more frequent; both types occur primarily in adults. The relative frequency of distribution of spinal tumors by histology is shown in Table 27-2.[5]

PREVENTION AND EARLY DETECTION

There is no known method for prevention of spinal cord tumors. Early detection relies on careful neurologic examination and consideration of the possibility of a spinal cord tumor in the differential diagnosis. Because the median duration of symptoms before diagnosis for spinal cord ependymomas and astrocytomas is 2 to 4 years, earlier detection should be an achievable goal.

PATHOLOGY, MOLECULAR BIOLOGY, BIOLOGIC CHARACTERISTICS, AND PATHWAYS OF SPREAD

Approximately 15% to 25% of spinal tumors involve the cervical spine, including the foramen magnum; 50% to 55% involve the thoracic spinal canal; and 25% to 30% involve the lumbosacral spine. Spinal tumors are typically classified according to extradural or intradural location. Intradural tumors either arise within the spinal cord (intramedullary) or outside of it (extramedullary)[6] (Fig. 27-1). Approximately 70% of intradural tumors are extramedullary and 30% are intramedullary.

Table 27-1 Incidences of Primary Neural Axis Tumors

Category	Incidence*
Benign	6.3
Malignant	7.7
Male	14.2
Female	13.9
White	14.3
Black	9.9
Hispanic	10.8

*All numbers are per 100,000 person-years.

Table 27-2 Distribution of Primary Spinal Cord Tumors by Histology

Histology	Incidence
Tumors of glial origin	23%
Astrocytoma	7-11%
Ependymoma	13-15%
Meningioma	25-46%
Schwannoma	22-30%
Vascular lesions	6%
Chordoma/chondrosarcoma	4%
Other miscellaneous tumors	3-4%

Data from Preston-Martin S: Descriptive epidemiology of primary tumors of the spinal cord and spinal meninges in Los Angeles County, 1972-1985. Neuroepidemiology 9:106-111, 1990; and Sloof JL: Primary Intramedullary Tumors of the Spinal Cord and Filum Terminale. Philadelphia, WB Saunders, 1964.

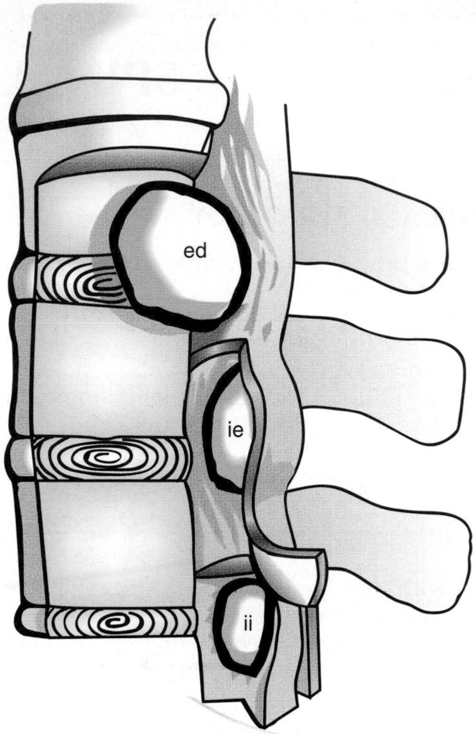

Figure 27-1 Location within the spinal column. ed, extradural; ie, intradural extramedullary; ii, intradural intramedullary. (From Shiff D: Principles of Neuro-oncology. McGraw-Hill, New York, New York, 2005.)

Table 27-3 Anatomic Distribution of Spinal Tumors by Histologic Diagnosis

Extradural	Intradural Extramedullary	Intradural Intramedullary
Chondroblastoma	Ependymoma, myxopapillary type	Astrocytoma
Chordoma	Epidermoid	Ependymoma
Chondrosarcoma	Lipoma	Ganglioglioma
Hemangioma	Meningioma	Hemangioblastoma
Lipoma	Neurofibroma	Hemangioma
Lymphoma	Paraganglioma	Lipoma
Meningioma	Schwannoma	Medulloblastoma
Metastasis		Neuroblastoma
Neuroblastoma		Neurofibroma
Neurofibroma		Oligodendroglioma
Osteoblastoma		Teratoma (mature)
Osteochondroma		
Osteosarcoma		
Sarcoma		
Vertebral hemangioma		

The diversity of primary spinal axis tumors partly results from the diversity of phenotypically distinct cells capable of transformation into tumors.[7] The genetic and molecular bases of spinal cord tumors are not yet well understood.[8] Table 27-3 classifies spinal axis tumors by histology and location. Intradural extramedullary schwannoma (neurilemmoma) and meningioma are the most common intradural tumors, although occasionally they may present as extradural tumors. Other intradural extramedullary tumors include chordomas, epidermoids, and intradural drop metastases of intracranial primary tumors such as medulloblastomas. The most common intramedullary tumors are those that are derived from glial precursors: 40% are ependymomas; the next most common are the astrocytomas of low to intermediate grade; these are followed in frequency by less common histologies.

The predominant mode of spread of primary tumors is by direct extension. Spread along the subarachnoid space with spinal or cranial involvement of the meninges may also occur. Upward spread is seen with some spinal cord tumors and is discussed later.[9] One should not always assume that the spinal cord tumor found on imaging is the primary lesion. Supratentorial tumors that show a tendency toward leptomeningeal

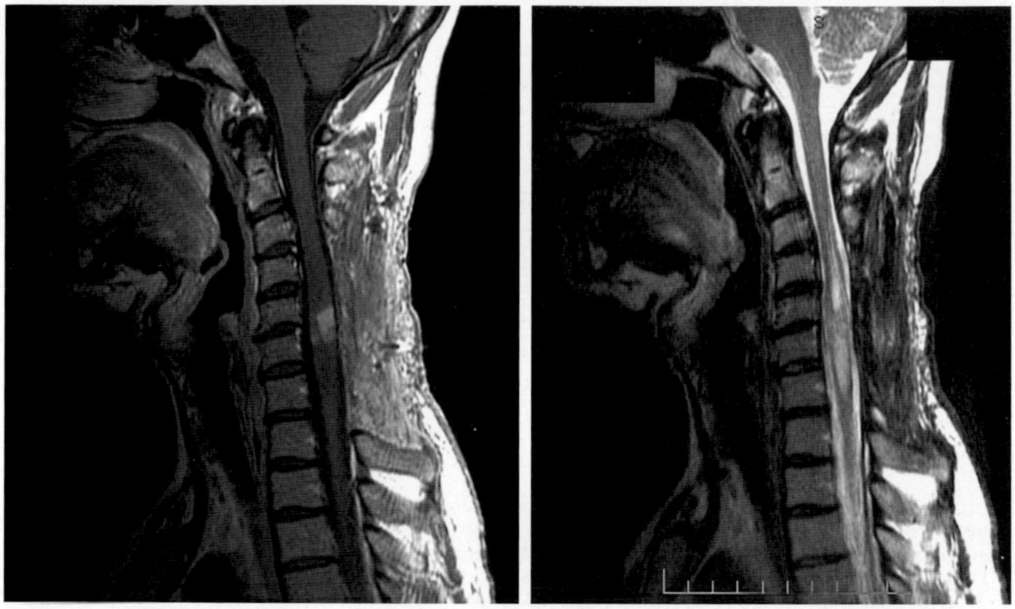

Figure 27-2 A pseudotumor, mimicking a neoplastic lesion, is shown in a sagittal-view, T1-weighted MR image with contrast *(left)* and in a T2-weighted image *(right)*.

metastases include 1.2% of glioblastomas and 1.5% of anaplastic gliomas.[10] Thus, imaging of the entire craniospinal axis is often necessary.

Nonneoplastic Lesions Mimicking Spinal Cord Tumors

Various nonneoplastic conditions may mimic spinal cord tumors (Fig. 27-2). These may include (in alphabetical order) acute transverse myelitis, *Angiostrongylus cantonensis* infection, infectious meningitis, intradural disc hernia, pseudotumor, sarcoidosis, and tuberculosis.[11-16]

CLINICAL MANIFESTATIONS, PATIENT EVALUATION, AND STAGING

The clinical presentation of tumors of the spinal axis is a function of the local anatomy[6] (Figs. 27-3 and 27-4). Within the spinal canal there exists a well-defined extradural space containing epidural fat and blood vessels. The extradural space communicates with adjacent extraspinal compartments via the intervertebral foramina. A spinal cord tumor produces local and distal symptoms and signs; the latter reflect involvement of motor and sensory long tracts within the spinal cord. These allow localization of the level of the lesion based on clinical findings.[6] However, the clinical presentation of a spinal tumor rarely indicates if it is extradural or intradural.

Location

Intramedullary

Tumors in this location can cause a characteristic neurologic syndrome.[6] Early on, decreased temperature and pain sensation occurs in the dermatomes of the spinal segments occupied by the tumor and two or three segments caudal to the lesion. Other sensory modalities are not diminished while the tumor is confined to the central cord. This "dissociated" sensory loss is rarely seen with extramedullary tumors. Additionally, weakness and atrophy are early findings in the myotomes of the corresponding cord segments involved by tumor. As the tumor grows transversely, reflexes produced at the level of the tumor disappear, spastic paralysis with hyperreflexia develops below the lesion. Eventually all sensory modalities are affected. Cervical tumors can produce Horner's syndrome by interrupting unilateral autonomic pathways.

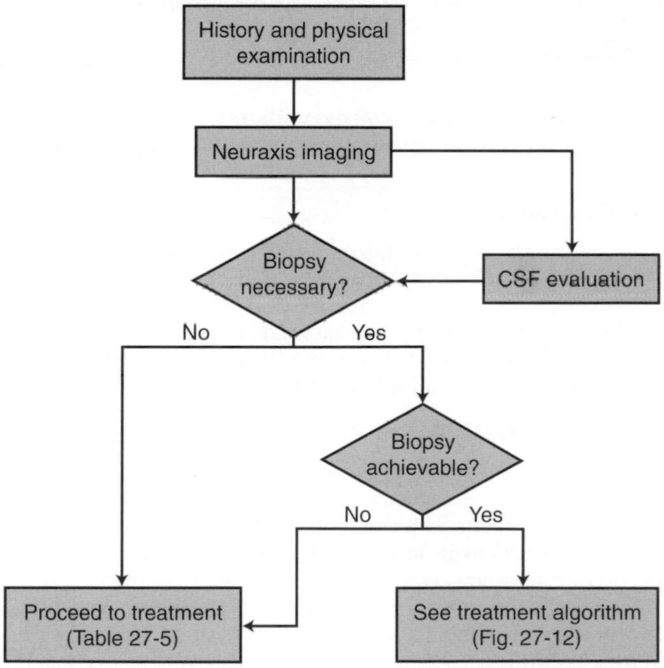

Figure 27-3 **Diagnostic algorithm for primary spinal cord tumors.** CSF, cerebrospinal fluid.

Conus Medullaris

Lesions can produce several symptoms including saddle anesthesia, acute urinary retention, incontinence of bowel and bladder, and impotence. If the lesion remains confined to the conus, it will not cause paralysis of the lower limbs and the ankle reflexes are preserved. More commonly, tumors originating in the conus are diagnosed when they have enlarged enough to cause signs characteristic of intramedullary tumors.

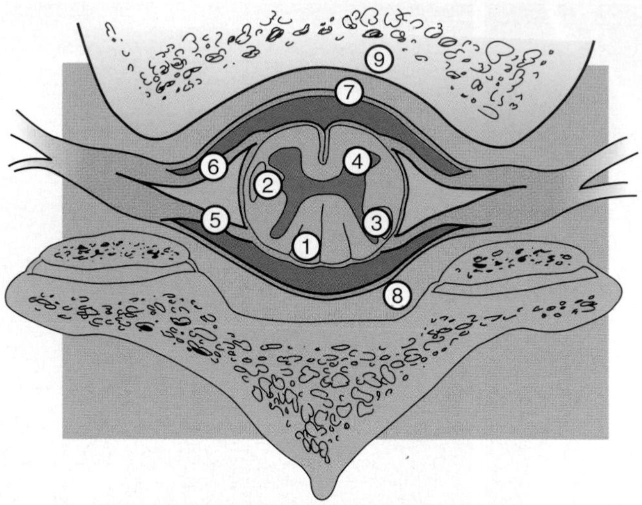

Figure 27-4 Spinal cord anatomy 1. Posterior column 2. Lateral spinothalamic tract 3. Lateral corticospinal tract 4. Anterior horn cells 5. Dorsal root 6. Ventral root 7. Dura 8. Epidural space 9. Vertebral body. (Adapted from Netter FH, Freidberg SR, Baker RA: Disorders of spinal cord, nerve root and plexus. *In* Netter FH, Jones HR Jr, Dingle RV [eds]: The Ciba Collection of Medical Illustrations, vol 1. Nervous System, part II. West Caldwell, NJ, Ciba-Geigy, 1986, pp 181-189. Copyright 1983. Novartis. Reprinted with permission from The Netter Collection of Medical Illustrations, vol. 1, Part II. Illustrated by Frank H. Netter, M.D. All rights reserved.)

These findings can also be mixed with those caused by growth of the tumor in the direction of the cauda equina, such as radicular pain.

Cauda Equina

Lesions can cause radicular pain in the thigh, weakness, and atrophy of muscles including the glutei, hamstrings, gastrocnemius, and the anterior tibialis. Saddle anesthesia, absent ankle reflexes, impotence, urinary urgency or acute retention, and constipation are also commonly seen. Depending upon the location of the lesion, other reflexes may be affected.

Sign or Symptom

Flaccid weakness, atrophy, fasciculations, and reduced deep tendon reflexes are seen in corresponding myotomes with involvement of the anterior horn cells and the ventral roots (lower motor neuron lesions).[6] A tumor involving the lateral corticospinal tracts can cause weakness, spasticity, hyperreflexia, and an extensor plantar response (Babinski's sign). Motor weakness and spasticity are seen with tumors above the conus medullaris. Weakness and flaccidity are seen with tumors below the conus because they compress the peripheral nerve roots of the cauda equina. A tumor restricted to the conus should not cause weakness, although one also involving the cauda equina or the lumbar enlargement of the spinal cord will do so.

Sensory impairment often helps to localize the level of the tumor based on loss of dermatome function, although the upper level of impaired long tract function may be several segments below the actual tumor (Fig. 27-5). A lesion involving the lateral spinothalamic tract causes numbness, paresthesias, and decreased temperature sensation over the contralateral limb or trunk below the lesion. This produces the classic finding of a sensory level, which is best demonstrated with a pin, a large metal or cold object to test temperature (cold) sensation, and observation for absence of perspiration. A lesion in the posterior column causes an ataxic or tabetic gait. Standing posture is affected with the eyes closed (Romberg's sign). Paresthesias can occur below the level of the lesion.

Since pain and temperature pathways cross over in the spinal cord and proprioceptive and motor pathways do not, a unilateral spinal cord lesion can result in ipsilateral paralysis and proprioceptive loss as well as contralateral pain-temperature loss below the level of the lesion. Because light touch travels in two pathways, one that crosses in the spinal cord (spinothalamic tract) and one that does not (posterior columns), it is usually spared in unilateral lesions. This combination of findings is known as the Brown-Séquard syndrome.

Both bladder and bowel symptoms can result from a spinal cord tumor. Bladder symptoms include hesitancy, dribbling, incontinence, urgency with incontinence, or acute retention. Loss of bladder control is seen early in the presentation of tumors in or below the conus and later in tumors above the conus. If the bowel is affected, constipation occurs more frequently than incontinence. Cord lesions above L1 can lead to impotence or reflex priapism. Lesions involving S2-4 may produce loss of erection and ejaculation ability. Decreased genital sensation can occur from lesions affecting the S2 nerve roots.

Pain from spinal canal tumors is caused by nerve root compression, by bone destruction, or, more subtly, by pressure on the dura or by deafferentation. The pain may thus be radicular, midline, or central. Radicular pain is secondary to involvement of the posterior roots and is typically described as shooting pain in a dermatomal distribution. The nerve can be compressed inside or outside the dura. Midline spinal pain causes discomfort localized to the area of the tumor and is thought to arise from pain sensitive structures in the dura and extradural tissues. Characteristically, pain is more severe in extradural lesions. Sometimes with spinal cord compression, a dull or burning pain, more widespread than segmental spinal or radicular pain, occurs. This type of pain, while relatively rare, has numerous designations including central pain, causalgia, and deafferentation pain. It involves a limb or trunk below the lesion. Pain is the most common presenting symptom in patients with sacrococcygeal tumors. Headaches may be caused by elevated intracranial pressure, which is unusual in patients with primary spinal cord tumors, with the exception of large tumors involving the foramen magnum. It can be caused by upward seeding of the tumor or by the development of carcinomatous meningitis from malignant tumors.

Neuroimaging

Magnetic resonance imaging (MRI) is the diagnostic study of choice in the evaluation of intramedullary and extramedullary spinal cord lesions. A complete description of the fundamentals of MRI is beyond the scope of this chapter. Most spinal cord tumors enhance with contrast, the most common exception being World Health Organization (WHO) grade II gliomas. On MRI, edema appears as an area of low-signal intensity on T1-weighted images and high-signal intensity on T2-weighted images. Tumor infiltration may be differentiated from edema by suppression of CSF signal using fluid-attenuated inversion recovery sequences (FLAIR) sequences.[17] MR spectroscopy may help to differentiate tumor from spinal cord necrosis by evaluating the regional distribution of chemicals associated with energy metabolism in the tumor.[18-21]

Tumor and Cerebrospinal Fluid Markers

Examination of cerebrospinal fluid (CSF) may occasionally be useful for differential diagnosis and for monitoring of thera-

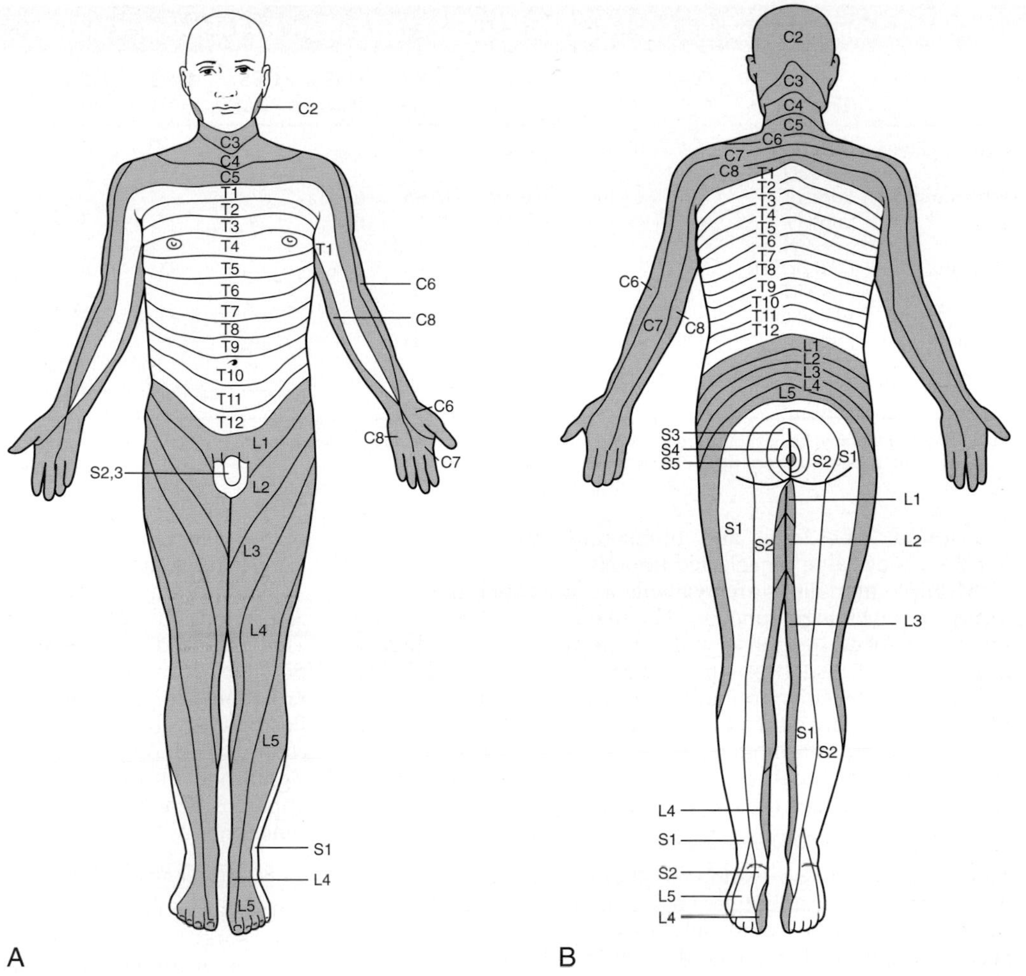

Figure 27-5 Dermatomes shown in the front (**A**) and the back (**B**). C, cervical; T, thoracic; L, lumbar; S, sacral. (Adapted from Netter FH, Freidberg SR, Baker RA: Disorders of spinal cord, nerve root, and plexus. *In* Netter FH, Jones HR Jr, Dingle RV [eds]: The Ciba Collection of Medical Illustrations, vol 1. Nervous System, part II. West Caldwell, NJ, Ciba-Geigy, 1986, pp 181-189; Keegan JJ, Garrett FD: The segmental distribution of cutaneous nerves in the limbs of man. Anat Rec 102:409, 1948.)

peutic response. Because of the risk of herniation due to increased intracranial pressure, neuroimaging studies should precede lumbar puncture. When obstruction of CSF flow occurs due to tumor expansion, patients can develop hydrocephalus; thus, one should be especially wary of performing a lumbar puncture in a patient with a spinal cord tumor who presents with a headache.[22]

CSF examination is especially useful in the management of tumors that may seed the subarachnoid space and spread via the CSF, such as medulloblastoma and ependymoma. The appearance of xanthochromic CSF, due to high protein content, with an absence of erythrocytes is characteristic of spinal cord tumors obstructing the subarachnoid space and producing stasis of the CSF in the caudal thecal sac. The CSF is examined for malignant cells (cytology), protein, and glucose. A high protein concentration with normal glucose levels and normal cytology is seen in spinal cord tumors—although if the tumor has seeded the meninges, sugar may be low and cytology malignant.

PRIMARY THERAPY

General Principles of Surgery

Surgery has traditionally been the mainstay of therapy for spinal cord tumors.[23-26] As modern diagnostic and therapeutic technology, such as MRI, the operating microscope, microsurgical tools, and intraoperative neurophysiology, have become available, more aggressive surgical intervention has become a more prevalent treatment strategy.[27] This section discusses general principles of surgery for these lesions depending on anatomic location within the spinal cord. The outcome of surgery and its role in multidisciplinary management are described in the sections for each individual type of tumor. Table 27-4 provides an overview of the outcomes of the most common spinal cord tumors by treatment modality.

Surgical Planning

Neuroimaging is the basis for preoperative planning of the surgical approach. MRI obtained both before and after the administration of intravenous gadolinium-based contrast agents is the most sensitive modality for detecting tumor and delineating tumor from reactive changes such as a syrinx. Computed tomography (CT) scans are most useful for delineating bony anatomy, acute blood, and intratumoral calcifications. Spinal angiography is occasionally necessary to distinguish spinal cord tumors from vascular malformations such as dural arteriovenous malformations, which may mimic them clinically and on MRI.

Surgery Techniques, Postoperative Management, and Complications

The use of the operating microscope is essential for spinal cord tumor surgery. The availability of other surgical adjuncts, including image-guided navigation systems, intraoperative

Table 27-4 Outcomes of the Most Common Spinal Cord Tumors by Treatment Modality

	Treatment	OS_3 (%)	OS_5 (%)	OS_{10} (%)	CSS_5 (%)	CSS_{10} (%)	CSS_{15} (%)	DFS_5 (%)	DFS_{10} (%)	DFS_{15} (%)	LC_3 (%)	LC_5 (%)	LC_{10} (%)	Overall LC (%)
Low grade glioma	GTR or STR + XRT	—	57-88	52-83	—	—	—	38-44	10-26	—	—	—	—	31-100
Ependymoma	Surgery	—	67-100	68-100	69-96	62-93	—	—	—	—	—	—	—	95-100
	Surgery + XRT	—	67-100	67-100	69-97	62	46	59	59	—	—	—	—	88-100
Meningioma	GTR or STR + XRT	—	—	—	—	—	—	93	80	68	—	—	—	94-99
	STR alone							63	45	9	—	—	—	—
Chordoma	Surgery + XRT	88-97	75-80	54	—	—	—				67-71	40-75	54	—
Chondrosarcomas		—	—	90	—	—	—	36-72	84	—	—	—	—	97

XRT, radiation therapy; OS, overall survival; CSS, cause-specific survival; DFS, disease-free survival; LC, local control; GTR, gross total resection; STR, subtotal resection. The numbers in subscript denote the number of years.

ultrasound, CO_2 laser, and ultrasound surgical aspirator (CUSA), is of value for selected tumors.

Multiple modalities are available for intraoperative monitoring of physiologic function. The most commonly used are sensory evoked response and electromyography, whereas motor evoked response is more difficult to monitor reliably as it is more sensitive to paralytic agents used in anesthesia. Electromyography is of particular use for cauda equina and foramen magnum tumors where monitoring of the extremity musculature, the anal sphincter, and sometimes the urinary sphincter can reduce the risk of postoperative deficits.

Surgery of Intradural Extramedullary Tumors

Meningiomas and schwannomas (neurilemmomas) occur in the intradural extramedullary spinal compartment.[28] Most of these tumors can be completely resected with curative intent because the normal spinal cord is not invaded by tumor.[29]

Surgery of Intramedullary Tumors

The most common intramedullary tumors are ependymomas and astrocytomas. Modern series advocate maximum safe resection of intramedullary spinal tumors. The ability to resect these tumors completely varies widely from less than 10% to as high as 86%, depending on histology.[30-39] The majority of completely resectable lesions are WHO grade I because higher grades are defined by their infiltrative potential.[35,40-58] The gross total resection rates for ependymomas range from 19% to 100%, whereas 0% to 43% of astrocytomas are resectable. For infiltrative astrocytomas, the role of surgery is most frequently limited to biopsy for diagnosis. Laminectomy offers limited functional benefit by decompressing the spinal cord in the case of bulky, infiltrative tumors. Functional postoperative outcomes may be excellent in selected cases, with the majority of patients (72% to 79%) experiencing either improvement or stabilization of their preoperative presenting symptoms, often after transient postsurgical worsening.[30,31,38,39,54,59-61] The incidence of total, permanent postoperative paralysis is reported at 1%.[27] Paralysis is often the result of unpredictable, sporadic vascular events.

Intramedullary tumors are almost always approached through a laminectomy exposure with the patient in the prone position.[27] After the dura is opened, a longitudinal myelotomy is made over the widened region of the spinal cord, where imaging demonstrates the closest approximation of the tumor to the surface and the incision is deepened several millimeters until the tumor surface is reached. Infiltrative tumors with poorly defined dissection planes cannot be removed completely and therefore biopsy for diagnosis is often the safest course of action. When there is an exophytic component to the tumor, maximum safe debulking is typically performed.

Both intramedullary and extramedullary tumors can be associated with a CSF-filled syrinx dilating the central canal. The preferred treatment is tumor removal. If this is not possible, even modest shrinkage of the tumor as a result of radiation can stabilize or even reduce the size of a syrinx. Postoperatively, a syrinx can form from scarring in the central canal. A syrinx drainage procedure may not result in a significant improvement in neurologic function, and the apparent benefit is stabilization or slowing of the decline in function.

Postoperative Management

Corticosteroids are routinely administered before, during, and after surgery to minimize edema of the spinal cord. Intravenous or oral dexamethasone or high-dose intravenous methylprednisolone is most often the agent of choice. Once maximum symptom resolution has occurred, usually approximately 7 days after beginning high-dose glucocorticoids, tapering steroids as rapidly as possible without resultant symptomatic worsening minimizes the chance for and the extent of the numerous serious side effects of these agents.

Complications of Surgery

In patients who are neurologically intact before surgery, the incidence of significant acute morbidity is generally below 5% for extramedullary tumors and is as low as 5% for carefully selected patients with intramedullary tumors.[27,62] Spinal deformities, including scoliosis and kyphosis, as well as infection and CSF leakage, can occur.[62-67] The development of postlaminectomy spinal deformities represents a serious postoperative complication, occurring in up to 40% of pediatric and adolescent patients, and may be observed as soon as 8 months postoperatively.[68]

General Principles of Radiation Therapy

The intent of radiation therapy in the treatment of spinal cord tumors is to improve local control, possibly increase survival, and improve neurologic function.[69-71] Outcomes of radiation therapy and its role in multidisciplinary management are described in the sections for each individual type of tumor. Because of the potential for growth and developmental side effects, the use of radiation therapy in children and infants with spinal cord tumors is controversial. Some authors do not recommend postoperative radiation therapy, suggesting that observation with close imaging follow-up and re-resection at the time of second occurrence is a better approach.[30,72] With this strategy, radiation therapy may be avoided or used only for children with multiply recurrent tumors.

Chemotherapy: General Principles

The efficacy of chemotherapy agents may be limited by the intact blood–nervous system barrier. Regional drug delivery may be in the form of intra-CSF therapy, intra-arterial infusion, and intratumoral therapy.[73] Extramedullary spinal tumors gain their blood supply from meningeal blood vessels that are significantly more permeable than those of the brain, and chemotherapy may be of more use for these tumors. Drugs with some efficacy in treating primary CNS malignancies[74] and that are thought to cross the blood-brain barrier have been used in the treatment of malignant glial tumors of the spinal cord; however, no clear benefit from the use of chemotherapy has been demonstrated thus far.[46,75-83]

Combined Modality Therapy: By Histology

Astrocytoma

General Background

Astrocytomas represent approximately 7% to 11% of all primary spinal tumors. They are the most common intramedullary spinal cord tumors and comprise 35% to 45% of all reported cases. The median age at presentation is approximately 35.[22,35,40,70] There does not appear to be a difference in the age of presentation between low- and high-grade tumors.[35] In children, 75% to 90% of intramedullary spinal cord tumors are astrocytomas and 85% to 95% of these are low-grade, fibrillary, or juvenile pilocytic astrocytomas (Fig. 27-6). Less than 10% of pediatric and 25% of adult spinal cord astrocytomas are malignant.[27,30-32,34,35,38,40,59,84-90]

Motor weakness is the most common presenting symptom in astrocytomas, occurring in up to 87% of patients. The median time from onset of symptoms to diagnosis ranges from 6 months to 2 years.[35,40,51,61,68,69,71] In general, high-grade astrocytomas tend to have a shorter prodrome (median duration, 1.6 to 7 months) than low-grade tumors (median duration of 2 years).[22,35,38] Tumor dissemination by spread along the subarachnoid space is reported in up to 58% of patients with high-grade astrocytomas.[22,91] Approximately 1% of WHO grade III/IV spinal cord astrocytomas have multifocal disease at presentation.[10]

Prognostic Factors

The most significant prognostic factors in patients with primary spinal cord astrocytomas are tumor histology, grade, and performance status.[30,32,36,47,49,70,89,92] High histopathologic grade is typically associated with a high risk of mortality and short median survival time. The 10-year overall survival rate of patients with pilocytic astrocytomas is 81%, in contrast to 15% for patients with diffuse fibrillary astrocytic tumors.[51] For patients with WHO grade I/II spinal cord astrocytomas, the 5-year survival rates are 69% to 89%, but they are only 0% to 33% for WHO grade III/IV lesions[69-71]; the latter have a median survival time of approximately 6 months.[22] Other factors thought to be prognostic include: young age (younger than 18 years live the longest, whereas those older than 40 years of age do poorly); the pattern of failure (local versus disseminated, the latter developing in approximately 60% of all patients with high-grade tumors) and duration of symptoms prior to diagnosis (<6 months versus >6 months, with short duration doing worse).[36,42,44,84,93,94] In most authors' series, neither extent of resection nor adjuvant radiation therapy appears to be prognostic[27,42,44,47,48,51,70] although this is controversial and approaches statistical significance in some series.[50,51,70]

Treatment and Outcomes

Surgery The treatment of choice for intramedullary astrocytomas is complete excision of the tumor, providing this can be accomplished without neurologic compromise. Otherwise, an incomplete excision is typically performed for grade I lesions, and biopsy alone is the surgical strategy for the nonexophytic component of an infiltrative glioma. Gross total resection (GTR) is typically extremely difficult to achieve due to the infiltrative nature of all but the pilocytic lesions, with most authors reporting between 0% and 50% likelihood of GTR for spinal cord astrocytoma.[33,36,37,40,41,44,45,48,50,70,95,96]

In patients with favorable prognostic factors (low-grade histology, good performance status, and young age), observation with serial imaging studies, reserving radiation therapy for local recurrence, is an appropriate management option, particularly for young children.[27,88] In the remainder of patients, adjuvant radiation therapy is usually recommended.[30,35,36,41,89,92]

Radiation Therapy Patients who undergo subtotal resection or biopsy of a low-grade glioma often receive subsequent radiation therapy, because progression of tumor in the spinal cord may lead to significant neurologic impairment. With intracerebral low-grade glioma, randomized trials have demonstrated that radiation therapy does not alter survival but increases the disease-free interval.[97] There does not appear to be a dose response between 45 and 64.8 Gy for cerebral low-grade glioma,[98,99] and in the treatment of spinal cord astrocytoma, doses have traditionally been based on the experience with cerebral tumors.[98-101]

The overall outcomes are similar for patients with low-grade gliomas of the spinal cord treated by either gross total resection or subtotal resection/biopsy followed by radiation therapy, with most series reporting overall survival rates at 5

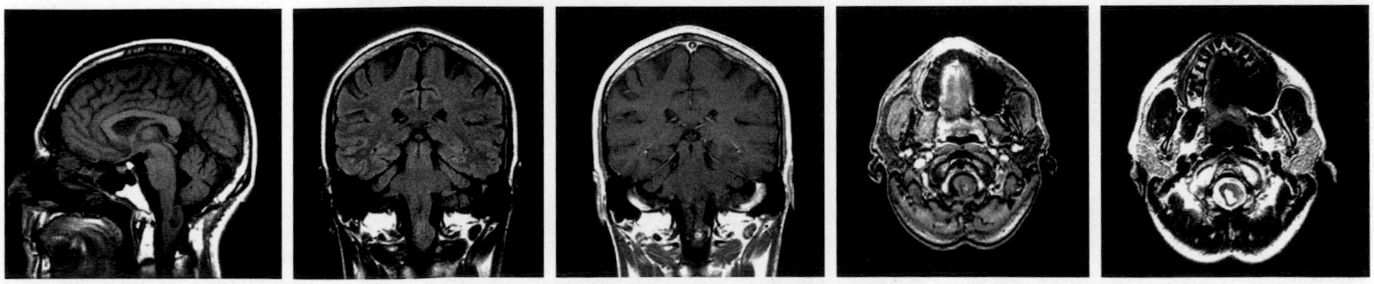

Figure 27-6 MRI of an upper cervical spine pilocytic (WHO grade I) astrocytoma. Shown are *(left to right)* sagittal-view, T1-weighted; coronal-view, fluid-attenuated inversion recovery (FLAIR); coronal-view, T1-weighted with contrast; axial-view, T1-weighted, spoiled gradient-recalled (SPGR) with contrast; and axial-view, T2-weighted images.

and 10 years in the ranges of 57% to 88% and 52% to 83%, respectively, and disease-free survival rates of 38% to 44% and 26% at 5 and 10 years, respectively. Overall, long-term local control rates range from 31% to 100%.[42,44,45,49-51,70,89,102] A comparison of survival and local control rates is shown in Table 27-4.

With high-grade tumors in adults and children, median survival time is quite poor (4 to 10 months) despite surgery and radiation therapy; approximately two thirds of patients die of both local and disseminated disease.[22,43,48,51,70,94,103,104] One small series suggested a survival benefit for patients with high-grade tumors treated with craniospinal axis irradiation.[105]

Chemotherapy Data specific to adjuvant chemotherapy (after surgery and/or radiation therapy) for spinal cord astrocytomas are scant and composed mostly of small retrospective series.[75,77,78,94,106] In two small trials, children with high-grade spinal astrocytoma had a 5-year progression-free survival of 46% to 50% and a 5-year overall survival of 54% to 88% when chemotherapy was given either in the adjuvant setting or at time of relapse.[78,94] Overall, while there is no clear evidence of a difference in outcomes with or without chemotherapy for spinal cord tumors, chemotherapy is usually given for patients with malignant astrocytoma.[74]

Ependymoma

General Background

These glial tumors are approximately equal in incidence to astrocytomas.[62] The mean age at presentation for patients with ependymoma is 30 to 39 years of age. They are more common in adults than in children[35,56,89,107-109] and in males than in females.[53,56,71,107,109-112] The median duration of symptoms prior to presentation is 2 to 4 years.[35,40,54,96,110,112] Two thirds occur in the lumbosacral regions, 40% from the filum terminale[54,107-108,112] (Fig. 27-7). Because of the propensity of these tumors for seeding the craniospinal axis, CSF evaluation and craniospinal MRI are favored for patients diagnosed with ependymoma. It is also important to note that 11% of patients with intracranial ependymomas have documented spinal metastases, so imaging of the brain may be indicated to rule out a primary brain tumor[113] (Fig. 27-8).

Most tumors are low grade.[32,40,55,89,107] Most intradural-extramedullary ependymomas are myxopapillary and are often amenable to complete surgical resection if they are not multifocal.[110,114-117] Late failures may occur more than 4 years after curative surgery, particularly with the myxopapillary subtype, so long-term follow-up is warranted.[112,118-120] Myxopapillary ependymomas often progress slowly and cause more mild than expected neurologic deficits as a function of size.

Pathology

Ependymomas arise from ependymal cells and typically occur in the central canal of the spinal cord, the filum terminale, and white matter adjacent to a ventricular surface.[121] They are either low-grade tumors or anaplastic tumors that are more likely to disseminate via the CSF. Myxopapillary ependymomas are low-grade tumors that typically occur in the lumbosacral region (filum terminale), are well differentiated, and are often encapsulated[112,117,122] but can seed the CSF,[123] typically going to the thecal sac.[117] Some series have included ependymoblastomas; however, these are primitive neuroectodermal tumors (PNETs), which have a high propensity to disseminate throughout the CNS and therefore should be considered in the medulloblastoma-PNET family of tumors.[124]

Prognostic Factors

Multiple factors have been reviewed in the literature as being prognostic for local recurrence and survival. Factors prognostic for a favorable outcome include age (patients <40 years of age), location (lumbosacral spine), histologic subtype (myxopapillary, although not all authors agree[110]), grade of the tumor (WHO grade I), extent of surgical resection (gross total or subtotal resection versus biopsy only), and good preoperative function.[53,55,56,108,117,125-127] Some authors believe that the volume of residual disease appears to correlate with a worse outcome after radiation therapy,[108,127,128] whereas other authors have found no differences in outcomes when comparing complete excision to subtotal resection followed by radiation therapy.[55,126] Myxopapillary subtypes appear to be associated with a favorable prognosis perhaps because of the ease of resection due to their anatomic location.[53] Overall 5-year sur-

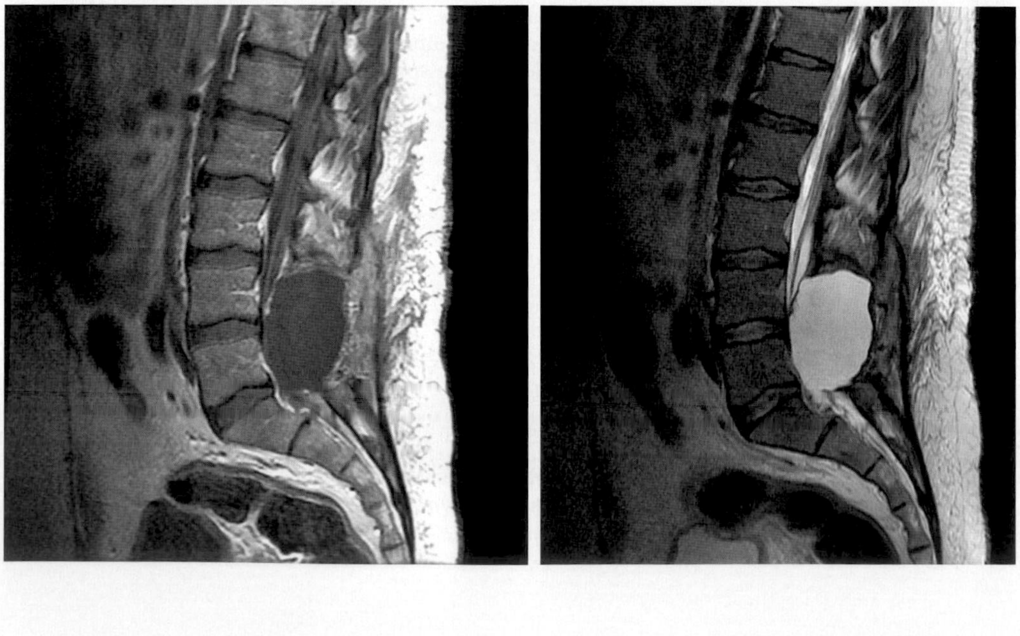

Figure 27-7 MRI of a sacral ependymoma. Shown are T1-weighted with contrast *(left)* and T2-weighted sagittal *(right)* images.

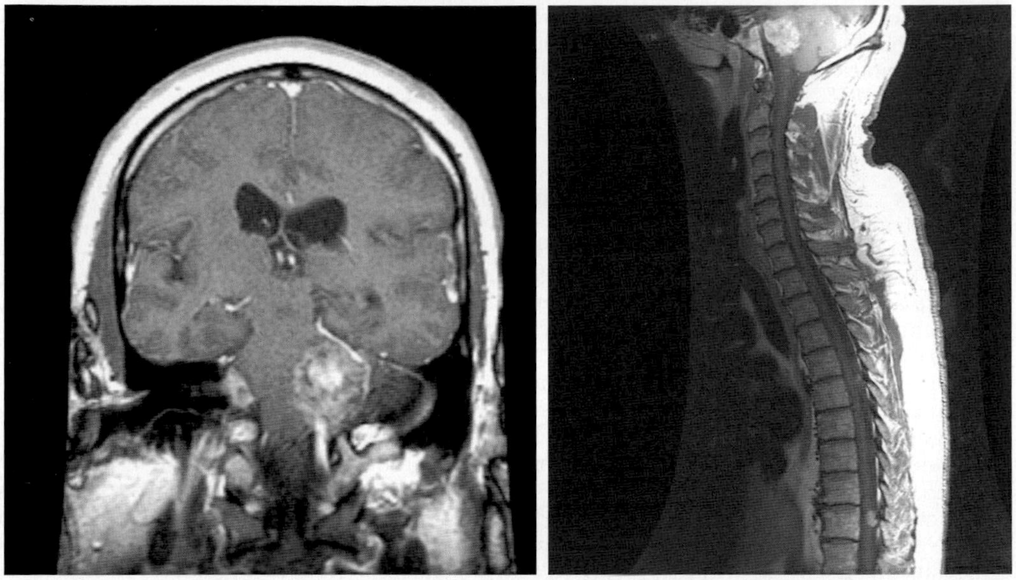

Figure 27-8 MRI of a myxopapillary ependymoma with drop metastases. Shown are T1-weighted, coronal-view *(left)* and sagittal-view *(right)* images, both with contrast.

vival for the myxopapillary subtype and for WHO grade I tumors is 97% to 100%, and 5-year disease-specific survival is 97%.[125,126]

Therapy and Outcomes

Surgery The goal of surgery is gross total resection. Every attempt should be made to remove myxopapillary tumors as a whole as opposed to piecemeal, due to the risk of seeding including upward seeding to the cranial nerves. The potential for cure may increase the severity of a hopefully transient deficit that surgeon and patient may be willing to incur and illustrates the importance of prospective multidisciplinary management of these tumors. Typically, complete resection is achievable in 79% to 100% of modern series[39,41,52,54,56,58,59,96] Some authors report complete resection rates as low as 19% to 50%, but these tend to be older series or those with a significant number of high-grade tumors.[33,35,40,53,108]

Five- and 10-year overall survival rates for all spinal cord ependymomas are 67% to 100% and 68% to 100%, respectively[34,40,55-57,108,125,126] Disease-specific survival rates at 5 and 10 years are 69% to 96% and 62% to 93%, respectively.[35,53,89] Local control rates after gross total resection are 95% to 100%.[32,52,56] Myxopapillary subtypes may be associated with a favorable prognosis because of their relative ease of resection.

Radiation Therapy Postoperative radiation therapy appears to improve local control in patients with subtotally resected ependymomas,[40,53,108,110,129] for all high-grade lesions, and for patients with craniospinal axis dissemination (positive CSF or MRI). In most series, the outcome for subtotal resection followed by radiation therapy appears to be similar to that of complete excision. Typically, the dose given to the tumor bed is 49 to 56 Gy while the craniospinal axis (if indicated) receives 30 to 36 Gy.[52,55,57,125] Low-grade lesions with low risk of seeding are typically treated with limited fields to 50.4 to 55.8 Gy in 1.8-Gy daily fractions. In patients with tumors at high risk of seeding, when pretreatment CSF cytology studies reveal malignant cells, or if the spinal MRI scan shows evidence of leptomeningeal disease, the craniospinal axis should be treated to 36 Gy in 1.5- to 1.8-Gy daily fractions. Subsequently, the primary tumor site is boosted to a total dose of 50.4 to 55.8 Gy. If gross leptomeningeal spread is evident, the craniospinal axis dose should be 39.6 Gy (1.8 Gy/fraction) or 40.5 Gy (1.5 Gy/fraction), with the same boost dose to primary as previously discussed.

In those patients undergoing incomplete resection followed by radiation therapy, overall survival rates at 5 and 10 years are 67% to 100% and 67% to 100%, respectively.[55-57,125,126] Cause-specific survival rates at 5, 10, and 15 years for all tumors are 69% to 93%, 62% to 93%, and 46%, respectively.[53,89] By tumor grade, cause-specific survival rates at 5 years are 87% to 97% for myxopapillary and low-grade lesions and 27% to 71% for high-grade tumors.[125,126] Disease-free survival rates at 5 and 10 years are 59% and 59%, respectively.[53] Local control rates are 88% to 100%.[52,55,57,126,130]

Chemotherapy There is no strong body of evidence thus far demonstrating that the addition of chemotherapy to radiotherapy improves the outcome.[76,79-83] A single trial of etoposide for recurrent spinal ependymoma has shown a median response duration of 15 months with a median survival time of 16 months.[80] Patients who were responders had a median survival of 20 months, whereas those who did not respond only lived 4 months; the results approached statistical significance. Pediatric patients with anaplastic ependymoma or ependymoblastoma are routinely given chemotherapy.[131,132] Further clinical research in this area is necessary.

Meningioma

General Background

Spinal meningiomas make up only 8% of all meningiomas[133] but 25% to 46% of all spinal neoplasms.[64,65,133,134] They tend to occur in females 3 to 7 times more commonly than in males.[63,65,133-137] Most patients are over the age of 40 with the mean age at diagnosis of 49 to 63 years.[136,137] The incidence appears to be bimodal, with the first peak being in the third decade of life and a second larger peak seen after age 50, especially in the sixth and seventh decades of life.[136,137] In younger patients, 13% have neurofibromatosis type 2.[137] Younger patients (<50 years of age) also have a recurrence rate of 23% versus 5% in older patients,[137] although not all authors agree that young age in and of itself carries a worse prognosis.[133]

The most common site is in the thoracic region, accounting for 55% to 80%, while cervical lesions make up approximately one third of all lesions.[64,65,133,135-139] The incidence by location varies with age: before age 50, 39%, 56%, and 5% occur in the cervical, thoracic, and lumbar spine, respectively; over age 50, 16%, 80%, and 5% occur in the cervical, thoracic, and lumbar spine, respectively.[137]

Treatment and Outcomes

Surgery The mainstay of treatment of spinal meningiomas is surgical resection. Meningiomas in most patients can be removed through a posterior (laminectomy) approach, because they are commonly lateral or anterolateral, and even the more anteriorly placed tumors cause enough lateral displacement of the spinal cord to allow access for resection without traction on the spinal cord. If the tumor is located anterior to the spinal cord, it may require an anterior approach including corpectomy with arthrodesis. Anteriorly situated meningioma are sometimes unresectable because of their encasement of the anterior spine or their location at the foramen magnum of a vertebral artery.[29]

Functional improvement of neurologic deficits is seen in 66% to 100% of patients.[63,64,135,136,139] Complete resection is achievable in 82% to 100% of cases with a 1% to 6% late local failure rate.[64,65,139] With subtotal resection, late local recurrence rates range from 17% to 100%.[63-65] Local failures take place even decades after surgery. After complete resection, recurrence-free rates at 5, 10, and 15 years are 93%, 80%, and 68%, respectively, and after subtotal resection, recurrence-free rates at 5, 10, and 15 years are 63%, 45%, and 9%, respectively.[133] Thus, the necessity for life-long follow-up cannot be overemphasized. Because local failure rates in the spine are higher with subtotal resection, some authors recommend radiation therapy (see later).

Radiation Therapy and Chemotherapy The role of radiation therapy is not well understood due to the small number of cases reported in the literature, and most clinicians extrapolate from the data on irradiation of intracranial meningiomas.[136,139,140] The expected outcome of radiation therapy is long-term stabilization of disease.[141] Patients who undergo complete resection should be observed. Even those with subtotally resected disease who either have improvement of their neurologic status or are asymptomatic postoperatively can be closely followed. When patients are irradiated, the dose delivered is typically 52.2 to 54 Gy, based on the data from the treatment of intracranial meninigoma.[141] Single-fraction spinal stereotactic radiosurgery must be considered investigational at this time.[142] Hydroxyurea chemotherapy may also be of benefit in stabilizing postradiation disease progression.[143]

Chordoma

General Background

Chordomas are slowly growing neoplasms thought to be remnants of the embryonic notochord.[7] They make up approximately 4% of spinal tumors: 24% to 35% arise in the region of the base of skull (but in some series as many as 17% are thought to have originated in the cervical spine), 11% to 15% are known as chordomas of the mobile spine and arise in the true vertebral region (usually lumbar), and 50% to 58% in the sacrococcygeal region.[144-150] Most chordomas occur during the fourth decade of life with a 2:1 male-to-female ratio,[151] although sacrococcygeal chordomas tend to arise in the fifth and sixth decades.[152-156] Median survival is 6 years.[147]

Prognostic Factors

Several prognostic factors have been identified. Location is prognostic for survival,[157] with overall 5-year survival rates of 66% for sacrococcygeal tumors and 50% for vertebral lesions. Overall, 14% to 39% of patients develop metastases at a median of 5 years, most commonly to the lungs.[145-147,153,158-161] The incidence of metastases varies by location of the primary tumor: 26% to 44% of patients with sacrococcygeal lesions develop metastatic disease (usually to the thecal sac), whereas 61% of those with vertebral primaries can metastasize, typically in a caudal direction. In some series, skull base lesions have rarely been reported to metastasize.[147,153,154] Gender may also be prognostic: 5- and 8-year local control rates are 81% and 75% for men and 65% and 17% for women, respectively.[162,163] The prognostic importance of age is controversial: in some series, children have a higher incidence of metastases[164]; in other series, patients over the age of 52 years have a worse local control rate.[144] Finally, residual microscopic disease after resection (either tumor spillage or positive margins) increases the risk of local relapse to 60% to 64% from 25% to 28% after a gross total resection.[155-165]

Treatment and Outcomes

While en bloc gross total resection has traditionally been advocated for these lesions, it is rarely possible. As such, most patients undergo subtotal resection or biopsy, followed by radiation therapy. In most series, patients have been treated with conventional photon radiation therapy, typically to doses of 55 to 70 Gy in 2-Gy fractions, with 5-year actuarial survival rates of 38% to 58%.[146,147,151,153-155,166,167] While radiation therapy prolongs the disease-free interval,[151] the majority of tumors still recur unless they have also undergone complete resection[147,151] and local progression is the most common cause of death. In one older series, the local control rate of sacrococcygeal tumors was 0% with either surgery or radiation therapy as monotherapy but 40% when the two were combined.[146]

Some treatment series using conventional photon radiation therapy suggest that local control rates improve with increasing radiation doses. With doses of less than 40, greater than 48, less than 50, and greater than 55 Gy, 5-year disease-free survival rates are approximately 0%, 13%, 31%, and 41%, respectively.[153,167] However, not all authors have found that increased dose improves outcome.[168]

In order to improve the therapeutic ratio when treating residual or recurrent disease, most authors now advocate a combination of photon and charged particle therapy (typically protons).[144,157,169-174] When patients are treated either immediately after maximum resection or at the time of recurrence, with median doses of 65 to 76 Gy-equivalent using charged particle radiation therapy (with or without photons), local control rates at 3, 5, and 10 years are 67% to 71%, 40% to 75%, and 54%, respectively, with overall survival rates at 3, 5, and 10 years at 88% to 97%, 75% to 80%, and 54%, respectively.[144,158,169,171,175] There is no known role for chemotherapy.

Radiosurgery has also been used in the treatment of residual and recurrent cervical spine chordoma. A mean dose of 19 Gy in a single fraction prescribed at the tumor margin resulted in a 4-year local control rate of 80% without neurologic sequelae in one series.[176] The experience with interstitial irradiation is minimal, and this modality has fallen out of favor with the advent of charged particle therapy and radiosurgery.[177-179]

Chondrosarcoma

General Background

Primary chondrosarcoma of the spine is a rare, slowly growing tumor thought to originate from primitive mesenchymal cells or from the embryonal rests of the cranial cartilaginous matrix.[7] Spinal chondrosarcomas are slightly more common in men than in women[180,181] The mean and median ages of presentation are 45 and 51 years, respectively.[181-183] Of the axial skeleton chondrosarcomas, 33% occur in the mobile spine, most often in the thoracic region.[182,183] Another 33% arise in the sacrum.[184]

Patients with spinal chondrosarcomas typically have a 25% to 54% overall long-term survival rate.[180,182,183,185,186] Adverse prognostic factors include positive surgical margins, high tumor grade, and older patient age.[184,186] From 12% to 19% of lesions may be grade 4 tumors,[184,186] which carry a poor prognosis with an overall survival rate of only 14% at 3 years, a median survival time of 2.7 years, and a 75% to 86% incidence of metastases.[184,186]

Treatment and Outcomes

Surgical resection is the mainstay of treatment of these lesions. Overall survival rates after any degree of resection are 55% to 72%, 67%, and 63% at 5, 10, and 15 years, respectively.[183,184] Median survival time is typically 6 years, with local control rates ranging from 36% to 72%.[182-184,186] Patients with gross total resection have a better outcome than those with subtotal resection. After complete resection, the local control rate is 97%, with a 90% 10-year overall survival rate and an 84% disease-free survival rate.[184] Many chondrosarcomas have indolent courses, but others behave more aggressively. Radiation therapy after incomplete resection has been shown to lengthen the disease-free interval from 16 to 44 months in one series.[182] Chemotherapy has not been shown to improve outcomes.[181,182]

Other Miscellaneous Tumors

Chloroma

Spinal canal chloroma (granulocytic sarcoma) is defined as an extramedullary localized tumor mass of blasts of the granulocytic lineage.[187-190] This tumor can arise during the course of acute myeloid leukemia (AML) or myelodysplastic syndrome (MDS) synchronic with initial diagnosis or as relapse but also as an isolated tumor without any signs of medullar involvement. Spinal chloromas can occasionally precede the development of systemic disease by weeks to years. Spinal complications of chloromas, such as cord compression secondary to epidural tumor or cauda equina syndrome, have been described but are uncommon. The median age at presentation is 22 years, with a 7.8 : 1 male-to-female ratio. The thoracic spine is most commonly involved (73%), followed by the lumbar (34%), sacral (23%), and cervical (5%) regions. Multiple noncontiguous areas of involvement are found in 18% of patients.

Eighty percent of patients present with pain (generalized, localized, or radicular), with half of these reporting back pain. Sixty-six percent of patients present with motor deficits, ranging from lower-extremity weakness (34%) to paraplegia (30%). Numbness is reported in 27% of patients. Disturbance of bladder or bowel function is seen in 27% of patients.

The most effective treatment appears to be multimodality therapy coupled with early diagnosis. Options include surgical decompression, intravenous and/or intrathecal chemotherapy, radiation therapy at doses of 20 to 30 Gy, or any combination of these treatments. Patient survival ranges from 18 days to 9.5 years after diagnosis. In a review of the literature, no clear relationship could be found between specific treatment modality and survival.[187] Those receiving systemic therapy soon after diagnosis experienced the longest disease-free episodes, however.

Epidermoid Tumor

Epidermoid tumors are rare tumors of male preponderance, most commonly found in the lumbosacral region.[121] Complete surgical excision is usually curative. Incompletely excised tumors may recur, but due to their slow growth, this may take several years.

Hemangioblastoma

General Background

Intramedullary hemangioblastomas are slowly growing vascular tumors composed of endothelial and stromal components and account for 3% to 13% of all intramedullary spinal tumors.[7,191,192] The median age of presentation is 36 years for sporadic lesions, while patients with von Hippel-Lindau syndrome (VHLS) typically present a decade earlier and have multiple tumors.[193] The male-to-female ratio is 1.8 : 1.[193]

In the spinal cord, some authors report that 70% to 80% occur as sporadic isolated lesions,[194,195] whereas other authors describe 80% of spinal cord hemangioblastomas as arising together with multiple cerebellar and retinal lesions as part of VHLS (Fig. 27-9). In patients with VHLS, 51% of all neuraxis lesions are located in the spinal cord and only 29% are com-

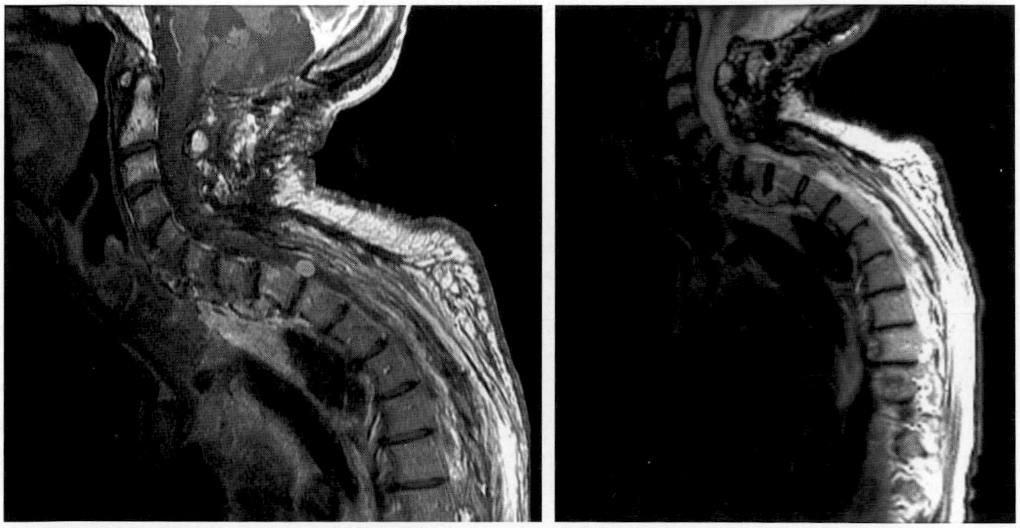

Figure 27-9 MRI of a spinal hemangioblastoma with an associated syrinx in the setting of von Hippel-Lindau syndrome. Shown are T1-weighted with contrast *(left)* and T2-weighted *(right)* sagittal-view images.

pletely intramedullary, with the remainder having an extramedullary component[196]; 56% present in the cervical spine, with another 40% arising in the thoracic spine.[193,196] In the setting of VHLS, 83% of patients present with hypesthesia, 65% with weakness, 65% with gait ataxia, 52% with hyperreflexia, 17% with pain, and 14% with incontinence.[197]

Multiple CNS hemangioblastomas are diagnostic of VHLS. Multiply recurrent hemangioblastoma may also raise the suspicion of VHLS. Patients with isolated spinal hemangioblastoma should be screened for other manifestations of VHL by ophthalmologic evaluation, brain MRI, and abdominal CT scanning to rule out retinal and cranial hemangioblastoma and renal tumors, respectively.

Prognostic Factors

Factors prognostic for favorable outcome (defined as improvement or stabilization of neurologic function) are minimal or no preoperative neurologic deficits, lesions smaller than 0.5 cm^2, dorsally located lesions, and total surgical removal of the lesion.[196,198] Progressive syringomyelia is a negative prognostic factor with respect to preservation of neurologic function and is often recalcitrant to treatment attempts.

Treatment and Outcomes

Surgical resection is the mainstay of treatment for symptomatic lesions. Hemangioblastomas are extremely vascular tumors occurring in the spinal intramedullary compartment. The dorsal location of most of these lesions and the commonly associated cyst help to simplify the removal as the cyst provides a safe route to approach the tumor. Removal of enhancing tumor is satisfactory to prevent reaccumulation of the cyst; the remainder of the cyst wall may, therefore, be left intact. Tumor margins are addressed first and feeding arteries are coagulated. Then the tumor is dissected and removed en bloc. After surgical resection, 41% to 68% of patients experience improvement of neurologic function and another 32% to 84% have stabilization of their preoperative function.[192,193,196] While single-fraction stereotactic radiosurgery is an option for cerebellar hemangioblastoma,[199] it has not been properly evaluated for spinal hemangioblastoma due to concerns regarding the radiation tolerance of the spinal cord.

Lipoma

Primary spinal lipomas are benign, congenital, intradural-extramedullary lesions located in the cervicothoracic region and account for approximately 1% of all spinal cord tumors.[200-205] The classic presentation is that of a slow ascending spastic monoparesis or paraparesis with rapid late deterioration. Early surgical decompression is mandatory for preservation of existing neurologic function,[48,202,205] but complete surgical debulking is almost impossible due to their infiltrative nature.[48,200,201] There is no known role for radiation therapy or chemotherapy.

Lymphoma

Primary spinal cord lymphomas are uncommon lesions. Only 4% of lymphomas are primary epidural tumors,[206] of which 90% are of B-cell origin[207] (Fig. 27-10). Typically, lymphomas involving the spinal cord are seen in the context of primary CNS non-Hodgkin's lymphoma, with 27% having positive CSF findings and 16% eventually developing into leptomeningeal disease involving the spine.[208]

If the initial presentation is one of spinal cord compression, management is similar to that of other metastatic tumors described later, although rapid responses may be seen with steroids, chemotherapy, and radiation therapy to a median dose of 38 Gy.[207] Lengthy administration of preoperative steroids may result in disappearance of the tumor by the time of surgery (the "ghost-tumor" effect).[209-212] Otherwise, their management is similar to that of cerebral non-Hodgkin's lymphoma.[213] After decompressive laminectomy, subtotal tumor resection, and spinal irradiation, the local control rate is 60%, with a median duration of survival of 42 months.[207]

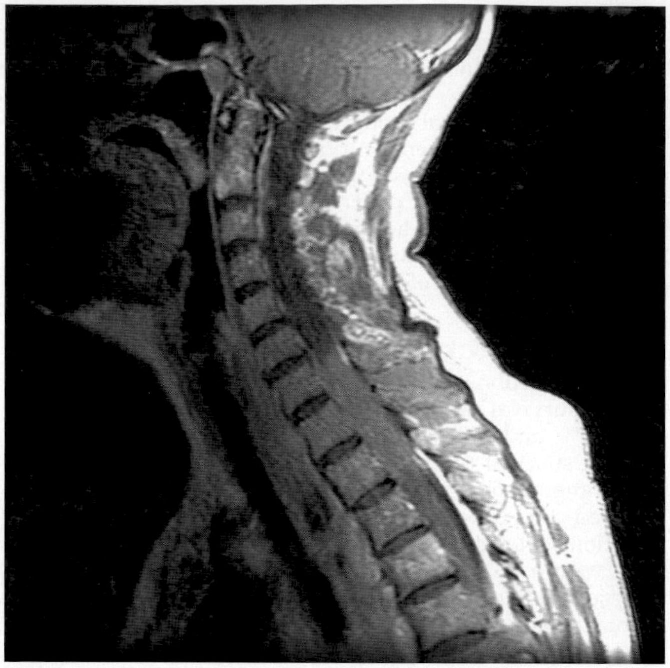

Figure 27-10 MRI of a lymphoma involving the bone and spinal cord. Shown is a sagittal-view, T1-weighted image with contrast.

Melanoma

Primary spinal melanoma must be distinguished from nonmalignant melanotic schwannoma. Primary nerve root melanomas have a prognosis more favorable than melanomas arising in other locations.[214]

Neurocytoma

Central neurocytoma has been reported to arise in the spine.[215-217] In the past, it may have often been mistaken for spinal oligodendroglioma. Staining for synaptophysin and neuro-specific enolase allows this tumor to be reliably distinguished. As in the brain, its behavior is variable. Because this tumor arises centrally in the spinal cord, observation or radiation may be primary management strategies with resection reserved for those with progressive neurologic deficits.

Sarcoma

General Background

Primary sarcomas of the spinal cord are exceedingly rare, accounting for 0.7% of all central nervous system malignancies; 5.6% of these are found in the spinal canal.[218] Malignant fibrous histiocytoma represents the most common histologic diagnosis,[218] arising from the nerve roots of the cauda equina, the spinal cord, or spinal blood vessels.[219]

Treatment and Outcomes

Surgical debulking and postoperative radiation therapy to approximately 60 Gy in 1.8- to 2.0-Gy fractions represents the typical treatment approach described in the literature.[218,219] The

5-year survival rate of patients with high-grade lesions is significantly worse at 28% than the 83% reported with low-grade lesions. The role of chemotherapy is not known.[220]

Schwannoma

Spinal schwannoma may present simultaneously in both the spinal canal and the thoracic cavity. These dumbbell-shaped tumors are typically benign and may involve the spinal cord and spinal nerves via the neural foramina. Surgical resection is the treatment of choice.[66,221,222] Schwannomas arise from spinal rootlets (most often the dorsal rootlets) and may grow along the nerve root in a dumbbell fashion through a neural foramen. Thus, resection requires removal of sections of the involved rootlets.[29] Only 3% of these tumors are malignant,[223] in which case adjuvant radiation therapy has been used. Outcomes are mixed.[222,223]

Teratoma

True intramedullary teratoma is an extremely rare tumor, with only nine cases reported in the literature. Early surgical resection is recommended to preserve neurologic status. Because teratomas may adhere to the functional neural tissue of the spinal cord with no dissection plane, complete resection is often not possible. Low-grade histopathology predominates, so the symptomatic recurrence of incompletely resected mature teratomas is often slow and may eventually require a second surgical procedure.[224] Radiation therapy is generally reserved for multiply recurrent, subtotally resected disease.

Vertebral Hemangioma

General Background

Vertebral hemangiomas are benign growths of endothelial origin typically located in the thoracic and upper lumbar spine. They are the most common benign spinal column tumors with an incidence of approximately 11%.[225] Because vertebral body hemangiomas are most frequently stable over long periods of time, some authors consider them to be nonneoplastic. Growth causing progressive symptoms has been documented. Only 1% to 2% of patients develop clinically significant pain. New-onset back pain followed by subacute progression of a thoracic myelopathy, typically over a period of 4 to 5 months, is the most common presentation for patients with neurologic deficit.[226] These tumors also occasionally cause root and cord compression syndromes. A preoperative diagnosis of compressive VH can be made in 65% of plain-film and 80% of CT examinations, whereas asymptomatic vertebral hemangioma is much more easily recognized with this imaging combination.[227]

Treatment and Outcomes

Treatment is initiated only when progressive symptoms, including focal pain or progressive neurologic deficit, develop. Historically, standard treatment consisted of surgical removal of the lesion. Endovascular embolization of these very vascular growths may also provide pain control. Vertebroplasty has high reported rates of success. The local control rate at 3 years is 70%. In those patients who experience regrowth of the lesion, 90% have recurrence within the first 2 years.[228]

Radiation therapy is an effective treatment alternative. A meta-analysis demonstrated that a total dose of 30 Gy given in 2-Gy fractions resulted in a 57% complete and 32% partial improvement of pain.[225] A second, smaller analysis showed an apparent dose response. Patients treated with the biologic equivalent 36 to 44 Gy in 2-Gy fractions had significantly better complete pain relief than those treated with 20 to 34 Gy (82% versus 39%, respectively).[229]

LOCALLY ADVANCED DISEASE AND PALLIATION

The principles of treatment are the same for patients with more locally advanced disease and palliation as for definitive treatment. Because of the severity of symptoms related to lack of control of spinal cord tumors, in most cases the dose should not be substantially decreased, although this may be a consideration with very large fields. End-stage patients requiring palliation of pain and mass effect are typically treated based on the general principles of palliative management, and the reader is referred to the corresponding topic chapter.

TECHNIQUES OF IRRADIATION

Definitions of Treatment Volumes and Reporting of Dose

Treatment planning is based on three-dimensional volumes of interest described by the International Commission on Radiation Units and Measurements (ICRU).[230,231] Gross tumor volume (GTV) represents the grossly visible disease burden.[231] Typically, this is the T1-enhancing abnormality on MRI or nonenhancing tumor seen on T2 or FLAIR images. If there is no residual abnormality after a surgical resection, the tumor resection cavity is defined to be the GTV. Surrounding edema is not considered part of the GTV. Clinical target volume (CTV) is the T2 or FLAIR abnormality (which does include edema) on MRI, as well as any areas potentially containing microscopic disease.[231] Suggested definitions of and doses to be delivered to GTV and CTV are given in Table 27-5 by histologic diagnosis.

The planning target volume (PTV) adds a dosimetric margin that takes into account variations in size, shape, and position of the CTV in relation to anatomic reference points, as well as uncertainties in daily treatment setup and physiologic variations that are difficult or impossible to control, such as (potential) fluctuations in the mass effect from cord edema that may occur over the course of treatment.[231] The target is usually considered to be appropriately treated if the PTV is enclosed within the 95% to 105% isodose lines. For plans emphasizing homogeneous dose delivery, the ICRU recommends that no more than 20% of the PTV should exceed 110% of the prescription dose.[230,231] However, because the spinal cord is exquisitely sensitive to both total dose and dose per fraction (Table 27-6), these factors must also be taken into consideration when deciding how much heterogeneity of dose is tolerable.

Organs at risk (OARs) are critical normal structures whose radiation sensitivity and proximity to the CTV may significantly influence the prescribed dose and the treatment-planning strategy. These typically include the thyroid and salivary glands, esophagus, lungs, heart, stomach, small bowel, liver, kidneys, bladders, ovaries, testicles, and uninvolved portions of the spinal cord itself.

Treatment Techniques

The most common treatment approaches include a single posterior field (PA), opposed lateral fields, a PA field with opposed laterals, and oblique wedge-pair fields.[51,232] They are typically designed to treat the CTV and GTV.

For tumors in the cervicothoracic region, a split-beam approach is often used. The central axis is placed just above the shoulders. Opposed lateral fields are used to treat the upper spine, while a PA field is used for the area of the spine below. Tumors in the thoracic region are often treated with a three-field approach using a PA field and opposed lateral

Table 27-5 Suggested Definitions of ICRU Volumes Based on MRI and Dose Ranges (in Gy) Delivered to Volumes

Diagnosis	Definition of Initial Treatment Field (CTV)	Dose to CTV	Definition of Final Field (GTV)	Dose to GTV	Dose to Craniospinal axis (if indicated)
WHO grade I glioma	NA	NA	Enhancing tumor (T1 + C) 1-cm margin	45-50.4 Gy	NA
WHO grade II glioma	Enhancing tumor (T1 + C) Edema (T2/FLAIR) 2-cm margin	45 Gy	Enhancing tumor (T1 + C) 2-cm margin	50.4-54 Gy	NA
WHO grade III/IV glioma	Enhancing tumor (T1 + C) Edema (T2/FLAIR) 2-cm margin	45-50.4 Gy	Enhancing tumor (T1 + C) 2-cm margin	55.8-59.4 Gy	Leptomeningeal spread on MRI: 30-39.6 Gy Bulky disease: 55.8-59.4 Gy
Ependymoma	Enhancing tumor (T1 + C) Edema (T2/FLAIR) 2-cm margin	45 Gy	Enhancing tumor (T1 + C) 2-cm margin	50.4-55.8 Gy	Negative CSF: 30 Gy Positive CSF: 36 Gy Leptomeningeal spread on MRI: 39.6 Gy Bulky disease: 54 Gy
Meningioma, benign/atypical	NA	NA	Enhancing tumor (T1 + C) 1-cm margin	52.2-55.8 Gy	NA
Meningioma, malignant	Enhancing tumor (T1 + C) Edema (T2/FLAIR) 2-cm margin	45-50.4 Gy	Enhancing tumor (T1 + C) 2-cm margin	55.8-59.4 Gy	NA
Chordoma	Enhancing tumor (T1 + C) Tumor bed 2-cm margin	50 Gy	Enhancing tumor (T1 + C) 2-cm margin	60-70 Gy	NA
Chondrosarcoma	Enhancing tumor (T1 + C) Tumor bed 2-cm margin	50 Gy	Enhancing tumor (T1 + C) 2-cm margin	60-70 Gy	NA
Sarcoma	Enhancing tumor (T1 + C) Tumor bed Surgical track, including scar 2-cm margin	50 Gy	Enhancing tumor (T1 + C) 2 cm margin	60-70 Gy	NA
Vertebral hemangioma	Enhancing vascular lesion Entire involved vertebral body ≥1-cm margin	NA	NA	36-45 Gy	NA
Metastasis	Enhancing tumor (T1 + C) Tumor bed Surgical track, including scar One vertebral body above and below	30-37.5 Gy	NA	NA	NA

GTV, gross tumor volume; CTV, clinical target volume; +C, with contrast.

beams. In the lumbar region, care must be taken to minimize dose to the kidneys; a four-field approach using AP/PA and opposed lateral beams with the AP/PA beams preferentially weighted may be useful. Comparison of differing treatment setups by means of dose-volume histograms (as described earlier) is strongly recommended.

Certain neoplasms, such as medulloblastomas and other primitive neuroectodermal tumors, some ependymomas, and some germ cell tumors, require treatment to the entire craniospinal axis (Fig. 27-11). Several modifications of this approach are used in clinical practice.[233] Patients may be treated in the supine or prone position, often in an immobi-

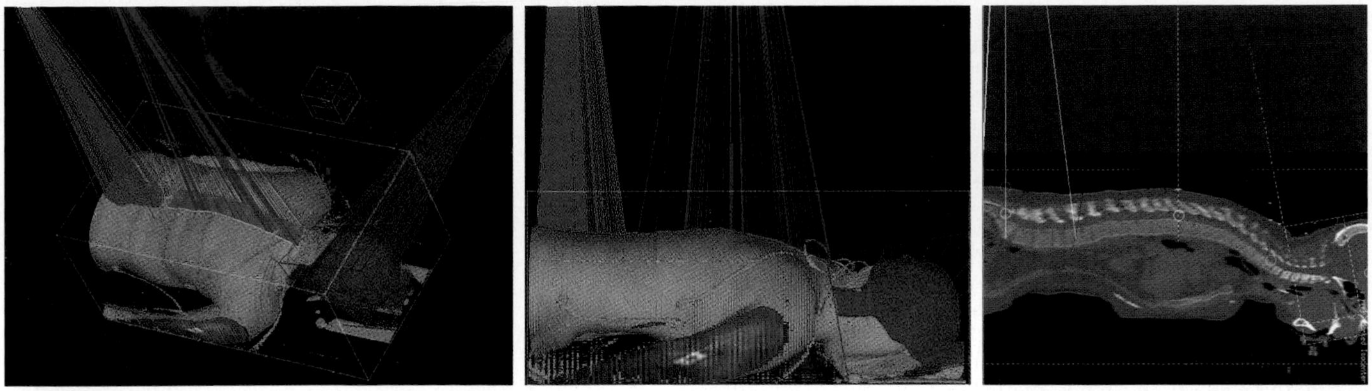

Figure 27-11 Two- and three-dimensional treatment planning images of craniospinal-axis radiation therapy. Patients are treated in the supine or prone position, and an immobilization cast often is used to ensure positional reproducibility. Intracranial contents and the upper one or two segments of the cervical cord are treated through opposed lateral fields. Customized blocks protect the normal head and neck tissues from the primary radiation beam. The spine is treated through one or two posterior fields.

Table 27-6 Fractionation Schemes With a 5% Risk of Radiation-Induced Spinal Cord Myelopathy

Dose per Fraction (Gy)	No. of Fractions	Total Dose (Gy)
2	29	58
3	13	39
3.3	11	33
4	7	28
5	5	25
10	1	10

lization cast to ensure daily positional reproducibility. The intracranial contents, including the upper one or two segments of the cervical cord, are treated through opposed lateral fields. Customized blocks protect the normal head and neck tissues from the primary radiation beam. The spine is treated through one or two posterior fields, depending on the size of the patient. In one method, the collimator for the lateral cranial fields is angled to match the divergence of the upper border of the adjacent spinal field, and the treatment couch is angled so that the inferior border of the cranial field is perpendicular to the superior edge of the spinal field. Alternatively, one may dispense with collimator and couch angles by calculating appropriate gaps. The gap is calculated so that the 50% isodose lines meet at the level of the anterior spinal cord. All junction lines are moved 0.5 to 1.0 cm every 8 to 10 Gy to avoid overdosing or underdosing segments of the cord. This is accomplished by shortening the inferior margin of the lateral cranial fields, symmetrically lengthening the superior and inferior margins of the posterior spine field, and shortening the cranial margin of the caudal spinal field; a fixed block is placed at the inferior margin of the caudal spinal field to keep the lower margin of the irradiated volume at the same location.

Intensity-modulated radiation therapy (IMRT) is a treatment delivery method that may be used to further optimize the dose distribution. There are two aspects of treatment that theoretically may benefit from the use of IMRT. First, because multiple critical sensitive organs are located near the spinal cord, one may reason that improved dose distribution should allow the dose to these structures to be minimized. Second, because most spinal cord tumors typically recur locally, IMRT should allow the exploration of anatomic/biologic treatment planning and delivery in order to optimize different doses to different cell populations within heterogeneous volumes.[234] The use of IMRT is under investigation at multiple institutions.

Stereotactic radiosurgery (SRS) of spinal cord lesions remains experimental at this time.[235,236] The limiting factor is the dose per fraction that can be safely delivered to the normal spinal cord (see Table 27-6). Progress combining "live" tumor imaging[237] with stereotactic repositioning[238] makes single-fraction SRS or fractionated SRT a promising field of research.

Selecting Radiation Therapy Doses

Table 27-5 gives an overview of the typical doses delivered to the ICRU volumes by diagnosis. Details and references are given in the sections for each individual diagnosis.

Tolerance of the Spinal Cord and Lumbosacral Nerve Roots

A dose of 45 to 50.4 Gy in 25 to 28 fractions over 5 to 5.5 weeks usually is considered to be safe, with the risk of myelopathy being less than 1%, well below the steep portion of the dose-response curve.[239,240] It is estimated that with conventionally fractionated irradiation (1.8 to 2.0 Gy per fraction, five fractions per week), at 5 years the incidence of myelopathy is 5% for doses in the range of 57 to 61 Gy (tolerance dose $TD_{5/5}$) and 50% for doses of 68 to 73 Gy ($TD_{50/5}$).[239] There is no convincing evidence that the cervical and thoracic cord differ in their radiosensitivity, and there appears to be little change in tolerance with variations in the length of cord irradiated.[239] Table 27-6 shows a range of isomorbid fractionation schemes, all of which carry a 5% risk of radiation myelopathy.[240-245] A single dose of 10 Gy to the optic chiasm carries approximately a 5% risk of visual impairment, and this may hold true for the spinal cord, based on early data from small retrospective series evaluating spinal radiosurgery.[246,247]

The tolerance of the lumbosacral nerve roots appears to be somewhat higher than that of the spinal cord. Most series report a 0% complication rate if patients are treated to doses of 70 Gy (or equivalent) as long as fraction sizes are kept at or below 2 Gy.[153,158,248]

Complications of Treatment

Radiation myelopathy may present as a transient early delayed or as a late delayed reaction. Transient radiation myelopathy is clinically manifested by momentary, electrical shock–like paresthesias or numbness radiating from the neck to the extremities, precipitated by neck flexion (Lhermitte's sign).[249] The syndrome typically develops 3 to 4 months after treatment and spontaneously resolves over the following 3 to 6 months without therapy. It is attributed to transient demyelination caused by radiation-induced inhibition of myelin-producing oligodendroglial cells in the irradiated spinal cord segment.[249-251]

Irreversible radiation myelopathy usually is not seen earlier than 6 to 12 months after completion of treatment. Typically, half of the patients who develop radiation-induced myelopathy in the cervical or thoracic cord region will do so within 20 months of treatment and 75% of the cases occur within 30 months.[252] It is thought to be multifactorial, involving demyelination and white matter necrosis ultimately due to oligodendroglial cell depletion and microvascular injury.

The signs and symptoms are typically progressive over several months, but acute onset of plegia over several hours or a few days is possible. The diagnosis of radiation myelopathy is one of exclusion that first requires a history of radiation therapy in doses sufficient to result in injury. The region of the irradiated cord must lie slightly above the dermatome level of expression of the lesion, the latent period from the completion of treatment to the onset of injury must be consistent with that observed in radiation myelopathy, and local tumor progression must be ruled out. There are no pathognomonic laboratory tests or imaging studies that conclusively diagnose radiation myelopathy. MRI findings include swelling of the spinal cord with hyperintensity on the T2-weighted images with or without areas of contrast enhancement.[251,253]

There is no known consistently effective treatment for radiation myelitis.[254,255] The probability of dying from radiation myelopathy is approximately 70% in cervical lesions and 30% with thoracic spinal cord injury.[256]

Radiation side effects in children include growth abnormalities, such as decreased vertebral height, kyphosis, and scoliosis.[257] Secondary malignancies, including bone or soft tissue sarcomas and glioblastoma multiforme, have been reported after irradiation of spinal cord tumors.[129,258,259]

Treatment Toxicity Scoring

Several toxicity-scoring systems are in use. The most commonly accepted are the National Cancer Institute's Common Terminology Criteria for Adverse Events (NCI CTCAE), version 3, and the Late Effects Toxicity Scoring of the EORTC, known as the LENT/SOMA scale (Late Effects on Normal Tissues, with four components: Subjective, Objective, Management, and Analytical).[260,261]

TREATMENT ALGORITHMS, CHALLENGES, AND FUTURE POSSIBILITIES

Treatment Algorithm

Primary tumors of the spinal cord are uncommon lesions. Much of the literature groups these tumors together by location (intramedullary versus extramedullary) when reporting outcomes. However, spinal cord tumors clearly behave differently depending on histology, and this needs to be taken into account when making management decisions. Nonetheless, the primary treatment for most spinal cord tumors continues to be surgical resection, with radiation therapy recommended for those patients in whom a complete resection cannot be achieved and for those at high risk of recurrence. The role of chemotherapy in the management of spinal cord tumors remains unclear. A general simplified treatment algorithm is shown (Fig. 27-12).

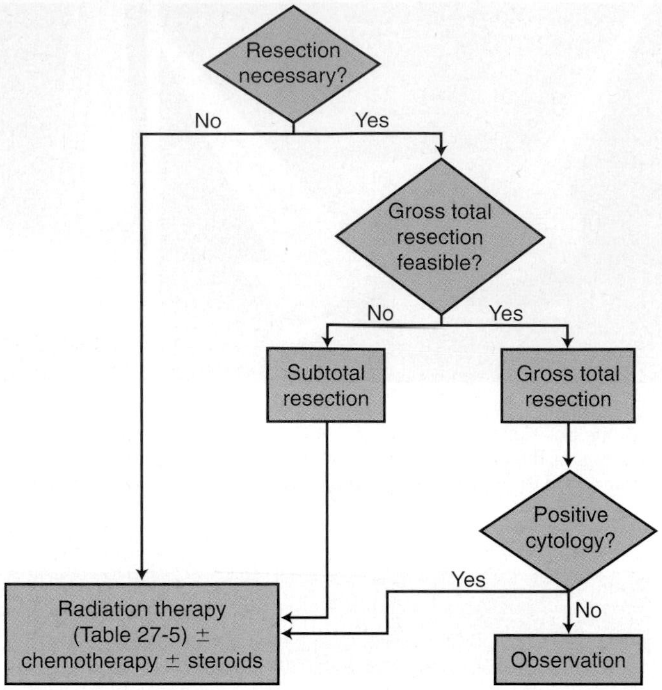

Figure 27-12 Treatment algorithm for the general management of primary spinal tumors. Details about the histologic diagnosis and radiation therapy are provided in the text and Table 27-5.

Future Possibilities

The most significant future advances one may anticipate are the possibility of noninvasively obtaining an accurate tissue diagnosis of a suspicious spinal cord lesion and accurately measuring treatment response. To this extent, novel magnetic resonance contrast agents could serve as biochemical reporters of various cellular function.[262] These newer contrast agents could be tailored to report on the physiologic status or metabolic activity of biological systems: enzyme-activated agents correlate developmental biological events with gene expression; calcium-activated agents can measure intracellular signal transduction; pH-activated agents provide a blood oxygen level–dependent (BOLD) signal that might be used for noninvasive mapping of human nervous system function; and T2-activated agents can detect specific oligonucleotide sequences. These agents of interest are under investigation in the setting of primary brain tumor treatment, and it remains to be seen how the results will be applied to spinal cord therapy.

REFERENCES

1. National Cancer Institute, DCCPS Surveillance Research Program Cancer Statistics Branch: Surveillance, Epidemiology, and End Results (SEER) Program. SEER*Stat Database: Incidence—SEER 9 Regs Public-Use, Nov 2002 Sub (1973-2000).
2. Central Brain Tumor Registry of the United States: 2002-2003 Primary Brain Tumors in the United States. Statistical Report 1995-1999 Years Data Collected. Chicago, CBTRUS, 2003.
3. Connoly ES: Spinal cord tumors in adults. *In* Winn RH (ed): Youmans' Neurological Surgery. Philadelphia, WB Saunders, 1982, p 3196.
4. Sasanelli F, Beghi E, Kurland LT: Primary intraspinal neoplasms in Rochester, Minnesota, 1935-1981. Neuroepidemiology 2:156-163, 1983.

5. Preston-Martin S: Descriptive epidemiology of primary tumors of the spinal cord and spinal meninges in Los Angeles County, 1972-1985. Neuroepidemiology 9:106-111, 1990.
6. Mumenthaler M: Diseases affecting mainly the spinal cord. *In* Mumenthaler M (ed): Neurology, 3rd ed. New York, Thieme Medical Publishers, 1990, pp 181-232.
7. International Agency for Research on Cancer: World Health Organization Classification of Tumours: Pathology and Genetics: Tumours of the Nervous System, 2nd ed. Lyon, Oxford University Press, 2000.
8. Parsa AT, Fiore AJ, McCormick PC, et al: Genetic basis of intramedullary spinal cord tumors and therapeutic implications. J Neurooncol 47:239-251, 2000.
9. Hardison HH, Packer RJ, Rorke LB, et al: Outcome of children with primary intramedullary spinal cord tumors. Childs Nerv Syst 3:89-92, 1987.
10. Choucair AK, Levin VA, Gutin PH, et al: Development of multiple lesions during radiation therapy and chemotherapy in patients with gliomas. J Neurosurg 65:654-658, 1986.
11. Aydin MV, Ozel S, Sen O, et al: Intradural disc mimicking a spinal tumor lesion. Spinal Cord 42:52-54, 2004.
12. Dhiwakar M, Buxton N: Acute transverse myelitis mimicking an intramedullary neoplasm. Br J Neurosurg 18:72-73, 2004.
13. Petjom S, Chaiwun B, Settakorn J, et al: *Angiostrongylus cantonensis* infection mimicking a spinal cord tumor. Ann Neurol 52:99-101, 2002.
14. Yukawa Y, Kato F: Isolated spinal cord sarcoidosis mimicking an intramedullary tumor. J Spinal Disord 12:530-533, 1999.
15. Fouladi M, Heideman R, Langston JW, et al: Infectious meningitis mimicking recurrent medulloblastoma on magnetic resonance imaging. Case report. J Neurosurg 91:499-502, 1999.
16. Kilic G, Blankstein J, Kadanoff R: Vertebral tuberculosis presenting with elevated CA-125 and weight loss mimicking ovarian malignancy; case report. Eur J Gynaecol Oncol 24:561-562, 2003.
17. Essig M, Metzner R, Bonsanto M, et al: Postoperative fluid-attenuated inversion recovery MR imaging of cerebral gliomas: initial results. Eur Radiol 11:2004-2010, 2001.
18. Li BS, Movsas B, Babb JS, et al: Quantifying injury to the brain from radiation therapy (RT) with whole brain N-acetylaspartate (WBNAA) proton magnetic resonance spectroscopy (1H-MRS). Int J Radiat Oncol Biol Phys 48:299-300, 2000.
19. Pirzkall A, Larson DA, McKnight TR, et al: MR-spectroscopy results in improved target delineation for high-grade gliomas. Int J Radiat Oncol Biol Phys 48:115, 2000.
20. McKnight TR, dem Bussche MH, Vigneron DB, et al: Histopathological validation of a three-dimensional magnetic resonance spectroscopy index as a predictor of tumor presence. J Neurosurg 97:794-802, 2002.
21. Bourland JD, Shaw EG: The evolving role of biological imaging in stereotactic radiosurgery. Technol Cancer Res Treat 2:135-139, 2003.
22. Cohen AR, Wisoff JH, Allen JC, et al: Malignant astrocytomas of the spinal cord. J Neurosurg 70:50-54, 1989.
23. Gowers WR, Horsley V: A case of tumour of the spinal cord. Removal and recovery. Med Chir Trans 53:377-428, 1888.
24. Eiselsberg AV, Ranzi E: Über die chirurgische Behandlung der Hirn- und Rückenmarkstumoren. Arch Klin Chir 102:309-468, 1913.
25. Elsberg CA, Beer E: The operability of intramedullary tumors of the spinal cord. A report of two operations with remarks upon the extrusion of intraspinal tumors. Am J Med Sci 142:636-647, 1911.
26. Wood EH, Berne AS, Taveras JM: The value of radiation therapy in the management of intrinsic tumors of the spinal cord. Radiology 63:11-24, 1954.
27. Jallo GI, Freed D, Epstein F: Intramedullary spinal cord tumors in children. Child Nerv Syst 19:641-649, 2003.
28. el Mahdy W, Kane PJ, Powell MP, et al: Spinal intradural tumours: part I—extramedullary. Br J Neurosurg 13:550-557, 1999.
29. McCormick PC, Stein BM: Spinal cord tumors in adults. *In* Youmans JR (ed): Neurological Surgery: A Comprehensive Reference Guide to the Diagnosis and Management of Neurosurgical Problems, 4th ed. Philadelphia, Elsevier, 1996, pp 3111-3114.
30. Constantini S, Miller DC, Allen JC, et al: Radical excision of intramedullary spinal cord tumors: surgical morbidity and long-term follow-up evaluation in 164 children and young adults. J Neurosurg 93:183-193, 2000.
31. Zileli M, Coskun E, Ozdamar N, et al: Surgery of intramedullary spinal cord tumors. Eur Spine J 5:243-250, 1996.
32. Goh KY, Velasquez L, Epstein FJ: Pediatric intramedullary spinal cord tumors: is surgery alone enough? Pediatr Neurosurg 27:34-39, 1997.
33. Lunardi P, Licastro G, Missori P, et al: Management of intramedullary tumours in children. Acta Neurochir (Wien) 120:59-65, 1993.
34. Abdel-Wahab M, Corn B, Wolfson A, et al: Prognostic factors and survival in patients with spinal cord gliomas after radiation therapy. Am J Clin Oncol 22:344-351, 1999.
35. Shirato H, Kamada T, Hida K, et al: The role of radiotherapy in the management of spinal cord glioma. Int J Radiat Oncol Biol Phys 33:323-328, 1995.
36. Rodrigues GB, Waldron JN, Wong CS, et al: A retrospective analysis of 52 cases of spinal cord glioma managed with radiation therapy. Int J Radiat Oncol Biol Phys 48:837-842, 2000.
37. Weiner HL, Freed D, Woo HH, et al: Intra-axial tumors of the cervicomedullary junction: surgical results and long-term outcome. Pediatr Neurosurg 27:12-18, 1997.
38. Cristante L, Herrmann HD: Surgical management of intramedullary spinal cord tumors: functional outcome and sources of morbidity. Neurosurgery 35:69-74, 1994.
39. Xu QW, Bao WM, Mao RL, et al: Aggressive surgery for intramedullary tumor of cervical spinal cord. Surg Neurol 46:322-328, 1996.
40. Hulshof MC, Menten J, Dito JJ, et al: Treatment results in primary intraspinal gliomas. Radiother Oncol 29:294-300, 1993.
41. Nishio S, Morioka T, Fujii K, et al: Spinal cord gliomas: management and outcome with reference to adjuvant therapy. J Clin Neurosci 7:20-23, 2000.
42. Sandler HM, Papadopoulos SM, Thornton AF Jr, et al: Spinal cord astrocytomas: results of therapy. Neurosurgery 30:490-493, 1992.
43. Santi M, Mena H, Wong K, et al: Spinal cord malignant astrocytomas. Clinicopathologic features in 36 cases. Cancer 98:554-561, 2003.
44. Bouffet E, Pierre-Kahn A, Marchal JC, et al: Prognostic factors in pediatric spinal cord astrocytoma. Cancer 83:2391-2399, 1998.
45. Rossitch E Jr, Zeidman SM, Burger PC, et al: Clinical and pathological analysis of spinal cord astrocytomas in children. Neurosurgery 27:193-196, 1990.
46. Merchant TE, Nguyen D, Thompson SJ, et al: High-grade pediatric spinal cord tumors. Pediatr Neurosurg 30:1-5, 1999.
47. Innocenzi G, Salvati M, Cervoni L, et al: Prognostic factors in intramedullary astrocytomas. Clin Neurol Neurosurg 99:1-5, 1997.
48. Kim MS, Chung CK, Choe G, et al: Intramedullary spinal cord astrocytoma in adults: postoperative outcome. J Neurooncol 52:85-94, 2001.
49. Lee HK, Chang EL, Fuller GN, et al: The prognostic value of neurologic function in astrocytic spinal cord glioma. Neurooncology 5:208-213, 2003.
50. Przybylski GJ, Albright AL, Martinez AJ: Spinal cord astrocytomas: long-term results comparing treatments in children. Childs Nerv Syst 13:375-382, 1997.
51. Minehan KJ, Shaw EG, Scheithauer BW, et al: Spinal cord astrocytoma: pathological and treatment considerations. J Neurosurg 83:590-595, 1995.
52. Lee TT, Gromelski EB, Green BA: Surgical treatment of spinal ependymoma and post-operative radiotherapy. Acta Neurochir (Wien) 140:309-313, 1998.
53. Whitaker SJ, Bessell EM, Ashley SE, et al: Postoperative radiotherapy in the management of spinal cord ependymoma. J Neurosurg 74:720-728, 1991.
54. McCormick PC, Torres R, Post KD, et al: Intramedullary ependymoma of the spinal cord. J Neurosurg 72:523-532, 1990.
55. McLaughlin MP, Marcus RB, Jr. Buatti JM, et al: Ependymoma: results, prognostic factors and treatment recommendations. Int J Radiat Oncol Biol Phys 40:845-850, 1998.

56. Hanbali F, Fourney DR, Marmor E, et al: Spinal cord ependymoma: radical surgical resection and outcome. Neurosurgery 51:1162-1172, 2002.
57. Kochbati L, Nasr C, Frikha H, et al: [Primary intramedullary ependymomas: retrospective study of 16 cases]. Cancer Radiother 7:17-21, 2003.
58. Ohata K, Takami T, Gotou T, et al: Surgical outcome of intramedullary spinal cord ependymoma. Acta Neurochir (Wien) 141:341-346, 1999.
59. Hejazi N, Hassler W: Microsurgical treatment of intramedullary spinal cord tumors. Neurol Med Chir (Tokyo) 38:266-271, 1998.
60. Fowler JF, Bentzen SM, Bond SJ, et al: Clinical radiation doses for spinal cord: the 1998 international questionnaire. Radiother Oncol 55:295-300, 2000.
61. Cooper PR: Outcome after operative treatment of intramedullary spinal cord tumors in adults: intermediate and long-term results in 51 patients. Neurosurgery 25:855-859, 1989.
62. Constantini S, Allen JC, Epstein F: Pediatric and adult primary spinal cord tumors. *In* Black PM, Loeffler JS (eds): Cancer of the Nervous System. Cambridge, Blackwell Publishers, 1997, pp 637-649.
63. Klekamp J, Samii M: Surgical results of spinal meningiomas. Acta Neurochir Suppl (Wien) 65:77-81, 1996.
64. Levy WJ Jr, Bay J, Dohn D: Spinal cord meningioma. J Neurosurg 57:804-812, 1982.
65. Solero CL, Fornari M, Giombini S, et al: Spinal meningiomas: review of 174 operated cases. Neurosurgery 25:153-160, 1989.
66. Seppala MT, Haltia MJ, Sankila RJ, et al: Long-term outcome after removal of spinal schwannoma: a clinicopathological study of 187 cases. J Neurosurg 83:621-626, 1995.
67. Sim FH, Svien HJ, Bickel WH, et al: Swan-neck deformity following extensive cervical laminectomy. A review of twenty-one cases. J Bone Joint Surg Am 56:564-580, 1974.
68. Reimer R, Onofrio BM: Astrocytomas of the spinal cord in children and adolescents. J Neurosurg 63:669-675, 1985.
69. Jyothirmayi R, Madhavan J, Nair MK, et al: Conservative surgery and radiotherapy in the treatment of spinal cord astrocytoma. J Neurooncol 33:205-211, 1997.
70. Huddart R, Traish D, Ashley S, et al: Management of spinal astrocytoma with conservative surgery and radiotherapy. Br J Neurosurg 7:473-481, 1993.
71. Kopelson G, Linggood RM, Kleinman GM, et al: Management of intramedullary spinal cord tumors. Radiology 135:473-479, 1980.
72. Epstein F, Epstein N: Surgical treatment of spinal cord astrocytomas of childhood. A series of 19 patients. J Neurosurg 57:685-689, 1982.
73. Weingart J, Brem H, Grossman SA, et al: Gliadel followed by radiotherapy for newly diagnosed malignant glioma: safety results, pathologic findings, and survival. Int J Radiat Oncol Biol Phys 48:256, 2000.
74. Stewart LA: Chemotherapy in adult high-grade glioma: a systematic review and meta-analysis of individual patient data from 12 randomised trials. Lancet 359:1011-1018, 2002.
75. Hassall TE, Mitchell AE, Ashley DM: Carboplatin chemotherapy for progressive intramedullary spinal cord low-grade gliomas in children: three case studies and a review of the literature. Neuro-oncology 3:251-257, 2001.
76. Robertson PL, Zeltzer PM, Boyett JM, et al: Survival and prognostic factors following radiation therapy and chemotherapy for ependymomas in children: a report of the Children's Cancer Group. J Neurosurg 88:695-703, 1998.
77. Fort DW, Packer RJ, Kirkpatrick GB, et al: Carboplatin and vincristine for pediatric primary spinal cord astrocytomas [abstract]. Childs Nerv Syst 14:484, 1998.
78. Doireau V, Grill J, Zerah M, et al: Chemotherapy for unresectable and recurrent intramedullary glial tumours in children. Brain Tumours Subcommittee of the French Society of Paediatric Oncology (SFOP). Br J Cancer 81:835-840, 1999.
79. Evans AE, Anderson JR, Lefkowitz-Boudreaux IB, et al: Adjuvant chemotherapy of childhood posterior fossa ependymoma: cranio-spinal irradiation with or without adjuvant CCNU, vincristine, and prednisone: a Childrens Cancer Group study. Med Pediatr Oncol 27:8-14, 1996.
80. Chamberlain MC: Etoposide for recurrent spinal cord ependymoma. Neurology 58:1310-1311, 2002.
81. Goldwein JW, Leahy JM, Packer RJ, et al: Intracranial ependymomas in children. Int J Radiat Oncol Biol Phys 19:1497-1502, 1990.
82. Levin VA, Edwards MS, Gutin PH, et al: Phase II evaluation of dibromodulcitol in the treatment of recurrent medulloblastoma, ependymoma, and malignant astrocytoma. J Neurosurg 61:1063-1068, 1984.
83. Goldwein JW, Glauser TA, Packer RJ, et al: Recurrent intracranial ependymomas in children. Survival, patterns of failure, and prognostic factors. Cancer 66:557-563, 1990.
84. Epstein FJ, Farmer JP: Pediatric spinal cord tumor surgery. Neurosurg Clin N Am 1:569-590, 1990.
85. McCormick PC, Stein BM: Intramedullary tumors in adults. Neurosurg Clin N Am 1:609-630, 1990.
86. Guidetti B, Mercuri S, Vagnozzi R: Long-term results of the surgical treatment of 129 intramedullary spinal gliomas. J Neurosurg 54:323-330, 1981.
87. Stein BM: Surgery of intramedullary spinal cord tumors. Clin Neurosurg 26:529-542, 1979.
88. Mottl H, Koutecky J: Treatment of spinal cord tumors in children. Med Pediatr Oncol 29:293-295, 1997.
89. Linstadt DE, Wara WM, Leibel SA, et al: Postoperative radiotherapy of primary spinal cord tumors. Int J Radiat Oncol Biol Phys 16:1397-1403, 1989.
90. Miller DC: Surgical pathology of intramedullary spinal cord neoplasms. J Neurooncol 47:189-194, 2000.
91. Chun HC, Schmidt-Ullrich RK, Wolfson A, et al: External beam radiotherapy for primary spinal cord tumors. J Neurooncol 9:211-217, 1990.
92. McLaughlin MP, Buatti JM, Marcus RB Jr, et al: Outcome after radiotherapy of primary spinal cord glial tumors. Radiat Oncol Investig 6:276-280, 1998.
93. Merchant TE, Nguyen D, Thompson SJ, et al: High-grade pediatric spinal cord tumors. Pediatr Neurosurg 30:1-5, 1999.
94. Allen JC, Aviner S, Yates AJ, et al: Treatment of high-grade spinal cord astrocytoma of childhood with "8-in-1" chemotherapy and radiotherapy: a pilot study of CCG-945. Children's Cancer Group. J Neurosurg 88:215-220, 1998.
95. Merchant TE, Nguyen D, Thompson SJ, et al: High-grade pediatric spinal cord tumors. Pediatr Neurosurg 30:1-5, 1999.
96. Fornari M, Pluchino F, Solero CL, et al: Microsurgical treatment of intramedullary spinal cord tumours. Acta Neurochir Suppl (Wien) 43:3-8, 1988.
97. Karim AB, Afra D, Cornu P, et al: Randomized trial on the efficacy of radiotherapy for cerebral low-grade glioma in the adult: European Organization for Research and Treatment of Cancer Study 22845 with the Medical Research Council study BRO4: an interim analysis. Int J Radiat Oncol Biol Phys 52:316-324, 2002.
98. Karim AB, Maat B, Hatlevoll R, et al: A randomized trial on dose-response in radiation therapy of low-grade cerebral glioma: European Organization for Research and Treatment of Cancer (EORTC) Study 22844. Int J Radiat Oncol Biol Phys 36:549-556, 1996.
99. Shaw E, Arusell R, Scheithauer B, et al: Prospective randomized trial of low- versus high-dose radiation therapy in adults with supratentorial low-grade glioma: initial report of a North Central Cancer Treatment Group/Radiation Therapy Oncology Group/Eastern Cooperative Oncology Group Study. J Clin Oncol 20:2267-2276, 2002.
100. Walker MD, Strike TA, Sheline GE: An analysis of dose-effect relationship in the radiotherapy of malignant gliomas. Int J Radiat Oncol Biol Phys 5:1725-1731, 1979.
101. Chang CH, Horton J, Schoenfeld D, et al: Comparison of postoperative radiotherapy and combined postoperative radiotherapy and chemotherapy in the multidisciplinary management of malignant gliomas. A joint Radiation Therapy Oncology Group and Eastern Cooperative Oncology Group study. Cancer 52:997-1007, 1983.
102. Cervoni L, Salvati M, Celli P, et al: Gliomas of the conus medullaris. Tumori 82:249-251, 1996.
103. Epstein FJ, Farmer JP, Freed D: Adult intramedullary astrocytomas of the spinal cord. J Neurosurg 77:355-359, 1992.

104. Merchant TE, Nguyen D, Thompson SJ, et al: High-grade pediatric spinal cord tumors. Pediatr Neurosurg 30:1-5, 1999.
105. Ciappetta P, Salvati M, Capoccia G, et al: Spinal glioblastomas: report of seven cases and review of the literature. Neurosurgery 28:302-306, 1991.
106. Merchant TE, Nguyen D, Thompson SJ, et al: High-grade pediatric spinal cord tumors. Pediatr Neurosurg 30:1-5, 1999.
107. Chigasaki H, Pennybacker JB: A long follow-up study of 128 cases of intramedullary spinal cord tumours. Neurol Med Chir (Tokyo) 10:25-66, 1968.
108. Sgouros S, Malluci CL, Jackowski A: Spinal ependymomas—the value of postoperative radiotherapy for residual disease control. Br J Neurosurg 10:559-566, 1996.
109. Fine MJ, Kricheff II, Freed D, et al: Spinal cord ependymomas: MR imaging features. Radiology 197:655-658, 1995.
110. Shaw EG, Evans RG, Scheithauer BW, et al: Radiotherapeutic management of adult intraspinal ependymomas. Int J Radiat Oncol Biol Phys 12:323-327, 1986.
111. Di Marco A, Griso C, Pradella R, et al: Postoperative management of primary spinal cord ependymomas. Acta Oncol 27:371-375, 1988.
112. Mork SJ, Loken AC: Ependymoma: a follow-up study of 101 cases. Cancer 40:907-915, 1977.
113. Marks JE, Adler SJ: A comparative study of ependymomas by site of origin. Int J Radiat Oncol Biol Phys 8:37-43, 1982.
114. Clover LL, Hazuka MB, Kinzie JJ: Spinal cord ependymomas treated with surgery and radiation therapy. A review of 11 cases. Am J Clin Oncol 16:350-353, 1993.
115. Rivierez M, Oueslati S, Philippon J, et al: [Ependymoma of the intradural filum terminale in adults: 20 cases]. Neurochirurgie 36:96-107, 1990.
116. Schiffer D, Chio A, Giordana MT, et al: Histologic prognostic factors in ependymoma. Childs Nerv Syst 7:177-182, 1991.
117. Sonneland PR, Scheithauer BW, Onofrio BM: Myxopapillary ependymoma. A clinicopathologic and immunocytochemical study of 77 cases. Cancer 56:883-893, 1985.
118. Chan HS, Becker LE, Hoffman HJ, et al: Myxopapillary ependymoma of the filum terminale and cauda equina in childhood: report of seven cases and review of the literature. Neurosurgery 14:204-210, 1984.
119. Schweitzer JS, Batzdorf U: Ependymoma of the cauda equina region: diagnosis, treatment, and outcome in 15 patients. Neurosurgery 30:202-207, 1992.
120. Stein BM: Intramedullary spinal cord tumors. Clin Neurosurg 30:717-741, 1983.
121. Russell DS, Rubinstein LJ: Pathology of Tumors of the Nervous System. Philadelphia, Lippincott Williams & Wilkins, 1998.
122. Kline MJ, Kays DW, Rojiani AM: Extradural myxopapillary ependymoma: report of two cases and review of the literature. Pediatr Pathol Lab Med 16:813-822, 1996.
123. Rezai AR, Woo HH, Lee M, et al: Disseminated ependymomas of the central nervous system. J Neurosurg 85:618-624, 1996.
124. Vanuytsel L, Brada M: The role of prophylactic spinal irradiation in localized intracranial ependymoma. Int J Radiat Oncol Biol Phys 21:825-830, 1991.
125. Waldron JN, Laperriere NJ, Jaakkimainen L, et al: Spinal cord ependymomas: a retrospective analysis of 59 cases. Int J Radiat Oncol Biol Phys 27:223-229, 1993.
126. Schild SE, Nisi K, Scheithauer BW, et al: The results of radiotherapy for ependymomas: the Mayo Clinic experience. Int J Radiat Oncol Biol Phys 42:953-958, 1998.
127. Cervoni L, Celli P, Fortuna A, et al: Recurrence of spinal ependymoma. Risk factors and long-term survival. Spine 19:2838-2841, 1994.
128. Healey EA, Barnes PD, Kupsky WJ, et al: The prognostic significance of postoperative residual tumor in ependymoma. Neurosurgery 28:666-671, 1991.
129. Garcia DM: Primary spinal cord tumors treated with surgery and postoperative irradiation. Int J Radiat Oncol Biol Phys 11:1933-1939, 1985.
130. Wen BC, Hussey DH, Hitchon PW, et al: The role of radiation therapy in the management of ependymomas of the spinal cord. Int J Radiat Oncol Biol Phys 20:781-786, 1991.
131. Duffner PK, Horowitz ME, Krischer JP, et al: Postoperative chemotherapy and delayed radiation in children less than three years of age with malignant brain tumors. N Engl J Med 328:1725-1731, 1993.
132. Grill J, Le Deley MC, Gambarelli D, et al: Postoperative chemotherapy without irradiation for ependymoma in children under 5 years of age: a multicenter trial of the French Society of Pediatric Oncology. J Clin Oncol 19:1288-1296, 2001.
133. Mirimanoff RO, Dosoretz DE, Linggood RM, et al: Meningioma: analysis of recurrence and progression following neurosurgical resection. J Neurosurg 62:18-24, 1985.
134. Helseth A, Mork SJ: Primary intraspinal neoplasms in Norway, 1955 to 1986. A population-based survey of 467 patients. J Neurosurg 71:842-845, 1989.
135. Namer IJ, Pamir MN, Benli K, et al: Spinal meningiomas. Neurochirurgia (Stuttg) 30:11-15, 1987.
136. Gezen F, Kahraman S, Canakci Z, et al: Review of 36 cases of spinal cord meningioma. Spine 25:727-731, 2000.
137. Cohen-Gadol AA, Zikel OM, Koch CA, et al: Spinal meningiomas in patients younger than 50 years of age: a 21-year experience. J Neurosurg 98:258-263, 2003.
138. Calogero JA, Moossy J: Extradural spinal meningiomas. Report of four cases. J Neurosurg 37:442-447, 1972.
139. Roux FX, Nataf F, Pinaudeau M, et al: Intraspinal meningiomas: review of 54 cases with discussion of poor prognosis factors and modern therapeutic management. Surg Neurol 46:458-463, 1996.
140. Schiebe ME, Hoffmann W, Kortmann RD, et al: Radiotherapy in recurrent malignant meningiomas with multiple spinal manifestations. Acta Oncol 36:88-90, 1997.
141. Goldsmith BJ, Wara WM, Wilson CB, et al: Postoperative irradiation for subtotally resected meningiomas. A retrospective analysis of 140 patients treated from 1967 to 1990. J Neurosurg 80:195-201, 1994.
142. Ryu SI, Chang SD, Kim DH, et al: Image-guided hypo-fractionated stereotactic radiosurgery to spinal lesions. Neurosurgery 49:838-846, 2001.
143. Schrell UM, Rittig MG, Anders M, et al: Hydroxyurea for treatment of unresectable and recurrent meningiomas. II. Decrease in the size of meningiomas in patients treated with hydroxyurea. J Neurosurg 86:840-844, 1997.
144. Noel G, Habrand JL, Jauffret E, et al: Radiation therapy for chordoma and chondrosarcoma of the skull base and the cervical spine. Prognostic factors and patterns of failure. Strahlenther Onkol 179:241-248, 2003.
145. Chetiyawardana AD: Chordoma: results of treatment. Clin Radiol 35:159-161, 1984.
146. Saxton JP: Chordoma. Int J Radiat Oncol Biol Phys 7:913-915, 1981.
147. Sundaresan N, Galicich JH, Chu FC, et al: Spinal chordomas. J Neurosurg 50:312-319, 1979.
148. Mabrey RE: Chordoma: a study of 150 cases. Am J Cancer 25:501-517, 1935.
149. Birrell JH: Chordomata: a review of nineteen cases of chordomata including five vertebral cases. Aust N Z J Surg 22:258-267, 1953.
150. Dahlin DC, Maccarty CS: Chordoma. Cancer 5:1170-1178, 1952.
151. Klekamp J, Samii M: Spinal chordomas—results of treatment over a 17-year period. Acta Neurochir (Wien) 138:514-519, 1996.
152. O'Neill P, Bell BA, Miller JD, et al: Fifty years of experience with chordomas in southeast Scotland. Neurosurgery 16:166-170, 1985.
153. Fuller DB, Bloom JG: Radiotherapy for chordoma. Int J Radiat Oncol Biol Phys 15:331-339, 1988.
154. Rich TA, Schiller A, Suit HD, et al: Clinical and pathologic review of 48 cases of chordoma. Cancer 56:182-187, 1985.
155. Kaiser TE, Pritchard DJ, Unni KK: Clinicopathologic study of sacrococcygeal chordoma. Cancer 53:2574-2578, 1984.
156. Bethke KP, Neifeld JP, Lawrence W Jr: Diagnosis and management of sacrococcygeal chordoma. J Surg Oncol 48:232-238, 1991.
157. Benk V, Liebsch NJ, Munzenrider JE, et al: Base of skull and cervical spine chordomas in children treated by high-dose irradiation. Int J Radiat Oncol Biol Phys 31:577-581, 1995.
158. Schoenthaler R, Castro JR, Petti PL, et al: Charged particle irradiation of sacral chordomas. Int J Radiat Oncol Biol Phys 26:291-298, 1993.

159. Chetty R, Levin CV, Kalan MR: Chordoma: a 20-year clinicopathologic review of the experience at Groote Schuur Hospital, Cape Town. J Surg Oncol 46:261-264, 1991.
160. Markwalder TM, Markwalder RV, Robert JL, et al: Metastatic chordoma. Surg Neurol 12:473-478, 1979.
161. Higinbotham NL, Phillips RF, Farr HW, et al: Chordoma. Thirty-five-year study at Memorial Hospital. Cancer 20:1841-1850, 1967.
162. Suit HD, Goitein M, Munzenrider J, et al: Definitive radiation therapy for chordoma and chondrosarcoma of base of skull and cervical spine. J Neurosurg 56:377-385, 1982.
163. Terahara A, Niemierko A, Goitein M, et al: Analysis of the relationship between tumor dose inhomogeneity and local control in patients with skull base chordoma. Int J Radiat Oncol Biol Phys 45:351-358, 1999.
164. Borba LA, Al Mefty O, Mrak RE, et al: Cranial chordomas in children and adolescents. J Neurosurg 84:584-591, 1996.
165. Ozaki T, Hillmann A, Winkelmann W: Surgical treatment of sacrococcygeal chordoma. J Surg Oncol 64:274-279, 1997.
166. Magrini SM, Papi MG, Marletta F, et al: Chordoma—natural history, treatment and prognosis. The Florence Radiotherapy Department experience (1956-1990) and a critical review of the literature. Acta Oncol 31:847-851, 1992.
167. Romero J, Cardenes H, la Torre A, et al: Chordoma: results of radiation therapy in eighteen patients. Radiother Oncol 29:27-32, 1993.
168. Cummings BJ, Hodson DI, Bush RS: Chordoma: the results of megavoltage radiation therapy. Int J Radiat Oncol Biol Phys 9:633-642, 1983.
169. Hug EB, Loredo LN, Slater JD, et al: Proton radiation therapy for chordomas and chondrosarcomas of the skull base. J Neurosurg 91:432-439, 1999.
170. Slater JM, Slater JD, Archambeau JO: Proton therapy for cranial base tumors. J Craniofac Surg 6:24-26, 1995.
171. Munzenrider JE, Liebsch NJ: Proton therapy for tumors of the skull base. Strahlenther.Onkol 175(Suppl 2):57-63, 1999.
172. Austin-Seymour M, Munzenrider JE, Goitein M, et al: Progress in low-LET heavy particle therapy: intracranial and paracranial tumors and uveal melanomas. Radiat Res Suppl 8:S219-S226, 1985.
173. Noel G, Habrand JL, Mammar H, et al: Combination of photon and proton radiation therapy for chordomas and chondrosarcomas of the skull base: the Centre de Protontherapie D'Orsay experience. Int J Radiat Oncol Biol Phys 51:392-398, 2001.
174. Berson AM, Castro JR, Petti P, et al: Charged particle irradiation of chordoma and chondrosarcoma of the base of skull and cervical spine: the Lawrence Berkeley Laboratory experience. Int J Radiat Oncol Biol Phys 15:559-565, 1988.
175. Castro JR, Linstadt DE, Bahary JP, et al: Experience in charged particle irradiation of tumors of the skull base: 1977-1992. Int J Radiat Oncol Biol Phys 29:647-655, 1994.
176. Chang SD, Martin DP, Lee E, Adler JR Jr: Stereotactic radiosurgery and hypofractionated stereotactic radotherapy for residual or recurrent cranial base and cervical chordomas. Neurosurg Focus 10, 2001.
177. Kumar PP, Good RR, Skultety FM, et al: Local control of recurrent clival and sacral chordoma after interstitial irradiation with iodine-125: new techniques for treatment of recurrent or unresectable chordomas. Neurosurgery 22:479-483, 1988.
178. Gutin PH, Leibel SA, Hosobuchi Y, et al: Brachytherapy of recurrent tumors of the skull base and spine with iodine-125 sources. Neurosurgery 20:938-945, 1987.
179. Bernstein M, Gutin PH: Interstitial irradiation of skull base tumours. Can J Neurol Sci 12:366-370, 1985.
180. Camins MB, Duncan AW, Smith J, et al: Chondrosarcoma of the spine. Spine 3:202-209, 1978.
181. Sim FH, Frassica FJ, Wold LE: Chondrosarcoma of the spine: Mayo Clinic experience. *In* Sundaresan N, Schmidek HH, Schiller AL, et al (eds): Tumors of the Spine: Diagnosis and Clinical Management. Philadelphia, WB Saunders, 1990, pp 155-162.
182. York JE, Berk RH, Fuller GN, et al: Chondrosarcoma of the spine: 1954 to 1997. J Neurosurg 90:73-78, 1999.
183. Shives TC, McLeod RA, Unni KK, et al: Chondrosarcoma of the spine. J Bone Joint Surg Am 71:1158-1165, 1989.
184. Bergh P, Gunterberg B, Meis-Kindblom JM, et al: Prognostic factors and outcome of pelvic, sacral, and spinal chondrosarcomas: a center-based study of 69 cases. Cancer 91:1201-1212, 2001.
185. Ozaki T, Hillmann A, Lindner N, et al: Chondrosarcoma of the pelvis. Clin Orthop Relat Res Apr 337:226-239, 1997.
186. Sheth DS, Yasko AW, Johnson ME, et al: Chondrosarcoma of the pelvis. Prognostic factors for 67 patients treated with definitive surgery. Cancer 78:745-750, 1996.
187. Mostafavi H, Lennarson PJ, Traynelis VC: Granulocytic sarcoma of the spine. Neurosurgery 46:78-83, 2000.
188. Ugras S, Cirak B, Karakok M, et al: Spinal epidural granulocytic sarcoma (chloroma) in a non-leukemic child. Pediatr Int 43:505-507, 2001.
189. Fiegl M, Rieger C, Braess J, et al: Isolated epidural chloroma with translocation t(15;17) successfully treated with chemotherapy and all-trans-retinoic acid. Br J Haematol 122:688-689, 2003.
190. Landis DM, Aboulafia DM: Granulocytic sarcoma: an unusual complication of aleukemic myeloid leukemia causing spinal cord compression. A case report and literature review. Leuk Lymphoma 44:1753-1760, 2003.
191. Ho VB, Smirniotopoulos JG, Murphy FM, et al: Radiologic-pathologic correlation: hemangioblastoma. AJNR Am J Neuroradiol 13:1343-1352, 1992.
192. Cristante L, Herrmann HD: Surgical management of intramedullary hemangioblastoma of the spinal cord. Acta Neurochir (Wien) 141:333-339, 1999.
193. Roonprapunt C, Silvera VM, Setton A, et al: Surgical management of isolated hemangioblastomas of the spinal cord. Neurosurgery 49:321-327, 2001.
194. Neumann HP, Eggert HR, Weigel K, et al: Hemangioblastomas of the central nervous system. A 10-year study with special reference to von Hippel-Lindau syndrome. J Neurosurg 70:24-30, 1989.
195. Browne TR, Adams RD, Roberson GH: Hemangioblastoma of the spinal cord. Review and report of five cases. Arch Neurol 33:435-441, 1976.
196. Lonser RR, Weil RJ, Wanebo JE, et al: Surgical management of spinal cord hemangioblastomas in patients with von Hippel-Lindau disease. J Neurosurg 98:106-116, 2003.
197. Wanebo JE, Lonser RR, Glenn GM, et al: The natural history of hemangioblastomas of the central nervous system in patients with von Hippel-Lindau disease. J Neurosurg 98:82-94, 2003.
198. Lee DK, Choe WJ, Chung CK, et al: Spinal cord hemangioblastoma: surgical strategy and clinical outcome. J Neurooncol 61:27-34, 2003.
199. Jawahar A, Kondziolka D, Garces YI, et al: Stereotactic radiosurgery for hemangioblastomas of the brain. Acta Neurochir (Wien) 142:641-644, 2000.
200. Dyck P: Intramedullary lipoma. Diagnosis and treatment. Spine 17:979-981, 1992.
201. Kodama T, Numaguchi Y, Gellad FE, et al: Magnetic resonance imaging of a high cervical intradural lipoma. Comput Med Imaging Graph 15:93-95, 1991.
202. Lee M, Rezai AR, Abbott R, et al: Intramedullary spinal cord lipomas. J Neurosurg 82:394-400, 1995.
203. Kujas M, Sichez JP, Lalam TF, et al: Intradural spinal lipoma of the conus medullaris without spinal dysraphism. Clin Neuropathol 19:30-33, 2000.
204. Timmer FA, van Rooij WJ, Beute GN, et al: Intramedullary lipoma. Neuroradiology 38:159-160, 1996.
205. Razack N, Jimenez OF, Aldana P, et al: Intramedullary holocord lipoma in an athlete: case report. Neurosurgery 42:394-396, 1998.
206. Chahal S, Lagera JE, Ryder J, et al: Hematological neoplasms with first presentation as spinal cord compression syndromes: a 10-year retrospective series and review of the literature. Clin Neuropathol 22:282-290, 2003.
207. Lyons MK, O'Neill BP, Kurtin PJ, et al: Diagnosis and management of primary spinal epidural non-Hodgkin's lymphoma. Mayo Clin Proc 71:453-457, 1996.
208. Ishikawa H, Hasegawa M, Tamaki Y, et al: Comparable outcomes of radiation therapy without high-dose methotrexate for patients with primary central nervous system lymphoma. Jpn J Clin Oncol 33:443-449, 2003.

209. Heckmann JG, Druschky A, Kern PM, et al: ["Ghost and mimicry-tumor"—primary CNS lymphoma]. Nervenarzt 71:305-310, 2000.
210. Vaquero J, Martinez R, Rossi E, et al: Primary cerebral lymphoma: the "ghost tumor." Case report. J Neurosurg 60:174-176, 1984.
211. Gray RS, Abrahams JJ, Hufnagel TJ, et al: Ghost-cell tumor of the optic chiasm. Primary CNS lymphoma. J Clin Neuroophthalmol 9:98-104, 1989.
212. Coca A, Goday A, Font J, et al: Primary cerebral lymphoma: the "ghost tumor." J Neurosurg 61:202-203, 1984.
213. DeAngelis LM, Seiferheld W, Schold SC, et al: Combination chemotherapy and radiotherapy for primary central nervous system lymphoma: Radiation Therapy Oncology Group Study 93-10. J Clin Oncol 20:4643-4648, 2002.
214. Schneider F, Putzier M: Primary leptomeningeal melanoma. Spine 27:E545-E547, 2002.
215. Tatter SB, Borges LF, Louis DN: Central neurocytomas of the cervical spinal cord. Report of two cases. J Neurosurg 81:288-293, 1994.
216. Tatter SB, Borges LF, Louis DN: Correction: central neurocytomas of the cervical spinal cord. J Neurosurg 82:706, 1995.
217. Martin AJ, Sharr MM, Teddy PJ, et al: Neurocytoma of the thoracic spinal cord. Acta Neurochir (Wien) 144:823-828, 2002.
218. Oliveira AM, Scheithauer BW, Salomao DR, et al: Primary sarcomas of the brain and spinal cord: a study of 18 cases. Am J Surg Pathol 26:1056-1063, 2002.
219. Merimsky O, Lepechoux C, Terrier P, et al: Primary sarcomas of the central nervous system. Oncology 58:210-214, 2000.
220. Sarcoma Meta-analysis Collaboration: Adjuvant chemotherapy for localised resectable soft-tissue sarcoma of adults: meta-analysis of individual data. Lancet 350:1647-1654, 1997.
221. Konno S, Yabuki S, Kinoshita T, et al: Combined laminectomy and thoracoscopic resection of dumbbell-type thoracic cord tumor. Spine 26:E130-E134, 2001.
222. Shadmehr MB, Gaissert HA, Wain JC, et al: The surgical approach to "dumbbell tumors" of the mediastinum. Ann Thorac Surg 76:1650-1654, 2003.
223. Seppala MT, Haltia MJ: Spinal malignant nerve-sheath tumor or cellular schwannoma? A striking difference in prognosis. J Neurosurg 79:528-532, 1993.
224. Hejazi N, Witzmann A: Spinal intramedullary teratoma with exophytic components: report of two cases and review of the literature. Neurosurg Rev 26:113-116, 2003.
225. Heyd R, Strassmann G, Filipowicz I, et al: [Radiotherapy in vertebral hemangioma]. Rontgenpraxis 53:208-220, 2001.
226. Fox MW, Onofrio BM: The natural history and management of symptomatic and asymptomatic vertebral hemangiomas. J Neurosurg 78:36-45, 1993.
227. Cross JJ, Antoun NM, Laing RJ, et al: Imaging of compressive vertebral haemangiomas. Eur Radiol 10:997-1002, 2000.
228. Djindjian M, Nguyen JP, Gaston A, et al: Multiple vertebral hemangiomas with neurological signs. Case report. J Neurosurg 76:1025-1028, 1992.
229. Rades D, Bajrovic A, Alberti W, et al: Is there a dose-effect relationship for the treatment of symptomatic vertebral hemangioma? Int J Radiat Oncol Biol Phys 55:178-181, 2003.
230. Wambersie A, Landberg T: International Commission on Radiation Units and Measurements, Inc. ICRU Report 62: Prescribing, Recording and Reporting Photon Beam Therapy (Supplement to ICRU Report 50). Journal of the ICRU 62 1999. Bethesda, MD, Nuclear Technology Publishing.
231. International Commission on Radiation Units and Measurements, Inc. ICRU Report 50, Prescribing, Recording, and Reporting Photon Beam Therapy 50 1993. Bethesda, MD, Nuclear Technology Publishing.
232. Michalski JM: Spinal canal. *In* Leibel SA, Phillips TL (eds): Textbook of Radiation Oncology. Philadelphia, WB Saunders, 1998, pp 860-875.
233. Shiu AS, Chang EL, Ye JS, et al: Near simultaneous computed tomography image-guided stereotactic spinal radiotherapy: an emerging paradigm for achieving true stereotaxy. Int J Radiat Oncol Biol Phys 57:605-613, 2003.
234. Stieber VW, Munley M: Central nervous system tumors. *In* Mundt AJ, Roeske JC (eds): Intensity-Modulated Radiation Therapy: A Clinical Perspective. Ontario, BC Decker, 2004.
235. Yin FF, Ryu S, Ajlouni M, et al: A technique of intensity-modulated radiosurgery (IMRS) for spinal tumors. Med Phys 29:2815-2822, 2002.
236. Ryu SI, Chang SD, Kim DH, et al: Image-guided hypo-fractionated stereotactic radiosurgery to spinal lesions. Neurosurgery 49:838-846, 2001.
237. Jaffray DA, Siewerdsen JH, Wong JW, et al: Flat-panel cone-beam computed tomography for image-guided radiation therapy. Int J Radiat Oncol Biol Phys 53:1337-1349, 2002.
238. Blomgren H, Lax I, Naslund I, et al: Stereotactic high dose fraction radiation therapy of extracranial tumors using an accelerator. Clinical experience of the first thirty-one patients. Acta Oncol 34:861-870, 1995.
239. Schultheiss TE, Kun LE, Ang KK, et al: Radiation response of the central nervous system. Int J Radiat Oncol Biol Phys 31:1093-1112, 1995.
240. Marcus RB Jr, Million RR: The incidence of myelitis after irradiation of the cervical spinal cord. Int J Radiat Oncol Biol Phys 19:3-8, 1990.
241. Macbeth FR, Wheldon TE, Girling DJ, et al: Radiation myelopathy: estimates of risk in 1048 patients in three randomized trials of palliative radiotherapy for non-small cell lung cancer. The Medical Research Council Lung Cancer Working Party. Clin Oncol (R Coll Radiol) 8:176-181, 1996.
242. Wara WM, Phillips TL, Sheline GE, et al: Radiation tolerance of the spinal cord. Cancer 35:1558-1562, 1975.
243. Cohen L, Creditor M: An iso-effect table for radiation tolerance of the human spinal cord. Int J Radiat Oncol Biol Phys 7:961-966, 1981.
244. Niewald M, Feldmann U, Feiden W, et al: Multivariate logistic analysis of dose-effect relationship and latency of radiomyelopathy after hyperfractionated and conventionally fractionated radiotherapy in animal experiments. Int J Radiat Oncol Biol Phys 41:681-688, 1998.
245. Ang KK, Jiang GL, Feng Y, et al: Extent and kinetics of recovery of occult spinal cord injury. Int J Radiat Oncol Biol Phys 50:1013-1020, 2001.
246. Leber KA, Bergloff J, Pendl G: Dose-response tolerance of the visual pathways and cranial nerves of the cavernous sinus to stereotactic radiosurgery. J Neurosurg 88:43-50, 1998.
247. Benzil DL, Saboori M, Mogilner AY, et al: Safety and efficacy of stereotactic radiosurgery for tumors of the spine. J Neurosurg 101 (Suppl 3):413-418, 2004.
248. Pieters RS, O'Farrell D, Fullerton B: Cauda equina tolerance to radiation therapy [abstract]. Int J Radiat Oncol Biol Phys 36:359, 1996.
249. Esik O, Csere T, Stefanits K, et al: A review on radiogenic Lhermitte's sign. Pathol Oncol Res 9:115-120, 2003.
250. Okada S, Okeda R: Pathology of radiation myelopathy. Neuropathology 21:247-265, 2001.
251. Nieder C, Ataman F, Price RE, et al: Radiation myelopathy: new perspective on an old problem. Radiat Oncol Investig 7:193-203, 1999.
252. Schultheiss TE, Higgins EM, El Mahdi AM: The latent period in clinical radiation myelopathy. Int J Radiat Oncol Biol Phys 10:1109-1115, 1984.
253. Wang PY, Shen WC, Jan JS: MR imaging in radiation myelopathy. AJNR Am J Neuroradiol 13:1049-1055, 1992.
254. Feldmeier JJ, Lange JD, Cox SD, et al: Hyperbaric oxygen as prophylaxis or treatment for radiation myelitis. Undersea Hyperb Med 20:249-255, 1993.
255. Liu CY, Yim BT, Wozniak AJ: Anticoagulation therapy for radiation-induced myelopathy. Ann Pharmacother 35:188-191, 2001.
256. Schultheiss TE, Stephens LC, Peters LJ: Survival in radiation myelopathy. Int J Radiat Oncol Biol Phys 12:1765-1769, 1986.
257. Mayfield JK: Postradiation spinal deformity. Orthop Clin North Am 10:829-844, 1979.
258. Nadeem SQ, Feun LG, Bruce-Gregorios JH, et al: Post radiation sarcoma (malignant fibrous histiocytoma) of the cervical spine following ependymoma (a case report). J Neurooncol 11:263-268, 1991.

259. Rappaport ZH, Loven D, Ben Aharon U: Radiation-induced cerebellar glioblastoma multiforme subsequent to treatment of an astrocytoma of the cervical spinal cord. Neurosurgery 29:606-608, 1991.
260. CTEP and NCI. Common Terminology Criteria for Adverse Events v3.0 (CTCAE). NIH, 2003. NIH Available at http://ctep.cancer.gov.
261. Pavy J-J, Denekamp J, Letschert J, et al: Late effects toxicity scoring: the SOMA scale. Int J Radiat Oncol Biol Phys 31:1043-1047, 1995.
262. Meade TJ, Taylor AK, Bull SR: New magnetic resonance contrast agents as biochemical reporters. Curr Opin Neurobiol 13:597-602, 2003.
263. Sloof JL: Primary Intramedullary Tumors of the Spinal Cord and Filum Terminale. Philadelphia, WB Saunders, 1964.
264. Nieder C, Milas L, Ang KK: Tissue tolerance to reirradiation. Semin Radiat Oncol 10:200-209, 2000.
265. McCunniff AJ, Liang MJ: Radiation tolerance of the cervical spinal cord. Int J Radiat Oncol Biol Phys 16:675-678, 1989.
266. Schultheiss TE: The radiation dose response of the human cervical spinal cord [abstract]. Int J Radiat Oncol Biol Phys 45:174, 1999.
267. Niewald M, Feldmann U, Feiden W, et al: Multivariate logistic analysis of dose-effect relationship and latency of radiomyelopathy after hyperfractionated and conventionally fractionated radiotherapy in animal experiments. Int J Radiat Oncol Biol Phys 41:681-688, 1998.
268. Jeremic B, Djuric L, Mijatovic L: Incidence of radiation myelitis of the cervical spinal cord at doses of 5500 cGy or greater. Cancer 68:2138-2141, 1991.

CHAPTER 28

ORBITAL, OCULAR, AND OPTIC NERVE TUMORS

Kathryn McConnell Greven and Craig M. Greven

INCIDENCE

There are 2200 estimated cases of primary ocular tumors annually.

The most frequent primary tumor is ocular melanoma; the second most frequent primary tumor is retinoblastoma.

BIOLOGIC CHARACTERISTICS

Characteristics vary with specific histologic type.

STAGING EVALUATION

For melanoma, Collaborative Ocular Melanoma Study size criteria are used, and for orbital lymphoma, Ann Arbor staging is used. Ocular rhabdomyosarcomas and retinoblastomas are discussed in Chapters 65 and 68.

PRIMARY THERAPY

For melanoma, plaque radiation is used for small and intermediate-size lesions, and enucleation is used for large lesions or eyes with poor vision.

For lymphoma, orbital radiation is used for low-grade lymphoma, and chemotherapy with or without radiation is used for high-grade lymphoma.

ADJUVANT THERAPY

Adjuvant therapy and outcomes vary with tumor type and extension.

LOCALLY ADVANCED DISEASE

Treatment approach and outcomes vary with specific tumor type.

PALLIATION

Irradiation is effective treatment for advanced primary or metastatic disease; chemotherapy/hormonal treatment is used for some metastatic tumors.

Based on the incidence rates from the Surveillance, Epidemiology and End Results Program of the National Cancer Institute, the American Cancer Society estimated that approximately 2200 new cases of all types of primary ocular and orbital malignancy were diagnosed in the United States in 2002.[1] This demonstrates the rarity of ocular malignancies. Uveal melanoma is the single most common malignancy of the eye and orbit and makes up nearly 70% of all malignancies of these tissues.[1] Radiation is used in the management of many ocular and orbital malignancies, as well as in the management of several benign ocular processes. Understanding the pathophysiology and results from radiation treatment can guide treatment recommendations.

Complicating the assessment of treatment of ocular cancer is the real possibility that therapy itself may result in loss of vision or loss of an eye. Understanding the radiation tolerances and sequelae from radiation is vital for estimating the vision-related quality of life following treatment.

ETIOLOGY AND EPIDEMIOLOGY

Eyelid Skin Cancers

Basal and squamous cell carcinomas of the periorbital skin (nasal bridge, medial canthus, and eyelid) most frequently occur on the lower eyelid and medial canthus. Patients with sun exposure and who are immunosuppressed have increased incidence of these cancers.

Choroid Melanoma

Uveal melanoma is the most common primary malignant intraocular neoplasm.[1] It is believed to arise from melanocytes of the uveal tract and in the United States occurs in approximately 1500 patients per year.[1,2] Uveal melanomas are more common in lightly pigmented persons and are infrequent in nonwhite races. The average age at the time of diagnosis is 60 years in most large series,[2-4] and it occurs with equal frequency in men and women. The tumors are rarely bilateral. Factors proposed as increasing the risk for the development of uveal melanoma are prolonged sustained sunlight exposure[5,6] and lighter-colored irises.[5,6] Certain diseases may predispose to melanoma, including xeroderma pigmentosum, which is an inherited disorder of DNA repair; oculodermal melanocytosis,[7] in which the ocular surface and the uveal tract are hyperpigmented; and the dysplastic nevus syndrome. There are some reports implying a possible rare genetic predisposition, although most melanomas occur as sporadic tumors.

Retina

Retinoblastomas are discussed in Chapter 68.

Optic Nerve

Meningioma

Optic nerve sheath meningiomas may be primary and arise from the meningothelial cap cells of arachnoid villi, and they can develop anywhere along the course of the optic nerve from globe to prechiasmal intracisternal optic nerve. They may be unilateral, bilateral, or multifocal. Patients with type 2 neurofibromatosis are predisposed to have bilateral or multifocal lesions.[8] Meningiomas from other locations can also involve the optic nerve.

Optic nerve sheath meningiomas are more common in women. Dutton's meta-analysis estimates a female preponderance of 61%.[9] The typical age is 40 years. Bilateral cases appear to have an earlier mean age of onset.

Glioma

Optic nerve gliomas account for 1% to 5% of intracranial gliomas and 4% of orbital tumors. They occur most frequently in children, with 75% in the first decade and 90% in the first two decades of life.[10] Approximately 25% of patients with optic gliomas also have type 1 neurofibromatosis. These tumors are increasingly being seen as markers of enhanced risk in patients and their families for the subsequent development of central nervous system tumors.[11]

Orbit

In a recent report of 1264 consecutive patients with orbital masses, 33% of patients had malignant lesions. Rhabdomyosarcoma was the most common malignancy in children, representing 3% of all orbital masses, and lymphoma was the most common malignancy in older patients, representing 10% of cases.[12] Metastatic breast cancer comprised 4% of these lesions.

Rhabdomyosarcoma

Rhabdomyosarcomas are discussed in Chapter 65.

Lacrimal Gland

Lacrimal gland tumors are rare. The gender distributions are equal and the ages of the patients range from 10 to 73 years (mean age, 46 years).[13] The majority of these lesions are malignant, with adenoid cystic carcinoma and mucoepidermoid cancer being the two most frequent. Benign pleomorphic adenomas also occur.

Lymphoma

Primary orbital lymphomas are rare and account for less than 1% of all lymphomas diagnosed.[14] Lymphomas in the orbit can occur anteriorly in the conjunctival tissues or in the retrobulbar region. Patients with other sites of lymphoma can also present with eye involvement in the course of their disease.

Primary intraocular lymphoma (PIOL) may have malignant lymphoid cells involving the retina, vitreous, or optic nerve head, with or without concomitant central nervous system (CNS) involvement. The incidence of PIOL has been increasing in the past 15 years, and it has been observed in both immunocompetent and immunocompromised people.[15] The cause of this increased incidence is unknown. This is a disease of persons in their 50s and 60s, occurring more often in men than women.

Metastatic Tumors

The most common tumor to metastasize to the orbit is from breast cancer.[12] Other orbital metastases have been reported to occur from neuroblastoma, lung cancer, renal cell cancer, and prostate cancer.

Similarly, choroidal metastases are most frequently of breast cancer origin, followed by lung cancer. In one report of 420 patients, the uveal metastasis came from a primary cancer of the breast in 196 (47%), lung in 90 (21%), gastrointestinal tract in 18 (4%), kidney in 9 (2%), skin in 9 (2%), prostate in 9 (2%), and other cancers in 16 (4%).[16]

Benign Ocular Conditions

Pterygium

A pterygium is a benign growth of fibrovascular tissue on the cornea. These lesions may become red and inflamed, encroach on the visual axis, or just be a cosmetic issue for patients.

The majority of them are located nasally and occur in patients aged 20 to 50.[17] They are more commonly encountered in warm, dry climates or in patients who are chronically exposed to outdoor elements or smoky and dusty environments. Ultraviolet light exposure appears to be the most significant factor in the development of pterygia. Heredity may also be a factor.

Pterygia represent a degeneration of the conjunctival stroma with replacement by thickened, tortuous elastotic fibers.[18] Activated fibroblasts in the leading edge of the pterygium invade and fragment Bowman's layer. Pterygium development resembles actinic degeneration of the skin.

Pseudotumor

Orbital pseudotumor or idiopathic orbital inflammatory syndrome (IOIS) is a nonspecific inflammatory process of unknown etiology that may mimic orbital lymphoma.[19] Because the disease mimics infectious or neoplastic processes, these must be ruled out. Autoimmune disease, endocrinopathies, and granulomatous processes must be excluded, as well as local infection with secondary involvement of the orbit, such as sinusitis and subperiosteal abscess. The diagnosis of pseudotumor is vague and remains one of exclusion.

The etiology is unknown but several theories have been proposed. The response to steroids and immunosuppressive drugs suggests an autoimmune disorder. A fibroproliferative disorder has been suggested. Aberrant wound healing provoked by infection or autoimmune disease has also been postulated.

The term "pseudolymphoma" has been advocated for the diagnosis of reactive lymphoid hyperplasia. Unfortunately, the literature includes reports of patients with biopsied and unbiopsied lesions, as well as reactive lymphoid hyperplasia and the more nonspecific inflammatory lesions when reporting the outcome of treatment. For this reason, the term "pseudotumor" refers to any idiopathic inflammatory lesion of the orbit.

Graves' Ophthalmopathy

The pathogenesis of Graves' ophthalmopathy is believed to be an autoimmune disease in which activated T-lymphocytes invade the orbit and stimulate glycosaminoglycan production in fibroblasts, resulting in tissue edema, lymphocyte infiltration, and marked enlargement of the extraocular muscles.[20] Because lymphocytes and fibroblasts are sensitive to radiation, retrobulbar irradiation has been advocated as a logical method of treatment. The ophthalmopathy typically goes through three phases—progression, followed by stabilization and, perhaps, some improvement. Residual signs of ophthalmopathy after the disease has reached a plateau are believed likely to be the result of fibrosis and other tissue changes rather than persistent inflammation amenable to radiation.

Macular Degeneration

Age-related macular degeneration (AMD) is the leading cause of blindness in patients older than 65 years.[21] The progressive loss of central vision results in the majority of patients from an atrophic process involving the retinal epithelium and choriocapillaris in the macula, which is classified as dry AMD. The wet form of AMD is an exudative process with subretinal neovascularization. Wet AMD generally progresses to destructive disciform scarring of the macula, and fibrovascular scars involving the choroid and sensory retina. Patients develop poor visual acuity.

PREVENTION AND EARLY DETECTION

Because of the rarity of all ocular tumors, no prevention or early detection methods have been developed for most tumor types. However, in children born into a family with known retinoblastoma, early and careful ophthalmologic evaluation is warranted. Genetic counseling and evaluation of the siblings of patients with retinoblastoma are important, given the high hereditary likelihood.[22] Finally, after the diagnosis of unilateral retinoblastoma, routine evaluation of the uninvolved eye is indicated because of the increased risk of contralateral disease (see Chapter 68).

BIOLOGIC CHARACTERISTICS AND MOLECULAR BIOLOGY

Ocular Melanoma

Biologic characteristics that have been determined to help predict outcomes in patients with ocular melanoma are tumor cell type, tumor size, tumor location, and extension of the tumor outside the sclera.[23] Cell type is discussed in the pathology section of this chapter, with spindle cell tumors having a better survival than epithelioid cell tumors. Many tumors are treated by means other than enucleation, and because biopsy is rarely performed, cell type is often unknown.

Survival is adversely affected by increased size of the uveal melanoma. Although the earlier literature had various size classifications, the Collaborative Ocular Melanoma Study (COMS) has established the standard size classification.[24-26] Small melanomas are 1 to 3 mm thick and less than 16 mm in the largest tumor dimension. Medium-sized melanomas are 3 to 8 mm thick and less than 16 mm in the largest tumor dimension, and large choroidal melanomas are more than 8 mm thick or greater than 16 mm in the largest tumor dimension (Table 28-1).

Prognosis is also affected by the location of the anterior tumor margin. Tumors located anterior to the equator of the eye in the anterior choroid or ciliary body have a worse prognosis than those tumors located more posteriorly.[23] Extraocular extension of a uveal melanoma has poor prognostic implications.[24]

Orbital Lymphoma

The biology of these tumors varies with the histologic classification within the Revised European-American Lymphoma system or the Working Formulation.[27,28] Stage and histologic type of the tumor play the most significant roles in outcome for orbital lesions.

Primary intraocular lymphoma is believed to be a subset of primary central nervous system lymphoma. It is usually a diffuse large B-cell non-Hodgkin's lymphoma or may be T-cell lymphoma. Because pathologic diagnosis can be difficult, flow cytometry can be done to demonstrate monoclonal populations of B-lymphocytes. Immunohistochemistry has also been used to demonstrate expression of BCL-6 and MUM1.[29] These two markers have been revealed in systemic diffuse large B-cell lymphoma. Molecular analysis detecting immunoglobulin gene rearrangements and ocular cytokine levels showing elevated interleukin (IL)-10, with a ratio of IL-10 to IL-6 greater than 1.0, are helpful adjuncts for the diagnosis of intraocular lymphoma.[14,30]

Table 28-1 Various Other Definitions of Choroidal Melanoma Size

Size	Measurement
Small	1.5-2.4 mm height and 5-16 mm diameter
Medium	2.5-10 mm height and <16 mm diameter
Large	>10 mm height and >16 mm diameter

Orbital Pseudotumor

Histopathology varies, and attempts to refine and subdivide patients have been advocated. The histopathologic spectrum of idiopathic orbital inflammation is typically nondiagnostic and diverse, ranging from the typical diffuse polymorphous infiltrate to the atypical granulomatous inflammation, tissue eosinophilia, and infiltrative sclerosis. One report suggested dividing this condition into three principal types: lymphoid, granulomatous, and sclerosing types.[31] Several authors have endorsed the exclusion of reactive lymphoid hyperplasia and defined pseudotumor as a mixed inflammatory infiltrate with fibrosis of varying degrees.[19]

Immunologic cytochemical staining, polymerase chain reaction, and flow cytometry are all helpful for demonstrating surface membrane or cytoplasmic markers that correspond to a lymphoma. Polyclonal distributions are associated with pseudolymphoma.

PATHOLOGY AND PATHWAYS OF SPREAD

Skin Cancers

Basal cell cancers are seen in 90% of patients, followed by squamous cell cancers in 10%. For patients with squamous cell cancer, regional lymph nodes have been reported in as many as 24% of patients.[32] Lymph node involvement is more common for larger tumors, recurrent tumors, and those with perineural invasion. Patients with recurrent lesions or perineural invasion may have tumor cells spread more peripherally than clinically apparent. This may require wider radiation treatment fields. Tumors located in the embryologic fusion planes of the face have been found to be more deeply infiltrating. This area around the medial canthus may affect the depth of treatment necessary for successful outcome.

Ocular Melanoma

Uveal melanomas arise from melanocytes that are of neuroectodermal origin. Melanoma cells have large nuclear to cytoplasmic ratio, prominent or multiple nucleoli, and frequent mitotic figures. Tumor cells are generally classified as being of two types: spindle cells and epithelioid cells.[33] Spindle cells have a fusiform shape and less pronounced atypia, while epithelioid cells are larger, more ovoid in shape with more anaplastic characteristics. Uveal melanomas are classified as spindle cell melanomas if they are composed of only spindle cells, mixed cell melanomas if they contain both spindle and epithelioid cells, and epithelioid cell melanomas if they contain predominantly or exclusively epithelioid cells. Occasionally, the cells within the melanoma undergo necrosis and are classified as necrotic melanomas.

The prognosis for survival is more favorable in spindle cell melanoma, intermediate in mixed cell tumors, and poorest in epithelioid or necrotic melanoma. Other negative prognostic indicators include largest tumor dimension, tumor thickness, and location of the anterior tumor margin.[33] Melanomas tend to be slow growing tumors, but the rate of growth can be quite variable. More rapidly growing tumors, which have a worse prognosis, tend to be anaplastic and composed of epithelioid cells.

At the time of diagnosis, most posterior uveal melanomas are confined inside the sclera of the eye. Extraocular extension of the melanoma can occur through emissary canals, through which normal ocular structures like vessels and nerves enter and exit the sclera, and generally not by atrophy or thinning of the sclera. Extraocular extension is classified as microscopic and gross (visible on gross inspection). The presence of extraocular extension occurs in 8% to 14% of eyes harboring a melanoma and is associated with a worse prognosis.[34]

Metastatic disease occurs in less than 3% of patients at the time of initial diagnosis. The most common sites of involvement include hematogenous spread to the liver and the lung. More unusual sites of spread include bone, skin and subcutaneous tissue, and brain and spinal cord. Lymph node involvement did occur in 10% of metastatic deaths within the COMS.[35]

Choroidal Metastasis

The most common pathology is adenocarcinoma from the breast or non–small cell lung cancer. The majority of patients have other sites of metastatic disease. Disease extent can be localized to the choroid. The average number of lesions seen in the choroid in one large series was two.[16] In this situation, involvement of the opposite choroid can occur in as many as 50% of patients. Orbital metastases can occur and are typically unilateral.

Orbital/Ocular Lymphoma

A wide range of non-Hodgkin's lymphomas has been described involving the orbit and globe. In patients with orbital lymphomas, most of the lesions are of B-cell origin and classified as low or intermediate grade by the Working Formulation.[36] Intraocular lymphomas are usually of intermediate or high grade.[15]

The pattern of spread in low-grade lymphomas is similar to its counterparts in the rest of the body, with a risk of distant sites of involvement. Intraocular lymphomas tend to disseminate into or be a component of disease within the CNS and therefore carry a more ominous prognosis.

Orbital Meningioma

Meningiomas spread along paths of least resistance, remaining confined to the subarachnoid or intradural space of the intraorbital optic nerve. The tumor may invade dura, adjacent orbital tissue, muscle, bone, and globe. These tumors may traverse the optic canal and affect the intracranial segment of the optic nerve or adjacent structures. Orbital meningiomas have histologic features similar to those of intracranial meningioma. The majority of lesions demonstrate concentric formations of spindle or ovoid cells, meningothelial with sheets of polygonal cells separated by vascular trabeculae.[37]

Lacrimal Gland Tumors

Pathology is typically adenoid cystic cancer, followed by mucoepidermoid cancer and adenocarcinoma. Outcome seems to be related to the presence of necrosis, hemorrhage, perineural invasion, and high mitotic count.[38]

Optic Nerve Glioma

In the pediatric form of the disease, the cell of origin for optic nerve gliomas is unknown. Optic nerve gliomas are classified as grade I astrocytomas (pilocytic astrocytoma) in the World Health Organization (WHO) classification of gliomas, are slow growing, and do not tend to metastasize.[39] Development of optic nerve gliomas occurs in stages, from generalized hyperplasia of glial cells in the nerve to complete disorganization with loss of neural landmarks within the nerve and nerve sheath. A reactive meningeal hyperplasia may be incited, making it difficult to distinguish from a perioptic meningioma.

In pediatric patients with optic nerve glioma, 10% to 38% have type 1 neurofibromatosis (NF-1), and 15% to 40% of children with NF-1 have an optic glioma.[40] When bilateral, the lesions are pathognomonic for NF-1.

In the adult form of the disease, the optic nerve gliomas are more likely to be diffusely infiltrative including astrocytoma (WHO grade II), anaplastic astrocytoma (WHO grade III), or glioblastoma multiforme (WHO grade IV).[41] Nuclear atypia, mitoses, endothelial proliferation, and necrosis are potential histologic features.

CLINICAL MANIFESTATIONS, PATIENT EVALUATION, AND STAGING

The diagnostic algorithm for ocular, orbital, and lid tumors is given in Figure 28-1.

Skin Cancers

Patients should be evaluated for lymph node involvement with physical exam of the parotid, facial, and neck node areas. Symptoms of pain or sensory changes may indicate perineural invasion. MRI of the skull base may detect enlargement of the affected nerves.

Ocular Melanoma

At the time of presentation, patients with uveal melanomas may be asymptomatic or complain of visual symptoms such as flashes of light, floaters, decreased visual acuity, or a visual field defect. Those who have visual symptoms typically have a more posteriorly located tumor, a large tumor, or an

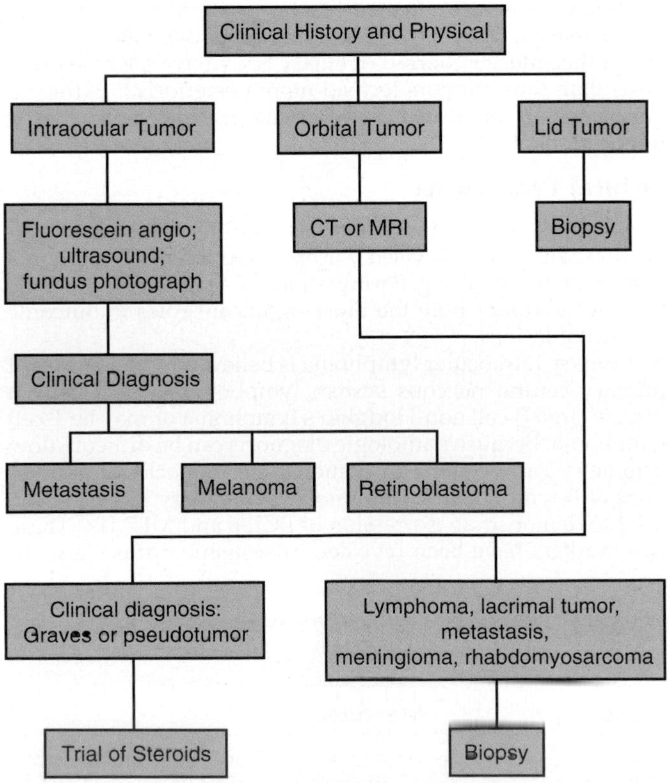

Figure 28-1 Diagnostic algorithm for ocular, orbital, and lid tumors.

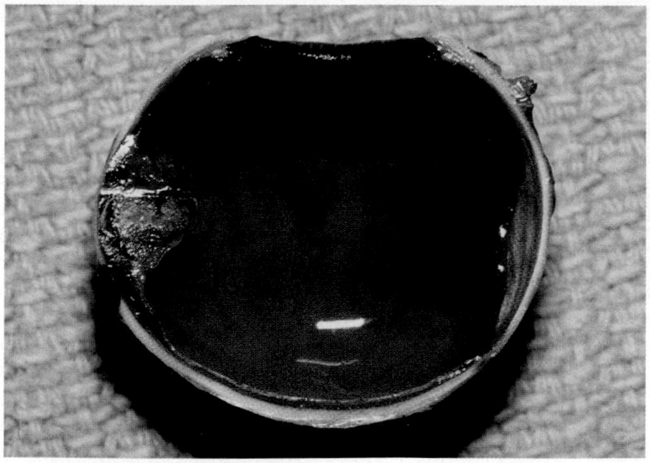

Figure 28-2 Photograph of a melanoma in the cross section of a globe.

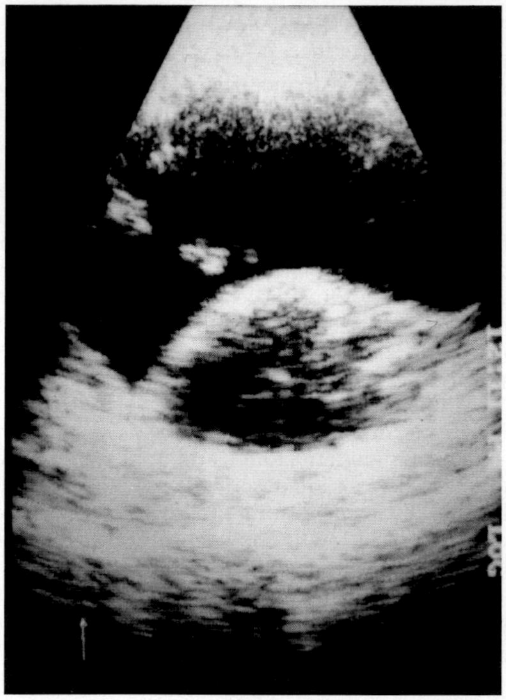

Figure 28-3 Ultrasound scan of a dome-shaped tumor.

associated retinal detachment leading to a visual field deficit. Rarely, pain and redness are presenting symptoms, occurring in large or necrotic tumors that have associated inflammation.

The diagnosis of melanoma is based primarily on ophthalmoscopic appearance and ancillary testing. The tumor typically appears as a unilateral, solitary, elevated, dark brown or gray, variable pigmented, dome-shaped mass (Fig. 28-2). Orange pigment (lipofuscin) often is on the surface of the tumor and is thought to represent increased metabolic activity.[42] Retinal detachment may be present and is more likely in larger tumors.

The initial ophthalmologic work-up includes fundus photography, fluorescein angiography, and ultrasonography of the globe (Fig. 28-3). These tests facilitate making a correct diagnosis and are also useful in following the lesions for growth or regression after treatment. In a large prospective trial, 645 of 647 patients who underwent enucleation for melanoma were found to have diagnostic accuracy. Two of the patients had adenocarcinoma.[24] In eyes with opaque media secondary to cataract or vitreous hemorrhage, ultrasonography of the globe and MRI of the orbits can allow an accurate diagnosis. Biopsy of a lesion suspicious for an ocular melanoma is used only in cases of diagnostic uncertainty. In patients requiring biopsy, histopathology and immunohistochemistry can be useful in confirming the diagnosis.

In order to assess disease extent, a general history and physical examination should be performed with attention directed to skin lesions, weight loss, lungs, and liver. History of a prior malignancy would indicate the possibility of a metastatic lesion in the eye rather than a primary melanoma. The most frequent site of metastasis for melanoma is the liver, so work-up generally includes liver enzyme levels. Elevated levels will prompt evaluation with radiographic imaging. This approach was recently reported to have a low sensitivity but high specificity and predictive value.[43] Other sites of metastatic disease include the lung, and imaging with chest CT scan is most accurate for early detection of disease. The COMS report of sites of metastasis from melanoma demonstrated that sites included liver (91%), lung (28%), and bone (18%).[43] Melanomas of the iris rarely metastasize. Brain is an infrequent site of metastasis and was discovered in only 4% of patients at the time of death.[44]

Ocular Metastasis

Patients with uveal metastasis from breast cancer presented to ophthalmologists with visual symptoms in 93% of cases. Of 264 patients with uveal metastasis, 225 (85%) had choroidal metastasis, 8 (3%) had iris metastasis, 2 (<1%) had ciliary body metastasis, and 29 (11%) had metastasis in multiple uveal sites. Asymptomatic metastases were detected in 56% of the opposite eye.[45]

Patients with orbital tumors more often present with diplopia, ocular motility disorder, and proptosis. Lesions are usually unilateral.[46] Metastatic disease may be detected in a high proportion of the patients who present with this entity.

Orbital Lymphoma

Orbital lymphomas can involve the soft tissues and present as a palpable mass. Proptosis, diplopia, and inflammation can also be present. Conjunctival lymphomas are erythematous and present as a visible and palpable mass that is sometimes referred to as salmon colored. Patients should be evaluated for systemic disease with routine staging for a lymphoma work-up, including imaging of the chest, abdomen, and pelvis. Full nodal examination with assessment of symptoms including weight loss, fevers, and night sweats should be included. Bone marrow examination should be performed. CT scans of the orbit can be used to delineate the extent of retrobulbar and soft tissue involvement.

PIOL is one of the most challenging intraocular tumors to diagnose. Cytologic examination of vitreal aspirates remains the gold standard for exclusion of neoplastic disease in patients with idiopathic uveitis.[14] Patients with primary vitreous involvement should also have CSF examination and MRI of the brain and meninges. Eighty percent of patients with primary vitreous involvement have bilateral involvement.

Staging is done using the Ann Arbor staging system.[47] A localized orbital lymphoma would be stage IeA.

Optic Nerve Meningioma

Patients typically present with visual loss, afferent papillary defect, color vision disturbance, visual field defect, proptosis, and optic disc edema. Ophthalmoscopic examination may reveal optic nerve head swelling, macular edema, nerve pallor, or choroidal folds. Optic disc swelling may also be observed. MRI is the procedure of choice for diagnosis of these lesions. Lesions appear slightly hypointense to brain and optic nerve tissue on T1-weighted images with fat suppression and gadolinium contrast. Thin CT scans may reveal regular or irregular thickening of the nerve sheath meninges. The nerve may appear normal in size or smaller as the result of circumferential compression or atrophy. Calcification has been described in 30% of patients and is associated with slower growth.[48] Differential diagnosis includes sarcoid, demyelinating optic neuritis, orbital inflammatory disease, schwannoma, lymphoma, hemangiopericytoma, and optic nerve metastasis.

Usually these lesions are described as slow growing. Visual loss will generally occur in untreated eyes over a period of 5 to 10 years.[49] Rapid growth has been observed during pregnancy, which may be mediated by hormone receptors.[50] Other tumors have demonstrated rapid visual loss even in the absence of radiographic enlargement.

Optic Nerve Gliomas

Of optic pathway gliomas, 10% to 20% are confined to the orbit, with the remainder involving the intracranial compartment.[10] MRI is the preferred method for evaluation of optic pathway glioma. Both the intraorbital lesion and its intracranial extent can be effectively characterized on MRI. When evaluating the orbit, gadolinium-enhanced T1-weighted images with fat saturation are effective at defining the extent of adult optic glioma. Intracranially, MRI provides superior evaluation of the optic nerve, chiasm, tracts, geniculate body, and optic radiation compared with CT.

Orbital Pseudotumors

Patients present with proptosis, decreased ocular motility, soft tissue edema, and pain. Decreased visual acuity is not unusual. The condition may be unilateral or bilateral.[51] CT scan may reveal a unilateral focal or more diffuse mass. One review documented infiltration of the retrobulbar fat in 76%, enlargement of the extraocular muscles in 57%, thickening of the optic nerve/sheath complex in 38%, contrast enhancement in 95%, and proptosis in 71%.[52]

Intracranial extension is unusual but has been documented in up to 8.8%.

Biopsy is recommended whenever possible to ensure accuracy of diagnosis. Lymphoma, metastatic carcinoma, and sarcomas may be ruled out by a biopsy.

Lacrimal Gland Tumors

Most patients presented with an orbital mass and pain. A mass is frequently appreciated on examination. Biopsy can frequently be accomplished with fine needle aspiration. CT scan of the orbit should be performed to determine extent.

Graves' Ophthalmopathy

Signs and symptoms of Graves' ophthalmopathy include bilateral exophthalmia, extraocular muscle dysfunction, diplopia, blurred vision, eyelid and periorbital edema, chemosis, lid lag and retraction, and compressive optic neuropathy. Imaging with CT scan of the orbit will demonstrate changes consistent with enlargement of extraocular muscles, which are usually symmetrical.

PRIMARY AND ADJUVANT THERAPY

Eyelid Skin Cancers

In general, treatment with surgical excision is preferred. Surgical treatment may depend on the skill of the reconstructive surgeon. A large report of patients treated with Mohs surgery for basal cell cancer revealed a 0% recurrence following treatment for a newly diagnosed basal cell cancer, with a 7% recurrence for those treated with recurrent basal cell cancer.[55] Another report for patients with squamous cell cancer demonstrated recurrence of 3% at 5 years following Mohs surgery.[56]

If surgery is not feasible because of associated functional and cosmetic problems, treatment with radiation has been very successful for patients with either histology.[57] In a series of more than 1000 patients with eyelid tumors treated with radiation, Fitzpatrick and colleagues[58] noted a 5-year local control rate of 95% (basal cell, 1009 of 1062 [95%]; squamous cell, 97 of 104 [93%]).

Ocular Melanoma

The primary therapy for posterior uveal melanomas depends on many factors. Ocular factors involved in the primary treatment modality chosen include size of the tumor, location of the tumor, the presence or absence of extraocular extension of the tumor, visual function in the involved eye, and visual function in the patient's fellow eye. Systemic factors important in management decisions include age of the patient, presence or absence of metastatic disease, and general health of the patient.

Observation without treatment is a modality used for melanomas that are small and have dormant characteristics. Patients managed by this strategy are often asymptomatic and have the lesion picked up on routine ocular examination. Another subset of patients who may be managed by observation includes elderly patients with severe systemic health problems or with short life expectancy. In these situations, the treating physician and patient must weigh the risks of treatment (loss of vision and possible tumor dissemination) against the risks of withholding treatment with growth of the tumor and subsequent increased risk of metastatic disease. The COMS found that 21% of small melanomas managed initially by observation had grown by two years with 31% having grown by 5 years.[26]

Enucleation has been the standard of care for the treatment of choroidal melanoma since the nineteenth century. Enucleation requires disinsertion of the extraocular muscles from the sclera, with removal of the entire globe with a long segment of optic nerve. It is the treatment of choice for very large tumors, for eyes that are blind and/or painful, or where the tumor has invaded or is contiguous with the optic nerve. An increase in death rate at 2 years following enucleation has been reported, supporting the proposal that enucleation may help to disseminate tumor cells (Zimmerman-McLean hypothesis), but this remains controversial with no strong evidence to support its validity.[59] Although all eyes with uveal melanoma can be treated by enucleation, the obvious morbidity of immediate and permanent loss of the eye and of vision prompted the development of other techniques to treat these neoplasms.

Photocoagulation, transpupillary thermotherapy, and local resection have been used for treating selected patients.[60] Transpupillary thermotherapy is probably the most common management for small melanomas and has produced excellent control in selected patients. Local resection is most appropriate for anterior tumors involving the ciliary body. Appropri-

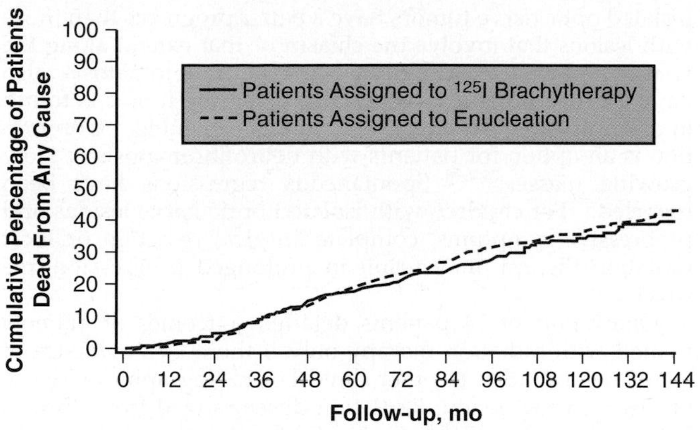

Figure 28-4 Cumulative proportion of patients who died by time after enrollment. The *red dashed line* indicates patients treated with primary enucleation, and the *solid blue line* represents patients treated by brachytherapy with ^{125}I plaques.

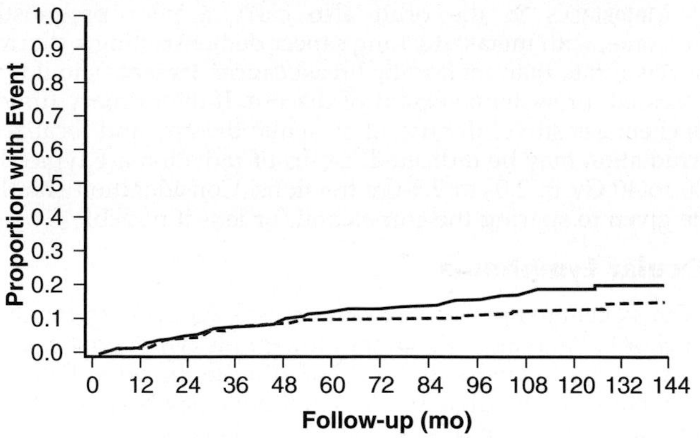

Figure 28-5 Cumulative proportion of all patients undergoing enucleation *(solid blue line)* and those with only local treatment failure *(dashed red line)* after ^{125}I brachytherapy.

ate use of these techniques in the treatment of choroidal melanomas remains investigational.

Radiation therapy in the management of uveal melanomas has revolutionized the treatment of this ocular malignancy. The principal advantage of radiation in the management of these tumors is that the globe is spared, salvaging the eye and useful vision in many patients. Two main modalities of treatment are used: episcleral plaque radiotherapy and charged particle therapy. In episcleral plaque therapy, tumors up to 18 mm in diameter and 8 to 10 mm thick may be treated, whereas with charged particle therapy tumors up to 24 mm in diameter and 12 mm in height have been treated.

A randomized multicenter trial (COMS) enrolled 1317 patients with medium-size melanomas to treatment with enucleation or with brachytherapy with ^{125}I plaques. This study demonstrated equivalent 5-year overall survival rates of 81% in both arms (Fig. 28-4).[24] Visual acuity was found to decrease over time in a proportion of eyes treated with brachytherapy. Vision was 20/200 or worse in 43% of eyes. The risk of vision loss was associated with a history of diabetes, thick tumors, tumors close to or beneath the macula, tumors with secondary retinal detachments, and tumors that were not dome shaped. Five years after plaque therapy, enucleation was necessary in 10% of patients because of tumor growth and in 3% of patients secondary to complications such as radiation-induced ischemia.[61] Complications leading to enucleation increased over time and consisted mainly of pain and/or loss of visual acuity[62] (Fig. 28-5).

Charged particle radiotherapy is a more uncommon technique for treating uveal melanoma. With this technique, tantalum rings are sutured to the external sclera at the margins of the tumor for localization, and charged particles (either protons or helium ions) are delivered in four or five equivalent fractions over a 7-day period. The standard target dose is 50 to 70 Gy. An advantage of charged particle therapy is the relatively uniform dose of radiation delivered to the entire tumor and the sharp reduction in dose outside the treated area.[62] The treatment algorithm is given in Figure 28-6.

Newer techniques like stereotactic radiosurgery and gamma knife radiotherapy are being used at some centers. However, no long-term data are available on efficacy or complication rates.

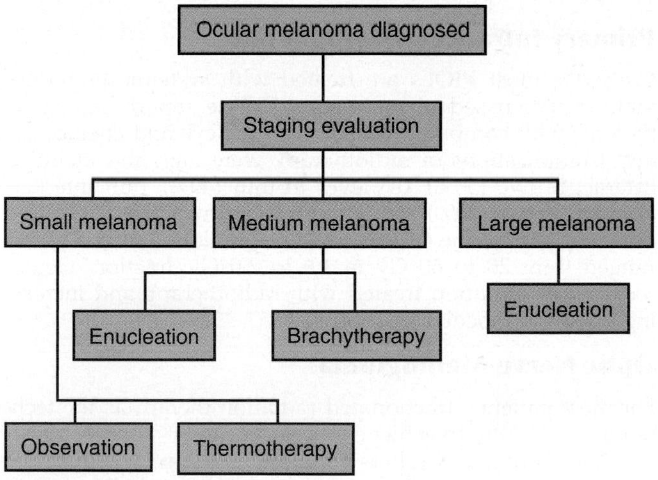

Figure 28-6 Treatment algorithm for ocular melanoma.

Ocular Metastasis

Choroidal metastases are very sensitive to radiation treatment, but overall survival is poor. In one study, external beam radiotherapy was used in 137 patients with uveal metastasis (52%), providing tumor control in 116 patients (85%) at a mean follow-up of 21 months. Using Kaplan-Meier estimates, survival rates of all patients with uveal metastasis from breast cancer was 65% at 1-year, 34% at 3-year, and 24% at 5-year follow-up.[45]

In 1994, a prospective study of the German Cancer Society was initiated to examine the results of a standardized radiation therapy for choroidal metastases with 40 Gy in 20 fractions.[63] With a median follow-up of 5.8 months (1 to 44 months), 41 of 50 patients were dead. The median survival of all patients was 7 months, and for patients with breast cancer, 10 months. Of the 50 symptomatic eyes, visual acuity increased two or more lines in 36% (18 of 50 eyes), was stabilized in 50% (25 of 50 eyes), and decreased in 14% (7 of 50 eyes). No patient with asymptomatic metastasis (n = 15 eyes) developed ocular symptoms during follow-up. No patient with unilateral tumor and unilateral irradiation developed contralateral metastasis. Severe side effects, possibly related to tumor progression, occurred in three eyes (5%).

Metastases to the orbit also carry a poor prognostic outcome, with metastatic lung cancer demonstrating a shorter survival rate than metastatic breast cancer. Patients should be assessed for systemic extent of disease. If the primary tumor is chemosensitive, the use of systemic therapy and localized irradiation may be indicated. Doses of radiation are typically 30 to 40 Gy in 2.0- to 2.5-Gy fractions. Consideration should be given to sparing the cornea and/or lens if possible.

Ocular Lymphoma

With systemic disease, chemotherapy is the primary therapy of choice. Patients with solitary low-grade lymphoma can be successfully treated with local radiation to the orbit. Patients who have intermediate-grade lymphoma may best be treated with a combination of systemic chemotherapy and radiation. Radiation should be considered if response of disease in the orbit is not complete. Doses to the orbit or conjunctiva range from 20 to 36 Gy in 10 to 18 fractions in most series, with 89% to 100% local control rates. Complications were thought to be acceptable with these doses.[64-67] Cataract formation was common without lens shielding.[64]

Primary Intraocular Lymphoma

Currently, most PIOLs are treated with systemic high-dose methotrexate-based chemotherapy.[68] One report treated 10 patients with combined radiation to the eye and chemotherapy. Complications of radiotherapy were high and included cataract in five (50%), dry eyes in four (40%), punctate keratopathy in two (20%), radiation retinopathy in two (20%), and optic atrophy in one (10%).[69] Doses of radiation in this report ranged from 20 to 60 Gy in 1.6 to 2.0 Gy/fraction. Ocular recurrences are often treated with radiotherapy and increasingly with intraocular methotrexate.

Optic Nerve Meningioma

For most patients, fractionated radiation therapy is the technique most likely to achieve long-term preservation of visual function. Turbin and others[50] studied 59 patients with visual loss at presentation. These patients were divided into four groups: observation, surgery, radiation, or surgery and radiation. Only the group treated with radiation alone did not have significant visual loss at the time of follow-up. Other series with shorter durations of follow-up have reported stable or improved vision in the majority of patients treated with more modern radiation delivery techniques.[70-73] More precise delivery of radiation to smaller volumes of tissue will reduce the amount of normal tissue exposed to radiation. These techniques involve better immobilization for reproducibility of treatment, CT treatment planning for better tumor localization, and conformal beam arrangements for optimizing treatment planning.

Treatment is usually initiated as soon as a decline in visual acuity or fields is documented. Tumor enlargement on scan even without loss of vision may provide an indication for radiotherapy. It is advised to treat these lesions with tight margins. Dose per fraction should be no more than 1.8 Gy with total doses of 50 to 54 Gy.[74] Complications can include radiation retinopathy, optic neuropathy, cataract formation, or dry eye depending on the volume of normal tissue and dose gradients. Some authors have expressed concerns when treating a patient with diabetes because of potential vascular complications associated with radiation.

Optic Nerve Glioma

Treatment options should be considered not only to improve survival but also to stabilize visual function. Children with isolated optic nerve tumors have a better prognosis than those with lesions that involve the chiasm or that extend along the visual pathway.[75-77] Children with neurofibromatosis also have a better prognosis, especially when the tumor is found in asymptomatic patients at the time of screening.[75] Observation is an option for patients with neurofibromatosis or slow growing masses.[75,76,78] Spontaneous regressions have been reported.[79] For children with isolated optic nerve lesions and progressive symptoms, complete surgical resection or local radiation therapy may result in prolonged progression-free survival.[75]

One report of 24 patients detailed outcomes of patients treated with radiation therapy only if there was evidence of visual deterioration or other clinical or radiographic evidence of disease progression. Radiation doses ranged from 4500 to 5660 cGy (median, 5400 cGy) in 1.8 Gy/fraction with up to a 17-year follow-up period (median, 6 years). The 6-year actuarial freedom from disease progression and overall 6-year survival are 88% and 100%, respectively. Visual improvement or stabilization was seen in 21 (91%) patients after radiation. A high incidence of endocrine abnormalities is reported, with 15 of the 18 patients evaluated after treatment showing growth hormone deficiency.[80] Treatment with chemotherapy has been used in order to avoid surgery or radiation. One study treated 50 patients with progressive gliomas with carboplatin on a phase II POG study. Objective responses were found in 30% of patients.[81]

Orbital Pseudotumor

Treatment for this condition is usually recommended because of clinical symptoms and decreased visual function. Nonradiotherapeutic options include the use of steroids with recommended doses of 60 to 100 mg of daily prednisone for at least 1 week. Surgical treatment has included local resection or orbital decompression. Finally, immunosuppressive therapy with Cytoxan, Imuran, or methotrexate has been advocated for aggressive or refractory lesions. These lesions have also been demonstrated to be radioresponsive. Radiation is typically used for patients who fail to respond to medical management, patients who are intolerant of steroids, or those who have a rapidly aggressive course.

The radiation treatment technique varies based on the anatomic extent of the lesion. Orbital imaging is important to verify the extent of the lesion. Typical presentations include unilateral or bilateral anterior pseudotumor, or unilateral or bilateral retrobulbar disease. Patients with anterior lesions may be treated with an anterior direct electron beam that includes the lesion with a margin that is determined by the beam penumbra. Central lens shielding may be accomplished with either a lead-mounted contact lens or a hanging lens block. Low-energy electrons have significant skin sparing and bolus may be necessary to increase the surface dose.

Patients with unilateral retrobulbar lesions are usually treated with a photon wedged-pair technique. Donaldson and colleagues[82] suggested treatment with a central eye bar to shield the lens in each field. However, low-dose regions in the retrobulbar area do result from this technique. Bilateral retrobulbar lesions are treated with opposed lateral fields with a half beam block used to spare the anterior segment of the eye if it is uninvolved (Fig. 28-7).

Total doses are typically 20 Gy delivered in 2-Gy fractions. One report of nine patients treated with initial total doses of 3 Gy noted that five of these patients required further irradiation for durable control of orbital disease.[83] Local control rates range from 74% to 100% for doses of 380 to 3600 cGy.[51,82-84]

Lacrimal Gland Tumors

Primary therapy is surgical resection with adjuvant radiation as needed for close surgical margins, perineural invasion, or adenoid cystic histology. Even with aggressive treatment, local recurrence was high following surgery and radiation for adenoid cystic histology.[85]

Graves' Disease

Peterson and others[86] reported results in 311 patients treated with orbital irradiation, with 80% showing improvement of soft-tissue symptoms; 75% showing improvement in corneal signs; 61% and 52% having improved extraocular dysfunction and proptosis, and 41% to 71% having improved visual acuity. After irradiation, 76% were able to discontinue corticosteroid therapy.

A randomized controlled double-blinded trial treated 42 patients with EBRT to one eye and sham therapy to the other eye.[87] Six months later, the therapies were reversed. There was no apparent benefit for the orbit that received initial radiation. This study has been criticized because the patient characteristic included patients who had onset of symptoms ranging from 0.2 years up to 16 years' duration and may have included patients who had a more fibrotic reaction that would have been more stable compared with an inflammatory process.

A more recent controlled trial randomized 44 patients to orbital irradiation and 44 to sham irradiation. After 12 months, 52% of irradiated patients had improvement compared with 27% of sham-irradiated patients.[88]

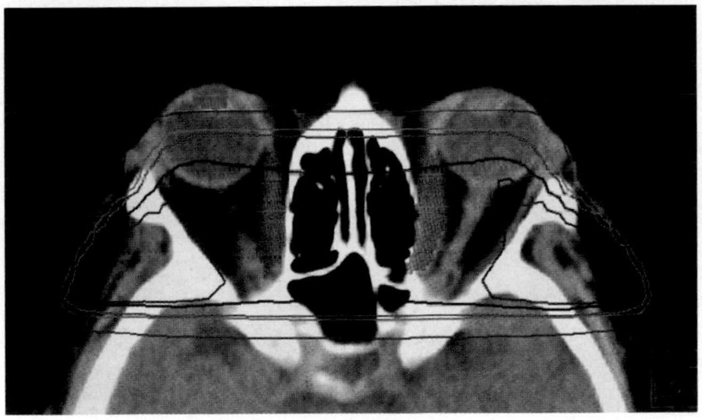

Figure 28-7 Bilateral treatment plan for Graves' disease.

Long-term follow-up suggests that orbital irradiation is safe, with a similar incidence of cataract formation to the corticosteroid group but with a possibly increased risk of retinopathy for diabetic patients.[89] Orbital radiation is typically used in the setting of symptomatic Graves' ophthalmopathy that is difficult to control with steroids, for patients with poor tolerance to steroids, or for patients for whom surgical orbital decompression has failed.

Pterygia

Treatment for these lesions involves surgical excision with removal of the fibrous tissue down to the level of Tenon's capsule. Free conjunctival flaps may be grafted over the bare sclera. Recurrence rates have varied between 20% and 68% with surgery alone.[90-92] Postoperative adjuvant therapy with radiation, topical thiotepa, mitomycin-C, or other antimetabolic agents may diminish the chance of recurrence.

Multiple retrospective studies have been published that used radiation with beta emitters started within 24 hours of surgery (Table 28-2). Doses range from 10 to 60 Gy given in one to six fractions.[93-97] There does not appear to be a dose-response curve. Recurrence rates are more common for pterygia, which are recurrent after initial surgery. Complication rates are low, but instances of scleral necrosis, cataract induction, corneal thinning, symblepharon, cataract, and corneal ulceration have been described. These are much more common in patients who have been reirradiated.[97] Treatment of multiple fields with possible dose overlap may be responsible for some of these complications as well.[97]

A randomized trial treated 96 patients with a single dose of 2500 cGy using ^{90}Sr ophthalmic applicator or sham radiation within 24 hours of surgery. Crude control rates of 93% versus 33% were observed and no serious complications were observed.[98]

Macular Degeneration

Effective therapeutic management is lacking for these patients. In the 1990s, there was increasing interest in investigating the effects of ionizing radiation, which has the potential to destroy vascular tissue and prevent neovascularization. The rationale for using local irradiation for choroidal neovascular membrane is based on the radiosensitivity of proliferating endothelial cells, reduction in the inflammatory response, and possible occlusion of aberrant vessels.

Various dose schedules have been given ranging from 10 to 24 Gy, with fractionation of 200 to 400 cGy. Several small

Table 28-2 Radiation Treatment Following Resection of Pterygia

Author, Year	No. of Patients	Recurrence (%)	Dose/No. of Fractions
Monteiro-Grillo et al, 2000[93]	94 Primary 63 Recurrent	5.4 19	30 Gy/3 or 60 Gy/6
[94]Nishimura Y, 2000	490	11.8	50 Gy/4-5
Paryani et al, 1994[95]	149 Recurrent 500 New	 1.7	 60 Gy/6
Wilder et al, 1992[96]	258	12	24 Gy/3
Dusenbery et al, 1992[97]	36	29	24 Gy/2-4
Jurgenliemk-Schulz et al, 2004[98]	86	7	25 Gy/1

series suggested stabilization of vision and even improvement in vision. However, follow-up times were short.

Other studies do not have such optimistic results. A prospective trial on 95 eyes treated with 10 to 36 Gy did not reveal an effect of dose, and decrease in visual acuity was not prevented.[99] Another group compared a historical group of patients treated with interferon with those who had been treated with radiation therapy. Radiation did not prevent vision loss.[100] Another report of 69 patients followed for at least 1 year who received 16 Gy in eight fractions failed to show any influence on vision or reading ability.[101] A randomized controlled trial from the Netherlands treated 34 patients with 24 Gy in four fractions compared with a control group. The time until vision decreased by at least three lines was prolonged.[102] A large prospective multicenter trial from Germany randomly assigned 205 patients to treatment or observation. Radiation did not prevent visual loss in this trial.[103] At this time, there is little information that justifies treatment of AMD outside of a clinical study.

LOCALLY ADVANCED DISEASE AND PALLIATION

Ocular Melanoma

Patients with large choroidal melanoma are usually treated with enucleation. The COMS enrolled 1003 patients to a study that randomized them to either enucleation or enucleation preceded by external beam radiation (20 Gy).[25] Patients receiving preoperative radiation had no significant difference in 5-year survival. The 5-year all-cause mortality rate for large melanomas was 40%. There was no difference in local control between the two groups.

Orbital Lymphoma

Radiation to the orbit can provide effective palliation for patients with widespread systemic disease or locally advanced disease. Even in patients who have received prior irradiation, local disease progression that is resulting in progressive visual loss or symptoms can be considered.

TECHNIQUES OF IRRADIATION

Plaque Irradiation

Multiple different isotopes have been used for plaque therapy, including cobalt 60, gold 198, palladium 103, ruthenium 106, iodine 125, and iridium 192. The largest experience is with iodine 125. This isotope carries the advantage of low-energy gamma rays and therefore decreased shielding and dose to distant structures. Ruthenium 106 is a beta emitter that has few shielding concerns, but it has a penetration of only a short distance, which may limit its application.

A variety of plaque applicators have been used for ocular melanomas, but the most common ones used are the ones developed for the COMS (Fig. 28-8). This plaque allows shielding of the posterior and lateral structures with a gold shield. A plaque that allows at least a 2-mm margin circumferentially around the tumor should be selected. Placement of the seeds within the applicator varies depending on the height of the tumor. The prescription point should be the apex of the tumor or 5 mm, whichever is greater. A scleral thickness of 1 mm is added to the apical height. In the COMS, a total dose of 85 Gy was used and delivered to the apex of the tumor at a dose rate between 0.5 and 1.25 Gy/hr.

The plaque is placed by the ophthalmologist by marking the boundary of the tumor base with a surgical marking pencil or light cautery that can be seen when the tumor is transilluminated (Fig. 28-9). The plaque is then centered over the marks. Plaque placement may require detachment of the recti muscles. The plaque is then sutured to the sclera (Fig. 28-10). Good placement can be confirmed with ultrasonic evaluation of the eye. Occasionally, the melanoma is located adjacent to the optic nerve. The use of a notched plaque may allow better dosimetry and coverage of the tumor in this situation.

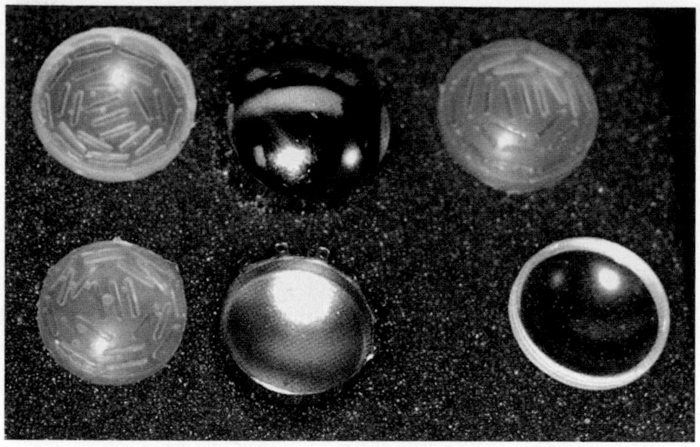

Figure 28-8 The plaque applicator was developed for the Collaborative Ocular Melanoma Study.

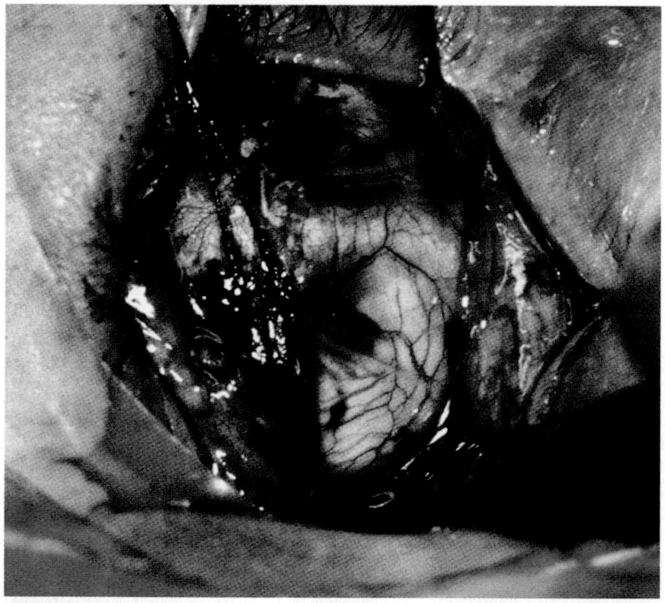

Figure 28-9 The ophthalmologist uses a surgical marking pen on the sclera, and the plaque is then centered over the marks.

Principal complications of radiotherapy to the eye include cataract, radiation retinopathy, and optic neuropathy. Radiation effects on the retina and optic nerve can be potentiated by the presence of systemic vascular diseases like hypertension and diabetes mellitus and often result in loss of useful vision. The proximity of the tumor to critical visual structures like the optic nerve and macula is predictive of long-term visual prognosis.

Skin

Treatment of skin lesions close to the eye can be difficult. The close proximity of normal structures must be balanced with

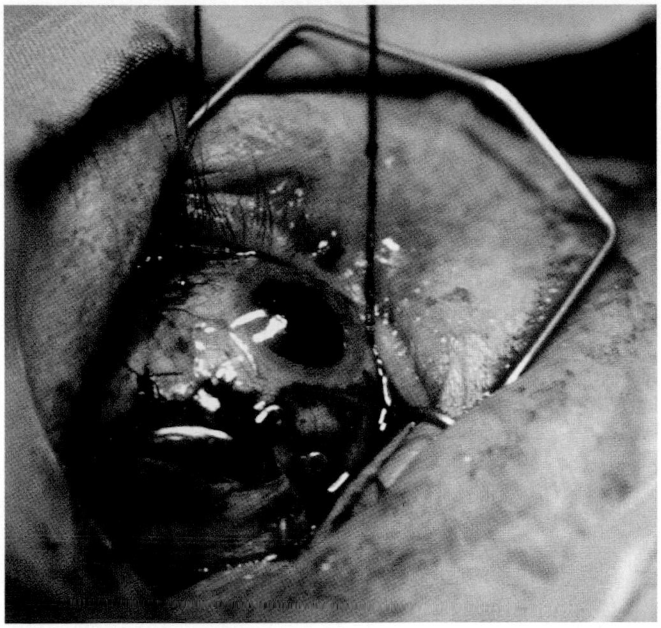

Figure 28-10 The plaque is sutured to the sclera.

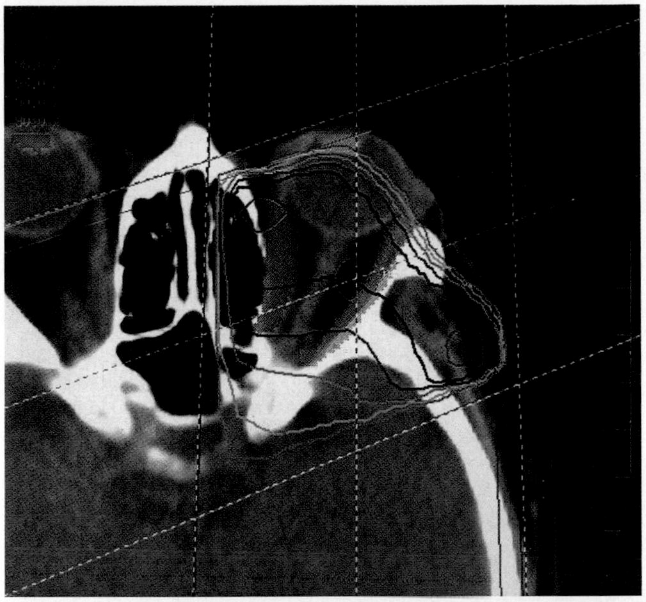

Figure 28-11 Unilateral orbit treatment plan.

the dosimetric constraints that are present with electrons. Most of the data supporting the use of radiation therapy came from series using kilovoltage x-ray beams. However, this type of x-ray equipment is no longer widely available. Electrons have a larger penumbra and area of beam constriction laterally, necessitating larger treatment fields than kilovoltage. One report demonstrated higher corneal doses with electrons compared with kilovoltage (doses were 2 to 4 times higher).[118] Also, the 95% isodose area was 32% wider with kilovoltage than with 6-MeV electrons.[118] Tungsten eye shields may provide better shielding of anterior eye structures than lead for 9-MeV electrons.[119]

After the patient is immobilized, the tumor volume should be outlined followed by design of the treatment field based on margin felt necessary to encompass the tumor, beam penumbra, and setup uncertainties. Depth of treatment should be determined with attention to perineural invasion, location near an embryologic fusion plane, and size of the lesion.

Unilateral

Treatment of one eye may be necessary for patients with choroidal or orbital metastasis or orbital lymphomas. This field arrangement is designed to limit the radiation to the opposite eye. Typically, a wedged pair technique is used if the entire orbit needs to be treated. CT planning can assist with location of the normal optic structures and the tumor volume that is to be included in the field (Fig. 28-11). Three-dimensional treatment planning may enable more treatment conformity around the structure to be treated and decrease normal tissue sequelae.

Bilateral

Treatment of both eyes is usually done with opposed lateral fields. If it is possible to spare the lens, the central axis of the beam can be placed at the location of the lens (5 mm behind the anterior globe). A split beam technique is used to block the anterior structures if possible. Treatment of Graves' disease, bilateral choroidal metastasis, and bilateral lymphomas are treated in this manner (see Fig. 28-7).

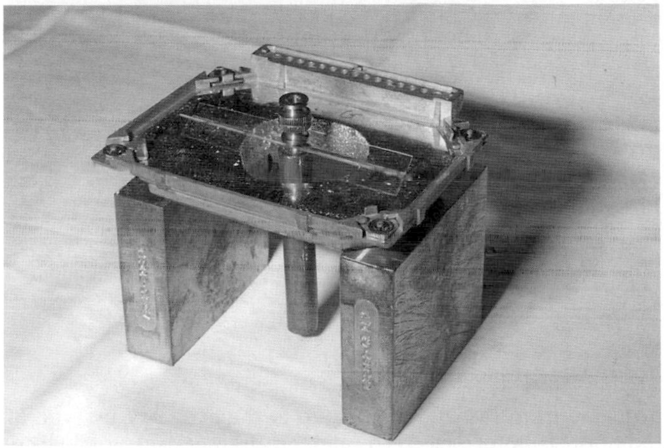

Figure 28-12 Apparatus used for the hanging block technique.

Anterior

Involvement of the conjunctiva may require treatment to the anterior structures alone. This can be accomplished with electron fields directed en face to the globe. Central lens shielding can be accomplished with a hanging block at which the patient is instructed to look (Fig. 28-12). En face electrons can be used with a lead contact lens if electrons not more than 6 meV are used[118] (Fig. 28-13).

Intensity-Modulated Radiation Therapy

Techniques using three-dimensional treatment planning and intensity-modulated radiation therapy may be advantageous for treating optic nerve meningiomas or gliomas. All critical structures of the eye should identified and appropriate dose constraints applied. Patient immobilization is crucial along with CT simulation (Fig. 28-14).

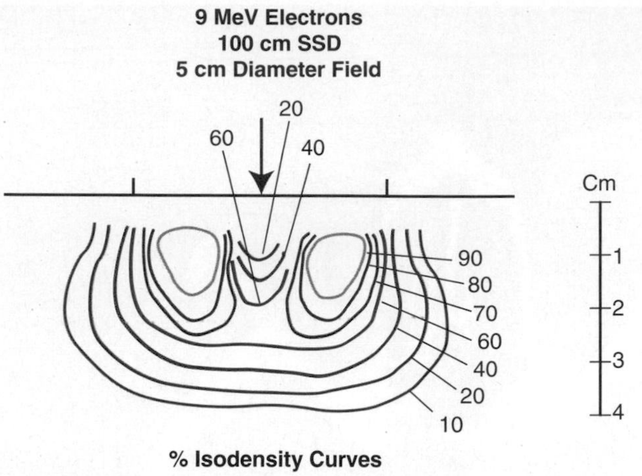

Figure 28-13 Electron cloud generated with the contact lens technique.

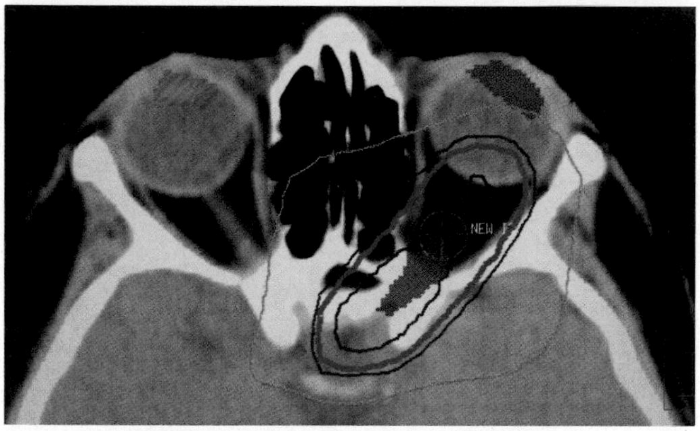

Figure 28-14 Unilateral treatment plan for an optic meningioma.

Tolerance Issues

Sequelae from radiation exposure to the eye vary by type of radiation (photon, electron, and brachytherapy), total dose, radiation fraction size, and part of the eye included in the radiation exposure. Unrelated medical conditions such as diabetes, hypertension, and collagen vascular diseases can affect the radiation tolerance of structures in the eye. Systemic chemotherapy or steroids can enhance radiation toxicity or contribute to additional symptoms.

The most sensitive structure in the eye is the lens, which is located directly behind the pupil. The germinal layer of the lens is located at the equator and is the layer most sensitive to irradiation. These cells undergo mitotic division, elongate, lose their nuclei, and migrate posteriorly to the center of the lens. This posterior migration and proliferation of the lens epithelial cells reduce lens clarity, causing a cataract, and often some degree of visual loss. Therefore, a radiation cataract usually presents first as a posterior subcapsular opacification. The latency and frequency of lens opacities are a function of radiation dose.

In most human studies, total fractionated doses under 500 cGy have not produced visually significant lens opacities. Merriam and Focht[106] reported cataract formation using fractionated radiation doses of 150 to 200 cGy to a total dose of 1200 cGy. When single-dose total-body irradiation was used, cataracts developed in 80% of survivors; the incidence decreased to 20% when fractionated irradiation was given to a total dose of 1300 cGy.[107] Reduction of dose to the lens may be possible with customized lens shields, pencil beam lead blocks, or more complex treatment planning with intensity-modulated radiation therapy. Lens extraction for cataract development can correct the vision in an otherwise functioning eye following radiation.

Other anterior structures in the globe include the cornea and conjunctiva. The conjunctiva is a mucous membrane of nonkeratinized squamous epithelium with goblet cells overlying a thin substantia propria.[108] It covers the inner surface of the eyelid and outer surface of the eye, extending to the peripheral cornea. The cornea is composed of nonkeratinized stratified squamous epithelium. Its outermost surface is composed of irregular microvilli made optically smooth by the precorneal tear film. The basal cells are attached to Bowman's layer, which is made up of randomly dispersed collagen fibrils that may become opacified by scar tissue. The stroma, which makes up 90% of the total corneal thickness, is composed of fibroblasts and collagen lamellae.

Acute effects of fractionated radiotherapy include injection and erythema of the conjunctiva with irritation that is usually self-limited. Fractionated doses of radiation to a total dose above 40 to 50 Gy to the cornea can produce edema with punctate keratitis.[109] Management consists of aggressive lubrication, patching, and antibiotic drops. Recurrent corneal erosions may progress to ulceration and infection leading to either opacification or perforation. Ulcerations of the cornea have been reported with fractionated radiation to doses above 40 Gy.[64,109] Similarly, ulceration, telangiectasias, and keratinization can develop in the conjunctiva.

The eyelid skin is the thinnest in the body. The lids contain sebaceous, serous, and apocrine glands, which contribute to the tear film. There are puncta on the medial lid margins that form the opening to the nasolacrimal drainage system. Transient effects of eyelash loss and erythema occur at 30 to 40 Gy with conventional fractionation, while permanent lash loss occurs at doses above 50 Gy.[111] Scarring and fibrosis can develop at doses above 50 Gy, which can result in ectropion or entropion of the lid as well as stenosis of the eyelid puncta.

There are several structures necessary for adequate tear film production, which include the lacrimal gland, goblet cells, meibomian glands, and accessory lacrimal glands. Dry eye syndrome can result from injury to any component of the tear film. Symptoms include burning, decreased vision, excessive tearing, and a foreign body sensation. Examination reveals corneal changes ranging from keratitis to corneal scarring and opacification. One report described 19% of patients who received doses less than or equal to 45 Gy in 25 fractions developing a dry eye syndrome compared with 100% for doses above or equal to 57 Gy in 30 fractions.[112] Severe keratitis sicca can lead to corneal ulceration and perforation of the globe. Prevention of lacrimal damage requires consideration of the location of the lacrimal gland when designing fields for radiation delivery.[113]

The sclera covers the posterior 80% of the globe. It is largely avascular and consists of collagen fibrils, fibroblast, and ground substance. It is very resistant to radiation and can withstand doses over 150 Gy that are delivered with plaque radiotherapy used to treat choroidal melanomas. Scleral thinning and ulceration are unusual complications of high doses of radiation.[114]

The retina consists of an extensive network of neural, glial, and vascular elements. The blood supply to the outer layers of the retina is via the choriocapillaries. The inner retinal layers are supplied by the branches of the central retinal artery, of which the largest branches are the temporal and nasal arcades. Pathology involving the region within the temporal arcades is more visually significant than that occurring elsewhere. Radiation retinopathy is caused by occlusive microangiopathy manifest by cotton wool spots, microaneurysms, telangiectasias, hemorrhages, macular edema, exudates, neovascularization, vitreous hemorrhage, and pigment changes. Visual symptoms secondary to radiation retinopathy depend on the area of the retina that is affected. A history of diabetes, collagen vascular disease, hypertension, and treatment with chemotherapy predisposes patients to radiation-induced injury.[115] In one report, radiation retinopathy was not observed at doses below 45 Gy in 25 fractions but increased steadily above this dose.[115] (Patients also seemed to be at increased risk if they were treated with doses per fraction greater than or equal to 1.9 Gy.[115]) The estimated tolerance for retinal damage is very steep with a tolerance dose of 5% risk at 5 years (TD 5/5) of 45 Gy and TD 50/5 of 65 Gy.[116]

Optic nerve injury occurs secondary to ischemia. Damage begins with perivascular lymphocyte cuffing, loss of endothelial cells, hyalinization, with fibrosis, thrombosis, and infarction of neural tissue. Optic nerve injury presents with painless monocular loss of vision. Fractionation is quite important in the development of optic nerve injury. Of patients who were treated to a total dose of 45 to 50 Gy and received a daily fraction size of more than 250 cGy, 18% developed visually significant changes, while those patients who received fractions below 250 cGy did not develop optic neuropathy.[117] Stereotactic radiosurgery that delivers large fraction sizes can cause optic neuropathy with single doses of 800 cGy, although tiny volumes to high doses have been given without toxicity.[118] With conventional fractionation, the TD 5/5 of the optic nerve is considered to be 60 Gy.[119]

TREATMENT ALGORITHM, CONCLUSIONS AND FUTURE POSSIBILITIES

The COMS has made a significant contribution in the understanding and the treatment of choroidal melanoma, which is the most common primary intraocular malignancy. Future investigations may shed light on the role of charged particle therapy and optimize patient selection for additional therapy. By understanding and incorporating ocular anatomy and physiology with more directed treatment techniques, a better therapeutic ratio may be expected with the use of radiation for patients with ocular pathology. Finally, advances in molecular biology and immunohistochemistry may lead to better insight into disease processes and patient selection for treatment.

REFERENCES

1. American Cancer Society: Cancer Facts and Figures. Atlanta, American Cancer Society, 2002.
2. Singh AD, Topham A: Incidence of uveal melanoma in the United States: 1973. Ophthalmology 110:956, 2003.
3. Egan KM, Seddon JM, Glynn RJ, et al: Epidemiologic aspects of uveal melanoma. Surv Ophthalmol 32:239, 1988.
4. Iskovitch J, Ackerman C, Andrew H, et al: An epidemiologic study of posterior uveal melanomas in Israel, 1961. Int J Cancer 61:291, 1995.
5. Seddon JM, Gragoudas ES, Glynn RJ, et al: Hot factors, UV radiation, and risk of uveal melanoma: a case-controlled study. Arch Ophthalmol 108:1274-1280, 1990.
6. Tucker MA, Shields JS, Hartge P, et al: Sunlight exposure as a risk factor for intraocular melanoma. N Engl J Med 313:789, 1985.
7. Singh AD, De Potter Patrick, Fijal BA, et al: Lifetime prevalence of uveal melanoma in white patients with oculo(dermal) melanocytosis. Ophthalmology 105:195, 1998.
8. Spencer WH: Primary neoplasms of the optic nerve and its sheaths: clinical features and current concepts of pathogenetic mechanisms. Trans Am Ophthalmol Soc 70:490, 1972.
9. Dutton JJ: Optic nerve gliomas and meningiomas. Neurol Clin 1:163, 1991.
10. Hollander MD, FitzPatrick M, O'Connor SG, et al: Optic gliomas. Radiol Clin North Am 37:59, 1999.
11. Walker D: Recent advances in optic nerve glioma with a focus on the young patient. Curr Opin Neurol 16:657, 2003.
12. Shields JA, Shields CL, Scartozzi R: Survey of 1264 patients with orbital tumors and simulating lesions: the 2002 Montgomery Lecture, part 1. Ophthalmology 111:997-1008, 2004.
13. Esmaeli B, Ahmadi MA, Youssef A, et al: Outcomes in patients with adenoid cystic carcinoma of the lacrimal gland. Ophthal Plast Reconstr Surg 20:22, 2004.
14. Chan CC, Buggage RR, Nussenblatt RB: Intraocular lymphoma. Curr Opin Ophthalmol 13:411, 2002.
15. Schabel M: Epidemiology of primary CNS lymphoma. J Neurooncol 43:199, 1999.
16. Shields CL, Shields JA, Gross NE, et al: Survey of 520 eyes with uveal metastases. Ophthalmology 104:1265, 1997.
17. Coroneo MT, Di Girolamo N, Wakefield D: The pathogenesis of pterygia. Curr Opin Ophthalmol 10:282, 1999.
18. Dushku N, John MK, Schultz GS, Reid TW: Pterygia pathogenesis: corneal invasion by matrix metalloproteinase expressing altered limbal epithelial basal cells. Arch Ophthalmol 119:695, 2001.
19. Mombaerts I, Goldschmeding R, Schlingemann RO, Koornneef L: What is orbital pseudotumor? Surv Ophthalmol 41:66, 1996.
20. Zobian J, Maus M: Thyroid-related ophthalmology. Curr Opin Ophthalmol 9:105, 1998.
21. Bressler NM, Bressler SB, Fine SL: Age-related macular degeneration. Surv Ophthalmol .32:375, 1998.
22. Smith BJ, O'Brien JM: The genetics of retinoblastoma and current diagnostic testing. J Pediatr Ophthalmol Strabismus 33:120, 1996.
23. Diener-West M, Hawkins BS, Markowitz JA, Schachat AP: A review of mortality from choroidal melanoma. II. A meta-analysis of 5-year mortality rates following enucleation: 1966 through 1988. Arch Ophthalmol 110:245, 1992.
24. The Collaborative Ophthalmology Study Group: The Collaborative Ocular Melanoma Study randomized trial of iodine-125 brachytherapy for choroidal melanoma, III: initial mortality findings. COMS report No. 18. Arch Ophthalmol 119:969, 2001.
25. Collaborative Ocular Melanoma Study Group: The Collaborative Ocular Melanoma Study randomized trial of pre-enucleation radiation of large choroidal melanoma, II: initial mortality findings. COMS report No. 10. Am J Ophthalmol 125:779, 1998.
26. Collaborative Ocular Melanoma Study Group: Mortality in patients with small choroidal melanoma. COMS report No. 4. Arch Ophthalmol 115:886, 1997.
27. Simon R, Durrleman S, Hoppe RT, et al: The Non-Hodgkins Lymphoma Pathologic Classification Project: long-term follow-up of 1153 patients with non-Hodgkins lymphomas, Ann Intern Med 109:939, 1988.
28. Harris N, Jaffe ES, Stein H, et al: A revised European-American classification of lymphoid neoplasms: a proposal from the International Lymphoma Study Group. Blood 84:1361, 1994.
29. Harris NL, Stein H, Coupland SE, et al: New approaches to lymphoma diagnosis. Hematology (Am Soc Hematol Educ Progr) 94:194-200, 2001.
30. Wolf LA, Reed GF, Buggage RR, et al: Vitreous cytokine levels. Ophthalmology 110:426, 2003.
31. Fujii H, Fugisada H, Kondo T, et al: Orbital Pseudotumor: Histopathological Classification and Treatment. Basel, Ophthalmologica, 1985.
32. Faustina M, Diba R, Ahmadi MA, et al: Patterns of regional and distant metastasis in patients with eyelid and periocular squamous cell carcinoma. Ophthalmology 111:1930, 2004.
33. McLean IW, Saraiva VS, Burnier MN Jr: Pathological and prognostic features of uveal melanomas. Can J Ophthalmol 39:343, 2004.

34. Singh AD, Shields CL, Shields JA: Prognostic factors in uveal melanoma. Melanoma Res 11:255, 2001.
35. The Collaborative Ocular Melanoma Study Group: Assessment of metastatic disease status at death in 435 patients with large choroidal melanoma in the Collaborative Ocular Melanoma Study (COMS). COMS report 15. Arch Ophthalmol 119:670, 2001.
36. Bessell EM, Henk JM, Wright JE, et al: Orbital and conjunctival lymphoma. treatment and prognosis. Radiother Oncol 13:237, 1988.
37. Saeed P, Rootman J, Nugent RA, et al: Optic nerve sheath meningiomas. Ophthalmology 110:2019, 2003.
38. Tellado MV, McLean IW, Specht CS, Varga J: Adenoid cystic carcinomas of the lacrimal gland in childhood and adolescence. Ophthalmology 104:1622, 1997.
39. Dutton JJ: Optic nerve gliomas and meningioma. Neurol Clin 9:163, 1991.
40. Czyzyk E, Jozwiak S, Roszkowski M, Schwartz RA: Optic pathway gliomas in children with and without neurofibromatosis. J Child Neurol 18:471, 2003.
41. Dutton JJ: Gliomas of the anterior visual pathway. Surv Ophthalmol 38:427, 1994.
42. Font RL, Simmerman, LE, Armaly MF: The nature of orange pigment over a choroidal melanoma: histochemical and microscopic observations. Arch Ophthalmol 91:359, 1974.
43. Diener-West M, Reynolds SM, Agugliaro DJ, et al: Screening for metastasis from choroidal melanoma: the Collaborative Ocular Melanoma Study Group Report 23. J Clin Oncol 22:2438, 2004.
44. The Collaborative Ocular Melanoma Study Group: Assessment of metastatic disease status at death in 435 patients with large choroidal melanoma in the Collaborative Ocular Melanoma Study (COMS). COMS report 15. Arch Ophthalmol 119:670, 2001.
45. Demirci H, Shields CL, Chao AN, Shields JA: Uveal metastasis from breast cancer in 264 patients. Am J Ophthalmol 136:264, 2003.
46. Demirci H, Shields CL, Shields JA, et al: Orbital tumors in the older adult population. J Clin Ophthalmol 109:243, 2002.
47. Carbone PP, Kaplan HS, Musshoff K: Report of the Committee on Hodgkin's Disease Staging Classification. Cancer Res 31:1860-1861, 1971.
48. Saeed P, Rootman J, Nugent RA, et al: Optic nerve sheath meningiomas. Ophthalmology 110:2019-2030, 2003.
49. Egan RA, Lessell S: A contribution to the natural history of optic nerve sheath meningiomas. Arch Ophthalmol 120:1505-1508, 2002.
50. Turbin RE, Thompson CR, Kennerdell JS, et al: A long-term visual outcome comparison in patients with optic nerve sheath meningioma managed with observation, surgery, radiotherapy, or surgery and radiotherapy. Ophthalmology 109:890, 2002.
51. Lanciano R, Fowble B, Sergott RC, et al: The results of radiotherapy for orbital pseudotumor. Int J Radiat Oncol Biol Phys 18:407, 1990.
52. Flanders AE, Mafee MF, Rao VM, et al: CT characteristics of orbital pseudotumors and other orbital inflammatory processes. J Comput Assist Tomogr 13:40, 1989.
53. Clifton AG, Borgstein RL, Moseley IF, et al: Intracranial extension of orbital pseudotumor. Clin Radiol 45:23, 1992.
54. Enzmann DR, Donaldson SS, Kriss JP: Appearance of Graves' disease on orbital computed tomography. J Comput Assist Tomogr 3:815, 1979.
55. Malhotra R, Huilgol SC, Huynh NT, Selva D: The Australian Mohs database, part II: periocular basal cell carcinoma outcome at 5-year follow-up. Ophthalmology 111:631, 2004.
56. Malhotra R, James CL, Selva D, et al: The Australian Mohs database: periocular squamous carcinoma. Ophthalmology 111:617, 2004.
57. Leshin B, Yeatts P, Anscher M, et al: Management of periocular basal cell carcinoma: Mohs' micrographic surgery versus radiotherapy. Surv Ophthalmol 38:193, 1993.
58. Fitzpatrick PJ, Thompson GA, Easterbrook WM, et al: Basal and squamous cell carcinoma of the eyelids and their treatment by radiotherapy. Int J Radiat Oncol Biol Phys 10:449, 1984.
59. Singh AD, Rennie IG, Kivela T, et al: The Zimmerman-McLean-Foster hypothesis: 25 years later. Br J Ophthalmol 88:962, 2004.
60. Augsberger JA, Damato BE, Bornfield N: Uveal melanoma. *In* Yanoff M, Duker JS (eds): Ophthalmology, 2nd ed. St. Louis, Mosby, 2004, p 1053.
61. Jampol LM, Moy CS, Murray TG, et al: The COMS Randomized Trial of Iodine 125 Brachytherapy for Choroidal Melanoma, IV. Local treatment failure and enucleation in the first 5 years after brachytherapy. COMS Report No. 19. Ophthalmology 109:2197-2206, 2002.
62. Wilson MW, Hungerford JL: Comparison of episcleral plaque and proton beam radiation therapy for the treatment of choroidal melanoma. Ophthalmology 106:1579-1587, 1999.
63. Wiegel T, Bottke D, Kreusel KM, et al. German Cancer Society: external beam radiotherapy of choroidal metastases—final results of a prospective study of the German Cancer Society (ARO 95-08). Radiother Oncol 64:13, 2002.
64. Bolek TW, Moyses HM, Marcus RB, et al: Radiotherapy in the management of orbital lymphoma. Int J Radiat Oncol Biol Phys 44:31, 1999.
65. Dunbar SF, Linggood RM, Doppke KP, et al: Conjunctival lymphoma: results and treatment with a single anterior electron field. A lens sparing approach. Int J Radiat Oncol Biol Phys 19:249, 1990.
66. Smitt MC, Donaldson SS: Radiotherapy is successful treatment for orbital lymphoma. Int J Radiat Oncol Biol Phys 26:59, 1991.
67. Letschert JGJ, Gonzales DG, et al: Results of radiotherapy in patients with stage I orbital non-Hodgkin's lymphoma. Radiother Oncol 22:36, 1991.
68. Hormigo A, DeAngelis LM: Primary ocular lymphoma: clinical features, diagnosis, and treatment. Clin Lymphoma 4:22, 2003.
69. Hoffman PM, McKelvie P, Hall AJ, et al: Intraocular lymphoma: a series of 14 patients with clinicopathological features and treatment outcomes. Eye 17:513, 2003.
70. Narayan S, Cornblath WT, Sander HM, et al: Preliminary visual outcomes after three-dimensional conformal radiation therapy for optic nerve sheath meningioma. Int J Radiat Oncol Biol Phys 56:537, 2003.
71. Andrews DW, Faroozan R, Yang BP, et al: Fractionated stereotactic radiotherapy for the treatment of optic nerve sheath meningiomas: preliminary observations of 33 optic nerves in 30 patients with historical comparison to observation with or without prior surgery. Neurosurgery 51:890, 2002.
72. Narayan S, Cornblath WT, Sandler HM, et al: Preliminary visual outcomes after three-dimensional conformal radiation therapy for optic nerve sheath meningioma. Int J Radiat Oncol Biol Phys 5:537, 2003.
73. Moyer PD Golnik KC, Breneman J: Treatment of optic nerve sheath meningioma with three-dimensional conformal radiation. Am J Ophthalmol 129:694, 2000.
74. Turbin RE, Pokorny K: Diagnosis and treatment of orbital optic nerve sheath meningioma. Cancer Control 11:334, 2004.
75. Jenkin D, Angyalfi S, Becker L, et al: Optic glioma in children: surveillance, resection, or irradiation? Int J Radiat Oncol Biol Phys 25:215, 1993.
76. Sovalic JJ, Grigsby PW, Shepard MJ, et al: Radiation therapy for gliomas of the optic nerve and chiasm. Int J Radiat Oncol Biol Phys 18:927, 1990.
77. Tao ML, Barnes PD, Billett AL, et al: Childhood optic chiasm gliomas: radiographic response following radiotherapy and long-term clinical outcome. Int J Radiat Oncol Biol Phys 39:579, 1997.
78. Packer RJ, Ater J, Allen J, et al: Carboplatin and vincristine chemotherapy for children with newly diagnosed progressive low-grade gliomas. J Neurosurg 86:747, 1997.
79. Schmandt SM, Packer RJ, Vezina LG, et al: Spontaneous regression of low-grade astrocytomas in childhood. Pediatr Neurosurg 32:132, 2000.
80. Pierce SM, Barnes PD, Loeffler JS, et al: Definitive radiation therapy in the management of symptomatic patients with optic glioma. Survival and long-term effects. Cancer 65:45, 1990.
81. Mahoney DH Jr, Cohen ME, Friedman HS, et al: Carboplatin is effective therapy for young children with progressive optic pathway tumors: a Pediatric Oncology Group phase II study. Neuro-oncology 2:213, 2000.

82. Donaldson SS, McDougall IR, Egbert PR, et al: Treatment of orbital pseudotumor by radiation therapy. Int J Radiat Oncol Biol Phys 6:79, 1980.
83. Notter M, Kern TH, Forrer A, et al: Radiotherapy of pseudotumor orbitae. Front Radiat Ther Oncol 30:180, 1997.
84. Austin Seymoour MM, Donaldson SS, Egbert PR, et al: Radiotherapy of lymphoid disease of the orbit. Int J Radiat Oncol Biol Phys 11:371, 1985.
85. Esmaeli B, Ahmadi MA, Youssef A, et al: Outcomes in patients with adenoid cystic carcinoma of the lacrimal gland. Ophthal Plast Reconstr Surg 20:22, 2004.
86. Peterson IA, Kriss JP, McDougall IR, et al: Prognostic factors in the radiotherapy of Graves' ophthalmopathy. Int J Radiat Oncol Biol Phys 19:259, 1990.
87. Gorman CA, Garrity JA, Fatourechi V, et al: A prospective randomized, double-blinded controlled study of orbital radiotherapy for Graves' ophthalmopathy. Ophthalmology 108:1523-1534, 2001.
88. Prummel MF, Terwee CB, Gerding MN, et al: A randomized controlled trial of orbital radiotherapy versus sham irradiation in patients with mild Graves' ophthalmopathy. J Clin Endocrinol Metab 89:15, 2004.
89. Wakelkamp IM, Tan H, Saeed P, et al: Orbital irradiation for Graves' ophthalmopathy: is it safe: a long-term follow-up study. Ophthalmology 111:1557, 2004.
90. Cameron ME: Pterygium Throughout the World. Springfield, IL, Charles C Thomas, 1965.
91. Bahrassa F, Datta R: Postoperative beta radiation treatment of pterygium. Int J Radiat Oncol Biol Phys 9:679, 1983.
92. Youngson RM: Recurrence of pterygium after excision. Br J Ophthalmol 56:120, 1972.
93. Monteiro-Grillo I, Gaspar L, Monteiro-Grillo M, et al: Postoperative irradiation of primary or recurrent pterygium: and sequelae. Int J Radiat Oncol Biol Phys 48:865, 2000.
94. Nishimura Y, Nakai A, Yoshimasu T, et al: Long-term results of fractionated strontium-90 radiation therapy for pterygia. Int J Radiat Oncol Biol Phys 46:137, 2000.
95. Paryani SB, Scott WP, Wells JW, et al: Management of pterygium with surgery and radiation therapy. North Florida Pterygium Study Group. Int J Radiat Oncol Biol Phys 28:101, 1994.
96. Wilder RB, Buatti JM, Kittelson JM, et al: Pterygium treated with excision and postoperative beta irradiation. Int J Radiat Oncol Biol Phys 23:533, 1992.
97. Dusenbery KE, Alul IH, Holland EJ, et al: Beta irradiation of recurrent pterygia: results and complications. Int J Radiat Oncol Biol Phys 24:315, 1992.
98. Jurgenliemk-Schulz IM, Hartman LJ, Roesink JM, et al: Prevention of pterygium recurrence by postoperative single-dose beta-irradiation: a prospective randomized clinical double-blind trial. Int J Radiat Oncol Biol Phys 59:1138, 2004.
99. Tholen AM, Meister A, Bernasconi PP, Messmer EP: Radiotherapy for choroidal neovascularization (CNV) in age-related macular degeneration (AMD). Klin Monastbl Augenheilkd 216:112, 2000.
100. Spaide RF, Guyer DR, McCormick B, et al: External beam radiation therapy for choroidal neovascularization. Ophthalmology 105.24, 1998.
101. Gripp S, Stammen J, Petersen C, et al: Radiotherapy in age-related macular degeneration. Int J Radiat Oncol Biol Phys 52:489, 2002.
102. Bergink GJ, Hoyng CB, van-der-Maazen RW, et al: A randomized controlled clinical trial on the efficacy of radiation therapy in the control of subfoveal choroidal neovascularization in age-related macular degeneration: radiation versus observation. Graefes Arch Clin Exp Ophthalmol 236:321, 1998.
103. Holz FG, Engenhart-Cabillic R, Unnebrink K, et al: A prospective, randomized, double-masked trial on radiation therapy for neovascular age-related macular degeneration. Ophthalmology 106:2239-2247, 1999.
104. Amdur RJ, Kalbaugh KJ, Ewald LM, et al: Radiation therapy for skin cancer near the eye: kilovoltage x-rays versus electrons. Int J Radiat Oncol Biol Phys 23:767, 1992.
105. Shiu AS, Tung SS, Gastorf RJ, et al: Dosimetric evaluation of lead and tungsten eye shields in electron beam treatment. Int J Radiat Oncol Biol Phys 35:599, 1996.
106. Merriam GR, Focht EF: A clinical study of radiation cataracts and the relationship to dose. AJR Am J Roentgenol 77:759, 1957.
107. Deeg HJ, Fluornoy N, Sullivan K, et al: Cataracts after TBI and marrow transplantation: a sparing effect of dose fractionation. Int J Radiat Oncol Biol Phys 10:957-964, 1984.
108. Gordon KB, Char DH, Sagerman, RH: Late effects of radiation on the eye and ocular adnexa. Int J Radiat Oncol Biol Phys 31:1123-1139, 1995.
109. Merriam GR Jr: The effects of B-irradiation on the eye. Radiology 66:240, 1956.
110. Kwok SK, Ho PC, Leung SF, et al: An analysis of the incidence and risk factors of developing severe keratopathy in eyes after megavoltage external beam radiation. Ophthalmology 105:2051, 1998.
111. Fitzpatrick PJ, Thompson GA, Easterbrook WM, et al: Basal and squamous cell carcinoma of the eyelids and their treatment by radiotherapy. Int J Radiat Oncol Biol Phys 10:449, 1984.
112. Parson JT, Bova FJ, Fitzgerald CR, et al: Severe dry-eye syndrome following external beam irradiation. Int J Radiat Oncol Biol Phys 30:775, 1994.
113. Metcalfe P, Chapman A, Arnold A, et al: Intensity-modulated radiation therapy: not a dry eye in the house. Australas Radiol 48:35, 2004.
114. Brady LW, Shields J, Augusburger J, et al: Radiation tolerance of normal tissues. Front Radiat Ther Oncol 23:238, 1989.
115. Parsons JT, Bova FJ, Fitzgeral CR, et al: Radiation retinopathy after external-beam irradiation: analysis time-dose factors. Int J Radiat Oncol Biol Phys 30:765, 1994.
116. Emami B, Lyman J, Brown A, et al: Tolerance of normal tissue to therapeutic irradiation. Int J Radiat Oncol Biol Phys 21:109, 1991.
117. Harris JR, Levene MB: Visual complications following irradiation for pituitary adenomas and craniopharyngiomas. Radiation 120:167-171, 1976.
118. Stafford SL, Pollock BE, Leavitt JA, et al: A study on the radiation tolerance of the optic nerves and chiasm after stereotactic radiosurgery. Int J Radiat Oncol Biol Phys 55:1177, 2003.
119. Parsons JT, Bova FJ, Fitzgerald CR, et al: Radiation optic neuropathy after megavoltage external-beam irradiation: analysis of time-dose factors. Int J Radiat Oncol Biol Phys 30:755, 1994.

PART B

HEAD AND NECK TUMORS

Overview

K. Kian Ang

Although representing about 4% of cancers, a variety of neoplasms with diverging natural histories arise in the relatively small body region of the head and neck, which is essential for basic physiologic functions and critical for a person's appearance, expression, and social interactions. Depending on the site, size, and pattern of spread, head and neck cancers can cause various degrees of structural deformities and functional handicaps, compromising comfort and social integration. Treatments of head and neck tumors can induce additional mutilations and malfunctions, worsening quality of life. Consequently, head and neck cancers are challenging to manage.

Knowledge of the basic principles of oncology and expertise in patient assessment and in individual specialties are essential for staging workup of patients and for proper treatment selection. Integrated interdisciplinary collaborations among surgical, radiation, medical, and dental oncologists and interactions between oncologists with pathologists, radiologists, reconstructive surgeons, nurses, and other health care personnel are essential ingredients for optimal management and rehabilitation of head and neck cancer patients. Well-functioning coordinated care is essential to yield the highest complication-free cure rate with maximal functional and cosmetic outcome. Close collaborations among radiation oncologists, dosimetrists, medical physicists, radiotherapists, and oncology nurses are important to deliver quality radiotherapy.

Laboratory research and clinical investigations have yielded important results since the publication of the first edition of Clinical Radiation Oncology. Such long-term investment in cancer research has come to fruition for certain cancers. After increasing for decades, the mortality rate from most cancers in the United States has decreased since 1975.[1] Many advances have been achieved in the understanding of the biology, natural history, and treatment of head and neck cancers.

This summary highlights a few interesting and evolving concepts and recent findings of clinical interest in the carcinogenesis, biology, and treatment of head and neck cancers. Site-specific issues are discussed in the following chapters.

MOLECULAR BIOLOGY AND ECOGENETICS

The molecular tumor progression model was initially proposed by Fearon and Vogelstein.[2] This model states that tumors progress by activation of oncogenes and inactivation of tumor suppressor genes (TSGs), each producing a growth advantage for a clonal population of cells, and that specific genetic events usually occur in a distinct order (i.e., multistep carcinogenesis) that is not necessarily the same for each tumor.

For head and neck carcinomas, Califano and associates[3] described a preliminary tumor progression model using allelic loss or imbalance as a molecular marker for oncogene amplification or TSG inactivation. They identified *CDKN2A* (formerly designated *p16*; 9p21), *TP53* (17p), and *RB1* (13q) as candidate TSGs, and *CCND1* (cyclin D1 gene; 11q13) as a candidate proto-oncogene. The results of this work support the initial observations of the colorectal molecular progression model in that clonal genetic changes occur early in the histopathologic continuum of tumor progression. About one third of histopathologically benign squamous hyperplasia already consists of a clonal population of cells with shared genetic anomalies characterizing head and neck cancer. Identification of such early events facilitates discovery of genetic alterations associated with further transformation and aggressive clinical behavior. With further validation, this knowledge will contribute greatly to the development of screening strategies, focusing on earlier steps of the estimated 10 or more genetic alterations required to generate an invasive tumor phenotype and to the conception of early pharmacologic or genetic therapy approaches.

Tobacco and alcohol exposure have long been recognized as the dominant risk factor in head and neck carcinogenesis. Although their consumption was estimated to account for approximately three fourths of oral and pharyngeal carcinomas in the United States,[4] neoplasms develop in only a small fraction of exposed individuals. This intriguing information raised the notion of the contribution of genetic susceptibility or predisposition and other cofactors (e.g., viral infection) to carcinogenesis. The potential pathways are thought to include genetic polymorphism influencing environmental carcinogen absorption and detoxification, individual sensitivity to carcinogen-induced genotypic alterations, and so on. These ideas can now be tested properly because of progress in molecular biology concepts and assay methodology. The ability to identify smokers at high risk for the development of cancer, for example, has important practical clinical implications, such as in selecting individuals for more aggressive screening programs or for enrollment in intensive chemoprevention trials (discussed later).

RECEPTOR TYROSINE KINASES

Intensive research efforts sparked by the characterization of epidermal growth factor receptor (EGFR, also known as HER1 or ERBB1) in the late 1970s generated insights into the structures and functions of *receptor tyrosine kinases* (RTKs) and their roles in the ligand-mediated signaling pathways governing proliferation, differentiation, survival, and other key cellular processes.

More than 2 decades after initial characterization of the EGFR, it is known that RTKs are highly related in structure and domain arrangements despite their unique biologic roles. This class of receptors comprises 58 members distributed among 20 subfamilies (reviewed by Gschwind and colleagues[5]). The EGFR-mediated signaling and its deregulation in pathogenesis and as the target of therapeutic intervention of human tumors have also been reviewed.[6,7] Its value as a prognostic-predictive biomarker and as a target of therapeutic intervention in head and neck carcinoma is addressed in "Biomarkers and Molecular Targeting."

Deregulation of the *RET* gene–encoded transmembrane RTK plays an important role in the pathogenesis of papillary and medullary thyroid cancer (reviewed by Santoro and coworkers[8]). The *RET* gene is located in the pericentromeric region of the short arm of chromosome 10. Alternative splicing of the *RET* product results in two protein isoforms: RET9 and RET51. *RET* is an example that a single gene can induce different types of cancer depending on the mutation. The genetic characteristics of papillary thyroid carcinomas (PTC), the most common thyroid neoplasm, are chromosomal inversions or translocations leading to several types of combinations of intracellular kinase-coding RET domain with heterologous genes, producing the *RET/PTC* chimeric oncogenes. In vitro and in vivo irradiation was found to induce the formation of a RET/PTC1[9] rearrangement, and RET/PTC rearrangements have been found in more than 60% of post-Chernobyl accident PTCs.[10] These findings contribute to the understanding of the pathogenesis of radiation-induced thyroid carcinoma.

In contrast to rearrangement observed in PTC, germline point mutations in *RET* cause three types of related dominantly inherited cancer syndromes: multiple endocrine neoplasia type 2A (MEN2A), MEN2B, and familial medullary thyroid carcinoma (FMTC).[11-13] Most *RET* mutations in MEN2A and FMTC affect cysteine in the extracellular cysteine-rich domain (i.e., codon 634 [particularly C634R] in MEN2A) or are evenly distributed among various cysteines in FMTC. Mutations in the kinase domain have also been observed. The most common mutation in MEN2B is M918T in the kinase domain. Somatic mutations of V804, M918, and E768 occur in about one half of sporadic MTC.[11-14] Functionally, RET cysteine mutants form covalent dimers leading to constitutive kinase activity, whereas the M918T mutation causes a change in the substrate specificity.[15]

VIRAL CAUSES

Nasopharyngeal carcinoma (NPC) has been an excellent model for studying viral causes of human cancer. Although the association between Epstein-Barr virus (EBV) and NPC has been recognized for about 4 decades, significant progress in this field has been made only more recently. For example, the EBV genome was characterized (reviewed by Liebowitz[16]) and found to consist of a linear, 172-kb, double-stranded DNA having five unique sequences, separated by four internal repeats along with two terminal repeats. The DNA circularizes by homologous recombination at random locations within terminal repeats in the nucleus of infected cells. The length of terminal repeat is therefore specific for each infected cell, and this is the basis for clonality assay, which may be useful in determining the putative primary tumor in patients presenting with nodal metastasis from an unknown source. The genome encodes several families of proteins, such as early antigens (EAs), EB nuclear antigens (EBNAs), and latency membrane proteins (LMPs). Many of these proteins control viral behavior and affect cell proliferation regulatory mechanisms, and they are thought to play a role in transformation and carcinogenesis and to influence tumor response to therapy. EBNA-1 regulates viral genome replication during cell division and was found to induce growth and dedifferentiation of an EBV(−) NPC cell line[17] LMP-1 seems to alter growth of epithelial cells, induce well-differentiated squamous carcinomas from human epithelial cell–line transfectants, and is associated with BCL2 expression in tumors.[18,19]

More work has been done on the molecular genetics of NPC. Many NPCs were found to have deletions of the short arm or some regions of the short arm of chromosomes 3 and 9, suggesting the possibility of the existence of TSGs in these regions.[20,21] For example, some studies[22,23] revealed that the combined frequency for chromosome 3p and 9p (bearing *CDKN2A* and *RASSF1A*) losses in the normal nasopharyngeal epithelium among southern Chinese in Hong Kong, a population at high risk for NPC, was 82.6%, compared with 20% in the low-risk populations. In contrast, latent EBV infection was detected only in high-grade nasopharyngeal dysplasia or NPC. Consequently, it was postulated that the abnormal genetic changes in chromosomes 3p and 9 predispose nasopharyngeal cells to sustain latent EBV infection, and this combination promotes a cascade of events leading to malignancy. One study revealed that in patients with nonmetastatic NPC, the plasma level of EBV DNA, particularly when assayed after completion of therapy, is a robust prognostic biomarker (see "Biomarkers and Molecular Targeting").

The causal relationship between human papillomaviruses (HPVs) and some human neoplasms has been established, particularly for carcinoma of the uterine cervix. Most cervical cancers contain integrated HPV DNA, most commonly of high-risk types HPV-16 and HPV-18.[24] Cell culture studies clearly demonstrated that the high-risk HPVs can transform and immortalize epithelial cells from the cervix, foreskin, and oral cavity.[25-27] In contrast, HPV-6 and HPV-11, associated more often with benign lesions, do not possess this capability.[28,29] Expression of *E6* and *E7* open reading frames of HPV-16 or HPV-18 genome is sufficient for immortalization.[30,31]

The potential role of HPV in head and neck carcinogenesis has attracted attention (reviewed by Herrero[32]). Carcinomas of the tonsil, oral tongue, and floor of mouth were found to have a relatively high prevalence of HPV DNA.[33-35] A high proportion of verrucous carcinomas, rare locally invasive carcinomas with papillomatous morphology, is associated with HPV.[36,37] Verrucous carcinomas of the larynx predominantly contain HPV-6, HPV-11, or HPV-16 or related DNA.[36,38] The evidence for the role of HPVs in carcinogenesis of tonsillar carcinomas is increasing because these tumors contain HPV DNA in most of the cells and express readily detectable levels of HPV RNA.[39] In a series of 253 patients, Gillison and colleagues[40] detected HPV in 25% of tumors, with HPV-16 present in 90% of the positive neoplasms. HPV presence was most common in oropharyngeal carcinoma, occurring in individuals with no history of smoking and alcohol consumption, having basaloid subtype without *TP53* mutation. Laboratory data showing that transcriptionally active, integrated HPV-16 DNA persisted in an oral carcinoma cell line having features indistinguishable from those of the primary tumor[41] provide strong evidence for an active role of HPV in carcinogenesis.

Understanding HPV infection and the mechanisms of HPV-induced malignant conversion is essential for developing strategies for preventing HPV infection and virus-associated carcinogenesis, such as blocking expression of its E6 and E7 proteins.

TREATMENT OF RELATIVELY, LOCALLY ADVANCED CANCERS

Refinement in surgical resection-reconstructive techniques and advances in radiation therapy planning and delivery technology yield good outcomes for most patients with early-stage head and neck cancers. Unfortunately, for more locally advanced cancers, the current standard therapy consisting of surgical resection and preoperative or postoperative irradiation achieves poor results in terms of disease control or preservation of organ function, or both. Consequently, there has been continuous search for better treatment approaches. This quest and the simplicity of clinical evaluation and well-characterized pattern of relapse make head and neck carcinomas ideal models for testing the relative efficacy of novel therapy concepts and modalities. For example, most clinical radiobiologic investigations have been conducted in patients with head and neck cancers.

Clinical Radiobiology: Fractionation Schedules

Radiobiologic concepts derived from more than 2 decades of integrated laboratory and clinical investigations led to the conception of two classes of new fractionation schedules for the treatment of head and neck cancers. These altered fractionation regimens are referred to as *hyperfractionation* and *accelerated fractionation* schedules. Hyperfractionation exploits the difference in fractionation sensitivity between tumors and normal tissues manifesting late morbidity. In contrast, accelerated fractionation attempts to reduce tumor proliferation as a major cause of radiation therapy failure. Although there are many permutations in accelerating radiation treatment, the existing schedules can be conceptually grouped into two categories: pure and hybrid accelerated fractionation regimens, depicting the absence and presence of concurrent changes in other fractionation parameters, respectively.

These radiobiologically sound fractionation regimens have been extensively tested in patients with intermediate and advanced head and neck carcinomas, mainly of the oropharynx. This line of clinical research is nearing conclusion. Results of the completed phase III clinical trials have been reviewed,[42,43] and the results and conclusions are briefly reviewed here.

Hyperfractionation

The clinical trial results, most notably those of the European Organization for Research on Treatment of Cancer (EORTC), show a moderate (10% to 15%) but consistent improvement in the local control of T2-3N0-1 oropharyngeal carcinomas.[44] The incidence of late toxicity with a 10% to 15% total dose increment delivered twice daily in smaller than the standard fraction sizes was within the range observed with conventional fractionation schedules, although none of the studies was designed to test equivalency of late morbidity.

Accelerated Fractionation

The trial results indicate that mucosal toxicity limits the magnitude of overall time reduction to at most 2 weeks without decreasing the total dose. With *pure accelerated* fractionation (no or minimal change in the total dose and fraction size relative to conventional schedule), delivery of 10 fractions per week (Vancouver trial[45]) induced very severe acute mucositis. Administration of continuous daily irradiation without a weekend break (Gliwice trial[46]) caused severe late effects, which were thought to be consequential.

With *hybrid accelerated* fractionation, delivery of three fractions of 1.6 Gy per day, separated by an approximate 6-hour interval, without reduction of the total dose (EORTC trial[47]) increased late complications such as soft tissue fibrosis, peripheral neuropathy, and myelopathy. Based on the repair kinetic data obtained from experimental spinal cord and skin models and from human skin, these late morbidities can be ascribed in part to the occurrence of compounding incomplete cellular repair of sublethal injury. A 12-Gy total dose reduction (as in continuous hyperfractionated, accelerated radiation therapy [CHART][48]) seemed more than sufficient to offset the compounding incomplete repair associated with the delivery of three fractions per day and thereby resulted in a lesser severity in a number of late complications, including skin telangiectasia, mucosal ulceration, and laryngeal edema. However, CHART did not improve tumor control in patients with a variety of locally advanced head and neck carcinomas. This study showed that it is possible to substitute radiation dose by overall time reduction and, thereby, provide indirect evidence for the importance of tumor clonogenic proliferation in determining local cure by radiation. Theoretically, this regimen should benefit a subset of patients with very rapidly proliferating tumors. Based on subset analyses, the investigators postulated that this subgroup might be those with T3-4, well-differentiated carcinomas of the larynx. This study warrants further analysis.

A pure accelerated fractionation regimen by delivering 6 fractions per week (Danish trial[49]) and a hybrid variant by concomitant boost (Radiation Therapy Oncology Group [RTOG] trial[50]) yielded improved local control rates of locally advanced head and neck cancers without increasing the morbidity. The Danish trial (DAHANCA 7) randomized a total of 1485 patients eligible for primary irradiation alone to receive 66 to 68 Gy in 33 to 34 fractions given in 5 or 6 fractions per week. The compliance rate to therapy regimens was high. The incidence of acute severe mucositis and dysphagia was higher in patients receiving 6 fractions per week, but there was no difference in the incidence of late edema or fibrosis. The 5-year actuarial locoregional control rates in 1476 evaluable patients were 70% and 60% for accelerated and conventional regimens, respectively (P = .0005). The benefit for acceleration resulted primarily from improvement in primary tumor control.

The RTOG randomized trial 90-03 compared the relative efficacy of three altered fractionation regimens with the standard 70 Gy in 35 fractions over 7 weeks.[50] The test radiation schedules were hyperfractionation (81.6 Gy in 68 fractions over 7 weeks, with 1.2 Gy given twice daily), split-course accelerated fractionation (67.2 Gy in 42 fractions of 1.6 Gy twice daily over 6 weeks, including a 2-week break), and concomitant boost regimen (72 Gy in 42 fractions over 6 weeks, with 1.8 Gy daily for 3.6 weeks and 1.8 Gy [large field] plus 1.5 Gy [boost field], 6 hours apart, for 2.4 weeks). Analysis of results for the 1073 patients enrolled showed that concomitant boost and hyperfractionation regimens yielded significantly higher locoregional control rates than those of standard fractionation. The split-course accelerated regimen did not improve locoregional control rates over the standard fractionation regimen. The acute mucosal reactions were more severe in patients receiving altered fractionation regimens, but there was no difference in the complication rates at 6, 12, 18, and 24 months after therapy.

Conclusions

More than 2 decades of intensive clinical investigations on altered fractionation schedules have produced conceptually interesting and clinically important findings. Trials addressing hyperfractionation show that this biologically sound regimen yields a moderate but consistent improvement in locoregional control of moderate or advanced head and neck squamous cell carcinoma, with no observed increase in late toxicity.

The results of accelerated fractionation indicate that acute mucosal toxicity limits the magnitude of overall time reduction to at most 2 weeks and that late complications resulting from compounding incomplete repair compromise delivery of 3 fractions of 1.6 Gy per day without total dose reduction. However, acceleration of radiation therapy by delivering 6 fractions per week and by concomitant boost yielded significantly improved local tumor control rates relative to standard fractionation without increasing the morbidity in the treatment of predominantly locally advanced carcinomas. These two types of regimens are conceptually similar in that radiation therapy duration is shortened by 1 week without reducing the total radiation dose or introducing an interruption.

All in all, well-organized clinical trials enrolling more than 6000 patients to test the relative efficacy of various altered fractionation regimens have generated important data. Radiobiologically, the trial results demonstrated the existence of differential fractionation sensitivity between head and neck carcinomas and late-responding normal tissues and firm evidence that tumor clonogenic proliferation is a major obstacle to curing advanced head and neck cancers with fractionated radiation therapy. Clinically, the results of these trials call for changing radiation therapy practice for the treatment of moderate or advanced head and neck carcinomas. Because the magnitudes of therapeutic gain achieved with hyperfractionation (6 fractions per week) and a concomitant boost regimen are similar, the economic and logistic considerations determine the choice of the new standard treatment. For reasons of cost, resource use, and patient convenience, many centers have adopted the relatively simple concomitant boost regimen as the standard radiation therapy for patients with intermediate-stage head and neck carcinomas and those with locally advanced cancers not eligible for protocol studies or choosing to receive irradiation alone.

The data open the challenge for conceiving creative approaches to integrate altered fractionation regimens with cytotoxic or biologic agents to further improve the therapy outcome. Several concepts have been tested or are undergoing preclinical and clinical testing.

Combination of Radiation with Chemotherapy

Sequential versus Concurrent Radiation Chemotherapy Combination

Most combined irradiation-chemotherapy regimens tested have evolved empirically by administering drugs found to have some activity against tumors of interest in a dose and time sequence known to be tolerated in a single modality therapy setting. Meta-analyses of available data of randomized trials in head and neck cancer undertaken a few years ago showed that despite a high initial response rate, multiagent chemotherapy given before radiation treatment (neoadjuvant setting) has a small impact on the locoregional control and survival rates.[51] Concurrent irradiation and chemotherapy yielded an almost 10% higher survival rate relative to irradiation alone.[52] Unfortunately, the complication rates of combined regimens are also higher than those of radiation therapy only.[52]

The Meta-Analysis of Chemotherapy on Head and Neck Cancer (MACH-NC) Collaborative Group undertook an extensive meta-analysis. The project investigators obtained updated patient data of 63 randomized trials enrolling a total of 10,741 patients. This study revealed tremendous heterogeneity in eligibility criteria and results between studies exploring chemotherapy for patients with nonmetastatic head and neck carcinoma, which made a simple conclusion on the role of chemotherapy difficult. Nonetheless, the analysis revealed a small statistically significant benefit with the addition of chemotherapy to locoregional therapy, which consists of a 4% improvement in survival at 2 and 5 years. The benefit primarily reflected the favorable effect of concurrent and alternating irradiation and chemotherapy, resulting in an 8% overall improvement in survival. However, the greatest heterogeneity was also seen in these groups. The study authors conclude that concurrent chemoradiation should remain experimental, particularly when toxicity and cost-benefit ratio are taken into account in addition to survival.[53]

Results of many published phase III trials[54-60] confirm the finding of meta-analyses that chemotherapy given concurrently with irradiation yields better locoregional control and survival rates than irradiation alone in patients with locally advanced head and neck squamous cell carcinoma (HNSCC). Two trials have also shown the benefit of concurrent irradiation and chemotherapy given in postoperative adjuvant setting.[61,62]

The combined irradiation-chemotherapy regimen most extensively tested is the combination of conventionally fractionated radiation therapy (70 Gy in 35 fractions over 7 weeks) with cisplatin. In earlier trials, cisplatin was given in a dose of 100 mg/m^2, administered during weeks 1, 4, and 7 of radiation therapy (approximately one third of patients were not able to tolerate the last dose). The systemic and mucosal toxicities of such a high-dose, intermittent cisplatin regimen are rather severe. There are four trials showing locoregional control or survival benefit of alternative cisplatin regimens, such as five doses of 20 mg/m^2 over 5 consecutive days or four doses of 25 mg/m^2 over 4 sequential days during weeks 1, 4, and 7,[63,64] weekly fixed doses of 50 mg during the 7- to 9-week course of postoperative radiation therapy,[65] or 6 mg/m^2/day for 5 days each week during the 7-week course of radiation therapy.[60]

Unfortunately, recording and reporting of the late morbidity of combined irradiation and chemotherapy have not been sufficiently consistent and systematic.[66] A thorough report of the long-term results of a French cooperative group (GORTEC) trial reveals that the late complication rate of the combination of radiation with concurrent carboplatin and fluorouracil was significantly higher than that of radiation alone.[57] Because of the lack of adequate reporting, controversy still exists about whether the late toxicity of the combination of standard irradiation with 100 mg/m^2 of cisplatin given every 3 weeks may be higher than irradiation alone. It is hoped that longer and more complete follow-up data on late morbidities will be reported in the future. Despite this uncertainty, many oncologists consider 100 mg/m^2 of cisplatin given during weeks 1, 4, and 7 of conventionally fractionated radiation therapy as the standard of care for patients with locally advanced head and neck carcinomas who are found to be medically fit to receive chemotherapy.

Principles for Optimizing Combination of Radiation with Systemic Therapy

A clear understanding of the therapy objective is essential for designing a logical combined-therapy regimen. The purpose for combining radiation and systemic therapy in the treatment of neoplastic diseases can be to eliminate hematogenous micrometastases that have occurred before initiation of locoregional therapy or to improve the probability of eradicating primary tumors and involved regional nodes. Depending on the pattern of failure, one or both objectives may be desirable in given clinical settings. The primary objective determines the choice of the agents and the timing of drug administration relative to irradiation. If the main aim is to reduce the probability of metastatic relapse, it is logical to select least toxic agents with proven antitumor activity and administer irradiation and systemic therapy sequentially, rather than concurrently, to minimize direct drug-radiation interactions that may increase normal tissue toxicity within the radiation portals. If the major purpose is to increase local tumor control, it is logical to select drugs based on mechanisms of action and administer systemic therapy concurrently with irradiation to maximize drug-radiation interactions. In the latter scenario, therapeutic benefit occurs only when the combined therapy enhances tumor response more than it increases normal-tissue toxicity.

Analysis of the data of randomized trial RTOG 90-03 on altered fractionations for locally advanced head and neck carcinomas enrolling more than 1000 patients, 60% of whom had stage IV disease, revealed that locoregional relapse is the predominant pattern of failure. Overall, the actuarial locoregional tumor recurrence rate was close to 50%, compared with less than 20% for distant metastasis.[50] Consequently, for the time being, effort should preferentially focus on developing combined therapy aiming at improving locoregional control for patients with advanced head and neck squamous cell carcinoma. The finding that concurrent irradiation and systemic therapy improved outcome but that sequential combined therapy did not improve outcome is consistent with this first principle. Such confirmation should be taken into account in the design of future trials.

Despite 3 decades of clinical research, many scientific questions related to combinations of irradiation and chemotherapy are still not answered. These include whether cisplatin has benefit when added to altered fractionation, whether newer cytotoxic agents have higher efficacy, and whether neoadjuvant chemotherapy can further improve the outcome of concurrent irradiation and chemotherapy. Factors to be taken into account in selecting agents for combination with radiation include mechanisms of drug-radiation interaction, pharmacodynamic characteristics, and clinical activity in inducing tumor response in a single-modality therapy setting. A large number of laboratory studies have been undertaken to optimize the combination of radiation with chemotherapy, particularly using newer cytotoxic and biologic agents such as taxanes, inhibitors of growth factor receptor signaling pathways, and so on.

HIGH-PRECISION RADIOTHERAPY

Advances in computerized radiation therapy planning and delivery technology offered the possibility of conforming irradiation to an irregular tumor target volume (i.e., conformal radiation therapy).[67] It is feasible to reduce radiation dose to more of the critical normal tissues surrounding the tumor without compromising dose delivery to the intended target volume, resulting in a reduction in morbidity. Reduced toxicity permits escalation of the radiation dose or combining irradiation with intensive chemotherapy, each of which has the prospect of improving head and neck squamous cell carcinoma control. Basic expertise in anatomy, imaging, and patterns of tumor spread are vital for clinical application of precision radiation therapy.

Precision radiation therapy can be accomplished by the use of an array of x-ray beams individually shaped to conform to the projection of the target, which is referred to as three-dimensional conformal radiation therapy (3D-CRT). Technology is also available to modify the intensity of the beams across the irradiated field as an added degree of freedom to enhance the capability of conforming dose distributions in three dimensions. This irradiation technique is called *intensity-modulated radiation therapy* (IMRT). A proton beam offers even a higher magnitude of normal tissue sparing, which is more desirable for the treatment of skull base neoplasms, pediatric cancers, and other tumors.

The roles of 3-D CRT and particularly IMRT in reducing morbidity and perhaps improving control of squamous cell carcinoma through radiation dose escalation are being tested in a number of medical centers. Results already reveal that it is effective in sparing parotid glands from receiving a high radiation dose and thereby diminishes radiation-induced permanent xerostomia in selected patients.[68]

Single-institution studies testing the role of IMRT in the management of NPC and oropharyngeal cancers have yielded exciting results. In patients with NPC, IMRT was given alone or, for locally advanced stages, in combination with chemotherapy consisting of concurrent cisplatin and adjuvant cisplatin plus 5-fluorouracil.[69] In a series of 67 patients with a median follow-up of 31 months, the 4-year estimates of local progression-free, locoregional progression–free, distant metastasis–free, and overall survival rates were 98%, 97%, 66%, and 88%, respectively. The worst acute toxicity was grade 1-2 in 51 (76%), grade 3 in 15 (22%), and grade 4 in 1 (2%) patients. The worst late morbidity was grade 1 in 20 (30%), grade 2 in 15 (22%), grade 3 in 7 (10%), and grade 4 in 1 (2%) patients. Xerostomia was less pronounced than after 3D-CRT and decreased with time. At 3 months after IMRT, 8% had no dry mouth, 28% had grade 1 xerostomia, and 64% had grade 2 xerostomia. Of the 41 patients evaluated at 2 years, 66% had no dry mouth, 32% had grade 1 xerostomia, and only 1 patient had grade 2 xerostomia.

In a series of 74 patients with oropharyngeal carcinoma reported by Chao and coworkers,[70] 14 received IMRT alone, 17 had IMRT combined with cisplatin-based chemotherapy, and 43 underwent surgery followed by postoperative IMRT. With a median follow-up of 33 months, the 4-year estimates of locoregional control, distant metastasis–free, disease-free survival, and overall survival rates were 87%, 90%, 81%, and 87%, respectively. Grade 1 and 2 cases of late xerostomia were reported for 32 and 9 patients, respectively. Late skin toxicity occurred in 3 (2 grade 1 and 1 grade 2), mucositis in 3 (all grade 1), and trismus in 3 patients.

Inspired by encouraging single-institution data, a number of multi-institutional trials addressing the role of IMRT in the treatment of head and neck carcinomas (e.g., RTOG trial 0022 for early-stage oropharyngeal carcinoma and trial 0225 for NPC) have been launched. The results will be available in the future.

More developments are needed to fully benefit from this sophisticated technology. Areas needing improvement to refine margins of coverage include topographic and biologic tumor imaging to better define target volumes and quantification of day-to-day anatomic variations occurring during the course of radiation therapy due to motion and changes in tumor and normal tissue volume.

Although results of IMRT and particle therapy are encouraging, the observation that most recurrences originated from the high-dose region indicates that radiation dose escalation alone will improve outcome only for a subset of patients. Further advances in the treatment of solid tumors will likely come through application of newer knowledge about tumor biology, as exemplified by translational research addressing the role of epidermal growth factor receptor in tumor progression and as a target for therapeutic intervention.

BIOMARKERS AND MOLECULAR TARGETING

Progress in searching for useful markers for early detection of tumor, estimation of tumor burden, prediction of response to therapy, and monitoring disease progression has been slow. A prototypical marker is prostate-specific antigen (PSA), which proved to be quite useful for screening for and prognostic grouping and monitoring of therapy response of prostate carcinoma. Unfortunately, equivalent markers have yet to be identified for most other solid tumors. However, some studies of head and neck carcinomas have generated optimism.

Review of literature data up to a few years ago identified TP53, epidermal growth factor receptor (EGFR) and one of its ligands, transforming growth factor-α (TGF-α), and cyclin D1 as promising prognostic biomarkers for HNSCC.[71-73] A few studies[74-76] corroborated the prognostic value of EGFR. Our own study using HNSCC specimens of patients enrolled in a phase III trial of the RTOG[50] and randomized to receive standard irradiation,[76] for example, revealed no correlation between EGFR expression and T stage, N status, American Joint Committee on Cancer (AJCC) stage grouping, and recursive partitioning analysis (RPA) classes[77] (r = –.07 to .17). However, patients with more than median EGFR-expressing tumors, as measured using an image analysis–based immunohistochemical (IA-IHC) assay, were found to have significantly lower overall and disease-free survival rates because of a significantly higher locoregional relapse rate. Multivariate analysis showed that EGFR expression was a strong, independent predictor of survival and of locoregional relapse.

A completed follow-up study, using a validation set of patients enrolled into the same trial, revealed high reproducibility of the IA-IHC assay and confirmed the absence of correlation between EGFR expression and tumor stage and other clinical prognostic variables (r = –.20 to .18). The results validated our previous finding that higher tumor EGFR expression predicted worse survival, disease-free survival, and locoregional relapse, with hazard ratios of 1.97, 2.15, and 3.12, respectively. However, the questions of whether EGFR predicts for the risk for metastasis and whether EGFR is a marker for tumor clonogen proliferation have not been resolved.

Recognition of the importance of ERBB family tyrosine kinase receptors in co-regulating cell proliferation, death, and angiogenesis led to development of several strategies targeting the EGFR signaling pathway for cancer treatment. Two of these strategies—a monoclonal antibody (e.g., cetuximab) and small-molecule kinase inhibitors (e.g., gefitinib, erlotinib)—have gone through various stages of preclinical and clinical development for several types of cancers. Several reviews summarize the status of these clinical investigations.[6,7,76,78] Randomized trials of treatment for colorectal adenocarcinoma[79] and HNSCC[80] showed that cetuximab given in combination with irinotecan or cisplatin yielded higher objective response rates (23% and 26%, respectively) than chemotherapy alone. However, the higher response rates to combined therapies have not translated into improved overall survival relative to monotherapy. Two phase III trials enrolling patients with NSCLC showed that gefitinib did not improve response rate or survival when added to cisplatin-gemcitabine or carboplatin-paclitaxel doublets.[81,82]

In contrast to the results of combinations of EGFR antagonists with chemotherapy, data of the combination of cetuximab with radiation therapy in patients with locally advanced HNSCC are impressive. A completed international phase III trial (IMCL CP02-9815) revealed that compared with irradiation alone, adding cetuximab to radiation resulted in a significant improvement in overall survival and locoregional control rates without increasing mucositis or dysphagia.[83] These findings validate the notion that selective enhancement of tumor response leading to durable locoregional control can be achieved by "designer drugs" targeting a specific molecular pathway.

Progress has been made in identifying prognostic markers in patients with NPC. The study of Chan and associates[84] showed in a series of 170 patients that the post-treatment plasma level of Epstein-Barr virus (EBV) DNA was strongly correlated with progression-free and overall survival, more so than the pretreatment titer. For example, the relative risk for NPC recurrence was 11.9 (95% CI, 5.53 to 25.43) for patients with post-treatment EBV DNA titer, compared with 2.5 (1.14 to 5.70) for patients with higher pretreatment EBV DNA. The positive and negative predictive values for recurrence for higher post-therapy EBV DNA were 83% (58% to 98%) and 98% (76% to 89%), respectively. When validated in larger series, this marker would be useful in identifying high-risk patients for testing more aggressive therapy and monitoring their response to treatment.

PREVENTION OF HEAD AND NECK CANCERS

The concept of *field cancerization* was first described by Slaughter and associates in 1953[85] and has long been validated by clinical data. This evolving notion describes diffuse subcellular injury to epithelium, resulting from interactions between prolonged carcinogen exposure and individuals' genetic profiles, rendering the whole anatomic field at risk for developing invasive cancers through stepwise, progressive accumulation of genetic alterations. It follows that an individual who develops and survives an upper aerodigestive cancer is at a higher risk (i.e., susceptible) for forming a second primary tumor (SPT) in the same anatomic field during the ensuing years. The field cancerization and multistep carcinogenesis concepts form the basis for research on cancer chemoprevention.

Results of relatively large series revealed that patients cured of their first head and neck cancer had more than 20% projected lifetime risk of development of SPT. The estimated annual SPT development rate ranged from 4% to 6% for at least 8 years after the diagnosis of the first cancer.[86,87] SPT is the leading cause of death in patients with early head and neck cancers.[88]

This patient population has served as a model for addressing the efficacy of *adjuvant chemoprevention* regimens. Initial trial testing the role of *cis*-retinoic acid in preventing SPT had yielded encouraging results.[89] Unfortunately, a large, multi-institutional, randomized trial did not confirm its benefit (unpublished data).

Leukoplakia and erythroplakia carry increased risk for transformation into squamous carcinomas. This patient subset has been used as a model to test *chemoprevention of malignant transformation*. The weaknesses of this model are that the natural history of leukoplakia is rather variable, with spontaneous improvement occurring in many cases, and that the malignant transformation rate at 8 years may vary from 18% to 36%, depending on the degree of dysplasia observed histologically.[90] Consequently, large series and prolonged follow-up studies are required to properly test the efficacy of a given primary chemoprevention strategy.

Identification of key genetic changes resulting in development of malignant clones and markers of multistep carcinogenesis will aid in selecting patients with the highest risk for enrollment into chemoprevention trials and thereby in reducing the required sample size. Markers can also serve as intermediate, surrogate end points for assessing the efficacy of chemoprevention regimens, and thereby, shortening the length of the required follow-up.

SUMMARY

It has been exciting and gratifying to participate in laboratory research and clinical trials on head and neck cancer during the past 2 decades. Advances in molecular biology techniques opened new research avenues yielding new concepts or knowledge, such as multistep tumor progression model, genetic susceptibility to environmental carcinogen-induced tumorigenesis, processes of virus-induced changes in cellular behavior, and factors and mechanisms governing cellular and tissular radiation response. Some of the wisdom gained has already found applications in developing novel therapy strategies that have completed or are undergoing preclinical and clinical testing. Examples include altered fractionation regimens, mechanism- or molecular-oriented combined therapy modalities, and conformal radiation therapy. The basic and translational research efforts have paid off in that the head and neck cancer mortality rate in the United States has declined since the inception of record keeping. For example, the annual death rate for men due to oral cavity and pharyngeal cancers in the United States decreased by an average of 1.9% and 3% between 1975 and 1993 and between 1993 and 2001, respectively.[1]

It is likely that the pace of discovery will increase in the coming years. Sensitive methods for detecting occult tumor foci for screening and staging purposes will be developed, and new approaches in characterizing the genetic profile of cancers will accurately depict their individual virulence, predict therapy response, and guide treatment selection. Optimism about developing rational novel therapy strategies aimed at specific molecular targets to prevent malignant transformation or reverse malignant phenotype is also increasing. The insights and new technologies gained from further research should have a sizable impact in reducing the mortality rate caused by head and neck cancers.

The accelerated pace of new discoveries and the large number of research directions make it increasingly complex to determine what constitutes the standard therapy for a variety of patient subsets. When several treatment options can yield approximately the same locoregional tumor control rate, other determinants to be taken into account in selecting the treatment of choice include cosmetic and functional outcome, acute and long-term morbidity (quality of life), resource use (cost), physician expertise, and patient convenience.

REFERENCES

1. Jemal A, Clegg LX, Ward E, et al: Annual report to the nation on the status of cancer, 1975-2001, with a special feature regarding survival. Cancer 101:3-27, 2004.
2. Fearon ER, Vogelstein BA: A genetic model for colorectal tumorigenesis. Cell 61:759-767, 1990.
3. Califano J, van der Riet P, Westra W, et al: Genetic progression model for head and neck cancer: implications for field cancerization. Cancer Res 56:2488-2492, 1996.
4. Blot WJ, McLaughlin JK, Winn DM, et al: Smoking and drinking in relation to oral and pharyngeal cancer. Cancer Res 48:3282-3287, 1988.
5. Gschwind A, Fischer OM, Ullrich A: The discovery of receptor tyrosine kinases: targets for cancer therapy. Nat Rev Cancer 4:361-370, 2004.
6. Mendelsohn J, Baselga J: Status of epidermal growth factor receptor antagonists in the biology and treatment of cancer. J Clin Oncol 21:2787-2799, 2003.
7. Ang KK, Andratschke NH, Milas L: Epidermal growth factor receptor and response of head-and-neck carcinoma to therapy. Int J Radiat Oncol Biol Phys 58:959-965, 2004.
8. Santoro M, Melillo RM, Carlomagno F, et al: Minireview: RET: normal and abnormal functions. Endocrinology 145:5448-5451, 2004.
9. Mizuno T, Iwamoto KS, Kyoizumi S, et al: Preferential induction of RET/PTC1 rearrangement by x-ray irradiation. Oncogene 19:438-443, 2000.
10. Williams D: Cancer after nuclear fallout: Lessons from the Chernobyl accident. Nat Rev Cancer 2:543-549, 2002.
11. Eng C, Clayton D, Schuffenecker I, et al: The relationship between specific RET proto-oncogene mutations and disease phenotype in multiple endocrine neoplasia type 2. International RET mutation consortium analysis. JAMA 276:1575-1579, 1996.
12. Brandi ML, Gagel RF, Angeli A, et al: Consensus: guidelines for diagnosis and therapy of MEN type 1 and type 2. J Clin Endocrinol Metab 86:5658-5671, 2001.
13. Machens A, Niccoli-Sire P, Hoegel J, et al: Early malignant progression of hereditary medullary thyroid cancer. N Engl J Med 349:1517-1525, 2003.
14. Bugalho MJ, Domingues R, Sobrinho L: Molecular diagnosis of multiple endocrine neoplasia type 2. Expert Rev Mol Diagn 3:769-777, 2003.
15. Santoro M, Carlomagno F, Romano A, et al: Activation of RET as a dominant transforming gene by germline mutations of MEN2A and MEN2B. Science 267:381-383, 1995.
16. Liebowitz D: Nasopharyngeal carcinoma: the Epstein-Barr virus association. Semin Oncol 21:376-381, 1994.
17. Sheu LF, Chen A, Meng CL, et al: Enhanced malignant progression of nasopharyngeal carcinoma cells mediated by the expression of Epstein-Barr nuclear antigen 1 in vivo. J Pathol 180:243-248, 1996.
18. Nicholson LJ, Hopwood P, Johannessen I, et al: Epstein-Barr virus latent membrane protein does not inhibit differentiation and induces tumorigenicity of human epithelial cells. Oncogene 15:275-283, 1997.
19. Murray PG, Swinnen LJ, Constandinou CM, et al: BCL-2 but not its Epstein-Barr virus-encoded homologue, BHRF1, is commonly expressed in posttransplantation lymphoproliferative disorders. Blood 8287:706-711, 1996.
20. Choi PHK, Suen MWM, Path MRC, et al: Nasopharyngeal carcinoma: genetic changes, Epstein-Barr virus infection, or both. Cancer 72:2873-2878, 1993.
21. Huang DP, Lo KW, van Hasselt CA, et al: A region of homozygous deletion on chromosome 9p21-22 in primary nasopharyngeal carcinoma. Cancer Res 54:4003-4006, 1994.
22. Chan ASC, To KF, Lo KW, et al: High frequency of chromosome 3p deletion in histologically normal nasopharyngeal epithelia from southern Chinese. Cancer Res 60:5365-5370, 2000.
23. Chan ASC, To KF, Lo KW, et al: Frequent chromosome 9P losses in histologically normal nasopharyngeal epithelia from southern Chinese. Int J Cancer 102:300-303, 2002.
24. Zur house H, Schneider A: The role of papillomaviruses in human anogenital cancer. *In* Salzman NP, Howley PM (eds): The Papovaviridae, vol 2. New York, Plenum Publishing, 1987.
25. Woodworth CD, Bowden PE, Doniger J, et al: Characterization of normal human exocervical epithelial cells immortalized in vitro by papillomavirus types 16 and 18 DNA. Cancer Res 48:4620-4628, 1988.
26. Kaur P, McDougall JK: Characterization of primary human keratinocytes transformed by human papillomavirus type 18. J Virol 62:1917-1924, 1988.
27. Park NH, Min BM, Li SL, et al: Immortalization of normal human oral keratinocytes with type 16 human papillomavirus. Carcinogenesis 12:1627-1631, 1991.
28. Schlegel R, Phelps WC, Zhang YL: Quantitative keratinocyte assay detects two biological activities of human papillomavirus DNA and identifies viral types associated with cervical carcinoma. EMBO J 7:3181-3187, 1988.
29. Pecoraro G, Morgan D, Defendi V: Differential effects of human papillomavirus type 6, 16, and 18 DNAs on immortalization and transformation. Proc Natl Acad Sci U S A 86:563-567, 1989.

30. Barbosa MS, Schlegel R: The E6 and E7 genes of HPV-18 are sufficient for inducing two-stage in vitro transformation of human keratinocytes. Oncogene 4:1529-1532, 1989.
31. Munger K, Phelps WC, Bubb V, et al: The E6 and E7 genes of the human papillomavirus type 16 together are necessary and sufficient for transformation of primary human keratinocytes. J Virol 63:4417-4421, 1989.
32. Herrero R: Human papillomavirus and cancer of the upper aerodigestive tract. J Natl Cancer Inst Monogr 31:47-51, 2003.
33. Brachman DG, Graves D, Vokes E, et al: Occurrence of p53 gene deletions and human papilloma virus infection in human head and neck cancer. Cancer Res 52:4832-4836, 1992.
34. Ogura H, Watanabe S, Fukushima K, et al: Human papillomavirus DNA in squamous cell carcinoma of the respiratory and upper digestive tracts. Jpn J Clin Oncol 23:221-225, 1993.
35. Brandwein M, Zeitlin J, Nuovo GJ, et al: HPV detection using "hot start" polymerase chain reaction in patients with oral cancer: a clinicopathological study of 64 patients. Mod Pathol 7:720-727, 1994.
36. Brandsma JL, Steinberg BM, Abramson AL, et al: Presence of human papillomavirus type 16 related sequences in verrucous carcinoma of the larynx. Cancer Res 46:2185-2188, 1986.
37. Noble-Topham SE, Fliss DM, Hartwick WJ: Detection and typing of human papillomavirus in verrucous carcinoma of the oral cavity using the polymerase chain reaction. Arch Otolaryngol Head Neck Surg 119:1299-1302, 1993.
38. Fliss DM, Noble-Topham SE, McLachlin M, et al: Laryngeal verrucous carcinoma: a clinicopathologic study and detection of human papillomavirus using polymerase chain reaction. Laryngoscope 104:146-152, 1994.
39. Snijders PJ, Cromme FV, van den Brule AJ, et al: Prevalence and expression of human papillomavirus in tonsillar carcinomas, indicating a possible viral etiology. Intl J Cancer 51:845-850, 1992.
40. Gillison ML, Koch WM, Capone RB, et al: Evidence for a causal association between human papillomavirus and a subset of head and neck cancers. J Natl Cancer Inst 92:709-720, 2000.
41. Steenbergen R, Hermsen M, Walboomers J, et al: Integrated human papillomavirus type 16 and loss of heterozygosity at 11q22 and 18q21 in an oral carcinoma and its derivative cell line. Cancer Res 55:5465-5471, 1995.
42. Nguyen LN, Ang KK: Radiotherapy for cancer of the head and neck: altered fractionation regimens. Lancet Oncol 3:693-701, 2002.
43. Bernier J, Bentzen SM: Altered fractionation and combined radiochemotherapy approaches: pioneering new opportunities in head and neck oncology. Eur J Cancer 39:560-571, 2003.
44. Horiot JC, LeFur RN, Guyen T, et al: Hyperfractionation versus conventional fractionation in oropharyngeal carcinoma: final analysis of a randomized trial of the EORTC cooperative group of radiotherapy. Radiother Oncol 25:231-241, 1992.
45. Jackson SM, Weir LM, Hay JH, et al: A randomised trial of accelerated versus conventional radiotherapy in head and neck cancer. Radiother Oncol 43:39-46, 1997.
46. Skladowski K, Maciejewski J, Golen M, et al: Randomized clinical trial on 7-day continuous accelerated irradiation (CAIR) of head and neck cancer—report on 3-year tumor control and normal tissue toxicity. Radiother Oncol 55:93-102, 2000.
47. Horiot JC, Bontemps P, van den Bogaert V, et al: Accelerated fractionation (AF) compared to conventional fractionation (CF) improved head and neck cancers: results of the EORTC 22851 randomized trial. Radiother Oncol 44:111-121, 1997.
48. Dische S, Saunders M, Barrett A, et al: A randomised multicentre trial of CHART versus conventional radiotherapy in head and neck cancer. Radiother Oncol 44:123-136, 1997.
49. Overgaard J, Hansen HS, Specht L, et al: Five compared with six fractions per week of conventional radiotherapy of squamous-cell carcinoma of head and neck: DAHANCA 6 and 7 randomised controlled trial. Lancet 362:933-940, 2003.
50. Fu KK, Pajak TF, Trotti A, et al: A radiation therapy oncology group (RTOG) phase III randomized study to compare hyperfractionation and two variants of accelerated fractionation to standard fractionation radiotherapy for head and neck squamous cell carcinomas: first report of RTOG 9003. Int J Radiat Oncol Biol Phys 48:7-16, 2000.
51. Munro AJ: An overview of randomised controlled trials of adjuvant chemotherapy in head and neck cancer. Br J Cancer 71:83-91, 1995.
52. El-Sayed S, Nelson N: Adjuvant and adjunctive chemotherapy in the management of squamous cell carcinoma of the head and neck region. A meta-analysis of prospective and randomised trials. J Clin Oncol 14:838-847, 1996.
53. Pignon JP, Bourhis J, Domenge C, et al: Chemotherapy added to locoregional treatment for head and neck squamous-cell carcinoma: three meta-analyses of updated individual data. Lancet 355:949-955, 2000.
54. Adelstein DJ, Li Y, Adams GL, et al: An Intergroup phase III comparison of standard radiation therapy and two schedules of concurrent chemoradiotherapy in patients with unresectable squamous cell head and neck cancer. J Clin Oncol 21:92-98, 2003.
55. Al-Sarraf M, LeBlance M, Shanker PG, et al: Chemoradiotherapy versus radiotherapy in patients with advanced nasopharyngeal cancer: phase III randomized intergroup study 0099. J Clin Oncol 16:1310-1317, 1998.
56. Forastiere AA, Goepfert H, Maor M, et al: Concurrent chemotherapy and radiotherapy for organ preservation in advanced laryngeal cancer. N Engl J Med 349:2091-2098, 2003.
57. Denis F, Garaud P, Bardet E, et al: Late toxicity results of the GORTEC 94-01 randomized trial comparing radiotherapy with concomitant radiochemotherapy for advanced-stage oropharynx carcinoma: comparison of LENT/SOMA, RTOG/EORTC, and NCI-CTC scoring systems. Int J Radiat Oncol Biol Phys 55:93-98, 2003.
58. Wendt TG, Grabenbauer GG, Rodel CM, et al: Simultaneous radiochemotherapy versus radiotherapy alone in advanced head and neck cancer: a randomized multicenter study. J Clin Oncol 16:1318-1324, 1998.
59. Brizel DM, Albers ME, Fisher SR, et al: Hyperfractionated irradiation with or without concurrent chemotherapy for locally advanced head and neck cancer. N Engl J Med 338:1798-1804, 1998.
60. Jeremic B, Shibamoto Y, Milicic B, et al: Hyperfractionated radiation therapy with or without concurrent low-dose daily cisplatin in locally advanced squamous cell carcinoma of the head and neck: a prospective randomized trial. J Clin Oncol 18:1458-1464, 2000.
61. Bernier J, Domenge C, Ozsahin M, et al: Postoperative irradiation with or without concomitant chemotherapy for locally advanced head and neck cancer. N Engl J Med 350:1945-1952, 2004.
62. Cooper JS, Pajak TF, Forastiere AA, et al: Postoperative concurrent radiotherapy and chemotherapy for high-risk squamous-cell carcinoma of the head and neck. N Engl J Med 350:1937-1944, 2004.
63. Huguenin P, Beer KT, Allal A, et al: Concomitant cisplatin significantly improves locoregional control in advanced head and neck cancers treated with hyperfractionated radiotherapy. J Clin Oncol 22:4665-4673, 2004.
64. Wee J, Tan EH, Tai BC, et al: Phase III randomized trial of radiotherapy versus concurrent chemoradiotherapy followed by adjuvant chemotherapy in patients with AJCC/UICC (1997) stage 3 and 4 nasopharyngeal cancer of the endemic variety. Proc Am Soc Clin Oncol 23:487, 2004.
65. Bachaud J-M, Cohen-Jonathan E, Alzieu C, et al: Combined postoperative radiotherapy and weekly cisplatin infusion for locally advanced head and neck carcinoma: final report of a randomized trial. Int J Radiat Oncol Biol Phys 36:999-1004, 1996.
66. Trotti A, Bentzen SM: The need for adverse effects reporting standards in oncology clinical trials. J Clin Oncol 22:19-22, 2004.
67. Verhey LJ: Comparison of three-dimensional conformal radiation therapy and intensity-modulated radiation therapy systems. Semin Radiat Oncol 9:78-98, 1999.
68. Eisbruch A, Ten Haken RK, Kim HM, et al: Dose, volume, and function relationships in parotid salivary glands following conformal and intensity-modulated irradiation of head and neck cancer. Int J Radiat Oncol Biol Phys 45:577-587, 1999.
69. Lee N, Xia P, Quivey JM, et al: Intensity-modulated radiotherapy in the treatment of nasopharyngeal carcinoma: an update of the UCSF experience. Int J Radiat Oncol Biol Phys 53:12-22, 2002.

70. Chao KSC, Ozyigit G, Blanco AI, et al: Intensity-modulated radiation therapy for oropharyngeal carcinoma: impact of tumor volume. Int J Radiat Oncol Biol Phys 59:43-50, 2004.
71. Smith BD, Haffty BG: Molecular markers as prognostic factors for local recurrence and radioresistance in head and neck squamous cell carcinoma. Radiat Oncol Invest 7:125-144, 1999.
72. Salesiotis AN, Cullen KJ: Molecular markers predictive of response and prognosis in the patient with advanced squamous cell carcinoma of the head and neck: evolution of a model beyond TNM staging. Curr Opin Oncol 12:229-239, 2000.
73. Quon H, Liu FF, Cummings BJ: Potential molecular prognostic markers in head and neck squamous cell carcinomas. Head Neck 23:147-159, 2001.
74. Maurizi M, Almadori G, Ferrandina G, et al: Prognostic significance of epidermal growth factor receptor in laryngeal squamous cell carcinoma. Br J Cancer 74:1253-1257, 1996.
75. Grandis J, Melhem M, Gooding W, et al: Levels of TGF-α and EGFR protein in head and neck squamous cell carcinoma and patient survival. J Natl Cancer Inst 90:824-832, 1998.
76. Ang KK, Berkey BA, Tu X, et al: Impact of epidermal growth factor receptor expression on survival and pattern of relapse in patients with advanced head and neck carcinoma. Cancer Res 62:7350-7356, 2002.
77. Cooper J, Farnum N, Asbell S, et al: Recursive partitioning analysis of 2,105 patients treated in RTOG studies of head and neck cancer. Cancer 77:1905-1911, 1996.
78. Harari PM, Huang S-M: Combining EGFR inhibitors with radiation or chemotherapy: will preclinical studies predict clinical results? Int J Radiat Oncol Biol Phys 58:976-983, 2004.
79. Cunningham D, Humblet Y, Siena S, et al: Cetuximab monotherapy and cetuximab plus irinotecan in irinotecan-refractory metastatic colorectal cancer. N Engl J Med 351:337-345, 2004.
80. Burtness B, Li Y, Flood W, et al: Phase III trial of cisplatin + placebo versus cisplatin + C225, a monoclonal antibody directed to the epidermal growth factor receptor: an Eastern Cooperative Group trial. Presented at the AACR-NCI-EORTC International Conference on Molecular Targets and Cancer Therapeutics, Boston, MA, 2003.
81. Giaccone G, Herbst RS, Manegold C, et al: Gefitinib in combination with gemcitabine and cisplatin in advanced non-small-cell lung cancer: a phase III trial—INTACT 1. J Clin Oncol 22:777-784, 2004.
82. Herbst RS, Giaccone G, Schiller JH, et al: Gefitinib in combination with paclitaxel and carboplatin in advanced non-small-cell lung cancer: a phase III trial—INTACT 2. J Clin Oncol 22:785-794, 2004.
83. Bonner JA, Giralt J, Harari PM, et al: Cetuximab prolongs survival in patients with locoregionally advanced squamous cell carcinoma of head and neck: a phase III study of high dose radiation therapy with or without cetuximab. Proc Am Soc Clin Oncol 23:488, 2004.
84. Chan ATC, Lo YMD, Zee B, et al: Plasma Epstein-Barr virus DNA and residual disease after radiotherapy for undifferentiated nasopharyngeal carcinoma. J Natl Cancer Inst 94:1614-1619, 2002.
85. Slaughter DP, Southwick HW, Smejkal W: "Field cancerization" in oral stratified squamous epithelium: clinical implications of multicentric orgin. Cancer 6:963-968, 1953.
86. Cooper JS, Pajak TF, Rubin P, et al: Second malignancies in patients who have head and neck cancer: incidence, effect on survival and implications based on the RTOG experience. Int J Radiat Oncol Biol Phys 17:449-456, 1989.
87. Vokes EE, Weichselbaum RR, Lippman SM, et al: Head and neck cancer. N Engl J Med 328:184-193, 1993.
88. Lippman SM, Hong WK: Second malignant tumors in head and neck squamous cell carcinoma: the overshadowing threat for patients with early stage disease. Int J Radiat Oncol Biol Phys 17:691-694, 1989.
89. Hong WK, Lippman SM, Itri LM, et al: Prevention of second primary tumors with isotretinoin in squamous-cell carcinoma of the head and neck. N Engl J Med 323:795-801, 1990.
90. Silverman SJ, Gorsky M, Lozada F: Oral leukoplakia and malignant transformation: a follow-up study of 257 patients. Cancer 53:563-568, 1984.

CHAPTER 29

ORAL CAVITY CANCER

Russell W. Hinerman, Robert L. Foote, Pamela L. Sandow,
and William M. Mendenhall

INCIDENCE

In 2006, there were an estimated 22,040 new cases and 5320 estimated deaths.

BIOLOGIC CHARACTERISTICS

The natural history of oral cavity carcinoma depends on its anatomical site, histologic type, and stage of the tumor.

STAGING EVALUATION

Physical examination is performed to determine the location and extent of the primary tumor and to assess for presence and extent of nodal involvement.

Computed tomography is performed to determine extent (particularly deep invasion), to detect bone invasion (computed tomography plus panoramic radiography), and to assess regional lymph nodes. For retromolar trigone lesions, magnetic resonance imaging is useful to assess muscle invasion. Chest radiography is used to detect pulmonary metastases. The routine use of positron emission tomography is not recommended.

PRIMARY THERAPY

For early lesions (T1 and early T2), single-modality surgery or radiation therapy (RT) can achieve excellent local control and survival in most oral cavity sites (85% to 90%). Treatment choice is predicated on function and treatment side effects.

For moderately advanced lesions (large T2 and early T3), most lesions are treated with RT alone or with surgery plus irradiation with moderate local control (60% to 80%).

LOCALLY ADVANCED OR RECURRENT DISEASE

For locally advanced disease (large T3 or T4), combined RT plus surgery or RT plus concomitant chemotherapy is indicated in most sites because single-modality disease control is poor (30% or less).

For locally recurrent cancers after surgery alone salvage with surgery followed by postoperative RT, RT with or without chemotherapy, or palliative RT is indicated.

For locally recurrent cancers after definitive RT alone or combined with chemotherapy, surgical salvage, palliative chemotherapy, or supportive care is indicated.

PALLIATION

Moderate-dose palliative RT, 30 Gy in 10 fractions over 2 weeks or 14 Gy in 4 fractions over 2 days, to be repeated after 2 to 3 weeks, is indicated.

The estimated number of newly diagnosed oral cancers in 2006 is 22,040.[1] The estimated number of deaths is 5320. Approximately 5490 males and 4790 females will be diagnosed with squamous cell carcinoma of the floor of mouth in 2006, making it the most common oral cavity cancer.[1] The estimated number of deaths from this disease is 1870.

The oral cavity consists of the lip, floor of mouth, oral tongue (the anterior two thirds of the tongue), buccal mucosa, upper and lower gingiva, hard palate, and retromolar trigone. The frequency of involvement of various locations is shown in Table 29-1.[2] After a general discussion of etiology and epidemiology, issues relative to the various subsites will be presented separately. A discussion of dental care before and after radiation therapy (RT) is included.

ETIOLOGY AND EPIDEMIOLOGY

Oral cavity cancer is predominantly a disease of middle-aged men who use tobacco and alcohol. Approximately 95% of carcinomas appear after age 45, with an average age of 60.[2] The use of tobacco in any form is associated with an increased risk of oral cancer.[3-6] Some evidence suggests that patients with oral cavity cancer who continue to smoke during RT have poorer outcomes.[7] The risk of tobacco-related cancers of the upper aerodigestive tracts declines among ex-smokers after 5 years and may approach the same risk of nonsmokers after 10 years of abstention.[8] Although the effects of alcohol and tobacco in inducing cancers of the upper aerodigestive tract seem to be additive, the risk of alcohol consumption without tobacco use is unclear. Some studies indicate a slightly increased risk with alcohol use in the absence of tobacco, while others show no apparent increased risk.[6,9-17]

Acquired immune deficiency syndrome (AIDS) is associated with squamous cell carcinoma, particularly in patients younger than 40.[18] Human papillomavirus (HPV), marijuana smoking, betel quid, and the beverage "mate" have also been implicated as causative agents in the formation of squamous cell carcinomas of the upper aerodigestive tract.[19-25] Oral cancers have increased among relatively young women who have never consumed alcohol or smoked. The reason for this is unclear.[26]

Smokeless tobacco (snuff) can promote carcinomas of the buccal gingival sulcus, which is diagnosed most often in older, white women living in the southeastern United States. Carcinoma of the buccal mucosa is also associated with chewing tobacco. It is commonly seen in the southeastern United States, with a male-to-female ratio of 3 or 4:1.[27] Leukoplakia is seen with oral carcinoma in approximately 15% of cases.[28]

Persons with a "Scotch-Irish" complexion (red hair and blue eyes) and/or prolonged exposure to sunlight are most susceptible to lip carcinoma.[29,30] In one series, 82% of persons with lip cancer were previous or present tobacco smokers.[31] Pipe smoking is an alleged risk factor, but this has not been substantiated by most studies. Lip cancer is often associated

Table 29-1 Distribution of Oral Cavity Cancer: 14,253 Cases

Site	Percentage
Lower lip	38
Tongue	22
Floor of mouth	17
Gingiva	6
Palate	6
Retromolar trigone	5
Upper lip	4
Buccal mucosa	2

Data from Krolls SO, Hoffman S: Squamous cell carcinoma of the oral soft tissues: a statistical analysis of 14,253 cases by age, sex, and race of patients. J Am Dent Assoc 92:571, 1976.

with poor dental hygiene or edentulous patients.[31,32] Lip trauma and a history of alcohol abuse are also related factors.[29,31] Most cases appear after age 40, but approximately 10% occur before age 40 and a few before age 30. This disease is uncommon in blacks.

PREVENTION AND EARLY DETECTION

This information is of major importance for patients with oral cavity cancers and is covered in the Part B Overview, "Head and Neck Tumors," by K. Kian Ang; it will not be reiterated here.

ORAL CARE

A complete oral examination should be performed on all patients, whether dentate or edentulous, prior to irradiating any portion of the mandible or maxilla. It is important that the radiation oncologist inform the dentist of the anticipated RT treatment plan, including dose and location of the RT fields. In order to make appropriate pretherapy recommendations, the dentist should be familiar with possible post-RT complications, such as caries and osteoradionecrosis. There is a lifelong risk of impaired healing that can lead to osteoradionecrosis, especially when teeth are extracted from hypovascularized and hypocellular bone.[33] Therefore, one objective of the pretherapy oral evaluation is to determine whether teeth in the proposed irradiated area can be reasonably maintained in a healthy state for the remainder of the patient's life.

Medical, dental, and psychosocial issues that impact future dental health should be assessed at the pretherapy evaluation. The patient's compliance, motivation for daily oral hygiene procedures, dental awareness, and access to dental care are predictors of dental health. A panoramic radiograph, intraoral radiographs, and hard and soft tissue examinations should be performed to identify high dental risk factors such as deep caries, nonrestorable teeth, root tips, bony pathology, endodontically treated teeth, periapical and pulpal pathology, and nonfunctional teeth. Teeth exhibiting periodontal disease should be evaluated to determine their long-term prognosis. Some prognostic factors for poor periodontal health include probing depths more than 6 mm, gingival recession, furcation involvement, or mobility.[34,35] In light of the numerous reported cases of progression of gingival recession and periodontal disease after RT, it may be difficult to assess the longevity of each tooth.[36]

To reduce the future risk of osteoradionecrosis, teeth with high dental risk factors should be removed prior to receiving doses more than 55 Gy.[34] Whether extraction of teeth with moderate disease is indicated remains controversial. If the patient has poor resistance to dental disease or an unwillingness to perform routine dental care or fluoride applications, pretherapy extraction of moderately diseased teeth may be justified. A healing time of 14 to 21 days is recommended after extraction, prior to the initiation of RT.[33] Extraction should be accomplished as atraumatically as possible, with alveoloplasty to remove sharp, bony projections. The dentist should coordinate dental appointments with the radiation oncologist to minimize the delay in cancer therapy.

Denture adjustments, smoothing edges of sharp teeth, dental cleaning, and oral hygiene instruction can be accomplished at the pretherapy dental visit. Ill-fitting dentures that irritate mucosal surfaces should be worn with caution during RT. Daily disinfection of dental prostheses is recommended.

Impressions for custom fluoride trays can be made prior to or within the first 2 weeks of RT. Patients who receive RT to major salivary glands are at lifelong risk for rampant caries. Daily use of 0.4% stannous or 1.1% sodium fluoride gel for 5 minutes, in custom trays, is imperative as long as natural teeth remain. Patients should be advised to refrain from rinsing, eating, or drinking for 30 minutes after fluoride application. The dentist and radiation oncologist should consistently promote proper oral hygiene and use of fluoride throughout the posttreatment years.

Clinical practice guidelines for the treatment of cancer therapy–induced oral mucositis have been published.[37] RT-induced mucositis cannot be prevented; however, excellent oral hygiene can reduce the risk of oral infections. Supersoft toothbrushes and mild toothpastes are available for patients to facilitate proper oral hygiene during and after RT.

Consultation with the radiation oncologist is required prior to postirradiation extraction of teeth or invasive procedures that involve the exposure of irradiated bone. Preextraction and postextraction hyperbaric oxygen therapy may be indicated to promote healing of extraction or surgical sites.

Patients should be closely monitored for possible late effects of RT to oropharyngeal regions. Trismus, xerostomia, caries, and oral candidiasis can persist or occur at any time after treatment is completed.

MOLECULAR BIOLOGY

A discussion of the molecular biology of head and neck cancers is found in Part B: Head and Neck Overview, preceding this chapter.

LIP

Anatomy

The lips are composed of the orbicularis oris muscle, which surrounds the mouth and is covered externally by skin and internally by mucous membrane. The upper and lower lips are attached to the gingiva by raised folds of mucous membrane called the labial frenula. The vascular supply is from the superior and inferior labial branches of the facial arteries. The sensory nerve of the upper lip is the infraorbital nerve; the mental nerve provides sensory innervation for the lower lip.

Lymph vessels from both lips drain into the submandibular lymph nodes. In addition, lymph from the central part of the lower lip drains into the submental lymph nodes. The submental nodes drain either to the submandibular lymph nodes or to the jugulo-omohyoid node. The submandibular lymph nodes drain to the deep cervical chain of lymph nodes.[38]

Pathology and Patterns of Spread

The most common neoplasms are moderately to well-differentiated squamous cell carcinomas; approximately 5% are poorly differentiated.[39] Basal cell carcinomas usually arise on the skin above or below the lip and invade the vermilion border, but they rarely arise from the vermilion border.[40] Squamous cell carcinomas start on the vermilion of the lower lip and, less commonly, on the upper lip. The commissure is rarely the site of origin. Leukoplakia is a common problem on the lower lip and may precede carcinoma by many years.[28]

Early lesions can initially invade adjacent skin and the orbicularis oris muscle. Advanced lesions can invade the adjacent commissures of the lip and buccal mucosa, the skin and wet mucosa of the lip, the adjacent mandible, and eventually the mental nerve. The incidence of perineural invasion is approximately 2%.[41] Lymph node involvement at presentation occurs in approximately 5% to 10% of patients. An additional 5% to 10% of patients with a clinically negative neck subsequently develop lymph node metastases. The risk of lymph node involvement increases with depth of invasion, poor differentiation, larger lesions, invasion of the commissure, and recurrence after prior treatment.[40,32]

Hendricks and associates[42] from the Mayo Clinic reported the following incidence of positive cervical lymph nodes by T stage: T1, 2%; T2, 9%; and T3, 30%. The overall incidence of adenopathy was 19% when the commissure was involved.[39] De Visscher and colleagues[43] reported a nodal recurrence rate of 5.4% after primary surgical resection in 184 patients with squamous cell carcinoma of the lower lip. Ninety-three percent were stage I at presentation.

Clinical Manifestations and Staging

Carcinoma of the lip usually presents as a slowly enlarging exophytic lesion with an elevated border. Occasionally, there is minor bleeding. Erythema of the adjacent skin may suggest dermal lymphatic invasion. Anesthesia or paresthesia of the skin indicates perineural invasion.[44]

The American Joint Committee on Cancer (AJCC) staging for lip cancer applies to lesions arising from the vermilion surface[45] (Table 29-2).

Table 29-2 American Joint Committee on Cancer: Oral Cavity Primary Tumor Staging

Stage	
TX	Primary tumor cannot be assessed
T0	No evidence of primary tumor
Tis	Carcinoma in situ
T1	Tumor 2 cm or less in greatest dimension
T2	Tumor more than 2 cm but not more than 4 cm in greatest dimension
T3	Tumor more than 4 cm in greatest dimension
T4 (lip)	Tumor invades through cortical bone, inferior alveolar nerve, floor of mouth, or skin of face, i.e., chin or nose
T4 (oral cavity)	Tumor invades through cortical bone into deep (extrinsic) muscle of tongue (genioglossus, hyoglossus, palatoglossus, and styloglossus), maxillary sinus, or skin of face
T4b	Tumor involves masticator space, pterygoid plate, or skull base and/or encases internal carotid artery

From the American Joint Committee on Cancer: Lip and oral cavity. In: Greene FL, Page DL, Fleming ID, et al (eds): AJCC Cancer Staging Manual, 6th ed. New York, Springer, 2004, pp 23-32.

Early lip cancers rarely require diagnostic imaging. Locally advanced, deeply infiltrating, or recurrent carcinomas may benefit from a computed tomography (CT) scan or panoramic radiograph to evaluate possible bony invasion and regional nodal spread.

Treatment

Early Lesions (<2.0 cm)

The majority of these lesions can be surgically excised with primary closure as an outpatient procedure. Surgery is satisfactory if the lip commissure does not need to be resected, and if the resulting aperture of the oral cavity permits the insertion of dentures. Postoperative RT is recommended for positive margins or perineural invasion.[41,46,47]

Tumors that should be treated with RT include those involving a commissure in order to obtain better cosmesis and improved local control.[48-50] The uncommon, poorly differentiated lesions are also preferably treated by RT in order to cover a more generous treatment volume and the first echelon lymph nodes. An algorithm for treatment planning is shown in Figure 29-1.

Moderately Advanced Lesions (2 to 4 cm)

The length of the lower lip is approximately 7 cm. Removal of greater than half of the lower lip with simple closure produces a poor cosmetic and functional result so that a reconstructive procedure is usually necessary. In these cases, RT has the advantage of a better functional and cosmetic result. Traditionally, the reconstructed lip may look normal in a photograph, but may lack sensory and motor innervation as well as elasticity. However, numerous published articles attest to improvements in the functional and cosmetic results of various reconstructive surgical procedures.[51-56]

Stranc and colleagues[48] studied lip function in 37 patients after surgery (19 cases) or RT (18 cases) and compared them with normal controls. Compared with surgery, RT produced better preservation of lip sensation, intercommissural distance, and elasticity. Inadequate lip seal was observed in 2 of 18 patients (11%) after RT compared with 8 of 19 patients (42%) treated surgically.

Teichgraeber and Larson reviewed the M. D. Anderson Hospital experience for patients with lip cancer involving the commissure. Of the 22 patients with T2 lesions who were treated with surgery, 10 patients (45%) had recurrence. There are no data for commissure involvement treated with RT, but the relative ease of RT and the cosmetic and functional results lead us to recommend RT for lesions exhibiting this pattern of spread.

Locally Advanced Lesions (>4 cm)

Large lesions without bone or nerve invasion are generally managed initially with definitive RT, with surgery reserved for salvage. Lesions with bony or nerve invasion are managed by resection and postoperative RT.[47] Erythema of the skin adjacent to the lesion may indicate dermal lymphatic involvement; wide-field irradiation is recommended followed by consideration of surgical resection depending on the response to RT.

Management of the Neck

Regional lymphatics are not electively treated for T1 and T2 lesions unless commissure involvement is present.[40] Patients with advanced (>4 cm), poorly differentiated, and/or recurrent tumors often require elective neck treatment.[40,58] Other factors associated with an increased risk of nodal spread include perineural invasion, maximal thickness more than 6 mm, or low p27Kip1 protein expression.[59] The decision to

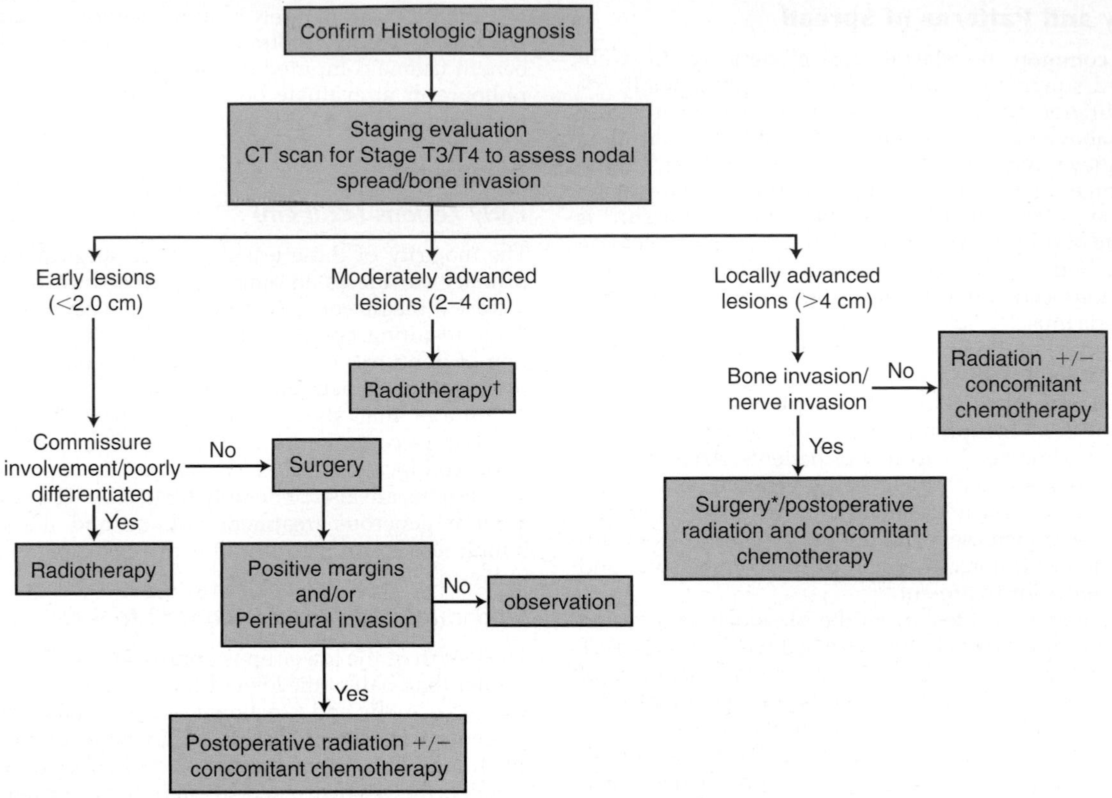

Figure 29-1 **Treatment algorithm for de novo lip cancer.** *Treat neck with surgical dissection or radiotherapy.[42] † Treat neck if the tumor is poorly differentiated or there is dermal or commissural involvement.[39,40]

use elective neck irradiation or elective neck dissection depends on the modality selected for treatment of the primary tumor.

Results

T1-T3 Lesions

INTERSTITIAL WITH OR WITHOUT EXTERNAL BEAM RADIATION

Jorgensen and associates[60] reviewed 869 patients with squamous cell carcinoma who were treated with an interstitial radium implant alone; 90% of the lesions were less than 2 cm in size. The local recurrence and survival rates are shown in Table 29-3; 99% of the primary tumors were ultimately controlled with RT alone or combined with salvage surgery. Thirty-eight percent of patients with T3 tumors who developed a local recurrence developed lymph node metastases. Only 4% of patients died of lip cancer. Twenty-nine complications arose, of which two were bone necrosis.

Pierquin and colleagues[61] reported on 50 patients with carcinoma of the lower lip treated with brachytherapy. Only one local recurrence (2%) was observed.

McKay and Sellers[39] reviewed 2854 patients; 92% were initially treated with brachytherapy and external beam radiation (EBRT). The primary lesion was controlled in 84% of the cases; 8% were salvaged later for an overall local control rate of 92%. Regional control was achieved in 58% of patients who presented with positive nodes. However, the ultimate rate of neck control was only 35% when neck nodes appeared at a later date. The cause-specific and absolute 5-year survival rates were 89% and 65%, respectively.

Table 29-3 **Lip Carcinoma Treated With Interstitial Radiotherapy (N = 869 Patients)**

Stage	Local Recurrence (5 y)	Survival (5 y)
T1	7.4%	99.5%
T2	12.7%	97.4%
T3	26.4%	81.4%

Data from Jorgensen K, Elbrond O, Andersen AP: Carcinoma of the lip. A series of 869 patients. Acta Otolaryngol (Stockh) 75:312-313, 1973.

Tombolini and associates[62] reported on 57 patients with squamous cell carcinoma of the lower lip treated with low-dose-rate brachytherapy alone. Patients with clinically positive neck nodes received external RT to the involved side of the neck. International Union Against Cancer (UICC) T stages were T1 in 27 cases (47%), T2 in 20 cases (35%), and T3 in 10 cases (18%). The 5-year local control rate was 90%.

Orrechia and colleagues[63] treated 47 patients with T1 (n = 21) and T2 (n = 26) lip cancers with iridium-192 brachytherapy. The 5- and 10-year actuarial disease-free survival rates were 92% and 85%, respectively.

Guinot and associates[64] treated 39 patients with lip carcinoma using high dose rate brachytherapy twice daily to total doses ranging from 40.5 to 45 Gy and observed a 3-year local control rate of 88%. Acute and chronic reactions were similar to those observed after low dose rate brachytherapy.

Petrovich and associates[65] reported on 250 patients with lip cancer treated with RT; half were treated with brachytherapy

Table 29-4 **Carcinoma of the Lip—University of Michigan (N = 279 Patients)***

Extent of Primary Lesion	No. of Patients	Local Recurrence	5-Y Survival Cause-Specific	Absolute
<1 cm	85	10.6%	100%	76%
1-3 cm	154	9.1%	92%	71%
>3 cm	29	20.7%	71%	52%
Bone invasion	11	90.9%	50%	45%

*Treated by radiotherapy, 47%; treated by surgery, 53%.
Modified from Baker SR, Krause CJ: Carcinoma of the lip. Laryngoscope 90:19-27, 1980.

and the remainder with EBRT. Two hundred forty-seven patients (99%) had squamous cell carcinomas and 240 patients (96%) had lower lip carcinomas. The incidence of lymph node metastasis was 9%. Eleven percent experienced recurrences after RT and half were salvaged; 18 patients (7%) died of lip cancer. Moderately advanced tumors and those with tumors near the commissures were best treated with EBRT.

External Beam Radiation or Surgery

Babington and colleagues[47] reported on 130 patients with lip carcinoma; 75% had T1 tumors. Initial treatment consisted of surgery (39%), RT (48%), or both (13%). Close (≤2 mm) or positive margins were observed in 27% of those treated surgically. The 2-year relapse-free survival rates were 82% and 54% after RT and surgery, respectively ($p < .001$). The recurrence rate after surgery was significantly higher for those with close or positive margins.

Baker and Krause[31] reported on 279 patients treated with either RT (47%) or surgery (53%) at the University of Michigan (Table 29-4). There was no difference in the 5-year cause-specific survival rates between the two groups. Patients with positive regional nodal metastases had a 5-year cause-specific survival rate of 29%. Regional lymph node metastases developed in 31% of those treated for locally recurrent lesions, indicating the need for elective neck treatment for this subset of patients.

De Visscher and colleagues[43] treated 184 patients with squamous cell carcinoma of the lower lip surgically; 93% had stage I cancers. The local and regional recurrence rates were 4.9% and 5.4%, respectively.

Mohs Surgery

Mohs and Snow[66] reported on 1148 patients with squamous cell carcinomas of the lower lip treated with microscopically controlled surgery. The 5-year local control rates were 94.2% for those with T1 lesions and 59.6% for patients operated on for T2 lesions. The 5-year local control rates were 96.3% for well to moderately differentiated tumors compared with 66.7% for those with poorly differentiated cancers.

Holmkvist and Roenigk[67] reported on 50 consecutive patients with squamous cell carcinoma of the lip treated with Mohs micrographic surgery (MMS). Four patients (8%) experienced a recurrence; all were successfully salvaged with additional MMS. The average time to recurrence after the initial MMS was 2.5 years. Hruza[68] also reported a relatively long interval between MMS and initial recurrence, with 20% of recurrences developing after 5 years.

T4 Lesions

Cancers that present with bone or nerve involvement are usually treated with a combination of surgery and EBRT. There are limited data pertaining to the local control rates after RT or surgery alone, ranging from 0% to 74%[39,64]; therefore, combined treatment is usually recommended. Byers and associates[41] observed that 80% of patients with histologically proven perineural invasion developed cervical node metastases. Eight of 25 patients (32%) in their series who presented with either perineural invasion, tumors larger than 3 cm, or regional metastases died of disease.

The postoperative EBRT portals should include the primary site as well as the regional lymphatics (submandibular, submental, and jugulo-omohyoid lymph nodes). The low neck is usually treated to doses sufficient for subclinical disease, and frequently higher in patients with positive nodes. Total dose ranges from 60 to 70 Gy, at 2.0 Gy per once-daily fraction to the primary site, depending on the pathologic findings. Higher doses with altered fractionation schemes (e.g., 7440 cGy at 120 cGy/fraction twice daily), as well as concomitant chemotherapy should be considered in patients with positive margins or other high-risk factors.

Recurrent Lesions

Cross and colleagues[32] reported on 563 patients treated with surgery for recurrent lip cancer. The prognosis was particularly poor for those with high-grade tumors, of whom 16.7% were salvaged, compared with 31.8% and 42.9% for those with well and moderately differentiated cancers, respectively. Holmkvist and Roenigk[67] reported on four patients treated with MMS; all four were salvaged.

Techniques of Irradiation

External beam RT is usually delivered with either orthovoltage x-rays or electron beam. The electron beam energy depends on the tumor thickness. Lead shields are placed behind the lip to limit the dose to the oral cavity and mandible. Orthovoltage fractionation schedules range from 40 to 45 Gy in 3 to 4 weeks for smaller lesions, and 50 to 55 Gy in 4 to 6 weeks for moderately advanced lesions. The dose is increased 10% to 15% for electron beam RT to account for differences in the relative biological effectiveness. Orthovoltage x-rays are preferred if available; because the maximum dose is at the surface and there is less beam constriction compared with electron beam.

An appositional field with a margin of 1 to 1.5 cm is sufficient for most small to moderately advanced lesions if orthovoltage irradiation is used. The field borders are determined by bimanual palpation. Because of beam constriction, 2.0- to 2.5-cm margins are necessary if an electron beam is used. A lead shield is used to collimate the beam at the skin/lip surface.

Brachytherapy may be used as the sole treatment or in conjunction with EBRT. Implantation is usually performed under local anesthesia using ^{192}Ir sources and a single-plane plastic tube technique. The sources are arranged horizontally 10 to 12 mm apart with crossing sources on the lateral aspects of the implant. Three to five horizontal sources are used depending on the size of the lesion. The advantage of the plastic tube

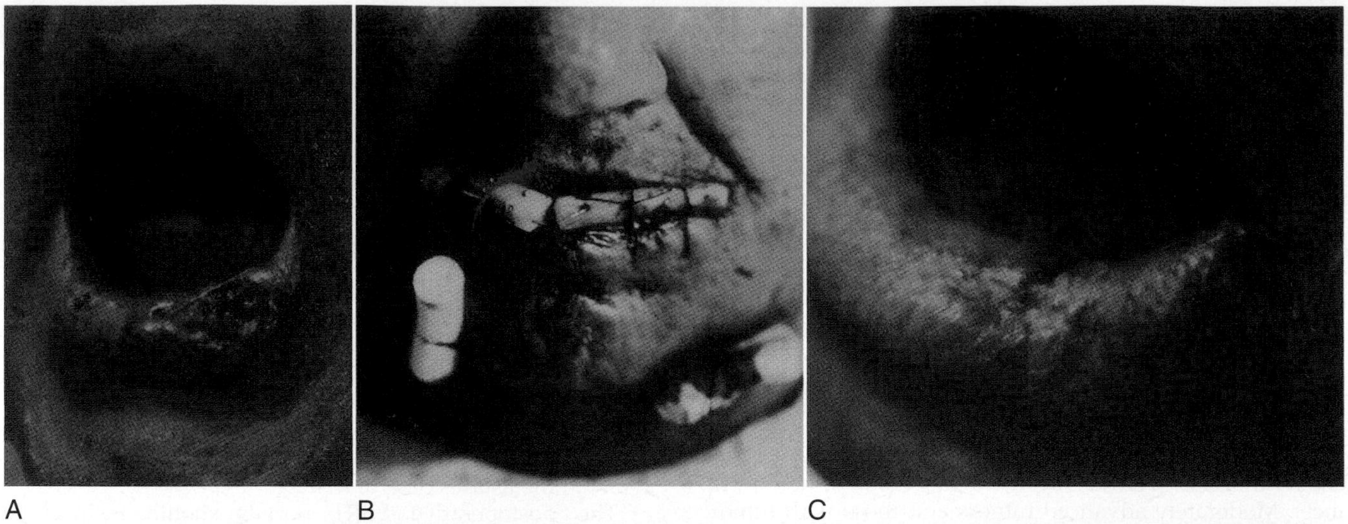

Figure 29-2 **A,** A 65-year-old man had a T2N0 squamous cell carcinoma of the left lower lip and a T1N0 lesion on the right. The left-sided lesion measured 2.5 × 2.0 × 1.5 cm. Radiation therapy was elected because of the functional deficit likely to result from excision of the larger lesion. The man received 30 Gy over 2 weeks, 3 Gy/fraction, of 250 kV (0.5 mm Cu). **B,** A single-plane cesium needle implant with double crossing was used. A chin pack was used to anchor the gingivolabial pack in place. A gauze pack was sewn into the gingivolabial gutter to displace the radium from the mandible and upper lip. The implant added 35 Gy at 0.5 cm. **C,** At 2 years and 5 months, there was no evidence of disease and the lip had completely healed.

technique is that the volume of the implant is more easily adapted to the extent of the tumor and the commissure is readily included, if necessary. Alternatively, cesium needles mounted in a nylon bar may be used (Fig. 29-2). The sources are spaced 1 cm apart and the dose is specified 0.5 cm from the plane of the implant. A gauze roll is placed between the lip and gum to increase the distance between the radioactive sources and the alveolar ridge. The recommended dose is 60 Gy at a dose rate of 0.4 to 0.5 Gy per hour for an implant alone. Large infiltrative lesions may be first treated with EBRT, 30 Gy at 2.5 Gy/fraction to shrink the tumor, followed by interstitial brachytherapy boost to deliver an additional 35 to 40 Gy. Treatment of lip cancer with high-dose-rate (HDR) interstitial needles is advocated by some.[64]

T3 and T4

Low-volume T3 cancers may be treated with primary RT, preferably combining EBRT to the primary lesion and neck followed by a brachytherapy boost. EBRT is administered with parallel-opposed fields, including the lip lesion and the level 1 and 2 lymph nodes[69] (Fig. 29-3). A cork is placed in the mouth to displace the maxilla and upper lip and reduce the volume of normal tissues included in the fields. A separate anterior field is used to treat the level 3 and 4 lymph nodes with a tapered midline block over the larynx. The supraclavicular lymph nodes are at low risk and are not included in the fields. Both sides of the neck are treated with RT because it is unlikely that T3 and T4 primary lesions would be well lateralized.

The junction between the parallel-opposed fields and the low-neck field is at the thyroid notch. The dose fractionation schedule used varies from 38.4 Gy at 1.6 Gy twice daily to 50 Gy at 2 Gy/fraction once daily, followed by a brachytherapy boost. Low-energy photons such as 4-MV or 6-MV beams are recommended.

High-volume T3 and T4 cancers are unlikely to be cured with RT alone and are better treated with surgery and postoperative RT. RT fields are similar to those used to treat patients with RT alone. Petroleum jelly gauze bolus is placed over incisions to ensure the surface dose is adequate. The fields are extended to the skull base along the course of the third division of cranial nerve V if perineural invasion is present. The dose depends on the surgical margins: negative (R0), 60 Gy; microscopically positive (R1), 66 Gy; and gross residual disease (R2), 70 Gy. Patients are treated once daily at 2 Gy/fraction, 5 days a week, in a continuous course. Consideration should be given to using an altered fractionation schedule to reduce the overall treatment time for patients with positive margins and/or extensive perineural invasion.

Complications

After RT, there is gradual atrophy of the irradiated tissues. The irradiated lip must be protected from sun exposure by use of hats and ultraviolet protectants. Because the anterior teeth and gingiva are protected by lead shields when radiation is given by EBRT, radiation caries, bone exposure, and osteoradionecrosis are uncommon.

Fitzpatrick[70] reported a 3.3% incidence of late complications that required surgical intervention. Orrechia and colleagues[63] observed a 10.6% incidence of mucosal necrosis after RT for 47 T1 and T2 lip cancers treated with ^{192}Ir brachytherapy. The risk of late complications increased with dose, dose per fraction, and volume.

FLOOR OF MOUTH

Anatomy

The floor of the mouth is a semilunar space overlying the mylohyoid and hyoglossus muscles, extending from the inner surfaces of the mandibular alveolar ridge to the ventral surface of the oral tongue. Its posterior boundary is the base of the anterior tonsillar pillar; it is bisected anteriorly by the frenulum of the tongue. The mylohyoid muscle arises from the mylohyoid ridge of the mandible and is the muscular floor of the oral cavity. The posterior insertion is at the level of the third molars.

The submandibular glands lie along the body of the mandible. The inferior aspect of the gland extends below the

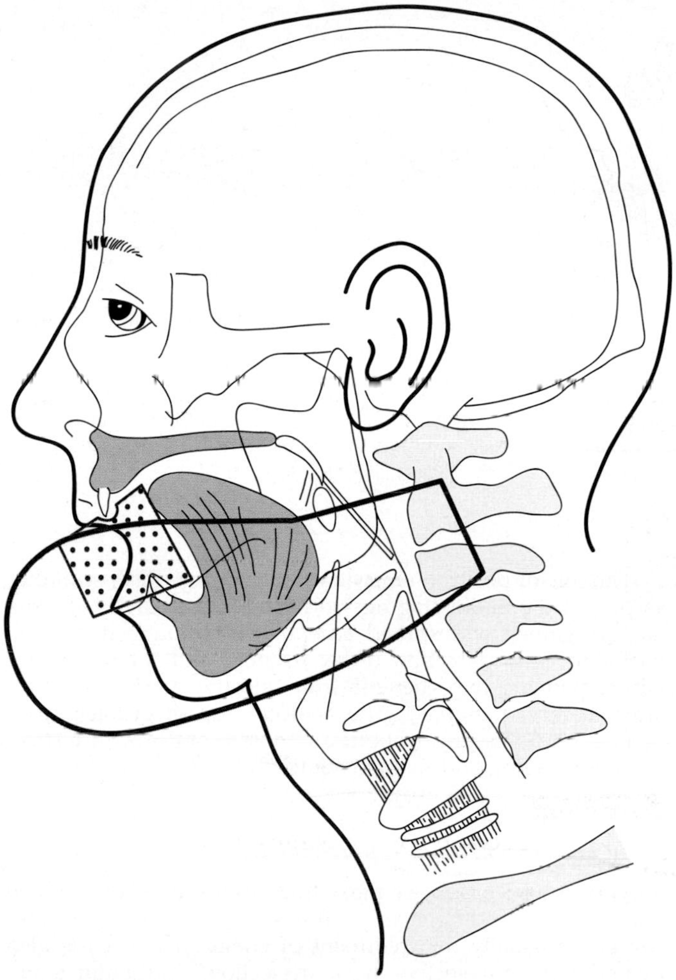

Figure 29-3 Parallel-opposed fields used to treat a carcinoma of the lower lip in conjunction with the level 1 and level 2 lymph nodes. (Adapted from Mendenhall WM: Radiotherapy for cancer of the lip: Treatment technique. *In* Werning JW [ed]: Oral Cancer. New York, Thieme Publishing, 2005.)

inferior edge of the mandibular arch; part of the gland is superficial to the mylohyoid muscle. The submandibular gland is palpable as a soft mass over the posterior portion of the mylohyoid muscle when the muscle is tensed by forcing the tip of the tongue against the maxillary incisor teeth.

The submandibular duct (Wharton's duct) is approximately 5 cm long and arises from the portion of the gland that lies between the mylohyoid and hyoglossus muscles. The duct passes deep and then superficial to the lingual nerve and exits in the anterior floor of the mouth near the midline.

The sublingual glands are the smallest of the major salivary glands and are the most deeply situated. Each lies in the floor of the mouth between the mandible and the genioglossus muscle.

The first echelon nodes for the floor of mouth are the submandibular lymph nodes that may be stratified into preglandular, intraglandular, and postglandular groups. Lymph may also drain into the submental nodes. These lymph nodes eventually drain to the jugulo-omohyoid node.[71]

The lingual nerve is a branch of the mandibular nerve and provides the sensory innervation to the floor of the mouth. It enters the mouth between the medial pterygoid muscle and the ramus of the mandible and passes anteriorly under the oral mucosa medial to the third mandibular molar.

Table 29-5 Floor of Mouth Carcinomas: Correlation of Primary Tumor Thickness With Neck Failure*

Thickness (mm)	T1 N0	T2 N0
.1-1.5	1/38 (3%)	0/19
1.6-3.5	1/5 (20%)	3/7 (43%)
≥3.6	7/11 (64%)	2/4 (50%)

*No. of treatment failures/total No. of patients.

Modified from Mohit-Tabatabai MA, Sobel HJ, Rush BF, Mashberg A: Relation of thickness of floor of mouth stage I and II cancers to regional metastasis. Am J Surg 152:351-353, 1986. Copyright 1986, with permission from Excerpta Medica, Inc.

The hypoglossal nerve (cranial nerve XII) is the motor nerve of the tongue. It passes anterior to the inferior aspect of the hyoglossus muscle and then to the lateral aspect of the genioglossus muscle. Injury to the hypoglossal nerve results in paralysis and atrophy of the ipsilateral oral tongue. The tongue deviates to the paralyzed side upon protrusion because of the unopposed contralateral genioglossus muscle.

Pathology and Patterns of Spread

The majority of floor of mouth neoplasms are squamous cell carcinomas; most are moderately differentiated. Adenoid cystic and mucoepidermoid carcinomas arise from the minor salivary glands and account for 2% to 3% of floor of mouth malignancies. Most floor of mouth carcinomas are located in the anterior midline adjacent to Wharton's ducts. Extension toward the gingiva and periosteum occurs early and frequently. Small to moderate-size lesions (T1 and T2) are associated with metastases to the ipsilateral regional lymph nodes in 15% to 38% of cases, depending on the size and depth of invasion of the primary tumor.[72-75]

Mohit-Tabatabai and associates[76] reviewed 84 patients with squamous cell carcinoma of the floor of the mouth and concluded that lesion thickness was related to the probability of subclinical cervical metastases in clinically node-negative (N0) patients (Table 29-5). Based on these data, elective neck treatment is recommended for any patient with a primary lesion more than 1.5 mm thick.[76] Histologic grade and configuration of the primary lesion did not have a statistically significant correlation with subsequent development of neck node metastases. The reported incidence of recurrence in the untreated clinically negative neck varies from 20% to 35%.[73,77-80] Histologic grade and vascular and perineural invasion have been implicated as predictors of lymph node spread.[81]

The distribution of clinically positive neck nodes at diagnosis is shown in Figure 29-4,[82] and the distribution of pathologically positive nodes after elective neck dissection in 62 patients with carcinoma of the floor of the mouth is shown in Figure 29-5.[83] The incidence of positive lymph nodes was 19% for those with T1 or T2 lesions and 26% for patients with T3 or T4 cancers.

Clinical Manifestations, Patient Evaluation, and Staging

Floor of mouth carcinomas usually present as slightly elevated mucosal lesions with well-defined borders. A background of leukoplakia may be present. The lesions are often diagnosed by a dentist or physician during a routine physical examination.

T1 and T2 tumors may be noted initially when the patient feels a lump in the floor of the mouth with the tip of his or her

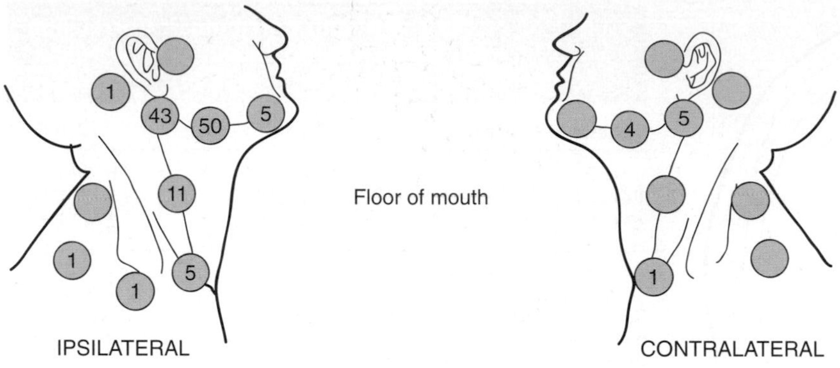

N_0	N_1	N_{2A}	N_{2B}	N_{3A}	N_{3B}	N_1–N_3 / Total
179	38	4	17	9	11	79 / 258=30.5%

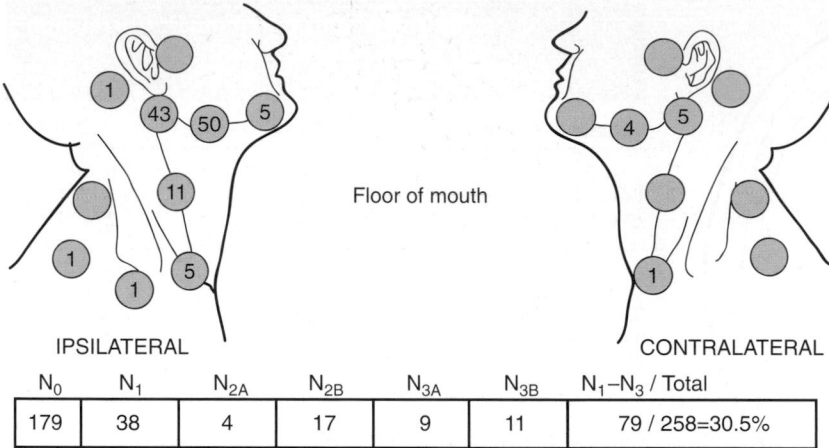

Figure 29-4 Carcinoma of the floor of the mouth: nodal distribution on admission to the M. D. Anderson Hospital, 1948 to 1965. (Adapted from Lindberg RD: Distribution of cervical lymph node metastases from squamous cell carcinoma of the upper respiratory and digestive tracts. Cancer 29:1448, 1972.)

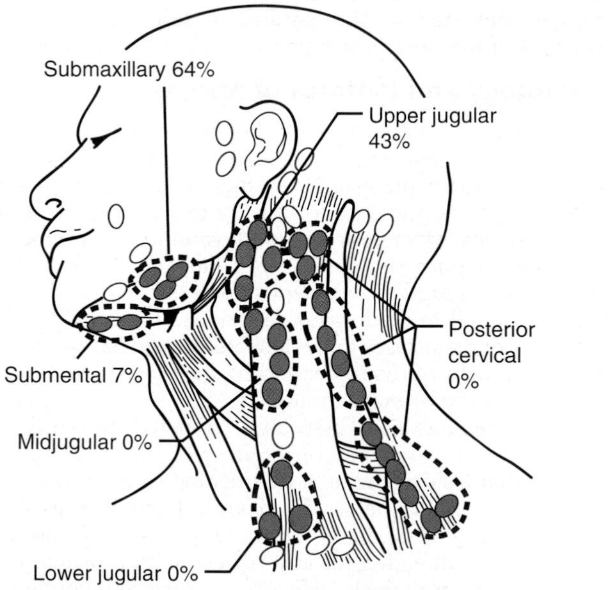

Figure 29-5 Distribution of involved neck nodes in the N0 neck after elective dissection in 62 patients with carcinoma of the floor of the mouth. (Adapted from Byers RM, Wolf PF, Ballantyne AJ: Rationale for elective modified neck dissection. Head Neck Surg 10:162, 1998.)

tongue. Advanced lesions tend to produce pain, bleeding, foul breath, loose teeth, and change in speech due to fixation of the tongue. Bimanual palpation is necessary to accurately determine the extent of induration and degree of fixation to the periosteum. Extensive lesions may exhibit invasion into the soft tissues of the neck or skin.

The AJCC staging system[45] (see Table 29-2) is based on tumor size and invasion of adjacent structures such as bone or soft tissue of the neck. Radiographic studies may facilitate staging with reference to the status of the mandible and teeth, the deep extent of the tumor, and the evaluation of the regional lymph nodes. CT should be done in essentially all patients. The mandible may be evaluated by panoramic radiography, dental films, and CT. Magnetic resonance imaging (MRI) is useful to evaluate marrow space invasion and perineural involvement.[84]

The role of positron emission tomography (PET) scanning as part of the initial staging work-up for oral cavity cancers has not gained widespread acceptance, although it may be useful in early detection of recurrences and for predicting which patients may benefit from elective neck dissection after chemoradiation.[85-89] The anatomic detail gleaned from PET/CT fusion seems to hold the most promise with respect to tumor staging and management.[90,91]

Treatment

Early Lesions (T1 and Superficial T2)

Surgery and RT produce equal cure rates for these lesions. The risk of RT-induced bone and soft tissue necrosis is significant; surgery is usually the treatment of choice. The neck is also treated with an elective neck dissection,[92] although some advocate observation of the neck in select patients with clinically negative nodes (cN0).[93] A treatment algorithm is shown in Figure 29-6.

Sentinel lymph node biopsy is being investigated for possible use in oral cavity cancers.[94,95] A study showed that this procedure was less sensitive for floor of mouth cancers (80%) compared with other oral sites (100%).[96]

Some patients present after excisional biopsy of the primary tumor. If the margins are either close or involved and if there is no evidence of visible or palpable residual tumor, an interstitial implant alone to the primary site is a good alternative provided that the depth of invasion is less than 1.5 mm. Reexcision may not be feasible because the surgeon does not know exactly what to remove. An additional advantage of RT is the ability to treat a larger area. Six patients were treated in this manner at the M. D. Anderson Hospital,[97] and seven patients were treated at the University of Florida.[98] All had disease locally controlled and none of the patients developed regional lymph node metastases. Conversely, Sessions and colleagues[93] have recommended reexcision rather than RT if close or positive margins are found on permanent sections.

Moderately Advanced Lesions (Large T2 and Exophytic T3)

Infiltrative lesions with fixation or tethering to inner tables of the mandible are best treated by excision with resection of the periosteum with or without a rim of mandible.[99] Postoperative RT is indicated for patients with close (≤5 mm) or positive margins, perineural invasion, and/or lymphatic space invasion.[100]

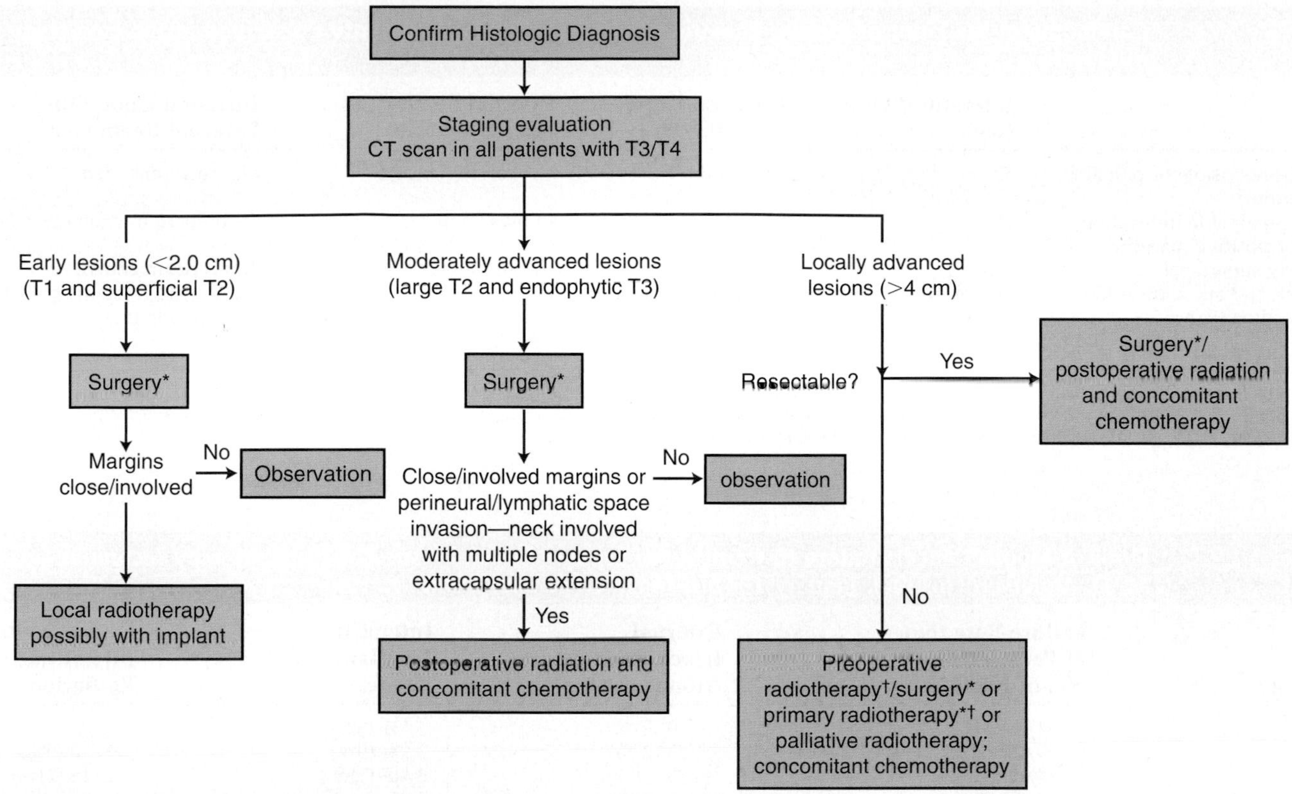

Figure 29-6 **Treatment algorithm for de novo floor of mouth cancer.** *Treat neck with dissection or radiotherapy in any patient with a primary lesion larger than 1.5 mm thick.[76] †May use concomitant chemotherapy.[204]

One common indication for adjuvant RT is the inability of the surgeon to obtain adequate margins of resection, because this often leads to local recurrence,[99,101-103] even if immediate reexcision is performed.[104] Jacobs and colleagues[105] and Laramore and colleagues[106] reported a large intergroup study where adjuvant postoperative EBRT (60 Gy) was administered for locally advanced cancers. They found that the relapse rate was 11% in patients with satisfactory margins and 26% in those with unsatisfactory margins. Unsatisfactory margins tend to reflect a higher residual tumor burden; it may be prudent to deliver a higher dose of postoperative RT. At the University of Florida, patients with involved margins receive hyperfractionated RT to increase the dose given to the primary site while attempting to minimize the potential late morbidity.[100,107]

Lapeyre and associates[108] reported on 36 patients with oral tongue or floor of mouth carcinomas treated with brachytherapy after resection with close or positive margins. Local control was 88.5% at 2 years. Grade 2 to 3 chronic sequelae were seen in 3 of 19 patients (16%) with floor of mouth cancers. Raybaud-Diogene and colleagues[109] reported that the local relapse rate after RT alone was very high among patients with oral cavity cancers if their tumors exhibited both a high level of *p53* expression and a low level of *ki-67* expression. The authors concluded these patients may be better treated by surgery with postoperative RT or combined chemotherapy/RT rather than RT alone.

The neck should be electively dissected if it is clinically negative. If there are multiple positive nodes or extracapsular extension, postoperative RT is indicated.[46,100,110] Based on the latest results of the EORTC and RTOG trials, concomitant chemotherapy is generally recommended as well in high-risk postoperative settings.

Locally Advanced Lesions (Endophytic T3 and T4)

Patients with locally advanced floor of mouth cancers are treated with surgery followed by postoperative RT. In some cases, preoperative RT can be used for unresectable tumors. Patients with extensive tongue invasion with fixation or extension into the soft tissues of the neck, as well as those with massive neck disease, can be treated with palliative RT (30 Gy in 10 fractions or 14 Gy in 4 fractions over 2 days, to be repeated after 2 to 3 weeks).

Concomitant Postoperative Chemoradiation

The issue of whether concomitant chemotherapy is beneficial when administered with postoperative RT for head and neck cancer was recently addressed by two randomized trials (RTOG 9501 and EORTC 22931). Each of these showed an improvement in locoregional control and disease-free survival when cisplatin (100 mg/M^2) was given on days 1, 22, and 43 of the RT regimen.[111,112] Prior to that, two publications showed a similar benefit using concomitant chemoradiation, although an earlier review of the RTOG 9501 data that appeared in abstract form was inconclusive.[113-115] Severe acute effects are seen more frequently with chemoradiation compared with postoperative RT alone.[111,112]

Results

Outcomes after RT alone vary with the stage of disease and treatment technique. The RT schedules used at the University of Florida are shown in Table 29-6.[116] EBRT alone results in

Table 29-6 Carcinoma of the Floor of Mouth: Radiation Therapy Schedules Currently Prescribed at the University of Florida

	Interstitial Only (Gy)	Intraoral Cone Only (Gy)	External Beam Plus Interstitial (Gy)	Intraoral Cone Plus External Beam (Gy)
TX—no visible or palpable tumor	55	45 over 3 wk	Not recommended	Not recommended
TX—palpable induration or positive margins	65	55 over 4 wk	45 plus 25	15-18 in 10 fractions plus 50
Early superficial	60-65	45 over 3 wk	Not recommended	Not recommended
Early, 1-3 cm, induration	Not recommended	Not recommended	45 plus 25-30	15-24 in 10 fractions plus 45
Locally advanced	Not recommended	Not recommended	74.4-76.8 (1.2 twice a day) EBRT plus cisplatin	Not recommended

EBRT, external beam radiation therapy; TX, status postexcisional biopsy.
Modified from Million PR, Cassisi NJ, Clark JR: Cancer of the head and neck. In: DeVita VT Jr, Hellman S, Rosenberg SA (eds): Cancer: Principles and Practice of Oncology, 3rd ed. Philadelphia, JB Lippincott, 1989, pp 488-590.

Table 29-7 Floor of Mouth Cancer: Failure to Control the Primary Lesion Versus Radiation Therapy Technique—M. D. Anderson Hospital, January 1948 Through December 1968

Stage	Failure Rate (No. of Failures/Total No. of Patients)	External Irradiation Alone	Interstitial Irradiation Alone	External plus Interstitial Radiation
T1	1/49 (2%)	0/10	1/31 (3%)	0/8
T2	9/77 (11.5%)	5/23 (22%)	3/34 (9%)	1/20 (5%)
T3	14/60 (23%)	9/25 (36%)	3/17 (18%)	2/18 (11%)
T4	19/24 (79%)	13/16 (81%)	2/4	4/4

Data from Chu A, Fletcher GH: Incidence and causes of failures to control by irradiation the primary lesions in squamous cell carcinomas of the anterior two-thirds of the tongue and floor of mouth. Am J Roentgenol Radium Ther Nucl Med 117:502-508, 1973.

Table 29-8 Floor of Mouth Carcinoma: 5-Year Cause-Specific Survival Rates Versus Treatment Modality and cTNM Stages: Washington University (N = 227)

Treatment	All Stages (N = 227)	Stage I (n = 58)	Stage II (n = 51)	Stage III (n = 54)	Stage IV (n = 64)
Local resection	76.2%	81.2%	50.0%	100%	.0%
Composite resection	62.5%	25.0%	100%	100%	53.9%
RT	43.2%	41.7%	33.3%	33.3%	53.9%
Local resection and RT	60.9%	75.0%	41.7%	100%	100%
Composite resection and RT	54.9%	94.4%	75.9%	35.0%	40.0%
Significance level	$P = .158$	$P = .0032$	$P = .059$	$P = .0045$	$P = .401$

RT, radiation therapy.
*Significant $P < .05$ by χ^2/Fisher's exact test.
From Sessions DG, Spector GJ, Lenox J, et al: Analysis of treatment results for floor-of-mouth cancer. Laryngoscope 110(10 Pt 1):1764-1772, 2000.

lower local control rates compared with brachytherapy alone or combined with EBRT.[117] The M. D. Anderson experience with RT alone is depicted in Table 29-7.[118] The failure rates range from 2% for T1 lesions to 23% and 79% for T3 and T4 lesions, respectively. For T2 and T3 lesions, brachytherapy with or without EBRT appears to result in better local control than EBRT alone.

Sessions and colleagues[93] described 280 patients who were treated with surgery alone, RT alone, or combined surgery and RT. Tumor stages were T1 (106 patients); T2 (107 patients); T3 (40 patients); and T4 (27 patients). The local recurrences rate was 41%. The 5-year cause-specific survival rates by treatment modality are shown in Table 29-8.

Wadsley and associates[119] reported on 29 patients with oral tongue (n = 21) or floor of mouth (n = 8) carcinomas treated with ^{192}Ir brachytherapy at the Royal Berkshire Hospital; 7 patients (24%) experienced a local recurrence.

One hundred sixty patients with T1 (79 patients) and T2 (81 patients) floor of mouth cancers were treated at the Institut Gustave-Roussy with low-dose-rate ^{192}Ir brachytherapy.[120] One hundred twenty-seven patients had a clinically negative neck and 33 patients (21%) had N1 neck disease. Patients with T2 and/or N1 lesions underwent a neck dissection. With a minimum follow-up of 9 years, local control rates were 93% for T1 cancers and 88% for T2 tumors.

Table 29-9 **Floor of Mouth Carcinoma: Initial and Ultimate Local Control Rates*: University of Florida (N = 194 patients)**

T Stage	Radiation Therapy Alone	Surgery Alone	Surgery and Radiation Therapy
T1			
Initial	32/37 (86%)	9/10 (90%)	1/1 (100%)
Ultimate	35/37 (94%)	9/10 (90%)	1/1 (100%)
T2			
Initial	25/36 (69%)	9/12 (75%)	7/7 (100%)
Ultimate	31/36 (86%)	10/12 (83%)	7/7 (100%)
T3			
Initial	11/20 (55%)	†	9/9 (100%)
Ultimate	13/20 (65%)	†	9/9 (100%)
T4			
Initial	2/5 (40%)	1/2 (50%)	5/8 (63%)
Ultimate	2/5 (40%)	1/2 (50%)	5/8 (63%)

*Grouped by initial treatment to the primary site. Forty-seven patients were excluded from local control analysis because they died within 2 years of treatment with the primary site continuously disease free.

†No patients in category.

From Rodgers LW Jr, Stringer SP, Mendenhall WM, et al: Management of squamous cell carcinoma of the floor of mouth. Head Neck 15:16-19, 1993.

Pernot and colleagues[121] reported 207 patients with floor of mouth carcinomas treated with EBRT and ^{192}Ir brachytherapy (105 patients) or brachytherapy alone (102 patients). Tumor stages were 41% for Tl; 48%, T2; 8%, T3; 2%, T4; and 1%, Tx. Neck stages were 83% for NO; 12%, Nl; 3%, N2; and 2%, N3. The 5-year local control rates were 97%, 72%, and 51% for Tl, T2, and T3 tumors, respectively. The 5-year cause-specific survival rates were T1, 88%; T2, 47%; and T3, 36%.

Rodgers and associates[122] reviewed 194 patients treated at the University of Florida. Patients with advanced lesions (T3, T4) had lower control rates when treated with RT or surgery alone compared with those treated with combined surgery and RT (Table 29-9). The 5-year cause-specific survival rates were stage I, 96%; stage II, 70%; stage III, 67%; and stage IVA, 44%.

Techniques of Irradiation

Because of the proximity of the gingival ridge, which is vulnerable to high-dose RT–induced soft tissue injury or osteoradionecrosis, the floor of the mouth has a lower RT tolerance than other portions of the oral cavity. Therefore, pre- and post-RT oral care is critical.

T1 and T2 Cancers

Patients with superficial (≤4 mm thick), well-differentiated squamous cell carcinoma of the floor of mouth may be treated either with brachytherapy alone or, when accessible, with intraoral cone RT. Brachytherapy is not feasible if the tumor abuts or extends onto the mandibular alveolar ridge, because of the risk of a bone exposure. Brachytherapy may be performed using rigid cesium needles mounted in a customized template or with iridium using the plastic tube technique. The rigid needles are preferable because, although the needles are active, the implant can be accomplished rapidly because the needles are mounted in a rigid template[123,124] (Figs. 29-7 and 29-8). An additional advantage of this technique is that the geometry of the implant is optimal and dosimetry can be obtained before the implant. The vertical needles are spaced approximately 1 cm apart with a crosser to ensure adequate surface dose. The implant is anchored in place by a suture placed through the submentum into the floor of mouth.

Intraoral cone RT is administered with either orthovoltage x-rays or electrons. Orthovoltage x-rays are preferred because there is less beam constriction and the surface dose is higher. Before each treatment, it is necessary for the radiation oncologist to verify the position of the tumor relative to the intraoral cone.[125] Because a small volume of tissue is included in the intraoral cone field, the dose per fraction may be increased to 2.5 to 3.0 Gy once daily.

Cancers thicker than 4 mm and those that are poorly differentiated have an increased risk of subclinical disease in the regional nodes. The first echelon nodes for the floor of mouth

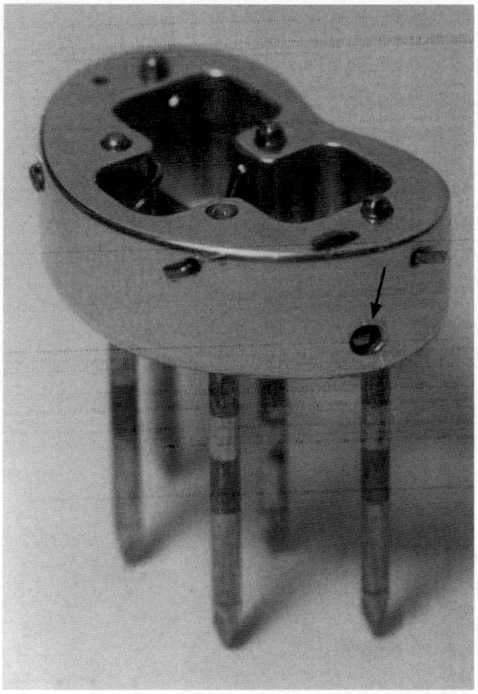

Figure 29-7 Custom-made implant device for stage T1-2 cancers of the floor of the mouth. Notice the single crossing needle through the center of the device (*arrows*). The device is now machined from nylon, and cesium needles have replaced the radium needles. (Adapted from Marcus RB Jr, Million RR, Mitchell TA: A preloaded, custom-designed implantation device for stage T1-T2 carcinoma of the floor of mouth. Int J Radiat Oncol Biol Phys 6:112, 1980.)

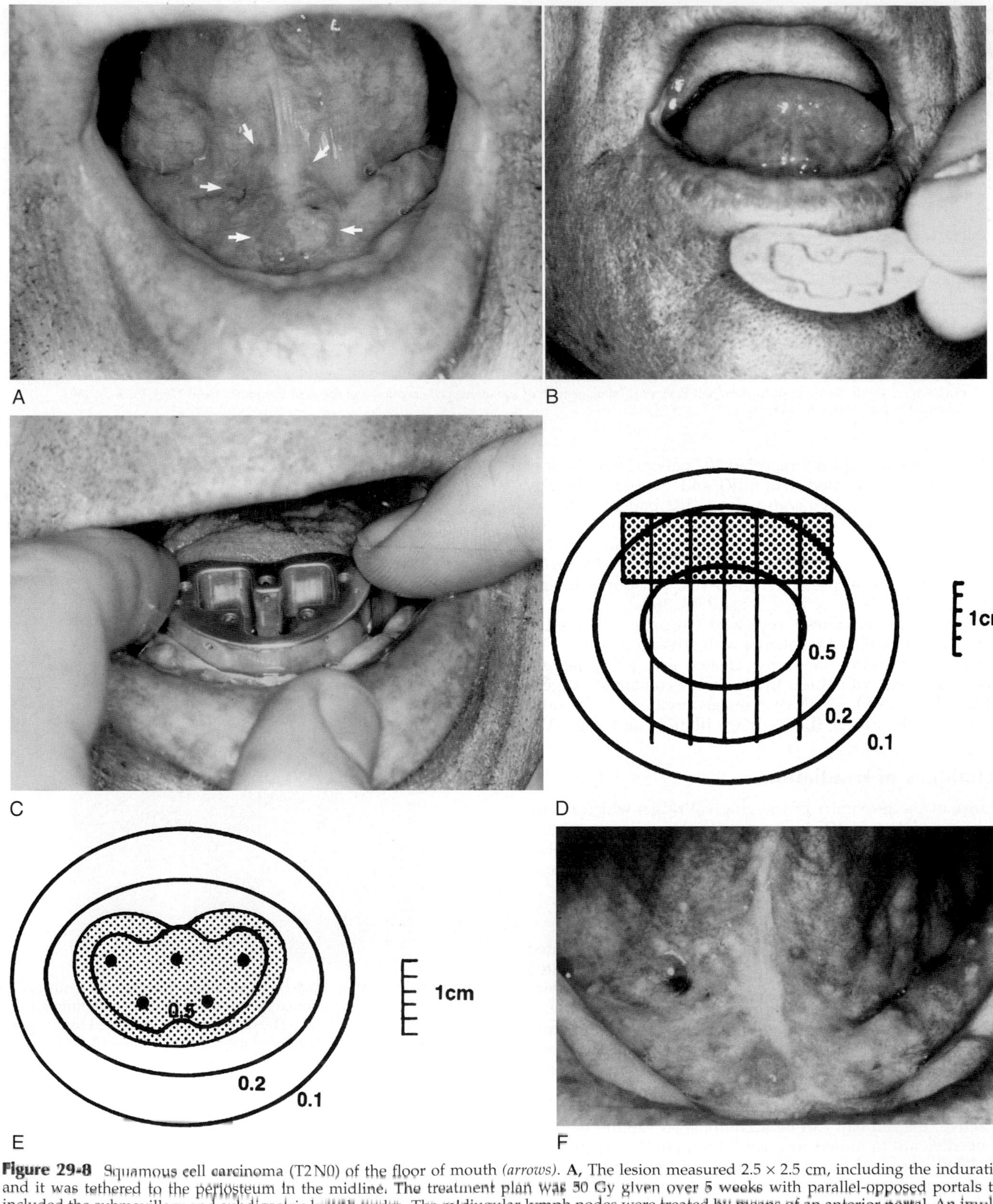

Figure 29-8 Squamous cell carcinoma (T2N0) of the floor of mouth *(arrows)*. **A,** The lesion measured 2.5 × 2.5 cm, including the induration, and it was tethered to the periosteum in the midline. The treatment plan was 50 Gy given over 5 weeks with parallel-opposed portals that included the submaxillary and subdigastric lymph nodes. The midjugular lymph nodes were treated by means of an anterior portal. An implant was planned to add 15 Gy. **B,** A cardboard template used for the design of the radium needle holder. **C,** Implant in position. The device was secured with two sutures from the submental skin. There were five 2.0-cm active-length, full-intensity needles without crossing. **D,** Sagittal isodose distribution. The 0.5-Gy/h isodose line was selected for specification at dose, and the implant remained in place for 30 hours. The *stippled area* represents the implant device. **E,** Midplane isodose distribution. The 0.5-Gy/h isodose line is approximately 1 mm outside the needles. The highest dose rate to the anterior lingual gingiva would be about 0.30 to 0.35 Gy/h or at least 4.5 Gy lower than the minimum tumor dose. **F,** The patient was free of disease at 4 years 8 months and had no complications. (From Million RR, Cassisi NJ, Mancuso AA: Oral cavity. *In* Million RR, Cassisi NJ (eds): Management of Head and Neck Cancer: A Multidisciplinary Approach, 2nd ed. Philadelphia, JB Lippincott, 1994, pp 321-400.)

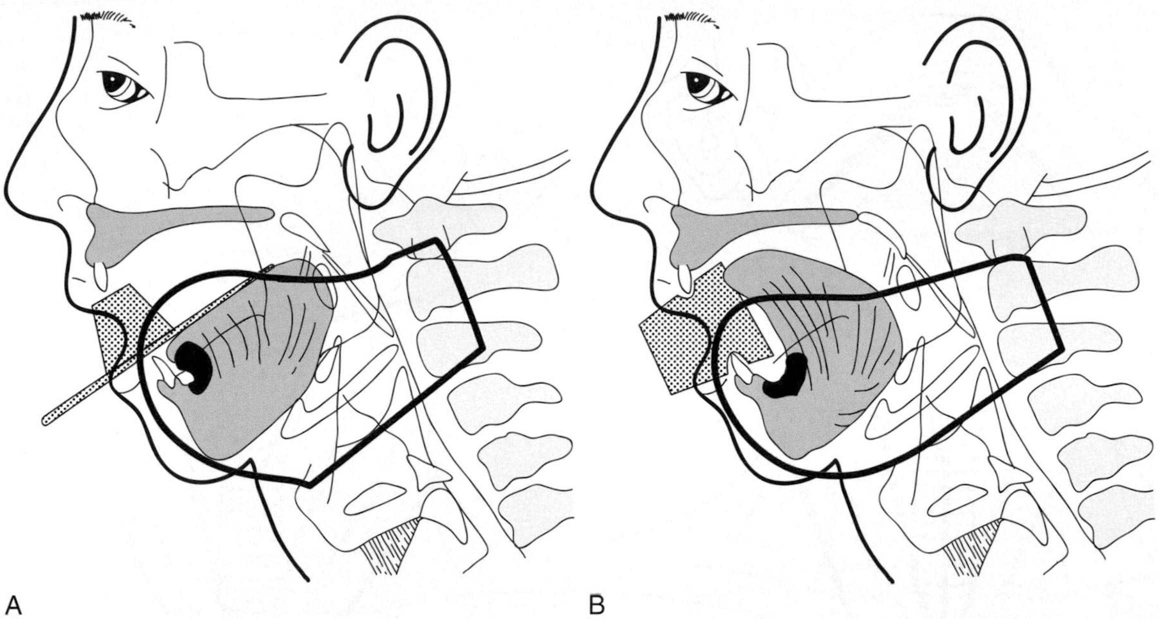

Figure 29-9 **A,** Portal for the treatment of carcinoma of the floor of the mouth with tongue invasion. The tongue is depressed into the floor of the mouth with a tongue blade and cork. **B,** Portal for irradiation of limited anterior floor of the mouth carcinoma without tongue invasion. Two notches are cut on a cork so it can be held in the same position between the patient's upper and lower incisors during every treatment session. The tip of the tongue is displaced from the treatment field. The anterior border of the field covers the full thickness of the mandibular arch. The lower field edge is at the thyroid cartilage, ensuring adequate coverage of the submandibular lymph nodes. The superior border is shaped so that much of the oral cavity, oropharynx, and parotid glands are out of the portal. The minimum tumor dose is specified at the primary site (i.e., not along the central axis of the portal) with the aid of computer dosimetry. (Adapted from Parsons JT, Mendenhall WM, Moore GJ, Million RR: Radiotherapy of tumors of the oral cavity. *In* Thawley SE, Panje WR, Batsakis JG, Lindberg RD (eds): Comprehensive Management of Head and Neck Tumors, 2nd ed. Philadelphia, WB Saunders, 1999, pp 695-719.)

are the level 1 and level 2 nodes. EBRT is delivered with either 4-MV or 6-MV x-rays using parallel-opposed fields that encompass the primary tumor as well as the first echelon nodes. A cork is placed in the mouth to displace the maxilla and upper lip out of the fields[69] (Fig. 29-9). The external beam fields are treated to 46 Gy in 23 fractions once daily or 38.4 Gy at 1.6 Gy/fraction twice daily. Brachytherapy follows the EBRT if that is the technique selected to boost the tumor. If intraoral cone RT is selected to boost the tumor, it precedes the EBRT so the extent of the tumor can be optimally defined and because it may be difficult to place the cone after EBRT because of patient discomfort. The total dose ranges from 65 to 70 Gy.

The low neck is irradiated with an anterior field, using 4-MV or 6-MV x-rays to 50 Gy in 25 fractions or 40.5 Gy in 15 fractions. The latter schedule is preferred if treatment to the upper neck is to be completed in less than 25 fractions. A tapered midline block is used to shield the larynx. The junction between the parallel-opposed fields and the low neck field is at the thyroid notch[126] (Fig. 29-10).

T3 and T4 Cancers

The likelihood of cure without a major complication after primary RT is low. If patients are treated with curative intent, postoperative RT is combined with resection of the primary tumor and a neck dissection. The fields are similar to those described for patients treated with RT alone. The superior border of the field is extended to the skull base if there are multiple positive nodes and/or extracapsular extension. The portals are reduced off the spinal cord at 44 to 46 Gy and, if necessary, the neck posterior to the reduced fields may be irradiated with 8- to 10-MeV electrons. Petroleum jelly gauze bolus is placed on the incision to ensure an adequate surface dose. Patients with negative margins generally receive 60 Gy at 2 Gy/fraction. Altered fractionation should be considered for patients with positive margins and for those with a greater than 6-week interval between surgery and initiation of postoperative RT. The preferred schedule at the University of Florida is 74.4 Gy at 1.2 Gy/fraction administered twice daily in a continuous course over 6.5 weeks, usually with concomitant cisplatin.

An occasional patient may present with an incompletely resectable tumor, usually because of fixed neck disease. In this event, RT precedes surgery in an effort to render the tumor resectable. Approximately 46 to 50 Gy is delivered to the primary tumor and both sides of the neck followed by a reduction and a boost to the area limiting resection to 60 to 70 Gy.

Patients with advanced disease and a remote chance of cure are treated with palliative intent. The dose fractionation schedules used at the University of Florida are 20 Gy in 2 fractions with a 1-week interfraction interval or 30 Gy in 10 fractions over 2 weeks.

Complications

A limited soft tissue necrosis may develop in the floor of the mouth, usually at the site of the original lesion. These ulcers are painful and usually respond to local anesthetic measures (Xylocaine), antibiotics, and time. If the ulceration develops on the gingiva, the underlying mandible may be exposed. It is recommended to discontinue dentures, apply a local anesthetic and administer antibiotics. Data suggest that pentoxifylline, 400 mg three or four times daily, may be beneficial in this setting and may reduce late RT-induced fibrosis.[127-129] The mechanism of injury is not entirely clear, although tumor necrosis factor-α and fibroblast growth factor 2 have been shown to be abnormally elevated in irradiated tissues and

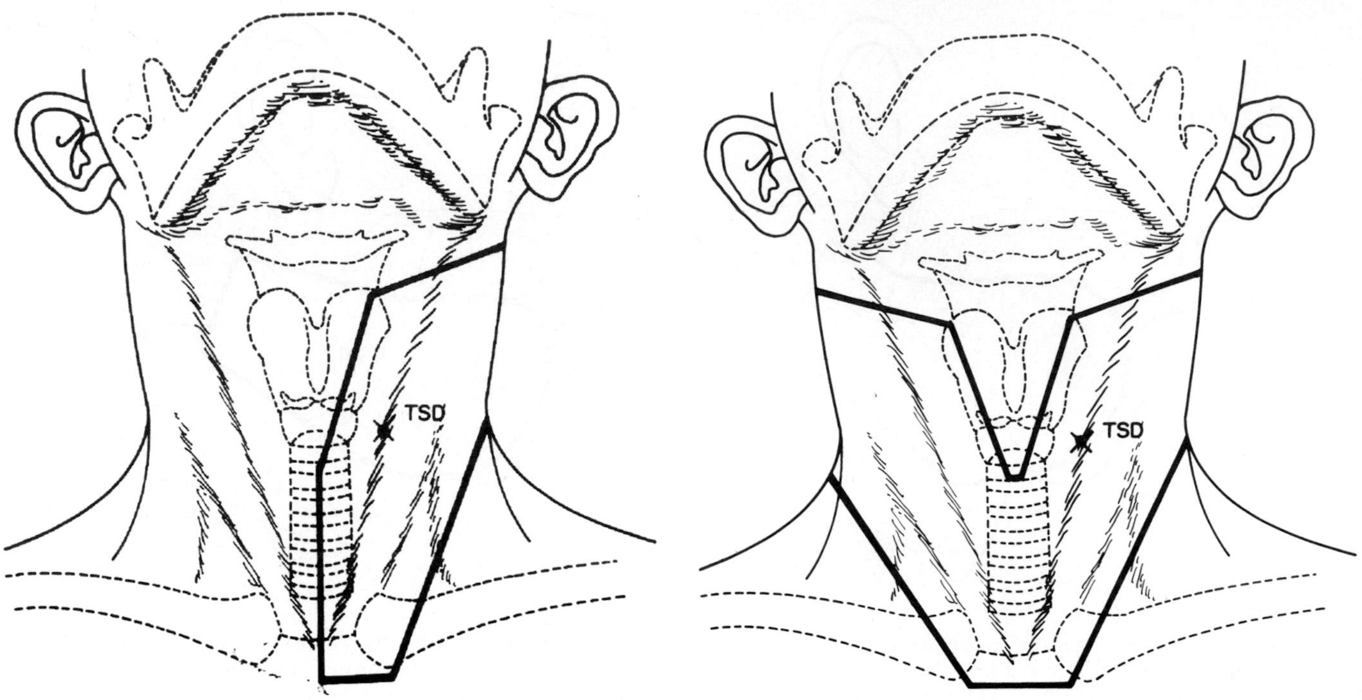

A B

Figure 29-10 **A,** Portal used to irradiate the ipsilateral neck. In patients with N0 disease, the nodes in the lateral supraclavicular fossa are at very low risk for disease spread and are not irradiated electively. **B,** Fields for bilateral radiation therapy of the N0 neck. The larynx shield should be carefully designed. Because the internal jugular vein lymph nodes lie adjacent to the posterolateral margin of the thyroid cartilage, the shield cannot cover the entire cartilage without producing a low-dose area in these nodes. A common error in the treatment of the lower neck is to extend the low neck portal laterally out to the shoulders, encompassing lateral supraclavicular lymph nodes that are at negligible risk while partially shielding the high-risk midjugular lymph nodes with a large rectangular laryngeal block. The inferior extent of the shield is at the cricoid cartilage or first or second tracheal ring. The shield must be tapered because the nodes tend to lie closer to the midline as the lower neck is approached. (From Parsons JT, Mendenhall WM, Million RR: Radiotherapy of tumors of the oropharynx. *In* Thawley SE, Panje WR, Batsakis JG, Lindberg RD (eds): Comprehensive Management of Head and Neck Tumors, ed 2. Philadelphia, WB Saunders, 1999, pp 861-875.)

may mediate RT fibrovascular injury.[128] If the soft tissue or bone necrosis progresses, hyperbaric oxygen and surgical debridement may be necessary.[130,131] Eighteen of 194 patients (9%) treated at the University of Florida developed severe complications[122] (Table 29-10).

Sessions and colleagues[93] reported on 280 patients treated with surgery alone and/or RT. They observed late RT complications in 41% of patients treated by EBRT and brachytherapy, most of which appeared within 1 year of treatment. Surgical complications included infection (5%), wound slough (9.6%), orocutaneous fistula (6.1%), carotid artery exposure/blowout (1.1%), and delayed fatality (1.4%). Fifty-eight percent of these complications were related to the use of combined surgery and external RT.

Bone necrosis was seen in 18% of patients treated with brachytherapy for T1-T2 floor of mouth cancers at the Institut Gustave-Roussy; 2.5% were severe.[120]

Table 29-10 **Carcinoma of the Floor of the Mouth: Treatment Complications (N = 194 Patients)**

Initial Treatment	Patients With Severe* Complications	Patients With Mild to Moderate† Complications
Radiotherapy alone	6/117 (5%)	49/117 (42%)
Surgery alone	6/36 (17%)	3/36 (8%)
Surgery and radiotherapy‡	6/41 (15%)	8/41 (20%)

*Postoperative complications (myocardial infarction, pulmonary embolism, etc.), wound infection or dehiscence, fistula formation, or osteoradionecrosis requiring hospitalization or surgical intervention.

†Small bone exposure, soft tissue necrosis, or minor infection. Osteoradionecrosis or surgical wound complication requiring outpatient therapy only.

‡Preoperative or postoperative.

From Rodgers LW Jr, Stringer SP, Mendenhall WM, Parsons JT, Cassisi NJ, Million RR: Management of squamous cell carcinoma of the floor of mouth. Head Neck 15:16 19, 1993. Copyright © 1993 John Wiley & Sons, Inc.

ORAL TONGUE

Anatomy

The tongue is located in the floor of the mouth and, at rest, fills most of the oral cavity. It is involved with mastication, taste, and oral cleansing; but its main functions are propelling food into the pharynx when swallowing, and forming words when speaking.

The sulcus terminalis divides the tongue into the oral and pharyngeal portions; the oral portion consists of the anterior two thirds of the tongue. The tongue is attached to the floor of the mouth by the frenulum. The circumvallate papillae are the largest taste buds; they are 1 to 2 mm in diameter and lie anterior to the sulcus terminalis. The oral tongue consists of four muscles: the genioglossus, hyoglossus, styloglossus, and palatoglossus. They all originate outside the tongue and insert into it, and their function is to move the tongue. There are four intrinsic muscles of the tongue that alter the shape of the tongue.

The muscles and mucous membranes of the tongue have separate nerve supplies. The hypoglossal nerve (cranial nerve XII) is the motor nerve of the tongue. It descends from the medulla and exits through the hypoglossal canal, from whence it passes laterally between the internal jugular vein and internal and external carotid arteries to curve anteriorly and enter the tongue. It passes anteriorly on the inferior aspect of the hyoglossus muscle and then to the lateral aspect of the genioglossus muscle. Injury of the hypoglossal nerve results in paralysis and eventual atrophy of the ipsilateral tongue.

The lingual nerve, which is a branch of the mandibular division of cranial nerve V, is the sensory nerve for the oral tongue. For special sensations such as taste, the anterior two thirds of the tongue is supplied by the chorda tympani branch of the facial nerve (cranial nerve VII). The chorda tympani joins the lingual nerve and runs anteriorly in its sheath. The blood supply to the tongue is from the lingual artery; two lingual veins accompany the lingual artery. The deep lingual vein begins at the tip of the tongue and runs posteriorly in the median plane.

The tongue has a submucosal plexus of lymph vessels. There are three routes of lymphatic drainage from the oral tongue: the tip of the tongue drains to the submental lymph nodes; lymph from the lateral aspects of the tongue drains to the submandibular lymph nodes and from there into the deep cervical lymph nodes; and lymph from the medial tongue drains directly to the inferior deep cervical lymph nodes. Lymphatic drainage is unilateral; drainage to the contralateral lymphatics is unlikely.

Pathology and Patterns of Spread

Ninety-five percent of oral tongue cancers are squamous cell carcinomas. Leukoplakia is also common.[132,133] Verrucous carcinoma and minor salivary gland tumors occur infrequently.

Nearly all squamous cell carcinomas occur on the lateral and ventral surfaces of the tongue. Anterior-third (tip) lesions are usually diagnosed early. Middle-third lesions often invade the musculature of the tongue and subsequently extend into the lateral floor of mouth. Posterior-third lesions grow into the musculature of the tongue, floor of mouth, anterior tonsillar pillar, base of tongue, glossotonsillar sulcus, and the mandible.

The distribution of clinically positive neck node metastases on presentation is shown in Figure 29-11.[82] Forty-five percent of patients with cancers of the oral tongue have clinically positive nodes at diagnosis; 5% are bilateral. Byers and associates[83] reported a 19% incidence of subclinical disease for T1N0 and T2N0 lesions and 32% for T3N0 to T4N0 cancers after elective neck dissection. Ozeki and colleagues[134] have reported three cases with metastases to the lingual lymph nodes.

Clinical Manifestations, Patient Evaluation, and Staging

Patients with oral tongue carcinomas usually present with a sense of tongue irritation or of a mass in the tongue. Deep infiltration may affect speech and swallowing. Advanced ulcerative lesions are often associated with a foul odor and pain.

Palpation of the tongue and floor of mouth, visual examination, and assessment of tongue mobility will help define the extent of the primary tumor. CT and, to a lesser extent MRI, is useful for defining the deep extent of larger primary tumors and to assess the neck. The staging system is depicted in Table 29-2.[45]

Treatment

A treatment algorithm is shown in Figure 29-12.

Early Lesions (T1 and Superficial T2)

Surgery and RT are equally effective in controlling small oral tongue cancers. Superficial well-defined lesions can be cured using resection alone with good functional results.[135-137] Postoperative RT is recommended for close or positive margins,[103,138] multiple positive neck nodes, vascular space invasion, extracapsular extension, or perineural invasion.[46,100] Although the risk of a significant RT complication is low, surgery is the preferred treatment in the authors' institution because of a lower risk of bone exposure or soft tissue necrosis that may persist for months or years after RT.

Patients are treated with definitive RT if they decline surgery or are at high risk for operative complications.[139] RT

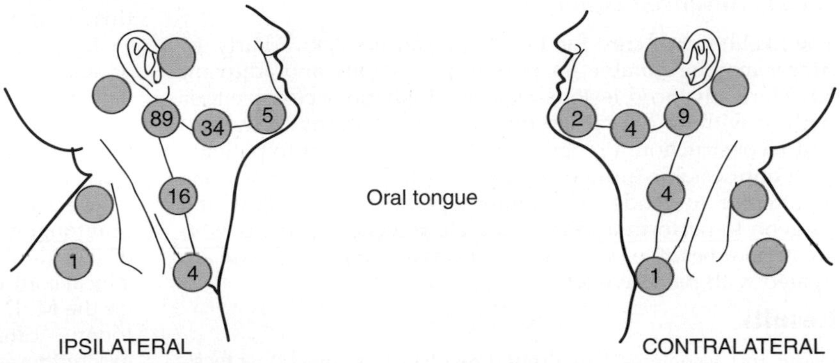

N_0	N_1	N_{2A}	N_{2B}	N_{3A}	N_{3B}	N_1–N_3 / Total
197	40	9	32	8	16	105 / 302=35%

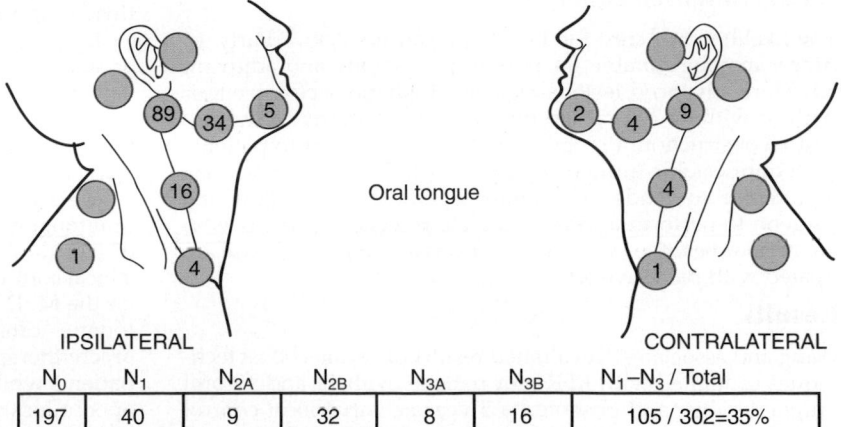

Figure 29-11 Carcinoma of the oral tongue: nodal distribution on admission to the M. D. Anderson Hospital from 1948 to 1965. (Adapted from Lindberg RD: Distribution of cervical lymph node metastases from squamous cell carcinoma of the upper respiratory and digestive tracts. Cancer 29:1448, 1972.)

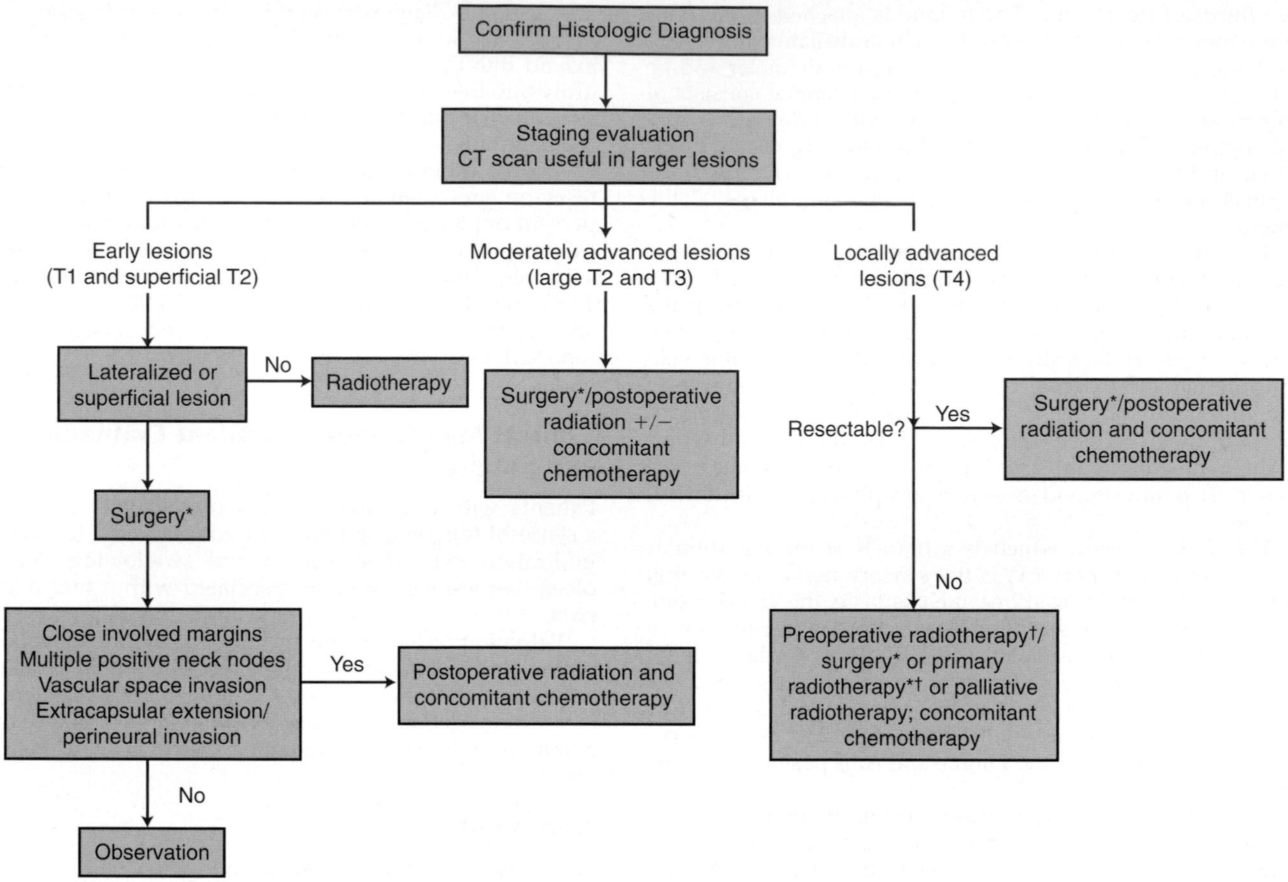

Figure 29-12 Treatment algorithm for de novo oral tongue cancer. *Treat with neck dissection or radiotherapy for primary tumors more than 2 mm thick.[135] †May use concomitant chemotherapy.

for early-stage oral tongue carcinoma can be given with EBRT combined with an interstitial implant or an intraoral cone boost, or with an interstitial implant alone.[118,140-142] The results of EBRT alone are suboptimal.

Moderately Advanced Lesions (Large T2 and T3)

Moderately advanced primary cancers are managed by partial glossectomy followed by postoperative RT. Preoperative RT is rarely used because it is easier for the surgeon to define the extent of the tumor in the unirradiated patient and because the risk of postoperative complications is higher.

Locally Advanced Lesions (T4)

The likelihood of cure for T4 tongue cancers is low. Early T4 cancer may be suitable for partial glossectomy and adjuvant RT. More advanced lesions require a total glossectomy either with or without a total laryngectomy (to prevent aspiration) and reconstruction. Preoperative RT can be given to patients with unresectable tumors, giving at least 50 Gy in 25 fractions to attempt to render the tumor operable or to allow the surgeon to perform a more complete resection. Patients who are in poor health or who also have advanced neck disease are treated with palliative RT.

Results

Wang and associates[143] evaluated results of various boost techniques combined with EBRT for patients with T1 and T2 oral tongue lesions, and observed a 5-year actuarial local control rate of 54% after an interstitial implant, 50% after intraoral cone orthovoltage RT, and 86% after intraoral cone electron beam. The reason that local control was better after electron beam intraoral cone boost compared with orthovoltage intraoral cone is unclear. Compared with interstitial implantation, intraoral cone RT is associated with a lower dose to the mandible and does not require anesthesia or hospitalization. It may also be associated with fewer complications. Physicians at Massachusetts General Hospital give 3.0 Gy/fraction for 8 to 9 daily fractions with intraoral electron beam RT (5 fractions per week) followed immediately by EBRT with 1.6 Gy twice daily for 12 days.[143] The patient is given a 1.5- to 2-week split and resumes RT to an external beam dose of 51.4 Gy; the total dose is approximately 75 Gy.

Intraoral cone RT with orthovoltage x-rays is preferred at the University of Florida.[124] Patients usually receive 3.0 Gy/fraction with intraoral cone treatment for 7 to 9 days for a total of 21 to 27 Gy followed by EBRT to 30 Gy in 10 once-daily fractions or 32 Gy at 1.6/fraction twice daily over 2 weeks to the primary site and neck.

Brachytherapy may also be combined with EBRT to treat oral tongue cancer.[136,141,144,145] Patients treated at the University of Florida with EBRT followed by an interstitial implant had a local control rate of 83%.[139] Wendt and colleagues[145] reported on the M. D. Anderson experience with T1N0 and T2N0 oral tongue carcinomas in which patients underwent either brachytherapy alone or combined with EBRT. Of eight patients who were treated with EBRT alone, five (63%) developed a local recurrence. Six of 18 patients (33%) treated with interstitial therapy failed at the primary site. In those patients treated with a combination of EBRT and brachytherapy, the 2-year local control rate was 92% for those treated with EBRT doses less than 40 Gy combined with a moderately high brachytherapy dose, compared with 65% for patients who received EBRT doses of 40 Gy or more with a lower brachytherapy dose.[145] A review of the pertinent literature supports the efficacy of the brachytherapy[117] (Table 29-11).

Subclinical disease in the neck nodes is common in patients with oral tongue cancer. Matsuura and colleagues[146] stressed the importance of elective treatment to the neck, especially as tumor thickness increases. In their experience, patients with tumor thickness of 8 mm or more were at an increased risk of nodal failure in the clinically negative neck. Wendt and colleagues[145] also showed the importance of elective therapy to the clinically negative neck. Failure in the neck occurred in 44% of patients receiving no elective neck RT; 27% of the failures were in patients receiving less than 40 Gy compared with an 11% failure rate for those who received 40 Gy or more. Byers and associates[147] recommended elective treatment to the clinically negative neck in patients with T2-T4 primary tumors. Haddadin and colleagues[148] observed that patients with T2 tongue carcinomas had a significantly better outcome after an elective neck dissection compared with those who were followed with salvage reserved until development of a regional failure (75% versus 39% 5-year survival rates, respectively). Based on a review of the Memorial Sloan-Kettering Cancer Center experience, Spiro and colleagues[135] recommended that elective neck therapy be given for primary tumors exceeding 2 mm in thickness because the risk of cervical metastasis approached 40% in this cohort of patients. O-Charoenrat and associates[149] found that increasing tumor thickness predicted for occult cervical node metastasis and poor outcomes in patients with stage I/II oral tongue squamous cell carcinoma treated at the Royal Marsden Hospital. Univariate analysis of disease-free survival showed poorer outcomes for patients older than 60 years ($p = .0423$) and with tumors thicker than 5 mm ($p = .0067$). The impact of tumor thickness on outcome ($p = .005$) was also appreciated in a multivariate analysis. They recommended elective neck treatment for tumors more than 5 mm thick. The use of sentinel lymph node biopsy and PET scanning may alter the treatment paradigm as more experience is gained in their use for oral cavity cancers.[150]

Fein and colleagues[139] compared the results and complications of treatment with RT and/or surgery for squamous cell carcinoma of the oral tongue. The control rates for RT alone or surgery alone or in combination with RT were the same for stage T1 and T2 lesions; combined modality treatment resulted in higher cure rates for T3 and T4 tumors (Table 29-12). In an analysis of patients with T1 and T2 lesions, those receiving less than 30 Gy of EBRT plus an interstitial implant had a better outcome than those receiving surgery plus or minus postoperative RT[139] (Table 29-13). For patients receiving

Table 29-11 Local Control of Oral Tongue Carcinoma as a Function of Radiation Modality Used

Reference	E + I vs E	I vs E	E + I vs I
Chu and Fletcher[118]	E + I > E	I > E	No difference
Fu and coworkers[141]	E + I > E	I > E	E + I < I*
Horiuchi and Adachi[140]	E + I > E	I > E	E + I > I†
Lees[142]	E + I > E	I > E	No difference
Mendenhall and coworkers[117]	—	—	E + I < I‡

E, external beam irradiation; I, interstitial irradiation; vs, versus.

External beam plus more than 40 Gy radium produced significantly better results than external beam plus less than 40 Gy radium.

*Local control alone not reported by T stage.

†Difference noted primarily in T3 and T4 lesions.

‡T2 lesions.

Adapted from Mendenhall WM, Van Cise WS, Bova FJ, et al: Analysis of time-dose factors in squamous cell carcinoma of the oral tongue and floor of mouth treated with radiation therapy alone. Int J Radial Oncol Biol Phys 7:1005-1011, 1981.

Table 29-12 Oral Tongue Carcinoma: Probability of Local Control at 2 Years According to T Stage and Treatment Method—University of Florida

	Local Control, % (No. of Patients)		
T Stage	Radiation Alone*	Surgery Alone or Combined With Radiation	*P* Value
T1	79 (18)	76 (17)	.76
T2	72 (48)	76 (19)	.86
T3	45 (29)	82 (24)	.03
T4	0 (10)	67 (5)	.08

Note: Numbers in parentheses indicate number of patients in each subset.

*Radiation alone or followed by a neck dissection.

Adapted from Fein DA, Mendenhall WM, Parsons JT, et al: Carcinoma of the oral tongue: a comparison of results and complications of treatment with radiotherapy and/or surgery. Head Neck 16:358-365, 1994. Copyright © 1994 John Wiley & Sons, Inc.

Table 29-13 Oral Tongue Carcinoma: 5-Year Cause-Specific Survival Versus Treatment and Stage Grouping (N = 279)

Treatment	All Stages (N = 279)	Stage I (n = 95)	Stage II (n = 85)	Stage III (n = 65)	Stage IV (n = 34)
Local resection	73%*	71.4%	86.7%	33.3%	—
Composite resection	60.9%	100%	62.5%	57.1%	40%
Radiotherapy	46%	75%	58.8%	25%	11.1%
Local resection and radiotherapy	65.4%	81%	50%	71.4%	—
Composite resection and radiotherapy	43.8%	100%	66.7%	33.3%	30%
Significance level	$P = .002$	$P = .770$	$P = .230$	$P = .225$	$P = .559$

*Significant at $P < .05$ by χ^2/Fisher's exact test.

From Sessions DG, Spector GJ, Lenox J, et al: Analysis of treatment results for oral tongue cancer. Laryngoscope 112:616-625, 2002.

RT alone, a dose of 1.6 Gy/fraction is given twice daily to 32 Gy followed immediately by an interstitial implant for an additional 35 to 40 Gy. This technique decreases the overall treatment time and avoids the large dose per fraction associated with 30 Gy in 10 fractions over 2 weeks.[139]

Chao and associates[138] reported on 55 patients with stage T1 and T2 lesions treated with surgery and postoperative RT. Thirty-nine patients received EBRT alone and 16 patients had an interstitial implant as part of the treatment. By adding an interstitial implant for patients with positive margins, the local control was equivalent to that observed for patients with negative margins treated with EBRT alone.

Sessions and colleagues[136] reported on 332 patients with oral tongue cancer treated with surgery and/or RT at Washington University. Tumor stages at presentation were T1, 116 patients; T2, 128 patients; T3, 71 patients; and T4, 17 patients. Local recurrences occurred in 34%, and 31% sustained a neck recurrence. The 5-year cause-specific survival rates versus treatment group for 279 of the 332 patients are shown in Table 29-13.

Techniques of Irradiation

T1 and T2 Cancers

Reduction of overall treatment time is key to the successful treatment of oral tongue carcinomas with RT alone. Patients with well-differentiated carcinomas that are 4 mm or less are optimally treated with brachytherapy alone (Fig. 29-13). Interstitial implantation may be accomplished using rigid cesium needles mounted in a bar or with iridium using the plastic tube technique. Rigid cesium needles mounted in a bar are difficult to position because of the length of the needles unless the lesion is relatively superficial. The plastic tube technique is preferred. The total dose varies from 65 to 70 Gy over 5 to 7 days.

Although intraoral cone RT has been used successfully to treat oral tongue cancers, it is often difficult to immobilize the lesion so that setup reproducibility may be problematic. If treatment with an intraoral cone is chosen, the cone is positioned so that the tumor is treated with a 1-cm margin. The intraoral cone therapy should be done before external beam treatment because of better tolerance and because the lesion can be clearly defined. Orthovoltage x-rays or electron beam may be used. If electrons are used, a beam spoiler or bolus is necessary to ensure an adequate surface dose. Additionally, a larger margin is necessary due to beam constriction compared with orthovoltage RT.

Patients who have poorly differentiated carcinomas, as well as those with 5 mm or more depth of invasion, should be treated with a combination of EBRT and brachytherapy. Parallel-opposed fields include the primary tumor as well as the level 1 and 2 lymph nodes. A cork and tongue block displaces the tongue inferiorly and the maxilla superiorly to minimize the amount of normal tissue included in the portals (Fig. 29-14). The fields are weighted 3:2 to the side of the tumor and either 30 Gy in 10 fractions once daily or 32 to 38.4 Gy at 1.6 Gy/fraction twice daily is delivered over 2 to 2.5 weeks with 4-MV or 6-MV x-rays. Although ^{60}Co is an ideal beam for treatment of patients with oral cavity cancers, it is not available in most clinics. The level 3 and 4 nodes are included in an anterior field as previously described. After EBRT, 35 to 40 Gy is added with an interstitial implant.

T3 and T4

Patients with T3 and T4 oral tongue carcinomas are difficult to cure with RT alone. The ability to adequately encompass the primary tumor with an interstitial implant is difficult for all but the occasional patient with a favorable low-volume T3 cancer. The risk of a major complication, such as a soft tissue necrosis and/or bone necrosis, is high after successful RT. Therefore, most patients are treated with surgery and postoperative RT. As for other sites, dose depends on margin status: Patients with negative margins generally receive 60 Gy at 2 Gy/fraction. Altered fractionation should be considered for patients with positive margins and/or for those with multiple risk factors or a greater than 6-week interval between surgery and initiation of postoperative RT. At our institution, the preferred schedule is 74.4 Gy at 1.2 Gy/fraction administered twice daily in a continuous course over 6.5 weeks. Concomitant cisplatin is also recommended for high-risk situations.

Radiotherapy portals are designed to include the primary tumor and both sides of the neck. The initial fields extend to the skull base to include the retropharyngeal nodes if the cervical nodes are involved. Petroleum jelly gauze bolus is placed on the incisions to ensure an adequate surface dose.

Patients with incompletely resected T3 and T4 carcinomas have a poor prognosis and are treated with RT from 74.4 to 76.8 Gy at 1.2 Gy/fraction twice daily over 6.5 weeks with concomitant chemotherapy. Patients are evaluated for resection of residual primary tumor (nidusectomy) versus an interstitial implant. Nidusectomy is preferred because of the high risk of necrosis associated with the addition of brachytherapy. Patients who have advanced, unfavorable oral tongue cancers and who are unsuitable for aggressive treatment are treated with palliative RT consisting of either 30 Gy in 10 fractions over 2 weeks or 14 Gy in 4 fractions over 2 days, to be repeated after 2 to 3 weeks.

Complications

After RT, patients may complain of a sensitive tongue, even after the mucosa appears to have healed. Taste tends to reappear from 1 to 3 months after treatment; because of xerostomia, taste perception is less sensitive than it was before RT.

Small, self-limited soft tissue necroses are fairly common. If these occur, recurrent cancer must be ruled out. If the lesion is thought to be necrotics, conservative treatment is instituted. The patient is examined frequently and broad-spectrum antibiotics such as tetracycline are initiated as well as pentoxifylline.[128,129,151] Viscous lidocaine can be applied to the ulcer for local analgesia. Hyperbaric oxygen treatment is indicated for larger progressive necroses that do not respond to conservative management.[152] Surgery is used as a last resort for large persistent necroses that are often associated with bone necrosis.[153]

Osteoradionecrosis occurs infrequently; the onset varies from 1 month to many years after RT.[154] It is more common in patients receiving higher doses per fraction and/or with tumor invading the bone.[155] If a patient has dentures, the dentures must be removed or altered by the dentist to avoid trauma to areas of exposed bone; healing may require many months. Management is similar to that for soft tissue necroses. RT-induced xerostomia is common and is related to the volume of salivary tissue irradiated and the radiation dose. Patients who are treated with brachytherapy or intraoral cone RT without EBRT usually retain salivary function.

Oral pilocarpine has been advocated by some for xerostomia.[156,157] Pilocarpine exercises a broad spectrum of pharmacologic effects, including increasing the secretions of exocrine glands, most notably the salivary glands. In a multicenter, randomized, double-blind, placebo-controlled trial published in 1993, pilocarpine produced a clinically significant benefit.[158]

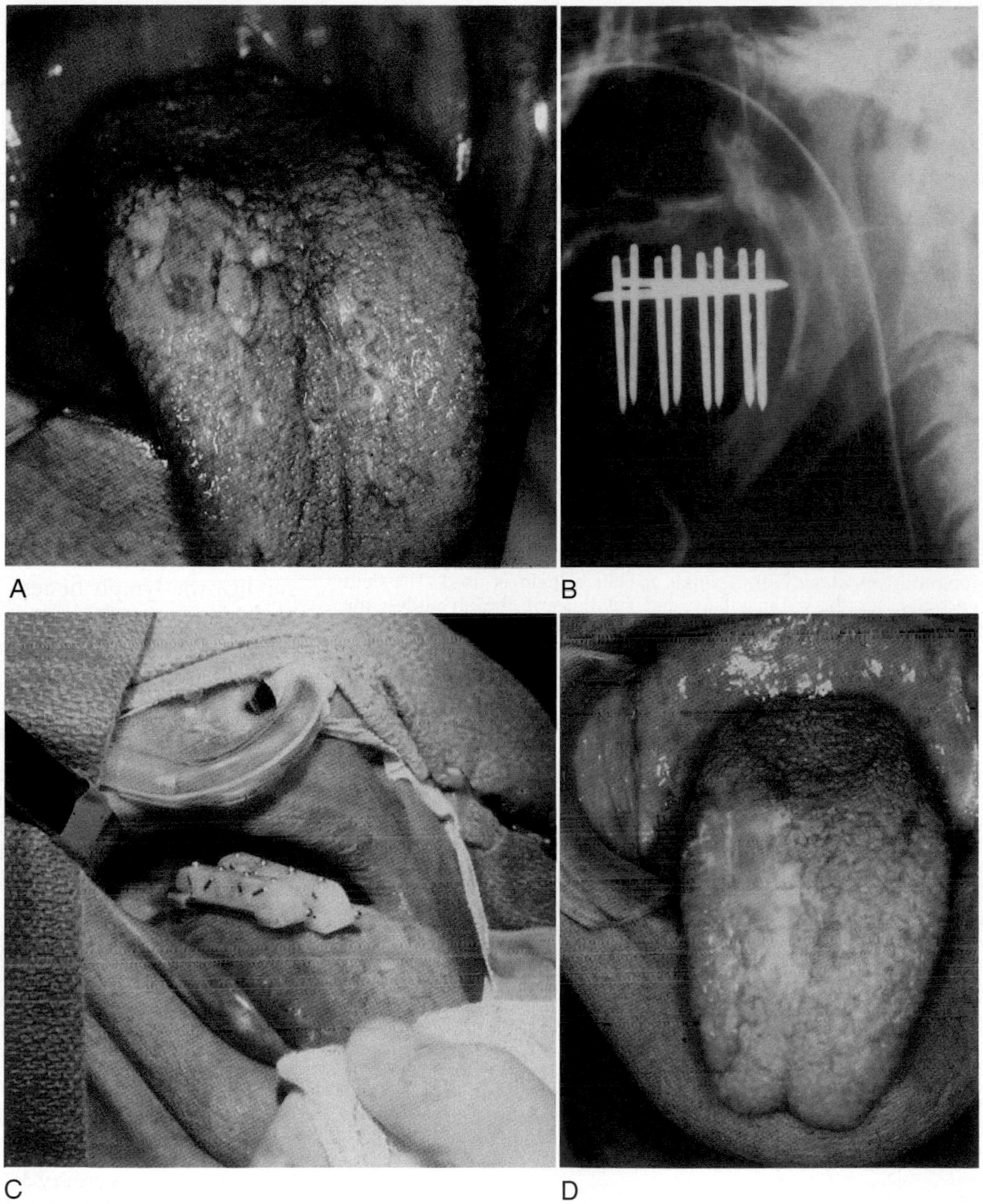

Figure 29-13 A 51-year-old man presented with a 3-month history of a painful sore on the right dorsum of the tongue. The lesion measured 3 × 2 cm and extended to near the midline. Biopsy revealed squamous cell carcinoma (T2N0). The treatment plan included using opposed lateral portals to deliver 30 Gy (^{60}Co) over 2 weeks and using a radium needle implant for delivering 45 Gy. **A,** Squamous cell carcinoma on the dorsum of the oral tongue. **B,** Radiogra of radium needles in a patient. The needles were mounted in a nylon bar. There were two crossing needles in the lateral bar and one crossing needle in the medial bar. The nylon holder assisted in maintaining the active portion of the needles above the lesion to give an adequate dose to the dorsum of the tongue. **C,** Radium implant in place. **D,** Complete healing at 3 months. There was no evidence of disease at 8 years. (**C,** From Hinerman RW et al: Radiation therapy in the management of the oral cavity cancer. *In* Werning JW (ed): Oral Cancer. New York, Thieme Publishing, 2005.)

However, its efficacy has been questioned by the outcomes of recent randomized trials.[159,160] The recommended dose is 5 mg, 3 to 4 times a day. The time interval necessary to achieve optimal results is 8 to 12 weeks.

Amifostine has been used more recently in an effort to lessen the untoward effects of RT. It can be administered either intravenously or subcutaneously.[161,162] The latter is generally felt to be more convenient and associated with less toxicity.[163] A full course of treatment with amifostine is quite expensive. This fact, coupled with its potential to cause nausea and skin reactions, has limited its acceptance in some centers.

At the University of Florida, the severe complication rate for 65 patients treated with surgery alone or in combination with RT for oral tongue cancer was evaluated. The findings are compared with the severe complication rate for 105 patients patients treated with RT alone in Table 29-14.[139]

Sessions and colleagues[136] reported major treatment complications in 21 of 270 patients (12.8%), most of which occurred in those receiving composite resection and RT. Complications associated with RT included orocutaneous fistula (6 of 224 [2.7%]), flap necrosis (1 of 224 [0.4%]), carotid hemorrhage (1 of 224 [0.4%]), xerostomia (7 of 224 [3.1%]), trismus (5 of 224 [2.2%]), radiation caries (3.1%), soft tissue ulcer (22 of 224 [9.8%]), bone necrosis (14 of 224 [6.2%]), and dysphagia (3 of 224 [1.3%]).[136]

BUCCAL MUCOSA

Anatomy

The lateral walls of the oral cavity are formed by the cheeks. The buccal mucosa is composed of the inner lining of the cheeks. It is contiguous with the lips and has the same structure. The muscle of the cheek is the buccinator. The buccal fat pad is superficial to the fascia covering the buccinator muscle and gives the cheeks a rounded contour.

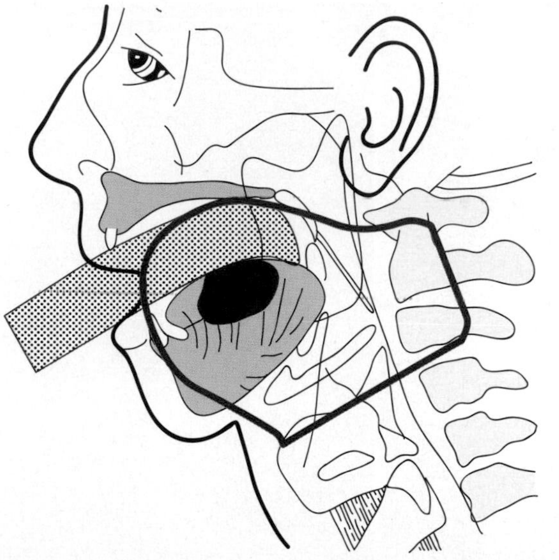

Figure 29-14 Well-lateralized squamous cell carcinoma of the oral tongue (neck stage N0). A single ipsilateral field is used. The field encompasses the submaxillary and subdigastric lymph nodes; the entire width of the vertebral body is included to ensure adequate posterior coverage of the subdigastric lymph nodes. Stainless steel pins usually are inserted into the anterior-most and posterior-most aspects of the lesion to aid in localizing the cancer on the treatment planning (simulation) roentgenogram and to confirm coverage by the interstitial implant. For lesions smaller than 2.0 cm in diameter, the low neck is not irradiated (unless the histology is poorly differentiated squamous cell carcinoma). The larynx is excluded from the radiation field. When possible, the anterior submental skin and subcutaneous tissues are shielded to reduce submental edema and late development of fibrosis. The upper border is shaped to exclude most of the parotid gland. An intraoral lead block *(stippled area)* shields the contralateral mucosa. The block is coated with beeswax to prevent a high-dose effect on the adjacent mucosa resulting from scattered low-energy electrons from the metal surface. The usual preinterstitial tumor dose is 32 Gy, using 1.6 Gy/fraction in a twice-daily fractionation schedule. For larger lesions that extend near the midline, treatment is applied by means of parallel-opposed portals with no intraoral lead block. (Adapted from Parsons JT, Mendenhall WM. Million RR: Radiotherapy of tumors of the oral cavity. *In* Thawley SE, Panje WR, Batsakis JG, Lindberg RD (eds): Comprehensive Management of Head and Neck Tumors, vol 1, 2nd ed. Philadelphia, WB Saunders, 1999, pp 695-719.)

Table 29-14 Oral Tongue Carcinoma: Severe Complications (N = 170 Patients)

T Stage	Radiation Alone*	Surgery Alone or Combined With Radiation	*P* Value
T1	1/18 (6%)	1/17 (6%)	.74
T2	6/48 (13%)	3/19 (16%)	.50
T3	1/29 (3%)	7/24 (29%)	.01
T4	1/10 (10%)	2/5 (40%)	.24
Overall	9/105 (9%)	13/65 (20%)	.03

*Radiation alone or followed by planned neck dissection.

Reprinted from Fein DA, Mendenhall WM, Parsons JT, et al: Carcinoma of the tongue: a comparison of results and complications of treatment with radiotherapy and/or surgery. Head Neck 16:358-365, 1994.

Branches of the maxillary and mandibular nerves (cranial nerves VII and VIII) provide sensory innervation to the skin, cheek, and the mucous membranes lining the cheeks. The facial nerve (cranial nerve VII) provides motor innervation to the muscles of the cheeks and lips. The lips and cheeks function together as an oral sphincter propelling food into the oral cavity. If the facial nerve is paralyzed, food tends to accumulate within the cheek along the affected side so that saliva and food dribble out of the corner of the mouth.

Pathology and Patterns of Spread

The majority of tumors originating from the buccal mucosa are low-grade squamous cell carcinomas that are frequently associated with leukoplakia. Verrucous carcinomas are observed more frequently in the buccal mucosa than in other parts of the oral cavity.[164,165]

Early lesions tend to be discrete, exophytic, mucosal growths. Advanced tumors tend to be ulcerated and are often associated with muscle invasion. Lesions that involve the lower gum may invade the mandible. Advanced lesions may extend to the soft tissues of the cheek.

The first echelon lymphatics are the submandibular and subdigastric lymph nodes. The incidence of positive nodes at diagnosis ranges from 9% to 31%; the risk of subclinical disease is 16%.[166] Bilateral cervical node metastases is very unusual. Advanced cancers have a higher propensity (60%) for lymph node metastases.[164]

Clinical Manifestations and Staging

Although pain tends to be minimal, even when the lesion is large, posterior extension may result in involvement of the lingual or dental nerves, which may cause pain referred to the ear. Extension behind the pterygomandibular raphe into the pterygoid muscles or into the buccinator and masseter muscles may cause trismus. Intermittent bleeding may occur when the lesions are irritated by chewing.

CT imaging can be used to evaluate the deep extension of the lesion, to detect bone invasion, and to assess the parotid and facial nodes.[84] The AJCC staging system is depicted in Table 29-2.[45]

Treatment

Early Lesions (T1 and Superficial T2)

The preferred treatment for patients with carcinoma of the buccal mucosa is surgery. RT alone is used to treat patients by default in the uncommon situation where surgery is not feasible. Patients with T1 and T2 cancers may be treated with a combination of EBRT and an interstitial implant.[164] A treatment algorithm is shown in Figure 29-15.

Moderate to Locally Advanced Cancers (Large T2, T3, and T4)

Superficial T2 and T3 cancers may be treated with RT; however, if there is deep muscle invasion, the cure rates after RT are poor.[167-169] The preferred treatment for patients with large T3 and T4 cancers is resection of the primary tumor in conjunction with a neck dissection followed by postoperative RT. Patients who are not surgical candidates are treated with EBRT and concomitant chemotherapy. Although it would be desirable to include brachytherapy as part of the treatment, the likelihood of adequately encompassing an advanced tumor with an interstitial implant is remote, and so these patients are treated with EBRT to 76.8 Gy in 64 twice-daily fractions over 6.5 weeks. The concomitant chemotherapy regimen that is used most often at our institution is once-weekly cisplatin, 30 mg/M^2.

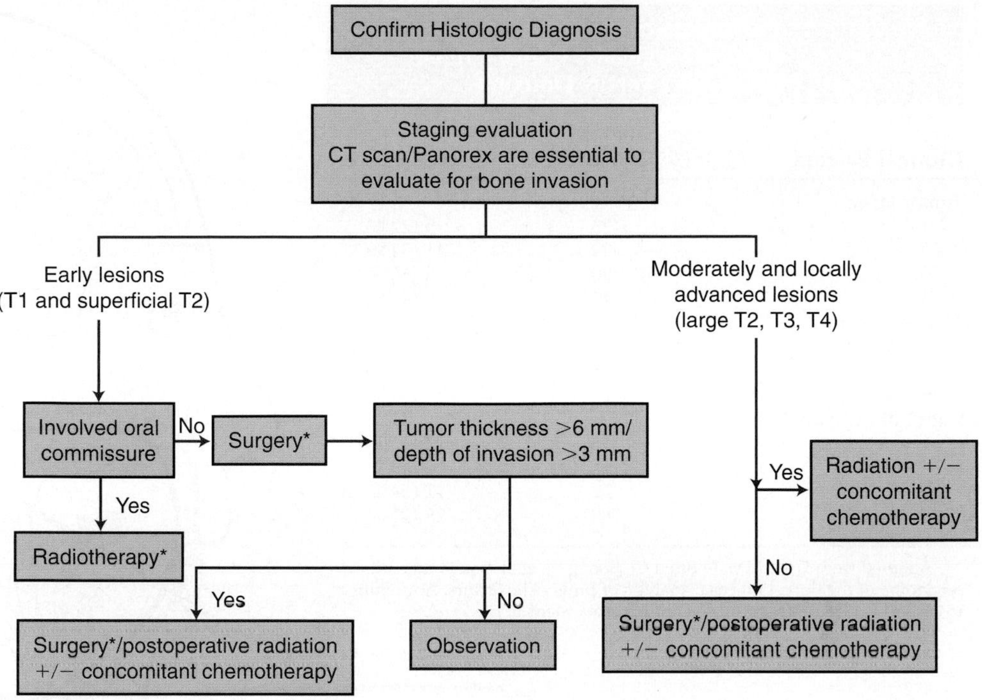

Figure 29-15 Treatment algorithm for de novo buccal mucosa cancer. *Treat neck with radiotherapy or neck dissection for T2-T4 tumors.[164-166]

The management of verrucous carcinomas is controversial because of the perceived risk that the tumor may become more aggressive if it recurs after RT. However, there is little evidence in the literature to support this theory.[170] Many tumors that recur after treatment (surgery, RT, or chemotherapy) are biologically more aggressive. It is reasonable to treat these lesions with RT if surgery is not feasible.[171] The dose is essentially the same as that prescribed for other squamous cell carcinomas. Wang[172] reported a series of patients with verrucous carcinoma treated with RT; the results were comparable to those for patients treated for squamous cell carcinoma.

Results

Five-year disease-free survival rates after RT range from 50% to 60%, depending on the stage of the primary lesion and the presence or absence of lymph node metastases.[79,165,172] Ash[79] reviewed the outcomes of 374 patients; 97% were initially treated with RT. The primary lesion was controlled in 52% of the patients; only 25% of advanced lesions were controlled. Nair and associates[173] evaluated the role of RT in the management of carcinomas of the buccal mucosa; RT was either administered with an interstitial implant consisting of 65 Gy over 6 days (45 patients), continuous course EBRT consisting of 52.5 Gy in 15 fractions over 19 days or 60 Gy in 25 fractions over 33 days (139 patients), or as planned split-course EBRT consisting of 35 Gy in 15 fractions over 19 days—3-week split—25 Gy in 10 fractions over 12 days (46 patients). The split-course technique tended to be used in elderly patients or for those with massive tumors. The results are shown in Table 29-15. Relapse at the primary site increased with T stage.

Urist and colleagues[174] reviewed results of 105 patients with squamous cell carcinomas of the buccal mucosa treated by resection of the primary tumor and neck dissection (Table 29-16). In a multivariate analysis, tumor thickness greater than 6 mm was the only significant prognostic factor. Depth of invasion greater than 3 mm was also highly significant but only in the univariate analysis.

Table 29-15 Results of Radiotherapy in Cancer of the Buccal Mucosa: Site of Failure Versus Stage

UICC Stage	Primary Failure, No. (%)	Nodal Failure, No. (%)	Total Failure, No. (%)
T1N0	0/13 (0)	0/13 (0)	0/13 (0)
T2N0	13/49 (27)	7/49 (14)	18/49 (37)
T3N0	15/49 (31)	1/49 (2)	15/49 (31)
T4N0	6/12 (50)	1/12 (8)	7/12 (58)
Any T and N1	51/94 (54)	48/94 (51)	55/94 (59)
Any T and N3	12/17 (71)	15/17 (88)	14/17 (82)

From Nair MK, Sankaranerayanen R, Padmanabhan TK: Evaluation of the role of radiotherapy in the management of carcinoma of the buccal mucosa. Cancer 61:1326-1331, 1988. Copyright © 1988 American Cancer Society. Reprinted by permission of Wiley-Liss, Inc., a subsidiary of John Wiley & Sons, Inc.

Diaz and colleagues[168] reported on 119 patients with buccal mucosal carcinomas treated at the M. D. Anderson Cancer Center. Eighty-four were treated with surgery alone (71%), while 22 received postoperative RT and 13 received preoperative RT. None were treated with RT alone. Thirty-eight patients (32%) experienced local recurrences. Five-year survival rates by T stage were T1, 79%; T2, 65%; T3, 56%; and T4, 69%. Muscle invasion, Stensen's duct involvement, and extracapsular spread of involved nodes were significantly associated with decreased survival.[168]

Chhetri and associates[175] reported on 27 patients treated with surgery at the University of California at Los Angeles School of Medicine. Treatment consisted of surgery alone in 15 patients, surgery followed by RT in 6 patients, and surgical salvage for RT failure in 6 patients. The 5-year survival rates were stage I, 100%; stage II, 45%; stage III, 67%; and stage IV,

Table 29-16 **Carcinoma of the Buccal Mucosa Treated Surgically: Primary Tumor Parameters Versus Outcome**

Clinical Factors	No. of Patients	Recurrence
Tumor stage		
T1	23	5 (22%)
T2	32	11 (34%)
T3	20	6 (30%)
T4	14	6 (43%)
Thickness (mm)		
<3	18	4 (22%)
3-5.9	26	6 (23%)
≥6	26	14 (54%)
Depth of invasion (mm)		
<1	13	2 (15%)
1-2.9	18	6 (33%)
≥3	22	12 (54%)
Total cases	89	28 (31%)

Adapted from Urist MM, O'Brien CJ, Soong SJ, et al: Squamous cell carcinoma of the buccal mucosa: analysis of prognostic factors. Am J Surg 154:411-414, 1987. With permission of Excerpta Medica, Inc.

78%. The locoregional recurrence rates were stage I, 0%; stage II, 27%; stage III, 44%; and stage IV, 0%, respectively. The 5-year actuarial survival rates were 80% after surgery and 82% after surgery and postoperative RT. Of patients who underwent surgical salvage after RT failure, none were cured.

Fang and colleagues[176] reported on 57 patients with buccal mucosal carcinoma treated with surgery and postoperative RT. Stage distribution was stage II, 6 patients; stage III, 21 patients; and stage IV, 30 patients. Total dose area ranged from 45 Gy to 68.4 Gy (median, 61.2 Gy). Eighteen patients (32%) sustained a local recurrence. The 3-year cause-specific survival rate was 62%.

Techniques of Irradiation

T1 and T2

The patient is immobilized in the supine position with an aquaplast face mask. EBRT is administered with an ipsilateral field arrangement that includes the primary lesion and the level 1 and 2 lymph nodes. The anterior and superior borders of the field should be at least 2 cm from the borders of the primary tumor. The posterior border should be at the posterior aspect of the spinous processes if the nodes are to be irradiated; the inferior border is at the thyroid notch. The oral commissures and lips are shielded if possible to reduce the acute effects. Patients may be treated with either a "wedge pair" of 6-MV x-ray beams or an en face "mixed beam" of 6-MV x-rays and electrons (Fig. 29-16). The electron energy used in the mixed beam technique varies depending on the depth of the tumor. Because of the steep falloff of the electron beam at depth, it is preferable to risk overshooting rather than underdosing the deep extent of the tumor and to use higher electron beam energies such as 15-MeV or 20-MeV beams. The RT dose fractionation schedule is 38.4 Gy at 1.6 Gy/fraction, twice daily. The ipsilateral low neck is treated with en face 6-MV x-ray field matched at the level of the thyroid notch.

If possible, a portion of the treatment should be given with intraoral cone irradiation or an interstitial implant to minimize the high dose volume and reduce the overall treatment time. Interstitial implantation is accomplished using ^{192}Ir via the

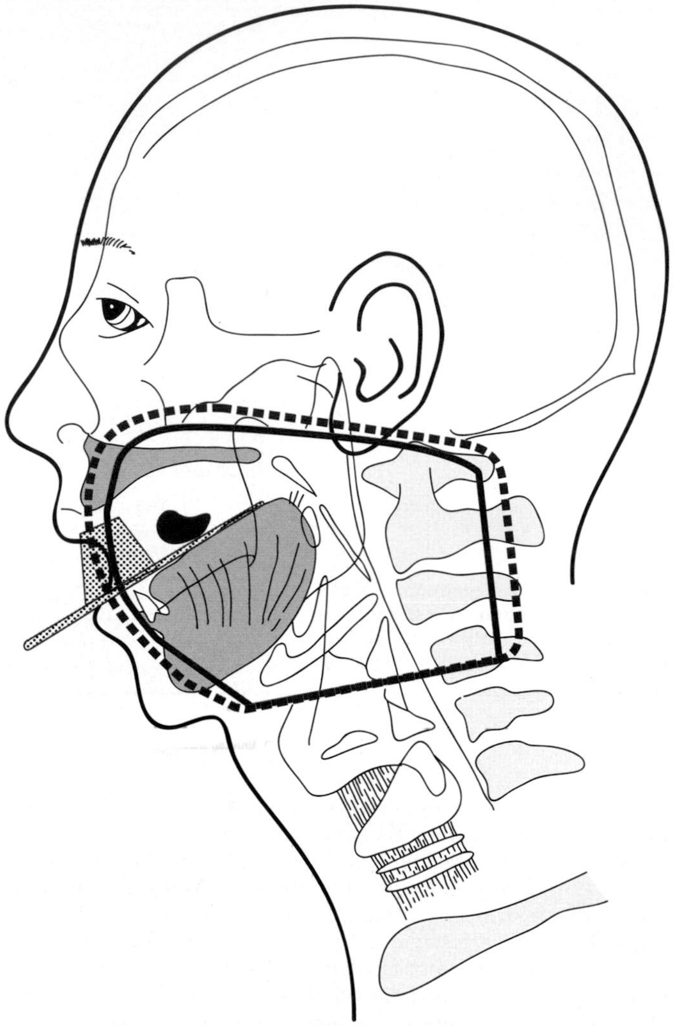

Figure 29-16 Buccal mucosa cancer treated with a mixed beam of ipsilateral en face 6-MV x-rays *(solid line)* and electrons *(dotted line)*. The electron field is 1 cm larger in all dimensions because of beam constriction, except where it matches the anterior low neck field at the thyroid notch. (Adapted from Mendenhall WM: Radiotherapy treatment technique. Cancer of the buccal mucosa. *In* Werning JW (ed): Oral Cancer. New York, Thieme Medical Publishers, 2005.)

plastic tube technique. The implant consists of a single plane of three to five horizontal tubes spaced 10 to 12 mm apart with crossing tubes at either end of the horizontal tubes. Ribbons containing ^{192}Ir seeds are afterloaded into the tubes to deliver approximately 30 to 35 Gy at 10 to 12 Gy/day specified at 5 mm from the plane of the sources.

T3 and T4

Well-lateralized tumors may be treated with the ipsilateral field arrangement as previously described. Patients with significant tumor extension toward the midline are treated with parallel-opposed fields weighted 3:2 toward the side of the lesion. Field reductions occur at 40.8 to 45.6 Gy and at 60 Gy. The low neck is treated with an anterior field with a 6-MV x-ray beam to 50 Gy in 25 fractions once daily. Thereafter, part or all of the low neck may be boosted depending on the presence and location of clinically positive neck nodes.

For postoperative RT, the RT target volume includes the primary tumor bed and ipsilateral submandibular and subdigastric nodes. Patients with positive ipsilateral nodes should be considered for RT to both sides of the neck. Patients with tumor stage T2 or higher, tumor thickness more than 6 mm, or depth of invasion more than 3 mm have a greater than 30% risk of local recurrence and should be treated with postoperative RT.[174]

Patients with advanced cancers unsuitable for aggressive therapy are treated with palliative RT. The fractionation scheme is either 20 Gy in 2 fractions with a 1-week interfraction interval or 30 Gy in 10 fractions over 2 weeks.

Complications

The buccal mucosa tolerates high-dose RT with a low risk of late complications. Trismus may develop if the muscles of mastication receive high doses of RT.

GINGIVA

Anatomy

The gingiva is composed of fibrous tissue covered by mucous membrane that is firmly attached to the periosteum of the alveolar processes of the mandible and maxilla. The lower gingiva includes the mucosa covering the mandible from the gingival-buccal gutter to the origins of the mobile mucosa on the floor of the mouth. There are no minor salivary glands in the mucous membranes of the alveolar ridges. The gingiva receives sensory innervation from the nerves supplying the teeth that are branches of V2 and V3 (buccal, infraorbital, greater palatine, and mental nerves).

Pathology and Patterns of Spread

Squamous cell carcinomas are most common, usually arise from the posterior portion of the mandibular gingiva, and are often associated with leukoplakia. Verrucous carcinomas may also occur, usually on the lower gingiva.

Squamous cell carcinomas of the mandibular gingiva may invade the underlying bone, retromolar trigone, adjacent buccal mucosa, and floor of the mouth. Byers and associates[177] reported that 22% had associated leukoplakia, 36% had mandibular invasion, and 5% had perineural involvement. Bone invasion usually starts because there is no complete bony barrier in the edentulous portion of the mandible. The lingual and buccal plates are relatively resistant to tumor penetration. Tumor entry through the mental, mandibular, and other small foramina tend to occur in less than 10% of patients.[178]

Metastatic spread occurs first to the submandibular and upper internal jugular lymph nodes. Byers and colleagues[177] reported 16% clinically positive nodes at diagnosis; contralateral lymph node involvement was found in only 3% of cases. Subclinical lymph node disease has been reported in 17% to 19% of cases.[177] The incidence of involved lymph nodes was 12% for T1 and T2 lesions and 13% for T3 and T4 stage cancers.[83] The distribution of positive lymph nodes after elective neck dissection is shown in Figure 29-17.[83]

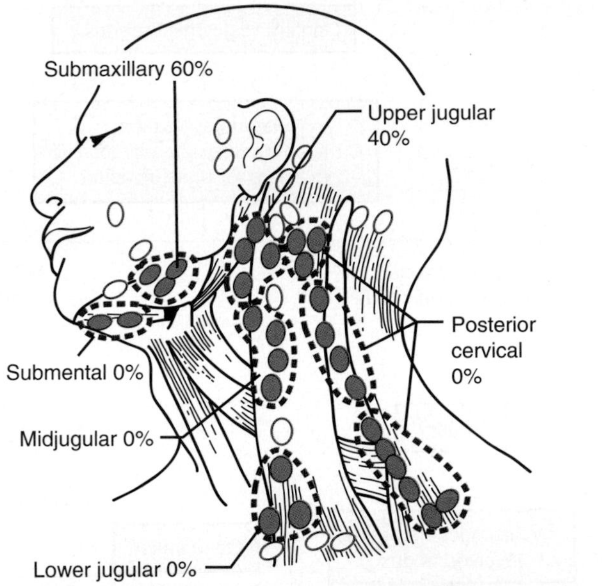

Figure 29-17 Carcinoma of the gingiva: distribution of involved lymph nodes after elective modified neck dissection for patients with a clinically negative neck. (Adapted from Byers RM, Wolff PF, Ballantyne AJ: Rationale for elective modified neck dissection. Head Neck Surg 10:163, 1988.)

Clinical Manifestations and Staging

The patient with squamous cell carcinoma of the gingiva may first present to the dentist with ill-fitting dentures, pain, loose teeth, or a sore that will not heal. Intermittent bleeding and pain may occur when the lesion is traumatized. Invasion of the inferior dental nerve may produce paresthesia or anesthesia of the lower lip.

Because bone invasion compromises the results of RT, careful radiographic examination of the mandible with panoramic radiograph, dental x-rays, and CT scan is essential. The AJCC staging system is shown in Table 29-2.[45]

Treatment

Early Lesions (T1 and Superficial T2)

The majority of these lesions are managed by surgery. Small lesions may be removed by transoral resection; however, rim resection is necessary in most cases. When direct bone invasion is present, removal of a segment of the mandible (segmental mandibulectomy) or maxilla is required. A treatment algorithm is shown in Figure 29-18.

Moderate to Locally Advanced Lesions (Large T2, T3, and T4)

Large lesions may require a hemimandibulectomy or partial maxillectomy.[179] Because of the likelihood of the local invasion through or along the subperiosteal lymphatics, RT is often indicated after resection to eradicate microscopic disease at the margins, to sterilize subclinical disease in the cervical lymph nodes, and thus improve the likelihood of cure.[46] Postoperative RT is also indicated in the presence of perineural invasion, multiple positive nodes, or extranodal extension.[100] Concomitant chemotherapy during EBRT is also recommended in the postoperative setting, as outlined elsewhere in this chapter.

Results

Cady and Catlin[179] reviewed 606 patients with squamous cell carcinoma of the gingiva treated by surgery. The survival rate was 43% for patients with mandibular gingival lesions and 40% for those with maxillary alveolar ridge cancers. Soo and coworkers[180] reviewed a 20-year experience with squamous carcinoma of the gums in 347 patients treated at the Memorial Sloan-Kettering Cancer Center. Sixty-four percent of patients presented with a clinically negative neck (N0). Ninety-seven percent of patients were treated surgically. The 5-year cause-specific survival rate was 54%. Advanced clinical stage (stages III and IV), prior dental extractions, bone invasion, and involvement of surgical margins were predictive of a lower survival rate on univariate analysis. Clinical stage was

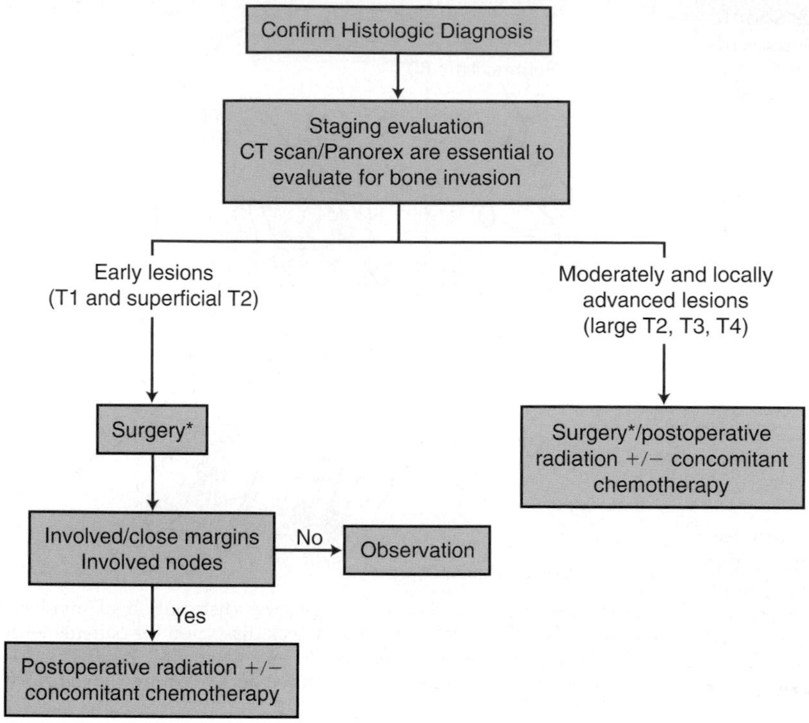

Figure 29-18 Treatment algorithm for de novo gingival cancer. *Treat neck with neck dissection.[83,177]

the only significant predictor of survival on multivariate analysis.

Byers and associates[177] reported a 5-year survival rate of 43% for patients with squamous cell carcinoma of the mandibular gingiva. Fifty-one of these patients were treated with surgery that included resection of bone in 28 patients with early lesions. Only 1 of 28 patients developed a recurrence. Segmental mandibulectomy and neck dissection were used for 23 patients with advanced disease; there were no local failures. Postoperative RT was given for close margins, nerve invasion, or extensive nodal metastases. For those treated with surgery and postoperative RT, control above the clavicles was achieved in 95% of patients.

Overholt and coworkers[181] retrospectively reviewed results of 155 patients treated surgically for carcinoma of the mandibular gingiva. Decreased local control was observed for primary lesions larger than 3 cm (p = .021) and persistently positive surgical margins (p = .027). Survival was adversely affected by advanced T stage (p = .001), positive initial and final surgical margins (p = .004), mandibular invasion (p = .014), and cervical metastases (p < .001). Local control and survival were not affected by extent of mandibular resection, tumor extension beyond the mandibular gingiva, recent dental extractions in the region of the primary, perineural invasion, or histologic grade.

Patients treated with RT alone for T3 and T4 lesions have 5-year survival rates ranging from 30% to 40%.[166,177,182] Wang[172] reported a 78% control rate for patients with T1 lesions and 27% for those with T2 cancers after treatment with RT alone. Fayos[183] reported a 50% local control rate after RT alone for lesions with early bone invasion and a 25% local control rate after RT alone for those with extensive invasion.

Techniques of Irradiation

T1 and T2

Patients who are not deemed to be surgical candidates are treated with RT. Small lesions may be treated by intraoral cone RT combined with EBRT. Interstitial implant has no place in the management of this disease because of the proximity of the bone and the high risk of osteoradionecrosis.

External radiation may be administered with either an ipsilateral en face combination of 4-MV or 6-MV x-rays and electrons or with two 4-MV or 6-MV x-ray beams arranged in a "wedge pair" (Fig. 29-19). The latter technique is preferred because it is possible to vary the depth of the target volume more precisely, and underdosing the medial extent of the tumor is less likely. Lesions that exhibit significant extension onto the soft palate or into the tongue (unusual for a T1 or T2 tumor) would be treated with parallel-opposed fields weighted 3:2 to the side of the tumor. The doses used are from 60 to 65 Gy over 6 to 6.5 weeks for T1, and 70 Gy over 7 weeks or 74.4 Gy in 62 fractions twice daily for T2 tumors. The low neck is treated with an anterior 4-MV or 6-MV x-ray field matched at the thyroid notch and receives 50 Gy in 25 fractions.

T3 and T4

Patients with T3 and T4 carcinomas have a relatively low chance of cure with RT alone and are optimally treated with surgery and postoperative RT. The postoperative dose varies with the margins: Patients with negative margins generally receive 60 Gy at 2 Gy/fraction. Altered fractionation is considered for patients with positive margins and for those with multiple risk factors and/or prolonged surgery-to-RT interval. At our institution, the preferred schedule is 74.4 Gy at 1.2 Gy/fraction administered twice daily in a continuous course over 6.5 weeks. As with other sites, concomitant cisplatin is also recommended for high-risk situations.

Patients are treated with parallel-opposed portals that include the primary tumor and upper neck nodes (Fig. 29-20). The fields are weighted 3:2 toward the side of the tumor. The anterior low neck is treated with an en face 6-MV x-ray field matched at the level of the thyroid notch. Petroleum jelly gauze bolus is placed on the incisions to ensure an adequate

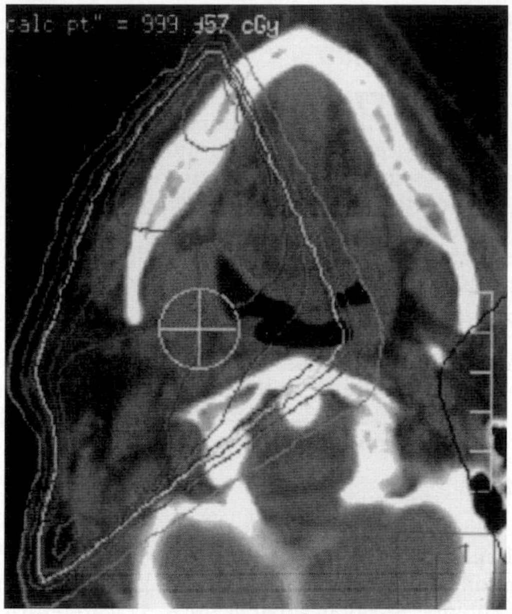

Figure 29-19 Patient with an early-stage carcinoma of the retromolar trigone. Radiotherapy is delivered with two 6-MV x-ray beams using a wedge-pair arrangement. (Adapted from Mendenhall WM: Radiotherapy treatment technique. Cancer of the maxillary alveolar ridge and retromolar trigone. *In* Werning JW (ed): Oral Cancer. New York, Thieme Publishing, 2005.)

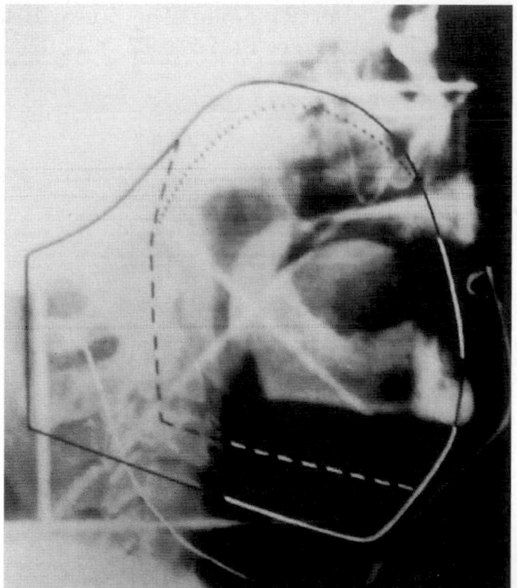

Figure 29-20 Typical portal for irradiation after hemimandibulectomy, partial maxillectomy, and radical neck dissection for pathologic T4N0 retromolar trigone lesion. Field reductions made at 45 Gy *(dashed line)* and 60 Gy *(dotted line)*. (Adapted from Mendenhall WM: Radiotherapy treatment technique. Cancer of the maxillary alveolar ridge and retromolar trigone. *In* Werning JW (ed): Oral Cancer. New York, Thieme Publishing, 2005.)

surface dose. Fields are reduced off of the spinal cord at approximately 45 Gy. An electron beam may be used to irradiate the posterior strips if additional RT to these sites is indicated after off-cord reduction.

Patients who are not suitable for surgery are treated with twice-daily RT to 76.8 Gy in 64 fractions over 6.5 weeks combined with concomitant chemotherapy. The field arrangements are similar to those previously described. We routinely exclude the spinal cord at 40 Gy if chemotherapy is used concomitantly. Patients who are unsuitable for aggressive treatment receive moderate-dose palliative RT: 30 Gy in 10 fractions over 2 weeks or 14 Gy in 4 fractions over 2 days, to be repeated after 2-3 weeks.

For postoperative cases, radiation portals include the adjacent segment of the mandible or maxilla. The entire hemimandible or hemimaxilla from the distal neural foramen to the pterygopalatine ganglion must be treated when perineural invasion is present. The low neck must be irradiated if involved nodes are present or if the primary tumor is advanced. Postoperative RT doses range from 60 to 75 Gy at 1.8 to 2.0 Gy/day. If the resection margins are positive, 74.4 Gy at 1.2 Gy/fraction, twice daily with a minimum 6-hour interfraction interval, is used at our institution. Cisplatin is administered concomitantly, based on the results of randomized data from the RTOG and EORTC.[111,112]

Complications

Surgical complications include orocutaneous fistulas and bone exposure. The complications of RT include dental caries, soft tissue necrosis, and osteoradionecrosis. The risk is greatest for more advanced lesions.

RETROMOLAR TRIGONE

Anatomy

The small triangular surface posterior to the third mandibular molar, overlying the ascending ramus, is called the retromolar trigone. Beneath the mucosa of the retromolar trigone is the pterygomandibular raphe, which is attached to the pterygoid hamulus on the posterior mylohyoid ridge of the mandible. It serves as the insertion of the buccinator, orbiculus oris, and superior constrictor muscles. Behind the pterygomandibular raphe (between the medial pterygoid muscle and the ascending ramus of the mandible) is the pterygomandibular space, which contains the lingual and dental nerves. There is a small fat pad between the pterygoid muscle group and the mandibular foramen through which the mandibular nerve passes before it enters the alveolar canal. The subdigastric lymph nodes are the first echelon nodes for the retromolar trigone.

Pathology and Patterns of Spread

The vast majority of these tumors are squamous cell carcinomas. The primary tumor may spread to the adjacent buccal mucosa, anterior tonsillar pillar, mandibular gingiva, and mandible. Posterior spread to the pterygomandibular space and medial pterygoid muscle may occur. Invasion of the periosteum may occur early. Byers and associates[184] reported a 25% incidence of bone invasion at diagnosis.

The incidence of clinically positive ipsilateral nodes on presentation is 39%, and the risk of subclinical disease in the cervical lymph nodes is approximately 25%.[184] The distribution of positive nodes after an elective neck dissection is shown in Figure 29-21.[83]

Clinical Manifestations and Staging

Retromolar trigone cancers tend to produce pain that may be referred to the external auditory canal and preauricular area. Invasion of the pterygoid muscles can produce trismus and is better demonstrated by MRI than by CT.[84] CT scan of the head and neck (and MRI in selected cases) is useful for determining the deep extent of the primary tumor bone invasion and presence of positive neck nodes. The staging system is depicted in Table 29-2.

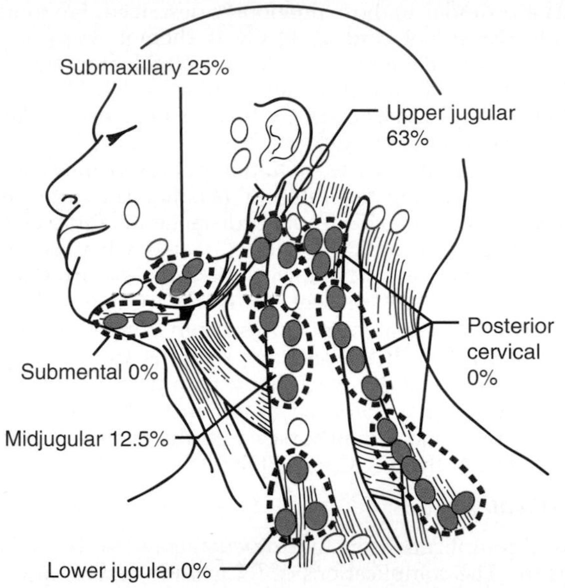

Figure 29-21 Carcinoma of the retromolar trigone: distribution of involved lymph nodes after elective modified neck dissection for patients with a clinically negative neck. (Adapted from Byers RM, Wolf PF, Ballantyne AJ: Rationale for elective modified neck dissection. Head Neck Surg 10:163, 1988.)

Treatment

Early Lesions (T1 and T2)

Local control rates for T1 and T2 lesions are similar following surgery or RT.[184] If the tumor extends to the tonsillar pillar, soft palate, or buccal mucosa and an extensive resection is required, RT is selected. If possible, intraoral cone irradiation should be used for a portion of the treatment. Small lesions without detectable bone invasion can be resected with removal of the periosteum or a rim resection of the mandible. A treatment algorithm is shown in Figure 29-22.

Locally Advanced Lesions (T3 and T4)

Superficial T3 lesions can be treated by RT. Locally advanced cancers (especially those with evidence of bony invasion) require a segmental mandibulectomy followed, in almost all cases, by postoperative RT.

Results

Lo and colleagues[185] reported on a series of patients treated with RT at the M. D. Anderson Hospital (Table 29-17). Patients with retromolar trigone cancers were grouped with those having anterior tonsillar pillar lesions. Local control varied from 70% to 76% after RT for those with T1, T2, and T3 cancers. Salvage surgery resulted in ultimate local control rates varying from 92% to 100%.

Huang and associates[186] reported on 65 patients treated for retromolar trigone cancer at Washington University (St. Louis). The 5-year disease-free survival rates were 90% after preoperative RT and surgery, 63% after surgery and postoperative RT, and 31% after RT alone. The 5-year disease-free survival rates by T stage were T1, 76%; T2, 50%; T3, 72%; and

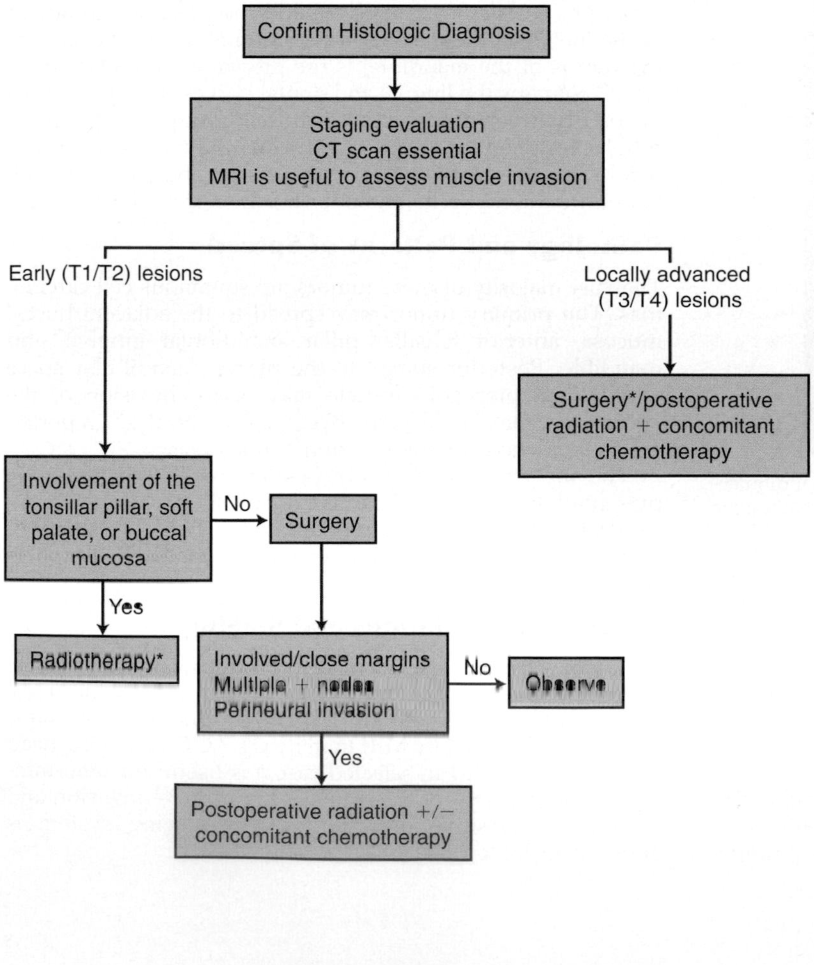

Figure 29-22 **Treatment algorithm for de novo retromolar trigone cancer.** *Treat neck with radiotherapy or neck dissection.[182]

Table 29-17 **Local Control Rates after Radiotherapy: Anterior Faucial Pillar-Retromolar Trigone—M. D. Anderson Hospital**

Stage	Local Control	Treatment of Primary Failure	No. of Patients Salvaged	Ultimate Control Rate
T1	12/17 (71%)	Surgery (5)*	5/5	17/17 (100%)
T2	57/81 (70%)	No treatment (2) Surgery (21) Surgery + RT (1)	19/24†	76/81 (94%)
T3	19/25 (76%)	Surgery (5) Surgery + chemotherapy (1)	4/6†	23/25 (92%)
T4	3/5	Surgery (1) Chemotherapy (1)	1/2†	4/5

RT, radiation therapy.
*Numbers in parentheses indicate number of patients.
†Five T2 patients, one T3 patient, and one T4 patient died within 2 years with no evidence of local disease.
Adapted from Lo K, Fletcher GH, Byers RM, et al: Results of irradiation in the squamous cell carcinomas of the anterior faucial pillar-retromolar trigone. Int J Radiat Oncol Biol Phys 13:969-974, 1987.

T4, 54%. The 5-year disease-free survival rates by N stage were N0, 69%; N1, 56%; and N2, 26%. The locoregional recurrence rates were 10% (1 of 10) after preoperative RT and surgery, 23% (9 of 39) after surgery and postoperative RT, and 44% (7 of 16) after RT alone. Factors that significantly influenced disease-free survival on multivariate analysis were treatment modality (p = .002) and N stage (p = .012); for locoregional control, treatment modality (p = .046); and for distant metastasis, N stage (p = .002).

Kowalski and coworkers[187] reported on 114 patients who underwent an extended "commando" operation between 1960 to 1991 for carcinoma of the retromolar trigone. Sixty-six patients received postoperative RT (median, 50 Gy). Tumor stages were T1, 5 patients; T2, 44 patients; T3, 24 patients; T4, 28 patients; and Tx, 13 patients. Forty-one patients (36%) experienced a recurrence at one or more sites: local, 31 (27%); dissected neck, 9 (22%); contralateral neck, 3 (7%); and distant, 7 (17%). The 5-year overall survival rates by T stage were T1, 80.0%; T2, 57.8%; T3, 46.5%; T4, 65.2%, and overall, 55.3%.

Byers and associates[184] reported on 110 patients with squamous carcinoma of the retromolar trigone who were treated at the M. D. Anderson Hospital from 1965 to 1977 and followed for at least 5 years. Seventy patients had T1 and T2 tumors, and 77 patients had a clinically negative neck. Sixty patients received either surgery alone (n = 46) or combined with preoperative or postoperative RT (n = 14). Fifty patients were treated with RT alone. Failure at the primary site occurred in 7 of 60 patients (12%) treated surgically and in 8 of 50 patients (16%) of patients treated with RT alone.

Antoniades and coworkers[188] reported on 31 patients treated surgically for carcinoma of the retromolar trigone-anterior faucial pillar; 90% of patients received postoperative RT (51 to 58 Gy). The 3-year locoregional recurrence rate was 44.8%.

Techniques of Irradiation

Treatment techniques for retromolar trigone cancers are similar to those discussed in the preceding section on gingival cancers.

Complications

Thirty percent of the patients reported by Lo and coworkers[185] developed some degree of bone exposure, but only nine patients (5.6%) required a segmental mandibulectomy. The probability of bone exposure was not found to be dose related. Huang and associates[186] reported on 65 patients treated for retromolar trigone cancer and observed complications that included bone necrosis, soft tissue necrosis, and severe trismus, occurring in 12% after surgery and postoperative RT, 11% after RT alone, and none after preoperative RT and surgery. Kowalski and coworkers[187] observed complications in 51.8% of 114 patients who underwent an extended "commando" operation between 1960 to 1991; 21 patients (18.4%) had a wound infection.

HARD PALATE

Squamous cell carcinoma of the hard palate is relatively rare. In a series of about 5000 patients with oral cavity cancers, only 25 patients (0.5%) had squamous cell carcinoma of the hard palate.[189] In a similar study, carcinoma of the hard palate represented 3% of all oral cavity carcinomas.[190] The male-to-female rate is approximately 1:1. For both males and females, the peak incidence tends to occur in the seventh decade, with over 98% of patients over the age of 40.[191]

Anatomy

The palate forms the roof of the oral cavity and the floor of the nasal cavity. The anterior two thirds, or bony part of the palate, is called the hard palate and is formed by the palatine processes of the maxilla and the horizontal plates of the palatine bones. Anteriorly and laterally, the hard palate is bounded by the maxillary alveolar ridge and gingiva. Posteriorly, the hard palate is contiguous with the soft palate. The hard palate is covered by a mucous membrane overlying the periosteum. Deep to the mucosa are the secreting palatine glands. The incisive foramen is posterior to the maxillary central incisors; the nasopalatine nerves pass through this foramen.

The greater palatine foramina are medial to the third maxillary molars; the greater palatine vessels and nerves emerge from this foramen. The greater palatine nerve innervates the gingiva, mucous membrane, and glands of the hard palate. The nasopalatine nerve innervates the mucous membrane of the anterior part of the hard palate. Because of the rich blood supply from the greater palatine artery, the incidence of osteoradionecrosis and soft tissue necrosis is lower than that reported for the mandible.[192]

Pathology and Patterns of Spread

Malignant tumors of the hard palate are most often adenoid cystic carcinomas and mucoepidermoid carcinomas arising from minor salivary glands. Squamous cell carcinoma is relatively uncommon. Kaposi's sarcoma and melanomas may also originate on the hard palate.[191]

Most squamous cell carcinomas originate on the gingiva and spread secondarily to the hard palate. Perineural invasion occurs via the greater palatine foramen. The risk of positive lymph nodes is 13% to 24% at diagnosis.[193-195] The incidence of subclinical disease in the cervical lymphatics is 22%.[79]

Clinical Manifestations, Patient Evaluation, and Staging

Patients with squamous cell carcinomas of the hard palate may first present to the dentist with either ill-fitting dentures, pain, loose teeth, or a sore that will not heal. Intermittent bleeding and paresthesias may also occur.

Imaging of the hard palate is primarily with CT and occasionally supplemented with MRI. Imaging of the neck nodes must include the facial and retrozygomatic nodes.[84] Facial nodes are best assessed by bimanual examination, particularly in patients with dental fillings. If the lesion is an adenoid cystic carcinoma, it is essential to search for perineural spread. The AJCC staging system is shown in Table 29-2.[45]

Treatment

Surgery is the usual initial treatment for most lesions; postoperative RT is indicated for patients with more extensive cancers. The role of primary RT in the management of hard palate carcinomas is ill defined. If the lesion has a large surface area and is superficial, RT can be used as initial treatment. However, most patients are treated with surgery because the underlying bone is often involved and, in that scenario, RT is unlikely to be effective.[196] Postoperative RT is indicated for close or involved margins, perineural or vascular invasion, multiple involved nodes, extracapsular extension, or bone invasion.[100] Dose and fractionation recommendations are similar to those given for other sites. A treatment algorithm is shown in Figure 29-23.

Malignant salivary gland tumors of the hard palate are often treated by a combination of surgery and postoperative RT, particularly if they are high grade. Low-grade minor salivary gland carcinomas can be treated by surgery alone if negative margins can be achieved. Some malignant minor salivary gland tumors have been successfully controlled by high-dose RT alone.[197]

Results

Shibuya and colleagues[198] reported the RT results for malignant lesions of the hard palate; the 5-year survival rate for those with squamous cell carcinomas was approximately 45%. For patients with minimal bone invasion and clinically negative neck, the 5-year survival was 75%. Data from the University of Virginia are presented in Table 29-18 for 41 patients treated with surgery, RT or both.[199]

Yorozu and colleagues[200] reported on 31 patients treated with EBRT at the Christie Hospital between 1990 and 1997. Twenty-six received RT alone and five were treated postoperatively for positive surgical margins. The 5-year local and ultimate local control rates after salvage surgery were 53% and 69%, respectively. Survival was 48% for patients with squamous carcinomas and 63% for those with minor salivary gland carcinomas. T stage was the only significant predictor of 5-year local control: 80% for T1 and T2 lesions and 24% for T3 and T4. The only significant predictor for survival was N stage.

Tran and coworkers[201] reported on 38 patients treated for salivary gland tumors of the palate at the University of California at Los Angeles. Twenty-three of 38 tumors were on the hard palate; adenoid cystic carcinoma was the most common histology. Twenty-five patients received surgery alone; 13 were treated with surgery and postoperative RT. The local control rates were comparable for the two groups of patients (88% and 85%, respectively).

Kovalic and associates[202] reported on 13 patients with carcinoma of the hard palate treated at Washington University. Histologies included adenoid cystic carcinoma, 9 patients; squamous cell carcinoma, 3 patients; and mucoepidermoid carcinoma, 1 patient. T stages were T1, 1 patient; T2, 5 patients;

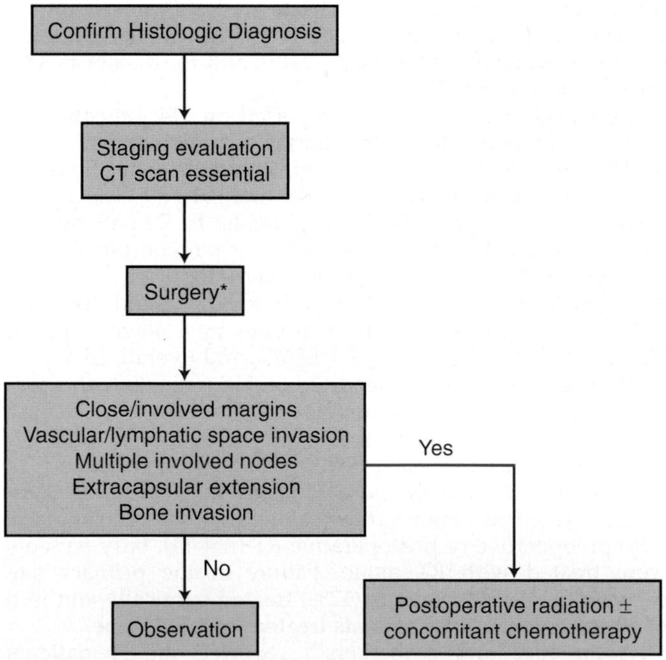

Figure 29-23 Treatment algorithm for de novo hard palate cancer. *Treat neck with neck dissection.[79,193-195]

Table 29-18 Hard Palate Malignancies Treated by Surgery, Radiotherapy, or Both: 5- and 10-Year Survival Rates

Histology	5-Y Absolute	Cause-Specific	10-Y Absolute	Cause-Specific
Squamous cell carcinoma	10/26 (38%)	10/17 (59%)	8/23 (35%)	8/15 (53%)
Salivary gland tumors				
Adenocarcinoma	5/7 (71%)	5/7 (71%)	3/6 (50%)	3/5 (60%)
Adenoid cystic carcinoma	3/3	3/3	1/2	1/1
Malignant mixed tumor	5/5	5/5	1/4	1/1

From Chung CK, Johns ME, Cantrell RW, Constable WC: Radiotherapy in the management of primary malignancies of the hard palate. Laryngoscope 90:576-584, 1980.

T3, 3 patients; and T4, 4 patients. All had a clinically negative neck. Ten patients received excision and postoperative RT; three patients were treated with RT alone. The 10-year actuarial disease-free survival and local control rates were 77% and 92%, respectively.

Fifty patients were treated surgically at the University of Cincinnati and included 25 patients with squamous cell carcinomas, 11 with adenoid cystic carcinomas, 6 with adenocarcinomas, and 8 with miscellaneous histologies.[203] The 5-year survival rates by histology were squamous carcinoma, 76%; adenoid cystic carcinoma, 90%; and overall, 85%. The 10-year survival rate for adenoid cystic carcinomas fell to 75%, consistent with their tendency to develop late recurrences.

Most relapses are found at the primary site. Evans[191] reported a 53% incidence of isolated primary site failure. The incidence of recurrence in the cervical nodes was 30%; failure involving both the primary site as well as the cervical lymph nodes was 10%. No patient treatment failed with results of distant metastases only. Seven percent of the patients' treatment failed in both distant and locoregional sites.

The risk of development of metachronous carcinomas is high. In the University of Virginia's experience, 28% of the patients developed a metachronous primary carcinoma during their lifetime and 13% developed a third, fourth, or fifth carcinoma. The oral cavity was the most common site for metachronous cancers.[193]

Techniques of Irradiation: Hard Palate and Maxillary Alveolar Ridge

T1 and T2

The preferred initial treatment for patients with T1 and T2 carcinomas of the hard palate is surgery. RT is used by default to treat the occasional patient who is not a surgical candidate. Most of these lesions are not well lateralized, consequently, RT is administered with parallel-opposed fields encompassing the primary tumor with a margin of 2 cm or less. A cork and tongue block is placed in the mouth to displace the tongue, mandible, and lower lip inferiorly and to reduce the amount of normal tissue included in the fields (Fig. 29-24A). These

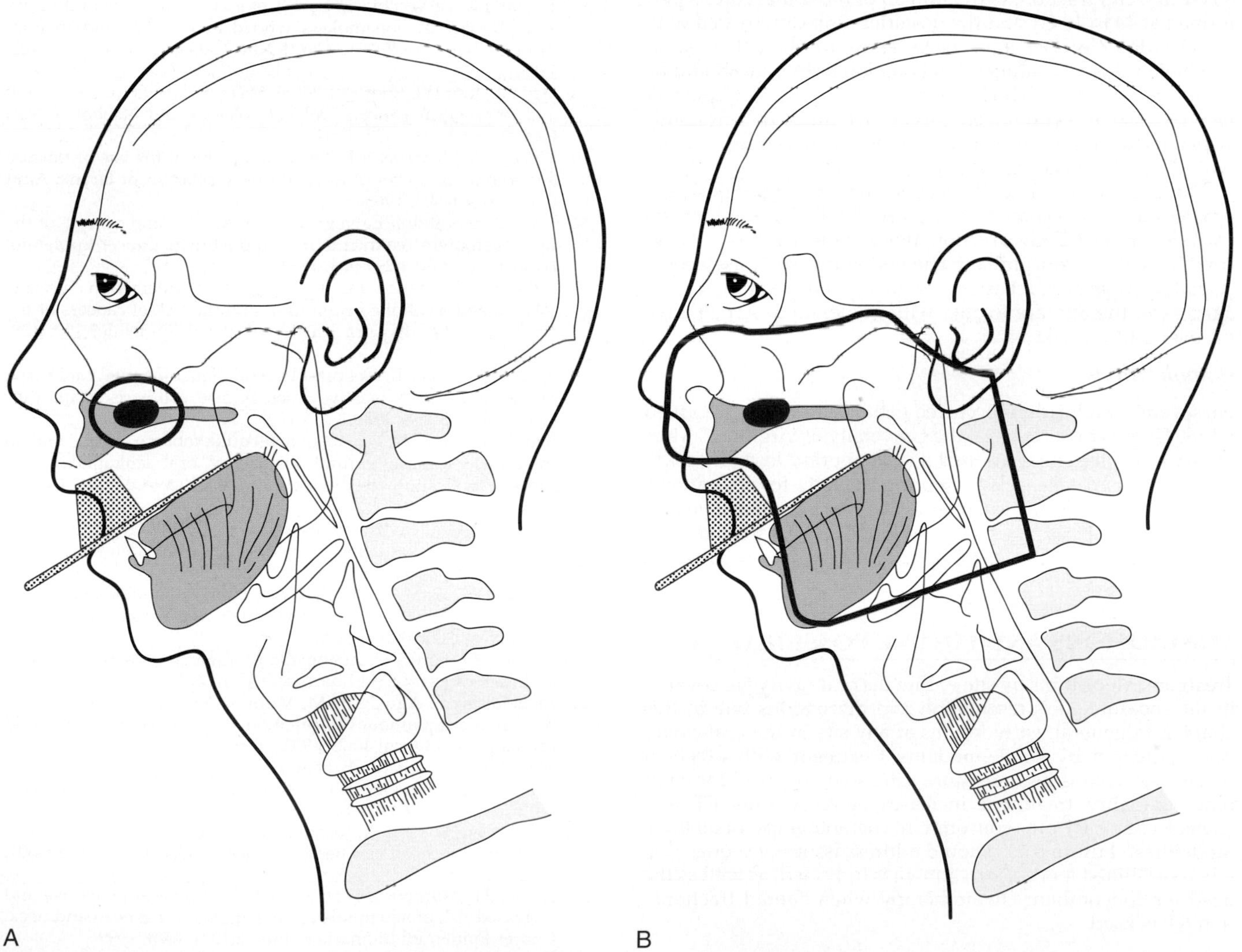

Figure 29-24 **A,** Early-stage hard palate carcinomas. Parallel-opposed 6-MV x-ray fields include the tumor with a 2-cm margin. A cork and tongue block displace the tongue and mandible inferiorly to minimize the amount of normal tissue included in the fields. **B,** Advanced hard palate carcinoma. Portals include the primary tumor and upper neck nodes. The superior margin of the portals is extended to include V_2 to the skull base. (Adapted from Mendenhall WM: Radiotherapy treatment technique. Cancer of the maxillary alveolar and hard palate. *In* Werning JW (ed): Oral Cancer. New York, Thieme Publishing, 2005.)

lesions are not amenable to brachytherapy, so patients are treated with EBRT alone. The likelihood of cure with RT alone, even for early-stage lesions, is relatively low so that an altered fractionation technique should be used. We prefer hyperfractionated RT and treat from 74.4 to 76.8 Gy at 1.2 Gy/fraction, twice daily, over 6 to 6.5 weeks. The fields are extended to include the regional lymph nodes (level 1 and 2) for patients with aggressive, poorly differentiated cancers (see Fig. 29-24B). The disadvantage of irradiating the regional lymph nodes is the acute toxicity of the treatment is significantly increased. Fields are reduced at 45.6 Gy in 38 fractions to limited portals that adequately encompass the primary cancer. The low neck is irradiated with an interior field that abuts the primary fields at the level of the thyroid notch and receives 50 Gy in 25 fractions over 5 weeks.

T3 and T4

Patients with T3 and T4 cancers are optimally treated with surgery and postoperative RT using fields encompassing the primary tumor and regional lymph nodes as previously described. Postoperative RT is initiated within 6 weeks of surgery. Patients with negative margins generally receive 60 Gy at 2 Gy/fraction. Reduction off of the spinal cord is performed at 44 to 46 Gy and the posterior strips are treated with 8- to 10-MeV elections if it is necessary to irradiate these areas to a higher dose. An altered fractionation technique should be considered for those who have positive margins, multiple risk factors, and/or a prolonged surgery-RT interval.[100] Systemic cisplatin chemotherapy is usually administered concomitantly with RT in the postoperative setting.[111,112]

Patients with T3 and T4 cancers who are not surgical candidates have a low chance of cure with RT. Patients are treated to 76.8 Gy at 1.2 Gy/fraction twice daily over 6.5 weeks combined with concomitant chemotherapy such as weekly cisplatin 30 mg/M^2. Patients who are not candidates for aggressive therapy are treated with moderate-dose palliative RT over 1 to 2 weeks.

Complications

No severe complications occurred in the patients who received RT (60 Gy in 5 to 6 weeks) at the University of Virginia.[199] Most patients developed xerostomia and temporary loss of taste.[193]

Yorozu and colleagues[200] reported results for 31 patients treated with EBRT at the Christie Hospital between 1990 and 1997. Twenty-six received RT alone and five were treated postoperatively for positive surgical margins; necrosis occurred in one patient.

CONCLUSIONS AND FUTURE POSSIBILITIES

Treatment algorithms by site within the oral cavity are covered in the separate site presentation and discussions within this chapter. In general, early lesions at any site in the oral cavity can be treated by single-modality treatment with excellent results. As lesions become more extensive, the need for combined-modality treatment increases (surgery plus RT and chemotherapy, RT plus concomitant chemotherapy, or all three modalities). Future trials should address issues of sequencing when combined modality treatment is indicated, as well as the need for concomitant chemotherapy when altered fractionation RT is used.

REFERENCES

1. Jemal A, Siegel E, Ward E, Murray T, et al: Cancer statistics, 2006. CA Cancer J Clin 56:106-130, 2006.
2. Krolls SO, Hoffman S: Squamous cell carcinoma of the oral soft tissues: a statistical analysis of 14,253 cases by age, sex, and race of patients. J Am Dent Assoc 92:571-574, 1976.
3. Taybos G: Oral changes associated with tobacco use. Am J Med Sci 326:179-182, 2003.
4. Kulkarni V, Saranath D: Concurrent hyperthermethylation of multiple regulatory genes in chewing tobacco associated oral squamous cell carcinomas and adjacent normal tissues. Oral Oncol 40:145-153, 2004.
5. Sham AS, Cheung LK, Jim LJ, et al: The effects of tobacco use on oral health. Hong Kong Med J 9:271-277, 2003.
6. Znaor A, Brennan P, Gajalakshmi V, et al: Independent and combined effects of tobacco smoking, chewing and alcohol drinking on the risk of oral, pharyngeal and esophageal cancers in Indian men. Int J Cancer 105:681-686, 2003.
7. Browman GP, Wong G, et al: Influence of cigarette smoking on the efficacy of radiation therapy in head and neck cancer. N Engl J Med 328:159-163, 1993.
8. Wynder EL: The epidemiology of cancers of the upper alimentary and upper respiratory tracts. Laryngoscope 88:50-51, 1978.
9. Castellsague X, Quintana MJ, Martinez MC, et al: The role of type of tobacco and type of alcoholic beverage in oral carcinogenesis. Int J Cancer 108:741-749, 2004.
10. Johnson N. Tobacco use and oral cancer: a global perspective. J Dent Educ 65:328-339, 2001.
11. Talamini R, La Vecchia C, Levi F, et al: Cancer of the oral cavity and pharynx in nonsmokers who drink alcohol and in nondrinkers who smoke tobacco. J Natl Cancer Inst 90:1901-1903, 1998.
12. Day GL, Blot WJ, Shore RE, et al: Second cancers following oral and pharyngeal cancers: role of tobacco and alcohol. J Natl Cancer Inst 86:131-137, 1994.
13. Vincent RG, Marchetta F: The relationship of the use of tobacco and alcohol to cancer of the oral cavity, pharynx or larynx. Am J Surg 106:501-505, 1963.
14. Franceschi S, Bidoli E, Negri E, et al: Alcohol and cancers of the upper aerodigestive tract in men and women. Cancer Epidemiol Biomarkers Prev 3:299-304, 1994.
15. Schlecht NF, Franco EL, Pintos J, et al: Interaction between tobacco and alcohol consumption and the risk of cancers of the upper aero-digestive tract in Brazil. Am J Epidemiol 150:1129-1137, 1999.
16. Spitz MR, Fueger JJ, Goepfert H, et al: Squamous cell carcinoma of the upper aerodigestive tract. A case comparison analysis. Cancer 61:203-208, 1988.
17. Shiu MN, Chen TH: Impact of betel quid, tobacco and alcohol on three-stage disease natural history of oral leukoplakia and cancer: implication for prevention of oral cancer. Eur J Cancer Prev 13:39-45, 2004.
18. Wang CC: Oral cavity. *In* Perez CA, Brady LW (eds): Principles and Practice of Radiation Oncology, ed 2. Philadelphia, JB Lippincott, 1992, pp 672-690.
19. McKaig RG, Baric RS, Olshan AF: Human papillomavirus and head and neck cancer: epidemiology and molecular biology. Head Neck 20:250-265, 1998.
20. Hashibe M, Ford DE, Zhang ZF: Marijuana smoking and head and neck cancer. J Clin Pharmacol 42:103S-107S, 2002.
21. Zienolddiny S, Aguelon AM, Mironov N, et al: Genomic instability in oral squamous cell carcinoma: relationship to betel-quid chewing. Oral Oncol 40:298-303, 2004.
22. Mork J, Lie AK, Glattre E, et al: Human papillomavirus infection as a risk factor for squamous cell carcinoma of the head and neck. N Engl J Med 344:1125-1131, 2001.
23. Goldenberg D, Golz A, Joachims HZ: The beverage mate: a risk factor for cancer of the head and neck. Head Neck 25:595-601, 2003.
24. Zhang ZF, Morgenstern H, Spitz MR, et al: Marijuana use and increased risk of squamous cell carcinoma of the head and neck. Cancer Epidemiol Biomarkers Prev 8:1071-1078, 1999.
25. Chen PC, Kuo C, Pan CC, et al: Risk of oral cancer associated with human papillomavirus infection, betel quid chewing, and cigarette smoking in Taiwan—an integrated molecular and epidemiological study of 58 cases. J Oral Pathol Med 31:317-322, 2002.

26. Mashberg A, Samit A: Early diagnosis of asymptomatic oral and oropharyngeal squamous cancers. CA Cancer J Clin 45:328-351, 1995.
27. McGuirt WF: Snuff dipper's carcinoma. Arch Otolaryngol 109:757-760, 1983.
28. Shklar G: The oral cavity, jaws, and salivary glands. *In* Robbins S (ed): Pathologic Basis of Disease, ed 3. Philadelphia, WB Saunders, 1984, pp 783-784.
29. Perea-Milla Lopez E, Minaro-Del Moral RM, Martinez-Garcia C, et al: Lifestyles, environmental and phenotypic factors associated with lip cancer: a case-control study in southern Spain. Br J Cancer 88:1702-1707, 2003.
30. Vaness M: Lip cancer: important management issues. Australas J Dermatol 42:30-32, 2001.
31. Baker SR, Krause CJ: Carcinoma of the lip. Laryngoscope 90:19-27, 1980.
32. Cross JE, Guralnick E, Daland EM: Carcinoma of the lip. A review of 563 case records of carcinoma of the lip at the Pondville Hospital. Surg Gynecol Obstet 81:153-162, 1948.
33. Marx RE, Johnson RP: Studies in the radiology of osteoradionecrosis and their clinical significance. Oral Surg Oral Med Oral Pathol 64:379-390, 1987.
34. Schiodt M, Hermund NU: Management of oral disease prior to radiation therapy. Support Care Cancer 10:40-43, 2002.
35. Meraw SJ, Reeve CM: Dental considerations and treatment of the oncology patient receiving radiation therapy. J Am Dent Assoc 129:201-205, 1998.
36. Epstein JB, Corbett T, Galler C, et al: Surgical peridontal treatment in the radiotherapy-treated head and neck cancer patient. Spec Care Dentist 14:182-187, 1994.
37. Rubenstein EB, Peterson DE, Schubert M, et al: Clinical practice guidelines for the prevention and treatment of cancer therapy-induced oral and gastrointestinal mucositis. Cancer 100:2026-2046, 2004.
38. Rouviére H: Anatomy of the Human Lymphatic System, Tobias MJ (trans). Ann Arbor, Edwards Brothers, 1938, pp 1-28, 77-78.
39. MacKay EN, Sellers AH: A statistical review of carcinoma of the lip. Can Med Assoc J 90:670-672, 1964.
40. Wurman LH, Adams GL, Meyerhoff WL: Carcinoma of the lip. Am J Surg 130:470-474, 1975.
41. Byers RM, O'Brien J, Waxler J: The therapeutic and prognostic implications of nerve invasion in cancer of the lower lip. Int J Radiat Oncol Biol Phys 4:215-217, 1978.
42. Hendricks JL, Mendelson BC, Woods JE: Invasive carcinoma of the lower lip. Surg Clin North Am 57:837-844, 1977.
43. de Visscher JG, van den Elsaker K, Grond AJ, et al: Surgical treatment of squamous cell carcinoma of the lower lip: evaluation of long-term results and prognostic factors—a retrospective analysis of 184 patients. J Oral Maxillofac Surg 56:814-820, 1998.
44. Petrovich Z, Kuisk H, Tobochnik N, et al: Carcinoma of the lip. Arch Otolaryngol 105:187-191, 1979.
45. American Joint Committee on Cancer: Lip and oral cavity. *In* Greene FL, Page DL, Fleming ID, et al (eds): AJCC Cancer Staging Manual, ed 6. New York, Springer, 2004, pp 23-32.
46. Amdur RJ, Parsons JT, Mendenhall WM, et al: Postoperative irradiation for squamous cell carcinoma of the head and neck: an analysis of treatment results and complications. Int J Radiat Oncol Biol Phys 16:25-36, 1989.
47. Babington S, Veness MJ, Cakir B, et al: Squamous cell carcinoma of the lip: is there a role for adjuvant radiotherapy in improving local control following incomplete or inadequate excision? A N Z J Surg 73:621-625, 2003.
48. Stranc MF, Fogel M, Dische S: Comparison of lip function: surgery vs radiotherapy. Br J Plast Surg 40:598-604, 1987.
49. Huynh NT, Veness MJ: Basal cell carcinoma of the lip treated with radiotherapy. Australas J Dermatol 43:15-19, 2002.
50. Harrison LB: Applications of brachytherapy in head and neck cancer. Semin Surg Oncol 13:177-184, 1997.
51. Wei FC, Tan BK, Chen IH, et al: Mimicking lip features in free-flap reconstruction of lip defects. Br J Plast Surg 54:8-11, 2001.
52. Zilinsky I, Winkler E, Weiss G, et al: Total lower lip reconstruction with innervated muscle-bearing flaps: modification of the Webster flap. Dermatol Surg 27:687-691, 2001.
53. Liu J, Okutomi T, Cao Z, et al: Modified labial tissue sliding flaps for repairing large lower lip defects. J Oral Maxillofac Surg 59:887-891, 2001.
54. Ergun SS: Reconstruction of the labiomental region with local flaps. Dermatol Surg 28:863-865, 2002.
55. Ozdemir R, Ortak T, Kocer U, et al: Total lower lip reconstruction using sensate composite radial forearm flap. J Craniofac Surg 14:393-405, 2003.
56. Chang KP, Lai CS, Tsai CC, et al: Total upper lip reconstruction with a free temporal scalp flap: long-term follow-up. Head Neck 25:602-605, 2003.
57. Teichgraeber JF, Larson DL: Some oncologic considerations in the treatment of lip cancer. Otolaryngol Head Neck Surg 98:589-592, 1988.
58. Vartanian JG, Carvalho AL, de Araujo Filho MJ, et al: Predictive factors and distribution of lymph node metastasis in lip cancer patients and their implications on the treatment of the neck. Oral Oncol 40:223-227, 2004.
59. Rodolico V, Barresi E, Di Lorenzo R, et al: Lymph node metastasis in lower lip squamous cell carcinoma in relation to tumour size, histologic variables and p27Kip1 protein expression. Oral Oncol 40:92-98, 2004.
60. Jorgensen K, Elbrond O, Andersen AP: Carcinoma of the lip. A series of 869 patients. Acta Otolaryngol (Stockh) 75:312-313, 1973.
61. Pierquin B: Basic techniques of endocuriethrapy. *In* Pierquin B, Wilson JF, Chassagne D (eds): Modern Brachytherapy. New York, Masson, 1987, pp 69-79.
62. Tombolini V, Bonanni A, Valeriani M, et al: Brachytherapy for squamous cell carcinoma of the lip. The experience of the Institute of Radiology of the University of Rome "La Sapienza." Tumori 84:478-482, 1998.
63. Orecchia R, Rampino M, Gribaudo S, et al: Interstitial brachytherapy for carcinomas of the lower lip. Results of treatment. Tumori 77:336-338, 1991.
64. Guinot JL, Arribas L, Chust ML, et al: Lip cancer treatment with high dose rate brachytherapy. Radiother Oncol 69:113-115, 2003.
65. Petrovich Z, Parker RG, Luxton G, et al: Carcinoma of the lip and selected sites of head and neck skin. A clinical study of 896 patients. Radiother Oncol 8:11-17, 1987.
66. Mohs FE, Snow SN: Microscopically controlled surgical treatment for squamous cell carcinoma of the lower lip. Surg Gynecol Obstet 160:37-41, 1985.
67. Holmkvist KA, Roenigk RK: Squamous cell carcinoma of the lip treated with Mohs micrographic surgery: outcome at 5 years. J Am Acad Dermatol 38:960-966, 1998.
68. Hruza GJ: Mohs micrographic surgery local recurrences. J Dermatol Surg Oncol 20:573-577, 1994.
69. Parsons JT, Mendenhall WM, Moore GJ, Million RR: Radiotherapy of tumors of the oral cavity. *In* Thawley SE, Panje WR, Batsakis JG, Lindberg RD (eds): Comprehensive Management of Head and Neck Tumors, ed 2, vol 1. Philadelphia, WB Saunders, 1999, pp 695-719.
70. Fitzpatrick PJ: Cancer of the lip. J Otolaryngol 13:32-36, 1984.
71. Rouviére H: Anatomy of the Human Lymphatic System, Tobias MJ (trans). Ann Arbor, Edwards Brothers, 1938, pp 44-56.
72. Harrold CC Jr: Management of cancer of the floor of the mouth. Am J Surg 122:487-493, 1971.
73. Teichgraeber JF, Clairmont AA: The incidence of occult metastases for cancer of the oral tongue and floor of the mouth: treatment rationale. Head Neck Surg 7:15-21, 1984.
74. Lindberg RD: Site of first failure in head and neck cancer. Cancer Treat Symp 2:21-31, 1983.
75. Strong EW: Site of treatment failure in head and neck cancer. Cancer Treat Symp 2:5-20, 1983.
76. Mohit-Tabatabai MA, Sobel HJ, Rush BF, Mashberg A: Relation of thickness of floor of mouth stage I and II cancers to regional metastasis. Am J Surg 152:351-353, 1986.
77. Campos JL, Lampe I, Fayos JV: Radiotherapy of carcinoma of the floor of the mouth. Radiology 99:677-682, 1971.
78. Crissman JD, Gluckman J, Whiteley J, Quenelle D: Squamous-cell carcinoma of the floor of the mouth. Head Neck Surg 3:2-7, 1980.
79. Ash CL: Oral cancer: a twenty-five year study. Am J Roentgenol Radium Ther Nucl Med 87:417-430, 1962.

80. Million RR: Elective neck irradiation for TxNo squamous carcinoma of the oral tongue and floor of mouth. Cancer 34:149-155, 1974.
81. Woolgar JA, Scott J: Prediction of cervical lymph node metastasis in squamous cell carcinoma of the tongue/floor of mouth. Head Neck 17:463-472, 1995.
82. Lindberg R: Distribution of cervical lymph node metastases from squamous cell carcinoma of the upper respiratory and digestive tracts. Cancer 29:1446-1449, 1972.
83. Byers RM, Wolf PF, Ballantyne AJ: Rationale for elective modified neck dissection. Head Neck Surg 10:160-167, 1988.
84. Mancuso AA, Harnsberger HR, Dillon WP: Oropharynx, oral cavity, and floor of mouth. *In* Grayson TH (ed): Workbook for MRI and CT of the Head and Neck, ed 2. Baltimore, Williams & Wilkins, 1989, pp 151-170.
85. Wong WL, Chevretton EB, McGurk M, et al: A prospective study of PET-FDG imaging for the assessment of head and neck squamous cell carcinoma. Clin Otolaryngol 22:209-214, 1997.
86. Kubota K, Yokoyama J, Yamaguchi K, et al: FDG-PET delayed imaging for the detection of head and neck cancer recurrence after radio-chemotherapy: comparison with MRI/CT. Eur J Nucl Med Mol Imaging 31:590-595, 2004.
87. Anzai Y, Carroll WR, Quint DJ, et al: Recurrence of head and neck cancer after surgery or irradiation: prospective comparison of 2-deoxy-2-[F-18] fluoro-D-glucose PET and MR imaging diagnoses. Radiology 200:135-141, 1996.
88. Rogers JW, Greven KM, McGuirt WF, et al: Can post-RT neck dissection be omitted for patients with head-and-neck cancer who have a negative PET scan after definitive radiation therapy? Int J Radiat Oncol Biol Phys 58:694-697, 2004.
89. Yao M, Graham MM, Hoffman HT, et al: The role of post-radiation therapy FDG PET in prediction of necessity for post-radiation therapy neck dissection in locally advanced head-and-neck squamous cell carcinoma. Int J Radiat Oncol Biol Phys 59:1001-1010, 2004.
90. Greven KM: Positron-emission tomography for head and neck cancer. Semin Radiat Oncol 14:121-129, 2004.
91. Schoder H, Yeung HW, Gonen M, et al: Head and neck cancer: clinical usefulness and accuracy of PET/CT image fusion. Radiology 231:65-72, 2004.
92. Dias FL, Kligerman J, Matos de Sa G, et al: Elective neck dissection versus observation in stage I squamous cell carcinomas of the tongue and floor of the mouth. Otolaryngol Head Neck Surg 125:23-29, 2001.
93. Sessions DG, Spector GJ, Lenox J, et al: Analysis of treatment results for floor-of-mouth cancer. Laryngoscope 110:1764-1772, 2000.
94. Ross GL, Soutar DS, MacDonald DG, et al: Improved staging of cervical metastases in clinically node-negative patients with head and neck squamous cell carcinoma. Ann Surg Oncol 11:213-218, 2004.
95. Hoft S, Maune S, Muhle C, et al: Sentinel lymph-node biopsy in head and neck cancer. Br J Cancer 91:124-128, 2004.
96. Ross GL, Soutar DS, MacDonald DG, et al: Sentinel node biopsy in head and neck cancer: preliminary results of a multicenter trial. Ann Surg Oncol 11:690-696, 2004.
97. Ange DW, Lindberg RD, Guillamondegui OM: Management of squamous cell carcinoma of the oral tongue and floor of mouth after excisional biopsy. Radiology 116:143-146, 1975.
98. Mendenhall WM, Parsons JT, Stringer SP, et al: Radiotherapy after excisional biopsy of carcinoma of the oral tongue/floor of the mouth. Head Neck 11:129-131, 1989.
99. Nason RW, Sako K, Beecroft WA, et al: Surgical management of squamous cell carcinoma of the floor of the mouth. Am J Surg 158:292-296, 1989.
100. Hinerman RW, Mendenhall WM, Morris CG, et al: Postoperative irradiation for squamous cell carcinoma of the oral cavity: 35 year experience. Head Neck 26:984-994, 2004.
101. Looser KG, Shah JP, Strong EW: The significance of "positive" margins in surgically resected epidermoid carcinomas. Head Neck Surg 1:107-111, 1978.
102. Lee JG: Detection of residual carcinoma of the oral cavity, oropharynx, hypopharynx, and larynx: a study of surgical margins. Trans Am Acad Ophthalmol Otolaryngol 78:49-53, 1974.
103. Scholl P, Byers RM, Batsakis JG, et al: Microscopic cut-through of cancer in the surgical treatment of squamous carcinoma of the tongue. Prognostic and therapeutic implications. Am J Surg 152:354-360, 1986.
104. Byers RM, Bland KI, Borlase B, Luna M: The prognostic and therapeutic value of frozen section determinations in the surgical treatment of squamous carcinoma of the head and neck. Am J Surg 136:525-528, 1978.
105. Jacobs JR, Ahmad K, Casiano R, et al: Implications of positive surgical margins. Laryngoscope 103:64-68, 1993.
106. Laramore GE, Scott CB, Al-Sarraf M, et al: Adjuvant chemotherapy for resectable squamous cell carcinomas of the head and neck: report on Intergroup Study 0034. Int J Radiat Oncol Biol Phys 23:705-713, 1992.
107. Parsons JT, Million RR: Radiation therapy of tumors of the oral cavity. *In* Thawley SE, Panje WR, Batsakis JG, Lindberg RD (eds): Comprehensive Management of Head and Neck Tumors, vol 1. Philadelphia, WB Saunders, 1987, pp 516-535.
108. Lapeyre M, Hoffstetter S, Peiffert D, et al: Postoperative brachytherapy alone for T1-2 N0 squamous cell carcinomas of the oral tongue and floor of mouth with close or positive margins. Int J Radiat Oncol Biol Phys 48:37-42, 2000.
109. Raybaud-Diogene H, Fortin A, Morency R, et al: Markers of radioresistance in squamous cell carcinomas of the head and neck: a clinicopathologic and immunohistochemical study. J Clin Oncol 15:1030-1038, 1997.
110. Mendenhall WM, Million RR, Cassisi NJ: Squamous cell carcinoma of the head and neck treated with radiation therapy: the role of neck dissection for clinically positive neck nodes. Int J Radiat Oncol Biol Phys 12:733-740, 1986.
111. Bernier J, Domenge C, Ozsahin M, et al: Postoperative irradiation with or without concomitant chemotherapy for locally advanced head and neck cancer. N Engl J Med 350:1945-1952, 2004.
112. Cooper JS, Pajak TF, Forastiere AA, et al: Postoperative concurrent radiotherapy and chemotherapy for high-risk squamous cell carcinoma of the head and neck. N Engl J Med 350:1937-1944, 2004.
113. Bachaud JM, Cohen-Jonathan E, Alzieu C, et al: Combined postoperative radiotherapy and weekly cisplatin infusion for locally advanced head and neck carcinoma: final report of a randomized trial. Int J Radiat Oncol Biol Phys 36:999-1004, 1996.
114. Bernier J, Domenge C, Eschwege F, et al: Chemo-radiotherapy, as compared with radiotherapy alone, significantly increases disease-free and overall survival in head and neck cancer patients after surgery: results of EORTC Phase III Trial 22931 [abstract]. Int J Radiat Oncol Biol Phys 51:1, 2001.
115. Cooper JS, Pajak TF, Forastiere AA, et al: Postoperative concurrent radiochemotherapy in high-risk SCCA of the head and neck: initial report of RTOG 9501/Intergroup Phase III trial [abstract]. Am Soc Clin Oncol 2002.
116. Million RR, Cassisi NJ, Clark JR: Cancer of the head and neck. *In* DeVita VT Jr, Hellman S, Rosenberg SA (eds): Cancer: Principles and Practice of Oncology, ed 3. Philadelphia, JB Lippincott, 1989, pp 488-580.
117. Mendenhall WM, Van Cise WS, Bova FJ, Million RR: Analysis of time-dose factors in squamous cell carcinoma of the oral tongue and floor of mouth treated with radiation therapy alone. Int J Radiat Oncol Biol Phys 7:1005-1011, 1981.
118. Chu A, Fletcher GH: Incidence and causes of failures to control by irradiation the primary lesions in squamous cell carcinomas of the anterior two-thirds of the tongue and floor of mouth. Am J Roentgenol Radium Ther Nucl Med 117:502-508, 1973.
119. Wadsley JC, Patel M, Tomlins CD, Gildersleve JQ: Iridium-192 implantation for T1 and T2a carcinoma of the tongue and floor of mouth: retrospective study of the results of treatment at the Royal Berkshire Hospital. Br J Radiol 76:414-417, 2003.
120. Marsiglia H, Haie-Meder C, Sasso G, et al: Brachytherapy for T1-T2 floor-of-the-mouth cancers: the Gustave-Roussy Institute experience. Int J Radiat Oncol Biol Phys 52:1257-1263, 2002.
121. Pernot M, Hoffstetter S, Peiffert D, et al: Epidermoid carcinomas of the floor of mouth treated by exclusive irradiation: statistical

study of a series of 207 cases. Radiother Oncol 35:177-185, 1995.
122. Rodgers LW Jr, Stringer SP, Mendenhall WM, et al: Management of squamous cell carcinoma of the floor of the mouth. Head Neck 15:16-19, 1993.
123. Marcus RB Jr, Million RR, Mitchell TP: A preloaded, custom-designed implantation device for stage T1-T2 carcinoma of the floor of mouth. Int J Radiat Oncol Biol Phys 6:111-113, 1980.
124. Million RR, Cassisi NJ, Mancuso AA: Oral cavity. *In* Million RR, Cassisi NJ (eds): Management of Head and Neck Cancer: A Multidisciplinary Approach, ed 2. Philadelphia, JB Lippincott, 1994, pp 321-400.
125. Million RR, Cassisi NJ: General principles for treatment of cancers in the head and neck: radiation therapy. *In* Million RR, Cassisi NJ (eds): Management of Head and Neck Cancer: A Multidisciplinary Approach. Philadelphia, JB Lippincott, 1984, pp 77-90.
126. Parsons JT, Mendenhall WM, Moore GJ, Million RR: Radiotherapy of tumors of the oropharynx. *In* Thawley SE, Panje WR, Batsakis JG, Lindberg RD (eds): Comprehensive Management of Head and Neck Tumors, ed 2, vol 1. Philadelphia, WB Saunders, 1999, pp 861-875.
127. Delanian S, Lefaix JL: Complete healing of severe osteoradionecrosis with treatment combining pentoxifylline, tocopherol and clodronate. Br J Radiol 75:467-469, 2002.
128. Okunieff P, Augustine E, Hicks JE, et al: Pentoxifylline in the treatment of radiation-induced fibrosis. J Clin Oncol 22:2207-2213, 2004.
129. Aygenc E, Celikkanat S, Kaymakci M, et al: Prophylactic effect of pentoxifylline on radiotherapy complications: a clinical study. Otolaryngol Head Neck Surg 130:351-356, 2004.
130. King GE, Scheeetz J, Jacob RF, Martin JW: Electrotherapy and hyperbaric oxygen: promising treatments for postradiation complications. J Prosthet Dent 62:331-334, 1989.
131. Engelmeier RL, King GE: Complications of head and neck radiation therapy and their management. J Prosthet Dent 49:514-522, 1983.
132. Braakhuis BJ, Leemans CR, Brakenhoff RH: A genetic progression model of oral cancer: current evidence and clinical implications. J Oral Pathol Med 33:317-322, 2004.
133. Ishii J, Fujita K, Munemoto S, Komori T: Management of oral leukoplakia by laser surgery: relation between recurrence and malignant transformation and clinicopathological features. J Clin Laser Med Surg 22:27-33, 2004.
134. Ozeki S, Tashiro H, Okamoto M, Matsushima T: Metastasis to the lingual lymph node in carcinoma of the tongue. J Maxillofac Surg 13:277-281, 1985.
135. Spiro RH, Huvos AG, Wong GY, et al: Predictive value of tumor thickness in squamous cell carcinoma confined to the tongue and floor of the mouth. Am J Surg 152:345-350, 1986.
136. Sessions DG, Spector GJ, Lenox J, et al: Analysis of treatment results for oral tongue cancer. Laryngoscope 112:616-625, 2002.
137. Hicks WL Jr, North JH Jr, Loree TR, et al: Surgery as a single modality therapy for squamous cell carcinoma of the oral tongue. Am J Otolaryngol 19:24-28, 1998.
138. Chao KS, Emami B, Akhileswaran R, et al: The impact of surgical margin status and use of an interstitial implant on T1, T2 oral tongue cancers after surgery. Int J Radiat Oncol Biol Phys 36:1039-1043, 1996.
139. Fein DA, Mendenhall WM, Parsons JT, et al: Carcinoma of the oral tongue: a comparison of results and complications of treatment with radiotherapy and/or surgery. Head Neck 16:358-365, 1994.
140. Horiuchi J, Adachi T: Some considerations on radiation therapy of tongue cancer. Cancer 28:335-339, 1971.
141. Fu KK, Ray JW, Chan EK, Phillips TL: External and interstitial radiation therapy of carcinoma of the oral tongue. A review of 32 years' experience. AJR Am J Roentgenol 126:107-115, 1976.
142. Lees AW: The treatment of carcinoma of the anterior two-thirds of the tongue by radiotherapy. Int J Radiat Oncol Biol Phys 1:849-858, 1976.
143. Wang CC: Radiotherapeutic management and results of T1N0, T2N0 carcinoma of the oral tongue: evaluation of boost techniques. Int J Radiat Oncol Biol Phys 17:287-291, 1989.
144. Inoue T, Fuchihata H, Wada T, Shigematsu Y: Local prognosis after combined external and interstitial radiation therapy for carcinoma of the tongue. Acta Radiol Ther Phys Biol 15:315-320, 1976.
145. Wendt CD, Peters LJ, Delclos L, et al: Primary radiotherapy in the treatment of stage I and II oral tongue cancers: importance of the proportion of therapy delivered with interstitial therapy. Int J Radiat Oncol Biol Phys 18:1287-1292, 1990.
146. Matsuura K, Hirokawa Y, Fujita M, et al: Treatment results of stage I and II oral tongue cancer with interstitial brachytherapy: maximum tumor thickness is prognostic of nodal metastasis. Int J Radiat Oncol Biol Phys 40:535-539, 1998.
147. Byers RM, El-Naggar AK, et al: Can we detect or predict the presence of occult nodal metastases in patients with squamous cell carcinoma of the oral tongue? Head Neck 20:138-144, 1998.
148. Haddadin KJ, Soutar DS, Oliver RJ, et al: Improved survival for patients with clinically T1/T2, N0 tongue tumors undergoing a prophylactic neck dissection. Head Neck 21:517-525, 1999.
149. O-Charoenrat P, Pillai G, Patel S, et al: Tumour thickness predicts cervical nodal metastases and survival in early oral tongue cancer. Oral Oncol 39:386-390.2003.
150. Civantos FJ, Gomez C, Duque C, et al: Sentinel node biopsy in oral cavity cancer: correlation with PET scan and immunohistochemistry. Head Neck 25:1-9, 2003.
151. Aygenc E, Celikkanat S, Bilgili H, et al: Pentoxifylline effects on acute and late complications after radiotherapy in rabbit. Otolaryngol Head Neck Surg 124:669-673, 2001.
152. Jereczek-Fossa BA, Orecchia R: Radiotherapy-induced mandibular bone complications. Cancer Treat Rev 28:65-74, 2002.
153. Coffin F: The incidence and management of osteoradionecrosis of the jaws following head and neck radiotherapy. Br J Radiol 56:851-857, 1983.
154. Fujita M, Hirokawa Y, Kashiwado K, et al: An analysis of mandibular bone complications in radiotherapy for T1 and T2 carcinoma of the oral tongue. Int J Radiat Oncol Biol Phys 34:333-339, 1996.
155. Glanzmann C, Gratz KW: Radionecrosis of the mandibula: a retrospective analysis of the incidence and risk factors. Radiother Oncol 36:94-100, 1995.
156. Mosqueda-Taylor A, Luna-Ortiz K, Irigoyen-camacho ME, et al: Effect of pilocarpine hydrochloride on salivary production in previously irradiated head and neck cancer patients. Med Oral 9:204-211, 2004.
157. Taylor SE: Efficacy and economic evaluation of pilocarpine in treating radiation-induced xerostomia. Expert Opin Pharmacother 4:1489-1497, 2003.
158. LeVeque FG, Montgomery M, Potter D, et al: A multicenter, randomized, double-blind, placebo-controlled, dose-titration study of oral pilocarpine for treatment of radiation-induced xerostomia in head and neck cancer patients. J Clin Oncol 11:1124-1131, 1993.
159. Warde P, O'Sullivan B, Aslanidis J, et al: A phase III placebo-controlled trial of oral pilocarpine in patients undergoing radiotherapy for head-and-neck cancer. Int J Radiat Oncol Biol Phys 54:9-13, 2002.
160. Gornitsky M, Shenouda G, Sultanem K, et al: Double-blind randomized, placebo-controlled study of pilocarpine to salvage salivary gland function during radiotherapy of patients with head and neck cancer. Oral Surg Oral Med Oral Pathol Oral Radiol Endod 98:45-52, 2004.
161. Kouloulias VE, Kouvaris J, Kokakis JD, et al: Impact on cytoprotective efficacy of intermediate interval between amifostine administration and radiotherapy: a retrospective analysis. Int J Radiat Oncol Biol Phys 59:1148-1156, 2004.
162. Komaki R, Lee JS, Milas L, et al: Effects of amifostine on acute toxicity from concurrent chemotherapy and radiotherapy for inoperable nonsmall-cell lung cancer: report of a randomized comparative trial. Int J Radiat Oncol Biol Phys 58:1369-1377, 2004.
163. Rades D, Fehlauer F, Bajrovic A, et al: Serious adverse effects of amifostine during radiotherapy in head and neck cancer patients. Radiother Oncol 70:261-264, 2004.
164. Conley J, Sadoyama JA: Squamous cell cancer of the buccal mucosa. A review of 90 cases. Arch Otolaryngol 97:330-333, 1973.

165. Bloom ND, Spiro RH: Carcinoma of the cheek mucosa. A retrospective analysis. Am J Surg 140:556-559, 1980.
166. MacComb WS, Fletcher GH, Healey JE: Intra-oral cavity. *In* MacComb WS, Fletcher GH (eds): Cancer of the Head and Neck. Baltimore, Williams & Wilkins, 1967, pp 89-151.
167. Vegers JW, Snow GB, van der Waal I: Squamous cell carcinoma of the buccal mucosa. A review of 85 cases. Arch Otolaryngol 105:192-195, 1979.
168. Diaz EM Jr, Holsinger FC, Zuniga ER, et al: Squamous cell carcinoma of the buccal mucosa: one institution's experience with 119 previously untreated patients. Head Neck 25:267-273, 2003.
169. Dixit S, Vyas RK, Toparani RB, et al: Surgery versus surgery and postoperative radiotherapy in squamous cell carcinoma of the buccal mucosa: a comparative study. Ann Surg Oncol 5:502-510, 1998.
170. Koch BB, Trask DK, et al: National survey of head and neck verrucous carcinoma: patterns of presentation, care and outcome. Cancer 92:110-120, 2001.
171. Jyothirmayi R, Sankaranarayanan R, Varghese C, et al: Radiotherapy in the treatment of verrucous carcinoma of the oral cavity. Oral Oncol 33:124-128, 1997.
172. Wang CC: Radiation Therapy for Head and Neck Neoplasms: Indications, Techniques and Results. Littleton, MA, John Wright-PSG, 1983.
173. Nair MK, Sankaranarayanan R, Padmanabhan TK, Madhu CS: Oral verrucous carcinoma. Treatment with radiotherapy. Cancer 61:458-461, 1988.
174. Urist MM, O'Brien CJ, Soong SJ, et al: Squamous cell carcinoma of the buccal mucosa: analysis of prognostic factors. Am J Surg 154:411-414, 1987.
175. Chhetri DK, Rawnsley JD, Calcaterra TC: Carcinoma of the buccal mucosa. Otolaryngol Head Neck Surg 123:566-571, 2000.
176. Fang FM, Leung SW, Huang CC, et al: Combined-modality therapy for squamous carcinoma of the buccal mucosa: treatment results and prognostic factors. Head Neck 19:506-512, 1997.
177. Byers RM, Newman R, Russell N, Yue A: Results of treatment for squamous carcinoma of the lower gum. Cancer 47:2236-2238, 1981.
178. McGregor AD, MacDonald DG: Routes of entry of squamous cell carcinoma to the mandible. Head Neck Surg 10:294-301, 1988.
179. Cady B, Catlin D: Epidermoid carcinoma of the gum. A 20-year survey. Cancer 23:551-569, 1969.
180. Soo KC, Spiro RH, King W, et al: Squamous carcinoma of the gums. Am J Surg 156:281-285, 1988.
181. Overholt SM, Eicher SA, Wolf P, Weber RS: Prognostic factors affecting outcome in lower gingival carcinoma. Laryngoscope 106:1335-1339, 1996.
182. Lampe I: Radiation therapy of cancer of the buccal mucosa and lower gingiva. Am J Roentgenol Ther Nucl Med 73:628-638, 1955.
183. Fayos JV: Carcinoma of the mandible. Results of radiation therapy. Acta Radiol Ther Phys Biol 12:378-386, 1973.
184. Byers RM, Anderson B, Schwarz EA, et al: Treatment of squamous carcinoma of the retromolar trigone. Am J Clin Oncol 7:647-652, 1984.
185. Lo K, Fletcher GH, Byers RM, et al: Results of irradiation in the squamous cell carcinomas of the anterior faucial pillar-retromolar trigone. Int J Radiat Oncol Biol Phys 13:969-974, 1987.
186. Huang CJ, Chao KS, Tsai J, et al: Cancer of retromolar trigone: long-term radiation therapy outcome. Head Neck 23:758-763, 2001.
187. Kowalski LP, Hashimoto I, Magrin J: End results of 114 extended "commando" operations for retromolar trigone carcinoma. Am J Surg 166:374-379, 1993.
188. Antoniades K, Lazaridis N, Vahtsevanos K, et al: Treatment of squamous cell carcinoma of the anterior faucial pillar-retromolar trigone. Oral Oncol 39:680-686, 2003.
189. New GB, Hallberg OE: The end results of the treatment of malignant tumors of the palate. Surg Gynecol Obstr 73:520-524, 1941.
190. Chierici G, Silverman S Jr, Forsythe B: A tumor registry study of oral squamous carcinoma. J Oral Med 23:91-98, 1968.
191. Evans JF, Shah JP: Epidermoid carcinoma of the palate. Am J Surg 142:451-455, 1981.
192. Barker GJ, Barker BF, Gier RE: Oral Management of the Cancer Patient: A Guide for the Health Care Professional. Kansas City, MO, The Curators of the University of Missouri, 1981.
193. Chung CK, Rahman SM, Lim ML, Constable WC: Squamous cell carcinoma of the hard palate. Int J Radiat Oncol Biol Phys 5:191-196, 1979.
194. Eneroth CM, Hjertman L, Moberger G: Squamous cell carcinomas of the palate. Acta Otolaryngol (Stockh) 73:418-427, 1972.
195. Martin H: Tumors of the palate (benign and malignant). Arch Surg 44:599-635, 1942.
196. Ratzer ER, Schweitzer RJ, Frazell EL: Epidermoid carcinoma of the palate. Am J Surg 119:294-297, 1970.
197. Ellis ER, Million RR, Mendenhall WM, et al: The use of radiation therapy in the management of minor salivary gland tumors. Int J Radiat Oncol Biol Phys 15:613-617, 1988.
198. Shibuya H, Horiuchi JI, Suzuki S, et al: Oral carcinoma of the upper jaw. Results of radiation treatment. Acta Radiol Oncol 23:331-335, 1984.
199. Chung CK, Johns ME, Cantrell RW, Constable WC: Radiotherapy in the management of primary malignancies of the hard palate. Laryngoscope 90:576-584, 1980.
200. Yorozu A, Sykes AJ, Slevin NJ: Carcinoma of the hard palate treated with radiotherapy: a retrospective review of 31 cases. Oral Oncol 37:493-497, 2001.
201. Tran L, Sadeghi A, Hanson D, et al: Salivary gland tumors of the palate: the UCLA experience. Laryngoscope 97:1343-1345, 1987.
202. Kovalic JJ, Simpson JR: Carcinoma of the hard palate. J Otolaryngol 22:118-120, 1993.
203. Truitt TO, Gleich LL, Huntress GP, Gluckman JL: Surgical management of hard palate malignancies. Otolaryngol Head Neck Surg 121:548-552, 1999.
204. Bourhis J, Pignon JP, Designé L, et al: Meta-analysis of chemotherapy in head and neck cancer (MACH-NC): (1) loco-regional treatment vs. same treatment + chemotherapy. [abstract]. Proc Annu Meet Am Soc Clin Oncol 386a, 1998.

CHAPTER 30

OROPHARYNGEAL CANCER

William H. Morrison, Adam S. Garden, and K. Kian Ang

INCIDENCE

The estimated incidence of oral cavity and pharynx cancers in men in the United States for 2006 was 20,180 new cases, with no breakdown by location in the oral cavity and pharynx.

BIOLOGIC CHARACTERISTICS

Patients with squamous carcinomas of the oropharynx have an approximately 70% incidence of nodal involvement at presentation.

Distant metastases occur in approximately 15% of patients who present with nodal involvement.

Squamous carcinomas of the oropharynx are radiosensitive tumors.

STAGING EVALUATION

Staging entails a history and physical examination, computed tomography (CT) or magnetic resonance imaging (MRI) of the head and neck, a chest radiograph, and routine blood cell counts and serum chemistries.

Chest CT should be obtained in patients who have advanced nodal disease. Additional workup may be indicated for further evaluation of specific clinical findings.

PRIMARY THERAPY AND RESULTS

The preferred treatment for patients with T1 and T2 oropharyngeal squamous carcinomas is radiation therapy. Parotid-sparing techniques, such as intensity-modulated radiation therapy, should be used in most patients.

Concurrent chemoradiation is appropriate for patients with T3 or T4 primary tumors and those with N3 or fixed nodal disease.

Patients who present with multiple nodes and small primary tumors are candidates for protocols designed to eradicate systemic micrometastases.

Neck dissection can be performed before or after the course of radiation therapy. Patients are selected for neck dissections before radiation therapy if they require general anesthesia for dental extractions and if nodal disease is sufficiently advanced that a neck dissection will likely be indicated for management. Postirradiation therapy neck dissections are indicated for patients who do not have a complete response to a full course of radiation therapy. These dissections are performed approximately 6 to 8 weeks after completion of radiation therapy.

ADJUVANT THERAPY

Several phase III trials and a large meta-analysis have demonstrated that concurrent chemotherapy can enhance the radiation response in locally advanced head and neck cancers, leading to improved local and regional control. Approximately 40% of the patients enrolled on these trials had oropharyngeal carcinomas.

The best results have been obtained using cisplatin-based concurrent therapy. In some of the phase III trials testing concurrent chemotherapy, survival improvement has also been demonstrated.

LOCALLY ADVANCED DISEASE

Patients with locally advanced, resectable squamous carcinomas can be treated with surgery and postoperative radiation therapy.

Preoperative radiation therapy can be given to patients with locally advanced, unresectable tumors in an effort to render the tumors resectable.

The morbidity of large resections is substantial, especially for tongue base and soft palate tumors.

Alternately, these patients can be entered into clinical trials investigating the role of irradiation combined with chemotherapy and targeted biologic agents.

PALLIATION

Patients with far-advanced, incurable oropharyngeal carcinoma may benefit from a short course of palliative radiation therapy.

The oropharynx consists of the base of the tongue, tonsillar region, soft palate, and lateral and posterior oropharyngeal walls (Fig. 30-1). These structures play an essential role in swallowing and speech. Neoplasms arising in the oropharynx can impede these functions by infiltrating the musculature, obstructing the cavity, or causing pain. In the United States, the 2006 estimated incidence of new cases of oral cavity and pharynx cancers occurring in men was 20,180.[1] Treatments administered to cure the disease can cause further structural deformity and functional impairment. Radiation therapy, in some cases enhanced with concurrent chemotherapy, is generally preferred for the management of early to moderately advanced–stage oropharyngeal tumors. Tumoricidal doses can be given with a relatively high likelihood of preserving swallowing and speech.

Carcinomas of the oropharynx have served as a good model for investigating the radiobiology of human tumors. Squamous carcinomas of the oropharynx usually are radiosensitive. Because these tumors are readily accessible to examination, staging and therapeutic response evaluations can be accurately performed. A large body of time-dose–fractionation data has been obtained from studying the response of oropharyngeal tumors to irradiation.[2-4] Approximately 40% of patients enrolled on phase III trials investigating the role of chemoirradiation compared with irradiation alone had oropharyngeal tumors. In recent years, the oropharynx has

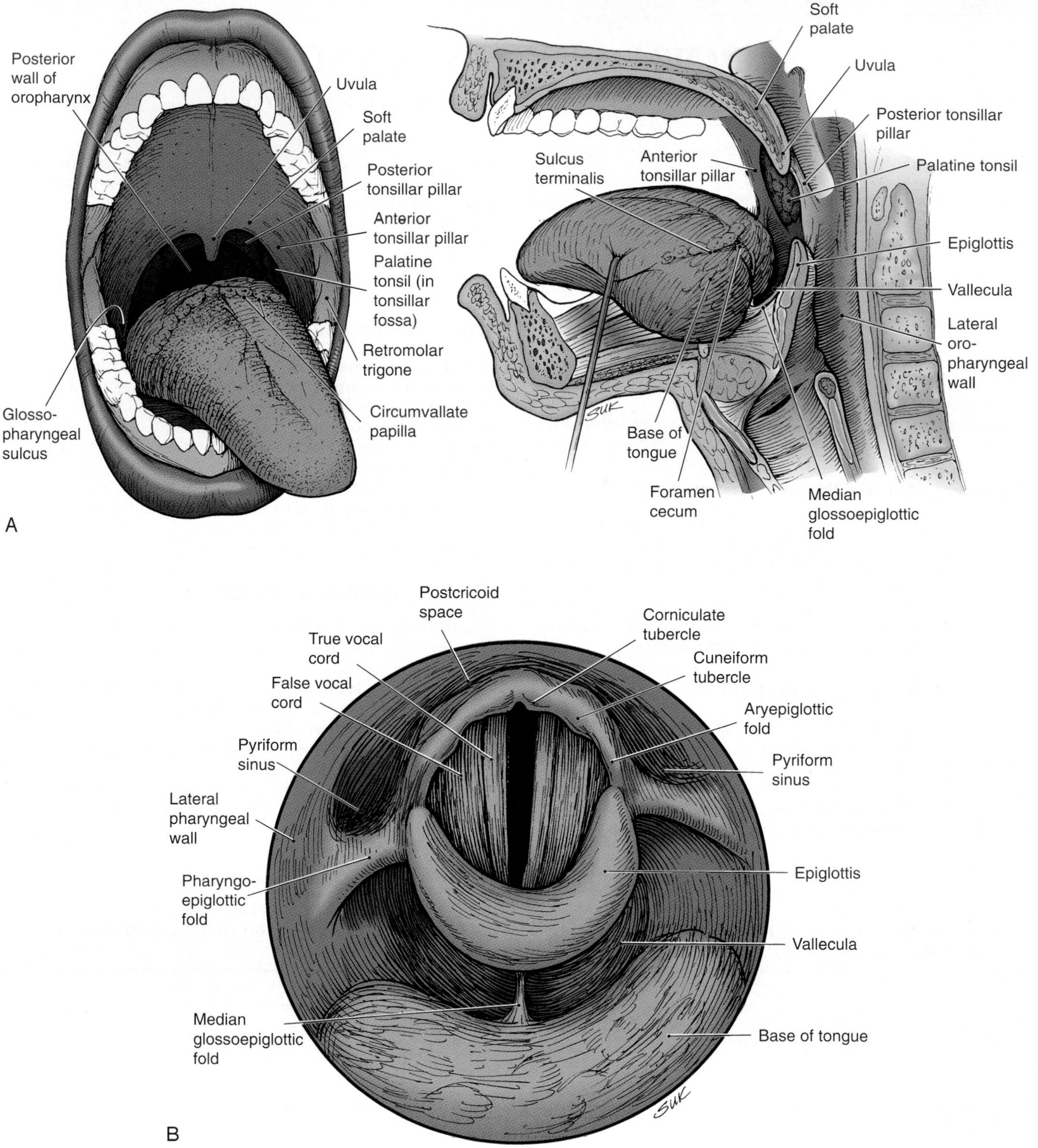

Figure 30-1 Normal anatomy of the oropharynx. **A,** Anterior view and lateral view of the oropharynx with left lateral structures removed. **B,** Oropharynx as viewed through a fiberoptic endoscope.

been an important testing site for parotid-sparing irradiation techniques.

ETIOLOGY AND EPIDEMIOLOGY

Squamous carcinoma of the oropharynx commonly affects patients older than 50 years with a prolonged history of tobacco or heavy alcohol abuse. However, approximately 20% of patients with the disease are younger and have no association with these common risk factors. Research has focused on whether their disease might have a viral origin, with the most frequently identified inciting agent being human papillomavirus 16 (HPV-16).

The association between HPV-16 and oropharyngeal carcinoma, particularly tonsil carcinoma, has been identified by several investigators. Li and colleagues at the Sydney Head and Neck Cancer Institute evaluated 86 tonsil carcinomas for HPV with polymerase chain reaction (PCR) techniques.[5] Evidence of HPV was detected in 46%, and 90% of those cases were positive for HPV-16. Patients with HPV-associated tumors had a significantly improved survival outcome. At the Mayo Clinic, Strome and colleagues[6] studied 52 patients with tonsil cancer. The HPV genome was detected in 46% by PCR. Clinically, HPV-associated carcinomas were identified more often in younger patients than HPV-negative tumors. The consensus of opinion is that HPV-associated tonsil carcinomas occur more often in younger patients who do not have the typical risk profile of smoking and alcohol abuse. Their disease tends to respond better to therapy.[7]

PREVENTION AND EARLY DETECTION

Smoking and, to a lesser degree, heavy alcohol ingestion promote induction of these tumors. Most patients with oropharyngeal squamous carcinomas are smokers. Discontinuing these habits decreases the patient's risk for oropharyngeal carcinoma. Do and collaborators[8] found that patients who continue to smoke after treatment of their index cancer have a twofold increase in the risk of developing a second primary tumor. Patients who ingest more than 14 alcoholic drinks per week after treatment of their index cancer have a 50% increase in the risk for second primary tumors.[8]

Medical personnel can easily visualize most carcinomas of the tonsil and soft palate. Early diagnosis requires identification of the neoplastic cause of a patient's sore throat or other suspicious symptoms. Some soft palate carcinomas manifest as superficial erythema only or as erythema with slightly raised nodules or plaques. Carcinomas of the base of the tongue generally are not visible by simple inspection. For patients who present with soreness in the region of the posterior tongue, an indirect examination and palpation of the base of the tongue should be performed.

BIOLOGIC CHARACTERISTICS AND MOLECULAR BIOLOGY

Ang and coworkers[9] studied the impact of epidermal growth factor receptor (EGFR) expression on survival and pattern of relapse in 155 patients with squamous carcinoma of the head and neck that were treated on Radiation Therapy Oncology Group (RTOG) protocol 90-03. Of the patients studied, 53% had oropharyngeal carcinoma. EGFR expression was not correlated with disease stage at presentation or other known prognostic factors. The overall survival and locoregional control rates of patients whose tumors had high levels of EGFR expression were significantly lower (P = .0006 and P = .003, respectively) than those of patients who had lower levels of tumor EGFR expression. The rate of distant metastases was similar in the two groups. These results were confirmed by Ang in an (unpublished) analysis of patients treated on the concomitant boost arm of RTOG protocol 90-03.

PATHOLOGY AND PATHWAYS OF SPREAD

Approximately 95% of oropharyngeal tumors are squamous cell carcinomas. In patients who have prolonged exposure to tobacco and alcohol, wide areas of mucosal damage along the aerodigestive tract may develop, which is often clinically evident in premalignant form as leukoplakia or erythroplasia (Fig. 30-2). Eventually, this field defect may lead to development of second primary squamous carcinomas, occurring synchronously or metachronously. The annual rate of development of second tumors in head and neck squamous carcinoma is estimated to be 4% to 7%.[8] Malignant transformation is much more likely to develop from erythroplakic mucosal changes than from leukoplakia.

One variant of squamous carcinoma that occurs in the oropharynx is basaloid squamous carcinoma.[10] This is a squamous carcinoma that has cytomorphologic resemblance to the solid variant of adenoid cystic carcinoma. The clinical course of the patients in the series reported[11] seems to be more aggressive than that of the standard squamous carcinoma.

Less common epithelial neoplasms originating in the oropharynx are minor salivary gland tumors[12] and squamous carcinoma with lymphoid stroma (formerly known as lymphoepithelioma).[13] Malignant lymphomas occasionally occur in the Waldeyer ring of the oropharynx.

Pathways of Spread

The route of spread of oropharyngeal cancer varies somewhat with the subsites. Knowledge of the anatomy of the subsites facilitates insight into the pathways of spread.

Tongue Base

The tongue base is the posterior, vertical component of the tongue, and it includes the valleculae. It starts behind the lingual sulcus terminalis and ends at the glossopharyngeal sulcus laterally and at the junction between valleculae and the base of the lingual epiglottis inferiorly. The tongue base contains numerous submucosal lymphoid follicles, which gives the surface an irregular appearance. This lymphoid tissue can enhance on a CT scan with contrast, a radiologic

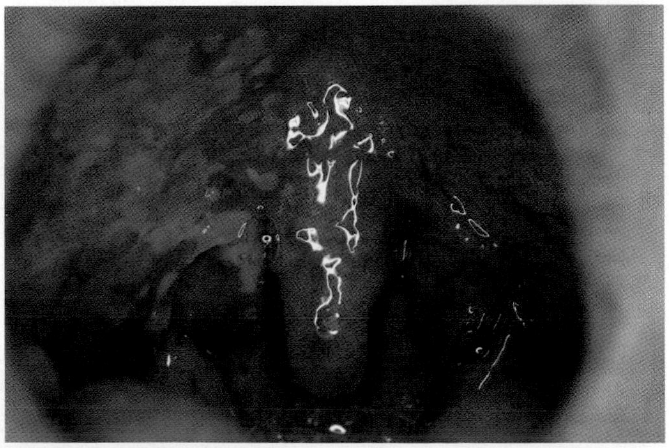

Figure 30-2 The right soft palate has superficial leukoplakia, which on biopsy showed severe squamous cell dysplasia without any invasive carcinoma. The patient presented with a synchronous squamous cell carcinoma of the epiglottis.

appearance that may be confused with tumor. The base of the tongue can also enhance on ^{18}F-fluorodeoxyglucose positron emission tomography (FDG-PET) scans, particularly in young patients.

The base of the tongue has a different embryologic origin than the oral tongue. The main sensory innervation of the tongue base is from the lingual branch of the glossopharyngeal nerve. The motor innervation of the tongue, including the base, is through the hypoglossal nerve. The main lymphatic drainage pathway is to the jugular chain of nodes.

An early-stage tongue base tumor manifests locally as an exophytic tumor growing out from the tongue or as a superficial mucosal tumor. In more advanced stages, the tumors can have a prominent submucosal infiltrative or an ulcerative component (Fig. 30-3A) that invades into the intrinsic tongue muscles. At a later stage, tongue base tumors can extend anteroinferiorly through the intrinsic tongue muscles to invade the extrinsic muscles, causing tongue deviation or impairing mobility (see Fig. 30-3B); spread laterally through the glossopharyngeal (glossopalatine) sulcus to the inferior tonsillar fossa and pharyngeal wall; or grow inferiorly into the larynx, hypopharynx, and pre-epiglottic space. Very advanced tongue base tumors can extend into the soft tissues of the neck or uncommonly invade the mandible.

The incidence of nodal involvement at diagnosis in patients referred to M. D. Anderson Cancer Center (MDACC) between 1948 and 1965 was 78%.[14] Figure 30-4 shows the distribution of nodal disease in 185 patients with tongue base carcinoma. Bilateral nodal disease occurred in 29% of patients, which is as expected for a tumor arising in a midline structure with rich lymphatic networks. In a series of patients with no palpable lymphadenopathy who underwent neck dissections at the Mayo Clinic, the incidence of subclinical nodal involvement was 44%.[15]

Tonsillar Region

The tonsillar region contains the palatine tonsil, which is located between the anterior and posterior tonsillar (faucial) pillars. The palatine tonsil has a surface mucosa of stratified squamous epithelium overlying lymphatic nodules. A fibrous capsule forms the lateral surface of the tonsil, and underneath this capsule are the superior pharyngeal constrictor muscle, the parapharyngeal space, the pterygoid muscles, and the mandible. The internal carotid is located approximately 2 cm lateral and posterior to the tonsil in the parapharyngeal space. The sensory innervation of the tonsil is from the middle and posterior palatine branches of the maxillary nerve.

Tumors originating in the tonsillar fossa can grow as an exophytic mass into the pharyngeal air space, particularly in early-stage presentations. More often, these tumors spread medially into the soft palate (Fig. 30-5), anteriorly into the anterior tonsillar pillar and retromolar trigone, across the glossopalatine sulcus into the tongue base, posteriorly to the posterior tonsillar pillar and lateral pharyngeal wall, laterally into the parapharyngeal space and pterygoid muscles, superiorly into the nasopharynx, and inferiorly into the piriform sinus. Invasion of the tongue base can impair tongue mobility, and infiltration of the pterygoid muscles can cause trismus. Very advanced cancers can extend directly into the neck, encase the carotid artery, or erode the mandible cortex.

The pattern of local extension for 160 patients referred to MDACC between 1968 and 1979 is shown in Table 30-1.[15] In this series, nodal disease was present at diagnosis in 69% of patients. Figure 30-6 shows the sites of nodal involvement in these patients.[15] In a series of patients with no palpable lymphadenopathy who underwent neck dissections at the Mayo Clinic between 1970 and 1988, the incidence of subclinical nodal involvement was 32%.[16]

Soft Palate

The soft palate consists of five muscles (i.e., levator veli palatini, tensor veli palatini, uvular, palatoglossus, and palatopharyngeus) covered with stratified squamous epithelium on the oral surface and most of the nasal surface. The soft palate has an important role in speech and swallowing. It closes off the nasopharynx during swallowing to prevent nasal reflux and

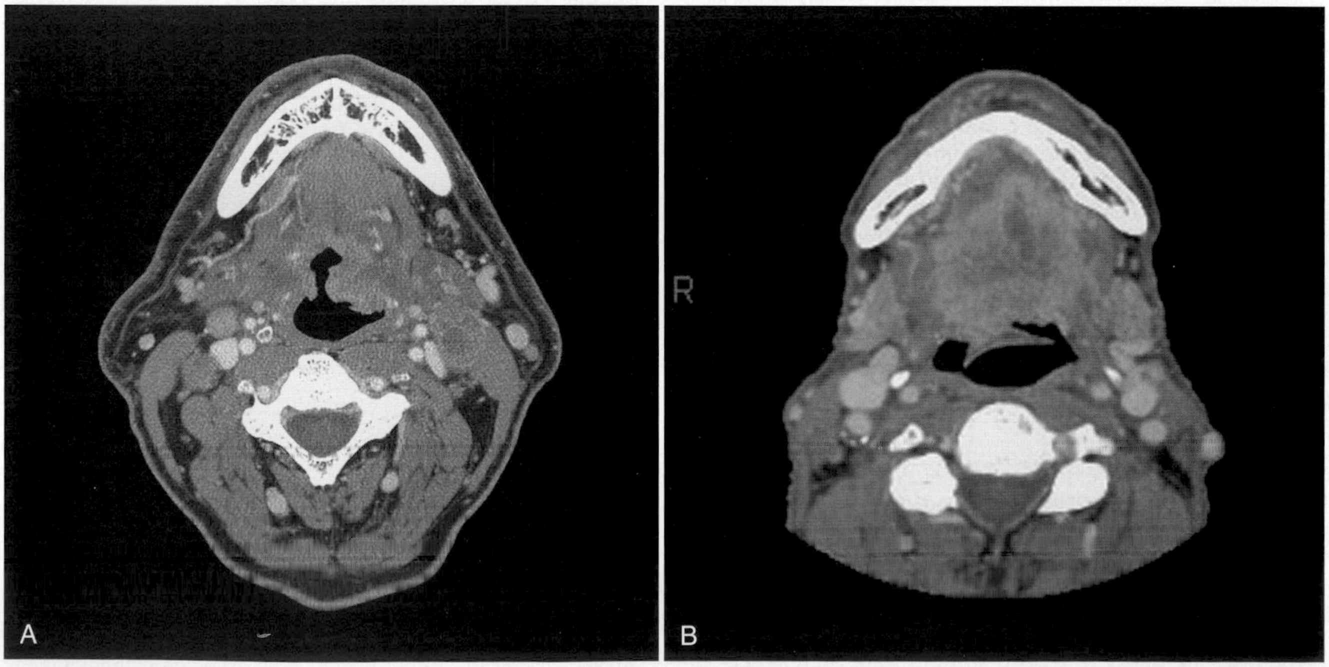

Figure 30-3 **A,** CT demonstrates an ulcerative carcinoma of the base of the tongue. The ulcer is surrounded by a rim of enhancing tumor. **B,** CT shows an infiltrative base of the tongue carcinoma that is invading the extrinsic tongue muscles and fixing the tongue.

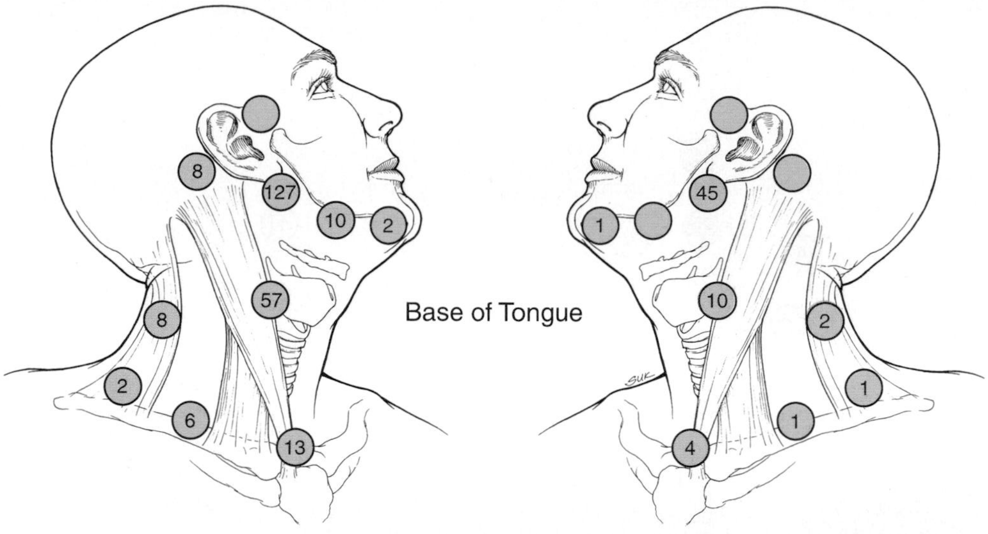

N₀	N₁	N₂A	N₂B	N₃A	N₃B	N₁–N₃ / Total
41	30	21	26	14	53	144 / 185 = 78%

Figure 30-4 Distribution of positive nodes in patients with squamous cell carcinoma of the base of the tongue on presentation to M. D. Anderson Cancer Center, 1948 to 1965. (Data from Lindberg RD: Distribution of cervical lymph node metastases from squamous cell carcinoma of the upper respiratory and digestive tracts. Cancer 29:1446, 1972, with permission.)

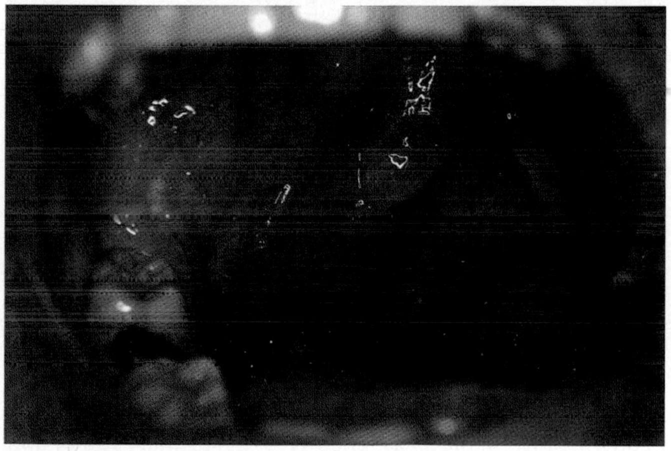

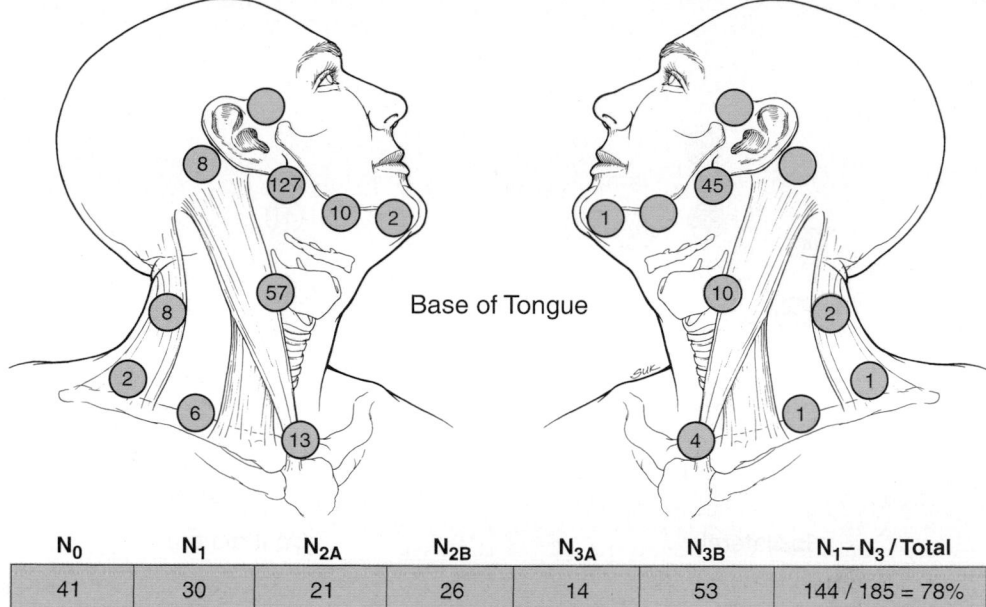

Figure 30-5 Exophytic squamous cell carcinoma of the tonsil. The tumor is growing submucosally along the soft palate and into the pharyngeal airspace without showing evidence of highly infiltrative or ulcerative features.

Table 30-1 Sites of Local Extension for 160 Patients Seen at M. D. Anderson Cancer Center (1968-1979) with Carcinoma of the Tonsil

Site	Percentage of Patients
Tonsil and pillars only	23
Base of tongue	38
Lateral pharyngeal wall	31
Soft palate	23
Retromolar trigone	10
Oral tongue	4
Posterior pharyngeal wall	3
Buccal mucosa	3
Lateral floor of mouth	2
Pterygoid muscles	2
Mandibular or maxillary bone	1

Data from Remmler D, Medina JE, Byers RM, et al: Treatment of choice for squamous carcinoma of the tonsillar fossa. Head Neck Surg 7:206-211, 1985.

during phonation to produce certain sounds. The lesser palatine nerve, a branch of the maxillary nerve, provides sensory innervation to the soft palate. The tensor veli palatini muscle is innervated by the mandibular nerve through the branch to the medial pterygoid muscle. The other soft palate muscles receive innervation by the contribution of the vagus nerve to the pharyngeal plexus.

Almost all soft palate tumors arise on the oral surface. Early tumors tend to grow superficially along mucosal surfaces and often appear as regions of erythroplasia with indistinct borders. The erythroplasia may be multifocal. More advanced tumors extend off of the soft palate; common routes of spread are down the anterior tonsillar pillars (Fig. 30-7), into the tonsillar fossa and pharyngeal wall, and anteriorly onto the hard palate. Locally advanced tumors are not as common as in other oropharyngeal sites.

Figure 30-8 shows the sites of nodal involvement in 80 patients with soft palate carcinoma who were seen at MDACC between 1948 and 1965.[15] The frequency of nodal involvement at diagnosis was 40%, which was lower than the incidences for tongue base and tonsillar region cancers.

Oropharyngeal Wall

The lateral and posterior oropharyngeal walls consist of squamous epithelium overlying the superior and middle pharyngeal constrictor muscles. Located behind the posterior pharyngeal wall epithelium are the retropharyngeal space, longus capitis and longus colli muscles, the prevertebral fascia, and the vertebral bodies.

Tumors of the posterior oropharyngeal wall usually grow anteriorly into the pharyngeal cavity and posteriorly into the prevertebral muscles. However, invasion through the prevertebral fascia and into the vertebral bodies rarely occurs. Tumors of the lateral pharyngeal wall extend anteriorly and posteriorly along the mucosa and parapharyngeal space, can grow as exophytic masses into the pharyngeal cavity, and in

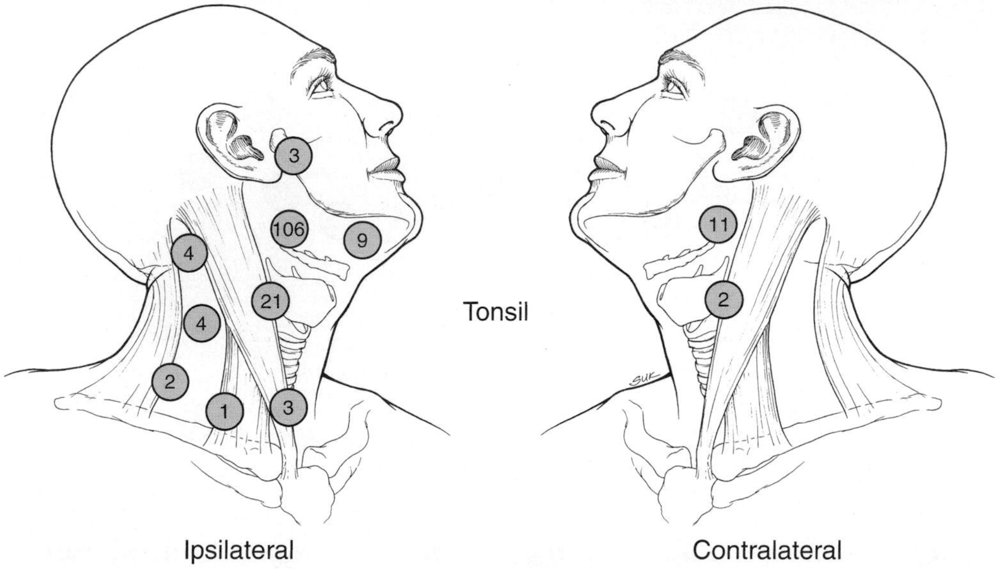

Figure 30-6 Distribution of positive nodes in patients with squamous cell carcinoma of the tonsil on presentation to M. D. Anderson Cancer Center, 1968 to 1979. (Data from Remmler D, Medina JE, Byers RM, et al: Treatment of choice for squamous carcinoma of the tonsillar fossa. Head Neck Surg 7:206-211.)

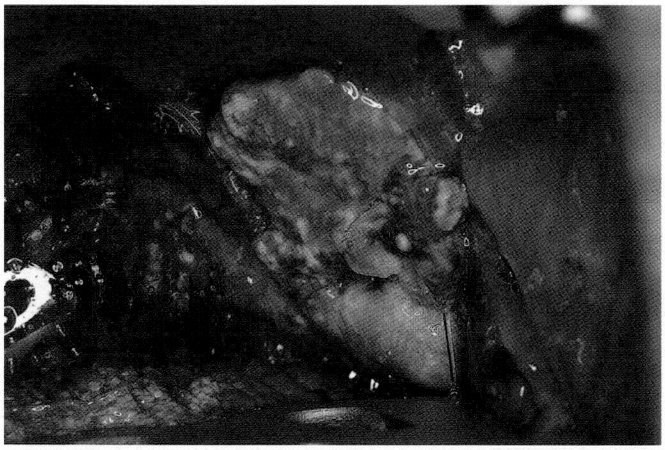

Figure 30-7 Plaquelike squamous cell carcinoma of the left soft palate involved the entire uvula, spread into the right soft palate, and extended into the tonsillar fossa and tonsillar pillar. The tumor was not thick, was mobile on examination, and did not have highly infiltrative features.

advanced stages, can directly invade the neck. A CT image of an oropharyngeal wall tumor is shown in Figure 30-9. The incidence of nodal involvement in patients referred to MDACC with oropharyngeal wall squamous carcinomas was 57%.[17]

CLINICAL MANIFESTATIONS, PATIENT EVALUATION, AND STAGING

Oropharyngeal tumors are relatively asymptomatic in the early stages. Pain, which can be local or radiate to the ear, is a common first symptom. The initial sign of disease is often an asymptomatic neck mass located in the jugulodigastric region. Tongue base carcinomas generally cannot be visualized directly, which may lead to a delay in diagnosis. Patients with advanced-stage disease can present with trismus, necrotic odor, odynophagia, dysphagia, and dysarthria.

Table 30-2 Diagnostic Evaluation for Orophargngeal Cancer

History
Physical examination, including fiberoptic endoscopy
Complete blood cell count, routine serum chemistry tests
Pathologic biopsy
Chest radiograph
CT or MRI of head and neck
Lung CT for T3 to T4 primary tumor stages or for N2 or N3 nodal disease

Patient Evaluation

Physical examination includes assessment of the local extent of the primary tumor and the presence and location of lymphadenopathy (Table 30-2). The size of the primary tumor and nodal disease should be measured, because this is the basis of the American Joint Committee on Cancer (AJCC) staging system for oropharyngeal cancer.[18] Impairment of tongue protrusion in the anterior or lateral direction is a sign of root of tongue involvement. Trismus, a consequence of infiltration of the pterygoid muscles, is documented by measuring the distance between upper and lower incisors or alveolar ridges in edentulous patients. Indirect examination should be performed to detect tumor extension into the larynx or piriform sinus. This finding has a crucial impact on the portal field arrangement. Documentation of the anterior tumor border in relation to the position of radiopaque anatomic structures, such as the retromolar trigone, hard palate, and various teeth, is useful for radiation portal design. All borders of the tumor must be determined precisely, particularly if conformal therapy with intensity-modulated radiation therapy (IMRT) is planned.

Aside from complete history and physical examination, staging workup includes a chest radiograph, complete blood cell count, and routine serum chemistry studies (see Table 30-2). Contrast-enhanced CT and MRI are essential in defining the anatomic extensions of the primary and nodal disease; nodal disease that is not evident on physical examination may be detected by these imaging techniques. Imaging can demon-

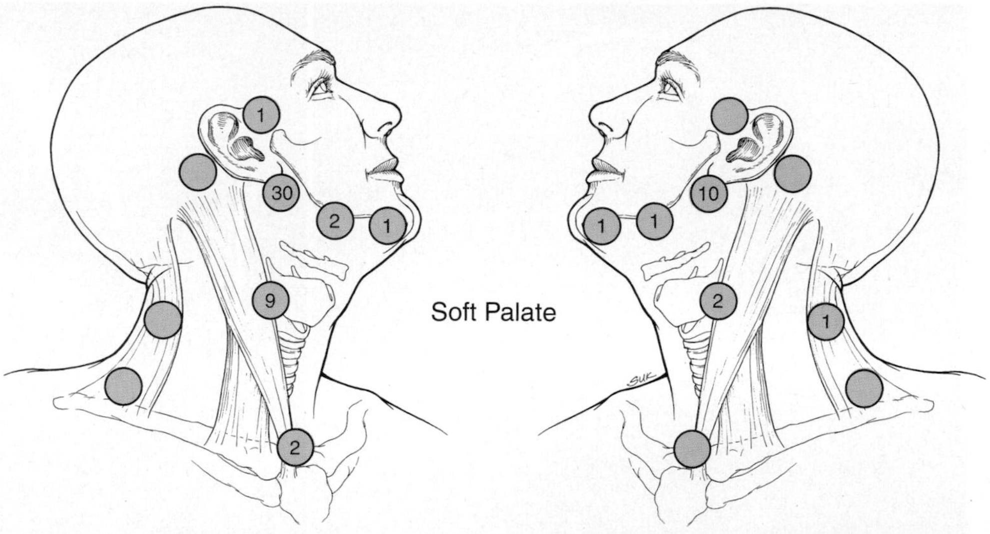

N_0	N_1	N_{2A}	N_{2B}	N_{3A}	N_{3B}	N_1-N_3 / Total
45	12	2	4	4	13	35 / 80 = 44%

Figure 30-8 Distribution of positive nodes in patients with squamous carcinoma of the soft palate on presentation to M. D. Anderson Cancer Center, 1948 to 1965. (Data from Lindberg RD: Distribution of cervical lymph node metastases from squamous cell carcinoma of the upper respiratory and digestive tracts. Cancer 29:1446, 1972, with permission.)

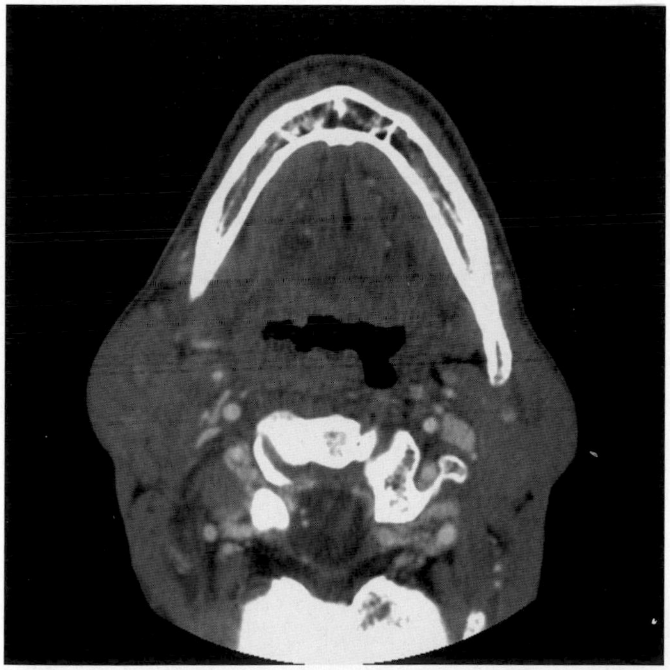

Figure 30-9 CT of a patient with a posterior oropharyngeal wall squamous cell carcinoma demonstrates that the tumor extends to the right lateral oropharyngeal wall. Deep extension into the prevertebral muscles has not occurred.

strate the presence of retropharyngeal nodes (Fig. 30-10A), invasion into the pterygoid muscles (see Fig. 30-10B), and the extent of base of tongue invasion. At MDACC, CT is the standard modality used for staging oropharyngeal patients. MRI is occasionally used to provide improved definition of fascial planes (Fig. 30-11). For patients who present with advanced-stage disease, CT of the lung is a reasonable approach because it is a more sensitive test than a chest radiograph in detecting lung metastases. Other tests are obtained as indicated by the clinical findings. The ability of PET scanning to detect occult systemic metastases that cannot be identified with standard CT imaging is being studied.[19]

Many patients present with asymptomatic subdigastric lymphadenopathy, which should be appropriately evaluated if indicated by the clinical situation. On CT, malignant nodes associated with oropharyngeal tumors often appear cystic. These nodes should not be confused with benign branchial cleft cysts. The preferable method to biopsy an oropharyngeal node is by fine-needle aspiration, with ultrasound guidance if the node is not palpable. Excisional nodal biopsy often causes scarring in the operative bed, which can be indistinguishable from tumor on imaging and physical examination. Determining whether the surgeon resected all of an early-stage nodal presentation or just biopsied a node can be difficult. Excisional nodal biopsy complicates treatment planning. Patients can also present with advanced nodal presentations, with features such as matting, fixation, and extension through the skin.

Patients who present with malignant jugulodigastric or, less commonly, midcervical nodes and no clear primary tumor may have an oropharyngeal primary. Examination under anesthesia should be performed with biopsy of suspicious mucosal sites of the head and neck. Early-stage tongue base cancers may have the appearance of mucosal erythema, hypervascularity, or slight thickening of the mucosa without being a component of an obvious mass. Manipulation of the base of the tongue during the examination under anesthesia may cause bleeding, which can serve as a sentinel sign of an occult base of tongue primary tumor. Subtle asymmetry of the tonsils can result from a small tonsil tumor. Ipsilateral tonsillectomy is often performed if the tumor is suspected to be originating in the oropharynx. The role of PET in detecting occult primary oropharyngeal carcinomas is being investigated at many medical centers.[19]

Staging

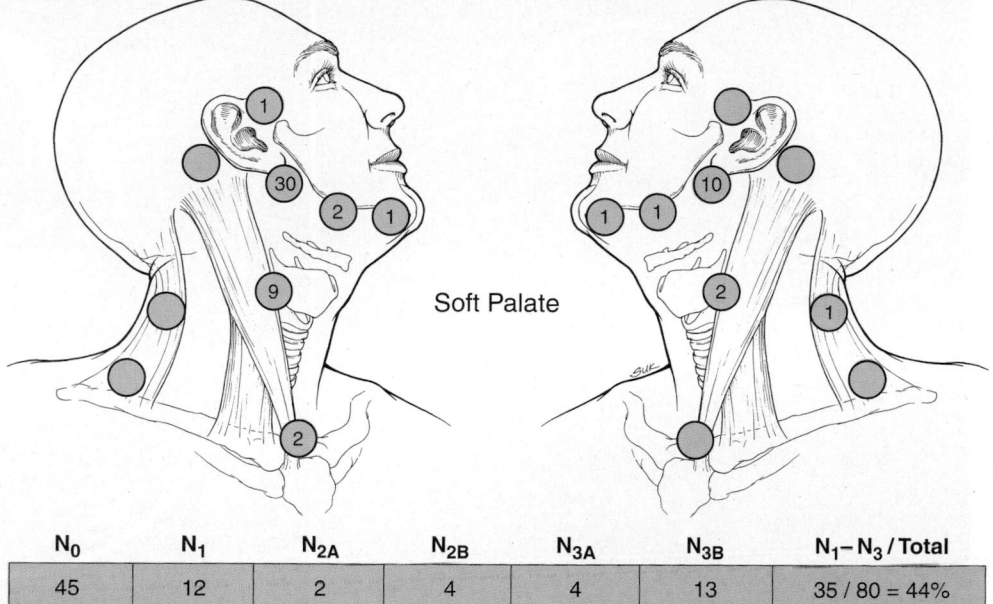

The 2002 AJCC staging system for oropharyngeal carcinomas, which is a clinical staging system, is shown in Table 30-3.[18] All available information obtained before initiation of definitive

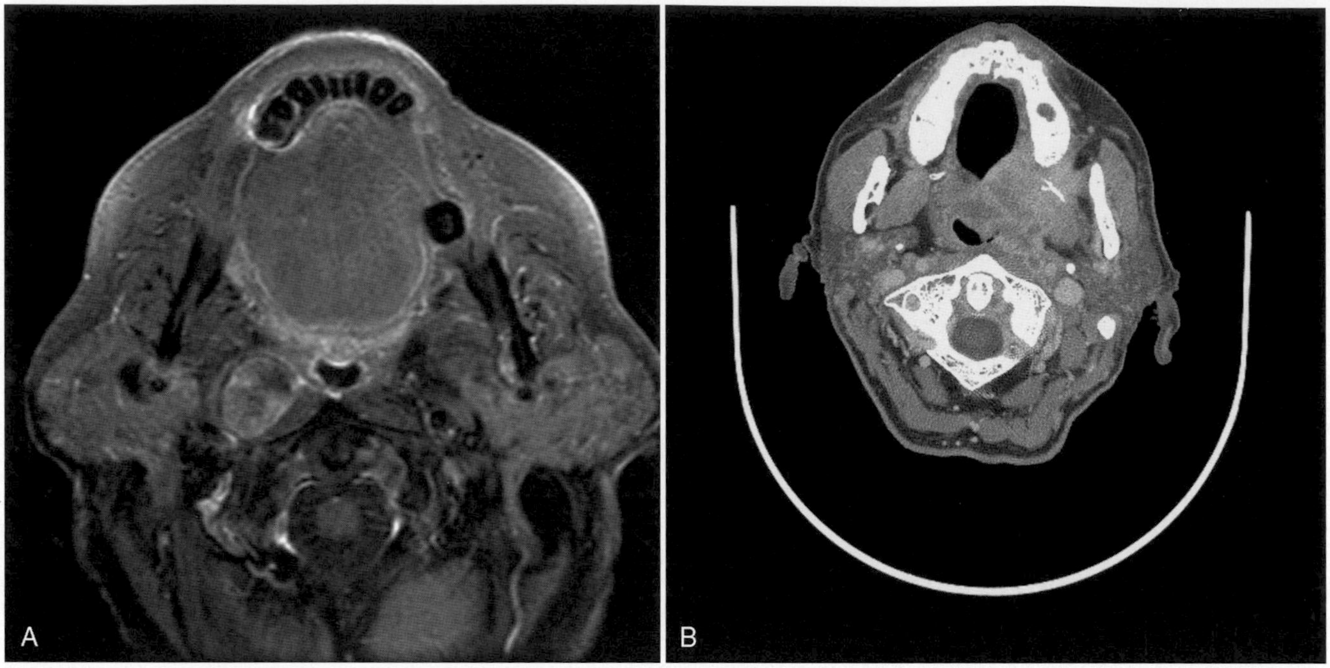

Figure 30-10 **A,** MRI shows a large, right retropharyngeal lymph node in a patient with tongue base cancer. **B,** CT demonstrates an infiltrative tonsil carcinoma directly invading the pterygoid muscles and causing trismus.

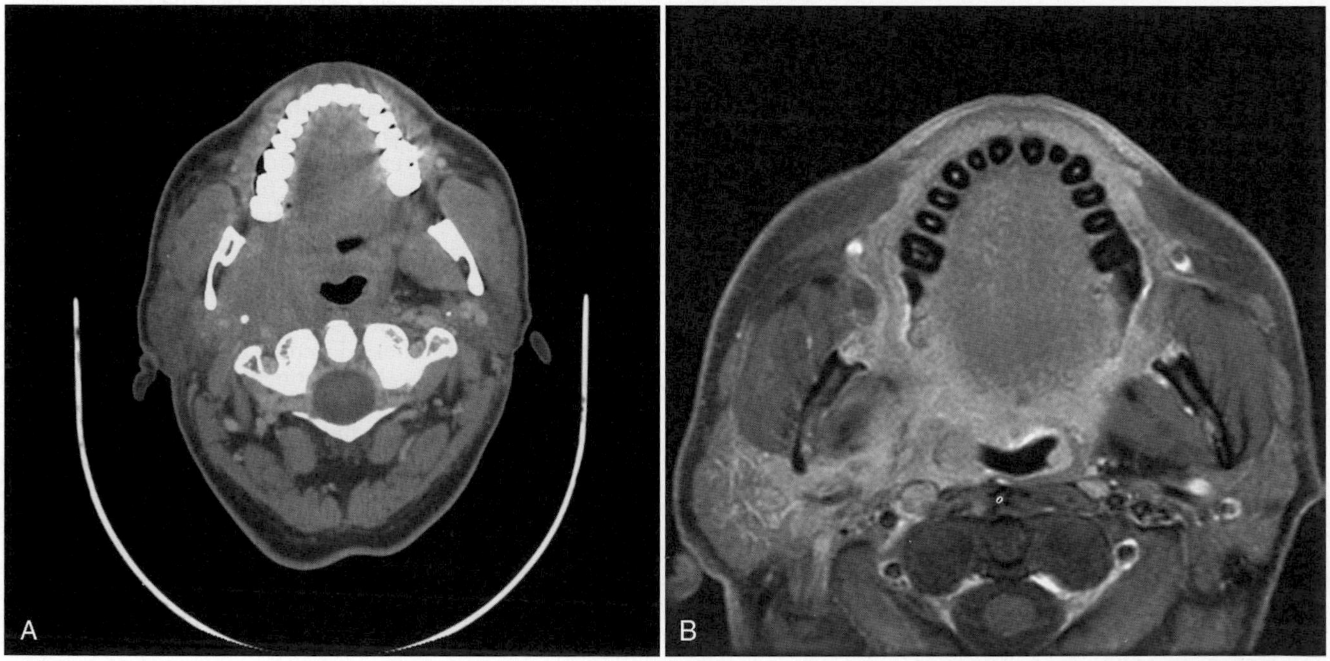

Figure 30-11 **A,** CT of a patient with a T4N2c tonsil carcinoma shows diffuse involvement of the tonsil, pterygoid muscles, parapharyngeal space, and prevertebral muscles. **B,** MRI of the same patient shows improved definition of the involved structures and tissue planes. A right-sided retropharyngeal node is evident, and prevertebral musculature does not appear to be involved with tumor. The lateral pterygoid muscle appears to be less diffusely infiltrated than on CT.

treatment that contributes to the accuracy of disease assessment, including CT, MRI, and ultrasound findings, can be used to stage the disease.

The distinction among TI, T2, and T3 tumors is based on primary tumor size. In the current staging system, T4 lesions have been divided into T4a (resectable) and T4b (unresectable). Tumors are classified as T4a on the basis of invasion into the following adjacent structures: larynx, deep or extrinsic muscles of the tongue, medial pterygoid muscle, hard palate, or mandible. T4b tumors invade the lateral pterygoid muscle, pterygoid plates, lateral nasopharynx, or skull base or encase the carotid artery. Stage IV has been divided into IVA and IVB, based on whether the disease is T4a or T4b or whether the patient has N2 or N3 nodal disease.

Table 30-3 TNM Definitions and Stage Grouping for Oropharyngeal Carcinomas

Primary Tumor (T)	Regional Lymph Nodes (N)
TX: Primary tumor cannot be assessed	NX: Regional lymph nodes cannot be assessed
T0: No evidence of primary tumor	N0: No regional lymph node metastasis
Tis: Carcinoma in situ	N1: Metastasis in a single ipsilateral lymph node, 3 cm or less in its greatest dimension
T1: Tumor 2 cm or less in its greatest dimension	N2: Metastasis in a single ipsilateral lymph node, more than 3 cm but not more than 6cm in it greatest dimension, or in multiple ipsilateral lymph nodes, none more than 6 cm in the greatest dimension, or in bilateral or contralateral lymph nodes, none more than 6 cm in the greatest dimension
T2: Tumor more than 2 cm but not more than 4 cm in its greatest dimension	N2a: Metastasis in a single ipsilateral lymph node more than 3 cm but not more than 6 cm in greatest dimension
T3: Tumor more than 4 cm in its greatest dimension	N2b: Metastasis in multiple ipsilateral lymph nodes, none more than 6 cm in the greatest dimension
T4a: Tumor invades the larynx, deep/extrinsic muscle of tongue, medial pterygoid, hard palate, or mandible	N2c: Metastasis in bilateral or contralateral lymph nodes, none more than 6 cm in its greatest dimension
T4b: Tumor invades lateral pterygoid muscle, pterygoid plates, lateral nasopharynx, or skull base or encases carotid artery	N3: Metastasis in a lymph node more than 6 cm in its greatest dimension

Stage Grouping for Tumors of the Oropharynx and Hypopharynx

Stage 0	Tis	N0	M0
Stage I	T1	N0	M0
Stage II	T2	N0	M0
Stage III	T3	N0	M0
	T1	N1	M0
	T2	N1	M0
	T3	N1	M0
Stage IVA	T4a	N0	M0
	T4a	N1	M0
	T1	N2	M0
	T2	N2	M0
	T3	N2	M0
	T4a	N2	M0
Stage IVB	T4b	Any N	M0
	Any T	N3	M0
Stage IVC	Any T	Any N	M1

Green F, Page D, Fleming I, et al: Pharynx (including base of tongue, soft palate and uvula). *In* American Joint Committee on Cancer (eds): Cancer Staging Manual, 6th ed. New York, Springer, 2002, pp 31-46.

The T4 classification is based on invasion of local tumor into adjacent structures. The flaw of such a system is that a small favorable tumor can invade an adjacent site and be upstaged to T4. For example, a small tumor in the vallecula can spread into the lingual surface of the epiglottis and be upstaged to T4. We think that for the system to have any meaning, minor clinical extensions to the listed structures should not upstage a patient's disease to a T4 classification. For a tumor to be T4, invasion of the pterygoid muscles should be extensive enough to cause some evidence of trismus. Mere extension of soft palate tumors onto the adjacent hard palate should not upstage a patient to T4. Tumor invasion into the deep or extrinsic muscles of the tongue is a difficult clinical determination, because the boundary of the deep muscles cannot be seen or palpated on examination. Tumors that cause significant tongue deviation on protrusion or cause tongue fixation can be assumed to be invading the deep tongue muscles. Base of tongue tumors that significantly involve the deep tongue muscles can usually be palpated through the posterolateral floor of mouth gutter. Staging of nodal disease using the AJCC system is relatively straightforward based on nodal size, number, and location.

PRIMARY THERAPY

General Principles of Treatment

The goal of treatment is to maximize the control rate while minimizing functional impairment and other morbidities. The choice of treatment depends on the stage and site of the disease. Modifications of treatment technique, including altered fractionation and IMRT, have been shown to improve outcomes by reducing treatment-related morbidity.

Influence of Stage and Site of Disease

Early-stage oropharyngeal carcinomas (T1, T2, N0-1 disease) can be treated by radiation therapy or surgery (often with the addition of postoperative radiation therapy, as indicated by the pathologic findings) with the expectation of achieving similar local and regional control rates. Consequently, treatment selection is based on the anticipated functional and cosmetic outcome and the need for and extent of nodal therapy. For example, surgery is an option for the treatment of small and superficial tumors of the anterior faucial pillars or tonsillar fossa, particularly when resection can be done through a transoral approach and the likelihood of obtaining tumor-free resection margins is high. If standard portals are being used, radiation therapy is also suitable for the treatment of most T1-2N0-1 carcinomas of the tonsillar region with minimal extension onto the soft palate or other midline structures because a high local and regional control rate can be achieved with unilateral irradiation without producing permanent xerostomia. If IMRT is used, most patients with early-stage oropharyngeal carcinomas can be treated with the expectation of retaining adequate salivary flow. Radiation therapy is preferred for the treatment of small tonsil tumors that extend onto the soft palate and for almost all soft palate tumors because resection of portions of the soft palate will impair swallowing. Tumors involving midline oropharyngeal structures should be treated with bilateral irradiation. At MDACC, almost all early-stage oropharyngeal squamous carcinomas are treated with radiation therapy.

Intermediate-stage carcinomas (i.e., larger T2, nonextensive T3, or N2-3 disease) are preferably treated by primary radiation therapy with or without chemotherapy because most patients undergoing surgical treatment ultimately receive postoperative radiation therapy for the presence of multiple positive nodes, extranodal extension, or close resection margins. Resection of intermediate-stage carcinomas often causes some loss of normal tissue function. The approaches to management of nodal disease are presented later.

Locally advanced infiltrative primary tumors (i.e., larger, infiltrative T3 and T4) can be treated with composite primary resection, nodal dissection, and postoperative irradiation with or without chemotherapy. Large tissue deficits can be reconstructed with microvascular free flaps, which makes these procedures more cosmetically acceptable. However, because of the severe functional loss that occurs when large oropharyngeal carcinomas are resected, most patients are treated with irradiation and concurrent systemic therapy.

Treatment Duration and Altered Fractionation Schedules

Several studies have documented an inverse correlation between treatment duration and local control in patients with oropharyngeal carcinoma. Bataini and colleagues[20] performed a multivariate analysis of the data of 465 patients with carcinoma of the tonsillar region who were treated at the Institut Curie between 1958 and 1976. They found that T stage and radiotherapy duration, as a continuous variable, had a highly significant correlation with local control (both at the $P < .0001$ level). When stratified by T stage, treatment duration was inversely correlated with the local control of T3 ($P = .002$) and T4 tumors ($P = .04$).

Withers and colleagues,[4,21] at nine institutions in North America and England, investigated the effectiveness of various fractionation schemes in the treatment of 676 patients with tonsil carcinoma irradiated with external beam photons alone between 1976 and 1985. Fractionation schedules used varied between 51 Gy in 16 fractions and 75 Gy in 37 fractions. The mean treatment duration was 37 days and ranged from 20 to 56 days in 90% of the patients. Treatment parameters that significantly correlated with local control were total dose, treatment duration, and whether nodal disease was present. For a constant treatment duration, local control probability increased by nearly 2% for every 1 Gy increment in total dose. For a constant total dose, the local control probability decreased by 1% per day of treatment prolongation, presumably due to accelerated regrowth of surviving tumor clonogens during therapy. The estimated extra dose that must be given to compensate for each day of treatment prolongation was in the range of 0.5 to 0.7 Gy per day. Fraction size by itself was not an independent prognostic factor for tumor control. Patients with nodal disease had worse local control rates than node negative patients ($P < .02$). After accounting for the significant variables studied, the dose-response curves for tumor control were still shallow, suggesting that additional causes for response heterogeneity exist for these tumors.

Withers and collegues[4,21] also studied the late (>3 months) normal tissue complications that occurred in these 676 patients. Higher total dose correlated with a higher incidence of bone, muscle, and mucosal complications. For a given total dose, larger fraction size was associated with an increased risk of bone and muscle (but not mucosal) complications. There was an inverse relationship between treatment duration and mucosal complications. Field size correlated significantly with the incidence of mandibular complications. Mucosal complications occurred earlier in follow-up than bone or muscle complications. Withers and coworkers[4,21] concluded that the radiobiologic characteristics of bone and muscle were similar to the characteristics of other late-responding tissues, whereas late complications in mucosa had radiobiologic parameters similar to those of acutely responding tissues.

Overgaard and associates[22] evaluated the impact of treatment duration in a phase III trial of head and neck squamous carcinomas. In this Danish trial, 1476 patients were randomized to receive 5 or 6 fractions of 2 Gy per week. The total dose was 66 to 68 Gy, except for T1 glottic patients, who received 62 Gy. Median overall treatment durations were 39 days (group receiving 6 fractions/week) and 46 days (group receiving 5 fractions/week). Of the patients enrolled, 62% had larynx cancer, and 29% had pharyngeal tumors. Overall 5-year local control rates were 76% and 64% for the 6 and 5 fractions/week groups, respectively ($P = .0001$). Acute morbidity was increased in the accelerated treatment arm but uniformly resolved within 3 months after the initiation of therapy. Rates of late toxicity were the same for both groups. By shortening the treatment duration, local control was improved without any increase in late toxicity.

The benefit of using *altered fractionation schedules* for treating head and neck squamous carcinoma was evaluated in the Radiation Oncology Group protocol 90-03.[23] Sixty percent of the patients on the trial had oropharyngeal carcinoma. Patients were randomized to receive standard fractionation (70 Gy in 35 fractions over 7 weeks), hyperfractionation (81.6 Gy in 68 fractions over 7 weeks), split-course accelerated fractionation (67.2 Gy in 42 fractions of 1.6 Gy twice daily over 6 weeks, with a split after 38.4 Gy), or accelerated fractionation with concomitant boost (72 Gy in 42 fractions over 6 weeks). On the concomitant-boost schedule, patients receive 54 Gy in 1.8-Gy fractions over 6 weeks to a field that includes known disease and sites of suspected subclinical disease. The boost field, which includes only clinically evident disease, is given as a second daily fraction of 1.5 Gy for 12 fractions (18 Gy total) with at least a 6-hour interfraction interval during the last 2.5 weeks of treatment. The 1113 patients were randomized on the four arms of the trial. Patients treated with hyperfractionation and concomitant boost fractionation had significantly better locoregional control ($P = .045$ and $P = .054$, respectively) than patients who were treated with standard fractionation. No significant difference in overall survival was found between the four trial arms. All three altered fractionation groups had higher rates of acute side effects compared with standard fractionation, but these acute reactions resolved within 3 months of completing therapy. No significant increase in late complications was seen in the altered fractionation arms. The concomitant boost fractionation schedule was thought to be the preferred schedule for patients being treated with radiotherapy alone, because it requires 26 fewer fractions than hyperfractionation.

Intensity-Modulated Radiation Therapy

The treatment technique of choice for delivering external beam radiation therapy for most patients with oropharyngeal carcinoma is IMRT. Partial sparing of the function of one or both parotid glands is achievable in most cases without compromising tumor coverage. With proper knowledge of anatomy and pattern of tumor spread, the radiation dose can be focused with some precision on the desired target, and partial sparing of normal tissue can be achieved, sometimes even in the targeted gland. Patients who have nodal disease that extends posteriorly around the lateral aspect of the vertebral bodies and patients with posterior pharyngeal wall disease with similar posterolateral extension will have improved tumor coverage if IMRT is used.

Integration of Treatment of Primary Tumor and Nodal Disease

Three strategies are used to manage patients with resectable nodal disease whose primary tumor is being treated with definitive radiation therapy (alone or with concurrent chemotherapy): radiation therapy followed by neck dissection only for patients with persistent nodal masses 6 weeks after completing radiation therapy, neck dissection followed by radiation therapy, or planned neck dissection after radiation therapy regardless of disease response.

The strategy used for most patients at MDACC is to treat patients initially with irradiation (alone or with concurrent chemotherapy) and perform a neck dissection only for residual disease that is present 6 to 8 weeks after the completion of therapy. However, if extensive dental extractions are necessary before radiation therapy, it is reasonable to perform a neck dissection under the same general anesthesia. Patients selected for preradiotherapy neck dissections usually have nodes that are 5 cm or larger, which increases the probability that the patient will require a neck dissection after radiation therapy. This strategy is being used at MDACC less often than in the past, because many patients with larger nodes have complete responses to irradiation and can avoid neck dissection.

Patients who are treated with a planned neck dissection regardless of response to irradiation often have nodal disease located near the brachial plexus low in level IV (below the cricoid cartilage) and in the supraclavicular fossa. After it traverses between the anterior and medial scalene muscles, the brachial plexus is located relatively superficial in the lateral supraclavicular fossa; boost treatment with an electron beam energetic enough to treat the nodal disease in many cases also irradiates some of the plexus. If the brachial plexus will receive doses of more than 64 Gy in the field required for nodal treatment, it is preferable to give a lower radiation dose and follow this with a postirradiation neck dissection. In this scenario, the treatment to the supraclavicular fossa and low neck are terminated at 60 Gy, and a neck dissection is performed approximately 6 weeks later.

Treatment Policies by Subsite

Tonsillar Region Carcinomas

Radiation therapy is the preferred treatment for T1 and T2 tonsillar region carcinomas in many centers; for most T3 carcinomas, concurrent chemotherapy is given as a radiation enhancer. Unilateral irradiation designed to avoid permanent xerostomia has been increasingly used in the treatment of T1-2N0-1 carcinomas of the tonsillar fossa with at most minor extension onto the soft palate. With IMRT, the function of the contralateral parotid and submandibular glands can be spared. More advanced stages are treated with coverage that includes the bilateral neck nodes at risk. In selected cases, boost dose to the primary tumor extension into the base of the tongue, which is often slower to regress than the tonsillar fossa component of the tumor, is delivered by interstitial therapy for an additional dose of 15 to 20 Gy.[24] The implant should be performed within 2 weeks after completing external beam therapy.

The standard therapy for T4b tumors is surgery and comprehensive postoperative radiation therapy. Preoperatively, the surgeon must rule out extension of tumor to unresectable structures including the carotid, nasopharynx, and skull base. Depending on the anatomic extensions of the primary tumor, various normal tissue structures must be resected, including variable extents of mandible, soft palate, pterygoid muscles, and tongue. The role of organ-preserving therapy with chemoirradiation is being actively investigated, and almost all patients at MDACC are being treated on nonsurgical protocols.

Tongue Base Carcinomas

Most centers regard definitive radiation therapy using IMRT as the treatment of choice for T1 and T2 tongue base carcinomas. For T3 tongue base carcinomas, concurrent chemoradiation is usually given to enhance the tumor response. Lymph nodes on both sides of the neck are treated in all patients because the primary tumors are situated at or close to midline and have a high propensity for bilateral nodal spread. In selected cases, boost dose to the primary tumor or supplemental dose to slowly regressing tumors is delivered using interstitial brachytherapy (Fig. 30-12).

The traditional therapy for T4 resectable tumors is surgery and postoperative irradiation. However, this often requires a laryngectomy to prevent aspiration and the patient will frequently have severe dysphagia, partly due to loss of propulsive force of the tongue base. Increasingly, these patients are being treated with combinations of systemic therapy and irradiation on clinical trials with the goal of organ preservation.

Soft Palate Carcinomas

Early-stage soft palate tumors often have indistinct borders and are associated with other areas of erythroplasia. Consequently, surgeons can have difficulty achieving negative surgical margins if they attempt to perform a small excision on tumors with vague clinical borders. Surgical excision of all but the smallest soft palate carcinomas will cause velopharyngeal incompetence resulting in nasal regurgitation and speech dysfunction that cannot be adequately corrected with prosthetic devices. Radiation therapy is generally considered the treatment of choice.

In well-delineated, accessible T1 and T2 tumors, the boost phase of treatment can be delivered by an intraoral cylindric applicator using orthovoltage radiation. The boost dose, in the range of 15 to 18 Gy in 5 or 6 fractions, is generally administered before external beam radiation therapy, while the tumor can be clearly visualized. A patient's tolerance of the applicator is better if it is used before mucositis develops. Use of the intraoral applicator is most feasible for edentulous patients, because more space is present to insert the applicator. Boosting soft palate tumors with interstitial brachytherapy is routinely performed in selected European centers.[25,26]

Concurrent chemoradiation is the preferred treatment for T3 and T4 tumors. An exception is for patients whose tumors are stage T3 on length criteria but who have superficial tumors with low volumes.

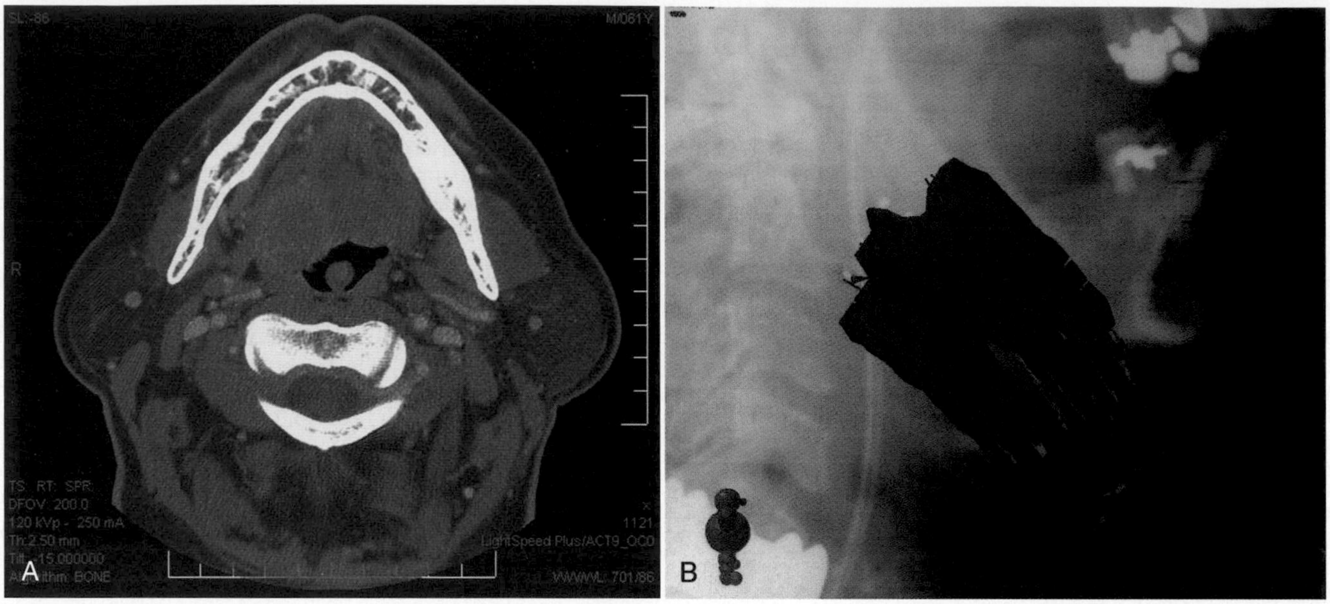

Figure 30-12 **A,** A 62-year-old man presented in August 2004 with a firm, T2N0 squamous carcinoma in the right base of the tongue. He was treated with intensity-modulated radiation therapy using a concomitant boost fractionation schedule to 72 Gy in 40 fractions over 6 weeks. Ten days after completing treatment, he continued to have a significant, palpable tongue mass, and a decision was made to perform an interstitial implant on the 14th posttreatment day. Under direct palpation, the initial three catheters were placed 1 cm apart in a coronal-plane row, positioned 1 cm behind the mass. Three more coronal rows, 1 cm apart, of three catheters were placed moving anteriorly until the persistent mass was encompassed three dimensionally. A total of 12 catheters was used. **B,** The treatment goal was to deliver a 15-Gy boost using iridium 192, dosed at 70 cGy per hour. The isodose cloud, generated using BrachyVision software, shows the volume of tissue *(red)* that received 15 Gy. The patient had no evidence of disease and was functioning well and without complications in December 2005.

Oropharyngeal Wall Carcinomas

Radiation therapy with chemotherapy enhancement for locally advanced stages is the preferred treatment for oropharyngeal wall tumors. Because the posterior pharyngeal wall is immediately adjacent to the prevertebral fascia and muscles, it is usually not possible to resect tumors of the posterior oropharyngeal wall with a wide margin, except for very small, superficial tumors. Surgical access to the posterior and lateral pharyngeal wall is more technically complex than access to more anteriorly located oropharyngeal structures.

Treatment Results

The results of treatment using radiation therapy or surgery for early-stage carcinomas are described in the following sections, including outcomes using IMRT in patients with short-term follow-up. The results for locally advanced carcinomas focus on patients treated with two different approaches: surgery with postoperative radiotherapy and chemoirradiation.

Results Using Intensity-Modulated Radiation Therapy for Early-Stage Oropharyngeal Carcinomas

Most reports of the results of treating head and neck cancer with IMRT group all head and neck sites together when reporting outcome. Three reports focus on the results of treating the oropharynx only.

Chao and associates[27] described the outcome of treatment of oropharyngeal carcinoma with IMRT at Washington University. Seventy-four patients were treated; 43 were given postoperative IMRT, and 31 were treated definitively. The primary tumors were T1 and T2 in 55% of cases; 84% had nodal disease. The mean dose to patients being treated definitively was 70 Gy given in 35 fractions over 7 weeks; postoperative patients were given 66 Gy in 2-Gy fractions over 6.6 weeks. The mean parotid dose was reported to be 18.6 Gy. Chemotherapy was given to 17 patients, mostly concurrently with the IMRT. Ten locoregional recurrences (crude rate of 13%) were reported at a median follow-up of 13 months. The study authors concluded that IMRT was effective treatment in these patients and had a favorable toxicity profile.

Garden and colleagues[28] described outcomes for 54 patients with TX, T1, or T2 oropharyngeal carcinomas treated with IMRT at MDACC by June 2002. Nodal disease was present in 45 patients, and concurrent chemotherapy was given to 7 of these patients; 4 of the 7 had N3 nodal disease. The most common fractionation schedule, used in 72% of patients, was 66 Gy given in 30 fractions over 6 weeks to the primary tumor and nodal disease and 54 Gy to subclinical sites. Another schedule used for four patients with larger T2 tumors was concomitant boost (72 Gy in 40 fractions over 6 weeks). Acute toxicity was similar to that seen with parallel-opposed fields and similar fractionation, and as expected, the mean parotid dose was markedly reduced. At a median follow-up interval of 13 months, the locoregional control rate was 91%. The actuarial 2-year relapse-free and overall survival rates were 86% and 89%, respectively. Although not specifically measured, parotid function was improved compared with what would be expected with parallel-opposed field treatment.

By September 2003, 130 patients with oropharynx tumors had been treated with IMRT at MDACC. (A. Garden, personal communication, 2006). Most patients had tonsillar or tongue base carcinoma. Neck dissections were performed as needed 6 weeks after the completion of radiation therapy. The median follow-up period was 30 months. There were 21 TX, 47 T1, 46 T2, 11 T3, and 5 patients with T4 tumors. The 3-year actuarial local control rate and overall survival rate for all patients were 95% and 93%, respectively. The series is being analyzed for a full report.

De Arruda and coworkers[29] reported results at Memorial Sloan-Kettering Cancer Center (MSKCC) using IMRT to treat 50 patients with oropharyngeal carcinoma. The tumors were T1 and T2 in 66% of the patients; 82% of patients had nodal disease. Concurrent chemotherapy was used in 86%, usually consisting of single agent cisplatin. Median follow-up was 18 months. The most common fractionation schedule used was 70 Gy given in 33 fractions over 6.6 weeks, with doses of 59.4 Gy and 54 Gy given to regions of high-risk and low-risk subclinical disease in the same field. The 2-year actuarial local control rate was 98%, and the regional control rate was 88%. Ten patients underwent neck dissection for persistent nodal masses, and only one patient had pathologic nodal disease. The incidence of RTOG grade 2 late toxicity was 33%. Three patients had esophageal strictures that required dilatation. Saliva output was improved with an increasing time interval from the completion of therapy. The investigators, who included some prominent surgeons at MSKCC, concluded that IMRT is an ideal therapy for oropharyngeal cancer in terms of effectiveness and tolerability. Acute toxicities were manageable, and the focused sparing of the parotids was thought to enable a better quality of life for the patients after treatment.

IMRT has become the standard of care for oropharyngeal cancer at MDACC because of the excellent locoregional control rates achieved and the obvious improvement in parotid function. Parallel-opposed fields are used only for frail patients who cannot tolerate the longer duration of daily therapy required for IMRT and for an occasional patient whose tumor is so extensive that significant parotid sparing cannot be achieved.

Treatment Results for T1 and T2 Oropharyngeal Carcinoma Using Standard Fields

The results of treatment with radiation for T1N0 and T2N0 squamous carcinoma of the oropharynx at MDACC were reported by Selek and associates in 2004.[30] Between 1970 and 1998, 175 patients were treated. Seventy-one percent of the tumors were classified as T2, and the remaining tumors were classified as T1 or TX. The two most common treatment schedules were standard daily fractionation to a median dose of 66 Gy given in 33 fractions over 6.6 weeks (85 patients) and concomitant boost fractionation in a dose of 72 Gy given in 42 fractions over 6 weeks (73 patients). The 5-year actuarial local control rates for T1/TX and T2 disease were 92% and 81%, respectively. The local control rate for each subsite within the oropharynx did not vary significantly. The 5-year actuarial regional control rate was 93%. Surgical salvage was successful in 11 of 34 patients who had a local or regional recurrence. The 5-year actuarial distant metastasis rate was 8%. Grade 4 complications included mucous membrane ulceration (9 patients), and bone necrosis and exposure (7 patients). Nine patients had esophageal strictures that required dilatation.

The 5-year and 10-year actuarial overall survival rates were 70% and 43%, respectively, and the 5-year and 10-year disease-free survival rates were 85% and 79%, respectively. The disappointing rate of 10-year survival partly resulted from the frequent occurrence of second primary tumors, which developed in 29% of the patients. Eighty-six percent of the second tumors were in the upper aerodigestive tract, and the development of second primary tumors was strongly correlated with active smoking and heavy alcohol consumption. The development of secondary upper aerodigestive tract malignancies with the index cancer controlled caused a significant decrement in survival compared with patients who remained free of cancer.

Because of the high rate of development of esophageal stricture that was observed, the treatment technique for the standard supraclavicular field was changed at MDACC. Formerly, the supraclavicular field was treated to 50 Gy in 25 fractions specified at maximum depth with no midline shielding inferior to the larynx block. In recent years, a midline block has been placed in the supraclavicular field after 40 Gy to shield the esophagus; after introducing this modification, esophageal stricture has essentially been eliminated as a complication of neck radiation.

Garden and associates[31] analyzed the subset of patients with T1 and T2 oropharyngeal carcinoma who presented to MDACC with regional adenopathy between 1975 and 1998. These tumors are stage III and IV according to the AJCC staging system, and concurrent systemic therapy commonly is recommended for these patients with advanced-stage disease. Irradiation alone was used to treat 299 patients with this clinical presentation. The 5-year actuarial local control rates for T1/TX and T2 tumors were 99% and 85%, respectively. The 5-year actuarial regional control rates for patients with NX, N1, and N2 disease were 100%, 93%, and 91%, respectively; patients with N3 disease presentations had a 5-year regional control rate of 76%. Focusing on the N2 subclassifications, the 5-year actuarial regional control rates for N2a, N2b, and N2c disease were 94%, 89%, and 89%, respectively. For patients who remained in local control, the 5-year actuarial regional control rates for N1, N2a, N2b, N2c, and N3 disease were 97%, 95%, 88%, 95%, and 82%, respectively. The actuarial 5-year locoregional control rates for T1/TX and T2 disease were 95% and 79%, respectively.

Patients who remained in locoregional control had an actuarial 5-year distant metastatic rate of 17%. For patients with NX, N1, and N2a presentations, the 5-year actuarial distant metastatic rate was 10%, but for N2b, N2c, and N3 disease, the 5-year distant metastatic rate was 26%, 21%, and 43%, respectively.

Garden and colleagues concluded that patients with small primary tumors and NX, N1, and N2a presentations would not significantly benefit from further treatment intensification with concurrent chemotherapy. However, patients with more advanced nodal disease have a moderate incidence of distant metastases and require treatment strategies that are designed to counteract this pattern of disease relapse.

The radiation treatment techniques for regional disease have dramatically improved since the initial 1.5 decades of Garden's study. Before the early 1990s at MDACC, the skin-match technique used for the neck junction was geometrically imperfect. If the junction had been placed through an N3 node, a region of underdosage would have occurred in the node. This may partially explain the high rate of regional recurrence in N3 nodes in this historical study.

Treatment Results by Subsite Using Standard Fields

In this section, we present the data of relatively large historical series organized by control of primary tumor (by disease subsites, tumor stage, and radiation therapy strategies), management of nodal disease, and incidence of distant metastasis. The available data on prognostic factors as well as concurrent chemotherapy and radiation are also briefly summarized.

Tongue Base Carcinomas

External Beam Radiation

Some results that have been reported using radiotherapy to treat tongue base carcinomas are shown in Table 30-4. Accord-

Table 30-4 Local Control Rates Reported for Treatment of Squamous Carcinoma of the Tongue Base

Study	Institution	T1 (%)	T2 (%)	T3 (%)	T4 (%)	Comments
Spanos et al[32]	MDACC	91	71	78	52	1954-1971, varied once-daily fractionation
Foote et al[33]	University of Florida	89	90	81	36	Once-daily fractionation
Wang[34]	MGH	87	74	28	17	Once-daily fractionation
Weber et al[68]	MDACC	100	86	59	44	Interstitial boosts in 14 (8%); once-daily fractionation
Wang[34]	MGH	90	84	64	28	Accelerated split course
Mak et al[69]	MDACC	100 (3/3)	98	76	0 (0/1)	Concomitant boost results; 5-yr actuarial rates
Mendenhall et al[70]	Florida	96	91	81	38	Once-daily fractionation: 31% Hyperfractionation: 69%
Harrison et al[36]	MSKCC	87	93	82	100 (2/2)	External + interstitial; 5-yr actuarial rates

MDACC, M.D. Anderson Cancer Center; MGH, Massachusetts General Hospital; MSKCC, Memorial Sloan-Kettering Cancer Center.

ing to data published by Spanos and colleagues (MDACC),[32] Foote and coworkers (University of Florida),[33] and Wang (Massachusetts General Hospital [MGH]),[34] radiation delivered in standard daily 2-Gy fractions yields about 90% control rate for T1 tongue base tumors. The dose per fraction and total dose used varied somewhat among series, but the results were similar. For T2 tumors, the local control rates ranged from 70% to 90%. A wide range of local control rates have been reported for T3 tumors; this may be due in part to heterogeneity of patient selection, because there is no upper size limit to the T3 classification.

Complications after once-daily fractionation have included bone (mandible) exposure, soft tissue necrosis, and dysphagia. Foote and associates[33] reported a 4% incidence of moderate to severe bone exposure and a 7% incidence of moderate soft tissue necrosis. The main complication in the large series reported from MDACC in 1976 was mandibular exposure and necrosis.[32] The incidence of mandibular exposure that healed with conservative management was 5%, and an additional 3% of patients required resection of the mandible. Mendenhall and colleagues,[35] reporting results of a series in which the patients were treated predominantly with hyperfractionation, observed that 4% experienced severe late complications. These complications included severe dysphagia requiring a permanent gastrostomy (2%) and osteonecrosis (1%).

External Beam and Brachytherapy

High local and regional control rates can also be achieved using a combination of external beam radiation therapy and brachytherapy boost. Harrison and colleagues[36] described 68 patients who were treated with this approach at Memorial Sloan-Kettering Cancer Center (MSKCC); 48 patients (71%) had tumors classified as T1 and T2. Patients were considered unsuitable candidates for brachytherapy if their disease extended below the hyoid bone, eroded the mandible, or involved the epiglottis. Patients were treated with 50 to 54 Gy of external beam radiation therapy to the primary site and upper neck followed by 20- to 30-Gy boost to the primary tumor using an ^{192}Ir implant. The 5-year actuarial local control rates for T1, T2, and T3 tumors were 87%, 93%, and 82%, respectively. The 5-year actuarial regional control rate was 96%. Complications, including soft tissue ulceration, mandibular osteonecrosis, and bleeding at the time of catheter removal, occurred in 19% of the cases. Similar results for patients with tongue base carcinoma treated with external beam radiation and brachytherapy have been reported from Stanford University[37] and from Long Beach Memorial Medical Center.[38]

With the high control rates that are being reported with IMRT, altered fractionation schedules and concurrent chemoirradiation, the use of brachytherapy in the management of tongue base carcinoma has declined, because it requires a significant operation for the patient with no clear benefit in results.

Surgery Alone for Early-Stage Tumors

Foote and colleagues[14] reported a series of 55 patients with tongue base carcinomas who were treated with surgery alone at the Mayo Clinic between 1971 and 1986. During this era at Mayo Clinic, the surgeons were largely opposed to irradiating this subset of patients, including postoperative radiotherapy. The surgical procedure used was a partial glossectomy, which included a partial or complete laryngectomy in 11 patients. The crude rates of local control by T classification were 77% for T1, 81% for T2, and 75% for T3. The crude rate of regional control and disease control above the clavicles was 56% and 49%, respectively. Additional surgery to manage complications was necessary in 16 patients to treat fistulas and abscess formations (n = 8), osteomyelitis with bone necrosis (n = 6), pectoralis myocutaneous flap failure (n = 2), and hemorrhage (n = 2). Five patients required permanent gastrostomy tubes. The surgical mortality rate was 4%. The locoregional control rate using a surgery-alone approach appears to be worse in this experience than that achievable with radiation therapy, and the complication rate was substantial.

Combination of Surgery and Radiation Therapy

Extensive (>6 cm), infiltrative T3 and T4 tumors of the base of the tongue generally have low control rates when treated with radiotherapy alone, and they have therefore been treated with a combination of surgery and postoperative radiotherapy. De los Santos and coworkers[39] reported a series of 51 patients with advanced base of tongue carcinoma who were treated with surgery and postoperative radiotherapy at MDACC between 1980 and 1997. Ninety percent of the patients had T3 (21 patients) or T4 (23 patients) tumors. The surgical procedure, besides a glossectomy, included laryngectomy in 51% and mandibulectomy in 35%. The median radiotherapy dose was 63 Gy. The 5-year actuarial locoregional control rate was 74%, and the distant metastatic rate at 5 years was 35%. Although patients were not formally assessed, various degrees of swallowing deficits occurred in 21 patients; this is not surprising, given the significance of the propulsive force of the base of the tongue during swallowing.

Treatment with surgery and postoperative radiotherapy resulted in a reasonably high locoregional control rate for these patients with advanced-stage disease, but functional problems were very significant. For this reason, these patients are being treated on clinical trials of irradiation and concurrent chemotherapy at MDACC.

Tonsillar Fossa Carcinomas

M. D. Anderson Cancer Center Series of External Beam Radiation Therapy

The data of 150 patients treated at MDACC with 2-Gy fractionation between 1968 and 1983 were reported by Wong and associates.[40] The mean tumor doses were 64, 68, and 70 Gy for T1, T2, and T3 tumors, respectively. Boosts were usually given through ipsilateral reduced fields, most frequently with a combination of high-energy electrons and photons. A planned neck dissection was performed on 26 patients approximately 6 weeks after completing radiation. The local control rates after radiation therapy for T1, T2, and T3 tumors were 94%, 79%, and 58%, respectively (Table 30-5). The ultimate local control rates after surgical salvage were 100%, 85%, and 60% for T1, T2, and T3 tumors, respectively. The regional control rate, calculated after excluding patients who had a local recurrence, was 96%. Seventeen severe complications in 14 patients consisted of bone necrosis requiring mandibular resection ($n = 7$), soft tissue necrosis ($n = 4$), trismus ($n = 5$), and cranial nerve palsies ($n = 1$). These patients all received doses of more than 67.5 Gy. Most patients received one-field irradiation per day and 2:1 weighting during this era. This technique increases the dose per fraction received by the ipsilateral normal tissues.

Ninety-eight patients (41 with T2 tumors and 57 with T3 tumors) with intermediate-stage tonsil carcinoma have been treated with the concomitant boost fractionation schedule at MDACC using standard fields. The 5-year actuarial local control rates for T2 and selected T3 tumors were 86% and 83%, respectively (Morrison WH, unpublished data).

Other Series of External Beam Radiation

Over a 33-year interval, 400 patients with squamous carcinoma of the tonsillar region were treated at the University of Florida.[35] Hyperfractionation to a median dose of 76.8 Gy was used in 60% of the patients; the other 40% of the patients were treated with standard fractionation. In addition to the external beam radiotherapy, 27% of the patients received a brachytherapy boost of 10 to 15 Gy, usually into the base of the tongue component of the tumor. Planned neck dissections were performed on 125 patients after completing radiotherapy. The local control rates for T1, T2, T3, and T4 primary tumors were 83%, 81%, 74%, and 60%, respectively. When anterior tonsillar pillar cases were excluded, the local control rates for the T1, T2, T3, and T4 tonsillar fossa and posterior tonsillar pillar tumors were 90%, 88%, 66%, and 58%, respectively. Nineteen patients developed severe late complications, with the most common being osteonecrosis necessitating a segmental mandibulectomy (8 patients), and swallowing difficulty requiring a permanent gastrostomy (6 patients).

Bataini and associates[20] reported a series of 465 patients with squamous carcinoma of the tonsillar region who were treated almost exclusively with external beam radiation therapy at the Institut Curie. The mean radiation dose given for T1, T2, T3, and T4 tumors was 65 Gy, 65 Gy, 67 Gy, and 68 Gy, respectively. The local control rates reported for T1, T2, T3, and T4 tumors were 89%, 84%, 63%, and 43%, respectively. The study authors reported that tumors of the tonsillar fossa had higher local control rates than tumors originating in other sites of the tonsillar region, with a significance level of $P < .01$. Both the series from the University of Florida and the Institut Curie concluded that patients with anterior tonsillar pillar tumors have worse local control rates than patients with tonsillar fossa tumors.

Moderate-Dose External Beam Radiation with Brachytherapy Boost

Several French investigators have reported good results treating tonsil cancer with external beam radiation therapy to doses in the range of 45 to 50 Gy followed by an interstitial brachytherapy boost. Pernot and others[25] reported a series of 343 patients with velotonsillar carcinomas who were treated with external beam to 50 Gy in 5 weeks followed by a brachytherapy boost of 20 to 30 Gy. Local control rates for T1, T2, and T3 tumors were 89%, 85%, and 67%, respectively. Mazeron and coworkers[41,42] treated 69 patients with T1 and T2 tonsil tumors with external beam radiation therapy to 45 Gy followed by a 30-Gy interstitial boost. Local recurrence developed in only 2 of the 69 patients.

Soft Palate Carcinomas

External Beam Radiation

Table 30-6 shows some results that have been reported with various treatment approaches. At the Institut Curie[43] 146 patients with soft palate carcinoma were treated with external beam alone (71%) or an intraoral applicator followed by external beam (29%). The mean total dose and treatment duration were 68 Gy and 45 days, respectively. The 5-year actuarial local

Table 30-5 Local Control Rates for Patients with Squamous Carcinoma of the Tonsil Treated with Standard 2-Gy Fractionation at M. D. Anderson Cancer Center between 1968 and 1983*

All Patients		Evaluable Patients†			
Tumor Stage	*Local Control after RT (%)*	*Local Control after RT (%)*	*Salvage Surgery*	*Local Control after Surgery*	*Ultimate Local Control (%)*
T1	16/17 (94)	15/16 (94)	1	1/1	16/16 (100)
T2	48/59 (81)	41/52 (79)	6	3/6	44/52 (85)
T3	44/66 (67)	30/52 (58)	10	1/10	31/52 (60)
T4	5/8 (63)	3/6 (50)	1	0/1	3/6 (50)
Total	113/150 (75)	89/126 (71)	18	5/18	94/126 (75)

*The study period was July 1968 to December 1983; analysis was completed in December 1986.

†Twenty-four patients who died within 2 years from the date of irradiation without local failure are excluded from the analysis of local control. Length of follow-up after salvage ranges from 26 to 162 months.

RT, radiation therapy.

Data from Wong C, Ang KK, Fletcher GH, et al: Definitive radiotherapy for squamous cell carcinoma of the tonsillar fossa. Int J Radiat Oncol Biol Phys 16:657-662, 1989.

Table 30-6 Local Control of Soft Palate Tumors Treated with Radiation Therapy

Study	Fractionation Schedule	Tumor Control Rates* T1	T2	T3	T4
Keus et al,[43] Netherlands Cancer Institute	Once daily	92%	67%	58%	37%
Lindberg and Fletcher,[56] MDACC	Once daily	100%	88%	77%	83%
Wang,[34] MGH (1970-1994)		96%	81%	55%	24%
Fein et al,[71] University of Florida	Every day	81% (9/11)	65% (13/20)	50% (5/10)	25% (1/4)
Mazeron et al,[45] Henry Mondor Hospital	Once daily†	93% (13/14)	87% (20/23)	—	—
Fein et al,[71] University of Florida	Twice daily	— 1/1	100% (10/10)	60% (6/10)	0/3
Wang,[34] MGH	Accelerated split course	91%	79%	68% (T3 + T4)	—
Morrison WH*, MDACC	Concomitant boost	— 2/2	95% (21/22)	65% (13/20)	—
Erkal et al,[44] University of Florida	53% once daily, 47% twice daily	86%	91%	67%	36%

MDACC, M.D. Anderson Cancer Center; MGH, Massachusetts General Hospital.
*Unpublished data.
†Patients received interstitial irradiation.

control rates are shown in Table 30-6. As predicted, patients who were given boost doses by the intraoral cylinder had less normal tissue complications. For T3 and T4 tumors, the control rates did not increase when doses were escalated from 60 to 75 Gy; however, doses were sometimes increased when there was residual disease at the completion of the initially planned dose. The study authors recommended limiting the external beam radiation doses to at most 70 Gy to minimize complications.

Erkal and colleagues[44] reported on 107 patients with soft palate carcinoma who were treated with radiation therapy at the University of Florida between 1965 and 1996. Radiation boosts were given with an intraoral applicator using orthovoltage in 29 patients and with interstitial therapy in 8 patients. Standard daily fractionation and hyperfractionation were used in 53% and 47% of the treatment courses, respectively. The median dose given by the intraoral applicator was 15 Gy given in 3-Gy fractions. The median doses and treatment duration used for once-daily fractionation and hyperfractionation were 65 Gy over 48 days and 76.8 Gy over 46 days, respectively. Actuarial 5-year local control rates for T1, T2, T3, and T4 carcinomas were 86%, 91%, 67%, and 36%, respectively. Patients who had prolonged overall treatment duration had worse local control (P = .0002). Thirty-six patients had 51 second primary tumors

Brachytherapy

Several groups, mostly from France, achieved good results treating soft palate tumors with interstitial irradiation, usually in combination with external beam therapy. Mazeron and colleagues[45] reported treatment to a mean external beam dose of 47 Gy and a mean brachytherapy dose of 31 Gy. The crude local control rates for T1 and T2 tumors were 93% and 87%, respectively. The incidence of soft tissue necrosis was low, and complications could usually be managed conservatively. An additional six patients with small tumors were treated with interstitial therapy alone, and all achieved local control. At the Institut Gustave-Roussy,[26] 43 patients who had early-stage soft palate carcinoma were treated with interstitial irradiation with or without external beam irradiation. All 34 patients with T1 tumors achieved local control, and the actuarial local control rate of all patients was 92%.

Oropharyngeal Wall Carcinomas

Standard Fractionated and Concomitant Boost Radiotherapy

Hull and coworkers[46] reported a series of 148 patients treated for squamous carcinoma of the pharyngeal wall between 1964 and 2000 at the University of Florida. The epicenters of the tumors were in the hypopharyngeal wall and the oropharyngeal wall in 63% and 37%, respectively. Most patients were treated with hyperfractionation to 76.8 Gy. Eleven patients also received chemotherapy. The local control rates after radiotherapy for T1, T2, T3, and T4 tumors were 93%, 82%, 59%, and 50%, respectively. The ultimate local control rate for T2 patients, including those patients who were successfully salvaged after local disease recurrence, was 87%. On multivariate analysis, the locoregional control rates were significantly better for oropharyngeal carcinomas than hypopharyngeal carcinomas (P = .02) and for patients treated with hyperfractionation (P = .0009).

Twenty-six patients (T2: 15 patients, T3: 11 patients) with intermediate-stage oropharyngeal wall carcinoma have been treated with the concomitant boost schedule at MDACC. Standard three-field technique was used, with the posterior field border slightly anterior to the posterior aspect of the vertebral body. The 5-year actuarial local control rates for the T2 and T3 tumors were 93% and 82%, respectively (Morrison WH, unpublished data).

LOCALLY ADVANCED DISEASE AND PALLIATION

Concurrent with or without Adjuvant Chemotherapy

Bourhis and colleagues updated the Meta-Analysis of Chemotherapy in Head and Neck Cancer (MACH-NC) database by adding data from 24 randomized trials conducted between 1994 and 2000.[47] The question addressed in the meta-analysis is whether patients benefit from the addition of chemotherapy to radiation therapy. The meta-analysis includes data from 87 phase III trials and more than 16,000 patients treated between 1965 and 2000. Fifty trials focused on the role of concurrent chemotherapy. The oropharynx was the most common primary site, with oropharyngeal tumors occurring in 37% of the patients.

Patients who received concurrent chemotherapy on the trials had a 5-year actuarial survival benefit of 8% ($P < .0001$) compared with patients treated with irradiation alone. Overall survival at 5 years was 27% in the radiotherapy patients and 35% in the concurrent chemoradiation group. The magnitude of the benefit for concurrent chemotherapy was the same among patients who were treated between 1965 and 1993 and between 1994 and 2000, but the heterogeneity of the patients was less in the more recent trials. Results did not vary significantly by tumor site, but younger patients benefited more than older patients, particularly those older than 70 years.

Patients who received concurrent cisplatinum, with or without other agents, derived the most benefit. Patients who were treated with concurrent cisplatinum alone had a survival benefit of 11%. Data from the meta-analysis and other recently completed phase III trials have established concurrent cisplatinum-based chemotherapy as standard treatment for locally advanced head and neck carcinomas.

Of the recent phase III trials involving concurrent chemotherapy, the trial performed by the French Head and Neck Oncology and Radiotherapy Group (GORTEC)[48] is of particular interest because it focused specifically on oropharyngeal carcinoma. In this trial, 222 patients with stage III or IV oropharyngeal carcinoma were randomized to receive 70 Gy in 7 weeks or the same radiation regimen with three cycles of concurrent carboplatin and 5-fluorouracil (5-FU) given during the first, fourth, and seventh week. Locoregional control was achieved in 48% of the combined-modality group and 25% of the radiotherapy alone group ($P = .002$). The actuarial 5-year overall survival was 22% in the combined treatment arm compared with 16% in the radiotherapy arm ($P = .05$). The incidence of distant metastases was the same in both arms. The rates of grade 3 and 4 complications at 5 years were evaluated by the RTOG/EORTC scale for late effects assessment and other tools and were 56% for the combined modality arm and 30% for the radiotherapy alone patients ($P = .12$). Only a few of the original patients were alive at 5 years and available for assessment of late toxicity. The investigators concluded that concurrent chemotherapy given for locally advanced oropharyngeal carcinoma increased the locoregional control and survival rates without statistically significantly increasing the severe late complication rates. The study authors assessed late toxicity rates using different scoring systems, and they found that the late complication rates vary, depending on which toxicity scale is used.[48]

The disadvantage of concurrent chemotherapy is that it increases acute in-field and systemic toxicity, including enhancement of mucositis and suppression of bone marrow function. The mortality rate, during and within 1 month after treatment, is increased with concurrent chemoirradiation. Concurrent chemotherapy probably increases late effects, although this has not been conclusively demonstrated. Only patients with locally or regionally advanced disease should receive chemotherapy concurrently with radiation. Patients with local or regional advanced disease are considered at MDACC to have T3 and T4 oropharyngeal tumors, as are those with fixed lymph nodes, especially if nodes are N3. An occasional patient who has a significantly infiltrative or ulcerative T2 tumor may also be considered for concurrent chemotherapy. High rates of local control can be achieved with irradiation alone for T1 and most T2 oropharyngeal tumors if appropriately dose-intense radiotherapy is delivered. Dose intensification with concurrent chemotherapy is also not necessary for the treatment of mobile nodes because residual nodal masses can be removed surgically after the completion of radiation therapy.

The RTOG is enrolling stage III and IV patients in a phase III protocol (0522) in which all head and neck patients entered receive concurrent chemotherapy with cisplatin and accelerated fractionation by a concomitant boost schedule. Patients on the experimental arm of the trial will receive concurrent cetuximab (C225). Patients are eligible for concurrent chemotherapy if their stage is T2 N2-3 M0 or T3-4 any N M0. The investigators specifically exclude patients from the trial who have T1-2 N1 or T1 N2-3 disease, because they considered radiation therapy alone with neck dissection to be suitable treatment for these patients. Patients with small primary tumors (TX, T1, and T2) and N2 disease have high local and regional control rates when treated with irradiation alone, as demonstrated by Garden and associates,[31] and therefore would not be the target candidates for this phase III trial.

Nodal disease, particularly when it extends into the lower neck, is a predictor for distant metastases.[49] The RTOG 91-11 trial, a larynx carcinoma study, did show that distant metastases can be significantly reduced by concurrent chemotherapy. However, strategies to combat this pathway of spread usually focus on neoadjuvant or adjuvant chemotherapy. Higher doses of chemotherapy can be delivered when it is not given concurrently with radiation, and, theoretically, this should enhance the control rate of distant micrometastases. Some phase III trials of neoadjuvant chemotherapy have shown that chemotherapy can reduce the distant metastatic rate,[50] but this has not translated into a survival benefit in these trials.

Nevertheless, new trials of neoadjuvant chemotherapy testing innovative approaches are worth pursuing. Haraf and colleagues[51] published the results of a phase II trial conducted at the University of Chicago testing a brief course of induction chemotherapy followed by concurrent chemoradiation in patients with stage IV head and neck cancer. The neoadjuvant chemotherapy regimen was six cycles of weekly carboplatin and paclitaxel. The 3-year actuarial distant metastatic rate was only 5%. At MDACC, a study has been initiated to test a neoadjuvant regimen using a similar course of six cycles of weekly carboplatin and paclitaxel to which weekly cetuximab is added. This is followed by appropriate locoregional therapy, which can include concurrent chemoradiation if indicated.

Concurrent Cetuximab

Bonner and coworkers[52] investigated in a phase III study whether blocking the EGFR receptor with concurrent cetuximab could improve the outcomes of patients with locoregionally advanced head and neck carcinoma who were being treated with high-dose irradiation. Of the 424 patients enrolled, 60% had oropharyngeal carcinoma. Patients were treated with standard fractionation, hyperfractionation, or the concomitant boost fractionation schedule with or without cetuximab. The 3-year survival rates were 55% in the patients who received cetuximab versus 45% in those who did not ($P = .05$). The rate of acute mucositis was not increased by cetuximab. Among those who received cetuximab, 34% developed a grade 3 or 4 maculopapular skin reaction, but the rash typically resolved when the antibody was discontinued. The investigators concluded that the addition of cetuximab to radiation therapy prolongs overall survival without significantly increasing toxicity. Because of this favorable therapeutic ratio, many investigators, including the RTOG, are incorporating

EGFR-blocking antibodies into the treatment regimens of clinical trials.

Control of Nodal Disease

The treatment policy for regional disease from oropharyngeal cancer varies among institutions. A strategy formerly used at the MSKCC before the IMRT era for patients with base of tongue carcinoma and palpable nodes was to perform systematic postirradiation planned neck dissections.[53] In these patients, the primary tumor and neck lymphatics were initially treated with external beam radiation to 54 Gy given in 1.8-Gy fractions. Nodal disease was further irradiated with an electron beam to 60 Gy. The primary tumor received boost dose using an interstitial implant, and patients underwent a modified radical neck dissection during the same anesthesia. In a series of 50 patients, 70% were found to have pathologically negative neck dissection specimens. Patients who presented with advanced nodal stage had similar rates of complete pathologic response as patients with more limited nodal disease. The 5-year actuarial rate of regional control was 96%. Morbidity from neck dissection after this radiation dose was minimal. The investigators thought that this treatment policy might lead to overtreatment of some patients. However, the strategy of giving 60 Gy followed by neck dissection is particularly beneficial when significant nodal disease is present in the low neck, because high radiation doses given to the region of the brachial plexus could cause a plexopathy.

The nodal treatment strategy at MDACC follows three pathways. Patients who will receive general anesthesia for extensive dental extractions and who probably will require a neck dissection after radiotherapy (usually with nodal disease ≥5 cm at presentation) often undergo neck dissection before radiation therapy. An occasional patient with extensive nodal disease caudal to the cricoid level and overlying the brachial plexus is treated to 60 Gy, followed 6 weeks later by a planned neck dissection. The other patients are treated initially with definitive irradiation. Reassessment of these patients is performed with a clinical examination and CT scan approximately 6 weeks after completing radiotherapy. Patients who have a complete clinical and radiologic response are observed. Deciding what constitutes a complete response on CT can be a difficult clinical judgment, because most patients have some remaining nonenhancing nodal tissue evident on CT imaging as a residual of the original disease. Further assessment is often performed with an ultrasound examination and fine-needle aspiration of nodes that persist but do not enhance on CT and are less than 1.5 cm in diameter. If the result of needle aspiration is pathologically negative, the patient is usually observed, and no dissection is performed. Patients who have persistent nodal masses larger than 1.5 cm or persistent tumor on needle aspiration undergo a focused modified neck dissection consisting of removal of the residual mass and immediately surrounding nodes. The neck dissection should be limited in nature, because postirradiation neck dissection after high-dose irradiation causes significant neck fibrosis. The role of PET scan performed 2 months after the completion of radiation in assessing whether persistent nodal masses contain viable tumor is being studied by many investigators.[19,54]

An analysis of an MDACC series of patients treated between 1984 and 1993 with the concomitant boost schedule[55] revealed that 17 patients who underwent preradiotherapy neck dissections had slightly larger nodes at presentation than 75 patients who were treated initially with radiotherapy (median nodal size, 4 versus 3 cm, respectively). Four (23%) of the 17 patients who were initially treated with neck dissection had a regional recurrence. Of 75 patients who were initially treated with radiotherapy, 13 underwent a planned neck dissection for persistent nodal masses; nodal size at presentation was larger than 3 cm in 12 of the 13 patients. None of these 13 patients developed regional recurrence. The remaining 62 patients achieved a complete response in the neck and, therefore, did not undergo neck dissection. Subsequent nodal recurrence occurred in 7 (11%) of these 62 patients, of whom only 3 (5%) had an isolated regional relapse.

There was no difference in nodal control between the different oropharyngeal subsites and no relationship between initial nodal size and the risk of subsequent neck failure. The actuarial 2-year probability of neck control was 87% for patients who had initial nodal size smaller than 3 cm, compared with 85% in those who had initial nodes larger than 3 cm. However, the probability of obtaining a complete response to radiotherapy was less in those patients who presented with larger initial node size. It was concluded that neck dissection could be omitted in patients whose nodes are included in the high-dose volume and who respond completely to treatment. Significant improvements in treatment delivery have occurred since 1993, and ultrasound-guided fine-needle aspiration allows for more accurate assessment of nodal response after the completion of irradiation.

Garden and colleagues[28] analyzed the neck disease outcome of 80 oropharyngeal patients with small primary tumors who presented with nodal disease and who were treated with IMRT at MDACC. Nodal staging distribution was 22 N1, 17 N2a, 27 N2b, 2 N2c, and 12 NX tumors. Median follow-up was 17 months. Twenty-six patients had neck dissections after radiotherapy for persistent nodal masses, and only five patients (19%) had pathologic evidence of disease. The other 54 patients were thought to have a complete response and were observed. Three patients had regional recurrences. The actuarial 2-year regional control rate was 93%.

The current strategy at MDACC with a three-field technique (see "Techniques of Irradiation") is to treat nodes 2 cm in diameter or larger with radiation to a dose of 69 to 72 Gy in 6 weeks using the concomitant boost fractionation schedule. Smaller palpable nodes are treated to doses between 66 and 69 Gy, depending on their size. The nodal disease, when located in the upper jugular region, can often be encompassed in the field treating the primary tumor, especially when oblique boost fields are used. When boosting nodes located outside of the primary tumor fields, attempts are made to exclude as much of the mucosal surfaces as possible by using electron beam or anterior or posterior directed photon fields with the midline mucosal surfaces blocked. When these midneck photon fields are used, the volume of the midneck that is treated to high dose is limited by giving at least 6 Gy with an appositional electron field that encompasses the nodal disease while excluding most of the neck.

For patients with small primary tumors and nodal disease who are treated with IMRT, the fractionation schedule used at MDACC is 66 Gy in 30 fractions over 6 weeks to the primary tumor and positive nodes. If a node is larger than 1.5 cm, an electron boost is delivered to the node for 2 fractions so that the final nodal dose is 70 Gy given in 32 fractions. Larger primary tumors are treated at MDACC with 70 Gy given in 33 fractions or the concomitant boost fractionation schedule, and nodal disease larger than 1.5 cm receives the same dose as the primary tumor.

Reirradiation

Full-dose reirradiation of head and neck tumors was widely considered to be a futile exercise in the past. However, investigations at some academic centers have demonstrated that between 10% and 20% of selected patients who are reirradiated can be 5-year survivors.

The University of Chicago has recently published their long-term outcomes of 115 patients treated with chemotherapy and reirradiation for recurrent and second primary squamous carcinomas.[56] The re-treatment series included 30 patients with oropharyngeal carcinoma. The reirradiation was for clinically evident disease in 57% and postoperative in 43%. The median lifetime total radiation dose was 131 Gy, and the median reirradiation dose was 65 Gy. The patients were treated on seven consecutive chemotherapy protocols with different drugs. The 3-year actuarial survival rate was 22%. On multivariate analysis, significant factors for overall survival were reirradiation dose ($P < .001$), having surgery before reirradiation ($P < .002$), and receiving concurrent cisplatin, paclitaxel, or gemcitabine ($P < .017$). Patients who received 58 Gy or more had a 3-year overall survival rate of 30%, and those who received less than 58 Gy had a 3-year overall survival rate of 6%. Grade 4 or 5 complications included carotid hemorrhage in 6 patients, osteoradionecrosis in 13 patients, and myelopathy and peripheral neuropathy in 1 patient each. The investigators concluded that full-dose reirradiation with concurrent chemotherapy is a viable treatment option offering long-term survival potential for selected patients with recurrent or second primary head and neck cancer.

Similar results were reported by De Crevoisier and associates[57] from the Institut Gustave Roussy. In this series, 169 patients were reirradiated. The median cumulative dose of the two irradiations was 120 Gy. The actuarial 5-year overall survival rate was 9%. The incidence and severity of late toxicity was markedly increased compared with that observed after the first irradiation. In multivariate analysis, the volume of the second irradiation was the only factor significantly associated with the risk of death from toxicity ($P = .01$).

These and other studies have shown that reirradiation given concurrently with chemotherapy does have some curative potential. It is worth offering to selected patients who have no other therapeutic option.

Distant Metastasis

In analyzing the outcome of a series of 751 patients with oropharyngeal carcinomas treated with radiotherapy at MDACC between 1960 and 1974, Lindberg[58] found that distant metastasis was the first site of disease relapse in 7.7% of the patients. The crude incidence of distant metastases was 2% for patients with stage I, II, or III disease and 13% for those with stage IV disease. In the RTOG 90-03 study,[23] in which 62% of the patients had oropharynx cancer and 31% had T4 primary tumors, the actuarial 2-year incidence of distant metastases was 17%.

Al-Othman and coworkers[49] analyzed the distant metastasis rate of 873 patients who were treated with definitive radiotherapy at the University of Florida. The number of patients who had tonsil, base of tongue, and soft palate tumors was 246, 166, and 42, respectively. The 5-year rate of distant metastasis–free survival (DMFS) in the 873 patients was 86%. Patients with base of tongue and tonsil primary tumors each had 5-year DMFS rates of 86%, and patients with soft palate tumors had a 98% rate of DMFS. Some factors that predicted a highly significant increase in the distant metastasis rate ($P < .0001$) on multivariate analysis included increasing T stage, the presence of lower neck nodal disease, and recurrent head and neck disease. Other significant factors predicting a higher distant metastasis rate were increasing N stage ($P < .006$) and male gender ($P = .03$). The median time to develop distant metastases was 12 months, and the median survival after the diagnosis of distant metastases was 4 months.

TECHNIQUES OF IRRADIATION

Primary Radiation Therapy: Treatment Setup and Portal Arrangement

T1-2, N0-1, and Limited N2 Tonsillar Fossa Carcinoma

Unilateral irradiation encompassing the primary tumor and ipsilateral nodes for early-stage cancer of the tonsillar region is used in many centers. A series of 228 patients with tonsillar region carcinomas who were treated with unilateral irradiation at Princess Margaret Hospital was reported by O'Sullivan and colleagues in 2001.[59] T1 and T2 tumors were present in 84% of the patients. The primary tumors were located in the tonsillar fossa in 150 patients, anterior tonsillar pillar in 73, and posterior tonsillar pillar in 5. The N stages were N0, N1, and N2-3 in 58%, 25%, and 17%, respectively. Patients were treated predominantly with unilateral wedge-pair technique. Only 8 patients (3%) experienced contralateral nodal relapse; in patients whose primary tumors were locally controlled, the contralateral nodal recurrence rate was 1.7%. No contralateral nodal recurrences occurred in patients who had T1 tumors or in patients who presented with N0 neck disease. The authors recommended unilateral radiation for tonsillar region carcinomas with at most minor extension (1 cm) onto the soft palate or the mucosa of the base of the tongue.

A series of 155 patients with tonsillar carcinoma who were treated with unilateral irradiation was reported from the Vancouver Cancer Center.[60] The incidence of contralateral nodal recurrence was 2.6%.

In a surgical series from the Mayo Clinic,[16] 56 patients, 45 (80%) of whom had T1-2 tumors, were treated with surgical procedures that did not include contralateral neck dissection. Six patients (11%) experienced contralateral nodal recurrence.

Given these data, ipsilateral treatment is reasonable with the goal of minimizing morbidity, particularly xerostomia, for patients with tonsillar fossa carcinoma confined to the tonsil or extending to the anterior tonsillar pillar, lateral pharyngeal wall, or minimally onto the soft palate. A typical primary tumor that was treated with unilateral irradiation is shown in Figure 30-13.

Unilateral irradiation of the primary tonsillar tumor and upper neck can be done with wedge-pair photon beam technique or preferably with IMRT. The planning target volume (PTV) of the treatment field should encompass the primary tumor with at least 1.5-cm margins, including adjacent components of the ipsilateral pterygoid muscles, the ipsilateral upper neck nodes, and the ipsilateral retropharyngeal nodes anterior to C1. The subclinical dose extends into the retromolar trigone region. An intraoral stent is used to push the tongue out of the high-dose region as much as possible. The dose to the contralateral submandibular gland and parotid gland, as well as the ipsilateral parotid gland, can be minimized if IMRT is used. Figure 30-14 shows some dose distributions of a patient who was treated with ipsilateral radiation using IMRT.

Other Oropharyngeal and More Advanced Tonsil Carcinomas

Comprehensive irradiation encompassing the primary tumor and bilateral neck nodes is recommended for all stages of tongue base, soft palate, and oropharyngeal wall carcinomas and for more advanced stages of tonsillar fossa carcinomas.

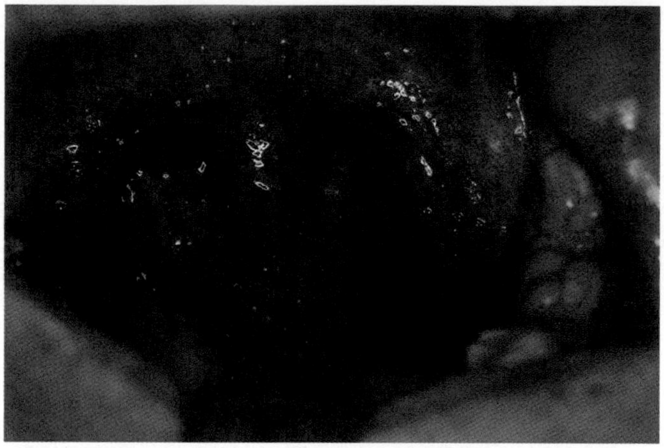

Figure 30-13 A 48-year-old man presented with a tonsil tumor and an ipsilateral, 4-cm, subdigastric node in February 2005. He was treated with unilateral irradiation using intensity-modulated radiation therapy because his tumor was confined to the tonsillar fossa and did not have significant medial extension to the soft palate or base of the tongue.

IMRT has become the preferred technique for treating these patients. The opposed lateral field technique is still used and is discussed subsequently.

Intensity-Modulated Radiation Therapy

Essential steps to successful IMRT treatment include reproducible patient immobilization, accurate tumor localization using physical examination findings and high-quality imaging, appropriate delineation of target volumes and attention to dose distribution and fractionation within the field.

Extended thermoplastic masks can be used to accomplish patient immobilization. A tongue-depressing stent is used for patients with base of tongue carcinomas to separate the tongue base from the superior structures of the oropharynx. For patients with soft palate carcinoma, a tongue-depressing stent is used to displace the soft palate from the tongue base. Tongue-displacing stents can be used in patients with tonsil cancer who do not have tumor extension into the tongue base. Shoulder straps are sometimes necessary to depress the shoulders out of the horizontal upper neck fields.

The radiation oncologist planning IMRT fields must precisely localize the tumor. Information is gathered from the physical examination, which should include fiberoptic endoscopy, and from imaging studies, which can include CT, MR, PET (investigationally),[19] and ultrasound. The ultrasound is sometimes supplemented with fine-needle aspiration if it can help answer an important clinical question. The examiner also should notice whether the tumor is exophytic with distinct borders to palpation or infiltrative with diffuse borders. The infiltrative tumor requires a wider margin (Fig. 30-15).

Contrast-enhanced diagnostic images should be reviewed to supplement the physical examination in determining the location of nodal involvement and extent of the primary tumor. Necrosis in a cervical node is considered diagnostic of malignant nodal involvement, as is nodal size greater than 1.5 cm in level II and 1 cm in levels III, IV, and V. The measurement should be made along the short axis of the node to avoid having too many false positive interpretations. Invasion of tumor out of lymph nodes and into the adjacent cervical tissues should be identified. Imaging of the primary tumor should assess for extension into contiguous structures.

The two logical options for IMRT planning are to treat the oropharynx and entire neck in one large field or to use a mono-isocentric match technique and use two fields.[61] If two fields are used, the inferior border of the primary tumor must be considered in junction placement. If the inferior border of the tumor extends into the hypopharynx or larynx, the junction should be lowered such that there is 1.5- to 2-cm clearance between the tumor and the field junction. If the location of the primary tumor allows for junction placement above the arytenoid cartilages, it is preferable to treat the lower neck with an anterior larynx block because the dose under the larynx block to the arytenoids, vocal cords, and cricopharyngeus muscle will be negligible. The dose to the larynx, even when specified as an avoidance structure, is considerably higher when treating the whole neck with IMRT using the current software.

At MDACC, the two-field approach has been consistently used if the junction between the upper neck and the supraclavicular fields can be placed above the shoulders. The junction is placed without regard to whether it traverses through nodal disease. With current treatment-planning software, the IMRT and supraclavicular isodose distributions can be displayed on one plan, and the dose through the junction can be observed. We have not observed nodal recurrences attributable to this junction technique.

The target volume is drawn from knowledge of the gross tumor volume and understanding of the pattern of spread in the various sites. Tumors of each subsite have their own particular spread characteristics that are incorporated in the tumor outlining process. Tumor outlining is not as simple as assigning a standard margin in all directions from the gross tumor volume (GTV). For example, posterior pharyngeal wall tumors only rarely involve the vertebral body, so a smaller margin can be assigned in that direction if imaging confirms that there is no suspicion of vertebral body invasion.

Clinical judgment is the key to successful IMRT planning. Rather than focus on GTVs, clinical target volumes (CTVs), and PTVs, it is preferable to specify what dose is required to what volume to control the disease. The following questions should be contemplated before the dose volumes are drawn:

1. Where *exactly* is the primary tumor and malignant adenopathy and with what certainty can the tumor anatomy be defined?
2. What dose-fractionation schedule, with or without chemotherapy, will optimize the therapeutic ratio in this specific case?
3. How close to the tumor can the margins be drawn in a specific case without a risk of missing known tumor? Can the descending dose volumes around the high-dose region covering the primary tumor be used to treat immediately adjacent tissues possibly containing subclinical tumor extensions?
4. What are the sites of potential subclinical spread that will require the dose necessary to control subclinical disease?
5. What are the consequences to the normal tissues of delivering the specified dose? What are the consequences of having excessive dose in the target volumes to the underlying normal tissue?

Drawing tumor volumes and normal tissue avoidances is such a subjective process that describing margin dimensions in centimeters underestimates the cognitive process required. The tumor dose volume must be sagaciously determined after integrating all available information, and the resultant margin

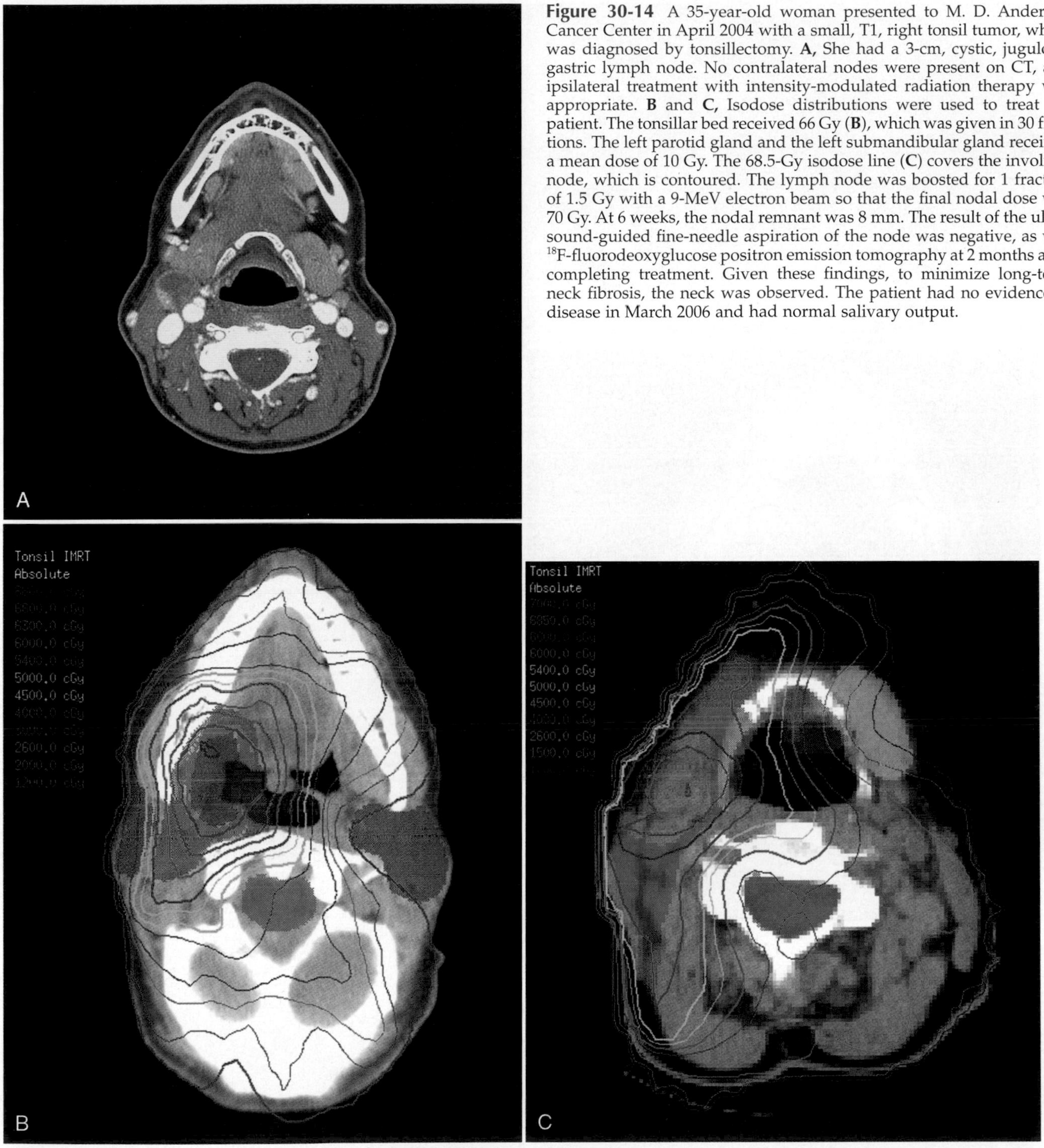

Figure 30-14 A 35-year-old woman presented to M. D. Anderson Cancer Center in April 2004 with a small, T1, right tonsil tumor, which was diagnosed by tonsillectomy. **A,** She had a 3-cm, cystic, jugulodigastric lymph node. No contralateral nodes were present on CT, and ipsilateral treatment with intensity-modulated radiation therapy was appropriate. **B** and **C,** Isodose distributions were used to treat the patient. The tonsillar bed received 66 Gy (**B**), which was given in 30 fractions. The left parotid gland and the left submandibular gland received a mean dose of 10 Gy. The 68.5-Gy isodose line (**C**) covers the involved node, which is contoured. The lymph node was boosted for 1 fraction of 1.5 Gy with a 9-MeV electron beam so that the final nodal dose was 70 Gy. At 6 weeks, the nodal remnant was 8 mm. The result of the ultrasound-guided fine-needle aspiration of the node was negative, as was ^{18}F-fluorodeoxyglucose positron emission tomography at 2 months after completing treatment. Given these findings, to minimize long-term neck fibrosis, the neck was observed. The patient had no evidence of disease in March 2006 and had normal salivary output.

around the tumor should be appropriate for the clinical presentation.

Tonsillar Fossa

Irradiating the tonsillar fossa causes fewer functional consequences than irradiating the tongue base or soft palate because it does not have significant motor function. Tumors of the tonsillar fossa may have submucosal spread to the anterior or posterior tonsillar pillar. For tonsillar fossa tumors, the treatment policy at MDACC is to irradiate the whole tonsillar region. The target for high-dose coverage for tumors centrally located in the tonsillar fossa includes at least the lateral pharyngeal wall, the tonsillar fossa, and the anterior tonsillar pillar. The minimum field length used extends from the lower aspect of the maxillary tuberosity to the tip of the epiglottis for early-stage tumors and to the hyoid for more advanced disease. The anterior border for the subclinical dose extends to the retromolar trigone. Coverage of the parapharyngeal

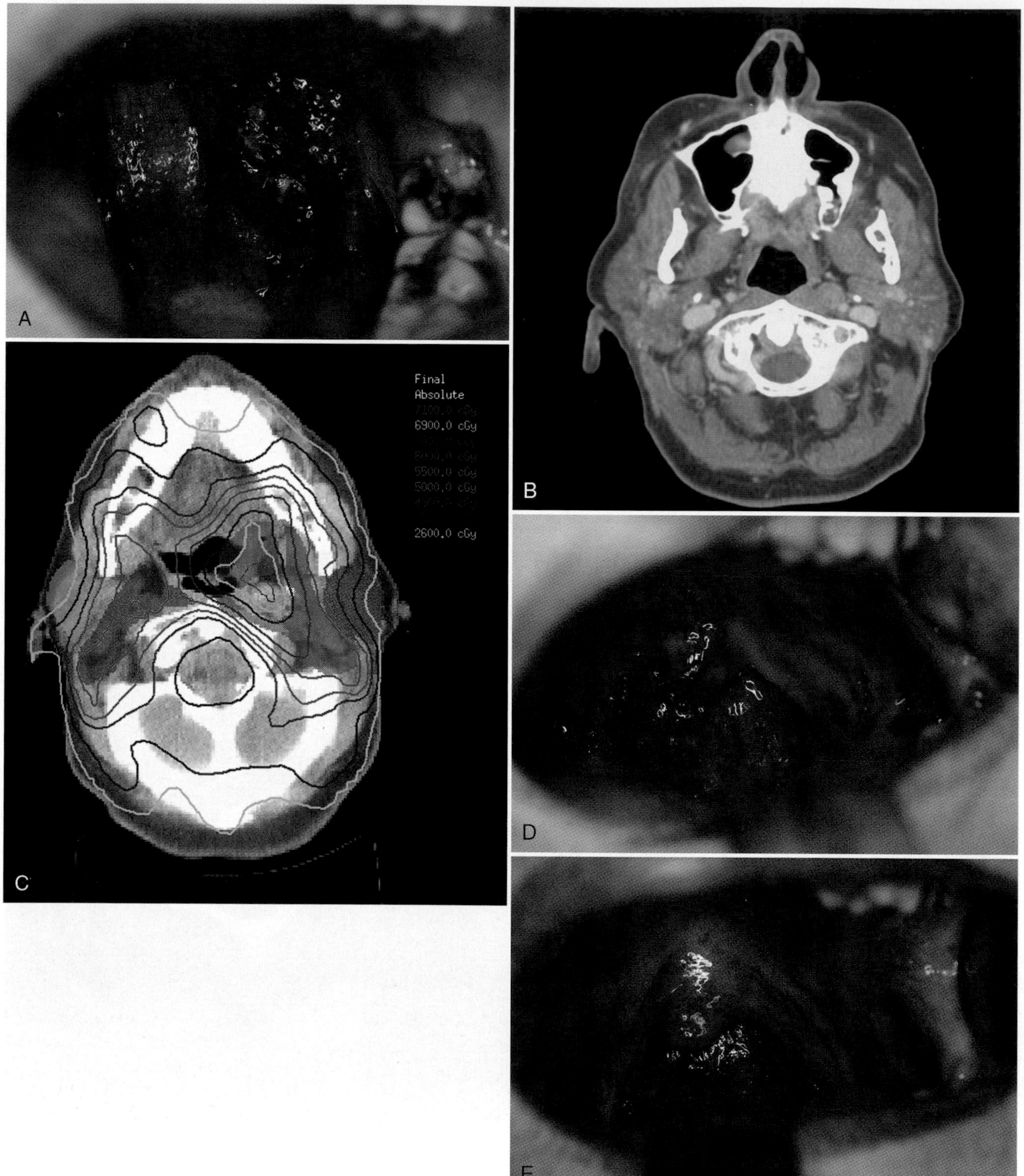

Figure 30-15 **A,** A 64-year-old woman presented in January 2004 with an exophytic, well-demarcated squamous cell carcinoma of the tonsil. **B,** CT showed a left lateral retropharyngeal node (node of Rouviere) anterior to the C1 vertebral body. Her tumor was staged T2N1. **C,** The treatment plan was to give 66 Gy in 30 fractions to the retropharyngeal node and the primary tumor. The 66-Gy line covers the planning target volume, and the 69-Gy line encompassed the tumor and nodal disease without margin. At this level, parotid sparing is suboptimal, but it was substantial more superiorly. After 48 Gy, the tumor was no longer evident. **D,** Photograph taken after 62 Gy shows the complete response and foci of confluent mucositis on the soft palate. **E,** Photograph taken 7 months after the completion of treatment shows the mucosa to be healed and relatively normal in appearance. The patient had no evidence of disease and was doing well in November 2005. Her salivary flow improved in the 1.5 years since she completed treatment and is now reported to be 85% of normal.

space and at least some of the adjacent pterygoid muscles is included in all cases; the extent of pterygoid muscle treated for subclinical spread increases with advancing T stage. If there is no clear extension of tumor into the parapharyngeal space, the pterygoid region can be treated to a lower dose than the GTV. The maxillary tuberosity and the retromolar trigone are useful anatomic landmarks for planning, because both can be precisely localized on physical examination and imaging.

On physical examination, if the tumor is clearly located more than 1.5 cm below the maxillary tuberosity, a lower dose can be assigned to the tuberosity region itself. Extensions of disease onto the soft palate can be localized with some precision on inspection and palpation; the PTV around the soft palate extension should be 1 cm past the known disease. Other adjacent sites, such as the nasopharynx, tongue base, lateral pharyngeal wall, pterygoid muscles, parapharyngeal space, mandible, piriform sinus, and larynx, are evaluated clinically for evidence of neoplasm. Local tumor extensions are covered with a margin of 1 to 1.5 cm. With IMRT, a volume of declining but significant dose surrounds the region of prescribed dose, and the lower dose provides some wider coverage of subclinical disease extensions. For eccentrically located tonsil tumors, the PTV should be 1 to 1.5 cm past the known tumor.

Coverage of the neck is discussed subsequently. An example of treatment of an advanced tonsil carcinoma is shown in Figure 30-16.

Base of Tongue

The base of the tongue is preferably treated with a custom-fabricated tongue-depressing stent. However, some patients cannot tolerate this device because of excessive gag reflex or saliva buildup during the long treatment session. Other patients may allow the tongue to prolapse behind the stent, which may be a more comfortable position when severe mucositis is present. This change in position of the tongue is evident on the port films, and the patient must be instructed to reproduce the position of the tongue during simulation.

For early-stage base of tongue carcinomas, the temptation to draw too small a margin anteriorly should be avoided, especially because the tongue is a mobile structure. For superficial base of tongue tumors that are only vaguely palpable or have been removed by excisional biopsy, the field should be specified so that the full dose is delivered 2 cm anterior to the mucosa. If the tumor is well localized on one side of the tongue base, a lower dose can be given to the contralateral side.

For more extensive tongue base neoplasms, the anterior and lateral borders can be palpated and observed on imaging. The high-dose region of the coverage should be located approximately 1.0 to 1.5 cm anterior and lateral to the tumor. If the margins of the tongue base carcinoma are difficult to pinpoint on imaging and examination, delineation of a wider PTV may be necessary. The hypopharynx and larynx, including the pre-epiglottic space, are evaluated clinically to determine if the disease extends inferior to the hyoid. If not, the field junction can be placed above the arytenoids cartilages. If one piriform sinus is involved, it can be targeted without giving a high dose to the contralateral laryngohypopharynx. An example of a patient treated for a T3N2b ulcerative base of tongue carcinoma is shown in Figure 30-17.

Soft Palate

For soft palate tumors, the boost dose is given by an intraoral applicator when feasible. The IMRT field usually includes the tumor with a 1.0- to 1.5-cm margin if the tumor borders are distinct on physical examination and the tumor can be identified on the planning CT scan. The uvula, which can be localized on examination and by imaging, is a useful reference point. Soft palate carcinomas commonly are superficially spreading and have vague borders, in which case a wider margin of coverage is necessary. Both sides of the neck and the retropharyngeal nodes are targeted in the IMRT fields. An example of a patient treated for soft palate carcinoma is shown in Figure 30-18.

Oropharyngeal Wall

Oropharyngeal wall tumors may extend posteriorly around the paravertebral muscles. These extensions can be easily encompassed in an IMRT field. The borders of the tumor can usually be determined by integrating the findings on physical examination and imaging. Given the midline nature of these tumors, both sides of the neck are irradiated.

Intensity-Modulated Radiation Planning for the Upper Neck and Retropharyngeal Nodes

The Danish Head and Neck Cancer (DAHANCA), European Organization for Research and Treatment of Cancer (EORTC), GORTEC, National Cancer Institute of Canada (NCIC), and RTOG have produced a consensus statement for the delineation of the CTV in the N0 neck of patients with head and neck squamous cell carcinoma.[62] Diagrams of the location of nodal beds have been published for all levels of the neck. For neck nodes in levels II and V, they recommend treating cranially up to the level of the caudal edge of the lateral process of C1. The consensus opinion is that the retropharyngeal nodes should be treated to the level of the jugular fossa bilaterally, unless unilateral treatment is being delivered. The consensus group did not recommend that parapharyngeal nodes be included in the elective nodal coverage.

Eisbruch and colleagues[63] at the University of Michigan treated 133 non-nasopharyngeal head and neck patients with squamous carcinoma using conformal radiation techniques. All patients were determined to be clinically node negative in the contralateral neck. Sixty percent of the patients had oropharyngeal carcinoma, 55% were treated postoperatively, and 86% of the patients had ipsilateral neck metastases. The contralateral neck was uniformly treated superiorly to the anatomic landmark where the digastric muscle crosses the jugular vein. No relapse occurred in the contralateral neck superior to this level. The study authors concluded that it is not necessary to treat the uninvolved contralateral neck more cranially than their landmark, which is slightly more caudal than the consensus recommendation.

The issue of the cranial border of coverage is important, because parotid sparing can be increased if the more caudal coverage is adequate. More data would be useful to further elucidate how much superior coverage is needed in the contralateral neck.

The RTOG for protocol 0522 has issued guidelines for IMRT target volumes around locally advanced tumors that illustrate the complexity of the planning process. The treatment goal using IMRT and chemotherapy is to deliver 70 Gy in 35 fractions over 6 weeks to PTV_1. The subclinical dose to PTV_2 is 56 Gy at 1.6 Gy per fraction. However, when desired, a CTV_{int} can be defined, and it is treated to the dose range of 59.5 to 63 Gy. They recommend defining a GTV and surrounding this with a CTV_1 and CTV_2 located 1 and 2 cm around the GTV, respectively. CTV_2 is also used to define dose to subclinical nodal sites. When the tumor is infiltrative or when the tumor border is ill defined, they recommend adding a CTV_{int} that is slightly larger than CTV_1. Around this, they recommend a PTV with a minimum margin of 0.5 cm to compensate for variability in treatment setup.

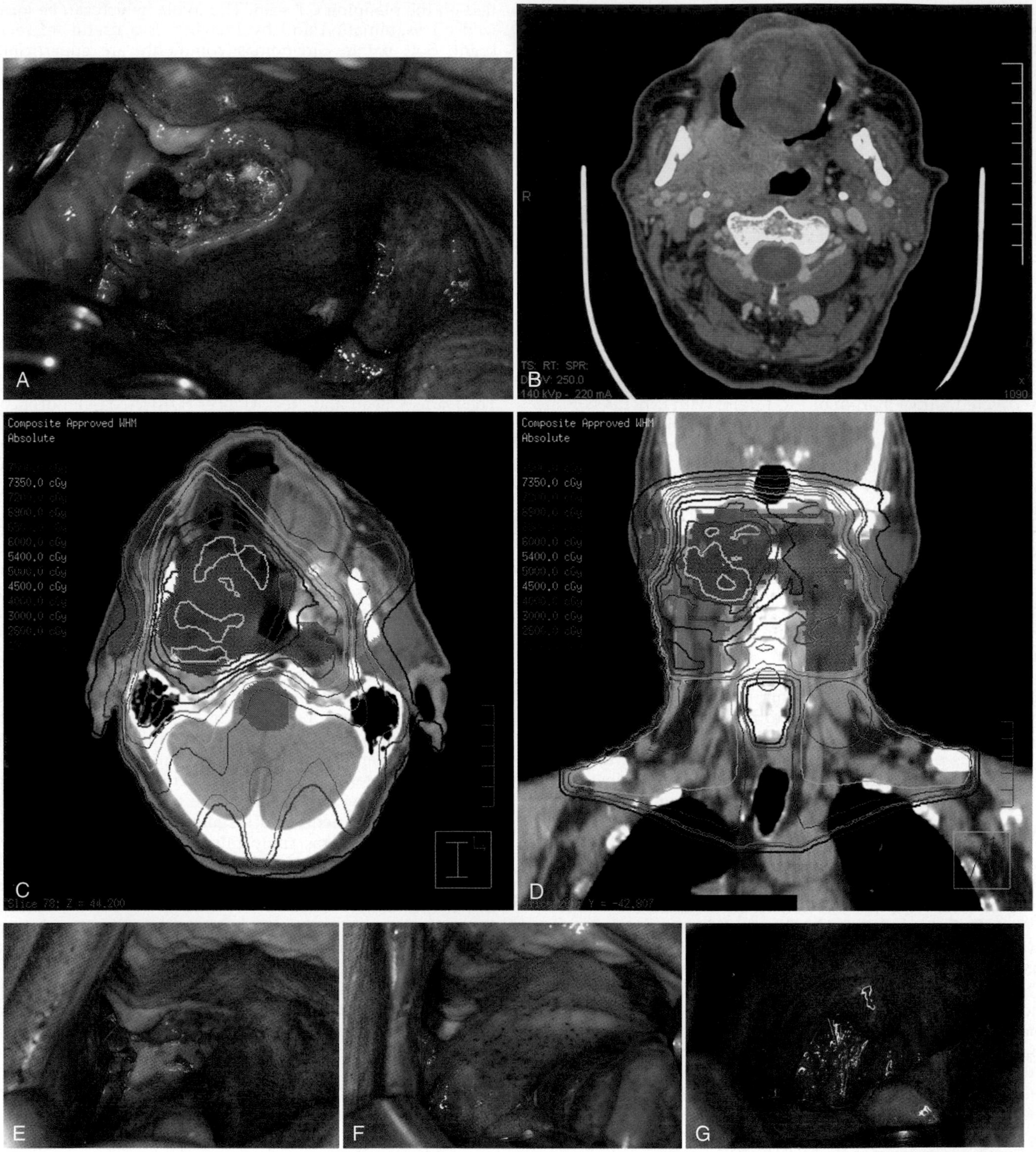

Figure 30-16 **A,** A 76-year-old white man presented in July 2005 with advanced squamous cell carcinoma of the tonsil. The tumor is seen to be displacing the uvula to the left. **B,** CT through the tumor demonstrates that the right parapharyngeal space is obliterated and the right pterygoid muscles are invaded, which caused mild trismus. The tumor was staged T3N0 and dispositioned to receive concurrent chemoradiation with weekly carboplatin and taxol. **B** and **C,** The radiation strategy was a concomitant boost fractionation schedule to 72 Gy in 40 fractions over 6 weeks. The isodose plans are shown in the transverse (**C**) and coronal (**D**) planes. On the transverse plane, the tumor volume demonstrated on the diagnostic CT scan is covered by the 72-Gy isodose line. Regions of potential subclinical extension are encompassed by the 69-Gy line. On the coronal plane, approximately 70% of the parotid is receiving less than 26 Gy. **E,** Photograph of the area after 30.4 Gy given in 16 fractions. The tumor has responded significantly, and the patient has developed an erythematous mucositis in the midline of the soft palate and some "tumoritis" in the clinical tumor. **F,** Appearance of the oropharynx on the last day of treatment shows that the tumor has resolved, and a diffuse confluent mucositis is evident. **G,** The photograph was taken 5 weeks after the completion of chemoradiation. The tumor had completely resolved, and the severe mucositis had mostly healed, with the mucosa continuing to have some moderate erythema. The patient was free of disease when seen in March of 2006.

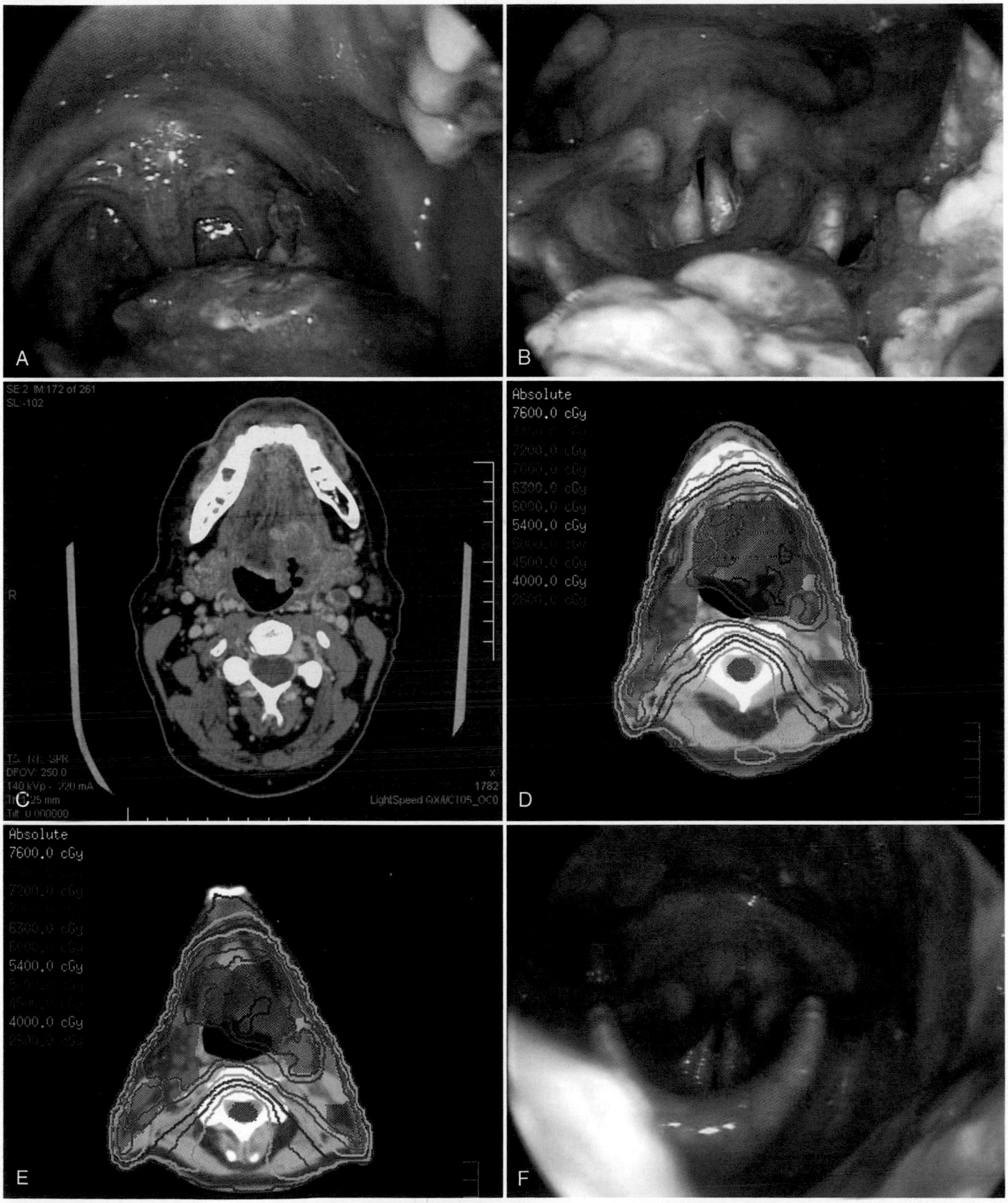

Figure 30-17 A 48-year-old man presented in June 2005 with an invasive, ulcerative T3 N2b base of the tongue carcinoma and associated severe pain. **A,** The tumor can be seen growing along the superior surface of the base of the tongue and oral tongue and extending onto the tonsillar fossa. **B,** The tumor had an ulcerative, necrotic appearance at the base of the tongue. **C,** On CT, the ulcer with surrounding tumor can be seen in the base of the tongue. On palpation, the tumor extended anteriorly in the tongue and was palpable through the floor of the mouth gutter to a coronal plane distance of 1 cm in front of the retromolar trigone. The patient was treated with two cycles of cisplatin at a dose of 100 mg/m^2, given 3 weeks apart concurrently with radiation using a concomitant boost fractionation schedule (72 Gy in 40 fractions over 6 weeks). **D** and **E,** The isodose plans are shown. The gross tumor volume of the tongue base tumor was covered by the 72-Gy line, and the necrotic nodes in the clinical target volume *(yellow)* received a minimum of 71 Gy. By the end of the third week of treatment, the patient had an approximately 75% regression of the tumor. **F,** Photograph taken in November 2005 of the tongue base 6 weeks after completing treatment. The patient had no evidence of disease with still-resolving mucositis and gastrostomy dependence due to tongue pain. This was expected to resolve during follow-up.

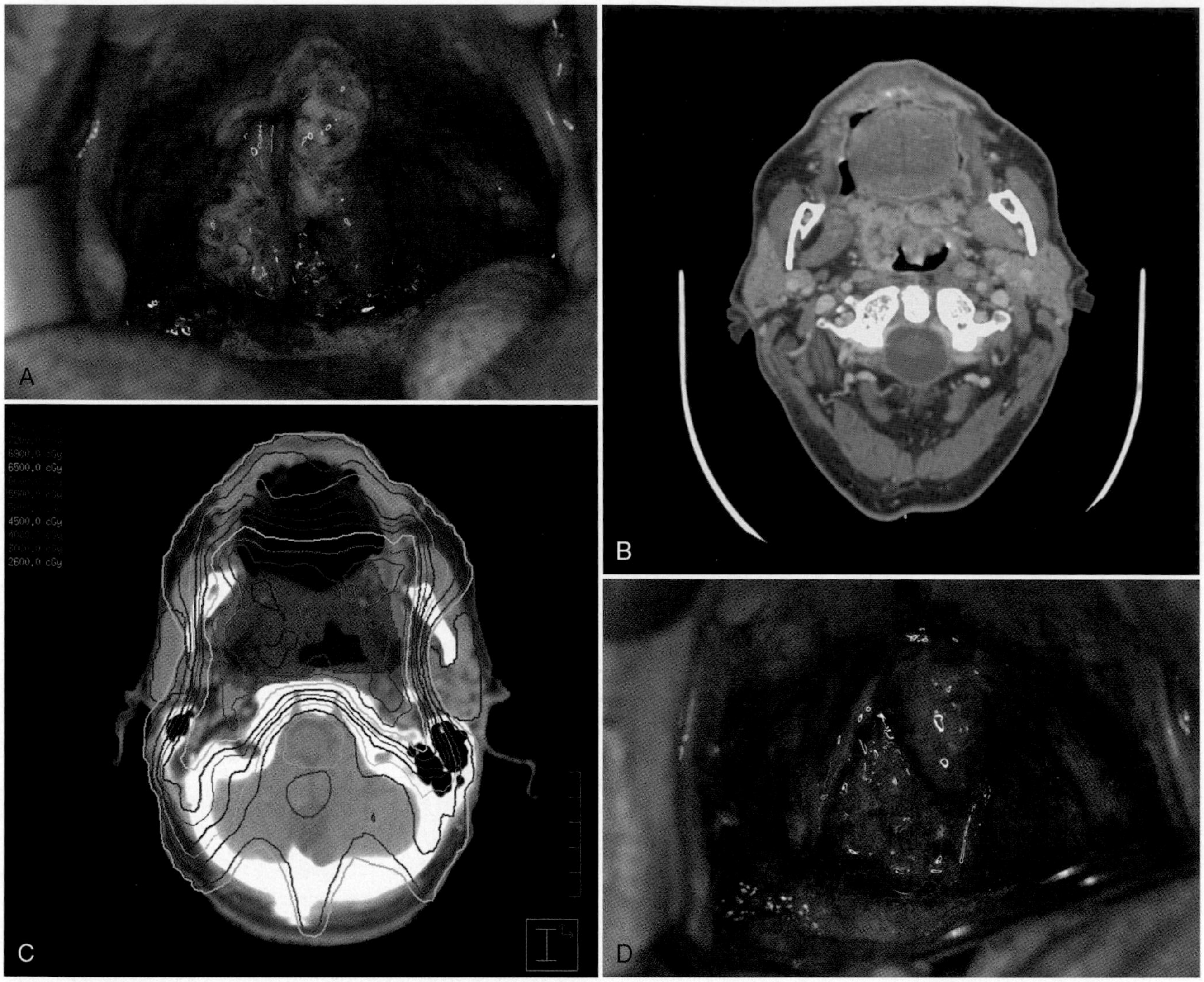

Figure 30-18 **A,** A 58-year-old man presented in August 2005 with an ulcerative squamous cell carcinoma that involved the entire soft palate and extended into both tonsillar fossae, on the right more than the left. Some necrosis of the right soft palate can be seen. **B,** CT confirms transpalatal involvement. The tumor was staged T3N0 and dispositioned to be treated with concurrent cisplatin at a dose of 100 mg/m^2, given every 3 weeks with a concomitant boost fractionation schedule to 72 Gy in 40 fractions over 6 weeks. A tongue-depressing stent was used to exclude the tongue from the higher doses. **C,** The treatment plan shows coverage of the clinical tumor by the 72-Gy isodose line. Significant parotid sparing was achieved. **D,** A photograph in September 2005, taken during the last week of treatment, showed that the patient's tumor had resolved and that he had some perforations of his soft palate due to tumor regression. These will be reassessed when he returns for follow-up evaluation.

For protocol 0522, the RTOG recommends limiting the mean dose to at least one parotid gland to 26 Gy; alternatively, at least 20 cc of the combined volume of both parotid glands should receive less than 20 Gy, or at least 50% of one gland should receive less than 30 Gy. They recommend limiting the dose to the larynx to less than 45 Gy whenever feasible, as well as limiting the dose to the brachial plexus to 60 Gy in patients with level IV nodes.

Delineating GTVs, CTVs, and PTVs requires judgment about the relative benefit and toxicity of delivering specific doses to malignant and normal tissues. The radiation oncologist must assess the final treatment plan and feel confident that the tumor is covered with a reasonable but not excessive margin. This assessment is preferably performed with the tumor outlining turned off, so that only the image of the tumor itself and the radiation doses are evident. At this juncture in the planning process for difficult cases, reexamining the patient may further clarify whether the dose coverage is appropriate.

Attention should be focused on the mean dose and on the minimum and maximum doses. If the focus of the planning is to have the minimum dose cover the entire PTV, the mean dose is often considerably higher, which may lead to excessive complications.

Dose-Fractionation Schedules Used with Intensity-Modulated Radiation Therapy

Two schedules have been tested by the RTOG for tumors of the head and neck. For early-stage oropharyngeal carcinomas on RTOG protocol 0022, 66 Gy in 30 fractions over 6 weeks was given to regions of gross disease. Regions of the neck deemed to be at intermediate risk received 60 Gy in 30 fractions, and subclinical disease regions were treated to 54 Gy in 30 fractions.

The RTOG also was investigating giving 70 Gy in 33 fractions over 6.6 weeks for tumors of the nasopharynx on RTOG protocol 0225. Subclinical disease regions received 59.4 Gy in 33 fractions. Most of the patients on this study were also treated with concurrent cisplatin chemotherapy. At MDACC, we have used this schedule on patients with more locally advanced oropharyngeal disease if they are receiving concurrent chemotherapy. For subclinical regions in patients who are receiving chemotherapy, the subclinical dose used at MDACC has been 57 Gy in 33 fractions. In this setting, the dose per fraction for subclinical disease is 1.73; because this is a lower dose per fraction than the standard 1.8 to 2 Gy and is given over a longer treatment duration, the total dose used for subclinical disease was increased to 57 Gy (relative to the RTOG dose of 54 Gy in 30 fractions for subclinical disease).

At MDACC, some patients with intermediate-stage oropharyngeal carcinoma are also being treated with IMRT using a modification of the concomitant boost fractionation schedule. The rationale for using this schedule is based on the superior local control seen on RTOG 90-03 when accelerated fractionation was compared with standard fractionation. Patients are treated with 54 Gy in 30 fractions to areas of subclinical disease; in the same IMRT field, the clinical tumor receives 57 Gy. The boost is given in the last 2 weeks of treatment as a second daily fraction with a 6-hour interfraction interval. The boost dose to the clinically evident disease is 15 Gy in 10 fractions. The tumor receives 72 Gy in 40 fractions over 6 weeks. The results indicate that tumor control and acute mucositis rates are similar to those seen when the concomitant boost fractionation schedule is used to treat conventional fields.

Standard Technique

The standard technique continues to be an effective field arrangement for patients who have advanced tumors. It is also useful for patients who cannot tolerate the prolonged immobilization required for IMRT. Another indication is for postoperative patients who have bilateral level II neck dissections and operative beds that extend to the mastoid tips bilaterally. In that situation, parotid-sparing technique with IMRT is technically difficult to achieve.

Parallel-Opposed Lateral Fields for Primary and Upper Neck Nodes

Parallel-opposed lateral fields can be used to treat the primary tumor with 2 cm margins. The most frequently used photon beam is 6 MV because higher beam energies may underdose superficial nodal disease. The superior border of the initial portals should be high enough to cover the retropharyngeal nodes and high jugular nodes approaching the jugular fossa, especially in patients with advanced nodal disease. The ipsilateral pterygoid muscles should be treated in patients with tonsil carcinoma. The anterior border is determined by the extent of the primary tumor, and for tonsil tumors it always should be anterior to the retromolar trigone. The posterior border is just behind the spinous processes or more posteriorly in the presence of large posterior cervical nodal masses. The inferior border, which matches the anterior lower neck field, is placed above the arytenoid cartilages, unless a more inferior border is necessary to encompass extension of the primary tumor into the laryngeal or hypopharyngeal region. In patients who have cervical adenopathy extending inferior to the arytenoid level, an asymmetric jaw match is generally done through the nodal disease to avoid unnecessary irradiation of the larynx and cricopharyngeal muscles. The isocenter is placed just above the arytenoids, and the lateral primary fields and low-neck field are matched using an asymmetric jaw mono-isocentric technique.

Large upper jugular nodal disease often will be located in the junction between the photon field and the posterior cervical electron portals if horizontal off-cord fields are used. The coverage of upper jugular nodal disease may be improved by using oblique off-cord and boost fields, angled to prevent transection of the nodal disease. An oblique angle is selected that can provide a 1-cm margin behind the nodal mass (Fig. 30-19). Parallel-opposed oblique beam angles of 20 to 35 degrees above and below the horizontal often are necessary to achieve this goal.

If there are large nodes on one side of the neck and smaller nodes on the contralateral side, an oblique beam angle is chosen through which the larger nodes are fully encompassed in the photon field. If the contralateral smaller nodes are located posterior to the oblique photon field or are transected by it, these nodes can have the dose boosted with a matching oblique electron beam field located posterior to the oblique photon fields.

Tumors of the Posterior Pharyngeal Wall

Because of the proximity of the tumor to the spinal cord, it is particularly challenging to treat tumors of the posterior pharyngeal wall. Using CT or MRI, the anatomic relationships of the tumor, vertebral body, and spinal cord should be assessed. In many cases, the posterior border of the off-cord field needs to be only millimeters in front of the posterior aspect of the vertebral body. In situations where the tumor extends in a posterolateral direction along the lateral aspect of the vertebral body, coverage of the tumor may be improved by using shallow oblique fields or intensity-modulated radiotherapy. Multiple portal films need to be taken to assure that the setup is accurate.

Anterior Field: Middle and Low Neck Nodes

An anterior photon field is used for treatment of the middle and lower neck nodes and the supraclavicular fossa bilaterally. Involved nodal disease located in the middle or lower neck can receive boost dose through an appositional electron portal or glancing anteroposterior fields, or both, depending on the size and location of the nodes.

Boost Fields: Primary or Nodal Disease

The boost dose to the primary tumor and involved upper neck nodes is usually administered through external beam irradiation using photons, electrons of appropriate energy, or a combination of both. A supplemental boost dose of 15 Gy by interstitial implant can be administered to selected patients with residual tongue base disease after completion of the planned external beam dose. Patients are selected to receive an interstitial boost if their clinical rate of tumor regression is deemed to be inadequate. The decision to deliver boost dose by brachytherapy must be made sufficiently early so that the total duration of treatment is not overly prolonged.

Patients with base of tongue carcinoma may have an improved set up if a tongue depressing stent is used. During the boost phase of treatment in patients with tongue base tumors, the use of a stent often can make it possible to exclude various amounts of the superior oropharynx and oral cavity.

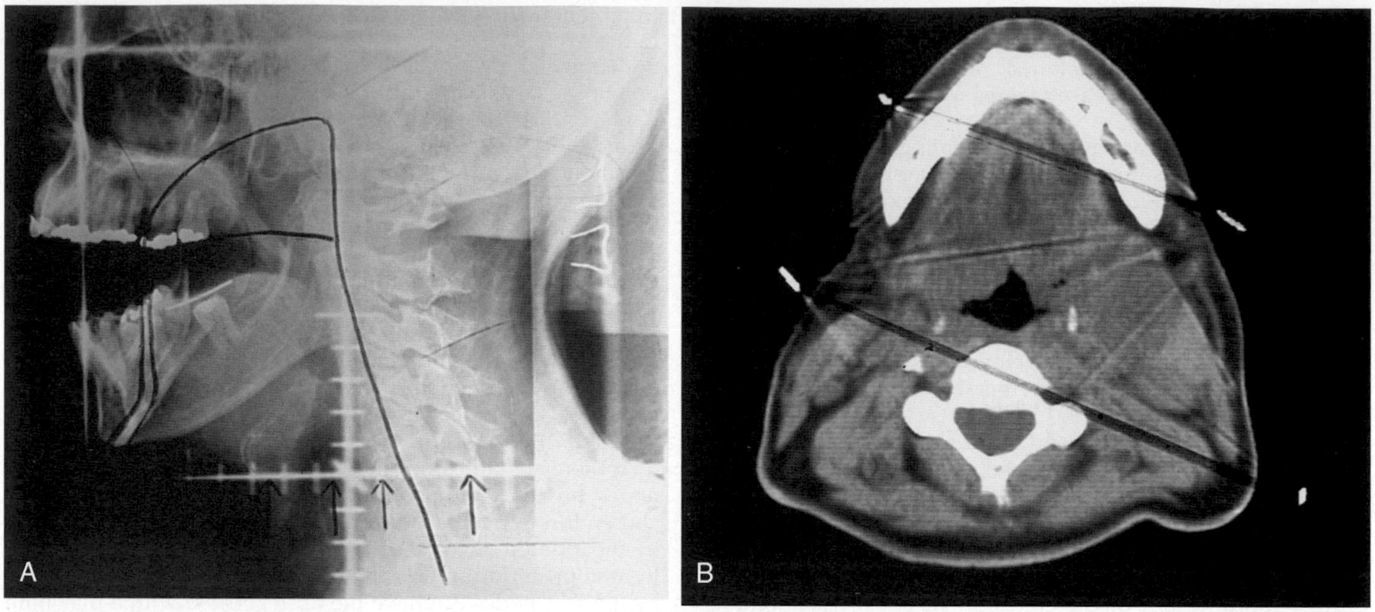

Figure 30-19 **A,** The patient presented with a T2N2c carcinoma of the base of the tongue. During the off-cord phase of the treatment, oblique fields angled 25 degrees above and below the horizontal were used to improve the coverage of the nodal disease. **B,** CT demonstrates the anterior and posterior borders of the oblique off-cord fields. The field was designed so that the beam edge is located 1 cm posterior to the nodal disease.

External Radiotherapy Dose-Fractionation Schedules

A conventionally fractionated regimen delivering 2-Gy fractions, 5 fractions per week, to a total dose of 66 Gy given over 6.5 weeks yields a control rate of 90% or higher for T1 carcinomas of the oropharynx, and it is therefore considered the standard radiotherapy regimen. With this fractionation schedule, the recommended dose for elective nodal irradiation is 50 Gy in 25 fractions and that for therapeutic irradiation of palpable involved nodes ranges from 64 to 70 Gy in 32 to 35 fractions, depending on the nodal size.

The concomitant boost fractionation schedule is used for patients with T2 oropharyngeal carcinomas who are treated outside of a protocol study setting. The recommended dose to the primary tumor is 69 to 72 Gy given in 40 to 42 fractions over 6 weeks, with the smaller tumors receiving the lower dose. With proper supportive care, the need for prolonging treatment beyond 6 weeks due to acute mucosal reactions can be limited to no more than 2% of patients. It is no longer considered ethical to introduce planned treatment interruption to reduce acute toxicity. Patients with T3 oropharyngeal carcinomas are generally treated with concurrent chemoradiation.

Some phase III protocols[64,65] compared 70 Gy in 35 fractions over 7 weeks to the same radiation regimen with concurrent high-dose cisplatin (100 mg/m^2 on days 1, 22, and 43) and showed the superiority of the combined regimen. This established the regimen of 70 Gy in 2-Gy fractions as the standard concurrent chemoirradiation schedule to be used with high-dose cisplatin. In the H0129 study, the RTOG asked whether concomitant boost fractionation was superior to standard fractionation when used in the chemoirradiation setting. Patients were randomized between the two fractionation schedules in the setting of receiving cisplatin (100 mg/m^2 every 3 weeks). This study has closed to accrual, and the results should be available in the near future. The new RTOG study (0522) for advanced head and neck cancer is using accelerated fractionation with concurrent cisplatin in both arms of the trial.

Postoperative Radiotherapy

Treatment Setup and Portal Arrangement

The general technique for postoperative radiotherapy is similar to that of primary external beam radiation. The initial target volume covers the entire surgical bed and all nodal areas of the neck at risk, and the boost volume encompasses areas that harbored known disease. The disease anatomy and extent of surgery (scar or flap) determine the portal borders. The need to deliver adequate dose to the surgical scar and subcutaneous tissues in the postoperative setting is illustrated in Figure 30-20.

IMRT or lateral opposed photon fields are used for treating the primary tumor and upper neck nodes and a matching anterior photon field is used to cover the middle and lower neck. The location of the lower border of the lateral fields is determined predominantly by the extent of the primary disease. It is desirable to place this border above the arytenoids to avoid irradiating the larynx; a midline-shielding block can be placed in the anterior low-neck field to exclude the larynx and esophageal inlet from the beam. The skin and subcutaneous tissue over the larynx, if part of the surgical bed, are irradiated with low energy electrons.

Dose-Fractionation Schedules

When given in 2-Gy fractions, a dose of 56 Gy is administered to the operative bed and 60 Gy to regions of potentially high clonogenic density, such as areas of positive margins, multiple positive nodes, and extracapsular extension. Higher doses may be needed in selected patients, such as those who have tumor resected off of the carotid artery or those with gross residual disease after surgery.

Phase III trials of the RTOG[64] and the EORTC[66] have shown that chemotherapy with cisplatin, when given concurrently

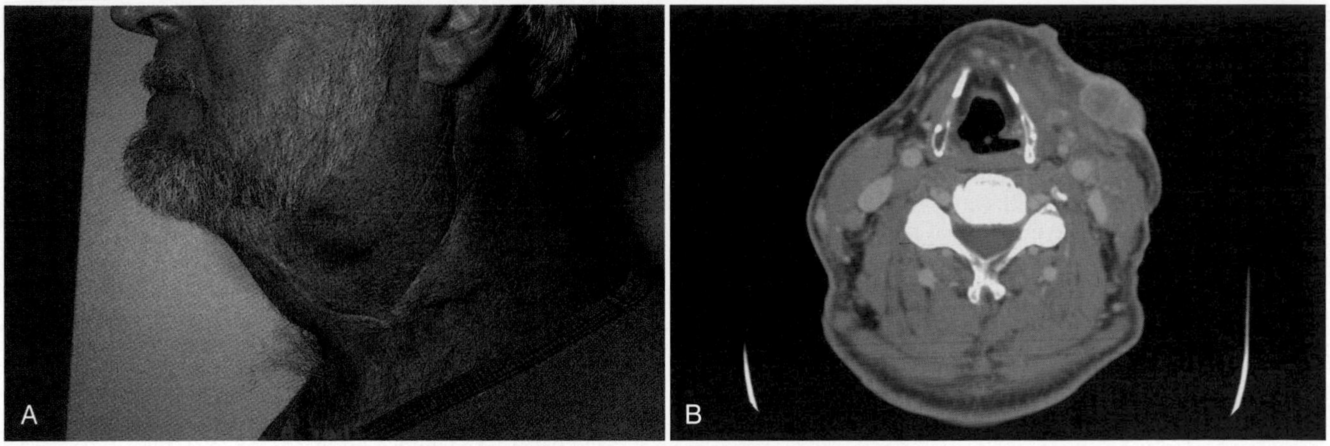

Figure 30-20 A 49-year-old man presented in April 2004 to M. D. Anderson Cancer Center after a modified radical left neck dissection and tonsil biopsy had been done for a T1 N3 squamous carcinoma of the left tonsil. He refused further treatment. **A** and **B,** He returned in June 2005 with scar and subcutaneous recurrences in the left neck. This case illustrates the importance of using a bolus in postoperative patients who are treated with high-energy photons (>4 MV) to increase the dose delivered to the surgical scar and subcutaneous tissues.

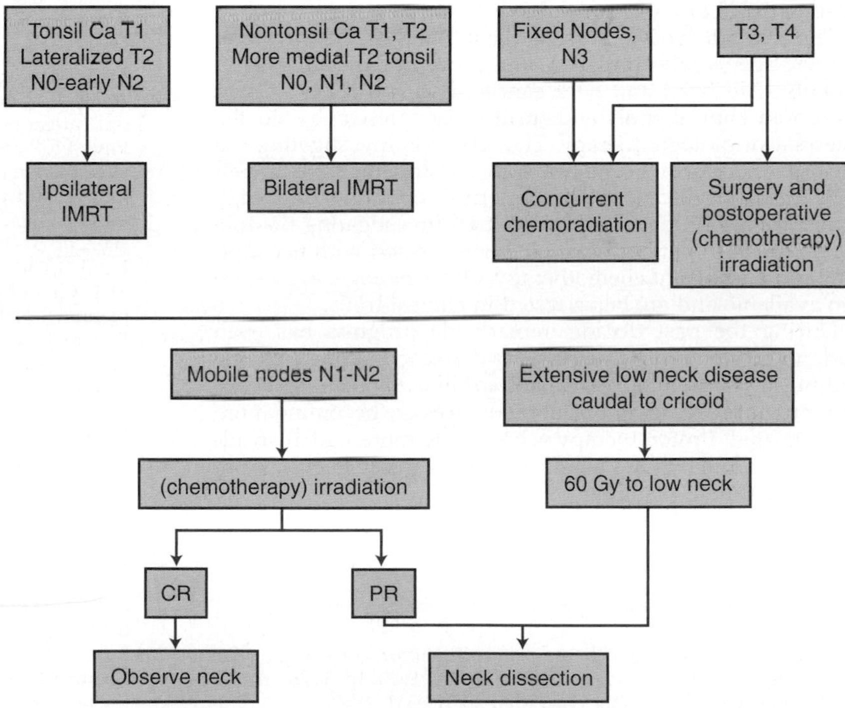

Figure 30-21 Treatment algorithm for the primary tumor and regional nodes in oropharyngeal carcinoma. Indications for concurrent chemoradiation include local or regionally advanced disease (T3 or T4 primary; N3 or fixed nodes). Cetuximab may become an option when approved by the FDA.

with postoperative irradiation, can improve the rate of local and regional control in patients with locally advanced head and neck cancer. The EORTC trial also showed improvement in survival for the patients treated with chemotherapy and irradiation. On the RTOG phase III study, 42% of the patients randomized had oropharynx carcinoma. Patients were eligible if they had two or more involved nodes, extracapsular extension, or microscopically involved mucosal margins of resection. Patients were treated with 60 to 66 Gy, with or without cisplatin. The 2-year rates of local control were 72% and 82% for the radiotherapy and combined therapy arms, respectively ($P = .01$). Concurrent cisplatin chemotherapy with irradiation is reasonable to give in the postoperative setting when high-risk features are present.

Reirradiation

Reirradiation given concurrently with chemotherapy does have some curative potential and is worth offering to patients who have no other therapeutic option (see "Locally Advanced Disease and Palliation"). Results appear to be best in patients who can be treated to limited fields with moderately high doses of reirradiation (in the University of Chicago series, patients did better with retreatment doses of 58 Gy or more).

Patients preferably should have a good performance status and healthy appearing irradiated tissues. Severe toxicity occurs frequently but not invariably.

Palliation of Local and Regional Disease

Oropharyngeal carcinomas are radiosensitive tumors, and they respond to standard palliative regimens such as 30 Gy in 10 fractions. This regimen will cause significant mucositis, which may not be desirable in terminal patients. At MDACC, some patients who have a short life expectancy are treated with 14 Gy in 4 fractions, given over 2 days. This regimen can be repeated every 3 to 4 weeks for three cycles to a total of 42 Gy. The third cycle is given off the spinal cord. The advantage of this regimen is that it does not induce mucositis to any degree.

TREATMENT ALGORITHM, CHALLENGES, AND FUTURE POSSIBILITIES

A treatment algorithm of our preferred approach to the primary tumor and regional nodes is shown in Figure 30-21. With increasing T stage, the transition from unimodality to multimodality treatment is shown. Concurrent chemoradiation is preferred for patients with T3 or T4 primary tumors and those with N3 or fixed nodal disease.

The cetuximab trial[52] demonstrated that the combination of biologic agents with radiation could improve the survival of patients with head and neck cancer. This result has ignited interest in clinical trials and further basic research into the potential of biologic therapy. The RTOG is investigating the role of cetuximab in the definitive and postoperative treatment of head and neck cancer. The Eastern Cooperative Oncology group has also initiated a phase II trial investigating the role of cetuximab in patients who are being treated with neoadjuvant and concurrent chemotherapy. Other biologic agents are also available and are being tested in clinical trials.

During the past decade, remarkable progress has been made in radiation dose delivery, and research along this line continues. The technology of standard linear accelerators continues to improve. Immobilization devices are becoming more sophisticated. Proton therapy is becoming more widely available in the United States, which will make possible even more precise treatment planning.

REFERENCES

1. Jemal A, Siegel R, Ward E, et al: Cancer statistics, 2006. Cancer J Clin 56:106-130, 2006.
2. Courtard H: Roentgen therapy of epitheliomas of the tonsillar region, hypopharynx, and larynx from 1920 to 1926. Am J Roentgenol Radium Ther Nucl Med 28:313-331, 1932.
3. Fletcher G, MacComb WS, Chau PM, Farnsley WG: Comparison of medium voltage and supervoltage roentgen therapy in the treatment of oropharynx cancers. Am J Roentgenol Radium Ther Nucl Med 81:375-401, 1959.
4. Withers H, Peters LJ, Taylor JM, et al: Local control of carcinoma of the tonsil by radiation therapy: an analysis of patterns of fractionation in nine institutions. Int J Radiat Oncol Biol Phys 33:549-562, 1995.
5. Li W, Thompson CH, O'Brien CJ, et al: Human papillomavirus positivity predicts favourable outcome for squamous carcinoma of the tonsil. Int J Radiat Oncol Biol Phys 106:553-558, 2003.
6. Strome S, Savva A, Brissett AE, et al: Squamous cell carcinoma of the tonsils: a molecular analysis of HPV associations. Clin Cancer Res 8:1093-1100, 2002.
7. Ringstrom E, Peters E, Hasegawa M, et al: Human papillomavirus type 16 and squamous cell carcinoma of the head and neck. Clin Cancer Res 8:3187-3192, 2002.
8. Do KA, Johnson MM, Doherty DA, et al: Second primary tumors in patients with upper aerodigestive tract cancers: joint effects of smoking and alcohol (United States). Cancer Causes Control 14:131-138, 2003.
9. Ang K, Berkey BA, Tu X, et al: Impact of epidermal growth factor receptor expression on survival and pattern of relapse in patients with advanced head and neck carcinoma. Cancer Res 62:7350-7356, 2002.
10. Klijanienko J, el-Naggar A, Ponaio-Prion A, et al: Basaloid squamous carcinoma of the head and neck. Immunohistochemical comparison with adenoid cystic carcinoma and squamous cell carcinoma. Arch Otolaryngol Head Neck Surg 119:887-890, 1993.
11. Luna M, el-Naggar A, Parichatikanond P, et al: Basaloid squamous carcinoma of the upper aerodigestive tract. Cancer 66:537-542, 1990.
12. Garden A, Weber RS, Ang KK, et al: Postoperative radiation therapy for malignant tumors of minor salivary glands. Outcome and patterns of failure. Cancer 73:2563-2569, 1994.
13. Dubey P, Ha CS, Ang KK, et al: Nonnasopharyngeal lymphoepithelioma of the head and neck. Cancer 82:1556-1562, 1998.
14. Lindberg R: Distribution of cervical lymph node metastases from squamous cell carcinoma of the upper respiratory and digestive tracts. Cancer 29:1446-1449, 1972.
15. Foote R, Olsen KD, Davis DL, et al: Base of tongue carcinoma: patterns of failure and predictors of recurrence after surgery alone. Head Neck 15:300-307, 1993.
16. Foote R, Schild SE, Thompson WM, et al: Tonsil cancer. Patterns of failure after surgery alone and surgery combined with postoperative radiation therapy. Cancer 73:2638-2647, 1994.
17. Meoz-Mendez RT, Fletcher GH, Guillamondegui OM, Peters LJ: Analysis of the results of irradiation in the treatment of squamous cell carcinomas of the pharyngeal walls. Int J Radiat Oncol Biol Phys 4:579-585, 1978.
18. Green F, Page DL, Fleming ID, et al: Pharynx (including base of tongue, soft palate and uvula). *In* American Joint Committee on Cancer: AJCC Cancer Staging Manual, 6th ed. New York, Springer, 2002, pp 31-46.
19. Frank S, Chao KS, Schwartz DL, et al: Technology insight: PET and PET/CT in head and neck tumor staging and radiation therapy planning. Nat Clin Pract Oncol 2:526-533, 2005.
20. Bataini J, Asselain B, Jaulerry C, et al: A multivariate primary tumour control analysis in 465 patients treated by radical radiotherapy for cancer of the tonsillar region: clinical and treatment parameters as prognostic factors. Radiother Oncol 14:265-277, 1989.
21. Withers H, Peters LJ, Taylor JM, et al: Late normal tissue sequelae from radiation therapy for carcinoma of the tonsil: patterns of fractionation study of radiobiology. Int J Radiat Oncol Biol Phys 33:563-568, 1995.
22. Overgaard J, Hansen HS, Specht L, et al: Five compared with six fractions per week of conventional radiotherapy of squamous-cell carcinoma of head and neck: DAHANCA 6 and 7 randomised controlled trial. Lancet 362:933-940, 2003.
23. Fu KK, Pajak TF, Trotti A, et al: A Radiation Therapy Oncology Group (RTOG) phase III randomized study to compare hyperfractionation and two variants of accelerated fractionation to standard fractionation radiotherapy for head and neck squamous cell carcinomas: first report of RTOG 90-03. Int J Radiat Oncol Biol Phys 48:7-16, 2000.
24. Gwozdz JT, Morrison WH, Garden AS, et al: Concomitant boost radiotherapy for squamous carcinoma of the tonsillar fossa. Int J Radiat Oncol Biol Phys 39:127-135, 1997.
25. Pernot M, Malissard L, Taghian A, et al: Velotonsillar squamous cell carcinoma: 277 cases treated by combined external irradiation and brachytherapy—results according to extension, localization, and dose rate. Int J Radiat Oncol Biol Phys 23:715-723, 1992.
26. Esche BA, Hale CM, Gerbaulet AP, et al: Interstitial and external radiotherapy in carcinoma of the soft palate and uvula. Int J Radiat Oncol Biol Phys 15:619-625, 1988.
27. Chao KS, Ozyigit G, Blanco AI, et al: Intensity-modulated radiation therapy for oropharyngeal carcinoma: impact of tumor volume. Int J Radiat Oncol Biol Phys 59:43-50, 2004.

28. Garden A, Morrison WH, Rosenthal DI, et al: Intensity modulated radiation therapy (IMRT) for metastatic cervical adenopathy from oropharynx carcinomas. Int J Radiat Oncol Biol Phys 60:S318, 2004.
29. de Arruda FF, Puri DR, Zhung J, et al: Intensity-modulated radiation therapy for the treatment of oropharyngeal carcinoma: the Memorial Sloan-Kettering Cancer Center experience. Int J Radiat Oncol Biol Phys 64:363-373, 2006.
30. Selek U, Garden AS, Morrison WH, et al: Radiation therapy for early-stage carcinoma of the oropharynx. Int J Radiat Oncol Biol Phys 59:743-751, 2004.
31. Garden A, Asper JA, Morrison WH, et al: Is concurrent chemoradiation the treatment of choice for all patients with stage III or IV head and neck carcinoma? Cancer 100:1171-1178, 2004.
32. Spanos WJ, Shukovsky L, Fletcher G: Time, dose, and tumor volume relationships in irradiation of squamous cell carcinomas of the base of the tongue. Cancer 37:2591-2599, 1976.
33. Foote RL, Parsons JT, Mendenhall WM, et al: Is interstitial implantation essential for successful radiotherapeutic treatment of base of tongue carcinoma? Int J Radiat Oncol Biol Phys 18:1293-1298, 1990.
34. Wang C: Radiation Therapy for Head and Neck Neoplasms. New York, Wiley-Liss, 1997.
35. Mendenhall W, Amdur RJ, Stringer SP, et al: Radiation therapy for squamous cell carcinoma of the tonsillar region: a preferred alternative to surgery? J Clin Oncol 18:2219-2225, 2000.
36. Harrison L, Lee HJ, Pfister DG, et al: Long term results of primary radiotherapy with/without neck dissection for squamous cell cancer of the base of tongue. Head Neck 20:668-673, 1998.
37. Gibbs I, Le QT, Shah RD, et al: Long-term outcomes after external beam irradiation and brachytherapy boost for base-of-tongue cancers. Int J Radiat Oncol Biol Phys 57:489-494, 2003.
38. Puthawala AA, Syed AM, Eads DL, et al: Limited external beam and interstitial 192 iridium irradiation in the treatment of carcinoma of the base of the tongue: a ten year experience. Int J Radiat Oncol Biol Phys 14:839-848, 1988.
39. De los Santos J, Buchholtz TA: Surgery and post-operative radiation therapy for advanced squamous cell carcinoma of the base of tongue. Cancer J Clin 6:411, 2000.
40. Wong C, Ang KK, Fletcher GH, et al: Definitive radiotherapy for squamous cell carcinoma of the tonsillar fossa. Int J Radiat Oncol Biol Phys 16:657-662, 1989.
41. Mazeron JJ, Lunischi A, Marinello G, et al: Interstitial radiation therapy for squamous cell carcinoma of the tonsillar region: the Creteil experience (1971-1981). Int J Radiat Oncol Biol Phys 12:895-900, 1986.
42. Mazeron J, Noel G, Simon J: Head and neck brachytherapy. Semin Radiat Oncol 12:95-108, 2002.
43. Keus RB, Pontvert D, Brunin F, et al: Results of irradiation in squamous cell carcinoma of the soft palate and uvula. Radiother Oncol 11:311-317, 1988.
44. Erkal HS, Serin M, Amdur RJ, et al: Squamous cell carcinomas of the soft palate treated with radiation therapy alone or followed by planned neck dissection. Int J Radiat Oncol Biol Phys 50:359-366, 2001.
45. Mazeron J, Belkacemi Y, Simon JM, et al: Place of iridium 192 implantation in definitive irradiation of faucial arch squamous cell carcinomas. Int J Radiat Oncol Biol Phys 27:251-257, 1993.
46. Hull M, Morris CG, Tannehill SP, et al: Definitive radiotherapy alone or combined with a planned neck dissection for squamous cell carcinoma of the pharyngeal wall. Cancer 98:2224-2231, 2003.
47. Bourhis J, Amand C, Pignon J: Update of MACH-NC (Meta-Analysis of Chemotherapy in Head & Neck Cancer) database focused on concomitant chemoradiotherapy. J Clin Oncol 22(Suppl 14):5505, 2004.
48. Denis F, Garaud P, Bardet E, et al: Final results of the 94-01 French Head and Neck Oncology and Radiotherapy Group randomized trial comparing radiotherapy alone with concomitant radiochemotherapy in advanced-stage oropharynx carcinoma. J Clin Oncol 22:69-76, 2004.
49. Al-Othman MO, Morris CG, Hinerman RW, et al: Distant metastases after definitive radiotherapy for squamous cell carcinoma of the head and neck. Head Neck Surg 25:629-633, 2003.
50. Adelstein D: Induction chemotherapy in head and neck cancer. Hematol Oncol Clin North Am 13:689-698, 1999.
51. Haraf D, Rosen FR, Stenson K, et al: Induction chemotherapy followed by concomitant TFHX chemoradiotherapy with reduced dose radiation in advanced head and neck cancer. Clin Cancer Res 9:5936-5943, 2003.
52. Bonner JA, Harari PM, Giralt J, et al: Radiotherapy plus cetuximab for squamous-cell carcinoma of the head and neck. N Engl J Med 354:567-578, 2005.
53. Lee H, Zelefsky MJ, Kraus DH, et al: Long-term regional control after radiation therapy and neck dissection for base of tongue carcinoma. Int J Radiat Oncol Biol Phys 38:995-1000, 1997.
54. Porceddu SV, Jarmolowski E, Hicks RJ, et al: Utility of positron emission tomography for the detection of disease in residual neck nodes after (chemo) radiotherapy in head and neck cancer. Head Neck Surg 27:175-181, 2005.
55. Peters LJ, Weber RS, Morrison WH, et al: Neck surgery in patients with primary oropharyngeal cancer treated by radiotherapy. Head Neck 18:552-559, 1996.
56. Salama JK, Vokes EE, Chmura SJ, et al: Long-term outcome of concurrent chemotherapy and reirradiation for recurrent and second primary head-and-neck squamous cell carcinoma. Int J Radiat Oncol Biol Phys 64:382-391, 2006.
57. De Crevoisier R, Bourhis J, Domenge C, et al: Full-dose reirradiation for unresectable head and neck carcinoma: experience at the Gustave-Roussy Institute in a series of 169 patients. J Clin Oncol 16:3556-3562, 1998.
58. Lindberg R, Fletcher G: The role of irradiation in the management of head and neck cancer: analysis of results and causes of failure. Tumori 64:313-325, 1978.
59. O'Sullivan B, Warde P, Grice B, et al: The benefits and pitfalls of ipsilateral radiotherapy in carcinoma of the tonsillar region. Int J Radiat Oncol Biol Phys 51:332-343, 2001.
60. Jackson SM, Hay JH, Flores AD, et al: Cancer of the tonsil: the results of ipsilateral radiation treatment. Radiother Oncol 51:123-128, 1999.
61. Dabaja B, Salehpour MR, Rosen I, et al: Intensity-modulated radiation therapy (IMRT) of cancers of the head and neck: comparison of split-field and whole-field techniques. Int J Radiat Oncol Biol Phys 63:1000-1005, 2005.
62. Gregoire V, Levendag P, Ang KK, et al: CT-based delineation of lymph node levels and related CTVs in the node-negative neck: DAHANCA, EORTC, GORTEC, NCIC, RTOG consensus guidelines. Radiother Oncol 73:383-384, 2003.
63. Eisbruch A, Marsh LH, Dawson LA, et al: Recurrences near base of skull after IMRT for head-and-neck cancer: implications for target delineation in high neck and for parotid gland sparing. Int J Radiat Oncol Biol Phys 59:28-42, 2004.
64. Cooper J, Ang K: Concomitant chemotherapy and radiation therapy certainly improves local control. Int J Radiat Oncol Biol Phys 61:7-9, 2005.
65. Forastiere AA, Goepfert H, Maor M, et al: Concurrent chemotherapy and radiotherapy for organ preservation in advanced laryngeal cancer. N Engl J Med 349:2091-2098, 2003.
66. Bernier J, Domenge C, Ozsahin M, et al: Postoperative irradiation with or without concomitant chemotherapy for locally advanced head and neck cancer. N Engl J Med 350:1945-1952, 2004.
67. Remmler D, Medina JE, Byers RM, et al: Treatment of choice for squamous carcinoma of the tonsillar fossa. Head Neck Surg 7:206-211, 1985.
68. Weber RS, Gidley P, Morrison WH, et al: Treatment selection for carcinoma of the base of the tongue. Am J Surg 160:415-419, 1990.
69. Mak A, Morrison WH, Garden AS, et al: Base-of-tongue carcinoma: treatment results using concomitant boost radiotherapy. Int J Radiat Oncol Biol Phys 33:289-296, 1995.
70. Mendenhall WM, Stringer SP, Amdur RJ, et al: Is radiation therapy a preferred alternative to surgery for squamous cell carcinoma of the base of tongue? J Clin Oncol 18:35-42, 2000.
71. Fein DA, Lee WR, Amos WR, et al: Oropharyngeal carcinoma treated with radiotherapy: a 30-year experience. Int J Radiat Oncol Biol Phys 34:289-296, 1996.

CHAPTER 31

NASOPHARYNGEAL CARCINOMA

Roger Ove, Robert L. Foote, and James A. Bonner

INCIDENCE

In the United States, nasopharyngeal carcinoma is uncommon, occurring at a rate of 0.2 to 0.5 case/100,000 people.

In contrast, in southern China and Hong Kong, the incidence is 25 to 50/100,000, and among the Inuit in Alaska and Greenland, the rate is 15 to 20/100,000.

BIOLOGY

A potential link between Epstein-Barr virus (EBV) and nasopharyngeal cancer was first described more than 30 years ago; advances in molecular biology have advanced understanding of this association. The rate of positive EBV serology is higher with nonkeratinizing or poorly differentiated versus well-differentiated lesions, and EBV DNA is detected less frequently in patients with keratinizing squamous cell carcinomas.

STAGING EVALUATION

Physical examination and workup for nasopharyngeal cancer includes detailed palpation of neck nodes, flexible nasopharyngoscopy with biopsy, computed tomography with or without magnetic resonance imaging of the head and neck, complete blood count, chemistry panel, and chest radiography. Positron emission tomography should be considered.

PRIMARY THERAPY

Treated with radiotherapy as a single modality, patients with nasopharyngeal carcinoma have a similar 10-year survival rate in the United States, Denmark, and Hong Kong—34%, 37%, and 43%, respectively.

Advancing technology promises to allow better optimization of radiotherapy, improving target coverage and minimizing morbidity.

The Intergroup study 0099 showed an advantage to the addition of concurrent plus adjuvant chemotherapy for stage III and IV disease, with a survival advantage at 3 years (78% versus 48%, $p = .005$).[1] The advantage of concurrent chemotherapy for advanced disease is now well established, although the benefit of adjuvant chemotherapy remains unclear.

LOCALLY RECURRENT OR PERSISTENT DISEASE

For persistent or recurrent nodal disease, surgical resection is the preferred treatment if technically possible, but recurrent disease at the site of the primary lesion is difficult to approach surgically.

Reirradiation for recurrent disease appears to be most effective in patients with a prolonged disease-free interval (DFI) and at a high reirradiation dose. In one series, patients with a DFI of greater than 24 months had a 5-year survival rate of 66% versus 13% for those with a DFI of 24 months or less; in patients receiving a dose of 60 Gy or more versus 60 Gy or less, the 5-year survival rate was 45% versus 0%.

Advances in clinical and basic research have led to a better understanding of the carcinogenesis of nasopharyngeal carcinoma and to better treatment of this condition; however, such advances have also raised many new questions about this disease. This chapter provides an overview of the current understanding of etiologic factors, such as Epstein-Barr virus (EBV), and the present diagnostic and therapeutic interventions for nasopharyngeal carcinoma. Therapeutic controversies are highlighted, and the data relevant to controversial issues are reviewed to guide treating physicians in applying clinical data to individual patients.

ETIOLOGY AND EPIDEMIOLOGY

Nasopharyngeal carcinoma is an uncommon tumor in the United States, where the incidence is approximately 0.2 to 0.5 case/100,000 people.[3] In comparison, the incidence is considerably greater in southern China and Hong Kong (25 to 50/100,000) and among the Inuit residing in Alaska and Greenland (15 to 20/100,000). The incidence of nasopharyngeal cancer is also higher in other parts of southeast Asia (Taiwan, Vietnam, and Thailand), the Philippines, Malaysia, and in some Mediterranean and North African populations (8 to 12/100,000). These areas of increased incidence of nasopharyngeal cancer are considered endemic areas, and the incidence outside endemic areas is much lower and more often associated with tobacco use.

Several geographic-specific etiologic factors have been implicated in the incidence variations throughout the world. The high consumption of salted fish in southern China and Hong Kong has been implicated as a possible etiologic factor for nasopharyngeal carcinoma in these areas.[4,5] It has been suggested that various macromolecular lignins associated with these foods in southern China (and perhaps other areas such as Alaska) may activate EBV,[6] which has also been identified as a probable etiologic factor in nasopharyngeal carcinoma.[7,8] Studies by Bouvier and colleagues[6] involved the fractionation of harissa, a homemade spice mixture used in Tunisia on various foods, including salted fish. Harissa was separated into various macromolecular fractions by column chromatography. The lignin-containing complexes extracted from harissa induced the EBV promoter in Raji cells.[6] The possibility that these environmental factors are important in the etiology of nasopharyngeal carcinomas is further supported by the finding that incidence rates decrease for successive generations of people who originally emigrated from southern China to California.[9]

Other potential environmental etiologic factors that have been associated with nasopharyngeal carcinoma include alcohol consumption and exposure to dust, fumes, formaldehyde, and cigarette smoke.[10,11] Cigarette smoke and alcohol have long been associated with many other head and neck carcinomas, but their association with nasopharyngeal carcinoma has been controversial. Some studies have suggested that alcohol consumption and cigarette use were not associated with nasopharyngeal carcinoma.[10-12] Nam and associates[11] conducted a case-control study using a National Mortality Follow-Back Survey based on death certificates and found that cigarette smoking and alcohol consumption are independent statistically significant risk factors for nasopharyngeal carcinoma. The increased risk of nasopharyngeal carcinoma with heavy smoking (adjusted for alcohol consumption) was threefold, and an excess risk of 80% was demonstrated for heavy alcohol consumption (adjusted for cigarette use).

PREVENTION AND EARLY DETECTION

The nasopharynx cannot be visualized externally, and tumors of this area often present after they have eroded into a vital structure and produce a presenting symptom. The association of EBV and nasopharyngeal cancer has led some investigators to hypothesize that serologic screening (EBV titer) may be useful in certain high-risk populations to identify groups of patients who might benefit from frequent nasopharyngeal exams.[13] In a study from China of 338,868 patients who underwent serologic screening for EBV titer, 9367 persons had immunoglobulin (Ig)A antibodies to EBV. Of these 9367 patients, 306 were positive for IgA to EBV early antigen. Nasopharyngeal cancer was detected in 113 of the 9367 patients (1.2%) and in 63 of the 306 (20.5%). Most of the tumors (>85%) were early-stage lesions. Serologic EBV IgA screening is currently being used in endemic areas.

In addition to EBV serologic screening as a means of early detection and possible prevention of advanced-stage disease, several environmental and genetic predisposing factors are being explored as possible markers that could identify groups of patients at high risk for nasopharyngeal cancer.[14] Real-time polymerase chain reaction (PCR) techniques show promise as screening tools for nasopharyngeal cancer.[15] EBV DNA detection—in particular, detection of EBV nuclear antigen—eliminates many false-positives and improves the sensitivity and specificity of EBV IgA serologic screening.[16] A retrospective analysis of blood samples from patients with disease relapse from previous clinical trials indicates that EBV nuclear antigen screening by PCR would have led to earlier detection of distant failure but, because of the quality of current imaging, would not have significantly affected detection of local recurrences.[17] Real-time PCR screening for EBV LMP1 (latent membrane protein 1) in nasopharyngeal swabs has also been shown to be a promising screening tool for high-risk populations, with a sensitivity of 87% and specificity of 98%.[18] These techniques are likely to replace serum IgA screening in endemic areas and have a promising role in screening for relapse in EBV-positive patients.[19] The further study of other environmental and genetic markers may lead to the identification of patient populations that could benefit from screening or chemoprevention.[14]

Chemoprevention has been tested extensively in patients with a prior diagnosis of head or neck malignancy, because second primary tumors in the respiratory and digestive tracts are common in that population.[20-23] Hong and others[20] conducted a prevention trial for patients with head and neck carcinoma after curative surgery, radiotherapy, or both. Patients were randomly assigned to receive 1 year of 13-*cis*-retinoic acid (isotretinoin) as a chemoprevention agent (see Khuri and associates[14] for discussion of the biology) or placebo. The treated group had significantly fewer second primary tumors (4%) than the placebo group (24%) ($p = .005$); however, there was no difference in survival or incidence of relapse between the two groups. In addition, the chemopreventive effect appeared to abate after 3 years; the incidence of second primary tumors was similar in the 2 groups after 3 years.[20]

The results of the trial by Hong and colleagues[20] were not confirmed by a controlled trial of 316 patients by Bolla and associates,[22] in which patients were randomly assigned to 2 years of etretinate (a retinoic acid similar to isotretinoin) at a maintenance dosage of 25 mg/d. Subsequently, a large intergroup effort was mounted, and 1302 patients with previously treated head and neck malignancies were randomly assigned to receive 3 years of isotretinoin or placebo.[23] Because of unacceptable toxicity seen with higher doses of isotretinoin (100 to 200 mg/m^2 [≈ 150 to 400 mg total]) in prior studies, the dosage was decreased to 30 mg/d in this trial. No difference was seen in the occurrence of second primary tumors (4.7% in both arms), which was the primary end point of the study.[24] A decrease in local recurrence was seen, however, and 13-*cis*-retinoic acid remains a topic of investigation.

The issue of whether retinoids or other chemopreventive agents should be used in the setting of premalignant lesions of the oral cavity has been considered, and many trials have suggested that retinoids can induce considerable responses in oral leukoplakia.[25,26] Toxicity has been a limiting issue in these trials, however. It will be important to determine whether these chemoprevention strategies, developed for leukoplakia, can be extrapolated to prevention of nasopharyngeal cancer in subgroups of patients at high risk for such malignancies.

Blockade of cyclooxygenase-2 (COX-2) has also shown some promise as a chemopreventive strategy, and COX-2 inhibitors were recently the topic of investigation for various malignancies including head and neck cancer.[27] A phase II study at Fox Chase Cancer Center evaluated a 3-month course of celecoxib in patients with biopsy-proved dysplastic or hyperplastic leukoplakia, with results pending. A study of patients with leukoplakia at the M. D. Anderson Cancer Center (MDACC) compared chemoprevention with celecoxib, EKB-569 (an epidermal growth factor receptor–tyrosine kinase inhibitor), or both drugs in combination. The results are not yet published. Most recent COX-2 inhibitor cancer prevention trials have been closed, except in very high-risk settings such as familial polyposis, because of the increased rate of cardiovascular events seen in a few of the celecoxib and rofecoxib prevention trials.

PATHOLOGY, ANATOMY, AND PATHWAYS OF SPREAD

Malignancies of the nasopharyngeal area are generally carcinomas (90%), with lymphomas comprising approximately 5% of lesions.[28] The pathologic type has been grouped into three major categories by the World Health Organization (WHO)[29]: WHO type 1, keratinizing squamous cell carcinoma; WHO type 2, nonkeratinizing squamous cell carcinoma; and WHO type 3, poorly differentiated carcinoma or lymphoepithelioma.

Keratinizing squamous cell carcinomas histologically appear well differentiated with intercellular bridges. These WHO type 1 lesions comprise approximately 20% of carcino-

Table 31-1 **Treatment Results of Studies in Three Diverse Locations**

	Sanguineti et al[31]	Johansen[32]	Lee et al[33]
Location	United States (MDACC)	Denmark	Hong Kong
Study size	$N = 378$	$N = 167$	$N = 5037$
Histology, No. or % of patients			
WD	5	8%	0.3%*
MD	36	5%	
PD	109	87%	
SCC	193		
NS	43		
LymE	154		
Undifferentiated			99.7%
Unk	31		
N0, % of patients	21	25	39
Primary treatment	60.2-72 Gy	57-68 Gy/1.8-2.0 Gy/d	65 Gy†
Neck treatment	Yes	Yes	906 of 1290 N0 patients not treated
Primary control, %	66 (10 y)	67 (10 y)	87 (initial CR)
Nodal control, %	83 (10 y)	86 Overall, 60 if not irradiated	87 (initial CR)
Survival, %	48 (5 y)	37 (10 y)	52 (initial CR)
Complications	(See Table 31-6)	Xerostomia Edema Dysphagia Skin fibrosis/necrosis Osteonecrosis Radiation myelitis	9% Neurologic damage 7% Significant functional disturbance (soft tissue necrosis) 1% Death

CR, complete response; LymE, lymphoepithelioma; MD, moderately differentiated; MDACC, M. D. Anderson Cancer Center; NS, not specified; NO, node negative; PD, poorly differentiated; SCC, squamous cell carcinoma; Unk, unknown; WD, well differentiated.

*WD or nonkeratinizing.

†Median equivalent dose using time and dose fractionation (TDF) tables. Large (>2 Gy) fraction sizes were often used.

mas.[29,30] WHO type 2 lesions (30% to 40% of carcinomas) lack well-defined squamous cell characteristics but continue to show a "pavement stone pattern," characteristic of squamous cell histology.[29] WHO type 3 carcinomas, or undifferentiated lymphoepitheliomas (40%-50%), are characterized by a lymphoplasmacytic infiltrate; cytologically the cells appear uniform, with round to oval nuclei and prominent nucleoli.[29] The frequency of the different histologic types varies with geographic area (Table 31-1).

Anatomy and Pathways of Spread

The nasopharynx is a musculofascial tube that connects the nasal cavity and oropharynx. The anatomic borders of the nasopharynx are (1) anteriorly, the posterior nasal apertures and nasal septum; (2) posteriorly, the pharyngeal mucosa; (3) superiorly, the pharyngeal mucosa and body of sphenoid; and (4) inferiorly, the oropharynx. The lateral wall of the nasopharynx contains the pharyngeal opening of the auditory tube. The medial cartilaginous extension of the auditory tube forms a protrusion from the lateral wall of the nasopharynx at the superior and posterior aspects of the opening of the auditory tube. This protrusion with its overlying mucosa creates the torus tubarius. Just posterior to the torus tubarius lies the pharyngeal fossa, or the fossa of Rosenmüller, which is formed by the junction of the lateral and posterior walls of the nasopharynx (Fig. 31-1).

The superior wall of the nasopharynx warrants review; extension of tumors superiorly often leads to invasion of structures, the symptoms of which are typical of the initial clinical presentation of patients. The sphenoid bone lies superior to the mucosa and pharyngobasilar fascia of the nasopharynx. Several cranial nerves exit the base of skull in this area. Critical foramina housed in the sphenoid include the superior orbital fissure (cranial nerves III, IV, V [ophthalmic division], and VI), the foramen rotundum (cranial nerve V [maxillary division]), the foramen ovale (cranial nerve V [mandibular division]), and the foramen spinosum (recurrent branch of cranial nerve V [mandibular division]). The foramen lacerum is formed by the junction of the sphenoid and temporal bones. The internal carotid artery passes over the superior opening of the foramen lacerum but does not traverse through the foramen. The nerve of the pterygoid canal and the meningeal branch of the ascending pharyngeal artery course through the foramen lacerum. Deep to the mucosa of the superior aspect of the lateral wall of the nasopharynx lies the superior pharyngeal constrictor muscle. Beyond this muscle lie cranial nerves IX, X, and XI, which exit the base of the skull from the jugular foramen in the temporal bone, and cranial nerve XII, which exits the base of the skull through the hypoglossal canal of the temporal bone.

The sensory innervation is shown in Figure 31-1D. The maxillary division of the trigeminal nerve supplies the upper nasopharynx, the posterior part of the nasal cavity, and most of the palate and upper gums of the oral cavity. The general sensory branches of the lingual and pharyngeal branches of the glossopharyngeal nerve supply the sensory innervation of the lower part of the nasopharynx, the posterior third of the tongue, and part of the soft palate and oropharynx.

Understanding the anatomic relationships of the nasopharynx and adjacent structures is important to correctly diagnose patients with nasopharyngeal carcinoma. The importance of superior extension into the sphenoid bone of the base of skull is exemplified by the fact that cranial nerves can be involved at presentation. The frequency of involvement of cranial nerves has been described in two large series.[31,34] Cranial nerves VI and V are the most commonly involved. These nerves traverse the sphenoid bone and can be involved when

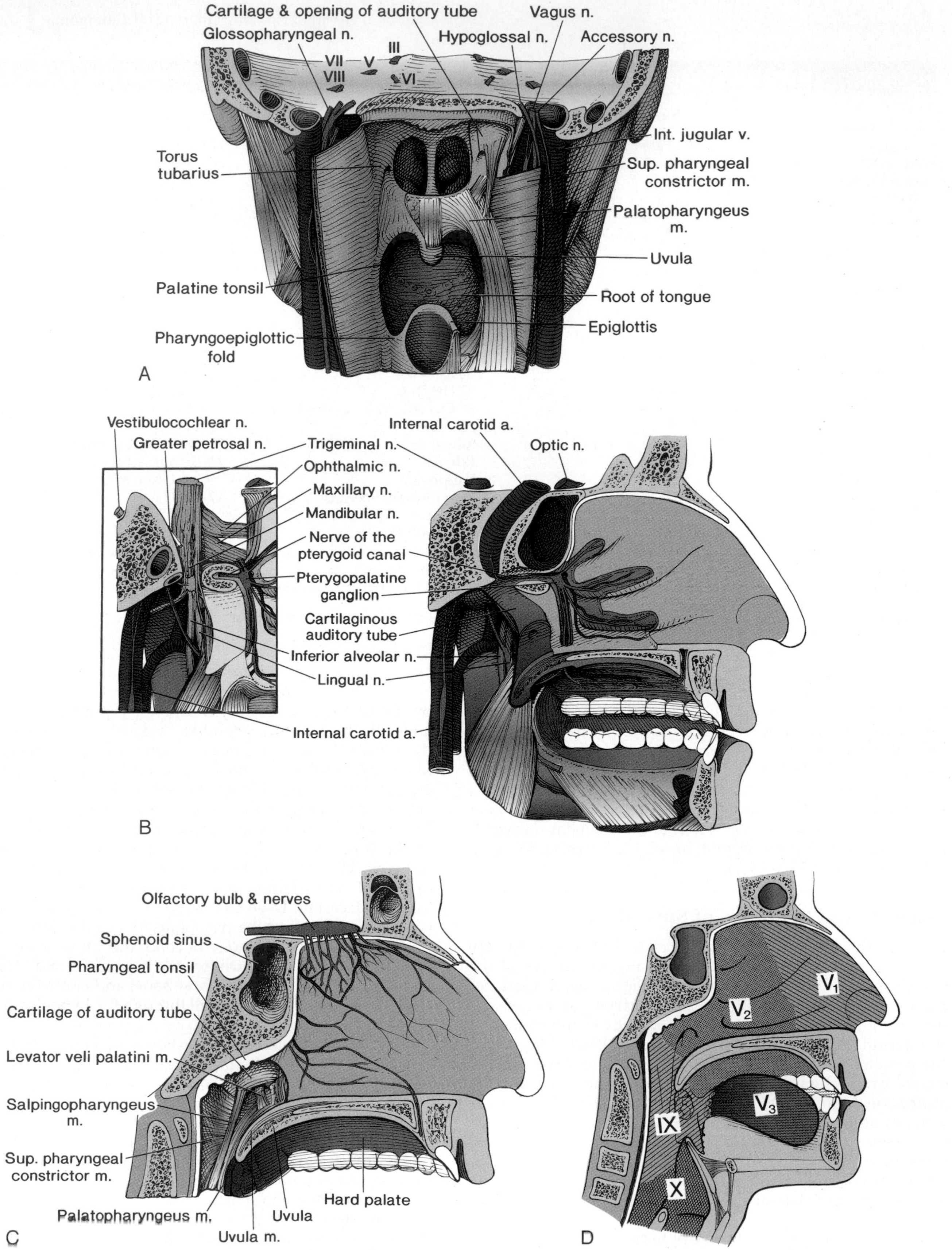

Figure 31-1 Anatomic relationships of the structures of the nasopharynx and adjacent structures. **A,** Coronal section through the center of the nasopharynx, with a view of lateral structures. **B,** Sagittal section through the nasopharynx lateral to midline, with a view of the lateral relationships of the nasopharynx *(inset)*. **C,** Sagittal section through the nasopharynx, with a view of the anterior and adjacent structures. **D,** Sensory innervation of the nasopharynx. Roman numerals refer to cranial nerves. a., artery; Int., internal; m., muscle; n., nerve; Sup, superior; v., vein; V_1, ophthalmic division of trigeminal nerve; V_2, maxillary division of trigeminal nerve; V_3, mandibular division of trigeminal nerve. (**A–C,** Adapted from Clemente CD: Anatomy: A Regional Atlas of the Human Body. Philadelphia, Lea & Febiger, 1975; **D,** adapted from Pernkopf E: *In* Ferner H [ed]: Atlas of Topographical and Applied Human Anatomy, 2nd ed. Baltimore, Urban & Schwarzenberg, 1980.)

tumors erode superiorly through bone. Tumors of the nasopharynx can also gain access to the cranial nerves of the base of skull by eroding superiorly through the foramen lacerum, which is bordered superiorly by the internal carotid artery (see Fig. 31-1B).

Lateral extension of nasopharyngeal carcinomas can lead to erosion of the medial opening of the auditory tube and the medial pterygoid plate and can involve cranial nerves IX, X, XI, and XII (see Fig. 31-1B and C). Lateral extension can lead to involvement of the carotid artery and internal jugular vein.

Lymph node involvement is common; 65% to 80% of patients present with clinically involved cervical neck nodes. The upper posterior cervical and subdigastric lymph nodes are commonly involved. The published frequency of involvement of these areas in two large series[31,34] is presented later in "Clinical Manifestations."

BIOLOGICAL CHARACTERISTICS AND MOLECULAR BIOLOGY

The potential etiologic link between EBV and nasopharyngeal carcinoma was first described more than 30 years ago[35]; however, advances in molecular biology have shed further light on this association. Earlier work explored the clinical utility of serologic evaluation of antibodies to the viral capsid antigen and the diffuse component of the early antigen in patients with nasopharyngeal carcinoma. Anti–viral capsid antigen IgA was detected in 80% to 85% of patients with nasopharyngeal cancers,[36,37] but this finding was uncommon in patients with carcinomas of other head and neck sites. An association between decreasing antibody titers and response to therapy also suggested that antibody titers could be used to assess a patient's prognosis.[38] Neel and Taylor,[39] in a prospective study of a North American population, did not confirm this association, but they did report a higher rate of EBV-positive serologic results for patients with nonkeratinizing or poorly differentiated lesions.

The cellular and humoral immune response to various EBV-associated antigens is a topic of investigation, and these measures of immune response appear to have a bearing on prognosis. Failure to mount an appropriate immune response to EBV may contribute to the development of nasopharyngeal carcinoma, and mutations in the viral antigens may decrease the host immune response. A restricted pattern of EBV antigens is presented in nasopharyngeal cancer, unlike other EBV-associated diseases in which immunotherapy has been more successful.[40] The primary latent antigens include EBV nuclear antigen and latent membrane proteins. In a staging system proposed by Neel and Taylor,[41] additional prognostic separation could be obtained by taking into account the antibody-dependent cellular cytotoxicity (ADCC) titer. High ADCC titers were correlated with improved survival. The ADCC assay appears to measure the IgG response, which is a cytotoxic response to latent membrane antigen. High IgA (viral capsid response) may block the IgG response and prevent its beneficial cytotoxic activity. Therefore, low levels of ADCC correlate with poor prognosis.[8] Allogeneic cytotoxic T cells to various EBV antigens have been developed and show some promise for treating locally recurrent nasopharyngeal carcinoma.[42]

Studies of other antibodies to EBV have found a significant association between tumors with high EBV titers (e.g., nonkeratinizing squamous cell carcinomas [WHO type 2] and poorly differentiated tumors [WHO type 3]) and poor prognosis. For example, high titers of antibodies to the EBV replication activator (ZEBRA) have been associated with a high risk of distant spread.[43] Somewhat paradoxically, keratinizing squamous cell carcinomas (WHO type 1), which generally are associated with low or zero EBV titers, have been associated with a poorer prognosis than type 2 or 3 tumors.[41] Further work is needed to determine whether these biological markers can help to assess the risk of local and distant spread and so direct therapeutic interventions.

The detection rate of EBV infection in patients with nasopharyngeal carcinoma has been the subject of debate, much of which probably stems from variability in the sensitivity of different assays. Investigators have focused on the assessment of EBV in tumor cells in addition to serologic evaluation of human plasma. Previous serologic studies suggested that higher titers may be present in undifferentiated tumors than in nonkeratinizing carcinomas and that even lower titers are present in keratinizing squamous cell carcinomas.[7,39] Using the Southern blot technique, Raab-Traub and others[44] showed the presence of EBV in all three histologic variants of nasopharyngeal carcinoma, but the EBV copy number was lowest in keratinizing squamous cell carcinomas. In subsequent studies, EBV DNA was detected less frequently in tumor specimens from keratinizing squamous cell carcinoma than in the less differentiated histologic variants.[45-47] In a study by Murono and associates,[48] EBV DNA was not detected by PCR in any of the 5 keratinizing squamous cell tumors but was detected in 13 of 13 undifferentiated tumors, and in situ hybridization for EBV-encoded small RNAs was positive in 30 of 32 nonkeratinizing carcinomas. These results may be clinically useful; therapeutic interventions may eventually be tailored to account for risk factors based on biological marker profiles.

In addition to environmental factors, the potential association of various genetic factors and nasopharyngeal cancer is a topic of current investigation. Earlier work implicated a disease susceptibility gene linked to the human leukocyte antigen (HLA) region, which has been associated with the increased incidence of nasopharyngeal carcinoma in southern China.[49] Simons and associates[50] originally described an association in Chinese patients with nasopharyngeal carcinoma and the HLA-A2 antigen with a deficit of the second antigen at the second locus (B locus). Later Simons and coworkers[51] reported on 110 Chinese patients in Singapore with nasopharyngeal carcinoma and hypothesized that the new B-locus antigen (Sin 2) may be associated with the tumor. Various other cytogenetic abnormalities have been reported. Deletions of the short arm of chromosome 3 (3p25, 3p14)[29] and of chromosome 9 (9p21-22)[52] have been associated with nasopharyngeal carcinoma. These findings may lead to a greater understanding of the genetic basis of nasopharyngeal carcinomas and the interplay of environmental factors with these genetic factors.

CLINICAL MANIFESTATIONS, PATIENT EVALUATION, AND STAGING

Clinical Manifestations

As mentioned, nasopharyngeal carcinoma is rare in the United States and is not often suspected as a possible cause of a patient's early symptoms. In addition, the list of possible early symptoms of nasopharyngeal carcinomas includes many symptoms that could have more common causes. In a series of 378 patients from the MDACC,[31] the presenting symptoms included neck mass in 41%, hearing loss, ear drainage, or otalgia in 27%, nasal bleeding or obstruction in 21%, cranial nerve deficits in 8%, and other nonspecific symptoms in 8%. Investigators from Washington University noted that the typical presentation involved multiple symptoms.[34] In this series of 143 patients, presenting symptoms included otitis in 43%, throat pain in 39%, nasal obstruction in 37%, a neck mass in 35%, nasal bleeding in 29%, cranial nerve involvement in 24%, and trismus or other symptoms in 5%.

Similar to these data, most series have shown that neck masses, obstructive ear symptoms, and cranial nerve deficits are common presenting symptoms for nasopharyngeal carcinoma. In the Washington University series,[34] 66% of patients were found to have ipsilateral neck masses and 28% had contralateral neck masses on examination, although only 35% of patients had reported a neck mass as the reason for seeking medical advice. Of the patients with clinically involved neck disease, 60% had enlarged ipsilateral subdigastric lymph nodes, and 32% had enlarged ipsilateral posterior cervical chain nodes. The most frequently involved cranial nerves in the series were cranial nerve VI in 15% of patients, V in 7.7%, and VIII, X, and XII in 5.6% each.

In the series from MDACC,[31] the posterior cervical lymph nodes were most commonly enlarged (54% of patients), followed by the subdigastric nodes (49% of patients). The midjugular and midposterior groups were involved in 24% and 22% of patients, respectively. The low jugular lymph nodes, low posterior cervical lymph nodes, and supraclavicular lymph nodes were involved in 10%, 13%, and 10% of patients, respectively. Similar to the series from Washington University, cranial nerve VI was the most frequently involved nerve (6% of cases).

Patient Evaluation

The initial evaluation of patients with nasopharyngeal carcinoma should include a history and physical examination, with special attention to the level of nodal involvement (if any). It is helpful to diagram the clinically involved lymph nodes in the neck because it can be helpful when the radiotherapy boost is considered.

Patients should undergo flexible fiberoptic nasopharyngoscopy to determine the involvement of mucosal surfaces. A diagram of these findings should also be made. Biopsy of the primary lesion should be attempted first. If this procedure gives indeterminate results, a needle biopsy of a potentially involved lymph node should be taken.

Computed tomography (CT) and magnetic resonance imaging (MRI) of the head and neck are useful in the evaluation of both erosion of tumor into the bony structures of the base of skull and retropharyngeal and cervical lymphadenopathy. Although the same information is often provided by CT and MRI, some investigations have suggested that MRI may be more useful in delineating soft-tissue invasion outside the nasopharynx and the extent of retropharyngeal lymph node involvement, whereas CT may be most useful in delineating skull base erosion.[53,54] The usefulness of CT and MRI are dependent on the expertise of both the radiologist and the clinician. It appears that the two tests may be complementary in certain settings, but current recommendations stop short of routinely using both tests in each patient.

Positron emission tomography (PET) can be useful for situations in which other imaging is unclear, particularly in the evaluation of possible recurrence after radiotherapy. PET can be ambiguous if performed within 6 months of radiotherapy, however.[55] PET and other functional imaging methods may also be useful for radiotherapy planning.[56]

The completion of diagnostic evaluation involves acquiring routine complete blood counts, chemistry panel, and a chest radiograph. Further evaluation of possible metastases should be done on the basis of the clinical presentation of the patient (see Fig. 31-8A).

Staging

Staging and the prognostic significance of the staging of nasopharyngeal carcinoma are complex. After a pathologic assessment has been made, the work-up or evaluation leads to a clinical stage (Table 31-2). Clinical staging has been a matter of controversy. The previous American Joint Committee on Cancer (AJCC) classifications (1977 and 1992) for head and neck malignancies often resulted in a stage III or IV grouping for most nasopharyngeal malignancies because of the high incidence of clinically involved neck disease.[59,62]

Several studies[60,63] showed that the Ho staging system[64] may result in superior prognostic separation of patient groups compared with the 1977 AJCC system or the 1967 Uniform International Committee on Cancer (UICC) system. These investigators cited the high incidence of lymph node involvement in patients with nasopharyngeal carcinoma, and the Ho system separates patients into prognostic groups (stages) based on the level of lymph node involvement (see Table 31-2).[60,63] Similar to the previous 1977 AJCC system, the 1992 AJCC system included some patients with N1 disease in stage III, but the patients with nodal involvement and metastasis outside the neck were all grouped together into stage IV. In the Ho system, nodal involvement appears in stage II, and patients with supraclavicular metastases are represented in a separate stage IV (see Table 31-2). In 1997, the AJCC system incorporated some of the aspects of the Ho system,[57] and these changes remain in place in the current system.[58] In 1992, Chinese physicians adopted an independent system similar to the Ho system.[61]

The current AJCC system has been shown to be superior to both the previous AJCC system and the Ho system.[65,66] Further refinement may lead to improvement in risk stratification, because among T4 patients, intracranial invasion or involvement of the orbit or cranial nerves leads to a worse prognosis.[65]

A staging system proposed by Neel and Taylor[41] takes into account numerous symptoms and tumor characteristics. Through regression analysis of data on 182 patients, various prognostic groups were developed which resulted in greater prognostic separation of patients than in the 1977 AJCC system.[41] Neel and Taylor's[41] system has not been compared with the current AJCC system. In their report, additional prognostic separation was afforded by taking into account the ADCC titer of each patient, with worse survival in patients with low IgG responses.[41] Detailed understanding of the interplay of a patient's immune system and the molecular biology of a clonal population of tumor cells may eventually form the basis for more accurate stratification of risk. At present, several measures of biological activity, including viral titers, gene expression, and measures of host immune response, are under investigation and may have a role in future biological staging systems. As has been done in the setting of other malignancies, the use of biological assays in the assessment of risk will likely become more comprehensive, using the technology of microarrays to profile gene expression on a genomic scale.[67]

PRIMARY THERAPY

Traditionally, the nasopharyngeal area has not been easy to examine without fiberoptic technology and has been difficult to approach surgically. Surgical exposure of the area and resection of tumors with adequate tumor margins have long been

Table 31-2 Comparison of Staging Systems

Classification	SYSTEM Current and 1997 AJCC[57,58]	1992 AJCC[59]	Ho Staging[60]	Ma et al[61]
T1	Confined to nasopharynx	1 Subsite	Confined to nasopharynx	Confined to nasopharynx
T2	Soft tissue invasion a: Without parapharyngeal extension b: With parapharyngeal extension	>1 Subsite	Nasal fossa, oropharynx, muscle, or nerves below base of skull	Nasal cavity, oropharynx, soft palate, cervical prevertebral soft tissue, parapharyngeal anterior to the SO* line
T3	Bony or paranasal sinus extension	Nasal cavity and/or oropharynx involvement	a: Bone involvement below base of skull b: Involves base of skull c: Cranial nerves d: Orbits, laryngopharynx, or infratemporal fossa	Posterior to SO* line, either anterior or posterior cranial nerves, skull base, pterygoid plates, pterygopalatine fossa
T4	Intercranial extension, or cranial nerve or infratemporal fossa, hypopharynx, or orbital involvement	Invades adjacent structure	—	Both anterior and posterior cranial nerves, paranasal sinuses, cavernous sinus, orbit, infratemporal fossa, C1 or C2
N1	Unilateral, ≤6 cm	Single ipsilateral ≤3-cm node	Upper neck above thyroid notch	Mobile nodes <4 cm above hyoid
N2	Bilateral, ≤6 cm	a: Single ipsilateral >3 cm, ≤6 cm b: Multiple ipsilateral nodes all ≤6 cm c: Bilateral or contralateral nodes all ≤6 cm	Below thyroid notch above line joining end of clavicle and superior margin of trapezius	Nodes below hyoid or 4-7 cm
N3	a: >6-cm node b: Supraclavicular involvement	>6-cm node	Supraclavicular or skin involvement	Supraclavicular, fixed, skin involvement, or >7 cm
M1	—	Metastases	Metastases	Metastases
Stage I	T1 N0 M0	T1 N0 M0	T1 N0	T1 N0 M0
Stage II	A: T2a N0 M0 B: T1 N1 M0 T2 N1 M0 T2a N1 M0 T2b N0 M0 T2b N1 M0	T2 N0 M0	T2 and/or N1	T2 N0-1 M0 or T1-2 N1 M0
Stage III	T1 N2 M0 T2a N2 M0 T2b N2 M0 T3 N0-2 M0	T3 N0 M0 T1-3 N1 M0	T3 and/or N2	T3 N0-2 M0 or T1-3 N2 M0
Stage IV	A: T4 N0-2 M0 B: Any T N3 M0 C: Any T any N M1	T4 N0-1 M0 Any T N2 M0 Any T N3 M0 Any T any N M1	N3 (any T)	A: T4 N0-3 M0 or T1-4 N3 M0 B: M1
Stage V	—	—	M1	—

*The SO (stylo-occipital) line extends from the styloid process to posterior edge of the occipital foramen.

challenging.[68] For these reasons, primary surgical intervention fell out of favor in the 1950s, and primary treatment has generally consisted of radiotherapy alone and, more recently, radiotherapy with chemotherapy.

Single-Modality Therapy

Although histologic presentations of nasopharyngeal tumors vary throughout the world, with more undifferentiated tumors found in southern China and Hong Kong, the 10-year survival rates for patients treated with radiation therapy alone in the United States (MDACC),[31] Denmark,[68] and Hong Kong[33] are similar—34%, 37%, and 43%, respectively (see Table 31-1). The rate from the Hong Kong study may be somewhat inflated because many patients had early-stage disease (39% node negative) and few patients with WHO type 1 histology (0.3%) were present in the series.[33] However, elevation of EBV titers has been correlated with a poor prognosis,[43] and higher titers would be expected in Hong Kong, an endemic area. The North American and European populations have a greater percentage of WHO type 1 than type 2 or 3 patients, however, and the prognosis for type 1 disease has been poorer than for type 2 or 3.[41] Therefore, comparison of groups from various parts of the world is difficult, and our understanding of the role of EBV and histologic classifications is incomplete. Still, some general statements can be made.

The MDACC series elucidated the long-term outcome in a large population of patients treated with radiotherapy alone.[31] Using the 1992 AJCC staging system (see Table 31-2), they found that advanced T stage, squamous histology, and cranial nerve deficits were predictive of poor prognosis for local control in univariate and multivariate analyses. Five-year local control rates for T1, T2, T3, and T4 stages were 93%, 79%, 68%, and 53%, respectively. These results illustrate the good tumor control that can be achieved with radiotherapy alone for early-stage lesions but demonstrate the need to explore multimodality options for more advanced lesions.

Altered Versus Standard Fractionation With or Without Chemotherapy

The use of altered fractionation regimens has been explored in several trials during the past few years. The U.S. Intergroup study 0099[1] used once-daily radiation treatments with or without chemotherapy. Some groups have begun to treat patients with nasopharyngeal cancer on twice-daily regimens, which have led to local control improvements in other sites such as the oropharynx.[69]

Only one randomized trial addressing the role of twice-daily versus once-daily irradiation for head and neck cancer has included tumors of the nasopharynx.[70] Sanchiz and colleagues'[70] large trial included 892 patients (852 evaluable patients) with advanced head and neck cancers (T3-4 N0-3 M0 by UICC staging). The patients were randomly assigned to once-daily irradiation (group A), twice-daily irradiation (group B), and once-daily irradiation with 5-fluorouracil (5-FU) (group C). The trial included 92 patients with nasopharyngeal cancer. No differences were seen in median duration of response or overall survival between groups B and C; however, when either group B or C was compared individually with group A, there were significant improvements in both measures. Further work will be necessary to determine the role of twice-daily irradiation and the role of chemotherapy in patients with nasopharyngeal carcinoma and the role of chemotherapy in the context of altered fractionation irradiation. The complications associated with these treatments will become better defined as these studies mature.

Combined-Modality Therapy: Irradiation Plus Chemotherapy

The randomized trial of Sanchiz and associates[70] serves as an introduction for using chemotherapy in nasopharyngeal cancer, although only a small number of patients with nasopharyngeal cancer were included. As mentioned, the optimal method of delivering fractionated irradiation, either once or twice daily, with chemotherapy is unknown.

Brizel et al[71] reported a small randomized trial comparing twice-daily irradiation (1.25 to 75 Gy) to twice-daily irradiation (1.25 to 70 Gy) with concurrent cisplatin and 5-FU treatment. This trial included 121 patients with locally advanced (T3 and T4) squamous cell carcinoma of all head and neck sites (including some nasopharyngeal carcinomas). With a median follow-up of 41 months, locoregional control at 3 years was 70% for the combined-modality arm versus 44% for irradiation alone ($p = .01$). The actuarial survival at 3 years was 55% for the combined-modality arm versus 34% for irradiation alone ($p = .07$). Mucositis appeared to be more prevalent in the combined-modality arm; 45% of patients required feeding tubes compared with 28% in the irradiation-alone arm. However, the severe late complications of soft-tissue necrosis or osteoradionecrosis were uncommon and similar in both arms—three patients in the irradiation group and five in the combined-modality group. Further follow-up will be of interest with regard to late complications.

Several groups have conducted phase III trials specific to nasopharyngeal primary tumors (instead of a wide array of head and neck cancers) that compared chemotherapy plus irradiation versus irradiation alone[1,61,72-78] (Table 31-3). Several well-performed retrospective series have addressed this question (see Table 31-3). The studies listed in Table 31-3 are separated based on whether chemotherapy was sequential or concurrent with radiotherapy.

The Intergroup study 0099 showed a dramatic improvement in survival with combined-modality treatment.[1] The trial was closed at a planned interim analysis (October 1995) after review of the preliminary results by the Data Safety and Monitoring Committee for the Southwest Oncology Group, and the results are shown in Table 31-3. Patients treated with standard irradiation received 70 Gy to gross disease in daily fractions of 1.8 to 2.0 Gy. Patients enrolled in the combined-modality arm received 100 mg/m^2 of cisplatin on days 1, 22, and 43 of irradiation and cisplatin (80 mg/m^2) and 5-FU (1000 mg/m^2) on days 1 to 4 every 3 weeks for three courses after irradiation. The marked statistically significant improvement in both disease-free and overall survival ($p = .001$) in the combined-modality arm is in contrast to several other randomized trials documented in Table 31-3. However, the other trials typically used neoadjuvant chemotherapy before irradiation in the combined-modality treatments, whereas the Intergroup study used initial concomitant cisplatin and irradiation in the combined-modality arm followed by maintenance 5-FU and cisplatin. This is the same strategy that has resulted in positive disease control and survival results for many gastrointestinal malignancies (e.g., rectal, gastric, and esophageal).

The International Nasopharynx Cancer Study Group trial (sequential chemotherapy) showed a statistically significant improvement ($p < .01$) in disease-free survival but not overall survival for patients receiving the combined-modality treatment.[72] Treatment-related deaths, possibly related to

Table 31-3 Major Chemotherapy/Radiotherapy Randomized Trials

Study (No. of Patients)	Stage	Randomization	Disease-Free Survival, 2 y	*p* Value	Overall Survival, 2 y	*p* Value
Sequential chemoradiation						
International Nasopharynx Cancer Study Group[72] (*N* = 339)	Any TN ≥ 2M0 by UICC, 1987	• 70 Gy/7 wk • Bleomycin/epirubicin/cisplatin ×3 (d 1, 21, and 42), followed by 70 Gy/7 wk	40% 54%	<.01	60% 63%	NS
Chan et al[73] (*N* = 82)	Ho system[60] stage N3 or any nodes ≥4 cm	• Irradiation alone • Cisplatin/5-FU ×2, followed by irradiation, followed by cisplatin/5-FU ×4	72% 68%	NS	81% 80%	NS
Asian-Oceanic Clinical Oncology Association Nasopharynx Cancer Study Group[74] (*N* = 334)	Ho system[60] stage T3 or N2-3 or any nodes ≥3 cm	• 70 Gy/7 wk • Epirubicin/cisplatin ×3 (d 1, 21, and 42), followed by 70 Gy/7 wk	42% (3 y) 48% (3 y)	NS	71% (3 y) 78% (3 y)	NS
Ma et al[61] (*N* = 449)	Ma et al[61] stage III or IV	• 68-72 Gy/7-8 wk • Cisplatin/bleomycin/5 followed by 68-72 Gy 7-8 wk	49% (5 y) 59% (5 y)	.05	56% (5 y) 63% (5 y)	.11
Concurrent chemoradiation						
Intergroup study 0099[1] (*N* = 150)	AJCC 1992 stage III: T3N0; T1-3N1M0 AJCC 1992 stage IV: T4N0-1; any TN2-3M0	• 70 Gy/7-8 wk • 70 Gy/7-8 wk with cisplatin, followed by 3 cycles of cisplatin/5-FU	24% (3 y) 69% (3 y)	<.001	47% (3 y) 78% (3 y)	.005
Wee et al[75] (*N* = 220)	AJCC 1997 stage III or IV; WHO type 2 or 3	• 70 Gy/7 wk • 70 Gy/7 wk with cisplatin, followed by 3 cycles of cisplatin/5-FU	62% 76%	NS	77% 85%	.02
Chan et al[76,77] (*N* = 350)	Ho system[60] stage N2-3 or any nodes ≥4 cm	• 70 Gy/7 wk • 70 Gy/7 wk with cisplatin	52% (5 y) 62% (5 y)	NS	59% (5 y) 72% (5 y)	.05
Lee et al[78] (*N* = 348)	AJCC T1-4N2-3M0; WHO type 2 or 3	• >66 Gy/7-8 wk • >66 Gy/7-8 wk with cisplatin, followed by 3 cycles of cisplatin/5-FU	61% 69%	.24	79% 78%	.76
Nonrandomized matched-pair study						
Geara et al[79] (*N* = 122)	Stage IV (97%) Stage III (3%)	• Irradiation alone • Cisplatin/5-FU ×3, followed by irradiation	42% (5 y) 64% (5 y)	.02	48% (5 y) 69% (5 y)	.01

AJCC, American Joint Committee on Cancer; 5-FU, 5-fluorouracil; NS, not stated; UICC, Uniform International Committee on Cancer; WHO, World Health Organization.

bleomycin, eliminated any overall survival advantage that may have otherwise been seen. A similar trial by the Asian-Oceanic Clinical Oncology Association,[74,80] with the omission of bleomycin but retaining the sequential design, compared irradiation alone with combined treatment with three cycles of epirubicin and cisplatin followed by irradiation. The results showed no benefit with the addition of neoadjuvant chemotherapy.[74,80] The effect of histologic differences between the Intergroup 0099 trial and the other trials is not easily determined because of geographic differences and differences in reporting.

Several trials from endemic regions with negative results of chemoradiation suggest the possibility of a differing biology in undifferentiated tumors. However, study design of the trials has varied, with neoadjuvant chemotherapy historically being used in the international trials[61,72-74] versus concurrent chemoradiation in the Intergroup study 0099.

The results of the Intergroup 0099 trial were confirmed for endemic disease, supporting the benefit of concurrent chemoradiation for WHO type 2 and 3 disease. The preliminary results of this trial, conducted by the National Cancer Center of Singapore, showed a promising survival advantage (p = .02) and a decrease in distant metastases (p = .03), with slightly improved disease-free survival (p = .1).[75] A randomized trial from Hong Kong of concurrent weekly cisplatin chemotherapy, without adjuvant or neoadjuvant therapy, versus irradiation alone also showed an improvement in overall survival for endemic cases.[76,77] However, the preliminary results of a similar endemic trial by the Hong Kong Nasopharyngeal Study Group, comparing radiotherapy alone with the Intergroup 0099 combined-modality regimen, show only a local control benefit to the combination regimen.[78] Further follow-up may clarify the issue.

Many additional trials have been performed exploring combination chemotherapy and radiotherapy for nasopharyngeal carcinoma. A meta-analysis combined the results of 78 randomized trials, the results of which support an improvement in overall survival and disease-free survival with concurrent chemoradiation, without clear evidence of a positive role for adjuvant or neoadjuvant chemotherapy.[81]

LOCALLY RECURRENT OR PERSISTENT DISEASE

Surgical Management

Surgical resection is the preferred treatment for persistent or recurrent lymph node involvement in the neck. However, surgical management of recurrent nasopharyngeal cancer at the primary site is hampered by the same factors that make surgery at this site difficult as a primary treatment, such as difficulties in obtaining adequate exposure and obtaining adequate surgical margins.[68,82-84] If surgery is attempted, several different approaches—transpalatal, transmaxillary, or transmandibular—may be used to gain access to the nasopharynx.

The technical aspects of these surgical approaches are described in detail in a study by Hsu and associates,[82] in which 24 patients had surgical resection of recurrent nasopharyngeal carcinoma (after one to three courses of irradiation to doses of 60 to 190 Gy). For this group of patients, the median survival had not been reached at the median follow-up of 18 months. Of these 24 patients, 14 were alive at the time of the report, with survival times of 8 to 50 months after surgery. Of these 14 patients, 11 were without evidence of recurrence. The recurrent lesions were staged by the AJCC staging system, and the authors made their assessments of the best approach for various lesions as shown in Table 31-4. The transmandibular approach was useful for cases in which surgical resection of an ipsilateral cervical relapse was also planned. Resection of parapharyngeal involvement of the anteromedial area of the internal carotid also could be accomplished through a transmandibular approach, but involvement of the lateral pterygoid muscle was a contraindication to surgery. Generally, surgical approaches to the treatment of recurrent nasopharyngeal carcinoma are controversial, and the literature contains only scattered anecdotal information. However, surgical resection may offer a reasonable disease-free period in certain well-selected cases without cranial nerve involvement.

Reirradiation

The retreatment of nasopharyngeal carcinoma with irradiation after prior irradiation is well documented and has been summarized by Cmelak et al[85] and others[2,82,86-94] (Table 31-5). Wang[2] reported on 51 previously irradiated patients treated for recurrent disease at Massachusetts General Hospital. The actuarial

Table 31-4 Surgical Approaches to Recurrent Nasopharyngeal Carcinoma as Proposed by Hsu and Colleagues[82]

Retreatment Stage	Subsite	Approach	Morbidity	Results
T1	Posterosuperior	Transpalatal	Minimal	Excellent
	Lateral	Transmaxillary	Moderate	Excellent
T2	>1 Subsite	Transmaxillary	Moderate	Good
T3	Nasoethmoid	Transmaxillary	Moderate	Good
	Oropharynx	Transmandibular	Moderate to severe	Fair
	Parapharynx	Transmandibular	Moderate to severe	Fair
T4	Skull base	Transmaxillary	Moderate	Palliative
	Cranial nerve	No indication		

Table 31-5 Results of Reirradiation for Locally Recurrent Nasopharyngeal Carcinoma

Study	No. of Patients	Dose, Gy	Local Control, No. (%)	5-y Survival, %	Major Complications, %
Fu et al (1975)[86]	42	12-63	5 (12)	41	9
Hoppe et al (1976)[87]	13	42-60	3 (23)	13	NR
McNeese and Fletcher (1981)[88]	30	40-65	10 (33)	2	NR
Yan et al (1983)[89]	162	30-70	23 (14)	18	29
Wang (1987)[2]	13	<60	NR	0	8
	48	≥60	—	45	—
Chen et al (1989)[90]	61	40-81	NR	14.8	NR
Lee et al (1993)[91]	706	57	209 (30)	NR	24

NR, not reported.

5-year survival for the 38 patients who received 60 Gy or greater (combination of external beam and implant) was 45% compared with 0% for the 13 patients who received less than 60 Gy. Also, reirradiation was more effective in patients who had a prolonged disease-free interval before the recurrence. The actuarial 5-year survival for patients with a disease-free interval greater than 24 months after initial treatment was 66% and only 13% for patients with a disease-free interval of less than 24 months. The report noted that "a few patients experienced minimal sloughing of the irradiated nasopharynx with fetid odor."[2] One patient had complete loss of the sphenoid sinus base with reepithelialization. Multiple cranial nerve palsies developed in 1 patient who survived for more than 20 years after reirradiation, and trismus and fibrosis of the soft palate developed in another patient. In the Massachusetts General Hospital experience, 60 Gy was generally delivered as an initial 40 Gy in 20 fractions through small external beam fields, followed by 20 Gy in 2 applications of 10 Gy by intracavitary cesium (Fig. 31-2).[82] Other brachytherapy applicators, similar in many ways to this cesium applicator, have allowed for the use of multiple iridium line sources.

Radiosurgery has been used to treat recurrent nasopharyngeal lesions after prior irradiation.[85,95,96] A Stanford University group reported on the use of radiosurgery in 12 patients with locally recurrent nasopharyngeal cancer.[85] All of the lesions had volumes less than or equal to 55 cm^3. The 12 patients with recurrent nasopharyngeal carcinoma had previously received primary radiotherapy consisting of 58.2 to 79.2 Gy, delivered at times ranging from 6 to 96 months before the recurrence. The patients received radiosurgery doses of 15 to 20 Gy (median, 18 Gy), and 7 of the 12 had local control at a median follow-up of 17 months. The dose to the optic nerve, optic chiasm, brainstem, and cavernous sinus was less than 8 Gy if the recurrence did not directly involve these structures. One patient had facial nerve palsy. Results from this series are consistent with others, and local control for recurrent disease treated in this manner is approximately 50% at 2 years.[85,95,96]

Radiosurgical treatment of these recurrent lesions is a promising approach because the technique allows for rapid fall-off of the radiation dose outside of the tumor volume and near critical structures that surround this anatomical area. Radiosurgery has also been explored as a component of primary treatment for nasopharyngeal cancer.[97]

Intensity-modulated radiotherapy (IMRT) is also well suited to this task. Preliminary reirradiation results with this method are promising.[98]

Combination chemotherapy and radiotherapy is being used increasingly for treatment of recurrent disease after primary radiotherapy.[99-102] In general, the late morbidity of these regimens is less severe than would be expected, given that reirradiation doses are comparable to the original radiotherapy doses.[101,102] Multiple chemoradiotherapy regimens have been explored, often incorporating hyperfractionation and, in some cases, split-course therapy. Chemotherapy agents commonly used include cisplatin, 5-FU, and hydroxyurea, and acute toxicity can be substantial. In general, these reirradiation trials have included few nasopharyngeal cases. Historically, reirradiation without chemotherapy, possibly including brachytherapy, has given better results for nasopharyngeal cases than for other sites.[99] However, it is reasonable to extrapolate the results of combination

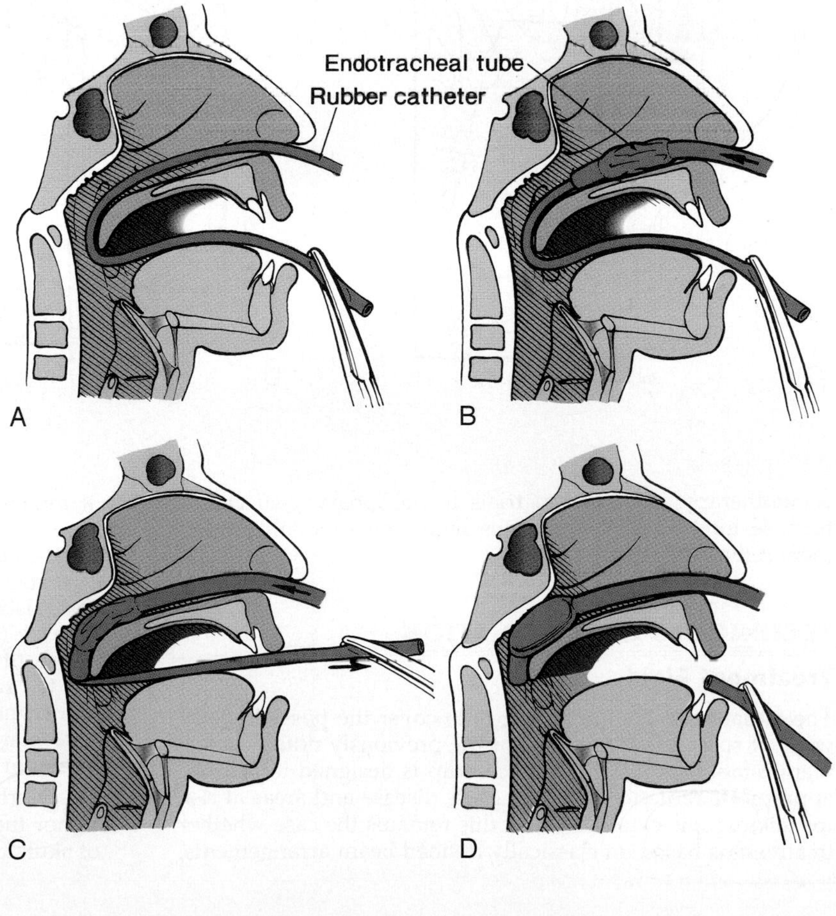

Figure 31-2 Use of brachytherapy to treat the nasopharynx. Two pediatric endotracheal tubes are placed in the nasopharynx (often guided into place by a rubber catheter) by using a source carrier. Dummy sources are initially placed such that they are at the free edge of the soft palate and uvula posteriorly and behind the posterior wall of the maxillary sinus anteriorly. The treatment is then prescribed to the 0.5-cm point below the vault mucosa at midline. (Adapted from Wang CC: Radiation Therapy for Head and Neck Neoplasms: Indications, Techniques, and Results, 2nd ed. Chicago, Year Book, 1990, p 274).

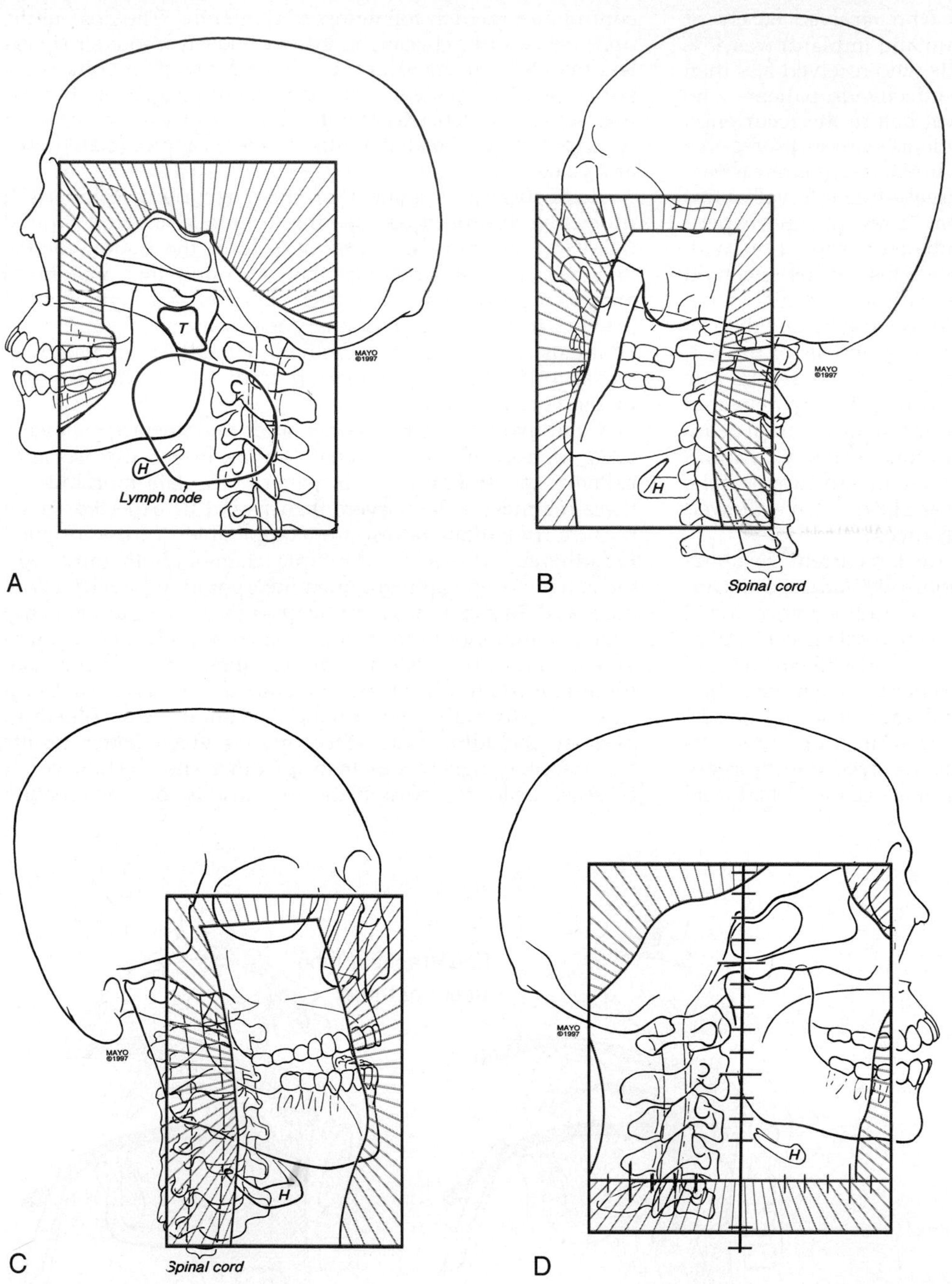

Figure 31-3 **A–C,** Pituitary shielding technique to treat a T2 nasopharyngeal cancer. The initial fields were opposed lateral fields **(A),** followed by oblique fields **(B** and **C),** with an electron field (not shown) to treat the contralateral neck. **D,** The base of the skull is included in the treatment of a T3 nasopharyngeal cancer. H, hyoid bone; T, primary tumor. (**A–D,** Courtesy of the Mayo Foundation, Rochester, MN.)

chemotherapy reirradiation trials to nasopharyngeal cancer because long-term salvage rates with single-modality treatment remain relatively low.

TECHNIQUES OF IRRADIATION

Treatment Fields

The radiation fields are arranged to cover the possible pathways of spread that account for the previously noted clinical manifestations (Fig. 31-3). Field setup is designed to provide appropriate radiation doses to gross disease and areas at risk for microscopic extension, and this remains the case whether treatment is based on classically defined beam arrangements, or if modern techniques such as intensity modulation and inverse planning are used. The Intergroup study 0099 (see Table 31-3) provides a structure for general irradiation guidelines that can be modified on the basis of individual tumor characteristics.[1] This trial included patients with stage III and IV disease (there was a downward stage migration starting with the fifth edition of the *AJCC Staging Manual*). In this study, the radiation field arrangements for treatment of the nasopharynx and upper neck have called for treatment with opposed lateral fields and have been designated as follows (with minor modifications):

1. Superiorly: the field margin should be at least 2 cm beyond tumor that is visible on the head CT and include the base of skull and sphenoid sinus.

2. Posteriorly: the field should allow 2 cm of margin beyond the mastoid process. The posterior margin may extend further to allow at least a 1.5-cm margin on enlarged nodes.
3. Anteriorly: the field should include the posterior third of the maxillary sinus and nasal cavity. This anterior border can be modified to accommodate adequate margin (2 cm) for tumors with anterior extension.
4. Inferiorly: the lower field margin is at the thyroid notch to allow sparing of the larynx by a central block on the anterior lower neck field which is matched to these lateral fields.

The lower neck is generally treated with an anterior field with a central larynx block that extends inferiorly to the cricoid. This lower neck field is matched to the lower edge of the lateral fields and, thus, the larynx block also prevents the spinal cord from receiving an excessive dose due to possible overlap of the lateral fields and anterior field. The lower neck field should extend inferiorly to the level of the lower border of the clavicle at the sternoclavicular joint. If the neck disease dictates that opposed anterior-to-posterior (AP-PA) fields are required for the lower neck treatment, it is sometimes convenient to set the isocenter at the level of the match between the upper lateral fields and the lower AP-PA fields. Thus, the lower portion of the field can be blocked (beam-splitting technique) while treatment is given to the upper lateral fields; similarly, the upper half of the field can be blocked during the treatment of the lower AP-PA fields. The point of beam splitting can be feathered (moved superiorly or inferiorly .5 to 1.0 cm) every 10 to 15 Gy, to decrease the potential consequences of unintentional field overlap. Feathering is important if the distribution of disease precludes the use of a larynx block or other means of safeguarding the spinal cord from unintentional field overlap. Boosting gross disease in the lower neck may require oblique fields to cover the target volumes and respect spinal cord tolerance.

Radiotherapy Dose

With the Intergroup study 0099 as a general guideline for doses,[68] the primary head and neck fields should be treated at a dose of 40 Gy (1.8 to 2.0 Gy/d) before the placement of spinal cord block (see Fig. 31-3). The treatment then proceeds to 50 Gy, with the newly blocked posterior neck portion of the field treated with electron fields. Electron energies should be determined by CT simulation and treatment planning to allow adequate treatment of the posterior neck with minimal dose to the spinal cord. After 50 Gy, the fields are reduced to include a margin of 1.5 to 2.0 cm around the primary and any enlarged lymph nodes (>1 cm on CT of the neck). This reduced field arrangement is treated to a dose of 66 Gy; consideration can be given for a second reduction around gross disease to a final dose of 70 Gy.

Possible Field Modifications

The above borders for radiation treatment serve as a general guideline for patients with nasopharynx cancer (see Fig. 31-3). The general guidelines must be modified for each patient, taking into account the distribution of disease and structures at risk for radiation morbidity.

For example, there has been considerable debate about the practice of treating the entire base of skull with margin (to a dose that would potentially eradicate microscopic disease) in all patients, because this would require treatment of the pituitary to a dose of 45 to 50 Gy in all patients. Sham and others[103] studied a group of 152 patients with no evidence of erosion of the base of skull or sphenoid and no extension of disease to the nasal fossa and ethmoid sinuses (generally AJCC T1 and T2 lesions). These patients were randomly assigned to receive "standard therapy," including margin on the base of skull and inclusion of the pituitary, or to a modified technique that shielded the pituitary and the anterior part of the hypothalamus. At a median follow-up of 31.5 months, tumor control was not different between the two groups. However, symptomatic neuroendocrine complications occurred in 8 of 71 patients in the standard-field group, versus 0 of 81 in the modified-field group. Of the eight patients with neuroendocrine complications, two had secondary hypothyroidism, one had oligomenorrhea with increased prolactin levels, and five had temporal lobe necrosis.

The techniques used by Sham and associates[103] are worth noting. Approximately 25% of patients were treated with a three-field technique comprised of two lateral wedged fields and an anterior field that delivered 3.5 Gy 3 times per week to 59.5 Gy. In patients who did not have a pituitary shield, a substantial portion of the inferior temporal lobes received 80% to 100% of this dose. For patients with a pituitary shield, the pituitary received 30% of this dose, and most of the inferior temporal lobes were excluded from the fields. The other patients (approximately 75%) were treated with opposed lateral fields that delivered 2.5 Gy 4 times a week to a total dose of 40 Gy, followed by a boost of 21 Gy in six fractions, using the above-noted three-field technique. Again, in patients without pituitary shielding, the pituitary received the full dose, and pituitary shielding reduced the dose to 10%. The temporal lobes also received a higher total dose at a higher dose per fraction in patients without a pituitary shield, in comparison with shielded patients.

A follow-up editorial to the article by Sham and colleagues[103] called for even greater use of the pituitary shield.[104] Cheng and others[104] reported a series of 24 patients with T1 to T3 tumors in which pituitary shielding was used in 21 patients. The tumors were treated with opposed lateral fields, generally to a dose of 72 Gy in 36 fractions. After a median follow-up of 26 months, primary tumor control for the 24 patients was 100%, including the 21 who had the pituitary shielded. These data support excluding the pituitary from the initial fields for early-stage lesions (T1 and T2 lesions); however, further work will be necessary to determine which advanced lesions can undergo treatment with pituitary shielding.

Radiotherapy Boost Techniques and Normal Tissue Tolerance

Various techniques have been used to treat the final target volume to full dose. The MDACC group analyzed various techniques with respect to treatment-related complications (Tables 31-1 and 31-6).[31] In their experience, patients were generally treated with opposed lateral fields, including the primary site and upper neck (lower neck treated with an anterior field), to a dose of 45 Gy. Subsequently, the primary site was treated with one of three techniques: oblique fields, opposed lateral fields (generally high-energy beams), or a single central field. The single central field technique was used more frequently during the first and second of three time periods: 1954-1971, 1972-1982, and 1983-1992. During the latest time period, opposed lateral fields were used almost exclusively. The use of three-dimensional (3D) conformal techniques to optimize the final boost portion of treatment has not been shown to lead to a decrease in complications.[105,106]

The incidence and types of complications of irradiation for nasopharyngeal cancer at MDACC between 1954 and 1992 are listed in Table 31-6. The actuarial frequency of grade 3 to 5

Table 31-6 Serious Complications of Radiotherapy Alone for Nasopharyngeal Carcinoma in 378 Patients

Complication	RTOG Grade 3	4	5	Total
Connective tissues				
Skin/mucosal ulcers	—	3	1	4
Fibrosis	13	3	—	16
Trismus	11	—	—	11
Bone	3	7	—	10
Larynx	1	1	—	2
Endocrine				
Pituitary	9	13	—	22
Thyroid	3	7	—	10
Nervous system				
Brain	2	2	—	4
Cranial nerve	3	8	6	17
Spinal cord	2	2	5	9
Hearing loss	10	—	—	10
Total	57	46	12	115

RTOG, Radiation Therapy Oncology Group.
From Sanguineti G, Geara FB, Garden AS, et al: Carcinoma of the nasopharynx treated by radiotherapy alone: determinants of local and regional control. Int J Radiat Oncol Biol Phys 37:985-996, 1997.

complications was 16%, 19%, and 29% at 5, 10, and 20 years, respectively. However, the actuarial frequency of grade 3 to 5 complications at 10 years decreased steadily over the above-noted three consecutive time periods: 14%, 10%, and 5%, respectively. Of nine severe spinal cord injuries, eight occurred in the early time period (1954-1971). In univariate analysis, the frequency of moderate to severe complications was dependent on treatment technique. The actuarial incidence of moderate to severe complications at 10 years was 58% for the single central field technique compared with 12% and 25% for oblique fields and opposed lateral fields, respectively ($p < .001$). It should be noted that patients treated with oblique and opposed lateral fields were treated in more recent periods, and the decreased frequency of complications may also be related to the use of custom blocking and CT treatment planning. However, use of oblique and opposed lateral fields is generally accepted and has been shown to have acceptable tolerance.

Other investigators have reported the frequency of complications attributed to radiation treatment (see Table 31-1), but these retrospective reviews have usually reported complication rates in general terms. The use of conformal techniques for the final boost portion of radiotherapy could potentially decrease the risk of complications, but this has not been shown to be the case. Conformal techniques are associated with a 25% incidence of grade 3 to 4 morbidity, including hearing loss, trismus, dysphagia, chronic sinusitis, and cranial neuropathy.[105] This result has led to an interest in delivering the full course of therapy with intensity modulation.[105-108]

When treating lesions with base of skull involvement, it is important to consider the potential for optic neuropathy. A University of Florida review of 106 patients receiving treatment encompassing the optic nerves reported no optic nerve damage at doses less than 59 Gy.[109] However, for nerves that received more than 60 Gy, daily fractionation regimens appeared to affect the frequency of optic nerve damage. Specifically, patients who received more than 60 Gy and daily fractions of more than 1.9 Gy had a 47% incidence of optic nerve injury, compared with 11% for patients treated with daily fractions of less than 1.9 Gy. It is important to be aware of these data when counseling patients about the potential for these injuries.

Intensity Modulation

In the 1970s and 1980s, it was becoming clear that advancing technology would make it possible to optimize radiotherapy by deriving the set of optimal incident stationary and moving beams from a desired dose distribution.[110,111] These techniques deliver a set of beamlets of varying weights, with the weights chosen to optimally conform the resulting distribution of dose to a target.[112,113] More generally, the optimization can be performed to optimize biological or physical objective functions, based on minimizing complications and maximizing tumor-control probabilities.[114] The technique of optimizing beam delivery with inverse planning has become known as IMRT for historical reasons, although typically beam intensity is not modulated.

Target movement places a potential limitation on the applicability of IMRT. Movement during beam delivery could lead to the unintentional overlap of beamlets, or possibly lead to untreated portions of target volume. For this reason, IMRT is currently used in situations where motion is minimal or can be controlled for with gating techniques. The head and neck is an area where target motion can be controlled reasonably well with immobilization devices, and for this reason much of the early work on IMRT centered on head and neck cancer. IMRT is particularly applicable to the nasopharynx, in that several critical structures are in close proximity to the target, and because the incidence of morbidity with conventional radiotherapy techniques is high.

Several institutions have shown a potential dosimetric improvement for IMRT over conventional techniques and 3D conformal techniques in the setting of nasopharyngeal cancer.[106,115-118] Several single-institution series have shown the efficacy of IMRT for head and neck cancer in general[119] and for the nasopharynx in particular,[107] and a phase II trial has been initiated through the Radiation Therapy Oncology Group (RTOG). Preservation of salivary function by sparing at least 1 parotid gland has been a primary objective of head and neck IMRT,[120] and objective measurement of salivary output is incorporated into the current phase II RTOG nasopharynx IMRT trial (RTOG 0225).

The ability to tailor dose to a desired distribution allows the simultaneous delivery of different fractionation schemes to different portions of the target. The primary target can be hypofractionated and conventional fractionation can be delivered to subclinical neck disease,[121] or conventional fractionation can be applied to the target while delivering doses of less than 1.8 Gy to the secondary targets.[119,122] The RTOG 0225 trial uses a conservative integration of the boost, with 2.12 Gy is delivered to the planning target volume (PTV) while 1.8 Gy is delivered to the subclinical PTV, both over 33 fractions. The PTV receives a total dose of 70 Gy, and 59.4 Gy is delivered to the retropharyngeal lymph nodes, neck levels I through V, the clivus, skull base, pterygoid fossae, parapharyngeal space, inferior sphenoid sinus, and the posterior nasal cavity and maxillary sinuses. A total dose of 50.4 Gy is delivered to the supraclavicular nodes. This regimen is based on promising single-institution experience from University of California, San Francisco, reporting on 67 patients with nasopharyngeal cancer treated with IMRT.[107] The 4-year actuarial local control was 97% and locoregional control was 98%, with median follow-up of 31 months. Long-term xerostomia was minimal at 2 years, with 66% of the patients having no xerostomia (grade 0), and no grade 2 or higher late xerostomia. Failures that did occur tended to arise in areas that were recognized as high risk and treated appropriately, rather than from marginal misses near the parotid gland or other structures intentionally spared.[119,123] PET and other functional imaging techniques have the potential to improve selection of appropriate therapy and improve technical delivery of radiotherapy.[56]

Figure 31-4 illustrates a dosimetric comparison of IMRT and the conventional technique for a sample patient treated in the RTOG 0225 trial. The conventional ports used for the comparison are shown in Figure 31-5. Considerable sparing of normal tissue, in particular the parotid glands, is achieved with IMRT, and there is better coverage of the base of skull than can be achieved with lateral fields. Figure 31-6 shows the dose volume histograms for this case, again comparing conventional technique with IMRT. Seven coplanar nonopposed fields were used with a 0.5-cm multileaf collimator using sliding window technique, optimized with a gradient inverse planning engine. In principle, the same results achieved with IMRT can be achieved with 3D conformal technique, the only fundamental difference being that IMRT is inverse planned (optimized). However, in practice, the time required to obtain equivalent results with forward-planned 3D conformal technique is prohibitive to the point that, in a practical sense, the two methods are very different. Figure 31-7 illustrates the dosimetry of a reirradiation case, a situation in which the critical need to spare normal structures makes IMRT techniques essential.

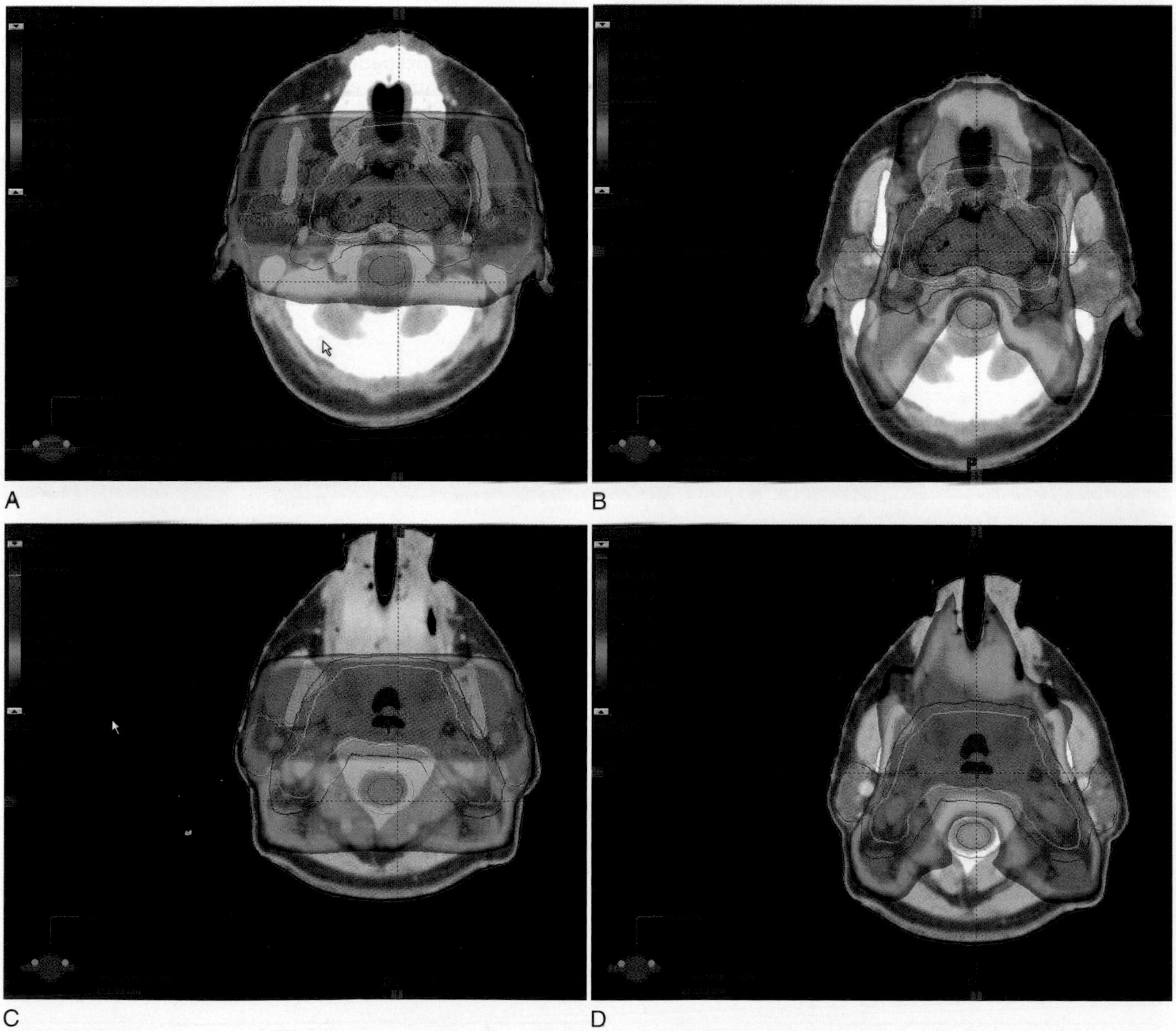

Figure 31-4 Dose-colorwash comparison of coverage on a representative patient with T2b N0 M0 nasopharyngeal cancer treated in the RTOG 0225 intensity-modulated radiation therapy (IMRT) trial. (For comparison, Figure 31-5 illustrates the conventional lateral ports used.) Computed tomography cuts are shown at the level of the pterygoid plates for the conventional technique **(A)** and for IMRT **(B)**. The level of the uvula is shown for conventional radiotherapy **(C)** and IMRT **(D)**. The conventional plan is a composite of comprehensive head and neck fields with a boost to the primary lesion. Sparing of the parotid glands is the primary benefit of IMRT in this case. For the IMRT plan, 7 coplanar, nonopposed fields were used with a 0.5-cm multileaf collimator using a sliding-window technique, optimized with a gradient inverse planning algorithm.

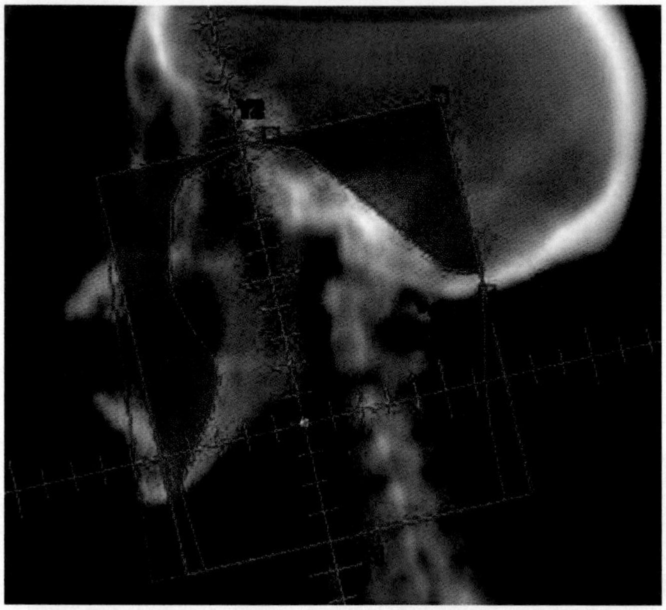

Figure 31-5 Digitally reconstructed radiograph of the conventional ports used in the comparison of IMRT, with conventional therapy illustrated (see Figs. 31-4 and 31-6). The posterior neck was blocked and treated with electrons at 40 Gy, and the boost treated the primary tumor with margins using 15-MV photons.

TREATMENT ALGORITHM, CONCLUSIONS, AND FUTURE POSSIBILITIES

A preferred diagnostic and treatment algorithm for patients with nasopharyngeal carcinoma is illustrated in Figure 31-8. With early-stage disease, irradiation alone with once-daily fractionation generally yields excellent local control results. For locally advanced disease (nonmetastatic stage IIb, III, or IV in the current AJCC staging system), concomitant chemotherapy and radiotherapy results are encouraging, and entry of patients into further trials testing combined-modality treatment is indicated. Once-daily versus twice-daily fractionation is also being evaluated with these patients. The advancement in radiotherapy optimization and the integration of functional imaging with radiotherapy planning promise improvement in both tumor control and decreased morbidity of treatment.

Several investigators have reported novel methods of delivering chemotherapy or chemotherapy and radiation combinations for patients with nasopharyngeal carcinoma (Table 31-7). Further exploration of novel combinations of chemotherapy and radiation are warranted.[79,124-128]

ACKNOWLEDGMENT

We thank Kim Dempsey for assistance in preparing this chapter.

Table 31-7 Alternative Chemotherapy Regimens for Nasopharyngeal Carcinoma

Study	Patients	Regimen	Results
Cooper et al[124]	Technically respectable but advanced laryngeal, base of tongue, piriform sinus, or nasopharyngeal carcinoma ($N = 65$)	Cisplatin 20 mg/m²/d, 5-FU 800 mg/m²/d, leucovorin 500 mg/m²/d; continuous infusion for 96 h on days 1 and 28, followed by irradiation on day 56 with concomitant cisplatin (100 mg/m²)	Median follow-up, 21.1 mo 85% with grade 3/4 mucositis 1 death on treatment Seven of 9 nasopharyngeal CA cases free of disease
Chi et al[125]	Nasopharyngeal CA; 12 metastatic or recurrent, 14 locally advanced	Paclitaxel 175 mg/m²/3 h every 3 wk × 2	Response rate, 33% Mild peripheral neurotoxicity, 19%
Siu et al[126]	21 patients with locally advanced nasopharyngeal CA, 18 recurrent cases; 51 metastatic cases	Cyclophosphamide, doxorubicin, cisplatin, methotrexate, and bleomycin; variable number of cycles; subsequent radiotherapy	86% PR or CR (1 patient) to chemotherapy among locally advanced cases 40% PR, recurrent cases Frequent mucositis and myelosuppression
Ma et al[127]	32 patients; 29 were WHO type 2, most had received prior chemotherapy	18 treated with gemcitabine, 14 with gemcitabine and cisplatin; regimen repeated every 28 days	34% response to gemcitabine 64% response to gemcitabine and cisplatin 48% 1-y survival Myelosuppression was dose limiting

CA, carcinoma; CR, complete response; 5-FU, 5-fluorouracil; PR, partial response; WHO, World Health Organization.

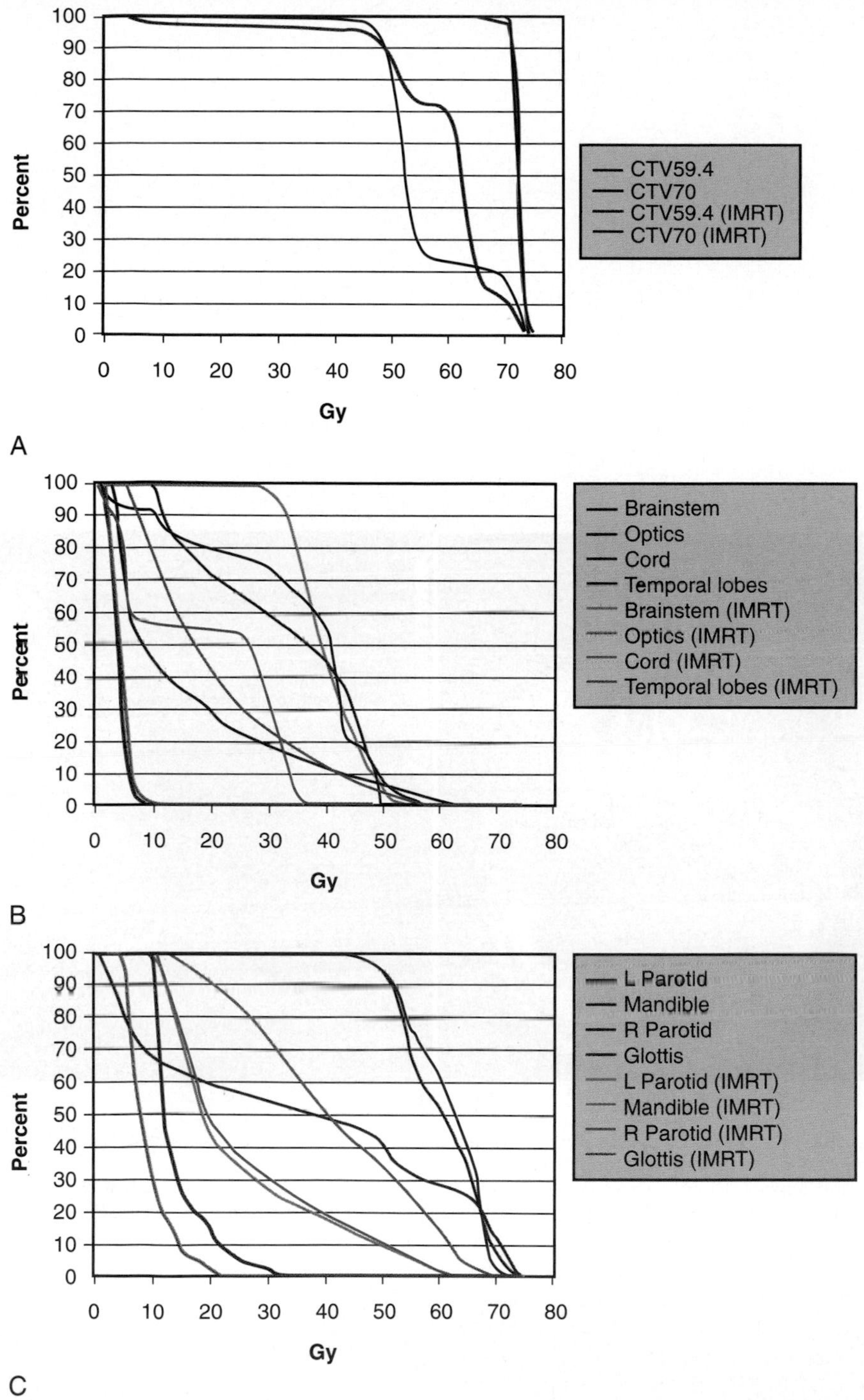

Figure 31-6 Dose-volume histograms (DVHs) for the patient in Figures 31-4 and 31-5, comparing intensity modulated radiation therapy (IMRT) with the conventional technique. Substantial gains can be made with IMRT in terms of target coverage and sparing of normal tissue. **A,** Target coverage. Differences in the CTV59.4 (clinical target volume to be covered by 59.4 Gy) target coverage reflect the relatively high dose given to subclinical risk areas in the RTOG 0225 trial, with much of this target volume intentionally prescribed a dose of 50.4 Gy in the conventional plan. A conventional anterior low-neck field was used in the IMRT plan, with a midline block over the spinal cord and larynx in that region that blocked a portion of the CTV59.4, a portion that was not included in the optimization but that was included in the DVH. The DVH for central nervous system (CNS) structures **(B)** and other normal structures **(C)** are also shown. Greater relative sparing of CNS structures by IMRT was seen for patients with higher-stage tumors.

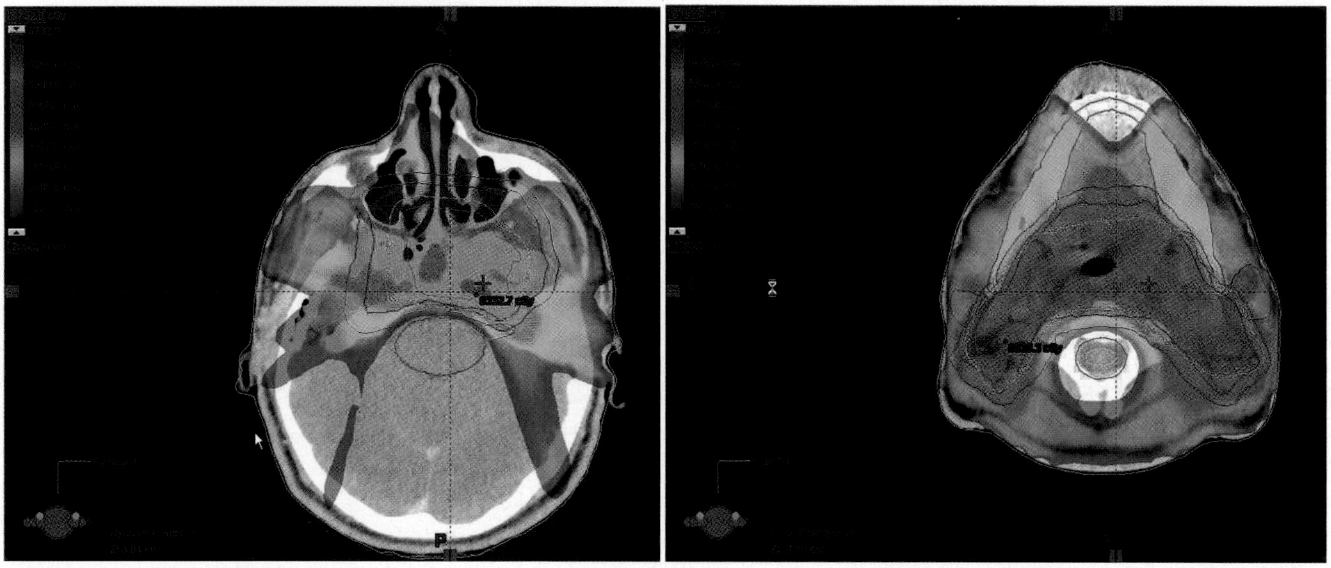

A B

Figure 31-7 Dose-colorwash pattern illustrating radiotherapy coverage near the base of skull for a case of recurrent nasopharyngeal cancer, in which IMRT was used to minimize reirradiation risk to normal structures. The colorwash ranges between 20 Gy and the maximum dose. **A,** The tolerance of the brainstem and temporal lobes places constraints on the dosimetry of the base of skull. **B,** The tolerance of the mandible and spinal cord constrain the neck coverage. The IMRT technique used was similar to that in another case (see Figs. 31-4 and 31-5) but with 9 coplanar, nonopposed fields.

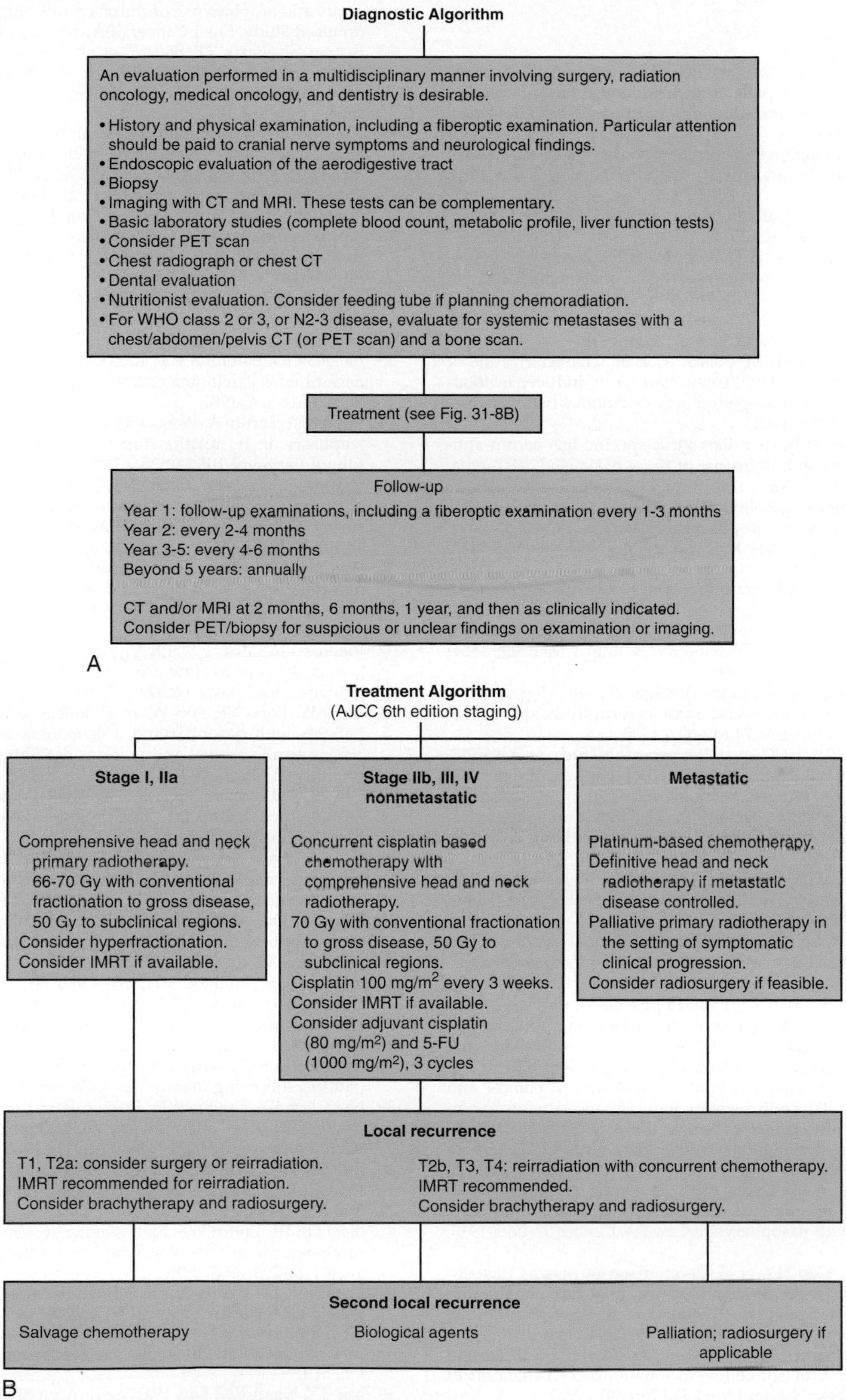
Diagnostic Algorithm
An evaluation performed in a multidisciplinary manner involving surgery, radiation oncology, medical oncology, and dentistry is desirable.
• History and physical examination, including a fiberoptic examination. Particular attention should be paid to cranial nerve symptoms and neurological findings.
• Endoscopic evaluation of the aerodigestive tract
• Biopsy
• Imaging with CT and MRI. These tests can be complementary.
• Basic laboratory studies (complete blood count, metabolic profile, liver function tests)
• Consider PET scan
• Chest radiograph or chest CT
• Dental evaluation
• Nutritionist evaluation. Consider feeding tube if planning chemoradiation.
• For WHO class 2 or 3, or N2-3 disease, evaluate for systemic metastases with a chest/abdomen/pelvis CT (or PET scan) and a bone scan.
Treatment (see Fig. 31-8B)
Follow-up
Year 1: follow-up examinations, including a fiberoptic examination every 1-3 months
Year 2: every 2-4 months
Year 3-5: every 4-6 months
Beyond 5 years: annually
CT and/or MRI at 2 months, 6 months, 1 year, and then as clinically indicated.
Consider PET/biopsy for suspicious or unclear findings on examination or imaging.
A
Treatment Algorithm
(AJCC 6th edition staging)
Stage I, IIa
Comprehensive head and neck primary radiotherapy.
66-70 Gy with conventional fractionation to gross disease, 50 Gy to subclinical regions.
Consider hyperfractionation.
Consider IMRT if available.
Stage IIb, III, IV nonmetastatic
Concurrent cisplatin based chemotherapy with comprehensive head and neck radiotherapy.
70 Gy with conventional fractionation to gross disease, 50 Gy to subclinical regions.
Cisplatin 100 mg/m2 every 3 weeks.
Consider IMRT if available.
Consider adjuvant cisplatin (80 mg/m2) and 5-FU (1000 mg/m2), 3 cycles
Metastatic
Platinum-based chemotherapy.
Definitive head and neck radiotherapy if metastatic disease controlled.
Palliative primary radiotherapy in the setting of symptomatic clinical progression.
Consider radiosurgery if feasible.
Local recurrence
T1, T2a: consider surgery or reirradiation.
IMRT recommended for reirradiation.
Consider brachytherapy and radiosurgery.
T2b, T3, T4: reirradiation with concurrent chemotherapy.
IMRT recommended.
Consider brachytherapy and radiosurgery.
Second local recurrence
Salvage chemotherapy
Biological agents
Palliation; radiosurgery if applicable
B

Figure 31-8 Nasopharyngeal carcinoma diagnostic (A) and treatment (B) algorithms for the management of nasopharyngeal carcinoma based on the 6th edition of the American Joint Committee on Cancer (AJCC) staging system. Patients with stage IIb disease would have been stage III or IV when many of the chemoradiation trials were performed and are therefore included as patients with locally advanced disease. Intensity-modulated radiation therapy (IMRT) is generally recommended if available, and if not, other techniques, such as pituitary shielding, oblique boost fields, and the use of radioprotectors (amifostine), may be appropriate to decrease morbidity. In the case of local failure, reirradiation is a consideration if the time to recurrence exceeds 6 months. In elderly patients or in patients with multiple medical problems or poor performance status, concurrent chemotherapy should be used with caution. Such patients are not well represented in clinical trials, and meta-analysis of chemoradiation trials suggests less clinical benefit from chemotherapy. CT, computed tomography; 5-FU, 5-fluorouracil; MRI, magnetic resonance imaging; PET, positron emission tomography; WHO, World Health Organization.

REFERENCES

1. Al-Sarraf M, LeBlanc M, Giri PG, et al: Chemoradiotherapy versus radiotherapy in patients with advanced nasopharyngeal cancer: phase III randomized Intergroup study 0099. J Clin Oncol 16:1310-1317, 1998.
2. Wang CC: Re-irradiation of recurrent nasopharyngeal carcinoma: treatment techniques and results. Int J Radiat Oncol Biol Phys 13:953-956, 1987.
3. Yu MC: Nasopharyngeal carcinoma: epidemiology and dietary factors. IARC Sci Publ 105:39-47, 1991.
4. Yu MC, Ho JH, Lai SH, et al: Cantonese-style salted fish as a cause of nasopharyngeal carcinoma: report of a case-control study in Hong Kong. Cancer Res 46:956-961, 1986.
5. Ho JH, Huang DP, Fong YY: Salted fish and nasopharyngeal carcinoma in southern Chinese. Lancet 2:626, 1978.
6. Bouvier G, Hergenhahn M, Polack A, et al: Characterization of macromolecular lignins as Epstein-Barr virus inducer in foodstuff associated with nasopharyngeal carcinoma risk. Carcinogenesis 16:1879-1885, 1995.
7. Henle G, Henle W: Epstein-Barr virus-specific IgA serum antibodies as an outstanding feature of nasopharyngeal carcinoma. Int J Cancer 17:1-7, 1976.
8. Neel HB III, Pearson GR, Taylor WF: Antibodies to Epstein-Barr virus in patients with nasopharyngeal carcinoma and in comparison groups. Ann Otol Rhinol Laryngol 93(5 Pt 1):477-482, 1984.
9. Buell P: The effect of migration on the risk of nasopharyngeal cancer among Chinese. Cancer Res 34:1189-1191, 1974.
10. Henderson BE, Louie E, SooHoo Jing J, et al: Risk factors associated with nasopharyngeal carcinoma. N Engl J Med 295:1101-1106, 1976.
11. Nam JM, McLaughlin JK, Blot WJ: Cigarette smoking, alcohol, and nasopharyngeal carcinoma: a case-control study among U.S. whites. J Natl Cancer Inst 84:619-622, 1992.
12. Lin TM, Chen KP, Lin CC, et al: Retrospective study on nasopharyngeal carcinoma. J Natl Cancer Inst 51:1403-1408, 1973.
13. Deng H, Zhao Z, Zhang Z: Serologic screening on nasopharyngeal cancer in 338,868 persons in 21 cities and counties of Guangxi Region, China [Chinese]. Zhonghua Yu Fang Yi Xue Za Zhi 29:342-343, 1995.
14. Khuri FR, Lippman SM, Spitz MR, et al: Molecular epidemiology and retinoid chemoprevention of head and neck cancer. J Natl Cancer Inst 89:199-211, 1997.
15. Lo YM, Chan LY, Lo KW, et al: Quantitative analysis of cell-free Epstein-Barr virus DNA in plasma of patients with nasopharyngeal carcinoma. Cancer Res 59:1188-1191, 1999.
16. Leung SF, Tam JS, Chan AT, et al: Improved accuracy of detection of nasopharyngeal carcinoma by combined application of circulating Epstein-Barr virus DNA and anti-Epstein-Barr viral capsid antigen IgA antibody. Clin Chem 50:339-345, 2004.
17. Hong RL, Lin CY, Ting LL, et al: Comparison of clinical and molecular surveillance in patients with advanced nasopharyngeal carcinoma after primary therapy: the potential role of quantitative analysis of circulating Epstein-Barr virus DNA. Cancer 100:1429-1437, 2004.
18. Hao SP, Tsang NM, Chang KP: Screening nasopharyngeal carcinoma by detection of the latent membrane protein 1 (LMP-1) gene with nasopharyngeal swabs. Cancer 97:1909-1913, 2003.
19. Shao JY, Li YH, Gao HY, et al: Comparison of plasma Epstein-Barr virus (EBV) DNA levels and serum EBV immunoglobulin A/virus capsid antigen antibody titers in patients with nasopharyngeal carcinoma. Cancer 100:1162-1170, 2004.
20. Hong WK, Lippman SM, Itri LM, et al: Prevention of second primary tumors with isotretinoin in squamous-cell carcinoma of the head and neck. N Engl J Med 323:795-801, 1990.
21. Benner SE, Pajak TF, Lippman SM, et al: Prevention of second primary tumors with isotretinoin in patients with squamous cell carcinoma of the head and neck: long-term follow-up. J Natl Cancer Inst 86:140-141, 1994.
22. Bolla M, Lefur R, Ton Van J, et al: Prevention of second primary tumours with etretinate in squamous cell carcinoma of the oral cavity and oropharynx:results of a multicentric double-blind randomised study. Eur J Cancer 30A:767-772, 1994.
23. Benner SE, Pajak TF, Stetz J, et al: Toxicity of isotretinoin in a chemoprevention trial to prevent second primary tumors following head and neck cancer. J Natl Cancer Inst 86:1799-1801, 1994.
24. Khuri F, Lee JJ, Lippman SM, et al: Isotretinoin effects on head and neck cancer recurrence and second primary tumors [abstract]. Prog Proc Am Soc Clin Oncol. 22:90, 2003.
25. Hong WK, Endicott J, Itri LM, et al: 13-*cis*-retinoic acid in the treatment of oral leukoplakia. N Engl J Med 315:1501-1505, 1986.
26. Lippman SM, Batsakis JG, Toth BB, et al: Comparison of low-dose isotretinoin with beta carotene to prevent oral carcinogenesis. N Engl J Med 328:15-20, 1993.
27. Lin DT, Subbaramaiah K, Shah JP, et al: Cyclooxygenase-2: a novel molecular target for the prevention and treatment of head and neck cancer. Head Neck 24:792-799, 2002.
28. Batsakis JG, Solomon AR, Rice DH: The pathology of head and neck tumors: carcinoma of the nasopharynx, Part 11. Head Neck Surg 3:511-524, 1981.
29. Vasef MA, Ferlito A, Weiss LM: Nasopharyngeal carcinoma, with emphasis on its relationship to Epstein-Barr virus. Ann Otol Rhinol Laryngol 106:348-356, 1997.
30. Shanmugaratnam K, Chan SH, de-The G, et al: Histopathology of nasopharyngeal carcinoma: correlations with epidemiology, survival rates and other biological characteristics. Cancer 44:1029-1044, 1979.
31. Sanguineti G, Geara FB, Garden AS, et al: Carcinoma of the nasopharynx treated by radiotherapy alone: determinants of local and regional control. Int J Radiat Oncol Biol Phys 37:985-996, 1997.
32. Johansen LV, Mestre M, Overgaard J: Carcinoma of the nasopharynx: analysis of treatment results in 167 consecutively admitted patients. Head Neck 14:200-207, 1992.
33. Lee AW, Poon YF, Foo W, et al: Retrospective analysis of 5037 patients with nasopharyngeal carcinoma treated during 1976-1985: overall survival and patterns of failure. Int J Radiat Oncol Biol Phys 23:261-270, 1992.
34. Perez CA, Devineni VR, Marcial-Vega V, et al: Carcinoma of the nasopharynx: factors affecting prognosis. Int J Radiat Oncol Biol Phys 23:271-280, 1992.
35. Old LJ, Boyse EA, Oettgen HF, et al: Precipitating antibody in human serum to an antigen present in cultured Burkitt's lymphoma cells. Proc Nat Acad Sci 56:1699-1704, 1966.
36. Sam CK, Prasad U, Pathmanathan R: Serological markers in the diagnosis of histopathological types of nasopharyngeal carcinoma. Eur J Surg Oncol 15:357-360, 1989.
37. Pearson GR, Weiland LH, Neel HB III, et al: Application of Epstein-Barr virus (EBV) serology to the diagnosis of North American nasopharyngeal carcinoma. Cancer 51:260-268, 1983.
38. Henle W, Ho JH, Henle G, et al: Nasopharyngeal carcinoma: significance of changes in Epstein-Barr virus-related antibody patterns following therapy. Int J Cancer 20:663-672, 1977.
39. Neel HB III, Taylor WF: Epstein-Barr virus-related antibody: changes in titers after therapy for nasopharyngeal carcinoma. Arch Otolaryngol Head Neck Surg 116:1287-1290, 1990.
40. Straathof KC, Bollard CM, Rooney CM, et al: Immunotherapy for Epstein-Barr virus-associated cancers in children. Oncologist 8:83-98, 2003.
41. Neel HB III, Taylor WF: New staging system for nasopharyngeal carcinoma: long-term outcome. Arch Otolaryngol Head Neck Surg 115:1293-1303, 1989.
42. Comoli P, De Palma R, Siena S, et al: Adoptive transfer of allogeneic Epstein-Barr virus (EBV)-specific cytotoxic T cells with in vitro antitumor activity boosts LMP2-specific immune response in a patient with EBV-related nasopharyngeal carcinoma. Ann Oncol 15:113-117, 2004.
43. Yip TT, Ngan RK, Lau WH, et al: A possible prognostic role of Immunoglobulin-G antibody against recombinant Epstein-Barr virus BZLF-1 transactivator protein ZEBRA in patients with nasopharyngeal carcinoma. Cancer 74:2414-2424, 1994.
44. Raab-Traub N, Flynn K, Pearson G, et al: The differentiated form of nasopharyngeal carcinoma contains Epstein-Barr virus DNA. Int J Cancer 39:25-29, 1987.

45. Chang YS, Tyan YS, Liu ST, et al: Detection of Epstein-Barr virus DNA sequences in nasopharyngeal carcinoma cells by enzymatic DNA amplification. J Clin Microbiol 28:2398-2402, 1990.
46. Niedobitek G, Agathanggelou A, Barber P, et al: P53 overexpression and Epstein-Barr virus infection in undifferentiated and squamous cell nasopharyngeal carcinomas. J Pathol 170:457-461, 1993.
47. Dictor M, Siven M, Tennvall J, et al: Determination of nonendemic nasopharyngeal carcinoma by in situ hybridization for Epstein-Barr virus EBER1 RNA: sensitivity and specificity in cervical node metastases. Laryngoscope 105(4 Pt 1):407-412, 1995.
48. Murono S, Yoshizaki T, Tanaka S, et al: Detection of Epstein-Barr virus in nasopharyngeal carcinoma by in situ hybridization and polymerase chain reaction. Laryngoscope 107:523-526, 1997.
49. Lu SJ, Day NE, Degos L, et al: Linkage of a nasopharyngeal carcinoma susceptibility locus to the HLA region. Nature 346:470-471, 1990.
50. Simons MJ, Wee GB, Day NE, et al: Immunogenetic aspects of nasopharyngeal carcinoma: I. differences in HL-A antigen profiles between patients and control groups. Int J Cancer 13:122-134, 1974.
51. Simons MJ, Wee GB, Goh EH, et al: Immunogenetic aspects of nasopharyngeal carcinoma: IV. Increased risk in Chinese of nasopharyngeal carcinoma associated with a Chinese-related HLA profile (A2, Singapore 2). J Natl Cancer Inst 57:977-980, 1976.
52. Golovleva I, Birgander R, Sjalander A, et al: Interferon-alpha and p53 alleles involved in nasopharyngeal carcinoma. Carcinogenesis 18:645-647, 1997.
53. Olmi P, Fallai C, Colagrande S, et al: Staging and follow-up of nasopharyngeal carcinoma: magnetic resonance imaging versus computerized tomography. Int J Radiat Oncol Biol Phys 32:795-800, 1995.
54. Chua DT, Sham JS, Kwong DL, et al: Retropharyngeal lymphadenopathy in patients with nasopharyngeal carcinoma: a computed tomography-based study. Cancer 79:869-877, 1997.
55. Peng N, Yen S, Liu W, et al: Evaluation of the effect of radiation therapy to nasopharyngeal carcinoma by positron emission tomography. Clin Positron-Imaging 3:51-56, 2000.
56. Nishioka T, Shiga T, Shirato H, et al: Image fusion between 18FDG-PET and MRI/CT for radiotherapy planning of oropharyngeal and nasopharyngeal carcinomas. Int J Radiat Oncol Biol Phys 53:1051-1057, 2002.
57. Fleming ID, Cooper JS, Henson DE, et al: AJCC Cancer Staging Manual: American Joint Committee on Cancer, 5th ed. Philadelphia, Lippincott-Raven, 1997.
58. Greene FL, Page DL, Fleming ID, et al: AJCC Cancer Staging Manual, 6th ed. New York: Springer-Verlag, 2002.
59. Beahrs OH, Henson DE, Hutter RVP, et al (eds): Manual for Staging of Cancer: American Joint Committee on Cancer, 4th ed. Philadelphia, Lippincott, 1992.
60. Teo PM, Leung SF, Yu P, et al (eds): A comparison of Ho's, International Union Against Cancer, and American Joint Committee stage classifications for nasopharyngeal carcinoma. Cancer 67:434-439, 1991.
61. Ma J, Mai HQ, Hong MH, et al: Results of a prospective randomized trial comparing neoadjuvant chemotherapy plus radiotherapy with radiotherapy alone in patients with locoregionally advanced nasopharyngeal carcinoma. J Clin Oncol 19:1350-1357, 2001.
62. American Joint Committee on Cancer Staging and End-Results Reporting: Manual for Staging of Cancer. Chicago, American Joint Committee, 1977.
63. Ho JH: Stage classification of nasopharyngeal carcinoma: a review. IARC Sci Publ 20:99-113, 1978.
64. Ho JH: Nasopharyngeal carcinoma (NPC). Adv Cancer Res 15:57-92, 1972.
65. Au JS, Law CK, Foo W, et al: In-depth evaluation of the AJCC/UICC 1997 staging system of nasopharyngeal carcinoma: prognostic homogeneity and proposed refinements. Int J Radiat Oncol Biol Phys 56:413-426, 2003.
66. Cooper JS, Cohen R, Stevens RE: A comparison of staging systems for nasopharyngeal carcinoma. Cancer 83:213-219, 1998.
67. Chung CH, Bernard PS, Perou CM: Molecular portraits and the family tree of cancer. Nat Genet 32 (Suppl):533-540, 2002.
68. Wilson CP: The approach to the nasopharynx. Proc Res Soc Med 44:353-358, 1950.
69. Horiot JC, Le Fur R, Schraub S, et al: Status of the experience of the EORTC cooperative group of radiotherapy with hyperfractionated and accelerated radiotherapy regimens. Sem Radiat Oncol 2:34-37, 1992.
70. Sanchiz F, Milla A, Torner J, et al: Single fraction per day versus two fractions per day versus radiochemotherapy in the treatment of head and neck cancer. Int J Radiat Oncol Biol Phys 19:1347-1350, 1990.
71. Brizel DM, Albers ME, Fisher SR, et al: Hyperfractionated irradiation with or without concurrent chemotherapy for locally advanced head and neck cancer. N Engl J Med 338:1798-1804, 1998.
72. Preliminary results of a randomized trial comparing neoadjuvant chemotherapy (cisplatin, epirubicin, bleomycin) plus radiotherapy vs. radiotherapy alone in stage IV(=N2, M0) undifferentiated nasopharyngeal carcinoma: a positive effect on progression-free survival. International Nasopharynx Cancer Study Group. VUMCA I trial. Int J Radiat Oncol Biol Phys 35:463-469, 1996.
73. Chan AT, Teo PM, Leung TW, et al: A prospective randomized study of chemotherapy adjunctive to definitive radiotherapy in advanced nasopharyngeal carcinoma. Int J Radiat Oncol Biol Phys 33:569-577, 1995.
74. Chua DT, Sham JS, Choy D, et al: Preliminary report of the Asian-Oceanian Clinical Oncology Association randomized trial comparing cisplatin and epirubicin followed by radiotherapy versus radiotherapy alone in the treatment of patients with locoregionally advanced nasopharyngeal carcinoma. Asian-Oceanian Clinical Oncology Association Nasopharynx Cancer Study Group. Cancer 83:2270-2283, 1998.
75. Wee J, Tan EH, Tai BC, et al: Phase III randomized trial of radiotherapy versus concurrent chemotherapy followed by adjuvant chemotherapy in patients with AJCC/UICC (1997) stage 3 and 4 nasopharyngeal cancer of the endemic variety [abstract]. Prog Proc Am Soc Clin Oncol 22 (Suppl):487, 2004.
76. Chan AT, Teo PM, Ngan RK, et al: Concurrent chemotherapy-radiotherapy compared with radiotherapy alone in locoregionally advanced nasopharyngeal carcinoma: progression-free survival analysis of a phase III randomized trial. J Clin Oncol 20:2038-2044, 2002.
77. Chan AT, Ngan RK, Teo PM, et al: Final results of the phase III randomized study of concurrent weekly cisplatin-RT versus RT alone in locoregionally advanced nasopharyngeal carcinoma (NPC) [abstract]. Prog Proc Am Soc Clin Oncol 22 (Suppl):492, 2004.
78. Lee AW, Lau WH, Tung SY, et al: Prospective randomized study on therapeutic gain achieved by addition of chemotherapy for T1-4N2-3M0) nasopharyngeal carcinoma (NPC) [abstract]. Prog Proc Am Soc Clin Oncol 22 (Suppl):488, 2004.
79. Geara FB, Glisson BS, Sanguineti G, et al: Induction chemotherapy followed by radiotherapy versus radiotherapy alone in patients with advanced nasopharyngeal carcinoma: results of a matched cohort study. Cancer 79:1279-1286, 1997.
80. Chua DT, Sham JS, Wei WI, et al: Control of regional metastasis after induction chemotherapy and radiotherapy for nasopharyngeal carcinoma. Head Neck 24:350-360, 2002.
81. Thephamongkhol K, Zou J, Browman G, et al: Chemoradiotherapy versus radiotherapy alone for nasopharyngeal carcinoma: a meta-analysis of 78 randomized controlled trials (RCTs) from English and non-English databases [abstract]. Prog Proc Am Soc Clin Oncol 22 (Suppl):91, 2004.
82. Hsu MM, Ko JY, Sheen TS, et al: Salvage surgery for recurrent nasopharyngeal carcinoma. Arch Otolaryngol Head Neck Surg 123:305-309, 1997.
83. Fee WE Jr, Gilmer PA, Goffinet DR: Surgical management of recurrent nasopharyngeal carcinoma after radiation failure at the primary site. Laryngoscope 98:1220-1226, 1988.
84. Fee WE Jr, Roberson JB Jr, Goffinet DR: Long-term survival after surgical resection for recurrent nasopharyngeal cancer after

radiotherapy failure. Arch Otolaryngol Head Neck Surg 117:1233-1236, 1991.

85. Cmelak AJ, Cox RS, Adler JR, et al: Radiosurgery for skull base malignancies and nasopharyngeal carcinoma. Int J Radiat Oncol Biol Phys 37:997-1003, 1997.
86. Fu KK, Newman H, Phillips TL: Treatment of locally recurrent carcinoma of the nasopharynx. Radiology 117:425-431, 1975.
87. Hoppe RT, Goffinet DR, Bagshaw MA: Carcinoma of the nasopharynx: eighteen years' experience with megavoltage radiation therapy. Cancer 37:2605-2612, 1976.
88. McNeese MD, Fletcher GH: Retreatment of recurrent nasopharyngeal carcinoma. Radiology 138:191-193, 1981.
89. Yan JH, Hu YH, Gu XZ: Radiation therapy of recurrent nasopharyngeal carcinoma: report on 219 patients. Acta Radiol Oncol 22:23-28, 1983.
90. Chen WZ, Zhou DL, Luo KS: Long-term observation after radiotherapy for nasopharyngeal carcinoma (NPC). Int J Radiat Oncol Biol Phys 16:311-314, 1989.
91. Lee AW, Law SC, Foo W, et al: Retrospective analysis of patients with nasopharyngeal carcinoma treated during 1976-1985: survival after local recurrence. Int J Radiat Oncol Biol Phys 26:773-782, 1993.
92. Wang CC, Busse J, Gitterman M: A simple afterloading applicator for intracavitary irradiation of carcinoma of the nasopharynx. Radiology 115:737-738, 1975.
93. Feehan PE, Castro JR, Phillips TL, et al: Recurrent locally advanced nasopharyngeal carcinoma treated with heavy charged particle irradiation. Int J Radiat Oncol Biol Phys 23:881-884, 1992.
94. Goffinet DR: Treatment of recurrent nasopharyngeal cancer by radiation therapy. Head Neck Cancer 3:455-463, 1993.
95. Xiao J, Xu G, Miao Y: Fractionated stereotactic radiosurgery for 50 patients with recurrent or residual nasopharyngeal carcinoma. Int J Radiat Oncol Biol Phys 51:164-170, 2001.
96. Chua DT, Sham JS, Kwong PW, et al: Linear accelerator-based stereotactic radiosurgery for limited, locally persistent, and recurrent nasopharyngeal carcinoma: efficacy and complications. Int J Radiat Oncol Biol Phys 56:177-183, 2003.
97. Le QT, Tate D, Koong A, et al: Improved local control with stereotactic radiosurgical boost in patients with nasopharyngeal carcinoma. Int J Radiat Oncol Biol Phys 56:1046-1054, 2003.
98. Lu TX, Mai WY, Teh BS, et al: Initial experience using intensity-modulated radiotherapy for recurrent nasopharyngeal carcinoma. Int J Radiat Oncol Biol Phys 58:682-687, 2004.
99. Chmura SJ, Milano MT, Haraf DJ: Reirradiation of recurrent head and neck cancers with curative intent. Semin Oncol 31:816-821, 2004.
100. Spencer S, Wheeler R, Peters G, et al: Phase 1 trial of combined chemotherapy and reirradiation for recurrent unresectable head and neck cancer. Head Neck 25:118-122, 2003.
101. Spencer SA, Harris J, Wheeler RH, et al: RTOG 96-10: reirradiation with concurrent hydroxyurea and 5-fluorouracil in patients with squamous cell cancer of the head and neck. Int J Radiat Oncol Biol Phys 51:1299-1304, 2001.
102. Kao J, Garofalo MC, Milano MT, et al: Reirradiation of recurrent and second primary head and neck malignancies: a comprehensive review. Cancer Treat Rev 29:21-30, 2003.
103. Sham J, Choy D, Kwong PW, et al: Radiotherapy for nasopharyngeal carcinoma: shielding the pituitary may improve therapeutic ratio. Int J Radiat Oncol Biol Phys 29:699-704, 1994.
104. Cheng SH, Jian JJ, Huang AT: Comments on "Radiotherapy for nasopharyngeal carcinoma: shielding the pituitary may improve therapeutic ratio." Int J Radiat Oncol Biol Phys 31:682-683, 1995.
105. Wolden SL, Zelefsky MJ, Hunt MA, et al: Failure of a 3D conformal boost to improve radiotherapy for nasopharyngeal carcinoma. Int J Radiat Oncol Biol Phys 49:1229-1234, 2001.
106. Hunt MA, Zelefsky MJ, Wolden S, et al: Treatment planning and delivery of intensity-modulated radiation therapy for primary nasopharynx cancer. Int J Radiat Oncol Biol Phys 49:623-632, 2001.
107. Lee N, Xia P, Quivey JM, et al: Intensity-modulated radiotherapy in the treatment of nasopharyngeal carcinoma: an update of the UCSF experience. Int J Radiat Oncol Biol Phys 53:12-22, 2002.
108. Xia P, Fu KK, Wong GW, et al: Comparison of treatment plans involving intensity-modulated radiotherapy for nasopharyngeal carcinoma. Int J Radiat Oncol Biol Phys 48:329-337, 2000.
109. Parsons JT, Bova FJ, Fitzgerald CR, et al: Radiation optic neuropathy after megavoltage external-beam irradiation: analysis of time-dose factors. Int J Radiat Oncol Biol Phys 30:755-763, 1994.
110. Brahme A: Optimization of stationary and moving beam radiation therapy techniques. Radiother Oncol 12:129-140, 1988.
111. Cormack AM: A problem in rotation therapy with X rays. Int J Radiat Oncol Biol Phys 13:623-630, 1987.
112. Gustafsson A, Lind BK, Brahme A: A generalized pencil beam algorithm for optimization of radiation therapy. Med Phys 21:343-356, 1994.
113. Mackie TR, Holmes T, Swerdloff S, et al: Tomotherapy: a new concept for the delivery of dynamic conformal radiotherapy. Med Phys 20:1709-1719, 1993.
114. Soderstrom S, Gustafsson A, Brahme A: The clinical value of different treatment objectives and degrees of freedom in radiation therapy optimization. Radiother Oncol 29:148-163, 1993.
115. Lee N, Xia P, Fischbein NJ, et al: Intensity-modulated radiation therapy for head-and-neck cancer: the UCSF experience focusing on target volume delineation. Int J Radiat Oncol Biol Phys 57:49-60, 2003.
116. Munter MW, Debus J, Hof H, et al: Inverse treatment planning and stereotactic intensity-modulated radiation therapy (IMRT) of the tumor and lymph node levels for nasopharyngeal carcinomas: description of treatment technique, plan comparison, and case study. Strahlenther Onkol 178:517-523, 2002.
117. Sultanem K, Shu HK, Xia P, et al: Three-dimensional intensity-modulated radiotherapy in the treatment of nasopharyngeal carcinoma: the University of California-San Francisco experience. Int J Radiat Oncol Biol Phys 48:711-722, 2000.
118. Verhey LJ: Comparison of three-dimensional conformal radiation therapy and intensity-modulated radiation therapy systems. Semin Radiat Oncol 9:78-98, 1999.
119. Chao KS, Ozyigit G, Tran BN, et al: Patterns of failure in patients receiving definitive and postoperative IMRT for head-and-neck cancer. Int J Radiat Oncol Biol Phys 55:312-321, 2003.
120. Eisbruch A, Ten Haken RK, Kim HM, et al: Dose, volume, and function relationships in parotid salivary glands following conformal and intensity-modulated irradiation of head and neck cancer. Int J Radiat Oncol Biol Phys 45:577-587, 1999.
121. Butler EB, Teh BS, Grant WH III, et al: SMART (simultaneous modulated accelerated radiation therapy) boost: a new accelerated fractionation schedule for the treatment of head and neck cancer with intensity modulated radiotherapy. Int J Radiat Oncol Biol Phys 45:21-32, 1999.
122. Chao KS, Low DA, Perez CA, et al: Intensity-modulated radiation therapy in head and neck cancers: the Mallinckrodt experience. Int J Cancer 90:92-103, 2000.
123. Dawson LA, Anzai Y, Marsh L, et al: Patterns of local-regional recurrence following parotid-sparing conformal and segmental intensity-modulated radiotherapy for head and neck cancer. Int J Radiat Oncol Biol Phys 46:1117-1126, 2000.
124. Cooper DL, DiStasio S, Son YH, et al: Induction chemotherapy with cisplatin, 5-FU and leucovorin followed by concomitant cisplatin and radiation in patients with larynx, pyriform sinus, base of tongue and nasopharyngeal tumors [abstract]. Prog Proc Am Soc Clin Oncol 16:399a, 1997.
125. Chi KH, Chan WK, Chao Y, et al: Phase II study of paclitaxel therapy for chemotherapy-naïve advanced nasopharyngeal carcinoma (NPC) [abstract]. Prog Proc Am Soc Clin Oncol 16:398a, 1997.
126. Siu LL, Czaykowski PM, Tannock IF: Phase I/II study of the CAPABLE regimen for patients with poorly differentiated carcinoma of the nasopharynx. J Clin Oncol 16:2514-2521, 1998.
127. Ma BB, Tannock IF, Pond GR, et al: Chemotherapy with gemcitabine-containing regimens for locally recurrent or metastatic nasopharyngeal carcinoma. Cancer 95:2516-2523, 2002.
128. Chi KH, Chang YC, Guo WY, et al: A phase III study of adjuvant chemotherapy in advanced nasopharyngeal carcinoma patients. Int J Radiat Oncol Biol Phys 52:1238-1244, 2002.

CHAPTER 32

LARYNX AND HYPOPHARYNX CANCER

Adam S. Garden, William H. Morrison, and K. Kian Ang

INCIDENCE

Larynx and hypopharynx cancers account for about one third of all head and neck neoplasms, affecting about 15,000 Americans per year.

BIOLOGIC CHARACTERISTICS

Prognosis for all tumors is primarily dependent on extent of disease, although it is also influenced by the anatomic site of origin.

Glottic tumors have the lowest incidence of metastases, as they more commonly present with earlier staged lesions and the true cords do not have a rich lymphatic supply compared to supraglottic and hypopharyngeal neoplasms. Hypopharyngeal cancers have a relatively high metastatic rate among head and neck cancers.

STAGING EVALUATION

Staging includes history, complete head and neck examination including indirect and direct laryngoscopy, contrast-enhanced computed tomography and/or magnetic resonance scans of the head and neck region, blood chemistry, and chest x-ray.

PRIMARY THERAPY

Early-stage disease can be treated with a single modality, either surgery or radiation.

Reported cure rates range from 65% to 95% and are dependent primarily on the bulk of disease.

ADJUVANT THERAPY

High cure rates have not justified adjuvant therapies for early-stage disease.

Chemoprevention remains an area of active research for this group at high risk for second primary tumors.

LOCALLY ADVANCED DISEASE

The concept of larynx preservation has been validated as an option for patients with T3 disease.

Concurrent chemoradiation has been demonstrated to improve the larynx preservation rate compared to radiation alone or treatment with neoadjuvant chemotherapy, and the latter has been demonstrated to not compromise survival compared to laryngectomy. Approximate 5-year survival rates for these patients are 50% to 55%.

For elderly patients in whom the toxicity of chemotherapy is a concern, radiation alone is a valid alternative for patients desiring larynx preservation.

Surgery remains the mainstay for very advanced, but resectable disease (stage T4a), with adjuvant postoperative radiation used for patients at high risk for local regional failure.

Concurrent chemoradiation is advocated for patients with inadequate margins or extranodal or soft tissue disease extension. Local control rates for this group range from 60% to 90%, but 5-year survival rates are between 20% and 40%.

PALLIATION

Palliative therapies are dependent on prior therapies received and disease location and extent. Radiation, chemotherapy, or surgery are all used but are individualized.

Management of cancers of the larynx is a special challenge for head and neck oncologists. It is a disease that even in advanced stages has a relatively high cure rate if managed appropriately. Because of the high cure rates of this disease, it has become the paradigm of the concept of organ preservation in oncologic patient management. Curing the patient is not the only consideration in the management of this disease. Voice preservation and avoidance of tracheal stoma are important priorities.

In previous decades, surgery, radiation, or a combination of the two therapies were used and individualized to best meet these end points. Both modalities have improved over the years in eradicating the disease and preserving function. Newer, more technically sophisticated voice-conserving surgical procedures have been developed. Similarly, radiation oncologists have grown in their understanding of the influences of dose, treatment duration, and field placement to improve the results in managing these diseases. Important improvements in defining disease extent, by both physical examination with fiberoptic laryngoscopy and radiological images obtained with computerized tomography (CT) and magnetic resonance imaging (MRI), have allowed for better selection of the appropriate therapy for an individual patient. Systemic therapies have been incorporated into the management of these diseases, thus increasing the options in trying to cure patients with this disease while maintaining function.

Carcinomas of the hypopharynx are often considered together with carcinomas of the larynx, as the anatomy of the hypopharynx is essentially created by the location of the voice box in the throat. Hypopharyngeal tumors frequently involve the larynx and vice versa. In these situations, it is one's best guess whether the epicenter of a large tumor is laryngeal or hypopharyngeal. It is therefore not unexpected that the concept of voice preservation also applies to the management of cancers of the hypopharynx. The pharynx is also involved in glutition, and issues of preservation of swallowing are also important in the management of these tumors.

While immediately adjacent to the larynx and thus having similar management concerns to laryngeal carcinoma, hypopharyngeal cancers typically have different natural histories compared to cancers arising in their laryngeal neighbor. At diagnosis, hypopharyngeal tumors have much higher rates of spread beyond the primary tumor, so even with successful local treatment, survival rates tend to be worse than other cancers of the head and neck.

Primary tumors of the hypopharynx also tend to present in locally advanced stages. However, local therapies have improved in recent years. Surgical grafting techniques have been developed to replace the pharyngeal tissues resected and allow the patient a better swallowing mechanism. Without these techniques, larger hypopharyngeal lesions would be unresectable. Improved control with altered radiation schedules may allow preservation of the larynx and pharynx for intermediate-stage lesions. Adding systemic agents may also allow for organ preservation and help with the problem of distant disease prevalent in cancers of this site.

EPIDEMIOLOGY AND ETIOLOGY

Larynx cancer occurs in roughly 12,000 Americans per year, accounting for approximately one quarter to one third of all head and neck cancer cases. However, mortality due to larynx cancer is relatively low. About 4200 deaths per year in the United States are attributed to larynx cancer.

Larynx cancer remains predominantly a disease affecting older men. However, due to the increase of smoking among women, there has been a narrowing of the gender gap. Data from the Surveillance, Epidemiology, and End Results (SEER) program (1998-2002)[1] estimated an overall incidence of 3.8 cases per 100,000 people per year. Comparisons reveal case incidences of 6.7 versus 1.5 in males and females, respectively. The incidence for all Americans over the age of 65 is 30.2 cases per 100,000 people. There is a higher incidence among blacks than among whites.

Tobacco use is strongly associated with the development of larynx cancer, with the highest risk among active heavy smokers and an intermediate risk among ex-smokers.[2,3] Over 95% of patients with larynx cancer have a history of tobacco use.[4] Cigar and pipe smoking have also been associated with larynx cancer,[3] but studies on this issue have been more controversial.[2,5,6]

Alcohol use is also associated with larynx cancer but is believed to act synergistically with tobacco rather than independently. It is unusual to see larynx cancer in nonsmoking patients with alcohol abuse histories.[6] A history of heavy alcohol use is more strongly associated with supraglottic and hypopharyngeal cancers.[3,7] Likewise, occupational exposures to asbestos,[3,8,9] mustard gas, nickel, soot, and tars have been linked to larynx cancer, but generally a tobacco use history is also present.[10] Several authors have evaluated the influence of diet on the development of larynx cancer and have found, while controlling for tobacco and alcohol use, a higher incidence among patients with vitamin- and nutrient-deficient diets.[5,11,12]

Attention has been directed at the influence of gastroesophageal reflux disease (GERD) on laryngeal diseases, including carcinomas. Three separate studies[13-15] have described cohorts of nonsmoking patients with GERD and larynx cancer. Bacciu and coworkers[16] compared 36 consecutive patients with no history of tobacco and alcohol consumption who developed laryngeal carcinoma to a group of 125 lifetime nonsmokers who were cancer free. They found a much higher prevalence of GERD among the patients with larynx cancer. It is believed that chronic irritation on the larynx from acid may predispose these patients to cancer. It is thought that if this cancer is seen in nonsmokers, the influence of GERD on the development of larynx cancer in smokers and alcohol users (who are at higher risk for GERD) may be very significant.

Human papillomavirus (HPV) has been causally linked to multiple cancers, including head and neck cancers,[17,18] particularly cancers of the tonsil. HPV has also been demonstrated to be associated with laryngeal cancers, although studies are in general retrospective and the reported prevalence rates vary widely. The evidence for HPV having a role in laryngeal cancer is less obvious than in other malignancies, and its interaction with other carcinogens such as tobacco is unclear. As in cervical cancer in women and tonsillar cancer, HPV 16 is the most common variant noted.

Hypopharyngeal cancers are less common than laryngeal tumors. The estimated incidence in the United States is 2500 cases per year. Etiologic risk factors are similar to those for laryngeal tumors,[11] with a predominance among men and older individuals. It is closely linked to tobacco and alcohol use, and the ties to heavy alcohol use seem stronger than those for larynx cancer.

PREVENTION AND EARLY DETECTION

Prevention

The primary preventive methods taken to eliminate malignancies of the upper aerodigestive tract have come from public awareness that tobacco and alcohol are the major causative agents of these cancers. National public health measures have been directed at diminishing the prevalence of smoking and drinking. Over the next 15 years, a byproduct of these policies may be a decline in the incidence of laryngeal and hypopharyngeal carcinomas.

While government policies have been directed at diminishing carcinogenic etiologic agents for the general population, investigators have tried to identify high-risk groups in whom more direct measures can be taken. The major group identified consists of patients who have been cured of a cancer of the upper aerodigestive tract,[19-22] particularly patients who have smoking or alcohol use histories.[23] The incidence of second primary cancers of the upper aerodigestive tract ranges from 10% to 30%. The locations of these second cancers are evenly divided between the lungs, esophagus, and head and neck mucosal sites, including the larynx and hypopharynx.[23]

The high incidence of new cancers in this patient population has led investigators to develop programs designed to diminish the occurrence of second primary tumors. Hong and associates[24] studied 13-*cis*-retinoic acid as a possible agent to prevent new cancers in patients with a history of head and neck malignancy. A randomized trial showed a 14% versus 31% incidence of second primary tumors in patients who received a relatively high dose of 13-*cis*-retinoic acid versus placebo.[25] The RTOG in 2002 completed accrual to a trial testing chemoprevention with 13-*cis*-retinoic acid in a multi-institutional setting. Over 1100 patients with stage I or II cancer were accrued. Preliminary results have not demonstrated a benefit to low-dose isotretinoin but have demonstrated that continued smoking does contribute to an increased rate of malignancies.[26] Papadimitralopoulou and colleagues investigated α-tocopherol, interferon-α, and isotretinoin in patients with laryngeal dysplasia and reported a 50% complete response rate at 12 months.[27] A companion study suggested low chromosome polysomy appeared to predict response and be used as a screening tool.[28]

Early Detection

Similar to the issues surrounding prevention, early detection of laryngeal and hypopharyngeal cancers centers on targeting the population at highest risk for developing these carcinomas. Cancers of the larynx and hypopharynx affect roughly 15,000 Americans a year and therefore is not a large enough health problem to warrant screening of the general population. Some investigators have studied the role of screening a more focused population such as tobacco users who work at high-risk occupations and question the value of screening even a more limited population.[29] However, Prout and colleagues[30] argue that a primary care practitioner can, as part of a general evaluation, inquire about hoarseness in a patient from an at-risk population. If a positive response is obtained, the patient can be referred to an otolaryngologist for appropriate evaluations. The laryngeal carcinoma detection rate in this situation ranges between 3% and 4%.[30,31]

PATHOLOGY, BIOLOGY, AND PATHWAYS OF SPREAD

Pathology

The majority of laryngeal and hypopharyngeal cancers are squamous cell carcinomas. Laryngeal carcinomas are usually well differentiated. As patients with laryngeal tumors often present with early-stage disease, it is common to see a spectrum of pathologic tissue changes, ranging from premalignant atypia or dysplasia to carcinoma in situ (CIS) and superficially invasive carcinomas, within the larynx.

CIS is a pathologic entity representing carcinomatous changes confined to the thickened epithelium without breaching the lamina propria. The clinical appearance of CIS is a white or grayish-white thickening of the mucosa. Penetration through the basement membrane makes the diagnosis of invasive carcinoma. Invasive tumor may be missed if biopsy samples are too small or too superficial for proper histologic evaluation.

Less frequently, the larynx and hypopharynx can give rise to variants of squamous cell carcinoma. The most common of these cancers is verrucous carcinoma, accounting for approximately 4% of all larynx cancers.[32] They are classically slow-growing tumors with a gross warty appearance. A less common variant with numerous nomenclatures is squamous cell carcinoma with spindle cell features. As its name implies, along with typical squamous cells, carcinoma cells are spindle cells. The significance of these spindle cells is the subject of debate, as theories range from these cells being a benign reactionary process with little clinical significance to highly malignant elements with adverse outcome.[33] Molecular evidence suggests the sarcomatoid carcinoma evolves from the conventional epithelium-type component and the sarcomatoid component has a malignant nature.[34] Grossly, they can often present as large polypoid lesions that sometimes act as ball valves in the larynx. Basaloid squamous cell carcinoma and lymphoepithelioma of non-nasopharyngeal origin are rare tumors seen in numerous head and neck mucosal sites, including the larynx and hypopharynx.

The remaining 5% of larynx cancers are composed of neoplasms more commonly found in other locations. Salivary gland cancers, neuroendocrine tumors[35] (including small cell carcinomas), sarcomas, and lymphomas have all been reported in the literature.[36]

Pathways of Spread—Primary Site and Regional Lymphatics

Larynx

The larynx is divided into three regions: the supraglottis, glottis, and subglottis. The supraglottic larynx lies above the level where the mucosa of the upper surface of the true vocal cords turns upward to form the lateral wall of the ventricle. It consists of the false vocal cords, arytenoids, aryepiglottic folds, and infrahyoid and suprahyoid epiglottis. The glottic region by definition includes the true vocal cords and extends 0.5 cm inferiorly, and the subglottic region extends from there to the superior aspect of the trachea (Fig. 32-1).

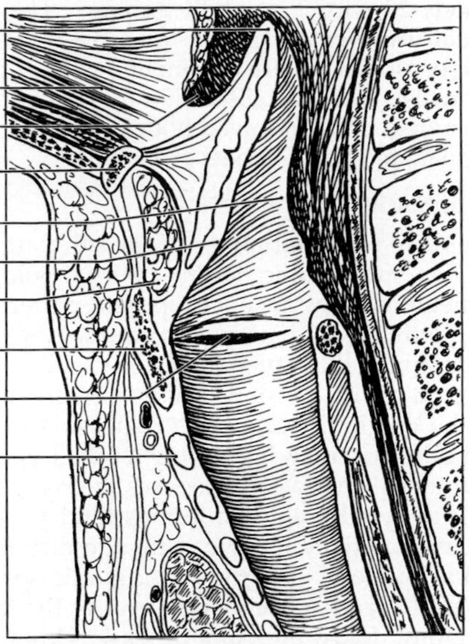

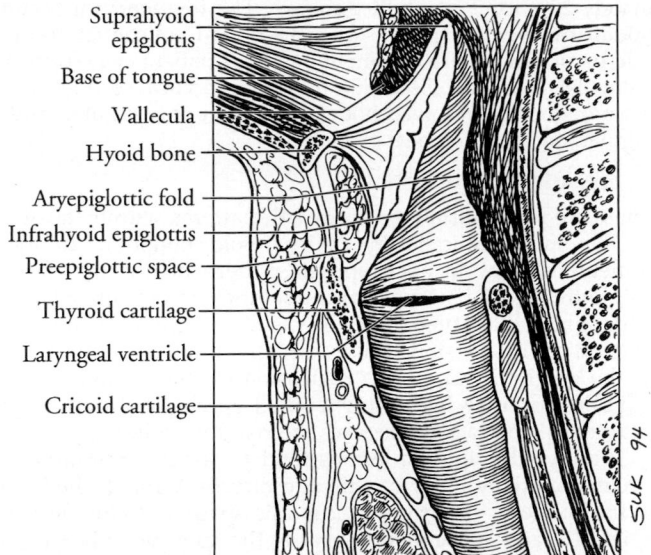

Figure 32-1 Anatomy of the larynx and its subdivisions.

Primary glottic cancers are about three times more common than supraglottic carcinomas, whereas subglottic carcinomas are extremely rare (about 2% of larynx cancers). At diagnosis, nearly two thirds of patients with larynx cancer have their disease confined to the laryngeal structures and less than 10% present with distant metastases. The patterns of spread, presentations, and management of cancers arising from these three subsites are very different.

GLOTTIS

Most glottic lesions arise on the free margin and upper surface of the anterior two thirds of the true cord. These tumors tend to grow slowly and remain confined to the mucosa of the true cords. Eventually they will spread superiorly or inferiorly onto the mucosa of the supraglottic or subglottic structures. Some tumors may grow outward, in an exophytic fashion, leading to voice changes and subsequently respiratory obstruction. Invasion into the intrinsic musculature and joints of the larynx decreases vocal cord mobility and ultimately causes vocal cord fixation. Noteworthy is that tumor bulk alone can cause impaired mobility. Less commonly, infiltration of the recurrent laryngeal nerve may also cause impairment of mobility.

Infiltrative tumors will breach into the paraglottic and preepiglottic spaces. These spaces lie between the external frame of the larynx (thyroid-cricoid cartilages and hyoid bone) and the internal components of the larynx (epiglottis, muscles, and ligaments) and are filled with fat and hence offer little resistance to infiltration. From these spaces, infiltrative tumors may break through ligaments above or below the thyroid cartilage into the neck or may invade the cartilage directly.

The mucosa of the true vocal cords has a sparse lymphatic supply. Thus, glottic carcinomas have a low propensity for lymphatic spread. The incidence of lymphadenopathy at diagnosis is approximately 5% for T1 and T2 lesions and approximately 20% for T3 and T4 tumors.[37] The frequency of occult nodal involvement is also low. Byers and colleagues found microscopic nodal involvement in 9 of 57 patients who underwent elective nodal dissection for T3 or T4 vocal cord lesions; most frequently involved nodes were the upper jugular, mid-jugular, and paratracheal groups.[38]

Supraglottis

There are some variations of growth patterns within subsites of the supraglottic larynx. Suprahyoid epiglottic tumors sometimes grow in an exophytic pattern off the tip of the epiglottis, causing no symptoms until they become quite large. Other times, they spread inferiorly, infiltrating and eroding the epiglottis. These lesions can eventually autoamputate the tip of the epiglottis. Complete regression of these tumors after radiotherapy may leave only a small epiglottic stump. Such anatomical aberration increases the risk for aspiration.

Infrahyoid epiglottic lesions tend to spread anteriorly or circumferentially. They can invade directly through the base of the epiglottis into the preepiglottic space, onto the lingual epiglottis, and subsequently invade the vallecula, pharyngoepiglottic folds, and tongue base. Other times, they spread onto the aryepiglottic folds, usually spreading from their midline position in both directions to involve both folds, producing a horseshoe-like appearance. They then spread either inferiorly onto the false vocal cords or over the aryepiglottic folds onto the piriform sinuses.

Lesions originating on the aryepiglottic folds can spread in all directions, that is, anteromedially onto the epiglottis, posteriorly to the arytenoids, inferiorly to the false cords, or laterally into the piriform sinus. Similar to lesions of the false vocal cords, they have variable growth patterns but often are infiltrative with easy access to the paraglottic space. They can frequently involve the cricoarytenoid joints or the musculature of the larynx, impairing mobility.

The primary difference between supraglottic cancers and true glottic cancers is the likelihood of developing cervical nodal metastases. At diagnosis, 55% of patients with supraglottic cancers have clinically involved lymph nodes. Lymphatic vessels in the supraglottic larynx collect in channels that pass through the piriform sinuses to drain to nodes along the jugular chain, particularly the upper and mid jugular lymph nodes. Lee and coworkers[39] reported on the data of a subgroup of patients with intermediate-stage disease who underwent supraglottic laryngectomy with neck dissections. One third of patients had palpable nodes on presentation, and nearly an additional third of patients had pathologic nodal involvement.

Subglottis

Subglottic tumors spread inferiorly to the trachea, extend through the cricothyroid membrane into the neck, or directly invade the cricoid cartilage. Superiorly they almost always involve the undersurface of the true glottis, and from a staging perspective, it is sometimes difficult to differentiate between a tumor truly originating from the subglottis and a glottic tumor with significant subglottic extension.

Hypopharynx

The hypopharynx is the inferior portion of the three divisions of the pharynx (Fig. 32-2). It extends from the hyoid bone superiorly to the cricoid inferiorly. Valleculae, pharyngoepiglottic fold, and lateral projections of aryepiglottic folds are considered the superior border separating hypopharynx from oropharynx. Inferiorly, the hypopharynx ends at the cervical esophageal inlet. The hypopharynx is subdivided into three components: the pharyngeal walls, the piriform sinus, and the postcricoid pharynx. The hypopharyngeal walls are a continuation of the lateral and posterior oropharyngeal walls. The pair of piriform sinuses is created by the invagination of the larynx into the hypopharynx. They are conical in shape (more truly pear shaped, hence the derivation of its name). Each sinus (or recess) consists of three walls. The medial wall is essentially the lateral aspect of the larynx; superiorly, it becomes the aryepiglottic fold. The lateral wall is a continuation of the lateral wall of the oropharynx. Anteriorly, the medial and lateral walls converge to form the narrow anterior wall. Superior is the base or vestibule formed by the rim of the three walls. Inferiorly, the three walls merge to form the apex.

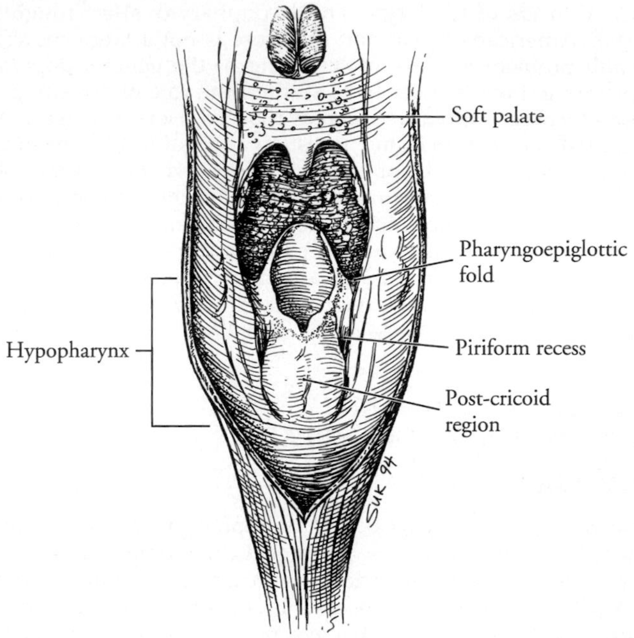

Figure 32-2 Anatomic relationship of the hypopharynx to the pharyngeal axis.

The postcricoid pharynx begins superiorly at the level of the arytenoids and ends inferiorly at the esophagus. The posterior larynx makes its anterior border, and posteriorly it again is a continuation of the posterior pharyngeal wall.

Hypopharyngeal cancers also commonly present with nodal metastases. Lindberg[40] reported a 75% incidence of nodal metastases in patients presenting to the M. D. Anderson Cancer Center (MDACC) with hypopharyngeal tumors. Levels II and III nodes were most frequently involved and bilateral lymphadenopathy was seen in 15% of patients. These tumors also have access to deep jugular and retropharyngeal lymph nodes.

Piriform Sinus Tumors

Piriform sinus tumors account for 70% of cancers originating in the hypopharynx. Tumors originating from the medial wall of the piriform sinus behave similarly to supraglottic tumors arising from the aryepiglottic folds, and it is often difficult to know the true origin of some of these lesions. Posteriorly, there is little to impede tumor extension into the postcricoid space or crossing from the ipsilateral arytenoid to the contralateral arytenoid. Lateral wall tumors also have few barriers to growth. They can extend medially along the mucosa to involve the posterior hypopharyngeal wall or anteromedially to involve the other two walls of the piriform sinus. Inferiorly, they have quick access to the apex and usually extend deep to the sinus submucosally to involve other adjacent structures, including the thyroid and cricoid cartilages, or directly into the thyroid gland. It is not uncommon to see advanced tumors from this location that have direct soft tissue extension into the neck. These tumors can also extend into the cervical esophagus, primarily through submucosal routes, making a true definition of disease extent extremely difficult. They can also behave similarly to more classic esophageal tumors with extensive spread along lymphatic spaces and with skip lesions.

Hypopharyngeal Wall Tumors

Tumors originating from the hypopharyngeal walls are less common. As early presentations are infrequent, it is unusual to see a lesion confined to and clearly originating from the lateral or posterior hypopharyngeal wall. Hypopharyngeal wall tumors frequently spread along the walls to involve either the posterior or lateral oropharyngeal walls. Posterior wall tumors can also invade the prevertebral tissues, or even more deeply to the bones of the cervical spine.

Postcricoid Tumors

Postcricoid tumors are the least common hypopharyngeal tumors. They almost always present in advanced stages. They can extend laterally into one or both piriform sinuses, or directly invade laryngeal structures.

Pathways of Spread—Distant Metastases

The incidence of distant metastases from cancers of the head and neck and specifically laryngeal and hypopharyngeal is low and is generally thought to be less than 10%. An often-referenced study by Crile in 1906[41] reported an incidence of 1% distant metastases in 4500 patients with epidermoid cancers of the head and neck. In subsets of patients with head and neck squamous cell cancers, patients with glottic tumors usually have the lowest rates of distant metastases, whereas patients with hypopharyngeal carcinomas often have the highest rates.

Merino and colleagues[42] analyzed the incidence of distant disease in over 5000 patients with head and neck squamous cell carcinomas treated from 1948 through 1967. Among patients with control of disease above the clavicle, the incidence of distant failure was 1%, 13%, and 23% for patients with carcinomas of the true vocal cords, supraglottic larynx, and hypopharynx, respectively. Similarly, Marks and associates[43] found that 23% of patients with piriform sinus cancers developed distant metastases, with a higher rate among patients who underwent total laryngectomies as part of their therapy. The incidence of metastases is associated with stage, as the clinical incidence of metastases is approximately 20% in patients with stage IV disease.

The sites of presentation of distant metastases are similar for cancers of the larynx and hypopharynx.[42] The lungs are the most common site and are the first site of presentation in nearly 60% of patients. Bones are the next most common site, as 20% of patients with distant disease develop osseous metastases. Liver metastases are common in autopsy studies, but clinical liver metastases develop in only 10% of patients with hematogenous spread of disease from the larynx and hypopharynx.[44] Spread to mediastinal lymph nodes, the brain, or other organs is very uncommon.

MOLECULAR BIOLOGY

The critical events of carcinogenesis and tumor progression occurring at a molecular level have been heavily studied over several decades. Paradoxically, as our knowledge of molecular tumor biology increases, the complexity of tumorigenesis at this level also appears to increase. This is in part due to the realization that laryngeal and hypopharyngeal tumors, while developing in a "single" site, represent a heterogeneous group of neoplasms. Investigators have found genotypic markers, either chromosomal rearrangements, or the presence of an oncogene, tumor suppressor gene, or other markers, but have only found them in some varying percentage of laryngeal and hypopharyngeal tumors.

A general view is that tumorigenesis of head and neck malignancies occurs due to a combination of factors. Carcinogen exposure (primarily tobacco) results in genetic damage. However, not all smokers develop cancer. The genetic damage in individuals varies based on the degree of exposure of the offending agent as well as the individual's inherent sensitivity to genetic damage. The latter can be tested indirectly in individuals using an assay quantifying chromosomal breakage induced by in vitro exposure to bleomycin. Patients with upper aerodigestive tract malignancies were compared with healthy controls. Mutagen-sensitive individuals had a higher likelihood of having a cancer, and mutagen-sensitive smokers were at the highest risk.[45]

A field of mucosa is placed at risk for developing carcinoma by the exposure and sensitivity described above, but it requires a number of events to develop a frank cancer. The concept of field cancerization was first described in 1953 by Slaughter and associates.[46] They found widespread microscopic abnormalities in "normal" mucosa adjacent to tumor obtained from resected specimens. These abnormalities ranged from hyperplasia to areas of carcinoma both invasive and in situ away from the known resected cancer. Califano and colleagues[47] proposed a genetic progression model in which the local clinical phenomenon of field cancerization involves the expansion and migration of clonally related preneoplastic cells.

The molecular events leading to the development of carcinomas are believed to occur by a multistep process and have been described for other cancers.[48] This theory is applicable to head and neck cancers and appears consistent with the pathologic findings of field cancerization. Genotypic alterations in histologically normal epithelium adjacent to invasive carcinomas have been described. Voravud and coworkers[49] found increased chromosomal polysomies in normal mucosa of smokers with invasive carcinomas but not in mucosa of healthy non-smoking volunteers. The most frequent findings in premalignant tissue are deletions of one of the two alleles at chromosomes 3p and 9p21.[50] These regions harbor tumor suppressor genes and thus may be involved with malignant transformation. It has also been observed that telomerase is activated in head and neck squamous carcinoma and dysplasia and may be an early event in the tumorigenic process.[50]

p53 is a tumor suppressor gene. A mutation in *p53* is regarded as the most common related genetic change in human cancers.[51] The normal p53 protein has a short half-life, so its detection is thought to represent *p53* mutation. Shin and colleagues[52] found *p53* expression in normal tissue and premalignant lesions adjacent to head and neck tumors but not in normal tissues from normal control patients. Numerous investigators have found overexpression of p53 protein in laryngeal carcinomas, typically in approximately half the tumors studied.[52,53] Alterations in *p53* are thought to be an important step early in the carcinogenic process but not a necessary step for all laryngeal and hypopharyngeal tumors. The finding of this protein in laryngeal specimens is also unclear, as while there are diverging study results, most investigators have not found a prognostic value to the finding of p53 protein in larynx tumor specimens.[53-56]

Other cellular changes in laryngeal carcinogenesis involve epidermal growth factor receptor (EGFR), cyclin D1, and p16. Weichselbaum and colleagues[57] described elevations in EGFR expression in head and neck tumor cell lines. In an analysis of premalignant and malignant head and neck tumor specimens, EGFR levels correlated with increasing severity of dysplasia.[58] Furthermore, Shin and colleagues[59] found elevated EGFR levels in premalignant tissues but dramatic upregulation in invasive carcinoma specimens. EGFR was amplified in DNA from 29% of sampled hypopharyngeal cancers, and it is overexpressed in at least 80% of head and neck cancers. This overexpression has been demonstrated to be an independent prognosticator in head and neck cancer.[58]

CLINICAL MANIFESTATIONS, PATIENT EVALUATION, AND STAGING

Clinical Manifestations

Hoarseness is the main presenting symptom in patients with *glottic carcinoma*. Patients with neglected advanced disease can also present with airway obstruction, pain, or dysphagia. Recurrent laryngeal nerve involvement may cause local pain or referred otalgia.

Patients with *supraglottic cancers* have differing symptomatology depending on the location of the primary lesion. Patients with false vocal cord lesions can present with hoarseness, whereas patients with epiglottic tumors can have voice changes often referred to as a supraglottic or "hot potato" voice. Patients can also present with throat pain or referred otalgia and sometimes dysphagia. On rare occasions, patients may present with an asymptomatic neck metastasis. Similar to glottic cancers, advanced tumors can cause airway obstruction and direct extension into the neck.

Patients with *hypopharyngeal cancer* usually present with throat pain with or without referred otalgia. Other symptoms include varying degree of dysphagia, ranging from the sensation of food "hanging up" in the throat to inability to swallow solids. Weight loss develops frequently in these patients who often have malnutrition and poor performance status. Hoarseness occurs with larynx invasion impairing vocal cord mobility. Due to the very high incidence of nodal involvement, patients with hypopharyngeal cancer can occasionally present with asymptomatic neck masses.

Patient Evaluation

Laryngeal Cancer

Clinical evaluation of laryngeal cancer includes indirect laryngoscopy with a mirror that is frequently supplemented by fiberoptic endoscopy (Table 32-1). Similar to other tumors in the head and neck, the examiner assesses the tumor size, morphology, infiltration (defect, distortion) of adjacent structures, and vocal cord mobility. It is important to palpate the base of the tongue to determine direct invasion from the supraglottic larynx and to look for indirect signs of preepiglottic space invasion such as fullness of the vallecula or ulceration of the infrahyoid epiglottis. A direct laryngoscopy is often the final step in evaluation. It is needed to further outline the disease extent and, in particular, to obtain biopsy specimens for tissue diagnosis.

Examination of the neck is important to detect lymphadenopathy or direct tumor extension manifesting as tenderness of the thyroid cartilage or the presence of a subcutaneous mass. Firm fullness over the thyroid notch is suggestive for preepiglottic space involvement.

Radiologic studies are indicated when there is suspicion for deep infiltration. CT (Fig. 32-3) or MRI is useful for the assessment of the preepiglottic space, tongue base, paraglottic region, and subglottis (which is sometimes difficult to evaluate from above with the mirror or fiberoptic scope). These images may help differentiate direct primary tumor extension to the soft tissue of the neck from nodal involvement. Anterior commissure lesions may have subtle thyroid cartilage invasion only detectable by CT.

Table 32-1 Evaluation of Patients With Suspected Laryngeal or Hypopharyngeal Cancer

Medical history
Physical examination
Directed examination of oral tissues, neck.
Fiberoptic laryngopharyngoscopy
Chest radiography
Thin-slice CT or MRI of the larynx
Direct laryngoscopy and biopsy of the primary tumor
*Optional examinations**
CT chest
PET scan
Barium swallow

*In patients with more advanced disease, these tests may augment the work-up for metastatic disease; PET scan and Barium studies may help better define the inferior extent of advanced hypopharyngeal cancers.

Hypopharyngeal Cancer

Evaluation of hypopharyngeal tumors is similar to that of larynx cancers. As these lesions are typically advanced, it is not uncommon to palpate disease in the neck by direct extension. The thyroid click may be lost due to anterior displacement of the larynx by a posteriorly located (particularly postcricoid) lesion. Phonation may provide better visualization of the piriform sinus on indirect mirror and fiberoptic examination. If unsuccessful, a Valsalva maneuver may open the sinus. Deep infiltrative lesions in the apex may be hard to see but are suspected by either pooling of secretions or arytenoid edema. Assessment of laryngeal mobility is important in medial wall lesions as they can invade directly into the laryngeal framework. In addition to CT (Fig. 32-4), a barium swallow is helpful in defining the inferior tumor extent.

Staging

Larynx

Tumors are staged using the American Joint Committee for Cancer TNM system (see Table 32-2).[60] The system is currently in its sixth iteration, most recently revised in 2002. The system stages larynx cancer primary tumors (T) by sites of extension and cord mobility but not size. For glottic tumors, stage T1 is disease limited to the vocal cord(s). The AJCC staging system further divides T1 glottic tumors into T1a for tumors confined to one true vocal cord and T1b for tumors involving both vocal cords. In general, this subdivision is more useful for communication and may influence the treatment decision (i.e., limited surgery versus radiation) but does not have a strong impact on prognosis. T2 glottic tumors have either supraglottic or subglottic extension, and/or impaired mobility. While not defined by the AJCC, T2 glottic lesions can be subdivided into T2a for normal mobility and T2b for impaired mobility. This subdivision is not uniformly used, however, as there is no general agreement that treatment outcomes differ among the substages.

Two significant revisions have been made to the sixth edition of the staging system. Historically, the definition of T3

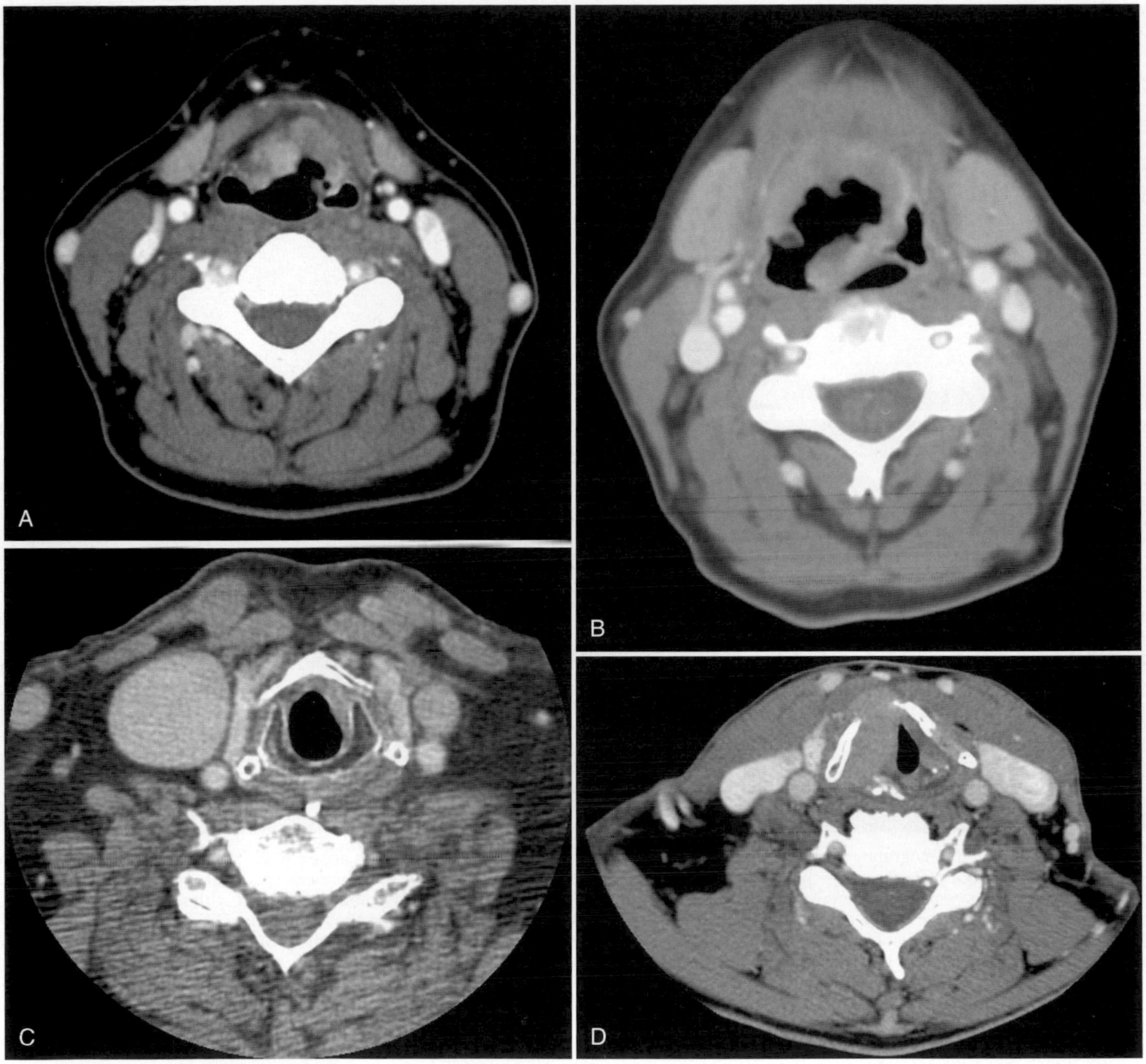

Figure 32-3 Computed tomography images of laryngeal cancers. **A,** Cancer of the supraglottis invades the preepiglottic space *(left)*. **B,** Cancer of the epiglottis with direct extension into the base of the tongue. **C,** Cancer of the true vocal cord with subglottic extension *(left)*. **D,** T4 laryngeal cancer, with destruction of the cartilage and invasion of the anterior strap muscles.

glottic disease has been fixation of the vocal cord. The most recent edition expands on this definition and includes paraglottic space invasion or minor thyroid cartilage invasion. Previous editions had defined T4 disease as invasion *through* the thyroid cartilage, but a common misinterpretation was to include any thyroid cartilage invasion into the T4 category. The new definition was made to clarify this point. The significance of this distinction is in the era of larynx preservation (see later); many still believe that the presentation of invasion through the cartilage into the extralaryngeal tissues precludes a nonsurgical approach, but patients presenting with minimal invasion into the inner cortex may have disease suitable for larynx preservation.

The second modification is the subdivision of T4 disease. For head and neck cancers in general, the new manual has subdivided stage T4 into resectable (T4a) and unresectable (T4b) categories. Thus, glottic cancer T4a disease has been defined as tumor that invades through the thyroid cartilage and/or invades tissues beyond the larynx (e.g., trachea, soft tissues of neck including deep extrinsic muscle of the tongue, strap muscles, thyroid, or esophagus), and T4b is tumor invading prevertebral space, encasing carotid artery, or invading mediastinal structures.

The staging of supraglottic cancers requires the division of the supraglottis into five subsites: the suprahyoid epiglottis, infrahyoid epiglottis, aryepiglottic folds, arytenoids, and ventricular bands (false cords). T1 disease is disease confined to one subsite (with normal vocal cord mobility). T2 disease invades more than one adjacent subsite, or region outside the supraglottis (mucosa of base of tongue, vallecula, or medial

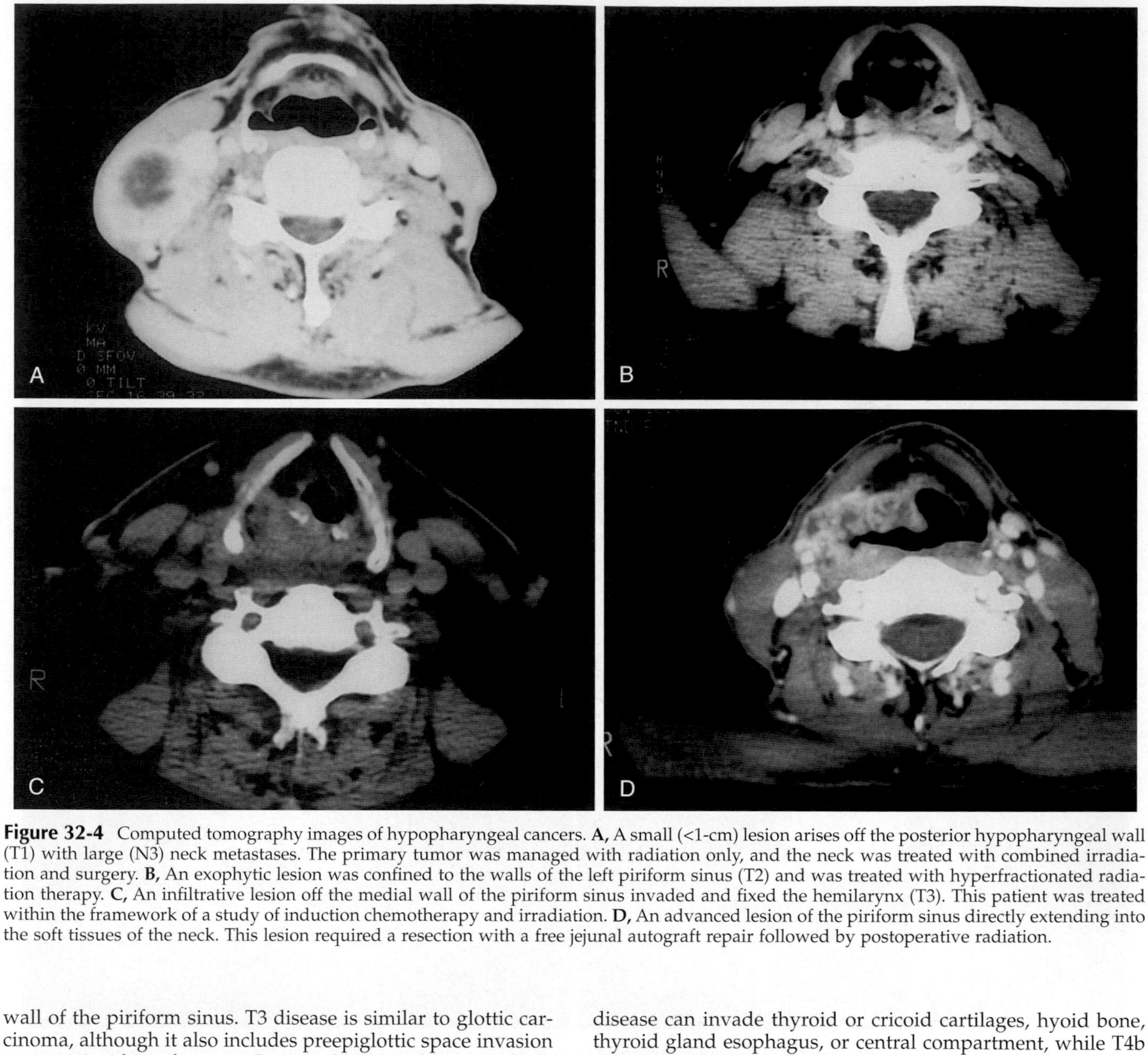

Figure 32-4 Computed tomography images of hypopharyngeal cancers. **A,** A small (<1-cm) lesion arises off the posterior hypopharyngeal wall (T1) with large (N3) neck metastases. The primary tumor was managed with radiation only, and the neck was treated with combined irradiation and surgery. **B,** An exophytic lesion was confined to the walls of the left piriform sinus (T2) and was treated with hyperfractionated radiation therapy. **C,** An infiltrative lesion off the medial wall of the piriform sinus invaded and fixed the hemilarynx (T3). This patient was treated within the framework of a study of induction chemotherapy and irradiation. **D,** An advanced lesion of the piriform sinus directly extending into the soft tissues of the neck. This lesion required a resection with a free jejunal autograft repair followed by postoperative radiation.

wall of the piriform sinus. T3 disease is similar to glottic carcinoma, although it also includes preepiglottic space invasion or postcricoid involvement. Last, in the new edition, the definition of T4 supraglottic cancer is the same as that for glottic cancer with subdivisions into resectable and unresectable (T4a and T4b) categories.

Hypopharynx

T staging for hypopharyngeal tumors is also based on sites of involvement and larynx motion (an indirect measurement of disease extension). The previous edition (fifth) had a significant modification to also include size of the tumor in staging. This change addressed a major deficiency in prior systems, as the older systems tended to understage hypopharynx tumors relative to other head and neck mucosal cancers. The hypopharyngeal T staging still does not reflect morphology, which remains an important criterion for selection of local therapies, as exophytic tumors in this site are usually selected more frequently than infiltrative lesions for organ preserving therapies. The sixth edition made one additional modification. As described for laryngeal cancers, a resectable T4a and unresectable T4b categories were defined. T4a hypopharyngeal disease can invade thyroid or cricoid cartilages, hyoid bone, thyroid gland esophagus, or central compartment, while T4b disease invades prevertebral fascia, encases carotid artery, or involves mediastinal structures.

Regional Staging

The nodal (N) staging is uniform for all head and neck cancer including laryngeal and hypopharyngeal tumors. No changes were made in the sixth edition. Table 32-2 summarizes the details of T and N stages for laryngeal (glottic and supraglottic) and hypopharyngeal cancers.

PRIMARY THERAPY

Early Carcinomas

T1 and T2 Glottic Tumors

The management of early glottic carcinomas is controversial and is often determined by the preferences and expertise of the attending physicians. Oncologists advocate either radiation or voice preserving partial laryngectomy. Large published series have for all practical purposes demonstrated equivalent

Table 32-2 AJCC (2002) Staging of Laryngeal and Hypopharyngeal Cancers

GLOTTIS	
Tis	Carcinoma in situ
T1	Tumor limited to the vocal cord(s) with normal mobility
T2	Tumor extends to supraglottis and/or subglottis and/or with impaired cord mobility
T3	Tumor limited to the larynx with vocal cord fixation and/or invades paraglottic space and/or minor thyroid cartilage erosion
T4a	Tumor invades through the thyroid cartilage, and/or invades tissues beyond the larynx
T4b	Tumor invades prevertebral space, encases carotid artery, or invades mediastinal structures
SUPRAGLOTTIS	
Tis	Carcinoma in situ
T1	Tumor limited to one subsite of the supraglottis with normal vocal cord mobility
T2	Tumor invades mucosa of more than one subsite of the supraglottis or glottis or adjacent site outside the glottis, without fixation of the larynx
T3	Tumor limited to the larynx with vocal cord fixation and/or invades any of the following: the preepiglottic space, the postcricoid area and/or minor thyroid cartilage erosion
T4a	Tumor invades through the thyroid cartilage, and/or invades tissues beyond the larynx
T4b	Tumor invades prevertebral space, encases carotid artery, or invades mediastinal structures
HYPOPHARYNX	
T1	Tumor limited to one subsite of hypopharynx, and 2 cm or less in greatest dimension.
T2	Tumor invades more than one subsite of hypopharynx or an adjacent site, or measures between 2 and 4 cm in greatest dimension, without fixation of hemilarynx.
T3	Tumor measures greater than 4 cm or with fixation of hemilarynx
T4a	Tumor invades thyroid/cricoid cartilage, hyoid bone, thyroid gland, esophagus, or central compartment soft tissue
T4b	Tumor invades prevertebral fascia, encases carotid artery, or involves mediastinal structures
NODAL INVOLVEMENT (N)	
Nx	Nodes cannot be assessed
N0	No clinically positive node
N1	Single clinically positive ipsilateral node 3 cm or less in diameter
N2	Single clinically positive ipsilateral node more than 3 cm, but not more than 6 cm in diameter or multiple clinically positive ipsilateral or bilateral or contralateral nodes, none more than 6 cm in diameter
N2a	Single clinically positive ipsilateral node more than 3 cm, but not more than 6 cm in diameter
N2b	Multiple clinically positive ipsilateral nodes, none more than 6 cm in diameter
N2c	Bilateral or contralateral lymph node, none more than 6 cm in greatest dimension
N3	Metastases in a lymph node more than 6 cm in greatest dimension
STAGE GROUPINGS	
Stage I	T1, N0, M0
Stage II	T2, N0, M0
Stage III	T3, N0, M0
	T1-3, N1
Stage IVA	T4a, N0-1, M0
	T1-4a, N2, M0
Stage IVB	T4b, N0-3, M0
	T1-4b, N3, M0
Stage IVC	T1-4, N0-3, M1

Used with permission of the American Joint Committee on Cancer (AJCC), Chicago, Illinois. The original source for this material is the AJCC Cancer Staging Handbook, ed 6, 2002, edited by Greene F, Page D, Fleming I, et al. New York: Springer-Verlag, pp. 33-57.

control rates with surgery (excision, cordectomy, or hemilaryngectomy) and radiation. There has not been a true comparative study between these two modalities, and it is highly unlikely that a prospective trial will be performed.

There are several difficulties in comparing the results of various treatment options. Nearly all series are retrospective single institutional studies. It is thus difficult to ascertain if small differences in control rates between series are real. Mendenhall and colleagues[61] address this issue by defining the surgical procedure that would have been recommended in their irradiated patients. They found that the surgical treatment option would have required total laryngectomy, rather than partial voice-conserving procedures, in 10% of patients with T1 disease and 55% of those with T2 disease. However, the supracricoid laryngectomy, a procedure that removes an entire circumferential portion of the larynx, and subsequently reconstitutes the larynx, has largely been developed during the past decade.[62] Many patients described by Mendenhall and coworkers in 1993 deemed suitable only for total laryngectomy may now be managed with this voice-preserving surgery.

In general, *T1 tumors* can be treated effectively with laser excision,[63] laryngofissure,[64] partial laryngectomy,[65,66] or radiation. Table 32-3 summarizes the results of radiotherapy. Local control rates of radiotherapy range from 85% to 95%, and ultimate control rates after salvage surgery for recurrences are greater than 95%. Surgical salvage for the uncommon local relapse often requires a total laryngectomy, but an occasional patient can have a lesion amenable to a voice-conserving partial laryngectomy.[67-71]

An important factor in selecting therapy for individual patients is the anticipated voice quality after therapy. Unfortunately, studies comparing voice quality between laser excision and radiation have yielded conflicting conclusions.

Table 32-3 Results of Radiation for T1 Carcinomas of the True Vocal Cords

First Author, Year	No. of Patients	Local Control	Salvage
Harwood, 1979[97]	333	86% (5-y A)	ND
Fletcher, 1980[109]	332	89% c	84% c
Lustig, 1984[150]	342	90% (3-y A)	ND
Olszewski, 1985[151]	137	80% c	82% c
Hendrickson, 1985[152]	364	90% c	ND
Pellitteri, 1991[153]	113	93% c	75% c
Akine, 1991[141]	154	89% c	94% c
Schwaab, 1994[71]	194	86% c	89% c
Wang, 1996[80]	665	93% (5-y A)	98% (5-y DSS)
Klintenberg, 1996[154]	129	90% c	75% c
Yu, 1997[144]	126	79% c	88% c
Le, 1997[85]	315	84% c	83% c
Warde, 1998[155]	449	91% T1a 82% T1b (5-y A)	ND
Mendenhall, 2001[86]	291	94% T1a 93% T1b (5-y A)	58% c

A, actuarial; c, crude; DSS, disease-specific survival; ND, no data.

Table 32-4 Results of Radiation for T2 N0 Glottic Carcinomas

First Author, Year	No. of Patients	Local Control	Salvage
Van den Boegart, 1983[156]	83	76% c	65% c
Lustig, 1984[150]	109	78% (3-y A)	ND
Kelly, 1984[157]	53	76% c	58% c
Hendrickson, 1985[152]	76	73% c	50% c
Karim, 1987[77]	156	78% (5-y A)	92%
Mendenhall, 1988[158]	108	75% c	74% c
Wiggenraad, 1990[81]	71	76% c	65% c
Howell-Burke, 1990[78]	114	68% c	76% c
Barton, 1992[159]	327	69% (5-y A)	ND
Schwaab, 1994[71]	65	66% c	55% c
Wang, 1996[80]	237	71-77% (5-y A)	84-92% (5-y DSS)
Klintenberg, 1996[154]	94	74% c	38% c
Le, 1997[85]	83	67% c	74% c
Warde, 1998[155]	230	69% (5-yY A)	ND

A, actuarial; c, crude; DSS, disease-specific survival; ND, no data.
Data given for T2a and T2b separately.

Hirano and associates[72] concluded in their analysis that hoarseness and incomplete glottic closure were more frequently seen in patients treated with laser. McGuirt and colleagues[73] had physicians, patients, and speech pathologists compare voice quality of patients who received radiotherapy or laser excision for early glottic cancer. They concluded that patients treated with limited excisions of tumors of the mid-cord had equivalent quality compared to those receiving radiotherapy. Using computerized assisted voice analysis, Harrison and associates[74] demonstrated that the majority of their patients irradiated for early vocal cord cancer maintained excellent voices. Mittal and colleagues[75] reported a cost savings with radiation compared to hemilaryngectomy and believed this should be an important component in treatment decisions if other important criteria are equivalent.

The outcome of radiotherapy for *T2 cancers* is, as expected, less favorable than that for T1 tumors. Local control rates range from 65% to 80%, and ultimate control rate is about 90% (Table 32-4). The wider range in the reported local control rates can, at least in part, be ascribed to a considerable heterogeneity of presentations within this stage, that is, varying from a superficial tumor spilling into the ventricle to a more bulky lesion transgressing the paraglottic space and impairing motion.

Oncologists have searched for prognostic determinants in this group of patients. Several reports showed that impairment in cord mobility adversely affects tumor control by radiotherapy (Table 32-5). Some physicians favor a hemilaryngectomy, if feasible, for T2b tumors.[65,66,76] However, Karim and colleagues[77] did not find impaired cord mobility to result in a worse outcome and attributed this observation to prescribing higher radiation doses to patients with such tumor feature. Similarly, a report from MDACC did not show a relationship between mobility and outcome, but some patients were treated with altered fractionated schedules that were theorized to have a therapeutic advantage.[78] An update of this report reinforced the lack of impact of mobility on prognosis, independent of fractionation.[79] This was contrary to the finding of Wang, who found that twice-daily radiation improved local control of T2 tumors with normal mobility but not those with impaired mobility.[80]

Several studies were also undertaken to assess the influence of impaired cord mobility on the success rate of salvage surgery for patients who developed recurrences. Schwaab and

Table 32-5 **Control of T2 Glottic Cancer as a Function of Cord Mobility**

First Author	No. of Patients (T2a/T2b)	Local Control T2a	T2b	Statistics
Harwood[160]	156/80	80% (5-y A)	52% (5-y A)	$p < .001$
Van den Boegart[156]	33/28	62%	65%	NS
Karim[77]	111/45	75-80%*	71-82%	NS
Kelly[157]	37/16	91%	50%	$p < .001$
Wiggenraad[81]	50/21	78%	71%	NS
Pellitteri[153]	34/14	80%	57%	Not given
Schwaab[71]	53/12	64%	75%	Not given
Wang[80]	145/72	77% (5-y A)	71% (5-y A)	$p = .16$
Klintenberg[154]	76/18	75% (5-y A)	60% (5-y A)	$p = .02$ NS (MV)
Le[85]	60/23	79% (5-y A)	40% (5-y A)	$p = .02$ (MV)
Mendenhall[86]	146/82	80% (5-y A)	72% (5-y A)	$p = .0003$* (MV)
Garden[79]	116/114	74% (5-y A)	70% (5-y A)	$p = .37$ (MV)

A, actuarial; NS, not significant; MV, multivariate.
*T1 patients included in stage analysis.

coworkers[71] noted difficulties in attempting salvage on a small cohort of patients presenting with T2b tumors (although, surprisingly, the initial control rate of T2b tumors in this series was better than that of T2a lesions). Wiggenraad and colleagues[81] reported ultimate control rates of 98% for T2a and 76% for T2b tumors ($p < .05$). Other groups, however, have reported equivalent ultimate local control rates for tumors with normal or impaired cord mobility.[71,79,82] Ang and Peters[83] suggested that the timeliness of diagnosis and the extent of surgery rather than the initial disease presentation might account for the difference in the salvage results.

Anterior commissure involvement was considered a potential prognostic factor because it may carry an increased risk for unsuspected thyroid cartilage invasion. However, this feature was not found to be a prognostic determinant in most recent series. Sessions and associates[84] found that anterior commissure involvement was more frequently associated with larger tumors, and it was the extent of disease rather than commissure involvement per se that impacted on outcome. Le and associates[85] found, in a multivariate analysis, that patients with anterior commissure involvement had a poorer local control rate but concluded that these patients also had a larger tumor burden and sometimes unsuspected subglottic disease. Modern high-resolution imaging techniques can detect clinically unsuspected thyroid cartilage invasion and eliminate the clinical significance of anterior commissure involvement.

Based on biologic rationale, it has been attempted to improve the control rate of T2 glottic carcinoma by increasing the total dose through hyperfractionation.[78] Two large retrospective studies have since been reported and both have suggested a trend ($p > .05$ but $< .1$) toward improved control with twice-daily treatments.[79,86] Mendenhall and coworkers[86] compared 182 patients treated with once-daily or twice-daily treatment and reported the following 5-year actuarial local control rates: T2a, 82% and 83%, respectively, and T2b, 71% and 69%, respectively. The authors contemplated that the advantages of hyperfractionation were mitigated by selection bias. Garden and colleagues[79] analyzed 230 patients, of whom 89 were treated with twice-daily fractionation. Local control rates were 79% and 67%, respectively, for patients treated with twice-daily or once-daily schedules. The authors hypothesized that while there may be a benefit to twice-daily treatment, the data more strongly favored higher daily dose as a more important treatment factor, as those patients treated with less than 2 Gy/day had control rates of 59% compared to an 80% central rate for those treated with greater than 2 Gy/day. The RTOG has completed accrual to a randomized trial designed to address this issue, but the results are still pending.

Carcinoma In Situ

Controversies of management even exist for carcinoma in situ (CIS) of true vocal cords. While not all lesions progress to invasive cancer, Hintz and colleagues[87] reported that with a watchful waiting policy nearly two thirds of patients developed invasive cancer that was not always suitable to voice-preserving therapies. Ferlito and coworkers polled otolaryngologists and found practices of management ranging from post biopsy observation, vocal cord stripping, cordectomy, open partial laryngectomy, to primary radiation.[88]

Primary radiotherapy is an effective treatment for CIS of the larynx. However, conservative surgical approaches such as microexcision, laser ablation,[89,90] or vocal cord stripping[91] are considered sufficient for the initial treatment of CIS. Repeated biopsies, strippings, or laser excisions may be counterproductive and lead to worsening of quality of voice. Radiotherapy is usually reserved for recurrences or for diffuse lesions that are not suitable for limited surgery as the first therapy.

The local control rates reported in modern series of patients with CIS treated with radiation ranges from 70% to 100% and are similar to rates described for invasive T1 disease (Table 32-6). It should be recognized that, due to limited biopsy sampling, many radiation series may include patients with unrecognized invasive disease. For example, nearly one third of the series of Pene and Fletcher diagnosed with CIS had clinical T2 disease.[92] The majority of patients developing recurrent laryngeal CIS undergo salvage surgery, most often with total laryngectomy, although some series have reported salvage with voice-preserving surgery.[93,94] Although control rates after irradiation are similar to those reported for early invasive disease, recurrences in patients with CIS take longer to manifest. Most series report median times to failure of greater than 2 years but the majority recur within 5 years of treatment.[87,92,94-97]

T1, T2, and Selected T3 Supraglottic Tumors

Similar to glottic cancer, the optimal management of supraglottic carcinomas is still being debated. Confounding the issue even more here is the necessity to manage the neck lymphatics in addition to the primary tumor. As presented earlier, nearly one third of patients with early- to intermediate-stage

Table 32-6 Results of Radiation for Carcinoma In Situ of the True Vocal Cords

First Author, Year	No. of Patients	Local Control	Salvage
Pene, 1976[92]	86	85%	92%
Sung, 1979[95]	21	90%	100%
Harwood, 1979[97]	45	90%	ND
Kalter, 1987[161]	62	100%	—
Fernberg, 1989[162]	40	90%	ND
Macleod, 1990[94]	20	70%	67%
Smitt, 1993[93]	29	93%	100%
Small Jr., 1993[163]	21	95%	0%
Wang, 1996[80]	60	92% A	98% u
Spayne, 2001[164]	67	98% A	100% u
Garcia-Serra, 2002[165]	30	88% A	100% u

A, actuarial (5-y) data; ND, no data; u, ultimate local control (5-y actuarial).

Table 32-7 Comparison of Once-Daily Versus Twice-Daily Fractionated Radiation for T2-3 Supraglottic Carcinomas

First Author, Institution	Stage	Once-Daily % Control	Twice-Daily % Control
Garden, MDACC[79,147]	T2-3a	76% (2-y A) (n = 98, 76%—T2)	80% (2-y A) (n = 102, 57%—T2)
Hinerman, UF[106]	T2	80% (crude) (n = 44)	89% (crude) (n = 65)
	T3	30% (crude) (n = 10)	66% (crude) (n = 77)
Wang, MGH[80]	T2	61% (5-y A) (n = 85)	83% (5-y A) (n = 126)
	T3	56% (5-y A) (n = 47)	71% (5-y A) (n = 136)

A, actuarial; MDACC, M.D. Anderson Cancer Center; MGH, Massachusetts General Hospital; UF, University of Florida.

supraglottic neoplasms present with palpable cervical lymphadenopathy,[40,98] and another third have subclinical nodal involvement detected by elective neck dissections.[99]

Voice-preserving treatment options for early- and intermediate-stage tumors are supraglottic laryngectomy or primary radiotherapy.[39,65,68,100-103] Local control rates in most surgical series range from 80% to 90%. Bocca and colleagues from Milan[101] reported a local control rate of 85% in one of the largest series of over 400 patients with predominantly T2 tumors. Of note is that postoperative radiation is often given to many patients undergoing partial laryngectomy. Common indications are presence of multiple nodes, extracapsular spread of nodal disease, and close or positive surgical margins. For example, 50 of 60 (83%) patients who underwent supraglottic laryngectomy at MDACC from 1974 to 1987 had indications for postoperative radiation.[39] The leading complication of supraglottic laryngectomy is aspiration, which can be morbid in heavy smokers (the majority of patients) with chronic pulmonary disease. Although preliminary data of endoscopic removal of early supraglottic lesions have been reported recently,[104,105] more experience is needed to determine its relative value.

Most surgical series selected middle-aged men who are medically fit for supraglottic laryngectomy. Hinerman and colleagues[106] analyzed 274 patients treated with primary radiation at the University of Florida and retrospectively grouped these patients into three groups: suitable for conservation surgery, anatomically suitable but medically unsuitable, and anatomically unsuitable. Using 1998 AJCC criteria, they reported that 45% of T1 patients, 36% of T2 patients, and 14% of T3 patients were suitable. Only 14% of T1 patients were anatomically unsuitable, compared to 46% and 68% of T2 and T3 patients, respectively. Of note, results with radiation for all their patients were dependent on T stage but were not dependent on suitability for conservation surgery. Similar to glottic carcinomas, the development of the supracricoid laryngectomy would alter the balance of patients with T2 and T3 patients thought to be anatomically unsuitable for conservative procedure. In a small series, Laccourreye and coworkers[107] reported on 19 patients treated with supracricoid laryngectomy. This cohort had disease in the infrahyoid epiglottis and was not suitable for more traditional conservative procedures.

In 1974, Bataini and colleagues[108] published an overall locoregional control rate of 76% for a relatively large series of patients with T1-2N0-2 supraglottic carcinomas treated with radiotherapy alone. Subsequent series reported control rates of 84% to 100% for T1 tumors.[80,109,110] Table 32-7 summarizes the outcome of radiotherapy in T2 and favorable T3 lesions. Fletcher[109] obtained a local control rate of 76% in this subset of patients by escalating the total dose of the conventional daily irradiation to 70 Gy. Application of an altered fractionation regimen during the past decade appears to have resulted in a trend toward further improvement in the local control.[80,98,110] In the DAHANCA randomized fractionation trials, the benefit of accelerated treatment for head and neck cancer in general was most noticeable in the subgroup of patients with supraglottic cancers.[111]

The impact of clinically positive nodal disease on local control has been evaluated in several series. Wall and colleagues[112] found the presence of lymphadenopathy was associated with a significantly lower local control rate. Similarly, Wang and coworkers describe a marked worsening of local control in node-positive patients. The 5-year actuarial local control rate obtained with accelerated fractionation was 86% in patients with no adenopathy as opposed to 46% in patients with N2-3 disease.[113] In contrast, Freeman and colleagues did not find an association between local control and the presence of lymph nodes.[114]

The potential impact of tumor volume, estimated by CT measurements, on the results of radiotherapy was addressed by Freeman and associates[115] in patients with T3 supraglottic tumors. They found a control rate of 83% for tumors of less than 6 cm^3 tumors compared to 46% for tumors of greater than 6 cm^3. This latter group may be more suitable for surgery, particularly if voice-conserving surgery is feasible. Kraas and coworkers[116] also studied tumor volume measurements, and while their threshold was 8 cm^3, the concept of increasing tumor volume predicting worse outcome with radiation was validated in a separate cohort.

Comparative studies have been undertaken in an attempt to delineate therapy recommendations for different subsets of patients. Fein and colleagues[103] analyzed the University of Florida experience and concluded that radiotherapy yielded a local control rate equivalent to that obtained by conservative surgery but was associated with a lower complication rate. Robbins and colleagues[100] from the MDACC compared the outcome of patients who underwent supraglottic laryngectomy with that of patients who received radiotherapy for tumors judged suitable for partial laryngectomy. They found a better tumor control rate in the surgically treated group, but the incidence of morbidity due to chronic aspiration was rather high. This finding contributed to the development of the current treatment policy at this institution. Briefly, supraglottic laryngectomy, with postoperative radiotherapy when indicated, is recommended for medically fit patients with bulky, infiltrative tumors T2-3 tumors (e.g., invasion into the false cords or infrahyoid epiglottis). Radiotherapy is selected for patients with either smaller or exophytic lesions (T2 or favorable T3) or patients with bulky lesions who are medically unfit for voice conserving surgery.

T1 and T2 Hypopharyngeal Tumors

Although uncommon, these tumors can be treated with radiotherapy. Because of the high propensity for neck metastases, it is not unusual to see patients with small-volume primary disease suitable for radiation but with large neck disease that requires multimodality treatment. In this situation, the options are to irradiate primary tumor and neck nodes to high doses and dissect the residual neck mass about 6 weeks after radiation, or to perform a neck dissection followed by definitive radiotherapy to the primary tumor and adjunctive radiation to the neck. The latter approach is frequently recommended to patients who need to undergo dental extractions requiring a delay in initiation of radiation.[117]

Some results with primary radiotherapy for early-stage hypopharynx lesions are shown in Table 32-8. Compared to historical control data, local control rates seem to have improved with the use of hyperfractionated regimens. For example, analysis of MDACC data revealed actuarial local control rates of 86% for hyperfractionation (35 patients) and 63% for conventional fractionation (23 patients).[118] Similarly, for stage T2 piriform sinus primaries, Amdur and coworkers[119] reported local control in 89% of patients treated with twice-a-day radiation compared to 73% for those treated only once per day (p = .09). While it is believed that hyperfractionation has improved the results, it should be realized that refinements in radiation technique, including customized cerrobend portal shaping, more generous coverage of the posterior route of spread, and the use of 6-MV x-rays with smaller penumbra, may all have contributed to the improvement of outcome. In addition, it is difficult to discern whether the rather subjective patient selection criteria have changed over the years and what impact this has on the results. Superficial and exophytic tumors, particularly in the vestibule, tend to be selected for primary radiotherapy, whereas infiltrative tumors of similar stage, especially in the apex, are chosen for multimodality treatment.

Management of Squamous Carcinoma Variants

Verrucous Carcinoma

Verrucous carcinoma is generally a well-differentiated, slow-growing, wart-like lesion. This tumor has a reputation for its relative radioresistance and a tendency for converting to a highly anaplastic neoplasm following radiation.[32] However, no firm data are available to support this belief. A 5-year control rate of 59% was achieved in a series of 43 patients treated with radiotherapy at the Princess Margaret.[120] The majority of these patients had early-stage disease, although over half were stage T2. The surgical salvage rate for radiation recurrences was high and only one patient died of the disease. Therefore, it is reasonable to treat patients with early verrucous carcinoma with radiation if the surgical option is a total laryngectomy. However, those with well-lateralized early tumors may be better suited for conservative surgery.

Table 32-8 **Results of Radiation Alone for Early (T1-2) Squamous Cell Carcinoma of the Hypopharynx**

First Author, Institution	Site	Stage (No. of Patients)	Control
Vandenbrouck, IGR, 1987[166]	Piriform sinus	T1 (19)	90%
		T2 (39)	78% (crude rate at 6 wk; 17% of patients subsequently recurred)
Amdur, UF, 2001[119]	Piriform sinus	T1 (22)	90% (5-y A)
		T2 (79)	80% (5-y A)
Garden, MDACC, 1996[118]	All hypopharynx	T1 (18)	89% (crude)
		T2 (46)	77% (crude)
Wang, MGH, 1997[127]	All hypopharynx	T1 (24)	74% (5-y A)
		T2 (51)	76% (5-y A)

A, actuarial; IGR, Institut Gustave-Rousy; MDACC, M. D. Anderson Cancer Center; MGH, Massachusetts General Hospital; UF, University of Florida.

Sarcomatoid Carcinoma

Sarcomatoid carcinoma of the larynx has a similar reputation for radioresistance and for dedifferentiation after radiation. In a review of 28 iradiated patients with T1-2 glottic sarcomatoid carcinoma, we found a 5-year actuarial control rate of 89%, which is similar to that obtained for ordinary squamous cell carcinoma.[121] Although the control rate for seven patients with T2 tumor was only 57%, all patients with recurrences could undergo salvage surgery and only one patient died of the disease.

Neuroendocrine Carcinoma

Neuroendocrine carcinomas of the head and neck are extremely uncommon. They can be subgrouped into three categories. The most common is small cell undifferentiated carcinoma. Moderately differentiated and well-differentiated tumors have also been described and are sometimes referred to as atypical and typical carcinoids, respectively. The latter is extremely rare. The behavior of these three subtypes is similar to their more common counterpart in the lung.

In a report[122] describing the results of patients presenting with nonsinonasal neuroendocrine cancer, we found that the majority of patients (65%) presented with laryngeal or hypopharyngeal disease. Radiation was very effective for local regional control, but most patients succumb to distant metastases. The addition of chemotherapy appeared to decrease the risk of distant failure and translated into improved survival. Our current policy is to recommend neoadjuvant chemotherapy, typically with cisplatin and VP-16 followed by radiation to the primary and lymphatics. Concurrent chemoradiation is offered to patients who have initial large primary disease or have suboptimal response to chemotherapy alone.

LOCALLY ADVANCED CARCINOMAS

These tumors have been traditionally managed with total laryngectomy with or without postoperative radiotherapy. It had been believed that while primary radiotherapy can preserve the larynx for some patients, this approach generally results in a lower survival rate than surgery does. Series describing radiation alone tended to be small, retrospective, and influenced by patient selection bias, so they were not generally accepted despite reporting results similar to surgery.

While it remains debatable whether induction chemotherapy has a role in the management of head and neck cancer, it was randomized trials using induction therapy that popularized the concept of larynx preservation. This led to the RTOG/Intergroup phase III trial 91-11, which randomized patients between three approaches: radiation alone, induction chemotherapy and local treatment based on response, and concurrent chemoradiation (see later).[123] This study added to our knowledge of the role of combined modality (concurrent chemotherapy and radiation) treatment and gave further validity to nonsurgical approaches for advanced larynx cancers.

Although tremendous advances have been made in laryngeal preservation, progress has also been made in rehabilitation of the postlaryngectomy patient. In particular, the popularity of tracheoesophageal hands-free speech has been a tremendous boon for patients. Thus, while RTOG/Intergroup 91-11 demonstrated that high larynx preservation rates can be achieved with concurrent chemotherapy and radiation, patients with large-volume T4 disease were not eligible for this approach and are still usually referred for surgery and postoperative radiation. While it may be debated whether equivalent cancer control rates can be achieved with nonsurgical approaches for very advanced larynx and hypopharynx disease, many of these patients have such vast destruction of their laryngeal structure that it would be unlikely to retain good laryngeal function even after successful therapy. In particular, this problem makes these patients at high risk of aspiration. Thus, a laryngectomy with rehabilitation may offer them a better quality of life than larynx preservation.

Randomized trials evaluating concurrent chemoradiation in the post–head and neck surgical setting have recently been reported. For patients deemed to be at high risk of locoregional recurrence, both the EORTC and RTOG/Intergroup[124,125] demonstrated that radiation and chemotherapy improve locoregional control compared to radiation alone. The definitions of high risk were different in the two studies. Approximately 30% to 40% of patients in both studies had laryngeal or hypopharyngeal cancers. Table 32-9 summarizes and contrasts the findings of these two important trials.

T3 Glottic Cancer

Most series of primary radiotherapy for *T3 glottic tumors* are relatively small. Table 32-10 summarizes the available data. Initial control rates range from 44% to 70%. Various twice-a-day fractionation schedules were found to control disease in approximately two thirds of patients.[126,127] In a comparative study, Bryant and colleagues[128] found that the disease-specific survival rate of patients treated with radiation and surgical salvage was not significantly different from that of patients who underwent surgery and, occasionally, postoperative radiation. They noted, however, that the control rate of patients requiring an emergency tracheotomy before radiotherapy was

Table 32-9 Comparison of the EORTC and RTOG/Intergroup "High-Risk" Postoperative Radiation With or Without Concurrent High-Dose Cisplatin Trials

	No. of Patients	Patient No. by Primary Site Control	Exp	Median Follow-up	Locoregional Failure Rates Control	Exp	Grade 3 Adverse Effects Control	Exp
EORTC 22931[124]	334							
Larynx		38	37	60 mo	31%	18%	21%	41%
Hypopharynx		34	34		$p = .007$*		$p = .001$	
RTOG/Intergroup[125]	459							
Larynx		44	42	46 mo	28%	18%	34%	77%
Hypopharynx		26	15		$p = .01$†		$p < .001$	

*EORTC 5-y actuarial rate.
†RTOG 2-y actuarial rate.
Exp, experimental.

Table 32-10 Results of Radiation Alone for T3 Glottic Cancer

First Author, Year	No. of Patients	Local Control	% Salvage
Lustig, 1984[150]	47	65% (3-y A)	ND
Hendrickson 1985[152]	39	56%	47%
Lundgren, 1988[167]	141	44%	59%
Croll, 1989[168]	30	70%	66%
Terhaard, 1991[169]	104*	53% (3-y A)	53%
Tennvall, 1993[170]	26*	50%	70%
Bryant, 1995[128]	55	55%	ND
Wang, 1996[80]	65	57% (5-y A)	75%
Pameijer, 1997[171]	42	62%	ND

A, actuarial; DSS, disease-specific survival; ND, no data.
*Includes all larynx.

very low (18%). Mendenhall and colleagues[126] also found similar disease-free and overall survival rates between patients treated with radiotherapy and those treated with total laryngectomy (occasionally with postoperative radiation). The success rate of salvage surgery for radiation recurrences is on average 50% but decreases with increasing initial disease extent.

Bulky Supraglottic Cancer

Most patients with *bulky, infiltrative T3 supraglottic primary tumors* (often with vocal cord fixation) have been treated with total laryngectomy with or without postoperative radiotherapy. Clinical trials addressing the role of neoadjuvant chemotherapy have enrolled predominantly this subset of patients.[129-131] The Veterans Affairs study,[129] for example, randomized patients to either surgery at the outset (standard therapy arm) or neoadjuvant chemotherapy with the responders receiving radiation and the nonresponders undergoing surgery. This trial showed that no difference in survival and larynx preservation was achieved in a substantial number of patients. However, this trial did not answer the important question of whether induction chemotherapy was more beneficial than radiation alone.

Subsequently, the RTOG/Intergroup trial 91-11 tested differing larynx preservation approaches.[123] Induction chemotherapy was the control arm, and radiation alone or combined with concurrent cisplatin were two experimental arms. The results of this trial addressed several issues. Survival rates were equivalent for all three approaches. Locoregional control and larynx preservation were superior with concurrent chemoradiation. Induction chemotherapy was not significantly better than radiation alone.

The addition of chemotherapy did increase the toxicity of treatment, principally acute toxicity. The suspected grade 5 toxicity rate in patients receiving concurrent chemoradiation was 5%, and the total rate of severe toxic effects was 20% in patients receiving chemotherapy. However, preliminary assessment of late dysphagia did not reveal an increased rate of swallowing difficulties in any treatment approach at 2 years, with all three arms reporting dysphagia rates ranging from 14% to 16%.[123]

T4 Larynx Cancer

Patients with *T4 glottic and supraglottic tumors* are best treated with total laryngectomy and radiation. The larynx preservation clinical trials testing neoadjuvant chemotherapy have not yielded encouraging results for patients with T4 disease.[129,131] Only 10% of the RTOG-Intergroup trial cohort had "T4" disease, most likely with minimal thyroid cartilage invasion that has been downstaged by the criteria of the current AJCC classification. In addition, many patients with large bulky disease often will be left with dysfunctional larynges, leading to aspiration if the therapy is successful in eradicating the tumors.

In addition to general indications of postoperative radiation in head and neck cancers (i.e., close or positive margins, multiple nodes, extracapsular spread of nodal disease, or extension of the primary lesion into the soft tissues of the neck), post total laryngectomy radiotherapy is also recommended when thyroid/cricoid cartilage invasion and extensive subglottic disease are present or emergency tracheotomy is performed before radiotherapy. In a series of Klein and Fletcher,[132] stomal recurrence occurred in 13 of 54 patients (24%) with radiological evidence of subglottic disease who did not receive postoperative radiotherapy. None of these patients was salvaged. Yuen and coworkers[133] analyzed the data of patients with T3 and T4 glottic lesions and found that surgery alone achieved locoregional control in 90% of patients without adverse features listed above compared to 73% of those with some of the adverse features; with surgery and postoperative radiation locoregional control was obtained in 46 of 50 patients (92%). In patients with stage IV supraglottic cancer, Goepfert and colleagues reported a 2-year determinate control rate of 37% for surgery alone as opposed to 63% for combined surgery and postoperative radiotherapy.[134]

Locally Advanced Hypopharynx Cancer

Surgery is the treatment of choice for patients with *T3-4 hypopharyngeal cancer*, but adjuvant adjuvant radiation is almost always indicated. Vandenbrouck and colleagues[135] performed a randomized trial comparing preoperative and postoperative radiation in the treatment of hypopharyngeal tumors. They reported a statistically better 5-year survival rate in patients treated postoperatively (56%) compared to those treated preoperatively (20%). Table 32-11 lists the results of postoperative radiotherapy. Analyzing a series of patients treated between 1949 and 1976, El Badawi and coworkers found that patients who received surgery and radiation had significantly higher local control and 5-year survival rates than those who underwent surgery alone.[136] Frank and colleagues[137] found that, despite having higher stages, patients who received postoperative irradiation had only a 14% locoregional failure rate compared to 57% in those treated with surgery only. When adjusted for confounding variables, particularly the stage discrepancy, they also found that patients receiving postoperative irradiation had an improvement in overall survival.

The issue of larynx preservation in hypopharyngeal cancer has been addressed in an European Multi-institutional (EORTC) Phase III trial.[138] Similar to the trial of Veterans Affairs in the United States for larynx cancer, the EORTC compared induction chemotherapy, followed by radiation or

Table 32-11 Results of Postoperative Radiation for Piriform Sinus Tumors

First Author, Year	No. of Patients	Failure Above Clavicle	Actuarial Survival
El Badawi, 1982[136]	125	14 (11%)	40% (5-y)
Mendenhall, 1987[172]	65	32 (49%)	28% (5-y)
Vandenbrouck, 1987[166]	199	35 (18%)	33% (5-y)
Frank, 1994[137]	35	5 (14%)	55% (3-y†)
Slotman, 1994[173]	32	5 (16%)	22% (5-y)
Lefebvre, 1996[138]	94*	25 (27%)	43% (5-y)

*Intent to treat—only 89 patients received postoperative irradiation.
†Estimated from curve.

surgery depending on the response, with immediate total laryngectomy and partial pharyngectomy. The 5-year actuarial voice preservation rate was 35% in patients receiving chemotherapy and there was no difference in the survival rate among the two arms.

Patients with locally advanced hypopharynx cancer may be suitable for therapy with concurrent chemoradiation. These patients have often been included in trials in which the eligibility has been broad and included patients with locally advanced cancers of multiple head and neck sites.[139,140] In most studies, as a subgroup, hypopharyngeal cancers represent a minority of patients. These studies have demonstrated an advantage to concurrent chemoradiation, and none of the studies has suggested that this general conclusion does not apply to locally advanced hypopharyngeal cancers. With regard to organ preservation for patients with locally advanced hypopharynx cancer, the same principles used for patient selection of larynx cancer should be applied.

TECHNIQUES OF IRRADIATION

Primary Radiotherapy

T1-2 N0 Glottic Carcinomas

T1-2 N0 glottic carcinomas are treated with a pair of small, lateral, opposed photon fields that encompass only the larynx proper (Fig. 32-5). In patients with a short neck, a 5- to 10-degree inferior tilt may be necessary to avoid irradiation through the shoulders. Other techniques include anterior wedged pairs or a four-field technique as described by Wang.[80] For T1 lesions the field is centered on the true vocal cord and extends at or above the top of the thyroid notch superiorly to the lower edge of the cricoid cartilage inferiorly and from the anterior margin of the vertebral bodies posteriorly to approximately 1-cm fall-off anteriorly. The superior and inferior borders are adjusted for T2 lesions that extend out of the glottis. When there is subglottic disease at least one tracheal ring must be included in the fields. Typical field sizes range from 25 cm^2 (5 × 5 cm) to 36 cm^2 (6 × 6 cm). Harwood and associates[97] reported better results with larger fields but acknowledged that at the time they used a free setup that likely accounted for some cases of geographic misses.

It is proper to use cobalt-60 gamma rays for treating glottic cancer, as higher-energy beams (6 MV or greater) may underdose the anterior commissure region, particularly in thin patients. Most radiation oncology centers nowadays no longer have cobalt-60 units, and thus rely on linear accelerators. Local control rates of over 90% have been obtained for T1 lesions treated with 6 MV photons.[141,142] Sombeck and colleagues performed a dosimetric comparison between cobalt-60 and 6-MV beams and found a similar dose distribution except for the most anterior tissues (3 mm below the surface) where underdosing occurred with the 6-MV beam.[143] Consequently, these authors cautioned against using the 6-MV beam for anterior commissure lesions. However, advocates of 6-MV photons for glottic cancer recommend either using tissue equivalent bolus material for build-up or using a beam spoiler for thin patients or patients with anterior lesions.[142]

A contour or CT plan is obtained to evaluate the dose distribution and determine the need for wedges (Fig. 32-6). Fifteen- or 30-degree wedges are often used and improve the dose distribution to the vocal cord, particularly for mid and posterior lesions. Treating without wedges results in a less homogeneous distribution, but this may be advantageous for anterior lesions where the built-in dose differential (5% to 10%) is desirable. Unilateral lesions can be treated by unequally weighting (e.g., 3:2) the fields favoring the side of the lesion.

Radiation doses range from 60 to 70 Gy given in 2-Gy fractions. In general, a dose of 60 Gy is given to patients with no obvious clinical disease after stripping, 66 Gy to those with bulky T1, and 68 to 70 Gy to patients with T2 lesions. Most centers deliver 2 Gy per day, five fractions a week. Several studies evaluating the importance of dose per fraction principally for T1 disease show that 2 Gy per fraction yields better control rates than 1.8 Gy per treatment (Table 32-12). Some centers even advocate the use of larger fraction sizes.[144] As described above, there are strong suggestions from multiple studies that for T2 lesions, 1.2 Gy fractions of twice-daily radiation to 74.4 to 79 Gy are appropriate. If hyperfractionation is not feasible, daily fractions of greater than 2 Gy per day result in superior outcomes to smaller daily doses.

Radiation treatment of early glottic cancers with small fields rarely induces severe complications. Fletcher and Goepfert[109] described a 1% crude incidence of late edema in patients treated from 1962 through 1979. An analysis of late complications in 230 patients with T2 tumors revealed a 4% incidence of severe complications.[79] The complications were five cases of dysfunctional larynx and/or chondronecrosis requiring tracheotomy, one case of reversible laryngeal edema, and four cases of postoperative complications related to salvage.

T3 N0 Glottic, T1-3 Supraglottic, T any N Glottic, or Hypopharynx

T3N0 glottic and T1-3N0 supraglottic carcinomas are treated with parallel, opposed, lateral portals covering the primary tumor and the subdigastric and midjugular lymph nodes. A matching anterior portal (with superior midline block to prevent overlap on the spinal cord) encompassing the lower jugular and supraclavicular lymph nodes is also used (Figs. 32-7 to 32-9). *Hypopharyngeal cancers* and larynx carcinomas with nodal involvement are treated with larger lateral portals covering the primary disease and the upper and midjugular nodes (under the insertion of the sternocleidomastoid muscle) and a matching anterior portal encompassing lower jugular and supraclavicular lymph nodes. For hypopharyngeal tumors, the inferior border must cover the entire piriform sinus

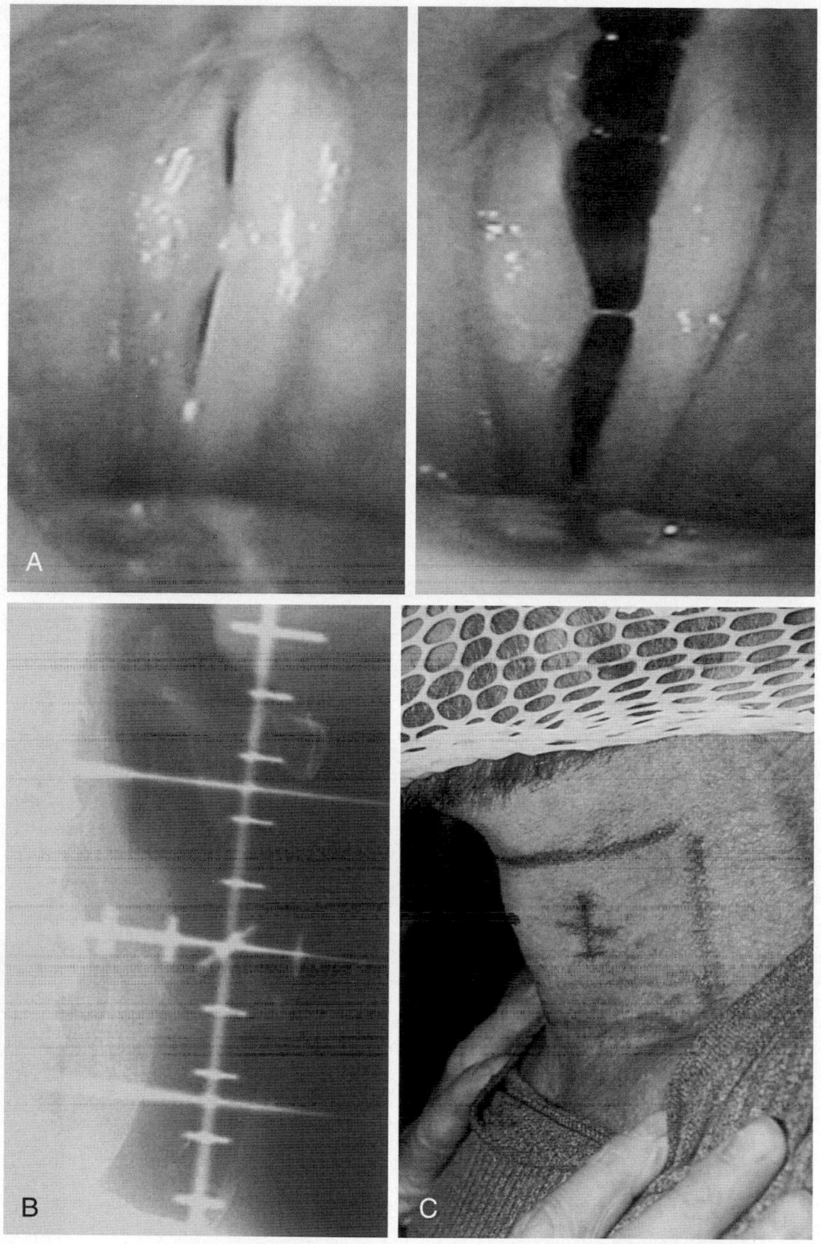

Figure 32-5 **A,** T1 glottic cancer. **B,** Simulation radiograph of a 5 × 5 cm field covering the glottis only for treatment of an early glottic tumor. **C,** Field for a T1 glottic cancer is outlined on the patient's skin.

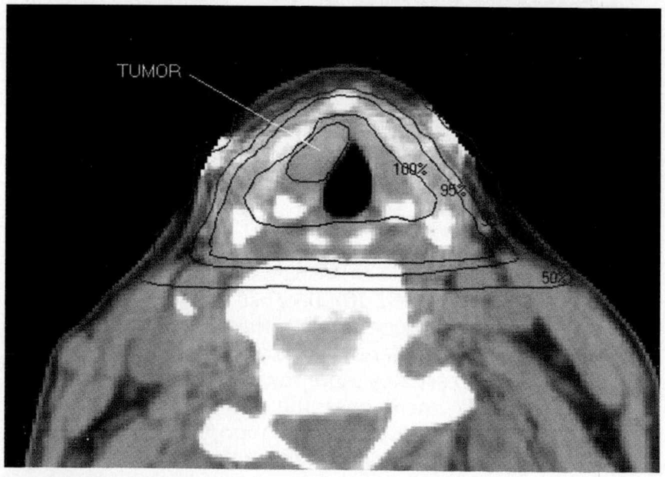

Figure 32-6 Dosimetry of parallel-opposed fields for early glottic carcinoma. Parallel-opposed, 5 × 5 cm fields were used with 30-degree wedges (heel anterior).

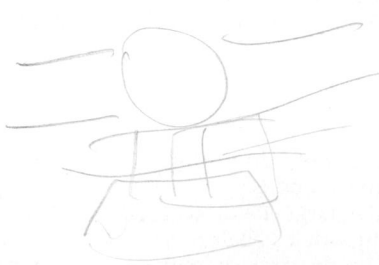

Table 32-12 Results of Radiation for T1 Glottic Tumors by Fraction Size

First Author, Year	No. of Patients	Control Rate by Fraction Size	*p* Value
Schwaibold, 1988[174]	56	1.8 Gy: 75% 2.0 Gy: 100%	<.01
Mendenhall, 1988[175]	75	2.0-2.2 Gy: 88% 2.25-2.3 Gy: 96%*	None
Kim, 1992[176]	85	1.8 Gy: 79% 2.0 Gy: 96%	.05
Rudoltz, 1993[177]	91	2.0 Gy: 62% ≥2.0 Gy: 87%	.006
Ricciardelli, 1994[178]	42	1.8 Gy: 70% 2.0 Gy: 100%	<.01
Yu, 1997[144]	126	2.0 Gy: 66% 2.25-2.5 Gy: 84%	.03
Burke, 1997[179]	100†	<2.0 Gy: 44% ≥2.1 Gy: 92%	<.01
Le, 1997[85]	315	<1.8 Gy: 79% ≥1.8 Gy: 81-94%	.05‡

*Control in patients receiving > 60 Gy.
†Includes T1 and T2 patients.
‡Tested continuous variable.

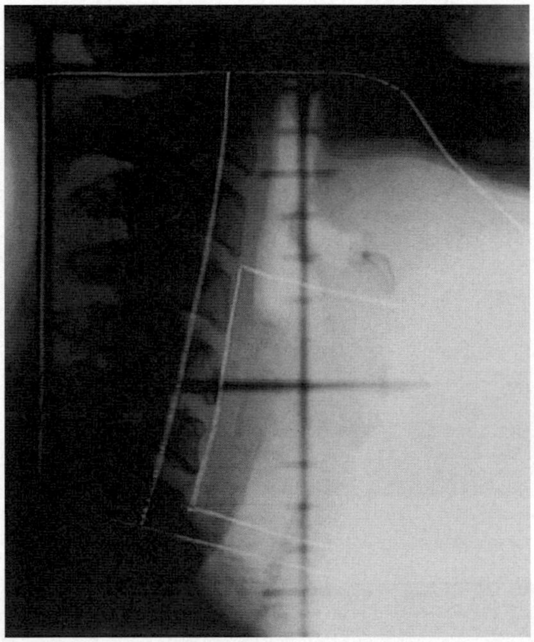

Figure 32-7 This 55-year-old man had squamous cell carcinoma of the right true vocal cord. The entire cord was involved, and there was subglottic extension. The cord was fixed, and the patient's disease was staged as T3 N0 M0. He received 70 Gy in 35 fractions with the shrinking fields shown and has been without disease for 30 months after therapy.

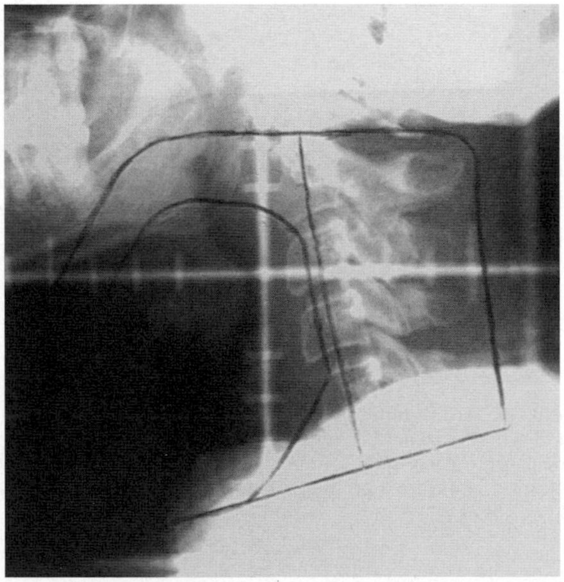

Figure 32-8 A 57-year-old woman presented with right otalgia and had a biopsy-proven squamous cell carcinoma of the epiglottis with extension of disease onto the aryepiglottic fold. The staging was T2 N0 M0, and she received 76.8 Gy at 1.2 Gy per fraction to the fields shown. She remains without evidence of disease.

including the apex (Fig. 32-10). Because of the posterior location of the majority of these tumors, the off–spinal cord fields extend slightly more posteriorly than for other head and neck primaries. This necessitates more frequent portal verification. It is important to encompass the retropharyngeal lymph nodes generously in patients with hypopharyngeal tumors. However, supraglottic lesions invading the medial wall of the piriform sinus only do not necessitate wide coverage of the retropharyngeal nodes.

The initial large field, on-cord radiation can be accomplished with either cobalt-60 gamma rays or 6-MV photons depending on the neck diameter and the depth of the nodes. It is preferable to irradiate thick patients and those with deep-seated neck nodes with 6-MV beams. The off-cord and boost irradiations are administered with 6-MV beam with delivery of supplemental dose to the posterior cervical nodes overlying the spinal cord with proper electron beams.

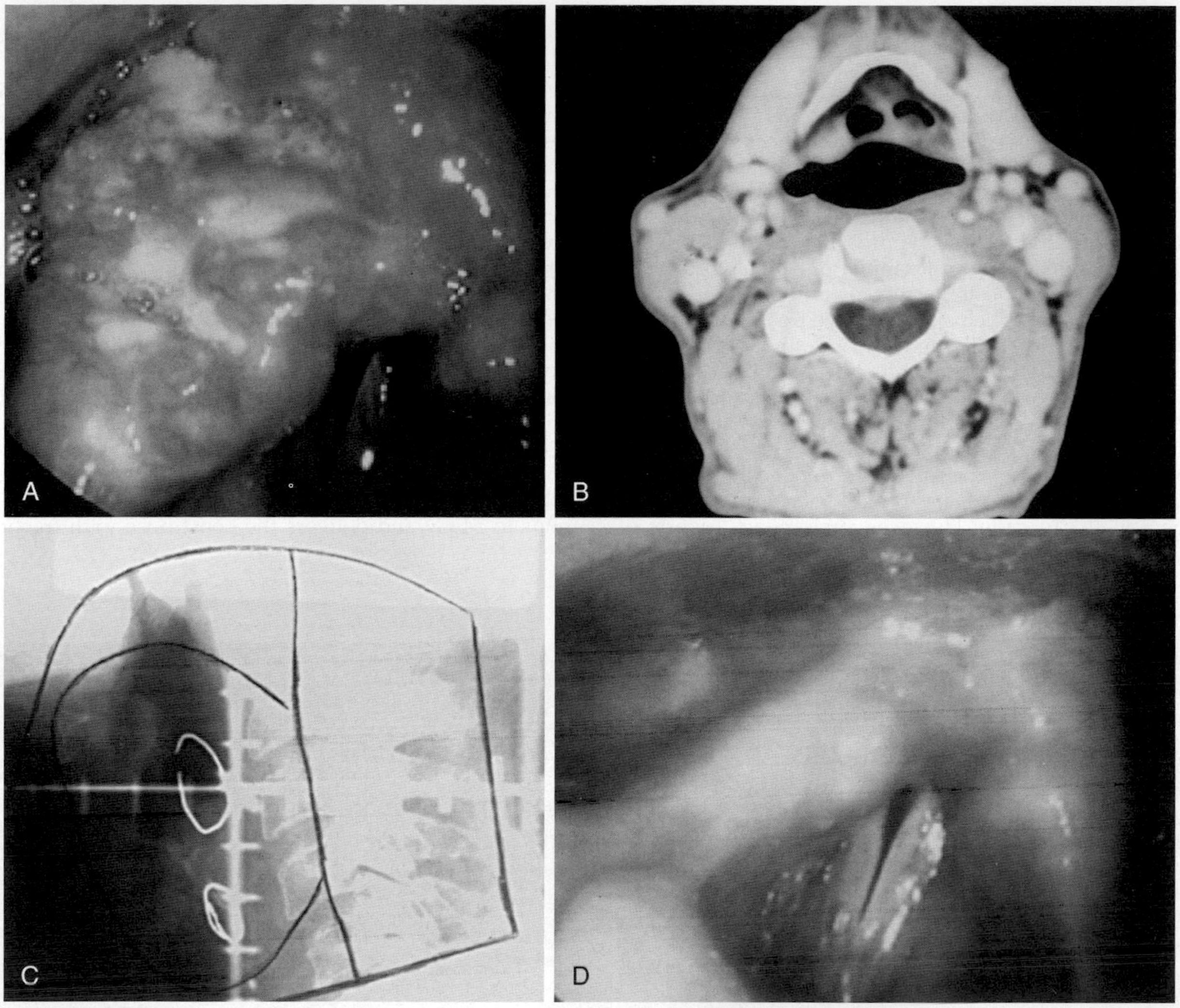

Figure 32-9 **A,** A 65-year-old woman presented with a bulky, exophytic squamous cell carcinoma of the right aryepiglottic fold. **B,** Two affected midjugular lymph nodes were detected on examination. **C,** She received hyperfractionated radiation to the fields shown. **D,** She had no evidence of disease 9 years later.

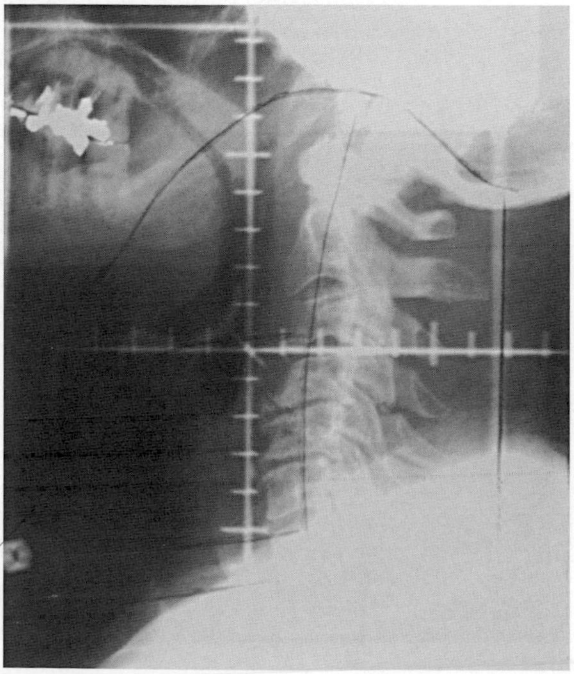

Figure 32-10 This 74-year-old man had a biopsy-proven squamous cell carcinoma arising from the medial wall of the right piriform sinus. The lesion was 1 cm in diameter. The patient's disease was staged T1N0M0. He received 66 Gy in 33 fractions. The initial fields included draining lymphatics and retropharyngeal nodes; an off–spinal cord reduction was made at 42 Gy, and the large fields continued to 50 Gy. A final reduction was made to the total dose. The patient remained without evidence of disease until his death 8 years later.

The use of "angled-down" or caudally oriented beams was described several decades ago. This technique has an advantage when the patient has a short neck. The rapid and recent developments in three-dimensional planning with either tissue compensators or step-and-shoot techniques to correct for dose heterogeneity have led to an increasing popularity in this approach. When using this technique we prefer treating the initial on-spinal cord fields with small (10-degree) posterior tilts in addition to the caudal tilts on the beams. This helps to minimize treatment through the shoulders. Typically, though, the off–spinal cord fields are treated without posterior tilts to minimize concerns regarding the electron matches in the posterior cervical regions. An example of this beam arrangement is shown in Figure 32-11.

Treatment of head and neck cancer with intensity-modulated radiation (IMRT) has rapidly increased during the early part of this decade. However, preliminary reports of IMRT have focused on treatment of nasopharynx and oropharynx cancer. In trials reporting more general head and neck results, the percentage of patients with laryngeal or hypopharyngeal cancers is extremely low.[145,146] The advantages of this modality remain theoretical for these diseases. However, particularly for hypopharyngeal cancers or patients with extensive nodal disease, the appeal of IMRT for potentially reducing xerostomia exists. An example of selected target delineation and isodose distributions for a patient with advanced supraglottic cancer is shown in Figure 32-12.

Patients with T1 disease usually receive daily 2-Gy fractions to 64 to 68 Gy and those with T2-3 lesions receive either daily 2-Gy fractions to 70 Gy, although preferably are treated with either hyperfractionated twice-daily radiation with fraction size of 1.2 Gy to 76.8 Gy or, alternatively, are treated with an accelerated schedule such as concomitant boost. This latter schedule treats patients to their large fields with 1.8-Gy fractions to 54 Gy and delivers the boost dose with fraction size

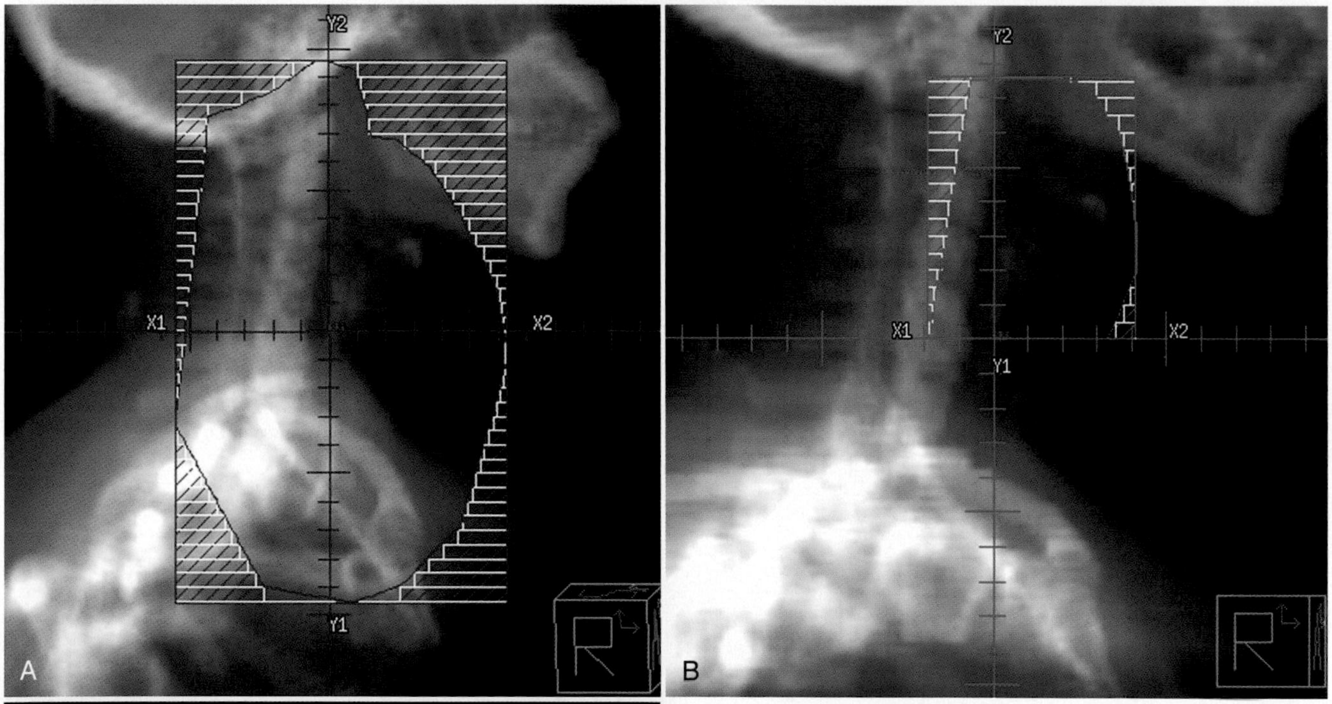

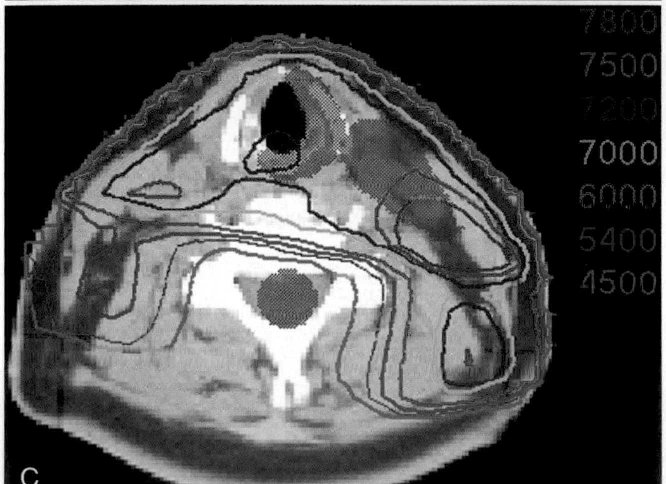

Figure 32-11 A 49-year-old woman with biopsy-proven stage T4N2b hypopharyngeal cancer is treated with irradiation. **A,** The initial treatment portals are right and left caudally and posteriorly oriented fields. **B,** After off–spinal cord reduction, the boost fields are parallel-opposed right anterior and left posterior oblique fields. **C,** A representative isodose distribution is shown.

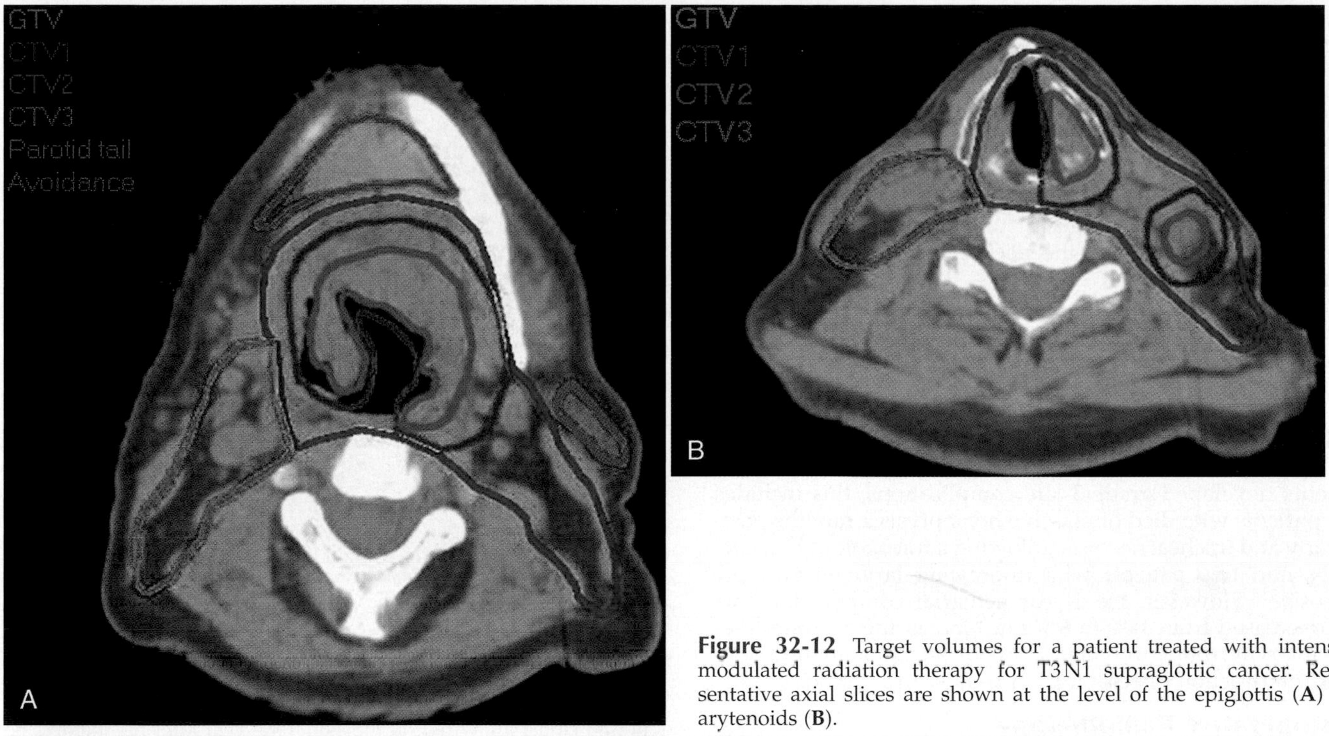

Figure 32-12 Target volumes for a patient treated with intensity-modulated radiation therapy for T3N1 supraglottic cancer. Representative axial slices are shown at the level of the epiglottis (**A**) and arytenoids (**B**).

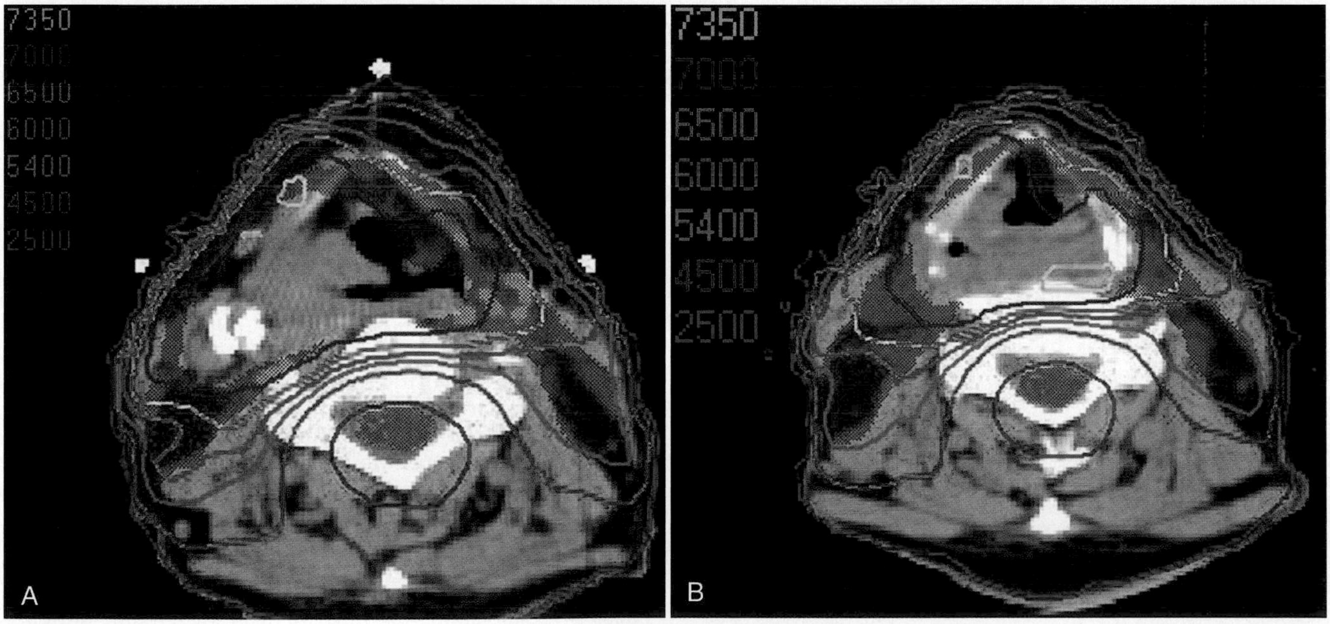

Figure 32-13 Isodose distributions on axial CT images of a patient with T3 carcinoma of the hypopharynx treated with concurrent chemotherapy and intensity-modulated radiation therapy. Representative slices through the vestibule (**A**) and apex (**B**) of the piriform sinus are shown. The high-dose target volume for gross disease and the margin (CTV1) is transparent so the underlying tumor can be visualized. CTV1 was planned to 70 Gy, and CTV2 *(blue)* was planned to 50 Gy. Treatment was planned with two sequential plans so that both targets would be fractionated at 2 Gy per fraction.

of 1.5 Gy/fraction during the last 2.5 weeks as a second daily fraction to bring the total dose to gross disease to 72 Gy delivered in 6 weeks. Portal size is reduced to encompass the gross primary disease with 1- to 2-cm margins after reaching an elective dose of 50 Gy (2-Gy fractions) to 54 (1.8-Gy fractions) or 55.2 Gy (1.2-Gy fractions) (Fig. 32-13).

Two common strategies applied for the treatment of involved nodes are to administer preoperative dose to the nodes followed by nodal dissection 4 to 6 weeks after completion of radiation or to irradiate the nodes to the same dose as the primary tumor and perform nodal dissection only in patients with incomplete regression. The advantage of the second strategy is that a neck dissection can be avoided in the majority of patients who achieve a complete response. The disadvantage is that patients who do need surgery have a more difficult procedure, often requiring a tracheotomy due to the high doses the tissues received. As mentioned above, occasionally in patients presenting with small primary lesions but large adenopathy who need full mouth dental extraction, nodal dissection may be performed during the same anesthesia. Subsequently, the primary tumor can be treated with definitive radiation while the neck receives adjuvant postoperative radiation.

Because of larger radiation volume, radiotherapy of supraglottic and hypopharyngeal tumors induces a higher complication rate than treatment of early stage glottic carcinomas. Mendenhall and associates[110] have reported a 6% severe acute and late complication rate in 211 patients receiving primary radiotherapy for supraglottic carcinomas. In a series of 236 patients treated with hyperfractionation at MDACC, 21 patients developed grade 3 late complications; this includes two patients who died of massive hemoptysis 2 months posttherapy and tracheal necrosis following a tracheotomy, respectively, and two patients who underwent laryngectomy for necrosis.[147] However, the 3-year actuarial complication rate has decreased from 14% to 8% since increasing the interfraction interval from 4 to 6 hours. We currently maintain the 6-hour interfraction interval for twice-daily irradiation.

Postoperative Radiotherapy

The technique for postoperative radiotherapy is similar to that of primary radiation. Briefly, initial fields cover the operative and tumor bed. Patients with adverse features requiring postoperative radiation are at increased risk for stomal failure. Patients are typically treated with a three-field technique, two lateral-opposed fields and an anterior low-neck portal (Fig. 32-14). The inferior borders of the lateral fields are in close proximity or even include the superior aspect of the stoma. The stoma itself is included in the anterior low-neck field. Occasionally it is complicated to find the ideal location for the match due to the stomal location. Caudally oriented fields as described above will often provide a simple solution for this problem and obviate concerns regarding matching through the stoma or needing to block the stoma for safety reasons.

The operative bed is treated to 57.6 Gy and areas of increased risk are boosted to 63 Gy given in 1.8-Gy fractions[148] or 56 Gy and 60 Gy, respectively, given in 2-Gy fractions. No dose reduction is applied for patients who have had free jejunal autograft reconstruction, as no significant complications have been observed in a series of 29 patients treated to these doses.[149] The dose delivered to surgically undisturbed elective sites is 50 to 54 Gy. The stoma is treated to 50 Gy, and boosted only if there was extensive paratracheal or soft tissue extension in the region of the stoma.

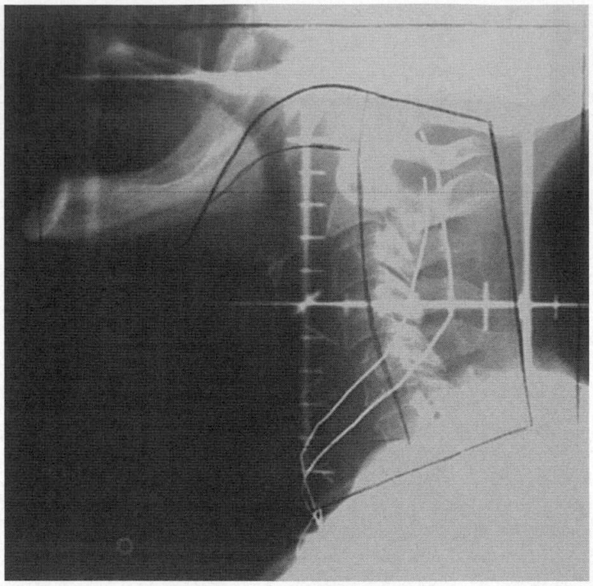

Figure 32-14 A 46-year-old man was diagnosed with squamous cell carcinoma of the right piriform sinus. He underwent a laryngopharyngectomy with jejunal autograft for repair. The tumor was 6 cm in the largest dimension, and it had invaded the soft tissues of the neck. He received postoperative radiation of 60 Gy to the fields shown. The scar and stoma are wired on the skin. One year after his therapy, he developed pulmonary metastases and died with metastatic disease.

TREATMENT ALGORITHM, CONTROVERSIES, CHALLENGES, AND FUTURE POSSIBILITIES

Treatment Algorithm

Stage Tis, T1, T2 tumors—These tumors nearly always can be treated with a single modality—either voice-sparing surgery or radiation.

Infiltrative T2 hypopharyngeal tumors may be considered similar to T3 disease.

Stage T3—Options include either total laryngectomy (with pharyngectomy for hypopharyngeal primary) or a voice-preservation approach. Concurrent cisplatin and radiation has been demonstrated to result in higher rates of larynx preservation than neoadjuvant chemotherapy or radiation alone and is usually the treatment of choice, although it does have a modest toxicity profile. Radiation alone is an option for selected patients who may desire larynx preservation but are deemed medically unsuitable for chemotherapy.

Stage T4—Surgery with adjuvant postoperative radiation management remains the treatment of choice. Patients considered to have high-risk features (inadequate surgical margins or soft tissue spread of disease) may require concurrent chemoradiation in the adjuvant postoperative setting. Highly selected T4 patients may be treated similar to T3 disease using concurrent chemoradiation in an attempt at larynx preservation.

Stage N1—If radiation is used for treating the primary, surgery is reserved for residual mass. If surgery is chosen for primary treatment, then neck dissection is performed and radiation is used if there is extracapsular extension.

Stage N2-N3—Combined surgery and radiation is used for the neck disease and sequencing chosen based on the preferred modality for treatment of the primary.

Stage M1—Systemic therapies are used for patients with good performance status; local therapies are provided for palliation if required.

A treatment algorithm for laryngeal and hypopharyngeal cancer is shown in Figure 32-15.

Controversies, Challenges, and Future Possibilities

The past two to three decades have seen seminal trials performed to maximize gains to preserve the larynx in patients requiring treatment for laryngeal and hypopharyngeal carcinoma. Ultimately, the concept of larynx preservation was vaguely defined. Trials designed with a primary end point of

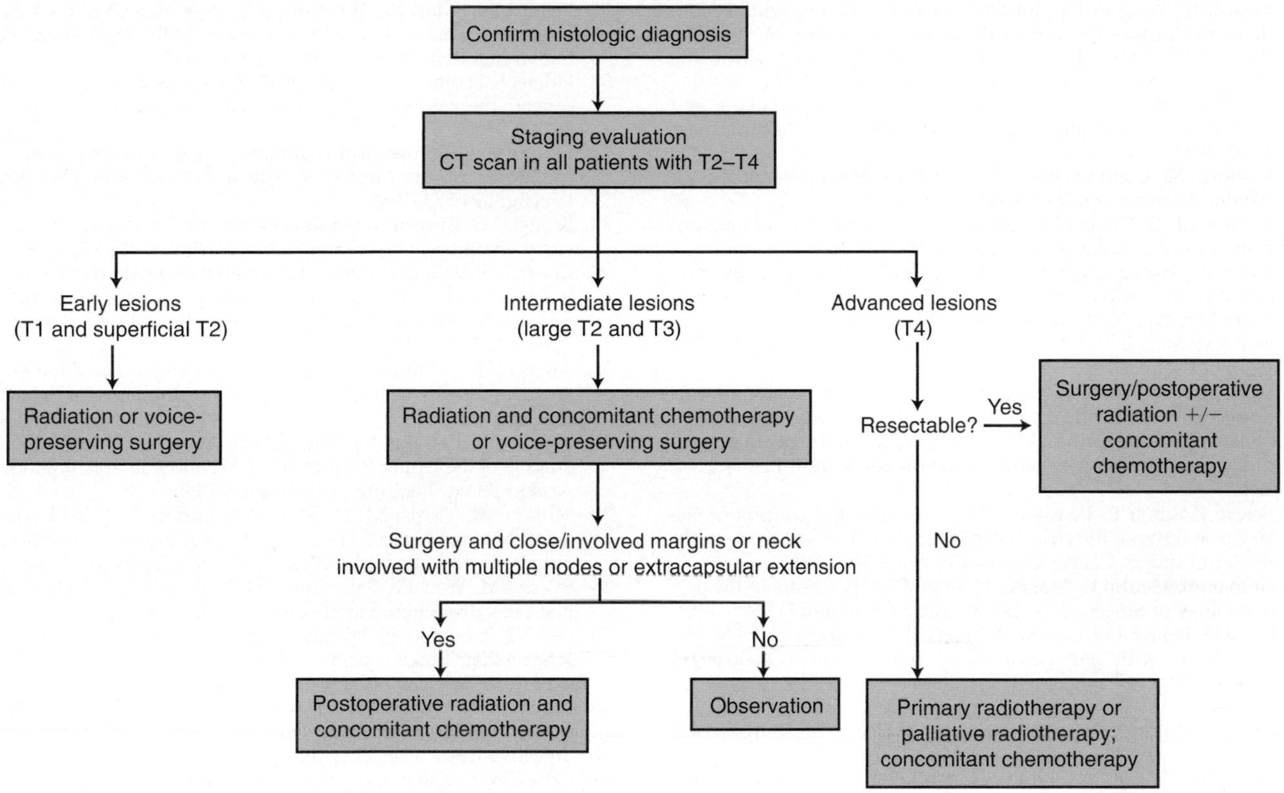

Figure 32-15 **Treatment algorithm for patients with cancer of the larynx or hypopharynx.**

an intact larynx ignored the multiple functions in addition to voice that the larynx provided, particularly swallowing functions (at least with regards to the primary end points). Thus, while in 2004 it can be proclaimed that high-dose cisplatin delivered concurrently with radiation is the standard of care for managing advanced larynx cancer, this conclusion should be accompanied with caveats.

Future directions depend on both our continued understanding of the disease and a better understanding of the impact our therapies have on the laryngopharyngeal structures and how alterations from either disease or therapy impact quality of life. To date, several decades of investigations have not necessarily improved survival rates but have made assumptions that we have improved quality of life in our patients, as we have preserved the larynx in many patients that otherwise would have been treated with laryngectomy. What is required is developing treatments with less toxicity or better prediction models of either the efficacy (with regard to the cancer) of varying treatments in specific individuals or the impact a treatment will have in an individual with regard to function.

In cancer therapy in general, there has been great interest in targeted therapy with the use of biologic agents. In head and neck cancer, the EGFR has been attractive as a target, and preliminary results with concurrent radiation and EGFR blockade have been interesting in terms of potential enhancement of radiation response without an increase in tissue toxicity. In patients who have high levels of EGFR with larynx cancer, this approach has great theoretical appeal in lieu of concurrent radiation and chemotherapy. Future directions in larynx cancer may actually have a deintensification of therapy for selected patients in whom an effective therapy can be selected with less toxicity.

Additional directions will be in better understanding which patients will, after effective tumoricidal therapy, have a functioning larynx and which patients will be subject to chronic aspiration or swallowing dysfunction. The full integration of speech and swallowing assessments prior to treatment disposition is becoming a critical component in the treatment selection process.

Laryngeal carcinoma (and, to a lesser extent, hypopharyngeal carcinoma) is a curable disease. Great challenges remain, though. We still need to understand which subgroups still do not benefit from their selected therapies and have disease relapse and determine if we can further improve survival rates by selecting the appropriate treatment in these patients. In the remaining patients who can be cured, we need to determine the least toxic approaches and continue to explore second primary cancer prevention, as the development of less curable malignancies remains an obstacle to prolonged survival in this patient population.

REFERENCES

1. Ries LAG, Eisner MP, Kosary CL, et al (eds): SEER Cancer Statistics Review, 1997-2002. Bethesda, MD, National Cancer Institute, 2005.
2. Wydner EL: Toward the prevention of laryngeal cancer. Laryngoscope 85:1190, 1975.

3. Muscat JE, Wydner EL: Tobacco, alcohol, asbestos, and occupational risk factors for laryngeal cancer. Cancer 69:2244, 1992.
4. Wydner EL, Bross IJ, Day E: Epidemiological approach to the etiology of cancer of the larynx. JAMA 160:1384, 1956.
5. Freudenheim JL, Graham S, Byers TE, et al: Diet, smoking and alcohol in cancer of the larynx: a case-control study. Nutr Cancer 17:33, 1992.
6. Rothman KJ, Cann CI, Flanders WD, Fried MP: Epidemiology of laryngeal cancer. Epidemiol Rev 2:195, 1980.
7. Wydner EL, Stellman SD: Comparative epidemiology of tobacco-related cancers. Cancer Res 37:4608, 1977.
8. Burch JD, Howe GR, Miller AB, Semenciw R: Tobacco, alcohol, asbestos, and nickel in the etiology of cancer of the larynx: a case-control study. J Natl Cancer Inst 67:1219, 1981.
9. Stell PM, McGill T: Asbestos and laryngeal cancer. Lancet 2:416, 1973.
10. Merletti F, Heseltine E, Saracci R, et al: Target organs for carcinogenicity of chemicals and industrial exposures in humans: a review of results in the IARC monographs on the evaluation of the carcinogenic risk of chemicals to humans. Cancer Res 44:2244, 1984.
11. Esteve J, Riboli E, Pequignot G, et al: Diet and cancers of the larynx and hypopharynx: the IARC multi-center study in southwestern Europe. Cancer Causes Control 7:240, 1996.
12. Graham S, Mettlin C, Marshall J, et al: Dietary factors in the epidemiology of cancer of the larynx. Am J Epidemiol 113:675, 1981.
13. Freije JE, Beatty TW, Campbell BH, et al: Carcinoma of the larynx in patients with gastroesophageal reflux. Am J Otolaryngol 17:386, 1996.
14. Morrison MD: Is chronic gastroesophageal reflux a causative factor in glottic carcinoma? Otolaryngol Head Neck Surg 99:370, 1988.
15. Ward PH, Hanson DG: Reflux as an etiologic factor of carcinoma of the laryngopharynx. Laryngoscope 98:1195, 1988.
16. Bacciu A, Mercante G, Ingegnoli A, et al: Effects of gastroesophageal reflux disease in laryngeal carcinoma. Clin Otolaryngol Allied Sci 29:545, 2004.
17. Syrjanen S: Human papillomavirus (HPV) in head and neck cancer. J Clin Virol 32(Suppl 1):S59, 2005.
18. Hobbs C, Birchall M: Human papillomavirus infection in the etiology of laryngeal carcinoma. Curr Opin Otolaryngol Head Neck Surg 12:88, 2004.
19. Cooper JS, Pajak TF, Rubin P, et al: Second malignancies in patients who have head and neck cancer: incidence, effect on survival and implication based on the RTOG experience. Int J Radiat Oncol Biol Phys 17:449, 1989.
20. Fijuth J, Mazeron JJ, Le Pechoux C, et al: Second head and neck cancers following radiation therapy of T1 and T2 cancers of the oral cavity and oropharynx. Int J Radiat Oncol Biol Phys 24:59, 1992.
21. Gluckman JL, Cissman JD, Donegan JO: Multicentric squamous cell carcinoma of the upper aerodigesive tract. Head Neck Surg 3:90, 1980.
22. Tepperman BS, Fitzpatrick PJ: Second respiratory and upper digestive tract cancers after oral cancer. Lancet 2:547, 1981.
23. Schwartz LH, Ozsahin M, Zhang GN, et al: Synchronous and metachronous head and neck carcinomas. Cancer 74:1933, 1994.
24. Hong WK, Lippman SM, Itri LM, et al: Prevention of second primary tumors with isotretinoin in squamous-cell carcinoma of the head and neck. N Engl J Med 323:795, 1990.
25. Benner SE, et al: Prevention of second primary tumors with isotretinoin in patients with squamous cell carcinoma of the head and neck: long-term follow-up. J Natl Cancer Inst 86:140, 1994.
26. Rhee J, Khuri F, Shin D: Advances in chemoprevention of head and neck cancer. Oncologist 9:302, 2004.
27. Papadimitrakopoulou V, Clayman G, Shin D, et al: Biochemoprevention for dysplastic lesions of the upper aerodigestive tract. Arch Otolaryngol Head Neck Surg 125:1083, 1999.
28. Papadimitrakopoulou V, Liu D, Mao L, et al: Biologic correlates of a biochemoprevention trial in advanced upper aerodigestive tract premalignant lesions. Cancer Epidemiol Biomarkers Prev 11:1605, 2002.
29. Fishinger J, Mlacak B: The usefulness of screening in the early detection of laryngeal cancer. Acta Otolaryngol 527:150, 1997.
30. Prout MN, Sidari JN, Witzburg RA, et al: Head and neck cancer screening among 4611 tobacco users older than forty years. Otolaryngol Head Neck Surg 116:201, 1997.
31. Hoare T, Thomson HG, Proops DW: Detection of early laryngeal cancer: the case for early specialist assessment. J R Soc Med 86:390, 1993.
32. Ferlito A: Diagnosis and treatment of verrucous squamous cell carcinoma of the larynx: a critical review. Ann Otol Rhinol Laryngol 94:575, 1985.
33. Brodsky G: Carcino (pseudo)sarcoma of the larynx: the controversy continues. Otolaryngol Clin North Am 17:185, 1984.
34. Choi H, Sturgis E, Rosenthal D, et al: Sarcomatoid carcinoma of the head and neck: molecular evidence for evolution and progression from conventional squamous cell carcinomas. Am J Surg Pathol 27:1216, 2003.
35. Gnepp DR: Small cell neuroendocrine carcinoma of the larynx. A critical review of the literature. J Otorhinolaryngol Relat Spec 53:210, 1991.
36. Hyams VJ, Batsakis JG, Michaels L: Atlas of Tumor Pathology: Tumors of the Upper Respiratory Tract and Ear. Washington, DC, Armed Forces Institute of Pathology, 1988.
37. Million RR, Cassisi NJ, Mancuso AA: Larynx. *In* Cassisi NJ, et al (eds): Management of Head and Neck Cancer: A Multidisciplinary Approach, 2nd ed. Philadelphia, JB Lippincott, 1994.
38. Byers RM, Wolf PF, Ballantyne AJ: Rationale for elective modified neck dissection. Head Neck Surg 10:160, 1988.
39. Lee NK, Goepfert H, Wendt CD: Supraglottic laryngectomy for intermediate stage cancer: U.T. M. D. Anderson Cancer Center experience with combined therapy. Laryngoscope 100:831, 1990.
40. Lindberg RD: Distribution of cervical lymph node metastases from squamous cell carcinoma of the upper respiratory and digestive tracts. Cancer 29:1446, 1972.
41. Crile CW: Excision of cancer of the head and neck. JAMA 47:1780, 1906.
42. Merino OR, Lindberg RL, Fletcher GH: An analysis of distant metastases from squamous cell carcinoma of the upper respiratory and digestive tracts. Cancer 40:145, 1977.
43. Marks JE, Kurnik B, Powers WE, Ogura JH: Carcinoma of the pyriform sinus: an analysis of treatment results and patterns of failure. Cancer 41:1008, 1978.
44. Distant metastases from head and neck squamous cancer: the role of adjuvant chemotherapy. *In* Hong WK, Weber RS (eds): Head and Neck Cancer: Basic and Clinical Aspects. Boston, Kluwer Academic Publishers, 1995, p 243.
45. Spitz MR, Fueger JJ, Halabi S, et al: Mutagen sensitivity in upper aerodigestive tract cancer: a case-control analysis. Cancer Epidemiol Biomarkers Prev 2:329, 1993.
46. Slaughter DP, Southwick HW, Smejkal W: Field cancerization in oral stratified squamous epithelium: Clinical implications of multicentric origin. Cancer 6:963, 1953.
47. Califano J, van der Riet P, Westra W, et al: Genetic progression model for head and neck cancer: implications for field cancerization. Cancer Res 56:2488, 1996.
48. Vogelstein B, Fearon ER, Hamilton SR, et al: Genetic alterations during colorectal tumor development. N Engl J Med 319:523, 1988.
49. Voravud N, Shin DM, Ro JY, et al: Increased polysomies of chromosomes 7 and 17 during head and neck multistage tumorigenesis. Cancer Res 53:2874, 1993.
50. Mao L, Hong W, Papadimitrakopoulou V: Focus on head and neck cancer. Cancer Cell 5:311, 2004.
51. Hollstein ML, Sidransky D, Vogelstein B, Harris C: p53 mutations in human cancers. Science 253:49, 1991.
52. Shin DM, Kim J, Ro JY, et al: Activation of p53 gene expression in premalignant lesions during head and neck tumorigenesis. Cancer Res 54:321, 1994.
53. Salam MA, Crocker J, Morris A: Over-expression of tumour suppressor gene p53 in laryngeal squamous cell carcinomas and its prognostic significance. Clin Otolaryngol 20:49, 1995.
54. Shin DM, Lee JS, Lippman SM, et al: p53 expressions. predicting recurrence and second primary tumors in head and neck squamous cell carcinoma. J Natl Cancer Inst 88:519, 1996.
55. Bradford CR, Zhu S, Wolf GT, et al: Overexpression of p53 predicts organ preservation using induction chemotherapy and

radiation in patients with advanced laryngeal cancer. Otolaryngol Head Neck Surg 113:408, 1995.
56. Nadal A, Campo E, Pinto J, et al: p53 expression in normal, dysplastic, and neoplastic laryngeal epithelium. Absence of a correlation with prognostic factors. J Pathol 175:181, 1995.
57. Weichselbaum R, Dunphy E, Beckett M, et al: Epidermal growth factor receptor gene amplification and expression in head and neck cancer cell lines. Head Neck 11:437, 1989.
58. Grandis J, Tweardy D: Elevated levels of transforming growth factor alpha and epidermal growth factor receptor messenger RNA are early markers of carcinogenesis in head and neck cancer. Cancer Res 53:3579, 1993.
59. Shin DM, Ro JY, Hong WK, Hittelman WN: Dysregulation of epidermal growth factor receptor expression in premalignant lesions during head and neck tumorigenesis. Cancer Res 54:3153, 1994.
60. Greene F, Page D, Fleming I, et al (eds): AJCC Cancer Staging Manual, 6th ed. New York, Springer-Verlag, 2002.
61. Mendenhall WM, Parsons JT, Stringer SP, et al: Radiotherapy alone or combined with neck dissection for T1-T2 carcinoma of the pyriform sinus: an alternative to conservation surgery. Int J Radiat Oncol Biol Phys 27:1017, 1993.
62. Ferlito A, Silver C, Howard D, et al: The role of partial laryngeal resection in current management of laryngeal cancer: a collective review. Acta Otolaryngol 120:456, 2000.
63. Strong MS: Laser excision of carcinoma of the larynx. Laryngoscope 85:1286, 1975.
64. Sessions D, Maness G, McSwain B: Laryngofissure in the treatment of carcinoma of the vocal cord. Laryngoscope 75:490, 1964.
65. Soo KC, Shah JP, Gopinath KS, et al: Analysis of prognostic variables and results after supraglottic partial laryngectomy. Am J Surg 156:301, 1988.
66. Laccourreye O, Weinstein G, Brasnu D, et al: Vertical partial laryngectomy: a critical analysis of local recurrence. Ann Otol Rhinol Laryngol 100:68, 1991.
67. Biller HF, Barnhill FR Jr, Ogura JH, Perez CA: Hemilaryngectomy following radiation failure for carcinoma of the vocal cords. Laryngoscope 80:249, 1970.
68. Laccourreye O, Weinstein G, Naudo P, et al: Supracricoid partial laryngectomy after failed laryngeal radiation therapy. Laryngoscope 106:495, 1996.
69. Lavey RS, Calcaterra TC: Partial laryngectomy for glottic cancer after high-dose radiotherapy. Am J Surg 162:341, 1991.
70. Rothfield RE, Johnson JT, Myers EN, Wagner RL: Hemilaryngectomy for salvage of radiation therapy failures. Otolaryngol Head Neck Surg 103:792, 1990.
71. Schwaab G, Mamelle G, Lartigau E, et al: Surgical salvage treatment of T1/T2 glottic carcinoma after failure of radiotherapy. Am J Surg 168:474, 1994.
72. Hirano M, Hirade Y, Kawasaki H: Vocal function following carbon dioxide surgery for glottic carcinoma. Ann Otol Rhinol Laryngol 94:232, 1985.
73. McGuirt WF, Blalock D, Koufman JA, et al: Comparative voice results after laser resection or irradiation of T1 vocal cord carcinoma. Arch Otolargol Head Neck Surg 120:951, 1994.
74. Harrison LB, Solomon B, Miller S, et al: Prospective computer-assisted voice analysis for patients with early stage glottic cancer: a preliminary report of the functional result of laryngeal irradiation. Int J Radiat Oncol Biol Phys 19:123, 1990.
75. Mittal B, Rao DV, Marks JE, Ogura JH: Comparative cost analysis of hemilaryngectomy and irradiation for early glottic carcinoma. Int J Radiat Oncol Biol Phys 9:407, 1983.
76. Biller HF, Ogura JH, Pratt LL: Hemilaryngectomy for T2 glottic cancers. Arch Otolaryngol 93:238, 1971.
77. Karim ABMF, Kralendonk JH, Yap LY, et al: Heterogeneity of stage II glottic carcinoma and its therapeutic implications. Int J Radiat Oncol Biol Phys 13:313, 1987.
78. Howell-Burke D, Peters LJ, Goepfert H, Oswald MJ: T2 glottic cancer. Arch Otolargol Head Neck Surg 116:830, 1990.
79. Garden A, Forster K, Wong P, et al: Results of radiotherapy for T2N0 glottic carcinoma: does the "2" stand for twice-daily treatment? Int J Radiat Oncol Biol Phys 55:322, 2003.
80. Wang CC: Carcinoma of the larynx. *In* Radiation Therapy for Head and Neck Neoplasms. New York, Wiley-Liss, 1997, p 221.
81. Wiggenraad RG, Terhaard CH, Horidjik GJ, Ravasz LA: The importance of vocal cord mobility in T2 laryngeal cancer. Radiother Oncol 18:321, 1990.
82. Fein DA, Mendenhall WM, Parsons JT, Million RR: T1-T2 squamous cell carcinoma of the glottic larynx treated with radiotherapy: a multivariate analysis of variables potentially influencing local control. Int J Radiat Oncol Biol Phys 25:605, 1993.
83. Ang KK, Peters LJ: Vocal cord cancer: 2B worse than not 2B? Radiother Oncol 18:365, 1990.
84. Sessions D, Ogura J, Fried M: The anterior commissure in glottic carcinoma. Laryngoscope 85:1624, 1974.
85. Le QX, Fu KK, Kroll S, et al: Influence of fraction size, total dose, and overall time on local control of T1-T2 glottic carcinoma. Int J Radiat Oncol Biol Phys 39:115, 1997.
86. Mendenhall W, Amdur R, Morris C, Hinerman R: T1-T2N0 squamous cell carcinoma of the glottic larynx treated with radiation therapy. J Clin Oncol 19:4029, 2001.
87. Hintz BL, Kagan AR, Nussbaum H, et al: A watchful waiting policy for in situ carcinoma of the vocal cords. Arch Otolaryngol 107:746, 1981.
88. Ferlito A, Polidoro F, Rossi M: Pathological basis and clinical aspects of treatment policy in carcinoma in situ of the larynx. J Laryngol Otol 95:141, 1981.
89. McGuirt WF, Browne JD: Management decisions in laryngeal carcinoma in situ. Laryngoscope 101:125, 1991.
90. Wolfensberger M, Dort JC: Endoscopic laser surgery for early glottic carcinoma: a clinical and experimental study. Laryngoscope 100:1100, 1990.
91. Maran AG, Mackenzie IJ, Stanley RE: Carcinoma in situ of the larynx. Head Neck Surg 7:28, 1984.
92. Pene F, Fletcher GH: Results in irradiation of the in situ carcinoma of the vocal cord. Cancer 37:2586, 1976.
93. Smitt MC, Goffinet DR: Radiotherapy for carcinoma-in-situ of the glottic larynx. Int J Radiat Oncol Biol Phys 28:251, 1994.
94. MacLeod PM, Daniel F: The role of radiotherapy in in-situ carcinoma of the larynx. Int J Radiat Oncol Biol Phys 18:113, 1990.
95. Sung DI, Chang CH, Harisiadis L, Rosenstein LM: Primary radiotherapy for carcinoma in situ and early invasive carcinoma of the glottic larynx. Int J Radiat Oncol Biol Phys 15:467, 1979.
96. Elman AJ, Goodman M, Wang CC, et al: In situ carcinoma of the vocal cords. Cancer 43:2422, 1979.
97. Harwood AR, Hawkins NV, Rider WD, Bryce DP: Radiotherapy of early glottic cancer—I. Int J Radiat Oncol Biol Phys 5:473, 1979.
98. Wendt CW, Peters LJ, Ang KK, et al: Hyperfractionated radiotherapy in the treatment of squamous cell carcinomas of the supraglottic larynx. Int J Radiat Oncol Biol Phys 17:1057, 1989.
99. Levendag P, Vikram B, Sessions R: The problem of neck relapse in early stage supraglottic cancer: results of different treatment modalities for the clinically negative neck. Int J Radiat Oncol Biol Phys 13:1621, 1987.
100. Robbins KT, Davidson W, Peters LJ, Goepfert H: Conservation surgery for T2 and T3 carcinomas of the supraglottic larynx. Arch Otolaryngol Head Neck Surg 114:421, 1988.
101. Bocca E, Pignataro O, Oldini C: Supraglottic laryngectomy: 30 years of experience. Ann Otol Rhinol Laryngol 92:14, 1983.
102. Burstein FD, Calcaterra TC: Supraglottic laryngectomy: series report and analysis of results. Laryngoscope 95:833, 1985.
103. Fein DA, Nichols RC Jr, Lee WR, et al: T2-T3 carcinoma of the supraglottic larynx: a comparison of surgery and radiotherapy. Radiat Oncol Investig 2:237, 1995.
104. Steiner W: Results of curative laser microsurgery of laryngeal carcinomas. Am J Otolaryngol 14:116, 1993.
105. Zeitels SM, Koufman JA, Davis RK, Vaughan CW: Endoscopic treatment of supraglottic and hypopharynx cancer. Laryngoscope 104:71, 1994.
106. Hinerman R, Mendenhall W, Amdur R, et al: Carcinoma of the supraglottic larynx: treatment results with radiotherapy alone or with planned neck dissection. Head Neck 24:456, 2002.
107. Laccourreye O, Brasnu D, Merite-Drancy A, et al: Cricohyoidopexy in selected infrahyoid epiglottic carcinomas presenting with pathological preepiglottic space invasion. Arch Otolaryngol Head Neck Surg 119:881, 1993.

108. Bataini JP, Ennuyer A, Poncet P, Ghossein NA: Treatment of supraglottic cancer by radical high dose radiotherapy. Cancer 33:1253, 1974.
109. Fletcher GH, Goepfert H: Larynx and hypopharynx. *In* Fletcher G (ed): Textbook of Radiotherapy, 3rd ed. Philadelphia, Lea & Febiger, 1980, p 330.
110. Mendenhall WM, Parsons JT, Mancuso AA, et al: Radiotherapy for squamous cell carcinoma of the supraglottic larynx: an alternative to surgery. Head Neck 18:24, 1996.
111. Overgaard J, Hansen H, Specht L, et al: Five compared with six fractions per week of conventional radiotherapy of squamous-cell carcinoma of head and neck: DAHANCA 6 and 7 randomised controlled trial. Lancet 362:1588, 2003.
112. Wall TJ, Peters LJ, Brown BW, et al: Relationship between lymph nodal status and primary tumor control probability in tumors of the supraglottic larynx. Int J Radiat Oncol Biol Phys 11:1895, 1985.
113. Wang CC, Nakfoor BM, Spiro IJ, Martins P: Role of accelerated fractionated irradiation for supraglottic carcinoma: assessment of results. Cancer J Sci Am 3:88, 1997.
114. Freeman DE, Mendenhall WM, Parsons JT, Million RR: Does neck stage influence local control in squamous cell carcinomas of the head and neck? Int J Radiat Oncol Biol Phys 23:733, 1992.
115. Freeman DE, Mancuso AA, Parsons JT, et al: Irradiation alone for supraglottic larynx carcinoma: can CT findings predict treatment results? Int J Radiat Oncol Biol Phys 19:485, 1990.
116. Kraas J, Underhill T, D'Agostino RJ, et al: Quantitative analysis from CT is prognostic for local control of supraglottic carcinoma. Head Neck 23:1031, 2001.
117. Byers RM, Clayman GK, Guillamondegui O, et al: Resection of advanced cervical metastasis prior to definitive radiotherapy for primary squamous carcinomas of the upper aerodigestive tract. Head Neck 14:133, 1992.
118. Garden AS, Morrison WH, Clayman GL, et al: Early squamous cell carcinoma of the hypopharynx: outcomes of treatment with radiation alone to the primary disease. Head Neck 18:317, 1996.
119. Amdur R, Mendenhall W, Stringer S, et al: Organ preservation with radiotherapy for T1-T2 carcinoma of the pyriform sinus. Head Neck 23:353, 2001.
120. O'Sullivan B, Warde P, Keane T, et al: Outcome following radiotherapy in verrucous carcinoma of the larynx. Int J Radiat Oncol Biol Phys 32:611, 1995.
121. Ballo MT, Garden AS, El-Naggar AK, et al: Radiation therapy for early stage (T1-T2) sarcomatoid carcinoma of true vocal cords: outcomes and patterns of failure. Laryngoscope 108:760, 1998.
122. Barker JL Jr, Glisson BS, Garden AS, et al: Management of nonsinonasal neuroendocrine carcinomas of the head and neck. Cancer 98:2322, 2003.
123. Forastiere A, Goepfert H, Maor M, et al: Concurrent chemotherapy and radiotherapy for organ preservation in advanced laryngeal cancer. N Engl J Med 349:2091, 2003.
124. Bernier J, Domenge C, Ozsahin M, et al: Postoperative irradiation with or without concomitant chemotherapy for locally advanced head and neck cancer. N Engl J Med 350:1945, 2004.
125. Cooper J, Pajak T, Forastiere A, et al: Postoperative concurrent radiotherapy and chemotherapy for high-risk squamous-cell carcinoma of the head and neck. N Engl J Med 350:1937, 2004.
126. Mendenhall WM, Parsons JT, Stringer SP, et al: Stage T3 squamous cell carcinoma of the glottic larynx: a comparison of laryngectomy and irradiation. Int J Radiat Oncol Biol Phys 23:725, 1992.
127. Wang CC: Carcinoma of the hypopharynx. *In* Radiation Therapy for Head and Neck Neoplasms. New York, Wiley-Liss, 1997, p 205.
128. Bryant GP, Poulsen MG, Tripcony L, Dickie GJ: Treatment decision in T3N0M0 glottic carcinoma. Int J Radiat Oncol Biol Phys 31:285, 1995.
129. The Department of Veterans Affairs Laryngeal Cancer Study Group: Induction chemotherapy plus radiation compared with surgery plus radiation in patients with advanced laryngeal cancer. N Engl J Med 324:1685, 1991.
130. Pfister D, Strong E, Harrison L: Larynx preservation with combined chemo and radiotherapy in advanced head and neck cancer. J Clin Oncol 9:830, 1991.
131. Shirinian MH, Weber RS, Lippman SM, et al: Laryngeal preservation by induction chemotherapy plus radiotherapy in locally advanced head and neck cancer: the M. D. Anderson Cancer Center experience. Head Neck 16:39, 1994.
132. Klein R, Fletcher GH: Evaluation of the clinical usefulness of radiological findings in squamous cell carcinomas of the larynx. AJR Am J Roentgenol 92:43, 1964.
133. Yuen A, Medina J, Goepfert H, Fletcher G: Management of stage T3 and T4 glottic carcinomas. Am J Surg 148:467, 1984.
134. Goepfert H, Jesse RH, Fletcher GH, Hamberger A: Optimal treatment for the technically resectable squamous cell carcinoma of the supraglottic larynx. Laryngoscope 85:14, 1975.
135. Vandenbrouck C, Sancho H, Le Fur R, et al: Results of a randomized clinical trial of preoperative irradiation versus postoperative in treatment of tumors of the hypopharynx. Cancer 39:1445, 1977.
136. El Bawadi SA, Goepfert H, Fletcher GH, et al: Squamous cell carcinoma of the pyriform sinus. Laryngoscope 92:357, 1982.
137. Frank JL, Garb JL, Kay S, et al: Postoperative radiotherapy improves survival in squamous cell carcinoma of the hypopharynx. Am J Surg 168:476, 1994.
138. Lefebvre JL, Chevalier D, Luboinski B, et al: Larynx preservation in pyriform sinus cancer: preliminary results of a European Organization for Research and Treatment of Cancer phase III trial. EORTC Head and Neck Cancer Cooperative Group. J Natl Cancer Inst 88:890, 1996.
139. Brizel D, Albers M, Fisher S, et al: Hyperfractionated irradiation with or without concurrent chemotherapy for locally advanced head and neck cancer. N Engl J Med 338:1798, 1998.
140. Adelstein D, Li Y, Adams G, et al: An Intergroup phase III comparison of standard radiation therapy and two schedules of concurrent chemoradiotherapy in patients with unresectable squamous cell head and neck cancer. J Clin Oncol 21:92, 2003.
141. Akine Y, Tokit N, Ogino T, et al: Radiotherapy of T1 glottic cancer with 6 MeV x-rays. Int J Radiat Oncol Biol Phys 20:1215, 1991.
142. Foote RL, Grado GL, Buskirk SJ, et al: Radiation therapy for glottic cancer using 6-MV photons. Cancer 77:381, 1996.
143. Sombeck MD, Kalbaugh KJ, Mendenhall WM, et al: Radiotherapy for early vocal cord cancer: a dosimetric analysis of 60Co versus 6 MV photons. Head Neck 18:167, 1996.
144. Yu E, Shenouda G, Beaudet MP, Black MJ: Impact of radiation therapy fraction size on local control of early glottic carcinoma. Int J Radiat Oncol Biol Phys 37:587, 1997.
145. Chao KSC, Ozygit G, Tran BN, et al: Patterns of failure in patients receiving definitive and postoperative IMRT for head-and-neck cancer. Int J Radiat Oncol Biol Phys 55:312, 2003.
146. Dawson LA, Anzai Y, Marsh L, et al: Patterns of local-regional recurrence following parotid-sparing conformal and segmental intensity-modulated radiotherapy for head and neck cancer. Int J Radiat Oncol Biol Phys 46:1117, 2000.
147. Garden AS, Morrison WH, Ang KK, Peters LJ: Hyperfractionated radiation in the treatment of squamous cell carcinomas of the head and neck: a comparison of two fractionation schedules. Int J Radiat Oncol Biol Phys 31:493, 1995.
148. Peters LJ, Goepfert H, Ang KK, et al: Evaluation of the dose for postoperative radiation therapy of head and neck cancer: first report of a prospective randomized trial. Int J Radiat Oncol Biol Phys 26:3, 1993.
149. Cole CJ, Garden AS, Frankenthaler RA, et al: Postoperative radiation of free jejunal autografts in patients with advanced cancer of the head and neck. Cancer 75:2356, 1995.
150. Lustig RA, MacLean CJ, Hanks GE, Kramer S: The patterns of care outcome studies: results of the national practice in carcinoma of the larynx. Int J Radiat Oncol Biol Phys 10:2357, 1984.
151. Olszewski SJ, Vaeth JM, Green JP, et al: The influence of field size, treatment modality, commissure involvement and histology in the treatment of early vocal cord cancer with irradiation. Int J Radiat Oncol Biol Phys 11:1333, 1985.
152. Hendrickson FR: Radiation therapy treatment of larynx cancers. Cancer 55:2058, 1985.
153. Pellitteri PK, Kennedy TL, Vrabec DP, et al: Radiotherapy—the mainstay in the treatment of early glottic carcinoma. Arch Otolaryngol Head Neck Surg 117:297, 1991.

154. Klintenberg C, Lundgren J, Adell G, et al: Primary radiotherapy of T1 and T2 glottic carcinoma: analysis of treatment results and prognostic factors in 223 patients. Acta Oncologica 35(Suppl 8): 81, 1996.
155. Warde P, O'Sullivan B, Bristow R, et al: T1/T2 glottic cancer managed by external beam radiotherapy: the influence of pre-treatment hemoglobin on local control. Int J Radiat Oncol Biol Phys 41:347, 1998.
156. Van den Bogaert W, Ostyn F, van der Schueren E: The significance of extension and impaired mobility in cancer of the vocal cord. Int J Radiat Oncol Biol Phys 9:181, 1983.
157. Kelly MD, Hahn SS, Spaulding CA, et al: Definitive radiotherapy in the management of stage I and II carcinomas of the glottis. Ann Otol Rhinol Laryngol 98:235, 1989.
158. Mendenhall WM, Parsons JT, Stringer SP, et al: T1-T2 vocal cord carcinoma: a basis for comparing the results of radiotherapy and surgery. Head Neck Surg 10:373, 1988.
159. Barton MB, Keane TJ, Gadalla T, Maki E: The effect of treatment time and treatment interruption on tumor control following radical radiotherapy of laryngeal cancer. Radiotherapy Oncology 23:137, 1992.
160. Harwood AR, Beale FA, Cummings BJ, et al: T2 glottic cancer: an analysis of dose-time-volume factors. Int J Radiat Oncol Biol Phys 7:1501, 1981.
161. Kalter PO, Lubsen H, Delemarre JFM, Snow GB: Squamous hyperplasia of the larynx (a clinical follow-up study). J Laryngol Otol 101:579, 1987.
162. Fernberg JO, Ringborg U, Silfversward C, et al: Radiation therapy in early glottic cancer. Analysis of 177 consecutive cases. Acta Otolaryngol 108:478, 1989.
163. Small W Jr, Mittal BB, Brand EN, et al: Role of radiation therapy in the management of carcinoma in situ of the larynx. Laryngoscope 103:663, 1993.
164. Spayne J, Warde P, O'Sullivan B, et al: Carcinoma-in-situ of the glottic larynx: results of treatment with radiation therapy. Int J Radiat Oncol Biol Phys 49:1235, 2001.
165. Garcia-Serra A, Hinerman R, Amdur R, et al: Radiotherapy for carcinoma in situ of the true vocal cords. Head Neck 24:390, 2002.
166. Vandenbrouck C, Eschwege F, De La Rochefordiere A, et al: Squamous cell carcinoma of the pyriform sinus: retrospective study of 351 cases treated at the Institut Gustave-Rousy. Head Neck Surg 10:4, 1987.
167. Lundgren JAV, Gilbert RW, Van Nostrand AWP, et al: T3N0M0 glottic carcinoma: a failure analysis. Clin Otolaryngol 13:455, 1988.
168. Croll GA, Gerritsen GJ, Tiwari RM, Snow GB: Primary radiotherapy with surgery in reserve for advanced laryngeal carcinoma: results and complications. Eur J Surg Oncol 15:350, 1989.
169. Terhaard CHF, Karim ABMF, Hoogenraad WJ, et al: Local control in T3 laryngeal cancer treated with radical radiotherapy, time dose relationship: the concept of nominal standard dose and linear quadratic model. Int J Radiat Oncol Biol Phys 20:1207, 1991.
170. Tennvall J, Wennerberg J, Willen R, et al: T3N0 glottic carcinoma: DNA S-phase as a predictor of the outcome after radiotherapy. Acta Otolaryngol 113:220, 1993.
171. Pameijer FA, Mancuso AA, Mendenhall WM, et al: Can pre-treatment computed tomography predict local control in T3 squamous cell carcinoma of the glottic larynx treated with definitive radiotherapy? Int J Radiat Oncol Biol Phys 37:1011, 1997.
172. Mendenhall WM, Parsons JT, Devine JW, et al: Squamous cell carcinoma of the pyriform sinus treated with surgery and/or radiotherapy. Head Neck Surg 10:88, 1987.
173. Slotman BJ, Kralendonk JH, Snow GB, et al: Surgery and postoperative radiotherapy and radiotherapy alone in T3-T4 cancers of the pyriform sinus. Treatment results and patterns of failure. Acta Oncol 33:55, 1994.
174. Schwaibold F, Scariato A, Nunno M, et al: The effect of fraction size on control of early glottic cancer. Int J Radiat Oncol Biol Phys 14:451, 1988.
175. Mendenhall WM, Parsons JT, Million RR, Fletcher GH: T1-T2 squamous cell carcinoma of the glottic larynx treated with radiation therapy: relationship of dose-fractionation factors to local control and complications. Int J Radiat Oncol Biol Phys 15:1267, 1988.
176. Kim RY, Marks ME, Salter MM: Early-stage glottic cancer: importance of dose fractionation in radiation therapy. Radiology 182:273, 1992.
177. Rudoltz MS, Benammar A, Mohiuddin M: Prognostic factors for local control and survival in T1 squamous cell carcinoma of the glottis. Int J Radiat Oncol Biol Phys 26:767, 1993.
178. Ricciardelli EJ, Weymuller EA Jr, Koh WJ, et al: Effect of radiation fraction size on local control rates for early glottic carcinoma. Arch Otolaryngol Head Neck Surg 120:737, 1994.
179. Burke LS, Greven KM, McGuirt WT, et al: Definitive radiotherapy for early glottic carcinoma: prognostic factors and implications for treatment. Int J Radiat Oncol Biol Phys 38:37, 1997.

CHAPTER 33

SINONASAL CANCER

Anesa Ahamad, Ian J. Bristol, Adam S. Garden, and K. Kian Ang

INCIDENCE AND EPIDEMIOLOGY

Sinonasal cancers comprise less than 1% of all malignant neoplasms. Approximately half arise in the maxillary sinus (55%), with the remaining divided equally between nasal cavity (23%) and ethmoid sinus (20%). Primary sphenoid sinus and frontal sinus cancer are very rare (1% each). It can be difficult to determine the site of origin of locally advanced tumors.

A number of sinonasal cancers are relatively more common in people engaged in certain occupations, such as carpenters, sawmill personnel, and nickel workers.

BIOLOGIC CHARACTERISTICS

The natural history of sinonasal cancer depends on the anatomic site, the histologic type, and the stage of the tumor. A clear understanding of their clinicopathologic features contributes to establishing the diagnosis, especially if immunohistochemistry is used.

Relatively little is known about the molecular biology of these rare neoplasms that contributes in understanding the natural history or guiding therapy decision.

STAGING EVALUATION

Staging includes a thorough history, complete head and neck examination, contrast-enhanced MRI of the head and neck region, blood chemistry, and chest radiographs. T-stage classification of nasal cavity tumors has recently been added to the AJCC staging system.

PRIMARY THERAPY

Radiotherapy is generally selected for the treatment of T1 and small T2 carcinomas of the nasal vestibule and anterior nasal fossa and yields high locoregional control rates with good cosmetic results. Radiation also yields an excellent control rate for stage A esthesioneuroblastoma.

Surgery by itself is effective in curing T1 nasal fossa and maxillary sinus carcinomas.

ADJUVANT THERAPY

A combination of surgery and radiotherapy (usually given in postoperative setting) is recommended for the management of more advanced resectable cancers.

The role of neoadjuvant combination chemotherapy in conjunction with surgery, radiotherapy, or both in improving locoregional control or in reducing the extent of surgery (leading to better functional and cosmetic outcome) is being addressed in clinical studies.

LOCALLY ADVANCED DISEASE AND PALLIATION

Radiotherapy can yield local control in patients with locally advanced carcinomas who are medically unfit for undergoing extensive resection or in occasional patients with inoperable tumors.

Concurrent chemotherapy is increasingly used with definitive radiotherapy in the management of inoperable tumors on the basis of improved results in other head and neck sites.

Radiation therapy or chemotherapy can be given to reduce symptoms for most patients with locally advanced inoperable cancer.

The nasal cavity and paranasal sinus tumors are discussed together because they are often diagnosed in locally advanced stage and involve multiple structures. They may even extend to the adjacent orbit, anterior and middle cranial fossa, infratemporal fossa, pterygopalatine fossa, and nasopharynx.

The nasal cavity is divided into three regions: nasal vestibule, nasal cavity proper, and olfactory region.[1] The paranasal sinuses (frontal, ethmoidal, sphenoidal, and maxillary) are air-filled outgrowths of the nasal cavity into the respective cranial bones. Secretions from these sinuses drain through meati of the lateral nasal walls.

Sinonasal neoplasms comprise less than 1% of cancers but present a difficult therapeutic challenge because they are often diagnosed at advanced stages. Clinical experience is limited due to their rarity. Surgery and radiotherapy are complicated because these tumors are often located close to multiple critical structures (the eye, brain, optic nerves and chiasm, brainstem, and cranial nerves). Aesthetic considerations argue for less radical surgical resection and delivery of adjuvant radiation treatment or consideration of definitive radiotherapy.

The treatment outcome of patients with carcinoma of the maxillary and ethmoid sinuses has improved progressively with most therapy modalities over each of the past five decades.[2] Advances have been made in methods of extirpation including skull base surgery, reconstruction, and highly conformal radiotherapy techniques that enable avoidance of adjacent critical normal tissues.

This chapter focuses on epithelial neoplasms originating in the nasal cavity or paranasal sinuses. Other histologic types such as sarcomas, lymphomas, and plasmacytomas are discussed in their respective chapters.

ETIOLOGY AND EPIDEMIOLOGY

Cancers of the nasal cavity and paranasal sinuses are uncommon neoplasms, with fewer than 4500 Americans diagnosed per year.[3] The incidence is about 0.75 per 100,000 individuals.[4] Tumors of the maxillary sinus are twice as frequent as those of the nasal cavity and ethmoid sinus, and neoplasms of the frontal and sphenoid sinuses are extremely rare. Sinonasal neoplasms occur twice as frequently in men as in women. These tumors are more frequently diagnosed in some regions outside the United States, such as Japan and South Africa.[5]

The etiologic factors are unclear in most patients diagnosed with sinonasal carcinomas. A number of sinonasal cancers are relatively more common in people engaged in certain occupations or exposed to some chemical compounds.[4-9] Squamous cell carcinoma of the nasal cavity develops more often in nickel workers.[5] Adenocarcinoma of the nasal cavity and ethmoid sinus, for instance, occurs more frequently in carpenters and sawmill workers who are exposed to the dust of mainly hard and exotic woods.[6-9] However, synthetic wood, binding agents, and glues may also be involved as cocarcinogens.[6]

Cigarette smoking is reported to increase the risk of nasal cancer, with a doubling of risk among heavy or long-term smokers and a reduction in risk after long-term cessation. After adjustment for smoking, a significant dose-response relation was also noted between alcohol drinking and risk of nasal cancer.[7]

Maxillary sinus carcinoma was associated with a radioactive thorium-containing contrast material, thorium dioxide (Thorotrast), used for radiographic study of the maxillary sinuses.[4,6] Occupational exposure in the production of chromium, mustard gas, isopropyl alcohol, and radium also increases the risk for sinonasal carcinomas.[4]

PREVENTION AND EARLY DETECTION

In general, carpenters, sawmill workers, and workers involved in the production of nickel, chromium, mustard gas, isopropyl alcohol, and radium should use appropriate face masks to reduce occupational exposure to potential carcinogens. Individuals in these professions who develop persistent nasal or sinus symptoms should see an otolaryngologist for evaluation.

PATHOLOGY, BIOLOGY, AND PATHWAYS OF SPREAD

The clinical disease course and prognosis depend on the anatomic site, the histologic type, and the stage of the tumor.

Nasal Vestibule

The nasal vestibules are the two entry points into the nasal cavity. Each is a triangle-shaped space situated in front of the limen nasi and defined *laterally* by the alae, *medially* by the membranous septum, the distal end of the cartilaginous septum, and columella, and *inferiorly* by the adjacent floor of the nasal cavity. The nasal vestibule is covered by skin and, therefore, lesions at this location are essentially squamous cell skin cancers[10] but may occasionally be basal cell carcinoma,[11] sebaceous carcinoma,[12] melanoma,[13] or non-Hodgkin's lymphoma.[14]

Nasal vestibule carcinomas can spread by invasion of the upper lip, gingivolabial sulcus, premaxilla, or nasal cavity. Vertical invasion may result in septal (membranous or cartilaginous) perforation or alar cartilage destruction. Lymphatic spread from nasal vestibule carcinomas is usually to the ipsilateral facial (buccinator and mandibular) and submandibular nodes. Large lesions extending across the midline may spread to the contralateral facial or submandibular nodes. The average incidence of nodal metastasis at diagnosis is around 5%.[15-19] Without elective lymphatic treatment, about 15% of patients develop nodal relapse.[15-18] Hematogenous metastasis is rare in nasal vestibule carcinomas.[17] Examples of nasal vestibule tumors are shown in the photographs and magnetic resonance (MR) images in Figures 33-1 and 33-2.

Nasal Cavity and Ethmoid Air Cells

The *nasal cavity proper* (nasal fossa) begins at the limen nasi anteriorly, ends at the choana posteriorly, and extends from the hard palate inferiorly to the base of the skull superiorly. The lateral walls consist of thin bony structures that have three shell-shaped projections (superior, middle, and inferior conchae or turbinates) into the nasal cavity. The septum divides the nasal cavity into right and left halves. The olfactory nerves penetrate the cribriform plate and innervate the roof of the nasal cavity, superior nasal concha, and the upper third of the septum. This portion of the nasal cavity is referred to as the *olfactory region*. The remaining part of the cavity, the respiratory region, contains orifices connecting the nasal cavity with the paranasal sinuses. The superior meatus connects the nasal cavity with the posterior ethmoid cells, the middle meatus with the anterior and middle ethmoid cells and the frontal sinus, and the inferior meatus with the nasolacrimal duct. The sphenoid sinus drains into the nasal cavity through an opening in the anterior wall.

The *ethmoid sinuses* comprise several small cavities, called *ethmoid air cells*, within the ethmoidal labyrinth located below the anterior cranial fossa and between the nasal cavity and the orbit.[18] They are separated from the orbital cavity by a thin, porous bone called the *lamina papyracea* and from the anterior cranial fossa by a portion of the frontal bone, the *fovea ethmoidalis*. The ethmoidal sinuses are divided into anterior, middle, and posterior groups of air cells. The middle ethmoidal cells open directly into the middle meatus. The anterior cells may drain indirectly into the middle meatus via the infundibulum. The posterior cells open directly into the superior meatus.

Neoplasms originating in the respiratory region of the nasal cavity and ethmoid cells are squamous cell carcinoma, adenocarcinoma, and adenoid cystic carcinoma. Carcinoma may arise from inverted papilloma.

The pattern of contiguous spread of carcinomas varies with the location of the primary lesion. Tumors arising in the upper nasal cavity and ethmoid cells extend to the orbit through the lamina papyracea and to the anterior cranial fossa via the cribriform plate, or they grow through the nasal bone to the subcutaneous tissue and skin. Lateral wall primaries invade the maxillary antrum, ethmoid cells, orbit, pterygopalatine fossa, and nasopharynx. Primaries of the floor and lower septum may invade the palate and maxillary antrum. Spreading may also occur through perineural spaces. Such mode of extension is best recognized in adenoid cystic carcinomas.

Lymphatic spread of respiratory region primaries is uncommon. Of the University of Texas M. D. Anderson Cancer Center (MDACC) series of 51 patients, only one had palpable subdigastric lymphadenopathy at diagnosis. This patient had a stage III poorly differentiated carcinoma of the lateral wall. Of the 36 patients who did not receive elective lymphatic irradiation, 2 (6%) experienced subdigastric nodal relapse. Hematogenous dissemination is rare in this disease. In the MDACC series, for example, distant metastasis to bone, brain, or liver occurred in 4 of 51 patients.[20]

The *olfactory region* is located at the roof of the nasal cavity. It represents a narrow strip demarcated by the lamina cribrosa and the adjoining septum and lateral walls. The olfactory region is the site of origin of esthesioneuroblastoma and, occasionally, adenocarcinomas.

Esthesioneuroblastoma is a tumor of neural crest origin first reported by Berger and Luc in 1924 as esthesioneuroepi-

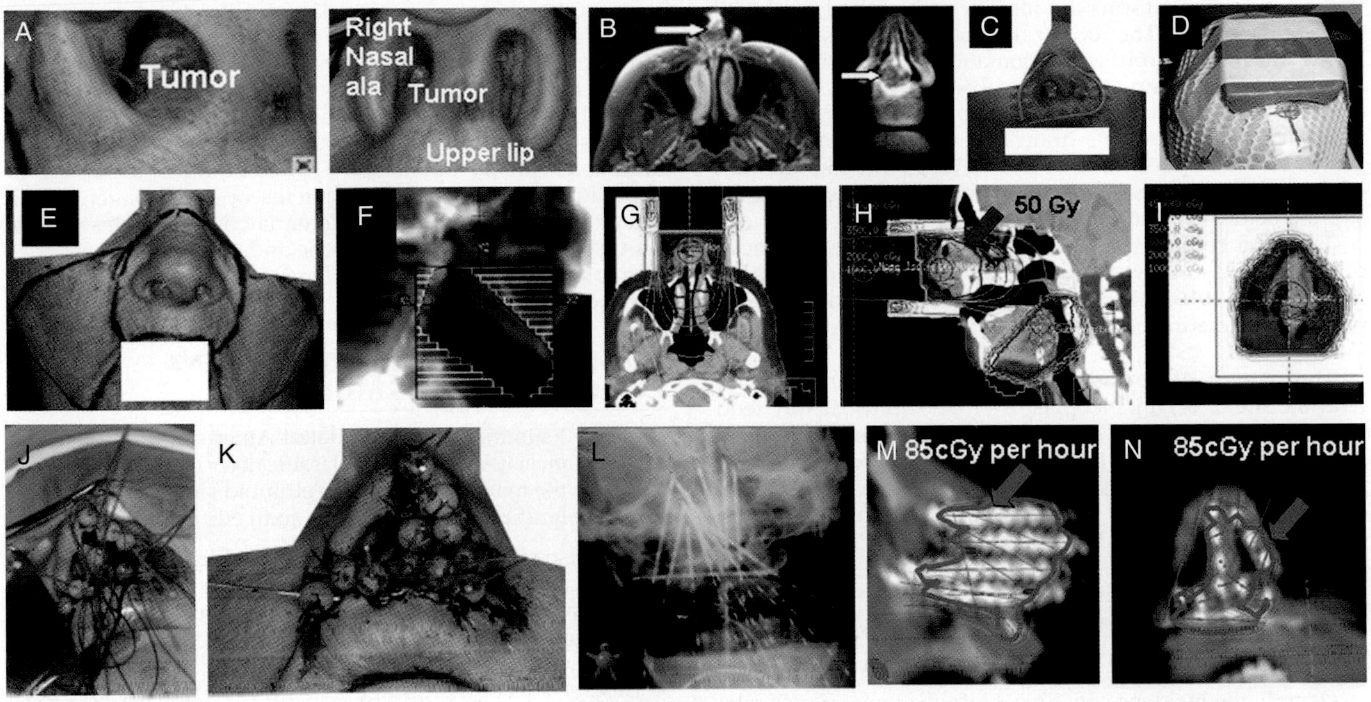

Figure 33-1 T2N0 carcinoma of tumor of the left and right nasal septum, vestibules, and columella, which was treated with external beam radiation therapy and brachytherapy boost. **A,** Photograph of the tumor. **B,** In the transverse and coronal magnetic resonance images, the *arrow* points to the tumor. **C,** Setup at simulation with the tentative field wired and bolus in the nostrils. **D,** Beeswax bolus in situ over the region of custom immobilization, which is cut out to allow wax contact with skin. **E,** "Mustache" fields for irradiation of facial and buccal lymph nodes. **F,** Radiograph of the lateral photon field that encompasses level II nodes. **G–I,** Isodose distribution of the plan for the initial 50 Gy. The *red isodose line* represents 50 Gy. **J,** Needle placement for a brachytherapy boost of an additional 25 Gy at 85 cGy per hour. **K,** Positions of needles, with the left nasal ala apposed to the septum by two additional sutures to close the air gap of the left nostril for optimal dosimetry. **L,** Anteroposterior radiograph taken in the operating room. **M and N,** Sagittal and transverse sections of the final brachytherapy plan, which shows that the 85 cGy/h line adequately covers the tumor volume *(green line).*

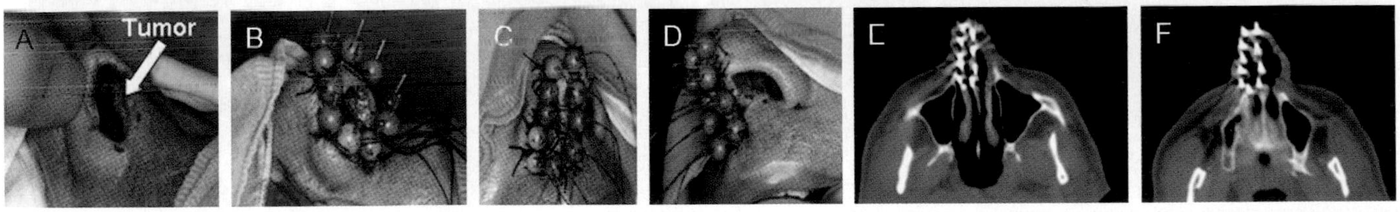

Figure 33-2 **A,** A 2.5-cm squamous cell carcinoma (T2N0) located on the right side of the columella. **B–D,** The entry points are shown for the hollow stainless steel needles that are inserted for afterloading with low-dose-rate iridium 192 interstitial implants. **E and F,** Needle positions are seen on CT images. A dose of 60 Gy was administered at 68 cGy per hour (total treatment time was 90.6 hours).

thelioma olfactif.[21] It has been given a variety of other names, including *olfactory neuroblastoma,* and *esthesioneurocytoma.* Esthesioneuroblastoma constitutes approximately 3% of all intranasal neoplasms. About 250 cases were reported in the literature between 1924 and 1990.[22] A typical histologic feature of esthesioneuroblastoma is that of a tumor comprised of round, oval, or fusiform cells containing neurofibrils with pseudorosette formation and diffusely increased microvascularity.[23] Perivascular palisading of cells can be observed in the absence of pseudorosette formation.

Esthesioneuroblastoma may be mistaken for any other "small round-cell tumor": a group of aggressive malignant tumors composed of relatively small and monotonous undifferentiated cells. It includes Ewing's sarcoma, peripheral neuroepithelioma (also referred to as primitive neuroectodermal tumor or extraskeletal Ewing's), peripheral neuroblastoma ("classic-type"), rhabdomyosarcoma, desmoplastic small round-cell tumor, lymphoma, leukemia, small-cell osteosarcoma, small-cell carcinoma (either undifferentiated or neuroendocrine), olfactory neuroblastoma, cutaneous neuroendocrine carcinoma (Merkel-cell carcinoma), small-cell melanoma, and mesenchymal chondrosarcoma. Their clinical presentations often overlap but clinicopathologic features and immunohistochemistry may help in differentiation.

The route of contiguous spread of esthesioneuroblastomas is similar to that of ethmoid carcinomas. The incidences of lymph node involvement and distant metastasis at diagnosis were 11% and 1%, respectively.[24]

Maxillary Sinus

Maxillary sinuses, the largest of the paranasal sinuses, are pyramid-shaped cavities located in the maxillae.[19] The base of the maxillary sinus forms the inferior part of the lateral wall of the nasal cavity. The roof of the maxillary sinus is formed by the floor of the orbit, which contains the infraorbital canal, and the floor is composed of the alveolar process. The apex extends toward, and frequently into, the zygomatic bone. Maxillary sinus secretions drain into the middle meatus via the hiatus semilunaris through an aperture in the superior part of its base. Ohngren's line divides maxillary sinuses into the suprastructures and infrastructures.

The most common maxillary sinus cancers are squamous cell carcinoma, followed by adenoid cystic carcinoma. Other histologic types are adenocarcinoma, mucoepidermoid carcinoma, undifferentiated cancers, and, occasionally, malignant melanoma.

The pattern of spread of maxillary sinus cancer varies with the site of origin. Neoplasms of the suprastructure tend to extend into the nasal cavity, nasopharynx, ethmoid cells, inferior or medial wall of the orbit, orbital contents, pterygopalatine fossa, masticator space, infratemporal fossa, base of the skull, parasellar region and cavernous sinus, and middle cranial fossa, as shown in Figure 33-3A. Tumors of the infrastructure extend to the palate, alveolar process, gingivobuccal sulcus, soft tissue of the cheek, nasal cavity, masseter muscle, pterygopalatine space, and pterygoid fossa. It is sometimes difficult to differentiate from tumors extending from the upper alveolus and hard palate.

Overall, the incidence of clinical lymphadenopathy is relatively uncommon at diagnosis.[25] Only 6 (8%) of the MDACC series of 73 patients had palpable lymphadenopathy at diagnosis. The incidence of nodal spread, however, varies with the histologic type, that is, 5 (17%) of 29 patients with squamous cell and poorly differentiated carcinomas versus 1 (4%) of 27 patients with adenocarcinoma, adenoid cystic carcinoma, and mucoepidermoid carcinoma. The incidence of subclinical disease as reflected in the rate of nodal relapse in patients who did not receive elective neck treatment also varies with histologic type, that is, 9 (38%) of 24 patients with squamous cell and poorly differentiated carcinomas versus 2 (8%) of 26 patients with adenocarcinoma, adenoid cystic carcinoma, and mucoepidermoid carcinoma. The cumulative incidence of nodal involvement (gross and microscopic) for patients with squamous cell and poorly differentiated carcinomas is thus about 30%. Ipsilateral subdigastric and submandibular nodes are most frequently involved. Hematogenous spread is rather uncommon.

CLINICAL MANIFESTATION, PATIENT EVALUATION, AND STAGING

Table 33-1 summarizes the updated American Joint Committee on Cancer (AJCC) TNM classification (sixth edition) for cancer of the maxillary sinus, the ethmoid sinus, and the nasal cavity.[26] Significant updates in the sixth edition are as follows:

- The nasoethmoid complex is described by two regions: the nasal cavity proper and the ethmoid sinuses.
- The nasal cavity is divided into four subsites (vestibule, septum, floor, and lateral wall), and the ethmoid sinuses into two subsites (right and left).
- Descriptions of the T staging of ethmoid tumors have been added.
- T4 maxillary sinus tumors are divided into T4a (resectable) and T4b (unresectable).

There was no official AJCC staging for nasal carcinomas before the publication of the sixth edition of the AJCC Cancer Staging Manual.[26] Therefore, the University of Florida (UF) staging

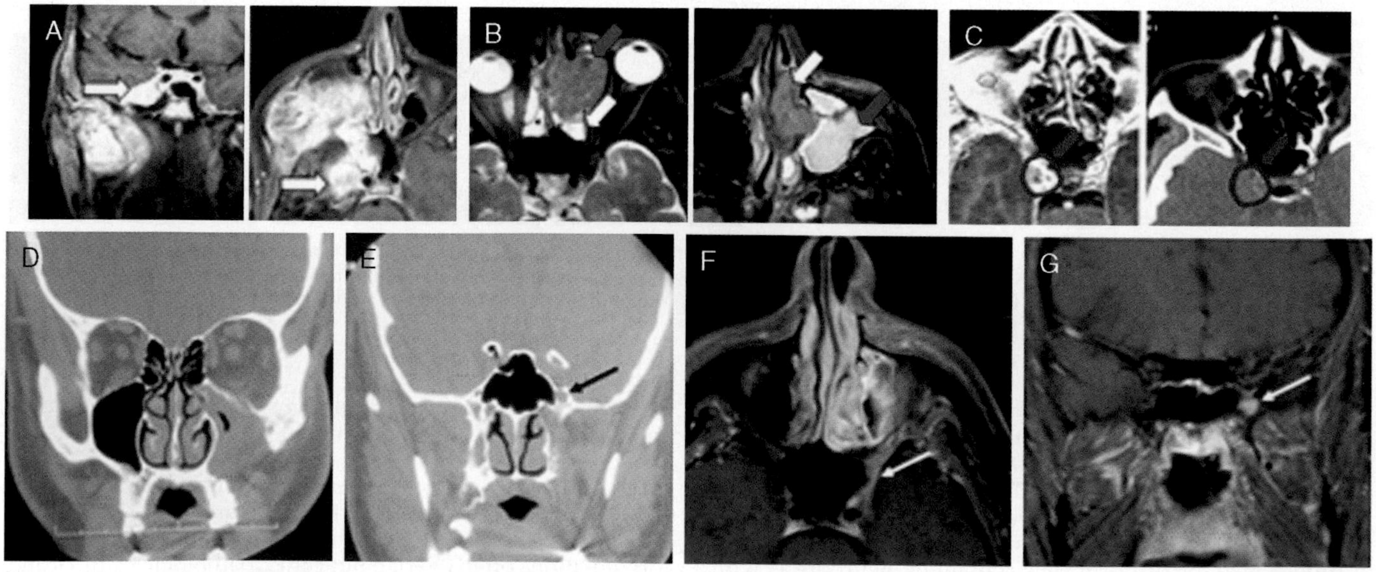

Figure 33-3 **A,** Middle cranial fossa extension *(arrows)* from a tumor centered in the right maxilla and masticator space. There is extension through the lateral and posterior walls of the right maxillary sinus superiorly through the floor of the right middle cranial fossa to the cavernous sinus. Meckel's cave is compressed. **B,** MRI reveals the difference between secretions *(white arrows)* and tumor *(green arrows)* in the sinus. **C,** Fusion of MRI with planning CT demonstrates tumor in the cavernous sinus on MRI *(orange arrow)*, which is not clearly seen on the CT image. **D–G,** MRI shows perineural invasion in a 46-year-old man after a Caldwell-Luc procedure, at which time sarcomatoid carcinoma was resected from the left maxillary sinus. Repeat imaging showed perineural tumor spread along the maxillary division (V_2) of the left trigeminal nerve. **D,** Coronal CT with a bone window shows postoperative changes in the left maxillary sinus. **E,** More posteriorly, MRI shows enlargement of the left foramen rotundum *(arrow)*. Axial **(F)** and coronal **(G)**, fat-suppressed, postcontrast, T1-weighted MR images show excessive enhancement representing tumor within foramen rotundum *(arrows)*. (**D–G,** Courtesy of Lawrence E. Ginsberg, MD, Department of Diagnostic Radiology, M. D. Anderson Cancer Center, Houston, TX.)

Table 33-1 Nasal Cavity and Paranasal Sinuses TNM Staging Classification by the American Joint Committee on Cancer[26]

PRIMARY TUMOR (T)	
Maxillary Sinus	
TX:	Primary tumor cannot be assessed
T0:	No evidence of primary tumor
Tis:	Carcinoma in situ
T1:	Tumor limited to maxillary sinus mucosa with no erosion or destruction of bone
T2:	Tumor causing bone erosion or destruction including extension into the hard palate and/or the middle of the nasal meatus, except extension to the posterior wall of maxillary sinus and pterygoid plates
T3:	Tumor invades any of the following: bone of the posterior wall of maxillary sinus, subcutaneous tissues, floor or medial wall of orbit, pterygoid fossa, ethmoid sinuses
T4a:	Tumor invades anterior orbital contents, skin of cheek, pterygoid plates, infratemporal fossa, cribriform plate, sphenoid or frontal sinuses
T4b:	Tumor invades any of the following: orbital apex, dura, brain, middle cranial fossa, cranial nerves other than maxillary division of trigeminal nerve (V_2), nasopharynx, or clivus
Nasal Cavity and Ethmoid Sinus	
TX:	Primary tumor cannot be assessed
T0:	No evidence of primary tumor
Tis:	Carcinoma in situ
T1:	Tumor restricted to any one subsite, with or without bony invasion
T2:	Tumor invading two subsites in a single region or extending to involve an adjacent region within the nasoethmoidal complex, with or without bony invasion
T3:	Tumor extends to invade the medial wall or floor of the orbit, maxillary sinus, palate, or cribriform plate
T4a:	Tumor invades any of the following: anterior orbital contents, skin of nose or cheek, minimal extension to anterior cranial fossa, pterygoid plates, sphenoid or frontal sinuses
T4b:	Tumor invades any of the following: orbital apex, dura, brain, middle cranial fossa, cranial nerves other than (V_2), nasopharynx, or clivus
REGIONAL LYMPH NODES (N)	
NX:	Regional lymph nodes cannot be assessed
N0:	No regional lymph node metastasis
N1:	Metastasis in a single ipsilateral lymph node, ≤3 cm in greatest dimension
N2:	Metastasis in a single ipsilateral lymph node, >3 cm but ≤6 cm in greatest dimension, or in multiple ipsilateral lymph nodes, ≤6 cm in greatest dimension, or in bilateral or contralateral lymph nodes, ≤6 cm in greatest dimension
N2a:	Metastasis in a single ipsilateral lymph node >3 cm but ≤6 cm in greatest dimension
N2b:	Metastasis in multiple ipsilateral lymph nodes, ≤6 cm in greatest dimension
N2c:	Metastasis in bilateral or contralateral lymph nodes, ≤6 cm in greatest dimension
N3:	Metastasis in a lymph node more than 6 cm in greatest dimension
	In clinical evaluation, the actual size of the nodal mass should be measured, and allowance should be made for intervening soft tissues. Most masses over 3 cm in diameter are not single nodes but confluent nodes or tumors in soft tissues of the neck. There are 3 stages of clinically positive nodes: N1, N2, and N3. The use of subgroups a, b, and c is not required but recommended. Midline nodes are considered homolateral nodes.
DISTANT METASTASIS (M)	
MX:	Distant metastasis cannot be assessed
M0:	No distant metastasis
M1:	Distant metastasis
AJCC STAGE GROUPINGS	
Stage 0:	Tis N0 M0
Stage I:	T1 N0 M0
Stage II:	T2 N0 M0
Stage III:	T3 N0 M0 or T1-3 N1 M0
Stage IVA:	T4a N0-1 M0 or T1-4a N2 M0
Stage IVB:	T4b any N M0 or any T N3 M0
Stage IVC:	Any T any N M1

system (stages I to III) has been used. The correlation between the UF and the T-classification by the criteria of the sixth edition AJCC Staging Systems is approximately as follows:

- Stage I represents tumors confined to nasal fossa equivalent to T1 and T2.
- Stage II represents tumors with extension to adjacent sites: paranasal sinuses, skin, orbit, pterygomaxillary fossa, and nasopharynx equivalent to T3 and small T4a
- Stage III represents tumor extension beyond adjacent structures equivalent to T4.

Imaging plays a crucial role in the staging of sinonasal tumors. MR imaging (MRI) and computed tomography (CT) scans are complementary and provide most of the staging information. MRI is superior at detecting direct intracranial or perinueral spread as shown in Figure 33-3A and 33-D to 33-3G. T2-weighted MRI can be helpful in differentiating tumor (low signal) from obstructed secretions (bright) as illustrated in Figure 33-3B. CT is superior for early cortical bone erosion or extension at the cribriform plate or orbital walls. Fusion of MRI with planning CT scans is useful in delineating tumor not visible on CT (Fig. 33-3C). MRI or positron emission tomography (PET) fusion with planning CT is also useful when induction chemotherapy is given where the prechemotherapy images facilitate the accurate mapping of the initial volume of gross tumor for more precise target delineation.

Certain typical features may provide clues to the nature of the tumors in this region. Slowly progressive lesions tend to deform instead of destroy bony structures. Intermediate-grade tumors can deform surrounding bone with additional sclerosis. Lymphomas tend to permeate bone without frank destruction while carcinomas and sarcomas infiltrate and destroy adjacent bones.

Nasal Vestibule

Small carcinomas of the nasal vestibule usually present as asymptomatic plaques or nodules, often with crusting and scabbing. Advanced lesions may extend to adjacent structures, such as upper nasal septum, upper lip, philtrum, skin of nose, nasolabial fold, hard palate, buccogingival sulcus, etc. Deep muscle and bone and nerve involvement may cause pain accompanied by bleeding or ulceration. Large ulcerated lesions may become infected, leading to severe tenderness that hinders complete clinical assessment. The contiguous spread is best assessed by bimanual palpation and examination through a nasal speculum or fiberoptic telescope after mucosal decongestion and topical anesthesia. Early buccinator and submandibular nodal involvement are also best detected by bimanual palpation. Staging of nasal vestibule carcinoma is by the TNM classification system for the skin. However, other staging systems have been utilized in reporting data.[27-29]

Nasal Cavity and Ethmoid Air Cells

Carcinoma

The presenting symptoms and signs of *nasal fossa* tumors are similar to those associated with nasal polyps, that is, chronic unilateral nasal discharge, ulcer, obstruction, anterior headache, and intermittent nosebleeds. This similarity often leads to delays in diagnosis. Other symptoms and signs include nasal ulcer, tenderness, facial swelling, or pain.[13] Invasion of the orbital cavity may produce palpable medial orbital mass, proptosis, and diplopia; obstruction of the nasolacrimal duct causes epiphora; involvement of the olfactory region may produce anosmia and expansion of the nasal bridge; and extension through the cribriform plate results in frontal headache.

The presenting symptoms and signs of *ethmoid cell* tumors are sinus ache and referred pain to the nasal or retrobulbar region, subcutaneous nodule at the inner canthus, nasal obstruction and discharge, diplopia, and proptosis.

Physical assessment should include examination of the nasal cavity and nasopharynx with a fiberoptic telescope after mucosal decongestion and topical anesthesia, evaluation of cranial nerves (particularly cranial nerves III, IV, V, and VI), and palpation of the nose bridge, cheek, and medial orbital cavity. CT and/or MRI is essential to determine the disease extent and invasion of adjacent structures (e.g., orbital cavity and anterior cranial fossa).

Staging of nasal cavity tumors has been issued for the first time by the American Joint Committee on Cancer (AJCC)[26] (see Table 33-1). Previously, the classification system proposed by the University of Florida has been used.[30] The correlation between these two systems is shown earlier.

Primary tumors of the lateral wall and floor tend to be diagnosed in more advanced stages. Of the patients referred to the MDACC between 1969 and 1985, 3 (21%) of 14 patients with septal lesions versus 20 (65%) of 31 patients with lateral wall or floor primaries had disease extension beyond the nasal cavity (stages II and III).[20]

Esthesioneuroblastoma

Because of the rarity of esthesioneuroblastoma, the natural history was not well known. A literature review of 97 patients reported between 1969 and 1977[24] found that the age distribution is bimodal, with a first peak incidence occurring between 11 and 20 years and a second higher peak incidence between 51 and 60 years. There is a slight preponderance for women.

The most common presenting symptoms are nasal obstruction and epistaxis. Anosmia can precede diagnosis by many years.[31] Other symptoms are related to contiguous disease extension into the orbit (proptosis, visual field defects, orbital pain, epiphora), paranasal sinuses (medial canthus mass, facial swelling), anterior cranial fossa (headache), and manifestation of inappropriate antidiuretic hormone secretion.

Physical evaluation and recommended staging workup procedures for esthesioneuroblastoma are similar to those for nasal fossa tumors. The commonly used staging system, proposed by Kadish and coworkers,[23] is as follows:

- Stage A: disease confined to the nasal cavity
- Stage B: disease confined to the nasal cavity and one or more paranasal sinuses
- Stage C: disease extending beyond the nasal cavity and the paranasal sinuses, including involvement of the orbit, the base of the skull or intracranial cavity, cervical lymph nodes, or distant metastasis

The stage distribution of the 97 patients reviewed by Elkon and associates[24] at diagnosis is 30% stage A, 42% stage B, and 28% stage C. Of the 22 patients who had stage C disease, 9 had orbital involvement, 6 had invasion of the cribriform plate or cranial fossa, 11 had palpable neck nodes, and only 1 had distant metastasis. Of 8 patients treated at MDACC over the past 3.5 years, 1 was in stage B and 7 were in stage C.

Maxillary Sinus

Maxillary cancers are usually diagnosed at advanced stages. Of the 73 patients referred to MDACC for treatment between 1969 and 1985, for example, symptoms and signs related to extension to the premaxillary region (facial swelling, pain, or paresthesia of the cheek) occurred in 26 (36%). Symptoms due to tumor spread to the nasal cavity (e.g., epistaxis, nasal discharge or obstruction) or oral cavity (e.g., ill-fitting denture, alveolar or palatal mass, or unhealed tooth socket after extraction) occurred in 20 (27%) and 19 (26%), respectively. Five patients (7%) presented with symptoms and signs of orbital invasion such as proptosis, diplopia, impaired vision, or orbital pain.[25]

Physical examination should include assessment of the oral and nasal cavities, palpation of the cheek, evaluation of the eye movement and function, and assessment of the trigeminal nerve, particularly the branches of the maxillary division (infraorbital, anterior superior alveolar, posterior superior alveolar, and greater palatine nerves). Numbness of the incisor teeth and upper lip, however, can result from biopsy through a Caldwell-Luc procedure. CT and/or MRI are essential to determine the disease extent and the invasion of adjacent structures (e.g., orbital cavity, infratemporal, pterygopalatine, and anterior cranial fossae).

The T stage description by the 2002 AJCC staging system is shown in Table 33-1[26] and is based on clinical and radiologic evidence of involvement of various adjoining anatomic structures.

PRIMARY THERAPY

Nasal Vestibule

Radiotherapy is generally preferred for carcinoma of the nasal vestibule because of better cosmetic outcome; surgery often results in loss of a major portion of the nose. Depending on the location and size of the primary lesion, radiation treatment can be accomplished by external irradiation, brachytherapy, or a combination of both. Cartilage invasion per se is not a contraindication for radiation therapy since the risk of necrosis is low with fractionated irradiation.[32] Surgery can yield a high control rate with excellent cosmetic results in selected small, superficial lesions. Rare cases of large primaries with extensive tissue destruction and distortion are best managed by resection in combination with preoperative or postoperative radiotherapy. Experienced prosthodontists can design custom-made nasal prostheses for large defects. Smaller defects can be reconstructed by a rotational or advancement flap.

Between 1967 and 1984, 32 patients with newly diagnosed squamous cell carcinoma of the nasal vestibule received definitive radiotherapy at MDACC.[18] Eleven patients with small, localized lesions received local treatment with interstitial brachytherapy and 21 patients received external beam irradiation to the primary disease only (n = 7) or primary lesion and draining lymphatics (n = 14). Local control was achieved in 11 of 11 patients treated with brachytherapy and 20 of 21 patients managed with teletherapy, resulting in an overall primary control rate of 97%. None of the 11 patients with well-delineated small lesions treated with brachytherapy developed nodal recurrence. Neck node relapse occurred in four of nine patients who received external beam irradiation to the primary lesion (in two patients also to the facial lymphatics). In contrast, none of 12 patients who received local treatment with elective neck node irradiation developed nodal failure.

Table 33-2 summarizes the results of five series of patients treated by radiotherapy.[17,18,28,33,34] Patients received brachytherapy, external beam irradiation, or a combination. A number of conclusions can be derived from these data sets. First, brachytherapy or external beam irradiation cures, on average, about 90% of nasal vestibule lesions smaller than 2 cm. Second, when sufficient radiation dose is administered, external beam irradiation can control 70% to 80% of 2- to 4-cm tumors. Third, occult nodal spread is extremely rare in lesions smaller than 2 cm but can be as high as about 40% in larger primary tumors. Finally, the incidence of severe late complications is low with proper radiation technique and fractionation schedule.

An overall local control of 93% was found on analysis of irradiation of 1676 carcinomas of the skin of the nose and nasal vestibule performed by the Groupe Européen de Curietherapie in France.[11] Local control was dependent on tumor size (<2 cm, 96%; 2 to 3.9 cm, 88%; ≥4 cm, 81%), site (external surface, 94%; vestibule, 75%), and recurrent tumors versus new tumors (88% versus 95%). Local control was independent of histology for tumors less than 4 cm, but for those larger than

Table 33-2 Reported Local and Regional Control Rates of Nasal Vestibule Carcinomas Treated by Definitive Radiotherapy

Institution	Local Control	Nodal Control	Late Complications
University of Texas M. D. Anderson Cancer Center[18]	Brachytherapy: 11/11 Teletherapy: 20/21 (95%) Total: 31/32 (97%)	Small lesions: 11/11 Large lesions: ELR: 12/12 (100%) No ELR: 5/9 (56%) Total: 28/32 (88%)	Osteonecrosis (at area of hot spot): 1 Nosebleeds: 1
University of Florida[33]	Brachytherapy: 9/9 Teletherapy: 8/11 (73%) Combination: 12/16 (75%) Total: 29/36 (81%)	ELR: 3/3 No ELR: 23/27 (85%); 4 relapses were salvaged. Total: 26/30** (87%)	Transient soft tissue necrosis after implants: 4 Nasal stenosis: 1
Rotterdam Radiotherapy Institute[34]	≤1.5 cm (n = 15): 72%* >1.5 cm (n = 17): 50%* <54 Gy†: 37%* ≥54 Gy†: 82%*	Details not presented	Details not presented
Princess Margaret Hospital[17]	<2 cm (n = 34): 97%* ≥2 cm (n = 16) and size not recorded (n = 6): 57%* • <55 Gy/5 wk: 30% • ≥55 Gy/5 wk: 82%	No ELR: 51/54 (94%) (2 patients presented with nodes)	Osteonecrosis: 2 (1 resulting in fistula) Nasal stenosis: 2 Massive epistaxis: 1
VU University Medical Center, Amsterdam (Johannes A. Langendijk et al)[28]	Overall: 79% (ultimate local control: 95%) <1.5 cm (n = 32): 83% (ultimate: 94%) ≥1.5 cm (n = 24): 74% (ultimate: 96%)	Routine ELR to the mustache region 2-y regional control rate: 87% (6 of 7 neck relapses were salvaged) Ultimate regional control rate at 5 y was 97%	Rhinorrhea: 45% Nasal dryness: 39% Epistaxis: 15% Adhesions: 4% Skin necrosis in 3 patients (all in IDR brachytherapy group) Post–radiation therapy RT sarcoma in the nasal vestibule in 1 patient

ELR, elective lymphatic radiation; IDR: intermediate-dose-rate of 2.7 Gy/h (range, .7-7.1 Gy), median dose per fraction of IDR brachytherapy was 15 Gy (range, 3.2-26 Gy). The total dose of IDR brachytherapy was 16 Gy (range, 8-40 Gy).

*5-y Actuarial rates.

†2.5-3 Gy/fraction.

‡Eligible for 2-y follow-up.

4 cm, basal cell carcinomas were more frequently controlled than squamous cell carcinomas. There were few complications (necrosis, 2%). The local control rate with surgery was approximately 90%.

Nasal Cavity and Ethmoid Air Cells

Carcinoma

Radiotherapy and surgery are effective in curing stage I lesions of the respiratory region. The choice of therapy depends on the size and location of the tumor and the anticipated cosmetic outcome. Posterior nasal septum lesions are generally treated by surgery. In contrast, interstitial brachytherapy (^{192}I wire implant) is an excellent treatment option for small anteroinferior septal lesions (1.5 cm) to avoid partial removal of the anterior nasal septum. It is preferable to treat lateral wall lesions extending to the ala nasi with external irradiation for cosmetic reasons.

Stage II and operable stage III neoplasms are best treated with surgery. In most cases, postoperative irradiation is indicated.

Nasal Cavity—M. D. Anderson Cancer Center Experience

Between 1969 and 1985, 51 patients with carcinomas of the nasal cavity proper were referred to MDACC, of whom 45 received curative treatment and were followed for 2.8 to 16.8 years (median, 11 years).[20] Eighteen patients were treated with radiotherapy only (interstitial brachytherapy in 5 and external beam therapy in 13 patients), and 27 received surgery and postoperative radiotherapy. The site of origin was nasal septum in 14 patients and the lateral wall or floor of the cavity in 31 patients. All 14 lesions of the nasal septum were squamous cell carcinomas. Of the 31 nonseptal nasal fossa tumors, 16 were squamous cell carcinomas, 9 were adenocarcinomas, 5 were adenoid cystic carcinomas, and 1 was undifferentiated cancer.

Table 33-3 shows the pattern of failure in this series of patients. All 14 patients with carcinoma of the nasal septum had the disease controlled (10 after initial therapy and 4 after salvage therapy). Nine of 31 patients with lesions of the lateral wall and floor died of the disease, 5 of uncontrolled local disease, 2 of distant metastases, and 2 of both. The disease-specific survival rates at 5 and 10 years were 83% and 80%, respectively. The corresponding overall survival rates were 69% and 58%, respectively.

These results[20] indicate that the prognosis of patients with nasal cavity carcinoma was better than that of patients with maxillary sinus cancer treated during the same era (see later). This finding is supported by a systematic review of 154 articles published from 1960 to 1998 with 16,396 patients with carcinoma of the nasal cavity and paranasal sinuses.[1] The survival of patients with nasal cavity cancer was consistently better than that of maxillary sinus cancer. For example, among patients treated during the decade of the 1990s, the overall survival of patients with nasal cavity cancer was 66% ± 15% versus 45% ± 11% for patients with maxillary sinus cancer.

Nasal Cavity—Comparative Outcome by Series

Table 33-4 summarizes the results of relatively large series focusing on nasal fossa tumors. Locoregional control rates range from 60% to 80%.[20,35-37] The incidence of isolated regional recurrence in patients who did not receive elective nodal treatment was approximately 5% in the MDACC series. Treatment morbidity was proportional to disease extent, which dictates the magnitude of surgical resection and the target volume of radiotherapy. Most frequent complications were soft tissue necrosis, nasal stenosis, and visual impairment (see Table 33-4).

Nasal Cavity—Comparative Outcome by Histology, Stage, and Pathologic Features

The data on 783 of a total of 981 cases of nasal cavity cancer extracted from the Surveillance, Epidemiology and End Results (SEER) database from 1988 through 1998 were analyzed.[38] Squamous cell carcinoma was the most common tumor type (49.3%), followed by esthesioneuroblastoma (13.2%). More than half of the cases presented with a small primary tumor (T1), and only 5% had positive nodes at diagnosis. Overall mean (median) survival was 76 (81) months, with an overall 5-year survival rate of 56.7%. On multivariate analysis, male gender, increasing age, T stage, N stage, and poorer tumor grade adversely affected survival independently ($p < .05$). Radiotherapy was administered in 50.5% of patients and also independently predicted poorer survival ($p = .03$), which is likely due to selection of patients with poor prognostic features, such as perineural invasion, positive margins, or poor performance status (medically unfit for surgery) for radiotherapy. The median and 5-year survivals by histology, T stage, and differentiation are shown in Table 33-5.[38]

Ethmoid Cells—M. D. Anderson Cancer Center Experience

Between 1969 and 1985, 17 patients with carcinomas of the ethmoid cells were referred to MDACC for treatment. Nine patients received definitive radiotherapy and eight underwent surgical resection preceded (two patients) or followed (six patients) by radiation. None of the patients received elective nodal treatment.

At the last follow-up, 11 patients had no evidence of disease, 4 patients developed local recurrence, and 2 patients

Table 33-3 Pattern of Failure of Nasal Cavity Carcinomas

Relapse	No. of Patients	LR	N	LR + DM	DM Only
After initial therapy					
Septum	14	2	2	0	0
Lateral and floor	31	9	0	1	2
After salvage therapy					
Septum	4	0	0	0	0
Lateral and floor	5	1	0	1	0

DM, distant metastasis; LR, local recurrence; N, nodal relapse.

Modified from Ang KK, Jiang GL, Frankenthaler RA, et al: Carcinomas of the nasal cavity. Radiother Oncol 24:163-168, 1992.

Table 33-4 **Outcome of Patients With Nasal Cavity Cancers of Various Histologies Treated by Radiation, Surgery, or Both**

Institution	Treatment	Survival	Late Complications
University of Texas M. D. Anderson Cancer Center[20]	Radiotherapy only: 18 patients Radiation + surgery: 2 patients Surgery + radiation: 25 patients	5-y actuarial: 75% All 14 nasal septum lesions and 22/31 tumors of lateral wall and floor were controlled	Radiation-induced blindness: 2 patients Surgical blindness: 2 patients Maxilla necrosis: 2 patients Stenosis/perforation: 3 patients
Roswell Park Memorial Institute*[35]	Radiotherapy only: 30 patients Surgery only: 13 patients Surgery + radiation: 14 patients	5-y actuarial: 67% Patients with WDSCC had the best outcome	Not presented
University of Puerto Rico*[36]	Radiotherapy only: 34 patients Surgery only: 6 patients	5-y overall: 56%	Not presented
Mallinckrodt Institute of Radiology*[37]	Radiotherapy only: 28 patients Radiation + surgery: 18 patients Surgery + radiation: 10 patients	5-year actuarial: 52% Survival not significantly affected by histology Neck relapse occurred in 10/52 N0 patients	Complications (soft tissue necrosis, cataract, synechiae, otitis media) requiring surgery: 5 patients

WDSCC, well-differentiated squamous cell carcinoma.
*Includes patients with nasal vestibule carcinomas.

Table 33-5 **Treatment Results of the Nasal Cavity Cancer From the Analysis of the Surveillance, Epidemiology, and End Results Database for 1988 Through 1998**

Tumor Type	5-y Survival, %
Adenocarcinoma	49.0
Adenoid cystic carcinoma	59.1
Melanoma	22.1
Other tumors	59.5
Sarcoma	78.0
Squamous cell carcinoma	61.6
Esthesioneuroblastoma	63.6
SNUC	49.5
Overall	56.7
Classification	**5-y Survival, %**
T	
T1	66.4
T2	51.8
T3	45.6
T4	40.2
N	
N0	62.3
N1	28.4
N2	NA
N3	NA
Not assigned	
GRADE	
Well differentiated (I)	75.3
Moderately differentiated (II)	61.9
Poorly differentiated (III)	47.6
Undifferentiated (IV)	36.8
Not assigned	NA

NA, not applicable; SNUC, sinonasal undifferentiated carcinomas.
*Because of rounding, percentages may not total 100.
From Bhattacharyya N: Cancer of the nasal cavity: survival and factors influencing prognosis. Arch Otolaryngol Head Neck Surg 128:1079-1083, 2002.

had distant metastasis (1 of these 2 patients experienced regional relapse that was subsequently controlled by nodal dissection and postoperative radiotherapy). The 5-year actuarial local control, overall survival, and relapse-free survival rates of this group of patients were 70%, 55%, and 61%, respectively. Treatment complications were vision impairment (three patients), frontal lobe necrosis (two patients), bone necrosis (one patient), and nasal stenosis (one patient).

Esthesioneuroblastoma

Literature Review

Because of the low incidence of esthesioneuroblastoma, it is not possible to define the optimal therapy by prospective studies. In a review of case reports of patients treated before 1977 (Table 33-6), Elkon and colleagues[24] found that single-modality therapy, radiotherapy or surgery, yields a greater than 90% ultimate locoregional control rate for stage A lesions (although a number of patients had to undergo salvage therapy for local or regional relapse after initial treatment). The optimal therapy for stage B disease is unclear, partly because this stage represents a heterogeneous patient group. A combination of surgery and radiotherapy may have a slight advantage for this patient subset. For patients with stage C lesions, the evidence suggests better results with the combination of surgery and radiotherapy. The available data do not justify routine elective nodal treatment since the incidence of isolated nodal relapse is less than 15%.

Table 33-6 summarizes the literature data of patients with esthesioneuroblastoma treated by various modalities between 1969 and 1977.[24] Only 1 of 24 patients with stage A tumors died of the disease (neck node recurrence and lung metastasis). The prognosis of patients with stage B disease is also excellent. The locoregional recurrence rate of patients with stage B tumors after initial therapy is not higher than that of patients with stage A lesions, but salvage therapy has been less successful. Overall, 30% of patients with stage B tumor died of the disease.

About 60% of patients with stage C tumors died of the disease and most patients succumbed to local tumor progression. Distant metastasis is not a prominent pattern of failure

Table 33-6 **Treatment Results of Esthesioneuroblastoma by Stage and Therapy Modality**

Kadish Stage	Therapy	Local Recurrence	Nodal Relapse	Salvage by Subsequent RT or S	Distant Metastasis	Died of Disease
A (n = 24)	RT	2/5	1/5	3/3	0/5	0/5
	S	4/9	1*/9	4/4	0/9	0/9
	S + RT	1/10	2/10	2/2	1†/10	1/10
	All	7/24 (29%)	4/24 (17%)	9/9	1/24 (4%)	1/24 (4%)
B (n = 33)	RT	1/7	2/7	0/1	0/7	3/7
	S	3/6	0/6	1/2	0/6	2/6
	S + RT	5/20	1/20	3/4	3/20	5/20
	All	9/33 (27%)	3/33 (9%)	4/7	3/33 (9%)	10/33 (30%)
C (n = 21)	RT	3/5	0/5	0/0	1/5	4/5
	S	0/1	0/1	0/0	0/1	0/1
	S + RT‡	6/15	1/15	1/1	1/15	8/15
	All	9/21 (43%)	1/21 (5%)	1/1	2/21 (10%)	12/21 (57%)

RT, radiotherapy; S, surgery.
*Along with local recurrence.
†Along with nodal relapse.
‡Site of relapse not specified in 2 patients.
Modified from Elkon D, Hightower SI, Lim ML, et al: Esthesioneuroblastoma. Cancer 44:1087-1094, 1979.

(10%), even in locoregionally advanced esthesioneuroblastoma.

Eight patients were treated at MDACC over the past 3.5 years with surgery and adjuvant radiotherapy using intensity modulated radiotherapy to 60 Gy. One patient had stage B disease and 7 had stage C, of whom 5 had intracranial extension. There were no local recurrences and 1 nodal recurrence was salvaged surgically. All eight are alive with no evidence of disease.

The adverse impact of poor tumor differentiation established previously has been validated by retrospective pathological studies[39] as well as the analysis of the SEER database from 1988 through 1998 (see Table 33-5).[38]

Comparative Series

Spaulding and colleagues[31] reported one of the largest single-institution retrospective series, consisting of 25 patients treated at the University of Virginia Medical Center from 1959 through 1986 followed for 2 years after therapy. There had been a gradual evolution of treatment with progressive introduction of craniofacial resections, complex field megavoltage radiation, and, for stage C disease, the addition of chemotherapy. Therefore, patients were divided into two groups, based on treatment era, for comparative analysis. Although the series is relatively small, this analysis revealed two interesting findings: (1) extensive craniofacial resection does not appear to confer a major advantage over wide local excision for patients with stage B lesions; and (2) the addition of chemotherapy to craniofacial resection and radiotherapy for patients with stage C tumors may yield a higher disease-specific survival.

Analysis of 72 sinonasal neuroendocrine tumors treated at MDACC between 1982 and 2002 included a spectrum of histologies: esthesioneuroblastoma (ENB, 31 patients), sinonasal undifferentiated carcinoma (SNUC, 16 patients), neuroendocrine carcinoma (NEC, 18 patients), and small cell carcinoma (SmCC, 7 patients). The overall survival at 5 years was 93.1% for patients with ENB, 62.5% for SNUC, 64.2% for NEC, and 28.6% for SmCC (p = .0029; log-rank test). The local control rate at 5 years also was superior for patients with ENB (96.2%) compared with patients who had SNUC (78.6%), NEC (72.6%), or SmCC (66.7%) (p = .04). The regional failure (RF) rate at 5 years was 8.7% for patients with ENB, 15.6% for SNUC, 12.9% for NEC, and 44.4% for SmCC. The corresponding distant metastasis rates were 0.0% for ENB, 25.4% for SNUC, 14.1% for NEC, and 75.0% for SmCC. ENB had excellent local and distant control rates with local therapy alone.[40]

Among the 783 cases of nasal cavity cancer extracted from the SEER database, 103 (13.2%) were esthesioneuroblastoma. The median survival was 88 months, and 5-year survival was 63.6%.[38]

Maxillary Sinus

T1 or T2 tumors of the infrastructure can be cured by surgery alone, which may be limited to a partial maxillectomy. However, most of these tumors present at fairly advanced stages and the combination of surgery and radiotherapy, usually given postoperatively, is considered standard treatment. The results of radical surgical excisions such as craniofacial resection, total maxillectomy, or orbital exenteration have improved over the past decades, especially with aggressive plastic reconstructive techniques. Nonetheless, these operations still carry significant morbidity.

Analyses of the SEER database revealed that the treatment outcome of patients with maxillary sinus carcinomas have improved over the last four decades.[1] The overall survival of the decades of the 1960s, 1970s, 1980s, and 1990s was 26% ± 13%, 31% ± 8%, 39% ± 14%, and 45% ± 11% respectively (p = .02). However, treatment outcome is still poor, and less than 55% of patients survive longer than 5 years despite radical surgery (Table 33-7).[25,41-46] Local recurrence at the primary site and distant metastasis are the most common patterns of treatment failure.

Postoperative Radiotherapy

The available literature data reveal that the combination of surgery and irradiation yields a 53% to 78% 5-year local control rate and a 39% to 64% 5-year survival rate.[27-36] These rates are better than those achieved with surgery or radiotherapy alone (see later). The results with the combination of surgery and radiotherapy have also improved over the past four decades, with overall survival in the 1960s, 1970s, 1980s, and 1990s being 33% ± 18%, 42% ± 15%, 54% ± 15%, and 56% ± 13% ($p < .001$).[1]

The data from 73 patients with carcinomas of the maxillary sinus who received postoperative radiotherapy at MDACC between 1969 and October 1985 were analyzed in 1989. The T stage distribution by the AJCC system was 3 T1, 16 T2, 32 T3, and 22 T4. Only six patients had palpable nodal disease at diagnosis. All patients underwent partial or radical maxillectomy followed by radiotherapy delivered through a wedge-pair or three-field technique. The radiation doses ranged from 50 to 60 Gy, except in three patients who received lower doses. Elective nodal irradiation was given to 17 patients.[25]

The findings of the retrospective analysis can be briefly summarized as follows: (1) local recurrence and distant metastasis were the major pattern of relapse (Table 33-8) and causes of death; (2) nodal relapse rate without elective lymphatic irradiation was higher than 30% in patients with squamous cell and undifferentiated carcinomas (Table 33-9); (3) local recurrence rate increased with T stage and was significantly higher in the 42 patients with evidence of perineural invasion in the primary tumor than in the 29 patients without it (36% versus 10%) (Table 33-10); and (4) major complications occurred predominantly during the earlier part of the study period when large wedge-pair portals were used, radiation was administered in doses higher than 2 Gy/fraction, and significant dose heterogeneity existed within the target volume (Table 33-11).

Based on these observations, the following modifications in the treatment policy were introduced in August 1989: (1) to design radiation portals to encompass the base of the skull, including the gasserian ganglion, more generously in patients with evidence of perineural invasion and those with adenoid cystic carcinoma; (2) to deliver elective irradiation to the ipsilateral upper neck nodes in patients with T2 to T4 squamous cell or undifferentiated carcinoma; and (3) to use measures to improve dose distribution within the target volume, such as a water-filled balloon to reduce the size of the air cavity.

A reanalysis was undertaken to assess how these changes in treatment policy have affected outcome in postoperative maxillary sinus patients. This retrospective study included patients with maxillary sinus carcinoma who received postoperative radiotherapy between 1969 and 2002 at MDACC. Of a total of 147 patients, 90 (group A) received treatment before and 57 (group B) after the implementation of the revised treatment policy. Group A had proportionately fewer

Table 33-7 Outcome of Patients With Locally Advanced Cancer of the PNS Treated With Combined Surgery and Radiation Therapy

Study	Year	No. of Patients	5-y Survival	Local Recurrence	Distant Metastasis
Lavertu et al[41]	1989	54	38%	52%	—
Spiro et al[42]	1989	105	38%	49%	15%
Zaharia et al[43]	1989	149	36%	43%	—
Paulino et al[44]	1998	48	47%	46%	17%
Le et al[45]	1999	97	34%	54%	34%
Myers et al[46]	2002	141	52%	56%	33%
Jiang et al[25]	1991	67*	53%†	24%	27%

*Node-negative patients.
†5-y relapse-free survival.

Table 33-8 Pattern of Failure in 73 Patients With Maxillary Sinus Carcinomas

Relapse Pattern	L	N	L + N	DM	L + DM	N + DM
After initial therapy	10	10	1	8	3	1
After salvage therapy	11	0	1	11	4	1

DM, distant metastasis; L, local recurrence; N, nodal relapse.
Modified from Jiang GL, Ang KK, Peters LJ, et al: Maxillary sinus carcinomas: natural history and results of postoperative radiotherapy. Radiother Oncol 21:193-200, 1991.

Table 33-9 Incidence of Nodal Metastasis by Histologic Type*

Histology	No. of Patients Presenting With Neck Nodes (%)	No. of Patients Who Developed Nodal Recurrence (%)
Squamous cell carcinoma	5/23 (22%)	6/18 (33%)
Undifferentiated tumor	0/6	3/6 (50%)
Adenocarcinoma	1/6	1/5
Adenoid cystic carcinoma	0/19	1/19 (5%)
Mucoepidermoid carcinoma	0/2	0/2

Modified from Jiang GL, Ang KK, Peters LJ, et al: Maxillary sinus carcinomas: natural history and results of postoperative radiotherapy. Radiother Oncol 21:193-200, 1991.
*Excludes 17 patients who received elective neck irradiation.

Table 33-10 Influence of Disease and Therapy Variables on the Treatment Outcome for 73 Patients With Maxillary Sinus Tumors

Variable	No. of Patients	DISEASE CONTROL, 5-Y, % Local	Nodal	DM	SURVIVAL, 5-Y, % RFS	DSS
PATHOLOGIC T STAGE*						
T1 + 2	12	91	71	17	64	75
T3	28	77	80	25	57	69
T4	29	65	93	37	44	59
N STAGE						
N0	67	74	84	27‡	53	66‡
N1-2	6	67	82	48†	33	33
HISTOLOGY						
Squamous cell carcinoma	36	62	86	17‡	49	53
Undifferentiated	9	89	67	50	53	42
Adenocarcinoma	6	80	67	39	42	60
Adenoid cystic carcinoma	20	82	94	31	60	84
Mucoepidermoid	2	(2/2)	(2/2)	(0/2)	(2/2)	(2/2)
NERVE INVASION*						
No	29	90‡	86	20	74‡	78
Yes	42	64	80	36	37	57
MARGIN OF RESECTION*						
Negative	54	74	86	17	58	66
Positive	17	77	76	32	38	66
ELECTIVE NODAL RADIATION						
No	50	77	80	31§	51	58
Yes	17	61	100	0	61	68

*Excluding patients whose pathological reports were not complete.
†Including 11 patients who did not receive elective neck treatment and developed nodal recurrence.
‡Significant at .05 level.
DM, distant metastasis; DSS, disease-specific survival; RFS, relapse-free survival.
Modified from Jiang GL, Ang KK, Peters LJ, et al: Maxillary sinus carcinomas: natural history and results of postoperative radiotherapy. Radiother Oncol 21:193-200, 1991.

Table 33-11 Type and Incidence of Treatment Complications Occurring in 73 Patients

Type of Side Effects	Patients No. (%)	Latent Period: Range in Months After Radiotherapy
Ipsilateral blindness*	13 (30)	1-36
Bilateral blindness	4 (5)	13-36
Brain necrosis	5 (7)	5-73
Bone necrosis requiring	4 (5)	1-17
debridement	2 (3)	17, 74
Soft tissue necrosis/fistula	9 (12)	0-4
Trismus	3 (4)	60-72
Pituitary insufficiency	3 (4)	3-48
Hearing loss		

*Assessed in 44 patients who did not undergo ipsilateral enucleation.
Modified from Jiang GL, Ang KK, Peters LJ, et al: Maxillary sinus carcinomas: natural history and results of postoperative radiotherapy. Radiother Oncol 21:193-200, 1991.

patients with squamous cell carcinoma (53% versus 72%) than Group B but more patients with adenoid cystic (28% versus 14%) and undifferentiated histologies (10% versus 3.5%). Presence of perineural invasion was proportionately higher in group A (53% versus 21%) but group B had a greater proportion of patients with unknown perineural status (15% versus 2%). The two groups were balanced with regard to age, gender, T and N stage, margin status, radiation dose, and treatment time.

With a mean follow-up of 97 months in group A and 52 months in group B, there were no statistically significant differences in 5-year local control (76% versus 68%), regional control (83% versus 81%), distant metastases (29% versus 17%), recurrence-free survival (51% versus 54%), and overall survival (52% versus 61%) between the two groups. Recurrence within the primary site and distant metastasis remained significant contributors to mortality, accounting for over 50% of all deaths in the entire group.

In accord with the change in treatment policy to cover the base of skull in patients with evidence of perineural invasion, the association between local recurrence and presence of perineural invasion no longer remained significant for patients in group B. Prior to this change, 77% of the patients who recurred at the primary site also had perineural invasion (p = .01). Following the increase in radiation portals, only 22% of those patients recurring in the primary site also had perineural invasion (NS; 56% without neural invasion, 22% with unspecified status). It remains unclear at present as to why this finding did not translate into an improvement in local control.

In the entire subgroup of patients with N0 squamous and undifferentiated carcinomas, patients receiving elective neck irradiation (n = 45) had significantly better 5-year regional control (92% versus 63%; p = .0004) than those patients not receiving elective neck irradiation (n = 38). This effect also translated into an improvement in 5-year relapse-free survival (67% with elective treatment versus 42% without; p = .01). These findings held true when the patients in group A (n = 31) with N0 squamous and undifferentiated carcinomas who had not received elective neck irradiation were compared with the patients in group B (n = 26) who had received ipsilateral neck treatment as per institutional policy change (5-year regional control of 64% of group A versus 87% for group B, p = .03; 5-year relapse-free survival of 41% for group A versus 67% for group B, p = .03).

The most striking difference between the two groups as a consequence of treatment policy change was in the incidence of severe complications. Of the entire group of 147 patients late complications occurred in 58 of 90 patients in group A (64.4%) whereas only 13 occurred in the 57 group B patients (22.8%), a notable decrease in late side effects after implementation of these changes.

LOCALLY ADVANCED DISEASE AND PALLIATION

Primary Radiotherapy

Patients with locally advanced inoperable tumors or who are unfit for surgery are often treated with primary radiotherapy. Compilation of literature data reveals that primary radiotherapy yields a 22% to 39% 5-year local control rate and a 22% to 40% 5-year survival rate.[1,47-53] The results with radiotherapy as the primary modality have also improved over the past four decades, with overall survival in the 1960s, 1970s, 1980s, and 1990s being 21% ± 13%, 19% ± 17%, 28% ± 20%, and 33% ± 18% (p = .048).[2]

Chemotherapy—Neoadjuvant, Concurrent

Chemotherapy is used in several ways:

1. Neoadjuvant chemotherapy followed by either surgery and postoperative radiotherapy, or followed by definitive radiotherapy if inoperable, or radiotherapy and limited surgery.
2. Concurrent chemotherapy is increasingly used with definitive radiotherapy in the management of inoperable tumors on the basis of improved results in other head and neck sites.

The sequence and agents used vary with the tumor type, tumor extent, and medical comorbidity of individual patients. The data suggest that concurrent chemotherapy is more effective than neoadjuvant chemotherapy in improving local control.

Neoadjuvant Chemotherapy

Neoadjuvant chemotherapy in addition to standard radiotherapy failed to demonstrate any therapeutic advantage over radiation alone in a matched-control study from Seoul, Korea, comparing standard radiotherapy versus neoadjuvant chemotherapy and radiation.[54] Thirty-four patients with inoperable maxillary squamous cell cancer were treated with three cycles of neoadjuvant chemotherapy (cisplatin and a 5-day continuous infusion of 5-fluorouracil with or without intravenous vinblastine) followed by radiotherapy (66 Gy to 75 Gy; median, 70 Gy). The outcomes were compared with those for 34 patients treated with radiation alone who were matched for age, sex, performance status, tumor grade, and stage and local extent of tumor. Despite a higher response rate to neoadjuvant chemotherapy, the relapse rate and patterns of treatment failure were not influenced by the addition of neoadjuvant chemotherapy. Radiation-induced late complications occurred equally in both treatment groups. After a median follow-up of 48 months, there was no significant difference in 5-year actuarial survival or disease-free survival between the two treatment groups. Both groups had a 65% rate of local recurrence. The 5 year survival rate was 32% after radiotherapy alone and 30% after neoadjuvant chemotherapy followed by radiotherapy.

Neoadjuvant chemotherapy is still occasionally used for patients with extensive inoperable tumors to reduce tumor volume. Reducing the tumor size may be helpful in permitting removal of tumor even if this is only a limited resection or debulking procedure. If the tumor remains unresectable following induction chemotherapy or the patient is medically inoperable, the reduction in tumor volume may also prove useful in radiotherapy planning. For example, evagination of tumor superiorly into the brain or adjacent to the optic apparatus may shrink to yield a postchemotherapy tumor volume that may be boosted to full radiotherapy dose, whereas the prechemotherapy tumor volume may be given an intermediate dose, which will result in less severe late neurologic and visual complications.

Neoadjuvant Chemotherapy Plus Concurrent Chemoradiation

Neoadjuvant chemotherapy followed by surgical resection plus adjuvant concurrent chemoradiation produced excellent long-term outcome in a subgroup analysis from the University of Chicago Hospitals.[55] Promising rates with respect to local control, overall survival, and disease-free survival were achieved in 15 patients with locoregionally advanced paranasal sinus cancer treated with induction chemotherapy (three cycles of cisplatin and 5-fluorouracil), surgery, and concomitant chemoradiotherapy (hydroxyurea and 5-fluorouracil in a week-on, week-off sequence and median total radiotherapy dose of 60 Gy (range, 45 to 74 Gy). The 10-year overall survival, disease-free survival, and local control rates were 56%, 73%, and 79%, respectively.

Concurrent Chemoradiation

Concurrent chemotherapy and radiotherapy using accelerated fractionation (concomitant boost radiotherapy) produced surprisingly good local control and survival in a prospective study from Memorial Sloan-Kettering Cancer Center.[56] Among 82 patients with unresectable cancers of the head and neck, 12 had T4 paranasal sinus cancer. Patients received 70 Gy in 6 weeks using a concomitant-boost technique with cisplatin (100 mg/m^2) given on days 1 and 22 of radiotherapy. Three-year local control rates for T4 paranasal sinus cancer was 78% and 3-year survival rate was 42%.

Concurrent cisplatin (single agent) or carboplatin chemotherapy is often used during external beam radiation to treat patients with newly diagnosed unresectable squamous cell carcinoma. This may be given after induction chemotherapy. The addition of chemotherapy enhances acute toxicity such as mucosal and cutaneous toxicity in addition to the toxicity of chemotherapy.

Concurrent etoposide (VP-16) plus cisplatin (or carboplatin) is used during radiation to treat patients with sinonasal undifferentiated, poorly differentiated carcinoma, or neuroendocrine carcinoma. This may be given following neoadjucant chemotherapy with the same agents to reduce tumor bulk and systemic spread.

Chemotherapy is not routinely given concurrently with radiation for patients with esthesioneuroblastoma. Local therapy alone with surgery and postoperative radiotherapy[40] yields excellent results at 5 years with regard to both overall survival (93.1%) and local control rate (96.2%). Concurrent chemotherapy during radiation may be considered in inoperable cases.

Palliation

The symptoms of incurable sinonasal cancer are particularly distressing. Multidisciplinary input is required even with very advanced cases, because palliation may involve limited surgery, radiotherapy, chemotherapy, investigational studies, or best supportive care. The morbidity of each modality has to be balanced with the benefit to symptom control and improvement in quality of life. Attention is required to

- The control of pain and discomfort as a first priority
- Communication of the incurable status of the tumor
- Psychological effect of incurable status
- Impact of disfigurement and dysfunction that are frequently present
- Collaboration with caregivers, social services, and home and hospice care

Chemotherapy is often single agent or investigational. If radiation therapy is given, concurrent chemotherapy may be added. Larger dose per fraction is the usual practice for palliative cases in order to reduce the duration of treatment. If concurrent chemotherapy is added, consideration may be given to treating at 2 Gy/fraction to avoid severe acute effects.

Treatment with radiotherapy or chemotherapy is often effective in reduction of tumor bulk to provide relief of symptoms such as disfiguring masses, proptosis, discomfort or neuropathic pain, headache, epistaxis or other bleeding, nasal obstruction or discharge, and trismus.

TECHNIQUES OF IRRADIATION

Nasal Vestibule

Target Volume

For small, delineated, well-differentiated carcinoma measuring up to 1.5 cm, small fields with a 1- or 2-cm margin are appropriate. The initial target volume for all poorly differentiated tumors and well-differentiated primaries larger than 1.5 cm without palpable lymphadenopathy encompasses both nasal vestibules with at least 2- or 3-cm margins around the primary tumor (wider margins for infiltrative tumor) and bilateral facial ("Manchu mustache area"),[57] submandibular, and subdigastric nodes (see Fig. 33-1E). When lymph node involvement is present at diagnosis, the lower neck nodes are also irradiated.

For postoperative radiotherapy, the initial target volume includes the operative bed plus a 1- to 1.5-cm margin and the elective nodal regions. The volume is reduced off the nondissected nodal regions after 50 Gy (25 fractions) to deliver an additional 6 Gy to the surgical bed. At 56 Gy, a final conedown is done to include the preoperative tumor bed to administer 4 Gy, with the total dose being 60 Gy. If there are positive margins or a very limited excision was done, this final conedown is given with 10 Gy (total dose, 66 Gy).

Setup, Field Arrangement, and Dose Fractionation Schedule

BRACHYTHERAPY

Brachytherapy for small lesions is accomplished by ^{192}Ir wire implant or, in selected cases, by intracavitary ^{192}Ir mold. Hollow needles for afterloading are inserted under general anesthesia, which allows good exposure of the tumor as well as protection of the airway in the event of bleeding from the vascular Kiesselbach's plexus on the anterior nasal septum or from posterior hemorrhages originating from larger vessels near the sphenopalatine artery, behind the middle turbinate. Implantation of a T2 squamous cell carcinoma of the columella is shown in Figures 33-1 and 33-2. The recommended doses for low dose rate brachytherapy have evolved empirically and range from 60 to 65 Gy delivered over 5 to 7 days. An example of needle placement is shown in Figure 33-2.

Brachytherapy boosts may be given to T1 or T2 nasal vestibule tumors following initial larger field external beam radiotherapy. At 50 Gy, the patient is assessed, and if there is good reduction of tumor volume, a boost of 20 to 25 Gy may be administered in about 2 days by low-dose-rate brachytherapy.

High-dose-rate (HDR) brachytherapy has also been utilized as a boost. A custom mold of the nasal vestibule is fabricated and tumor is marked in the mold. Two to four plastic tubes with a 1.0-cm spacing are inserted in the mold alongside the tumor. In the case of tumors of the lateral part of the vestibule, two catheters are placed on the inner aspects of the nasal vestibule. In the case of medially localized tumors, catheters are placed on both sides of the vestibule. Following an external beam dose of 50 Gy in 4 weeks, HDR brachytherapy is delivered in week 6. The dose per fractions is 3 Gy (twice a day) to a total dose of 18 Gy specified at the center of the tumor. With a median overall treatment time (EBRT and brachytherapy) of 36 days, this technique yielded a 2-year local control of 86% and ultimate locoregional control of 100%.[28]

EXTERNAL BEAM IRRADIATION

The technique for external beam irradiation is illustrated in Figure 33-1 (nasal vestibule) and Figure 33-4 (nasal cavity). The patient lies supine and is immobilized with the head positioned (usually slightly flexed) such that the anterior surface of the maxilla is parallel to the top of the couch. This setup allows irradiation of the primary lesion through a vertical appositional field, usually with a combination of electrons and photons in a ratio of approximately 4:1. The position is maintained with a custom made head and neck mask. Skin collimation is used to reduce the penumbra of the electron field and, thereby, protect adjacent structures such as the, nasolacrimal duct and eye. Custom fabricated bolus material (beeswax) is applied to reduce the obliquity of the incident electrons at the sloping surface contour of the nose and to fill the nares for electron beam treatment portion to improve dose homogeneity as shown in Figures 33-1 and 33-4. Additional bolus material may be inserted into the nasal cavity as shown in Figures 33-1 and 33-4. The bolus is removed for photon treatments to achieve skin sparing of the skin of the dorsum and the nasal tip. The depth of the lesion is carefully assessed in order to select the appropriate energy.

The right and left facial lymphatics are irradiated with appositional fields, which require an approximately 15-degree gantry rotation to the respective side, each abutting the appositional primary lesion electron portal and the upper neck fields. Hinge angles of more than 30 degrees between the primary and nodal fields results in unacceptable hot spots at the junction region deep to the match-line. Abutting field junctions can be moved two times during treatment to minimize dose heterogeneity. The submandibular and subdigastric nodes are treated with lateral parallel-opposed photon fields with the posterior edge placed well anterior to the spinal cord as shown in Figure 33-1I.

The external beam radiation schedule for irradiating lesions of up to 1.5 cm with a combination of electrons and photons is 50 Gy in 25 fractions plus 10 to 16 Gy in 5 to 8 fractions boost (prescribed at 90% isodose line). Larger lesions to be treated by external beam alone receive 50 Gy in 25 fractions plus 16 to 20 Gy in 8 to 10 fractions boost. Alternatively, when accessible, it is reasonable to deliver a boost dose of 20 to

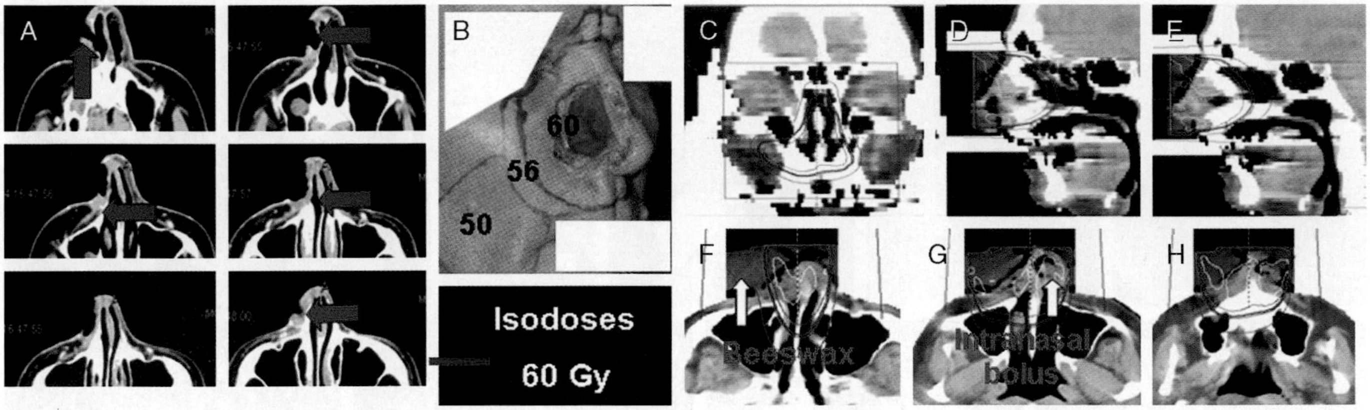

Figure 33-4 Adjuvant radiotherapy for a recurrent squamous cell carcinoma of the nasal cavity after partial rhinectomy. **A,** CT images show a small amount of tissue with heterogeneous enhancement. The patient had a complete resection, and pathologic analysis demonstrated invasion of bone, but the surgical section margins were negative. **B,** Fields were drawn at simulation before placing the beeswax bolus and intranasal bolus. The ipsilateral facial lymphatics (i.e., mustache field), the surgical bed with a wide margin (including the residual portion of his nostril and nasal septum), and the tumor bed with a 1.5-cm margin received 50 Gy, 56 Gy, and 60 Gy, respectively, with all doses given in 2-Gy fractions. The nostril was treated using 20-MeV electrons, and the mustache field was treated with 9-MeV electrons. A second set of skin collimation was fabricated for the reduced boost field. A wax bolus to compensate for surface obliquity was used for the whole treatment. An additional bolus was placed in the nostrils to reduce the perturbation of the electron beam with the air cavity and the air bone interfaces. **C–H,** Dose distributions.

Table 33-12 Target Volumes for Radiotherapy of Paranasal Sinuses Using IMRT

PRIMARY RADIOTHERAPY		
Target	**Description**	**Dose (33-35 Fractions)**
GTV	Gross tumor volume (represents prechemotherapy volume)	66-70 Gy
CTV_1 (primary CTV)	GTV + 1.0-1.5 cm	66-70 Gy
CTV_2 (intermediate dose CTV)	Primary CTV + 1.0-1.5 cm	59-63 Gy
CTV_3 (elective CTV)	Nodal volumes, nerve tract, and base of skull margin	56-57 Gy
ADJUVANT (POSTOPERATIVE RADIOTHERAPY)		
Target	**Description**	**Dose (30 Fractions)**
CTV_{HR} (high-risk CTV)	Sites of suspected positive margins, gross macroscopic residual tumor	66-70 Gy
CTV_1 (primary CTV)	Primary tumor bed with 1.0- to 1.5-cm margin	60 Gy
CTV_2 (intermediate dose)	Surgical bed	56 Gy
CTV_3 (low dose CTV)	Tract of V2 if there is perineural invasion, additional skull base margin, elective nodal volume if indicated	54 Gy

25 Gy in about 2 days by low-dose-rate brachytherapy (see earlier).

The schedule for elective nodal irradiation is 50 Gy in 25 fractions. Palpable nodes are given a boost to a total dose of 66 to 70 Gy in 33 to 35 fractions, depending on the size.

Nasal Cavity and Ethmoid Air Cells

Target Volume

The technique for primary or postoperative external beam radiotherapy of nasal cavity tumors depends on the depth of the tumor. For tumors located less than 3.5 to 4.0 cm from the skin of the nose, an electron beam technique may be used, as 20-MeV electrons will provide coverage up to 5 cm in depth. A margin of at least 1cm deep to the posterior edge has to be included in the full dose volume. The technique is described above as for nasal vestibule carcinoma and illustrated in Figure 33-4. CT-based treatment planning is necessary for accurate target localization and dose calculation.

Intensity modulated radiotherapy (IMRT) is recommended for tumors of the nasal cavity where the target volume extends greater than 5 cm depth or for tumors of the ethmoid sinus as shown in Figure 33-5. This technique delivers the desired dose to the target volume while minimizing the dose to critical organs such as cornea, lens, lacrimal glands, retina, optic nerve, optic chiasm, brain, and brainstem.

For postoperative radiotherapy the primary clinical target volume (CTV) descriptions are given in Table 33-12. CTV_1 consists of the primary tumor bed with 1.0- to 1.5-cm margins of normal tissue. A boost subvolume consisting of high-risk region (sites of positive margins, gross macroscopic residual tumor) to be treated to higher dose may be outlined. A secondary CTV_2 includes the entire operative bed. For ethmoid sinus tumors, the frontal sinus, maxillary sinus and sphenoid sinus may be explored during surgery, and these areas are included as part of the operative bed. The bony orbit is part of the operative bed when orbital exenteration is performed due to tumor invasion (Fig. 33-6). A third CTV may be delin-

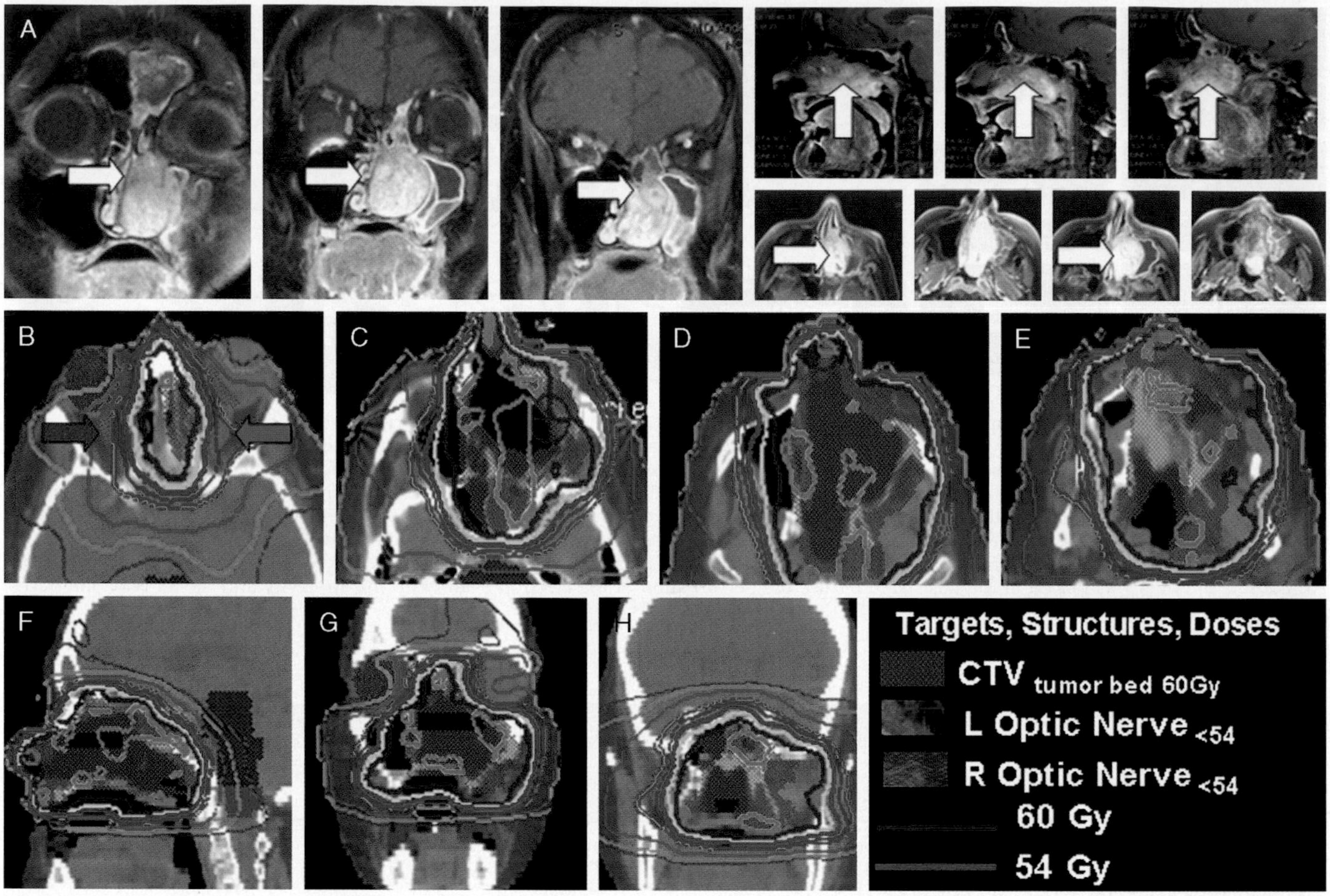

Figure 33-5 Adjuvant radiotherapy for a large tumor of the left nasal cavity after gross total resection with negative margins. **A,** In preoperative MRI, the *white arrows* indicate the primary tumor. **B–E,** Dose distributions at transverse sections. The depth of the target volume precludes the use of an electron beam. The proximity of the target volume to the optic chiasm, brainstem, eyes, and optic nerves (*arrow* in **B**) motivates the use of intensity-modulated radiation therapy. The dose limit for the chiasm and the contralateral optic nerve was set at 54 Gy, and the limit for the ipsilateral optic nerve was set at 56 Gy. **F–H,** Sagittal and coronal dose distributions.

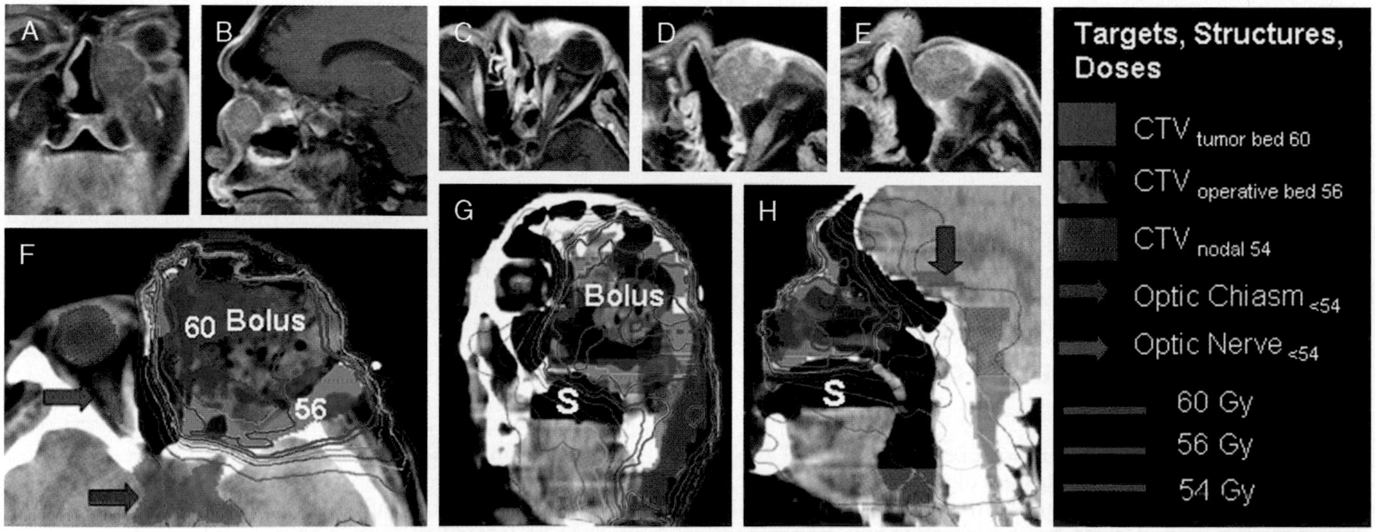

Figure 33-6 The patient underwent partial rhinectomy and septectomy for a nasal cavity carcinoma. One year later, disease recurred with an irregular, fungating mass measuring 4.5 × 3.5 × 0.7 cm, which was removed en bloc with clear margins by a medial maxillectomy. **A–E,** Follow-up MRI showed a 2.3 × 2.3 cm, enhancing soft tissue mass centered in the superior portion of the nasolacrimal duct and invading the medial inferior portion of the left orbit, displacing the globe laterally and involving the medial portion of the left inferior oblique muscle. The patient underwent left suprastructure maxillectomy with left orbital exenteration and removal of medial cheek skin. All margins were clear. Final pathologic analysis revealed an invasive schneiderian squamous cell carcinoma infiltrating the skeletal muscle. **F–H,** The intensity-modulated radiation therapy plan demonstrates target coverage and sparing of the optic nerve and chiasm. Notice the bolus material filling the orbital defect. S indicates the position of an intraoral stent used to depress the tongue.

eated to encompass the tract of V2 to the foramen rotundum if there is extensive perineural invasion (see Table 33-12).

For primary radiotherapy using IMRT, the gross tumor volume (GTV) plus 1- to 1.5-cm margin of normal appearing tissue is considered the CTV_1 to receive the full dose of 66 to 70 Gy. In patients receiving induction chemotherapy, this represents the pre-chemotherapy volume. Other secondary CTV include the rest of the involved sinus and region around the primary target to an intermediate dose (59 to 63 Gy), the tracts of nerves if there is perineural invasion, and elective nodal regions to a lower dose (56 to 57 Gy) (see Table 33-12).

For three-dimensional conformal radiotherapy (3-D CRT), the target volumes consist of the primary tumor with 2- to 3-cm margins for the initial portals and with 1- or 2-cm margins for the boost fields. The initial target volume for postoperative radiotherapy consists of the surgical bed with 1- or 2-cm margins, depending on the surgical pathology findings and the proximity of critical structures. The boost volume consisted of areas at higher risk for recurrence such as the regions of close or positive section margin or extensive perineural invasion.

For small anteroinferior septal lesions, brachytherapy can be accomplished by a single-plane implant of the lesion with about 2-cm margins. Elective neck irradiation is not given routinely even in patients with large tumors.

Setup and Field Arrangement

For target volumes less than 5 cm deep, an electron technique similar to the techniques for nasal vestibule carcinomas as described above is used. Treatment devices include lead skin collimation to obtain a sharp penumbra as well as bolus material in the nasal cavity, postoperative defects and on skin scars. An intraoral stent is used to depress the tongue, provide a patent airway, and aid in immobilization. Tungsten internal eye-shields may be used if the target volume approaches the orbits. An example is shown in Figures 33-1 and 33-4.

For external beam irradiation, the patient is immobilized in a supine position with the head positioned such that the hard palate is perpendicular to the treatment table. Metal-containing shielding devices are not placed on the skin during simulation because of their perturbation of CT images. Other devices and bolus are positioned, scars are marked with thin radiopaque wires, and transverse CT images are obtained from the vertex to the upper mediastinum.

For IMRT the patient is immobilized in a supine position with the head positioned such that the hard palate is perpendicular to the treatment table. Rigid immobilization is necessary including using special head and shoulder thermoplastic masks, which extend down to the upper thorax. The shoulders may be additionally depressed and fixed using wrist straps tethered to a foot-board. Target volumes are delineated as described above.

Multiple gantry angles are utilized either based on class solutions or using beam optimization algorithms. Non-coplanar beams may be preferred in some cases. An example of an 11-field non-coplanar arrangement is shown in Figure 33-7. The beam angle selections are based on the same principles as for three-dimensional conformal therapy: (1) preference for the shortest path to the target; (2) avoidance of direct irradiation of the critical structures (e.g., avoid beam segments entry through the contralateral eye after ipsilateral exenteration); and (3) use of as large beam separation as possible.

Inverse planning is usually done and multiple iterations (trials) may be necessary to ensure that the following are accomplished: (1) targets are covered; (2) normal tissue constraints are acceptable; and (3) dose is relatively homogenous. The dose calculations should include heterogeneity corrections because of the significant amount of air and bone of the sinuses. The radiation oncologist must work closely with the physicist and dosimetrist to ensure adherence to dose constraint. Figure 33-8 shows an example of a rejected plan and the reoptimized plans. Multiple "trial and error" iterations may be necessary. Note that the criteria for rejecting the plan may not be evident from the dose-volume histogram.

For 3-D CRT, anterior oblique wedge-pair photon fields are most suited for lesions located in the anterior lower half of the nasal cavity. Opposed-lateral fields may be applied to treat tumors at the posterior part of the nasal fossa, provided the ethmoid cells are not involved. The optic pathway can be excluded from the radiation fields with this setup. For primaries of the upper nasal cavity and ethmoidal air cells, a three-field setup allows coverage of the ethmoid cells without delivering high doses to the optic apparatus (Fig. 33-9).

CT-based treatment planning is necessary to select beam and wedge angles (usually 45 to 60 degrees) and the relative loading of the fields. It is also needed to evaluate the dose to critical structures such as brain, brainstem, and optic structures.

Dose Fractionation Schedule

The dose schedule of low dose rate brachytherapy is 60 to 65 Gy over 5 to 7 days. The external beam schedule for definitive radiotherapy is 50 Gy in 25 fractions plus 16 to 20 Gy in 8 to 10 fractions boost, depending on the size of the lesion, and for postoperative adjunctive radiotherapy is 54 Gy in 27 fractions plus 6 to 12 Gy in 3 to 6 fractions boost, depending on the risk factors such as close or positive surgical margins and perineural invasion. The dose regimens for primary or adjunctive radiotherapy using IMRT are summarized in Table 33-12.

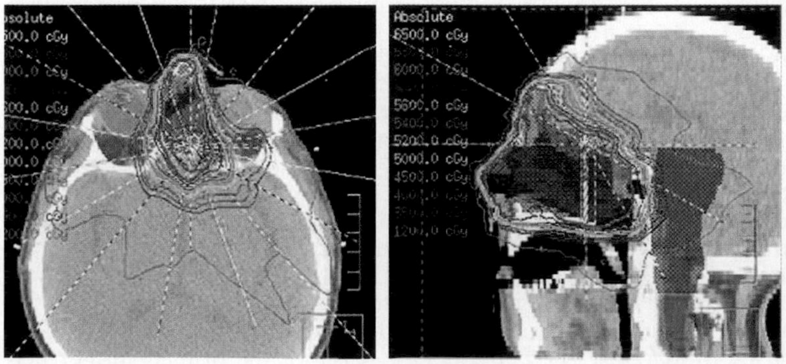

Non-coplanar beam orientation

Beam	Couch	Gantry	Beam	Couch	Gantry
1	000	220	7	000	100
2	000	260	8	000	140
3	000	300	9	090	030
4	000	340	10	300	355
5	000	010	11	090	345
6	000	060			

Figure 33-7 An example of non-coplanar beam arrangement for irradiation of an ethmoid sinus cancer. Beams 9, 10, and 11 are non-coplanar.

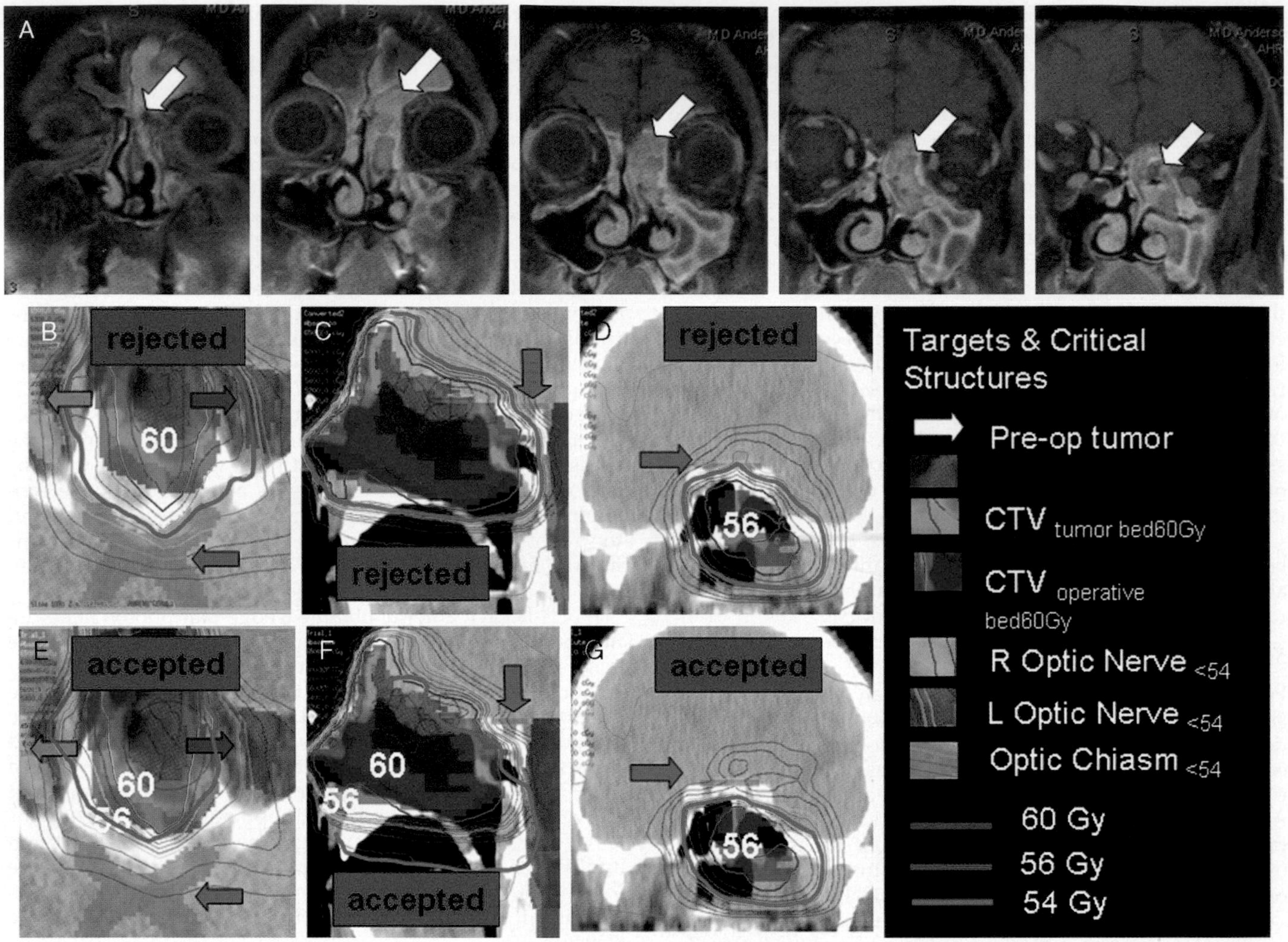

Figure 33-8 Plan evaluation and acceptance. **A,** Diagnostic MRI shows a left-sided, invasive, poorly differentiated, nasoethmoid carcinoma measuring 5 × 4 × 1.2 cm and invading the bone but not the overlying dura mater. After resection, the goal was to deliver a dose of 60 Gy in 30 fractions to the tumor bed and 54 Gy to the operative bed using intensity-modulated radiation therapy. **B–D,** The plan was rejected because the 54-Gy isodose line *(pink)* was very close to the optic nerves and chiasm *(arrow)*. **E–G,** The optimized plan was accepted. This information cannot be gleaned from the dose-volume histogram. The dosimetry on each image should be inspected.

Maxillary Sinus

Target Volume

Delineation of target volumes of *postoperative radiotherapy* is based on compilation of four sources of information (see Table 33-12). These are pretreatment physical examination, pretreatment imaging, intraoperative findings (tumor extension relative to critical structures such as orbital wall, cribriform plate, cranial verve foramina, etc., and ease of resection), and outcome of histologic examination (e.g., positive margin, perineural invasion).

IMRT is the preferred treatment method as it generally yields better dose distribution in terms of tumor coverage and normal tissue sparing than three-dimensional conformal technique. For postoperative radiotherapy, CTV_1 consists of the primary tumor bed with 1.0- to 1.5-cm margin of normal tissue. CTV_2 encompasses the entire operative bed including the bony orbit after exenteration and the ethmoid, frontal, and/or sphenoid sinuses if explored during surgery. A third CTV may be delineated to encompass the tract of V2 to the foramen rotundum if there is extensive perineural invasion as shown in Figure 33-10. CTV_{HR} (see Table 33-12) may be outlined, which encompasses sites of positive margins, gross macroscopic residual tumor where a higher dose may be delivered. Examples of an IMRT plan for postoperative radiotherapy are shown in Figure 33-11 (an infrastructure tumor), Figure 33-10 (a recurrent infrastructure tumor receiving repeat irradiation), and Figure 33-6 (a suprastructure tumor after resection including orbital exenteration).

For primary radiotherapy using IMRT, the prescription doses are 66 to 70 Gy to the gross tumor volume (GTV), prechemotherapy GTV for those receiving systemic treatment, plus a 1- to 1.5-cm margin of normal appearing tissue (CTV_1), 59 to 63 Gy to other secondary clinical target volumes such as the rest of the involved sinus and wider region around the primary target, and 56 to 57 Gy to the tracts of nerves if there is perineural invasion and elective nodal regions (see Table 33-12). An example of an IMRT plan for primary radiotherapy of a sinonasal undifferentiated carcinoma is shown in Figure 33-12.

For postoperative radiotherapy using 3-D CRT, the initial target volume consists of the operative bed with 1- to 2-cm margins. The boost field consists of the primary tumor bed and areas at higher risk for recurrence such as the regions of

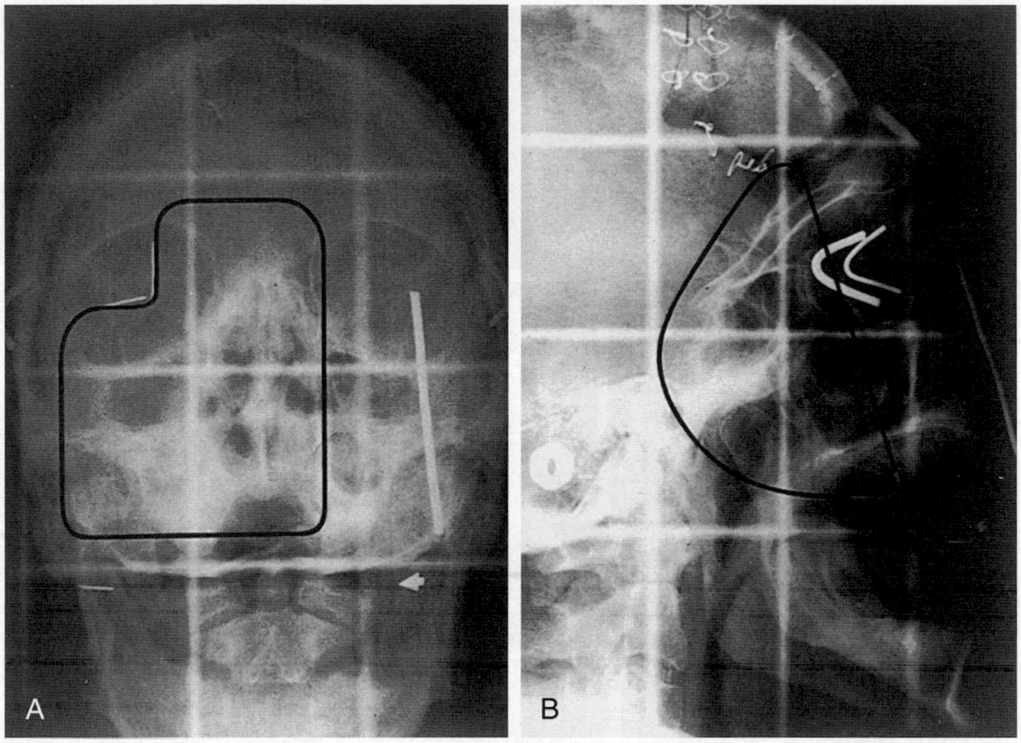

Figure 33-9 A 56-year-old man sought medical attention because of nasal stuffiness and pressure discomfort below the right eye. A polypoid mass was removed from the right nasal cavity, which was diagnosed as an adenocarcinoma. CT revealed a tumor in the right ethmoid sinuses and the upper part of the right nasal cavity. The floor of the right orbit was involved. The tumor was resected through a craniofacial approach. The right antrum and the sphenoid sinus were inspected and found free of gross disease, but the mucosal lining was removed. Pathologic examination revealed an adenocarcinoma in the ethmoid sinuses spreading to the mucosa of the nasal septum. The surgical bed was treated with an anterior field **(A)** and right **(B)** and left lateral fields using 6-MV photons. The lateral orbital canthi, external auditory canals, oral commissures, and position of the cornea of the right eye were marked at simulation. The thick, straight wire indicated the slope of the face. A dose of 56 Gy was delivered to the isocenter in 28 fractions. (From Ang KK, Kaanders JHAM, Peters LJ [eds]: Radiotherapy for Head and Neck Cancers: Indications and Techniques. Philadelphia, Lea & Febiger, 1994.)

close or positive resection margin or extensive perineural invasion. Adjunctive radiation of the lymphatic bed is administered to patients who undergo therapeutic nodal dissection if multiple nodes are involved and/or there is presence of extracapsular extension. Elective radiation of the ipsilateral submandibular and subdigastric nodes is given to patients with squamous cell or poorly differentiated carcinoma.

Setup, Field Arrangement, and Dose Fractionation Schedule

The patient is immobilized in a supine position with the head slightly hyperextended to bring the floor of the orbit parallel to the axis of the anterior field. Such position allows irradiation of the entire orbital floor while sparing most of the cornea and most of the globe. An intraoral stent is used to open the mouth and depress the tongue out of the radiation fields. Following palatectomy, the stent can be designed to hold a water-filled balloon to obliterate the large air cavity in the surgical defect to improve dose homogeneity. Orbital exenteration defect is also filled directly with a water-filled balloon to decrease the dose delivered to the temporal lobe. Proper marking of the lateral canthi, oral commissures, external auditory canals, and external scar facilitates target volume delineation.

IRRADIATION OF THE PRIMARY TUMOR OR SURGICAL BED

The principles of target delineation and plan evaluation for IMRT of the maxillary sinus cancer are the same as those described above for nasal cavity and ethmoid tumors. The dose and fractionation are summarized in Table 33-12.

For 3-D CRT, a three-field technique, consisting of an anterior portal and right and left lateral fields, is used for tumors involving the suprastructure or extending to the roof of the nasal cavity and ethmoid cells (Fig. 33-13). The lateral fields may have a 5-degree posterior tilt and 60-degree wedges. The relative loading varies from 1:0.15:0.15 to 1:0.07:0.07, depending on the tumor location and photon energy. For the initial target volume, the superior border of the anterior portal is above the crista galli to encompass the ethmoids and, in the absence of orbital invasion, at the lower edge of the cornea to cover the orbital floor; the inferior border is 1 cm below the floor of the sinus and the medial border is 1 to 2 cm, or further when necessary, across the midline to cover the contralateral ethmoidal extension; the lateral border is 1 cm beyond the apex of the sinus or falling off the skin. The superior border of the lateral portals follows the contour of the floor of the anterior cranial fossa, the anterior border is behind the lateral bony canthus parallel to the slope of the face, the posterior border should at least cover the pterygoid plates, and the inferior border corresponds to that of the anterior portal. The boost volume encompasses the tumor bed while sparing the optic pathway.

Anterior and ipsilateral wedge-pair (usually 45-degree wedges) photon fields are used for tumors of the infrastructure with no extension into the orbit or ethmoids. If necessary, the lateral portal can have a 5-degree inferior tilt to avoid beam divergence into the contralateral eye. In general, for the initial

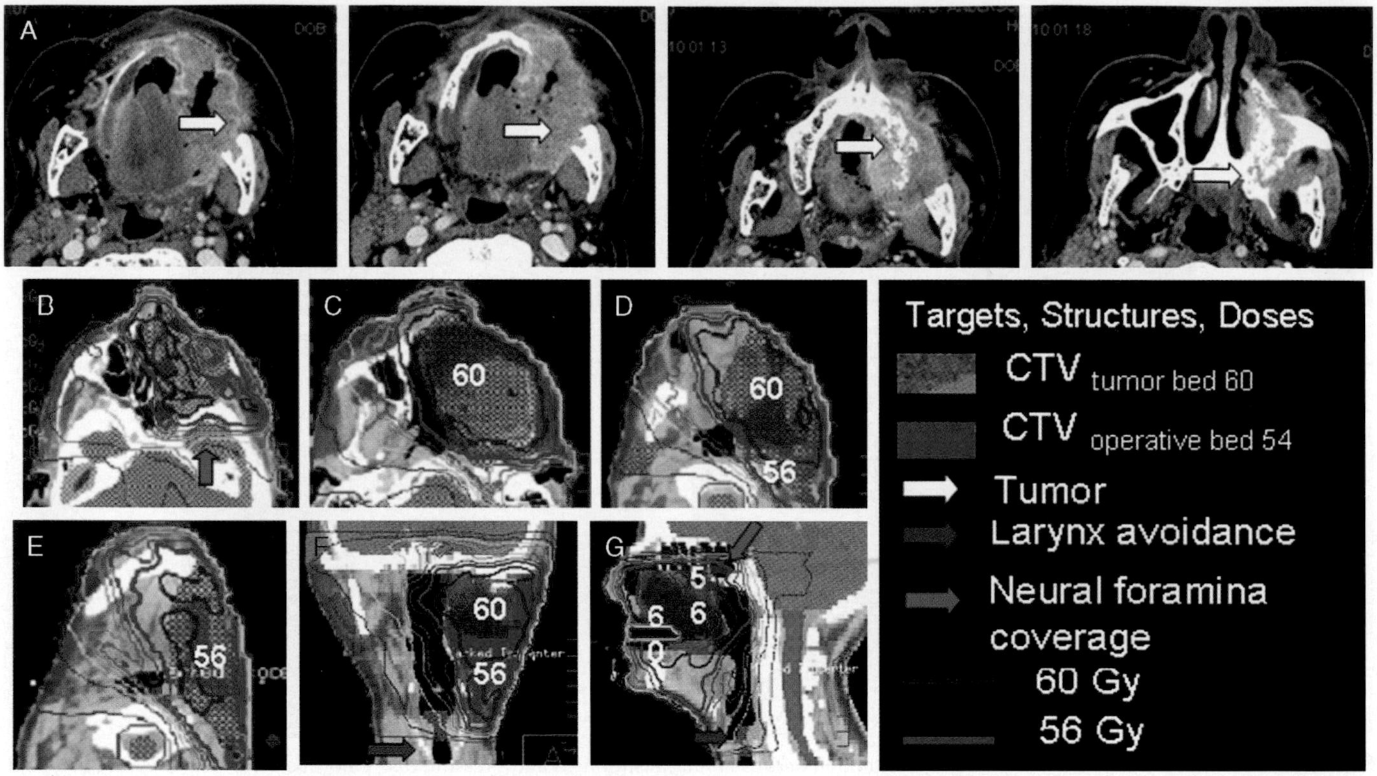

Figure 33-10 A 60-year-old woman had primary radiation therapy in 1999 to a total dose of 66.6 Gy for a left buccal cancer. In 2004, she developed a recurrence centered on the left side of the hard palate and left maxillary alveolar ridge, involving the left buccal mucosa and retromolar trigone, with gross destruction of the mandible and maxilla and the floor of the left maxillary sinus **(A)**. She underwent salvage surgery, which identified poorly differentiated squamous carcinoma with negative margins and found involvement of lymphovascular space and obvious invasion of the infraorbital nerve. She had adjuvant radiotherapy to 60 Gy using intensity-modulated radiation therapy with concurrent chemotherapy. **B–G,** Isodose distributions. The 54-Gy target volume encompasses the floor of the orbit and foramen rotundum at the base of the skull because of perineural invasion *(pink arrow)*, and the larynx was outlined for avoidance *(orange arrows)*.

target volume, the superior border of the anterior portal is just above the floor of the orbit but below the cornea; the inferior border is 1 cm below the floor of the sinus, the medial border is 1 to 2 cm across the midline, and the lateral border is 1 cm beyond the apex of the sinus or falling off when the tumor extends into the soft tissue of the cheek. The superior and inferior borders of the lateral field are the same as the anterior portal, the anterior border is in front of the anterior wall, and the posterior border is behind the pterygoid plates.

Lateral-opposed photon fields are preferred for tumors of the infrastructure spreading across midline through the hard palate. If necessary, the fields can be slightly oblique (5-degree inferior tilt from the ipsilateral side and 5-degree superior tilt from the contralateral side) to avoid irradiating the contralateral eye. In addition, the isocenter is placed at the level of the orbital floor and the upper half of the fields is shielded (half beam) to prevent exposure of the eyes by beam divergence. The field borders are similar to the lateral field described earlier.

The eye and the optic pathways are of particular concern. With three-dimensional conformal techniques, it is generally possible to shield the cornea in patients with limited involvement of the medial or inferior orbital wall to avoid keratitis. If the tumor invades the orbital cavity without necessitating orbital exenteration, care should be taken to avoid irradiation of the lacrimal gland to prevent xerophthalmia. It is important to exclude the contralateral optic nerve and optic chiasm from the volume that receives more than 54 Gy in 27 fractions to prevent bilateral blindness. For tumors extending through the posterior ethmoid cells to about the optic chiasm, the risk-benefit of delivering a dose of up to 60 Gy should be discussed with the patient.

Treatment of the Neck

Ipsilateral upper neck treatment is accomplished through a lateral appositional electron field (usually 12 MeV). The superior border of the field slopes up from the horizontal ramus of the mandible anteriorly to match the inferior border of the primary portal posteriorly; a small triangle over the cheek can be left untreated (except when there is involvement of the soft tissues of the cheek, where a triangular electron field is added); and the anterior border is just behind the oral commissure, the posterior border is at the mastoid process, and the inferior border is at the thyroid notch (above the arytenoids).

Bilateral neck treatment in patients presenting with extensive nodal involvement requires proper field matching. This can be accomplished by treating both the primary tumor bed and the upper neck with half-blocked photon beams. With this technique, the central axes of the primary fields and the opposed-lateral upper neck fields all are placed in the plane of the inferior border of the maxillary fields (i.e., usually 1 cm below the floor of the maxillary sinus); an independent collimator jaw (if not available, a beam-splitter block) is then used to shield the caudal half of maxillary fields and the cephalad half of neck fields. The junction line between the primary and the neck fields is moved during the course of treatment to

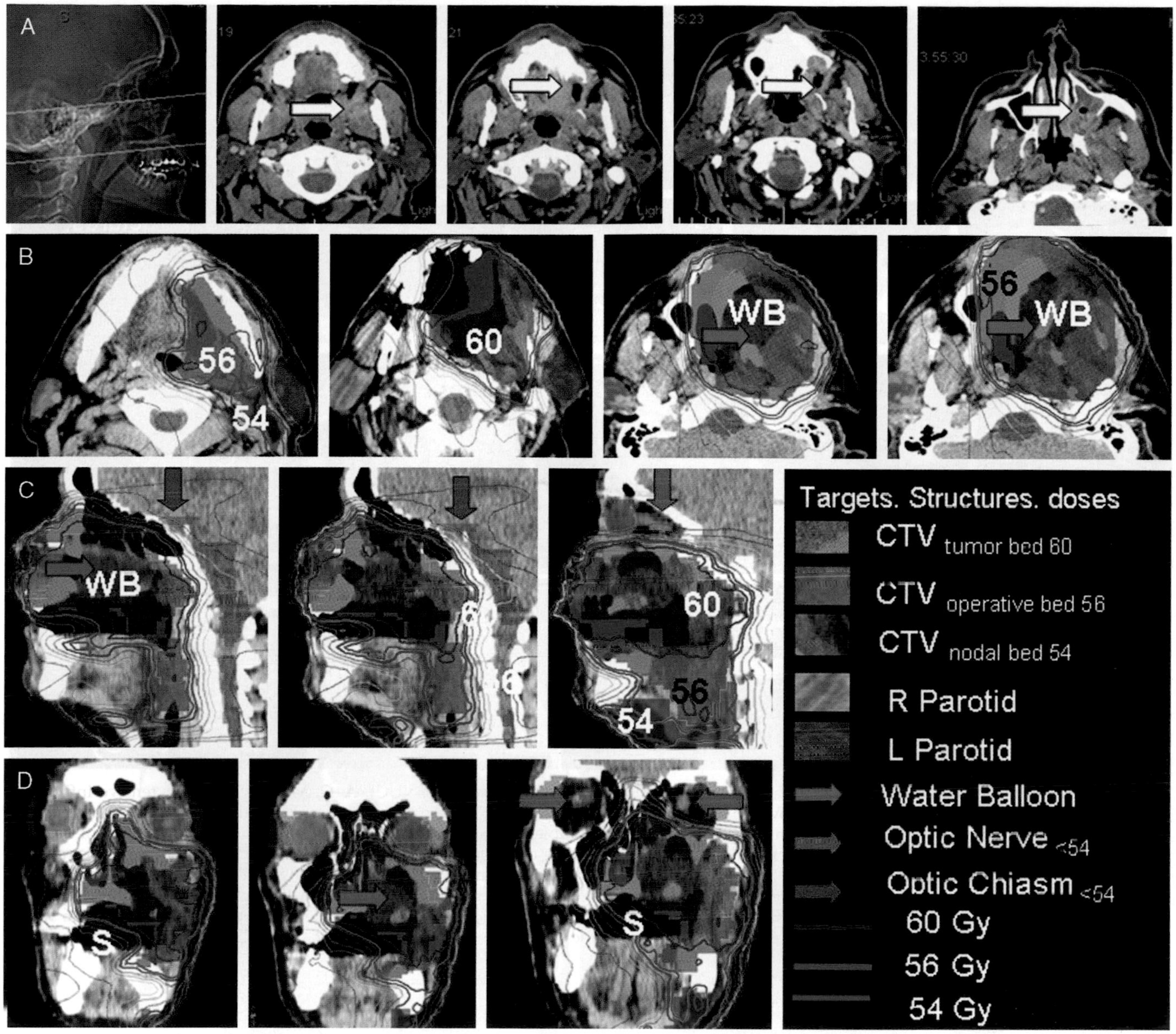

Figure 33-11 Adjuvant radiotherapy for a large, destructive T4N0 squamous cell carcinoma centered in the left hard palate and inferior maxilla, with extension up into the left descending pterygoid canal. **A,** Tumor *(white arrows)* is demonstrated in the base of the pterygoid plates, left pterygoid musculature, and floor of the left maxillary sinus, along with destruction of the left maxillary alveolar ridge and the left soft palate. The tumor extent was confirmed at resection, and pathologic analysis showed perineural invasion (PNI). **B–D,** Transverse, sagittal, and coronal images show the dose distribution using intensity-modulated radiation therapy. The 54-Gy target volume encompasses the floor of the orbit and foramen rotundum at the base of the skull because of PNI. *Pink arrows* point to a water balloon used to fill the space to provide scatter and reduce dose heterogeneity.

smooth the dose in this region. Portal reduction is made after about 42 Gy and the posterior cervical areas are irradiated with abutting electron fields to the desired dose. The mid and lower neck areas are irradiated with an anterior appositional photon field matched to the inferior border of opposed-lateral upper neck fields.

Dose Fractionation

Table 33-12 summarizes the dose regimens for IMRT. With 3-D CRT techniques, the dose for *postoperative radiotherapy* at 2 Gy/fraction is 50 Gy to elective nodes, 56 Gy to the operative bed, 60 Gy to the tumor bed (negative resection margins), and 66 Gy to positive margins. The recommended total dose to the tumor volume for *primary radiotherapy* at 2 Gy/fraction is 66 to 70 Gy. As mentioned earlier, the contralateral optic nerve and chiasm are excluded from the field after a dose of 50 to 54 Gy. This goal is accomplished by one or two (i.e., after 50 Gy and 54 Gy, respectively) portal reductions. When the primary lesion invades structures adjacent to the optic chiasm, such as posterior ethmoid cells and sphenoid sinus, a dose of up to 60 Gy to the chiasm may carry a higher therapeutic ratio (potentially higher control probability with a relative low risk for visual impairment) and thus may be acceptable after clear discussion of the therapy rationale with the patient.

Table 33-13 Side Effects That May Result from a Combination of Tumor, Surgery, and Radiotherapy in Patients With Paranasal Sinus Cancers

Vestibulocochlear	Vestibular dysfunction, persistent otitis, tinnitus, hearing impairment
Ophthalmologic (lacrimal gland, eyes, lens, optic nerves, and chiasm)	Retinopathy, xerophthalmia, keratopathy, cataracts, visual impairment
Neurologic (brain, brainstem, spinal cord, temporal lobe)	Neurocognitive impairment, cranial neuropathy, myelopathy, brain necrosis
Endocrine (pituitary gland, hypothalamus, thyroid gland if neck irradiated)	Multiple endocrine dysfunction: hyperprolactinemia, syndromes associated with decreased GH, FSH, LH, T_4, TSH, ACTH, and their downstream hormones
Oral (major salivary glands, oral mucosa, mandible and temporomandibular joint)	Xerostomia, dental caries, dysgeusia, mandible exposure, and necrosis, trismus
Connective tissue complications (oral cavity, soft palate musculature, pharynx, larynx, skin and subcutaneous tissues, skull bones)	Soft tissue necrosis, skin changes, persistent lymphedema, subcutaneous fibrosis, cartilage necrosis, nasal dryness, choanal stenosis, swallowing and voice dysfunction, bone necrosis

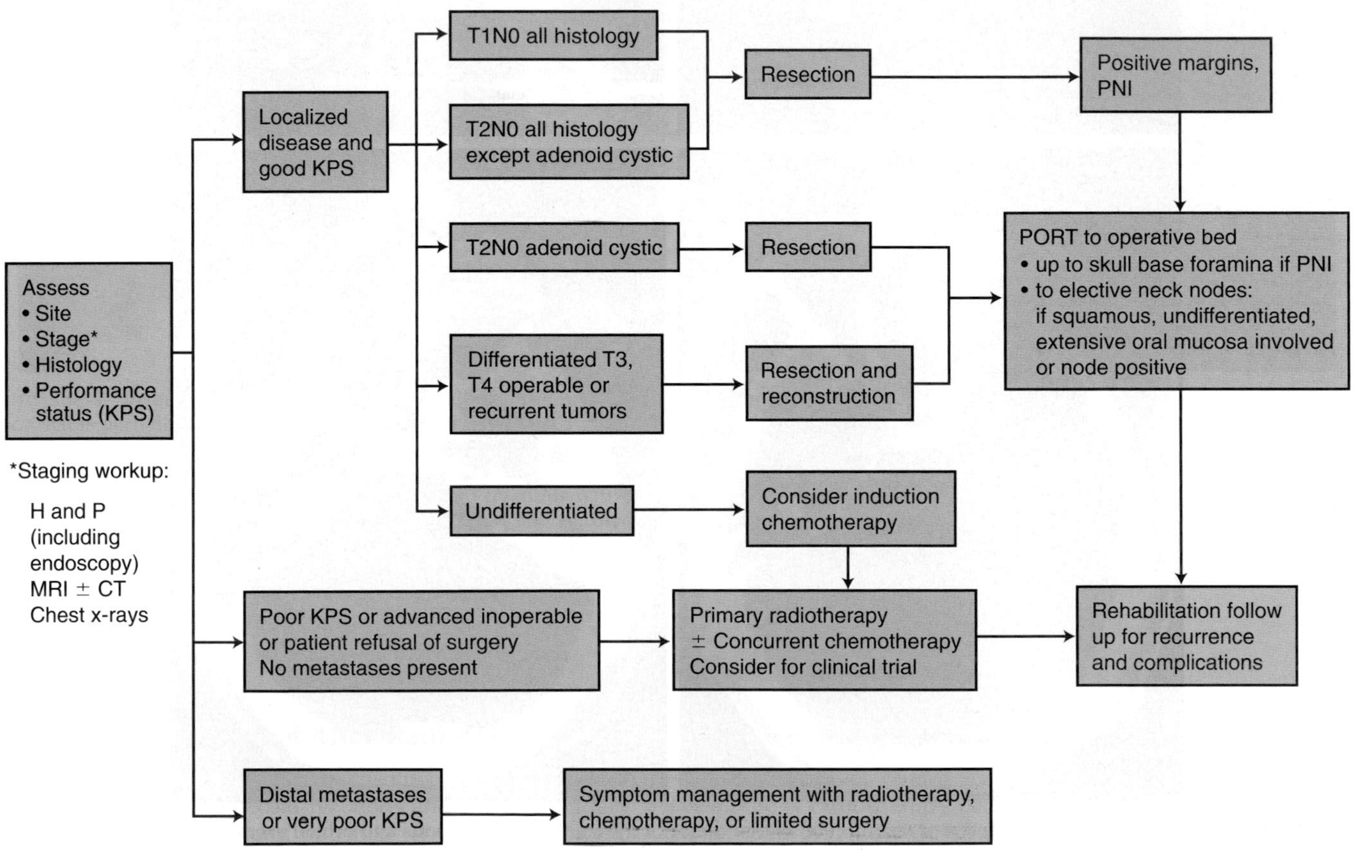

Figure 33-14 Diagnostic algorithm, staging workup, and treatment algorithm for patients with maxillary sinus carcinomas. CT, computed tomography; H&P, histologic and pathologic examinations; KPS, Karnofsky performance score; MRI, magnetic resonance imaging; PNI, perineural invasion.

Maxillary Sinus Carcinomas

Figure 33-14 summarizes the treatment algorithm based on tumor stage, type, resectability, and performance status. Stage I lesions can be effectively controlled by surgery alone. Stage II and III neoplasms are generally treated by a combination of surgery and radiotherapy. Selected patients having high risk for anesthesia can be treated with radiotherapy alone with good outcome.

New Therapy Directions and Clinical Studies

Surgical Techniques

Craniofacial resection and plastic reconstruction surgical techniques provide better access for complete tumor resection, particularly of neoplasms extending to the skull base, while preserving some functionally important structures. Orbital floor reconstruction affords preservation of the eye.

Table 33-14 Treatment Algorithms for Cancer of the Nasal Vestibule, Nasal Cavity, and Ethmoid Sinus

Site/Extent	Preferred Treatment	Comments
NASAL VESTIBULE		
Small tumors	Brachytherapy	Suited for septal lesions
Larger tumors	EBRT	Suited for nasal floor tumors
Advanced tumors	Surgery + EBRT	—
NASAL CAVITY/ETHMOIDS		
Stage I (A)	Surgery or EBRT	Based on expected esthetic outcome
Stage II (B), III (C)	Surgery + EBRT ± chemotherapy	EBRT ± chemotherapy if high risk for anesthesia

EBRT, external beam radiotherapy.

Conformal Radiotherapy

Technical innovations in radiotherapy, specifically IMRT and proton beams, enable better coverage to a greater target volume while reducing the dose to critical adjacent normal tissues. Once the reduction of normal tissue complications is clearly demonstrated and adequate expertise and experience is obtained, consideration may be given to escalation of radiation dose to increase local control rates.

Another notable advance is the ability to attempt definitive irradiation of advanced inoperable tumors involving the skull base, cavernous sinus, and intracranial extradural space. This may not be otherwise considered because of proximity to the optic chiasm, optic nerves, brainstem, and brain. In our recent experience with IMRT, tumors have been controlled in at least six patients with advanced inoperable tumors involving the skull base including two patients with frank intracranial extension.

Chemoradiotherapy

The efficacy of new cytotoxic drugs is being assessed in neoadjuvant settings where tumor regression is used as a marker of sensitivity. Ongoing and planned clinical studies will address questions such as the role and sequencing of chemotherapy, whether surgery can be reduced or avoided altogether in complete responders, and so on.

Unfortunately, because of the rarity of the disease, it will take many years to assess the relative value of these new developments in improving the overall outcome of patients with sinonasal cancers.

ACKNOWLEDGMENTS

The authors thank Cynthia Holt for administration assistance; Armando DeLaMora, Bryan Mason, Christopher L. Spicer, James E. Kanke, Khoi N. Vu, Pei-Fong Wong, and Samuel Tung for dosimetry and physics support; and Leah M. Theriot as a team member.

REFERENCES

1. Fletcher GH: Nasal and paranasal sinus carcinoma. *In* Fletcher GH (ed): Textbook of Radiotherapy. Philadelphia, Lea & Febiger, 1980, pp 408-425.
2. Dulguerov P, Jacobsen MS, Allal AS, et al: Nasal and paranasal sinus carcinoma: are we making progress? A series of 220 patients and a systematic review. Cancer 92:3012-3029, 2001.
3. Boring CC, Squires TS, Tong T: Cancer statistics. CA Cancer J Clin 43:7-26, 1993.
4. Roush GC: Epidemiology of cancer of the nose and paranasal sinuses. Head Neck Surg 2:3-11, 1979.
5. Torjussen W, Solberg LA, Hgetviet AC: Histopathological changes of nasal mucosa in nickel workers: a pilot study. Cancer 44:963-974, 1979.
6. Schwaab G, Julieron M, Janot F: Epidemiology of cancers of the nasal cavities and paranasal sinuses Neurochirurgie 43:61-63, 1997.
7. Zheng W, McLaughlin JK, Chow WH, et al: Risk factors for cancers of the nasal cavity and paranasal sinuses among white men in the United States. Am J Epidemiol 138:965-972, 1993.
8. Acheson ED, Hadfield EH, Macbeth RG: Carcinoma of the nasal cavity and accessory sinuses in woodworkers. Lancet 1:311-312, 1967.
9. Acheson ED, Cowdell RH, Hadfield E, et al: Nasal cancer in woodworkers in the furniture industry. Br Med J 2:587-596, 1968.
10. Goepfert H, Guillamondegui OM, Jesse RH, et al: Squamous cell carcinoma of nasal vestibule. Arch Otolaryngol Head Neck Surg 100:8-10, 1974.
11. Mazeron JJ, Chassagne D, Crook J, et al: Radiation therapy of carcinomas of the skin of nose and nasal vestibule: a report of 1676 cases by the Groupe Européen de Curietherapie. Radiother Oncol 13:165-173, 1988.
12. Murphy J, Bleach NR, Thyveetil MJ: Sebaceous carcinoma of the nose: multi-focal presentation? Laryngol Otol 118:374-376, 2004.
13. Prasad ML, Patel SG, Busam KJ: Primary mucosal desmoplastic melanoma of the head and neck. Head Neck 26:37, 2004.
14. Su K, Xu J, Qiao M, et al: CT characters of primary nasal non-Hodgkin lymphoma Lin Chuang Er Bi Yan Hou Ke Za Zhi 17:261-263, 2003.
15. Bars G, Visser AG, van Andel JG: The treatment of squamous cell carcinoma of the nasal vestibule with interstitial iridium implantation. Radiother Oncol 4:121-125, 1985.
16. McNeese MD, Chobe R, Weber RS, et al: Carcinoma of the nasal vestibule: treatment with radiotherapy. Cancer Bull 41:84-87, 1989.
17. Wong CS, Cummings BJ, Elhakim T, et al: External irradiation for squamous cell carcinoma of the nasal vestibule. Int J Radiat Oncol Biol Phys 12:1943-1946, 1986.
18. Chobe R, McNeese MD, Weber R, et al: Radiation therapy for carcinoma of the nasal vestibule. Otolaryngol Head Neck Surg 98:67-71, 1988.
19. Moore KL: Clinically Oriented Anatomy. Baltimore, Williams & Wilkins, 1985.
20. Ang KK, Jiang GL, Frankenthaler RA, et al: Carcinomas of the nasal cavity. Radiother Oncol 24:163-168, 1992.
21. Beitler JJ, Fass DE, Brenner HA, et al: Esthesioneuroblastoma: is there a role for elective neck treatment? Head Neck 13:321-326, 1991.
22. Goldsweig HG, Sundaresan N: Chemotherapy of recurrent esthesioneuroblastoma: case report and review of the literature. Am J Clin Oncol 13:139-143, 1990.
23. Kadish S, Goodman M, Wine CC: Olfactory neuroblastoma: a clinical analysis of 17 cases. Cancer 37:1571-1576, 1976.
24. Elkon D, Hightower SI, Lim ML, et al: Esthesioneuroblastoma. Cancer 44:1087-1094, 1979.
25. Jiang GL, Ang KK, Peters LJ, et al: Maxillary sinus carcinomas: natural history and results of postoperative radiotherapy. Radiother Oncol 21:193-200, 1991.
26. Nasal cavity and paranasal sinuses. *In* American Joint Committee on Cancer: AJCC Cancer Staging Manual, 6th ed. New York, Springer, 2002, pp 59-67.
27. Wang CC: Treatment of carcinoma of the nasal vestibule by irradiation. Cancer 38:100-106, 1976.

28. Langendijk JA, Poorter R, Leemans CR, et al: Radiotherapy of squamous cell carcinoma of the nasal vestibule. Int J Radiat Oncol Biol Phys 59:1319-1325, 2004.
29. Evensen JF, Jacobsen AB, Tausjo JE: Brachytherapy of squamous cell carcinoma of the nasal vestibule. Acta Oncol 35(Suppl 8): 87-92, 1996.
30. Parsons JT, Mendenhall WM, Mancuso AA, et al: Malignant tumors of the nasal cavity and ethmoid and sphenoid sinuses. Int J Radiat Oncol Biol Phys 14:11-22, 1988.
31. Spaulding CA, Kranyak MS, Constable WC, et al: Esthesioneuroblastoma: a comparison of two treatment eras. Int J Radiat Oncol Biol Phys 15:581-590, 1988.
32. Million RR: The myth regarding bone or cartilage involvement by cancer and the likelihood of cure by radiotherapy. Head Neck Surg 11:30-40, 1989.
33. McCollough WM, Mendenhall NP, Parsons JT, et al: Radiotherapy alone for squamous cell carcinoma of the nasal vestibule: management of the primary site and regional lymphatics. Int J Radiat Oncol Biol Phys 26:73-79, 1993.
34. Mak ACA, van Andel JG, van Woerkom-Eijkenboom WMH: Radiation therapy of carcinoma of the nasal vestibule. Eur J Cancer 16:81-85, 1980.
35. Badib AO, Kurohara SS, Webster JH, et al: Treatment of cancer of the nasal cavity. AJR Am J Roentgenol 106:824-830, 1969.
36. Bosch A, Vallecillo L, Frias Z: Cancer of the nasal cavity. Cancer 37:1458-1463, 1976.
37. Hawkins RB, Wynstra JH, Pilepich MV, et al: Carcinoma of the nasal cavity—results of primary and adjuvant radiotherapy. Int J Radiat Oncol Biol Phys 15:1129-1133, 1988.
38. Bhattacharyya N: Cancer of the nasal cavity: survival and factors influencing prognosis. Arch Otolaryngol Head Neck Surg 128:1079-1083, 2002.
39. Miyamoto RC, Gleich LL, Biddinger PW, et al: Esthesioneuroblastoma and sinonasal undifferentiated carcinoma: impact of histological grading and clinical staging on survival and prognosis. Laryngoscope 110:1262-1265, 2000.
40. Rosenthal DI, Barker JL Jr, El-Naggar AK, et al: Sinonasal malignancies with neuroendocrine differentiation: patterns of failure according to histologic phenotype. Cancer 101:2567-2573, 2004.
41. Lavertu P, Roberts JK, Kraus DH, et al: Squamous cell carcinoma of the paranasal sinuses: the Cleveland Clinic experience 1977-1986. Laryngoscope 99:1130-1136, 1989.
42. Spiro JD, Soo KC, Spiro RH: Squamous carcinoma of the nasal cavity and paranasal sinuses. Am J Surg 158:328-332, 1989.
43. Zaharia M, Salem LE, Travezan R, et al: Postoperative radiotherapy in the management of cancer of the maxillary sinus. Int J Radiat Oncol Biol Phys 17:967-971, 1989.
44. Paulino AC, Marks JE, Bricker P, et al: Results of treatment of patients with maxillary sinus carcinoma. Cancer 83:457-465, 1998.
45. Le QT, Fu KK, Kaplan M, et al: Treatment of maxillary sinus carcinoma: a comparison of the 1997 and 1977 American Joint Committee on cancer staging systems. Cancer 86:1700-1711, 1999.
46. Myers LL, Nussenbaum B, Bradford CR, et al: Paranasal sinus malignancies: an 18-year single institution experience. Laryngoscope 112:1964-1969, 2002.
47. Beale FA, Garrett PG: Cancer of paranasal sinus with particular reference to maxillary sinus cancer. J Otolaryngol 12:377-382, 1983.
48. Bush SE, Bagshaw MA: Carcinoma of the paranasal sinuses. Cancer 50:154-158, 1982.
49. Sakai S, Hohki A, Fuchihata H, et al: Multidisciplinary treatment of maxillary sinus carcinoma. Cancer 52:1360-1364, 1983.
50. St-Pierre S, Baker S: Squamous cell carcinoma of the maxillary sinus. Head Neck Surg 5:508-513, 1983.
51. Amendola BE, Eisert D, Hazra TA, et al: Carcinoma of the maxillary antrum: surgery or radiation therapy? Int J Radiat Oncol Biol Phys 7:743-746, 1981.
52. Frich JC: Treatment of advanced squamous carcinoma of the maxillary sinus by irradiation. Int J Radiat Oncol Biol Phys 8:1453-1459, 1982.
53. Olmi P, Cellai E, Chiavacci A, et al: Paranasal sinuses and nasal cavity cancer: different radiotherapeutic options, results, and late damages. Tumori 72:589-595, 1986.
54. Kim GE, Chang SK, Lee SW, et al: Neoadjuvant chemotherapy and radiation for inoperable carcinoma of the maxillary antrum: a matched-control study. Am J Clin Oncol. 23:301-308, 2000.
55. Lee MM, Vokes EE, Rosen A, et al: Multimodality therapy in advanced paranasal sinus carcinoma: superior long-term results. Cancer J Sci Am 5:219-223, 1999.
56. Harrison LB, Raben A, Pfister DG, et al: A prospective phase II trial of concomitant chemotherapy and radiotherapy with delayed accelerated fractionation in unresectable tumors of the head and neck. Head Neck 20:497-503, 1998.
57. Ang KK, Kaanders JHAM, Peters LJ (eds): Radiotherapy for Head and Neck Cancers: Indications and Techniques. Philadelphia, Lea & Febiger, 1994.

CHAPTER 34

SALIVARY GLAND CANCER

Robert L. Foote, Kerry D. Olsen, James A. Bonner, and Jean E. Lewis

INCIDENCE

The overall incidence in the general population is about 0.9 to 4.0 new cases per 100,000 population per year.

BIOLOGIC CHARACTERISTICS

Prognostic factors relate to histology, grade, primary tumor size and extent, lymph node involvement, gender, and age.

DNA ploidy, proliferating cell nuclear antigen levels, Ki-67 proliferation antigen levels, *c-erbB-2/neu* oncogene expression, p53 oncoprotein expression, and epidermal growth factor receptor and transforming growth factor-α overexpression may be independent prognostic factors.

STAGING EVALUATION

Staging includes a thorough history and physical examination, chest radiography, contrast-enhanced computed tomography scan and/or magnetic resonance imaging of the head and neck region, positron emission tomography scan, and liver function tests.

PRIMARY THERAPY

Surgical resection is the primary therapy of resectable major and minor salivary gland cancers. Cure rates of 85% or higher are achieved only with early lesions (low grade, favorable histologic features, small size, and negative lymph nodes).

Small cancers, typically arising within minor salivary glands in cosmetically or functionally critical areas, can be treated with primary irradiation with moderate success in the patient who refuses surgery.

ADJUVANT THERAPY

Such therapy is indicated on the basis of failure patterns and survival results with surgery alone (high incidence of local-regional relapse) when high-grade, aggressive histologic features, large primary tumor, perineural spread, and/or lymph node metastases are present.

Irradiation reduces locoregional relapse and may improve survival.

LOCALLY ADVANCED DISEASE

Intraoperative irradiation (electron beam or brachytherapy) combined with external irradiation produces long-term survival in 50% to 60% of patients in nonrandomized trials.

Control of local and regional disease can be obtained in a significant proportion of patients with high-dose altered-fractionation external irradiation, low- to moderate-dose external irradiation combined with hyperthermia, external irradiation combined with brachytherapy, or neutron beam therapy.

PALLIATION

Multiple drug chemotherapy regimens have response rates of 22% to 100%, the duration of which is several months with no effect on survival.

The salivary glands are composed of two main groups: major (parotid, submandibular, and sublingual) and minor (hundreds of small submucosal glands lining the mucosa of the upper aerodigestive tract). Approximately 50% of the minor salivary glands are located within the oral cavity on the hard palate. Other common minor salivary gland sites include the buccal mucosa, oropharynx, nasal cavity, and paranasal sinuses.

ETIOLOGY AND EPIDEMIOLOGY

The causes of salivary gland cancer are unknown. Reports consistently suggest etiologic associations with nutritional deficiencies, exposure to ionizing radiation, ultraviolet exposure, genetic predisposition, history of previous cancer of the skin of the face, occupational exposure, viral infection, alcohol use, hair dye use, and higher educational attainment.[1-6]

A high incidence has been reported in the Arctic Inuit, who have a low intake of vitamins A and C; in adults irradiated to the head and neck region for benign conditions (tinea capitis, acne, infected tonsils) during childhood; in the population within the southern district of the Surveillance, Epidemiology, and End Results (SEER) studies (ultraviolet exposure) in certain families (parotid cancer); in whites with Epstein-Barr virus infection (undifferentiated carcinomas of the parotid gland and malignant mixed tumors); and in survivors of the atomic bombs in Hiroshima and Nagasaki. Radiation-induced malignant salivary gland tumors may occur with higher frequency in the minor salivary glands. The latent period for development of radiation-induced cancers varies from 10 to 25 years. Most salivary gland cancers have no obvious cause.

Malignant tumors of the salivary glands account for less than 0.3% of all cancers and 7% of head and neck cancers diagnosed in North America each year. The overall incidence in the general population is about 0.9 to 4.0 new cases per 100,000 population per year. The incidence is equivalent in males and females. The average age of patients with malignant tumors is 53 to 55 years. Tumors of minor salivary gland origin are uncommon before age 20 and are rare before age 10. Female patients with carcinoma of the major salivary glands have an incidence of breast cancer 8 times higher than that of the general population.

Parotid gland cancers account for 80% to 90% of all malignant salivary gland tumors. Parotid gland cancers are 10 times more common than submandibular and minor salivary gland cancers and are 100 times more common than sublingual gland cancers. From 15% to 33% of all parotid gland tumors are malignant, and most (88%) arise within the superficial lobe. Fifty percent or more of all submandibular gland tumors, most (80%) sublingual gland tumors, and 65% to 88% of minor salivary gland tumors are malignant. Parotid gland tumors in children are more likely to be malignant compared with these tumors in adults (57% versus 15% to 25%).

PREVENTION AND EARLY DETECTION

Because malignant salivary gland tumors are so uncommon and because no etiologic factors have been proven, no specific recommendations regarding prevention or early detection can be made with confidence. Exposure to unnecessary ionizing radiation and ultraviolet light should be avoided. A well-balanced diet including several generous servings of fresh fruits or vegetables each day seems prudent. Abstinence from alcohol and hair dye use should be considered. People with a family history of parotid cancer or a history of exposure to ionizing radiation or skin cancer involving the face should undergo a thorough head and neck examination on a regular basis. Any persistent mass in the parotid, submandibular, sublingual, or oral cavity region should be brought to the attention of a physician.

PATHOLOGY AND PATHWAYS OF SPREAD

The histologic types of malignant salivary gland tumors[7,8] are shown in Table 34-1. The reserve cell system of the intercalated and excretory duct is thought to be the site of origin of most cancers.

The spread of most malignant salivary gland tumors is by local infiltration and perineural extension. These tumors can infiltrate the gland and adjacent structures, invade nerves, and grow along nerve sheaths. A malignant tumor can invade adjacent structures such as skin, muscle, and bone. Deep-lobe parotid tumors can invade the parapharyngeal space, skull base, and cranial nerves. Minor salivary cancers of the floor of mouth or sublingual gland are characterized by extensive local infiltration with invasion of muscle, bone, cartilage, nerves, and blood vessels. Hematogenous spread is more common than regional lymph node metastases for both major and minor salivary gland cancers.

Distant metastases are common and can occur late in the natural history of the disease. Distant metastases most commonly involve the lungs, bones, and liver. About 25% of patients with minor salivary gland cancers develop distant metastases. Distant metastases develop in as many as 50% of patients with adenoid cystic carcinoma.

The incidence of regional lymph node metastasis varied with the histologic features, primary tumor stage at presentation, site of origin, and grade. The incidence of lymph node metastasis for minor salivary gland cancers depends on the histologic features and the density of lymphatics at the site of origin. Cancers arising within the oropharynx or nasopharynx have about a 60% incidence of lymph node metastasis compared with 5% to 10% for hard palate and paranasal sinus sites. Minor salivary gland cancers arising within the tongue and floor of mouth have an approximately 40% incidence of lymph node metastasis; those arising within the gingiva have a 20% incidence of lymph node metastasis; and nasal cavity, buccal mucosa, and lip cancers have a 15% incidence or less. Table 34-2 outlines the incidence of lymph node metastases at initial diagnosis by site, grade, T stage, size, and facial nerve paralysis.[9-11]

The lymphatics of the parotid gland drain to the intraparotid, paraparotid, subparotid, tail of parotid, submandibular, upper jugular, subdigastric, middle and low jugular, and posterior triangle lymph nodes. The lymphatics of the submandibular gland drain to the adjacent submandibular nodes and then to the subdigastric node and high and middle jugular nodes. When indicated, modified or selective neck dissection needs to encompass all potential sites of disease in the patient with parotid and submandibular gland cancers (levels I to III). The lymphatics of the sublingual gland include the submandibular lymph nodes and the deep internal jugular chain.

Table 34-1 Classification of Malignant Salivary Gland Tumors

Carcinoma ex pleomorphic adenoma
Adenoid cystic carcinoma
Mucoepidermoid carcinoma
Adenocarcinoma (NOS)
Acinic cell carcinoma
Squamous cell carcinoma
Myoepithelial carcinoma
Cystadenocarcinoma
Small cell carcinoma
Polymorphous low-grade adenocarcinoma
Epithelial myoepithelial carcinoma
Clear cell carcinoma (NOS)
Basal cell adenocarcinoma
Salivary duct carcinoma
Carcino-sarcoma
Metastasizing pleomorphic adenoma
Large cell undifferentiated carcinoma
Lymphoepithelial carcinomas
Other rare histologic subtypes include malignant sebaceous tumors, mucinous adenocarcinoma, oncocytic carcinoma, and sialoblastoma. In addition, metastatic tumors, hematolymphoid tumors, and sarcomas may involve the salivary glands.

Classification from Barnes L, Eveson J, Reichart PA, Sidransky D (eds): World Health Organization Classification of Tumors. Pathology and Genetics of Tumors of the Head and Neck. Lyon, IARC Press, 2005.

BIOLOGIC CHARACTERISTICS AND MOLECULAR BIOLOGY

Histologic Subtype

The biologic behavior of these tumors depends on histologic subtype. Most carcinomas can be separated into two main groups: low grade and high grade. Low-grade cancers are more likely to simulate benign neoplasms in their clinical presentation; they infrequently metastasize and can usually be adequately treated with relatively conservative resection. High-grade tumors are aggressive; they present with symptoms of pain and/or palsy, are more likely to be fixed, have palpable adenopathy, frequently metastasize, and often require radical surgery and adjuvant radiation therapy to achieve local regional control.[12]

Most acinic cell cancers are typically slow-growing, low-grade cancers that arise within the parotid gland and may invade contiguous structures such as bone, nerve, skin, and blood vessels. The local recurrence rate is approximately 30% to 44% after parotidectomy and can occur late (30 years) in the natural history of the disease.[13] The incidence of lymph node metastases is 16%, and the rate of distant metastases is 15% to 19%. Distant metastases can occur late in the natural history and most commonly involve the lungs. Poor prognostic features include the following: pain or fixation; gross invasion; and microscopic features of desmoplasia, atypia, or increased mitotic activity.[13] Bilateral parotid gland involvement occurs in 3% of patients. Dedifferentiated acinic cell carcinomas are

Table 34-2 **Incidence of Lymph Node Metastases at Initial Diagnosis by Site, Grade, T Stage, Size, and Facial Nerve Paralysis**

	Clinically Positive (%)	Clinically and/or Pathologically Positive (%)	Elective Neck Dissection Revealing Occult Metastases (%)	Clinically Negative Developing Delayed Neck Metastases (%)
SITE				
Parotid	16-25	—	9	8
Submandibular/sublingual	8-44	—	21	8
Minor		—	—	10
Palate	16			
Sinuses or nasal	15			
Tongue	42			
Cheek or lips	15			
Gingiva	21			
Floor of mouth	41			
Larynx	67			
Tonsil	65			
Pharynx	0			
Adenoid cystic	14			
Mucoepidermoid	30			
Adenocarcinoma	24-28			
Malignant mixed	38			
Acinic cell	0			
Small cell	50			
GRADE				
Low	—	2	7	—
Intermediate	—	16	7	—
High	20-40	34	15-49	—
T STAGE				
T1-T2	—	—	7	—
T3	—	—	16	—
T4	—	—	24	—
SIZE				
<4 cm	—	—	17	—
≥4 cm	—	—	61	—
FACIAL NERVE PARALYSIS	—	>60	—	—

Data from Armstrong JG, Harrison LB, Thaler HT, et al: Indications for elective treatment of the neck in cancer of the major salivary glands. Cancer 69:615-619, 1992; Byers RM, Jesse RH, Guillamondegui ON, Luna MA: Malignant tumors of the submaxillary gland. Am J Surg 126:458-463, 1973; and Spiro RH, Koss LG, Hajdu SI, Strong EW: Tumors of minor salivary origin: a clinical pathologic study of 492 cases. Cancer 31:117-129, 1973.

highly malignant, are widely invasive, and metastasize early in the disease process.[14,15]

Mucoepidermoid carcinomas most commonly involve minor salivary glands of the palate and the parotid gland. These carcinomas appear to be associated with exposure to ionizing radiation. Mucoepidermoid carcinomas arising within minor salivary glands present with lymph node metastases in 30% of cases. Low-grade mucoepidermoid carcinomas tend to be slow-growing tumors that rarely aggressively invade local structures. The incidence of local or regional recurrence is 15%. These tumors rarely spread hematogenously. High-grade mucoepidermoid carcinomas are locally aggressive, with a local-regional recurrence rate of 60%. They commonly spread to regional lymph nodes (44% to 50%) and produce distant metastases in approximately 33%. Important prognostic factors for mucoepidermoid carcinomas arising within the oral cavity include grade and size (>2 cm).[16] Patients with mucoepidermoid carcinoma of the parotid gland appear to do well with few recurrences (5% to 6%) when treated with adequate parotidectomy and appropriate neck dissection independent of tumor grade and stage.[17]

Malignant mixed tumors (carcinoma ex pleomorphic adenoma) arise from preexistent benign mixed tumors (pleomorphic adenoma). They can exhibit aggressive local behavior, present with regional lymph node metastases in 25% to 38% of cases, and produce distant metastases, most commonly involving the lung, in 26% to 32% of cases. Adenocarinoma and salivary duct carcinoma are the most common histologic subtypes of carcinoma ex pleomorphic adenoma. They commonly recur locally after surgical removal (23%) and frequently metastasize to regional lymph nodes (56%). Distant metastasis can occur in 44% of cases. Most patients will die of the disease (55%), with 5-year overall survival of 30%. Important prognostic factors include tumor size, grade, and clinical and pathologic stage.[18]

Adenoid cystic carcinomas have a variable growth rate at the primary tumor site and can have a high incidence of late local recurrences, particularly when these tumors arise from a minor salivary gland. The biologic behavior also depends on histologic grade, with high-grade (predominantly solid type) tumors having a distinctly worse prognosis. Perineural invasion is a characteristic finding diagnosed histologically in 50%

of cases. Facial nerve paresis may be present in patients with parotid gland involvement at initial presentation. The cancer can extend both centrally and peripherally along the nerve. Extension through the skull base with intracranial growth has been well documented. Growth along the nerve has been shown to have "skip" areas of involvement and noninvolvement, so that a negative nerve margin does not guarantee a final negative margin. Adenoid cystic carcinoma can also grow along haversian systems of bone without showing gross bone destruction. Adenoid cystic carcinomas are relatively more common in submandibular glands and minor salivary glands. They uncommonly metastasize to regional lymph nodes (less than 20%, 7.5% at initial diagnosis). However, adenoid cystic carcinomas frequently metastasize systemically (40% to 50%), and the lungs are the most commonly involved site.

Salivary duct carcinomas are aggressive cancers with a high rate of lymph node metastases (42% to 73%). Perineural and lymphatic invasion are common. Distant metastasis is the most common pattern of failure. The prognosis is dismal.[19,20]

Adenocarcinomas are primarily high-grade malignant tumors with frequent lymph node metastases (27% to 36%) and distant metastases involving bone and lungs. In contrast, polymorphous low-grade adenocarcinomas are less common and behave less aggressively. They tend to arise from minor salivary glands within the oral cavity. Neurotropism is identified frequently. Complete surgical resection is associated with excellent long-term tumor control (97.6%) and survival.[21]

Undifferentiated carcinomas are highly malignant. Approximately one third are associated with benign mixed tumors (i.e., carcinoma ex pleomorphic adenoma). Fifty percent develop regional lymph node metastases.

Primary squamous cell carcinomas of the parotid gland behave aggressively. Approximately 50% to 60% present with lymph node metastases. Forty percent of patients with these tumors are found to have occult lymph node metastasis at the time of surgery. Deep fixation and facial nerve paralysis are poor prognostic features.[22]

Ploidy, Proliferation Indices, and Molecular Factors

DNA ploidy patterns have been evaluated in adenoid cystic carcinoma and in tumors with other histologic patterns.[23-26] Aneuploid tumors were found to be more advanced and to have a higher frequency of solid architecture, higher S-phase values, higher recurrence rates, worse survival, higher incidence of lymph node metastasis, higher incidence of nerve invasion, higher incidence of intravascular extension, higher grade, and higher stage than diploid tumors. These associations were not confirmed in acinic cell carcinoma.[27]

PCNA levels have been determined using the monoclonal antibody PC10. Patients with adenoid cystic carcinoma had a higher incidence of distant metastasis and shorter disease-free and overall survival when the PCNA level was greater than 15% versus less than 15%.[28,29] In patients with mucoepidermoid carcinomas of the parotid gland, the risk of death from cancer was 5% when the PCNA level was less than 7%, compared with a 48% risk of death with a PCNA level of 7% or higher.[30] Expression of PCNA has been shown to correlate with poor prognosis in mucoepidermoid carcinoma arising from various sites within the head and neck region.[31]

The Ki-67 proliferation antigen and *c-erbB-2/neu* oncogene expressions have been evaluated in minor salivary gland cancers arising in the palate.[32] Overexpression of the *c-erbB-2/neu* oncogene was discovered in 38% of the cancers and was associated with aggressive tumor behavior. Multivariate analysis confirmed that overexpression was an independent prognostic factor for survival. High levels of Ki-67 proliferation antigen are present in 26% of minor salivary gland cancers of the palate. This finding is associated with higher tumor grades and low survival rates on univariate analysis but not on multivariate analysis. Expression of Ki-67 has been correlated with a poor survival in patients with mucoepidermoid carcinoma.[31] Similarly, when MIB-1 is used as a measure of cell proliferation, levels greater than 10% are associated with poor survival.[33]

Expression of the p53 oncoprotein has been detected in 67% of malignant tumors of the salivary glands. Moderate or high levels of expression were associated with more advanced and larger primary tumors than low or no expression. Moderate or high levels of expression were also associated with presentation with signs of local aggressiveness, regional lymph node metastases, high incidence of distant metastases, and low disease-free and overall survival. Expression of the p53 oncoprotein appears to be an independent prognostic factor on univariate and multivariate analysis.[31,34] Expression of erbB-2, erbB-3, epidermal growth factor receptor (EGFR), and transforming growth factor (TGF)-α may have a role in the development and progression of mucoepidermoid carcinoma.[35] This finding may have therapeutic implications with the recent development of clinically effective EGFR inhibitors.

The foregoing results regarding proliferative indices and molecular biology are derived mainly from single-institution reports with relatively few cases. In the absence of validation, no conclusive data to date are available on the clinical utility of performing these studies routinely.

CLINICAL MANIFESTATIONS, PATIENT EVALUATION, AND STAGING

Clinical Manifestations by Site

Presenting symptoms and signs depend on histologic features, tumor grade, and site of origin. Most *malignant parotid tumors* present as a painless, rapidly enlarging mass. A more indolent growth rate that suddenly changes to rapid enlargement motivates a patient to seek medical evaluation. Facial nerve involvement manifested as facial weakness is uncommon (2% to 14%). Only 10% of patients complain of pain or numbness on presentation. Occasionally, locally advanced cancer can present with intractable pain and cranial neuropathy resulting from skull base involvement. Deep-lobe cancers, which account for approximately 12% of all parotid cancers, can produce dysphagia, sore throat, earache (referred) or the sensation of a "plugged" ear, trismus, headache, and facial nerve paresis. On physical examination, deep-lobe tumors can appear as a submucosal mass in the soft palate or lateral pharyngeal wall in the rare case in which the retromandibular portion of the deep lobe enters the parapharyngeal space. If the tumor extends into the retrostyloid portion of the parapharyngeal space, cranial nerves IX, X, XI, and XII may become involved. Pain can occur from involvement of the auriculotemporal branch of the third division of the fifth cranial nerve.

Submandibular gland cancers present as a mass with occasional mild pain. As the cancer enlarges, cranial nerves V, VII (marginal branch), and XII can be involved (14%).

Minor salivary gland cancers have a varied presentation because of their diverse location. Most of these tumors arise within the oral cavity or oropharynx and present as a submucosal, painless lump with indolent growth. Cancers arising within the nasal cavity or paranasal sinuses commonly present with facial pain and nasal obstruction. Laryngeal tumors present with a change in voice or hoarseness. Perineural involvement can manifest as pain, nerve paresis, and/or paresthesia.

Patient Evaluation

The evaluation of the patient with a malignant salivary gland tumor includes a thorough history and physical examination, with particular attention to symptoms and signs associated with local tumor extension, regional adenopathy, and distant metastases. Computed tomography (CT) scanning and magnetic resonance imaging (MRI) can be complementary in evaluating tumor depth and local extension. MRI can be particularly useful in evaluating cancer of the deep parotid lobe, parotid cancer contours, vascular structures, and perineural spread. MRI may yield images superior to those of CT for submandibular and minor salivary gland cancers because of the multiplanar capability and improved tissue contrast. It is not necessary to perform CT or MRI in patients with small, discrete, freely mobile cancers, especially tumors involving the superficial lobe of the parotid gland. Screening tests for regional nodal metastasis and distant metastases include liver function studies (aspartate aminotransferase, alkaline phosphatase, lactate dehydrogenase), chest radiography, and PET scanning for high-grade aggressive histologies. Table 34-3 summarizes the evaluation procedures for patients with malignant salivary gland tumors.

Fine-needle aspiration of the mass can confirm the diagnosis of malignancy in the majority of patients and can be particularly helpful when a patient is not a surgical candidate, when the patient presents with metastatic disease, and in preparing the patient for surgery.[36-39] Experience is important for establishing tissue diagnosis by fine-needle aspiration. The definitive diagnostic procedure is surgical resection of the tumor; therefore, a fine-needle aspiration cytologic examination negative for malignancy does not alter the initial management plan. A negative or benign finding does not exclude malignancy. For accurate diagnosis in these cases, excision of the gland is done with pathologic study of frozen sections, which requires expertise. The appropriate surgical procedure is then performed. An incisional or excisional biopsy should be avoided because it is associated with a higher rate of local recurrence, requires wide local excision of the scar, and may risk harm to critical structures such as the facial nerve.

Staging

The current American Joint Committee on Cancer staging system for major (parotid, submandibular, and sublingual) salivary gland cancers is shown in Table 34-4.[40] The primary

Table 34-3 Patient Evaluation for Malignant Salivary Gland Tumors

GENERAL
History
Physical examination

RADIOGRAPHIC STUDIES
Chest radiograph
CT scan of the head and neck with contrast *or*
MRI of the head and neck with contrast
PET scan for high-grade aggressive histologies

LABORATORY STUDIES
Liver function tests (lactate dehydrogenase, alkaline phosphatase, aspartate aminotransferase)

Table 34-4 American Joint Committee on Cancer Staging of Parotid, Submandibular, and Sublingual Gland Cancers

PRIMARY TUMOR (T)	
TX	Primary tumor cannot be assessed
T0	No evidence of primary tumor
T1	Tumor ≤ 2 cm in greatest dimension without extraparenchymal extension
T2	Tumor > 2 cm but < 4 cm in greatest dimension without extraparenchymal extension
T3	Tumor > 4 cm and/or tumor having extraparenchymal extension
T4a	Tumor invades skin, mandible, ear canal, and/or facial nerve
T4b	Tumor invades skull base and/or pterygoid plates and/or encases carotid artery
REGIONAL LYMPH NODES (N)	
NX	Regional lymph nodes cannot be assessed
N0	No regional lymph node metastasis
N1	Metastasis in a single ipsilateral lymph node, ≤ 3 cm in greatest dimension
N2	Metastasis in a single ipsilateral lymph node, > 3 cm but < 6 cm in greatest dimension; or in multiple ipsilateral lymph nodes, none > 6 cm in greatest dimension; or in bilateral or contralateral lymph nodes, none > 6 cm in greatest dimension
N2a	Metastasis in a single ipsilateral lymph node > 3 cm but < 6 cm in greatest dimension
N2b	Metastasis in multiple ipsilateral lymph nodes, none > 6 cm in greatest dimension
N2c	Metastasis in bilateral or contralateral lymph nodes, none >6 cm in greatest dimension
N3	Metastasis in a lymph node >6 cm in greatest dimension
DISTANT METASTASIS (M)	
MX	Distant metastasis cannot be assessed
M0	No distant metastases
M1	Distant metastases
STAGE GROUPING	
Stage I	T1 N0 M0
Stage II	T2 N0 M0
Stage III	T3 N0 M0
	T1 N1 M0
	T2 N1 M0
	T3 N1 M0
Stage IVA	T4a N0 M0
	T4a N1 M0
	T1 N2 M0
	T2 N2 M0
	T3 N2 M0
	T4a N2 M0
Stage IVB	T4b any N M0
	Any T N3 M0
Stage IVC	Any T any N M1

Used with permission of the American Joint Committee on Cancer (AJCC), Chicago, Illinois. The original source for this material is the AJCC Cancer Staging Handbook, 6th edition (2002), published by Springer-Verlag, New York.

tumor stage is based on size, clinical and/or macroscopic extraparenchymal extension, and resectability with clear margins. The nodal staging system is the same as for other head and neck cancer sites. The International Union Against Cancer revised their salivary gland staging system in 1997. The revised staging system has been validated.[41]

No formal staging system exists for malignant minor salivary gland cancers. Some clinicians choose to use the system for major salivary glands, whereas others use the staging system for squamous cell carcinomas arising from the same site. It is more common to use the staging system for squamous cell carcinomas. Significant local extension or lymph node metastasis is associated with a poor prognosis.

PRIMARY THERAPY

Surgical Techniques and Issues

The general approach to treatment depends on histologic features and grade. The mainstay of treatment for major and minor salivary gland cancers is surgical resection.

Parotid cancers are typically resected by superficial parotidectomy because most tumors involve the superficial lobe. In most cases, the deep lobe is also removed, but the decision to remove the deep lobe depends on location, extent, and histology. The facial nerve is generally preserved unless it is clearly involved with tumor. Resection of surrounding soft tissue, muscle, or bone is indicated only when the tumor directly extends into these structures. Cancers that involve the skull base and/or the deep lobe of the parotid gland with extension into the parapharynx may require skull base procedures.

No standard guidelines exist for sacrifice of the facial nerve when resecting malignant parotid gland tumors. Most surgeons agree that when the nerve is grossly encased or involved with cancer, resection is indicated. However, resection of the facial nerve results in serious disability because of the crucial role that facial movement plays in articulation, mastication, emotional expression, and socialization. Corneal exposure, ulceration, and blindness are potential severe complications associated with facial nerve damage from tumor involvement or surgical resection. Tarsorrhaphy or placement of a gold weight in the upper eyelid may be needed to help protect the eye. Nerve grafting can recover facial function in the majority of patients 2 to 13 months postoperatively. Alternatively, reconstruction methods are available to provide suspension and static support of the paralyzed face. Additional surgical complications include loss of sensation in the ear lobe and gustatory sweating (Frey's syndrome), which occurs in 5% to 25% of cases.

Dissection of the submandibular triangle is indicated for *submandibular gland cancers*. If the primary cancer directly involves the lingual and/or hypoglossal nerves or a portion of the mandible, the surgeon may need to sacrifice these structures.

The surgical approach to *minor salivary gland cancers* depends on the site of origin, tumor extent, and histologic features. Conservative resection to obtain negative margins but to minimize cosmetic and functional morbidity is the surgical goal. Minor salivary gland cancers located in the hard palate can be excised with conservative surgical procedures if these tumors are small. Partial palatectomy or formal maxillectomy may be necessary for advanced cancers. Rehabilitation of the defect can be accomplished with a prosthetic obturator or microvascular free tissue transfer (rectus abdominis).

Neck dissection is indicated for patients with palpable adenopathy or a high-grade primary cancer with aggressive histologic features and a high risk of subclinical nodal metastases.

Exceptions to Primary Surgery

Exceptions to surgical resection as the initial treatment procedure include patients who are medically inoperable, patients who refuse surgery, and patients with distant metastases, unresectable cancers, minor salivary gland cancers in inaccessible locations (nasopharynx or sphenoid sinus), and major or minor salivary gland cancers in which surgical resection would result in significant and unacceptable functional or cosmetic deficits. As discussed in the next section on locally advanced disease and palliation, radiation therapy alone can result in long-term tumor control and survival in a significant number of patients.

Adjuvant Irradiation: Indications

The indications for postoperative, adjuvant radiation therapy are listed in Table 34-5. For small, low-grade cancers of the major or minor salivary glands, surgical resection is adequate treatment. Because salivary gland cancers are so uncommon, no phase III clinical trials have been performed comparing surgery alone with surgery combined with postoperative, adjuvant radiation therapy. Most series are retrospective, covering several decades and comparing modern staging and treatment techniques to older standards. Improvements in surgical and irradiation techniques have occurred during the study periods. Few retrospective studies have included appropriate or detailed statistical analyses.

Major Salivary Gland Cancers

Table 34-6 summarizes the treatment results from five modern series comparing surgery with surgery and postoperative, adjuvant radiation therapy for malignant *major salivary gland cancers*. These five series provide evidence that the addition of postoperative radiation therapy, when indicated, improves both local control and survival in patients with major salivary gland cancers.

The series from Memorial Sloan-Kettering Cancer Center (MSKCC) in New York is particularly noteworthy.[42] The authors performed a matched-pair analysis to evaluate the effectiveness of postoperative radiation therapy. There did not appear to be an advantage to the routine use of postoperative radiation therapy for most patients with stage I and II cancers, particularly for patients with low-grade histologic types. These investigators found that postoperative radiation therapy significantly improved survival and local tumor

Table 34-5 Indications for Postoperative, Adjuvant Radiation Therapy for Major and Minor Malignant Salivary Gland Tumors

Close surgical margins (deep lobe parotid tumors, facial nerve sparing)
Microscopically positive margins
High-grade cancer
Involvement of skin, bone, nerve (gross invasion or extensive perineural involvement) and tumor extension beyond the capsule of the gland with periglandular and soft tissue invasion
Lymph node metastases
Large tumors requiring radical resection
Tumor spillage during operation
Recurrent cancer
Gross residual or unresectable/inoperable cancer

Table 34-6 Results of Surgery Alone and Combined Surgery and Postoperative External Irradiation for Malignant Salivary Gland Tumors

Institution (reference)	No. of Patients	Median Follow-up (y)	Prognostic Factors	Disease Outcomes, 5-y (%) Local Control S	Local Control S + RT	Survival S	Survival S + RT
MSKCC (42)	92	S: 10.5	Stage I/II	79	91	96	82 (det.)
		S + RT: 5.8	Stage III/IV	17	51	9.5	51 (det.)
				$P = .14$		$P = .015$	
			Positive nodes	40	69	19	49 (det.)
			(LRC)	$P = .05$		$P = .015$	
			High-grade	44	63	28	57 (det.)
Johns Hopkins (43)	87	—	All patients	58	92	59	75 (det.)
				$P = .001$		$P = .01$	
MDACC (44)	155	7.5	All patients	58	86	50-56*	66-72*
PMH (45)	271	10	All patients	—	—	60	75 (CSS)
						$P = .039$	
						29	68 (RFS)
						$P = .0005$	
MGH (46)	62	5.5	All patients	—	95	—	77 (DFS)

*Survival varies by presence of high-grade or perineural invasion.
CSS, cause specific survival; det., determinate; DFS, disease-free survival; LRC, locoregional control; MDACC, M. D. Anderson Cancer Center; MGH, Massachusetts General Hospital; MSKCC, Memorial Sloan-Kettering Cancer Center; PMH, Princess Margaret Hospital; RFS, relapse-free survival; S, surgery alone; S + RT, surgery and postoperative radiation therapy.

control for patients with stage III and IV disease ($P = .015$ and .14, respectively) and for patients with lymph node metastases ($P = .015$ and .05, respectively). A trend toward improved local control and survival was noted when postoperative radiation therapy was administered for high-grade cancers. However, the small number of patients included in the study may have precluded the discovery of additional subsets of patients who may benefit from adjuvant radiation therapy.

The study from the Johns Hopkins Hospital in Baltimore, although not prospective or a matched-pair analysis, did include a multivariate statistical analysis that identified important prognostic factors.[43] Facial nerve paresis, undifferentiated histologic features, male gender, and skin invasion were all significantly associated with a poor outcome. The addition of postoperative radiation therapy was associated with significantly improved survival ($P = .01$) and local tumor control ($P = .001$).

The group from M. D. Anderson Cancer Center (MDACC) found that patients with high-grade tumors and perineural invasion had statistically significant better locoregional control when they were treated with surgery and postoperative radiation therapy than did those who underwent surgery alone (86% versus 58%).[44] This group's multivariate analysis revealed that the presence of histologically positive cervical nodes, site (deep versus superficial lobe), and tumor size were the most important predictors of locoregional recurrence. Postoperative radiation therapy had a positive influence on survival in patients with high-grade cancers and in the presence of perineural invasion, but the improvement was not statistically significant. The multivariate analysis revealed that the four most important factors for survival were histologic grade, presence of cervical nodes, tumor size, and nerve invasion.

The multivariate analysis performed by the authors from Princess Margaret Hospital revealed that tumor size and the presence of regional lymph node metastases were the two most significant factors predicting cause-specific survival.[45] The multivariate analysis revealed that tumor size, presence of regional lymph node metastases, age, and histologic features were significant predictive factors for cause-specific survival. Patients treated with combined surgery and postoperative radiation therapy enjoyed a significantly improved relapse-free (68% versus 29%, $P = .0005$) and cause-specific survival rate (75% versus 60%, $P = .039$) compared with patients treated with surgery alone.

The report from Massachusetts General Hospital (MGH) in Boston did not contain a group of patients treated with surgery alone.[46] Nevertheless, the authors report an impressive 95% 5-year local tumor control rate and 77% 5-year disease-free survival rate using combined surgery and postoperative radiation therapy in patients with advanced malignant parotid gland tumors.

A review by the Dutch Head and Neck Oncology Cooperative Group of 565 malignant salivary gland (major and minor) tumors found that postoperative radiation therapy improved locoregional control ($P = .0005$). In multivariable analysis, local control was also predicted by clinical T stage, bone invasion, site, and resection margin. Regional control was predicted by N stage and facial nerve paralysis in addition to treatment. The relative risk with surgery alone, compared to surgery plus postoperative radiation therapy, was 9.7 for local recurrence and 2.3 for regional recurrence. Distant metastases were independently correlated with T and N stage, sex, perineural invasion, histologic type, and clinical skin involvement. Overall survival depended on age, sex, T and pathologic N stage, site, and skin and bone invasion.[47]

Table 34-7 summarizes local tumor control and survival by type of treatment for patients with *submandibular gland cancers*. The group from Princess Margaret Hospital reported improved locoregional tumor control (69% versus 30%, $P < .05$) and relapse-free survival (52% versus 27%, $P > .1$) with the addition of postoperative radiation therapy to surgical resection.[48] In the series from the MDACC, patients with soft tissue extension, perineural invasion, and adenoid cystic carcinoma had improved locoregional tumor control, but not survival.[49] Historically, patients treated with surgery alone had about a 50% locoregional control rate. Patients treated with surgery and postoperative radiation therapy have an 88% actuarial

Table 34-7 Results of Surgery and Surgery With Postoperative, Adjuvant Radiation Therapy for Malignant Tumors of the Submandibular Gland

Institution (Reference)	No. of Patients	Minimum Follow-up	Prognostic Factor	Local Control (%) S	Local Control (%) S + RT	Survival, 5-y (%) S	Survival, 5-y (%) S + RT
PMH (48)	91	—	All patients	*5 y* 30 *P* < .05 (LRC)	69	60 27 *P* > .1	65 (CSS) 52 (RFS)
MDACC (49)	86	24 mo	All patients	—	—	71	60
			Soft tissue extension	*Crude* 48 *P* < .034	85	—	—
			Perineural invasion	62	92	—	—
			Adenoid cystic carcinoma with soft tissue and perineural invasion	29 *P* < .01	100	—	—

CSS, cause-specific survival; LRC, locoregional control; MDACC, M. D. Anderson Cancer Center; PMH, Princess Margaret Hospital; RFS, relapse-free survival; S, surgery alone; S + RT, surgery and postoperative adjuvant radiation therapy.

Table 34–8 Results of Surgery and Surgery With Postoperative, Adjuvant Radiation Therapy for Malignant Minor Salivary Gland Tumors

Institution (Reference)	No. of Patients	Median Follow-up	Treatment	Local Control (%)	Survival (5-y) (%)
MSKCC (11)	434	—	S	53 (crude)	42 44.5 determinate
MDACC (53)	160	110 mo	S + RT	96 (5-y)	81
UF (57)	87	Minimum 2 y	S + RT	87.5 (crude)	63–100 cause-specific 56–100 overall 50–93 relapse-free
			RT	51.3 (crude)	38–90 cause-specific 39–82 overall 25–73 relapse-free
Stanford (54)	54	7.8 y	S + RT	88 (10-y)	81 10-y cause specific 63 10-y overall

MDACC, M. D. Anderson Cancer Center; MSKCC, Memorial Sloan-Kettering Cancer Center; RT, radiation therapy; S, surgery; UF, University of Florida.

locoregional control rate at 10 years. Important prognostic factors included soft tissue invasion or extraglandular extension, lymph node metastases, adenocarcinoma and high-grade histology, and treatment during the earlier years of the study.[50] Indications for postoperative radiation therapy at the Netherlands Cancer Institute include advanced stage, clinical skin and/or soft tissue invasion, lymph node involvement, and perineural growth.[51]

Sublingual gland cancers are rare, comprising 0.5% of all salivary gland tumors.[52] Most are adenoid cystic, mucoepidermoid, or adenocarcinoma. Local recurrences are uncommon (3 of 18, 17%) and overall survival can be prolonged (median, 74 months). Postoperative radiation therapy is indicated in patients with high-stage, high-grade tumors or when there is concern about the adequacy of resection.[52]

Minor Salivary Gland Cancers

Table 34-8 summarizes the treatment results for malignant *minor salivary gland* tumors. Local control and survival in four major series are presented by treatment method.

In the series from MSKCC, more than 90% of the patients were treated with surgery alone.[11] In the 224 patients who underwent initial treatment at MSKCC, the crude local control rate was 53%, and the determinate 5-year survival was 44.5%.

A series of 160 patients from the MDACC were all treated with surgery and postoperative radiation therapy. When the MDACC and MSKCC results are compared, local control appears to be improved to 96% at 5 years, and survival is improved to 81% at 5 years with the addition of postoperative radiation therapy.[53] The MDACC authors found that paranasal sinus involvement was statistically associated with an increased risk of local treatment failure. In addition, a prolonged interval between surgery and the start of adjuvant radiation therapy was associated with a significantly increased risk of local and distant treatment failure. The authors recommended that radiation therapy be started as soon as possible after surgery.

The Stanford University series included 54 patients. All except two patients were treated with postoperative radiation therapy. The 5-year actuarial local control rate was 91%. Only three patients developed recurrent nodal disease within the neck. The 5-year rate of freedom from distant metastasis was 86%. The 5-year cause-specific and overall survival rates were 84% and 75%, respectively. Important prognostic factors for tumor control, distant metastasis, and survival were T stage, surgical margins, primary site, N stage, and histology.[54] Additional important prognostic factors include bone involvement, sex, type of surgery, and soft tissue and vascular invasion.[55,56]

The authors from the University of Florida reported similar results with the use of surgery and postoperative radiation therapy, with local tumor control rates of 87.5% (crude) and cause-specific survival rates of 63% to 100%, depending on tumor stage.[57] A multivariate analysis found that local tumor control was significantly affected by tumor stage and treatment type (combined surgery and postoperative radiation therapy was better than radiation therapy alone). Tumor stage was also a significant predictor of cause-specific survival and freedom from relapse. Rates of freedom from relapse were higher for patients who received combined surgery and postoperative radiation therapy.

Adjuvant or Elective Neck Irradiation: Indications and Results

Patients who present with clinically positive lymph node metastases undergo neck dissection followed by postoperative radiation therapy. Patients with clinically negative neck lymph nodes but who are at high risk of occult lymph node metastases based on histologic subtype and grade should undergo elective neck dissection (followed by postoperative radiation therapy if occult metastases are pathologically confirmed) or elective neck irradiation if indications exist for treating the primary tumor site.

Patients with major salivary gland cancers who are at high risk of occult lymph node metastases were defined by Armstrong and associates from MSKCC.[9] The authors studied 474 previously untreated patients. Clinically positive nodes were present in 14%. Clinically occult, pathologically positive nodes occurred in 12%. Multivariate analysis revealed that primary tumor size and grade predicted occult lymph node metastases. Tumors of 4 cm or more in size had a 20% risk of occult metastases compared with a 4% risk with smaller tumors ($P < .00001$). High-grade tumors (regardless of histologic type) had a 49% risk of occult metastases compared with a 7% risk for intermediate-grade or low-grade tumors ($P < .00001$). Elective neck dissection in patients with large (>4 cm) and/or high-grade tumors appears appropriate. Additional indications for elective neck dissection may include facial nerve involvement, extraglandular extension, and severe desmoplasia.[58,59]

The authors from MSKCC have analyzed the anatomic distribution of occult metastases discovered by elective neck dissection in patients with parotid cancers. If the dissection had been limited to the parotid gland and level II, occult disease would not have been detected in 25% of the patients with occult nodal metastasis. The latter patients had skip metastases to levels III or IV without involvement of periparotid or level II nodes. By failing to extend the dissection to include level III, metastases would have been missed in 10%. The MSKCC authors also analyzed the anatomic distribution of occult metastases discovered by elective neck dissection in patients with submandibular gland cancers. A dissection incorporating levels I, II, and III would have detected all cases of occult disease. The authors recommended elective neck dissection or elective neck irradiation incorporating at least levels I, II, and III when the primary cancer is large or of high grade. Elective contralateral neck dissection or irradiation is not necessary even when ipsilateral lymph node metastases are present.[60,61]

For patients with malignant minor salivary gland tumors, node involvement occurs most often in patients with small cell carcinoma (50%), malignant mixed tumors (38.4%), mucoepidermoid carcinoma (30.3%), and adenocarcinomas (24.3% to 28.3%). The risk of lymph node metastases is also higher for anatomic sites with a high lymphatic density such as the tongue (42.2%), gingiva (20.7%), floor of mouth (41.2%), larynx (66.7%), and tonsil (64.6%).[11] Elective neck dissection or elective neck irradiation should be strongly considered in patients with minor salivary gland tumors of large size, of high-risk histologic features, of high grade, or of high-risk (rich lymphatic) primary tumor site.

LOCALLY ADVANCED DISEASE AND PALLIATION

Intraoperative Irradiation

Intraoperative irradiation has been administered after maximal tumor resection in patients with locally advanced primary or recurrent cancers who have close, microscopically positive or grossly positive margins. This method has been followed by conventional external irradiation. Long-term tumor control and survival with acceptable morbidity have been reported.

The Methodist Hospital of Indiana began a treatment program for locally advanced primary or locally recurrent salivary gland malignant tumors using surgical resection and intraoperative electron beam irradiation in 1982.[62] Thirty patients with T3 or T4 cancers with a minimum follow-up of 2 years have been treated with maximal resection plus intraoperative electron beam irradiation. Most cancers originated in the major salivary glands, including 20 parotid cancers and 3 submandibular cancers. Minor salivary gland cancers were treated at a variety of sites including the oral cavity and oropharynx (three cases), nasopharynx, and maxilla (four cases). Histologic types included mucoepidermoid carcinoma, adenoid cystic carcinoma, adenocarcinoma, malignant mixed tumors, and acinic cell carcinoma. Prior radiation therapy had been given to eight patients with a dose range of 50 to 72 Gy. Attempts were made to preserve the facial nerve, when possible, at the time of resection. If the nerve was involved with gross disease, it was sacrificed. Close surgical margins were obtained in 20 cases, 8 had microscopically positive margins, and 2 had gross residual cancer. A single fraction of 10 to 20 Gy was administered intraoperatively using 5- to 9-MeV electrons.

The 5-year locoregional control rate in the Methodist Hospital series of intraoperative electron beam irradiation was 74%, and the 5-year overall survival was 57%. Locoregional tumor control was significantly affected by margin status and prior irradiation. The survival was also adversely affected by margin status. Eight intact nerves, most commonly facial nerves, were within the intraoperative electron beam radiation therapy field. No clinical dysfunction had developed at the time of the report.

Neutron or Photon Irradiation, Hyperthermia

Table 34-9 summarizes the treatment results in patients with inoperable, recurrent, and unresectable major and minor salivary gland cancers. The Radiation Therapy Oncology Group and the Medical Research Council performed a randomized phase III clinical trial comparing conventional photon and/or electron radiation therapy with fast neutron radiation therapy.[63] Although the local tumor control rate was significantly improved with the use of neutrons, the neutron group had a higher incidence of distant metastases and no improvement in survival. In addition, the incidence of severe and life-threatening long-term treatment-related morbidity was greater in patients treated with neutrons. A similar experience has been reported for the treatment of adenoid cystic carcinomas with a neutron beam.[64] These findings, combined with the limited number of institutions with neutron beam capabilities, dampened the enthusiasm for neutron beam therapy. Never-

Table 34-9 Radiation Therapy Treatment Results for Inoperable, Recurrent, and Unresectable Major and Minor Malignant Salivary Gland Tumors

Institution (reference)	No. of Patients	Median Follow-up (mo)	Treatment	Local Control (%)	Survival
RTOG/MRC (63)	25	Minimum 76	NBT PRT/EBT	56% (LRC) 17% (LRC) *P* = .009	15% 10 y overall 25% 10 y overall
MGH (67)	24	—	AFRT	100% (5 y, parotid cancers) 78% (5 y, minor)	65% (5 y, parotid) 93% (5 y, minor)
Stanford (69)	4	36	RT + HT	3/4	29-60 mo

AFRT, altered fractionation radiation therapy; EBT, conventional electron beam therapy; HT, hyperthermia; LRC, locoregional control; MGH, Massachusetts General Hospital; MRC, Medical Research Center; NBT, neutron beam therapy; PRT, conventional photon radiation therapy; RT, radiation therapy; RTOG, Radiation Therapy Oncology Group.

theless, a large, uncontrolled single-institution study reported impressive tumor control and survival rates with 10% severe or life-threatening long-term toxicity (grade 3 and 4) using neutron beam therapy in advanced salivary gland neoplasms. Favorable prognostic variables included early stage, minor salivary sites, lack of skull base invasion, no prior radiation therapy, and prior surgical resection.[65] Carbon ion radiation therapy may provide similar tumor control as the neutron beam with less late effects.[66-68]

Photon radiation alone or in conjunction with hyperthermia has also been evaluated for the treatment of locally advanced disease. Wang and Goodman,[69] from Massachusetts General Hospital, reported results using high-dose, accelerated hyperfractionated photon beam therapy in patients with inoperable and unresectable major and minor salivary gland cancers. Promising long-term local tumor control rates and survival were achieved in a series of 24 patients. Mendenhall[70] reported that a significant proportion of patients with incompletely resected adenoid cystic carcinoma can experience long-term tumor control (43% at 10 years) and overall survival (42% at 10 years) with the use of aggressive primary photon radiation therapy without surgical resection.

In patients with recurrent, previously irradiated cancers, the combination of low-dose to moderate-dose external irradiation and hyperthermia has also been evaluated. Significant palliation of local symptoms was reported by Barnett and associates, from Stanford University in Stanford, California.[71]

In summary, neutron beam therapy and high-dose conventional or altered fractionation photon therapy can produce at least meaningful palliation in a significant proportion of patients with inoperable, recurrent, and unresectable major and salivary gland cancers. Significant 5-year survival has also been reported with conventional or altered fractionation photon therapy.

Chemotherapy

The role of chemotherapy has not been defined in malignant major and minor salivary gland cancers. Single agents such as 5-fluorouracil, hydroxyurea, methotrexate, cisplatin, bleomycin, doxorubicin, and cyclophosphamide have shown limited response rates. A combination of cyclophosphamide, doxorubicin, and cisplatin have shown response rates of 22% to 100%, and complete response rates of 0% to 40% lasting 5 to 9 months in patients with adenoid cystic carcinomas.[72-75] A Northern California Oncology Group study found a response rate of 35% with a combination of cisplatin, doxorubicin, and 5-fluorouracil.[76] A study from the Mayo Clinic revealed a 38% response rate using cisplatin-based chemotherapy for recurrent and advanced salivary gland cancers. This seemed to provide some palliation but had no significant effect on survival.[72] Systemic chemotherapy, therefore, plays a minor palliative role.

Retrospective review in one single institution suggested improved disease-free survival in high-risk patients treated with cisplatin-based concurrent postoperative radiation therapy and chemotherapy.[77]

Future studies should evaluate chemotherapy given concomitantly with postoperative, adjuvant radiation therapy or primary radiation therapy in patients with adverse features. In addition, the role of maintenance (adjuvant) chemotherapy should be evaluated after concomitant chemotherapy and radiation therapy.[78] Hormonal and biologic therapy (EGFR inhibitors) await the development of effective and acceptably toxic agents.

TECHNIQUES OF IRRADIATION

Parotid Gland Cancers

The postoperative radiation therapy target volume for parotid cancers should include the parotid bed only for low-grade cancers with indications for local irradiation but no lymph node involvement. The target volume should include the parotid bed and ipsilateral neck in patients with high-grade cancers, recurrent cancers, and/or lymph node metastases. With gross invasion of the facial nerve, generous coverage of the facial canal to the geniculate ganglion is indicated. A boost can be given to the tumor bed for close or positive surgical margins.

Combined Photon Electron Beam Technique

For parotid cancers involving the superficial lobe or the deep lobe in thin patients in whom the target volume is 5 cm or less deep, a combination of photons and electrons can be used. An intraoral stent containing Cerrobend can be fabricated to shield the posterior oral tongue and the contralateral oral mucosa (Fig. 34-1).[79] The scar and the lateral canthus of the ipsilateral orbit are marked with wire during simulation. The patient is immobilized using a thermoplastic face mask in the open neck or supine position. Additional immobilization can be obtained using an Accuform by MED-TEC to conform to the occiput, neck, and shoulders. The ipsilateral ear should be flattened against the mastoid process to minimize dose inhomogeneity caused by electron perturbation. Similarly, the external auditory canal is filled with water or wet gauze (at body temperature) before each electron treatment.

An appositional (open neck position) or lateral (supine position) field is used to cover the parotid bed and upper neck

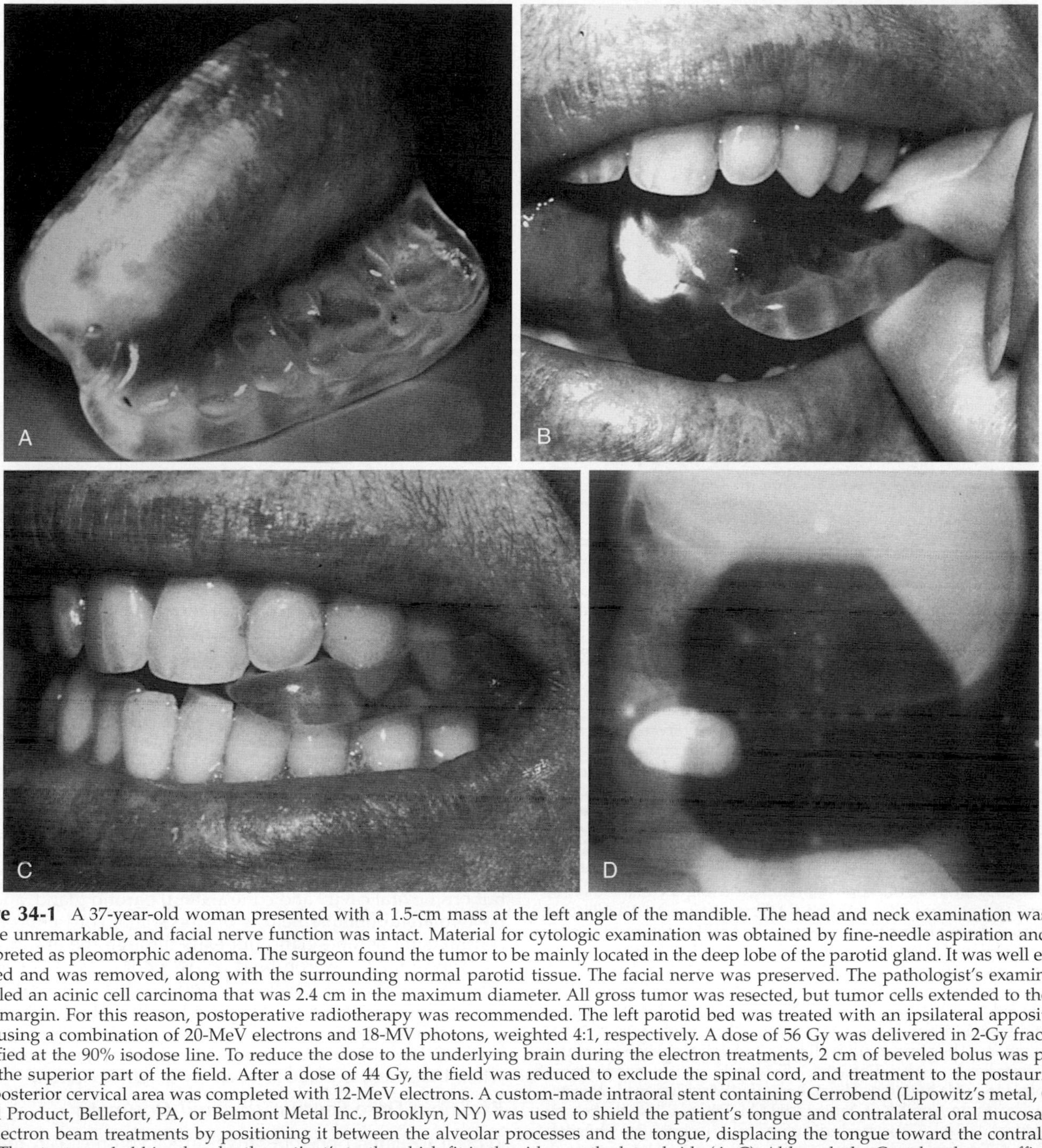

Figure 34-1 A 37-year-old woman presented with a 1.5-cm mass at the left angle of the mandible. The head and neck examination was otherwise unremarkable, and facial nerve function was intact. Material for cytologic examination was obtained by fine-needle aspiration and was interpreted as pleomorphic adenoma. The surgeon found the tumor to be mainly located in the deep lobe of the parotid gland. It was well encapsulated and was removed, along with the surrounding normal parotid tissue. The facial nerve was preserved. The pathologist's examination revealed an acinic cell carcinoma that was 2.4 cm in the maximum diameter. All gross tumor was resected, but tumor cells extended to the surgical margin. For this reason, postoperative radiotherapy was recommended. The left parotid bed was treated with an ipsilateral appositional field using a combination of 20-MeV electrons and 18-MV photons, weighted 4:1, respectively. A dose of 56 Gy was delivered in 2-Gy fractions, specified at the 90% isodose line. To reduce the dose to the underlying brain during the electron treatments, 2 cm of beveled bolus was placed over the superior part of the field. After a dose of 44 Gy, the field was reduced to exclude the spinal cord, and treatment to the postauricular and posterior cervical area was completed with 12-MeV electrons. A custom-made intraoral stent containing Cerrobend (Lipowitz's metal, Cerro Metal Product, Bellefort, PA, or Belmont Metal Inc., Brooklyn, NY) was used to shield the patient's tongue and contralateral oral mucosa from the electron beam treatments by positioning it between the alveolar processes and the tongue, displacing the tongue toward the contralateral side. The stent was held in place by the patient's teeth, which fit in the ridge on the lateral side (**A–C**). Although the Cerrobend was sufficiently thick to reduce the transmitted dose to approximately 10% when treating with electrons, it would have increased the dose directly behind the stent when treating with high-energy photons because of the forward scatter of secondary electrons. When the patient was treated with photons, a duplicate stent without the lead alloy was used to maintain the treatment field geometry. Because 80% of the dose was delivered by electrons, there was still significant protection of the tongue and contralateral oral mucosa to prevent mucositis in these areas. The intraoral stent was used for shielding the tongue and contralateral oral mucosa during ipsilateral radiation treatment for a parotid gland tumor. **A,** Lateral view. The flange on the lateral side of the stent contains occlusal registration. **B,** Stent insertion. **C,** Device in treatment position. **D,** Port film showing the position of the stent in relation to the radiation field. (From Kaanders JHAM, Fleming TJ, Ang KK, et al: Devices valuable in head and neck radiotherapy. Int J Radiat Oncol Biol Phys 23:639-645, 1992.)

nodes. The field borders include the zygomatic arch or higher, as indicated by tumor extension or scars superiorly. Anteriorly, the anterior edge of the masseter muscle is identified. Inferiorly, the thyroid notch is used. The field extends posteriorly just behind the mastoid process (Fig. 34-2).[79]

Radiation is delivered with a combination of electrons and photons, with the ratio and energy determined by computerized dosimetry and CT scan planning. An off-cord reduction is made to limit the spinal cord dose to 45 Gy, and the posterior portion of the neck is supplemented using lower-energy

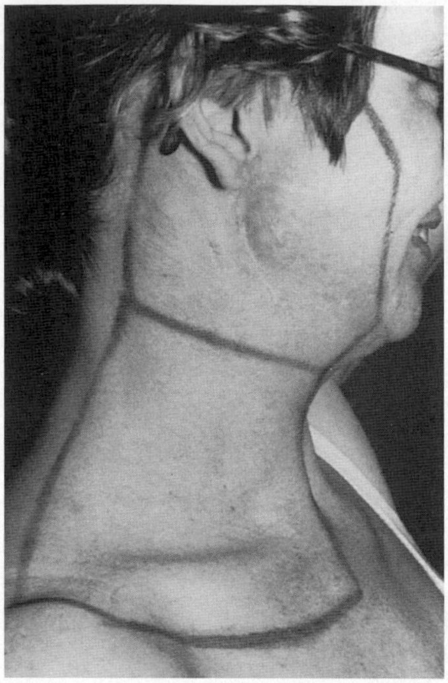

Figure 34-2 A 39-year-old woman presented with a 4-month history of right parotid swelling. She underwent surgical exploration. The surgeon found a large mass extending from the base of the skull to the subdigastric muscle inferiorly. This lesion was dissected from the facial nerve and was removed in two major pieces. Pathologic examination showed a pleomorphic adenoma. Five months later, the patient presented with a recurrent nodule in the upper posterior cervical region. This was excised and was also found to contain pleomorphic adenoma. Four months after the second intervention, a small induration was palpated at the posterior auricular region. Fine-needle aspiration showed carcinoma. The patient was then referred to the M. D. Anderson Cancer Center. Review of the slides revealed carcinoma ex pleomorphic adenoma in the specimens of the first and second surgical procedures. Physical examination on referral revealed no palpable gross disease and intact facial nerve function. It was decided to deliver postoperative radiotherapy to the parotid bed and upper neck with a lateral appositional field using a combination of electrons and photons (20 MeV and 6 MV, respectively). An intraoral stent was used to protect the mucosa of the oral tongue and the contralateral oral cavity, and a water bolus was used to fill the external auditory canal. The middle and lower neck nodes on the ipsilateral side were treated with a separate electron field. The tumor bed received a dose of 60 Gy in 30 fractions prescribed at the 90% isodose line, and the middle and lower neck areas were given a dose of 50 Gy in 25 fractions. The patient did well until 1 year later, when brain and lung metastases were detected. Treatment with combination chemotherapy was initiated. The patient died of widespread metastatic disease. (From Ang KK, Kaanders JHAM, Peters LJ: Radiotherapy for Head and Neck Cancers: Indications and Techniques. Philadelphia, Lea & Febiger, 1994, p 110.)

electrons. Another field reduction is made after 60 Gy in 30 fractions to deliver a boost dose when indicated. If the anterior edge of the field is close to the eye, skin collimation is applied, and the beam may be angled 5 to 10 degrees posteriorly. Beveled bolus, the thickness of which is determined by computerized dosimetry and CT scan planning, is placed in the superior portion of the field to reduce the dose to the temporal lobe. An appositional electron field or anteroposterior (AP) photon field is used to treat the middle and lower neck nodes when indicated.

Careful and detailed treatment planning must be used when using high-energy electrons and bolus. A phantom dosimetric study revealed a number of significant discrepancies between the measured and predicted dose when using this technique.[80] Measured doses were seen to exceed predicted doses by up to 23% in the temporal lobe region. Underpredictions of dose were found behind the mandible and in the nasal cavity. Overpredictions of dose by the planning algorithm of up to 22% were observed along the oropharynx. Some of these discrepancies were found to relate to underestimation of the dose in the fall-off region. Other errors were attributable to the difficulties in predicting dose at density interfaces. Localized overpredictions and underpredictions of this magnitude must be accounted for by the clinician prescribing treatment in terms of possible late effects of the temporal lobe and the dose specification point.

Oblique Wedged-Pair Technique

Anterolateral and posterolateral oblique photon fields are used for deep-seated tumors or when the facial canal is part of the target volume (Fig. 34-3).[79] The patient is immobilized using a Vac-Lok bag and thermoplastic face mask in an open neck or supine position with the head hyperextended to move the orbits out of the radiation fields.

Two simulations are required for this technique if a dedicated CT simulator is not available. (This is no longer necessary with a CT simulator as digitally reconstructed radiographs [DRRs] can be used.) The first simulation involves the marking of critical normal tissues and selecting a provisional isocenter for orthogonal reference films and CT scan treatment planning. The scar and both inferior orbital rims are marked with wire. The provisional isocenter is placed at the center of the square defined by the zygomatic arch, anterior edge of the masseter, thyroid notch, and mastoid, and halfway between the skin surface and the lateral oropharyngeal wall. A CT scan is obtained in the treatment position, and the target volume and critical normal structures are contoured on representative cuts. Field sizes and shapes, oblique field angles, and wedge thicknesses are determined using computerized dosimetry and a CT- or MRI-based treatment planning system. The setup parameters are subsequently reproduced at the second simulation (the anterolateral oblique field is on the spinal cord but off the oral cavity and contralateral parotid gland, and the posterolateral oblique field is off the spinal cord and off the contralateral parotid gland but exits through the oral cavity). An appositional electron field or AP photon field is used to treat the middle and lower neck nodes when indicated.

No off-cord reduction is required for the oblique wedged-pair technique because the posterolateral field is off the spinal cord for the entire treatment. A field reduction for a boost dose, when indicated, is made after 60 Gy is administered.

Radiation Dose Specification and Dosimetry

Typical ipsilateral postoperative target volumes can tolerate 2.0 Gy fractions to 60 Gy. (Tolerance is generally fine with ipsilateral therapy.) Surgically disturbed areas receive 60 Gy in 30 fractions. Areas at high risk because of incomplete resection receive 66 to 70 Gy in 33 to 35 fractions. The dose for elective neck irradiation is 50 Gy in 25 fractions. Typical dosimetric plans are shown in Figures 34-4 and 34-5. The oblique wedged-pair technique (see Fig. 34-4) generally gives fairly homogeneous dose distributions in the tumor volumes with hot spots of 105% to 110%, spinal cord doses of 46% to 62%, cerebellar doses of 47% to 105%, and contralateral parotid gland doses of 0% to 18%. The mixed electron-photon beam technique (see Fig. 34-5) using a single appositional field also gives a reasonably homogeneous dose distribution with hot spots of 110% to 125%, spinal cord doses of 28% to 42%, and contralateral parotid gland doses of 20% to 31%.[81]

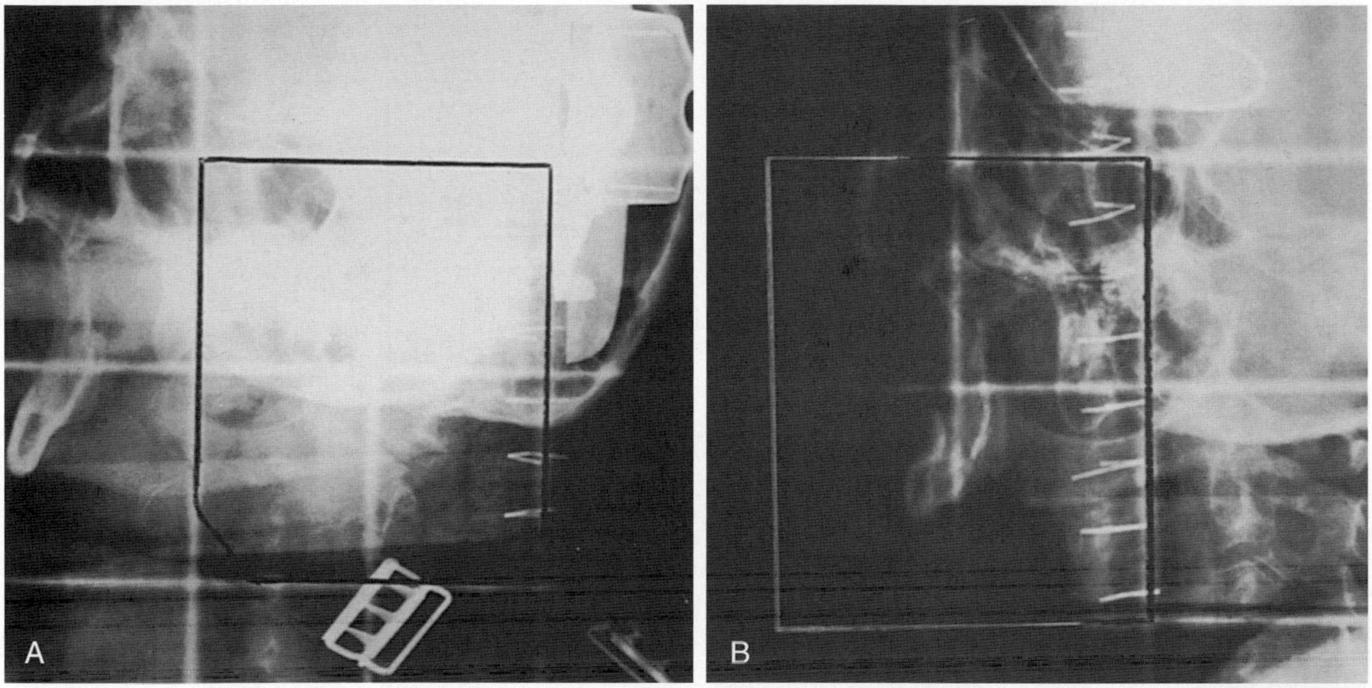

Figure 34-3 **A and B,** A 46-year-old woman presented with a 1-year history of intermittent left facial swelling and left parietal headache. Physical examination of the parotid region and of the other areas of the head and neck was unremarkable. The facial nerve was intact. However, CT showed a soft tissue mass in the deep lobe of the parotid gland. The patient underwent a total parotidectomy with sparing of the facial nerve. The tumor was removed from beneath the facial nerve with some difficulty. Pathologic examination revealed a pleomorphic adenoma measuring 3.5 × 3 × 2.5 cm. The deep margin of resection was positive. Two intraparotid lymph nodes and 16 periparotid nodes, removed to gain access to the parotid, were all free of tumor. It was decided to treat this patient with postoperative radiotherapy because of the difficult and incomplete resection. The target volume extended to 6 cm from the surface, which was too deep for the highest available electron energy (20 MeV), and treatment with wedged-pair fields was elected. A total dose of 50 Gy was delivered to the 95% isodose line in 25 fractions. This therapy was well tolerated. Follow-up examination 2.5 years later showed no evidence of local recurrence. However, a nodule was identified at the inferomedial quadrant of the patient's right breast. Fine-needle aspiration of this lesion revealed ductal carcinoma. The patient is undergoing treatment for breast cancer. (From Ang KK, Kaanders JHAM, Peters LJ: Radiotherapy for Head and Neck Cancers: Indications and Techniques. Philadelphia, Lea & Febiger, 1994, p 111.)

Customized, shaped Cerrobend blocks are fabricated or multileaf collimators are used to minimize dose to uninvolved normal critical structures.

Submandibular Gland Cancers

For submandibular gland cancers, the initial target volume includes the surgical bed for low-grade cancers with indications for postoperative radiation therapy. The target volume includes the surgical bed and entire ipsilateral neck for high-grade cancers and cancers with lymph node metastases. When perineural invasion is present but limited to focal involvement of small, unnamed nerves, the fields are enlarged by 2 to 3 cm, but no effort is made to treat the nerve pathways comprehensively. If named nerves are involved (lingual or hypoglossal), their course is traced and treated to the base of the skull. A boost dose can be given to the tumor bed if indicated.

Ipsilateral irradiation is sufficient for most patients. This technique can be accomplished with either a mixture of electrons and photons or an oblique wedged pair similar to that used in parotid cancers. Opposed anteroposterior-posteroanterior or opposed tangential fields can also be used, depending on optimal tumor coverage given the tumor extent and the desire to avoid irradiation of uninvolved normal structures. The patient is immobilized in the open neck or supine position using a thermoplastic face mask and Accu-Form by MED-TEC. The scar and oral commissures are wired.

If an appositional electron field is used, it encompasses the tumor bed and upper neck nodes. The superior border extends from the oral commissure sloping up to cover the ascending ramus of the mandible just short of the temporomandibular joint. The field is extended up to the base of the skull when there is gross perineural invasion. The anterior field edge is determined by the extent of surgery. The oral commissure, lip, and skin of the chin are shielded when possible. The inferior field edge is located at the thyroid notch and the posterior field edge is located just behind the mastoid process. An off-cord reduction is made to limit the spinal cord dose to 45 Gy, and a posterior neck strip is supplemented with lower-energy electrons. An appositional electron field or AP photon field is used to treat the middle and lower neck nodes, when indicated.

If oblique wedged-pair, opposed AP-PA, or opposed tangential fields are used, two simulations and CT scan treatment planning are required as in parotid cancers if a dedicated CT simulator is not available (Fig. 34-6).[79] The dose guidelines are the same as for parotid gland cancers. Figure 34-7 displays the dosimetry from a treatment plan.

Minor Salivary Gland Cancers

The initial target volume for minor salivary gland cancers includes the primary tumor or surgical bed for small or low-

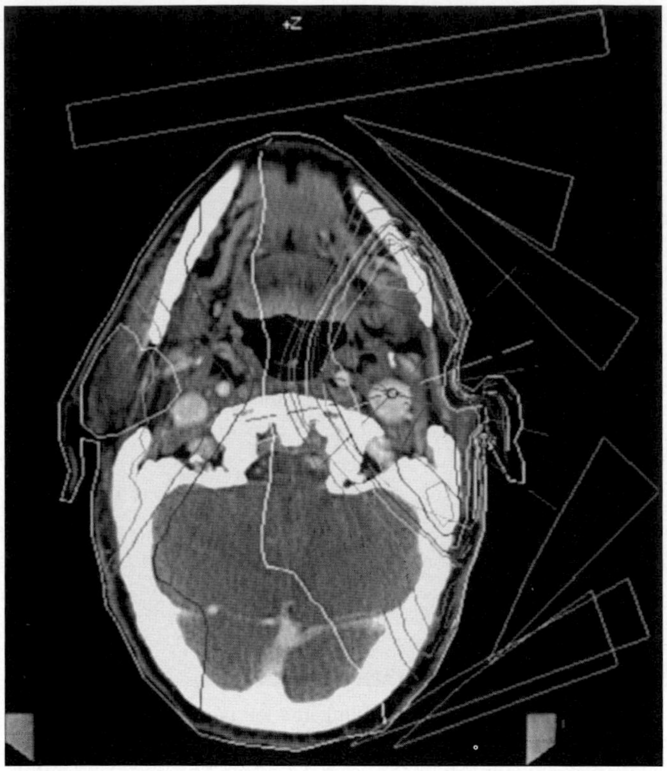

Figure 34-4 Dosimetry for the oblique wedged-pair technique.

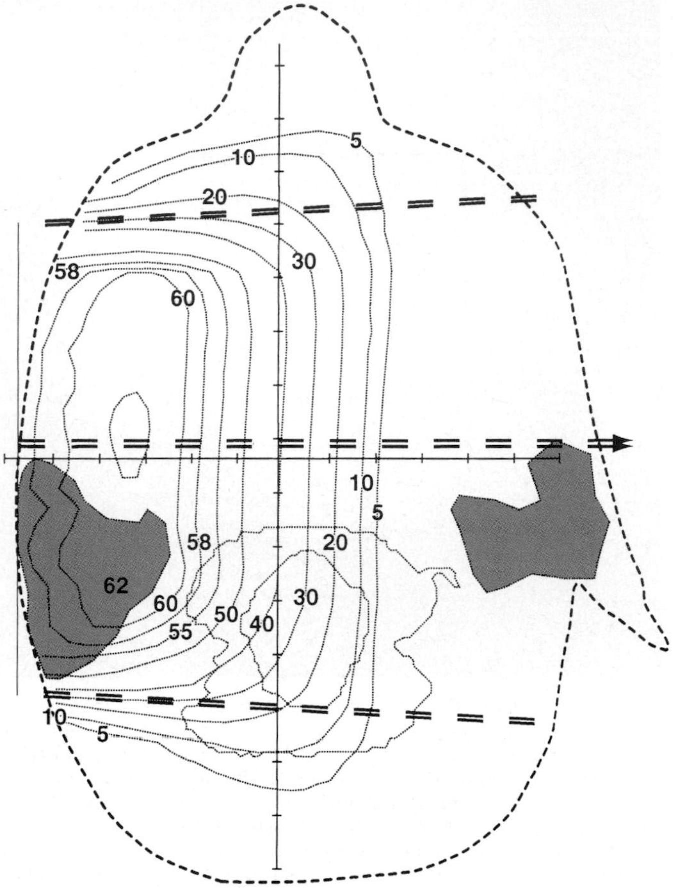

Figure 34-5 Dosimetry for the combined photon-electron beam technique.

grade cancers with indications for radiation therapy. The primary tumor or surgical bed and lymph nodes are included in the target volume for high-grade cancers and cancers with lymph node metastases. Elective neck treatment varies with histologic features, grade, and anatomic site of the primary cancer. The boost volume includes the primary tumor or tumor bed when indicated. The setup and field arrangement vary with the anatomic site of the primary lesion and follow the general guidelines of squamous cell carcinomas of the upper aerodigestive tract, as described throughout this head and neck cancer section. Dose guidelines are the same as for parotid and submandibular gland cancers. Specialized boost techniques such as intraoral cone or interstitial or intracavitary implant are site specific.

Intensity-Modulated Radiation Therapy

The use of intensity-modulated radiation therapy (IMRT) may be preferred in selected patients with malignant salivary gland tumors. Indications would include perineural involvement of named nerves (facial, trigeminal, hypoglossal, lingual) requiring treatment of the proximal nerve to the brainstem while attempting to spare the contralateral salivary glands, eyes, temporal lobes and brainstem. In the elective setting, subclinical intracranial disease in the cavernous sinus, adjacent to the brainstem or within the petrous bone, can be treated at 1.8 Gy per fraction while higher risk areas in the original tumor bed and/or high risk neck can be treated at 2.0 Gy per fraction. Positive distal nerve margins may also be an indication for IMRT. The entire course of the nerve can be treated distally while sparing critical normal structures such as the lacrimal gland and eye. Figure 34-8 is an example of an IMRT plan.

Side Effects of Treatment

Acute side effects of radiation therapy are site dependent. In general, mild to moderate skin erythema and oral mucositis are common.

Patients with parotid gland cancers develop xerostomia in 41% of cases (much of it is low grade and surgically induced; 59% have no xerostomia, 15% have mild xerostomia, 22% have moderate xerostomia, and 4% have severe xerostomia). Thirteen percent of patients complain of pain in the jaw. Additional chronic complications include numbness of the skin and muscle spasms in 4%, dry ear in 20%, persistent and repeated ear infections in 4%, hearing deficits in 4%, perforation of the tympanic membrane in 2%, hair loss in 4%, painful tongue in 2%, and dry eye in 2%. Hypoplasia of the mandible and skull is a concern when treating the pediatric population. Radiation-induced cancers and osteoradionecrosis are rare.[46]

Complications related to the treatment of minor salivary gland cancer are site dependent. Bone exposure or osteoradionecrosis can occur in 10% to 15% of patients. Minor bone complications occur in approximately 6%, moderate complications occur in 3%, and severe complications requiring surgical resection or resulting in mandibular fractures occur in about 4%; soft tissue necrosis is rare.[57] Patients irradiated for cancers involving the nasal cavity, paranasal sinuses, or nasopharynx can develop a transient central nervous system syndrome (8%), panhypopituitarism (3%), and unilateral blindness (16%).[57] Decreased hearing occurs in approximately 50%.[53]

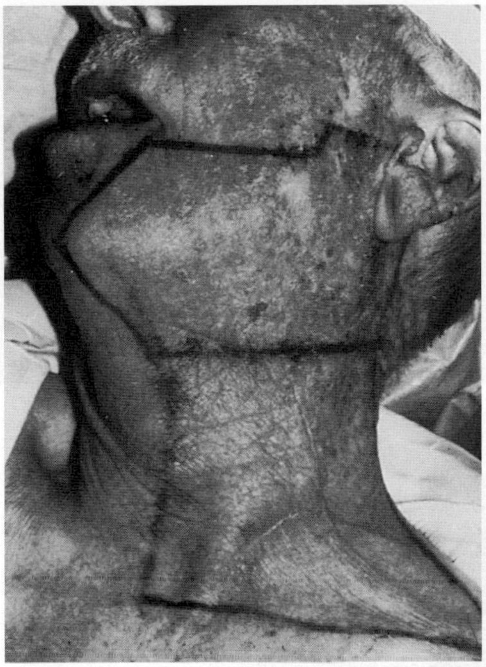

Figure 34-6 An 82-year-old man noticed an asymptomatic mass in the left submandibular area and sought medical attention immediately. On examination, he was found to have a 3-cm, left submandibular mass. This mass was resected, along with a left modified neck dissection. Pathologic examination revealed an adenoid cystic carcinoma in the submandibular gland measuring 2.5 × 2 × 2 cm with perineural invasion. One of the eight lymph nodes (a subdigastric node) in the specimen contained metastatic disease. The lingual and hypoglossal nerves were free of gross tumor invasion. Postoperative radiotherapy was delivered through a left lateral appositional field encompassing the tumor bed, the proximal extension of the nerves at risk, and the upper portion of the neck. A combination of 20-MeV electrons and 6-MV photons was used, weighted 4:1. A dose of 50 Gy was delivered in 25 fractions, after which the field was reduced to administer a booster of 10 Gy in 5 fractions to the tumor bed. The middle and lower neck nodes were treated with a separate 9-MeV electron field to a dose of 50 Gy in 25 fractions. This therapy was well tolerated. The patient died of intercurrent disease a year after completion of treatment. (From Ang KK, Kaanders JHAM, Peters LJ: Radiotherapy for Head and Neck Cancers: Indications and Techniques. Philadelphia, Lea & Febiger, 1994, p 114.)

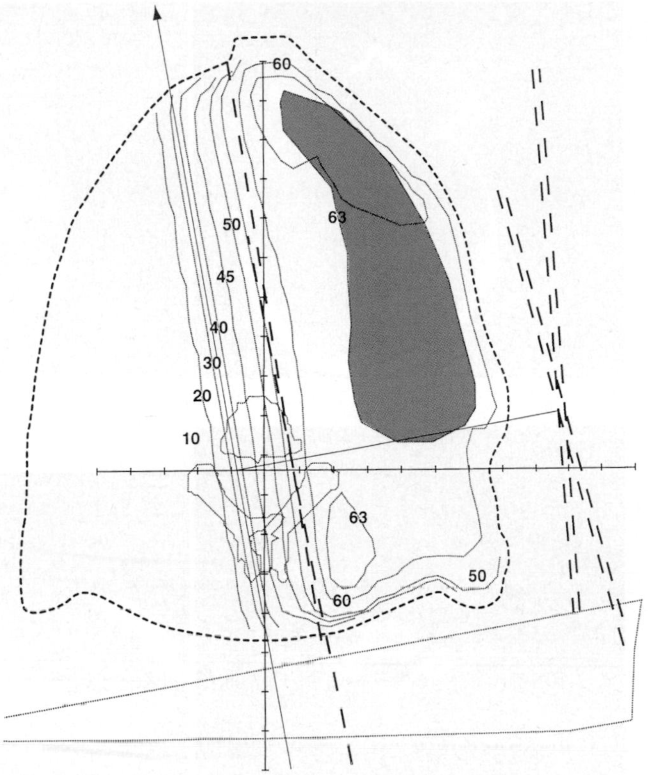

Figure 34-7 Dosimetry for submandibular gland cancer.

The incidence and severity of acute mucositis and xerostomia and chronic xerostomia and loss of taste may be reduced with the use of the radioprotector amifostine. Reported results of one small ($n = 39$) and one large ($n = 315$) randomized clinical trial suggested that amifostine significantly reduces one or both of these acute and chronic effects of radiation therapy without a detrimental effect on tumor control or survival.[82,83]

Nerve Grafts Versus Timing of Irradiation

When a facial nerve cable graft has been placed, the clinician walks a fine line between delaying the onset of radiation therapy, when indicated, to improve the success rate of the cable nerve graft and yet not delaying the radiation therapy to the extent that the patient has a higher risk of local relapse. Controlled experimental animal studies and some studies in humans suggest that regeneration of nerve following crush injuries, transection and repair or reconstruction with isografts is not adversely affected by the administration of radiation therapy.[84,85] McGuirt and associates reported 12 patients with facial nerve cable grafts who underwent irradiation.[86] Nine patients had long-term evaluation. All nine had return of some function 2 to 9 months postoperatively. Seven had moderate to excellent return to function. These investigators reported that this finding is similar to that in patients who do not receive radiation therapy who have a 70% rate of return of function. Brown and colleagues studied 52 patients with neoplasms involving the parotid gland. Cable facial nerve grafts were performed in 50 and 2 underwent direct anastomosis. Twenty-eight of the 52 patients received postoperative radiation therapy. The median time interval between nerve grafting and the onset of radiation therapy was 5.1 weeks. The median dose of radiation therapy administered was 60 Gy. The patients receiving postoperative radiation therapy were more likely to have pathologic nerve invasion by tumor and more extensive nerve resection. The median follow-up was 10.6 years.

There was no difference in functional outcome (House-Brackmann facial grading system) between the irradiated and nonirradiated graft patients. Median time to best facial nerve function after surgery was longer in the irradiated patients (13.1 versus 10.8 months), but this difference was not statistically significant. Whether radiation therapy was delivered less than 6 weeks after nerve grafting or more than 6 weeks had no impact on achievement of a functional facial nerve. Negative prognostic factors for achieving a functional facial nerve were the presence of preoperative facial nerve palsy, duration of preoperative palsy, and age greater than 60 years.[87] In general, radiation therapy should be started as soon as possible after surgical treatment, ideally within 4 to 6 weeks. Most cable nerve grafts function adequately after radiation therapy, especially in young patients. Cable grafts are not as successful in older patients.

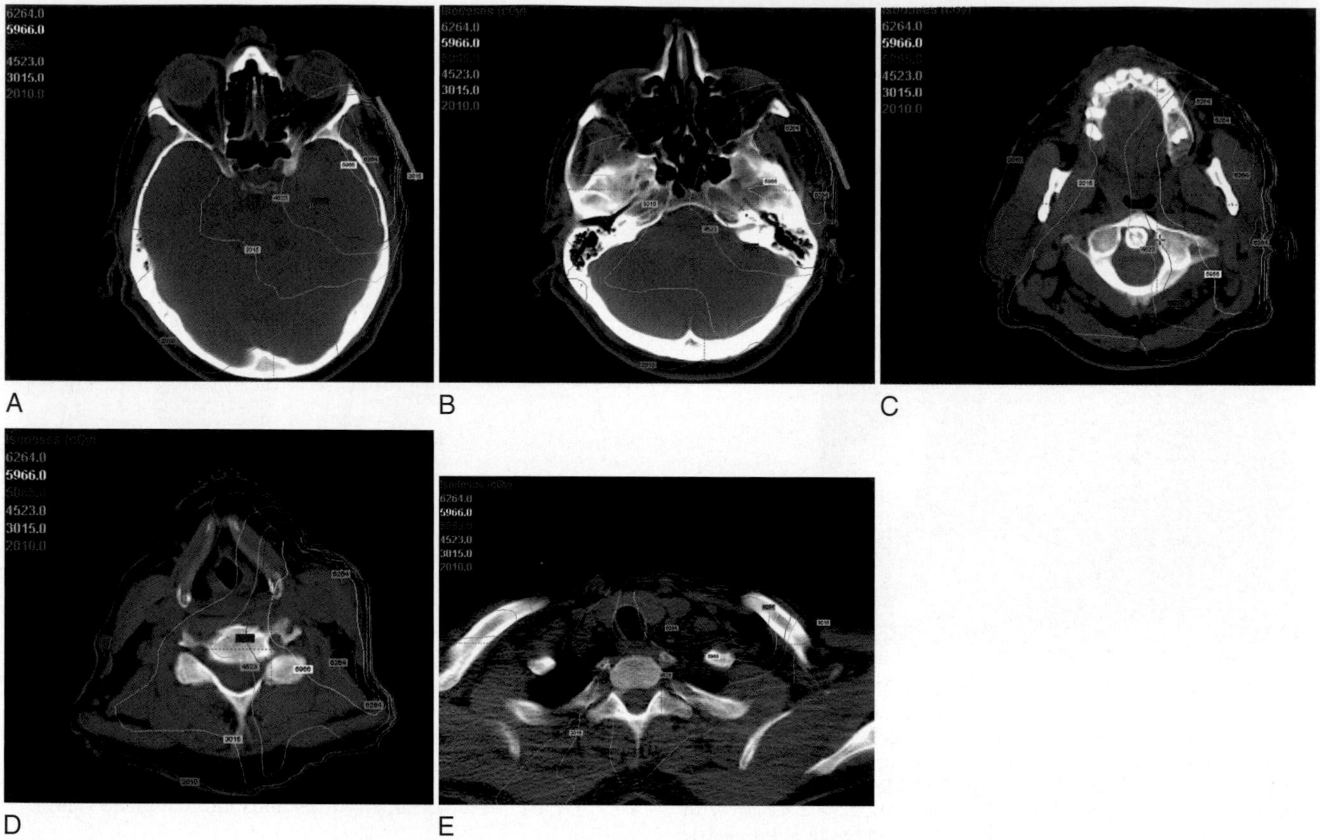

Figure 34-8 A 65-year-old man presented with left facial weakness. There was no palpable mass on examination, but MRI revealed an irregular, 2.0-cm maximum diameter mass in the left parotid gland just lateral to the condylar neck and posterior to the masseter muscle. Fine-needle aspiration was positive for carcinoma of the non–small cell type. Results of a chest radiograph and serum chemistries were normal. He underwent a left total parotidectomy with sacrifice of the upper division of the facial nerve, left upper neck dissection, facial nerve interpositional graft with microvascular neurorrhaphy, left direct brow lift, left gold weight implant, and left inferior lid canthoplasty. At surgery, the tumor was found to extensively involve the deep lobe of the parotid gland, invade muscle, and invade the entire upper division of the facial nerve. The pathologic review revealed grade 4 adenocarcinoma forming a 2.2-cm mass in the deep lobe of the parotid. There was extensive perineural invasion, including the upper facial and lower ocular nerves. After multiple repeat excisions of the deep, posterior and distal nerve margins, all final surgical margins were uninvolved. All lymph nodes removed from the pretragal, external jugular, and jugulodigastric regions were uninvolved. Postoperative radiation therapy was recommended because of the high-grade, aggressive histology; deep lobe involvement; and invasion of muscle and nerve with close distal nerve and deep margins. A customized neck rest was fabricated using Mold Care. The patient was immobilized using a combination of Aquaplast (head) and Bear Claw (shoulders). CT simulation was performed. A dose of 50.4 Gy in 28 fractions of 1.8 Gy each was prescribed to a planning target volume (PTV1) encompassing the ipsilateral neck nodes (levels II to V, parapharyngeal, retropharyngeal), the parotid bed with a 2-to 3-cm margin, and the course of the facial nerve from the brainstem through the petrous portion of the temporal bone and out into the periphery of the upper face and lower ocular muscles. A dose of 59.36 Gy in 28 fractions of 2.12 Gy each was prescribed to a PTV2, encompassing the same volume as PTV1 but excluding the brainstem, petrous bone, and temporal lobe. Inverse planning, 8-field, sliding window intensity-modulated radiation therapy was used to plan and deliver the prescribed dose. Phantom measurements confirmed that the dose delivered was within 0.6% of the dose calculation. The dose of 50.4 Gy was delivered to 99.8% of PTV1; 59.36 Gy was delivered to 95.3% of PTV2; and 65.6 Gy (110%) treated 0.24% of PTV2. The maximum brain dose was 61.21 Gy, with 2.24% of the brain receiving 56 Gy or more. The maximum brainstem dose was 49.05 Gy. The maximum spinal cord dose was 45 Gy (mean dose, 39.7 Gy). The contralateral submandibular gland received 28.3-Gy maximum, with a mean dose of 22.4 Gy. The contralateral parotid gland received 35.79 Gy maximum, with a mean dose of 22.58 Gy. The contralateral inner and middle ear received a mean dose of 25.12 Gy, and the maximum was 33.81 Gy. The ipsilateral eye received a maximum dose of 43.01 Gy, with a mean dose of 20.68 Gy. The oral cavity received a mean dose of 40.15 Gy, with a maximum of 62.82 Gy. The maximum esophageal dose was 62.03 Gy, with a mean dose of 43.54 Gy. The maximum laryngeal dose was 56.33 Gy, with a mean of 32.17 Gy. **A,** Dosimetry at the level of the eyes. **B,** Dosimetry at the level of the petrous bone. **C,** Dosimetry at the level of the contralateral parotid and oral cavity. **D,** Dosimetry at the level of the midneck and larynx. **E,** Dosimetry at the level of the lower neck.

TREATMENT ALGORITHM, CONCLUSIONS, AND FUTURE POSSIBILITIES

Table 34-10 summarizes treatment recommendations for malignant major and minor salivary gland cancers. Complete surgical resection is the mainstay of treatment. Postoperative adjuvant locoregional external beam radiation therapy is added when clinical, surgical, and/or pathologic factors predict a high risk of recurrence.

Despite adjuvant irradiation, a significant risk of local recurrence still exists in advanced T stage and high-grade cancers, and a significant risk of regional recurrence and distant metastases exists in patients with advanced N stage

Table 34-10 **Treatment Algorithm for Malignant Major and Minor Salivary Gland Cancers**

Clinical Situation	Standard Therapy	Proposed Clinical Trial
Complete resection, adjuvant therapy	Postoperative, adjuvant EBRT when indicated (see Table 34-5)	Intergroup trial of surgical resection plus postoperative adjuvant EBRT versus surgical resection plus postoperative, adjuvant EBRT with concomitant and maintenance chemotherapy
Locally advanced (primary or recurrent; unresectable or resected but residual)	1. High-dose conventional photon irradiation, including altered fractionation, brachytherapy, and intraoral cone boost 2. Maximal surgical resection, IOERT or brachytherapy and conventional EBRT 3. Neutron beam therapy	1. Neoadjuvant chemotherapy followed by resection (with or without IOERT or brachytherapy), EBRT with concomitant and maintenance chemotherapy 2. High-dose conventional or altered fractionation EBRT with concomitant and maintenance chemotherapy
Locally recurrent, prior irradiation	Low- to moderate-dose EBRT plus hyperthermia Palliative chemotherapy	3. Carbon ion therapy

EBRT, external beam irradiation; IOERT, intraoperative electron beam irradiation.

disease. The role of adjuvant concomitant and maintenance chemotherapy in this situation ideally should be tested in controlled clinical trials. Cisplatin-based regimens have produced significant response rates in patients with unresectable or metastatic disease and could be tested concomitantly with EBRT (low dose daily, moderate dose weekly, or high dose every 21 days) and as adjuvant therapy. Newer agents such as paclitaxel (Taxol) and gemcitabine could be evaluated. Promising results in squamous cell carcinomas of the upper aerodigestive tract with these regimens and targeted biologic agents should encourage investigation in malignant salivary gland tumors.[88-95]

When the disease is so advanced as to be unresectable with negative margins, treatment options include high-dose conventional or altered fractionation photon irradiation, neutron beam irradiation, carbon ion therapy, or maximal surgical debulking plus intraoperative electron beam irradiation or intraoperative high-dose rate brachytherapy followed by or preceded by conventional or altered fractionation external beam radiation therapy with or without concomitant and maintenance chemotherapy. Locoregional recurrence rates and the development of distant metastasis are substantial in this group of patients.

Controlled clinical trials should be developed to evaluate neoadjuvant, concomitant, and maintenance chemotherapy in the patient with unresectable disease. Neoadjuvant chemotherapy could be used in an attempt to obtain a response adequate for surgical resection, followed by adjuvant concomitant EBRT and chemotherapy and maintenance chemotherapy. Intraoperative electron beam irradiation, intraoperative high-dose rate brachytherapy, or afterloading brachytherapy could be used for patients with close or positive tumor margins. An alternative arm in a clinical trial would be planned preoperative concomitant chemoradiation, followed by maximal resection, intraoperative irradiation for close or positive margins, and maintenance chemotherapy. Advances using neoadjuvant, concomitant, and maintenance chemotherapy and/or targeted biologic agents in resectable and unresectable squamous cell carcinomas of the upper aerodigestive tract could be used as models for unresectable salivary gland cancers.[88-95]

REFERENCES

1. Spitz MR, Fueger JJ, Goepfert H, Newell GR: Salivary gland cancer: a case-control investigation of risk factors. Arch Otolaryngol Head Neck Surg 116:1163-1166, 1990.
2. Albeck H, Bentzen J, Ockelmann HH, et al: Familial clusters of nasopharyngeal carcinoma and salivary gland carcinomas in Greenland natives. Cancer 72:196-200, 1993.
3. Gallo O, Santucci M, Calzorlari A, Storchi OM: Epstein-Barr virus (EBV) infection and undifferentiated carcinoma of the parotid gland in Caucasian patients. Acta Otolaryngol (Stockh) 114:572-575, 1994.
4. Zheng R, Dahlstrom KR, Wei Q, Sturgis EM: Gamma radiation-induced apoptosis, G2 delay, and the risk of salivary and thyroid carcinomas—a preliminary report. Head Neck 26:612-618, 2004.
5. Beal KP, Singh B, Kraus D, et al: Radiation-induced salivary gland tumors: a report of 18 cases and a review of the literature. Cancer J 9:467-471, 2003.
6. Pinkston JA, Cole P: Incidence rates of salivary gland tumors: results from a population-based study. Otolaryngol Head Neck Surg 120:834-840, 1999.
7. Seifert G: Histological typing of salivary gland tumours. *In* International Histological Classification of Tumours, 2nd ed. Berlin, Springer, 1991.
8. Seifert G, Sobin LH: The World Health Organization's histological classification of salivary gland tumors: a commentary on the second edition. Cancer 70:379-385, 1992.
9. Armstrong JG, Harrison LB, Thaler HT, et al: Indications for elective treatment of the neck in cancer of the major salivary glands. Cancer 69:615-619, 1992.
10. Byers RM, Jesse RH, Guillamondegui ON, Luna MA: Malignant tumors of the submaxillary gland. Am J Surg 126:458-463, 1973.
11. Spiro RH, Koss LG, Hajdu SI, Strong EW: Tumors of minor salivary origin: a clinical pathologic study of 492 cases. Cancer 31:117-129, 1973.
12. Kane WJ, McCaffrey TV, Olsen KD, Lewis JE: Primary parotid malignancies: a clinical and pathologic review. Arch Otolaryngol Head Neck Surg 117:307-315, 1991.
13. Lewis JE, Olsen KD, Weiland LH: Acinic cell carcinoma: clinicopathologic review. Cancer 67:172-179, 1991.
14. Stanley RJ, Weiland LH, Olsen KD, Pearson BW: Dedifferentiated acinic cell (acinous) carcinoma of the parotid gland. Otolaryngol Head Neck Surg 98:155-161, 1988.

15. Hoffman HT, Karnell LH, Robinson RA, et al: National Cancer Data Base report on cancer of the head and neck: acinic cell carcinoma. Head Neck 21:297-309, 1999.
16. Olsen KD, Devine KD, Weiland LH: Mucoepidermoid carcinoma of the oral cavity. Otolaryngol Head Neck Surg 89:783-791, 1981.
17. Boahene DKO, Olsen KD, Lewis JE, et al: Mucoepidermoid carcinoma of the parotid gland. The Mayo Clinic experience. Arch Otolaryngol Head Neck Surg 130:849-856, 2004.
18. Olsen KD, Lewis JE: Carcinoma ex pleomorphic adenoma: a clinicopathologic review. Head Neck 23:705-712, 2001.
19. Lewis JE, McKinney BC, Weiland LH, et al: Salivary duct carcinoma: clinicopathologic and immunohistochemical review of 26 cases. Cancer 77:223-230, 1996.
20. Hosal AS, Fan C, Barnes L, Myers EN: Salivary duct carcinoma. Otolaryngol Head Neck Surg 129:720-725, 2003.
21. Castle JT, Thompson LDR, Frommelt RA, et al: Polymorphous low grade adenocarcinoma. A clinicopathologic study of 164 cases. Cancer 86:207-219, 1999.
22. Gaughan RK, Olsen KD, Lewis JE: Primary squamous cell carcinoma of the parotid gland. Arch Otolaryngol Head Neck Surg 118:798-801, 1992.
23. Luna MA, El-Naggar A, Batsakis JG, et al: Flow cytometric DNA content of adenoid cystic carcinoma of submandibular gland. Arch Otolaryngol Head Neck Surg 116:1291-1296, 1990.
24. Tytor M, Gemryd P, Wingren S, et al: Heterogeneity of salivary gland tumors studied by flow cytometry. Head Neck 15:514-521, 1993.
25. Tytor M, Gemryd P, Grenko R, et al: Adenoid cystic carcinoma: significance of DNA ploidy. Head Neck 17:319-327, 1995.
26. Franzen G, Norgård S, Boysen M, et al: DNA content in adenoid cystic carcinomas. Head Neck 17:49-55, 1995.
27. Timon CI, Dardick I, Panzarella T, et al: Acinic cell carcinoma of salivary glands: prognostic relevance of DNA flow cytometry and nucleolar organizer regions. Arch Otolaryngol Head Neck Surg 120:727-733, 1994.
28. Kim KH, Chung PS, Rhee CS, Kim WH: The manifestation of proliferating cell nuclear antigen in adenoid cystic carcinoma. Arch Otolaryngol Head Neck Surg 120:1221-1225, 1994.
29. Cho K, Lee S, Lee Y: Proliferating cell nuclear antigen and c-erbB-2 oncoprotein expression in adenoid cystic carcinomas of the salivary glands. Head Neck 21:414-419, 1999.
30. Frankenthaler RA, El-Naggar AK, Ordonez NG, et al: High correlation with survival of proliferating cell nuclear antigen expression in mucoepidermoid carcinoma of the parotid gland. Otolaryngol Head Neck Surg 111:460-466, 1994.
31. Pires FR, de Almeida OP, de Araujo VC, Kowalski LP: Prognostic factors in head and neck mucoepidermoid carcinoma. Arch Otolaryngol Head Neck Surg 130:174-180, 2004.
32. Giannoni C, El-Naggar AK, Ordonez NG, et al: c-erbB-2/neu oncogene and Ki-67 analysis in the assessment of palatal salivary gland neoplasms. Otolaryngol Head Neck Surg 112:391-398, 1995.
33. Norberg-Spaak L, Dardick I, Ledin T: Adenoid cystic carcinoma: use of cell proliferation, bcl-2 expression, histologic grade, and clinical stage as predictors of clinical outcome. Head Neck 22:489-497, 2000.
34. Gallo O, Franchi A, Bianchi S, et al: p53 oncoprotein expression in parotid gland carcinoma is associated with clinical outcome. Cancer 75:2037-2044, 1995.
35. Gibbons MD, Manne U, Carroll WR, et al: Molecular differences in mucoepidermoid carcinoma and adenoid cystic carcinoma of the major salivary glands. Laryngoscope 111:1373-1378, 2001.
36. Wong DSY, Li GKH: The role of fine-needle aspiration cytology in the management of parotid tumors: a critical clinical appraisal. Head Neck 22:469-473, 2000.
37. Bartels S, Talbot JM, DiTomasso J, et al: The relative value of fine-needle aspiration and imaging in the preoperative evaluation of parotid masses. Head Neck 22:781-786, 2000.
38. Postema RJ, van Velthuysen MLF, van den Brekel MWM, et al: Accuracy of fine-needle aspiration cytology of salivary gland lesions in the Netherlands Cancer Institute. Head Neck 26:418-424, 2004.
39. Zbaren P, Nuyens M, Loosli H, Stauffer E: Diagnostic accuracy of fine-needle aspiration cytology and frozen section in primary parotid carcinoma. Cancer 100:1876-1883, 2004.
40. Greene FL, Page DL, Fleming ID, et al: American Joint Committee on Cancer Staging Manual, 6th ed. New York, Springer-Verlag, 2002, pp 69-74.
41. Numata T, Muto H, Shiba K, et al: Evaluation of the validity of the 1997 International Union Against Cancer TNM classification of major salivary gland carcinoma. Cancer 89:1664-1669, 2000.
42. Armstrong JG, Harrison LB, Spiro RH, et al: Malignant tumors of major salivary gland origin: a matched-pair analysis of the role of combined surgery and postoperative radiation therapy. Arch Otorhinolaryngol Head Neck Surg 116:290-293, 1990.
43. North CA, Lee DJ, Piantadosi S, et al: Carcinoma of the major salivary glands treated by surgery or surgery plus postoperative radiotherapy. Int J Radiat Oncol Biol Phys 18:1319-1326, 1990.
44. Frankenthaler RA, Luna MA, Lee SS, et al: Prognostic variables in parotid gland cancer. Arch Otorhinolaryngol Head Neck Surg 117:1251-1256, 1991.
45. Theriault C, Fitzpatrick PJ: Malignant parotid tumors: prognostic factors and optimum treatment. Am J Clin Oncol 9:510-516, 1986.
46. Spiro IJ, Wang CC, Montgomery WW: Carcinoma of the parotid gland. Cancer 71:2699-2705, 1993.
47. Terhaard CHJ, Lubsen H, Van der Tweel I, et al: Salivary gland carcinoma: independent prognostic factors for locoregional control, distant metastases, and overall survival: results of the Dutch Head and Neck Oncology Cooperative Group. Head Neck 26:681-693, 2004.
48. Bissett RJ, Fitzpatrick PJ: Malignant submandibular gland tumors: a review of 91 patients. Am J Clin Oncol 11:41-51, 1988.
49. Weber RS, Byers RM, Petit B, et al: Submandibular gland tumors: adverse histologic factors and therapeutic implications. Arch Otolaryngol Head Neck Surg 116:1055-1060, 1990.
50. Storey MR, Garden AS, Morrison WH, et al: Postoperative radiotherapy for malignant tumors of the submandibular gland. Int J Radiat Oncol Biol Phys 51:952-958, 2001.
51. Vander Poorten VLM, Balm AJM, Hilgers FJM, et al: Prognostic factors for long term results of the treatment of patients with malignant submandibular gland tumors. Cancer 85:2255-2264, 1999.
52. Spiro RH: Treating tumors of the sublingual glands, including a useful technique for repair of the floor of the mouth after resection. Am J Surg 170:457-460, 1995.
53. Garden AS, Weber RS, Ang KK, et al: Postoperative radiation therapy for malignant tumors of minor salivary glands: outcome and patterns of failure. Cancer 73:2563-2569, 1994.
54. Le Q, Birdwell S, Terris DJ, et al: Postoperative irradiation of minor salivary gland malignancies of the head and neck. Radiother Oncol 52:165-171, 1999.
55. Lopes MA, Santos GC, Kowalski LP: Multivariate survival analysis of 128 cases of oral cavity minor salivary gland carcinomas. Head Neck 20:699-706, 1998.
56. Vander Poorten VLM, Balm AJM, Hilgers FJM, et al: Stage as major long term outcome predictor in minor salivary gland carcinoma. Cancer 89:1195-1204, 2000.
57. Parsons JT, Mendenhall WM, Stringer SP, et al: Management of minor salivary gland carcinomas. Int J Radiat Oncol Biol Phys 35:443-454, 1996.
58. de Brito Santos IR, Kowalski LP, de Araujo VC, et al: Multivariate analysis of risk factors for neck metastases in surgically treated parotid carcinomas. Arch Otolaryngol Head Neck Surg 127:56-60, 2001.
59. Bhattacharyya N, Fried MP: Nodal metastasis in major salivary gland cancer. Predictive factors and effects on survival. Arch Otolaryngol Head Neck Surg 128:904-908, 2002.
60. Harrison L, Armstrong J, Spiro R, et al: Postoperative radiation therapy for major salivary gland malignancies. J Surg Oncol 45:52-55, 1990.
61. King J, Fletcher G: Malignant tumors of the minor salivary glands. Radiology 100:001-004, 1971.
62. Garrett P, Rate W, Hamaker R, et al: Surgical resection and intraoperative radiation therapy (IORT) for advanced or recurrent salivary gland malignancies. *In* Fourth International Symposium on Intraoperative Radiation Therapy, Munich, Germany, 1992, pp 199-202.
63. Laramore GE, Krall JN, Griffin TW, et al: Neutron versus photon irradiation for unresectable salivary gland tumors: final report of

an RTOG-MRC randomized clinical trial. Int J Radiat Oncol Biol Phys 27:235-240, 1993.
64. Huber PE, Debus J, Latz D, et al: Radiotherapy for advanced adenoid cystic carcinoma: neutrons, photons or mixed beam? Radiother Oncol 59:161-167, 2001.
65. Douglas JG, Koh W, Austin-Seymour M, Laramore GE: Treatment of salivary gland neoplasms with fast neutron radiotherapy. Arch Otolaryngol Head Neck Surg 129:944-948, 2003.
66. Schulz-Ertner D, Nikoghosyan A, Jakel O, et al: Feasibility and toxicity of combined photon and carbon ion radiotherapy for locally advanced adenoid cystic carcinomas. Int J Radiat Oncol Biol Phys 56:391-398, 2003.
67. Mizoe JE, Tsujii H, Kamada T, et al: Dose escalation study of carbon ion radiotherapy for locally advanced head-and-neck cancer. Int J Radiat Oncol Brol Phys 60:358-364, 2004.
68. Schulz-Ertner D, Nikoghosyan A, Thilmann C, et al: Results of carbon ion radiotherapy in 152 patients. Int J Radiat Oncol Biol Phys 58:631-640, 2004.
69. Wang CC, Goodman M: Photon irradiation of unresectable carcinomas of salivary glands. Int J Radiat Oncol Biol Phys 21:569-576, 1991.
70. Mendenhall WM, Morris CG, Amdur RJ, et al: Radiotherapy alone or combined with surgery for adenoid cystic carcinoma of the head and neck. Head Neck 26:154-162, 2004.
71. Barnett TA, Kapp DS, Goffinet DR: Adenoid cystic carcinoma of the salivary glands: management of recurrent, advanced, or persistent disease with hyperthermia and radiation therapy. Cancer 65:2648-2656, 1990.
72. Creagan E, Woods J, Rubin J: Cisplatin-based chemotherapy for neoplasms arising from salivary glands and contiguous structures in the head and neck. Cancer 62:2313-2319, 1988.
73. Kaplan M, Johns M, Cantrell R: Chemotherapy for salivary gland cancer. Otolaryngol Head Neck Surg 95:167-170, 1986.
74. Suen J, Johns M: Chemotherapy for salivary gland cancer. Laryngoscope 92:235-239, 1982.
75. Dreyfuss AI, Clark JR, Fallon BG, et al: Cyclophosphamide, doxorubicin, and cisplatin combination chemotherapy for advanced carcinoma of salivary gland origin. Cancer 60:2869, 1987.
76. Venook A, Tseng A Jr, Meyers F: Cisplatin, doxorubicin, and 5-fluorouracil chemotherapy for salivary gland malignancies: a pilot study of the Northern California Oncology Group. J Clin Oncol 5:951-955, 1987.
77. Hocwald E, Korkmaz H, Yoo GH, et al: Prognostic factors in major salivary gland cancer. Laryngoscope 111:1434-1439, 2001.
78. Airoldi M, Gabriele AM, Gabriele P, et al: Concomitant chemoradiotherapy followed by adjuvant chemotherapy in parotid gland undifferentiated carcinoma. Tumori 87:14-17, 2001.
79. Ang KK, Garden AS: Radiotherapy for Head and Neck Cancers: Indications and Techniques. Philadelphia, Lippincott Williams & Wilkins, 2002.
80. Ostwald PM, Cooper SG, Denham JW, Hamilton CS: Dosimetry of high energy electron therapy to the parotid region. Radiother Oncol 33:148-156, 1993.
81. Lee DJ, Duhon M, North C, Lam WC: Radiotherapy treatment planning for parotid tumors. Int J Radiat Oncol Biol Phys 19:244-245, 1990.
82. Büntzel J, Küttner K, Fröhlich D, et al: Selective cytoprotection with amifostine in concurrent radiochemotherapy for head and neck cancer. Ann Oncol 9:505-509, 1998.
83. Sauer R, Wannenmacher M, Brizel D, et al: Randomized phase III trial of radiation (RT) ± Ethyol (amifostine) in patients with head and neck cancer. Int J Radiat Oncol Biol Phys 39:234, 1997.
84. Myckatyn TM, Brenner M, Mackinnon SE, et al: Effects of external beam radiation in the rat tibial nerve after crush, transection and repair, or nerve isograft paradigms. Laryngoscope 114:931-938, 2004.
85. Reddy PG, Arden RL, Mathog RH: Facial nerve rehabilitation after radical parotidectomy. Laryngoscope 109:894-899, 1999.
86. McGuirt WF, Welling DB, McCabe BF: Facial nerve function following irradiated cable grafts. Laryngoscope 99:27-34, 1989.
87. Brown PD, Eshleman JS, Foote RL, Strome SE: An analysis of facial nerve function in irradiated and unirradiated facial nerve grafts. Int J Radiat Oncol Biol Phys 48:737-743, 2000.
88. Jeremic B, Shibamto Y, Stanisavljevic B, et al: Radiation therapy alone or with concurrent low-dose daily either cisplatin or carboplatin in locally advanced unresectable squamous cell carcinoma of the head and neck: a prospective randomized trial. Radiother Oncol 43:29-37, 1997.
89. Brizel DM, Albers ME, Fisher SR, et al: Hyperfractionated irradiation with or without concurrent chemotherapy for locally advanced head and neck cancer. N Engl J Med 338:1798-1804, 1998.
90. Al-Sarraf M, LeBlanc M, Shanker Giri PG, et al: Chemo-radiotherapy versus radiotherapy in patients with advanced nasopharyngeal cancer: Phase III Randomized Intergroup Study 0099. J Clin Oncol 16:1310-1317, 1998.
91. Bernier J, Domenge C, Ozsahin M, et al: Postoperative irradiation with or without concomitant chemotherapy for locally advanced head and neck cancer. N Engl J Med 350:1945-1952, 2004.
92. Forastiere AA, Goepfert H, Maor M, et al: Concurrent chemotherapy and radiotherapy for organ preservation in advanced laryngeal cancer. N Engl J Med 349:2091-2098, 2003.
93. Lefebvre JL, Chevalier D, Luboinski B, et al: Larynx preservation in pyriform sinus cancer: preliminary results of a European Organization for Research and Treatment of Cancer Phase III trial. J Natl Cancer Inst 88:890-899, 1996.
94. Zakotnik B, Smid L, Budihna M, et al: Concomitant radiotherapy with mitomycin C and bleomycin compared with radiotherapy alone in inoperable head and neck cancer: final report. Int J Radiat Oncol Biol Phys 41:1121-1127, 1998.
95. Bonner JA, Harari PM, Giralt J, et al: Cetuximab prolongs survival in patients with locoregionally advanced squamous cell carcinoma of head and neck: a phase III study of high dose radiation therapy with or without cetuximab [abstract 5507]. Annu Proc Am Soc Clin Oncol 23:489s, 2004.

CHAPTER 35

THYROID CANCER

Ian D. Hay and Ivy A. Petersen

INCIDENCE

The incidence of thyroid cancer is 0.5 to 10 cases per 100,000 people in the general population. An estimated 30,180 cases occur annually in the United States.

Carcinomas are of follicular or parafollicular cell (C cell) origin, and 95% are well differentiated.

BIOLOGIC CHARACTERISTICS

Prognostic factors include patient age, histology, grade, tumor size, neoplastic extent, and completeness of initial surgical resection.

Reliable prognostic scoring systems permit accurate outcome prediction.

Only a small minority of thyroid carcinoma patients is at risk for cause-specific mortality.

STAGING EVALUATION

Staging includes the patient's history, physical examination of the neck, fine-needle aspiration, biopsy, ultrasound neck examination, and a chest radiograph.

Additional studies may include vocal cord examination, chest computed tomography, isotopic bone scanning, and ^{18}F-fluorodeoxyglucose positron emission tomography with computed tomography (fused PET/CT).

PRIMARY THERAPY

Surgical resection is the primary therapy for resectable, well-differentiated thyroid carcinomas. Most are treated by near-total or total thyroidectomy with excision of involved regional nodes. Cause-specific survival rates exceed 90% at 20 years.

ADJUVANT THERAPY

Thyroxine-suppressive therapy of thyroid-stimulating hormone is standard postoperative management of papillary and follicular cancers.

Radioactive iodine therapy is used for distant metastasis, unresectable or residual papillary thyroid carcinoma, and most cases of follicular thyroid carcinoma or Hürthle cell carcinoma.

External beam radiation is reserved for selected patients with locally advanced disease and with high-risk surgical pathologic features or those with recurrent or metastatic disease nonresponsive to radioactive iodine therapy.

UNDIFFERENTIATED TUMORS AND PALLIATIVE THERAPY

Anaplastic cancer is preferably treated by resection, external beam irradiation, and chemotherapy.

Thyroid lymphomas typically are diffuse, large cell lymphomas of B-cell origin. These tumors are best controlled with combination chemotherapy (cyclophosphamide, hydroxydaunomycin, Oncovin (vincristine), and prednisone) and local irradiation.

Thyroid tumors are the most common endocrine neoplasms. They usually manifest as anterior neck nodules, which in most cases can be localized to the thyroid gland by palpation. Most nodules are benign hyperplastic (or colloid) nodules, but 5% to 20% of nodules coming to medical attention are true neoplasms: benign follicular adenomas or carcinomas of follicular or parafollicular cell (C cell) origin. Differentiating true neoplasms from hyperplastic nodules and distinguishing benign from malignant tumors are major diagnostic challenges for clinical endocrinologists. High-resolution ultrasound studies assessing large groups of normal volunteers have suggested that the prevalence of incidentally discovered nodular thyroid disease in healthy adults is more than 60%.[1] In the United States during 2006, however, only 30,180 new cases of thyroid cancer were expected.[2] Given that the prevalence of clinical thyroid cancer in most populations is much less than 1%, most of the so-called thyroid incidentalomas must be benign.[3]

In the current era, when patients are increasingly being advised on the advantages of self-examination to detect cancer at an early stage, the finding of a palpable mass in such a superficial and visibly obvious location as the thyroid gland can be disconcerting. Accordingly, the patient is likely to seek prompt medical evaluation. Fortunately, at the conclusion of an appropriate investigation, the patient can usually be reassured that the nodule is benign. If the discovered lesion proves to be suspicious for malignancy, the patient can be advised that the management of typical thyroid cancer is effective[4] and usually consists of surgical resection,[5] followed by medical therapy[6] and regular postoperative surveillance.[7] In the 1990s, a degree of consensus was achieved with regard to the initial evaluation of nodular thyroid disease[8,9] and the management of differentiated thyroid cancer,[10,11] but important biologic and clinical questions remain unanswered.[12-14]

From a radiation oncologic standpoint, the follicular cell–derived cancer (FCDC) of the thyroid has some historic interest. In 1940, Hamilton and associates at the University of California, San Francisco, first reported evidence of uptake of radioactive iodine (RAI) in FCDC.[15] In 1942 at Columbia University, Keston and colleagues[16] gave a patient with an iodophilic femoral metastasis a 10-mCi therapeutic dose of RAI. Since that time, RAI therapy has become the primary treatment for iodophilic distant metastases in the papillary or follicular histologic type of FCDC.[17] The concept of radioiodine remnant ablation (RRA) to "complete" a thyroidectomy in FCDC, derived from pioneering work by Blahd and colleagues at the University of California, Los Angeles, in the late 1950s,[18] has been increasingly employed in the routine management of FCDC.[19] The use of external beam radiation therapy (EBRT) in managing thyroid cancer has its origin in the 1960s,[20] and since then, its role generally has been restricted to the treatment of advanced locoregional FCDC, but it has also been employed as primary therapy in the management of two rare malignancies: undifferentiated (anaplastic) thyroid carcinoma and primary malignant lymphoma of the thyroid.[21] In this chapter, we discuss the more common FCDC, but where indicated, the less common tumors derived from nonfollicular cell origin are considered.

ETIOLOGY AND EPIDEMIOLOGY

The annual incidence of thyroid cancer is between 0.5 and 10 per 100,000 people in the general population in most countries, and a global estimate suggested a total of 87,000 new cases worldwide each year.[22] Clinical thyroid malignancy is relatively uncommon, accounting for only about 2% of human malignancies.[2,23] Nonetheless, thyroid cancers in 2006 will account for 94% of endocrine malignancies in the United States.[2] It was estimated by the American Cancer Society that 1500 patients with thyroid cancer would die during 2006, accounting for 63% of deaths from endocrine malignancies.[2]

Most of these thyroid cancers are derived from follicular epithelium. In most countries, incidence rates for papillary thyroid carcinoma (PTC) generally exceed those for follicular thyroid carcinoma (FTC), and either is far more common than the usually lethal anaplastic (undifferentiated) thyroid carcinoma.[24,25] Very similar data on the frequency of the various histologic types are contained in three large series of more than 97,000 cases of thyroid cancer reported from the United States and Japan.[26-28] These data are summarized in Table 35-1.

Anaplastic carcinomas and FTCs tend to be relatively more common in endemic goiter areas, and a number of case-control studies have strongly suggested that dietary iodine content is responsible for the increased incidence rates in these areas.[29] This hypothesis is supported by the fact that dietary iodine supplementation has been shown to increase the relative proportion of PTC and to decrease the frequency of FTC.[30]

PTC and FTC are more than twice as common in women as men and tend to occur much more commonly in middle age and later, although patients with PTC are somewhat younger than those with FTC.[24,25] The female preponderance of patients with FCDC has led to speculation about the role of estrogens as a risk factor. Other putatively estrogen-dependent tumors, particularly breast cancer, and thyroid cancer occur more frequently in the same individual than expected by chance.[31] Case-control studies have suggested a correlation between pregnancy, a high estrogen state, and the onset of thyroid cancer.[32] Others have suggested that pregnancy per se, rather than the associated estrogen levels, may be associated with increased thyroid cancer risk.[33] On balance, the role of female sex hormones as a risk factor for thyroid cancer development must still be considered unresolved.

The most firmly established risk factor for thyroid cancer development is prior exposure to ionizing radiation, particularly to the head and neck region during childhood. This used to be a common problem in some exposed populations in Japan and the Pacific during the 1960s and 1970s in the aftermath of atomic bomb use at the end of World War II and in areas exposed to atmospheric nuclear bomb tests during the 1950s and 1960s.[34,35] In most other countries, radiation treatments for benign medical conditions, such as acne vulgaris, thymic enlargement, tinea capitis, or inflammatory connective tissue disorders, contributed to rising numbers of patients with thyroid cancer.[36,37] These practices have largely been abandoned, and radiation exposure as a risk factor has ceased to be of significant importance in most countries.[37] Exceptions are areas of high natural background radiation, patients who have undergone radiation therapy for malignant conditions,[38] and wherever radioactive contamination of the environment from military or civilian sources is a notable problem, particularly in a number of countries in the southern part of the former Soviet Union that were heavily contaminated in the wake of the Chernobyl nuclear reactor accident.[39] The contamination in parts of Belarus and Ukraine was significant and prolonged, and there is mounting clinical evidence that this has led to increased rates of thyroid malignancies, often of an unexpectedly aggressive nature.[40-42] In the United States, it has been disclosed that a significant segment of the U.S. population was exposed to radioiodine during a series of nuclear bomb explosions at the Nevada test site in the 1950s.[43] Predictions of excess relative risk of thyroid cancer vary but may prove to be significant. However, it is impossible to determine whether individual thyroid cancers arose as a result of radiation exposure or as sporadic events.[43]

Although most cases of thyroid cancer are sporadic occurrences, a small proportion of thyroid cancers may be familial, and in the case of C cell–derived malignancy, medullary thyroid carcinoma (MTC) may be associated with the multiple endocrine neoplasia (MEN) type 2 (MEN-2) syndrome and its associated adrenal medullary tumors (pheochromocytomas). In patients with the MEN-2a syndrome, a strong and typical family history can often be obtained. PTC may also be associated with other nonthyroid malignancies and with premalignant conditions such as Cowden's syndrome and familial adenomatous polyposis coli (i.e., Gardner's syndrome).[44] Several cases of familial PTC have been described.[45] No such distinct associations exist for FTC, but aggregation of FTC cases in families with dyshormonogenesis has been described.[46]

PREVENTION AND EARLY DETECTION

Most thyroid cancers are sporadic and not obviously caused by an avoidable environmental agent. Prevention of thyroid malignancy usually is therefore impossible.

Early detection of nodular thyroid disease is generally achieved by careful neck palpation in the course of routine physical examinations. High-resolution ultrasonography can

Table 35-1 Frequency of Various Histologic Types of Thyroid Cancers Diagnosed During 1973 to 1995

Study	Papillary *N* (%)	Follicular *N* (%)	Medullary *N* (%)	Anaplastic *N* (%)
SEER program of the NCI, 1973-1991[26]	11,857 (76%)	2,660 (17%)	516 (3%)	251 (2%)
Japanese Society of Thyroid Surgery, 1977-1995[27]	22,307 (80%)	3,320 (12%)	369 (1%)	489 (2%)
National Cancer Data Base, 1985-1995[28]	42,686 (79%)	8,349 (15%)	1,928 (4%)	893 (2%)

readily detect impalpable thyroid nodules less than 1 cm in diameter. However, there is no evidence that population screening for nodular thyroid disease using ultrasound imaging is warranted because 70% to 90% of diagnosed thyroid malignancies are of the papillary histologic type. In such incidentally discovered papillary tumors, 85% to 90% are deemed low risk and are associated with mortality rates close to those predicted by actuarial curves and comparable to those for nonmelanoma skin cancer.

In contrast, early detection of the often more aggressive, familial MTC is possible when there is evidence within the family of an inherited mutation of the *RET* proto-oncogene in the pericentromeric region of the short area of chromosome 10. Such mutations have been found in more than 90% of familial MTC cases, and since the successful cloning and sequencing of the *RET* gene, asymptomatic members of affected families can be tested for the presence of a mutation at this locus.[47] A positive test result obviates the need for any further testing. The present recommendation for persons shown to harbor the mutation is to undergo prophylactic total thyroidectomy, which completely prevents the development of the invariably multicentric MTC associated with these conditions.[48] If such a mutation is found in infancy, the current practice is to perform a total thyroidectomy when the child is between 5 and 7 years old.[49]

PATHOLOGY AND PATHWAYS OF SPREAD

Most thyroid cancers are well-differentiated tumors derived from follicular cells. PTC accounts for 40% to 90% of cases, whereas 15% to 40% are classified as FTC, which includes the so-called oxyphilic or Hürthle cell variant. Anaplastic thyroid cancer (ATC), also derived from the follicular cell, is the least common FCDC, typically constituting 1% to 5% of most series. The frequency of the C cell–derived MTC depends somewhat on the diligence with which reporting centers pursue the early diagnosis of patients with familial MTC and MEN-2, but it may account for 2% to 8% of thyroid cancers. Nonepithelial thyroid tumors include sarcomas, malignant hemangioendotheliomas, and malignant lymphomas. Lymphomas may involve the thyroid as the only manifestation of the disease or as part of a systemic disease; such tumors may rarely complicate Hashimoto's (autoimmune) chronic lymphocytic thyroiditis, which in the United States is the most common cause of goiter and noniatrogenic hypothyroidism. Bloodborne metastases to the thyroid are not uncommon at autopsy in patients with widespread malignancy, but they rarely cause clinically detectable thyroid enlargement.

PTC most often occurs in patients between 30 and 50 years old; the mean age at diagnosis is about 45 years. Most primary tumors are 1 to 4 cm in diameter; the average is about 2 to 3 cm in the greatest dimension. Ninety-five percent are classified on the basis of degree of differentiation as histologic grade 1 (of 4); 80% of primary PTC tumors are assessed to be DNA diploid by flow cytometry.[50] Extrathyroidal invasion of adjacent soft tissues is present in about 15% (range, 5% to 34%) at primary surgery, and about one third of PTC patients have clinically evident lymphadenopathy at presentation.[51] About 35% to 50% of excised neck nodes have histologic evidence of involvement, and in patients 17 years of age or younger, nodal involvement may be present in up to 90%.[52] The primary disease is confined to the neck in 93% to 99% of PTC patients at diagnosis.[50,51] Spread to superior mediastinal nodes is usually associated with extensive neck nodal involvement. Distant metastases are diagnosed in only 1% to 7% of patients with PTC before or within 30 days of primary treatment.[50,53]

FTC occurs in older patients, and the mean age in most studies is more than 50 years, about 10 years older than for typical PTC.[25,54] Women affected by FTC outnumber men by more than 2 to 1. FTC patients rarely (4% to 6%) have clinically evident lymphadenopathy at presentation.[55] In most series, the average tumor size in FTC is larger than in PTC.[54] When tumor grading is performed, higher-grade tumors are more common than with PTC.[54] DNA aneuploidy is present in about 60% of FTC tumors and in up to 90% of patients with oxyphilic or Hürthle cell variant tumors.[25,56] Direct extrathyroidal extension into adjacent soft tissues does not occur in the common "minimally invasive" FTC, but it is not unusual in the rare patient with "widely invasive" FTC. Between 5% and 20% of patients with FTC may have distant metastases at presentation, and the most common sites of distant spread are lung and bone.[25,57]

MTC arises from the C cells of the thyroid rather than the follicular epithelium; secretes a characteristic hormone, calcitonin; is frequently associated with one or more paraendocrine manifestations; and provides an early biochemical signal (i.e., hypersecretion of calcitonin) that permits its early detection, treatment, and cure.[58] The tumor occurs in sporadic and familial forms, with the latter making up about 20% of the total. The familial variety usually appears at a younger age, is almost invariably bilateral, is less likely to have associated cervical metastases at presentation, and has a better prognosis.[40] Most importantly, the familial variety is preceded by a premalignant C cell hyperplasia that can be cured by total thyroidectomy.[59]

ATC is the least common FCDC and typically constitutes less than 5% of most reported series.[60] It usually occurs after the age of 60 years, and it is only slightly more common in women than men (1.3 to 1.5 : 1). It is highly malignant, rapidly invading adjacent structures and metastasizing throughout the body. Pathologic examination of biopsied tumor may reveal evidence of PTC or FTC, which may represent a precursor of the ATC. Thorough sampling may be necessary to detect residual well-differentiated thyroid tissue. On histologic examination, the tumor is usually composed of atypical cells that exhibit numerous mitoses and form a variety of patterns. Spindle-shaped cells and multinucleated giant cells usually predominate, but in a third histologic pattern described as squamoid, the cells are undifferentiated but retain an epithelial appearance. Formerly, it was thought that there was a small cell ATC, but most of these tumors have been classified as malignant thyroid lymphomas.

BIOLOGIC CHARACTERISTICS, PROGNOSTIC FACTORS, AND STAGING

It has long been recognized that prognosis in thyroid cancer largely depends on the age of the patient, the histology of the tumor, and the anatomic extent of disease at presentation. Although head and neck cancer is staged entirely on the basis of anatomic extent, thyroid cancer staging is unique in that the histologic diagnosis and the age of the patient are included because of their prognostic importance.

The sixth edition of the TNM staging scheme for thyroid carcinoma, approved in 2002 by the International Union Against Cancer[61] and by the American Joint Committee on Cancer (AJCC),[62] is presented in Table 35-2. The primary tumor status is defined in this scheme on the basis of the size of the primary lesion (diameter in centimeters) and the presence of extrathyroidal extension. A T1 tumor is 2 cm or smaller and limited to the thyroid. A T2 tumor is between 2.1 and 4.0 cm in diameter and limited to the thyroid. A T3 tumor is larger than 4 cm and limited to the thyroid or any tumor with

Table 35-2 American Joint Committee on Cancer Stage Groupings for Thyroid Carcinoma

Stage*	PAPILLARY OR FOLLICULAR Age < 45 y	Age 45 or Older	MEDULLARY Any Age	ANAPLASTIC Any Age
I	M0	T1 N0 M0	T1 N0 M0	—
II	M1	T2 N0 M0	T2 N0 M0	—
III	—	T3 N0 M0	T3 N0 M0	—
		T1-3 N1a M0	T1-3 N1a M0	—
IVA	—	T4a N0-1a M0	T4a N0-1a M0	T4a Any N M0
		T1-4a N1b M0	T1-4a N1b M0	
IVB	—	T4b Any N M0	T4b Any N M0	T4b Any N M0
IVC	—	AnyT Any N M1	AnyT Any N M1	AnyT Any N M1

*T-stage definition: T1—greatest dimension 2 cm or less, limited to the thyroid; T2—more than 2 cm but not more than 4 cm, limited to the thyroid; T3—more than 4 cm, limited to thyroid or any tumor with minimal extra thyroid extension; T4a—Tumor of any size extending beyond the thyroid capsale to invade subcutaneous soft tissues, larynx, trachea, esophagus, or recurrent laryngeal nerve; T4b—Tumor invades prevertebral fascia or encases carotid artery or mediastinal vessels.

Data from Sobin LH, Wittekind CH, for the International Union Against Cancer: TNM Classification of Malignant Tumours, 6th ed. New York, Wiley-Liss, 2002; Shah JP, Kian K, Forastiere A, et al, for the American Joint Committee on Cancer: AJCC Cancer Staging Manual, 6th ed. New York, Springer-Verlag, 2002.

minimal extrathyroidal extension (i.e., to sternothyroid muscles or perithyroid soft tissues). A T4a tumor extends beyond the thyroid capsule and invades subcutaneous soft tissue, larynx, trachea, esophagus, or recurrent laryngeal nerve, whereas a T4b tumor invades prevertebral fascia or encases carotid artery or mediastinal vessels.

When tumor spreads to lymph nodes, it is classified as N1. N1a refers to metastasis in level VI (i.e., pretracheal and paratracheal lymph nodes, including prelaryngeal and delphian nodes), whereas N1b describes metastasis to other unilateral, bilateral, or contralateral cervical or superior mediastinal lymph nodes. M1 refers to presence of distant metastasis involving nonregional lymph nodes, internal organs, or bones. To make this TNM information clearer, several of these TNM descriptions can be grouped together into stages I through IV. For the sixth edition of the TNM/AJCC staging system, the grouping for MTC is the same as for PTC or FTC in patients older than 45 years, whereas all patients with ATC are considered as stage IV, reflecting the poor prognosis of this type of cancer.

For patients younger than 45 years with a diagnosis of PTC or FTC, the TNM stage is I (any T any N M0) if there is no distant spread and stage II (any T any N M1) if there are distant metastases beyond the neck or upper mediastinal lymph nodes. For patients with MTC or who are 45 years or older with PTC or FTC, the 6th edition of TNM staging system is somewhat more complicated than before.

In patients with PTC or FTC who are 45 years of age or older, stage I (T1 N0 M0) cancers are 2 cm or smaller and have not spread to lymph nodes or distant sites. Stage II (T2 N0 M0) cancers are more than 2 cm in diameter but not bigger than 4 cm, and they are localized to the thyroid. Stage III (T3 N0 M0 or T1-3 N1a M0) encompasses tumors larger than 4 cm or with minimal extrathyroidal extension and those of any size that have spread to central neck nodes.

In former TNM/AJCC classifications, stage IV referred only to patients who had distant spread, but the latest edition defines these patients as IVC (any T any N M1), and the designation of IVA and IVB define more aggressive tumors that have not spread to distant sites. The IVB stage (T4b any N M0) refers to the rather unusual situation of a tumor that has grown back to the spine (i.e., prevertebral fascia) or into nearby large blood vessels (i.e., carotid artery or mediastinal vessels). The new IVA stage (T1-4a N0-1b M0) was formerly considered to be stage III, and it encompasses locally invasive

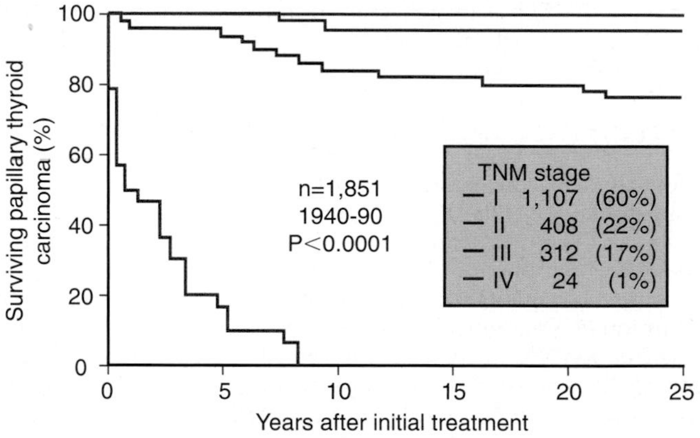

Figure 35-1 Cause-specific survival according to pathologic TNM stage for a cohort of 1851 patients with papillary thyroid carcinoma treated at the Mayo Clinic from 1940 to 1990. The numbers in parentheses are the percentages of patients in each pathologic TNM stage grouping. (From Larsen PR, Davies TF, Hay ID: The thyroid gland. *In* Wilson JD, Foster DW, Kronenberg HM, Larsen PR [eds]: Williams Textbook of Endocrinology, 9th ed. Philadelphia, WB Saunders, 1998, pp 389-515.)

T4a tumors (i.e., with or without nodal involvement [any N]) and node-positive N1b tumors (i.e., of any size but localized or showing only minimal extrathyroidal extension [T1-3]).

Because of significant differences in the tumor biology displayed by the four principal types of thyroid carcinomas, the remainder of this discussion of tumors is divided according to histologic type.

Papillary Carcinoma

Most PTC patients present with localized, node-negative disease.[28,50] Patients 45 years old or older with nodal metastases or extrathyroidal extension account for less than 20% of cases.[50] Only about 1% to 3% of older PTC patients present with distant metastases. Figure 35-1 demonstrates cause-specific survival according to pathologic TNM (pTNM) stage in a cohort of 1851 patients who underwent surgical treatment at Mayo Clinic during 1940 to 1990.[63]

Three types of tumor relapse may occur with PTC: postoperative regional nodal metastasis, local recurrences, and postoperative distant metastases. Local recurrence has been defined as "histologically confirmed tumor occurring in the resected thyroid bed, thyroid remnant, or other adjacent tissues of the neck (excluding lymph nodes)" after complete surgical removal of the primary tumor.[64] Nodal or distant spread is considered postoperative if the metastases are discovered within 180 days or 30 days, respectively. In a cohort of 1408 patients with PTC who did not have initial distant metastases and who underwent complete surgical resection of their primary tumors during treatment at Mayo Clinic from 1945 to 1985, relapse rates at nodal, local, and distant sites were 9%, 6%, and 5%, respectively, after 25 years of follow-up.[50] In a larger cohort of 1851 PTC patients treated from 1940 to 1990 at Mayo, the cause-specific survival rates at 5, 10, and 20 postoperative years were 98%, 96%, and 95%, respectively.[64] Of those with lethal PTC, 20% of deaths occurred within the first year after diagnosis, and 80% of the deaths occurred within 10 postoperative years.[50,65]

Only a fraction (≈15%) of PTC patients are liable for relapse of disease, and even fewer (≈5%) have a lethal outcome.[50,51] The exceptional patient who experiences an aggressive course tends to relapse early, and the rare fatalities usually occur within 5 to 10 years of initial diagnoses.[51,52,65] Multivariate analyses have been used to identify variables predictive of cause-specific mortality.[66-69] Increasing patient age and presence of extrathyroidal invasion are independent prognostic factors in all such studies.[66-69] The presence of initial distant metastases and large size of the primary tumor are also significant variables in most studies,[66,68] and some groups[26,28,50,66,67] have reported that histopathologic grade (i.e., degree of differentiation) is an independent variable. The completeness of initial tumor resection (i.e., postoperative status) is also a predictor of mortality.[50,69] The presence of initial neck nodal metastasis, although relevant to future nodal relapse, does not apparently influence cause-specific mortality.[50,51,69]

From a multivariate analysis of more than 14,200 patient-years of experience, a prognostic scoring system was devised, and named the AGES system after five independent variables: patient's *a*ge, tumor *g*rade, tumor *e*xtent (e.g., local invasion, distant metastasis), and tumor *s*ize.[50,66] With the use of such a scoring system, 86% of PTC patients were in the minimal-risk group (AGES score < 4), and they had a cause-specific mortality rate of only 1%.[50] In contrast, patients with AGES scores of 4+ (i.e., high-risk group is 14% of the total) had a 20-year cause-specific mortality rate of 40%. Based on the description of the Mayo Clinic–derived AGES system,[66] Cady and Rossi, working at the Lahey Clinic, devised a simplified version of the AGES system, which they called the AMES multifactorial system.[70] The AMES system disregarded tumor grade because this information was not readily available to them, but they took advantage of the other four variables, *a*ge, *m*etastasis, *e*xtent, and *s*ize. The details of Cady and Rossi's AMES system are shown in Table 35-3. Of Cady and Rossi's 1961 to 1980 cohort of patients, 89% were deemed low risk and had a death rate of 1.8%, outcome results virtually identical to those defined by the AGES prognostic scores.[50,66]

Although the AGES scheme had the potential for universal application, some academic centers could not include the differentiation variable (tumor grade [G]) because their surgical pathologists did not recognize higher-grade PTC tumors.[71] Accordingly, another prognostic scoring system for predicting PTC mortality rates was devised with the use of candidate variables that included completeness of primary tumor resection but excluded histologic grade.[69] Cox model analysis and stepwise variable selection led to a final prognostic model that included five variables: *m*etastasis, *a*ge, *c*ompleteness of resection, *i*nvasion, and *s*ize (MACIS). The final score was defined as MACIS = 3.1 (if age is 39 years or less) or 0.08 × age (if age is 40 years or more), +0.3 × tumor size (in centimeters), +1 (if tumor not completely resected), +1 (if locally invasive), +3 (if distant metastases are present). As illustrated by Figure 35-2, the MACIS scoring system permitted identification of patient groups with a broad range of risk of death from PTC. Twenty-year cause-specific survival rates for patients with MACIS scores of less than 6, 6 to 6.99, 7 to 7.99, and 8+ were 99%, 84%, 56%, and 24%, respectively. When cumulative mortality from all causes of death was considered, approximately 85% of PTC patients (who had AGES scores < 4 or MACIS scores < 6) experienced no excess mortality over rates predicted for control subjects.[50,66,69]

Table 35-3 Classification of Risk Group Categories According to the AMES System

Low risk
1. Younger patients (males < 41 y; females < 51 y), no distant metastasis
2. Older patients with (a) minor tumor capsule involvement *and* (b) primary cancers < 5 cm in diameter *and* (c) no distant metastasis

High risk
1. All patients with distant metastasis
2. All older patients with (a) major tumor capsule involvement *or* (b) primary cancers 5 cm or greater in diameter

Data from Cady B, Rossi R: An expanded view of risk-group definition in differentiated thyroid carcinoma. Surgery 104:947-953, 1988.

Follicular Carcinoma

When more than 75% of cells in an FTC exhibit Hürthle cell or oncocytic features, the tumor is classified as a Hürthle cell carcinoma (HCC), oncocytic carcinoma, or oxyphilic variant FTC.[25] Most patients with FTC or HCC present with tumors 2 cm or larger and confined to the neck. Patients 45 years or older with nodal metastases or extrathyroidal extension account for only about 4% to 7% of FTCs and 8% to 10% of HCCs.[28,63] Unlike PTC patients, among whom only 1% to 3% present with distant metastases, about 4% to 6% of HCC and

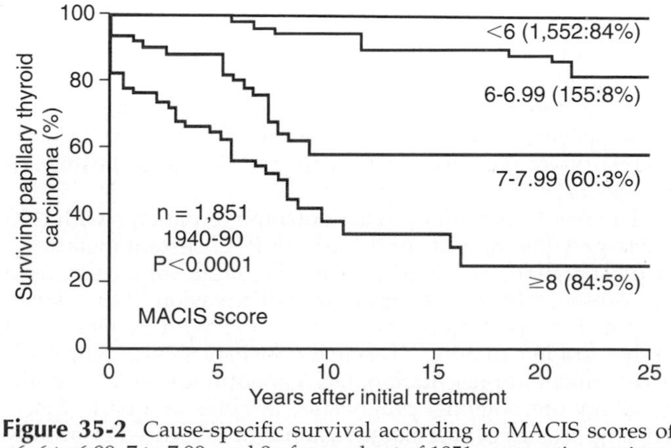

Figure 35-2 Cause-specific survival according to MACIS scores of <6, 6 to 6.99, 7 to 7.99, and 8+ for a cohort of 1851 consecutive patients with papillary thyroid carcinoma (PTC) undergoing initial treatment at the Mayo Clinic from 1940 to 1990. The numbers in parentheses are the numbers and percentages of patients with PTC in each of the four risk groups. (From Larsen PR, Davies TF, Hay ID: The thyroid gland. *In* Wilson JD, Foster DW, Kronenberg HM, Larsen PR [eds]: Williams Textbook of Endocrinology, 9th ed. Philadelphia, WB Saunders, 1998, pp 389-515.)

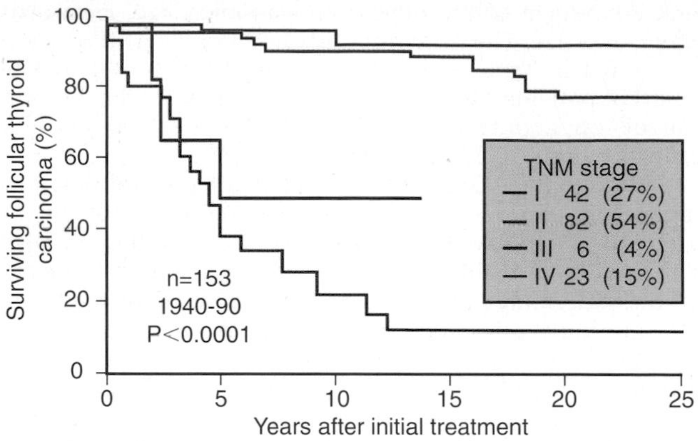

Figure 35-3 Cause-specific survival according to pathologic TNM stages for a cohort of 153 patients with nonoxyphilic follicular thyroid carcinoma treated at the Mayo Clinic from 1940 to 1990. The numbers in parentheses are the percentages of patients in each pathologic TNM stage grouping. (From Larsen PR, Davies TF, Hay ID: The thyroid gland. *In* Wilson JD, Foster DW, Kronenberg HM, Larsen PR [eds]: Williams Textbook of Endocrinology, 9th ed. Philadelphia, WB Saunders, 1998, pp 389-515.)

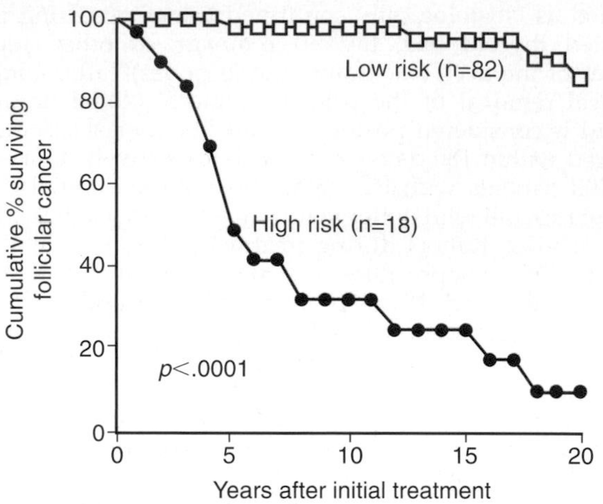

Figure 35-4 Cause-specific survival among 100 patients with nonoxyphilic follicular thyroid carcinoma treated at the Mayo Clinic from 1946 to 1970 and plotted by high-risk and low-risk categories. High risk is characterized by two or more of the following factors: age older than 50 years, marked vascular invasion, and metastatic disease at the time of initial diagnosis. (From Brennan MD, Bergstralh EJ, van Heerden JA, et al: Follicular thyroid cancer treated at Mayo Clinic, 1946 through 1970: initial manifestations, pathologic findings, therapy, and outcome. Mayo Clin Proc 66:11-19, 1991.)

7% to 15% of nonoxyphilic FTC patients have distant metastases at the time of initial diagnosis.[25,28,63] Figure 35-3 demonstrates cause-specific survival according to pTNM stage in a cohort of 153 patients with nonoxyphilic FTC surgically treated at Mayo Clinic from 1940 to 1990.[63]

Nodal metastases are rare in typical FTC, and nodal relapse rates at 10 and 20 postoperative years are 1% and 2%, respectively. About 6% of patients with HCC have nodal involvement at presentation,[55] but at 20 and 30 years after primary surgery, 18% and 24% of these patients have nodal relapse.[25] When relapse at neck or distant sites is considered, patients with HCC have the highest rates of tumor relapse after 10 or 20 years. Local recurrences account for most of these postoperative events, because the numbers of distant metastases in patients with HCC are comparable with those found in nonoxyphilic FTC (i.e., about 20% after 20 postoperative years).[25]

Cause-specific mortality rates vary with the presenting TNM stage for patients with FTC or HCC. The death rates tend to parallel the curves for development of distant metastases. In 5 decades of Mayo Clinic experience, the mortality rate for FTC initially exceeded that of HCC, but by 20 and 30 postoperative years, there were no significant differences in cause-specific survival rates between FTC and HCC,[25] with both survival rates about 80% at 20 and 70% at 30 postoperative years.

The risk factors that predict outcome of patients with FTC are largely the same as for those with PTC: distant metastases at presentation, increased patient age, large tumor size, and the presence of local (extrathyroidal) invasion.[25] To a lesser degree, increased mortality is associated with male sex and higher-grade tumors. Vascular invasiveness, lymphatic involvement at presentation, DNA aneuploidy, and oxyphilic histology are potential prognostic variables unique to FTC.[25] The importance of vascular invasion is underscored by a study showing that FTC patients with minimal capsular invasion and no evidence of vascular invasion had 0% cause-specific mortality after 10 years of postoperative follow-up.[72]

Prognostic scoring systems for FTC allow stratification of patients into high- and low-risk categories.[25,73] A multivariate analysis at the Mayo Clinic found that distant metastases, patient age greater than 50 years, and marked vascular invasion predicted a poor outcome.[54] As illustrated by Figure 35-4, if two or more of these factors are present, the 5-year survival rate is only 47%, and the 20-year survival rate is 8%. If only one of these factors is present, the 5-year survival rate is 94%, and the 20-year survival rate is 86%.[54]

Systems developed to predict outcomes for PTC or FTC have been applied to patients with FTC. Specifically, Cady and Rossi's AMES risk-group categorization has proved useful in FTC.[28,70] From a multivariate analysis of 228 patients with FTC treated at Sloan-Kettering, the independent adverse prognostic factors were identified as age older than 45 years, Hürthle cell histologic type, extrathyroidal extension, tumor size exceeding 4 cm, and the presence of distant metastasis.[74] The prognostic importance in FTC of histologic grade has also been confirmed[74,75] by the Sloan-Kettering group, who have included this factor in their assignment of risk groups to low-, intermediate-, and high-risk categories, with 20-year survival rates of 97%, 87%, and 49%, respectively.[74] The AGES and MACIS prognostic scoring systems, originally developed for PTC, have also been successfully applied to FTC.[76,77] It therefore appears that scoring systems used in PTC can be cautiously applied in FTC as long as some of the unique features of this tumor, such as vascular invasiveness and the remarkable significance of DNA aneuploidy in HCC, are considered.[25]

Medullary Carcinoma

In reported studies of treated MTC, the proportion of patients with intrathyroidal node-negative tumors of 2 cm in diameter or smaller (TNM stage I) varies, depending on the number of familial cases detected by biochemical testing or DNA screening. The number of patients who present with TNM stage I MTC varies from 5% to 25%, with the lower numbers representing the older series. Between 25% and 50% present with positive neck nodes; the proportion of patients presenting with distant metastases usually exceeds the proportion with PTC but is typically less than with FTC. Stage IV cases constitute 3% to 10% of most MTC series. Figure 35-5 illustrates cause-specific survival according to pTNM stage in a cohort

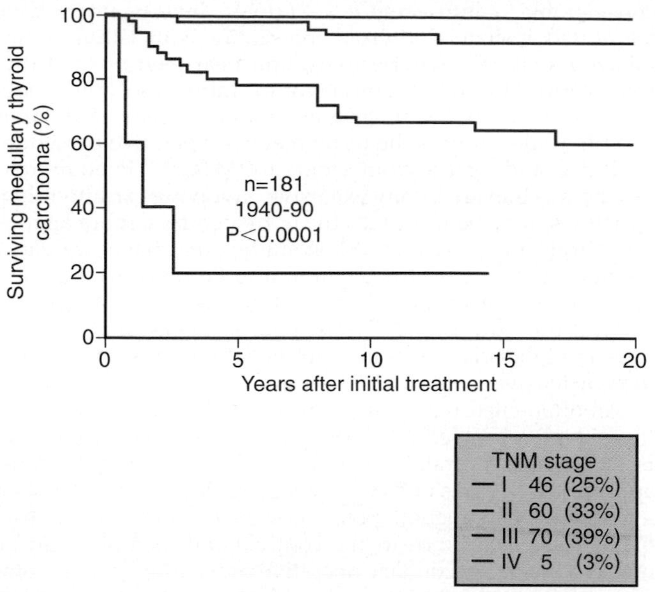

Figure 35-5 Cause-specific survival according to pathologic TNM stage for a cohort of 181 patients with medullary thyroid carcinoma treated at the Mayo Clinic from 1940 to 1990. The numbers in parentheses are the percentages of patients in each pathologic TNM stage grouping. (From Larsen PR, Davies TF, Hay ID: The thyroid gland. *In* Wilson JD, Foster DW, Kronenberg HM, Larsen PR [eds]: Williams Textbook of Endocrinology, 9th ed. Philadelphia, WB Saunders, 1998, pp 389-515.)

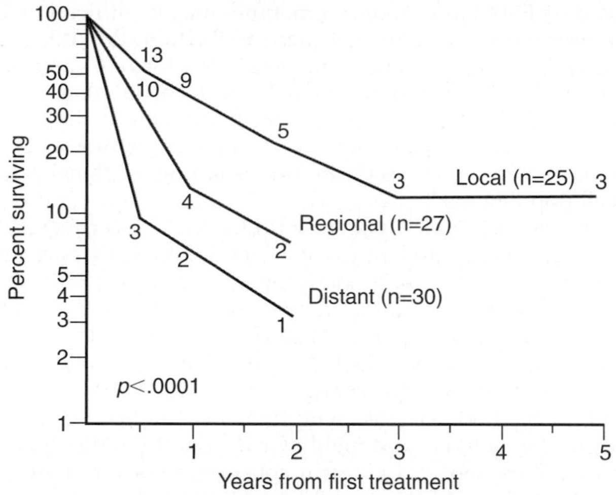

Figure 35-6 Survival to death from anaplastic thyroid cancer is plotted by extent of disease at presentation. Notice the logarithmic scale of the ordinate. (From Nel CJ, van Heerden JA, Goellner JR, et al: Anaplastic carcinoma of the thyroid: a clinicopathological study of 82 cases. Mayo Clin Proc 60:51-58, 1985.)

of 181 patients with MTC surgically treated at Mayo Clinic from 1940 to 1990.[63]

Other prognostic factors relevant to outcome in MTC include age at diagnosis, male gender, vascular invasion, calcitonin immunoreactivity, amyloid staining, presence or absence of postoperative gross residual disease, and abnormal postoperative plasma calcitonin levels.[78-80] In a multivariate analysis from Toronto, only the presence of extrathyroidal invasion and postoperative gross residual disease were significant in the prediction of cause-specific survival.[80] In another multivariate study from Mayo Clinic, however, the only factors remaining in the final Cox model were pTNM stages III or IV disease, negative Congo red staining for amyloid, and postoperative gross residual disease.[79] Based on these three independent prognostic variables, a scoring system was devised to define four risk groups with 10-year mortality rates varying from 5% to 100%.[79]

Anaplastic Carcinoma

Patients with ATC have a very poor prognosis, and survival beyond 1 year is very uncommon. There is no real use for an elaborate staging system for these patients, although distant and lymphatic spread at presentation, advanced age, and extremely poor differentiation have been identified as factors that make an already grim picture worse.[60,81] Figure 35-6 shows survival curves for 82 patients with ATC, stratified by extent of disease at presentation.[60]

CLINICAL MANIFESTATIONS AND PATIENT EVALUATION

At initial assessment, most patients with thyroid cancer have a palpable neck mass, which may represent the primary intrathyroidal tumor or metastatic regional lymphadenopathy. In some patients, however, the tumor may be clinically occult, and the impalpable lesion may first be recognized on high-resolution neck imaging[3] or during the course of a neck exploration for presumed benign thyroid disease. In patients with a family history of MTC or MEN-2 syndrome, the finding of a *RET* oncogene mutation (identical to the proband) or abnormal calcitonin (or stimulated calcitonin) levels, or both, may necessitate elective prophylactic thyroidectomy in a patient who may prove to have early MTC visible only under the surgical pathologist's microscope.[48,49]

Rarely do features of the history and physical examination provide convincing evidence for a diagnosis of thyroid malignancy.[82] The diagnosis of thyroid cancer necessitates pathologic confirmation from cytologic or histologic material. It is generally recognized that fine-needle aspiration (FNA) biopsy is the most effective method available of preoperatively distinguishing between benign and malignant thyroid nodules.[8,9] All cancer diagnoses, however, should be verified by careful examination of histologic material after surgical excision of affected tissues.[82] This approach is particularly relevant to the problem of the cellular follicular lesions described by cytologists as "suspicious" for follicular or Hürthle cell neoplasm. The diagnosis of FTC or HCC depends on the demonstration of invasion of the thyroid capsule or the adjacent blood vessels (i.e., angioinvasion), a process that typically necessitates careful evaluation of serial sections from the excised specimen for the presence or absence of such microinvasion. Even if FTC or HCC is apparently excluded at intraoperative frozen section, the resected specimen must be carefully reviewed in multiple sections from paraffin-embedded material.[25]

FNA biopsy can usually allow a confident diagnosis of PTC, which typically represents more than 75% of clinically recognized thyroid cancers in most contemporary series.[50] Some authorities claim that the characteristic nuclear abnormalities diagnostic for PTC may be best seen in cytologic preparations from an FNA biopsy specimen, rather than in frozen sections or in paraffin-embedded histologic material. MTC may be readily diagnosed by FNA biopsy, but in equivocal cases, amyloid stained by Congo red or immunoperoxidase labeling of intracytoplasmic calcitonin may allow a definitive preoperative diagnosis.[58] ATC may often be diagnosed by FNA biopsy, but it sometimes may be difficult to distinguish from carcinoma metastatic to the thyroid.[60] When the biopsy specimen is found to be suspicious for ATC, immunostaining for thyroglobulin can help confirm the diagnosis of ATC. An FNA diagnosis of thyroid lymphoma is difficult to make, and verification may necessitate examination of open biopsy material and specific immunostaining for clonal B- and T-cell populations.[82]

The evaluation of a patient with thyroid cancer requires a thorough history and physical examination with particular attention to signs and symptoms associated with local (extrathyroidal) invasion, involvement of regional (neck) nodes, and distant spread. Historical features suggesting a possible thyroid cancer include growth of a thyroid nodule over weeks or months; changes in speaking, breathing, or swallowing; and systemic symptoms of malignancy, such as weight loss, fatigue, and night sweats. On thyroid palpation, typical signs may include firm consistency of the dominant nodule, irregular shape, and fixation to underlying or overlying tissues. Evidence of suspicious regional lymphadenopathy may be present in up to one third of patients with PTC and MTC, but it is absent in most patients with FTC.

Patients with thyroid cancer are typically euthyroid, and when measured, the serum-sensitive thyroid-stimulating hormone (TSH) level is usually within normal limits. FNA biopsy can provide a confident diagnosis of PTC, MTC, and usually ATC. Diagnosing follicular cancer preoperatively remains a problem, because capsule or vascular invasion cannot be demonstrated in cytologic material. When FCDC is suspected and the decision is made for surgical exploration, it is often advisable to draw blood for a baseline serum thyroglobulin. This thyroid-specific protein can be used as a tumor marker to assess the efficacy of future therapies. Similarly, for patients with MTC, baseline measurements of calcitonin and carcinoembryonic antigen may permit a more accurate subsequent assessment of tumor control.

A preoperative vocal cord examination may permit the demonstration of unilateral vocal cord paralysis, which may raise suspicion about pressure or invasion of the ipsilateral recurrent laryngeal nerve. Particularly with PTC, MTC, and HCC, in which initial nodal involvement is common, a high-resolution, real-time ultrasound examination of the neck can provide a surgeon with valuable information regarding the extent of disease within the thyroid gland and in adjacent regional lymph nodes. With extensive nodal disease or suspected locally invasive thyroid cancer, examination of the lower central neck with computed tomography (CT) may delineate the presence of an intraluminal tumor or demonstrate more subtle evidence of tracheal or esophageal involvement with invasive disease. A high-resolution spiral CT scan of the chest or a whole-skeleton isotopic bone scan is not routinely performed before initial neck exploration, but it can be useful postoperatively to exclude metastases in mediastinum, lung, or bone, especially in patients without gross residual disease but with persistently elevated tumor markers.

Scanning with RAI has little role to play in the preoperative evaluation of thyroid malignancy. However, a postoperative whole-body scan has become the gold standard for identification of iodophilic distant metastasis in patients with PTC or FTC.[82]

PRIMARY THERAPY

Surgery

Surgery is the standard primary treatment for differentiated thyroid cancers, but the extent of initial surgery is an area of considerable controversy.[82-84] Various investigators have advocated ipsilateral thyroid lobectomy with isthmectomy, bilateral subtotal thyroidectomy, and near-total or total thyroidectomy. Most institutions favor the initial resection of both lobes of the thyroid. Clinical guidelines promote near-total or total thyroidectomy as the recommended operative procedure for FCDC and total thyroidectomy for MTC.[82-84] Even thyroid carcinomas that are locally extensive, involving extrathyroidal structures, may be most effectively treated by a more aggressive surgical approach.[85,86] Most studies that have evaluated the impact of surgical treatment in thyroid cancers have compared total or near-total thyroidectomy with less aggressive surgical procedures.[64,66,87] These reports suggest that survival rates in higher-risk cases are significantly improved after the more extensive surgery.[64,88-90]

An often-cited reason for removing all or nearly all of the thyroid gland is reducing the risk of future recurrence of FCDC in the contralateral thyroid lobe. This may be most appropriate in cases of PTC, in which multicentricity is not an infrequent phenomenon. Some, however, claim that a subsequent local recurrence in the contralateral lobe also can be managed with a secondary operative procedure.[91] Such "completion" thyroidectomies carry a higher morbidity, except in the hands of highly skilled surgeons.[64,92] One advantage of initial resection of the entire gland is the subsequent ability to follow serum thyroglobulin levels and to more easily perform meaningful radioiodine scanning.[7] Whole-body scans may be difficult to interpret in the setting of residual thyroid remnant, as would be found after unilateral or bilateral subtotal resection.

In addition to the initial resection of the thyroid, the question of the extent of neck node removal remains controversial. When clinically evident nodal metastases are identified by palpation or ultrasound examination, surgical removal is performed. The role of prophylactic or prognostic lymph node dissections is unclear.[55] For patients undergoing total or near-total thyroidectomy, removal of the central compartment lymph nodes does not add significantly to the morbidity of the procedure and should be included routinely with the primary resection. Modified radical neck dissection is indicated for gross nodal metastases found before or during surgery, and it may improve the outcome of older PTC patients with larger tumors or evidence of extrathyroidal invasion.[93,94] The advantage of total thyroidectomy over a near-total thyroidectomy may be nonexistent or limited to patients with more advanced malignancies.[64,66,95] The use of more limited surgery, such as unilateral total lobectomy, is probably only appropriate for a selected population of low-risk patients, such as those with papillary microcarcinoma.[82,84,96]

Adjuvant Therapy

Thyroid Hormone

Postoperative thyroid suppression therapy for FCDC is based on administration of supraphysiologic oral doses of levothyroxine. This mode of therapy has been widely used for more than 40 years, and it is assumed that suppression of endogenous TSH deprives TSH-dependent differentiated FCDC cells of an important growth-promoting influence. Traditionally, the goal of thyroxine therapy has been complete suppression of pituitary TSH secretion, as indicated by undetectable levels of serum TSH when measured in sensitive immunometric assays. Uncertainty surrounds the level to which the serum TSH level must be suppressed to maximize benefit while avoiding potential long-term complications.[97] A retrospective study[98] reported that a more stringent degree of TSH suppression (0.05 to 0.1 mU/L) was associated with a decreased incidence of tumor relapse. In a study of 1019 patients with FCDC, thyroid hormone therapy was associated with a "small, but apparently real" improvement in survival: 98.6% versus 85% adjusted 20-year survival rate.[99]

With the increasing availability of sensitive TSH assays, meticulous titration of the level of TSH suppression has become possible. If patients with FCDC are deemed, on the basis of scoring or staging systems,[62,69,70] to be at high risk for relapse or mortality, or if they have persistent or recurrent carcinoma that cannot be eradicated by surgical, RAI, or other therapeutic measures, the goal would be to maintain the TSH level below 0.1 mU/L or possibly closer to 0.01 mU/L with thyroxine suppression. In most patients with PTC who would be classified as low risk by prognostic scoring systems,[66,69,70,75] it is generally accepted that the degree of TSH suppression would be less stringent, and the goal for basal serum TSH should be in the readily detectable, barely subnormal range of 0.1 to 0.4 mU/L.[63,82,95]

Radioactive Iodine Therapy

Similar to the use of thyroid hormone for TSH suppression, the concept of adjuvant RAI therapy originated from treatment approaches to metastatic thyroid carcinoma and was also based on an equally compelling physiologic premise. Because most FCDC cells retain some architectural and functional features of normal thyrocytes, iodine trapping and sometimes organification may be preserved in the tumors. It therefore seemed appropriate to take advantage of this by trying to eradicate microscopic residual postoperative tumor foci with RAI.

RRA has been defined as "the destruction of residual macroscopically normal thyroid tissue after surgical thyroidectomy."[95] Typically, RRA is used to complete the initial therapy in a patient whose FCDC has been completely resected (i.e., no gross residual disease is reported at the conclusion of the primary neck exploration). RRA is a procedure that is offered to patients with FCDC who have undergone "potentially curative" surgical treatment, and it should not be confused with RAI therapy, in which larger doses of ^{131}I are used in an attempt to destroy persistent neck disease or distant metastatic lesions.[82,95]

Proponents of RAI describe at least three advantages for this adjunctive therapy. First, by being actively trapped by normal thyroid cells, RAI is believed to destroy occult microscopic carcinoma cells within the thyroid remnant. Second, the later detection of persistent or recurrent disease, particularly in the neck by RAI scanning, is facilitated by the destruction of remaining normal tissue. Third, the performance of RRA is thought to increase the value of serum thyroglobulin measurement during follow-up. This last benefit has convinced many physicians to even consider RRA in patients with FCDC who are, by prognostic scoring or staging, deemed to be at low risk for tumor relapse or cause-specific mortality.[19,97] Others, however, have not advocated RRA in these low-risk patients because of a lack of evidence of improved outcome.[94,95,97,98]

Investigators have reported benefit and a lack of benefit from the use of RAI.[50,88-90,94-96,97,99] It is not clear from these reports whether outcome is necessarily improved with the routine use of RAI in the initial therapy of all patients with differentiated thyroid carcinoma, largely because of difficulties obtaining a comparable control group and the potential for selection biases, which may account for the outcomes reported. Sawka and colleagues systematically reviewed 1543 English references to determine whether RRA decreases the risk of thyroid cancer-related death or relapse after bilateral thyroidectomy for PTC or FTC. In 18 cohort studies not adjusted for prognostic factors or interventions, the benefit of RRA in decreasing the thyroid cancer–related mortality and any relapse by 10 years was inconsistent among centers. However, pooled analyses suggested a statistically significant treatment effect of RRA in terms of 10-year outcomes for locoregional recurrence (relative risk of 0.31) and distant metastases (absolute decrease in risk 3%). The conclusion of their meta-analysis was that RRA might be beneficial in decreasing relapse of well-differentiated thyroid cancer; however, they said that "the incremental benefit of remnant ablation in low-risk patients treated with bilateral thyroidectomy and thyroid hormone suppressive therapy is unclear."

Use of prognostic scoring schemes may help to define a population at significant risk for relapse and who are therefore more appropriate for consideration of remnant ablation. For example, at Mayo Clinic, patients with PTC who have MACIS scores above 6.0 or are found to have persistent elevation of serum thyroglobulin levels after 6 to 8 postoperative weeks are considered for an ablative procedure. Use of such a scheme is applicable only if the patient undergoes a near-total or total thyroidectomy. If the goal is to minimize the use of RAI, more extensive surgery such as near-total or total thyroidectomy is more appropriate in the low-risk population. However, if RAI is planned, more extensive surgery may not give any advantage. In the high-risk population, the use of RAI in addition to more aggressive surgery appears warranted.[94,98,100]

After determining the need for remnant ablation, the question of dose after the primary surgical procedure is also an important consideration. In the United States, low-dose regimens of less than 30 mCi have been used when the amount of residual thyroid tissue is small. Higher doses of 75 to 150 mCi may be appropriate when microscopic residual is present or when the initial scan suggests an unsuspected metastatic site. Use of low-dose RAI in such a patient may decrease the ability of the tumor to subsequently concentrate sufficient radioiodine and therefore should be avoided.

Further treatment with RAI ideally should reflect the local or distant uptake of iodine in residual differentiated thyroid cancer tissue. Adequate ability of the thyroid cancer cells to concentrate the radioiodine is variable, and this approach may not be appropriate in all patients. Patients with FTC may concentrate RAI better than those with PTC.[99] In a multicenter Canadian study, Simpson and associates reviewed the outcomes of more than 1500 patients with PTC or FTC[99] and studied 321 patients who were treated with RAI. The use of RAI resulted in significantly improved local control in patients with microscopic residual disease. Cause-specific survival was also significantly better for PTC patients with microscopic residual disease who received RAI. Most of the patients received only thyroid remnant ablation doses (range 50 to 125 mCi), but total (cumulative) therapeutic doses given in one to seven treatments ranged from 75 to as high as 1000 mCi.

The definitive role of RAI therapy continues to evolve.[100] Multiple studies have suggested that it be used routinely in high-risk patients. Although the definition of high risk varies, most investigators favor using RAI in patients with large tumors or extensive extrathyroidal invasion, as well as in patients with incompletely resected disease or distant metastases. Robbins and Schlumberger[100] are recommending RRA for "any individual with a carcinoma larger than 1.5 cm or with a thyroid carcinoma of any size with obvious lymph node involvement, extrathyroidal extension, or multicentricity." The clinical guidelines proposed by the American Association of Clinical Endocrinologists (AACE), the American Thyroid

Association (ATA), and the National Cancer Centers Network (NCCN) should allow some greater uniformity of treatment approach.[10,82,83]

External Beam Radiation Therapy

The appropriate application of EBRT in PTC and FTC is controversial and therefore not uniformly used.[101,102] A better understanding of prognostic factors that are specific to local recurrence may help identify an appropriate population of patients who would be candidates for EBRT. Unfortunately, most prognostic schemes consider only the overall risk of relapse and cause-specific survival. Historically, indications for irradiation have included residual macroscopic or microscopic disease, extrathyroidal extension, multiple lymph node involvement, Hürthle cell histology, older age of patients, large tumor size, and residual disease that does not take up radioiodine. Several investigators have retrospectively reviewed their experience with EBRT and suggested improved local control or survival benefit, or both.[99,103-105] Unfortunately, the patient populations in these studies are not uniform with respect to other treatments that also effect local control, making interpretation difficult.

Most series support the use of adjuvant irradiation for patients with microscopic residual disease or narrow surgical margins of resection. An early Canadian study of follicular and papillary carcinomas evaluated the role of EBRT according to completeness of surgical resection.[103] Table 35-4 is a synopsis of these findings. Although the overall numbers are small, they suggest that patients with surgically narrow or microscopically positive margins may benefit from the addition of EBRT in moderate doses. These results were achieved with minimal morbidity. A larger synopsis of 13 Canadian institutions where EBRT was used predominantly in patients with high-risk features, such as extrathyroidal invasion, high-grade malignancies, and older age, revealed a significant improvement in local control for patients who had microscopically positive or narrow surgical margins.[101] In this study, the overall survival of PTC patients with presumed or microscopic residual was significantly improved with the addition of adjuvant EBRT. These improvements were seen with or without the use of RAI. Results from Germany for patients with pathologic T4 disease (based on the older staging system) with or without lymph node involvement also suggest a benefit from EBRT with respect to local control and distant failure rates, especially in patients older than 40 years.[105] In a review from Princess Margaret Hospital in Toronto of 207 patients with microscopic residual, the addition of EBRT did not significantly improve the cause-specific survival nor the local control ($P = .38$ and $P = .14$, respectively).[106]

Table 35-4 Local Recurrence of PTC and FTC at Princess Margaret Hospital by Method of Treatment

Extent of Disease	Surgery Alone *N*	%	EBRT *N*	%	RAI *N*	%
No residual disease	11/24	46	1/11	9	1/5	20
Probable residual	5/9	56	1/22	5	1/10	10
Microscopic residual	1/1	—	0/16	0	1/4	25

EBRT, external beam radiation therapy; FTC, follicular thyroid carcinoma; PTC, papillary thyroid carcinoma; RAI, radioactive iodine.

Data from Simpson WJ, Carruthers JS: The role of external irradiation in the management of papillary and follicular thyroid cancer. Am J Surg 1365:457-463, 1978.

Benker and associates described 932 patients with differentiated thyroid malignancies and found no overall survival benefit with the addition of external beam irradiation.[107] On subset analysis, however, patients older than 40 years with T3 or T4 disease experienced an improved survival that approached statistical significance ($P = .09$). All patients in this series received thyroxine-suppressive therapy and RAI.

The role of EBRT in the setting of gross residual disease has been evaluated by multiple investigators, with a wide range of outcomes. A study from the Royal Marsden Hospital showed complete response in 37% of patients and partial response in an additional 25%.[108] The Princess Margaret Hospital study had 33 patients with macroscopic disease treated with EBRT with or without RAI; the 5-year local recurrence-free rate was 62%.[106] Tubiana from Institut Gustav-Roussy evaluated 97 patients with macroscopic residual based on the surgeon's clinical assessment.[104] Local recurrence after EBRT was only 15%, compared with 32% in a similar surgical category without postoperative irradiation. None of these patients received RAI. With the ability to deliver higher doses of EBRT using techniques such as intensity-modulated radiation therapy (IMRT), it may be feasible to give higher doses than were used in these studies and perhaps increase the long-term control of disease in this difficult patient population.

Although the definitive role of EBRT for differentiated thyroid carcinoma remains controversial, retrospective data support its use in a selected population of patients who have microscopic or presumed microscopic residual cancer. The only randomized trial evaluating the role of EBRT was initiated in 2000 in patients with pathologic T4 N0-1 M0 disease after surgical resection and ablative ^{131}I.[109] The study closed due to inadequate accrual in March 2003 despite acceptable toxicity.[110] The study authors indicated that at early follow-up, there are lower than expected recurrence rates in the non-treatment arm. The improvements in surgical management of these patients and the appropriate application of radioiodine therapy may have accounted for the decreased recurrence and mortality rates compared with historical studies.

The use of EBRT for patients with differentiated thyroid cancer needs to be carefully tailored to the specific patient and applied after use of RAI. Changes in the staging of locally advanced thyroid cancers in 2002 by categorizing minimal extrathyroidal extension as T3 disease and creating two T4 categories should help further delineate the highest-risk population. In the clinical setting of T4b disease, it is unlikely that complete surgical resection can be achieved, and use of adjuvant EBRT in addition to RAI appears to help control gross disease. Improved surgical techniques and aggressive use of RAI in the other high-risk populations, as delineated by the aforementioned prognostic scoring systems, are diminishing the need for adjuvant EBRT. However, for patients with locally recurrent disease, care must be taken to consider early use of EBRT as a component of treatment.

Chemotherapy

The role of chemotherapy in the treatment of differentiated thyroid carcinoma is limited. Most agents have low response rates. The most active single agent reported in the treatment of thyroid cancers is doxorubicin. Other active agents that have been reported include cisplatin, carboplatin, and etoposide (VP-16).

The Eastern Cooperative Oncology Group (ECOG) reported the only randomized study of the use of chemotherapy in advanced thyroid cancer.[111] Patients with locally advanced or metastatic FTC, PTC, MTC, and ATC were eligible. In this study, the patients were randomized to chemotherapy with doxorubicin (Adriamycin) alone or doxorubicin with cisplatin. Of the 84 eligible patients, the investigators reported a complete response rate of 6% and a partial response rate of 15%. Eight (23%) of 35 patients with advanced differentiated thyroid carcinomas sustained a partial or complete response to the chemotherapy. Overall, there was no advantage to the combination-drug regimen over doxorubicin alone. All five complete responders were in the combination arm, however.

THYROID LYMPHOMA AND ANAPLASTIC CARCINOMA

Because 98% to 99% of thyroid cancers are well differentiated, and most are FCDC, the primary treatment for these tumors is surgical; adjuvant therapy consists mainly of thyroid hormone suppression and, in selected cases, RAI or EBRT. The most common poorly differentiated tumors of the thyroid, lymphoma and ATC, are treated quite differently from the well-differentiated FCDC and MTC. For that reason, these two tumors and their treatment plans are considered separately.

Primary Thyroid Lymphoma

Because of the development of immunocytochemical staining, this distinct entity has become more accurately recognized.[112] Most thyroid lymphomas are diffuse, large B-cell lymphomas (DLBCLs), but significant numbers are in the category of lymphomas known as mucosa-associated lymphoid tissue (MALT) lymphomas or mixed tumors containing elements of DLBCL and MALT. Rarely, other types of lymphoma, including follicular lymphomas and Hodgkin's lymphomas, have been reported.[112,113] Thyroid lymphomas usually manifest with a rapidly enlarging mass that is sometimes associated with respiratory and esophageal symptoms. These lymphomas typically occur in middle- to older-aged women and are often associated with chronic thyroiditis.[112,113] MALT lymphomas have a more indolent natural history, whereas the DLBCLs tend to be more aggressive.

An early review by Doria and colleagues before the widespread use of immunohistochemical staining suggests that the distant failure rate with thyroid lymphomas was seen primarily in the non-MALT population.[114] Their review included 211 patients in 11 series and showed an 11% distant relapse rate for the MALT lymphoma group, compared with 45% for the localized non-MALT patients. This suggests that local therapy alone in the DLBCL patients is inadequate and that systemic therapy is warranted.

Surgery has only a diagnostic role in the management of thyroid lymphomas, and this role is diminishing with the increasing accuracy of FNA.[115] Some investigators contend that surgery can indicate prognostic information, influence treatment options, and improve outcome.[113,116-118] They assert that the use of surgery may obviate the need for chemotherapy in some patients or identify a population requiring local therapy only. One investigator reported five patients with MALT lymphoma or small lymphocytic lymphoma treated with surgery alone who had no relapses.[113] Surgery may have a palliative role in selected patients with obstructive symptoms.[119] In the absence of prospective or randomized data, the improved outcome of patients who are able to undergo resection may indicate only selection of a favorable subgroup and not provide clear evidence of survival advantage associated with the surgery itself, nor does it eliminate the consideration of irradiation or chemotherapy. The infiltrative nature of this disease can lend itself to a higher rate of surgical complications involving the parathyroid glands and recurrent laryngeal nerves. Some investigators have failed to show any advantage to more aggressive surgery, provided the patient receives adequate irradiation with or without chemotherapy.[120,121]

The use of irradiation alone in the treatment of thyroid lymphomas has been reported by multiple institutions.[116,120-124] The reports indicate that the overall survival rate for patients with Ann Arbor stage I and II disease varies between 40% and 93%. Patients with stage I disease have a better outcome. Some of these reports indicate improved outcome with neck and mediastinal irradiation over neck treatment alone.[120,125-127] Others have not found this association.[116,118] In one report of 27 patients treated with irradiation alone or in combination with chemotherapy, all four local failures occurred in patients treated solely with irradiation.[124]

The role of irradiation alone in the treatment of thyroid lymphomas is limited, and given the randomized clinical data for DLBCL with combined chemoradiation, irradiation as the sole treatment modality should be given only when chemotherapy is not feasible or tolerated. With the increased risk of distant relapse reported by Doria and coworkers, survival was improved with the use of systemic chemotherapy in addition to local irradiation.[114] Other study authors have concluded that chemotherapy improves the outcome in these patients.[115,122]

Two large prospective randomized studies have evaluated the use of combined-modality therapy in thyroid lymphomas. Studies by ECOG and Southwestern Oncology Group (SWOG) evaluated the use of CHOP chemotherapy (cyclophosphamide, hydroxydaunomycin, Oncovin [vincristine], prednisone) with or without involved-field irradiation for stage I or II non-Hodgkin's lymphomas, including thyroid lymphomas.[128,129] The number of thyroid lymphoma patients enrolled in these studies is not published, but 18% of the patients in the ECOG study had stage IE disease (i.e., disease confined to one extranodal site). Both studies indicated a survival benefit for combined-modality therapy. Doses of 30 Gy were used in the ECOG study after eight cycles of CHOP chemotherapy, except when there was only a partial response to chemotherapy. In that circumstance, a dose of 40 Gy was delivered using standard fractionation. In the SWOG study, the combined-modality arm received only three cycles of CHOP along with 40 to 55 Gy. The overall survival at 6 years in the ECOG study was 84% for combined-modality therapy, compared with 70% with chemotherapy alone ($P < .05$).[128] Further data from this study await publication. The SWOG report estimated an 82% overall survival rate compared with 72% for CHOP alone ($P = .02$).[129] Based on these randomized studies, it appears that the use of combined-modality therapy offers the most appropriate management of this disease process.

Further improvement in outcomes for DLBCLs has been demonstrated with the addition of monoclonal antibodies, especially rituximab, to combination chemotherapy.[130,131] Other immunologic and radiolabeled agents are being evaluated. Radiation fields should be considered involved fields covering the thyroid region and local nodes. This would include the superior mediastinum, low cervical pretracheal, internal jugular, and supraclavicular nodal sites.

There is minimal information about the use of chemotherapy alone in this particular site.[132] The data from the SWOG and ECOG studies demonstrate a high response rate with CHOP chemotherapy alone. Given the locally aggressive nature of this extranodal site and the bulky disease that can extend into the mediastinum, however, the use of combined-modality therapy is preferable over chemotherapy alone.

Anaplastic Thyroid Carcinoma

The treatment of ATC is a frustrating problem because of the rapidly progressive nature of this disease and its high fatality rate. Most patients are women presenting in the sixth to seventh decade of life, typically with a mass rapidly enlarging over a short time interval. Symptoms of hoarseness, dyspnea, dysphagia, and pain are common in this form of thyroid malignancy. Persistent or recurrent local disease is often the cause of death. Distant metastases are present in almost one half of the patients at presentation.

The optimal role of surgery has not been well defined. Surgery may be accomplished initially in some patients, but this probably reflects the selection of a favorable population of patients.[133] The M. D. Anderson Cancer Center reported that more extensive surgery by itself did not provide a survival advantage.[81] Overall, most patients present with unresectable or metastatic disease, and the initial surgery in these situations is primarily for diagnostic purposes. However, in most reports, the only long-term survivors were patients who had undergone surgical resection.[133,135-138] For this reason, surgery should be strongly considered as a component of treatment. Surgery has been performed before or after irradiation, chemotherapy, or both.[81,139] The sequence of surgery relative to radiation and chemotherapy may be primarily a reflection of the extent of disease at time of patient presentation to the treating physicians.[140]

Radiation has been used in the treatment of these advanced tumors, but because of the high metastatic rate and high rate of local failure with irradiation alone, the use of chemotherapy in addition to irradiation is warranted.[141] Multiple studies have investigated the use of multimodality therapy.[134-136,139] The use of hyperfractionated irradiation has been examined because of the rapid proliferation rate of these malignancies.[134,136,139,142] A wide variety of approaches has been reported, but most studies use doxorubicin-based chemotherapy given concurrently with local irradiation.[128,134,135,143]

A Swedish group reported two hyperfractionated radiation protocols with weekly doxorubicin followed by surgery.[139] Although not a randomized study, the local control rate was significantly improved in the accelerated hyperfractionated group, with 28 of 39 patients obtaining local control ($P = .004$). Of the 40 patients able to undergo surgery 33 (83%) had no local failures. In this study, the accelerated irradiation correlated with local control despite the required surgery. The poor median survival times of 4.5 and 2 months in the accelerated hyperfractionated groups was attributed to the high rate of distant metastases.

A prospective study of multimodality therapy from France has shown early promise.[143] Surgical resection was used in 24 of 30 patients. Doxorubicin plus cisplatin chemotherapy was delivered before and after accelerated hyperfractionated irradiation. At a median follow-up of 45 months, 8 of the 30 patients were alive and had no evidence of disease. Most of the 20 tumor-related deaths were attributed to metastatic disease.

In a report of the National Cancer Institute's Surveillance, Epidemiology, and End Results database, the only factors predicting for lower cause-specific mortality were age younger than 60 years, intrathyroidal tumor, and combined use of surgery and irradiation.[144] However, the overall cause-specific mortality rate was 80.7% at 1 year. The use of multimodality therapy, including surgery, irradiation, and chemotherapy, is appropriate and offers the best chance for long-term survival, but more active systemic agents need to be found to significantly improve survival.

TECHNIQUES OF IRRADIATION

Treatment of the thyroid and the regional lymph nodes is challenging because of the contour of the body and the potential extension of disease to the upper mediastinum and involvement of lymph nodes in the neck and mediastinum. Historically, several approaches have been reported for the initial extended fields, including a single anterior electron field,[106] an anterior field with a posterior supplemental field for the mediastinum, and even lateral fields.[104]

For optimal treatment in an adjuvant setting or for locoregional recurrent disease, the field extends from the angle of the mandible down to the tracheal bifurcation, encompassing the thyroid bed and the lymph nodes of the neck and upper mediastinum. When treating for palliation, it is reasonable to consider treating only the tumor or thyroid bed region. Treatment planning should incorporate the use of CT or magnetic resonance imaging (MRI) to evaluate the dose distribution because of the variability of the body contours involved. The use of IMRT has allowed for more elegant treatment of this disease site compared with conventional and three-dimensional treatment planning (Fig. 35-7). IMRT improves the minimum and mean dose to the planning tumor volume and significantly reduces the dose to the spinal cord.[145,146] This is true for treatment of the thyroid tumor bed or the thyroid region and locoregional nodal sites.

The radiation dose used in the postoperative setting for microscopic residual should be 60 Gy in 6 to 6.5 weeks. The necessary dose in some centers, however, has been suggested to be adequate at 40 Gy given over 3 to 3.5 weeks.[103] If feasible, the dose should be delivered using a shrinking-field technique, giving the nodal regions 45 to 50 Gy in conventional fractionation and boosting the thyroid bed to the 60-Gy level. For known gross residual disease, a dose escalation to 68 to 70 Gy is reasonable. One retrospective study from the United Kingdom suggested a possible dose-response effect above 50 Gy for patients treated with curative intent.[102] The use of higher doses without added morbidity may be feasible with IMRT.

TREATMENT ALGORITHM, CONCLUSIONS AND FUTURE POSSIBILITIES

Treatment Algorithm

The initial approach to a potentially malignant thyroid mass is to obtain an FNA biopsy. This technique permits the identification of a population of patients with definite cancer or for whom there is a high degree of suspicion for malignancy. At initial operation (i.e., open biopsy, thyroid lobectomy, and near-total or total thyroidectomy), the surgeon can assess tumor size, determine the presence or absence of gross local invasion or regional lymph nodal metastasis, and define the postoperative status (i.e., presence or absence of gross residual disease). The surgical pathologist can identify the degree of tumor differentiation (i.e., histologic grade), the tumor histologic type, and if requested, the DNA ploidy.

Typically, FCDC is treated by near-total or total thyroidectomy unless the primary tumor is 1 cm or less in diameter. MTC is treated by total thyroidectomy, whereas ATC and lymphoma probably require only an open biopsy for diagnosis verification. Postoperatively, all patients undergoing more than a lobectomy require thyroid hormone therapy, but only patients with high-risk FCDC receive TSH-suppressive doses of thyroxine.

Knowledge of the patient's age, cell type, pTNM stage, and postoperative status permits classification of patients into

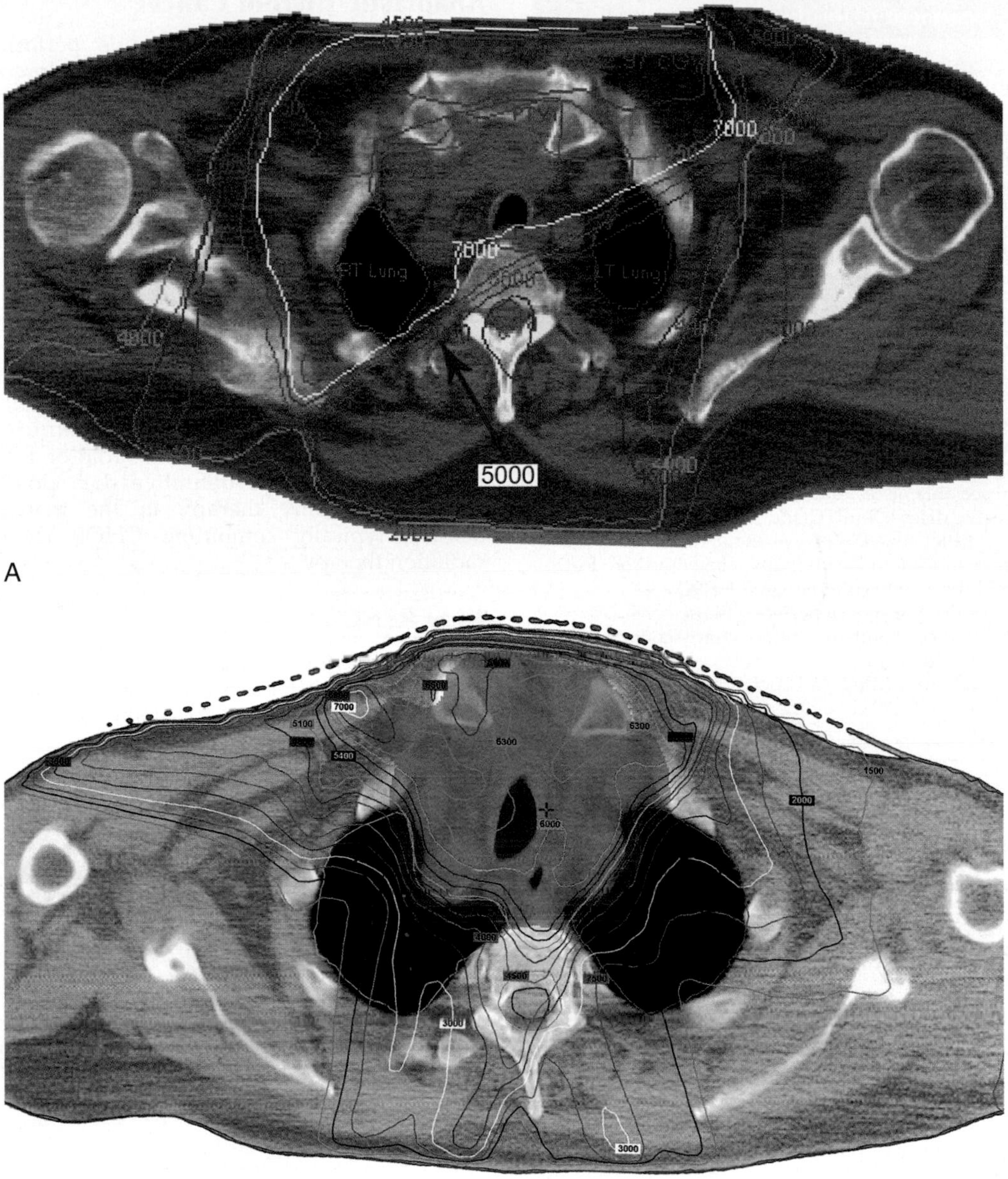

A

B

Figure 35-7 **A,** Three-dimensional treatment planning isodose curves for a patient with locally recurrent and progressive PTC, deemed unresectable. Treatment uses anteroposterior fields followed by oblique fields to left neck for a total dose of 70 Gy. **B,** IMRT treatment plan for a patient with resected recurrent Hürthle cell carcinoma. Treatment uses 9 IMRT fields delivering 60 Gy to central-low neck and 54 Gy to lateral upper neck and mediastinum.

risk groups, which may influence the selection of subsequent postoperative adjuvant therapy. The treatment of patients with different tumor histologies is outlined in the following paragraphs and summarized as four steps in the accompanying treatment algorithm (Table 35-5).

Papillary Thyroid Carcinoma, Follicular Thyroid Carcinoma, and Hürthle Cell Carcinoma

FCDC patients with documented distant metastases (e.g., lung, bone) at presentation undergo RAI scanning 6 to 8 weeks postoperatively and are treated with ^{131}I therapy; the dose depends on the extent of metastases and avidity for RAI. Subsequent repeat whole-body scans are performed at 3- to 6-month intervals until no further uptake is observed in the neck or distant sites. Serum thyroglobulin levels are obtained before RAI therapy and are closely monitored while on and off thyroxine to gauge progress in terms of tumor control.

Patients with unresectable or resected but residual FCDC are typically given the opportunity of whole-body scan and possible RAI therapy. If a whole-body scan reveals no significant uptake after therapy, a course of EBRT is considered.

Patients 45 years or older with locally invasive disease usually are given RAI therapy. Some authorities consider the addition of EBRT, especially if serum thyroglobulin levels continue to be elevated despite apparently adequate treatment with RAI.

Controversy continues regarding the role of remnant ablation in patients with intrathyroidal or node-positive PTC. Use of the AGES, AMES, or MACIS prognostic classifications may

Table 35-5 Treatment Algorithm

Step I	*Initial neck exploration/thyroid resection* FCDC: usually near-total or total thyroidectomy MTC: total thyroidectomy ATC: open biopsy or subtotal thyroidectomy Lymphoma: usually only open biopsy Lymph nodes: removal in FCDC and MTC; modified radical neck dissection for involved lateral nodes
Step II	*Thyroid hormone therapy* Replacement doses for MTC, ATC, lymphoma TSH-suppressive doses for FCDC, except microcarcinoma
Step III	*Outcome prediction by risk-group classification* Gauged according to age, stage, histologic type, and cancer type-specific scoring systems (e.g., AMES, MACIS)
Step IV	*Patient selection for RAI therapy, EBRT, chemotherapy, or combinations* FCDC: RAI therapy indicated for distant spread, unresectable or residual neck tumor, possibly invasive disease in PTC and most cases of FTC or HCC; EBRT for local or metastatic tumor nonresponsive to RAI therapy; almost no role for chemotherapy in differentiated FCDC MTC: residual or recurrent neck disease considered for EBRT; octreotide or chemotherapy considered for palliation only ATC: postbiopsy EBRT and concurrent chemotherapy Lymphoma: CHOP chemotherapy and radiation therapy

AMES system, uses variables of (patient) age, metastasis, (tumor) extent, and (tumor) size; ATC, anaplastic thyroid cancer; CHOP, cyclophosphamide, hydroxydaunomycin, Oncovin (vincristine), prednisone; EBRT, external beam radiation therapy; FCDC, follicular cell–derived cancer; FTC, follicular thyroid carcinoma; HCC, Hürthle cell carcinoma; MACIS system: uses variables of metastasis, age, completeness of resection, invasion, and size; MTC, medullary thyroid carcinoma; PTC, papillary thyroid carcinoma; RAI, radioactive iodine; TSH, thyroid-stimulating hormone.

permit a more selective use of RAI. In general, most patients with FTC or HCC undergo postoperative whole-body scans and are considered candidates for RAI therapy. This may be an overaggressive position because the prognosis is excellent for minimally invasive FTC after surgery alone and HCC usually does not avidly uptake RAI.

Medullary Thyroid Carcinoma

Because MTC may be bilateral and multicentric and because nodal metastases are common at presentation, most authorities recommend an initial surgical approach of total thyroidectomy, central compartment node removal, and possible modified radical neck dissection if the lateral neck is involved with disease. There is no role for TSH-suppressive or RAI therapy in this condition. Recurrent disease in the neck or mediastinum is typically treated by repeat surgical exploration. EBRT may have a limited role in local control if disease becomes unresectable, and it can be usefully employed in the treatment of osseous metastases, especially when vertebral deposits threaten the spinal cord. Combination chemotherapy has been used in stage IV MTC, as has subcutaneous octreotide therapy. These treatments have not been demonstrated to improve cause-specific survival in disseminated, symptomatic MTC.

Anaplastic Thyroid Cancer

Usually, only an open biopsy is performed at surgery when this disease is first diagnosed. More extensive initial resection should be considered if it can be achieved without significant morbidity. Most patients with ATC are given EBRT postoperatively, and many are given the option of considering concurrent chemotherapy. There is no generally approved efficacious chemotherapeutic program available to patients with ATC.

Primary Thyroid Lymphoma

In contrast to the outlook for ATC, much greater optimism is expressed in managing primary thyroid lymphomas. There has been a gradual shift from subtotal thyroidectomy to open biopsy and even FNA biopsy in diagnosing this condition. Recognition of the probably systemic nature of the disease led initially to an acceptance of the role of EBRT to neck and regional nodes. More definitive data point to the use of combined-modality therapy in the management of this disease, typically combining CHOP chemotherapy with radiation therapy.

REFERENCES

1. Bruneton JN, Balu-Maestro C, Marcy PY, et al: Very high frequency (13 MHz) ultrasonographic examination of the normal neck: detection of normal lymph nodes and thyroid nodules. J Ultrasound Med 13:87-90, 1994.
2. Jemal A, Siegel R, Ward E, et al: Cancer statistics, 2006. CA Cancer J Clin 56:106-130, 2006.
3. Tan GH, Gharib H: Thyroid incidentalomas: management approaches to nonpalpable nodules discovered incidentally on thyroid imaging. Ann Intern Med 126:226-231, 1997.
4. Mazzaferri EL: Impact of initial tumor features and treatment selected on the long-term course of differentiated thyroid cancer. Thyroid Today 18:1-13, 1995.
5. Tezelman S, Clark OH: Current management of thyroid cancer. Adv Surg 28:191-221, 1995.
6. Dulgeroff AJ, Hershman JM: Medical therapy for differentiated thyroid carcinoma. Endocr Rev 15:500-515, 1994.
7. Pacini F, Elisei R, Fugazzola L, et al: Post-surgical follow-up of differentiated thyroid cancer. J Endocrinol Invest 18:165-166, 1995.
8. Mazzaferri EL: Management of a solitary thyroid nodule. N Engl J Med 328:553-559, 1993.
9. Feld S, Garcia M, Baskin HJ, et al: AACE clinical practice guidelines for the diagnosis and management of thyroid nodules. Endocr Pract 2:78-84, 1996.
10. Cooper DS, Doherty GM, Haugen BR, et al: Management guidelines for patients with thyroid nodules and differentiated thyroid cancer. Thyroid 16:109-141, 2006.
11. Schlumberger M: Papillary and follicular thyroid carcinoma. N Engl J Med 338:297-306, 1998.
12. De Groot LJ: Long-term impact of initial and surgical therapy on papillary and follicular thyroid cancer. Am J Med 97:499-500, 1994.
13. Solomon BL, Wartofsky L, Burman KD: Current trends in the management of well-differentiated papillary thyroid carcinoma. J Clin Endocrinol Metab 81:323-339, 1996.
14. Wartofsky L: Management of patients with scan negative, thyroglobulin positive differentiated thyroid carcinoma. J Clin Endocrinol Metab 83:4195-4203, 1998.
15. Hamilton JG, Soley MH, Eichorn KB: Deposition of radioactive iodine in human thyroid tissue. Univ Calif Publ Pharmacol 1:330-346, 1940.
16. Keston AS, Bali RP, Frantz VK, et al: Storage of radioactive iodine in a metastasis from thyroid carcinoma. Science 95:362-366, 1942.
17. Freitas JE: Treatment of thyroid carcinoma with radioiodine. Curr Concept Diag Nucl Med 3:8-29, 1986.

18. Blahd WH, Nordyke RD, Bauer FK: Radioactive iodine (^{131}I) in the postoperative treatment of thyroid cancers. Cancer 13:745-753, 1960.
19. Sweeney DC, Johnston GS: Radioiodine therapy for thyroid cancer. Endocrinol Metab Clin North Am 24:803-839, 1995.
20. Sheline GE, Galante M, Lindsay S: Radiation therapy in the control of persistent thyroid cancer. Am J Roentgenol Radium Ther Nucl Med 97:923-930, 1966.
21. Brierley JD, Tsang RW: External radiation therapy in the treatment of thyroid malignancy. Endocrinol Metab Clin North Am 25:141-157, 1996.
22. Parkin DM, Pisani P, Ferlay J: Global cancer statistics. CA Cancer J Clin 49:33-64, 1999.
23. Robbins J, Merino MJ, Boice JD Jr, et al: Thyroid cancer: a lethal endocrine neoplasm. Ann Intern Med 115:133-147, 1991.
24. Ain KB: Papillary thyroid carcinoma. Endocrinol Metab Clin North Am 24:711-760, 1995.
25. Grebe SKG, Hay ID: Follicular thyroid cancer. Endocrinol Metab Clin North Am 24:761-801, 1995.
26. Gilliland FD, Hunt WC, Morris DM, et al: Prognostic factors for thyroid carcinoma: a population-based study of 15,698 cases from the Surveillance, Epidemiology and End Results (SEER) Program 1973-1991. Cancer 79:564-573, 1997.
27. Ebihara S, Saikawa M: Survey and analysis of thyroid carcinoma by the Japanese Society of Thyroid Surgery. Thyroidol Clin Exp 10:89-95, 1998.
28. Hundahl SA, Fleming ID, Fremgen AM, et al: A National Cancer Database report on 53,856 cases of thyroid carcinoma treated in the U.S., 1985-1995. Cancer 83:2638-2648, 1998.
29. Williams ED, Doniach I, Bjarnason O, et al: Thyroid cancer in an iodide rich area: a histopathological study. Cancer 39:215-222, 1977.
30. Harach HR, Williams ED: Thyroid cancer and thyroiditis in the goitrous regions of Salta, Argentina, before and after iodine prophylaxis. Clin Endocrinol 43:701-706, 1995.
31. McTiernan A, Weiss NS, Daling JR: Incidence of thyroid cancer in women in relation to known or suspected risk factors for breast cancer. Cancer Res 47:292-295, 1987.
32. Ron E, Kleinerman RA, Boice JD, et al: A population-based case-control study of thyroid cancer. J Natl Cancer Inst 79:1-12, 1987.
33. Kravdal O, Glattre E, Haldorsen T: Positive correlation between parity and incidence of thyroid cancer: new evidence based on complete Norwegian birth cohorts. Int J Cancer 49:831-836, 1991.
34. Hamilton TE, van Belle G, LoGerfo JP: Thyroid neoplasia in Marshall Islanders exposed to nuclear fallout. JAMA 258:629-636, 1987.
35. Prentice RL, Kato H, Yoshimoto K, et al: Radiation exposure and thyroid cancer incidence among Hiroshima and Nagasaki residents. Natl Cancer Inst Monogr 62:207-212, 1982.
36. Schneider AB, Recant W, Pinsky SM, et al: Radiation-induced thyroid carcinoma: clinical course and results of therapy in 296 patients. Ann Intern Med 105:405-412, 1986.
37. Mahta MP, Goetowski PG, Kindella TJ: Radiation-induced thyroid neoplasms, 1920 to 1987: a vanishing problem? Int J Radiat Oncol Biol Phys 16:1471-1475, 1989.
38. McHenry C, Jarosz H, Calundra D, et al: Thyroid neoplasia following radiation therapy for Hodgkin's lymphoma. Arch Surg 122:684-686, 1987.
39. Nikiforov Y, Gnepp DR: Pediatric thyroid cancer after the Chernobyl disaster: pathomorphologic study of 84 cases (1991-92) from the Republic of Belarus. Cancer 74:748-766, 1994.
40. Robbins J: Lessons from Chernobyl: the event, the aftermath fallout: radioactive, political, social. Thyroid 7:180-192, 1997.
41. Becker DV, Robbins J, Beebe GW, et al: Childhood thyroid cancer following the Chernobyl accident: a status report. Endocrinol Metab Clin North Am 25:197-211, 1995.
42. Nikiforov YE, Fagin JA: Radiation induced thyroid cancer in children after the Chernobyl accident. Thyroid Today 21:1-11, 1998.
43. Hundahl SA: Review: National Cancer Institute report on iodine-131 exposure from fallout following Nevada atmospheric nuclear bomb tests. CA Cancer J Clin 48:285-298, 1998.
44. Farid NR, Shi Y, Kou M: Molecular basis of thyroid cancer. Endocr Rev 15:202-232, 1994.
45. Houlston RS, Stratton MR: Genetics of non-medullary thyroid cancer. Q J Med 88:685-693, 1995.
46. Cooper DS, Axelrod L, DeGroot LJ, et al: Congenital goiter and the development of metastatic follicular carcinoma with evidence for a leak of non-hormonal iodine: clinical, pathological, kinetic and biochemical studies and a review of the literature. J Clin Endocrinol Metab 52:294-306, 1981.
47. Ledger GA, Khosla S, Lindor NM, et al: Genetic testing in the diagnosis and management of multiple endocrine neoplasia type II. Ann Intern Med 122:118-126, 1995.
48. Wells SA, Chi DD, Toshima K, et al: Predictive DNA testing and prophylactic therapy in patients at risk for multiple endocrine neoplasia type 2A. Ann Surg 120:1377-1381, 1994.
49. Wohlik N, Cote GJ, Evans DB, et al: Application of genetic screening to the management of medullary thyroid carcinoma and multiple endocrine neoplasia type 2. Endocrinol Metab Clin North Am 25:1-15, 1996.
50. Hay ID: Papillary thyroid carcinoma. Endocrinol Metab Clin North Am 19:545-576, 1990.
51. McConahey WM, Hay ID, Woolner LB, et al: Papillary thyroid cancer treated at the Mayo Clinic, 1946 through 1970: initial manifestations, pathologic findings, therapy and outcome. Mayo Clin Proc 61:978-996, 1986.
52. Zimmerman D, Hay ID, Gough IR, et al: Papillary thyroid carcinoma in children and adults: long-term follow-up of 1,039 patients conservatively treated at one institution during three decades. Surgery 104:1157-1166, 1988.
53. Dinneen SF, Valimaki MJ, Bergstralh EJ, et al: Distant metastases in thyroid carcinoma: 100 cases observed at one institution during 5 decades. J Clin Endocrinol Metab 80:2041-2045, 1995.
54. Brennan MD, Bergstralh EJ, van Heerden JA, et al: Follicular thyroid cancer treated at the Mayo Clinic, 1946 through 1970: initial manifestations, pathologic findings, therapy, and outcome. Mayo Clin Proc 66:11-19, 1991.
55. Grebe SKG, Hay ID: Thyroid cancer nodal metastases: biologic significance and therapeutic considerations. Surg Oncol Clin N Am 5:43-63, 1996.
56. Hay ID: Cytometric DNA ploidy analysis in thyroid cancer. Diagn Oncol 1:181-185, 1991.
57. Ruegemer JJ, Hay ID, Bergstralh EJ, et al: Distant metastases in differentiated thyroid carcinoma: a multivariate analysis of prognostic variables. J Clin Endocrinol Metab 63:960-967, 1988.
58. Moley JF: Medullary thyroid cancer. Surg Clin N Am 75:405-420, 1995.
59. Lips CJM, Landsvater RM, Hoppener JWM, et al: Clinical screening as compared with DNA analysis in families with multiple endocrine neoplasia type 2A. N Engl J Med 331:828-835, 1994.
60. Nel CJ, van Heerden JA, Goellner JR, et al: Anaplastic carcinoma of the thyroid: a clinicopathologic study of 82 cases. Mayo Clin Proc 60:51-58, 1985.
61. Sobin LH, Wittekind CH, for the International Union Against Cancer: TNM Classification of Malignant Tumours, 6th ed. New York, Wiley-Liss, 2002.
62. Shah JP, Kian K, Forastiere A, et al, for the American Joint Committee on Cancer: AJCC Cancer Staging Manual, 6th ed. New York, Springer-Verlag, 2002.
63. Larsen PR, Davies TF, Hay ID: The thyroid gland. *In* Wilson JD, Foster DW, Kronenberg HM, Larsen PR (eds): Williams Textbook of Endocrinology, 9th ed. Philadelphia, WB Saunders, 1998, pp 389-515.
64. Grant CS, Hay ID, Gough IR, et al: Local recurrence in papillary thyroid carcinoma: is extent of surgical resection important? Surgery 104:954-962, 1988.
65. Smith SA, Hay ID, Goellner JR, et al: Mortality from papillary thyroid carcinoma: a case-control study of 56 lethal cases. Cancer 62:1381-1390, 1988.
66. Hay ID, Grant CS, Taylor WF, et al: Ipsilateral lobectomy versus bilateral lobar resection in papillary thyroid carcinoma: a retrospective analysis of surgical outcome using a novel prognostic scoring system. Surgery 102:1088-1095, 1987.
67. Simpson WJ, McKinney SE, Carruthers JS, et al: Papillary and follicular thyroid cancer: prognostic factors in 1,578 patients. Am J Med 83:474-488, 1987.

68. Shah JP, Loree TR, Dharker D, et al: Prognostic factors in differentiated carcinoma of the thyroid gland. Am J Surg 164:658-661, 1992.
69. Hay ID, Bergstralh EJ, Goellner JR, et al: Predicting outcome in papillary thyroid carcinoma: development of a reliable prognostic scoring system in a cohort of 1,779 patients surgically treated at one institution during 1940 through 1989. Surgery 114:1050-1058, 1993.
70. Cady B, Rossi R: An expanded view of risk-group definition in differentiated thyroid carcinoma. Surgery 104:947-953, 1988.
71. DeGroot LJ, Kaplan EL, Straus FH, et al: Does the method of management of papillary thyroid carcinoma make a difference in outcome? World J Surg 18:123-130, 1994.
72. van Heerden JA, Hay ID, Goellner JR, et al: Follicular thyroid carcinoma with capsular invasion alone: a non-threatening malignancy. Surgery 112:1130-1136, 1992.
73. Mueller-Gaertner HW, Brzac HT, Rehpenning W: Prognostic indices for tumor relapse and tumor mortality in follicular thyroid carcinoma. Cancer 67:1903-1908, 1991.
74. Shaha AR, Loree TR, Shah JP: Prognostic factors and risk group analysis in follicular carcinoma of the thyroid. Surgery 118:1131-1138, 1995.
75. Loree TR: Therapeutic implications of prognostic factors in differentiated carcinoma of the thyroid gland. Semin Surg Oncol 11:246-255, 1995.
76. D'Avanzo A, Ituarte P, Treselar P, et al: Prognostic scoring systems in patients with follicular thyroid cancer: a comparison of different staging systems in predicting the patient outcome. Thyroid 14:453-458, 2004.
77. Davis NL, Bugis JD, McGregor GI, et al: An evaluation of prognostic scoring systems in patients with follicular thyroid cancer. Am J Surg 170:476-480, 1995.
78. Gharib H, McConahey WM, Tiegs RD, et al: Medullary thyroid carcinoma: clinicopathologic features and long-term follow-up of 65 patients treated during 1946 through 1970. Mayo Clin Proc 67:934-940, 1992.
79. Pyke CM, Hay ID, Goellner JR, et al: Prognostic significance of calcitonin immunoreactivity, amyloid staining, and flow cytometric DNA measurements in medullary thyroid carcinoma. Surgery 110:964-970, 1991.
80. Brierley J, Tsang R, Simpson WJ, et al: Medullary thyroid cancer: analyses of survival and prognostic factors and the role of radiation therapy in local control. Thyroid 6:305-310, 1996.
81. Venkatesh YS, Ordonez NG, Schultz PN, et al: Anaplastic carcinoma of the thyroid: a clinicopathologic study of 121 cases. Cancer 66:321-328, 1990.
82. American Association of Clinical Endocrinologists: AACE/AAES medical/surgical guidelines for clinical practice: management of thyroid carcinoma. Endocr Pract 7:202-230, 2001.
83. Mazzaferri E: NCCN thyroid carcinoma practice guidelines. Oncology 13:391-442, 1999.
84. Singer PA, Cooper DS, Daniels GH, et al: Treatment guidelines for patients with thyroid nodules and well-differentiated thyroid cancer. Arch Intern Med 156:2165-2172, 1996.
85. Friedman M, Danielzadeh JA, Caldarelli DD: Treatment of patients with carcinoma of the thyroid invading the airway. Arch Otolaryngol Head Neck Surg 120:1372-1381, 1994.
86. Ballantyne AJ: Resections of the upper aerodigestive tract for locally invasive thyroid cancer. Am J Surg 168:636-639, 1994.
87. Hay ID, Grant CS, Bergstralh EJ, et al: Unilateral total lobectomy: is it sufficient surgical treatment for patients with AMES low-risk papillary thyroid carcinoma? Surgery 124:958-966, 1998.
88. De Groot LJ, Kaplan EL, McCormick M, et al: Natural history, treatment, and course of papillary thyroid carcinoma. J Clin Endocrinol Metab 71:414-424, 1990.
89. Samaan NA, Schultz RN, Hickey RC, et al: The results of various modalities of treatment of well differentiated thyroid carcinomas: a retrospective review of 1599 patients. J Clin Endocrinol Metab 75:714-720, 1992.
90. Mazzaferri EL, Jhiang SM: Long-term impact of initial surgical and medical therapy of papillary and follicular thyroid cancer. Am J Med 97:418-428, 1994.
91. Cady B: Our AMES is true: how an old concept still hits the mark: or, risk group assignment points the arrow to rational therapy selection in differentiated thyroid cancer. Am J Surg 174:461-468, 1997.
92. DeGroot LJ, Kaplan EL: Second operations for "completion" of thyroidectomy in treatment of differentiated thyroid cancer. Surgery 110:936-939, 1991.
93. Noguchi S, Murakami N, Yamashita H, et al: Papillary thyroid carcinoma: modified radical neck dissection improves prognosis. Arch Surg 133:276-280, 1998.
94. Sanders LE, Cady B: Differentiated thyroid cancer: reexamination of risk groups and outcome of treatment. Arch Surg 133:419-425, 1998.
95. Grebe SKG, Hay ID: Follicular cell-derived thyroid carcinomas. Cancer Treat Res 89:91-140, 1997.
96. Hay ID, McConahey WM, Goellner JR: Managing patients with papillary thyroid carcinoma: insights gained from the Mayo Clinic experience of treating 2,512 consecutive patients during 1940 through 2000. Trans Am Clin Climatol Assoc 113:241-260, 2002.
97. Sawka AM, Thephamongkhol K, Brouwers M, et al: Clinical review 170. A systemic review and metaanalysis of the effectiveness of radioactive iodine remnant ablation for well-differentiated thyroid cancer. J Clin Endocrinol Metab 89:3668-3676, 2004.
98. Schlumberger M, Hay ID: Use of radioactive iodine in patients with papillary and follicular thyroid cancer: towards a selective approach. J Clin Endocrinol Metab 83:4201-4203, 1998.
99. Simpson WJ, Panzarella I, Carruthers JS, et al: Papillary and follicular thyroid cancer: impact of treatment in 1578 patients. Int J Radiat Oncol Biol Phys 14:1063-1071, 1988.
100. Robbins RJ, Schlumberger MJ: The evolving role of I-131 for the treatment of differentiated thyroid carcinoma. J Nucl Med 46:28-37S, 2005.
101. Eichhorn W, Tabler H, Lippold R, et al: Prognostic factors determining long-term survival in well-differentiated thyroid cancer: an analysis of four hundred eighty-four patients undergoing therapy and aftercare at the same institution. Thyroid 13:949-958, 2003.
102. Ford D, Giridharan S, McConkey C, et al: External beam radiotherapy in the management of differentiated thyroid cancer. Clin Oncol (R Coll Radiol) 15:337-341, 2003.
103. Simpson WJ, Carruthers JS: The role of external irradiation in the management of papillary and follicular thyroid cancer. Am J Surg 1365:457-463, 1978.
104. Tubiana M, Haddad E, Schlumberger M, et al: External radiotherapy in thyroid cancers. Cancer 55:2062-2071, 1985.
105. Farahati J, Reiners C, Stuschke M, et al: Differentiated thyroid cancer: impact of adjuvant external radiotherapy in patients with perithyroidal tumor infiltration. Cancer 77:177-180, 1996.
106. Tsang RW, Brierley JD, Simpson WJ, et al: The effects of surgery, radioiodine, and external radiation therapy on the clinical outcome of patients with differentiated thyroid carcinoma. Cancer 82:375-388, 1998.
107. Benker G, Olbricht T, Reinwein D, et al: Survival rates in patients with differentiated thyroid carcinoma: influence of postoperative external radiotherapy. Cancer 65:1517-1520, 1990.
108. O'Connell MEA, A'Hern RP, Harmer CL: Results of external beam radiotherapy in differentiated thyroid carcinoma: a retrospective study from the Royal Marsden Hospital. Eur J Cancer 30A:733-739, 1994.
109. Biermann M, Pixberg MK, Schuck A, et al: Multicenter study differentiated thyroid carcinoma: diminished acceptance of adjuvant external beam radiotherapy. Nuklearmedizin 9:244-250, 2003.
110. Schuck A, Bierman M, Pixberg MK, et al: Acute toxicity of adjuvant radiotherapy in locally advanced differentiated thyroid carcinoma. Strahlenther Onkol 179:832-839, 2003.
111. Shimaoka K, Schoenfeld DA, De Wys WD, et al: A randomized trial of doxorubicin versus doxorubicin plus cisplatin in patients with advanced thyroid carcinoma. Cancer 56:2155-2161, 1985.
112. Derringer GA, Thompson LDR, Frommelt RA, et al: Malignant lymphoma of the thyroid gland: a clinicopathologic study of 108 cases. Am J Surg Pathol 24:623-639, 2000.

113. Thieblemont C, Mayer A, Dumontet C, et al: Primary thyroid lymphoma is a heterogeneous disease. J Clin Endocrinol Metab 87:105-111, 2002.
114. Doria R, Jekel JF, Cooper D: Thyroid lymphoma: the case for combined modality therapy. Cancer 73:200-206, 1994.
115. Matsuzuka F, Miyauchi A, Katayama S, et al: Clinical aspects of primary thyroid lymphoma: diagnosis and treatment based on our experience of 119 cases. Thyroid 3:93-99, 1993.
116. Tupchong L, Hughes F, Harmer CL, et al: Primary lymphoma of the thyroid gland: clinical features, prognostic factors, and results of treatment. Int J Radiat Oncol Biol Phys 12:1813-1821, 1986.
117. Rosen IB, Sutcliffe SB, Gospodarowicz MK, et al: The role of surgery in the management of thyroid lymphoma. Surgery 104:1095-1099, 1988.
118. Junor EJ, Paul J, Reed NS: Primary non-Hodgkin's lymphoma of the thyroid. Eur J Surg Oncol 18:313-321, 1992.
119. Sippel RS, Gauger PG, Angelos P, et al: Palliative thyroidectomy for malignant lymphoma of the thyroid. Ann Surg Oncol 9:907-911, 2002.
120. Blair TJ, Evans RG, Buskirk SJ, et al: Radiotherapeutic management of primary thyroid lymphoma. Int J Radiat Oncol Biol Phys 11:365-370, 1985.
121. Logue JP, Hale RJ, Stewart AL, et al: Primary malignant lymphoma of the thyroid: a clinicopathologic analysis. Int J Radiat Oncol Biol Phys 22:929-933, 1992.
122. Tsang R, Gospodarowicz M, Sutcliffe S, et al: Non-Hodgkin's lymphoma of the thyroid gland: Prognostic factors and treatment outcome. Int J Radiat Oncol Biol Phys 27:594-604, 1993.
123. Vigliotti A, Kong JS, Fuller LM, et al: Thyroid lymphomas stages IE and IIE: comparative results for radiotherapy only, combination chemotherapy only, and multimodality treatment. Int J Radial Oncol Biol Phys 12:1807-1812, 1986.
124. DiBiase SJ, Grigsby PW, Guo C, et al: Outcome analysis for stage IE and IIE thyroid lymphoma. Am J Clin Oncol 27:178-184, 2004.
125. Burke JS, Butler JJ, Fuller LM: Malignant lymphomas of the thyroid: a clinicopathologic study of 35 patients including ultrastructural observations. Cancer 39:1587-1602, 1977.
126. Souhami L, Simpson W, Carruthers J: Malignant lymphoma of the thyroid gland. Int J Radiat Oncol Biol Phys 6:1143-1147, 1980.
127. Harrington KJ, Michalaki VJ, Nutting CM, et al: Management of non-Hodgkin's lymphoma of the thyroid: the Royal Marsden Hospital experience. Br J Radiol 78:405-410, 2005.
128. Horning SJ, Weller E, Kim K, et al: Chemotherapy with or without radiotherapy in limited-stage diffuse aggressive non-Hodgkin's lymphoma: Eastern Cooperative Oncology Group study 1484. J Clin Oncol 22:3032-3038, 2004.
129. Miller TP, Dahlberg S, Cassady JR, et al: Chemotherapy alone compared with chemotherapy plus radiotherapy for localized intermediate- and high-grade non-Hodgkin's lymphoma. N Engl J Med 339:21-26, 1998.
130. Coiffier B, Lepage E, Briere J, et al: CHOP chemotherapy plus rituximab compared with CHOP alone in elderly patients with diffuse large B-cell lymphoma. N Engl J Med 346:235-242, 2002.
131. Mounier N, Briere J, Gisselbrecht C, et al: Rituximab plus CHOP (R-CHOP) overcomes bcl-2 associated resistance to chemotherapy in elderly patients with diffuse large B-cell lymphoma (DLBCL). Blood 101:4279-4284, 2003.
132. Leedman PJ, Sheridan WP, Downey WF, et al: Combination chemotherapy as single modality therapy for stage 1E and IIE thyroid lymphoma. Med J Aust 152:40-43, 1990.
133. McIver B, Hay ID, Giuffrida DF, et al: Anaplastic thyroid carcinoma: a 50-year experience at a single institution. Surgery 130:1029-1034, 2001.
134. Kim JH, Leeper RD: Treatment of anaplastic giant and spindle cell carcinoma of the thyroid gland with combination Adriamycin and radiation therapy: a new approach. Cancer 52:954-963, 1983.
135. Schlumberger M, Parmentier C, Delisle MJ, et al: Combination therapy for anaplastic giant cell thyroid carcinoma. Cancer 67:564-566, 1991.
136. Tallroth E, Wallin G, Lundell G, et al: Multimodality treatment in anaplastic giant cell thyroid carcinoma. Cancer 60:1428-1431, 1987.
137. Sugino K, Ito K, Mimura T, et al: The important role of operations in the management of anaplastic thyroid carcinoma. Surgery 131:245-248, 2002.
138. Goutsouliak V, Hay JH: Anaplastic thyroid cancer in British Columbia 1985-1999: a population-based study. Clin Oncol 17:75-87, 2005.
139. Tennvall J, Lundell G, Wahlberg P, et al: Anaplastic thyroid carcinoma. Br J Cancer 86:1848-1853, 2002.
140. Besic N, Auersperg M, Us-Krasovec M, et al: Effect of primary treatment on survival in anaplastic thyroid carcinoma. Eur J Surg Oncol 27:260-264, 2001.
141. Levendag PC, De Porre PM, van Putten WL: Anaplastic carcinoma of the thyroid gland treated by radiation therapy. Int J Radiat Oncol Biol Phys 26:125-128, 1993.
142. Simpson WJ: Anaplastic thyroid carcinoma: a new approach. Can J Surg 23:25-31, 1980.
143. De Crevoisier R, Baudin E, Bachelot A, et al: Combined treatment of anaplastic thyroid carcinoma with surgery, chemotherapy, and hyperfractionated accelerated radiotherapy. Int J Radiat Oncol Biol Phys 60:1137-1143, 2004.
144. Kebebew E, Greenspan FS, Clark OH, et al: Anaplastic thyroid carcinoma: treatment outcome and prognostic factors. Cancer 103:1330-1335, 2005.
145. Nutting CM, Convery DJ, Cosgrove VP, et al: Improvements in target coverage and reduced spinal cord irradiation using intensity-modulated radiotherapy (IMRT) in patients with carcinoma of the thyroid gland. Radiother Oncol 60:173-180, 2001.
146. Posner MD, Quivey JM, Akazawa PF, et al: Dose optimization for the treatment of anaplastic thyroid carcinoma: a comparison of treatment planning techniques. Int J Radiat Oncol Biol Phys 48:475-483, 2000.

CHAPTER 36

UNKNOWN HEAD AND NECK PRIMARY SITE

William M. Mendenhall, Anthony A. Mancuso, and Douglas B. Villaret

INCIDENCE

Approximately 3% of head and neck squamous cell carcinomas metastasize to the neck from an unknown head and neck primary site.

BIOLOGIC CHARACTERISTICS

They are similar to head and neck mucosal squamous cell carcinomas with known primary sites.

STAGING EVALUATION

Evaluation includes history and physical examination, computed tomography of the head and neck, chest radiography, direct laryngoscopy with ipsilateral tonsillectomy, and directed biopsies. Optional studies include chest computed tomography and positron emission tomography.

PRIMARY THERAPY AND RESULTS

Therapy consists of neck dissection and/or radiotherapy (RT) to involved neck and RT to oropharynx and nasopharynx if RT is indicated for treatment of neck disease. The 5-year survival is approximately 50%.

ADJUVANT THERAPY

Concomitant cisplatin chemotherapy is administered for advanced N2 and N3 neck disease.

LOCALLY ADVANCED DISEASE

RT is administered to the oropharynx, nasopharynx, and both sides of the neck with concomitant chemotherapy followed by evaluation for a neck dissection.

PALLIATION

Moderate-dose RT (30 Gy/10 fractions or 20 Gy/2 fractions with a 1-week interfraction interval) is administered to the involved neck.

In a small percentage of patients with squamous cell carcinoma metastatic to the cervical lymph nodes, the primary lesion cannot be found, even after an extensive evaluation. Patients with metastatic adenopathy in the upper neck have a good prognosis when treated aggressively, compared with those with metastatic lymph nodes in the level IV nodes or supraclavicular fossa.[1] The latter group is more likely to have a primary lesion located below the clavicles and the probability of cure is remote. The majority of patients have either squamous cell carcinoma or poorly differentiated carcinoma. Those with adenocarcinoma almost always have a primary lesion below the clavicles, although if the nodes are located in the upper neck, one must exclude a salivary gland, thyroid, or parathyroid primary tumor.

This chapter addresses the management of patients presenting with squamous cell or poorly differentiated carcinoma in the upper or middle neck. Squamous cell carcinoma presenting in a parotid area lymph node is almost always metastatic from a cutaneous primary site and will not be addressed.[2]

DIAGNOSTIC EVALUATION

Patients should be evaluated with a thorough physical examination including careful evaluation of the head and neck by multiple examiners. A needle biopsy of the lymph node should be performed; fine-needle aspiration (FNA) is preferred to a biopsy because it is less traumatic, and there is a lower likelihood of seeding tumor cells along the needle track.[3-7] Evaluation of the neck node biopsy for Epstein-Barr virus (EBV) DNA, via polymerase chain reaction, may be useful in detecting a nasopharyngeal primary tumor in geographic areas where this malignancy is prevalent.[8] After chest roentgenography, computed tomography (CT) or magnetic resonance imaging (MRI) of the head and neck is performed to detect an unknown primary lesion arising from the mucosa of the head and neck. Our preference has been to use CT initially and to follow with MRI only in cases with equivocal findings where MRI might yield additional useful information. A complete blood count is obtained to evaluate the patient for anemia, which may reduce the likelihood of locoregional control after irradiation alone. A chest CT should be considered for patents with N3 neck disease, as well as those with N2B to N2C disease and bulky adenopathy in the lower neck, to assess the lungs for pulmonary metastases.[9] The recommended diagnostic evaluation[10] is depicted in Table 36-1.

Preliminary evidence suggested that fluorodeoxyglucose (FDG) single-photon emission computed tomography (SPECT) or positron emission tomography (PET) scans may identify primary lesions that would not otherwise be identifiable.[11] Theoretically, tumor cells have a higher metabolic rate than normal tissues and, therefore, take up more FDG so that they appear "hot" on a PET or SPECT scan. If an FDG-SPECT or PET scan is obtained as part of the workup, it should be performed before panendoscopy so that any suspicious areas of increased uptake can be biopsied. Limited data pertaining to the usefulness of FDG-SPECT and FDG-PET scans suggest these procedures may identify the primary site in a relatively small subset of patients.[12-14] The FDG-SPECT scan was the sole procedure that correctly identified the occult primary site in only 1 of 24 patients (4%) at our institution (Table 36-2).[12] Currently, FDG-PET scans are not routinely obtained at our institution as part of diagnostic evaluation of these patients.

Direct endoscopy and examination using anesthesia are performed with directed biopsies of the nasopharynx, tonsils, base of tongue, and piriform sinuses and of any abnormalities noted on CT or MRI or suspicious mucosal lesions observed during endoscopy.

A subset of patients will have the primary tumor site discovered at direct laryngoscopy. The likelihood of discovering the primary site is related to whether or not a suspected (but not definite) primary site is discovered on physical examination and/or radiographic evaluation (Table 36-3).[12] The majority of suspected primary sites are detected by pretreatment radiographic workup as opposed to physical examination.

An ipsilateral[12,15] tonsillectomy should be performed in patients who have not had a prior tonsillectomy and who have adequate lymphoid tissue remaining in the tonsillar fossa. Although some authors recommend a bilateral tonsillectomy,[16] the likelihood of finding the primary site in the contralateral tonsil for patients with ipsilateral neck nodes is probably quite low. Lapeyre and colleagues[15] reported 87 patients who were evaluated between 1969 and 1992 and underwent a unilateral tonsillectomy; 26% of patients were found to have a tonsillar cancer. Thirty-four of 130 patients who were evaluated at the University of Florida underwent a tonsillectomy at the time of direct laryngoscopy; the primary site was detected in the tonsil in 12 patients (35%).[12] The likelihood of detecting the primary site was related to whether there were suspicious findings on physical examination and/or radiographic evaluation (see Table 36-3).[12]

Fifty-eight primary head and neck cancers were found in 56 of 130 patients (43%) in the University of Florida series. The

Table 36-1 Diagnostic Workup

GENERAL
History
Physical examination
Careful examination of the neck and supraclavicular regions
Examination of oral cavity, pharynx, and larynx (indirect laryngoscopy with a flexible endoscope)

RADIOGRAPHIC STUDIES
Chest roentgenogram
Computed tomography and/or magnetic resonance imaging scans of head and neck (special attention to nasopharynx, pharynx, and larynx)

LABORATORY STUDIES
Complete blood cell count
Blood chemistry profile

DIRECT ENDOSCOPY AND DIRECTED BIOPSIES
Nasopharynx, both tonsils, base of tongue, both piriform sinuses, and any suspicious or abnormal mucosal areas
Ipsilateral tonsillectomy
Fine-needle aspirate or core needle biopsy of the cervical node

From Mendenhall WM, Parsons JT, Mancuso AA, et al: Head and neck: management of the neck. *In* Perez CA, Brady LW (eds). Principles and Practice of Radiation Oncology, 3rd ed. Philadelphia, JB Lippincott, 1998, pp 1135-1156.

Table 36-2 Biopsy-Proved Primary Site Versus ^{18}F-fluorodeoxyglucose (FDG) Single-Photon Emission Computed Tomography (SPECT) Findings (No. of Patients With Biopsy-Proved Primary Site/No. of Patients Having FDG-SPECT Study)

Patient Group	FDG-SPECT∅	FDG-SPECT⊕
PE∅/RAD∅	No data	1/5*
PE⊕ and/or RAD⊕	2/4	6†/15* (40%)
Total	2/4	7/20 (35%)

*p = .4058.
†Two of six patients had a positive FDG-SPECT, a negative head and neck CT, and suggestive findings on physical examination.
FDG/SPECT∅, no evidence of a primary site; FDG-SPECT⊕, findings suggestive of a primary site; PE∅/RAD∅, no evidence of a primary site on physical examination or radiographic studies; PE⊕ and/or RAD⊕, findings suggestive of a primary site on physical examination, radiographic studies (CT and/or magnetic resonance imaging), or both.
From Mendenhall WM, Mancuso AA, Parsons JT, et al: Diagnostic evaluation of squamous cell carcinoma metastatic to cervical lymph nodes from an unknown head and neck primary site. Head Neck 20:739-744, 1998[12] (Table 2, p 742).

Table 36-3 Biopsy-Proved Primary Site Versus Physical and Radiographic Findings and Number of Panendoscopies (No. of Patients With Biopsy-Proved Primary Site/No. Patients Evaluated)*

Patient Group	No. of Panendoscopies 1	2	3	Total Patients
PE∅/RAD∅	6/34 (18%)	0/7	1/1	7/42 (17%)
PE∅/RAD⊕	19/34 (56%)	9/21 (43%)	1/1	29†/56 (52%)
PE⊕/RAD∅	4/6	1/3	No data	5/9 (56%)
PE⊕/RAD⊕	11/16 (69%)	4/7	No data	15‡/23 (65%)
Total	40/90 (44%)	14/38 (37%)	2/2	56/130 (43%)

*Significance levels: 7/42 versus 34/65, p = .00023; 7/42 versus 15/23, p = .00012; 34/65 versus 15/23, p = .20413.
†One of 29 patients had a positive FDG-SPECT scan and a negative CT of the head and neck; the remaining 28 patients had a positive CT and/or MR scan.
‡Two of 15 patients had a positive FDG-SPECT scan and a negative CT of the head and neck; the remaining 13 patients had a positive CT and/or MR scan.
PE∅, no suggestive findings on physical examination; PE⊕, suggestive of a primary site, but not definitely positive; RAD∅, no suggestive findings on radiographic studies; RAD⊕, radiographic studies suggestive of primary site.
From Mendenhall WM, Mancuso AA, Parsons JT, et al: Diagnostic evaluation of squamous cell carcinoma metastatic to cervical lymph nodes from an unknown head and neck primary. Head Neck 20:739-744, 1998[12] (Table 1, p 741).

primary sites included tonsillar fossa, 25 patients (45%); base of tongue, 23 (41%); pyriform sinus, 5 (9%); posterior pharyngeal wall, 2 (4%); lateral pharyngeal wall, 1 (2%); vallecula, 1 (2%); and lingual surface of the suprahyoid epiglottis, 1 (2%). Most of the primary cancers detected are in the tonsillar fossa or base of tongue, which is in contrast to earlier reports, where a significant number of primary sites were found in the nasopharynx and hypopharynx.[7,17,18] The reason for the decreased likelihood of detecting cancers in these sites may be that they are found on physical examination with fiberoptic endoscopy and on radiographic evaluation. In contrast, it is still very difficult to discern a small primary cancer hidden in the lymphoid tissue of the tonsillar fossa or tongue base.

Treatment Techniques

Treatment options range from treatment of the involved neck alone with a neck dissection and/or radiotherapy to irradiation of the suspected primary site and both sides of the neck followed by evaluation for a planned neck dissection.[19,20] Although treatment of the potential mucosal primary site and contralateral neck appears to reduce the risk of a locoregional recurrence, the impact on survival is modest at best. Therefore, patients with a single positive node without extracapsular extension may be treated with a neck dissection alone and followed closely provided that the neck was not violated with an open procedure prior to surgery.[21-23]

If radiotherapy is indicated to treat the involved neck, we usually irradiate the nasopharynx and oropharynx, as well as both sides of the neck (Fig. 36-1A).[1] Although it may be tempting to irradiate the involved neck alone or combined with radiotherapy to the ipsilateral mucosal sites deemed to be at risk, the base of tongue is a midline structure that probably harbors the undetected primary site as often as the tonsillar fossa, so it has been our policy to treat the entire oropharynx. Failure to do so is likely associated with an increased risk of a locoregional recurrence and further radiotherapy would be complicated by the initial treatment.[24] It is not necessary to irradiate the oral cavity unless the patient has submandibular adenopathy, in which case we either do a neck dissection and observe the patient or irradiate the oral cavity and oropharynx. At one time, it was our policy to irradiate the larynx and hypopharynx, but because the likelihood of a primary tumor in these sites is low, and because the morbidity of irradiating these areas is significant, we modified our technique several years ago. It could be argued that the nasopharynx should also be eliminated from the primary treatment portals. However,

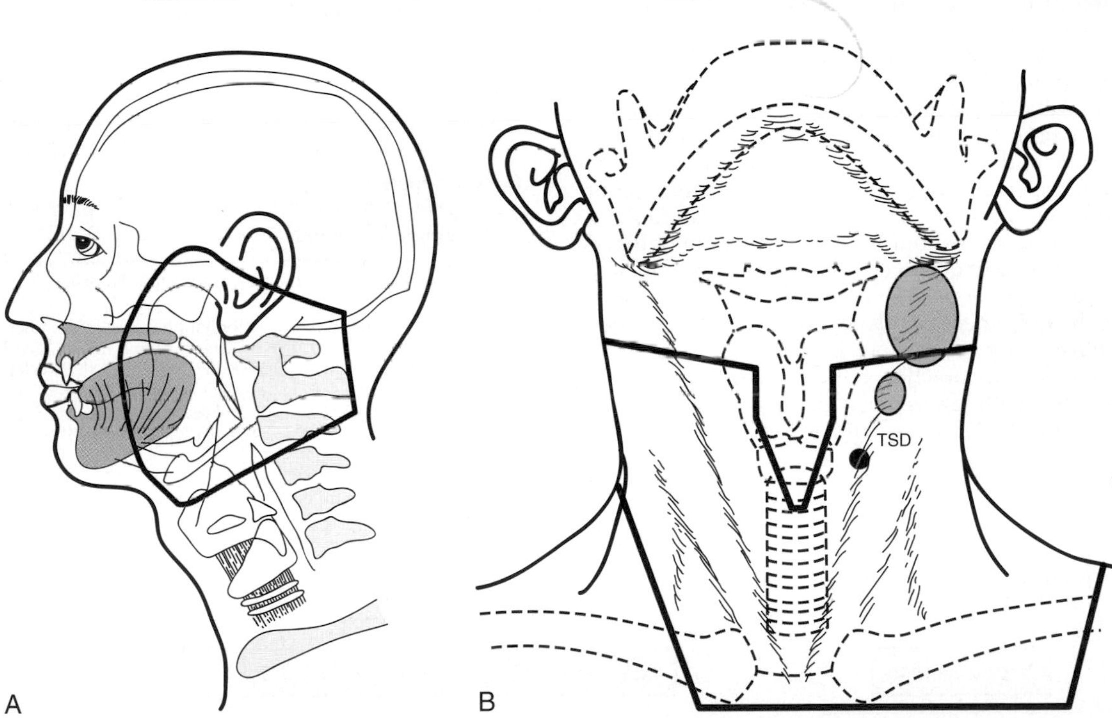

Figure 36-1 **A,** Radiation treatment technique for carcinoma from an unknown primary site. Superiorly, the portal treats the nasopharynx and the jugular and spinal accessory lymph nodes to the base of the skull. The posterior border is behind the spinous process of C2. The inferior border is at the thyroid notch. Anteroinferiorly, the skin and subcutaneous tissues of the submentum are shielded, except in the case of advanced neck disease. The anterior tongue margin is set to obtain a 2-cm margin on the base of the tongue and tonsillar fossa, as well as the nasopharynx. One portal reduction is shown (reduction off the spinal cord). **B,** Fields for bilateral lower neck radiotherapy. The larynx shield should be carefully designed. Because the internal jugular vein lymph nodes lie adjacent to the posterolateral margin of the thyroid cartilage, the shield cannot cover the entire thyroid cartilage without producing a low-dose area in these nodes. A common error in the treatment of the lower neck is to extend the low neck portal laterally out to the shoulders, encompassing lateral supraclavicular lymph nodes that are at negligible risk while partially shielding the high-risk midjugular lymph nodes with a large rectangular laryngeal block. The inferior extent of the shield is at the cricoid cartilage or first or second tracheal ring; the shield must be tapered because the nodes tend to lie closer to the midline as the lower neck is approached. Lateral borders of the low-neck portals are set to cover only the lymph nodes in the root of the neck when the risk of low-neck disease on that side is small (i.e., stage N0 or N1 disease). If there are clinically positive lymph nodes in the lower neck or if major disease exists in the upper neck, the lateral border of the low-neck field is widened on that side to cover the entire supraclavicular region out to the junction of the trapezius muscle with the clavicle. (**A,** From Mendenhall WM, Mancuso AA, Amdur RJ, et al: Squamous cell carcinoma metastatic to the neck from an unknown head and neck primary site. Am J Otolaryngol 22:264, 2001; B, from Million RR, Cassisi NJ, Mancuso AA, et al. Management of the neck for squamous cell carcinoma. *In* Million RR, Cassisi NJ [eds]: Management of Head and Neck Cancer: A Multidisciplinary Approach, 2nd ed. Philadelphia, Lippincott Williams & Wilkins, 1994, p 135.)

the incidence of positive retropharyngeal nodes is relatively high in patients presenting with advanced neck disease[25] so that the portals must include the skull base (jugular foramen and retropharyngeal nodes) and at least part of the nasopharynx. It is our belief that a modest increase in the size of the portals to adequately irradiate the nasopharynx does not significantly increase morbidity.

Patients are treated with parallel-opposed fields at 1.8 Gy/fraction to a midline dose of 64.8 Gy with reduction off the spinal cord at 45-Gy tumor dose (see Fig. 36-1B).[26] The lower neck is treated through a separate en face anterior field. Treatment is administered with Co^{60}, 4-MV x-rays, or 6-MV x-rays. Dosimetry is obtained at the level of the central axis (which usually corresponds to the oropharynx) and the nasopharynx. The dose to the nasopharynx is usually 3 to 5 Gy lower than the central axis. Patients with advanced, fixed adenopathy undergo a boost to the involved part of the neck using anteroposterior wedged beams to a total dose in the range of 70 to 75 Gy. Concomitant chemotherapy should be considered for patients with advanced N2 and N3 neck disease. Our preference is to use weekly cisplatin (30 mg/m^2) or low-dose weekly carboplatin and paclitaxel.[27]

Treatment of the neck depends on the extent and location of the adenopathy. Patients with N1 and early N2B neck disease located in the high-dose fields may be treated with irradiation alone if the nodes have resolved completely.[28-31] Similarly, if the patient has undergone an excisional biopsy of a single positive node, the neck may be treated with radiation alone with a 95% likelihood of neck control.[32] Patients undergo a CT scan of the neck 1 month after completing radiotherapy at our institution, and the decision whether to proceed with neck dissection depends on the likelihood that viable tumor remains in the neck.[33] The criteria used for determining whether a neck dissection should be performed are outlined in Table 36-4.[33] Because the likelihood of cure is low if a regional recurrence develops in a clinically positive neck after treatment with radiotherapy alone, we usually proceed with a modified neck dissection if the risk of residual disease exceeds 5%.[34] In practice, patients with N2-N3 neck disease and those with gross neck disease after an open neck biopsy usually undergo a planned neck dissection after radiation therapy.[30,35] The treatment algorithm is depicted in Figure 36-2.

RESULTS

A total of 136 patients were treated at the M. D. Anderson Hospital between 1968 and 1992 and had a median duration of follow-up of 8.7 years.[36] Both sides of the neck and potential head and neck mucosal primary sites were irradiated. A mucosal head and neck cancer developed in 14 patients (10%); 6 of the 14 cancers were located in unirradiated sites. Recurrent disease in the neck developed in 12 patients (9%). The 5-year cause-specific survival rate was 74%.

Table 36-4 Univariate Analysis: Frequency of Positive Surgical Specimen in 113 Heminecks in Relation to Variables on Computed Tomography Findings

Variables	Negative Specimen	Positive Specimen	p (χ^2)
Size of lymph nodes*			
≤15 mm	41 (78.8%)	11 (21.2%)	.015
>15 mm	35 (57.4%)	26 (42.6%)	
Focal defect†			
No (grade 0 or 1)	34 (97.1%)	1 (2.9%)	.001
Yes (grade 2, 3, or 4)	42 (53.8%)	36 (46.2)	
Capsular rupture‡			
No (grade 0 or 1)	42 (87.5%)	6 (12.5%)	.001
Yes (grade 2, 3, or 4)	34 (52.3%)	31 (47.7%)	

*Largest dimension of the largest lymph node in each hemineck on axial images.
†Highest grade of focal defect of lymph nodes in each hemineck.
‡Highest grade of capsular rupture of lymph nodes in each hemineck.
From Ojiri H, Mendenhall WM, Stringer SP, et al: Post-RT CT results as a predictive model for the necessity of planned post-RT neck dissection in patients with cervical metastatic disease from squamous cell carcinoma. Int J Radiat Oncol Biol Phys 52:420-428, 2002[40] (Table 5, p 425).

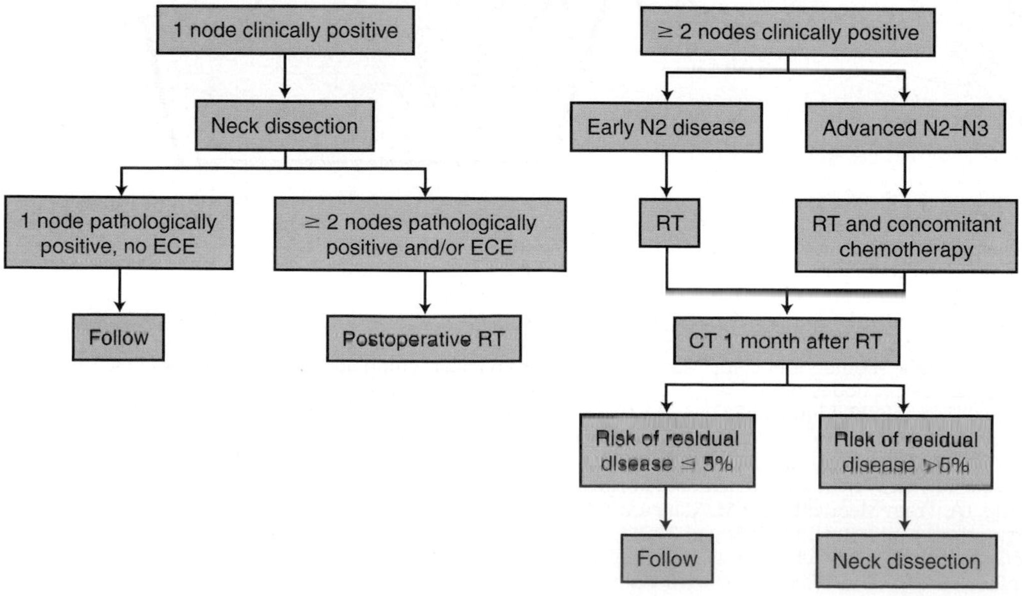

Figure 36-2 Treatment algorithm. ECE, extracapsular extension; RT, radiotherapy; CT, computed tomography.

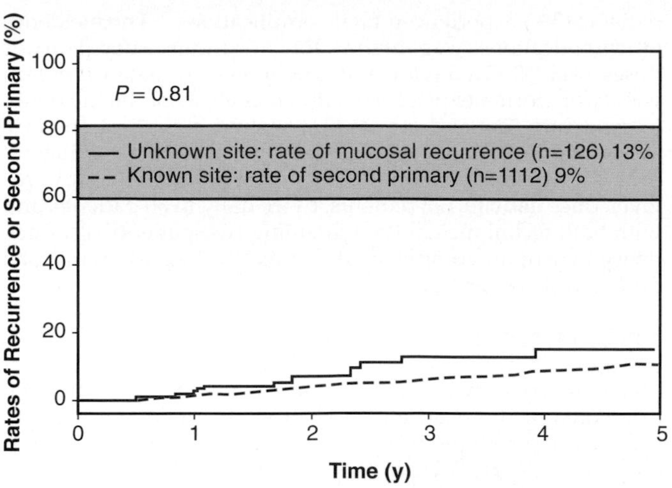

Figure 36-3 The rate of developing carcinomas in head and neck mucosal sites for patients treated for carcinomas with an unknown head and neck mucosal site compared with the rate for developing metachronous carcinomas in head and neck mucosal sites for patients treated for carcinomas with a known head and neck mucosal site. (From Erkal HS, Mendenhall WM, Amdur RJ, et al: Squamous cell carcinomas metastatic to cervical lymph nodes from an unknown head-and-neck mucosal site treated with radiation therapy alone or in combination with neck dissection. Int J Radiat Oncol Biol Phys 50:58, 2001.)

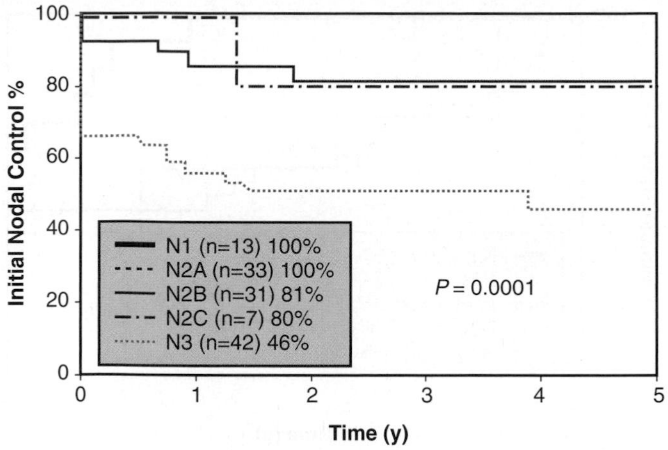

Figure 36-4 Nodal control rates according to N stage after initial treatment. (From Erkal HS, Mendenhall WM, Amdur RJ, et al: Squamous cell carcinomas metastatic to cervical lymph nodes from an unknown head-and-neck mucosal site treated with radiation therapy alone or in combination with neck dissection. Int J Radiat Oncol Biol Phys 50:58, 2001.)

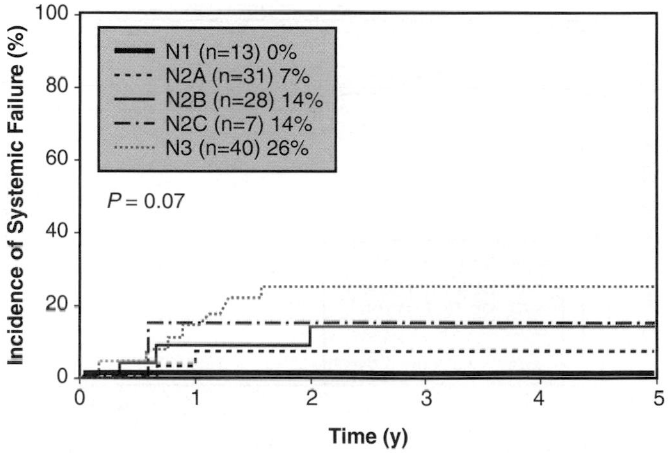

Figure 36-5 Distant metastases rates according to N stage after treatment. (From Erkal HS, Mendenhall WM, Amdur RJ, et al: Squamous cell carcinomas metastatic to cervical lymph nodes from an unknown head-and-neck mucosal site treated with radiation therapy alone or in combination with neck dissection. Int J Radiat Oncol Biol Phys 50:59, 2001.)

The incidence of subsequent mucosal primary lesions was compared by Erkal and coworkers[37] for patients with a known primary site and a series of 126 patients treated for an unknown primary site at the University of Florida. The incidence for both groups was similar at 5 years, suggesting either that mucosal irradiation significantly reduced the risk of primary site failure or that patients with unknown primary sites have a much lower risk of a second primary head and neck cancer developing subsequently (Fig. 36-3).[37] The 5-year absolute and cause-specific survival rates for the 126 patients with an unknown primary were 47% and 67%, respectively. The 5-year outcomes stratified by stage are shown in Figures 36-4 through 36-7.[37]

Reddy and Marks[24] reported 52 patients treated to the neck alone (16 patients) or to the neck and potential head and neck primary sites (36 patients). Failure in the head and neck mucosa occurred in 44% of those who underwent treatment to the neck alone, compared with 8% in those who underwent irradiation of the head and neck mucosa ($p = .0005$). The 5-year survival rates were similar for the two treatment groups.

Grau and colleagues[38] reported 273 patients treated with curative intent at five cancer centers in Denmark between 1975 and 1995 with surgery alone (23 patients), radiotherapy to the ipsilateral neck alone or combined with surgery (26 patients), and radiotherapy to the neck and head and neck mucosa alone or combined with surgery (224 patients). The ipsilateral oropharynx unintentionally received some irradiation in patients treated to the ipsilateral neck alone, depending on the treatment technique.[38] The 5-year rates of freedom from failure in the head and neck mucosa were as follows: surgery alone, 45%; radiotherapy with or without surgery to the ipsilateral neck, 77%; and radiotherapy to the head and neck mucosa with or without surgery, 87%. Failure in the oropharynx, particularly the base of tongue, was the most common location of mucosal site failure.

Complications

The main complication of radiation therapy for patients treated for an unknown head and neck primary tumor is xerostomia. Intensity-modulated radiation therapy (IMRT) may be used to reduce the dose to the contralateral parotid gland so long as the patient does not have bilateral clinically positive neck nodes. It is difficult to limit the dose to the parotid if there are positive nodes in the same side of the neck without risking underdosing the adenopathy and increasing the risk of a marginal miss. The risk of bone exposure, radiation myelitis, and/or radiation-induced malignancy is very low.

The complications of neck irradiation include subcutaneous fibrosis and lymphedema of the larynx and submentum. The latter complications may be minimized by sparing an anterior strip of skin when designing the parallel-opposed

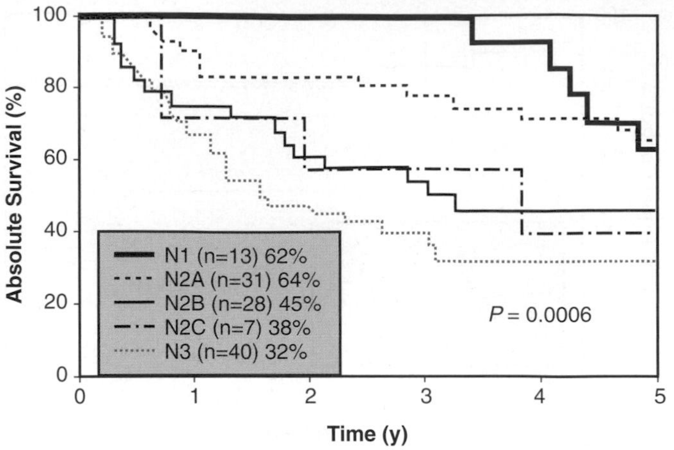

Figure 36-6 Absolute survival rates according to N stage after treatment. (From Erkal HS, Mendenhall WM, Amdur RJ, et al: Squamous cell carcinomas metastatic to cervical lymph nodes from an unknown head-and-neck mucosal site treated with radiation therapy alone or in combination with neck dissection. Int J Radiat Oncol Biol Phys 50:59, 2001.)

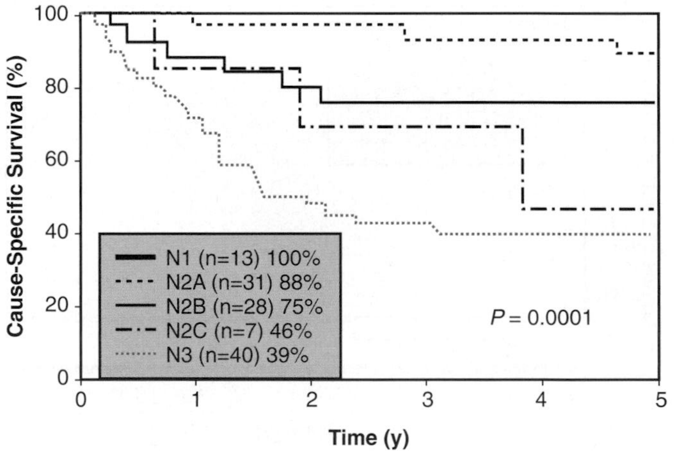

Figure 36-7 Cause-specific survival rates according to N stage after treatment. (From Erkal HS, Mendenhall WM, Amdur RJ, et al: Squamous cell carcinomas metastatic to cervical lymph nodes from an unknown head-and-neck mucosal site treated with radiation therapy alone or in combination with neck dissection. Int J Radiat Oncol Biol Phys 50:60, 2001.)

lateral portals used to encompass the primary lesion. This will also reduce the risk of desquamation, particularly in patients who receive concomitant chemotherapy. A 5-mm-wide midline block in the en face low-neck field may also diminish the likelihood of postirradiation edema. The probability of complications is directly related to radiation dose and volume.

Complications of neck dissection include hematoma, seroma, lymphedema, wound infection, wound dehiscence, chyle fistula, damage to cranial nerves VII, X, XI, and XII, carotid exposure, and carotid rupture. The incidence of complications after neck dissection is probably higher when the operation follows a course of radiation therapy.

The incidence of postoperative complications in a series of 143 patients treated with radiation to the primary lesion and neck followed by unilateral neck dissection was 23%.[30] Seventeen patients (12%) required a second operation and four patients (3%) experienced fatal complications.[30] The incidence of complications was higher for maximum subcutaneous doses over 60 Gy. Taylor and coworkers[39] updated the University of Florida experience with an analysis of the incidence of moderate (2+) and severe (3+) wound complications in a series of 205 patients who underwent a planned unilateral neck dissection after radiation therapy. Radiation therapy was given once daily in 123 patients, twice daily in 80 patients, and with both techniques in the remaining two patients. The incidence of wound complications tended to increase with total dose and dose per fraction.

CONCLUSION

The diagnostic evaluation of patients with squamous cell carcinoma of the head and neck from an unknown primary site includes multiple head and neck examinations by experienced examiners, FNA of the neck node, CT from the skull base to the clavicles, direct laryngoscopy and biopsies, and an ipsilateral tonsillectomy. The primary site will be detected in approximately 40% of patients and will be located in the oropharynx in over 80% of patients. The management of these patients is controversial. Treatment usually includes irradiation of both sides of the neck and the potential mucosal primary sites. The likelihood of 5-year survival is approximately 50% and is related to the extent of disease in the neck.

ACKNOWLEDGMENT

The authors thank the research support staff of the Department of Radiation Oncology for their help in statistics, editing, and manuscript preparation.

REFERENCES

1. Mendenhall WM, Mancuso AA, Amdur RJ, et al: Squamous cell carcinoma metastatic to the neck from an unknown head and neck primary site. Am J Otolaryngol 22:261-267, 2001.
2. DelCharco JO, Mendenhall WM, Parsons JT, et al: Carcinoma of the skin metastatic to the parotid area lymph nodes. Head Neck 20:369-373, 1998.
3. McGuirt WF, McCabe BF: Significance of node biopsy before definitive treatment of cervical metastatic carcinoma. Laryngoscope 88:594-597, 1978.
4. Parsons JT, Million RR, Cassisi NJ: The influence of excisional or incisional biopsy of metastatic neck nodes on the management of head and neck cancer. Int J Radiat Oncol Biol Phys 11:1447-1454, 1985.
5. Ellis ER, Mendenhall WM, Rao PV, et al: Incisional or excisional neck-node biopsy before definitive radiotherapy, alone or followed by neck dissection. Head Neck 13:177-183, 1991.
6. Robbins KT, Cole R, Marvel J, et al: The violated neck: cervical node biopsy prior to definitive treatment. Otolaryngol Clin North Am 94:605-610, 1986.
7. Martin H, Morfit HM: Cervical lymph node metastasis as the first symptom of cancer. Surg Gynecol Obstet 76:133-159, 1944.
8. Macdonald MR, Freeman JL, Hui MF, et al: Role of Epstein-Barr virus in fine-needle aspirates of metastatic neck nodes in the diagnosis of nasopharyngeal carcinoma. Head Neck 17:487-493, 1995.
9. Al-Othman MOF, Morris CG, Hinerman RW, et al: Distant metastases after definitive radiotherapy for squamous cell carcinoma of the head and neck. Head Neck 25:629-633, 2003.
10. Mendenhall WM, Parsons JT, Mancuso AA, et al: Head and neck: management of the neck. *In* Perez CA, Brady LW (eds): Principles

and Practice of Radiation Oncology, 3rd ed. Philadelphia, Lippincott-Raven, 1998, pp 1135-1156.

11. Mukherji SK, Drane WE, Mancuso AA, et al: Occult primary tumors of the head and neck: detection with 2-[F-18] fluoro-2-deoxy-D-glucose SPECT. Radiology 199:761-766, 1996.
12. Mendenhall WM, Mancuso AA, Parsons JT, et al: Diagnostic evaluation of squamous cell carcinoma metastatic to cervical lymph nodes from an unknown head and neck primary site. Head Neck 20:739-744, 1998.
13. Greven KM, Keyes JW Jr, Williams DW III, et al: Occult primary tumors of the head and neck. Lack of benefit from positron emission tomography imaging with 2-[F-18]fluoro-2-deoxy-D-glucose. Cancer 86:114-118, 1999.
14. Safa AA, Tran LM, Rege S, et al: The role of positron emission tomography in occult primary head and neck cancers. Cancer J Sci Am 5:214-218, 1999.
15. Lapeyre M, Malissard L, Peiffert D, et al: Cervical lymph node metastasis from an unknown primary: is a tonsillectomy necessary? Int J Radiat Oncol Biol Phys 39:291-296, 1997.
16. McQuone SJ, Eisele DW, Lee D-J, et al: Occult tonsillar carcinoma in the unknown primary. Laryngoscope 108:1605-1610, 1998.
17. Fletcher GH, Jesse RH, Healey JE Jr, Thoma GW Jr: Oropharynx. *In* MacComb WS, Fletcher GH (eds): Cancer of the Head and Neck. Baltimore, Williams & Wilkins, 1967, pp 179-212.
18. Jones AS, Cook JA, Phillips DE, et al: Squamous carcinoma presenting as an enlarged cervical lymph node. Cancer 72:1756-1761, 1993.
19. Coster JR, Foote RL, Olsen KD, et al: Cervical nodal metastasis of squamous cell carcinoma of unknown origin: indications for withholding radiation therapy. Int J Radiat Oncol Biol Phys 23:743-749, 1992.
20. Weir L, Keane T, Cummings B, et al: Radiation treatment of cervical lymph node metastases from an unknown primary: an analysis of outcome by treatment volume and other prognostic factors. Radiother Oncol 35:206-211, 1995.
21. Olsen KD, Caruso M, Foote RL, et al: Primary head and neck cancer. Histopathologic predictors of recurrence after neck dissection in patients with lymph node involvement. Arch Otolaryngol Head Neck Surg 120:1370-1374, 1994.
22. Huang DT, Johnson CR, Schmidt-Ullrich R, Grimes M: Postoperative radiotherapy in head and neck carcinoma with extracapsular lymph node extension and/or positive resection margins: a comparative study. Int J Radiat Oncol Biol Phys 23:737-742, 1992.
23. Mendenhall WM, Amdur RJ, Hinerman RW, et al: Postoperative radiation therapy for squamous cell carcinoma of the head and neck. Am J Otolaryngol 24:41-50, 2003.
24. Reddy SP, Marks JE: Metastatic carcinoma in the cervical lymph nodes from an unknown primary site: results of bilateral neck plus mucosal irradiation vs. ipsilateral neck irradiation. Int J Radiat Oncol Biol Phys 37:797-802, 1997.
25. McLaughlin MP, Mendenhall WM, Mancuso AA, et al: Retropharyngeal adenopathy as a predictor of outcome in squamous cell carcinoma of the head and neck. Head Neck 17:190-198, 1995.
26. Million RR, Cassisi NJ, Mancuso AA, et al: Management of the neck for squamous cell carcinoma. *In* Million RR, Cassisi NJ (eds): Management of Head and Neck Cancer: A Multidisciplinary Approach, 2nd ed. Philadelphia, JB Lippincott, 1994, pp 75-142.
27. Mendenhall WM, Riggs CE, Amdur RJ, et al: Altered fractionation and/or adjuvant chemotherapy in definitive irradiation of squamous cell carcinoma of the head and neck. Laryngoscope 113:546-551, 2003.
28. Peters LJ, Weber RS, Morrison WH, et al: Neck surgery in patients with primary oropharyngeal cancer treated by radiotherapy. Head Neck 18:552-559, 1996.
29. Johnson CR, Silverman LN, Clay LB, Schmidt-Ullrich R: Radiotherapeutic management of bulky cervical lymphadenopathy in squamous cell carcinoma of the head and neck: is postradiotherapy neck dissection necessary? Radiat Oncol Investig 6:52-57, 1998.
30. Mendenhall WM, Million RR, Cassisi NJ: Squamous cell carcinoma of the head and neck treated with radiation therapy: the role of neck dissection for clinically positive neck nodes. Int J Radiat Oncol Biol Phys 12:733-740, 1986.
31. Mendenhall WM, Parsons JT, Stringer SP, et al: Squamous cell carcinoma of the head and neck treated with irradiation: management of the neck. Semin Radiat Oncol 2:163-170, 1992.
32. Mack Y, Parsons JT, Mendenhall WM, et al: Squamous cell carcinoma of the head and neck: management after excisional biopsy of a solitary metastatic neck node. Int J Radiat Oncol Biol Phys 25:619-622, 1993.
33. Ojiri H, Mancuso AA, Mendenhall WM, Stringer SP: Lymph nodes of patients with regional metastases from head and neck squamous cell carcinoma as a predictor of pathologic outcome: size changes at CT before and after radiation therapy. Am J Neuroradiol 23:1012-1018, 2002.
34. Mendenhall WM, Villaret DB, Amdur RJ, et al: Planned neck dissection after definitive radiotherapy for squamous cell carcinoma of the head and neck. Head Neck 24:1012-1018, 2002.
35. Brizel DM, Prosnitz RG, Hunter S, et al: Necessity for adjuvant neck dissection is setting of concurrent chemoradiation for advanced head-and-neck cancer. Int J Radiat Oncol Biol Phys 58:1418-1423, 2004.
36. Colletier PJ, Garden AS, Morrison WH, et al: Postoperative radiation for squamous cell carcinoma metastatic to cervical lymph nodes from an unknown primary site: outcomes and patterns of failure. Head Neck 20:674-681, 1998.
37. Erkal HS, Mendenhall WM, Amdur RJ, et al: Squamous cell carcinomas metastatic to cervical lymph nodes from an unknown head-and-neck mucosal site treated with radiation therapy alone or in combination with neck dissection. Int J Radiat Oncol Biol Phys 50:55-63, 2001.
38. Grau C, Johansen LV, Jakobsen J, et al: Cervical lymph node metastases from unknown primary tumours: results from a national survey by the Danish Society for Head and Neck Oncology. Radiother Oncol 55:121-129, 2000.
39. Taylor JMG, Mendenhall WM, Parsons JT, Lavey RS: The influence of dose and time on wound complications following post-radiation neck dissection. Int J Radiat Oncol Biol Phys 23:41-46, 1992.
40. Ojiri H, Mendenhall WM, Stringer SP, et al: Post-RT CT results as a predictive model for the necessity of planned post-RT neck dissection in patients with cervical metastatic disease from squamous cell carcinoma. Int J Radiat Oncol Biol Phys 52:420-428, 2002.

CHAPTER 37

MANAGEMENT OF THE NECK

Vincent Grégoire, Thierry Duprez, Benoit Lengelé and Marc Hamoir

Assessment and treatment of regional lymph nodes (LNs) in the neck are of utmost importance in the management of patients with head and neck squamous cell carcinoma (SCC). The philosophy of treatment of the neck has evolved over the past decades. Radiation oncologists and head and neck surgeons progressively realized that extensive treatments were associated with more morbidity but not always with a better oncologic outcome than less extensive procedures. Today, a comprehensive approach of the treatment of the neck needs to be multidisciplinary, taking into account the quality of life of the patients but without jeopardizing cure and survival. A better understanding of the patterns of LN metastasis promoted the use of not only selective dissection but also selective irradiation in selected patients. Concepts are still evolving, for example, with the sentinel LN biopsy (SNB), for which the exact role is under evaluation.

In this chapter, only the management of the neck for oral cavity, oropharyngeal, hypopharyngeal, and laryngeal SCC is discussed.

ANATOMY OF THE LYMPHATIC SYSTEM OF THE NECK

The head and neck region has a rich network of lymphatic vessels draining from the base of the skull through the jugular nodes, the spinal accessory nodes, and the transverse cervical nodes to the venous jugulosubclavian confluent or the thoracic duct on the left side and the lymphatic duct on the right side.[1,2] A comprehensive anatomic description of this network was made by Rouvière more than 50 years ago.[1] The whole lymphatic system of the neck is contained in the celluloadipose tissue delineated by aponeurosis enveloping the muscles, the vessels, and the nerves (Fig. 37-1). The lymphatic drainage is mainly ipsilateral, but structures like the soft palate, the tonsils, the base of the tongue, the posterior pharyngeal wall, and especially the nasopharynx have bilateral drainage. On the other hand, sites such as the true vocal cord, the paranasal sinuses, and the middle ear have few or no lymphatic vessels at all.

The nomenclature of head and neck LNs has been complicated by various confusing synonyms that are still in use in major textbooks and articles. Several expert bodies have proposed the adoption of systematic classifications aimed at standardizing the terminology. Following the description by Rouvière, the TNM atlas proposed a terminology, dividing the head and neck LNs into 12 groups.[3] In parallel to this classification, the Committee for Head and Neck Surgery and Oncology of the American Academy for Otolaryngology–Head and Neck Surgery has been working on a classification (the so-called Robbins classification), dividing the neck into six levels including eight node groups.[4] This classification is based on the description of a level system that has been used for a long time by the Head and Neck Service at the Memorial Sloan-Kettering Cancer Center (MSKCC).[5] As one of the objectives of the Robbins classification was to develop a standardized system of terminology for neck dissection procedures, only the LN groups routinely removed during neck dissection were considered. The terminology proposed by Robbins was recommended by the UICC.[6] A comparison between the TNM and the Robbins terminology is shown in Table 37-1. The major advantage of the Robbins classification over the TNM terminology is the definition of the boundaries of the node levels. The delineation of these boundaries is based on anatomic structures such as major blood vessels, muscles, nerves, bones, and cartilage that are easily identifiable by the surgeon during neck dissection procedures. The orientation of these anatomic boundaries refers to a patient lying in a supine position with his neck in a surgical position, that is, in hyperextension, to better individualize the anatomic structures.

Level Ia is a unique median region that contains the submental nodes. The LNs are located in a triangular region limited anteriorly by the platysma muscle, posteriorly by the mylohyoid muscles, cranially by the symphysis of the mandible, caudally by the hyoid bone, and laterally by the anterior belly of the digastric muscle. The medial limit of level Ia is virtual, as the region continues into the contralateral level Ia. Nodes in level Ia drain the skin of the chin, the mid lower lip, the tip of the tongue, and the anterior floor of the mouth. Level Ia is at greatest risk for harboring metastases from cancer arising from the floor of the mouth, the anterior oral tongue, the anterior mandibular alveolar ridge, and the lower lip.

Level Ib contains the submandibular nodes. It is located within the boundaries of the anterior and posterior belly of the digastric muscle, the stylohyoid muscle, and the body of the mandible. It is limited anteriorly by the stylohyoid muscle, posteriorly by a vertical plane defined by the spinal accessory nerve (SAN), medially (deeply) by the anterior belly of the digastric muscle, and laterally (superficially) by the basilar border of the mandible. Cranially, it is limited by the basilar border of the mandible, and caudally, by the posterior belly of the digastric muscle. The submandibular nodes receive efferent lymphatics from the submental LNs, the medial canthus, the lower nasal cavity, the hard and soft palate, the maxillary and mandibular alveolar ridges, the cheek, the upper and lower lips, and most of the anterior tongue. Nodes in level Ib are at risk for developing metastases from cancers of the oral cavity, anterior nasal cavity, soft tissue structures of the midface, and the submandibular gland.

Level II contains the upper jugular LNs located around the upper one third of the internal jugular vein (IJV) and the upper spinal accessory nerve (SAN). It extends from the level of the skull base to the carotid bifurcation (surgical landmark) or the caudal border of the body of the hyoid bone (clinical landmark). Level II is limited cranially by the insertion of the posterior belly of the digastric muscle to the mastoid, caudally by the caudal border of the body of the hyoid bone, anteriorly by the stylohyoid muscle, posteriorly by the posterior edge of the sternocleidomastoid muscle (SCM), medially by the carotid artery and the paravertebral muscles (levator scapulae and splenius capitis), and laterally by the SCM and the platysma. Level II is further subdivided into two compartments. The LNs located anterior to a vertical plane defined by the upper third of the SAN are included in level IIa, whereas the LNs

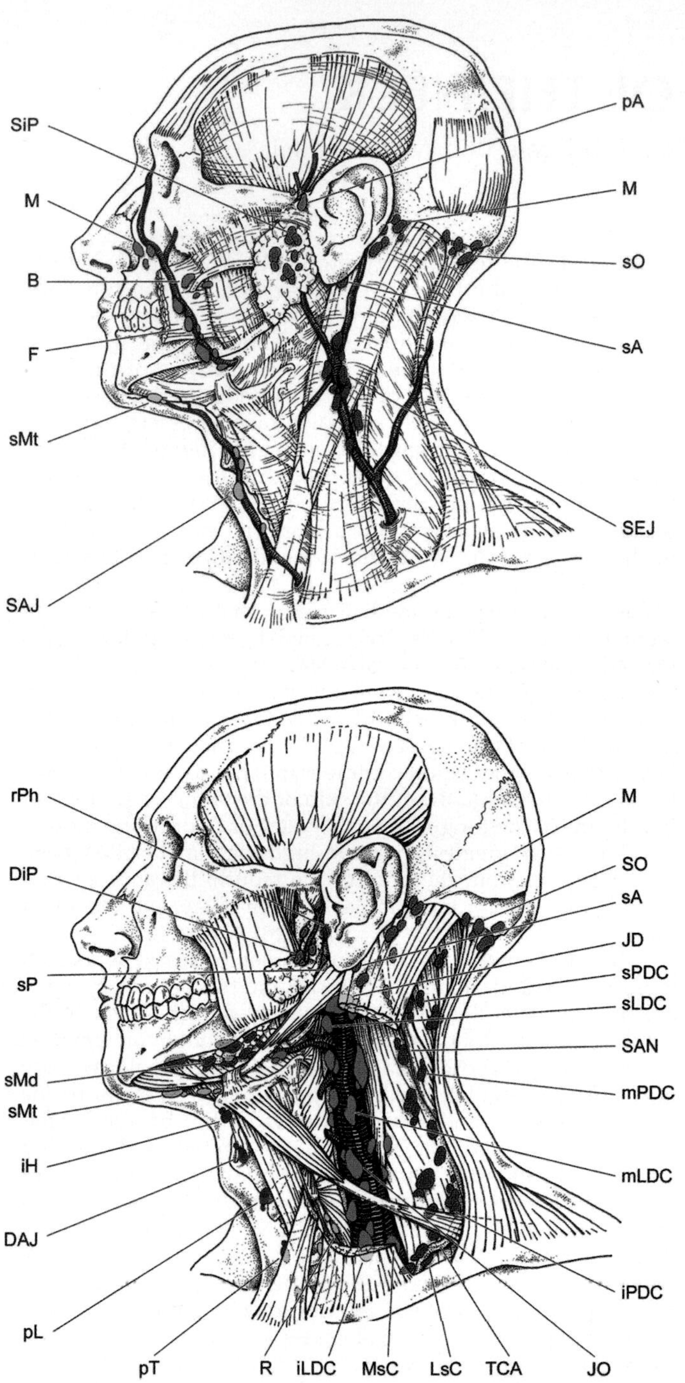

Figure 37-1 Lymphatic nodes of the head and neck. Lateral view of the superficial and deep node groups of the cervicocephalic region. B, buccal nerve; DAJ, deep anterior jugular nerve; DiP, deep intraparotid nerve; F, facial nerve; iH, infrahyoid nerve; JD, jugulodigastric nerve (Kütner's nerve); JO, jugulo-omohyoid nerve (Poirier's nerve); LDC, superior (s), middle (m), and inferior (i) lateral deep cervical nerves; LsC, lateral supraclavicular nerve; M, malar nerve; MsC, medial supraclavicular nerve; PDC, superior (s), middle (m), and inferior (i) posterior deep cervical nerves; M, mastoid nerve; pA, preauricular nerve; pL, prelaryngeal nerve; pT, pretracheal nerve; R, recurrent nerve; SAJ, superficial anterior jugular nerve; sA, subauricular nerve; SEJ, superficial external jugular nerve; SiP, superficial intraparotid nerve; sMd, submandibular nerve; sMt, submental nerve; sO, suboccipital nerve; sP, subparotid nerve; rPh, retropharyngeal nerve. (Adapted from Grégoire V, Scalliet P, and Ang KK: Clinical Target Volumes in Conformal and Intensity Modulated Radiation Therapy. A Clinical Guide to Cancer Treatment. New York, Springer-Verlag, 2003.)

located posterior to the SAN are included in level IIb. Level II receives efferent lymphatics from the face, the parotid gland, and the submandibular, submental, and retropharyngeal nodes. Level II also directly receives the collecting lymphatics from the nasal cavity, the pharynx, the larynx, the external auditory canal, the middle ear, and the sublingual and submandibular glands. The nodes in level II are therefore at greatest risk for harboring metastases from cancers arising from the nasal cavity, oral cavity, nasopharynx, oropharynx, hypopharynx, larynx, and the major salivary glands. Level IIb is more likely associated with primary tumors arising in the oropharynx or nasopharynx and less frequently involved in tumors of the oral cavity, larynx, or hypopharynx.

Level III contains the middle jugular LNs located around the middle third of the IJV. It is the caudal extension of level II. It is limited cranially by the caudal border of the body of the hyoid bone, and caudally by a plane where the omohyoid muscle crosses the IJV (surgical landmark) or by the caudal border of the cricoid cartilage (clinical landmark). The anterior limit is the lateral edge of the sternohyoid muscle, and the posterior limit is the posterior border of the SCM. Laterally, level III is limited by the SCM and medially by the internal carotid artery and the paraspinal muscles. Level III contains a highly variable number of LNs and receives efferent lymphatics from levels II and V and some efferent lymphatics from the retropharyngeal, pretracheal, and recurrent laryngeal nodes. It collects the lymphatics from the base of the tongue, tonsils, larynx, hypopharynx, and thyroid gland. Nodes in level III are at greatest risk for harboring metastases from cancers of the oral cavity, nasopharynx, oropharynx, hypopharynx, and larynx.

Level IV includes the lower jugular LNs located around the inferior third of the IJV from the caudal limit of level III to the clavicle caudally. The anterior and posterior limits are the same as for level III, i.e., the lateral border of the sternohyoid muscle and the posterior edge of the SCM, respectively. Laterally, level IV is limited by the SCM and medially by the internal carotid artery and the paraspinal muscles. Level IV contains a variable number of nodes and receives efferent lymphatics primarily from levels III and V, some efferent lymphatics from the retropharyngeal, pretracheal, and recurrent laryngeal nodes, and collecting lymphatics from the hypopharynx, larynx, and thyroid gland.[1] Level IV nodes are at high risk for harboring metastases from cancers of the hypopharynx, larynx, and cervical esophagus.

Level V includes the LNs of the posterior triangle group. This group includes the LNs located along the lower part of the SAN and the transverse cervical vessels. Level V is limited cranially by the convergence of the SCM and the trapezius muscles, caudally by the clavicle, anteriorly by the posterior border of the SCM, and posteriorly by the anterior border of the trapezius muscle. Laterally, level V is limited by the platysma muscle and the skin and medially by the splenius capitis, levator scapulae, and scaleni (posterior, medial, and anterior) muscles. Level V is currently subdivided into levels Va and Vb. The distinction between the upper posterior triangle (level Va) and the lower posterior triangle (level Vb) allows LN involvement of the lower two thirds of the SAN chain to be differentiated from that of the transverse cervical vessel chain.[7,8] A horizontal plane defined by the caudal edge of the cricoid cartilage separates these two compartments. It should be pointed out that the demarcation between the posterior end of level IIb and the uppermost part of level Va has still not been clearly defined. The American Academy for Otolaryngology–Head and Neck Surgery defined the posterior boundary of level IIb as the posterior border of the SCM and the apex of the convergence of the SCM and the trapezius muscles as

Table 37-1 **Comparison of the TNM Atlas Terminology and the Robbins Classification of the Lymph Nodes of the Neck**

TNM Atlas for Lymph Nodes of the Neck		Robbins Classification	
Group Number	*Terminology*	*Level*	*Terminology*
1	Submental nodes	Ia	Submental group
2	Submandibular nodes	Ib	Submandibular group
3	Cranial jugular nodes	II	Upper jugular group
4	Medial jugular nodes	III	Middle jugular group
5	Caudal jugular nodes	IV	Lower jugular group
6	Dorsal cervical nodes along the spinal accessory nerve	V	Posterior triangle group
7	Supraclavicular nodes	V	Posterior triangle group
8	Prelaryngeal and paratracheal nodes	VI	Anterior compartment group
9	Retropharyngeal nodes	—	—
10	Parotid nodes	—	—
11	Buccal nodes	—	—
12	Retroauricular and occipital nodes	—	—

the cranial boundary of level Va. However, the uppermost part of level Va contains superficial occipital LNs and, inconsistently, one subfascial LN close to the occipital attachment of the SCM.[1]

These LNs collect lymphatics from the occipital scalp and the postauricular and nuchal regions. They are not involved in the drainage of head and neck cancers except for skin tumors. Consequently, Hamoir proposed to subdivide the level Va into two sublevels: the apex of level V or level Vas (superior) and level Vai (inferior).[9] The border between level Vas and level Vai should be the lower two thirds of the SAN. From a radiologic point of view, a horizontal plane defined by the upper edge of the body of the hyoid bone appears to be a reliable landmark to separate the two sections. Dissection of the apex (level Vas) seems not required in mucosal head and neck SCC. It should only be considered in skin cancer of the posterior scalp and posterior neck. Level V receives efferent lymphatics from the occipital and postauricular nodes as well as those from the occipital and parietal scalp, the skin of the lateral and posterior neck and shoulder, the nasopharynx, and the oropharynx (tonsils and base of the tongue). Level V LNs are at high risk for harboring metastases from cancers of the nasopharynx and oropharynx. Nodes in level Va are more often associated with primary cancers of the nasopharynx, the oropharynx, or the cutaneous structures of the posterior scalp, whereas those in level Vb are more commonly associated with tumors arising in the thyroid gland.

Level VI, also called the anterior compartment group, contains the LNs located in the visceral space: the pretracheal and paratracheal nodes, the precricoid (Delphian) node, and the perithyroid nodes including the LNs along the recurrent laryngeal nerves. It is limited cranially by the hyoid bone, caudally by the suprasternal notch and laterally by the medial border of both carotid sheaths. Level VI receives efferent lymphatics from the thyroid gland, the glottic and subglottic larynx, the hypopharynx, and the cervical esophagus. These nodes are at high risk for harboring metastases from cancers of the thyroid gland, the glottic and subglottic larynx, the apex of the piriform sinus, and the cervical esophagus.

IMAGING OF THE NECK

Available armamentarium for imaging workup of the metastatic cervical LNs includes computed tomography (CT), magnetic resonance imaging (MRI), ultrasonography (US), and positron emission tomography (PET).[10] Nodal imaging is mandatory in pretreatment work-up because clinical assessment of nodal status in patients with a thick and/or small neck have low sensitivity and because deep-located nodes remain inaccessible in all patients.[11]

CT and MRI are standard cross-sectional imaging modalities through which anatomic "slices" covering the whole neck and depicting the contours and the internal structure of the nodes are obtained (Figs. 37-2 and 37-3). Higher spontaneous contrast between fatty and nonfatty tissues may appear as an advantage of MRI over CT. Multiplanar capability of MRI has been for two decades the advantage of the technique since its introduction in clinical use in the early 1980s. However, the multirow detector technology and the spiral acquisition modality implemented on new-generation CT systems have boosted the image multiplanar reformatting capabilities of CT, which now equal those of MRI. Major criteria for nodal malignancy using CT and/or MRI include the size of the nodes (a short axis longer than 10 mm) and the presence of a central necrosis (hypodensity on CT images; hypointensity on T1-weighted and hyperintensity on T2-weighted MR images). Central necrosis is well highlighted by intravenous contrast agent perfusion by enhancing nodal areas with arterial blood supply on both CT and MR images (see Figs. 37-2A and 37-3C). However, the two techniques share common weaknesses: the inability to detect micrometastatic deposits within normal-sized nodes (false-negative results) and the risk for inappropriate classification of malignancy in nodes that are enlarged by benign reactive changes (false-positive results). Thus far, neither MR nor CT gives a perfect diagnostic accuracy for nodal metastatic work-up. It has been shown in a large series of patients that the two techniques have an almost similar and unsatisfactory performance.

Ultrasonography (US) has long been regarded as a low-cost, widely available, and innocuous alternative to CT/MRI with the additional advantages of color Doppler flow-encoded vascular architecture depiction and of fine-needle aspiration guidance. Time demands and operator skill requirements are limiting factors. Moreover, the technical difficulties of fusing two-dimensional (2D) US data and three-dimensional (3D) CT/MRI data for radiation therapy (RT) planning are unsolved. In addition, US detects nodal necrosis less efficiently than CT and MRIs,[13] and deeply located nodes may be poorly accessible to the technique.

Multiple research ways are now being explored to improve the diagnostic accuracy of MRI: experimental lymphophilic

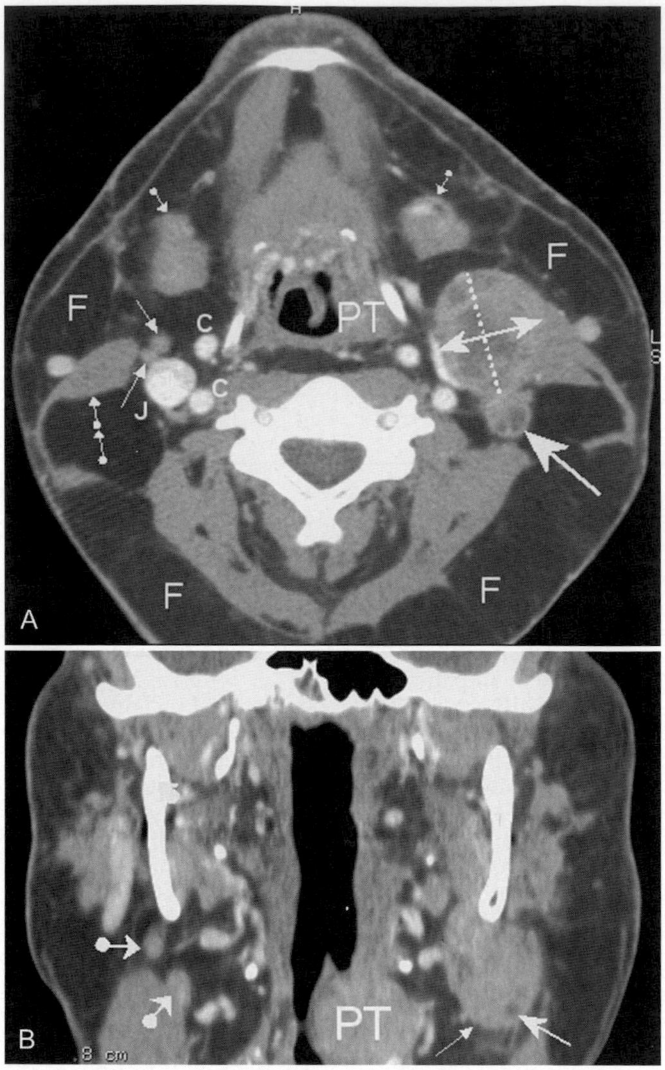

Figure 37-2 CT nodal display in a patient with left oropharyngeal squamous cell carcinoma (SCC). **A,** Native contrast-enhanced slice in the axial transverse plane using multi-slice multi-row detector (MSMD) spiral acquisition technique. Hypodense fatty (F) environment allows clear delineation of the neck structures. Left oropharyngeal SCC (PT) is present. Abnormal nodes are seen within the left level II, with anterior adenomegaly (long axis of 26 mm shown as *dotted line;* short transverse axis of 18 mm is shown between the *double-ended arrow*) and a posterior, normal-sized node showing necrotic hypodensity *(thick arrow)*. Normal-sized contralateral nodes are indicated *(thin arrows)*. Observe the isodensity of the submandibular glands *(ball-arrowhead)* and of the muscles *(double ball-arrowhead)*. Jugular veins (J) and carotid arteries (C) are strongly opacified at this early second phase of biphasic iodinated contrast agent perfusion. Notice the lamination of the left internal jugular vein by adenomegaly. **B,** Reformatted image in the coronal plane from the same three-dimensional data set shows the primary tumor (PT), left metastatic adenomegaly, and contralateral, normal-sized nodes *(ball-arrowhead)*. Observe the irregularities of the inferior aspect of the enlarged node, suggesting extranodal spread *(thin arrow)* and hypodense foci corresponding to necrotic areas within adenomegaly *(thick arrow)*. (Courtesy of E. Coche, MD, PhD.)

Table 37-2 American Joint Committee on Cancer Staging for Neck Node Metastasis

Stage	Definition
Nx	Regional lymph nodes cannot be assessed
N0	No regional lymph node metastasis
N1	Metastasis in a single ipsilateral node, ≤3 cm in greatest dimension
N2a	Metastasis in a single ipsilateral node, >3 cm but ≤6 cm in greatest dimension
N2b	Metastasis in multiple ipsilateral nodes, ≤6 cm in greatest dimension
N2c	Metastasis in bilateral or contralateral nodes, ≤6 cm in greatest dimension
N3	Metastasis in a lymph node >6 cm in greatest dimension

From Greene FL, Page DL, Fleming ID, et al: AJCC Cancer Staging Handbook, 6th ed. Heidelberg, Springer, 2002.

contrast agents, magnetization transfer imaging (MTI), free water diffusion-weighted imaging (DWI), magnetic resonance spectroscopy (MRS), and bolus tracking perfusion-weighted imaging (PWI).[14-16] Many believe that molecular imaging probes targeting either specific membrane antigens or metabolic pathways of the tumor cells could be the definitive contributor to perfect diagnostic accuracy in nodal metastatic workup, in which case MRI and PET will be competitors.

PET, using fluorodeoxyglucose (FDG) as tracer, has evolved into the most available technique for "metabolic imaging" by enhancing foci of increased glucose uptake. However, the restricted diagnostic accuracy of PET alone requires the coregistration of PET information on anatomic CT or MR images (see Fig. 37-4).[17] In addition to the research for dedicated tissue-specific MR contrast agents, that for PET radiopharmaceutical tracers allowing the assessment of hypoxia, angiogenesis, apoptosis, and receptor status is the second main field of research in oncology imaging.[18] The detection of tumor recurrences in previously treated primary sites by anatomic imaging modalities is unsatisfactory because extensive unspecific posttherapeutic changes may mask small foci of neoplastic recurrence.[19] On the other hand, very promising data have been reported with the use of FDG-PET in this setting.[20] Similar concepts apply to nodal metastases, and one may speculate that molecular and metabolic imaging methods will also become standard in nodal relapse detection. The key imaging concept for the radiation oncologist's day-to-day practice is the capability to superimpose PET/MRI metabolic/molecular mapping onto CT/MRI anatomic images to improve the delineation of the target for RT.[21] PET-CT and PET-MRI fusion are the founding paradigms that have now emerged into the clinical routine (Figs. 37-3 and 37-4).[22]

STAGING

The sixth edition (2002) of the American Joint Committee on Cancer (AJCC) staging for neck node metastasis is presented in Table 37-2.[23] This classification does not apply to nasopharyngeal, thyroid, or skin cancers. In comparison with the fourth (1987) or fifth (1998) edition, the only modification is the possibility to use a descriptor for nodal metastasis located below (L) or above (U) the lower border of the cricoid cartilage. The use of this descriptor will not influence the nodal staging. The classification for nodal staging does apply irrespective of the modality used for the neck assessment, that is, clinical examination or imaging. The routine use of CT or MRI and, in expert hands, US, is recommended especially to assess nodes not clinically identifiable (e.g., retropharyngeal, intraparotid, or superior mediastinal nodes) or in patients for whom clinical palpation of the neck is less sensitive (e.g., thick

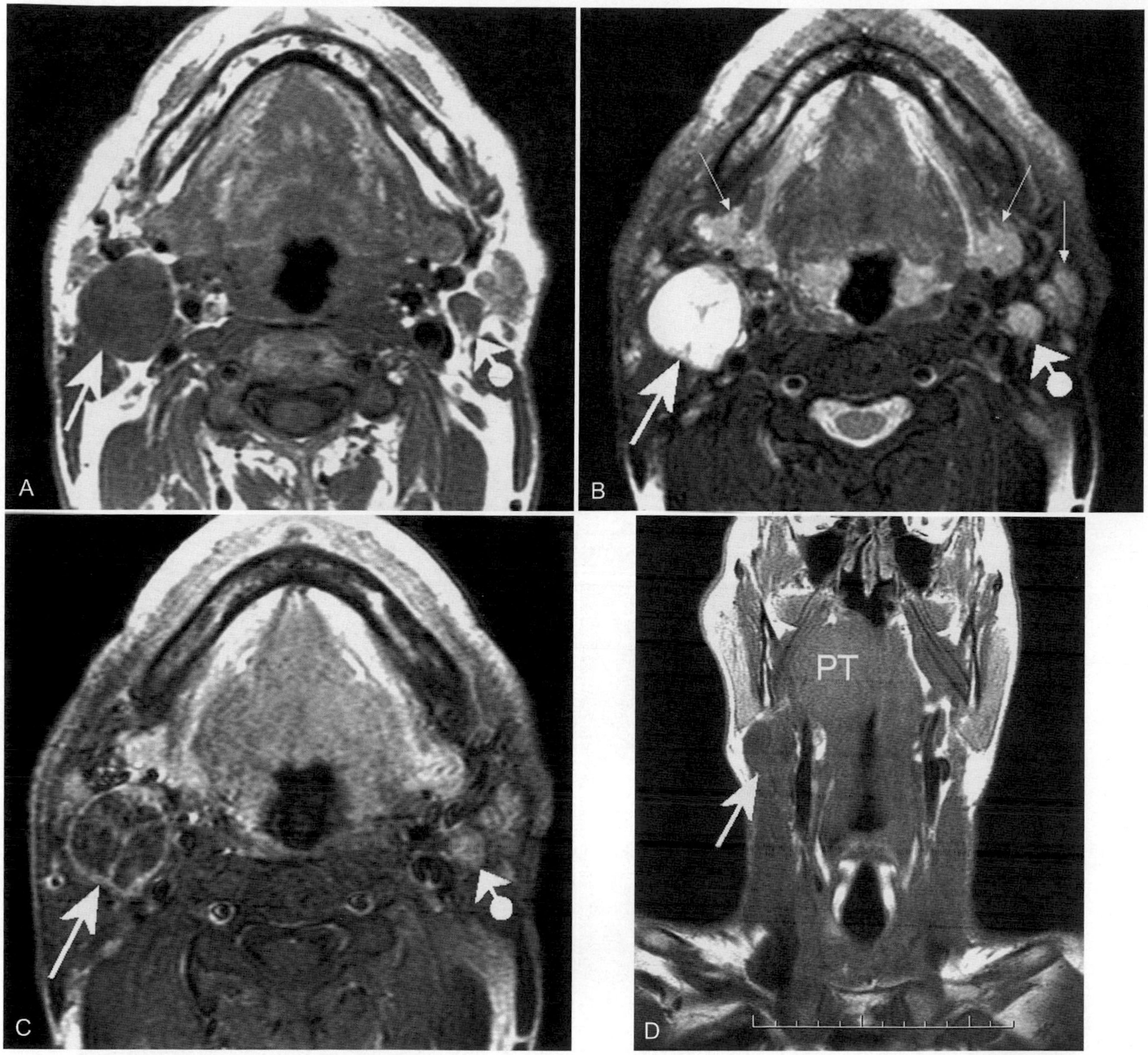

Figure 37-3 Magnetic resonance nodal display in a patient with right oropharyngeal squamous cell carcinoma (SCC). **A,** Transverse, unenhanced, T1-weighted spin-echo (SE) image showing a left level II hypointense necrotic adenomegaly *(arrow)* with a normal contralateral node in level II *(ball-arrowhead)*. **B,** Transverse, T2-weighted fast spin-echo (FSE) image with fat suppression option in a similar slice location discloses strong hyperintensity of the necrotic node due to fluid-like content *(arrow)* compared with the normal contralateral node, which displays the usual intermediate to high signal intensity *(ball-arrowhead)*. Observe the almost similar signal intensity of the normal node and of the parotid and submandibular glands *(thin arrows)*. **C,** Transverse, contrast-enhanced, T1-weighted SE image with fat suppression option in a similar slice location as in **A** and **B** shows only peripheral ring-like enhancement of the margin of the necrotic adenomegaly *(arrow)*. The normal contralateral node enhances slightly and homogeneously *(ball-arrowhead)*. **D,** Coronal-view, precontrast, T1-weighted MR image shows a primary tumor (PT) and hypointense necrotic adenomegaly *(arrow)*.

or small neck).[24] Last, it should be emphasized that the Nx classification only applies when the neck was not assessed or could not be assessed.

INCIDENCE AND DISTRIBUTION OF NECK NODE METASTASIS

Clinical and Radiologic Assessment

The metastatic spread of head and neck tumors into the cervical LNs is rather consistent and follows predictable pathways, at least in the neck that has not been violated by previous surgery or RT. In Table 37-3, the frequency of metastatic LNs is expressed as a percentage of node-positive patients.[25,26]

The frequency of neck node metastases and the distribution of clinically involved nodes depend to a major extent on the primary tumor site. Typically, hypopharyngeal tumors have the highest propensity for nodal involvement, which occurs in 70% of cases. Cranial and anterior tumors (e.g., oral cavity tumors) mainly drain into levels I, II, and III, whereas more caudally located tumors (e.g., laryngeal tumors) mainly

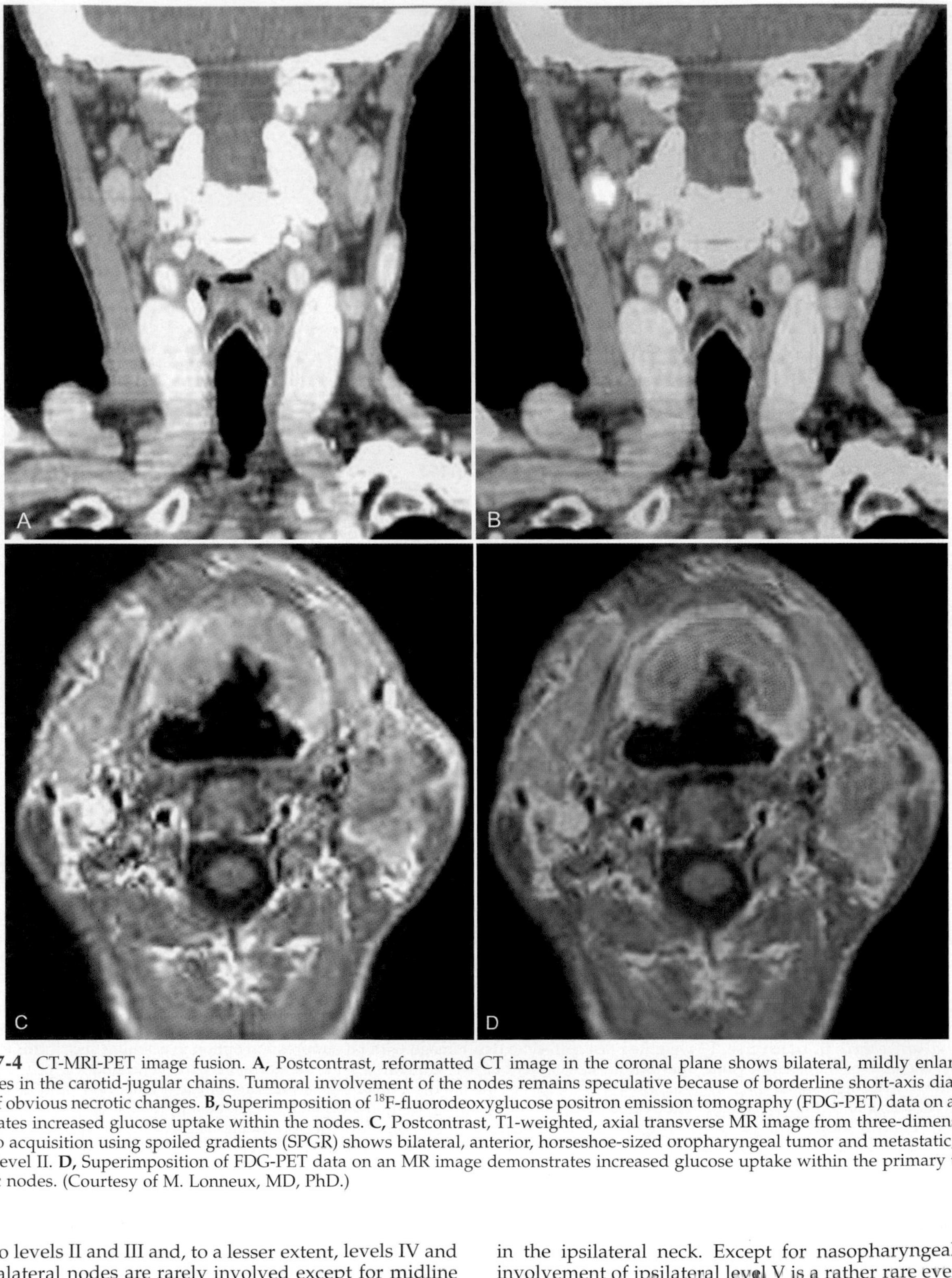

Figure 37-4 CT-MRI-PET image fusion. **A,** Postcontrast, reformatted CT image in the coronal plane shows bilateral, mildly enlarged metastatic nodes in the carotid-jugular chains. Tumoral involvement of the nodes remains speculative because of borderline short-axis diameter and absence of obvious necrotic changes. **B,** Superimposition of ^{18}F-fluorodeoxyglucose positron emission tomography (FDG-PET) data on a CT image demonstrates increased glucose uptake within the nodes. **C,** Postcontrast, T1-weighted, axial transverse MR image from three-dimensional gradient-echo acquisition using spoiled gradients (SPGR) shows bilateral, anterior, horseshoe-sized oropharyngeal tumor and metastatic, left-sided nodes in level II. **D,** Superimposition of FDG-PET data on an MR image demonstrates increased glucose uptake within the primary tumor and metastatic nodes. (Courtesy of M. Lonneux, MD, PhD.)

drain into levels II and III and, to a lesser extent, levels IV and V. Contralateral nodes are rarely involved except for midline tumors or tumors in those sites where bilateral lymphatic drainage has been reported, such as the soft palate, base of the tongue, and pharyngeal wall. Even in these tumors, the incidence of contralateral involvement is much lower, reaching, for example, in base of the tongue tumors with clinically positive nodes, 31% in contralateral level II compared with 73% in ipsilateral level II (data not shown). Interestingly, node distribution follows the same pattern in the contralateral neck as in the ipsilateral neck. Except for nasopharyngeal tumors, involvement of ipsilateral level V is a rather rare event, occurring in less than 1% of all oral cavity tumors, in less than 10% of all oropharyngeal and laryngeal tumors, and in about 15% of all hypopharyngeal tumors. It almost never occurs in contralateral level V.

Metastatic LN involvement in the neck depends on the size of the primary tumor, increasing with the T stage. In the series reported by Bataini and associates,[25] 44% of patients with a T1 tumor had clinical LN involvement; this increased to 70% for

Table 37-3 Distribution of Clinical Metastatic Neck Nodes from Oral Cavity and Pharyngolaryngeal Squamous Cell Carcinomas

Tumor Site	Patients with N+	DISTRIBUTION* OF METASTATIC LYMPH NODES PER LEVEL (PERCENTAGE OF THE NODE-POSITIVE PATIENTS) I	II	III	IV	V	Other†
Oral cavity (n = 787)	36%	42/3.5	79/8	18/3	5/1	1/0	1.4/0.3
Oropharynx (n = 1479)	64%	13/2	81/24	23/5	9/2.5	13/3	2/1
Hypopharynx (n = 847)	70%	2/0	80/13	51/4	20/3	24/2	3/1
Supraglottic larynx (n = 428)	55%	2/0	71/21	48/10	18/7	15/4	2/0

*Ipsilateral/contralateral.
†Parotid, buccal nodes.
Modified from Lindberg R: Distribution of cervical lymph node metastases from squamous cell carcinoma of the upper respiratory and digestive tracts. Cancer 29:1446-1449, 1972; Bataini JP, Bernier J, Asselain B, et al: Primary radiotherapy of squamous cell carcinoma of the oropharynx and pharyngolarynx: tentative multivariate modelling system to predict the radiocurability of neck nodes. Int J Radiat Oncol Biol Phys 14:635-642, 1988.

Table 37-4 Incidence of Retropharyngeal Lymph Nodes in Oral Cavity and Pharyngolaryngeal Primary Tumors

Authors	Primary Site	INCIDENCE OF RETROPHARYNGEAL LYMPH NODES (PERCENTAGE OF THE TOTAL NUMBER OF PATIENTS) Overall	N0 Neck*	N+ Neck†
McLaughlin[140]	Oropharynx			
	Pharyngeal wall	18/93 (19%)	6/37 (16%)	12/56 (21%)
	Soft palate	7/53 (13%)	1/21 (5%)	6/32 (19%)
	Tonsillar fossa	16/176 (9%)	2/56 (4%)	14/120 (12%)
	Base of tongue	5/121 (4%)	0/31 (0%)	5/90 (6%)
	Hypopharynx (pyriform sinus or postcricoid area)	7/136 (5%)	0/55 (0%)	7/81 (9%)
	Supraglottic larynx	4/196 (2%)	0/87 (0%)	4/109 (4%)
	Nasopharynx	14/19 (74%)	2/5 (40%)	12/14 (86%)
Chua[141]	Nasopharynx	106/364 (29%)	21/134 (16%)	85/230 (37%)
Chong[142]	Nasopharynx	Not stated	Not stated	59/91 (65%)

*Clinically negative nodes in levels I-V.
†Clinically positive nodes in levels I-V.

patients with T4 lesions. There are, however, no data suggesting that the relative distribution of involved neck levels varies with the T stage.

Retropharyngeal LNs represent a special entity inasmuch as they are usually not clinically detectable. The incidence of retropharyngeal LN involvement can thus only be estimated from series in which CT or MRI of the retropharynx has been systematically performed as part of the diagnostic procedure. Retropharyngeal node involvement occurs in primary tumors arising from (or invading) the mucosa of the occipital and cervical somites, such as the nasopharynx, the pharyngeal wall, and the soft palate (Table 37-4). Interestingly, the incidence of retropharyngeal LNs is higher in patients in whom involvement of other neck node levels has also been documented. However, in clinically N0 patients with nasopharyngeal tumors and, to a lesser extent, in patients with pharyngeal wall tumors, the incidence of retropharyngeal nodes is still significant, between 16% and 40%. Also, as already described for the other LN levels, involvement depends on the T stage and is typically lower for T1 tumors. Accurate figures are, however, not available.

Pathologic Lymph Node Metastases

The distribution of pathologic LN metastasis in patients with primaries of the oral cavity, oropharynx, hypopharynx, and larynx can be derived from retrospective series where a systematic radical neck node dissection was proposed as part of the initial treatment procedures.[27-30] In essence, retrospective series are biased regarding patient and treatment selection, but these series from the Head and Neck Department at MSKCC are the largest and most consistent data ever published on that matter. The results of these retrospective studies are shown in Tables 37-5 to 37-8. The data are presented in terms of the number of neck dissections with positive LNs divided by the total number of neck dissection procedures and expressed as a percentage. Most patients (>99% for the N0 neck patients and 95% for the N+ neck patients) only had unilateral treatment and no distinction between the ipsilateral and contralateral neck was made.

Overall, metastatic disease was detected in 33% of the prophylactic neck dissections and in 82% of the therapeutic neck dissections. In these series, the overall sensitivity and specificity of the clinical examination thus reached 85% and 62%, respectively. As already observed with the pattern of clinical metastatic LNs, the distribution of pathologically confirmed metastatic LNs depended on the primary tumor site. Typically, in clinically N0 patients, metastatic LNs were observed in levels I to III for oral cavity tumors and in levels II to IV for oropharyngeal, hypopharyngeal, and laryngeal tumors. This pattern of node distribution is similar to that determined from the clinical palpation of the neck. It should be noted that the

Table 37-5 Incidence of Pathologic Lymph Node Metastasis in Squamous Cell Carcinomas of the Oral Cavity

	Distribution of Metastatic Lymph Nodes per Level (Percentage of the Neck Dissection Procedures)										
	Prophylactic RND (192 Patients; 192 Procedures)						Therapeutic (Immediate or Subsequent) RND (308 Patients; 323 Procedures)				
Tumor Site	No. of RNDs	I	II	III	IV	V	No. of RNDs	I	II	III	IV	V
Tongue	58	14%	19%	16%	3%	0%	129	32%	50%	40%	20%	0%
Floor of mouth	57	16%	12%	7%	2%	0%	115	53%	34%	32%	12%	7%
Gum	52	27%	21%	6%	4%	2%	52	54%	46%	19%	17%	4%
Retromolar trigone	16	19%	12%	6%	6%	0%	10	50%	60%	40%	20%	0%
Cheek	9	44%	11%	0%	0%	0%	17	82%	41%	65%	65%	0%
Total	192	20%	17%	9%	3%	1%	323	46%	44%	32%	16%	3%

RND, radical neck dissection.
Modified from Shah JP: Patterns of cervical lymph node metastasis from squamous carcinomas of the upper aerodigestive tract. Am J Surg 160:405-409, 1990.

Table 37-6 Incidence of Pathologic Lymph Node Metastasis in Squamous Cell Carcinomas of the Oropharynx

	Distribution of Metastatic Lymph Nodes per Level (Percentage of the Neck Dissection Procedures)										
	Prophylactic RND (47 Patients; 48 Procedures)						Therapeutic (Immediate or Subsequent) RND (157 Patients; 165 Procedures)				
Tumor Site	No. of RNDs	I	II	III	IV	V	No. of RNDs	I	II	III	IV	V
Base of tongue + vallecula	21	0%	19%	14%	9%	5%	58	10%	72%	41%	21%	9%
Tonsillar fossa	27	4%	30%	22%	7%	0%	107	17%	70%	42%	31%	9%
Total	48	2%	25%	19%	8%	2%	165	15%	71%	42%	27%	9%

RND, radical neck dissection.
Modified from Candela FC, Kothari K, Shah JP: Patterns of cervical node metastases from squamous carcinoma of the oropharynx and hypopharynx. Head Neck 12:197-203, 1990.

Table 37-7 Incidence of Pathologic Lymph Node Metastasis in Squamous Cell Carcinomas of the Hypopharynx

	Distribution of Metastatic Lymph Nodes per Level (Percentage of the Neck Dissection Procedures)										
	Prophylactic RND (24 Patients; 24 Procedures)						Therapeutic (Immediate or Subsequent) RND (102 Patients; 104 Procedures)				
Tumor Site	No. of RNDs	I	II	III	IV	V	No. of RNDs	I	II	III	IV	V
Pyriform sinus	13	0%	15%	8%	0%	0%	79	6%	72%	72%	47%	8%
Pharyngeal wall	11	0%	9%	18%	0%	0%	25	20%	84%	72%	40%	20%
Total	24	0%	12%	12%	0%	0%	104	10%	75%	72%	45%	11%

RND, radical neck dissection.
Modified from Candela FC, Kothari K, Shah JP: Patterns of cervical node metastases from squamous carcinoma of the oropharynx and hypopharynx. Head Neck 12:197-203, 1990.

Table 37-8 Incidence of Pathologic Lymph Node Metastasis in Squamous Cell Carcinomas of the Larynx

	Distribution of Metastatic Lymph Nodes per Level (Percentage of the Neck Dissection Procedures)										
	Prophylactic RND (78 Patients; 79 Procedures)						Therapeutic (Immediate or Subsequent) RND (169 Patients; 183 Procedures)				
Tumor Site	No. of RNDs	I	II	III	IV	V	No. of RNDs	I	II	III	IV	V
Supraglottic larynx	65	6%	18%	18%	9%	2%	138	6%	62%	55%	32%	5%
Glottic larynx	14	0%	21%	29%	7%	7%	45	9%	42%	71%	24%	2%
Total	79	5%	19%	20%	9%	3%	183	7%	57%	59%	30%	4%

RND, radical neck dissection.
Modified from Candela FC, Shah J, Jaques DP, et al: Patterns of cervical node metastases from squamous carcinoma of the larynx. Arch Otolaryngol Head Neck Surg 116:432-435, 1990.

T stage distribution was different in the various groups. Of patients with laryngeal tumors, 54% (42 of 79) had T3-4 tumors (mainly supraglottic) compared to 27% (52 of 192), 25% (6 of 24), and 17% (8 of 47) in patients with oral cavity, hypopharyngeal and oropharyngeal tumors, respectively. Such a difference in T stage presumably explains the high incidence of microscopic node metastases in the larynx group.

When considering the patients who underwent therapeutic neck dissection, the pattern of metastatic node distribution was similar to that observed in clinically N0 patients, with the difference that significant pathologic infiltration of an additional nodal level was typically observed—level IV for oral cavity tumors and levels I and V for oropharyngeal, hypopharyngeal, and, to a lesser extent, laryngeal tumors. Overall, this observation illustrates the gradual infiltration of node levels in the neck. This concept is well illustrated by the prevalence of metastases in level V. In the MSKCC series, the prevalence of pathologic infiltration in level V was quite low, averaging 3% in 1,277 neck dissections in patients with oral cavity, oropharyngeal, hypopharyngeal, and laryngeal tumors.[31] It peaked at 11% for hypopharyngeal tumors with pathologically positive nodes (see Table 37-7). A thorough analysis of level V infiltration showed that for all tumor sites pooled together, infiltration of level V without metastases in levels I to IV was observed in only one patient (0.2%). This patient had a hypopharyngeal tumor. Infiltration in level V remained below 1% when a single pathologically confirmed positive node was also observed in levels I to III but reached 16% when a single pathologically confirmed positive node was also observed in level IV. When more than one level was infiltrated, the probability of level V involvement progressively increased, reaching 40% when levels I to IV were all involved. The pattern of involvement of level I is also a good illustration of the concept of gradual node infiltration. In the MSKCC series, pathologic involvement of level I was found in only 2% of clinical N0 patients with oropharyngeal tumors (see Table 37-6) and was not observed in clinical N0 patients with hypopharyngeal tumors (see Table 37-7). On the other hand, in patients with clinically positive nodes, metastases in level I were reported in 15% and 10% of patients with oropharyngeal and hypopharyngeal tumors, respectively.

Incidence of "Skip Metastases" in the Neck

"Skip metastases" are those metastases that bypass the orderly progression from one level to a contiguous level, such as from level I to level II and from level II to level III. Depending on their frequency, "skip metastases" in patients clinically staged N0 may have a profound implication on the therapeutic management of the neck. In the series from the MSKCC, 8 of 343 clinically N0 patients (2.5%) developed "skip metastases."[30] Seven of these patients had oral cavity tumors that metastasized in levels IV or V only. One patient had a laryngeal tumor. These low figures are in good agreement with a rate of neck failure outside the dissected levels of 3% (2 of 64) observed in pathologically N0 patients treated at the same institution by supraomohyoid neck dissection.[32] The majority of these patients had tumors of the oral cavity. None of them received postoperative RT, as they were all free of metastases. Byers carefully evaluated the frequency of "skip metastases" in 270 patients primarily treated by surgery at the M. D. Anderson Cancer Center from 1970 to 1990 for SCC of the oral tongue.[33] Of these patients, 12 had metastases in level III only, 9 had metastases in level IV only, and 2 had metastases in level IIb (i.e., nodes that are far enough posterior to the IJV). In addition, in 90 of the patients who were pathologically N0 after selective neck dissection (SND) of levels I to III and who did not receive postoperative RT, 9 subsequently developed recurrence in level IV. Altogether (levels IIb, III, and IV), the frequency of skip metastases reached 12% (32 of 270). If one excludes the "skip metastases" in level IIb and III, the frequency reached only 7.0% (18 of 270).

Incidence and Pattern of Node Distribution in the Contralateral Neck

There are very few data available on the pattern of pathologic node distribution in the contralateral neck. Bilateral neck dissection was only performed when the surgeon considered that there was a high risk of contralateral node involvement, for example, tumors of the oral cavity or the oropharynx reaching or extending beyond the midline or hypopharyngeal and supraglottic tumors. Obviously, in such cases, bilateral radical neck dissection was never performed, so that an accurate estimate of the pattern of node involvement in levels I to V of the contralateral neck is not possible. Furthermore, in almost every study, data on both sides of the neck were pooled for presentation. Kowalski[34] presented data on 90 patients who underwent bilateral supraomohyoid neck dissection, and in whom the pattern of node distribution in each side of the neck was reported separately. The majority of these patients had SCC of the lip or the oral cavity. In the ipsilateral neck, pathologic infiltration in levels I, II, and III reached 20%, 15%, and 15%, respectively. In the contralateral neck, corresponding values reached 13%, 11%, and 0%, respectively. These figures are in good agreement with data on clinical node distribution showing that both sides of the neck exhibited a similar pattern of node distribution but with a lower incidence in the contralateral neck.

Foote and colleagues[35] reported the rate of contralateral neck failure in a limited series of 46 clinically N0 patients with base of the tongue tumors treated by some form of glossectomy and ipsilateral neck dissection. None of these patients received postoperative RT. Ten patients (22%) had contralateral neck recurrence, and the most common sites were in levels II, III, and IV. It appears that in two of these patients, recurrence was also observed at the primary site. The development of delayed contralateral neck metastases was not related to the clinical or pathologic extent of the base of the tongue tumor. O'Sullivan and associates[36] reported a retrospective series of 228 patients with tonsillar carcinoma who were treated on the primary tumor and the ipsilateral neck only with RT. The vast majority of these patients had T1-2 and N0-1 disease. Contralateral recurrence in the neck was only observed in eight patients (2%), including five patients with local recurrence as well. None of these neck failures occurred in the 133 N0 patients. Although not significant due to the small number of events, involvement of midline structure (i.e., soft palate and base of tongue) appeared to be a prognostic factor for contralateral neck recurrence. Similar results were reported in a series of 101 node-negative tonsil carcinoma (mainly T1-3) cases treated unilaterally.[37] Only two neck recurrences were observed in the contralateral neck.

RECOMMENDATIONS FOR THE SELECTION OF THE TARGET VOLUMES IN THE NECK

The data presented indicate that metastatic LN involvement of primary SCC of the oral cavity, pharynx, and larynx typically follows a predictive pattern. Both data on clinical and pathologic neck node distribution and on neck recurrence after selective dissection procedures support the concept that not all the neck node levels should be treated as part of the initial management strategy of head and neck primaries of squamous cell origin.[38,39] One should bear in mind, however, that the data on which such a concept is based have come from retrospective series, and thus may include possible bias (e.g., patient selection, series from preimaging area, and so on) that could limit its validity.

Tables 37-9 to 37-12 present recommendations for the selection of the target volumes in the neck for pharyngolaryngeal SCCs. These guidelines can be applied irrespective of the treatment modality, that is, surgery and RT. The discussion of the choice between these two modalities is beyond the objective of this chapter but should be considered relative to the neck stage, the treatment option for the primary tumor, the performance status of the patient, and the institutional policy agreed upon by a multidisciplinary head and neck tumor board.

For clinically N0 patients with head and neck SCC of the oral cavity, oropharynx, hypopharynx, and larynx, selective treatment of the neck is appropriate.[32,39,40] Typically, levels I to III should be treated for oral cavity tumors and levels II to IV for oropharyngeal, hypopharyngeal, and laryngeal tumors. Robbins[7] suggested that elective treatment of level IIb is probably not necessary for clinically N0 patients with a primary tumor of the oral cavity, larynx, or hypopharynx. On the other hand, Byers and associates[33] suggested that level IV be included in the treatment of the mobile tongue due to the high incidence (10%) of skip metastases. Retropharyngeal nodes should be treated in tumors of the posterior pharyngeal wall. For subglottic tumors, tumors with subglottic or transglottic extension, or hypopharyngeal tumors with esophageal extension, level VI nodes should also be included in the treatment volume.

As proposed by Byers,[40] similar guidelines could also be recommended for N1 patients without radiologic evidence of extracapsular infiltration. However, when an involved LN is located at the boundary with a level which has not been selected in the target volume, it has been recommended to

Table 37-9 Recommendations for Selection of the Target Volume in the Neck for Oral Cavity Tumors

Nodal Stage (AJCC 2002)	Levels to Be Included in the CTV: Ipsilateral Neck	Contralateral Neck
N0-N1 (in level I, II or III)	I, II,* III + IV†	I, II,* III + IV†
N2a-N2b	I, II, III, IV, V‡	I, II,* III + IV for anterior tongue tumor
N2c	According to N stage on each side of the neck	According to N stage on each side of the neck
N3	I, II, III, IV, V ± adjacent structures according to clinical and radiologic data	I, II,* III + IV for anterior tongue tumor

*Level IIb could be omitted for N0 patients.
†For anterior tongue tumor and for any tumor with extension to the oropharynx, e.g., anterior tonsillar pillar, tonsillar fossae, base of tongue.
‡Level V could be omitted if only levels I-III are involved.

Table 37-10 Recommendations for Selection of the Target Volume in the Neck for Oropharyngeal Tumors

Nodal Stage (AJCC 2002)	Levels to Be Included in the CTV: Ipsilateral Neck	Contralateral Neck
N0-N1 (in level II, III, or IV)	(Ib)*-II-III-IV + RP† for posterior pharyngeal wall tumor	II-III-IV + RP† for posterior pharyngeal wall tumor
N2a-N2b	Ib, II, III, IV, V + RP†	II-III-IV + RP† for posterior pharyngeal wall tumor
N2c	According to N stage on each side of the neck	According to N stage on each side of the neck
N3	I, II, III, IV, V + RP† ± adjacent structures according to clinical and radiologic data	II-III-IV + RP† for posterior pharyngeal wall tumor

*Any tumor with extension to the oral cavity, e.g., retromolar trigone, mobile tongue, inferior gum, oral side of anterior tonsillar pillar.
†Retropharyngeal nodes.

Table 37-11 Recommendations for Selection of the Target Volume in the Neck for Hypopharyngeal Tumors

Nodal Stage (AJCC 2002)	Levels to Be Included in the CTV: Ipsilateral Neck	Contralateral Neck
N0	II*-III-IV + RP† for post. phar. wall tumor + VI for apex of pirif. sinus or esophageal extension	II*-III-IV + RP† for post. phar. wall tumor + VI for esophageal extension
N1-N2a-N2b	Ib, II, III, IV, V + RP + VI for pirif. sinus or esophageal extension	II*-III-IV + RP† for post. phar. wall tumor + VI for esophageal extension
N2c	According to N stage on each side of the neck	According to N stage on each side of the neck
N3	I, II, III, IV, V + RP + VI pirif. sinus or for esophageal extension ± adjacent structures according to clinical and radiologic data	II*-III-IV + RP† for post. phar. wall tumor + VI for esophageal extension

*Level IIb could be omitted for N0 patients.
†Retropharyngeal nodes.
post. phar., posterior pharyngeal; pirif., piriform.

Table 37-12 **Recommendations for Selection of the Target Volume in the Neck for Laryngeal Tumors (T1 N0 Glottic Carcinoma Excluded)**

Nodal Stage (AJCC 2002)	Levels to Be Included in the CTV: Ipsilateral Neck	Contralateral Neck
N0-N1 (in level II, III, or IV)	II*-III-IV + VI for transglottis or subglottis extension	II*-III-IV + VI for transglottis or subglottis extension
N2a-N2b	II, III, IV, V + VI for transglottis or subglottis extension	II*-III-IV + VI for transglottis or subglottis extension
N2c	According to N stage on each side of the neck	According to N stage on each side of the neck
N3	Ib, II, III, IV, V + VI for transglottis or subglottis extension ± adjacent structures according to clinical and radiologic data	II*-III-IV + VI for transglottis or subglottis extension

*Level IIb could be omitted for N0 patients.

extend the selection to include the adjacent level.[41] Typically, this will only apply for oropharyngeal tumors with a single LN in level II at the boundary with level Ib or for an oral cavity tumor with an N1 node in level III at the boundary with level IV.

For patients with multiple nodes (N2b), the available data suggest that adequate treatment should include levels I to V. Level I could, however, be omitted for laryngeal tumors, and level V for oral cavity tumors with neck involvement limited to levels I to III. Prophylactic treatment of the retropharyngeal nodes should be systematically performed for oropharyngeal and hypopharyngeal tumors. As for N0 patients, level VI nodes should also be treated for subglottic tumors, tumors with subglottic or transglottic extension, or hypopharyngeal tumors with esophageal extension. For patients with nodes in the upper neck (i.e., upper level II), it has been proposed to extend the upper limit of the target volume to include the retrostyloid space.[41] Similarly, the subclavicular fossae should also be included in the target volume in case of lower neck involvement, that is, level IV or Vb nodes.[41]

There are no data available on the distribution of pathologic metastatic neck nodes in patients presenting with a single ipsilateral large node (N2a or N3) or with bilateral or contralateral nodes (N2c). For patients with a single large node, in the absence of data, it appears safe not to recommend selective treatment. For N3 patients, the type of treatment of the neck is likely to be also dictated by the local extension of the node into the adjacent structures (e.g., paraspinal muscles, parotid gland, blood vessels). For N2c patients, one proposal is to consider each side of the neck separately, such as selective treatment in both sides for a small single node in each side, selective treatment for a small single node in one side, and more extensive treatment in the other side in the case of multiple nodes.

Prophylactic treatment of the contralateral N0 neck is still in the gray zone and is likely to be based on clinical judgment rather than on strong scientific evidence. Typically, patients with midline tumors or tumors originating from or extending to a site that has bilateral lymphatic drainage (e.g., base of the tongue, vallecula, posterior pharyngeal wall) are thought to benefit from bilateral neck treatment, whereas well-lateralized tumors (e.g., the lateral border of the tongue, retromolar trigone, tonsillar fossa) can be spared contralateral treatment. It has also been reported in tumors of the pharynx and larynx that the risk of contralateral neck metastases increased with involvement of the ipsilateral neck.[42] Putting all these data together, one could recommend restricting the treatment to the ipsilateral neck for tumors of the lower gum (not approaching the midline), lateral floor of the mouth, lateral border of the mobile tongue, upper gum, cheek, retromolar trigone, tonsillar fossa (without extension to the base of the tongue, soft palate, posterior pillar), and lateral wall of the piriform sinus. In the other situations, where prophylactic contralateral neck treatment is recommended, the selection of the node levels to be treated should follow similar rules to those for the ipsilateral neck.

In principle, a similar approach should apply for the definition of the node levels to be irradiated postoperatively. However, if one agrees on the selection criteria for postoperative RT (i.e., capsular rupture, patients with a metastatic node over 3 cm in diameter or with more than one metastatic node), irradiation of levels I to V will typically be performed. As for primary RT, the retrostyloid space and the subclavicular fossae should be included in the target volume depending on the location of the metastatic nodes.[41] For laryngeal tumors, level I could be omitted. For oral cavity tumors, postoperative irradiation of level V could be omitted in the case of metastatic nodes located in level I and/or II only. Retropharyngeal and paratracheal nodes should be treated as mentioned earlier.

NECK NODE DISSECTION PROCEDURES AND SENTINEL NODE BIOPSY

In 1991, based on the definition of the neck level, the Committee for Head and Neck Surgery and Oncology of the American Academy for Otolaryngology–Head and Neck Surgery made several recommendations for the neck dissection terminology. The main objectives of such recommendations were to develop a standardized terminology limited to the use of few defined procedures where the lymphatic and nonlymphatic structures removed are unambiguously described. Such recommendations had to correlate with the biology of neck metastases and meet the standards of oncologic principles. The goal of each type of neck dissection is to remove the lymphatic structures (nodes and vessels) that are poorly individualized in the fatty tissue of the neck. When oncologically sound, some or all nonlymphatic structures of the neck, such as the IJV, SAN, SCMs, and submandibular glands may be preserved. Since the 1991 classification, revisions have recently been proposed; the current neck dissection terminology and definitions are summarized in Table 37-13.[7,8,43,44]

Radical neck dissection (RND), previously considered as the standard basic procedure, is defined as the resection of LN levels I to V, including removal of the SCMs, IJV, and SAN.

Modified radical neck dissection (MRND) refers to the removal of all LNs routinely resected by the RND but sparing

Table 37-13 **Classification of Neck Dissection: Definitions and Terminology**

Type of Neck Dissection	Lymph Node Levels Resected	Nonlymphatic Structures Removed
Radical neck dissection	I, II, III, IV, V	SCM, IJV, SAN
Modified radical neck dissection	I, II, III, IV, V	Preservation of one or more of the following: SCM, IJV, SAN
Selective neck dissection	Preservation of one or more of the following: I, II, III, IV, V. Parentheses are used to denote levels or sublevels removed, e.g., SND (I-IV)	None
Extended neck dissection	Resection of one or more or additional lymph node group not routinely removed by the radical neck dissection, e.g., parapharyngeal, paratracheal	Resection of one or more nonlymphatic structures not routinely routinely removed by the radical neck dissection, e.g., carotid artery, hypoglossal nerve, overlying skin

IJV, internal jugular vein; SAN, spinal accessory nerve; SCM, sternocleidomastoid muscle.
Adapted from Robbins KT: Classification of neck dissection: current concepts and future considerations. Otolaryngol Clin North Am 31:639-656, 1998.

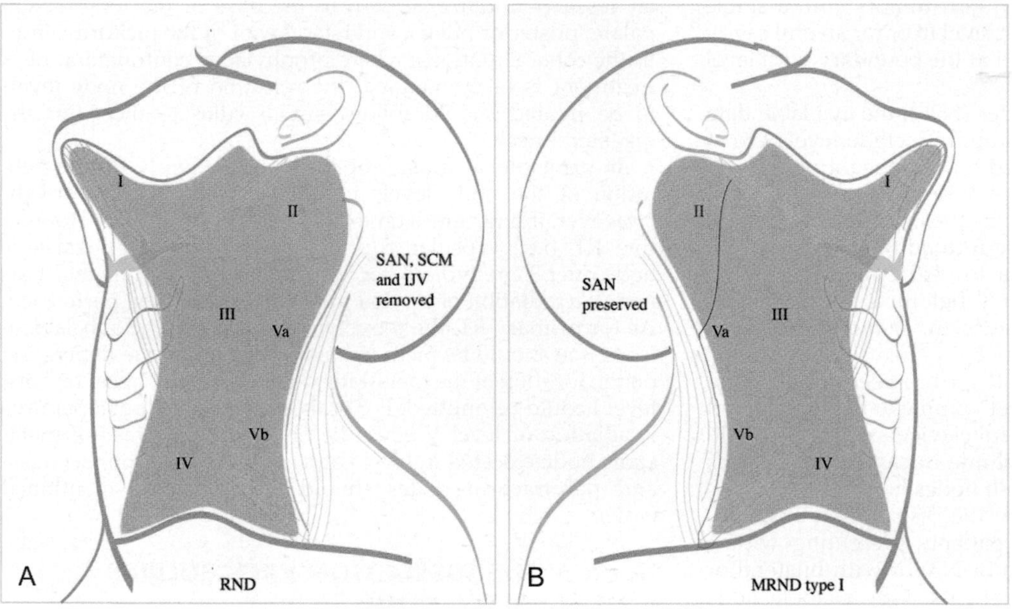

Figure 37-5 Lymph node levels and nonlymphatic structures removed in radical neck dissection (**A**) and modified radical neck dissection type I (**B**). In radical neck dissection for level I to V, the spinal accessory nerve (SAN), the sternocleidomastoid muscle (SCM), and the internal jugular vein (IJV) are resected. In a modified radical neck dissection type I for level I to V, the SCM and the IJV are resected. The SAN is preserved.

one or more of the nonlymphatic structures (SAN, IJV, and SCMs) usually removed during RND (Fig. 37-5). Medina[45] subclassified the MRND into three types: MRND type I preserves the SAN only; MRND type II preserves the SAN and the SCMs; and MRND type III preserves the SAN, the SCMs, and the IJV. Type III is also called by European authors "functional neck dissection" as first described by Suarez[46] and popularized by Bocca and associates.[47,48] However, in their classic description, the submandibular gland was not removed.

SND consists of dissection in which there is preservation of one or more LN levels routinely resected in RND (Fig. 37-6). To avoid confusion in the terminology of the different subtypes of SND, the 2002 revision of the ND classification decided to exclude "named" NDs (e.g., supraomohyoid ND, posterolateral ND) and proposed that the term SND be followed by the node levels or sublevels removed, in parentheses (e.g., SND [I to III]).[43]

Extended RND (ERND) is defined by the removal of one or more additional LN groups (e.g., parapharyngeal, paratracheal LNs) or nonlymphatic structures (e.g., carotid artery, paraspinal muscles, pneumogastric nerve), or both, nonroutinely resected by the RND. Any additional structure(s) removed should be identified in parentheses.

A promising method to detect occult micrometastases in the neck is the lymphoscintigraphy associated with the SLNB. The concept is based on the identification of the primary echelon of lymphatic drainage followed by the harvest of the SLN within this basin or basins only, assuming that if the SLN or SLNs are negative, there is no need for a comprehensive neck dissection. The technique was initially proposed for the detection of LN invasion in cutaneous melanoma, and thereafter in various sites.[49-51] SLNB of cervical LNs was introduced as a diagnostic minimally invasive procedure, able to predict more accurately the nodal status in node-negative patients with oral or oropharyngeal SCC.[52] Lymphoscintigraphy and SLNB not only offer the ability to stage the neck disease but also provide information on the presence of atypical basins or lymphatic flow that is not predictable and would typically not be addressed by an SND.[53]

The routine use of SNB for head and neck SCC remains limited, as its role remains inadequately defined in terms of therapeutic efficacy, standardization of the procedure, and

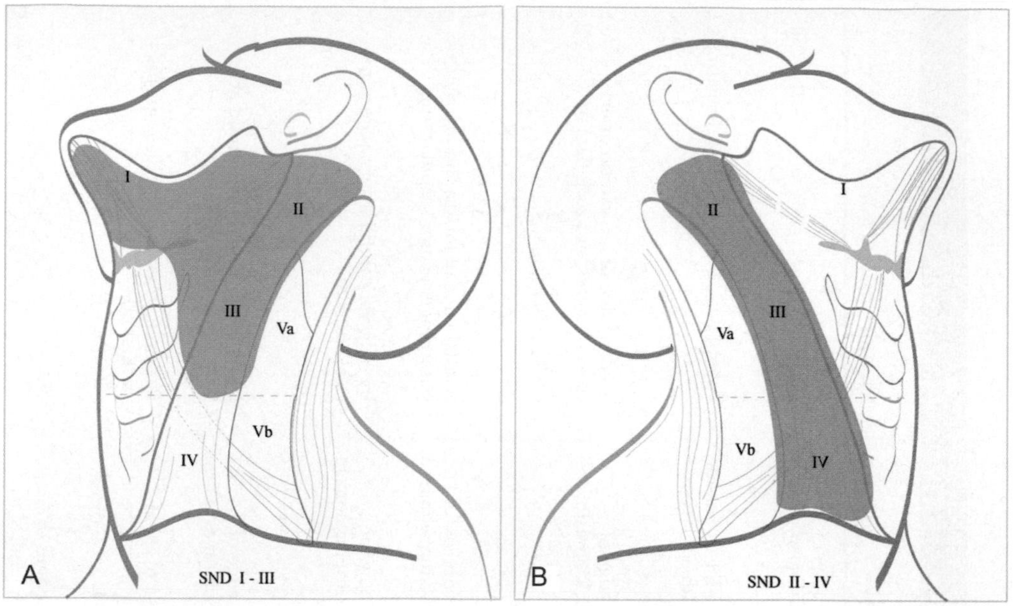

Figure 37-6 Examples of selective neck dissection (SND). In SND I to III or supraomohyoid neck dissection (**A**), only levels I, II, and III are removed. In SND II to IV or lateral neck dissection (**B**), only levels II, III, and IV are removed.

quality of life in comparison with an SND, SNB should not be considered as a standard of care and therefore should only be considered as an investigational technique to be performed within the framework of clinical trials.[54] Multi-institutional trials are ongoing to confirm the validity of this technique.[55]

NECK NODE DELINEATION AND IRRADIATION TECHNIQUES

Delineation of the Clinical Target Volume

Several authors have proposed recommendations for the delineation of the neck node levels.[44,56-59] It is beyond the scope of this chapter to compare them all. In the radiation oncology community, however, the so-called Brussels and Rotterdam guidelines have emerged as those most widely used.[56-58] Detailed comparison of these guidelines reveals a few important discrepancies, preventing uniform target volume delineation in the neck among radiation oncologists. A critical review of the two proposals was undertaken in collaboration with representatives of the major European and North American clinical cooperative groups to generate an international set of guidelines for the delineation of the neck node levels in the node-negative neck.[60] The correspondence between these guidelines and neck dissection procedures was further validated.[61] Last, a few amendments were recently proposed to take into account the specific situation of the node-positive and the postoperative neck.[41,62]

The consensus guidelines for the delineation of levels I to VI and the retropharyngeal LNs are presented (Table 37-14 and Fig. 37-7). It should be emphasized that the volumes delineated in this Figure correspond to the clinical target volume (CTV), and hence do not include margins for organ motion or setup inaccuracy. The boundaries refer to a patient lying supine with the head in a "neutral" position. The terms "cranial" and "caudal" refer to structures closer to the cephalic and pedal ends, respectively. The terms "anterior" and "posterior" were chosen to be less confusing than the terms "ventral" and "dorsal," respectively.

It is beyond the scope of this section to discuss in depth the various boundaries of all the node levels. The reader is referred to the original publication.[60] We would like to draw attention to a few specific issues. The upper limit of level II was set at the caudal edge of the lateral process of the first vertebra, which is an easier landmark than the insertion of the posterior belly of the digastric muscle to the mastoid, which is the surgical landmark. For the caudal limit of level IV, it was proposed to arbitrarily set the caudal limit of level IV 2 cm cranially to the cranial edge of the sternoclavicular joint, as the dissection of level IV typically does not go all the way down to the clavicle and definitely never reaches the medial portion of the clavicle at the level of the sternoclavicular joint. The cranial limit of level V (i.e., the base of skull) that was commonly accepted and depicted has been questioned. Hamoir and colleagues[9] challenged the necessity to treat the uppermost part of level Va in mucosal head and neck SCC. They proposed to divide the level Va into two sublevels: level Vas (superior) and level Vai (inferior), using the lower two thirds of the SAN as the cranial limit of level V. From a radiologic point of view, a horizontal plane crossing the cranial edge of the body of the hyoid bone appears as a reliable landmark to separate level Vas and Vai. For the caudal limit of level V, it appears from critical examination of neck dissection procedure that surgeons never dissect the neck further down than the cervical transverse vessels. It was thus agreed to set the caudal limit of level V at CT slices encompassing the cervical transverse vessels.

Last, as the dissection of level V does not extend all the way to the anterior edge of the trapezius muscle, it was proposed to use a virtual line joining the anterolateral border of both trapezius muscles as the posterior limit of level V. The retropharyngeal space is bounded anteriorly by the pharyngeal constrictor muscles, and posteriorly by the prevertebral fascia. For the sake of simplicity and consistency, it was proposed to use the fascia below the pharyngeal mucosa as the anterior limit, and the prevertebral muscles (longus colli and longus capitis) as the posterior limit. Typically, retropharyngeal nodes are divided into a medial and a lateral group. The medial group is an inconsistent group that consists of one or two LNs intercalated in or near the midline, and it was proposed that it could be omitted from the delineation of the retropharyngeal CTV.[63]

As already discussed, in some clinical situations, it was proposed to extend the delineation of the "standard" neck

Table 37-12 **Consensus Guidelines for the Radiologic Boundaries of the Neck Node Levels**

Level	Anatomic Boundaries: Cranial	Caudal	Anterior	Posterior	Lateral	Medial
Ia	Geniohyoid m., plane tangent to basilar edge of mandible	Plane tangent to body of hyoid bone	Symphysis menti, platysma m.	Body of hyoid bone	Medial edge of ant. belly of digastric m.	NA*
Ib	Mylohyoid m., cranial edge of submandibular gland	Plane through central part of hyoid bone	Symphysis menti, platysma m.	Posterior edge of submandibular gland	Basilar edge/innerside of mandible, platysma m., skin	Lateral edge of ant. belly of digastric m.
IIa	Caudal edge of lateral process of C1	Caudal edge of the body of hyoid bone	Post. edge of submandibular gland; ant. edge of int. carotid artery; post. edge of post. belly of digastric m.	Post. border of int. jugular vein	Medial edge of sternocleidomastoid m.	Medial edge of int. carotid artery, paraspinal (levator scapulae) m.
IIb	Caudal edge of lateral process of C1	Caudal edge of the body of hyoid bone	Post. border of int. jugular vein	Post. border of the sternocleidomastoid m.	Medial edge of sternocleidomastoid m.	Medial edge of int. carotid artery, paraspinal (levator scapulae) m.
III	Caudal edge of the body of hyoid bone	Caudal edge of cricoid cartilage	Posterolateral edge of the sternohyoid m.; ant. edge of sternocleidomastoid m.	Post. edge of the sternocleidomastoid m.	Medial edge of sternocleidomastoid m.	Int. edge of carotid artery, paraspinal (scalenius) m.
IV	Caudal edge of cricoid cartilage	2 cm cranial to sternoclavicular joint	Anteromedial edge of sternocleido-mastoid m.	Post. edge of the sternocleidomastoid m.	Medial edge of sternocleidomastoid m.	Medial edge of internal carotid artery, paraspinal (scalenius) m.
V	Cranial edge of body of hyoid bone	CT slice encompassing the transverse cervical vessels†	Post. edge of the sternocleidomastoid m.	Anterolateral border of the trapezius m.	Platysma m., skin	Paraspinal (levator scapulae, splenius capitis) m.
VI	Caudal edge of body of thyroid cartilage‡	Sternal manubrium	Skin; platysma m.	Separation between trachea and esophagus§	Medial edges of thyroid gland, skin, and anteromedial edge of sternocleidomastoid m.	NA
Retropharyngeal	Base of skull	Cranial edge of the body of hyoid bone	Fascia under the pharyngeal mucosa	Prevertebral m. (longus colli, longus capitis)	Medial edge of the internal carotid artery	Midline

*Midline structure lying between the medial borders of the anterior bellies of the digastric muscles.

†For NPC, the reader is referred to the original description of the UICC/AJCC 1997 edition of Ho's triangle. In essence, the fatty planes below and around the clavicle down to the trapezius muscle.

‡For paratracheal and recurrent nodes, the cranial border is the caudal edge of the cricoid cartilage.

§For pretracheal nodes, trachea and anterior edge of cricoid cartilage.

m = muscle; post = posterior; ant = anterior; int = internal; NA = not available.

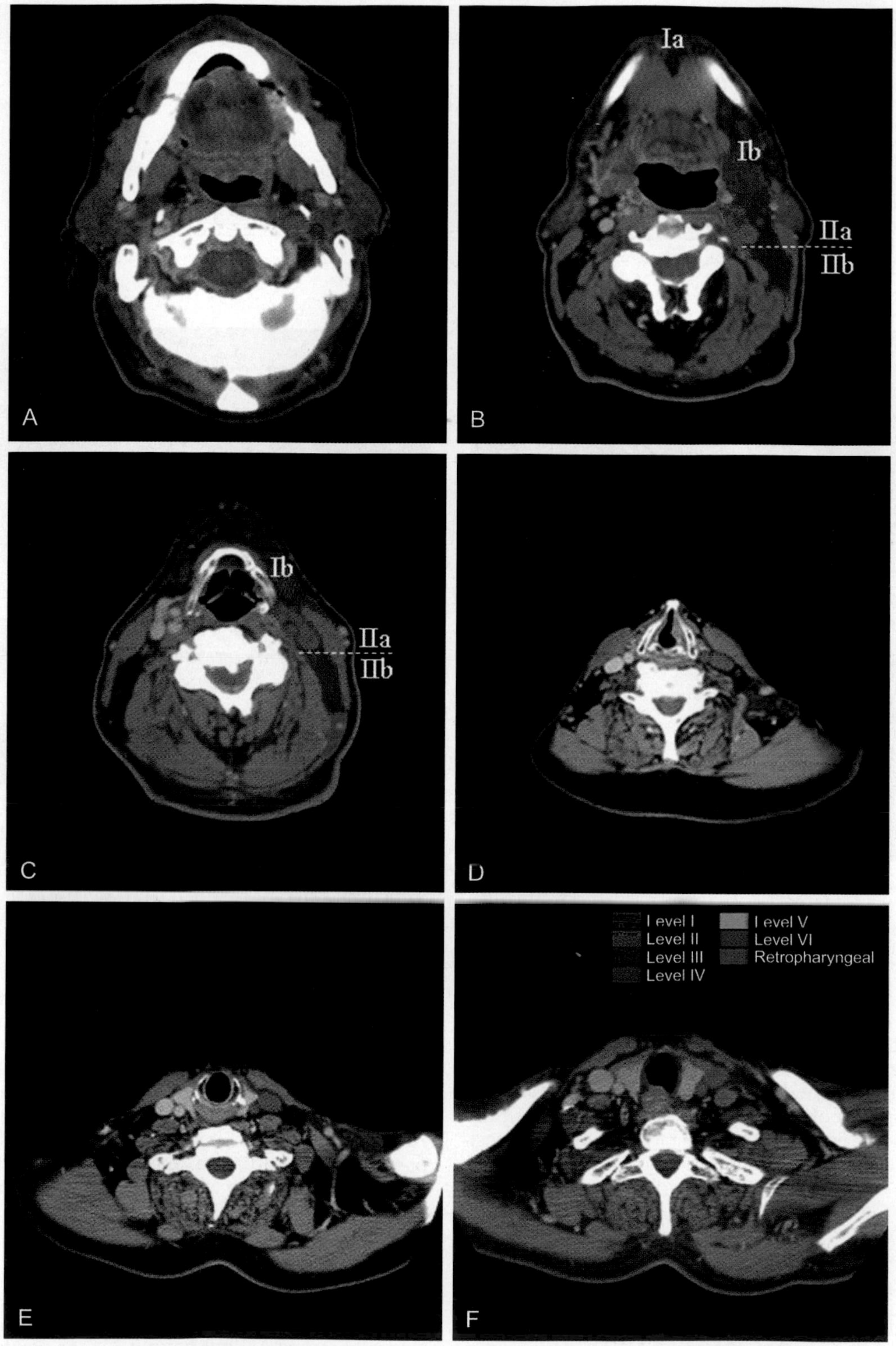

Figure 37-7 CT of a patient with a T1N0M0 glottic squamous cell carcinoma (see tumor in **D**). The examination was performed on a dual-detector spiral CT (Elscint Twin, Haifa, Israel) using a slice thickness of 2.7 mm, an interval reconstruction of 2 mm, and a pitch of 0.7. Contrast was injected intravenously at a rate of 2 mL/s, with a total amount of 100 mL. Sections were taken at the level of the bottom edge of C1 (**A**), upper edge of C3 (**B**), mid-C4 (**C**), bottom edge of C6 (**D**), bottom edge of C7 (**E**), and mid-D1 (**F**). Neck node levels were drawn on each CT slice using the radiologic boundaries detailed in Table 37-14. Each node level corresponds to the clinical target volume and does not include any security margin for organ motion or set-up inaccuracy.

Table 37-15 Boundaries of the Retrostyloid Space and the Subclavicular Fossae

Space	Cranial	Caudal	Anterior	Posterior	Lateral	Medial
Retrostyloid space	Base of skull	Upper limit of level II	Retrostyloid muscles	Vertebral body/base of skull	Deep lobe of parotid	Lateral edge of the RP nodes
Subclavicular fossae	Lower border of level IV/Vb	Sterno-clavicular joint	SCM, skin, clavicle	Anterior edge of posterior scalenus muscle/rib/lung apex	Lateral edge of medial scalenus muscle	Thyroid gland/trachea

PP, parapharyngeal; RP, retropharyngeal; SCM, sternocleidomastoid muscle.

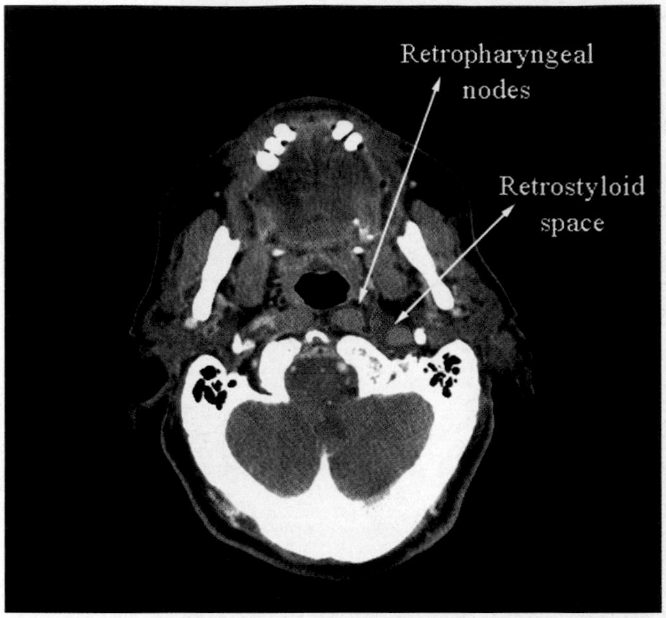

Figure 37-8 CT section at the level of the base of the skull. The image was acquired as explained in Figure 37-7. The delineated areas correspond to the clinical target volume and do not include any security margin for organ motion or set-up inaccuracy.

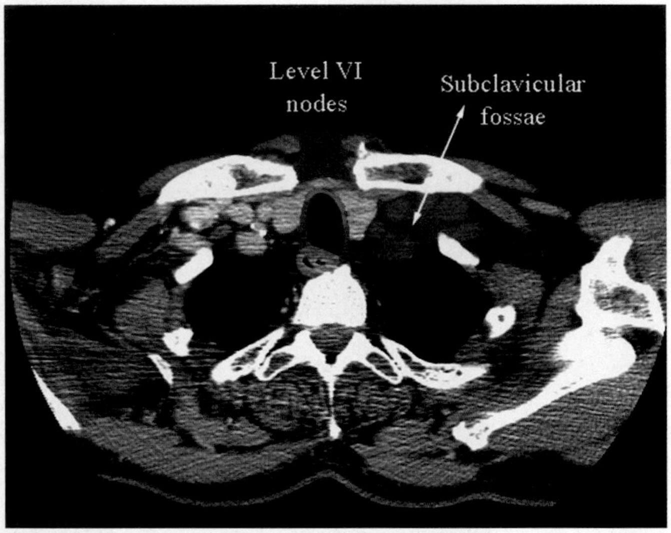

Figure 37-9 CT section at the level of the subclavicular area, 10 mm above the sternoclavicular joint. The image was acquired as explained in Figure 37-7. The delineated areas correspond to the clinical target volume and do not include any security margin for organ motion or set-up inaccuracy.

node levels to include the retrostyloid space and/or the subclavicular fossae. The anatomic boundaries of these spaces are presented in Table 37-15 and illustrated in Figures 37-8 and 37-9. In case of suspicion of extracapsular extension, it was proposed to include the entire SCM in the target volume, at least in the entire invaded level.[41] Another proposal was to adopt a 1-cm margin around the gross tumor volume (GTV) to take into account the microscopic spread outside of the nodes.[62] This proposal would typically apply for the delineation of the therapeutic nodal CTV.

Irradiation Techniques

With the use of 3D conformal radiotherapy (3D-CRT) and intensity modulated radiation therapy (IMRT), there is no standard recipe anymore on how to set up the field sizes and borders according to bony landmarks. Instead, the irradiation technique should be selected and adapted so that the entire planning target volume (PTV) receives the prescribed dose within the adopted dose-volume constraints and in full respect of the ICRU recommendations. It should be mentioned that a new ICRU report is in preparation aiming at updating the present recommendations on dose prescription, specification, and reporting for 3D-CRT and IMRT.

The dose prescription depends on various factors, such as prophylactic versus therapeutic irradiation, the use of combined modality treatment, planned neck node dissection, postoperative irradiation, and so on, which is beyond the scope of this section for comprehensive review. Typically, for primary RT, a prophylactic dose on the order of 50 Gy in about 2 Gy/fraction over 5 weeks and a therapeutic dose on the order of 70 Gy in about 2 Gy/fraction over 7 weeks is prescribed. For postoperative irradiation, depending on the risk factors, doses will range from 60 to 64 to 66 Gy, in 2-Gy fractions over 6 to 6.5 weeks.

CONTROL OF THE N0 NECK

It is generally recommended to perform prophylactic treatment of the neck in patients with primary head and neck SCC clinically staged N0 but having 20% or greater probability of occult LN metastases.[64] Elective neck dissection and elective neck irradiation are equally effective in controlling the N0 neck. The choice between these two procedures generally depends on the treatment modality chosen for the primary tumor, which in turn mainly depends on the institutional policy. However, the basic rule that should govern the choice between surgery and RT is to favor the use of a single modality treatment if possible, avoiding overtreatment. For example, for a T1 or a T2N0 supraglottic larynx, typically, a supraglot-

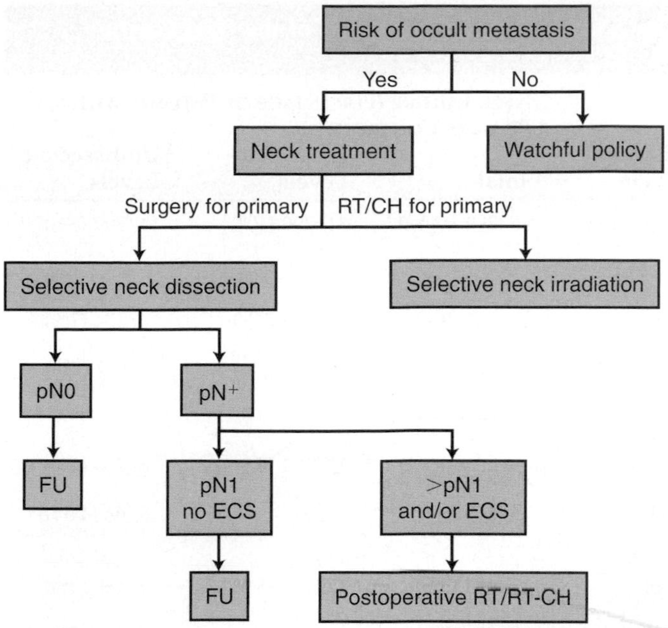

Figure 37-10 Treatment algorithm for the clinically negative neck (N0). ECS, extracapsular spread; FU, follow-up; RT, radiotherapy; RT-CH, concomitant chemoradiotherapy.

tic laryngectomy with a selective neck node dissection and primary RT of the larynx and the neck are equally effective therapeutic options. For such disease stage, the need for postoperative RT is indeed quite low. Conversely, for a T3N0 supraglottic larynx, a conservative treatment approach with primary RT or concomitant chemoradiotherapy should be favored, because of the necessity of postlaryngectomy RT and the nonsuperiority of the surgical approach (Fig. 37-10).

Neck Control after Neck Node Dissection

SND has become more widely used despite some concerns that it may not be as effective as more comprehensive neck dissection, such as an MRND. Anticipating the conclusions that could be drawn from the MSKCC data with regard to the extent of the neck dissection, several groups have been performing SND since the 1950s.[32,34,40,65-74] Such selective neck procedures were initially proposed for clinically node-negative patients and later extended to clinically node-positive patients. These studies are biased, as the patients treated by a selective procedure were probably highly selected with regard to the tumor site, tumor stage, and nodal status. In addition, in the majority of these patients, postoperative RT was usually performed in the presence of high-risk features for primary tumor or neck recurrence, such as resection, multiple node involvement, large node infiltration, or extracapsular spread. It is likely that the irradiated field encompassed those node levels that were not dissected but that could be at risk for microscopic infiltration.

Originally, SND was typically considered as a method to accurately stage the neck but without impact on regional control and survival. A retrospective review of 359 patients with T1-2N0 SCC of the oral cavity and oropharynx treated at the University of Pittsburgh showed significant improvement in regional control, disease-free survival, and regional recurrence-free survival for the group of patients who underwent an SND along with primary tumor excision when compared with another group of patients who only had excision of the primary.[68] It should be noted that the group of patients who underwent an SND were three times more likely to receive postoperative RT, most likely because of identification of adverse prognostic factors on the pathologic specimen. In a prospective randomized trial comparing MRND and SND I to III (supraomohyoid), for clinically node-negative patients with T2-4 tumors of the oral cavity, the Brazilian Head and Neck Cancer Study Group was not able to demonstrate any difference either in the 5-year actuarial overall survival or in the rate of neck failure.[65] Postoperative RT was delivered in case of positive margin of the primary tumor and/or positive LNs. However, this study is biased by the fact that patients included in the SND group and found to have a positive LN (on frozen section) during the neck dissection were offered an MRND.

With these limitations in mind, in some of these studies, the level of the neck recurrence was reported allowing an estimate of the failure rate in the neck inside and outside the dissected levels (Table 37-16). In most of these studies, neck recurrence was reported only in patients with the primary tumor controlled, thus excluding neck recurrence as a result of reseeding from the recurrent primary. In summary, after SND I to III or SND II to IV, the rate of neck failure in nondissected levels was low, typically below 10%. Consequently, SND can be considered as the optimal procedure to manage surgically the N0 neck in patients with a high risk of occult LN metastasis.

Neck Control after Radiotherapy

Table 37-17 presents the percentage of neck recurrences in large retrospective series of pharyngolaryngeal SCCs treated with conventional fractionated RT.[75-77] Some of the patients reported in those series were treated in the late 1950s, and thus the data must be interpreted with caution owing to the likelihood of large uncertainties on the absolute dose calculation and dose distribution. Altogether, the neck control reached more than 92% after RT. After salvage surgery, the ultimate neck control reached a range of 94% to 100%. As expected, because of the high probability of regional control obtained with standard fractionation regimens, altered fractionation regimens or combined chemoradiotherapy does not improve the neck control.[78,79] All these studies were performed using 2D irradiation techniques, that is, with target volumes extending typically from the base of the skull to the clavicles.

With the introduction of 3D-CRT and IMRT and selective neck irradiation, one important issue is the potential risk of geographic miss outside of the irradiated volumes. Eisbruch and associates[80] reported a series of 135 patients treated bilaterally from 1994 to 2002 with 3D-CRT or IMRT for primary tumors mainly located in the oropharynx (n = 80) and without node metastasis on the contralateral neck. Of these, 73 patients received postoperative RT, but none had neck node dissection on the contralateral neck. On the contralateral neck, the CTV included typically level II to IV and the retropharyngeal LNs. For the contralateral level II, the upper limit was set at the junction between the posterior belly of the digastric muscle and the jugular vein. The median prophylactic dose was 50.4 Gy with fraction of 1.8 or 2 Gy. With a median follow-up of 30 months (range, 6 to 105 months), 15 patients had a regional recurrence (of these, 6 had also a primary tumor recurrence), 11 on the ipsilateral side and 4 on the contralateral side. Only 1 of the 15 patients presented a retropharyngeal node recurrence marginal to the CTV. Using a similar treatment philosophy, Bussels and colleagues[81] did not report any recurrence on the ipsilateral N0 neck treated with parotid-sparing 3D-CRT

Table 37-16 **Neck Failure after Selective Neck Dissection for Squamous Cell Carcinomas of the Oral Cavity, Oropharynx, Hypopharynx, and Larynx**

Authors	Site	Clinical Stage (AJCC 1980)	Dissected Levels	Neck Failure (Percentage of Patients with Primary Controlled) Total	Dissected Levels	Undissected Levels
Byers, 1988[66]	Oral cavity, oropharynx, hypopharynx, larynx	T1-4N0	I, I-III, II-IV, I-V	45/299 (15%)*	31/299 (10%)	14/299 (5%)†
Byers, 1985[40]	Oral cavity, oropharynx	T1-4N0-3	I-III	21/234 (9%)	16/234 (7%)	5/234 (2%)
Byers, 1999[67]	Oral cavity, oropharynx, hypopharynx, larynx	T1-4N0-1-2b	I, I-III, I-IV II-IV	37/517 (7%)	26/517 (5%)	11/517 (2%)
Byers, 1999[67]	Oral cavity, oropharynx	T1-4N0-1-2b	I-III, I-IV	19/284 (6.5%)	13/284 (4.5%)	6/284 (2%)
Brazilian[65] HNCSG 1998	Oral cavity	T2-4N0	I-III‡	6/64 (9%)	3/64 (4.5%)	3/64 (4.5%)§
Duvvuri, 2004[68]	Oral cavity, oropharynx.	T1-2N0	I-III	17/180 (9.5%)	12/180 (6.5%)¶	5/180 (3%)
Pellitteri, 1997[72]	Oral cavity + oropharynx,	T1 T4 N0-3 T1-4N0-3	I-III/I-IV	7/42 (17%)	2/42 (5%)	5/42 (12%)**
	Hypopharynx + larynx	T1-4 N0-3	II-IV	1/25 (4%)	1/25 (4%)	0/25 (0%)
Pitman, 1997[73]	Oral cavity orohypopharynx, larynx	T1-4N0 T1-4N0	I-III/I-IV II-IV	5/142 (3.5%)	5/142 (3.5%)	0/142 (0%)
Spiro, 1988[32]	Oral cavity, oropharynx, larynx	T1-4N0-1	I-III	12/107 (11%)	5/107 (4.5%)	7/107 (6.5%)
Spiro, 1996[74]	Oral cavity, oropharynx (98%)	T1-4N0-1-2a-2b	I-III	16/296 (5.5%)	8/296 (2.7%)	8/296 (2.7%)

HNCSG, Head and Neck Cancer Study Group.
*Patients treated by surgery alone.
†Six of these patients had failure on the contralateral undissected neck.
‡Part of a randomized study comparing radical modified versus supraomohyoid neck dissection.
§One of these patients had failure on the contralateral undissected neck.
¶Including one neck failure of unknown location.
**Three of these patients had failure on the contralateral undissected neck.

Table 37-17 **Neck Failure after Primary Radiotherapy for Node-Negative Patients**

Authors	Primary Tumor Site	No. of Patients (Study Period)	Dose/Overall Treatment Time	Control of the Neck After Radiotherapy	After Salvage Surgery
Bernier and Bataini[75]	Oropharynx, hypopharynx, larynx	611 (1958-1974)	45-55 Gy 4.5-5.5 wk	93%	Not stated
Johansen[77]	Oropharynx, hypopharynx, larynx	1324 (1963-1991)	57-72 Gy 6-9 wk*	92% at 10 y	94% at 10 y
Alpert[76]	Supraglottic larynx	98 (1971-1998)	50 Gy/5 wk	96.7%	100%

*Including 28% of patients with a split course.

in a series of 72 patients with oral cavity and pharyngolaryngeal SCC. Chao and associates[82] also looked at the pattern of recurrence in a series of 126 patients treated postoperatively (n = 74) or primarily (n = 52) for head and neck SCC by IMRT from 1997 to 2000. In this series, the lower neck (below the thyroid notch) was treated with a "traditional" anterior field. With a median follow-up of 26 months, 17 (13%) recurrences were observed. Six of these patients had recurrence outside of the target volumes, of which only one was in the lower neck of an N0 patient.

CONTROL OF THE N1-3 NECK

Neck Control after Surgery Alone

The surgical management of the N1 neck is controversial (Fig. 37-11). Traditionally, a comprehensive neck dissection (RND and MRND) has been the surgical standard for patients presenting with neck disease. Andersen and associates[83] reported that the rates of regional recurrences in the dissected neck following RND or MRND type I for N1 or N2 disease were similar. Selective procedures have, however, gained popularity. In the retrospective study by Byers and colleagues,[67] including 517 SND procedures mainly for patients with N0 or N1 neck disease, 50 patients were finally staged pN1. Of these patients, 36 received postoperative RT for the presence of risk factors on either the tumor or nodal site, and only 1 (3%) presented with a regional recurrence. Without RT despite the presence of risk factors, 5 of 14 patients (36%) had neck failure. In a large retrospective review of 296 SNDs I to III, Spiro and colleagues[74] reported a rate of regional failure of 6.5% in patients staged with a pathologically positive neck. Most patients with pathologically invaded LNs had postoperative RT. With the inherent limitation of retrospective studies, it appears that SND for patients with limited neck disease is a safe procedure, providing that postoperative RT is given in presence of risk factors for regional relapse.

Despite use of aggressive single and combined treatment protocols, patients with advanced metastatic neck disease still have poor prognosis because of high risk of regional failure and distant metastases.[84,85] However, the concept of less than radical procedure has gained acceptance even in advanced regional disease. Khafif and associates[86] reported the results of 118 patients with N2-3 disease, treated with RND or MRND and was not able to find any difference in overall survival between the two groups. The recurrence rate in the MRND group increased significantly in comparison with the group of patients treated with standard RND (52% versus 33%), but some MRND procedures were not really comprehensive. In a study comparing RND and MRND (type I) in 212 patients with stages N2 and N3, the MSKCC group reported an overall 86% 5-year neck control rate and 61% 5-year actuarial survival rate.[83] No difference was found between the two groups. Adjuvant postoperative RT enhances regional control but does not seem to significantly improve survival.[87] Investigators of the Royal Prince Alfred Hospital in Sydney, Australia reported the outcome of 181 patients who had 233 neck dissections for N2-3 disease (163 ERND, RND, or MRND, and 70 SND).[88] Postoperative RT to the neck was given in 82% of the patients. At 5 years, the control of disease in the treated neck was achieved in 86%. Adjuvant RT significantly improved neck control (p = .004) but did not alter survival.

The utility of ERND depends on whether acceptable control rates are attainable without prohibitive morbidity. Shaha[89] described the results on 40 patients staged N2-3 treated by ERND combined with postoperative RT. The regional control reached a rate of 70% at 2 years, with one perioperative death. The morbidity of ERND depends on the additional structure or structures resected. If a common carotid artery is removed, the perioperative mortality ranges from 6% to 58%.[90,91] However, when the structures sacrificed are of no major neurovascular significance (e.g., parotid gland LNs, paraspinal muscles), the additional morbidity is minimal.

Neck Control after Primary Radiotherapy

The lower probability of regional control of the positive neck with RT already has been documented by several retrospective series.[75,77,92] In a series of 1646 patients with SCC of the oropharynx and pharyngolarynx from the Institut Curie in Paris, the 3-year regional control probability was 98%, 90%, 88%, and 71% for N0, N1, N2, and N3 (AJCC 1976 classification), respectively.[75] The nodal size was an even more discriminating factor with nodal failure of 6%, 14%, and 39% for nodes below 3 cm, between 4 and 7 cm, and more than 7 cm, respectively.[92] In this series, 75% of the neck nodes were, however, treated by a form of concomitant boost approach with total dose in the range of 70 to 85 Gy in 5 to 6 weeks. In the series of 458 node-positive patients with SCC of the larynx and pharynx treated at Aarhus University Hospital from 1963 to 1991, the 5-year neck node control reached 68%, 68%, and 56% for N1, N2, and N3 UICC 1982 stage, respectively.[77]

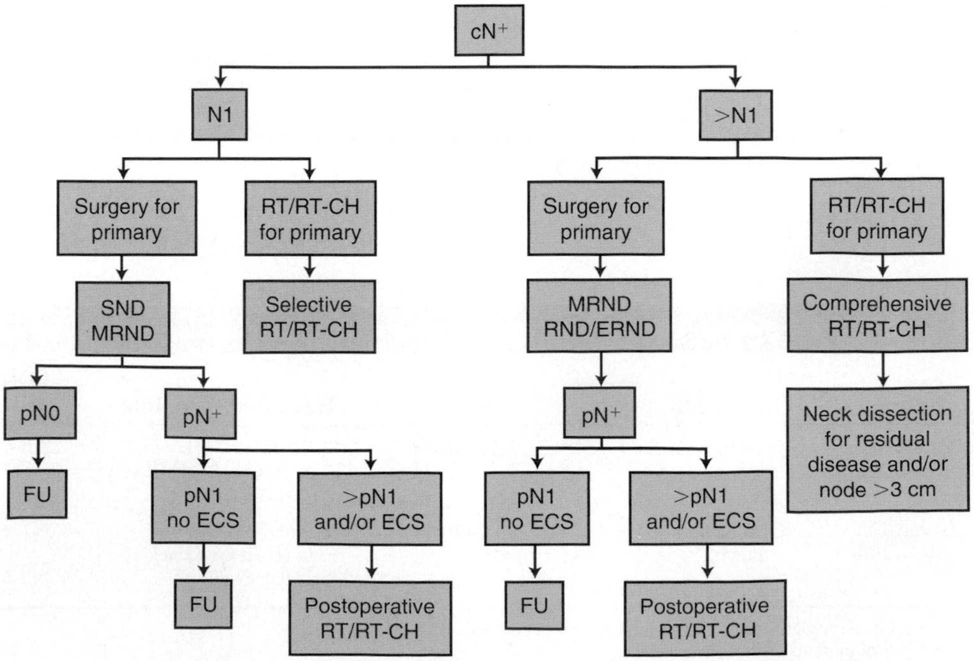

Figure 37-11 Treatment algorithm of the clinically positive neck. ECS, extracapsular spread; ERND, extended radical neck dissection; FU, follow-up; MRND, modified radical neck dissection; RND, radical neck dissection; RT, radiotherapy; RT-CH, concomitant chemoradiotherapy; SND, selective neck dissection.

A key issue in the management of the positive neck by RT is whether these rather poor results are improved by hyperfractionated or accelerated regimens or by concomitant chemoradiotherapy. In randomized studies comparing a standard fractionated regimen to an altered fractionated regimen, no improvement was observed between the two arms (Table 37-18).[93-95] In the European Organization for Research and Treatment of Cancer (EORTC) 22791, only N0 or N1 neck patients were included, and because of the very good control of the neck in the standard arm, it was not surprising that the hyperfractionated regimen did not bring any benefit.[93] In the DAHANCA 6 and 7 trials, no significant regional improvement was observed with the accelerated regimen in the node-positive patients.[94] Similarly, despite a benefit in overall survival, the Toronto trial did not observe any increase in the control of the neck with an accelerated hyperfractionated regimen.[95] Contrary to results achieved with altered fractionation regimens, concomitant chemoradiotherapy regimens appear to have an impact on the control of the neck (Table 37-19).[96,97] In the study of Calais, all neck stages were analyzed together. However, because 75% of the patients were node positive, it is very unlikely that the 12% improvement results only from a beneficial effect on the N0 patients. In the study of Lavertu, which included fewer patients, the improvement in node control was observed for all positive neck stages.

Indications for Postoperative Irradiation and Postoperative Chemoirradiation

The benefit of postoperative RT in head and neck SCC has progressively emerged in the 1970s and 1980s as a standard of care for patients at high risk of locoregional relapse after surgery.[98-101] Prognostic indicators for locoregional relapse after surgery have been progressively identified including the primary disease site, the surgical margins at the primary site, the presence of perineural invasion, the number of metastatic LNs, and the presence of extracapsular rupture.[102,103] Based on the clustering of these pathologic factors, the M.D. Anderson Cancer Center proposed to stratify the patients into three risk categories, conditioning the need for postoperative irradiation (Table 37-20).[104] In the absence of any risk factor, the need of postoperative RT could not be demonstrated. Patients with extracapsular rupture or a combination of two or more risk factors were identified as being at high risk of locoregional relapse, and for those patients, a randomized study demonstrated the benefit of a radiation dose of 63 Gy (in 35 fractions) compared to 57.6 Gy (in 32 fractions). For patients with only one risk factor other than extracapsular rupture, a dose of 57.6 Gy was demonstrated as optimal. A subsequent study from the same group further validated the use of these categories of risk factors and also individualized the time between surgery and the start of postoperative RT and the total treatment time (from surgery to the end of RT) as additional risk factors.[105] In this study, it was also demonstrated that patients with high risk of relapse benefited from an accelerated treatment (63 Gy in 5 weeks versus 63 Gy in 7 weeks) in terms of both locoregional control and survival.

With the need to further improve the locoregional control after surgery and postoperative RT, few trials combining postoperative concomitant chemotherapy and RT were reported in the 1990s.[106,107] Although positive in favor of the combined approach, these studies did not really influence the pattern of

Table 37-18 Probability of Neck Node Control after Altered Fractionated Regimens

Authors	Primary Tumor Site	Stage	Treatment Schedule	Control of the Neck Std. Arm	Exp. Arm
Horiot[93] EORTC 22791 (N = 325)	Oropharynx	T2-3 N0-1 M0	Std: 70 Gy/35 f/7 wk Exp: 80.5 Gy/70 f/7 wk	N0: 93% at 5 y N1: 90% at 5 y	N0: 93% at 5 y N1: 90% at 5 y
Overgaard[94] DAHANCA 6 and 7 (N = 1476)	Oral cavity, pharynx, supraglottic larynx	Stage I-IV	Std: 62-68 Gy/6-7 wk Exp: 62-68 Gy/5-6 wk	N^-: 68% N^+: 44%	N^-: 77%*† N^+: 52%*‡
Cummings[95] (N = 331)	Oropharynx, hypopharynx, larynx	Stage III-IV	Std: 51 Gy/20 f/4 wk Exp: 58 Gy/40 f/4 wk	All stage: 71% at 5 y	All stage: 68%§ at 5 y

F, fraction; Std, standard; exp, experimental.
*Locoregional control.
†Odds ratio (95% CI): .65 (.50-.85).
‡Odds ratio (95% CI): .72 (.49-1.05).
§$p = .80$.

Table 37-19 Probability of Neck Node Control after Concomitant Chemoradiotherapy

Authors	Primary Tumor Site	Stage	Treatment Schedule	Control of the Neck Std. Arm	Exp. Arm
Calais[96] (n = 222)	Oropharynx	Stage III-IV*	Std: 70 Gy/7 wk Exp: 70 Gy/7 wk + Carbo-5-FU ×3	All stage: 69%	All stage: 81%
Lavertu[97] (n = 100)	Oral cavity, pharynx, larynx	Stage III-IV†	Std: 65-72 Gy/7 wk Exp: 65-72 Gy/7 wk + CDDP-5-FU ×2	N1: 6/10 (60%) N2-3: 13/27 (48%)	N1: 8/8 (100%) N2-3: 17/26 (65%)

Carbo, carboplatin; 5FU, 5-fluorouracil; CDDP, cisplatin.
*75% of patients were node positive.
†71% of patients were node positive.

care of patients primarily treated with surgery. The European Organization for Research and Treatment of Cancer (EORTC) and the Radiation Therapy Oncology Group (RTOG) conducted similarly designed studies aiming at assessing the benefit of postoperative RT (60 to 66 Gy) combined with cisplatin (100 mg/m^2) given on days 1, 22, and 43 for patients with a variety of risk factors but slightly different between the two trials.[108,109] In the EORTC study, a highly statistically significant benefit in favor of the combined treatment was observed for both locoregional control and overall survival (Table 37-21). In the RTOG study, the benefit in locoregional control probability did not translate into a statistically significant difference in survival. Combined-modality treatment did not decrease the incidence of distant metastasis in any of these studies. In both studies, the concomitant use of chemotherapy significantly enhanced the acute local toxicity of RT and only half the patients could actually receive the full treatment as planned. A meta-analysis of these two studies demonstrated a statistically significant benefit of combined chemoradiotherapy but only in patients presenting with positive surgical margins and/or extracapsular spread, that is, patients with the highest risk of relapse after surgery.[110] For the other patients, RT alone can still be considered as a standard of care.

Table 37-20 Prognostic Factors for Locoregional Relapse after Surgery

Moderate Risk	High Risk
Positive margin at the primary (R1) or close margin (<5 mm)	Extracapsular spread (ECS)
Primary tumor in the oral cavity	A combination of two or more of the moderate risk factors
Perineural invasion	
Two or more invaded lymph nodes	
Two or more invaded node levels	
Invaded node(s) more than 3 cm in diameter	
More than 6 weeks between surgery and start of RT	

From Peters LJ, Goepfert H, Ang KK, et al: Evaluation of the dose for postoperative radiation therapy of head and neck cancer: first report of a prospective randomized trial. Int J Radiat Oncol Biol Phys 26:3-11, 1993.

Indications for Postradiotherapy Neck Node Dissection

Advances in (chemo)radiation for advanced head and neck carcinoma have demonstrated that organ preservation was feasible without compromising disease-free survival and overall survival.[111,112] This strategy has led to controversial issues concerning the role of node dissection following RT or chemoradiation for patients with N2-3 disease at initial diagnosis. Residual neck mass may be present in as much as 30% to 50% of patients after completion of chemoradiotherapy. For those patients, irrespective of the neck stage, there seems to be a consensus in the literature favoring an immediate neck node dissection, because of the very low probability of achieving neck control with salvage surgery when recurrence develops.[113] Whether a neck dissection should be proposed to all patients with N2-3 disease at diagnosis or only to those without a complete response is still a matter of debate.[114-117] This controversy seems to be fueled by the difficulty of assessing the residual neck disease after organ-preservation protocol. In this respect, the use of FDG-PET scanning has gained some interest. In a study including 41 patients treated with definite RT (with or without concomitant chemotherapy), a negative post-RT PET was highly correlated with a negative pathologic finding after neck node dissection or fine-needle aspiration or with the absence of neck relapse (negative predictive value of 100% for a maximum standardized uptake values (SUV) <3.0).[118] In another study including 24 patients staged with FDG-PET after induction chemotherapy followed by chemoradiotherapy, the negative predictive value of PET reached only 73%.[119] Further prospective studies are thus needed to validate the use of PET to assess the need for post (chemo)radiation neck node dissection. In the meantime, balancing the benefit with the increased morbidity of post (chemo)radiation surgery, evidence suggests that neck node dissection be restricted to those patients with a noncomplete response after organ-preservation protocol.

LATE COMPLICATIONS AFTER NECK TREATMENT

Complications of Neck Node Dissection

In addition to medical complications inherent to any surgical procedure, neck dissection may potentially be associated with some specific perioperative complications and late complications or sequelae. The description of perioperative complications is beyond the scope of this chapter. Readers interested in such topics will find detailed information in a textbook dedicated to head and neck surgery.[120]

Table 37-21 Efficacy of Concomitant Chemotherapy and Postoperative Radiotherapy

			LR Control		Overall Survival	
Authors	Site	Regimen	RT	RT-CH	RT	RT-CH
Bernier[108] (N = 334)	Oral cavity, oropharynx, hypopharynx, larynx	66 Gy (6.5 w) vs 66 Gy (6.5 w) + CDDP (100 mg/m^2) d 1, d 22, d 43	69% at 5 y	82% at 5 y*	40% at 5 y	53% at 5 y†
Cooper[109] (N = 416)	Oral cavity, oropharynx, hypopharynx, larynx	60-66 Gy (6-6.5 wk) vs 60-66 Gy (6-6.5 wk) + CDDP (100 mg/m^2) d 1, d 22, d 43	72% at 2 y	82% at 2 y‡	56% at 2 y	64% at 2 y§

CDDP, cisplatin; CH, chemotherapy; RT, radiation therapy.
*p = .007 (Gray's test).
†p = .02 (log-rank test).
‡p = .01 (Gray's test).
§p = .19 (log-rank test).

Recognized complications after neck dissection include numbness and/or burning of the neck and ear, neck pain, shoulder discomfort, neck tightness, lower lip weakness, and cosmetic disfigurement. In 2001, Shah proposed a neck dissection–specific quality-of-life (QOL) questionnaire used in a series of patients who had undergone neck dissection as part of their treatment.[121] Some of these patients had been previously treated by chemotherapy (25%) or RT (50%). Neck tightness and shoulder discomfort had the greatest effect on QOL. Advanced tumor stage, often requiring more radical surgery and use of chemotherapy or RT, was associated with a worse QOL after neck dissection. Overall, QOL after neck dissection tends to improve with time.[121]

The most noticeable sequela induced by SAN resection is the decreased ability to abduct the shoulder above 90 degrees. We should, however, be aware that any type of neck dissection may result in impairment of shoulder function.[122] Studies reported that preservation of the SAN in MRND and SND was associated with a better QOL and fewer shoulder disorders at both short and long term.[121] Using the University of Washington QOL questionnaire, the Liverpool group reported that little morbidity associated with shoulder dysfunction was observed following a unilateral level I to III or I to IV neck dissection in comparison with patients undergoing primary surgery without a neck dissection.[123] However, unilateral neck dissection extending to level V and bilateral SND (I to III or I to IV) were associated with statistically significantly worse shoulder dysfunction. Adjuvant RT seemed to have a detrimental effect on shoulder dysfunction, whether or not the patient had a unilateral SND. In another series, assessment of patients who underwent neck dissection with or without RT at least 1 year previously revealed that neck pain was present in one third of the patients, shoulder pain was present in 37%, and loss of sensation was reported in 65% of the patients (related to the number of dissected levels and to RT).[124] A prospective study on objective assessment after treatment concluded that adjuvant RT had no effect on shoulder joint function and that shoulder disability was inevitable in all types of neck dissections, whether the SAN was spared or not. However, shoulder function was better after SND and MRND than after RND, but electromyographic findings were similar after either RND or MRND/SND.[125] The benefit of postoperative physical therapy has been stressed, and it should be started in the early postoperative period after all types of neck dissections.[126]

Complications of Neck Irradiation

Late complications after head and neck irradiation were discussed in the previous chapters. In the following section, only specific complications arising in the soft tissues of the neck will be reviewed. They mainly concern subcutaneous fibrosis, thyroid dysfunction, and carotid artery stenosis. Typically, late complication probability depends on the total dose, the dose per fraction, the time interval between fractions, the volume of normal tissue that received a high dose, and the use of concomitant chemotherapy and/or biologic modifier.

The probability of grade 3-4 (RTOG late morbidity scale) subcutaneous fibrosis in the neck is rather low after standard RT. From randomized studies performed in the 1990s, it can be estimated at around 3%.[96,127-129] After accelerated or hyperfractionated treatments, no increase in grade 3-4 subcutaneous toxicity was observed, providing that enough time was left between fractions.[128] Indeed, in an EORTC trial with only a 4-hour interfraction time, a 50% risk of fibrosis was documented at 5 years after treatment.[130] After concomitant chemoradiotherapy, randomized trials reported a substantial increase in late skin morbidity reaching figures around 10%.[96]

Clinically indolent hypothyroidism has been reported in patients irradiated on the lower neck with a frequency of up to 24%.[131,132] The majority of patients usually develop hypothyroidism within 1 year posttreatment. Postoperative RT, especially after laryngeal surgery, including partial thyroidectomy, has been shown to be a risk factor. Yearly thyroid function testing (i.e., thyroid-stimulating hormone level) is advised in the follow-up of patients irradiated to the neck.

Carotid artery stenosis after neck irradiation has been reported by several authors, but very few studies have investigated the incidence, disease patterns, and risk factors. Matched control Doppler US examinations have reported significant carotid stenosis in 30% to 50% of patients previously irradiated to the neck.[133] Compared to the general population, a relative risk of stroke of 5.6 has been reported in patients previously irradiated to the neck.[134] This relative risk was further increased for patients older than 60 years and with follow-up longer than 10 years. Increased attention to the clinical signs of carotid stenosis together with proper management of the other risk factors (e.g., diabetes, hypertension, hypercholesterolemia, smoking, obesity) should contribute to decrease the incidence of stroke and neurologic sequelae in this patient population.

All the published data on late complications are from the pre-IMRT era. With the use of modern RT technique, a major reduction in late complications is anticipated mainly through a reduction in the volume of normal tissue irradiated at high dose and a reduction of the "uncontrolled" hot spot within or outside of the PTV. The introduction of IMRT has, however, raised the controversial concern of an increased risk of radiation-induced secondary neoplasm since a larger volume of normal tissue might be irradiated at lower dose in comparison with standard 2D techniques. Also, the delivery of a specified dose to the isocenter from modulated fields requires a longer beam time compared to the same dose delivered with a nonmodulated field. The IMRT treatment plan then results in an increase in the number of monitor units by a factor of 2 to 3, increasing the dose outside the boundary of the primary collimator as a result of leakage and scattered radiation.[135] As a consequence, the total body dose received is substantially increased. It is estimated that an additional 0.5% of surviving patients will develop a secondary malignancy as a result of an increased volume of normal tissue receiving a small radiation dose. This number needs to be added to the 0.25% of surviving patients who subsequently develop a radiation-induced malignancy. In all, it is thus estimated that about 0.75% of surviving patients are expected to develop a secondary malignancy as a result of the switch to IMRT, which is approximately twofold greater than the incidence observed following more conventional RT.[136] Whatever the contribution of IMRT in the induction of secondary cancers may be, we should bear in mind that even if IMRT increases the probability of locoregional control and the potential for increased cause-specific survival, this group of patients will suffer from comorbidities and increased risk for a second primary associated with their lifestyle. This may decrease the relative importance of radiation-induced secondary malignancies.

MANAGEMENT OF THE RECURRENT NECK

Whether treated by RT, surgery, or the combination of both, the prognosis of patients with recurrence in the neck remains abysmal. Recurrent neck disease is quite invariably associated with unfavorable prognostic factors. Extracapsular spread is almost always reported and multiple LNs levels are frequently involved.[137] Neck recurrences are often unresectable, due to involvement of the wall of the common carotid artery or the internal carotid artery, the paraspinal muscles, and the cranial nerves. Even when salvage surgery is attempted, the inability to achieve a complete resection with clear margins is generally the rule.

Very few studies have specifically addressed the problem of recurrent neck disease following curative treatment in HNSCC. Godden retrospectively reviewed the charts of 35 patients with recurrent neck disease.[137] More than 80% of patients had primary surgery and the remainders were treated with RT. Fifty percent of the patients treated with primary surgery had postoperative RT. Eighteen patients had a neck dissection at initial presentation. The recurrence was managed by neck dissection in 25 patients, and among them, 18 had postoperative RT. Ten (29%) were considered as inoperable. Of the 18 patients who had an initial neck dissection, 9 (50%) recurred in level II, previously cleared. Neck recurrence seemed to be more related to residual disease after the first neck dissection. This surprisingly high rate of level II recurrence stresses the necessity of an adequate training for surgeons performing neck dissection procedures. In this series, the ultimate control of the neck was only obtained in 5 of the 35 patients and the 4-year overall survival did not exceed 20%.

The likelihood of successful salvage treatment in patients who experienced neck recurrence after primary RT is very low. Bernier and Bataini[75] reviewed 116 patients with isolated nodal failure after RT alone for oropharyngeal, hypopharyngeal, and laryngeal carcinoma. Fourteen patients had salvage neck dissection and 18 were reirradiated on the neck. Only one patient (1%) was successfully salvaged. The University of Florida reviewed the medical records of 51 patients who experienced recurrent disease occurring in the neck only.[138] Only 18 patients (35%) underwent salvage treatment, chemotherapy alone in 4 patients, chemotherapy and neck dissection in 1 patient, neck dissection alone in 11 patients, and neck dissection with postoperative RT in 2 patients. After salvage treatment, all patients had relapse of disease (locally, regionally, or distantly). Control of the neck at 5 years was 9% for the group who underwent salvage treatment, which was similar to the rate of neck control for the whole population. For the whole group of patients, absolute and cause-specific survival reached 10% at 5 years for both end points. However, at 3 years, patients who received salvage treatment had absolute and cause-specific survival rates of 44%. In comparison, none of the 33 remaining patients was alive at 3 years.

Some institutions have evaluated salvage treatment with aggressive combined modality approaches that include low-dose reirradiation (preoperative or postoperative with or without concurrent chemotherapy) combined with an attempt at gross resection plus intraoperative irradiation (IORT) with either electrons (IOERT) or high dose rate brachytherapy (HDR-IORT).[139] Although the series involve small numbers of patients, early results suggest potential improvements in both locoregional control and survival when compared with standard salvage approaches, and further evaluation is warranted.

Summary

The majority of patients with regional recurrence are unable to undergo salvage treatment, and when salvage treatment with standard approaches (surgical resection, external beam radiation) is attempted, control of the neck remains poor. Salvage neck dissection alone should be restricted to patients with limited recurrence in the neck.

REFERENCES

1. Rouvière H: Anatomie Humaine Descriptive Et Topographique, 6th ed. Paris, Masson et Cie, 1948, pp 226-230.
2. Vidic B, Suarez-Quian C: Anatomy of the head and neck. *In* Harrison LB, Sessions RB, Ki Hong W (eds): Head and Neck Cancer. A Multidisciplinary Approach. Philadelphia, Lippincott-Raven, 1998, pp 79-114.
3. Spiessl B, Beahrs OH, Hermanek P, et al: TNM Atlas. Illustrated Guide to the TNM/pTNM Classification of Malignant Tumours, 3rd ed, 2nd rev. Berlin/Heidelberg/New York, Springer, 1992.
4. Robbins KT, Medina JE, Wolfe GT, et al: Standardizing neck dissection terminology. Official report of the Academy's Committee for Head and Neck Surgery and Oncology. Arch Otolaryngol Head Neck Surg 117:601-605, 1991.
5. Shah JP, Strong E, Spiro RH, et al: Surgical grand rounds. Neck dissection: current status and future possibilities. Clin Bull 11:25-33, 1981.
6. Hermanek P, Henson DE, Hutter RVP, Sobin LH (eds): TNM Supplement. A Commentary on Uniform Use. Berlin/Heidelberg/New York, Springer, 1993.
7. Robbins KT: Classification of neck dissection: current concepts and future considerations. Otolaryngol Clin North Am 31:639-656, 1998.
8. Robbins KT: Integrating radiological criteria into the classification of cervical lymph node disease. Arch Otolaryngol Head Neck Surg 125:385-387, 1999.
9. Hamoir M, Desuter G, Gregoire V, et al: A proposal for redefining the boundaries of level V. Is dissection of the apex of level V necessary in mucosal cell carcinoma of the head and neck? Arch Otolaryngol Head Neck Surg 128:1381-1383, 2002.
10. Coche EE, Duprez T, Lonneux M: Imaging the lymph nodes: CT, MRI, and PET. *In* Grégoire V, Scaillet P, Ang K (eds): Clinical Target Volumes in Conformal and Intensity Modulated Radiation Therapy. New York, Springer-Verlag, 2002, pp 37-67.
11. Ishikawa M, Anzai Y: MR imaging of lymph nodes in the head and neck. Neuroimaging Clin N Am 14:679-694, 2004.
12. Curtin HD, Ishwaran H, Mancuso AA, et al: Comparison of CT and MR imaging in staging of neck metastases. Radiology 207:123-130, 1998.
13. King AD, Tse GMK, Ahuja AT, et al: Necrosis in metastatic neck nodes: diagnostic accuracy of CT, MR imaging, and US. Radiology 230:720-726, 2004.
14. Star-Lack JM, Adalsteinsson E, Adam MF, et al: In vivo 1H MR spectroscopy of human head and neck lymph node metastasis and comparison with oxygen tension measurements. AJNR Am J Neuroradiol 21:183-193, 2000.
15. Fischbein NJ, Noworolski SM, Henry RG, et al: Assessment of metastatic cervical adenopathy using dynamic contrast-enhanced MR imaging. AJNR Am J Neuroradiol 24:301-311, 2003.
16. Sumi M, Sakihama N, Sumi T, et al: Discrimination of metastatic cervical lymph node with diffusion-weighted MR imaging in patients with head and neck cancer. AJNR Am J Neuroradiol 24:1627-1634, 2003.
17. Schroder H, Yeung HW, Gonen M, et al: Head and neck cancer: clinical usefulness and accuracy of PET-CT image fusion. Radiology 231:65-72, 2004.
18. Torabi M, Aquino SL, Harishinghani MG: Current concepts in lymph node imaging. J Nucl Med 45:1509-1518, 2004.
19. Van de Wiele C, Versijpt J, Dierckx RA, et al: Tc-99m-labelled HL91 versus CT and biopsy for the visualization of tumor recurrence of squamous head and neck carcinoma. Nucl Med Commun 22:269-275, 2001.
20. Lonneux M, Lawson G, Ide C, et al: Positron emission tomography with fluorodeoxyglucose for suspected head and neck tumor recurrence in the symptomatic patient. Laryngoscope 110:1493-1497, 2000.
21. Daisne JF, Duprez T, Weynand B, et al: Tumor volume in pharyngolaryngeal squamous cell carcinoma: comparison at CT, MR imaging, and FDG PET and validation with surgical specimen. Radiology 233:93-100, 2004.

22. Schwartz DL, Ford E, Rajendran J, et al: FDG-PET/CT imaging for preradiotherapy staging of head-and-neck squamous cell carcinoma. Int J Radiat Oncol Biol Phys 61:129-136, 2005.
23. Greene FL, Page DL, Fleming ID, et al: AJCC Cancer Staging Handbook, 6th ed. Heidelberg, Springer, 2002.
24. O'Sullivan B, Shah J: New TNM staging criteria for head and neck tumors. Semin Surg Oncol 21:30-42, 2003.
25. Bataini JP, Bernier J, Brugere J, et al: Natural history of neck disease in patients with squamous cell carcinoma of the oropharynx and pharyngolarynx. Radiother Oncol 3:245-255, 1985.
26. Lindberg R: Distribution of cervical lymph node metastases from squamous cell carcinoma of the upper respiratory and digestive tracts. Cancer 29:1446-1449, 1972.
27. Candela FC, Kothari K, Shah JP: Patterns of cervical node metastases from squamous carcinoma of the oropharynx and hypopharynx. Head Neck 12:197-203, 1990.
28. Candela FC, Shah J, Jaques DP, et al: Patterns of cervical node metastases from squamous carcinoma of the larynx. Arch Otolaryngol Head Neck Surg 116:432-435, 1990.
29. Shah JP, Candela FC, Poddar AK: The patterns of cervical lymph node metastases from squamous carcinoma of the oral cavity. Cancer 66:109-113, 1990.
30. Shah JP: Patterns of cervical lymph node metastasis from squamous carcinomas of the upper aerodigestive tract. Am J Surg 160:405-409, 1990.
31. Davidson BJ, Kulkarny V, Delacure MD, et al: Posterior triangle metastases of squamous cell carcinoma of the upper aerodigestive tract. Am J Surg 166:395-398, 1993.
32. Spiro JD, Spiro RH, Shah JP, et al: Critical assessment of supraomohyoid neck dissection. Am J Surg 156:286-289, 1988.
33. Byers RM, Weber RS, Andrews T, et al: Frequency and therapeutic implications of "skip metastases" in the neck from squamous carcinoma of the oral tongue. Head Neck 19:14-19, 1997.
34. Kowalski LP, Magrin J, Waksman G, et al: Supraomohyoid neck dissection in the treatment of head and neck tumors. Survival results in 212 cases. Arch Otolaryngol Head Neck Surg 119:958-963, 1993.
35. Foote RL, Olsen KD, Davis DL, et al: Base of tongue carcinoma: patterns of failure and predictors of recurrence after surgery alone. Head Neck 15:300-307, 1993.
36. O'Sullivan B, Warde P, Grice B, et al: The benefits and pitfalls of ipsilateral radiotherapy in carcinoma of the tonsillar region. Int J Radiat Oncol Biol Phys 51:332-343, 2001.
37. Jackson SM, Hay JH, Flores AD, et al: Cancer of the tonsil: the results of ipsilateral radiation treatment. Radiother Oncol 51:123-128, 1999.
38. Byers RM: Neck dissection: concepts, controversies, and technique. Semin Surg Oncol 7:9-13, 1991.
39. Clayman GL, Frank DK: Selective neck dissection of anatomically appropriate levels is as efficacious as modified radical neck dissection for elective treatment of the clinically negative neck in patients with squamous cell carcinoma of the upper respiratory and digestive tracts. Arch Otolaryngol Head Neck Surg 124:348-352, 1998.
40. Byers RM: Modified neck dissection. A study of 967 cases from 1970 to 1980. Am J Surg 150:414-421, 1985.
41. Grégoire V, Hamoir M, Levendag P, et al: Proposal for the delineation of the nodal CTV in the node-positive and the post-operative neck. Radiother Oncol, 2006 (in press).
42. Marks JE, Devineni VR, Harvey J, et al: The risk of contralateral lymphatic metastases for cancers of the larynx and pharynx. Am J Otolaryngol 13:34-39, 1992.
43. Robbins KT, Clayman G, Levine PA, et al: Neck dissection classification update: revisions proposed by the American Head and Neck Society and the American Academy of Otolaryngology-Head and Neck Surgery. Arch Otolaryngol Head Neck Surg 128:751-758, 2002.
44. Som PM, Curtin HD, Mancuso AA: An imaging-based classification for the cervical nodes designed as an adjunct to recent clinically based nodal classifications. Arch Otolaryngol Head Neck Surg 125:388-396, 1999.
45. Medina JE: A rational classification of neck dissections. Otolaryngol Head Neck Surg 100:169-176, 1989.
46. Suarez O: El problema de las metastasis linfaticas y alejadas del cancer de laringe e hipofaringe. Rev Otorinolaringol 23:83-89, 1963.
47. Bocca E, Pignataro O: A conservation technique in radical neck dissection. Ann Otol Rhinol Laryngol 76:975-987, 1967.
48. Bocca E, Pignataro O, Sasaki CT: Functional neck dissection. A description of operative technique. Arch Otolaryngol Head Neck Surg 106:524-527, 1980.
49. Morton DL, Wen DR, Wong JH, et al: Technical details of intraoperative lymphatic mapping for early stage melanoma. Arch Surg 127:392-399, 1992.
50. Pan D, Narayan D, Ariyan S: Merkel cell carcinoma: five case reports using sentinel lymph node biopsy and a review of 110 new cases. Plast Reconstr Surg 110:1259-1265, 2002.
51. Veronesi U, Paganelli G, Viale G, et al: A randomized comparison of sentinel-node biopsy with routine axillary dissection in breast cancer. N Engl J Med 349:546-553, 2003.
52. Shoaib T, Soutar DS, MacDonald DG, et al: The accuracy of head and neck carcinoma sentinel lymph node biopsy in the clinically N0 neck. Cancer 91:2077-2083, 2001.
53. Pitman KT, Johnson JT, Brown ML, et al: Sentinel lymph node biopsy in head and neck squamous cell carcinoma. Laryngoscope 112:2101-2113, 2002.
54. Ferlito A, Rinaldo A, Robbins KT, et al: Changing concepts in the surgical management of the cervical node metastasis. Oral Oncol 39:429-435, 2003.
55. Ross GL, Soutar DS, Gordon MacDonald D, et al: Sentinel node biopsy in head and neck cancer: preliminary results of a multicenter trial. Ann Surg Oncol 11:690-696, 2004.
56. Gregoire V, Coche E, Cosnard G, et al: Selection and delineation of lymph node target volumes in head and neck conformal radiotherapy. Proposal for standardizing terminology and procedure based on the surgical experience. Radiother Oncol 56:135-150, 2000.
57. Nowak PJ, Wijers OB, Lagerwaard FJ, et al: A three-dimensional CT-based target definition for elective irradiation of the neck. Int J Radiat Oncol Biol Phys 45:33-39, 1999.
58. Wijers OB, Levendag PC, Tan T, et al: A simplified CT-based definition of the lymph node levels in the node negative neck. Radiother Oncol 52:35-42, 1999.
59. Martinez-Monge R, Fernandes PS, Gupta N, et al: Cross-sectional nodal atlas: a tool for the definition of clinical target volumes in three-dimensional radiation therapy planning. Radiology 211:815-828, 1999.
60. Grégoire V, Levendag P, Ang KK, et al: CT-based delineation of lymph node levels and related CTVs in the node-negative neck: DAHANCA, EORTC, GORTEC, NCIC, RTOG consensus guidelines. Radiother Oncol 69:227-236, 2003.
61. Levendag P, Grégoire V, Hamoir M, et al: Intraoperative validation of CT-based lymph nodal levels, sublevels IIA and IIB: is it of clinical relevance in selective radiation therapy? Int J Radiat Oncol Biol Phys 62:690-699, 2005.
62. Apisarnthanarax S, Elliott D, El Naggar AK, et al: Determining optimal clinical target volume margins in head and neck cancer based on microscopic extracapsular extension of metastatic neck nodes. Int J Radiat Oncol Biol Phys 64:678-683, 2006.
63. Bussels B, Hermans R, Rijnders A, Van den Bogaert W: Retropharyngeal nodes in squamous cell carcinoma of the oropharynx: implications for target volume delineation. Radiother Oncol 73(Suppl 1):S179, 2004.
64. Weiss MH, Harrison LB, Isaacs RS: Use of decision analysis in planning a management strategy for the stage N0 neck. Arch Otolaryngol Head Neck Surg 120:699-702, 1994.
65. Brazilian Head and Neck Cancer Study Group: Results of a prospective trial on elective modified radical classical versus supraomohyoid neck dissection in the management of oral squamous carcinoma. Am J Surg 176:422-427, 1998.
66. Byers RM, Wolf PF, Ballantyne AJ: Rationale for elective modified neck dissection. Head Neck Surg 10:160-167, 1988.
67. Byers RM, Clayman GL, McGill D, et al: Selective neck dissections for squamous carcinoma of the upper aerodigestive tract: patterns of regional failure. Head Neck 21:499-505, 1999.
68. Duvvuri U, Simental AA Jr, D'Angelo G, et al: Elective neck dissection and survival in patients with squamous cell carcinoma of

the oral cavity and oropharynx. Laryngoscope 114:2228-2234, 2004.
69. Jesse RH, Ballantyne AJ, Larson D: Radical or modified neck dissection: a therapeutic dilemma. Am J Surg 136:516-519, 1978.
70. Lingeman RE, Helmus C, Stephens R, et al: Neck dissection: radical or conservative. Ann Otol 86:737-744, 1977.
71. Medina JE, Byers RM: Supraomohyoid neck dissection: rationale, indications, and surgical technique. Head Neck 11:111-122, 1989.
72. Pellitteri PK, Robbins KT, Neuman T: Expanded application of selective neck dissection with regard to nodal status. Head Neck 19:260-265, 1997.
73. Pitman KT, Johnson JT, Myers EN: Effectiveness of selective neck dissection for management of the clinically negative neck. Arch Otolaryngol Head Neck Surg 123:917-922, 1997.
74. Spiro RH, Morgan GJ, Strong EW, et al: Supraomohyoid neck dissection. Am J Surg 172:650-653, 1996.
75. Bernier J, Bataini JP: Regional outcome in oropharyngeal and pharyngolaryngeal cancer treated with high dose per fraction radiotherapy. Analysis of neck disease response in 1646 cases. Radiother Oncol 6:87-103, 1986.
76. Alpert TE, Morbidini-Gaffney S, Chung CT, et al: Radiotherapy for the clinically negative neck in supraglottic laryngeal cancer. Cancer J 10:335-338, 2004.
77. Johansen LV, Grau C, Overgaard J: Nodal control and surgical salvage after primary radiotherapy in 1782 patients with laryngeal and pharyngeal carcinoma. Acta Oncol 43:486-494, 2004.
78. Nakfoor BM, Spiro IJ, Wang CC, et al: Results of accelerated radiotherapy for supraglottic carcinoma: a Massachusetts General Hospital and Massachusetts Eye and Ear Infirmary experience. Head Neck 20:379-384, 1998.
79. Dische S, Saunders M, Barrett A, et al: A randomised multicentre trial of CHART versus conventional radiotherapy in head and neck cancer. Radiother Oncol 44:123-136, 1997.
80. Eisbruch A, Marsh LH, Dawson LA, et al: Recurrences near base of skull after IMRT for head-and-neck cancer: implications for target delineation in high neck and for parotid gland sparing. Int J Radiat Oncol Biol Phys 59:28-42, 2004.
81. Bussels B, Maes A, Hermans R, et al: Recurrences after conformal parotid-sparing radiotherapy for head and neck cancer. Radiother Oncol 72:119-127, 2004.
82. Chao KS, Ozyigit G, Tran BN, et al: Patterns of failure in patients receiving definitive and postoperative IMRT for head-and-neck cancer. Int J Radiat Oncol Biol Phys 55:312-321, 2003.
83. Andersen PE, Shah JP, Cambronero E, et al: The role of comprehensive neck dissection with preservation of the spinal accessory nerve in the clinically positive neck. Am J Surg 168:499-502, 1994.
84. Merino OR, Lindberg RD, Fletcher GH: An analysis of distant metastases from squamous cell carcinoma of the upper respiratory and digestive tracts. Cancer 40:145-151, 1977.
85. Carew JF, Singh B, Shah JP: Cervical lymph nodes. *In* Shah JP, Johnson NW, Batsakis JG, Dunitz M (eds): Oral Cancer. New York, Thieme Medical Publishers, 2003, pp 215-249.
86. Khafif RA, Gelbfish GA, Asase DK, et al: Modified radical neck dissection in cancer of the mouth, pharynx, and larynx. Head Neck 12:476-482, 1990.
87. Shah JP: Cervical lymph node metastases—diagnostic, therapeutic, and prognostic implications. Oncology (Huntingt) 4:61-69, 1990.
88. Clark J, Li W, Smith G, Shannon K, et al: Outcome of treatment for advanced cervical metastatic squamous cell carcinoma. Head Neck 27:87-94, 2005.
89. Shaha AR: Extended neck dissection. J Surg Oncol 45:229-233, 1990.
90. Brennan JA, Jafek BW: Elective carotid artery resection for advanced squamous cell carcinoma of the neck. Laryngoscope 104:259-263, 1994.
91. Maves MD, Bruns MD, Keenan MJ: Carotid artery resection for head and neck cancer. Ann Otol Rhinol Laryngol 101:778-781, 1992.
92. Bataini JP, Bernier J, Asselain B, et al: Primary radiotherapy of squamous cell carcinoma of the oropharynx and pharyngolarynx: tentative multivariate modelling system to predict the radiocurability of neck nodes. Int J Radiat Oncol Biol Phys 14:635-642, 1988.
93. Horiot JC, Le Fur R, N'Guyen T, et al: Hyperfractionation versus conventional fractionation in oropharyngeal carcinoma: final analysis of a randomized trial of the EORTC cooperative group of radiotherapy. Radiother Oncol 25:231-241, 1992.
94. Overgaard J, Hansen HS, Specht L, et al: Five compared with six fractions per week of conventional radiotherapy of squamous-cell carcinoma of head and neck: DAHANCA 6 and 7 randomised controlled trial. Lancet 362:933-940, 2003.
95. Cummings B, O'Sullivan B, Keane T, et al: 5-Year results of 4 week/twice daily radiation schedule: the Toronto Trial [abstract]. Radiother Oncol 56:S8, 2000.
96. Calais G, Alfonsi M, Bardet E, et al: Randomized trial of radiation therapy versus concomitant chemotherapy and radiation therapy for advanced-stage oropharynx carcinoma. J Natl Cancer Inst 91:2081-2086, 1999.
97. Lavertu P, Bonafede JP, Adelstein DJ, et al: Comparison of surgical complications after organ-preservation therapy in patients with stage III or IV squamous cell head and neck cancer. Arch Otolaryngol Head Neck Surg 124:401-406, 1998.
98. Nisi KW, Foote RL, Bonner JA, et al: Adjuvant radiotherapy for squamous cell carcinoma of the tongue base: improved local-regional disease control compared with surgery alone. Int J Radiat Oncol Biol Phys 41:371-377, 1998.
99. Lundahl RE, Foote RL, Bonner JA, et al: Combined neck dissection and postoperative radiation therapy in the management of the high-risk neck: a matched-pair analysis. Int J Radiat Oncol Biol Phys 40:529-534, 1998.
100. Vikram B, Strong EW, Shah JP, et al: Failure in the neck following multimodality treatment for advanced head and neck cancer. Head Neck Surg 6:724-729, 1984.
101. Dixit S, Vyas RK, Toparani RB, et al: Surgery versus surgery and postoperative radiotherapy in squamous cell carcinoma of the buccal mucosa: a comparative study. Ann Surg Oncol 5:502-510, 1998.
102. Amdur RJ, Parsons JT, Mendenhall WM, et al: Postoperative irradiation for squamous cell carcinoma of the head and neck: an analysis of treatment results and complications. Int J Radiat Oncol Biol Phys 16:25-36, 1989.
103. Parsons JT, Mendenhall WM, Stringer SP, et al: An analysis of factors influencing the outcome of postoperative irradiation for squamous cell carcinoma of the oral cavity. Int J Radiat Oncol Biol Phys 39:137-148, 1997.
104. Peters LJ, Goepfert H, Ang KK, et al: Evaluation of the dose for postoperative radiation therapy of head and neck cancer: first report of a prospective randomized trial. Int J Radiat Oncol Biol Phys 26:3-11, 1993.
105. Ang KK, Trotti A, Brown BW, et al: Randomized trial addressing risk features and time factors of surgery plus radiotherapy in advanced head-and-neck cancer. Int J Radiat Oncol Biol Phys 51:571-578, 2001.
106. Haffty BG, Son YH, Sasaki CT, et al: Mitomycin C as an adjunct to postoperative radiation therapy in squamous cell carcinoma of the head and neck: results from two randomized clinical trials. Int J Radiat Oncol Biol Phys 27:241-250, 1993.
107. Bachaud JM, Cohen-Jonathan E, Alzieu C, et al: Combined postoperative radiotherapy and weekly cisplatin infusion for locally advanced head and neck carcinoma: final report of a randomized trial. Int J Radiat Oncol Biol Phys 36:999-1004, 1996.
108. Bernier J, Domenge C, Ozsahin M, et al: Postoperative irradiation with or without concomitant chemotherapy for locally advanced head and neck cancer. N Engl J Med 350:1945-1952, 2004.
109. Cooper JS, Pajak TF, Forastiere AA, et al: Postoperative concurrent radiotherapy and chemotherapy for high-risk squamous-cell carcinoma of the head and neck. N Engl J Med 350:1937-1944, 2004.
110. Bernier J, Cooper J, Pajak T, et al: Defining risk levels in locally advanced head and neck cancers: a comparative analysis of concurrent postoperative radiation plus chemotherapy trials of the EORTC (#22931) and RTOG (#9501). Head Neck 27:843-850, 2005.
111. Forastiere AA, Goepfert H, Maor M, et al: Concurrent chemotherapy and radiotherapy for organ preservation in advanced laryngeal cancer. N Engl J Med 349:2091-2098, 2003.

112. Lefebvre JL, Lartigau E: Preservation of form and function during management of cancer of the larynx and hypopharynx. World J Surg 27:811-816, 2003.
113. Mendenhall WM, Villaret DB, Amdur RJ, et al: Planned neck dissection after definitive radiotherapy for squamous cell carcinoma of the head and neck. Head Neck 24:1012-1018, 2002.
114. Narayan K, Crane CH, Kleid S, et al: Planned neck dissection as an adjunct to the management of patients with advanced neck disease treated with definitive radiotherapy: for some or for all? Head Neck 21:606-613, 1999.
115. Stenson KM, Haraf DJ, Pelzer H, et al: The role of cervical lymphadenectomy after aggressive concomitant chemoradiotherapy: the feasibility of selective neck dissection. Arch Otolaryngol Head Neck Surg 126:950-956, 2000.
116. Clayman GL, Johnson CJ 2nd, Morrison W, et al: The role of neck dissection after chemoradiotherapy for oropharyngeal cancer with advanced nodal disease. Arch Otolaryngol Head Neck Surg 127:135-139, 2001.
117. McHam SA, Adelstein DJ, Rybicki LA, et al: Who merits a neck dissection after definitive chemoradiotherapy for N2-N3 squamous cell head and neck cancer? Head Neck 25:791-798, 2003.
118. Yao M, Graham MM, Hoffman HT, et al: The role of post-radiation therapy FDG PET in prediction of necessity for post-radiation therapy neck dissection in locally advanced head-and-neck squamous cell carcinoma. Int J Radiat Oncol Biol Phys 59:1001-1010, 2004.
119. McCollum AD, Burrell SC, Haddad RI, et al: Positron emission tomography with 18F-fluorodeoxyglucose to predict pathologic response after induction chemotherapy and definitive chemoradiotherapy in head and neck cancer. Head Neck 26:890-896, 2004.
120. Medina JE, Houck JR, O'Malley BB: Management of cervical lymph nodes in squamous cell carcinoma. *In* Harrison LB, Sessions RB, Ki Hong W (eds): Head and Neck Cancer. A Multidisciplinary Approach. Philadelphia, Lippincott-Raven, 1998, pp 353-378.
121. Shah S, Har-El G, Rosenfeld RM: Short-term and long-term quality of life after neck dissection. Head Neck 23:954-961, 2001.
122. Leipzig B, Suen JY, English JL, et al: Functional evaluation of the spinal accessory nerve after neck dissection. Am J Surg 146:526-530, 1983.
123. Laverick S, Lowe D, Brown JS, et al: The impact of neck dissection on health-related quality of life. Arch Otolaryngol Head Neck Surg 130:149-154, 2004.
124. van Wilgen CP, Dijkstra PU, van der Laan BF, et al: Morbidity of the neck after head and neck cancer therapy. Head Neck 26:785-791, 2004.
125. Erisen L, Basel B, Irdesel J, et al: Shoulder function after accessory nerve-sparing neck dissections. Head Neck 26:967-971, 2004.
126. Blessing R, Mann W, Beck C: How important is preservation of the accessory nerve in neck dissection? Laryngol Rhinol Otol (Stuttg) 65:403-405, 1986.
127. Lee DJ, Cosmatos D, Marcial VA, et al: Results of an RTOG phase III trial (RTOG 85-27) comparing radiotherapy plus etanidazole with radiotherapy alone for locally advanced head and neck carcinomas. Int J Radiat Oncol Biol Phys 32:567-576, 1995.
128. Fu KK, Pajak TF, Trotti A, et al: A Radiation Therapy Oncology Group (RTOG) phase III randomized study to compare hyperfractionation and two variants of accelerated fractionation to standard fractionation radiotherapy for head and neck squamous cell carcinomas: first report of RTOG 9003. Int J Radiat Oncol Biol Phys 48:7-16, 2000.
129. Trotti A: Toxicity in head and neck cancer: a review of trends and issues. Int J Radiat Oncol Biol Phys 47:1-12, 2000.
130. Horiot JC, Bontemps P, van den Bogaert W, et al: Accelerated fractionation (AF) compared to conventional fractionation (CF) improves loco-regional control in the radiotherapy of advanced head and neck cancers: results of the EORTC 22851 randomized trial. Radiother Oncol 44:111-121, 1997.
131. Kumpulainen EJ, Hirvikoski PP, Virtaniemi JA, et al: Hypothyroidism after radiotherapy for laryngeal cancer. Radiother Oncol 57:97-101, 2000.
132. Sinard RJ, Tobin EJ, Mazzaferri EL, et al: Hypothyroidism after treatment for nonthyroid head and neck cancer. Arch Otolaryngol Head Neck Surg 126:652-657, 2000.
133. Abayomi OJ: Neck irradiation, carotid injury and its consequences. Oral Oncol 40:872-878, 2004.
134. Dorresteijn LD, Kappelle AC, Boogerd W, et al: Increased risk of ischemic stroke after radiotherapy on the neck in patients younger than 60 years. J Clin Oncol 20:282-288, 2002.
135. Williams BC, Hounsella R: X-ray linkage considerations for IMRT. Br J Radiol 74:98-102, 2001.
136. Hall EJ, Wuu CS: Radiation-induced second cancers: the impact of 3D-CRT and IMRT. Int J Radiat Oncol Biol Phys 56:83-88, 2003.
137. Godden DR, Ribeiro NF, Hassanein K, et al: Recurrent neck disease in oral cancer. J Oral Maxillofac Surg 60:748-753, 2002.
138. Mabanta SR, Mendenhall WM, Stringer SP, et al: Salvage treatment for neck recurrence after irradiation alone for head and neck squamous cell carcinoma with clinically positive neck nodes. Head Neck 21:591-594, 1999.
139. Foote RL, Garrett P, Rate W, et al: IORT for head and neck cancer. *In* Gunderson LL, Willett CG, Harrison LB, Calvo FA (eds): Intraoperative Irradiation: Techniques and Results. Totowa, NJ, Humana Press, 1999, pp 471-497.
140. McLaughlin MP, Mendenhall WM, Mancuso AA, et al: Retropharyngeal adenopathy as a predictor of outcome in squamous cell carcinoma of the head and neck. Head Neck 17:190-198, 1995.
141. Chua DTT, Sham JST, Kwong DLW, et al: Retropharyngeal lymphadenopathy in patients with nasopharyngeal carcinoma. A computed tomography-based study. Cancer 79:869-877, 1997.
142. Chong VF, Fan YF, Khoo JB: Retropharyngeal lymphadenopathy in nasopharyngeal carcinoma. Eur J Radiol 21:100-105, 1995.

CHAPTER 38

CUTANEOUS CARCINOMA

K. Kian Ang and Randal S. Weber

✓INCIDENCE

Basal and squamous cell carcinomas of the skin are the most common cancers in the United States. One in five Americans will develop a skin cancer during his or her lifetime.

BIOLOGIC CHARACTERISTICS

The natural history of skin cancers varies extensively with the histologic type. It ranges from an indolent course with a very high cure rate (e.g., basal cell carcinomas) to the aggressive course of virulent tumors with high mortality rates (e.g., Merkel cell carcinomas).

✓STAGING EVALUATION

Staging includes a thorough history, physical examination, and when indicated, blood chemistry tests, chest radiographs, and contrast-enhanced computed tomography or magnetic resonance imaging, or both.

PRIMARY THERAPY

Surgical resection is the primary therapy for most skin cancers. The indications for postoperative irradiation include positive surgical margins, perineural spread, invasion of bone or cartilage, and extensive skeletal muscle infiltration.

Primary radiation therapy is preferable for the treatment of basal and squamous carcinomas on and around the nose, lower eyelids, and ears, because it usually yields better functional and cosmetic results than surgery.

ADJUVANT THERAPY

Patient subsets with tumors having a high incidence of occult nodal spread (e.g., Merkel cell carcinoma) may benefit from elective nodal dissection or irradiation.

No effective systemic adjuvant therapy is available for skin carcinomas.

LOCALLY ADVANCED DISEASE AND PALLIATION

Surgery and irradiation constitute the standard treatment for locally advanced but resectable tumors.

Radiation therapy can yield local control in some patients with locally advanced carcinomas that are inoperable or in a few patients with unresectable tumors. Radiation can be given to reduce symptoms for most patients with advanced inoperable cancer or metastatic masses.

Cutaneous basal and squamous cell carcinomas are the most common malignant neoplasms in the United States. More than 1 million new cases of basal and squamous cell skin cancers were expected to be diagnosed in 2005.[1] They most frequently affect persons with fair complexions and those with outdoor occupations. Skin cancers may be disfiguring in certain locations, but fortunately, they are rarely lethal. The frequency of basal cell carcinoma is four times that of cutaneous squamous cell carcinoma. Basal cell cancers tend to be more indolent, and they rarely metastasize.

Uncommon skin neoplasms include Merkel cell carcinoma and adnexal cancers. Merkel cell carcinoma, also known as primary cutaneous neuroendocrine carcinoma or trabecular carcinoma of the skin, is a rare tumor that was originally described by Toker in 1972.[2] Sebaceous gland carcinoma accounts for less than 1% of all skin neoplasms.[3] Eccrine or sweat gland carcinoma is rare, estimated to account for less than 0.01% of malignant epithelial neoplasms of the skin,[4] and apocrine carcinoma is even less common. Etiologic and epidemiologic data on Merkel cell and adnexal carcinomas are scarce. Likewise, knowledge on prevention and early detection is scanty, and no official staging systems are available for these rare skin neoplasms.

ETIOLOGY AND EPIDEMIOLOGY

The main etiologic factor for cutaneous carcinoma is sun exposure in individuals whose skin is susceptible to the carcinogenic effect of ultraviolet light.[5] Other etiologic factors for skin carcinoma include exposure to chemical carcinogens (e.g., arsenic, tar, anthracene, crude paraffin oil), chronic irritation or inflammation, and ionizing radiation. The incidence of cutaneous squamous cell carcinomas is greatly increased in individuals with defective immune function, including chronic lymphocytic leukemia and iatrogenic immunosuppression in organ transplant recipients.

A number of genetic syndromes are associated with a higher incidence of skin carcinoma. Individuals with xeroderma pigmentosum are prone to developing basal cell carcinoma and squamous cell carcinoma at a very young age because of defective repair of ultraviolet light–induced DNA damage.[6] These patients usually die in their early 20s from disseminated squamous cell carcinoma or melanoma. The basal cell nevus syndrome is a genetic form of basal cell carcinoma inherited through an autosomal dominant gene.[7] Persons with epidermodysplasia verruciformis tend to develop nodules of squamous cell carcinoma within large verrucous plaques in the third and fourth decades of life.[8]

PREVENTION AND SCREENING

The incidence of skin cancer allows researchers to assess the impact of preventive and screening measures, because most cancers are caused by ultraviolet light exposure. A panel of the American College of Preventive Medicine (ACPM) performed a thorough medical literature search and review and issued practice policy statements with regard to skin cancer prevention, as summarized by Hill and Ferrini.[9] Recommended preventive measures to reduce skin cancer include avoidance of sunlight exposure (particularly limiting time spent outdoors between 10 AM and 3 PM) and wearing protective physical barriers, such as hats and clothing. If sun exposure cannot be limited because of occupational, cultural, or other factors, the use of sunscreens that are opaque or that block ultraviolet A and B radiation is recommended. The ACPM recommends discussion of sun avoidance and sun protection measures with children and teenagers.

The ACPM also recommends periodic screening, consisting of a total cutaneous examination and a 2- to 3-minute visual inspection by adequately trained physicians of the entire integument of high-risk individuals or through mass screening. Risk factors include family history of skin cancer, fair skin, multiple nevi, and a history of other skin cancers.

CLINICAL MANIFESTATIONS, PATHOBIOLOGY, AND PATHWAYS OF SPREAD

Basal Cell Carcinoma

Clinical Presentation and Pathology

Basal cell carcinoma is most commonly found on the head and neck region, where it may manifest as an asymptomatic nodule, a pruritic plaque, or a bleeding sore that characteristically waxes and wanes.[10,11] Multiple synchronous lesions may be present. Approximately one third of the patients treated for basal cell carcinomas developed at least one more basal cell cancer.[12] Careful evaluation of the sun-exposed skin areas should be part of the follow-up examination.

Basal cell carcinoma manifests as a number of variants, and each has distinctive clinical and histologic features and a characteristic natural history. The characteristics of commonly occurring types are briefly summarized. Nodular-ulcerative basal cell carcinoma, also referred to as rodent ulcer, is the most frequently observed variety. This type of skin cancer begins as a papule that develops central umbilication, progressing to central ulceration as the lesion grows. The margins of the lesion appear pearly (i.e., pale and translucent) and contain enlarged capillaries. A histologic feature of the rodent ulcer is the presence of large islands of monomorphous basaloid cells in various sizes and shapes that are embedded in a fibroblastic stroma in the dermis. The basaloid cells have large, oval hyperchromatic nuclei; scant cytoplasm; and no intercellular bridges. The peripheral cell layer of the aggregate frequently shows palisading, whereas central cells are less organized. Nodular-ulcerative basal cell carcinoma may show various degrees of pigmentation (i.e., blue, brown, or black), depending on the number of melanocytes present in the lesion, and it may be difficult to differentiate clinically from malignant melanoma.[13] Biopsy may be required for establishing the correct diagnosis.

Superficial basal cell carcinoma presents as red, scaly macules with indistinct margins, usually located on the trunk. It enlarges into a crusted, erythematous patch without induration that may be difficult to differentiate clinically from solar keratosis, psoriasis, squamous cell carcinoma in situ, or extramammary Paget's disease. Histologic examination shows multiple foci of buds of neoplastic cells with peripheral palisading originating from the undersurface of the epidermis.[13]

Morphea-form (serpiginous) and sclerosing basal cell carcinomas appear as single, flat, indurated, ill-defined macules. The lesions generally have a smooth and shiny surface that becomes depressed as it grows into a plaque. Histologically, it is characterized by the presence of small groups and narrow strands of basaloid cells embedded in a dense, fibrous connective tissue; there is little peripheral palisading.[13]

Infiltrative basal cell carcinoma has an opaque, yellowish appearance and blends subtly with the surrounding skin.[14] Histologically, the lesion is characterized by poorly circumscribed, spiky cell aggregates in the superficial portion and the main bulk, consisting of strands of neoplastic cells infiltrating the reticular dermis and subcutis.

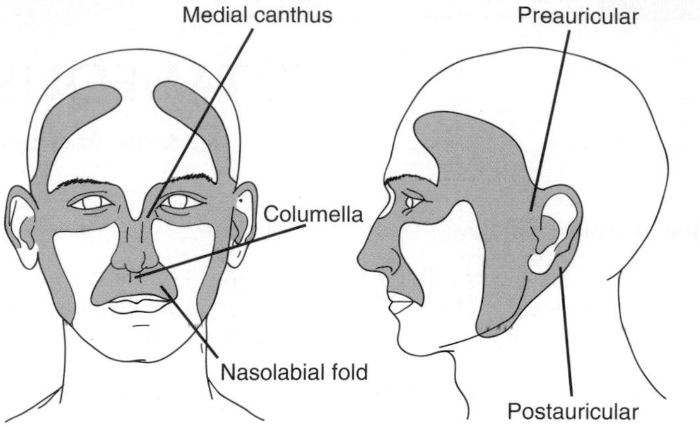

Figure 38-1 Diagram of the H zone. Especially problematic areas are the medial canthus, glabella, nasolabial folds, and the periauricular region.

Terebrant carcinoma is a variant that presents as a small ulcerated tumor, most commonly in so-called H zone (Fig. 38-1) of the periauricular region, glabella, medial canthus, nose, nasolabial region, and columella.[15] The extent of tumors in this region is frequently underestimated, leading to inadequate surgical excision and a higher rate of local recurrence. Histologic examination usually reveals extensive infiltration of deeper structures by small nests of undifferentiated basal cells. This type of lesion may invade the orbit, nose, and maxilla, resulting in significant deformity. It should be readily recognized and treated promptly.

Biology and Pattern of Spread

The biologic behavior of basal cell carcinomas varies with the histologic type. The superficial basal cell carcinoma may remain stable for a long period or enlarge gradually over a number of years to become a nodular-ulcerative variant. The nodular-ulcerative basal cell carcinomas grow slowly over many years by peripheral and deep invasion, particularly along embryonal fusion planes, and perineural spread. Morphea-form, infiltrative, and terebrant basal cell carcinomas are more aggressive variants that spread through peripheral extension and infiltration of deeper structures. Perineural or neurotropic spread in basal cell carcinoma is rare, occurring in only 0.1% of patients, and it generally occurs in the setting of recurrent disease or after irradiation failure. The most common cranial nerves affected are V and VII.

Basal cell carcinomas rarely spread to the regional lymph nodes or distant organs. The overall incidence of metastasis is less than 0.01%.[16] Two thirds of metastases are found in the regional lymphatics, and as many as 20% involve bone, lung, and liver.[17] Distant spread is usually preceded by regional metastasis. Regional disease typically develops with large, ulcerated lesions in the head and neck region that have recurred after repeated surgery and radiation.[18]

Squamous Cell Carcinoma

Clinical Presentation and Pathology

Squamous cell carcinoma arises from keratinocytes of the epidermis. This type of skin cancer most commonly develops from skin exhibiting solar damage. Actinic keratosis is generally a precursor lesion. Less frequently, squamous cell carcinoma occurs from other preexisting skin lesions such as arsenical keratosis, a thermal burn scar, or a chronic ulcer. Rarely, it arises from normal-appearing skin.[13]

Clinically, squamous cell carcinoma in situ (i.e., Bowen's disease) manifests as a soft, erythematous, scaly, circumscribed patch. Superficial carcinoma manifests as a scaly, crusted plaque or ulcer with a verrucous or papillated border, and infiltrating squamous cancer manifests as a firm, ulcerated mass with an elevated nodular border.

Microscopically, squamous cell carcinoma is composed of strands and sheets of atypical keratinocytes. It is referred to as squamous cell carcinoma in situ when atypical keratinocytes are confined to the epidermis. Superficial squamous cell carcinoma represents atypical keratinocyte proliferation confined to the upper reticular dermis, whereas infiltrating squamous cell carcinoma denotes disease extension into and beyond the lower reticular epidermis.

Histologically, squamous cell carcinoma is graded as well, moderately, or poorly differentiated, based on the magnitude of cellular polymorphism, keratinization, and mitosis. The spindle cell variant mimics other skin tumors such as amelanotic melanoma and may require a panel of immunohistochemical studies for complete characterization.

Biology and Pattern of Spread

Squamous cell carcinoma usually has a more aggressive course than basal cell carcinoma. Carcinoma in situ evolves gradually into superficial carcinoma, although in some cases, it may stay dormant for several years. Untreated, it progresses further into an infiltrating type, which invades the surrounding and underlying structures. The rate of progression depends on the degree of cellular differentiation.

The incidence of regional and distant metastases is higher for squamous cell carcinoma than for basal cell carcinoma. At the time of diagnosis, metastatic spread is present in approximately 2% of patients with squamous cell carcinoma. However, up to 10% may eventually develop regional metastasis.[19] Factors determining the likelihood of metastasis include anatomic site, duration and size of the lesion, depth of dermal invasion, and degree of differentiation.[20,21] Regional and distant metastases occur more frequently in the presence of perineural invasion that occurs in approximately 7% of patients.[22] Squamous cell carcinoma arising from normal-appearing skin seems to invade more rapidly and have a higher incidence of metastasis than that developing in sun-damaged skin.[22]

Merkel Cell Carcinoma

Clinical Presentation and Pathology

Merkel cell carcinoma manifests as a firm, painless, pink-red dermal nodule or plaque, most frequently on the head or neck and extremities of individuals older than 60 years. The median size of the primary lesion at diagnosis is less than 2 cm, and the overall incidence of nodal involvement at presentation is approximately 20%.[23]

The cell of origin of this neoplasm is believed to be the dermal neurotactile cell arising from the neural crest described by Merkel.[24] The lesion usually involves the reticular dermis and subcutaneous tissues, with minimal extension to the papillary dermis and sparing of the epidermis. Vascular and lymphatic permeation are common. Ultramicroscopically, the neoplastic cells exhibit cytoplasmic extensions and small, uniform, membrane-bound neurosecretory granules.[25] Several immunohistochemical markers have been identified in Merkel cell carcinoma. The neoplastic cells stain most consistently with polyclonal antisera to neuron-specific enolase and calcitonin, monoclonal antibody to neurofilament, and cytokeratin.[26-28]

Biology and Pattern of Spread

The results of many retrospective studies show that Merkel cell carcinoma has an aggressive course characterized by propensity for contiguous spread, reflected in high local recurrence rates after wide surgical excision, and a high incidence of nodal involvement and hematogenous dissemination.[23,29-32] Assessment of pattern of failure in a series of 54 patients treated at the University of Texas M.D. Anderson Cancer Center (MDACC) revealed overall local and regional relapse rates of 35% and 67%, respectively. Distant metastases occurred in 32 (59%) patients. The median time to relapse after surgical resection was 4.9 months, and 91% of relapses occurred within the first year. One patient died of uncontrolled primary disease, and 32 patients died of distant metastases. The 5-year freedom from relapse and survival rates in this series were 19% and 30%, respectively.[23]

Adnexal Carcinoma

Sebaceous Carcinoma

Clinical Presentation and Pathology

Sebaceous carcinoma arises most commonly from the sebaceous glands of the ocular adnexa, the meibomian glands in the tarsus or glands of Zeis at the lid margin, and the caruncle. Extraocular locations, in decreasing frequency, are the head and neck region, trunk and extremities, and external genitalia.[33-36]

Histologically, these carcinomas are composed of dermal-based lobules and cords of tumor cells, with various degrees of sebaceous differentiation and infiltration into the surrounding tissues. Differentiated cells contain foamy or vacuolated slightly basophilic cytoplasm, whereas less differentiated cells contain more deeply basophilic cytoplasm. Clinical and pathologic features indicative of poor prognosis include size of primary lesion (>1 cm is associated with 50% mortality rate), vascular and lymphatic invasion, poor sebaceous differentiation, highly infiltrative growth pattern, and intraepithelial carcinomatous changes in the overlying epithelia.[37]

For malignant neoplasms of the eyelids, sebaceous carcinomas are second only to basal cell carcinomas in frequency and second only to malignant melanoma in lethality.[37] The most common location of ocular sebaceous carcinomas is the upper eyelid, followed by the lower eyelid and caruncle. Sebaceous carcinomas predominantly affect individuals older than 60 years. There is a slight preponderance in women. These lesions present clinically as slow-growing, nontender, deep-seated, firm nodules. Often, they produce a chalazion or manifestations suggesting inflammatory processes, such as conjunctivitis, blepharitis, or tarsitis. Small primary tumors may be overlooked until orbital invasion or spread to preauricular or cervical nodes occurs.

The differential diagnosis includes sebaceous adenoma and basal cell carcinoma with sebaceous differentiation (i.e., basosebaceous epithelioma).[38,39] Distinction between basosebaceous epithelioma and sebaceous carcinoma is important because of the difference in the biologic behavior.

Biology and Pattern of Spread

Sebaceous carcinoma behaves more aggressively than squamous cell carcinomas, with a propensity for nodal and hematogenous spread. Of the 104 patients registered by the Ophthalmic Pathology of the Armed Forces Institute of Pathology, 23 patients (22%) experienced local recurrence once, and 11 patients developed local relapse two or more times. Twenty-three patients died of metastatic disease.[37] The mortality rate was 41% in a series of 100 patients, with meibomian carcinomas followed for 1 to 20 years.[40]

Eccrine Carcinoma

Clinical Presentation and Pathology

Eccrine carcinoma arises most frequently in the skin of the head and neck or the extremities and presents as painless papules or nodules that grow slowly.[33] This type of neoplasm is usually diagnosed in individuals between 50 and 70 years old.[39]

Histologically, eccrine or sweat gland carcinoma resembles carcinomas of the breast, bronchus, and kidney and therefore may be difficult to differentiate from cutaneous metastases.[33,41] Histologic variants reported include ductal eccrine carcinoma, mucinous eccrine carcinoma, porocarcinoma, syringoid eccrine carcinoma, clear cell carcinoma, and microcystic adnexal carcinoma.[39,42-46]

Biology and Pattern of Spread

Eccrine carcinoma also has a more aggressive behavior than basal and squamous cell carcinomas. For instance, in a series of 14 patients who underwent surgical excision with free microscopic margins, 11 developed at least one local recurrence, and 5 failed at regional nodes or distant sites. One patient died of uncontrolled local relapse, and four died of distant metastatic disease 2 months to 10 years after diagnosis.[39]

Apocrine Carcinoma

Apocrine carcinoma arises most commonly from apocrine glands of the axilla, but it can originate from apocrine glands of the vulva and eyelids and from ceruminal glands of the external auditory canal.[47-49] It presents clinically as a red-purple, single or multinodular, firm or cystic dermal mass in elderly individuals. Because of the rarity, the natural history of apocrine carcinoma is not well known. Nodal and distant spread has been reported.[48]

PATIENT EVALUATION AND STAGING

General Approach

Clinical evaluation of skin cancers consists of inspection and palpation of the involved area and the regional lymph nodes. Symptoms suggesting perineural spread, such as pain, tingling, and hypesthesia, should be specifically sought from the patient. Up to 60% of patients with perineural spread may be asymptomatic. A crawling sensation on the skin known as formication suggests sensory nerve involvement. The most common primary sites associated with perineural extension are the frontozygomatic and infraorbital regions. Facial nerve involvement is usually preceded by muscle fasciculations and followed by frank paralysis.

Imaging studies (i.e., chest radiographs, computed tomography [CT], or magnetic resonance imaging [MRI]) should be obtained as indicated. Lymph node metastasis and bone involvement are best assessed with contrast-enhanced CT scan acquired with soft tissue and bone windows. MRI with and without contrast enhancement and fat suppression should be obtained for all patients in whom perineural spread is suspected.

Staging of Basal and Squamous Cell Carcinomas

Official staging systems are available for basal and squamous cell carcinomas. There has been no recent change in the American Joint Committee on Cancer (AJCC) tumor, nodes, and metastasis (TNM) staging system (Table 38-1), which is based primarily on clinical findings. In case of multiple simultaneous tumors, it is recommended that the tumor with the highest T category be specified and the number of separate tumors be indicated in parentheses. By these criteria, the stage of a patient presenting with five simultaneous skin cancers, the largest of which is 3 cm in diameter without extradermal extension, is T2.[5]

Table 38-1 American Joint Committee on Cancer Staging System for Carcinoma of the Skin (Excluding Eyelid, Vulva, and Penis)

PRIMARY TUMOR (T)	
TX	Primary tumor cannot be assessed
T0	No evidence of primary tumor
Tis	Carcinoma in situ
T1	Tumor 2 cm or less in diameter
T2	Tumor more than 2 cm but not more than 5 cm in greatest dimension
T3	Tumor more than 5 cm in greatest dimension
T4	Tumor invades deep extradermal structures (i.e., cartilage, skeletal muscle, or bone)
REGIONAL LYMPH NODES (N)	
NX	Regional lymph nodes cannot be assessed
N0	No regional lymph node metastasis
N1	Regional lymph node metastasis
DISTANT METASTASIS (M)	
MX	Distant metastasis cannot be assessed
M0	No distant metastasis
M1	Distant metastasis

American Joint Committee on Cancer Staging Manual, 6th ed. Springer, New York, 2002.

PRIMARY THERAPY AND RESULTS

Carcinoma

Primary Tumor

The general strategy for treatment of the primary lesion is the same for basal and squamous cell carcinomas. A variety of approaches are available for the management of cutaneous carcinomas, including curettage and electrodesiccation, Mohs' micrographic surgery, cryotherapy, surgical resection, and primary radiation therapy.

Literature data reveal that with proper case selection, these procedures are equally effective in curing most skin cancers. The choice of treatment for individual patients therefore is determined by factors such as the site and size of lesion, anticipated functional and cosmetic results, treatment time and cost, patient age, occupation, and general condition. For instance, carcinomas in the H zone or embryonic fusion planes tend to have extensive local spread, and treatment techniques that ensure wide marginal coverage should be selected for such lesions.

Overall, surgical modalities are preferred for most patients. Simple procedures can yield a high probability of disease control for those with small lesions. Composite resection is, however, necessary for patients with extensive tumor (Fig. 38-2). Younger patients who have years of exposure to sunlight are also better managed by surgery than by radiation therapy. In a number of clinical conditions, postoperative radiation therapy may be beneficial.

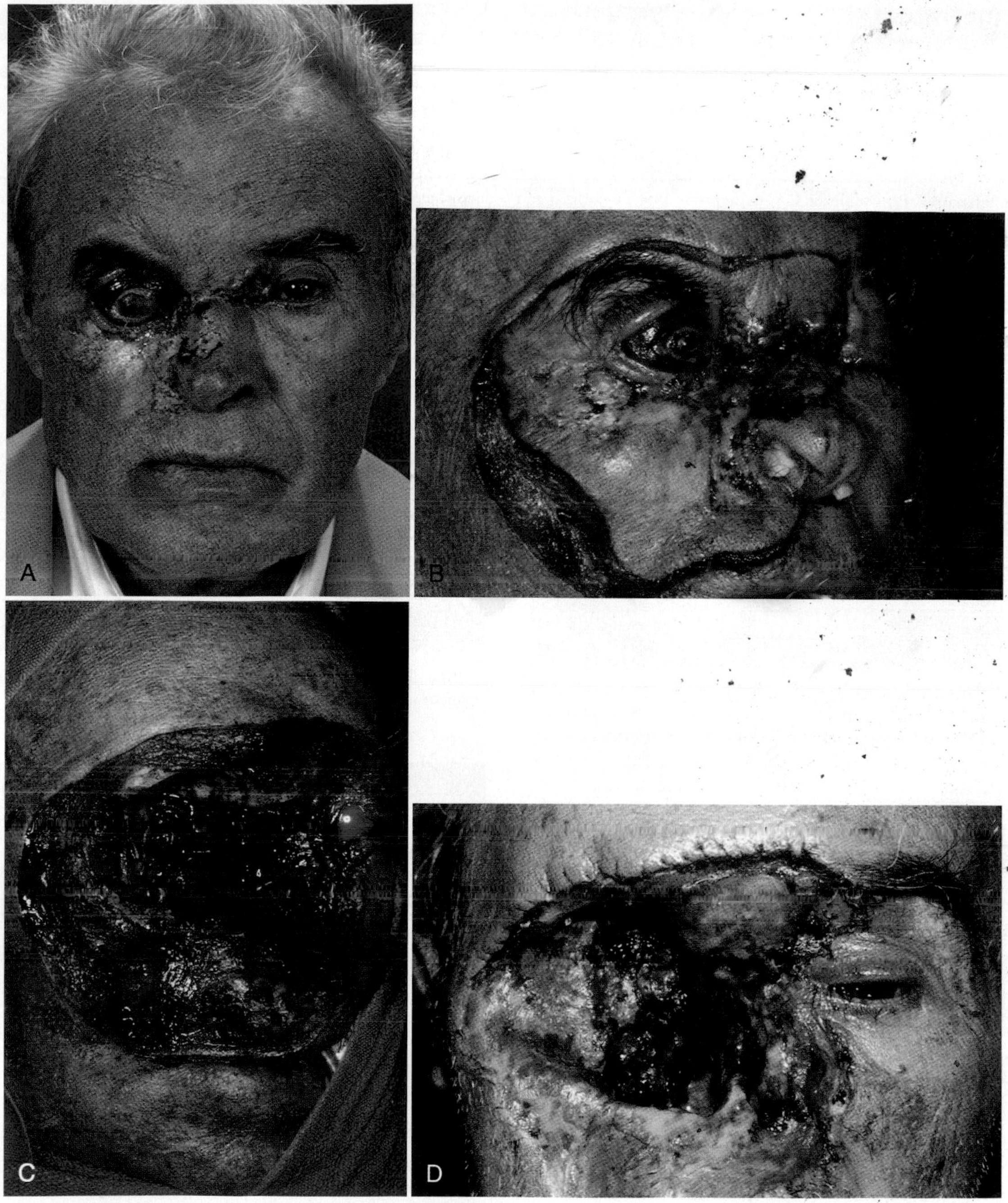

Figure 38-2 **A,** An elderly male with a neglected morphea-form basal cell carcinoma. The patient has no sight in the right eye because of tumor invasion, and the left eye is in jeopardy because of tumor encroachment. **B** and **C,** Radical resection, including right orbital contents, nose, and midfacial structures. **D,** Postoperative appearance with skin graft resurfacing. The patient will be fitted for a prosthesis. The left orbit and vision have been preserved.

The indications for postoperative radiation include positive surgical margins, perineural spread, invasion of bone and cartilage, lymph node metastasis, and extensive skeletal muscle infiltration. A relative indication for postoperative radiation therapy is poorly differentiated histology, because this tumor has a higher risk for local recurrence and is often associated with other adverse histologic findings. Relevant information, including size, depth of invasion, differentiation, presence or absence of perineural invasion, and margin status, should be obtained from the pathologist.

Primary radiation therapy is most often indicated for lesions on and around the nose, lower eyelids, and ears, where it yields better functional and cosmetic results than surgery. Extensive lesions of the cheek, lip, and oral commissures that may require full-thickness resection may be better irradiated.

The overall local control rate of all sizes and types of cutaneous carcinoma treated with various therapy modalities is about 90%. In a large series of patients treated with different strategies, the 5-year recurrence rates were 19.8% for curettage

Table 38-2 Control Rates of Carcinomas of the Eyelid Treated with Radiotherapy

Histology	Previously Untreated	Recurrent	Total	Five-Year Local Control
Basal cell carcinoma	686	376	1062	1009/1062 (95%)
Squamous cell carcinoma	62	42	104	97/104 (92%)
Total	748	418	1166	1106/1166 (95%)

Data from Fitzpatrick PJ, Thompson GA, Easterbrook WM, et al: Basal and squamous cell carcinoma of the eyelids and their treatment by radiotherapy. Int J Radiat Oncol Biol Phys 10:449-454, 1984.

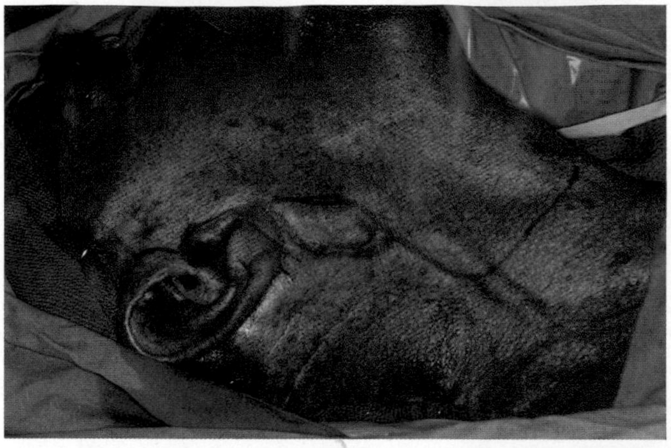

Figure 38-3 Lymph node relapse occurred in a patient 1 year after excision of a postauricular squamous cell carcinoma. The planned incision allows for dissection of the parotid and cervical nodal basins.

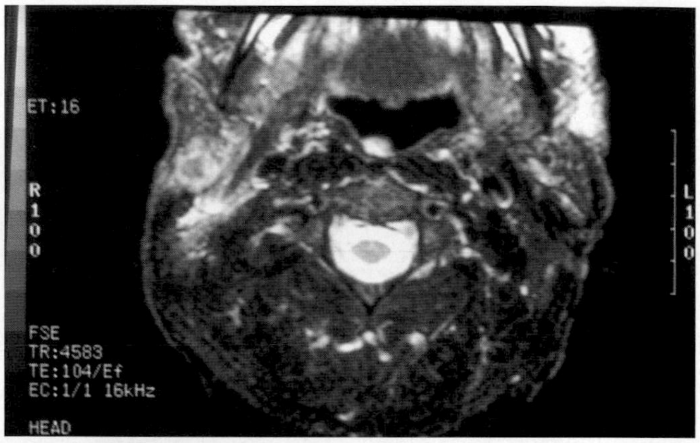

Figure 38-4 Magnetic resonance imaging demonstrates metastatic disease in the tail of the parotid and upper neck.

and electrodesiccation, 9.3% for radiation therapy, and 8.9% for surgical excision.[10] The author attributed the high recurrence rate for curettage and electrodesiccation to the fact that residents in training executed this procedure most frequently. Physician expertise is essential in obtaining good results.

The overall control rate of more than 1000 patients with eyelid tumors treated with radiation therapy is higher than 90% (Table 38-2).[50] The size of the primary lesion appears to be the major determinant for local control after radiation therapy. The 10-year control rates of a series of 646 patients with carcinomas of the eyelid, pinna, nose, and lip treated by radiation were 98% for tumors 2 cm or smaller, 79% for lesions of 2 to 5 cm, and 53% (at 8 years) for carcinomas larger than 5 cm.[51] For tumors of the same size, the control rate appears to be slightly higher for basal cell carcinoma than for squamous cell carcinoma (e.g., 97% versus 91% for lesions smaller than 1 cm and 87% versus 76% for tumors of 1 to 5 cm).[52] Although the initial cosmetic result after irradiation therapy is excellent, over time, fibrosis and soft tissue atrophy may become apparent. For this reason, irradiation is usually not recommended for patients under 50 years of age.

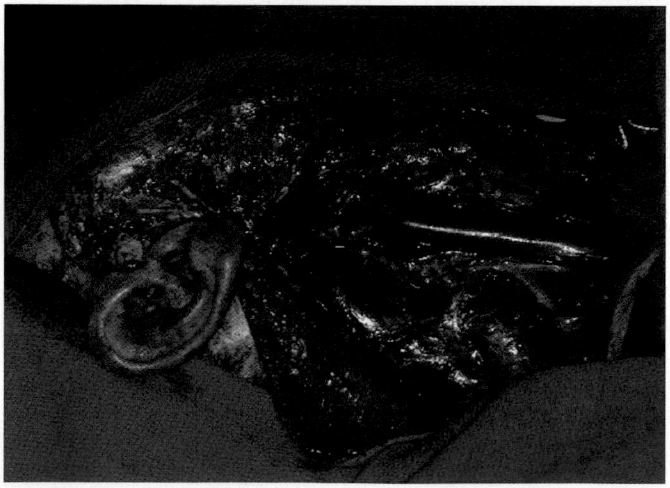

Figure 38-5 Surgical bed after superficial parotidectomy and modified radical neck dissection. The facial nerve and the internal jugular vein have been preserved. The patient received postoperative radiation therapy and remained free of disease 4 years postoperatively.

Regional Nodes

Elective nodal treatment is not indicated for cutaneous basal or squamous carcinomas because of the low incidence of lymphatic spread. Exceptions are large infiltrative-ulcerative squamous cell carcinomas and recurrent carcinomas after previous surgery.

The choice of treatment for patients who present with nodal disease depends on the type of therapy selected for the primary lesion and the size of the node. In general, a combination of surgery and radiation therapy is indicated when a nodal mass is larger than 3 cm or in the presence of extracapsular extension (Figs. 38-3 to 38-5). Taylor and colleagues[53] reported on 37 patients treated with surgery and postoperative radiation therapy for lymph node metastasis to the parotid region from skin carcinomas. The overall regional control rate was 89%, which was superior to single-modality therapy in these high-risk patients. All four recurrences occurred in patients with positive surgical margins and clinical evidence of facial nerve involvement.

Merkel Cell Carcinoma

The initial treatment for Merkel cell carcinoma is usually surgery to establish tissue diagnosis. The role of radiation in the management of Merkel cell carcinoma has been evaluated since the early 1980s because of poor results obtained with surgery alone.

Several studies have demonstrated the radiosensitivity of Merkel cell carcinoma.[23,28,54-56] In the series of Pacella and associates,[28] local control was achieved in 35 of 36 fields irradiated in 19 patients; gross disease was present in 23 of the fields. Similarly, in-field control was obtained in 30 of 31 patients treated at the MDACC. However, marginal recurrence occurred in three patients.[23] This observation indicates the necessity to irradiate a wide margin of adjacent dermis and subcutaneous tissues.

Since 1982, as the natural history of Merkel cell carcinoma became better understood, elective postoperative locoregional irradiation was given to five of six patients referred to the MDACC after local excision. The primary tumor bed and the draining lymphatics were irradiated with electron beams to cumulative doses of 50 to 55 Gy and 45 to 55 Gy (administered in 2 to 2.5 Gy per fraction), respectively. None of these patients experienced local or regional recurrences during a minimum follow-up period of 3 years. More patient accrual is necessary to determine the value of combined treatment in patients with Merkel cell carcinoma. The available data are insufficient for a detailed analysis of radiation dose response. It appears that in-field recurrence is rare after a total dose of 50 Gy administered in 2 to 2.5 Gy per fraction.

Data on the response of Merkel cell carcinoma to cytotoxic agents are emerging.[57-59] The most active drugs are doxorubicin, cyclophosphamide, and vincristine. Response of metastatic deposits to multiagent therapy can be dramatic, but unfortunately, it is frequently of short duration.

The treatment policy for Merkel cell carcinoma at MDACC can be summarized as follows. Surgical excision of the primary lesion followed by elective irradiation of the surgical bed with generous margins and the draining lymphatics is recommended for patients presenting with localized disease. The excision margin need not be wide, and elective nodal dissection is not done because of routine use of postoperative irradiation. Given the radiosensitivity of Merkel cell carcinoma, patients at high surgical risk are treated with primary radiation to a higher dose. For patients presenting with regional adenopathy, our practice is to perform therapeutic nodal dissection, along with local excision followed by irradiation of the surgical bed and draining lymphatics, although primary irradiation is a reasonable alternative. Patients with a large primary tumor and particularly those presenting with adenopathy are also considered for investigational chemotherapy regimens.

Adnexal Carcinoma

The standard treatment of sebaceous carcinoma is wide local excision and therapeutic nodal dissection if lymphadenopathy is present. The role of adjunctive therapeutic modalities has not been explored systematically. On general principles, postoperative irradiation is indicated when the surgical section margins are positive or close, multiple lymph nodes are involved, or extracapsular nodal extension is present.

For eccrine and apocrine carcinomas, wide excision of the primary lesion is accepted as the standard treatment in patients with no lymphadenopathy at diagnosis. Postoperative radiation therapy to the surgical bed with 2- to 3-cm margins is indicated, particularly for eccrine carcinoma, because of the high incidence of local recurrence after surgery alone. The role of elective treatment of regional lymphatics is controversial in this rare disease. Treatment for patients with palpable lymphadenopathy consists of wide local excision, lymph node dissection, and postoperative irradiation to the primary and nodal bed.

LOCALLY ADVANCED DISEASE AND PALLIATION

Radiation therapy administered to total doses of 60 to 70 Gy (depending on the tumor size, location, and the anticipated toxicity) can yield local control in some patients with locally advanced carcinomas. Lee and coworkers[60] reported a 5-year local control rate of 67% in 33 patients with previously untreated T4 skin carcinomas given radiation therapy to doses of 60 to 75 Gy over 6 to 8 weeks. Bone invasion or perineural spread was found to reduce the likelihood of local control in this small series of patients.

Radiation can reduce symptoms for most patients with advanced inoperable cancer or metastatic disease. The recommended dose-fractionation schedule depends on the tumor's location and patient's life expectancy. The most frequently used regimens include 30 Gy in 10 fractions over 2 weeks for skeletal or cerebral metastasis and 45 to 50 Gy in 18 to 25 fractions over 4 to 5 weeks for patients with tumor deposits in the proximity of critical structures (e.g., axillary or ilioinguinal region) but otherwise having a reasonable life expectancy.

TECHNIQUES OF IRRADIATION

Carcinoma

Primary radiation therapy yields an excellent disease control rate with very good functional and cosmetic results for lesions around the nostril, lower eyelids, auricles, and lips. Patients who are poor surgical risks or those with large lesions are sometimes best treated with radiation therapy. Proper planning and execution of radiation therapy are essential to obtain uncomplicated disease control.

Target Volume

The target volume of radiation is determined by the size of the lesion and the type of growth (i.e., infiltrative lesions require more generous coverage). Typically, the treatment field encompasses the visible or palpable tumor and 1 to 2 cm of normal-appearing skin. Margins may be tighter when treating areas close to the eye or when the primary lesion is smaller than 1 cm. More generous margins are appropriate for lesions with ill-defined borders. In this situation, the field size may be reduced after delivering a dose sufficient to sterilize potential microscopic contiguous extension.

In some patients, almost exclusively those with squamous cell carcinoma presenting with small lymphadenopathy or advanced primary lesions, the initial field encompasses the primary lesion and the regional lymphatics. The portal volume is subsequently reduced to cover the areas of gross disease with adequate margins.

In patients receiving postoperative irradiation for pathologically proven lymph node metastasis or perineural invasion, the initial portal encompasses the primary tumor bed, the regional lymphatics, or the potential route of perineural spread. The portal is then coned down to cover the involved nodal basin (e.g., involved intraparotid nodes).

Setup, Field Arrangement, and Dose Fractionation Schedule

Patients are best immobilized in a position that gives optimal access to irradiate the tumor to ensure daily reproducibility.

Preferably, the position is such that the plane of the skin to be treated is horizontal to facilitate the placement of lead shield for skin collimation. Radiation is delivered through an appositional field, in most cases using orthovoltage x-rays (usually 75 to 150 kVp) or electrons (usually 6 to 12 MeV). The energy of x-rays or electrons is chosen based on the thickness of tissues to be treated. This is critical when using electrons, the energy of which should be selected such that the 90% isodose line including surface bolus is a few millimeters deeper than the base of the lesion. The treatment distance for x-rays also depends on the thickness of the lesion. A 23-cm focus skin distance (FSD) cone is proper for superficial tumors, but a 50-cm FSD open field with skin collimation is preferable for thicker lesions to avoid a large dose gradient across the lesion. The FSD for electrons is usually 100 cm.

Several techniques and devices are helpful in minimizing radiation exposure to the surrounding normal tissues and obtaining the desired dose distribution. A lead cut-out is used for portal shaping, conforming to the geometry of the lesion by skin collimation (Fig. 38-6). The overall size of the cut-out should be large enough so that the cone or collimator setting for electron beams is at least 4 × 4 cm for reliable dosimetry.

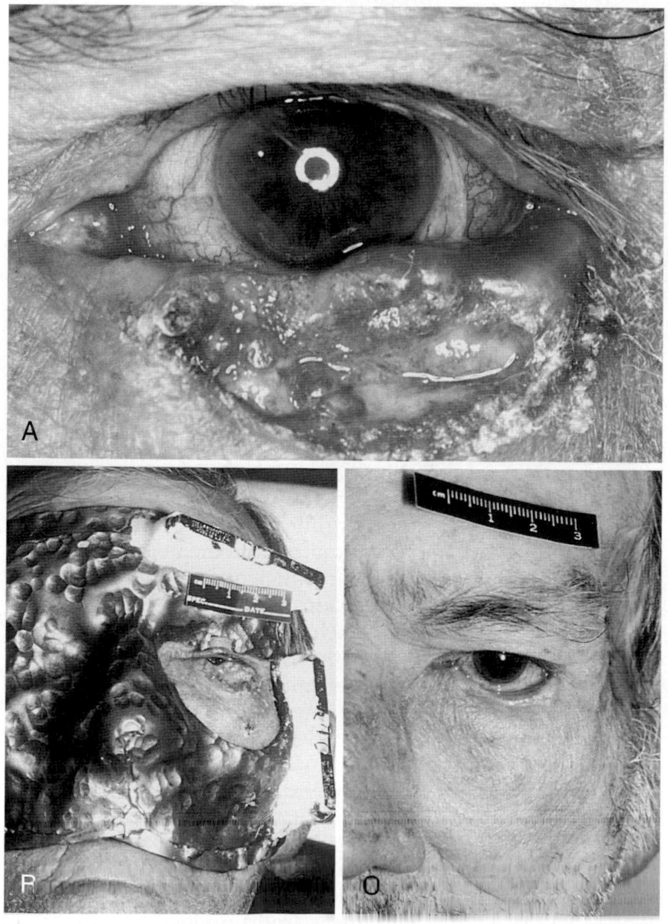

Figure 38-6 **A,** A 79-year-old man presented with a relatively large squamous cell carcinoma of the left lower eyelid, causing epiphora. **B,** He received radiation with an electron beam shaped by lead cutout skin collimation treatment to a dose of 58 Gy, prescribed to D_{90}, in 26 fractions. **C,** He was free of disease and complications more than 5 years after treatment.

Skin bolus or a Perspex scatter plate is used when treatment is given with electrons to ensure full surface dose. Additional shielding can be applied to protect tissues from exit radiation. For example, an internal eye shield is inserted when treating an eyelid lesion with orthovoltage x-rays or electrons of 8 MeV or less (Fig. 38-7). It is important to calibrate commercially available eye shields individually with respect to their electron-attenuating properties, because transmission through these shields can be considerable, even for a nominal 6-MeV beam. A customized stent containing Cerrobend is used to shield the gum when treating a lip cancer.

Several fractionation schedules have been used and were found to be effective in curing primary cutaneous carcinomas. In general, more protracted treatment gives the best cosmetic results. The recommended radiation regimen for individual patients depends on the size and site of the lesion. For most skin cancers, a dose of 40 Gy in 10 fractions, 45 Gy in 15 fractions, or 50 Gy in 20 fractions is an appropriate and effective regimen. If the patient is in poor general condition, hypofractionation (e.g., 32 Gy in 4 fractions or a single dose of 20 Gy) may be used. For large lesions close to the eye, however, maximum tolerance is obtained with 60 to 70 Gy in 30 to 35 fractions.

The dose for treatment with x-rays is specified at the maximal depth dose (D_{max}). The dose for irradiation with electrons is prescribed at 90%. Prescription of electron doses at 90% versus D_{max} for x-rays allows for the relative biologic effectiveness difference between the two beam qualities.

Patients with positive nodes usually receive radiation in 2-Gy fractions because of the large treatment volume (Fig. 38-8). Similarly, postoperative radiation is delivered in 2 Gy per fraction.

Merkel Cell and Adnexal Carcinoma

Target Volume

The target volume for Merkel cell carcinoma consists of surgical bed with margins of 4 to 5 cm, except when the lesion is situated at or close to critical structures (e.g., optic apparatus) and the draining lymphatics. For Merkel cell carcinoma of the head and neck region, the whole ipsilateral neck is irradiated.

The target volume for adnexal carcinoma consists of surgical bed with margins of 2 to 3 cm and, depending on the site and size of the primary tumor, the draining lymphatics.

Setup, Field Arrangement, and Dose Fractionation Schedule

The general principles of patient setup and portal arrangement are as outlined in the basal and squamous cell carcinoma section. As primary treatment, radiation is administered, preferably with electrons, in 2-Gy fractions to cumulative dose of 46 to 50 Gy for elective irradiation, plus a boost dose of 10 Gy in 5 fractions to the gross disease. A cumulative dose of 66 Gy may be recommended for the treatment of bulky, inoperable primary tumors.

Irradiation regimens used for adnexal carcinoma are 60 Gy given in 30 fractions or 63 Gy given in 35 fractions, depending on the site and target volume. The portal is generally reduced to encompass areas of known gross disease after 50 Gy or 54 Gy, respectively.

Patient Care during and after Radiation Therapy

A tumoricidal dose of radiation generally produces moist desquamation of the skin. The irradiated skin area should be protected from heat, cold, sunlight, friction, disinfectants, and other sources of irritation to avoid additional tissue injury.

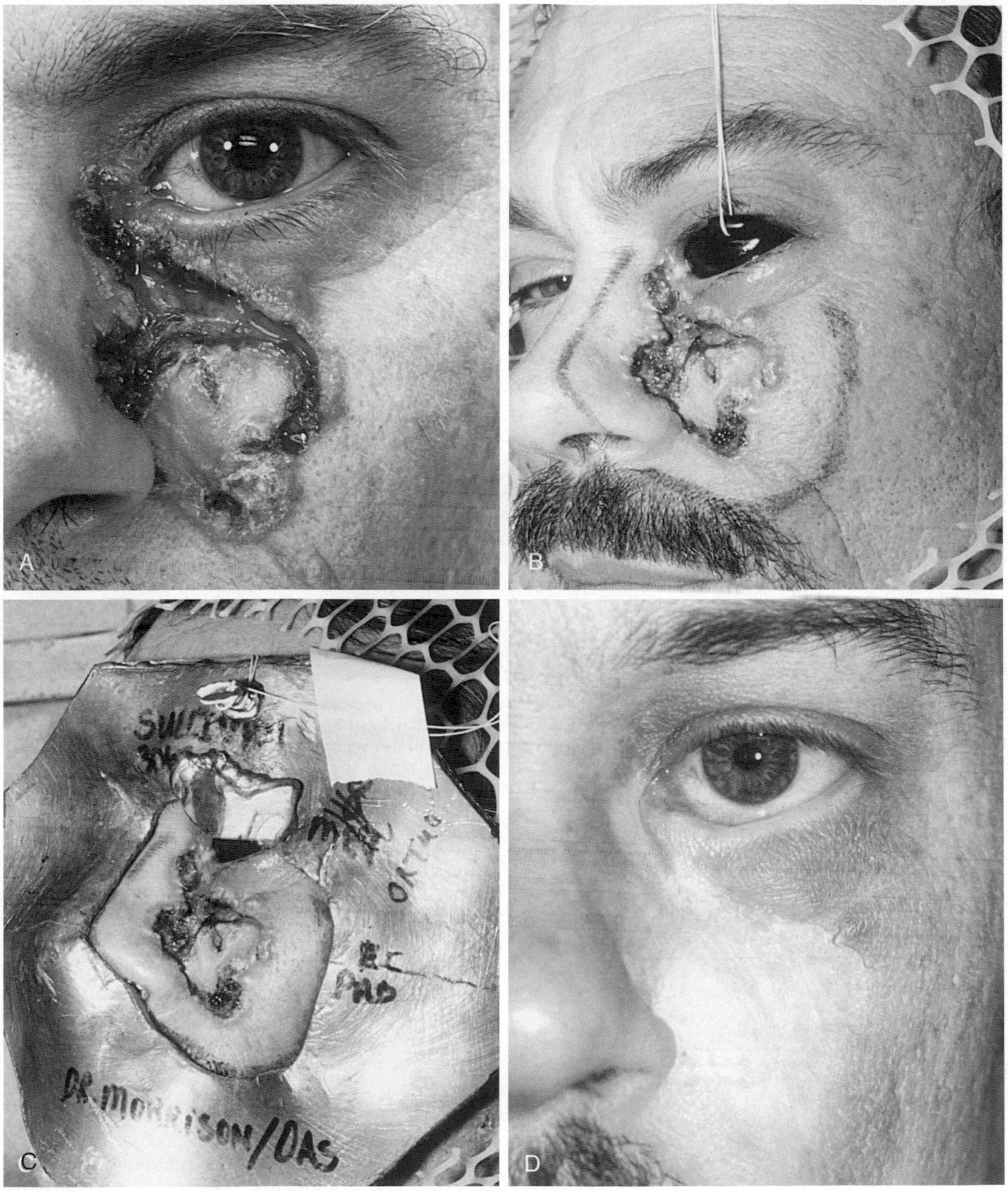

Figure 38-7 **A,** A 37-year-old man presented with a basal cell carcinoma of the left cheek that had been neglected for 6 years. The tumor extended to the medial canthus and the nose. **B** and **C,** He received radiation treatment initially with 250 kVp and with an internal eye shield and custom lead mask to a dose of 42 Gy in 22 fractions, followed by a 9-MeV electron beam to an additional dose of 22 Gy in 11 fractions. **D,** He had no evidence of disease and good eyelid function 3 years after therapy.

After moist desquamation occurs, the area should be cleaned with 1% hydrogen peroxide to prevent secondary infection. Patients are instructed to use sun blocks over the irradiated area after completion of treatment.

Patients should also be informed about the specific acute and late side effects of treatment, such as mucositis of the nasal passages and upper lip, nasal dryness, synechiae (when treating nostril lesions), and conjunctivitis and loss of eyelashes (when treating eyelid cancers). After treatment involving the lacrimal canaliculi, irrigation of the ducts during the healing phase helps to prevent synechiae.

Regular follow-up examinations include evaluation of the treated area for late complications and search for new lesions. New tumors develop in one third of the treated patients.

Late side effects include hypopigmentation, hyperpigmentation, telangiectasis, and skin atrophy. Skin retraction at the lower eyelid may result in ectropion. These are rarely serious after properly administered irradiation.

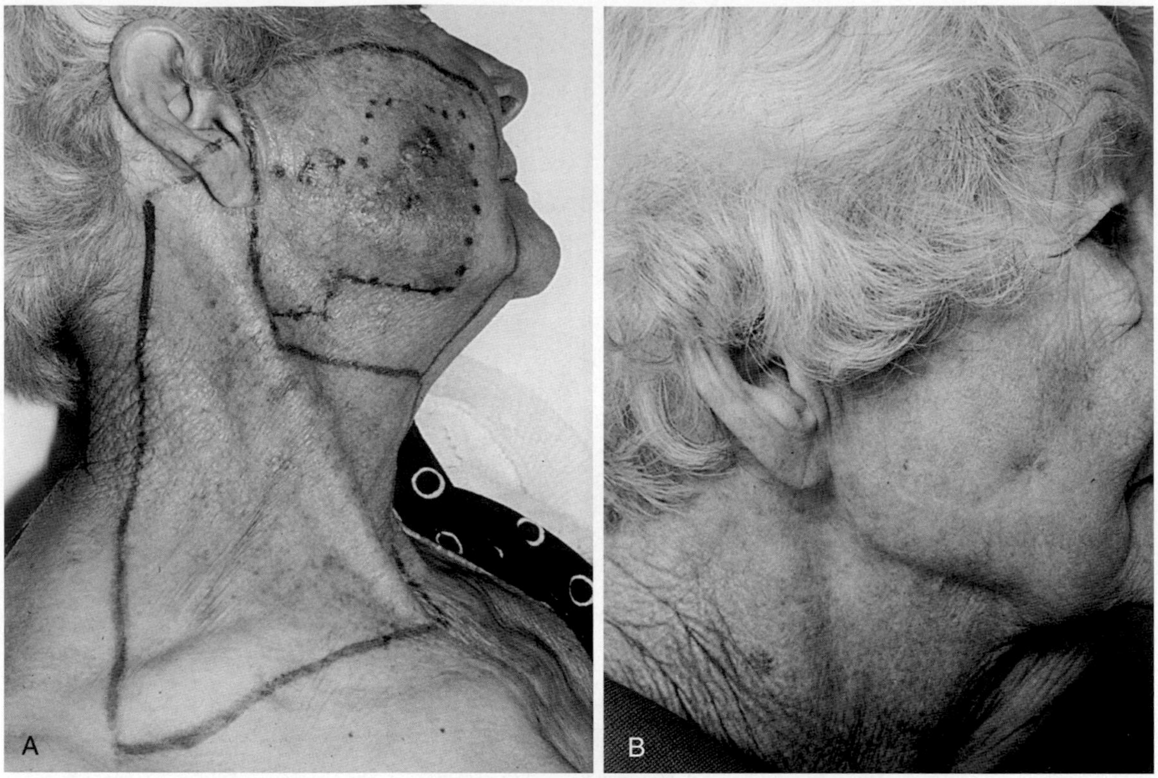

Figure 38-8 An 86-year-old woman with a history of chronic lymphocytic leukemia and excision of multiple skin cancers presented with a 3-cm, rapidly growing, ulcerated squamous cell carcinoma of the right cheek with a 1-cm hard right subdigastric lymphadenopathy. **A,** She received a dose of 54 Gy in 27 fractions to the cheek and submandibular and subdigastric nodes with a 13-MeV electron beam and 50 Gy in 25 fractions with a 9-MeV electron beam to the remaining ipsilateral neck nodes. The primary tumor and palpable node received a boost dose of 12 Gy in 6 fractions and 16 Gy in 8 fractions, respectively, given as second daily fractions twice each week (i.e., concomitant boost technique). **B,** This therapy yielded local regional tumor control with good cosmetic outcome. The patient subsequently underwent treatment for other skin cancers and died, most likely of chronic lymphocytic leukemia, 6 years later.

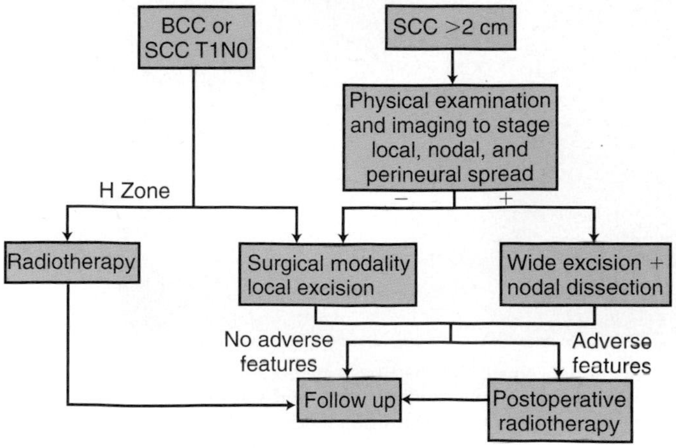

Figure 38-9 Diagnostic and treatment algorithm for cutaneous basal and squamous cell carcinoma.

DIAGNOSTIC AND TREATMENT ALGORITHMS

Basal and Squamous Cell Carcinomas (BCC and SCC)

Figure 38-9 illustrates the diagnostic and treatment algorithm. The choice of treatment for individual patients is determined by factors such as the site and size of lesion, the anticipated functional and cosmetic results, treatment time, and therapy cost. Surgical modalities are preferred for most patients with resectable tumors, but radiation therapy can yield better functional and cosmetic results for lesions of the nose, lower eyelids, and ears. A combination of surgery and irradiation is indicated in larger tumors or those with perineural spread, invasion of bone or cartilage, extensive skeletal muscle infiltration, or nodal metastasis.

Merkel Cell and Adnexal Carcinoma

A combination of surgery and elective or adjunctive irradiation is recommended for most patients with Merkel cell and adnexal carcinomas. The role of chemotherapy for the treatment of Merkel cell carcinoma needs to be further defined. Some institutions prefer to give several cycles of systemic chemotherapy before and after treatment of the locoregional component of disease in view of the high incidence of metastases.

REFERENCES

1. Jemal A, Murray T, Ward E, et al: Cancer statistics, 2005. CA Cancer J Clin 55:10-30, 2005.
2. Toker C: Trabecular carcinoma of the skin. Arch Dermatol 105:107-110, 1972.
3. Urban FH, Winkelmann RK: Sebaceous malignancy. Arch Dermatol 84:63-72, 1961.
4. Tulenko JF, Conway H: An analysis of sweat gland tumors. Surg Gynecol Obstet 121:343-348, 1965.

5. Eastcott DF: Epidemiology of skin cancer in New Zealand. Natl Cancer Monogr Inst 10:141-151, 1963.
6. Cleaver JE: Defective repair replication of DNA in xeroderma pigmentosum. Nature 218:652-656, 1968.
7. Anderson DE, Taylor WB, Falls HF, et al: The nevoid basal cell carcinoma syndrome. Am J Hum Genet 19:12-22, 1967.
8. Lutzner MA: Epidermodysplasia verruciformis: an autosomal recessive disease characterized by viral warts and skin cancer. A model for viral oncogenesis. Bull Cancer (Paris) 65:169-182, 1978.
9. Hill L, Ferrini RL: Skin cancer prevention and screening: summary of the American College of Preventive Medicine's practice policy statements. CA Cancer J Clin 48:232-235, 1998.
10. Kopf AW: Computer analysis of 3531 basal cell carcinomas of the skin. J Dermatol 6:267-281, 1979.
11. Rahbari H, Mehregan AH: Basal cell epitheliomas in usual and unusual sites. J Cutan Pathol 6:425-431, 1979.
12. Robinson JK: Risk of developing another basal cell carcinoma: a 5-year prospective study. Cancer 60:118-120, 1987.
13. Patterson JAK, Geronemus RG: Cancers of the skin. *In* DeVita VT, Hellman S, Rosenberg SA (eds): Cancer Principles & Practice of Oncology, 3rd ed. Philadelphia, JB Lippincott, 1989, pp 1469-1498.
14. Siegle RJ, MacMillan J, Pollack S: Infiltrative basal cell carcinoma: a nonsclerosing subtype. J Dermatol Surg Oncol 12:830-836, 1986.
15. Battle RJV, Patterson TJS: The surgical treatment of basal-celled carcinoma. Br J Plast Surg 13:118-135, 1960.
16. Paver K, Poyzer K, Burry N, et al: The incidence of basal cell carcinomas and their metastases in Australia and New Zealand. Aust J Dermatol 14:53, 1973.
17. Cannon JR, Schneidman DW: Recent developments in adnexal pathology. *In* Moschella SL (ed): Dermatology Update: Reviews for Physicians. New York, Elsevier, 1982, pp 217-252.
18. Soffer D, Gomori JM, Seigal T, et al: Intracranial meningiomas after high-dose irradiation. Cancer 63:1514-1519, 1989.
19. Epstein E, Epstein NN, Bragg K, et al: Metastases from squamous cell carcinomas of the skin. Arch Dermatol 97:245-251, 1968.
20. Friedman HI, Cooper PH, Wanebo HJ: Prognostic and therapeutic use of microstaging of cutaneous squamous cell carcinoma of the trunk and extremities. Cancer 56:1099-1105, 1985.
21. Immerman SC, Scanlon EF, Christ M, et al: Recurrent squamous cell carcinoma of the skin. Cancer 51:1537-1540, 1983.
22. Fukamizu H, Inoue K, Matsumoto K, et al: Metastatic squamous-cell carcinomas derived from solar keratosis. J Dermatol Surg Oncol 11:518-522, 1985.
23. Morrison WH, Peters LJ, Silva EG, et al: The essential role of radiation therapy in securing locoregional control of Merkel cell carcinoma. Int J Radiat Oncol Biol Phys 19:583-591, 1990.
24. Merkel F: Tastzellen und Tastkoerperchen bei den haushieren und beim Menschen. Arch Mikr Anat 11:636-652, 1875.
25. Silva EG, Mackay B, Goepfert H, et al: Endocrine carcinoma of the skin (Merkel cell carcinoma). Pathol Ann 19:1-30, 1984.
26. Bonfiglio TA: Neuroendocrine carcinoma of the skin: diagnostic and management considerations. Int J Radiat Oncol Biol Phys 14:1321-1322, 1988.
27. Drijkoningen M, De Wolf-Peeters C, Van Limbergen E, et al: Merkel cell tumor of the skin: an immunohistochemical study. Hum Pathol 17:301-307, 1986.
28. Pacella J, Ashby M, Ainslie J, et al: The role of radiotherapy in the management of primary cutaneous neuroendocrine tumors (Merkel cell or trabecular carcinoma): experience at the Peter MacCallum Cancer Institute (Melbourne, Australia). Int J Radiat Oncol Biol Phys 14:1077-1084, 1988.
29. Bourne RG, O'Rourke MG: Management of Merkel cell tumour. Aust N Z J Surg 58:971-974, 1988.
30. Hitchcock CL, Bland KI, Laney RG, et al: Neuroendocrine (Merkel cell) carcinoma of the skin. Its natural history, diagnosis and treatment. Ann Surg 207:201-207, 1988.
31. Meland NB, Jackson IT: Merkel cell tumor: diagnosis, prognosis, and management. Plast Reconstr Surg 77:632-638, 1986.
32. Sibley RK, Dehner LP, Rosai J: Primary neuroendocrine (Merkel cell?) carcinoma of the skin I. A clinicopathologic and ultrastructural study of 43 cases. Am J Surg Pathol 9:95-108, 1985.
33. Civatte J, Tsoitis G: Adnexal skin carcinomas. *In* Andrade R, Gumport SL, Popkin GL, et al (eds): Cancer of the Skin, vol 2. Philadelphia, WB Saunders, 1976, pp 1045-1068.
34. Rulon DB, Helwig EB: Cutaneous sebaceous neoplasms. Cancer 33:82-102, 1974.
35. Oppenheim AR: Sebaceous carcinoma of the penis. Arch Dermatol 117:306-307, 1981.
36. Batsakis JG, Littler ER, Leahy MS: Sebaceous cell lesions of the head and neck. Arch Otolaryngol 95:151-157, 1972.
37. Rao NA, Hidayat AA, McLean IW, et al: Sebaceous carcinomas of the ocular adnexa: a clinicopathologic study of 104 cases, with five-year follow-up data. Hum Pathol 13:113-122, 1982.
38. Boniuk M, Zimmerman LE: Sebaceous carcinoma of the eyelid, eyebrow, caruncle and orbit. Trans Am Acad Opthalmol Otolaryngol 72:619-642, 1968.
39. Wick MR, Goellner JR, Wolfe JT, et al: Adnexal carcinomas of the skin. II Extraocular sebaceous carcinomas. Cancer 56:1163-1172, 1985.
40. Ni C, Kuo P: Meibomian gland carcinoma. A clinicopathological study of 156 cases with long-period follow-up of 100 cases. Jpn J Ophthalmol 23:388-401, 1979.
41. Berg JW, McDivitt RW: Pathology of sweat gland carcinomas. Pathol Ann 3:123-144, 1968.
42. Mishima Y, Morioka S: Oncogenic differentiation of the intraepidermal eccrine sweat duct: eccrine poroma, poroepithelioma and porocarcinoma. Dermatologica 138:238-250, 1969.
43. Lipper S, Peiper SC: Sweat gland carcinoma with syringomatous features: a light microscopic and ultrastructural study. Cancer 44:157-163, 1979.
44. Mendoza S, Helwig EB: Mucinous (adenocystic) carcinoma of the skin. Arch Dermatol 103:68-78, 1971.
45. Liu Y: The histogenesis of clear cell papillary carcinoma of the skin. Am J Pathol 25:93-99, 1949.
46. Nickoloff BJ, Fleischmann HE, Carmel J, et al: Microcystic adnexal carcinoma: immunohistologic observations suggesting dual (pilar and eccrine) differentiation. Arch Dermatol 122:290-294, 1986.
47. Pawlowski A, Haberman HF, Menon IA: Junctional and compound pigmented nevi induced by 9,10-demethyl, benzanthracene in skin of albino guinea pigs. Cancer Res 36:2813-2821, 1976.
48. Kripke ML, Fisher MS: Immunologic parameters of ultraviolet carcinogenesis. J Natl Cancer Inst 57:211-215, 1976.
49. Crombie IK: Variation of melanoma incidence with latitude in North America and Europe. Br J Cancer 40:774-781, 1979.
50. Fitzpatrick PJ, Thompson GA, Easterbrook WM, et al: Basal and squamous cell carcinoma of the eyelids and their treatment by radiotherapy. Int J Radiat Oncol Biol Phys 10:449-454, 1984.
51. Petrovich Z, Parker RG, Luxton G, et al: Carcinoma of the lip and selected sites of head and neck skin. A clinical study of 896 patients. Radiother Oncol 8:11-17, 1987.
52. Lovett RD, Perez CA, Shapiro SJ, et al: External irradiation of epithelial skin cancer. Int J Radiat Oncol Biol Phys 19:235-242, 1990.
53. Taylor BW Jr, Brant TA, Mendenhall NP, et al: Carcinoma of the skin metastatic to parotid area lymph nodes. Head Neck 13:427-433, 1991.
54. O'Brien PC, Denham JW, Leong AS: Merkel cell carcinoma: a review of behaviour patterns and management strategies. Aust N Z J Surg 57:847-850, 1987.
55. Cotlar AM, Gates JO, Gibbs FA: Merkel cell carcinoma: combined surgery and radiation therapy. Am Surg 52:159-164, 1986.
56. Pilotti S, Rikle F, Bartoli C, et al: Clinicopathologic correlations of cutaneous neuroendocrine Merkel cell carcinoma. J Clin Oncol 6:1863-1873, 1988.
57. Feun LG, Savaraj N, Legha SS, et al: Chemotherapy for metastatic Merkel cell carcinoma. Review of the M.D. Anderson Hospital's experience. Cancer 62:683-685, 1988.
58. Wynne CJ, Kearsley JH: Merkel cell tumor: a chemosensitive skin cancer. Cancer 62:28-31, 1988.
59. Grosh WW, Giannone L, Hande KR, et al: Disseminated Merkel cell tumor. Treatment with systemic chemotherapy. Am J Clin Oncol 10:227-230, 1987.
60. Lee WR, Mendelhall WM, Parsons JT, et al: Radical radiotherapy for T4 carcinoma of the skin of the head and neck: a multivariate analysis. Head Neck 15:320-324, 1993.

CHAPTER 39

MALIGNANT MELANOMA

Matthew T. Ballo and K. Kian Ang

INCIDENCE

The incidence of melanoma continues to rise faster than that of any other cancer. In 2006, an estimated 62,190 new cases of melanoma will be diagnosed in the United States, and there will be approximately 8000 deaths.

BIOLOGIC CHARACTERISTICS

Sun exposure is clearly associated with the development of cutaneous melanoma. Inherited mutations may also play a role in some cases.

The natural history of melanoma is characterized by early, stepwise dissemination from primary to regional lymph nodes and then to distant sites.

The primary determinants of survival are primary thickness (measured in millimeters), presence or absence of primary ulceration, status of regional lymph nodes, and the site of distant disease.

STAGING EVALUATION

For evaluating localized disease, a thorough history and physical examination can suffice. For patients with nodal spread, staging evaluation should include a serum level of lactate dehydrogenase, contrast-enhanced computed tomography, and consideration of magnetic resonance imaging of the brain, which should be routine for patients with distant metastases.

PRIMARY THERAPY

Treatment of primary melanoma that is less than 1 mm thick is wide local excision alone. Sentinel lymph node biopsy is generally recommended for any lesion that is 1 mm thick or larger or if ulceration or Clark level IV or V invasion exists in a thinner lesion. If the sentinel node is not involved, the patient may be observed, but if it is involved, complete lymph node dissection should follow.

If complete lymph node dissection is not possible because of medical comorbidities, irradiation is preferred to observation.

ADJUVANT THERAPY

For patients at risk for nodal spread in whom sentinel lymph node biopsy will not alter subsequent management because of medical comorbidities, regional irradiation (i.e., elective irradiation) is preferred to observation.

Indications for postdissection nodal irradiation (i.e., therapeutic irradiation) are nodal extracapsular extension, lymph nodes measuring 3 cm or more in the widest diameter, at least four involved lymph nodes, and recurrent nodal disease after previous dissection for pathologically involved lymph nodes.

Adjuvant systemic interferon-alpha-2b improves relapse-free survival and may improve overall survival for patients with thick, localized melanoma and those with nodal metastases.

LOCALLY ADVANCED DISEASE AND PALLIATION

Irradiation reduces symptoms in more than 80% of patients with inoperable disease or metastatic masses.

Malignant melanoma remains a surgically treated disease, and most patients with early-stage disease are cured by simple excision of the primary lesion. By the time growth of the primary reaches a few millimeters, however, the risk of nodal and distant spread increases rapidly, and the role of adjuvant irradiation and systemic therapy takes on increasing importance. As for many diseases, irradiation is often recommended as an adjuvant to surgical dissection of locally advanced disease or as a palliative treatment of distant metastases. However, the acceptance of irradiation as part of a standard treatment algorithm for patients with melanoma has been slow and marred by controversy.

In the early 1930s, when categorizing tumor radiosensitivity gained widespread acceptance, melanoma was considered to be categorically radioresistant. This belief was perpetuated by popular textbooks of the time until laboratory data showed that the reputed radioresistance of melanoma might reflect a broad shoulder in the low-dose portion of the cell survival curve. The data suggested that melanoma cells might be more sensitive to radiation delivered as a large dose per fraction (i.e., hypofractionation regimen). Although a randomized trial performed by the Radiation Therapy Oncology Group (RTOG) did not confirm clinical superiority for hypofractionation in a heterogeneous group of patients receiving palliative radiation therapy, these types of regimens are favored by clinicians specializing in melanoma radiation therapy.[1] Retrospective reviews of clinical experiences have suggested that the hypofractionated regimens are effective and can be safely delivered in a short period of time to a group of patients for whom survival is ultimately dictated by the risk of distant metastasis.[2]

Although hypofractionated irradiation has been shown to be effective in several clinical settings, the perceived risk of distant metastatic disease and concern over the rate of long-term radiation-related toxicity often precludes its use, regardless of effectiveness. In this chapter, we present the rates of local failure, regional failure, distant failure, and long-term treatment-related toxicity for patients with melanoma and provide data supporting the use of irradiation in a defined group of patients. Only by balancing the competing risks of failure and treatment-related toxicity can physicians appropriately integrate radiation therapy into the management of patients with malignant melanoma.

ETIOLOGY AND EPIDEMIOLOGY

There will be an estimated 62,190 new cases of cutaneous malignant melanoma in 2006, or 4% of all newly diagnosed cancers.[3] Although the incidence of malignant melanoma more than doubled between 1975 and 2000, new cases of melanoma are being diagnosed earlier in the course of the disease because of increased public awareness, and the mortality rate has steadily decreased.[3] The reason for the rise in incidence has not been explained. The number of deaths due to melanoma in 2005 was approximately 8000.

Several lines of evidence link sun or ultraviolet (UV) radiation exposure to the development of cutaneous melanoma.[4,5] There is a higher incidence of melanoma in populations living in areas of high ambient sunlight, among sun-sensitive people, on sun-exposed body sites, in populations with high sun exposure, and among people with other sun-related skin conditions.[6,7] The development of melanoma may also be reduced by protection of the skin against sun exposure.[6]

Analysis of patients with familial clustering of melanoma has identified two genes, *CDKN2A* and *CDK4,* that confer increased susceptibility to melanoma development.[8] Although only a small percentage of patients with melanoma has a mutation in *CDKN2A*, carriers of this mutation have an almost 70% chance of developing melanoma by the age of 80 years.[9,10]

The presence of an increasing number of nevi also represents a well-accepted risk factor for the development of melanoma.[11] Whether the type of nevi (i.e., common, atypical, or dysplastic) is also important or merely reflects the degree of previous sun-related damage remains controversial.

PREVENTION AND EARLY DETECTION

Advocates of early detection and screening programs generally assume that early detection and treatment will significantly impact mortality and quality of life, particularly in melanoma, for which the association between tumor thickness and survival is well documented. Unfortunately, there are no randomized clinical trials to support routine screening of the general population. In the United States, routine screening of high-risk populations is still generally recommended, and educational efforts have been directed to clinicians and the public to promote early recognition of suspicious skin lesions. Recognized signs of melanoma include the ABCDs of early diagnosis: A, asymmetry; B, border irregularity; C, color variation; and D, a diameter greater than 6 mm.

A panel of the American College of Preventive Medicine (ACPM) performed a thorough review of the medical literature and issued a practice policy statement regarding skin cancer prevention.[12] Recommended preventive measures include avoidance of sunlight exposure—particularly limiting time spent outdoors between 10 AM and 3 PM—and wearing protective physical barriers such as hats and clothing. If sun exposure cannot be limited because of occupational, cultural, or other factors, the use of sunscreens that are opaque or that block ultraviolet A and B radiation is recommended.

The ACPM recommends periodic separate or mass screening for high-risk individuals, consisting of a total cutaneous examination and a 2- to 3-minute visual inspection of the entire integument by adequately trained physicians. Risk factors include a family history of skin cancer, fair skin, multiple nevi, and a history of other skin cancers.

CLINICAL MANIFESTATIONS, PATHOBIOLOGY, AND PATHWAYS OF SPREAD

Clinical Presentation and Pathology

Primary cutaneous melanoma may develop in or adjacent to one of the precursor lesions (e.g., lentigo maligna, dysplastic nevus) or in normal skin, and it can manifest clinically in four major growth patterns.[13] The most prevalent variant is superficial spreading melanoma, which constitutes approximately 70% of cases.[14,15] This growth pattern can occur at any age after puberty and affects women more frequently than men. Superficial spreading melanoma often arises in a junctional nevus, where it first appears as a deeply pigmented area, progressing gradually to a flat induration, generally over several years. There are often patches of amelanotic areas within the lesion thought to result from focal regression. As the lesion grows, the surface and perimeter may become irregular. Histologically, it is characterized by a prominent intraepidermal proliferation of malignant melanocytes. The malignant cells resemble the cells of Paget's disease; hence, this pattern is called *pagetoid melanoma.*[16] The malignant cell may be confined to the lower portion of the epidermis or may spread up into the granular cell layer of the epidermis, which is frequently hyperplastic. As the lesion enlarges, clusters of malignant cells invade into the dermis and subcutaneous tissues.

Nodular melanoma is the second most common variant, comprising 15% to 25% of cases.[14,15] Nodular melanoma develops more frequently de novo on the trunk, head, or neck of middle-aged individuals. In contrast to superficial spreading melanoma, the nodular variant affects men more than women. It manifests as a raised or dome-shaped, blue-black lesion, which is usually darker than superficial spreading melanoma. Approximately 5% of nodular variants manifest as nonpigmented, fleshy nodules, and therefore this type of lesion is called *amelanotic melanoma.* Histologically, nodular melanoma is characterized by an expansile nodule centered at the papillary dermis, with little or no epidermal component, composed of epithelioid cells. Spindle cells, small epithelioid cells, and mixtures of cells may be present. Deeper invasion of the dermis and subcutis occurs as the lesion grows.

Lentigo maligna melanoma constitutes less than 10% of malignant melanoma.[15,17] This variant occurs most frequently on the face or neck of white women older than 50 years, and it arises from a precursor lesion of melanoma in situ called *lentigo maligna* (i.e., Hutchinson's melanotic freckle).[18] It manifests as a relatively large (>3 cm), flat, tan-colored (with different shades of brown) lesion that often has been present for more than 5 years. The border becomes irregular as the lesion enlarges. Histologically, invasive tumor is usually composed of spindle-like cells. These cells may be embedded in a fibrous stroma (i.e., desmoplastic pattern) or may form fascicles displaying neural features and infiltrating endoneural and perineural structures of the cutaneous nerves.[18,19]

Acral lentiginous melanoma occurs characteristically on the palms or soles or beneath nail beds.[20-22] The relative frequency of acral lentiginous melanoma varies substantially with race. It represents about 5% of melanomas in whites and 35% to 60% of melanomas in dark-skinned individuals.[23,24] Most acral lentiginous melanomas occur on the foot sole in individuals older than 60 years. They generally start as tan or brown stains and evolve over a period of years to reach an average diameter of 3 cm before diagnosis is established.[21,22] Histologically, early-stage acral lentiginous melanoma is composed of large, highly atypical, pigmented cells along the dermoepidermal junction in an area of hyperplastic epidermis. At the invasive stage, infiltrating cells may be epithelioid or spindle shaped.[19] Sometimes, infiltration to deeper structures occurs, predominantly through the eccrine ducts.[16]

Biology and Pattern of Spread

Superficial spreading and lentigo maligna melanomas generally grow slowly over many years (i.e., radial growth phase). Left untreated, however, these lesions gradually invade the dermis and subcutis (i.e., vertical growth phase) and acquire metastatic potential. Acral lentiginous melanomas and particularly nodular melanomas have a shorter natural history, with rapid progression to the vertical growth pattern.

Previously, two microstaging systems were used. The Breslow system classifies lesions by the vertical thickness between the granular layer of the epidermis and the deepest part of invasion, measured with an ocular micrometer. In ulcerated lesions, measurements are made from the surface to the deepest part.[25] The Clark method categorizes lesions into five groups by the level of dermal or subcutis invasion: level I, confined to the epidermis; level II, invasion to the papillary dermis; level III, invasion to the papillary-reticular dermal interface; level IV, invasion to the reticular dermis; and level V, invasion to the subcutaneous tissue.[14] Of the two systems, tumor thickness is more accurate in predicting outcome, although level of invasion remains prognostic for patients with lesions less than 1.0 mm thick.[26]

In an analysis of 17,600 patients with melanoma, several clinical and histologic variables were found to be of prognostic value, and they formed the basis for an updated American Joint Committee on Cancer (AJCC) staging system (Table 39-1).[26,27] For patients without clinical evidence of nodal spread, primary thickness and ulceration were the most important prognostic features. The 10-year melanoma-specific mortality rate increased proportionally as the thickness of the primary increased (Fig. 39-1), and the survival of patients with ulcerated primary lesions diminished to a level equivalent to that of patients with thicker primary lesions that were not ulcerated (Fig. 39-2).[26] There was a significantly inferior 10-year disease-specific survival rate according to site of the primary lesion (i.e., worse for trunk, head, and neck than

Table 39-1 American Joint Committee on Cancer Staging System for Melanoma of the Skin, 2002

PRIMARY TUMOR (T)

TX	Primary tumor cannot be assessed (e.g., shave biopsy, regressed melanoma)
T0	No evidence of primary tumor
Tis	Melanoma in situ
T1	Melanoma ≤1.0 mm thick, with or without ulceration
T1a	Melanoma ≤ 1.0 mm thick and level II or III, no ulceration
T1b	Melanoma ≤ 1.0 mm thick and level IV or V, or with ulceration
T2	Melanoma 1.01-2 mm thick with or without ulceration
T2a	Melanoma 1.01-2 mm thick, no ulceration
T2b	Melanoma 1.01-2 mm thick, with ulceration
T3	Melanoma 2.01-4 mm thick, with or without ulceration
T3a	Melanoma 2.01-4 mm thick, no ulceration
T3b	Melanoma 2.01-4 mm thick, with ulceration
T4	Melanoma greater than 4.0 mm thick, with or without ulceration
T4a	Melanoma > 4.0 mm thick, no ulceration
T4b	Melanoma > 4.0 mm thick, with ulceration

REGIONAL LYMPH NODES (N)

NX	Regional lymph nodes cannot be assessed
N0	No regional lymph node metastasis
N1	Metastasis in one lymph node
N1a	Clinically occult (microscopic) metastasis
N1b	Clinically apparent (macroscopic) metastasis
N2	Metastasis in two or three regional nodes or intralymphatic regional metastasis without nodal metastases
N2a	Clinically occult (microscopic) metastasis
N2b	Clinically apparent (macroscopic) metastasis
N2c	Satellite or in-transit metastasis without nodal metastasis
N3	Metastasis in four or more regional nodes, or matted metastatic nodes, or in-transit metastasis or satellite(s) with metastasis in regional node(s)

DISTANT METASTASIS (M)

MX	Distant metastasis cannot be assessed
M0	No distant metastasis
M1	Distant metastasis
M1a	Metastasis to skin, subcutaneous tissues, or distant lymph nodes
M1b	Metastasis to lung
M1c	Metastasis to all other visceral sites or distant metastasis at any site associated with elevated serum lactate dehydrogenase (LDH)

CLINICAL STAGE GROUPING

Stage 0	Tis	N0	M0
Stage IA	T1a	N0	M0
Stage IB	T1b	N0	M0
	T2a	N0	M0
Stage IIA	T2b	N0	M0
	T3a	N0	M0
Stage IIB	T3b	N0	M0
	T4a	N0	M0
Stage IIC	T4b	N0	M0
Stage III	Any T	N1	M0
	Any T	N2	M0
	Any T	N3	M0
Stage IV	Any T	Any N	M1

PATHOLOGIC STAGE GROUPING

Stage 0	Tis	N0	M0
Stage IA	T1a	N0	M0
Stage IB	T1b	N0	M0
	T2a	N0	M0
Stage IIA	T2b	N0	M0
	T3a	N0	M0
Stage IIB	T3b	N0	M0
	T4a	N0	M0
Stage IIC	T4b	N0	M0
Stage IIIA	T1-4a	N1a	M0
	T1-4a	N1a	M0
Stage IIIB	T1-4b	N1a	M0
	T1-4b	N2a	M0
	T1-4a	N1b	M0
	T1-4a	N2b	M0
	T1-4a/b	N2c	M0
Stage IIIC	T1-4b	N1b	M0
	T1-4b	N2b	M0
	Any T	N3	M0
Stage IV	Any T	Any N	M1

Balch CM, Buzaid AC, Soong SJ, et al: Final version of the American Joint Committee on Cancer staging system for cutaneous melanoma. J Clin Oncol 19:3635-3648, 2001.

extremity), gender (i.e., worse for male than female patients), and age (i.e., worse for older than younger patients).[26]

For patients with documented nodal metastases, the most important prognostic feature was the number of involved lymph nodes, but primary tumor ulceration and burden of nodal disease (microscopic versus macroscopic) remained of prognostic significance on multivariate analysis (Table 39-2).[26] Patients with skin, subcutaneous, and distant lymph node metastases fared better than those with visceral metastases.[26]

PATIENT EVALUATION AND STAGING

Suggested staging guidelines for patients with melanoma are shown in Table 39-3. Clinical evaluation of patients with melanoma consists of inspection and palpation of the involved area of skin and the regional lymph nodes. Patients with primary lesions 1 mm thick or larger are generally staged at the time of wide local excision with sentinel lymph node biopsy. Patients with thinner lesions may still be at risk of nodal disease and may benefit from sentinel lymph node biopsy if the primary is ulcerated, associated with satellitosis, or is Clark level IV or V. Imaging studies (i.e., chest, abdomen and pelvis computed tomography [CT] or brain magnetic resonance imaging [MRI]) should be obtained as indicated by the result of immunohistochemical examination of the sentinel node. If the sentinel node is involved, CT of the lungs, abdomen, and pelvis is warranted as a baseline evaluation.[28]

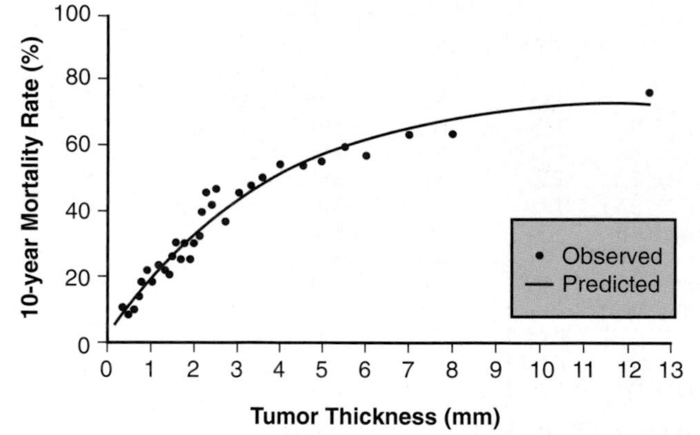

Figure 39-1 Observed and predicted 10-year mortality rate of 15,320 patients with clinically localized melanoma based on the mathematical model $f(t) = 1 - 0.988\ e\ (-211\ lt + 0.009\ t^2)$, which is derived from the melanoma database of the American Joint Committee on Cancer (AJCC). T is the measured thickness (mm), and $f(t)$ is the 10-year melanoma-specific mortality rate ($P < .0001$). (From Balch CM, Soong S, Gershenwald JE, et al: Prognostic factors analysis of 17,600 melanoma patients: validation of the American Joint Committee on Cancer melanoma staging system. J Clin Oncol 19:3622-3634, 2001.)

Chest radiography plays little or no role in the initial management of patients with localized disease. MRI of the brain is indicated for patients with multiple or clinically palpable nodal metastases and for all patients with documented distant disease.

PRIMARY THERAPY AND RESULTS

Primary Tumor

Standard treatment for localized melanoma (stages I and II) is wide local excision. Wide local excision is a therapeutic intervention, but it also establishes tissue diagnosis and provides accurate microstaging. Five randomized trials have examined the appropriate width of excision for primary melanoma.[29-33] The recommended skin margins are 1 cm for lesions less than 1 mm thick and 2 cm for 1 mm or thicker melanomas.[33,34]

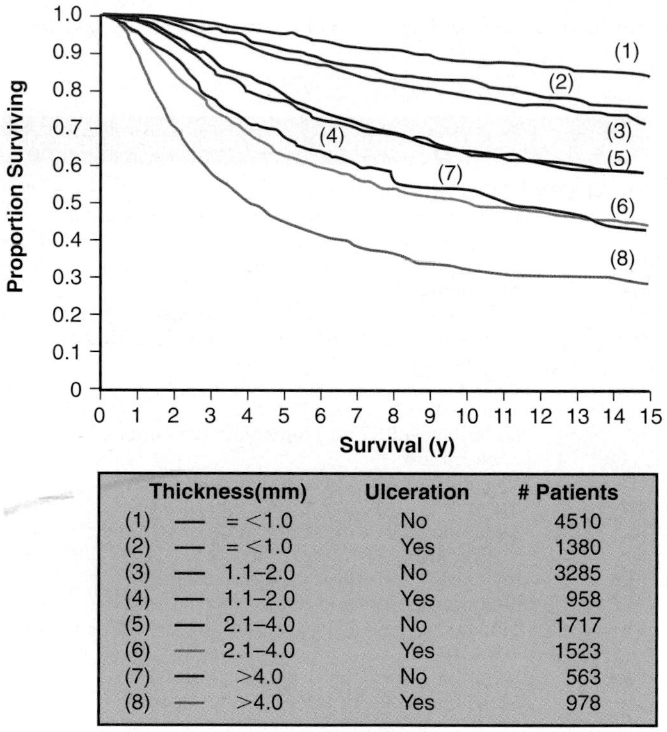

Figure 39-2 Survival curves for 14,914 patients with localized melanoma stratified by melanoma thickness and presence or absence of ulceration. The correlation of the subgroups used for defining melanoma TNM staging with melanoma-specific survival is significant ($P < .0001$). (From Balch CM, Soong S, Gershenwald JE, et al: Prognostic factors analysis of 17,600 melanoma patients: validation of the American Joint Committee on Cancer melanoma staging system. J Clin Oncol 19:3622-3634, 2001.)

Table 39-2 Five-Year Survival Rates for Patients with Stage III (Nodal Metastases) Disease Stratified by Number of Metastatic Nodes, Ulceration, and Tumor Burden

	Microscopic Nodal Disease (No. Involved)						Macroscopic Nodal Disease (No. Involved)					
	1 Node		2-3 Nodes		>3 Nodes		1 Node		2-3 Nodes		>3 Nodes	
Melanoma Ulceration	% ± SE	No.	% ± SE	No.	% ± SE	No.	% ± SE	No.	% ± SE	No.	% ± SE	No.
Absent	69 ± 3.7	252	63 ± 5.6	130	27 ± 9.3	57	59 ± 4.7	122	46 ± 5.5	93	27 ± 4.6	109
Present	52 ± 4.1	217	50 ± 5.7	111	37 ± 8.8	46	29 ± 5.0	98	25 ± 4.4	109	13 ± 3.5	104

Balch CM, Soong SJ, Gershenwald JE, et al: Prognostic factors analysis of 17,600 melanoma patients: validation of the American Joint Committee on Cancer melanoma staging system. J Clin Oncol 19:3622-3634, 2001.

Sentinel lymph node biopsy is recommended according to the aforementioned criteria (see "Patient Evaluation and Staging"). This procedure provides accurate nodal staging, but it should be followed by nodal irradiation (see "Regional Nodes") or formal lymph node dissection if the sentinel node is involved. The rate of nodal spread according to primary thickness is shown in Table 39-4; it is less than 5% for lesions 0.75 mm or smaller, 10% for lesions 0.76 to 1.50 mm, 20% for lesions 1.51 to 4.0 mm, and 30% to 50% for lesions larger than 4.0 mm.[35-46]

Radiation therapy is not indicated as definitive management of primary malignant melanoma. An exception to this rule is large facial lentigo maligna melanoma for which wide surgical resection may require extensive reconstruction. In a series of 25 patients treated at the Princess Margaret Hospital with primary radiation therapy and followed for a period of 6 months to 8 years (median, 2 years), local control was achieved in 23 patients (92%).[47] The median time to complete regression of lesions was 8 months, and some lesions took 2 years to disappear. Radiation treatment was delivered with orthovoltage x-rays (100 to 250 KeV), and regimens used were 35 Gy in 5 fractions over 1 week for lesions smaller than 3 cm, 45 Gy in 10 fractions over 2 weeks for primaries of 3 to 4.9 cm, and 50 Gy in 15 to 20 fractions over 3 to 4 weeks for tumors 5 cm or larger.

Radiation is rarely recommended as an adjuvant to wide local excision. Local recurrence in the five randomized trials examining margin width for primary lesions ranged from less than 1% to 8% of patients.[29-33] Although high-risk features such as primary thickness greater than 4 mm, head or neck primary site, and primary ulceration or satellitosis have been reported to significantly increase the risk of local recurrence, few series report recurrence rates much higher than 15% (Table 39-5).[31,48-59]

Table 39-3 Staging Guidelines and Diagnostic Algorithm

Disease Presentation	Workup
Primary lesion <1.0 mm, and Clark level II-III, and not ulcerated	History and physical examination*
Primary lesion ≥1.0 mm, or Clark level IV-V, or ulcerated	History and physical examination* Sentinel lymph node biopsy
Microscopic nodal metastases	History and physical examination* Chest radiograph and serum lactate dehydrogenase level Further imaging if warranted
Macroscopic nodal metastases	History and physical examination* Serum lactate dehydrogenase level CT imaging of chest, abdomen, pelvis CT imaging of head and neck if primary above clavicles Consider brain MRI Further imaging if warranted
Distant metastases	History and physical examination* Chest radiograph and serum lactate dehydrogenase level CT imaging of chest, abdomen, pelvis CT imaging of head and neck if primary above clavicles Brain MRI Further imaging if warranted

*Attention to comprehensive skin and nodal basin examination.

Table 39-5 Local Recurrence Rates after Surgery Alone for Primary Tumor According to High-Risk Pathologic Characteristics

Characteristic	Rate (%)	References
Breslow thickness ≥4 mm	6 to 14	34, 48-52
Head and neck location	5 to 17	31, 48, 49, 51, 53-57
Ulceration	10 to 17	31, 34, 49, 51
Satellitosis	14 to 16	58, 59
Desmoplastic histology	23 to 48	60-67

Adapted from Ballo MT, Ang KK: Radiotherapy for cutaneous malignant melanoma: rationale and indications. Oncology 18:99-107, 2004.

Table 39-4 Percentage of Patients with Positive Sentinel Lymph Nodes by Primary Melanoma Thickness

	Patients (%) by Tumor Thickness (mm)							
Study	*≤0.75*	*0.76-1.5*	*1.51-4*	*>4*	*≤1*	*1.01-2*	*2.01-4*	*>4*
Krag et al[35]	4	3	22	27	—	—	—	—
Joseph et al[36]	0	7	18	30	—	—	—	—
Mraz-Gernhard et al[37]	—	—	22	28	—	—	—	—
Haddad et al[38]	0	15	19	29	—	—	—	—
Gershenwald et al[39]	5	5	19	34	—	—	—	—
Statius Muller et al[40]	0	15	26	57	—	—	—	—
Bachter et al[41]	—	7	21	44	—	—	—	—
Blumenthal et al[42]	—	9	64	27	—	—	—	—
Caprio et al[43]	2	4	17	39	—	—	—	—
Vuylsteke et al[44]	—	—	—	—	6	16	34	55
McMasters et al[45]	—	—	—	—	—	15	30	45
Rousseau et al[46]	—	—	—	—	4	12	28	44
Weighted average (%)	1	7	21	33	4	14	29	45

From Bonnen MD, Ballo MT, Myers JN, et al: Elective radiotherapy provides regional control for patients with cutaneous melanoma of the head and neck. Cancer 100:383-389, 2003.

One variant of melanoma, the desmoplastic subtype, is clearly associated with an increased rate of local recurrence. These tumors typically manifest in elderly patients with a predilection for head and neck sites, and they are associated with perineural invasion. Recurrence rates as high as 50% have been reported after wide local excision alone (see Table 39-5).[60-67] An analysis by Vongtama and colleagues included 44 patients with desmoplastic melanoma and reported recurrence rates of 48% (21 of 44 patients) without irradiation and 0% (0 of 14 patients) with irradiation.[66] The investigators' recommendations for adjuvant irradiation included all desmoplastic melanomas, but particularly those with locally recurrent disease, Clark level IV or greater, and cases in which excision with wide margins would compromise function or cosmetic outcome.

Regional Nodes

Elective Nodal Treatment

The role of elective nodal therapy at the time of wide local excision of the primary has been disputed extensively. Advocates of elective lymph node dissection (ELND) argue that melanoma progresses in a stepwise fashion from primary to regional nodes and then to distant sites, whereas opponents suggest that positive regional lymph nodes are only indicators of systemic spread. Results of an early nonrandomized study by the Sydney Melanoma Unit involving 1319 patients suggested that ELND improved the survival of patients with intermediately thick melanomas (0.76 to 4 mm).[68] Four prospective phase III trials, however, have not confirmed these results. The first trial, conducted by the World Health Organization (WHO) Melanoma Group, randomized 553 patients to receive wide local excision and ELND or wide local excision and delayed therapeutic lymphadenectomy (i.e., lymph node dissection only if regional nodes became clinically detectable), and results showed no difference in the survival rates for the two groups.[69] A smaller trial, performed at the Mayo Clinic, showed results similar to those of the WHO group.[70]

An Intergroup Melanoma Surgical Trial enrolled 740 patients with clinically localized melanomas of 1.0 to 4.0 mm and revealed no significant difference in overall 10-year survival between patients randomized to receive ELND or observation (77% versus 73%; $P = .12$). Significant differences in overall survival rates were observed, however, in subsets of patients as old as 60 years (81% with ELND versus 74% with observation; $P = .03$), particularly when they had nonulcerative tumors (84% versus 77%; $P = .03$) and had melanomas 1 to 2 mm thick (86% versus 80%; $P = .03$).[71] A second WHO Melanoma Trial enrolled patients with trunk melanomas thicker than 1.5 mm to ELND or delayed dissection at the time of regional recurrence. This trial demonstrated a trend toward improved survival in the immediate-dissection arm ($P = .09$).[72]

Although the latter two trials have been used to argue the benefits of ELND for subgroups of patients with melanoma, the controversy has been essentially superseded by the practice of sentinel lymph node biopsy (SLNB) with selective lymph node dissection. This diagnostic procedure involves injection of the primary site with a dye and radiotracer-tagged colloid that localizes to the first draining lymph node or nodes after a short period of time. These nodes are then removed, serially sectioned, and examined with immunohistochemical staining techniques. Patients without involved lymph nodes are spared a comprehensive lymph node dissection.

The surgical community has embraced SLNB with selective lymph node dissection as a replacement to ELND, despite no reported therapeutic benefits in terms of overall survival. This choice depends on several lines of reasoning.[73,74] The status of the sentinel lymph node is a powerful predictor of subsequent survival and provides prognostic information to the patient, it identifies patients with early regional lymph node metastases that might benefit from nodal dissection as a way of avoiding advanced regional recurrence, and it identifies patients who may be candidates for investigational systemic therapy trials.

Although the standard approach to patients with early-stage melanoma is SLNB with selective dissection, there are some patients with significant medical comorbidities for whom detailed prognostic information is of little relevance and enrollment in a clinical trial is unlikely. For these patients, elective nodal irradiation is superior to observation, which places the patients at unnecessary risk of regional recurrence.[75] In a retrospective analysis from the M.D. Anderson Cancer Center, Bonnen and colleagues reviewed 157 patients with stage I or II cutaneous melanoma of the head and neck who received elective regional irradiation instead of lymph node dissection after wide local excision of the primary site.[76] Indications for regional irradiation included primary thickness of 1.5 mm or greater or Clark level IV or V disease. There were 15 regional failures (89% regional control at 10 years) despite an estimation that 33 to 40 patients had microscopically involved regional nodes (based on data from Table 39-4). Six percent of patients required medical care for a clinically significant complication, with moderate hearing loss being the most common complaint (5 patients). Although elective nodal irradiation suffers from the same limitations as ELND, it can effectively provide regional control to patients at risk for regional recurrence while avoiding surgical dissection.

Therapeutic Nodal Approaches

For most patients, nodal dissection results in more than an 80% likelihood of regional control. For patients with certain clinicopathologic features, however, the surgical literature suggests recurrence rates as high as 80% and therefore a need for additional regional therapy. Although nodal extracapsular extension remains the strongest predictor of subsequent regional recurrence after surgery alone, several series have reported elevated recurrence rates if at least four lymph nodes are involved, the lymph nodes measure at least 3 cm in diameter, they are located in the cervical basin, or they are detected during a therapeutic dissection (as opposed to elective dissection or at the time of sentinel lymph node biopsy (SLNB).[77-82] Although less well described in literature, nodal recurrence after previous dissection for involved regional nodes also places the patient at increased risk of subsequent recurrence. Patients with one of these six clinicopathologic features have a 30% to 50% rate of subsequent regional recurrence after nodal dissection alone (Table 39-6).

There are substantial retrospective data supporting the effectiveness of regional irradiation for patients with one of the aforementioned high-risk features. Recurrence rates after adjuvant irradiation range from 5% to 20%, compared with the much higher range seen without adjuvant irradiation (compare Tables 39-6 and 39-7).[80,83-92]

Tolerance to adjuvant radiation therapy is generally excellent. Most patients receiving comprehensive neck irradiation experience transient parotid swelling after the first radiation fraction that typically lasts 1 day. For most sites, brisk erythema with patches of moist skin desquamation, particularly within the axilla and the groin, are common. Late radiation-related complications are distinctly uncommon, except for thinning of the subcutaneous fat with mild or moderate fibrosis. Clinically significant extremity lymphedema (requiring some form of medical management such as a compressive

Table 39-6 Regional Recurrence Rates after Surgery Alone for Nodal Disease According to High-Risk Pathologic Characteristics

Nodal Characteristic	Study (Year)	Recurrence Rate (%)
Extracapsular extension	Calabro et al[77] (1989)	28*
	Lee et al[78] (2000)	63*
	Monsour et al[79] (1993)	54
	Shen et al[80] (2000)	31*
≥4 involved lymph nodes	Calabro et al[77] (1989)	17 to 33*
	Lee et al[78] (2000)	46 to 63
	Miller et al[81] (1992)	53*
Lymph node ≥ 3 cm	Lee et al[78] (2000)	42 to 80
	Shen et al[80] (2000)	14
Cervical lymph node location	Bowsher et al[82] (1986)	33
	Lee et al[78] (2000)	43*
	Monsour et al[79] (1993)	50
Therapeutic dissection	Byers[54] (1986)	50
	O'Brien et al[56] (1991)	34
	Lee et al[78] (2000)	36
	Shen et al[80] (2000)	20

*Significant on multivariate analysis.

Table 39-7 Regional Recurrence Rates after Surgery and Radiotherapy for Regionally Advanced Nodal Disease

Study (Year)	Rate (%)	Indication for Adjuvant Radiation Therapy
Burmeister et al[83] (1995)	12	ECE
O'Brien et al[84] (1997)	18	ECE, number of LN
Corry et al[85] (1999)	20	ECE, number of LN, recurrent disease
Fenig et al[86] (1999)	16	ECE, number of LN
Shen et al[80] (2000)	14	ECE, recurrent disease
Morris et al[87] (2000)	5	"Bulky" LN disease
Cooper et al[88] (2001)	16	ECE, positive margins, recurrent disease
Fuhrmann et al[89] (2001)	15	ECE, number of LN
Ballo et al[90] (2002)	6	ECE, number of LN, large LN size, recurrent disease
Ballo et al[91] (2003)	13	ECE, number of LN, large LN size, recurrent disease
Ballo et al[92] (2004)	5*	ECE, number of LN, large LN size, recurrent disease

*In-basin nodal recurrence.
ECE, extracapsular extension; LN, lymph nodes.

sleeve or physical therapy) occurs in a minority of patients, but it can be problematic. It is more common after groin dissection than after cervical or axillary dissection, and it appears to moderately increase further in the setting of adjuvant irradiation, particularly for patients with locally advanced groin metastases (Table 39-8).[82,90-97] In one series examining the timing of lymphedema, however, one half of the patients had developed lymphedema before starting adjuvant groin irradiation.[92] This suggested that the higher rate of lymphedema was to some extent a consequence of locally advanced disease and its surgical treatment and not due solely to the irradiation. In this same series, there was a correlation between body mass index (BMI) and the development of chronic lymphedema, suggesting that patient factors need to be incorporated into rational treatment guidelines.[92]

Distant Disease and Adjuvant Systemic Therapy

A great amount of resources has been directed toward developing effective systemic therapy for patients with melanoma. Although surgical resection with selective use of adjuvant irradiation results in satisfactory local and regional control for most patients, even thin melanomas have significant metastatic potential. Most research initiatives have focused on interferon alfa-2b (IFN), vaccines, or combinations of both. European investigators have examined the role of low-dose IFN therapy, and U.S. investigators have focused primarily on high-dose regimens. Three randomized Eastern Cooperative Oncology Group (ECOG) trials support the use of adjuvant IFN for patients with T4 primary disease and those with nodal metastases from melanoma.[98-100]

The first trial (ECOG 1684) enrolled 287 patients with primary melanomas thicker than 4 mm without palpable nodes, lymph node metastasis detected at elective lymph node dissection, clinically palpable regional lymph node with primary melanoma of any stage, or regional lymph node recurrence at any interval after appropriate surgery for primary melanoma of any depth.[98] This prospective study revealed a significant prolongation of relapse-free survival (5-year actuarial rate, 37% versus 26%; $P = .002$) and overall survival (5-year actuarial rate, 46% versus 37%; $P = .02$) associated with high-dose IFN therapy (i.e., intravenous administration five times per week for 4 weeks, then subcutaneous administration three times per week for 48 weeks). The overall benefit

Table 39-8 **Clinically Significant Lymphedema According to Site of Regional Disease and Treatment**

Nodal Basin	Surgery Alone* Study (Year)	Rate (%)	Surgery and Radiation* Study (Year)	Rate (%)
Cervical	Urist et al[93] (1983)	0	Ballo et al[90] (2002)	0
	Wrightson et al[94] (2003)	0	Burmeister et al[97] (2002)	0
Axilla	Urist et al[93] (1983)	1	Ballo et al[91] (2003)	16
	Wrightson et al[94] (2003)	5	Burmeister et al[97] (2002)	7
	Bowsher et al[82] (1986)	3		
Groin	Bowsher et al[82] (1986)	18	Burmeister et al[97] (2002)	45
	Karakousis et al[95] (1994)	10	Ballo et al[92] (2004)	27
	Hughes et al[96] (2000)	19		
	Wrightson et al[94] (2003)	32		

*Clinically significant lymphedema required some form of medical management (e.g., compressive device or physical therapy).

of treatment in this trial was correlated with the tumor burden and the presence of microscopic nonpalpable and palpable regional lymph node metastases. The benefit of therapy with IFN was greatest among recipients with palpable regional nodal metastases or nodal recurrences.

The second trial (ECOG 1690) compared high-dose IFN for 1 year or low-dose IFN for 2 years versus observation.[99] Intention-to-treat analysis revealed 5-year relapse-free survival rates of 44% and 40% for the high-dose and low-dose IFN arms, respectively, compared with 35% in the observation arm ($P = .05$ for high-dose IFN versus observation and $P = .17$ for low-dose IFN versus observation). Most of the benefit was observed for patients with two to three involved lymph nodes. For overall survival, there was no difference demonstrated for the three treatment arms (52%, 53%, and 55% for high-dose IFN, low-dose IFN, and observation, respectively).

The third trial (ECOG 1694) compared high-dose IFN with a ganglioside GM_2 melanoma vaccine.[100] After 880 patients were randomized to one of the treatment arms, an interim analysis indicated inferiority of the ganglioside vaccine with respect to relapse-free survival and overall survival. In subgroup analysis, however, the beneficial effects of IFN were seen only in the patients with T4N0 disease and not those with nodal disease.

Debate over the merits of routine IFN therapy has focused on the inconsistent subgroup analysis findings and concerns about the toxicity of IFN.[101] In ECOG 1684 and 1690, node-positive patients benefited most from adjuvant IFN, whereas only the node-negative patients benefited in ECOG 1694. Advocates of IFN argue that the subgroups analyzed in the individual trials were too small to detect real differences in survival and that the relative benefits of interferon are consistent across all subgroups of patients. IFN toxicity was evaluated using a quality of life–adjusted survival analysis.[102] This determined that although the high-dose IFN group was essentially trading 8.9 months of time without disease recurrence for 5.8 months of severe IFN-related toxicity, the time without disease recurrence was valued more than the time with toxicity.

Frequently observed regression of primary melanoma and even occasionally metastatic disease has suggested an important role for the immune system. This has fueled a longstanding search for active vaccine therapies against melanoma.[103] A large, retrospective study from John Wayne Cancer Center compared 935 patients with nodal metastases who received a polyvalent melanoma vaccine (Canvaxin, CancerVax Corp., Carlsbad, CA) with 1667 patients with similar disease who were observed or treated with chemotherapy, bacille Calmette-Guérin (BCG) vaccine, or some other vaccine formulation.[104] After controlling for the impact of known prognostic factors and date of treatment, the polyvalent melanoma vaccine was found to be associated with higher 5-year overall survival. Confirmation of this finding awaits results of a randomized trial comparing the polyvalent vaccine plus BCG with placebo plus BCG.

LOCALLY ADVANCED DISEASE AND PALLIATION

Irradiation can reduce symptoms for more than 80% of patients with advanced inoperable or metastatic disease. The recommended dose-fractionation schedule depends on the tumor's location and the patient's life expectancy. The most frequently used regimens are 30 Gy given in 10 fractions over 2 weeks for skeletal or multiple cerebral metastasis, 36 Gy in 12 fractions for pathologic fracture of extremity bones (after internal fixation), 50 Gy in 25 fractions for solitary metastases after resection or radiosurgery (brain), and 36 Gy in 6 fractions over 3 weeks (twice each week) for dermal or subcutaneous melanoma masses or for neck node metastasis. Conventional fractionation schedules may always be considered if tumor lies near critical structures.

TECHNIQUES OF IRRADIATION

Target Volume

Adjuvant irradiation for primary melanoma should encompass the primary site scar with a 3- to 4-cm margin, depending on the anatomic site and surrounding critical structures.

The target volume for patients receiving elective nodal irradiation for head and neck primary sites includes the primary lesion, preauricular and postauricular lymph nodes (for high facial and scalp primaries), and the ipsilateral levels I through V lymph nodes, including the ipsilateral supraclavicular fossa (Fig. 39-3). For patients receiving therapeutic nodal irradiation for one of the aforementioned high-risk nodal features, the target volume is essentially the same, except that the primary tumor bed is irradiated only if regional relapse occurred less than 1 year after excision of the primary disease.

For axillary nodal metastases, radiation fields include the axillary levels I through III lymph nodes (Fig. 39-4). The supraclavicular fossa and low cervical lymph nodes may be included if there is bulky high axillary disease.

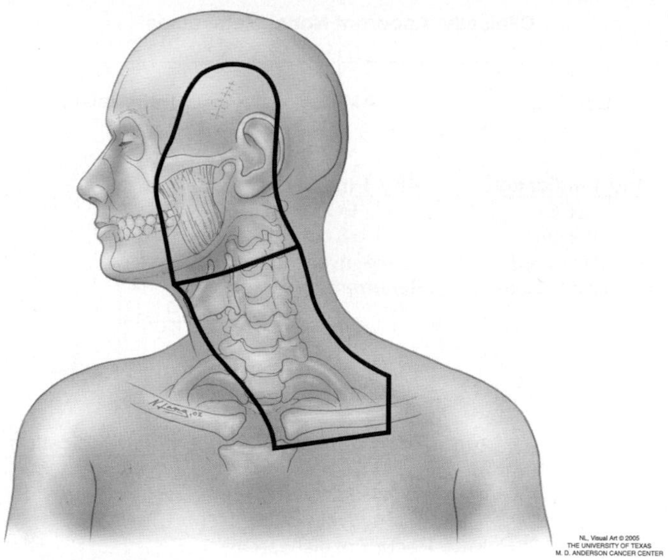

Figure 39-3 Typical external beam radiation treatment field for a patient with cervical lymph node metastases. A similar field is used for a patient requiring elective irradiation. (Courtesy of NL Visual Art © 2005, The University of Texas M.D. Anderson Cancer Center, Houston, Texas.)

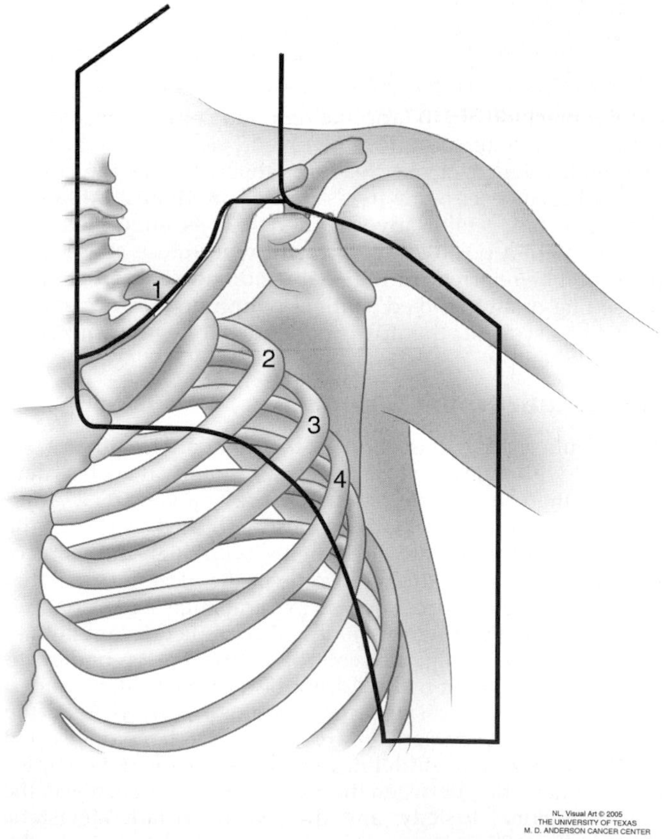

Figure 39-4 Typical external beam radiation treatment field for a patient with axillary lymph node metastases. Numbers correspond to the ribs. The upper border of the field typically ends at the superior aspect of the clavicle, but the cervical lymph nodes may be irradiated if clinically involved or if level III axillary lymph nodes are involved. (Courtesy of NL Visual Art © 2005, The University of Texas M.D. Anderson Cancer Center, Houston, Texas.)

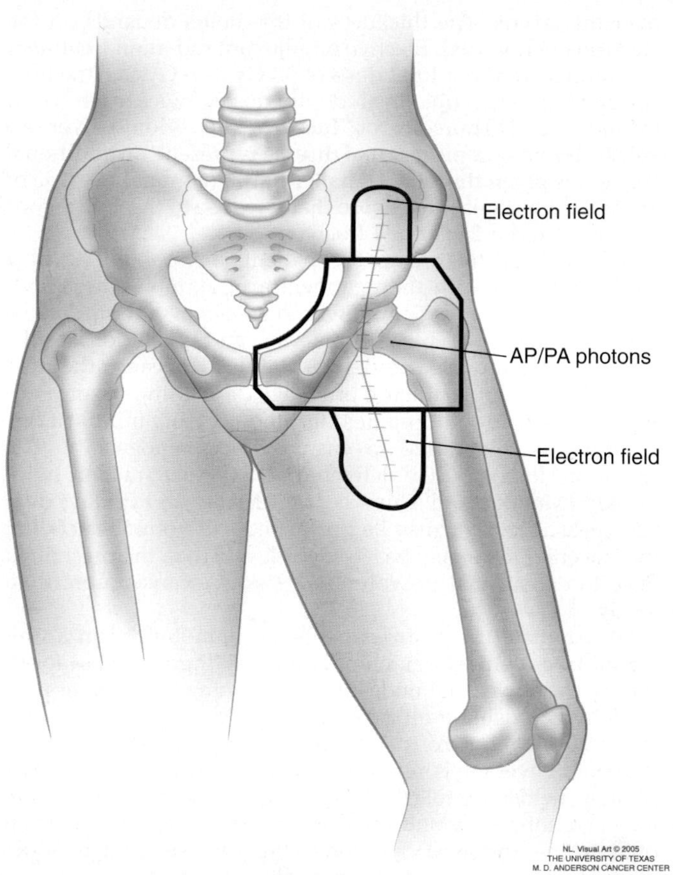

Figure 39-5 Typical external beam radiation field for a patient with groin lymph node metastases. (Courtesy of NL Visual Art © 2005, The University of Texas M.D. Anderson Cancer Center, Houston, Texas.)

At a minimum, fields for groin lymph node metastases cover the nodal regions that have pathologically confirmed nodal disease and always include the entire surgical scar (Fig. 39-5). Judgment must be used regarding elective irradiation of adjacent nodal regions (i.e., external iliac coverage in the setting of confirmed inguinal disease) because of concern about the increased toxicity associated with groin irradiation, particularly for obese patients. Unlike the cervical or axillary regions, where electrons and flashing photon fields, respectively, generally deliver a full dose to the skin, special attention must be paid to delivering a full dose to the groin scar.

Setup, Field Arrangement, and Dose-Fractionation Schedule

For patients with cervical disease, an open neck position provides access to the primary site and parotid and cervical lymphatics, and it allows treatment delivery with electrons of appropriate energy. Lesions of frontal, temporal, and preauricular areas; the auricle; and the cheek are usually treated with two or three fields, depending on the distance between the primary and parotid nodes. A 6- to 9-MeV electron field superiorly can cover the primary site, and an adjoining 9-MeV electron field is used to irradiate the parotid and lower neck nodes. The junctions between the fields are moved (0.5 to 1.0 cm) after the second and fourth treatment to improve dose homogeneity. A tissue-equivalent bolus is placed over a line connecting the lateral canthus and the mastoid tip to spare the temporal lobe, and an additional piece of bolus may be placed over the larynx. The thickness of this bolus depends on the electron energy used. Elective or adjuvant radiation treatment is administered to a total dose of 30 Gy at 6 Gy per fraction, specified at D_{max} (maximal depth dose), twice each week (Monday and Thursday or Tuesday and Friday) over 2.5 weeks. If microscopic residual disease is present, an additional fraction is given through a smaller portal (cumulative dose of 36 Gy). Care is taken to ensure that the dose to the spinal cord does not exceed 24 Gy in 4 fractions.

For axillary treatment, the patient is immobilized in a supine position with the treatment arm akimbo. Laser lines that include the upper and lower torso ensure a reproducible treatment setup. Typically, anterior and posterior 18-MV photon fields are used to deliver the dose. Because the field size often precludes the use of wedges, a missing-tissue compensator or field-within-a-field technique (using multileaf collimators) is imperative to ensure dose homogeneity. The radiation dose is 30 Gy delivered at 6 Gy per fraction twice weekly (Monday and Thursday or Tuesday and Friday) over 2.5 weeks. The dose may be prescribed to a volume such that the isocenter dose may be 3% to 6% lower than the prescribed dose to ensure that no volume of tissue receives more than 33 Gy.

To irradiate the groin, patients are immobilized in a unilateral frog-leg position, eliminating any inguinal skin folds. If only the superficial nodes require coverage, treatment may be delivered using a mixed-beam technique (4 fractions with 16- or 20-MeV electrons and 1 fraction with 18-MV photons). If deeper coverage is required, anterior and posterior 18-MV photon fields are used. Lower-energy electron fields are matched superiorly and inferiorly to cover the full extension of the scar. If the 18-MV photon technique is selected, a tissue-equivalent bolus is used over the scar, and the dose is weighted anteriorly. A dose of 30 Gy is delivered at 6 Gy per fraction, twice each week (Monday and Thursday or Tuesday and Friday) over 2.5 weeks. Appropriate reductions are made to limit the small-bowel dose to 24 Gy.

Patient Care during and after Radiation Therapy

Patients are informed of the specific acute side effects of treatment, such as mucositis and parotiditis after irradiation of the cervical basin and moist desquamation after irradiation of the axilla or groin. After moist desquamation occurs, cleaning the area with 1% hydrogen peroxide to prevent secondary infection is recommended.

Regular follow-up examinations include evaluation of the treated area for late complications and a search for potential recurrence. The most common late side effects include hypopigmentation, hyperpigmentation, telangiectasia, and skin and subcutaneous tissue atrophy. After cervical irradiation, monitoring for subclinical hypothyroidism and the signs and symptoms of hearing loss, although relatively uncommon, is essential. Acute lymphedema is managed early and aggressively with physical therapy and compressive devices to avoid chronic lymphedema.

TREATMENT ALGORITHMS AND CLINICAL TRIALS

Elective Nodal Treatment

SLNB has obviated routine elective treatment of the draining lymphatics of patients with thick primary melanomas. Although retrospective studies of elective irradiation have verified the effectiveness of this approach, SLNB with complete lymph node dissection has become accepted as the standard of care. However, for patients whose medical comorbidities preclude SLNB (and the required comprehensive dissection if the sentinel node is involved), elective nodal irradiation is favored over observation, which reduces the risk of regional recurrence with its associated morbidity. Although this approach is still investigational, it is suggested that patients with a positive SLNB result who refuse subsequent dissection be referred for regional irradiation. Observation in the setting of an involved sentinel lymph node is not appropriate, and systemic therapy is not a substitute for completing regional therapy.

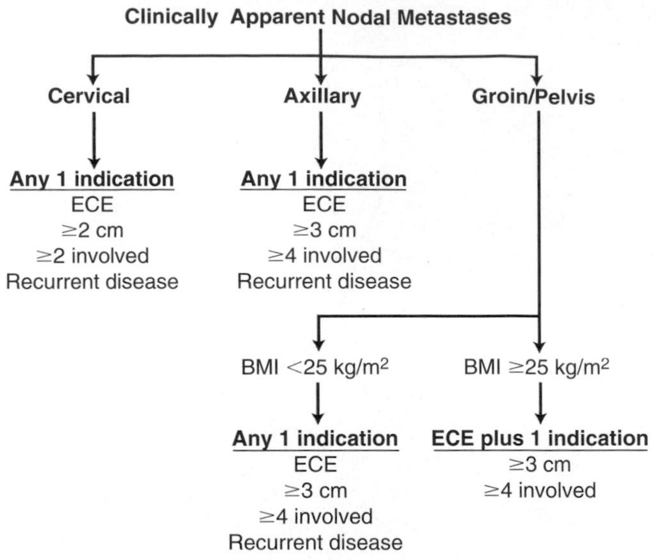

Figure 39-6 The M.D. Anderson treatment algorithm for patients with nodal metastases from melanoma. Typically, the threshold for irradiating patients with cervical lymph node metastases is lower than for those with inguinal lymph node metastases, for which the risk of long-term lymphedema is higher. BMI, body mass index; ECE, extracapsular extension.

Therapeutic Nodal Approaches

Therapeutic nodal dissection is the standard treatment for patients with lymph node metastases, and available data support the use of systemic, high-dose adjuvant IFN. Adjuvant postoperative irradiation is also indicated to reduce the regional recurrence rate in patients with high-risk clinicopathologic features. Although some of the same features that predict regional failure, such as extracapsular extension and number of involved lymph nodes, also predict distant failure, the importance of regional control should not be underestimated, and irradiation should not be systematically avoided because the risk of distant metastasis is perceived to be too high. At M.D. Anderson Cancer Center, we have developed radiation treatment guidelines that account for the complex clinical interaction between the risk of regional recurrence, the risk of regional toxicity, and the risk of distant metastatic disease (Fig. 39-6). For patients with cervical disease, the threshold for irradiation may be lowered to include those with at least two involved lymph nodes or those with tumors measuring at least 2 cm in diameter. For patients with groin metastases, the threshold may be raised so that combinations (two or more) of the high-risk features must be present before adjuvant irradiation is given.

REFERENCES

1. Sause WT, Cooper JS, Rush S, et al: Fraction size in external beam radiation therapy in the treatment of melanoma. Int J Radiat Oncol Biol Phys 12:1839-1842, 1986.
2. Ballo MT, Ang KK: Radiation therapy for malignant melanoma. Surg Clin N Am 83:323-342, 2003.
3. Jemal A, Siegal R, Ward E, et al: Cancer statistics, 2006. CA Cancer J Clin 56:106-130, 2006.
4. Beral V, Evans S, Shaw H, et al: Cutaneous factors related to the risk of malignant melanoma. Br J Dermatol 109:165-172, 1983.
5. Gellin GA, Kopf AW, Garfinkel L: Malignant melanoma. A controlled study of possibly associated factors. Arch Dermatol 99:43-48, 1969.
6. English DR, Armstrong BK, Kricker A, et al: Sunlight and cancer. Cancer Causes Control 8:271-283, 1997.
7. Tucker MA, Goldstein AM: Melanoma etiology: where are we? Oncogene 22:3042-3052, 2003.
8. Hussussian CJ, Struewing JP, Goldstein AM, et al: Germline p16 mutations in familial melanoma. Nat Genet 8:15-21, 1994.
9. Aitken J, Welch J, Duffy D, et al: CDKN2A variants in a population-based sample of Queensland families with melanoma. J Natl Cancer Inst 3:446-452, 1999.
10. Bishop DT, Demanais F, Goldstein AM, et al: Geographical variation in the penetrance of CDKN2A mutation in melanoma. J Natl Cancer Inst 94:894-903, 2002.
11. Bliss JM, Ford D, Swerdlow AJ, et al: Risk of cutaneous melanoma associated with pigmentation characteristics and freckling: systematic overview of 10 case controlled studies. The International Melanoma Analysis Group (IMAGE). Int J Cancer 62:367-376, 1995.
12. Hill L, Ferrini RL: Skin cancer prevention and screening: Summary of the American College of Preventive Medicine's practice policy statements. CA Cancer J Clin 48:232-235, 1998.
13. Gruber SB, Barnhill RL, Stenn KS, et al: Nevomelanocytic proliferations in association with cutaneous melanoma: a multivariate analysis. J Am Acad Dermatol 21:773-780, 1989.
14. Clark WH, Ainsworth AM, Bernardino EA: The developmental biology of primary human malignant melanomas. Semin Oncol 2:83-103, 1975.
15. McGovern VJ, Murad TM: Pathology of melanoma: an overview. *In* Balch CM, Milton GW (eds): Cutaneous Melanoma: Clinical Management and Treatment Results Worldwide. Philadelphia, JB Lippincott, 1985, pp 29-53.
16. Barnhill RL, Mihm MC: Histopathology of malignant melanoma and its precursor lesions. *In* Balch CM, Houghton AN, Milton GW, et al (eds): Cutaneous Melanoma. Philadelphia, JB Lippincott, 1992, pp 234-263.
17. Urist MM, Balch CM, Soong SJ: Head and neck melanoma in 534 clinical stage I patients: a prognostic factor analysis and results of surgical treatment. Ann Surg 200:769-775, 1984.
18. Clark WH, Mihm MC: Lentigo maligna and lentigo-maligna melanoma. Am J Pathol 55:39-67, 1969.
19. Reed RJ: The pathology of human cutaneous melanoma. *In* Malignant Melanoma I. The Hague, Martinus Nijhoff, 1983, pp 85-116.
20. Arrington JH, Reed RJ, Ichinose H, et al: Plantar lentiginous melanoma: a distinctive variant of human cutaneous malignant melanoma. Am J Surg Pathol 1:131-143, 1977.
21. Coleman WP, Loria PR, Reed RJ, et al: Acral lentiginous melanoma. Arch Dermatol 116:773-776, 1980.
22. Krementz ET, Feed RJ, Coleman WP, et al: Acral lentiginous melanoma. A clinicopathologic entity. Ann Surg 195:632-645, 1982.
23. Seiji M, Takahashi M: Acral melanoma in Japan. Hum Pathol 13:607-609, 1982.
24. Reintgen DS, McCarty KM, Cox E, et al: Malignant melanoma in black American and white American populations: a comparative review. JAMA 248:1856-1859, 1982.
25. Breslow A: Thickness, cross-sectional areas and depth of invasion in the prognosis of cutaneous melanoma. Ann Surg 172:902-908, 1970.
26. Balch CM, Soong S, Gershenwald JE, et al: Prognostic factors analysis of 17,600 melanoma patients: validation of the American Joint Committee on Cancer melanoma staging system. J Clin Oncol 19:3622-3634, 2001.
27. Balch CM, Buzaid AC, Soong S, et al: Final version of the American Joint Committee on Cancer staging system for cutaneous melanoma. J Clin Oncol 19:3635-3648, 2001.
28. Buzaid AC, Tinoco L, Ross MI, et al: Role of computed tomography in the staging of patients with local-regional metastases of melanoma. J Clin Oncol 13:2104-2108, 1995.
29. Veronesi U, Cascinelli N, Adamus J, et al: Thin stage I primary cutaneous malignant melanoma. Comparison of excision with margins of 1 or 3 cm [Erratum: N Engl J Med 325:292, 1991]. N Engl J Med 318:1159-1162.
30. Cohn-Cedermark G, Rutqvist LE, Andersson R, et al: Long term results of a randomized study by the Swedish Melanoma Study Group on 2-cm versus 5-cm resection margins for patients with cutaneous melanoma with a tumor thickness of 0.8-2.0 mm. Cancer 89:1495-1501, 2000.
31. Balch CM, Soong S, Smith T, et al: Long-term results of a prospective surgical trial comparing 2 cm versus 4 cm excision margins for 740 patients with 1-4 mm melanomas. Ann Surg Oncol 8:101-108, 2001.
32. Khayat D, Rixe O, Martin G, et al: Surgical margins in cutaneous melanoma (2 cm versus 5 cm) for lesions measuring less than 2.1-mm thick. Long-term results of a large European multicentric phase III study. Cancer 97:1941-1946, 2003.
33. Thomas JM, Newton-Bishop J, A'Hern R, et al: Excision margins in high-risk malignant melanoma. N Engl J Med 350:757-766, 2004.
34. Heaton KM, Sussman JJ, Gershenwald JE, et al: Surgical margins and prognostic factors in patients with thick (>4 mm) primary melanoma. Ann Surg Oncol 5:322-328, 1998.
35. Krag DN, Meijer SJ, Weaver DL, et al: Minimal-access surgery for staging of malignant melanoma. Arch Surg 130:654-658, 1995.
36. Joseph E, Brobeil A, Glass F, et al: Results of complete lymph node dissection in 83 melanoma patients with positive sentinel nodes. Ann Surg Oncol 5:119-125, 1998.
37. Mraz-Gernhard S, Sagebiel RW, Kashani-Sabet M, et al: Prediction of sentinel lymph node micrometastasis by histological features in primary cutaneous malignant melanoma. Arch Dermatol. 134:983-987, 1998.
38. Haddad FF, Stall A, Messina J, et al: The progression of melanoma nodal metastasis is dependent on tumor thickness of the primary lesion. Ann Surg Oncol 6:144-149, 1999.
39. Gershenwald JE, Thompson W, Mansfield PF, et al: Multi-institutional melanoma lymphatic mapping experience: the prognostic value of sentinel lymph node status in 612 stage I and II melanoma patients. J Clin Oncol 17:976-983, 1999.
40. Statius Muller MG, Borgstein PJ, Pijpers R, et al: Reliability of the sentinel node procedure in melanoma patients: analysis of failures after long-term follow-up. Ann Surg Oncol 7:461-468, 2000.
41. Bachter D, Michl C, Büchels H, et al: The predictive value of the sentinel lymph node in malignant melanomas. Recent Results Cancer Res 58:129-136, 2001.
42. Blumenthal R, Banic A, Brand CU, et al: Morbidity and outcome after sentinel lymph node dissection in patients with early-stage malignant cutaneous melanoma. Swiss Surg 8:209-214, 2002.
43. Caprio MG, Carbone G, Bracigliano A, et al: Sentinel lymph node detection by lymphoscintigraphy in malignant melanoma. Tumori 88:S43-S45, 2002.
44. Vuylsteke RJ, van Leeuwen PA, Statius Muller MG, et al: Clinical outcome of stage I/II melanoma patients after selective sentinel lymph node dissection: long-term follow up results. J Clin Oncol 21:1057-1065, 2003.
45. McMasters KM, Wong SL, Edwards MJ, et al: Factors that predict the presence of sentinel lymph node metastasis in patients with melanoma. Surgery 130:151-156, 2001.
46. Rousseau DL, Ross MI, Johnson MM, et al: Revised American Joint Committee on Cancer staging criteria accurately predict sentinel lymph node positivity in clinically node-negative melanoma patients. Ann Surg Oncol 10:569-574, 2003.
47. Harwood AR: Conventional fractionated radiotherapy for 51 patients with lentigo maligna and lentigo maligna melanoma. Int J Radiat Oncol Biol Phys 9:1019-1021, 1983.

48. Urist MM, Balch CM, Soong S, et al: The influence of surgical margins and prognostic factors predicting the risk of local recurrence in 3445 patients with primary cutaneous melanoma. Cancer 55:1398-1402, 1985.
49. Ames FC, Balch CM, Reintgen D: Local recurrence and their management. *In* Balch CM, Houghton AN, Milton GW, et al (eds): Cutaneous Melanoma. Philadelphia, JB Lippincott, 1992, pp 287-294.
50. Roses DF, Harris MN, Rigel D, et al: Local and in-transit metastases following definitive excision for primary cutaneous malignant melanoma. Ann Surg 198:65-69, 1983.
51. Karakousis CP, Balch CM, Urist MM, et al: Local recurrence in malignant melanoma: long-term results of the multiinstitutional randomized surgical trial. Ann Surg Oncol 3:446-452, 1996.
52. Ng AK, Jones WO, Shaw JH: Analysis of local recurrence and optimizing excision margins for cutaneous melanoma. Br J Surg 88:137-142, 2001.
53. Neades GT, Orr DJ, Hughes LE, et al: Safe margins in the excision of primary cutaneous melanoma. Br J Surg 80:731-733, 1993.
54. Byers RM: The role of modified neck dissection in the treatment of cutaneous melanoma of the head and neck. Arch Surg 121:1338-1341, 1986.
55. Loree TR, Spiro RH: Cutaneous melanoma of the head and neck. Am J Surg 158:388-391, 1989.
56. O'Brien CJ, Coates AS, Petersen-Schaefer K, et al: Experience with 998 cutaneous melanomas of the head and neck over 30 years. Am J Surg 162:310-314, 1991.
57. Fisher SR, O'Brien CJ: Head and neck melanoma. *In* Balch CM, Houghton AN, Sober AJ, Soong S (eds): Cutaneous Melanoma. St Louis, Quality Medical Publishing, 1998, pp 163-174.
58. Kelly JW, Sagebiel RW, Calderon W, et al: The frequency of local recurrence and microsatellites as a guide to reexcision margins for cutaneous malignant melanoma. Ann Surg 200:759-763, 1984.
59. Leon P, Daly JM, Synnestvedt M, et al: The prognostic implications of microscopic satellites in patients with clinical stage I melanoma. Arch Surg 126:1461-1468, 1991.
60. Egbert B, Kempson R, Sagebiel R: Desmoplastic malignant melanoma: a clinicohistopathologic study of 25 cases. Cancer 62:2033-2041, 1988.
61. Beenken S, Byers R, Smith JL, et al: Desmoplastic melanoma. Arch Otolaryngol Head Neck Surg 115:374-379, 1989.
62. Smithers BM, McLeod GR, Little JH: Desmoplastic melanoma: patterns of recurrence. World J Surg 16:186-190, 1992.
63. Calson JA, Dickersin GR, Sober AJ, et al: Desmoplastic neurotropic melanoma: a clinicopathologic analysis of 28 cases. Cancer 75:478-494, 1995.
64. Quinn MJ, Crotty KA, Thompson JF, et al: Desmoplastic and desmoplastic neurotropic melanoma: experience with 280 patients. Cancer 83:1128-1135, 1998.
65. Payne WG, Kearney R, Wells K, et al: Desmoplastic melanoma. Am Surg 67:1004-1006, 2001.
66. Vongtama R, Safa A, Gallardo D, et al: Efficacy of radiation therapy in the local control of desmoplastic malignant melanoma. Head Neck 25:423-428, 2003.
67. Jaroszewski DE, Pockaj BA, DiCaudo DJ, et al: The clinical behavior of desmoplastic melanoma. Am J Surg 182:590-595, 2001.
68. Milton GW, Shaw HM, McCarthy WH, et al: Prophylactic lymph node dissection in clinical stage I cutaneous malignant melanoma: results of surgical treatment in 1319 patients. Br J Surg 69:108-111, 1982.
69. Veronesi U, Adamus J, Bandiera DC, et al: Delayed regional lymph node dissection in stage I melanoma of the skin of the lower extremities. Cancer 49:2420-2430, 1982.
70. Sim FH, Taylor WF, Pritchard DJ, et al: Lymphadenectomy in the management of stage I malignant melanoma: a prospective randomized study. Mayo Clin Proc 61:697-705, 1986.
71. Balch CM, Soong S, Ross MI, et al: Long-term results of a multi-institutional randomized trial comparing prognostic factors and surgical results for intermediate thickness melanomas (1.0-4.0 mm). Ann Surg Oncol 7:87-97, 2000.
72. Cascinelli N, Morabito A, Santinami M, et al: Immediate or delayed dissection of regional nodes in patients with melanoma of the trunk: a randomised trial. Lancet 351:793-796, 1998.
73. Doubrovsky A, de Wilt JH, Scolyer RA, et al: Sentinel node biopsy provides more accurate staging than elective lymph node dissection in patients with cutaneous melanoma. Ann Surg Oncol 11:829-836, 2004.
74. McMasters KM: What good is sentinel lymph node biopsy for melanoma if it does not improve survival? Ann Surg Oncol 11:810-812, 2004.
75. Ang KK, Peters LJ, Weber RS, et al: Postoperative radiotherapy for cutaneous melanoma of the head and neck region. Int J Radiat Oncol Biol Phys 30:795-798, 1994.
76. Bonnen MD, Ballo MT, Myers JN, et al: Elective radiotherapy provides regional control for patients with cutaneous melanoma of the head and neck. Cancer 100:383-389, 2003.
77. Calabro A, Singletary SE, Balch CM: Patterns of relapse in 1001 consecutive patients with melanoma nodal metastases. Arch Surg 124:1051-1055, 1989.
78. Lee RJ, Gibbs JF, Proulx GM, et al: Nodal basin recurrence following lymph node dissection for melanoma: implications for adjuvant radiotherapy. Int J Radiat Oncol Biol Phys 46:467-474, 2000.
79. Monsour PD, Sause WT, Avent JM, et al: Local control following therapeutic nodal dissection for melanoma. J Surg Oncol 54:18-22, 1993.
80. Shen P, Wanek LA, Morton DL: Is adjuvant radiotherapy necessary after positive lymph node dissection in head and neck melanomas? Ann Surg Oncol 7:554-559, 2000.
81. Miller EJ, Synnestvedt M, Schultz D, et al: Loco-regional nodal relapse in melanoma. Surg Oncol 1:333-340, 1992.
82. Bowsher WG, Taylor BA, Hughes LE: Morbidity, mortality and local recurrence following regional node dissection for melanoma. Br J Surg 73:906-908, 1986.
83. Burmeister BH, Smithers BM, Poulsen M, et al: Radiation therapy for nodal disease in malignant melanoma. World J Surg 19:369-371, 1995.
84. O'Brien CJ, Petersen-Schaefer K, Stevens GN, et al: Adjuvant radiotherapy following neck dissection and parotidectomy for metastatic malignant melanoma. Head Neck 19:589-594, 1997.
85. Corry J, Smith JG, Bishop M, et al: Nodal radiation therapy for metastatic melanoma. Int J Radiat Oncol Biol Phys 44:1065-1069, 1999.
86. Fenig E, Eidelevich E, Njuguna E, et al: Role of radiation therapy in the management of cutaneous malignant melanoma. Am J Clin Oncol 22:184-186, 1999.
87. Morris KT, Marquez CM, Holland JM, et al: Prevention of local recurrence after surgical debulking of nodal and subcutaneous melanoma deposits by hypofractionated radiation. Ann Surg Oncol 7:680-684, 2000.
88. Cooper JS, Chang WS, Oratz R, et al: Elective radiation therapy for high-risk malignant melanoma. Cancer J 7:498-502, 2001.
89. Fuhrmann D, Lippold A, Borrosch F, et al: Should adjuvant radiotherapy be recommended following resection of regional lymph node metastases of malignant melanomas? Br J Dermatol 144:66-70, 2001.
90. Ballo MT, Strom EA, Zagars GK, et al: Adjuvant irradiation for axillary metastases from malignant melanoma. Int J Radiat Oncol Biol Phys 52:964-972, 2002.
91. Ballo MT, Bonnen MD, Garden AS, et al: Adjuvant irradiation for cervical lymph node metastases from melanoma. Cancer 97:1789-1796, 2003.
92. Ballo MT, Zagars GK, Gershenwald JE, et al: A critical assessment of adjuvant radiotherapy for inguinal lymph node metastases from melanoma. Ann Surg Oncol 11:1079-1084, 2004.
93. Urist MM, Maddox WA, Kennedy JE, et al: Patient risk factors and surgical morbidity after regional lymphadenectomy in 204 melanoma patients. Cancer 51:2152-2156, 1983.
94. Wrightson WR, Wong SL, Edwards MJ, et al: Complications associated with sentinel lymph node biopsy for melanoma. Ann Surg Oncol 10:676-680, 2003.
95. Karakousis CP, Driscoll DL, Rose B, et al: Groin dissection in malignant melanoma. Ann Surg Oncol 1:271-277, 1994.
96. Hughes TM, A'Hern RP, Thomas JM: Prognosis and surgical management of patients with palpable inguinal lymph node metastases from melanoma. Br J Surg 87:892-901, 2000.

97. Burmeister BH, Smithers BM, Davis S, et al: Radiation following nodal surgery for melanoma: an analysis of late toxicity. ANZ J Surg 72:344-348, 2002.
98. Kirkwood JM, Strawderman MH, Ernstoff MS, et al: Interferon-alfa-2b adjuvant therapy of high-risk resected cutaneous melanoma: the Eastern Cooperative Oncology Group Trial EST 1684. J Clin Oncol 14:7-17, 1996.
99. Kirkwood JM, Ibrahim JG, Sondak VK, et al: High- and low-dose interferon alpha-2b in high-risk melanoma: first analysis of intergroup trial E1690/s9111/c9190. J Clin Oncol 18:2444-2458, 2000.
100. Kirkwood JM, Ibrahim JG, Sosman JA, et al: High-dose interferon alpha-2b significantly prolongs relapse-free and overall survival compared with the GM2-KLH/QS-21 vaccine in patients with resected stage IIB-III melanoma: results of intergroup trial E1694/S9512/C509801. J Clin Oncol 19:2370-2380, 2001.
101. Sabel MS, Sondak VK: Pros and cons of adjuvant interferon in the treatment of melanoma. Oncologist 8:451-458, 2003.
102. Cole BF, Gelber RD, Kirkwood JM, et al: Quality-of-life-adjusted survival analysis of interferon alpha-2b adjuvant treatment of high-risk resected cutaneous melanoma: an Eastern Cooperative Oncology Group study. J Clin Oncol 14:2666-2673, 1996.
103. Perales M, Wolchok JD: Melanoma vaccines. Cancer Invest 20:1012-1026, 2002.
104. Morton DL, Hsueh EC, Essner R, et al: Prolonged survival of patients receiving active immunotherapy with canvaxin therapeutic polyvalent vaccine after complete resection of melanoma metastatic to regional lymph nodes. Ann Surg 236:438-449, 2002.

PART C

THORACIC NEOPLASMS

Overview

L. Chinsoo Cho and Hak Choy

Primary thoracic cancers include lung cancer, esophageal carcinomas, thymomas, mesotheliomas, carcinoids, lymphomas, and tracheal tumors. In this overview, we consider developments in the diagnosis and treatment of non–small cell lung cancer (NSCLC), small cell lung cancer (SCLC), esophageal cancer, thymic tumors, and mesothelioma. Detailed reviews of these thoracic neoplasms are provided in the following chapters.

EPIDEMIOLOGY

Lung Cancer

Lung cancer is the most common thoracic neoplasm. In the United States alone, approximately 173,770 people were diagnosed with lung cancer and 160,440 patients died of it in 2004.[1] The median age of patients who present with lung cancer is 70 years.[2] Lung cancer is broadly divided into SCLC and NSCLC types.

NSCLC accounts for approximately 80% to 85% of cases, and SCLC accounts for 15% to 20% of cases. Fewer than 50% of patients with NSCLC have resectable disease on initial presentation. Approximately 25% of patients present with locally advanced disease, and they are commonly managed with radiation therapy with or without chemotherapy. Patients who present with locally advanced disease often have involvement of the regional lymph nodes without evidence of distant metastases.[2] Approximately 30% of patients with SCLC have limited-stage disease on presentation.[3]

Tobacco remains the most important cause of lung cancer.[4] Approximately 4 million people around the world die annually of tobacco-related diseases. This number is predicted to rise to 8.4 million by 2020.[5] From 1995 to 1999, smoking was implicated in 440,000 annual deaths in the United States. In 85% to 90% of cases, the lung cancer can be directly linked to tobacco exposure. An additional 10% to 15% of patients may have a history of exposure to second-hand smoke.[6,7] The risk of death correlates with the number of cigarettes smoked daily. The relative risk of dying may be as high as 22 for those smoking at least 30 cigarettes each day compared with nonsmokers.[8]

Esophageal Cancer

In 2004, an estimated 14,250 Americans were diagnosed with esophageal cancer, and most eventually die of their disease.[1] Patients with esophageal cancers often present with advanced-stage disease. Approximately 50% of the patients present with locally advanced disease, and another 30% to 40% present with systemic metastases.[9]

Esophageal carcinomas are often divided into squamous cell carcinoma and adenocarcinoma. Squamous cell carcinoma is common in parts of Asia, where environmental and dietary factors are implicated. Although the incidence of squamous cell carcinoma has remained stable in the United States, the incidence of esophageal adenocarcinoma has increased dramatically over the past several decades, surpassing squamous cell carcinoma as the most common esophageal cancer in the United States.[10]

Exposure to alcohol is an important factor in the development of esophageal squamous cell carcinoma.[11,12] Additional risk may accrue from exposure to tobacco products.[13,14] Nutritional deficits, often in conjunction with low economic status, may contribute to the risk of developing squamous cell carcinoma of the esophagus.

The prognosis is poor for patients with esophageal adenocarcinoma, with overall 5-year survival rates of approximately 5% to 12%.[1] Although esophageal adenocarcinoma was uncommon in the past, it now accounts for more than one half of esophageal cancers in the United States. Barrett's metaplasia caused by gastroesophageal reflux appears to be the precursor lesion of esophageal adenocarcinoma.[15] The incidence of adenocarcinoma from Barrett's esophagus has increased more rapidly than any other cancer in the United States.[16] Barrett's esophagus can develop after chronic gastroesophageal reflux, in which the normal squamous epithelium of the esophagus undergoes metaplastic change to the columnar epithelium. In addition to gastroesophageal reflux, other factors that contribute to the development of esophageal adenocarcinoma include smoking and obesity.[17,18] Esophageal adenocarcinoma more commonly affects whites than blacks, and it is significantly more common in men than women.[16]

Thymic Neoplasm

Most of the thymic neoplasms arise in the epithelial cells of the thymus. Thymomas, thymic carcinomas, and thymic carcinoids represent common neoplasms found in the thymus.[19] The precise incidence of thymoma in the United States is unknown. The incidence of thymoma in the United States is estimated to be 0.13 to 0.15 per 100,000 people.[20] The median age of patients with thymomas is older than 50 years, and thymomas are diagnosed equally in men and women.[21,22] Thymic carcinomas may account for between 5% and 36% of all thymic neoplasms,[23-25] and they are usually more aggressive than thymomas.[26] Thymic neoplasm also occurs in the elderly, but with a male predominance. Thymic carcinoids account for less than 5% of anterior mediastinal neoplasms.[27,28] Thymic carcinoids are more aggressive compared with carcinoids found in other locations in the body. For example, patients with thymic carcinoids have a higher rate of regional lymph node metastases on presentation.[26]

Pulmonary Carcinoid

Typical carcinoid, atypical carcinoid, large-cell neuroendocrine cancer, and SCLC represent the neuroendocrine lung tumors.[29] Pulmonary or bronchial carcinoid tumors are often low-grade malignant neoplasms that arise from the basal layer of the bronchial epithelium.[30] They are rare, and the clinical behavior depends on the histology. The respiratory tract is the second most common site for carcinoids, after the gastrointestinal tract. They are often centrally located and confined to the main or lobar bronchi.[31] The incidence of bronchopulmonary carcinoids in the United States is estimated to be 0.6 per 100,000 people.[32] Carcinoid tumor of the lung accounts for approximately 1% to 2% of all lung malignancies, and it occurs equally in men and women.[33]

Mesothelioma

The incidence of mesothelioma cases in the United States is estimated to be 10 cases per million people,[34] or approximately 3000 patients per year, and the rate is expected to rise to approximately 4000 cases per year by 2025. Prognosis remains poor despite multimodality treatment . Approximately 90% of mesothelioma can be attributed to prior occupational asbestos exposure. It occurs predominantly in men. However, asbestos exposure from a spouse or parent asbestos worker can be as significant as environmental asbestos exposure.

BIOLOGY

Lung Cancer

Lung cancer treatment has been traditionally divided according to histology alone. However, there are molecular distinctions between SCLC and subtypes of NSCLC.[35,36]

Squamous cell lung cancers may develop after sequential events that include hyperplastic, metaplastic, and dysplastic changes in the respiratory mucosa. Adenocarcinoma of the lung may arise after adenomatous hyperplasia.

Mutations of *kras* were one of the first mutations to be described in adenocarcinomas of the lung.[37] The *kras* mutations in NSCLC were found to correlate with poor prognosis and survival.[38,39]

Expression of cyclooxygenase-2 (COX-2),[40] death-associated protein kinase (DAPK),[41] and interleukin-8 (IL-8) mRNA have been associated with poor prognosis. Other factors that correlated with poor survival include overexpression of macrophage migration inhibitory factor,[42] hypermethylation of insulin-like growth factor–binding protein-3 (IGFBP-3), and low expressions of IL-10.[43]

Mutations in selective genes can lead to a malignant phenotype. A common genetic abnormality in SCLC and NSCLC is the loss of 3p.[44] Deletions in the short arm of chromosome 3 and inactivation of the retinoblastoma gene *(RB1)* are seen more commonly in SCLC.[45,46] Loss of heterozygosity on chromosomes 5, 9, 13, and 17 can be seen, as well as mutations and allelic loss of *TP53* (formerly *P53* or *p53*) and *RB1* tumor suppressor genes. The presence of *RAS* mutations and overexpression of *ERBB2* (also designated *HER2*, formerly *HER2/neu*) are markers for a worse prognosis in adenocarcinoma.[47] Point mutations in the *RAS* family of oncogenes are rarely observed in SCLC. The overexpression of the *MYC* oncogenes may be a relatively late event in the pathogenesis of SCLC.[48]

Esophageal Squamous Cell Cancer

Epidermal growth factor (EGF) is overexpressed in esophageal squamous cell carcinoma,[49] and its overexpression has been associated with poor prognosis.[50] Transforming growth factor-α (TGF-α) is another growth factor, and its overexpression is associated with poor survival of patients with esophageal carcinoma.[51] TGF-α protein is overexpressed in approximately 35% of esophageal squamous cell carcinomas.[51] Unlike other gastrointestinal tumors, *RAS* is rarely mutated in esophageal adenocarcinoma or squamous cell carcinoma. The significance of *MYC* overexpression is inconclusive in both types of esophageal cancers.[52]

The *TP53* mutation appears to precede the development of esophageal squamous cell carcinoma. *TP53* mutations are seen in up to 85% of esophageal squamous cell carcinomas and are often found in abnormal cells adjacent to these cancers.[52] Loss of chromosomes 2, 3, 13q, or X and gain of chromosome 19 are more frequently seen in esophageal squamous cell carcinoma.[53]

Esophageal Adenocarcinoma

Cell cycle transitions are regulated by cyclins and cyclin-dependent kinases (CDKs). Cyclin D1 (CDK4) regulates transitions in G1 by phosphorylating the retinoblastoma gene (RB1) that activates S-phase transition genes. CDKN2A (previously designated p16) promotes cell cycle arrest by preventing the association of CDK4 and cyclin D1. Allelic loss of *CDKN2A* may be one of the early events in the development of esophageal adenocarcinoma. It precedes aneuploidy, and it is seen more often than the loss of TP53 in Barrett's metaplasia.[54]

Mutations in *TP53* may be found in up to 95% of patients with esophageal adenocarcinomas.[55] It is associated with the development of aneuploidy and may be a precursor of esophageal adenocarcinoma.[54] TP53 can also promote sequestration of CDKs.[56] Loss of heterozygosity (LOH) of chromosomal regions is seen with formation and progression of cancer. LOH of the *RB1* (13q14.2) gene locus is seen in a significant proportion of patients with adenocarcinomas and metaplasia.[55]

Amplification of 7q21-22 and 17q12-21 is more commonly seen in adenocarcinoma than in squamous cell carcinoma.[17] Cyclin D1 and cyclin E have been implicated in the progression of premalignant cells to adenocarcinoma.[57] EGF and transforming growth factor-α (TGF-α) promote the proliferation of epithelial cells in the gastrointestinal tract. Overexpression of the EGF receptor (EGFR) has been associated with poor prognosis.[54] There is disagreement as to the prevalence of *ras* mutations in adenocarcinoma. Some have found that *ras* mutation is rare in adenocarcinoma.[58] However, a study reported *KRAS* (12p12) mutation to be present in up to 40% of patients.[59] Telomerase, which helps to maintain cellular immortality, appears to be important in the development of esophageal adenocarcinoma.[57]

Thymus Tumors

The cause of thymic neoplasm is unclear. Some of the environmental factors that contribute to the development of thymic neoplasms may include Epstein-Barr virus infection[60] and exposure to ionizing irradiation.[61] The translocation of chromosomes 15 and 19 has been observed in thymic carcinoma.[62] Benign thymoma has been associated with deletion of the short arm of chromosome 6.[63] Abnormalities in TP53, EGF, and EGFR may contribute to the development of thymoma.[64]

Thymic Carcinoma

Thymic carcinoma displays features that are similar to those of carcinoma arising in other body sites. It has a higher rate of capsular invasion, involvement of the regional lymph nodes, and systemic metastases compared with invasive thymomas.[65,66] Features of thymic carcinomas may include expression of high levels of EGFR,[67] vascular endothelial growth factor (VEGF), and basic fibroblast growth factor (bFGF).[68,69] CD70 positivity may serve as a marker for thymic carcinoma.[70] Unlike lung cancer, thymic carcinomas usually do not express transcription termination factor-1 (TTF1).[71]

Pulmonary Carcinoid

Although most pulmonary carcinoids are nonfunctional, some can secrete a variety of substances, which can lead to paraneoplastic syndromes, including carcinoid and Cushing's syndrome.[72] Although serotonin (5-hydroxytryptamine [5-HT]) is one of the common substances released by carcinoid tumors, others may include corticotropin, histamine, dopamine, substance P, neurotensin, prostaglandins, and kallikrein.[73-76]

Typical carcinoids usually display an indolent clinical course. However, atypical carcinoids have a higher rate of regional and systemic involvement on presentation.[77,78] The risk of regional nodal metastasis is approximately 30% to 57%,[79-81] and more than 20% of patients may present with distant metastasis.[79] In atypical carcinoids, there appears to be a higher rate of inactivation of the tumor suppressor gene *TP53*.[82,83] Grossly, the tumor is often firm with occasional foci of hemorrhage, and calcification may be present.[84] Most pulmonary carcinoids are typical carcinoids. Sometimes, it may be difficult to distinguish atypical carcinoids from SCLC without additional stains with immunohistochemical exmination.[85]

There is evidence to support a genetic component in the pathogenesis of pulmonary carcinoid tumors. Some of the atypical carcinoid cells express the retinoblastoma gene products and mutant TP53.[86] Most familial pulmonary carcinoids have been reported in patients with multiple endocrine neoplasia 1 (MEN1).[87-89] Other genetic alterations in lung carcinoids include losses of 3p, 5p, 9p, 10q, and 13q.[90]

STAGING AND WORKUP

Lung Cancer

As with other medical conditions, the workup begins with a careful history and physical examination. There should be an emphasis on the duration of symptoms and signs related to the thoracic neoplasm and the overall baseline medical condition of the patient.

The performance status is very important in determining prognosis. Weight loss of more than 10% is a poor prognostic indicator. Other factors associated with prognosis include lactate dehydrogenase (LDH), alkaline phosphatase, and serum sodium levels; white blood cell counts; loss of blood group antigens; and an inability to quit smoking.[91,92]

Patients with SCLC have higher rates of symptoms related to the lung cancer than those with NSCLC. The symptoms of SCLC and NSCLC often depend on the location and the extent of the disease involvement. Patients with SCLC can present with associated paraneoplastic syndromes of inappropriate secretion of antidiuretic hormone (SIADH), atrial natriuretic peptide (ANP) syndrome, and Cushing's syndrome.[93,94] Other syndromes may include myasthenia gravis–like Lambert-Eaton syndrome, which affects less than 5% of patients with SCLC. Many symptoms related to paraneoplastic syndromes improve with response to therapy for SCLC.[95]

The most common staging system for bronchogenic cancer uses the guidelines established by the International Union Against Cancer (UICC) and American Joint Committee on Cancer (AJCC).[96] Although this system has been widely adopted for staging patients with NSCLC, it is used less for patients with SCLC. It is more common to use the 1973 Veterans Administration Lung Cancer Study Group's Staging System for staging SCLC. It is imprecise and distinguishes disease extent with subjective terms such as *limited* and *extensive*.[97] The patient with limited-stage SCLC is often described as one with a "reasonable" radiation therapy portal to encompass the known disease. Investigators now require staging of SCLC patients with the standard tumor-node-metastasis (TNM) system.

The first diagnostic test for suspected thoracic neoplasm is usually a chest radiograph. This is usually followed by computed tomography (CT) of the chest and upper abdomen for staging of patients with lung and esophageal carcinoma. The overall accuracy of CT staging has been estimated to be between 39% and 100%.[98,99] For example, the sensitivity of the CT scan in correctly predicting a mediastinal node involvement is 60% to 70%. Unfortunately, approximately 20% of patients with clinically staged (c) cT1N0 and cT2N0 NSCLC have positive nodes found during mediastinoscopy.[100] There are no consistently reliable indicators of pathologic involvement. Cytologic or pathologic confirmation of the mediastinal lymph node status remains an important endeavor for patients who may qualify for curative surgery. Such information can aid in designing the radiation volume to direct higher dose to clearly involved lymph nodes. In patients with a histologic diagnosis of SCLC, there is rarely a need for invasive mediastinal staging because there is limited role for surgery.

Positron emission tomography (PET) uses tissue metabolic activity rather than size to determine the presence of tumor. Metabolically active sites show increased uptake of radiolabeled fluorinated glucose (^{18}F-fluorodeoxyglucose). Overall, PET scans are quite accurate in the staging of lung cancer. PET scans can assist in determining the disease extent and the treatment options.[101]

Bronchoscopy is done to study the endobronchial anatomy, and it often can assist in establishing a pathologic diagnosis.[102] Patients suspected of having esophageal involvement (cT4) should undergo esophagoscopy in addition to the previous studies. Similarly, patients with thoracic neoplasms should undergo pulmonary function testing to determine their ability to tolerate aggressive local therapy.

Esophageal Cancer

In evaluation of esophageal cancer, transesophageal ultrasound and CT have replaced esophageal barium studies. The current staging system is based on the pathologic depth of invasion rather than the length of esophageal involvement, despite the fact that many patients are not treated with primary surgical management. Endoscopic ultrasound correlates well with pathologic findings at the time of surgery.[103] The accuracy of endoscopic ultrasound in determining pathologic depth of invasion is approximately 90% and is more accurate than CT in evaluating early lesions and evaluating mediastinal nodes.[104] Patients with upper- and middle-third esophageal cancers may require bronchoscopy to evaluate possible airway invasion. PET scanning is very useful for

Table C-1 Masaoka Staging System for Thymoma

Stage	Criteria
I	Completely encapsulated macroscopically and no microscopic capsular invasion
II-1	Macroscopic invasion into surrounding fatty tissue or mediastinal pleura
II-2	Microscopic invasion into the capsule
III	Microscopic invasion into adjacent organs
IVA	Pleural or pericardial implants
IVB	Lymphatogenous or hematogenous metastasis

Table C-2 GETT Staging System for Thymoma

Stage	Criteria
IA	Encapsulated tumor, totally resected
IB	Macroscopically encapsulated tumor, totally resected, but the surgeon suspects mediastinal adhesions and potential capsular invasion
II	Invasive tumor, totally resected
IIIA	Invasive tumor, subtotally resected
IIIB	Invasive tumor, biopsy only
IVA	Supraclavicular metastasis or distant pleural implant
IVB	Distant metastasis

GETT, Groupe d'Etudes des Tumeurs Thymiques.

detection of disease extent (especially nodal and metastases) in these patients.

Thymic Tumors

In the workup of thymic tumors, particular attention should be given to detect signs and symptoms that suggest the presence of myasthenia gravis. Approximately 10% to 15% of patients with myasthenia gravis have thymoma, and 30% to 45% of patients with thymomas have myasthenia gravis.[105-108] The presence of myasthenia gravis does not appear to affect the long-term prognosis of patients with thymoma.[107] In the case of suspected Cushing's syndrome, the peak petrosal sinus to peripheral adrenocorticotropic hormone (ACTH) ratio and urinary cortisol level should be obtained. Serum alpha-fetoprotein (AFP) and β-human chorionic gonadotropin (β-hCG) levels should be obtained in young adult males to exclude nonseminomatous germ cell tumors.[109,110] Thymic carcinoids may also be associated with Cushing's syndrome, Eaton-Lambert syndrome, SIADH, and hypercalcemia.[111] Symptoms of classic carcinoid syndrome are rare in patients with thymic carcinoids.

Approximately 30% to 40% of patients with thymic neoplasms are found during a routine chest x-ray.[105] CT is the most valuable radiologic study in the workup of thymic tumors.[112] It can establish the initial clinical staging and response to treatment. Magnetic resonance imaging (MRI) has not been shown to be more accurate than the CT scan in assessing anterior mediastinal tumors.[113] The role of PET has not been established in the workup of thymic neoplasms. Most patients with thymic mass need a histologic diagnosis before initiation of definitive therapy. The risk of tumor spillage during biopsy remains uncertain.[114]

Thymomas histologically display epithelial and lymphatic cell types. They can be classified according to the degree of the epithelial and lymphatic cell combination. The neoplastic cells are the epithelial cells, but there is no consistent correlation between the histology of thymomas and their malignant potential or systemic syndromes. The degree of invasion of the capsule and adjacent tissues defines malignancy.[115] Thymomas may metastasize as local implants or pulmonary nodules, but they rarely metastasize to extrathoracic areas.[116] The Masaoka staging system[117] is used widely and is based on the anatomic extent of disease at the time of surgery. It emphasizes the extent of invasion of the capsule and the surrounding tissues. The Masaoka staging system is provided in Table C-1. The French Groupe d'Etudes des Tumeurs Thymiques (GETT) classification is a similar staging system, and it correlates well with the Masaoka system.[118] The GETT system is outlined in Table C-2.

Thymic carcinoma (type C) histology is cytologically not different from carcinomas in other sites. Thymic carcinomas often involve the pleura and locoregional lymph nodes. It can also develop distant metastases to the lungs, liver, brain, and bone.[119] Although a TNM-type staging system was proposed,[120] it is not widely accepted.

There are no environmental risk factors conclusively associated with the development of lung carcinoids.[121] Functioning carcinoids are diagnosed by demonstrating an increase in urinary excretion of the serotonin metabolite, 5-hydroxyindoleacetic acid (5-HIAA). Thyroid transcription factor-1 is expressed in 80% of metastatic pulmonary carcinoids but not in intestinal carcinoids.[122]

Most patients with pulmonary carcinoids are between the ages of 40 and 60 years at presentation.[123] These tumors are often located centrally within the tracheobronchial tree.[124] A few patients with pulmonary carcinoids present with asymptomatic peripheral lesions.[125]

Targeted radioactive octreotide or pentetreotide has been used to detect metastatic carcinoids.[126,127] Such targeted imaging against type 2 somatostatin receptors may be useful in 80% of carcinoids. Although the standard PET scans for carcinoids are not useful, PET with ^{64}Cu-TETA-octreotide as a tracer appears promising.[128] The AJCC lung staging system (TNM) is commonly used for lung carcinoids.

Mesothelioma

In patients with malignant pleural mesothelioma, a history of asbestos exposure should be investigated. A chest radiograph is a reasonable initial evaluation. Rib tenderness may indicate direct tumor extension, and sites of previous procedures (e.g., chest tubes) may harbor disease.

Although CT of the chest is the most commonly used staging tool, it often underestimates the extent of the disease. In particular, disease involvement of diaphragm, chest wall, and the contralateral mediastinal lymph nodes may be difficult to visualize. Additional invasive studies such as laparoscopy and peritoneal lavage may be indicated to document resectability. MRI may be slightly more accurate in predicting the extent of chest wall and diaphragm invasion. The AJCC staging system, which is based on the International Mesothelioma Interest Group (IMIG) staging system, is commonly used. There is no validated clinical staging system. Some of the important prognostic markers in malignant pleural mesothelioma include performance status, lymph node involvement, completeness of resection, and weight loss. Patients with sarcomatoid or mixed tumors have a worse prognosis than patients with epithelioid histology.

Thoracentesis and percutaneous fine-needle aspiration biopsy have a low diagnostic sensitivity.[129] Video-assisted thoracoscopic biopsy appears to be the most accurate means to establish a pathologic diagnosis. Mesothelioma may recur at previously placed thoracoscopy sites if they are not excised at the time of surgery. Previous thoracotomy for diagnosis may significantly compromise the chance for curative surgery.

NORMAL TISSUE TOXICITY CONSIDERATIONS

The spinal cord, lung, esophagus, and heart are the dose-limiting structures in radiation therapy for thoracic malignancy. It is critical to consider normal tissue toxicities related to thoracic irradiation planning. In general, functioning subunits of an organ may be arranged as an in-series or in-parallel structure. Normal tissue such as the lung is an example of an in-parallel structure in which critical numbers of functioning units must be damaged before the organ is impaired.[130] Organ failure occurs when functional subunits are damaged beyond a critical level. The gastrointestinal tract and spinal cord represent in-series structures in which a loss of a single functioning subunit may lead to organ impairment or development of clinical symptoms. The current grading systems for toxicities include the National Cancer Institute's Common Toxicity Criteria version 3.0. It is outlined in Table C-3, which focuses on the selected toxicities related to thoracic radiation therapy.

Normal Thoracic Tissue Toxicity of the Esophagus

The esophagus extends approximately from C6 to T12.[131] The esophagus is generally anterior to the spinal cord, and the distance between the two structures is greater toward the distal end of the esophagus. This separation is accentuated when the patient is prone. The esophagus is lined with squamous epithelium, a basal cell layer, submucosa, and a layer of striated muscle fibers, without a serosal layer. It is common for esophageal cancer to spread along the submucosal layer for several centimeters beyond any grossly detected abnormalities. The lack of a serosal layer allows easier lateral spread into periesophageal soft tissue.

Most upper esophageal carcinomas drain into the cervical, tracheoesophageal, and paratracheal nodes. Lower esophageal cancers generally drain into the lower thoracic and celiac nodal basins. Patients with lower esophageal cancer often require irradiation to the celiac axis, which can be visualized with a CT-based treatment planning system.

After fractionated radiation therapy in excess of 45 Gy, one of the common radiologic abnormalities is esophageal dysmotility. The abnormality may reveal incomplete peristaltic waves or contraction with an inability of the distal esophageal sphincter to relax. Esophageal dysmotility can be seen as early as a week after chemoradiotherapy or approximately 4 weeks after irradiation alone is administered.[132,133]

Early symptoms of acute esophagitis start usually in the second or third week of standard fractionated thoracic radiation therapy (1.8 to 2.0 Gy/day). Patients often complain of dysphagia, which progresses to odynophagia. Subsequently, persistent chest pain unrelated to swallowing may develop as the esophagitis progresses, and the patient may require intravenous hydration and parenteral nutrition. Acute esophagitis symptoms often persist for 1 to 6 weeks after completion of radiation therapy. Symptoms of late esophageal injury may occur 3 to 8 months after completion of radiation therapy. The symptoms of late esophageal injury may include dysphagia to solids due to esophageal stricture, and patients may require dilation of the esophagus.

Combined chemoradiotherapy increases the risk of severe (grade 3) acute esophagitis. The risk of severe esophagitis may be less than 5% when irradiation alone is used for lung cancer, but it can be close to 50% when gemcitabine is incorporated into the concurrent chemoradiotherapy regimen.[134]

The severity of acute esophagitis may be increased by the use of accelerated radiation therapy. The duration and the severity of esophagitis are increased when intense accelerated radiation therapy is administered. The length of the esophagus appears not to correlate with the development of severe esophagitis.[135]

The commonly accepted dose tolerance of the esophagus considers the length of the esophagus to be irradiated. The tolerance dose was derived from the review of the literature and from opinions of experienced radiation oncologists. The tolerance of the esophagus relates the total dose given in standard fractionation to the development of strictures and perforations. The $TD_{5/5}$ (tolerance dose) varies with the length of the esophagus irradiated, and it represents the 5% complication rate at 5 years. The $TD_{5/5}$ for the entire esophagus is 55 Gy, and it is 60 Gy for one third of the esophagus.[136]

Three-dimensional (3D) dosimetry has allowed a more precise calculation of the given dose to the esophagus. A maximal esophageal dose of more than 58 Gy was associated with development of grade 3 esophagitis.[137]

There are strategies to lower the rate of esophagitis in patients undergoing irradiation for thoracic malignancy. Intensity-modulated radiation therapy (IMRT) and 3D treatment optimization can substantially reduce the dose given to the esophagus. Use of the radioprotector amifostine has shown mixed results, and it cannot be routinely recommended as prevention against development of esophagitis.[138]

Normal Thoracic Tissue Toxicity of the Spinal Cord

The morbidity of thoracic spinal cord radiation injury is less than that of cervical spinal cord injury due to the general lower location of the injury within the spinal cord.[139] However, there is little pathologic difference in myelopathy between the two sites, and radiation myelitis remains a feared complication of spinal cord irradiation. Radiation myelopathy has been studied extensively in animals, but there are few clinical data regarding the incidence of thoracic radiation myelitis after standard fractionated treatment.[140] Demyelination, white matter necrosis, and malacia are commonly observed pathologic findings in radiation injury to the spinal cord. These processes are from direct damage of glial cells and the surrounding vasculature.[141]

The initial symptoms of radiation myelopathy may be nonspecific. Lhermitte's sign may precede the development of permanent radiation myelopathy by several months. However, Lhermitte's sign may occur at doses well below tolerance level, and it is independent of the development of radiation myelopathy.

Clinical signs may include paresthesias, lower extremity weakness, and a decrease in proprioception. Brown-Séquard syndrome, a positive Babinski sign, spasticity of extremities, pain, and hyperreflexia may be seen. The severity of symptoms does not appear to be related to the radiation dose. These symptoms suggest progressive and irreversible demyelinating disease. There is no effective treatment for total spinal cord transection.

The latency period for radiation myelopathy is usually more than 6 months from the completion of radiation.[142] Other medical conditions, including tumor progression, are excluded before considering radiation-induced myelopathy. The dosimetry and medical conditions that potentially reduce the radiation tolerance of the spinal cord must be considered. Pediatric patients and patients who receive concurrent chemotherapy generally have lower spinal cord radiation tolerance.

Table C-3 **Selected Scores of Toxicities Related to Treatment of Thoracic Malignancy: National Cancer Institute Common Toxicity Criteria Version 3.0**

Adverse Event	Toxicity Grade 1	2	3	4	5
Cardiac Arrhythmia	Mild	Moderate	Severe	Life-threatening	Death
Left ventricular diastolic dysfunction	Asymptomatic diagnostic finding; intervention not indicated	Asymptomatic, intervention indicated	Symptomatic CHF responsive to intervention	Refractory CHF, poorly controlled; intervention such as ventricular assist device or heart transplant indicated	Death
Left ventricular systolic dysfunction	Asymptomatic, resting EF <60-50%; SF <30-24%	Asymptomatic, resting EF <50-40%; SF <24-15%	Symptomatic, CHF responsive to intervention; EF <40-20% SF <15%	Refractory CHF or poorly controlled; EF <20%; intervention such as ventricular-assist device, ventricular reduction surgery, or heart transplantation indicated	Death
Pericarditis	Asymptomatic, ECG or physical examination (rub) changes consistent with pericarditis	Symptomatic, pericarditis (e.g., chest pain)	Pericarditis with physiologic consequences (e.g., pericardial constriction)	Life-threatening consequences; emergency intervention indicated	Death
Valvular heart disease	Asymptomatic, valvular thickening with or without mild valvular regurgitation or stenosis; treatment other than endocarditis prophylaxis not indicated	Asymptomatic, moderate regurgitation or stenosis by imaging	Symptomatic, severe regurgitation or stenosis; symptoms controlled with medical therapy	Life-threatening; disabling; intervention (e.g., valve replacement, valvuloplasty) indicated	Death
Esophagitis	Asymptomatic, pathologic, radiographic, or endoscopic findings only	Symptomatic, altered eating or swallowing (e.g., altered dietary habits, oral supplements); IV fluids indicated <24 h	Symptomatic, severely altered eating or swallowing (e.g., inadequate oral caloric or fluid intake); IV fluids, tube feedings, or TPN indicated ≥24 h	Life-threatening consequences	Death
Myelitis	Asymptomatic, mild signs (e.g., Babinski, Lhermitte)	Weakness or sensory loss not interfering with ADLs	Weakness or sensory loss interfering with ADLs	Disabling	Death
Pneumonitis	Asymptomatic, radiographic findings only	Symptomatic, not interfering with ADLs	Symptomatic, interfering with ADLs; O_2 indicated	Life-threatening; ventilatory support indicated	Death
Pulmonary fibrosis	Minimal radiographic findings(or patchy or bibasilar changes) with estimated radiographic proportion of total lung volume that is fibrotic <25%	Patchy or bibasilar changes with estimated radiographic proportion of total lung volume that is fibrotic of 25-50%	Dense or widespread infiltrates or consolidation with estimated radiographic proportion of total lung volume that is fibrotic <25%	—	—
Cough	Symptomatic, non-narcotic medication only indicated	Symptomatic, narcotic medication indicated	Symptomatic, significantly interfering with sleep or ADLs	—	—
Dyspnea	Dyspnea on exertion, but can walk 1 flight of stairs without stopping	Dyspnea on exertion but unable to walk 1 flight of stairs or 1 city block (0.1 km) without stopping	Dyspnea with ADLs	Dyspnea at rest; intubation or ventilator indicated	Death

ADLs, activities of daily living; CHF, congestive heart failure; ECG, electrocardiogram; EF, ejection fraction; IV, intravenous; SF, shortening fraction; TPN, total parenteral nutrition.

Findings of radiographic studies such as CT scans, MRI scans, and plain radiographs are most often unremarkable. There exists no definitive diagnostic tool to confirm radiation-induced myelopathy. Nerve conduction velocities may reveal slowed spinal conduction or complete blocks.[143]

The most widely accepted dose limit of the spinal cord is between 45 and 50 Gy in standard fractionation schedules. There is no significant report of radiation-induced myelopathy at these dose levels. For the cervical cord, the myelopathy rate is expected to be 1% with a total dose of 52 Gy in 2-Gy fractions. The myelopathy rate for the thoracic cord may be even lower.[141] Although chemotherapy can be neurotoxic, the additional risk of myelopathy from combining chemotherapy to radiation therapy remains uncertain. A total dose of 45 Gy with the spinal cord given with chemotherapy may be safe. Altered fractionation with 1.2 Gy twice daily with an interval of 4 to 6 hours between fractions to a total dose of 45 Gy appears to be safe for the cervical cord.[144]

It is generally prudent to wait 6 hours between fractions because of the uncertainties related to the repair kinetics. The precise amount of recovery and the duration of time required for repair of the given dose to the spinal cord are unknown. However, it is reasonable to assume that substantial recovery is several years after completing radiation therapy.[145]

Normal Thoracic Tissue Toxicity of the Lung

Exposure of normal lung to ionizing radiation can cause pneumonitis and pulmonary fibrosis. Clinical pneumonitis occurs in about 10% of patients treated for lung cancer and occurs typically 4 to 6 weeks after completion of thoracic radiation therapy, perhaps earlier after chemoradiotherapy. The influence of treatment factors on development of pneumonitis remains unclear, but dose, volume, and fractionation have been implicated.[146-149]

Radiation-induced lung injury classically has been divided into *acute* and *late* phases. The onset of acute pneumonitis occurs 1 to 4 months after completing radiation therapy. Symptoms may include shortness of breath, cough, and low-grade fever. The radiographic findings during the acute phase may be unremarkable. Medical conditions, including infection, cardiovascular disease, other pulmonary disease, and tumor recurrence, must be excluded. Radiation-induced pneumonitis is a diagnosis of exclusion. The acute phase responds well to 40 to 60 mg of prednisone given daily for several weeks, with a slow taper of steroids over another several weeks. The late phase consists of development of radiation-induced fibrosis with scarring of the irradiated lung. This may occur months to years after completing radiation therapy. Radiographic findings include fibrosis of the portion of the lung, and patients may remain asymptomatic. There is no direct correlation between the degree of radiographic abnormalities and clinical symptoms. Unusual pulmonary complications, such as bronchial stenosis and bronchial malacia, may follow a high dose of radiation.[150]

A decrease in the diffusion capacity is one indicator of damage to functional lung parenchyma[151] and pulmonary function testing usually shows greater abnormality in carbon monoxide diffusion capacity (DLCO) than inforced expiratory volume in 1 second (FEV_1).[141] The decrease in FEV_1 indicates development of bronchial obstruction after irradiation. CT scans reveal more detailed information regarding abnormal radiographic findings than a plain chest radiograph. CT findings of lung fibrosis may include pleural thickening and lung contraction.[141]

Dosimetric evaluation of the lung can be difficult to analyze. Most dose-volume histograms from the available treatment planning system assume equally distributed functioning lung subunits. For example, the process of ventilation and perfusion is more efficient at lung base. However, this information is difficult to convey in conventional dosimetric analysis. This lack of detailed understanding of the spatial differences in the location of the functioning subunits may produce unexpected clinical symptoms. Various parameters of the dosimetric evaluation have been used to predict lung toxicity after thoracic radiation therapy. One of the factors that determine radiation-induced pulmonary toxicity is the volume of normal lung that receives more than a certain dose. Graham and associates reported the risks of pneumonitis based on the volume of lung that receives more than 20 Gy (V20).[152]

The *latency period* represents a time interval between completion of radiation therapy and onset of clinical evidence of pneumonitis. During this period, complex subclinical molecular interactions occur before histopathologic or clinical changes. The pulmonary functioning subunits are composed of alveoli, type II pneumocytes, capillary bed, and vascular endothelial cells, and the target cells of radiation injury appear to be the type II pneumocytes found in the alveoli and the alveolar vascular endothelial cells.[153]

Histologic examination after radiation therapy often reveals exudation of proteinaceous material into the alveoli, desquamation of epithelial cells from the alveolar walls, interstitial edema, and the presence of inflammatory cells.[154] The mechanism of late injury, which includes progressive fibrosis, is not completely understood. After irradiation, the type II cells release surfactant and surfactant precursors.

The type II cells are also influenced by transforming growth factor-α (TGF-α) and TGF-β.[155] TGF-β is a potent regulator of cell growth and differentiation that stimulates connective tissue formation and promotes fibrosis by decreasing collagen degradation. Macrophages help to maintain surfactant equilibrium by processing surfactant released from type II cells. When the macrophage numbers decrease because of irradiation, the surfactant tends to accumulate in the alveolar space or is released to the systemic circulation through damaged endothelium. Macrophages play a role in protecting the lung from pneumonitis.[156]

When vascular endothelial cells are injured from radiation therapy, they secrete various cytokines and induce a proliferation of reactive cells. Macrophages, mononuclear cells, and helper T cells contribute to a proliferation of fibroblasts. TGF-β released from type II pneumocytes may directly influence stromal cells, which contribute to the formation of collagen.[156] Fibroblasts and infiltrating T lymphocytes also promote this activity.[157,158] TGF-β plays a critical role in the stimulation and prolonged activation of fibroblasts and premature terminal differentiation of this cell type.[156]

Patients with elevated TGF-β levels at the completion of radiation therapy may have a higher incidence of clinical pneumonitis than those with normal plasma TGF-β levels.[159] Attempts to improve the therapeutic ratio of treatment for patients with thoracic malignancies must address treatment efficacy and toxicity.

Cardiac Toxicity

Most of the cardiovascular toxicity data comes from long-term survivals of patients with Hodgkin's disease and breast cancer. Such data is lacking in patients with locally advanced lung cancer who have limited long-term survival. Multiple studies have shown that Hodgkin's disease patients are at higher risk for fatal myocardial infarction many years after mediastinal irradiation.[160] Although the total dose used to treat

Hodgkin's disease has been lowered over the years, it is unclear whether lower dose results in less risk of myocardial infarctions.

The volume of the heart exposed to radiation appears to affect the risk of myocardial infarction. This association is evident from studies of breast cancer survivors who have undergone irradiation of the right or left side of the chest.[161]

In patients with documented acute coronary obstruction, coronary artery bypass graft surgery may be better than percutaneous coronary angioplasty because left main coronary artery and ostial lesions are commonly seen. Emergency coronary bypass graft surgery after angioplasty complication may be more difficult due to mediastinal fibrosis.[162] There may be a transient decrease in the left ventricular ejection fraction shortly after completing mediastinal radiation therapy, but delayed ventricular dysfunctions are also observed.[163]

The type of cardiomyopathy appears to be related to the type of systemic chemotherapy given along with radiation therapy. Diastolic dysfunction is more common in patients who did not receive anthracyclines, whereas systolic dysfunction is more common in patients who received an anthracycline. Symptomatic heart failure is rare after irradiation alone, but subclinical changes such as perfusion defects are common.[164] Perfusion defects from likely microvascular damage may be seen on radionuclide scans 6 months after completing radiation therapy for left breast cancer.[165]

Pericarditis was a common toxicity seen after mediastinal radiation therapy in the past. The clinical symptoms consist of pleuritic chest pain, dyspnea, fever, and presence of friction rub on auscultation. Pericarditis is uncommon in the modern treatment setting in which the total dose and the volume of the heart irradiated are reduced.[166]

Acute pericarditis from radiation therapy is treated conservatively. A minority of patients requires treatment with anti-inflammatory drugs and diuretics. Chronic symptomatic pericardial effusion may require pericardiectomy to relieve symptoms and to prevent constrictive pericarditis.

The incidence of valvular heart disease may be increased after mediastinal irradiation. It is relatively commonly seen in persons who survive Hodgkin's disease and who received mediastinal radiation therapy. The threshold dose for development of valvular regurgitation appears to be approximately 30 Gy.[167] However, it remains unclear whether radiation exposure is a direct cause of the valvular disease. The incidence of serious conduction abnormalities appears to be low.

TREATMENT CONSIDERATIONS

Esophageal Cancer

There is no standard treatment for patients with esophageal cancer. A survey of the clinical practice by the U.S. Patterns of Care Study revealed diverse treatment modalities, including chemoradiation (54%), irradiation (20%), preoperative (13%) or postoperative (8%) chemoradiation, and preoperative (1%) or postoperative (4%) irradiation.[168] An analysis of 130 papers published between 1980 and 1988 showed that resectability improved from 40% to 60%, but the 5-year survival remained dismal.[169] Patients who undergo curative surgery generally have 5-year survival rates less than 25%.

The transthoracic approach (Ivor-Lewis esophagectomy) is the most commonly used surgical technique for esophageal cancer. This technique removes the tumor and periesophageal tissue through a right thoracotomy. Although periesophageal and lesser curvature lymph nodes are dissected, the mediastinal or upper abdominal lymph nodes are not removed. Transhiatal esophagectomy is a technique that avoids open thoracotomy. Instead, the esophagus is removed through combined cervical and abdominal incisions.[170] A more aggressive surgical technique, en bloc transthoracic esophagectomy, has been advocated to improve tumor control. This technique involves resection of the mediastinal contents and a two-field lymphadenectomy of the upper abdominal and thoracic lymph nodes.[171] Some investigators advocate an even more extensive three-field lymphadenectomy to remove the cervical lymph nodes.[172] The optimal surgical procedure for lower esophageal carcinomas is unclear. Two randomized studies and a meta-analysis indicated no significant difference in survival or postoperative complications between transthoracic or transhiatal approaches.[173-175]

It is reasonable to expect resectability rates of 60% to 70% with perioperative mortality rates of 2% to 10% after a curative resection. After curative surgery, local control rates can be 70% to 90%, and 5-year survival rates are approximately 20% to 40%. The 5-year survival rate after primary external beam radiation therapy alone is 0% to 10%.[176]

Many randomized trials of preoperative radiation therapy have been reported.[177-179] Only one trial that also administered chemotherapy showed an improvement in survival.[177] Other trials have failed to show benefit for preoperative irradiation alone. A meta-analysis of preoperative radiation did not show improvement in resectability or survival.[180] Preoperative irradiation alone has a minor role in the management of esophageal cancer.

Two randomized studies of postoperative irradiation failed to show improvement in local control.[181,182] Only one of the randomized, postoperative radiation therapy trials showed improvements in local control when patients without pathologic lymph node involvement received postoperative irradiation. Radiation therapy given before or after surgery is an inadequate treatment for patients with esophageal cancer.

Adenocarcinomas and squamous cell carcinomas of the esophagus have a propensity to disseminate early. To treat the potential subclinical metastases, chemotherapy has been combined with surgery or irradiation. A combination of cisplatin and 5-fluorouracil (5-FU) has resulted in pathologic complete response rates of approximately 20% to 25%. The risk of perioperative mortality is increased when chemotherapy is added to surgery.[183] Randomized trials of preoperative chemotherapy versus surgery alone have been reported.[183-187] Four of the six randomized trials showed no significant benefit. There were similar patterns of failure, and histology of the tumor did not affect prognosis. Although two of the trials suggested that preoperative chemotherapy might improve outcome, preoperative chemotherapy in cases of resectable esophageal carcinoma remains experimental.[184,187]

Three randomized trials from Japan studied the role of postoperative chemotherapy.[188-190] Two of the studies reported no significant benefit. The preliminary results from the third trial showed an overall survival benefit for node-positive patients.[189]

Many randomized trials have compared combined chemotherapy and irradiation with irradiation alone. The Radiation Therapy Oncology Group (RTOG 8501) administered cisplatin, 5-FU, and radiation therapy. Two additional cycles of chemotherapy were administered as consolidation therapy after the combined-modality treatment. The patients on the radiation-alone arm received 64 Gy, and the patients in the combined-modality arm received 50 Gy in 2-Gy fractions.[191] After it became clear that survival was significantly better in the combined-modality arm, the trial was closed early, with 123 patients on the study. Chemoradiation was associated with significantly higher acute toxicity. Only one half of the patients assigned to the combined-modality arm completed all four cycles of chemotherapy.[192]

Increasing the radiation dose to the tumor with higher doses of external beam irradiation or with brachytherapy after external beam irradiation or chemoradiation failed to improve the local control or survival.[193] Two cycles of cisplatin plus 5-FU with concurrent continuous external beam radiation therapy to a total dose of 50.4 Gy remains the nonsurgical standard chemoradiation therapy for the management of esophageal cancer.

Four randomized trials compared preoperative concurrent chemoradiation with surgery alone.[194-197] Urba and associates[194] observed a decrease in local recurrence, favoring preoperative chemoradiotherapy, without survival benefit. Walsh and colleagues[195] demonstrated significantly better survival when patients received preoperative cisplatin plus 5-FU and irradiation compared with surgery alone. Bosset and coworkers[196] reported a better local control when preoperative chemoradiotherapy was administered, but the overall survival was not improved. Burmeister and colleagues[197] also reported that preoperative cisplatin plus 5-FU with irradiation did not improve overall survival. Preoperative chemoradiation resulted in improvement of local control, but an overall survival benefit was not established.

Two trials randomized patients to receive chemoradiotherapy with or without subsequent surgery. The French FFCD 9102 trial[198] and the German Esophageal Cancer Study Group trial[199] found no significant difference in survival between patients who received preoperative chemoradiotherapy or chemoradiotherapy alone. Patients who respond to chemoradiotherapy may not benefit from surgery. However, surgery may benefit patients who have a poor response to preoperative chemoradiotherapy.

Although definitive chemoradiotherapy has not been directly compared with surgery, evidence from the previously mentioned trials suggests that 5-year survival may be equivalent. Surgery alone and chemoradiotherapy alone result in 5-year survival rates of approximately 20% to 27%. Surgery or chemoradiotherapy may be appropriate for patients who present with resectable disease. Salvage surgery should be considered for patients who have residual disease after chemoradiation.

Non–Small Cell Lung Cancer

Surgery is the best treatment for patients with early-stage NSCLC. Lobectomy remains the most effective treatment for many patients with stage I and II disease. Pneumonectomy increases the treatment-related morbidity and mortality. Wedge resection results in an increased rate of local recurrence.[200]

Although some lung cancers remain localized, most develop systemic metastases. There were very few complete responses with older chemotherapy combinations for NSCLC. However, platinum-based chemotherapy modestly improved survival.[201,202] A meta-analysis showed that postoperative administration of cisplatin-containing chemotherapy resulted in a nonsignificant lower risk of death. In a pivotal study by the International Adjuvant Lung Cancer Trial (IALT),[203] 1867 patients with stage I-III NSCLC received cisplatin-based chemotherapy or no chemotherapy after surgery. There was an absolute 5-year survival benefit of 4% ($P < .03$) for patients who received postoperative cisplatin-based chemotherapy. Age, gender, and performance status did not affect survival. An Eastern Cooperative Oncology Group (ECOG) study failed to show a local control or survival benefit of combining etoposide and cisplatin with radiation therapy (50.4 Gy) compared with irradiation alone administered postoperatively for patients with stage II or IIIA disease.[204]

Neoadjuvant chemotherapy has been shown to improve survival. Depierre and colleagues[205] showed that patients with stage I or II disease who received neoadjuvant chemotherapy had a survival advantage at 2 years. However, there was no significant benefit for patients with stage III disease from neoadjuvant chemotherapy. Clinical trials commonly restrict entry to patients who have ECOG performance status of 0 to 1. However, many patients present with poor performance status. There is little evidence to suggest that systemic therapy benefits this population. Modern chemotherapy for NSCLC may include gemcitabine, topoisomerase-2 inhibitors, taxanes, tirapazamine, and vinorelbine. These drugs often are administered with cisplatin or carboplatin for the treatment of advanced NSCLC to produce response rates between 17% and 35% and median survival times of 7 to 10 months.[206-208]

In addition to systemic chemotherapy, targeted therapy with inhibitors of EGFRs have been used to treat NSCLC. Although EGFR inhibitors such as gefitinib (Iressa) have been shown to be beneficial in patients who have failed systemic chemotherapy, there was no improvement in the outcome when gefitinib was combined with systemic chemotherapy.[209] VEGF inhibitors have been combined with chemotherapy for patients with NSCLC. The preliminary results showed an increased survival for patients who received a VEGF inhibitor along with chemotherapy. However, there was an increased risk for patients with squamous histology to develop fatal hemoptysis after administration of VEGF inhibitor.[210] Other targeted therapies under investigation include cetuximab and bevacizumab. Second-line chemotherapy for NSCLC includes docetaxel and pemetrexed (Alimta).[211,212]

The early RTOG 73-01 study suggested that 60 Gy was the optimal dose for NSCLC,[213] and this dose has been standard in subsequent clinical trials in the United States for decades. This dose resulted in only an 8% local control at 5 years. The traditional large radiation therapy portal limited the maximum dose that could be delivered safely. This irradiation technique often encompassed the gross tumor along with most of the mediastinal and supraclavicular lymph nodes. Few data exist to support extensive lymph nodal radiation therapy in patients with NSCLC. The rate of isolated failure in the lymph nodes is low. Supraclavicular lymph nodes or contralateral hilar lymph nodes are rarely dissected during a curative surgery. More centers in the United States use target volumes that include only the tumor and lymph nodes that measure more than 1 cm in diameter.[214,215]

For medically inoperable stage I NSCLC, definitive radiation therapy has yielded 5-year survival rates of about 20%, which is far lower than rates for surgery.[216,217] A promising phase I dose-escalation study of stereotactic radiosurgery conducted by Timmerman and colleagues reported a response rate of 87% and complete response rate of 27%. In patients who received 18 Gy per fraction for 3 fractions, there was no local recurrence.[218] Stereotactic radiosurgery for medically inoperable lung cancer is being tested in a phase II study sponsored by the RTOG.

Routine preoperative radiation therapy without chemotherapy is seldom used in the United States, and randomized trials have found no survival advantage from its use.[219] Postoperative irradiation is occasionally added to increase locoregional control. The relative indications for postoperative irradiation include positive surgical margins, positive mediastinal lymph nodes, or lesions that were T3 or T4 on presentation. The meta-analysis (PORT) of adjuvant irradiation in nine randomized trials suggested that patients with N0-1 involvement who received postoperative irradiation had lower survival rates than those who did not receive postoperative irradiation.[220] The meta-analysis included patients with stages I to III who might not have been recommended to receive irradiation in a contemporary setting. At 2 years, 55% of the patients who had surgery alone survived, compared with 48% of those who received postoperative irradiation. Although a large, retrospective study from the Mayo Clinic showed improved survival[221] after postoperative irradiation, routine postoperative radiation therapy remains controversial.

A landmark study by Dillman and associates of sequential chemotherapy followed by irradiation established a new standard for management of unresectable stage III NSCLC. This trial showed that two cycles of neoadjuvant cisplatin and vinblastine followed by irradiation (60 Gy) for stage III NSCLC patients with good performance status and less than 5% weight loss was superior to irradiation alone. The 7-year survival rates showed superiority of combined-modality therapy over thoracic irradiation alone (13% versus 6%).[222] A phase III Intergroup trial confirmed Dillman's results and reported a 5-year survival rate of 17% for the chemoradiotherapy arm versus 10% for the irradiation-alone arm.[223]

The proper sequencing of chemotherapy and irradiation has also been investigated, and concurrent chemotherapy and radiation therapy appear to be better than sequential therapy.[224,225] RTOG has reported[225] that the survival difference at 4 years was 21% versus 12%, in favor of the concurrent therapy ($P = .46$). Unfortunately, the grade 3/4 esophagitis was 25% with concurrent chemoradiotherapy and 4% with sequential treatment.

The role of surgery in stage III patients is unclear. A randomized, prospective trial of cisplatin plus etoposide and irradiation (45 Gy) followed by surgery versus cisplatin plus etoposide and irradiation (61 Gy) without surgery was reported by Albain and coworkers.[226] Progression-free survival was significantly better in the arm that incorporated surgery. There were more non–cancer-related deaths in the surgery arm. Patterns of failure were similar, and overall survival was not statistically different at 3 years, but a survival trend favoring surgery was observed at 3 years (38% versus 33%).

Small Cell Lung Cancer

In the past, the primary therapy for SCLC was combination chemotherapy. Recurrences after chemotherapy were common and often occurred in the area of the original disease. To investigate the role of radiation therapy, several trials compared chemotherapy with or without irradiation. Two meta-analyses based on randomized, prospective studies that compared chemotherapy alone with chemotherapy plus thoracic irradiation were published.[227,228] Both concluded that there was a 5% survival benefit for patients who received thoracic irradiation with chemotherapy. In addition to the improvement in survival, the local control was improved by 25% with radiation therapy.[228] A meta-analysis reviewed seven randomized trials published after 1985 that investigated the timing of thoracic irradiation in limited-stage SCLC. The results showed a 2-year survival benefit for patients who were started on radiation therapy within 9 weeks of initiation of chemotherapy. There was a 5.2% greater survival for patients who received irradiation early.[229] In some instances, it is appropriate to delay radiation therapy until after a few cycles of chemotherapy. These patients include those who present with massive tumors or those who have significant atelectasis for which irradiation on presentation may unreasonably compromise the pulmonary function.

SCLC responds relatively well to radiation therapy. Unlike NSCLC, the commonly prescribed total dose is less than 70 Gy given once each day. The National Cancer Institute of Canada (NCIC) conducted a trial in which patients were randomized between 25 and 37.5 Gy given in 2.5-Gy fractions.[230] The local failure rates were 80% and 69%, in favor of a higher dose of radiation. Most published trials reported the local tumor control rates between 58% and 85% with a total dose between 40 and 60 Gy given once each day, and a dose-response relationship in this range was not clearly seen.[231,232]

The intensity of therapy can be changed by altered radiation fractionation. Several promising studies led to the phase III Intergroup Trial 0096, which has since set the standard of care for patients with limited-stage SCLC. In this trial, patients were given a total of 45 Gy by once-daily (QD-RT) or twice-daily (BID-RT) fractionation. Radiation therapy on both study arms began with the first cycle of chemotherapy. There was a significant survival advantage for the BID-RT compared with QD-RT. The 5-year survival rates were 26% versus 16%, in favor of BID-RT. However, the rate of grade 3 esophagitis in the BID-RT arm was three times higher than that in the QD-RT arm.[233]

The North Central Cancer Treatment Group (NCCTG) published a trial that included SCLC patients who were initially treated with three cycles of etoposide plus cisplatin.[234] The patients without progression were randomized to etoposide plus cisplatin and QD-RT or BID-RT. Patients in the QD-RT arm were given 1.8 Gy per fraction to a total dose of 50.4 Gy, and the BID-RT arm consisted 1.5 Gy per fraction to 24 Gy, a 2.5-week break, and an additional 24 Gy. The 5-year survival rates of 21% and 22% were similar, but there was a higher rate of grade 3+ esophagitis with the BID-RT regimen.

The ability of a patient with limited SCLC to tolerate increasingly aggressive radiation therapy regimens with concurrent chemotherapy is in part related to the irradiated target volume. Investigators demonstrated tumor failures just beyond the margins of the thoracic radiation therapy fields when the fields were designed after a response to chemotherapy.[235] These reports supported the use of large treatment volumes that incorporated the tumor with a 2.0-cm margin, both hilar regions, the mediastinum from the thoracic inlet to at least the subcarinal region, and both supraclavicular regions. Such large volumes precluded a high-dose radiation therapy because of the substantial increase in toxicity. In recent years, the contralateral hilum and both supraclavicular regions have been excluded. The smaller portal volume, emphasizing the treatment of the primary tumor, appears not to increase the rate of marginal failure. The Mayo Clinic and NCCTG found that intrathoracic disease commonly recurred within the original irradiation field.[236] Southwest Oncology Group (SWOG) investigators found that targeting the postchemotherapy tumor volume instead of the tumor volume on presentation did not result in increased failure rates.[237]

Although cyclophosphamide/doxorubicin/vincristine (CAV) and etoposide/cisplatin (EP) combinations have similar efficacy,[238] etoposide plus cisplatin alone remains the widely accepted treatment for limited and extensive SCLC. This may reflect observations that cisplatin plus etoposide regimens produce less hematologic morbidity and equivalent efficacy.

The RTOG has investigated adding paclitaxel to etoposide plus cisplatin with BID-RT for patients with limited-stage SCLC. Preliminary results showed a 1-year survival rate of 83% and a median survival in excess of 30 months.[239]

The novel therapeutic agents for SCLC include mitumomab, a monoclonal antibody that stimulates an immunologic response to SCLC expressing GD3, erlotinib (OSI-774, Tarceva); and gefitinib (Iressa, ZD1839). These are being investigated in the treatment of SCLC. An inhibitor of VEGFR and EGFR, ZD6474, also is being investigated.

Although surgery is seldom used in the management of SCLC, the Veterans Administration Surgical Oncology Group reported that 5-year survival rates could be as high as 60% when patients underwent surgery followed by available chemotherapy in the 1970s.[240] However, a randomized trial of limited-stage SCLC by the Lung Cancer Study Group found no benefit for surgery after chemotherapy.[241] There is limited information regarding the role of surgical resection of intrathoracic recurrences. The role of surgical salvage of patients who fail chemoradiotherapy is unknown.

Prophylactic cranial irradiation (PCI) for patients with SCLC began in the 1970s, when a high rate of brain metastases was seen after successful treatment of the primary thoracic mass. One of the early ECOG trials demonstrated a reduction in brain metastases from 22% to 5% with the incorporation of PCI.[242] Unfortunately, confusion and controversies regarding the morbidity associated with PCI persisted for decades. A French trial randomized patients with limited-stage SCLC to PCI or no PCI after achieving a complete response to chemotherapy.[243] There was a statistically significant reduction in brain relapse rates by approximately 20% after PCI, with a nonsignificant trend toward improved survival at 2 years without significant central nervous system morbidity. A similar 20% reduction in relapse was demonstrated by a randomized, multicenter trial conducted in Great Britain for patients who received PCI after completion of chemotherapy.[244] The patients who received a PCI dose of 36.0 Gy in 18 fractions had the greatest benefit. A statistically significant survival benefit with PCI was not demonstrated. The British trial did not find substantial treatment-related central nervous system deficits. A meta-analysis of prospective randomized trials that compared PCI with no PCI after achieving a complete response showed a 5.4% greater 3-year survival for patients who received PCI ($P = .01$).[245]

Thymoma

Initial treatment of choice for thymic tumors is surgery. Adjuvant radiation or chemotherapy should be considered for patients at high risk for recurrence. Complete en bloc surgical resection is the treatment of choice for patients with resectable thymomas. The primary determinants of clinical outcome remain surgicopathologic staging, tumor size, histology, and extent of surgical resection. Radiation therapy is important in the management of incompletely resected or unresectable thymomas. Completely resected thymoma can lead to low recurrence and excellent survival rates.[246] Patients who present with symptoms of myasthenia gravis can benefit from thymectomy.[247]

Invasive thymoma should be removed as much as possible at the time of surgery. When complete resection is not possible, a debulking operation followed by postoperative radiation therapy can result in satisfactory long-term results.[107] Prospective, randomized data on the value of adjuvant radiation therapy are lacking. Most retrospective studies have demonstrated improvements in local tumor control and survival.[117,248,249] The recurrence rate after complete surgery of noninvasive stage I thymoma is low, and adjuvant postoperative radiation therapy is not indicated. In general, patients with Masaoka stage II disease do not benefit from post operative radiation therapy after complete resection.[250] An exception may be those with fibrous adhesions of the tumor to the pleura or microscopic invasion of the pleura, for which the recurrence rate can be as high as 36% without postoperative irradiation.[251]

Many sources of evidence support postoperative radiation therapy for stage III or IV disease. The local control rates after a complete resection and adjuvant radiation therapy range from 65% to 100% and are lower for radiation therapy after incomplete resection.[118,248,249,251,252] In contrast, Kondo and Monden reported a large multi-institutional, retrospective study of 1320 patients with stage II or III thymic epithelial tumors for whom no significant benefit of adjuvant irradiation after surgery was found.[26] Preoperative irradiation for patients who present with extensive disease produced response rates as high as 80%.[107,118,248]

Primary radiation therapy has been administered occasionally to patients with unresectable disease. Irradiation alone may result in approximately 65% local control and a 5-year survival rate of 40% to 50%.[252,253] There appears to be no significant difference in relapse rate or survival between patients undergoing biopsy and radiation therapy and those receiving subtotal resection and radiation therapy.[249] However, the most common approach for advanced thymomas is a combined-modality approach, and irradiation is rarely used alone. Salvage radiation therapy for patients with recurrent thymoma may achieve a 7-year survival rate of approximately 70%.[254]

In patients with advanced thymoma, combination chemotherapy can produce overall response rates up to 60%.[255] Cisplatin-containing regimens appear the most promising, and they are being investigated in an Intergroup trial.[256] The role of chemotherapy as adjuvant therapy after resection has not been established.

In summary, radiation therapy after complete surgical resection is not indicated for patients without tumor capsular extension. Incompletely resected thymoma may be controlled with external beam radiation therapy after maximal surgical debulking. Neoadjuvant chemotherapy may increase the chance for complete surgical resection in patients with locally advanced or unresectable disease at presentation.

Thymic Carcinoma

Similar to the treatment for thymomas, surgery remains the predominant treatment for patients with thymic carcinomas, which are treated similarly to carcinomas found in other body sites. Adjuvant radiation therapy is commonly administered after surgery.[257] There may be a trend toward improved survival and local control with adjuvant therapy, but it is difficult to demonstrate.[31,32] There are reports of promising 5-year overall survival rates of more than 50% for patients who received irradiation after surgery.[31,32,35] Neoadjuvant platinum-based chemotherapy can be considered for patients with marginally resectable cancer.

Thymic Carcinoids

Complete surgical resection is the preferred method of treatment for thymic carcinoids.[26] The recurrence rate can be as high as 64%, even after complete resection.[26] Irradiation or chemotherapy, or both, after complete resection may improve the rate of local control.[27] The long-term prognosis for patients with thymic carcinoids is often poor.

Pulmonary Carcinoids

Surgery is the primary treatment for typical and atypical pulmonary carcinoids, and the long-term results after complete resection are excellent.[79,257,258] Clinical symptoms such as flushing can be relieved with ondansetron, one of the 5-HT3 antagonists. Somatostatin analogues, inhibitors of neuropeptide release, relieve the symptoms of carcinoids by binding to somatostatin receptors.[259] Long-acting analogues of somatostatin such as octreotide and lanreotide are used to control diarrhea and flushing, and they have an approximately 70% chance of improving the symptoms.

Typical carcinoids do not require adjuvant therapy after curative resection.[77,260] Patients with a tumor greater than 3 cm in diameter, lymph node metastasis, atypical histology, or residual disease may benefit from radiation therapy.[77,261]

Tumor targeting with radioactive somatostatin analogues has been used in patients with carcinoids with inconclusive results.[262] Interferon-α, alone or in combination with octreotide, has resulted in symptomatic relief in some patients.[87,262,263] Chemotherapy results have been inconclusive at best, with a possible role for cisplatin and etoposide in patients with atypical carcinoids.[264-267] Radiation therapy may palliate some of the symptoms in patients with locally advanced or metastatic disease.[268] Adjuvant radiation therapy or systemic chemotherapy may be considered in high-risk patients.

Mesothelioma

Because mesothelioma usually involves the visceral and parietal pleural surfaces of the lung and extends into the pleural lined pulmonary fissures, it can be difficult to perform a complete resection without an extrapleural pneumonectomy (EPP). Most authorities consider EPP to be the surgery of choice for mesothelioma. However, recurrence rates can be high without adjunctive therapy. Modern treatment techniques may have local recurrence rates between 40% and 50% after combined-modality therapy. Sugarbaker and colleagues reported a local recurrence rate of 13% for patients treated with combined-modality therapy. Malignant pleural mesothelioma has a tendency to recur along the tracks of previous chest wall instrumentation,[269] and prophylactic irradiation such as electron fields to the sites of instrumentations may reduce such recurrences.

Chemotherapy for mesothelioma is at best moderately successful.[270] Malignant pleural mesotheliomas are usually incurable with irradiation alone.[271] One factor is the technical difficulty in administering an adequate dose to the desired target volume without causing unacceptable toxicities in normal tissues. Moving targets such as the diaphragm pose added challenge in sparing normal tissues such as the liver. One study[272] described the results of 22 patients treated with pleurectomy or decortication, intraoperative irradiation, and postoperative external beam radiation therapy. The external beam radiation therapy included 3D treatment and IMRT in some patients. Twelve patients also received chemotherapy (i.e., cyclophosphamide, doxorubicin, and cisplatin). The median survival was disappointing at 18 months. There exists no prospective, randomized trial to assist in treatment planning.

A large report described treatment results of 49 patients who underwent EPP.[273] Thirty-five patients received postoperative chemotherapy followed by irradiation.[273] The 3-year overall survival rate was 34%, although almost one third of the patients had local recurrences. Memorial Sloan-Kettering Cancer Center[274] also reported the treatment results of 54 patients who underwent EPP followed by radiation therapy. Irradiation was directed to the ipsilateral hemithorax. Thirteen percent of patients had locoregional recurrences. Another 40% of patients had peritoneal recurrence.

Incorporation of modern irradiation techniques such as IMRT after EPP has been reported from the M. D. Anderson Cancer Center.[275] The target volume was delineated using CT scans and surgical clips to cover the entire hemithorax, drain sites, ipsilateral mediastinum, and the insertion of the diaphragm. The 2-year survival rate was 62%, with no in-field failures. Although partial pleurectomy followed by postoperative irradiation may have less treatment-related morbidity, EPP followed by chemotherapy and irradiation appears to be significantly more effective in controlling the disease.

Radiation therapy can provide effective palliation for patients with malignant pleural mesothelioma. Most patients achieve significant relief of pain when a dose of more than 40 Gy is administered.[276]

REFERENCES

1. Jemal A, Tiwari RC, Murray T, et al: Cancer Statistics, 2004. CA Cancer J Clin 54:8-29, 2004.
2. National Cancer Institute: Surveillance, Epidemiology, and End Results (SEER) Program (http://seer.cancer.gov/csr/1975_2000/sections.html).
3. Warde P, Payne D: Does thoracic irradiation improve survival and local control in limited-stage small-cell carcinoma of the lung? A meta-analysis. J Clin Oncol 10:890-895, 1992.
4. Wynder EL: Tobacco as a cause of lung cancer: some reflections. Am J Epidemiol 146:687-694, 1997.
5. Giovino GA: Epidemiology of tobacco use in the United States. Oncogene 21:7326-7340, 2002.
6. Boffetta P, Agudo A, Ahrens W, et al: Multicenter case-control study of exposure to environmental tobacco smoke and lung cancer in Europe. J Natl Cancer Inst 90:1440-1450, 1998.
7. Blot WJ, McLaughlin JK: Passive smoking and lung cancer risk: what is the story now? J Natl Cancer Inst 90:1416-1417, 1998.
8. Garfinkel L, Stellman SD: Smoking and lung cancer in women: findings in a prospective study. Cancer Res 48:6951, 1988.
9. Kelsen D: Preoperative chemoradiotherapy for esophageal cancer. J Clin Oncol 19:283-285, 2001.
10. Devesa SS, Blot WJ, Fraumeni JF Jr: Changing patterns in the incidence of esophageal and gastric carcinoma in the United States. Cancer 83:2049-2053, 1998.
11. Tavani A, Negri E, Franceschi S, et al: Risk factors for esophageal cancer in lifelong nonsmokers. Cancer Epidemiol Biomarkers Prev 3:387-392, 1994.
12. Vaughan TL, Davis S, Kristal A, et al: Obesity, alcohol, and tobacco as risk factors for cancers of the esophagus and gastric cardia: adenocarcinoma versus squamous cell carcinoma. Cancer Epidemiol Biomarkers Prev 4:85-92, 1995.
13. Stoner GD, Rustgi AK: Biology of esophageal squamous-cell carcinoma. *In* Rustgi AK (ed): Gastrointestinal Cancers: Biology, Diagnosis, and Therapy. Philadelphia, Lippincott-Raven, 1995, pp 141-148.
14. Wynder EL, Bross IJ: A study of etiological factors in cancer of the esophagus. Cancer 14:389-413, 1961.
15. Reid BJ, Thomas CR Jr: Esophageal neoplasms. *In* Yamada T, Alpers DH, Owyang C, et al (eds): Textbook of Gastroenterology, 2nd ed. Philadelphia, JB Lippincott, 1995, pp 1256-1283.
16. Blot WJ, Devesa SS, Kneller RW, et al: Rising incidence of adenocarcinoma of the esophagus and gastric cardia. JAMA 265:1287, 1991.
17. Weiss MM, Kuipers EJ, Hermsen MA, et al: Barrett's adenocarcinomas resemble adenocarcinomas of the gastric cardia in terms of chromosomal copy number changes, but relate to squamous cell carcinomas of the distal oesophagus with respect to the presence of high-level amplifications. J Pathol 199:157-165, 2003.
18. Davis RD, Oldham HN, Sabiston DC: Primary cysts and neoplasms of the mediastinum: recent changes in clinical presentation, methods of diagnosis, management, and results. Ann Thorac Surg 44:229-237, 1987.
19. Mullen B, Richardson JD: Primary anterior mediastinal tumors in children and adults. Ann Thorac Surg 42:338-345, 1986.

20. Engels EA, Pfeiffer RM: Malignant thymoma in the United States: demographic patterns in incidence and associations with subsequent malignancies. Int J Cancer 105:546-551, 2003.
21. Batata MA, Martini N, Nuvos AG, et al: Thymomas: clinicopathologic features, therapy, and prognosis. Cancer 34:389, 1974.
22. LeGolvan DP, Abell MR: Thymomas. Cancer 39:2142, 1977.
23. Suster S, Rosai J: Thymic carcinoma. A clinicopathologic study of 60 cases. Cancer 67:1025-1032, 1991.
24. Hsu CP, Chen CY, Chen CL, et al: Thymic carcinoma. Ten years' experience in twenty patients. J Thorac Cardiovasc Surg 107:615-620, 1994.
25. Wick MR, Weiland LH, Scheithauer BW, et al: Primary thymic carcinomas. Am J Surg Pathol 6:613-630, 1982.
26. Kondo K, Monden Y: Therapy for thymic epithelial tumors: a clinical study of 1,320 patients from Japan. Ann Thorac Surg 76:878-884, 2003.
27. Economopoulos GC, Lewis JW, Lee MW, et al: Carcinoid tumors of the thymus. Ann Thorac Surg 50:58-61, 1990.
28. Moran CA, Suster S: Spindle-cell neuroendocrine carcinoma of the thymus: a clinicopathologic and immunohistochemical study of seven cases. Mod Pathol 12:587-591, 1999.
29. Travis WD, Linnoila RI, Tsokos MG, et al: Neuroendocrine tumors of the lung with proposed criteria for large-cell neuroendocrine carcinoma: an ultrastructural, immunohistochemical, and flow cytometric study of 35 cases. Am J Surg Pathol 15:529-553, 1991.
30. Mendonca C, Baptista C, Ramos M: Typical and atypical lung carcinoids: clinical and morphological diagnosis. Microsc Res Tech 38:468-472, 1997.
31. Martini N, Zaman MB, Bains MS, et al: Treatment and prognosis in bronchial carcinoids involving regional lymph nodes. J Thorac Cardiovasc Surg 107:1-6, discussion 6-7, 1994.
32. Modlin IM, Lye KD, Kidd M: A 5-decade analysis of 13,715 carcinoid tumors. Cancer 97:934-959, 2003.
33. Godwin JD 2nd: Carcinoid tumors: an analysis of 2,837 cases. Cancer 36:560-569, 1975.
34. Connelly RR, Spirtas R, Myers MH, et al: Demographic patterns for mesothelioma in the United States. J Natl Cancer Inst 78:1053-1060, 1997.
35. Wistuba II, Mao L, Gazdar AF: Smoking molecular damage in bronchial epithelium. Oncogene 21:7298-7306, 2002.
36. Nacht M, Dracheva T, Gao Y, et al: Molecular characteristics of non-small cell lung cancer. Proc Natl Acad Sci U S A 98:15203-15208, 2001.
37. Rodenhuis S, van de Wetering ML, Mooi WJ, et al: Mutational activation of the K-ras oncogene. A possible pathogenic factor in adenocarcinoma of the lung. N Engl J Med 317:929-935, 1987.
38. Mitsudomi T, Steinberg SM, Oie HK, et al: Ras gene mutations in non-small cell lung cancers are associated with shortened survival irrespective of treatment intent. Cancer Res 51:4999-5002, 1991.
39. Graziano SL, Gamble GP, Newman NB, et al: Prognostic significance of K-ras codon 12 mutations in patients with resected stage I and II non-small-cell lung cancer. J Clin Oncol 17:668-675, 1999.
40. Khuri FR, Wu H, Lee JJ, et al: Cyclooxygenase-2 overexpression is a marker of poor prognosis in stage I non-small cell lung cancer. Clin Cancer Res 7:861-867, 2001.
41. Tang X, Khuri FR, Lee JJ, et al: Hypermethylation of the death-associated protein (DAP) kinase promoter and aggressiveness in stage I non-small-cell lung cancer. J Natl Cancer Inst 92:1511-1516, 2000.
42. Tomiyasu M, Yoshino I, Suemitsu R, et al: Quantification of macrophage migration inhibitory factor mRNA expression in non-small cell lung cancer tissues and its clinical significance. Clin Cancer Res 8:3755-3760, 2002.
43. Soria JC, Moon C, Kemp BL, et al: Lack of interleukin-10 could predict poor outcome in patients with stage I non-small-cell lung cancer. Clin Cancer Res 9:1785-1791, 2003.
44. Testa JR: Chromosome alterations in human lung cancer. *In* Pass HI, Mitchell JB, Johnson DH, Turrisi AT (eds): Lung Cancer: Principles and Practice. Philadelphia, Lippincott-Raven, 1996, pp 55-71.
45. Hibi K, Takahashi T, Yamakawa K, et al: Three distinct regions involved in 3p deletion in human lung cancer. Oncogene 7:445-449, 1992.
46. Harbour JW, Lai SL, Whang-Peng J, et al: Abnormalities in structure and expression of the human retinoblastoma gene in SCLC. Science 241:353-357, 1988.
47. Harpole DH Jr, Marks JR, Richards WG, et al: Localized adenocarcinoma of the lung: oncogene expression of erbB-2 and p53 in 150 patients. Clin Cancer Res 1:659-664, 1995.
48. Gazdar A: The molecular and cellular basis of human lung cancer. Anticancer Res 13:261-268, 1994.
49. Lu SH, Hsieh LL, Luo FC, et al: Amplification of the EGF receptor and c-myc genes in human esophageal cancers. Int J Cancer 42:502-505, 1988.
50. Mukaida H, Toi M, Hirai T, et al: Clinical significance of the expression of epidermal growth factor and its receptor in esophageal cancer. Cancer 68:142-148, 1991.
51. Iihara K, Shiozaki H, Tahara H, et al: Prognostic significance of transforming growth factor-alpha in human esophageal carcinoma: implication for autocrine proliferation. Cancer 71:2902-2909, 1993.
52. Lam AK: Molecular biology of esophageal squamous cell carcinoma. Crit Rev Oncol Hematol 33:71-90, 2000.
53. Varis A, Puolakkainen P, Savolainen H, et al: DNA copy number profiling in esophageal Barrett adenocarcinoma: comparison with gastric adenocarcinoma and esophageal squamous cell carcinoma. Cancer Genet Cytogenet 127:53-58, 2001.
54. Beilstein M, Silberg D: Cellular and molecular mechanisms responsible for progression of Barrett's metaplasia to esophageal carcinoma. Gastroenterol Clin North Am 31:461-479, 2002.
55. Jenkins GJ, Doak SH, Parry JM, et al: Genetic pathways involved in the progression of Barrett's metaplasia to adenocarcinoma. Br J Surg 89:824-837, 2002.
56. Shinohara M, Aoki T, Sato S, et al: Cell cycle-regulated factors in esophageal cancer. Dis Esophagus 15:149-154, 2002.
57. Souza RF, Morales CP, Spechler SJ: A conceptual approach to understanding the molecular mechanisms of cancer development in Barrett's oesophagus [review]. Aliment Pharmacol Ther 15:1087-1100, 2001.
58. Casson AG, Mukhopadhyay T, Cleary KR, et al: Oncogene activation in esophageal cancer. J Thorac Cardiovasc Surg 102:707-709, 1991.
59. Galiana C, Lozano JC, Bancel B, et al: High frequency of Ki-ras amplification and p53 gene mutations in adenocarcinomas of the human esophagus. Mol Carcinog 14:286-293,1995.
60. Patton DP, Ribeiro RC, Jenkins JJ, et al: Thymic carcinoma with a defective Epstein-Barr virus encoding the BZLF1 transactivator. J Infect Dis 170:7-12, 1994.
61. Jensen MO, Antonenko D: Thyroid and thymic malignancy following childhood irradiation. J Surg Oncol 50:206-208, 1992.
62. Lee ACW, Kwong YL, Fu KH, et al: Disseminated mediastinal carcinoma with chromosomal translocation (15:19). Cancer 72:2273-2276, 1993.
63. Herens C, Radermecker M, Servais A, et al: Deletion (6)(p22p25) is a recurrent anomaly of thymoma: report of a second case and review of the literature. Cancer Genet Cytogenet 146:66-69, 2003.
64. Hayashi Y, Ishii N, Obayashi C, et al: Thymoma: tumour type related to expression of epidermal growth factor (EGF), EGF-receptor, p53, v-erb B and ras p21. Virchows Arch 426:43-50, 1995.
65. Jung KJ, Lee KS, Han J, et al: Malignant thymic epithelial tumors: CT-pathologic correlation. AJR Am J Roentgenol 176:433-439, 2001.
66. Zhang Z, Cui Y, Li B, et al: Thymic carcinoma (report of 14 cases). Chin Med Sci J 12:252-255, 1997.
67. Henley JD, Koukoulis GK, Loehrer PJ Sr: Epidermal growth factor receptor expression in invasive thymoma. J Cancer Res Clin Oncol 128:167-170, 2002.
68. Fukai I, Masaoka A, Hashimoto T, et al: Cytokeratins in normal thymus and thymic epithelial tumors. Cancer 71:99-105, 1993.
69. Oyama T, Osaki T, Mitsudomi T, et al: P53 alteration, proliferating cell nuclear antigen, and nucleolar organizer regions in thymic epithelial tumors. Int J Mol Med 1:823-826, 1998.
70. Hishima T, Fukayama M, Hayashi Y, et al: CD70 expression in thymic carcinoma. Am J Surg Pathol 24:742-746, 2000.

71. Fukai I, Masaoka A, Hashimoto T, et al: The distribution of epithelial membrane antigen in thymic epithelial neoplasms. Cancer 70:2077-2081, 1992.
72. Mendonca C, Baptista C, Ramos M: Typical and atypical lung carcinoids: clinical and morphological diagnosis. Microsc Res Tech 38:468-472, 1997.
73. Feldman JM, O'Dorisio TM: Role of neuropeptides and serotonin in the diagnosis of carcinoid tumors. Am J Med 81:41-48, 1986.
74. Sandler M, Karim SM, Williams ED: Prostaglandins in amine-peptide-secreting tumours. Lancet 2:1053-1054, 1968.
75. Skrabanek P, Cannon D, Kirrane J, et al: Substance P secretion by carcinoid tumours. Irish J Med Sci 147:47-49, 1978.
76. Lucas KJ, Feldman JM: Flushing in the carcinoid syndrome and plasma kallikrein. Cancer 58:2290-2293, 1986.
77. Kaplan B, Stevens CW, Allen P, et al: Outcomes and patterns of failure in bronchial carcinoid tumors. Int J Radiat Oncol Biol Phys 55:125-131, 2003.
78. Thomas CF Jr, Tazelaar HD, Jett JR: Typical and atypical pulmonary carcinoids: outcome in patients presenting with regional lymph node involvement. Chest 119:1143-1150, 2001.
79. Fink G, Krelbaum T, Yellin A, et al: Pulmonary carcinoid: presentation, diagnosis, and outcome in 142 cases in Israel and review of 640 cases from the literature. Chest 119:1647-1651, 2001.
80. Marty-Ane CH, Costes V, Pujol JL, et al: Carcinoid tumors of the lung: do atypical features require aggressive management? Ann Thorac Surg 59:78-83, 1995.
81. Smolle-Juttner FM, Popper H, Klemen H, et al: Clinical features and therapy of "typical" and "atypical" bronchial carcinoid tumors (grade 1 and grade 2 neuroendocrine carcinoma). Eur J Cardiothorac Surg 7:121-124, discussion 125, 1993.
82. Sugio K, Osaki T, Oyama T, et al: Genetic alteration in carcinoid tumors of the lung. Ann Thorac Cardiovasc Surg 9:149-154, 2003.
83. Lohmann DR, Fesseler B, Putz B, et al: Infrequent mutations of the p53 gene in pulmonary carcinoid tumors. Cancer Res 53:5797-5801, 1993.
84. Kennedy A: The diagnosis of pulmonary carcinoid tumours. Br J Dis Chest 73:71-80, 1979.
85. Crapanzano JP, Zakowski MF: Diagnostic dilemmas in pulmonary cytology. Cancer 93:364-375, 2001.
86. Laitinen KL, Soini Y, Mattila J, et al: Atypical bronchopulmonary carcinoids show a tendency toward increased apoptotic and proliferative activity. Cancer 88:1590-1598, 2000.
87. Oberg K: Carcinoid tumors: molecular genetics, tumor biology, and update of diagnosis and treatment. Curr Opin Oncol 14:38-45, 2002.
88. Debelenko LV, Brambilla E, Agarwal SK, et al: Identification of MEN1 gene mutations in sporadic carcinoid tumors of the lung. Hum Mol Genet 6:2285-2290, 1997.
89. Thakker RV: Multiple endocrine neoplasia—syndromes of the twentieth century. J Clin Endocrinol Metab 83:2617-2620, 1998.
90. Onuki N, Wistuba II, Travis WD, et al: Genetic changes in the spectrum of neuroendocrine lung tumors. Cancer 85:600-607, 1999.
91. Albain KS, Crowley JJ, LeBlanc M, et al: Determinants of improved outcome in small cell lung cancer: an analysis of the 2,580-patient Southwest Oncology Group database. J Clin Oncol 8:1563-1574, 1990.
92. Souhami RL, Bradbury I, Geddes OM, et al: Prognostic significance of laboratory parameters measured at diagnosis in small cell carcinoma of the lung. Cancer Res 45:2878-2882, 1985.
93. List AF, Hainsworth JD, Davis BV, et al: The syndrome of inappropriate secretion of antidiuretic hormone (SIADH) in small cell lung cancer. J Clin Oncol 4:1191-1198, 1986.
94. Dimopoulos MA, Fernandez JF, Samaan NA, et al: Paraneoplastic Cushing's syndrome as an adverse prognostic factor in patients who die early with small cell carcinoma of the lung. Am J Med 77:851-857, 1984.
95. Patel AM, Davila DG, Peters SG: Paraneoplastic syndromes associated with lung cancer. Mayo Clin Proc 68:278-287, 1993.
96. American Joint Committee on Cancer (AJCC): Manual for Staging of Cancer, 6th ed. Philadelphia, JB Lippincott, 2002, pp 189-204.
97. Stahel RA, Ginsberg R, Havermann K, et al: Staging and prognostic factors in small cell lung cancer: a consensus. Lung Cancer 5:119-126, 1989.
98. Quint LE, Francis IR, Wahl RL, et al: Imaging of lung cancer. *In* Pass F II, Mitchell JB, Johnson DH, Turrisi AT (eds): Lung Cancer: Principles and Practice. Philadelphia, Lippincott-Raven, 1996, pp 437-470.
99. van Overhagen H, Becker CD: Diagnosis and staging of carcinoma of the esophagus and gastroesophageal junction, and detection of postoperative recurrence, by computed tomography. *In* Meyers MA (ed): Neoplasms of the Digestive Tract: Imaging, Staging, and Management. Philadelphia, Lippincott-Raven, 1998, pp 31-48.
100. De Leyn P, Vansteenkiste J, Cuypers P, et al: Role of cervical mediastinoscopy in staging of non-small cell lung cancer without enlarged mediastinal lymph nodes on CT scan. Eur J Cardiothorac Surg 12:706-712, 1997.
101. Kamel EM, Zwahlen D, Wyss MT, et al: Whole-body (18)F-FDG PET improves the management of patients with small cell lung cancer. J Nucl Med 44:1911-1917, 2003.
102. Shure D: Transbronchial biopsy and needle aspiration. Chest 95:1130-1138, 1989.
103. Tio TK: Diagnosis and staging of esophageal carcinoma by endoscopic ultrasound. *In* Meyers MA (ed): Neoplasms of the Digestive Tract: Imaging, Staging, and Management. Philadelphia, Lippincott-Raven, 1998, pp 61-70.
104. Gress FG, Savides TJ, Sandler A, et al: Endoscopic ultrasonography, fine-needle aspiration biopsy guided by endoscopic ultrasonography, and computed tomography in the preoperative staging of non-small cell lung cancer: a comparison study. Ann Intern Med 127:604-612, 1997.
105. Detterbeck FC, Parsons AM: Thymic tumors. Ann Thorac Surg 77:1860-1869, 2004.
106. Morgenthaler TI, Brown LR, Colby TV, et al: Thymoma. Mayo Clin Proc 68:1110-1123, 1993.
107. Maggi G, Casadio C, Cavallo A, et al: Thymoma: results of 241 operated cases. Ann Thorac Surg 51:152-156, 1991.
108. Drachman DB: Myasthenia gravis. N Engl J Med 330:1797-1810, 1994.
109. Hoffman OA, Gillespie DJ, Aughenbaugh GL, et al: Primary mediastinal neoplasms (other than thymoma). Mayo Clin Proc 68:880-891, 1993.
110. Shields TW: Primary tumors and cysts of the mediastinum. *In* Shields TW (ed): General Thoracic Surgery. Philadelphia, Lea & Febiger, 1983, p 927.
111. Wick MR, Rosai J: Neuroendocrine neoplasms of the mediastinum. Semin Diagn Pathol 8:35-51, 1991.
112. Baron RL, Lee JK, Sagel SS, Levitt RG: Computed tomography of the abnormal thymus. Radiology 142:127-134, 1982.
113. Casamassima F, Villari N, Fargnoli R, et al: Magnetic resonance imaging and high-resolution computed tomography in tumors of the lung and the mediastinum. Radiother Oncol 11:21-29, 1988.
114. Shih DF, Wang JS, Tseng HH, et al: Primary pleural thymoma. Arch Pathol Lab Med 121:79-82, 1997.
115. Eng TY, Fuller CD, Jagirdar J, et al: Thymic carcinoma: state of the art review. Int J Radiat Oncol Biol Phys 59:654-664, 2004.
116. Lewis JE, Wick MR, Scheithauer BW, et al: Thymoma: a clinicopathologic review. Cancer 60:2727-2743, 1987.
117. Masaoka A, Monden Y, Nakahara K, Tanioka T: Follow-up study of thymomas with special reference to their clinical stages. Cancer 48:2485-2492, 1981.
118. Cowen D, Richaud P, Mornex F, et al: Thymoma: results of a multicentric retrospective series of 149 non-metastatic irradiated patients and review of the literature. FNCLCC trialists. Federation Nationale des Centres de Lutte Contre le Cancer. Radiother Oncol 34:9-16, 1995.
119. Lee JD, Choe KO, Kim SJ, et al: CT findings in primary thymic carcinoma. J Comput Assist Tomogr 15:429-433, 1991.
120. Tsuchiya R, Koga K, Matsuno Y, et al: Thymic carcinoma: proposal for pathological TNM and staging. Pathol Int 44:505-512, 1994.
121. Beasley MB, Thunnissen FB, Brambilla E, et al: Pulmonary atypical carcinoid: predictors of survival in 106 cases. Hum Pathol 31:1255-1265, 2000.

122. Oliveira AM, Tazelaar HD, Myers JL, et al: Thyroid transcription factor-1 distinguishes metastatic pulmonary from well-differentiated neuroendocrine tumors of other sites. Am J Surg Pathol 25:815-819, 2001.
123. Modlin IM, Sandor A: An analysis of 8305 cases of carcinoid tumors. Cancer 79:813-829, 1997.
124. Schrevens L, Vansteenkiste J, Deneffe G, et al: Clinical-radiological presentation and outcome of surgically treated pulmonary carcinoid tumours: a long-term single institution experience. Lung Cancer 43:39-45, 2004.
125. Soga J, Yakuwa Y: Bronchopulmonary carcinoids: an analysis of 1,875 reported cases with special reference to a comparison between typical carcinoids and atypical varieties. Ann Thorac Cardiovasc Surg 5:211-219, 1999.
126. Musi M, Carbone RG, Bertocchi C, et al: Bronchial carcinoid tumours: a study on clinicopathological features and role of octreotide scintigraphy. Lung Cancer 22:97-102, 1998.
127. Kaltsas G, Korbonits M, Heintz E, et al: Comparison of somatostatin analog and meta-iodobenzylguanidine radionuclides in the diagnosis and localization of advanced neuroendocrine tumors. J Clin Endocrinol Metab 86:895-902, 2001.
128. Anderson CJ, Dehdashti F, Cutler PD, et al: 64Cu-TETA-octreotide as a PET imaging agent for patients with neuroendocrine tumors. J Nucl Med 42:213-221, 2001.
129. Renshaw AA, Dean BR, Antman KH, et al: The role of cytologic evaluation of pleural fluid in the diagnosis of malignant mesothelioma. Chest 111:106-109, 1997.
130. Marks LB: The impact of organ structure on radiation response. Int J Radiat Oncol Biol Phys 34:1165-1171, 1996.
131. Patti MG, Gantert W, Way IW: Surgery of the esophagus: anatomy and physiology. Surg Clin North Am 77:959-970, 1997.
132. Goldstein HM, Rogers LF, Fletcher GH, Dodd GD: Radiological manifestations of radiation-induced injury to the normal upper gastrointestinal tract. Radiology 117:135-140, 1975.
133. Werner-Wasik M, Scott C, Curran WJ Jr, Byhardt R: Correlation between acute esophagitis and late pneumonitis in patients (pts) with locally advanced non-small cell lung cancer (LANSCLC) receiving concurrent thoracic radiotherapy (RT) and chemotherapy: a multivariate analysis of the Radiation Therapy Oncology Group (RTOG) database [abstract 1192]. Proc Am Soc Clin Oncol 21:299a, 2002.
134. Vokes EE, Leopold KA, Herndon JE, et al: A randomized phase II study of gemcitabine or paclitaxel or vinorelbine with cisplatin as induction chemotherapy and concomitant chemoradiotherapy for unresectable stage III non-small cell lung cancer (NSCLC) [abstract]. Proc Am Soc Clin Oncol 18:459a, 1999.
135. Werner-Wasik M, Pequignot E, Leeper D, et al: Predictors of severe esophagitis include use of concurrent chemotherapy, but not the length of irradiated esophagus: a multivariate analysis of patients with lung cancer treated with non-operative therapy. Int J Radiat Oncol Biol Phys 48:689-696, 2000.
136. Emami B: Three-dimensional conformal radiation therapy in bronchogenic carcinoma. Semin Radiat Oncol 6:92-97, 1996.
137. Singh AK, Lockett MA, Bradley JD: Predictors of radiation-induced esophageal toxicity in patients with non-small cell lung cancer treated with three-dimensional conformal radiotherapy. Int J Radiat Oncol Biol Phys 55:337-341, 2003.
138. Movasa B, Scott C, Langer C, et al: Phase III study of amifostine in patients with locally advanced non-small cell lung cancer (NSCLC) receiving chemotherapy and hyperfractionated radiation (chemo/HfxRT): Radiation Therapy Oncology Group (RTOG) 98-01 [abstract 2559]. Proc Am Soc Clin Oncol 22:636, 2003.
139. Schultheiss TE, Stephens LC, Peters LJ: Survival in radiation myelopathy. Int J Radiat Oncol Biol Phys 12:1765-1769, 1986.
140. Lambert PM: Radiation myelopathy of the thoracic spinal cord in long-term survivors treated with radical radiotherapy using conventional fractionation. Cancer 41:1751-1760, 1978.
141. Werner-Wasik M, Yu X, Marks LB, Schultheiss TE: Normal-tissue toxicities of thoracic radiation therapy: esophagus, lung, and spinal cord as organs at risk. Hematol Oncol Clin N Am 18:131-160, 2004.
142. Schultheiss TE, Higgins EM, El-Mahdi AM: The latent period in clinical radiation myelopathy. Int J Radiat Oncol Biol Phys 10:1109-1115, 1984.
143. Dorfman LJ, Donaldson SS, Gupta PR, Bosley TM: Electrophysiologic evidence of subclinical injury to the posterior columns of the human spinal cord after therapeutic radiation. Cancer 50:2815-2819, 1982.
144. Marcus RG, Million RR: The incidence of myelitis after irradiation of the cervical spinal cord. Int J Radiat Oncol Biol Phys 19:3-8, 1990.
145. Ang KK, Jiang GL, Feng Y, et al: Extent and kinetics of recovery of occult spinal cord injury. Int J Radiat Oncol Biol Phys 50:1013-1020, 2001.
146. Movsas B, Raffin TA, Epstein AH, et al: Pulmonary radiation injury. Chest 111:1061-1076, 1997.
147. Roach M III, Gandara DR, Yuo H-S, et al: Radiation peritonitis following combined-modality therapy for lung cancer: analysis of prognostic factors. J Clin Oncol 13:2606-2612, 1995.
148. Rubin P, Casarett GW: Clinical Radiation Pathology, vol 1. Philadelphia, WB Saunders, 1968, pp 423-470.
149. Byhardt RW, Martin L, Pajak TF, et al: The influence of field size and other treatment factors on pulmonary toxicity following hyperfractionated irradiation for inoperable non-small cell lung cancer (NSCLC)—analysis of a Radiation Therapy Oncology Group (RTOG) protocol. Int J Radiat Oncol Biol Phys 27:537-544, 1993.
150. Maguire PD, Marks LB, Sibley GS, et al: 73.6 Gy and beyond: hyperfractionated, accelerated radiotherapy for non-small-cell lung cancer. J Clin Oncol 19:705-711, 2001.
151. Abratt RP, Bezwoda WR, Goedhals L, et al: Weekly gemcitabine with monthly cisplatin: effective chemotherapy for advanced non-small cell lung cancer. J Clin Oncol 15:744-749, 1997.
152. Graham MV, Purdy JA, Emami B, et al: Clinical dose-volume histogram analysis for pneumonitis after 3D treatment for NSCLC. Int J Radiat Oncol Biol Phys 45:323-329, 1999.
153. Abratt RP, Morgan GW, Silvestri G, Wilcox P: Pulmonary complications of radiotherapy. Clin Chest Med 25:167-177, 2004.
154. Travis EL, Harley RA, Fenn JO, et al: Pathologic changes in the lung following single and multifraction irradiation. Int J Radiat Oncol Biol Phys 2:475-490, 1977.
155. Rubin P, Johnston CJ, Williams JP, et al: A perpetual cascade of cytokines postirradiation leads to pulmonary fibrosis. Int J Radiat Oncol Biol Phys 33:99-109, 1995.
156. Rodemarm HP, Bamberg M: Cellular basis of radiation-induced fibrosis. Radiother Oncol 35:83-90, 1995.
157. Sempowski GD, Chess PR, Phipps RP: CD40 is a functional activation antigen and B7-independent T cell costimulatory molecule on normal human lung fibroblasts. J Immunol 158:4670-4677, 1997.
158. Fries KM, Sempowski GD, Gaspari AA, et al: CD-40 expression by human fibroblasts. Clin Immunol Immunopathol 77:42-51, 1995.
159. Anscher M, Kong F, Andrews K, et al: Plasma transforming growth factor β-1 as a predictor of radiation pneumonitis. Int J Radiat Oncol Biol Phys 41:1029-1036, 1998.
160. Hancock SL, Tucker MA, Hoppe RT: Factors affecting late mortality from heart disease after treatment for Hodgkin's disease. JAMA 270:1949-1955, 1993.
161. Paszat LF, Mackillop WJ, Groome PA: Mortality from myocardial infarction following postlumpectomy radiotherapy for breast cancer: population-based study in Ontario, Canada. Int J Radiat Oncol Biol Phys 43:755-762, 1999.
162. Hicks GL Jr: Coronary artery operation in radiation-associated atherosclerosis: long-term follow-up. Ann Thorac Surg 53:670-674, 1992.
163. Cameron EH, Lipshultz SE, Tarbell NJ: Cardiovascular disease in long-term survivors of pediatric Hodgkin's disease. Prog Pediatr Cardiol 8:139-144, 1998.
164. Adams MJ, Lipshultz SE, Schwartz C, et al: Radiation-associated cardiovascular disease: manifestations and management. Semin Radiat Oncol 13:346-356, 2003.
165. Hardenbergh PH, Munley MT, Bentel GC: Cardiac perfusion changes in patients treated for breast cancer with radiation

therapy and doxorubicin: preliminary results. Int J Radiat Oncol Biol Phys 49:1023-1028, 2001.
166. Stewart JR, Fajardo LF: Radiation-induced heart disease: an update. Prog Cardiovasc Dis 27:173-194, 1984.
167. Lund MB, Ihlen H, Voss BM: Increased risk of heart valve regurgitation after mediastinal radiation for Hodgkin's disease: an echocardiographic study. Heart 75:591-595, 1996.
168. Coia LR, Minsky BD, John MJ, et al: The evaluation and treatment of patients receiving radiation therapy for carcinoma of the esophagus: results of the 1992-1994 Patterns of Care Study. Cancer 85:2499-2505, 1999.
169. Muller JM, Erasmi H, Stelzner M, et al: Surgical therapy of oesophageal carcinoma. Br J Surg 77:845-857, 1990.
170. Chu KM, Law SY, Fok M, et al: A prospective randomized comparison of transhiatal and transthoracic resection for lower-third esophageal carcinoma. Am J Surg 174:320-324, 1997.
171. Skinner DB: En bloc resection for neoplasms of the esophagus and cardia. J Thorac Cardiovasc Surg 85:59-71, 1983.
172. Isono K, Ochiai T, Okuyama K, et al: The treatment of lymph node metastasis from esophageal cancer by extensive lymphadenectomy. Jpn J Surg 20:151-157, 1990.
173. Hulscher JB, Tijssen JG, Obertop H, et al: Transthoracic versus transhiatal resection for carcinoma of the esophagus: a meta-analysis. Ann Thorac Surg 72:306-313, 2001.
174. Goldminc M, Maddern G, Le Prise E, et al: Oesophagectomy by a transhiatal approach or thoracotomy: a prospective randomized trial. Br J Surg 80:367-370, 1993.
175. Chu KM, Law SY, Fok M, et al: A prospective randomized comparison of transhiatal and transthoracic resection for lower-third esophageal carcinoma. Am J Surg 174:320-324, 1997.
176. Okawa T, Kita M, Tanaka M, et al: Results of radiotherapy for inoperable locally advanced esophageal cancer. Int J Radiat Oncol Biol Phys 17:49-54, 1989.
177. Nygaard K, Hagen S, Hansen HS, et al: Pre-operative radiotherapy prolongs survival in operable esophageal carcinoma: a randomized, multicenter study of pre-operative radiotherapy and chemotherapy. The second Scandinavian trial in esophageal cancer. World J Surg 16:1104-1110, 1992.
178. Arnott SJ, Duncan W, Kerr GR, et al: Low dose preoperative radiotherapy for carcinoma of the oesophagus: results of a randomized clinical trial. Radiother Oncol 24:108-113, 1992.
179. Wang M, Gu XZ, Yin WB, et al: Randomized clinical trial on the combination of preoperative irradiation and surgery in the treatment of esophageal carcinoma: report on 206 patients. Int J Radiat Oncol Biol Phys 16:325-327, 1989.
180. Arnott SJ, Duncan W, Gignoux M, et al: Preoperative radiotherapy in esophageal carcinoma: a meta-analysis using individual patient data (Oesophageal Cancer Collaborative Group). Int J Radiat Oncol Biol Phys 41:579-583, 1998.
181. Fok M, Sham JS, Choy D, et al: Postoperative radiotherapy for carcinoma of the esophagus: a prospective, randomized controlled study. Surgery 113:138-147, 1993.
182. Teniere P, Hay JM, Fingerhut A, et al: Postoperative radiation therapy does not increase survival after curative resection for squamous cell carcinoma of the middle and lower esophagus as shown by a multicenter controlled trial. French University Association for Surgical Research. Surg Gynecol Obstet 173:123-130, 1991.
183. Kelsen DP, Ginsberg R, Pajak T, et al: Chemotherapy followed by surgery compared with surgery alone for localized esophageal cancer. N Engl J Med 339:1979-1984, 1998.
184. Kok TC, Lanschot JV, Siersema PD, et al: Neoadjuvant chemotherapy in operable esophageal squamous cell cancer: final report of a phase III multi-center randomized control trial [abstract]. Proc Am Soc Clin Oncol 16:277, 1997.
185. Roth JA, Pass HI, Flanagan MM, et al: Randomized clinical trial of preoperative and postoperative adjuvant chemotherapy with cisplatin, vindesine, and bleomycin for carcinoma of the esophagus. J Thorac Cardiovasc Surg 96:242-248, 1988.
186. Schlag P: Randomized trial of preoperative chemotherapy in squamous cell cancer of the esophagus. CAO Esophageal Cancer Study Group [in German]. Chirurgie 63:709-714, 1992.
187. Medical Research Council Oesophageal Cancer Working Group: Surgical resection with or without preoperative chemotherapy in oesophageal cancer: a randomised controlled trial. Lancet 359:1727-1733, 2002.
188. Japanese Esophageal Oncology Group (JCOG): A comparison of chemotherapy and radiotherapy as adjuvant treatment to surgery for esophageal carcinoma. Chest 104:203-220, 1993.
189. Lizuka T, Isono K, Watanabe H, et al: A randomized trial comparing surgery to surgery plus postoperative chemotherapy for localized squamous carcinoma of the thoracic esophagus: The Japan Clinical Oncology Group (JCOG) study [abstract]. Proc Am Soc Clin Oncol 17:282, 1998.
190. Ando N, Iizuka T, Ide H, et al: A randomized trial of surgery alone vs surgery plus postoperative chemotherapy with cisplatin and 5-fluorouracil for localized squamous carcinoma of the thoracic esophagus: the Japan Clinical Oncology Group study (JCOG 9204) [abstract]. Proc Am Soc Clin Oncol 18:269a, 1999.
191. Al-Sarraf M, Martz K, Herskovic A, et al: Progress report of combined chemoradiotherapy versus radiotherapy alone in patients with esophageal cancer: an intergroup study. J Clin Oncol 15:277-284, 1997.
192. Cooper JS, Guo MD, Herskovic A, et al: Chemoradiotherapy of locally advanced esophageal cancer: long-term follow-up of a prospective randomized trial (RTOG 85-01). Radiation Therapy Oncology Group. JAMA 281:1623-1627, 1999.
193. Minsky BD, Pajak TF, Ginsberg RJ, et al: INT 0123 (Radiation Therapy Oncology Group 94-05) phase III trial of combined-modality therapy for esophageal cancer: high-dose versus standard-dose radiation therapy. J Clin Oncol 20:1167-1174, 2002.
194. Urba SG, Orringer MB, Turrisi A, et al: A randomized trial of preoperative chemoradiation versus surgery alone in patients with locoregional esophageal carcinoma. J Clin Oncol 19:305-313, 2001.
195. Walsh TN, Noonan N, Hollywood D, et al: A comparison of multimodal therapy and surgery for esophageal adenocarcinoma. N Engl J Med 335:462-467, 1996.
196. Bosset JF, Gignoux M, Triboulet JP, et al: Chemoradiotherapy followed by surgery compared with surgery alone in squamous-cell cancer of the esophagus. N Engl J Med 337:161-168, 1997.
197. Burmeister BH, Smithers BM, Fitzgerald L, et al: A randomized phase III trial of preoperative chemoradiation followed by surgery (CR-S) versus surgery alone (S) for localized resectable cancer of the esophagus [abstract 518]. Proc Am Soc Clin Oncol 21:130a, 2002.
198. Bedenne L, Michel P, Bouche O, et al: Randomized phase III trial in locally advanced esophageal cancer: radiochemotherapy followed by surgery versus radiochemotherapy alone (FFCD 9102) [abstract]. Proc Am Soc Clin Oncol 21:130a, 2002.
199. Stahl M, Stuschke M, Lehmann N, et al: Chemoradiation with and without surgery in patients with locally advanced squamous cell carcinoma of the esophagus. J Clin Oncol 23:2310-2317, 2005.
200. Ginsberg RJ, Rubinstein IV: Randomized trial of lobectomy versus limited resection for T1 N0 non-small cell lung cancer. Lung Cancer Study Group. Ann Thorac Surg 60:615-622, 1995.
201. Gandara DR, Chansky K, Albain KS, et al: Consolidation docetaxel after concurrent chemoradiotherapy in stage IIIB non-small-cell lung cancer: phase II Southwest Oncology Group study S9504. J Clin Oncol 21:2004-2010, 2003.
202. Non-Small Cell Lung Cancer Collaborative Group: Chemotherapy in non-small cell lung cancer: a meta-analysis using updated data on individual patients from 52 randomised clinical trials. BMJ 311:899-909, 1995.
203. The International Adjuvant Lung Cancer Trial Collaborative Group: Cisplatin-based adjuvant chemotherapy in patients with completely resected non-small-cell lung cancer. N Engl J Med 350:351-360, 2004.
204. Keller SM, Adak S, Wagner H, et al: A randomized trial of postoperative adjuvant therapy in patients with completely resected II or IIIA non-small-cell lung cancer. N Engl J Med 343:1217-1222, 2000.
205. Depierre A, Milleron B, Moro-Sibilot D, et al: Preoperative chemotherapy followed by surgery compared with primary surgery in resectable stage I (except T1N0), II, and IIIA non-small-cell lung cancer. J Clin Oncol 20:247-253, 2002.

206. Schiller JH, Harrington D, Belani CP, et al: Comparison of four chemotherapy regimens for advanced non-small-cell lung cancer. N Engl J Med 346:92-98, 2002.
207. Kosmidis P, Mylonakis N, Nicolaides C, et al: Paclitaxel plus carboplatin versus gemcitabine plus paclitaxel in advanced non-small-cell lung cancer: a phase III randomized trial. J Clin Oncol 20:3578-3585, 2002.
208. Kelly K, Crowley J, Bunn PA Jr, et al: Randomized phase III trial of paclitaxel plus carboplatin versus vinorelbine plus cisplatin in the treatment of patients with advanced non-small-cell lung cancer: a Southwest Oncology Group trial. J Clin Oncol 19:3210-3218, 2001.
209. Herbst RS, Giaccone G, Schiller JH, et al: Gefitinib in combination with paclitaxel and carboplatin in advanced non-small-cell lung cancer: a phase III trial-INTACT2. J Clin Oncol 22:785-794, 2004.
210. DeVore RF, Fehrenbacher L, Herbst RS, et al: A randomized phase II trial comparing RhuMab VEGF (recombinant humanized monoclonal antibody to vascular endothelial cell growth factor) plus carboplatin/paclitaxel (CP) to CP alone in patients with stage IIIB/IV NSCLC [abstract 1896]. Proc Am Soc Clin Oncol 19:485a, 2000.
211. Fossella FV, DeVore R, Kerr RN, et al: Randomized phase III trial of docetaxel versus vinorelbine or ifosfamide in patients with advanced non-small cell lung cancer previously treated with platinum-containing chemotherapy regimens. The TAX 320 Non-Small Cell Lung Cancer Study Group. J Clin Oncol 18:2354-2362, 2000.
212. Hanna NH, Shepherd FA, Foselta FV, et al: Randomized phase III study of pemetrexed vs docetaxel in patients with non-small cell lung cancer previously treated with chemotherapy. J Clin Oncol 22:1589-1597, 2004.
213. Perez CA, Bauer M, Edelstein S, et al: Impact of tumor control on survival in carcinoma of the lung treated with irradiation. Int J Radiat Oncol Biol Phys 12:539-547, 1986.
214. Robertson JM, Ten Haken RK, Hazuka MB, et al: Dose escalation for non-small cell lung cancer using conformal radiation therapy. Int J Radiat Oncol Biol Phys 37:1079-1085, 1997.
215. Graham MV, Purdy JA, Emami B, et al: 3-D conformal radiotherapy for lung cancer: the Washington University experience. Front Radiat Ther Oncol 29:188-198, 1996.
216. Morita K, Fuwa N, Suzuki Y, et al: Radical radiotherapy for medically inoperable non-small cell lung cancer in clinical stage I: a retrospective analysis of 149 patients. Radiother Oncol 42:31-36, 1997.
217. Sibley GS, Jamieson TA, Marks LB, et al: Radiotherapy alone for medically inoperable stage I non-small cell lung cancer: the Duke experience. Int J Radiat Oncol Biol Phys 40:149-154, 1998.
218. Timmerman RD, Papiez L, McGarry R, et al: Extracranial stereotactic radioablation: results of a phase I study in medically inoperable stage I non-small cell lung cancer. Chest 124:1946-1955, 2003.
219. Warram J: Preoperative irradiation of cancer of the lung: final report of a therapeutic trial. A Collaborative Study. Cancer 36:914-925, 1975.
220. Postoperative Radiotherapy (PORT) Meta-analysis Trialists Group: Postoperative radiotherapy in non-small cell lung cancer: systematic review and meta-analysis of individual patient data from nine randomised controlled trials. Lancet 352:257-263, 1998.
221. Sawyer TE, Bonner JA, Gould PM, et al: Effectiveness of postoperative irradiation in stage IIIA non-small cell lung cancer according to regression tree analyses of recurrence risks. Ann Thorac Surg 64:1402-1407, 1997.
222. Dillman RO, Herndon J, Seagren SL, et al: Improved survival in stage III non-small-cell lung cancer: seven-year follow-up of cancer and leukemia group B (CALGB) 8433 trial. J Natl Cancer Inst 88:1210-1215, 1996.
223. Sause WT, Scott C, Tayjor S, et al: Radiation Therapy Oncology Group (RTOG) 88-08 and Eastern Cooperative Oncology Group (ECOG) 4588: preliminary results of a phase III trial in regionally advanced, unresectable non-small cell lung cancer. J Natl Cancer Inst 87:198-205, 1995.
224. Furuse K, Fukuoka M, Kawahara M, et al: Phase III study of concurrent versus sequential thoracic radiotherapy in combination with mitomycin, vindesine, and cisplatin in unresectable stage III non-small-cell lung cancer. J Clin Oncol 17:2692-2699, 1999.
225. Curran W, Scott CB, Langer CJ, et al: Long-term benefit is observed in a phase III comparison of sequential vs. concurrent chemoradiation for patients with unresectable stage III NSCLC: RTOG 9410 [abstract 2499]. Proc Am Soc Clin Oncol 22:621, 2003.
226. Albain KS, Scott CB, Rusch VR, et al: Phase III comparison of concurrent chemotherapy plus radiotherapy (CT/RT) and CT/RT followed by surgical resection for stage IIIA (pN2) non-small cell lung cancer (NSCLC): initial results from intergroup trial 0139 (RTOG 93-09) [abstract 2497]. Proc Am Soc Clin Oncol 22:621, 2003.
227. Pignon JP, Arriagada R, Ihde D: Meta-analysis of small-cell lung cancer. N Engl J Med 327:1618-1624, 1992.
228. Warde P, Payne D: Does thoracic irradiation improve survival and local control in limited-stage small-cell carcinoma of the lung? A meta-analysis. J Clin Oncol 10:890-895, 1992.
229. Fried DB, Morris DE, Hensing TA, et al: Timing of thoracic radiation therapy in combined modality therapy for limited-stage small cell lung cancer: a meta-analysis [abstract O-70]. Lung Cancer 41(Suppl 2):23, 2003.
230. Coy P, Hodson I, Payne D, et al: The effect of dose of thoracic irradiation on recurrence in patients with limited stage small cell lung cancer: initial results of a Canadian multicenter randomized trial. Int J Radiat Oncol Biol Phys 14:219-226, 1988.
231. Lichter AS, Turrisi AT: Small cell lung cancer: the influence of dose and treatment volume on outcome. Semin Radiat Oncol 5:44-49, 1995.
232. Komaki R, Shin DM, Glisson BS, et al: Interdigitating versus concurrent chemotherapy and radiotherapy for limited small cell lung cancer. Int J Radiat Oncol Biol Phys 31:807-811, 1995.
233. Turrisi A, Kim K, Blum R, et al: Twice-daily compared with once-daily thoracic radiotherapy in limited small cell lung cancer treated concurrently with cisplatin and etoposide. N Engl J Med 340:265-271, 1999.
234. Schild SE, Bonner JA, Shanahan TG, et al: Long-term results of a phase III trial comparing once-daily radiotherapy with twice-daily radiotherapy in limited stage small-cell lung cancer. Int J Radiat Oncol Biol Phys 59:943-951, 2004.
235. Mira JG, Livingston RB: Evaluation and radiotherapy implications of chest relapse patterns in small cell lung carcinoma treated with radiotherapy-chemotherapy: study of 34 cases and review of the literature. Cancer 46:2557-2565, 1980.
236. Liengswangwong V, Bonner JA, Shaw EG, et al: Limited-stage small cell lung cancer: patterns of intrathoracic recurrence and the implications for thoracic radiotherapy. J Clin Oncol 12:496-502, 1994.
237. Kies MS, Mira JG, Crowley JJ, et al: Multimodal therapy for limited small cell lung cancer: a randomized study of induction combination chemotherapy with or without thoracic radiation in complete responders, and with wide-field versus reduced-field radiation in partial responders. A Southwest Oncology Group study. J Clin Oncol 5:592-600, 1987.
238. Roth BJ, Johnson DH, Einhorn LH: Randomized study of cyclophosphamide plus doxorubicin plus vincristine versus etoposide plus cisplatin versus alternation of these two regimens in extensive small cell lung cancer: a phase II study of the Southeastern Cancer Study Group. J Clin Oncol 10:282-291, 1992.
239. Ettinger D, Seiferheld W, Abrams R, et al: Cisplatin (P) , etoposide (E), paclitaxel (T) and concurrent hyperfractionated thoracic radiotherapy (TRT) for patients (Pts) with limited disease (LD) small cell lung cancer (SCLC): preliminary results of RTOG 96-09 [abstract 1917]. Proceedings of the meeting of American Society of Clinical Oncology, New Orleans, LA. J Clin Oncol 19:490a, 2000.
240. Shields TW, Higgins GA, Matthews MJ, et al: Surgical resection in the management of small cell lung cancer. J Thorac Cardiovasc Surg 84:481-488, 1982.
241. Lad T, Piantadosi S, Thomas P, et al: A prospective randomized trial to determine the benefit of surgical resection of residual disease following response of small cell lung cancer to combination chemotherapy. Chest 106:320-323, 1994.

242. Gregor A: Prophylactic cranial irradiation in small cell lung cancer: is it ever indicated? Oncology 12:19-24, 1998.
243. Arriagada R, LeCahvalier T, Borie F, et al: Prophylactic cranial irradiation for patients with small cell lung cancer in complete remission. J Natl Cancer Inst 87:183-190, 1995.
244. Gregor A, Cull A, Stephens RJ, et al: Effects of prophylactic irradiation for patients with small cell lung cancer in complete response [abstract]. Eur J Cancer 31A:S19, 1995.
245. Auperin A, Arriagada R, Pignon JP, et al, for the Prophylactic Cranial Irradiation (PCI) Overview Collaborative Group: Prophylactic cranial irradiation for patients with small-cell lung cancer in complete remission. N Engl J Med 342:476-484, 1999.
246. Yagi K, Hirata T, Fukuse T, et al: Surgical treatment for invasive thymoma, especially when the superior vena cava is involved. Ann Thorac Surg 61:521-524, 1996.
247. Venuta F, Rendina EA, De Giacomo T, et al: Thymectomy for myasthenia gravis: a 27-year experience. Eur J Cardiothorac Surg 15:621-625, 1999.
248. Curran WJ Jr, Kornstein MJ, Brooks JJ, et al: Invasive thymoma: the role of mediastinal irradiation following complete or incomplete surgical resection. J Clin Oncol 6:1722-1727, 1988.
249. Urgesi A, Monetti U, Rossi G, et al: Role of radiation therapy in locally advanced thymoma. Radiother Oncol 19:273-280, 1990.
250. Mangi AA, Wright CD, Allan JS, et al: Adjuvant radiation therapy for stage II thymoma. Ann Thorac Surg 74:1033-1037, 2002.
251. Haniuda M, Miyazawa M, Yoshida K, et al: Is postoperative radiotherapy for thymoma effective? Ann Surg 224:219-224, 1996.
252. Jackson MA, Ball DL: Postoperative radiotherapy in invasive thymoma. Radiother Oncol 21:77-82, 1991.
253. Thomas CR, Wright CD, Loehrer PJ: Thymoma: state of the art. J Clin Oncol 17:2280-2289, 1999.
254. Urgesi A, Monetti U, Rossi G, et al: Aggressive treatment of intrathoracic recurrences of thymoma. Radiother Oncol 24:221-225, 1992.
255. Giaccone G, Ardizzoni A, Kirkpatrick A, et al: Cisplatinum and etoposide combination chemotherapy for locally advanced or metastatic thymoma. A phase II study of the European Organization for Research and Treatment of Cancer Lung Cancer Cooperative Group. J Clin Oncol 14:814-820, 1996.
256. Loehrer PJ, Jiroutek M, Aisner S, et al: Combined etoposide, ifosfamide, and cisplatinum in the treatment of patients with advanced thymoma and thymic carcinoma: an intergroup trial. Cancer 91:2010-2015, 2001.
257. Filosso PL, Rena O, Donati G, et al: Bronchial carcinoid tumors: surgical management and long-term outcome. J Thorac Cardiovasc Surg 123:303-309, 2002.
258. Terzi A, Lonardoni A, Falezza G, et al: Sleeve lobectomy for non-small cell lung cancer and carcinoids: results in 160 cases. Eur J Cardiothorac Surg 21:888-893, 2002.
259. Kubota A, Yamada Y, Kagimoto S, et al: Identification of somatostatin receptor subtypes and an implication for the efficacy of somatostatin analogue SMS 201-995 in treatment of human endocrine tumors. J Clin Invest 93:1321-1325, 1994.
260. Beasley MB, Thunnissen FB, Brambilla E, et al: Pulmonary atypical carcinoid: predictors of survival in 106 cases. Hum Pathol 31:1255-1265, 2000.
261. Carretta A, Ceresoli GL, Arrigoni G, et al: Diagnostic and therapeutic management of neuroendocrine lung tumors: a clinical study of 44 cases. Lung Cancer 29:217-225, 2000.
262. Granberg D, Eriksson B, Wilander E, et al: Experience in treatment of metastatic pulmonary carcinoid tumors. Ann Oncol 12:1383-1391, 2001.
263. Oberg K, Astrup L, Eriksson B, et al: Guidelines for the management of gastroenteropancreatic neuroendocrine tumours (including bronchopulmonary and thymic neoplasms). Acta Oncol 43:617-625, 2004.
264. Oberg K, Eriksson B: The role of interferons in the management of carcinoid tumours. Br J Haematol 79:74-77, 1991.
265. Bukowski RM, Johnson KG, Peterson RF, et al: A phase II trial of combination chemotherapy in patients with metastatic carcinoid tumors. A Southwest Oncology Group Study. Cancer 60:2891-2895, 1987.
266. Engstrom PF, Lavin PT, Moertel CG, et al: Streptozocin plus fluorouracil versus doxorubicin therapy for metastatic carcinoid tumor. J Clin Oncol 2:1255-1259, 1984.
267. Moertel CG, Hanley JA: Combination chemotherapy trials in metastatic carcinoid tumor and the malignant carcinoid syndrome. Cancer Clin Trials 2:327-334, 1979.
268. Schupak KD, Wallner KE: The role of radiation therapy in the treatment of locally unresectable or metastatic carcinoid tumors. Int J Radiat Oncol Biol Phys 20:489-495, 1991.
269. Van Ooijen B, Eggermont AMM, Wiggers T: Subcutaneous tumor growth complicating the positioning of Denver shunt and intrapleural Port-a-Cath in mesothelioma patients. Eur J Surg Oncol 18:638-640, 1992.
270. Stewart DJ, Edwards JG, Smythe WR, et al: Malignant pleural mesothelioma—an update. Int J Occup Environ Health 10:26-39, 2004.
271. Muers MF, Rudd RM, O'Brien ME, et al, for the British Thoracic Society Mesothelioma Group: BTS randomised feasibility study of active symptom control with or without chemotherapy in malignant pleural mesothelioma: ISRCTN 54469112. Thorax 59:144-148, 2004.
272. Lee TT, Everett DL, Shu HK, et al: Radical pleurectomy/decortication and intraoperative radiotherapy followed by conformal radiation with or without chemotherapy for malignant pleural mesothelioma. J Thorac Cardiovasc Surg 124:1183-1189, 2002.
273. Baldini EH, Recht A, Strauss GM, et al: Patterns of failure after trimodality therapy for malignant pleural mesothelioma. Ann Thorac Surg 63:334-338, 1997.
274. Kutcher GJ, Kestler C, Greenblatt D, et al: Technique for external beam treatment for mesothelioma. Int J Radiat Oncol Biol Phys 13:1747-1752, 1987.
275. Ahamad A, Stevens CW, Smythe WR, et al: Promising early local control of malignant pleural mesothelioma following postoperative intensity modulated radiotherapy (IMRT) to the chest. Cancer J 9:476-484, 2004.
276. Gordon W, Antman KH, Greenberger JS, et al: Radiation therapy in the management of patients with mesothelioma. Int J Radiat Oncol Biol Phys 8:19-25, 1982.

CHAPTER 40

SMALL CELL LUNG CANCER

Steven E. Schild and Walter J. Curran, Jr.

INCIDENCE

Almost 35,000 Americans are diagnosed with small cell lung cancer (SCLC) each year. This represents 15% to 20% of all cases of bronchogenic carcinoma.

PATHOLOGY AND PATHWAYS OF SPREAD

The 2004 World Health Organization classification system describes two variants: small cell carcinoma and combined small cell carcinoma. The latter includes SCLC cells and any of the histologic types of non–small cell lung cancer (NSCLC).

BIOLOGIC CHARACTERISTICS

Several genetic mutations frequently observed in SCLC tumors are often distinguishable from those seen in NSCLC cases. These include deletions in the short arm of chromosome 3 in 80% of cases, inactivation of the retinoblastoma gene in 90% of cases, and *TP53* mutations in more than 80%.

Neuroendocrine products such as neuron-specific enolase and gastrin-releasing peptide are secreted by SCLC tumors more commonly than by NSCLC lesions.

CLINICAL MANIFESTATIONS, PATIENT EVALUATION, AND STAGING

The International Union Against Cancer system is recommended for use in staging SCLC, but the 1973 Veterans Administration distinction of extensive stage versus limited stage is commonly employed. This system relies on the ability to include all known disease within a reasonable radiation field for patients with limited-stage disease.

PRIMARY THERAPY

The standard management of limited-stage SCLC (L-SCLC) disease is platinum-based chemotherapy given concurrently with thoracic radiation therapy (TRT). Total radiation doses range from 40 to 55 Gy in most trials. A large, randomized, prospective trial demonstrated a survival advantage for twice-daily accelerated hyperfractionated radiation therapy over standard once-daily radiation therapy.

TECHNIQUES OF IRRADIATION

Most current clinical protocols for L-SCLC employ the involved-field technique of TRT, in which the target volume includes the known extent of the primary tumor and malignant lymphadenopathy, with one additional nodal station. Large fields, including more extensive elective nodal irradiation, are discouraged.

TREATMENT ALGORITHMS

The algorithm for SCLC includes adequate staging. If a patient is diagnosed as having limited-stage disease and has adequate vigor to undergo combined-modality therapy, he or she should receive aggressive twice-daily TRT to 45 Gy with concurrent platinum-based chemotherapy for four cycles.

If a patient achieves a complete response and is in remission on restaging, prophylactic cranial radiation therapy should be recommended.

If a patient is diagnosed with extensive-stage disease, primary therapy consists of platinum-based therapy and irradiation for symptomatic or nonresponding sites. Prophylactic cranial radiation therapy also should be offered in the setting of complete response and complete remission after chemotherapy.

Bronchogenic carcinoma is divided into two distinct entities: small cell lung cancer (SCLC) and non–small cell lung cancer (NSCLC), and these categories have distinguishing clinical, biologic, and histologic features. During 2004, lung cancer was diagnosed in an estimated 173,770 patients and caused an estimated 169,440 deaths in the United States.[1] Between 15% and 20% of patients with lung cancer have SCLC, and of these, 30% have limited-stage disease.[2] Few patients have International Union Against Cancer (UICC) stage I disease at diagnosis. The median age of patients diagnosed with lung cancer is 70 years.[3] The natural history of untreated SCLC includes rapid tumor progression, with a median survival of 2 to 4 months.[4] Until the late 1960s, physicians did not differentiate the management of SCLC from that of NSCLC, and clinical trials in the 1970s continued to include both types of lung cancer. It was recognized that most patients with SCLC had poor survival after surgery or irradiation, or both, with little apparent survival benefit derived from either therapy. The major breakthrough occurring in the late 1960s was the recognition that SCLC tumors were more responsive to chemotherapy than NSCLC tumors.[5] Since then, the standard of care for SCLC patients has included systemic therapy in addition to locoregional therapy.

PATHOLOGY AND PATHWAYS OF SPREAD

The 2004 World Health Organization classification defined SCLC as "a malignant epithelial tumor consisting of small cells with scant cytoplasm, ill-defined cell borders, finely granular nuclear chromatin, and absent or inconspicuous nucleoli." The cells are round, oval, and spindle shaped. Nuclear molding is prominent. Necrosis is extensive, and the mitotic count is high. SCLC occurs in two variant forms: small cell carcinoma and combined small cell carcinoma. The latter type includes SCLC cells and any of the histologic types of NSCLC.[6]

BIOLOGIC CHARACTERISTICS AND MOLECULAR BIOLOGY

A number of genetic mutations are observed in SCLC tumors that frequently involve tumor suppressor genes.[7] The most

Table 40-1 Molecular Abnormalities in Lung Cancer

Molecular Abnormality	SCLC (%)	NSCLC (%)
RAS mutation	<1	30-40
MYC amplification	30	10
EGFR expression	NR	40-80
ERBB2 (HER2) overexpression	10	30
KIT (SCFR) coexpression	70	15
BCL2 expression	95	35
TP53 mutation	75-100	50
RB1 deletion (loss of RB1 protein)	90	20
CDKN2A (p16) inactivation	<1	70
COX2 expression	NR	70
3p deletion	90	50
VEGF expression	>100-fold variation	
Matrix metalloproteinase (gelatinase)	50	65
Neuropeptides	90	NR

CDKN2A, cyclin-dependent kinase inhibitor 2A gene (formerly designated *p16*); COX, cyclooxygenase; EGFR, epidermal growth factor receptor; NSCLC, non–small cell lung cancer; NR, not reported; SCFR, stem cell factor receptor; SCLC, small cell lung cancer; *RB1*, retinoblastoma gene; VEGF, vascular endothelial growth factor; 3p, deletion in the short arm of chromosome 3 in the 3p14-23 region.

Adapted from Dye GK, Adjei AA: Novel targets for lung cancer therapy. Part I. J Clin Oncol 20:2881-2894, 2002.

common mutations are a deletion in the short arm of chromosome 3 in the 3p14-23 region (>80% of SCLC cases), inactivation of the retinoblastoma gene *(RB1)* on chromosome 13 (90%), and mutations of the *TP53* tumor suppressor gene on the short arm of chromosome 17 (>80%) (Table 40-1). There has been tremendous progress in understanding the relationship of these abnormalities and the events leading from normal bronchial epithelium to invasive carcinoma.

The chromosome 3 genetic deletions have been observed in dysplastic and preneoplastic changes, and they have been most convincingly demonstrated as the known genetic mutation associated with the transformation of precancerous lesions into carcinoma. Evidence indicates that the critical deletion in SCLC and many other malignancies may occur in a fragile portion of chromosome 3 (3p14.2) known as the *FHIT* gene deletion.[8,9] Inactivation of the *RB1* gene most likely results in a loss of control of growth. It is believed that a functional *RB1* gene maintains the G_1/S cell cycle boundary in check and that its inactivation results in uncontrolled growth.[10] The *TP53* mutations specific to SCLC have also been observed in preneoplastic lesions, and they appear to most closely resemble *TP53* mutations observed in other malignancies for which tobacco is a known carcinogen. It is likely that the mutation of *TP53* in SCLC tumors impairs the ability of tumor cells to undergo apoptosis in response to anticancer therapy.[11] Another growth regulator, which is overexpressed in 95% of SCLC tumors, is the product of *BCL2*. It is believed that this overexpression interferes with the tumor's apoptotic response to therapy.[12] There are ongoing research efforts to develop therapies that target the tumor-specific biologic lesions.

In many NSCLC specimens studied, point mutations in the *RAS* family of oncogenes have been observed.[13] These mutations are rarely observed in SCLC specimens, but amplification and overexpression of the *MYC* family of oncogenes and gene products commonly are observed, particularly *MYC* (formerly designated c-*Myc*), *MYCN* (formerly N-*Myc*), and *MYCL1* (formerly L-*Myc*). It appears that abnormalities are more often observed in recurrent tumors, tumors with variant rather than classic SCLC histology, and tumors with a more aggressive and unfavorable prognosis. This has led to the hypothesis that the overexpression of the *MYC* gene products is a relatively late event in the pathogenesis of SCLC.[14]

Another biologic feature that distinguishes SCLC from NSCLC is the more common expression of neuroendocrine markers in SCLC. These markers include enzymes such as neuron-specific enolase and L-dopa decarboxylase, peptide hormones such as gastrin-releasing peptide and arginine vasopressin, and surface markers such as neural cell adhesion molecule (NCAM). The two peptide hormones meet the criteria of autocrine growth factors, which require the cellular production of a growth-promoting protein—for which the producing cell has functional receptors. In the case of gastrin-releasing peptide, there is clear evidence that it is produced and secreted by many SCLC cells and then attaches to its cellular membrane receptors, thereby stimulating further cellular growth.[15] Murine monoclonal antibodies have been developed against the gastrin-releasing peptide and are undergoing clinical testing.[16] Such an antibody could potentially block this autocrine growth cycle function.

CLINICAL MANIFESTATIONS, PATIENT EVALUATION, AND STAGING

The presentation of patients with SCLC differs somewhat from those with NSCLC. These differences include fewer cases of SCLC diagnosed by imaging of asymptomatic patients; a shorter time from first thoracic symptoms to life-threatening symptoms; and the occasional manifestation of SCLC with paraneoplastic symptoms. The signs and symptoms of SCLC or NSCLC depend on the location and bulk of the primary tumor, adenopathy, and metastatic disease. Because of the high frequency of nodal involvement in SCLC cases, patients frequently present with symptoms such as dyspnea, dysphagia, hoarseness, and superior vena cava syndrome. As with NSCLC, many SCLC patients present with other thoracic symptoms, including cough, hemoptysis, chest pain, and weight loss.

SCLC is the most common solid tumor to have a number of associated paraneoplastic syndromes. Several of these are endocrinologic and neurologic. The most common endocrinologic abnormality is the syndrome of inappropriate secretion of antidiuretic hormone (SIADH). This condition results from the excessive secretion of ADH from tumor tissue, leading to severe hyponatremia with resultant hypo-osmolality. SIADH occurs in 11% to 46% of SCLC patients and typically resolves after response to anticancer therapy.[17] Two less common endocrinologic syndromes are atrial natriuretic peptide (ANP) syndrome, which can produce hyponatremia, natriuresis, and hypotension, and ectopic adrenocorticotropic hormone (ACTH) production syndrome, resulting in Cushing's syndrome. ANP syndrome occurs in about 15% of SCLC cases and responds to therapy, whereas ACTH syndrome occurs in 5% of cases and is associated with a poor prognosis.[18]

The neurologic syndromes associated with SCLC include Lambert-Eaton syndrome, cerebellar degeneration syndrome, encephalomyelitis, sensory neuropathy, and cancer-associated retinopathy. Each of these is observed in 5% of all SCLC patients. Patients with Lambert-Eaton syndrome present with myasthenia gravis–like symptoms of proximal myopathy, autonomic dysfunction, and hyporeflexia. Like many paraneoplastic syndromes, this condition is improved with response to anticancer therapy, although there can be symp-

Table 40-2 **Syndromes Associated with Small Cell Lung Cancer**

Syndrome	Manifestation(s)	Frequency (%)	Correctable with Therapy
SIADH	Hyponatremia, hypo-osmolality	11-46	Yes
ANP syndrome	Hyponatremia, hypotension, natriuresis	15	Yes
Ectopic ACTH production	Cushingoid symptoms	5	Rarely
Lambert-Eaton syndrome	Myasthenia gravis–like symptoms	<5	Yes
Cerebellar degeneration syndrome	Cerebellar symptoms	<5	Rarely
CAR	Visual loss	<5	Rarely

ACTH, adrenocorticotropic hormone; ANP, atrial natriuretic peptide; CAR, cancer-associated retinopathy; SIADH, syndrome of inappropriate antidiuretic hormone secretion.

tomatic responses to antimyasthenia therapies.[19] The other neurologic syndromes are thought to be primarily autoimmune phenomena, and they respond poorly to cancer therapy.[20,21] Table 40-2 summarizes these SCLC-associated syndromes.

SCLC can be diagnosed by means of histology or cytology. In most cases, a diagnosis can be obtained by sputum expectoration or bronchoscopic technique. Frequently, transthoracic fine-needle aspiration is required and, less frequently, mediastinoscopy or thoracotomy. Cytologic techniques have improved sufficiently that bronchoscopic brush technique can usually distinguish SCLC from NSCLC, as can the needle aspirate from a transthoracic needle. After the diagnosis of SCLC is established, there is no need for additional invasive mediastinal staging, as there sometimes is for NSCLC, because of the limited role of surgical resection in management.

The UICC/American Joint Commission on Cancer (AJCC) published its most recent staging system for bronchogenic cancer in 2002.[22] This system has been universally adopted for staging patients with NSCLC, but it is less frequently employed for SCLC. Instead, the 1973 Veterans Administration Lung Cancer Study Group's staging system, which distinguishes between limited and extensive SCLC, is more commonly used, despite its considerable imprecision.[23] The initial definition of limited disease was an extent of intrathoracic disease that can be encompassed within a "reasonable" radiation field. Such a vague definition allows for many interpretations, which have ranged from patients with ipsilateral pleural effusions and contralateral mediastinal, supraclavicular, and hilar adenopathy to those without effusions and with ipsilateral adenopathy. Investigators have recognized the dangers of variable interpretations, and recent North American cooperative group trials require staging of SCLC patients with the standard TNM system before study entry.

Approximately two thirds of SCLC patients have extensive-stage or stage IV disease at presentation. This rate has increased from approximately 50% in the 1970s and 1980s, in part due to the greater sensitivity of screening techniques for metastatic disease. One of the principal goals of staging is to distinguish stages I through III from stage IV disease. This evaluation typically includes contrast-enhanced computed tomography (CT) of the thorax and upper abdomen, bone scan, and CT or magnetic resonance imaging (MRI) of the brain. Serum studies can include a complete blood cell count with a differential cell count and a complete chemistry screening panel. Bone marrow aspirates and biopsies have been advocated by some investigators. If all of these investigations confirm that the patient has limited-stage SCLC (L-SCLC), the patient should also undergo pulmonary function testing to confirm his or her ability to tolerate aggressive thoracic radiation therapy (TRT). Positron emission tomography (PET) scans are quite accurate in the staging of SCLC. PET can aid in the choice of appropriate therapy because of more accurate staging of disease and in radiation therapy planning by better identifying the target.[24]

Investigators should be cautioned regarding the influence of better staging techniques on the interpretation of survival results. If, for example, many patients previously believed to have L-SCLC are upstaged to the extensive-disease category because of more sensitive staging, it is likely that their inclusion in the extensive-disease group and their exclusion from the L-SCLC category will improve survival rates in both groups. This effect, known as the *Will Rogers phenomenon,* was first described in oncology for patients with SCLC, and it is based on the quotation, "When the Okies left Oklahoma and moved to California, they raised the average IQ in both states." One method of reducing the statistical distortions of the Will Rogers phenomenon (i.e., stage migration) is to compare survival outcome of entire populations rather than on a stage-by-stage basis. The best method of controlling for this effect is to perform randomized trials.

There have been several efforts to identify prognostic factors other than staging as a means to better select patients for specific therapies. As with many malignancies, good performance status, young age, and female gender are associated with better prognosis, and these have been verified in large, multivariate analyses.[25-27] Among available laboratory tests, elevated lactate dehydrogenase (LDH) serum levels were most commonly associated with a poor prognosis, and hyponatremia and low albumin levels were found in several studies to be independent adverse prognostic factors. The metastatic site found to be most unfavorable was the liver. Although such studies are valuable in understanding a disease, they are confounded by the extent and quality of imaging evaluation, available therapies, and selection of variables tested. Risk categories created by two British groups include prognostic factors such as performance status and several laboratory tests such as those for LDH, alkaline phosphatase, and sodium levels.[26,27]

PRIMARY THERAPY

Limited-Stage Small Cell Lung Cancer

Decisions regarding optimal therapy of patients with L-SCLC must consider a patient's pulmonary and cardiac fitness, ability to tolerate specific chemotherapeutic agents, history of malignancies and their treatment, age, and performance status. Because the diagnosis of limited-stage disease by definition implies the potential ability to receive an aggressive course of TRT, such treatment should be feasible. The issues discussed in the following sections have generally been studied in trials involving patients with ambulatory performance status, no prior anticancer therapy, and acceptable organ (i.e., pulmonary, cardiac, renal, and hepatic) function. How these principles can be applied to patients not meeting those criteria should be determined on an individual basis.

Although performance status is an important prognostic factor for SCLC patients, a decline in performance status may be related to factors other than the malignancy. With the help of pulmonary physicians or other caregivers, a patient suffering from treatable conditions such as bronchitis, pneumonia, or an exacerbation of chronic obstructive lung disease can improve his or her performance status before the initiation of therapy. Such an improvement may increase the likelihood of tolerating and benefiting from aggressive multimodality therapy. Recent weight loss among patients with a lung malignancy is usually considered a symptom of cancer-related cachexia that is reversible only with a response to anticancer therapy. However, there can be more easily reversible causes of weight loss among these patients, including problems with dentition or dentures, oral candidiasis, thoracic pain requiring analgesia, or gastroesophageal reflux. Management of these problems is likely to improve a patient's tolerance of therapy.

Thoracic Irradiation

After the demonstration in the late 1960s of activity for several chemotherapeutic agents and the poor prognosis of patients treated with surgery or irradiation, or both, multiagent chemotherapy became the primary therapy for all stages of SCLC.[28,29] Unfortunately, recurrence inevitably followed the response to chemotherapy, and these relapses were most frequent in areas of previous disease. This pattern of failure led investigators to re-examine the use of radiation therapy for L-SCLC. In modern practice, radiation therapy and chemotherapy have central roles in the treatment of L-SCLC.[30,31]

A series of randomized trials have compared chemotherapy alone with chemotherapy plus TRT.[32-35] In 1992, two meta-analyses were published regarding the role of TRT in addition to chemotherapy.[2,35] They were based on randomized, prospective studies that compared chemotherapy alone with chemotherapy plus TRT. Pignon and colleagues[35] reported a 3-year survival rate of 14.3% with combined-modality therapy and 8.9% with chemotherapy alone (P = .001). This 5.4% difference in 3-year survival was identical to the 5.4% difference in 2-year survival (P < .001) reported by Warde and Payne.[2] Although 5.4% may seem rather small, this difference represented a 61% increase in the 3-year survival rate of 8.9% achieved with chemotherapy alone.[35] The intrathoracic tumor control was improved by 25.3% in the radiation therapy arms.[2]

Sequencing and Timing of Thoracic Radiation Therapy and Chemotherapy

Chemotherapy and TRT have been delivered concurrently, sequentially, or in an alternating manner. Potential advantages of concurrent delivery include the shorter overall treatment time, an increase in overall treatment intensity, and potential anticancer synergism between the various therapies. Disadvantages include the heightened risk of toxicity and the inability to assess the antitumor response rate of the chemotherapy alone. The Japanese Clinical Oncology Group performed a phase III trial in which L-SCLC patients were randomized to sequential TRT or concurrent TRT. All 231 patients received four cycles of etoposide plus cisplatin (EP) every 3 weeks (sequential arm) or 4 weeks (concurrent arm) and were randomized to receive TRT during the first cycle of chemotherapy in the concurrent arm or after the fourth cycle in the sequential arm. TRT consisted of 45 Gy given in 1.5-Gy fractions twice daily over 3 weeks. Concurrent TRT yielded better survival than sequential TRT (P = .097). The median survival time was 19.7 months in the sequential arm and 27.2 months in the concurrent arm of the study. The 5-year survival rate for patients treated sequentially was 18.3%, compared with 23.7% for those treated concurrently. Hematologic toxicity was more severe for patients enrolled in the concurrent arm. However, severe esophagitis was infrequent in both arms, occurring in 9% of the patients in the concurrent arm and 4% in the sequential arm. The study authors concluded that the findings strongly suggested that concurrent therapy was more effective for the treatment of L-SCLC than sequential therapy.[36]

Multiple randomized trials have addressed the issue of timing of TRT during programs of concurrent chemotherapy and TRT. In the trial conducted by the Cancer and Leukemia Group B (CALGB) from 1981 to 1984, 426 L-SCLC patients were treated with cyclophosphamide (C), etoposide (E) or doxorubicin (A), and vincristine (V) and randomized to no radiation therapy (arm 1), radiation therapy starting during cycle 1 of chemotherapy (arm 2), or radiation therapy starting during cycle 4 (arm 3).[32] TRT in both arms was 50 Gy delivered over 6 weeks. There was a survival advantage favoring arms 2 and 3 over the no-irradiation arm, and the best results were achieved in arm 3 (P = .0099). The 5-year survival rates were 3% for chemotherapy alone, 7% for early irradiation, and 13% for delayed radiation therapy. One criticism of this trial is that the doses of chemotherapy in arm 2 are intentionally reduced to lessen the risk of heightened toxicity during concurrent TRT early in the chemotherapy program.

A National Cancer Institute of Canada trial compared TRT (40 Gy in given 15 fractions over 3 weeks) applied during cycle 2 versus cycle 6 of an alternating-chemotherapy regimen that included cyclophosphamide, doxorubicin, and vincristine (CAV) and EP.[37] A survival advantage was seen for the patients randomized to cycle 2 radiation therapy, with median survival times of 16 versus 12 months and 4-year survival rates of 25% versus 15% (P = .008).

James and coworkers[38] reported an English study of early versus late TRT. The 325 L-SCLC patients were randomized to early TRT with the second course of chemotherapy or to late TRT with the sixth course of chemotherapy. The chemotherapy was identical in each arm and included six cycles of CAV that alternated with EP. The TRT dose was 40 Gy given in 15 fractions over 3 weeks. Prophylactic cranial irradiation (PCI) was given to responding patients. Median survival times and 3-year survival rates were 13.5 months and 16% with arly TRT versus 15.1 months and 20% with late TRT (P = .18).[38]

Thus conflicting results have been reported regarding the timing of TRT. However, a meta-analysis[39] does help make sense of the contradictory data. This study analyzed randomized trials published after 1985 and addressed the timing of TRT relative to chemotherapy in L-SCLC. Early TRT was initiated less than 9 weeks after starting chemotherapy and late TRT more than 9 weeks. Seven trials (N = 1524 patients) met the inclusion criteria and were included in the analysis. The relative risk of survival for early TRT compared with late TRT for all studies was 1.17 (95% confidence interval [CI], 1.02 to 1.35; P = .03), indicating an increased 2-year survival for early TRT compared with late TRT patients. This translated to a 5.2% (95% CI, 0.6% to 9.7%; P = .03) improvement in the 2-year survival for early TRT. This small but significant improvement in 2-year survival for early TRT was similar in overall magnitude to the benefit of adding TRT or PCI to chemotherapy.[39]

It appears that the therapeutic window of opportunity for TRT to optimally improve survival is early during the chemotherapy. There may be reasons to delay the initiation of concurrent TRT for some patients with very large tumors, very limited pulmonary function, or postobstructive atelectasis. In all three instances, more normal lung may be spared by irradiating the tumors after a favorable response to a few cycles of chemotherapy.

Thoracic Radiation Therapy Dose

SCLC is considered a relatively radioresponsive malignancy because the low doses of TRT previously used produced encouraging responses. Total TRT doses for L-SCLC have ranged from 25 to 30 Gy in 10 fractions in the 1970s to up to 60 Gy in 30 to 33 fractions in recent years. Doses in the lower end of this range may have been acceptable when chemotherapy was less effective and disseminated disease occurred earlier in the course of disease. Improvements in systemic therapy have increased the need for aggressive TRT regimens that produce more durable responses. It was estimated by Choi and Carey that the risk of intrathoracic tumor recurrence at total doses of 40 Gy or less was 80%,[40] and this was confirmed in a National Cancer Institute of Canada trial in which patients with L-SCLC were randomized between 25 Gy in 10 fractions and 37.5 Gy in 15 fractions.[41] The 2-year actuarial rates of local failure were 80% and 69%, respectively.

The most commonly administered doses of TRT range from 45 to 54 Gy in 1.8- to 2.0-Gy daily fractions. Although a radiation dose response can be well demonstrated for tumor control below 40 Gy, it is difficult to conclusively establish a relationship between radiation dose and tumor control in the range between 40 and 60 Gy in standard fractionation. Most randomized and nonrandomized trials estimate rates for local tumor control in this dose range as between 58% and 85%.[42-45] A single-institution trial from Yale–New Haven Hospital reported a local tumor control rate of 96% with a total radiation dose in excess of 60 Gy.[46] The CALGB conducted a phase I dose escalation of standard fractionation and found that a dose higher than 70 Gy was the maximal tolerated dose with the given assumptions with respect to irradiation field definitions and chemotherapy employed.[47] That trial was not designed to detect a difference in tumor control rates, but it demonstrated that doses higher than the usual range of L-SCLC doses could be tested in subsequent trials. There is inadequate information available to recommend total TRT doses in once-daily fractionation. The randomized trial summarized in the following section illustrates, however, the inadequate tumor control achieved with daily intermediate dose TRT.

Altered Fractionation

Another means of intensifying therapy is the use of altered radiation fractionation. For L-SCLC patients, most altered fractionation strategies have employed twice-daily fractionation, with fraction sizes of 1.1 to 1.8 Gy and total doses of 40 to 54 Gy. Most regimens have tested the principle of accelerated hyperfractionation (AHF), in which a twice-daily regimen allows the delivery of a standard total radiation dose over a shortened period. Such a regimen should benefit patients with rapidly growing tumors such as SCLC with a small shoulder and a steep slope on its radiobiologic cell survival curve.

Several encouraging pilot studies led to the development of a national Intergroup Trial testing the concept that AHF radiation therapy could contribute to improved tumor control for L-SCLC patients. The experimental regimen was 45.0 Gy in 1.5-Gy fractions delivered twice daily beginning on day 1 of a four-cycle regimen of EP. The interfraction interval was 6 to 8 hours, and the elapsed treatment time was 19 to 21 days. This regimen was piloted by Turrisi and colleagues in 23 patients, resulting in a median survival time of 25 months and a 5-year survival rate of 36%.[48] A subsequent multi-institution phase II trial of the same regimen conducted by the Eastern Cooperative Oncology Group (ECOG) resulted in a 2-year survival rate of 36%.[49] These results were considered sufficiently promising to launch a phase III trial (Intergroup Trial 0096) in 1988. A total of 419 patients were randomized between the regimens of 45.0 Gy in 1.8-Gy fractions delivered daily (QD-TRT arm) and 45.0 Gy in 30 fractions of 1.5 Gy delivered twice daily (BID-TRT arm). In both arms, the TRT began on day 1 of a four-cycle course of EP. There was a significant survival advantage for the BID-TRT patients compared with the QD-TRT patients, with 5-year survival rates of 26% and 16%, respectively (P = .04). The intrathoracic tumor failure rate was 36% for the BID-TRT arm and 52% for the QD-TRT arm (P = .06). The principal difference in toxicity was a higher rate of grade 3 esophagitis in the BID-TRT arm (27% versus 11%; P < .001).[50] This study confirms the principle that intensification of TRT beyond standard RT can improve local control and survival (Table 40-3). This trial has altered the standard of care for L-SCLC patients in the United States.

Table 40-3 Intergroup 0096 Study Comparing Once- with Twice-Daily Thoracic RT for L-SCLC Patients Treated with Concurrent Cisplatin and Etoposide

Characteristic	Arm 1 (once-daily)	Arm 2 (twice-daily)	*P* Value
Number of patients	206	211	—
Median survival time (mo)	19	23	—
2-year survival rate	41%	47%	—
5-year survival rate	16%	26%	.04
Failure-free survival rate	24%	29%	.10
Local failure rate	52%	36%	.06
Simultaneous local and distant failure rate	23%	6%	.005
Grade 3 esophagitis rate	11%	27%	<.001

L-SCLC, limited-stage small cell lung cancer; RT, radiation therapy.

The North Central Cancer Treatment Group (NCCTG) performed a trial (89-20-52) that has been incorrectly interpreted as contradicting the findings of the Intergroup Trial 0096. The findings of these studies provide complementary information regarding BID-TRT. The NCCTG trial included 310 patients with L-SCLC initially treated with three cycles of EP.[51] Subsequently, the 261 patients without significant progression were randomized to two cycles of EP plus QD-TRT (50.4 Gy in 28 fractions) or split-course BID-TRT (24 Gy in 16 fractions, a 2.5-week break, and 24 Gy in 16 fractions). Patients then received a sixth cycle of EP followed by PCI. The median survival times and 5-year survival rates from randomization were 20.6 months and 21% for patients who received QD-TRT and 20.6 months and 22% for those who received BID-TRT (P = .68). There were no significant differences in the rates of intrathoracic failure or distant failure between the treatment arms.

There was no significant difference in the overall rates of grade 3 or greater toxicity. Grade 3+ esophagitis (P = .05) was more common in the BID-TRT arm, as was grade 5 toxicity, which occurred in 4 (3%) of 130 patients who received BID-TRT, compared with 0 (0%) of 131 patients who received QD-TRT (P = .04).

The results of these two randomized, prospective studies comparing QD-TRT with BID-TRT for L-SCLC led to the conclusion that continuous-course BID-TRT is better than QD-TRT, but split-course BID-TRT is not. This finding has precedence and is identical to the findings regarding twice-daily radiation therapy for head and neck cancer. The Radiation Therapy Oncology Group (RTOG) conducted a phase III randomized trial (RTOG 9003) enrolling patients with locally advanced squamous cell carcinomas of the head and neck and compared various radiation therapy regimens. Patients treated in the two arms of continuously administered, twice-daily radiation therapy had better locoregional control than those treated with split-course, twice-daily radiation therapy or standard-dose, once-daily radiation therapy. This study also found that continuously administered, twice-daily radiation therapy was better than once-daily radiation therapy but that split-course, twice-daily irradiation was not.[52]

Treatment Volumes and Normal Tissue Considerations

The ability of a patient with L-SCLC to tolerate increasingly aggressive radiation therapy regimens and higher total doses during concurrent chemotherapy is in part related to selection of the irradiated target volume.[42] In the early 1980s, both CALGB and Southwest Oncology Group (SWOG) investigators demonstrated poorer survival when patients were not treated with the recommended large fields employing elective nodal irradiation.[53,54] Mira and Livingston also demonstrated tumor failures just beyond the margins of the TRT fields when the fields were designed after a response to chemotherapy.[55] These reports further supported the need for generous TRT fields. As an example of such a field, the radiation therapy target volume for a patient with a tumor in the left upper lobe with ipsilateral hilar and mediastinal adenopathy may include only the tumor itself with a 2.0-cm margin, both hilar regions, the mediastinum from the thoracic inlet to at least the subcarinal region, and both supraclavicular regions. Such large fields were in part responsible for the acceptance of a moderate total radiation dose as appropriate for treating SCLC, because the large volume irradiated precluded a substantial increase in dose.

In the 1980s and 1990s, there emerged evidence that defining a smaller target volume for irradiation did not adversely influence tumor control in patients receiving concurrent cisplatin-containing chemotherapy. The fields employed in Intergroup Trial 0096 for such a patient confined the high-dose volume to the tumor with a 1.5-cm margin, the ipsilateral hilum, and the mediastinum from the thoracic inlet to the subcarinal region. The contralateral hilum and both supraclavicular regions were excluded, and the regions requiring therapy were treated with a reduced margin. These treatment recommendations have been widely adopted in subsequent clinical trials.

There is growing evidence that using a smaller radiation target volume does not adversely influence tumor control rates and that regions just beyond the reduced target volume are not frequent sites of relapse. Liengswangwong and colleagues studied L-SCLC patients from the Mayo Clinic and NCCTG with intrathoracic recurrence and found all recurrences within the TRT high-dose volume, regardless of whether patients were irradiated to the prechemotherapy or postchemotherapy volume.[56] A similar conclusion was made by Kies and coworkers from SWOG; they found no recurrence rate difference between patients randomized to receive wide-field (prechemotherapy target volume) or reduced-field (postchemotherapy target volume) TRT.[57] Brodin and associates from Uppsala also found that most (86%) intrathoracic recurrences occurred "in field," suggesting an inadequate dose rather than inadequate fields.[58] All these reports support the concept advocated by Lichter and Turrisi[42] that reductions in target volumes do not compromise patient outcome and may allow for higher TRT doses to be delivered (Fig. 40-1).

Smaller volumes have the advantage of further sparing of the surrounding normal tissues of the lung, esophagus, heart, spinal cord, and bone marrow. Optimal sparing is important and may decrease the morbidity and mortality from therapy. We compiled the toxicity data of the 263 patients treated on NCCTG 89-20-52, which included concurrent chemotherapy plus BID-TRT or QD-TRT. The most common type of toxicity was hematologic; 90% of patients had grade 3+ hematologic toxicity, and 43% had grade 4+ hematologic toxicity. Forty-seven percent of patients had grade 3+ nonhematologic toxicities, and 11% had grade 4+ nonhematologic toxicities. Nausea, vomiting, and esophagitis were the most common nonhematologic toxicities. Grade 3+ esophagitis was more common (P = .05) when BID-TRT (12%) was compared with QD-TRT (5%). Fatal (grade 5) toxicity occurred in four patients (2%) and resulted from pneumonitis in three patients and infection in one patient.[51]

Radiation-induced toxicity is related to dose-volume parameters. Graham and associates reported that the risk of grade 2+ pneumonitis was 0% when the V20 (i.e., percentage of pulmonary volume irradiated to more than 20 Gy) was less than 22%, 7% when the V20 was 22% to 31%, 13% when the V20 was 32% to 40%, and 36% when V20 was more than 40%.[59] It is generally accepted that the spinal cord can safely receive 45 to 50 Gy in 1.8- to 2.0-Gy fractions. In most BID-TRT regimens employing 1.5-Gy fractions, the spinal cord is limited to 36 to 37 Gy without incident.[51] When using the Intergroup 0096 regimen, the oblique off-cord fields can be used for the second daily treatment for the last 8 to 10 treatments. The $TD_{5/5}$ (toxic dose to 5% of patients in 5 years) was estimated at 60 Gy for one third of the heart, 45 Gy for two thirds of the heart, and 40 Gy for the entire heart.[60] Esophagitis is related to the dose of radiation, the volume of esophagus irradiated, the fractionation schema, and the timing of chemotherapy. Of the patients in the Intergroup Trial 0096 who received BID-TRT, 32% had grade 3 or worse esophagitis, compared with 16% for those who received QD-TRT (P = .001). This arm of the trial included concurrent chemotherapy plus BID-TRT. Although esophagitis is uncomfortable and can lead to significant dehydration and the possible need for frequent intravenous hydration, these factors should not be used as reasons to deny fit patients BID-TRT, because their best chance for survival may depend on it.

Chemotherapy Selection and Dosing

The selection of chemotherapeutic agents to combine with TRT for patients with L-SCLC is largely based on trials of multiagent regimens used for extensive-stage SCLC (E-SCLC). The first generation of therapies for E-SCLC included alkylating agents such as cyclophosphamide. Subsequently, doxorubicin, an anthracycline, was added to multiagent regimens that produced improved results. The standard chemotherapeutic regimen for E-SCLC and L-SCLC in the United States is the two-drug regimen of EP. This regimen was first studied in SCLC in the late 1970s,[61] and its efficacy in treating E-SCLC is comparable to the previously used standard of CAV.[62] The

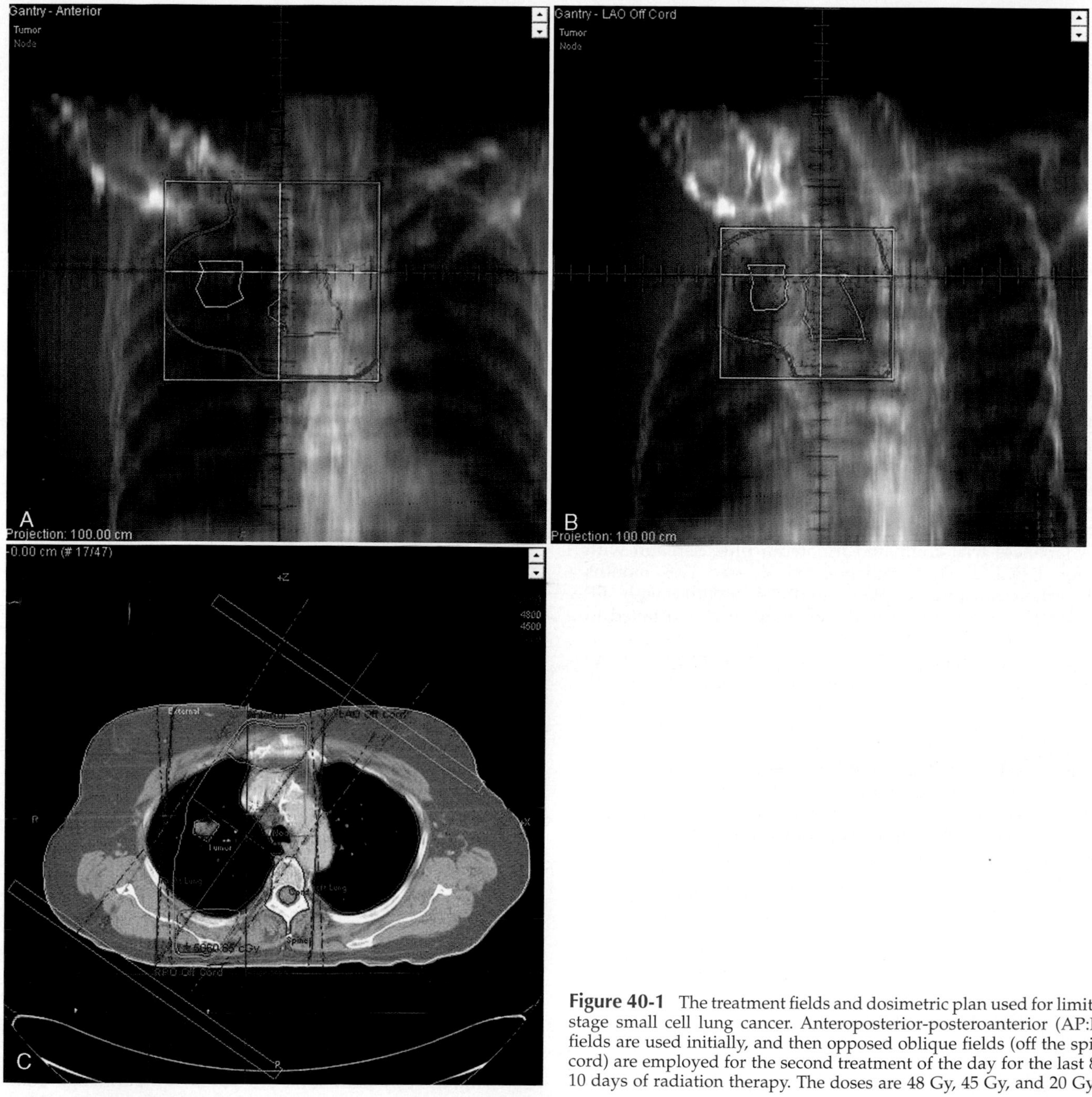

Figure 40-1 The treatment fields and dosimetric plan used for limited-stage small cell lung cancer. Anteroposterior-posteroanterior (AP:PA) fields are used initially, and then opposed oblique fields (off the spinal cord) are employed for the second treatment of the day for the last 8 to 10 days of radiation therapy. The doses are 48 Gy, 45 Gy, and 20 Gy.

wide acceptance of this regimen over CAV mainly results from its more manageable toxicity profile and the ability to stop therapy after four rather than six cycles. The concept of alternating cycles of regimens such as EP and CAV was conceptually attractive, and at least one randomized trial demonstrated a survival benefit for E-SCLC patients with alternating regimens compared with either regimen alone.[63] Despite this finding, EP alone is the standard U.S. chemotherapeutic regimen for E-SCLC and L-SCLC patients. A particularly popular regimen in Europe is cyclophosphamide, doxorubicin, and etoposide, in part because of its ease of outpatient administration and its lack of platinum-related nephrotoxicity.[64]

SWOG was the first group to report a completed trial of concurrent TRT with EP for L-SCLC. This trial reported a median survival time of 17.5 months and a 4-year survival rate of 30%, which appeared superior to the previously reported results with TRT combined with CAV and other non–platinum-containing regimens.[65] The pulmonary, cardiac, and cutaneous risks of combining EP with TRT were believed to be lower than with CAV or other anthracycline-containing regimens. Additional promising results were subsequently reported from groups at the University of Pennsylvania,[48] the National Cancer Institute,[66] and ECOG[49] with TRT and EP, and they were confirmed in the Intergroup Trial 0096.[50] No randomized trial has demonstrated the superiority of TRT and EP over any other regimen for L-SCLC, including CAV and TRT. It remains uncertain to what extent stage migration contributed to the apparent improvement in survival of L-SCLC patients from the early 1980s to the mid-1990s.

Newer Agents

Because even standard doses of EP chemotherapy are not as myelosuppressive as CAV or other SCLC regimens, investigators have tested the addition of a third agent to this regimen. The alkylating agent ifosfamide has been added to EP and was demonstrated in one randomized trial to improve survival of patients with E-SCLC.[67] This result has not been found in at least one RTOG phase II study of L-SCLC patients.[68] Paclitaxel, a tubulin toxin, has been added to EP for treating E-SCLC, with encouraging phase II results.[69] The RTOG has investigated adding paclitaxel to EP (EPT) plus BID-TRT for L-SCLC. Preliminary results of a phase II trial have produced a 1-year survival rate of 83% and a median survival in excess of 30 months. The three-drug regimen and concurrent TRT appears to produce better survival (with similar toxicity) than EP and concurrent TRT in patients with L-SCLC. The preliminary report from this study stated that a phase III study comparing concurrent TRT with EPT or EP in patients with L-SCLC is planned.[70]

A Japanese trial compared irinotecan plus cisplatin with EP for E-SCLC. The median survival was 12.8 months with irinotecan plus cisplatin and 9.4 months with EP (P = .002).[71] An American trial was performed and failed to confirm these findings.[72]

Several chemotherapeutic agents have demonstrated activity against SCLC for which further investigation is warranted. These include the vinca alkaloid vinorelbine, the topoisomerase II inhibitors topotecan and irinotecan, the nucleotide analogue gemcitabine, and other taxane derivatives, including docetaxel.[73-76] There has been acceptance in the United States that it is ethical and appropriate that regimens containing new agents first be tested in newly diagnosed E-SCLC patients.[77] Agents are typically tested with TRT for L-SCLC only after promising results are obtained among E-SCLC patients.

TARGETED THERAPY AND SMALL CELL LUNG CANCER

Surface antigens overexpressed in SCLC that are potential targets for immunotherapy include gangliosides (i.e., GM_2, GD_2, 9-0-acetyl GD_3, and fucosyl-GM_1 [FUC-GM1]). Mitumomab (BEC2) is a monoclonal antibody that mimics the GD_3 antigen by stimulating an immunologic response to SCLC expressing GD_3. Bacille Calmette-Guerin (BCG) vaccine is used as an adjuvant for stimulating the production of antibodies.[78] A phase III trial (EORTC 08971) of chemoradiation followed by a placebo or BCG plus GD_3 was performed in L-SCLC without finding a benefit for the vaccine.

Erlotinib (OSI-774, Tarceva) and gefitinib (Iressa, ZD1839) are orally administered, small molecules that function as EGFR tyrosine kinase inhibitors (EGFR TKI). Gefitinib has activity as a salvage treatment for advanced NSCLC, and it has been approved by the U.S. Food and Drug Administration for use in treating recurrent NSCLC. The most common side effects of the TKIs include an acneiform rash and diarrhea. Gefitinib is being used in a phase II trial as second-line therapy for E-SCLC. ZD6474 (Zactima) is a TKI that inhibits VEGFR and EGFR.[79] A phase II SCLC trial is being performed by the National Cancer Institute of Canada using ZD6474. Patients with SCLC who have achieved a partial response or better will be randomized to therapy with ZD6474 or placebo.

Activation of the KIT receptor tyrosine kinase (RTK) can result from a mutant ligand-independent activation or an autocrine loop created by overexpression of its ligand, stem cell factor. Activation of this pathway has been found in up to 70% of SCLCs. Imatinib mesylate (Gleevec) inhibits KIT RTK and other tyrosine kinases and is being used in trials for treating SCLC. Many other targeted therapies are in development and will be assessed in upcoming trials.

Role of Surgery

The use of surgical resection as primary management of SCLC was abandoned in the 1970s, when poor survival rates were reported and few complete resections were achieved.[80] Several indications for surgical intervention have been evaluated since then, including the management of patients with N0 or N1 lesions with surgical resection followed by chemotherapy or chemoradiation, the resection of residual disease after chemotherapy or chemoradiation, and the role of surgical salvage of intrathoracic recurrences of SCLC. This section briefly reviews each of those issues.

In a report by the Veterans Administration Surgical Oncology Group that was published in 1982, the 5-year survival rates for patients with resected T1N0, T1N1, and T2N0 SCLC lesions were 60%, 31%, and 28%, respectively.[81] All of these patients received the chemotherapy available in the 1970s postoperatively. A SWOG protocol enrolled 15 SCLC patients to undergo surgical resection followed by chemoradiation and found this group to have a better 2-year survival rate than a cohort of matched patients treated nonoperatively in other SWOG trials (45% versus 14%).[82] Ichinose and colleagues reported on 112 SCLC patients who underwent surgical resection and were then randomized between two chemotherapy regimens.[83] Although the chemotherapy regimens produced comparable outcomes, the 3-year survival rates were encouraging for all enrolled patients: 65% for N0 disease, 52% for N1 disease, and 29% for N2 disease. Each of these three reports suggests that for the rare SCLC patients with N0 or N1 disease, surgical resection followed by chemotherapy produces survival results that may be superior to any available nonoperative approaches. The role of postoperative TRT in addition to chemotherapy in this setting remains uncertain. A pattern-of-failure study of patients with completely resected SCLC receiving postoperative chemotherapy alone would help clarify this issue.

At least four studies have evaluated the role of surgical resection of patients with L-SCLC after initial chemotherapy. In the three phase II trials conducted at Vanderbilt and the University of Toronto and on a multi-institutional basis, a postchemotherapy pathologic N0 status or a pathologic complete response was associated with long-term survival.[84-86] A randomized trial was conducted by the Lung Cancer Study Group in which L-SCLC patients achieving a partial or complete response to chemotherapy were randomized between resection and no resection.[87] There was no survival difference between the arms, with a 2-year survival rate of 20% in both arms (P = .55). Based on this trial and on the proven survival benefit of concurrent TRT, adjuvant surgery after chemotherapy is not recommended.

There is limited information regarding the role of surgical resection of intrathoracic recurrences. Shepherd and coworkers from the University of Toronto described 28 patients with L-SCLC who underwent salvage surgery after a partial response to chemotherapy or for subsequent progressive disease.[88] Ten of the 28 patients had NSCLC elements in their specimen. Their 5-year survival rate from the date of surgical salvage was 23%. There is only anecdotal information on surgical salvage of patients initially treated with chemotherapy and TRT.

Prophylactic Cranial Irradiation

PCI was initially introduced into practice in the 1960s for patients with acute lymphoblastic leukemia and who were at high risk for failure in the central nervous system (CNS).[89] PCI was first tested for patients with SCLC in the 1970s, following the recognition that brain metastases were common. The blood-brain barrier prevents the penetration of most chemotherapeutic agents, leaving the brain as a sanctuary site for relapse. The first trials demonstrated a substantial reduction in brain metastases, with one randomized trial of more than 200 patients conducted by ECOG revealing a decrease from 22% to 5%.[90] Unfortunately, at the same time, a number of long-term survivors of SCLC were recognized to have various neurologic abnormalities, including dementia, and many of these patients had received PCI.[91,92] The lack of prospective evidence linking PCI to these changes and the uncertainty about the optimal total PCI dose and fractionation and the optimal time of delivery contributed to a confused and controversial status for PCI.

Two large, randomized trials have evaluated the therapeutic benefit and neurotoxicity of PCI for SCLC patients after a response to initial therapy. In two French trials coordinated to run parallel (PCI 85 and PCI 88), a total of 505 patients were randomized between PCI and no PCI after a complete response to chemotherapy.[93] Most patients received 24.0 Gy in 8 fractions of 3.0 Gy each. There was a highly significant reduction in overall and isolated brain relapse rates favoring the PCI-containing arms (40% versus 59% and 39% versus 57%, respectively; $P < .0001$) and a nonsignificant trend toward improved survival at 2 years (31% versus 27%; $P = .10$). There was a slight increase in clinical asymptomatic imaging abnormalities, but no significant CNS morbidity was reported.

Gregor and associates reported a 314-patient multicenter trial conducted in the United Kingdom (UK02) that randomized L-SCLC patients in remission after completion of chemotherapy between PCI and no PCI.[94] Forty percent of the PCI patients received 30.0 Gy in 10 fractions, and other regimens ranged from 8 Gy in 1 fraction to 36.0 Gy in 18 fractions. At the 2-year follow-up evaluation, a reduction in brain relapse was seen for the PCI arm from 52% to 29% ($P = .0002$). The advantage was greatest for the patients receiving the higher PCI doses, particularly 36.0 Gy in 18 fractions. There was also a nonsignificant trend in overall survival outcome favoring the PCI arm ($P = .14$). Detailed neuropsychometric testing of PCI patients and controls failed to demonstrate a substantial treatment-related deficit. There was, however, substantial impairment of function in up to 40% of patients before PCI, suggesting that factors other than PCI may contribute to neurologic dysfunction in SCLC patients. Table 40-4 summarizes the French and UK trials.

In addition to TRT, PCI has been shown to positively influence survival in patients who achieve a complete response. Auperin and coworkers published a meta-analysis that included data from seven randomized, prospective studies that compared PCI with no PCI after a complete response was achieved.[95] As in the TRT meta-analyses, the 3-year survival rate of 20.7% was 5.4% better for those who received PCI compared with 15.3% for those who did not receive PCI ($P = .01$). Although 5.4% appears small, it does reflect a 35% increase in 3-year survivors. A statistically significant PCI dose-response effect was observed for the risk of brain recurrence but not survival rates. Neurotoxicity was not evaluated in this analysis.[95]

Based on available data, it is recommended that SCLC patients achieving a complete or near-complete response to initial therapy should be evaluated for PCI because PCI appears to significantly improve survival. Optimizing the dose-fractionation scheme is being investigated in a large, international, phase III trial. Commonly employed dose-fractionation patterns for PCI include 8 3-Gy fractions to a total of 24 Gy and 15 to 18 2-Gy daily fractions to total doses of 30 to 36 Gy.

MANAGEMENT OF METASTATIC AND RECURRENT DISEASE

Extensive-Stage Small Cell Lung Cancer

Approximately two thirds of all SCLC patients have extensive-stage disease. E-SCLC can vary from intrathoracic primary tumor and nodal disease only that is not amenable to a reasonable TRT field to multiple sites of extrathoracic metastases. The most common sites of extrathoracic metastases are the liver, bone, brain, and adrenal glands. The initial management of most patients with newly diagnosed extensive-stage disease is four or more cycles of platinum-based chemotherapy. A Japanese trial compared irinotecan plus cisplatin with EP in treating extensive SCLC.[71] The median survival was significantly improved for patients who received irinotecan plus cisplatin ($P = .002$).[71] However, this was not confirmed in an American trial.[72]

Irradiation has utility in treating E-SCLC. One role for radiation therapy is the palliation of bulky intrathoracic disease causing airway compromise, hemoptysis, postobstructive pneumonia, or superior vena cava syndrome. Although the role of irradiation is less clear in patients with E-SCLC than those with L-SCLC, there may be a benefit for delivering radiation therapy in the initial management of some patients with E-SCLC. Jeremic and coworkers reported the results of a

Table 40-4 Randomized Trials of Prophylactic Cranial Irradiation for Small Cell Lung Cancer

Trial	PCI dose	Outcome	Finding	Significance
PCI 85 and 88 (Arriagada et al[93])	24 Gy/8 fractions (Most)	Fewer brain metastases with PCI	41% vs. 59%	$P < .0001$
		Fewer isolated brain metastases with PCI	39% vs. 57%	$P < .0001$
		2-year survival rate not different	31% vs. 27%	$P = .1$
UK02 (Gregor et al[94])	36 Gy/18 fractions	Fewer brain metastases with PCI	29% vs. 52%	$P = .0002$
	24 Gy/12 fractions	PCI dose response 24-36 Gy		
	30 Gy/10 fractions	No neuropsychometric testing differences		
	8 Gy/1 fraction			

PCI, prophylactic cranial irradiation.

randomized prospective study that evaluated EP chemotherapy with or without BID-TRT and concurrent daily carboplatin plus etoposide (CE) in patients with E-SCLC.[96] Patients initially received three cycles of CE, and those with a complete response at distant sites and a partial response or complete response in the chest received BID-TRT (54 Gy in 36 fractions) with CE, followed by two cycles of EP or four cycles of EP alone. Patients who received TRT had significantly better survival than those who did not (median survival, 17 versus 11 months; 5-year survival, 9.1% versus 3.7%, respectively; $P = .041$).[96]

Bonner and associates performed a pilot study that included seven cycles of a six-drug combination.[97] PCI and TRT were given during the chemotherapy. After the seven cycles, patients received 6 Gy of upper hemibody irradiation, followed by 8 Gy to the lower hemibody. Despite considerable toxicity, the median survival time and 5-year survival rate were 11.5 months and 16%. Hemibody irradiation is not used in many institutions. However, irradiation of the sites of initial disease may be helpful, because failures after chemotherapy alone generally occur in the sites of original disease, and irradiation may lower the risk of such recurrences. With improved imaging techniques such as PET combined with CT (fused PET/CT), it is possible to precisely locate all sites of disease accurately, allowing focal irradiation of sites of metastases. This approach may spare enough marrow to allow the relatively safe delivery of aggressive multiagent chemotherapy.

Patients with brain metastases at diagnosis require cranial irradiation in their initial management, usually concurrently with the first or second cycle of chemotherapy. The whole-brain radiation therapy (WBRT) doses most commonly used for brain metastases range from 30.0 Gy in 10 fractions to 37.5 Gy in 15 fractions. One particular subgroup of E-SCLC patients has disease limited only to the chest and brain. This group may benefit from the use of chemotherapy, WBRT, and TRT. Kochhar and colleagues identified 30 such patients who initially received cisplatin-based chemotherapy and concomitant WBRT consisting of 36 to 48 Gy.[98] Subsequently, 22 patients also received TRT. The median survival of the entire group was 14 months. The results of this study suggested that the outcome of treating E-SCLC patients with the brain as the sole site of distant metastases at initial diagnosis is similar to that of L-SCLC patients. Patients who received TRT tended to have a longer median survival (16 months) than those who did not receive TRT or who received it at the time of local disease progression (12 months) ($P = .3$).[98]

Other sites of E-SCLC involvement may merit palliation radiation therapy for effective symptom management. These include painful or weight-bearing bony lesions, painful adrenal metastases, or soft tissue masses. Because SCLC is frequently a chemotherapy-responsive disease, there is a greater tendency to rely on chemotherapy in the palliative management of metastases than for other solid tumors. It is important to recognize the potential benefits of integrating radiation therapy with chemotherapy.

Management of Recurrent Small Cell Lung Cancer

The prognosis for any patient suffering a recurrence of SCLC is grave, regardless of the site of relapse. Although responses to second-line chemotherapy occur, they usually are short lived and often precede rapid tumor progression. Palliative or salvage radiation or reirradiation can be of substantial benefit to such patients, with a higher likelihood of palliative benefit than observed with most solid tumors.

TREATMENT ALGORITHM, CONTROVERSIES, AND CLINICAL TRIALS

A proposed treatment algorithm for patients with SCLC is shown in Figure 40-2.

Limited-Stage Disease and Good Performance Status

Management of patients with SCLC depends on disease stage and the patient's medical fitness. For patients with good performance status and limited-stage disease (clinical stages I to IIIB, excluding those with a malignant pleural effusion), the recommended management is concurrent TRT with platinum-based chemotherapy. The most widely accepted management protocol in the United States includes four cycles of EP chemotherapy, with BID-TRT beginning early (<90 days from the beginning of chemotherapy). The BID-TRT is delivered in 1.5-Gy fractions with an interfraction interval of at least 6 hours to a total dose of 45.0 Gy, with 8 to 10 of the 30 fractions sparing the spinal cord. This recommendation is based on the Intergroup Trial 0096 reported by Turrisi and colleagues.[50] For patients with huge tumors, postobstructive pneumonia, or atelectasis, there may be value in delaying initiation of TRT until a later cycle of chemotherapy.

Limited-Stage Disease in Special Populations: The Elderly and Patients with a Lower Performance Status

Treatment in fit elderly patients (>70 years of age) can be carried out in a manner similar to fit younger individuals. NCCTG 89-20-52 included 263 patients with L-SCLC and an

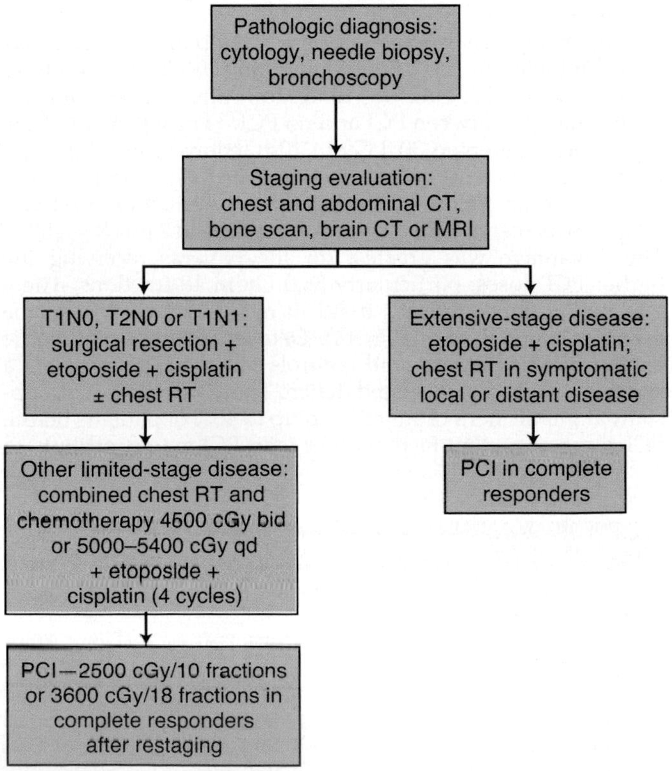

Figure 40-2 Treatment algorithm for small cell lung cancer. CT, computed tomography; MRI, magnetic resonance imaging; PCI, prophylactic cranial irradiation; RT, radiation therapy.

ECOG performance status of less than 2 who were randomized to QD-TRT or split-course BID-TRT. The outcomes of the 209 (79%) younger patients (<70 years old) were compared with the 54 (21%) elderly patients (≥70 years old). The overall incidence of grade 3 or grade 4 toxicity was not significantly greater among elderly patients. One specific toxicity, grade 4+ pneumonitis, occurred in 0% of those younger than 70 years and in 6% of older patients ($P = .008$). Although hematologic toxicity was not significantly worse in those older than 70 years, it was significantly worse in patients older than 65 years compared with younger individuals ($P = .03$). Grade 5 toxicity occurred in 3 (5.6%) of 54 patients older than 70 years and in 1 (0.5%) of 209 younger individuals ($P = .03$). Death was caused by pneumonitis in the three elderly patients and infection in the patient younger than 70 years. The 2-year and 5-year survival rates were 48% and 22%, respectively, for the younger patients, compared with 33% and 17% for the older patients ($P = .14$). Survival was not significantly worse for older individuals. Fit elderly patients with L-SCLC can receive combined-modality therapy if carefully monitored, with a reasonable expectation of 5-year survival.[99]

Patients with lower performance status tolerate the aggressive BID-TRT and platinum-based therapy more poorly than those whose performance status is good. However, there is still a likely benefit to concurrent chemoradiation for these patients, particularly if their reduced functional status is primarily due to their tumor burden. One reasonable option is to deliver QD-TRT in 1.8-Gy fractions to 50 to 54 Gy, while sparing the spinal cord above 45 Gy. This therapy can be delivered beginning with the first or second cycle of platinum-based chemotherapy.

Extensive-Stage Disease

Initial management of extensive-stage disease involves primary chemotherapy, with radiation therapy reserved for brain metastases, bulky and symptomatic intrathoracic disease, and symptomatic bony or visceral metastatic sites. Patients with a good performance status and low-volume metastatic disease may benefit from an aggressive regimen of chemotherapy and TRT at the time of initial management.

Prophylactic Cranial Irradiation

PCI should be considered for any SCLC patient who has achieved a complete response or near-complete response by all evaluable disease after initial management with chemotherapy or chemoradiation and who has no evidence of disease progression elsewhere.

Controversies and Clinical Trials

Issues likely to be the subject of clinical trials over the next several years include the benefit of BID-TRT versus higher-total-dose QD-TRT; the value of new systemic agents in the management of L-SCLC; and the optimal dose-fractionation regimen for PCI.

Although the benefit of twice-daily versus standard irradiation to 45 Gy has been demonstrated, no randomized, prospective studies have compared twice-daily radiation therapy with a higher total dose of daily radiation therapy. Such regimens are being evaluated in pilot studies by the CALGB, ECOG, and SWOG. A phase III trial is being planned to compare various TRT fractionation schemes.

Several new agents are being evaluated for the treatment of extensive disease and limited disease as substitutes for cisplatin and etoposide. They include conventional chemotherapeutic drugs and newer targeted agents.[100]

REFERENCES

1. Jemal A, Tiwari R, Murray T, et al: Cancer Statistics, 2004. CA Cancer J Clin 54:8-29, 2004.
2. Warde P, Payne D: Does thoracic irradiation improve survival and local control in limited-stage small-cell carcinoma of the lung? A meta-analysis. J Clin Oncol 10:890-895, 1992.
3. National Cancer Institute, Surveillance, Epidemiology, and End Results (SEER) Program: http://seer.cancer.gov/statfacts/html/lungb.html
4. National Cancer Institute: http://www.cancer.gov/cancertopics/pdq/treatment/small-cell-lung/healthprofessional
5. Green RA, Humprey E, Close H, et al: Alkylating agents in bronchogenic carcinoma. Am J Med 49:360-367, 1969.
6. Travis WD, Brambill E, Harris CC, Muller-Hermelink HK (eds): World Health Organization Classification of Tumors, Pathology, and Genetics: Tumors of the Lung, Pleura, Thymus, and Heart. Lyon, IARC Press, 2004.
7. Dye GK, Adjei AA: Novel targets for lung cancer therapy. Part I. J Clin Oncol 20:2881-2894, 2002.
8. Hibi K, Takahashi T, Yamakawa K, et al: Three distinct regions involved in 3p deletion in human lung cancer. Oncogene 7:445-449, 1992.
9. Sozzi G, Veroneses ML, Negrini M, et al: The FHIT gene at 3p14.2 is abnormal in lung cancer. Cell 85:17-26, 1996.
10. Harbour JW, Lai SL, Whang-Peng J, et al: Abnormalities in structure and expression of the human retinoblastoma gene in SCLC. Science 241:353-357, 1988.
11. Gazdar AF: Molecular markers for the diagnosis and prognosis of lung cancer. Cancer 69:1592-1599, 1992.
12. Ben-Ezra JM, Kornstein MJ, Grimes MM, et al: Small cell carcinomas of the lung express Bcl-2 protein. Am J Pathol 145:1036-1040, 1994.
13. Slebos RJO, Kribbalaar RE, Dadesic O, et al: *K-ras* oncogene activation as a prognostic marker in adenocarcinoma of the lung. N Engl J Med 323:561-565, 1990.
14. Gazdar A: The molecular and cellular basis of human lung cancer. Anticancer Res 13:261-268, 1994.
15. Kelly MJ, Linnoila RI, Avis IL, et al: Antitumor activity of a monoclonal antibody directed against gastrin-releasing peptide in patients with small cell lung cancer. Chest 112:256-261, 1997.
16. Johnson BE, Kelly MJ: Autocrine growth factors and neuroendocrine markers in the development of small cell lung cancer. Oncology 12(Suppl 1):11-14, 1998.
17. List AF, Hainsworth JD, Devis BV, et al: The syndrome of inappropriate secretion of antidiuretic hormone (SIADH) in small cell lung cancer. J Clin Oncol 4:1191-1198, 1986.
18. Dimopoulos MA, Fernandez JF, Samaan NA, et al: Paraneoplastic Cushing's syndrome as an adverse prognostic factor in patients who die early with small cell carcinoma of the lung. Am J Med 77:851-857, 1984.
19. Patel AM, Davila DG, Peters SG: Paraneoplastic syndromes associated with lung cancer. Mayo Clin Proc 68:278-287, 1993.
20. De La Monte SM, Hutchins GM, Moore GW: Paraneoplastic syndromes and constitutional symptoms in prediction of metastatic behavior of small cell carcinoma of the lung. Am J Med 77:851-857, 1984.
21. Marchioli CC, Graziano SL: Paraneoplastic syndromes associated with small cell lung cancer. Chest Surg Clin North Am 7:65-80, 1997.
22. American Joint Committee on Cancer (AJCC): Manual for Staging of Cancer, 6th ed. Philadelphia, JB Lippincott, 2002, pp 189-204.
23. Stahel RA, Ginsberg R, Havermann K, et al: Staging and prognostic factors in small cell lung cancer: a consensus. Lung Cancer 5:119-126, 1989.
24. Kamel EM, Zwahlen D, Wyss MT, et al: Whole-body (18)F-FDG PET improves the management of patients with small cell lung cancer. J Nucl Med 44:1911-1917, 2003.
25. Albain KS, Crowley JJ, LeBlanc M, et al: Determinants of improved outcome in small cell lung cancer: an analysis of the 2,580-patient Southwest Oncology Group database. J Clin Oncol 8:1563-1574, 1990.

26. Souhami RL, Bradbury I, Geddes OM, et al: Prognostic significance of laboratory parameters measured at diagnosis in small cell carcinoma of the lung. Cancer Res 45:2878-2882, 1985.
27. Cerny T, Blair V, Anderson H, et al: Pretreatment prognostic factors and scoring system in 407 small cell lung cancer patients. Int J Cancer 39:146-149, 1987.
28. Edmondson JH, Lagakos SW, Selawry OS, et al: Cyclophosphamide and CCNU in the treatment of inoperable small cell carcinoma and adenocarcinoma of the lung. Cancer Treat Rep 60:925-932, 1976.
29. Lowenbraun S, Bartolucci A, Smalley RV, et al: The superiority of combination chemotherapy over single-agent chemotherapy in small cell lung carcinoma. Cancer 44:406-413, 1979.
30. Souhami RI, Geddes DM, Spiro SG, et al: Radiotherapy in small cell cancer of the lung treated with combination chemotherapy: a controlled trial. Br J Med 288:1643-1646, 1984.
31. Byhardt RW, Cox JD, Holoye PY, et al: The role of consolidation irradiation in combined-modality therapy of small cell carcinoma of the lung. Int J Radiat Oncol Biol Phys 8:1271-1276, 1982.
32. Perry M, Eaton WC, Propert KJ, et al: Chemotherapy with or without radiation therapy in limited small cell lung cancer. N Engl J Med 316:912-918, 1987.
33. Bunn PA, Lichter AS, Makuch RW, et al: Chemotherapy alone or chemotherapy with chest radiation therapy in limited-stage small cell lung cancer. Ann Intern Med 106:655-662, 1987.
34. Perez CA, Krauss S, Bartolucci AA, et al: Thoracic and elective brain irradiation with concomitant or delayed multiagent chemotherapy in the treatment of localized small cell carcinoma of the lung: a randomized prospective study by the Southeastern Cancer Study Group. Cancer 47:2407-2413, 1981.
35. Pignon JP, Arriagada R, Ihde D: Meta-analysis of small-cell lung cancer. N Engl J Med 327:1618-1624, 1992.
36. Takada M, Fukuoka M, Kawahara M, et al: Phase III study of concurrent versus sequential thoracic radiotherapy in combination with cisplatin and etoposide for limited-stage small-cell lung cancer: results of the Japan Clinical Oncology Group study 9104. J Clin Oncol 20:3054-3060, 2002.
37. Murray N, Coy P, Pater JL, et al: The importance of timing of thoracic irradiation in the combined-modality treatment of limited-stage small cell lung cancer. J Clin Oncol 11:336-344, 1993.
38. James LE, Spiro S, O'Donnell MK, et al: A randomised study of timing of thoracic irradiation in small cell lung cancer-study 8 [abstract O-69]. Lung Cancer 41(Suppl 2):23, 2003.
39. Fried DB, Morris DE, Hensing TA, et al: Timing of thoracic radiation therapy in combined modality therapy for limited-stage small cell lung cancer: a meta-analysis [abstract O-70]. Lung Cancer 41(Suppl 2):23, 2003.
40. Choi N, Carey R: Importance of radiation dose in achieving improved locoregional tumor control in limited stage small cell lung carcinoma: an update. Int J Radiat Oncol Biol Phys 17:307-310, 1989.
41. Coy P, Hodson I, Payne D, et al: The effect of dose of thoracic irradiation on recurrence in patients with limited stage small cell lung cancer: initial results of a Canadian multicenter randomized trial. Int J Radiat Oncol Biol Phys 14:219-226, 1988.
42. Lichter AS, Turrisi AT: Small cell lung cancer: the influence of dose and treatment volume on outcome. Semin Radiat Oncol 5:44-49, 1995.
43. Papac RJ, Son Y, Bien R, et al: Improved local control of thoracic disease in small cell lung cancer with higher dose thoracic irradiation and cyclic chemotherapy. Int J Radiat Oncol Biol Phys 13:993-998, 1987.
44. Shank B, Scher H, Hilaris BS, et al: Increased survival with high-dose multifield radiotherapy and intensive chemotherapy in limited small cell carcinoma of the lung. Cancer 56:2771-2778, 1985.
45. Komaki R, Shin DM, Glisson BS, et al: Interdigitating versus concurrent chemotherapy and radiotherapy for limited small cell lung cancer. Int J Radiat Oncol Biol Phys 31:807-811, 1995.
46. Armstrong J, Shank B, Scher H, et al: Limited small cell lung cancer: do favorable short-term results predict ultimate outcome? Am J Clin Oncol 14:285-290, 1991.
47. Choi N, Herndon J, Rosenman J, et al: Phase I study to determine the maximum tolerated dose of radiation in standard and accelerated twice-daily radiotherapy schedules with concurrent chemotherapy for limited stage small lung cancer: CALGB 8837 [abstract]. Proc Am Soc Clin Oncol 14:363, 1995.
48. Turrisi AT, Glover DJ, Mason B, et al: Concurrent twice-daily multifield radiotherapy and platinum-etoposide chemotherapy for limited small-cell lung cancer: update 1987 [abstract]. Proc Am Soc Clin Oncol 6:172, 1987.
49. Johnson DH, Turrisi AT, Chang AY, et al: Alternating chemotherapy and twice-daily thoracic radiotherapy in limited small cell lung cancer: a pilot study of the Eastern Cooperative Oncology Group. J Clin Oncol 11:879-884, 1993.
50. Turrisi A, Kim K, Blum R, et al: Twice-daily compared with once-daily thoracic radiotherapy in limited small cell lung cancer treated concurrently with cisplatin and etoposide. N Engl J Med 340:265-271, 1999.
51. Schild SE, Bonner JA, Shanahan TG, et al: Long-term results of a phase III trial comparing once-daily radiotherapy with twice-daily radiotherapy in limited stage small-cell lung cancer. Int J Radiat Oncol Biol Phys 59:943-951, 2004.
52. Fu KK, Pajak TF, Trotti A, et al: A Radiation Therapy Oncology Group (RTOG) phase III randomized study to compare hyperfractionation and two variants of accelerated fractionation to standard fractionation radiotherapy for head and neck squamous cell carcinomas: first report of RTOG 9003. Int J Radiat Oncol Biol Phys 48:7-16, 2000.
53. Eaton W, Maurer H, Glicksman A, et al: The relationship of infield recurrences to prescribed tumor dose in small cell carcinoma of the lung [abstract]. Int J Radiat Oncol Biol Phys 7:1223, 1981.
54. White J, Chen R, McCracken J, et al: The influence of radiation therapy quality control on survival, response, and sites of relapse in oat cell carcinoma of the lung: preliminary report of a SWOG study. Cancer 50:1084-1090, 1982.
55. Mira JG, Livingston RB: Evaluation and radiotherapy implications of chest relapse patterns in small cell lung carcinoma treated with radiotherapy-chemotherapy: study of 34 cases and review of the literature. Cancer 46:2557-2565, 1980.
56. Liengswangwong V, Bonner JA, Shaw EG, et al: Limited-stage small cell lung cancer: patterns of intrathoracic recurrence and the implications for thoracic radiotherapy. J Clin Oncol 12:496-502, 1994.
57. Kies MS, Mira JG, Crowley JJ, et al: Multimodal therapy for limited small cell lung cancer: a randomized study of induction combination chemotherapy with or without thoracic radiation in complete responders; and with wide-field versus reduced-field radiation in partial responders. A Southwest Oncology Group study. J Clin Oncol 5:592-600, 1987.
58. Brodin O, Rikner G, Steinholtz L, et al: Local failure in patients treated with radiotherapy and multidrug chemotherapy for small cell lung cancer. Acta Oncol 29:739-746, 1990.
59. Graham MV, Purdy JA, Emami B, et al: Clinical dose-volume histogram analysis for pneumonitis after 3D treatment for NSCLC. Int J Radiat Oncol Biol Phys 45:323-329, 1999.
60. Emami B, Lyman J, Brown A, et al: Tolerance of normal tissue to therapeutic irradiation. Int J Radiat Oncol Biol Phys 21:109-122, 1991.
61. Sierocki JS, Hilaris BS, Hopfan S, et al: *Cis*-dichlorodiammine-platinum (II) and VP-16-213: an active induction regimen for small cell carcinoma of the lung. Cancer Treat Rep 63:1593-1597, 1979.
62. Roth BJ, Johnson DH, Einhorn LH: Randomized study of cyclophosphamide plus doxorubicin plus vincristine versus etoposide plus cisplatin versus alternation of these two regimens in extensive small cell lung cancer: a phase II study of the Southeastern Cancer Study Group. J Clin Oncol 10:282-291, 1992.
63. Fukuoka M, Furuse K, Saijo N: Randomized trial of cyclophosphamide, doxorubicin, and vincristine versus cisplatin and etoposide versus alternation of these regimens in small cell lung cancer. J Natl Cancer Inst 83:855-861, 1991.
64. Postmus P, Smit EF: Small cell lung cancer: is there a standard therapy? Oncology 12(Suppl 2):25-30, 1998.
65. MacCracken JD, Janaki LM, Crowley JJ, et al: Concurrent chemotherapy/radiotherapy for limited small-cell lung carci-

noma: a Southwest Oncology Group study. J Clin Oncol 8:892-898, 1990.
66. Johnson BE, Salem C, Nesbitt J, et al: Limited stage small cell lung cancer treated with concurrent BID chest radiotherapy and etoposide/cisplatin followed by chemotherapy selected by in vitro drug sensitivity testing. Proc Am Assoc Clin Oncol 10:240, 1991.
67. Loehrer P, Ansari R, Gonin R, et al: Cisplatin plus etoposide with and without ifosfamide in extensive stage small cell lung cancer: a Hoosier Oncology Group study. J Clin Oncol 13:2494-2499, 1995.
68. Glisson B, Scott C, Komaki R, et al: Cisplatin, ifosfamide, prolonged oral etoposide, and concurrent accelerated hyperfractionated thoracic radiotherapy for patients with limited small cell lung cancer: results of a phase II trial [abstract]. Lung Cancer 18(Suppl 1):89, 1997.
69. Ettinger DS, Finkelstein DM, Sarma RP, et al: Phase II study of paclitaxel in patients with extensive stage small cell lung cancer: an Eastern Cooperative Oncology Group study. J Clin Oncol 13:1430-1435, 1995.
70. Ettinger D, Seiferheld W, Abrams R, et al: Cisplatin (P) , etoposide (E), paclitaxel (T) and concurrent hyperfractionated thoracic radiotherapy (TRT) for patients (Pts) with limited disease (LD) small cell lung cancer (SCLC): preliminary results of RTOG 96-09 [abstract 1917]. Proceedings of the meeting of the American Society of Clinical Oncology (ASCO), New Orleans, LA. J Clin Oncol 19:490a, 2000.
71. Noda K, Nishiwaki Y, Kawahara M, et al: Irinotecan plus cisplatin compared with etoposide plus cisplatin for extensive small-cell lung cancer. N Engl J Med 346:85-91, 2002.
72. Hanna NH, Einhorn L, Sandler A, et al: Randomized, phase III trial comparing irinotecan/cisplatin (IP) with etoposide/cisplatin (EP) in patients with previously untreated, extensive-stage small cell lung cancer (SCLC). Abstract 7004. Proceedings of the Annual Meeting of ASCO, 2005.
73. Masuda N, Fukuoka M, Kusunoki Y, et al: CPT-11: a new derivative of camptothecin for the treatment of refractory or relapsed small cell lung cancer. J Clin Oncol 10:1225-1229, 1992.
74. Smyth JF, Smith IE, Seesa C, et al: Activity of docetaxel (Taxotere) in small cell lung cancer. Eur J Cancer 30A:1058-1060, 1994.
75. Abratt R, Bezwoda WR, Goedhals W, et al: Weekly gemcitabine with monthly cisplatin: effective chemotherapy for advanced non-small cell lung cancer. J Clin Oncol 15:744-749, 1997.
76. Evans WK, Radwi J, Tomiak E, et al: Oral etoposide and carboplatin: effective therapy for elderly patients with small cell lung cancer. Am J Clin Oncol 18:149-155, 1995.
77. Ettinger DS: Evaluation of new drugs in untreated patients with small cell lung cancer: its time has come [comment]. J Clin Oncol 8:374-377, 1990.
78. Giaccone G, Debruyne C, Felip E, et al: Phase III study of BEC2/BCG vaccination in limited disease small cell lung cancer (LD-SCLC) patients, following response to chemotherapy and thoracic irradiation (EORTC 08971, the SILVA study). Abstract 7020. Proceedings of the Annual Meeting of ASCO, 2004.
79. Carlomagno F, Vitagliano D, Guida T, et al: ZD6474, an orally available inhibitor of KDR tyrosine kinase activity, efficiently blocks oncogenic RET kinases. Cancer Res 62:284-290, 2002.
80. Fox W, Scadding JG: Medical Research Council comparative trial of surgery and radiotherapy for primary treatment of small-celled or oat-celled carcinoma of the bronchus: ten-year follow-up. Lancet 2:63-65, 1973.
81. Shields TW, Higgins GA, Matthews MJ, et al: Surgical resection in the management of small cell lung cancer. J Thorac Cardiovasc Surg 84:481-488, 1982.
82. Friess GG, McCracken JD, Troxell MJ, et al: Effect of initial resection of small cell carcinoma of the lung: a review of Southwest Oncology Group study 7628. J Clin Oncol 3:964-968, 1985.
83. Ichinose Y, Hara N, Ohta M, et al: Comparison between resected and irradiated small cell lung cancer in patients in stage I through IIIa. Ann Thorac Surg 53:95-100, 1992.
84. Prager RL, Foster JM, Hainsworth JM, et al: The feasibility of adjuvant surgery in limited stage small cell carcinoma: a prospective evaluation. Ann Thorac Surg 38:622-625, 1984.
85. Shepherd FA, Ginsberg RJ, Patterson GA, et al: A prospective study of adjuvant surgical resection after chemotherapy for limited small cell lung cancer: a University of Toronto Lung Oncology Group study. J Thorac Cardiovasc Surg 97:177-186, 1989.
86. Baker RR, Ettinger DS, Ruckdeschel JD: The role of surgery in the management of selected patients with small cell cancer of the lung. J Clin Oncol 5:697-702, 1987.
87. Lad T, Piantadosi S, Thomas P, et al: A prospective randomized trial to determine the benefit of surgical resection of residual disease following response of small cell lung cancer to combination chemotherapy. Chest 106:320-323, 1994.
88. Shepherd FA, Ginsberg R, Patterson GA, et al: Is there ever a role for salvage operations in limited small cell lung cancer? J Thorac Cardiovasc Surg 101:196-200, 1991.
89. Bleyer WA, Poplack DG: Prophylaxis and treatment of leukemia in the central nervous system and other sanctuaries. Semin Oncol 12:131-148, 1985.
90. Gregor A: Prophylactic cranial irradiation in small cell lung cancer: is it ever indicated? Oncology 12:19-24, 1998.
91. Johnson BE, Becker B, Geoff WB, et al: Neurologic, neuropsychologic, and computed cranial tomography scan abnormalities in 2- to 10-year survivors of small cell lung cancer. J Clin Oncol 3:1659-1667, 1985.
92. Catane R, Schwade JG, Varr I, et al: Follow-up neurologic evaluation in patients with small cell lung carcinoma treated with prophylactic cranial irradiation and chemotherapy. Int J Radiat Oncol Biol Phys 7:105-109, 1981.
93. Arriagada R, LeCahvalier T, Borie F, et al: Prophylactic cranial irradiation for patients with small cell lung cancer in complete remission. J Natl Cancer Inst 87:183-190, 1995.
94. Gregor A, Cull A, Stephens RJ, et al: Effects of prophylactic irradiation for patients with small cell lung cancer in complete response [abstract]. Eur J Cancer 31A:S19, 1995.
95. Auperin A, Arriagada R, Pignon JP, et al, for the PCI Overview Collaborative Group: Prophylactic cranial irradiation for patients with small-cell lung cancer in complete remission. N Engl J Med 342:476-484, 1999.
96. Jeremic B, Shibamoto Y, Nikolic N, et al: Role of radiation therapy in the combined-modality treatment of patients with extensive disease small-cell lung cancer: a randomized study. J Clin Oncol 17:2092-2099, 1999.
97. Bonner JA, Eagan RT, Liengswangwong V, et al: Long term results of a phase I/II study of aggressive chemotherapy and sequential upper and lower hemibody radiation for patients with extensive stage small cell lung cancer. Cancer 76:406-412, 1995.
98. Kochhar R, Frytak S, Shaw EG: Survival of patients with extensive small-cell lung cancer who have only brain metastases at initial diagnosis. Am J Clin Oncol 20:125-127, 1997.
99. Schild SE, Stella, PJ, Brooks B, et al: The results of combined modality therapy for limited stage small cell lung cancer in the elderly [abstract 7043]. Proc Am Soc Clin Oncol 23:624, 2004.
100. Bunn PA, Shepherd FA, Sandler A, et al: Ongoing and future trials of biologic therapies in lung cancer. Lung Cancer 41, S175-S186, 2003.

CHAPTER 41

NON–SMALL CELL LUNG CANCER

Henry Wagner, Jr.

EPIDEMIOLOGY/PATHOLOGY

An estimated 173,770 new cases and 160,440 deaths from lung cancer occurred in the United States in 2004. The relative mortality rate of almost 90% is strikingly greater than that of other common tumors, such as breast, prostate, or colorectal cancer. U.S. incidence and death rates have begun to decline for white men but are stable or rising for other demographic groups. An increasing percentage of newly diagnosed lung cancer patients are exsmokers.

Three histologic types, squamous cell carcinoma, adenocarcinoma (including bronchioalveolar), and large cell undifferentiated carcinoma, constitute non–small cell lung cancer (NSCLC). About 20% to 25% of lung cancers are undifferentiated small cell carcinomas (SCLCs). The relative incidence of SCLC has decreased in recent decades for reasons not well understood.

BIOLOGIC CHARACTERISTICS

Changes in structure or expression in a variety of oncogenes and tumor suppressor genes have been described in NSCLC and in premalignant tissues in lung exposed to carcinogens. The sequence by which these changes occur during carcinogenesis is not well understood. Genomic and proteomic profiling of lung cancer is adding to and may supplant anatomic staging, particularly in identifying patients with early-stage disease at high risk for systemic recurrence who may benefit from systemic adjuvant therapy.

STAGING

NSCLC is staged using the TNM system. Combined positron emission tomography and computed tomography (PET/CT) is the best single test for evaluation of the primary tumor; regional lymph nodes; upper abdominal organs, including liver and adrenals; and most of the skeleton. False-positive rates of 20% to 30% dictate that patients not be denied potentially curative treatment solely on the basis of radiographic findings without histologic confirmation. In patients lacking symptoms, bone scans and imaging of the central nervous system by CT or magnetic resonance imaging have low true-positive yields for patients with stage I or II disease, but positive yields are more common for patients with stage IIIA and B disease and should be obtained before submitting these patients to the rigors of combined-modality therapy.

PRIMARY THERAPY FOR EARLY-STAGE DISEASE

Resection by lobectomy or pneumonectomy with thorough sampling or formal dissection of hilar and mediastinal nodes is the preferred therapy for patients with clinical stage IA to IIB NSCLC. Patients with medical contraindications to surgery should be offered radiation therapy (with or without chemotherapy) with curative intent. Stereotactic radiotherapy has shown considerable promise in the management of these patients, producing local control in some series rivaling that of surgical resection.

ADJUVANT THERAPY

Postoperative irradiation of the ipsilateral hilum and the mediastinum reduces the risk of local recurrence in patients with resected node-positive NSCLC. A small survival benefit for patients with N2 disease has been suggested by several trials, but it remains controversial and inadequately tested in prospective trials. Postoperative radiation therapy is not routinely indicated for patients with N0 or N1 disease. Several large phase III trials and meta-analyses have shown a significant survival benefit for adjuvant chemotherapy using platinum-containing regimens (North America and Europe) or tegafur and uracil (Japan), and such therapy should be offered after resection to patients of good performance status. For patients with primarily resectable but poor-prognosis disease (stages IIB to IIIA), the role of neoadjuvant therapy with chemotherapy or chemoradiation is being investigated. For patients with more advanced mediastinal disease (N2-3, selected T4N0 with direct mediastinal invasion), adjuvant surgery after induction chemotherapy or chemoradiation and definitive chemoradiation are acceptable options.

UNRESECTABLE LOCALLY ADVANCED DISEASE

Combinations of radiation therapy and sequential or concurrent chemotherapy are superior to radiotherapy alone. Accelerated fractionation regimens also have shown some benefit. The optimal combination and sequence of surgery, radiation therapy, and chemotherapy for patients with stage IIIA and IIIB disease are subjects of active clinical investigation. With conventional radiation dose and fractionation regimens, concurrent chemoradiation gives better median and long-term survival than the sequential use of these modalities. Patients with stage IIIB (without malignant pleural or pericardial effusions) or unresectable IIIA disease are treated nonsurgically with irradiation combined with chemotherapy, with a 10% to 20% expectation of long-term survival for patients in good clinical condition.

PALLIATION

External beam radiation therapy effectively palliates symptoms of cough, hemoptysis, dyspnea, and chest pain arising from the primary tumor, nodal metastases, or tumor metastatic to bone or brain. Hypofractionated regimens are effective, well tolerated, and considerate of the limited life expectancy of many of these patients. Endobronchial irradiation or photodynamic therapy can offer palliation to patients with obstruction or hemoptysis. Endobronchial stents are another option for relief of airway obstruction, particularly in patients who have already received high-dose radiation therapy. In addition to extending the survival of patients with metastatic disease who have good performance status, chemotherapy can relieve symptoms and improve quality of life.

Lung cancer killed an estimated 160,440 men and women in the United States in 2004, more than colon, breast, prostate, and pancreatic cancer combined.[1] More than 80% of cases are caused by habitual or environmental exposure to tobacco smoke.[2] This clear-cut origin makes lung cancer a disease better suited to prevention than treatment. The reduction of lung cancer deaths in U.S. white men over the past 2 decades results more from the decrease of cigarette smoking after the publication of the U.S. Surgeon General's report in 1964 than the real but modest advances in the effectiveness of therapy.

Although the results of current therapy are disappointing, they must not be met by nihilism. Small improvements in therapy help many individuals, comparable in years of life saved to the modest benefit seen with adjuvant therapy of patients with other common tumors, such as breast or colon cancer. Although reduction of lung cancer incidence by avoidance of tobacco use is the most efficient strategy for reducing lung cancer deaths, optimization of current therapeutic modalities of surgery, irradiation, and chemotherapy is clearly worthwhile. Even if all current smokers quit now, their previous carcinogen exposure would lead to another million or more cases of lung cancer. Although primary and secondary forms of prevention are the best long-term strategies to reduce deaths from lung cancer, the need for effective treatment will continue in the foreseeable future.

The key to improved treatment outcomes for patients with lung cancer is the planned integration of all appropriate diagnostic and treatment modalities by a team whose members are interested in lung cancer and its treatment, well versed in the application of the appropriate modalities, and able to combine them without undue bias regarding their effectiveness.[3,4] Although major gaps remain in our knowledge about the most appropriate treatment, and clinical experience and preferences are valid, there is no room for the expert in a single modality who is unaware of what other modalities can bring to the treatment of his or her patients. Multidisciplinary evaluation of patients and planning of their treatment is the gold standard for this approach. The development of advocacy groups such as Alliance for Lung Cancer Advocacy, Support, and Education (ALCASE) that understand and demand such treatment approaches and their endorsement by groups such as the American Academy of Chest Physicians should hasten their becoming the standard of practice, much as happened previously for patients with breast and prostate cancers.

ETIOLOGY AND EPIDEMIOLOGY

More than 80% of cases in the present worldwide epidemic of lung cancer can be attributed to the carcinogens in tobacco smoke. Habitual and environmental exposures are clearly linked to lung cancer at levels ranging from descriptive epidemiology, to the appearance of characteristic patterns of oncogene and tumor suppressor gene mutations in smokers, to measurement of tobacco-associated carcinogens in the urine of individuals exposed to second-hand smoke.[5-8] Hecht and associates showed that nonsmokers, when exposed to side stream smoke in concentrations comparable to those found in a smoky bar, excreted metabolites of tobacco-specific carcinogens in their urine, providing experimental support for second-hand environmental carcinogenesis.[9,10] Pipe and cigar smokers have lower lung cancer rates than cigarette smokers, but these habits are far from innocuous, particularly in former cigarette smokers, who often continue to inhale.

The risk of lung cancer is related to the daily amount smoked and duration of smoking, leading to the term *pack-years* as a unit of smoking exposure. When individuals quit smoking, their risk of lung cancer declines, although several reports indicate a transiently increased risk during the first year, suggesting that some smokers quit in response to ill-defined symptoms or a sense of malaise associated with their undiagnosed lung cancer. Although the risk decreases over at least a decade, it remains higher than that of individuals who never smoked.[11-13] Examination of the respiratory epithelium of former smokers years after quitting shows persistence of telltale patterns of chromosomal loss and mutation or loss of oncogenes and tumor suppressor genes.[14,15] Once initiated, the process of lung carcinogenesis can proceed without continued smoke exposure. Although this raises a caution about the immediate benefits of smoking cessation in reducing lung cancer deaths, the proper interpretation is that it is better not to start smoking rather than that it is too late to quit. Although not falling to unity, the cancer risk clearly declines, and the risk of cardiovascular disease due to smoking declines even faster.

Past epidemiologic efforts have successfully indicted tobacco smoking as the major cause of lung cancer through the overall correlation between exposure and risk. Current efforts are devoted to better understanding the molecular determinants of risk that are distal to smoke exposure, including metabolic activation of procarcinogens, degradation and excretion of carcinogens, accurate repair of damaged DNA (or apoptotic execution of cells harboring DNA damage), and other less well understood mechanisms that result in the development of lung cancer in some heavy smokers.[16-20] Although no single genetic abnormality has been clearly implicated in causing lung cancer, there is considerable epidemiologic evidence for an inherited component of risk, particularly for cases of lung cancer diagnosed in younger individuals.[21] One candidate hypothesis is that carcinogenesis by cigarette smoke occurs in part through substances produced in the host from precursors in smoke. Individual variability in metabolic pathways leading to production and elimination or inactivation of these substances may produce differences in exposure to such carcinogens at a cellular level in two individuals with identical smoking histories. This hypothesis has been extensively investigated for a family of enzymes involved in oxidative metabolism of many xenobiotics, using the antihypertensive drug debrisoquin as a marker of enzyme activity. Polymorphisms at several loci are well described in human populations, and initial studies suggested that these correlated with the risk of development of lung cancer. Later studies that have analyzed genotype and phenotype have failed to confirm a significant correlation.[22-29] Although it appears that this particular metabolic marker is not a good predictor of lung cancer risk, this does not invalidate the hypothesis that the molecular exposure to carcinogens is a function of the introduction of foreign substances and their internal conversion to active or inactive metabolites. Other enzyme systems involved in drug metabolism, including glutathione transferase, are being investigated for their possible role in the individual and population variations in lung cancer incidence.[30,31]

In addition to tobacco smoke, many other substances have been implicated in causing lung cancer. Several industrial chemicals, particularly the chloromethyl ethers, have been associated with lung cancer. Exposure to asbestos and tobacco smoke produces lung cancer more frequently than either exposure alone. Exposure to inhaled radioactive substances by uranium miners or by individuals living in areas with high endogenous radon levels also increases risk.

Variations in DNA repair play a major role in the development of some malignancies (e.g., colorectal). Their role in lung carcinogenesis is less clear. Spitz and colleagues observed that lymphocytes from individuals with lung or head and neck cancers are more prone to develop DNA damage when exposed to a variety of mutagens than normal lymphocytes, perhaps reflecting a shift in the balance between damage induction and damage repair.[32,33]

Smokers with significant chronic obstructive lung disease (COLD) are at significantly higher risk for lung cancer than individuals with similar smoke exposure without COLD.[34,35] It is not known whether this reflects a common behavioral cause (e.g., deeper smoke inhalation, longer smoke retention) in these individuals or there are differences in metabolism of components of tobacco smoke that increase the risk for COLD and lung cancer.

The respiratory epithelium has a total surface area about the size of a tennis court. It may be divided functionally and pathologically into three zones. From the trachea through the major bronchi, the normal lining is made of squamous cells with interspersed neuroendocrine cells, which appear most commonly at airway bifurcations. Terminal alveoli are lined predominantly with type I and type II pneumocytes. Intermediate bronchi and bronchioles show a transition between squamous and adenomatous lining cells and a corresponding mixture of tumor types. The exposure of this large organ to a common set of inhaled toxins sets in process a widespread set of molecular and subsequent morphologic changes. Slaughter, who first observed this phenomenon in patients with multiple primary tumors of the head and neck, referred to it as *field cancerization*.[36] Auerbach described similar widespread changes in the lungs of smokers with lung cancer, and Saccomano described a pattern of progressive degrees of cytologic atypia leading to frankly invasive carcinoma.[37,38] The practical consequence of this is that patients who develop one neoplasm of the upper aerodigestive tract (i.e., head, neck, lung, and esophagus), if treated successfully, remain at substantial risk for developing a second or subsequent primary tumor. For patients with resected stage I non–small cell lung cancer (NSCLC), this risk is on the order of 2% to 3% per year for at least 10 years after treatment of the first cancer.[39-41] It can sometimes be difficult to distinguish second primary tumors from local recurrences or metastases; differences in histology, location, and presence of adjacent mucosal abnormalities have been proposed as criteria. The availability of several oncogene markers may allow for molecular fingerprinting by characteristic mutations at such sites as *KRAS* or *TP53* (which are known to have different mutational spectra in different parts of the aerodigestive tract), although it may still sometimes be difficult to distinguish between separate primary tumors and clonal variation of a metastasis and most cells in its primary tumor.

Lung cancer has been reported in a number of patients with human immunodeficiency virus (HIV) infection, and there is debate about the role of such infection, directly or indirectly through immunosuppression, in its cause. Lung cancer is not reported in particularly high incidence in individuals otherwise immunosuppressed, such as after organ transplantation. HIV-positive individuals with lung cancer tend to be younger than other patients with lung cancer, almost always have a history of heavy tobacco use, tend to present with advanced-stage disease (80% stage III and IV), show a predominance of adenocarcinomas, and have a poorer prognosis, even for those presenting with early-stage disease.[42-45] It is not clear whether HIV infection is an independent risk factor for the development of lung cancer or is strongly correlated with other risk factors such as early start of cigarette smoking, or both. The tolerance of these patients to treatment, particularly to aggressive chemoradiotherapy, may be compromised by limited hematologic reserve and development of severe mucositis during and after radiation therapy. Care must be taken to balance therapeutic aggressiveness and tolerance. HIV-infected individuals with resected early-stage NSCLC are at very high risk for relapse and warrant very close follow-up, but the role of adjuvant therapy in this population is unknown.

MOLECULAR BIOLOGY OF LUNG CANCER

The variety of cell types, the difficulty in obtaining serial biopsies of preneoplastic bronchial epithelium, and scarcity of good animal models of lung carcinogenesis induced by chronic cigarette smoke exposure have made this a difficult disease in which to study the molecular events of carcinogenesis. Although a large number of genetic changes have been identified in lung cancers and cell lines derived from them, the role of these in the pathogenesis of lung cancer is less well understood than in colorectal cancer, for which clear sequential development has been described.[46,47]

The morphologic and clinical differences between small cell carcinoma (SCLC) and NSCLC are reflected in decidedly different patterns of oncogene and tumor suppressor genes in these two disease families. Although there are no absolute differences or characteristic mutations for either type in the way that the *BCR-ABL* translocation is relatively pathognomonic of chronic myeloid leukemia, some molecular abnormalities frequent in one histologic type are rare in another, and vice versa.

RAS

The *RAS* oncogene family contains three members, *HRAS* (formerly designated H-*ras*), *KRAS* (formerly K-*ras*), and *NRAS* (formerly N-*ras*), which encode membrane-associated proteins involved in mediation of signals arising from binding of ligands to extracellular receptors by the cytosolic kinase cascade to nuclear transcription factors.[48] Mutation in several specific sites, including codons 12, 13, and 61, lead to constitutive activation of these signaling pathways independent of ligand binding.[49] In lung cancer, mutations are commonly seen in *KRAS* but not other members of the family. They are most frequently seen in adenocarcinoma but are also seen in other NSCLC histologies.[50] The presence of mutated *RAS* genes has been an adverse prognostic factor in resected and advanced lung cancer in most series in which this has been assessed.[51] *RAS* mutations are rare in SCLC, and when detected, they may represent an admixture of NSCLC elements or the development of an intermediate SCLC line.[52]

MYC

The *MYC* gene products are nuclear transcription factors. Structural mutations are not reported in lung cancer, but amplification of copy number and overexpression are common in SCLC and uncommon in NSCLC. Amplification has been more commonly reported in cell lines derived from patients with clinically resistant tumors after chemotherapy, but the role of *MYC* amplification in de novo drug resistance is uncertain.[53-57]

TP53

Abnormalities in *TP53* function through deletion or mutation of the gene *(TP53)* are among the most common genetically induced changes in human malignancies.[58] Mutations are reported in a high frequency in lung cancer, about 50% of NSCLCs and 90% of SCLCs. The exact frequencies of *TP53* abnormalities have varied somewhat with the techniques used to detect them.[59,60] The normal *TP53* gene-encoded product plays several key roles in determining cellular response to genetic damage, particularly whether cells enter growth arrest or apoptosis. There have been conflicting reports about the prognostic implications of abnormal TP53 function in lung cancer. For a number of chemotherapeutic agents and ionizing radiation, cells lacking normal TP53 function are resistant to apoptotic cell death, although the effect on overall cell survival is controversial.[60-62] Because *TP53*-knockout mice are viable, it is clear that there exist alternate pathways of detecting and responding to DNA damage and initiating apoptosis.

RB1

The *RB1* gene-encoded product is a nuclear protein that undergoes cyclic phosphorylation and dephosphorylation during the cell cycle under the control of G_1 cyclins.[63,64] The RB1 protein regulates E2F transcription factor activation. Absence of normal function occurs in most SCLCs but only in about 10% of NSCLC lines examined.[65-67]

CDKN2A

Normally, CDKN2A (previously designated p16) regulates transcription through phosphorylation of the RB1 protein. Abnormalities of CDKN2A function are reported in a reciprocal fashion to those of RB1; they are common in NSCLC and rare in SCLC. Because either of these abnormalities can allow uncontrolled transcriptional activation through E2F, it is not surprising that they are not commonly found together.[68] Although mutations in either are common in lung cancer, these mutations have not been correlated with prognosis.

Growth Factors

Abnormalities in normal autocrine growth factor signaling pathways have been proposed as a common mechanism for the dysregulated cell growth in cancer. In lung cancer, several clear examples of this have been demonstrated to exist and have become targets for possible therapeutic intervention.

Epidermal Growth Factor Receptor and ERBB2/HER2

The epidermal growth factor receptor (EGFR) mediates a number of signaling pathways critical for cell growth, survival, and response to cytotoxins, including ionizing radiation and several chemotherapeutic agents. It is overexpressed in a variety of malignancies, and overexpression has been correlated with poorer clinical outcome and resistance to radiation. Clinical attempts to target this pathway have included monoclonal antibodies targeted to the extracellular domain of the receptor (C225, ABX) and low-molecular-weight compounds that bind the ATP site and inhibit the tyrosine kinase activity of the receptor. About 10% of patients with NSCLC have mutations involving the ATP-binding pocket of the EGFR, which gives rise to more prolonged signaling activity in response to ligands such as epidermal growth factor (EGF) or transforming growth factor-β (TGF-β) and causes them to bind these inhibitors more tightly.[69-71] Patients whose tumors have these mutations are likely to have significant objective responses to treatment with these compounds, but it is postulated that patients with wild-type, overexpressed EGFR are more likely to show a response of growth restraint but not regression. The relative importance of mutation and overexpression of EGFR in predicting outcome of treatment with low-molecular-weight tyrosine kinase inhibitors such as erlotinib is a subject of controversy and active clinical research.

Overexpression ERBB2 (also designated HER2/NEU) is common in NSCLC, particularly adenocarcinoma, and it is correlated with decreased survival of patients with resected disease.[72,73] Compared with the overexpression of HER2 seen in cancer of the breast, the degree of overexpression is typically much less, with few lung cancer patients showing 3+ staining by immunohistochemistry. Trials of monoclonal antibodies directed against HER2 in NSCLC have shown relatively little activity whether used alone or in combination with cytotoxic chemotherapy.

In addition to overexpression of wild-type HER2, activating point mutations have been described in a number of patients with NSCLC.[74] These patients, about 5% of all with NSCLC or 15% of those with adenocarcinoma, may be more sensitive to therapies directed against HER2-mediated signaling and warrant particular with these agents.

Gastrin-related peptide (GRP) is the mammalian analogue of bombesin, the amphibian peptide that was first described as an autocrine regulatory factor. It is normally expressed in neuroendocrine cells in the central nervous system (CNS), the gut, and fetal lung. Its expression is increased in histologically normal lung exposed to chronic damage such as cigarette smoke.[75] Detectable GRP secretion is found in most SCLC and about 10% to 20% of NSCLC lines, many of which show other evidence for neuroendocrine derivation. SCLC cells possess high-affinity GRP receptors, and provision of exogenous GRP in cell culture stimulates growth.[76] Monoclonal antibodies raised against GRP inhibit SCLC growth in vitro and in vivo in animal models in nude mice.[77] Human trials of these antibodies have been conducted with some regressions reported, but logistic difficulties in antibody production have limited this approach.[78]

KIT

The KIT receptor and its ligand (i.e., stem cell factor or Steele factor) represent a potential autocrine loop present in about 15% of SCLCs. Because of the potent effects of the drug imatinib in inhibiting mutant KIT in gastrointestinal stromal tumors, this agent has been investigated in SCLC, unfortunately with little evidence of activity. These trials were conducted without the requirement of KIT being overexpressed, and it is not clear that overexpression, as distinct from specific point mutations, is sufficient for druggability of this target.

EARLY DETECTION AND PREVENTION

The poor survival of most patients diagnosed with symptomatic lung cancer has prompted numerous efforts to diagnose the disease in asymptomatic individuals. In the United States, the National Cancer Institute (NCI) sponsored several trials in the 1970s that compared active screening using a chest radiograph and sputum cytology with "routine" medical care that often included an annual chest radiograph.[79,80] These studies showed an increased detection of earlier stage disease in the screened populations, with higher rates of resectability, but there was not a measurable improvement in overall survival. This led to recommendations from the American Cancer Society to abandon routine screening for lung cancer by the methods used and in the populations studied (warranted by the data) and to an unwarranted pessimism about early diagnosis in general.

Since the time of these trials, important demographic and technologic changes have occurred. Lung cancer is increasingly a disease of women, who have taken up cigarette smoking in growing numbers.[81] Lung cancer has increasingly become a disease of former smokers. Several large centers have reported that more than one half of their lung cancer patients are former (i.e., more than 1 year since cessation) rather than current smokers.[82] This change has key implications for therapeutic interventions and in the possibility of enlisting this population, who have already demonstrated a high degree of motivation by quitting smoking, in studies of early detection and chemoprevention.

COMPUTED TOMOGRAPHY–BASED SCREENING STUDIES

The availability of fast high-resolution computed tomography (CT) has prompted a new round of screening trials.[83] Several groups have demonstrated that CT is more sensitive in detecting pulmonary nodules in asymptomatic individuals than chest radiography. The percentage of detected nodules ultimately proved to be cancerous has varied considerably between different series, in part due to the background frequency of conditions such as endemic fungal infections that may give rise to benign pulmonary nodules. Most series have shown a shift to earlier stage at diagnosis for screened patients compared with historical controls, which is potentially a marker for improved survival. However, others have argued that screening-detected tumors are likely to have a different and more indolent biology than other tumors and that only prospective trials can convincingly show whether CT screening reduces overall or tumor-specific mortality.

CYTOLOGIC AND MOLECULAR SCREENING

Advances in molecular technology offer the promise of detecting malignant changes in exfoliated cells well before morphologic changes appear. Tockman has shown that in monoclonal antibody staining using sera developed against SCLC and NSCLC lines, sputum cells showing atypia could predict which patients were going to develop frank malignancy with a lead time of about 2 years.[84,85] This technique is being studied further in a prospective trial of patients who have undergone resection of a stage I NSCLC and are at high risk for local recurrence and development of a second primary lung cancer. Mao reported similar findings using probes for mutations of *KRAS* and *TP53* genes.[86] Mills also reported detection of *KRAS* mutations in fluid obtained at bronchioalveolar lavage.[87] These findings, reported initially in retrospective pilot trials, are being validated in large, prospective trials seeking to detect second malignancies in patients curatively resected for their first lung cancers. Examination of the bronchial epithelium reveals multiple areas of dysplasia and carcinoma in many of these patients at the time of their initial diagnosis, and the risk of a second invasive malignancy is about 3% per year.

One reasonable interpretation of the results of the NCI-sponsored early-detection trials is that although they were successful in detecting disease earlier than would have been done without screening, this "early" disease was still quite advanced in terms of the natural history of the disease. Key events such as the ability of tumor cells to metastasize, induce angiogenesis, and develop resistance to chemotherapeutic agents were likely to have occurred earlier in their history. Recognition of the long promotion period in the development of lung cancer suggests that a more fruitful approach would be to detect intermediate points in this process, to screen for carcinogenesis instead of cancer.[88]

Autofluorescence bronchoscopy by Xillix and other systems has been used to examine the tracheobronchial tree and look for early neoplastic or preneoplastic lesions.[89] This approach complements that of CT screening, which primarily detects peripheral lesions and has poor sensitivity for small endobronchial lesions.

The increasing understanding of epithelial carcinogenesis as a process rather than an event has identified several candidate biomarkers for early detection strategies. Mulshine has classified such markers in several categories[90]:

- Tissue-specific products such as carcinoembryonic antigen or surfactant for which there are known polymorphisms
- Differentiation markers (i.e., blood group and other carbohydrate antigens)
- Positive or negative growth regulators (e.g., bombesin)

Several groups have described detection of circulating tumor-derived DNA fragments in patients with a variety of malignancies. Screening these for mutations known to be common in lung cancer (e.g., *RAS* codon 63 mutations) or characteristic patterns of DNA methylation represents another potentially useful strategy.[91,92] These and other potential molecular markers for screening and early detection have been reviewed and are areas of active investigation, but none is ready for widespread adoption.[93] Long-term trials of therapeutic interventions with serial monitoring of these and other candidate markers will be needed to confirm their predictive value and to investigate whether their expression is an integral feature of lung carcinogenesis or an epiphenomenon.

CHEMOPREVENTION

Several classes of compounds have been investigated as potential agents for chemoprevention of lung cancer.[94] Epidemiologic data suggest that the incidence of lung cancer is higher in populations with low dietary intake of retinoids and carotenoids. Deficiencies of these agents can lead to squamous metaplasia in animal models. Provision of exogenous vitamin A to animals that have developed metaplasia or atypia can lead to morphologic normalization of the epithelium. Retinoids can also reduce the rate of development of carcinoma after exposure of respiratory epithelium to acute doses of a number of carcinogens. At a cellular level, retinoids bind to members of several families or nuclear receptors (i.e., transcription factors) and influence cell differentiation, maturation, and senescence. The role of specific retinoids in these processes and possible tissue and species differences in retinoid effects remain under investigation.

Several trials of retinoids have been conducted in patients at high risk for lung cancer. Hong and associates randomized patients with treated cancers of the head and neck to 13-*cis*-retinoic acid or placebo and found that although the recurrence rates of the initial lesion were unchanged, the treated group had a significantly reduced incidence of second primary tumors, particularly of the head, neck, lung, and esophagus.[95,96] Pastorino and coworkers conducted a similar trial in resected patients lung cancer using retinoyl palmitate and observed fewer second primaries and a borderline improvement in overall survival.[97] However, larger, prospective, confirmatory trials testing isotretinoin or retinyl palmitate and *N*-acetylcysteine have failed to confirm the initial promise of earlier trials.[41,98] To further complicate matters, several trials of β-carotene as a chemopreventive agent have observed increased rates of cancer in populations of individuals who continue to smoke.[99]

The epidemiologic correlation between reduced consumption of foods rich in carotenoids and an increased risk of lung cancer in smokers and the laboratory data showing a protective effect of β-carotene against lung carcinogenesis led to two large chemoprevention trials.[100-103] In Finland, a trial of placebo versus β-carotene or α-tocopherol (i.e., vitamin E), or both, showed increased rates of and death from lung cancer in subjects receiving β-carotene.[104] Participants in this trials were predominantly actively smoking males. In the United States, a trial of β-carotene (CARET trial) was closed prematurely when interim analysis also showed an increased incidence of lung cancer in the treated arm.[105] The increased risk of lung cancer incidence and death of lung cancer persisted even after further administration of β-carotene was discontinued.[106,107] Although the popular interpretation of these trials has been negative, they offer clear proof of the principle that human lung carcinogenesis is a dynamic process amenable to pharmacologic manipulation. They also reinforce the basic principle that clever ideas must be tested in careful trials before becoming standard of practice. No agent has yet been recognized and confirmed as an effective chemopreventive agent for lung, head, or neck cancers, and an untreated control group remains appropriate and essential for future trials.

Selenium is a trace mineral whose presence in the soil varies considerably with geography. It is a required cofactor for a number of important enzymes, and selenium deficiency in animals can produce premalignant changes. Epidemiologic studies have suggested correlation between low dietary intake and cancer of a number of sites. With these considerations in mind, Clark and colleagues performed a trial of selenium versus placebo in subjects with a history of multiple skin cancers, with a reduction in subsequent skin cancers as the designed trial outcome.[108] Such a reduction was not seen, but it was observed that the number of cases of lung cancer in the treated group was one half of that in the control group. Because multiple secondary comparisons were made in the trial, this observation might reflect chance, and a confirmatory trial to compare selenium with placebo in patients with resected stage I NSCLC is being coordinated by the Eastern Cooperative Oncology Group (ECOG).

One limitation of the chemoprevention trials is that the candidate agents were administered systemically, with the attendant toxicities associated with this approach. An approach of delivering agents directly to the bronchial epithelium, where the smoke went and where carcinogenesis occurs, is appealing and is being explored with the development of agents deliverable by aerosol.[109]

PATHOLOGY AND PATHWAYS OF SPREAD

The outcome of an individual case of lung cancer is a function of the histology and stage of the disease and the status of the host. Host factors are of major importance in lung cancer as reflections of tumor burden not yet demonstrable by imaging techniques and as a reflection of the individual's ability to withstand the morbidity of treatment. In patients with lung cancer, physiologic function is frequently impaired, in part due to the advanced age of many patients (median age of diagnosis is in the seventh decade) and the frequency of other illnesses, such as chronic obstructive pulmonary disease and cardiac disease, that are also tobacco related.

Lung cancer is divided into two major histologic subgroups: SCLC and the combination of squamous cell carcinoma, adenocarcinoma, and large cell undifferentiated carcinoma considered collectively as NSCLC. Although there are some differences in the behavior of these subtypes of NSCLC in early-stage disease, these distinctions are largely lost with more advanced disease. In the past, SCLC and NSCLC were viewed as quite different diseases, but there is increasing convergence in modern therapeutic approaches with the understanding that both are usually disseminated diseases that manifest with substantial bulk disease in the chest, for which successful treatment requires systemic and locoregional therapies.

In addition to cell type and anatomic stage, a variety of molecular prognostic factors have been proposed to provide further prognostic or predictive information in lung cancer (Table 41-1). These include measures of cell proliferation (e.g., S-phase fraction, proliferating-cell nuclear antigen [PCNA], Ki-67, potential doubling time [T_{pot}]), mutated or overexpressed oncogenes and or tumor suppressor genes (e.g., *KRAS*, *TP53*, *ERBB2* [*HER/NEU*], *BCL2*), cell surface antigens (i.e., blood type antigens and their precursors), and induction of angiogenesis. Most of these have been proposed on the basis of small series of patients treated in a nonuniform fashion, and they often are based on univariate rather than multivariate analysis. Proper validation of these will require prospective study in large series of patients staged, treated, and followed in a uniform fashion.[110] It is likely that patterns of expression of multiple markers as assessed by genomic or proteomic analysis will more successfully predict prognosis, as has been shown for breast cancer and intermediate grade lymphomas. Small series have reported the success of such profiling in lung adenocarcinomas but large validation series in uniformly patient groups are awaited.[111] Such profiling may also be useful in determining those patients at greatest risk for specific patterns of metastatic spread, such as to the brain, for whom particular targeted adjuvant therapies such as prophylactic cranial irradiation may be more appropriate than in an unselected population.

Lung cancer spreads through regional lymphatic vessels within the lung to the hilar and paratracheal nodes, which drain to the supraclavicular fossae and, to a lesser degree, the upper abdomen (Fig. 41-1). The patterns of nodal spread are partially predictable on the basis of tumor size, histology, and proximity to central airways. Involvement most often begins with intrapulmonary nodes, extends centrally to the hilum, and then extends to the mediastinum. However, noncontiguous "skip" metastases are well described. Although nodal involvement can usually be detected by preoperative CT scan-

Table 41-1 Proposed Nonstage Prognostic Factors for Non–Small Cell Lung Cancer

Tumor volume
Number of nodal sites
Clinically evident nodal involvement
Extranodal extension
Immunohistochemical detection of nodal metastases
Histology
Grade
Ploidy
Proliferating-cell nuclear antigen (PCNA) staining
Ki-67 staining
Bromodeoxyuridine (BRDU) labeling
KRAS mutation
3p deletion
TP53 mutation
TP53 protein overexpression
Angiogenesis (microvessel density)
Vascular endothelial growth factor (VEGF) overexpression
Epidermal growth factor receptor (EGFR) overexpression and/or mutation
ERBB2 (HER/NEU) oncogene expression and/or mutation
Blood group A expression
H, Ley, and Leb blood group antigen expression

Adapted from Wagner H, Bonomi P: Preoperative and postoperative therapy for non–small cell lung cancer. *In* Roth JA, Ruckdeschel JC, Weisenburger TH (eds): Thoracic Oncology. Philadelphia, WB Saunders, 1995, pp 147-163.

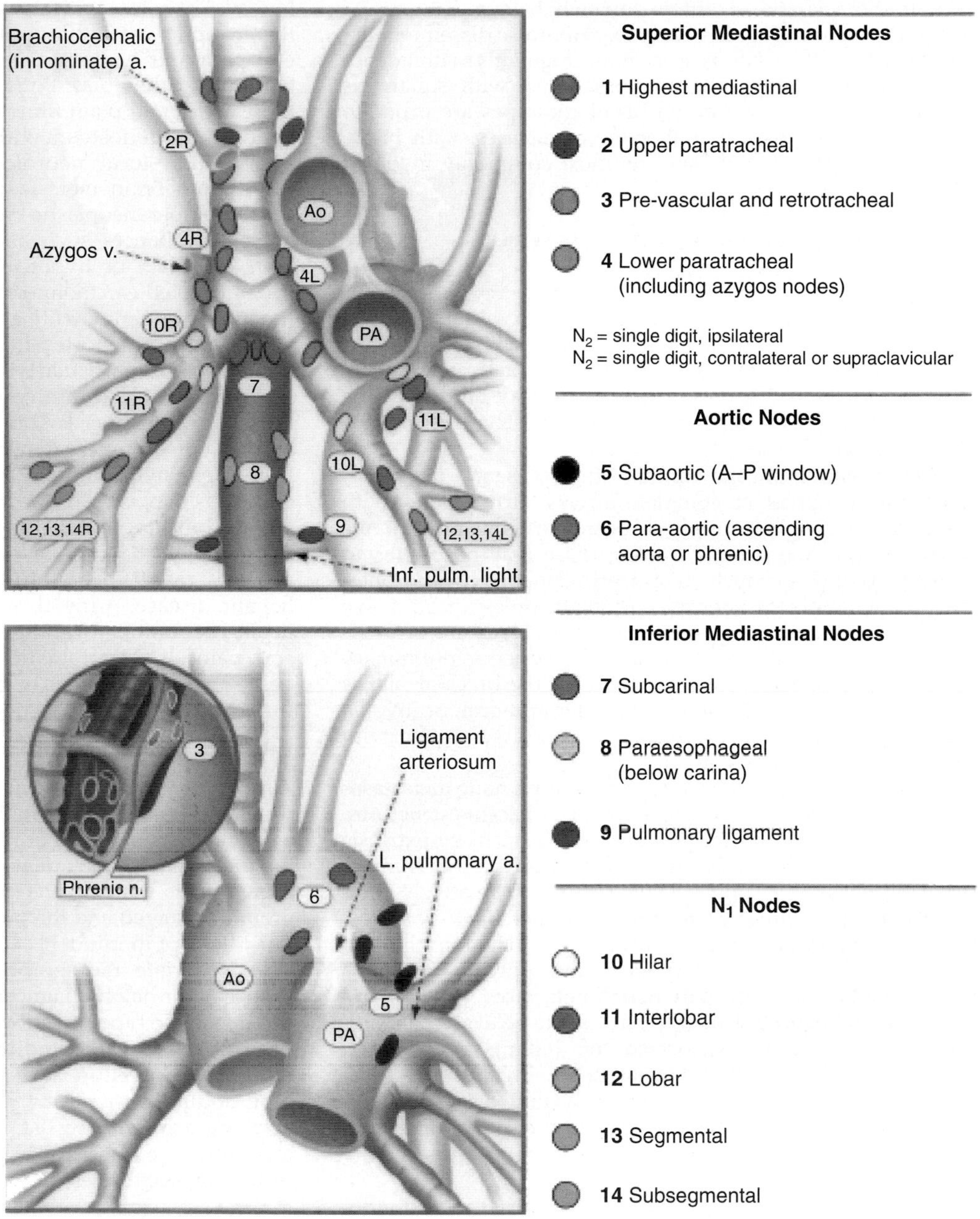

Figure 41-1 Map of intrathoracic lymph node stations. Single-digit stations (1 to 9) are N2 nodes; double-digit stations (10 to 14) are N1 nodes. (From Mountain C: Revisions in the international system for staging lung cancer. Chest 111:1710-1717, 1997.)

ning, even for T1 primary tumors, the incidence of clinically unsuspected nodal metastases can be as high as 15% to 20% for peripheral adenocarcinomas.[112,113] Treatment approaches that do not include surgical removal or radiotherapeutic treatment of hilar or mediastinal nodes should keep these numbers in mind.

Hematogenous dissemination is common and usually is associated with nodal involvement, although about 20% of patients with resected T1 N0 lesions will relapse in distant sites. Nodes which appear normal on routine histology, when examined by immunohistochemical staining for epithelial antigens, contain tumor cells in 15% to 25% of cases.[113] Occult bone marrow metastases in resected rib at the time of thoracotomy are also found by this method, including patients without any evidence of nodal disease.[114] It appears that nodal and hematogenous spread, which usually is associated, may occur independently. Although some have reported artifacts in the methodology used in these studies and the occasional presence of epithelial cells in normal lymph nodes, it is generally agreed that routine histologic examination of nodes underestimates the true frequency of metastatic involvement.[115]

Although nodal drainage is primarily to ipsilateral nodes, the left upper lobe drains commonly to contralateral paratracheal nodes as well as to nodes in the anterior mediastinum.[116] Direct involvement of the visceral and parietal pleura by peripheral tumors puts the pleural space at risk for involvement. The true frequency of this is not well known, nor is its clinical significance or appropriate therapeutic response. Several series have reported that intraoperative pleural lavage detects tumor cells in about 10% of patients and that their survival is markedly worse than that of patients with tumors of otherwise similar stage with cytologically negative lavage.[117,118]

Extrathoracic spread differs somewhat among the major histologic types of NSCLC. Early extrathoracic dissemination, particularly to the CNS, is seen more frequently with adenocarcinoma and large cell carcinoma than with squamous cell carcinoma.[119] However, all histologic types are prone to early and widespread extrathoracic metastases, with brain, bone, liver, adrenal, and lung the most commonly involved sites.

CLINICAL MANIFESTATIONS, PATIENT EVALUATION, AND STAGING

Most patients diagnosed with lung cancer present with symptomatic disease, it is the uncommon patient who is diagnosed from detection of an unsuspected mass on a chest x-ray obtained for other purposes. Symptoms may be due to the primary tumor, its nodal and systemic metastases, or to paraneoplastic syndromes.

Central endobronchial tumors often present with symptoms due to partial or complete airway obstructions, with symptoms of cough, hemoptysis, postobstructive pneumonia, or dyspnea. In the chronic smoker, these may not represent new symptoms so much as exacerbation of baseline ones. Peripheral tumors are often asymptomatic unless they involve the chest wall and produce pain from involvement of intercostal nerves. Tumors that involve the superior pulmonary sulcus may directly involve branches of the brachial plexus with pain and weakness in the shoulder and arm, or involve the sympathetic trunk producing Horner's syndrome with ipsilateral ptosis, miosis, and anhidrosis.

Symptoms produced from regional lymph node metastases are usually due to compression of adjacent structures. Although complete obstruction of main bronchi by extrinsic compression is uncommon, this occurs more readily in more distal airways. The superior vena cava is a relatively thin-walled, low-pressure system, and it is vulnerable to compression with significant clinical consequences. The intrathoracic course of the recurrent laryngeal and phrenic nerves is vulnerable to compression by nodal metastases. Patients presenting with hoarseness or who have a fixed elevated hemidiaphragm should be suspected of having such nodal involvement. Recurrent laryngeal nerve involvement occasionally may be detected radiographically by asymmetry of vocal cord glucose uptake on positron emission tomography (PET), with the paretic cord having reduced activity (Fig. 41-2).

Lung cancer can metastasize to a wide variety of extrathoracic sites and produce diverse symptoms. The most frequent symptoms of distant metastatic disease are bone pain and neurologic symptoms from brain metastases. These are not, however, absolute indicators of metastatic disease. Pulmonary hypertrophic osteoarthropathy typically presents with bilateral pain and tenderness in the legs, which are often most tender over the tibias. Bone scan will show diffuse uptake in these areas, and plain films usually show a characteristic elevation of the periosteum without involvement of cortical bone.

Although focal neurologic symptoms most commonly result from brain metastases, CNS symptoms may also be caused by paraneoplastic cerebellar degeneration or to metabolic disturbances such as hyponatremia (most commonly seen in SCLC) or hypercalcemia (most commonly seen in squamous cell carcinoma). Nonspecific deceases in cognitive function compared with age and gender matched controls have also been reported in patients with lung cancer before any treatment, particularly in SCLC.[120]

Liver metastases are common but usually asymptomatic unless quite advanced. Abnormalities in liver function studies are uncommon unless there has been extensive destruction of liver parenchyma, although alkaline phosphatase and bilirubin levels may be elevated by small-volume hepatic or nodal disease blocking the common hepatic duct. Elevation of the lactate dehydrogenase level is a poor prognostic sign, but it probably reflects overall tumor burden more than specifically hepatic disease. Adrenal metastases are quite common, particularly at autopsy but rarely symptomatic unless quite large and painful. Symptomatic adrenal hypofunction has been described but is decidedly uncommon.

Radiographic Procedures in Staging

As with any other medical test, radiographic staging procedures should be used primarily when their results will lead to a change in choice of therapy. A secondary role is in defining homogeneous groups of patients for clinical research. When used in this manner, the possibility of differences between groups so staged and the more general population of patients must be kept in mind.

Appropriate radiographic procedures for patients with suspected or newly diagnosed lung cancer depend in part on the histologic type of cancer and on the therapeutic options. The otherwise healthy individual who presents for an elective orthopedic procedure and is found to have a 2-cm peripheral lung nodule without any other abnormalities on chest radiography, combined PET/CT of the chest, and routine laboratory studies (e.g., complete blood cell count, chemistry profile including electrolytes, renal, and hepatic function) is unlikely to have any useful information found with further testing. At the other end of the spectrum, the patient who presents with limiting cardiopulmonary disease, substantial recent weight loss, poor performance status, new bone pain and a

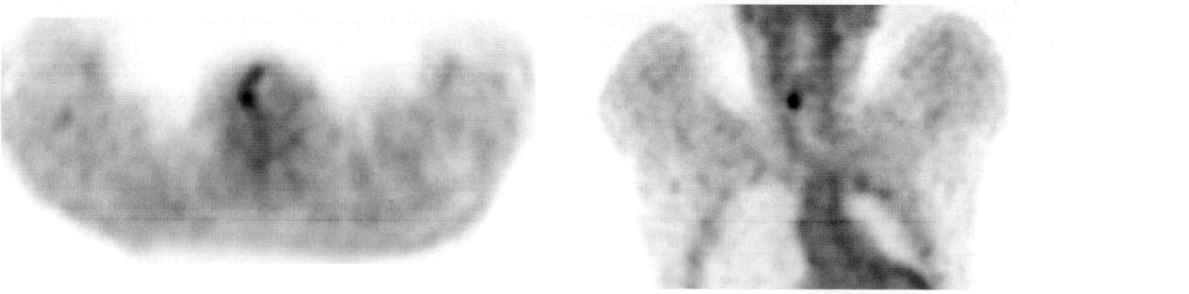

Figure 41-2 This patient presented with dyspnea and hoarseness and had a large squamous cell carcinoma of the left mainstem bronchus, directly invading the mediastinum at the level of the anteroposterior window. The PET scan shows physiologic uptake of ^{18}F-fluorodeoxyglucose in the normal right vocal cord and a lack of uptake in the left vocal cord, which was paralyzed due to involvement of the recurrent laryngeal nerve. Direct visualization of the cords confirmed this interpretation.

large hilar mass requires only an efficient choice of the least invasive means of obtaining a tissue diagnosis and choice of appropriate palliative therapy. Delineation of all sites of metastatic disease in such a setting is an expensive and wasteful application of resources that does not often lead to changes in care.

Evaluation of the primary tumor is generally best accomplished by CT scanning enhanced with intravenous contrast.[121] This will optimally be done with a spiral scanner which can rapidly obtain multiple contiguous scans through the chest without registration artifacts and with greatly reduced motion artifacts compared with conventional scanning. The parameters of contrast enhancement (dose, infusion rate, and site of infusion [left side preferred to visualize vessels crossing in the anterior mediastinum]) can make a large difference in the quality of information obtained. It is important to examine the chest using lung and mediastinal window settings.

In general, imaging of the primary tumor by magnetic resonance imaging (MRI) is neither better nor worse than by CT. No particular signal characteristics have been shown to reliably distinguish tumor from normal tissue or areas of atelectasis or fibrosis. Because of its greater facility at obtaining high resolution images in multiple planes, however, MRI has been preferred for certain specific situations, such as evaluation of invasion of the chest wall (although chest pain is the most specific indicator of this), extension of tumor into the mediastinum, and involvement of vascular and neural structures in the lung apex by superior sulcus tumors.[122] The development of rapid, high-resolution multislice CT scanners capable of volumetric reconstructions may return this modality to the one of choice for these situations.

Staging of the Mediastinum

Combined PET/CT is the radiographic method of choice for evaluation of the mediastinum.[121,123] The false-positive and false-negative rates are about 20%, however, and this should be considered when planning therapy. In most cases, histologic confirmation or nodal involvement suspected on radiographic grounds should be done before making decisions regarding the choice of potentially curative treatment. The increasing accessibility of mediastinal nodes to biopsy under guidance of CT or of endoesophageal or endobronchial ultrasound makes this a simple, minimally invasive procedure for most patients, with the use of the more invasive procedures of mediastinoscopy or anterior sternotomy (i.e., Chamberlain procedure) reserved for a minority of patients.[124,125] It is important to recognize that diagnostic radiologists are neither uniform nor necessarily precise in their description of the appearance and nature of mediastinal nodes. In some cases, a patient is said to have "mediastinal adenopathy" with the implication of unresectable N2 disease, although what has been shown by CT is the presence of several 1-cm nodes. The distribution of size of mediastinal nodes in normal individuals easily includes this range, and of nodes 1.5 cm in the greatest dimension, about 20% will be histologically benign. The percentage of such false-positive results is even higher among patients with obstructing endobronchial lesions or extrinsic bronchial obstruction from hilar nodes and postobstructive infection. In a patient who is otherwise a good operative candidate, the histologic involvement of such nodes should always be confirmed by biopsy before treatment decisions are made. When normal-size nodes are histologically positive, disease is usually intranodal and technically resectable. It remains unresolved whether these patients are better served by initial resection and postoperative adjuvant therapy or detection of these N2 nodes by preoperative mediastinoscopy or mediastinotomy and treatment with neoadjuvant therapy before resection.

Although there was initially great hope that MRI might be superior to CT in differentiating benignly enlarged from malignant mediastinal nodes, this has not been the case. CT, with its better spatial resolution and greater freedom from motion artifact, is the superior modality for imaging of the mediastinum. MRI does have a role in evaluation of lesions that involve the lung apex (and possibly the brachial plexus) and medial lesions that abut the vertebrae and may invade the neural foramina. Such involvement precludes resection and poses a risk for spinal cord compression, and its delineation has important implications for planning treatment.

Several reports have suggested that PET with ^{18}F-fluorodeoxyglucose (FDG-PET) may have good sensitivity and specificity in detecting mediastinal nodal involvement and diseases in extrathoracic metastatic sites.[126-132] PET has greater sensitivity and specificity than CT, but it is still imperfect. Nodes that appear involved by PET or CT should be biopsied for confirmation of their status when such information will lead to alterations in clinical management, particularly when deciding whether to consider resection. If a negative PET scan is being considered to avoid performing mediastinoscopy, it is important to require that the primary tumor show good uptake, that there not be a central primary whose uptake could obscure small nodes, and that a dedicated PET scanner be used.[133] FDG-PET has also been studied for evaluating response to preoperative chemotherapy or chemoradiation and for distinguishing between viable tumor and fibrosis in patients who have received radiation or chemotherapy, or both, in assessing local disease control in patients treated nonoperatively.[134-142]

Evaluation for Extrathoracic Metastases

The liver and adrenals are common sites of metastasis for SCLC and NSCLC and are well imaged by CT and PET. Although metastases to the adrenals are common, so are adenomas, and the distinction between these may require biopsy in the patient who is otherwise a good candidate for curative resection. Routine bone scans are of limited value. Many patients have abnormal bone scans due to benign degenerative diseases. The likelihood of detecting occult metastatic disease in patients without focal symptoms or elevation in alkaline phosphatase levels is low.

The use of total-body PET scanning has been advocated as a cost-effective replacement for CT scans of the liver and adrenals and radionuclide bone scanning and may well be a reasonable replacement for these. Because the typical PET scan does not image the brain, it will not replace MRI for this purpose. The typical PET or fused PET/CT scan does not image the entire skeleton, typically omitting the calvarium and the distal portions of the arms and legs.

Clinically occult involvement of the CNS, especially in patients with SCLC, adenocarcinoma, and large cell carcinoma, is more common, especially in patients with involvement of mediastinal nodes. Although scanning of the brain is probably not indicated for patients with stage IA disease, for which the probability of involvement is about 5%, for patients with N2 disease, it is in the range of 15% to 20% with high-resolution gadolinium-enhanced MRI (Wagner, unpublished data). For patients being considered for aggressive chemoradiotherapy with or without surgery, the finding of CNS metastases will lead to major changes in therapy, and scanning is warranted. We do not routinely scan patients with extrathoracic metastatic disease to look for CNS disease in the absence of symptoms, but we instead inquire carefully for early symptoms and scan at that time.

The role of CNS imaging in the patient with stage IB-II disease is controversial. Although the false-positive rate of CT and MRI is low and few patients would wrongly be excluded from surgery, the true-positive rate is also low, making this an uninformative test for most patients. However, in some series, 10% of patients with stage I-II NSCLC without neurologic symptoms had metastases demonstrated on enhanced CT.[143] Such a frequency of involvement probably warrants more common CNS imaging as part of routine staging, particularly considering the cost and morbidity of a thoracotomy, which would most likely be futile in the face of brain metastases.

TNM Stage Grouping

NSCLC is staged according to the principles of the tumor-node-metastasis (TNM) system. The International Staging System as outlined by Mountain in 1986 has been the standard for reporting treatment results since that time.[144] The broad outlines of this system are clearly valid. However, several areas emerged that indicated the need for modification of this system, and several revisions were implemented in 1997.[145,146]

The TNM staging system generally is used for patients with NSCLC, and it is reasonably predictive of outcome, particularly for patients treated surgically (Tables 41-2 and 41-3). This system does not deal well with anatomic prognostic factors important for nonsurgical treatment.

The distinction between T2 and T3 lesions based on their proximity to the carina is of little importance in radiotherapeutic treatment. Although bulky central mediastinal disease may be difficult to treat while adequately protecting the esophagus and spinal cord, this is more commonly caused by nodal disease than tumor extending proximally along the mainstem bronchus.

Tumor bulk is not considered as an independent prognostic factor. It is taken into account only in the 3-cm demarcation between T1 and T2 lesions, but a 1-cm lesion involving the visceral pleura is T2, and a 2.9-cm lesion surrounded by lung parenchyma is T1. It might be expected that the smaller T2 lesion would be more readily controlled by radiation therapy than the larger T1 lesion, and available data are in agreement with this expectation. Data from several institutions support the hypothesis that tumor volume, independent of stage, is prognostic for local control in and survival of patients with NSCLC treated with radiation or chemoradiation therapy.[147-151] Such volumetric measurements can be performed using commercially available radiation therapy planning software, although standardization of technique is important to reduce interobserver variability.[152]

There are several reports that size is an important predictor of prognosis within the clinical T1 N0 group, with particular importance in predicting microscopic involvement of hilar and mediastinal lymph nodes.[153] This is relevant to treatment strategies that try to reduce the extent of resection or limit the radiation target volume by eliminating elective nodal irradiation in these patients. Data suggest that only patients with lesions smaller than 1 cm in diameter have a risk of nodal involvement below 10%.

Several of the old TNM stage groups have considerable heterogeneity in outcome.[154] This is true to some degree for patients with stage I disease, where the survival of patients with T1 N0 M0 disease (≈ 80%) is strikingly better than that of patients with T2 N0 M0 disease (≈ 60%). It is in the current stage group III that the heterogeneity and need for subgrouping is greatest. This was partially recognized by Mountain, who divided the grouping into IIIA (i.e., no invasion of the mediastinum or involvement of contralateral mediastinal or supraclavicular nodes, no pleural effusion) and IIIB (i.e., with one or more of the previous characteristics). In retrospect, this

Table 41-2 International Staging System: TNM Classification

Category	Definition
T1	A tumor that is 3 cm or less in its greatest dimension, surrounded by lung or visceral pleura and without radiographic or bronchoscopic evidence of invasion proximal to a lobar bronchus
T2	A tumor more than 3 cm in its greatest dimension or a tumor of any size that invades the visceral pleura or has associated atelectasis or obstructive pneumonitis extending to the hilar region. At bronchoscopy, the proximal extent of demonstrable tumor must be within a lobar bronchus or at least 2 cm distal to the carina. Any associated atelectasis or obstructive pneumonitis must involve less than an entire lung.
T3	A tumor of any size with direct extension into the chest wall (including superior sulcus), diaphragm, or the mediastinal pleura or pericardium without involving the heart, great vessels, trachea, esophagus, or vertebral body, or a tumor in the main bronchus within 2 cm of the carina without involving the carina
T4	A tumor of any size with invasion of the mediastinum or involving the heart, great vessels, trachea, esophagus, vertebral body or carina or the presence of a malignant pleural effusion
N0	No demonstrable metastases to regional lymph nodes
N1	Metastases to ipsilateral peribronchial or hilar lymph nodes, including direct extension
N2	Metastases to ipsilateral mediastinal or subcarinal lymph nodes
N3	Metastases to contralateral mediastinal lymph nodes, contralateral hilar lymph nodes, and ipsilateral or contralateral scalene or supraclavicular lymph nodes
M0	No distant metastases
M1	Distant metastasis; specify sites

Data from Mountain C: A new international staging system for lung cancer. Chest 89(Suppl):225-233, 1986; Mountain C: Revisions in the international system for staging lung cancer. Chest 111:1710-1717, 1997.

Table 41-3 Stage Grouping and TNM Categories

Stage	TNM Categories
Stage Ia	T1 N0 M0
Stage Ib	T2 N0 M0
Stage IIa	T1 N1 M0
Stage IIb	T2 N1 M0, T3 N0 M0
Stage IIIA	T3 N1 M0, T1-3 N2 M0
Stage IIIB	T4 N0-3 M0, T1-4 N3 M0
Stage IV	Any T any N M1

Data from Mountain C: Revisions in the international system for staging lung cancer. Chest 111:1710-1717, 1997.

has separated a group of patients (IIIA), some of whom are treated surgically, can undergo complete resection, and have a reasonable favorable prognosis (especially T3 N1 M0), from those who have unresectable disease and are often treated palliatively. If we consider instead patients with IIIA and IIIB NSCLC who are treated nonsurgically with radical radiotherapy or chemoradiation, the survival differences are much less striking.[155]

Although the modifications introduced to the staging system are modest steps in the right direction, they have failed to deal adequately with a number of the issues that pertain to surgical and nonsurgical therapy. The number of lymph node stations involved, as well as whether their involvement is microscopic or macroscopic, has also been found to be of prognostic significance in patients with resected stage IIIA disease.[156]

Practical treatment decisions for patients with stage IIIA and IIIB NSCLC are often made along the following lines:[157]

T1-3 N2a M0: Involvement of a single mediastinal nodal station is discovered at mediastinoscopy or mediastinotomy or at thoracotomy. The nodal capsule is not breached. In some institutions, these patients have disease resected and then are given adjuvant postoperative therapy; others are given preoperative therapy.

T1-3 N2b M0: There is involvement of multiple mediastinal nodal stations with potentially resectable disease. Current trials compare chemoradiotherapy or chemotherapy as preoperative regimens.

T1-3 N2c M0: There is bulky involvement of mediastinal nodes (e.g., seen on a chest radiograph), possibly with superior vena caval compression. Disease is not likely to be resectable, even with preoperative therapy, but the patient is a candidate for definitive chemoradiotherapy.

T4a NX M0: Central T4 or N3 disease can all be encompassed within a reasonable radiation therapy portal. These patients should be considered for definitive chemoradiotherapy.

T4b NX M0: Disease extent includes malignant pleural effusion. Because all known disease cannot be irradiated to a tumoricidal dose, these patients should be treated as patients with stage IV disease, with irradiation used to treat or prevent local symptoms.

Several other groups have proposed different revisions to the current staging system. Based on the European Lung Cancer working Party data on patients receiving chemoradiation, Berghmans proposed separating patients with T3-4 N3 M0 from other factors that better predicted survival than the usual IIIA versus IIIB disctinction.[158] Andre, looking at patients with resected stage III NSCLC, some of whom had received induction chemotherapy, found that the number of lymph node levels and clinically detectable nodal metastases (cN2) were adverse prognostic factors.[156] The International Association for the Study of Lung Cancer (IASLC) is conducting a major project to develop new staging classifications for patients with NSCLC treated by multimodality therapy.

MEDICAL CONSIDERATIONS FOR SURGICAL RESECTION: CARDIOPULMONARY EVALUATION

Before undergoing surgery, patients must undergo careful cardiopulmonary evaluation to determine their ability to tolerate the operative procedure and the expected reduction in lung function after resection.[159] Patients with any history of cardiac disease, such as hypertension, angina, congestive failure, or prior myocardial infarction, should be carefully evaluated most often including a stress test along with stress radionuclide angiography. Patients in whom coronary artery calcification can be seen on CT scan should be similarly evaluated.[157,160-162]

Pulmonary function evaluation should routinely include determination of lung volumes and flow rates, diffusing capacity, and arterial blood gasses. Recommended minimal values for these parameters are shown in Table 41-4, and reflect the fact that patients with borderline function may tolerate a lobectomy but not a pneumonectomy. Some patients with poor baseline pulmonary function due to extensive bullous disease and poor lung compliance may have improvement in function after combined resection of the tumor and pulmonary dead space.

Patients not meeting criteria for lobectomy should be considered for lesser resections (i.e., wedge or segmental resection) if these appear capable of obtaining negative margins. Although the Lung Cancer Study Group (LCSG) trial, which randomized patients with T1 N0 M0 NSCLC between lobectomy and more conservative resection, showed significantly better local control for lobectomy, there was not a significant difference in survival.[163] The role of limited excision followed by radiation therapy to the tumor bed, either planned or if margins are found to be close or involved on final pathologic review, is not known and is being studied in a prospective phase II trial conducted by the Cancer and Leukemia Group B (CALGB) and ECOG. Because the radiation doses required for local control of even microscopic disease exceed the tolerance of normal lung tissue, it is not clear whether this strategy, which has been quite successful in organs such as breast

Table 41-4 Preoperative Evaluation of Pulmonary Function

Test	Desirable Value	Comment
FEV_1	Predicted postop. value ≥ 700 mL	Should obtain regional ventilation and perfusion scans and calculate predicted postoperative FEV_1 in borderline cases
FEV_1/FVC	>50%	—
P_{CO_2}	<50 mm Hg	—
DLCO	60% of predicted	—
$\dot{V}O_2max$	10 mL/kg/min	Values ≥ 15 mL/kg/min predict low surgical morbidity. Those > 10 but < 15 are borderline and the patient's overall clinical status needs to be considered carefully.

DLCO, diffusing capacity of the lung for carbon dioxide; FEV_1, forced expiratory volume in 1 second; FVC, forced vital capacity; P_{CO_2}, partial pressure of carbon dioxide; $\dot{V}O_2max$, maximum oxygen consumption.

Data from Beckles M, Spiro S, Colice G, Rudd R: The physiologic evaluation of patients with lung cancer being considered for resectional surgery. Chest 123(Suppl 1):105s-114s, 2003.

and gastrointestinal tract, which are not called on to perform their normal physiologic functions after irradiation, will be successful in the lung.

Sometimes, a patient referred to the radiation oncologist for definitive radiation therapy appears to be a reasonable surgical candidate. Such situations require an honest but tactful discussion of the issues with the patient and the referring physician (usually a pulmonologist or a general surgeon) and occasionally the suggestion of referral to another surgeon, preferably a cardiothoracic surgeon with particular expertise and interest in lung cancer, for a second opinion. In this setting, the difference in experience between a surgeon who specializes in treating thoracic malignancies and a general thoracic surgeon may be significant, and the best interests of the patient must be kept in view.

PRIMARY THERAPY

Early-Stage Disease

Surgery is the most effective treatment for patients with technically resectable NSCLC of stage IA through IIB. The role of surgery for patients with IIIA disease is controversial. Several points arise from consideration of the survival of patients with surgically resected disease and the patterns of failure for those with disease that recurs.

- Overall 5-year survival for the most favorable patients, those with small T1 N0 M0 lesions, approaches 80%, which is not far from what is seen for women with early-stage breast cancer.[164] This clearly refutes the common impression of lung cancer as an intrinsically incurable disease and more correctly focuses attention on issues of early detection.
- Most of treatment failures are due to systemic metastases rather than locoregional failure (Table 41-5).
- Many patients with compromised pulmonary function can be managed surgically, if they undergo careful perioperative care.[165]
- Complication rates depend on patient (age, physiologic status), disease (e.g., extent of required resection), and technical (e.g., surgical expertise) factors.[166]

Definitive Radiation Therapy

There are many single-institution reports of results of definitive radiation therapy for patients with stage I or II NSCLC who refuse surgery or are thought to be inoperable for medical reasons (Table 41-6). There is considerable variation in radiotherapy techniques and outcomes. Much of this variation undoubtedly arises from different local institutional definitions of "medical unresectabilty," with institutions that consider many patients with borderline disease to be unresectable, improving the apparent results of their surgical and radiotherapeutic series by the Will Rogers effect (i.e., stage migration).[167] However, several general conclusions may be drawn from these series:

1. Some patients with locally confined disease are curable with definitive radiotherapy. Unresectable is not synonymous with incurable.
2. Survival of clinically staged patients treated with radical radiation therapy is inferior to that of surgically staged patients treated surgically.
3. Survival of these patients decreases with increasing T stage, tumor size (within T stage), and clinical involvement of hilar lymph nodes.
4. Even for the most favorable patients, local control has been poor.
5. Even for favorable patients, distant metastases are a common cause of death.

These observations suggest several strategies that may improve treatment outcomes. The combination of radiation therapy with systemic chemotherapy in an attempt to reduce distant relapse or to improve local control is a logical approach to explore, particularly as the toxicity of current chemotherapeutic regimens has decreased. Radiotherapeutic parameters are another fertile ground for clinical trials. Sibley reviewed 10 reports of definitive radiation therapy for patients with medically inoperable stage I NSCLC. About 15% of patients were long-term survivors, 25% died of intercurrent disease, 30% died of distant metastases, and 30% died of local failure. Neither time to local failure nor overall survival correlated with the treatment volume (i.e., primary tumor volume alone or prophylactic nodal irradiation), whereas the total tumor dose, in the range of 55 to 70 Gy, did correlate with outcome.[168] This strongly suggests that trials of escalation of the biologic effective dose (by increasing the total dose or decreasing overall time with an increased fraction size or multiple fractions per day) to a small target volume, typically that of the primary tumor with margins, are a logical approach to improve the radiotherapeutic management of these patients. Such an approach would not preclude combination with systemic treatment, although caution should be taken because of a possible increase in pneumonitis with concurrent chemoradiation.[169,170]

In addition to the use of conventionally fractionated radiation therapy for patients with medically inoperable NSCLC, a number of investigators have explored the use of hypofractionated high dose stereotactic irradiation for these patients (see Table 41-5). This was based initially on the experience with frame-based stereotactic irradiation developed for intracranial lesions. For treatment of intrathoracic lesions, frame-based and frameless systems have been used. Motion due to respiration presents a complicating factor not encountered in intracranial stereotactic treatment. Such motion is present in conventional large-field radiation treatment, but it is often accommodated by increasing field margins at the expense of treating increasing volumes of normal lung tissue. This is unacceptable for stereotactic large-fraction treatment. A number of approaches have been developed for minimizing respiratory motion through breath-hold and abdominal compression techniques, gating the beam on time to a particular phase of the respiratory cycle, or tracking the tumor or radiopaque fiducial markers implanted in it and adapting the target volume to the real time position of the tumor. All of these approaches are still in early development, but the reported results are quite promising and suggest that, at least for smaller T1 tumors (e.g., those likely to be detected by CT screening programs), the results of stereotactic radiotherapy may rival those of surgery for local control and survival (see Table 41-5). Until recently, the experience with such stereotactic approaches had been limited to single institutions, but the Radiation Therapy Oncology Group (RTOG) has launched a phase I/II trial of fractionated stereotactic radiotherapy for patients with medically inoperable stage I NSCLC using a regimen of three treatment fractions.

Adjuvant Therapy for Early-Stage Disease

Discussing the risks and benefits of adjuvant treatment with patients is often a difficult task. Telling a patient who is recovering from a major surgical procedure that he or she is at high risk for recurrence despite having had a complete resection, that adjuvant therapy designed to reduce this risk is of only modest benefit (typically making a difference in long-term survival for about 5% of patients), and that we are in a sense treating 20 patients to benefit one can be a daunting task. The statistical nuances of disease-free and overall survival curves

Table 41-5 **Reports of Stereotactic Radioablation of Lung Tumors: Primary Lung Cancers and Metastatic Lesions**

Study*	No. of Patients	Stage	Dose/ Fractions/ Time	Localization and Immobilization	Local Control	Survival	Comments
Timmerman et al[343]	44	T1-2N0	24-60 Gy 3 fractions 2 weeks	Stereotactic body frame	NS	NS	Phase I dose escalation trial; six local failures seen at lower dose range; no clinical MTD reached, although G2 pneumonitis seen for patients with larger (T2) tumors
Nagata et al[344]	55	T1-3N0	48 Gy 4 fractions 12 days	Stereotactic body frame	100% for T1-2 tumors	1 y: 95 T1, 95 T2 2 y: 92 T1, 82 T2	Worst toxicity: G2 pneumonitis
Onishi[345]	40	T1-2N0	60 Gy 10 fractions 5 days (bid)	Breath-hold	2 y: 94%	2 y: 63% 2 y cause specific: 75%	Single-institution study using combined CT scan-Linac gantry; no toxicity >G2
Onishi et al[346]	241	153 T1N0 88 T2N0	18-75 Gy 1-22 fractions	Varies among institutions	Local recurrence in 10.4%	3 y: 56% 3 y cause specific: 71.8%	Multi-institution study using a variety of treatment techniques and dose schedules; may include some patients from other series listed here; pneumonitis ≥G3 in 2.1%
Harada et al[347]	25	T1-2N0	35-48 Gy 4 fractions 1 week	Real-time tumor tracking and machine gating	1 y: 77%	1 y: 83%	G2 pneumonitis in 24%
Niibe et al[348]	22	T1-2 (≤5 cm)	59.5-75 Gy 3-4 Gy/fraction 25-38 days	NS	1 y: 92.3% 2 y: 83.1% 3 y: 83.1%	1 y: 100% 2 y: 83.3% 3 y: 55.6%	G2 pneumonitis in 10%
Hof et al[349]	10	T1-2N0	19-26 Gy Single fraction	Stereotactic body frame	1 y: 88.9% 2 y: 71.1%	1 y: 80% 2 y: 64%	5 patients failed with DM, 1 with NM 3 patients developed pneumothoraces requiring chest tube placement after placement of fiducial marker in tumor
Whyte et al[350]	23	T1-2N0 or metastatic	15 Gy Single fraction	Breath-holding for 9 patients Real-time tumor tracking and machine gating for 14 patients	NS	NS	
Fukumoto et al[351]	22	T1-2N0M0	48-60 Gy 8 fractions 2 weeks	Free-breathing. PTV based on CT scans at full inspiration and full expiration in addition to free breathing	94% for 17 patients with minimum 24-mo follow-up	Lung cancer–specific survivals: 1 y: 94% 2 y: 73%	No clinical radiation-related side effects or significant changes in VC, FEV_1, TLC, or DLCO; radiographic fibrosis in all; 5 patients have died with DM and 6 of intercurrent disease; 3 failed in regional nodes (also DM)

*When series have included patients with primary lung cancer and pulmonary metastases, data are reported for primary tumors only when they were available separately.

DLCO, diffusing capacity of the lung for carbon dioxide; DM, distant metastases; FEV_1, forced expiratory volume in 1 second; G2, grade 2; G3, grade 3; MTD, maximum tolerated dose; NM, nodal metastases; NS, not stated; PTV, planning target volume; TLC, total lung capacity; VC, vital capacity.

Table 41-6 Radical Radiation Therapy for Patients with Medically Inoperable Non–Small Cell Lung Cancer

Study	No. of Patients	Clinical Stage	2-Year Survival (%)	5-Year Survival (%)	Local Failure (%)
Morrison et al[324]	28	Operable	14	6 (4 y)	NA
Smart[325]	40	Operable	≈ 50	22	NA
Coy and Kennelly[326]	141	T1-3NX	31	11	45‡
Cooper et al[327]	72	T1-3N0-1	NA	6	NA
Haffty et al[328]	43	T1-2N0-1	60	21	39
Noordijk et al[329]	50	T1-2N0	56	16	70
Zhang et al[330]	44	T1-2N0-2	≈ 55	32	27
Talton et al[331]	77	T1-3N0	36	17	NA
Sandler et al[332]	77	T1-2NX	30	≈ 10	56
Ono et al[333]	38	T1N0	68	42	NA
Dosoretz et al[334,335]	152	T1-3N0-1	40	10	70
	44§	T1N0-1	≈ 60	≈ 60	30
Hayakawa et al[336]	17	Stage I	75	31	NA
	47	Stage II	44	22	NA
Rosenthal et al[337]	62	T1-2N1	33	12	60
Kaskowitz et al[338]	53	T1-2N0	43	6	55
Graham et al[339]	103	T1-2N0-1	35	14	NA
	35§	T1N0-1	NA	29	NA
Gauden et al[340]	347	T1-2N0	NA	27	NA
Sibley et al[168,341]	141	Stage I	39	13	42
Furuta et al[342]	32	Stage I-II	40	16	NA

Includes some patients with small cell carcinoma.
Includes some patients with proximal unresectable T3 lesions.
Data from autopsies of 31 patients (22% of series), of whom 14 had locoregional disease, 17 had disseminated disease, and 6 had no evidence of disease.
Subset of entire series.

can escape many patients. The format in which data are presented (i.e., whether the effect of an adjuvant treatment is expressed as a hazard ratio, a relative survival difference, or an absolute survival difference) can make a substantial difference in its acceptability to patients.[171,172]

Postoperative Radiation Therapy

Several retrospective series published in the 1960s claimed that postoperative irradiation of mediastinal and hilar nodes improved survival of patients with resected NSCLC, particularly if they had nodal metastases.[173-176] This issue has been investigated in several prospective trials which, although methodologically flawed, provide a consensus answer that survival is minimally if at all improved, but local failure is probably reduced with such treatment.

A meta-analysis of 2128 patients treated in nine randomized trials of postoperative radiation therapy concluded that this treatment was associated with a highly significant increase in the risk of death (Fig. 41-3).[177] Overall the risk ratio was 1.21 (P = .001). The study authors concluded that postoperative radiation therapy as used in these studies was detrimental and should not be used, at least for the time being. It is important to recognize that there are several significant differences between the treatment administered in a number of the trials included in this meta-analysis and current practice patterns in the United States. First, a substantial portion of the patients included in this study, 562 of 2128, had stage I disease without demonstrated nodal metastases. There has never been a strong case favoring the postoperative irradiation of these patients and little suggestion from patterns of their failure after surgery that such treatment would be beneficial (Table 41-7). One fourth of the patients in this analysis stood to gain little from treatment. Second, the details of treatment, including preoperative staging, surgical technique, and radiation dose and dose delivery, differed substantially from current practice. Several of the trials required or allowed daily fraction sizes in excess of 2.0 Gy, with the Medical Research Council (MRC) trial using 2.6 Gy/day and the Slovenian trial using 3.0 Gy/day. The larger fraction sizes would be expected to produce an increase in acute and late complications compared with slower fractionation. Seven of the nine trials also allowed the use of ^{60}Co treatment beams, with their poorer depth-dose characteristics than higher energy accelerator beams, and only one study included CT-based treatment planning. Compared with current standards of treatment, the likelihood is great that postoperative radiation therapy would lead to excess deaths from cardiac and pulmonary damage. In a meta-analysis that included patients with little chance of benefit of treatment this approach would likely result in an overall survival detriment. It is notable that in this meta-analysis the increase in risk of death was most marked in those patients with stage I disease and was not significant for patients with N2 disease. This is consistent with, but does not prove, a potential benefit for properly delivered irradiation for patients with resected N2 disease.

The Postoperative Radiotherapy (PORT) Meta-analysis Group has updated their analysis with the inclusion of one additional trial.[178] The overall conclusions that PORT was detrimental for patients with stage I or II NSCLC and that there were no clear evidence for benefit or detriment for patients with stage III N2 disease were not altered. However, results and updates of several other recent trials were not included in this analysis.[179-181]

Phlips reported on the results of postoperative therapy given over two time periods, one with ^{60}Co therapy and a later one with high energy photons.[182] For stage and demographically comparable patient groups, the 5-year survival rate was 8% for those treated with ^{60}Co but 30% for those treated on linear accelerators with CT-based treatment planning. Less cardiac and pulmonary toxicity was reported in the more recent patient group. Schraube reported calculated complication probabilities for patients receiving postpneumonectomy

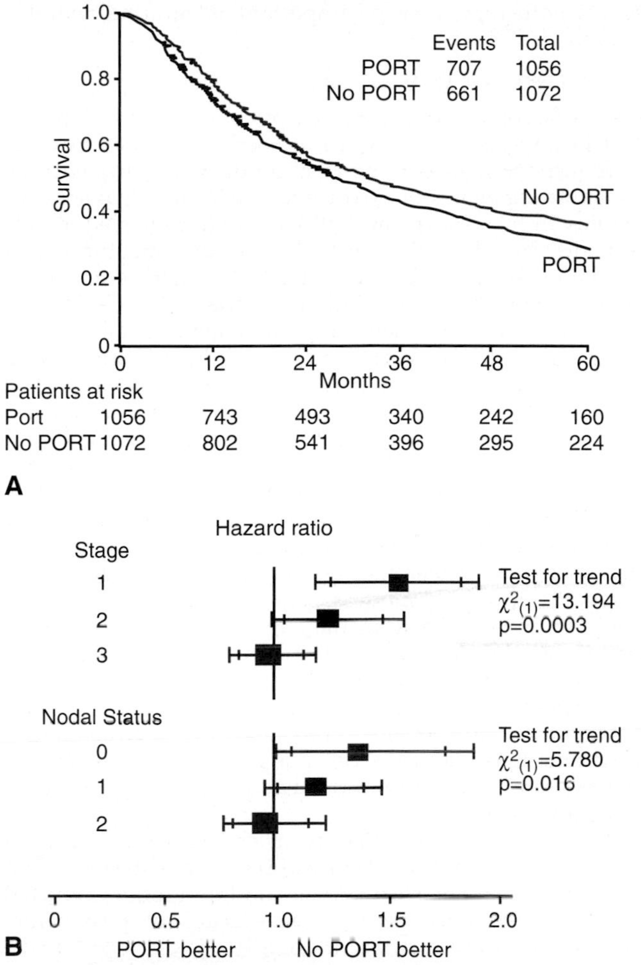

Figure 41-3 **A,** The overall survival curves for all patients analyzed show a significant deleterious effect of postoperative radiation therapy (PORT) on survival. **B,** This deleterious effect varies strongly with extent of local disease (expressed as stage group or N stage), with the hazard function not overlapping with unity for patients with stage groups 1 or N0 disease. (From Burdett S, Stewart L: Postoperative radiotherapy in non-small-cell lung cancer: update of an individual patient data meta-analysis. Lung Cancer 47:81-83, 2005.)

radiation therapy delivered using two-dimensional or three-dimensional treatment planning.[183] For equivalent physical doses to the mediastinal nodal target volume, the biologic mean dose to lung and heart and the associated normal tissue complication probabilities were considerably lower with three-dimensional treatment planning. Machtay compared the rates of death from intercurrent disease (DID) for patients who had received adjuvant postoperative radiation therapy.[184] They observed a 4-year actuarial risk of 13.5%, which was minimally but not significantly greater than the 10% expected. The total radiation dose was strongly associated with the risk of DID: 2% for doses less than 54 Gy and 17% for 54 Gy and higher doses. Wakelee performed a retrospective analysis of DID in the INT 0115 trial, which compared PORT with or without concurrent chemotherapy with cisplatin and etoposide (VP-16) against that expected based on U.S. vital statistics.[185] The actuarial rates of DID at 4 years were 12.3 for irradiation and 13.7 for irradiation plus chemotherapy (not significant) and no higher than expected given the age and smoking status of the treated patients.

If the trials in the PORT meta-analysis failed to demonstrate a survival benefit for patients with N2 disease because this benefit was counterbalanced by excess deaths due to complications of the radiation therapy as given and modern radiation therapy is less toxic as the described studies suggest, a trial conducted now might well show a survival benefit. Because even with nontoxic therapy, this benefit would be relatively small (on the order of a 5% to 10% gain in absolute survival), any trial attempting to demonstrate a difference will require a large number of patients (approximately 2000) to minimize the risk of type 2 error.

Evidence from several institutions indicates that locoregional failure is increasingly common with a higher number of involved N2 nodes, and that induction chemotherapy followed by surgery gives inadequate control of mediastinal disease.[186-189]

The CALGB initiated a phase III trial of PORT in patients with resected N2 disease in an attempt to answer this question. Patients received four cycles of adjuvant chemotherapy with carboplatin plus paclitaxel and then were randomly assigned to observation or mediastinal irradiation. Accrual to the trial was slow, and it was closed having accrued only 40 patients.[190] Median failure-free survival time was 15.6 months

Table 41-7 Rates and Patterns of Relapse Following Resection of Non–Small Cell Lung Cancer

Study	Stage	Histology	No. of Patients	Survival (y)	Chest Only (%)	Distant Only (%)
Feld et al[352]*	T1 N0	NSCLC	162	NS	9	17
	T2 N0	NSCLC	196	NS	11	30
	T1 N1	NSCLC	32	NS	9	22
Pairolero et al[353]	T1 N0	NSCLC	170	71% (5)	6	15
	T2 N0	NSCLC	158	59% (5)	6	23
	T1 N1	NSCLC	18	33% (5)	28	39
Thomas and Rubinstein[354*†]	T1 N0	Squamous cell	226	≈ 85%	5	7
	T1 N0	Nonsquamous	346	≈ 65%	9	17
Martini et al[316†‡]	T1-2 N1	Squamous cell	93	44%	16	31
	T1-2 N1	Adenocarcinoma	114	34%	8	54
	T2-3 N2	Squamous cell	46	≈ 30% (5)	13	52
	T2-3 N2	Nonsquamous	103	≈ 30% (5)	17	61

*First site of relapse only.
†Relapse rates include patients relapsing in multiple sites.
‡Some patients received postoperative radiation and/or chemotherapy.
NSCLC, non–small cell lung cancer; NS, not specified.
From Wagner H, Bonomi P: Preoperative and postoperative therapy for non–small cell lung cancer. *In* Roth JA, Ruckdeschel JC, Weisenburger TH (eds): Thoracic Oncology. Philadelphia, WB Saunders, 1995, pp 147-163.

for the nonirradiated patients and 25.9 months for those receiving mediastinal irradiation. Failure-free and overall survival at 1 year were 60% and 70%, respectively, on the observation arm and 56% and 72% on the irradiation arm. None of these differences reached statistical significance. The premature closure of this trial rendered it highly underpowered to detect an effect of reasonable but clinically worthwhile magnitude, and its negative results do not exclude such a possible benefit.

A difficult clinical situation that is most commonly seen in referral centers is the question of postoperative radiation therapy for a patient without proven mediastinal lymph node involvement but whose surgery did not adequately sample or dissect the mediastinum. This is most often encountered in patients who have undergone, for one reason or another, a conservative resection such as wedge excision or segmentectomy rather than lobectomy. It is also more common with general thoracic surgeons than oncologic specialists. CT scans done postoperatively may show one or more somewhat enlarged mediastinal nodes, but this may reflect tumor or postoperative infection or inflammation. The use of PET in this setting has been explored by Roberts and colleagues, who suggested that it might be helpful in directing when to give and when to withhold further therapy.[140]

At present postoperative radiation therapy cannot be recommended on the basis of demonstrably improved survival, but should be considered in selected patients at high risk of local recurrence, particularly when there is involvement of multiple nodal stations or extracapsular tumor spread.

The role of prophylactic cranial irradiation (PCI) in patients with NSCLC has been less well evaluated than in SCLC. Three reported randomized trials of PCI in patients with NSCLC failed to show any survival benefit, but none of them included patients with early-stage, resected disease or even patients thought to be in complete remission after definitive radiation therapy (with or without chemotherapy).[191-193] One retrospective series reported benefit for PCI in patients with stage III NSCLC treated with an aggressive chemoradiation regimen. The earlier group of patients who did not receive PCI had a CNS failure rate of 46% (13 of 28) compared with 9% (4 of 47) of a subsequent group who received PCI.[194] Others have also reported high CNS relapse rates for aggressively treated patients with stage IIIA/B NSCLC (Table 41-8). As control of local and extrathoracic metastatic tumor improve the potential benefit of PCI will increase, but it cannot be considered standard at this time. The RTOG is conducting a phase III trial of PCI in patients with stage IIIA/B NSCLC who have completed all other planned therapy, which may include various combinations of surgery, radiation therapy, and chemotherapy. The primary end point of the trial is survival, and the sample size required to show the desired 20% improvement is 1058 patients. As is the case for patients with SCLC, attention to details of PCI dose and fractions, as well as timing relative to chemotherapy, may be important in limiting neurologic toxicity.[120,195,196]

Postoperative Chemotherapy

Early trials of postoperative therapy for patients with resected NSCLC failed to show significant benefit for such treatment. In retrospect, many of these were conducted with agents, such as alkylating agents or doxorubicin, with minimal antitumor activity in this disease, and all were underpowered to detect a modest but clinically worthwhile improvement in survival on the order of 5%. Because of a lack of consensus and the small size of many of the individual trials, the NSCLC Meta-analysis Group conducted a meta-analysis of all published randomized trials comparing observation with adjuvant chemotherapy.[197] Although no overall benefit was seen, the results were distinctly different by type of chemotherapy regimen. Older alkylating agent–based regimens significantly worsened survival by 5%, whereas cisplatin-based regimens gave a 5-year survival improvement of 5%, which approached statistical significance ($P = .08$). Although there was considerable heterogeneity of stage, surgical procedure, and planned and delivered chemotherapy, this result suggested that chemotherapy with modest activity for metastatic disease could improve survival in the adjuvant setting, as had been previously demonstrated in breast and colorectal cancers. It was believed that differences between the older and newer drug regimens likely reflected greater intrinsic activity of the newer drugs and an improved ability to deliver adequate dose-time schedules because of aggressive and effective supportive care (e.g., better antiemetics, improved management of neutropenia).

Several large trials of adjuvant chemotherapy have been reported in full or abstract since publication of the meta-analysis (Table 41-9). The North American Intergroup conducted a large trial designed to test the efficacy of postoperative chemotherapy in patients with completely resected N1 and N2 NSCLC.[198] After extensive discussion of trial design, a two-arm comparison of postoperative radiation therapy with or without concurrent chemotherapy (cisplatin and etoposide) was adopted. The use of postoperative irradiation in both arms was designed to optimize local control, potentially increasing the ability to detect an effect of chemotherapy on systemic metastases. It was also believed that a comparison of two adjuvant regimens rather than treatment versus observation would be more acceptable to both patients and physicians. This trial (INT 0115), which enrolled 488 patients, showed no trend or significant difference in survival for the two arms, regardless of whether all 488 entered patients or 368 eligible and evaluable patients were considered. Multivariate analysis showed no benefit of the chemotherapy used in this study (i.e., four cycles of cisplatin and etoposide beginning concurrently with the start of irradiation) for any clinical subset of patients. Concurrent chemoradiation therapy also

Table 41-8 Central Nervous System Relapse in Patients with Locally Advanced Non–Small Cell Lung Cancer

Study	Stage	No. of Patients	CNS Failure (Crude Risk)	Median Survival (mo)
Choi et al[322]	T1-3pN2		30%	25
Stuschke et al[194]	T1-4pN2	28	46%	20
Albain et al[355]	pN2-3 or T4		21%	15
Andre et al[356]	cN2		22%	NA
Law et al[357]	IIIA/B or IV	32	28%	20

c, clinical; NA, no data available; p, pathologic.

Table 41-9 Adjuvant Chemotherapy Trials

Study/Trial	No. of Patients	Stage	Regimen	5-Year Survival	*P* Value
Keller et al[198]/Intergroup Trial (INT) 0115	488	IIA-IIIA (N1-2)	RT/DDP/VP16		NS
			RT		
Scagliotti et al[199]/Adjuvant Lung Project Italy (ALPI)	1209	IA-IIIA	MMC/VBL/DDP	HR 0.96	NS
			OBS		
Arriagada et al[200]/International Adjuvant Lung Cancer Trial (IALT)	1867	IA-IIIB	DDP/X	44.4	<.03
			OBS	40.4	
Strauss et al[203]/Cancer and Leukemia Group B (CALGB) 9633	344	IB	CBP/PTX	71 (4 y)	.028
			OBS	59	
Winton et al[201]/National Cancer Institute of Canada (NCIC)	482	IB-II (T3 N0)	DDP/VNB	69 (3 y)	.011
			OBS	54	
National Cancer Institute of the United States Intergroup JBR.10 Trial					
Kato et al[358]/Japan Lung Cancer Research Group on Postsurgical Adjuvant	716	IA	Oral UFT	89	NS
			OBS	90	
Chemotherapy (JLCRG)	263	IB	Oral UFT	85	.005
			OBS	74	

CBP, carboplatin; DDP, cisplatin; HR, hazard ratio; MMC, mitomycin C; NS, not specified; OBS, observation; UFT, tegafur and uracil; VNB, vinorelbine; VP16, etoposide; X, etoposide, vinblastine, vindesine, or vinorelbine.

failed to improve local mediastinal control, compared with radiation therapy alone.

The Adjuvant Lung Project Italy (ALPI) enrolled 1209 patients with resected stage IA-IIIA NSCLC to a randomization between observation and chemotherapy with mitomycin, vindesine, and cisplatin.[199] Forty-three percent of patients also received postoperative irradiation (after chemotherapy if this was given). There was a survival trend favoring the chemotherapy arm that did not reach statistical significance.

The International Adjuvant Lung Cancer Trial (IALT) is the largest trial of adjuvant chemotherapy in lung cancer that has been conducted.[200] The trial was planned to study 3000 patients, but it closed after enrolling 1867 patients because of declining accrual and evidence of a significant difference between the arms on interim analysis. Patients were randomized between observation and adjuvant chemotherapy that used cisplatin and an institutional choice of second agents (i.e., etoposide, vindesine, vinblastine, or vinorelbine). Radiation therapy could be given (by institutional policy) after chemotherapy. There was an overall absolute improvement in the 5-year survival rate of 4% (44.4% versus 40.4%), which was highly significant, was present for all stage groups, and was seen whether patients also received postoperative mediastinal irradiation (not a randomized variable in this trial but done according to institutional preference). Although this trial showed a clear benefit in survival for adjuvant chemotherapy, it did not provide information on patterns of failure. To facilitate rapid accrual of a large number of patients to the trial, which was key in demonstrating the primary survival end point, the amount of data collected on patients was limited. Restricting the amount of information collected at randomization and during follow-up facilitated enrollment, as in previous trials.

Two other trials have demonstrated the strong, positive effects of adjuvant chemotherapy. The National Cancer Institute of Canada Cancer Treatment Group (NCIC-CTG) randomized patients with resected stage IB-IIIA NSCLC to observation or adjuvant chemotherapy with cisplatin and vinorelbine. They found a rather large and significant improvement in overall survival: 69% versus 54%.[201] Despite the availability of effective antiemetic regimens, compliance with this adjuvant chemotherapy regimen was not very good; only about 50% of patients completed all four cycles of this regimen, with variations by age, gender, extent of surgery, and nationality.[202] That this was a randomized trial with a no-treatment option may have contributed to the poor compliance, with patients making the choice between known toxicity and possible benefit. With survival benefits for adjuvant chemotherapy not reasonably well established, patients may find the same regimens that were difficult to tolerate when their benefits were uncertain much more tolerable. The CALGB randomized patients with resected T2 N0 M0 NSCLC to observation or adjuvant therapy with carboplatin plus paclitaxel. The result of this trial was also strongly positive, with 71% versus 59% survival at 4 years.[203]

Hotta and associates published a meta-analysis of trials of adjuvant chemotherapy limited to those trials reported after the Collaborative Group meta-analysis published in 1995.[204] Eleven trials and 5716 patients were analyzed. They excluded trials in which the randomization was between postoperative radiation therapy and chemoradiation (e.g., INT 0115). With the exception of several Japanese trials using only tegafur and uracil (UFT), the chemotherapy was cisplatin plus a variety of other agents, mostly vinca alkaloids or etoposide. A significant survival improvement (hazard ratio = 0.872; $P = .001$) was seen overall, and in subset analysis, this held for the cisplatin-containing chemotherapy and for UFT. The latter results are not well understood in view of the rather low response rates (6.3%) seen with UFT in the setting of metastatic disease.[205] Hamada also analyzed six published Japanese trials of UFT adjuvant chemotherapy with a highly significant improvement in 5-year overall survival (absolute magnitude of 5%; $P = .01$).[206]

Although there are sufficient data to establish adjuvant chemotherapy as standard for most patients with resected NSCLC, with the exception of patients with T1 N0 M0 disease, there are few data on the ability of this therapy to reduce the high rates of local recurrence seen in some patient subgroups. With the failure of CALGB 9734 to accrue adequate numbers of patients, the question of adjuvant radiation in combination with or after adjuvant chemotherapy for patients with N2 disease remains unresolved.

Potentially Resectable Disease: Stages IIIA and IIIB

Preoperative Treatment for Patients with Resectable Non–Small Cell Lung Cancer

Several trials conducted in the 1960s showed that for patients with initially resectable lung cancers, preoperative radiation therapy did not improve survival, and for those with initially unresectable disease, it improved resectability without any effect on survival.[207-209] Surgical complications, particularly bronchopleural fistulas, were increased. The approach was largely discarded until recently, when the flurry of trials of preoperative chemotherapy or chemoradiotherapy prompted renewed interest in preoperative radiation therapy. Unlike the trials of the 1960s, these have used strict criteria for resectability, surgical staging of the mediastinal nodes, and modern attention to radiation therapy planning. Two small, randomized, phase II trials have been reported from the CALGB and the LCSG.[210,211] Both studies randomized patients with unresectable stage IIIA/B NSCLC between preoperative radiation therapy followed by surgery or preoperative chemotherapy followed by surgery. Postoperative treatment was not specified in the LCSG trial but included radiation therapy to varying doses depending on tumor status at time of resection in the CALGB trial. Table 41-10 shows the results of these two trials, as well as those of several other randomized trials which compared immediate resection to induction chemotherapy followed by surgery for patients with stage IIIA NSCLC.[212-215] Results of the trials reported by Roth and Rosell were significantly positive, and the trials were closed early because of survival differences seen on interim analysis, but the LCSG, Japan Clinical Oncology Group (JCOG), and CALGB trials failed to show any difference in survival or resectability between preoperative radiation therapy, a strategy which might improve local but not systemic control, and preoperative chemotherapy. The trial by Depierre included patients with stages IB through IIIB, and although it demonstrated a survival benefit for patients with stage IB and IIA/B disease, it did not show a significant difference for patients with stage IIIA disease. Because all of these studies were small, there is no clear consensus on the optimal management of patients with operable stage IIIA NSCLC at this time. In the United States, most centers advocate the use of preoperative treatment with chemotherapy or chemoradiation, but whether this is superior to resection and postoperative therapy remains unclear, although a number of theoretical considerations ranging from better patient tolerance to earlier treatment of occult systemic disease favor the preoperative approach.

The Bimodality Lung Oncology Team (BLOT), an outgrowth of the LCSG, investigated preoperative therapy in patients with clearly resectable stage IB and II NSCLC using carboplatin and paclitaxel for two or three cycles. Despite a disappointingly low overall pathologic complete response rate of only 5%, 2- and 3-year survival rates compared very favorably with those of historical controls. The data were sufficiently encouraging to warrant a prospective trial coordinated by the Southwest Oncology Group (SWOG, S9900) comparing surgery alone to induction chemotherapy for patients with stage IB through IIIA disease. Unlike the original BLOT trial, pathologic assessment of the mediastinum was not required. The accrual goal of this trial was over 600 patients, and it was closed early in 2004 because of declining accrual. Since it opened, the positive results of the Depierre trial for preoperative chemotherapy (at least for patients with stage IB and II disease) and the positive IALT trial for adjuvant postoperative chemotherapy for all stages made the randomization on S9900 unappealing. Results of the approximately 400 patients entered on this trial are anticipated.

It is unlikely that it will be possible in the United States to conduct a large, multicenter, prospective trial of neoadjuvant chemotherapy in a well-staged group of patients, and we may be left without a scientifically rigorous answer to this question. For patients with resectable NSCLC, preoperative irradiation should not be considered standard treatment. Patients with more extensive stage IIIA and IIIB disease, who are at the border of technical resectability, should be considered for entry on trials investigating the role of surgery after induction treatment with chemotherapy alone or chemoradiation.

The role of surgery in patients with more than minimal stage IIIA and IIIB disease has remained controversial. A very small RTOG/ECOG trial of induction chemotherapy followed by radiation therapy or surgery found no difference but was inadequately powered.[216] The North American Intergroup

Table 41-10 Randomized Phase II and Phase III Trials of Neoadjuvant Therapy in Patients with Stage IIIA/IIIB Non–Small Cell Lung Cancer

Study	Therapy	No. of Patients	Median Survival (mo)	2- to 3-Year Survival
Pass et al[212]	ST	14	15.6	23*
	PE→ST	12	28.7	50
Rosell et al[359]	ST	30	8	0*
	MIP→ST	29	26	29
Roth et al[213]	ST	32	11	15*
	CEP→ST	28	64	56
Wagner et al[360] (Lung Cancer Study Group)	MVP→ST	24	12	≈ 30†
	RT→ST	25	12	≈ 30
Elias et al[210] (Cancer and Leukemia Group B)	PE→ST→PE→RT	23	23	NA
	RT→ST	24	19	NA
Depierre et al[361]	ST	(167)	NR	21‡
	MIP→ST			28
Ichinose[380]	ST	(62)	16	25‡
	PU→ST		10	8

*Three-year survival.
†Two-year survival.
‡Five-year survival.
CEP, cyclophosphamide, etoposide, and cisplatin; MIP, mitomycin C, ifosfamide, and cisplatin; MVP, mitomycin C, vinblastine, and cisplatin; NA, data not available; NR, not reported; PE, cisplatin and etoposide; RT, radiation therapy; ST, surgery.

Trial INT 0139 which randomized patients with pathologic N2 disease to definitive chemoradiation (cisplatin/etoposide concurrent with 61 Gy) or concurrent preoperative chemoradiation to 45 Gy, showing better disease-free but not overall survival with the inclusion of surgery, has not resolved this question for many.[217] Advocates of surgery argue that better exclusion of patients at poor risk for surgery would have shown an overall survival benefit, whereas partisans of nonsurgical treatment promote the technologic improvements in radiation therapy planning and delivery since the time of this trial. Although the current RTOG trial for these patients includes surgery in both treatment arms, this decision has come about as much because of investigator fatigue as compelling data.

The German Lung Cancer Cooperative Group trial of preoperative CT or CT plus radiation therapy showed no progression-free or overall survival benefit to the irradiation-containing arm.[218] However, postoperative irradiation was given to the patients in the arm not receiving preoperative treatment. The overall resectability rate in the trial was low, only about 50%, in a population that was composed of about two thirds of patients with stage IIIB disease. By including radiation therapy in both arms, the issue becomes one of timing rather than amount of treatment, and the similarity in overall outcome is perhaps not surprising.

Betticher reported 90 patients with stage IIIA N2 NSCLC preoperative given induction chemotherapy with cisplatin and docetaxel of whom 75 were resected, with 59 R_0 resections (i.e., microscopically negative margins).[219] The overall median survival was 27.6 months and 33 months for resected patients. Among patients with resected disease, 38 had relapsed (10 local, 10 local plus distant, and 18 distant only). The new RTOG neoadjuvant trial takes the Betticher regimen and adds radiation therapy in one arm to determine whether preoperative radiation therapy in this setting improves local control. Unlike the German trial discussed earlier, patients not receiving preoperative irradiation will also not receive it postoperatively unless the resection was known to be incomplete.

Several trials have found that those patients faring best after preoperative treatment with chemotherapy or chemoradiation have been those with pathologic sterilization of mediastinal nodes, but not necessarily of the primary tumor. If sterilization of mediastinal lymph nodes is a useful criterion in selecting patients for surgery, how can this best be assessed preoperatively? CT is not particularly helpful, and it is not clear that early PET scanning, done to allow resection within 4 to 6 weeks after neoadjuvant therapy, can discriminate between dead or dying cells or radiation-induced inflammatory changes at this early point.

Unresectable Stage IIIA/IIIB Disease

Patients with stage III NSCLC have a poor prognosis for two reasons, frequent dissemination of tumor leading to early death from distant metastases, and poor local control. The frequency of distant failure, together with reports of good early response of local disease to radiation therapy, with short follow-up, led for a time to the belief that the systemic problem was the greater one. There are few prospective data on the dependence of local control and survival of patients with NSCLC on radiation dose. In the 1980s, it was believed by many authorities that local control could be achieved in about one half of patients treated to doses to 60 Gy given in 30 fractions over 6 weeks. However, the data on which an assumption was based (RTOG 73-01) indicated failure of progression rather than long-term control.[220] Patients were randomized to 40, 50, or 60 Gy given as a continuous course with 2 Gy per day and to a fourth arm of 40 Gy given by split course (i.e., 20 Gy in 5 fractions, a 2-week break, repeated dosage). The 50- and 60-Gy arms showed modest improvement in local control and survival compared with the 40-Gy split or continuous arms, but this advantage was lost after 2 years. The lack of durable benefit for the higher doses may be due to the fact that local control was poor with even the highest doses and to the lack of CT treatment planning and use of posterior spinal cord blocks. Patterns of failure in this trial were reported in terms of crude risk of clinically detected local failure: 33% with 60 Gy and 44% to 49% with 40 Gy. It is incorrect to assume that local control is achieved in 67% of patients with 60 Gy. That this greatly overestimated local control was clearly demonstrated by Le Chevalier, who reported actuarial local control, assessed radiographically and bronchoscopically, for patients treated with definitive radiation therapy alone or preceded and followed by chemotherapy with cyclophosphamide, cisplatin, chloroethylcyclohexylnitrosourea (CCNU), and vindesine. For both arms, the local control rate was very poor, only 17% to 20% at 1 year and falling to about 10% at 4 years.[221-224] It was clear that oncologists could not rest with the belief that standard radiation therapy provided adequate local control and that the only theater of clinical research was the use of chemotherapy to suppress distant metastases. In addition to its necessity for cure, local control of disease is also important for quality of life, because even patients dying of systemic disease are benefited if they can avoid the complications of local disease progression, such as airway obstruction with dyspnea or postobstructive infection, hemoptysis, compression of mediastinal structures such as the superior vena cava, phrenic or recurrent laryngeal nerves, or pain from chest wall invasion.

Several strategies have been investigated to improve local control. One approach uses chemotherapeutic agents or biologic response modifiers in conjunction with radiation, and several of these appear to be effective. Another involves surgery following induction therapy with chemotherapy, radiation therapy, or both, a strategy that is being investigated in the phase III trials discussed in the preceding section. Strategies involving modification of radiation time dose and fractionation have also been explored, falling into the general categories of accelerated hyperfractionation and classic hyperfractionation.

INTEGRATION OF RADIATION THERAPY AND CHEMOTHERAPY

The use of irradiation and chemotherapy together can take several distinct strategies. The physician can try to achieve additive cytotoxicity, treating the known local disease with radiation therapy and the local and systemic disease with chemotherapy. Such an approach is epitomized by the use of chemotherapy before local treatment with radiation or surgery. This strategy may allow greater sparing of normal tissue by virtue of smaller radiation target volumes or lesser resections performed of the postchemotherapy tumor volume. Another approach is to administer radiation and chemotherapy concurrently in the hope of shortening the overall time of treatment and avoid delay of starting either modality. This appears to have a bit more acute toxicity (myelosuppression and esophagitis), and its superiority to sequential therapy is unproved. Both approaches showed superiority to radiation therapy as a sole modality in prospective trials conducted in the 1980s (Tables 41-11 and 41-12).

The success of concurrent and sequential combinations of radiation therapy and chemotherapy compared with radiation therapy as a single modality prompted the direct comparison

Table 41-11 Stage IIIA-IIIB Non–Small Cell Lung Cancer: Major Phase III Sequential Chemoradiation Trials

Study	No. of Patients	Stage	Radiation Therapy	Chemotherapy	Median Survival (mo)	2-Year Survival (%)	Comments
Dillman et al[362,363]	77 78	IIIA/B	60 Gy 60 Gy	— VBL/DDP	9.6 13.7	13 (2) 26 (2)*	Survival difference persists to 5 years (17% vs. 6%)
Le Chevalier et al[222,223]	177 176	IIIA/B	65 Gy 65 Gy	— VDS/DDP/CTX/CCNU	NR NR	14 (2) 21 (2)*	No difference in local control for two arms; only 15% and 17% at 1 year assessed bronchoscopically.
Sause et al[234,364]	452	IIIA/B	60 Gy 60 Gy 69.6 Gy (bid)	— VBL/DDP —	11.4 13.8 12.3	19 32* 24	Difference between induction chemotherapy and bid RT arms decreased beyond 3 years; both remained slightly superior to standard RT.

*Statistically superior to control arm

CCNU, cyclohexylchloromethylnitrosourea; CTX, cyclophosphamide; DDP, cisplatin; NR, not reported; RT, radiation therapy; VBL, vinblastine; VDS, vindesine.

Table 41-12 Stage IIIA-IIIB Non–Small Cell Lung Cancer: Phase III Radiation versus Concurrent Chemoradiation Trials

Study	No. of Patients	Stage	Radiation Therapy (Gy)	Chemotherapy	Median Survival (mo)	2-Year Survival (%)	Comments
Schake-Koning et al[365]	108 102 98	Inoperable	55 55 55	— DDP q wk DDP q d	— — —	13 19 26	 NS $P = .009$ compared with RT alone. Local control also improved, $P = .003$
Trovo et al[366]	88 85		45 45	— DDP q d	44 43	— —	NS
Blanke et al[367]	111 104	Locally advanced	60-65 60-65	— DDP q 21 days	11 10.5	11 19	
Jeremic et al[368]	61 52 56	Nonresectable	64.8 bid 64.8 bid 64.8 bid	— CBP/VP16 q wk CBP/VP16 weeks 1, 3, 5	8 18 13	6.6 (3 y) 23 (3 y) 16 (3 y)	Patients not selected for favorable performance status; survival signif. improved for weekly chemotherapy versus none ($P = .0027$)
Jeremic et al[369]	66 65	Stage III	69.6 bid 69.6 bid	— CBP/VP16 q d	14 22	9 (4 y) 23 (4 y)	Improved local control without effect on distant failure

CBP, carboplatin; DDP, cisplatin; NS, not specified; RT, radiation therapy; VP16, etoposide.

of these approaches. At least six randomized trials comparing the sequential and concurrent use of chemotherapy and radiation therapy for patients with stage IIIA/B NSCLC have been reported (Table 41-13). Although all trials addressed the same general question of sequencing, they differed in many details. In some trials, different chemotherapy regimens were used in the two arms. The number of cycles of induction chemotherapy used before the start of radiation therapy ranged from two to four. It is not clear in all trials whether the prechemotherapy or postchemotherapy tumor volume was taken as the gross tumor volume or whether, if the prechemotherapy volume was to be used, the treatment planning was completed before the start of chemotherapy.

The overall tendency, although one not reaching statistical significance in most of these small trials, is for better results with concurrent rather than sequential combination of irradiation and chemotherapy. An alternate interpretation is that the overall treatment time is key, and that this is shorter in these concurrent regimens. With protraction of the overall treatment time, accelerated repopulation of the tumor, which may have begun during chemotherapy, may outpace the ability of daily fractionated radiation to kill remaining tumor clonogens.

Table 41-13 Chemoradiation Sequencing in Non-Small Cell Lung Cancer: Randomized Trials

Study/Trial	No. of Patients	Chemotherapy Regimen	Radiation Dose (Gy)	Median Survival (mo)	Actuarial Survival (%)	Statistics	Comments
Furuse[370]	314	MVP	56 SEQ 56 CON	13 17	9 19 (2 y)	$P = .04$	Improved local control in concurrent arm despite split-course RT
Curran[371] (RTOG)	400	VP	63 SEQ 63 CON	14.6 17.1	18 26 (3 y)	$P = .04$	Third arm with concurrent bid RT and DDP/VP16 was not statistically superior to sequential arm
Pierrl[372] (GLOT)	212	NP EP/NP	66 SEQ 66 CON	13.9 15.6	24 36 (2 y)	NS	Different chemotherapy regimens in the two arms
Zotoukal[373]	102	NP	60 SEQ 60 CON	13 20.4	—	$P = .02$	RT delayed until after 4 cycles of chemotherapy in in sequential arm
Choy[374] (LAMP)	178	TC	63 SEQ 63 CON	13 17.2	31 35 (2 y)	NS	Randomized phase II trial without planned comparison between arms

MVP, Mitomycin C/vindesine/cisplatin; VP, vinblastine/cisplatin; NP, vinorelbine/cisplatin; TC, paclitaxel/carboplatin; PE/NP, cisplatin/etoposide during RT; Navelbine/cisplatin after RT; NS, not specified.

Data from the U.K. Continuous Hyperfractionated Accelerated Radiation Therapy (CHART) trial and ECOG 2597 are consistent with this hypothesis that shortening overall treatment time may be clinically important. The median survival for the ECOG sequential chemotherapy followed by accelerated irradiation arm was 20.3 months, which is similar to what has been reported in multiple series using concurrent therapy.

The CALGB has reported a trial comparing induction chemotherapy with carboplatin and paclitaxel followed by concurrent chemoradiation with initial concurrent therapy. Unlike the LAMP trial, this was planned as a phase III comparison. This large cooperative group trial failed to confirm the earlier phase II results, with somewhat disappointing median survival times of 11.4 months for the initial concurrent regimen and 14 months for induction followed by concurrent therapy ($P = .154$).[225]

The SWOG conducted a phase II trial of consolidation with docetaxel rather than additional cycles of cisplatin plus etoposide after concurrent irradiation with cisplatin plus etoposide. Median survival was 26 months, and the 3-year survival rate was 37%. In the prior trial with cisplatin plus etoposide, consolidation values were 15 months and 17%.[226] This is a striking difference, but it does represent two studies done at different times, with potentially different staging, patient allocation, and treatment planning. A proposal from SWOG to perform a proper phase III trial was disallowed by the Cancer Therapy Evaluation Program (CTEP) of the NCI.

Radiation Dose and Fractionation

In North America, standard radiation dose and fractionation for potentially curative treatment of patients with unresectable NSCLC has generally been 1.8 to 2.0 Gy per fraction, with one fraction per day, 5 days per week, to a total dose of 60 to 65 Gy. Such a low total dose has been recognized as unlikely to achieve a high rate of local control, but simple dose escalation was for many years believed to be limited by acute and late toxicity to normal tissues. Several series have challenged this assumption by using conformal treatment planning and quantitative evaluation of doses to various normal tissues. Some of these trials have also limited the target volume by eliminating elective nodal irradiation.[149,227] Others have treated more traditional elective volumes, at least to doses of 50 Gy or so for possible microscopic disease.[228] These trials have clearly demonstrated the feasibility of dose escalation substantially above what had been previously believed limiting, to at least 74 to 78 Gy. Retrospective review suggests improvement in clinical outcome, particularly in patients with bulky disease, with such higher doses.[229] Whether such doses will truly result in better local control and survival when used as a component of combined-modality therapy remains to be evaluated in prospective trials.

The use of altered fractionation schedules is another way in which to try to exploit differences between tumor and normal tissues in the fraction-size dependence of their radiation sensitivity.[230] Several variations on standard fractionation have been proposed and evaluated (Table 41-14):

- *Hyperfractionation*: The use of small dose fractions given two or more times each day allows a higher total dose to be delivered within the tolerance of late effects to normal tissues. This spares late-reacting normal tissues more than acutely reacting tissues.
- *Accelerated fractionation*: Reduction of the overall treatment time lessens the effects of tumor cell proliferation during radiation therapy, increasing the probability of local control for a given dose.
- *Concomitant boost*: Another approach to rapid proliferation during treatment is to begin with conventional fractionation but accelerate with twice-daily treatment during the last 2 or 3 weeks of treatment. Data suggest that, during a course of treatment, stem cell proliferation accelerates after about 4 weeks.
- *Continuous hyperfractionated accelerated radiation therapy*: In a combination of the previous two methods, fraction size is decreased but overall time significantly shortened, typically by treating with three fractions per day.

Table 41-14 **Phase III Trials of Altered Fractionation in Treating Non–Small Cell Lung Cancer**

Study	Regimen	No. of Patients	Stage	MST (mo)	%S1	%S2	%S3	%S5	Comments
Sause et al[234,235]	60 Gy/30 Fx/6 wk CF 69.6 Gy HF	149 151	II-III favorable	11.4 12.2	46 51	19 24	9 14	5 6	Third arm with this regimen plus induction chemotherapy
Fu et al[237]	64 Gy CF 69.6 Gy HF	51 54	I-IIIB	— —	32 53	9 13	— —	— —	Significant survival advantage for subset of patients with stage I-IIIA
Kagami et al[375]	65 Gy CF 71.5 Gy HF	18 18	Unresectable	— —	— —	31 50	0 22	— —	Large difference but marginally significant because of small trial size ($P = 0.07$)
Bonner et al[236]	60 Gy/30 Fx/6 wk 30 Gy/20 Fx/2 wk 2-wk break 30 Gy/20 Fx/2 wk	34 38	IIIA/B ECOG PS 0-2 Weight loss <10%	8.6 11.6	≈ 35 ≈ 50	≈ 20 ≈ 25	— —	— —	Trial terminated early because of results of other trials favoring addition of chemotherapy; third arm with this regimen plus concurrent chemotherapy
Saunders et al[240,241]	60 Gy/30 Fx/6 wk 54 Gy/36 Fx/2 wk	225 338	Unresectable for medical reasons or stage (198 stage I-II), ECOG PS 0-1	≈ 12 ≈ 16	55 63	20 29	≈ 13 ≈ 20	— —	Overall survival difference $P = .004$; survival benefit seen for squamous but not nonsquamous histologies
Belani et al[244]	 57.6 Gy/36 Fx/2.5 wk	141	IIIA/B	14.9 20.3		34 44	14 24		Patients received two cycles of induction chemotherapy with carboplatin/paclitaxel before radiation therapy; differences did not reach statistical significance. Trial had planned to accrue 360 patients but was closed because of slow accrual. Of 141 patients entered to induction chemotherapy step, 119 were randomized between the two radiation therapy schedules.

%S*n* = percent surviving at *n* years; ≈, estimated from published survival curve; CF, conventional fractionation; Fx, fractions; HF, hyperfractionation; MST, median survival time (months).

In addition to these regimens, many other variations have been proposed and tested to some degree. Some regimens that have had some popularity, although the rational for their use is questionable, are those that give accelerated fractionation in two courses with an intervening treatment break. Although the weekly dose rate during the weeks of treatment is increased, when the break is taken into account, the overall rate of dose delivery is often no or only minimally greater than with conventional fractionation.

Hyperfractionation

The RTOG has conducted a series of trials exploring the use of altered fractionation in NSCLC.[231,232] The first group-wide trial (81-08) evaluated acute toxicity of several radiation dose levels using fractions of 1.2 Gy given 4 to 6 hours apart. Dose to the initial large volume encompassing known and electively treated tissues was always 50.4 Gy, whereas the dose to known disease was increased from 50.4 to 60, 69.6, and 74.4 Gy. This was a dose-seeking and toxicity study, but comparison of the group of patients treated to 69.6 Gy with contemporaneous controls from other RTOG trials (78-11 and 79-17) suggested a late survival benefit (8.3 ± 4.0% versus 5.6 ± 1.5% survival at 5 years). After this, RTOG 83-11 increased the total dose in two sequential randomizations from 60 to 79.2 Gy.[233] Late toxicities were similar in all arms, and overall survival did not differ among arms. However, when a favorable subset of patients, identified retrospectively by the CALGB criteria of good performance status and minimal weight loss, was analyzed, the 69.6-Gy arm appeared superior to other arms and to patients treated to 60 Gy in 6 weeks on other RTOG trials (13 months on median survival time (MST), with 1- and 2-year survival rates of 56% and 29%, compared with 9 months on RTOG 83-21, with rates of 35% and 10%, respectively). The higher-dose arms did not show this benefit, nor were they associated with greater toxicity, which might have offset a better therapeutic effect.

An Intergroup RTOG/ECOG trial made two comparisons: conventional radiation therapy alone or preceded by induction chemotherapy (as in CALGB 8433) and, as a third arm, the 69.6-Gy, twice-daily regimen, which had been the most favorable dose level in prior RTOG trials. It confirmed the CALGB demonstration of benefit for induction chemotherapy, with a statistically significant difference between this and standard radiation therapy alone.[234,235] The twice-daily arm was numerically superior to daily fractionation but the survival curve differences did not reach statistical significance.

The North Central Cancer Treatment Group conducted a trial of similar design.[236] Instead of using a continuous twice-daily regimen, they used a split-course regimen of 1.5 Gy given twice daily for 20 fractions over 2 weeks, a 2-week break, and another 1.5 Gy given in 20 fractions. The total dose was 60 Gy in 20 fractions, but the overall time was no shorter than with conventional fractionation. This was compared with standard fractionation of 60 Gy in 30 fractions over 6 weeks. A third arm combined the twice-daily, split-course regimen with concomitant cisplatin plus etoposide chemotherapy. Accrual to this trial was slow, and it was closed short of the planned sample size. The results trend toward favoring the twice-daily arm (with or without chemotherapy) for freedom from progression and survival. For patients with nonsquamous histology, survival was significantly improved ($P = .02$). In the North Central Cancer Treatment Group (NCCTG) trial, freedom from local progression was better for the twice-daily regimen with or without concomitant chemotherapy, although this did not quite reach statistical significance ($P = .06$).[236]

Fu and associates reported a trial in which 109 patients with stage I-IIIB NSCLC were randomized between a standard daily regimen of 63.9 Gy and a twice-daily regimen of 69.6 Gy.[237] The English abstract of this paper, published in Chinese, states that although the two arms did not differ for the entire group, in a subgroup of patients with stage I-IIIA disease (number not specified), there ware significant benefits for local control and survival for the twice-daily arm (2-year survival, 32% versus 6%; local control, 28% versus 13%).

Stuschke and Thames combined the data from the trials reported by Sause, Fu, and Kagami, and found that the P value for the pooled data was 0.02.[238] For local control in the two trials in which this had been reported (Fu and Kagami), the pooled P value was 0.09. Although favoring hyperfractionation, such retrospective meta-analyses cannot substitute for the design and conduct of primary trials of sufficient statistical power.

Secondary analyses of several of the previous trials have identified a number of factors associated with outcome. In RTOG 83-01, 11% of patients had significant treatment interruptions (for a variety of reasons). When compared with those completing treatment in the planned time, survival at 2 and 5 years was significantly less for those with treatment interruption (24% versus 13% at 2 years; 10% versus 3% at 5 years).[239] However, the length of treatment was not determined randomly and may reflect other prognostic factors. Survival differences, like the benefit for hyperfractionation, were seen only for the subset of patients with good performance status and minimal weight loss.

Accelerated Fractionation: CHART, HART, and CHARTWEL Regimens

In the United Kingdom, Saunders and colleagues compared an accelerated regimen called continuous hyperfractionated accelerated radiation therapy (CHART) with a conventional regimen of 60 Gy in 30 fractions in a mixed group of patients who had locally advanced (stage IIIA/IIIB) or medically unresectable (stage I or II) disease. The CHART regimen consisted of 54 Gy given in 36 fractions over 12 consecutive days (weekends included). The interfraction interval was 6 hours, which necessitated an extended treatment day. About 80% of patients on this trial had squamous cell carcinoma. Results show a survival advantage (30% versus 20% at 2 years; $P < .001$) for the CHART regimen, with local control also significantly improved.[240,241] Modifications of this regimen that have modestly increased total dose, shortened interfraction interval to 4 hours, and omitted weekend treatments (CHARTWEL in the United Kingdom and HART in the United States) have reported similar encouraging results in phase II trials.[242,243]

ECOG conducted a trial of HART compared with standard daily fractionation in patients with stage IIIA and IIIB NSCLC.[244] Patients received two cycles of induction chemotherapy with carboplatin and paclitaxel and were then randomized to conventional radiation therapy or HART. The study was designed to look for an improvement in median survival from 14 to 21 months, but it was closed before completing planned accrual due to slow patient entry. The results, a median survival of 21 months on the HART arm and 13 months on the standard arm, are provocative, but the difference did not reach statistical significance.

Physical Considerations in Fractionation Trials

The previously discussed trials evaluating radiation dose and fractionation were done during the 1980s and 1990s, in an era when routine CT scanning and three-dimensional planning were not uniformly employed. There was often considerable uncertainty and error about the extent of disease and the adequacy of its coverage by the treatment beams, particularly with the use of lateral and oblique beams used to spare the spinal cord. If a different proportion of the total dose is administered through anteroposterior-posteroanterior (AP-PA) and oblique beam arrangements in the two fractionation regimens and the rate of tumor miss is greater for oblique than for AP-PA beams, it is reasonable to expect a difference in local control based on technique that is independent of any difference due to fractionation. Even in trials incorporating fairly straightforward patient eligibility criteria and irradiation technique requirements, errors in staging and field size or placement are commonly in the range of 15%.[245] Because more complex (and likely more error-prone) techniques were typically used in the hyperfractionated regimens that gave a higher total dose, the net effect might have been to mask a possible biologic benefit of the higher-dose regimen. Possible benefits of fractionation might have been underestimated or missed entirely. Possible solutions to this involve the following:

- Retrospective assessment of the adequacy of tumor coverage in three dimensions has been reported by Boxwala and colleagues for the CALGB 8433 trial.[246] This latter approach is labor intensive, and although it has demonstrated substantial error rates in this trial, it is probably not worth doing routinely now that three-dimensional planning is required from the start in new trials.
- More accurate determination of tumor volume and treatment planning probably require three-dimensional treatment planning and conformal treatment delivery.
- At least for the purpose of a phase III trial, identical beam arrangements and weightings should be required for the conventional and investigational (total dose or fractionation) arms. The dose per fraction or number of fractions, or both, would differ between arms. The drawback to this approach is that it could require nonoptimal beam arrangements for one of the arms to meet the constraints of the other.

Evaluation of Local Control

Most trials of altered fractionation have attempted to evaluate patterns of failure to determine whether there is a difference in local control. It must be kept in mind, however, that assessing local control in irradiated NSCLC is difficult for a number of reasons:

- Difficulty in distinguishing between recurrence and fibrosis
- Variable assessment of local control after relapse in other sites
- High rate of early death from systemic relapse and intercurrent disease

Some of these difficulties can be dealt with statistically through methods such as reporting failures in terms of competing risks, and PET scanning may be useful in distinguishing scar from tumor.[126,134,247,248] Current estimates of postirradiation local control should be considered approximations at best.

RADIATION TECHNIQUES IN DEFINITIVE AND ADJUVANT THERAPY

Positioning and Immobilization

Patients are generally positioned supine during treatment, with the torso supported and partially immobilized using custom devices such as Alpha Cradles or VacLoc bags or using adjustable wingboards. Positioning the arms above the head allows for more options using lateral or oblique beam angles, but care must be taken to allow the arms to fit in the gantry (typically 70 or 80 cm) of CT scanners used for image acquisition. Prone positioning may seem appealing for patients with tumors located posteriorly in the chest, but it usually results in greater motion of intrathoracic structures with respiration. In the absence of more formal respiratory arrest (deep breathing and breath-hold) or respiratory gating techniques, patients should be instructed in quiet, steady respiration during treatment and planning.

Definition of Target Volume

Traditional treatment volumes for patients with stage IIIA/B NSCLC have been based on principles of covering the known volume of the primary tumor and its nodal metastases and on the "elective" irradiation of nodal echelons at risk for microscopic involvement.[249] This initial volume was treated to a dose appropriate for microscopic disease, usually in the range of 45 to 50 Gy, and then areas of known disease were boosted to a total of 60 to 65 Gy. Such an approach typically treated large amounts of normal tissue, including lung, heart, and spinal cord, to a moderately high dose. More current approaches that restrict the target volume to known disease and try to avoid the transit of opposed beams through normal tissue can produce dose distributions that better conform to the target volume but that may treat larger volumes of normal tissue, albeit to lower dose.[250-253] Figures 41-4 and 41-5 show isodose curves and dose-volume histograms for a patient with a T3N0M0 squamous cell carcinoma of the left lung for two different treatment plans, one with and the other without elective nodal irradiation. The development of appropriate dose-volume–effect nomograms, with and without chemotherapy, for clinically important normal tissues, including lung, esophagus, heart, and spinal cord, is an active area of clinical development.[254]

As larger target volumes are treated, it becomes more difficult to limit doses to normal tissue tolerances, and there is a reciprocal relation between the volume of the target and the dose to which it can be safely treated. The spinal cord, because of its intolerance of damage to even a short section, is probably an exception to this dose-volume relationship. Late esophageal stricture formation probably falls in this category as well, because even a short length of stricture can be quite symptomatic, but it is of less clinical importance because of the ease and effectiveness of esophageal dilatation. If we wish to improve local control by increasing radiation dose, it follows that we need to consider reducing target volume. Several trials have demonstrated the feasibility of such an approach and the impossibility of major dose escalations when large target volumes are used.[149,255-258]

The use of FDG-PET scanning to aid in radiation therapy planning for NSCLC, as a separate study or as combined dual imaging with CT, has been reported in several series.[259-270] Significant changes in planned target volumes have been reported in about one third of patients. Two general types of field change have been made, inclusion of normal-sized lymph nodes showing avid FDG uptake and probable tumor involvement and exclusion of lung densities not showing glucose uptake, which are presumed to be atelectatic rather than tumor. The validity of these changes awaits outcome studies. There are also considerable technical issues to resolve, including issues of tumor motion during image acquisition for CT (seconds), PET, minutes, and treatment (fractions of minutes per beam), which are being studied through various approaches to respiratory immobilization (e.g., breath-holding, automatic breathing control, abdominal

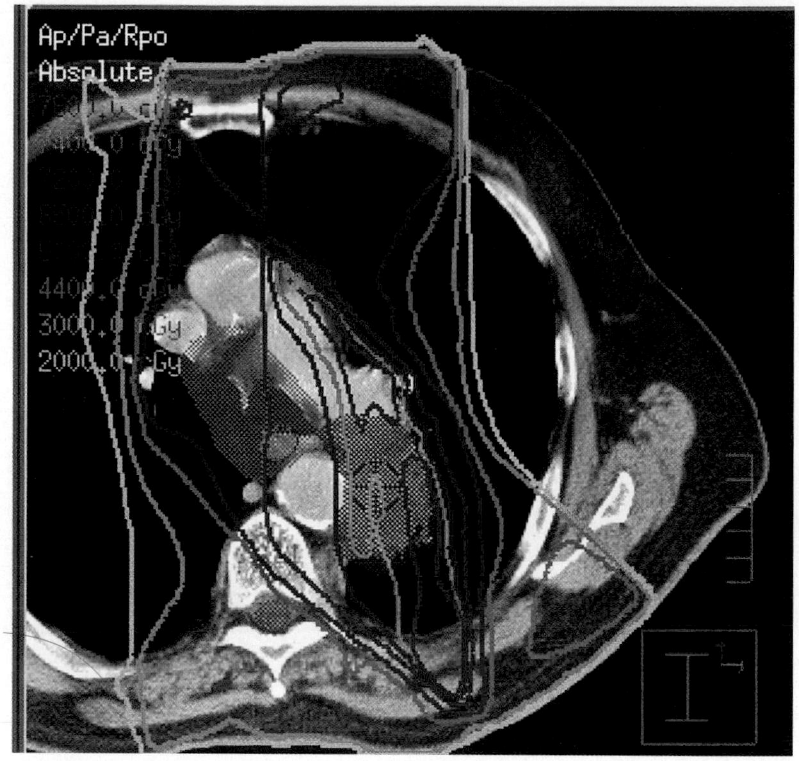

A

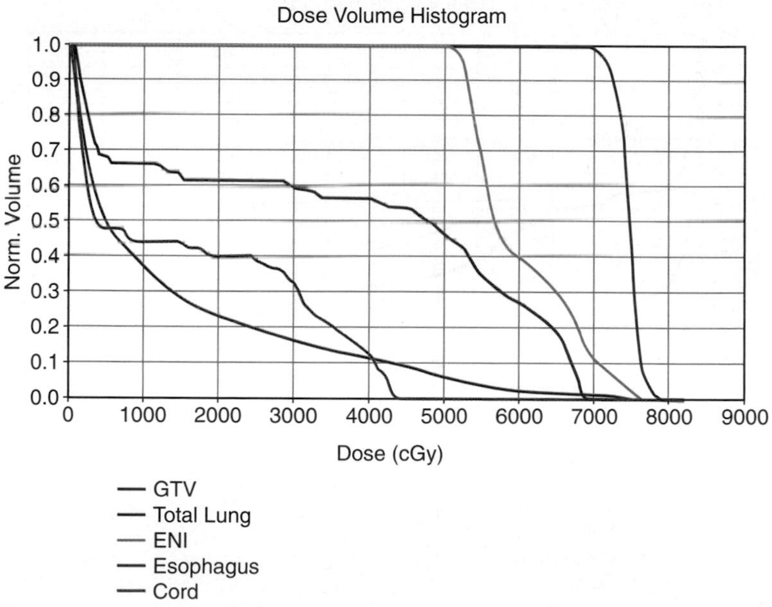

B

Figure 41-4 Isodose curves (**A**) and dose-volume histogram (**B**) for a patient with T3N0M0 non–small cell lung cancer being treated with definitive chemoradiation. This plan was designed to deliver 74 Gy to areas of known disease and 50 Gy to possible sites of lymph node drainage in the mediastinum. The lung V20 was 27%, and the maximum cored dose was 46 Gy.

compression) or gating treatment delivery to the patient's free breathing, as discussed earlier for stereotactic treatment.

Beam Energy

The preferred beam energy used to treat patients with lung cancer has gone through several changes. The wide availability of high-energy photon beams (>15 MV) and their superior isodose distributions in homogeneous phantoms, particularly lower cord dose in AP-PA treatment of the thorax, made them the modality of choice for some time. More careful dosimetry has indicated that in regions of electronic disequilibrium, as seen in going from low-density lung to higher-density tumor, they can lead to significant underdosing of tumor cells at such interfaces or of microscopic extensions of tumor into lung.[271,272] This problem is reduced but not eliminated, particularly for small fields, with lower photon energies (6 to 10 MV), and these are making a return to favor. With multiple-beam conformal and intensity-modulated radiation therapy (IMRT) plans, there is little reason to use higher energies.

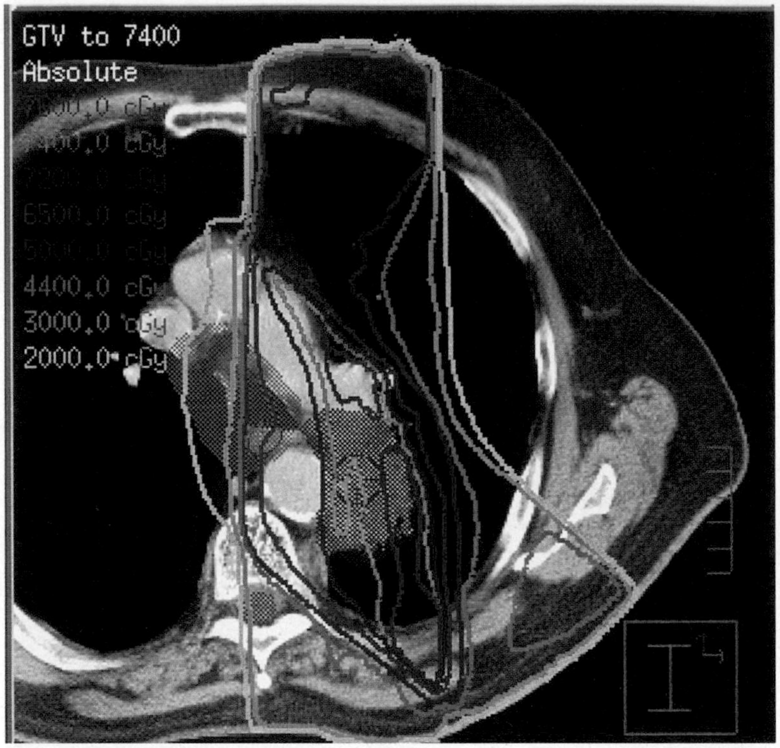

A

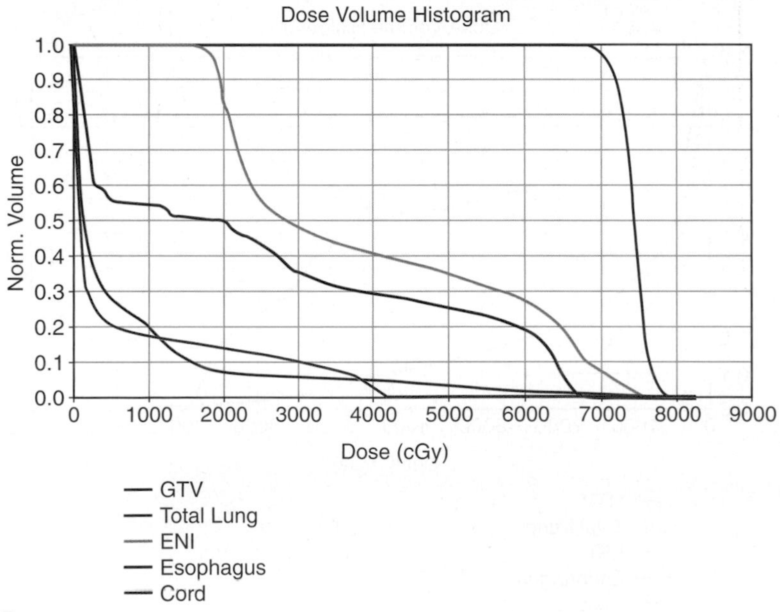

B

Figure 41-5 Isodose curves (**A**) and dose-volume histogram (**B**) for a patient with a T3N0M0 non–small cell lung cancer being treated with definitive chemoradiation. This plan was designed to deliver 74 Gy to areas of known disease without intentional irradiation of elective nodal drainage sites. The lung V20 was 9%, and maximum cord dose was 42 Gy. Elective nodal regions, although not intentionally targeted, received a non-negligible dose for microscopic disease with 40% of the potential elective nodal irradiation, primarily the ipsilateral paratracheal region, receiving 40 Gy or more.

Choice of Beam Direction

Traditional two-dimensional treatment-planning schemes typically treated the tumor and regional nodes with opposed anterior and posterior portals until the spinal cord tolerance was approached and then switched to lateral or oblique beam angles, sparing the cord. During both phases of treatment, substantial volumes of lung were treated to a relatively uniform dose that exceeded lung tolerance in the first phase and often neared or exceeded it in the second. The general planning optimization sought to accept these high doses but attempted to limit the volume of normal lung receiving them. An alternative approach, whose implementation is facilitated by modern treatment planning systems, is to avoid the use of opposed beams entirely, increasing the total number of beams used and, in some cases, using non-coplanar beams. The net result of these strategies is to increase the volume of lung receiving some radiation dose but to keep this well below lung tolerance, except in the immediate vicinity of the tumor. Particularly when the target volume is kept small, a higher degree of heterogeneity of dose (e.g., hot spots) can be accepted within the target volume if this allows better sparing of normal tissue. These considerations, although valid for all patients with lung cancer, are particularly important for those who are unable to undergo resection because of poor pulmonary function.[251,273,274] Some groups are also exploring the possibility of optimizing beam placement through relatively nonfunctional portions of lung (e.g., those involved with extensive bullous disease or postobstructive atelectasis) and minimizing dose to functional lung parenchyma.[275,276]

TOXICITY OF THORACIC IRRADIATION AND COMBINED-MODALITY THERAPY

Treatment of patients with aggressive multimodality therapy requires attention to and management of a variety of acute and chronic toxicities.[277] These involve local anatomic toxicities such as esophagitis and pneumonitis and systemic considerations such as cytopenias. Acute toxicities during radiation therapy may compromise the ability of patients to complete aggressive regimens without interruption, and late effects limit the total dose that can be given. The acute and late toxicities pose obstacles to increasing radiation dose in lung cancer treatment.

Risk factors for radiation pneumonitis include radiation dose and lung volume treated and considerations of the patient's baseline pulmonary function.[278] Patients with lower lobe tumors are more likely to have pneumonitis, probably because of the greater lung volume treated.[279] Although the effect of most chemotherapeutic agents on pneumonitis is not well defined, there is an increased risk associated with the use of mitomycin C, gemcitabine, and CPT-11 (irinotecan).[253,280-282]

Management of patients with moderately severe radiation pneumonitis symptomatic with cough and dyspnea has generally included suppression of cough with codeine or Tessalon and the use of oral corticosteroids such as prednisone in doses of 20 to 60 mg/day to reduce acute inflammation and in the hope of decreasing late fibrosis. Some investigators have reported the use of inhaled rather than oral corticosteroids as prophylactic treatment.[283] The reduction in systemic symptoms afforded by this approach is appealing, and it warrants further study.

Esophagitis is common in patients who receive concurrent radiation therapy and chemotherapy or accelerated radiation therapy regimens. Management with a soft diet, use of topical analgesics such as lidocaine or diphenhydramine, and systemic narcotics helps but does not entirely relieve symptoms. Particularly in patients treated with curative intent, the presence of moderate to severe acute esophagitis should prompt aggressive supportive therapy, including enteral or parenteral feeding when indicated, rather than a treatment interruption, which jeopardizes local control. Acute esophagitis is a common toxicity with hyperfractionated and accelerated regimens, particularly when concurrent chemotherapy is also used. It is often the acute dose-limiting toxicity and is a common reason for patients to request treatment interruptions. Toxicity requiring narcotic analgesics or intravenous fluid support is seen in 20% to 30% of patients, clearly more than with conventional fractionation.

Amifostine, a thioester that is actively taken up by normal tissues but enters most tumor cells only by passive diffusion, can protect normal tissues to some degree against radiation mucositis and the renal and bone marrow toxicity of chemotherapeutic agents such as cisplatin.[284-286] Preliminary results of a phase III trial enrolling patients with head and neck cancers demonstrate a delay in time of onset and reduction in maximal severity of oral mucositis, and phase II data for lung cancer are similarly promising.[287] However, a phase III trial with concurrent irradiation, carboplatin, and paclitaxel failed to demonstrate statistically significant differences in objective measures of esophagitis and only borderline differences in patient self-assessment by diary.[288]

Myelitis is the most dreaded complication of thoracic irradiation, but it is rare with current radiotherapeutic techniques. The tolerance dose ($TD_{5/5}$) for the thoracic spinal cord has been estimated at about 50 Gy, but it may be higher than this. With the use of multiple fractions per day, however, repair of damage is not complete in 6 hours, and the total cord dose should be lowered for twice- or thrice-daily regimens, because several cases of transverse myelitis were reported in early trials of thoracic irradiation given three times daily.[240]

Late normal tissue effects of radiation have until recently been thought to be irreversible. Changes in our understanding of fibrosis have indicated that this is a dynamic process, undergoing continued tissue remodeling long after irradiation, and have raised hopes that fibrosis may be reversed after the fact by disruption of ongoing cytokine cascades.[289-294]

Attempts to improve the therapeutic ratio of treatment for patients with stage III NSCLC must address treatment efficacy and toxicity. Efforts to adopt new uniform criteria for reporting acute and late toxicities, shown in Table 41-15, should facilitate these efforts. Mornex and coworkers reviewed the issues of late effects reporting and clinical research and proposed an agenda for future trials.[295] These considerations are of great importance so long as the clinical gains achieved with even aggressive treatments are often modest.

INTEGRATION OF MOLECULAR TARGETED AGENTS WITH RADIATION THERAPY

Identification of radioresistant cells in human tumors has led to several approaches to sensitize them while not altering the radiation response of normal tissues. Tumor cells may be resistant for reasons of local environment (e.g., hypoxia) or because of genetic changes (e.g., mutations in *TP53* or *KRAS*). Past strategies have looked largely to reverse environmental hypoxia without great success, but some newer agents show promise. Several approaches that exploit specific tumor genetic changes are being explored.[296,297]

Epidermal Growth Factor Receptor Inhibitors

Exposure of cells to ionizing radiation induces phosphorylation of EGFR and activation of its kinase activity in much the same fashion as binding of ligands such as EGF or TGF-α. This leads to activation of several signaling cascades with resultant increased cellular proliferation, decreased apoptosis, and effects on angiogenesis and DNA repair.[298-302] Inhibition of these processes through anti-EGFR monoclonal antibodies, expression of a dominant-negative truncated version of EGFR, or low-molecular-weight compounds that bind to the ATP site of EGFR and block its kinase activity result in significant radiosensitization of a number of cell lines in vitro and in vivo.[298,303,304] A completed phase III trial comparing radiation therapy with or without the anti-EGFR antibody C225 in patients with squamous cell carcinoma of the head and neck, which commonly overexpresses EGFR, has demonstrated clinically significant improvements in local control and survival.[305] Similar trials using monoclonal antibodies and the low-molecular-weight tyrosine kinase inhibitors (TKIs) erlotinib and gefitinib are being conducted. Although several groups have shown that objective regressions of NSCLC in response to treatment with these TKIs occur almost exclusively in patients with specific point mutations in the ATP-binding region, which are present in only a minority of patients, it is not clear that such mutations are required

Table 41-15 Common Toxicity Criteria of Particular Importance in Lung Cancer

Toxicity	Grade 1	Grade 2	Grade 3	Grade 4	Grade 5
Cough	Symptomatic, only non-narcotic medication indicated	Symptomatic, narcotic medication indicated	Symptomatic and significantly interfering with sleep or ADLs	—	Death
Dyspnea	Dyspnea on exertion but can walk one flight of stairs without stopping	Dyspnea on exertion but unable to walk one flight of stairs or one city block (0.1 km) without stopping	Dyspnea with ADLs	Dyspnea at rest; intubation/ventilator indicated	Death
Pneumonitis	Asymptomatic, radiographic findings only	Symptomatic, not interfering with ADLs	Symptomatic, interfering with ADLs; O_2 indicated	Life threatening; ventilatory support indicated	Death
Esophagitis	Asymptomatic pathologic, radiographic, or endoscopic findings only	Symptomatic; altered eating/swallowing (e.g. altered dietary habits, oral supplements), IV fluids indicated <24 hours	Symptomatic and severely altered eating/swallowing (e.g., inadequate caloric or fluid intake); IV fluids, tube feedings, or TPN indicated ≥24 h	Life-threatening consequences	Death

ADLs, activities of daily living; IV, intravenous; TPN, total parenteral nutrition.
Data from Common Toxicity Criteria: Cancer Therapy Evaluation Program, Version 3.0, 2003.

for response to monoclonal antibodies that target the extracellular domain of the receptor or for radiosensitization by TKIs.[69-71]

Gadolinium Texaphyrin

There has long been interest in the use of porphyrins as tumor selective cytotoxins. The texaphyrins are ring-expanded porphyrins in which a variety of metal ions can be inserted. With gadolinium as the central ion the compound (motexafin gadolinium) is highly electron affinic, producing highly reactive π-radical cations after ionizing radiation. Selectivity for tumor cells derives from preferential accumulation in tumor tissue, and initial animal and human studies have not shown significant sensitization of normal tissues. These compounds have two potential advantages over previous electron-affinic sensitizers such as the nitroimidazoles. They sensitize oxic and hypoxic tumor cells, and the paramagnetic gadolinium ion acts as an MRI contrast agent, allowing localization of the compound and monitoring of its persistence in tumor tissue.[306] Motexafin gadolinium has shown some promise in a subset of patients with brain metastases from lung cancer in one phase III trial, and a confirmatory trial is nearing completion.[307] The compound is also being investigated in conjunction with thoracic irradiation for SCLC and NSCLC.

PALLIATION OF LOCAL AND SYSTEMIC DISEASE

Most patients with lung cancer have symptoms of their intrathoracic disease. Radiation therapy has long been the mainstay of treatment for such patients, with relatively high rates of palliation for irritative or obstructive symptoms and for hemoptysis, with poorer results for symptoms of nerve compression such as recurrent laryngeal and phrenic paralysis (Table 41-16). In the United States, common radiotherapeutic practice has been to treat such patients to doses of 30 to 35 Gy in 10 to 15 fractions over 2 to 3 weeks. In the United Kingdom, several randomized trials conducted by the MRC have compared such schedules with more abbreviated regimens of 17 Gy in 2 fractions 1 week apart or a single fraction of 10 Gy, with equally good palliation of symptoms and survival and toxicity no greater than with more fractionated treatment (Table 41-17). Such schedules are particularly attractive for patients who may otherwise have to travel substantial distances or remain hospitalized for their radiation therapy. They provide good symptom management while limiting the use of medical resources and reducing disruption of the schedules of the patients and their caregivers. For patients with better performance status, however, more fractionated schedules have resulted in modest improvements in survivals compared with one- or two-fraction schedules.[308,309]

The most common sites of locally symptomatic metastases of NSCLC are bone and brain. These can be palliated in most patients with relatively brief courses of irradiation, typically 2 weeks in the United States and 2 fractions in the United Kingdom (see Table 41-15). In appropriate situations, consideration of resection of solitary CNS metastases or orthopedic stabilization of metastases to weight-bearing bones should be considered. For patients with one to three CNS metastases, stereotactic radiosurgery in addition to whole-brain radiation therapy (WBRT) improves radiographic and clinical response and improves survival for patients with a single metastatic lesion.[310] It has been suggested that for these patients, WBRT can be omitted in their initial management and used only if needed subsequently, without a detrimental effect on survival.[311,312] A concern with this strategy is that the risk of subsequent CNS events is rather high in these patients, about 30% to 60%, and the psychological morbidity of multiple brain metastases and their treatment may be substantial. The American College of Surgeons Oncology Group (ACOSOG) attempted to conduct a prospective trial of stereotatic radiosurgery alone or followed by WBRT in patients with one to three metastases, but this trial was closed because of poor accrual.

In past years, the role of chemotherapy for palliation of specific symptoms was thought to be inferior to irradiation. Trials of new chemotherapeutic regimens have typically reported response rates of measurable disease and survival but rarely reported palliation of specific symptoms or effects of treatment on quality of life. Several trials have addressed these issues

Table 41-16 Management of Local Expressions of Systemic Metastatic Disease

Syndrome	Presentation	Management
Brain metastases	Headache; nausea and/or vomiting; altered mental status; focal motor, sensory, or cerebellar deficits; focal or generalized seizures	Corticosteroids; whole-brain irradiation. Consider resection or radiosurgery of oligometastatic disease in patients whose other sites of disease are controlled or indolent. Avoid prophylactic anticonvulsants that are ineffective and have their own potential toxicities. Caution patients about driving.
Spinal cord compression	Back pain (early); motor or sensory deficits, loss of sphincter control (late)	Emergency evaluation by contrast-enhanced MRI; high-dose corticosteroids; local radiation and/or surgical decompression
Pleural effusion	Dyspnea; chest pain	Thoracentesis and pleurodesis with doxycycline, bleomycin, or talc
Pericardial effusion	Dyspnea; syncope	Emergency evaluation by cardiac ultrasound to exclude atrial collapse; pericardiocentesis or pericardiectomy. Avoid diuretics.
Superior vena cava obstruction	Dyspnea; facial and neck swelling; distention of superficial chest wall veins	Corticosteroids; mediastinal irradiation? Concurrent chemotherapy if good performance status
Bone metastases	Pain; may be asymptomatic	Analgesics, radiation therapy. Consider prophylactic orthopedic intervention for weight-bearing bones.

Table 41-17 Palliation of Symptoms of Non–Small Cell Lung Cancer with External Beam Irradiation or with Multiagent Chemotherapy

	Percentage of Patients with Symptom Palliated				
Symptom	Standard RT (24-30 Gy in 6-10 Fractions)*	17 Gy in 2 Fractions (1st trial/2nd trial)*	1 Fraction of 10 Gy*	EDAM/MMC/VBL†	DDP/MMC/VBL‡
Cough	56	65/48	56	23/10	40
Hemoptysis	86	81/75	72	5/0.3	100
Chest Pain	80	75/59	72	21/10	44
Anorexia	64	68/45	55	NA	NA
Depression	57	72/NA	NA	NA	NA
Anxiety	66	71/NA	NA	NA	NA
Breathlessness	57	66/41	43	22/15	66

DDP, cisplatin; EDAM, edatrexate; MMC, mitomycin C; NA, data not available; RT, radiation therapy; VBL, vinblastine.

Trial 1 compared standard RT with 17 Gy in 2 fractions; Trial 2 compared 17 Gy in 2 fractions with a single fraction.

*Data from Bleehen N: Inoperable non–small cell lung cancer (NSCLC): a Medical Research Council randomized trial of palliative radiotherapy with two fractions or ten fractions. Br J Cancer 63:265-270, 1991; Bleehen N, Girling D, Machin D, Stephens R: A Medical Research Council (MRC) randomised trial of palliative radiotherapy with two fractions or a single fraction in patients with inoperable non–small-cell lung cancer (NSCLC) and poor performance status. Br J Cancer 65:934-941, 1992.

†Data from Kris M, Gralla R, Potanovich L, et al: Assessment of pretreatment symptoms and improvement after EDAM + mitomycin + vinblastine (EMV) in patients with inoperable non–small cell lung cancer (NSCLC) [abstract 883]. Proc Am Soc Clin Oncol 1990;9:299. Scores are not percentage of patients improved, but rather median symptom severity (0 = least, 100 = most) before and after chemotherapy.

‡Data from Tummarello D, Graziano F, Isidori P, et al: Symptomatic, stage IV, non–small cell lung cancer (NSCLC): response, toxicity, performance status change, and symptom relief in patients treated with cisplatin, vinblastine, and mitomycin C. Cancer Chemother Pharmacol 3:249-253, 1995.

and have shown that with a number of platinum-containing chemotherapy regimens, the rates of clinical improvement and symptomatic palliation were about twice as great as the rates of objective response (see Table 41-15). This suggests that for patients with widely metastatic disease and good performance status, an initial trial of chemotherapy should be offered, with radiation therapy reserved for nonresponding lesions. Radiation should also be employed early in patients with metastases to weight bearing bones, impending spinal cord compression, or caval or major airway obstruction. Because of the increased risk of neutropenic sepsis in patients with lobar or mainstem bronchus obstruction, attempts to open such obstructed airways with external beam or endobronchial irradiation, laser excision, or stent placement are desirable before chemotherapy.

A comparison of data from SWOG 0003 and the Japanese Four-Arm Cooperative Study suggests that there are clinically significant ethnic differences in chemotherapy tolerance. These trials had generally similar outcomes, except for 1-year survival, but despite a lower dose of paclitaxel in the Japanese trial (200 versus 225 mg/m^2), there was twice the incidence of neutropenia in the Japanese populations.[313] Data also were available for population variations in the rate of glucuronidation of irinotecan metabolites among different racial and ethnic groups. What in the past had been puzzling differences between national trials may be pointing toward the development of metabolically individualized treatment regimens.

CONTROVERSIES

The past several decades have seen the clear demonstration of modest survival improvements for patients with locally advanced NSCLC when treated with careful combination of currently available radiation and chemotherapy. They have also provided a number of new tools for tumor imaging and radiation dose delivery that hold the promise of allowing us to escalate tumor dose with manageable normal tissue toxicity and determining whether this dose increase results in improved local control and survival. The increased knowledge of and ability to manipulate tumor genetics introduce a wide variety of new therapeutic approaches. Several reasonable guidelines for stage-specific therapy may be proposed based on good-quality evidence from prospective clinical trials (Table 41-18). We are chastened to admit, however, that there remain a number of basic questions about the roles of radiation therapy that have not been answered or often well addressed by clinical research:

1. Should elective nodal irradiation be reduced or eliminated for early-stage patients, in whom the probability of nodal disease is low, or in patients with bulky primary disease which is not likely to be controlled with current chemoradiation? Is there an intermediate subgroup of patients with a reasonable probability of primary tumor control and substantial risk of regional nodal metastases for whom elective nodal treatment improves survival?
2. Will systemic adjuvant chemotherapy effective against occult M1 disease also eradicate microscopic nodal disease?
3. Is the superiority of concurrent to sequential combinations of radiation and chemotherapy the result primarily of selective radiosensitization or of a shortening of overall treatment time? If it is overall time rather than concurrency that is the critical factor, alternate strategies to shorten time while not exposing tissues to overlapping toxicities of concurrent treatment, such as induction chemotherapy followed by accelerated radiation or rapidly interdigitated therapy (e.g., radiation therapy during the week with chemotherapy on the weekend), are worthy of investigation.
4. What is the role of surgical resection in patients with advanced IIIA and IIIB disease? The North American Intergroup Trial INT 0139, showing better disease-free but not overall survival with the inclusion of surgery, has not resolved this question for many. Advocates of surgery argue that better exclusion of patients at poor operative risk would have shown an overall survival benefit, whereas partisans of nonsurgical treatment point to the technologic improvements in radiation therapy planning and delivery since the time of this trial. Although the current RTOG trial for these patients includes surgery in both treatment arms, this choice has come about as much because of investigator fatigue as compelling data. If sterilization of mediastinal lymph nodes is a useful criterion in selecting patients for surgery, how can this best be assessed preoperatively?

Table 41-18 Recommended Therapy for Good-Risk Patients with Non–Small Cell Lung Cancer

Clinical Stage	Therapy*	Comments
T1 N0 M0	Resection (usually lobectomy)	If pathologic N0, no adjuvant therapy is indicated. Should be considered for trials of early detection and chemoprevention
T2 N0 M0	Resection (usually lobectomy)	Postoperative adjuvant chemotherapy†
T1-2 N1 M0	Resection (consider preoperative chemotherapy)	Postoperative adjuvant chemotherapy†
T3 N0-1 M0	Resection (consider preoperative chemotherapy)	Postoperative adjuvant chemotherapy†
T1-3 N2 M0	Resection followed by adjuvant chemotherapy ± mediastinal irradiation‡	Single N2 node found at intraoperative mediastinoscopy
T1-3 N2 M0	Induction chemotherapy or chemoradiotherapy and resection or definitive chemoradiotherapy	Multiple N2 nodes or single node with extranodal extension identified prior to thoracotomy
T1-3 N3 M0	Definitive chemoradiotherapy	Chemoradiotherapy clearly superior to standard radiation therapy alone; local control remains poor. With conventional fractionation, use concurrent rather than sequential chemoradiation.
T4 N1-3 M0	Definitive chemoradiotherapy	Consider preoperative radiochemotherapy and resection for patients with T4 N0 M0 lesions, especially those of the superior sulcus.§
T1-4 N 0-3 M1	Symptomatic palliative treatment with radiation and/or chemotherapy	Consider more aggressive therapy for primary and metastatic disease, including resection for patients with T1-3 N0 M1 lesions with a solitary lesion in the brain or adrenal, particularly if responsive to initial chemotherapy.

*Good-risk patients are characterized by adequate cardiopulmonary function, ECOG PS ≤1, weight loss ≤5%. Patients not meeting these criteria may still be suitable for therapy but should be evaluated with particular care.

†Regimens with demonstrated efficacy in this setting include cisplatin or carboplatin and a second agent such as etoposide, vinorelbine, paclitaxel, docetaxel, or gemcitabine.

‡Adjuvant postoperative radiation to the mediastinum, if given, should be carefully planned to avoid excessive cardiac and pulmonary treatment and limited to a dose of 45 to 50 Gy (1.8 to 2.0 fractions) with a possible boost to a small field if there is known extracapsular extension or adherence of nodal metastases to adjacent unresected structures.

§For preoperative chemoradiation, radiation doses in the range of 45 to 50 Gy are best established using concurrent chemotherapy with cisplatin/etoposide or carboplatin/paclitaxel.

Will increasing radiation dose to the mediastinum to increase the rate of sterilization of mediastinal nodes translate to an increase in survival even though it does not affect systemic disease?
5. Are there meaningful differences in survival between preoperative and postoperative chemotherapy when combined with surgery for patients with clearly resectable disease? If survival is similar, are there other differences (e.g., logistics, toxicity, the ability to obtain a biologic assessment of chemotherapy effectiveness if it is given preoperatively) that sway the preference in one direction or the other, or is this a matter of institutional or individual preference?
6. Does close follow-up benefit patients with NSCLC after surgical or nonsurgical therapy? There is marked variation in current clinical practice after curative resection.[314] Most recurrences are detected clinically; patients with asymptomatic recurrences are most commonly detected by routine chest radiographs or CT. Although there is some time gained for these patients, overall survival did not seem significantly affected, and close follow-up does not clearly improve survival.[315] This does not preclude real benefits as perceived by the patients to know that they remain under medical care. The high rate of second primary lung cancers in these patients is also a strong argument for close surveillance.[316,317]
7. How is local tumor control best evaluated in patients not undergoing surgical resection? Several investigators have demonstrated that assessment based on CT measurement of tumor size, whether evaluated unidimensionally as in the Response Evaluation Criteria in Solid Tumors (RECIST), traditional bidimensional measurements, or volumetric assessment does not correlate particularly well with clinical outcome.[318] Assessment by ^{18}FDG-PET scanning has correlated better with end points such as pathologic response at surgery or survival, but postirradiation inflammatory changes and infection may also result in persistently increased FDG uptake.[134,138,141,319-322]

CONCLUSIONS

The past several years have seen modest progress in the treatment of patients with NSCLC, particularly in the combination of local and systemic modalities of treatment. Staging has become more accurate with the introduction of ^{18}FDG-PET scanning, and although this does not improve treatment per se, it allows a better match between a patient's real extent of disease and the treatment recommended for it. Adjuvant chemotherapy for most resected patients (excluding T1 N0 M0) has demonstrated a survival benefit of similar magnitude to those seen with other adult solid tumors such as breast or colorectal cancer.

Better imaging and treatment planning technologies for radiation therapy, including the beginnings of serious consideration that lung tumors are moving targets, herald a new era of treatment precision and the ability to explore dose escalation in a far more meaningful fashion than was previously possible. As more effective systemic treatment agents are introduced, we may reasonably expect modest gains in survival. This progress is real, can be achieved with acceptable cost, and should be made widely available to patients with unresectable disease.[323] These gains should not blind us to the fact that prevention of this disease is far better than its treatment, and that detection and treatment of early-stage disease is far better than the best chemoradiation for advanced disease. Basic research and clinical trials assessing smoking prevention and cessation, chemoprevention, and early detection in smokers and the growing population of former smokers who remain at high risk for lung cancer must remain high priorities to produce a major reduction in deaths from this disease.

ACKNOWLEDGMENT

In memory of Robert Ginsburg, MD, who was a friend, teacher, and pioneer in the multidisciplinary management of patients with cancer of the lung.

REFERENCES

1. Jemal A, Murray T, Ward E, et al: Cancer Statistics, 2005. CA Cancer J Clin 55:10-30, 2005.
2. Alberg A, Samet JM: Epidemiology of lung cancer. Chest 123:21S-49S, 2003.
3. Alberts W, Bepler G, Hazelton T, et al: Practice organization. Chest 123:332S-337S, 2003.
4. Wells F: Lung cancer, 10. Delivering a lung cancer service in the 21st century. Thorax 58:996-997, 2003.
5. Boyle P, Maissonneuve P: Lung cancer and tobacco smoking. Lung Cancer 12:167-181, 1995.
6. Denissenko M, Pao A, Tang M, Pfeifer G: Preferential formation of benzo[a]pyrene adducts at lung cancer mutational hotspots in p53. Science 274:430-432, 1996.
7. Foiles P, Murphy S, Peterson L, et al: DNA and hemoglobin adducts as markers of metabolic activation of tobacco-specific carcinogens. Cancer Res 52:2698s-2701s, 1992.
8. Mao L, Lee J, Kurie J, et al: Clonal genetic alterations in the lungs of current and former smokers. J Natl Cancer Inst 89:857-862, 1997.
9. Hecht S: Environmental tobacco smoke and lung cancer: the emerging role of carcinogen biomarkers and molecular epidemiology. J Natl Cancer Inst 86:1369-1370, 1994.
10. Hecht S, Carmella S, Murphy S, et al: A tobacco-specific lung carcinogen in the urine of men exposed to cigarette smoke. N Engl J Med 329:1543-1546, 1993.
11. Lubin J, Blot W: Lung cancer and smoking cessation: patterns of risk [editorial]. J Natl Cancer Inst 85:422-423, 1993.
12. Lubin J, Blot W, Berrino F, et al: Modifying risk of developing lung cancer by changing habits of cigarette smoking. BMJ 288:1953-1956, 1984.
13. US Department of Health and Human Services: The health benefits of smoking cessation. A report of the Surgeon General. DHHS publication no. (CDC) 90-8416. Washington, DC, US Government Printing Office, 1990.
14. Gazdar A, Hung J, Walker L, et al: Extensive areas of dysplasia and aneuploidy of the entire bronchial mucosal tract accompanies non-small cell lung cancers (NSCLC) and provides evidence for the field cancerization theory [abstract 1114]. Proc Am Soc Clin Oncol 12:334, 1993.
15. Carbone D: The biology of lung cancer. Semin Oncol 24:388-410, 1997.
16. Lynch H, Kimberling W, Markvicka S, et al: Genetics and smoking-associated cancers. Cancer 57:1640-1646, 1986.
17. Mulvihill J, Bale A: Ecogenetics of lung cancer: genetic susceptibility in the etiology of lung cancer. *In* Mizell C, Correa P (eds): Proceedings of the International Lung Cancer Update Conference, New Orleans, Louisiana. Deerfield Beach, FL, Verlag Chernie International, 1984, pp 141-152.
18. Sellers T, Chen P-L, Potter J, et al: Segregation analysis of smoking associated malignancies: evidence for mendelian inheritance. Am J Med Genet 52:308-314, 1994.
19. Sellers T, Elson R, Atwood L, Rothschild H: Lung cancer histologic type and family history of cancer. Cancer 69:86-91, 1992.
20. Wiest J, Franklin W, Drabkin H, et al: Genetic makers for early detection of lung cancer and outcome measures for response to chemoprevention. J Cell Biochem Suppl 28-29:64-73, 1997.

21. Kreuzer M, Kreienbrock L, Gerken M: Risk factors for lung cancer in young adults. Am J Epidemiol 147:1028-1037, 1998.
22. Benitez J, Ladero J, Jara C, et al: Polymorphic oxidation of debrisoquine in lung cancer patients. Eur J Cancer 27:158-161, 191.
23. Caporaso N, Tucker M, Hoover R, et al: Lung cancer and the debrisoquine metabolic phenotype. J Natl Cancer Inst 82:1264-1272, 1990.
24. Kaisary A, Smith P, Jaczq E, et al: Genetic predisposition to bladder cancer: ability to hydroxylate debrisoquine and mephenytoin as risk factors. Cancer Res 47:5488-5493, 1987.
25. Law M, Hetzel M, Idel J: Debrisoquine metabolism and genetic predisposition to lung cancer. Br J Cancer 59:686-687, 1987.
26. Speirs C, Murray S, Davies D, et al: Debrisoquine oxidation phenotype and susceptibility to lung cancer. Br J Clin Pharmacol 29:101-109, 1990.
27. Christensen P, Gotzsche P, Brosen K: The sparteine/debrisoquine (CYP2D6) oxidation polymorphism and the risk of lung cancer: a meta-analysis. Eur J Clin Pharmacol 51:389-393, 1997.
28. Agundez J, Martinez C, Ladero J, et al: Debrisoquin oxidation genotype and susceptibility to lung cancer. Clin Pharmacol Ther 55:10-14, 1994.
29. Caporaso N, Hayes R, Dosemeci M, et al: Lung cancer risk, occupational exposure, and the debrisoquine metabolic phenotype. Cancer Res 49:3675-3679, 1989.
30. Vineis P, Caporaso N: Tobacco and cancer: epidemiology and the laboratory. Environ Health Perspect 103:156-160, 1995.
31. Brockmoller J, Kerb R, Drakoulis N, et al: Genotype and phenotype of glutathione S-transferase class mu isozymes mu and psi in lung cancer patients and controls. Cancer Res 53:1004-1011, 1993.
32. Spitz M, Hsu T: Mutagen sensitivity as a marker of cancer risk. Cancer Detect Prev 18:299-303, 1994.
33. Spitz M, Hsu T, Wu X, et al: Mutagen sensitivity as a biological marker of lung cancer risk in African Americans. Cancer Epidemiol Biomarkers Prev 4:99-103, 1995.
34. Islam S, Schottenfeld D: Declining FEV_1 and chronic productive cough in cigaret smokers: a 25-year prospective study of lung cancer incidence in Tecumseh, Michigan. Cancer Epidemiol Biomarkers Prev 3:289-298, 1994.
35. Tockman M, Anthonisen N, Wright E, et al: Airways obstruction and the risk for lung cancer. Ann Intern Med 106:512-518, 1987.
36. Slaughter D, Southwick H, Smejkal W: "Field cancerization" in oral stratified squamous epithelium: clinical implications of multicentric origin. Cancer 6:963-968, 1953.
37. Auerbach O, Gere J, Forman J, et al: Changes in the bronchial epithelium in relation to smoking and cancer of the lung. N Engl J Med 256:97-104, 1957.
38. Saccomanno G, Auerbach A, Kuschner M, et al: A comparison between the localization of lung tumors in uranium miners and in nonminers from 1947 to 1991. Cancer 77:1278-1283, 1996.
39. Neugut A, Sherr D, Robinson E, et al: Differences in histology between first and second primary lung cancer. Cancer Epdemiol Biomarkers Prev 1:109-112, 1992.
40. Richardson G, Tucker M, Venzon D, et al: Smoking cessation significantly reduces the risk of second primary cancer in long-term cancer-free survivors of small cell lung cancer (SCLC) [abstract 1080]. Proc Am Soc Clin Oncol 12:326, 1993.
41. Lippman S, Lee J, Karp D, et al: Randomized phase III intergroup trial of isotretinoin to prevent second primary tumors in stage I non-small-cell lung cancer. J Natl Cancer Inst 93:605-618, 2001.
42. Karp J, Profeta G, Marantz P, et al: Lung cancer in patients with acquired immunodeficiency syndrome. Chest 103:410-413, 1993.
43. Sridhar K, Flores M, Raub WJ, Saldana M: Lung cancer in patients with human immunodeficiency virus infection compared with historic control subjects. Chest 102:1704-1708, 1992.
44. Vaccher E, Tirelli U, Spina M, et al: Lung cancer in 19 patients with HIV infection [letter]. Ann Oncol 4:8506, 1993.
45. Vyzula R, Remick S: Lung cancer in patients with HIV infection. Lung Cancer 15:325-340, 1996.
46. Vogelstein B, Kinzler K: Colorectal cancer and the intersection between basic and clinical research. Cold Spring Harb Symp Quant Biol 59:517-521, 1994.
47. Sanchez-Cespedes M: Dissecting the genetic alterations involved in lung carcinogenesis. Lung Cancer 40:111-121, 2003.
48. Khosravi-Far R, Der C: The ras signal transduction pathway. Cancer Metastasis Rev 13:67-89, 1994.
49. Barbacid M: Ras genes. Annu Rev Biochem 56:779-827, 1987.
50. Rodenhuis S, Slebos R, Boot A, et al: Incidence and possible clinical significance of K-ras oncogene activation in adenocarcinoma of the human lung. Cancer Res 48:5738-5741, 1988.
51. Slebos R, Kibbelaar R, Dalesio O, et al: K-ras oncogene activation as a prognostic marker in adenocarcinoma of the lung. N Engl J Med 323:561-565, 1990.
52. Mabry M, Nakagawa T, Nelkin BD: v-Ha-ras oncogene insertion: a model for tumor progression of human small cell lung cancer. Proc Natl Acad Sci U S A 85:6523-6527, 1988.
53. Funka K, Steinholtz L, Nou E, et al: Increased expression of N-myc in human small-cell lung cancer biopsies predicts lack of response to chemotherapy and poor prognosis. Am J Clin Pathol 88:216-220, 1987.
54. Johnson B, Idhe D, Makuch R, et al: Myc family oncogene amplification in tumor cell lines established from small cell lung cancer patients and its relationship to clinical status and course. J Clin Invest 79:1629-1634, 1987.
55. Johnson B, Makuch R, Simmons A, et al: Myc family DNA amplification in small cell lung cancer patients' tumors and corresponding cell lines. Cancer Res 48:5163-5166, 1988.
56. Mizushima Y, Kashii T, Kobayashi M: Effect of cisplatin exposure on the degree of N-myc amplification in small cell lung carcinoma cell lines with N-myc amplification. Oncology 53:417-421, 1996.
57. Takahashi T, Obata Y, Sekido Y, et al: Expression and amplification of myc gene family in small cell lung cancer and its relation to biological characteristics. Cancer Res 49:2683-88, 1989.
58. Lane D: P53, guardian of the genome. Nature 358:15-16, 1992.
59. Carbone DP, Mitsudomi T, Rusch V, et al: P53 protein overexpression, but not gene mutation, is predictive of significantly shortened survival in resected non-small cell lung cancer (NSCLC) patients [abstract 1112]. Proc Am Soc Clin Oncol 12:334, 1993.
60. Pai H, Rochon L, Clark B, et al: Overexpression of p53 protein does not predict local-regional control or survival in patients with early-stage squamous cell carcinoma of the glottic larynx treated with radiotherapy. Int J Radiat Oncol Biol Phys 41:37-42, 1998.
61. Lee J, Bernstein A: P53 mutations increase resistance to ionizing radiation. Proc Natl Acad Sci U S A 90:5742-5746, 1993.
62. Jung M, Notario V, Dritschilo A: Mutations in the p53 gene in radiation-sensitive and -resistant human squamous carcinoma cells. Cancer Res 52:6390-6393, 1992.
63. Buchkovich K, Duffy L, Harlow E: The retinoblastoma protein is phosphorylated during specific phases of the cell cycle. Cell 58:1097-1105, 1989.
64. Ewen M: The cell cycle and the retinoblastoma protein family. Cancer Metastasis Rev 13:45-66, 1994.
65. Reissmann PT, Koga H, Takahashi R: Inactivation of the retinoblastoma gene in non-small cell lung cancer. Proc Am Assoc Cancer Res 31:318, 1990.
66. Yokota J, Akiyama T, Fung Y-K: Altered expression of the retinoblastoma (RB) gene in small-cell carcinoma of the lung. Oncogene 3:471-475, 1988.
67. Carbone D, Minna J: The molecular genetics of lung cancer. Adv Intern Med 37:153-171, 1992.
68. Shapiro G, Edwards C, Kobzik L, et al: Reciprocal Rb inactivation and p16INK4 expression in primary lung cancers and cell lines. Cancer Res 55:505-509, 1995.
69. Lynch TJ, Bell D, Sordella R, et al: Activating mutations in the epidermal growth factor receptor underlying responsiveness of non-small cell lung cancer to gefitinib. N Engl J Med 350:2129-2139, 2004.
70. Paez J, Janne P, Lee J, et al: EGFR mutations in lung cancer: correlation with clinical response to gefitinib. Science 304:1497-1500, 2004.
71. Pao W, Miller V, Zakowski M, et al: EGF receptor gene mutations are common in lung cancers from "never smokers" and are associated with sensitivity of tumors to gefitinib and erlotinib. Proc Natl Acad Sci U S A 101:13306-13311, 2004.

72. Kern J, Schwartz D, Nordberg J, et al: P185neu expression in human lung adenocarcinomas predicts shortened survival. Cancer Res 50:5184-5187, 1990.
73. Weiner D, Nordberg J, Robinson R, et al: Expression of the neu gene-encoded protein (P185neu) in human non-small cell carcinomas of the lung. Cancer Res 50:421-425, 1990.
74. Stephens P, Hunter C, Bignell G, et al: Intragenic EBBB2 kinase mutations in tumours. Nature 431:525-526, 2004.
75. Aguayo S, Kane M, King T Jr: Increased levels of bombesin-like peptides in the lower respiratory tract of asymptomatic cigarette smokers. J Clin Invest 84:1105-1113, 1989.
76. Cuttitta F, Carney DN, Mulshine J, et al: Bombesin-like peptides can function as autocrine growth factors in human small-cell lung cancer. Nature 316:823-826, 1985.
77. Mulshine J, Magnani J, Linnoila R: Clinical applications of monoclonal antibodies in solid tumors. *In* Devita V, Hellman S, Rosenberg S (eds): Principles and Practices of Biotherapy. Philadelphia, JB Lippincott, 1991, pp 563-588.
78. Kelley M, Avis I, Linnoila R, et al: Complete response in a patient with small cell lung cancer (SCLC) treated on a phase II trial using a murine monoclonal antibody (2A11) directed against gastrin releasing peptide (GRP) [abstract 1133]. Proc Am Soc Clin Oncol 12:339, 1993.
79. Berlin N, Buncher C, Fontana R, et al: National Cancer Institute Cooperative Lung Cancer Detection Program: results of initial screen (prevalence) early lung cancer detection—introduction. Am Rev Respir Dis 130:545-549, 1984.
80. Melamed M, Flehinger B, Zaman M, et al: Detection of true pathologic stage I lung cancer in a screening program and the effect on survival. Cancer 41:1182-1187, 1981.
81. Gritz E: Lung cancer: now, more than ever, a feminist issue. CA Cancer J Clin 43:197-199, 1993.
82. Strauss G, DeCamp M, Dibiccaro E, et al: Lung cancer diagnosis is being made with increasing frequency in former smokers [abstract]. Proc Am Soc Clin Oncol 14:1106, 1994.
83. Diederich S, Wormanns D: Impact of low-dose CT on lung cancer screening. Lung Cancer 45(Suppl 2):S13-S19, 2004.
84. Tockman M, Erozan Y, Gupta P, et al: The early detection of second primary lung cancers by sputum immunostaining. Chest 106(Suppl):385s-390s, 1994.
85. Tockman M, Gupa P, Myers J, et al: Sensitive and specific monoclonal antibody recognition of human lung cancer antigen on preserved sputum cells. J Clin Oncol 6:1685-1693, 1988.
86. Mao L, Hruban R, Boyle J, et al: Detection of oncogene mutations in sputum precedes diagnosis of lung cancer. Cancer Res 54:1634-1637, 1994.
87. Mills N, Fishman C, Scholes J, et al: Detection of k-ras oncogene mutations in bronchoalveolar lavage fluid for lung cancer diagnosis. J Natl Cancer Inst 87:1056-1060, 1995.
88. Sporn M: Carcinogenesis and cancer: different perspectives on the same disease. Cancer Res 51:6215-6218, 1991.
89. Stanzel F: Fluorescent bronchoscopy: contribution for lung cancer screening? Lung Cancer 45(Suppl 2):S29-S37, 2004.
90. Mulshine J, Linnoila R, Treston A, et al: Candidate biomarkers for application as intermediate end points of lung carcinogenesis. J Cellular Biochem 16G:183-186, 1992.
91. Zochbauer-Muller S, Fong K, Virmani A, et al: Aberrant promoter methylation of multiple genes in non-small cell lung cancers. Cancer Res 61:249-255, 2001.
92. Belinsky S, Palmisano W, Gilliland F, et al: Aberrant promoter methylation in bronchial epithelium and sputum from current and former smokers. Cancer Res 62:2370-2377, 2002.
93. Kennedy T, Hirsch F: Using molecular markers in sputum for the early detection of lung cancer: a review. Lung Cancer 45(Suppl 2):S21-S27, 2004.
94. Van Zandwijk N, Hirsch F: Chemoprevention of lung cancer: current status and future prospects. Lung Cancer 42:S71-S79, 2003.
95. Hong W, Lippman S, Itri L, et al: Prevention of second primary tumors with isotretinoin in squamous-cell carcinoma of the head and neck. N Engl J Med 323:795-800, 1990.
96. Hong W, Lippman S, Hittelman W, Lotan R: Retinoid chemoprevention of aerodigestive cancer: from basic research to the clinic. Clin Cancer Res 1:677-686, 1995.
97. Pastorino U, Infante M, Maioli M, et al: Adjuvant treatment of stage I lung cancer with high-dose vitamin A. J Clin Oncol 11:1216-1222, 1993.
98. van Zandwijk N, Dalesio O, Pastorino U, et al: EUROSCAN, a randomized trial of vitamin A and *N*-acetylcysteine in patients with head and neck cancer or lung cancer. The European Organization for Research and Treatment of Cancer Head and Neck and Lung Cancer Cooperative Groups. J Natl Cancer Inst 92:977-986, 2000.
99. Omenn G: Chemoprevention of lung cancer: the rise and demise of beta-carotene. Annu Rev Public Health 19:73-99, 1998.
100. Menkes M, Comstock G, Vuilleumier J, et al: Serum beta-carotene, vitamins A and E, selenium, and the risk of lung cancer. N Engl J Med 315:1250-1254, 1986.
101. Peto R, Doll R, Buckley J, et al: Can dietary beta-carotene materially reduce cancer rates? Nature 290:201-208, 1981.
102. Stich H, Rosin M, Vallejera M: Reduction with vitamin A and beta-carotene administration of proportion of micronucleated buccal mucosal cell in Asian Betel nut and tobacco chewers. Lancet 1:1204-1206, 1984.
103. Ziegler RG, Mason RJ, Sternhagen A: Dietary carotene and vitamin A and risk of lung cancer among white men in New Jersey. J Natl Cancer Inst 73:1429-1435, 1984.
104. The effect of vitamin E and beta carotene on the incidence of lung cancer and other cancers in male smokers. The Alpha-Tocopherol, Beta Carotene Cancer Prevention Study Group. N Engl J Med 330:1029-1035, 1994.
105. Omenn G, Goodman G, Thornquist M, et al: Effects of a combination of beta carotene and Vitamin A on lung cancer and cardiovascular disease. N Engl J Med 334:1150-1155, 1996.
106. Duffield-Lillico A, Begg C: Reflections on the landmark studies of β-carotene supplementation. J Natl Cancer Inst 96:1729-1731, 2004.
107. Goodman G, Thornquist M, Balmes J, et al: The beta-carotene and retinol efficacy trial: incidence of lung cancer and cardiovascular disease mortality during 6-year follow-up after stopping β-carotene and retinol supplements. J Natl Cancer Inst 96:1743-1750, 2004.
108. Clark L, Combs G, Turnbull B, et al: Effects of selenium supplementation for cancer prevention in patients with carcinoma of the skin. JAMA 276:1956-1963, 1996.
109. Mulshine J, Neckers L: Epithelial-directed drug delivery: influence of formulation and delivery devices. Lung Cancer 46:387-392, 2004.
110. Greatens T, Niehans G, Rubins J, et al: Do molecular markers predict survival in non-small-cell lung cancer? Am J Respir Crit Care Med 157(Pt 1):1093-1097, 1998.
111. Chen G, Gharib T, Wang, H, et al: Protein profiles associated with survival in lung adenocarcinoma. Proc Natl Acad Sci U S A 100:13537-13542, 2003.
112. Asamura H, Nakayama H, Kondo H, et al: Lymph node involvement, recurrence, and prognosis in resected small, peripheral, non-small cell lung carcinomas. J Thorac Cardiovasc Surg 111:1125-1134, 1996.
113. Chen Z-L, Perez S, Holmes E, et al: Frequency and distribution of occult micrometastases in lymph nodes of patients with non-small cell carcinoma. J Natl Cancer Inst 85:493-498, 1993.
114. Pantel K, Izbicki J, Passlick B, et al: Frequency and prognostic significance of isolated tumour cells in bone marrow of patients with non-small-cell lung cancer without overt metastases. Lancet 347(9002):649-653, 1996.
115. Izbicki J, Passlick B, Hosch SB, et al: Mode of spread in the early phase of lymphatic metastasis in non-small-cell lung cancer: significance of nodal micrometastasis. J Thorac Cardiovasc Surg S112:623-630, 1996.
116. Baird A: The pathways of lymphatic spread of carcinoma of the lung. Br J Surg 52:868-872, 1965.
117. Arnau Obrer A, Canto Armengod A, Martin Diaz E, et al: [Prognostic value of positive cytology found in pleural lavage of patients with cancer of the lung. Prospective study. Valor pronostico de la citologia positiva hallada en el lavado pleural de pacientes con cancer de pulmon. Estudio prospectivo. Arch Bronconeumol 32:321-326, 1996.

118. Buhr J, Berghauser K, Gonner S, et al: [Intrapulmonary tumor cell dissemination and intraoperative pleural lavage as prognostic factors in bronchial carcinoma]. Intrapulmonale Tumorzellausbreitung und intraoperative Pleuralavage als Prognosefaktoren beim Bronchialkarzinom. Zentralb Chir 121:90-95, 1996.
119. Matthews M, Kanhouwa S, Pickren J, et al: Frequency of residual and metastatic tumor in patients undergoing curative surgical resection for lung cancer. Cancer Chemother Rep 4(Pt 3):63-67, 1973.
120. Komaki R: Neuropsychological functioning of patients with small cell lung cancer before and shortly following prophylactic cranial irradiation: evidence for pre-existing cognitive impairments [abstract 1084]. Proc Am Soc Clin Oncol 12:327, 1993.
121. Silvestri G, Tanoue L, Margolis M, et al: The noninvasive staging of non-small cell lung cancer—the guidelines. Chest 123(Suppl): 147S-156S, 2003.
122. Broderick L, Tarver R, Conces DJ: Imaging of lung cancer: old and new. Semin Oncol 24:411-418, 1997.
123. Toloza E, Harpole L, McCrory D: Noninvasive staging of non-small cell lung cancer: a review of the current evidence. Chest 123:137S-146S, 2003.
124. Detterbeck F, DeCamp M, Kohman L, Silvestri G: Invasive staging: the guidelines. Chest 123:167S-175S, 2003.
125. Toloza E, Harpole L, Detterbeck F, et al: Invasive staging of non-small cell lung cancer: a review of the current evidence. Chest 123:157S-166S, 2003.
126. Duhaylongsod F, Lowe V, Patz EJ, et al: Detection of primary and recurrent lung cancer by means of F-18 fluorodeoxyglucose positron emission tomography (FDG-PET). J Thorac Cardiovasc Surg 110:130-139, 1995.
127. Guhlman A, Storck M, Kotzerke J, et al: Lymph node staging in non-small cell lung cancer: evaluation by [18F]FDG positron emission tomography (PET). Thorax 52:438-441, 1997.
128. Patz EJ, Lowe V, Goodman P, et al: Thoracic nodal staging with PET imaging with 18F-FDG in patients with bronchogenic carcinoma. Chest 108:1617-1621, 1995.
129. Steinert H, Hauser M, Allemann F, et al: Non-small cell lung cancer: nodal staging with FDG PET versus CT with correlative lymph node mapping and sampling. Radiology 202:441-446, 1977.
130. Sasaki M, Ichiya Y, Kuwabara Y, et al: The usefulness of FDG positron emission tomography for the detection of mediastinal lymph node metastases in patients with non-small cell lung cancer: a comparative study with x-ray computed tomography. Eur J Nucl Med 23:741-747, 1996.
131. Hicks R, Kalff V, Mac Manus M, et al: ^{18}F-FDG PET provides high-impact and powerful prognostic stratification in staging newly diagnosed non-small cell lung cancer. J Nucl Med 42:1596-1604, 2001.
132. Vansteenkiste J, Stroobants S, De Leyn P, et al: Mediastinal lymph node staging with FDG-PET scan in patients with potentially operable non-small cell lung cancer: a prospective analysis of 50 cases. Chest 112:1480-1486, 1997.
133. Vansteenkiste J: FDG-PET for lymph node staging in NSCLC: a major step forward but beware of the pitfalls. Lung Cancer 47:151-153, 2005.
134. Choi N, Hamberg L, Hunter GJ, et al: Assessment of therapy response with positron emission tomography (PET) and glucose analogue 2-[18F]-fluoro-2-deoxy-D-glucose in lung cancer [abstract]. Proc Am Soc Clin Oncol 15:1138, 1996.
135. Ichiya Y, Kuwabara Y, Sasaki M, et al: A clinical evaluation of FDG-PET to assess the response in radiation therapy for bronchogenic carcinoma. Ann Nucl Med 10:193-200, 1996.
136. Watanabe A, Shimokata K, Saka H, et al: Evaluation of therapeutic effect on lung cancer by F-fluoro-2-deoxy-D-glucose (FDG) positron emission tomography (PET) [abstract 1151]. Proc Am Soc Clin Oncol 12:343, 1993.
137. Hoekstra C, Hoekstra O, Stroobants S, et al: Methods to monitor response to chemotherapy in non-small cell lung cancer with ^{18}F-FDG PET. J Nucl Med 43:1304-1309, 2002.
138. Vansteenkiste J, Stroobants S, Hoekstra C, et al: ^{18}Fluoro-2-deoxyglucose positron emission tomography (PET) in the assessment of induction chemotherapy (IC) in stage IIIa-N2 NSCLC: a multicenter prospective study [abstract 1250]. Proc Am Soc Clin Oncol 20:313, 2001.
139. Kostakoglu L, Goldsmith S: 18F-FDG PET evaluation of the response to therapy for lymphoma and for breast, lung, and colorectal carcinoma. J Nucl Med 44:224-239, 2003.
140. Roberts K, MacManus M, Hicks R, et al: PET imaging for suspected residual tumour or thoracic recurrence of non-small cell lung cancer after pneumonectomy. Lung Cancer 47:49-57, 2005.
141. Lowe V, Hebert M, Anscher M, et al: Serial evaluation of increased chest wall F-18 fluorodeoxyglucose (FDG) uptake following radiation therapy in patients with bronchogenic carcinoma. Clin Positron Imag 1:185-191, 1998.
142. Hicks R, MacManus M, Matthews J, et al: Early FDG-PET imaging after radical radiotherapy for non-small cell lung cancer: inflammatory changes in normal tissues correlate with tumor response and do not confound therapeutic response evaluation. Int J Radiat Oncol Biol Phys 60:412-418, 2004.
143. Ferrigno D, Bucheri G: Cranial computed tomography as a part of the initial staging procedures for patients with non-small cell lung cancer. Chest 106:1025-1029, 1994.
144. Mountain C: A new international staging system for lung cancer. Chest 89(Suppl):225-233, 1986.
145. Mountain C: Revisions in the international system for staging lung cancer. Chest 111:1710-1717, 1997.
146. Mountain C, Dresler C: Regional lymph node classification for lung cancer staging. Chest 111:1718-1723, 1997.
147. Bradley J, Ieumwananonthachai N, Purdy J, et al: Gross tumor volume, critical prognostic factor in patients treated with three-dimensional conformal radiation therapy for non-small-cell lung carcinoma. Int J Radiat Oncol Biol Phys 52:49-57, 2002.
148. Etiz D, Marks L, Zhou S-M, et al: Influence of tumor volume on survival in patients irradiated for non-small-cell lung cancer. Int J Radiat Oncol Biol Phys 53:835-846, 2002.
149. Martel M, Strawderman M, Hazuka M, et al: Volume and dose parameters for survival of non-small cell lung cancer patients. Radiother Oncol 44:23-29, 1997.
150. Popple R, Ove R, Shen S: Tumor control probability for selective boosting of hypoxic subvolumes, including the effect of reoxygenation. Int J Radiat Oncol Biol Phys 54:921-927, 2002.
151. Willner J, Baier K, Caragiani E, et al: Dose, volume, and tumor control predictions in primary radiotherapy of non-small-cell lung cancer. Int J Radiat Oncol Biol Phys 52:382-389, 2002.
152. Bowden P, Fisher R, MacManus M: Measurement of lung tumor volumes using three dimensional computer planning software. Int J Radiat Oncol Biol Phys 53:566-573, 2002.
153. Port J, Kent M, Korst R, et al: Tumor size predicts survival within stage IA non-small cell lung cancer. Chest 124:1828-1833, 2003.
154. Green M, Lilenbaum R: Stage IIIA category of non-small-cell lung cancer: a new proposal. J Natl Cancer Inst 86:586-588, 1994.
155. Curran W, Staford P: Lack of apparent difference in outcome between clinically staged IIIA and IIIB non-small-cell lung cancer treated with radiation therapy. J Clin Oncol 8:409-415, 1990.
156. Andre F: Survival of patients with resected N2 non-small cell lung cancer: evidence for a subclassification and implications. J Clin Oncol 18:2981-2989, 2000.
157. Ruckdeschel J, Wagner H, Robinson L: Locally advanced lung cancer: controversies in management. Adv Oncol 12:22-28, 1996.
158. Berghmans T, Lafitte J, Thiriaux J, et al: Survival is better predicted with a new classification of stage III unresectable non-small cell lung carcinoma treated by chemotherapy and radiotherapy. Lung Cancer 45:339-348, 2004.
159. Beckles M, Spiro S, Colice G, Rudd R: The physiologic evaluation of patients with ling cancer being considered for resectional surgery. Chest 123(Suppl 1):105s-114s, 2003.
160. Ali M, Ewer M: Preoperative cardiopulmonary evaluation of patients undergoing surgery for lung cancer. 32:100-104, 1980.
161. Gass G, Olsen G: Preoperative pulmonary function testing to predict postoperative morbidity and mortality. Chest 89:127-135, 1986.
162. Morice R: Preoperative evaluation of the patients with lung cancer. *In* Roth J, Cox J, Hong W (eds): Lung Cancer, 2nd ed. Malden, MA, Blackwell Science, 1998, pp 73-86.

163. Ginsberg R, Rubenstein L: Randomized trial of lobectomy versus limited resection for T1N0 non-small cell lung cancer. Lung Cancer Study Group. Ann Thorac Surg 60:615-623, 1995.
164. Naruke T, Gota T, Tsuchiya R, Suemasu K: Prognosis and survival in resected lung carcinoma based on the new international staging system. J Thorac Cardiovasc Surg 96:440-447, 1998.
165. Walsh G, Morice R, Putnam J, et al: Resection of lung cancer is justified in high-risk patients selected by exercise oxygen consumption. Ann Thorac Surg 58:740-711, 1994.
166. Ginsberg R, Hill L, Eagan R, et al: Modern day operative mortality for surgical resection in lung cancer. J Thorac Cardiovasc Surg 86:654-658, 1983.
167. Feinstein A, Sosin D, Wells C: Stage migration and new diagnostic techniques as a source of misleading statistics for survival in cancer. N Engl J Med 312:1604-1608, 1985.
168. Sibley G: Radiotherapy for patients with medically inoperable stage I nonsmall cell lung carcinoma: smaller volumes and higher doses—a review. Cancer 82:433-438, 1998.
169. Goor C, Scallier P, van Meerbeak J, et al: A phase II study combining gemcitabine and radiotherapy in stage III NSCLC [abstract]. Ann Oncol 7:101, 1996.
170. Reckzeh B, Merte H, Pfluger KH, et al: Severe lymphocytopenia and interstitial pneumonia in patients treated with paclitaxel and simultaneous radiotherapy for non-small-cell lung cancer. J Clin Oncol 14:1071-1076, 1996.
171. Chao C, Studts J, Abell T, et al: Adjuvant chemotherapy for breast cancer: how presentation of recurrence risk influences decision making. J Clin Oncol 21:4299-4305, 2003.
172. Wieand H: Is relative risk reduction a useful measure for patients or families who must choose a method of treatment? J Clin Oncol 21:4263-4264, 2003.
173. Choi N, Grillo H, Gardiello M, et al: Basis of new strategies in postoperative radiotherapy of bronchogenic carcinoma. Int J Radiat Oncol Biol Phys 6:31-35, 1980.
174. Chung C, Stryker J, O'Neill M, Demuth W: Evaluation of adjuvant postoperative radiotherapy for lung cancer. Int J Radiat Oncol Biol Phys 8:1877-1880, 1992.
175. Green N, Kurohara S, George F, Crews Q: Postresection irradiation for primary lung cancer. Radiology 116:405-407, 1975.
176. Kirsch M, Sloan H: Mediastinal metastasis in bronchogenic carcinoma: influence of postoperative irradiation, cell type and location. Ann Thorac Surg 33:459-463, 1982.
177. Postoperative radiotherapy in non-small cell lung cancer: systematic review and meta-analysis of individual patient data from nine randomised trials. PORT Meta-analysis Trialists Group. Lancet 352:257-263, 1998.
178. Burdett S, Stewart L: Postoperative radiotherapy in non-small-cell lung cancer: update of an individual patient data meta-analysis. Lung Cancer 47:81-83, 2005.
179. Dautzenberg B, Arriagada R, Chammard A, Jarema A, et al: A controlled study of postoperative radiotherapy for patients with completely resected nonsmall cell lung carcinoma. Cancer 86:265-273, 1999.
180. Feng Q, Wang M, Wang L, et al: A study of postoperative radiotherapy in patients with non-small cell lung cancer: a randomized trial. Int J Radiat Oncol Biol Phys 47:925-929, 2000.
181. Mayer R, Smolle-Juettner F-M, Szolar D, et al: Postoperative radiotherapy in radically resected non-small cell lung cancer. Chest 112:954-959, 1997.
182. Phlips P, Rocmans P, Vanderhoef P, et al: Postoperative radiotherapy after pneumonectomy: impact of modern treatment facilities. Int J Radiat Oncol Biol Phys 27:525-529, 1993.
183. Schraube P, Kampen M-U, Oetzel D, et al: The impact of 3-D radiotherapy planning after a pneumonectomy compared with a conventional treatment set-up. Radiother Oncol 37:65-70, 1995.
184. Machtay M, Lee J, Shrager J, et al: Risk of death from intercurrent disease is not excessively increased by modern postoperative radiotherapy for high-risk resected non-small cell lung carcinoma. J Clin Oncol 19:3912-3917, 2001.
185. Wakelee H, Stephenson P, Keller S, et al: Post-operative radiotherapy (PORT) or chemoradiotherapy (CPORT) following resection of stages II and IIIA non-small cell lung cancer does not increase the expected risk of death from intercurrent disease (DID). Lung Cancer 48:389-397, 2005.
186. Taylor N, Liao Z, Stevens C, et al: Postoperative radiotherapy increases locoregional control of patients with stage IIIA non-small-cell lung cancer treated with induction chemotherapy followed by surgery. Int J Radiat Oncol Biol Phys 56:616-625, 2003.
187. Bonner J: The role of postoperative radiotherapy for patients with completely resected nonsmall cell lung carcinoma: seeking to optimize local control and survival while minimizing toxicity. Cancer 86:195-196, 1999.
188. Sawyer T, Bonner J, Gould P, et al: Effectiveness of postoperative irradiation in stage IIIA non-small cell lung cancer according to regression tree analysis of recurrence risk. Ann Thor Surg 64:1402-1407, 1997.
189. Sawyer T, Bonner J, Gould P, Lang C, Li H: Tumor and patient characteristics that are predictive of subclinical nodal involvement in patients with non-small cell lung cancer (NSCLC) without nodal enlargement on pre-operative chest CT. Proc Am Radium Soc 23:39, 1998.
190. Perry M, Kohman L, Bonner J, et al: A phase III study of surgical resection and chemotherapy (paclitaxel/carboplatin) (CT) with or without adjuvant radiotherapy (RT) for resected stage III non-small cell lung cancer (NSCLC) [abstract O-183]: CALGB 9734. Lung Cancer 23:S55, 2004.
191. Cox J, Petrovich Z, Paig C, et al: Prophylactic cranial irradiation in patients with inoperable carcinoma of the lung. Cancer 42:1135-1140, 1978.
192. Mira J, Miller T, Crowley J: Chest irradiation (RT) vs. chest RT + chemotherapy +/− prophylactic brain RT in localized non-small cell lung cancer: a Southwest Oncology Group randomized study. Int J Radiat Oncol Biol Phys 19(Suppl 1):145, 1990.
193. Russell A, Pajak T, Selim H, et al: Prophylactic cranial irradiation for lung cancer patients at high risk for development of cerebral metastases: results of a prospective randomized trial conducted by the Radiation Therapy Oncology Group. Int J Radiat Oncol Biol Phys 21:637-643, 1991.
194. Stuschke M, Eberhardt W, Pottgen C, et al: Prophylactic cranial irradiation in locally advanced non-small cell lung cancer after multimodality treatment: long-term follow-up and investigation of late neuropsychologic effects. J Clin Oncol 17:2700-2709, 1999.
195. Turrisi A: Brain irradiation and systemic chemotherapy for small-cell lung cancer: dangerous liaisons [editorial? J Clin Oncol 8:196-199, 1990.
196. Le Chevalier T, Arriagada R: Small cell lung cancer and prophylactic cranial irradiation (PCI): perhaps the question is not who needs PCI but who wants PCI? Eur J Cancer 33:17-19, 1997.
197. Chemotherapy in non-small cell lung cancer: meta-analysis using updated data on individual patients from 52 randomised clinical trials. Non-small Cell Lung Cancer Collaborative Group. Br Med J 311:899-909, 1995.
198. Keller S, Adak S, Wagner H, et al: A randomized trial of postoperative adjuvant therapy in patients with completely resected stage II or IIIa non-small-cell lung cancer. N Engl J Med 343:1217, 2000.
199. Scagliotti G, Fossati R, Torri V, et al, for the Adjuvant Lung Project Italy/European Organization for Research Treatment of Cancer–Lung Cancer Cooperative Group Investigators: randomized study of adjuvant chemotherapy for completely resected stage I, II, or IIIA non-small cell lung cancer. J Natl Cancer Inst 95:1453-1461, 2003.
200. Arriagada R, Bergman B, Dunant A, et al, for the International Adjuvant Lung Cancer Trial (IALT) Group: Cisplatin-based adjuvant chemotherapy in patients with completely resected non-small-cell lung cancer. N Engl J Med 350:351-360, 2004.
201. Winton T, Livingston R, Johnson D, et al, for the National Cancer Institute of Canada Clinical Trials Group; National Cancer Institute of the United States Intergroup JBR 10 Trial Investigators: A prospective randomized trial of adjuvant vinorelbine (VIN) and cisplatin (CIS) in completely resected stage IB and II non-small cell lung cancer (NSCLC) Intergroup JBR 10 [abstract 7018]. Proc Am Soc Clin Oncol 22:621, 2004.
202. Alam N, Shepherd F, Winton T, et al: Compliance with post-operative adjuvant chemotherapy in non-small cell lung cancer. An analysis of National Cancer Institute of Canada and intergroup trial JBR.10 and a review of the literature. Lung Cancer 47:385-394, 2005.

203. Strauss G, Herndon J, Maddaus M, et al: Randomized clinical trial of adjuvant chemotherapy with paclitaxel and carboplatin following resection in stage IB non-small cell lung cancer: report of Cancer and Leukemia Group B (CALGB) protocol 9633 [abstract 7019]. Proc Am Soc Clin Oncol 22:621, 2004.
204. Hotta K, Matsou K, Ueoka H, et al: Role of adjuvant chemotherapy in patients with resected non-small cell lung cancer: reappraisal with a meta-analysis of randomized controlled trials. J Clin Oncol 22:3860-3867, 2004.
205. Keicho N, Saijo N, Shinkaig T, et al: Phase II study of UFT in patients with advanced non-small cell lung cancer. Jpn J Clin Oncol 16:143-146, 1986.
206. Hamada C, Ohta M, Wada H, et al: Survival benefit of oral UFT for adjuvant chemotherapy after completely resected non-small-cell lung cancer. Proc Am Soc Clin Oncol 22:7002, 2004.
207. Bloedorn F, Cowley R, Cuccia C, et al: Preoperative irradiation in bronchogenic carcinoma. Am J Roentgenol Radium Ther Nucl Med 92:77-87, 1964.
208. Kirscher P: Lung cancer: preoperative radiation therapy and surgery. N Y State J Med 81:339-342, 1981.
209. Warram J: Preoperative irradiation of cancer of the lung: final report of a therapeutic trial. Cancer 36:914-925, 1975.
210. Elias A, Herndon J, Kumar P, et al: A phase III comparison of "best local-regional therapy" with or without chemotherapy (CT) for stage IIIA T1-3N2 non-small cell lung cancer (NSCLC): preliminary results [abstract]. Proc Am Soc Clin Oncol 16:1611, 1997.
211. Wagner H Jr, Lad T, Piantadosi S: Randomized phase II evaluation of preoperative radiation therapy and preoperative chemotherapy with mitomycin-C, vinblastine, and cisplatin in patients with technically unresectable stage IIIA and IIIB non-small-cell lung cancer. Chest 7(Suppl):157, 1991.
212. Pass H, Pohrebnia H, Steinberg S, et al: Randomized trial of neoadjuvant therapy for lung cancer: interim analysis. Ann Thorac Surg 53:992-998, 1992.
213. Roth J, Fossella F, Komaki R, et al: A randomized trial comparing preoperative chemotherapy and surgery with surgery alone in resectable stage III non-small cell lung cancer. J Natl Cancer Inst 86:673-680, 1994.
214. Roth J, Atkinson E, Fossella F, et al: Long-term follow-up of patients enrolled in a randomized trial comparing perioperative chemotherapy and surgery with surgery alone in stage IIIA non-small-cell lung cancer. Lung Cancer 21:1-6, 1998.
215. Rossell R, Codina J, Camps C, et al: A randomized trial comparing preoperative chemotherapy plus surgery with surgery alone in patients with non-small cell lung cancer. N Engl J Med 330:23-32, 1994.
216. Johnstone D, Byhardt R, Ettinger D, Scott C: Phase III study comparing chemotherapy and radiotherapy with preoperative chemotherapy and surgical resection in patients with non-small cell lung cancer with spread to mediastinal nodes(N2); final report of RTOG 89-01. Radiation Therapy Oncology Group. Int J Radiat Oncol Biol Phys 54:365-369, 2002.
217. Albain K, Scott C, Rusch V, et al: Phase III comparison of concurrent chemotherapy plus radiotherapy (CT/RT) and CT/RT followed by surgical resection for stage IIIA (pN2) non-small cell lung cancer: initial results from intergroup trial 0139 (RTOG 93-09) [abstract 2497]. Proc Am Soc Clin Oncol 22:621, 2003.
218. Thomas M, Macha H, Ukena D, et al: Cisplatin etoposide (PE) followed by twice-daily chemoradiation (hfRT/CT) versus PE alone before surgery in stage III non-small cell lung cancer: a randomized phase III trial of the German Lung Cancer Cooperative Group (GLCCG) [abstract 7004]. Proc Am Soc Clin Oncol 22:618, 2004.
219. Betticher D, Hsu Smitz S, Totsch M, et al: Mediastinal lymph node clearance after docetaxel-cisplatin neoadjuvant chemotherapy is prognostic of survival in patients with stage IIIA pN2 non-small-cell lung cancer: a multicenter phase II trial. J Clin Oncol 21:1752-1759, 2003.
220. Perez C, Pajak T, Rubin P, et al: Long-term observations of the patterns of failure in patients with unresectable non-oat cell carcinomas of the lung treated with definitive radiotherapy. Cancer 59:1874-1881, 1987.
221. Arriagada R, LeChevalier T, Quoix E, et al: Chemotherapy effect on locally advanced non-small cell lung carcinoma: a randomized study on 353 patients. Proceedings of the 32nd annual ASTRO meeting, 1990. Int J Radiat Oncol Biol Phys 19(Suppl 1):195, 1990.
222. Le Chevalier T, Arriagada R, Quoix E: Impact of chemotherapy (CT) on survival of locally advanced non-small cell lung cancer (NSCLC): results of a randomized study in 353 patients. Lung Cancer 7:159, 1991.
223. Le Chevalier T, Arriagada R, Tarayre M, et al: Significant effect of adjuvant chemotherapy on survival in locally advanced non-small-cell lung cancer. J Natl Cancer Inst 84:58, 1992.
224. Le Chevalier T, Arriagada R, Quoix E, et al: Radiotherapy alone versus combined chemotherapy and radiotherapy in unresectable non-small cell lung carcinoma. Lung Cancer 10:S239-S244, 1994.
225. Vokes E, Herndon J, Kelley M, et al: Induction chemotherapy followed by concomitant chemoradiotherapy (CT/XRT) versus CT/XRT alone fro regionally unresectable non-small cell lung cancer (NSCLC): initial analysis of a randomized phase III trial. Proc Am Soc Clin Oncol 22:7005, 2004.
226. Gandara D, Chansky K, Albain K, et al: Consolidation docetaxel after concurrent chemoradiotherapy in stage IIIB no-small-cell lung cancer: phase II Southwest Oncology Group study S9504. J Clin Oncol 21:2004-2010, 2003.
227. Rosenzweig K, Yorke E, Jackson A, et al: Results of a phase I dose escalation trial in operable non-small cell lung cancer [abstract]. Int J Radiat Oncol Biol Phys 57:5417-5418, 2003.
228. Rosenman J, Halle J, Socinski M, et al: High-dose conformal radiotherapy for treatment of stage IIIA/IIIB non-small cell lung cancer: technical issues and results of a phase I/II trial. Int J Radiat Oncol Biol Phys 54:348-356, 2002.
229. Regnan R, Rosenzweig K, Venkatraman E, et al: Improved local control with higher doses of radiation in large-volume stage III no-small cell lung cancer. Int J Radiat Oncol Biol Phys 60:741-747, 2004.
230. Ang K, Thames H, Peters L: Altered fractionation schedules. *In* Perez C, Brady L (eds): Principles and Practice of Radiation Oncology. Philadelphia, Lippincott-Raven, 1997, pp 119-142.
231. Byhardt R: The evolution of Radiation Therapy Oncology Group (RTOG) protocols for nonsmall cell lung cancer. Int J Radiat Oncol Biol Phys 32:1513-1525, 1995.
232. Byhardt R: Hyperfractionation. *In* Pass H, Mitchell J, Johnson D, Turrisi A (eds): Lung Cancer: Principles and Practice. Philadelphia, Lippincott-Raven, 1996, pp 711-719.
233. Cox J, Azarnia N, Byhardt R, et al: A randomized phase I/II trial of hyperfractionated radiation therapy with total doses of 60.0 Gy to 79.2 Gy: possible survival benefits with >69.6 Gy in favorable patients with stage III radiation therapy oncology group non-small-cell lung carcinoma: report of the radiation therapy oncology group 83-11. J Clin Oncol 8:1543-1555, 1990.
234. Sause W, Scott C, Taylor S, et al: Radiation Therapy Oncology Group (RTOG) 88-08 and Eastern Cooperative Oncology Group (ECOG) 4588; preliminary results of a phase III trial in regionally advanced, unresectable, non-small cell lung cancer. J Natl Cancer Inst 87:198-205, 1995.
235. Sause W, Kolesar P, Taylor SI, et al: Final results of phase III trial in regionally advanced unresectable non-small cell lung cancer: Radiation Therapy Oncology Group, Eastern Cooperative Oncology Group, and Southwest Oncology Group. Chest 117:358-364, 2000.
236. Bonner J, McGinnis WL, Stella P, et al: The possible advantage of hyperfractionated thoracic radiotherapy in the treatment of locally advanced nonsmall cell lung carcinoma: results of a North Central Cancer Treatment Group phase III study. Cancer 82:1037-1048, 1998.
237. Fu S, Jiang G, Wang L: Hyperfractionated irradiation for non-small-cell lung cancer: a phase III clinical trial [in Chinese]. Chung Hua Chung Liu Tsa Chih 16:306-309, 1994.
238. Stuschke M, Thames H: Hyperfractionated radiotherapy of human tumors: overview of the randomized clinical trials. Int J Radiat Oncol Biol Phys 37:259-267, 1997.
239. Cox J, Pajak T, Asbell S, et al: Interruptions of high-dose radiation therapy decrease long-term survival of favorable patients with unresectable non-small cell carcinoma of the lung: analysis

of 1244 cases from 3 radiation therapy oncology group (RTOG) trials. Int J Radiat Oncol Biol Phys 27:493-498, 1993.
240. Saunders M, Dische S, Barrett A, et al: Randomised multicentre trials of CHART vs conventional radiotherapy in head and neck and non-small-cell lung cancer: an interim report. CHART Steering Committee. Br J Cancer 73:1455-1462, 1996.
241. Saunders M, Dische S, Barrett A, et al: Continuous hyperfractionated accelerated radiotherapy (CHART) versus conventional radiotherapy in non-small-cell lung cancer: a randomised multicentre trial. Lancet 350:161-165, 1997.
242. Mehta M, Tannehill S, Martin L, et al: ECOG 4593: phase II hyperfractionated accelerated radiotherapy (HART) for non-small cell lung cancer (NSCLC): early results and RT quality assurance (QA) [abstract]. Lung Cancer 18(Suppl 1):481, 1997.
243. Saunders M, Lyn E, Pigott K, et al: Dose escalation study using CHARTWEL (continuous hyperfractionated accelerated radiotherapy weekendless) in non-small cell lung cancer [abstract]. Lung Cancer 18(Suppl 1):482, 1997.
244. Belani C, Wang W, Johnson D, et al: Induction chemotherapy followed by standard thoracic radiotherapy vs. hyperfractionated accelerated radiotherapy for patients with unresectable stage IIIA & B non-small cell lung cancer: phase III study of the Eastern Cooperative Oncology Group (ECOG 2597) [abstract]. Proc Am Soc Clin Oncol 22:622, 2003.
245. Schaake-Koning C, Kirkpatrick A, Kroger R, et al: The need for immediate monitoring of treatment parameters and uniform assessment of patient data in clinical trials. A quality control study of the EORTC and lung cancer cooperative groups. Eur J Cancer 27:615-619, 1991.
246. Boxwala A, Rosenman J: Retrospective reconstruction of three dimensional treatment plans from two dimensional planing data. Int J Radiat Oncol Biol Phys 28:1009-1015, 1994.
247. Inoue T, Kim E, Komaki R: Detecting recurrent or residual lung cancer with FDG-PET. J Nucl Med 36:788-793, 1995.
248. Patz E, Lowe V, Hoffman J, et al: Persistent or recurrent bronchogenic carcinoma: detection with PET and 2-[F-18]-2-deoxy-D-glucose. Radiology 191:379-382, 1994.
249. Perez C, Stanley K, Grundy G, et al: Impact of irradiation technique and tumor extent in tumor control and survival of patients with unresectable non-oat-cell carcinoma of the lung. Cancer 50:1091-1099, 1982.
250. Armsrong J: Target volume definition for three-dimensional conformal radiation therapy of lung cancer. Br J Radiol 71:587-594, 1998.
251. Derycke S, van Duyse B, de Gersem W, et al: Non-coplanar beam intensity modulation allows large dose escalation in stage III lung cancer. Radiother Oncol 45:253-261, 1997.
252. Graham M, Jain N, Kahn M, et al: Evaluation of an objective plan-evaluation model in the three dimensional treatment of nonsmall cell lung cancer. Int J Radiat Oncol Biol Phys 34:469-474, 1996.
253. Turrisi AI: Its about time, or is it volume, fractionation, or technique? Int J Radiat Oncol Biol Phys 36:753-755, 1996.
254. Ten Haken R, Balter J, Martel M, et al: Tissue inhomogeneity in the thorax: implications for 3-D treatment planning. Front Radiat Ther Oncol 29:180-187, 1996.
255. Armstrong J, Zelefsky M, Leibel S, et al: Strategy for dose escalation using 3-dimensional conformal radiation therapy for lung cancer. Ann Oncol 6:693-697, 1995.
256. Emami B, Graham M: Three-dimensional conformal radiotherapy in bronchogenic carcinoma. *In* Pass H, et al (eds): Lung Cancer: Principles and Practices. Philadelphia, Blackwell Scientific, 2000.
257. Graham M, Purdy J, Emami B, et al: 3-D conformal radiotherapy for lung cancer. The Washington University experience. Front Radiat Ther Oncol 29:188-198, 1996.
258. McGibney C, Holmberg O, McCLean B, et al: The potential impact of 3-D conformal radiotherapy (3DCRT) on continuous hyperfractionated accelerated radiotherapy (CHART) for NSCLC [abstract]. Lung Cancer 18(Suppl 1):486, 1997.
259. Cai J, Chu J, Recine D, et al: CT and PET image registration and fusion in radiotherapy treatment planning using the chamfer-matching method. Int J Radiat Oncol Biol Phys 43:883-891, 1999.
260. Dizendorf E, Baumert B, von Schulthess G, et al: Impact of whole-body ^{18}F-FDG PET on staging and managing patients for radiation therapy. J Nucl Med 44:24-29, 2003.
261. Erdi YE, Rosenzweig KE, Erdi AK, et al: Radiotherapy treatment planning for patients with non-small cell lung cancer using positron emission tomography (PET). Radiother Oncol 62:51-60, 2002.
262. Giraud P, Grahek D, Montravers F, et al: CT and (18)F-deoxyglucose (FDG) image fusion for optimization of conformal radiotherapy of lung cancers. Int J Radiat Oncol Biol Phys 49:1249-1257, 2001.
263. Hicks R, MacManus M: 18F-FDG PET in candidates for radiation therapy: is it important and how do we validate its impact? J Nucl Med 44:30-32, 2003.
264. Mah K, Caldwell C, Ung Y, et al: The impact of 18FDG-PET on target and critical organs in CT-based treatment planning of patients with poorly defined non-small-cell lung carcinoma: a prospective study. Int J Radiat Oncol Biol Phys 52:339-350, 2002.
265. Nestle U, Walter K, Schmidt S, et al: 18F-deoxyglucose positron emission tomography (FDG-PET) for the planning of radiotherapy in lung cancer: high impact on patients with atelectasis. Int J Radiat Oncol Biol Phys 44:593-597, 1999.
266. Skalski J, Wahl R, Meyer C: Comparison of mutual information-based warping accuracy for fusing body CT and PET by 2 methods: CT mapped onto PET emission scan versus CTC mapped onto PET transmission scan. J Nucl Med 43:1184-1187, 2002.
267. Tomlinson S, Russo S, Bourland J: Radiation treatment planning with positron emission tomography (PET) imaging for lung cancer alters computed tomographic (CT)-defined tumor and treatment volumes [abstract 2228]. Int J Radiat Oncol Biol Phys 51(Suppl):S343-S344, 2002.
268. Cai J, Chu JC, Recine D: CT and PET lung image registration and fusion in radiotherapy treatment planning using the chamfer matching method. Int. J. Radiation Oncology 43:883-891, 1999.
269. Erdi Y, Rosenzweig K, Erdi A: Radiotherapy treatment planning for patients with non small cell lung cancer using positron emission tomography (PET). Radiother Oncol 62:51-60, 2002.
270. Bradley J, Thorstad WL, Mutic S, et al: Impact of FDG-PET on radiation therapy volume delineation in non-small cell lung cancer. Int J Radiat Oncol Biol Phys 59:78-86, 2004.
271. Saitoh H, Fujisaki T, Sakai R, et al: Dose distribution of narrow beam irradiation for small lung tumor. Int J Radiat Oncol Biol Phys 53:1380-1387, 2002.
272. Johnson H, Schreiber E, Cullip T, Rosenman J: Significant underdosing of small tumors or portions of tumor in lung cancer treatment [abstract 1072]. Int J Radiat Oncol Biol Phys 54:S201, 2002.
273. Derycke S, De Gersem W, Van Duse B, De Neve W: Conformal radiotherapy of stage III non-small cell lung cancer: a class solution involving non-coplanar intensity modulated beams. Int J Radiat Oncol Biol Phys 41:771-777, 1998.
274. Derycke S, de Gersem W, van Duyse B, et al:. Intensity-modulated radiotherapy in stage III nonsmall cell lung cancer: a planning study comparing 6 MV and 25 MV photons. *In* Mornex F, van Houte P (eds): Treatment Optimization for Lung Cancer: From Classical to Innovative Procedures. Paris, Elsevier, 1998, pp 89-97.
275. Marks L, Spencer D, Sherouse G, et al: The role of three-dimensional functional lung imaging in radiation treatment planning: the functional dose-volume histogram. Int J Radiat Oncol Biol Phys 33:65-75, 1995.
276. Marks L, Munley M, Spencer D, et al: Quantification of radiation-induced regional lung injury with perfusion imaging. Int J Radiat Oncol Biol Phys 38:399-409, 1997.
277. Edelman M, Suntharalingam M, Krasna M: The management of the patient undergoing combined modality therapy for locally advanced non-small cell lung cancer. Curr Treat Options Oncol Cancer 4:45-53, 2003.
278. Lind P, Marks L, Hollis D, et al: Receiver operating characteristic curves to assess predictors of radiation-induced symptomatic lung injury. Int J Radiat Oncol Biol Phys 54:340-347, 2002.
279. Yamada M, Kudoh S, Hirata K, et al: Risk factors for pneumonitis following chemoradiotherapy for lung cancer. Eur J Cancer 34:71-75, 1998.

280. Hazuka M, Turrisi AR, Martel M, Ten Haken R, et al: Dose-escalation in non-small cell lung cancer (NSCLC) using conformal 3-dimensional radiation treatment planning (3DRTP): Preliminary results of phase I study [meeting abstract]. Proc Am Soc Clin Oncol 13:1, 1994.
281. Oetzel D, Schraube P, Hensley F, et al: Estimation of pneumonitis risk in three dimensional treatment planning using dose-volume histogram analysis. Int J Radiat Oncol Biol Phys 33:455-460, 1995.
282. Roach M 3rd, Gandara DR, Yuo HS, et al: Radiation pneumonitis following combined modality therapy for lung cancer: analysis of prognostic factors. J Clin Oncol 13:2606-2612, 1995.
283. Pagel J, Mohorn M, Kloetzer K, et al: [The inhalation versus systemic prevention of pneumonitis during thoracic irradiation]. Strahlenther Onkol 174:25-29, 1998.
284. Buntzel J, Kuttner R, Russell L, et al: Selective cytoprotection by amifostine in the treatment of head and neck cancer with simultaneous chemoradiotherapy [abstract]. Proc Am Soc Clin Oncol 16:1400, 1997.
285. Kemp G, Rose P, Lurain J, et al: Amifostine pretreatment for protection against cyclophosphamide and cisplatin-induced toxicities: results of a randomized controlled trial in patients with advanced ovarian cancer. J Clin Oncol 14:2101-2112, 1996.
286. Sauer R, Wannenmacher M, Brizel M, et al: Randomized phase III trial of radiation (RT) ± Ethyol (Amifostine) in patients with head and neck cancer [abstract]. Int J Radiat Oncol Biol Phys 39:234, 1997.
287. Tannehill S, Mehta M, Larson M, et al: Effect of amifostine on toxicities associated with sequential chemotherapy and radiation therapy for unresectable non-small cell lung cancer: results of a phase II trial. J Clin Oncol 15:2850-2857, 1997.
288. Werner-Wasik M, Scott C, Mousas B, et al: Amifostine as mucosal protectant in patients with locally advanced non-small cell lung cancer (NSCLC) receiving intensive chemotherapy and thoracic radiotherapy (RT): results of the Radiation Therapy Oncology Group (RTOG) 98-01 study [abstract 152]. Int J Radiat Oncol Biol Phys 57(Suppl 2):S216, 2003.
289. Border W, Noble N: Transforming growth factor beta in tissue fibrosis. N Engl J Med 19:1286-1292, 1994.
290. Connor T, Roberts A, Sporn M, et al: Correlation of fibrosis and transforming growth factor-β type 2 in the eye. J Clin Invest 83:1661-1666, 1989.
291. Anscher MS, Peters W, Reisenbichler H, et al: Transforming growth factor beta as a predictor of liver and lung fibrosis after autologous bone marrow transplantation for advanced breast cancer. N Engl J Med 328:1592-1598, 1993.
292. Rodemann H, Bamberg M: Cellular basis of radiation-induced fibrosis. Radiother Oncol 35:83-90, 1995.
293. Rubin P, Johnston C, Williams J, et al: A perpetual cascade of cytokines postirradiation leads to pulmonary fibrosis. Int J Radiat Oncol Biol Phys 33:99-109, 1995.
294. Trotti A: Toxicity antagonists in cancer therapy. Curr Opin Oncol 9:569-578, 1997.
295. Mornex F: Lung tolerance and toxicity to radiation. *In* Mornex F, van Houte P (eds): Treatment Optimization for Lung Cancer: from Classical to Innovative Procedures. Paris, Elsevier, 1998, pp 117-124.
296. Blanke K, Rudoltz M, Kao G, et al: The molecular regulation of apoptosis and implications for radiation oncology. Int J Radiat Biol 71:455-466, 1997.
297. Muschel R, McKenna W, Bernhard E: Cell cycle checkpoints and apoptosis: potential for improving radiation therapy. Vitam Horm 54:1-25, 1997.
298. Sartor C: Mechanisms of disease: radiosensitization by epidermal growth factor receptor inhibitors. Nat Clin Pract 1:80-87, 2004.
299. Schmidt-Ullrich R, Contessa J, Lammering G, et al: ERBB receptor tyrosine kinases and cellular radiation responses. Oncogene 22:5855-5865, 2003.
300. Baumann M, Krause M: Targeting the epidermal growth factor in radiotherapy: radiobiological mechanisms, preclinical and clinical results. Radiother Oncol 72:257-266, 2004.
301. Harari P, Huang S-M: Combining EGFR inhibitors with radiation or chemotherapy: will preclinical studies predict clinical results? Int J Radiat Oncol Biol Phys 58:976-983, 2004.
302. Ochs J: Rationale and clinical basis for combining gefitinib (Iressa, ZD1839) with radiation therapy for solid tumors. Int J Radiat Oncol Biol Phys 58:941-949, 2004.
303. She Y, Lee F, Chen J, et al: The epidermal growth factor receptor tyrosine kinase inhibitor ZD1839 selectively potentiates radiation response of human tumors in nude mice, with a marked improvement in therapeutic index. Clin Cancer Res 9:3773-3778, 2003.
304. Williams K, Telfer B, Wedge S: ZD1839 ('Iressa'), a specific oral epidermal growth factor receptor-tyrosine kinase inhibitor, potentiates radiotherapy in a human colorectal cancer xenograft model. Br J Cancer 86:1157-1161, 2002.
305. Bonner J, Harari PM, Gia HJ, et al: Cetuximab prolongs survival in patients with locoregionally advanced carcinoma of head and neck: a phase III study of high dose radiation therapy with or without cetuximab [abstract 5507]. Proc Am Soc Clin Oncol 22:621S, 2004.
306. Rosenthal D, Becerra C, Nurenberg P: Phase I study of gadolinium texaphyrin as an MRI contrast and radiosensitizer [abstract]. Proc Am Soc Clin Oncol 15:1663, 1996.
307. Mehta M, Rodrigus P, Terhaard CH, et al: Survival and neurologic outcomes in a randomized trial of motexafin gadolinium and whole-brain radiation therapy in brain metastases. J Clin Oncol 21:2529-2536, 2003.
308. Hoskin P: Palliative radiotherapy for non-small-cell lung cancer: which dose? Clin Oncol 17:59-60, 2005.
309. Erridge S, Gaze M, Price A, et al: Symptom control and quality of life in people with lung cancer: a randomized trial of two palliative radiotherapy schedules. Clin Oncol 17:61-67, 2005.
310. Andrews D, Scott C, Sperduto P, et al: Whole brain radiation therapy with or without stereotactic radiosurgery boost for patients with one to three brain metastases: phase III results of the RTOG 9508 randomised trial. Lancet 363:1665-1672, 2004.
311. Noel G, Medioni J, Valery C-A, et al: Three irradiation treatment options including radiosurgery for brain metastases from primary lung cancer. Lung Cancer 41:333-343, 2003.
312. Sneed P, Suh J, Goetsch S, et al: A multi-institutional review of radiosurgery alone vs. radiosurgery with whole brain radiotherapy as the initial management of brain metastases. Int J Radiat Oncol Biol Phys 53:519-526, 2002.
313. Gandara D, Ohe Y, Kubota K, et al: Japan-SWOG common arm analysis of paclitaxel/carboplatin in advanced stage non-small cell lung cancer (NSCLC): a model for prospective comparison of cooperative group trials. Proc Am Soc Clin Oncol 22:7007, 2004.
314. Naunheim K, Virgo K, Coplin M, et al: Clinical surveillance testing after lung cancer operations. Ann Thorac Surg 60:1612-1616, 1995.
315. Walsh G, O'Connor M, Willis K, et al: Is follow-up of lung cancer patients after resection medically indicated and cost-effective. Ann Thorac Surg 60:1563-1572, 1995.
316. Martini N, Bains M, Burt M, et al: Incidence of local recurrence and second primary tumors in resected stage I lung cancer. J Thorac Cardiovasc Surg 109:120-129, 1995.
317. Rocco P, Antkowiak J, Takita H, et al: Long-term outcome after pneumonectomy for nonsmall cell lung cancer. J Surg Oncol 61:278-280, 1996.
318. Werner-Wasik M, Xiao Y, Pequignot E, et al: Assessment of lung cancer response after nonoperative therapy: tumor diameter, bidimensional product, and volume, a serial CT scan-based study. Int J Radiat Oncol Biol Phys 51:56-61, 2001.
319. MacManus M, Hicks R, Matthews J, et al: Positron emission tomography is superior to computed tomography scanning for response assessment after radical radiotherapy or chemoradiotherapy in patients with non-small-cell lung cancer. J Clin Oncol 21:1285-1292, 2003.
320. Kubota K, Yamada S, Ishiwata K, Ito T: Positron emission tomography for treatment evaluation and recurrence detection compared with CT in long-term follow-up cases of lung cancer. Clin Nucl Med 17:877-881, 1992.
321. Venugopal P, Ali A, Patel S, et al: Positron emission tomography (PE) scan as a predictor of response following combined modal-

ity chemo-radiotherapy for stage III non-small cell lung cancer (NSCLC) patients [abstract]. Proc Am Soc Clin Oncol 15:1239, 1995.
322. Choi N, Fischman A, Niemierko A, et al: Dose-response relationship between probability of pathologic tumor control and glucose metabolic rate measured with FDG PET after preoperative chemoradiotherapy in locally advanced non-small-cell lung cancer. Int J Radiat Oncol Biol Phys 54:1024-1035, 2002.
323. Evans W, Will B, Berthelot J-M, Earle C: Cost of combined modality interventions for stage III non-small cell lung cancer. J Clin Oncol 15:3038-3048, 1997.
324. Morrison R, Deeley T, Cleland W: The treatment of carcinoma of the bronchus: a clinical trial to compare surgery and supervoltage radiotherapy. Lancet 1:683, 1963.
325. Smart J: Can lung cancer be cured by irradiation alone? JAMA 195:158-159, 1966.
326. Coy P, Kennelly G: The role of curative radiotherapy in the treatment of lung cancer. Cancer 45:698; 1980.
327. Cooper J, Pearson F, Todd T, et al: Radiotherapy alone for patients with operable carcinoma of the lung. Chest 87:289-292, 1985.
328. Haffty B, Goldberg N, Gerstley J, et al: Results of radical radiation therapy in clinical stage I, technically operable non-small cell lung cancer. Int J Radiat Oncol Biol Phys 15:69-73, 1988.
329. Noordijk E, Poest C, Hermans J, et al: Radiotherapy as an alternative to surgery in elderly patients with resectable lung cancer. Radiother Oncol 13:83-89, 1988.
330. Zhang H, Yin W, Yang Z: Curative radiotherapy of early operable non-small-cell lung cancer. Radiother Oncol 14:89-94, 1989.
331. Talton B, Constable W, Kersh C: Curative radiotherapy in non-small cell carcinoma of the lung. Int J Radiat Oncol Biology Phys 19:15-21, 1990.
332. Sandler H, Curran W, Turrisi A: The influence of tumor size and pre-treatment staging on outcome following radiation therapy alone for stage I non-small cell lung cancer. Int J Radiat Oncol Biology Phys 19:9-13, 1991.
333. Ono R, Egawa S, Suemasu K, et al: Radiotherapy in inoperable stage I lung cancer. Jpn J Clin Oncol 21:125-128, 1991.
334. Dosoretz D, Katin M, Blitzer P, et al: Radiation therapy in the management of medically inoperable carcinoma of the lung: results and implications for future treatment strategies. Int J Radiat Oncol Biol Phys 24:3-9, 1992.
335. Dosoretz D, Galmarini D, Rubenstein J, et al: Local control in medically inoperable lung cancer: an analysis of its importance in outcome and factors determining the probability of tumor eradication. Int J Radiat Oncol Biol Phys 27:507-516, 1993.
336. Hayakawa K, Mitsuhashi N, Furuta M, et al: High-dose radiation therapy for inoperable non-small cell lung cancer without mediastinal involvement (clinical stage N0, N1). Strahlenther Onkol 172:489-495, 1996.
337. Rosenthal S, Curran WJ, Herbert S, et al: Clinical stage II non-small cell lung cancer treated with radiation therapy alone. The significance of clinically staged ipsilateral hilar adenopathy. Cancer 70:2410-2417, 1992.
338. Kaskowitz B, Graham M, Emami B, et al: Radiation therapy alone for stage I non-small cell lung cancer. Int J Radiat Oncol Biol Phys 27:517, 1993.
339. Graham M, Gebski V, Langlands A: Radical radiotherapy for early non-small cell lung cancer. Int J Radiat Oncol Biol Phys 31:261-266, 1995.
340. Gauden S, Ramsay J, Tripcony L: The curative treatment by radiotherapy alone of stage I non-small-cell carcinoma of the lung. Chest 108:1278-1282, 1995.
341. Sibley G, Jamieson T, Marks L, et al: Radiotherapy alone for medically inoperable stage I non-small-cell lung cancer: the Duke experience. Int J Radiat Oncol Biol Phys 40:149-154, 1998.
342. Furuta M, Hayakawa K, Katano S, et al: Radiation therapy for stage I-II non-small cell lung cancer in patients aged 75 years and older. Jpn J Clin Oncol 26:95-98, 1996.
343. Timmerman R, Papiez L, McGarry R, et al: Results of a phase I study in medically inoperable stage I non-small cell lung cancer. Chest 124:1946-1955, 2003.
344. Nagata Y, Negoro Y, Aoki Y, et al: Clinical outcomes of 3-D conformal hypofractionated single high dose radiotherapy for one or two lung tumors using a stereotactic body frame. Int J Radiat Oncol Biol Phys 52:1041-1046, 2002.
345. Onishi H: Stereotactic three dimensional (3-D) conformal multiple dynamic arc radiotherapy for stage I non-small cell lung cancer using a linear accelerator unified with self-moving CT scanner and patient's self-breath and beam control technique [abstract 2589]. Proc Am Soc Clin Oncol 22:644, 2003.
346. Onishi H, Nagata Y, Shirato H, et al: Stereotactic hypofractionated high-dose irradiation for patients with stage I non-small cell lung carcinoma: clinical outcomes in 241 cases of a Japanese multi-institutional study [abstract 30]. Int J Radiat Oncol Biol Phys 27(Suppl 1):57:S142, 2003.
347. Harada T, Shirato H, Ogura S, et al: Real-time tumor tracking radiation therapy (RTRT) for stage I non-small cell lung cancers (NSCLCs) [abstract 2591]. Proc Am Soc Clin Oncol 22:644, 2003.
348. Niibe Y, Karasawa M, Shibuya M, et al: Prospective study of three-dimensional radiation therapy (3D-CRT) using middle fraction size for small-sized lung tumor in elderly patients [abstract 2702]. Proc Am Soc Clin Oncol 22:672, 2003.
349. Hof H, Herfarth K, Munter M, et al: Stereotactic single-dose radiotherapy of stage I non-small cell lung cancer (NSCLC). Int J Radiat Oncol Biol Phys 56:335-341, 2003.
350. Whyte RI, Crownover R, Murphy MJ, et al: Stereotactic radiosurgery for lung tumors: preliminary report of a phase I trial. Ann Thorac Surg 75:1097-1101, 2003.
351. Fukumoto S, Shirata H, Shimzu S: Small-volume image-guided radiotherapy using hypofractionated, coplanar, and noncoplanar multiple fields for patients with inoperable stage I nonsmall cell lung carcinomas. Cancer 95:1546-1553, 2002.
352. Feld R, Rubinstein L, Weisenberg T, et al: Sites of recurrence in resected stage I non-small cell lung cancer: a guide for future studies. J Clin Oncol 2:1352-1358, 1985.
353. Pairolero P, Williams D, Bergstralh M, et al: Post-surgical stage I bronchogenic carcinoma: morbid implications of recurrent disease. Ann Thorac Surg 38:331-338, 1984.
354. Thomas P, Rubinstein L: Cancer recurrence after resection: T1N0 non-small cell lung cancer. Lung Cancer Study Group. Ann Thorac Surg 49:242-247, 1990.
355. Albain K, Crowley J, Turrisi AI, et al: Concurrent cisplatin, etoposide, and chest radiotherapy in pathologic stage IIIB non-small-cell lung cancer: a Southwest Oncology Group phase II study. J Clin Oncol 20:3454-3460, 2002.
356. Andre F, Grunenwald D, Pujol J, et al: Patterns of relapse of N2 nonsmall-cell lung carcinoma in patients treated with pre-operative chemotherapy. Should prophylactic cranial irradiation be considered? Cancer 91:2394-2400, 2001.
357. Law A, Daly B, Madsen M, et al: High incidence of isolated brain metastases (CNS mets) following complete response (CR) in advanced non-small cell lung cancer (NSCLC): a new challenge [abstract]. Lung Cancer 18(Suppl 1):248, 1997.
358. Kato H, Ichinose Y, Ohta M, et al, for the Japan Lung Cancer Research Group on Postsurgical Adjuvant Chemotherapy (JLCRG): A randomized trial of adjuvant chemotherapy with uracil-tegafur for adenocarcinoma of the lung. N Engl J Med 350:1713-1721, 2004.
359. Rosell R, Gomez-Codina J, Camps C, et al: A randomized trial comparing preoperative chemotherapy plus surgery with surgery alone in patients with non-small cell lung cancer. N Engl J Med 330:153-158, 1994.
360. Wagner H, Lad T, Piantadosi S, Ruckdeschel J: Randomized phase 2 evaluation of preoperative radiation therapy and preoperative chemotherapy with mitomycin, vinblastine, and cisplatin in patients with technically unresectable stage IIIA and IIIB non-small cell cancer of the lung: LCSG 881. Chest 106(Suppl):348s-354s, 1994.
361. Depierre A, Milleron B, Moro-Sibilot D, et al: Preoperative chemotherapy followed by surgery compared with primary surgery in resectable stage I (except T1N0), II, and IIIa non-small-cell lung cancer. J Clin Oncol 20:247-253, 2002.
362. Dillman R, Seagren S, Propert K, et al: A randomized trial of induction chemotherapy plus high-dose radiation versus radiation alone in stage III non-small cell lung cancer. N Engl J Med 940-945, 1990.

363. Dillman R, Herndon J, Seagren S, et al: Improved survival in stage III non-small cell lung cancer: seven year follow-up of Cancer and Leukemia Group B (CALGB) 8433 trial. J Natl Cancer Inst 88:1210-1215, 1996
364. Sause W, Kolesar P, Taylor S, et al: Five-year results; phase III trial of regionally advanced unresectable non-small cell lung cancer, RTOG 8808, ECOG 4588, SWOG 8992 [abstract 1743]. Proc Am Clin Soc Oncol 17:453, 1998.
365. Schaake-Koning C, Van Den Bogert W, Dalesio O, et al: Effects of concomitant cisplatin and radiotherapy in inoperable non-small-cell lung cancer. N Engl J Med 326:524-530, 1992.
366. Trovo M, Zanelli G, Minatel E, et al: Radiotherapy versus radiotherapy enhanced by cisplatin in stage III non-small cell lung cancer. Int J Radiat Oncol Biol Phys 24:573-574, 1992.
367. Blanke C, Ansari R, Mantravadi R, et al: Phase III trial of thoracic irradiation with or without cisplatin for advanced unresectable non-small-cell lung cancer: a Hoosier Oncology Group protocol. J Clin Oncol 13:1425-1429, 1995.
368. Jeremic B, Shibamoto Y, Acimovic L, Djuric L: Randomized trial of hyperfractionated radiotherapy with or without concurrent chemotherapy for stage III non-small cell lung cancer. J Clin Oncol 13:452-458, 1995.
369. Jeremic B, Shibamoto Y, Acimovic L, Milisavljevic S: Hyperfractionated radiation therapy with or without concurrent low-dose daily carboplatin/etoposide for stage III non-small-cell lung cancer: a randomized study. J Clin Oncol 4:1065-1070, 1996.
370. Furuse K, Fukuoka M, Kawahara K, et al: Phase III study of concurrent versus sequential thoracic radiotherapy in combination with mitomycin, vindesine, and cisplatin in unresectable stage III non-small-cell lung cancer. J Clin Oncol 17:2692-2699, 1999.
371. Curran W, Scott C, Langer C, et al: Long-term benefit is observed in a phase III comparison of sequential vs. concurrent chemoradiation for patients with unresected stage III NSCLC: RTOG 9410 [abstract 621]. Proc Am Soc Clin Oncol l22:621, 2003.
372. Pierre F, Maurice P, Gilles R, et al: A randomized phase III trial of sequential chemo-radiotherapy versus concurrent chemoradiotherapy in locally advanced non-small cell lung cancer (NSCLC) (GLOT-GFPC NPC 95-01 study) [abstract 1246]. Proc Am Soc Clin Oncol 20:512, 2001.
373. Zatloukal P, Petruzelka L, Zemanova M, et al: Concurrent versus sequential radiochemotherapy with vinorelbine plus cisplatin (V-P) in locally advanced non-small-cell lung cancer. A randomized phase II study [abstract 1159]. Proc Am Soc Clin Oncol 21:290, 2002.
374. Choy H, Curran W, Scott C, et al: Preliminary report of Locally Advanced Multimodality Protocol (LAMP): ACR 427: a randomized phase II study of three chemo-radiation regimens with paclitaxel, carboplatin, and thoracic radiation therapy (TRT) for patients with locally advanced non-small cell lung cancer (LA-NSCLC) [abstract 1160]. Proc Am Soc Clin Oncol 21:291, 2002.
375. Kagami Y, Nishio M, Narimatsu N, et al: Prospective randomized trials comparing hyperfractionated radiotherapy with conventional radiotherapy in stage III nonsmall cell lung cancer. Nippon Igaku Hoshasen Gakkai Zasshi 52:1452-1455, 1992.
376. Bleehen N: Inoperable non-small cell lung cancer (NSCLC): a Medical Research Council randomized trial of palliative radiotherapy with two fractions or ten fractions. Br J Cancer 63:265-270, 1991.
377. Bleehen N, Girling D, Machin D, Stephens R: A Medical Research Council (MRC) randomised trial of palliative radiotherapy with two fractions or a single fraction in patients with inoperable non-small-cell lung cancer (NSCLC) and poor performance status. Br J Cancer 65:934-941, 1992.
378. Kris M, Gralla R, Potanovich L, et al: Assessment of pretreatment symptoms and improvement after EDAM + mitomycin + vinblastine (EMV) in patients with inoperable non-small cell lung cancer (NSCLC) [abstract 883]. Proc Am Soc Clin Oncol 9:299, 1990.
379. Tummarello D, Graziano F, Isidori P, et al: Symptomatic, stage IV, non-small cell lung cancer (NSCLC): response, toxicity, performance status change, and symptom relief in patients treated with cisplatin, vinblastine, and mitomycin C. Cancer Chemother Pharmacol 3:249-253, 1995.
380. Ichinose Y, Tsuchiya R, Kate H: Randomized trial of chemotherapy followed by surgery for stage IIIA non-small cell lung cancer; The Japan Clinical Oncology Group (lung cancer surgical study group). [9209 Abstract] Lung Concer 29:173, 2000.

CHAPTER 42

CANCER OF THE ESOPHAGUS

A. William Blackstock

EPIDEMIOLOGY AND PATHOLOGY

An estimated 14,520 Americans were diagnosed with esophageal cancer in 2005, and more than 90% of them will die of their disease. The incidence of distal esophageal and gastroesophageal adenocarcinomas has drastically increased over the past 10 to 15 years.

The predominant histologies are squamous cell carcinoma and adenocarcinoma.

BIOLOGIC CHARACTERISTICS

Major prognostic factors are local tumor extent, nodal involvement, and distant metastases.

STAGING EVALUATION

Staging should include a history and physical examination, complete blood cell count, liver chemistries, computed tomography of the chest and upper abdomen, barium swallow, and endoscopy with biopsy. The use of ^{18}F-fluorodeoxyglucose positron emission tomography has become more routine.

PRIMARY THERAPY

Surgical resection is the primary therapy for early-stage disease. Cure rates of 60% to 80% are achieved for the rare patients found to have node-negative, organ-confined disease.

For patients with locally advanced disease, primary radiation therapy, surgical resection alone, and concurrent chemotherapy or neoadjuvant chemoradiation followed by resection result in a 20% to 30% cure rate.

PALLIATION AND BRACHYTHERAPY

With complete response rates of 25% to 35% observed in most combined-modality studies, the use of irradiation and concurrent chemotherapy for palliation of obstruction or bleeding is appropriate.

The addition of intraluminal brachytherapy with chemotherapy or external beam radiation therapy, or both, is most often used for palliation.

The diagnosis and management of esophageal cancer are the focus of considerable clinical investigation. Advances in operative and postoperative management and in rational applications of multimodality therapy have resulted in a significant improvement in outcome for patients with localized disease. In this chapter, I review changes in the histologic composition of esophageal cancers and explain how they relate to tumor biology and epidemiologic factors. Discussion follows about the evolving impact of ^{18}F-fluorodeoxyglucose positron emission tomography (FDG-PET) for the staging of esophageal cancer, the rationale for novel combined-modality approaches in the treatment of esophageal cancer, the results of clinical trials testing single-modality and combined-modality therapies, and the use of palliative therapies for noncurative disease. Clinical conditions and techniques unique to esophageal cancer are presented, including the management of patients with tracheoesophageal fistula and the usefulness of intraluminal brachytherapy. The chapter concludes with a summary of the data, synopsis of treatment recommendations, and discussion of several important clinical trials in progress.

ETIOLOGY AND EPIDEMIOLOGY

Esophageal cancer is a highly aggressive neoplasm. In 2005, an estimated 14,520 Americans were diagnosed with esophageal cancer; about one half had adenocarcinoma histology, and more than 90% were expected to die of their disease.[1] Approximately one half of patients with esophageal cancer present with locally advanced disease,[2] and they have a 5-year survival rate of less than 30% after surgical resection or multimodality therapy. Esophageal cancer represents one of the few cancers for which survival has not improved substantially over the past 25 years.[1] The incidence of adenocarcinoma of the distal esophagus and gastroesophageal junction is increasing in Western countries, but squamous cell carcinoma remains dominant in underdeveloped parts of the world.[3] Data from the Surveillance Epidemiology, and End Results (SEER) program of the National Cancer Institute (1973-1998) demonstrate that in the United States, the incidence of adenocarcinoma among white men is still rising (7.8%/year), with the same trend observed for white women (6.48%/year), Hispanic men (3.91%/year), and Hispanic women (9.4%/year).[4] The incidence of squamous cell carcinoma has been steadily declining among white men and women and among African American women since 1973, with the incidence showing a dramatic and significant decline in African American men beginning in 1992.[5] In general, the incidence of adenocarcinomas has risen two to three times the previously reported rates for African American men and women. Data reported by Hesketh in a review of the New England tumor registries show that the incidence of adenocarcinoma has increased even when tumors located at the esophagogastric junction are excluded.[6] Table 42-1 reflects recent changes in the prevalence of adenocarcinoma of the esophagus over the span of several decades. Pohl and colleagues provide compelling data to counter a number of suggested possibilities for the recent increase in adenocarcinomas of the esophagus.[7] Extracting information from the National Cancer Institute's SEER database (1973-2001), the investigators found no evidence for histologic reclassification of esophageal squamous cancers or anatomic reclassification of adenocarcinomas of the gastric cardia (i.e., the incidence of adenocarcinoma of the gastric cardia did not fall but instead increased as that of

Table 42-1 Incidence of Adenocarcinoma of the Esophagus

Study	Study Interval	Adenocarcinoma (%)
Smithers[148]	1936-1951	7.3
Hesketh et al/ Conn. Register[6]	1983-1986	22.9
Birgisson et al[149]	1987-1994	73.5
Steyerberg et al[10]	1991-1999	52

esophageal adenocarcinomas rose). There is no explanation for the predominant increase in adenocarcinomas seen in white men.[8,9]

Esophageal cancer is more common in men than women; of the more than 14,000 estimated cases of esophageal cancer diagnosed in the United States in 2005, approximately 11,000 occurred in men.[1] Esophageal cancer is the sixth leading cause of cancer death among men in the United States. African American men are more likely to present with advanced or metastatic disease, resulting in a survival rate that is one half that for white men.[1] Provocative data from Steyerberg and coworkers[10] suggest that the underuse of potentially curative surgery may in part explain the poorer survival observed for African American patients with locally advanced disease; in a population-based analysis the study authors observed that once corrected for treatment received, there was no difference in survival between white patients and black patients. It has been postulated that the increased incidence and mortality observed in African American patients is a reflection of socioeconomic status and dietary risk factors, not ethnicity. Data from Brown and coworkers[11] support a correlation between an increased rate of squamous cancers in African American men with known risk factors. In this population-based, case-control study, there appeared to be a risk for developing esophageal cancer in African American patients beyond what could be attributed to alcohol and tobacco use.[11] The reasons for the apparent racial difference in risk from the same level of alcohol and tobacco use could be associated in part with increased mutations in the *TP53* gene in esophageal cancers found in African Americans, as reported by Baron and associates.[12]

PREVENTION AND EARLY DETECTION

Barrett's esophagus is a precursor lesion for esophageal adenocarcinoma, although most Barrett's lesions do not proceed to carcinoma. Adenocarcinomas and squamous cancers of the esophagus overexpress the cyclooxygenase-2 (COX-2) enzyme.[13,14] More relevant to chemoprevention strategies are data from Shamma and associates demonstrating that COX-2 expression correlated with the proliferative activity in dysplastic (precancerous) lesions of the esophagus.[15] In this study, the COX-2 level was found to be increased in a stepwise fashion with the transition from normal esophagus to low-grade dysplasia to high-grade dysplasia. These data suggest that COX-2 is involved in the early stages of carcinogenesis and that interruptions in the dysplasia-carcinoma sequence could prove to be an important part of a chemoprevention strategy. Precancerous lesions of the esophagus have also been shown to overexpress the proteins TP53, CCND1 (also called cyclin D1), and CDKN2A (previously designated p16).[16-18]

Although families with Barrett's have been described, most cases are sporadic and believed to be caused by chronic gastroesophageal reflux. Suleiman and colleagues postulate that the use of pharmaceutical agents for the treatment of gastroesophageal reflux (antisecretory agents and therapies to relax the lower esophageal sphincter) is related to the recent increase in the incidence of Barrett's lesion–associated adenocarcinomas.[19] These treatment strategies are effective in resolving the symptoms associated with gastroesophageal reflux, but they may preclude the surveillance required for the detection and management of Barrett's esophagus. Additional risk factors for adenocarcinoma of the esophagus include cigarette smoking, with the risk increasing with duration and intensity of smoking; obesity; and reduced consumption of fruits and vegetables.[20]

There are additional studies, as reviewed by Maley and colleagues, further defining the complexity of these types of studies.[21] The neoplastic progression in Barrett's esophagus is associated with a process of genomic instability associated with widespread loss of heterozygosity, point mutations, alterations in microsatellite alleles (shifts), and epigenetic changes, including hypermethylation of promotor regions.[21] Although our molecular understanding of the premalignant conditions associated with Barrett's esophagus and esophageal dysplasia continues to expand, the incorporation of this information into chemoprevention efforts is still being investigated.

Because of the strong association of Barrett's esophagus with esophageal adenocarcinoma, there has been substantial interest in how to use this information to detect and perhaps prevent early cancerous lesions. The supposition is that the rapidly increasing incidence in Barrett's lesions reflects an increased incidence of gastroesophageal reflux disease, which may be related to the increased incidence of obesity in the population. The dysplastic epithelium associated with Barrett's can be screened endoscopically and treated to prevent cancer progression. Alternatively, it can be treated when it progresses to high-grade dysplasia or early cancer. The difficulty is that there is no good treatment for Barrett's lesions, and some approaches (e.g., phototherapy) may treat only superficial dysplasia, leaving behind higher-grade, deep dysplastic lesions.

MOLECULAR CHARACTERISTICS OF ESOPHAGEAL CANCER

Epidermal Growth Factor Receptor

Epidermal growth factor receptor (EGFR) overexpression, partially accounted for by gene amplification, is found in up to 80% of esophageal squamous cell carcinomas and esophageal adenocarcinomas, as well as their precursor lesions, such as squamous dysplasia and Barrett's esophagus.[22-24] Significant differences in EGFR expression have been reported among histologic subtypes, generally with higher EGFR expression in squamous cell carcinoma than in adenocarcinoma. Several clinical studies of esophageal cancer have correlated EGFR tumor overexpression with patient survival (Table 42-2). Gibson and coworkers, in a study of 54 patients receiving preoperative chemoradiation, evaluated pretreatment EGFR expression using an EGFR immunoreactive score (EGFR-IRS).[24] Using a univariate analysis with EGFR-IRS coded as a continuous variable, each 1-unit increase in EGFR-IRS resulted in a 14% decrease in survival. When adjusted for all other clinical covariates, only the lower EGFR-IRS remained a significant predictor of survival.

TP53 Mutations

Mutations in the *TP53* gene occur in up to 80% of primary tumors of the esophagus. The mutations for squamous tumors

Table 42-2 **EGFR Expression in Esophageal Cancer and Outcome**

Study	Patient Samples	Method of Analysis	EGFR Tumor Expression Correlates with Survival
Lui et al[150]	97	Immunohistochemistry	Yes
Gibson et al[24]	54	Immunohistochemistry	Yes; $P = .009$
Wilkinson et al[151]	38	Immunohistochemistry	Trend; $P = .06$
Inada et al[152]	40	Immunohistochemistry	Yes; $P < .05$

EGFR, epidermal growth factor receptor.

(i.e., mutations at A-T base pairs) are very different from the mutations usually seen in adenocarcinomas.[25] Data from Montesano and colleagues indicate that the mutations common to squamous tumors are correlated with smoking.[26] Mutations in *TP53* are an early event in the carcinogenic process in the Barrett's mucosa, high-grade dysplasia, and esophageal adenocarcinoma sequence. In data from Coggi and coworkers, *TP53* mutations in exons 5 to 8 were detected in 53% of 74 esophageal cancers studied.[27] There was no concordance between *TP3* mutations and accumulation of the TP53 protein, nor were the mutations in *TP53* independently predictive of clinical outcome. In vitro data from investigators at Cornell evaluating the sensitivity of esophageal adenocarcinoma cell lines to chemotherapeutic agents (i.e., 5-fluorouracil [5-FU], mitomycin C, and cisplatinum [cisplatin]) showed that wild-type TP53 protein levels increased after treatment with each of the agents by posttranslational and translational processes. These investigators also confirmed a positive correlation with drug sensitivity and the increased expression of wild-type TP53 compared with a negative in vitro sensitivity effect for deficient TP53 expression or expression of mutated TP53.[28]

Vascular Endothelial Growth Factor and Cyclooxygenase-2

Vascular endothelial growth factor (VEGF) messenger RNA expression levels were evaluated in specimens of Barrett intestinal metaplasia, dysplasia, adenocarcinoma, and matching normal squamous esophageal tissues.[29] Expression levels were significantly increased in adenocarcinoma compared with normal squamous mucosa or intestinal metaplasia. VEGF levels were also significantly higher in cancer compared with dysplastic tissues. Microvessel density was generally higher in adenocarcinomas compared with the preneoplastic Barrett tissues. These data suggest a role for these angiogenic factors in the development of esophageal cancer.

Kulke and colleagues,[30] in a study of 46 patients with esophageal cancer receiving preoperative chemoradiation followed by surgical resection, observed that preoperative chemotherapy and irradiation induced expression of COX-2 in stromal cells and induced VEGF expression in tumor and stromal cells. Pretreatment VEGF expression, however, did not correlate with treatment response, whereas COX-2 expression correlated with treatment response only in the subset of patients with squamous cell carcinoma, although patients whose tumors expressed high levels of VEGF and COX-2 tended to have shorter overall survival times.

Other Molecular Targets

Additional molecular targets include cyclin D1 (CCND1), a cell cycle–regulating protein involved in the G_1 to S transition. Overexpression of cyclin D1 has been observed in approximately 30% to 40% of esophageal adenocarcinomas and squamous cell carcinomas.[31]

Inactivation of *CDKN2A*, a tumor suppressor gene, occurs in a significant number of esophageal cancers.[32] Restoring CDKN2A expression appears to markedly inhibit the proliferation and tumorigenicity of esophageal cancers.[28]

EGFR, TP653, CCND1, and CDKN2A represent only a few of the potential molecular targets for directing therapies. These and other examples of gene amplification or suppression and abnormal protein expression should be pursued in future clinical studies.

PATHOLOGY AND PATHWAYS OF SPREAD

The predominant histologies in esophageal cancer are squamous cell carcinoma and adenocarcinoma. Chronic esophagitis is thought to be a precursor for the development of squamous cell cancer.[33] Limited prospective data indicate that more than 30% of patients known to have severe esophagitis related to alcohol and smoking exposures will develop invasive cancers. Data reported by Auerbach and collegaues,[34] who examined esophageal autopsy specimens from two cohorts of men (smokers versus nonsmokers), revealed that in the nonsmokers, no specimen exhibited in situ cancer, whereas only 6.6% of the cases reviewed showed atypical nuclei. An almost 2% incidence of in situ disease and a 79.8% incidence of atypical nuclei were observed for specimens taken from previous smokers.[34] Other environmental factors associated with the development of squamous cell cancers include exposure to nitrates and potentially carcinogenic nitrosamines, asbestos fibers, and water contaminated with petroleum products. Thermal injury resulting from the ingestion of hot beverages has also been implicated in the development of squamous cancers of the esophagus.[35,36] An array of possible environmental and dietary risks are under investigation, as are potential molecular pathogenic factors.[37] Data from several laboratories have implicated genital-mucosal strains of human papillomaviruses (HPV-16 and HPV-18) as risk factors for the development of cancers of the esophagus.[38,39]

Approximately 20% of esophageal squamous tumors involve the upper "cervical" esophagus, and 50% are found in the middle esophagus, defined as the segment of esophagus from the aortic arch to the inferior pulmonary vein and usually representing the segment at 25 to 32 cm from the incisors. The remaining 30% of squamous tumors are found in the distal esophagus (33 to 42 cm). In contrast, more than 90% of adenocarcinomas are found in the distal esophagus and gastroesophageal junction. Other malignant histologies are unusual but include adenosquamous, mucoepidermoid, adenoid cystic, and malignant tumors with endocrine differentiation (small cell). In a histologic review of 77 patients treated with esophagectomy for early-stage disease, Holscher and associates found little difference between the overall rate of submucosal spread and lymph node metastasis for squamous and adenocarcinomas.[40] In a review of 349 surgically resected patients by Dumont and associates, no difference in survival could be correlated with histologic subtype, supporting the findings of other groups.[41,42]

CLINICAL MANIFESTATIONS, PATIENT EVALUATION, AND STAGING

Table 42-3 lists the most common clinical symptoms associated with esophageal cancer at presentation. More than 90% of patients present with progressive and worsening dysphagia, often resulting in significant weight loss. Other findings include odynophagia, chest pain, cough, and fever associated with possible respiratory fistula, hoarseness associated with tumor involvement of the recurrent laryngeal nerve, and melena from intraluminal bleeding. Recommended staging tests are outlined in Table 42-4.

The utility of fluorodeoxyglucose positron emission tomography (FDG-PET) for staging in esophageal cancer continues to evolve. Sihvo and colleagues, in an analysis of 55 esophageal cancer patients, found that adding FDG-PET to standard staging techniques improved the detection of occult metastatic disease.[43] Flanagan and coworkers, in a series of 36 patients, observed that FDG-PET detected computed tomography (CT)–negative metastatic disease in 5 (14%) patients with locally advanced esophageal cancer.[44] Block and associates compared FDG-PET with CT-based staging in 58 patients with esophageal cancer and found that FDG-PET was more sensitive for detecting micrometastatic disease.[45] Luketich and colleagues, in a study of 91 patients, also found FDG-PET (84%) was more sensitive than CT (63%) for detecting distant disease.[46] Flamon and coworkers, in a prospective study of 74 patients with esophageal cancer or cancers of the gastroesophageal junction, observed that FDG-PET had a greater accuracy compared with CT and endoscopic ultrasound (EUS)[47]; the addition of FDG-PET resulted in an upstaging of 11 patients (15%) from M0 to M1. In a meta-analysis reported by van Westreenen and coworkers,[48] FDG-PET showed limited sensitivity (0.51) and reasonable (0.81) specificity for the detection of locoregional metastases. This was improved for detecting distant lymphatic and hematogenous metastasis, with a sensitivity and specificity of 0.67 and 0.97, respectively.[48] Taken in total, these data are compelling and have resulted in the increasing use of FDG-PET for the routine staging of patients with esophageal cancer.

The esophagus is a hollow tube approximately 25 cm long that extends from the pharynx to the stomach and consists of three parts: the cervical, thoracic, and distal esophagus. The cervical esophagus lies just left of the midline behind the larynx and trachea. The upper portion of the thoracic esophagus passes behind the tracheal bifurcation (i.e., carina) and left mainstem bronchus, and the lower thoracic esophagus runs behind the left atrium. The distal esophagus is an area approximately 6 to 8 cm long that merges into the gastroesophageal junction.

In the esophagus, mucosal lymphatics merge with a submucosal plexus, which then merge with lymphatic channels in the muscularis. These channels communicate with an extensive network of cooperating lymphatics that extend throughout the esophagus. The lymphatics of the esophagus follow arteries and mainly course longitudinally and eventually drain into nodal groups as caudal as the internal jugular and as cephalad as the celiac lymph nodes. The nodal groups at risk for involvement in cancers of the cervical esophagus include the supraclavicular and right upper paratracheal nodes. In contrast, for gastroesophageal tumors, the nodes at risk include the pulmonary ligament, paracardial, left gastric, common hepatic, splenic, and celiac nodes.

The esophagus lacks a serosal surface and is separated from adjacent structures only by a loose connective tissue, the adventitia. The adventitia provides little barrier to local spread, and as a consequence, tracheoesophageal and esophagobronchial fistula develops in 5% to 10% of patients with cancer of the esophagus.

The tumor-node-metastasis (TNM) staging system for esophageal cancer is shown in Table 42-5. The designation for regional nodes (M1a versus M1b) is based on the location of the primary tumor and involved regional nodes. As reflected in the staging, patients with regional or celiac axis lymphadenopathy should not necessarily be considered to have metastatic disease. Some difficulties have arisen because this is a surgical staging system, and many patients are now treated initially without resection, making accurate staging impossible. Esophageal cancers are staged according to the depth of invasion and the presence of regional lymph nodes. Diagnostic tools relevant to determining locoregional stage include endoscopic ultrasound, and thoracoscopic staging. Hiele and associates, in a prospective review, found that preoperative EUS reflected an accurate T stage for 59% of patients subsequently taken to surgery and an accuracy of 82% for patients with transmural tumor extension.[49] Natsugoe and colleagues found the accuracy of EUS to be 87% for detecting mediastinal nodal disease.[50] The Cancer and Leukemia Group B (CALGB), in a multi-institutional trial of thoracoscopic staging, found thoracoscopic determination of tumor penetration and lymph node staging to be accurate in 88% of patients later taken to resection. The accuracy of overall staging further improved with concomitant laparoscopic lymph node staging.[51] The precise role of EUS or thoracoscopic staging is not well defined, and the results often do not impact on clinical management. These studies were done before the common use of PET scans, and the incremental value of routine thoracoscopy and laparoscopy is now probably small.

Cancers confined to the epithelium and muscularis mucosa and without nodal involvement are considered stage I and II tumors. In a clinicopathologic review of 165 patients with esophageal cancer treated with resection only, Holscher and

Table 42-3 Presenting Signs and Symptoms of Esophageal Cancer

Anorexia
Chest pain
Cough
Dysphagia
Odynophagia

Table 42-4 Staging Tests for Esophageal Cancer

Chest radiograph
Barium swallow
Computed tomography (CT) of chest and upper abdomen
^{18}F-fluorodeoxyglucose positron emission tomography (FDG-PET)
Bone scan/head CT or magnetic resonance imaging (MRI)*
Blood chemistry (e.g., complete blood cell count, liver function tests)

*If clinically indicated.

Table 42-5 TNM Staging of Esophageal Cancer

PRIMARY TUMOR	
TX	Primary tumor cannot be assessed
T0	No evidence of primary tumor
Tis	Carcinoma in situ
T1	Tumor invades lamina propria or submucosa
T2	Tumor invades muscularis propria
T3	Tumor invades adventitia
T4	Tumor invades adjacent structures
REGIONAL LYMPH NODES	
NX	Regional nodes cannot be assessed
N0	No regional lymph node metastasis
N1	Regional lymph node metastasis
DISTANT METASTASIS	
MX	Distant metastasis cannot be assessed
M0	No distant metastasis
M1	Distant metastasis
	Tumors of the lower thoracic esophagus
	M1a: Metastasis in celiac lymph nodes
	M1b: Other distant metastasis
	Tumors of the midthoracic esophagus*
	M1a: Not applicable
	M1b: Nonregional lymph nodes and/or other distant metastasis
	Tumors of the upper thoracic esophagus
	M1a: Metastasis in cervical nodes
	M1b: Other distant metastasis
STAGE GROUPINGS	
Stage 0	Tis N0 M0
Stage I	T1 N0 M0
Stage IIA	T2 N0 M0, T3 N0 M0
Stage IIB	T1 N1 M0, T2 N1 M0
Stage III	T3 N1 M0, T4 any N M0

*For tumors of midthoracic esophagus, use only M1b because these tumors with metastases in nonregional lymph nodes have equally poor prognoses as those with metastases in other distant sites.

From Greene FL, Page DL, Fleming ID, et al (eds), for the American Joint Committee on Cancer: AJCC Cancer Staging Manual, 6th ed. New York, Springer, 2002.

colleagues observed a 0% rate of lymph node metastases in patients with disease confined to the mucosa, compared with 18% for tumors with submucosal spread.[52] The overall 5-year survival reported for patients with node-negative disease was 63%. Tumors invading the adventitia or surrounding structures have a worse outcome than more limited disease, and there is usually associated nodal involvement.

PRIMARY THERAPY

Single-Modality Therapy

Surgery

In 1913, Dr. Franz Torek used a transpleural approach to perform the first successful resection of an esophageal carcinoma.[53] He concluded that the patient "feels very happy with her (external) rubber esophagus." With improvements in anesthesia, subsequent surgeons used mainly a transthoracic approach with primary esophagogastric anastomosis, and in 1933, Ohsawa reported extended survival in 8 of 20 patients who underwent resection.[54] In 1938, Adams and Phemister were the first Western surgeons to successfully adopt the Japanese transthoracic technique. The results of these studies, however, revealed a discouraging 5-year survival rate of 5% to 10%.[55]

Despite recent advances in surgical and anesthetic techniques, the overall results with surgery alone have produced only modest improvements in outcome. Moertel reviewed 18 surgical series involving 4109 patients treated with resection and found an overall 5-year survival rate of 9.6% (range, 3% to 20%).[56] A review of more recently published surgical series reveals slightly more encouraging results, but there has been careful patient selection in some of these trials. Mariette and colleagues, in a series of 179 patients with stage 0-II esophageal cancer treated with surgery alone between 1982 and 2002, observed an overall actuarial survival rate at 5 years of 59%. The investigators reported that no long-term survivors were observed among a subset of patients with locally advanced disease.[57]

Analysis of surgical pathology shows that a significant number of patients present with disease involving the regional lymph nodes and that such involvement results in a worse outcome. Of 156 patients evaluated by Frunberger and coworkers, 53% had nodal disease at surgery.[58] Sun and coworkers found that of 474 operable patients, 211 (44.5%) had involved regional lymph nodes at the time of surgery.[59] The overall survival rate for the entire group was 31%, but only 13% of patients with nodal disease were alive at 5 years, compared with 44% of patients with node-negative disease. Similar results have been reported by Collard and colleagues; the 5-year survival after surgery alone fell from 57% for node-negative patients to 15% for patients with positive nodes.[60] Holscher and associates, in an evaluation of 165 patients treated with an en bloc esophagectomy, found that no patient with greater than 30% regional nodal tumor involvement was alive at 5 years, compared with a 45% survival rate for patients with less than 30% nodal disease.[60]

These data indicate that many in the limited cohort of patients who present without regional nodal involvement will do well with surgery alone. Equally important, however, is that patients found to have nodal disease at the time of resection are rarely treated successfully with surgery alone. Unfortunately, our diagnostic tools for determining regional nodal status are not very sensitive, and a significant percentage of patients with esophageal cancer will present with locally advanced, node-positive tumors. Despite its modest success, surgical resection remains the standard of care for the treatment of early-stage esophageal cancer.

There are two standard surgical approaches for resecting tumors in patients with potentially curable disease. The transthoracic resection, or Ivor-Lewis procedure, allows better access to lesions in the upper two thirds of the esophagus and complete visualization of the esophagus. For distal tumors, this approach also allows resection of a greater proximal margin and placement of the anastomosis higher in the chest, which is thought to result in fewer anastomotic leaks and less postoperative reflux. The initial laparotomy is performed for exploring the abdomen for distant disease and mobilization of the stomach. The second and sometimes third thoracotomy incisions are for exposure and dissection of the esophagus. After the tumor is resected, the stomach is pulled through the hiatus for an intrathoracic anastomosis.

Orringer and others have reintroduced the transhiatal procedure as an alternative to the transthoracic approach.[156] The advantages for this technique include eliminating the morbidity associated with a thoracotomy by performing the operation through a laparotomy and left neck incision. The esophagus is removed by blunt dissection, and continuity is re-established with a cervical esophagogastric anastomosis.

There are no definitive data to suggest one technique is superior to another. Fok, in a review of 210 patients treated with a transthoracic resection ($n = 172$) or a transhiatal ($n = 38$)

Table 42-6 Response to Single-Agent Chemotherapy for Esophageal Cancer

Drug	No. of Patients	CR/PR (%)	Median Duration of Response (mo)*
Cisplatinum[153,154]	47	38%	2-3
5-Fluorouracil[155]	26	15%	1-5
Methotrexate[155]	26	12%	3
Vindesine[157]	71	27%	4
Mitomycin C[153]	51	27%	3-4
Paclitaxel[158]	52	32%	4
Etoposide[159]	26	19%	4
Irinotecan[160]	13	22%	4
Tarceva[161]	20	15%	NS
Gefitinib[162]	34	9%	NS

*Response as determined by radiographic or endoscopic methods, or both.

CR, complete response; NS, not significant; PR, partial response.

Table 42-7 Response to Combination-Agent Chemotherapy for Esophageal Cancer

Combination	No. of Patients	Overall Response (%)*
Cisplatinum + bleomycin[163]	61	15
Cisplatinum + vindesine + bleomycin[164]	68	53
Taxol + cisplatinum[165]	20	40
5-Fluorouracil + cisplatinum + doxorubicin[166]	21	33
Cisplatinum + etoposide[167]	73	48
5-Fluorouracil + cisplatinum[168]	88	35
Bleomycin + doxorubicin[169]	16	19
Irinotecan + cisplatinum[114]	35	57
Gemcitabine + cisplatinum[170]	36	41
Gemcitabine + irinotecan[171]	61	Not significant

*Response as determined by radiographic or endoscopic methods, or both.

resection, reported an increased incidence of tumor perforation (18%) and injuries to the recurrent laryngeal nerve (13%) after the transhiatal approach.[61] In a retrospective study of 238 patients, Pac and colleagues observed increased wound infections, pneumothorax, and in-hospital mortality for patients treated with a transthoracic resection.[62] In contrast, Stark and coworkers observed increased respiratory complications and in-hospital mortality after a transhiatal resection.[63] In a limited randomized study reported by Chu and colleagues, 39 patients with cancers involving the lower third of the esophagus were randomized to transhiatal versus transthoracic resection.[64] There were no differences in overall complications or operative mortality rates, and median survival times were similar: 16 months in the transthoracic group and 13.5 months in the transhiatal cohort. The transthoracic technique was the preferred operation because it allowed for superior tumor exposure and better lymph node dissection. Rentz and associates used the Veterans Administration National Surgical Quality Improvement Program to prospectively analyze risk factors for morbidity and mortality in 945 patients undergoing transthoracic esophagectomy or transhiatal esophagectomy from 1991 to 2000.[65] There were no differences in recorded preoperative variables between the groups. Overall mortality was 10.0% (56 of 562) for transthoracic esophagectomy and 9.9% (38 of 383) for transhiatal esophagectomy ($P = .983$). Morbidity occurred in 47% (266 of 562) of patients after transthoracic esophagectomy and in 49% (188 of 383) of patients after transhiatal esophagectomy ($P = .596$). These findings are consistent with the results of a meta-analysis reported by Hulscher and coworkers, who observed that the 5-year survival rate with surgery alone was approximately 20% after transthoracic and transhiatal resections.[66]

Chemotherapy

It has been observed in several autopsy series that esophageal cancer has a distant failure rate of greater than 70%. A large number of chemotherapy agents have been evaluated for response in cancer of the esophagus (Table 42-6), but unfortunately, the response rates remain very low, with only about 20% of patients having an objective response to a variety of single agents. Combination chemotherapeutic regimens have shown a higher response rate; the best responses were seen in patients receiving combinations with cisplatinum (Table 42-7). Although the increased response rate has been gratifying, the duration of response has been short and comparable to that seen with single-agent chemotherapy. Drugs under intense investigation include oxaliplatin, irinotecan, and gemcitabine in combination with cisplatinum and the anti-EGFR agents erlotinib (Tarceva) and gefitinib (Iressa).

Radiation Therapy

The early results for curative radiation therapy alone were poor. The initial application of irradiation in the management of esophageal cancer involved brachytherapy. Exner described his brachytherapy techniques in 1909, not long after the discovery of x-rays,[67] and Guisez, using radium bougies, reported a 5-year survival rate of 1%.[68] As the use of external beam irradiation became more common, the limitations of brachytherapy in curative therapy led to its use primarily for palliation.

Early attempts to cure esophageal cancer with radical irradiation were generally restricted to patients with middle and upper esophageal lesions, whereas lesions of the distal esophagus were managed with surgical resection. In the 1950s, Buschke reported a 5-year survival rate of 5% for patients with lesions of the middle esophagus treated with irradiation, similar to the surgical results being reported at that time.[69]

For several reasons, the results of primary radiation therapy alone in the treatment of clinically localized esophageal cancer are poor: a 2-year survival rate of approximately 10% to 20% and 5-year survival rate of approximately 5% (Table 42-8). Several autopsy studies of untreated patients who died shortly after their diagnosis (it was presumed that the extent of tumor found at autopsy reflected the tumor burden at diagnosis) demonstrated that most patients had metastatic disease at presentation. Data pooled from four studies showed that 9% to 27% of patients had local disease only, whereas 50% to 89% of patients had local and distant disease.[70]

Evaluating the ability of irradiation as a single modality to control tumor locally, Aisner and colleagues reviewed the literature to examine the patterns of failure after irradiation alone and reported a local failure rate of 50% to 91% after doses greater than 5000 cGy and a distant failure rate of 23% to 66%.[71] In a later report, John and coworkers reviewed 35 patients treated with radiation alone and reported a locoregional recurrence rate of 77% after 5600 to 6100 cGy delivered

Table 42-8 Results with Irradiation Alone in the Treatment of Esophageal Cancer

Study	Study Interval	No. of Patients	5-Year Survival (%)
Hussey et al[172]	1945-1975	69	10
Newaishy et al[173]	1956-1974	444	9
Van Houtte[174]	1962-1972	81	3
Applequist et al[175]	1965-1974	50	4
Lewinsky et al[176]	1966-1971	85	4
Petrovich et al[177]	1963-1986	137	2
Girinsky et al[178]*	1986-1993	88	6 at 3 y

*Some patients received chemotherapy.

Table 42-9 Results of Randomized, Prospective Trials of Preoperative Irradiation for Esophageal Cancer

Study	Year	No. of Patients	Radiation Dose (cGy)	5-Year Survival (%)
Launois et al[179]	1981	67	4000	9.5
		57	Control	11.5
Huang et al[79]	1986	83	4000	45.5
		77	Control	25.0
Gignoux et al[81]	1987	102	3300	16
		106	Control	10
Nygaard et al[180]*	1992	108	3500	21
			Control	9
Arnott et al[181]	1992	176	2000	9
			Control	17

*Three-year survival data.

with standard fractionation.[72] Herskovic and colleagues found failures within the radiation field in 52% of patients treated to 6400 cGy.[73] Even in patients treated with relatively modern techniques using moderately high doses of radiation, local and distant failures constitute major clinical problems. This is not surprising because local control of most large solid tumors (>3 cm) cannot be obtained with high probability when using radiation doses in the range of 6000 cGy.

Early attempts to improve local control and survival combined irradiation and surgery. At Memorial Sloan-Kettering from 1956 through 1966, 85 patients were treated with preoperative irradiation and surgery, with 47 patients ultimately going on to resection. The overall crude 5-year survival rate was 6%, and the median survival time was 14 months. No tumor was seen in the surgical specimen in 7 (14%) of the tumors resected.[74] Nakayama and associates reported one of the largest series of a planned multistage program. After staging laparotomy and gastrostomy and after the patients' nutritional status was improved, a course of preoperative irradiation to 2000 to 2500 cGy in 4 to 5 fractions was followed by total esophagectomy. Intestinal continuity was fully established 6 to 12 months later. The investigators initially reported a 3-year survival rate of 27% for the patients treated with combined therapy, 22% for those treated with surgery alone, and 6% for irradiation alone,[75] but updated data showed a 5-year survival rate of 13% for the combined-modality cohort.[76] Akakura and colleagues reported the results of a preoperative regimen of 5000 to 6000 cGy given over 5 to 6 weeks and followed by a one-stage surgical resection and reanastomosis. The 5-year survival rate was 25%, compared with 14% for patients treated at his institution with surgery alone over the same period.[77] These studies were all retrospective reviews and did not allow direct comparisons of treatments.

In 1981, Launois reported the results of a prospective, randomized trial of 124 patients treated with surgery alone or with irradiation (4000 cGy delivered over 8 to 12 days) plus surgery 8 days after the completion of irradiation. The overall 5-year survival rates were not different: 9.5% for the irradiation and surgery group and 11.5% for patients treated with surgery alone.[78] In 1986, Huang and coworkers reported 160 highly selected patients with early-stage disease who were randomized in a prospective trial of 4000 Gy given preoperatively versus surgery alone. The 5-year survival rate was greater for the group that received combined-modality therapy: 45% versus 25%.[79] In 1989, however, an update concluded that the preoperative regimen offered no survival benefit.[80] The European Organization for Research and Treatment of Cancer (EORTC) randomized 208 patients to a regimen of preoperative irradiation (3300 cGy in 8 to 12 fractions) followed in 8 days with surgical resection as opposed to surgery alone. The investigators found no statistically significant difference in survival between the groups: 16% for the combined-modality arm and 10% for the irradiation-only arm.[81] Table 42-9 summarizes the results of external beam irradiation alone followed by surgical resection.

In collected series, even though approximately 15% of patients treated with preoperative irradiation had no tumor in the specimen at the time of resection, the result did not always translate into improved overall survival. Unlike the local failure rates of 50% to 91% seen with irradiation alone, the combination of irradiation and surgery resulted in a local failure rate of 20% to 58%. The modest improvements in local control have not resulted in significant improvements in overall survival, and there is little enthusiasm for the routine use of regimens employing only radiation therapy and surgery.

In the setting of curative therapy for esophageal cancer and in light of the positive results observed with multimodality therapies (discussed later), irradiation alone or preoperative radiation therapy should be restricted to patients who are medically unable to receive combined-modality therapy.

Combined-Modality Therapy

Chemoradiotherapy

In the past decade, numerous single institutions and cooperative groups have investigated the use of concurrent chemotherapy and radiation therapy as definitive treatment or as preoperative therapy for patients with localized esophageal cancer. It is not known whether the benefits of combined-modality therapy in esophageal cancer result more from an additive effect of two partially effective modalities or a synergism exists between the two therapies. However, a significant body of information suggests that chemotherapeutic agents such as 5-FU, cisplatinum, mitomycin C, gemcitabine, and taxol have a greater than additive effect when used in combination with radiation therapy. Most studies testing the safety and efficacy of multimodality therapy have used these agents and in a concurrent schedule. The mechanisms of the interactions between radiation and these chemotherapeutic agents are complex and not entirely understood. Because of the uncertainty of these interactions, it seems sensible to use both modalities with treatment schemes and at drug dose levels that are optimal when used alone rather than relying on a synergistic effect. The use of concurrent radiation therapy and chemotherapy in esophageal cancer is modeled primarily on the successful use of combined-modality therapy with 5-FU and mitomycin C in carcinomas of the anal canal.

Sequential Chemotherapy and Radiation

The usefulness of sequential chemotherapy followed by a course of definitive radiation therapy alone has been evaluated on a limited scale. Izquierdo and associates, in a study of 25 patients treated with sequential cisplatinum and bleomycin chemotherapy for three courses followed by a definitive thoracic irradiation, reported a 52% partial response rate and 16% complete response rate determined by CT and endoscopy. Although 64% of patients reported an improvement in dysphagia, the 1- and 4-year survival rates were a disappointing 20% and 8%, respectively.[82] Valerdi and colleagues, in an evaluation of two cycles of induction cisplatinum, vindesine, and bleomycin chemotherapy followed by definitive radiation therapy, also found a discouraging 15% overall survival rate at 5 years.[83] A phase II sequential study reported by Sharma and coworkers, which tested multiple cycles of 5-FU and cisplatinum followed by a definitive course of radiation (60 Gy), was equally disappointing; only one patient had a complete response (8%), and the median survival time was a dismal 39 weeks.[84] This approach has generated relatively little interest because it does not take advantage of the probable benefit of chemotherapy and irradiation given in combination.

Induction or Concurrent Chemotherapy and Radiation

Several investigators have tested the use of induction chemotherapy followed by a course of definitive irradiation delivered concurrently with chemotherapy. Stahl and associates, in a phase II study of 90 patients with locally advanced esophageal cancer, reported their results with three cycles of induction 5-fluorouracil, leucovorin, etoposide, and cisplatinum followed by irradiation to 40 Gy and concurrent cisplatinum plus etoposide. Of the 72 evaluable patients, 44 underwent resection, with a pathologic complete response rate of 22%. Unfortunately, the operative mortality rate was 15%. The median survival time for evaluable patients was 17 months, and the overall 3-year survival was 33%.[85] Minsky and associates, in a study of 45 patients with locally advanced disease, evaluated three cycles of induction 5-FU and cisplatinum followed by two additional cycles of chemotherapy delivered concurrently with irradiation to 64.8 Gy. Although the median survival time was an encouraging 20 months, six patients died of treatment-related toxicity.[86,87] The lack of benefit seen with neoadjuvant chemotherapy before surgical resection makes it less likely that neoadjuvant chemotherapy before concurrent chemoradiation therapy will be successful.

Twice-Daily Chemoradiation

Building on the encouraging data reported using twice-daily radiation therapy in other tumor sites, investigators have studied its usefulness in esophageal cancer. Kikuchi and colleagues, in a study reported in 1991 of 60 patients receiving twice-daily concomitant boost radiation therapy alone, observed a 5-year, cause-specific survival rate of 31.5%.[88] The study authors suggest the encouraging 5-year survival rate was related to improved local tumor control with the twice-daily regimen. In a retrospective analysis, Zhao and coworkers reported the feasibility of late-course accelerated hyperfractionated irradiation for early-stage esophageal carcinoma. All patients (n = 56) were treated with conventional fractionation during the first two thirds of the treatment to a dose of 41.4 Gy in 5 weeks. This was followed by a 2-week course of twice-daily irradiation (1.5 Gy per fraction) using reduced fields, for a cumulative dose of 67 to 70 Gy. The investigators observed an encouraging 5-year local control rate of 85%.[89] Girvin and associates, in a limited study of 29 patients, used twice-daily preoperative irradiation plus concurrent 5-FU, cisplatinum, and vinblastine, and they observed a remarkable complete response rate of 79%. Fifteen patients remained alive at a mean of 28 months.[90] However, data from a larger series using a similar concurrent 5-FU and cisplatinum and twice-daily irradiation regimen did not confirm the findings of Girvin and associates. For a cohort of 74 patients, Adelstein and colleagues observed a complete response rate of 27% and an operative mortality rate of 18%.[91]

Yu and associates reported their results with an alternating chemotherapy and twice-daily irradiation treatment schedule: cisplatinum and 5-FU delivered during weeks 1, 4, and 7 and the radiation therapy (1.8 to 2.0 Gy) delivered twice daily on weeks 2, 5, and 8, for a total radiation dose of 60 Gy. Of the 24 patients with esophageal cancer entered on the study, 7 died of acute toxicity.[92] Although a local tumor control rate of 94% was reported, the use of 1.8- to 2.0-Gy fractions delivered twice daily with chemotherapy carries significant toxicity. The use of concurrent chemotherapy and twice-daily irradiation shows promise but should be restricted to further investigation in the setting of a controlled clinical trial.

Concurrent Chemotherapy and Radiation

Table 42-10 reports the results of several nonrandomized trials employing concomitant chemotherapy and irradiation for the definitive treatment of esophageal cancer. Generally, the most successful treatment regimens have combined 5-FU (given by infusion) with mitomycin C or cisplatinum. Data reported from Wayne State employing a 5-FU plus cisplatinum regimen given concurrently with radiation therapy (5000 cGy) resulted in a median survival time of 19 months.[93] For patients treated with the same chemotherapy regimen but given a radiation dose of 3000 cGy, the median survival was 9.8 months, suggesting a dose-response effect. In a phase II trial reported by Coia and colleagues, 57 patients were treated with curative intent to 6000 cGy combined with 5-FU (1 $g/m^2/24$ h) as a continuous 4-day infusion during the first and fifth weeks of

Table 42-10 **Results from Combined Chemotherapy and Radiotherapy as Primary Therapy for Patients with Esophageal Cancer**

Study	No. of Patients	Radiation Dose (cGy)	Chemotherapy	Median Survival (mo)	2-Year Survival (%)
Kavanagh[112]	45	6000-6400	5-FU or VP-16, CDDP or Carbo	18	27
Seitz[182]	35	4000	5-FU, CDDP	17	45
Keane[183]	35	4500-5000	5-FU, MMC	NS	28
Hukku[184]	34	3000	5-FU, CDDP	NS	38
Podolsky[185]	30	4100-5000	5-FU, CDDP, MMC	11	29
Herskovic[93]	22	5000	5-FU, CDDP	19.5	36
Herskovic[93]	39	3000	5-FU, CDDP	9.8	20

5-FU, 5-fluorouracil; Carbo, carboplatin; CDDP, *cis*-diamminedichloroplatinum (cisplatinum); MMC, mitomycin C; NS, not significant; VP-16, etoposide.

Table 42-11 **Randomized Studies Comparing Radiation Alone with Combined Irradiation and Chemotherapy for Esophageal Cancer**

Study	No. of Patients	Radiation Dose (cGy)	Chemotherapy	2-Year Survival (%)
Araujo et al[95]	28	5000	Control	22
	31	5000	5-FU, MMC, Bleo	38
Sischy et al[96]*	62	6000	Control	12
	65	6000	MMC, 5-FU	30
Roussel et al[186]	69	4500	Control	31 at 1 y
	75	5600	MTX	35 at 1 y
Herskovic et al[73]	60	6400	Control	10
	61	5000	5-FU, CDDP	38

*Some patients went to resection.
5-FU, 5-fluorouracil; Bleo, bleomycin; CDDP, *cis*-diamminedichloroplatinum (cisplatinum); MMC, mitomycin C; MTX, methotrexate.

irradiation and mitomycin C (10 mg/m^2) on day 2, resulting in a median survival of 18 months and a 3-year survival rate of 29%.[94]

Subsequent randomized data (Table 42-11) from other investigators have shown benefit in patients treated with concurrent therapy. Araujo randomly assigned 59 patients to irradiation alone (50 Gy in 2.0-Gy daily fractions) versus the same dose of radiation delivered concurrently with 5-FU as a continuous infusion for 72 hours, mitomycin C, and bleomycin. The local complete response rate was 58% for irradiation alone versus 75% for the irradiation and chemotherapy group, and the overall 5-year survival rates were 6% and 16%, respectively.[95] Sischy and colleagues reported preliminary data from a study that randomized patients to 6000 cGy of radiation or to 6000 cGy with concurrent bolus mitomycin C and two cycles of infusional 5-FU. A median survival and 2-year survival advantage was observed in the combined-modality arm of the trial: 14.9 months versus 9.3 months and 30% versus 12%, respectively.[96]

The most important contemporary trial is that of Herskovic and colleagues (RTOG 85-01).[73] One hundred and twenty-one patients were randomized to 5000 cGy with concurrent chemotherapy with 5-FU (1000 mg/m^2 for 4 days) and cisplatinum (75 mg/m^2) or to irradiation with 6400 cGy alone. At 5 years, 27% of the combined-modality patients were alive, compared with none of the patients in the irradiation-only group. The median survival time for the combined-modality arm was 14.1 months, compared with 9.3 months for irradiation alone.[97] These results are important because they demonstrate a survival advantage with the combined-modality therapy and show that the survival advantage cannot be obtained by simply increasing the radiation dose, as might be the case if chemotherapy were acting as a pure radiation sensitizer.

The improvement in survival in the combination trials previously discussed is related in part to an improvement in local control. Tables 42-12 and 42-13 show the crude patterns of failure from several chemoradiation trials. These data suggest that combined-modality therapy produced a shift in the pattern of failure, from a local failure rate of 50% to 90% for irradiation alone to 20% to 50% with combined-modality therapy. Data from the Araujo randomized trial showing a survival advantage for patients treated with concurrent therapy also revealed a difference in local control; the local only failure rate was 74% for the irradiation-only group versus 46.5% for patients treated with irradiation and concurrent chemotherapy.[95] Herskovic and coworkers reported a crude local persistence or recurrence rate of 44% for patients treated with chemoradiation versus 64% for the irradiation-alone group.[73] The 2-year actuarial local failure rate was reduced from 68% to 43% and distant metastases from 70% to 25% with combined-modality therapy.

In an attempt to improve on the results of the Herskovic trial, the Intergroup 0122 phase II trial was designed to intensify the chemotherapeutic and radiation doses of the combined-modality arm of RTOG 85-01. The combined-modality regimen was modified as follows. The 5-FU continuous infusion was increased from 4 to 5 days; the total number of cycles of chemotherapy was increased from four to five cycles; three cycles of full-dose neoadjuvant 5-FU plus cisplatinum were delivered before the start of combined-modality therapy; and the radiation dose was increased from 5000

Table 42-12 Patterns of Failure after Concurrent Chemotherapy and Irradiation for Esophageal Cancer

Study	No. of Patients	Local (%)	Local and Distant (%)	Distant (%)
Kavanaugh et al[112]	45	24	20	18
Chan[187]	21	24	18	43
Coia et al[94]	57	25	23	16
Herskovic et al[93]	22	32 (5000 cGy)	18	23
Herskovic et al[93]	39	67 (3000 cGy)	18	3
Total	184	34.4	19.4	20.6

Table 42-13 Patterns of Failure from Randomized Studies of Therapy for Esophageal Cancer

Study	No. of Patients	Therapy	Local (%)	Distant (%)
Herskovic et al[73]	121	RT	64	70
		RT + Chemo	44	25
Araujo et al[95]	59	RT	74	13
		RT + Chemo	46.5	18
Minsky et al[98]	236	50-Gy RT + Chemo	52	
		64-Gy RT + Chemo	56	

Chemo, chemotherapy; RT, radiation therapy.

to 6480 cGy. The response, locoregional control, and survival rates for INT 0122 were similar to those reported in the combined-modality arm of RTOG 85-01. However, the incidence of treatment-related mortality was higher (9% versus 2%). Because of this unexpected increase in the mortality rate, this neoadjuvant treatment regimen was not pursued. Nonetheless, because the higher radiation dose was well tolerated and did not seem to be the cause of the higher mortality rate, it was used in the high-dose arm (64.8 Gy) of the subsequent randomized trial. In the Intergroup 0123 study, patients were randomized to receive combined-modality therapy consisting of four monthly cycles of 5-FU (1000 mg/m^2/24 h for 4 days), and cisplatinum (75 mg/m^2 bolus on day 1) with concurrent radiation to 64.8 Gy or to the same chemotherapy schedule but with the radiation dose limited to 50.4 Gy. Unfortunately, the trial was stopped after an interim analysis.[98] For the 218 eligible patients, there was no significant difference in median survival (13.0 versus 18.1 months), 2-year survival (31% versus 40%), or locoregional failure (56% versus 52%) between the high-dose and standard-dose treatment arms, respectively. Although 11 treatment-related deaths occurred in the high-dose arm compared with 2 in the standard-dose arm, 7 of the 11 deaths were patients who had received 50.4 Gy or less. The reason for the lack of benefit in the high-dose arm is unclear. When comparing the high-dose and low-dose arms, there was a significant prolongation of treatment time because of toxicity breaks when correcting for the number of radiation treatments and a significantly lower actual dose of 5-FU as a percentage of protocol dose.

An important concern regarding the use of combined-modality therapy is treatment toxicity. In the Wayne State series, 5 of 20 patients required hospitalization for intravenous hydration and nutritional support, and 38% developed pulmonary compromise (thought to result from bleomycin plus irradiation) that required corticosteroids.[93] The overall radiation dose appears to be important, as reflected in data from Sauter and colleagues.[99] In a study of 30 patients receiving concurrent chemotherapy and radiation (60 Gy), only 67% were able to complete the radiation as planned, and only 18 of the 30 patients were able to proceed to resection.[99] Coia and coworkers reported a 56% incidence of moderate to severe acute toxicities, and the RTOG 85-01 found side effects were severe in 44% and life threatening in 20% of patients in the combined-modality arm, compared with 25% and 3%, respectively, in the irradiation-only group.[73,94,100] Most of the toxicity was hematologic, along with significant reactions (i.e., esophagitis and stomatitis) in the oral cavity, pharynx, and esophagus. Although only 1 of 61 patients in the combined-modality group died of acute toxicity, only 50% of patients completed all four cycles of chemotherapy.

Although the magnitude of the benefit obtained with irradiation and concurrent 5-FU infusion and cisplatinum or mitomycin C is unclear, there seems little doubt that this combination represents a therapeutic advance over single-modality radiation therapy or chemotherapy. The optimal regimen has not been established. A radiation dose of 5000 cGy combined with infusional 5-FU (1000 mg/m^2/day for 4 days) and cisplatinum (100 mg/m^2), with the drugs given twice during radiation therapy, remains a reasonable standard.

Neoadjuvant or Adjuvant Chemotherapy and Surgery

A treatment approach being tested for a variety of solid tumors is the use of chemotherapy before surgery or chemoradiation. The rationale for this approach includes the early treatment of subclinical distant disease while the primary is also being treated, administering the drug when the patient can best tolerate the toxicities. In addition to improving local and distant control, it may also identify patients who can respond to additional chemotherapy for control of minimal residual disease.

Although a number of studies evaluating preoperative chemotherapy have demonstrated good response rates, only a few randomized studies have been reported. Roth and associates randomized 39 patients to surgery only or to preoperative cisplatinum, vindesine, and bleomycin chemotherapy.[101] The response rate to chemotherapy was 47%. There was no difference in survival, although patients who responded to chemotherapy had a median survival of more than 20 months, compared with 8.6 months for nonresponders.[101] A similar result from a randomized study of 147 patients reported by

Law and associates did not observe a survival advantage for patients receiving preoperative chemotherapy compared with surgery alone (median survival of 16.8 versus 13 months, respectively).[102] Kok and colleagues reported the results of a phase III randomized trial comparing neoadjuvant chemotherapy followed by surgery versus surgery alone.[103] Of the 160 operable patients entered, 64 patients received induction chemotherapy with two cycles of cisplatinum plus etoposide, and an equal number had resection. With a median follow-up of 15 months, the median survival time for patients receiving induction therapy was 18.5 months, compared with 11 months for patients going straight to resection.[103]

The most robust experience comes from the Medical Research Council Oesophageal Cancer Working Party.[104] In this study, 802 previously untreated patients with resectable esophageal cancer were randomized to receive two 4-day cycles, 3 weeks apart, of cisplatinum (80 mg/m^2) plus fluorouracil (1000 mg/m^2) daily by continuous infusion for 4 days, followed by surgery (n = 400) or surgery alone (n = 402). Overall survival was better in the chemotherapy-treated patients (hazard ratio = 0.79; 95% CI, 0.67 to 0.93; P = .004). The median survival was 16.8 months for patients randomized to chemotherapy and 13.3 months for the surgery-alone group. The 2-year survival rate of 43% was also improved for patients randomized to chemotherapy, compared with 34% for the surgery-only patients.

A striking contrast is provided by the data from Kelsen and coworkers from the Intergroup trial.[105] Four hundred sixty-seven patients were entered into this randomized trial comparing surgery alone versus induction chemotherapy (three cycles of cisplatinum plus 5-FU chemotherapy) followed by surgery in patients with operable disease. With a median follow-up of 55.4 months, there were no significant differences between the two groups in median survival: 14.9 months for the patients who received preoperative chemotherapy and 16.1 months for those who underwent immediate surgery (P = .53). At 1 year, the survival rate was 59% for those who received chemotherapy and 60% for those who had surgery alone; at 2 years, the survival rates were 35% and 37%, respectively.

The utility of postoperative chemotherapy (alone) has also been studied in a limited fashion. Armanios and associates, in a multicenter phase II trial, evaluated four cycles of adjuvant paclitaxel and cisplatinum chemotherapy in 59 patients with resected cancers of the distal esophagus, gastroesophageal junction, or gastric cardia.[106] All patients had locally advanced disease and margin-negative resections. Most patients (84%) were able to complete all four cycles of the chemotherapy with moderate toxicity. The reported 42% 3-year survival rate was encouraging, but with most patients (76%) eventually failing at distant sites, this study confirms the need for more effective systemic agents. In a randomized trial reported by Ando and colleagues, 242 patients with squamous cell carcinoma of the esophagus, after transthoracic esophagectomy with lymphadenectomy, were randomized to observation or to two courses of cisplatinum plus 5-FU chemotherapy.[107] Although an improvement in the 5-year disease-free survival rate was seen for patients receiving the adjuvant chemotherapy (55% versus 45%), the slight improvement in overall survival was not statistically significant (61% versus 52%). These results were not different from those observed in a 205-patient phase III trial showing no benefit with the addition of adjuvant cisplatinum plus vindesine chemotherapy to surgery.[108] Because of these conflicting data, the recommendation is for patients to receive neoadjuvant or adjuvant chemotherapy only as part of a clinical trial.

Preoperative Chemoradiation Therapy

The Southwestern Oncology Group (SWOG) and the Radiation Therapy Oncology Group (RTOG), based on pilot study data from Wayne State, performed two very similar phase II trials using concurrent chemotherapy and irradiation followed by planned resection. A total of 113 patients with initially resectable tumors received treatment with an infusional 5-FU and cisplatinum chemotherapy regimen with concurrent irradiation to a total dose of 3000 cGy. At the completion of the preoperative regimen, only 63% of the tumors remained resectable. The median survival time was 12 months, with 16% of patients alive at 3 years.[109] Of the 41 patients entered on a similar RTOG preoperative trial of concurrent irradiation and 5-FU plus cisplatinum, 7.5% were alive at 3 years.[110] The data from the University of Michigan and Duke are more positive, with 34% and 27% of patients, respectively, alive at 5 years.[111,112] The results from several nonrandomized trials employing cisplatinum and 5-FU–based preoperative chemoradiation strategies are shown in Table 42-14.

The next generations of chemoradiation trials attempted to incorporate more novel chemotherapeutic agents. Choi and colleagues, in a phase II study of irradiation and concurrent

Table 42-14 Results from Surgical Resection after Combined Irradiation and Chemotherapy for Esophageal Cancer

Study	No. of Patients	Radiation Dose (cGy)	Chemotherapy	2-Year Survival	Median Survival
Bates et al[116]	35	4500	5-FU, CDDP	22 mo	47%
Forastiere et al[188]	47	4400	5-FU, CDDP	31.3 mo	58%
Kavanaugh et al[112]	58	4500	5-FU or VP-16, CDDP or Carbo	37%	18 mo
Gignoux et al[81]	119	3750	CDDP	56.5 at 18 mo	NS
Bidoli et al[189]	34	3000	5-FU, CDDP	38%	NS
Seydel et al[110]	41	3000	5-FU, CDDP	15%	13 mo
Poplin et al[109]	71	3000	5-FU, CDDP	28%	
Stewart et al[190]	68	3000	5-FU, CDDP, VP-16/Leu	51%	NS
Urba et al[191]	69	4500 bid	Paclitaxel, CDDP	50%	24 mo
Meluch et al[192]	129	4400	Paclitaxel, 5-FU	47%	22 mo
Ajani et al[193]	43	45 Gy, CPT-11/CDDP	Paclitaxel, 5-FU, CDDP	42%	22.1 mo
Khushalani et al[115]	38	50.4	Oxaliplatin/5-FU	NS	NS

Carbo, carboplatin; CDDP, *cis*-diamminedichloroplatinum (cisplatinum); CPT-11, irinotecan; 5-FU, 5-fluorouracil; Leu, leucovorin; NS, not significant; VP-16, etoposide.

cisplatinum, 5-fluorouracil, and paclitaxel in 46 patients, observed a pathologic complete response rate of 45% for the 40 patients able to undergo resection.[113] The overall median survival time was 34 months, with 37% of patients alive at 5 years. The RTOG is evaluating in a randomized, phase II study the combination of irradiation and paclitaxel plus cisplatinum chemotherapy. Ilson and coworkers reported that the combination of cisplatinum and irinotecan possesses activity in this setting.[114] A 57% response rate was seen in 35 patients with metastatic or advanced esophageal cancer. The median duration of response was 4.2 months, and the toxicity was mild. This regimen is being investigated in combination with irradiation by the CALGB.

Data reported by Khushalani and associates suggest that a course of preoperative oxaliplatin at a dose of 85 mg/m^2 given on days 1, 15 and 29 concurrently with protracted venous infusion of 5-FU at a dose of 180 mg/m^2 given on days 8 to 42 with irradiation (50.4 Gy) is an active regimen in locally advanced esophageal cancer.[115] Thirty-eight patients received therapy: 22 with stage IV disease and 16 with stage II and III disease. Thirty-six patients completed the first cycle, and 24 patients completed the second cycle. The combined-modality therapy was well tolerated, but toxicity prevented dose escalation. Eleven cases of grade 3 and two cases of grade 4 clinical toxicities were observed in eight patients. After the first cycle, 29 patients (81%) had no clinical evidence of cancer in the esophageal mucosa. Thirteen patients underwent an operation with curative intent; five patients (38%) exhibited pathologic complete responses. The study authors conclude that oxaliplatin administered with protracted venous infusion [PVI] 5-FU and radiation therapy is safe, tolerable, and seems effective for the treatment of esophageal cancer. This regimen is being investigated by the SWOG.

Data reported from the University of North Carolina revealed an encouraging disease-free survival of 33 months and overall 3-year survival rate of 36% in a cohort of 35 patients receiving preoperative chemoradiation. The study found the use of preresection esophagogastroduodenoscopy was not useful for determining tumor response; although 77% of patients were reported to have had a clinical complete response preoperatively, 41% of these patients had residual tumor in the pathologic specimen.[116] The inaccuracy of endoscopy, further confirmed in a study from Roswell Park,[117] in discerning response after preoperative chemoradiation is important because it suggests that a strategy of initial chemoradiation therapy with surgery saved for patients who do not have a complete clinical response may not be successful. Whether PET is a better indicator of complete response needs to be determined.

Compared with historical unimodality series, failures locally and distantly have markedly improved with the advent of multimodality therapy (Table 42-15). In general, preoperative irradiation and chemotherapy result in a 30% to 50% rate of no pathologic evidence of tumor at the time of resection (Table 42-16). This finding predicts a favorable outcome. In the SWOG study, patients who had no evidence of disease at the time of surgery, compared with all patients who had a resection, had a projected 3-year survival of 45% versus 14%, and a median survival of 32 versus 14 months. Data from the University of North Carolina showed that the median survival for patients found to have no evidence of disease at resection was 37 months, compared with 13 months for patients with residual tumor. For patients who had no evidence of disease at the time of surgery in the Michigan series, the median survival was 70 months, compared with 29 months for all patients taken to resection. Although survival was higher in patients who had no disease in the surgical specimen in the University of Michigan and University of North Carolina series, some long-term survivors were patients with residual disease, suggesting that the addition of surgery, at least in a subset of patients, can produce additional cures after chemoradiation therapy.

Despite the encouraging results from the preoperative chemoradiation therapy studies, it is still unclear whether this approach is superior to surgery alone (Table 42-17). In a nonrandomized study of preoperative chemoradiation and

Table 42-15 Patterns of Failure for Surgical Resection after Concurrent Chemotherapy and Irradiation for Esophageal Cancer

Study	No. of Patients	Local (%)	Local and Distant (%)	Distant (%)
Herskovic et al[93]	50	36	38	16
MacFarlane et al[194]	22	0	38	16
Forastiere et al[41]	43	2	5	28
Kavanagh et al[112]	57	14	10	29

Table 42-16 Pathologic Findings after Preoperative Irradiation and Chemotherapy for Esophageal Cancer

Study	No. of Patients	pCR (5)	Radiation Dose (cGy)	Chemotherapy
Parker[195]	33	33%	30	5-FU, MMC
Seydel et al[110]	41	19.6%	30	5-FU, CDDP
Herskovic et al[93]	50	24%	30	5-FU, CDDP
Gignoux et al[81]	101	24%	37.5	CDDP
Forastiere et al[41]	43	24%	37.5-45	5-FU, CDDP, Vinb
Bates et al[116]	32	50%	45	5-FU, CDDP
Kavanaugh et al[112]	72	42%	45	5-FU or VP-16, CDDP or Carbo
Hoff[196]	51	21%	30	5-FU, CDDP

Carbo, carboplatin; CDDP, *cis*-diamminedichloroplatinum (cisplatinum); 5-FU, 5-fluorouracil; MMC, mitomycin C; pCR, pathologic complete response; Vinb, vinblastine; VP-16, etoposide.

Table 42-17 **Randomized Trials of Chemoradiation plus Surgery versus Surgery Alone for Esophageal Cancer**

Study	No. of Patients	Treatment	3-Year Median Survival	Significance
Urba et al[119]	50	S	16%	*P* = .15
	50	Chemo-RT-S	30%	
Walsh et al[120]	55	S	6%	*P* = .01
	58	Chemo-RT-S	32%	
Bosset et al[121]	139	S	37%*	*P* = .78
	143	Chemo-RT-S	39%*	
Burmeister et al[197]	256	S	19 mo	*P* = .38
		Chemo-RT-S	22 mo	

*Approximate 3-year survival determined from the survival curve.
Chemo, chemotherapy; RT, radiation therapy; S, surgery.

surgery versus surgery alone, Vogel reported an overall survival advantage for patients receiving multimodality therapy; 36% were alive at 5 years, compared with 11% of those receiving surgery alone.[118] Randomized data from Urba and coworkers, in a study of patients receiving preoperative concurrent chemoradiation compared with surgery alone, demonstrated an overall non–statistically significant survival advantage for patients in the multimodality arm: 30% were alive at 3 years, compared with 16% in the surgery-only arm.[119] Walsh and colleagues, in a randomized study of patients treated with two 5-day courses of 5-FU given on weeks 1 and 6 and cisplatinum with concurrent (4000 cGy) irradiation delivered before surgery compared with surgery alone, the reported (actuarial) survival data favored patients receiving combined-modality therapy; 32% were alive at 3 years, compared with 6% of the surgery-only group.[120] In contrast, a randomized study reported by Bosset and coworkers discerned no survival advantage for patients receiving preoperative chemoradiation versus surgery alone. This study, however, used a unique irradiation and chemotherapy schedule; irradiation was delivered by a split course, and over the span of 2 weeks, a total dose of 3700 cGy was delivered in 3.7-Gy daily fractions. The chemotherapy consisted of cisplatinum given before each week of irradiation. Patients were taken to surgery 2 to 4 weeks after completing the preoperative regimen.[121] The lack of benefit and increased toxicity observed for the combined-modality arm may have been predicted with the application of large radiation fractions, the inclusion of a planned treatment break, an inadequate recovery period between the preoperative therapy and surgery, and the use of single-agent chemotherapy. A meta-analysis of more than 1000 patients enrolled in nine randomized trials evaluated preoperative chemoradiation versus surgery alone and revealed a survival odds ratio at 3 years (0.66) in favor of patients receiving preoperative therapy.[122]

Because the Intergroup trial testing preoperative chemoradiation therapy versus surgery alone was abandoned before completion due to poor accrual, it is not likely U.S. studies will discern whether preoperative chemoradiation followed by surgery is superior to surgery alone.

Preoperative Chemoradiation Versus Definitive Chemoradiation

Bedenne and associates reported the results of a study comparing preoperative chemoradiation followed by surgery versus definitive chemoradiation.[123] In this randomized phase III trial, patients with locally advanced esophageal cancer received two cycles of induction 5-FU plus cisplatinum with radiation therapy delivered by standard fractionation (4600 cGy in 4.5 weeks) or as split-course therapy. Patients were then randomized to surgical resection or to completion of the definitive chemoradiation to 6100 cGy. Of the initial cohort of 455 patients, 259 were randomized. The reported 2-year survival rates and median survival times were not different: 34% and 17.7 months for patients in the preoperative arm versus 40% and 19.3 months for patients randomized to definitive chemoradiation (P = .56). Because these data have been reported only in abstract form, the results should be interpreted with caution. In a related German study, patients with locally advanced squamous carcinoma of the esophagus received induction chemotherapy followed by randomization to chemoradiotherapy (4000 cGy) followed by surgery (arm A) or to definitive chemoradiotherapy (arm B).[124] Analysis of the 172 randomized patients (86 patients per arm) showed overall survival to be equivalent; survival at 3 years was 31% for patients randomized to arm A and 24% for patients treated on arm B (P = .02).

A study from the Minnie Pearl Cancer Research Network reflects the difficulties associated with studies that randomize patients away from a surgical intervention.[125] Patients with locally advanced esophageal cancer were randomized to receive a course of preoperative chemoradiation followed by surgery or completion of the definitive chemoradiation. In this study, 194 patients were entered, but only 57 proceeded with the treatment to which they were randomized. When all patients were considered, survival was similar; the 3-year survival for patients (n = 91) undergoing resection was 35%, compared with 31% for patients (n = 50) receiving definitive chemoradiation. The data taken in aggregate suggest that the result with definitive chemoradiation is comparable to that with treatment strategies that incorporate preoperative chemoradiation and surgery.

PALLIATION AND SPECIAL TOPICS

Oncologists can achieve palliation with radiation therapy alone by using external beam doses ranging from 3000 cGy in 2 weeks to 5000 to 6000 cGy over 6 weeks (Table 42-18). Wara reported 103 patients who completed 5000 to 6000 cGy, with 89% having symptomatic improvement and 66% maintaining relief for 2 months or more. The average duration of palliation was 6.0 months. Dysphagia usually improved near the end of therapy, and almost all patients reported an arrest of their previous symptom progression.[126] Caspers found a 70.5% improvement in dysphagia, with 54% of patients able to eat solids until death.[127] Langer reported that dysphagia was improved in 60% of 51 patients treated to doses above 5000 cGy.[128] Coia and associates evaluated the swallowing function in 120 patients receiving concurrent chemotherapy and irradiation. Improvement in dysphagia was reported for

Table 42-18 **Results of Palliative Radiation Therapy with and without Chemotherapy for Esophageal Cancer**

Study	No. of Patients	Radiation Dose (Gy)	Chemotherapy	Palliation of Dysphagia (%)
Langer et al[128]	44	50-60	None	55
Albertsson et al[198]	67	<45	None	55
	43	>45	None	65
Wara et al[126]	169	50-60	None	67
Petrovich et al[177]	133	55	None	52
Whittington et al[199]	165	50-60	5-FU/MMC	87
Kavanagh et al[112]	143	44-60	CDDP/Carbo/VP-16/5-FU	71
RANDOMIZED				
Herskovic et al[73]	121	64	None	66
		50	5-FU/CDDP	58
Roussel et al[186]	170	56.2	None	78*
		56.2	MTX	71

*Control group.
Carbo, carboplatin; CDDP, *cis*-diamminedichloroplatinum (cisplatinum); 5-FU, 5-fluorouracil; MMC, mitomycin C; MTX, methotrexate; VP-16, etoposide.

88% of patients, with a median time to improvement of 2 weeks.[100] In the cohort of 25 patients who survived a year, all were able to tolerate soft or solid foods. Similarly encouraging results have been reported by Urba and colleagues; 59% of patients receiving chemotherapy and split-course radiation therapy who presented with dysphagia were able to achieve durable relief of their symptoms.[129] Aggressive concurrent irradiation and chemotherapy potentially increases morbidity in patients with incurable disease and a limited life span, but it may offer a more effective means of palliation.

Unfortunately, benign strictures can result from irradiation of esophageal cancers, resulting in a worsening of symptoms. O'Rourke and colleagues described a 30% incidence of benign stricture in a series of 80 patients treated with irradiation alone, which usually developed 4 to 6 weeks after therapy.[130] This is not inconsistent with the 17% reported by Beatty and coworkers.[131] For 25 patients treated with concurrent irradiation and chemotherapy, Coia and associates observed a 12% incidence of benign strictures that responded to one to two dilatations.[100]

Tracheoesophageal Fistula

In cases of malignant fistulas between the esophagus and the airway, treatment with irradiation should be discontinued according to the literature. In general, excision, bypass, or intubation has been recommended in an attempt to prevent further contamination of the airway. The median survival after these limited measures can be as brief as 6 to 10 weeks, with the procedures themselves resulting in a mortality rate of 10% to 32%.[132]

The development of a malignant fistulous tract between the esophagus and airway (trachea or bronchus) is not uncommon because of the anatomic location of the two structures. Most fistulas involve the trachea, but they can also involve a mainstem, lobar, or segmental bronchus. Involvement of the trachea with tumor can lead to fistula formation during irradiation because of necrosis of the tumor or the natural progression of the disease. The middle-third lesions are most commonly involved. It is estimated that the incidence of this complication is 5% to 10% of all patients with esophageal cancer.

Many oncologists accept that irradiation of a fistula worsens the condition because healing may be compromised by the radiation. Burt and colleagues found the survival for patients with an untreated fistulous tract to be 4% at 6 months and 1% at a year, compared with 15% and 5%, respectively, if treated with irradiation.[133] Yamado and coworkers reported 14 patients with fistulas from esophageal cancer who were treated with primary irradiation. Closure of the fistula occurred in 5 of 8 patients whose fistulas developed before or during irradiation. In two of these cases, the closure was long term.[134] For patients who developed fistulas during irradiation, resolution or closure was less likely. Gschossmann and associates described 10 patients with fistulas treated with irradiation at the Mayo Clinic and reported a median survival of 4.8 months.[135] The investigators stated that the severity of the fistulas did not increase with therapy. Data are accumulating on the safe use of chemotherapy with or without irradiation in managing patients with a tracheoesophageal fistula. Malik and coworkers observed an objective response and closure of the fistulas in two patients treated with chemoradiation and concluded that the presence of a fistula should not exclude a patient from receiving combined-modality therapy.[136]

It is difficult to determine whether aggressive combined-modality therapy will increase treatment-related morbidity in patients who present with airway-esophageal fistulas or develop them shortly after starting therapy. After the diagnosis of a fistulous tract into the airway is documented and the process is stabilized, proceeding with planned curative therapy for selected patients with localized disease is recommended.

Brachytherapy

For the treatment of esophageal cancer, intracavitary irradiation (i.e., brachytherapy) has been used for palliation. With the advent of remote afterloading techniques, continued improvements in endoscopy, and the use of high dose rate brachytherapy, interest has been renewed in intracavitary treatment alone or in combination with external beam irradiation and chemotherapy as a means of palliation or cure. The poor prognosis associated with esophageal cancer treated with irradiation results in part from the difficulty of achieving local control. Because of the position of the esophagus in the chest and its proximity to vital structures, it is not possible to increase the dose of external beam irradiation without increasing the risk of injury to neighboring organs. The use of intracavitary radiation therapy might allow us to increase safely the radiation dose to the tumor in the esophageal wall and thereby improve local control.

The results of high dose rate intracavitary radiation used as a local boost have been encouraging but limited. Sur and colleagues reported the results of 50 patients randomized to external beam radiation therapy alone that delivered 5500 cGy in 15 fractions or to 3500 cGy delivered by external beam irradiation followed by a high dose rate intracavitary boost totaling 1200 cGy in two 600-cGy sessions. Local control at 1 year was better for patients receiving brachytherapy, as was survival: 71% versus 38% and 78% versus 44%, respectively. Although no difference was observed in the development of strictures or fistulas, radiation-induced ulcerations were more common in the patients receiving intracavitary radiation therapy (32% versus 12%).[137] Hishikawa similarly observed improvement in local control and survival after combining external beam and intracavitary therapy and found an increase in treatment-related complications, including esophageal ulceration (90%), fistula (19%), and stricture formation (25%).[138,139]

Beitler and associates reported the results for 12 patients in a phase II study evaluating the use of concurrent chemotherapy, external and intraluminal irradiation, and surgery. None of the first eight patients was able to go on to resection, due to excessive toxicity.[140] Gaspar and colleagues, in a phase I/II study of external beam irradiation, brachytherapy, and chemotherapy, also reported significant toxicity with a comparable regimen.[141] Patients received 50-Gy external beam therapy, followed 2 weeks later with intraluminal therapy consisting of 5-Gy high dose rate brachytherapy on weeks 8, 9 and 10 or low dose rate brachytherapy (20 Gy) delivered on week 8. Cisplatinum plus 5-FU chemotherapy was given on weeks 1, 5, 8, and 11. Life-threatening toxicity was observed in 26% of patients, and four patients died of treatment-related toxicity. Treatment-related fistulas developed in 14% of patients, and the study authors urged extreme caution in combining external beam therapy with intraluminal therapy concurrent with chemotherapy.

In an attempt to discern the potential role of high dose rate brachytherapy delivered concurrently with chemotherapy in the setting of preoperative therapy, Peddada and colleagues observed a disappointing complete response rate of 13% and a 2-year survival rate of 33%.[142] The investigators concluded that high dose rate brachytherapy alone in conjunction with chemotherapy was inadequate for locoregional control and that such a regimen must be supplemented with external beam therapy. The optimal intracavitary dose and fractionation schemes have not been defined. Until the advantages and techniques of intracavitary therapy given with external beam become clear, their combined role in the curative management of patients remains experimental. The inability of brachytherapy to effectively treat extraesophageal spread of disease is a significant impediment to its use in the curative setting.

Several small series have demonstrated that intracavitary irradiation in the appropriately selected patient is a safe and effective method of palliation. Harvey reviewed 22 patients treated with 2000 cGy in three fractions of low dose rate brachytherapy or with 1250 cGy in one fraction of high dose rate brachytherapy and found that both modalities resulted in an equally effective palliation of dysphagia.[143] Accelerated treatments are especially suitable for patients in poor physical condition or with short life expectancy and thereby unlikely to complete a full course of external beam irradiation. Fleischmann and coworkers reported 90% resolution of dysphagia and acceptable morbidity in patients treated with intracavitary brachytherapy.[144] Similarly, Sur achieved 100% relief of dysphagia in nine patients treated with high dose rate brachytherapy but found that multiple applications were sometimes necessary.[137] Data reported by Gava and colleagues showed that the use of intraluminal brachytherapy in conjunction with chemotherapy or external beam irradiation resulted in superior palliation compared with brachytherapy alone: 89%, 88%, and 71%, respectively.[145] There was no apparent increase in treatment-related morbidity when two modalities were used. The incidence of stricture and fistula formation increased with brachytherapy fraction size: 9.5% for fractions less than 500 cGy, 20% between 500 and 800 cGy, and 38% at fractions larger than 800 cGy. The effectiveness of intraluminal brachytherapy, whether using a low dose rate or high dose rate, is well established. The use of high dose rate brachytherapy is attractive in that the palliative effect can often be seen rapidly and after a single intraluminal application.

When using intraluminal brachytherapy in esophageal cancer, the biology of the disease and the physics of brachytherapy must be considered. Esophageal tumors are rarely confined to the mucosa or the muscular wall and generally extend outside the walls of the esophagus, and they have a high incidence of nodal spread. The physics of brachytherapy are such that the dose is primarily delivered within a radius of approximately 1 cm from the applicator. It is unlikely that this approach can offer effective curative treatment for most esophageal carcinomas because of inadequate dose delivered to most of the tumor. It may, however, be useful for palliation when central disease is producing the symptoms and can be effectively treated with brachytherapy.

TECHNIQUES OF RADIATION THERAPY

Irradiation of esophageal cancer presents a challenge to radiation oncologists because these tumors are situated deeply in the mediastinum and are surrounded by several vital structures. The mucosa of the esophagus is mostly squamous epithelium, and the acute mucosal reaction can be substantial. Acute odynophagia and dysphagia are common, usually developing 10 to 14 days after the initiation of therapy. The esophagitis is self-limited, but without nutritional support, the acute mucosal reaction may force a delay in completing treatment.

Portions of the upper airway, trachea, bronchi, lung parenchyma, and pleura are unavoidably irradiated during therapy. The pulmonary parenchyma is highly susceptible to radiation injury, with clinical lung damage reported at total fractionated doses in the range of 2000 cGy. However, the likelihood of clinical injury is strongly related to the baseline pulmonary status of the patient and to the amount of lung in the radiation field. It is not uncommon for patients with esophageal cancer to have chronic obstructive lung disease, which affects the amount of normal lung that can be safely irradiated. The risk of permanent lung injury and late pneumonitis is also volume related.

If the heart is irradiated, complications involving the pericardium and the myocardium can result. Irradiation of the pericardium can result in acute and chronic pericarditis. The former is an uncommon complication of thoracic irradiation that usually develops within the first year after treatment. It is often associated with viral infections, which makes diagnosis difficult. Although it has been reported at doses in the range of 2000 to 4000 cGy, acute pericarditis generally occurs with substantially higher doses. Chronic pericarditis typically develops more than 1 year after treatment and is related to the volume of pericardium treated.

Irradiation of the myocardium can result in an interstitial fibrosis that decreases cardiac function. This phenomenon is also related to the volume of irradiated heart and a total dose that exceeds 4200 cGy. Data have associated irradiation of the myocardium with an acceleration of coronary arteriosclerosis and sudden cardiac death in young persons. Because most patients with esophageal cancer are older and have a limited prognosis, myocardial injury is not a significant clinical problem.

Other rare complications of esophageal irradiation include the risk of rib fractures, damage to the brachial plexus, and spinal cord injury, which is potentially the most devastating side effect. In general, it is safe to treat the spinal cord with radiation alone to a cumulative dose of 4500 cGy delivered in standard 170- to 200-cGy single daily fractions.

The difficulty in controlling esophageal tumors with irradiation is related to the frequent extension of tumor through the thin esophageal wall, the involvement of vital mediastinal structures (including large vessels and the trachea), and the threat of perforation; the frequent spread of tumor through submucosal lymphatics, ultimately involving long segments of the esophagus; the spread of tumor to regional lymph nodes; the presence of metastatic disease in a high percentage of patients (occult or clinically apparent); and the generally poor nutritional status of patients at presentation. Esophageal tumors can extend submucosally in the cephalocaudad direction for a significant distance from the primary tumor. In 1962, Miller reported a 15% incidence of longitudinal microscopic tumor spread more than 6 cm from the primary lesion, and the incidence of regional nodal disease was approximately 40% to 70%[146]; in an autopsy series reported by Bloedorn, nodal disease was present in 70%.[147]

For lesions of the cervical esophagus, radiation fields must take into account tumor spread into mediastinal, supraclavicular, and low anterior cervical lymph nodes. The supraclavicular nodes usually are electively treated in patients with high thoracic tumors, but not those with middle or distal thoracic tumors. Although there is a significant incidence of involvement of the celiac axis lymph nodes, little information supports routine treatment of this nodal group without evidence of tumor involvement.

The typical radiation field extends approximately 5 cm above and below gross tumor, with a field width of approximately 8 cm (Fig. 42-1). The size of the tumor dictates the exact field width needed to obtain adequate mediastinal nodal coverage and to adequately cover the primary tumor mass. Over 4 to 5 weeks, patients treated for cure with radiation alone receive approximately 4000 cGy in 1.8- to 2.0-Gy daily fractions with anteroposterior treatment fields. The dose is limited to this level to prevent overdose to the spinal cord, which usually receives a higher dose per fraction than the esophagus. The treatments then continue, avoiding the spinal cord, with oblique or lateral fields to a total dose of 4500 to 6000 cGy. Careful consideration must be given to the dose and volume of lung irradiated so as not to exceed tolerance. It is difficult to use higher doses of radiation because of the limited tolerance of the esophagus and surrounding normal structures. High-energy radiation beams are crucial for adequate dose delivery. When irradiation is used concurrently with sensitizing chemotherapy without surgery, the recommended total dose is of 5000 to 6000 cGy.

FUTURE POSSIBILITIES AND A TREATMENT ALGORITHM

Until recently, patients with esophageal cancer were allowed little optimism because treatment successes were rare. Although surgery alone remains the standard of care in the management of localized esophageal cancer, oncologists must consider the mounting data on combined-modality approaches. Today, the treatment of this disease requires a multimodality approach by the surgeon, radiation oncologist, and medical oncologist and a clear understanding of the interactions and toxicities associated with these modalities. The results using combined irradiation and 5-FU plus cisplatinum–based chemotherapy as definitive therapy or in the preoperative setting are encouraging but require further confirmation with multi-institutional, phase III trials when combined with surgery, because although local control has improved, the effect on survival has not been well demonstrated. The significant morbidity associated with multimodality therapy also must be considered. The evolving role of newer chemotherapeutic agents such as paclitaxel, oxaliplatin, and the molecularly targeted compounds and attempts at altering radiation schedules and doses are being studied. The optimal combinations of chemotherapy, irradiation, and surgery are being actively investigated.

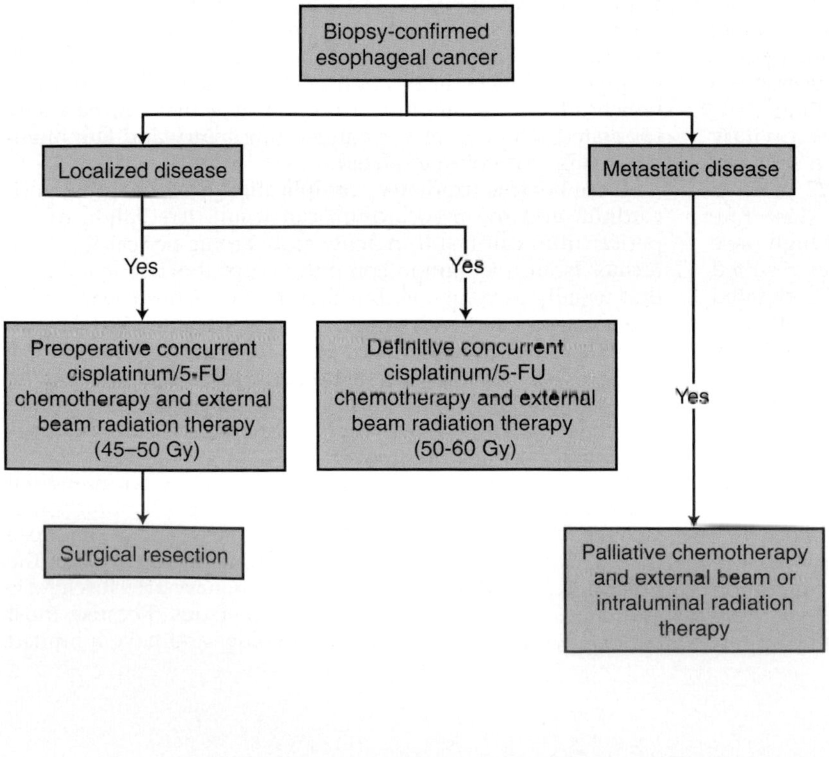

Figure 42-1 Treatment algorithm for newly diagnosed esophageal cancer. 5-FU, 5-fluorouracil.

REFERENCES

1. Jemal A, Murray T, Ward E, et al: Cancer statistics, 2005. CA Cancer J Clin 55:10-30, 2005.
2. Kelsen D: Preoperative chemoradiotherapy for esophageal cancer. J Clin Oncol 19:283-285, 2001.
3. Parkin DM, Bray F, Ferlay J, et al: Global cancer statistics, 2002. CA Cancer J Clin 55:74-108, 2005.
4. Younes M, Henson DE, Ertan A, et al: Incidence and survival trends of esophageal carcinoma in the United States: racial and gender differences by histological type. Scand J Gastroenterol 37:1359-1365, 2002.
5. Kubo A, Corley DA: Marked multi-ethnic variation of esophageal and gastric cardia carcinomas within the United States. Am J Gastroenterol 99:582-588, 2004.
6. Hesketh PJ, Clapp RW, Doos WG, et al: The increasing frequency of adenocarcinoma of the esophagus. Cancer 64:526-530, 1989.
7. Pohl H, Welch HG: The role of overdiagnosis and reclassification in the marked increase of esophageal adenocarcinoma incidence. J Natl Cancer Inst 97:142-146, 2005.
8. Blot WJ, Devesa SS, Kneller RW, et al: Rising incidence of adenocarcinoma of the esophagus and gastric cardia. JAMA 265:1287-1289, 1991.
9. Devesa SS, Blot WJ, Fraumeni JF Jr: Changing patterns in the incidence of esophageal and gastric carcinoma in the United States. Cancer 83:2049-2053, 1998.
10. Steyerberg EW, Earle CC, Neville BA, et al: Racial differences in surgical evaluation, treatment, and outcome of locoregional esophageal cancer: a population-based analysis of elderly patients. J Clin Oncol 23:510-517, 2005.
11. Brown LM, Hoover RN, Greenberg RS, et al: Are racial differences in squamous cell esophageal cancer explained by alcohol and tobacco use? J Natl Cancer Inst 86:1340-1345, 1994.
12. Baron PL, Gates CE, Reed CE, et al: P53 overexpression in squamous cell carcinoma of the esophagus. Ann Surg Oncol 4:37-45, 1997.
13. Wilson KT, Fu S, Ramanujam KS, et al: Increased expression of inducible nitric oxide synthase and cyclooxygenase-2 in Barrett's esophagus and associated adenocarcinomas. Cancer Res 58:2929-2934, 1998.
14. Katja CZ, Mario S, Artur-Aron W, et al: Cyclooxygenase-2 expression in human esophageal carcinoma. Cancer Res 59:198-204, 1999.
15. Shamma A, Yamamoto H, Doki Y, et al: Up-regulation of cyclooxygenase-2 in squamous carcinogensis of the esophagus. Clin Can Res 6:1229-1238, 2000.
16. Casson AG, Mukopadhyay T, Cleary KR, et al: p53 gene mutations in Barrett's epithelium and esophageal cancer. Cancer Res 51:4495-4499, 1991.
17. Arber N, Lightdale C, Rotterdam H, et al: Increased expression the cyclin D1 gene in Barrett's esophagus. Cancer Epidemiol Biomarkers Prev 5:457-459, 1996.
18. Barrett MT, Sanchez CA, Galipeau PC, et al: Allelic loss of 9p21 and mutation of the CDKN2/p16 gene develop as early lesions during neoplastic progression in Barrett's esophagus. Oncogene 13:1867-1873, 1996.
19. Suleiman UL, Harrison M, Britton A, et al: H2-receptor agonist may increase the risk of cardio-oesophageal adenocarcinoma: a case-control study. Eur J Cancer Prev 9:185-191, 2000.
20. Engel LS, Chow WH, Vaughan TL, et al: Population attributable risks of esophageal and gastric cancers. J Natl Cancer Inst 95:1404-1413, 2003.
21. Malay CC, Galipeau PC, Li X, et al: Selective advantageous mutations and hitchhikers in neoplasms: p16 lesions are selected in Barrett's esophagus. Cancer Res 64:3414-3427, 2004.
22. Itakura Y, Sasano H, Shiga C, et al: Epidermal growth factor receptor overexpression in esophageal carcinoma. An immunohistochemical study correlated with clinicopathologic findings and DNA amplification. Cancer 74:795-804, 1994.
23. Yacoub L, Goldman H, Odze RD: Transforming growth factor-alpha, epidermal growth factor receptor, and MiB-1 expression in Barrett's-associated neoplasia: correlation with prognosis. Mod Pathol 10:105-112, 1997.
24. Gibson MK, Abraham SC, Wu TT, et al: Epidermal growth factor receptor, p53 mutation, and pathological response predict survival in patients with locally advanced esophageal cancer treated with preoperative chemoradiotherapy. Clin Cancer Res 9:6461-6468, 2003.
25. Montesano R, Hollstein M, Hainaut P: Genetic alterations in esophageal cancer and their relevance to etiology and pathogenesis: a review. Int J Cancer 69:225-235, 1996.
26. Montesano R, Hollstein M, Hainaut P: Molecular etiopathogenesis of esophageal cancers. Ann Ist Super Sanita 32:73-84, 1996.
27. Coggi G, Bosari S, Roncalli M, et al: P53 protein accumulation and p53 gene mutation in esophageal carcinoma. A molecular and immunohistochemical study with clinicopathologic correlations. Cancer 79:425-432, 1997.
28. Schrump DS, Chen A, Consuli U, et al: Inhibition of esophageal cancer proliferation by adenoviral-mediated delivery of p16INK4. Caner Gene Ther 51:5766-5769, 1996.
29. Lord RV, Park JM, Wickramasinghe K, et al: Vascular endothelial growth factor and basic fibroblast growth factor expression in esophageal adenocarcinoma and Barrett esophagus. J Thorac Cardiovasc Surg 125:246-253, 2003.
30. Kulke MH, Odze RD, Mueller JD, et al: Prognostic significance of vascular endothelial growth factor and cyclooxygenase 2 expression in patients receiving preoperative chemoradiation for esophageal cancer. J Thorac Cardiovasc Surg 127:1579-1586, 2004.
31. Jiang W, Kahn SM, Tomita N, et al: Amplication and expression of the human cyclin D gene in esophageal cancer. Cancer Res 52:2980-2983, 1992.
32. Barrett MT, Galipeau PC, Sanchez CA, et al: Determination of the frequency of loss of heterozygosity in esophageal adenocarcinoma by cell sorting, whole genome amplication and microsatellite polymorphisms. Oncogene 12:1873-1878, 1996.
33. Gore RM: Esophageal cancer. Radiol Clin North Am 35:243-263, 1997.
34. Auerbach O, Stout AP, Hammond EC, et al: Histologic changes in esophagus in relation to smoking habits. Arch Environ Health 11:4-15, 1965.
35. Sons HU: Etiologic and epidemiologic factors of carcinoma of the esophagus. Surg Gynecol Obstet 165:183-190, 1987.
36. Stellman JM, Stellman SD: Cancer and the work place. CA Cancer J Clin 46:70-92, 1996.
37. Meltzer SJ: The molecular biology of esophageal carcinoma. Recent Results Cancer Res 142:1-8, 1996.
38. Togowa K, Rustigi A: Human papillomavirus DNA sequences in esophagus squamous cell carcinoma. Gastroenterology 107:128-136, 1994.
39. He D, Zhang DK, Lam KY, et al: Prevalence of HPV infection in esophageal squamous cell carcinoma in Chinese patients and its relationship to the p53 mutation. Int J Cancer 72:959-964, 1997.
40. Holscher AH, Bollschweiler E, Schneider PM, et al: Prognosis of early esophageal cancer. Comparison between adeno and squamous cell carcinoma. Cancer 76:178-186, 1995.
41. Forastiere AA, Orringer MB, Perez-Tamayo C, et al: Preoperative chemoradiation followed by transhiatal esophagectomy for carcinoma of the esophagus: final report. J Clin Oncol 11:1118-1123, 1993.
42. Dumont P, Wihlm JM, Roeslin N, et al: Results of surgery of esophageal cancer. Analysis of a series of 349 cases based on resection methods. Ann Chir 47:773-783, 1993.
43. Sihvo EI, Rasanen JV, Knuuti MJ, et al: Adenocarcinoma of the esophagus and the esophagogastric junction: positron emission tomography improves staging and prediction of survival in distant but not in locoregional disease. J Gastrointest Surg 8:988-996, 2004.
44. Flanagan FL, Dehdashti F, Siegel BA, et al: Staging of esophageal cancer with 18F-fluorodeoxyglucose positron emission tomography. AJR Am J Roentgenol 168:417-424, 1997.
45. Block MI, Patterson GA, Sundaresan RS, et al: Improvement in staging of esophageal cancer with the addition of positron emission tomography. Ann Thorac Surg 64:770-776, discussion 776-777, 1997.
46. Luketich JD, Friedman DM, Weigel TL, et al: Evaluation of distant metastases in esophageal cancer: 100 consecutive positron

emission tomography scans. Ann Thorac Surg 68:1133-1136, discussion 1136-1137, 1999.
47. Flamen P, Lerut A, Van Cutsem E, et al: Utility of positron emission tomography for the staging of patients with potentially operable esophageal carcinoma. J Clin Oncol 18:3202-3210, 2000.
48. van Westreenen HL, Westerterp M, Bossuyt PM, et al: Systematic review of the staging performance of 18F-fluorodeoxyglucose positron emission tomography in esophageal cancer. J Clin Oncol 22:3805-3812, 2004.
49. Hiele M, De Leyn P, Schurmans P, et al: Relation between endoscopic ultrasound findings and outcome of patients with tumors of the esophagus or esophagogastric junction. Gastrointest Endosc 45:381-386, 1997.
50. Natsugoe S, Yoshinaka H, Morinaga T, et al: Ultrasonographic detection of lymph-node metastasis in superficial carcinoma of the esophagus. Endoscopy 28:674-679, 1996.
51. Krasna MJ, Reed CE, Jaklitsch MT, et al: Thoracoscopic staging of esophageal cancer: a prospective, multiinstitutional trial. Cancer and Leukemia Group B Thoracic Surgeons. Ann Thorac Surg 60:1337-1340, 1995.
52. Holscher AH, Bollschweiller E, Bumm R, et al: Prognostic factors of resected adenocarcinoma of the esophagus. Surgery 118:845-855, 1995.
53. Torek F: The first successful case of resection of the thoracic portion of the oesphagus for carcinoma. Surg Gynecol Obstet 16:614-617, 1913.
54. Ohsawa T: The surgery of the esophagus. Arch Jpn Chir 10:605, 1933.
55. Adams W, Phemister D: Carcinoma of the lower thoracic esophagus: report of successful resection and esophagogastrostomy. J Thoracic Surg 7:621-632, 1938.
56. Moertel CG: Carcinoma of the esophagus: is there a role for surgery? The case against surgery. Am J Dig Dis 23:735-736, 1978.
57. Mariette C, Piessen G, Balon JM, et al: Surgery alone in the curative treatment of localised oesophageal carcinoma. Eur J Surg Oncol 30:869-876, 2004.
58. Frunberger L, Kraus B, Dworak O: Distribution of lymph nodes and lymph node metastasis in esophageal carcinoma. Zentralb Chir 121:102-105, 1996.
59. Sun K, Zhang R, Zhang D, et al: Prognostic significance of lymph node metastasis in surgical resection of esophageal cancer. Chin Med J 109:89-92, 1996.
60. Collard JM, Otte JB, Reynaert MS, et al: Extensive lymph node clearance for cancer of the esophagus or cardia: merits and limits in reference to 5 year absolute survival. Hepatogastroenterology 42:619-627, 1995.
61. Fok M, Siu KF, Wong J: A comparison of transhiatal and transthoracic resection for carcinoma of the thoracic esophagus. Am J Surg 158:414-419, 1989.
62. Pac M, Basoglu A, Kocak H, et al: Transhiatal versus transthoracic esophagectomy for esophageal cancer. J Thorac Cardiovasc Surg 106:205-209, 1993.
63. Stark SP, Romberg MS, Pierce GE, et al: Transhiatal versus transthoracic esophagectomy for adenocarcinoma of the distal esophagus and cardia. Am J Surg 172:478-481, 1996.
64. Chu KM, Law SY, Fok M, et al: A prospective randomized comparison of transhiatal and transthoracic resection for lower-third esophageal carcinoma. Am J Surg 174:320-324, 1997.
65. Rentz J, Bull D, Harpole D, et al: Transthoracic versus transhiatal esophagectomy: a prospective study of 945 patients. J Thorac Cardiovasc Surg 125:1114-1120, 2003.
66. Hulscher JB, Tijssen JG, Obertop H, et al: Transthoracic versus transhiatal resection for carcinoma of the esophagus: a meta-analysis. Ann Thorac Surg 72:306-313, 2001.
67. Exner A: Veber die Behandlung von Oesophagus Karzinomen mit Ardiumstrahlen. Wien Klin Wochenschr 17:514, 1904.
68. Guisez J: Présentation de malades soignés par la radiumtherapie pour cancer de l'oesophage. Bull Mem Soc Med Hôp Paris 47:908-912, 1931.
69. Buschke F: Surgical and radiological results in the treatment of esophageal carcinoma. AJR Am J Roentgenol 71:9-21, 1954.
70. Kelsen D: Neoadjuvant therapy for gastrointestinal cancers. Oncology 7:25-32, 1993.
71. Aisner JF, Forastiere AA, Aroney R: Patterns of recurrence for cancer of the lung an esophagus. Cancer Treat Symp 2:87-105, 1983.
72. John MF, Flam MS, Mowry P, et al: Radiotherapy alone and chemoradiation for nonmetastatic esophageal carcinoma. A critical review of chemoradiation. Cancer 63:2397-2403, 1989.
73. Herskovic AMK, al-Sarraf M, Leichman L, et al: Combined chemotherapy and radiotherapy compared with radiotherapy alone in patients with cancer of the esophagus. N Engl J Med 326:1593-1598, 1992.
74. Goodner JT: Surgical and radiation treatment of cancer of the thoracic esophagus. AJR Am J Roentgenol 105:523-528, 1969.
75. Nakayama K, Orihata H, Yamaguchi K: Surgical treatment combined with preoperative concentrated irradiation for esophageal cancer. Cancer 20:778-788, 1967.
76. Isono K, Onoda S, Ishikawa T, et al: Studies on the causes of deaths from esophageal carcinoma. Cancer 49:2173-2179, 1982.
77. Akakura I, Nakamura Y, Kakegawa T, et al: Surgery of carcinoma of the esophagus with preoperative radiation. Chest 57:47-57, 1970.
78. Launois B, DeLarue D, Campion JP, et al: Preoperative radiotherapy for carcinoma of the esophagus. Surg Gynecol Obstet 153:690-692, 1981.
79. Huang G, Gu X, Wang I: Experience with combined preoperative irradiation and surgery for carcinoma of the esophagus. Gann Monogr Cancer Res 31:159-164, 1986.
80. Wang LJ, Huang GJ: Combined preoperative irradiation and surgery versus surgery alone for carcinoma of the midthoracic esophagus: a prospective randomized study in 360 patients (abstract). Presented at the Fourth World Congress of the International Society for Diseases of the Esophagus. Rennes, France, 1989.
81. Gignoux M, Rousell A, Paillot B: The value of preoperative radiotherapy in esophageal cancer: results of a study of the EORTC. World J Surg 11:426-432, 1987.
82. Izquierdo MA, Marcuello E, Gomez de Segura G, et al: Unresectable nonmetastatic squamous cell carcinoma of the esophagus managed by sequential chemotherapy (cisplatin and bleomycin) and radiation therapy. Cancer 71:287-292, 1993.
83. Valerdi JJ TM, Illarramendi JJ, Domininguez MA, et al: Neoadjuvant chemotherapy and radiotherapy in locally advanced esophageal carcinoma: long-term results. Int J Radiat Oncol Biol Phys 27:843-847, 1993.
84. Sharma D, Krasnow SH, Davis EB, et al: Sequential chemotherapy and radiotherapy for squamous cell esophageal carcinoma. Am J Clin Oncol 20:151-153, 1997.
85. Stahl M, Wilke H, Fink U, et al: Combined preoperative chemotherapy and radiotherapy in patients with locally advanced esophageal cancer. Interim analysis of a phase II trial. J Clin Oncol 14:829-837, 1996.
86. Minsky BD, Neuberg D, Kelsen DP, et al: Neoadjuvant chemotherapy plus concurrent chemotherapy and high-dose radiation for squamous cell carcinoma of the esophagus: a preliminary analysis of the phase II Intergroup Trial 0122. J Clin Oncol 14:149-155, 1996.
87. Minsky BD, Neuberg D, Kelsen DP, et al: Final report of Intergroup Trial 0122 (ECOG PE-289, RTOG 90-12): Phase II trial of neoadjuvant chemotherapy plus concurrent chemotherapy and high-dose radiation for squamous cell carcinoma of the esophagus. Int J Radiat Oncol Biol Phys 43:517-523, 1999.
88. Kikuchi Y: Study on clinical application of multiple fractions per day radiation therapy with concomitant boost technique for esophageal cancer [in Japanese]. Hokkaido Igaku Zasshi 68:537-556, 1993.
89. Zhao KL, Wang Y, Shi XH: Late course accelerated hyperfractionated radiotherapy for clinical T1-2 esophageal carcinoma. World J Gastroenterol 9:1374-1376, 2003.
90. Girvin GW, Matsumoto GH, Bates DM, et al: Treating esophageal cancer with combination of chemotherapy, radiation and excision. Am J Surg 169:557-559, 1995.
91. Adelstein DJ, Rice TW, Becker M, et al: Use of concurrent chemotherapy, accelerated fractionation radiation, and surgery for patients with esophageal carcinoma. Cancer 80:1011-1020, 1997.

92. Yu L, Vikram B, Malamud S, et al: Chemotherapy rapidly alternating with twice-a-day accelerated radiation therapy in carcinomas involving the hypopharynx or esophagus: an update. Cancer Invest 13:567-572, 1995.
93. Herskovic A, Leichman L, Lattin P, et al: Chemo/radiation with and without surgery in the thoracic esophagus: the Wayne State experience. Int J Radiat Oncol Biol Phys 15:655-662, 1988.
94. Coia LR, Engstrom PF, Paul AR, et al: Long term results of infusional 5-FU, mitomycin C, and radiation as primary management of esophageal carcinoma. Int J Radiat Oncol Biol Phys 20:29-36, 1991.
95. Araujo C, Souhami L, Gil R, et al: A randomized trial comparing radiation therapy versus concomitant radiation therapy and chemotherapy in carcinoma of the thoracic esophagus. Cancer 67:2258-2261, 1991.
96. Sischy B, Ryan L, Haller D, et al: Interim report of EST 1282 phase III protocol for the evaluation of combined modalities in the treatment of patients with carcinoma of the esophagus, stage I and II [abstract]. Proc Am Soc Clin Oncol 9:105, 1990.
97. al-Sarraf M, Martz K, Herskovic A, et al: Progress report of combined chemoradiotherapy versus radiotherapy alone in patients with esophageal cancer: an intergroup study. J Clin Oncol 15:277-284, 1997.
98. Minsky BD, Pajak TF, Ginsberg RJ, et al: INT 0123 (Radiation Therapy Oncology Group 94-05) phase III trial of combined-modality therapy for esophageal cancer: high-dose versus standard-dose radiation therapy. J Clin Oncol 20:1167-1174, 2002.
99. Sauter ER, Coia LR, Keller SM: Pre-operative high dose radiation and chemotherapy in adenocarcinoma of the esophagus and esophagogastric junction. Ann Surg Oncol 1:5-10, 1994.
100. Coia L, Soffen E, Schultheiss T, et al: Swallowing function in patients with esophageal cancer treated with concurrent radiation and chemotherapy. Cancer 71:281-286, 1993.
101. Roth JA, Pass HI, Flanagan MM, et al: Randomized clinical trial of pre-operative and post-operative adjuvant chemotherapy with cisplatin, vindesine, and bleomycin for carcinoma of the esophagus. J Thorac Cardiovasc Surg 96:242-248, 1988.
102. Law S, Fok M, Chow S, et al: Preoperative chemotherapy versus surgical therapy alone for squamous cell carcinoma of the esophagus: a prospective randomized trial. J Thorac Cardiovasc Surg 114:210-217, 1997.
103. Kok TC, Lanschot J, Siersema PD, et al: Neoadjuvant chemotherapy in operable esophageal squamous cell cancer: final report of a phase III multi-center randomized controlled trial [abstract]. Proc Am Soc Clin Oncol 16:277a, 1997.
104. Medical Research Council Oesophageal Cancer Working Group: Surgical resection with or without preoperative chemotherapy in oesophageal cancer: a randomised controlled trial. Lancet 359:1727-1733, 2002.
105. Kelsen DP, Ginsberg R, Pajak TF, et al: Chemotherapy followed by surgery compared with surgery alone for localized esophageal cancer. N Engl J Med 339:1979-1984, 1998.
106. Armanios M, Xu R, Forastiere AA, et al: Adjuvant chemotherapy for resected adenocarcinoma of the esophagus, gastro-esophageal junction, and cardia: phase II trial (E8296) of the Eastern Cooperative Oncology Group. J Clin Oncol 15:4495-4499, 2004.
107. Ando N, Iizuka T, Ide H, et al: Surgery plus chemotherapy compared with surgery alone for localized squamous cell carcinoma of the thoracic esophagus: a Japan Clinical Oncology Group Study—JCOG9204. J Clin Oncol 15:4592-4596, 2003.
108. Ando N, Iizuka T, Kakegawa T, et al: A randomized trial of surgery with and without chemotherapy for localized squamous carcinoma of the thoracic esophagus: the Japan Clinical Oncology Group Study. J Thorac Cardiovasc Surg 114:205-209, 1997.
109. Poplin E, Fleming T, Leichman L, et al: Combined therapies for squamous cell carcinoma of the esophagus, a Southwest Oncology Group Study (SWOG-8037). J Clin Oncol 5:622-628, 1990.
110. Seydel HG, Leichman L, Byhardt R, et al: Preoperative radiation and chemotherapy for localized squamous cell carcinoma of the esophagus: a RTOG Study. Int J Radiat Oncol Biol Phys 14:33-35, 1988.
111. Forastiere A, Orringer MB, Perez-Tamayo C, et al: Concurrent chemotherapy and radiation therapy followed by transhiatal esophagectomy for local-regional cancer of the esophagus. J Clin Oncol 8:119-127, 1990.
112. Kavanagh B, Ancher M, Leopold K, et al: Patterns of failure following combined modality therapy or esophageal cancer, 1984-1990. Int J Radiat Oncol Biol Phys 24:633-642, 1992.
113. Choi N, Park SD, Lynch T, et al: Twice-daily radiotherapy as concurrent boost technique during two chemotherapy cycles of adjuvant chemoradiotherapy for resectable esophageal carcinoma: mature results of a phase II study. Int J Radiat Oncol Biol Phys 60:111-122, 2004.
114. Ilson DH, Saltz L, Enzinger P, et al: Phase II trial of weekly irinotecan plus cisplatin in advanced esophageal cancer. J Clin Oncol 17:3270-3275, 1999.
115. Khushalani NI, Leichman CG, Proulx G, et al: Oxaliplatin in combination with protracted-infusion fluorouracil and radiation: report of a clinical trial for patients with esophageal cancer. J Clin Oncol 20:2844-2850, 2002.
116. Bates BA, Detterbeck FC, Bernard SA, et al: Concurrent radiation therapy and chemotherapy followed by esophagectomy for localized esophageal carcinoma. J Clin Oncol 14:156-163, 1996.
117. Shaukat A, Mortazavi A, Demmy T, et al: Should preoperative, post-chemoradiotherapy endoscopy be routine for esophageal cancer patients? Dis Esophagus 17:129-135, 2004.
118. Vogel SB, Mendenhall WM, Sombeck MD, et al: Downstaging of esophageal cancer after pre-operative radiation and chemotherapy. Ann Surg 221:685-693, 1995.
119. Urba SG, Orringer MB, Turrisi A, et al: Randomized trial of preoperative chemoradiation versus surgery alone in patients with locoregional esophageal carcinoma. J Clin Oncol 19:305-313, 2001.
120. Walsh TN, Noonan N, Hollywood D, et al: A comparison of multimodal therapy and surgery for esophageal adenocarcinoma. N Engl J Med 335:462-467, 1996.
121. Bosset JF, Gignoux M, Triboulet JP, et al: Chemoradiotherapy followed by surgery compared with surgery alone in squamous cell cancer of the esophagus. N Engl J Med 337:161-167, 1997.
122. Urschel JD, Vasan H: A meta-analysis of randomized controlled trials that compared neoadjuvant chemoradiation and surgery to surgery alone for resectable esophagus cancer. Am J Surg 185:538-543, 2003.
123. Bonnetain F, Bouche O, Michel P, et al: A comparative longitudinal quality of life study using the Spitzer quality of life index in a randomized multicenter phase III trial (FFCD 9102): chemoradiation followed by surgery compared with chemoradiation alone in locally advanced squamous resectable thoracic esophageal cancer. Ann Oncol 17:827-834, 2006.
124. Stahl M, Stuschke M, Lehmann N, et al: Chemoradiation with and without surgery in patients with locally advanced squamous cell carcinoma of the esophagus. J Clin Oncol 23:2310-2317, 2005.
125. Gray JR, Hainsworth JD, Meluch AA, et al: Concurrent paclitaxel/carboplatin/infusional 5-FU/radiation therapy (RT) with or without subsequent esophageal resection in patients with localized esophageal cancer: a Minnie Pearl Cancer Research Network [abstract 4018]. Proc Am Soc Clin Oncol 24, 2005.
126. Wara WM, Mauch PM, Thomas AN, et al: Palliation for carcinoma of the esophagus. Radiology 121:717-720, 1976.
127. Caspers R, Welvaart K, Verkes R: The effect of radiotherapy on dysphagia and survival in patients with esophageal cancer. Radiother Oncol 12:15-23, 1988.
128. Langer M, Choi NC, Orlow E, et al: Radiation therapy alone or in combination with surgery in the treatment of carcinoma of the esophagus. Cancer 58:1208-1213, 1986.
129. Urba SG, Orringer MB, Iannettoni M, et al: Concurrent cisplatin, paclitaxel, and radiotherapy as preoperative treatment for patients with locoregional esophageal carcinoma. Cancer 98:2177-2183, 2003.
130. O'Rourke IC, Tiver K, Bull C, et al: Swallowing performance after radiation therapy for carcinoma of the esophagus. Cancer 61:2022-2026, 1988.
131. Beatty JD, DeBoer G, Rider WG: Carcinoma of the esophagus—pretreatment assessment, correlation of radiation treatment parameters with survival and identification and management of radiation treatment failure. Cancer 43:2254-2267, 1979.
132. Little AG, Ferguson MK, Demeester TR, et al: Esophageal carcinoma with respiratory tract fistula. Cancer 53:1322-1328, 1984.

133. Burt M, Diehl W, Martini N, et al: Malignant esophagorespiratory fistula: management options and survival. Ann Thorac Surg 52:1222-1228, 1991.
134. Yamado S, Takai Y, Ogawa Y, et al: Radiotherapy for malignant fistula to other tract. Cancer 64:1026-1028, 1989.
135. Gschossmann JM, Bonner JA, Foote RL, et al: Malignant tracheoesophageal fistula in patients with esophageal cancer. Cancer 72:1513-1521, 1993.
136. Malik SM, Krasnow SH, Wadleigh RG: Closure of tracheoesophageal fistulas with primary chemotherapy in patients with esophageal cancer. Cancer 73:1321-1323, 1994.
137. Sur RK, Singh DP, Sharma SC, et al: Radiation therapy of esophageal cancer: role of high dose rate brachytherapy. Int J Radiat Oncol Biol Phys 22:1043-1046, 1992.
138. Hishikawa Y, Kamikonya N, Tanaka S, et al: Esophageal stricture following high dose rate intracavitary irradiation for esophageal cancer. Radiology 159:715-716, 1986.
139. Hishikawa Y, Tanaka S, Miura T: Esophageal fistulae associated with intracavitary irradiation for esophageal carcinoma. Radiology 159:549-551, 1986.
140. Beitler JJ, Wadler S, Haynes H, et al: Phase II trial of chemotherapy, external and intraluminal radiation plus surgery for oesophageal cancer. Med Oncol 12:115-120, 1995.
141. Gaspar LR, Qian C, Kocha WI, et al: A phase I/II study of external beam radiation, brachytherapy and concurrent chemotherapy in localized cancer of the esophagus (RTOG 92-07): preliminary toxicity report. Int J Radiat Oncol Biol Phys 37:593-599, 1997.
142. Peddada AV, Harvey JC, Anderson PJ, et al: High dose rate intraluminal radiation in a combined modality treatment plan for carcinoma of the esophagus. J Surg Oncol 52:160-163, 1993.
143. Harvey JC, Fleishman EH, Bellotti JE, et al: Intracavitary radiation in the treatment of advanced esophageal carcinoma: a comparison of high dose rate vs. low dose rate brachytherapy. J Surg Oncol 52:101-104, 1993.
144. Fleischman EH, Kagan AR, Bellotti JE, et al: Effective palliation for inoperable esophageal cancer using intensive intracavitary radiation. J Surg Oncol 44:234-237, 1990.
145. Gava A, Fontan L, Bolner A, et al: High-dose-rate brachytherapy in esophageal carcinoma: the Italian experience. Radiol Med (Torino) 91:118-121, 1996.
146. Miller C: Carcinoma of thoracic oesophagus and cardia. A review of 405 cases. Br J Surg 49:507-522, 1962.
147. Bloedorn FG, Kasdorf H: Radiotherapy in squamous cell carcinoma of the esophagus. *In* Clark RL, Cumley RW, McCay JE, et al (eds): Oncology. Chicago, Year Book Medical Publishers, 1971, pp 111-120.
148. Smithers DW: Adenocarcinoma of the oesophagus. Thorax 11:257-267, 1956.
149. Birgisson S, Rice TW, Easley KA, et al: The lack of association between adenocarcinoma of the esophagus and gastric surgery: a retrospective study. Am J Gastroenterol 92:216-221, 1997.
150. Lui KE, Panchal AS, Santhanagopal A, et al: Epidermal growth factor stimulates proton efflux from chondrocytic cells. J Cell Physiol 192:102-112, 2002.
151. Wilkinson NW, Black JD, Roukhadze E, et al: Epidermal growth factor receptor expression correlates with histologic grade in resected esophageal adenocarcinoma. J Gastrointest Surg 8:448-453, 2004.
152. Inada S, Koto T, Futami K, et al: Evaluation of malignancy and the prognosis of esophageal cancer based on an immunohistochemical study (p53, E-cadherin, epidermal growth factor receptor). Surg Today 29:493-503, 1999.
153. Engstrom P, Lavin P, Lassen D: Evaluation of mitomycin and cisplatinum in advanced esophageal carcinoma. Cancer Treat Rep 67:709-711, 1983.
154. Davis S, Shanmugathasa M, Kessler W: *Cis*-dichorodiammine platinum (II) in the treatment of esophageal carcinoma. Cancer Treat Rep 64:709-711, 1980.
155. Ezdinli E, Gelber R, Desai D, et al: Chemotherapy of advanced esophageal carcinoma. Cancer 46:2149-2153, 1980.
156. Orringer MB, Marshall B, Iannettoni MD: Transhiatal esophagectomy: Clinical experience and refinements. Ann Surg 230:392-400, 1999.
157. Bezwoda W, Derman D: Treatment of advanced oesophageal cancer with vindesine [abstract]. Proceedings of the 13th International Cancer Congress. Volume 41, 1983.
158. Ajani JA, Ilson DH, Daugherty K, et al: Activity of taxol in patients with squamous cell carcinoma and adenocarcinoma of the esophagus. J Natl Cancer Inst 86:1086-1091, 1994.
159. Harstrick A, Bokemeyer C, Preusser P, et al: Phase II study of single-agent etoposide in patients with metastatic squamous-cell carcinoma of the esophagus. Can Chemother Pharmacol 29:321-322, 1992.
160. Muhr-Wilkenshoff F, Hinkelbein W, Ohnesorge I, et al: A pilot study of (CPT-11) as single-agent therapy in patients with locally advanced or metastatic esophageal carcinoma. Int J Colorectal Dis 18:330-334, 2003.
161. Tew WP, Shah M, Schwartz G, et al: Phase II trial of erlotonib for second-line treatment in advanced esophageal cancer [abstract]. Proc Am Soc Clin Oncol 10:247, 2005.
162. Janmaat ML, Gallegos-Ruiz MI, Rodriguez JA, et al: Predictive factors for outcomes in a phase II study of gefitinib in second-line treatment of advanced esophageal cancer patients. J Clin Oncol 24:1612-1619, 2006.
163. Kelsen DP, Cvitkovic E, Bains M: *Cis*-diammine II platinum II and bleomycin in the treatment of esophageal carcinoma. Cancer Treat Rep 62:1041-1046, 1978.
164. Kelsen K, Coonley C, Hilaris B: Cisplatinum, vindesine, and bleomycin combination chemotherapy of local-regional and advanced esophageal carcinoma. Am J Med 75:639-652, 1983.
165. Petrasch S, Welt A, Reinacher A, et al: Chemotherapy with cisplatin and paclitaxel in patients with locally advanced, recurrent or metastatic oesophageal cancer. Br J Cancer 78:511-514, 1998.
166. Grisselbrecht C, Calvo F, Mignot L: Fluorouracil, adriamycin, and cisplatinum combination chemotherapy of advanced esophageal carcinoma. Cancer 52:974-977, 1983.
167. Kok TC, Van der Gaast A, Dees J, et al: Cisplatin and etoposide in oesophageal cancer: a phase II study. Rotterdam Oesophageal Tumour Study Group. Br J Cancer 74:980-984, 1996.
168. Bleiberg H, Conroy T, Paillot B, et al: Randomised phase II study of cisplatin and 5-fluorouracil (5-FU) versus cisplatin alone in advanced squamous cell oesophageal cancer. Eur J Cancer 33:1216-1220, 1997.
169. Kolaric K, Maricic Z, Roth A, et al: Combination of bleomycin and adriamycin with and without radiation on the treatment of inoperable esophageal cancer. A randomized study. Cancer 45:2265-2273, 1980.
170. Kroep JR, Pinedo HM, Giaccone G, et al: Phase II study of cisplatin preceding gemcitabine in patients with advanced oesophageal cancer. Ann Oncol 15:230-235, 2004.
171. Williamson SK, McCoy SA, Gandara DR et al: Phase II trial of gemcitabine plus irinotecan in patients with esophageal cancer: a Southwest Oncology Group (SWOG) trial. Am J Clin Oncol 29:116-122, 2006.
172. Hussey DH, Barkley HT, Bloedorn FG: Carcinoma of the esophagus. *In* Fletcher GH (ed): Textbook of Radiotherapy. Philadelphia, Lea and Febiger, 1980, pp 688-703.
173. Newaishy GA, Read GA, Duncan W, et al: Results of radical radiotherapy of squamous cell carcinoma of the esophagus. Clin Radiol 33:347-352, 1982.
174. Van Houtte P: Radiotherapie du cancer l'oesophage. Acta Gastroenterol Belg 40:121-128, 1977.
175. Appelqvist O, Silvo J, Rissanen P: The results of surgery and radiotherapy in the treatment of small cell carcinomas of the thoracic oesophagus. Ann Clin Res 11:184-188, 1979.
176. Lewinsky BS, Annes GP, Mann SG: Carcinoma of the esophagus: an analysis of results and of treatment techniques. Radiol Clin North Am 44:192-204, 1975.
177. Petrovich Z, Langholz B, Formenti S, et al: Management of carcinoma of the esophagus: The role of radiotherapy. Am J Clin Oncol 14:80-86, 1991.
178. Girinsky T, Auperin A, Marsiglia H, et al: Accelerated fractionation in esophageal cancers: a multivariate analysis on 88 patients. Int J Radiat Oncol Biol Phys 38:1013-1018, 1997.
179. Launois B, DeLarue D, Campion JP, et al: Preoperative radiotherapy for carcinoma of the esophagus. Surg Gynecol Obstet 153:690-692, 1981.

180. Nygaard K, Hagen S, Hansen HS, et al: Pre-operative radiotherapy prolongs survival in operable esophageal carcinoma: a randomized, multicenter study of pre-operative radiotherapy and chemotherapy. The second Scandinavian trial in esophageal cancer. World J Surg 16:1104-1109, discussion 1110, 1992.
181. Arnott SJ, Duncan W, Kerr GR, et al: Low dose preoperative radiotherapy for carcinoma of the oesophagus: results of a randomized clinical trial. Radiother Oncol 24:108-113, 1992.
182. Seitz J, Giovannini M, Paduat-Cesana J, et al: Inoperable nonmetastatic squamous cell cancer of the esophagus managed by concomitant chemotherapy (5-fluorouracil and cisplatin) and radiation therapy. Cancer 66:214-219, 1990.
183. Keane TJ, Harwood AR, Elhakim T, et al: Radical radiation therapy with 5-fluorouracil and mitomycin C for oesophageal squamous cell cancer. Radiother Oncol 4:205-210, 1985.
184. Hukku S, Gernades P, Vasishta S, et al: Radiation therapy alone and in combination with bleomycin and 5-FU in advanced carcinoma of the esophagus. Indian J Med 26:131-136, 1989.
185. Podolsky WJ, Xavier AM, Wittlinger PS, et al: Radiotherapy alone and chemoradiation for non-metastatic esophageal carcinoma. Cancer 63:2397-2403, 1989.
186. Roussel A, Bleiberg H, Dalesio O, et al: Palliative therapy of inoperable oesphageal carcinoma with radiotherapy and methotrexate: final results of a controlled clinical trial. Int J Radiat Oncol Biol Phys 16:67-72, 1989.
187. Chan A, Wong A, Arthur K: Concomitant 5-fluorouracil infusion, mitomycin C and radical radiation therapy in esophageal squamous cell carcinoma. Int J Radiat Oncol Biol Phys 16:59-65, 1989.
188. Forastiere AA, Heitmiller RF, Lee DJ, et al: Intensive chemoradiation followed by esophagectomy for squamous cell and adenocarcinoma of the esophagus. Cancer J Sci Am 3:144-152, 1997.
189. Bidoli P, Spinazze S, Valente M, et al: Combined chemotherapy (CT)-radiotherapy (RT) ± esophagectomy (E) in squamous cell cancer of the esophagus (SCCE) [abstract]. Proc Am Soc Clin Oncol 9:110, 1990.
190. Stewart JR, Hoff SJ, Johnson DH, et al: Improved survival with neoadjuvant therapy and resection for adenocarcinoma of the esophagus. Ann Surg 218:571-576, 1993.
191. Urba SG, Orringer MB, Ianettonni M, et al: Concurrent cisplatin, paclitaxel, and radiotherapy as preoperative treatment for patients with locoregional esophageal carcinoma. Cancer 98:2177-2183, 2003.
192. Meluch AA, Greco FA, Gray JR, et al: Preoperative therapy with concurrent paclitaxel/carboplatin/infusional 5-FU and radiation therapy in locoregional esophageal cancer: final results of a Minnie Pearl Cancer Research Network phase II trial. Cancer J 9:251-260, 2003.
193. Ajani JA, Walsh G, Komaki R, et al: Preoperative induction of CPT-11 and cisplatin chemotherapy followed by chemoradiotherapy in patients with locoregional carcinoma of the esophagus or gastroesophageal junction. Cancer 100:2347-2354, 2004.
194. MacFarlane SD, Hill LD, Jolly PC, et al: Improved results of surgical treatment for esophageal and gastroesophageal junction carcinomas after preoperative combined chemotherapy and radiation. J Thorac Surg 95:415-423, 1988.
195. Parker EF, Gregorie HB, Prioleau WH, et al: Carcinoma of the esophagus—observations of 40 years. Ann Surg 195:618-623, 1982.
196. Hoff J, Stewart R, Sawyers L: Preliminary results with neoadjuvant therapy and resection for esophageal carcinoma. Ann Thorac Surg 56:282-286, 1993.
197. Burmeister BH, Smithers BM, Gebski V, et al: Surgery alone versus chemoradiotherapy followed by surgery for resectable cancer of the oesophagus: a randomised controlled phase III trial. Lancet Oncol 6:659-668, 2005.
198. Albertsson M, Ewers SB, Widmark H, et al: Evaluation of the palliative effect of radiotherapy for esophageal carcinoma. Acta Oncol 28:267-270, 1989.
199. Whittington R, Coia L, Haller D, et al: Adenocarcinoma of the esophagus and esophago-gastric junction: the effects of single and combined modalities on the survival and patterns of failure following treatment. Int J Radiat Oncol Biol Phys 19:593-603, 1990.

CHAPTER 43

UNCOMMON THORACIC TUMORS

Tony Y. Eng, Craig W. Stevens, David Rice, and Charles R. Thomas, Jr.

INCIDENCE

Approximately 0.13 to 0.15 cases of thymoma occur per 100,000 people in the United States each year. The most common tumor type occurs in the anterior mediastinum, accounting for 30% of anterior mediastinal lesions and 20% of all mediastinal tumors in adults.

Between 1 and 2 cases of carcinoid tumor occur per 100,000 people in the United States. The rate for bronchopulmonary carcinoids is 0.6 per 100,000.

The incidence for malignant pleural mesothelioma is 10 cases per million people. The incidence is increasing, and the disease is a significant clinical problem for patients exposed to asbestos.

BIOLOGIC CHARACTERISTICS

Thymomas are usually slow-growing tumors with an indolent natural history. Histologically benign, they are capable of local and regional invasion and have a marked tendency for local recurrence. The two most important prognostic factors are invasiveness and completeness of surgical resection.

Pulmonary carcinoids generally are nonfunctional, but they can secrete physiologically active substances, leading to paraneoplastic syndromes. Biologic behavior ranges from indolent to aggressive. Prognostic factors are atypical histology, nodal involvement, and the presence of symptoms at presentation.

Malignant pleural mesothelioma is aggressive, and local disease progression is the main cause of symptoms and death. It spreads by direct extension and seeding in the pleural space. Local recurrence is the most common cause of relapse.

STAGING EVALUATION

Patients with suspected thymoma require routine screening blood work and chemistries, chest radiograph, computed tomography (CT), and CT- or ultrasound-guided fine-needle aspiration biopsy of the mass. Bronchoscopy, video-assisted thoracic surgery, mediastinoscopy, or anterior thoracoscopy may help yield a diagnosis before resection.

Pulmonary carcinoid requires a similar workup. Transbronchial biopsy or CT- or ultrasound-guided fine-needle aspiration biopsy may establish the diagnosis preoperatively.

Patients with suspected mesothelioma should be asked about a history of asbestos exposure. CT of the chest is needed. Although thoracentesis, percutaneous fine-needle aspiration, or ultrasound-guided core biopsy may yield the diagnosis, the most accurate method is video-assisted thoracoscopic biopsy.

PRIMARY THERAPY

Complete en bloc surgical resection is the treatment of choice for all thymomas, regardless of invasiveness, except in rare advanced cases with extensive intrathoracic or extrathoracic metastasis.

Curative resection of localized primary lung carcinoids is the treatment of choice. Endoscopic laser ablation may be used to alleviate tumor obstruction, improve atelectasis, and reduce inflammation before resection.

Pleurectomy and extrapleural pneumonectomy are extensive surgical procedures for mesothelioma. Patients require careful assessment to ensure that the operation will be tolerated physiologically.

ADJUVANT THERAPY

Encapsulated, noninvasive, stage I thymomas do not require adjuvant postoperative radiation therapy. Radiation therapy is an effective adjuvant therapy for invasive thymomas.

Typical carcinoids usually do not require adjuvant therapy after resection. Certain symptoms, including flushing, can be relieved by pharmacologic agents. Adjuvant radiation therapy has been used in patients with large tumors (>3 cm), positive nodes, positive margins, atypical histology, residual disease, and inoperable disease.

For mesothelioma, high-dose postoperative radiation therapy can dramatically reduce ipsilateral thoracic failures. Postoperative irradiation should include the entire volume immediately adjacent to the pleural space, but it is technically difficult to deliver.

LOCALLY ADVANCED DISEASE

Preoperative adjuvant radiation therapy or primary radiation therapy alone has been advocated in thymoma patients with unresectable advanced disease. Chemotherapy may produce an improvement in overall survival. Chemoradiation may be appropriate for some patients with locally advanced unresectable malignant thymoma.

Radiation therapy has been used adjuvantly or to palliate symptoms from locally advanced or metastatic carcinoids.

Extrapleural pneumonectomy followed by irradiation may provide better local control of mesothelioma than surgery alone.

PALLIATION

Radiation therapy can provide effective palliation in patients with symptomatic metastatic or unresectable disease.

Primary thoracic tumors can originate from any intrathoracic organ or tissue, producing tumors such as lung cancer, lymphoma, esophageal neoplasms, mediastinal tumors (i.e., thymic, neurogenic, and germ cell tumors), cardiac malignancies, pulmonary or bronchial carcinoid tumors, mesothelioma, and tracheal tumors. Among the different thoracic tumors, lung cancer is by far the most common, and it is discussed in Chapters 40 and 41. This chapter focuses on the less common neoplasms: thymic tumors, pulmonary carcinoids, and mesothelioma.

THYMIC TUMORS

The thymus gland is a lobulated lymphoepithelial organ located in the anterior mediastinum. It is thought to function in T-lymphocyte differentiation and maturation. It slowly involutes and is largely replaced by adipose tissue during adulthood.[1] Although various tumors and cysts can arise in the thymus, tumors of the thymus are relatively uncommon.

Most thymic tumors arise in the epithelial cells of the thymus. They account for approximately 50% of anterior mediastinal masses.[2,3] The most common thymic tumors are thymoma, thymic carcinoma, and thymic carcinoids. Thymomas, 90% of which are found in the anterosuperior mediastinum, are commonly associated with myriad paraneoplastic syndromes. They are the most common tumor found in the anterior mediastinum.[2,4] Thymomas are associated with an exuberant lymphoid component composed of immature cortical thymocytes. Although they appear benign histologically, they may exhibit invasive behavior clinically.

Like thymomas, thymic carcinomas (i.e., type C thymomas) also arise in the thymic epithelium, but they have a higher propensity for capsular invasion and widespread metastases, especially those with features of high-grade malignancy. The histologic subtypes include clear cell carcinoma, sarcomatoid carcinoma, and anaplastic carcinoma. Low-grade thymic carcinomas (well-differentiated squamous cell carcinomas, basaloid carcinomas, and mucoepidermoid carcinomas) also exist. They are characterized by a relatively more favorable clinical course, with a lower incidence of local recurrence and metastasis.[5,6]

Thymic carcinoid tumors, also known as neuroendocrine tumors of the thymus, are rare, accounting for less than 5% of all neoplasms of the anterior mediastinum. They are thought to originate from endodermal cell (or foregut cellular) precursors. Unlike carcinoids in other locations, most thymic carcinoids are clinically aggressive. They often invade locally, and commonly metastasize to regional lymph nodes.[7] Approximately 50% of patients may develop endocrine abnormalities.[8]

Etiology and Epidemiology

The cause of thymic tumors is largely unknown. There is a reported association between Epstein-Barr virus (EBV) infection and tumors of the thymus. Defective viral genomes have been isolated in patients with lymphoepithelioma-like thymic carcinoma.[9,10] The diseases are more frequent in Far Eastern countries, where the incidence of EBV infection is higher.[11-13] Childhood thymus irradiation has been linked to the development of thymic tumors,[14] and familial cases have been reported, suggesting a possible relationship with cytogenetic abnormalities.[15,16] In patients with primary thymic carcinoid tumors, up to 30% were reported in the setting of multiple endocrine neoplasia (MEN) type 1 and 2.[17,18] Other studies have reported a distinctive chromosome abnormality involving translocation of fragments of chromosome 15 and 19 [t(15:19)(q15:p13)] in thymic carcinoma, often in young adults or pediatric patients with high-grade thymic carcinoma.[19-21] Deletion of the short arm of chromosome 6 is associated with benign thymomas.[22] However, the molecular mechanisms of thymic tumor oncogenesis are largely unknown. There are frequent recurrent aberrations involving chromosome 6 reported for patients with thymoma, suggesting the presence of several putative tumor suppressor genes on this chromosome that may contribute to the pathogenesis of thymoma.[23]

In a small study of 37 cases, most type A thymomas did not show any chromosomal aberration, whereas type B3 thymomas and thymic carcinoma (i.e., type C thymoma) showed partially shared genetic aberrations, including the loss of chromosome 6 and gain of 1q.[24] The loss of chromosome 6, on which the human leukocyte antigen (HLA) locus and some of the tumor suppressor genes have been identified, and gain of 1q, to which growth promoter genes have been mapped,[24-26] may play a role in tumorigenesis and pathogenesis of the paraneoplastic autoimmunity characteristics of thymoma. Such chromosomal aberrations have been implicated in a variety of human neoplasms.[27,28]

The true incidence of thymoma is unknown, and the annual incidence in the United States has not been well defined. The Surveillance, Epidemiology, and End Results (SEER) program reported a thymoma incidence of .13 to .15 per 100,000 people.[29,30] Although thymoma occurs infrequently, it is the most common tumor of the anterior mediastinum, representing approximately 30% of anterior mediastinal lesions and 20% of all mediastinal tumors in adults.[2-4,31-34] Thymomas are less common in children, accounting for approximately 15% of anterior mediastinal masses.[4] Most patients with thymoma are between the ages of 40 and 60 years, with a median age of 52 years and an equal overall gender ratio.[35-38] Thymic carcinomas are distinct from invasive thymomas pathologically and clinically and have a worse prognosis. They account for 5% to 36% of all thymic neoplasms.[39-42] The large difference in incidences from various studies reflects differences and changes in the pathologic classification of this rare tumor. Patients with thymic carcinoma are typically middle-aged or elderly, and there is a slight male predominance. Thymic carcinoids represent less than 5% of anterior mediastinum lesions[43,44] and typically affect middle-aged men.[5]

Prevention and Early Detection

Although a few small subgroups of cases are associated with thymus irradiation during childhood, EBV infection, or familial cytogenetic abnormalities, the etiologic factors for most thymic tumors are unknown, and there is no known mechanism for prevention. Thymomas are characterized by an indolent growth pattern with a tendency toward local invasion. Thymomas are associated with autoimmune disorders, particularly myasthenia gravis, in 30% to 45% of cases.[45,46] Most thymic tumors are discovered incidentally because of abnormalities observed on routine radiographs or during evaluation for myasthenia gravis. Approximately 10% to 15% of patients with myasthenia gravis have benign or malignant thymomas.[47-51] Thymic carcinomas and carcinoids are commonly detected incidentally. They are locally invasive and are found to have metastasized to regional lymph nodes and distant sites in up to 30% of patients at diagnosis.[7,40,52]

Biologic Characteristics and Molecular Biology

Thymomas are usually slow-growing tumors with an indolent natural history. Although histologically benign, they are capable of local and regional invasion and have a marked tendency for recurrence in the mediastinum and pleura. Intrathoracic recurrence can develop after complete surgical resection in up to 40% of those with invasive disease.[53] Late relapse is not uncommon.[48,54,55] Nodal and hematogenous metastases may occur but are rare.[34] An increased risk for second malignancies has been reported.[56-58]

Patients with thymoma may have dysregulation of the lymphocyte selection process associated with abnormal proliferation, autoimmunity, and immunodeficiency. Thymoma-associated autoimmune disease involves an alteration in circulating T-cell subsets.[59-61] Up to 70% of thymomas may be associated with paraneoplastic syndromes.[51] Various autoantibodies have been described.[62,63] In addition to T-cell defects, B-cell lymphopenia has been observed in thymoma-related immunodeficiency along with hypogammaglobulinemia (i.e., Good syndrome).[64,65]

Factors influencing the different biologic behavior of thymoma subtypes are poorly understood. Some pathologic features, such as altered expression of TP53 and BCL2,[66,67] counts of argyrophilic nucleolar organizer regions,[68,69] proliferating cell nuclear antigen, matrix metalloproteinases, and Ki-67 index,[68,70] are associated with biologic behavior, clinical stage, and prognosis.[71] There is a tendency for upregulation of adhesion and co-stimulatory molecules in thymoma.[72-75] Altered TP53 expression may be implicated in the initial stages of tumorigenesis, and increased expression of epidermal growth factor (EGF) and epidermal growth factor receptor (EGFR) may play a role in thymoma genesis.[76]

Thymic carcinomas possess overt features of malignancy similar to those of carcinoma arising in any other organ, with a higher propensity to capsular invasion and metastases than invasive thymomas. Associated paraneoplastic syndromes occasionally exist with well-differentiated lesions.[77,78] Most variants of thymic carcinoma are highly lethal, producing frequent metastases to regional lymph nodes, bone, liver, and lung.[79-81] Thymic carcinomas may express high levels of EGFR.[76,82,83] Tumor and serum levels of vascular endothelial growth factor (VEGF) and basic fibroblast growth factor (bFGF) can be elevated,[84,85] and correlations among such growth factors, angiogenesis, and invasiveness have been observed.[84,86] Thymic carcinoma has been associated with increased expression of epithelial membrane antigen, cytokeratin subtypes, and TP53 protein.[66,87-91] Increased expression of CD70 may serve as a marker for thymic carcinoma.[92] Other surface antigenic molecules, such as CD5 and CD99, have aberrant expression in thymic carcinoma.[93-95] Thymic carcinomas can be distinguished from lung carcinomas by negative expression of thyroid transcription factor-1 expression[87] and a distinctly different cytokeratin profile.[96]

Thymic carcinoids have a similar malignant clinical course with a poor prognosis, frequently worse than other midgut carcinoids. They may secrete peptides, amines, kinins, prostaglandins, or other substances. In a study of 80 patients with thymic carcinoids, 74% were male, 72% had related symptoms, 6% exhibited the Cushing syndrome, and 16% had other endocrine abnormalities.[97] Even after complete resection, the recurrence rates ranged between 36% and 87%.[7,97,98] Overall survival rates were only 28% and 10% at 5 and 10 years, respectively.

Pathology and Pathways of Spread

There is no consistent correlation between the histopathology of thymomas and their malignant potential.[38,99,100] However, an accurate histologic diagnosis is still crucial in patient management.

The classification of thymic tumors is controversial. Tumors with true malignant cytologic characteristics are usually considered to be thymic carcinomas rather than thymoma. Malignant thymoma refers to invasive thymoma, as defined macroscopically or microscopically, with typically "bland" cytologic characteristics of thymic epithelial cells admixed with mature lymphocytes. The term *invasive thymoma* should be used instead of malignant thymoma to denote its predilection for capsular invasion.

Grossly, thymomas are nodular, multilobulated, and firm. They may contain cystic spaces, calcification, or hemorrhage, and they may be neatly encapsulated, adherent to surrounding structures, or invasive. Thymomas generally display two cell types: epithelial and lymphatic. The neoplastic cells are the epithelial cells (Fig. 43-1). They are classified as predominantly epithelial, predominantly lymphocytic, mixed lymphoepithelial, or spindle cell type. Morphologically, these cells are rather large and may be round, oval, or spindle shaped with vesicular nuclei and small nucleoli. The cyto-

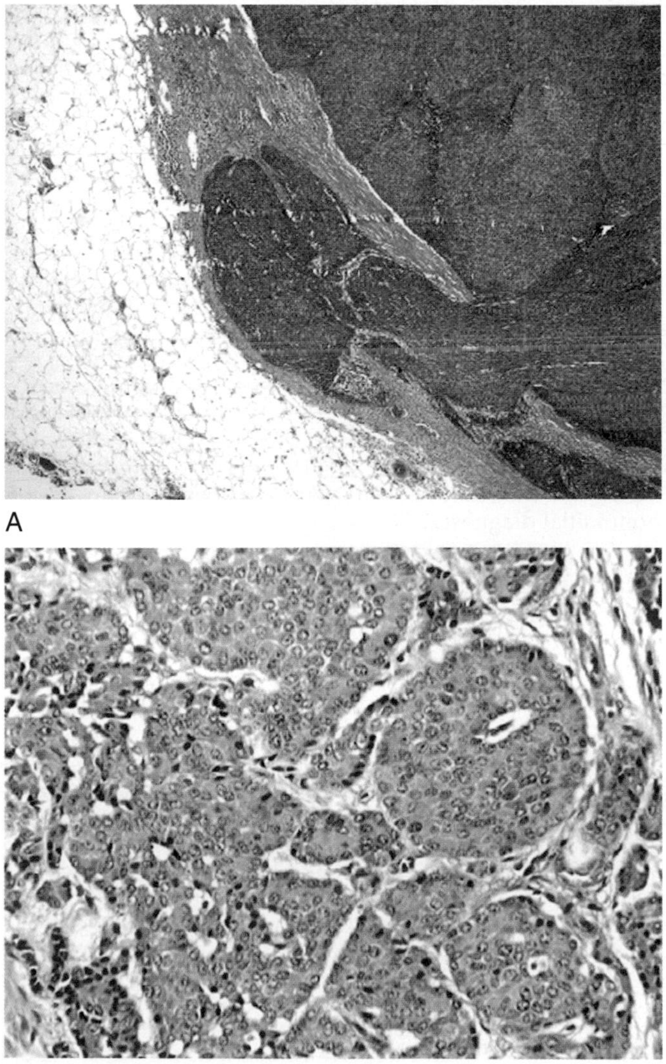

A

B

Figure 43-1 Lymphocyte-rich thymoma with dense lymphocytic cell population containing scattered larger epithelial cells with pale cytoplasm surrounding perivascular spaces. **A,** Low power (×100). **B,** High power (×400).

Disease Sites

plasm is often eosinophilic or amphophilic. The lymphocytic component is mostly made up of normal-appearing mature lymphocytes. Some of the other microscopic features that may be seen in thymomas include Hassall's corpuscles, keratinizing squamous epithelium, rosettes, glands, cysts, papillary structures, and germinal centers. Immunohistochemistry is often helpful in making the diagnosis. Thymomas typically are positively stained with a number of thymic epithelial markers, including cytokeratin, thymosin β3 and α1, and epithelial membrane antigen.

Thymic carcinoma histology is more diverse. It is cytologically malignant, and subtypes include keratinizing and nonkeratinizing squamous carcinomas, lymphoepithelioma-like carcinomas, clear cell carcinomas, sarcomatoid carcinomas, adenosquamous carcinomas, mucoepidermoid carcinomas, adenocarcinomas, and basaloid squamous cell carcinomas.[5] Their histologic appearances are not different from carcinomas in other sites.[101]

The histologic features of thymic carcinoid are identical to carcinoid tumors in other organs. Unlike thymomas, they are rarely encapsulated. Immunohistochemically, they may stain positively with CAM 5.2, low-molecular-weight cytokeratins, chromogranins, synaptophysin, and leucine-7.[97]

The predominant pattern of spread of thymomas is by direct invasion into adjacent organs. The degree of encapsulation and the invasion of adjacent tissues define malignancy for these tumors rather than the histologic appearance.[54] Approximately 50% of cases in surgical series are noninvasive.[2,35,36,38,53,102-106] Thymomas may metastasize as implants on pleural surfaces or pulmonary nodules, but they rarely metastasize to extrathoracic areas.[34] The most frequent area of dissemination is into the pleural cavity with resultant pleural plaques, diaphragmatic masses, and malignant pleural effusions. Invasion into the superior vena cava, brachiocephalic vein, lung, and pericardium may be observed.[107]

Thymic carcinomas invade locally, often involve the pleura and mediastinal nodes, and sometimes involve the cervical and axillary lymph nodes.[108] Distant metastases to the lungs, liver, brain, and bone also occur. Distant metastases to bone, liver, or skin occur in 30% to 40% of cases of thymic carcinoids,[8] and they may be seen in 70% of patients within 8 years from initial diagnosis.[109]

Clinical Manifestations, Patient Evaluation, and Staging

Approximately 30% to 40% of patients with thymomas, thymic carcinomas, or carcinoids are asymptomatic, and the tumor is usually found as an incidental finding on a chest radiograph.[34,37,46,110] Clinical symptoms vary greatly, but they are usually those of a mediastinal mass producing cough, chest pain, dyspnea, hoarseness, superior vena cava syndrome, and symptoms related to tumor hemorrhage.[5,111] Patients may also have dysphagia, fever, weight loss, and anorexia.

Some thymoma patients manifest symptoms caused by hormone production with resulting paraneoplastic syndromes; the most common is myasthenia gravis, which is seen in approximately 45% of patients.[46] Other syndromes are shown in Table 43-1.[4,46,51,54,112-115] Thymic carcinoids may also be associated with Cushing's syndrome, Eaton-Lambert syndrome, syndrome of inappropriate secretion of antidiuretic hormone (SIADH), and hypercalcemia,[8] but the classic carcinoid syndrome is rare. The causes of these syndromes remain obscure, although autoantibodies have been demonstrated, mostly in thymoma patients.[62,63,116]

Myasthenia gravis is an autoimmune disease characterized by the presence of antiacetylcholine receptor antibodies, which cause an acetylcholine receptor deficiency at the motor end plate. The disease is characterized by rapid exhaustion of voluntary muscular contractions, with a slow return to the normal state.[117,118] Patients with thymoma and myasthenia gravis may have an increased operative mortality rate, and most surgical deaths are attributed to myasthenia gravis crisis. Death of patients with thymoma and myasthenia gravis is commonly caused by complications of myasthenia gravis, whereas in patients without myasthenia gravis, death often is attributed to local progression of tumor.[48] The overall long-term prognosis does not appear to be adversely affected by the presence of myasthenia gravis.[48,104]

Table 43-1 Paraneoplastic Diseases Associated with Thymoma

Addison's disease	Myasthenia gravis
Carcinoid syndrome	Nephrotic syndrome
Chronic mucocutaneous candidiasis	Pancytopenia
Cushing's syndrome	Panhypopituitarism
DiGeorge syndrome	Pemphigus
Erythroid and neutrophil hypoplasia	Pernicious anemia
Hashimoto's thyroiditis	Polymyositis
Hyperparathyroidism	Polyneuritis
Hyperthyroidism	Red cell aplasia
Hypertrophic osteoarthropathy	Rheumatoid arthritis
Hypogammaglobulinemia	Sarcoidosis
Lambert-Eaton syndrome	Syndrome of inappropriate secretion of antidiuretic hormone (SIADH)
Lupus erythematosus	Sjögren's syndrome
Myocarditis polyarthropathy	Ulcerative colitis
Myotonic dystrophy	Whipple's disease
Myotonic dystrophy scleroderma	

Prognostic Factors

The two most important prognostic factors for thymoma are invasiveness (stage) and completeness of surgical resection.[35-37,102,119-121] Invasiveness is commonly used as the basis for designation as benign or malignant. Tumor size (>10 cm) and the presence of symptoms also have prognostic value.[34,122,123] Patients with complete or radical excision have significantly improved survival over those with subtotal resection or biopsy only.[120,124] Although almost all noninvasive thymomas can be totally resected, the ability to achieve a complete resection in invasive cases varies from 58% to 73%.[104,105,120] Older series reported a poor prognosis associated with myasthenia gravis,[35,36,106] but several modern series have failed to confirm this observation.[105,119,120,123,125-130] Myasthenia gravis may even confer a survival advantage because it may lead to earlier discovery of a small thymoma.[122,131,132] Moreover, with an increasing time interval after thymectomy, patients with myasthenia gravis have better improvement in symptoms.[133] Patients with autoimmune diseases such as red cell aplasia, hypogammaglobulinemia, and lupus erythematosus appear to have a poorer prognosis.[48,122,131,134]

Although degree of tumor invasiveness is strongly related to stage and prognosis of thymoma, there are data to support the prognostic significance of histology, independent of tumor stage.[125,135,136] The most widely accepted histologic classification is that proposed by Marino and Muller-Hermelink, who classified thymoma into cortical, mixed, and medullary types.[137] According to their data, cortical thymomas have a more aggressive course than medullary thymomas and are more likely to be associated with myasthenia gravis. Tumors that are mixed tend to have an intermediate prognosis.[138] The 10-year survival rates are approximately 100% for medullary, 76% for mixed, and 45% for cortical and well-differentiated thymomas.[138-141] In one series, no medullary and mixed thymomas (types A and AB) recurred, even though 30% had capsular invasion. Organoid and cortical thymomas (types B1 and B2) showed intermediate invasiveness and low but significant risk of late relapse, even with minimal invasion.[99] Likewise, the World Health Organization (WHO) classification based on histology has been shown to predict prognosis[136] (Table 43-2).

Table 43-2 World Health Organization Classification of Thymic Epithelial Tumors

Type	Pathologic Classification	Prognosis
A	Medullary thymoma Spindle-cell thymoma	Benign clinical course
AB	Mixed thymoma	
B1	Lymphocyte-rich thymoma Lymphocytic thymoma Predominately cortical thymoma Organoid thymoma	Moderately malignant clinical course
B2	Cortical thymoma	
B3	Epithelial thymoma Atypical thymoma Squamoid thymoma Well-differentiated thymic carcinoma	
C	Thymic carcinoma	Highly malignant clinical course

Associated paraneoplastic syndromes occasionally exist with well-differentiated thymic carcinomas.[77,78] However, clinical features have not proved useful as prognostic indicators for thymic carcinomas.[135] Similar to prognostic factors for thymomas, total resection and stage at presentation are important factors.[7]

Diagnostic Workup for Thymic Tumors

The diagnostic workup of a patient with an anterior mediastinal mass begins with a thorough history and physical examination. Particular focus should be given to detect subtle physical findings that may suggest the presence of myasthenia gravis. Routine screening blood work and chemistries should be obtained because they may give clues to the presence of associated syndromes. In the case of suspected Cushing's syndrome, the peak petrosal sinus to peripheral adrenocorticotropic hormone (P-ACTH) ratio and urinary cortisol level should be obtained. The differential diagnosis, in addition to thymic lesions, includes germ cell tumors, lymphomas, and thyroid proliferative disorders. Serum alpha-fetoprotein (AFP) and β-human chorionic gonadotropin (β-hCG) levels should be obtained in young men if the presence of nonseminomatous germ cell tumors is suspected.[142-144] Exclusion of extrathymic primaries is important because carcinomas and carcinoids are rare in the thymus and may represent metastases.

The chest radiograph often demonstrates a mass in the hilar region that may be mistaken for the heart border or pulmonary artery (Fig. 43-2). Computed tomography (CT) is one of the most valuable radiologic techniques in the evaluation and clinical staging of thymic tumors.[145,146] The size, contour, tissue density, and homogeneity of a mediastinal lesion can be defined, as well as its relation to or invasion of other mediastinal structures. Thymic tumors are usually well defined, round, or lobulated, and they vary in size and occasionally have calcification (Fig. 43-3). Pleural involvement may be seen

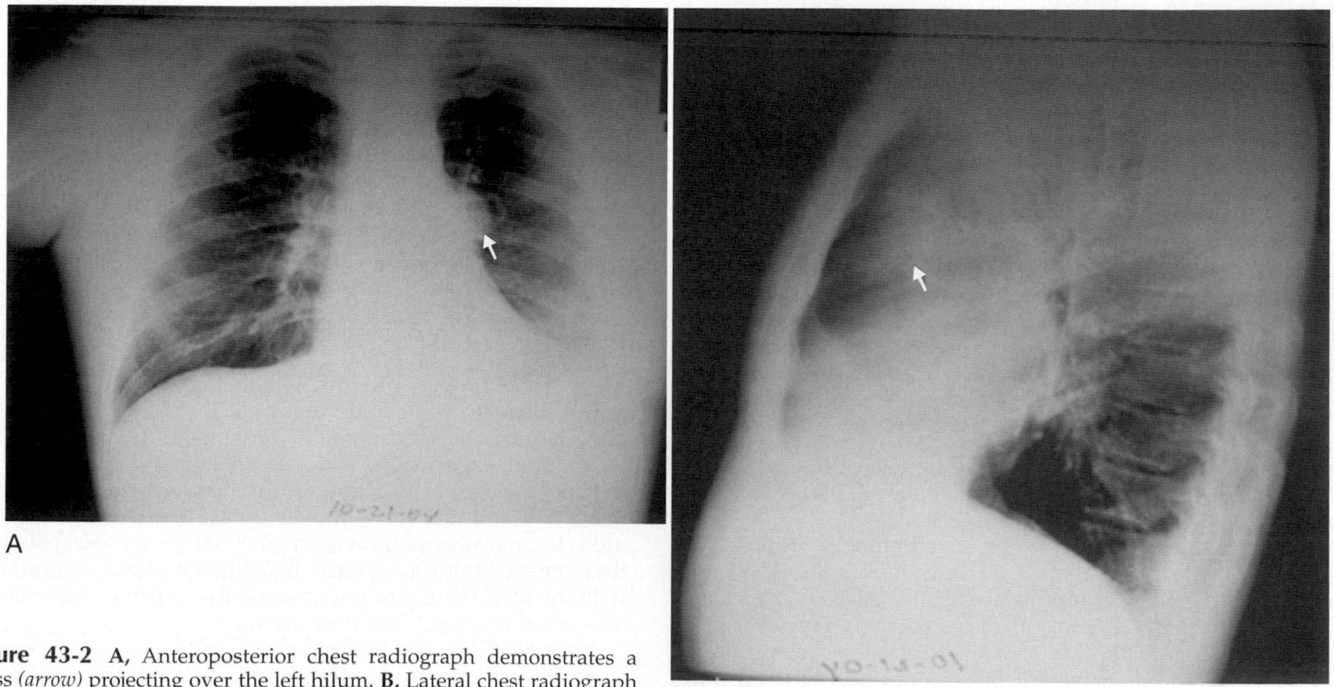

A B

Figure 43-2 **A,** Anteroposterior chest radiograph demonstrates a mass *(arrow)* projecting over the left hilum. **B,** Lateral chest radiograph confirms the location of the mass in the anterior mediastinum.

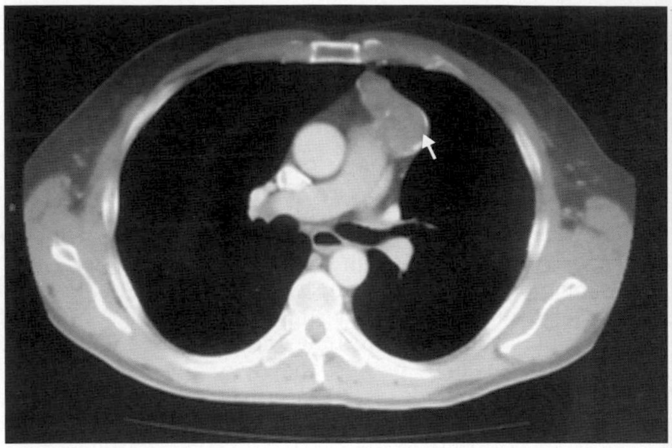

A

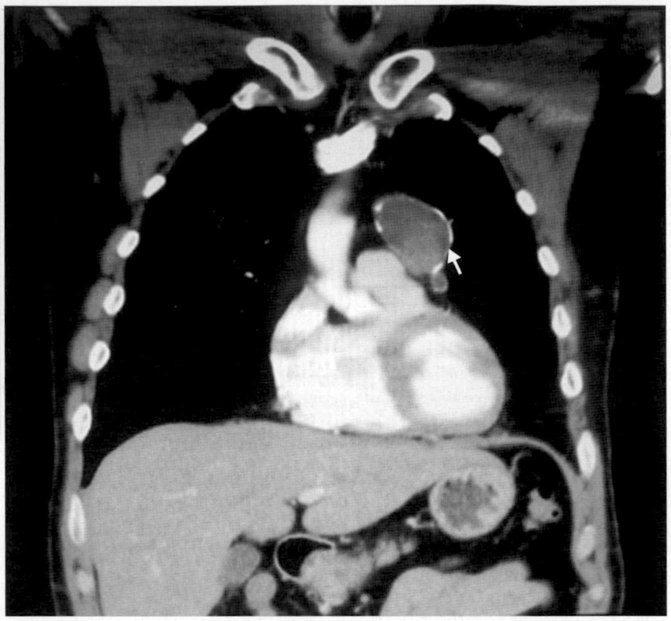

B

Figure 43-3 Computed tomography demonstrates a mass *(arrow)* with calcification in the anterior mediastinum. **A,** Axial view. **B,** Coronal view.

in advanced disease. In the absence of symptoms and signs, extensive radiographic imaging is unnecessary. Magnetic resonance imaging (MRI) has not been superior to CT.[147] The role of positron emission tomography (PET) has not been established, but early data suggests it can differentiate thymoma from thymic hyperplasia, and high uptake of fluorodeoxyglucose appears to correlate with the degree of tumor invasiveness.[148,149]

Patients presenting with a thymic mass need a histologic diagnosis before instituting definitive therapy. CT- or ultrasound-guided fine-needle aspiration biopsy of the mass may be performed to establish the diagnosis preoperatively.[150] Such procedures have a sensitivity and specificity of 87% to 90% and 88% to 100%, respectively, for thoracic neoplasms.[151] When larger tumor samples are required to distinguish between lymphoma and lymphoid-predominant thymoma, core-needle biopsy provides sufficient specimens with an overall sensitivity of 96% and specificity of 100%.[151] Bronchoscopy, video-assisted thoracic surgery, mediastinoscopy, or anterior thoracoscopy may help yield the diagnosis before resection, especially if enlarged lymph nodes are present.[143,152,153] The potential risk of breaching the capsule, leading to spillage and seeding of tumor cells during biopsy, has been debated and remains unsettled.[115,154,155]

Staging

Bergh and associates introduced the first clinical staging system for thymoma in 1978.[102] Their staging system was subsequently modified and refined by Masaoka and associates in 1981[120] and is the most widely used (Table 43-3). It is based on pathologic findings at time of surgery.

A separate, simplified staging paradigm was proposed by Suster and Moran.[156] Stage I includes lesions localized and encapsulated. Stage II lesions are locally invasive, and stage III lesions have nodal, visceral, or distant metastasis. A tumor-node-metastasis (TNM) type of staging system was proposed by Tsuchiya and associates,[157] but has not been proved clinically, and it is not widely accepted.

Table 43-3 Masaoka Staging System for Thymoma

Stage	Description
I	Macroscopically completely encapsulated with no microscopic detectable capsular invasion
II	Macroscopic invasion into surrounding mediastinal fatty tissue or mediastinal pleura or microscopic invasion into the capsule
III	Macroscopic invasion into surrounding organs (e.g., pericardium, great vessels, lung) or intrathoracic metastases, or both
IVA	Pleural or pericardial implants or dissemination
IVB	Lymphogenous or hematogenous metastases

Adapted from Masaoka A, Monden Y, Nakahara K, Tanioka T: Follow-up study of thymomas with special reference to their clinical stages. Cancer 48:2485-2492, 1981.

Treatment

Surgery for Thymoma

Surgery is the mainstay of therapy in resectable cases. However, adjuvant or neoadjuvant radiation therapy plays an important role in subtotally resected or unresectable cases. Many patients who present with symptoms of myasthenia gravis benefit from undergoing a thymectomy.[130] Consequently, surgical resection alone for stage II thymomas, in the hands of an experienced team, is a reasonable approach.[158,159] In general, surgical resection for thymoma carries low risks of morbidity and mortality; most surgical deaths can be attributed to myasthenia gravis crisis.[48] After an encapsulated thymoma without associated myasthenia gravis is removed without disturbing the integrity of the capsule, recurrences have been observed, but they are rare.[35,103,104,160]

Successful surgical treatment of locally invasive thymoma depends on the completeness of resection.[161] Consequently, the surgeon should remove as much of the lesion as possible, possibly to include an extended thymectomy.[162] However, resection of an involved phrenic nerve is controversial, and some surgeons advocate that both phrenic nerves should be left intact if both nerves are involved. When complete resection is not possible, a debulking operation should be considered, because good long-term results can be achieved when such surgery is followed by postoperative radiation therapy.[48] The surgeon should delineate the extent of the tumor, specify the areas of invasion, and identify the areas of positive or questionable margins and residual disease with metallic clips to assist future radiation therapy planning.

Radiation Therapy for Thymoma

Although the role of adjuvant irradiation for thymomas has never been tested in a prospective, randomized fashion, there is general agreement that radiation therapy is an effective adjuvant therapy for invasive thymomas,[163] and most retrospective studies have reported improvements in local tumor control and survival after adjuvant irradiation.[53,105,119-120,124,126] However, patients with encapsulated, noninvasive stage I thymoma do not require postoperative radiation therapy after complete resection because the recurrence rate is approximately 1% to 2%.[48,53,164]

For patients with Masaoka stage II disease, there is controversy about whether postoperative radiation therapy should be used for completely resected invasive thymomas. Although some studies showed no benefit from adjuvant radiation therapy,[158,159] the recurrence rates of completely resected invasive thymoma may approach 30%.[53,122] In cases with gross fibrous adhesions of the tumor to the pleura at the time of surgery or microscopic invasion of the pleura on histology, there is an increased risk for recurrence. Haniuda and colleagues found that patients with fibrous adhesion to the mediastinal pleura without microscopic invasion benefited most from postoperative radiation therapy.[165,166] The recurrence rates, with and without adhesion to the mediastinal pleura, were 36% and 0%, respectively. In another study by Monden and colleagues, patients with resected stage II thymoma had recurrence rates of 8% and 29%, respectively, with and without adjuvant radiation therapy.[56] Although postoperative radiation therapy decreases local recurrence, it does not appear to decrease the incidence of subsequent pleural dissemination that may occur outside of radiation fields. This may be a reflection of the natural pattern of spread of this disease, with pleural dissemination occurring before, during, or after the time of surgery. Extended irradiation to include the entire pleura significantly increases the normal tissue toxicity and is not routinely employed.

Locally Advanced Thymoma and Palliation

For patients with stage III/IV disease, the evidence supporting the use of postoperative radiation therapy is robust. Urgesi and colleagues reported no in-field recurrences in a study of 33 patients with completely resected stage III thymoma treated with postoperative irradiation.[119] Curran and associates reported a 53% 5-year actuarial mediastinal relapse rate with stage II and III patients after surgery alone, compared with 0% after total resection and irradiation and 21% after subtotal resection or biopsy and irradiation.[53] Similarly, in a study of 70 patients with Masaoka stage III/IV thymoma, the relapse rate for patients receiving postoperative radiation therapy was reduced from 50% to 20%, and most disease (80%) recurred outside of the irradiated field.[167]

Preoperative adjuvant radiation therapy has been advocated for unresectable or marginally resectable thymomas.[35,57,58,168] Several small studies assessing preoperative radiation therapy for extensive disease found a decrease in tumor burden at the time of surgery, with response rates as high as 80%, and described a theoretical decrease in the potential for tumor seeding during surgery.[48,53,169] These series demonstrated that preoperative irradiation facilitated total or subtotal resection of the invasive thymoma mass by reducing the tumor volume.[168]

Primary radiation therapy alone as the definitive treatment has been advocated in nonsurgical candidates or patients with unresectable advanced disease. In a study of 12 patients who presented with unresectable tumors and were treated with primary radiation therapy, 7 patients were alive 1 year 8 months to 5 years 1 month later.[170] Similar outcomes were reported for 31 patients with unresectable stage III or IV disease.[171] Five-year survival rates of 53% to 87% and 10-year survival rates of 44% were reported for patients with advanced thymoma receiving irradiation after biopsy only or incomplete resection.[172,173] Urgesi and associates reported the use of radiation therapy alone in 21 patients with intrathoracic recurrences of thymoma.[174] The 7-year survival rate of 70% was similar for those treated with irradiation alone and those treated with surgery and adjuvant therapy. However, the retrospective nature of these studies, small number of patients, differing amounts of clinical disease, and variations in radiation doses and techniques are significant confounding variables.

The role of preoperative and primary radiation therapy alone has fallen out of favor. Because of the improved response rates to chemotherapy, most patients with advanced disease are treated with a combined-modality approach.

Chemotherapy for Thymoma

In general, chemotherapy is reserved for locally advanced or metastatic disease. Numerous case reports and small series have reported antineoplastic activity for multiple and single agents in the treatment of patients with advanced thymoma.[175-191] However, there are no reported prospective, randomized trials comparing different chemotherapeutic agents.[192] Platinum-based regimens have commonly been used over the past decade, with response rates ranging between 24% and 100%, and response rates of more than 50% have been found consistently with the application of combination chemotherapy.[193] Some of the commonly employed active drugs are cisplatin, doxorubicin, and cyclophosphamide, with reported overall responses in excess of 50%.[194,195] In a study by Fornasiero and colleagues, 37 patients with stage III or IV thymoma were treated with cisplatin, doxorubicin, vincristine, and cyclophosphamide.[181] The overall response rate was 92%, and 43% were complete responses. Loehrer and associates studied 23 patients with localized but unresectable thymomas[194] treated with cisplatin, doxorubicin, and cyclophosphamide followed by radiation therapy. The overall objective response rate was 70%, with five complete responders. The estimated 5-year disease-survival rate was 54%, with a median survival of 93 months. Multivariate analysis demonstrated that chemotherapy was associated with an improvement in overall survival for patients with stage III and IV disease.

Combined-Modality Therapy for Thymoma

The role of chemotherapy as an adjuvant therapy after resection has not been established, but there is anecdotal evidence that combining chemotherapy with irradiation with or without surgery can be effective with acceptable toxicity in selected cases.[189,196-198] It has also been shown that neoadjuvant chemotherapy and then surgery, followed by additional chemotherapy and irradiation, may improve the resectability and survival of the patients with locally advanced disease.[196]

In a study by Macchiarini and colleagues,[189] all seven patients with stage III invasive thymoma treated with neoadjuvant cisplatin, epirubicin, and etoposide were able to undergo surgical resection. Four had complete resections, and three had incomplete resections. Shin and colleagues reported that 9 of 11 patients with unresectable stage III and IV thymoma were able to undergo complete resection after induction chemotherapy consisting of cyclophosphamide, doxorubicin, and cisplatin.[197] All nine patients were given additional postoperative radiation therapy and chemotherapy. Of these patients, seven were disease-free at a median follow-up of 43 months.

Results of Thymoma Treatment

There are no large prospective, randomized, phase III clinical trials to evaluate the efficacy of primary or adjuvant radiation therapy in patients with thymoma. The local control rates after a complete resection and adjuvant radiation therapy have ranged from 65% to 100%, and rates are lower for incomplete resection and radiation therapy.[53,119,124,165,169,170,173,197,199] Curran and coworkers reported a retrospective study of patients with stage II or III thymoma.[53] Twenty-six percent (20 of 78) of the patients treated with surgery alone developed local recurrences, compared with 5% (2 of 43) of similar patients who had received postoperative radiation therapy. There was no significant difference in relapse rate or survival between patients undergoing biopsy and radiation therapy and those having subtotal resection and radiation therapy. The investigators reported a 5-year actuarial mediastinal relapse of 53% for patients treated with total resection alone, compared with no relapses in patients who received postoperative irradiation after total resection. Contrary to most studies, Kondo and Monden reported a multi-institutional, retrospective study of 1320 patients with thymic epithelial tumors and found no significant difference in the recurrence between the surgery alone and surgery plus adjuvant irradiation groups with stage II or III thymoma.[7] This observation may reflect the fact that most of the patients underwent complete resection (100% with stage II, 85% with stage III disease), and as pointed out by the study authors, the recurrence rates they found were lower than in previous reports.

Postoperative radiation therapy has resulted in improved survival of patients with invasive thymomas after complete and incomplete resections.[192] In a study of 141 patients with thymoma, Nakahara and associates[105] reported a 5-year survival rate of 92% for patients with stage II and 88% for patients with stage III disease who were treated with postoperative irradiation. Patients undergoing radical surgery with complete resection before adjuvant radiation therapy often had substantially better local control and 5-year survival compared with those undergoing biopsy alone or limited tumor resection.[48,105,169,200]

After complete resection, invasive thymomas still tend to carry a poorer prognosis than noninvasive tumors.[36,192,201] Survival rates continue to fall with long-term follow-up, and 10-year survival rates may be considerably lower.[128] The 5- and 10-year survival rates for well-encapsulated thymomas without invasion are more than 90%, and for invasive thymomas, the rates range from approximately 30% to 70%.[53,102,105,106,119,120,128] The 5-year survival rates according to Masaoka stage are 83% to 100% for stage I, 86% to 98% for stage II, 68% to 89% for stage III, and 50% to 71% for stage IV.[7,120,202,203] The approximate 10-year survival rates are 80%, 78%, 47%, and 30%, and the 15-year rates are 78%, 73%, 30%, and 8% for stages I to IV, respectively.[203] Table 43-4 provides a summary of treatment results.

Anecdotal studies have demonstrated good local control of thymomas treated with primary irradiation. Of 23 patients treated with irradiation alone, 8 had complete regression, 10 had partial regression, and 5 had no regression of disease.[35] In a report by Marks and colleagues, tumor was controlled in all nine cases treated with megavoltage irradiation.[204] The average follow-up was 5.5 years (minimum, 30 months). Ariaratnam and associates observed tumor control in 8 of 11 patients with malignant thymoma with a minimum follow-up of 2 years.[205] Two of the three patients who died had received only 30 Gy in 3 weeks to the mediastinum. Overall, irradiation as monotherapy may result in approximately 65% local control and 40% to 50% 5-year survival.[172,173,192]

In patients with mostly advanced thymoma, the results of combination chemotherapy with or without surgery or irradiation are encouraging, with an overall response rate of approximately 60%.[181,183,195] All patients who achieved a pathologic complete response had received cisplatin-containing regimens. However, the impact of multimodality therapy on survival for these patients still needs confirmation, and these encouraging results are being evaluated in a prospective Intergroup study.[188]

Treatment of Thymic Carcinoma

Although the optimal treatment of thymic carcinoma is unclear, surgical extirpation remains the cornerstone of therapy, and in most published studies, surgery has been followed by adjuvant radiation therapy.[6,52,209-211] Because many series are gathered over decades, it has been difficult or impossible to control for the changes in pretreatment tumor imaging, surgical techniques, and thoracic radiation therapy planning and delivery, all of which may contribute to the inconsistent results in the literature. A prescriptive dose range has yet to be identified, with most studies using 40 to 70 Gy with a standard fractionation scheme (1.8 to 2.0 Gy per fraction). Although a survival benefit has not been seen, there is a trend toward improved survival and local control with adjuvant therapy.[6,210] No dose-related survival advantage has been established, although a relationship between dose and local control has been demonstrated.[212]

In a series of 26 patients treated with surgery and postoperative irradiation, Hsu and associates observed a 77% 5-year overall survival rate, with respective 82% and 66% survival rates for completely resected and subtotally resected cohorts.[210] With a median dose of 60 Gy (range, 40 to 70 Gy), an excellent 5-year local control rate of 91% was observed. For a cohort of 40 patients receiving definitive or adjuvant radiation therapy, Ogawa and associates reported an absence of local recurrence for those with complete resection and radiation doses greater than 50 Gy.[6] Kondo and Monden reported the largest retrospective, comparative study and found no statistically significant survival benefit from the addition of adjuvant irradiation to surgical resection, although the study authors stipulated that no definitive conclusions could be made regarding the role of adjuvant radiation therapy because of subgroup sample size limitations and the retrospective nature of the study.[7]

Although local control is increased with irradiation, a survival benefit remains to be demonstrated. For patients with any question of clinical resectability, neoadjuvant platinum-based chemotherapy is a reasonable treatment consideration.[213] Table 43-5 summarizes some of the treatment results of thymic carcinoma.

Treatment of Thymic Carcinoid

Complete surgical resection is the preferred method of treatment, although recurrence and distant metastases are

Table 43-4 Summary of Adjuvant Therapy Results of Thymoma

Study	Patients (Stage)	Irradiation Regimen	Radiation Dose (Gy)	Local Control (%)	5-Year Survival Rate (%)	Comments
Bretti et al[206] (2004)	43 (III) 20 (IVA)	Preop/postop ± chemo	24-30 preop 45-55 postop	—	Median PFS 59 (III) 21 (IVA)	Preop RT improved resection rate
Cowen et al[169] (1995)	13 (I) 46 (II) 58 (III) 32 (IVA)	Preop/postop ± chemo	22-50 preop 30-70 postop (median, 40-55)	78.5 (overall) 100 (I) 98 (II) 69 (III) 59 (IVA)	59.5 (DFS) (49.5% at 10 y)	Stage and extent of resection influenced local control and survival
Curran et al[53] (1988)	43 (I) 21 (II) 36 (III) 3 (IV)	Postop for II-IV	32-60	100 (II/III–total resection) 79 (II/III–subtotal resection or biopsy)	100 (I) (DFS) 58 (II) 53 (III)	No recurrence for stage I after surgery only; RT improved local control for stage II/III
Haniuda et al[165] (1992)	70 (II/III)	Postop	40-50	100 (IIp1)* 70 (III)	74 (II) 69 (III)	RT benefited patients with pleural adhesion, without microinvasion
Hug et al[207] (1990)	44 (II-IV)	Preop/postop	40 (median)	89 (II/III)	92 (II) 62 (III)	High failure rates in surgery-only patients
Jackson and Ball[173] (1991)	28 (II/III)	Postop (after biopsy or subtotal resection)	32-60 (mean, 42)	61	53 (OS) (44% at 10 y)	High RT complications of 11%, with 2 deaths
Kondo and Monden[7] (2003)	522 (I) 247 (II) 201 (III) 101 (IV)	± Postop ± Chemo	— 43.7 ± 7.7 (II) 45.4 ± 8.4 (III)	99.1 (I) 95.9 (II) 71.6 (III) 65.7 (IV)	100 (I) 98 (II) 89 (III) 71 (IV)	Largest study; no difference in recurrence ± RT in stage II and III patients; high complete resection rates
Latz et al[208] (1997)	10 (II) 14 (III) 19 (IV)	Postop ± chemo	10-72 (median, 50)	81	90 (II) 67 (III) 30 (IV)	Uncertain RT benefit for completely resected stage II
Mornex et al[200] (1995)	21 (IIIA) 37 (IIIB) 32 (IVA)	Preop and postop ± chemo	30-70 (median, 50)	86 (IIIA) 59 (IIIB/IVA)	64 (IIIA) 39 (IIIB)	Great impact of RT on local control; >50 Gy recommended for incomplete resection
Nakahara et al[105] (1988)	45 (I) 33 (II) 48 (III) 12 (IVA) 3 (IVB)	Postop (73% received RT)	30-50	—	100 (I) 91.5 (II) 87.8 (III) 46.6 (IV) 97.6 (complete resection) 68.2 (subtotal) 25 (biopsy)	Complete resection + RT resulted in best survival
Pollack et al[124] (1992)	11 (I) 8 (II) 10 (III) 7 (IV)	Postop; primary RT (22 patients)	50 (median)	59 (overall)	74 (I) 71 (II) 50 (III) 29 (IV)	Patients with incomplete resections did worse; multimodality treatment recommended for these patients
Urgesi et al[119] (1990)	59 (III) 18 (IVA)	Preop and postop	39.6-60	85-90	78 (III) (58% at 10 y)	Most relapses were out of RT fields

*Fibrous adhesion to the mediastinal pleura without microscopic invasion.
Chemo, chemotherapy; DFS, disease-free survival; OS, overall survival; preop, preoperatively; postop, postoperatively; PFS, progression-free survival; RT, radiation therapy; ±, with or without.

Table 43-5 **Summary of Thymic Carcinoma Treatment Results**

Study	No. of Patients	Treatment	RT Dose (Gy)	Local Control (%)	5-Year Overall Survival (%)	Comments
Blumberg et al[52] (1998)	43	TR/SR ± chemo/RT	—	52 (CR)	65 (35% at 10 y) 68 (TR) 62 (SR)	Masaoka stage was not prognostic but invasion of innominate vessel was.
Chang et al[211] (1992)	16	TR/SR/BX ± chemo/RT		77	31 (median, 30 mo)	Better survival was seen with squamous type.
Hsu et al[210] (2002)	26	TR/SR ± RT	40-70	91 (overall)	77 (overall) 82 (TR) 66 (SR)	Masaoka stage was prognostic; very good local control observed with surgery + RT.
Kondo and Monden[7] (2003)	186	TR/ST/BX ± chemo/RT	—	49 (TR)	50.5 (overall) 66.9 (TR) 30.1 (SR) 24.2 (BX) Subgroups: 72.2 (TR alone) 73.6 (TR + RT) 46.6 (TR + chemo/RT) 81.5 (TR + chemo)	Largest number of patients gathered from multiple institutions in Japan; total resection was the most important factor in survival; RT did not improve results for completely resected tumors.
Liu et al[214] (2002)	38	TR/SR/BX ± chemo/RT			27 (median, 24 mo)	Grade, stage, and resectability were predictors of survival.
Lucchi et al[213] (2001)	13	TR/SR ± chemo/RT	45-60	46 (overall)	61 (median, 38 mo)	100% objective tumor response with induction chemo, but small study
Nakamura et al[215] (2000)	10	BX + chemo ± RT	6-56	0	0 (median, 11 mo)	Poor survival for unresectable disease; median chemo response was only 6 mo.
Ogawa et al[6] (2002)	40	TR/SR/BX ± chemo/RT	10-70 (mean, 50)	100 (TR + RT)	38 (28% at 10 y)	Long-term study; better survival and local control with complete resection + RT (12/16 vs. 1/24).

BX, biopsy only or unresectable; chemo, chemotherapy; CR, complete response; DSS, disease specific survival; RT, radiation therapy; SR, subtotal resection or debulking; TR, total or complete resection; ±, with or without.

Adapted from Eng TY, Fuller CD, Jagirdar J, et al: Thymic carcinoma: state of the art review. Int J Radiat Oncol Biol Phys 59:654-664, 2004.

common.[7,216] In a study of 40 patients, the recurrence rate was 64%, even though 35 of the 40 patients had a complete resection,[7] and the 5-year survival was 84%. Despite a lack of conclusive evidence, incomplete resections followed by irradiation or chemotherapy, or both, may improve local control without significantly increased morbidity and mortality.[43,109,217-219] However, distant metastases occur in approximately 30% of the patients.[217] The long-term prognosis is poor, with an overall 5-year survival rate of 0% to 31%.[221,222]

Techniques of Irradiation

High-energy (>10-MV) x-rays usually are preferred for irradiation. A CT scan is indispensable for adequate treatment planning. Clips placed at the time of surgery denoting the extent of resection in completely resected tumors or outlining regions of residual disease are useful in guiding postoperative irradiation. The planning target volume (PTV) should include the gross tumor volume (GTV) and the thymus, if any, and tumor bed with a 1.5- to 2.0-cm margin. Depending on histology and surgical findings, areas of suspicious subclinical disease and regional lymphatics are commonly included. However, treatment of the entire mediastinal and supraclavicular nodal basin prophylactically is controversial because the pattern of failure has little similarity to lung cancer, and a higher normal tissue complication rate can be expected when large target volumes are used.[194,199,208,223]

Conventional port arrangements may include a single anterior port, two opposed anteroposterior ports (weighted 2:1 or 3:2), wedged-pair techniques, and other multiple-field arrangements. Given the advanced technical capabilities available, three-dimensional (3D) conformal therapy or intensity-modulated radiation therapy (IMRT) should be considered to provide dose homogeneity and allow better sparing of adjacent normal critical structures. Figure 43-4 shows a postoperative radiation therapy field with custom blocks covering the surgical tumor bed and involved upper mediastinum. Figure 43-5 shows a 3D conformal radiation treatment field with IMRT. The isodose lines more closely conform to the shape of the PTV. The risks of side effects depend on normal tissue tolerance, surrounding critical organs, prior treatments, radiation

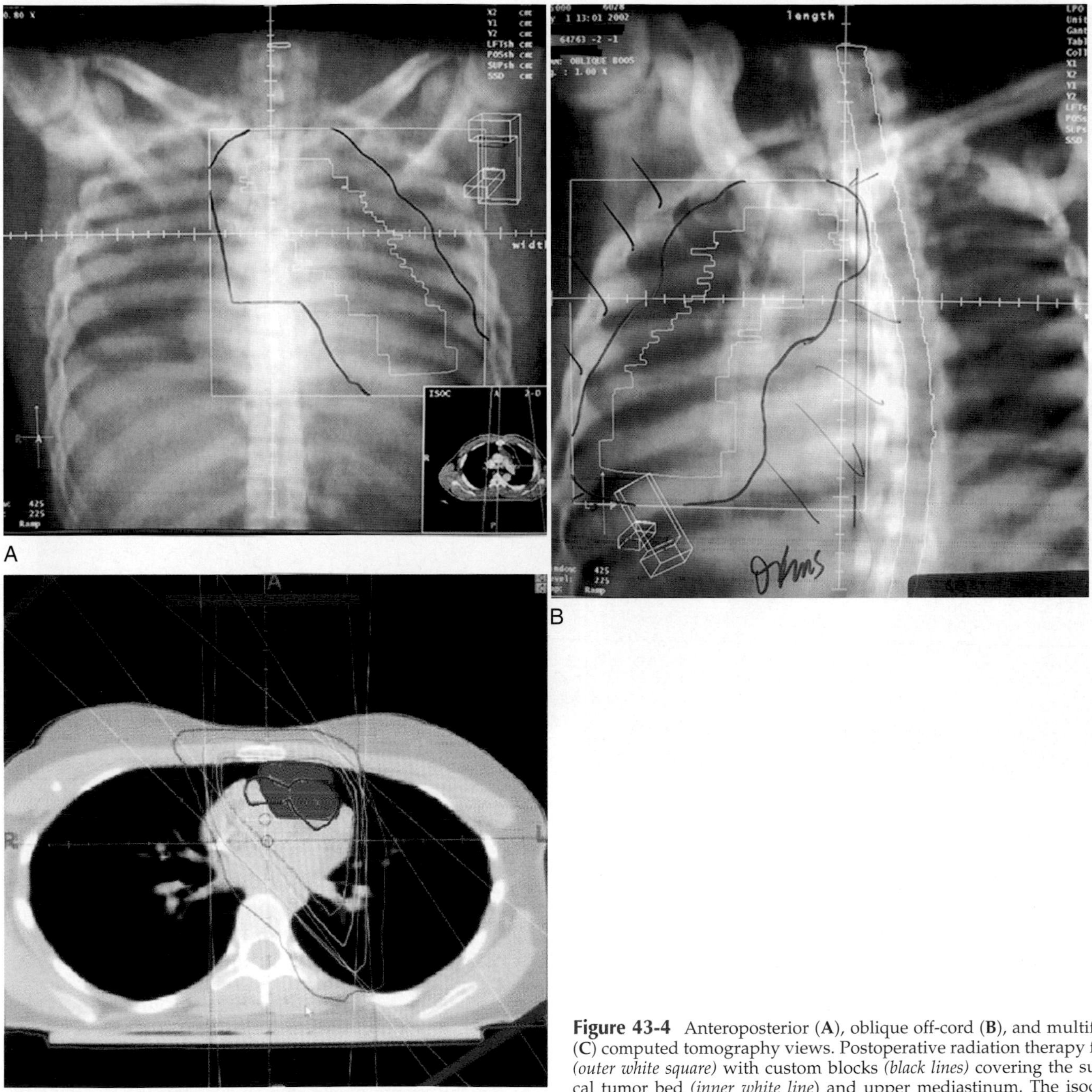

A

B

C

Figure 43-4 Anteroposterior (**A**), oblique off-cord (**B**), and multifield (**C**) computed tomography views. Postoperative radiation therapy field *(outer white square)* with custom blocks *(black lines)* covering the surgical tumor bed *(inner white line)* and upper mediastinum. The isodose lines cover the planning target volume *(orange)* very well.

dose, other concurrent therapies, and the general health of the patient.

Various dose and fractionation schemes for thymoma are reported in the literature.[192,224] Although one retrospective study did not find any relationship between radiation dose and local control,[169,212] others have found that radiation dose was a significant prognostic factor for local control, with good results reported when doses higher than 40 Gy were used for subclinical or microscopic disease.[200,225] Postoperative doses of 45 to 55 Gy given by conventional fractionation have been used effectively in most cases.[53,122,166,169,170,197,200,208] The dose to the spinal cord should be limited to 45 Gy using oblique mediastinal fields. For patients with gross residual disease after resection or unresectable disease, doses of 60 Gy or more probably are required,[124,171,200] but higher doses correlate with higher risks of complications.[226]

Treatment Algorithm and Controversies

The initial treatment for thymic tumors is surgery if the disease is resectable. Adjuvant irradiation or chemotherapy should be considered for patients with features indicating a high risk for recurrent disease and those with an unresectable or inoperable tumor. Optimal treatment must be customized, and the following guidelines should be considered:

1. Pathologic stage I-II thymoma (WHO type A, AB, B1, B2, B3) does not require adjuvant therapy after a complete thymectomy (R0 resection, negative margins).

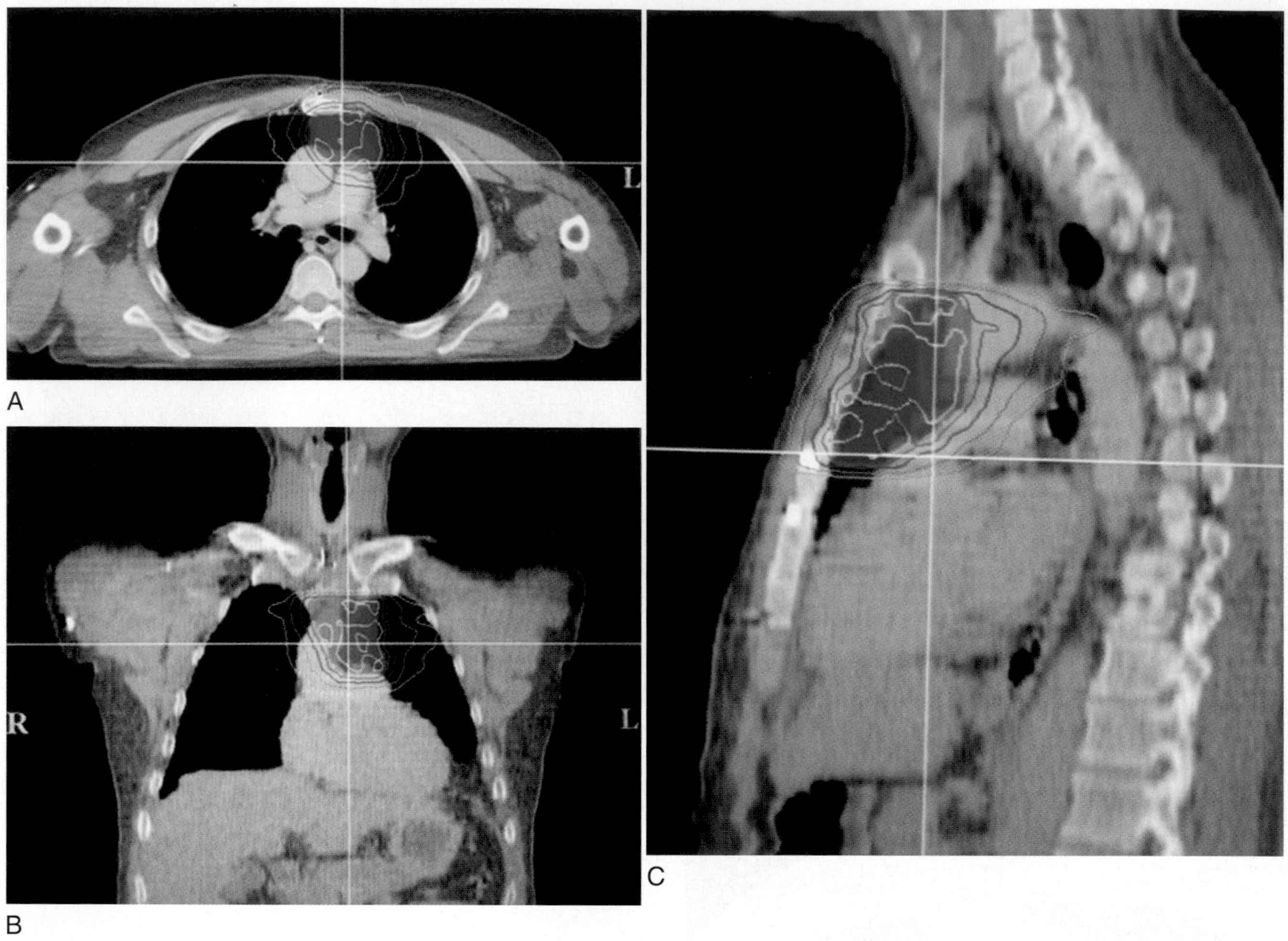

Figure 43-5 Axial (**A**), coronal (**B**), and sagittal (**C**) views for intensity-modulated radiation therapy. Isodose lines are closely conformal to the shape of planned target volume *(red)*.

2. Pathologic stage II thymoma (WHO type A, AB, B1, B2, B3) patients with less than a complete thymectomy (as outlined in no. 1) may benefit from postresection thoracic irradiation. A dose of 50 to 66 Gy (depending on the amount of residual disease) can usually be safely administered.
3. Pathologic stage II thymic carcinoma (WHO type C) can be treated with multimodality adjuvant therapy, which includes concomitant chemoradiotherapy with or without consolidation chemotherapy after a complete thymectomy (R0 resection, negative margins).
4. Pathologic stage III-IVA thymic neoplasms (WHO type A, AB, B1, B2, B3, C) are treated with multimodality adjuvant therapy (as outlined in no. 3) even after a complete thymectomy (R0 resection, negative margins).
5. Clinically unresectable stage III-IVA thymic neoplasms are treated with neoadjuvant chemoradiotherapy, followed by sequential thymectomy, postoperative thoracic irradiation, and consolidation chemotherapy.

PULMONARY CARCINOID TUMORS

Neuroendocrine lung tumors include typical carcinoid, atypical carcinoid, large cell neuroendocrine, and small cell lung carcinoma.[227] The term *carcinoid* ("karzinoide") was originally defined as a carcinoma-like lesion without malignant characteristics by Oberndorfer in 1907.[228] Pulmonary or bronchial carcinoid tumors are typically low-grade malignant neoplasms that arise from neuroendocrine cells of the amine precursor uptake and decarboxylation (APUD) system. These cells are the Kulchitsky (enterochromaffin) cells, which are located in the basal layer of bronchial epithelium.[229,230] Approximately, 25% of carcinoids are located in the respiratory tract, which is the second most common site after the gastrointestinal tract. Pulmonary carcinoids are frequently centrally located and confined to the main or lobar bronchi.[231] These tumors are rare, and their biologic behavior mostly depends on histology.

Etiology and Epidemiology

The cause of pulmonary carcinoid is unknown, and no environmental risk factors have been established. Carcinogens that are associated with lung cancer have not been consistently associated with pulmonary carcinoids,[232] although a few studies revealed a higher frequency of smokers with atypical carcinoids.[233-235] Some of the neoplastic cells express the retinoblastoma gene *(RB1)* products and mutant TP53, and they show occasional loss of heterozygosity, especially in atypical carcinoids.[236] Most familial pulmonary carcinoids have been reported in patients with MEN1. In cases of atypical and typical lung carcinoids, there is a characteristic allelic loss within the region 11q-13, which harbors the *MEN1* gene, a tumor suppressor gene.[237-241] Other frequently detected genetic alterations in lung carcinoids, especially atypical carcinoids, include losses of 3p, 5p, 9p, 10q, and 13q.[238,241]

The annual incidence of carcinoid tumors is 1 or 2 cases per 100,000 people in the United States.[232,242] For bronchopulmonary carcinoids, the reported incidence is 0.6 per 100,000.[243] Carcinoid tumor of the lung represents 1% to 2% of all lung malignancies, with an equal frequency of these tumors occurring in men and women,[232] and approximately 3500 new cases were reported in 2004.[244,245] Data from the SEER program of the National Cancer Institute have shown a trend of relative increase of pulmonary carcinoids.[232,243]

Prevention and Early Detection

There is no known preventive measure for pulmonary carcinoids. Carcinoids are detected like other space-occupying tumors. The most common findings on a chest radiograph include a hilar mass with occasional atelectasis. Functioning carcinoids are suspected on the basis of the symptoms and signs, and the diagnosis is confirmed by demonstrating increased urinary excretion of the serotonin metabolite 5-hydroxyindoleacetic acid (5-HIAA). Thyroid transcription factor-1 is expressed in 80% of metastatic pulmonary carcinoids but not in intestinal carcinoids, and it may be of value in the workup and diagnosis of pulmonary carcinoids.[246,247] Sometimes, localization of the tumor may require an extensive evaluation, including laparotomy. If hepatic involvement is suspected, a specific liver scan may be sufficient to demonstrate metastases.

Biologic Characteristics and Molecular Biology

Carcinoid tumors often occur sporadically and are thought to arise from neuroendocrine cells, which are present in a wide range of organs. The WHO classification of lung neuroendocrine tumors describes two different subtypes of carcinoids, typical and atypical carcinoids, with distinctive clinical behaviors and different prognoses.[244,248] Based on the criteria proposed by Travis and associates, the spectrum of neuroendocrine tumors also includes large cell neuroendocrine carcinoma and small cell lung carcinoma.[227,248]

Although most pulmonary carcinoids are nonfunctional, some have the ability to synthesize and secrete a variety of physiologically active substances, leading to paraneoplastic syndromes, including carcinoid syndrome, Cushing's syndrome, and acromegaly.[230] Serotonin (5-hydroxytryptamine [5-HT]) is one of the frequently encountered vasoactive substances released by carcinoid tumors. Other substances, including corticotropin, histamine, dopamine, substance P, neurotensin, prostaglandins, and kallikrein, have been reported.[249-254]

The biologic behavior of these tumors ranges from indolent to aggressive, depending on the histology. Although typical carcinoids have an indolent clinical course, atypical carcinoids behave more aggressively and commonly produce nodal (mediastinal nodes), regional, and distant metastases. The recurrence rates and stage at presentation frequently are higher. In atypical carcinoids, there is a high frequency of molecular alterations and inactivation of tumor suppressor genes, such as *TP53*, *RB1*, *CDKN2A* (previously designated *p16*), and *CDKN2D* (previously designated *p19*). The proliferation rates, as assessed by MIB-1 and Ki-67, are also higher than for typical carcinoids.[244,255,256]

Pathology and Pathways of Spread

Carcinoids are thought to be derived from different embryonic divisions of the gut and are classified accordingly. Foregut carcinoids are often found in the lungs, bronchi, and stomach, and midgut and hindgut tumors are typically seen in small and large intestines. Histologically, they may stain positive with silver or Grimelius stains, cytokeratin 7 and 11, neuron-specific enolase, synaptophysin, carcinoembryonic antigen, and chromogranin.[246,257,258] Microscopically, they are characterized by small, uniform cells and the presence of numerous membrane-bound, neurosecretory eosinophilic granules containing a variety of hormones and biogenic amines in the cytoplasm. Most pulmonary carcinoids (70% to 90%) are typical carcinoids or well-differentiated neuroendocrine tumors, which are characterized by small cells with well-rounded nuclei; atypical carcinoids (10% to 30%) or poorly differentiated neuroendocrine tumors, have malignant histologic features of increased nuclear atypia with high mitotic activity (>2 mitoses per 10 high-power fields), lymphovascular invasion, nuclear pleomorphism, and areas of necrosis.[248,257,259-261]

Sometimes, it is difficult to establish the specific diagnosis of carcinoid because of small biopsy samples or to differentiate atypical carcinoid from small cell lung carcinoma without immunohistochemical tests.[248,262-264] Well-differentiated carcinoids are often indolent, with a relatively low risk of nodal or distant metastasis of 3% to 15%.[245,260,265-267] Atypical carcinoid may have an aggressive clinical course, with frequent organ metastases.[236,268,269] The risk of nodal metastasis, frequently to mediastinal lymph nodes, is 30% to 57%.[245,270,271] Distant metastases occur in more than 20% of patients.[245] The most common sites of distant metastasis include liver, bone, adrenal, brain, skin, and soft tissue.[244,272-275]

Clinical Manifestations, Patient Evaluation, and Staging

Most patients with pulmonary carcinoids present in their 50s.[232,242,245,269] Carcinoids in children are rare.[276] Between 70% and 80% of these tumors are located centrally near the hilum within the tracheobronchial tree and produce a variety of clinical symptoms and neuroendocrine manifestations at the time of diagnosis.[277,278] Patients with peripheral lesions may be asymptomatic, and their lesions are often discovered incidentally.[279,280]

Patients present with recurrent pneumonia, cough, hemoptysis, or chest pain. Hyperparathyroidism may be seen. Carcinoids may produce various amines and polypeptides with corresponding signs and symptoms, often precipitated by emotion, food ingestion, or alcohol. The serotonin metabolite 5-HIAA, which is excreted in urine, acts on smooth muscle to produce bronchoconstriction or diarrhea, colic, and malabsorption. Histamine and bradykinin, through their vasodilator effects, cause flushing. The release of such vasoactive substances into the systemic circulation can cause the carcinoid syndrome, characterized by episodic flushing, typically of the head and neck; asthmatic wheezing; abdominal cramps with recurrent diarrhea resulting in malabsorption syndrome; and valvular heart disease, including right-sided endocardial fibrosis, leading to pulmonary stenosis and tricuspid regurgitation.[281] Lesions of the left side of the heart, which have been reported with bronchial carcinoids, are rare because serotonin is destroyed during passage through the lung. Some patients complain of decreased libido and impotence. However, the incidence of carcinoid syndrome or other paraneoplastic syndromes, including Cushing's syndrome and acromegaly, is usually no more than 3% to 5% of cases, and these syndromes mainly occur in patients with larger tumors (>5 cm) or

Table 43-6 **Presenting Symptoms in Patients with Pulmonary Carcinoids**

Symptoms	Schrevens et al[277] (n = 67)	Kaplan et al[268] (n = 144/62)*	Fink et al[245] (n = 142)
Cough		39%/45%	35%
Dyspnea, wheezes		17%/25%	41%†
Chest pain	7%	9%/18%	
Infection, fever	42%		
Weight loss		11%/20%	15%‡
Hemoptysis	21%	16%/12%	23%
Paraneoplastic syndromes	0%	1%/3%	<1%
Asymptomatic	24%		30%

*Typical/atypical groups.
†Bronchial obstruction, including dyspnea, pain, and pneumonitis.
‡Others include weight loss, weakness, nausea, and neuralgia.

metastatic disease.[248,249,260,265,270,278,282] Levels of hCG and pancreatic polypeptide are occasionally elevated.

Patients with a suspected lung mass require a thorough history and physical examination. Routine screening blood tests and chemistries may give clues to the presence of associated syndromes (Table 43-6). The differential diagnosis, in addition to bronchopulmonary carcinoid, includes lung carcinoma and metastasis from an extrapulmonary primary tumor. Conventional radiographs of the chest and comparison with older films are often helpful. CT and bronchoscopy are two of the most valuable diagnostic procedures. Up to 80% of carcinoids manifest with type 2 somatostatin receptors, and the receptors can be targeted by radioactive octreotide or pentetreotide. Somatostatin receptor scintigraphy with radiolabeled octreotide (^{111}In-octreotide) has demonstrated reliable uptake in primary tumors and been used to detect early recurrence.[283-285] The result of ^{18}F-fluorodeoxyglucose positron emission tomography (FDG-PET) is often negative.[234,286-288] PET with ^{64}Cu-TETA-octreotide as a tracer has been investigated in carcinoids.[289]

Transbronchial biopsy or CT- or ultrasound-guided fine-needle aspiration biopsy of the mass may establish the diagnosis preoperatively. Bronchoscopy, video-assisted thoracic surgery, or mediastinoscopy may help yield the diagnosis before resection, especially if enlarged lymph nodes are present.

The prognostic factors are atypical histology, nodal involvement, and the presence of symptoms at the time of presentation.[268-270,277,279,284] High mitotic rate, tumor size larger than 3.5 cm, and female gender have also been implicated as prognostic factors for patients with atypical pulmonary carcinoids.[233] There is no specific staging system for pulmonary carcinoids, and the American Joint Committee on Cancer (AJCC) lung cancer staging system (TNM) is commonly used.

Treatment

Primary Therapy

Curative resection is the treatment of choice.[244,272,290-292] After complete resection, the long-term results are generally excellent.[245,277,290,292] Conservative surgical resection, consisting of wedge or segmental resection is the preferred therapy for localized pulmonary carcinoids.[293,294] Patients with central lesions may require bronchial sleeve resection or sleeve lobectomy.[291] Endoscopic laser ablation may be used to alleviate tumor obstruction, improve atelectasis, and reduce inflammation before resection.[266] Intraoperative nodal evaluation should be performed, and if results are positive, complete nodal dissection is indicated. Because of higher rates of local recurrence in patients with atypical carcinoids, a more extensive surgical procedure, such as lobectomy or pneumonectomy with nodal dissection, should be considered.[244,272,290,295] However, patients may present with metastatic or unresectable disease, and curative resection is not obtainable. Debulking and other cytoreduction procedures may be of benefit in cases of gastrointestinal carcinoids,[296,297] but these procedures are of uncertain benefit for patients with pulmonary carcinoids.

Medical Treatment

Certain symptoms, including flushing, can be relieved by pharmacologic agents. Ondansetron, one of the specific 5-HT3 antagonists, provides sustained symptomatic relief in patients with carcinoid syndrome.[298] Somatostatin analogues are potent inhibitors of neuropeptide release and gut exocrine or endocrine function. These analogues are effective in relieving symptoms by binding to somatostatin receptors (mainly receptor 2),[299] which are present in approximately 80% of carcinoids, leading to inhibition of hormone secretion.[300,302] Octreotide and lanreotide, long-acting analogues of somatostatin, are the drugs of choice for controlling diarrhea and flushing. The response rate is about 70% for symptomatic improvement, and there is a more than 50% reduction in urinary 5-HIAA secretion, with a median duration of response of 12 months. Data suggest that these somatostatin analogues may have a direct antitumoral effect, with stabilization of tumor growth and reduction of tumor size in patients with carcinoids of various sites.[301,303]

Radiation Therapy

In general, typical carcinoids do not require adjuvant radiation therapy or chemotherapy after curative resection.[245,277,290,292,304] Martini and associates reported a study of 25 patients with node-positive bronchial carcinoids (12 typical and 13 atypical) and found no benefit from postoperative radiation therapy.[231] Recurrence and survival appeared to depend on cell type rather than nodal status. However, in another study of 163 patients (including three fourths of patients with typical carcinoids, most of which were N0), prognosis depended on the presence (N positive versus N negative) and extent (N1 versus N2) of nodal involvement, rather than histologic subtype.[305] In most studies, the role of adjuvant radiation therapy is unsettled because of the retrospective nature of studies and the small number of patients.[233,268,306] Although prospective, randomized data are lacking, adjuvant radiation therapy has been used in patients at high risk for locoregional recurrence, including those with large tumor size (>3 cm), positive nodes, positive margins, atypical histology, residual disease, and inoperable disease.[260,268,306,307]

Palliative radiation therapy can be considered in patients with metastatic typical or atypical pulmonary carcinoids. Tumor-targeted irradiation with radioactive somatostatin analogues (^{111}In-octreotide or ^{131}I-metaiodobenzylguanidine [^{131}I-MIBG]) has been used, often as second- or third-line therapy.[307-309] The results have been inconclusive, with occasional long-term survivors reported.

Chemotherapy

Unlike chemotherapy for patients with small cell lung cancer, systemic chemotherapy has produced only limited success in patients with metastatic carcinoid tumors.[307] Although no effective chemotherapeutic regimen has been established, aggressive treatment with adjuvant systemic chemotherapy is recommended in high-risk patients with stage III atypical or metastatic carcinoid.[270] Several trials have shown response rates of 21% to 33% with various combinations of doxorubicin, streptozocin, cyclophosphamide, etoposide, and fluorouracil in patients with metastatic carcinoids.[310-313] There was no significant difference in survival between treatment groups, and the side effects were substantial. Patients with atypical carcinoids treated with a combination of cisplatin and etoposide appear to have a higher response rate than patients on other regimens.

Locally Advanced Disease and Palliation

For patients with locally advanced or metastatic disease, surgery is generally limited to those whose metastases are confined to one site amenable to local resection, because aggressive debulking may enhance the outcome in terms of symptomatic relief.[296,314] Radiation therapy has been used successfully to palliate symptoms in patients with locally advanced or metastatic disease.[315] Local control and symptomatic relief can be achieved in most patients with 4000 to 5000 cGy. Endoscopic resection and laser photoablation have been used for palliation of symptoms.[266] Somatostatin analogues alone or in combination with chemotherapy or interferon-α may be considered for symptomatic treatment or tumor stabilization.[316]

Results of Therapy

In general, patients with typical carcinoid tumors treated with surgery alone have a very good outcome. However, patients with atypical pulmonary carcinoid tumors and regional lymph node metastases are at high risk for recurrent disease and have worse survival rates when they are treated with surgical resection alone.[269] The 5-year overall survival rate ranges from 78% to 100% for all resected pulmonary carcinoids, 90% to 100% for typical carcinoids, 25% to 69% for atypical carcinoids, and 18% to 38% for metastatic carcinoids.[245,260,265-267,269,271,272,279,317] The 10-year survival rates are 10% to 20% lower than the 5-year rates. Some of the published results are summarized in Table 43-7. Although the role of adjuvant radiation therapy as part of multimodality treatment is undefined, adjuvant irradiation may improve the outcome of high-risk patients with atypical carcinoid tumors, positive nodes, or positive margins.[275]

Techniques of Irradiation

The same general principles of thoracic irradiation apply to irradiation of pulmonary carcinoids. High-energy (>10-MV) x-rays are preferred with a CT scan for treatment planning. As in treating other tumors, surgical clips denoting the extent of resection or outlining regions of residual disease are useful in guiding postoperative irradiation. The PTV should include the gross or residual tumor volume and tumor bed with a 1.5- to 2.0-cm margin. Depending on histology and surgical findings, areas of suspicious subclinical disease and regional lymphatics are included. Treatment field arrangements may resemble the typical lung tumor fields. There are no consistent guidelines regarding dose and fractionation regimens in the literature. Postoperative doses of 45 to 58 Gy delivered in conventional fractionation of 1.8 to 2.0 Gy per day have been reported (see Table 43-7). For patients with gross residual or unresectable disease, a higher total dose may be justified as long as the dose to other critical structures does not exceed the tolerance of normal tissues.

Algorithm and Controversies

Surgery is the primary treatment for typical and atypical pulmonary carcinoids. Although conservative resection has resulted in low recurrence rates and excellent long-term survival for patients with well-differentiated pulmonary carcinoids, the adequacy of such resection in patients with atypical carcinoids has not been settled. More extensive surgical procedures, with higher treatment-related morbidity, have been advocated by some investigators.[270,319] Adjuvant radiation therapy or systemic chemotherapy may be considered even for patients with early-stage disease because of the high incidence of regional and distant failure.[268] Palliative irradiation should be considered for those with symptomatic disease.

MESOTHELIOMA

Malignant pleural mesothelioma (MPM) is an aggressive malignancy, and local disease progression is the main cause of symptoms and death. Disseminated disease is usually reported only very late in the course of MPM.[321,322] MPM spreads by direct extension and seeding throughout the pleural space, including fissures, diaphragmatic and pericardial surfaces, through the chest wall, and into the mediastinum, peritoneum, and lymph nodes. The major problem for patients with MPM is poor local disease control in the thorax. Aggressive surgery alone, even in carefully selected patients with early-stage disease, has not improved the 2-year survival rate of 10% to 33%.[323-325] Combined-modality treatment suggests improved local control and survival rates,[326-328] but local recurrence is still the most common site of first relapse.[329]

Even after extrapleural pneumonectomy (EPP), the diffuse nature of most malignant mesotheliomas and the manipulation of the exposed tumor during surgery put the entire ipsilateral chest wall, diaphragm insertion, pericardium, mediastinum, and bronchial stump at very high risk for local recurrence. The hemithorax and mediastinum have an irregular shape and are adjacent to critical structures, such as the spinal cord, liver, kidneys, esophagus, heart, and contralateral lung. Conventional irradiation of the hemithorax and mediastinum is limited by the ability of these organs to tolerate radiation[321,329,330] and by the total volume of tissue being irradiated.

Etiology and Epidemiology

MPM has an incidence of approximately 10 cases per million people per year in the United States.[331] The incidence has been increasing and represents a significant clinical problem in populations exposed to asbestos. The Center for Lung Cancer and Related Disorders estimates approximately 3000 new cases of MPM per year, with a peak incidence of approximately 4000 per year expected to occur in about 2025.

Table 43-7 **Treatment Results for Pulmonary Carcinoids**

Study	No. of Patients	Treatment	Radiation Dose (Gy)	Local Control	Survival	Comments
Wirth et al[320] (2004)	8 Typical 10 Atypical (advanced or metastatic)	4 Ch + RT 14 Ch (no surg)	46-54	22% (overall response)	20 mo MS	4/18 responded to Ch ± RT without surg (inoperable patients).
Beasley et al[233] (2000)	106 Atypical	Surg ± RT/Ch	Various (not stated)		61% 5 y OS 35% 10 y OS 28% 15 y OS	Higher mitotic rate, size ≥ 3.5 cm, female gender, presence of rosettes are independent variables (multivariate analysis) for worse survival.
Choi et al[275] (2004)	19 Atypical	15 Surg 3 Surg + RT/Ch 1 Ch + RT	54	89%	79% 3 y OS 41 mo MS 74% 3 y DSS	Adjuvant RT may improve those with positive margins or positive nodes.
Kaplan et al[268] (2003)	144 Typical 62 Atypical	129 Surg 12 Surg + RT/Ch 2 Ch + RT 35 Surg 19 Surg + RT/Ch 9 Ch + RT	Various (not stated)	92% at 5 y (surg, stage I) 77% at 5 y (surg, stage I)	79% 5 y DSS 63% 10 y DSS 39% 20 y DSS 60% 5 y DSS 37% 10 y DSS 28% 20 y DSS	Poor prognostic factors: male gender, high stage, symptoms at presentation, and age ≥60; 56/206 had second malignancies; atypical carcinoids had worse outcome.
Carretta et al[306] (2000)	36 Typical 3 Atypical 5 LCNEC	Surg ± RT/Ch	45-58		93% 5 y AS 70% 5 y AS	Patients with nodal metastases had worse outcome.
Schrevens et al[277] (2004)	59 Typical 8 Atypical	All surg	—		92% 5 y 67% 5 y (92% 5 y OS, 84% 10 y OS)	Independent prognostic factors were nodal status and pathology; size of primary did not correlate with nodal metastasis.
Fink et al[245] (2001)	128 Typical 14 Atypical	All surg (4 inoperable or refusal)	—		89% 5 y 82 % 10 y 75% 5 y 56% 10 y	Long-term results are excellent with typical carcinoids.
Ferguson et al[304] (2000)	109 Typical 26 Atypical	All surg	—		90% 5 y 70% 5 y	Early-stage tumors did well regardless of histology.
Mezzetti et al[318] (2003)	88 Typical 10 Atypical	All surg	—		92% 5 y OS 90% 10 y OS 71% 5 y OS 60% 10 y OS	Early stage (I) did well.

AS, actuarial survival; Ch, chemotherapy; DSS, disease-specific survival; LCNEC, large cell neuroendocrine carcinoma; MS, median survival; OS, overall survival; RT, radiation therapy; Surg, surgery.

Approximately 90% of mesothelioma cases can be attributed to prior asbestos exposure. This is typically an occupational exposure (e.g., construction, automotive brake repair, boiler work, shipbuilding), and it explains the approximately 90% male predominance. However, other sources of exposure may include a spouse or parent asbestos worker. Even a history of living near asbestos-using businesses, such as automotive shops (from brake linings) or cement manufacturers (which may have added asbestos), can increase the risk of mesothelioma. Patients from certain regions of the world (e.g., central Turkey, Western Australia) also have endogenous environmental asbestos exposure.

Clinical Evaluation and Staging

Dyspnea, chest pain, cough, and weight loss are common presenting symptoms of MPM. All patients should be asked about their history of asbestos exposure. MPM has a tendency to grow along tracks of previous chest tubes. All sites of previous instrumentation should be identified and examined for evidence of tumor seeding. Such chest wall progression may manifest as pain, a nodule, or an ulcer. Particularly when transthoracic extension is identified, the axillary and supraclavicular lymph nodes should be palpated for possible involvement. Sometimes, new scoliosis can occur because of ipsilateral lung volume loss.

Imaging

A chest radiograph should be used for initial evaluation. Careful attention should be paid to the presence of pleural effusions or calcified pleural plaques. Nodular irregularities often can be identified. Sites of rib tenderness should be evaluated for direct tumor extension, although chest pain is more often attributable to involvement of the endothoracic fascia.

CT of the chest is the mainstay of radiographic staging, but it often underestimates disease extent. Invasion of the diaphragm and chest wall invasion are difficult to detect in early cases. Miliary disease can be present on the undersurface of the diaphragm or peritoneum and remain undetected by modern imaging. MPM tends to manifest late in the disease course, often with large masses and pleural effusions. Pleural-based irregular masses are common, particularly in dependent regions of the pleural space. The interlobar fissures are also often involved. MPM can invade adjacent structures, such as the chest wall, mediastinum, great vessels, vertebral body, or heart. Mediastinal and hilar lymph nodes can be involved with tumor, but the pattern of spread is often different from that of non–small cell lung cancers. MPM spreads to the lower paraesophageal nodes (level 8), pulmonary ligament nodes (level 9), and diaphragmatic nodes much more commonly than lung cancers. Pericardial effusions and ascites can also be seen on CT, and they should be evaluated pathologically before any attempt at curative resection. The anteromedial extent of tumor, particularly extension across the midline, should be determined before surgery. Because surgery obliterates the costomediastinal space, the anterior pleural reflection cannot be accurately delineated on post-operative studies.

The utility of MRI in the staging of mesothelioma is controversial. MRI may slightly more accurately predict the extent of chest wall invasion. However, this finding should not necessarily preclude surgery, as long as the region of invasion can be removed with a limited chest wall resection. Invasion to the peritoneal surface of the diaphragm cannot always be appreciated without invasive staging. FDG-PET or PET/CT scanning has been applied to mesotheliomas[332] because they tend to avidly take up FDG.

Invasive Staging

Before beginning multimodality treatment, accurate preoperative staging is necessary. Unfortunately, preoperative assessment of mesothelioma tumor stage is less than ideal using current diagnostic imaging techniques. Although CT, PET, and MRI are reasonably accurate in defining tumor volume within the thorax and chest wall and in identifying sites of distant disease, they are less successful in determining tumor involvement at two critical sites: contralateral mediastinal nodal involvement and tumor invasion through the diaphragm. Tumor involvement at either site negates resection, and we therefore believe that an accurate assessment of these areas is necessary before performing EPP. All patients at our institution undergo pretreatment laparoscopy with peritoneal lavage and cervical mediastinoscopy. For patients who have significant weight loss, a percutaneous feeding jejunostomy tube is sometimes placed at the time of laparoscopy to allow nutritional supplementation. At the University of Texas M.D. Anderson Cancer Center, for 118 patients with MPM who were clinically and radiographically determined to have resectable disease, laparoscopy and peritoneal lavage revealed transdiaphragmatic or peritoneal involvement in 12 (11%) of 109 patients and mediastinoscopy identified positive contralateral nodes in 4 (4%) of 111 patients. Overall, 15 (13%) patients were identified with occult advanced disease and spared unnecessary EPP.

Staging

The AJCC staging system for mesothelioma is shown in Table 43-8 and is based on the International Mesothelioma Interest Group (IMIG) staging system. The staging systems are useful only after surgical staging, and no clinical staging system has been developed or validated.

Several important prognostic markers have been identified for MPM. Metastases to any nodal stations predict a worse outcome. However, unlike non–small cell lung cancer, it is not clear that mediastinal metastases reflect a worse prognosis than hilar or intrapulmonary nodal metastases. The completeness of resection also is prognostic. Patients with R1 or R2 resections have been reported to have a worse outcome in some series, but not in others.

Another poor prognostic marker is non-epithelioid histology. Patients with sarcomatoid or mixed tumors fare much worse than patients with epithelioid histology. Thrombocytosis and high levels of platelet-derived growth factor predict a worse outcome. Several reports suggest that serum levels of mesothelin are elevated in most patients at diagnosis and that they fall after surgery. Serum mesothelin may be a marker for tumor recurrence,[333] much like prostate-specific antigen (PSA) for prostate cancer.

Treatment

Surgery

Surgical Diagnosis

The diagnosis of mesothelioma can be difficult because of the relative rarity of the disease and the cytologic similarity to more common metastatic neoplasms, such as adenocarcinoma. Thoracentesis is often the first procedure performed to obtain diagnosis, but it has a diagnostic sensitivity of only 32%.[334] Percutaneous fine-needle aspiration biopsy similarly has low diagnostic sensitivity, although ultrasound-guided core-needle biopsy has been reported to improve accuracy.[335] The most accurate method of diagnosis is video-assisted thoracoscopic (VATS) biopsy. VATS provides a detailed visual inspection of the hemithorax, allowing any abnormal tissue to be biopsied. This technique enables the surgeon to obtain much larger quantities of tissue than can be obtained percutaneously, and it permits assessment of the degree of tumor involvement of the diaphragm, pericardium, and visceral pleura. Thoracoscopy should ideally be performed through a single port site placed through the sixth interspace and within the line of a possible future thoracotomy incision. Mesothelioma has a tendency to track along sites of chest wall violation, and tumor may recur at previously placed thoracoscopy port sites if they are not excised at the time of definitive surgery. Limiting the number of port sites at the time of VATS and placing the port sites where they are easily excised help to reduce local chest wall recurrence. When it is difficult to establish entrance into the pleural space, it is preferable to perform a limited open biopsy of the parietal pleura by extending the port site incision slightly, rather than to perform a formal thoracotomy. A thoracotomy performed for diagnosis significantly compromises potentially curative surgery.

Surgical Treatment

Pleurectomy. Pleurectomy for treatment of MPM has been advocated by many surgeons, although there is a growing consensus that it is less preferable for disease control than EPP. Local recurrences are significantly higher than after

Table 43-8 **TNM Staging of Mesothelioma**

PRIMARY TUMOR (T)	
TX	Primary tumor cannot be assessed
T0	No evidence of primary tumor
T1	Tumor involves ipsilateral parietal pleura, with or without focal involvement of visceral pleura
T1a	Tumor involves ipsilateral parietal pleura (mediastinal, diaphragmatic). No involvement of the visceral pleura
T1b	Tumor involves ipsilateral parietal pleura (mediastinal, diaphragmatic), with focal involvement of the visceral pleura
T2	Tumor involves any of the ipsilateral pleural surfaces with at least one of the following: • Confluent visceral pleural tumor (including fissure) • Invasion of diaphragmatic muscle • Invasion of lung parenchyma
T3	Tumor involves any of the ipsilateral pleural surfaces, with at least one of the following: • Invasion of the endothoracic fascia • Invasion into mediastinal fat • Solitary focus of tumor invading the soft tissues of the chest wall • Nontransmural involvement of the pericardium
T4	Tumor involves any of the ipsilateral pleural surfaces, with at least one of the following: • Diffuse or multifocal invasion of soft tissues of the chest wall • Any involvement of rib • Invasion through the diaphragm to the peritoneum • Invasion of any mediastinal organs • Direct extension to the contralateral pleura • Invasion into the spine • Extension to the internal surface of the pericardium • Pericardial effusion with positive cytology • Invasion of the myocardium • Invasion of the brachial plexus
REGIONAL LYMPH NODES (N)	
NX	Regional nodes cannot be assessed
N0	No regional lymph node metastasis
N1	Metastases in the ipsilateral bronchopulmonary and/or hilar lymph node(s)
N2	Metastases in the subcarinal lymph node(s) and/or the ipsilateral internal mammary or mediastinal lymph node(s)
N3	Metastases in the contralateral mediastinal, internal mammary, or hilar lymph node(s) and/or the ipsilateral or contralateral supraclavicular or scalene lymph node(s)
DISTANT METASTASIS (M)	
MX	Distant metastasis cannot be assessed
M0	No distant metastasis
M1	Distant metastasis
STAGE GROUPINGS	
I	T1 N0 M0
IA	T1a N0 M0
IB	T1b N0 M0
II	T2 N0 M0
III	T1-2 N1 M0 T1-2 N2 M0 T3 N0-2 M0
IV	T4 Any N M0 Any T N3 M0 Any T Any N M1
RESIDUAL TUMOR (R)	
RX	Presence of residual tumor cannot be assessed
R0	No residual tumor
R1	Microscopic residual tumor
R2	Macroscopic residual tumor

From Green FL, Page DI, Fleming ID, et al (eds), for the American Joint Committee on Cancer: AJCC Cancer Staging Manual, 6th ed. New York, Springer, 2002.

EPP. Because the ipsilateral lung is preserved by pleurectomy, the procedure is often preferred for patients with poor contralateral lung function. Unfortunately, mesothelioma usually involves the visceral and parietal pleural surfaces of the lung, and these extend into the pleura-lined pulmonary fissures. Cytoreduction is not as complete as that achieved with EPP. Because the lung and hemidiaphragm remain after pleurectomy, tumoricidal postoperative radiation therapy cannot be effectively administered. At our institution, we reserve pleurectomy for patients who cannot tolerate EPP because of diminished cardiopulmonary reserve.

Extrapleural Pneumonectomy. Most experts consider EPP to be the operation of choice for mesothelioma because it provides the maximum cytoreduction possible and allows adjunctive therapies such as chemoperfusion, photodynamic therapy, or hemithoracic radiation to be given without risk to the remaining vital organs. Without adjunctive therapy, EPP has been associated with recurrence rates as high as 80%, but with current multimodality techniques, studies have reported local recurrence rates between 40% and 50%. One study[336] reported a local recurrence rate of 13% (7 of 55) for patients treated with hemithoracic radiation to 54 Gy after EPP.

EPP is an extensive surgical procedure, and patients require careful assessment preoperatively to exclude the presence of locally advanced or distant disease (which would preclude resection) and meticulous cardiopulmonary screening to ensure that the operation can be tolerated physiologically. We perform EPP only after surgical staging of the mediastinum and abdomen (with washings). In general, patients should have adequate cardiac function (i.e., ejection fraction greater than 40% and no reversible ischemia on radionuclide imaging) and have an estimated postoperative FEV_1 value greater than 0.8 L/min, or 30% of predicted.

Chemotherapy

Chemotherapy for mesothelioma has not met with much success. Reviews[337,338] describe modest success with several chemotherapeutic agents. Reported response rates greater than 25% include the use of methotrexate (37%),[339] gemcitabine plus cisplatin (48%),[340] pemetrexed plus carboplatin (50%),[341] pemetrexed plus cisplatin (38%),[342] mitomycin plus cisplatin (26%),[343] raltitrexed plus oxaliplatin (26%),[344] and doxorubicin plus cisplatin (28%).[345]

Perhaps the most exciting development in chemotherapy for mesothelioma is the use of cisplatin plus the antifolate pemetrexed.[346] A total of 456 patients were randomized. Median survival was 12.1 months for the pemetrexed plus cisplatin arm and 9.3 months for cisplatin alone ($P = .020$). Toxicity was dramatically reduced by the addition of vitamin supplementation, but this did not influence the effectiveness of therapy. Time to progression was improved from 3.9 to 5.7 months by the addition of pemetrexed ($P = .001$). The response rate was 17% for cisplatin alone, compared with 41% for combined treatment.[341]

The British Thoracic Society performed a randomized trial to assess the possible role of chemotherapy in palliation.[347] For the trial, 242 patients were registered, and 109 were randomized to active symptom control (ASC) or one of two chemotherapy regimens (i.e., mitomycin C, vinblastine, and cisplatin or vinorelbine alone). They found that ASC with chemotherapy provided better palliation of chest pain and shortness of breath than ASC alone.

Rationale for Radiation

MPMs are almost impossible to cure with radiation therapy as a single modality. The tumors are large, and potential cure requires commensurately large radiation doses. The treatment volumes are very large, extending from the supraclavicular fossa to the insertion of the diaphragm, because the entire pleural space is at risk for recurrence, even the intrapulmonary fissures. The treatment volumes are very close to radiosensitive structures, such as the lung, kidney, liver, esophagus, and heart.

Although technical challenges remain, several lines of evidence suggest that radiation therapy can be effective in treating mesothelioma. First, mesothelioma cell lines are not particularly radioresistant in vitro, and they have radiosensitivities similar to non–small cell lung cancer.[348,349] Second, there is a clinically meaningful dose-response relationship for symptom palliation, such that doses greater than 40 Gy seem more effective than lower doses.[322] This dose-response relationship suggests that clinically significant cell killing results from modest radiation doses. Third, modest radiation doses can dramatically reduce the local MPM failure rate at thoracotomy or other instrumentation sites. These data demonstrate that irradiation can effectively kill mesothelioma cells in regions where the tumor burden is low. Because MPM is moderately radiosensitive, it follows that postoperative irradiation can be effective in preventing locoregional recurrence and potentially improve survival.

Curative Radiation Therapy

Radiation Therapy Alone

Irradiation alone is not the treatment of choice for MPM. The lung is very sensitive to irradiation, and the volume of lung irradiated above 20 Gy has been linked to pulmonary toxicity.

Sparing is difficult if the lung and diaphragm remain in place because of two problems. First, the fissures are bathed in pleural fluid and therefore with mesothelioma cells. Unfortunately, the intrapulmonary fissures are complex, three-dimensional structures surrounded by lung. Respiratory motion is the second and most important problem for the use of irradiation as the sole treatment modality. When the diaphragm is in place, there can be 2 to 3 cm of superoinferior motion, 1 to 2 cm of mediolateral motion along the mediastinum, and 1 to 1.5 cm of anterior chest wall motion. Expanding the PTV to account for this motion results in destruction of the liver in right-sided MPM, the most common side, and delivery of very high cardiac and bowel doses in left-sided cases. Radiation therapy without surgery is best considered a palliative treatment.

Radiation Therapy Combined with Surgery

Several groups have reported promising outcome for MPM patients treated with surgery and irradiation, with or without chemotherapy. Operative approaches have used pleurectomy or decortication or employed EPP.

Radiation Therapy after Pleurectomy or Decortication

Thirty-four patients with pathologically proven MPM were treated between 1982 and 1988 at the Helsinki University Central Hospital.[350,351] Twenty-nine patients had partial pleurectomy, and the others had only biopsy. Patients were irradiated with one of three schedules that delivered between 55 Gy and 70 Gy to the hemithorax, and significant pulmonary damage occurred in many patients. A similar study at the Memorial Sloan-Kettering Cancer Center[352] treated 41 patients with partial pleurectomy, and all had residual gross disease that was given a boost dose with permanent ^{125}I implantation at surgery. Photon and electron fields were combined to treat the superficial chest wall and spare the underlying lung. Radiation doses were 45 Gy to the pleural surface, but the dose to "most of the lung" was kept below 20 Gy. Local recurrence developed in 29 of 41 patients, with 22 having distant failures. Median time to local failure was 9 months. Radiation-related toxicity occurred in four patients (one each of radiation pneumonitis, symptomatic pulmonary fibrosis, pericardial effusion, and esophagitis), but the severity of toxicity was not described.

These results were updated with results for 105 patients treated with pleurectomy or decortication from 1976 to 1988.[321,323] Forty-one patients received external beam radiation treatment only, and 53 patients received external beam irradiation with an intraoperatively placed ^{125}I boost to gross disease. Median survival was 12.6 months, but 12 patients developed radiation pneumonitis, and 8 developed radiation pericarditis. The severity of these reactions and the degree of local control were not described.

One article[353] described the results of 24 patients treated with pleurectomy or decortication, intraoperative radiation therapy (IORT), and postoperative external beam radiation therapy. Fourteen patients were irradiated using 3D conformal radiation therapy, and IMRT was used to treat 10 patients. IORT was targeted mainly to the intrapulmonary fissures, pericardium, and diaphragm, with doses ranging from 5 to 15 Gy. The target volumes for the external beam treatments were not described, but the doses ranged from 30.1 to 48.8 Gy (median, 41.4 Gy). Twelve patients also received chemotherapy (i.e., cyclophosphamide, doxorubicin, and cisplatin). Despite the relatively early-stage disease, outcome was relatively poor, with a median overall survival of 18 months and progression-free survival of 12 months. Major complications included radiation pneumonitis in four patients, pericarditis in one, and esophageal stricture in one patient who had received previous radiation therapy to the esophagus. Tumor recurrence was "mostly locoregional" at sites of previous gross tumor. Only the number of IORT sites was predictive of overall survival, suggesting that higher external beam doses might be required for this approach to be widely used.

Pleurectomy or decortication followed by irradiation can reduce locoregional failure compared with historical controls. However, local failure is common, and survival is disappointing even when modern IMRT techniques are applied. Although overall median survival times in these pleurectomy or decortication studies tend to be about 2 years, carefully selected patients with early-stage disease treated with EPP can expect median survival times of more than 4 years.[326] Unfortunately, there are no prospective, randomized trials to guide therapy.

Radiation Therapy after Extrapleural Pneumonectomy

The first large report of combined-modality therapy that included EPP was described in 1997.[329] In this series, 49 patients underwent EPP. Four to six cycles of chemotherapy were given postoperatively, followed by irradiation in 35 patients. The target volumes, stage, and technique were not described. The prescribed dose was 30.6 Gy to the "hemithorax," followed by a boost to bring the dose to about 50 Gy. The criteria for boost and the locations, volumes, and techniques were not described. Sixteen irradiated patients had a "local" recurrence. However, of the patients with "abdominal" failures, five had a chest mass extending into the abdomen, two had ascites, and four had a "retroperitoneal mass." This latter fact is potentially important because the diaphragm is reconstructed much higher than the insertion of the diaphragm, "abdominalizing" the retroperitoneal posterior chest wall (Fig. 43-6). Failure to irradiate this region, which can occasionally be below the ipsilateral kidney, can result in apparent retroperitoneal recurrences. The true rate of locoregional failure was at least 21 of 49 and possibly as high as 25 of 49 cases. Despite this finding, the 3-year overall survival rate was 34%. Radiation-related morbidity was tolerable, including esophagitis[321] and thrombocytopenia.[323] No radiation pneumonitis was described, but five patients experienced "respiratory compromise," one of whom died of pneumonia. These data suggest that postoperative radiation therapy can reduce local recurrence and result in the long-term survival of well-selected patients.

Encouraging results have also been reported from Memorial Sloan-Kettering Cancer Center.[323] From 1995 to 1998, 54 patients underwent EPP followed by radiation therapy.[354] Two thirds of the patients had stage III disease. The target volume was described as the "hemithorax" and drain sites, and the inferior field edge "rarely" included the ipsilateral kidney. The treatment technique involved photon radiation to a dose of 54 Gy in 30 fractions. The spinal cord was shielded after 41.4 Gy, and the liver, heart, and stomach were appropriately shielded. The chest wall in the shielded regions was irradiated with matched electron fields so that the goal dose of 54 Gy could be more safely achieved. The median survival time was about 18 months. Only seven patients had local recurrences; two had only local recurrences. Another 22 patients had "peritoneal" or "ipsilateral visceral" recurrences. It is not clear whether any of these were in the radiation fields or whether some might have been marginal misses. It is critical to distinguish marginal failures (which require better definition of the clinical target volume [CTV]) from in-field failures (which require more dose or perhaps less inhomogeneity in dose).

The results of 28 patients treated with EPP followed by IMRT have been reported[355-357] by our group at the M.D. Anderson Cancer Center. Twenty-six had stage III disease, most had involved lymph nodes, and all patients required partial chest wall resection. During EPP, radiopaque surgical clips were placed at the insertion of the diaphragm, including the crus, and at the anteromedial pleural extension, which often crosses midline over the heart. The target volume included the entire hemithorax and all surgical clips, all sites of instrumentation, and the ipsilateral mediastinum. Boosts were given to any close or positive resection margins. All volumes were reviewed with the surgeon. The goal dose was 45 to 50 Gy to the hemithorax and 60 Gy to the boost volume. All irradiation was completed in 25 fractions. The 2-year overall survival rate was 62%. There were no in-field failures. Two marginal misses occurred, one near the crus and one across midline anterior to the heart. Major toxicities include nausea and vomiting, fatigue, and skin irritation. This series has been extended to 57 patients with EPP followed by IMRT to 45 or 50 Gy. There has been one failure within the prescribed dose, and three marginal failures (two in the first five patients). One fatal case of radiation pneumonitis occurred several weeks after completion of IMRT (unpublished observations). The 3-year disease-free survival rate was 45% for patients with lymph node–negative disease and epithelioid histology (about half of our patients). The 3-year disease-free survival rate for five patients with stage I disease treated with this technique was 100%.

An update of the Memorial Sloan-Kettering Cancer Center experience has been published regarding their radiation therapy technique and outcome.[358] Thirty-five patients underwent radiation therapy after EPP, with the goal of delivering 54 Gy in 30 fractions. The target volume was the ipsilateral hemithorax from the top of T1, ideally to the bottom of L2, and laterally to flash the skin. All drain sites were included. The medial field edge was the contralateral edge of the vertebral bodies if mediastinal lymph nodes were negative, otherwise the field was extended 1.5 to 2 cm beyond the contralateral edge of the vertebral bodies. For right-sided lesions, the liver and ipsilateral kidney were blocked. For left-sided lesions, the heart was blocked after 19.8 Gy. The blocked regions were boosted to the target dose with electrons. After 41.4 cGy, the medial field edge was moved to the ipsilateral edge of the vertebral bodies. Patients tolerate this therapy well, with the main toxicities being nausea, vomiting, and dysphagia.

The results of this study, however, were difficult to interpret. Local failure was documented in 13 of 35 patients, but in-field failures were not separated from marginal misses. It is not clear whether the pattern of failure results from inade-

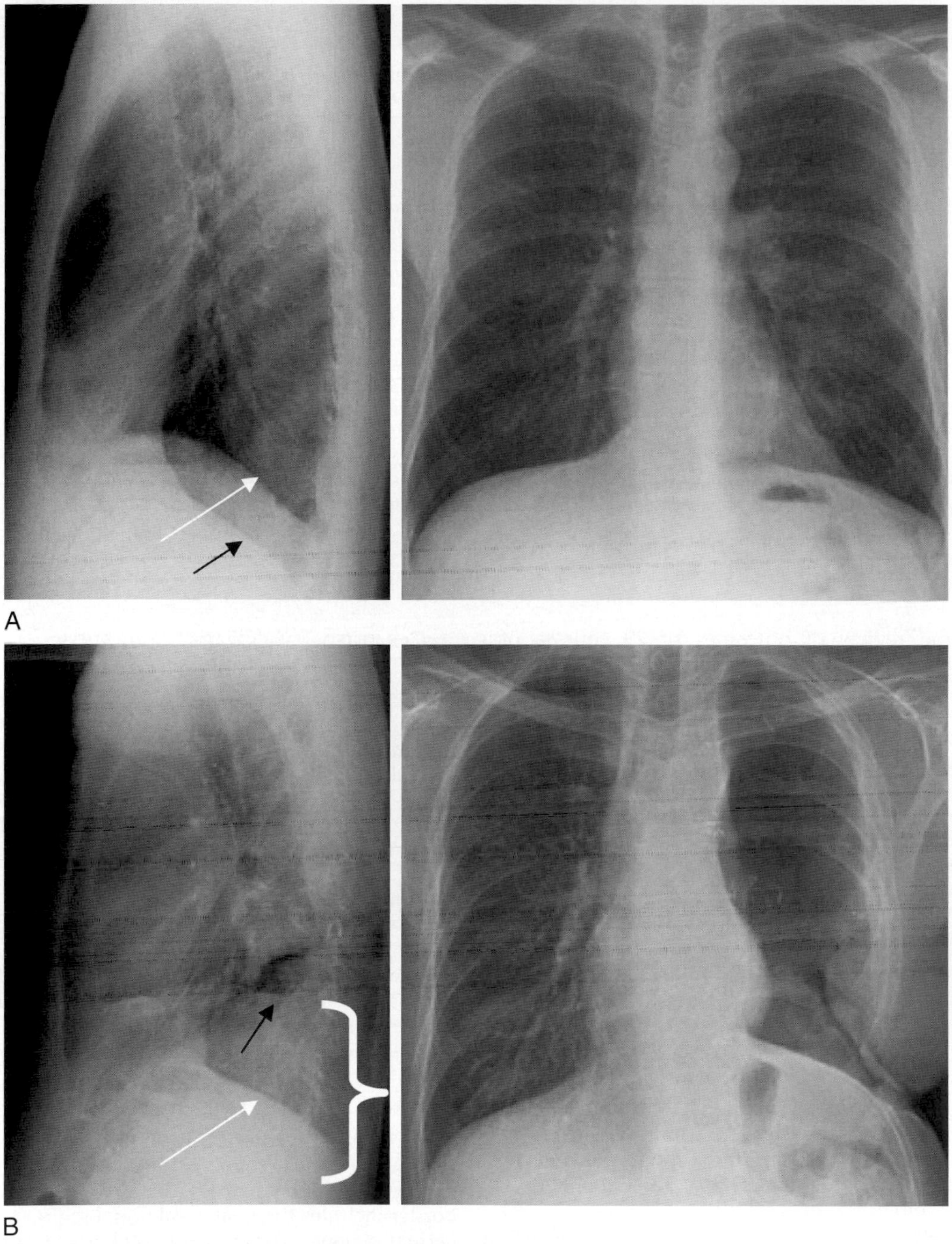

Figure 43-6 Extrapleural pneumonectomy (EPP) can abdominalize portions of the posterior costophrenic recess. **A,** A preoperative radiograph shows that the diaphragm on the contralateral side *(black arrow)* is higher than the ipsilateral hemidiaphragm *(white arrow)*. **B,** After EPP, the posterior insertion of the reconstructed hemidiaphragm *(white arrow)* is well above the now flattened, remaining hemidiaphragm *(black arrow)*. In this example, the posterior insertion of the diaphragm is about 15 cm higher than before surgery.

quate margins or inadequate dose. However, of the remaining 22 patients with local control, only 5 are disease free. Better systemic therapy is needed.

These data demonstrate several important points (Table 43-9). First, high-dose postoperative irradiation can dramatically reduce ipsilateral thoracic failures. Second, irradiation after pleural decortication results in a much higher rate of locoregional failure than irradiation after EPP. EPP with postoperative radiation therapy therefore seems preferable to less morbid but much less effective approaches. Third, true in-field failure needs to be well documented so that it can be explained. Fourth, postoperative irradiation is well tolerated. Fifth, postoperative radiation therapy changes the pattern of relapse so that distant metastases become more prevalent, requiring the integration of systemic therapy into the treatment regimen.

Palliative Radiation Therapy

Pain Control

Radiation can provide effective palliation for patients with MPM. A radiation dose-response relationship has been

Table 43-9 **Large Studies Combining Surgery with Postoperative Radiotherapy**

Study	Surgery	No. of Patients	Radiotherapy Dose (Gy)	Local Failure	Survival
Maasilta[351] (1991)	Pleurectomy	34	55-70	33% progression, but remainder with "stable" disease	12 mo median
Hilaris et al[352] (1984)	Pleurectomy	41	45 + implant	29/41	12.6 mo median
Lee et al[353] (2002)	Pleurectomy	24	41.4 (median) 5-15 IORT	"Most"	18 mo median
Baldini et al[329] (1997)	EPP	49	30.6 ≈20 boost	21/49	22 mo
Rusch et al[323] (1991)	EPP	55	54	7/55	Stage I Stage III
Ahamad et al[355] (2003)	EPP	28	45-50	0 2 marginal misses	Not yet reached (2 y OS 62%)
Yajnik et al[358] (2003)	EPP	35	54	13/35	Not reported
Weder et al[364] (2004)	Chemo + EPP	19	Selected volumes	8/13 (13 patients completed all therapy)	16.5 mo

Chemo, chemotherapy; EPP, extrapleural pneumonectomy; IORT, intraoperative radiation therapy; OS, overall survival.

reported after the review of outcomes of 29 courses of palliative external beam radiation therapy delivered to 17 patients with MPM.[322] Four of six patients treated with more than 40 Gy achieved significant relief of symptoms. Only one patient treated with lower doses achieved significant palliation of any symptom, and this was for a painful chest wall mass.

In another study,[359] 26 radiation therapy courses were reviewed for symptomatic improvement. Pain was improved in 13 of 18 cases, and the response was similar regardless of dose or fractionation (i.e., 20 Gy in 5 fractions or 30 Gy in 10 fractions). Although the sample size is small, palliation was achieved in about one half of cases in this very mixed patient group. The duration of response was not assessed in either study. These data demonstrate that symptoms from mesothelioma can usually be palliated effectively with brief courses of irradiation.

Drain Sites

Unlike most malignancies, MPM has a tendency to predictably recur along tracks of previous chest wall instrumentation.[360] One group hypothesized that local irradiation might prevent this type of painful tumor growth pattern.[361] Forty consecutive patients with pathologically proven MPM were randomized to immediate prophylactic irradiation to each site of instrumentation or to observation. Prophylactic treatment was 21 Gy in 3 fractions delivered using en face electron fields. The study authors found no subcutaneous MPM progression in the irradiated patients, but nodules developed in 8 (40%) of 20 of the untreated patients. Because such recurrences typically are painful, the investigators concluded that prophylactic irradiation was a safe and effective means of maintaining the patients' quality of life.

Techniques of Irradiation

Patient Immobilization and Setup

Two basic techniques have been described for post-EPP thoracic irradiation.[357,358] A description of the IMRT techniques for the postoperative treatment of MPM has been described.[355,357] This level of detail is required to ensure that the very complex target volumes can be identified and reproducibly treated for 5 weeks.

Computed Tomography Simulation

MPM tends to recur at sites of previous instrumentation, and all incision and drain sites should be included in the CTV. Laparoscopy or mediastinoscopy sites have not been included within the CTV as long as the mediastinoscopy was pathologically negative. Radiopaque wires mark the surgical incisions, and tissue equivalent bolus extends to 4 cm around the wires. Patients are immobilized supine on the CT simulator using a combination of a vacuum bag and an "extended wing board with T-bar handgrip" immobilization device used in conjunction with a headrest.

Because of the large target volume, the optimal scan slice thickness is 5 mm. This simplifies contouring and speeds dose calculations. The patient should be scanned from the middle neck to the anterior superior iliac spine. This low inferior border allows complete definition of both kidneys so that accurate dose-volume histograms can be constructed.

Target Volume Delineation

The ipsilateral mediastinum should be included in the target volume,[355,361,362] even for node-negative patients. The superior border should be placed at the thoracic inlet. The medial border includes the ipsilateral nodal regions, trachea and subcarinal regions,[357] or the vertebral body.[358] The posterior mediastinal structures behind the heart need not be included, because no failures in this region have been recorded (unpublished data) despite their omission from the CTV.[355]

The anteromedial pleural reflection is a potential problem for target volume delineation. As shown in Figure 43-7A, the medial pleural space sometimes can cross midline. This anatomic relationship can be lost after surgery (see Fig. 43-7B). When possible, this region should be marked intraoperatively with radiopaque clips. Alternatively, the medial extent of the pleura could be identified on preoperative CT scans, and this extent estimated on the treatment planning CT. This has been the site of a marginal miss in our series (see Fig. 43-7C, *arrow*).

The inferior border should be the insertion of the diaphragm. The location of this is quite variable, ranging from L1 to L4. Because of this variability, the diaphragm insertion should be marked by intraoperative placement of radiopaque

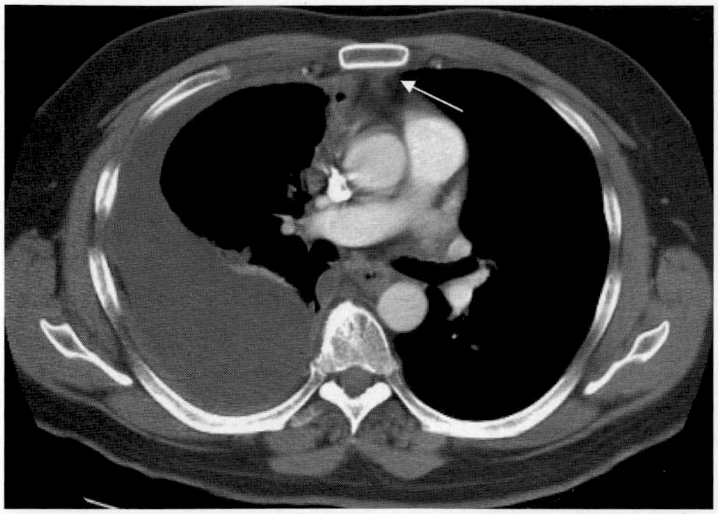

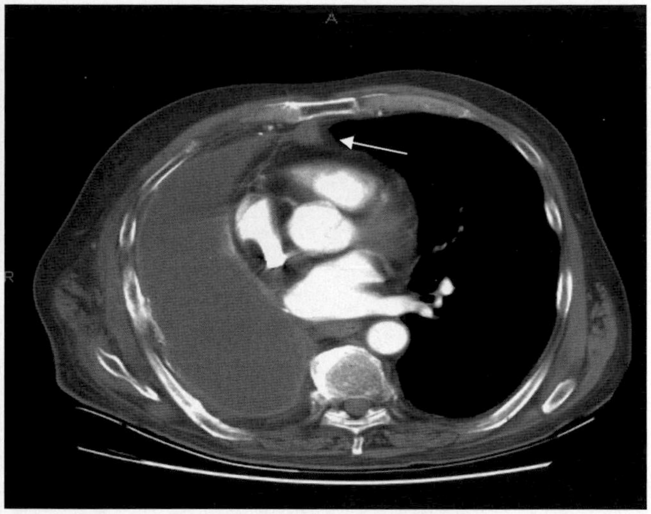

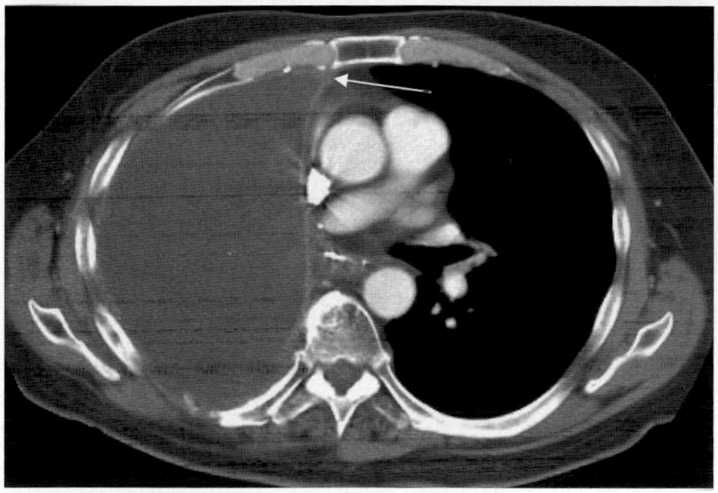

Figure 43-7 The costomediastinal sulcus can cross midline. **A,** Preoperatively, pleural thickening crosses the midline anteriorly *(arrow)*. **B,** This involvement is obliterated by extrapleural pneumonectomy, and the medial edge of the clinical target volume (CTV) was placed at the insertion of the rib *(arrow)*. **C,** Unfortunately, the tumor recurred immediately adjacent to the CTV *(arrow)* in a region that received less than 40 Gy.

clips[356] or by suturing the neodiaphragm in this location.[358] When the border of intrathoracic contents and abdominal contents is well marked, the radiation therapy margins can be maximally reduced. Because there can be great difficulty in differentiating liver from thoracic fluid, we have used radiopaque Gore-Tex patches for diaphragm reconstructions.

Another potential source of contouring error is the medial extent of the crus of the diaphragm, especially at its most inferior extent. The ipsilateral crus is usually very difficult to identify after surgery without clips. The best way to individualize the inferior edge of the target volume is with extensive intraoperative placement of radiopaque clips, with particular attention to the crus.

When the entire region is extensively clipped, a pattern such as that seen in Figure 43-8 emerges, with regions of potential pitfall highlighted. These potential problem areas include the anterior medial pleural reflection, the crus of the diaphragm, and the inferior aspect of the diaphragmatic insertion.

Treatment Planning

Three-Dimensional Conformal Radiation Therapy

The 3D conformal radiation therapy approach has been described best in two reports from the Memorial Sloan-Kettering Cancer Center.[354,358] The technique applies anteroposterior-posteroanterior beam geometry to the hemithorax using the volumes described previously as the CTV. For right-sided cases, an abdominal block is present throughout treatment, and the region is boosted with electrons at 1.53 Gy per day, which accounts for scatter under the block. For left-sided cases, the kidney and heart are blocked. The kidney block is present throughout treatment, and the heart block is added after 19.8 Gy. The spinal cord is shielded after 41.4 Gy in all cases. The goal dose to the target volume is 54 Gy in 30 fractions, with the dose calculated at midplane with equally weighted beams. Patients were treated with arms akimbo.

Treatment by this simple approach results in good coverage of most volumes at risk to the target dose of 54 Gy. Doses are very homogeneous within the regions at risk, although regions such as the crus, the pericardium, and the neodiaphragm may be difficult to treat. Radiosensitive structures such as the liver and heart can be spared quite well. Protection of the ipsilateral kidney is clearly better than with IMRT.

Intensity-Modulated Radiation Therapy

The target doses and the dose-volume limits for the critical structures are listed in Table 43-10. Treatment is delivered with

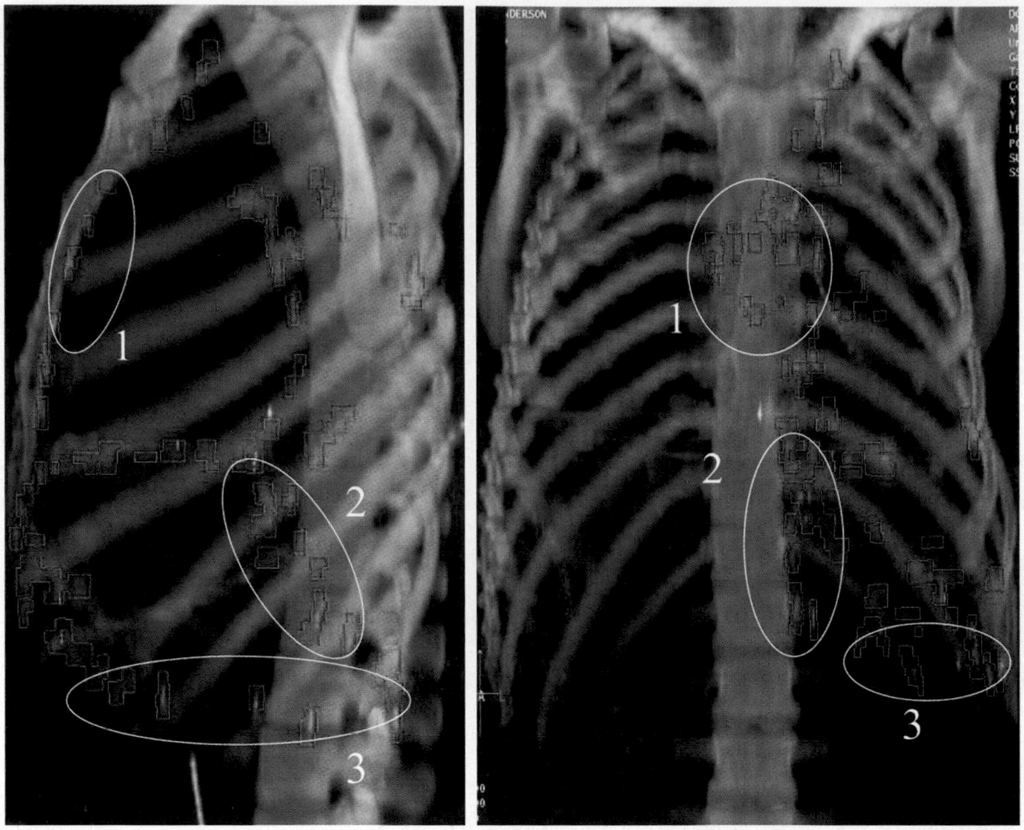

Figure 43-8 Potential problem areas for clinical target volume (CTV) determination. Three parts of the CTV are potentially difficult to discern without great care: the anteromedial pleural reflection of the sternopericardial recess (1), the inferior and medial extents of the crus of the diaphragm (2), and the inferior insertion of the diaphragm (3).

Table 43-10 Goal Dose or Constraint Dose of the Target or Organ

Target or Organ	Goal Dose or Constraint Dose
CTV	50 Gy in 25 fractions
bCTV	60 Gy in 25 fractions
Lung	<20% to receive >20 Gy and mean less than 9.5 Gy
Liver	<30% to receive >30 Gy
Contralateral kidney	<20% to receive >15 Gy
Heart	<50% to receive >45 Gy
Spinal cord	<10% to receive >45 Gy No portion to receive >50 Gy
Esophagus	<30% to receive >55 Gy

bCTV, boost clinical target volume; CTV, clinical target volume.

13 to 27 intensity-modulated fields using 8 to 11 gantry angles, typically with 100 segments per intensity-modulated field. Because patients have only one lung after EPP, the volumes of contralateral lung irradiated should be limited such that the mean lung dose is less than 9.5 Gy. With experience, the mean lung dose can be kept well under 8 Gy. This is consistent with the results of whole-lung irradiation.[363] All patients can be set up and treated within a 45-minute period. Our previous experience was with the Corvus planning system, but acceptable plans can be obtained with other planning systems such as Pinnacle and Eclipse (unpublished observations).

IMRT is more complicated and takes longer to deliver than 3D conformal radiation therapy, but very good coverage of the target can be achieved. As shown in Figure 43-9, the 50-Gy isodose line encompasses most of the CTV. Review of the dose-volume histogram for this case (Fig. 43-10) demonstrates that the target volume is well covered and the normal tissue constraints are met. The liver and contralateral lung are spared with this technique. In this patient, it was possible to spare the ipsilateral kidney because the organ was particularly low. The ipsilateral kidney usually receives a high dose because the CTV typically abuts its posterior edge. Adequate contralateral renal function is ensured by pretreatment renal scans. For left-sided lesions, the spleen is likely to receive a high radiation dose, and pneumococcal prophylaxis is recommended.

SUMMARY

A review of the limited patient studies (see Table 43-9) in MPM suggests that EPP followed by irradiation gives better local control than pleurectomy followed by irradiation in selected patients. Postoperative irradiation should include the entire volume immediately adjacent to the pleural space that is at highest risk for microscopic residual disease. This volume should include all sites of pleural reflection, the ipsilateral mediastinum, and the insertion of the diaphragm. The technique by which radiation is delivered (traditional or IMRT) is probably not as important as target volume delineation and coverage. Prospective trials integrating systemic therapy with EPP and postoperative irradiation are being conducted.

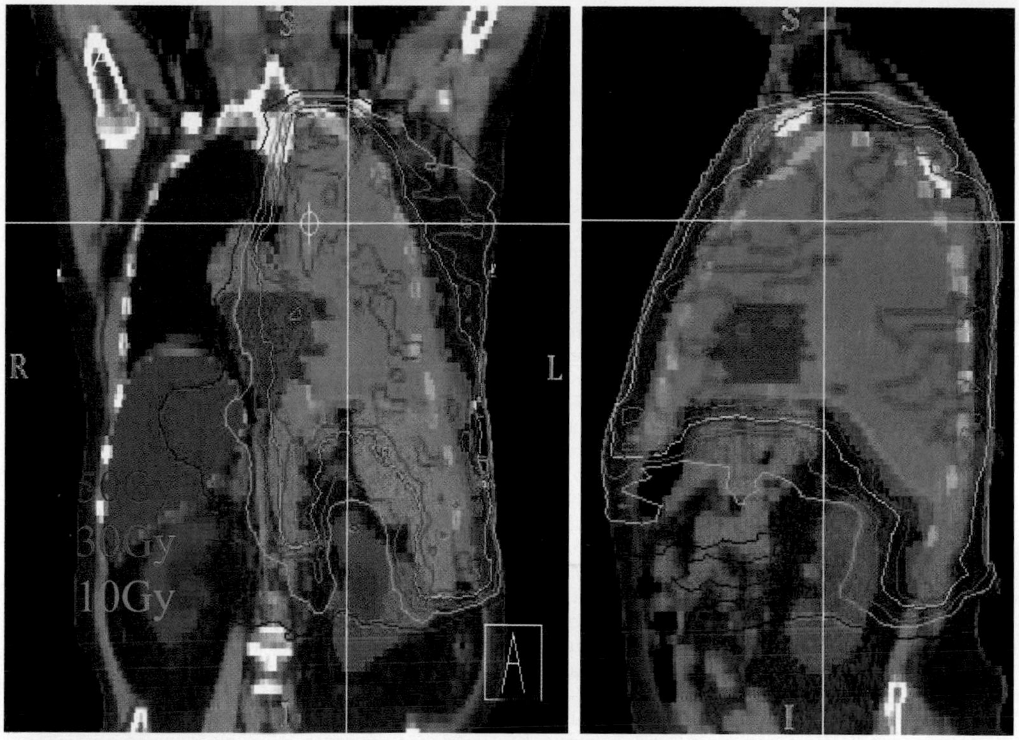

A B

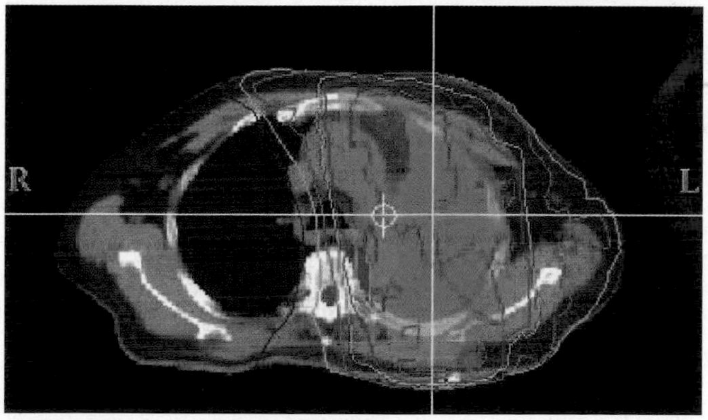

C

Figure 43-9 A–C, The dose distributions for intensity-modulated radiation therapy demonstrate good coverage of the clinical target volume (CTV) and the high-dose gradients achievable with this technique. The goal was 50 Gy to the CTV. The 50-, 30-, and 10-Gy isodose lines are shown in magenta, orange, green, and blue, respectively.

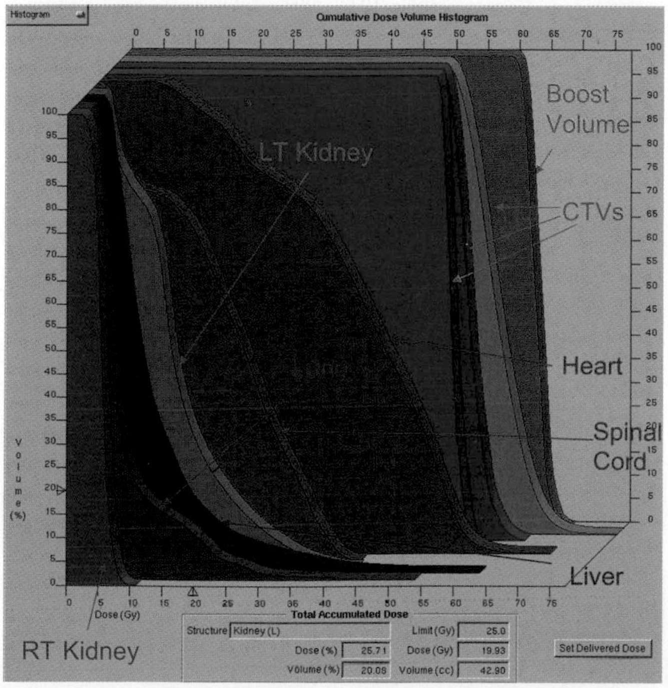

Figure 43-10 The dose-volume histogram demonstrates that coverage of the target volumes is adequate. The contralateral kidney was well below the goal dose, as was about 25% of the ipsilateral kidney. The mean lung dose was about 9.5 Gy. In this left-sided case, the heart dose was slightly higher than the goal dose (60% to 45 Gy, rather than 50%).

ACKNOWLEDGMENTS

We wish to thank the following people for their suggestions and contributions: Clifton Fuller, MD (Radiation Oncology Department, University of Texas Health Science Center at San Antonio), David Hussey (Radiation Oncology Department, University of Texas Health Science Center at San Antonio), Jaishree Jagirdar, MD (Pathology Department, University of Texas Health Science Center at San Antonio), and Cindy Scharfen (Redwood Regional Radiation Oncology Center).

REFERENCES

1. VonGaudecker B: Functional histology of the human thymus. Anat Embryol 183:1, 1991.
2. Davis RD, Oldham HN, Sabiston DC: Primary cysts and neoplasms of the mediastinum: recent changes in clinical presentation, methods of diagnosis, management, and results. Ann Thorac Surg 44:229-237, 1987.
3. Whooley BP, Urschel JD, Antkowiak JG, et al: Primary tumors of the mediastinum. J Surg Oncol 70:95-99, 1999.
4. Mullen B, Richardson JD: Primary anterior mediastinal tumors in children and adults. Ann Thorac Surg 42:338-345, 1986.
5. Ritter JH, Wick MR: Primary carcinomas of the thymus gland. Semin Diagn Pathol 16:18-31, 1999.
6. Ogawa K, Toita T, Uno T, et al: Treatment and prognosis of thymic carcinoma: a retrospective analysis of 40 cases. Cancer 94:3115-3119, 2002.
7. Kondo K, Monden Y: Therapy for thymic epithelial tumors: a clinical study of 1,320 patients from Japan. Ann Thorac Surg 76:878-884, 2003.
8. Wick MR, Rosai J: Neuroendocrine neoplasms of the mediastinum. Sem Diagn Pathol 8:35-51, 1991.
9. Leyvraz S, Henle W, Chahinian A, et al: Association of Epstein-Barr virus with thymic carcinoma. N Engl J Med 312:1296-1299, 1985.
10. Patton DP, Ribeiro RC, Jenkins JJ, et al: Thymic carcinoma with a defective Epstein-Barr virus encoding the BZLF1 transactivator. J Infect Dis 170:7-12, 1994.
11. Teoh R, McGuire L, Wong K, Chin D: Increased incidence of thymoma in Chinese myasthenia gravis: possible relationship with Epstein-Barr virus. Acta Neurol Scand 80:221-225, 1989.
12. Dimery IW, Lee JS, Blick M, et al: Association of Epstein-Barr virus with lymphoepithelioma of the thymus. Cancer 61:2475-2480, 1988.
13. McGuire LJ, Huang DP, Teoh R, et al: Epstein-Barr virus genome in thymoma and thymic lymphoid hyperplasia. Am J Pathol 131:385-390, 1988.
14. Jensen MO, Antonenko D: Thyroid and thymic malignancy following childhood irradiation. J Surg Oncol 50:206-208, 1992.
15. Lam WW, Chan FL, Lau YL, et al: Pediatric thymoma: unusual occurrence in two siblings. Pediatr Radiol 23:124-126, 1993.
16. Matani A, Dritsas C: Familial occurrence of thymoma. Arch Pathol 95:90-91, 1973.
17. Rosai J, Higa E, Davie J: Mediastinal endocrine neoplasm in patients with multiple endocrine adenomatosis: a previously unrecognized association. Cancer 29:1075-1083, 1972.
18. Teh BT, Zedenius J, Kytola S, et al: Thymic carcinoids in multiple endocrine neoplasia type 1. Ann Surg 228:99-105, 1998.
19. Kubonishi I, Takehara N, Iwata J, et al: Novel t(15:19)(q15;p13) chromosome abnormality in a thymic carcinoma. Cancer Res 51:3327-3328, 1991.
20. Lee ACW, Kwong YL, Fu KH, et al: Disseminated mediastinal carcinoma with chromosomal translocation (15:19). Cancer 72:2273-2276, 1993.
21. Kees UR, Mulcahy MT, Willoughby ML: Intrathoracic carcinoma in an 11-year-old girl showing a translocation t(15:19). Am J Pediatr Hematol Oncol 13:459-464, 1991.
22. Herens C, Radermecker M, Servais A, et al: Deletion (6)(p22p25) is a recurrent anomaly of thymoma: report of a second case and review of the literature. Cancer Genet Cytogenet 146:66-69, 2003.
23. Inoue M, Marx A, Zettl A, et al: Chromosome 6 suffers frequent and multiple aberrations in thymoma. Am J Pathol 161:1507-1513, 2002.
24. Zettl A, Ströbel P, Wagner K, et al: Recurrent genetic aberrations in thymoma and thymic carcinoma. Am J Pathol 157:257-266, 2000.
25. Abdollahi A, Roberts D, Godwin AK, et al: Identification of a zinc-finger gene at 6q25: a chromosomal region implicated in development of many solid tumors. Oncogene 14:1973-1979, 1997.
26. Miozzo M, Pierotti MA, Sozzi G, et al: Human TRK proto-oncogene maps to chromosome 1q32-q41. Oncogene 9:1411-1414, 1990.
27. Knuutila S, Bjorkqvist AM, Autio K, et al: DNA copy number amplifications in human neoplasms. Am J Pathol 16:1153-1169, 1995.
28. Knuutila S, Aalto Y, Autio K, et al: DNA copy number losses in human neoplasms. Am J Pathol 155:683-694, 1999.
29. Engels EA, Pfeiffer RM: Malignant thymoma in the United States: demographic patterns in incidence and associations with subsequent malignancies. Int J Cancer 105:546-551, 2003.
30. National Cancer Institute: Surveillance Epidemiology and End Results Program (SEER). 1990. www.cancer.gov
31. Azarow KS, Pearl RH, Zurcher R, et al: Primary mediastinal masses. A comparison of adult and pediatric populations. J Thorac Cardiovasc Surg 106:67-72, 1993.
32. Cohen AJ, Thompson L, Edwards FH, Bellamy RF: Primary cysts and tumors of the mediastinum. Ann Thorac Surg 51:378-384, 1991.
33. Strollo DC, Rosado-de-Christenson ML, Jett JR: Primary mediastinal tumors. Part I. Tumors of the anterior mediastinum. Chest 112:511-522, 1997.
34. Lewis JE, Wick MR, Scheithauer BW, Bernatz PE, et al: Thymoma: a clinicopathologic review. Cancer 60:2727-2743, 1987.
35. Batata MA, Martini N, Huvos AG, et al: Thymomas: clinicopathologic features, therapy, and prognosis. Cancer 34:389-396, 1974.
36. Bernatz PE, Khonsari S, Harrison EG, et al: Thymoma: factors influencing prognosis. Surg Clin North Am 4:885, 1973.
37. LeGolvan DP, Abell MR: Thymomas. Cancer 39:2142-2157, 1977.
38. Salyer WR, Eggleston JC: Thymoma: a clinical and pathological study of 65 cases. Cancer 37:229-249, 1976.
39. Suster S, Rosai J: Thymic carcinoma. A clinicopathologic study of 60 cases. Cancer 67:1025-1032, 1991.
40. Hsu CP, Chen CY, Chen CL, et al: Thymic carcinoma. Ten years' experience in twenty patients. J Thorac Cardiovasc Surg 107:615-620, 1994.
41. Wick MR, Weiland LH, Scheithauer BW, et al: Primary thymic carcinomas. Am J Surg Pathol 6:613-630, 1982.
42. Kuo TT, Chang JP, Lin FJ, et al: Thymic carcinomas: histopathological varieties and immunohistochemical study. Am J Surg Pathol 14:24-34, 1990.
43. Economopoulos GC, Lewis JW, Lee MW, et al: Carcinoid tumors of the thymus. Ann Thorac Surg 50:58-61, 1990.
44. Moran CA, Suster S: Spindle-cell neuroendocrine carcinoma of the thymus: a clinicopathologic and immunohistochemical study of seven cases. Mod Pathol 12:587-591, 1999.
45. Lara PN Jr: Malignant thymoma: current status and future directions. Cancer Treat Rev 26:127-131, 2000.
46. Detterbeck FC, Parsons AM: Thymic tumors. Ann Thorac Surg 77:1860-1869, 2004.
47. Morgenthaler TI, Brown LR, Colby TV, et al: Thymoma. Mayo Clin Proc 68:1110-1123, 1993.
48. Maggi G, Casadio C, Cavallo A, et al: Thymoma: results of 241 operated cases. Ann Thorac Surg 51:152-156, 1991.
49. Drachman DB: Myasthenia gravis. N Engl J Med 330:1797-1810, 1994.
50. Willcox N: Myasthenia gravis. Curr Opin Immunol 5:910-917, 1993.

51. Souadjian JV, Enriquez P, Silverstein MN, et al: The spectrum of diseases associated with thymoma. Coincidence or syndrome? Arch Intern Med 134:374-379, 1974.
52. Blumberg D, Burt ME, Bains MS, et al: Thymic carcinoma: current staging does not predict prognosis. J Thorac Cardiovasc Surg 115:303-309, 1998.
53. Curran WJ Jr, Kornstein MJ, Brooks JJ, et al: Invasive thymoma: the role of mediastinal irradiation following complete or incomplete surgical resection. J Clin Oncol 6:1722-1727, 1988.
54. Cohen DJ, Ronnigen LD, Graeber GM, et al: Management of patients with malignant thymoma. J Thorac Cardiovasc Surg 87:301-307, 1984.
55. Ruffini E, Mancuso M, Oliaro A, et al: Recurrence of thymoma: analysis of clinicopathologic features, treatment, and outcome. J Thorac Cardiovasc Surg 113:55-63, 1997.
56. Monden Y, Nakahara K, Ioka S, et al: Recurrence of thymoma: clinicopathological features, therapy, and prognosis. Ann Thorac Surg 39:165-169, 1985.
57. Sellors TH, Thackray AC, Thomson AD: Tumours of the thymus: a review of 88 operation cases. Thorax 22:193-220, 1967.
58. Weissberg D, Goldberg M, Pearson FG: Thymoma. Ann Thorac Surg 16:141-147, 1973.
59. Hoffacker V, Schultz A, Tiesinga JJ, et al: Thymomas alter the T-cell subset composition in the blood: a potential mechanism for thymoma-associated autoimmune disease. Blood 96:3872-3879, 2000.
60. Buckley C, Douek D, Newsom-Davis J, et al: Mature, long-lived CD4+ and CD8+ T cells are generated by the thymoma in myasthenia gravis. Ann Neurol 50:64-72, 2001.
61. Ströbel P, Helmreich M, Menioudakis G, et al: Paraneoplastic myasthenia gravis correlates with generation of mature naive CD4(+) T cells in thymomas. Blood 100:159-166, 2002.
62. Agarwala SS: Paraneoplastic syndromes. Med Clin North Am 80:173-184, 1996.
63. Mygland A, Vincent A, Newsom-Davis J, et al: Autoantibodies in thymoma-associated myasthenia gravis with myositis or neuromyotonia. Arch Neurol 57:527-531, 2000.
64. Tarr PE, Sneller MC, Mechanic LJ, et al: Infections in patients with immunodeficiency with thymoma (Good syndrome). Report of 5 cases and review of the literature. Medicine (Baltimore) 80:123-133, 2001.
65. Montella L, Masci AM, Merkabaoui G, et al: B-cell lymphopenia and hypogammaglobulinemia in thymoma patients. Ann Hematol 82:343-347, 2003.
66. Tateyama H, Eimoto T, Tada T, et al: P53 protein expression and p53 gene mutation in thymic epithelial tumors: an immunohistochemical and DNA sequencing study. Am J Clin Pathol 104:375-381, 1995.
67. Chen, FF, Yan JJ, Jin YT, et al: Detection of bcl-2 and p53 in thymoma: expression of bcl-2 as a reliable marker of tumor aggressiveness. Hum Pathol 27:1089-1092, 1996.
68. Tateyama H, Mizuno T, Tada T, et al: Thymic epithelial tumours: evaluation of malignant grade by quantification of proliferating cell nuclear antigen and nucleolar organizer regions. Virchows Arch A Pathol Anat 422:265-269, 1993.
69. Pich A, Chiarle R, Chiusa L, et al: Long-term survival of thymoma patients by histologic pattern and proliferative activity. Am J Surg Pathol 19:918-926, 1995.
70. Yang WI, Efird JT, Quintanilla-Martinez L, et al: Cell kinetic study of thymic epithelial tumors using PCNA (PC10) and Ki-67 (MIB-1) antibodies. Hum Pathol 27:70-76, 1996.
71. Takahashi E, Tateyama H, Akatsu H, et al: Expression of matrix metalloproteinases 2 and 7 in tumor cells correlates with the World Health Organization classification subtype and clinical stage of thymic epithelial tumors. Hum Pathol 34:1253-1258, 2003.
72. Marx AD, Schomig A, Schultz S, et al: Distribution of molecules mediating thymocyte-stroma-interactions in human thymus, thymitis and thymic epithelial tumors. Thymus 23:83-93, 1994.
73. Ruco LP, Paradiso P, Pittiglio M, et al: Tissue distribution of very late activation antigens-1/6 and very late activation antigen ligands in the normal thymus and in thymoma. Am J Pathol 142:765-772, 1993.
74. Schultz A, Greiner R, Nenninger D, et al: CD40 as a mediator of proliferation in normal and neoplastic thymic epithelium. Verh Dtsch Ges Pathol 80:21250-21255, 1996.
75. Willcox N, Harcourt G, Nagvekar N, et al: Antigen presentation by thymoma epithelial cells from myathenia gravis patients to potentially pathogenic T cells. J Neuroimmunol 56:65-76, 1995.
76. Hayashi Y, Ishii N, Obayashi C, et al: Thymoma: tumour type related to expression of epidermal growth factor (EGF), EGF-receptor, p53, v-erb B and ras p21. Virchows Arch 426:43-50, 1995.
77. Negron-Soto JM, Cascade PN: Squamous cell carcinoma of the thymus with paraneoplastic hypercalcemia. Clin Imaging 19:122-124, 1995.
78. Suzuki K, Tanaka H, Shibusa T, et al: Parathyroid-hormone-related-protein-producing thymic carcinoma presenting as a giant extrathoracic mass. Respiration 65:83-85, 1998.
79. Jung KJ, Lee KS, Han J, et al: Malignant thymic epithelial tumors: CT-pathologic correlation. AJR Am J Roentgenol 176:433-439, 2001.
80. Zhang Z, Cui Y, Li B, et al: Thymic carcinoma (report of 14 cases). Chin Med Sci J 12:252-255, 1997.
81. Shimosato Y, Kameya T, Nagai K, et al: Squamous cell carcinoma of the thymus. An analysis of eight cases. Am J Surg Pathol 1:109-121, 1977.
82. Henley JD, Koukoulis GK, Loehrer PJ Sr: Epidermal growth factor receptor expression in invasive thymoma. J Cancer Res Clin Oncol 128:167-170, 2002.
83. Gilhus NE, Jones M, Turley H, et al: Oncogene proteins and proliferation antigens in thymomas: increased expression of epidermal growth factor receptor and Ki67 antigen. J Clin Pathol 48:447-455, 1995.
84. Tomita M, Matsuzaki Y, Edagawa M, et al: Clinical and immunohistochemical study of eight cases with thymic carcinoma. BMC Surg 2:3-9, 2002.
85. Sasaki H, Yukiue H, Kobayashi Y, et al: Elevated serum vascular endothelial growth factor and basic fibroblast growth factor levels in patients with thymic epithelial neoplasms. Surg Today 31:1038-1040, 2001.
86. Tomita M, Matsuzaki Y, Edagawa M, et al: Correlation between tumor angiogenesis and invasiveness in thymic epithelial tumors. J Thorac Cardiovasc Surg 124:493-498, 2002.
87. Fukai I, Masaoka A, Hashimoto T, et al: The distribution of epithelial membrane antigen in thymic epithelial neoplasms. Cancer 70:2077-2081, 1992.
88. Fukai I, Masaoka A, Hashimoto T, et al: Cytokeratins in normal thymus and thymic epithelial tumors. Cancer 71:99-105, 1993.
89. Oyama T, Osaki T, Mitsudomi T, et al: P53 alteration, proliferating cell nuclear antigen, and nucleolar organizer regions in thymic epithelial tumors. Int J Mol Med 1:823-826, 1998.
90. Kuo TT, Chan JK: Thymic carcinoma arising in thymoma is associated with alterations in immunohistochemical profile. Am J Surg Pathol 22:1474-1481, 1998.
91. Hino N, Kondo K, Miyoshi T, et al: High frequency of p53 protein expression in thymic carcinoma but not in thymoma. Br J Cancer 76:1361-1366, 1997.
92. Hishima T, Fukayama M, Hayashi Y, et al: CD70 expression in thymic carcinoma. Am J Surg Pathol 24:742-746, 2000.
93. Hishima T, Fukayama M, Fujisawa M, et al: CD5 expression in thymic carcinoma. Am J Pathol 145:268-275, 1994.
94. Tateyama H, Eimoto T, Tada T, et al: Immunoreactivity of a new CD5 antibody with normal epithelium and malignant tumors including thymic carcinoma. Am J Clin Pathol 111:235-240, 1999.
95. Dorfman DM, Shahsafaei A, Chan JK: Thymic carcinomas, but not thymomas and carcinomas of other sites, show CD5 immunoreactivity. Am J Surg Pathol 21:936-940, 1997.
96. Fukai I, Masaoka A, Hashimoto T, et al: Differential diagnosis of thymic carcinoma and lung carcinoma with the use of antibodies to cytokeratins. J Thorac Cardiovasc Surg 110:1670-1675, 1995.
97. Moran CA, Suster S: Neuroendocrine carcinomas (carcinoid tumor) of the thymus. Am J Clin Pathol 114:100-110, 2000.
98. Fukai I, Masaoka A, Fujii Y, et al: Thymic neuroendocrine tumor (thymic carcinoid): a clinicopathologic study in 15 patients. Ann Thorac Surg 67:208-211, 1999.

99. Rosai J, Levine GD: Tumors of the thymus. *In* Atlas of Tumor Pathology, series 2, fascicle 34. Washington, DC, Armed Forces Institute of Pathology, 1976, pp 55-99.
100. Quintanilla-Martinez L, Wilkins EW, Choi N, et al: Thymoma. Cancer 74:606, 1994.
101. Eng TY, Fuller CD, Jagirdar J, et al: Thymic carcinoma: state of the art review. Int J Radiat Oncol Biol Phys 59:654-664, 2004.
102. Bergh NP, Gatzinsky P, Larsson S, et al: Tumors of the thymus and thymic region. I. Clinicopathological studies on thymomas. Ann Thorac Surg 25:91-98, 1978.
103. Fujimura S, Kondo T, Handen M, et al: Results of surgical treatment for thymoma based on 66 patients. J Thorac Cardiovasc Surg 93:708-714, 1987.
104. Maggi C, Giaccone G, Donadio M, et al: Thymomas: a review of 169 cases, with particular reference to results of surgical treatment. Cancer 58:765-776, 1986.
105. Nakahara K, Ohno K, Hashimoto J, et al: Thymoma: results with complete resection and adjuvant postoperative irradiation in 141 consecutive patients. J Thorac Cardiovasc Surg 95:1041-1047, 1988.
106. Wilkins EW Jr, Castleman B: Thymoma: a continuing survey at Massachusetts General Hospital. Ann Thorac Surg 28:252-256, 1978.
107. Akaogi E, Ohara K, Mitsui K, et al: Preoperative radiotherapy and surgery for advanced thymoma with invasion to the great vessels. J Surg Oncol 63:17-22, 1996.
108. Lee JD, Choe KO, Kim SJ, et al: CT findings in primary thymic carcinoma. J Comput Assist Tomogr 15:429-433, 1991.
109. Asbun HJ, Calabria RP, Calmes S, et al: Thymic carcinoid. Ann Surg 57:442-445, 1991.
110. Legg MA, Brady WJ: Pathology and clinical behavior of thymoma: a survey of 51 cases. Cancer 18:1131-1144, 1965.
111. Patterson GA: Thymomas. Semin Thorac Cardiovasc Surg 4:39-44, 1992.
112. Marchevsky AM, Kaneko M: Surgical Pathology of the Mediastinum. New York, Raven Press, 1984.
113. Chahinian A, Bhardwaj S, Meyer RJ, et al: Treatment of invasive or metastatic thymoma. Cancer 47:1752-1761, 1981.
114. LeBlanc J, Wood DE: Diagnosis of mediastinal tumors. *In* Wood DE, Thomas CR Jr (eds): Mediastinal Tumors: Update 1995. Medical Radiology-Diagnostic Imaging and Radiation Oncology. Heidelberg, Germany, Springer-Verlag, 1995, pp 1-10.
115. Wilkins EW, Grillo HC, Scannell JG, et al: Role of staging in prognosis and management of thymoma. Ann Thorac Surg 51:888-892, 1991.
116. Vincent A: Autoimmunity to acetylcholine receptors in myasthenia gravis. Biochem Soc Trans 19:180-183, 1991.
117. Drachman DB: Myasthenia gravis. N Engl J Med 298(Pat 1):136-143, 1978.
118. Vincent A, Palace J, Hilton-Jones D: Myasthenia gravis. Lancet 357:2122-2128, 2001.
119. Urgesi A, Monetti U, Rossi G, et al: Role of radiation therapy in locally advanced thymoma. Radiother Oncol 19:273-280, 1990.
120. Masaoka A, Monden Y, Nakahara K, Tanioka T: Follow-up study of thymomas with special reference to their clinical stages. Cancer 48:2485-2492, 1981.
121. Rea F, Marulli G, Girardi R, et al: Long-term survival and prognostic factors in thymic epithelial tumours. Eur J Cardiothorac Surg 26:412-418, 2004.
122. Blumberg D, Port JL, Weksler B, et al:Thymoma: a multivariate analysis of factors predicting survival. Ann Thorac Surg 60:908-914, 1995.
123. Pescarmona E, Rendina EA, Venuta F, et al: Analysis of prognostic factors and clinicopathological staging of thymoma. Ann Thorac Surg 50:534-538, 1990.
124. Pollack A, Komaki R, Cox JC, et al: Thymoma: treatment and prognosis. Int J Radiat Oncol Biol Phys 23:1037-1043, 1992.
125. Lardinois D, Rechsteiner R, Lang RH, et al: Prognostic relevance of Masaoka and Muller-Hermelink classification in patients with thymic tumors. Ann Thorac Surg 69:1550-1555, 2000.
126. McCart JA, Gaspar L, Inculet R, et al: Predictors of survival following surgical resection of thymoma. J Surg Oncol 54:233-238, 1993.
127. Murakawa T, Nakajima J, Kohno T, et al: Results from surgical treatment for thymoma: 43 years of experience. Jpn J Thorac Cardiovasc Surg 48:89-95, 2000.
128. Park HS, Shin DM, Lee JS, et al: Thymoma. Cancer 73:2491-2498, 1994.
129. Wilkins KB, Sheikh E, Green R, et al: Clinical and pathologic predictors of survival in patients with thymoma. Ann Surg 230:562-572, 1999.
130. Venuta F, Rendina EA, De Giacomo T, et al: Thymectomy for myasthenia gravis: a 27-year experience. Eur J Cardiothorac Surg 15:621-625, 1999.
131. Kohman LJ: Controversies in the management of malignant thymoma. Chest 112(Suppl):296S-300S, 1997.
132. Verstandig AG, Epstein DM, Miller WT Jr, et al: Thymoma: report of 71 cases and a review. Crit Rev Diagn Imaging 33:201-230, 1992.
133. El-Medany Y, Hajjar W, Essa M, et al: Predictors of outcome for myasthenia gravis after thymectomy. Asian Cardiovasc Thorac Ann 11:323-327, 2003.
134. Murakawa T, Nakajima J, Sato H, et al: Thymoma associated with pure red-cell aplasia: clinical features and prognosis. Asian Cardiovasc Thorac Ann 10:150-154, 2002.
135. Rios A, Torres J, Galindo PJ, et al: Prognostic factors in thymic epithelial neoplasms. Eur J Cardiothorac Surg 21:307-313, 2002.
136. Chen G, Marx A, Chen WH, et al: New WHO histologic classification predicts prognosis of thymic epithelial tumors: a clinicopathologic study of 200 thymoma cases from China. Am Cancer Soc 95:420-429, 2002.
137. Marino M, Muller-Hermelink H: Thymoma and thymic carcinoma: relation of thymoma epithelial cells to the cortical and medullary differentiation of thymus. Virchows Arch 407:119-149, 1985.
138. Ricci C, Rendina EA, Pescarmona E, et al: Correlation between histological type, clinical behavior and prognosis in thymoma. Thorax 44:455-460, 1989.
139. Ho FC, Fu KH, Lam SY, et al: Evaluation of a histogenetic classification for thymic epithelial tumours. Histopathology 25:21-29, 1994.
140. Tan PH, Sng IT: Thymoma: a study of 60 cases in Singapore. Histopathology 26:509-518, 1995.
141. Verley JM, Hollmann KH: Thymoma. A comparative study of clinical stages, histologic features, and survival in 200 cases. Cancer 55:1074-1086, 1985.
142. Hoffman OA, Gillespie DJ, Aughenbaugh GL, et al: Primary mediastinal neoplasms (other than thymoma). Mayo Clin Proc 68:880-891, 1993.
143. Shields TW: Primary tumors and cysts of the mediastinum. *In* Shields TW (ed): General Thoracic Surgery. Philadelphia, Lea & Febiger, 1983, p 927.
144. Dahlgren S, Sandstedt B, Sundstrom C: Fine needle aspiration cytology of thymic tumors. Acta Cytologica 27:1-6, 1983.
145. Baron RL, Lee JKT, Sagel SS: Computed tomography of the abnormal thymus. Radiology 142:127, 1982.
146. Levitt RG, Husband JE, Glazer HS: CT of primary germ cell tumors of the mediastinum. Am J Radiol 142:73-78, 1984.
147. Casamassima F, Villari N, Fargnoli R, et al: Magnetic resonance imaging and high-resolution computed tomography in tumors of the lung and the mediastinum. Radiother Oncol 11:21-29, 1988.
148. Kubota K, Yamada S, Kondo T, et al: PET imaging of primary mediastinal tumours. Br J Cancer 73:882-886, 1996.
149. Liu RS, Yeh SH, Huang MH, et al: Use of fluorine-18 fluorodeoxyglucose positron emission tomography in the detection of thymoma: a preliminary report. Eur J Nucl Med 22:1402-1407, 1995.
150. Shabb NS, Fahl M, Sabb B, et al: Fine-needle aspiration of the mediastinum: a clinical, radiologic, cytologic, and histologic study of 42 cases. Diagn Cytopathol 19:428-436, 1998.
151. Morrissey B, Adams H, Gibbs AR: Percutaneous needle biopsy of the mediastinum: review of 94 procedures. Thorax 48:632-637, 1993.
152. Cirino LM, Milanez de Campos JR, et al: Diagnosis and treatment of mediastinal tumors by thoracoscopy. Chest 117:1787-1792, 2000.

153. Demmy TL, Krasna MJ, Detterbeck FC, et al: Multicenter VATS experience with mediastinal tumors. Ann Thorac Surg 66:187-192, 1998.
154. Moran CA, Travis WD, Rosado-de-Christenson M, et al: Thymoma presenting as pleural tumors. Report of eight cases. Am J Surg Pathol 16:138-144, 1992.
155. Shih DF, Wang JS, Tseng HH, et al: Primary pleural thymoma. Arch Pathol Lab Med 121:79-82, 1997.
156. Suster S, Moran CA: Thymic carcinoma: spectrum of differentiation and histologic types. Pathology 30:111-122, 1998.
157. Tsuchiya R, Koga K, Matsuno Y, et al: Thymic carcinoma: proposal for pathological TNM and staging. Pathol Int 44:505-512, 1994.
158. Singhal S, Shrager JB, Rosenthal DI, et al: Comparison of stages I-II thymomas treated by complete resection with or without adjuvant radiation. Ann Thorac Surg 76:1635-1642, 2003.
159. Mangi AA, Wright CD, Allan JS, et al: Adjuvant radiation therapy for stage II thymoma. Ann Thorac Surg 74:1033-1037, 2002.
160. Reddy RHV, Shah R, Kumar B, et al: Recurrence of stage I thymoma in sternum, 13 years after 'complete' excision. Eur J Cardiothorac Surg 23:134-135, 2003.
161. Yagi K, Hirata T, Fukuse T, et al: Surgical treatment for invasive thymoma, especially when the superior vena cava is involved. Ann Thorac Surg 61:521-524, 1996.
162. Mussi A, Lucchi M, Murri L, et al: Extended thymectomy in myasthenia gravis: a team-work of neurologist, thoracic surgeon and anaesthesist may improve the outcome. Eur J Cardiothorac Surg 19:570-575, 2001.
163. Ohara K, Tatsuzaki H, Fuji H, et al: Radioresponse of thymomas verified with histologic response. Acta Oncologica 37:471-474, 1998.
164. Fehner RE: Recurrence of noninvasive thymomas. Cancer 23:1423-1427, 1969.
165. Haniuda M, Morimoto M, Nishimura H, et al: Adjuvant radiotherapy after complete resection of thymoma. Ann Thorac Surg 54:311-315, 1992.
166. Haniuda M, Miyazawa M, Yoshida K, et al: Is postoperative radiotherapy for thymoma effective? Ann Surg 224:219-224, 1996.
167. Gripp S, Hilgers K, Wurm R, et al: Thymoma: prognostic factors and treatment outcomes. Cancer 83:1495-1503, 1998.
168. Ohara K, Okumura T, Sugahara S, et al: The role of preoperative radiotherapy for invasive thymoma. Acta Oncol 29:425-429, 1990.
169. Cowen D, Richaud P, Mornex F, et al: Thymoma: results of a multicentric retrospective series of 149 non-metastatic irradiated patients and review of the literature. FNCLCC trialists. Federation Nationale des Centres de Lutte Contre le Cancer. Radiother Oncol 34:9-16, 1995.
170. Arakawa A, Yasunaga T, Saitoh Y, et al: Radiation therapy of invasive thymoma. Int J Radiat Oncol Biol Phys 18:529-534, 1990.
171. Ciernik IF, Meier U, Lutolf UM: Prognostic factors and outcome of incompletely resected invasive thymoma following radiation therapy. J Clin Oncol 12:1484-1490, 1994.
172. Ichinose Y, Ohta M, Yano T, et al: Treatment of invasive thymoma with pleural dissemination. J Surg Oncol 54:180-183, 1993.
173. Jackson MA, Ball DL: Postoperative radiotherapy in invasive thymoma. Radiother Oncol 21:77-82, 1991.
174. Urgesi A, Monetti U, Rossi G, et al: Aggressive treatment of intrathoracic recurrences of thymoma. Radiother Oncol 24:221-225, 1992.
175. Boston B: Chemotherapy of invasive thymoma. Cancer 38:49-52, 1976.
176. Campbell MG, Pollard R, Al-Sarraf M: A complete response of metastatic malignant thymoma to cis-platinum, doxorubicin and cyclophosphamide. Cancer 48:1315-1317, 1981.
177. Chahinian AP, Holland JF, Bhardwaj S: Chemotherapy for malignant thymoma. Ann Intern Med 99:736, 1983.
178. Daugaard G, Hansen HH, Rorth M: Combination chemotherapy for malignant thymoma. Ann Intern Med 99:189-190, 1983.
179. Dy C, Calvo F, Mindan J, et al: Undifferentiated epithelial-rich invasive malignant thymoma: complete response to cisplatinum, vinblastine, and bleomycin therapy. J Clin Oncol 6:536-542, 1988.
180. Evans WK, Thompson DM, Simpson WJ, et al: Combination chemotherapy in invasive thymoma: role of COPP. Cancer 46:1523-1527, 1980.
181. Fornasiero A, Daniele O, Ghiotto C, et al: Chemotherapy for invasive thymoma: a 13-year experience. Cancer 68:30-33, 1991.
182. Fornasiero A, Daniele O, Sperandio P, et al: Chemotherapy of invasive or metastatic thymoma: report of 11 cases. Cancer Treat Rep 68:1205-1210, 1984.
183. Giaccone G, Ardizzoni A, Kirkpatrick A, et al: Cisplatinum and etoposide combination chemotherapy for locally advanced or metastatic thymoma. A phase II study of the European Organization for Research and Treatment of Cancer Lung Cancer Cooperative Group. J Clin Oncol 14:814-820, 1996.
184. Green JD, Forman WH: Response of thymomas to steroids. Chest 65:114-116, 1974.
185. Highley MS, Underhill CR, Parnis FX, et al: Treatment of invasive thymoma with single agent ifosfamide. J Clin Oncol 17:2737-2744, 1999.
186. Hu E, Levine J: Chemotherapy of malignant thymoma: case report and review of the literature. Cancer 57:1101-1104, 1986.
187. Jaffrey IS: Response to maytansine in a patient with malignant thymoma. Cancer Treat Rep 64:193-194, 1980.
188. Loehrer PJ, Jiroutek M, Aisner S, et al: Combined etoposide, ifosfamide, and cisplatinum in the treatment of patients with advanced thymoma and thymic carcinoma: an intergroup trial. Cancer 91:2010-2015, 2001.
189. Macchiarini P, Chella A, Ducci F, et al: Neoadjuvant chemotherapy, surgery, and postoperative radiation therapy for invasive thymoma. Cancer 68:706-713, 1991.
190. Oshita F, Kasai T, Kurata T, et al: Intensive chemotherapy with cisplatinum, doxorubicin, cyclophosphamide, etoposide and granulocyte colony-stimulating factor for advanced thymoma or thymic cancer: preliminary results. Jpn J Clin Oncol 25:208-212, 1995.
191. Sickles EA, Belliveau RE, Wiernik PH: Primary mediastinal choriocarcinoma in the male. Cancer 33:1196-1203, 1974.
192. Thomas CR, Wright CD, Loehrer PJ: Thymoma: state of the art. J Clin Oncol 17:2280-2289, 1999.
193. Hejna M, Haberl I, Raderer M: Nonsurgical management of malignant thymoma. Cancer 85:1871-1884, 1999.
194. Loehrer PJ Sr, Chen M, Kim K, et al: Cisplatinum, doxorubicin, and cyclophosphamide plus thoracic radiation therapy for limited-stage unresectable thymoma: an intergroup trial. J Clin Oncol 15:3093-3099, 1997.
195. Loehrer PJ Sr, Kim K, Aisner SC, et al: Cisplatinum plus doxorubicin plus cyclophosphamide in metastatic or recurrent thymoma: final results of an intergroup trial. The Eastern Cooperative Oncology Group, Southwest Oncology Group, and Southeastern Cancer Study Group. Clin Oncol 12:1164-1168, 1994.
196. Venuta F, Rendina EA, Pescarmona EO, et al: Multimodality treatment of thymoma: a prospective study. Ann Thorac Surg 64:1585-1592, 1997.
197. Shin DM, Walsh GL, Komaki R, et al: A multidisciplinary approach to therapy for unresectable malignant thymoma. Ann Intern Med 129:100-104, 1998.
198. Goldel N, Boning L, Fredrik A, et al: Chemotherapy of invasive thymoma: a retrospective study of 22 cases. Cancer 63:1493-1500, 1989.
199. Krueger JB, Sagerman RH, King GA: Stage III thymoma: results of postoperative radiation therapy. Radiology 168:855-858, 1988.
200. Mornex F, Resbeut M, Richaud P, et al: Radiotherapy and chemotherapy for invasive thymomas: a multicentric retrospective review of 90 cases. The FNCLCC trialists. Federation Nationale des Centres de Lutte Contre le Cancer. Int J Radiat Oncol Biol Phys 32:651-659, 1995.
201. Penn CRH, Hope-Stone HF: The role of radiotherapy in the management of malignant thymoma. Br J Surg 59:533-539, 1972.
202. Whooley BP, Urschel JD, Antkowiak JG, et al: A 25-year thymoma treatment review. J Exp Clin Cancer Res 19:3-5, 2000.
203. Regnard JF, Magdeleinat P, Dromer C, et al: Prognostic factors and long-term results after thymoma resection: a series of 307 patients. J Thorac Cardiovasc Surg 112:376-384, 1996.
204. Marks RDJ, Wallace KM, Pettit HS: Radiation therapy control of nine patients with malignant thymoma. Cancer 41:117, 1978.

205. Ariaratnam LS, Kalnicki S, Mincer F, et al: The management of malignant thymoma with radiation therapy. Int J Radiat Oncol Biol Phys 5:77-80, 1979.
206. Bretti S, Berruti A, Loddo C, et al: Piemonte Oncology Network. Multimodal management of stages III-IVa malignant thymoma. Lung Cancer 44:69-77, 2004.
207. Hug E, Sobczak M, Choi N, et al: The role of radiotherapy in the management of invasive thymoma. Int J Radiat Oncol Biol Phys 19(Suppl 1):161-162, 1990.
208. Latz D, Schraube P, Oppitz U, et al: Invasive thymoma: treatment with postoperative radiation therapy. Radiology 204:859-864, 1997.
209. Takeda S, Sawabata N, Inoue M, et al: Thymic carcinoma: clinical institutional experience with 15 patients. Eur J Cardiothorac Surg 26:401-406, 2004.
210. Hsu HC, Huang EY, Wang CJ, et al: Postoperative radiotherapy in thymic carcinoma: treatment results and prognostic factors. Int J Radiat Oncol Biol Phys 52:801-805, 2002.
211. Chang HK, Wang CH, Liaw CC, et al: Prognosis of thymic carcinoma: analysis of 16 cases. J Formos Med Assoc 91:764-769, 1992.
212. Arriagada R, Bretel JJ, Caillaud JM, et al: Invasive carcinoma of the thymus. A multicenter retrospective review of 56 cases. Eur J Cancer Clin Oncol 20:69-74, 1984.
213. Lucchi M, Mussi A, Basolo F, et al: The multimodality treatment of thymic carcinoma. Eur J Cardiothorac Surg 19:566-569, 2001.
214. Liu HC, Hsu WH, Chen YJ, et al: Primary thymic carcinoma. Ann Thorac Surg 73:1076-1081, 2002.
215. Nakamura Y, Kunitoh H, Kubota K, et al: Platinum-based chemotherapy with or without thoracic radiation therapy in patients with unresectable thymic carcinoma. Jpn J Clin Oncol 30:385-388, 2000.
216. De Montpreville VT, Macchiarini P, Dulmet E: Thymic neuroendocrine carcinoma (carcinoid): a clinicopathologic study of fourteen cases. J Thorac Cardiovasc Surg 111:134-141, 1996.
217. Wang DY, Chang DB, Kuo SH, et al: Carcinoid tumours of the thymus. Thorax 49:33, 1994.
218. Lin FC, Lin CM, Hsieh CC, et al: Atypical thymic carcinoid and malignant somatostatinoma in type I multiple endocrine neoplasia syndrome: case report. Am J Clin Oncol 26:270-272, 2003.
219. Tiffet O, Nicholson AG, Ladas G, et al: A clinicopathologic study of 12 neuroendocrine tumors arising in the thymus. Chest 124:141-146, 2003.
220. Vietri F, Illuminati R, Guglielmi R, et al: Carcinoid tumors of the thymus gland. Eur J Surg 160:645-647, 1994.
221. Chaer R, Massad MG, Evans A, et al: Primary neuroendocrine tumors of the thymus. Ann Thorac Surg 74:1733-1740, 2002.
222. De Montpreville VT, Macchiarini P, Dulmet E: Thymic neuroendocrine carcinoma (carcinoid): a clinicopathologic study of fourteen cases. J Thorac Cardiovasc Surg 111:134-141, 1996.
223. Kersh CR, Eisert DR, Hazra TA: Malignant thymoma: role of radiation therapy in management. Radiology 156:207-209, 1985.
224. Johnson SB, Eng TY, Giaccone CG, et al: Thymoma: update for the new millennium. Oncologist 6:239-246, 2001.
225. Mayer R, Beham-Schmid C, Groell R, et al: Radiotherapy for invasive thymoma and thymic carcinoma. Clinicopathological review. Strahlenther Onkol 175:271-278, 1999.
226. Marcus RG, Million RR: The incidence of myelitis after irradiation of the cervical spinal cord. Int J Radiat Oncol Biol Phys 19:3-8, 1990.
227. Travis WD, Linnoila RI, Tsokos MG, et al: Neuroendocrine tumors of the lung with proposed criteria for large-cell neuroendocrine carcinoma: an ultrastructural, immunohistochemical, and flow cytometric study of 35 cases. Am J Surg Pathol 15:529-553, 1991.
228. Oberndorfer S: Karzinoide Tumoren des Dunndarms. Frankf Z Pathol 1:425-429, 1907.
229. Gould VE, Memoli V, Chejfec G, et al: The APUD cell system and its neoplasms: observations on the significance and limitations of the concept. Surg Clin North Am 59:93-108, 1979.
230. Mendonca C, Baptista C, Ramos M: Typical and atypical lung carcinoids: clinical and morphological diagnosis. Microsc Res Tech 38:468-472, 1997.
231. Martini N, Zaman MB, Bains MS, et al: Treatment and prognosis in bronchial carcinoids involving regional lymph nodes. J Thorac Cardiovasc Surg 107:1-6, discussion 6-7, 1994.
232. Godwin JD 2nd: Carcinoid tumors: an analysis of 2,837 cases. Cancer 36:560-569, 1975.
233. Beasley MB, Thunnissen FB, Brambilla E, et al: Pulmonary atypical carcinoid: predictors of survival in 106 cases. Hum Pathol 31:1255-1265, 2000.
234. Erasmus JJ, McAdams HP, Patz EF Jr, et al: Evaluation of primary pulmonary carcinoid tumors using FDG PET. AJR Am J Roentgenol 170:1369-1373, 1998.
235. Kayser K, Kayser C, Rahn W, et al: Carcinoid tumors of the lung: immuno- and ligandohistochemistry, analysis of integrated optical density, syntactic structure analysis, clinical data, and prognosis of patients treated surgically. J Surg Oncol 63:99-106, 1996.
236. Laitinen KL, Soini Y, Mattila J, et al: Atypical bronchopulmonary carcinoids show a tendency toward increased apoptotic and proliferative activity. Cancer 88:1590-1598, 2000.
237. Walch AK, Zitzelsberger HF, Aubele MM, et al: Typical and atypical carcinoid tumors of the lung are characterized by 11q deletions as detected by comparative genomic hybridization. Am J Pathol 153:1089-1098, 1998.
238. Onuki N, Wistuba II, Travis WD, et al: Genetic changes in the spectrum of neuroendocrine lung tumors. Cancer 85:600-607, 1999.
239. Dong Q, Debelenko LV, Chandrasekharappa SC, et al: Loss of heterozygosity at 11q13: analysis of pituitary tumors, lung carcinoids, lipomas, and other uncommon tumors in subjects with familial multiple endocrine neoplasia type 1. J Clin Endocrinol Metab 82:1416-1420, 1997.
240. Debelenko LV, Swalwell JI, Kelley MJ, et al: MEN1 gene mutation analysis of high-grade neuroendocrine lung carcinoma. Genes Chromosomes Cancer 28:58-65, 2000.
241. Lai SL, Brauch H, Knutsen T, et al: Molecular genetic characterization of neuroendocrine lung cancer cell lines. Anticancer Res 15:225-232, 1995.
242. Modlin IM, Sandor A: An analysis of 8305 cases of carcinoid tumors. Cancer 79:813-829, 1997.
243. Modlin IM, Lye KD, Kidd M: A 5-decade analysis of 13,715 carcinoid tumors. Cancer 97:934-959, 2003.
244. Hage R, de la Riviere AB, Seldenrijk CA, et al: Update in pulmonary carcinoid tumors: a review article. Ann Surg Oncol 10:697-704, 2003.
245. Fink G, Krelbaum T, Yellin A, et al: Pulmonary carcinoid: presentation, diagnosis, and outcome in 142 cases in Israel and review of 640 cases from the literature. Chest 119:1647-1651, 2001.
246. Cai YC, Banner B, Glickman J, et al: Cytokeratin 7 and 20 and thyroid transcription factor 1 can help distinguish pulmonary from gastrointestinal carcinoid and pancreatic endocrine tumors. Hum Pathol 32:1087-1093, 2001.
247. Oliveira AM, Tazelaar HD, Myers JL, et al: Thyroid transcription factor-1 distinguishes metastatic pulmonary from well-differentiated neuroendocrine tumors of other sites. Am J Surg Pathol 25:815-819, 2001.
248. Travis WD, Rush W, Flieder DB, et al: Survival analysis of 200 pulmonary neuroendocrine tumors with clarification of criteria for atypical carcinoid and its separation from typical carcinoid. Am J Surg Pathol 22:934-944, 1998.
249. Limper AH, Carpenter PC, Scheithauer B, et al: The Cushing syndrome induced by bronchial carcinoid tumors. Ann Intern Med 117:209-214, 1992.
250. Feldman JM: Increased dopamine production in patients with carcinoid tumors. Metab Clin Exp 34:255-260, 1985.
251. Feldman JM, O'Dorisio TM: Role of neuropeptides and serotonin in the diagnosis of carcinoid tumors. Am J Med 81:41-48, 1986.
252. Sandler M, Karim SM, Williams ED: Prostaglandins in amine-peptide-secreting tumours. Lancet 2:1053-1054, 1968.
253. Skrabanek P, Cannon D, Kirrane J, et al: Substance P secretion by carcinoid tumours. Irish J Med Sci 147:47-49, 1978.
254. Lucas KJ, Feldman JM: Flushing in the carcinoid syndrome and plasma kallikrein. Cancer 58:2290-2293, 1986.
255. Sugio K, Osaki T, Oyama T, et al: Genetic alteration in carcinoid tumors of the lung. Ann Thorac Cardiovasc Surg 9:149-154, 2003.

256. Lohmann DR, Fesseler B, Putz B, et al: Infrequent mutations of the p53 gene in pulmonary carcinoid tumors. Cancer Res 53:5797-5801, 1993.
257. Kulke MH, Mayer RJ: Carcinoid tumors. N Engl J Med 340:858-868, 1999.
258. Hasleton PS, Bostanci G: Pulmonary carcinoid and related tumours. Rocz Akad Med Bialymst 42(Suppl 1):28-42, 1997.
259. Garcia-Yuste M, Matilla JM, Alvarez-Gago T, et al: Prognostic factors in neuroendocrine lung tumors: a Spanish Multicenter Study. Spanish Multicenter Study of Neuroendocrine Tumors of the Lung of the Spanish Society of Pneumonology and Thoracic Surgery. Ann Thorac Surg 70:258-263, 2000.
260. McCaughan BC, Martini N, Bains MS: Bronchial carcinoids. Review of 124 cases. J Thorac Cardiovasc Surg 89:8-17, 1985.
261. Grote TH, Macon WR, Davis B, et al: Atypical carcinoid of the lung. A distinct clinicopathologic entity. Chest 93:370-375, 1988.
262. Crapanzano JP, Zakowski MF: Diagnostic dilemmas in pulmonary cytology. Cancer 93:364-375, 2001.
263. Nicholson SA, Ryan MR: A review of cytologic findings in neuroendocrine carcinomas including carcinoid tumors with histologic correlation. Cancer 90:148-161, 2000.
264. Thomas JS, Lamb D, Ashcroft T, et al: How reliable is the diagnosis of lung cancer using small biopsy specimens? Report of a UKCCCR Lung Cancer Working Party. Thorax 48:1135-1139, 1993.
265. Okike N, Bernatz PE, Woolner LB: Carcinoid tumors of the lung. Ann Thorac Surg 22:270-277, 1976.
266. Schreurs AJ, Westermann CJ, van den Bosch JM, et al: A twenty-five-year follow-up of ninety-three resected typical carcinoid tumors of the lung. J Thorac Cardiovasc Surg 104:1470-1475, 1992.
267. Torre M, Barberis M, Barbieri B, et al: Typical and atypical bronchial carcinoids. Respir Med 83:305-308, 1989.
268. Kaplan B, Stevens CW, Allen P, et al: Outcomes and patterns of failure in bronchial carcinoid tumors. Int J Radiat Oncol Biol Phys 55:125-131, 2003.
269. Thomas CF Jr, Tazelaar HD, Jett JR: Typical and atypical pulmonary carcinoids: outcome in patients presenting with regional lymph node involvement. Chest 119:1143-1150, 2001.
270. Marty-Ane CH, Costes V, Pujol JL, et al: Carcinoid tumors of the lung: do atypical features require aggressive management? Ann Thorac Surg 59:78-83, 1995.
271. Smolle-Juttner FM, Popper H, Klemen H, et al: Clinical features and therapy of "typical" and "atypical" bronchial carcinoid tumors (grade 1 and grade 2 neuroendocrine carcinoma). Eur J Cardiothorac Surg 7:121-124, discussion 125, 1993.
272. Scott WJ: Surgical treatment of other bronchial tumors. Chest Surg Clin North Am 13:111-128, 2003.
273. Rena O, Donati G, Casadio C, et al: Bronchial carcinoid tumors: surgical management and long-term outcome. J Thorac Cardiovasc Surg 123:303-309, 2002.
274. Skuladottir H, Hirsch FR, Hansen HH, et al: Pulmonary neuroendocrine tumors: incidence and prognosis of histological subtypes. A population-based study in Denmark. Lung Cancer 37:127-135, 2002.
275. Choi N, Mohiuddin M, Fidias P: Atypical carcinoids of the thorax. Proceedings of the 90th Radiological Society of North America Conference, Chicago, Nov 28-Dec 3, 2004.
276. Moraes TJ, Langer JC, Forte V, et al: Pediatric pulmonary carcinoid: a case report and review of the literature. Pediatr Pulmonol 35:318-322, 2003.
277. Schrevens L, Vansteenkiste J, Deneffe G, et al: Clinical-radiological presentation and outcome of surgically treated pulmonary carcinoid tumours: a long-term single institution experience. Lung Cancer 43:39-45, 2004.
278. Rosado de Christenson ML, Abbott GF, Kirejczyk WM, et al: Thoracic carcinoids: radiologic-pathologic correlation. Radiograph 19:707-736, 1999.
279. Harpole DH Jr, Feldman JM, Buchanan S, et al: Bronchial carcinoid tumors: a retrospective analysis of 126 patients. Ann Thorac Surg 54:50-54, discussion 54-55, 1992.
280. Soga J, Yakuwa Y: Bronchopulmonary carcinoids: an analysis of 1,875 reported cases with special reference to a comparison between typical carcinoids and atypical varieties. Ann Thorac Cardiovasc Surg 5:211-219, 1999.
281. Anderson AS, Krauss D, Lang R: Cardiovascular complications of malignant carcinoid disease. Am Heart J 134:693-702, 1997.
282. Lorcy Y, Perdu S, Sevray B, et al: Acromegaly due to ectopic GH-RH secretion by a bronchial carcinoid tumor: a case report. Ann Endocrinol 63(Pt 1):536-539, 2002.
283. Lamberts SW, Bakker WH, Reubi JC, et al: Somatostatin receptor imaging in vivo localization of tumors with a radiolabeled somatostatin analog. J Steroid Biochem Mol Biol 37:1079-1082, 1990.
284. Musi M, Carbone RG, Bertocchi C, et al: Bronchial carcinoid tumours: a study on clinicopathological features and role of octreotide scintigraphy. Lung Cancer 22:97-102, 1998.
285. Kaltsas G, Korbonits M, Heintz E, et al: Comparison of somatostatin analog and meta-iodobenzylguanidine radionuclides in the diagnosis and localization of advanced neuroendocrine tumors. J Clin Endocrinol Metab 86:895-902, 2001.
286. Marom EM, Sarvis S, Herndon JE 2nd, et al: T1 lung cancers: sensitivity of diagnosis with fluorodeoxyglucose PET. Radiology 223:453-459, 2002.
287. Squerzanti A, Basteri V, Antinolfi G, et al: Bronchial carcinoid tumors: clinical and radiological correlation. Radiol Med 104:273-284, 2002.
288. West WM: Image and diagnosis: carcinoid tumor of the lung. West Indian Med J 51:200-204, 2002.
289. Anderson CJ, Dehdashti F, Cutler PD, et al: ^{64}Cu-TETA-octreotide as a PET imaging agent for patients with neuroendocrine tumors. J Nucl Med 42:213-221, 2001.
290. Filosso PL, Rena O, Donati G, et al: Bronchial carcinoid tumors: surgical management and long-term outcome. J Thorac Cardiovasc Surg 123:303-309, 2002.
291. Terzi A, Lonardoni A, Falezza G, et al: Sleeve lobectomy for non-small cell lung cancer and carcinoids: results in 160 cases. Eur J Cardiothorac Surg 21:888-893, 2002.
292. Hurt R, Bates M: Carcinoid tumours of the bronchus: a 33 year experience. Thorax 39:617-623, 1984.
293. Stamatis G, Freitag L, Greschuchna D: Limited and radical resection for tracheal and bronchopulmonary carcinoid tumour. Report on 227 cases. Eur J Cardiothorac Surg 4:527-532, discussion 533, 1990.
294. Dusmet ME, McKneally MF: Pulmonary and thymic carcinoid tumors. World J Surg 20:189-195, 1996.
295. Ruggieri M, Scocchera F, Genderini M, et al: Therapeutic approach of carcinoid tumours of the lung. Eur Rev Med Pharmacol Sci 4:43-46, 2000.
296. Makridis C, Rastad J, Oberg K, et al: Progression of metastases and symptom improvement from laparotomy in midgut carcinoid tumors. World J Surg 20:900-906, discussion 907, 1996.
297. Nave H, Mossinger E, Feist H, et al: Surgery as primary treatment in patients with liver metastases from carcinoid tumors: a retrospective, unicentric study over 13 years. Surg 129:170-175, 2001.
298. Platt AJ, Heddle RM, Rake MO, et al: Ondansetron in carcinoid syndrome. Lancet 339:1416, 1992.
299. Kubota A, Yamada Y, Kagimoto S, et al: Identification of somatostatin receptor subtypes and an implication for the efficacy of somatostatin analogue SMS 201-995 in treatment of human endocrine tumors. J Clin Invest 93:1321-1325, 1994.
300. Reichlin S: Somatostatin. N Engl J Med 309:1495-1501, 1983.
301. *Ibid.*
302. Reubi JC, Kvols LK, Waser B, et al: Detection of somatostatin receptors in surgical and percutaneous needle biopsy samples of carcinoids and islet cell carcinomas. Cancer Res 50:5969-5977, 1990.
303. *Ibid.*
304. Ferguson MK, Landreneau RJ, Hazelrigg SR, et al: Long-term outcome after resection for bronchial carcinoid tumors. Eur J Cardiothorac Surg 18:156-161, 2000.
305. Cardillo G, Sera F, Di Martino M, et al: Bronchial carcinoid tumors: nodal status and long-term survival after resection. Ann Thorac Surg 77:1781-1785, 2004.

306. Carretta A, Ceresoli GL, Arrigoni G, et al: Diagnostic and therapeutic management of neuroendocrine lung tumors: a clinical study of 44 cases. Lung Cancer 29:217-225, 2000.
307. Granberg D, Eriksson B, Wilander E, et al: Experience in treatment of metastatic pulmonary carcinoid tumors. Ann Oncol 12:1383-1391, 2001.
308. Krenning EP, de Jong M, Kooij PP, et al: Radiolabelled somatostatin analogues for peptide receptor scintigraphy and radionuclide therapy. Ann Oncol 10 Suppl 2:S23-S29, 1999.
309. Filosso PL, Ruffini E, Oliaro A, et al: Long-term survival of atypical bronchial carcinoids with liver metastases, treated with octreotide. Eur J Cardiothorac Surg 21:913-917, 2002.
310. Oberg K, Eriksson B: The role of interferons in the management of carcinoid tumours. Br J Haematol 79(Suppl 1):74-77, 1991.
311. Bukowski RM, Johnson KG, Peterson RF, et al: A phase II trial of combination chemotherapy in patients with metastatic carcinoid tumors. A Southwest Oncology Group Study. Cancer 60:2891-2895, 1987.
312. Engstrom PF, Lavin PT, Moertel CG, et al: Streptozocin plus fluorouracil versus doxorubicin therapy for metastatic carcinoid tumor. J Clin Oncol 2:1255-1259, 1984.
313. Moertel CG, Hanley JA: Combination chemotherapy trials in metastatic carcinoid tumor and the malignant carcinoid syndrome. Cancer Clin Trials 2:327-234, 1979.
314. Que FG, Nagorney DM, Batts KP, et al: Hepatic resection for metastatic neuroendocrine carcinomas. Am J Surg 169:36-42, discussion 42-43, 1995.
315. Schupak KD, Wallner KE: The role of radiation therapy in the treatment of locally unresectable or metastatic carcinoid tumors. Int J Radiat Oncol Biol Phys 20:489-495, 1991.
316. Oberg K, Astrup L, Eriksson B, et al: Guidelines for the management of gastroenteropancreatic neuroendocrine tumours (including bronchopulmonary and thymic neoplasms). Acta Oncol 43:617-625, 2004.
317. Vadasz P, Palffy G, Egervary M, et al: Diagnosis and treatment of bronchial carcinoid tumors: clinical and pathological review of 120 operated patients. Eur J Cardiothorac Surg 7:8-11, 1993.
318. Mezzetti M, Raveglia F, Panigalli T, et al: Assessment of outcomes in typical and atypical carcinoids according to latest WHO classification. Ann Thorac Surg 76:1838-1842, 2003.
319. Chughtai TS, Morin JE, Sheiner NM, et al: Bronchial carcinoid—twenty years' experience defines a selective surgical approach. Surgery 122:801-808, 1997.
320. Wirth LJ, Carter MR, Janne PA, et al: Outcome of patients with pulmonary carcinoid tumors receiving chemotherapy or chemoradiotherapy. Lung Cancer 44:213-220, 2004.
321. Rusch VW: Pleurectomy/decortication and adjuvant therapy for malignant mesothelioma. Chest 103:382S-384S, 1993.
322. Gordon W, Antman KH, Greenberger JS, et al: Radiation therapy in the management of patients with mesothelioma. Int J Radiat Oncol Biol Phys 8:19-25, 1982.
323. Rusch VW, Piantadosi S, Holmes EC: The role of extrapleural pneumonectomy in malignant pleural mesothelioma: a Lung Cancer Study Group trial. J Thorac Cardiovasc Surg 102:1-9, 1991.
324. Butchart EG, Ashcroft T, Barnsley WC, Holden MP: Pleuropneumonectomy in the management of diffuse malignant mesothelioma of the pleura: experience with 29 patients. Thorax 31:15-24, 1976.
325. Jaklitsch MT, Grondin SC, Sugarbaker DJ: Treatment of malignant mesothelioma. World J Surg 25:210-217, 2001.
326. Sugarbaker DJ, Flores RM, Jaklitsch MT, et al: Resection margins, extrapleural nodal status, and cell type determine postoperative long-term survival in trimodality therapy of malignant pleural mesothelioma: results in 183 patients. J Thorac Cardiovasc Surg 117:54-65, 1999.
327. Huncharek M, Kelsey K, Mark EJ, et al: Treatment and survival in diffuse malignant pleural mesothelioma: a study of 83 cases from the Massachusetts General Hospital. Anticancer Res 16:1265-1268, 1996.
328. Calavrezos A, Koschel G, Husselmann H, et al: Malignant mesothelioma of the pleura. A prospective therapeutic study of 132 patients from 1981-1985. Klin Wochenschr 66:607-613, 1988.
329. Baldini EH, Recht A, Strauss GM, et al: Patterns of failure after trimodality therapy for malignant pleural mesothelioma. Ann Thorac Surg 63:334-338, 1997.
330. Bricout PB, Engler MJ: Computerized tomography scanning and the planning of high dose radiotherapy for pleural mesothelioma: a report of five patients. Int J Radiat Oncol Biol Phys 7:821-826, 1981.
331. Connelly RR, Spirtas R, Myers MH, et al: Demographic patterns for mesothelioma in the United States. J Natl Cancer Inst 78:1053-1060, 1997.
332. Steinert HC, Santos Dellea MM, Burger C, et al: Therapy response evaluation in malignant pleural mesothelioma with integrated PET-CT imaging. Lung Cancer 49(Suppl 1):S33-S35, 2005.
333. Robinson BW, Creaney J, Lake R, et al: Mesothelin-family proteins and diagnosis of mesothelioma. Lancet 362:1612-1616, 2003.
334. Renshaw AA, Dean BR, Antman KH, et al: The role of cytologic evaluation of pleural fluid in the diagnosis of malignant mesothelioma. Chest 111:106-109, 1997.
335. Heilo A, Stenwig AE, Solheim OP: Malignant pleural mesothelioma: US-guided histologic core-needle biopsy. Radiology 211:657-659, 1999.
336. Rusch VW, Rosenzweig K, Venkatraman E, et al: A phase II trial of surgical resection and adjuvant high-dose hemithoracic radiation for malignant pleural mesothelioma. J Thorac Cardiovasc Surg 122:788-795, 2001.
337. Kindler HL: Malignant pleural mesothelioma. Curr Treat Options Oncol 1:313-326, 2000.
338. Stewart DJ, Edwards JG, Smythe WR, et al: Malignant pleural mesothelioma—an update. Int J Occup Environ Health 10:26-39, 2004.
339. Solheim OP, Saeter G, Finnanger AM, et al: High-dose methotrexate in the treatment of malignant mesothelioma of the pleura. A phase II study. Br J Cancer 65:956-960, 1992.
340. Byrne MJ, Davidson JA, Musk AW, et al: Cisplatin and gemcitabine treatment for malignant mesothelioma: a phase II study. J Clin Oncol 17:25-30, 1999.
341. Calvert AH, Hughes AN, Calvert PM, et al: Alimta in combination with carboplatin demonstrates clinical activity against malignant mesothelioma in a phase I trial [abstract]. Proc Am Soc Clin Oncol 19:495a, 2000.
342. Reck M, Gatzemeier U: Pemetrexed-cisplatin combination in mesothelioma. Exp Rev Anticancer Ther 5:231-237, 2005.
343. Chahinian AP, Antman K, Goutsou M, et al: Randomized phase II trial of cisplatin with mitomycin or doxorubicin for malignant mesothelioma by the Cancer and Leukemia Group B. J Clin Oncol 11:1559-1565, 1993.
344. Fizazi H, Doubre H, Viala J, et al: The combination of raltitrexed ("tomudex") and oxaliplatin is an active regimen in malignant mesothelioma: results of a phase II study [abstract]. Proc Am Soc Clin Oncol 19:578a, 2000.
345. Berghmans T, Paesmans M, Lalami Y, et al: Activity of chemotherapy and immunotherapy on malignant mesothelioma: a systematic review of the literature with meta-analysis. Lung Cancer 38:111-121, 2002.
346. Vogelzang NJ, Rusthoven JJ, Symanowski J, et al: Phase III study of pemetrexed in combination with cisplatin versus cisplatin alone in patients with malignant pleural mesothelioma. J Clin Oncol 21:2636-2644, 2003.
347. Muers MF, Rudd RM, O'Brien ME, et al, for the British Thoracic Society Mesothelioma Group: BTS randomised feasibility study of active symptom control with or without chemotherapy in malignant pleural mesothelioma: ISRCTN 54469112. Thorax 59:144-148, 2004.
348. Hakkinen AM, Laasonen A, Linnainmaa K, et al: Radiosensitivity of mesothelioma cell lines. Acta Oncol 35:451-456, 1996.
349. Carmichael J, Degraff WG, Gamson J, et al: Radiation sensitivity of human lung cancer cell lines. Eur J Cancer Clin Oncol 25:527-534, 1989.
350. Maasilta P, Kivisaari L, Holsti LR, et al: Radiographic chest assessment of lung injury following hemithorax irradiation for pleural mesothelioma. Eur Respir J 4:76-83, 1991.
351. Maasilta P: Deterioration in lung function following hemithorax irradiation for pleural mesothelioma. Int J Radiat Oncol Biol Phys 20:433-438, 1991.

352. Hilaris BS, Nori D, Kwong E, et al: Pleurectomy and intraoperative brachytherapy and postoperative radiation in the treatment of malignant pleural mesothelioma. Int J Radiat Oncol Biol Phys 10:325-331, 1984.
353. Lee TT, Everett DL, Shu HK, et al: Radical pleurectomy/decortication and intraoperative radiotherapy followed by conformal radiation with or without chemotherapy for malignant pleural mesothelioma. J Thorac Cardiovasc Surg 124:1183-1189, 2002.
354. Kutcher GJ, Kestler C, Greenblatt D, et al: Technique for external beam treatment for mesothelioma. Int J Radiat Oncol Biol Phys 13:1747-1752, 1987.
355. Ahamad A, Stevens CW, Smythe WR, et al: Intensity-modulated radiation therapy: a novel approach to the management of malignant pleural mesothelioma. Int J Radiat Oncol Biol Phys 55:768-775, 2003.
356. Ahamad A, Stevens CW, Smythe WR, et al: Promising early local control of malignant pleural mesothelioma following postoperative intensity modulated radiotherapy (IMRT) to the chest. Cancer J 9:476-484, 2004.
357. Forster KM, Smythe WR, Starkschall G, et al: Intensity-modulated radiotherapy following extrapleural pneumonectomy for the treatment of malignant mesothelioma: clinical implementation. Int J Radiat Oncol Biol Phys 55:606-616, 2003.
358. Yajnik S, Rosenzweig KE, Mychalczak B, et al: Hemithoracic radiation after extrapleural pneumonectomy for malignant pleural mesothelioma. Int J Radiat Oncol Biol Phys 56:1319-1326, 2003.
359. Van Ooijen B, Eggermont AMM, Wiggers T: Subcutaneous tumor growth complicating the positioning of Denver shunt and intrapleural Port-a-Cath in mesothelioma patients. Eur J Surg Oncol 18:638-640, 1992.
360. Boutin C, Rey F, Viallat JR: Prevention of malignant seeding after invasive diagnostic procedures in patients with pleural mesothelioma. A randomized trial of local radiotherapy. Chest 108:754-775, 1995.
361. Sugarbaker DJ, Garcia JP: Multimodality therapy for malignant pleural mesothelioma. Chest 112(Suppl 4):272S-275S, 1997.
362. Rusch VW: Surgical techniques for pulmonary metastasectomy. Semin Thorac Cardiovasc Surg 14:4-9, 2002.
363. Della Volpe A, Ferreri AJ, Annaloro C, et al: Lethal pulmonary complications significantly correlate with individually assessed mean lung dose in patients with hematologic malignancies treated with total body irradiation. Int J Radiat Oncol Biol Phys 52:483-488, 2002.
364. Weder W, Kestenholz P, Taverna C, et al: Neoadjuvant chemotherapy followed by extrapleural pneumonectomy in malignant pleural mesothelioma. J Clin Oncol 22:3451-3457, 2004.
365. Green FL, Page DL, Fleming ID, et al (eds), for the American Joint Committee on Cancer: AJCC Cancer Staging Manual, 6th ed. New York, Springer, 2002.

PART D

GASTROINTESTINAL TUMORS

Overview

Joel E. Tepper and Leonard L. Gunderson

Gastrointestinal (GI) cancer continues to be a common health problem. Approximately 253,500 new cases of GI malignancy were estimated to occur in the United States in 2005.[1] Although colorectal tumors account for more than 50% of the cases in the United States, cancers of the esophagus, stomach, liver, and pancreas continue to occur with regularity and high mortality, and the incidence of hepatoma is increasing rapidly. Gastric and hepatic cancers are two of the most common causes of cancer incidence and death worldwide. Hereditary factors play a role in the etiology of GI cancer, and environmental toxins are causative agents in certain diseases. As these are a diverse group of tumors, the etiology, epidemiology, diagnosis, and treatment vary enormously between diseases and are discussed in the respective chapters.

A significant problem with many GI cancers relates to a delay in clinical presentation. Signs that give early warning of other types of cancer (e.g., pain or palpation of a mass) do not occur early in patients with GI cancers. For example, the severe back pain that can occur with pancreatic cancer is usually a manifestation of unresectability due to posterior tumor extension. Patients with alimentary tract GI cancers often present with symptoms of obstruction or gross hemorrhage, which may be associated with large primary tumors, high risk of metastasis, and a low chance of cure.

Physicians should search for early signs of GI cancer, educate their patients to be aware of certain symptoms in order to make earlier diagnoses, and perform screening procedures, as indicated. In general, the early warning signs include vague abdominal discomfort, unexplained weight loss, change in bowel habits, or new onset of anemia. Routine sigmoidoscopy and stool testing for occult blood are recommended screening procedures for colorectal cancer and have been shown to impact on outcome both by finding cancers at an early stage and by removing benign polyps before they have had a chance to progress to an invasive cancer. Colorectal cancers are one of the few cancer types where many tumors can actually be prevented, in this case by removing polyps when they are benign. Other tests such as routine contrast radiography, upper endoscopy, or cytologic analysis have yet to demonstrate cost effectiveness in the United States as a general screening procedure but may be appropriate for select high-risk populations. There is substantial interest in innovative approaches of screening such as molecular analyses of stool or bile that could be important in the future. There is also hope that proteomics may allow for a blood assay to determine patients with early cancers, but at the present time this is more hope than reality.

This overview discusses conceptual issues pertinent to a variety of GI cancers, with site-specific details covered in the disease site chapters. Topics covered here include epidemiology and prevention, biology, anatomy and pathway of tumor spread, staging, prognostic factors and patterns of relapse, treatment issues of surgery alone versus primary chemo/irradiation or trimodality treatment (surgery, radiation therapy, and chemotherapy), and tolerance of organs and structures that limit the radiation dose in the treatment of abdominal-pelvic GI cancers.

EPIDEMIOLOGY AND PREVENTION

It has long been known that colon and rectal cancers are related to dietary factors, and these tumors have thus been used as a model for cancer epidemiology. There is a strong association of these tumors with high fat and low fiber diets.[2] It has been argued as to whether high fat or low fiber is most important in the process of cancer development, or whether there are other nutrients associated with these diets that are most important. However, data now strongly suggest that neither high fat nor low fiber is critical, but rather the fact that high fat/low fiber diets tend to be low in folate[3,4] and perhaps other nutrients. Confirmation of this is critical in designing prevention strategies, as dietary supplementation with folate (or other nutrients) is far easier to implement than is a major change in the eating habits of the population. Other environmental factors, specifically exercise, are very important in colorectal carcinogenesis, suggesting that a lifestyle that is healthy for the heart is also beneficial in decreasing colorectal cancer incidence. The same strong dietary correlate with cancer formation is unfortunately not present for most other GI tract tumors. Smoking is a major risk factor primarily for esophageal cancer and, to a lesser extent, for pancreatic cancer.

Along with the dietary factors just described, there have been major epidemiologic changes in geographic location and histopathology for tumors of the esophagus, stomach, colon, and rectum, although the reason for these changes is largely unknown. The primary histopathology of esophageal cancer has changed rapidly from squamous cell carcinoma of the proximal and mid esophagus to adenocarcinomas of the distal esophagus, gastroesophageal junction, and proximal stomach. At many U.S. institutions, three fourths of all patients with esophageal cancer have distal esophageal adenocarcinomas, although this was a relatively rare entity only 20 to 30 years ago. The reasons for these changes are unknown but may be related to the increased incidence of Barrett's esophagus and esophageal reflux.[5] It has been postulated that the increased use of H_2 blockers has improved the symptomatology of patients with reflux but has not decreased the inflammatory response in the distal esophageal mucosa, thus leading to the formation of Barrett's lesions with metaplastic changes and subsequently esophageal cancer. The concomitant substantial increase in the incidence of proximal (cardia)gastric cancer suggests a similar etiology for both abnormalities and that the increased incidence of esophageal cancer is not just a misclassification of proximal gastric cancers as esophageal adenocarcinomas.[6]

At the same time that there has been an increased incidence of proximal gastric adenocarcinomas, the overall incidence of gastric cancer is decreasing. At the beginning of the 20th century, gastric cancer was the most common malignancy in the United States. Although it is still a common cause of cancer mortality, the incidence has decreased to where it is only the seventh most common cause of cancer death in the United States, although with a much higher incidence worldwide.[1] This change has been attributed to dietary modifications, although the exact cause is unknown.

In the large bowel, there has been a more gradual epidemiologic change with a higher percentage of tumors now located proximally in the right colon. Previously, the majority of colorectal cancers were located in the rectum, but now the majority are located in the right colon. Although screening for, and removal of, precancerous polyps in the rectum and sigmoid colon with sigmoidoscopy could be producing some of these changes, it is unlikely to be a major factor. Dietary changes are suspected but unproved as a cause.

There has also been a major increase in the incidence of hepatoma in the United States, although not nearly as high as its incidence worldwide. Some of the reasons for this are known, such as its strong association with hepatitis B and C virus infection. Although radiation oncologists have historically not had a major role in treatment of this disease, improvements in technology may allow for better radiation dose delivery and a greater use of radiation in selected clinical situations, especially for localized but unresectable hepatocellular carcinomas.

A major emphasis in the future will be to determine ways to prevent tumor formation or to find tumors early enough so that the risk of tumor mortality is minimized. There are now data to suggest strongly that one can utilize prevention strategies to decrease the incidence of colorectal cancers by screening and removal of polyps prior to their becoming malignant, thus interfering with the polyp-to-cancer sequence that occurs in the majority of colon and rectal cancers. Studies of patients screened with flexible sigmoidoscopy have demonstrated a markedly decreased incidence of cancer within reach of the sigmoidoscope but no decrease in areas that could not be effectively screened.[7,8] There are convincing data that demonstrate a value to regular screening stool guaiac studies in decreasing colorectal cancer mortality.[9,10] However, neither of these interventions is used widely enough to decrease the overall incidence of these diseases. Virtual colonoscopy, a CT-based radiographic examination, has generated a great deal of interest as a screening tool. However, the data do not yet support its widespread use and patients currently still need to do what many consider to be the worst part of an endoscopic procedure—the bowel preparation. Controlled studies are being performed to determine whether the bowel prep is necessary or whether deletion techniques can be used to exclude stool.

Screening approaches have also been considered for tumors of other sites in the GI tract, but cost-effective strategies have not been defined. The incidence of gastric cancer in the United States and many other Western countries is not high enough to justify the cost and morbidity of screening endoscopy for gastric or esophageal cancer, and radiographic studies such as CT scans are not sensitive enough to justify their use. If it were possible to define a very high risk group of patients, then perhaps screening could be used successfully. The one situation in the upper GI tract where screening may be useful at the present time is in patients with Barrett's esophagus, where the incidence of esophageal cancer is high and regular endoscopy, or elective surgery, may be justified.

Prevention strategies have been studied extensively, especially for colon and rectal cancers. There are a variety of agents that are thought to have potential as preventative agents for people at high risk. These include aspirin[11,12] and other nonsteroidal anti-inflammatory drugs (NSAIDs) and calcium.[13,14] The data are now quite convincing that the incidence of polyps can be decreased with the use of NSAIDs, presumably reflecting their activity as inhibitors of COX-2.[15] The finding of increased cardiovascular events in patients taking the selective COX-2 inhibitors will have a major impact on the use of these agents for cancer prevention.

BIOLOGY OF GASTROINTESTINAL CANCERS

Over the past decade an enormous amount of information has been gathered regarding the molecular correlates of GI carcinomas. As is true for other anatomic sites, there are a large number of molecular changes in most of these tumors, but most of the changes occur in only a relatively small subset of tumors. There is a wide spectrum of molecular abnormalities found with the entire spectrum of changes likely defining the genetic characteristics of the tumor. The specific molecular abnormalities will probably have a major effect on both the pace of disease progression and response of the tumor to therapy, but the relationship is clearly complex. Colorectal cancers are one of the best-studied adult solid tumor in this regard and illustrate the type of information that we are likely to obtain about other solid tumors. The molecular changes associated with GI tumors and the general issues related to carcinogenesis are beyond the scope of this introduction but are covered elsewhere in this book, as well as in multiple reviews.[16]

Although there are a large number of molecular changes observed in colorectal cancer, a few are most common. These include altered methylation, mutations of the *ras* oncogene, mutations in the *p53* tumor suppressor gene, mutations in a gene on the short arm of chromosome 18 (in an area referred to as the *DCC* gene [deleted in colon cancer]), and mutations in chromosome 5 in a region associated with the familial polyposis syndrome (FAP). Although there is clearly no orderly progression from one molecular change to another, there is a tendency for certain of these changes to occur early in the oncogenesis pathway. For example, changes in the *FAP* gene and altered methylation tend to occur early, while *p53* mutations tend to occur late.[17] As one probes deeply into the genome a very large number of abnormalities are being found, but many of these may be secondary to a generalized chromosomal instability. The significance of some types of molecular abnormalities is better understood. For example, microsatellite instability in colon cancer is associated with right-sided colon tumors but with an improved prognosis compared to those with no microsatellite instability. These tumors may also have altered chemosensitivity compared to tumors without microsatellite instability. Some investigators now classify colorectal cancer into those that either have microsatellite instability (15% of tumors) or chromosomal instability (85%), and this classification may help in the understanding of the management of these diseases.

An area of interest is the correlation of the known epidemiologic factors for cancer formation and the molecular abnormalities. For example, it is unknown how dietary changes are related to the observed molecular alterations.

Determining which dietary factors are of true importance and which dietary factors produce which molecular changes, and the mechanisms by which they do so, may be critical in designing effective prevention strategies.

For other tumors of the GI tract, the molecular correlates are not nearly as well established. Pancreatic cancer is unusual because approximately 90% of these tumors have a mutation in the *ras* oncogene,[18] and mutations in *p16, p53,* and *MADH4* are very common. The finding of abnormalities that are present in most cancers of a certain type produces exciting possibilities for detection, prevention, and therapy because it suggests that these mutational events may be required for cancer formation. In addition, even when a specific mutation is not present, an abnormality in that pathway may be required for carcinogenesis. However, the abnormality may be produced by one of many mutational events or even by gene silencing through altered methylation.

There is a major effort to develop pharmaceuticals that will block the function of critical pathways and thereby either inhibit tumor growth or kill the tumor. Many of the drugs that have been developed as pure molecular inhibitors for primary therapy do not seem to be very effective when used alone. However, most of these agents (EGFR or VEGF inhibitors, for example) have substantial radiation sensitization properties and may be very useful adjuncts to standard radiation therapy (see Chapter 5).

A great deal of interest exists in using DNA microarray data to improve prognostication and to define better which tumors would be best treated with which modalities. These studies are still in their early phases and require much additional work prior to routine clinical application.

ANATOMY AND PATHWAYS OF TUMOR SPREAD

Upper GI (stomach, pancreas, biliary tract) and colorectal cancers have anatomic similarities that lead to common patterns or pathways of tumor spread. The four common mechanisms of tumor spread for these sites include direct extension, lymphatic spread, blood-borne hematogenous metastases, and peritoneal seeding. Esophageal and anal cancers have no risk for peritoneal seeding because of anatomic location unless they extend to involve organs with access to the peritoneal cavity (e.g., stomach or upper rectum).

Direct extension of tumor that may lead to surgical unresectability due to fixation to or involvement of surrounding organs or structures is more common with upper GI cancers than with lower GI cancers. Within the triad of upper GI cancers, gastric cancers are most likely to be resectable at the time of diagnosis.

Lymphatic spread and nodal involvement are common at all GI sites. For the alimentary sites (esophagus, stomach, colorectum, anus), the risk is nonexistent for lesions limited to the mucosa. The risk increases with direct extension into the submucosa in view of the presence of submucosal lymphatics—especially prominent in the stomach and esophagus. The mechanism of tumor spread within submucosal and subserosal lymphatics can also lead to subclinical tumor spread 5 to 10 cm or more from the margin of the gross tumor for both esophageal and gastric cancers. For colorectal cancers, it is unusual to have subclinical tumor extension in the bowel wall for more than 1 to 1.5 cm beyond the gross tumor, but nodal spread can occur at more distant locations.

Hematogenous dissemination from GI cancers is usually to the liver or lungs. With esophageal, anal, and rectal cancers both sites are at risk. Gastric, colon, or pancreas cancers that do not extend beyond the wall/organ to involve other organs or structures have venous drainage via the portal circulation, placing the liver at primary risk for blood-borne metastases.

Peritoneal seeding can theoretically occur when a tumor extends to a free peritoneal surface. The finding of peritoneal seeding at initial surgical exploration is highest for gallbladder and pancreas cancers, is rare with low rectal cancers, and can sometimes be found with gastric, colon, bile duct, and upper (± mid) rectal cancers.

STAGING

The current TNM (tumor, lymph nodes, metastasis) staging system by the American Joint Committee on Cancer (AJCC) is the accepted staging system for GI cancers.[19] Portions of this system are compared in Table D-1 with a modification of the Astler-Coller rectal system (MAC) that has been used for all alimentary tract carcinomas. For gastric cancers, the pathologic examination of 10 to 15 nodes is not routine in many U.S. institutions, so the value of the N classification is uncertain (N1, metastases in 1 to 6 nodes; N2, metastases in 7 to 15 nodes; N3, metastases in >15 nodes). However, it appears that for both gastric and colorectal tumors the aggressiveness of lymph node staging (both by the surgeon in removing nodes and by the pathologist in evaluating nodes) is of enormous prognostic importance. Prognosis is much inferior for "N0" tumors when very few lymph nodes have been evaluated compared to when large numbers of nodes have been studied.[20] These variations by pathologist and by institution result in the phenomenon of both understaging and stage migration, which make it difficult to compare results by series.

Colorectal Cancers

The TNM system applies to both clinical and pathologic staging, defines the degree of primary tumor extension for lesions confined to and extending beyond the bowel wall, and defines node involvement by the number of nodes involved

Table D-1 Comparison of Staging Systems for Colorectal Adenocarcinoma

TNM[17]	Dukes	Modified Astler-Coller
I	A	
Tis, N0, M0		A
T1-2, N0, M0		B1
II	B	
T3-4a, N0, M0		B2
T4b, N0, M0		B3
III	C	
T1-2, N1-2, M0		C1
T3-4a, N1-2, M0		C2
T4b, N1-2, M0		C3
IV	D	
Any T, any N, M1*		D

T4 is preferably substaged as T4a and T4b.

*Lymph nodes beyond those encompassed by standard resection of the primary tumor and regional lymphatics (e.g., retroperitoneal nodes) are considered distant metastases.

Tis, carcinoma in situ; T1, tumor invades submucosa; T2, tumor invades muscularis propria; T3, tumor invades through the muscularis propria into the subserosa or into nonperitonealized pericolic or perirectal tissues; T4a, tumor perforates the visceral peritoneum; T4b, tumor (is adherent to) directly invades other organs or structures (surgical or pathologic definition); N0, no regional lymph node metastases; N1, metastasis in one to three pericolic or perirectal lymph nodes; N2, metastasis in ≥ four pericolic or perirectal lymph nodes; M0, no distant metastasis; M1, distant metastasis.

Table D-2 **Pooled Rectal Analysis: Impact of TN Stage on Survival, Postoperative Chemoradiation***

TN Stage	Overall Survival† No.	5 y (%)	*p* Value	Disease-Free Survival† No.	5 y (%)	*p* Value
T1-2 N1	225	81	.002	225	74	<.001
N2	180	69		180	62	
T3 N0	668	74		664	65	
N1	544	61	<.001	536	51	<.001
N2	663	48		659	38	
T4 N0	95	65		95	54	
N1	59	33	<.001	59	30	<.001
N2	84	38		84	30	

*NCCTG 794751, NCCTG 864751, U.S. GI Intergroup 0114.
†Unadjusted Kaplan-Meier estimates.
From Gunderson LL, Sargent DJ, Tepper JE, et al: Impact of T and N substage on survival and disease relapse in adjuvant rectal cancer: a pooled analysis. Int J Radiat Oncol Biol Phys 54:389, 2002.

Table D-3 **Pooled Rectal Analysis: Impact of TN Stage on Disease Relapse, Postoperative Chemoradiation**

TN Stage	Local Recurrence† No.	5 y (%)	*p* Value	Distant Metastases† 5 y (%)	*p* Value
T1-2 N1	225	6	.06	15	<.001
N2	180	8		26	
T3 N0	664	8		19	
N1	536	11	<.001	34	<.001
N2	659	15		45	
T4 N0	95	15		28	
N1	59	22	.48	39	.004
N2	84	19		50	

†Cumulative incidence rates.
From Gunderson LL, Sargent DJ, Tepper JE, et al: Impact of T and N substage on survival and disease relapse in adjuvant rectal cancer: a pooled analysis. Int J Radiat Oncol Biol Phys 54:389, 2002.

(N1, ≤3, N2, ≥4). The updated 2002 AJCC/UICC TNM classification should be used as the standard staging system (see Table D-1).

Improvements in the 2002 update of the AJCC system (sixth edition) include the addition of the terminology "adherence" to the definition of T4 lesions and the substaging of both stages II and III disease. The use of substages was based on differential survival and relapse rates found within TNM stages II and III colon and rectal cancer.

Subsequent pooled analyses of phase III North American rectal cancer adjuvant studies[21,22] have demonstrated the independent prognostic significance of each TN category of resected rectal cancer and the value of substaging (see Tables D-2 and D-3 and subsequent section on Prognostic Factors and Patterns of Relapse). The continued use of either Dukes stages A, B, or C or TNM stage I, II, or III without the benefit of substaging is insufficient, since patient prognosis is not accurately reflected. Data from the pooled analyses further demonstrated that patients with N2 disease have differential prognosis by T stage (see subsequent section). Accordingly, placement of all N2 patients within AJCC IIIC substage does not reflect the markedly different prognosis of N2 patients found in the rectal cancer pooled analyses.

Other Gastrointestinal Cancers

Staging of pancreatic, biliary, and esophageal cancers is less useful. The major factors defining therapy are whether the tumor is resectable, borderline resectable or locally unresectable and whether distant metastatic disease is present. As therapy becomes more sophisticated and treatment outcomes improve, we will likely be better able to use more precise staging information. The ability to evaluate stage more effectively preoperatively through PET scans (esophageal cancer) and endoscopic ultrasound (esophageal and gastric cancers) should be of benefit over the long term with regard to choice of treatment (single modality versus bimodality or trimodality) and sequencing of various modalities (preoperative, postoperative, or both).

PROGNOSTIC FACTORS AND PATTERNS OF RELAPSE

Adjuvant Colorectal

Survival and disease relapse after surgery with or without adjuvant treatment for colon and rectal cancer are a function of both degree of bowel wall penetration of the primary lesion and nodal status. Nodal involvement alone is not the most important pathologic factor that determines survival and relapse. In fact, as noted previously, the rectal cancer pooled analyses demonstrated the independent prognostic significance of each TN and NT stage of resected rectal cancer (N substage within T stage and T substage within N stage (Tables D-2 through D-5).[21,22]

Rectal Cancer Pooled Analysis No. 1

The intent of the first rectal cancer pooled analysis was to determine the rates of survival and disease control by TNM and MAC stage in three randomized North American rectal adjuvant studies.[21] Data were merged from 2551 eligible patients on NCCTG 79-47-51 ($N = 200$), NCCTG 86-47-51 ($N = 656$) and INT 0114 ($N = 1695$). All patients received postoperative radiation and 96% were randomized to receive concurrent and maintenance chemotherapy. Five-year follow-up was available in 94% of patients and 7-year follow-up in 84%.

Overall survival (OS) and disease-free survival (DFS) were dependent on both TN stage (see Tables D-2 and D-3) and NT stage (see Tables D-4 and D-5). Even among N2 patients (four or more positive lymph nodes), T-stage influenced 5-year OS (T1-2, 69%; T3, 48%; T4, 38%) (see Table D-5). Three risk groups of patients were defined: (1) intermediate, T3N0, T1-2 N1, (2) moderately high, T4N0, T1-2N2, T3N1, and (3) high, T3N2, T4N1, T4N2. For group 1, 5-year OS rates were 74% and 81% and 5-year DFS was 66% and 74%. With group 2, 5-year OS ranged from 61% to 69%, and for group 3, OS ranged from 33% to 48%. Cumulative incidence rates of local relapse (LR) and distant metastases (DMs) revealed similar differences by TN and NT stage as seen in the survival analyses.

Rectal Cancer Pooled Analysis No. 2

The objective of the second pooled analysis was to determine survival rates by TN stage and treatment method in five phase III North American rectal cancer postoperative adjuvant trials (Table D-6).[22] Data were merged from 3791 eligible patients on NCCTG 79-47-51 (*N* = 200), NCCTG 86-47-51 (*N* = 656), INT 114 (*N* = 1695), NSABP R01 (*N* = 544), or NSABP R02 (*N* = 696). Surgery alone was the treatment arm in 179 patients (R01). The remaining patients received adjuvant treatment with either irradiation (RT, *N* = 281; 79-47-51, R01), RT+ bolus chemotherapy (CT, *N* = 779; NCCTG, NSABP), RT+ protracted venous infusion CT (PVI CT, *N* = 325; 86-47-51), RT+ bolus CT (*N* = 1695; INT 114), or CT alone (*N* = 532; R01, R02).

Both OS and DFS were dependent on TN stage (3745 evaluable patients) and treatment method. For patients with intermediate risk lesions (T1-2N1, T3N0) adjuvant CT had 5-year OS of 85% and 84%. This was equivalent to results with RT + CT (T1-2N1, 78% to 83%; T3N0, 74% to 80%). However, 5-year DFS with S + CT were 78% (T1-2N1) and 69% (T3N0), indicating room for improvement. For moderately high-risk lesions (T1-2N2, T4N0, T3N1), 5-year OS ranged from 43% to 70% with CT and 44% to 80% with RT + CT. For high-risk lesions (T3N2, T4N1-2), 5-year OS ranged from 25% to 45% with CT and 29% to 57% with RT + CT.

Results by TN Stage

Patients with the best survival are those with the primary lesion confined to the bowel wall and uninvolved nodes (T1-2N0M0, TNM stage I) with an expected 5-year survival of about 90%. For such patients, distant relapse rates are about 10%, and local recurrence rates are 5% for colon cancers and less than 10% for rectal cancers.

Intermediate but still excellent results are found in patients with one high-risk feature, either primary tumor extension beyond the bowel wall (T3N0, TNM IIA) or confined to the wall, but with positive nodes (T0-2N1, TNM IIIA). Five-year

Table D-4 Pooled Rectal Analysis: Impact of NT Stage on Survival

NT Stage	Survival, 5 y Overall* No.	%	*p* Value	Disease-Free* No.	%	*p* Value
N0 T3	668	74	.046	664	66	.05
T4	95	65		95	54	
N1 T1-2	225	81		225	74	
T3	544	61	<.001	536	50	<.001
T4	59	33		59	30	
N2 T1-2	180	69		180	62	
T3	663	48	<.001	659	39	<.001
T4	84	38		84	30	

*Unadjusted Kaplan-Meier estimates.

Table D-5 Pooled Rectal Analysis: Impact of NT Stage on Disease Relapse

NT Stage	Disease Relapse, 5 y: Local Recurrence* No.	%	*p* Value	Distant Metastasis* %	*p* Value
N0 T3	664	8	.04	19	.04
T4	95	15		28	
N1 T1-2	225	6		15	
T3	536	11	.002	34	<.001
T4	59	22		39	
N2 T1-2	180	8		26	
T3	659	15	.14	45	<.001
T4	84	19		50	

*Cumulative incidence rates.

From Gunderson LL, Sargent DJ, Tepper JE, et al: Impact of T and N substage on survival and disease relapse in adjuvant rectal cancer: a pooled analysis. Int J Radiat Oncol Biol Phys 54:390, 2002.

Table D-6 Rectal Cancer Pooled Analysis—Survival and Relapse Rates by Stage of Disease

Risk for Relapse*	Stage TN	MAC	Survival, 5-y† OS	DFS	Relapse Local	Distant	Stage Dukes (New)	TNM
Low‡	T1-2N0	A,B1	~90	~90	≤5	~10	A	I
Intermediate	T1-2N1	C1	81	74	7	15	C	IIIA
	T3N0	B2	74	66	9	20	B	IIA
Moderately high	T1-2N2	C1	69	62	8	31	C	IIIC
	T4N0	B3	65	54	13	28	B	IIB
	T3N1	C2	61	50	12	37	C	IIIB
High	T3N2	C2	48	39	14	47	C	IIIC
	T4N1	C3	33	30	23	39	C	IIIB
	T4N2	C3	38	30	17	53	C	IIIC

*Data from rectal cancer pooled analysis.[21]
†Survival—unadjusted Kaplan-Meier estimates.
‡Data derived from prior publications, as low-risk patients were not eligible for the five phase III trials in the rectal cancer pooled analysis.
DFS, disease-free survival; OS, overall survival.
From Gunderson LL, Sargent DJ, Tepper JE, et al: Impact of T and N substage on survival and disease relapse in adjuvant rectal cancer: a pooled analysis. Int J Radiat Oncol Biol Phys 54:393, 2002.

survival rates can range from 75% to 80%.[21-23] Somewhat surprisingly, results may be slightly superior for T1-2N1 tumors than for those with T3N0 disease reflecting the independent prognostic importance of advanced T stage.

A moderately high risk of relapse is expected with either more advanced local or nodal disease (T4N0 [IIB], T3N1 [IIIB], T1-2N2 [IIIC]), reflecting overall a more advanced tumor. For node-negative patients with adherence to or invasion of surrounding organs or structures (T4N0), patients with a higher number of involved nodes (T1-2N2) or those with extension beyond the wall and one to three nodes positive (T3N1), 5-year survival expectancy is 60% to 70%. Overall relapse rates are similar for this group of patients (LR rates of 8% to 15% and distant relapse rate of 26% to 34% with adjuvant postoperative treatment in the initial rectal pooled analysis). For patients in the intermediate and moderately high-risk groups, biologic and other risk factors may have independent prognostic significance.

The poorest survival and highest relapse rates are found in patients with both high-risk factors of nodal involvement and tumor extension beyond the colonic or rectal wall (T3-4N1-2, TNM IIIB, IIIC). Five-year survival of these patients after resection plus adjuvant therapy is 30% to 50%. The rate of LR after surgery plus postoperative adjuvant treatment was 15% to 22% in the initial rectal pooled analysis, and the risk of DM was 39% to 50% (approximately double that of patients with a single risk factor). These data in total suggest that both the extent of the primary tumor and the extent of the nodal disease are independent prognostic factors and that both of them must be taken into consideration in designing appropriate therapy.

Adjuvant Gastric

As with other alimentary tract cancers, the two most important prognostic features are depth of invasion and lymph node involvement. Nodal involvement reduces survival and the number of positive nodes is of prognostic importance. However, if the primary lesion is confined to the gastric wall (T1 or T2) when nodes are involved, the prognosis at 5 years (40% survival) is similar to that of patients with T2N0 or T3N0 lesions (~50% 5-year survival) (see Chapter 44).

TREATMENT—SINGLE VERSUS COMBINED MODALITY

RT has a role as a component of primary therapy in most cancers of the GI tract. It is used as part of initial management for patients with locally advanced cancers of the esophagus, stomach, pancreas, colon, rectum, and anus in most U.S. institutions and for hepatobiliary cancer in some institutions.

Chemoradiation, 5-Fluorouracil Based

Although combined modality therapy with chemotherapy and radiation therapy is of great importance in many adult solid tumors, its use in treatment of GI tumors is substantial and of long duration. 5-Fluorouracil (5-FU) has been used as an anticancer therapy since the 1950s, and since the late 1960s, it has been used in combination with RT for GI tumors (concomitant ± maintenance) (Fig. D-1). Early studies of the combination were reported from the Mayo Clinic in the treatment of locally advanced pancreatic, gastric, and large bowel cancers.[24] Although modifications of this therapy have been developed, the use of concomitant 5-FU–based chemotherapy plus RT has remained standard therapy for treatment of selected patients with tumors at almost all sites in the GI tract. Although drugs such as cis-platinum or mitomycin C are used

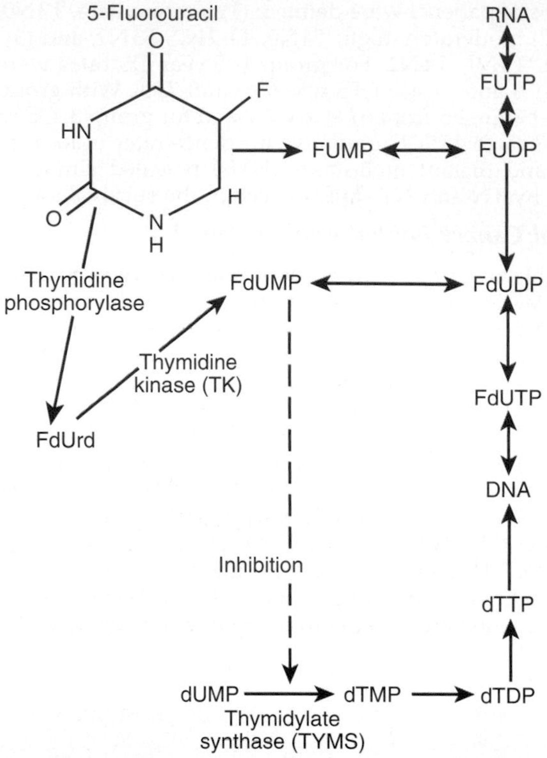

Figure D-1 5-Fluorouracil (5-FU) has, as its primary mode of action, conversion into fluorodeoxyuridine monophosphate (F-dUMP), which acts to inhibit the enzyme thymidylate synthase, which is necessary for production of DNA. 5-FU can also be converted into fluorouracil triphosphate (FUTP) and incorporated into RNA or into fluorodeoxyuridine triphosphate (FdUTP) and incorporated into DNA.

in combination with 5-FU in a number of these anatomic sites (especially esophagus and anus), they have not replaced 5-FU but are used in conjunction with 5-FU and radiation. There is now interest in the use of oral 5-FU analogs (capecitabine), with the hope that the oral formulation will make this treatment more acceptable to patients but it is unlikely to change the toxicity profile. 5-FU was essentially the only drug useful in colorectal and pancreatic cancer for decades, but gemcitabine has displaced 5-FU as the primary drug treatment in pancreatic cancer, and the combination of 5-FU and oxaliplatin or irinotecan is becoming routine in the chemotherapeutic management of colorectal cancer. All of these agents have substantial radiation-sensitizing properties, and their use in rectal cancer is being extensively explored. As mentioned, the use of EGFR or VEGF inhibitors as radiation sensitizers in a variety of sites in the GI tract, but especially in the rectum, has generated substantial interest.

While surgery remains the primary mode of curative treatment for gastric, pancreatic, and large bowel cancers, combined chemoradiation has become the primary treatment for anal cancer and may offer an equivalent option to surgery alone for patients with esophageal cancer. Although surgical techniques have continued to evolve, most prominently with the use of total mesorectal excision, therapy with surgery alone is unlikely to significantly improve further the survival rates for gastric, pancreatic, esophageal, and large bowel cancers. Adjuvant and neoadjuvant RT, chemotherapy, or both offer the best prospect for improving cure rates.

A large number of studies have been performed using the above strategies. With unresected esophageal cancers, combined chemoradiation has clearly improved disease control and 5-year survival over irradiation alone in phase 3 randomized trials.[25] It is unclear whether preoperative chemoradiation has improved survival compared to surgery alone, although it has improved local control. For resected high-risk rectal cancers, postoperative chemoradiation has improved local and distant disease control and DFS and OS compared to surgery alone or adjuvant irradiation control arms.[26,27] Preoperative irradiation has demonstrated improved local control and survival when compared to surgery alone for resectable rectal cancer in a large randomized trial from Sweden,[28] and a large German trial[29] has shown the superiority of preoperative chemoradiation over the same therapy delivered postoperatively. Adjuvant postoperative chemoradiation has resulted in improved local control and survival in some phase II and III trials for resected pancreatic cancer[30] and improved local control and survival for resected gastric cancers.[31,32] For resected node-positive colon cancers, adjuvant chemotherapy has produced improved DFS and OS compared to surgery alone. Postoperative chemoradiation has been evaluated in patients with resected high-risk colon cancers[33] and, although shown not in general use, may be of value in selected clinical situations, such as when microscopic residual disease remains (not truly an adjuvant setting). A preferred approach would be to use imaging to identify patients who would likely have marginal resection if surgery were the initial component of treatment (e.g., T4 lesion with adherence to surgically unresectable structure). In such patients, preoperative chemoradiation would preferably precede surgical resection. Finally, chemoradiation has replaced surgical resection as the primary treatment for anal carcinomas with surgical resection being reserved for salvage therapy. While these positive trials are exciting and encouraging, refinements in multimodality therapy will necessitate continued enrollment of patients in clinical trials to help develop the most effective combined modality treatment strategies for the future.

Chemoradiation, Non–5-Fluorouracil

For the first time in many years, there are a variety of new drugs that may supplement or supplant 5-FU in combination with radiation therapy in the treatment of GI cancers. These new drugs include gemcitabine, irinotecan, oxaliplatin, and oral 5-FU compounds.

Gemcitabine is the first drug developed in many years with single-drug activity against pancreatic cancer.[34] There are also good data demonstrating that gemcitabine has substantial radiation-sensitizing properties,[35] and clinical studies are proceeding in combination with radiation therapy for patients with both locally advanced and resected pancreatic cancer.[36] As gemcitabine is a potent radiation sensitizer, it needs to be used cautiously. Although this combination may have effectiveness in other sites in the GI tract, the lack of substantial gemcitabine activity when used alone in colon and rectal cancer makes its use for these diseases unlikely.

A number of other drugs have been developed with substantial activity in colon and rectal cancer, including the topoisomerase inhibitor CPT-11 (irinotecan) and the platinum compound oxaliplatin. Data exist to demonstrate radiation sensitization with CPT-11[37] and oxaliplatin.[38] Both of these drugs are being tested in combination with radiation therapy for patients with rectal cancer and appear to increase the rates of pathologic complete response when used with 5-FU and radiation in the preoperative setting in phase II trials.

There are a group of drugs that are oral analogs of 5-FU, although they have different specific mechanisms of action. Some of these drugs are 5-FU prodrugs, some act to inhibit the degradation of 5-FU either by direct or indirect inhibition of the degradation pathway, while others attempt to increase tumor selectivity, and yet others act as specific inhibitors of thymidylate synthase rather than the nonspecific action of 5-FU.[39] The major potential advantage of these compounds is in patient convenience and the elimination of infusion pumps for continuous infusion 5-FU administration. The toxicity spectrum of these agents does not differ substantially from that of conventional infusion 5-FU.

Capecitabine is the agent that has entered routine clinical use both alone as a chemotherapeutic agent and combined with radiation.[40] Capecitabine is delivered twice daily and, although serum levels are much flatter than for 5-FU, major variations in serum levels do exist. Thus, timing of radiation and capecitabine is likely to be important. We recommend taking capecitabine approximately one hour prior to the delivery of radiation therapy to maximize radiation sensitization. Capecitabine doses when used with concurrent radiation are substantially less than when used alone, typically 1650 mg/m^2/d delivered in two doses.

IRRADIATION TECHNIQUE AND TOLERANCE

Irradiation Field Definition

Because treatment tolerance to irradiation is usually a function of both dose and volume, proper definition of tumor and target volumes is of utmost importance. If patients are referred for primary or preoperative irradiation, the radiation oncologist can obtain the necessary imaging studies to define both the primary tumor and nodal areas at risk. If the patient is referred after complete resection, however, the radiation oncologist is dependent on the availability of pertinent preoperative imaging studies or placement of surgical clips at sites of tumor adherence or microscopic residual disease.

For unresected alimentary tract cancers (esophagus, stomach, colorectum, anus), the primary lesions and nodal areas at risk are best defined with a combination of contrast radiographs (upper GI for esophagus and stomach; barium enema including a cross-table lateral for colorectum ± anus) and CT (chest plus abdomen for esophagus, abdomen ± chest for gastric, abdomen and pelvis for colorectum and anus) ± transluminal ultrasound. This is the best imaging technique for determining T stage for esophagus, gastric, and rectal cancers prior to resection. The use of endoscopy to both define lesions and obtain biopsies has markedly reduced the use of contrast radiographs preoperatively, thus making it difficult to construct proper radiation fields if patients are referred after resection unless CT or MRI scans are obtained preoperatively. Improvements in CT and MRI technology are continuing to make these technologies the primary imaging modalities for most GI tumors and decreasing the importance of conventional imaging. However, there are some important structures (such as the anal verge) that are not well defined with cross-sectional imaging.

The need to rely on surgical clip placement for proper design of radiation fields is fraught with difficulty as demonstrated in a U.S. Intergroup colon adjuvant study evaluating the addition of irradiation to 5-FU leucovorin in high-risk patients.[33] Of the 94 evaluable patients randomized to receive chemotherapy plus irradiation, only 18 patients (19%) had clips placed by the surgeon to assist proper field design. Neither preoperative imaging nor clip placement was available to guide field design in 17% of patients. It is unlikely that the trial could hope to demonstrate a value of radiation with chemotherapy for resected high-risk colon cancers, because the fields may have been inappropriate in a substantial portion of patients.

For unresected biliary tract cancers, endoscopic retrograde cholangiopancreatography (ERCP), percutaneous transhepatic cholangiography (PTHC), and MRI or MRCP demonstrate the distal and proximal extent of disease most precisely. If transhepatic catheters have been placed at the time of PTHC, the radiation oncologist can reinject the catheter with contrast to reconstruct the ductal system and define target volumes. If stents have been placed at the time of ERCP, the relationship of the stent to ductal involvement as demonstrated on ERCP imaging films is used to define tumor and target volumes. MRI can also effectively image these tumors and is commonly used.

With unresected pancreatic cancers, abdominal CT or MRI best demonstrates tumor and nodal target volumes. If the tumor has been resected, postoperative CT or MRI of the abdomen can rule out liver metastases and define postoperative nodal volumes, and the preoperative CT and surgical clips can be used to define the tumor bed.

Conformal three-dimensional radiation therapy with CT-based treatment planning is recommended for the treatment of most, if not all GI cancer patients, and intensity modulated radiation therapy is being evaluated in some GI cancer sites. Although three-dimensional conformal techniques have been used extensively in the treatment of pancreatic, gastric, esophagus, and biliary tumors, they are used less commonly in the routine treatment of rectal and anal cancers as the targets are broad and reasonably well defined on routine radiographs with contrast. For patients with esophageal cancer, CT-based planning is useful in defining the mediolateral and anteroposterior extent of tumor but should be combined with contrast radiographs to determine the proximal and distal extent of the primary lesion. With gastric cancer patients, the proximal stomach or gastric remnant is best defined by a combination of contrast radiographs and CT, as CT alone underestimates the extent of the stomach. A caution in using CT planning for rectal cancer is that the precise location of the anal sphincter is best determined using simple techniques to mark the anal verge, and this margin is not well visualized on a CT scan without contrast.

Normal Tissue Tolerance

When irradiating the abdomen and pelvis, there are numerous normal structures that can be dose limiting and must be considered in treatment planning. These include the stomach, small intestine, spinal cord, large intestine, liver, and kidneys, in addition to the soft tissue in the abdomen. A full discussion of the tolerance of these structures is beyond the scope of this overview, but a brief review is given here.

Upper Gastrointestinal and Extrapelvic Colon Cancers

The tolerance of the liver is limiting when a substantial portion of the liver is included in the radiation field. The hepatic parenchyma is relatively sensitive to radiation, with total organ tolerance doses in the range of 30 Gy, using conventional fractionation (1.5 to 1.8 Gy), being near tolerance. The ability to tolerate higher doses to portions of the liver is primarily dependent on the volume of liver receiving high doses, since recovery of hepatic parenchyma is dependent on regeneration by the unirradiated liver. In an individual with normal baseline hepatic function, it is possible to irradiate approximately 50% to 60% of the liver to high doses without undue problems if the remainder of the liver remains untreated. If hepatic function is compromised, less parenchyma can be safely treated although an exact determination of the safe amount is not defined. Because it is possible to totally irradiate and destroy a portion of the liver without danger to the patient, there is essentially no limit to the dose that can be given to small portions of the liver, although biliary obstruction may be produced after very high doses to the major biliary radicals. Dawson and colleagues have conducted a series of elegant clinical trials that define hepatic tolerance better than has been done for most other organs.[41]

The tolerance of the kidney is conceptually similar to that of the liver in that irradiation of a portion of the kidney to high dose is well tolerated if the baseline renal function is good and if a significant portion of the remaining kidney is unirradiated to allow for hypertrophy (e.g., only 20% to 30% receives more than 20 Gy). It is important to be certain that the baseline renal function is adequate (by measuring creatinine clearance or by estimating the clearance from the creatinine level, age, sex, and weight using the Cockcroft formula) and that the contralateral kidney is functioning properly so that it can take over the renal function. The latter is best done with a functional renal scan (such as DSMA) which can provide the percentage of function from each kidney. Although the data on renal tolerance is fairly old, even moderate doses (in the range of 25 Gy) can produce substantial renal injury. Doses over 30 Gy are likely to produce major renal injury to the irradiated parenchyma. Studies suggest that clinically significant sequelae are unlikely after conventional abdominal irradiation if the above factors are taken into consideration.[42] Although it is possible to produce severe kidney injury with secondary renovascular hypertension, this is an uncommon event.

The stomach has generally been considered to be a radiation sensitive structure with ulcer formation occurring after doses greater than 45 to 50 Gy (1.8- to 2.0-Gy fractions), but precise gastric tolerance has not been well established. Although a large number of patients have received moderate to high doses of radiation therapy to the upper abdomen, this has usually been done for tumors that have a poor cure rate and for patients where survival of greater than 2 years is relatively unusual. The experience in the treatment of Hodgkin's disease clearly demonstrates gastric tolerance to doses of 45 Gy. When irradiating a portion of the stomach in the treatment of upper GI cancers one must minimize both the volume and dose to the stomach. It is of interest, however, that there are very little recent data describing gastric ulceration, suggesting that some of the old tolerance data may not be reliable. Mayo Clinic data in the treatment of bile duct cancers suggest that gastroduodenal tolerance is best if doses of 54 Gy or less (1.8-Gy fractions) are used, with a corresponding 10% or less rate of grade 3 or higher GI intolerance with external beam radiation therapy (EBRT) (±5-FU) with doses of 54 Gy or less versus a 30% to 40% rate with doses greater than 54 Gy.[43]

Tolerance of the pancreas to radiation therapy is not often discussed, but there is anecdotal evidence that both exocrine and endocrine dysfunction can result, although analyses are complicated by effects of the tumor and of surgery. It is appropriate for the radiation oncologist to consider the possibility of pancreatic dysfunction during patient follow-up.

Pelvic Gastrointestinal Cancers

The small bowel is the organ that has produced the most clinical problems after conventional radiation therapy in the pelvis. Moderate doses to the small bowel (50 Gy in 1.8- to 2.0-Gy fractions) will begin to cause clinically significant problems. It has been suggested that risk factors for injury include diabetes and hypertension as well as prior surgery, but these are not well substantiated. It is clear that volume of irradiated small bowel is also important, but it has not been well quantified as to how much bowel can be treated safely. When larger volumes are treated, small bowel obstruction is the most likely complication.[44] The obstructive episodes can be recurrent, and 50% of patients or more may require laparotomy for resolution. At surgery it is often not possible to resect the damaged small bowel, which is usually enveloped in a fibrotic mass, and a surgical bypass is often the treatment of choice. However, if the damaged bowel can be resected with low morbidity, that approach is optimal. Dissection of irradiated bowel in an attempt to free up all adhesions may result in enterotomy and later fistulas. Small bowel complications are most common when irradiating the pelvis, an area that has commonly been exposed to extensive surgery with associated adhesions and small bowel fixation. Although complications are less likely in the upper abdomen, they can still occur, and efforts should be made to minimize the volume of irradiated small bowel at all sites.

There are a number of manipulations that the radiation oncologist can use to minimize the amount of small bowel in a pelvic radiation field. The first action is to determine the location of the small bowel. This can be done by giving oral small bowel contrast at least 45 minutes before a radiographic imaging study, either conventional simulation or CT scan. With this information, the radiation oncologist can design fields that will minimize the volume of small bowel irradiated. It is also helpful to work with a surgeon who can perform surgical manipulations to move small bowel out of the pelvis. A number of techniques have been tried, including reperitonealization of the pelvic floor after abdominal-perineal resection, using a vascularized omental sling or pedicle to displace small bowel out of the pelvis, retroverting the uterus to act as a space-occupying device, and putting mesentery or a foreign body into the pelvis for the same purpose. In addition, during simulation, one can use bladder distension or displacement devices to shift small bowel out of the pelvis. Having the patient lay in the prone position on a false table top located at or superior to the radiation field ($\approx 9 \times 12$-cm opening) is one technique that has been effective for many patients. These techniques work to a varying extent on individual patients.[45] Small bowel being fixed in the pelvis is much less of a problem when patients are receiving preoperative radiation therapy for rectal cancer, a progressively more commonly used option. Whichever approach is taken, the treating physician must pay attention to the location of the small bowel and dose to the organ or risk significant complications.

There is less information on the tolerance of the large bowel (colon and rectum) to high radiation doses and much of the information available comes from irradiation of non-GI tumors, especially the prostate and cervix. There is very little information on the tolerance of the colon, partially because there has been very little high dose irradiation of the intraperitoneal or retroperitoneal colon. Rarely is the colon a dose-limiting structure. The rectum or portions thereof has been treated to doses of 65 to 70 Gy or higher for cervical, prostate, and anal cancer and for localized treatment of rectal cancers. It is clear that portions of the rectum can be treated to high doses with minimal late effects. The most obvious example of this is in the use of endocavitary radiation therapy of small rectal cancers. In this technique, doses of approximately 90 to 120 Gy have been delivered in four fractions. Although the rectal wall receives minimal dose from the first two fractions, because of rapid dose fall-off it receives full dose for the last one to two fractions. Late complications (bleeding, ulceration) occur in 10% to 15% of patients and only an occasional temporary diverting colostomy is needed, likely because of the ability of the rectal mucosa to be repopulated from surrounding normal tissue, and because the scarring is not over a large enough area to cause stricture formation.

However, when high doses of radiation are given to a substantial portion of the rectal circumference ((more than one half), the tolerance is much less. With circumferential irradiation, the dose to a 10-cm length of rectum is preferably limited to 60 Gy or less in 2-Gy fractions to prevent problems with bleeding, ulceration, and narrowing of the rectum. Even with partial organ radiation therapy, there have been significant problems with bleeding (10% to 15% incidence) reported at doses of approximately 72 Gy. While conservative treatment with bulk agents and steroid preparations can alleviate most situations, use of laser at time of endoscopy may be necessary to control bleeding. Difficult management problems are rare, but at the extreme can require surgical correction, usually a temporary diverting colostomy.

There is even less information available on anal tolerance. However, it is generally thought that doses higher than 55 to 60 Gy to the whole anal canal in conjunction with chemotherapy, as used in the treatment of anal cancer, have a risk of stricture formation. In the treatment of rectal cancer, one should try to minimize the amount of anus in the radiation field, as anal irradiation produces a large amount of acute morbidity, occasional stricture formation, or poor late functioning of the anus. There is clearly a significant risk of late morbidity in anorectal function that is not well defined but that can cause clustering and frequency of bowel movements with suboptimal control and intolerance to certain foods.[46] These effects are likely due at least partially to anal dysfunction, as well as poor rectal capacity from surgery or radiation. Minimizing radiation dose and volume and careful surgical techniques need to be used to minimize the risk of late effects.

Irradiation Boost Techniques

For completely resected, margin-negative GI cancers, adjuvant doses of irradiation (50 to 54 Gy) plus concomitant 5-FU–based chemotherapy are adequate to achieve local control in 85% to 90% of patients. For margin-positive or unresected GI cancers, the dose of irradiation required to achieve adequate local control would usually exceed normal tissue tolerance (e.g., >70 Gy in 1.8- to 2.0-Gy fractions). Therefore, the use of brachytherapy or intraoperative electron irradiation (IOERT) as a supplement to EBRT and chemotherapy after resection may improve local control in the treatment of locally advanced GI cancers.

The use of IOERT as a component of treatment for a variety of disease sites is discussed in Chapters 15, 44, 45, 46, and 47. IOERT plus EBRT (± 5-FU) and maximal resection appear to improve both local control and survival for locally unresectable and locally recurrent colorectal cancers.[47,48] With unresectable pancreatic cancers, the addition of IOERT to EBRT ± 5-FU improves local control but has no apparent impact on survival in view of high rates of relapse in the liver and peritoneal cavity.[49,50]

Brachytherapy has been used as a supplement to EBRT with biliary tract cancers.[38-40] There is a suggestion of improved survival in patients treated with both EBRT and brachytherapy compared with either alone (see Chapter 46), but phase III trials are unlikely in view of small patient numbers.

SUMMARY

Radiation therapy is now a part of the therapeutic approach in many patients with cancers of the GI tract, although mostly in patients with moderately advanced locoregional disease. In most of these sites the combination of radiation therapy and

5-FU–based chemotherapy is standard therapy, although cisplatin or mitomycin is used with 5-FU in tumors of the esophagus and anus. In many GI cancer sites, chemoradiation is used as an adjuvant to surgical resection because of the propensity of these tumors to recur locally and the difficulty in obtaining a wide resection margin, usually relating to the anatomic site. Careful attention to radiation therapy technique and respect for normal tissue tolerance are essential if local control is to be obtained without producing unacceptable normal tissue morbidity.

REFERENCES

1. Jemal A, Murray T, Ward E, et al: Cancer statistics, 2005. CA Cancer J Clin 55:10-30, 2005.
2. Palmer S, Bakshi K: Diet, nutrition and cancer. I. Interim dietary guidelines. J Natl Cancer Inst 70:1151, 1983.
3. Giovannucci E, Stampfer M, Colditz G, et al: Multivitamin use, folate, and colon cancer in women in the Nurses' Health Study. Ann Intern Med 129:517-524, 1998.
4. Fuchs CS, Giovannucci EL, Colditz GA, et al: Dietary fiber and the risk of colorectal cancer and adenoma in women. N Engl J Med 340:169-176, 1999.
5. Lagergren J, Bergstrom R, Lindgren A, et al: Symptomatic gastroesophageal reflux as a risk factor for esophageal adenocarcinoma. N Engl J Med 340:825-831, 1999.
6. Blot WJ, Devesa SS, Kneller RW, et al: Rising incidence of adenocarcinoma of the esophagus and gastric cardia. JAMA 265:1287-1289, 1991.
7. Selby J, Friedman G, Quesenberry C, et al: A case-control study of screening sigmoidoscopy and mortality from colorectal cancer. N Engl J Med 326:653-657, 1992.
8. Newcomb P, Norfleet R, Surawicz T, et al: Screening sigmoidoscopy and colorectal cancer mortality. J Natl Cancer Inst 1992:1572-1575, 1992.
9. Mandel JS, Bond JH, Church TR: Reducing mortality from colorectal cancer by screening for fecal occult blood. N Engl J Med 328:1365-1371, 1993.
10. Winawer S, Andrews M, Flehinger B: Progress report on controlled trial of fecal occult blood testing for the detection of colorectal neoplasia. Cancer 45:2959, 1980.
11. Sandler RS, Halabi S, Baron JA, et al: A randomized trial of aspirin to prevent colorectal adenomas in patients with previous colorectal cancer. N Engl J Med 348:883-890, 2003.
12. Baron JA, Cole BF, Sandler RS, et al: A randomized trial of aspirin to prevent colorectal adenomas. N Engl J Med 348:891-899, 2003.
13. Baron JA, Beach M, Mandel JS, et al: Calcium supplements for prevention of colorectal adenomas. N Engl J Med 340:101-107, 1999.
14. Muscat J, Stellman S: Nonsteroidal antiinflammatory drugs and colorectal cancer. Cancer 74:1847, 1994.
15. Koehne CH, Dubois RN: COX-2 inhibition and colorectal cancer. Semin Oncol 31:12-21, 2004.
16. Vogelstein B, Kinzler KW: Cancer genes and the pathways they control. Nat Med 10:789-799, 2004.
17. Vogelstein B, Fearon E, Hamilton S: Genetic alterations during colorectal-tumor development. N Engl J Med 319:525-532, 1988.
18. Almonguera C, Shibata D, Forrester K: Most human carcinomas of the exocrine pancreas contain mutant c-K-ras genes. Cell 53:549, 1988.
19. Greene FL, Page, DL, Fleming ID, et al: AJCC Cancer Staging Manual, 6th ed. New York, Springer, 2002.
20. Tepper JE, O'Connell MJ, Niedzwiecki D, et al: Impact of number of nodes retrieved on outcome in patients with rectal cancer. J Clin Oncol 19:157-163, 2001.
21. Gunderson LL, Sargent DJ, Tepper JE, et al: Impact of T and N substage on survival and disease relapse in adjuvant rectal cancer: a pooled analysis. Int J Radiat Oncol Biol Phys 54: 386-396, 2002.
22. Gunderson LL, Sargent DJ, Tepper JE, et al: Impact of T and N stage and treatment on survival and relapse in adjuvant rectal cancer: a pooled analysis. J Clin Oncol 22:1785-1796, 2004.
23. Greene FL, Stewart AK, Norton HJ: A new TNM staging strategy for node-positive (stage III) rectal cancer: an analysis of 5,988 patients. *In* Steven M, Grunberg M (eds): Thirty-Ninth Annual Meeting of the ASCO. Chicago, IL, American Society of Clinical Oncology, 2003, p 251.
24. Moertel CG, Childs DS, Reitemeier RJ: Combined 5-fluorouracil and supervoltage radiation therapy of locally unresectable gastrointestinal cancer. Lancet 2:865-867, 1969.
25. Herskovic A, Leichman I, Lattin P: Combined chemotherapy and radiotherapy compared with radiotherapy alone in patients with cancer of the esophagus. N Engl J Med 326:1593, 1992.
26. Douglass HO, Moertel CG, Mayer RJ: Survival after postoperative combination treatment of rectal cancer. N Engl J Med 315:1294, 1986.
27. Krook JE, Moertel CG, Gunderson L, et al: Effective surgical adjuvant therapy for high-risk rectal carcinoma. N Engl J Med 324:709-715, 1991.
28. Swedish Rectal Cancer Trial: Improved survival with preoperative radiotherapy in resectable rectal cancer. N Engl J Med 336:980-987, 1997.
29. Sauer R, Becker H, Hohenberger W, et al: Preoperative versus postoperative chemoradiotherapy for rectal cancer. N Engl J Med 351:1731-1740, 2004.
30. Gastrointestinal Tumor Study Group: Pancreatic cancer: adjuvant combined radiation and chemotherapy following curative resection. Arch Surg 120:899-903, 1985.
31. Hallissey MT, Dunn JA, Ward LC, et al: The second British Stomach Cancer Group trial of adjuvant radiotherapy or chemotherapy in resectable gastric cancer: five-year follow-up. Lancet 343:1309-1312, 1994.
32. Macdonald J, Smalley S, Benedetti J, et al: Chemoradiotherapy after surgery compared with surgery alone for adenocarcinoma of the stomach or gastroesophageal junction. N Engl J Med 345:725-730, 2001.
33. Martenson JA Jr, Willett CG, Sargent DJ, et al: Phase III study of adjuvant chemotherapy and radiation therapy compared with chemotherapy alone in the surgical adjuvant treatment of colon cancer: results of Intergroup protocol 0130. J Clin Oncol 22:3277-3283, 2004.
34. Burris HA 3rd, Moore MJ, Andersen J, et al: Improvements in survival and clinical benefit with gemcitabine as first-line therapy for patients with advanced pancreas cancer: a randomized trial. J Clin Oncol 15:2403-2413, 1997.
35. Lawrence TS, Chang EY, Hahn TM, et al: Radiosensitization of pancreatic cancer cell lines by 2′,2′-difluoro-2′-deoxycytinine. Int J Radiat Oncol Biol Phys 34:867-872, 1996.
36. Blackstock AW, Tepper JE, Niedzwiecki D, et al: Cancer and Leukemia Group B (CALGB) 89805: phase II chemoradiation trial using gemcitabine in patients with locoregional adenocarcinoma of the pancreas. Int J Gastrointest Cancer 34:107-116, 2003.
37. Omura M, Torigoe S, Kubota N: SN-38, a metabolite of the camptothecin derivative CPT-11, potentiates the cytotoxic effect of radiation in human colon adenocarcinoma cells grown as spheroids. Radiother Oncol 43:197-201, 1997.
38. Magne N, Fischel JL, Formento P, et al: Oxaliplatin-5-fluorouracil and ionizing radiation. Importance of the sequence and influence of p53 status. Oncology 64:280-287, 2003.
39. Humerickhouse RA, Schilsky RL: Thymidylate synthase inhibitors in clinical development. Cancer Ther 1:100-113, 1998.
40. Rodel C, Grabenbauer GG, Papadopoulos T, et al: Phase I/II trial of capecitabine, oxaliplatin, and radiation for rectal cancer. J Clin Oncol 21:3098-3104, 2003.
41. Dawson LA, Normolle D, Balter JM, et al: Analysis of radiation-induced liver disease using the Lyman NTCP model. Int J Radiat Oncol Biol Phys 53:810-821, 2002.
42. Willett C, Tepper J, Orlow E, et al: Renal complications secondary to radiation treatment of upper abdominal malignancies. Int J Radiat Oncol Biol Phys 12:1601-1604, 1986.
43. Buskirk SJ, Gunderson LL, Schild SE, et al: Analysis of failure after curative irradiation of extrahepatic bile duct carcinoma. Ann Surg 215:125-131, 1992.
44. Letschert JGJ, Lebesque JV, Aleman BMP, et al: The volume effect in radiation-related late small bowel complications: results of a clinical study of the EORTC Radiotherapy Cooperative Group in

patients treated for rectal carcinoma. Radiother Oncol 32:116-123, 1994.
45. Gallagher MJ, Brereton HD, Rostock RA, et al: A prospective study of treatment techniques to minimize the volume of pelvic small bowel with reduction of acute and late effects associated with pelvic irradiation. Int J Radiat Oncol Biol Phys 12:1565-1573, 1986.
46. Ooi BS, Tjandra JJ, Green MD: Morbidities of adjuvant chemotherapy and radiotherapy for resectable rectal cancer. Dis Colon Rectum 42:403-418, 1999.
47. Lindel K, Willett CG, Shellito PC, et al: Intraoperative radiation therapy for locally advanced recurrent rectal or rectosigmoid cancer. Radiother Oncol 58:83-87, 2001.
48. Gunderson LL, Nelson H, Martenson JA, et al: Locally advanced primary colorectal cancer: intraoperative electron and external beam irradiation +/− 5-FU. Int J Radiat Oncol Biol Phys 37:601-614, 1997.
49. Garton GR, Gunderson LL, Nagorney DM, et al: High-dose preoperative external beam and intraoperative irradiation for locally advanced pancreatic cancer. Int J Radiat Oncol Biol Phys 27:1153-1157, 1993.
50. Tepper J, Shipley W, Warshaw A, et al: The role of misonidazole combined with intraoperative radiation therapy in the treatment of pancreatic carcinoma. J Clin Oncol 5:579-584, 1987.

CHAPTER 44

STOMACH CANCER

Leonard L. Gunderson, Joel E. Tepper, and Felipe A. Calvo

INCIDENCE

For 2006, the predicted incidence of stomach cancer in the United States is 22,280 cases, and the predicted number of deaths is 11,430.

The site of origin is shifting in the United States as more proximal lesions are diagnosed.

BIOLOGIC CHARACTERISTICS

The main prognostic factors relate to local-regional tumor extent and include both nodal involvement and direct tumor extension beyond the gastric wall.

STAGING EVALUATION

Initial evaluation should include history and physical examination, complete blood count, chest film, liver chemistries, endoscopy with biopsy and ultrasonography (determine degree of direct tumor extension), and computed tomography (CT) of the abdomen (define extragastric disease).

Additional studies that may help define extent of disease include upper gastrointestinal (GI) imaging, CT chest (especially for gastroesophageal junction lesions) and laparoscopy (rule out peritoneal seeding or early liver metastasis).

PRIMARY THERAPY

Surgical resection is the primary therapy for resectable gastric cancers. Cure rates of 80% or higher are achieved with early lesions (nodes negative, confined to mucosa or submucosa), which are uncommon in the United States.

Extended D2 node dissection has not improved survival in randomized trials.

ADJUVANT THERAPY (CHEMOTHERAPY, RADIATION)

Adjuvant therapy is indicated on the basis of patterns of relapse and survival results with surgery alone (high incidence of local-regional relapse and distant metastases). Most Western trials of chemotherapy alone are negative for both single and multiple drugs; some recent trials are positive.

U.S. Intergroup phase III trial of 556 patients demonstrated a survival benefit for combined modality postoperative chemoradiation versus a surgery alone control arm (3-year relapse-free survival 48% versus 31%, $p = .001$; 3-year overall survival (OS) 50% versus 41%, $p = .005$). This approach is now viewed by many as the standard of care.

Preoperative radiation reduced local-regional relapse and improved OS in a Beijing phase III trial.

LOCALLY ADVANCED DISEASE

Both external beam radiation plus chemotherapy and intraoperative radiation result in long-term survival in 10% to 20% of patients in randomized and nonrandomized trials.

Neoadjuvant chemotherapy may increase resection rates, but the incidence of local-regional relapse is still high. Pathologic CR specimens are uncommon (0% to 9%).

PALLIATION

Multidrug chemotherapy regimens have response rates of 30% to 50%, but survival improvements are modest.

The ECF regimen of epirubicin, cisplatin, and 5-fluorouracil had improved response rates and survival when compared with the FAMTx combination of 5-fluorouracil, doxorubicin (Adriamycin), and high-dose methotrexate in a British phase III trial.

European phase III trials demonstrate improvement in quality and duration of life with palliative chemotherapy versus supportive care.

The primary therapy for resectable gastric cancer for patients who can tolerate the procedure is surgical resection. At the time of diagnosis, gastric cancers are localized and surgically resectable in approximately 50% of patients; however, regional nodal metastases or direct invasion of surrounding organs or structures is frequently encountered and precludes cure by surgery alone in many patients. For patients with lower risk lesions (confined to gastric wall, nodes negative; T1-2 N0 M0) adjuvant treatment is usually not recommended. Since both local and systemic relapses are common after resection of high-risk gastric cancers (beyond wall, nodes positive, or both; T3-4 N0, T any N1-3), adjuvant treatment is indicated for these patients. The results of phase III trials that demonstrate a survival benefit for postoperative chemoradiation versus surgery alone will be summarized and future trial designs will be discussed.

For patients with locally advanced disease that appears unresectable for cure, several treatment options appear to favorably impact disease control and survival. These include external beam radiation therapy (EBRT) plus concurrent chemotherapy, maximal resection plus intraoperative radiation therapy (IORT), and preoperative chemotherapy or chemoradiation.

In the setting of metastatic disease, there are many active chemotherapy agents that can produce meaningful response alone or in combination with other agents, but the duration of response is usually limited. Phase III trials demonstrate both a survival and quality of life benefit for multidrug chemotherapy versus best supportive care for patients with metastatic cancers.

EPIDEMIOLOGY AND ETIOLOGY

Epidemiology

In the United States, gastric cancer now ranks 14th in incidence among the major types of malignancy. Over the past 60 years, there has been a significant decline in the incidence of gastric cancer among both sexes in Western countries[1] (Fig. 44-1). In the United States, from 1930 to 1980, the incidence decreased from 38 to 10 (per 100,000) for men and from 30 to 5 (per 100,000) for women. In 2006, it is estimated that 22,280 new cases and approximately 11,430 deaths will occur.[2] The disease rarely occurs before the age of 40 years, but its incidence increases steadily thereafter and peaks in the seventh decade. African Americans, Hispanic Americans, and Native Americans are twice as likely to develop gastric cancer as are whites.[3] There has been a slight improvement in overall 5-year survival among U.S. patients: 11% (1900 to 1963), 15% (1974 to 1976), 18% (1980 to 1982), and 21% (1989 to 1994).[3]

Although gastric cancer incidence has decreased significantly in the United States, on a worldwide scale, gastric cancer has a very high incidence and is still a leading cause of cancer death.[2,4] Of the 45 countries in which age-adjusted death rates for gastric cancer were compared for 2000 (Fig. 44-2), the United States ranked 45th for both males and females.[2] Kyrgyzstan ranked first for both males (47.0 in 100,000) and females (18.9 in 100,000).

The site of origin within the stomach has changed in frequency in the United States over recent decades, with proximal lesions now being diagnosed and treated much more commonly than previously. The largest percentage of gastric cancers still arises within the antrum or distal stomach (≈ 40%), are least common in the body of the stomach (≈ 25%), and are of intermediate frequency in the fundus, cardia, and esophagogastric junction (≈ 35%). In 1930, most cases of gastric carcinoma originated in the distal stomach (body and antrum). The reduction in incidence of gastric cancer from 1930 to 1980 primarily is attributable to a decline in distal lesions.[5] Since the 1970s, there has been a steady rise in the incidence of adenocarcinoma of the gastroesophageal (GE) junction and proximal stomach. For both sites, the rate of increase during the 1970s and 1980s surpasses that of any other cancer, including melanoma, lung cancer, and non-Hodgkin's lymphoma.[6] Similar trends in the increased incidence of gastric cardia cancer have also been reported in Denmark, where rates were much higher in men, and in the United Kingdom, where rates were highest among those in higher socioeconomic classes.[7]

Etiology

While the precise etiology is unknown, environmental factors are likely to be important. The incidence of gastric cancer in first- and second-generation Japanese who have moved to the United States is much lower than in native Japanese citizens.[8] Studies of immigrant populations from Japan and Eastern Europe show that the risk of the disease declines markedly in the second and third generations.[9] The excess risk of first-generation immigrants is largely restricted to the intestinal type.[10] The risk of gastric cancer is inversely associated with socioeconomic status throughout the world,[11] and the marked decline in the incidence of gastric cancer in industrialized countries, including the United States, suggests that environmental factors play an important role. These may be related to poor nutrition, inadequate sanitation facilities, and substandard quality of food preservation.

Diets rich in fruits or vegetables are associated with a reduced risk of gastric cancer,[12] whereas diets containing abundant quantities of smoked, heavily salted, or poorly preserved foods are associated with an increased risk of this disease.[12,13] Excessive dietary salt has been associated with atrophic changes in the gastric mucosa.[14] Chronic atrophic gastritis and the associated abnormality, intestinal metaplasia, are most closely linked to the intestinal type of gastric adenocarcinoma. These lesions can progress to dysplasia and carcinoma.[15] The prevalence of atrophic gastritis and intestinal metaplasia is highest in regions of the world that have the highest rates of gastric cancer.[16]

It has been postulated that endogenous formation of *N*-nitroso compounds (amine or amides) can occur in the stomach when both an amino compound and a nitrating agent such as nitrate are present.[13] Anaerobic bacteria that colonize stomachs in which achlorhydria occurs can convert nitrates and nitrites to potentially carcinogenic nitroso compounds.[12]

Epidemiologic studies have demonstrated an association between *Helicobacter pylori* infection and risk of gastric cancer.[17] Serologic studies have reported that persons with *H. pylori* infection have a threefold to sixfold higher risk of distal gastric cancer than those without infection.[18,19] The exact role of *H. pylori* in gastric carcinogenesis is still to be determined, although infection is associated with the development of chronic atrophic gastritis and decreased acid production.[12] However, only a minority of infected patients develop gastric cancer, and data do not yet exist on the effect of treatment of the *H. pylori* infection on subsequent malignancy. Proximal gastric cancers (GE junction, cardia) do not appear to be related to either *H. pylori* infection, atrophic gastritis, or decreased acid production; it is possible that an inverse relationship exists.

In summary, the worldwide decline in distal, predominantly intestinal-type gastric adenocarcinoma may be the result of improved food handling (refrigeration and storage). In contrast, proximal (mostly diffuse-type) gastric cancer, which is equally prevalent in both high-risk and low-risk regions, is probably attributable to other, as yet unrecognized, factors.[20] There has been a dramatic increase in the incidence of gastroesophageal and gastric cardia carcinoma over the past few decades, similar to the increase in distal esophagus adenocarcinomas, suggesting that they may have similar etiologies. The exact role of *H. pylori* in gastric carcinogenesis remains to be defined.[14]

PREVENTION AND EARLY DETECTION

Early detection would markedly improve prognosis of gastric cancer, since surgical resection has a high cure rate with lesions limited to the mucosa or submucosa. In the United States, however, the incidence of early gastric cancer is less than 5% in most series. In Japan, whereas the incidence of carcinoma confined to the mucosa or submucosa was only 3.8% in the 1955 to 1956 period, by 1966 the incidence of early lesions had increased to 34.5% because of vigorous screening procedures (5-year survival rates of 90.9% in this cohort of patients).[21] The value of screening is evidenced by the 5-year survival rate of 53% for all gastric cancers in Japan versus 21% for the world.[4]

Although mass screening has been useful in Japan to detect early cancers, defined high-risk populations do not exist in the

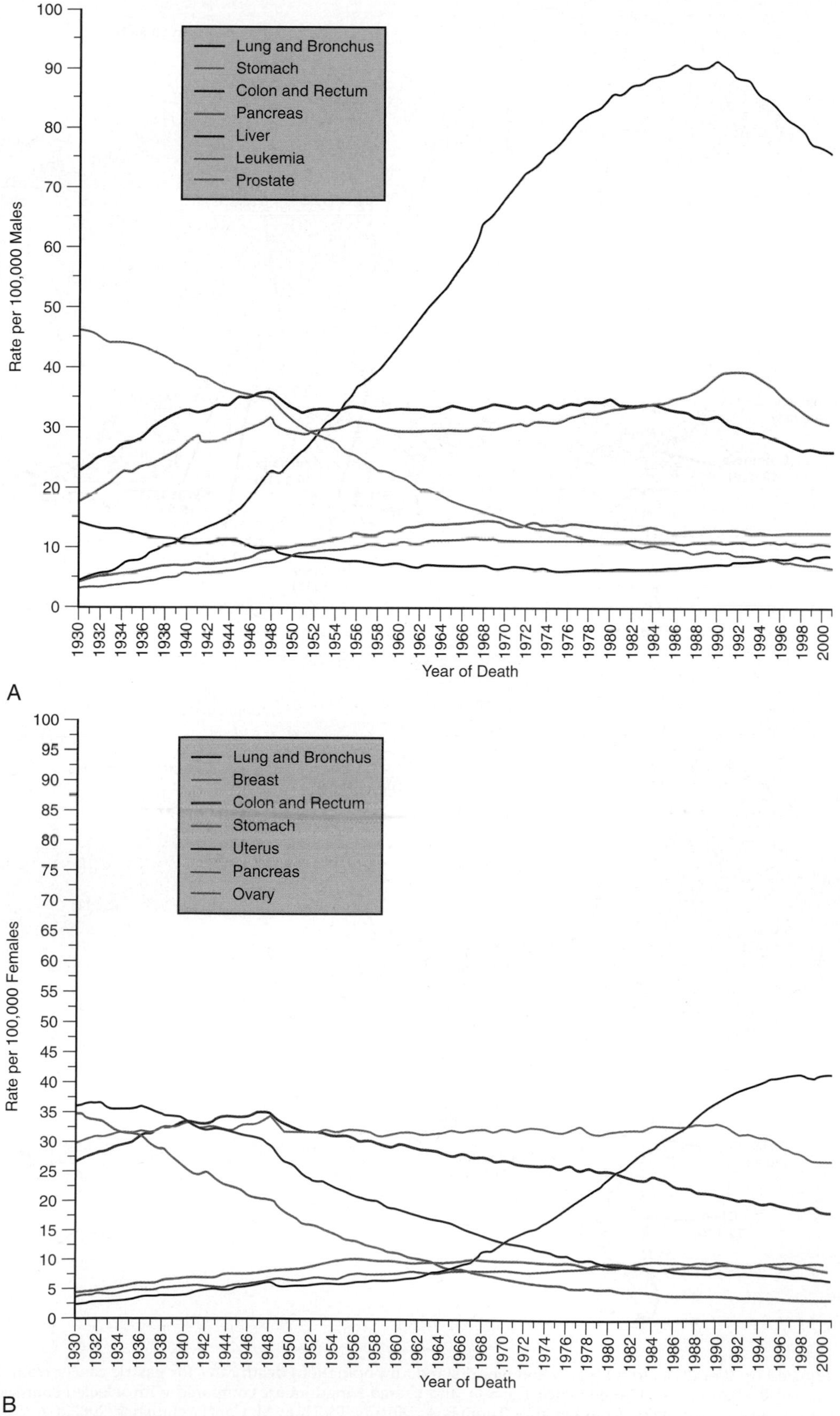

FIGURE 44-1 Age-adjusted (to U.S. 1970 standard population) cancer death rates in the United States from 1930 to 2001 in selected sites for males (**A**) and females (**B**). In females there is a steady decrease in death rates for stomach, breast, and colorectal cancers. From 1960 to 1998, a marked increase in death rates has occurred for lung cancer in females. For males, a similar decrease in death rates has occurred with gastric cancer. An increase in death rates for lung cancer existed in males from 1930 to 1990 with a continual decrease during the 1990's. (Redrawn from Jemal A, Murray T, Ward E, et al: Cancer statistics, 2005. CA Cancer J Clin 55:10-30, 2005.)

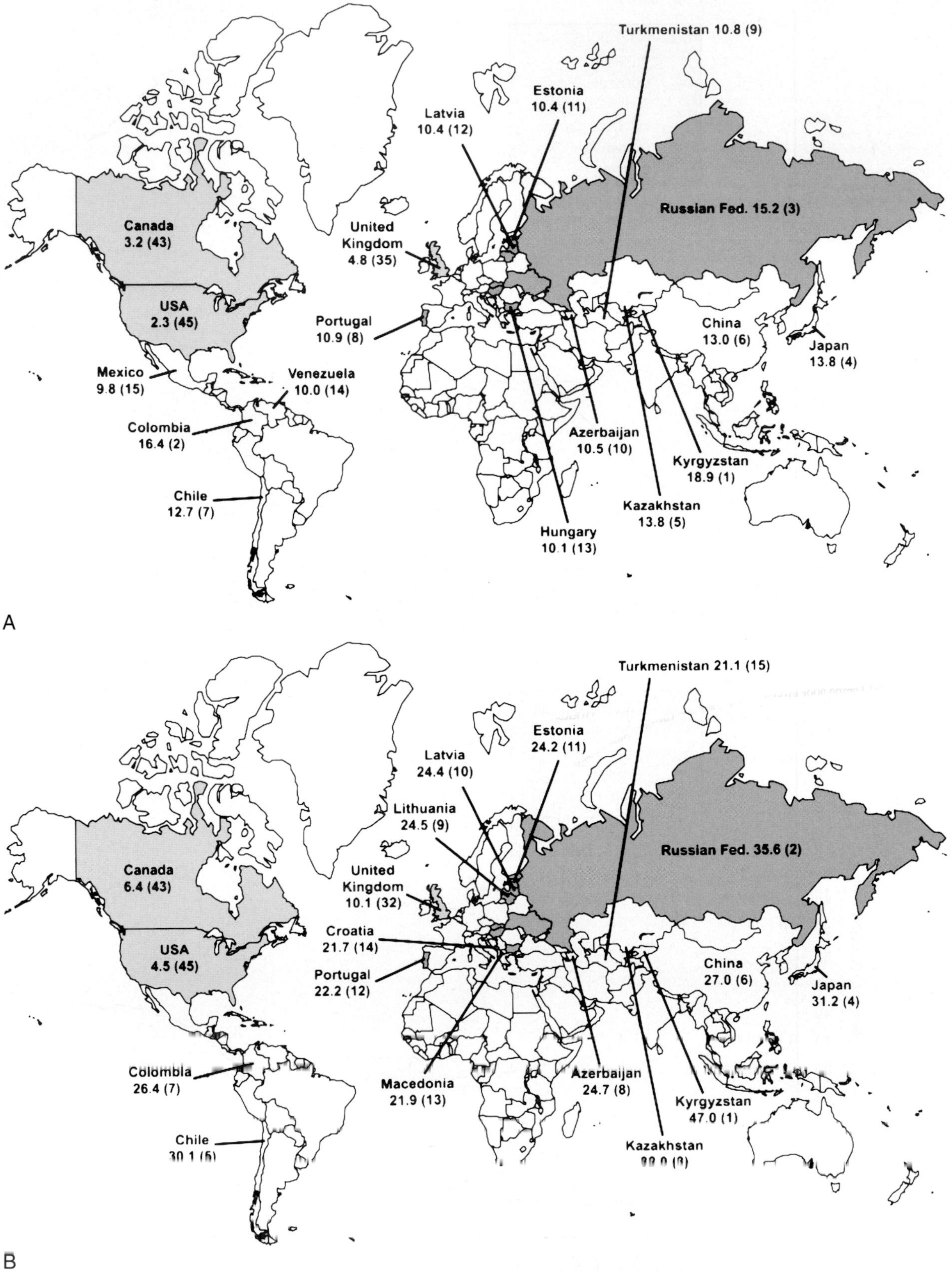

Figure 44-2 Age-adjusted (to World Health Organization world standard population) death rates for gastric cancer from 2000 in 45 countries for males (**A**) and females (**B**). Rates in the United States, Canada, and United Kingdom are compared with selected countries, including the 15 countries with the highest death rates. (Data from Jemal A, Thomas A, Murray T , Thun M: Cancer statistics, 2002. CA Cancer J Clin 52:23-47, 2002.)

United States to justify the expense of widespread screening. Individual practitioners should use upper gastrointestinal (UGI) series or preferably endoscopy to screen patients who have occupational or precursor risk factors or patients with persistent dyspepsia or gastroesophageal symptoms. It is not yet known whether screening of patients with *H. pylori* infection will be of value in achieving diagnosis of early gastric cancer, although treating *H. pylori* infection could reduce incidence.

Germline mutations in the *CDH-1* gene, which encodes the E-cadherin protein, have been recognized in families with hereditary diffuse gastric adenocarcinoma. Carriers of these mutations have a 70% lifetime risk of developing gastric cancer. Several reports of prophylactic gastrectomy have demonstrated the routine presence of microscopic intraepithelial carcinomas for patients having regular endoscopic surveillance with multiple random biopsies.[22-24] Early total gastrectomy has been recommended for this small patient population because of the lack of effective early tumor detection. Microscopic evaluation of the proximal and distal resection margins for complete removal of the gastric mucosa is necessary, since residual gastric mucosa can degenerate and result in a gastric cancer.[24]

BIOLOGIC CHARACTERISTICS AND MOLECULAR BIOLOGY

Prognostic Factors

The most valuable prognostic indicators relate to tumor extent. With either blood-borne metastasis or peritoneal seeding, cure is rare to nonexistent. Survival decreases with progressive direct tumor extension both within and beyond the wall of the stomach.[25-29] Lymph node involvement, per se, is not as important as the number and location of nodes.[26,30] Minimal lymph node involvement adjacent to the primary lesion is the most favorable.[31] The solitary finding of either involved lymph nodes or extension beyond the gastric wall is usually not as ominous as the presence of both.[26-30]

Tumor grade and gross and microscopic pathologic appearance of the primary malignancy appear to provide some prognostic information, but none of these factors is an independent prognostic variable relative to tumor stage. Prognosis is generally worse with higher-grade and diffuse-type carcinomas, which usually present with a higher stage of disease. Borrmann's type I and II carcinomas have a relatively favorable 5-year survival rate, whereas patients with type IV tumors (linitis plastica) have very poor prognosis.[31,32]

Prognostic factors recently evaluated in a British Study Group Trial included tumor size, macroscopic aspect, number of sites involved, wall invasion (pT), involvement of surgical resection limits, nodal stage, and histologic grade. Multivariate analyses established as prognostic features the depth of pT, nodal involvement, and surgical resection margins involvement.[33]

Some investigators have suggested that tumors of the gastric cardia may have different epidemiologic factors than cancers of the distal stomach[34,35] and may exhibit different tumor biology.[36] Prognosis appears worse for cardia lesions,[37,38] and flow cytometry reveals a greater incidence of aneuploidy when compared with tumors of the antrum and body.[39]

Molecular Biology

The molecular biology of gastric cancer reflects the heterogeneity of its causes and its histologic subtypes. Identification of the genetic and phenotypic variables existing among gastric cancers may lead to more directed therapeutic approaches and a more accurate prediction of clinical outcome. Changes that may affect the behavior of gastric tumor cells involve four major types of alterations. Loss of tumor-suppressor gene function, especially inactivation of the *p53* gene, certainly plays a critical role. The *p53* gene is located on the short arm of chromosome 17 and plays a key role in tumor suppression and cell-cycle regulation.[40] The *p53* gene puts a brake on DNA replication and triggers programmed cell death in response to DNA damage.[41] Loss of *p53* function is associated with the development of malignancy, impacts the effectiveness of chemotherapy and irradiation,[42,43] and predisposes cells to genetic instability. The latter is particularly important, since *p53* mutations typically occur early in carcinogenesis.[44]

A second major aberration affecting gastric epithelial cells is the impact of alterations in mismatch repair genes. Two such genes, *HMSH3* and *HMLH1*, on chromosomes 2 and 3, respectively, account for replication errors throughout the genome. Mutations in these genes are implicated in cancer family syndromes and hereditary nonpolyposis colorectal cancer (HNPCC), a syndrome associated with an increased tendency for the development of colorectal and gastric tumors.[45] Mutations in these genes generate genetic instability and have the potential to lead to further alterations in oncogenes.

Two proto-oncogenes, c-*met* and K-*sam*, are associated with scirrhous carcinoma of the stomach. The former encodes hepatocyte growth factor, which is a potent endogenous promoter of gastric epithelial cell growth.[46] Its overexpression correlates with tumor progression and metastasis.[47] The latter encodes a tyrosine kinase receptor family.[47] In scirrhous carcinoma, c-*met* and K-*sam* amplification may occur independently. There is a tendency for K-*sam* to be activated in women with gastric cancer younger than 40 years of age and c-*met* to be amplified in men older than 50 years of age.[48,49]

Flow cytometry provides valuable prognostic information for gastric cancer and may be an independent prognostic factor.[39] As noted previously, aneuploidy is associated with unfavorable tumor location such as the cardia[39,50] but is also associated with lymph node metastasis[50-52] and direct tumor extension.[28] Unfavorable DNA flow cytometry characteristics seem to relate to an unfavorable prognosis.[39, 50,51] In one series in which multivariate analysis of DNA ploidy was analyzed with other known prognostic factors such as stage, age, and sex, DNA ploidy carried statistically significant independent prognostic information.[52]

The presence of several peptides including estrogen receptor,[53] epidermal growth factor receptor,[54] and the erb-B2 protein[55] appears to affect prognosis adversely. The expression of epidermal growth factor receptor and high levels of epidermal growth factor correlate with a higher incidence of primary tumor infiltration, poor histologic differentiation, and linitis plastica. The pathophysiologic relationship between these peptide receptors and poor patient prognosis is not clear.

Modern molecular biology observations confirm the heterogeneity of human gastric cancer. Genetic alterations, detected and potentially associated with worse prognosis, included CD44 expression, telomerase reactivation, *p53* gene inactivation, dysfunction of repair genes such as *HMSH3* and *HMLH1*, overexpression of proto-oncogenes like *erb-B2*, *bcl-2*, c-*met*, and K-*sam*, estrogenic receptor expression, and presence of viral genome.[56] Gastric cancers with class II major histocompatibility complex antigen expression (HLA-DR) have a better prognosis, but the loss of expression is not an independent prognostic factor.[57]

PATHOLOGY AND PATHWAYS OF SPREAD

Pathology

Adenocarcinoma (ACA) histology accounts for 90% to 95% of all gastric malignancies, and the terms "gastric" and "stomach cancer" usually refer to such. Other histologies include lymphoma (usually unfavorable histology), leiomyosarcoma, carcinoid, adenoacanthoma, and squamous cell carcinomas.[58]

Gastrointestinal stromal tumors (GISTs) were previously classified as leiomyosarcomas but commonly arise in the stomach. GISTs need to be recognized, as their management (surgery alone or plus Gleevec) is distinctly different from ACA (surgery plus postoperative chemoradiation).

Gastric carcinomas have been categorized with regard to both microscopic and gross pathologic features. The Lauren classification system includes an intestinal type with improved prognosis (predominates in regions with high prevalence of gastric cancer) and a diffuse histologic type with poor prognosis (occurs more commonly in countries with low prevalence).[59] Diffuse carcinomas occur more often in young patients and develop throughout the stomach but especially in the cardia. Intestinal-type lesions are frequently ulcerative and occur in the distal stomach more commonly than the diffuse type. Grossly, gastric cancers can be categorized according to Borrmann's five types: I, polypoid or fungating; II, ulcerating lesions surrounded by elevated borders; III, ulceration with invasion of the gastric wall; IV, diffusely infiltrating (linitis plastica); and V, not classifiable.[60] The Japanese Research Society for Gastric Cancer has a classification system that divides lesions into protruded (I), superficial (II) (with elevated [IIa], flat [IIb], and depressed [IIc] subtypes), and excavated (III) types.[58]

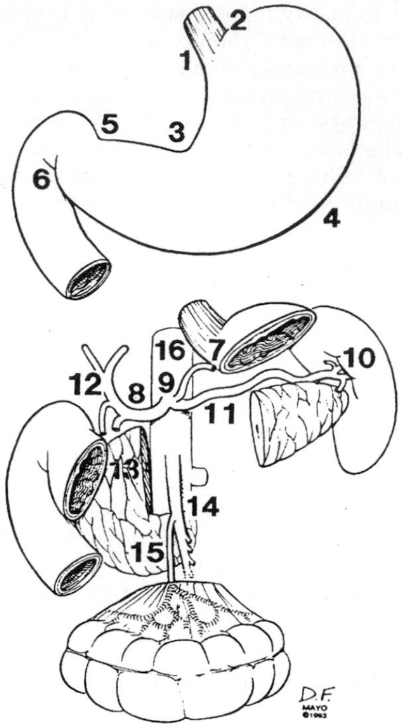

Figure 44-3 Classification and anatomic location of lymph node groups. 1, right paracardial; 2, left paracardial; 3, lesser curvature; 4, greater curvature; 5, suprapyloric; 6, infrapyloric; 7, left gastric artery; 8, common hepatic artery; 9, celiac artery; 10, splenic hilus; 11, splenic artery; 12, hepatic pedicle; 13, retropancreatic; 14, mesenteric root; 15, middle colic artery; 16, para-aortic. (By permission of Mayo Foundation for Medical Education and Research.)

Pathways of Spread

Direct Extension

The stomach is surrounded by organs and structures that can be involved by direct tumor extension when a lesion has spread beyond the gastric wall. These include the omenta, pancreas, diaphragm, transverse colon or mesocolon, duodenum, jejunum, spleen, liver, superior mesenteric and celiac vessels, abdominal wall, left adrenal gland, and kidney. Although adherence from inflammatory conditions can mimic direct extension of tumor, all adhesions between a gastric carcinoma and adjacent structures should be regarded as malignant, and en bloc resection of involved structures is preferred, if feasible.

Lymphatics

Abundant lymphatic channels are present within the submucosal and subserosal layers of the gastric wall. Microscopic or subclinical spread beyond the visible gross lesions (intramural spread) occurs commonly via the lymphatic channels. Frozen sections of the gastric resection margins should therefore be obtained intraoperatively to ensure that margins of resection are uninvolved microscopically. The submucosal lymphatic plexus is also prominent in the esophagus and the subserosal plexus in the duodenum, allowing both proximal and distal intramural tumor spread.

Because of the numerous pathways of lymphatic drainage in the stomach, it is difficult to perform a complete nodal dissection (Fig. 44-3). Although initial drainage is usually to lymph nodes along the lesser and greater curvatures (perigastric or N1 nodes using the Japanese Research Society for Gastric Cancer designation), primary nodal drainage includes nodes along all three branches of the celiac (left gastric, common hepatic, splenic) and the celiac itself (Japanese N2 nodes).[58] Node groups that are more distal include hepatoduodenal, peripancreatic, root of mesentery (Japan N3), periaortic, and middle colic (N4). When proximal gastric lesions extend into the distal esophagus, that nodal system is at risk.

Hematogenous Spread

For cancers that are limited to the gastric wall, venous drainage is primarily to the liver via the portal system, although spread can occur to virtually any organ. At initial exploration, liver involvement is found in up to 30% of patients, predominantly due to hematogenous metastases but sometimes because of direct tumor extension. When cancers extend proximally to involve the esophagus or extend posteriorly, the lung may be at risk for metastasis.

Peritoneal Involvement

Because the stomach is an intraperitoneal organ, peritoneal spread is feasible when a lesion extends beyond the gastric wall to a free peritoneal (serosal) surface. Peritoneal involvement may initially be a localized process limited by surrounding organs and ligaments (gastrohepatic, gastrosplenic, and gastrocolic), but is often a diffuse process.

CLINICAL MANIFESTATIONS, PATIENT EVALUATION, AND STAGING

Clinical Manifestations

Neither patient symptoms nor routine physical examination leads to an early diagnosis of gastric cancer. The most common presenting symptoms and signs are loss of appetite, abdominal discomfort, weight loss, weakness (due to anemia), nausea and vomiting, and melena. The duration of symptoms is less than 3 months in nearly 40% of the patients and longer than 1 year in only 20%.

Patient Evaluation

Positive physical examination findings are those of advanced disease. These may include an abdominal mass (representing the primary tumor, hepatic metastasis, or ovarian metastasis [Krukenberg tumor]); remote nodal metastasis (left supraclavicular [Virchow's node]; periumbilical [Sister Mary Joseph node]; or left axillary [Irish's node]), ascites, or a rectal shelf (peritoneal seeding).

The diagnosis of gastric cancer is usually confirmed by UGI endoscopy or radiographs (Table 44-1). Double-contrast radiographs may reveal small lesions limited to the superficial (inner) layers of the gastric wall. Endoscopy is now the preferred diagnostic study, as it allows direct tumor visualization, cytology, and histologic biopsy that yields the diagnosis in 90% or more of patients with exophytic lesions. Ulcerated cancers and linitis plastica lesions may be harder to diagnose endoscopically, but multiple biopsies and washings enhance the probability of accurate diagnosis. Endoscopic ultrasonography (EUS) has a high degree of accuracy in determining depth of tumor invasion prior to resection (i.e., does the lesion extend beyond the muscularis propria?) but is less accurate in detecting regional nodal metastasis.[61,62] Needle biopsies of suspicious nodes can be performed at the time of endoscopy with EUS. Although EUS may not affect therapy decisions with most current management approaches, the use of EUS may lead to selective management strategies based on tumor stage.

The abdominal extent of disease at laparoscopy or exploration is usually more extensive than is suggested on UGI films or endoscopy. Abdominal computed tomography (CT) is quite valuable in determining the abdominal extent of disease with regard to liver metastasis, involvement of celiac or periaortic nodes, or extragastric extension (may help determine which lesions extend to surgically unresectable structures) but is of little value in ruling out peritoneal seeding. Diagnostic laparoscopy allows visualization and biopsy of small peritoneal implants or surface liver metastases and aids in determining the extent of the primary tumor.

Distant (hematogenous) metastases should be ruled out with a chest radiograph and abdominal CT or liver ultrasonography. (CT is preferable to ultrasonography for the radiation oncologist because of the additional information concerning regional nodal status, extragastric extent of disease, and extension within the distal esophagus.) CT scans also provide valuable tumor localization information should irradiation be indicated. If a proximal gastric cancer extends to involve the esophagus, CT of the chest should be done to rule out involvement of mediastinal nodes or the lung parenchyma.

The value of laparoscopy in the staging of gastric cancer is still being defined. In 71 patients with CT criteria of resectable disease, 69 completed a laparoscopic evaluation.[63] Laparoscopy confirmed disease in 16 of the 17 patients with peritoneal metastasis (avoiding 12 laparotomies) and 1 of 3 patients with small liver metastases and negative CT scan. The combination of CT scan and laparoscopy staging information yielded a resectability rate of 93% for patients defined as potential candidates for curative gastric cancer surgery.

Treatment planning in gastric cancer patients could be improved by accurate preoperative classifications of depth of invasion (T category) and lymph node involvement (N category). A prospective study in 108 consecutive patients evaluated EUS, CT scan, and intraoperative surgical assessment for T and N classification.[64] Staging of the T category was correct with CT scan in 43% of the cases, 86% with EUS, and in 56% with intraoperative assessment. Staging of N1 and N2 lymph nodes was correct with CT in 51% of the cases, with EUS in 74%, and with intraoperative assessment in 54%. Advanced gastric tumors tended to be more accurately staged with CT; CT in general overstaged in T category and understaged the N category. Endoscopic ultrasound showed high and similar accuracy for all the T categories, although it also tended to understage N categories. Finally, intraoperative assessment was equally accurate for all N categories, but tended to overstage early T stages and to understage N categories.

Staging

The current TNM (tumor, lymph nodes, metastasis) staging system is depicted in Table 44-2.[65] The TNM system is now

Table 44-1 Diagnostic Algorithm—Gastric Cancer

Diagnostic Procedure	Diagnosis and Staging Capability	Recommend Routine Use
PRIMARY TUMOR/ REGIONAL NODES*		
Single-contrast upper GI (UGI)	Useful in detecting and defining primary lesions in stomach	Optional—consider along with double-contrast UGI study
Gastroscopy	Very accurate modality to detect and define primary lesion, ≈ 90% confirmation rate	Yes; use to confirm lesion detected in UGI series and to screen high risk patients
Ultrasound-endoscopy	Most accurate method of determining extension within and beyond gastric wall	Yes; biopsy node(s), if feasible
Double-contrast UGI	Useful in detecting early gastric cancers	Consider along with single-contrast
CT—abdomen + chest	Most valuable modality to determine degree of extragastric extension and distant metastases	Yes; include CT chest for GE junction cancers
METASTATIC TUMORS		
Chest films	Good for detecting metastases	Yes
Laparoscopy	May allow visualization of small serosal implants or liver metastases	Optional—recommended if plan preoperative chemotherapy or chemoradiation

*Laboratory studies: CBC, creatinine, liver function studies (alkaline phosphate, bilirubin, SGOT, LDH), albumin.

Table 44-2 **TNM Staging for Carcinoma of the Stomach**

Stage	T	N	M
O	Tis	0	0
IA	1	0	0
IB	1	1	0
	2	0	0
II	1	2	0
	2a/b	1	0
	3	0	0
IIIA	2a/b	2	0
	3	1	0
	4	0	0
IIIB	3	2	0
IV	4	1 to 3	0
	1 to 3	3	0
	Any	Any	0

[a]TNM definitions are as follows:
Tis: carcinoma in situ; intraepithelial tumor without invasion of the lamina propria.
T1: Tumor invades lamina propria or submucosa.
T2: Tumor invades the muscularis propria (T2a) or the subserosa (T2b).
T3: Tumor penetrates the serosa (visceral peritoneum) without invasion of adjacent structures.
T4: Tumor invades adjacent structures.
N0: No regional lymph node metastasis.
N1: Metastasis in 1-6 regional nodes.
N2: Metastasis in 7-15 regional nodes.
N3: Metastasis in more than 15 regional nodes.
[†]Metastasis to other intra-abdominal lymph nodes such as hepatoduodenal, retropancreatic, mesenteric, or para-aortic are considered distant metastasis within this system but are N3 or N4 in the Japanese Research Society Classification.
M0: no distant metastasis.
M1: distant metastasis.

acknowledged as the standard system for reporting outcomes in this disease.

Follow-up

Patients who are treated for gastric cancer should be followed for nutritional problems as well as disease relapse. Generally, patients are seen at 3- to 6-month intervals for the first 2 to 3 years and then less frequently. There are no agreed upon critical follow-up strategies, as curative salvage therapy for recurrent gastric cancer after trimodality therapy is unusual. However, it is reasonable to have endoscopy performed one or two times and to use periodic CT scans to detect intra-abdominal relapse. There are little data to suggest that early treatment of systemic metastases improves outcomes.

PRIMARY THERAPY

Surgical Method

Surgical excision of the gastric and nodal components of disease remains the primary therapy for all potentially curable gastric carcinomas. Most cancers can be removed with adequate margins by subtotal gastrectomy, and total gastrectomy is used only when mandated by proximal cancer location or disease extent. Routine total gastrectomy does not improve survival by providing wider margins and eliminating multicentric disease but does increase morbidity and mortality. Surgical resection alone is an excellent treatment for carcinomas limited to the mucosa or submucosa without nodal involvement (Tis or T1N0M0). Although these early gastric cancers occur with an incidence of over 30% in Japan, the incidence is still less than 5% in the United States and other Western countries. For the more invasive gastric carcinomas, surgical resection is indicated for 50% to 60% of patients at the time of disease presentation, but only 25% to 40% of patients will have potentially curative procedures.

While only one small prospective randomized trial has been performed with regard to extent of the gastric resection,[66] extensive experience exists with various different surgical procedures, and appropriate generalizations can be made. The preferred treatment for lesions arising in the body or antrum of the stomach is a radical distal subtotal resection. This removes approximately 80% of the stomach along with the first portion of the duodenum, the gastrohepatic and gastrocolic omenta, and the nodal tissue adjacent to the three branches of the celiac axis. Extensive or proximal cancers will require a total gastrectomy to achieve an adequate proximal gastric margin. However, total gastrectomy is not necessary when subtotal gastrectomy will provide a 5-cm clearance of the gross tumor.[67,68] The propensity for gastric carcinoma to spread via submucosal and subserosal lymphatics dictates the need for a 5-cm surgical resection margin of normal stomach beyond the visible lesion. It may be necessary to extend the resection to include some (or additional) esophagus or duodenum if frozen section pathologic evaluation of the surgical margins fails to confirm the adequacy of proximal and distal resection margins. If total gastrectomy is necessary, a splenectomy is sometimes performed particularly in gastric cancers of the proximal third of the stomach, and tumors of the body near the greater curvature. Cancers in these locations are more apt to metastasize to lymph nodes in the splenic hilum that cannot be completely excised without a splenectomy. Although the value of routine splenectomy has not been addressed in prospective randomized trials, retrospective Japanese and American data do not provide evidence of a survival benefit with the routine use of this procedure.[69,70]

Direct extension beyond the gastric wall should be treated with "en bloc" extended resection to achieve negative margins if a curative resection is contemplated. Common examples of local tumor extension include involvement of the body or tail of the pancreas (treated by distal pancreatectomy and splenectomy), invasion of the transverse mesocolon (often requires transverse colectomy), and involvement of the spleen (splenectomy) or left lobe of the liver (usually requires wedge resection with a 1-cm or wider clearance).

The optimal extent of lymph node dissection for gastric cancer remains controversial. Several studies have shown that the presence and extent of lymph node metastasis correlate with the depth of primary tumor invasion.[71-73] Although several nonrandomized clinical trials have suggested that extended lymphadenectomies may improve survival,[70,74-78] other nonrandomized[79,80] and randomized trials[81-87] have not demonstrated an advantage. A large multicenter phase III study in the Netherlands accrued 996 evaluable patients and provides additional objective data on the lack of value of extended lymphadenectomy in gastric carcinoma.[82] Among the 711 patients having curative resections, both morbidity and mortality were significantly higher with the more extensive nodal dissection.[83-85] A randomized study of 400 patients conducted by the Medical Research Council (MRC) in the United Kingdom has also demonstrated higher morbidity and mortality in the extended lymphadenectomy cohort.[86,87] No benefit in disease-free or overall survival was found in either the Dutch or British trials (Table 44-3). Any apparent survival benefit seen with the extended node dissection performed in Japan may be due to the phenomenon of a shift in stage rather than superior surgery. While most patients with five or more

Table 44-3 **Extent of Surgery: Randomized Trials of D1 Versus D2 Dissection**

Series	No. of Patients	5-Y Survival D1	5-Y Survival D2	Operative Mortality D1	Operative Mortality D2	P Value
Dutch[84,85]	711	45%	47%	4%	10%	<.05
MRC[86,87]*	400	35%	33%	6.5%	13%	<.05

*Defined D1 dissection as resection of AJCC nodes (those within 3 cm of primary tumor).
Both trials showed significantly increased morbidity and mortality with more extensive dissections.

lymph node metastases or with lymph node metastasis not adjacent to the primary tumor have a very poor outcome, extended lymph node dissection seems reasonable when it can be performed by experienced surgeons without significant additional surgical morbidity or mortality.[88,89]

Endoscopic laser surgery has been used in selected patients with early gastric cancer.[90] Small lesions (≤3 cm) that are pedunculated, do not invade the submucosa, and are well differentiated infrequently have lymph node metastasis (<5%). Nearly 75% of these select tumors can be completely removed endoscopically. While early gastric cancer may have a long natural history before progression, standard surgical resection rather than endoscopic removal is still preferable.[91] Irradiation plus chemotherapy should be considered as adjuvant therapy when the tumor is endoscopically treated.

Quality of life (QOL) after gastrectomy is being analyzed.[92,93] In a University of Heidelberg report of 104 patients, 12 months after gastrectomy, postoperative symptoms of heartburn or dumping in the group undergoing total gastrectomy with pouch reconstruction did not differ significantly from the group having only distal gastric resection.[94] In a recent prospective trial of 120 patients requiring total gastrectomy plus pouch who were randomized to two different types of reconstruction (jejunal interposition versus Roux-en-Y), there were no differences in food passage, body weight, or quality of life parameters.[95] However, for all patients there are significant QOL issues related to decreased absorption of fats, iron, and calcium, as well as the loss of intrinsic factor, and thus B12 deficiency. These losses need to be addressed with dietary supplements (iron, calcium), monitoring for osteoporosis, and possible monthly B12 injections.

Surgery Alone Survival Results

Overall survival with surgery alone remains poor, despite improved perioperative care that has resulted in a substantial decline in postoperative mortality.[96] A large review from Europe reported excellent 5-year survival for early gastric cancer patients (83%) but a marked diminution in survival for more invasive cancers (31% for tumors of the antrum, 24% for the midstomach, and 16% for the cardia).[97] Survival in excess of 90% has been achieved throughout the world with resection of lesions confined to the mucosa or submucosa.[98-102] In reports with lower 5-year survivals for the early lesions, most of the mortality is from noncancer causes.[99,103] For gastric cancers with deeper invasion or nodal involvement, survival decreases proportional to the degree of invasion or nodal involvement. When N1 or N2 nodes are involved, Western reports continue to show 5-year survivals of 10% to 30%,[104,105] whereas Japanese authors report 5-year survival of 25% to 60% (versus less than 10% with N3 or N4 involvement) (Table 44-4).[70] Although pathologic staging differences, different tumor biology, and more radical surgical extirpation have been proposed as explanations, the cause of the difference in U.S. and Japanese results with N1 or N2 disease remains uncertain. Even in the Orient, half of all patients with more

Table 44-4 **Comparison of 5-Year Survivals Following Surgery for Gastric Carcinoma**

Tumor Classification	Nodal Status	5-Year Survival (%) *Japan*	5-Year Survival (%) *United States*
T1	N0	90	90
T2	N0	60	52
T3	N0	30	47
T4	N0	5	15
—	N1	53	20
—	N2	26	10
—	N3	10	—
—	N4	3	—

Modified from Noguchi Y, Imada T, Matsumoto A, et al: Radical surgery for gastric cancer: a review of the Japanese experience. Cancer 64:2053, 1989. Copyright © 1989 American Cancer Society. Reprinted by permission of Wiley-Liss, Inc., a subsidiary of John Wiley & Sons, Inc.

invasive gastric cancer cannot survive their disease, a fact that underlies the need for new nonsurgical therapies. Results of phase III trials, to be discussed subsequently, demonstrate improvements in survival with the addition of adjuvant chemoradiation to surgical resection.

Relapse Patterns after "Curative Resection"

Local relapse or failure (LF) in the tumor bed and regional lymph nodes (RF) or distant failures (DF) via hematogenous (DM) or peritoneal (PS) routes are all common mechanisms of relapse after "curative resection" in clinical,[110-112] reoperative,[28] and autopsy[113-117] series. For lesions of the esophagogastric junction, both the liver and lungs are common sites of DM. With gastric lesions that do not extend to the esophagus, the initial site of DM is usually the liver, and many relapses could be prevented if an effective "abdominal" or liver therapy could be combined with treatment of the primary tumor and regional lymph nodes.

Local-regional failures occur commonly within the region of the gastric bed and nearby lymph nodes (Table 44-5 and Fig. 44-4). Tumor relapse in anastomoses, the gastric remnant, or the duodenal stump is also frequent. In a University of Minnesota reoperative analysis,[28,29] local-regional failure occurred as the only evidence of relapse in 29% of the 86 patients with relapse (23% of the 105 evaluable patients at risk) and as any component of failure in 88%. More extensive operative procedures including routine splenectomy, omentectomy, and radical lymph node dissection neither improved survival[118] nor decreased the incidence of LF-RF[28,29] in the reoperative analysis. Subsequent relapse within the scope of the initial node dissection occurred in a high percentage of the patients even when radical node dissections were performed (removal of N1 and N2 with or without N3 nodes)[29] (Table 44-6). These

Table 44-5 Gastric Cancer: Patterns of Locoregional Relapse in Clinical, Reoperation, and Autopsy Series

Failure Area	MGH[112] (Clinical) (n = 130)	U. Minn.[29] (Reoperation) (n = 105)	McNeer et al[114] (Autopsy) (n = 92)	Thomson and Robins[116] (Autopsy) (n = 28)
	Incidence—Any Component of Local or Regional Relapse (No. [%])			
Gastric bed	27 (21)	58 (55)	48 (52)	19 (68)
Anastomosis or stumps	33 (25)	28 (27)	55 (60)	15 (54)
Abdominal or stab wound	—	5 (5)	—	—
Lymph node(s)	11 (8)	45 (43)	48 (52)	—

Table 44-6 Extent of Gastrectomy and Node Dissection Versus Type of Local Regional Relapse: Reoperation Series

Operative Procedure‡	No. of Failures/ Total at Risk	Any Component of Local-Regional Relapse*: Gastric Bed N	(%)	Anastomosis or Stumps N	(%)	Abdomen or Stab Wound N	(%)	Nodes (LN) N	(%)
Subtotal gastrectomy	53/72	36	(50)	18	(25)	3	(4)	29	(40)
Method 1†	25/36	18	(50)	13	(36)	0	—	11	(31)
Method 2†	15/17	9	(53)	4	(24)	1	(6)	9	(53)
Method 3†	13/19	9	(47)	1	(5)	2	(11)	9	(47)
Total gastrectomy	27/33	20	(61)	8	(24)	2	(6)	15	(45)
Method 1†	0	—	—	—	—	—	—	—	—
Method 2†	14/15	10	(67)	5	(33)	1	(7)	11	(73)
Method 3†	13/18	10	(56)	3	(17)	5	(6)	4	(22)
Total	80/105‡	56	(53)	26	(25)	5	(5)	44	(42)

*Figures in parentheses represent percentage of patients at risk with complete follow-up.

†Method 1 (pre-1950): subtotal or total gastrectomy, greater omentectomy, regional node dissection; Method 2 (1950-1954): method 1 plus splenectomy, total omentectomy, additional node dissection regarding splenic, suprapancreatic, and central celiac axis; Method 3 (1954 on): methods 1 and 2 plus extension of node dissection to porta hepatis and pancreaticoduodenal (intent: total lymph node dissection of all primary node areas equivalent to current D2 or D3 dissection).

‡An additional 6 patients had a relapse; 80 of 86 were evaluable regarding both operative method and pattern of relapse.

Modified from MacDonald JS, Cohn I, Gunderson LL: Carcinoma of the stomach. *In* Devita V, Hellman S, Rosenberg S (eds): Principles and Practice of Oncology, 2nd ed. Philadelphia, Lippincott, 1985, pp 659-690.

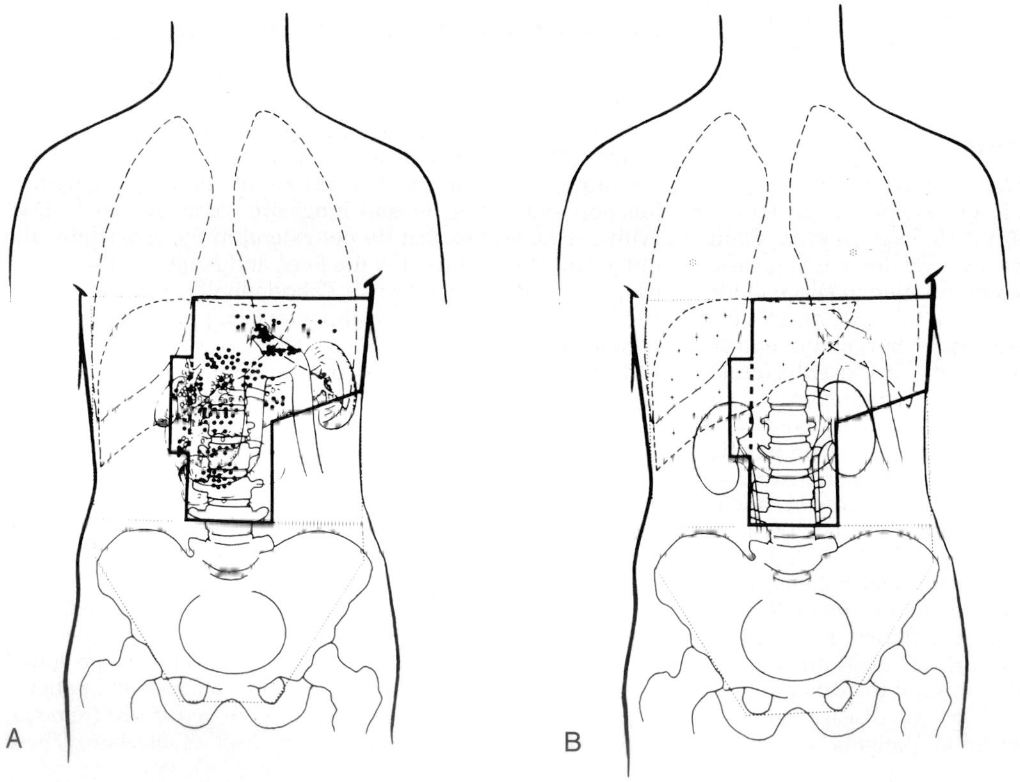

Figure 44-4 Patterns of failure in the University of Minnesota gastric cancer reoperative series with superimposed idealized irradiation fields (**A** and **B**) and relationship to dose-limiting organs or structures. •, Local failures in surrounding organs or tissues; ○, lymph node failures; *, lung metastases; +, liver metastases. (Modified from Gunderson LL, Sosin H: Adenocarcinoma of the stomach areas of failure in a reoperation series [second or symptomatic looks]: clinicopathologic correlation and implications for adjuvant therapy. Int J Radiat Oncol Biol Phys 8:1, 1982. Copyright 1982.)

data indicate the difficulty of performing a complete lymph node and lymphatic resection in this anatomic location.

Patterns of relapse by stage were analyzed in detail in a series of 130 patients who underwent resection with curative intent at the Massachusetts General Hospital (MGH).[112] Local-regional relapse occurred as any component of failure in 49 patients (38%) and as the sole failure in 21 (16% of 130 patients at risk and 24% of the 88 with disease progression). The incidence of local-regional relapse by stage was in excess of 35% for modified Astler-Coller stages B2 (T3 N0), B3 (T4 N0), C2 (T3 N1-3), and C3 (T4 N1-3). The sites at higher risk for local-regional relapse included the gastric bed (27 of 130 patients, 21%) and the anastomosis or gastric remnant (33 of 130 patients, 25%). The true incidence of gastric bed, regional lymph node, and peritoneal failures may be higher because this was neither a reoperative nor an autopsy series (see comparative findings in Table 44-4). Some additional information on patterns of relapse by stage exist in both the University of Minnesota reoperation analysis[28] and the University of Washington autopsy analysis.[117] Although patterns of relapse data are more accurate in such analyses, patient selection is biased.

All of these data suggest that the development of an effective therapy for local-regional disease as an adjuvant to surgery could potentially benefit at least 20% of patients. Effective systemic therapy is also essential to improve the outcome for resected high-risk gastric cancer patients in view of the risks of both intra-abdominal (liver and peritoneal) and extra-abdominal metastasis (lung, other).

Adjuvant Chemotherapy

The role of adjuvant chemotherapy in gastric cancer has been extensively studied over the past decades, being the first attempt to improve the prognosis of resected gastric cancer.[119-152] Results of randomized clinical trials of adjuvant single-agent chemotherapy, following curative resection in gastric cancer have generally not shown any survival benefit when compared with surgical resection alone.

Two phase III clinical trials evaluated the impact of FAM combination chemotherapy after curative surgery in resected high-risk gastric cancer.[119,120] Coombs and associates[119] included 315 patients, and no difference was observed in either overall survival (FAM 45% versus control 35%) or relapse rates (FAM 56% versus control 56%). In a Southwest Oncology Group (SWOG) study, no advantage to adjuvant treatment with FAM was reported, either.[120]

A Spanish trial compared high-dose mitomycin C following surgical resection (33 patients) versus surgery alone (37 patients).[121] This small trial showed a significant 5-year survival advantage ($p = .001$) in the group receiving chemotherapy (76% versus 30%), and a low rate of relapse in the treated arm (7 of 33 or 21% of the patients) versus the control arm (23 of 37 patients or 62%). This trial was extended to 134 patients with median follow-up of 8.75 years and still showed a survival advantage for postoperative mitomycin ($p = .025$). A subsequent randomized Spanish trial observed a significantly better 5-year survival for mitomycin plus ftorafur (67%) versus mitomycin alone (44%) in resected high-risk gastric cancer, suggesting a strong benefit in patients with node-negative and early stage.[122]

Neri and colleagues treated surgically resected, node-positive patients with the addition of adjuvant epirubicin, 5-FU, and leucovorin (68 patients) and compared them to 69 surgery alone control patients.[123] They noted an improvement in 5-year survival from 13% to 30% for those receiving adjuvant chemotherapy.

Adjuvant chemotherapy with FAM2, seven cycles, was compared with surgery alone in an EORTC (European Organization for Research and Treatment of Cancer) randomized phase II trial that included 314 patients with stage II and III gastric ACA.[125] Five-year survival was 70% for stage II, and 32% for stage III patients with no significant differences between groups. Toxicity was high with FAM2 but time to disease progression was significantly longer in this group. Disease-free survival increased to a borderline significant value. Similarly, an adjuvant FAM randomized trial done by the SWOG, failed to show improved survival results.[126]

The European Organization for Research and Treatment of Cancer (EORTC) and the International Collaborative Cancer Group (ICCG) conducted independent randomized phase III studies of either adjuvant FAMTX or FEMTX compared to surgery alone.[127] Both studies were closed when they failed to reach accrual after being open for 7 years. A pooled analysis of the two studies demonstrated that they both caused substantial toxicity but had no significant effect on overall survival, the primary end point of each study.

Meta-Analysis of Adjuvant Trials

Since many of the trials conducted to date have been underpowered to adequately assess potential differences between the control and treatment arms in regard to overall survival, six meta-analyses have been performed since 1990 to better assess the use of adjuvant chemotherapy.[129-133] The two most recent meta-analyses both showed a significant survival advantage to the use of chemotherapy following surgical resection of gastric cancer. Seventeen randomized clinical trials, involving 3118 patients, were included in the meta-analysis by Panzini and associates.[129] The pooled odds ratio was 0.72 (95% CI, 0.62-0.84). The meta-analysis by Janunger and coworkers included 21 randomized clinical trials, involving 3962 patients, a slightly larger and somewhat different group of studies.[130] The pooled odds ratio from this study was 0.84 (95% CI, 0.74-0.96). In a subanalysis, Western and Asian studies were assessed separately. The meta-analysis of the Western studies did not show a benefit to adjuvant therapy (pooled odds ratio of 0.96; 95% CI, 0.83-1.12), while the Asian studies did show evidence of benefit (pooled odds ratio of 0.58; 95% CI, 0.44-0.76). Both meta-analyses urged caution in interpreting the apparent positive results. Many of the individual trials had small numbers of patients, used chemotherapy regimens of limited efficacy, and had an inadequate trial design.

Adjuvant Irradiation

Irradiation has only been minimally evaluated as the sole adjuvant treatment following complete surgical resection in randomized phase III trials. Adjuvant EBRT reduced local-regional failures when compared with the surgery-alone control arm in the British adjuvant trial noted later, but no survival benefits were found.[148,153] While phase III trials from Japan[154,155] and China[156] suggest some survival benefit for IORT versus a surgery-alone control arm, the advantage was found only in subset analyses. Phase II studies combining EBRT and IORT are currently ongoing in Spain (Pamplona, Madrid) and Lyon, France.

Postoperative Adjuvant External Beam Irradiation

The British Stomach Cancer Group (BSCG) completed a prospectively randomized trial of surgery alone versus postoperative FAM or EBRT (45 Gy in 25 fractions ± 5-Gy boost).[153] A total of 436 patients were randomized and followed for a minimum of 12 months; arms were well balanced with regard to prognostic factors. No survival differences by treatment arm were seen (median, 15 months). However, local-regional failure was documented in only 15 of 153 patients (10%) in the adjuvant irradiation arm versus 39 of 145 (27%) in the surgery-alone arm, and 26 of 138 (19%) in the FAM group. Interpretation of the results is complicated by the inclusion of 93 patients with resection but gross residual disease and 78 patients (18%) with gross total resection but microscopically positive resection margins. Neither group of patients would be candidates for current gastric surgical adjuvant trials in the United States. In addition, nearly one third of the patients randomized to receive adjuvant treatment did not receive the assigned therapy. Of 153 patients randomized to the irradiation arm, only 104 (68%) received a dose of 40.5 Gy or more. Only 62% of the patients received six or more cycles of chemotherapy. The results in this study are similar to results seen in the adjuvant treatment of rectal cancer, in which adjuvant pre- and postoperative irradiation improve local control but do not increase patient survival unless combined with chemotherapy.

Preoperative Adjuvant External Beam Irradiation

Randomized trials testing preoperative irradiation have been performed in both Russia and China. All have reported a positive survival benefit when compared with surgery-alone control arms.

Three prospective randomized Russian trials have evaluated preoperative irradiation in potentially resectable gastric cancer.[157-159] The first trial randomly assigned 293 patients to receive either surgery alone, surgery after preoperative EBRT (20 Gy in four fractions), or surgery after the same EBRT plus daily hyperthermia. The survival rates at 3 and 5 years were improved in both irradiation arms compared with surgery alone, and the improvement with combined EBRT and hyperthermia was statistically significant at both 3 and 5 years.[157] The second trial compared preoperative EBRT (20 Gy) versus surgery alone in 279 patients. Three- and 5-year survival rates were increased, and no increase in operative morbidity was observed.[158] The third trial compared surgery alone versus preoperative EBRT (32 Gy with concomitant inhalation of oxygen) plus surgery. A survival advantage was observed with preoperative treatment, and the resection rate was increased by 17%.[159] There are some methodologic uncertainties with all three of these trials, and their applicability to Western gastric carcinoma is not clear.

A double-blind, randomized trial from Beijing, conducted from 1978 to 1989, compared a surgery-alone control arm (n = 199) with preoperative EBRT plus surgery (n = 171) for patients with ACA of the gastric cardia.[160] Irradiation was given with 8 MV photons or cobalt with AP-PA fields to a dose of 40 Gy in 20 fractions of 2 Gy over 4 weeks. Surgery was performed 2 to 4 weeks after completion of irradiation. The addition of preoperative EBRT produced downstaging of disease and improvements in radical resection rates (radical resection rates of 80% versus 62% with preoperative EBRT versus surgery alone).

Survival and local regional disease control were improved in the patients assigned to preoperative EBRT versus surgery alone. The 5- and 10-year survival rates were 30% versus 20% and 20% versus 13%, respectively (Fig. 44-5; p = .009 Kaplan-Meier log rank). The divergence in survival curves began in the first year of follow-up and persisted through 9 years. Local and regional disease control were also improved with combined modality treatment with local relapse rates of 39% versus 52% (p < .025) and regional node relapse rates of 39% versus 54% (p < .005). The rates of distant metastases were the same at 24% versus 25%. The improvements in survival and disease control (local-regional) were accomplished with no increase in treatment-related morbidity or mortality (operative mortality 0.6% versus 2.5% with or without preoperative EBRT; intra-thoracic leak rates were 1.8% and 4.2%, respectively).

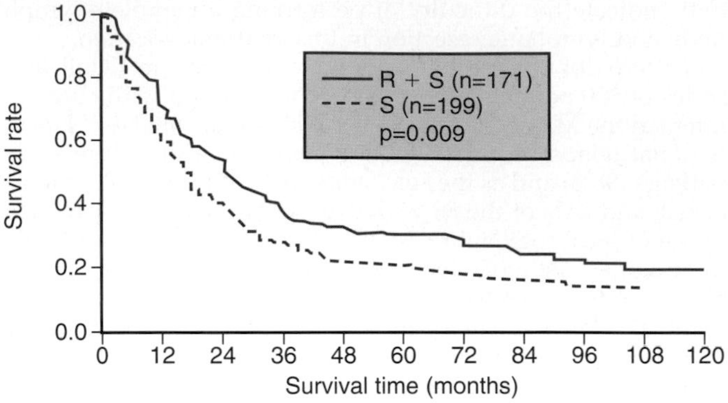

Figure 44-5 Overall survival rates in Beijing phase III randomized trial of surgery alone or plus preoperative external beam irradiation for adenocarcinoma of the gastric cardia. (From Zhang ZX, Gu XZ, Yin WB, et al: Randomized clinical trial combination on the preoperative irradiation and surgery in the treatment of adenocarcinoma of the gastric cardia [AGC]: report on 370 patients. Int J Radiat Oncol Biol Phys 42:931, 1998. Copyright 1998.)

In view of the survival advantage demonstrated for preoperative EBRT in four published trials from Russia and China, such approaches need to be evaluated further in U.S. and European study groups. As suggested by the authors from the Beijing trial, factors to be evaluated include radiation dose escalation to 45 to 50 Gy (1.8- to 2.0-Gy fractions) and the addition of chemotherapy (maintenance ± concomitant with EBRT).

Adjuvant Irradiation Plus Chemotherapy

Postoperative External Beam Irradiation Plus Chemotherapy

Phase II Trials

Phase II single-institution gastric cancer trials that showed promise for postoperative adjuvant chemoirradiation included series from MGH,[161] Israel (Hadassah),[162] Thomas Jefferson University Hospital (TJUH),[163,164] the University of Pennsylvania,[165] and Mayo Clinic.[166] Results are seen in Table 44-7. Gunderson and associates reported a median survival of 24 months and 4-year survival of 43% in 14 patients from MGH who had complete resection of tumors with extension beyond the wall, nodal involvement, or both.[161] Patients received postoperative EBRT (45 to 52 Gy, 1.8 Gy/d) plus concurrent 5-FU–based chemotherapy. Subsequent local-regional relapse was documented in 2 of 14 patients (14%) in contrast to a 42% incidence in similar high-risk patients treated with surgery alone at MGH.[112] In a gastric series from TJUH, 120 patients had surgical resection but were at high risk for relapse because of extension beyond the gastric wall, nodal metastases, or positive margins of resection.[163] Seventy patients had surgery alone and 50 received adjuvant therapy. Apparent improvements in local control as well as median and 5-year survival were noted with additional therapy. For patients with negative resection margins, 2-year local control with surgery

Table 44-7 Surgery ± Adjuvant Therapy for Resected Gastric Cancer (or Gastroesophageal [GE] Junction), Phase II Trials

Institution/Disease Site/Treatment	SURVIVAL Patient No.	SURVIVAL Median (mo)	Long-term* (%)	*p* Value	LOCAL-REGIONAL RELAPSE No.	(%)	*p* Value	Ref. No.
1. MGH (gastric)[112,161]								
a. Surgery alone[161]	110	—	38 (B2, B3) 15 (C1-3)	—	46	42	—	161
b. Postop EBRT + CT[112]	14	24	43 (4 yr)	—	2	14	—	112
2. TJUH (gastric)[163]								
a. Total group T3, T4, or N+	120							163
• Surgery alone	70	12	13		17/38	45	—	
• Postop CT, EBRT, both	50	19	17	<.05	13/36	36	—	
• Postop EBRT + CT	20 of 50	19	21		3/16	19	—	
b. T3/T4, N1/N2 (surg ± adjuv)	44, 30	9 vs 13	4 vs 22	.04	—	—	—	
3. U Penn (gastric or EG)*[165]								165
a. Surgery alone	40	16	31 (2 yr)	—	31	75	—	
b. Postop EBRT	17	15	50 (2 yr)	—	4	24	—	
c. Postop EBRT + CT	27	21	55 (2 yr)	—	4	15	—	
4. Mayo Clinic (gastric, EG)[166] Postop EBRT ± CT T3, T4 or N+	25	19	31 (4 yr)	—	5	20	—	166
5. TJUH (EG junction)†[164]	S / EBRT		S / EBRT					164
Surgery + EBRT + CT	37 / 18	12 vs 20	— / —	—		74 vs 36	.0014	
• T3, T4	— / —	—	11 / 14	—	—	87 vs 47	.0016	
• LN (–)	— / —	—	42 / 100	—	—	—	—	
• LN (+)	— / —	—	0 / 15	.001	—	97 vs 14	.0001	
6. U Navarre[178-180]								178-180
a. Surgery + EBRT	35	—	38	—	7	20		
b. Surgery + IORT + EBRT	27	—	41 (8 yr)	—	3	11		
7. H U Lyon (pT3 or N+)[182,183]								182, 183
a. Surgery	NA	—	28			42		
b. Surgery + IORT + EBRT	49	—	50			—		

*Long-term survival, 5 yr data unless specified;
†Mehta and Mohuidden, ASTRO abstract, IJROBP 30(1):272, 1994.
CT, chemotherapy; EBRT, external beam radiation; IORT, intraoperative radiation; N+, node positive; postop, postoperative; S, surgery. adjuv, adjuvant therapy.

alone was 55% versus 93% with adjuvant irradiation with or without chemotherapy ($p = .03$). For patients with T3 and T4 tumors and lymph node involvement, median survival was 9 months versus 13 months (surgery alone or plus adjuvant treatment), and 5-year survival was 4% versus 22% ($p = .03$). In a separate TJUH analysis of 55 patients with cancers of the GE junction, local relapse with surgery alone was 74% versus 36% in patients with adjuvant EBRT ± chemotherapy ($p = .0014$).[164] Survival trends for node-positive patients appeared better in patients who received adjuvant treatment (5-year survival 15% versus 0%, $p > .01$). In a University of Pennsylvania analysis, treatment intensification appeared to improve both disease control and survival. The incidence of local relapse with surgery alone was 75% (31 of 40) versus 24% with adjuvant irradiation (4 of 17) and 15% with adjuvant irradiation plus chemotherapy (4 of 27).[165] Five-year survival trends favored adjuvant chemoradiation over surgery alone at 55% versus 31%. In a retrospective Mayo analysis, 63 patients received postoperative EBRT ± 5-FU after resection of carcinoma of the stomach or GE junction.[166] Twenty-five of the 63 patients had complete resection with no residual disease but had high-risk factors for disease relapse (extension beyond gastric wall, 92% of the patients; involved nodes, 92%; both high-risk factors, 84%). Concurrent 5-FU ± leucovorin was given with EBRT in 84% of the 25 adjuvantly treated patients, but maintenance chemotherapy was given in only 20%. Locoregional control was achieved in 20 of the 25 (80%) with median survival of 19 months. Four-year survival was 31% in spite of the very poor prognostic factors in these 25 patients.

Phase III Trials—Mayo Clinic, U.S. GI Intergroup Trial

A prospective randomized trial was conducted at the Mayo Clinic and included 62 patients with poor prognosis completely resected gastric cancers (Table 44-8). Patients were randomized to either surgery alone or surgery followed by EBRT plus concomitant 5-FU (37.5 Gy in 24 fractions over 4 to 5 weeks; 5-FU, 15 mg/kg/d 1–3 by IV bolus).[167] A nonstratified, prerandomization scheme was used with a 2:3 ratio favoring treatment. Informed consent was requested only of the 39 patients randomized to treatment. Ten of the 39 refused further therapy and were observed. When analyzed by intent to treat, the adjuvant arm had statistically significant improvement in both relapse-free and overall survival (overall 5-year survival 23% versus 4%; $p < .05$). When patient outcome was compared by actual treatment received (29 adjuvant treatment, 33 surgery alone), 5-year survival still favored the adjuvant group (20% versus 12%), but the differences were not statistically significant. The 10 patients who refused assignment to adjuvant treatment had more favorable prognostic findings than the other two groups of patients. When the two groups with equally poor prognostic factors were compared, 5-year overall survival was 20% versus 4%, with an advantage to those receiving adjuvant treatment. When analyzed by treatment delivered, local-regional relapse was decreased with adjuvant treatment (54% incidence with surgery alone versus 39% with irradiation plus 5-FU).

Because of conflicting results in prior small phase III studies, a U.S. GI Intergroup trial (INT 0116) was initiated to evaluate postoperative combined 5-FU–based chemotherapy and irradiation to the gastric bed and regional nodes versus surgery only in resected but high-risk gastric cancer patients.[168] Patients eligible had completely resected ACA of the stomach or GE junction with complete penetration of the muscularis propria (T2-4N0) or involved nodes (T1-4N1-3). After an en-bloc resection, 556 patients were randomized to either surgery alone or postoperative combined modality therapy. This consisted of one 5-day cycle of 5-FU and leucovorin followed by concurrent chemoradiation (45 Gy in 25 fractions plus concurrent 5-FU and leucovorin, 4 d week 1, 3 d week 5) followed by two additional 5-day cycles of 5-FU and leucovorin given at 1-month intervals. Nodal metastases were present in 85% of patients. With median follow-up of 5 years, relapse-free survival at 3 years is 48% for adjuvant treatment and 31% for observation ($p = .001$); 3-year overall survival is 50% for treatment and 41% for observation ($p = .005$) (see Table 44-8). The median overall survival in the surgery-only group was 27 months, as compared with 36 months in the chemoradiation group. The median duration of relapse-free survival was 30 months in the chemoradiation group and 19 months in the surgery-only group (Fig. 44-6).

Patterns of relapse were based on the site of first relapse only and were categorized as local, regional, or distant. Local recurrence occurred in 29% of the patients who relapsed in the surgery-only group and 19% of those who relapsed in the chemoradiation patients. Regional relapse—typically abdominal carcinomatosis—was reported in 72% of those who relapsed in the surgery-only group and 65% of those who relapsed in the chemoradiation patients. Extra-abdominal distant metastases were diagnosed in 18% of those who relapsed in the surgery-only patients and 33% of those who

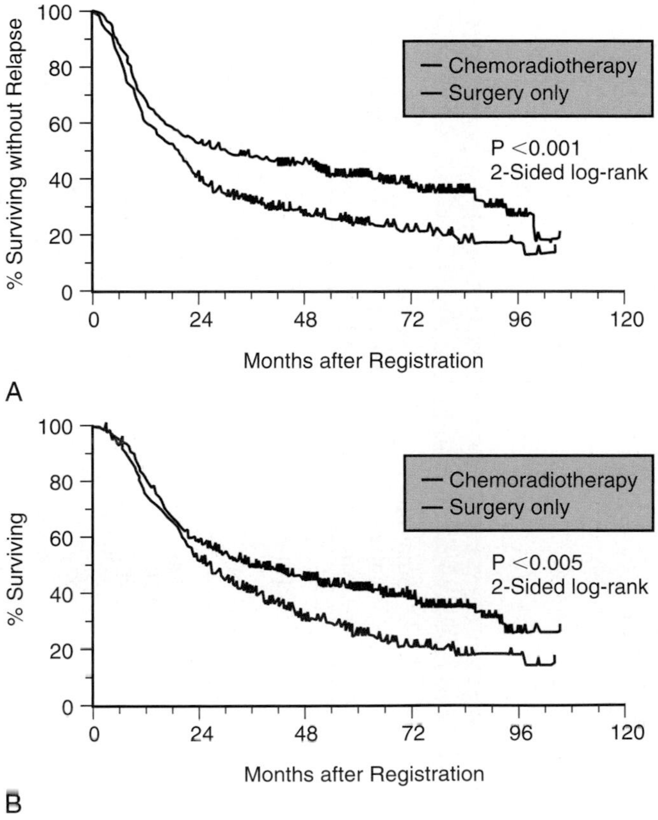

Figure 44-6 Relapse-free survival (RFS) (**A**) and overall survival (OS) (**B**) curves from the U.S. Gastrointestinal (GI) Intergroup phase III randomized trial (INT 0116) demonstrate a survival benefit for combined modality postoperative chemoradiation versus a surgery alone control arm. Patients had resected high-risk adenocarcinoma of the stomach or GE junction. (3-year RFS 48% versus 31%, p = 0.001; 3-year OS 50% versus 41%, p = 0.005). (From MacDonald JS, Smalley SR, Benedetti J, et al: Chemoradiotherapy after surgery compared with surgery alone for adenocarcinoma of the stomach or gastroesophageal junction. N Engl J Med 345:725-730, 2001)

Table 44-8 **Surgery ± Adjuvant Therapy for Resected Gastric Cancer (or Gastroesophageal [GE] Junction), Phase III Trials**

Series/Treatment Method	Patient No.	Survival			Local-Regional Relapse			Ref. No.
		Median (mo)	Long-term* (%)	*p* Value	No.	(%)	*p* Value	
1. British Stomach Group (3 yr)[148,153]		15						148, 153
a. Surgery alone	145	—	20	—	39	27	—	
b. Postop CT	138	—	19	—	26	19	—	
c. Postop EBRT	153	—	12	—	15	10	—	
2. Japan—Surgery ± IOERT[b154,155]	S IOERT 110 101		S IOERT					154, 155
a. Stage I	43 24	—	93 vs 87%	—	—	—	—	
b. Stage II	11 20	—	62 vs 84%	—	—	—	—	
c. Stage III	38 30	—	37 vs 62%	—	—	—	—	
d. Stage IV	18 27	—	0 vs 15%	—	—	—	—	
3. China—Surgery ± IOERT[†156]	100 100							156
a. Stage III (5 yr)	— —	—	30 vs 65%	<.01	—	—	—	
b. Stage III (8 yr)	— —	—	22 vs 52%		—	—	—	
4. Mayo Clinic[‡167]								167
a. Surgery alone	23	15	4	—	—	54	—	
b. Postop EBRT + 5-FU	39	24	23	.05	—	39	—	
5. China-Beijing[160]								160
a. Surgery alone	199	—	20		—	52	<.025	
b. Preop EBRT	171	—	30	.009	—	39		
6. U.S. GI Intergroup (INT 0116)[168]			(3-y)			RFS (3-y)		168
a. Surgery alone	275	27	41			31		
b. Postop EBRT + 5-FU Leucovorin	281	36	50	.005		48	.001	

*Long-term survival = 5-year data unless otherwise specified.
†Advantage to IOERT in subset analyses—Japan Stage II-IV, China Stage III (37% of patients).
‡Survival data based on intent to treat, relapse data on actual treatment.
CT, chemotherapy; EBRT, external beam radiation; IORT, intraoperative radiation; N+, node positive; postop, postoperative; S, surgery.

relapsed in the chemoradiation patients. Treatment was tolerable, with three toxic deaths (1%). Grade 3 and 4 toxicity occurred in 41% and 32% of cases, respectively.

The results of this large randomized phase III U.S. GI Intergroup trial demonstrate a clear survival advantage to the use of postoperative chemoradiation in resected high-risk patients.[168] Furthermore, the results strongly support the integration of postoperative chemoradiation into the routine care of patients with curatively resected high-risk carcinoma of the stomach and GE junction. This approach is now viewed by many as the standard of care in the United States.

Quality control (QC) of irradiation field design in INT 0116 was conducted during the cycle of chemotherapy given prior to the start of concurrent chemoirradiation.[169] The upfront QC provided the mechanism to correct most of the major or minor deviations (35% incidence) in field design prior to the start of treatment and resulted in only a 6.5% final major deviation rate. Utilization of upfront QC may have been a key factor in achieving a positive survival advantage for adjuvant chemoradiation.

Preoperative External Beam Radiation Therapy Plus Chemotherapy

Although no randomized trials testing preoperative EBRT plus chemotherapy for gastric cancer have yet been published, the Walsh and associates[170] trial for ACA of the esophagus and gastric cardia certainly has relevance. Patients were randomized to either immediate surgery (control arm) or preoperative EBRT plus 5-FU and cisplatin (40 Gy in 15 fractions; 5-FU, 15 mg/kg/d for 5 days weeks 1 and 6 as a continuous infusion or approximately 600 $mg/m^2/d$ for 5 days; cisplatin 75 mg/m^2 on the first day of each 5-FU infusion), followed by surgical resection 8 weeks after completion of EBRT plus chemotherapy. A highly significant difference in survival was observed with combined modality therapy (intent to treat: median survival 16 versus 11 months; 3-year survival, 32% versus 6%; $p = .01$; actual treatment: median survival 32 versus 11 months; $p = .001$; 3-year survival, 37% versus 7%; $p = .006$). Survival rates for the control group of patients were inferior to other historical data. A confirmatory Intergroup trial was attempted in North America for either esophagus or esophagogastric junction cancers (squamous or ACA); this was stopped due to poor accrual.

Summary: Adjuvant External Beam Irradiation Alone or Plus Chemotherapy

In summary, although chemotherapy alone has not demonstrated a convincing benefit as adjuvant therapy for gastric cancer, postoperative chemoradiation[168,169] has been demonstrated to be superior to surgery alone for resectable gastric and GE junction cancers in randomized phase III trials. There are also randomized phase III data to suggest a benefit to preoperative radiation that need to be confirmed.[166] Future preoperative irradiation trials should evaluate the addition of concurrent and maintenance chemotherapy. Postoperative chemoradiation trials are evaluating more aggressive chemotherapy both as concurrent and maintenance components of treatment.

Intraoperative Radiation Alone or Plus External Beam Radiation

The pioneer work of Abe at Kyoto University, Japan, in the 1970s, fostered a renewed interest in the old idea of irradiating tumor-bearing areas under direct vision during laparotomy. Although Abe's work triggered gastric IORT trials around the world, only a few investigators have favored the use of IORT as the only adjuvant treatment after surgical resection.[171-177] Most Western IORT protocols included the delivery of EBRT pre- or postoperatively and used IORT doses considerably lower than those advised by Abe, because of fear of severe toxicity.[176-187] This followed a tendency in the design of IORT trials in other anatomic locations, where IORT doses, in the range of 10 to 20 Gy, were combined with adjuvant EBRT doses of 45 to 50 Gy in 1.8- to 2.0-Gy fractions (Fig. 44-7).

Survival and Local-Regional Relapse Outcomes

Survival results of IORT (± EBRT) are reviewed in Table 44-9.

Intraoperative Radiation Alone

Ogata and colleagues reported a study from the Kochi Medical School, Japan, with 178 gastric cancer patients, JRS stages II through IV treated with surgery alone (120 patients) or surgery plus IORT (58 patients) from August 1983 to July 1992.[174] The patients were not randomized, but a surgery-alone group served as controls. In general, the IORT patients had more unfavorable features. The IORT results by stage (see Table 44-7) demonstrated a survival advantage in stages III and IV that was not statistically significant; the survival in stage II patients was surprisingly high but did not reach statistical significance.

Takahashi and Abe[155] reported results from a large Japanese trial in which 211 patients were randomized, on the basis of day of hospital admission, to receive surgery only or surgery plus IORT (28 to 35 Gy). Five-year survival rates for

Table 44-9 **Treatment Strategy and Results in IORT Clinical Series**

Series	No. Patients	IORT Dose (Gy)	EBRT Dose (Gy)	Local-Regional Relapse (%)	Survival
Ogata[174]	58	28-30	None	—	Stage II, 100% Stage III, 55% Stage IV, 12%
Sindelar[171]	15	20	None	31	10%, 5 y
Kramling[176,177]	54	28	None	12	55mo, mean
Calvo[178-180]	48	15	40-46*	11	39%, 5 y
Avizonis[182]	27	12.5-16.5	45*	37	47%, 2 y
Coquard[185]	30	12-15	46	25	44%, 5 y
Chambert[186]	21	15-20	28-46	33	32%, 5 y

*EBRT field derived from Univ. Minnesota reoperation data.
EBRT, external beam radiation; IORT, intraoperative radiation.

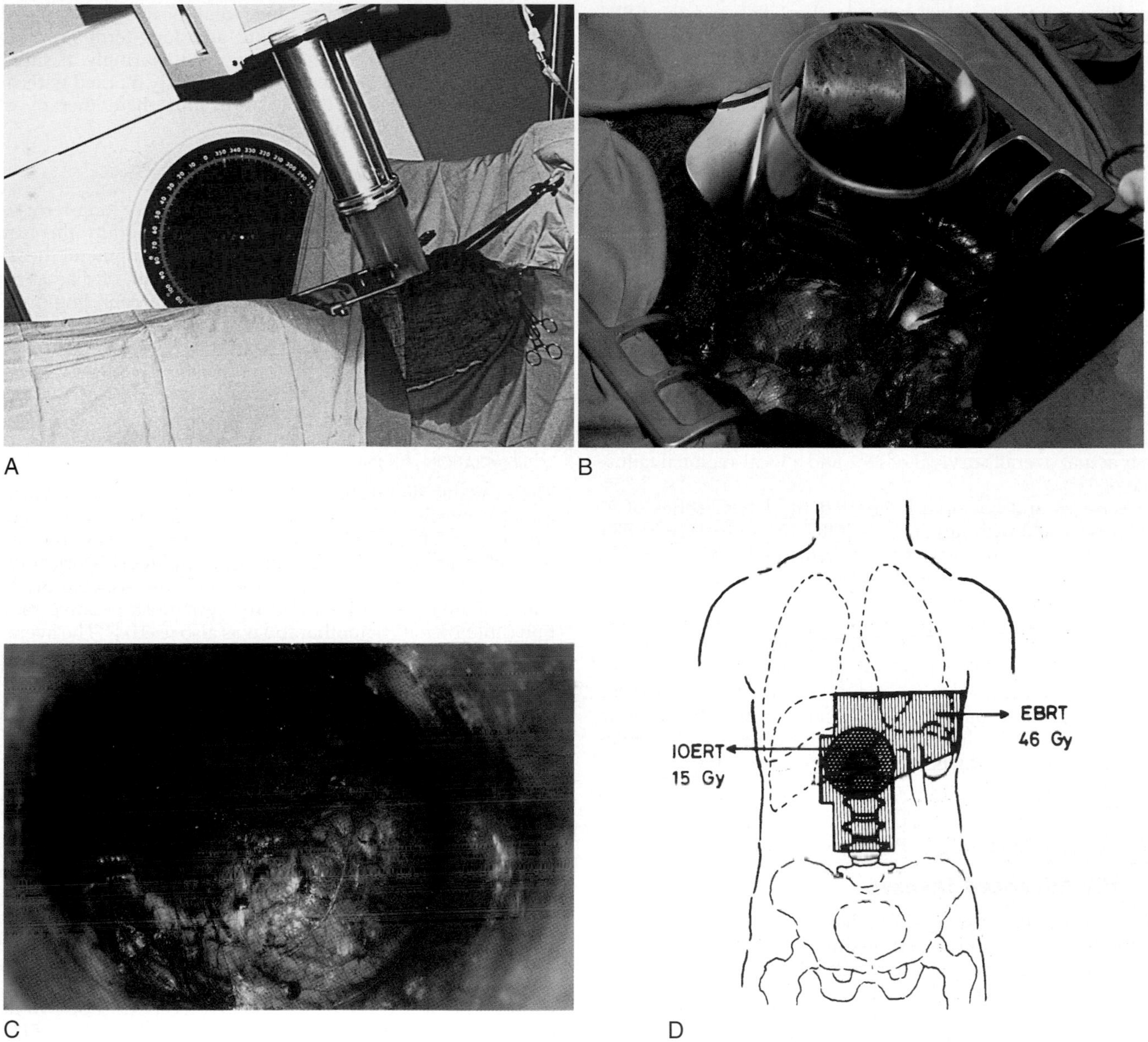

Figure 44-7 Intraoperative electron radiation (IOERT) procedure in a gastric cancer patient. **A,** View of the linear accelerator and electron beam Lucite applicator **B,** Applicator (9-cm diameter) positioned for treatment; visceral structures are mobilized from field. **C,** IOERT applicator beam's-eye view of the IOERT target volume: body of pancreas, celiac trunk, and peripancreatic nodal regions. **D,** Idealized artist's depiction of integration of the IOERT and external beam radiation (EBRT) treatment components.

Japanese stages II to IV were improved approximately 15% to 25% in the IORT group versus those treated with surgery alone (see Table 44-8; stage II, 84% versus 62%; stage III, 62% versus 37%; stage IV, 15% versus 0%). This magnitude of survival improvement correlates nicely with the approximately 20% of patients who fail only locoregionally after complete surgical resection. However, this method of randomization is susceptible to bias in treatment selection, and the trial failed to stratify for important prognostic factors.

In an analysis from Beijing, patients with stage III (serosal involvement or node-positive tumors) or stage IV (unresectable metastasis or adjacent organ involvement) disease were randomized to surgery alone or IORT (single dose, 25 to 40 Gy).[156] In the most recent report of 200 patients, a survival advantage with IORT was demonstrated for stage III patients (see Table 44-8; 65% versus 30% 5-year OS; 52% versus 22% 8-year OS; $p < .01$).

Intraoperative Versus External Beam Radiation

At the National Cancer Institute (NCI), Sindelar and associates[171] performed a small randomized trial of IORT versus EBRT following complete surgical resection that demonstrated improved local control with IORT but no survival benefit. The incidence of tumor bed recurrence was lower in the IORT versus control group, at 31% versus 80% ($p < .01$). The 5-year survival rate was 10% for 15 patients with resected gastric cancer stages III and IV treated with radical surgery plus IORT.[171] Median survival time for this subset of patients was 25 months. However, for the total group of patients, there were no differences in survival between the IORT and the EBRT arms. The median survival of the surgery + EBRT arm of 25 patients was 21 months, and the 5-year survival was 20%. No stage III or IV patient in the control group survived after a median follow-up of 7 years, whereas 3 out of 15 (20%) in the IORT group were alive with no evidence of disease (NED) at the time of the analysis ($p = .06$).

Intraoperative Plus External Beam Radiation

Calvo and coworkers described a 5-year survival of 39% and a local-regional failure rate of 10.4% in 48 patients treated with IORT plus EBRT in Pamplona.[178-181] This report included 16 patients with AJCC stages I and II and 8 patients with anastomotic or nodal recurrences. The proportion of patients with serosal involvement was 70% and of nodal involvement 56%. An update of the series by Martinez-Monge and colleagues[180] included only the 28 patients with serosal (89%) and/or lymph node involvement (63%) treated with IORT 15 Gy and EBRT 40 to 46 Gy in 1.8- to 2-Gy fractions. The update revealed a 10-year actual overall survival of 38% and a local-regional failure rate of 11%.

Avizonis and coworkers reported the RTOG series of 27 patients treated with surgery plus IORT 12.5 to 16.5 Gy ± EBRT 45 Gy.[182] Seventy percent of the patients had AJCC stages III and IV tumors. The 2-year OS was 47%, 2-year DFS 27% and median survival 19.3 months.

Gilly and associates reported on 45 patients treated in Lyon with surgical resection, IORT 15 Gy, and EBRT 44 Gy.[183] The 5-year survival rate for N1/N2+ patients was 51%. In the last update of the Lyon experience with 82 patients,[184] 8-year survival among the 49 patients with pT3 and/or pN+ treated with surgery plus IORT plus EBRT was 50% versus 28% in similar stage patients treated with surgery alone during the same time period.

LOCALLY ADVANCED DISEASE, PALLIATION

Locally Advanced Disease

The term *locally advanced disease* has different interpretations depending on the author and institution. For the purposes of this chapter, the term refers to cancers that the surgeon would not expect to resect with negative pathologic margins (i.e., unresectable for cure as determined at surgical exploration or as defined preoperatively with CT, endoscopy with ultrasonography, laparoscopy, or other studies). Other authors use the term to include lesions that are completely resected but have high-risk factors for local recurrence or distant metastasis (nodal involvement, extension beyond the gastric wall, or both).

Surgery

The extent of a surgical procedure must be tempered by the knowledge that cure is at best improbable. Patients with symptomatic obstruction, hemorrhage, and ulceration, and some with perforation, can be successfully relieved of symptoms by even limited gastric resection. Radical subtotal or total gastrectomy may be indicated in some patients whose lesions cannot be completely resected with negative pathologic margins in order to achieve symptomatic palliation. Results with total gastrectomy in advanced gastric cancer showed good quality of life when this procedure was indicated for bulky or proximal tumors, but symptom relief was less likely for patients with linitis plastica.[188] Although adjacent organ resection should be undertaken if all gross tumor can be removed, it is rarely justified if gross residual tumor (visible or palpable) would remain. Since total (or near total) gastrectomy has the risk of both acute and long-term morbidity (severe early satiety), it should be used sparingly. If sites of adherence or residual disease are judiciously marked with surgical clips, postoperative irradiation plus chemotherapy can be delivered with greater accuracy.

Irradiation ± Chemotherapy

Although some patients with no resection have long-term survival using irradiation alone or plus chemotherapy, this is not a viable alternative to surgical resection plus adjuvant therapy if that therapy is appropriate. The initial bulk of disease and the limited tolerance of the stomach and surrounding organs prevent a suitable therapeutic ratio between cure and complications. When locally unresectable disease is diagnosed preoperatively, preoperative chemoirradiation would preferably be delivered prior to an attempt at resection of all gross primary and lymph node disease.

Irradiation Alone

The available literature suggests that ACA of the stomach is radioresponsive. Wieland and Hymmen used 60 Gy when feasible (1.5 to 2.0 Gy daily) with 11% (9 of 82) 3-year and 7% (5 of 72) 5-year survival.[189] Takahashi compared historical controls with patients whose tumors were unresectable or who had palliative procedures and received postoperative radiation (unknown if chemotherapy was also used).[190] The average survival for irradiated patients was 9 to 10 months longer, with 74% 1-year (32 of 43) and 27% 2.5-year survival (12 of 43). Abe and Takahashi reported 15% 5-year survival with a single dose of IORT after resection (28 to 33 Gy) in a group of 27 patients with stage IV disease.[154,155] Three of the four long-term survivors had proven residual disease after maximal resection. In the same study, 18 stage IV patients were randomized to a surgery-alone control arm; the 5-year survival was 0%.

Irradiation Plus Chemotherapy

Most reports of combined irradiation and chemotherapy for gastric cancer involve patients with residual and unresectable disease, and most phase III trials in this setting show an advantage for combined modality treatment over single modality treatment. In a randomized series from the Mayo Clinic, 5-FU was used during the first 3 days of EBRT in half of the patients (EBRT, 35 to 37.5 Gy in 4 to 5 weeks; 5-FU 15 mg/kg for 3 days, week 1 of EBRT).[191,192] For the combined treatment group, mean and overall survival was improved (13 versus 5.9 months and 3 of 25 or 12% versus 0 of 23 for 5-year survival) (Table 44-10). In a randomized study by the GITSG,[193,194] the combination of EBRT and 5-FU followed by maintenance 5-FU plus MeCCNU resulted in statistically superior long-term survival when compared with 5-FU MeCCNU alone (3- and 4-year survivals of 18% versus 6% to 7%; $p < .05$). GITSG performed a second trial in which combined irradiation plus chemotherapy did not produce a survival advantage when compared with chemotherapy alone.[195] Since 46% of the patients on the combined arm either did not receive full-course EBRT or had a major deviation in the delivery of the EBRT, the results are difficult to interpret. In a randomized EORTC trial of EBRT with or without 5-FU, residual disease after resection was identified in 22 patients.[196] The three long-term survivors (14%) received both EBRT and 5-FU.

Data from nonrandomized single-institution or group analyses also suggest that the combination of EBRT and chemotherapy may have an impact on disease control and survival. In published series from the Mayo Clinic[197] and MGH,[161]

Table 44-10 Unresectable or Residual Gastric Cancer: Treatment Results

Group or Institution	Treatment Arms	EBRT Dose/ Schedule (Gy)	Chemotherapy	No. of Patients	Results (Failure Patterns) and Survival
RANDOMIZED					
Mayo Clinic[191,193]	EBRT ± 5-FU	35-40/9-12 Gy/wk	5-FU 15 mg/kg, d 1-3, wk 1 EBRT	48	Increased SR for EBRT + 5-FU with mean SR 13 vs. 5.9 mo and 3/25 (12%) vs. 0/23 5-y SR
GITSG[194,195]	CT ± EBRT	50/8 wk-2 wk split after 25/3 wk	5-FU 500 mg/m^2, d 1-3, wk 1 + 6 EBRT; 5-FU + MeCCNU maintenance vs. 5-FU + MeCCNU	90	Advantage in long-term SR with EBRT + CT at 18% vs. 7% ($p < .05$)
Japan[155,167]	Operation ± IORT*	IORT, 28-40	None	110 101 IORT	Increased 5-y SR for 27 patients with IORT + operation for stage IV disease vs. 18 patients with operation alone (15% vs. 0%)
NONRANDOMIZED					
MGH[178]	EBRT ± CT	45-55/5-6½ wk	5-FU 500 mg/m^2, 3 d wk 1 EBRT ± maintenance FAM or 5-FU, + MeCCNU	32†	Median SR res(m) 24 mo, res (g) 15 mo, unresected 14 mo; survival ≥30 mo, unresected 0%, residual after resection ≈10%
Mayo Clinic[185,203]	EBRT ± CT ± IOERT	45-54/5-6½ wk IOERT boost 13 patients	5-FU 500 mg/m^2, 3 d wk 1, 5 or 5-FU 400 mg/m^2, + leucovorin 20 mg/m^2	87	Median SR res(m) 17 mo, res(g) 9 mo, unresectable 12 mo; locally recurrent 10 mo; 4-y SR ≤ 9% res(m) and res(g), 18% unresectable or locally recurrent

*Treatment method based on date of hospitalization.
†An additional 14 had "curative resection" with high-risk LF: 40% 4-y actuarial SR with EBRT + CT.
CT, chemotherapy; EBRT, external beam irradiation; IORT, intraoperative irradiation; SR, survival; res(m), microscopic residual; res(g), gross residual; MGH, Massachusetts General Hospital; GITSG, Gastrointestinal Tumor Study Group. 5-FU, 5-fluorouracil; FAM, 5FU, Adriamycin, anitomycin-C.

long-term survival of 10% or more was demonstrated in patients who received EBRT plus chemotherapy following subtotal surgical resection with residual disease (MGH) or with unresectable lesions. In a University of Pennsylvania analysis of patients with unresected ACA of the esophagogastric junction or esophagus, local control was better with combined versus single modality treatment (irradiation, 1 of 23, or 4%; chemotherapy, 0 of 8; irradiation plus chemotherapy, 11 of 21, or 52%).[165] Median survival with the combined modality treatment was 10 months compared with 5 months for irradiation alone. In a Mayo Clinic-NCCTG dose escalation pilot study, EBRT was combined with 5-FU plus low-dose leucovorin (400 mg/m^2 and 20 mg/m^2, respectively for 3 to 4 days, week 1, or 1 plus 5 of irradiation).[198] Two of six patients with locally advanced gastric cancer were alive and disease free beyond 3 years.

Published analyses from both GITSG and MGH suggest an improvement in survival if partial resection with gross residual disease or gross total resection with microscopic residual can be accomplished. In the GITSG series 3-year survival was about 25% versus 10% in partially resected versus unresected patients.[193,194] In the MGH analysis, median survival with irradiation plus chemotherapy was 24 months for microscopic residual, 15 months with gross residual, and 14 months in unresected patients.[161] Four-year survival was 0% in unresected patients versus 10% in those with residual disease after maximal resection.

In a Mayo Clinic analysis of irradiation ± chemotherapy for gastric or GE junction cancers, an improvement in median survival was also suggested for patients with gross total resection but microscopic residual when compared with higher-risk subsets of patients.[199] In these analyses, the results of irradiation or chemoradiation were evaluated in 87 patients with either locally advanced primary or locally recurrent ACA of the stomach or esophagogastric junction treated from July 1980 through January 1996 at the Mayo Clinic. Of those with primary lesions, 28 had unresectable disease and 39 had resection but residual disease (microscopic, 28; gross, 11). An additional 21 presented with a local or regional relapse with no evidence of abdominal (liver, peritoneal) or extra-abdominal metastasis (lung, other). Chemotherapy with 5-FU (± leucovorin) was given during or following EBRT in 75% of the patients with microscopic residual disease and 92% of the other subgroups (concomitant with EBRT in 84%). An intraoperative electron irradiation (IOERT) supplement to EBRT was given in 13 patients. Median survival in primary cancer patients with microscopic residual was 16.7 months versus 9.6 months for patients with subtotal resection and gross residual or 12 months in those with unresectable disease. Patients who presented with local or regional relapse had a median survival of 10 months.

Prognostic factor analyses showed that long-term survival appeared slightly poorer in patients who had resection before irradiation or chemoirradiation in the Mayo Clinic analysis.[199]

Actual 4-year survival was 0% versus 9% in patients with gross residual after partial resection (1 of 11 patients alive NED 2 years after treatment), 9% in those with microscopic residual after gross total resection, and 18% in patients with unresectable primary or locally recurrent cancers. The survival trends may be a reflection of both treatment sequence and higher irradiation dose, since 12 of 13 patients with EBRT plus IOERT had unresectable primary or locally recurrent cancers. In the 21 patients with local or regionally recurrent cancers, irradiation dose greater than 54 Gy had a trend for improved survival (median survival 25.6 versus 5.5 months, $p = .06$). If patients with microscopic residual are excluded, an increase in the number of cycles of chemotherapy appeared to correlate with an improvement in median survival (<2 cycles, median 5.2 months versus 11.5 months with two or three cycles and 14.5 months with four or more cycles, $p = .014$).

Although problems with excess toxicity were encountered in the GITSG study,[193,194] such problems were minimal or nonexistent in the MGH series of 46 patients.[161] In the MGH series, shaped radiation portals and single fraction size of 1.8 Gy were used; 43 of 46 patients received both irradiation and chemotherapy.

Neoadjuvant Chemotherapy

The use of adjuvant preoperative (neoadjuvant) chemotherapy has been less well studied compared to adjuvant postoperative therapy. Due to the inability of adjuvant (postoperative) systemic therapy to prolong survival in surgically managed gastric cancer, several investigators have pursued the approach of neoadjuvant chemotherapy in an attempt to increase resectability and improve survival. These studies involve a mix of patients including those with clinically operable, "locally advanced" or unresectable lesions. Table 44-11 summarizes the results of these reports. All but one of these studies are phase II protocols.[200-214]

Unresectable

Wilke and colleagues examined the role of etoposide, Adriamycin, and cisplatin (EAP) in a group of 34 patients with laparotomy-determined unresectable stomach cancer.[200] This study was prompted by the promising results with this regimen in advanced disease (21% complete remission and 73% overall response rate).[215] Following exploratory laparotomy, patients were begun on EAP. Twenty patients (59%) who achieved clinical response went on to a second-look operation followed by two additional courses of chemotherapy. Fifteen patients (44%) out of the original cohort were able to have a resection and 5 patients were pathologic complete responders (15% of the original 34). Median survival in this phase II trial was 18 months for the entire study group. In an update of these data, results were reported in 21 patients who had total resection after EAP chemotherapy for locally unresectable disease.[216] Fourteen of 21 patients had relapsed, and 11 of 14 had a local regional component of disease (79% of relapses, 52% of group at risk).

Verschueren and associates evaluated 17 patients with unresectable gastric cancer.[201] Fifteen of them were defined as unresectable at laparotomy whereas two were deemed unresectable on the basis of CT imaging. After receiving up to four courses of sequential 5-FU and high-dose methotrexate, 13 patients (76%) underwent attempted resection. Although seven patients had resectable tumors (41%), local-regional relapse occurred in five of seven.

Locally Advanced

Two studies have tested the use of preoperative systemic treatment for patients with "locally advanced" stomach cancer. Ducreux and colleagues treated 30 patients with two or three cycles of cisplatin and 5-FU before surgery.[202] Twenty-eight (93%) patients subsequently underwent laparotomy, and 23 (77%) had their tumor resected; the pathologic response rate was not reported. Median survival was 16 months. Kang and colleagues randomized 107 patients with locally advanced gastric cancer to receive two or three cycles of EFP (etoposide, fluorouracil, Platinol) followed by surgery versus surgery alone.[203,204] Of the 53 patients randomized to preoperative treatment, 47 (89%) were explored, and 37 (70%) had a com-

Table 44-11 Neoadjuvant Therapy for Gastric Cancer

Author	Patients	Regimen	Response Rate (%)	Explored (%)	Resected (%)	Pathologic CR (%)	Median Survival (mo)
UNRESECTABLE							
Wilke[200]	34	EAP	68	59	44	15	18
Verschueren[201]	17	5-FU/MTX	NS	76	41	NS	14
BORDERLINE RESECTABLE, LOCALLY ADVANCED							
Ducreux[202]	30	5-FU/CDDP	50	93	77	0	16
Kang[203,204]	53	EAP	NS	89	70	7	43
	54	Control	—	100	61	0	30
RESECTABLE							
Ajani[206]	25	EFP pre/postop	24	100	72	0	15
Ajani[207]	48	EAP pre/postop	31	85	77	0	15.5
Kelsen[208,209]	56	FAMTX preop, ip5-FU/CDDP, IV 5-FU postop	51	89	61	0	15.3
Crookes, Leichman[210,211]	59	5-FU, LV, CDDP preop; IP FUDR, CDDP postop	54	95	68	9	52
Songun[213]	27	FAMTX	30	100	56	7	13.1
	29	Control	—	100	62	—	12.8

EAP, etoposide, Adriamycin, cisplatin; 5-FU, 5-fluorouracil; MTX, methotrexate; EFP, etoposide, 5-FU, cisplatin; CDDP, cisplatin; FAMTX, 5-FU, Adriamycin, high-dose methotrexate; CF, citrovorum factor (leucovorin); IP, intraperitoneal; ci, continuous infusion; Med, median; mo, months; NS, not stated; preop, preoperative; postop, postoperative.

plete resection. A complete pathologic response rate of 7% was noted. More patients were able to undergo a curative resection in the treated group when compared with surgery alone (70% versus 61%). Median survival was 43 versus 30 months in favor of neoadjuvant treatment, but this did not achieve statistical significance ($p = .114$).

Potentially Resectable

Ajani and colleagues reported two phase II studies of preoperative chemotherapy (EFP, EAP) in patients thought clinically to have potentially resectable disease.[206,207] Patients were treated with two or three cycles of EFP/EAP preoperatively plus an additional two or three cycles postoperatively if a positive response to neoadjuvant treatment could be detected. No pathologic complete responses were seen with either EFP ($n = 25$ patients) or EAP ($n = 48$ patients) and median survival was 15 and 15.5 months, respectively. The impressive results obtained with neoadjuvant EAP in Wilke and coworkers' study could not be reproduced in this group of patients who had potentially smaller tumor burdens.

Other investigators have examined the utility of combining preoperative chemotherapy and postoperative treatment with intraperitoneal chemotherapy in view of the high peritoneal failure rate following resection of gastric cancer.[208-211] Schwartz and colleagues[208,209] delivered three cycles of neoadjuvant FAMTx (sequential 5-FU and high-dose methotrexate followed by doxorubicin [Adriamycin)]) plus postoperative intraperitoneal (IP) 5-FU and cisplatin along with infusional 5-FU. No complete pathologic responses were observed. Leichman and colleagues[210,211] delivered two cycles of 5-FU, leucovorin, and cisplatin preoperatively, and two cycles of IP 5-FUDR and cisplatin postoperatively. In the updated report of 59 potentially resectable patients, 96% underwent exploration and 68% had complete resection.[211] The pathologic CR was only 9%, but median survival was about 52 months.

One of the few randomized trials to assess the potential benefit of preoperative chemotherapy to surgery alone in potentially resectable patients failed to show any benefit.[213] In this Dutch study, patients were randomized to either FAMTx followed by surgery or surgery alone. The study was closed early due to poor accrual, but analysis of the enrolled patients showed no benefit to rate of curative resectability, rate of relapse, or median survival.

Summary

The high response rates achieved with neoadjuvant chemotherapy are of interest, and this form of treatment will undoubtedly be the subject of further investigation. The roles of neoadjuvant systemic treatment in increasing resectability rates and improving survival in localized gastric cancer are unknown. While resectability rates seem higher than the median rate of 40% from several studies, the patients in the neoadjuvant studies were highly selected. Except for the two trials in which tumors were unresectable on the basis of exploratory laparotomy, the successful resection in these reports may not have been influenced by neoadjuvant chemotherapy. In general, pathologic complete response rates are low (≤15%), and no proof exists that primary lesions are made more resectable by such treatment. The impact of preoperative systemic treatment on survival is even less clear. The one randomized trial that has been reported shows a nonsignificant improvement in survival for neoadjuvant chemotherapy in borderline resectable locally advanced disease.[203,204] Newer technologies such as EUS may identify patients who will do poorly with standard therapy alone and would be reasonable candidates for adjuvant studies.[217]

In view of the high incidence of local-regional relapse in several series of patients whose tumors were resected after neoadjuvant chemotherapy for initially unresectable lesions, irradiation should be incorporated into the study design of future trials for patients with high-risk factors. Patients with unresectable lesions who do not respond to neoadjuvant chemotherapy may still respond to preoperative EBRT plus chemotherapy. The study by Walsh and colleagues compared preoperative 5-FU, cisplatin plus radiotherapy followed by surgery ($n = 58$) versus surgery alone ($n = 55$) in patients with adenocarcinoma of the esophagus and gastric cardia.[170] Pathologic complete response was found in 13 of 52 patients (25%) who had surgery after preoperative chemoradiation, and both median and long-term survival was improved with the preoperative treatment ($p = .01$). The positive trial by Walsh and colleagues, and high pathologic complete response rates in similar pilot studies with gastric cancer[218] led to a U.S. GI Intergroup confirmatory trial of neoadjuvant combined modality therapy in carcinoma of the esophagus and gastroesophageal junction. This was stopped due to inadequate accrual.

Palliation for Metastatic Disease

This section is limited to discussion of patients with hematogenous or peritoneal metastasis at time of disease presentation.

Surgery

Surgical intervention in the patient with metastatic gastric cancer requires sound judgment. The underlying health and function (performance status) of the patient, the estimated duration of patient survival, and the nature of the symptoms must all be taken into account before deciding to proceed with an operation. Resection for palliation is generally better than bypass or intubation in appropriately selected patients, leading to better symptomatic relief and often longer survival.[188] Obstructing lesions may be resected with excellent palliation, but endoluminal stents, endoscopic laser treatments, or gastrostomy tube placement should be considered for poor operative candidates.[219] While significant hemorrhage from an ulcerating or necrotic polypoid tumor may be temporarily controlled by endoscopic techniques, stabilization and urgent surgical intervention should be undertaken when appropriate. A perforated gastric cancer usually presents as an emergency and may be unrecognized preoperatively. Aggressive treatment with gastric resection should be carried out in the fit patient; pain control and hydration alone are preferable for the moribund or unfit patient.

Laser or Irradiation

If palliative resection is not indicated in symptomatic patients with metastases, laser treatment, stent placement, or a shortened course of EBRT with or without 5-FU could be used (37.5 Gy in 15 fractions over 3 weeks), to be followed by systemic treatment. Patients who have proximal lesions with esophageal obstruction may be candidates for laser or esophageal stents instead of irradiation. If either method is successful in overcoming obstruction, patients could proceed directly to treatment with chemotherapy.

Chemotherapy

Traditional chemotherapy agents with 20% or more response rates include doxorubicin,[220,221] cisplatin,[222] 5-FU,[223] etoposide,[224] and mitomycin C.[225] More recently a variety of chemotherapy drugs have shown promising response rates in advanced gastric cancer including taxotere (23%), irinotecan (23%), and paclitaxel (17% to 21%).[226-228] Complete remissions with single agent chemotherapy are exceedingly rare, and remission duration is usually 3 to 5 months. For patients with measurable disease, survival is usually only 3 to 6 months. Single-agent chemotherapy therefore offers little practical benefit to the patient.

Combination chemotherapy regimens, which almost universally incorporate a fluorinated pyrimidine, obtain reliable responses in 25% to 50% of patients. Combination chemotherapy regimens that have produced response rates of 30% to 45% include the following: the FAM regimen[225]; 5-FU + BCNU[229]; 5-FU + MeCCNU[230]; 5-FU + mitomycin C[221]; 5-FU + doxorubicin + MeCCNU (FAMe)[220,230]; 5-FU + doxorubicin + BCNU (FAB)[231]; 5-FU + doxorubicin + cisplatin (FAP)[232-234]; EAP[235]; FAMTx[234,236]; and etoposide, leucovorin, and 5-FU (ELF).[237] Most of the combination chemotherapy regimens report median survival of 5 to 7 months, which is similar to the survival of patients receiving single-agent chemotherapy. Many of the combinations that had promising activity in single institution evaluations were less active and more toxic in subsequent phase II and III trials.

Several trials have compared single-agent 5-FU with combination chemotherapy in advanced gastric cancer and have been unable to demonstrate improved survival for multiagent regimens. The NCCTG reported a prospective randomized phase III trial comparing 5-FU versus 5-FU + doxorubicin versus FAM. Overall responses were quite similar, and no differences were seen in survival.[238] A large Korean study randomized 324 patients to 5-FU, 5-FU plus cisplatin, or FAM. Responses were observed more often in the patients treated with 5-FU plus cisplatin, but overall survival was similar in all three treatment arms.[239] Others have reported similar problems in demonstrating improved survival for multiagent regimens in phase III trials.[240-241] Several trials have also used pharmacologic manipulation of 5-FU with leucovorin in gastric carcinoma in attempts to follow up on the apparent benefit that this combination achieved with colorectal carcinoma patients.[242] Responses varied between 11% and 50%, but median survival rates were almost identical to those of 5-FU alone at 5.5 months.

Many of the combination chemotherapy regimens, which achieved response rates of 30% to 50% in single-institution trials, have often failed to reproduce the initially high response rates when subjected to confirmatory trials. A case in point is the *EAP regimen*. The initial phase II trial reported overall response rates of 64% (complete and partial) and 21% (complete) and median survival of 9 months.[215] The studies that followed did not confirm such high response rates, and toxicity was sometimes substantial.[243]

The combination of 5-FU, doxorubicin, and methotrexate (FAMTx) was a widely used regimen in the 1990's. Klein first reported a 58% response rate for the combination in a phase II study.[244] The EORTC group performed a randomized phase II trial of FAM versus FAMTx in 213 patients with advanced measurable or nonmeasurable gastric cancer.[235] FAMTx was found to have a significantly superior response rate (41% versus 9%; $p < .0001$) and survival (median 42 versus 29 weeks; $p = .004$). The authors considered FAMTx the reference chemotherapy for future advanced gastric trials.

Kelsen and colleagues[236] randomly compared FAMTx and EAP for advanced disease in 60 patients. Response rates were similar, at 33% versus 20% (advantage to FAMTx; $p = .24$), and tolerance was better for FAMTx with a significantly higher toxic death rate for EAP. Accordingly, the trial was stopped.

In 1991, the combination of etoposide, leucovorin, and 5-FU (ELF) was introduced as an alternative to more aggressive regimens for patients with cardiac or poor medical conditions or advanced age.[245] It achieved a response rate of 53%, and a median survival time of 11 months. Multiple clinical trials have now evaluated the activity and tolerability of ELF, and have generally shown overall survival in the range of 8 to 10 months and response rates of about 30%.[246-248]

FAMTx has been compared to ELF and infusional 5-FU/cisplatin (FUP) in a phase III EORTC study. No apparent differences in response rates or survival have been demonstrated to date.[249]

A regimen combining epirubicin, cisplatin, and infusional 5-FU (ECF) was introduced by the Royal Marsden Hospital for patients with advanced esophagogastric adenocarcinoma. An overall response rate of 71% was obtained with a complete response rate of 12%.[250] A subsequent randomized phase III trial, which compared FAMTx with ECF, showed that ECF was associated with a superior response rate (45% versus 21%) and overall survival (median 9 versus 6 months).[251] In view of the promising results of this trial, ECF has become the standard regimen to which other regimens are compared.

The Italian Group for the Study of Digestive Tract Cancer reported an intensive, multiagent regimen including the most active agents in gastric cancer, cisplatin, epirubicin, leucovorin and 5-FU (PELF).[252] Administered weekly with growth factor support, this regimen produced an overall response rate of 62%, complete response rate of 17%, and a median survival time of 11 months. Investigators plan to test this regimen further in controlled studies.

Several recent phase II studies have evaluated non–5-FU–containing combinations. The response to combinations such as docetaxel and cisplatin, paclitaxel and cisplatin, and irinotecan and mitomycin C have been comparable to 5-FU–containing regimens.[253-255]

Supportive Care Versus Chemotherapy

In 1993 Murad and associates published results of a randomized trial where a modified FAMTx regimen was compared to best supportive care.[256] The trial was interrupted after entry of 22 patients, as the treated patients were enjoying a significantly better outcome. The next 18 patients were assigned directly to treatment. Median survival for all the treated patients was 10 months versus 3 months for the untreated controls ($p = .001$).

Pyrhonen and coworkers reported the results of 41 patients randomized to 5-FU, epirubicin, and methotrexate (FEMTx) plus vitamins A and E versus the same vitamins and best supportive care.[257] In FEMTx patients, 29% had an objective response and 33% had stable disease for greater than 2 months. In control patients, 20% had stable disease. Median time to progression (5.4 versus 1.7 months, $p = .0013$) and median survival (12.3 versus 3.1 months, $p = .0006$) both favored treatment with FEMTx.

Glimelius and colleagues recently studied, in a group of 61 patients with inoperable gastric cancer, the cost effectiveness of palliative therapy by randomly assigning patients to primary chemotherapy with ELF or 5-FU leucovorin versus best supportive care.[258] Improved or prolonged high quality of life was documented in patients receiving chemotherapy versus supportive care alone. Chemotherapy patients had a significantly longer median survival at 8 months versus 5 months ($p = .003$, adjusted) and QOL ($p < .05$) also favored the treated patients.

Park and colleagues performed a retrospective analysis of 409 patients with incurable gastric cancer in which 202 patients were treated with a modified FAM regimen and 207 were not treated.[259] The 1-year survival was 34.1% for patients treated with FAM versus 22.5% for the control group. Details on how treatment decisions were made were not in the report.

SUMMARY

The response rate of gastric cancers to combination chemotherapy is somewhat higher than other gastrointestinal malignancies. Patients who respond to therapy with acceptable tolerance have the potential of achieving symptomatic benefit from this palliative treatment. Nevertheless, aggressive combination regimens are costly, toxicity is sometimes formidable, and remissions are of short duration. If possible, all patients with disseminated gastric cancers should be considered for entrance into well-designed clinical trials.

IRRADIATION TECHNIQUE/TOLERANCE

The irradiation field should include unresected or residual tumor or the tumor bed plus major nodal regions (lesser and greater curvature; celiac axis including pancreaticoduodenal; suprapancreatic, splenic, and porta hepatis; paraesophageal with proximal lesions). The pattern of tumor bed and nodal failures in the reoperative series from the University of Minnesota is demonstrated in Figure 44-4A. This represents an idealized, shaped irradiation field that incorporates the areas of local-regional relapse.[28] For individual patients, this idealized field needs to be modified depending on the surgical or pathologic extent of disease (primary site, TN extent of disease) and the adjacency of tolerance organs or structures.[169,260,261] The tumor bed and nodal volumes are reconstructed with the aid of preoperative and postoperative imaging studies and surgical clip placement. In Figure 44-4B the idealized field is superimposed on the organs and structures that define irradiation tolerance.

Dose-limiting organs and structures in the upper abdomen are numerous (stomach, small intestine, liver, kidneys, and spinal cord). With properly shaped fields, doses of 45 to 50.4 Gy in 1.8- to 2.0-Gy fractions can be delivered to the stomach and small intestine with a 5% or less risk of severe toxicity.[260] In most patients a portion of both kidneys will be within the anteroposterior (AP:PA) treatment fields, but at least two thirds or three fourths of one kidney should be excluded (can include entirety of both kidneys to a dose of 20 Gy if necessary). For patients with GE junction, or proximal to mid gastric cancers (Figs. 44-8 to 44-12), one half to two thirds of the left kidney can often be spared as a result of accurate field definition, which is aided by pre- and postoperative imaging studies and surgical clip placement. The pancreatic-duodenal nodes can be included, if indicated, while sparing 75% to 90% of the right kidney. However, for distal gastric lesions with narrow or positive duodenal resection margins, the duodenal circumference may need to be included as target volume (Fig. 44-13). In such instances 50% or more of the right kidney is within the field, and two thirds to three fourths of the left kidney should be spared. Chronic renal problems are infrequent when these techniques are utilized.[262]

With preoperative or primary chemoradiation for GE junction or proximal gastric lesions, a 3- to 5-cm margin of distal esophagus should be within the irradiation field (see Fig. 44-9). If the lesion extends beyond the gastric wall with proximal lesions, a major portion of the left hemidiaphragm should be included. In either instance, Cerrobend blocks or multi-leaf collimators (MLC) should be used to decrease the volume of irradiated heart and other normal structures (see Fig. 44-9). Since doxorubicin (Adriamycin) may be a component of multidrug chemotherapy regimens, cardiac exclusion is important, when technically feasible. With postoperative irradiation of GE junction cancers (see Figs. 44-10 and 44-11), the irradiation field may include the anastomotic site and some or all of the remaining stomach. Postoperative fields will usually be larger than preoperative fields (see Fig. 44-9 versus Fig. 44-10) unless an involved field approach is chosen for select T3N0 patients (see Fig. 44-11). With unresectable *primary or locally recurrent* lesions at the level of the GE junction, moderate lateral extension on a preoperative CT is an indication for use of lateral or obliqued fields to decrease the volume of heart within the radiation field.

More routine use of multiple field techniques should be considered, when preoperative imaging exists to allow accurate reconstruction of target volumes (see Figs. 44-8 to 44-13). Single institution data suggest that multiple field arrangements may produce less toxicity.[166] When patients are treated preoperatively, paired lateral fields are combined with AP-PA fields to achieve improved dose homogeneity (see Fig. 44-9). Depending on the posterior extent of the gastric fundus, either obliqued or lateral fields can be used to deliver a 10 to 20 Gy component of radiation to spare spinal cord and kidney. Liver and kidney tolerance limits the use of lateral fields to 20 Gy or less for patients with gastric cancer; for patients with GE junction cancers, the contribution from lateral fields would preferably be limited to 10-15 Gy due to lung tolerance issues. With the wide availability of 3D conformal treatment-planning systems, it may be possible to target more accurately the high-risk volume and to use unconventional field arrangements and/or IMRT (intensity-modulated radiation therapy) to produce superior dose distributions. To accomplish this without marginal misses it will be necessary to both carefully define and encompass the various target volumes since target volumes that would be included in AP/PA fields may be missed with other field arrangements (oblique, lateral, non-coplanar).

In individual patients the idealized field needs to be modified depending on the surgical/pathologic extent of disease and site of the primary tumor.[260] The relative risk of nodal metastases at a specific nodal location is dependent on both the site of origin of the primary tumor and other factors including width and depth of invasion of the gastric wall. Tumors that originate in the proximal portion of the stomach and the GE junction have a higher propensity to spread to nodes in the mediastinum and pericardial region but a lower likelihood of involvement of nodes in the region of the gastric antrum, periduodenal area, and porta hepatis. Tumors that originate in the body of the stomach can spread to all nodal sites, but have the highest likelihood of spreading to nodes along the greater and lesser curvature, near the location of the primary tumor mass. Tumors that originate in the distal stomach have a high likelihood of spread to the periduodenal, peripancreatic, and porta hepatis nodes but a lower likelihood of spread to nodes near the cardia of the stomach, the periesophageal and mediastinal nodes, or splenic hilar nodes.[260] Any tumor originating in the stomach has a high propensity to spread to nodes along the greater and lesser curvature, although they are most likely to spread to those sites in close anatomic proximity to the primary tumor mass.

Guidelines for defining the clinical target volume for postoperative radiation fields have been developed by Tepper and Gunderson based on location and extent of the primary tumor (T-stage) and location and extent of known nodal involvement (N stage).[260] Table 44-12 presents general guidelines on the impact of T and N stages on inclusion of the remaining stomach (gastric remnant), tumor bed, and nodal sites, while

Continued

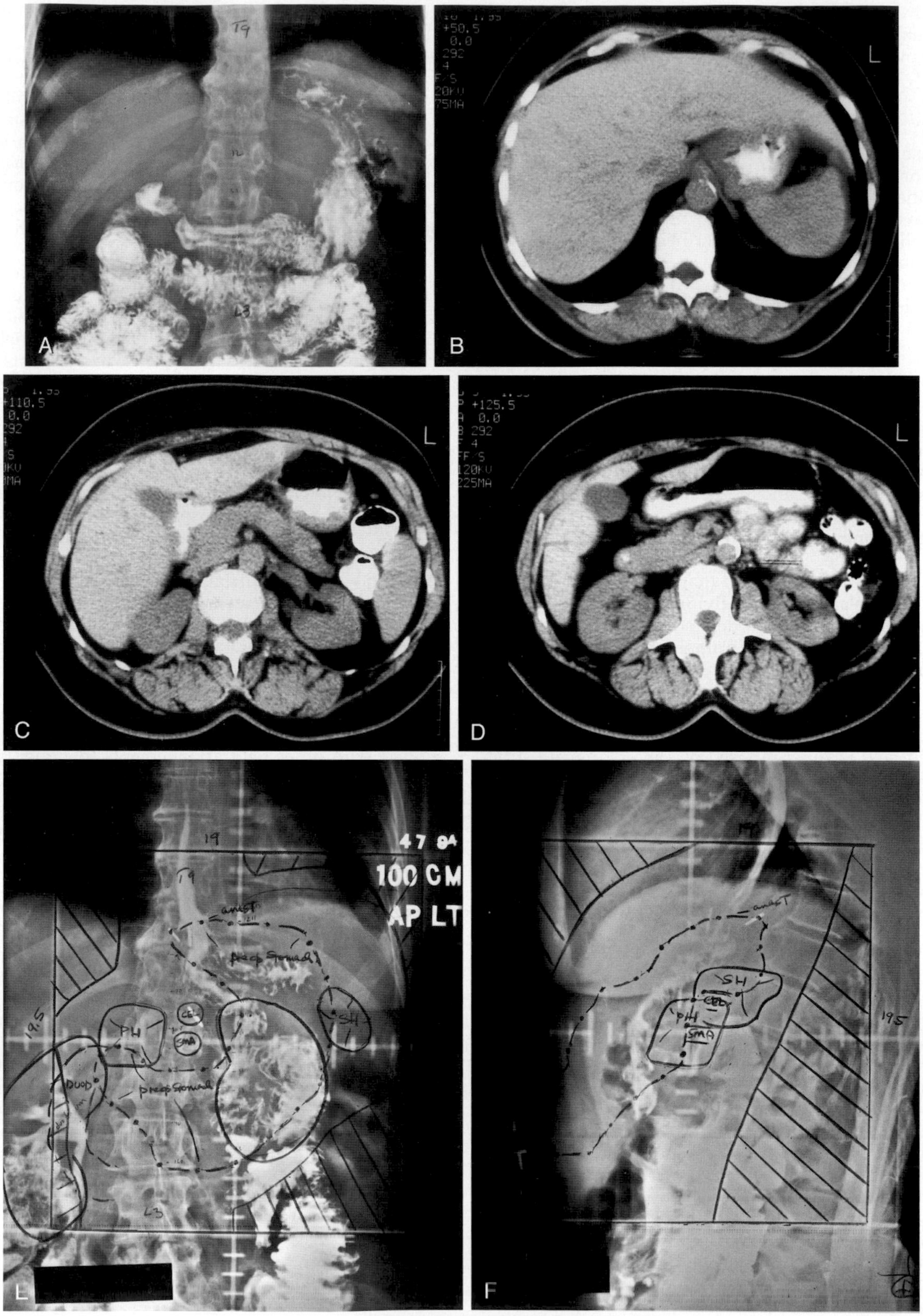

Figure 44-8 Postoperative radiation fields based on preoperative radiographs following complete resection of a proximal gastric cancer (T3, N2, M0); the patient was randomized to the irradiation plus chemotherapy arm on the U.S. GI Intergroup 0116 gastric adjuvant study. Tumor bed and target volumes were reconstructed using the preoperative upper GI (**A**) and CT (**B-D**). CT cuts demonstrated thickened gastric wall proximally (**B** and **C**) and normal thickness distally (**D**) as well as relationship of the stomach to surrounding organs including liver and spleen (**B**), liver, body and tail of pancreas, and splenic flexure (**C**), and head of pancreas (**D**). Anteroposterior-posteroanterior (AP-PA) irradiation field (**E**) with crosshatched blocks encompasses all of the left kidney but less than 20% of the right. Nodal groups at risk and preoperative gastric duodenal locations (- • - •) are demonstrated on the AP-PA and lateral (**F**) simulation fields. CEL, celiac; PH, porta hepatis; SH, splenic hilum; SMA, superior mesenteric artery. (From Gunderson LL, Donohue JH, Burch FA: Stomach. *In* Abeloff MD, Lichter AS [eds]: Clinical Oncology, 2nd ed. Philadelphia, Churchill Livingstone, 1999.)

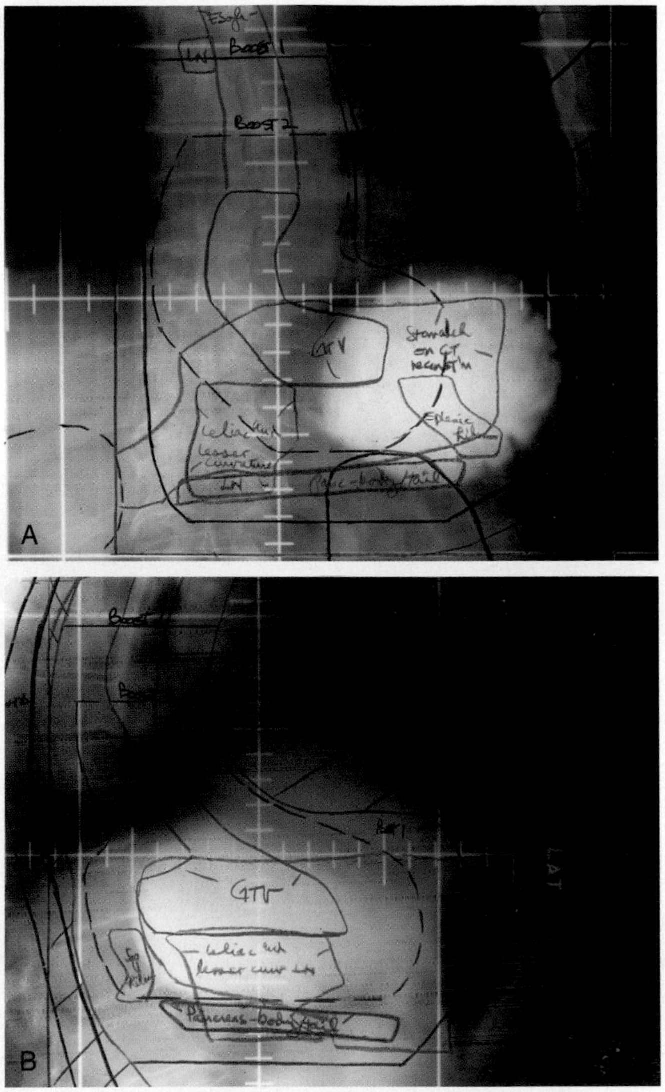

Figure 44-9 Patient is a 73-year-old male with T3N0 ACA of the gastroesophageal (GE) junction (see Table 44-13) who preferred primary chemoradiation treatment with surgery reserved for salvage, as indicated. Baseline PET scan and CT chest were negative for nodal or blood-borne metastases. Radiation fields were generated using treatment planning CT images and beam's eye reconstruction. The patient was treated with a four-field technique of AP/PA(**A**) and paired lateral fields (**B**). The initial fields included a ≥5 cm margin of uninvolved esophagus superiorly, ~ 5 cm margin of stomach in all directions and nodal groups including celiac artery and lesser curvature nodes, suprapancreatic (body/tail of pancreas) and splenic hilum. The patient received external beam irradiation (EBRT) plus one cycle of concurrent carboplatin/taxol and infusion 5-fluorouracil (5-FU) during the first week of EBRT, but did not receive further concurrent chemotherapy in view of intolerance. The extended fields received 39.6 Gy in 22 fractions (Fx) of 1.8 Gy; boost 1 received an additional 4.5 Gy in 3 Fx (total 45 Gy/25 Fx) and boost 2 received an additional 9 Gy in 5 Fx for a total dose of 54 Gy/30 Fx/6 weeks completing 28Oct04. There was no evidence of relapse on the basis of history, physical exam, imaging (CT chest/abdomen; PET scan) or endoscopy at the time of ongoing evaluation in Dec 2005.

Table 44-12 General Guidelines of Impact of T and N Stage on Inclusion of Remaining Stomach, Tumor Bed, and Nodal Sites within Radiation Fields

TN Stage	Remaining Stomach†	Tumor Bed	Nodes
T1-2 N0 (not into subserosa)	No	No	No
T2 N0 (into subserosa)*	Variable	Yes	No
T3 N0	Variable	Yes	No
T4 N0	Variable	Yes	Variable
T1-2 N+	Yes	No	Yes
T3-4 N+	Yes	Yes	Yes

*Posterior wall T2 N0 lesions that extend beyond muscularis propria in the proximal or distal stomach are at risk for local relapse. Patients with T1-2 N0 disease with close or positive surgical margins should be considered for treatment to the tumor bed.

†Inclusion of the remaining stomach is preferable in most patients if 2/3 of one kidney can be excluded. This is dependent on the extent of surgical resection and uninvolved margins (in cm).

Modified from Tepper JE, Gunderson LL: Radiation treatment parameters in the adjuvant postoperative therapy of gastric cancer. Semin Rad Oncol 12:187-195, 2002.

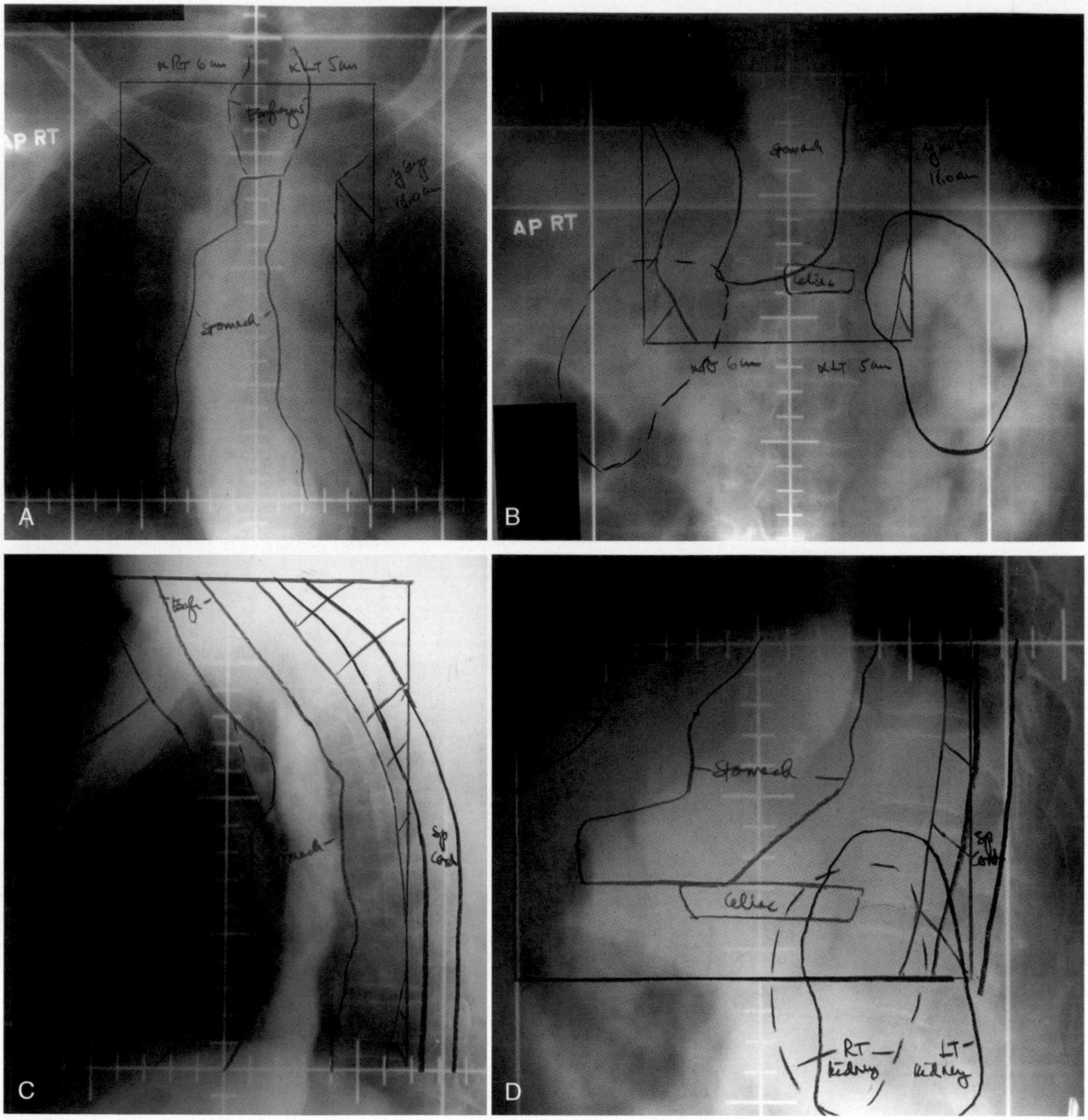

Figure 44-10 Radiation fields in a patient with a T2N1 adenocarcinoma (ACA) of the GE junction who had a transhiatal esophagectomy with cervical esophagogastrostomy (see table 44-13). Postoperative chemoradiation was recommended, and the patient was placed on the current phase III U.S. GI Intergroup trial. At the time of simulation, oral contrast medium was used to define the EG anastomosis at the thoracic inlet (**A** and **C**), the residual stomach within the mediastinum, and the duodenal sweep inferiorly (**B** and **D**). A combined treatment planning/diagnostic CT was obtained to define the celiac artery and dose-limiting structures including heart, lungs, spinal cord, kidneys, and liver. Irradiation fields were defined to include the distal cervical esophagus and supraclavicular nodes superiorly, the remaining stomach and perigastric nodes and nodal groups in the mediastinum and celiac axis (**A-D**). Lateral simulation films (**C** and **D**) demonstrate the ability to spare heart and spinal cord with appropriate use of blocks *(crosshatched blocks)*. The patient received 45 Gy/25Fx plus concurrent PVI 5-FU (200 $mg/m^2/24$ hours) in addition to systemic multidrug chemotherapy before and after concurrent chemoradiation.

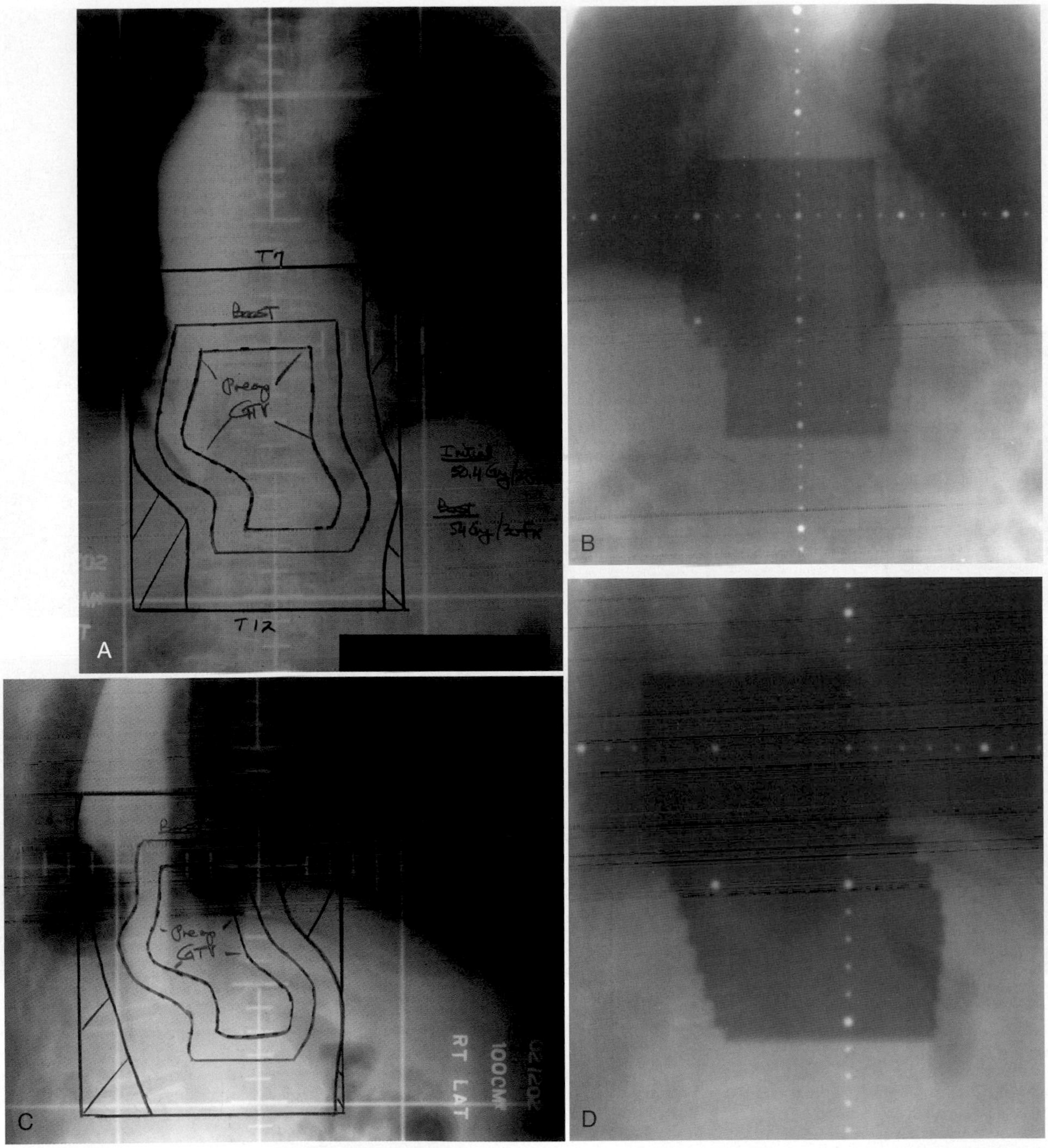

Figure 44-11 Radiation and port films on a 65-year-old patient with Ivor Lewis esophagogastrectomy (transthoracic plus abdominal approach) for a T3N0 ACA of the GE junction (see table 44-13). Postoperative chemoradiation, as per INT 0116 was recommended. Simulation films (**A, C**) were obtained with contrast in the remaining stomach, and a treatment planning CT was obtained for purpose of reconstructing tumor bed volumes. The patient was concerned about treatment-related morbidity, so the decision was made to treat with a more involved treatment field approach in view of pathologic findings of 12 negative nodes and adequate proximal and distal resection margins (~ 5cm). The involved fields included the tumor bed (preop GTV), as generated from preop CT imaging, but excluded the remaining stomach and nodal sites to decrease normal tissue morbidity. The initial AP-PA fields (**A, B**) included tumor bed with 3-cm supero inferior and 2-cm lateral margin to block edge (CTV/PTV). Lateral fields (**C, D**) were generated with an anterior margin of 2 cm to block edge and demonstrate sparing of heart and spinal cord. Initial fields were treated to 45 Gy/25 Fx; boost fields (**A, C**) received an additional 9 Gy/5Fx to GTV plus 1-cm margin to block edge (total 54Gy/30Fx completing April 22, 2002). The patient received 5-FU plus leucovorin before, during, and after EBRT as per INT 0116. He was NED and without symptoms at his 4-year post-treatment evaluation.

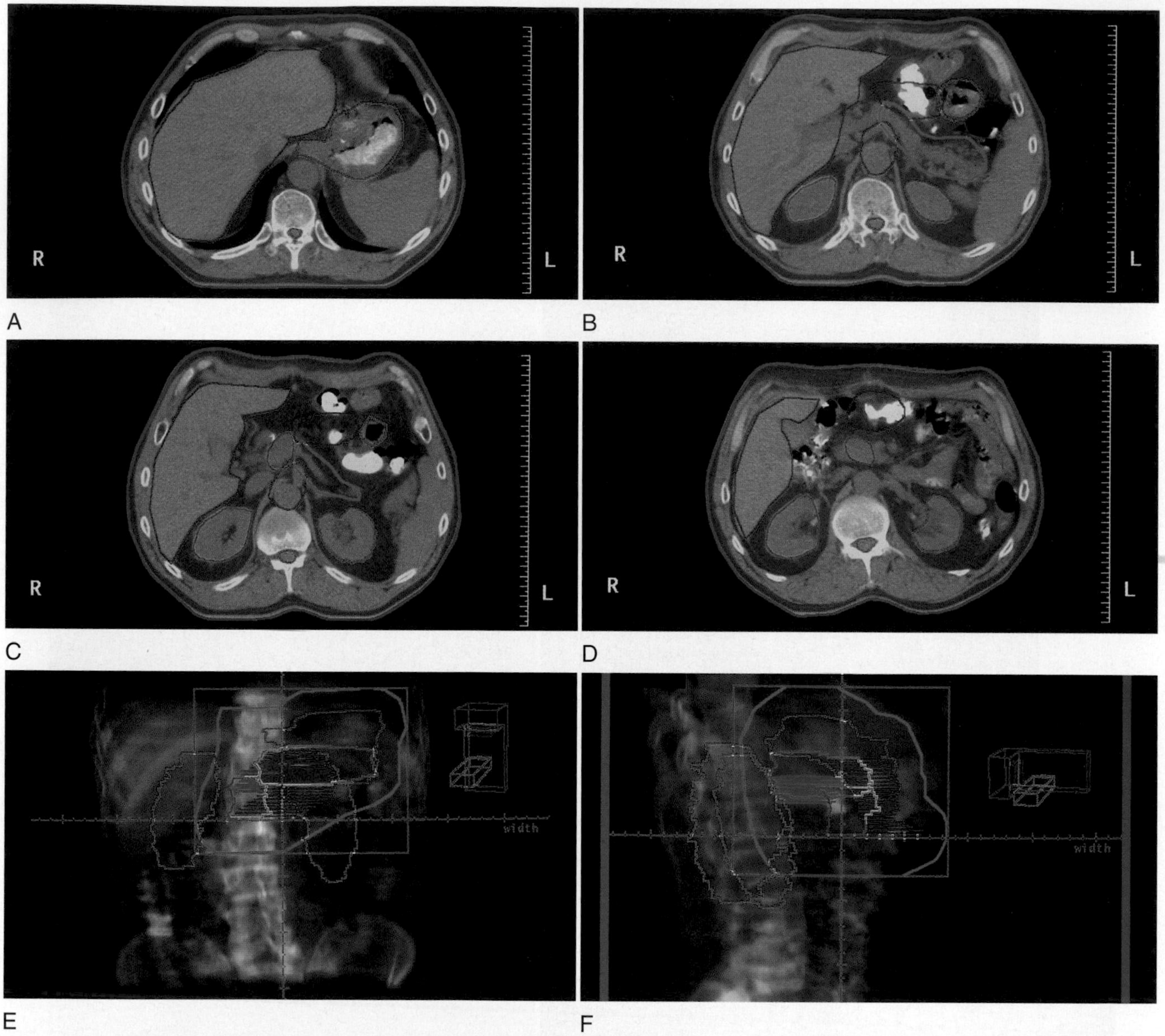

Figure 44-12 Optimized postoperative radiation fields for patient with T4N0 ACA of the posterior wall of the body of the stomach (middle third—see Table 44-14). CT simulation was performed and structures of interest were delineated based on pre- and postoperative CT imaging and operative/pathologic findings (**A-D**; tumor bed; gastric remnant; tolerance organs/structures—kidneys, liver, spinal cord). **A,** Gastric remnant and distal esophagus (yellow-green) are adjacent to liver (red-orange) and spleen. **B,** CT image demonstrates tumor bed (red), body/tail of pancreas (blue), celiac artery (orange), and kidneys (right—light blue; left—green). **C,** Head of pancreas (blue-green) and splenic artery/body of pancreas are shown at level of mid-kidney. **D,** Tumor bed and head of pancreas on more distal CT image.
Radiation fields were designed with the aid of digitally reconstructed radiographs (DRR, **E-F**) and a dose-volume histogram (DVH) was performed with regard to tolerance organs/structures (**G**). A four-field technique of AP/PA and paired lateral fields was selected (field margins in medium blue). The fields included the gastric remnant (yellow-orange), tumor bed (red), and nodal regions at risk based on sites of adherence of the primary lesion (celiac [blue-purple cross-hatched), suprapancreatic [body of pancreas—light blue], superior mesenteric, pancreatico-duodenal [head of pancreas, blue-green]). **E,** The AP/PA field includes ~ 2/3 of the left kidney and a portion of the left lobe of the liver but excludes most of the right kidney and the right lobe of the liver. **F,** The lateral field demonstrates exclusion of the spinal cord and posterior kidneys.

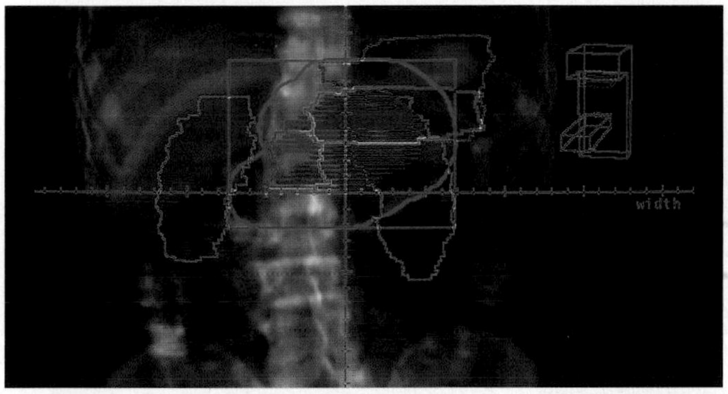

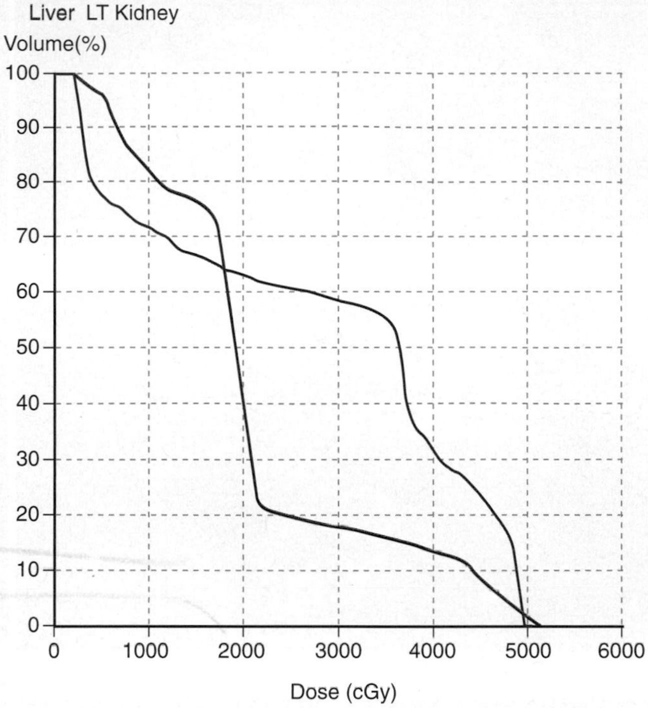

G

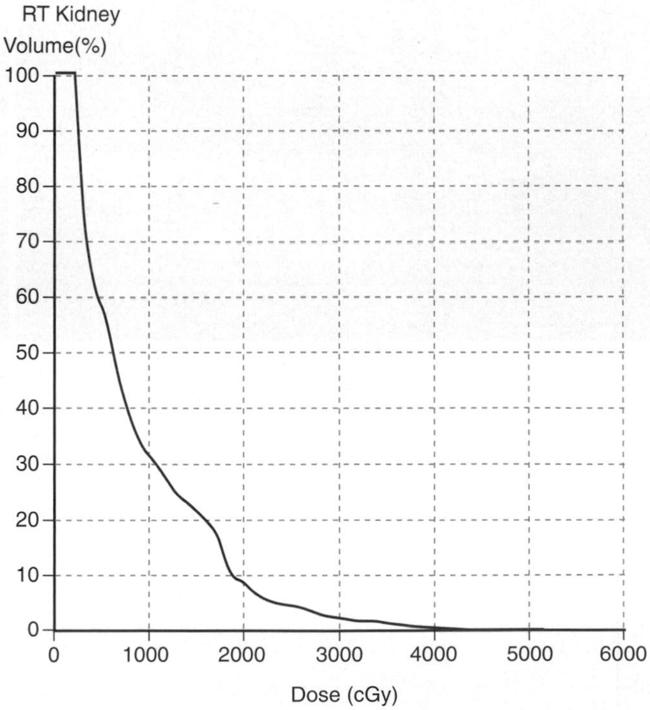

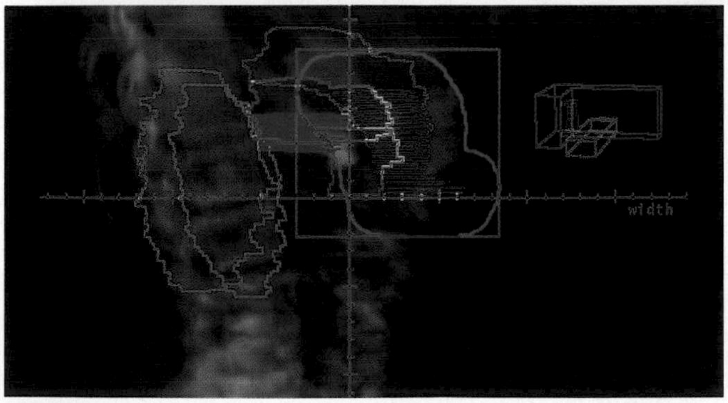

H

I

FIGURE 44-12—Cont'd **G, H**, AP/PA (**G**) and lateral (**H**) boost fields, **I**, DVH demonstrates a dose of 20 Gy to >60% of the left kidney versus less than 10% of the right kidney.

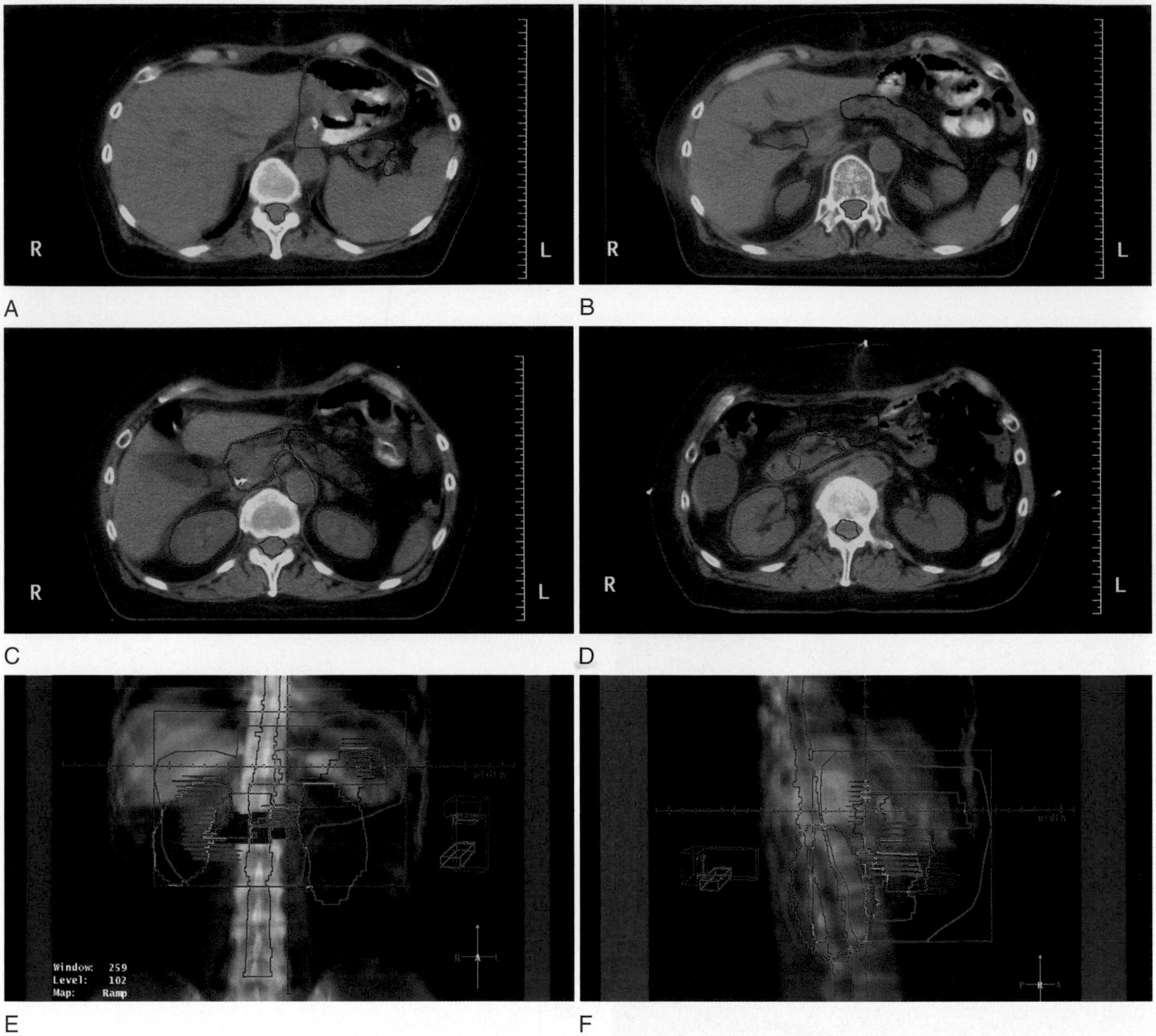

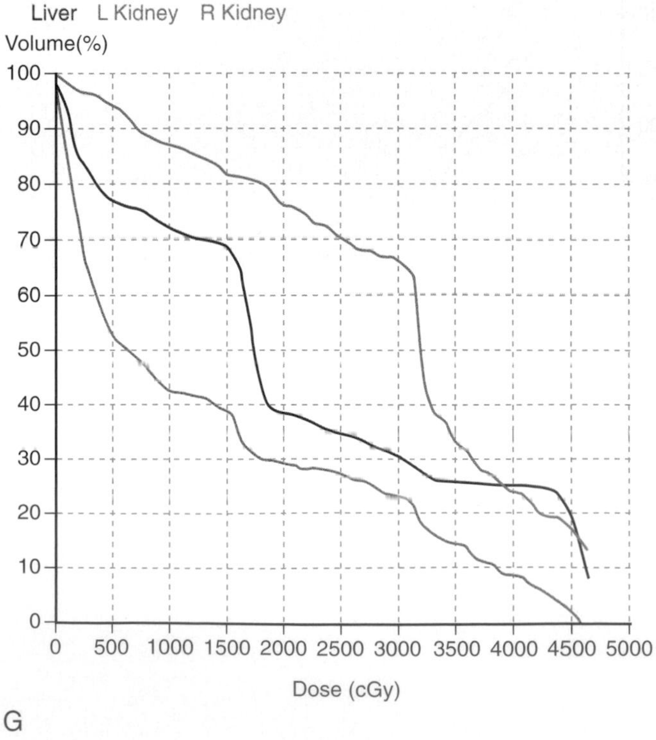

Figure 44-13 Optimized postoperative radiation fields for patient with T3N2 antral primary (distal third, see table 44-16). Structures of interest were delineated at time of CT simulation **(A–D)**. **A,** Gastric remnant (lavender) is demonstrated along with the body/tail of pancreas (red-orange), and splenic hilum (light green). **B,** Porta hepatis (blue-purple) and kidneys (left—yellow green, right—yellow orange) are delineated. **C,** Head of pancreas (yellow) and celiac versus superior mesenteric artery (light blue) are shown. **D,** Antral tumor bed (red) and duodenum (medium blue) are delineated. Irradiation fields were designed with the aid of DRR (**E,F**) and a dose volume histogram (DVH—**G**) was performed with regard to dose-limiting structures (liver, kidneys, spinal cord). A four-field technique of AP/PA and paired lateral fields was chosen (field margins shown in medium blue). Treatment fields include the gastric remnant, tumor bed, head of pancreas, first and second part of the duodenum (medium blue cross hatched), pertinent nodal volumes (perigastric, pancreaticoduodenal [head of pancreas], porta [blue blue-purple cross hatched], celiac, suprapancreatic [body/tail pancreas]) and the optional nodal volume of splenic hilum (light green cross hatched). **E,** AP/PA field (field margins exclude ~ 2/3 of the left kidney and include ~ 90% of the right kidney). Exclusion of optional splenic hilar nodes would not have allowed additional sparing of the left kidney in view of the adjacency of the gastric remnant and splenic hilum. **F,** Lateral field demonstrates exclusion of the spinal cord (turquoise) and substantial portions of both kidneys. **G,** The DVH, combining doses from all four fields, demonstrated that the dose volume of 20 Gy included ~ 30% of the left kidney versus ~ 75% of the right kidney. With regard to the liver, ~ 30% receives a dose of 30 Gy and ~25% receives a dose of 35 to 40 Gy.

Tables 44-13 to 44-16 present treatment guidelines based on TN stage for each of the four primary sites (GE junction, proximal, mid and distal stomach). In general, for patients with node-positive disease, there should be wide coverage of tumor bed, remaining stomach, resection margins, and nodal drainage regions. For node-negative disease, if there is a good surgical resection with pathologic evaluation of at least 10 to 15 nodes, and there are wide surgical margins on the primary tumor (at least 5 cm), treatment of the nodal beds is optional. Treatment of the remaining stomach should depend on a balance of the likely normal tissue morbidity and the perceived risk of local relapse in the residual stomach (see Fig. 44-11 versus Figs. 44-8, 44-9, 44-10, 44-12, and 44-13).

Nutritional Support (before, during, and after Chemoradiation)

Patients who have surgical resection for gastric cancer can have significant management problems. Postoperatively, especially after removal of more than three fourths of the stomach,

Table 44-13 Impact of Site of Primary Lesion and TN Stage on Irradiation Treatment Volumes: EG Junction (General Guidelines)

Site of Primary and TN Stage	Remaining Stomach‡	Tumor Bed Volumes‡	Nodal Volumes
EG junction*	If allows exclusion of 2/3 right kidney	T stage dependent	N stage dependent
T2 N0, invasion of subserosa	Variable, dependent on surgical pathologic findings†	Medial left hemidiaphragm; adjacent body of pancreas	None or perigastric, periesophageal§
T3 N0	Variable, dependent on surgical pathologic findings†	Medial left hemidiaphragm; adjacent body of pancreas	None or perigastric, periesophageal, mediast, celiac§
T4 N0	Preferable, dependent on surgical pathologic findings†	As for T3 N0 plus site(s) of adherence with 3-5 cm margin	Nodes related to site of adherence, ± perigastric, periesophageal, mediast, celiac
T1-2 N+	Preferable	Not indicated for T1, as above for T2 into subserosa	Periesophageal, mediast, prox perigastric, celiac
T3-4 N+	Preferable	As for T3 N0, T4 N0	As for T1-2 N+ and T4 N0

*Tolerance organs or structures: heart, lung, spinal cord, kidneys, liver.

†For tumors with wide (>5 cm) surgical margins confirmed pathologically, treatment of residual stomach is optional, especially if this would result in substantial increase in normal tissue morbidity.

‡Use preop imaging (CT, barium swallow), surgical clips, and postop imaging (CT, barium swallow).

§Optional node inclusion for T2-3 N0 lesions if adequate surgical node dissection (D2 dissection) and at least 10-15 nodes examined pathologically.

Modified from Tepper JE, Gunderson LL: Radiation treatment parameters in the adjuvant postoperative therapy of gastric cancer. Semin Rad Oncol 12:187-195, 2002.

Table 44-14 Impact of Site of Primary Lesion and TN Stage on Irradiation Treatment Volumes: Cardia/Proximal Third of Stomach (General Guidelines)

Site of Primary and TN Stage	Remaining Stomach†	Tumor Bed Volumes‡	Nodal Volumes
Cardia/prox third of stomach*	Preferred, but spare 2/3 of one kidney (usually right)	T stage dependent	N stage dependent
T2 N0, invasion of subserosa	Variable dependent on surg-path findings†	Medial left hemidiaphragm, adjacent body of pancreas (± tail)	None or perigastric§
T3 N0	Variable dependent on surgical pathologic findings†	Medial left hemidiaphragm, adjacent body of pancreas (± tail)	None or perigastric; optional: periesophageal, mediastinal, celiac§
T4 N0	Variable dependent on surgical pathologic findings†	As for T3 N0 plus site(s) of adherence with 3-5 cm margin	Nodes related to site of adherence, ± perigastric, periesophageal mediastinal, celiac
T1-2 N+	Preferable	Not indicated for T1, as above for T2 into subserosa	Perigastric, celiac, splenic, suprapancreatic, ± periesophageal, mediastinal, pancreaticoduodenal, porta hepatis¶
T3-4 N+	Preferable	As for T3 N0, T4 N0	As for T1-2 N+ and T4 N0

*Tolerance organs or structures: kidneys, spinal cord, liver, heart, lung.

†For tumors with wide (>5 cm) surgical margins confirmed pathologically, treatment of residual stomach is not necessary, especially if this would result in substantial increase in normal tissue morbidity.

‡Use preop imaging (CT, barium swallow), surgical clips, and postop imaging (CT, barium swallow).

§Optional node inclusion for T2-3 N0 lesions if adequate surgical node dissection (D2 dissection) and at least 10-15 nodes are examined pathologically.

¶Pancreaticoduodenal and porta hepatis nodes are at low risk if nodal positivity is minimal (i.e., 1-2 positive nodes with 10-15 nodes examined), and this region does not need to be irradiated. Periesophageal and mediastinal nodes are at risk if there is esophageal extension.

Modified from Tepper JE, Gunderson LL: Radiation treatment parameters in the adjuvant postoperative therapy of gastric cancer. Semin Rad Oncol 12:187-195, 2002.

Table 44-15 Impact of Site of Primary Lesion and TN Stage on Irradiation Treatment Volumes: Body/Middle Third of Stomach (General Guidelines)

Site of Primary and TN Stage	Remaining Stomach	Tumor Bed Volumes†	Nodal Volumes
Body/mid third of stomach*	Yes, but spare 2/3 of one kidney	T stage dependent	N stage dependent, spare 2/3 of one kidney
T2 N0, invasion of subserosa	Yes	Body of pancreas (± tail)	None or perigastric. Optional: celiac, splenic, suprapancreatic, pancreaticduodenal, porta hepatis‡
T3 N0	Yes	Body of pancreas (± tail)	None or perigastric; Optional: celiac, splenic, suprapancreatic, pancreatricduodenal, porta hepatis‡
T4 N0	Yes	As for T3 N0 plus site(s) of adherence with 3-5 cm margin	Nodes related to site of adherence ± perigastric, celiac, splenic, suprapancreatic, pancreaticduodenal, porta hepatis
T1-2 N+	Yes	Not indicated for T1	Pergastric, celiac, splenic, suprapancreatic, pancreaticduodenal, porta hepatis
T3-4 N+	Yes	As for T3 N0, T4 N0	As for T1-2 N+ and T4 N0

*Tolerance organs or structures: kidneys, spinal cord, liver.
†Use pre-op imaging (CT, barium swallow), surgical clips, and post-op imaging (CT, barium swallow).
‡Optional node inclusion for T2-3 N0 lesions if adequate surgical node dissection (D2 dissection) and at least 10-15 nodes examined pathologically.
Modified from Tepper JE, Gunderson LL: Radiation treatment parameters in the adjuvant postoperative therapy of gastric cancer. Semin Rad Oncol 12:187-195, 2002.

Table 44-16 Impact of Site of Primary Gastric Lesion and TN Stage on Irradiation Treatment Volumes: Antrum/Pylorus/Distal Third of Stomach (General Guidelines)

Site or Primary and TN Stage	Remaining Stomach†	Tumor Bed Volumes‡	Nodal Volumes
Pylorus/distal third of stomach*	Yes, but spare 2/3 of one kidney, usually left	T stage dependent	N stage dependent
T2 N0, invasion of subserosa	Variable, dependent on surgical pathologic findings†	Head of pancreas (± body), 1st and 2nd portion of duodenum	None or perigastric. Optional: pancreaticduodenal, porta hepatis, celiac, suprapancreatic§
T3 N0	Variable, dependent on surgical pathologic findings†	Head of pancreas (± body), 1st and 2nd portion of duodenum	None or perigastric. Optional: pancreaticduodenal, porta hepatis, celiac, suprapancreatic§
T4 N0	Preferable, dependent on surgical pathologic findings†	As for T3 N0 plus site(s) of adherence with 3-5 cm margin	Nodes related to site(s) of adherence ± perigastric, pancreaticduodenal, porta hepatis, celiac, suprapancreatic
T1-2 N+	Preferable	Not indicated for T1	Perigastric, pancreaticduodenal, porta hepatis, celiac, suprapancreatic. Optional: splenic hilum
T3-4 N+	Preferable	As for T3 N0, T4 N0	As for T1-2 N+ and T4 N0

*Tolerance organs or structures: kidneys, liver, spinal cord.
†For tumors with wide (>5 cm) surgical margins confirmed pathologically, treatment of residual stomach is optional if this would result in substantial increase in normal tissue morbidity.
‡Use preop imaging (CT, barium swallow), surgical clips, and postop imaging (CT, barium swallow).
§Optional node inclusion for T2-3N0 lesions if adequate surgical node dissection (D2 dissection) and at least 10-15 nodes examined pathologically.
From Tepper JE, Gunderson LL: Radiation treatment parameters in the adjuvant postoperative therapy of gastric cancer. Semin Rad Oncol 12:187-195, 2002.

maintaining adequate nutrition can be a major clinical problem. Placement of a feeding tube during surgery can be critical in getting the patient past the first 2 months postoperatively. Problems of early satiety are extremely common, and it is usually not feasible to start postoperative adjuvant therapy until the patient has stabilized any weight loss. This is facilitated by the use of a feeding jejunostomy.

During the course of *postoperative chemoradiation*, strict attention must also be paid to nutritional support. It is rare that a patient will manage with 3 meals per day; most need to eat five or six planned meals, often with nutritional supplements. Postoperative problems of dumping syndrome are fairly common, but are often not recognized by the treating physician. This is expressed by the enhanced gastrocolic reflex with clustered bowel movements in association with meals. What is not as well recognized is the reactive hypoglycemia that can occur in these patients, related to the rapid transit of the gastric contents into the small bowel, rapid absorption of glucose into the circulation and the associated insulin secretion. As there is no residual food in the stomach (as would normally occur), a reactive hypoglycemia occurs, typically 1.5 to 2 hours after meals. Proper patient awareness of this problem can alleviate many of the associated difficulties.

Many patients who receive *preoperative chemoradiation* (with plans to proceed to surgical resection) or *primary chemoradia-*

tion may also require parenteral or enteral hyperalimentation during treatment. Improvement in nutritional status may require stent placement during endoscopy, feeding jejunostomy, or PEG tube placement. Feeding jejunostomy may be preferable to PEG tube placement to preserve use of the stomach for reconstruction.

Nutritional problems can exist long term in these patients. The lack of acid production results in poor absorption of a number of minerals, but most importantly iron and calcium. The iron loss is usually noted because of the associated anemia, but the calcium malabsorption is not usually appreciated until many years later. Calcium supplementation (with calcium citrate, not calcium carbonate) will usually need to be life long, but iron requirements can be assessed during follow-up. Periodic bone densitometry is appropriate. Malabsorption of fat and other nutrients should also be observed. Loss of B12 absorptive capacity is well known after a total gastrectomy. However, the body typically has B12 stores to last for up to 3 years, so it is possible to observe the patient carefully to assess whether the patient will require lifelong B12 injections.

TREATMENT ALGORITHM, CHALLENGES, AND FUTURE POSSIBILITIES

Completely Resected Lesions

Early gastric cancer (lesions confined to the mucosa or submucosa) is a challenging diagnosis and the detection rate of early gastric cancer in both North America and Europe remains low (13%) even if open access gastroscopy is available.[263-267] Endoscopic resection of early gastric cancer is limited, at present, to lesions measuring up to 3 cm in diameter and to superficial submucosal invasion.[264]

Many patients with gross complete resection of their gastric cancer are not cured with surgery alone. The final results of the Dutch and British multicenter trials evaluating the value of extended lymphadenectomy demonstrated that the procedure increased morbidity but did not benefit survival. Since experienced surgeons can perform extended node dissection without significant additional surgical morbidity or mortality, use of the procedure is still reasonable in node-positive patients; however, existing studies do not define the optimal extent of surgical resection.

Patients with extended resection are still at high risk for local-regional and systemic relapse,[268] however, and should receive postoperative chemoradiation (see treatment algorithm by TNM extent, Fig. 44-14 and Table 44-17). The U.S. GI Intergroup trial tested combined modality postoperative chemoradiation versus a surgery-alone control arm in 556 patients and confirmed a survival advantage for chemoradiation.[168] Since D2 resections were not commonly performed as a component of surgery in the U.S. GI Intergroup Phase III trial, some have questioned whether chemoradiation would give added benefit following a D2 resection. A South Korean analysis evaluated the potential role of postoperative chemoradiation in a series of 990 patients with D2 resection for gastric cancer who had high risk for relapse.[271] Surgery alone was used in 446 patients and postoperative chemoradiation in 544 patients, using the GI Intergroup regimen of 45 Gy plus 5-FU leucovorin. Both disease control and survival were improved in patients who received trimodality treatment (5-yr OS 57 versus 51%, $p = 0.02$; 5-yr RFS, 54.5 vs 47.9%, $p = 0.016$; local-regional relapse; 14.9 versus 21.7%, $p = 0.005$). Five-year OS was consistently better in the trimodality versus surgery alone patients for each stage grouping.

The current U.S. GI Intergroup phase III randomized postoperative chemoradiation trial is testing 5-FU infusion versus bolus 5-FU leucovorin as the concurrent chemotherapy during EBRT, and ECF chemotherapy versus 5-FU leucovorin as the maintenance chemotherapy. A phase II trial tested the tolerance of the more aggressive infusion 5-FU and ECF regimen in a multicenter trial involving CALGB institutions and the Mayo Clinic.[269] The irradiation fields in both the phase II and successor phase III trials are based on optimized field design related to site of the primary lesion and TN stage of disease.[260]

On the basis of encouraging results with preoperative chemotherapy or chemoradiation for locally advanced or borderline resectable disease, future phase III studies should evaluate preoperative chemotherapy and preoperative chemoradiation for patients with potentially resectable lesions. A British phase III trial of surgery alone versus surgery plus neoadjuvant and postoperative ECF chemotherapy demonstrated a survival advantage with ECF chemotherapy.[271] The potential value of preoperative chemoradiation is supported by an analysis of the U.S. GI Intergroup phase III trial, testing preop chemoradiation versus surgery alone for patients with either esophagus or GE junction cancers (adenocarcinoma or squamous).[272] In spite of low accrual, patients radomized to trimodality treatment had a survival benefit (median, 54 mo versus 21.6 mo; 5-yr OS, 39% versus 16% ($p = 0.008$).

Locally Advanced Disease

For patients with locally advanced disease, it seems reasonable to build on existing positive treatment data (EBRT plus chemotherapy, IORT, preoperative chemotherapy, perioperative chemoirradiation) plus patterns of relapse information (see Fig. 44-14; Table 44-17). It would be of interest to merge these components of treatment.

If treatment were initiatedwith preoperative chemotherapy, patients with marginal gross total or subtotal resection with residual disease or complete resection but high-risk factors for relapse (beyond the gastric wall, nodes positive, or both) should be placed in studies that evaluate IORT, postoperative EBRT, or both in conjunction with concomitant and maintenance chemotherapy. For patients whose tumors are unresectable after preoperative chemotherapy but who still have localized tumor in the basis of preoperative staging (including laparoscopy) or exploratory laparotomy, EBRT plus concomitant chemotherapy should be given. Decisions regarding attempts at later resection with or without IORT could be individualized.

An alternate approach is to initiate treatment with preoperative chemoradiation followed by restaging, resection (with or without IORT), and postoperative maintenance chemotherapy. Questions to be addressed with this approach include whether to give several cycles of multiagent chemotherapy prior to initiating concomitant chemoradiation, how many cycles of chemotherapy to deliver, and which agents to give both with irradiation and in the systemic component of treatment.

Combinations of EBRT and new drugs should continue to be evaluated. This is best accomplished in the setting of locally advanced primary or locally recurrent cancers.

Metastatic Disease

Although newer combination chemotherapy regimens have produced better response rates than single agents, survival has not been dramatically enhanced. Clearly new drug regimens need to be tested in advanced gastric cancer. The topoisomerase I inhibitors and taxanes are presently being evaluated. Alternative approaches such as biologicals, gene therapy, angiogenesis, and metastasis inhibitors will also be evaluated in clinical trials. Given the limitations of chemotherapy, con-

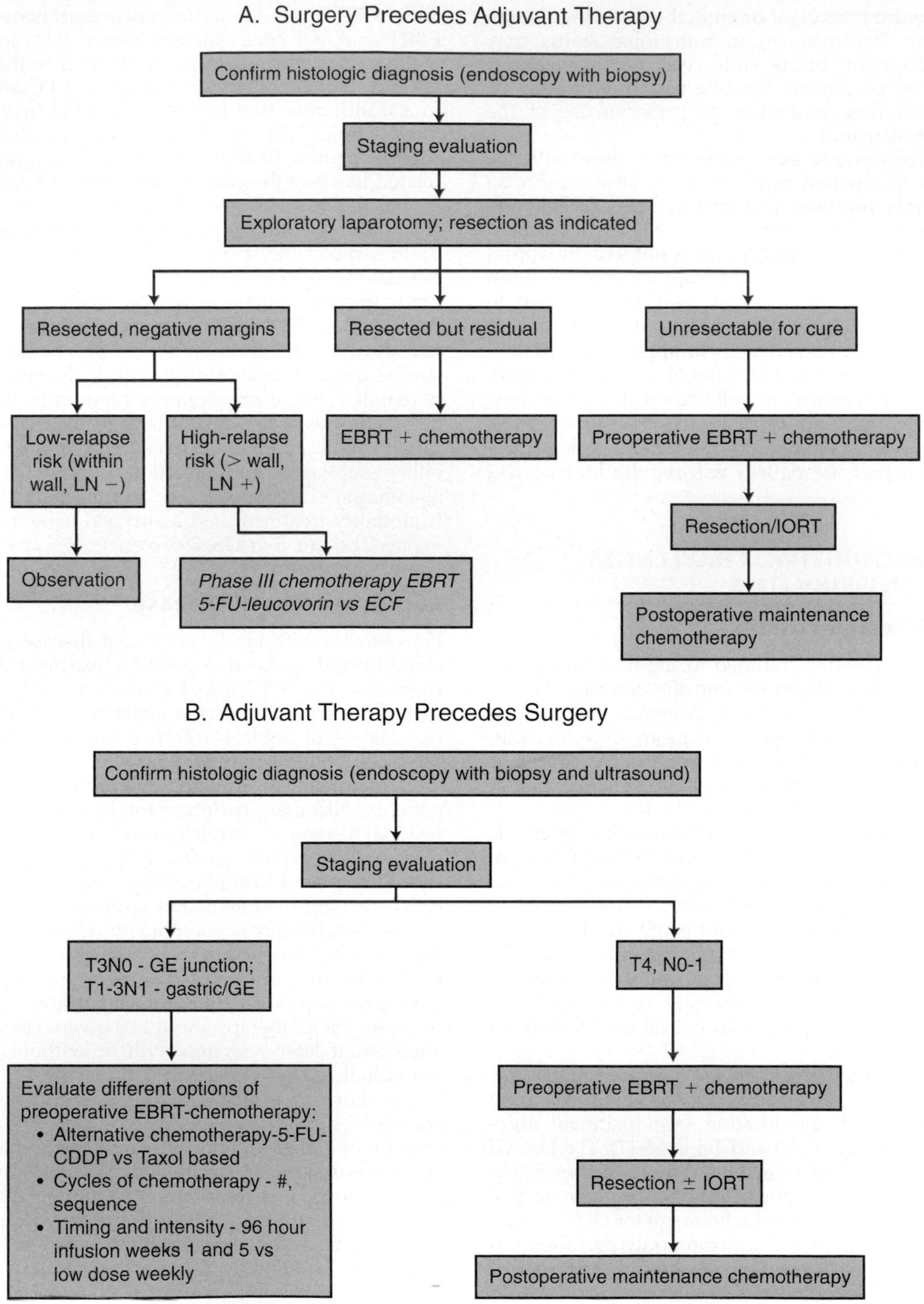

Figure 44-14 **Treatment algorithms for the patient with newly diagnosed gastric cancer.** EBRT, external beam radiation; ECF, epirubicin, cisplatin, 5-FU; IORT, intraoperative irradiation; LN−, lymph nodes negative; LN+, lymph nodes positive.

Table 44-17 **Treatment Algorithm: Gastric or GE Junction Cancer**

TNM Extent	Surgery	Irradiation (Alone or with Chemotherapy)	Chemotherapy (CT)
T1-2 N0 M0	Radical subtotal gastrectomy and regional nodes	Not routinely recommended; exception—posterior wall T2 N0 M0	NR
T1-2 N1-3 M0; T3 N0-3 M0	Radical subtotal and regional nodes	Postop chemo EBRT, 45-50 Gy; evaluate preop EBRT-CT, gastric; prefer preop EBRT-CT, GE junction*	5-FU/leucovorin bolus wk 1, 5—CCRT and maint; evaluate ECF in current U.S. GI Intergroup phase III
T4 N0-3 M0	Radical subtotal and regional nodes; attempt en bloc resection, involved organ(s)	Preop EBRT-CT, 45-50 Gy; attempt resection and IOERT	5-FU-leucovorin, bolus wk 1, 5; evaluate alternate CCRT including infusion 5-FU; evaluate other maint CT (ECF, other)
T any N any M1	Palliative if feasible	Palliative CCRT if indicated	MACT; ICT phase I, II, or III

*Prefer preop CRT for gastroesophageal (GE) junction cancers found to be T1-2 N1-3 M0 or T3 N0-3 M0 on EUS, as can usually design safer EBRT fields with preop CRT rather than postop CRT. If transhiatal resection is performed, keeping the reconstructed stomach in the mediastinal midline, postop CRT can be given more safely than if Ivor-Lewis resection is performed.

EBRT, external beam irradiation; IOERT, intraoperative electron irradiation; postop, postoperative; preop, preoperative; NR, not recommended; CCRT, concurrent chemoradiation; EBRT-CT, external beam irradiation + chemotherapy; MACT, multiagent chemotherapy; ICT, investigational chemotherapy clinical trials; maint, maintenance.

tinued evaluation of novel agents, either alone or in combination with chemotherapy, is indicated.

Treatment Algorithm by TNM Disease Extent

T1-2 N0 M0

Total surgical resection of the adenocarcinoma with a radical subtotal gastrectomy and reconstruction with gastrojejunostomy is recommended as standard treatment (see Table 44-17 and Fig. 44-14). Patients with posterior wall T2 N0 M0 lesions should be evaluated for postoperative adjuvant chemoradiation (see T1-2 N1-3 M0; T3 N0-3 M0).

T1-2 N1-3 M0; T3 N0-3 M0

Postoperative chemoradiation (CRT) is the preferred treatment. For GE junction cancers found to be T1-2 N1-3 M0 or T3 N0-3 M0 on EUS, preoperative CRT may be preferable, as one can usually design safer EBRT fields for preoperative CRT rather than postoperative CRT. If transhiatal resection is performed, keeping the reconstructed stomach in the mediastinal midline, postop CRT is facilitated.

T4 N0-3 M0

Preoperative chemoradiation followed by restaging, gross total resection (may include en bloc resection of adjacent organs), and intraoperative electron irradiation (IOERT) is recommended for potentially resectable T4 N0-3 lesions in institutions with that capability. Postoperative CRT has also been used for completely resected lesions. For locally unresectable T4 N0-3 M0 gastric cancers, preoperative or primary chemoradiation or multidrug chemotherapy can be used, preferably in the setting of controlled prospective clinical trials.

T any N any M1

Multidrug chemotherapy combinations are the preferred treatment for patients with metastatic cancers. Patients should be placed on controlled trials if available.

REFERENCES

1. Jemal A, Siegel R, Ward E, et al: Cancer statistics, 2006. CA Cancer J Clin 56:106-130, 2006.
2. Jemal A, Thomas A, Murray T, Thun M: Cancer statistics, 2002. CA Cancer J Clin 52:23-47, 2002
3. Wiggins CL, Becker TM, Key CR, et al: Stomach cancer among New Mexico's American Indians, Hispanic whites and non-Hispanic whites. Cancer Res 49:1595-1599, 1989.
4. Parkin DM, Pisani P, Ferlay J: Global cancer statistics. CA Cancer J Clin 49:33-64, 1999.
5. Blot WJ, Devesa SS, Kneller RW, et al: Rising incidence of adenocarcinoma of the esophagus and gastric cardia. JAMA 265:1287-1289, 1991.
6. Ries GA, Hanley BF, Edwards BK (eds): Cancer Statistics Review 1973-1987, vol. 90. Bethesda, MD, Department of Health and Human Services, NIH Publication, 1990, p 2789.
7. Powell J, McConkey CC: Increasing incidence of adenocarcinoma of the gastric cardia and adjacent sites. Br J Cancer 59:440-443, 1990.
8. Haenzel W, Kurihara M, Segi M, et al: Stomach cancer among Japanese in Hawaii. J Natl Cancer Inst 49:969-988, 1972.
9. Correa P, Cuello C, Duque E: Carcinoma and intestinal metaplasia of the stomach in Colombian migrants. J Natl Cancer Inst 44:297-306, 1970.
10. Fuchs CS, Mayer RJ: Gastric carcinoma. N Engl J Med 353:32-42, 1995.
11. You WC, Blot WJ, Chang YS, et al: Diet and high risk of stomach cancer in Shandong, China. Cancer Res 48:3518-3523, 1988.
12. Nomura A: Stomach cancer. *In* Schottenfeld D, Fraumeni JF Jr (eds): Cancer Epidemiology and Prevention. Oxford, United Kingdom, Oxford University Press, 1996, pp 707-724.
13. Wadström T: An update on *Helicobacter pylori*. Curr Opin Gastroenterol 11:69-75, 1995.
14. Neugut AI, Hayeh M, Howe G: Epidemiology of gastric cancer. Semin Oncol 23:281-291, 1996.
15. Correa P: Human gastric carcinogenesis: multistep and multifocal process. Cancer Res 52:6735-6740, 1992.
16. Correa P, Haenzel W, Cuello C, et al: Gastric precancerous process in a high-risk population: cross sectional studies. Cancer Res 50:4731-4736, 1990.

17. The Eurogast Study Group: An international association between *H. pylori* infection and gastric cancer. Lancet 341:1359-1362, 1993.
18. Nomura A, Stemmerman GN, Chyou PH, et al: *Helicobacter pylori* infection and gastric carcinoma among Japanese Americans in Hawaii. N Engl J Med 325:1132-1136, 1991.
19. Parsonnet J, Friedman GD, Vandersteen DP, et al: *Helicobacter pylori* infection and the risk of gastric carcinoma. N Engl J Med 325:1127-1131, 1991.
20. Levin B: Gastric cancer: new insights into epidemiology and etiology. ASCO Educational Book 1997, pp 273-274.
21. Prolla J, Kobayashi S, Kirsner J: Gastric cancer: some recent improvements in diagnosis based on the Japanese experience. Arch Intern Med 124:238, 1969.
22. Chun YS, Lindor NM, Smyrk TC, et al: Germline E-cadherin gene mutations. Is prophylactic total gastrectomy indicated? Cancer 92:181, 2001.
23. Huntsman DG, Carneiro F, Lewis FR, et al: Early gastric cancer in young, asymptomatic carriers of germ-line E-cadherin mutations. N Engl J Med 344:1904, 2001.
24. Lewis FR, Mellinger JD, Hayashi A, et al: Prophylactic total gastrectomy for familial gastric cancer. Surgery 130:612, 2001.
25. Thompson GB, van Heerden J, Sarr MC: Adenocarcinoma of the stomach: are we making progress? Lancet 342:713-718, 1993.
26. Dockerty MB: Pathologic aspects of primary malignant neoplasms of the stomach. *In* ReMine WH, Priestley JT, Berkson J (eds): Cancer of the Stomach. Philadelphia, WB Saunders, 1964, p 173.
27. Kennedy BJ: TNM classification for stomach cancer. Cancer 26:971, 1970.
28. Gunderson LL, Sosin H: Adenocarcinoma of the stomach areas of failure in a reoperation series (second or symptomatic looks): clinicopathologic correlation and implications for adjuvant therapy. Int J Radiat Oncol Biol Phys 8:1, 1982.
29. MacDonald JS, Cohn I, Gunderson LL: Carcinoma of the stomach. *In* Devita V, Hellman S, Rosenberg S (eds): Principles and Practice of Oncology, 2nd ed. Philadelphia, Lippincott, 1985, pp 659-690.
30. Nagatomo T, Mukarami E, Kondo K: Histologic criteria of serosal rupture and prognosis in gastric carcinoma. Cancer 29:180, 1969.
31. Dent DM, Werner ID, Novis B, et al: Prospective randomized trial of combined oncological therapy for gastric carcinoma. Cancer 44:385, 1979.
32. Tsukivama J, Akine Y, Kajiura Y, et al: Radiation therapy for advanced gastric cancer. Int J Radiat Oncol Biol Phys 15:123, 1988.
33. Yu CC, Levison DA, Dunn JA, et al: Pathological prognostic factors in the second British Stomach Cancer Group trial of adjuvant therapy in resectable gastric cancer. Br J Cancer 71:1106-1110, 1995.
34. MacDonald WC, MacDonald JB: Adenocarcinoma of the esophagus or gastric cardia. Cancer 60:33, 1987.
35. Meyers WC, Damiano RJ, Postlethwait RW, Rotolo FS: Adenocarcinoma of the stomach: changing patterns over the last 4 decades. Ann Surg 205:1, 1987.
36. Yamada Y, Kato Y: Greater tendency for submucosal invasion in fundic area gastric carcinomas than those arising in the pyloric area. Cancer 63:1757, 1989.
37. Fein R, Kelsen DP, Geller N, et al: Adenocarcinoma of the esophagus and gastroesophageal junction: prognostic factors and results of therapy. Cancer 56:2512, 1985.
38. Hartley LC, Evans E, Windsor CJ: Factors influencing prognosis in gastric cancer. Aust NZ J Surg 57:5, 1987.
39. Nanus DM, Kelsen DP, Niedzwiecki D, et al: Flow cytometry as a predictive indicator in patients with operable gastric cancer. J Clin Oncol 7:1105, 1989.
40. Finlay CA, Hinds PW, Levine AJ: The p53 proto-oncogene can act as a suppressor of transformation. Cell 57:1083-1093, 1989.
41. Lane DP: Worrying about p53. Curr Biol 2:581-583, 1989.
42. Kastan MB, Oyekwere O, Sidransky D, et al: Participation of p53 in the cell response to DNA damage. Cancer Res 51:6304-6311, 1991.
43. O'Connor PM, Jackman J, Jondle D, et al: Role of p53 tumor suppressor gene in cell cycle arrest and radiosensitivity of Burkitt's lymphoma cell lines. Cancer Res 53:4776-4780, 1993.
44. Fenoglio-Preiser CM, Noffsinger AE, Belli J, et al: Pathologic and phenotypic features of gastric cancer. Semin Oncol 23:292-306, 1996.
45. Lynch HT, Smyrk TC, Watson P, et al: Genetics, natural history, tumor spectrum and pathology of hereditary non-polyposis colon cancer: an updated review. Gastroenterology 10:1535-1549, 1993.
46. Takahashi M, Ota S, Shimada T, et al: Hepatocyte growth factor is the most potent endogenous stimulant of rabbit gastric epithelial cell proliferation and migration in primary culture. J Clin Invest 95:1994-2003, 1995.
47. Tahara E: Molecular mechanism of stomach carcinogenesis. J Cancer Res Clin Oncol 119:265-272, 1993.
48. Tahara E, Yokozaki H, Yasui W: Growth factors in gastric cancer. *In* Nishi M, Tahara E (eds): Gastric Cancer. Tokyo, Springer-Verlag, 1993, pp 209-217.
49. Fenoglio-Preiser CM: The effect of oncogenes on biology and prognosis of surgically resected gastric cancer. Educational Books, Am Soc Clin Oncol, 1997, pp 275-277.
50. Tushima K, Nagorney DM, Cha SS, Reiman HM: Correlation of DNA ploidy, histopathology, stage, and clinical outcome in gastric carcinoma. Surg Oncol 1:17, 1992.
51. Baba H, Korenaga D, Okamura T, et al: Prognostic significance of DNA content with special reference to age in gastric cancer. Cancer 63:1768, 1989.
52. Korenaga D, Okamura T, Saito A, et al: DNA ploidy is closely linked to tumor invasion, lymph node metastasis, and prognosis in clinical gastric cancer. Cancer 62:309, 1988.
53. Harrison JD, Morris DL, Ellis IO, et al: The effect of tamoxifen and estrogen receptor status on survival in gastric carcinoma. Cancer 64:1007, 1989.
54. Sugiyama K, Yomemura Y, Miyazaki I: Immunohistochemical study of epidermal growth factor and epidermal growth factor receptor in gastric carcinoma. Cancer 63:1557, 1989.
55. Yonemura Y, Ninimiya I, Ohoyama S, et al: Expression of C-erbB-2 oncoprotein in gastric carcinoma. Immunoreactivity for C-erbB-2 protein is an independent of poor short-term prognosis in patients with gastric carcinoma. Cancer 62:2914, 1991.
56. Hiton DA, West KP: An evaluation of the prognostic significance of HLA-DR expression in gastric carcinoma. Cancer 66:1154, 1990.
57. Tahara E, Semba S, Tahara H: Molecular biological observations in gastric cancer. Semin Oncol 23:307-315, 1996.
58. Japanese Research Society for Gastric Cancer: The general rules for the gastric cancer study in surgery and pathology: I. Clinical classification. Jpn J Surg 11:127, 1981.
59. Lauren P: The two histologic main types of gastric carcinomas: diffuse and so-called intestinal type carcinoma—an attempt at a histological classification. Acta Pathol Microbiol Scand 64:31, 1965.
60. Borrmann R: Geschwulste des Magens und Duodenums. *In* Henke F, Lanbarsch O (eds): Handbuch der Spaziellen Pathologischen Anatomie and Histologie, vol. 4. Berlin, Julius Springer, 1926.
61. Wang J-Y, Hsieh J-S, Juang Y-S, et al: Endoscopic ultrasonography for preoperative locoregional staging and assessment of resectability in gastric cancer. Clin Imaging 22:355, 1998.
62. Willis S, Truong S, Gribritz S et al: Endoscopic ultrasonography in the preoperative staging of gastric cancer. Accuracy and impact on surgical therapy. Surg Endosc 14:951, 2000.
63. Loury AM, Mansfield PF, Leach SD, et al: Laparoscopic staging for gastric cancer. Surgery 119:611-614, 1996.
64. Ziegler K, Sanft C, Zimmer T, et al: Comparison of computed tomography, endosonography, and intraoperative assessment in TN staging of gastric carcinoma. Gut 34:604-610, 1993.
65. Greene FL, Page DL, Fleming ID, et al: AJCC Cancer Staging Manual, 6th ed. New York, Springer-Verlag, 2002, p 99.
66. Robertson CS, Chung SCS, Woods SDS, et al: A prospective randomized trial comparing R1 subtotal gastrectomy with R3 total gastrectomy for antral cancer. Ann Surg 220:176-182, 1994.
67. Dupont JB Jr, et al: Adenocarcinoma of the stomach: review of 1497 cases. Cancer 41:941, 1978.

68. Serlin O, Keehn RJ, Higgins GA, et al: Factors related to survival following resection for gastric carcinoma. Cancer 40:1318, 1977.
69. Sugimachi K, Kodama Y, Kumashito R, et al: Critical evaluation of prophylactic splenectomy in total gastrectomy for stomach cancer. Gann 71:704, 1980.
70. Noguchi Y, Imada T, Matsumoto A, et al: Radical surgery for gastric cancer: a review of the Japanese experience. Cancer 64:2053, 1989.
71. Iriyama K, Asukawa T, Koike H, et al: Is extensive lymphadenectomy necessary for surgical treatment of intramucosal carcinoma of the stomach? Arch Surg 124:309, 1989.
72. Bolen T, Nakane Y, Okusa T, et al: Strategy for lymphadenectomy of gastric cancer. Surgery 105:585, 1989.
73. Maruyama K, Gunven P, Okabayashi K, et al: Lymph node metastases of gastric cancer: general pattern in 1931 patients. Ann Surg 210:596, 1989.
74. Douglas HO, Nava HR: Gastric adenocarcinoma: management of the primary disease. Semin Oncol 12:32, 1985.
75. Kodama Y, Sugimachi K, Soejima K, et al: Evaluation of extensive lymph node dissection for carcinoma of the stomach. World J Surg 5:241, 1981.
76. Okajima K: Surgical treatment of gastric cancer with specific reference to lymph node removal. Acta Med Okayama 31:369, 1977.
77. Shiu MH, Moore E, Sanders M, et al: Influence of the extent of resection on survival after curative treatment of gastric carcinoma. Arch Surg 122:1347, 1987.
78. Soja J, Ohyama S, Miyashita K, et al: A statistical evaluation advancement in gastric cancer surgery with special reference to the significance of lymphadenectomy for cure. World J Surg 12:398, 1988.
79. Kern KA: Gastric cancer: a neoplastic enigma. J Surg Oncol 1(Suppl):34-39, 1989.
80. Has CD, Mansfield CM, Leichman LP, et al: Combined nonsimultaneous radiation therapy and chemotherapy with 5-FU, doxorubicin and mitomycin for residual localized gastric adenocarcinoma. A Southwest Oncology Group pilot study. Cancer Treat Rep 67:421, 1983.
81. Dent DM, Madden MV, Price SK: Randomized comparison of R1 and R2 gastrectomy for gastric carcinoma. Br J Surg 75:110, 1988.
82. Sasako M, Maruyama K, Kinoshita T: Quality control of surgical technique in a multicenter, prospective, randomized, controlled study on the surgical treatment of gastric cancer. Jpn J Clin Oncol 22:41, 1992.
83. Burt AMG, Hermans J, Boon MC, et al: Evaluation of the extent of lymphadenectomy in a randomized trial of Western versus Japanese-type of surgery in gastric cancer. J Clin Oncol 12:417-422, 1994.
84. Bonnenkamp JJ, Songum I, Hermans J, et al: Randomized comparison of morbidity after D_1 and D_2 dissection for gastric cancer in 996 Dutch patients. Lancet 345:745-748, 1995.
85. Bonnenkamp JJ, Hermans J, Sasako M, Vande Velde CJH for the Dutch Gastric Cancer Group: Extended lymph node dissection for gastric cancer. N Engl J Med 340:908-914, 1999.
86. Cuschieri A, Fayers P, Fielding J, et al: Postoperative morbidity and mortality after D_1 and D_2 resections for gastric cancer: preliminary results of the MRC randomized controlled surgical trial. Lancet 347:995-999, 1996.
87. Cuschieri A, Weeden S, Fielding J, et al: Patient survival after D_1 and D_2 resections for gastric cancer: long-term results of the MRC randomized controlled surgical trial. Br J Cancer 79:1522, 1999.
88. de Aretxabala X, Konishi K, Yonemura Y, et al: Node dissection in gastric cancer. Br J Surg 74:770, 1987.
89. Smith JW, Shin MH, Kelsy L, Brennan MF: Morbidity of radical lymphadenectomy in the curative resection of gastric carcinoma. Arch Surg 126:1469, 1991.
90. Fukutomi H, Nakahara A: Endoscopic therapy of gastrointestinal cancer and its curability. Gan To Kagaku Ryoho 4:1132, 1988.
91. Adachi Y, Mori M, Sugimachi K: Persistence of mucosal gastric carcinomas for 8 and 6 years in two patients. Arch Pathol Lab Med 114:1046, 1990.
92. Bozzeti F, Bonfanti G, Castellani R, et al: Comparing reconstruction with Roux-en-Y to pouch following total gastrectomy. J Am Coll Surg 183:243-248, 1996.
93. Chareton B, Landen S, Manganas D, et al: Prospective randomized trial comparing Billroth I and II procedures for carcinoma of the gastric antrum. J Ann Coll Surg 183:190-194, 1996.
94. Buhl K, Lehnert T, Schlag P, et al: Reconstruction after gastrectomy and quality of life. World J Surg 19:558-564, 1995.
95. Fuchs KH, Thiede A, Engemam R, et al: Reconstruction of the food passage after total gastrectomy: randomized trial. World J Surg 19:698-706, 1995.
96. Macintyre DMC, Akoh JA: Improving survival in gastric cancer: review of operation mortality in English language publications from 1970. Br J Surg 68:773, 1981.
97. Heberer G, Teichmann RK, Kramling HJ, Gunther B: Results of gastric resection for carcinoma of the stomach: the European experience. World J Surg 12:374, 1988.
98. Green PH, O'Toole KM, Slonin D, et al: Increasing incidence and excellent survival of patients with early gastric cancer: expression in a United States Medical Center. Am J Med 85:658, 1988.
99. Itoh H, Oohata Y, Nakamura K, et al: Complete ten-year postgastrectomy follow-up of early gastric cancer. Am J Surg 158:14, 1989.
100. Endo M, Habu H: Clinical studies of early gastric cancer. Hepatogastroenterology 37:408, 1990.
101. de Dombral FT, Price AB, Thompson H, et al: The British Society of Gastroenterology early gastric cancer/dysplasia survey: an interim report. J Gut 3:115, 1990.
102. Gentsch HH, Grould H, Gerdl J: Results of surgical treatment of early gastric cancer in 113 patients. World J Surg 5:103, 1981.
103. Farley DR, Donohue JH, Nagorney DM, et al: Early gastric cancer. Br J Surg 79:539, 1992.
104. Majus WC, Damiano RJ Jr, Rotolo FS, et al: Adenocarcinoma of the stomach: changing patterns over the last four decades. Ann Surg 205:1, 1987.
105. Cady B, Rossi RL, Silverman ML, et al: Gastric adenocarcinoma: a disease in transition. Arch Surg 124:303, 1989.
106. Kim JP, Kim YW, Yang HK, et al: Significant prognostic factors by multivariate analyses of 3,926 gastric cancer patients. World J Surg 18:872-878, 1994.
107. Kajiyama Y, Tsurumaru M, Udagawa H, et al: Prognostic factors in adenocarcinoma of the gastric cardia: pathologic stage analysis and multivariate regression analysis. J Clin Oncol 15:2015-2021, 1997.
108. Jatzko GR, Lisborg PH, Denk H, et al: A 10-year experience with Japanese-type radical lymph node dissection for gastric cancer outside Japan. Cancer 76:1302-1312, 1995.
109. Bunt TMG, Bonnenkamp HJ, Hermans J, et al: Factors influencing the noncompliance and contamination in a randomized trial of "Western" (R1) versus "Japanese" (R2) types of surgery in gastric cancer. Cancer 73:1544-1551, 1994.
110. Nakamura K, Keyama T, Yao T, et al: Pathology and prognosis of gastric carcinoma: findings in 10,000 patients who underwent primary gastrectomy. Cancer 70:1030, 1992.
111. Papachristou DN, Fortner JG: Local recurrence of gastric adenocarcinomas after gastrectomy. J Surg Oncol 18:47, 1981.
112. Landry J, Tepper J, Wood W, et al: analysis of survival and local control following surgery for gastric cancer. Int J Radiat Oncol Biol Phys 19:1357, 1990.
113. Horn RC: Carcinoma of the stomach: autopsy findings in untreated cases. Gastroenterology 29:515, 1955.
114. McNeer G, Vandenberg H, Donn FY, Bowden LA: A critical evaluation of subtotal gastrectomy for the cure of cancer of the stomach. Ann Surg 134:2, 1957.
115. Stout AP: Pathology of carcinoma of the stomach. Arch Surg 46:807, 1943.
116. Thomson FB, Robins RE: Local recurrence following subtotal resection for gastric carcinoma. Surg Gynecol Obstet 91:341, 1952.
117. Wisbek WA, Becker EM, Russell AH: Adenocarcinoma of the stomach: autopsy observations with therapeutic implications for the radiation oncologist. Radiother Oncol 7:13, 1986.
118. Gilbertson VA: Results of treatment of stomach cancer: an appraisal of efforts for more extensive surgery and a report of 1,938 cases. Cancer 23:1305, 1969.
119. Coombs RC, Schein PS, Chilvers CE, et al: a randomized trial comparing adjuvant fluorouracil, doxorubicin, and mitomycin

with no treatment in operable gastric cancer. International Collaborative Cancer Group. J Clin Oncol 8:1362-1369, 1990.
120. Gagliano R, McCracken J, Chen T: Adjuvant chemotherapy with FAM in gastric cancer: a SWOG study. Proc Am Soc Clin Oncol 2:114, 1983.
121. Estape J, Grau J, Alcobendas F, et al: Mitomycin C as an adjuvant treatment to resected gastric cancer: a 20-year follow-up. Ann Surg 213:219-221, 1991.
122. Grau JJ, Estape J, Fuster J, et al: Randomized trial of adjuvant chemotherapy with mitomycin plus ftorafur versus mitomycin alone in resected locally advanced gastric cancer. J Clin Oncol 16:1036-1039, 1998.
123. Neri B, Cini G, Andreoli F, et al: Randomized trial of adjuvant chemotherapy versus control after curative resection for gastric cancer: 5-year follow-up. Br J Cancer 84:878, 2001.
124. Cirera L, Balil A, Batiste-Alentorn E, et al: Randomized clinical trial of adjuvant mitomycin plus tegafur in patients with resected stage III gastric cancer. J Clin Oncol 17:3810, 1999.
125. Lise M, Nitti D, Marchet A, et al: Final results of a phase II clinical trial of adjuvant chemotherapy with the modified fluorouracil, doxorubicin, and mitomycin regimen in resectable gastric cancer. J Clin Oncol 23:2757-2763, 1995.
126. MacDonald JS, Fleming TR, Peterson RF, et al: Adjuvant chemotherapy with 5-FU, Adriamycin, and mitomycin C (FAM) versus surgery alone for patients with locally advanced gastric adenocarcinoma: a Southwest Oncology Group Study. Ann Surg Oncol 2:488-494, 1995.
127. Wils J, Nitti D, Guimaraes dos Santos J, et al: Randomized phase III studies of adjuvant chemotherapy with FAMTX or FEMTX in resected gastric cancer. Pooled results of studies from the EORTC GI-group and the ICCG. Proc Am Soc Clin Oncol 21:131a, 2002.
128. Bajetta E, Buzzoni R, Mariani L, et al: Adjuvant chemotherapy in gastric cancer: 5-year results of a randomised study by the Italian Trials in Medical Oncology (ITMO) Group. Ann Oncol 13:299, 2002.
129. Panzini I, Gianni L, Fattori PP, et al: Adjuvant chemotherapy in gastric cancer: a meta-analysis of randomized trials and a comparison with previous meta-analyses. Tumori 88:21, 2002.
130. Janunger KG, Hafstrom L, Nygren P, et al: A systematic overview of chemotherapy effects in gastric cancer. Acta Oncol 40:309, 2001.
131. Gianni L, Panzini I, Tassinari D, et al: Meta-analyses of randomized trials of adjuvant chemotherapy in gastric cancer. Ann Oncol 12:1179, 2001.
132. Hermans J, Bonenkamp H: Meta-analysis of adjuvant chemotherapy in gastric cancer: a critical reappraisal. J Clin Oncol 12:878, 1994.
133. Earle CC, Maroun JA: Adjuvant chemotherapy after curative resection for gastric cancer in non-Asian patients: revisiting a meta-analysis of randomised trials. Eur J Cancer 35:1059, 1999.
134. Mari E, Floriani I, Tinazzi A, et al: Efficacy of adjuvant chemotherapy after curative resection for gastric cancer: a meta-analysis of published randomised trials. A study of the GISCAD (Gruppo Italiano per lo Studio dei Carcinomi dell'Apparato Digerente). Ann Oncol 11:837, 2000.
135. Serlin O, Wolkoff JS, Amadeo JM, Keehn RJ: Use of 5-fluorodeoxyuridine (FUDR) as an adjuvant to the surgical management of carcinoma of the stomach. Cancer 24:223, 1969.
136. Dixon WJ, Longmire WP, Holden J: Use of triethylenethiophosphoramide as an adjuvant to the surgical treatment of gastric and colorectal carcinoma: ten-year follow-up. Ann Surg 173:26, 1971.
137. The Gastrointestinal Tumor Study Group: Adjuvant chemotherapy following resection for gastric cancer. Cancer 49:1116, 1982.
138. Higgins GA, Amadeo JH, Smith DE, et al: Efficacy of prolonged intermittent therapy with combined 5-FU and methyl CCNU following resection for gastric carcinoma: Veterans Administration Surgical Oncology Group report. Cancer 52:1105, 1983.
139. Engstrom PF, Lavin PT, Douglas HO, Brunner KW: Postoperative adjuvant 5-FU and methyl CCNU therapy for gastric cancer patients: Eastern Cooperative Oncology Study Group 3275. Cancer 55:1868, 1985.
140. Italian Gastrointestinal Tumor Study Group: Adjuvant treatments following curative resection for gastric cancer. Br J Surg 75:1100, 1988.
141. Schlag P: Adjuvant chemotherapy in gastric cancer. World J Surg 11:473, 1987.
142. Hallissey MT, Dunn JA, Ward LC, et al: the Second British Stomach Cancer Group trial of adjuvant radiotherapy or chemotherapy in resectable gastric cancer: five-year follow-up. Lancet 343:1309-1312, 1989.
143. MacDonald JS, Gagliano R, Fleming T, et al: A phase II trial of FAM (5-fluorouracil, Adriamycin, and mitomycin C) chemotherapy versus control as adjuvant treatment for resected gastric cancer. Proc Am Soc Clin Oncol 11:488, 1992.
144. Estrada E, Lacave AJ, Valle M, et al: Methyl CCNU, 5-fluorouracil and Adriamycin (MeFA) as adjuvant chemotherapy in gastric cancer. Proc ASCO 7:358, 1988.
145. Krook JE, O'Connell MJ, Wieand HS, et al: A prospective, randomized evaluation of intensive-course 5-fluorouracil plus doxorubicin as surgical adjuvant chemotherapy for resected gastric cancer. Cancer 67:2454, 1991.
146. Hugier M, Destroyes JP, Baschet C, et al: Gastric carcinoma treated by chemotherapy after resection. A controlled study. Am J Surg 139:197, 1980.
147. Allum WH, Hallissey MT, Kelly KA: Adjuvant chemotherapy in operable gastric cancer. Five-year follow-up of first British Stomach Cancer Group trial. Lancet 1:571, 1989.
148. Jakesz R, Dittrich C, Funovics J, et al: The effect of adjuvant chemotherapy in gastric carcinoma is dependent on tumor histology: 5-year results of a prospective randomized trial. Recent results. Cancer Res 110:44, 1988.
149. Jakesz R, Bohnig HJ, Depisch D, et al: Failure of postoperative intraperitoneal cisplatin to prolong survival in patients operated for gastric carcinoma: a randomized trial. *In* Salmon SE (ed): Adjuvant Therapy of Cancer. vol. 6. Philadelphia, WB Saunders, 1990.
150. Carrato A, Diaz-Rubio E, Medrano J, et al: Phase III trial of surgery versus adjuvant chemotherapy with mitomycin C and tegafur plus uracil, starting within the first week after surgery for gastric carcinoma. Proc Am Soc Clin Oncol 14:198, 1995.
151. Neri B, De Leonardis V, Romano S, et al: Adjuvant chemotherapy after gastric resection in node-positive cancer patients: a multicenter randomized study. Br J Cancer 73:549-552, 1996.
152. Cirera L, Balil A, Batiste E, et al: Efficacy of adjuvant mitomycin C plus tegafur in stage III gastric cancer. Proc Am Soc Clin Oncol 16:986, 1997.
153. Allum WH, Hallissey MT, Ward LC, Hockey MS: A controlled prospective and randomized trial of adjuvant chemotherapy or radiotherapy in resectable gastric cancer: interim report. British Stomach Cancer Group. Br J Cancer 60:739, 1989.
154. Abe M, Takahashi M: Intraoperative radiotherapy: the Japanese experience. Int J Radiat Oncol Biol Phys 5:683, 1981.
155. Takahashi M, Abe M: Intraoperative radiotherapy for carcinoma of the stomach. Eur J Surg Oncol 12:247, 1986.
156. Chen G, Song S: Evaluation of intraoperative radiotherapy for gastric carcinoma: analysis of 247 patients. *In* Abe M, Takahashi M (eds): Proceedings of Third International IORT Symposium. Kyoto, Japan. New York, Pergamon Press, 1991, p 190.
157. Shchepotin IB, Evans SRT, Chorny V, et al: Intensive preoperative radiotherapy with local hyperthermia for the treatment of gastric carcinoma. Surg Oncol 3:37, 1994.
158. Talaev MI, Starinskii VV, Kovalev BN, et al: Results of combined treatment of cancer of the gastric antrum and gastric body. Vopr Onkol 36:1485, 1990.
159. Kosse VA: Combined treatment of gastric cancer using hypoxic radiotherapy. Vopr Onkol 36:1349, 1990.
160. Zhang ZX, Gu XZ, Yin WB, et al: Randomized clinical trial combination of preoperative irradiation and surgery in the treatment of adenocarcinoma of the gastric cardia (AGC): Report on 370 patients. Int J Radiat Oncol Biol Phys 42:929-934, 1998.
161. Gunderson LL, Hoskins B, Cohen AM, et al: Combined modality treatment of gastric cancer. Int J Radiat Oncol Biol Phys 9:965, 1983.
162. Gez E, Sulkes A, Yablonski-Peretz T, Weshler Z: Combined 5-fluorouracil (5-FU) and radiation therapy following resection of locally advanced gastric carcinoma. J Surg Oncol 31:139, 1986.

163. Regine WF, Mohuidden M: Impact of adjuvant therapy on locally advanced adenocarcinoma of the stomach. Int J Radiat Oncol Biol Phys 24:921, 1992.
164. Mehta K, Mohuidden M: Improved local control with adjunctive therapy for cancers of the gastroesophageal junction. Int J Radiat Oncol Biol Phys 30:272, 1994.
165. Whittington R, Coia L, Haller DG, et al: Adenocarcinoma of the esophagus and esophagogastric junction: the effects of single and combined modalities in the survival and patterns of failure following treatment. Int J Radiat Oncol Biol Phys 19:593, 1990.
166. Henning GT, Schild SF, Stafford SL, et al: Results of irradiation or chemoirradiation following resection of gastric adenocarcinoma. Int J Radiat Oncol Biol Phys 46:589-598, 2000.
167. Moertel CG, Childs DS, O'Fallon JR, et al: Combined 5-fluorouracil and radiation therapy as a surgical adjuvant for poor prognosis gastric carcinoma. J Clin Oncol 2:1249, 1984.
168. MacDonald JS, Smalley SR, Benedetti J, et al: Chemoradiotherapy after surgery compared with surgery alone for adenocarcinoma of the stomach or gastroesophageal junction. N Engl J Med 345:725, 2001.
169. Smalley SS, Gunderson L, Tepper J, et al: Gastric surgical adjuvant radiotherapy consensus report: rationale and treatment implementation. Int J Radiat Oncol Biol Phys 52:282, 2002.
170. Walsh TN, Noonan N, Hollywood D, et al: A comparison of multimodal therapy and surgery for esophageal adenocarcinoma. N Engl J Med 335:462-467, 1996.
171. Sindelar WF, Kinsella TJ, Tepper JE, et al: Randomized trial of intraoperative radiotherapy in carcinoma of the stomach. Am J Surg 165:178, 1993.
172. Abe M, Takahashi M, Yabumoto E, et al: Clinical experiences with intraoperative radiotherapy for locally advanced cancers. Cancer 45:40-48, 1980.
173. Abe M, Takahashi M, Ono K, et al: Japan gastric trials in intraoperative radiation therapy. Int J Radiat Oncol Biol Phys 15(6):1431-1433, 1998.
174. Ogata T, Araki K, Matsuura K, et al: A 10-year experience of intraoperative radiotherapy for gastric carcinoma and a new surgical method of creating a wider irradiation field for cases of total gastrectomy patients. Int J Radiat Oncol Biol Phys 32(2):341-347, 1995.
175. Farthmann EH, Kirchner R, Salm R, et al: Usefulness and limitations of preoperative radiotherapy in association with curative resection in the treatment of gastric cancer. Chirurgie 119/9:565-568, 1993-1994.
176. Kramling HJ, Grab J, Zaspel J, et al: Experimental study of vascular sequelae of combined upper abdominal intraoperative and external radiation therapy. *In* Vaeth J (ed): Intraoperative Radiation Therapy in the Treatment of Cancer. Front Radiat Ther Oncol 31:36-40, 1997.
177. Kramling HJ, Willich N, Cramer C et al: Results of IORT in the treatment of gastric cancer. ISIORT 2002 Proceedings; Abstract 4.3; Aachen, Germany.
178. Calvo FA, Henriquez I, Santos M, et al: Intraoperative and external beam radiotherapy in advanced resectable gastric cancer: technical description and preliminary results. Int J Radiat Oncol Biol Phys 17:183-189, 1989.
179. Calvo FA, Aristu JJ, Azinovic I, et al: Intraoperative and external radiotherapy in resected gastric cancer: updated report of a phase II trial. Int J Radiat Oncol Biol Phys 24(4):729-736, 1992.
180. Martinez-Monge R, Calvo FA, Azinovic I, et al: Patterns of failure and long-term results in high-risk resected gastric cancer treated with postoperative radiotherapy ± intraoperative electron boost. J Surg Oncol 66:24-29, 1997.
181. De Villa VH, Calvo FA, Bilbao JI: Arteriodigestive fistula: a complication associated with intraoperative and external beam radiotherapy following surgery for gastric cancer. J Surg Oncol 49(1):52-57, 1992.
182. Avizonis VN, Buzydlowski J, Lanciano R, et al: Treatment of adenocarcinoma of the stomach with resection, intraoperative radiotherapy and adjuvant external beam radiation: a phase II study from Radiation Therapy Oncology Group 85-04. Ann Surg Oncol 2(4):295-302, 1995.
183. Gilly FN, Gerard JP, Braillon G, et al: Intraoperative radiotherapy in gastric adenocarcinomas. Apropos of 45 cases. Ann Chir 47(3):234-239, 1993.
184. Gilly FN, Gerard JP, Braillon G, et al: Surgery, IORT and postoperative radiotherapy in the treatment of gastric cancer: the long term experience in Lyon. ISIORT 2002 Proceedings; Abstract 4.4; Aachen, Germany.
185. Coquard R, Ayzac L, Gilly FN, et al: Intraoperative radiation therapy combined with limited lymph node resection in gastric cancer: an alternative to extended dissection? Int J Radiat Oncol Biol Phys 39:1093-1098, 1997.
186. Chambert M, Schmitt T, Soglu M, et al: Intraoperative radiation therapy (IORT) for locally advanced gastric cancer. 6th International IORT Symposium and 31st San Francisco Cancer Symposium [Abstracts]. San Francisco, September 23-25, 1996.
187. Abe M, Nishimura Y, Shibamoto Y: Intraoperative radiation therapy for gastric cancer. World J Surg 19(4):544-547, 1995.
188. Monson JRT, Donohue JH, McIlrath DC, et al: Total gastrectomy for advanced cancer. A worthwhile palliative procedure. Cancer 68:1863, 1991.
189. Wieland C, Hymmen U: Megavoltage therapy for malignant gastric tumors. Strahlentherapie 40:20, 1970.
190. Takahashi T: Studies on preoperative and postoperative telecobalt therapy in gastric cancer. Nipon Acta Radiol 24:129, 1964.
191. Moertel CG, Childs DS Jr, Reitemeier RJ, et al: Combined 5-fluorouracil and supervoltage radiation therapy of locally unresectable gastrointestinal cancer. Lancet 2:865, 1969.
192. Holbrook MA: Radiation therapy. Current concepts in cancer. Gastric cancer: Treatment principles. JAMA 228:1289, 1974.
193. Schein PS, Novak J (for GITSG): Combined modality therapy (XRT-chemo) versus chemotherapy alone for locally unresectable gastric cancer. Cancer 49:1771, 1982.
194. Chevalier TL, Smith FP, Harter WK, Schein PS: Chemotherapy and combined modality therapy for locally advanced and metastatic gastric carcinoma. Semin Oncol 12:46, 1985.
195. The Gastrointestinal Tumor Study Group: The concept of locally advanced gastric cancer. Cancer 66:2324, 1990.
196. Bleiberg H, Goffin JC, Dalesie O, et al: Adjuvant radiotherapy and chemotherapy in resectable gastric cancer. Eur J Surg Oncol 15:535, 1989.
197. O'Connell MJ, Gunderson LL, Moertel CG, et al: A pilot study of intensive combined therapy for locally unresectable gastric cancer. Int J Radiat Oncol Biol Phys 11:1827, 1985.
198. Moertel CG, Gunderson LL, Malliard JA, et al: Early evaluation of combined fluorouracil and leucovorin as a radiation enhancer for locally unresectable, residual, or recurrent gastrointestinal carcinoma. J Clin Oncol 12:21, 1994.
199. Henning GT, Schild SF, Stafford SL, Gunderson LL: Results of irradiation or chemoirradiation for primary unresectable, locally recurrent or grossly incomplete resection of gastric adenocarcinomas. Int J Radiat Oncol Biol Phys 46:109-118, 2000.
200. Wilke H, Preusser P, Fink U, et al: Preoperative chemotherapy in locally advanced or non-resectable gastric cancer: a phase II study with etoposide, doxorubicin, and cisplatin. J Clin Oncol 7:1318, 1989.
201. Verschueren R, Willemse P, Sleijfer D, et al: Combined chemotherapeutic-surgical approach of locally advanced gastric cancer. Proc Am Soc Clin Oncol 7:355, 1988.
202. Ducreux M, Rougier P, Lasser P, et al: Neoadjuvant chemotherapy in locally advanced gastric carcinoma: does it increase long-term survival? Proc Am Soc Clin Oncol 12:670, 1993.
203. Kang YK, Choi DW, Kim CM, et al: the effect of neoadjuvant chemotherapy on the surgical outcome of locally advanced gastric adenocarcinoma: interim report of a randomized controlled arm. Proc Am Soc Clin Oncol 11:505, 1992.
204. Kang YK, Choi DW, Im YH, et al: A phase III randomized comparison of neoadjuvant therapy followed by surgery versus surgery for locally advanced stomach cancer. Proc ASCO 15:215, 1996.
205. Rougier PH, Mahjoubi M, Lasser PH, et al: Neoadjuvant chemotherapy in locally advanced gastric carcinoma—a phase II trial with combined continuous intravenous 5-fluorouracil and bolus cisplatin. Eur J Cancer 30A:1269-1275, 1994.

206. Ajani JA, Ota DM, Jessup JM, et al: Resectable gastric carcinoma. An evaluation of preoperative and postoperative chemotherapy. Cancer 68:1501, 1991.
207. Ajani JA, Mayer RJ, Ota DM, et al: Preoperative and postoperative combination chemotherapy for potentially resectable gastric carcinoma. J Natl Cancer Inst 85:1839, 1993.
208. Schwartz G, Kelsen D, Christman K, et al: A phase II study of neoadjuvant FAMTx (5-fluorouracil, Adriamycin, methotrexate) and postoperative intraperitoneal 5-FU and cisplatin in high risk patients with gastric cancer. Proc Am Soc Clin 12:572, 1993.
209. Kelsen D, Karpeh M, Schwartz G, et al: Neoadjuvant therapy of high risk gastric cancer: a phase II trial of preoperative FAMTx and postoperative intraperitoneal fluorouracil-cisplatin plus intravenous fluorouracil. J Clin Oncol 14:1818-1828, 1996.
210. Leichman L, Silberman H, Leichman CG: Preoperative systemic chemotherapy followed by adjuvant postoperative intraperitoneal therapy for gastric cancer: a University of Southern California pilot program. J Clin Oncol 10:1933, 1992.
211. Crookes P, Leichman GC, Leichman L, et al: Systemic chemotherapy for gastric carcinoma followed by postoperative intraperitoneal therapy. A final report. Cancer 79:1767-1775, 1997.
212. Fink U, Schumacher C, Stein HJ, et al: Preoperative chemotherapy for stage III-IV gastric carcinoma: feasibility, response and outcome after complete resection. Br J Surg 82:1248-1275, 1995.
213. Songun I, Keizer HJ, Hermans J, et al: Chemotherapy for operable gastric cancer: results of the Dutch randomised FAMTX trial. The Dutch Gastric Cancer Group (DGCG). Eur J Cancer 35:558, 1999.
214. Yano M, Shiozaki H, Inoue M, et al: Neoadjuvant chemotherapy followed by salvage surgery: effect on survival of patients with primary noncurative gastric cancer. World J Surg 26:1155, 2002.
215. Preusser P, Wilke H, Achterrath W, et al: Phase II study with the combination etoposide, doxorubicin, and cisplatin in advanced measurable gastric cancer. J Clin Oncol 7:1310-1317, 1989.
216. Wilke H, Preusser P, Fink U, et al: Neoadjuvant chemotherapy of primarily unresectable gastric cancer. *In* Proceedings of the International Conference on Biology and Treatment of Gastrointestinal Malignancies, Frankfurt, Germany, 1992.
217. Smith JW, Brennan MF, Botet JF, et al: Preoperative endoscopic ultrasound can predict the risk of recurrence after operation for gastric carcinoma. J Clin Oncol 11:2380, 1993.
218. Ajani JA, Mansfield PF, Janjan N, et al: Preoperative chemoradiation therapy in patients with potentially resectable gastric carcinoma: a multi-institutional pilot. Proc ASCO 17:283a, 1998.
219. Ell C, Hochberger J, May, et al: Coated and uncoated self-expanding metal stents for malignant stenosis in the upper GI tract: preliminary clinical experiences with wall stents. Am J Gastroenterol 89:1496-1500, 1994.
220. Gastrointestinal Tumor Study Group: Phase II-III chemotherapy studies in advanced gastric cancer. Cancer Treat Rep 63:1871, 1979.
221. Moertel CG, Lavin PT: Phase II-III chemotherapy studies in advanced gastric cancer. Cancer Treat Rep 63:1863, 1979.
222. Schein PS, Smith FP, Woolley PV, Ahlgren JD: Current management of advanced and locally unresectable gastric carcinoma. Cancer 50:2590, 1982.
223. Comis RL, Carter SK: Integration of chemotherapy into combined modality treatment of solid tumors. III. Gastric cancer. Cancer Treat Rev 1:221, 1974.
224. MacDonald JS, Havlin KA: Etoposide in gastric cancer. Semin Oncol 19:59, 1992.
225. MacDonald JS, Schein PS, Woolley PV, et al: 5-fluorouracil, mitomycin C and Adriamycin (FAM): a new combination chemotherapy program for advanced gastric carcinoma. Ann Intern Med 93:533, 1980.
226. Kelsen D: The use of chemotherapy in the treatment of advanced gastric cancer and pancreatic cancer. Semin Oncol 21 (suppl 7):58-66, 1994.
227. Sulkes A, Cavalli F, van Oosterom A, et al: Taxotere is active in advanced gastric carcinoma: Results of a phase II clinical trial. Eur J Cancer 23A (suppl 6):S101, 1993.
228. Kambe M, Wakui A, Nakao I, et al: A late phase II study of irinotecan (CPT-11) in patients with advanced gastric cancer. Proc Am Soc Clin Oncol 12:198, 1993.
229. Kovach JS, Moertel CG, Schutt AJ: A controlled study of combined 1.3-bis-2-chloroethyl-nitrosourea and 5-fluorouracil therapy for advanced gastric and pancreatic cancer. Cancer 33:563, 1974.
230. The Gastrointestinal Tumor Study Group: A comparative clinical assessment of combination of chemotherapy in the management of advanced gastric carcinoma. Cancer 49:1362, 1982.
231. Levi JA, Dalley DN, Aronev RS: Improved combination chemotherapy in advanced gastric cancer. Br Med J 2:1471, 1979.
232. Moertel CG, Rubin J, O'Connell MJ, et al: A phase II study of combined 5-fluorouracil, doxorubicin, and cisplatin in the treatment of advanced upper gastrointestinal adenocarcinomas. J Clin Oncol 4:1053, 1986.
233. Rougier P, Droz JP, Theodore C, et al: A Phase II trial of combined 5-fluorouracil plus doxorubicin plus cisplatin (FAP regimen) in advanced gastric carcinoma. Cancer Treat Rep 71:1301, 1987.
234. Woolley PV, Smith F, Estevez R: A phase II trial of 5-FU, Adriamycin, and cisplatin (FAP) in advanced gastric carcinoma. Proc Am Soc Clin 22:455, 1981.
235. Wils JA, Klein HO, Wagener DJT, et al: Sequential high-dose methotrexate and fluorouracil combined with doxorubicin—a step ahead in the treatment of advanced gastric cancer: a trial of the European Organization for Research and Treatment of Cancer. J Clin Oncol 9:827, 1991.
236. Kelsen D, Atiq O, Saltz L, et al: FAMTx versus etoposide, doxorubicin, and cisplatin: a random assignment trial in gastric cancer. J Clin Oncol 10:541-548, 1992.
237. Wilke H, Preusser P, Stahl M, et al: Etoposide, folinic acid, and 5-fluorouracil in carboplatin-pretreated patients with advanced gastric cancer. Cancer Chemother Pharmacol 29:83, 1991.
238. Cullinan S, Moertel CG, Fleming T, et al: A randomized comparison of 5-FU alone (F), 5-FU + Adriamycin (FA), and 5-FU + Adriamycin + mitomycin C (FAM) in gastric and pancreatic cancer. Proc Am Soc Clin Oncol 3:137, 1984.
239. Kim NK, Park YS, Heo DS, et al: A phase III randomized study of 5-fluorouracil and cisplatin versus 5-fluorouracil, doxorubicin, and mitomycin C versus 5-fluorouracil alone in the treatment of advanced gastric cancer. Cancer 71:3813, 1993.
240. Findlay M, Cunningham D: Chemotherapy of carcinoma of the stomach. Cancer Treat Rev 19:29, 1993.
241. Delasi V, Coconi G, Tonato M, et al: Randomized comparison of 5-FU alone or combined with carmustine, doxorubicin, and mitomycin (BAFM1) in the treatment of advanced gastric cancer: a phase III trial of the Italian Clinical Research Oncology Group (GOIRC). Cancer Treat Rep 70:481, 1986.
242. Machover D, Goldschmidt E, Chollet P, et al: Treatment of advanced colorectal and gastric adenocarcinomas with 5-fluorouracil and high-dose folinic acid. J Clin Oncol 4:685, 1986.
243. Wils JA: Perspectives in chemotherapy of advanced gastric cancer. Anti-Cancer Drugs 2:133, 1991.
244. Klein HO: Long-term results with FAMTx (5-fluorouracil, Adriamycin, methotrexate) in advanced gastric cancer. Anticancer Res 9:1025-1026, 1989.
245. Stahl M, Wilke H, Preusser P, et al: Etoposide, leucovorin and 5-fluorouracil (ELF) in advanced gastric carcinoma—final results of a phase II study in elderly patients or patients with cardiac risk. Onkologie 14:314-318, 1991.
246. Van Cutsem E, Filez L, Dewyspelaere J, et al: Etoposide, leucovorin and 5-fluorouracil in advanced gastric cancer: a phase II study. Anticancer Res 15:1079, 1995.
247. Chiou TJ, Tung SL, Hsieh RK, et al: Phase II study of the modified regimen of etoposide, leucovorin and 5-fluorouracil for patients with advanced gastric cancer. Jpn J Clin Oncol 28:318, 1998.
248. Au E, Koo WH, Tan EH, et al: a phase II trial of etoposide, leucovorin and 5-fluorouracil (ELF) in patients with advanced gastric cancer. J Chemother 8:300, 1996.
249. Wilke H, Wils J, Rougier P, et al: Preliminary analysis of a randomized phase III trial of FAMTx versus ELF versus cisplatin/FU in advanced gastric cancer. A trial of the EORTC Gastrointestinal Tract Cancer Cooperative Group and the AIO (Arbeitsgemeinschaft Internistische Onkologie). Proc ASCO 14:206, 1995.

250. Findlay M, Cunningham D, Scarffe JH, et al: A phase II study in advanced gastroesophageal cancer using epirubicin and cisplatin in combination with continuous infusion 5-fluorouracil (ECF). Ann Oncol 5:609-616, 1994.
251. Webb A, Cunningham D, Scarffe JH, et al: Randomized trial comparing epirubicin, cisplatin, and fluorouracil versus fluorouracil, doxorubicin, and methotrexate in advanced esophagogastric cancer. J Clin Oncol 15:261-267, 1997.
252. Cascinu S, Labianca R, Alessandroni P, et al: Intensive weekly chemotherapy for advanced gastric cancer using fluorouracil, cisplatin, epi-doxorubicin, 6s-leucovorin, glutathione, and filgrastim. A report from the Italian Group for the Study of Digestive Tract Cancer. J Clin Oncol 15:3313-3319, 1997.
253. Ridwelski K, Gebauer T, Fahlke J, et al: Combination chemotherapy with docetaxel and cisplatin for locally advanced and metastatic gastric cancer. Ann Oncol 12:47, 2001.
254. Kornek GV, Raderer M, Schull B, et al: Effective combination chemotherapy with paclitaxel and cisplatin with or without human granulocyte colony-stimulating factor and or erythropoietiu in patients with advanced gastric cancer. Br J Cancer 86:1858, 2002.
255. Yamao T, Shirao K, Matsumura Y, et al: Phase I-II study of irinotecan combined with mitomycin-C in patients with advanced gastric cancer. Ann Oncol 12:1729, 2001.
256. Murad AM, Santiago FF, Petroianu A, et al: Modified therapy with 5-fluorouracil, doxorubicin and methotrexate in advanced gastric cancer. Cancer 72:37, 1993.
257. Pyrhonen S, Kuitunen T, Nyandoto P, et al: Randomized comparison of fluorouracil, epidoxorubicin and methotrexate (FEMTX) plus supportive care with supportive care alone in patients with non-resectable gastric cancer. Br J Cancer 71:587, 1995.
258. Glimelius B, Ekstrom K, Hoffman K, et al: Randomized comparison between chemotherapy plus best supportive care with best supportive care in advanced gastric cancer. Ann Oncol 8:163, 1997.
259. Park JO, Chung HC, Cho JY, et al: Retrospective comparison of infusional 5-fluorouracil, doxorubicin, and mitomycin-C (modified FAM) combination chemotherapy versus palliative therapy in treatment of advanced gastric cancer. Am J Clin Oncol 20:484, 1997.
260. Tepper JE, Gunderson LL: Radiation treatment parameters in the adjuvant postoperative therapy of gastric cancer. Semin Rad Oncol 12:187-195, 2002.
261. Gunderson LL, Martenson JA: Gastrointestinal tract radiation tolerance. *In* Vaeth JM, Meyer JL (eds): Radiation Tolerance of Normal Tissues, vol. 23. Basel, Karger, 1989, p 277.
262. Willett CG, Tepper JE, Orlow EL, Shipley WU: Renal complications secondary to radiation treatment of upper abdominal malignancies. Int J Radiat Oncol Biol Phys 12:1601, 1986.
263. Surakovic Z, Bramble MG, Jones R, et al: Improving the detection rate of early gastric cancer requires more than open access gastroscopy: a five-year study. Gut 41:308-313, 1997.
264. Noda M, Kodama T, Atsumi M, et al: Possibilities and limitations of endoscopic resection for early gastric cancer. Endoscopy 29:361-365, 1997.
265. Kitamura K, Yamaguchi T, Nishida S, et al: Early gastric cancer mimicking advanced gastric cancer. Br J Cancer 75:1769-1773, 1997.
266. Seto Y, Nagawa H, Muto T: Impact of lymph node metastasis on survival with early gastric cancer. World J Surg 21:186-189, 1997.
267. Guadagni S, Catarci M, Kinoshita T, et al: Cause of death and recurrence after surgery for early gastric cancer. World J Surg 21:434-439, 1997.
268. Gunderson LL: Gastric cancer—patterns of relapse after surgical resection. Semin Rad Oncol 12:150-161, 2002.
269. Fuchs C, Fitzgerald TJ, Mamon H et al: Postoperative adjuvant chemoradiation for gastric or gastroesophageal adenocarcinoma using epirubicin, cisplatin and infusional 5-fluorouracil (ECF) before and after 5-FU and radiotherapy: a multicenter pilot study. ASCO abstract #1029. J Clin Oncol 22:257, 2003.
270. Kim S, Lim KH, Lee J, et al: An observational study suggesting clinical benefit for adjuvant postoperative chemoradiation in a population of over 500 cases after gastric resection with D2 nodal dissection for adenocarcinoma of the stomach. Int J Rad Onc Biol Phys 63:1279-1285, 2005.
271. Cunningham D, Allum WH, Stenning SP, et al: Perioperative chemotherapy in operable gastric and lower esophageal cancer: Final results of a randomized controlled trial (the MAGIC trial, ISRCTN93793971). ASCO Abstracts. J Clin Oncol 23:308, 2005.
272. Krasna M, Tepper JE, Niedzwiecki D, et al: Trimodality therapy is superior to surgery alone in esophageal cancer: results of CALGB 987. Gastrointestinal Cancer Symposium. Abstract #4, p 83, 2006.

CHAPTER 45

PANCREATIC CANCER

Ross A. Abrams and Julia Choo

INCIDENCE AND EPIDEMIOLOGY

The American Cancer Society estimated 33,730 new cases of pancreatic cancer and 32,300 pancreatic cancer deaths in the United States for 2006 (10th most common cancer in both men and women, 4th most common cause of cancer death in men, and 5th most common in women).

Incidence rates are highest in Western and industrialized countries; there are clear associations with cigarette smoking, high dietary fat intake, diabetes mellitus, and chronic pancreatitis.

BIOLOGIC CHARACTERISTICS AND MOLECULAR MECHANISMS

Prognosis is determined by resectability (5% to 25% of cases); surgical resection is a sine qua non for chance of cure.

Pathologic features related to prognosis include margin and nodal status, tumor size, differentiation, and DNA content.

The *TP16* tumor suppressor gene on chromosome 9p is inactivated in about 95% of pancreatic cancers.

Among oncogenes, the most frequently activated in pancreatic adenocarcinoma is *K-ras* (90%).

Molecular abnormalities may be used to define the precursors of infiltrating adenocarcinoma of the pancreas, to help characterize histologically ambiguous lesions, as the basis for new screening tests and as important epidemiologic tools.

STAGING EVALUATION

Staging should include history and physical examination, complete blood count, serum chemistries, and chest radiography or chest computed tomography (CT) and helical CT with contrast of the abdomen and pelvis.

For patients who present with apparently resectable pancreatic mass lesions, preoperative biopsy is not required for those proceeding directly to surgery. Biopsy to confirm diagnosis is required in anticipation of neoadjuvant therapy or for patients with locoregionally unresectable or metastatic disease. Possible biopsy approaches include CT or ultrasound guidance or at the time of endoscopic retrograde cholangiopancreatography.

CA 19-9 is of limited value as a screening tool, because it may be elevated by pancreatitis, poorly controlled diabetes, and/or obstruction of the pancreaticobiliary tree and may be falsely negative in patients lacking Lewis antigens. Nevertheless, when elevated due to pancreatic cancer, it is widely used to assist in following therapeutic response and disease course.

PRIMARY THERAPY

Surgery is the primary therapy for resectable pancreas cancers. Two-year survival rates range from 20% to 40% with surgery alone. Despite resection, local recurrence and/or distant metastases occur in up to 80% to 90% of patients. Dominant sites of relapse include liver, regional tissues and nodes, peritoneum, and lung.

ADJUVANT THERAPY (CHEMOTHERAPY, IRRADIATION)

On the basis of patterns of failure after surgery alone, adjuvant chemoradiation has been tested in both randomized and nonrandomized studies. Controversy exists as to the benefit of postoperative, adjuvant chemoradiation and available phase III randomized studies have not resolved this controversy.

LOCALLY ADVANCED DISEASE

External beam radiation therapy plus 5-fluorouracil chemotherapy doubles the median survival of patients with unresectable pancreas cancer, achieves a 2-year survival of 10% to 20%, and is effective in palliating symptoms of pain.

Chemoradiation, chemotherapy alone, intraoperative radiation therapy, and radioactive implants have been evaluated in this context. Therapeutic selection among these options seems to relate primarily to patient presentation and performance status, in conjunction with physician and institution preference.

PALLIATION, SUPPORT, AND CHEMOTHERAPY

Gastric and/or biliary bypass or stenting may be indicated to relieve obstruction. Average survival of patients with metastatic presentations in liver, lung, or peritoneum ranges from 3 to 6 months.

Best supportive care requires attention to medical issues before and during antineoplastic therapy for optimal intervention and opportunity for benefit. Important management issues typically include pain, nausea, depression, fat malabsorption, weight loss, hyperglycemia, susceptibility to dehydration, and jaundice.

Pancreatic adenocarcinoma remains a significant clinical challenge, as the natural history of the disease is characterized by early spread to regional lymphatics, liver, and peritoneal surfaces. The majority of patients have clinical or subclinical liver metastases at the time of diagnosis. Outcome appears to be determined primarily by the extent of evident disease and performance status at presentation. Patients with resectable tumors represent only 15% to 20% of those with pancreatic cancer, and although treatment is clearly curative in intent, this goal is infrequently achieved. Other than surgical resection, optimal treatment remains controversial.[1] Most (75% to 80%) pancreatic adenocarcinoma presents in the head, neck, and/or uncinate process (periampullary region), and data and results from these presentations form the basis for clinical management decisions. The data set for management decisions regarding presentations in the distal pancreatic body and tail is much less robust. The anatomic relationships of the pancreas are well illustrated in Figure 45-1.

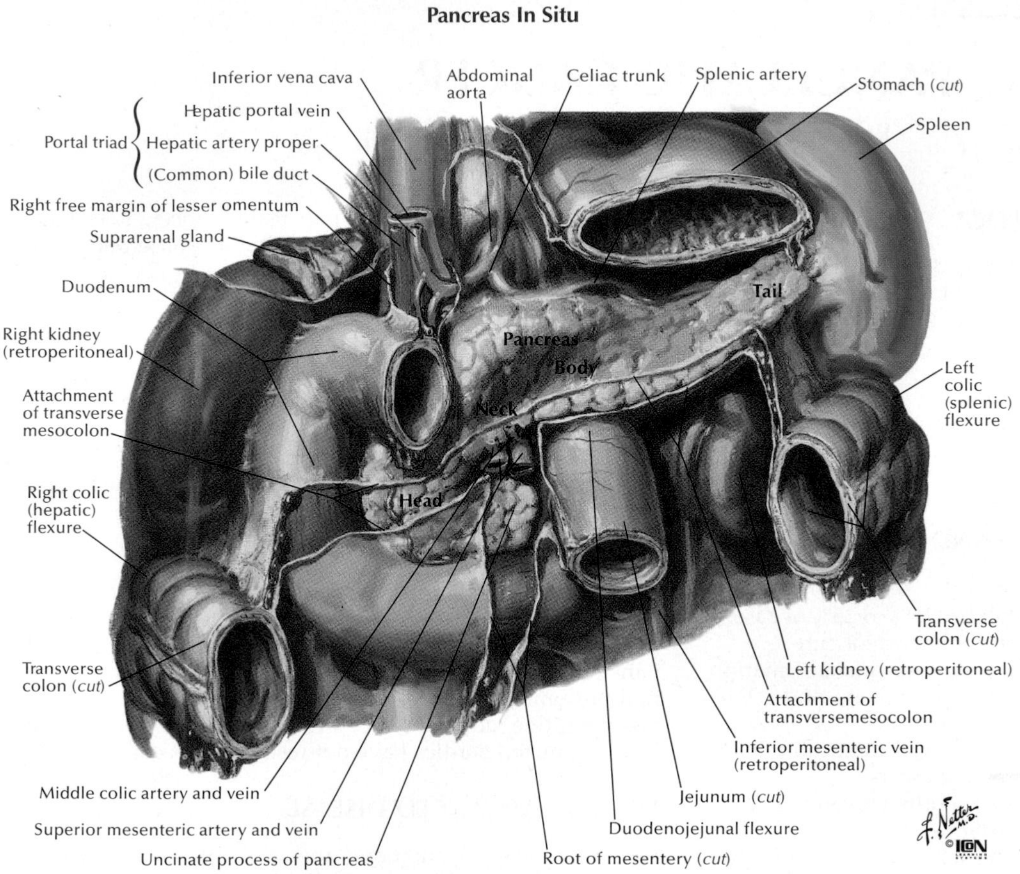

Figure 45-1 From Atlas of Human Anatomy by Frank H. Netter, MD, CIBA-GEIGY Corporation, West Caldwell, New Jersey, plate 279, 1992.

EPIDEMIOLOGY AND ETIOLOGY

Epidemiology

In 2006 there were an estimated 33,730 new cases of pancreatic carcinoma in the United States with slightly more cases in women than in men.[2] The number of deaths due to carcinoma of the pancreas was estimated to be nearly the same at 32,300. In the United States, it was anticipated that carcinoma of the pancreas would be the tenth most frequently diagnosed new cancer in men and women. In contrast, it was anticipated that carcinoma of the pancreas would be the fourth leading cause of cancer death in men (after lung and bronchus, prostate, and colon and rectum) and the fifth leading cause of cancer death in women (after lung and bronchus, breast, colon and rectum, and ovary). In the United States, the age-adjusted cancer death rates for this malignancy have been relatively constant in both men and women since roughly the 1970s.[2]

Most patients with pancreatic carcinoma present with advanced stage disease and only 14% of patients undergo resection with curative intent. About 75% to 80% of all pancreatic adenocarcinomas will present in the head, neck, or [illegible]cinate process of the pancreas (periampullary region), with [illegible]mainder roughly evenly divided between the body and [illegible] pancreas. Approximately 68% of cases will be diag-[illegible]nts 65 years of age or older. Patients undergo-[illegible]ction have a clear survival advantage as [illegible]ts not undergoing resection. The 1-, 2-, [illegible]f patients undergoing resection as com-[illegible]t undergoing resection are 48% versus [illegible], and 17% versus 6%, respectively.[3]

Etiology

Incidence rates of pancreatic cancer increase with age, and most cases occur in patients older than 60 years of age. Internationally, incidence rates are highest in Western and industrialized countries. All ethnic groups in the United States except Japanese Americans experience a high incidence of pancreas carcinoma.

Pancreatic cancer is clearly associated with cigarette smoking, dietary intake (higher risk with higher percentages of fat and meat in the diet), peptic ulcer surgery, diabetes mellitus, and chronic pancreatitis. Of these, the strongest association is with cigarette smoking. There is also an occupational association with the manufacture of 2-naphthylamine and benzidine and with those working with gasoline derivatives.[4] Although coffee consumption has sometimes been implicated in the occurrence of carcinoma of the pancreas, a review failed to confirm this association.[5]

There is an increased risk of developing pancreatic cancer, as well as other intra-abdominal malignancies, following radiation therapy to the abdomen for management of testicular malignancy, either seminoma or nonseminoma. The risk is noted as early as 10 years after management and continues to increase with time. For carcinoma of the pancreas, the observed to expected frequency is 2.21.[6]

An important development in our understanding of the etiology of pancreatic cancer is the recognition of familial pancreatic cancer.[7] Familial pancreatic cancer may occur in the absence of a recognizable clinical syndrome. As many as 10% of pancreatic cancers may be familial. Data from the National Familial Pancreas Tumor Registry have shown that the risk of cancer is 18-fold greater in first-degree relatives of familial pancreatic cancer cases (at least two first-degree relatives with pancreatic cancer in the family) than it is in first-degree relatives of sporadic pancreatic cancer cases (families in which there has been only one member with pancreatic cancer).[8] In addition, there are associations with other known syndromes such as the familial breast, ovarian, pancreas cancer syndrome associated with *BRCA2,* the familial pancreas cancer syndrome associated with *TP16* abnormalities, the Peutz-Jeghers polyposis gastrointestinal (GI) malignancy syndrome associated with mismatched repair genes, *LKB1/STK11,* and the hereditary nonpolyposis colon cancer (HNPCC) syndrome.

PREVENTION AND EARLY DETECTION

Although the above associations might permit identification of a patient population suitable for screening in the future, no simple, cost-effective test for the disease has been successful in establishing early diagnosis.[9] Potential imaging modalities for screening and early detection include computed tomography (CT) scan, magnetic resonance imaging (MRI), and endoscopic ultrasonography (EUS). For early detection, EUS may be the imaging modality of choice because it detects smaller pancreatic lesions than those detected with thin-section, dual-phase spiral CT. The accuracy of diagnosis of pancreatic cancer in patients with pancreatic masses suspected of having cancer is close to 100% for EUS and about 92% for dual-phase CT.[10] When combined with fine needle aspiration (FNA), EUS can provide a cytologic diagnosis of lesions as small as 2 to 5 mm not visualized by CT, US, or MRI. Endoscopic retrograde cholangiopancreatography (ERCP) is less likely to detect small tumors and is a relatively more invasive screening test due to the risk of developing pancreatitis (5% to 10%) but may be useful for detailed characterization of ductal abnormalities. Positron emission tomography (PET) may be useful in identifying otherwise occult metastases.

Serum carbohydrate antigen 19-9 (CA 19-9) is a tumor-associated antigen that is frequently elevated in patients with pancreatic adenocarcinoma.[11] It may also be elevated in biliary tract malignancies, some colon cancers, and non–cancer-related conditions such as pancreatitis, cholangitis, poorly controlled diabetes, and biliary obstruction due to benign causes (stones, strictures). Patients genetically lacking Lewis antigens may be incapable of producing CA 19-9. Nevertheless, CA 19-9 is often used to help monitor therapeutic response in patients with histologically proven pancreatic cancer who present with elevated levels.[12,13]

Biomarkers for early detection targeting are in development and include DNA-, RNA-, and protein-based approaches. DNA-based techniques aim to detect cancer-specific DNA alterations and methylation changes.[14] Analysis of pancreatic juice or fine needle aspirates may identify genes overexpressed at the RNA level in pancreatic cancers compared with normal pancreas.[15] Protein-based markers may also be overexpressed in pancreatic cancer patients compared with patients with other pancreatic diseases.[16]

BIOLOGIC CHARACTERISTICS AND MOLECULAR BIOLOGY

A number of studies have looked at DNA content and proliferative index in patients with pancreatic cancer. Bottger and associates[17] studied DNA content, tumor size, lymph node status, tumor stage, nuclear grade, and type of resection on outcomes in a series of 41 patients with adenocarcinoma of the pancreas. They observed that in univariate analysis, these factors had a significant ($p < .05$) association with outcome. However, in multivariate analysis, the most important predictors of outcome were the operative procedure (whether the tumor was resected to histologically negative margins) and the DNA content (whether the patient's tumor was tetraploid, having unfavorable prognostic implications). Similarly, Jorba and colleagues[18] found that among 73 patients undergoing pancreaticoduodenectomy for periampullary malignancies, 74% were diploid and 26% were aneuploid. In univariate analysis, there was a strong correlation between diploid status and long-term survival, with diploid cancer patients having a median survival of 30.1 months and aneuploid cancer patients having a median survival of 16 months. However, when tumor site (duodenum and ampulla versus bile duct and pancreas) and tumor size were taken into consideration, the effect of ploidy no longer produced a significant difference.

In contrast, Herrera and associates[19] failed to show a prognostic difference between patients with pancreatic cancer who had diploid tumors and those who had nondiploid tumors. Their study was performed on 62 paraffin-embedded specimens resected between 1951 and 1980 at the Mayo Clinic. They identified 19 patients surviving 3 or more years and 43 patients who died within 12 months of resection. In addition to not being able to show a survival advantage based on ploidy, they also failed to show a survival difference based on fraction of cells in S-phase or a difference of DNA index.

Pancreatic ductal adenocarcinoma is a genetic disease and a substantial amount of work has gone into defining its associated molecular biology. As summarized by Hruban,[20] cancer of the pancreas can now be viewed as a disease of acquired and inherited mutations involving a number of cancer-related genes. There are three types of such genes: tumor suppressor genes, oncogenes, and DNA mismatch repair genes. Tumor suppressor genes function to restrain cell proliferation. Oncogenes possess transforming properties when activated by mutation or amputation. DNA mismatch repair genes encode for proteins that correct errors that normally occur during DNA replication. All three types of potentially cancer-causing genes have been implicated in pancreatic cancer.

A number of suppressor genes have been found to play a role in the development of pancreatic cancer. A summary of the tumor suppressor genes in pancreatic cancer are listed in Table 45-1.[21] The *TP16* tumor suppressor gene on chromosome 9p is inactivated in approximately 95% of pancreatic cancers. The mechanism by which p16 inactivation promotes cell cycle progression is shown in Figure 45-2.[21]

The *TP53* gene located on chromosome 17p is inactivated in 50% to 70% of pancreatic cancers. The *DPC4* gene on chromosome 18q is inactivated in approximately 50% of pancreatic cancers. *DPC4* is now known as *SMAD4* and has been found to be of prognostic significance, with *SMAD4*-positive patients having improved survival over *SMAD4*-negative patients. Moreover, *SMAD4* positivity retains its prognostic significance in multivariate analysis adjusting for tumor size, lymph node involvement, margin status, and histologic differentiation.[22] The *BRCA2* gene is inactivated in 70% of pancreatic cancers. *BRCA2* is noteworthy because it represents mutation in the inherited germline in some cases. Additionally, *BRCA2* has been confirmed as the most common inherited genetic alteration associated with pancreatic cancer.[23]

Among oncogenes, the most frequently activated in pancreatic cancer is *K-ras*. Mutations convert the normal K-ras protein to an oncogene, causing the protein to become over-

Table 45-1 Tumor-Suppressor Genes in Pancreatic Cancer

Gene	Chromosome	Function	Percentage
Inactivated			
p16	9p	Cell cycle	40% HD 40% LOH and IM 15% Methylation
p53	17p	Cell cycle Apoptosis	50% to 75% LOH and IM
DPC4	18q	TGF β signaling	30% HD 20% LOH and IM
BRCA2	13q	DNA repair?	7% Germline IM
MKK4	17p	Apoptosis?	2% LOH and IM 2% HD

Hruban RH, Offerhaus JA, Kern, SE, et al: Tumor-suppressor genes in pancreatic cancer. J Hepatobiliary Pancreas Surg 5:383, 1998.

HD, homozygous deletion; IM, intragenic mutation; LOH, loss of heterozygosity.

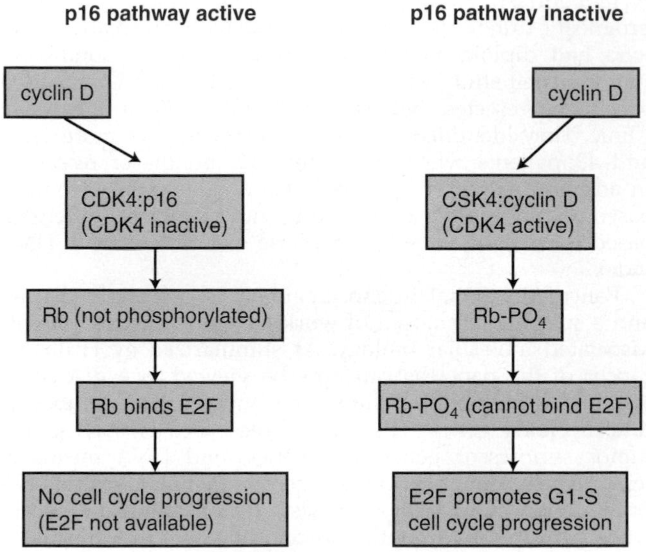

Figure 45-2 p16 inactivation promotes cell cycle progression. (Tascilar M, Skinner HG, Rosty C, et al: The SMAD4 protein and prognosis of pancreatic ductal adenocarcinoma. Clin Cancer Res 7:4115, 2001.)

active in transmitting the growth factor–initiated signals. *K-ras* activation is observed in 90% of pancreatic cancers.

Finally, abnormalities in DNA mismatch repair genes have been noted. A specific molecular phenotype called microsatellite instability, also identified in the HNPCC syndrome of colon cancer, has been found in 4% of pancreatic cancers and is associated with a unique morphologic appearance, the presence of wild-type (normal) *K-ras,* diploidy, and improved prognosis.[24]

These molecular abnormalities have several applications. They may be used to define the precursors of infiltrating adenocarcinoma of the pancreas or help characterize histologically ambiguous lesions. Moreover, they have the potential to form the basis for new screening tests for pancreatic neoplasia and subsequently, may serve as important epidemiologic tools.[20]

Just as specific genetic abnormalities have been associated with pancreatic cancer, karyotyping studies by Griffin and colleagues have shown consistent losses of chromosomes 18, 13, 12, 17, and 6.[25,26] This correlates well with the loss of the *DPC4* suppressor gene, which is known to reside on chromosome 18, and the loss of the tumor suppressor gene *TP53,* which is known to reside on chromosome 17.

There are consistent genetic and chromosome abnormalities identified with known associations of pancreatic carcinoma in families, such as the familial atypical multiple mole melanoma (FAMM) syndrome. Subsequently, there has been an increased interest in familial pancreatic carcinoma and investigators at Johns Hopkins Institutions have established a National Familial Pancreas Tumor Registry (NFPTR). As of 1998, over 150 families had been registered in which two or more first-degree relatives have been diagnosed with pancreatic cancer (familial cases). An additional 206 families had been registered in which only one family member had been diagnosed with pancreatic carcinoma (nonfamilial). An initial analysis revealed that the increased risk of pancreatic carcinoma in familial pancreatic cancer extended to second-degree relatives of the index case with 3.7% of 324 second-degree relatives of familial cases developing pancreatic cancer as compared with 0.6% of the 702 second-degree relatives of sporadic (nonfamilial) pancreatic cancers ($p < .001$).[28] In addition, there were other primary cancers that occurred in relatives of pancreatic cancer patients including breast, lung, and colon cancers. By July 2004, 1329 families had been enrolled in the NFPTR. In 528 of these families more than one first-degree relative (i.e., parent/child or siblings) had been diagnosed with pancreatic cancer and in 801 of these families a single member had been diagnosed with pancreatic cancer.[29] In an updated analysis, familial pancreatic cancer (FPC) kindreds were defined as kindreds having at least one pair of first-degree relatives with pancreatic cancer, and sporadic pancreatic cancer (SPC) kindreds as families without such an affected pair. Nineteen incident pancreatic cancers developed among 5179 individuals from 838 kindreds (at baseline, 370 FPC kindreds and 468 SPC kindreds). Of these 5179 individuals, 3957 had at least one first-degree relative with pancreatic cancer and contributed 10,538 person-years of follow-up. In this group, the observed-to-expected rate of pancreatic cancer was significantly elevated (Table 45-2) in members of FPC kindreds but not in the SPC kindreds.

PATHOLOGY AND PATHWAYS OF SPREAD

Pathology

Infiltrating ductal adenocarcinomas are the most common histologic type of malignant tumors of the exocrine pancreas, as shown in Figure 45-3. These malignant epithelial neoplasms show glandular or ductal differentiation, with most arising in the head of the pancreas.[30] Although ductal adenocarcinoma is the most common primary malignancy of the pancreas, accounting for approximately 75% of all primary nonen-

Table 45-2 Familial and Sporadic Pancreatic Cancer Rates

Kindred	Risk (95% Confidence Interval)
Familial (all)	9.0 (4.5-6.1)
Familial (3 first-degree relatives)	32.0 (10.2-74.7)
Familial (2 first-degree relatives)	6.4 (1.8-16.4)
Familial (1 first-degree relative)	4.6 (0.5-16.4)
Sporadic (0 first-degree relatives)	1.8 (0.22-6.4)
Spouse	2.4 (0.06-13.5)

Klein AP, Brune KA, Petersen GM, et al: Prospective risk of pancreatic cancer in familial pancreatic cancer kindreds. Cancer Res 64:2634, 2004.

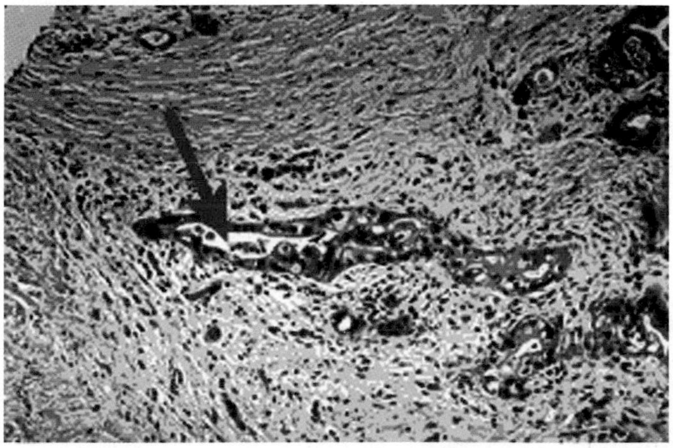

Figure 45-3 Pancreatic adenocarcinoma. When viewed under the microscope, cancerous cells can be seen that form small ducts. These cancers often cause scarring and inflammation (*arrow*). (Courtesy of Johns Hopkins Hospital Department of Pathology.)

docrine cancers in this organ, there are a number of other important epithelial malignancies arising in the pancreas that should be recognized because of their variant presentations and prognostic implications.[31]

Adenosquamous carcinoma is a rare histology that disseminates to lymphatics, perineural and perivascular pathways, and lymph nodes in the peritoneum much the same as is seen with standard adenocarcinoma of the pancreas. It may be seen after prior treatment with chemotherapy and radiation therapy.

Acinar cell carcinoma is also a rare histology in which 20% of cases may be associated with subcutaneous fat necrosis, a rash similar to erythema nodosum, peripheral eosinophilia, and polyarthralgias. These associated phenomena are a result of release of large amounts of lipase by the tumor.[32] These tumors typically present with large size and average dimension of 11 cm and occur in the head, body, and tail with frequencies of 60%, 30%, and 10%, respectively. Survival is not significantly superior to that seen with standard adenocarcinoma of the pancreas. Those patients presenting with large amounts of lipase production may have a less-than-average prognosis.

Giant cell carcinoma is a histology that accounts for approximately 5% of nonendocrine pancreatic cancers. These tumors also present as large sizes with an average of 11-cm diameter. These are very aggressive carcinomas with poor average survival and no 5-year survivors. Giant cell carcinoma with osteoclast-like giant cells is an extremely rare variant with an improved prognosis compared with giant cell carcinomas. These giant cells resemble the osteoclasts of resorbing bone.

The primary cystic, nonendocrine epithelial tumors are another type of pancreatic neoplasm. Only 5% to 15% of pancreatic cystic lesions are actually neoplastic, with the remaining nonneoplastic lesions including pseudocysts, congenital cysts, and retention cysts. The cystic neoplasms of the pancreas include serous and mucinous neoplasms. Most serous cystic neoplasms are serous cystadenomas, also known as microcystic adenomas and glycogen-rich cystadenomas. They occur more commonly in women with average age in the seventh decade.[33] These lesions may be large and patients with von Hippel-Lindau syndrome (familial cancer syndrome associated with clear cell renal cancer, cerebellar and spinal hemangioblastomas, pancreatic islet cell cancers, and other tumors) may be predisposed to develop serous cystadenomas. Most serous cystic neoplasms of the pancreas are benign.

In contrast, mucinous cystic neoplasms are more frequently malignant. These are also more common in women and are typically diagnosed in the fifth decade of life. Histologically, these lesions contain a mucin-positive, cloudy fluid and do not communicate with the main pancreatic duct.[34] Microscopic analysis reveals three types of mucinous cystic neoplasms: mucinous cystadenomas, borderline mucinous cystic neoplasms, and mucinous cystadenocarcinoma. It is generally thought that mucinous cystadenomas and borderline cystic neoplasms have the potential for progressing to overt malignancy and should be completely resected. Interestingly, mucinous cystadenocarcinomas are associated with a better prognosis than typical adenocarcinoma of the pancreas with roughly 50% of patients surviving 5 years.

Intraductal papillary mucinous neoplasms (IPMN) communicate with the main pancreatic duct system and are typically diagnosed in the seventh decade. They are associated with a good prognosis compared with more typical pancreatic malignancies.[35] A more aggressive variant is the papillary mucinous carcinoma where the histology displays significant cytologic and architectural atypia and/or overt invasion.

Solid and cystic papillary neoplasms are also known as Hamoudi tumors, occurring primarily in women in the third decade of life. Patients present with distention, discomfort, and/or pain. Typically, these tumors range in size from 5 to 15 cm in diameter. With surgical resection, most patients survive for many years, with metastases occurring rarely.

Other neoplasms that can be seen in the pancreas include pancreatoblastoma, a malignancy of childhood, acinar cyst adenocarcinoma—a rare variant of acinar cell carcinoma, and primary mesenteric mesenchymal tumors. Malignancies metastatic to the pancreas include primary tumors of the breast, lung, colon/rectum, stomach, and melanoma. Finally, lymphomas may compose 1% to 2% of all primary pancreatic neoplasms, with the most common type being diffuse large cell.

It has been well known that a precursor histology of intraepithelial neoplasia can be described in sites such as colon, cervix, and prostate. The precursor histology for pancreatic adenocarcinoma (PanIN) has now been well described.[36] These lesions have been named PanIN-1A and 1B, PanIN-2, and PanIN-3. They are often seen in association with invasive adenocarcinoma and have occasionally been observed to progress into invasive adenocarcinoma.

Pathways of Spread

The pancreas is a retroperitoneal organ that lies in close anatomic relationship to the stomach, duodenum, jejunum, kidneys, spleen, celiac trunk, superior mesenteric artery and vein, common bile duct, and portal vein. The main pancreatic duct is known as the duct of Wirsung, and the accessory pancreatic duct is known as the duct of Santorini. At the time of diagnosis, more than 85% of pancreas tumors will have extended into adjacent organs, lymph nodes, fat, or soft tissue, allowing early metastasis to regional and distant lymph nodes.[37]

Patterns of involvement in the regional lymphatics have long been well recognized. Frequently involved nodal sites include the posterior pancreaticoduodenal nodes, superior pancreatic head nodes, inferior pancreatic head nodes, superior pancreatic body nodes, and porta hepatic nodes.[38,39] There is also a relationship between para-aortic lymph node involvement and involvement of posterior pancreaticoduodenal nodes by direct interlymphatic communication[40] (Figure 45-4). Venous drainage of the pancreas is to the liver via the portal vein.

Patterns of failure following resection have been described with peritoneal relapse and hepatic metastases occurring in 42% and 62% of patients, respectively.[41-44] Although it is likely that the peripancreatic burden of disease has multiple direct lymphatic pathways to hepatic tissues, conventionally, hepatic involvement has been taken as a sign of systemic metastasis. The lung is the most frequently involved extra-abdominal organ.[37]

CLINICAL MANIFESTATIONS, PATIENT EVALUATION, AND STAGING

Cancer of the pancreas most often presents at an advanced stage at diagnosis. Most adenocarcinomas of the pancreas present in the periampullary region of the pancreas (head, neck, uncinate process). These patients typically present with symptoms of obstructive jaundice including pruritus, dark urine, clay-colored stools, and steatorrhea. They may also present with pain and gastric outlet obstruction. Approximately 15% to 20% of patients present with a new diagnosis of diabetes. In some cases, recent-onset depression and anxiety antedate the diagnosis of pancreatic cancer.

In contrast, tumors in the body or tail of the pancreas usually present when they are larger. For those tumors, jaundice is a late manifestation, and with body lesions, severe back pain is quite common. Tumors in the tail of the pancreas may have evidence of portal hypertension, upper GI bleeding, or splenomegaly.

Initial laboratory results may show an elevated serum bilirubin, alkaline phosphatase, and gamma glutamyl transpeptidase. In addition, the hepatic amino transferases may be increased in presenting patients. Although CA 19-9 has not proved useful as a marker for screening of pancreatic cancer, it has been used as a test to follow patients postoperatively. In general, increasing levels of CA 19-9 indicate

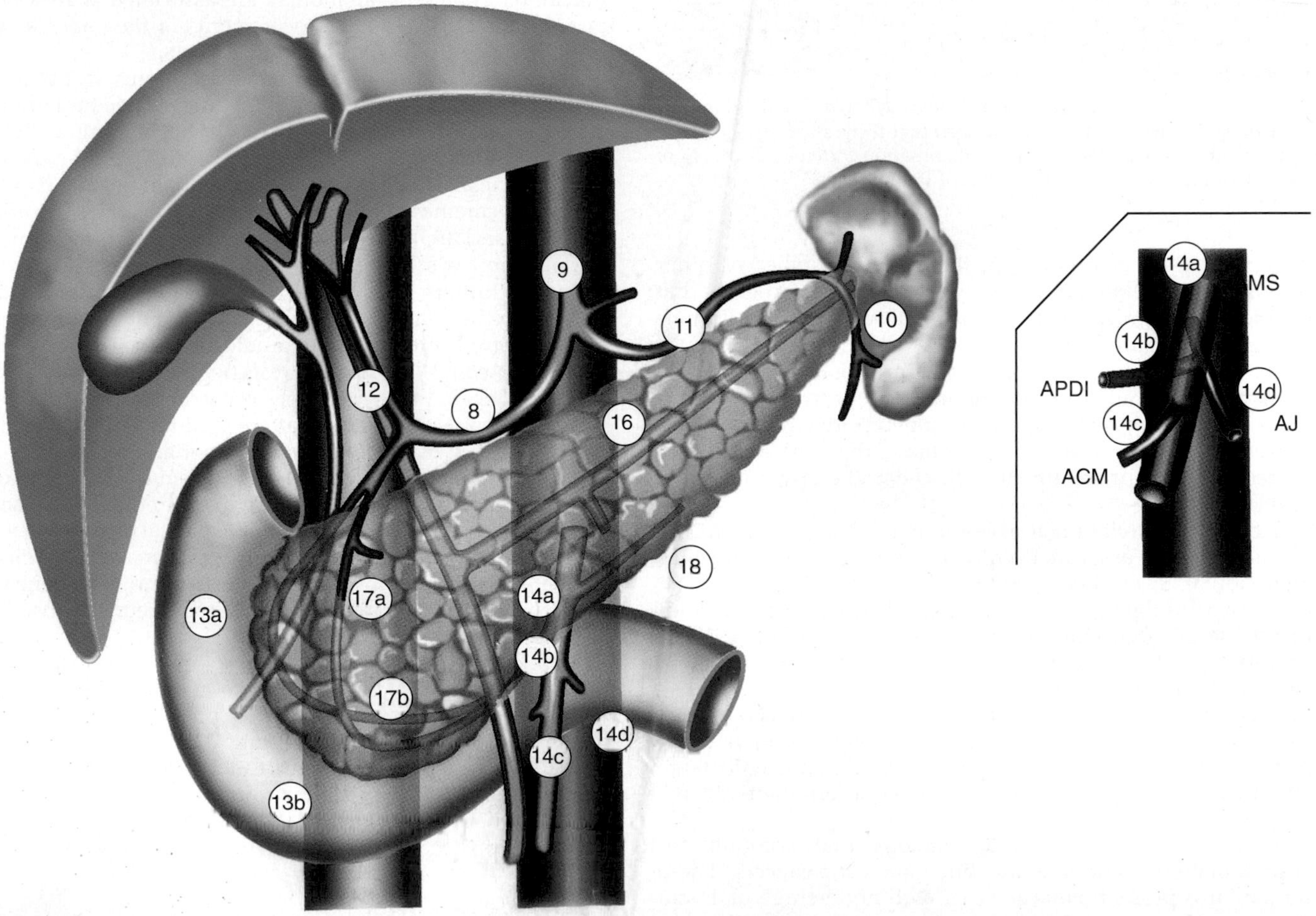

Figure 45-4 Classification of regional lymph nodes of the pancreas. *Inset*, subdivision of area 14. ACM, medial colic artery; AJ, jejunal artery; AMS, superior mesenteric artery; APDI, inferior pancreaticoduodenal artery. (From Cubilla AL, Fortner J, Fitzgerald PJ: Lymph node involvement in carcinoma of the head of the pancreas area. Cancer 41:880, 1978.)

progression of disease. Stable to declining levels of CA 19-9 are associated with a stable tumor burden and improved prognosis.[45]

Patient Evaluation

Assessment is guided by the patient's presenting symptoms, findings on history and physical exam, and initial laboratory results. US, CT scan, and ERCP are often included in the evaluation of patients with obstructive jaundice. With current spiral CT techniques combined with oral and intravenous contrast, pancreatic masses, pancreatic duct dilatation, local invasion, liver metastases, and vascular invasion of the great vessels are readily identified. ERCP is frequently used to obtain biopsy specimens, decompress the biliary tree, and localize the source of obstruction. Biliary obstruction can also be relieved by percutaneous and transhepatic cholangiography. Visceral angiography is selectively used based on concern regarding vascular invasion leading to unresectability. Laparoscopy is used in some institutions as a prelude to exploration. It appears that a tissue diagnosis by FNA prior to laparotomy is not necessary.[46]

Staging

The 2002 *AJCC Cancer Staging Handbook, Sixth Edition,* recognizes separate staging for carcinoma of the exocrine pancreas, carcinoma of the ampulla of Vater, carcinoma of the extrahepatic bile ducts, and carcinoma of the small intestine. Although there is a TNM staging system for pancreas cancer (Table 45-3), treatment and prognosis are defined by resectability and presence of distant metastatic disease, which most commonly involves the liver, peritoneum, or both.[47]

Pancreatic tumors staged as T1, T2, or T3 are generally considered to be resectable. Unresectable pancreatic tumors are those in which the tumor cannot be separated from the adjacent large arterial structures (celiac axis or superior mesenteric artery). The extent of resection also carries prognostic significance. A patient who has undergone an R0 complete resection with negative margins will have a better prognosis compared with a patient who has undergone an R1 or R2 resection with positive margins.[48]

Table 45-3 TNM Staging System for Pancreas Cancer

TX	Primary tumor cannot be assessed
T0	No evidence of primary tumor
Tis	Carcinoma in situ
T1	Tumor limited to the pancreas ≤2 cm in greatest dimension
T2	Tumor limited to the pancreas >2 cm in greatest dimension
T3	Tumor extends beyond the pancreas but without involvement of the celiac axis or the superior mesenteric artery
T4	Tumor involves the celiac axis or the superior mesenteric artery (unresectable primary tumor)
REGIONAL LYMPH NODES (N)	
NX	Regional lymph nodes cannot be assessed
N0	No regional lymph node metastasis
N1	Regional lymph node metastasis
DISTANT METASTASIS (M)	
MX	Distant metastasis cannot be assessed
M0	No distant metastasis
M1	Distant metastasis

PRIMARY THERAPY

Surgery

The classic operation for resection of a carcinoma of the head of the pancreas is a pancreaticoduodenectomy, also known as a Whipple procedure. In this operation, the gallbladder, common bile duct, second portion of the duodenum, and the head of the pancreas are resected along with either the postpyloric duodenum (pylorus-preserving pancreaticoduodenectomy) or the resection is continued proximally to include the distal stomach (classic pancreaticoduodenectomy). The regional lymph nodes are also resected. It appears well established that the pylorus-preserving pancreaticoduodenectomy improves GI function without compromise of oncologic management.[49-51] These two variants of surgical resection are shown in Figure 45-5.[52] Within the past two decades, the mortality of this operation has declined from approximately 20% to between 1% and 3% in major centers.[53-55]

It is important that the radiation oncologist understand the postsurgical anatomy. Examples of various types of anatomic connections are shown in Figure 45-6.[56] As illustrated, GI reconstruction after pancreaticoduodenectomy requires enteric, biliary, and pancreatic anastomoses. Although postoperative mortality is less than 3% at high-volume centers, the morbidity of pancreatectomy remains high, with pancreatic leak and infection, delayed gastric emptying, and pancreatic fistula among the most common complications.[57]

Surgical management of carcinoma of the body or tail of the pancreas requires a different orientation. Presenting symptoms such as jaundice or pain typically occur with larger and more locally advanced masses or evidence of overt metastatic disease. Even when explored, most patients at major centers were deemed unresectable when presenting with adenocarcinoma in the body or tail of the pancreas. If resectable, the operation performed is classically a distal pancreatectomy with en bloc splenectomy.

Prognostic Factors Associated with Results of Surgical Resection

Michelassi and colleagues[58] reported on their experience with 647 consecutive patients between 1946 and 1987 with tumors of the duodenum, ampulla, head of the pancreas, and distal common bile duct, including both resectable and nonresectable patients. The resectability rate varied from 16.5% for pancreatic adenocarcinoma to 89.3% for ampullary tumors. Among these 647 patients, there were 133 resections. Their data clearly show the importance of resection for any type of tumor presentation in the periampullary area with respect to 5-year survival. Evaluating only those patients with adenocarcinoma who underwent a curative intent resection and survived the perioperative period (n = 97), the following factors did not affect survival: tumor size, tumor differentiation, the presence of lymphovascular invasion, capillary invasion, perineural microinvasion, lymph node status, or type of procedure (pancreaticoduodenectomy versus total pancreatectomy). The authors analyzed relapse data and found that based on autopsy experience 29.4% of patients died with local recurrence alone, 23.5% died with distant metastasis alone, and 47.1% had both local and distant relapses.

Yeo and colleagues[59] have published two important papers that well summarize and describe the anticipated patient experience following surgery for periampullary malignancy. In their series of 650 consecutive pancreaticoduodenectomies in the 1990s, there were 443 patients resected for periampullary malignancy. Their data convincingly show the improved survival seen for duodenal and ampullary tumor as

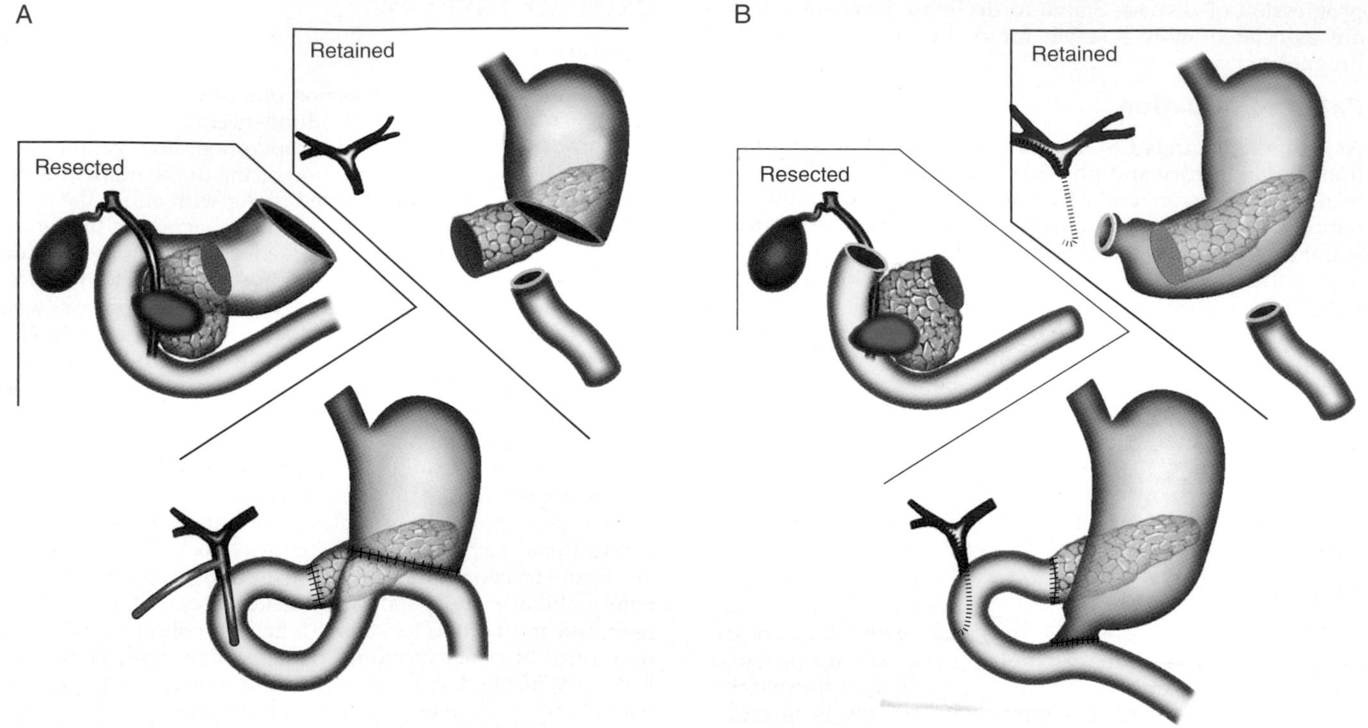

Figure 45-5 Classic pancreaticoduodenectomy **(A)** and pylorus-preserving pancreaticoduodenectomy **(B)**, showing the resected specimens, the structures retained, and one method of reconstruction by way of pancreaticojejunostomy and gastrojejunostomy. (From Yeo CJ, Cameron JL: The pancreas. *In* Hardy JD, ed: Hardy's Textbook of Surgery, 2nd ed. Philadelphia, JB Lippincott, 1988, pp. 717, 718.)

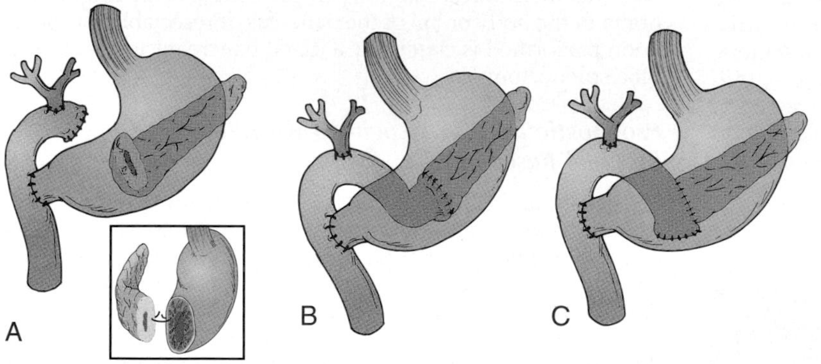

Figure 45-6 Schematic illustrations: **A,** pancreaticogastrostomy; **B,** end-to-end pancreaticojejunostomy; and **C,** end-to-side pancreaticojejunostomy. The inset details the location of the posterior gastrostomy. (From Yeo CJ, Cameron JL, Maher MM, et al: A prospective randomized trial of pancreaticogastrostomy versus pancreaticojejunostomy after pancreaticoduodenectomy. Ann Surg 222:580, 1995.)

opposed to pancreatic and distal common bile duct tumors. Moreover, in multivariate analysis, factors associated with improved survival are the absence of intraoperative blood loss greater than 700 mL, tumor site with duodenum and ampullary being better than bile duct and pancreas, tumor diameter of less than 3 cm as opposed to 3 cm or more, negative margins histologically, negative nodal status histologically, and having a well-differentiated tumor as opposed to a moderately or poorly differentiated tumor. Reoperation for complication was also significantly associated with decreased survival. Yeo and associates[60] further analyzed factors associated with long-term survival showing that negative nodal involvement is an important prognostic factor for any of the four periampullary sites. This series includes data on 242 patients operated from April 1990 though May 1992 (Fig. 45-7). In this group of patients, the median length of follow-up was 83 months for the 5-year survivors and 14 months for the patients surviving less than 5 years.

The importance of histologic differentiation, nodal involvement, and tumor size for patients with pancreatic adenocarcinoma has been demonstrated by Geer and Brennan[61] from Memorial Sloan-Kettering Cancer Center. The difference in survival at 36 months for well-differentiated tumors versus poorly differentiated tumors is roughly 50% and 10%, respectively. Less extreme but still highly significant differences are seen when comparing node-negative survivors versus node-positive survivors. At 36 months, the survivals were approximately 35% and 10%, respectively. In tumors smaller than or larger than 2.5 cm, the survival differences were 40% and 20%, respectively. This group[61a] has developed a nomogram based on data from 555 patients to predict outcome at 1, 2, or 3 years. The factors correlating with survival in their multivariate analysis are shown in Table 45-4. This nomogram can be downloaded from the web page of the Memorial Sloan-Kettering Cancer Center (www.mskcc.org).

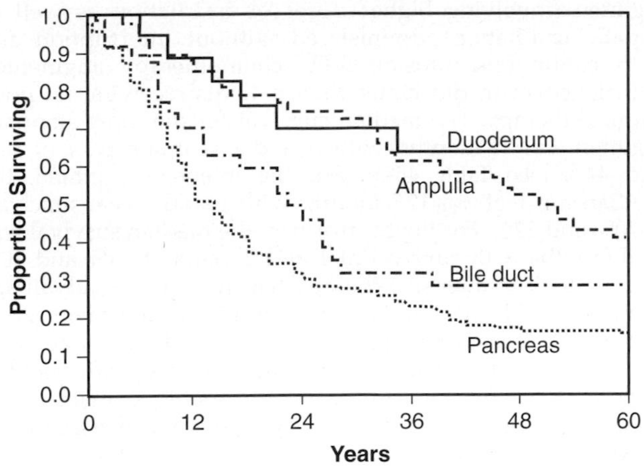

Figure 45-7 The tumor-specific actual 5-year survival curves for the cohort of 242 patients treated by pancreaticoduodenectomy for periampullary adenocarcinoma.

Table 45-4 Factors Correlating with Survival in Multivariate Analysis

Factor	*p* Value
Maximum tumor dimension	.001
No. of nodes positive	.001
Splenectomy required	.001
Differentiation	.002
Tumor located in head versus other pancreatic site	.006
Posterior margin status	.049

A second point to be emphasized was well demonstrated by Manabe and colleagues.[62] In a series of 17 cancers of the pancreas, all adenocarcinomas and all less than 2 cm in diameter, 41% of these patients had lymph node metastases, 24% capillary invasion, 24% retroperitoneal lymph node invasion, and 29% portal system involvement. It appears that in pancreatic cancer, small size does not necessarily equate with an early lesion.

Patterns of Failure after Surgical Resection

Tepper and colleagues[41] reported on 145 patients managed at the Massachusetts General Hospital (MGH) from 1963 to 1973. Of these patients, only 31 underwent radical surgery. Among these 31 patients, there were five operative deaths, leaving 26 for further analysis. Among these 26 patients, there were 13 or exactly 50% with either pathologically proven local recurrence or clinical evidence of local recurrence at the time of death from disease. In five patients, local status was unknown at the time of death. Four patients died of distant metastases without evidence of local recurrence.

Griffin and associates[42] did a more extensive analysis of patterns of failure after curative resection for pancreatic carcinoma. This analysis was on 36 patients undergoing resection with curative intent at the University of Kansas between 1977 and 1987. The 2- and 5-year survivals among these patients were 32% and 17%, respectively. The median survival was 11.5 months. Of all the patients who had failure, 100% had a component of failure within the intra-abdominal cavity. Seventy-three percent had a component of local failure, 42% had a component of peritoneal failure, and 62% had a component of hepatic failure. Extra-abdominal metastases were documented in only 27% of patients and never as the sole site of disease.

Foo and colleagues[63] described the outcome of 29 patients treated with radiotherapy following curative surgery for pancreatic cancer at the Mayo Clinic between 1974 and 1986. Their data suggested a significant increase in survival when adjuvant chemoradiation therapy was combined with surgery compared with surgery alone. Eighty-three percent of patients eventually relapsed. Among patients receiving chemotherapy and radiation, the chemotherapy was 5-fluorouracil (5-FU) and the radiation usually consisted of doses between 4500 and 5400 cGy. In contrast to the studies by Tepper and Griffin and coworkers,[41,42] there was only a 7% rate of local failure, although liver failure and peritoneal seeding remained high at 43%, with 61% of patients having a component of either liver or peritoneal relapse.

Kayahara and associates[43] reported on 45 patients undergoing curative resection of carcinoma of the head of pancreas between 1974 and 1991. Of these patients, 30 eventually relapsed. Documented at autopsy, patterns of failure included local recurrence in 80%, hepatic metastases in 66%, peritoneal dissemination in 53%, and lymph node relapse in 47%.

Finally, Willett and colleagues[64] analyzed patterns of failure after pancreaticoduodenectomy for periampullary carcinoma in 41 patients (surgery alone in 29 patients; adjuvant postoperative radiation in 12). They observed excellent local control of 88% with T stages of in situ disease, T1, or T2 compared with 44% for T3 or T4 local stages. Patients with lymph node positivity had a local control rate of 47% whereas patients with negative lymph nodes had a local control rate of 87%. Moderately differentiated tumors had a local control rate of 81% as compared with patients with poorly differentiated tumors with a 0% 5-year local control rate (3 patients). In the 17 surgery-alone patients who had high-risk features, as defined by the authors (tumor invading the pancreas, poorly differentiated, involved nodes, positive resection margins), the 5-year local control and survival were 50% and 38% respectively. For the 12 high-risk patients who received postoperative radiation alone or plus concurrent 5-FU, there was a trend toward improvement in 5-year local control (83% versus 50%) and survival (51% versus 38%), but this did not reach statistical significance in view of small patient numbers and the rate of distant metastasis. The observed patterns of failure in this analysis indicate the need for adjuvant interventions to address locoregional, peritoneal, and hepatic failure patterns.

Adjuvant Therapy with Chemotherapy and Radiation after Resection

PROSPECTIVE, RANDOMIZED TRIAL: GASTROINTESTINAL TUMOR STUDY GROUP

In 1974, the Gastrointestinal Tumor Study Group (GITSG) undertook a prospective, randomized trial of adjuvant 5-FU–based chemoradiotherapy compared with no adjuvant treatment.[65,66] This was a well designed trial that attempted to recruit patients with histologically negative margins of resection between 4 and 10 weeks postoperatively. However, only 49 patients were randomized into the study over an 8-year interval; moreover, 5 withdrew without being treated. The radiation was given as two courses of 2000 cGy in 10 fractions, each with a planned 2-week rest. Treatment fields did not exceed 20 × 20 cm and were given AP/PA. Shaping of fields was optional and 5-FU chemotherapy was given on the first 3 days of each half of the radiation therapy at a dose of 500 mg/m^2 as an IV bolus. Thirty-five percent of patients had tumor confined to the pancreas, 37% had contiguous invasion resected to clear margins, and 28% had nodal involvement.

Results showed that patients treated with combined chemoradiation therapy had improved survival ($p = .03$) compared with patients treated with surgery alone, with a median survival in the treatment group of 20 months versus 11 months in the control arm (Table 45-5). Two-year survival was 42% and 15%, respectively, and 5-year survival was 19% versus 5%. Prognostic factors including age, sex, type of resection, degree of cellular differentiation, initial performance status, location of tumor, and extent of tumor were evaluated. Performance status and extent of tumor were the only independently significant prognostic variables. The study was terminated prematurely because of poor accrual in spite of the long period of time during which it was open.

In an effort to partly address this issue, the GITSG registered an additional 30 patients in a nonrandomized fashion to receive the same adjuvant therapy. Results in these 30 patients essentially recapitulated the results of the treatment arm in the previous randomized study.[66] It was of interest to note that although the treatment produced relatively little toxicity, the local recurrence rate was between 30% and 50% in all patients regardless of whether they received adjuvant treatment and the incidence of hepatic metastases was between 40% and 50%. These results, while strongly suggesting a treatment effect, imply that the dose of radiation was too low to deal with the regional burden of disease present and the efficacy of 5-FU alone inadequate to sterilize disease outside the treatment fields for most patients.

RETROSPECTIVE AND PROSPECTIVE ADJUVANT CHEMORADIATION STUDIES

Past retrospective and prospective studies have confirmed the results of the GITSG. The retrospective data of Whittington and colleagues[67] lend credence to the need for combined modality adjuvant therapy. They reported on a series of 72 patients with pancreatic cancer managed surgically with curative intent between 1981 and 1989 at the Hospital of the University of Pennsylvania in three sequential treatment groups. The first group received surgery alone and the second group received postoperative radiation therapy with a few of these patients having received bolus 5-FU on the first 3 days of radiation and at the beginning of the fifth week of treatment with radiation. The last 20 patients reported received radiation therapy with 96-hour infusions of 5-FU on the first and fifth weeks of treatment. They observed a decrease in local recurrence from 85% in the patients treated with surgery only to 25% in the patients treated with radiation and infusional 5-FU (see Table 45-5). Inferior survival was noted with positive surgical margins. Among patients with negative resection margins, the 2-year survival was 41% for surgery alone, 33% for surgery plus radiation with or without bolus 5-FU, and 59% for surgery plus radiation with infusional 5-FU. More impressively, the 3-year survival was 22% for surgery alone, 11% for surgery plus radiation with or without bolus 5-FU, and 47% for patients receiving postoperative radiation with infusional 5-FU. Their work also emphasized the importance of nutritional support and the value of CT-based treatment planning.

The Johns Hopkins Hospital published results of a single-institution prospective but nonrandomized trial that was designed to evaluate survival benefit in patients with pancreatic cancer following surgical resection.[68] This report, involving 174 patients, demonstrated that patients receiving GITSG-style chemoradiotherapy with maintenance 5-FU truncated at 6 months (rather than 2 years), or a more intensive regimen (involving higher doses or irradiation as well as hepatic irradiation administered without interruption and with continuous infusion 5-FU chemotherapy augmented with leucovorin) did better than patients receiving no post-surgical therapy. The median survival for the more standard regimen was 21 months, with 1- and 2-year survivals of 80% and 44% (see Table 45-5). For the intensive regimen, the median survival was 17.5 months with 1- and 2-year survivals at 70% and 22%. For the control arm, the median survival was 13.5 months with survival at 1 and 2 years of 54% and 30% (Fig. 45-8). The intensive therapy had no survival advantage compared with the standard therapy group, but there was a statistically significant difference between the standard arm versus control ($p < .0002$). Multivariate analysis confirmed that prognostic factors for disease relapse included margin and lymph node status, tumor size (Fig. 45-9), and degree of differentiation.

The Stanford group published their experience of 52 patients with pancreatic cancer following surgical resection. Radiotherapy consisted of 45 Gy to the tumor bed and nodes in 1.8-Gy fractions with boost to a total of 54 Gy if surgical margins were positive. Chemotherapy was administered

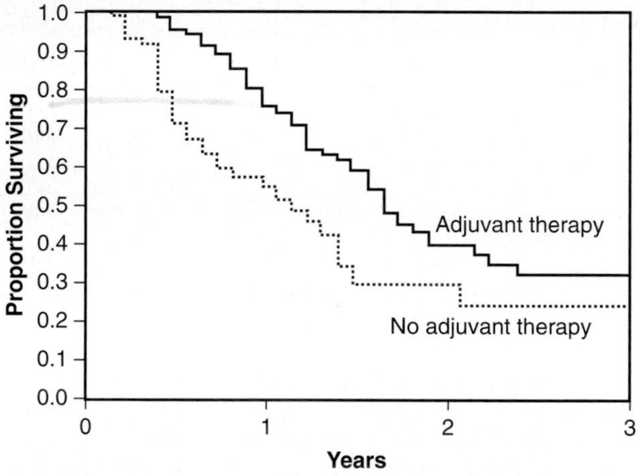

Figure 45-8 The actuarial survival curves for Johns Hopkius patients undergoing pancreaticoduodenectomy comparing patients receiving adjuvant therapy (n = 120) to those declining adjuvant therapy (n = 53; p = .003).

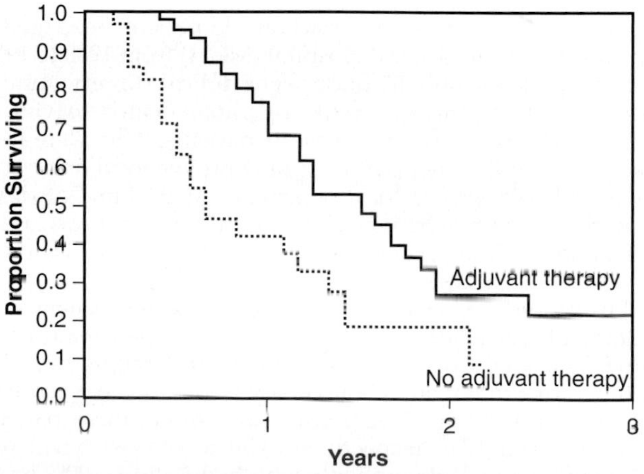

Figure 45-9 In patients with tumors of 3 cm (n = 97), the actuarial survival curves comparing those receiving adjuvant therapy (n = 69) to those declining adjuvant therapy (n = 28; p = .001).

Table 45-5 Adjuvant Radiation Therapy and Chemotherapy for Resected Ductal Adenocarcinoma of the Pancreas, Selected Series

Study	No.	RT Dose (Gy)	Chemotherapy	Median Survival (mo)	2 y (%)	5 y (%)	LR (%)	DM (%)
RANDOMIZED STUDIES								
GITSG (1985)[65]	22	Observation	Observation	11	15	5	33	52 (Liver)
	21	40 Split	Bolus 5-FU	20 ($p < .05$)	42	19	47	40 (Liver)
GITSG (1987)[66]	30	40 Split	Bolus 5-FU	18	43	—	55	45 (Liver)
EORTC (1999)[74]	54	Observation	Observation	12.6	23	10	—	—
	60	40 Split	CI 5-FU	17.1 ($p = .099$)	37	20	—	—
ESPAC-1 (2004)[75]	69	Observation	Observation	16.9	30	8	—	—
	73	40 Split	Concurrent bolus 5-FU	13.9	No adjuvant CTX	No adjuvant CTX	—	—
	72	40 Split	Concurrent bolus 5-FU; 5-FU/leucovorin	19.9	40 Adjuvant CTX	21 Adjuvant CTX	—	—
	75	Observation	Bolus 5-FU/leucovorin	21.6 $P = .009$, Adjuvant CTX			—	—
NONRANDOMIZED STUDIES								
Whittington et al, TJUH (1991)[67]	33	Observation	Observation	15	35	—	85*	23 (liver) 23 (PS)
	19	45-48.6 Negative margins 54-64 Positive margins	Bolus 5-FU	15	30	—	55	42 (liver) 21 (PS)
	20	45-48.6 Negative margins 54-63 Positive margins	CI 5-FU	16	43	—	25	25 (liver) 15 (PS)
Yeo et al, Johns Hopkins (1997)[68]	53	Observation	Observation	14	30	—	—	—
	120	>45	5-FU (bolus or CI)	20 ($p = .003$)	40	—	—	—
Picozzi et al, Virginia Mason (2003)[73]	53	45-54	5-FU, cisplatin, and IFN-α	46	53	—	—	—

CI, continuous infusion; CTX, chemotherapy; DM, distant metastases; 5-FU, 5-fluorouracil; IFN-α, interferon-α.; LR, locoregional recurrence; PS, peritoneal seeding; RT, radiation therapy; TJUH, Thomas Jefferson University Hospital; Neg, negative; Pos, positive.

*Incidence in 26 evaluable patients.

without break throughout radiation therapy and consisted of 5-FU, 200 to 250 mg/m^2/d. All patients were able to complete therapy without grade IV toxicities. With a median follow-up of 24 months, the median survival was 32 months.[69]

In an effort to enhance the activity of chemotherapy in pancreatic cancer, other agents have been examined in combination with 5-FU. Mitomycin-C (MMC) is an antitumor antibiotic with activity in several GI cancers including pancreatic cancer. The UCLA group has published their experience using MMC (10 mg/m^2 IV every 6 weeks) and 5-FU (200 mg/m^2/d administered via continuous infusion), in combination with leucovorin (30 mg/m^2 weekly) and dipyridamole (75 mg PO daily) in 38 patients with locally advanced pancreatic carcinoma.[70] There were 14 partial responders with one complete response. The median survival for all patients was 15.5 months, which is an improvement over historical data for locoregional advanced disease. This regimen has subsequently been applied to resected pancreatic cancer in combination with radiotherapy. The Hopkins group has presented data on 39 patients with pancreatic cancer following surgical resection treated with combined radiotherapy (50 Gy in 25 fractions with planned 2-week break after 25 Gy) and chemotherapy consisting of 5-FU (400 mg/m^2 days 1-3), MMC (10 mg/m^2 day 1), leucovorin (20 mg/m^2 days 1-3), and dipyridamole (75 mg PO QID days 0-4) administered on weeks 1 and 4. One month following combined chemoradiotherapy, patients received four additional cycles (4 months) of the same chemotherapy alone. At 12.6 months median follow-up, median survival was 16 months.[71]

The Virginia Mason Medical Center published their experience of 33 patients with resected pancreatic adenocarcinoma who received combined radiotherapy and chemotherapy. External beam radiotherapy was given to a dose of 45 to 54 Gy with standard fractionation and chemotherapy (5-FU 200 mg/m^2/d as continuous infusion, weekly cisplatin 30 mg/m^2 IV bolus, and interferon-α 3 million units SQ every other day) started with radiation therapy.[72] Following combined modality chemoradiotherapy, chemotherapy alone was administered (5-FU 200 mg/m^2/d as continuous infusion) in two 6-week courses during weeks 9 to 14 and 17 to 22. Of note, 13 of 17 patients randomized to the interferon-based chemoradiotherapy had positive lymph nodes compared with only 7 of 16 patients randomized to the GITSG-based chemoradiotherapy. There were significant grade III/IV GI toxicities including vomiting, mucositis, diarrhea, and GI bleeding in the interferon-based chemotherapy group, requiring hospitalization in 35% of patients. However, the majority of patients were still able to receive more than 80% of the planned therapy. The median overall survival and 2-year actuarial survival rates were 18.5 months and 54% for patients receiving GITSG-based chemoradiotherapy. In contrast, the median and 2-year survivals were more than 24 months and 84% respectively for the interferon-based chemoradiotherapy.

A follow-up study by the Virginia Mason group included 53 patients with resected pancreas cancer treated with similar interferon-based chemoradiotherapy. The clinical efficacy of this regimen remains encouraging, with a median survival of 46 months and a 2-year survival of 53% (see Table 45-5).[73]

The American College of Surgeons Oncology Group (ACOSOG) has initiated a multi-institutional phase II study of this interferon-based chemoradiation regimen in patients with pancreatic adenocarcinoma who have undergone resection. Patients will receive postoperative radiotherapy to 50.4 Gy with 1.8-Gy fractions given concurrently with 5-FU (175 mg/m^2 continuous infusion days 1-38), cisplatin (30 mg/m^2 IV weekly), and interferon-α (3 million units SQ every other day). This is followed by continuous infusion 5-FU for two cycles. Primary end points include overall survival, toxicity rate and severity, locoregional disease control, and distant disease control.

Prospective Randomized Chemoradiation Studies

The EORTC performed a multi-institutional, randomized trial in which 218 patients with periampullary cancers, including pancreatic adenocarcinoma, were randomized to receive surgery alone or surgery plus postoperative 5-FU–based chemoradiation.[74] The radiation dose and fractionation were the same as in the GITSG trial (40 Gy in split-course fashion over 6 weeks). There were two differences in the delivery of 5-FU compared with the GITSG study. Concurrent 5-FU during radiation was administered by continuous intravenous infusion, rather than bolus, during the first 3 days of each radiation sequence. Furthermore, no 5-FU was given after the concurrent chemoradiation. In the subset of 114 patients with pancreatic adenocarcinoma, patients in the chemoradiation arm ($n = 60$) had a median survival of 17.1 months versus 12.6 months in the pancreatectomy alone arm ($n = 54$). The 2-year overall survival (OS) rates for the two arms were 37% and 23%, respectively, and 5-year OS was 20% versus 10% ($p = .099$). There were no differences in locoregional recurrence rates, which were high with both surgery alone (37 of 103, 36% of patients at risk) and postoperative chemoradiation (34 of 104, 33% of patients at risk). The EORTC concluded that there was no demonstrable benefit from postoperative chemoradiation for the total group of patients but that survival trends favored adjuvant postoperative chemoradiation for the 114 patients with pancreatic cancer.

However, several aspects of the EORTC trial design, analysis, and interpretation warrant comment. Patients with T3 lesions were excluded and the pathologic basis for distinguishing between and including pancreatic and nonpancreatic periampullary lesions (which have different natural histories and prognoses than do pancreatic adenocarcinomas) was not made clear. Additionally, the adequacy of the retroperitoneal margin was not independently assessed, perhaps influencing the frequency of locoregional recurrence. Moreover, 20% of patients assigned to the chemoradiation arm never received that treatment (patient refusal, poor postoperative performance status, disease progression, etc.) but they were analyzed by intent-to-treat principles. Although this approach is statistically correct, one needs to consider that the chemoradiation group includes a sizable minority of patients who did not receive postoperative chemoradiation. Furthermore, unlike the GITSG trial, no chemotherapy was given after chemoradiation. Finally, the study lacked sufficient patient numbers to exclude a clinically significant 10% to 15% benefit from the addition of adjuvant chemoradiation to surgery. Thus, some investigators consider the EORTC trial to be an underpowered study that provides additional circumstantial evidence to support a role for postoperative chemoradiation.

An important trial for radiation oncologists to be aware of is the ESPAC-1 study,[75] which had a complex design (three separate but concurrent phase III trials) and was initiated to evaluate the independent effects of adjuvant chemotherapy and chemoradiation in 541 patients with grossly resected pancreas cancer. The study, with a 2 × 2 factorial design, randomized 285 patients with pancreatic adenocarcinoma into four arms: (1) observation; (2) concomitant chemoradiotherapy alone (20 Gy in 10 fractions over 2 weeks with 500 mg/m^2 5-FU IV bolus during the first 3 days of radiation therapy and then repeated after a planned 2-week break) followed by no additional chemotherapy; (3) chemotherapy alone (leucovorin 20 mg/m^2 bolus followed by 5-FU 425 mg/m^2 administered for 5 consecutive days repeated every 28 days for 6 cycles);

and (4) chemoradiotherapy followed by six cycles of adjuvant 5-FU leucovorin. Investigators were also allowed to randomize patients into two separate but concurrent trials testing one of the main treatment comparisons (adjuvant chemotherapy versus none—188 patients; adjuvant concurrent chemoradiation versus none—68 patients). Background therapy was allowed before patients were entered into the latter two trials, and radiation was given according to the standard of the individual institutions in all three trials. In the initial analysis,[76] a survival advantage for adjuvant chemotherapy was achieved only by merging data from the three separate randomized trials (median survival of 19.7 months in the 238 patients randomized to receive adjuvant chemotherapy versus median SR of 14 months in the 235 randomized to no adjuvant chemotherapy, $p = .005$). The latest analysis of the ESPAC-1 trial[75] analyzed only the patients randomized to the 2×2 factorial design ($n = 289$—no background therapy allowed). Patients randomized to receive adjuvant chemotherapy (two of the four arms, $n = 147$) had a survival advantage (2 year, 40% versus 30%; 5 year, 21% versus 8%; $p = .009$). Local recurrence was a component of relapse in 99 patients (34% of the 289 patients at risk, 63% of patients with relapse).

This trial has been reported as demonstrating a deleterious effect on survival for those patients who received 5-FU–based chemoradiotherapy. However, major concerns regarding the design and execution of this trial include more than one randomization scheme (three separate but concurrent phase III trials), patients were allowed to receive "background" therapy in addition to protocol therapy in two of the three trials, patients were not restaged after resection and before adjuvant therapy, and there were no quality assurance guidelines for the delivery of radiation (i.e., no section in the protocol on appropriate field design, no central audit of radiation fields) which is contrary to the routine in North American cooperative group trials.[77] ESPAC-1 was a trial of varying patient populations and the nature of the differences in the patients cannot be known. Thus, the validity of this analysis should be regarded with concern.

The completed Radiation Therapy Oncology Group (RTOG) 9704 trial will provide important insights into the comparative efficacy of 5-FU and gemcitabine administered before and after postoperative 5-FU–based chemoradiation. In this study, 518 patients with resected pancreatic cancer were treated with postoperative 5-FU–based chemoradiation (50.4 Gy in 28 fractions over 5.5 weeks plus concurrent protracted venous infusion of 5-FU). Patients were randomized to receive either 5-FU (250 $mg/m^2/d$) given as continuous infusion over 3 to 4 weeks or gemcitabine (1000 $mg/m^2/wk$) given for 3 of 4 weeks. Chemotherapy was given for a total of three cycles: one before chemoradiation and two cycles after chemoradiation. Patients were stratified by nodal status, tumor diameter, and margin positivity. This trial will provide important data on a variety of issues including (1) the role of gemcitabine versus infusional 5-FU after pancreaticoduodenectomy, (2) the ability to deliver continuous infusion 5-FU concurrently with a single course of standard-fractionation modern radiotherapy in a broad, multi-institutional setting, and (3) the prognostic significance of tumor size, nodal status, and margin positivity in the postoperative treatment of pancreatic cancer.

The ACOSOG has elected to test the Virginia Mason data in the cooperative group setting using CT-guided planning (three-dimensional conformal) and fields that were somewhat smaller than those conventionally utilized in the RTOG 9704 study. Radiotherapy volume is minimized to facilitate acute tolerance of the intensive chemotherapy regimen. The trial was designed to omit preoperative tumor bed coverage and includes just the regions at highest risk for local recurrence, namely the surgical margins and celiac as well as superior mesenteric artery/uncinate regions.

Neoadjuvant Strategies

In the mid to late 1980s, a number of institutions began considering the use of radiation therapy or chemotherapy as a planned, preoperative approach (neoadjuvant) for patients with apparently resectable, biopsy proven adenocarcinoma of the pancreas. In the early to mid 1990s, these results began to mature and a number of papers have described results in this context. Ishikawa and colleagues[78] reported on 54 consecutive patients, judged to be resectable, who either went directly to surgery ($n = 31$) or received 50 Gy of external beam radiotherapy to the region of the pancreatic head ($n = 23$). They found no difference in resectability, survival at 3 years, or survival at 5 years. There was a slight advantage to survival at 1 year to having preoperative radiotherapy. There was a decrease in the incidences of regional relapse during the first 1.5 postoperative years for patients undergoing preoperative radiotherapy.

Workers at the M.D. Anderson Cancer Center (MDACC) have published a series of papers regarding their experience with preoperative chemoradiation therapy for adenocarcinoma of the pancreas. Their described rationale for this approach is similar to that for neoadjuvant therapy in other contexts; namely, the increased efficacy of radiotherapy in well-oxygenated cells that have not been devascularized surgically, the expectation that radiation therapy prior to surgical exploration decreases the ability of treated tumor cells to disseminate or implant during and following laparotomy, and the expectation that patients who are destined to disseminate early will do so during the period of neoadjuvant therapy and thus be spared an operation that would have proved futile.[79] The authors reported on 28 patients managed with neoadjuvant therapy consisting of 5-FU as a continuous infusion of 300 $mg/m^2/d$ and conventionally fractionated irradiation to a total dose of 50.4 Gy. Of these patients, 5 disseminated prior to exploration, 23 were explored of whom 3 were found to have unsuspected metastatic disease, and an additional 3 were found to be unresectable. Thus, of their initial 28 patients, 17 underwent pancreaticoduodenectomy, with one perioperative death from myocardial infarction. This group updated their experience in 1996, describing results in 39 patients managed between September 1988 and April 1994. All patients received chemoradiotherapy and 5-FU was given continuously as described above. Thirty patients received 50.4 Gy as described above and nine patients received 30 Gy in 10 fractions. Thirty-three of these patients also received intraoperative electron beam radiotherapy. Six patients were not treated with intraoperative radiotherapy because of the need for vascular reconstruction. However, the authors noted that these six patients were from the earlier part of the experience and if managed later, they would have been treated with intraoperative radiotherapy.[80] With a median follow-up of 19 months, eight patients remained alive without evidence of disease and four patients were alive with evidence of disease. Twenty-seven patients had died, of whom 23 had died from pancreatic adenocarcinoma. There was one perioperative death and three late complications causing death. Among patients with disease relapse, 21% were locoregional and 79% were distant including lung, liver, and bone. Liver was the most frequent site of tumor relapse with 53% of patients having liver metastases as a component of treatment failure. Isolated local or peritoneal relapse occurred in only 11% of patients.

In 1997, workers from this same group reported on 142 patients managed from July 1990 though July 1995.[81] Although the institutional preference was for preoperative treatment, this was only performed for those patients in whom a diagnosis could be histologically established without laparotomy. Of 142 patients, 91 underwent neoadjuvant treatment after histologic documentation of tumor and 51 underwent laparotomy because tumor could not be documented preoperatively. Among those undergoing neoadjuvant therapy, 26% were found to have progressive disease on restaging following chemoradiation and prior to undergoing exploration. Of the remaining 67 patients, 52 underwent successful pancreaticoduodenectomy and 15 (22%) were found to have unresectable disease because of the presence of extrapancreatic disease or locally advanced primary tumor. Of the 52 patients who had resections, 41 had been prospectively enrolled in pilot studies of protocol-based preoperative chemoradiation. Among these 41 patients, 21 had received 50.4 Gy in 28 fractions and 14 had received 30 Gy in 10 fractions. Among 51 patients undergoing immediate laparotomy with planned postoperative adjuvant chemoradiation anticipated, 42 patients were found to have resectable disease, of whom 17 had adenocarcinoma of the periampullary region but not of the pancreas. Thus, there were 25 patients with pancreatic cancer who underwent resection for adenocarcinoma of the pancreas. Of these, 19 received postoperative adjuvant chemotherapy while 6 did not secondary to delayed recovery. Sixty-eight percent of all resected patients also received intraoperative radiotherapy. There was no difference in overall survival among patients treated with preoperative chemoradiation compared with those treated with postoperative chemoradiation. The incidence of local regional recurrence was 21% in patients receiving postoperative chemoradiation and 10% in those receiving preoperative chemoradiation. There was no evident difference in toxicity between the two approaches although the overall treatment time was significantly shorter in those patients receiving the 30 Gy/10-fraction approach as opposed to the 50.4 Gy/28-fraction approach.

Investigators at the Fox Chase Cancer Center in Philadelphia have also published a series of papers regarding neoadjuvant chemoradiation therapy for periampullary malignancy. Their approach has consisted of 50.4 Gy conventionally fractionated with 4-day infusions of 5-FU at 1000 mg/m^2 per day and bolus infusion of mitomycin-C, 10 mg/m^2 on the second day. In a report published in 1993, they described their initial experience with 31 patients of whom 24 had carcinoma of the head of the pancreas, 2 had carcinoma of the body of the pancreas, and 5 had carcinoma of the duodenum. They found the toxicity to be acceptable with one death from biliary sepsis and a resectability rate of 38% for pancreatic carcinoma and 80% for duodenal carcinoma.[82] This work was updated by Hoffman and associates[83,84] In the second of these reports, the authors described results in 34 patients with localized pancreatic cancer receiving the same treatment as already described. Nine of these patients did not have surgery: one refused, one died of cholangitis, and seven were found to have distant or unresectable local disease following the completion of neoadjuvant therapy. Of the 25 patients who underwent laparotomy, 11 were found to have unresectable disease due to hepatic or peritoneal dissemination and 3 had palliative pancreatectomies. Therefore, of the initial 34 patients, only 11 underwent surgery with curative intent, with 1 patient dying in the perioperative period. With a median follow-up of 33 months, the median survival was 45 months and the disease-free survival was 27 months in the patients who underwent potentially curative resection. In 1998, these workers reported on a comparison of their preoperative studies to 23 patients who were accrued sequentially following closure of their preoperative protocol. These patients were treated with postoperative chemoradiation, using the same radiation and chemotherapy dosing and scheduling as the preoperative regimen. They found that there was no difference in intraoperative management or length of postoperative stay. With preoperative therapy, there were fewer involved nodes and more patients with negative resection margins. After a median follow-up of 44 months, median survival was 20 months versus 25 months in the preoperative group compared with the postoperative group respectively. Local failure either alone or as a component of overall failure was the same in both groups at 16%. They concluded that both treatments were similar with respect to toxicity and benefit, but they noted that 22% of patients did not receive their intended postoperative therapy.[85]

Also in 1998, the results of this neoadjuvant approach as undertaken by the Eastern Cooperative Oncology Group (ECOG) were reported.[86] The treatment was essentially as described in the Fox Chase reports. However, the results were not especially encouraging. Twelve patients did not proceed to surgery (one due to death, one due to toxicity, three due to local progression, six due to distant metastases, and one due to intercurrent illness). Of the 41 patients undergoing surgery, 17 patients did not have curative resection (11 because of hepatic or peritoneal metastases and 6 from local extension that was unresectable). Among the 24 patients undergoing resection, the median survival was 15.7 months.

In aggregate to date, these results do not suggest a superior result for neoadjuvant therapy. However, it is clear that patients receiving neoadjuvant therapy are more likely to receive the chemoradiation than patients who undergo surgery first with anticipation of postoperative chemoradiation therapy. Nevertheless, there is no observed survival advantage between the two approaches.

LOCALLY ADVANCED (UNRESECTABLE) DISEASE AND PALLIATION

Palliative Surgery

Classically, a discussion of palliative surgery for periampullary carcinoma would imply hepaticojejunostomy, gastrojejunostomy, or both, to relieve biliary obstruction and gastric outlet obstruction. As summarized by Lillemoe and colleagues,[87] this type of operation can be performed with an in-hospital mortality rate of 2.5%, postoperative non–life-threatening morbidity of 37%, and a mean survival of 7.7 months. Several groups have looked at the role of palliative pancreaticoduodenectomy, that is, pancreaticoduodenectomy performed despite the surgeons' intraoperative realization that the final margins of resection are likely to be visibly positive. Lillemoe and colleagues looked at this issue in 64 consecutive patients undergoing surgery between 1986 and 1994, and compared the outcomes to 62 consecutive patients undergoing standard surgical palliation between 1986 and 1991. None of these patients had evidence of hepatic, serosal, or peritoneal dissemination. Patients undergoing palliative pancreaticoduodenectomy fared significantly better than patients undergoing palliative bypass ($p < .02$) with a 24-month survival of approximately 30% in the pancreaticoduodenectomy patients, versus less than 10% in the palliative bypass patients. However, the patients undergoing palliative pancreaticoduodenectomy who received postoperative chemoradiation therapy survived significantly longer than patients undergoing the same operation without adjuvant chemoradiotherapy. Similarly, patients undergoing bypass therapy who received postoperative radiation therapy survived significantly longer than patients undergoing bypass therapy without chemoradiation therapy. Similar results have been described by Ouchi and associates.[88]

Chemoradiotherapy for Unresectable Pancreatic Adenocarcinoma

For locoregionally unresectable disease, the GITSG has demonstrated that split course radiotherapy to a total dose of 40 to 60 Gy with bolus doses of 5-FU was superior to radiotherapy alone at a dose of 60 Gy (median SR from diagnosis at exploratory laparotomy of 5.5 months [60 Gy alone] versus 8.3 months [40 Gy + 5-FU] and 11.3 months [60 Gy + 5-FU]) (Table 45-6).[89] Subsequently, the GITSG demonstrated that combination chemotherapy with SMF (streptozocin, MMC, 5-FU) produced a significantly inferior survival result for patients with unresectable disease than 5-FU chemoradiotherapy to 54 Gy followed by SMF (median survival 42 weeks versus 32 weeks; 1-year survival 41% versus 19%, 2-year survival 18% versus none; radiotherapy group superior at all time points) (see Table 45-6).[90] The ability to give combined chemoradiotherapy, with either continuous or split course radiotherapy, to doses between 40 and 60 Gy combined with 5-FU, 5-FU and leucovorin, 5-FU and MMC, and 5-FU and cisplatin, with definite but acceptable toxicity has also been confirmed.[91-94] Conversion to operability was noted to occur rarely (10%), with pain relief occurring in the majority of patients. Treatment toxicity is related to treatment volume, total radiotherapy dose, radiotherapy fraction size, and the use or absence of a planned split, as well as to the intensity of the chemotherapy dosing. In patients with adequate nutrition and with hepatic and gastric obstruction absent or surgically relieved, toxicities, such as nausea and mucositis, are generally readily manageable.

There has been considerable interest in combining external beam radiation therapy (EBRT) with gemcitabine due to its clinical benefit in the metastatic setting and potent radiosensitizing properties. Blackstock and colleague examined in a phase I study gemcitabine (starting at 20 mg/m^2) twice weekly in combination with radiation therapy (total dose 50.4 Gy in 1.8-Gy fractions) in 19 patients with locally advanced pancreatic adenocarcinoma. Thrombocytopenia, neutropenia, and nausea/vomiting were dose-limiting toxicities. Of the 15 patients assessable for response, 3 partial responses were identified.[95] A dose of 40 mg/m^2 twice weekly in combination with radiotherapy to a total dose of 50.4 Gy was subsequently examined by the Cancer and Leukemia Group B (CALGB) in a phase II study of 39 patients with locally advanced pancreatic cancer. Following chemoradiotherapy, patients without disease progression received gemcitabine alone 1000 mg/m^2 weekly × 3 every 4 weeks for five additional cycles. Grade III/IV hematologic toxicity was significant and identified in 69% of patients. In addition, grade III/IV GI toxicity was identified in 41% of patients. The overall median survival was 8.2 months (see Table 45-6).[96]

The MDACC has published a corollary phase I study of 18 patients with locally advanced disease using rapid fractionation EBRT. Patients received dose escalation gemcitabine from 350 mg/m^2 to 500 mg/m^2 weekly × 7 with concurrent rapid fractionation 3000 cGy EBRT during the first two weeks of therapy. Hematologic and nonhematologic toxicities were significant in all three patient cohorts. There were eight responses (four minor and four partial). One of two patients who were subsequently explored had a curative resection. The recommended phase II testing dose of gemcitabine was 350 mg/m^2.[97]

The University of Michigan has described an alternative approach using standard doses of gemcitabine at 1000 mg/m^2 weekly × 3 every 4 weeks and administering radiation therapy as dose escalation beginning at 24 Gy (1.6-Gy in 15 fractions) in 37 patients with locally advanced disease. The majority of patients received additional chemotherapy following chemoradiotherapy at the discretion of the treating physician. Seventy-five percent of patients received at least 85% of planned gemcitabine. Two of six assessable patients experienced dose-limiting toxicity at the final planned radiation dose of 42 Gy in 2.8-Gy fractions. An additional two patients developed late GI toxicities at this dose level. Six patients were documented to have a partial response with a complete radiographic response in two patients. In addition, four patients with documented stable disease at the time of initial posttherapy evaluation experienced objective responses (two partial and two complete responses) with additional chemotherapy. Definitive resection was achieved in one of three surgically explored patients. With a median follow-up of

Table 45-6 Chemoradiation for Locally Unresectable Adenocarcinoma of the Pancreas

Study	No.	RT (Gy)	Chemotherapy	Median Survival (mo)	2-y Survival (%)	*p* Value
RANDOMIZED STUDIES						
Moertel et al, GITSG[89]	25	60 (Split)	—	5.5	1	
	83	40 (Split)	5-FU	8.3	10	<.01
	86	60 (Split)	5-FU	11.3	10	
GITSG[90]	24	—	SMF	8	19 (1 y)	
	24	54	5-FU/SMF	10.5	41 (1 y)	<.02
NONRANDOMIZED STUDIES						
Roldan et al, Mayo Clinic[112]	122	40-60*	Bolus 5FU	12.6	16	
Blackstock et al, CALGB[96]	39	50.4	Gemcitabine	8.2	5 (3 y)	NA
McGinn et al, University of Michigan[98]	37	24-42	Gemcitabine	11.6	8	NA
Martenson et al, NCCTG[100]	26	50.4	Gemcitabine/cisplatin	11.7	—	NA
Crane et al, MDACC[102]	61	30	CI 5-FU	9	28 (1 y)	0.19
	53	30	Gemcitabine	11	42 (1 y)	

CI, continuous infusion; 5-FU, 5-fluorouracil; MDACC, M.D. Anderson Cancer Center; NA, not applicable; RT, radiation therapy; SMF, streptozocin, mitomycin C, 5-fluorouracil.

*40- to 60-Gy split course or 45- to 54-Gy continuous.

22 months, median survival for the entire group was 11.6 months (see Table 45-6). The recommended phase II radiation dose was 36 Gy in 2.4-Gy fractions.[98]

Other chemotherapy agents have been added to gemcitabine combined with radiation therapy. The Eastern Cooperative Oncology Group (ECOG) published a phase I study of seven patients with locally advanced disease using combination chemotherapy consisting of radiation therapy to a maximum 59.4 Gy in 1.8-Gy fractions. 5-FU (200 mg/m^2/d as continuous infusion throughout radiation therapy) was administered with weekly gemcitabine dose escalation beginning at 100 mg/m^2. Due to dose-limiting toxicities seen in two of the first three patients, the study was amended to lower the initial dose of gemcitabine to 50 mg/m^2. However, dose-limiting toxicities were subsequently seen in 3 of 4 patients at the 50 mg/m^2 dose. Three of the five dose-limiting toxicities occurred at radiation doses less than 36 Gy and the study was subsequently closed.[99]

Gemcitabine has also been combined with cisplatin and radiation in published phase I trials, following up on promising preclinical synergistic data. A study based at the Mayo clinic gave twice-weekly gemcitabine and cisplatin for 3 weeks during radiation (50.4 Gy in 28 fractions) (see Table 45-6). Dose-limiting toxicities consisted of grade IV nausea and vomiting. The recommended phase II dose was gemcitabine 30 mg/m^2 and cisplatin 10 mg/m^2.[100] Another trial used strictly time-scheduled gemcitabine (days 2, 5, 26, and 33 after a weekly regimen was too toxic) and cisplatin (days 1 to 5 and 29 to 33) combined with radiation, with a recommended phase II dose of 20 mg/m^2 for cisplatin and 300 mg/m^2 for gemcitabine.[101] The response to chemoradiation allowed 10 of 30 initially unresectable patients to undergo surgery, with an R0 resection in nine cases and a CR in two cases.

Given the current published data, would 5-FU or gemcitabine be better suited to be used concurrently with radiation therapy for either resected or locally advanced disease? The MDACC retrospectively examined their database of 114 patients with locally advanced disease treated with combination radiation therapy (rapid-fractionation 30 Gy in 10 fractions) with either 5-FU continuous infusion 200 to 300 mg/m^2 (61 patients) or gemcitabine 250 to 500 mg/m^2 weekly x 7 (53 patients). Patients receiving gemcitabine developed significantly higher incidences of severe acute toxicity defined as toxicity requiring a hospital stay of more than 5 days, mucosal ulceration with bleeding, more than three-dose deletions of gemcitabine, or toxicity resulting in surgical intervention or death compared with those patients receiving 5-FU (23% versus 2%, $p < .0001$). Five of 53 patients treated with gemcitabine/radiation therapy subsequently underwent surgical resection compared with 1 of 61 patients treated with 5-FU/radiation therapy. However, with short median follow-up, median survival was similar (11 months versus 9 months, $p = .19$) (see Table 45-6).[102]

Because the benefit of chemoradiation is relatively modest, some oncologists recommend chemotherapy alone for locally advanced disease. Gemcitabine is the most commonly used agent, extrapolating from the metastatic disease setting. This is based on the randomized trial by Burris and colleagues, in which 26% of the study subjects had locally advanced disease, and showed that gemcitabine ameliorated symptoms and modestly improved survival compared with 5-FU.[103] The results for patients with locally advanced disease were not reported separately. An ECOG phase III trial comparing gemcitabine/radiation versus gemcitabine alone opened in April 2003 to examine this issue.

Locally Directed Therapy—IORT and Brachytherapy

Both intraoperative radiotherapy (IORT) and brachytherapy have been used in the setting of locally advanced disease (Table 45-7). Both modalities are aimed at improving locoregional control. Given the propensity of this disease to disseminate especially into the liver and adjacent peritoneum, what can be achieved overall for patients by the addition of either modality to EBRT and chemotherapy is not completely clear.

Mohiuddin and colleagues[104] reported on 81 patients with localized unresectable carcinoma of the pancreas managed at Thomas Jefferson using intraoperative iodine-125 implants, EBRT, and perioperative systemic chemotherapy. The radioactive iodine implant was designed to deliver a minimum peripheral dose up to 120 Gy over 1 year. Patients were also treated with 50 to 55 Gy of EBRT with systemic chemotherapy consisting of 5-FU, mitomycin, and occasionally CCNU. Implants were performed at laparotomy. There was a 5% mortality rate, a 34% acute morbidity rate with cholangitis, upper GI bleeding, and gastric outlet obstruction being the most

Table 45-7 Selected Trials for Locally Directed Therapy—Brachytherapy and Intraoperative Radiation Therapy

Study	No.	RT	Median Survival (mo)	2-y Survival (%)	Local Control (%)	Pain Relief (%)
BRACHYTHERAPY, LOCALLY UNRESECTABLE						
Mohiuddin et al, Thomas Jefferson[104]	81	^{125}I (120 Gy min peripheral dose) + EBRT (50 Gy) + chemo	12	21	71	—
Nori et al[105]	15	^{103}Pd (110 Gy matched peripheral dose) + EBRT (45 Gy) + chemo	10	0	—	83
IORT, LOCALLY UNRESECTABLE						
Tepper et al, RTOG[111]	51	IORT (20 Gy), EBRT (50.4 Gy) + chemo	9	9	—	—
Dobelbower et al, MCO[113]	26	IORT (12.5-30 Gy), EBRT (19.8-65 Gy)	10.5	—	80	92
Garton et al, Mayo Clinic[117]	27	Preop EBRT (50.4-54 Gy), IOERT (20 Gy)/chemo	14.9	27	78	—
IORT, ADJUVANT						
Zerbi et al, Italy[115]	43	IORT (12.5-20 Gy)	19	24	63	—

common. In addition, there was a 32% late morbidity rate with GI bleeding, cholangitis, and radiation enteritis being the most common late developments. Local control was obtained in 39 of 53 (71%) evaluable patients. Of 14 patients undergoing re-exploration more than six months following implantation, 86% showed extensive fibrosis and had negative biopsies from the region of the tumor. In eight patients undergoing autopsy, five (63%) were without evidence of locoregional tumor. Nevertheless, 52 of these 81 patients (62%) failed with intra-abdominal disease, primarily hepatic and peritoneal. With a minimum follow-up of 2 years, the median survival for the total group was 12 months, with 2- and 5-year survivals of 21% and 7%, respectively. For node-negative patients, the median survival was 13 months and the 2- and 5-year survivals were 27% and 8%, respectively. For patients with histologically involved lymph nodes, the median survival was 9 months, with 2- and 5-year survivals of 13% and 3%, respectively. Despite satisfactory local control in several patients, many centers would not be willing to accept this level of therapeutic intensity in a group of patients for whom management is ultimately primarily noncurative.

Nori and associates reported on a series of 15 patients undergoing similar management but using palladium-103 instead of iodine-125.[105] The implant was designed to provide a matched peripheral dose of 110 Gy. Patients also received EBRT of 4500 cGy over 4 1/2 weeks and chemotherapy of 5-FU and mitomycin C. Median survival was ten months (see Table 45-7) and the authors concluded that palladium-103 is an alternative to iodine-125 for interstitial brachytherapy for unresectable patients and that symptom relief appeared to occur somewhat faster. The study did not show any improvement in the median survival compared with iodine-125. A note of caution was raised by Raben and colleagues on the use of palladium brachytherapy for locally unresectable carcinoma of the pancreas. In their series of 11 patients, they found an unacceptably high complication rate including gastric outlet obstruction, duodenal perforation, and sepsis.[106] They did not find an improvement in median survival over other modalities and did not recommend this approach for further study.

The use of IORT using single-fraction electron beam treatment has been extensively studied.[107-109] In experienced hands, IORT can be given with acceptable morbidity. However, there are occasional reports of high complication rates.

Generally, IORT has been given in combination with EBRT in the range of 45 to 50.4 Gy in 25 to 28 fractions with 5-FU alone or 5-FU–based combination chemotherapy. As reviewed by Willett and associates,[110] the dose of IORT is generally in the range of 10 to 20 Gy (usually 20 Gy for patients with locally unresectable cancers; for those with resection after preoperative chemoradiation, the IORT dose varies from 10 to 12.5 Gy).

The RTOG reported on 51 patients with locally unresected nonmetastatic pancreatic cancer, and found a major postoperative complication rate of 12% and two patients with major morbidity leading to death. There was no obvious improvement in median survival (see Table 45-7).[111]

The combination of EBRT (±5-FU) plus IORT has resulted in an improvement in local control in series from both MGH and Mayo Clinic,[110,112] but this has not translated into an improvement in either median or 5-year survival. In a Mayo analysis of 159 patients by Roldan and coworkers,[112] the local control rate at one year was 82% for EBRT plus IORT (n = 37 patients) versus 48% for EBRT alone (n = 122 patients) and 2-year LC was 66% versus 20% (p = .0005). Median and 2-year survival were similar, however, with median SR of 13.4 versus 12.4 months (IORT versus none) and 2-year SR of 12% versus 16.5%. The lack of survival improvement was related to a high incidence of abdominal relapse in both groups of patients (IORT—54% with liver or peritoneal metastases versus 56% in non-IORT patients). An update of the MGH IOERT series is found in the chapter on intraoperative irradiation (see Chapter 15); 5-year SR of 7% (five survivors beyond 5 years).

Dobelbower and colleagues[113] have suggested that the greatest benefit results from combining IORT and EBRT when patients are being managed with palliative surgery (biliary and/or GI surgical bypass). This was also seen by Kawamura and associates.[114] Zerbi and colleagues[115] have suggested that the use of IORT as an adjuvant to resection decreases the risk of local recurrence. Mohiuddin and associates[116] have also reported excellent results with IORT in the management of unresectable pancreatic cancer, when combined with postoperative external beam chemoradiation.

In an attempt to improve patient selection and survival, a number of institutions have altered the sequencing of IORT and EBRT. Garton and colleagues[117] from the Mayo Clinic used EBRT alone or plus concurrent 5-FU preoperatively in 27 patients with localized, unresectable disease and then delivered IORT. Median survival from diagnosis was 14.9 months with 2-year SR of 27% and 5-year SR of 7% (see Table 45-7). Local control was achieved in 78% of patients, but 52% developed liver or peritoneal relapse.

Best Supportive Care

Care delivered in the context of locoregionally unresectable, periampullary pancreatic cancer is expected to be palliative. As such, one of the treatment options available includes best supportive care without specific antineoplastic intervention. The supportive care needs of patients with locoregionally advanced, periampullary pancreatic cancer can be substantial (Table 45-8). Attention to the management of these significant medical issues forms the foundation of excellent palliation and care, regardless of whether intervention with antineoplastic therapy (chemotherapy with or without radiotherapy) is selected. Moreover, adequate attention to the medical optimization of these needs before and during antineoplastic therapy is essential for optimal intervention and opportunity for benefit. Weight loss correlates closely with the inability to tolerate full-dose chemotherapy,[118] and patients are not well served when they receive systemic chemotherapy with unrelieved obstructive jaundice. Similarly, patients with incipient or fully expressed gastric outlet obstruction have difficulty tolerating intervention with irradiation to the upper abdomen because this is often associated with severe nausea, vomiting, and anorexia. Especially during the early phase of patient presentation and management, "best supportive care" should

Table 45-8 Common Supportive Care Needs: Patients with Locally Advanced Pancreatic Cancer

Nausea
Weight loss
Malabsorption, pancreatic enzyme insufficiency, lactose intolerance
Duodenal obstruction
Hyperglycemia
Dehydration, electrolyte abnormalities
Pain
Depression
Jaundice
Anxiety
Constipation
Anemia

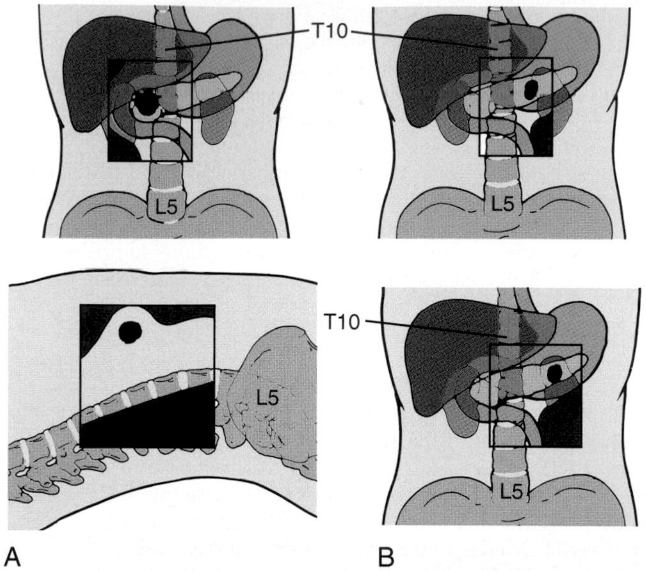

Figure 45-10 **A,** Schematic of anterior-posterior (AP) field, with blocking for pancreatic head lesion (*top*). Schematic of lateral field, with blocking (*bottom*). **B,** Schematic of AP field, with blocking for pancreatic body lesion (*top*). Schematic of AP field, with blocking, for pancreatic tail lesion (*bottom*). (From RTOG 97-04; Phase III study of pre- and post-chemoradiation gemcitabine for postoperative adjuvant treatment of resected pancreatic carcinoma.)

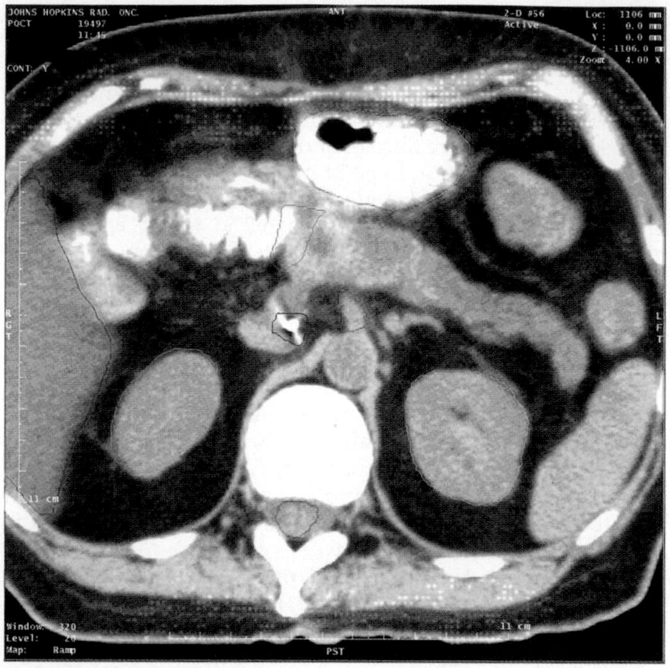

Figure 45-11 Example of localization of the pancreaticojejunostomy, superior mesenteric artery, and clip-on uncinate margin. (Courtesy of Ross A. Abrams, MD.)

not be a euphemism for a passive medical stance of minimal involvement and attention.

TECHNIQUES OF IRRADIATION

In the postoperative adjuvant setting for adenocarcinoma of the pancreas, the radiation therapy is generally given using three or four fields. High-energy photons (>10 MeV) are preferred, although low-energy megavoltage beams may be used. The classic volumes for treatment include the tumor bed, peripancreatic lymph nodes, and para-aortic lymph nodes between the eleventh thoracic vertebra and the third lumbar vertebra. The usual main challenge is to include these volumes without including unacceptable amounts of renal parenchyma. Therefore, precise kidney localization is essential.

Guidelines are illustrated for a classic four-field approach in Figure 45-10A and B. The information required to appropriately set these fields includes the preoperative CT scan to assess the location of the tumor before resection and a postoperative CT scan to confirm the absence of locally recurrent, persistent, or metastatic cancer, and to accurately localize the kidneys and other normal tissues plus nodal target volumes.

Significantly more treatment planning certainty can be accomplished with CT-based treatment planning (Fig. 45-11). This allows contouring of the hepaticojejunostomy, the pancreaticojejunostomy, the pancreatic remnant, the celiac axis, the superior mesenteric artery, and critical normal structures, such as liver, spinal cord, and kidneys. Preoperative tumor volumes can be superimposed on these volumes. The ability to visualize all of these relevant normal tissues and treatment planning volumes allows for enhanced flexibility in field placement, gantry angulation, and treatment planning.

For critical structure tolerance, the RTOG 9704 protocol offers some guidelines.[119] Efforts should be made to exclude the small bowel and liver as much as possible. The liver must not have greater than 60% of its volume receive greater than 30 Gy. The spinal cord dose is limited to less than 45 Gy by use of posterior blocking in the lateral fields. The equivalent of one kidney should receive 20 Gy or at least the equivalent of two thirds of one kidney must be spared from the radiotherapy fields. If only a single functioning kidney is present, at least two thirds of the functioning kidney must be excluded from any radiation port. For head lesions, 50% of the right kidney is often in the AP-PA fields and so two thirds of the left kidney should be shielded. For body or tail lesions, 50% of the left kidney is often in the AP-PA fields and so two thirds of the right kidney should be shielded.

In a standard simulation, it is virtually impossible to precisely localize the sites of surgical anastomoses. However, these sites represent potential areas of residual microscopic tumor either by direct or lymphatic extension. Care must be taken to allow for adequate margins that account for beam edge penumbra, daily setup variation, and respiratory or other physiologic movement.

Treatment planning considerations for locoregional unresectable tumors are similar but can be complicated by the size of the mass and by extension of gross tumor superiorly into the retrogastric region. Size can be a problem for avoiding excessive renal parenchyma exposure, and extension into the retrogastric area increases the amount of stomach, especially posterior antrum, that is treated. The importance of covering para-aortic lymph nodes has not been well studied. With the use of gemcitabine and other potent radiosensitizers with irradiation, it may become more important to not use large treatment volumes to avoid intestinal side effects.

The advent of intensity-modulated radiotherapy (IMRT) has sparked interest in the treatment of both resected and unresectable pancreatic adenocarcinomas. Two recent studies analyzed the use of IMRT to treat patients with malignancies of the pancreas.[120,121] The majority of patients received concurrent chemotherapy. The toxicity profile compared favorably with that of protocols based on continuous-infusion 5-FU or gemcitabine.[120] Compared with conventional RT, IMRT reduced the mean dose to the liver, kidneys, stomach, and small bowel.[121]

TREATMENT ALGORITHM, CONTROVERSIES, AND FUTURE POSSIBILITIES

A treatment algorithm for pancreatic carcinoma is provided in Figure 45-12.

For resectable disease, surgical therapy is clearly required for any chance at curing pancreatic cancer. However, controversies regarding effective adjuvant therapy remain debatable. From both retrospective and prospective studies, the considerable rates of local and distant relapse postoperatively dictate a natural consequence for using adjuvant chemoradiation if we strive for greater chance of cure. This finding was proved with the GITSG trial nearly 20 years ago but has not been confirmed with more recent phase III, randomized trials.

While the EORTC trial has been argued to be statistically underpowered, the ESPAC-1 trial has been criticized for nihilistically concluding that chemoradiotherapy has no role in the adjuvant therapy of resected pancreatic cancer.[122] Experts have challenged the ESPAC-1 trial for its lack of quality assurance monitoring, toxicity reporting, and nonadherence to the protocol, thus questioning the validity of the aforementioned conclusion.[122,123] If patterns of failure continue to show substantial rates of local and distant relapse, it would seem impossible to improve survival by discarding chemoradiation.

Future possibilities for improvement in survival for patients with locally advanced pancreas cancer need to involve more effective systemic or abdominal therapy and radiotherapy. The evaluation of high-dose preoperative irradiation plus simultaneous and maintenance chemotherapy is reasonable in both borderline and unresectable pancreas cancers in high performance status patients, if imaging and laparoscopy or laparotomy has ruled out peritoneal and liver metastases. For patients with marginal resection or locally unresectable disease, IOERT should be evaluated in conjunction with maintenance systemic therapy.

For patients in whom gross total resection of pancreatic cancer is feasible, the outcomes of RTOG 9704 have been awaited. The two-arm phase III postoperative adjuvant trial accrued 518 patients in a comparison of the efficacy of weekly gemcitabine versus continuous infusion 5-FU given as systemic chemotherapy before and after concurrent chemoradiation (infusion 5-FU). Updated results were presented at ASCO 2006.[124] In the 380 patients with pancreatic head lesions, survival was significantly improved in those randomized to receive gemcitabine versus 5-FU (median survival, 18.8 versus 16.7 months; 3-yr survival, 31% versus 21%; $p = .047$).

The most optimal rsults for patients with potentially curable pancreatic cancer (gross total resection with negative margins) will likely be achieved with trimodality treatment (surgery, chemotherapy, and radiation). The safest, most effective combination of all three components is yet to be determined. Future trials should address sequencing of the systemic components of treatment relative to the concurrent chemoradiation component with regard to giving several cycles of chemotherapy alone before starting concurrent chemoradiation. Moreovr, future treatment possibilities include molecular-based regimens utilizing gene targeting.[125] This approach is antibody-based, designed to target and kill pancreatic cancer cells.[124,125]

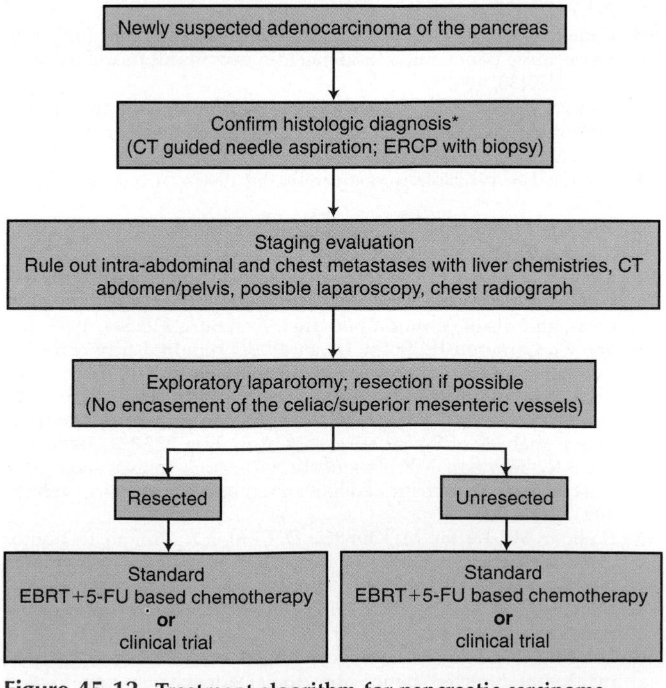

Figure 45-12 Treatment algorithm for pancreatic carcinoma. *Optional for patient going directly to surgery without neoadjuvant treatment.

REFERENCES

1. Brennan MF: Adjuvant therapy following resection for pancreatic adenocarcinoma. Surg Oncol Clin N Am 13:vii, 555, 2004.
2. Jamal A, Siegel R, Ward E, et al: Cancer statistics, 2006. CA Cancer J Clin 56:106-130, 2006.
3. Niederhuber JE, Brennan MF, Menck HR: The National Cancer Data Base Report on Pancreatic Cancer. Cancer 76:1671, 1995.
4. Warshaw AL, Fernandez-Del Castillo C: Pancreatic carcinoma. N Engl J Med 326:455, 1992.
5. Tavaria A, La Vecchia C: Coffee and Cancer: a review of epidemiologic studies, 1990-1999. Eur J Cancer Prev 9:241-256, 2000.
6. Travis LB, Curtis RE, Storm H, et al: The risk of second malignant neoplasms among long-term survivors of testicular cancer. J Natl Cancer Inst 89:1429, 1997.
7. Hilgers W, Kern SE: The molecular genetic basis of pancreatic adenocarcinoma. Genes Chromosomes Cancer 26:1, 1999.
8. Tersmette AC, Petersen GM, Offerhaus GJA, et al: Increased risk of incident pancreatic cancer among first-degree relatives of patients with familial pancreatic cancer. Clin Cancer Res 7:738, 2001.
9. Moossa AR, Gamagami RA: Diagnosis and staging of pancreatic neoplasms. Surg Clin North Am 75:871, 1995.
10. Legmann P, Vignaux O, Dousset B, et al: Pancreatic tumors: comparison of dual-phase helical CT and endoscopic sonography. AJR Am J Roentgenol 170:1315, 1998.
11. Ritts RE, Pitt HA: CA 19-9 in pancreatic cancer. Surg Oncol Clin N Am 7:93, 1998.
12. Abrams RA, Grochow LB, Chakravarthy A, et al: Intensified adjuvant therapy for pancreatic and periampullary adenocarcinoma: survival results and observations regarding patterns of failure, radiotherapy dose and CA19-9 levels. Int J Radiat Oncol Biol Phys 44:1039, 1999.
13. Montgomery RC, Hoffman JP, Riley LB, et al: Prediction of recurrence and survival by post-resection CA 19-9 values in patients with adenocarcinoma of the pancreas. Ann Surg Oncol 4:551, 1997.

14. Sato N, Fukushima N, Maitra A, et al: Discovery of novel targets for aberrant methylation in pancreatic carcinoma using high-throughput microarrays. Cancer Res 63:3735, 2003.
15. Iacobuzio-Donahue CA, Shen-Ong GL, Van Heek T, et al: Discovery of novel tumor markers of pancreatic cancer using global gene expression technology. Am J Pathol 160:1239, 2002.
16. Rosty C, Christa L, Kuzdzal S, Baldwin WM, et al: Identification of hepatocarcinoma-intestine-pancreas/pancreatitis-associated protein I as a biomarker for pancreatic ductal adenocarcinoma by protein biochip technology. Cancer Res 62:1868, 2002.
17. Bottger TC, Storkel S, Wellek S, et al: Factors influencing survival after resection of pancreatic cancer. Cancer 73:6372, 1994.
18. Jorba R, Jaurrieta E, Bernat R, et al: DNA ploidy and S+G2M fraction (proliferative index) as prognostic determinants in human periampullary cancer. Hepatogastroenterology 42:740, 1995.
19. Herrera MF, Van-Heerden JA, Katzman JA, et al: Evaluation of DNA nuclear pattern as a prognostic determinant in resected pancreatic adenocarcinoma. Ann Surg 215:120, 1992.
20. Hruban RH: Pancreatic cancer, 1999 update symposium. J Am Coll Surg 187:429, 1998.
21. Hruban RH, Offerhaus JA, Kern SE, et al: Tumor-suppressor genes in pancreatic cancer. J Hepatobiliary Pancreas Surg 5:383, 1998.
22. Tascilar M, Skinner HG, Rosty C, et al: The SMAD4 protein and prognosis of pancreatic ductal adenocarcinoma. Clin Cancer Res 7:4115, 2001.
23. Murphy KM, Brune KA, Griffin C, et al: Evaluation of candidate genes MAP2K, ACVR1B, and BRCA2 in familial pancreatic cancer: deleterious BRCA2 mutations in 17%. Cancer Res 62:3789, 2002.
24. Goggins RT, Murray T, Bolden S, et al: Pancreatic adenocarcinomas with DNA replication errors (RER+) are associated with wild type K-ras and characteristic histopathology. Am J Pathol 152:1501, 1998.
25. Griffin CA, Hruban RH, Morseberger L, et al: Consistent chromosome abnormalities and adenocarcinoma of the pancreas. Cancer Res 55:2394, 1995.
26. Griffin CA, Hruban RH, Long PP, et al: Chromosome abnormalities in pancreatic adenocarcinoma. Gene Chromosomes Cancer 9:93, 1994.
27. Hruban RH, Petersen GM, Ha PK, et al: Genetics of pancreatic cancer from genes to families. Surg Oncol Clin N Am 7:1, 1998.
28. Hruban RH, Petersen GM, Goggins M, et al: Familial pancreatic cancer. Ann Oncol 10:569, 1999.
29. Klein AP, Brune KA, Petersen GM, et al: Prospective risk of pancreatic cancer in familial pancreatic cancer kindreds. Cancer Res 64:2634, 2004.
30. Solcia E, Capella C, Kloppel G: Atlas of Tumor Pathology: Tumors of the Pancreas. 3rd series ed. Washington, DC: Armed Forces Institute of Pathology, 1997.
31. Wilentz RE, Hruban RH: Pathology of cancer of the pancreas. Surg Oncol Clin N Am 7:43, 1998.
32. Klimstra DS, Heffess CS, Oertel JE, et al: Acinar cell carcinoma of the pancreas. A clinicopathologic study of 28 cases. Am J Surg Pathol 16:815, 1992.
33. Compton CC: Serous cystic tumors of the pancreas. Semin Diagn Pathol 17:43, 1999.
34. Wilentz RE, Albores-Saavedra J, Zahurak M, et al: Pathologic examination accurately predicts prognosis in mucinous cystic neoplasms of the pancreas. Am J Surg Pathol 23:1320, 1991.
35. Adsay NV, Longnecker DS, Klimstra DS: Pancreatic tumors with cystic dilatation of the ducts: intraductal papillary mucinous neoplasms and intraductal oncocytic papillary neoplasms. Semin Diagn Pathol 17:16, 2000.
36. Wilentz RE, Hruban RH: Pathology of pancreatic cancer. *In* Cameron JL, ed: Pancreatic Cancer. Hamilton, Canada: BC Decker, 2001, pp 37-66.
37. Cubilla AL, Fortner J, Fitzgerald PJ: Pancreas cancer—duct cell adenocarcinoma: survival in relation to site, size, stage, and type of therapy. J Surg Oncol 10:465, 1978.
38. Cubilla AL, Fortner J, Fitzgerald PJ: Lymph node involvement in carcinoma of the head of the pancreas area. Cancer 41:880, 1978.
39. Nagai H, Kuroda A, Morioka Y: Lymphatic and local spread of T1 and T2 pancreatic cancer. Ann Surg 204:65, 1986.
40. Nagakawa T, Kobayashi H, Ueno K, et al: Clinical study of lymphatic flow to the para-aortic lymph nodes in carcinoma of the head of the pancreas. Cancer 73:1115, 1994.
41. Tepper J, Nardi G, Suit H: Carcinoma of the pancreas: review of MGH experience from 1963 to 1973. Analysis of surgical failure and implications for radiation therapy. Cancer 37:1519, 1976.
42. Griffin JF, Smalley SR, Jewell W, et al: Patterns of failure after curative resection of pancreatic carcinoma. Cancer 66:56, 1990.
43. Kayahara M, Nagakawa T, Ueno K, et al: An evaluation of radical resection for pancreatic cancer based on the mode of recurrence as determined by autopsy and diagnostic imaging. Cancer 72:2118, 1993.
44. Johnstone PA, Sindelar WF: Patterns of disease recurrence following definitive therapy of adenocarcinoma of the pancreas using surgery and adjuvant radiotherapy: correlation of a clinical trial. Int J Radiat Oncol Biol Phys 27:831, 1993.
45. Yeo TP, Hruban RH, Leach SD, et al: Pancreatic cancer. Curr Probl Cancer 26:176, 2002.
46. Sauter PK, Coleman J: Pancreatic cancer, a continuum of care. Semin Oncol Nursing 15:36, 1999.
47. American Joint Committee on Cancer: Exocrine pancreas. *In* Greene FL (ed): AJCC Staging Manual, 6th ed. New York, Springer, 2002, p. 161.
48. American Joint Committee on Cancer: Exocrine pancreas. *In* Greene FL (ed): AJCC Staging Manual, 6th ed. New York, Springer, 2002, p. 158.
49. Braash JW, Gagner M: Pylorus-preserving pancreaticoduodenectomy technical aspects. Langenbecks, Arch Surg 376:50, 1991.
50. Kozuschek W, Reith HB, Waleczek H, et al: A comparison of long-term results of the standard Whipple procedure and the pylorus-preserving pancreaticoduodenectomy. J Am Coll Surg 178:443, 1994.
51. Takao S, Aikou T, Shinchi H, et al: Comparison of relapse in long-term survival between pylorus-preserving and Whipple pancreaticoduodenectomy in periampullary cancer. Am J Surg 176:467, 1998.
52. Yeo CJ: Pylorus-preserving pancreaticoduodenectomy. Surg Oncol Clin N Am 7:143, 1988.
53. Yeo CJ, Cameron JL, Sohn TA, et al: Pancreaticoduodenectomy for cancer of the head of the pancreas, 201 patients. Ann Surg 221:721, 1995.
54. Cameron JL, Pitt HA, Yeo CJ, et al: One hundred and forty-five consecutive pancreaticoduodenectomies without mortality. Ann Surg 217:430, 1993.
55. Edis AJ, Kiernan PD, Taylor WF, et al: Attempted curative resection of ductal carcinoma of the pancreas. Review of the Mayo clinical experience. Mayo Clin Proc 55:531, 1980.
56. Yeo CJ: The Whipple procedure in the 1990's. Adv Surg 32:271, 1999.
57. Yeo CJ: Management of complications following pancreaticoduodenectomy. Surg Clin North Am 75:913, 1995.
58. Michelassi FM, Erroi F, Dawson PJ, et al: Experience with 647 consecutive tumors of the duodenum, ampulla, head of the pancreas, and distal common bile duct. Ann Surg 210:544, 1989.
59. Yeo CJ, Cameron JL, Sohn TA, et al: Six hundred fifty consecutive pancreaticoduodenectomies in the 1990's. Pathology, complications, and outcomes. Ann Surg 226:248, 1997.
60. Yeo CJ, Sohn A, Cameron JL, et al: Periampullary adenocarcinoma: analysis of 5-year survivors. Ann Surg 227:821, 1998.
61. Geer RJ, Brennan MF: Prognostic indicators for survival after resection of pancreatic adenocarcinoma. Am J Surg 165:68, 1993.
61a. Brennan MF, Kattan M, Klimstra D, Conlon K: Prognostic nomogram for patients undergoing resection for adenocarcinoma of the pancreas. Ann Surg 240:293, 2004.
62. Manabe T, Miyashita T, Ohshio G, et al: Small carcinomas of the pancreas. Cancer 62:135, 1988.
63. Foo ML, Gunderson LL, Nagorney DM, et al: Patterns of failure in grossly resected pancreatic ductal adenocarcinoma treated with adjuvant irradiation ± 5 fluorouracil. Int J Radiat Oncol Biol Phys 26:483, 1993.

64. Willett CG, Warshaw AL, Convery K, et al: Patterns of failure after pancreaticoduodenectomy for ampullary carcinoma. Surg Gynecol Obstet 176:33, 1993.
65. Kalser MH, Ellenberg SS: Pancreatic cancer: adjuvant combined radiation and chemotherapy following curative resection. Arch Surg 120:899, 1985.
66. Gastrointestinal Tumor Study Group: Further evidence of effective adjuvant combined radiation and chemotherapy following curative resection of pancreatic cancer. Cancer 59:2006, 1987.
67. Whittington R, Bryer MP, Haller DG, et al: Adjuvant therapy of resected adenocarcinoma of the pancreas. Int J Radiat Oncol Biol Phys 21:1137, 1991.
68. Yeo CJ, Abrams RA, Grochow LB, et al: Pancreaticoduodenectomy for pancreatic adenocarcinoma: postoperative adjuvant chemoradiation improves survival. Ann Surg 225:621, 1997.
69. Mehta VK, Fisher GA, Ford JM, at al: Adjuvant radiotherapy and concomitant 5-fluorouracil by protracted venous infusion for resected pancreatic cancer. Int J Radiat Oncol Biol Phys 48:1483, 2000.
70. Todd KE, Gloor B, Lane JS, et al: Resection of locally advanced pancreatic cancer after downstaging with continuous infusion 5-fluorouracil, mitomycin-C, leucovorin, and dipyridamole. J Gastrointest Surg 2:159, 1998.
71. Abrams RA, Grochow LB, Chakravarthy A, et al: Intensified adjuvant therapy for pancreatic and periampullary adenocarcinoma: survival results and observations regarding patterns of failure, radiotherapy dose, and CA 19-9 levels. Int J Radiat Oncol Biol Phys 44:1039, 1999.
72. Nukui Y, Picozzi VJ, Traverso LW: Interferon based adjuvant chemoradiation therapy improves survival after pancreaticoduodenectomy for pancreatic adenocarcinoma. Am J Surg 179:367, 2000.
73. Picozzi VJ, Kozarek RE, Jacobs AD, et al: Adjuvant therapy for resected pancreas cancer (PC) using alpha-interferon (IFN)-based chemoradiation: completion of a phase II trial. Proc ASCO 2003; 22:265, abstract 1061.
74. Klinkenbijl JH, Jeekel J, Sahmoud T, et al: Adjuvant radiotherapy and 5-fluorouracil after curative resection of cancer of the pancreas and periampullary region: phase III trial of the EORTC Gastrointestinal Tract Cancer Cooperative Group. Ann Surg 230:776, 1999.
75. Neoptolemos JP, Stocken DD, Friess H, et al: A randomized trial of chemoradiotherapy and chemotherapy after resection of pancreatic cancer. N Engl J Med 350:1200, 2004.
76. Neoptolemos JP, Stocken DD, Friess H, et al: Adjuvant chemoradiotherapy and chemotherapy in resectable pancreatic cancer: a randomized controlled trial. Lancet 358:1576, 2001.
77. Abrams RA, Lillemoe KD, Piantadosi S: Continuing controversy over adjuvant therapy of pancreatic cancer. Lancet 358:1565, 2001.
78. Ishikawa O, Ohigashi H, Imaoka S, et al: Is the long-term survival rate improved by preoperative irradiation prior to Whipple's procedure for adenocarcinoma of the pancreas head? Arch Surg 129:1075, 1994.
79. Evans DB, Byrd DR, Mansfield PF: Preoperative chemoradiotherapy for adenocarcinoma of the pancreas. Am J Clin Oncol 13:359, 1991.
80. Leach SD, Lee JE, Charnsangavej KR, et al: Survival following pancreaticoduodenectomy with resection of the superior mesenteric-portal vein confluence for adenocarcinoma of the pancreatic head. Br J Surg 85:611, 1996.
81. Spitz FR, Abbruzzese JL, Lee JE, et al: Preoperative and postoperative chemoradiation strategies in patients treated with pancreaticoduodenectomy for adenocarcinoma of the pancreas. J Clin Oncol 15:928, 1997.
82. Yeung RS, Weese JL, Hoffman JP, et al: Neoadjuvant chemoradiation in pancreatic and duodenal carcinoma—A phase II study. Cancer 72:2124, 1993.
83. Hoffman JP, Weese JL, Solin LJ, et al: A single institutional experience with preoperative chemoradiotherapy for stage I-III pancreatic adenocarcinoma. Am Surg 59:772, 1993.
84. Hoffman JP, Weese JL, Solin LJ, et al: A pilot study of preoperative chemoradiation for patients with localized adenocarcinoma of the pancreas. Am J Surg 169:71, 1995.
85. Pendurthi TK, Hoffman JP, Ross E, et al: Preoperative versus postoperative chemoradiation for patients with resected pancreatic adenocarcinoma. Am Surg 64:686, 1998.
86. Hoffman JP, Lipsitz S, Pisansky T, et al: Phase II trial of preoperative radiation therapy and chemotherapy for patients with localized, resectable adenocarcinoma of the pancreas: an Eastern Cooperative Oncology Group Study. J Clin Oncol 16:317, 1998.
87. Lillemoe K, Cameron J, Yeo C, et al: Pancreaticoduodenectomy—does it have a role in palliation of pancreatic cancer? Ann Surg 223:718, 1996.
88. Ouchi K, Sugawara T, Ono H, et al: Palliative operation for cancer of the head of pancreas: significance of pancreaticoduodenectomy and intraoperative radiation therapy for survival and quality of life. World J Surg 22:413, 1998.
89. Moertel CG, Frytak S, Hahn RG, et al: Therapy of locally unresectable pancreatic carcinoma: a randomized comparison of high dose (6000 rads) radiation alone, moderate dose radiation (4000 rads + 5-fluorouracil), and high dose radiation + 5-fluorouracil. Cancer 48:1705, 1981.
90. Gastrointestinal Tumor Study Group: Treatment of locally unresectable carcinoma of the pancreas: comparison of combined modality therapy (chemotherapy plus radiotherapy) to chemotherapy alone. J Natl Cancer Inst 80:751, 1988.
91. Flickinger J, Jawalekar K, Deutsch M, et al: Split course radiation therapy for adenocarcinoma of the pancreas. Int J Radiat Oncol Biol Phys 15:359, 1988.
92. Jeekel J, Treuniet-Donker AD: Treatment perspectives in locally advanced unresectable pancreatic cancer. Br J Surg 11:1332, 1978.
93. Bruckner HW, Kalnicki S, Dalton J, et al: Combined modality therapy increasing local control of pancreatic cancer. Cancer Invest 11:241, 1993.
94. Moertel C, Gunderson L, Mailliard J, et al: Early evaluation of combined fluorouracil and leucovorin as a radiation enhancer for locally unresectable, residual, or recurrent gastrointestinal carcinoma. J Clin Oncol 12:21, 1994.
95. Blackstock AW, Bernard SA, Richards F, et al: Phase I trial of twice weekly gemcitabine and concurrent radiation in patients with advanced pancreatic cancer. J Clin Oncol 17:2208, 1999.
96. Blackstock AW, Tempero MA, Niedzwiecki D, et al: Cancer and Leukemia Group B (CALGB) 89805: phase II chemoradiation trial using gemcitabine in patients with locoregional adenocarcinoma of the pancreas. Proc ASCO 20:15a, 2001.
97. Wolff RA, Evans DB, Gravel DM, et al: Phase I trial of gemcitabine combined with radiation for the treatment of locally advanced pancreatic adenocarcinoma. Clin Cancer Res 2246:2246, 2001.
98. McGinn CJ, Zalupski MM, Shureiqi I, et al: Phase I trial of radiation dose escalation with concurrent weekly full-dose gemcitabine in patients with advanced pancreatic cancer. J Clin Oncol 19:4202, 2001.
99. Talamonti MS, Catalano PJ, Vaughn DJ, et al: Eastern Cooperative Oncology Group phase I trial of protracted venous infusion fluorouracil plus weekly gemcitabine with concurrent radiation therapy in patients with locally advanced pancreas cancer: a regimen with unexpected early toxicity. J Clin Oncol 18:3384, 2000.
100. Martenson JA, Vigliotti APG, Pitot HC, et al: A phase I study of radiation therapy and twice-weekly gemcitabine and cisplatin in patients with locally advanced pancreatic cancer. Int J Radiat Oncol Biol Phys 55:1305, 2003.
101. Brunner TB, Grabenbauer GG, Klein P, et al: Phase I trial of strictly time-scheduled gemcitabine and cisplatin with concurrent radiotherapy in patients with locally advanced pancreatic cancer. Int J Radiat Oncol Biol Phys 55:141, 2003.
102. Crane CH, Abbruzzese JL, Evans DB, et al: Is the therapeutic index better with gemcitabine based chemoradiation than with 5-fluorouracil chemoradiation in locally advanced pancreatic cancer? Int J Radiat Oncol Biol Phys 52:1293, 2002.
103. Burris HA, Moore MJ, Andersen J, et al: Improvements in survival and clinical benefit with gemcitabine as first-line therapy for patients with advanced pancreas cancer: a randomized trial. J Clin Oncol 15:2403, 1997.
104. Mohiuddin M, Rosato F, Barbot D, et al: Long-term results of combined modality treatment with I-125 implantation for

carcinoma of the pancreas. Int J Radiat Oncol Biol Phys 23:305, 1992.
105. Nori D, Merimsky O, Osian AD, et al: Palladium-103: a new radioactive source in the treatment of unresectable carcinoma of the pancreas: a phase I-II study. J Surg Oncol 61:300, 1996.
106. Raben A, Mychalczak B, Brennan MF, et al: Feasibility study of the treatment of primary unresectable carcinoma of the pancreas with palladium-103 brachytherapy. Int J Radiat Oncol Biol Phys 25:351, 1996.
107. Gunderson LL, Tepper JE, Biggs DJ, et al: Intraoperative ± external beam irradiation. Curr Probl Cancer 7:1, 1983.
108. Gunderson LL, Nagorney DM, Martenson JA, et al: External beam plus intraoperative irradiation for gastrointestinal cancers. World J Surg 19:191, 1995.
109. Gunderson LL and Willett C: Pancreas and hepatobiliary tract cancer. *In* Perez CA, Brady LW (eds): Principles and Practice of Radiation Oncology, 3rd ed. Philadelphia, JB Lippincott, 1997, pp. 1467-1488.
110. Willett C, Daly W, Warshaw A, et al: CA 19-9 as an index of response to neoadjunctive chemoradiation therapy in pancreatic cancer. Am J Surg 172:350, 1996.
111. Tepper JE, Noyes D, Krall J, et al: Intraoperative radiation therapy of pancreatic carcinoma: a report of RTOG-8505. Int J Radiat Oncol Biol Phys 21:1145, 1991.
112. Roldan GE, Gunderson LL, Nagorney DM, et al: External beam versus intraoperative and external beam irradiation for locally advanced pancreatic cancer. Cancer 61:1110, 1988.
113. Dobelbower RR, Konski A, Merrick H, et al: Intraoperative electron beam radiotherapy (IOEBRT) for carcinoma of the exocrine pancreas. Int J Radiat Oncol Biol Phys 20:113, 1991.
114. Kawamura M, Kataoka M, Fuji T, et al: Electron beam intraoperative radiation therapy (EBIORT) for localized pancreatic carcinoma. Int J Radiat Oncol Biol Phys 23:751, 1992.
115. Zerbi A, Fossati V, Parolini D, et al: Intraoperative radiation therapy adjuvant to resection in the treatment of pancreatic cancer. Cancer 73:2930, 1994.
116. Mohiuddin M, Regine W, Stevens J, et al: Combined intraoperative radiation and perioperative chemotherapy for unresectable cancers of the pancreas. J Clin Oncol 13:2764, 1995.
117. Garton G, Gunderson L, Nagorney D, et al: High-dose preoperative external beam in intraoperative irradiation for locally advanced pancreatic cancer. Int J Radiat Oncol Biol Phys 27:1153, 1993.
118. Andreyev HJN, Norman AR, Oates J, et al: Why do patients with weight loss have a worse outcome when undergoing chemotherapy for gastrointestinal malignancies? Eur J Cancer 34:503, 1998.
119. A phase III study of pre and post chemoradiation 5-FU versus pre and post chemoradiation gemcitabine for postoperative adjuvant treatment of resected pancreatic adenocarcinoma, RTOG 97-04. www.RTOG.org
120. Ben-Josef E, Shields AF, Vaishampayan U, et al: Intensity-modulated radiotherapy (IMRT) and concurrent capecitabine for pancreatic cancer. Int J Radiat Oncol Biol Phys 50:454, 2004.
121. Milano MT, Chmura SJ, Garafalo MC, et al: Intensity-modulated radiotherapy in treatment of pancreatic and bile duct malignancies: toxicity and clinical outcome. Int J Radiat Oncol Biol Phys 59:445, 2004.
122. Koshy MC, Landry JC, Cavanaugh SX, et al: A challenge to the therapeutic nihilism of ESPAC-1. Int J Radiat Oncol Biol Phys 61:965, 2005.
123. Choti MA: Adjuvant therapy for pancreatic cancer—the debate continues. N Engl J Med 350:1249, 2004.
124. Regine WF, Winter KW, Abrams RA, et al: RTOG 9704, A phase III study of adjuvant pre- and post-chemo-irradiation 5-FU vs gemcitabine for resected pancreatic adenocarcinoma, ASCO Abstracts. J Clin Oncol 241:180S, 2006.
125. Gunderson LL, Haddock MG, Burch P, et al: Future role of radiotherapy as a component of treatment in biliopancreatic cancers. Ann Oncol 10(Suppl 4):S291, 1999.

CHAPTER 46

HEPATOBILIARY TUMORS

Edgar Ben-Josef and Theodore S. Lawrence

INCIDENCE

In 2006, the expected incidence in the United States is 27,080 cases with 19,460 deaths.

BIOLOGIC CHARACTERISTICS

Hepatocellular carcinoma is linked to chronic hepatitis B or C infections, liver cirrhosis, and aflatoxin ingestion. Gallbladder and biliary cancers may be related to cholelithiasis. The occurrence of intrahepatic cholangiocarcinoma is especially high in patients with primary sclerosing cholangitis.

STAGING EVALUATION

Work-up includes history and physical examination, complete blood count, liver chemistries, coagulation studies, and abdominal computed tomography or magnetic resonance scan. Evaluation of biliary tumors usually also includes a transhepatic or endoscopic retrograde cholangiogram. Examination for distant disease requires only a chest radiograph.

PRIMARY THERAPY

For all hepatobiliary tumors, the primary therapy is resection. Patients with resected hepatocellular carcinoma have a median survival of nearly 2 years and a 5-year survival rate of approximately 30%. Similar results are reported for extrahepatic cholangiocarcinoma. Five-year survival rates for gallbladder cancer vary from less than 10% to 30%.

ADJUVANT THERAPY

Although no randomized trials of adjuvant therapy have been performed, adjuvant radiation and chemotherapy are typically recommended for patients with high-risk features after resection.

LOCALLY ADVANCED DISEASE

Radiation has rarely been used for locally advanced intrahepatic disease because of concerns that radiation-induced liver disease would develop. Evidence suggests that long-term hepatic control may be obtained using high-dose radiation therapy, which can be given using three-dimensional radiation techniques, combined with hepatic arterial chemotherapy. Lower doses of radiation have been used with transcatheter arterial chemoembolization in Asia.

Unresectable extrahepatic cholangiocarcinomas may be treated using a combination of external beam radiation therapy and brachytherapy with or without 5-fluorouracil–based chemotherapy.

PALLIATION

Irradiation of the whole liver to 30 Gy can be palliative.

Hepatobiliary malignancies include hepatocellular carcinoma (HCC), gallbladder cancer, extrahepatic cholangiocarcinoma (EHCC), and intrahepatic cholangiocarcinoma (IHCC). HCC, already the fifth most common malignancy worldwide,[1] is increasing in incidence in the United States as a result of the hepatitis C epidemic.[2] A similar increase has been reported in the incidence of IHCC for reasons that are not known.[3] The primary therapy for all hepatobiliary tumors is resection, but only a minority of patients present with resectable disease. A number of therapies have been in use for these patients, including systemic and regional chemotherapy, chemoembolization, immunotherapy, and various ablative techniques. Today, the role of these modalities has not been defined and there is currently no accepted standard for the management of unresectable hepatic malignancies. Historically, radiotherapy has not played a significant role in the treatment of liver malignancies because of the low tolerance of the whole liver to radiation.[4,5] With the advent of three-dimensional conformal treatment planning, interest in the use of radiation for liver malignancies has increased. Modern-day techniques allow delivery of higher doses to the target lesions than had been previously possible, while minimizing dose to the noninvolved liver. At the same time, our understanding of the relationships between radiation dose and volume and the risk of radiation-induced liver disease (RILD) has improved considerably. These developments have led to a body of evidence that now exists in support of the use of radiotherapy for unresectable hepatobiliary cancer.

EPIDEMIOLOGY

Cancer of the hepatobiliary system is uncommon in the United States, accounting for only about 2% of new cancer cases.[6] Despite this infrequency, it was estimated that more people died in 2004 as a result of hepatobiliary cancer than of esophageal or rectal cancer. Hepatobiliary cancers occur primarily in the elderly; its incidence increases with age.[7] The most common hepatobiliary cancer is HCC, followed by gallbladder cancer, EHCC, and IHCC. Approximately one quarter of the cholangiocarcinomas occur at the bifurcation of the common hepatic duct and are known as hilar or Klatskin's tumors. Other cancers of the liver, such as carcinoid tumors, hepatoblastoma, angiosarcoma, and leiomyosarcoma are extremely rare. HCC and IHCC are three and two times more common in men than women, respectively, whereas gallbladder cancer is about three times more common in women, and EHCC occurs with approximately equal frequency.[5]

There is considerable variation in the incidence of HCC worldwide. In Asia, southeast Asia, and sub-Saharan Africa, HCC is between 15 and 100 times more common than in North America.[8] These areas also have a high incidence of chronic hepatitis B virus infection.[8,9] Carcinoma of the gallbladder also has shown substantial geographic variation, and incidence in some areas, such as northeastern Europe, is more than 20 times higher than in the United States.[10] Although EHCC has a fairly uniform incidence, IHCC is also more common in southeast Asia than in other parts of the world, presumably related to liver fluke infestation.

Considerable variation in the incidence of HCC is also observed in the United States. For example, HCC is 5 times more common in black men than white women.[7] Gallbladder cancer is 15 times more common among Native American women in New Mexico than in white women in the same state.[10] The other major types of hepatobiliary tumors are of approximately equal distribution or show a slight preponderance among whites.

ETIOLOGY

Hepatocellular Carcinoma

In Korea and Taiwan, approximately 90% of all patients with HCC are hepatitis B surface antigen (HBsAg) positive, and prospective studies have found that hepatitis B virus carriers have a 200-fold increase in relative risk for HCC.[8] Indeed, 90% of patients with HCC who are also HBsAg positive have viral DNA integrated into the host genome.[9] The greatest evidence of a causal relationship between hepatitis B infection and HCC development, however, is the observation that the incidence of childhood HCC in Taiwan has declined significantly since the institution of a nationwide vaccination program.[11]

The hepatitis C virus has also been implicated in the pathogenesis of HCC but with less incidence of coexistent cirrhosis and without evidence of host genome integration of the viral DNA.[8] These findings have suggested that an alternate mechanism may be in play, which does not involve either cirrhosis or host DNA alterations.

Cirrhosis without hepatitis infection probably accounts for more cases of HCC in the United States than hepatitis infections.[8,12] The development of HCC has been observed in a number of diseases, all of which share the endpoint of cirrhosis.[13]

Aflatoxin B is a toxic metabolite of fungi that can grow in stored grain and peanuts and has been linked with HCC development in some areas of Africa and Asia.[9] A reactive intermediate metabolite of aflatoxin B has been shown to selectively bind to guanine, which is excised and preferentially replaced with thymidine. This guanine-to-thymidine mutation is commonly found in the *TP53* (previously designated as *p53*) tumor suppressor gene in HCC, occurring in areas of high aflatoxin ingestion but is not found where aflatoxin levels are low.

Gallbladder Cancer

Epidemiologic studies have found that gallbladder cancer is more frequent in regions or among populations who have a high frequency of cholelithiasis.[10,14] However, whether the increased risk is related to a direct irritating effect of gallstones or to the presence of carcinogens in bile acids is unknown.[10,15] Additionally, the incidence rate of cancer in patients with calcified gallbladders has implied that any chronic inflammatory condition could lead to carcinogenesis.[16]

Cholangiocarcinoma

The development of cholangiocarcinoma has been epidemiologically linked to liver fluke infestation, hepatolithiasis, pyogenic cholangitis, congenital bile duct cysts, past exposure to thorium dioxide, typhoid carrier state, and ulcerative colitis.[8,17] Patients with primary sclerosing cholangitis also have an increased risk, with an incidence of cholangiocarcinoma of about 10%.[18] However, the cause of carcinogenesis in these settings is unclear. It is possible that EHCCs share a common pathway of carcinogenesis with gallbladder cancer, because the risk is lessened 10 years after cholecystectomy.[19]

PREVENTION AND EARLY DETECTION

The identification of patient groups at high risk for HCC and the poor results of therapy have made prevention and early detection strategies attractive.[20] The prevention of HCC by vaccination for hepatitis B has been supported by a review of the childhood HCC rates in Taiwan after introduction of a nationwide vaccination program.[11] Approximately 85% or more of infants in Taiwan have received hepatitis B vaccination since 1986 compared with none before 1984. On review, the incidence of HCC among 6- to 14-year-olds has significantly declined from 0.70 to 0.36 per 100,000, with corresponding reductions in mortality rates as well. Because the incidence of HCC peaks among people 50 to 60 years of age, it can be anticipated that reductions in HCC incidence will increase as the immunized population ages.

The early detection of HCC in endemic areas of hepatitis B has received considerable attention. One screening tool is the serum alpha-fetoprotein (AFP), which has been used in extensive population surveys in China, Taiwan, and South Africa and among Native Alaskans.[21] Unfortunately, even when screening was limited to people at high risk, the number of HCC cases detected was low. For example, a screening study in South Africa obtained AFP levels in more than 11,000 HBsAg-positive patients but found only 10 with HCC.[21] Similarly, in China, of about 2 million people who were screened with AFP, only 300 cases were found. Liver ultrasonography has also been pursued as a screening tool. Although ultrasonography may be superior to AFP,[21] it is more expensive.[20] Aside from cost issues, there is no evidence that current screening techniques can detect disease while it is still potentially curable.[22]

Given the increased risk of cholangiocarcinoma in patients with primary sclerosing cholangitis and ulcerative colitis, the difficulty obtaining a diagnosis of malignancy, and the lethality of the cancer when diagnosed, the finding that serum CA 19-9 may be useful for screening and early diagnosis is attractive.[23] There are no known preventive measures for the biliary tract cancers. Even though cholelithiasis is a risk factor for gallbladder cancer[10,14] and may also be related to extrahepatic bile duct cancers, there is no evidence to justify cholecystectomy as a preventive measure.[10,19]

PATHOLOGY AND PATTERNS OF SPREAD

Hepatocellular Carcinoma

Grossly, HCC can appear as expanding or spreading, depending on whether the margin is discrete or poorly defined, or as multifocal, with multiple tumors scattered throughout the liver without an obvious primary-to-secondary relationship.[24] The microscopic appearance of HCC resembles normal liver, both cytologically and by the characteristic plate-like growth. Nuclear grading is typically judged using a four-grade system, but for prognostic purposes cells are either low grade (grade 1 or 2) or high grade (grade 3 or 4).[25] Grade 1 tumors can be difficult to differentiate from adenomas or atypical hyperplastic nodules. Similarly, grade 4 tumors can resemble other anaplastic cancers and require special stains for further characterization.[13]

Hepatocellular carcinoma may locally invade the portal vein, hepatic vein, or diaphragm. Approximately one third of patients have regional disease at presentation, with metastases to the porta hepatic and celiac axis lymph node chains.[7] Intra-abdominal metastasis to the peritoneal lining or liver or extra-abdominal spread to the lungs is found in about one third of patients.[7] Metastasis to other sites, such as the brain or muscle, occurs infrequently.

Fibrolamellar carcinoma is a unique subtype of HCC that comprises about 5% of the cases in North America.[25] Fibrolamellar carcinoma has the longest survival of any of the HCC subtypes and is typically found in young women. Grossly, it is classified as an expanding, sclerosing tumor, characterized by septa of retracted collagenous structures radiating from a central region.[24] Cytologically, the tumor cells are large and polygonal, with a granular cytoplasm resulting from numerous mitochondria. The abundant fibrous stroma is characteristic and is arranged in parallel lamellae around nests, cords, and sheets of tumor cells.[13]

Gallbladder Cancer

Most gallbladder cancers are adenocarcinomas.[26] The gross appearance can vary from localized nodular growths to involvement of the entire organ.[27] Histologically, both grade and vascular invasion are of prognostic value.[26] Papillary adenocarcinoma is a variant histology which comprises about 6% of the total number of cases and has a much longer median survival. Mucinous carcinoma is another variant of adenocarcinoma, occurring in about 5% of cases and associated with perforation of the gallbladder.[27]

Direct liver invasion is frequent[16] and may be related to the thin wall and single muscular layer of the gallbladder, the presence of Rokitansky-Aschoff sinuses (which themselves can penetrate the muscle layer in cases of chronic cholecystitis), and the fact that the perimuscular connective tissue of the gallbladder is directly contiguous with the interlobular connective tissue of the liver.[26] Approximately 40% to 50% of patients will have distant metastases at presentation, usually to the liver or peritoneum.[16,26] Despite an increase in the number of cholecystectomies in recent years, driven mostly by the widespread adoption of laparoscopic techniques, the proportion of patients presenting with advanced disease has not declined.[28,29] Lymphatic spread to the cystic, pericholedochal, hilar, and celiac lymph nodes is found in 45% of patients.[16]

Cholangiocarcinoma

Biliary cancer is typically divided according to the site of origin into intrahepatic, extrahepatic, or hilar (Klatskin's tumors).[13] Grossly, biliary cancers are sclerotic, with a diffuse, firm, gray-white annular thickening of the duct.[30] Nearly all carcinomas of the biliary tree are mucin-producing adenocarcinomas with cell variation from cuboidal to columnar with prominent nucleoli. As with gallbladder cancer, the variant histology of papillary adenocarcinoma has a better prognosis.[31]

Cholangiocarcinoma typically spreads by direct extension along the biliary tree, although separate tumor nodules may represent either multifocal tumor development or metastatic deposits.[32] Direct invasion of adjacent organs is more common for intrahepatic and hilar tumors than for extrahepatic tumors.[7,31,33] Tumor involvement of the cystic, hilar, or celiac lymph nodes is found in 30% to 50% of patients.[7,16,33] The incidence of distant metastases is about 30%, with a lower incidence of peritoneal disease than for gallbladder cancer.[33]

BIOLOGIC CHARACTERISTICS AND MOLECULAR BIOLOGY

Molecular techniques have led to significant advances in delineating the process of hepatocarcinogenesis. Frequently, fragments of hepatitis B viral DNA can be found within the genome of the HCC,[8,9] leading to the hypothesis that viral integration activates oncogenes or interferes with tumor suppressor genes. In fact, the normal liver of patients with chronic hepatitis B infection will show viral DNA integration early in the course of the disease, suggesting that the HCC originated from clonal expansion of the affected hepatocytes.[34] Against these arguments, however, is the finding that the sites of viral DNA integration are not consistent and do not occur near any known oncogenes or tumor suppressor genes. Nor does the viral DNA itself contain any known oncogenes. Thus, if the integration of viral DNA is necessary for carcinogenesis, then the mechanism may be due to genomic instability from deletions and chromosomal rearrangement rather than specific oncogene activation or disruption of a tumor suppressor gene pathway.[34]

Hepatocarcinogenesis may not be due to one particular molecular change but related to the ability of the liver to respond to damage by regeneration. The continuous liver damage seen with chronic hepatitis or cirrhosis leads to increased turnover of hepatocytes. During normal hepatocyte regeneration, both proto-oncogene activation and inactivation of suppressor genes occur. Chronic liver damage leads to a nearly continuous cellular reproduction, which may allow carcinogenic molecular changes to accumulate without repair.[34] The observation of apparent stepwise progression of small HCC from regenerating nodules of liver cirrhosis supports this hypothesis.[35]

CLINICAL MANIFESTATIONS, PATIENT EVALUATION, AND STAGING

Symptoms and Signs

The typical presentation of a patient with hepatobiliary cancer depends on the site of origin. Patients with primary liver tumors, HCC or IHCC, frequently will complain of right upper abdominal or epigastric pain at presentation.[8,33,36,37] The pain is usually dull but may be sharp and severe with end-stage disease. Rarely, patients with HCC will complain of a sudden, sharp, severe pain related to acute bleeding into the tumor or rupture of the tumor with intra-abdominal bleeding. The patient may also be aware of an abdominal mass or increased girth related to ascites.

Cirrhosis is present in approximately 70% of patients with HCC.[12] Occasionally, patients with known cirrhosis will be evaluated because of an unexplained clinical deterioration. Jaundice is unusual with primary liver tumors and may be obstructive because of tumor compression of the biliary system or hepatocellular because of end-stage hepatic replacement with tumor.

In contrast to the primary liver tumors, patients with cholangiocarcinomas of the biliary hilum or distal biliary tree almost invariably present with jaundice.[33,36] Abdominal pain and the nonspecific complaints of weight loss, anorexia, fatigue, fever, and night sweats are common complaints of patients with either biliary or hepatic tumors. Patients with gallbladder cancer commonly complain of both abdominal pain and jaundice and may also have weight loss, anorexia, and fatigue but are usually undiagnosed before an attempted cholecystectomy.[16,38,39]

The most common physical finding in patients with primary hepatic tumors is hepatomegaly,[36,37] which is frequently tender. The liver is often smooth but may be nodular as a result of tumor or cirrhosis. Occasionally, patients with HCC may have a hepatic bruit because of the highly vascular nature of the tumor. Ascites is a particularly ominous finding because it represents either hepatic dysfunction resulting from cirrhosis or tumor replacement, Budd-Chiari syndrome from malignant invasion of the hepatic veins, or peritoneal spread of cancer.

Patients with EHCC or gallbladder cancer are usually jaundiced but can also have hepatomegaly or simply tenderness in the right upper quadrant. Although a mass may be palpable, patients with gallbladder cancer are typically thought to have benign disease until exploration and resection. In one review, only 41 of 143 patients with gallbladder cancer were suspected preoperatively of having a malignancy.[39]

Laboratory Studies

The goals of the work-up of patients with hepatobiliary malignancies are to define the extent of the tumor and to carefully assess liver function. Laboratory testing includes a complete blood count, routine biochemistry panel, and coagulation studies (Table 46-1). Serum CA 19-9 may have value as a tumor marker for cholangiocarcinoma.[23]

Serum AFP is a widely used tumor marker for HCC; normal values are 20 μg/L or less, and levels greater than 400 μg/L (4000 μg/L in patients with hepatitis) are considered diagnostic of HCC. There is some evidence that AFP levels are prognostic for patients with tumors 5 cm or smaller as well as those with more than 50% involvement of the liver.[40] The major difficulty using AFP is that elevations to levels between 20 and 400 μg/L may represent either an exacerbation of hepatitis or a small, curable HCC.[20,21] This observation has led to the recommendation that patients with known cirrhosis hepatitis and a rise in AFP undergo retesting in 1 to 3 months, after an exacerbation of hepatitis would be expected to have improved. Another difficulty is the false-negative rate, which occurs in 10% to 15% of patients with HCC, presumably because the tumor is either too anaplastic or too well differentiated to produce the protein.[20]

Patients with HCC also frequently have a history of hepatitis. Although hepatitis status does not appear to be prognostic,[12] response rates to chemotherapy were higher and toxicity was lower in hepatitis B– or C–negative patients in a trial of hepatic arterial chemotherapy.[41] Approximately 5% of patients with HCC have a paraneoplastic syndrome,[12] such as hypoglycemia, erythrocytosis, hypercalcemia, and hypercholesterolemia.[37]

Table 46-1 Diagnostic Evaluation for Hepatobiliary Cancers

GENERAL
History
Physical examination

LABORATORY STUDIES
Complete blood count
Biochemistry panel, including liver function studies
Coagulation studies (PT, PTT)
Serum CA 19-9 (if suspicious for cholangiocarcinoma)
AFP (if suspicious for hepatocellular carcinoma)
CEA (may be elevated for any hepatobiliary cancer)
Hepatitis studies (HBsAg, HBsAb, HBcAb, anti-HCV)

RADIOGRAPHIC STUDIES
Ultrasonography
Abdominal CT scan
Liver MRI/MRCP
Transhepatic or endoscopic cholangiography (if bile duct blockage is present)

AFP, alpha-fetoprotein; anti-HCV, antibody to hepatitis C virus; CEA, carcinoembryonic antigen; CT, computed tomography; HBcAb, hepatitis B core antibody; HBsAb, hepatitis B surface antibody; HBsAg, hepatitis B surface antigen; MRCP, magnetic resonance chalangiopancreatography; MRI, magnetic resonance imaging; PT, prothrombin time; PTT, partial thromboplastin time.

Radiographic Evaluation

The primary imaging modalities currently being used for characterizing the extent of liver tumors include ultrasonography (US), computed tomography (CT), and magnetic resonance imaging (MRI). Patients suspected of hepatic disease, whether IHCC or HCC, are typically first evaluated with US. Although findings of focal liver lesions are often nonspecific, advances such as the use of Doppler, contrast agents, and harmonic imaging have improved the usefulness of this examination.[42,43] Still, US may be limited by patient characteristics such as obesity, intestinal distention or scars, and it is very operator dependent. When evaluating for potential resection, MRI and CT are the dominant imaging modality because of their ability to display hepatic segmental anatomy, extent of hepatic disease and evaluate extrahepatic spread. The advent of spiral CT, and multislice spiral CT, has improved hepatic imaging considerably. With this new technology, spatial resolution has been improved; the acquisition time has been reduced so that liver imaging can be accomplished during one single breath hold; and thinner slices can be obtained, enabling multiplanar reformatting. State-of-the-art CT scanning involves acquisition of three contrast phases (arterial hepatic, portal venous, and equilibrium) that are very important for assessing lesion vascularity.[42] For instance, HCC is hypervascular and typically displays intense enhancement during the arterial-hepatic phase, whereas cholangiocarcinoma may display delayed enhancement.

CT scanning can also be performed after administration of contrast via an angiographically placed superior mesenteric artery catheter (CT arterial portography) or a hepatic artery catheter (CT hepatic arteriography). With the former, the bolus of contrast passes through the intestinal vasculature and collects in the portal vein, providing excellent contrast between normal liver and tumor (Fig. 46-1). CT arterial portography and CT hepatic arteriography are considered the most sensitive methods of detecting small liver cancers,[44,45] detecting lesions as small as 0.2 cm in diameter.[46] However, a high false-positive rate has limited their usefulness.[47]

MRI plays an important role in detection and characterization of liver tumors. Modern MRI protocols usually include parenchymal imaging with one or more types of contrast agents, MR angiography, and MR cholangiopancreatography (MRCP). The superior contrast resolution and inherent capability of multiplanar evaluation have made MRI the examination of choice for characterization of lesions in cirrhotic patients.[42,48]

In patients with biliary obstruction, MRCP has limited the role of transhepatic or endoscopic cholangiopancreatography to instances when drainage and decompression of the biliary system is required.[43] In addition to being noninvasive, the advantages of MRCP are its ability to define the extent of tumor not only within the intra- and extrahepatic bile ducts, but also provide information on the status of the portal vein and lymph nodes.

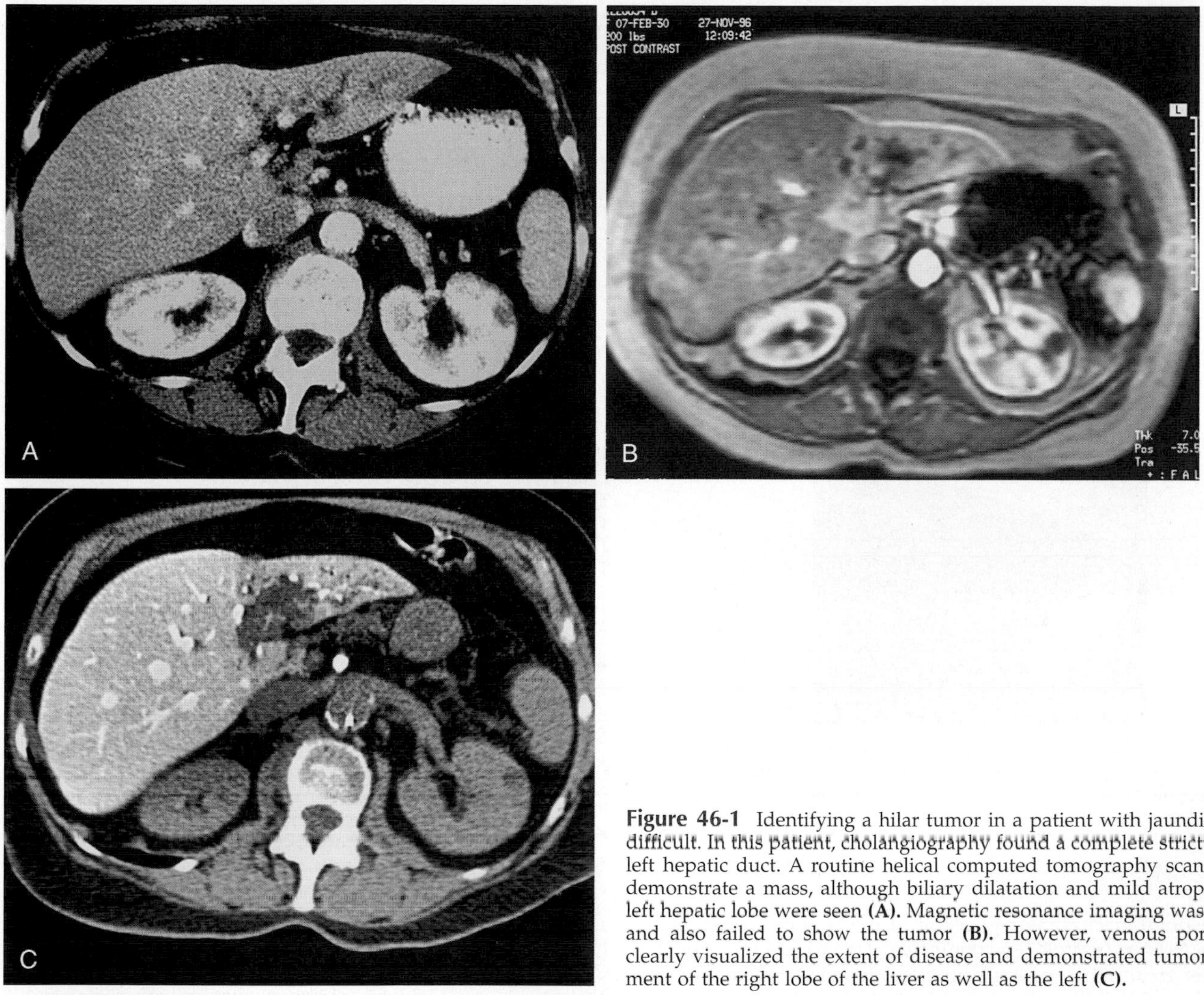

Figure 46-1 Identifying a hilar tumor in a patient with jaundice can be difficult. In this patient, cholangiography found a complete stricture of the left hepatic duct. A routine helical computed tomography scan failed to demonstrate a mass, although biliary dilatation and mild atrophy of the left hepatic lobe were seen **(A)**. Magnetic resonance imaging was obtained and also failed to show the tumor **(B)**. However, venous portography clearly visualized the extent of disease and demonstrated tumor involvement of the right lobe of the liver as well as the left **(C)**.

The usual appearance of an EHCC is a stricture at the site of involvement with dilatation of the biliary tract proximal to the stricture (Fig. 46-2). The tumor itself may extend for some distance along the biliary tract. One area of particular difficulty is distinguishing bile duct cancer from primary sclerosing cholangitis.[18] US, CT, and MRI of the abdomen frequently show only intrahepatic biliary dilatation (with or without hepatic atrophy) but no identifiable mass.[17]

Although ultrasonographic examination is frequently obtained in patients suspected of having gallbladder disease, the study is rarely diagnostic of gallbladder cancer.[38] Postoperative evaluation using CT scanning can be helpful in defining both residual disease and possible metastases.

Diagnosis

The National Comprehensive Cancer Network (NCCN) guidelines recommend a biopsy for patients suspected of having HCC when their AFP is 400 μg/L or less (4000 μg/L or less in patients with hepatitis). Fine-needle aspiration can also be used in patients with hepatic tumors to arrive at a diagnosis.[13] Cytologic efforts have found improved ability to confidently diagnose HCC on fine-needle aspiration by examining the nuclear-cytoplasmic ratio, trabecular pattern, and atypical naked hepatocytic nuclei.[49]

Establishing the diagnosis of cholangiocarcinoma can be difficult without exploration, presumably because of the large amount of sclerosis present. However, performing an incisional biopsy or curettage at the time of surgery should be avoided in view of an increased risk of peritoneal failure or wound implant with these procedures.[50] When only cytology is used, cancer can be confirmed in 50% to 90% of cases.[17,51]

Staging

The American Joint Committee on Cancer has defined separate TNM staging systems for hepatic tumors, including the IHCC, gallbladder, and EHCC tumors (Table 46-2).[52] The staging for both gallbladder cancer and EHCC tumors is primarily surgical, reflecting the role of resection.

PRIMARY THERAPY

Hepatocellular Carcinoma

Potentially curative treatments include partial hepatectomy, total hepatectomy with a liver transplant, and nonsurgical ablative therapies. As there are no controlled trials comparing these treatments, recommendations are based on nonrandomized cohort studies rather than on firm evidence. Resection

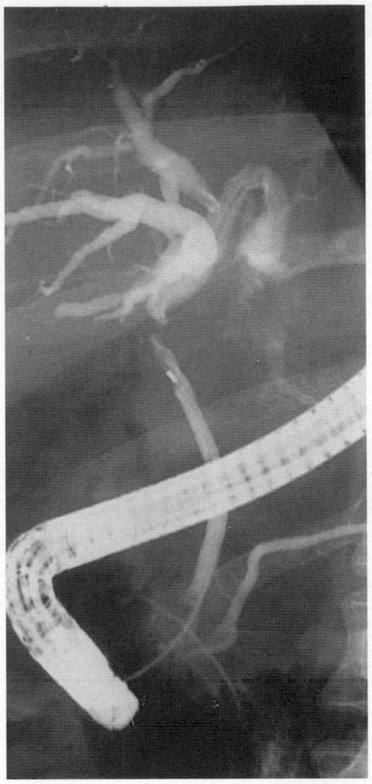

Figure 46-2 Endoscopic retrograde cholangiogram of a patient with a cholangiocarcinoma of the common hepatic duct. A stricture of the common hepatic duct can be seen proximal to the catheter, with dilatation of the intrahepatic biliary tree.

and transplantation appear to result in the best outcomes in well-selected candidates (5-year survival, 60% to 70%).[53-62] Percutaneous treatments provide good outcomes (5-year survival, 40% to 50%)[63-66] but generally inferior to those achieved with surgery. Exceptions to the latter might be patients with carcinoma in situ or single small tumors.

Resection

Hepatic resection is the treatment of choice for HCC in noncirrhotic patients in whom major resections can be accomplished with low rates of complications.[67] In contrast, among patients who have cirrhosis, strict selection criteria are required to avoid liver failure. State-of-the-art surgery is associated with operative mortality rates of 1% to 3% and 5-year survival rates of approximately 50%.[54] Approximately 70% of patients have tumor relapse.[67] Positive resection margins, microvascular invasion, poorly differentiated histology, and satellite lesions predict for relapse.[57,68] Adjuvant therapies have been attempted but their efficacy has not yet been established.

A review[69] of randomized controlled trials identified 13 trials with relapse or survival endpoints reported at 3 years or longer. Three studies involved predominantly systemic adjuvant chemotherapy; four involved predominantly hepatic artery–based chemotherapy or embolization; and six used other therapeutic modalities including adoptive immunotherapy, differentiation agents and hepatic artery infusion of iodine-131–labeled lipiodol. A therapeutic benefit in terms of disease-free or overall survival was noted in six trials, five of which involved modalities other than systemic or hepatic-artery chemotherapy or embolization. The authors concluded

Table 46-2 TNM Classification for Hepatobiliary Cancers

Classification	Description
PRIMARY TUMOR: LIVER AND INTRAHEPATIC CHOLANGIOCARCINOMA	
TX	Primary tumor cannot be assessed
T0	No evidence of primary tumor
T1	Solitary tumor without vascular invasion
T2	Solitary tumor with vascular invasion, or multiple tumors, none more than 5 cm
T3	Multiple tumors more than 5 cm or tumor involving a major branch of the portal or hepatic veins
T4	Tumors with direct invasion of adjacent organs other than the gallbladder or with perforation of the visceral peritoneum
PRIMARY TUMOR: GALLBLADDER	
TX	Primary tumor cannot be assessed
T0	No evidence of primary tumor
Tis	Carcinoma in situ
T1	Tumor invades lamina propria or muscle layer
T1a	Tumor invades lamina propria
T1b	Tumor invades muscle layer
T2	Tumor invades perimuscular connective tissue; no extension beyond serosa or into liver
T3	Tumor perforates the serosa (visceral peritoneum) and/or directly invades the liver and/or one other adjacent organ or structure, such as the stomach, duodenum, colon, or pancreas, omentum or extrahepatic bile ducts
T4	Tumor invades main portal vein or hepatic artery or invades multiple extrahepatic organs or structures
PRIMARY TUMOR: EXTRAHEPATIC CHOLANGIOCARCINOMA	
TX	Primary tumor cannot be assessed
T0	No evidence of primary tumor
Tis	Carcinoma in situ
T1	Tumor confined to the bile duct histologically
T2	Tumor invades beyond the wall of the bile duct
T3	Tumor invades the liver, gallbladder, pancreas, and/or unilateral branches of the portal vein (right or left) or hepatic artery (right or left)
T4	Tumor invades any of the following: main portal vein or its branches bilaterally, common hepatic artery, or other adjacent structures such as the colon, stomach, duodenum, or abdominal wall
REGIONAL LYMPH NODES	
NX	Regional lymph nodes cannot be assessed
N0	No regional lymph node metastasis
N1	Regional lymph node metastasis
DISTANT METASTASIS	
MX	Presence of distant metastasis cannot be assessed
M0	No distant metastasis
M1	Distant metastasis

Used with the permission of the American Joint Committee on Cancer (AJCC), Chicago, Illinois. The original source for this material is the AJCC Cancer Staging Handbook, 6th edition (2002) published by Lippincott-Raven Publishers, Philadelphia, Pennsylvania.

that systemic and hepatic-artery chemotherapy or chemoembolization have not been shown to improve overall or disease-free survival after resection of HCC. The other adjuvant modalities appeared more promising.

Liver Transplantation

The advantage of a total hepatectomy with orthotopic liver transplantation for patients with cirrhosis is that the entire organ is removed, thus taking all identifiable and nonidentifiable tumor as well as any premalignant disease. In addition, transplantation simultaneously addresses the underlying cirrhosis, replacing the diseased parenchyma with healthier liver. However, the widespread use of liver transplantation has been limited by the shortage of donor organs, the high cost of the procedure, and the high perioperative mortality rates, initially reported in the range of 10% to 25%.[8] The use of stricter selection criteria (one lesion smaller than 5 cm or up to three lesions smaller than 3 cm in diameter) has improved outcomes dramatically. Today, 5-year survival of 70% and relapse rates lower than 15% can be expected.[53,56-58,62]

Most centers advocate the use of chemotherapy, chemoembolization, percutaneous ablation, or a combination of these treatments while patients are on the waiting list. The value of these therapies is unknown.

Percutaneous Ablation

Only 30% of patients present with resectable HCC. For those with small unresectable lesions, percutaneous ablation is the most common option and may offer a chance for long-term survival.[64-66,70] Ablation can be accomplished by use of chemicals (alcohol, acetic acid) or by extreme temperature (radiofrequency, microwave, laser, and cryoablation). Percutaneous ethanol injection, not commonly used in the United States, has been reported to achieve responses of 90% to 100% in tumors smaller than 2 cm, 70% in those of 3 cm, and 50% in tumors of 5 cm in diameter.[64,65] Survival rates of 50% at 5 years have been reported in selected Child-Pugh class A patients with complete response.[63,64] Radiofrequency ablation applied percutaneously, laparoscopically, or during laparotomy can achieve similar objective responses as percutaneous ethanol injection but in fewer sessions.[71,72] The reported 5-year survival rates for radiofrequency ablation are 33% to 40%.[66,73] When interpreting these results, it is important to remember that these ablative techniques have not been studied, for the most part, in a rigorous controlled manner, and selection biases are common in most reports. In one randomized controlled trial comparing these two modalities no survival difference was identified, although radiofrequency ablation offered better local control.[71] In a review of 3670 patients treated by radiofrequency ablation, mortality was 0.5% and the complication rate 8.9%.[74] Subcapsular location and poorly differentiated histology have been implicated in needle-track seeding.[75] Cryoablation has fallen out of favor due to a high complication rate. Microwave and laser coagulation are still experimental.[70]

Intrahepatic Cholangiocarcinoma

Complete resection is the most effective treatment and the only potentially curative therapy. IHCCs are often large at presentation, and even with major hepatic resections (right or left hepatectomy or extended hepatectomy) few achieve negative margins. Median and 5-year survival after resection is 12 to 28 months and 22% to 36%, respectively.[76-82] Recognized predictors of poor survival are large tumor size, multiple tumors, vascular involvement, and positive resection margins. The negative prognostic value of lymph node involvement and macroscopic subtype (infiltrating periductal) is less well documented, and it is not known if lymph node dissection improves survival.[77,83]

Gallbladder Carcinoma

Resection is the only therapy with potential for cure for gallbladder carcinoma. However, most patients have unresectable disease and only 10% to 30% can be considered for surgery on presentation.

Depending on stage, surgical options include simple cholecystectomy; radical or extended cholecystectomy-involving removal of the gallbladder plus at least 2 cm of the gallbladder bed and dissection of lymph nodes from the hepatoduodenal ligament behind the second part of the duodenum, head of pancreas, and the celiac axis; radical cholecystectomy with liver (segmental or lobar) resection; radical cholecystectomy with extensive lymph node (para-aortic) dissection; and radical cholecystectomy with resection of bile duct or pancreaticoduodenectomy. Patients who were initially treated by laparoscopic cholecystectomy require additional resection of port sites.

Carcinoma Discovered by Laparoscopy or Open Cholecystectomy

Carcinoma of the gallbladder is discovered during or after cholecystectomy for benign disease in 1% to 2% of cases. In this setting, information about nodal involvement is usually not available and management depends on the depth of tumor invasion. If the tumor has invaded the muscularis propria (T1b and beyond), a radical cholecystectomy is recommended. Re-exploration may reveal residual tumor in 40% to 76% of cases[84-86] and regional lymph node metastases in 40% to 80% of patients; 20% have N2 level lymph node metastases.[87] Retrospective reports comparing survival after simple cholecystectomy and radical re-resection have suggested major benefit from the latter for tumors invading the muscularis propria or deeper.[85,86,88-90]

Gallbladder Carcinoma Identified Preoperatively

The surgical management of gallbladder carcinoma diagnosed preoperatively depends on the extent of the disease. Patients with organ-confined disease should have a radical cholecystectomy. The management of T3 and T4 disease has been more controversial, but it has become evident that cures are possible with radical surgery.[85,86,91-95] The role of more extensive surgery, including pancreaticoduodenectomy, right colectomy, and nephrectomy, has not been established. Para-aortic lymph node metastasis is present in 19% to 25% of patients with locally advanced disease[96] but para-aortic lymphadenectomy is not warranted.[97]

Adjuvant Therapy

Local failure after cholecystectomy for gallbladder cancer is common. In a review of the literature, 86% of patients dying within 5 years after surgery had a local recurrence.[98] Despite the publication of this observation more than 20 years ago, data on the role of adjuvant treatment with radiation or chemoirradiation are very limited.[99-101] Kresl and colleagues[101] reviewed the Mayo Clinic experience with adjuvant external-beam radiotherapy with concurrent bolus 5-FU. A total of 21 patients (12 with R0 resection, 5 with R1 resection, and 4 with R2 resection) received a median of 54 Gy to the tumor bed and regional lymphatics. For the whole cohort, 5-year survival and local control were 33% and 73%, respectively. These results appeared to be superior to historical controls.

Extrahepatic Cholangiocarcinoma

Tumors of the hilar area or common bile duct are typically treated with resection and reconstruction using a Roux-en-Y hepaticojejunostomy.[33,102] Tumors of the hilar area are resectable in approximately 14% to 40% of cases[102-104]; reported 5-year survival rates in resected patients range from 10% to 40%[33,105-112] and are substantially better after R0 resection. There is a strong association between performance of an en bloc partial hepatectomy and the rate of negative resection margins.[113] Tumors of the distal biliary tract are treated by pancreaticoduodenectomy, which can be performed in up to 90% of patients.[33] Survival rates are somewhat higher; 5-year survival rates range from 30% to 40%, and median survival is approximately 22 months.[114-117]

Adjuvant Therapy

Positive margins after resection are common for tumors of the hilar region, occurring in up to 85% of patients in one report,[106] and are a poor prognostic factor, with a 5-year survival rate of 9% versus up to 40% for those with negative margins.[33,115] Positive margins are less common in distal biliary tumors, probably because of the more radical resection possible in this area. Lymph node involvement is found in about 50% of resected patients.[33] The rate of local recurrence after complete resection has been reported to range from 25%[54] to 40%.[118]

The poor prognosis associated with pathologic invasion to the perimuscular connective tissue, hepatic invasion, and positive regional lymph nodes has been recognized for some time for both adenocarcinoma of the gallbladder and cholangiocarcinoma.[33,38,115] However, only recently has attention been directed to potentially important differences in biological behavior between the two entities.[119] In a detailed study of initial disease relapse in 156 patients, Jarnagin and colleagues[119] found a much greater tendency of cholangiocarcinoma to fail locally. The proportion of patients with a locoregional failure as the first site of failure was 59% and 15% for cholangiocarcinoma and gallbladder cancer, respectively. Multivariate analysis confirmed the independent predictive value of positive regional lymph node involvement, moderate/poor tumor differentiation, and a positive resection margin for relapse at any site; a diagnosis of cholangiocarcinoma was the only independent predictor of isolated locoregional recurrence.

The evaluation of adjuvant radiotherapy or chemoradiotherapy for cholangiocarcinoma has been very limited.[51,99-101,118,120-122] Adjuvant radiation was associated with a statistically significant survival benefit in a retrospective European Organization for Research and Treatment of Cancer (EORTC) report of 55 resected patients in which 52 had positive pathologic margins.[51,118] Postoperative irradiation was given in 38 patients, and 17 were treated with surgery alone. Irradiated patients had a median survival of 19 months versus 8 months for surgery alone. Survival at 2 and 3 years was 42% versus 18% and 31% versus 10%, respectively, favoring irradiated patients ($P = .0005$).

In a prospective, underpowered, nonrandomized trial of adjuvant radiation after resection at Johns Hopkins Hospital, 14 patients who elected radiation had no difference in survival duration or quality from 17 patients who elected observation.[122] The patterns of failure were not noted. A gross total resection was performed in 21 patients and partial resection in 10. No concurrent or adjuvant chemotherapy was given in the Johns Hopkins Hospital series.

Gerhards and colleagues[121] reviewed the University of Amsterdam experience with postoperative radiotherapy for resectable hilar cholangiocarcinoma. They retrospectively compared outcomes in 20 patients who received no adjuvant therapy, 41 patients who received external-beam radiotherapy with brachytherapy, and 30 patients who received external-beam radiotherapy alone. Median survival was significantly longer in patients who received postoperative radiotherapy than in patients who had surgery alone (24 months versus 8 months, $P < .01$). Interestingly, brachytherapy did not contribute to survival and was associated with a significantly higher complication rate. Still, the interpretation of these results is not straightforward, as the number of R0 resections in this series was low (14%). It is possible that the benefit suggested in this series is limited to patients who had not had a curative resection, and indeed the survival of patients who received postoperative radiation in this series is comparable to that of patients in other series who had an R0 resection and received no adjuvant therapy.[33,78,110-112]

Approximately one third of resected patients will be left with gross residual disease.[33] With the addition of radiation therapy, the median survival in this setting is about 13 months.[123]

Liver Transplant Alone or Plus Neoadjuvant Chemoradiation

Unfortunately, many patients present with disease that is unresectable with standard resection because of local extension or associated primary sclerosing cholangitis. The latter often have multifocal cholangiocarcinoma and are at an exceptionally high risk for developing additional tumors following standard resection. For these reasons, orthotopic liver transplantation has been proposed as an alternative to standard resection. Early experience with liver transplantation for cholangiocarcinoma has been disappointing, with 5-year survival of 2% to 23%.[124]

Rea and colleagues compared the Mayo Clinic experience with standard resection or transplantation preceded by neoadjuvant chemoradiation for perihilar cholangiocarcinoma.[125] The transplantation regimen consisted of neoadjuvant external-beam radiotherapy (45 Gy in 1.5-Gy fractions twice daily) with concurrent 5-fluorouracil followed by an intraluminal brachytherapy boost (20 to 30 Gy). Protracted venous infusion 5-FU was initiated with brachytherapy and continued until time of transplantation. An important part of the protocol was an exploratory laparotomy, performed after completion of the neoadjuvant treatment with routine biopsy of perihilar lymph nodes. Only patients with liver-confined disease and uninvolved lymph nodes remained eligible for the transplant. Of the 38 patients who underwent liver transplant after neoadjuvant chemoradiation, the 3- and 5-year actuarial survival is 82%. Survival in 26 patients who had standard resection at the Mayo Clinic during the same time period was 48% and 21% at 3 and 5 years, respectively.

LOCALLY ADVANCED DISEASE AND PALLIATION

Hepatocellular Carcinoma

Prognostic Factors

The prognosis for patients with unresectable primary liver tumors is poor. Death usually is due to hepatic dysfunction, gastrointestinal hemorrhage, or spontaneous bacterial peritonitis.[126] The high incidence of hepatic dysfunction, whether resulting from the tumor or from cirrhosis, has greatly limited the potential role of palliative liver radiation therapy, even though patients usually complain of pain.

A number of prognostic factors have been identified for patients with unresectable HCC. Albumin levels, AFP levels greater than 8.5, and portal vein obstruction were found to be independent negative predictors of survival on multivariate regression analysis of 314 patients, including 63 treated surgically.[12] The effects of treatment also have been shown to be dependent on the major prognostic features, such as the Child's class,[64] the AFP value,[127,128] the presence of serologic markers to hepatic B or C virus,[41] and the size of the tumor or presence of multiple tumors.[64] Large survival differences have been observed when these characteristics are present. For example, in a study of iodine-131 antiferritin, the median survival of patients who were AFP positive versus negative was 5 months and 10 months, respectively.[128] In a trial of hepatic arterial chemotherapy with an overall median survival of 15 months, patients who were hepatitis B or C reactive had a significantly worse survival (median, 7.5 months) and significantly greater incidence of treatment toxicity than those who were nonreactive.[41] Given these large effects of prognostic features, the selection bias inherent in any nonrandomized trial is great, and interpretation of the literature is more difficult.

Treatment Results

Medical treatments for unresectable HCC are generally ineffective.[129] A recent review of randomized controlled trials found no evidence for benefit from systemic chemotherapy.[130] In a large retrospective analysis of 314 patients with HCC, Stuart and colleagues[12] reported an overall median survival of 10 months but only 2 to 4 months in those who were untreated or received systemic chemotherapy alone. Other chemotherapy trials using Adriamycin or gemcitabine have reported median survivals of less than 4 months and 5 to 8 months, respectively.[131] Similarly disappointing were the results of a large randomized controlled trial[132] showing no benefit of tamoxifen over placebo.

Since hepatic neoplasms derive 80% of their blood supply from the hepatic artery,[133] higher concentrations of anticancer drugs can be delivered to the tumor by hepatic artery infusion than by the systemic intravenous route. Indeed, higher response and longer median survival rates have been reported with regional chemotherapy.[134] However, the only randomized controlled trial reported found a higher response rate in the hepatic arterial infusion group, but no significant difference in survival.[135]

Hepatocytes derive most of their oxygen via the portal vein. Thus, it is possible to obtain a pharmacologic benefit of chemotherapy by occluding the arterial supply without causing necrosis of the organ. Chemoembolization involves the administration of a chemotherapeutic agent via the hepatic artery with simultaneous embolization of the arterial supply using any of a number of substances such as Gelfoam, particulate polyvinyl alcohol, or metal coils.[136] Despite encouraging early reports, four of five randomized controlled trials comparing transcatheter arterial procedures to best supportive care have failed to demonstrate a survival advantage.[126,137-139] Only Llovet and colleagues[140] reported a 1-year survival advantage (24% versus 82%, $P = .009$) of arterial chemoembolization over best supportive care.

Intrahepatic Cholangiocarcinoma

In contrast to the large experience of various forms of treatment for HCC, few data are available on unresectable IHCC. Survival rates with or without treatment are poor; median survival is approximately 7 months with no 5-year survivors.[33,36] The results of liver transplant for IHCC are dismal,[84] and consequently IHCC is considered a contraindication even by the most aggressive proponents of this therapy.[85]

Radiation therapy studies have included trials of radiolabeled immunoglobulin combined with whole-liver radiation therapy and chemotherapy.[141] The tumor-bearing portions of the liver were treated with 3 Gy/day, four fractions per week, to a total dose of 21 Gy with concurrent doxorubicin and 5-FU. Approximately 1 month later, the patient received chemotherapy again, followed by the radiolabeled anti–carcinoembryonic antigen. Although the median survival rate was 10.1 months in this experience, higher than a previous study at the same institution, all 24 patients had died by 2 years. Patterns of failure were not provided.

Conformal Radiation Therapy for Hepatic Tumors

Developments in three-dimensional radiation therapy treatment planning have expanded the role of external-beam radiation therapy (EBRT) for patients with unresectable primary hepatobiliary malignancies. In a series of prospective controlled studies at the University of Michigan, doses well above the whole-liver tolerance dose have been delivered safely to focal lesions.[142-144] This was enabled by the development of a normal-tissue complication probability (NTCP) model that quantitatively described the relationship between dose and volumes irradiated and the probability of developing RILD[145] and by the use of conformal techniques. A phase I/II trial was conducted to test the safety of the model parameters and to begin to develop efficacy data at the maximum tolerated dose.[144] The radiation dose was individualized based on the volume of normal liver that could be spared. Each individual received the maximal possible dose associated with an estimated risk not exceeding 10% to 15%. The prescribed dose ranged from 40 Gy to 90 Gy (median, 60.75 Gy). Floxuridine (0.2 mg/kg/d) was delivered concurrently by continuous infusion through a hepatic arterial catheter. Subsequently, a phase II trial was conducted, the results of which have been recently updated. A total of 81 patients with HCC or cholangiocarcinoma have been accrued. With a median follow-up of 16 months (26 months in patients alive), 85% of patients had died. The median survival was 13 months in patients with cholangiocarcinoma and 15 months in patients with HCC. This was significantly higher than the anticipated rates of survival in historical controls. The total radiation dose was the most important predictor of survival in a multivariate analysis. The pattern-of-failure analysis revealed a tendency of these tumors to progress locally, with 61% of all failures occurring in the liver. Together, these findings underscored the need to develop even more intense liver-directed therapies.

The use of lower doses of radiation with transcatheter arterial chemoembolization (TACE) in unresectable HCC has been reported by Asian investigators.[146-149] Zeng and colleagues[147] reported on 203 patients who were treated with TACE, of whom 54 received EBRT as well. They excluded patients with severe cirrhosis, portal vein thrombus, lymph node involvement, or extrahepatic metastases. Selection for radiotherapy was mostly driven by unsatisfactory Lipiodol uptake or worsening of liver function after TACE. The planning target volume included the visible lesion on CT scan with 1.5-cm margins and the median dose was 50 Gy in 2-Gy fractions. In comparison with patients who received TACE alone, patients who received radiotherapy had superior response rates (76% versus 30.9%, $P < .001$) and median survival (20 months versus 14 months, $P = .026$).

Other reports are summarized in Table 46-3. In general, the objective responses were in the range of 50% to 90%, and median survival was 10 to 23 months. Considerable variability in patient selection and treatment details, as well as the nonprospective nature of these analyses, make the interpretation of these results difficult. Nevertheless, similar to the University of Michigan experience, a common finding was that radiotherapy dose was a major determinant of survival.

Table 46-3 **Results of Low- to Intermediate-Dose Radiotherapy With Transcatheter Arterial Chemoembolization in Unresectable Hepatocellular Carcinoma**

Study	Mean Tumor Size (range)	No. of Patients	Treatment	Median Survival (mo)
Li et al.[177]	8.5 cm (4-13)	45	TACE + 50.4 Gy	23
Zeng et al.[147]		54	TACE + 36-60 Gy	20
Seong et al.[146]	9.0 cm (6-12)	158	TACE + 48.2 ± 7.9 Gy	10
Guo et al.[149]	10.2 cm (5-18)	107	TACE + 25-55 Gy	18

TACE, transcatheter arterial chemoembolization.

Gallbladder Cancer

Patients with unresectable gallbladder cancer have a median survival of approximately 5 months and a 2-year survival rate of less than 5%.[26,38] Patients may be unresectable because of metastatic disease, extensive local involvement, or bulky nodal metastases with no difference in survival based on the reason for unresectability.[26,150] A large number of agents, including fluorouracil, mitomycin, methotrexate, etoposide, doxorubicin, and cisplatin, have been tested as single or combination therapies with little effect.[151-160] Short-lived partial responses lasting from weeks to several months have been observed in approximately 10% to 20% of cases. Although the combinations of cisplatin, epirubicin and 5-fluorouracil (CEF) and gemcitabine and cisplatin are associated with relatively high response rates of 32% to 40%[151,161] and 37% to 64%,[162,163] respectively, the impact of these regimens, or any chemotherapy, on survival is not known. Similarly, the efficacy of palliative radiotherapy for unresectable gallbladder cancer is unknown.

Extrahepatic Cholangiocarcinoma

Unresectable EHCC is typically located in the hilum; distal tumors are usually resectable. Most patients die from hepatic dysfunction resulting from biliary obstruction or cholangitis or both.[106] The median survival of patients treated palliatively is approximately 6 months, with 3-year survival rates of less than 10%.[31,33,104] Palliation can be performed either with a biliary enteric bypass at exploration[104] or nonsurgically, using transhepatic percutaneous drainage catheters or endoscopically placed indwelling biliary stents.[164] Cholangitis is frequent after both of these procedures, occurring in 26% to 47% of patients.[164] Complications related to the catheter are also common. In fact, most patients will require at least two exchanges, usually every 3 to 6 months, of either the percutaneous drainage catheter or endoprosthesis.[120] Septic deaths are reported in most series in which indwelling catheters or stents are left in place. Recurrent obstruction develops in 12% to 50% of patients, which can be due to progressive tumor growth or biliary sludge.[164]

Chemotherapy for unresectable cholangiocarcinoma is largely ineffective. An extensive review of 65 clinical trials of nonsurgical therapies failed to document a survival benefit of any such modality in patients with unresectable disease or in the adjuvant setting.[165]

External Beam Radiation Therapy With or Without Chemotherapy or Brachytherapy

The median survival of patients treated with EBRT to a total dose of 45 to 50 Gy, alone or with chemotherapy, has been reported to be 9 to 12 months. Long-term survival has been infrequent.[51,120]

Both IORT with electrons or brachytherapy and transcatheter brachytherapy have been used alone or in combination with EBRT to focally irradiate the bile duct to higher total doses. A summary of published reports is provided in Table 46-4. There is a considerable published experience with brachytherapy as a component of treatment; overall median survival rates range from 10 to 24 months and 3-year survival rates from 10% to 30%. In all reports that assess control, local failure is still common despite the high total dose of radiation therapy possible by including brachytherapy.[120] This finding may be related to the depth-dose characteristics of the single-line source, because the radiation dose is often calculated 0.5 to 1 cm from the catheter[120,166] even though unresectable biliary tumors are often larger than 2 cm in diameter.[124]

Although randomized studies have not been performed, it is possible that the combination of EBRT, brachytherapy, and 5-FU may be associated with improved survival. In a Mayo Clinic analysis of 24 patients with proximal extrahepatic bile duct carcinoma treated with EBRT and brachytherapy with or without 5-FU (9 patients), survival greater than 5 years was observed in 3 patients.[122] Two of the long-term survivors had received concurrent 5-FU with EBRT (i.e., long-term survival with trimodality treatment was 2 of 9, or 22%).[122] The intriguing Mayo Clinic results with transplant preceded by chemoradiation for bradytherapy were previously discussed.[125]

TECHNIQUES OF IRRADIATION

Dose-Limiting Organs

The major dose-limiting organ for any course of irradiation to the hepatobiliary system is the liver. Radiation-induced liver disease typically occurs 4 to 8 weeks after the completion of radiation therapy and clinically resembles veno-occlusive disease.[167] Patients complain of fatigue and may have vague right upper quadrant discomfort. They may have signs and symptoms of ascites, with rapid weight gain and increased girth. Laboratory studies show a large increase in alkaline phosphatase to 3 to 10 times normal and moderate elevations of the transaminases but little to no increase in bilirubin or lactic dehydrogenase (LDH) at first presentation. Evaluation includes an abdominal CT scan and paracentesis of the ascitic fluid to rule out recurrent disease. Of note, differentiation on CT scan of recurrent disease versus radiation change within the liver may be difficult. Although axial beam arrangements show typical straight-line borders between the liver and areas of radiation change, nonaxial beam arrangements can lead to poorly defined borders and can be confused with infiltrative recurrent disease.[168] Radiation-induced liver disease can be treated conservatively using diuretics and steroids, as with benign liver dysfunction, although some have suggested anticoagulation as well.

Table 46-4 Results of High-Dose Radiotherapy in Extrahepatic Bile Duct Cancers

Series/Treatment Method (Ref.)	No.	SURVIVAL Median (mo)	12 mo (%)	24 mo (%)	60 mo (%)	*P* Value
Iwasaki et al. (Japan)[178]						
Noncurative resection						
Alone	13	—	44	8	—	
Plus IORT	13	—	46	15	—	
Unresected						
Biliary drainage only	21	—	<5	—	—	
Plus IORT	6	—	33	17	—	
Mayo Clinic						
Unresected						
EBRT ± 5-FU[50]	11	12	55	—	—	
EBRT ± 5-FU + Ir-192[122]	24	12.8	67	19	14	
EBRT + 5-FU + Ir-192	9	13	67	22	22	
EBRT + Ir-192	15	12	67	16	8	
EBRT ± 5-FU + IOERT[179,180]	14	18.5	71	29	7	
EBRT/5FU/Ir-192 ± transplant[125,181,182]	71	60+	79	63	58	
EBRT/5FU/Ir-192 + transplant[125]	38	60+	92	92	82	
Standard resection ± EBRT/5FU[125]	26	34	82	70	21	
Thomas Jefferson University Hospital[183]	48	9	—	18	—	
No irradiation	24	5.5	—	17	—	
Irradiation + 5-FU ± Ir-192	24	12	—	30	—	<.05
<55 Gy	9	6	—	0	—	
>55 Gy	15	24	—	48	—	<.05
EORTC[51]						
Noncurative resection alone	17	8.3	36	18	—	
Noncurative resection plus EBRT	38	19	85	42	—	<.05
University of Heidelberg[120]	30	10	34	18	8	
EBRT + HDRB	21	7.9	38	5	0	
EBRT + HDRB + noncurative resection	9	12.1	64	32	32	<.05
University of Pittsburgh						
EBRT ± 5-FU ± resection[184]	55	9	32	10	—	
EBRT ± 5-FU + transplant	9/55	12	50	22	—	
EBRT + chemo; Bx or partial resection[185]	38*	14	60	20	0	
EBRT + chemo; Transplant or total resection	23*	60+	82	68	53.5	<.05

EBRT, external beam irradiation; IOERT, intraoperative electron irradiation; HDRB, high-dose rate brachytherapy; 5-FU, 5 fluorouracil; chemo, 5-FU/leucovorin/interferon alpha or paclitaxel.

*Biopsy, 34, subtotal resection, 4; orthotopic liver transplant, 17, other total resection, 6.

The risk for radiation-induced liver disease is highly dependent on the volume of liver irradiated.[145,168,169] Irradiation of the whole liver to a total dose of 30 Gy in 2-Gy fractions or less has little risk of a complication. The risk rises greatly above a dose of 33 Gy, and it has been estimated that at 42 Gy there is an approximately 50% risk for symptoms.[145,169] Partial liver volumes, however, can be irradiated to very high doses without clinically relevant toxicity. For example, trials from the University of Michigan using three-dimensional treatment planning have shown that approximately one third of the normal liver can tolerate up to 72.6 Gy.[145,169] In fact, sufficient data has accumulated in these trials to allow estimation of an individual's risk for complication based on the distribution of radiation dose within the liver.[145] While the use of concurrent hepatic arterial fluorodeoxyuridine was not found to increase the risk of radiation-induced liver disease, case reports suggest that previous alkylator therapy increases the chances of RILD.[167]

The other major dose-limiting organs within the upper abdomen are the kidneys, stomach, and small bowel. Kidney irradiation can especially be of concern when palliative whole-liver treatment is given, because opposed anteroposterior fields, which irradiate all or a major portion of the right kidney, are frequently used. If the patient has hepatomegaly, tangential fields may be required to avoid treating the entire left kidney. Even with tangential fields, the entire right kidney is frequently irradiated. Precautions, such as intravenous contrast or three-dimensional treatment planning, are required in this circumstance, to ensure that the left kidney is appropriately spared (if more than half of one kidney needs to receive 20 Gy or more, then no more than 10% of the other kidney can receive greater than 18 Gy).

The stomach and duodenum are of concern when techniques are used to irradiate the left lobe of the liver or the extrahepatic biliary tract to high doses. Of 128 University of Michigan patients with primary hepatobiliary malignancies treated on a phase II trial, with 40 to 90 Gy (1.5 Gy/fraction twice daily) 9 patients (7%) developed upper gastrointestinal bleeding. In that trial the maximum dose to the stomach or duodenum was not allowed to exceed 68 Gy. Although some authors suggested that a dose of 60 Gy to one third of the stomach will give a 5% risk of ulceration or perforation,[170] the Mayo Clinic data for biliary tract cancer suggest that the dose to stomach or duodenum needs to be 55 Gy or less for a 5% to 10% risk of severe gastrointestinal complications.[50] With doses of greater than 55 Gy with EBRT alone or combined with

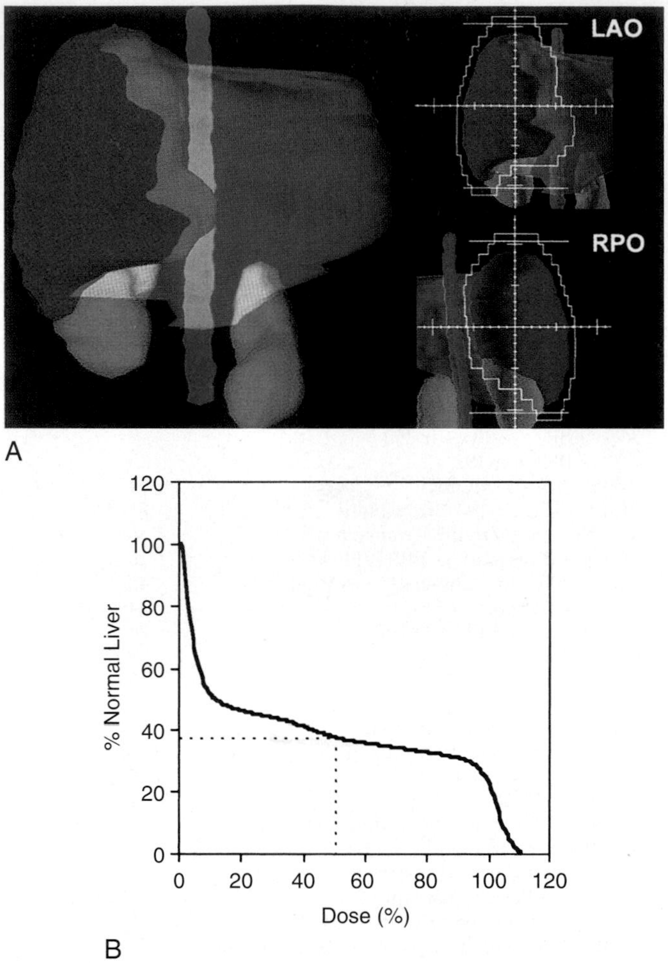

Figure 46-3 Three-dimensional treatment planning for a patient with an unresectable intrahepatic cholangiocarcinoma. **(A)** The solid-surface reconstruction of the target volume (red), liver (purple), kidneys (yellow), and spinal cord (green) was used to design treatment, using left anterior oblique (LAO) and right posterior oblique (RPO) fields, shown at right. **(B)** The dose-volume histogram for this beam arrangement demonstrated that a large volume of liver was excluded from the irradiated volume. (From McGinn CJ, Ten Haken RK, Ensminger WD, et al: Treatment of intrahepatic cancers with radiation doses based on a normal tissue complication probability model. J Clin Oncol 16:2246-2252, 1998.)

brachytherapy, the risk of severe gastrointestinal complications in the stomach or duodenum increased to 30% to 40% in the Mayo Clinic analysis.

Technique

Liver

Palliative liver irradiation may be indicated for both locally advanced hepatic tumors and metastatic disease. The appropriate dose and schedule for palliation was examined in a prospective, nonrandomized trial of more than 100 patients with symptomatic liver metastases.[171] Six different dose and fractionation options ranging from 21 Gy in 7 treatments to 25.6 Gy in 16 fractions were tested. Palliation of pain was achieved in 55% of patients, with no difference among the treatment regimens. Although radiation-induced liver disease was not reported with any of the dose fractionation options, the short median survival of this patient group and the problem distinguishing this complication from progressive disease make interpretation of this finding difficult. Field arrangements may include opposed anteroposterior or tangential approaches.

Irradiation of locally unresectable hepatic tumors to doses above the whole-liver tolerance requires three-dimensional treatment planning (Fig. 46-3).The gross tumor volume is typically defined as radiographically abnormal areas seen on the CT scan. The clinical target volume is defined as the gross tumor volume plus 1 cm based on surgical reports that at least a 1-cm resection margin is necessary for a successful partial hepatectomy.[9] The planning target volume includes the clinical target volume plus 0.5 cm for daily patient set-up variation and between 0.5 and 2.5 cm (determined under fluoroscopy) in the cranial-caudal dimension to account for liver motion resulting from breathing. The normal liver is defined as the gross tumor volume subtracted from the total liver volume. Using three-dimensional treatment planning, it has been possible to safely irradiate two thirds of the normal liver to 48 to 52.8 Gy and one third of the liver to 66 to 72.6 Gy (fraction size of 1.5 to 1.65 Gy twice daily with at least 4 hours' separation).[144,145,169]

Gallbladder and Extrahepatic Cholangiocarcinoma

In the case of gallbladder cancer, the treatment fields should be designed to include the gallbladder fossa, the hilar, and celiac lymph node–bearing areas (Fig. 46-4). Accurate definition of the gallbladder fossa can be difficult in the absence of preoperative CT scans or surgical clips placed at the time of resection. Doses in the range of 45 to 50 Gy (1.8- to 2-Gy fractions) for subclinical disease and 60 to 65 Gy for microscopically positive margins are probably appropriate, although caution must be exercised because irradiation of the gallbladder fossa can include large volumes of liver. Complex techniques, including three-dimensional non-coplanar, must be carefully evaluated.

The target volume for EHCC can require inclusion of large portions of normal liver, if the tumor is located in the hilum. In this case, the target volume may be extended between 3 to 5 cm within the liver to include subclinical spread along the biliary tree. Although more distal EHCC requires considerably less irradiation of the hepatic parenchyma, higher duodenal or distal gastric doses may be necessary. On the basis of Mayo Clinic tolerance data, if doses greater than 55 Gy are indicated for tumor control (i.e., unresectable or residual disease), three-dimensional treatment planning should be used to decrease normal tissue high-dose volumes.

Brachytherapy using both low-dose rate[122,166] and high-dose rate[120] techniques has frequently been used for EHCC. Usually, brachytherapy is given as a supplement to 45 to 50 Gy (1.8- to 2-Gy fractions) of EBRT. The external biliary drainage catheter is then used to gain access, and fluoroscopy helps to place a guide-wire in the treatment area (Fig. 46-5). In general, a boost dose of 15 to 20 Gy is prescribed to a radius of 0.5 to 1.0 cm from the brachytherapy catheter. Some authors suggested an evaluation of boost doses of 30 Gy to a 1-cm radius combined with 45 to 50 Gy EBRT (1.8-Gy fractions) depending on the disease location relative to the stomach and duodenum.[122]

TREATMENT ALGORITHM AND FUTURE DIRECTIONS

Figure 46-6 provides treatment algorithms for hepatobiliary cancers. A number of advances suggest avenues for

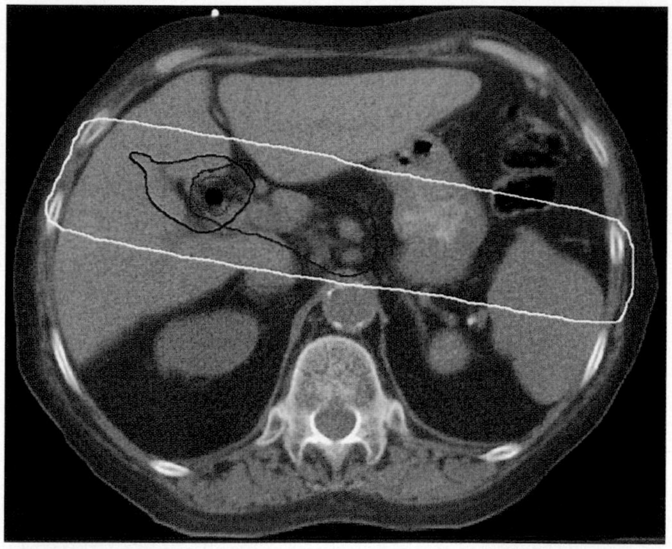

Figure 46-4 Treatment plan for a patient with a resected carcinoma of the gallbladder. The tumor did not penetrate through the gallbladder; however, the cystic duct margin of the specimen was positive, and a cystic lymph node contained metastatic disease. The target volumes were established as the draining regional lymph nodes including the celiac axis (red) and the common hepatic and common bile ducts (yellow). Opposed oblique fields were used to deliver an initial 50.4 Gy (volume shown in white), and an anterior wedge pair field arrangement was used to deliver a boost to 63 Gy (volume shown in blue).

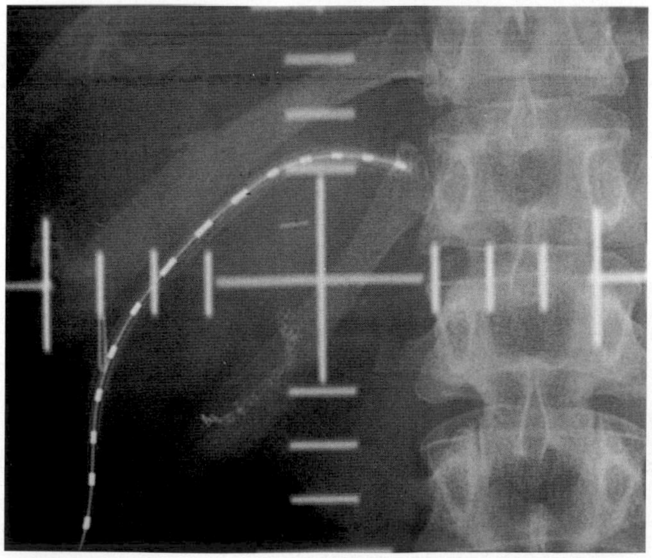

Figure 46-5 Brachytherapy planning film of a patient with cholangiocarcinoma, with dummy seeds loaded in the percutaneous catheter. The active length for brachytherapy was determined using a cholangiogram.

improving the results of the application of radiation to patients with intrahepatic cancers. As described, the use of three-dimensional treatment planning has already permitted the delivery of much higher doses of radiation for intrahepatic and gallbladder cancers than would have been possible using standard techniques. The addition of brachytherapy to EBRT with or without chemotherapy has done the same for EHCC. Further improvements in treatment may come from even better physical dose delivery and better tumor definition with improved imaging techniques.

Because evidence suggests that the dose of radiation that can be safely given depends on the volume of normal liver irradiated, it seems reasonable to investigate methods of decreasing the planning target volume (while preserving the clinical target volume). One approach could include elimination of the component of the planning target volume allotted for ventilation.[172] This could be accomplished by gating therapy; however, a simpler approach may be to use breath-holding techniques. It has been shown that performing treatment planning at end expiration takes a step in this direction, by decreasing the margin needed in the superior direction.[173] One method, called *active breathing control*, permits the margin for ventilatory movement to be eliminated without requiring modification of the treatment machine.[174] The target volume could also be reduced by improving the definition of the target volume with the use of better imaging.

Another method of improving the outcome of treatment for patients with intrahepatic cancer could include the more standard use of radiation sensitizers or radioprotectors. Today, most studies have used systemic 5-FU or hepatic arterial fluorodeoxyuridine. Other agents could be considered for concurrent systemic or hepatic arterial administration. The latter is particularly attractive for the treatment of intrahepatic tumors given that the dual blood supply of the liver permits the selective perfusion of tumors via the hepatic arterial circulation. Indeed, response rates as high as 50% have been reported with hepatic arterial infusion of fluorodeoxyuridine and mitomycin C[175] and with combinations of etoposide and cisplatin with 5-FU (EPF) or doxorubicin (EAP).[176] Making use of the same concepts, radioprotectors, such as amifostine, administered systemically or through the portal vein, could produce selective protection of the normal liver and thereby improve the therapeutic index.

Improved understanding of the disease underlying radiation-induced liver disease should ultimately permit toxicity of treatment to be decreased. Although advances in this area have been hampered by the lack of an animal model, data suggest that cytokines such as transforming growth factor β may at least participate in the process leading to veno-occlusive disease.

In summary, it seems likely that improvements in the outcome of treatment for patients with IHCC and EHCC can be obtained from a combination of better dose delivery using three-dimensional treatment planning and brachytherapy, more effective use of radiosensitizers, an evaluation of both chemical and biologic protectors of the normal liver, and improvements in imaging. In addition to these methods of safely increasing effective tumor dose without producing hepatic toxicity, future investigations need to address nonhepatic toxicities, which can sometimes limit the doses that can be delivered to patients with intrahepatic cancers.

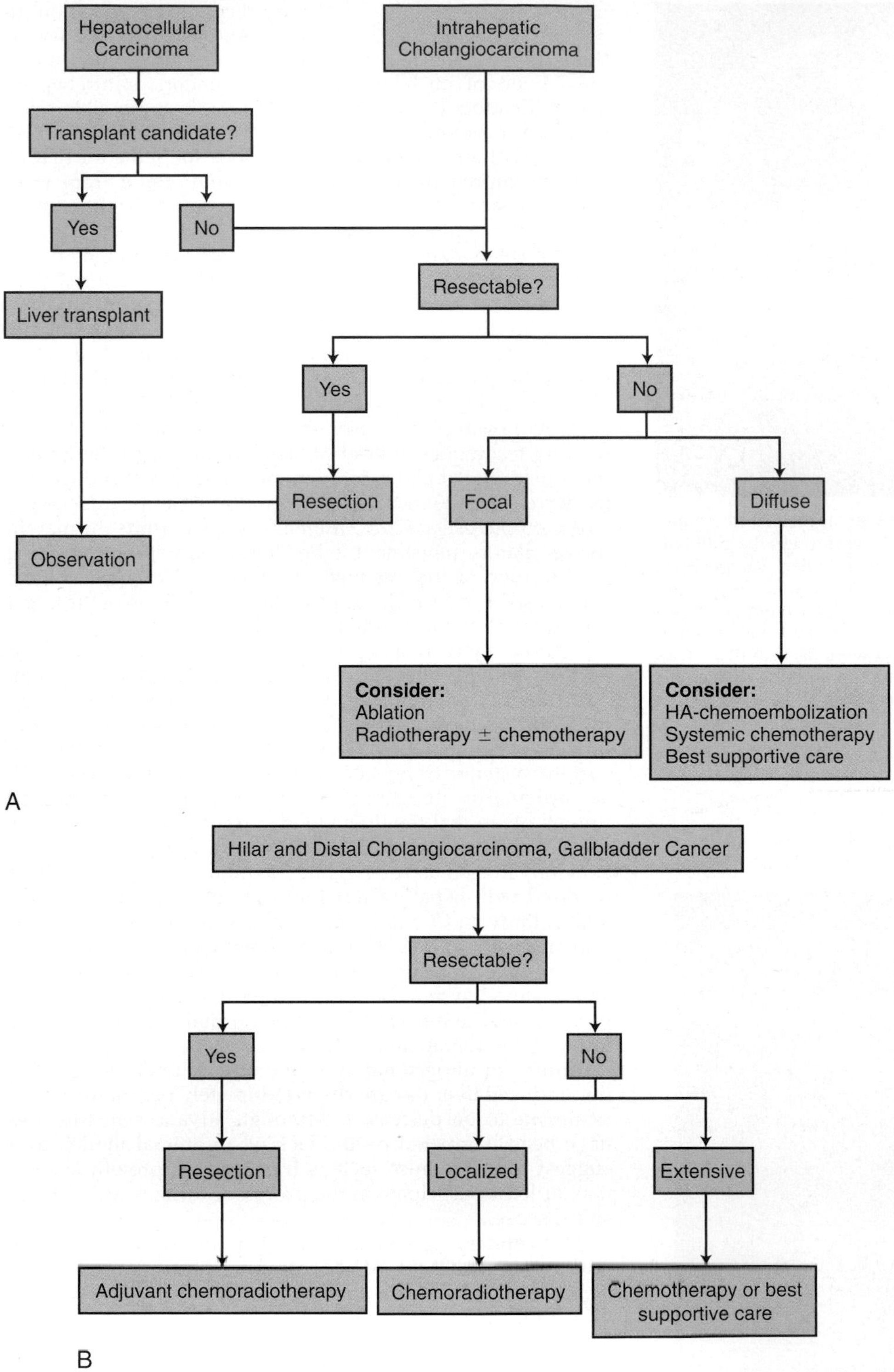

Figure 46-6 Treatment algorithms for a patient with hepatobiliary cancer.

REFERENCES

1. Parkin DM, et al: Estimating the world cancer burden: Globocan 2000. Int J Cancer 94:153, 2001.
2. El-Serag HB, et al: The continuing increase in the incidence of hepatocellular carcinoma in the United States: an update. Ann Intern Med 140:817, 2003.
3. Patel T: Increasing incidence and mortality of primary intrahepatic cholangiocarcinoma in the United States. Hepatology 33:1353, 2001.
4. Wharton JT, et al: Radiation hepatitis induced by abdominal irradiation with the cobalt 60 moving strip technique. Am J Roentgenol Radium Ther Nucl Med 117:73, 1973.
5. Ingold JA, Reed GB, Kaplan HS, Bagshaw MA: Radiation hepatitis. Am J Roentgenol Radium Ther Nucl Med 93:200, 1965.

6. American Cancer Society: Cancer Facts and Figures 2004. ACS, 2004.
7. Carriaga MT, Henson DE: Liver, gallbladder, extrahepatic bile ducts, and pancreas. Cancer 75(1 Suppl):171, 1995.
8. Nagorney DM, Gigot JF: Primary epithelial hepatic malignancies: etiology, epidemiology, and outcome after subtotal and total hepatic resection. Surg Oncol Clin N Am 5:283, 1996.
9. Khakoo SI, et al: Etiology, screening, and treatment of hepatocellular carcinoma. Med Clin North Am 80:1121, 1996.
10. Diehl AK: Epidemiology of gallbladder cancer: a synthesis of recent data. J Natl Cancer Inst 65:1209, 1980.
11. Chang MH, Chen CJ, Lai MS, et al: Universal hepatitis B vaccination in Taiwan and the incidence of hepatocellular carcinoma in children. Taiwan Childhood Hepatoma Study Group. N Engl J Med 336:1855, 1997.
12. Stuart KE, Anand AJ, Jenkins RL: Hepatocellular carcinoma in the United States. Prognostic features, treatment outcome, and survival. Cancer 77:2217, 1996.
13. Anthony P: Tumours and tumour-like lesions of the liver and biliary tract. *In* MacSween AP, Anthony PP, Scheuer PJ, et al: Pathology of the Liver. New York, Churchill Livingstone, 1994, p 635.
14. Zatonski WA, et al: Epidemiologic aspects of gallbladder cancer: a case-control study of the SEARCH Program of the International Agency for Research on Cancer. J Natl Cancer Inst 89:1132, 1997.
15. Strom BL, et al: Biochemical epidemiology of gallbladder cancer. Hepatology 23:1402, 1996.
16. Abi-Rached B, Neugut AI: Diagnostic and management issues in gallbladder carcinoma. Oncology (Huntingt) 9:19-24, 1995; discussion 24, 27, 30.
17. Van Leeuwen DJ, Huibregtse K, Tytgat GN: Carcinoma of the hepatic confluence 25 years after Klatskin's description: diagnosis and endoscopic management. Semin Liver Dis 10:102, 1990.
18. Rosen CB, Nagorney DM: Cholangiocarcinoma complicating primary sclerosing cholangitis. Semin Liver Dis 11:26, 1991.
19. Ekbom A, et al: Risk of extrahepatic bile duct cancer after cholecystectomy. Lancet 342:1262, 1993.
20. Regan LS: Screening for hepatocellular carcinoma in high-risk individuals. A clinical review. Arch Intern Med 149:1741, 1989.
21. Di Bisceglie AM, et al: NIH conference. Hepatocellular carcinoma. Ann Intern Med 108:390, 1988.
22. Colombo M, et al: Hepatocellular carcinoma in Italian patients with cirrhosis. N Engl J Med 325:675, 1991.
23. Nichols JC, et al: Diagnostic role of serum CA 19-9 for cholangiocarcinoma in patients with primary sclerosing cholangitis. Mayo Clin Proc 68:874, 1993.
24. Okuda K, Peters RL, Simson IW: Gross anatomic features of hepatocellular carcinoma from three disparate geographic areas. Proposal of new classification. Cancer 54:2165, 1984.
25. Nzeako UC, Goodman ZD, Ishak KG: Comparison of tumor pathology with duration of survival of North American patients with hepatocellular carcinoma. Cancer 76:579, 1995.
26. Henson DE, Albores-Saavedra J, Corle D: Carcinoma of the gallbladder. Histologic types, stage of disease, grade, and survival rates. Cancer 70:1493, 1992.
27. Weedon D: Diseases of the gallbladder. *In* MacSween AP, Scheuer PJ, et al: Pathology of the Liver. New York, Churchill Livingstone, 1994.
28. Malik IA: Clinicopathological features and management of gallbladder cancer in Pakistan: a prospective study of 233 cases. J Gastroenterol Hepatol 18:950, 2003.
29. Grobmyer SR, Lieberman MD, Daly JM: Gallbladder cancer in the twentieth century: single institution's experience. World J Surg 28:47, 2004.
30. Weinbren K, Mutum SS: Pathological aspects of cholangiocarcinoma. J Pathol 139:217, 1983.
31. Henson DE, Albores-Saavedra J, Corle D: Carcinoma of the extrahepatic bile ducts. Histologic types, stage of disease, grade, and survival rates. Cancer 70:1498, 1992.
32. Suzuki M, et al: The development and extension of hepatohilar bile duct carcinoma. A three-dimensional tumor mapping in the intrahepatic biliary tree visualized with the aid of a graphics computer system. Cancer 64:658, 1989.
33. Nakeeb A, et al: Cholangiocarcinoma. A spectrum of intrahepatic, perihilar, and distal tumors. Ann Surg 224:463, 1996; discussion 473.
34. Okuda K: Hepatocellular carcinoma: recent progress. Hepatology 15:948, 1992.
35. Sakamoto M, Hirohashi S, Shimosato Y: Early stages of multistep hepatocarcinogenesis: adenomatous hyperplasia and early hepatocellular carcinoma. Hum Pathol 22:172, 1991.
36. Altaee MY, et al: Etiologic and clinical characteristics of peripheral and hilar cholangiocarcinoma. Cancer 68:2051, 1991.
37. Kassianides C, Kew MC: The clinical manifestations and natural history of hepatocellular carcinoma. Gastroenterol Clin North Am 16:553, 1987.
38. Chao TC, Greager JA: Primary carcinoma of the gallbladder. J Surg Oncol 46:215, 1991.
39. Arnaud JP, et al: Primary carcinoma of the gallbladder—review of 143 cases. Hepatogastroenterology 42:811, 1995.
40. Nomura F, Ohnishi K, Tanabe Y: Clinical features and prognosis of hepatocellular carcinoma with reference to serum alphafetoprotein levels. Analysis of 606 patients. Cancer 64:1700, 1989.
41. Patt YZ, et al: Hepatic arterial infusion of floxuridine, leucovorin, doxorubicin, and cisplatin for hepatocellular carcinoma: effects of hepatitis B and C viral infection on drug toxicity and patient survival. J Clin Oncol 12:1204, 1994.
42. Braga L, Guller U, Semelka RC: Modern hepatic imaging. Surg Clin North Am 84:375, 2004.
43. Hann LE, et al: Diagnostic imaging approaches and relationship to hepatobiliary cancer staging and therapy. Semin Surg Oncol 19:94, 2000.
44. Hori M, et al: Sensitivity of double-phase helical CT during arterial portography for detection of hypervascular hepatocellular carcinoma. J Comput Assist Tomogr 22:861, 1998.
45. Murakami T, et al: Helical CT during arterial portography and hepatic arteriography for detecting hypervascular hepatocellular carcinoma. AJR Am J Roentgenol 169:131, 1997.
46. Li L, et al: CT arterial portography and CT hepatic arteriography in detection of micro liver cancer. World J Gastroenterol 5:225, 1999.
47. Li L, et al: Multi-phasic CT arterial portography and CT hepatic arteriography improving the accuracy of liver cancer detection. World J Gastroenterol 10:3118, 2004.
48. Taouli B, et al: Magnetic resonance imaging of hepatocellular carcinoma. Gastroenterology 127(5 Suppl 1):S144, 2004.
49. Cohen MB, et al: Cytologic criteria to distinguish hepatocellular carcinoma from nonneoplastic liver. Am J Clin Pathol 95:125, 1991.
50. Buskirk SJ, et al: Analysis of failure after curative irradiation of extrahepatic bile duct carcinoma. Ann Surg 215:125, 1992.
51. Gonzalez Gonzalez D, et al: Results of radiation therapy in carcinoma of the proximal bile duct (Klatskin tumor). Semin Liver Dis 10:131, 1990.
52. Greene FL, et al: American Joint Committee on Cancer Staging Manual, 6th ed. AJCC, 2002.
53. Bismuth H, Majno PE, Adam R: Liver transplantation for hepatocellular carcinoma. Semin Liver Dis 19:311, 1999.
54. Bruix J, Llovet JM: Prognostic prediction and treatment strategy in hepatocellular carcinoma. Hepatology 35:519, 2002.
55. Fong Y, et al: An analysis of 412 cases of hepatocellular carcinoma at a Western center. Ann Surg 229:790, 1999; discussion 799.
56. Jonas S, et al: Vascular invasion and histopathologic grading determine outcome after liver transplantation for hepatocellular carcinoma in cirrhosis. Hepatology 33:1080, 2001.
57. Llovet JM, Fuster J, Bruix J: Intention-to-treat analysis of surgical treatment for early hepatocellular carcinoma: resection versus transplantation. Hepatology 30:1434, 1999.
58. Mazzaferro V, et al: Liver transplantation for the treatment of small hepatocellular carcinomas in patients with cirrhosis. N Engl J Med 334:693, 1996.
59. Takayama T, et al: Early hepatocellular carcinoma as an entity with a high rate of surgical cure. Hepatology 28:1241, 1998.
60. Takayama T, et al: Adoptive immunotherapy to lower postsurgical recurrence rates of hepatocellular carcinoma: a randomised trial. Lancet 356:802, 2000.

61. Wayne JD, et al: Preoperative predictors of survival after resection of small hepatocellular carcinomas. Ann Surg 235:722, 2002; discussion 730.
62. Yao FY, et al: Liver transplantation for hepatocellular carcinoma: expansion of the tumor size limits does not adversely impact survival. Hepatology 33:1394, 2001.
63. Arii S, et al: Results of surgical and nonsurgical treatment for small-sized hepatocellular carcinomas: a retrospective and nationwide survey in Japan. The Liver Cancer Study Group of Japan. Hepatology 32:1224, 2000.
64. Livraghi T, et al: Hepatocellular carcinoma and cirrhosis in 746 patients: long-term results of percutaneous ethanol injection. Radiology 197:101, 1995.
65. Lencioni R, et al: Long-term results of percutaneous ethanol injection therapy for hepatocellular carcinoma in cirrhosis: a European experience. Eur Radiol 7:514, 1997.
66. Buscarini L, et al: Percutaneous radiofrequency ablation of small hepatocellular carcinoma: long-term results. Eur Radiol 11:914, 2001.
67. Bismuth H, Majno PE: Hepatobiliary surgery. J Hepatol 32(1 Suppl):208, 2000.
68. Nagasue N, et al: Incidence and factors associated with intrahepatic recurrence following resection of hepatocellular carcinoma. Gastroenterology 105:488, 1993.
69. Schwartz JD, et al: Neoadjuvant and adjuvant therapy for resectable hepatocellular carcinoma: review of the randomised clinical trials. Lancet Oncol 3:593, 2002.
70. Okada S: Local ablation therapy for hepatocellular carcinoma. Semin Liver Dis 19:323, 1999.
71. Lencioni RA, et al: Small hepatocellular carcinoma in cirrhosis: randomized comparison of radio-frequency thermal ablation versus percutaneous ethanol injection. Radiology 228:235, 2003.
72. Livraghi T, et al: Small hepatocellular carcinoma: treatment with radio-frequency ablation versus ethanol injection. Radiology 210:655, 1999.
73. Rossi S, et al: Percutaneous RF interstitial thermal ablation in the treatment of hepatic cancer. AJR Am J Roentgenol 167:759, 1996.
74. Mulier S, et al: Complications of radiofrequency coagulation of liver tumours. Br J Surg 89:1206, 2002.
75. Llovet JM, et al: Increased risk of tumor seeding after percutaneous radiofrequency ablation for single hepatocellular carcinoma. Hepatology 33:1124, 2001.
76. Inoue K, et al: Long-term survival and prognostic factors in the surgical treatment of mass-forming type cholangiocarcinoma. Surgery 127:498, 2000.
77. Weber SM, et al: Intrahepatic cholangiocarcinoma: resectability, recurrence pattern, and outcomes. J Am Coll Surg 193:384, 2001.
78. Pichlmayr R, et al: Surgical treatment of cholangiocellular carcinoma. World J Surg 19:83, 1995.
79. Jan YY, et al: Factors influencing survival after hepatectomy for peripheral cholangiocarcinoma. Hepatogastroenterology 43:614, 1996.
80. Casavilla FA, et al: Hepatic resection and transplantation for peripheral cholangiocarcinoma. J Am Coll Surg 185:429, 1997.
81. Madariaga JR, et al: Liver resection for hilar and peripheral cholangiocarcinomas: a study of 62 cases. Ann Surg 227:70, 1998.
82. Valverde A, et al: Resection of intrahepatic cholangiocarcinoma: a Western experience. J Hepatobiliary Pancreat Surg 6:122, 1999.
83. Isa T, et al: Predictive factors for long-term survival in patients with intrahepatic cholangiocarcinoma. Am J Surg 181:507, 2001.
84. de Aretxabala X, et al: Gallbladder cancer in Chile. A report on 54 potentially resectable tumors. Cancer 69:60, 1992.
85. Shirai Y, et al: Inapparent carcinoma of the gallbladder. An appraisal of a radical second operation after simple cholecystectomy. Ann Surg 215:326, 1992.
86. Bartlett DL, et al: Long-term results after resection for gallbladder cancer. Implications for staging and management. Ann Surg 224:639, 1996.
87. Fong Y, Heffernan N, Blumgart LH: Gallbladder carcinoma discovered during laparoscopic cholecystectomy: aggressive reresection is beneficial. Cancer 83:423, 1998.
88. de Aretxabala X, et al: Curative resection in potentially resectable tumours of the gallbladder. Eur J Surg 163:419, 1997.
89. Fong Y, Jarnagin W, Blumgart LH: Gallbladder cancer: comparison of patients presenting initially for definitive operation with those presenting after prior noncurative intervention. Ann Surg 232:557, 2000.
90. Yamaguchi K, Tsuneyoshi M: Subclinical gallbladder carcinoma. Am J Surg 163:382, 1992.
91. Nakamura S, et al: Aggressive surgery for carcinoma of the gallbladder. Surgery 106:467, 1989.
92. Onoyama H, et al: Extended cholecystectomy for carcinoma of the gallbladder. World J Surg 19:758, 1995.
93. Ogura Y, et al: Radical operations for carcinoma of the gallbladder: present status in Japan. World J Surg 15:337, 1991.
94. Matsumoto Y, et al: Surgical treatment of primary carcinoma of the gallbladder based on the histologic analysis of 48 surgical specimens. Am J Surg 163:239, 1992.
95. Donohue JH, et al: Carcinoma of the gallbladder. Does radical resection improve outcome? Arch Surg 125:237, 1990.
96. Fahim RB, et al: Carcinoma of the gallbladder: a study of its modes of spread. Ann Surg 156:114, 1962.
97. Kondo S, et al: Regional and para-aortic lymphadenectomy in radical surgery for advanced gallbladder carcinoma. Br J Surg 87:418, 2000.
98. Kopelson G, et al: The role of radiation therapy in cancer of the extra-hepatic biliary system: an analysis of thirteen patients and a review of the literature of the effectiveness of surgery, chemotherapy and radiotherapy. Int J Radiat Oncol Biol Phys 2:883, 1977.
99. Hanna SS, Rider WD: Carcinoma of the gallbladder or extrahepatic bile ducts: the role of radiotherapy. Can Med Assoc J 118:59, 1978.
100. Houry S, et al: Gallbladder carcinoma: role of radiation therapy. Br J Surg 76:448, 1989.
101. Kresl JJ, et al: Adjuvant external beam radiation therapy with concurrent chemotherapy in the management of gallbladder carcinoma. Int J Radiat Oncol Biol Phys 52:167, 2002.
102. Lillemoe KD: Current status of surgery for Klatskin tumors. Curr Opin Gen Surg 161:167, 1994.
103. Klempnauer J, et al: What constitutes long-term survival after surgery for hilar cholangiocarcinoma? Cancer 79:26, 1997.
104. Chao TC, Greager JA: Carcinoma of the extrahepatic bile ducts. J Surg Oncol 46:145, 1991.
105. Klempnauer J, et al: Resectional surgery of hilar cholangiocarcinoma: a multivariate analysis of prognostic factors. J Clin Oncol 15:947, 1997.
106. Cameron JL, et al: Management of proximal cholangiocarcinomas by surgical resection and radiotherapy. Am J Surg 159:91, 1990; discussion 97.
107. Su CH, et al: Factors influencing postoperative morbidity, mortality, and survival after resection for hilar cholangiocarcinoma. Ann Surg 223:384, 1996.
108. Hadjis NS, et al: Outcome of radical surgery in hilar cholangiocarcinoma. Surgery 107:597, 1990.
109. Jarnagin WR, et al: Staging, resectability, and outcome in 225 patients with hilar cholangiocarcinoma. Ann Surg 234:507, 2001; discussion 517.
110. Neuhaus P, et al: Extended resections for hilar cholangiocarcinoma. Ann Surg 230:808, 1999; discussion 819.
111. Kosuge T, et al: Improved surgical results for hilar cholangiocarcinoma with procedures including major hepatic resection. Ann Surg 230:663, 1999.
112. Nimura Y, et al: Hepatic segmentectomy with caudate lobe resection for bile duct carcinoma of the hepatic hilus. World J Surg 14:535, 1990; discussion 544.
113. Jarnagin WR, Shoup M: Surgical management of cholangiocarcinoma. Semin Liver Dis 24:189, 2004.
114. Wade TP, et al: Experience with distal bile duct cancers in US. Veterans Affairs hospitals: 1987-1991. J Surg Oncol 64:242, 1997.
115. Nagorney DM, et al: Outcomes after curative resections of cholangiocarcinoma. Arch Surg 128:871, 1993; discussion 877.
116. Fong Y, et al: Outcome of treatment for distal bile duct cancer. Br J Surg 83:1712, 1996.
117. Yeo CJ, et al: Six hundred fifty consecutive pancreaticoduodenectomies in the 1990s: pathology, complications, and outcomes. Ann Surg 226:248, 1997; discussion 257.

118. Fritz P, et al: Combined external beam radiotherapy and intraluminal high dose rate brachytherapy on bile duct carcinomas. Int J Radiat Oncol Biol Phys 29:855, 1994.
119. Jarnagin WR, et al: Patterns of initial disease recurrence after resection of gallbladder carcinoma and hilar cholangiocarcinoma: implications for adjuvant therapeutic strategies. Cancer 98:1689, 2003.
120. Foo ML, et al: External radiation therapy and transcatheter iridium in the treatment of extrahepatic bile duct carcinoma. Int J Radiat Oncol Biol Phys 39:929, 1997.
121. Gerhards MF, et al: Results of postoperative radiotherapy for resectable hilar cholangiocarcinoma. World J Surg 27:173, 2003.
122. Pitt HA, et al: Perihilar cholangiocarcinoma. Postoperative radiotherapy does not improve survival. Ann Surg 221:788, 1995; discussion 797.
123. Mahe M, et al: Radiation therapy in extrahepatic bile duct carcinoma. Radiother Oncol 21:121, 1991.
124. Shimoda M, et al: Liver transplantation for cholangiocellular carcinoma: analysis of a single-center experience and review of the literature. Liver Transpl 7:1023, 2001.
125. Rea DJ, Heimbach JK, Rosen CB, et al: Liver transplantation with neoadjuvant chemoradiation is more effective than resection for hilar cholangiocarcinoma. Ann Surg 242:451-461, 2005.
126. Groupe d'Etude et de Traitement du Carcinome Hepatocellulaire: A comparison of lipiodol chemoembolization and conservative treatment for unresectable hepatocellular carcinoma. N Engl J Med 332:1256, 1995.
127. Yamashita Y, et al: Prognostic factors in the treatment of hepatocellular carcinoma with transcatheter arterial embolization and arterial infusion. Cancer 67:385, 1991.
128. Stillwagon GB, et al: Prognostic factors in unresectable hepatocellular cancer: Radiation Therapy Oncology Group Study 83. Int J Radiat Oncol Biol Phys 20:65, 1991.
129. Mathurin P, et al: Review article: Overview of medical treatments in unresectable hepatocellular carcinoma—an impossible meta-analysis? Aliment Pharmacol Ther 12:111, 1998.
130. Simonetti RG, et al: Treatment of hepatocellular carcinoma: a systematic review of randomized controlled trials. Ann Oncol 8:117, 1997.
131. Fuchs CS, et al: A phase II trial of gemcitabine in patients with advanced hepatocellular carcinoma. Cancer 94:3186, 2002.
132. Chow PK, et al: High-dose tamoxifen in the treatment of inoperable hepatocellular carcinoma: a multicenter randomized controlled trial. Hepatology 36:1221, 2002.
133. Breedis C, Young G: The blood supply of neoplasms in the liver. Am J Pathol 30:969, 1954.
134. Yamashita T: Chemotherapy for advanced hepatocellular carcinoma: systemic chemotherapy or hepatic arterial infusion chemotherapy? J Gastroenterol 39:404, 2004.
135. Tzoracoleftherakis EE, et al: Intra-arterial versus systemic chemotherapy for nonoperable hepatocellular carcinoma. Hepatogastroenterology 46:1122, 1999.
136. De Maio E, et al: Transcatheter arterial procedures in the treatment of patients with hepatocellular carcinoma: a review of the literature. Crit Rev Oncol Hematol 46:285, 2003.
137. Pelletier G, et al: A randomized trial of hepatic arterial chemoembolization in patients with unresectable hepatocellular carcinoma. J Hepatol 11:181, 1990.
138. Madden MV, et al: Randomised trial of targeted chemotherapy with lipiodol and 5-epidoxorubicin compared with symptomatic treatment for hepatoma. Gut 34:1598, 1993.
139. Bruix J, et al: Transarterial embolization versus symptomatic treatment in patients with advanced hepatocellular carcinoma: results of a randomized, controlled trial in a single institution. Hepatology 27:1578, 1998.
140. Llovet JM, et al: Arterial embolisation or chemoembolisation versus symptomatic treatment in patients with unresectable hepatocellular carcinoma: a randomised controlled trial. Lancet 359:1734, 2002.
141. Stillwagon GB, et al: Variable low dose rate irradiation (131I-anti-CEA) and integrated low dose chemotherapy in the treatment of nonresectable primary intrahepatic cholangiocarcinoma. Int J Radiat Oncol Biol Phys 21:1601, 1991.
142. Robertson JM, et al: A phase I trial of hepatic arterial bromodeoxyuridine and conformal radiation therapy for patients with primary hepatobiliary cancers or colorectal liver metastases. Int J Radiat Oncol Biol Phys 39:1087, 1997.
143. McGinn CJ, et al: Treatment of intrahepatic cancers with radiation doses based on a normal tissue complication probability model. J Clin Oncol 16:2246, 1998.
144. Dawson LA, et al: Escalated focal liver radiation and concurrent hepatic artery fluorodeoxyuridine for unresectable intrahepatic malignancies. J Clin Oncol 18:2210, 2000.
145. Dawson LA, et al: Analysis of radiation-induced liver disease using the Lyman NTCP model. Int J Radiat Oncol Biol Phys 53:810, 2002.
146. Seong J, et al: Clinical results and prognostic factors in radiotherapy for unresectable hepatocellular carcinoma: a retrospective study of 158 patients. Int J Radiat Oncol Biol Phys 55:329, 2003.
147. Zeng ZC, et al: A comparison of chemoembolization combination with and without radiotherapy for unresectable hepatocellular carcinoma. Cancer J 10:307, 2004.
148. Li B, et al: Study of local three-dimensional conformal radiotherapy combined with transcatheter arterial chemoembolization for patients with stage III hepatocellular carcinoma. Am J Clin Oncol 26:e92, 2003.
149. Guo WJ, Yu EX: Evaluation of combined therapy with chemoembolization and irradiation for large hepatocellular carcinoma. Br J Radiol 73:1091, 2000.
150. Pradeep R, et al: Predictors of survival in patients with carcinoma of the gallbladder. Cancer 76:1145, 1995.
151. Ishii H, et al: Chemotherapy in the treatment of advanced gallbladder cancer. Oncology 66:138, 2004.
152. Harvey JH, Smith FP, Schein PS: 5-Fluorouracil, mitomycin, and doxorubicin (FAM) in carcinoma of the biliary tract. J Clin Oncol 2:1245, 1984.
153. Taal BG, et al: Phase II trial of mitomycin C (MMC) in advanced gallbladder and biliary tree carcinoma. An EORTC Gastrointestinal Tract Cancer Cooperative Group Study. Ann Oncol 4:607, 1993.
154. Okada S, et al: A phase II study of cisplatin in patients with biliary tract carcinoma. Oncology 51:515, 1994.
155. Patt YZ, et al: Phase II trial of cisplatin, interferon alpha-2b, doxorubicin, and 5-fluorouracil for biliary tract cancer. Clin Cancer Res 7:3375, 2001.
156. Patt YZ, et al: Phase II trial of intravenous fluorouracil and subcutaneous interferon alfa-2b for biliary tract cancer. J Clin Oncol 14:2311, 1996.
157. Jones DV Jr, et al: Phase II study of paclitaxel therapy for unresectable biliary tree carcinomas. J Clin Oncol 14:2306, 1996.
158. Sanz-Altamira PM, et al: A phase II trial of 5-fluorouracil, leucovorin, and carboplatin in patients with unresectable biliary tree carcinoma. Cancer 82:2321, 1998.
159. Pazdur R, et al: Phase II trial of docetaxel for cholangiocarcinoma. Am J Clin Oncol 22:78, 1999.
160. Penz M, et al: Phase II trial of two-weekly gemcitabine in patients with advanced biliary tract cancer. Ann Oncol 12:183, 2001.
161. Ellis PA, et al: Epirubicin, cisplatin and infusional 5-fluorouracil (5-FU) (ECF) in hepatobiliary tumours. Eur J Cancer 31A:1594, 1995.
162. Malik IA, et al: Gemcitabine and cisplatin is a highly effective combination chemotherapy in patients with advanced cancer of the gallbladder. Am J Clin Oncol 26:174, 2003.
163. Doval DC, et al: A phase II study of gemcitabine and cisplatin in chemotherapy-naive, unresectable gall bladder cancer. Br J Cancer 90:1516, 2004.
164. Lokich JJ, et al: Biliary tract obstruction secondary to cancer: management guidelines and selected literature review. J Clin Oncol 5:969, 1987.
165. Hejna M, Pruckmayer M, Raderer M: The role of chemotherapy and radiation in the management of biliary cancer: a review of the literature. Eur J Cancer 34:977, 1998.
166. Hayes JK Jr, Sapozink MD, Miller FJ: Definitive radiation therapy in bile duct carcinoma. Int J Radiat Oncol Biol Phys 15:735, 1988.
167. Lawrence TS, et al: Hepatic toxicity resulting from cancer treatment. Int J Radiat Oncol Biol Phys 31:1237, 1995.

168. Yamasaki SA, et al: High-dose localized radiation therapy for treatment of hepatic malignant tumors: CT findings and their relation to radiation hepatitis. AJR Am J Roentgenol 165:79, 1995.
169. Jackson A, et al: Analysis of clinical complication data for radiation hepatitis using a parallel architecture model. Int J Radiat Oncol Biol Phys 31:883, 1995.
170. Emami B, et al: Tolerance of normal tissue to therapeutic irradiation. Int J Radiat Oncol Biol Phys 21:109, 1991.
171. Borgelt BB, et al: The palliation of hepatic metastases: results of the Radiation Therapy Oncology Group pilot study. Int J Radiat Oncol Biol Phys 7:587, 1981.
172. Ten Haken RK, et al: Potential benefits of eliminating planning target volume expansions for patient breathing in the treatment of liver tumors. Int J Radiat Oncol Biol Phys 38:613, 1997.
173. Balter JM, et al: Uncertainties in CT-based radiation therapy treatment planning associated with patient breathing. Int J Radiat Oncol Biol Phys 36:167, 1996.
174. Balter JM, et al: Daily targeting of intrahepatic tumors for radiotherapy. Int J Radiat Oncol Biol Phys 52:266, 2002.
175. Atiq OT, et al: Treatment of unresectable primary liver cancer with intrahepatic fluorodeoxyuridine and mitomycin C through an implantable pump. Cancer 69:920, 1992.
176. Yodono H, et al: Arterial infusion chemotherapy for advanced hepatocellular carcinoma using EPF and EAP therapies. Cancer Chemother Pharmacol 31(Suppl):S89, 1992.
177. Li B, et al: Study of local three-dimensional conformal radiotherapy combined with transcatheter arterial chemoembolization for patients with stage III hepatocellular carcinoma. Am J Clin Oncol 26:e92, 2003.
178. Iwasaki Y, et al: The role of intraoperative radiation therapy in the treatment of bile duct cancer. World J Surg 12:91, 1988.
179. Gunderson LL, Garton GR, et al: Pancreas and bile duct cancer results of IORT. *In* Intraoperative Radiation Therapy. New York, Pergamon Press, 1991, p 212.
180. Monson JR, et al: Intraoperative radiotherapy for unresectable cholangiocarcinoma—the Mayo Clinic experience. Surg Oncol 1:283, 1992.
181. De Vreede I, et al: Prolonged disease-free survival after orthotopic liver transplantation plus adjuvant chemoirradiation for cholangiocarcinoma. Liver Transpl 6:309, 2000.
182. Gunderson LL, et al: Future role of radiotherapy as a component of treatment in biliopancreatic cancers. Ann Oncol 10(Suppl 4):291, 1999.
183. Alden ME, Mohiuddin M: The impact of radiation dose in combined external beam and intraluminal Ir-192 brachytherapy for bile duct cancer. Int J Radiat Oncol Biol Phys 28:945, 1994.
184. Flickinger JC, et al: Radiation therapy for primary carcinoma of the extrahepatic biliary system. An analysis of 63 cases. Cancer 68:289, 1991.
185. Urego M, Flickinger JC, Carr BI: Radiotherapy and multimodality management of cholangiocarcinoma. Int J Radiat Oncol Biol Phys 44:121, 1999.

CHAPTER 47

COLON CANCER

Brian G. Czito and Christopher G. Willett

EPIDEMIOLOGY AND ETIOLOGY

In 2006, it is estimated that 106,680 patients will be diagnosed with colon cancer and 55,170 deaths will occur in the United States.

Linkage between diet and environmental factors with colon cancer is supported by epidemiologic studies. Risk factors include advanced age, male sex, family history of colorectal cancer, increasing body mass index, low physical activity level, and red meat/processed meat consumption.

The site of origin is shifting in the United States, with a higher frequency of proximal tumors.

Adenomas are the precursor lesions, and polypectomy decreases the subsequent risk of malignancy.

BIOLOGIC CHARACTERISTICS AND PATHOLOGY

Most colon tumors are adenocarcinomas.

The most important prognostic factor is tumor extent, including extension through the bowel wall, nodal spread, and the presence of metastatic disease.

Approximately 10% of colorectal cancers arise in the setting of a hereditary syndrome. These syndromes are characterized by multiple adenomatous polyps (familial adenomatous polyposis) or nonpolypoid forms (hereditary nonpolyposis colorectal cancer). Inheritance is autosomal dominant.

Inflammatory bowel disease increases the risk of developing colon cancer.

STAGING EVALUATION

Staging should include history and physical examination, complete blood count, general chemistry panel (liver functions, creatinine), carcinoembryonic antigen (CEA), chest radiograph or computed tomography (CT) and CT of the abdomen/pelvis with colonoscopy or barium enema plus proctoscopy.

In advanced cases, ultrasonography, magnetic resonance imaging, or positron emission tomography may be helpful in assessing the extent of tumor spread outside the colon.

PRIMARY THERAPY

Resection is the principal therapy of primary and nonmetastatic colon cancers. This treatment modality results in mean 5-year survival rates of 97% (T1N0), 90% (T2N0), 78% (T3N0), 74% (T2N+), 63% (T4N0), 48% (T3N+), and 38% (T4N+).

ADJUVANT THERAPY

Adjuvant chemotherapy (5-fluorouracil [5-FU] with leucovorin) significantly improves survival rates of patients with nodal metastases by approximately 13% at 5 years in prospective randomized studies. 5-FU–based chemotherapy is the preferred regimen in the adjuvant setting.

Agents such as capecitabine and oxaliplatin may further benefit patients in the adjuvant setting and are under active investigation.

Retrospective studies from the Massachusetts General Hospital (MGH) and others have evaluated the role of adjuvant external beam radiation therapy (EBRT) in resected colon cancer. These studies found postoperative EBRT with or without 5-FU improved local control and disease-free survival for patients with resected stage T4N0 or T4N+ tumors versus historical rates with surgery alone.

An Intergroup randomized trial compared 12 months of adjuvant 5-FU/levamisole with or without tumor bed and nodal irradiation in T4N0-2 and select T3N1-2 patients. Results showed no overall survival or local control difference with the addition of radiation therapy. Interpretation of study results was handicapped by low accrual, high ineligibility rates, and low rates of preoperative imaging and surgical clip placement to assist radiation field design.

LOCALLY ADVANCED DISEASE

In a Mayo Clinic analysis of locally advanced disease, postoperative EBRT resulted in a 5-year actuarial local failure rate of 54% for patients with microscopic residual disease and 79% for patients with gross residual tumors. In patients receiving intraoperative electron irradiation (IOERT) and EBRT, local failure was observed in 11% of patients versus 82% of patients receiving EBRT only. The 5-year survival was 76% for patients receiving IOERT and EBRT, versus 26% for patients receiving EBRT alone.

Preoperative radiation therapy and chemotherapy followed by resection plus IOERT and maintenance chemotherapy should be considered for patients with locally advanced cancers (T4N0-2).

PALLIATION

For patients with metastatic disease, 5-FU and leucovorin have been given with partial response rates of 20% to 30%. The addition of newer agents (capecitabine, irinotecan, oxaliplatin, bevacizumab, cetuximab) has improved response rates and survival.

Palliative irradiation, often with 5-FU–based chemotherapy, is considered for patients with symptomatic metastatic disease.

The rationale for the adjuvant treatment of colon cancer stems from pattern of failure analyses of patients undergoing resection. Based on the finding of high rates of distant failure for patients with stage II and III colon tumors, investigators implemented treatment strategies employing systemic (chemotherapeutic) approaches. Early data prompted multicenter randomized prospective trials where survival was improved in patients with resected, "high-risk" colon cancer receiving adjuvant chemotherapy with 5-FU and leucovorin. Similarly, patterns of failure analyses have suggested that high locoregional failure rates occur in subsets of patients with resected colon cancer. This has stimulated investigation of adjuvant radiation with concurrent and maintenance chemotherapy. Although there is a compelling rationale for adjuvant radiation therapy with 5-FU–based chemotherapy for selected patients with resected high-risk colonic cancer, its efficacy has not been validated by a randomized prospective study. The benefit of adjuvant radiation therapy remains unclear. This chapter reviews the rationale for radiation therapy and 5-FU–based chemotherapy, as well as results, in patients with resected colon cancer.

ETIOLOGY AND EPIDEMIOLOGY

In 2006, the American Cancer Society estimated that 106,680 patients will be diagnosed with colon cancer and 55,170 deaths will occur from colon or rectal cancer.[1] Although this malignancy may be linked to chemical carcinogens within the bowel lumen, it is not established whether these are ingested, the result of chemical activation of substances in the fecal stream, or a bacterial byproduct.[2] Environmental and dietary factors have been established as contributing to colorectal cancer. Factors shown to increase the risk of developing this disease include increasing age, male sex, family history of colorectal cancer, increasing height, increasing body mass index, processed meat intake, excessive alcohol intake, and low folate consumption. Of these risk factors, only increasing age, male sex, and excessive alcohol use have been found to be associated with rectal cancer.[3] The value of consumption of fruits and vegetables in the prevention of colon and rectal cancer remains controversial, although studies have suggested that these associations may have been overstated.[4] Contemporary prospective and randomized data do not support a high fiber diet in the prevention of colorectal cancer.[5] Other studies have suggested that nonsteroidal anti-inflammatory drugs may serve in reducing colorectal cancer. The role of chemopreventive agents (carotenoids, aspirin, and other nonsteroidal anti-inflammatory drugs) in colorectal cancer is under active investigation.

PREVENTION AND EARLY DETECTION

Neoplastic polyps, including tubular adenomas, villous adenomas, and tubulovillous adenomas, are precursors of colon cancers. Most colorectal cancers arise from preexisting polyps.[6] Patients with neoplastic polyps should be considered at high risk for large bowel cancer, and polypectomy may reduce this risk. With the availability of the flexible colonoscope and endoscopic polypectomy, polyps can be removed at a premalignant stage and patients followed closely.

Screening

Because the cumulative lifetime risk of developing colorectal cancer in the United States is about 6%,[7] screening programs for the general population have been undertaken. The goal of screening is to detect preinvasive polyps or early invasive cancer. The presence of polyps increases the risk for cancer to approximately 15%. Data from programs in which proctoscopy is performed annually suggest that routinely scheduled polypectomy reduces the development of subsequent bowel cancer by 80% or more.[2] The American Cancer Society has recommended that screening should begin at age 50 in the average risk patient by either (1) annual fecal occult blood test and/or flexible sigmoidoscopy every 5 years, (2) double contrast barium enema every 5 years, or (3) colonoscopy every 10 years. Intensive surveillance is recommended for patients at high risk (patients with adenomatous polyps, history of colorectal cancer, first-degree relative diagnosed with colorectal cancer or adenomas, inflammatory bowel disease, or high risk due to family history or genetic testing). Computed tomography (CT) colonography and genetic fecal testing are being studied as potential screening tools. Although screening methods can detect colorectal cancer at an early stage, less than 40% of patients are diagnosed with early disease, likely reflecting low rates of disease awareness as well as the infrequency of screening in eligible candidates.[8]

BIOLOGIC CHARACTERISTICS AND MOLECULAR BIOLOGY

A detailed discussion of the biologic and genetic pathways of development of colorectal cancer is beyond the scope of this chapter. In brief, it has been established that the development of colon cancer is a multifactorial process, involving changes in many genes including both proto-oncogenes and tumor suppressor genes. Colorectal cancers appear to arise through inactivation of the tumor suppressor genes adenomatous polyposis coli *(APC)* and *P53* as well as mutations in the *ras* proto-oncogene.

Microsatellites are short-repeat DNA sequences, usually consisting of one to five nucleotides. Microsatellite "instability" is found in a majority of patients with hereditary nonpolyposis colorectal cancer (HNPCC), as well as in a minority of those with sporadic colorectal cancers. It has been shown that this instability occurs in patients with mutations in genes encoding enzymes that repair DNA replication errors. These defects in mismatch repair lead to high-frequency microsatellite instability. Studies have suggested that patients with tumors possessing a high frequency of microsatellite instability have a more favorable outcome and develop fewer metastases.[9] Further elucidation of the genetic pathways in the development of colorectal cancer remains an active area of investigation and may ultimately impact therapy of this disease.

PATHOLOGY AND PATHWAYS OF SPREAD

Tumors of the colon arise in the mucosa and are virtually all (>90%) adenocarcinomas. Other histologic types include squamous cell carcinoma, carcinoid, leiomyosarcoma, and lymphoma. Most grading systems classify adenocarcinoma as well, moderately, or poorly differentiated.

Large bowel tumors invade from mucosa through the bowel wall and beyond, with involvement of lymphatic channels and lymph nodes. Hematogenous spread can occur, primarily to the lung and liver. There is little propensity for colon cancer to spread longitudinally within the bowel wall, in contrast to esophageal or gastric cancers.

CLINICAL MANIFESTATION, PATIENT EVALUATION, AND STAGING

Colon cancer often produces minimal or no symptoms, emphasizing the need for screening programs in the general population. Many colon cancer symptoms are nonspecific, including changes in bowel habits, weakness, intermittent abdominal pain, nausea, and vomiting. The persistence of such symptoms and any evidence of iron deficiency anemia should be investigated.

The clinical presentation of colon cancer is determined largely by site of the tumor. Cancers of the right colon are often exophytic and commonly associated with iron deficiency anemia due to occult blood loss. During the past 20 years, the incidence of cancer of the right colon has increased and accounts for one third of large-bowel cancers. Many of these are diagnosed late.[2] Cancers of the left colon and sigmoid colon are often deeply invasive, annular, and accompanied by obstruction and rectal bleeding.

For patients undergoing resection, preoperative evaluation should include pathologic confirmation of adenocarcinoma, colonoscopy to evaluate extent of tumor and rule out synchronous primaries (occurring in 3% to 5%), and baseline blood counts with liver function tests and CEA levels. Patients should undergo abdominal and pelvic CT scan and chest radiography to evaluate extent of local regional disease, as well as the presence or absence of distant metastases. Positron emission tomography (PET) scan, magnetic resonance imaging (MRI), and ultrasound may be useful in evaluating patients with oligometastatic disease who may be appropriate candidates for resection of metastatic disease with curative intent. Figure 47-1 shows a diagnostic algorithm of the management of patients with potentially resectable colon cancer.

Prognostic factors influencing survival in colon cancer patients include depth of tumor invasion into and beyond the bowel wall, the number of involved regional lymph nodes, and the presence or absence of distant metastases. The tumor, node, metastasis (TNM) system of the American Joint Committee on Cancer can be used as a clinical (preoperative) or postoperative staging system (Tables 47-1 and 47-2).

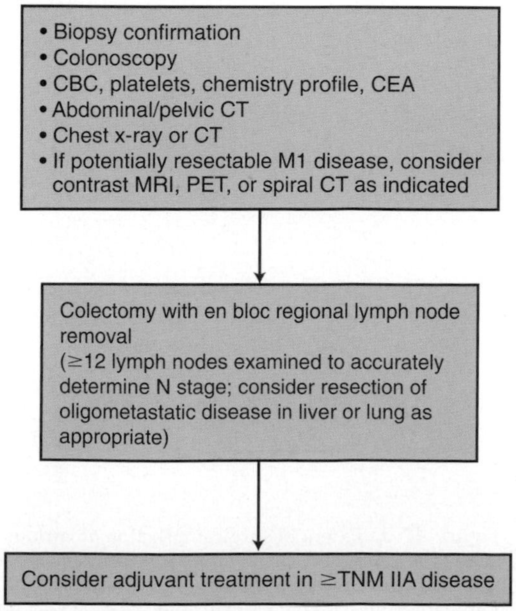
• Biopsy confirmation
• Colonoscopy
• CBC, platelets, chemistry profile, CEA
• Abdominal/pelvic CT
• Chest x-ray or CT
• If potentially resectable M1 disease, consider contrast MRI, PET, or spiral CT as indicated
Colectomy with en bloc regional lymph node removal
(≥12 lymph nodes examined to accurately determine N stage; consider resection of oligometastatic disease in liver or lung as appropriate)
Consider adjuvant treatment in ≥TNM IIA disease

Figure 47-1 **Diagnostic algorithm** of the management of patients with potentially resectable colon cancer.

Table 47-1 Colorectal TNM (Tumor, Node, Metastasis) Staging, 2002

PRIMARY TUMOR (T)	
TX	Primary tumor cannot be assessed
T0	No evidence of primary tumor
Tis	Carcinoma in situ: intraepithelial or invasion of lamina propria
T1	Tumor invades submucosa
T2	Tumor invades muscularis propria
T3	Tumor invades through the muscularis propria into the subserosa, or into nonperitonealized pericolic or perirectal tissues
T4	Tumor is adherent to or directly invades other organs or structures,* and/or perforates visceral peritoneum (includes invasion of other segments of colon)
REGIONAL LYMPH NODES (N)	
NX	Regional lymph nodes cannot be assessed
N0	No regional lymph node metastasis
N1	Metastasis in 1 to 3 regional lymph nodes
N2	Metastasis in 4 or more regional lymph nodes (Tumor nodules in the pericolonic adipose tissue without evidence of residual lymph node are classified as a regional lymph node metastases)
DISTANT METASTASIS (M)	
MX	Distant metastasis cannot be assessed
M0	No distant metastasis
M1	Distant metastasis

*Direct invasion in T4 includes invasion of other segments of the colorectum by way of the serosa, for example, invasion of the sigmoid by a carcinoma of the cecum. Tumor that is adherent to other organs or structures, macroscopically, is classified as T4. However, if no tumor is present in the adhesion, microscopically, the classification should be pT3.

From Colon and Rectum. North American Joint Committee on Cancer Staging Manual, 6th Ed. New York, Springer, 2002, 113-124.

Table 47-2 Stage Grouping of the American Joint Committee on Cancer

AJCC Stage	T	N	M	Dukes*	MAC*
0	Tis	N0	M0	—	—
I	T1	N0	M0	A	A
	T2	N0	M0	A	B1
IIA	T3	N0	M0	B	B2
IIB	T4	N0	M0	B	B3
IIIA	T1 T2	N1	M0	C	C1
IIIB	T3-4	N1	M0	C	C2/C3
IIIC	Any T	N2	M0	C	C1/C2/C3
IV	Any T	Any N	M1	—	D

*Dukes B is a composite of better (T3 N0 M0) and worse (T4 N0 M0) prognostic groups, as is Dukes C (Any T N1 M0 and Any T N2 M0). MAC is the modified Astler-Coller classification.

PRIMARY THERAPY

Surgery

Surgery remains the primary treatment for patients with colonic tumors. Resection with curative intent is possible in approximately 75% of patients.[2] Surgical resection of primary colon cancer is based on the anatomy and mechanisms by which this disease spreads. Adenocarcinomas of the colon may grow by direct extension into the lymphatics of the submucosa and bowel wall. To avoid cutting across tumor in intramural lymphatics, sufficient lengths of bowel must be resected proximal and distal to the primary cancer. Colon cancer often extends through the serosa into mesenteric lymphatics that run along the blood vessels draining into the portal watershed at the root of the mesentery. Resection includes removal of the major lymphatic drainage system in the mesentery. Because anatomic resections designed to include named blood vessels also include the draining lymphatics, the boundaries for resecting large bowel cancer are relatively uniform (Fig. 47-2). Right hemicolectomy, transverse colectomy, left hemicolectomy, and sigmoid resection are performed by adherence to surgical oncologic principles without major sacrifice of large bowel function.

Resection results in excellent cure rates for lesions limited to the bowel wall with negative nodes (average 5-year survival, 97% for T1N0; 85% to 90% for T2N0). With a single high-risk feature of extension beyond the colonic wall (T3-4 N0) or involved nodes (T0-2N+), 5-year survival with surgery falls to 65% to 75%, and adjuvant treatment is often indicated. When both high-risk features are present (T3-4N+), 5-year survival with surgery alone drops to approximately 50% (T3N+) and 35% (T4N+), and adjuvant treatment is usually advised.

Adjuvant Chemotherapy

Prospective randomized trials have shown that the addition of 5-FU and leucovorin improves survival for resected stage III patients.[10,11] This is now considered standard adjuvant therapy in these patients. Newer agents have been investigated and have shown potential benefit. Capecitabine, an oral 5-FU prodrug, has demonstrated similar overall and disease-free survival rates to 5-FU/leucovorin in patients with resected stage III colon cancer in a recent randomized trial.[12] Oxaliplatin is being investigated in the adjuvant treatment of resected colon cancer. A randomized study comparing 5-FU/leucovorin with 5-FU/leucovorin/oxaliplatin in resected stage II/III colon cancer patients showed improved disease-free survival in patients treated with oxaliplatin.[13] The efficacy of agents such as bevacizumab and cetuximab as adjuvant therapy is being investigated.

Adjuvant Irradiation with or without Chemotherapy

Rationale—Patterns of Relapse, Surgery Alone

Because of the documented efficacy of adjuvant chemotherapy and the perception by many oncologists that colonic (as opposed to rectal) cancer is much more likely to relapse distantly than locally, there has been little evaluation of the efficacy of postoperative irradiation with chemotherapy. The potential indications for adjuvant radiation therapy in colon cancer are based on analyses of patterns of failure following resection[14,15] (Table 47-3). Advanced stage predicts for local failure in both colon and rectal cancer; however, local failure in colon cancer also depends on anatomic origin. The ascending and descending colon are considered "anatomically immobile," and their close proximity to the retroperitoneal tissues often limits wide surgical resection (Fig. 47-3). Limitations in achieving satisfactory circumferential margins increase the risk of residual disease and consequently local failure. In contrast, the mid-sigmoid and mid-transverse colon are relatively "mobile" with a wide mesentery permitting the surgeon to obtain wide margins regardless of extent of disease invasion into the mesentery. Unless there is adjacent organ

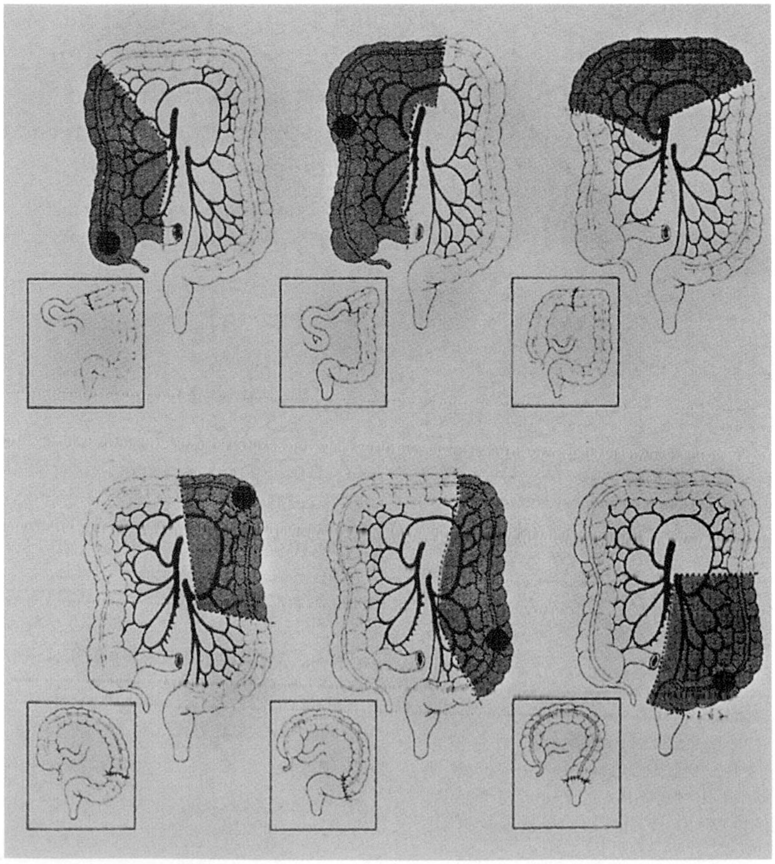

Figure 47-2 Extent of surgical resection at various colonic sites. The darkened circle represents primary disease site (anastomoses are shown in the *insets*). (From Shrock TR: Large intestine. *In* Way LW: Current Surgical Diagnosis and Treatment, 7th ed. Large Medical Publishers, Los Altos CA, 1985.)

Table 47-3 **Five-Year Actuarial Local Control and Relapse-Free Survival after Surgery Plus Postoperative Radiotherapy versus Surgery Alone, According to Stage—Massachusetts General Hospital**

TNM Stage	Surgery Alone No. of Patients	LC (%)	RFS (%)	Surgery Plus Postoperative Radiation No. of Patients	LC (%)	RFS (%)
T3 N0	163	90	78	23	91	72
T4 N0	83	69	63	54	93	79*
T3 N+	100	64	48	55	70	47
T4 N+	49	47	38	39	72	53*

*$p < .05$.
LC, local control; RFS, relapse-free survival.

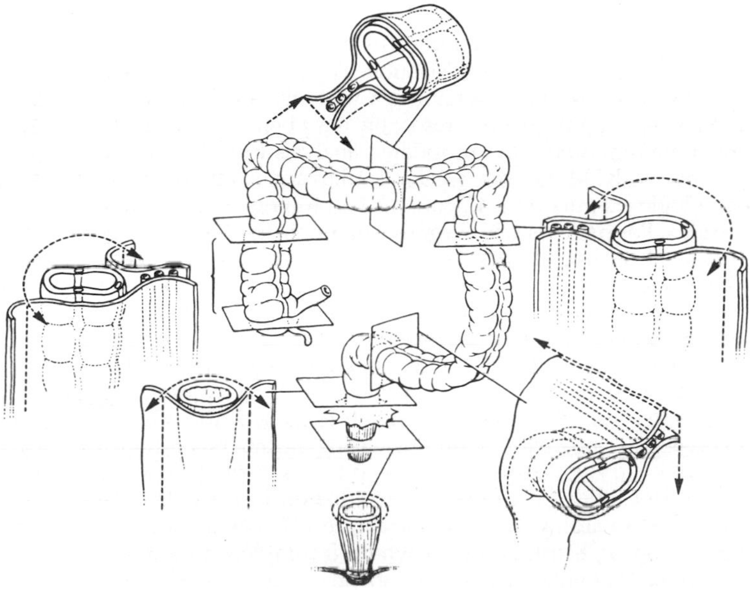

Figure 47-3 Idealized depiction of peritoneal relationships in the colon and rectum. The transverse and sigmoid colon are intraperitoneal, with a complete peritoneal covering (serosa) and mesentery. The ascending and descending colon are retroperitoneal, lack a true mesentery, and usually do not have a peritoneal covering posteriorly or laterally. The upper rectum begins above the peritoneal reflection and has peritoneum anteriorly and laterally. The lower half to two-thirds of the rectum is below the peritoneal reflection (infraperitoneal). (Reproduced with permission from Gunderson LL, O'Connell MJ: Postoperative chemotherapy/irradiation adjuvant strategy. *In* Cohen AF, Winawer SJ, Friedman MA, Gunderson LL, eds: Cancer of the Colon, Rectum, and Anus. New York, McGraw-Hill, 1995, Chapter 67, pp 631-645.)

adherence/invasion by tumor, local failure at these sites is uncommon. Local failure rates for cecal, hepatic/splenic flexure and proximal/distal sigmoid tumors are variable depending on the amount of mesentery present, tumor extension, and the adequacy of radial margins. When colon cancers adhere to or invade adjacent structures, local failure rates exceed 30% following surgery alone. Local failure occurs in patients with colonic tumors where there are anatomic constraints on radial resection margins, including tumors adherent to or invading adjacent structures.

Adjuvant Irradiation, Single Institution

Data evaluating the use of adjuvant radiation therapy in high-risk colon cancer patients had previously been limited to single-institution retrospective analyses.[16-19] To summarize, these studies have suggested that operative bed failures in high-risk patients undergoing resection alone are at least 30% and that the risk of local failure is reduced by the administration of adjuvant radiation therapy. These are discussed in detail below.

Massachusetts General Hospital

A report from the MGH evaluated outcomes in high-risk patients undergoing resection followed by adjuvant radiation therapy and compared these to a similar cohort of patients treated over the same period undergoing surgery only. Irradiated patients included those with T4 N0/N+, T3 N+ disease (excluding mid-sigmoid and mid-transverse colon) and T3 N0 patients with margins of less than 1 cm. A total of 171 patients received postoperative radiation, with 63 patients receiving concurrent chemotherapy, usually with bolus 5-FU (500 mg/m^2/d) for three consecutive days during the first and last weeks of radiation therapy. Radiation treatment was administered through parallel opposed or other multifield techniques to treat the tumor bed with an approximate 3- to 5-cm margin to a total dose of 45 Gy, followed by reduced fields to a total dose of 50.4 to 54 Gy. Draining nodes were included if thought to be at high risk for involvement. This cohort was compared to 395 patients with T3-4 N0/N+ tumors undergoing surgery alone during the same time period. Table 47-3 shows 5-year actuarial local control and relapse-free survival in the adjuvant group compared to patients undergoing surgery alone. Local control rates in T4 N0 and T4 N+ patients treated with radiation therapy were 93% and 72%, respectively, versus 69% and 47%, respectively, in patients undergoing surgery alone. Similarly, relapse-free survivals were 79% and 53%, respectively, in T4 N0/T4 N+ patients undergoing adjuvant radiation, versus 63% and 38%, respectively, in those undergoing surgery alone. No significant outcome differences were observed in patients with T3 N0 and T3 N+ lesions; however, there may be an element of selection bias in the radiation group given most patients were referred because of concerns of adequacy of local control following surgery alone. There was a trend toward improved local control in patients receiving 5-FU (Table 47-4). The rate of acute enteritis in patients receiving irradiation and 5-FU was 16% versus 4% in patients

Table 47-4 Five-Year Actuarial Local Control and Relapse-Free Survival of Adjuvantly Irradiated Patients Based on 5-Fluorouracil (5-FU) Administration—Massachusetts General Hospital

TNM Stage	WITHOUT 5-FU No. of Patients	LC (%)	RFS (%)	WITH 5-FU No. of Patients	LC (%)	RFS (%)
T3N0	16	87	69	7	100	80
T4N0	37	94	78	16	100	83
T3N+	41	69	48	14	70	43
T4N+	24	67	53	15	79	52

LC, local control; RFS, relapse-free survival.

undergoing irradiation only. This rate of enteritis is similar to data from studies of concurrent 5-FU and radiation therapy in rectal cancer. Late bowel complication rates were not increased by concomitant 5-FU administration. The conclusion was that patients with T4 tumors or tumors with abscess/fistula formation or margin-positive resection may benefit from postoperative radiation.[16] In an updated analysis from MGH, 152 patients with T4 tumors received adjuvant irradiation. On pathologic examination, 42 patients had tumors with positive margins. For patients with negative margins, the 10-year actuarial local control in T4N0 and T4N+ patients was 78% and 48%, respectively. In patients with node-negative tumors, the 10-year actuarial local control and relapse-free survival rates were 87% and 58%, respectively, compared to 65% and 33%, respectively, in patients with node-positive tumors. For patients with one involved lymph node, local control and relapse-free survival rates were similar to those without nodal involvement; however, with increasing numbers of nodes involved, survival steadily decreased.[19] Our current policy is to consider adjuvant tumor bed irradiation in patients with tumors (1) invading adjoining structures, (2) complicated by perforation or fistula, and (3) where incomplete excision is performed. Patients are generally given continuous 5-FU (225 mg/m^2/24 h) 5 days per week throughout the course of radiation therapy.

MAYO CLINIC

A report from the Mayo Clinic described a series of 103 patients receiving radiation therapy following surgery for locally advanced colon cancer.[18] Microscopic and gross residual disease was present in 18 and 35 patients, respectively. Over 90% of patients had T4N0/N+ disease. A median dose of 50.4 Gy was delivered through multifield techniques, and most patients received concurrent 5-FU–based chemotherapy. Eleven patients received an intraoperative "boost" of 10 to 20 Gy. Five-year actuarial overall local control was 40%. Patients with margin-negative tumors had a 5-year local control rate of 90%, compared to 46% for patients with microscopic residual tumor and 21% with gross residual tumor (Fig. 47-4). In patients with residual disease, local control rates in patients undergoing intraoperative boost were 89% compared to 18% in those undergoing external irradiation alone (Fig. 47-5). Similarly, 5-year survival rates were improved in patients undergoing margin-negative resection (66%) compared to those with microscopic residual (47%) or gross residual (23%) (Fig. 47-6). Patients undergoing intraoperative boost demonstrated improved survival (76% versus 26%) (Fig. 47-7).

UNIVERSITY OF FLORIDA

A report from the University of Florida of patients with locally advanced but completely resected colon cancers receiving adjuvant radiation reported a local control rate of 88%, similar to the 90% rate reported at the Mayo Clinic in patients who had completely resected tumors.[17] In addition, there

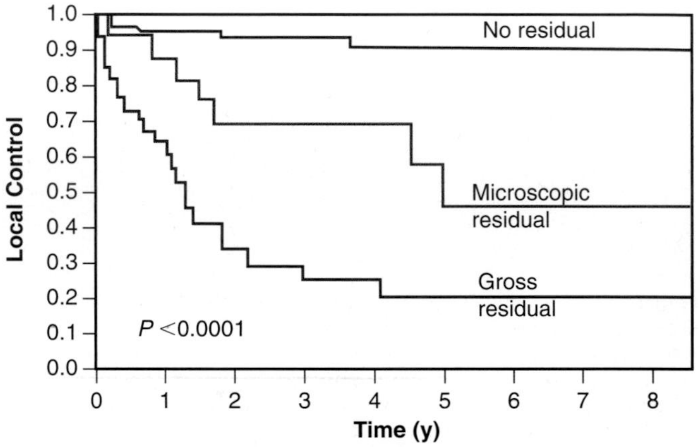

Figure 47-4 Local control by extent of residual disease following maximal resection in 103 Mayo Clinic colon cancer patients treated with external beam irradiation (EBRT) ± chemotherapy (concomitant ± maintenance) ± intraoperative electron irradiation (IOERT).

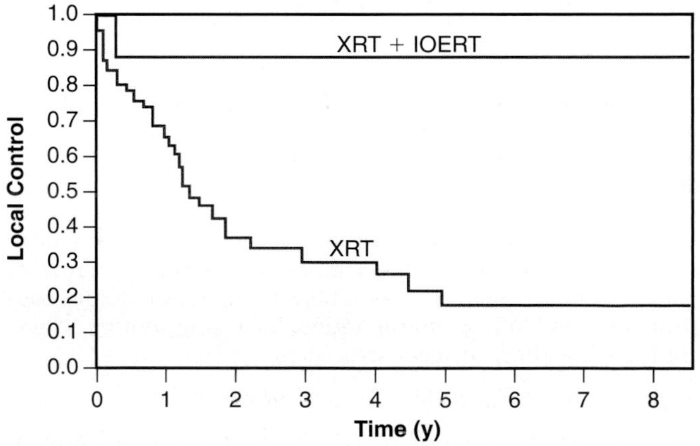

Figure 47-5 Local control by administration of IOERT following maximal resection in 103 Mayo Clinic colon cancer patients with residual disease treated with external beam irradiation (EBRT) ± chemotherapy (concomitant ± maintenance).

appeared to be a dose-response relationship to local control. The 5-year rate of local control was 96% for patients receiving 50 to 55 Gy versus 76% for patients receiving less than 50 Gy (p = .0095).

Phase III Intergroup Trial

To assess whether the addition of radiation therapy to adjuvant chemotherapy would result in superior survival and locoregional failure rates in resected, high-risk colon cancer

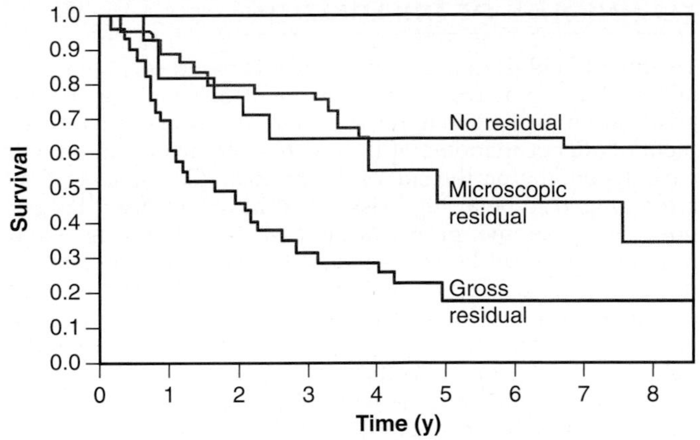

Figure 47-6 Survival results by amount of residual disease following maximal resection in a Mayo Clinic series of 103 patients with resected colon cancer treated with external beam irradiation (EBRT) ± chemotherapy (concomitant ± maintenance) ± intraoperative electron irradiation (IOERT).

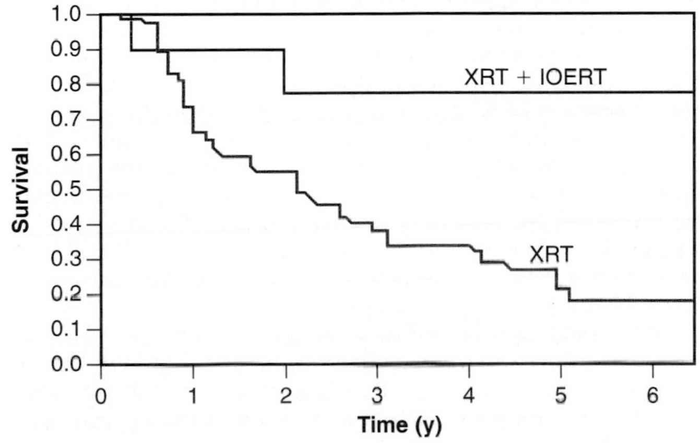

Figure 47-7 Survival results by intraoperative electron beam irradiation (IOERT) administration following maximal resection in a Mayo Clinic series of 103 patients with resected colon cancer treated with external beam irradiation (EBRT) ± chemotherapy (concomitant ± maintenance).

patients, U.S. Gastrointestinal Intergroup phase III trial was initiated in 1992. In this trial, patients with resected colon cancer were randomized to postoperative irradiation with 5-FU and levamisole versus 5-FU and levamisole alone. Eligibility criteria included margin-negative tumors with adherence to or invasion of surrounding structures (i.e, T4N0 or N+ disease, excluding peritoneal invasion) or tumors arising in the ascending or descending colon with metastatic regional nodes (T3N+). Patients were randomized to receive (1) weekly 5-FU combined with levamisole for 12 months' duration or (2) 5-FU and levamisole for 12 months with combined radiation therapy and chemotherapy beginning one month after the first 5-FU administration. The recommended total radiation dose was 45 Gy in 25 fractions over 5 weeks with an optional 5.4-Gy boost.

The initial trial accrual goal was 700 patients; however, the study was closed in 1996 due to poor accrual (222 patients; 189 evaluable). Total accrual was less than one third of initial goals, and statistical power to detect any differences between the groups was therefore decreased. No difference in overall or disease-free survival was seen between the two groups. Five-year overall survival of patients receiving chemotherapy only was 62% versus 58% for patients randomized to chemoirradiation ($p > .50$). Local recurrence rates were identical in both arms (18 patients each). Grade III/IV hematologic toxicity was higher in patients receiving radiation therapy.[20] Interpretation of study results was handicapped by decreased statistical power, high ineligibility rates, and lack of surgical clips and/or preoperative imaging to assist the definition of appropriate EBRT fields in a high percentage of patients. No definitive conclusions can be made regarding the efficacy of postoperative irradiation with 5-FU and levamisole based on this underpowered study with many flaws; however, this study provides no data supporting its routine use.

Adjuvant Hepatic and Whole Abdomen Irradiation

In addition to local failure, patterns of failure analyses have shown that hepatic metastases are common in patients with locally advanced colon carcinoma. As a result, investigators have examined the efficacy of hepatic irradiation following resection in high-risk patients. The only randomized, prospective trial evaluating adjuvant hepatic irradiation was performed by the Gastrointestinal Tumor Study Group (GITSG). Three hundred patients with resected, margin-negative Dukes B2/C colon cancer were randomized to observation only or adjuvant hepatic radiation with concurrent 5-FU given in bolus fashion week 1. Radiation was administered to the liver at 150 cGy per fraction to a total dose of 2100 cGy. Following hepatic irradiation, patients received further 5-FU. The combination of 5-FU and hepatic irradiation did not improve overall or disease-free survival.[21]

Relapse within the peritoneal cavity is also commonly observed in patients undergoing resection of locally advanced colon cancer. Investigators have reported outcomes and toxicities following adjuvant whole abdominal irradiation in high-risk patients. The Southwest Oncology Group (SWOG) reported the results of a pilot study evaluating 41 patients with resected T3N1-2M0 colon cancer treated with continuous infusion 5-FU (200 $mg/m^2/24$ h) with concomitant whole-abdominal irradiation. Patients received 30 Gy given at 1 Gy per fraction followed by a 16-Gy boost to the tumor bed at 1.6 Gy/fraction. Further 5-FU therapy was administered following completion of radiation. Five-year disease-free and overall survival estimates were 58% and 67%, respectively. Patients with tumors having more than 4 lymph nodes involved experienced 5-year disease-free and overall survival rates of 55% and 74%, respectively. Grade 3 and 4 toxicity was observed in 17% and 7% of patients, respectively. When compared to similarly staged patients from previous Intergroup trials treated with 5-FU/levamisole only, these survival results appeared favorable. The authors recommended that continuous infusion 5-FU and whole abdominal irradiation with tumor bed boost should be studied in a randomized trial.[22]

Estes and colleagues reported a pattern of failure analysis in patients with T3N+ colon cancer treated with 5-FU/levamisole chemotherapy only (Intergroup), combined chemotherapy/whole abdominal irradiation (SWOG), and patients undergoing surgery only from the previously described MGH study. Their analysis showed 5-FU/levamisole reduced the rates of lung metastases but was less effective at preventing local and peritoneal recurrence. In contrast, patients receiving whole abdominal irradiation with continuous 5-FU experienced a 12% tumor bed relapse rate, 22% hepatic relapse rate, and 15% peritoneal relapse rate, all of which were superior to the nonirradiated arms.[23] The use of whole abdominal irradiation should be considered investigational.

LOCALLY ADVANCED DISEASE AND PALLIATION

As previously described, the Mayo Clinic analyzed the results of 103 patients with advanced colonic carcinoma (microscopic or gross residual tumor [n = 53]; margin-negative tumors [n = 50]) treated by EBRT alohe or in conjunction with IOERT.[18] For patients with either microscopic or gross residual disease, local failure occurred in 11% receiving IOERT plus EBRT versus 82% of patients receiving EBRT only ($p = .02$) (see Fig. 47-5). The 5-year actuarial survival rate was 66% for patients with no residual disease, 47% for patients with microscopic residual disease, and 23% for patients with gross residual disease ($p = .0009$) (see Fig. 47-6). The 5-year survival rate in patients with residual disease was 76% for patients receiving IOERT and 26% for patients receiving EBRT alone ($p = .04$) (see Fig. 47-7).

For patients with metastatic disease, 5-FU–based chemotherapy is usually administered. Prospective randomized trials have shown that multiple agents improve survival in patients with metastatic colorectal cancer. Saltz and associates reported the results of a three-arm randomized trial comparing (1) irinotecan, 5-FU, and leucovorin (IFL), (2) 5-FU/leucovorin, or (3) irinotecan alone. Patients receiving IFL had an improved survival (median survival 14.8 months versus 12.6 months, $p = .04$) and response rate (39% versus 21%, $p < .001$) compared to 5-FU and leucovorin alone. The incidence of grade 3 or higher diarrhea was significantly higher with the three-drug regimen.[24] Hurwitz and colleagues reported a randomized trial comparing irinotecan, 5-FU and leucovorin with or without bevacizumab, a monoclonal antibody directed against vascular endothelial growth factor (VEGF). Median survival was significantly improved in the bevacizumab arm (median survival 20.3 months versus 15.6 months, $p < .001$). Additionally, response rates were improved in the bevacizumab-containing arm (45% versus 35%, $p = .004$).[25] Cunningham and associates randomized 329 patients with metastatic colorectal cancer refractory to irinotecan-based chemotherapy regimens to receive cetuximab (a monoclonal antibody directed against the epidermal growth factor receptor [EGFR]) or cetuximab with irinotecan. Response rates in patients receiving combination therapy were significantly higher (23% versus 11%, $p = .007$) as was median time to progression (4.1 versus 1.5 months, $p < .001$). No difference in survival was observed.[26] A study by Goldberg and colleagues randomized 795 patients with previously untreated, metastatic colorectal cancer patients to receive (1) irinotecan, 5-FU, and leucovorin; (2) oxaliplatin, 5-FU, and leucovorin; or (3) irinotecan and oxaliplatin. Patients receiving oxaliplatin, 5-FU, and leucovorin had an improved median survival compared to those receiving irinotecan, 5-FU, and leucovorin or irinotecan and oxaliplatin (19.5 months versus 15 months versus 17.4 months; $p < .05$ for oxaliplatin-containing regimens versus irinotecan-only regimen). Response rates in patients receiving 5-FU, leucovorin, and oxaliplatin were significantly higher than for those receiving irinotecan, 5-FU, and leucovorin or irinotecan with oxaliplatin (45% versus 31% versus 35%, $p < .05$).[27] Varying combinations of these drugs and other novel agents remain the focus of ongoing investigation in both the metastatic and nonmetastatic setting.

Palliative irradiation, sometimes in combination with 5-FU–based chemotherapy, is considered for patients with specific symptoms referable to metastatic disease—brain, bone, and other sites. The combination of radiation therapy and newer agents (capecitabine, irinotecan, oxaliplatin, bevacizumab, cetuximab) remains investigational.

TECHNIQUES OF IRRADIATION

Treatment field design in colon cancer is based on patterns of failure data. As is true in the treatment of rectal carcinoma, great care must be taken in the design of postoperative treatment of adenocarcinoma of the colon. Field arrangement will vary depending on the site of the primary disease as well as areas judged to be at high risk for local recurrence.[28] Patient positioning (supine, prone, decubitus) should be considered in planning. Small bowel is a dose-limiting structure, and it may be advantageous to position patients in the right or left decubitus position for at least a portion of their treatment, allowing displacement of the small bowel away from the treatment field. Immobilization devices may improve reproducibility. A small-bowel series may define small bowel volume within the treatment field. It may be useful to compare films in both the decubitus and supine positions to determine the actual amount of small bowel displacement. CT-based planning may facilitate defining the tumor bed and determining beam orientation, as well as estimating the volume of small bowel included within the treatment fields. As in other abdominal malignancies, a portion of one kidney may be irradiated. Unilateral renal irradiation results in minimal long-term clinical sequelae, assuming baseline function in the contralateral kidney is normal.[29]

The total radiation dose used in the adjuvant treatment of colon carcinoma depends on the amount of suspected residual disease and tolerance constraints of surrounding normal tissue. Generally, an initial dose of 45 Gy in 25 fractions of 1.8 Gy/fraction is delivered through larger fields to the primary tumor or tumor bed and at risk tissues. Reduced fields may be treated to 50 Gy if only a small portion of small bowel is included. For patients with T4 tumors, the general goal is to treat the tumor bed to a total dose of 54 to 60 Gy. Any treatment beyond 50 Gy mandates exclusion of all small bowel from the field. Spinal cord dose should be limited to 45 Gy. In addition, at least two thirds of one functional kidney should receive no more than 18 to 20 Gy and at least two thirds of the total liver volume should not receive more than 30 Gy. In a Mayo Clinic analysis, small bowel obstruction rates were lower when more than two treatment fields were used, and attempts should be made to implement multifield techniques, which may be aided by CT-based planning.[30]

Generally, the primary tumor site should be covered with a 4- to 5-cm margin proximally and distally with 3- to 4-cm margin medially and laterally to cover areas of potential residual disease. The nodal basins in the mesentery beyond surgical margins are usually not treated, as satisfactory margin clearance is obtained in these sites. An exception to this may be right colon tumors where both small bowel and right colon are supplied by ileocolic vessels, limiting the extent of resection. In some instances, treatment of the para-aortic nodes may be indicated, particularly with extensive retroperitoneal involvement by tumor. Treatment of proximal mesenteric nodes may be appropriate if nodes adjacent to the surgical or resection margin are involved. Figures 47-8 to 47-10 show actual and idealized radiation fields for varying colonic sites including cecum and descending colon, as well as sigmoid cancer. In many situations, it may be appropriate to exclude treatment of para-aortic nodal basins, based on operative and pathologic findings.

Because of improved survival seen in patients with rectal cancer treatment with concurrent radiation therapy and 5-FU chemotherapy, as well as survival benefit seen in node-positive colon cancer receiving 5-FU–based chemotherapy, adjuvant irradiation in patients with resected high-risk colon

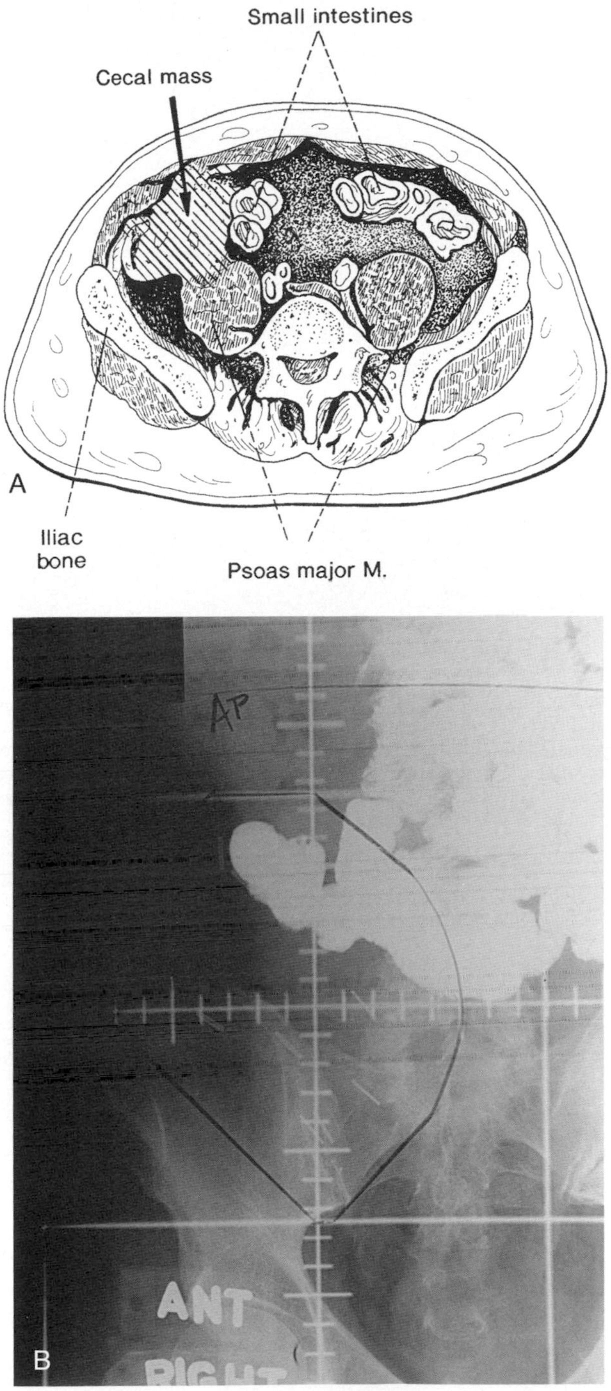

Figure 47-8 **A,** Patient with cecal mass adherent to the psoas muscle, as demonstrated on axial image of the abdomen. **B,** External beam irradiation fields through an anteroposterior-posteroanterior approach

cancer should be administered concurrently with 5-FU–based chemotherapy.

TREATMENT ALGORITHM, CONCLUSIONS, AND FUTURE POSSIBILITIES

Subsets of patients with colon cancer have local recurrence rates similar to patients with rectal cancer if surgery alone is undertaken. Because of encouraging pilot study results with postoperative irradiation with or without 5-FU for patients with resected high-risk colon cancers, and the positive results of 5-FU and levamisole in high-risk adjuvant colon cancer, an Intergroup randomized trial was undertaken, randomizing patients to 5-FU and levamisole or 5-FU and levamisole with tumor bed irradiation in patients at high risk for local recurrence following surgical resection. There was no benefit in survival in patients receiving adjuvant radiation therapy; however, interpretation of these results is handicapped by inadequate accrual and significant flaws that were previously discussed.

The value of adjuvant postoperative irradiation combined with systemic therapy for patients at high risk for local relapse is unlikely to ever be addressed in a definitive randomized trial. Treatment recommendations should be made on a case-by-case basis with existing data in the setting of an informed consent. A potential treatment algorithm for these patients is shown in Table 47-5 and reflects our personal preference.

The use of intraoperative irradiation as a supplement to EBRT in certain T4 tumors (i.e, those with uncertain margins) may also be appropriate. For patients with tumors adherent to or invading adjacent structures, the preferred treatment sequence would be preoperative EBRT plus 5-FU–based chemotherapy followed by resection with or without IOERT and postoperative systemic therapy, based on excellent results in preliminary IOERT reports from both U.S. and European institutions.[18,30-32] A similar approach would be reasonable for patients with locally recurrent cancers or with regional nodal relapse.[30,33-36]

Table 47-5 Treatment Algorithm: Approach to the Therapy of Colon Cancer

1. T1-2 N0*: complete resection.
2. T3 N0*: complete resection with consideration of adjuvant chemotherapy.
3. T4 N0*: complete resection with consideration of adjuvant chemotherapy; consider tumor bed/nodal irradiation with 5-FU–based chemotherapy.
4. T1-3 N+*: complete resection with consideration of adjuvant chemotherapy; for T3 N1 tumors arising in immobile bowel with narrow resection margins, consider tumor bed/nodal irradiation with 5-FU–based chemotherapy.
5. T4 N+*: complete resection followed by adjuvant chemotherapy; consider tumor bed/nodal irradiation with 5-FU–based chemotherapy.
6. Patients with fixed tumors: preoperative irradiation with 5-FU–based chemotherapy followed by resection with intraoperative irradiation (electrons or brachytherapy) and maintenance chemotherapy.
7. Patients undergoing subtotal resection: external beam irradiation with 5-FU–based chemotherapy with intraoperative irradiation (electrons or brachytherapy) and maintenance chemotherapy.

*TNM Stage—assumes M0 extent.

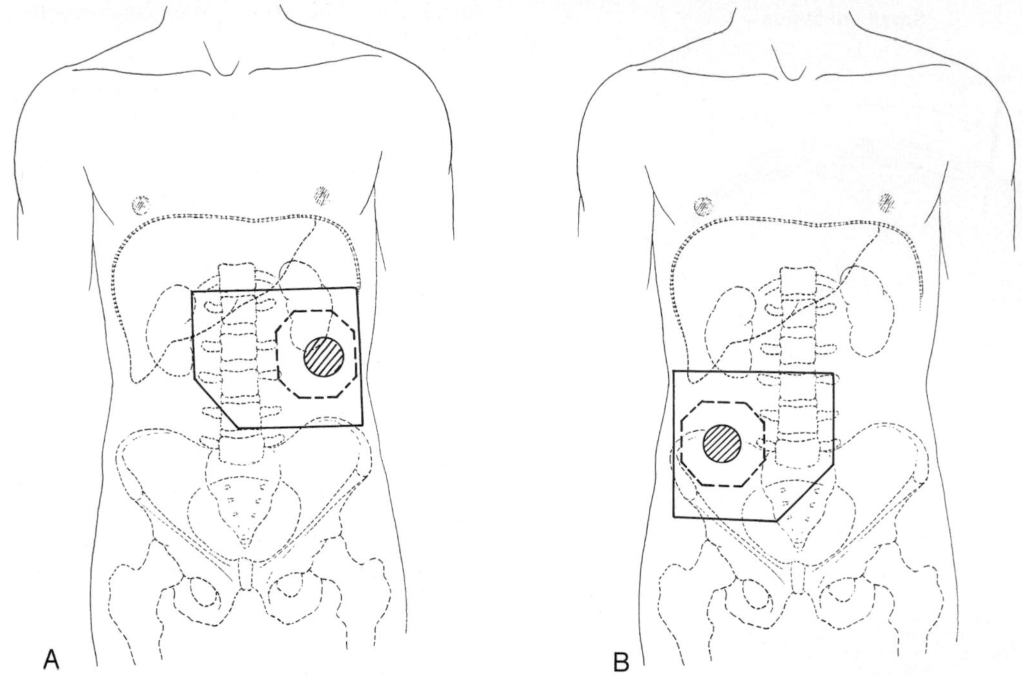

Figure 47-9 Idealized postoperative anteroposterior-posteroanterior irradiation fields of extrapelvic colon cancer (tumor bed and nodal regions). If treated preoperatively, lateral fields could be added based on imaging with CT abdomen and colon radiograph. **A,** Para-aortic nodes are at risk, in addition to tumor bed, due to tumor adherence to posterior abdominal wall with descending colon cancer. **B,** External and common iliac nodes are at risk, in addition to tumor bed, from proximal ascending colon cancer. (From Gunderson LL, Martenson JA, Smalley SR, Garton GR: Lower gastrointestinal cancer: rationale, results, and techniques of treatment. Front Radiat Ther Oncol 28:140-154, 1994; with permission from Karger, Basel.)

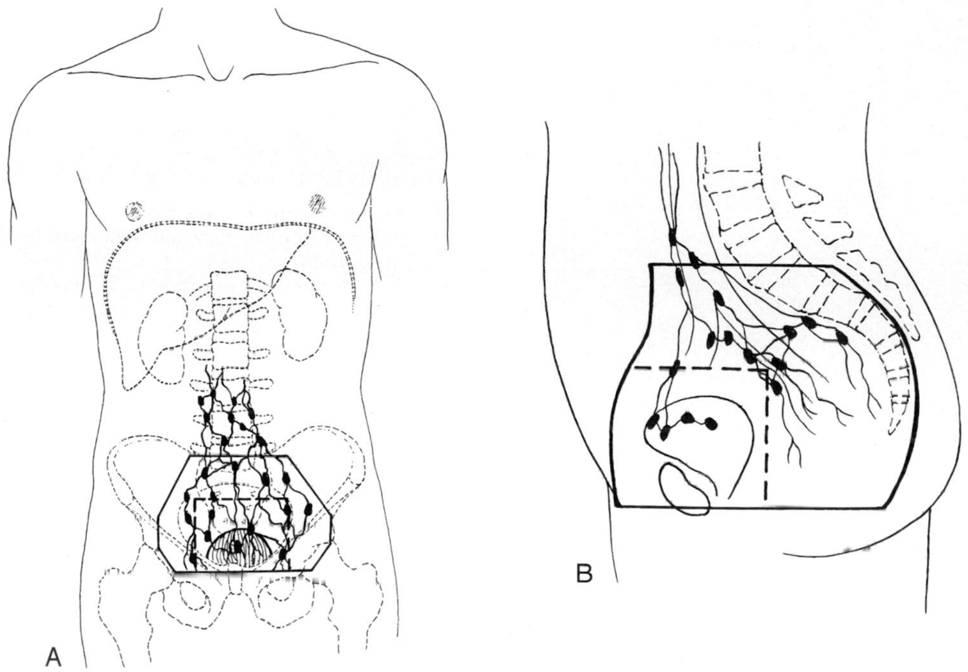

Figure 47-10 Idealized multiple-field preoperative or postoperative irradiation technique for a sigmoid colon cancer adherent to the bladder. Solid lines, large field; interrupted lines, boost field. **A,** Anteroposterior-posteroanterior. **B,** Paired laterals. (From Gunderson LL, Martenson JA, Smalley SR, Garton GR: Lower gastrointestinal cancer: rationale, results, and techniques of treatment. Front Radiat Ther Oncol 28:140-154, 1994; with permission from Karger, Basel.)

REFERENCES

1. Jemal A, Murray T, Ward E, et al: Cancer statistics, 2005. CA Cancer J Clin 55:10-30, 2005.
2. Steele G, Mayer R, Podolsky DK, et al: Cancer of the colon, rectum, and anus. *In* Cancer Manual, 9th ed. American Cancer Society, Massachusetts Division, 1996.
3. Wei EK, Govannucci E, Wu K: Comparison of risk factors for colon and rectal cancer. Int J Cancer 108:433-442, 2004.
4. Michaels KB, Govannucci E, Joshipura KJ, et al: Prospective study of fruit and vegetable consumption and incidence of colon and rectal cancers. J Natl Cancer Inst 92:1740-1752, 2000.
5. Gustin DM, Brenner DE: Chemoprevention of colon cancer: current status and future prospects. Cancer Metastases Rev 21:323-348, 2002.
6. Winawer SJ, Zauber AG, Ho MH, et al: Prevention of colorectal cancer by colonoscopic polypectomy. N Engl J Med 329:1977-1981, 1993.
7. Smith R, Cokkinides V, von Eschenbach A, et al: American Cancer Society guidelines for the early detection of cancer. CA Cancer J Clin 52:8-22, 2002.
8. Smith R, Cokkinides V, Eyre H: American Cancer Society guidelines for the early detection of cancer, 2004. CA Cancer J Clin 54:41-52, 2004.
9. Gryfe R, Kim H, Hsieh E, et al: Tumor microsatellite instability and clinical outcome in young patients with colorectal cancer. N Engl J Med 342:69-77, 2000.
10. Moertel CG, Fleming TR, MacDonald JS, et al: Levamisole and fluorouracil for adjuvant therapy of resected colon carcinoma. N Engl J Med 322:352-358, 1990.
11. O'Connell MJ, Mailliard JA, Kahn MJ, et al: Controlled trial of 5-FU and low-dose leucovorin given for 6 months as postoperative adjuvant therapy for colon cancer. J Clin Oncol 15:246-250, 1997.
12. Twelves C, Worg A, Nowacki M, et al: Capecitabine as adjuvant treatment for stage III colon cancer. N Engl J Med 352:2746-2748, 2005.
13. Andre' T, Boni C, Mounedji-Boudiaf L, et al: Oxaliplatin, fluorouracil and leucovorin as adjuvant treatment for colon cancer. N Engl J Med 350:2343-2351, 2004.
14. Willett CG, Tepper JE, Cohen AM, et al: Failure patterns following curative resection of colonic carcinoma. Ann Surg 200:685-690, 1984.
15. Gunderson LL, Sosin H, Levitt S: Extrapelvic colon—areas of failure in a reoperation series: implications for adjuvant therapy. Int J Radiat Oncol Biol Phys 11:731-741, 1985.
16. Willett C, Fung C, Kaufman D, et al: Postoperative radiation therapy for high-risk colon carcinoma. J Clin Oncol 11:1112-1117, 1993.
17. Amos EH, Mendenhall WM, McCarty PJ, et al: Postoperative radiotherapy for locally advanced colon cancer. Ann Surg Oncol 3:431-436, 1996.
18. Schild SE, Gunderson LL, Haddock MW, et al: The treatment of locally advanced colon cancer. Int J Radiat Oncol Biol Phys 37:51-58, 1997.
19. Willett C, Goldberg S, Shellito P, et al: Does postoperative radiation play a role in the adjuvant therapy of stage T4 colon cancer? Cancer J Sci Am 5:242-247, 1999.
20. Martenson JA, Willett CG, Sargent DJ, et al: A phase III study of adjuvant chemotherapy and radiation therapy compared with chemotherapy alone in the surgical adjuvant treatment of colon cancer: results of Intergroup Protocol 130. J Clin Oncol 22:3271-3283, 2004.
21. Gastrointestinal Tumor Study Group: Adjuvant therapy with hepatic irradiation plus 5-FU in colon carcinoma. Int J Radiat Oncol Biol Phys 21:1151-1156, 1991.
22. Fabian C, Giri S, Estes N, et al: Adjuvant continuous infusion 5-FU, whole abdominal radiation and tumor bed boost in high-risk stage III colon carcinoma: a Southwest Oncology Group Pilot Study. Int J Radiat Oncol Biol Phys 32:457-464, 1995.
23. Estes N, Giri S, Fabian C: Patterns of recurrence for advanced colon cancer modified by whole abdominal radiation and chemotherapy. Am Surg 62:546-550, 1996.
24. Saltz LB, Cox JV, Blanke C, et al: Irinotecan plus fluorouracil and leucovorin for metastatic colorectal cancer. N Engl J Med 343:905-914, 2000.
25. Hurwitz H, Fehrenbacher L, Novotny W, et al: Bevacizumab plus irinotecan, fluorouracil, and leucovorin for metastatic colorectal cancer. N Engl J Med 350:235-242, 2004.
26. Cunningham D, Humblet Y, Siena S, et al: Cetuximab monotherapy and cetuximab plus irinotecan in irinotecan-refractory metastatic colorectal cancer. N Engl J Med 351:337-345, 2004.
27. Goldberg RM, Sargent DJ, Morton RF, et al: A randomized controlled trial of fluorouracil plus leucovorin, irinotecan and oxaliplatin combinations in patients with previously untreated metastatic colorectal cancer. J Clin Oncol 22:23-30, 2004.
28. Gunderson LL, Martenson JA, Smalley SR, et al: Lower gastrointestinal cancer: rationale, results and techniques of treatment. *In* The Lymphatic System and Cancer. Front Radiat Ther Oncol 28:140-154, 1994.
29. Willett CG, Tepper JE, Orlow E, et al: Renal complications secondary to radiation treatment of upper abdominal malignancies. Int J Radiat Oncol Biol Phys 12:1601-1604, 1986.
30. Willett CG, Shellito PC, Tepper JE, et al: Intraoperative electron beam radiation therapy for primary locally advanced rectal and rectosigmoid carcinoma. J Clin Oncol 9:843-849, 1991.
31. Gunderson LL, Nelson H, Martenson J, et al: Locally advanced primary colorectal cancer. Intraoperative electron and external beam irradiation +/− 5-FU. Int J Radiat Oncol Biol Phys 37:601-614, 1997.
32. Rutten H, Klassen R, Martijn H, et al: IOEBRT in the treatment of locally advanced rectal cancer. Fourth International Conference of the International Society of Intraoperative Radiation Therapy. Miami, March 17-19, 2005.
33. Gunderson LL, Nelson H, Martenson J, et al: Intraoperative electron and external beam irradiation with or without 5-FU and maximal surgical resection for previously unirradiated locally recurrent colorectal cancer. Dis Colon Rectum 39:1380-1396, 1996.
34. Haddock MG, Gunderson LL, Nelson H, et al: Intraoperative irradiation for locally recurrent colorectal cancer in previously irradiated patients. Int J Radiat Oncol Biol Phys 49:1267-1274, 2001.
35. Haddock MG, Nelson H, Donahue J, et al: IORT as a component of salvage therapy for colo-rectal cancer patients with advanced nodal metastases. Int J Rad Oncol Biol Phys 56:966-973, 2003.
36. Rutten H, Gosens M, Klassen R, et al: The treatment of locally advanced rectal cancer with intraoperative election beam radiotherapy (IOEBRT). Fourth International Conference of the International Society of Intraoperative Radiation Therapy. Miami, March 17-19, 2005.

CHAPTER 48

RECTAL CANCER

Claus Rödel, Vincenzo Valentini, and Bruce D. Minsky

INCIDENCE

Colorectal cancer is the fourth most common form of cancer worldwide, with an estimated 800,000 new cases diagnosed each year, roughly 10% of all cancers.

In the United States, an estimated 41,930 new cases of rectal cancer were diagnosed in 2006 with 23,580 occurring in men and 18,350 occurring in women.

BIOLOGIC CHARACTERISTICS

The most important prognostic factor for overall survival is the pathologic extent of disease as determined by the degree of bowel wall penetration by the tumor, and the presence or absence of lymph node metastases or distant metastases (TNM stage).

Several biologic markers are now being prospectively evaluated in clinical trials to determine their prognostic utility.

STAGING EVALUATION

The pretreatment evaluation should include a careful history and physical examination. The primary imaging modalities to assess the extent of the primary tumor are endorectal ultrasound (ERUS), computed tomography, and magnetic resonance imaging. ERUS is the most accurate tool in predicting T stage of rectal cancers, and is the investigation of choice in selection of patients for potentially curative local excision (cT1 tumor), and/or for neoadjuvant treatment (cT3-4 tumors).

PRIMARY THERAPY

The primary therapy for potentially curative rectal cancer is surgery. Identification of radial microscopic lymphatic spread within the mesorectum has led to the common use of total mesorectal excision with improvement in local control rates compared with conventional surgery in nonrandomized series.

ADJUVANT THERAPY

There are two conventional adjuvant treatment approaches for clinically resectable rectal cancer—postoperative or preoperative. First is initial surgery, and if the tumor is pT3 and/or N1-2, this is followed by postoperative combined modality therapy.

Second, if the tumor is uT3-4 and/or N+, is preoperative combined modality therapy followed by surgery and postoperative systemic therapy. In the German Rectal Cancer phase III trial, which compared preoperative with postoperative combined modality therapy, patients who received preoperative therapy had a significant decrease in local failure, acute toxicity, chronic toxicity, and significant increase in sphincter preservation in the patients judged by the surgeon pretreatment to require an APR.

LOCALLY ADVANCED DISEASE

Most patients with primary or recurrent unresectable disease should receive preoperative combined modality therapy. Although 50% to 90% will be able to undergo a resection with negative margins, depending on the degree of tumor fixation, 24% to 55% still develop a local recurrence. The addition of intraoperative radiation decreases local recurrence.

Preoperative combined modality therapy regimens with novel chemotherapy regimens have appeared to increase the pathologic complete response rates compared with 5-fluorouracil.

PALLIATION

Pelvic radiation offers effective palliation. In most patients, it decreases pelvic pain and bleeding.

The treatment of rectal carcinoma is as variable as its clinical presentations. For example, it can present as an early tumor suitable for local excision, a locally advanced tumor that requires adjuvant therapy plus radical surgery, one invading an adjacent organ or structure with no evidence of distant metastases, or, last, as a tumor with distant metastases. Radiation therapy has a well-established role in the treatment of rectal cancer and is used in the definitive, adjuvant, neoadjuvant, and palliative settings. Identifying which patients may benefit from preoperative, postoperative, or intraoperative radiotherapy; whether or not to combine radiotherapy with concomitant chemotherapy; and which regimen should be used for the individual patient are questions undergoing active investigation.

ETIOLOGY AND EPIDEMIOLOGY

The etiology of colorectal cancer appears to be multifactorial and includes both environmental factors and a genetic component. Approximately 75% of colorectal cancers are sporadic, and 15% to 20% develop in those with either a positive family history or a personal history of colorectal cancer or polyps.[1,2] The remaining cases occur in people with certain genetic predispositions, such as hereditary nonpolyposis colon cancer (HNPCC) (4% to 7%) or familial adenomatous polyposis (FAP) (1%), or in people with inflammatory bowel disease, particularly chronic ulcerative colitis (1%).

The fundamental role of environmental factors is supported by data in migrant populations. Generally, migrants from low-incident regions in Africa and Asia to the high-incident regions of North America or Australia assume the incidence of the host country within one generation.[3] Specifically, a high-fat, low-fiber diet is implicated in the development of colorectal cancer. Conversely, the ingestion of a high-fiber diet appears to be partially protective against colorectal cancer. Fiber causes the formation of a soft, bulky stool that dilutes out carcinogens; it also decreases colonic transit time, allowing less time for carcinogenic substances to contact the mucosa. Other nutrients such as folate associated with high-fiber diets may be equally, or more, important. The more sedentary lifestyle in Western countries, cigarette smoking, and alcohol consumption also appear to be linked with the risk of colorectal neoplasia.

Most colorectal cancer arises from benign, adenomatous polyps lining the wall of the bowel. Those that grow to a large size (>2 cm) and have villous appearance or contain dysplastic cells are most likely to progress to cancer. This progression from adenoma to carcinoma is associated with an accumulation of genetic alterations, including activation of oncogenes and inactivation of tumor suppressor genes.[1] One of the early steps in this process is the interruption of the APC/β-catenin/TCF-4 pathway allowing unchecked cellular replication at the crypt surface.[4] This can occur in the germline of FAP patients with the second allele being inactivated somatically or in sporadic cancers for which both alleles are somatically inactivated. At least two pathways exist to develop colorectal cancer: chromosomal instability (CIN) and microsatellite instability (MSI).[5] CIN is the genetic reason for tumor formation in about 80% to 85% of colorectal cancer and the mechanism operative in FAP. It is typically coupled with mutations in K-*ras* and *TP53*, ultimately leading to loss of heterozygosity of *TP53* and malignant transformation. MSI is found in greater than 90% of HNPCC that carry a germline inactivation in DNA mismatch repair genes, but also in 15% of sporadic cancer, in which epigenetic hypermethylation silences gene transcription of *hMLH1*. With MSI, multiple frameshift mutations at microsatellite sequences occur, including those in exon coding sequences of the transforming growth factor β receptor II, the proapoptotic gene *BAX*, and DNA mismatch repair genes (*hMSH3* and *hMSH6*). Clinically, tumors with MSI are located more often in the right colon, tend to be diploid, exhibit a mucinous histology with a lymphoid reaction around the tumor, and have a more favorable stage-matched prognosis compared with nonMSI tumors.[6] Of the numerous molecular markers examined to date, MSI,[6,7] 18q,[7] thymidylate synthase,[8] and *TP53* overexpression[9] appear to have the most prognostic impact in colon cancer. Although they are not currently incorporated in the staging system, they should be noted.

Colorectal cancer is the fourth commonest form of cancer worldwide, with an estimated 800,000 new cases diagnosed each year, which accounts for roughly 10% of all cancers.[10] Globally, the colorectal cancer incidence per 100,000 in 1990 was 19.4 for men and 15.3 for women. High incidence rates are found in North America, Western Europe, and Australia (approximately 40 to 45 cases per 100,000 population), and intermediate rates in Eastern Europe (approximately 26 per 100,000), with the lowest rates found in Africa (approximately 3 to 8 per 100,000). Approximately two thirds of cases occur in the colon and one third in the rectum. In the United States, an estimated 41,930 new cases of rectal cancer will be diagnosed in 2006 with 23,580 occurring in men and 18,350 occurring in women.[11] Within the United States, little difference in incidence exists among whites, African Americans, and Asian Americans.

The occurrence of sporadic colorectal cancer increases continuously above the age of 45 to 50 years for both genders and peaks in the seventh decade. Subgroups of patients, including those with inherited syndromes, such as FAP, HNPCC, or hamartomatous polyposis conditions (e.g., Peutz-Jeghers syndrome), can experience colorectal cancer at a much earlier age, as can as patients with inflammatory bowel disease such as chronic ulcerative colitis.[12]

PREVENTION AND EARLY DETECTION

Primary Prevention

Primary prevention involves the identification and elimination of factors that cause or promote colorectal cancer or interfere with the adenoma-to-carcinoma cascade. Dietary and lifestyle approaches use higher fiber/lower fat components and increased physical activity to inhibit the carcinogenic process. Other dietary components, such as selenium, carotenoids, and vitamins A, C, and E, may also have protective effects by scavenging free oxygen radicals. Folic acid, a component of fresh fruits and green vegetables, supplies methyl groups necessary for nucleotide synthesis and gene regulation. Prospective studies generally support an inverse association between folate intake and colorectal cancer risk.[13] Chemopreventive strategies are based on population studies that strongly support an inverse relationship between use of nonsteroidal anti-inflammatory drugs, such as aspirin, sulindac, or selective cyclooxygenase (COX)-2 inhibitors, and the risk of colorectal adenomas or carcinomas.[14] COX-2 is overexpressed in more than 50% of adenomas and 80% to 85% of adenocarcinomas. Not all colorectal tumors follow the classic pattern of carcinogenesis from the polyp to cancer.

Screening for Early Detection

The process of malignant transformation from adenoma to carcinoma generally takes several years. The goal of screening is to prevent rectal cancer mortality through the detection and treatment of benign or premalignant lesions and curable-stage cancer.[15,16] For the average-risk population, screening should begin at age 50 and should follow one of the following five testing options: fecal occult blood testing every year, flexible sigmoidoscopy every 5 years, yearly fecal blood testing and flexible sigmoidoscopy every 5 years, double contrast barium enema every 5 years, and colonoscopy every 10 years. However, if polyps are found, colonoscopy should be performed every year until the patient is polyp free. Some individuals are at increased risk for colorectal cancer. For example, if there is an affected first-degree relative, a family history of FAP or HNPCC, or a personal history of adenomatous polyps, colorectal cancer, or chronic inflammatory bowel disease screening should begin earlier (age 40) and/or, more often than the average-risk group. In some settings such as a personal history of genetic predisposition, it should occur at an even younger age. Two promising but investigational approaches or screening tools include virtual colonoscopy and molecular stool testing.[17,18] The first employs virtual reality technology from cross-sectional CT or MRI scans, the second is based on the molecular detection of neoplasm-specific DNA from exfoliated cancer cells.

BIOLOGIC CHARACTERISTICS AND MOLECULAR BIOLOGY

The most important prognostic factor for overall survival is the pathologic extent of disease as determined by the degree of bowel wall penetration by the tumor and the presence or absence of lymph node metastases or distant metastases (TNM stage).[19] Tumor differentiation is also prognostically important, as poorly differentiated adenocarcinomas associate with lymph node metastases in more than 50% of cases, and also correlate with the likelihood of lymphatic and venous invasion.[20] An elevated carcinoembryonic antigen (CEA) level at the time of presentation has an adverse impact on survival independent of tumor stage.[21] If it is greater than 100, the patient has distant metastasis until proved otherwise. Detection of occult metastases in lymph nodes, blood, or bone marrow by molecular techniques may allow further refinement in pathologic staging. Molecular strategies added to more traditional histopathologic information may help in the future to identify patients in a lower stage whose tumors are likely to behave analogous to higher-stage lesions, and vice versa. Several biologic markers, including allelic loss of 18q, alteration in Kras, MSI, thymidylate synthase, thymidine phosphorylase, vascular endothelial growth factor (VEGF), epidermal growth factor receptor (EGFR), *TP21, TP27, bcl2, bax,* and *TP53,* among others, are being prospectively evaluated in clinical trials to determine their prognostic utility. However at the present time, the TNM staging system is the most reliable.

PATHOLOGY AND PATHWAYS OF SPREAD

Histopathology

The majority (>90%) of colorectal cancers are adenocarcinomas. Some adenocarcinomas have mucin which can be extracellular (colloid) or intracellular (signet ring cell). Colloid cancer, which occurs in 15% to 20% of adenocarcinomas, is not an independent prognostic factor whereas signet ring cell, which occurs in 1% to 2% of adenocarcinomas, is an independent poor prognostic factor for survival.[22,23] Other histologic types are rare and include carcinoid tumors,[24] leiomyosarcomas,[25,26] lymphoma,[27] and squamous cell cancers.[28] The grading system used for adenocarcinomas refers to the degree of differentiation. Some institutions use a three-grade system (well, moderate, poor), and others use a four-grade system. Despite substantial interobserver and intraobserver variability in tumor grading, poorly differentiated tumors have consistently been found to be associated with a worse prognosis in multivariate analysis.

Anatomy and Pathways of Spread

The rectum is approximately 15 cm in length. It is divided into three 5-cm segments in relation to the anal verge (upper third, middle third, and lower third). However, the actual rectal length and division into surgical segments reflect a variety of features such as height, body habitus, pelvic width, and curve of the sacral hollow. For treatment purposes, large bowel cancers that are located at or below the peritoneal reflection (rectosigmoid plus rectum) are collectively defined as rectal cancer. The anorectal ring is at the level of the puborectalis sling and levators, representing the pelvic floor from within the pelvis.

The anterior peritoneal reflection represents the point at which the rectum exits the peritoneal cavity and becomes retroperitoneal (approximately 12 to 15 cm from the anal verge). Below this level there is a mesorectal, or circumferential, resection margin all around the rectum. While distal intramural spread usually extends no more than a few millimeters beyond the grossly recognizable margin of the tumor, microscopic tumor nodules, so-called satellites, are found in the mesorectum predominantly in the radial direction, but also distal, a few centimeters from the lower tumor margin.[29] A layer of visceral fascia encloses both rectum and mesorectum and thus forms a separate compartment within the pelvis. With TME, this entire specimen is removed by sharp dissection. Patients entered in the postoperative U.S. adjuvant rectal trials were required to have tumors with the inferior aspect at or below the peritoneal reflection. For entry on preoperative trials, most use less than 12 cm from the anal verge for eligibility. However, the German trial allowed tumors as high as 16 cm.[30]

The major portion of the lymphatic drainage of the rectum passes along the superior hemorrhoidal arterial trunk toward the inferior mesenteric artery.[31] Only a few lymphatics follow the inferior mesenteric vein. The pararectal nodes above the level of the middle rectal valve drain exclusively along the superior hemorrhoidal lymphatic chain. Below this level (approximately 7 to 8 cm above the anal verge), some lymphatics pass to the lateral rectal pedicle. These lymphatics are associated with nodes along the middle hemorrhoidal artery, obturator fossa, and hypogastric and common iliac arteries. Extensive lymphatics are also present in women contiguous with the rectovaginal septum and in men along Denonvilliers' fascia.

The venous drainage of the upper rectum is to the inferior mesenteric vein via the superior hemorrhoidal and then to the portal system, whereas the lower rectum can, in addition, drain to the internal iliac veins and inferior vena cava. Therefore, either liver or lung metastases or both can occur with rectal cancers.

CLINICAL MANIFESTATIONS, PATIENT EVALUATION, AND STAGING

Clinical Manifestations

Rectal cancer is usually symptomatic prior to diagnosis. Common symptoms include gross red blood (mixed or covering stool, or by itself, sometimes accompanied by the passage of mucus), a change in bowel habits such as unexplained constipation, diarrhea, or reduction in stool caliber. Hemorrhoidal bleeding should always be a diagnosis of exclusion. Obstructing rectal cancers frequently present with diarrhea rather than constipation. In cases of locally advanced rectal cancer with circumferential growth and extensive transmural penetration, urgency, inadequate emptying, and tenesmus are seen. Urinary symptoms and buttock or perineal pain from posterior extension are grave signs. Sciatic pain is indicative of tumor invasion into the sciatic notch, and surgery will likely leave gross disease behind unless preceded by preoperative chemoradiation.

Patient Evaluation

The standard diagnostic algorithm for rectal cancer is seen in Table 48-1. The pretreatment evaluation of a patient with rectal cancer should include a careful history and physical examination. By digital rectal examination (the average finger can reach approximately 8 cm above the dentate line), tumors can be assessed for size, ulceration, and fixation to surrounding structures. This exam also permits evaluation of the patient's sphincter function, which is critical when determining whether a patient is a candidate for a sphincter-sparing procedure. Rigid proctosigmoidoscopy allows direct visualization of the lesion and provides an estimate of the size of the lesion and degree of obstruction. This procedure is used to obtain biopsy samples and gives an accurate measurement of the distance of the lesion from the anal verge. A complete evaluation of the large bowel, preferably by colonoscopy, should be done to rule out synchronous neoplasms.

Table 48-1 Diagnostic Algorithm for Rectal Cancer

History	Including family history of colorectal cancer or polyps
Physical Exam	Including assessment of size, minimum diameter of the lumen, mobility, distance from the anal verge, and cursory evaluation of sphincter function
Proctoscopy	Including assessment of mobility, minimum diameter of the lumen, and distance from the anal verge. Allows biopsy of the primary tumor
Colonoscopy or Barium Enema	To detect possible synchronous neoplasm (colonoscopy preferred)
Endorectal Ultrasound (US)	If considering a local excision or preoperative therapy
Pelvic CT or MRI	To assess the extent of the primary tumor and lymph node involvement (for the accuracy of transrectal ultrasound, CT, MRI for T and N staging see Table 48-2)
Chest X-ray and Abdominal CT	To detect possible metastatic disease
Abdominal MRI and Lung CT	To further investigate suspicious findings of chest X-ray and abdominal CT
CEA	To obtain baseline CEA level (a prognostic factor and important for follow-up)
CBC	Anemia secondary to bleeding

Table 48-2 Accuracy of Pelvic CT, MRI, and Endorectal Ultrasound (ERUS) for T and N Staging

	Accuracy (%)	Sensitivity (%)	Specificity (%)
T STAGE			
CT	73	78	63
ERUS	87	93	78
MRI	82	86	77
MRI with endorectal coil	84	89	79
N STAGE			
CT	66	52	78
ERUS	74	71	76
MRI	74	65	80
MRI with endorectal coil	82	82	83

Modified from Kwok and associates[228] and includes 83 studies from 1980-1998 with 4897 patients.

The primary imaging modalities to assess the extent of the primary tumor are ERUS, CT, and MRI. ERUS is the most accurate tool in predicting T stage of rectal cancers (Fig. 48-1 and Table 48-2). ERUS has been recommended as the investigation of choice in selection of potentially curative local excision as surgical management, which should be restricted to patients with cT1 tumors, as well as in selection of patients with cT3-4 tumors for neoadjuvant treatment.[31] Conversely, patients with cT1-T2 and N0 disease can be identified and selected for an initial surgical approach. This technique can result in understaging as well as overstaging. In the German CAO/ARO/AIO-94 study, 18% of patients in the immediate surgery arm, clinically staged by ERUS to have uT3 and/or N+ disease, had lymph node–negative tumors confined to the rectal wall (pT1-2) on pathologic assessment of the resected specimen.[30] This overstaging is likely due to the inflammatory process caused by the tumor but is also operator dependent. Endorectal coil MRI is an alternative to ERUS but does not appear to be superior to ERUS for T staging.[32]

Because of limited penetration by ERUS, invasion of larger tumors into adjacent organs and pelvic side walls is better evaluated by CT scan and pelvic surface MRI. The involvement of the anal sphincter and levator ani muscles cannot be easily seen on CT scans, whereas high-resolution MRI techniques using phased-array coils have led to better spatial resolution and have been shown to identify the anal sphincter, puborectalis, and particularly the mesorectal fascia. This latter finding is an important feature to predict negative circumferential margins between the tumor and the mesorectal fascia and, consequentially, the risk of local recurrence after TME surgery.[33,34]

The identification of positive lymph nodes is more difficult. Involvement is mainly assessed by size criteria (>1 cm), although enlarged lymph nodes are not pathognomonic of tumor involvement. Nodes less than 5 mm are commonly involved with cancer.[35] The overall accuracy in detecting positive lymph nodes with the above techniques is approximately 60% to 75% (see Table 48-2). The accuracy of MRI is similar to CT; however, it may be further enhanced with the use of superparamagnetic iron oxide particles.[36] Likewise, the accuracy of ERUS for the detection of involved perirectal lymph nodes may be augmented if combined with fine needle aspiration.[37] However, adequate clinical detection of lymph node involvement remains a challenge that is critically important with the increasing use of preoperative treatment strategies.

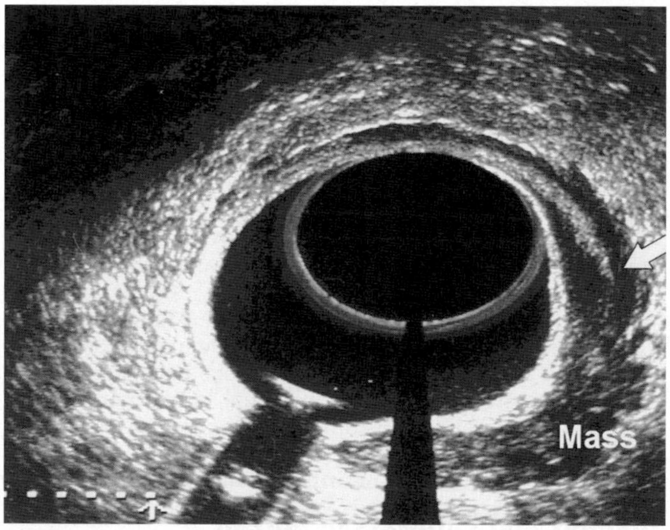

Figure 48-1 ERUS visualizes the rectal wall as alternating hyperechoic and hypoechoic layers of tissue. The first layer is the hyperechoic water-filled balloon or mucosal interface, which is bounded by the hypoechoic mucosa and muscularis mucosa, the hyperechoic submucosa, the hypoechoic muscularis propria, and, finally, the hyperechoic muscularis propria or perirectal fat interface. Depth of penetration is determined by identifying which of these layers is disrupted by the tumor. The figure shows a mass infiltrating beyond the muscularis propria (*thick arrow*) into the perirectal fat (*bright area in the lower part*), indicating a uT3 rectal tumor.

Screening for distant metastatic disease is commonly performed with CT and/or MRI. The major advantage of a positron emission tomography (PET) scan is to differentiate between recurrent tumor and scar tissue by measuring tissue metabolism of an injected glucose-based substance.[38,39] Scar tissue is inactive, whereas tumor generally is hypermetabolic. However, inflammatory masses are commonly positive with PET, which may decrease its utility. At the present time, PET is considered investigational for a routine preoperative metastatic workup.[40]

Staging

The first practical staging system was Dukes' classification.[41] This classified colorectal tumors from A to C, with stage A indicating penetration into but not through the bowel wall, stage B representing penetration through the bowel wall, and stage C representing involvement of lymph nodes, regardless of the extent of bowel wall penetration. However, it has since been modified by many authors, including Dukes, to reflect finer levels of penetration and nodal metastases and has been extended to include the colon as well as the rectum.

The Astler-Coller staging system allowed separation of wall penetration and nodal status. The Gunderson-Sosin modification of the Astler-Coller staging system subdivided T3 tumors into those with microscopic (B2m or C2m) or gross (B2m+g or C2m+g) penetration of tumor through the bowel wall.[42] It also defined tumors adherent to or invading an adjacent organ or structure as B3 if the nodes were negative and C3 if the nodes were positive. Several studies have analyzed both local failure and survival using the modified Astler-Coller staging system.[43] Most have confirmed the predictive capability of this staging system.

In 1988 the American Joint Committee on Cancer (AJCC) and the Union Internationale Contre le Cancer (UICC) proposed a joint TNM staging system. This was based on the fifth edition of the AJCC TNM staging system. The sixth edition of the AJCC TNM staging system is seen in Table 48-3.[44] There are four major changes from the fifth edition:

Table 48-3 AJCC TNM Staging System for Colorectal Cancer

PRIMARY TUMOR (T)

TX	Primary tumor cannot be assessed
T0	No evidence of primary tumor
Tis	Carcinoma in situ: intraepithelial or invasion of the lamina propria [1]
T1	Tumor invades submucosa
T2	Tumor invades muscularis propria
T3	Tumor invades through the muscularis propria into the subserosa, or into nonperitonealized pericolic or perirectal tissues
T4	Tumor is adherent to or directly invades other organs or structures, and/or perforates the visceral peritoneum. [2,3]

REGIONAL LYMPH NODES (N)

NX	Regional nodes cannot be assessed
N0	No regional lymph node metastasis
N1	Metastasis to 1-3 regional lymph nodes
N2	Metastasis to 4 or more regional lymph nodes

DISTANT METASTASIS (M)

MX	Distant metastasis cannot be assessed
M0	No distant metastasis
M1	Distant metastasis

	Stage Groupings*		
Stage	**T**	**N**	**M**
0	Tis	N0	M0
I	T1-2	N0	M0
IIA	T3	N0	M0
IIB	T4	N0	M0
IIIA	T1-2	N1	M0
IIIB	T3-4	N1	M0
IIIC	Tany	N2	M0
IV	Tany	Nany	M1

Prefix†	Reason
m	The presence of multiple primary tumors in a single site and is recorded in parentheses: pT(m)NM
y	When classification is performed during or following initial radiation and/or chemotherapy and is based on the amount of tumor present at the time of the examination, and not an estimate of tumor prior to therapy: ycTNM or ypTNM
r	Indicates recurrent tumor: rTNM
a	Indicates the stage at autopsy: aTNM

Lymphatic Vessel Invasion (L)

LX	Cannot be assessed
L0	No lymphatic vessel invasion
L1	Lymphatic vessel invasion present

Venous Invasion (V)

VX	Cannot be assessed
V0	No venous invasion
V1	Microscopic venous invasion present
V2	Macroscopic venous invasion present

1 = Tis includes cancer cells confined within the glandular basement membrane (intraepithelial) or lamina propria (intramucosal) with no extension through the muscularis mucosa into the submucosa.

2 = Direct invasion in T4 includes invasion of other segments of the colorectum by way of the serosa; for example, invasion of the sigmoid colon by a carcinoma of the cecum.

3 = Tumor that is adherent to other organs or structures, macroscopically, is classified as T4. However, if no tumor is present in the adhesion, microscopically, the classification should be pT3. The V and L substaging should be used to identify the presence or absence of vascular or lymphatic invasion.

*NOTE: A tumor nodule in the pericolonic adipose tissue of a primary carcinoma without histologic evidence of residual lymph node in the nodule is classified in the pN category as a regional lymph node metastasis if the nodule has the form and smooth contour of a lymph node. If the nodule has an irregular contour, it should be classified in the T category and also coded as V1 (microscopic venous invasion) or as V2 (if it was grossly evident), because there is a strong likelihood that it represents venous invasion.

†NOTE: Additional descriptors: Although they do not affect the stage grouping, additional prefixes are used which indicate the need for additional analysis.

From Greene FL, Page DL, Fleming ID, et al (eds): Colon and rectum. *In* AJCC Cancer Staging Manual, 6th ed. New York, Springer, 2002, pp 113-124.

1. A revised description of the anatomy of the colon and rectum that better delineates the data regarding the boundaries between the colon, rectum, and anus. Adenocarcinomas of the veriform appendix are classified with the TNM system but should be recorded separately.
2. Smooth metastatic nodules in the pericolic or perirectal fat are considered nodal metastasis. In contrast, irregularly contoured metastatic nodules in the peritumoral fat are considered vascular invasion and are coded as a subcategory of the T stage as V1 (microscopic vascular invasion) if microscopically visible or V2 (macroscopic vascular invasion) if grossly visible.
3. Stage group II is subdivided into IIA (T3 disease) and IIB (T4 disease).
4. Stage group III is subdivided into IIIA (T1-2 N1 M0 disease), IIIB (T3-4 N1 M0 disease), and IIIC (Tany N2 M0 disease).

The prognostic validity of subdividing stages II and III was supported by both the pooled analysis of Intergroup and NSABP postoperative trials[45] and the retrospective analysis of the American College of Surgeons National Cancer Database (NCDB).[46] The 5-year overall survival by stages IIIA, IIIB, and IIIC in the pooled analysis was 81%, 33% to 61% (T3 N1, 61%; T4 N1, 33%), and 52%, and in the NCDB, it was 55%, 35%, and 25%, respectively. The pooled analysis data suggest that all N2 patients should not be placed in stage IIIC, because 5-year survival for T1-2 N2 patients was 69%, and that for T4 N1 patients would fit better in stage IIIC, with 5-year overall survival of 33%.

There are also additional descriptors that, although they do not affect the stage grouping, do indicate cases needing separate analysis. The AJCC TNM staging system should be used routinely for staging and treatment purposes. Although CEA has prognostic importance, it was not added to the staging system.[19]

Clinical staging is designated as cTNM and is based on physical exam, radiologic imaging, endoscopy, biopsy, and laboratory findings. Pathologic staging is designated as pTNM and depends on data acquired clinically in addition to surgical and pathologic findings. Tumors that have recurred are designated with the r prefix. If there is uncertainty regarding the appropriate T, N, or M staging, the lower (less advanced) category should be used.

The role of the pathologist is critical to proper staging. At least 12 pelvic nodes would preferably be examined in order to obtain the most accurate pN stage.[47]

PRIMARY AND ADJUVANT THERAPY

Adjuvant Radiation Therapy (without Chemotherapy)

There are three general approaches in which radiation therapy alone has been used in the adjuvant treatment of resectable rectal cancer. These include postoperative, preoperative, and preoperative plus postoperative radiation therapy.

Postoperative Radiation

Until 1990, most patients in United States underwent surgery and, if needed, received postoperative radiation therapy. The primary advantage with this approach is pathologic staging. Despite advances in preoperative imaging techniques that allow more accurate patient selection, postoperative therapy remains the most common approach. The primary disadvantages include an increased amount of small bowel in the radiation field,[48] a potentially hypoxic postsurgical bed, and if the patient has undergone an abdominoperineal resection (APR), the radiation field must be extended to include the perineal scar.

Nonrandomized Trials

Nonrandomized data from the Massachusetts General Hospital (MGH)[49] and M. D. Anderson Cancer Center[50] reveal crude local failure rates of 4% to 31% in patients with stage pT3-4 N0 M0 disease and 8% to 53% in patients with stage pT3-4 N1-2 M0 disease who received 45 to 55 Gy. The MGH results of 261 patients who received postoperative radiation therapy reveal 5-year actuarial local control data by stage: pT3 N0 M0, 87%; pT4 N0 M0, 83%; pT1-2 N1-2 M0, 76%; pT3 N1-2 M0, 77%; and pT4 N1-2 M0, 23%.

Randomized Trials

There are five randomized trials examining the use of adjuvant postoperative radiation therapy alone in stages pT3 and/or N1-2 rectal cancer.[51-55] None has shown an improvement in overall survival. The series from Odense University is a two-arm trial comparing postoperative radiation therapy with surgery alone.[51] In one series, one of the arms included radiation plus chemotherapy (gastrointestinal tumor study group [GITSG])[52] or chemotherapy alone (NSABP R-01).[55] In the Mayo Clinic/NCCTG trial 79-47-51, there was no surgery-only control arm.[56] Two reveal a decrease in local failure; NSABP R-01 (16% versus 25%, $P = .06$)[55] and the Medical Research Council (21% versus 34%, $P = .001$).[54]

As discussed in the section on patterns of failure, local failure rates will depend on whether they are reported as first or cumulative failure. The randomized trials usually express failure as first site of failure as opposed to the nonrandomized trials, which express failure as cumulative failure. In the Mayo Clinic/NCCTG trial, the incidence of local failure as the first site of failure in node-positive patients was 25%.[56] More favorable local failure results (local failure as the first site of failure) were reported from the GITSG (18%)[52,57] and the NSABP (15%).[55]

In summary, postoperative radiation therapy decreases local failure. The only randomized trial that confirms this finding (with borderline significance) is from the NSABP. It should be noted that of the randomized trials that compare radiation therapy to a surgical control arm, the NSABP is the only trial in which the radiation therapy was delivered with a continuous course, full doses, and with "modern" techniques.

Preoperative Radiation

There are two approaches to preoperative therapy. The first, used most commonly in Northern Europe, and Scandinavia, is the intensive short course (25 Gy in 5 fractions). In contrast, most other investigators recommend standard course (50.4 Gy in 28 fractions) almost always combined with concurrent systemic chemotherapy. This approach is based on extrapolation of the significant improvement in local control and survival in patients with pT3 and/or N1-2 disease who receive adjuvant postoperative combined modality therapy.[58] The results of this approach are discussed next.

Gerard and colleagues advocate higher doses of radiation without chemotherapy. In their report of the Lyon R96-02 trial, 88 patients with cT2-3 rectal cancer received 39 Gy in 13 fractions to the pelvis and were randomized to observation or a boost with contact radiation to a total dose of 85 Gy.[59] A total of 23 were selected to receive postoperative chemotherapy. Patients who received the boost had a decrease in local failure (2% versus 7%) but no difference in 2-year disease-free survival (DFS) (92% versus 88%).

One clinical situation in which preoperative radiation therapy alone is recommended is when a patient has a distal uT2N0 tumor and refuses an APR. Although APR is the standard therapy, treatment with preoperative radiation followed by LAR and, if the pelvic nodes are positive, postoperative chemotherapy is an alternative. In a series of 26 patients with cT2N0 distal rectal cancer who refused APR, 77% underwent a sphincter-sparing operation.[60] The incidence of 5-year actuarial local failure was 15%, colostomy free, 80%, and overall, 89%. Overall, 75% of those undergoing a sphincter-sparing procedure had good/excellent bowel function.

The primary advantage of this approach is sphincter preservation. However, there are clear disadvantages. First, there is a chance of undertreatment, because approximately 50% of patients are downstaged from ypN+ to ypN0 after preoperative radiation and therefore, will not receive adjuvant chemotherapy. Although pretreatment MRI can help identify patients who may have positive circumferential margins,[33] neither MRI nor any other imaging modality or clinicopathologic factor can identify with a high degree of accuracy those patients with N+ disease. Second, there is the additional toxicity of pelvic radiation, which can adversely affect bowel, bladder, and sexual function.[61-65]

Intensive Short Course Preoperative Radiation

There are 12 modern randomized trials of preoperative radiation therapy (without chemotherapy) for clinically resectable rectal cancer.[66] All use low to moderate doses of radiation. Most of the trials showed a decrease in local recurrence, and in five of the trials, this difference reached statistical significance. Although in some trials a subset analysis revealed a significant improvement in survival, the Swedish Rectal Cancer Trial is the only one that reported a survival advantage for the total treatment group. Two meta-analyses report conflicting results. While both revealed a decrease in local recurrence, the analysis by Camma and associates[67] reported a survival advantage, whereas the analysis by the Colorectal Cancer Collaborative Group[68] did not.

The Swedish Rectal Cancer Trial is the only randomized trial of preoperative radiation therapy to report a significant improvement in survival. Patients with clinically resectable (T1-3) rectal cancer (N = 1168) were randomized to receive 25 Gy in 1 week followed by surgery 1 week later versus surgery alone.[69] Those who received preoperative radiation had a significant decrease in local recurrence (12% versus 27%; $P < .001$) as seen in Table 48-4 and a corresponding significant improvement in 5-year survival (58% versus 48%; $P = .004$), as seen in Table 48-5.

The most recent trial to report results was the Dutch CKVO 95-04 trial, which randomized 1805 patients with clinically resectable (cT1-3) disease to surgery alone (with a TME) or intensive short-course preoperative radiation followed by TME.[70] Although radiation significantly decreased local recurrence (8% versus 2%), there was no difference in 2-year survival (82%). With longer follow-up, 5-year local failure was higher with TME (12%) but significantly decreased to 6% with preoperative radiation.[71]

Even if future trials confirm a survival benefit, there are other equally important endpoints in rectal cancer that need to be addressed. These include acute toxicity, sphincter preservation and function, and quality of life. For example, acute toxicity in the Dutch CKVO 95-04 trial included 10% neurotoxicity, 29% perineal wound complications, and 12% postoperative leaks.[72] In the patients who developed postoperative leaks, 80% required surgery resulting in 11% mortality. A cost-benefit analysis of the Dutch CKVO trial suggested that even if survival is not changed with the addition of preoperative radiation, prevention of a local recurrence reduces long-term health care costs in those countries where it is used.[73]

The presence of a positive circumferential margin is an important negative prognostic sign. In the Dutch CKVO trial, 18% had positive circumferential margins. Although they received 50 Gy postoperatively, this did not compensate for positive margins.[74] Unfortunately, few centers in the United States perform the necessary pathologic examination to detect positive circumferential margins. Data from Beets-Tan and Beets[33] and others[75] suggest that MRI can identify patients who will have positive margins and can be used to better select patients for preoperative therapy.

It is not possible to accurately compare the local control and survival results of intensive short course radiation with conventional preoperative combined modality therapy. This is due to selection bias in favor of the series using short-course radiation. The conventional preoperative combined modality therapy regimens are limited to patients with uT3 and/or N+ disease, whereas most trials that use intensive short course preoperative radiation include patients with cT1-3 disease.

Table 48-4 Phase III Adjuvant Rectal Trials: Relapse with Preoperative or Preoperative Versus Postoperative Treatment

Sequence	Disease Relapse Rates Local Recurrence (%) Surgery	Preoperative	P	Distant Metastasis (%) Surgery	Preoperative	P
PREOPERATIVE (ALL STAGES)						
Rotterdam[249] — T_3, T_4	36	14	.08	45	32	NS
T_2	18	0	NS	26	45	NS
EORTC[250] — Curative	30	15	.003	25	25	.87
Total	35	20	.02	—	—	—
Swedish[69] — Curative	33	9	<.001	24	23	NS
Total	27	11	<.001	—	—	—
PREOPERATIVE VERSUS POSTOPERATIVE (ALL STAGES)						
Swedish (RT alone)[111]	—	13 vs 22 Adv to preop	.02	—	—	—
German (RT + 5-FU)[30]	—	6 vs 13 (5 y) Adv to preop	.006	—	36 vs 38 (5 y)	.84

Preop, preoperative; vs, versus; Adv, advantage.

Table 48-5 Phase III Adjuvant Rectal Trials: Survival with Preoperative and Postoperative Treatment

Sequence	Actuarial Survival Advantage Seen	Disease-free % (P value)	Overall % (P value)
PREOPERATIVE (ALL STAGES)			
Rotterdam[249] T_3, T_4	Preop RT vs surgery alone	Not given	50 vs 18 (.001)
T_2	None	Not given	62 vs 70 (NS)
EORTC[250] — Curative	Preop RT vs surgery alone	Not given	69 vs 59 (.08)
Total	None	56 vs 51 (.54)	52 vs 49 (.69)
Swedish[69] — Total	Preop RT vs surgery alone	—	58 vs 48 (.004)
PREOPERATIVE VERSUS POSTOPERATIVE (ALL STAGES)			
Swedish (RT alone)[111]	Preop = postop	Not given for total group	43 vs 37 (.43)
German (RT + chemo)[30]	Preop = postop	68 vs 65% (.32)	76 vs 74 (.8)
POSTOPERATIVE (5-Y ACTUARIAL DATA AND 2-TAILED *P* VALUES UNLESS OTHERWISE SPECIFIED)			
GITSG 7175[52]	ChemoRT vs surgery	70 vs 46 (.009)	58 vs 45 (.005, 1-tail)
NSABP R01[55]	Chemo vs surgery	41 vs 30 (.006)	53 vs 43 (.05)
Norwegian	RT/5-FU vs surgery	64 vs 46 (.01)	64 vs 50 (.05)
NCCTG/Mayo 794751[56]	Chemo/RT vs RT	59 vs 37 (.002)	58 vs 48 (.025)**
GITSG 7180[57] (3-y data)	RT/5-FU ± MeCCNU	68 vs 54 (.20)	75 vs 66 (.58)
NCCTG 864751[81] (4-y data)	RT/PVI 5-FU vs RT/bolus 5-FU	63 vs 53 (.01)	70 vs 60 (.005)
NSABP R02	ChemoRT vs Chemo No difference	~55% (.90) Estimate from figure	~ 65% (.89) Estimate from figure
U.S. GI Intergroup 0114[83]	RT/bolus 5-FU vs RT/5-FULV or 5-FULev No difference	54	64
Seoul, Korea[80] (4-y data)	ChemoRT– Chemo vs Chemo–ChemoRT	81 vs 70 (.04)	84 vs 82 (.387)
U.S. GI Intergroup 0144[82]	No difference	—	—

Chemo, chemotherapy; Chemo/RT, concurrent radiochemotherapy; 5-FU, 5-fluorouracil; Lev, levamisole; LV, leucovorin; preop, preoperative; postop, postoperative; RT, external beam irradiation; vs versus.

Preoperative plus Postoperative Radiation

This approach, also known as the "sandwich technique," includes a short preoperative course of radiation (5 to 15 Gy), followed by surgery, and in patients with pT3-4N1-2 disease, an additional 40 to 45 Gy postoperatively. This approach was developed in an era when imaging was inadequate to determine accurate preoperative extent of T and N disease. Accordingly, it was designed to combine the theoretical advantages of low dose preoperative radiation therapy (decreased tumor seeding) while reserving postoperative radiation therapy for those patients with pT3 and/or N1-2 disease. The results of this approach have been reported by a number of investigators.[76-78]

The Radiation Therapy Oncology Group (RTOG) presented the results of a randomized trial of 350 patients (87% with rectal cancer) who were randomized to 5 Gy preoperative versus surgery alone (RTOG 81-15).[78] Patients with stage pT3 and/or N1-2 disease received a minimum of 45 Gy postoperatively. No chemotherapy was delivered. With a minimum follow-up of 5 years, there were no differences in local failure, distant failure, or overall survival between the arms. A retrospective analysis of 155 patients treated at the Institut Gustave Roussy also revealed no advantage of the "sandwich technique" compared with preoperative radiation.[77] Since the benefits of preoperative therapy including downstaging and sphincter preservation require standard dose rather than low to intermediate doses of radiation, the RTOG randomized trial was negative, and improved preoperative imaging techniques have markedly improved selection criteria for patients who may benefit from preoperative adjuvant treatment, the "sandwich technique" should be abandoned.

Adjuvant Combined Modality Therapy

There are two conventional treatment approaches for clinically resectable rectal cancer. The first approach is initial surgery followed by postoperative combined modality therapy if the tumor is pT3 and/or N1-2.[58] The second is preoperative combined modality therapy followed by surgery if the tumor is uT3-4 and/or N+, and postoperative chemotherapy.[66]

Postoperative Therapy

The NCI Consensus Conference concluded in 1990 that combined modality therapy was the standard postoperative adjuvant treatment for patients with pT3 and/or N1-2 disease.[58] This recommendation was based on phase III trials that compared postoperative chemoradiation arms with control arms of either surgery alone (GITSG 7175)[52] or surgery plus postoperative radiation (Mayo/NCCTG 79-47-51)[56] and demonstrated improvements in both disease-free and overall survival (see Table 48-5).

The standard design in U.S. trials, to date, has been to deliver six cycles of chemotherapy with concurrent radiation during cycles 3 and 4. Although a randomized trial from South Korea reported by Lee and colleagues suggested that radiation should start with cycle 1 rather than cycle 3, optimal sequencing of postoperative combined modality therapy has not been tested in other countries.[80] In this trial of 303 patients, all patients had a TME resection and were to receive eight cycles of 5-fluorouracil (5-FU)/leucovorin (LV) at 4-week intervals plus 45 Gy in 25 fractions over 5 weeks. For patients randomized to start radiation and chemotherapy simultaneously, DFS was improved compared with patients who received two cycles of chemotherapy before starting concurrent chemoradiation (4-year DFS of 81% versus 70%, *P* = .04) (see Table 48-5). Although an interesting result, in view of the small size of the trial, and because a number of patients did not receive the treatment arm to which they were randomized, further data are needed before recommending a change in sequence.

The Intergroup (INT) 86-47-51 trial, coordinated by NCCTG, did not demonstrate an incremental benefit to MeCCNU when added to postoperative radiation plus concurrent and maintenance 5-FU. However, a 2 × 2 component of the study demonstrated a positive benefit for giving protracted venous infusion (PVI) 5-FU rather than interrupted bolus 5-FU concurrent with pelvic radiation. Patients randomized to receive PVI 5-FU (225 $mg/m^2/d$; 7 d/week or until intolerance) had improvements in disease control, DFS (4-year, 63% versus 53%, *P* = .01) and overall survival (4-year, 70% versus 60%; *P* = .005) (see Table 48-5).[81]

Before the positive results of 86-47-51 were available, the INT 0114 trial was developed to test four different arms of systemic bolus chemotherapy. All patients received concurrent chemoradiation with either bolus 5-FU alone or in combination with leucovorin. The trial had such rapid accrual that the trial was completed before the advantage of PVI 5-FU compared with bolus 5-FU alone had been demonstrated.

The INT 0114 4-arm trial randomized patients with pT3 and or N+ rectal cancer to postoperative radiation (RT) and bolus 5-FU with or without leucovorin, levamisole, or leucovorin plus levamisole. There was no significant difference in local control or survival among the four arms.[83] With longer follow-up, the study also revealed that local control and survival results continue to decrease after 5 years. With a median follow-up of 7.4 years, the 7-year local failure rate was 17% and the survival was 56% compared with 14% and 64%, respectively, at 5 years. Patients with high-risk (pT3N+ or T4) disease had a lower survival compared with those with lower-risk (pT1-2N+ or T3N0) disease (45% versus 70%). Further analysis of the INT 0114 trial has revealed that body mass is related to outcome and treatment-related toxicity[84] and both surgeons and hospitals with higher volumes of rectal cancer surgery have improved outcomes compared with those with lower volumes.[85]

The INT 0114 postoperative adjuvant rectal trial was designed to follow up on the positive results achieved with concurrent PVI 5-FU during radiation in trial 86-47-51.[82] Patients were randomized to three arms: arm 1 = bolus 5-FU—PVI 5-FU/RT—bolus 5-FU (the control arm from 86-47-51); arm 2 = PVI 5-FU—PVI 5-FU/RT—PVI 5-FU; and arm 3 = bolus 5-FU/LV/levamisole—bolus 5-FU/LV/levamisole/RT—bolus 5-FU/LV/levamisole. The lowest incidence of grade 3+ hematologic toxicity was seen in arm 2 (4%); however, there was no significant difference in local control or survival. Given these results, we recommend PVI 5-FU with radiation and either arm 1 or 2 is a reasonable choice. If arm 1 is chosen, we recommend the bolus chemotherapy segment should be the Roswell Park (weekly) rather than the Mayo Clinic regimen (monthly) given its more manageable acute toxicity profile.

Associated with the improvement in local control and survival with postoperative combined modality therapy is an increase in acute toxicity. For example, the incidence of grade 3+ toxicity in the combined modality arms of the GITSG 7175 and Mayo/NCCTG 79-47-51 trials was 25% to 50%. Furthermore, the percentages of patients finishing the prescribed six cycles of chemotherapy in those trials were only 65% and 50%, respectively.

Are There Patients Who Do Not Require Postoperative Adjuvant Therapy?

Although the 1990 NCI Consensus Conference recommended combined modality therapy for patients with pT3 and/or N1-2 disease,[58] retrospective data suggest that there may be a subset of patients with pT3N0 disease who may not require adjuvant therapy. Reports from the MGH[90] and Memorial Sloan-Kettering[91] have identified favorable subsets of patients with pT3N0 disease who, following surgery alone, had a 10-year actuarial local recurrence rate of less than 10%.

Data also exist from the Pooled Rectal Analysis, discussed previously, with regard to a more favorable prognosis for patients with T1-2N1 and T3N0 tumors.[45] In the pooled analysis of three phase III U.S. INT trials and two phase III NSABP trials, disease control and survival were analyzed as a function of stage. Radiation plus chemotherapy did not improve the overall survival achieved with chemotherapy alone in patients with stages pT3N0, T1-2N1 disease (5-year survival of 85% and 84% with surgery plus chemotherapy). However, for patients with T3N0 lesions, DFS was 69% with surgery plus chemotherapy and local failure was 11% (initial pattern of relapse).

Additional local control data are needed before recommending chemotherapy alone for this subset of patients. If the local control rates without radiation are acceptable, then patients with upper rectal cancers who undergo a total mesorectal excision, have at least 12 nodes examined, and have stage pT3N0 disease with an adequate radial resection margin likely do not need RT. The 4% to 5% benefit in local control with postoperative radiation may not be worth the risks, especially in women of reproductive age.

Preoperative Therapy

Preoperative therapy (most commonly combined modality therapy) has gained acceptance as a standard adjuvant therapy. The potential advantages of the preoperative approach include decreased tumor seeding, less acute toxicity, increased radiosensitivity due to more oxygenated cells, and enhanced sphincter preservation.[66] The primary disadvantage of preoperative radiation therapy is possibly overtreating patients with either early stage (pT1-2N0) or undetected metastatic disease. In the German CAO/ARO/AIO 94 trial, which used CT and transrectal ultrasound, 18% of patients were overstaged.[30]

Is Chemotherapy Necessary with Preoperative Radiation?

One retrospective[87] and two randomized[88,89] trials examine the question of whether chemotherapy improves the results of preoperative radiation in patients with cT3 rectal cancer. The EORTC 22921 is a four-arm randomized trial of preoperative 45 Gy with or without concurrent bolus 5-FU/leucovorin followed by surgery with or without 4 cycles of postoperative 5-FU/leucovorin.[88] The FFCD 9203 is a two-arm randomized trial also randomizing patients to preoperative 45 Gy with or without bolus 5-FU/leucovorin.[89] However, all patients received postoperative chemotherapy. Preliminary results of the EORTC trial reveal a significant increase in the rate of ypT0 (14% versus 5%, *P* = .0001) and ypN0 (27% versus 21%, *P* = .03) in those patients who receive radiation with concurrent chemotherapy versus preoperative radiation alone. A similar improvement in the pathologic complete response (pCR) rate was reported in the FFCD 9203 trial (10% versus 3%, *P* = .0005) but with an associated increase in grade 3+ toxicity (14% versus 2%, *P* = .00001). Local control and survival results are pending. Until the final results of these trials are available, radiation plus concurrent chemotherapy should remain the standard.

Sphincter Preservation with Preoperative Radiation

A major goal of preoperative therapy is sphincter preservation. From the viewpoint of sphincter preservation, the advantage of preoperative therapy is to decrease the volume of the primary tumor. When the tumor is located in close proximity to the dentate line, this decrease in tumor volume may allow the surgeon to perform a sphincter-conserving procedure that would not otherwise be possible. However, if the tumor directly invades the anal sphincter, sphincter preservation is unlikely even when a complete response is achieved.

One of the most important controversies with preoperative therapy is whether the degree of downstaging is adequate to enhance sphincter preservation. Furthermore, if preoperative RT is effective, what regimen (intensive short course versus conventional course) is preferred?

An analysis of 1316 patients treated in 2 previously published Scandinavian trials of intensive short course of radiation revealed that downstaging was most pronounced when the interval between the completion of radiation and surgery was at least 10 days.[92] In the Dutch CKVO 95-04 trial, where the interval was 1 week, there was no downstaging.[93] None of the other randomized trials of intensive short-course preoperative radiation addresses the issue of sphincter preservation and it is not an end point of the trials.

When the goal of preoperative therapy is sphincter preservation, conventional doses and techniques of radiation are recommended. These include multiple field techniques to a total dose of 45 to 50.4 Gy at 1.8 Gy/fraction. Surgery should be performed 4 to 7 weeks following the completion of radiation. Unlike the intensive short course of radiation regimen, this conventional design allows for two important events to occur. First is the recovery from the acute side effects of radiation and second is adequate time for tumor downstaging. Data from the Lyon R90-01 trial of preoperative radiation suggest that an interval of longer than 2 weeks following the completion of radiation increases the chance of downstaging.[94] Whether increasing the interval between the end of intensive short-course radiation and surgery to longer than 4 weeks will increase downstaging is not known. This question is being addressed in the ongoing Stockholm III trial.

Preoperative Prospective Clinical Assessment

The most accurate method by which to determine if preoperative therapy increases sphincter preservation is to perform a prospective clinical assessment. In this setting, the operating surgeon examines the patient prior to the start of preoperative therapy and declares the type of operation required. It should be noted that this assessment is based on an office examination and may not accurately reflect the assessment when the patient is relaxed under general anesthesia. The only method by which to account for this potential bias is to perform a randomized trial of preoperative versus postoperative therapy. The German CAO/ARO/AIO 94 randomized trial of preoperative versus postoperative combined modality therapy, which was stratified by surgeon, reported that this assessment is accurate in 80% of patients.

Clinical Experience with Sphincter Preservation

There are eight nonrandomized trials that have reported results in patients with clinically resectable rectal cancer who underwent a prospective clinical assessment by their surgeon prior to the start of preoperative therapy and were declared to need an APR. All used conventional doses and techniques of RT. Three used RT alone[60,94,95] and five used combined modality therapy.[30,96-99] The incidence of sphincter preservation was only 23% in the NSABP R-03 series[100] and 44% in the Lyon series.[94] In the remaining six series, it was approximately 70%.

A valid concern of surgeons is that in order to perform sphincter preservation in those patients who would otherwise require an APR, the distal resection margin may be suboptimal (<1 cm). Can preoperative therapy compensate for this? Retrospective data from Moore and associates reveal that with preoperative combined modality therapy, the 3-year local control rates were similar regardless of the margins being >2 cm, <2 cm, >1 cm, or <1 cm, providing they were negative.[101] Similar data have been reported from Kuvshinoff and colleagues.[98]

Sphincter preservation without good function is of questionable benefit. In a series of 73 patients who underwent surgery, Grumann and associates[102] reported that the 23 patients who underwent an APR had a more favorable quality of life compared with the 50 who underwent a low anterior resection.

Although preoperative combined modality therapy may adversely affect sphincter function,[63] the impact is most likely less than postoperative combined modality therapy.[103] In the four of eight preoperative series discussed earlier that report functional outcome, the majority (approximately 75%) have good to excellent sphincter outcome. Functional results continue to improve up to 1 year after surgery. Functional data from the German trial are pending. With careful techniques, it should not increase postoperative complications.[104]

In one series, the value of radical surgery in patients with T1-3 disease who had a biopsy-proven complete response was questioned.[105] In series limited to patients with cT3 disease who received preoperative therapy, radical surgery is still necessary to fully evaluate if a pathologic response has been achieved. Neither posttreatment ERUS[106,107] or physical exam (which is only 25% accurate)[108] is adequate. The use of PET scan[109,110] and diffusion MRI[75] as noninvasive measures of response is being investigated.

Preoperative Combined Modality Programs with Novel Agents

Chemotherapeutic agents such as capecitabine,[114] oxaliplatin,[115] and irinotecan,[116] as well as targeted therapies, such as bevacizumab[117] and cetuximab,[118] which have improved results of patients treated in the adjuvant and/or metastatic setting, are currently incorporated into phase I/II combined modality programs. Selected agents include UFT,[119] Tomudex,[120] oxaliplatin,[121-124] CPT-11,[125,126] Iressa,[128] bevacizumab,[129] and capecitabine[127,130] with pelvic RT. All suggest higher pCR rates compared with PVI 5-FU (Table 48-6). However, for some agents, with this increased pCR rate is an associated increase in acute toxicity. Phase III trials are needed to determine if these regimens offer an advantage compared with 5-FU–based combined modality therapy regimens.

Predicting the Response of the Primary Tumor

Although some series show no correlation,[131,132] most series suggest that there is improved outcome with increasing pathologic response to preoperative therapy.[108,133-138] Analysis of biopsies examining selected molecular markers such as *c-K-ras*,[139] thymidylate synthase,[140] p27kip1,[141] *p53*,[142] apoptosis,[143] DCC,[142] EGFR,[144,145] *p53*,[146] and Ki-67[147] have had varying success in helping to select patients who may best respond to preoperative therapy. Since all of the studies are limited retrospective trials and most do not examine multiple markers, the need for adjuvant therapy should still be based solely on

Table 48-6 **Selected Preoperative Combined Modality Therapy Using Novel Chemotherapeutic Agents**

Trial	Agents	% pCR	% Grade 3+ Toxicity
Sauer (German Trial)[30]	CI 5-FU	8*	27
Mehta[99]	FOLFIRI	37	21-28
Mitchell[229]		24	—
Mohiuddin (RTOG 0012)[126]		28	55
De Paoli[130]	Capecitabine	24	11
GERCOR[127]		24	10
Roedel[123]	CAPOX	19	8
SOCRATES[122]		31	22
Aschele[230]	FOLFOX	29	13
CALGB C89901[121]		25	

*CI 5-FU limited to weeks 1 and 5 of radiation.

T and N stage. Fortunately, the new intergroup rectal trials will prospectively collect tissues for these and other markers. In the future, molecular markers may help predict patients with lymph node–positive disease.

Preoperative Versus Postoperative Radiation with or without Chemotherapy

Four randomized trials of preoperative versus postoperative therapy for clinically resectable rectal cancer have been performed. The Uppsala trial used intensive short course radiation (5.5 Gy times 5) versus 60 Gy postoperatively with conventional fractionation.[111] The preoperative arm revealed a significant decrease in local failure (13% versus 22%); however, no difference in survival (43% vs 37%). The other three randomized trials were limited to patients with T3-4 disease, used conventional doses and techniques of RT and concurrent 5-FU–based chemotherapy and required a preoperative clinical assessment declaring the type of operation required. Two are from the United States (INT 0147, NSABP R0-3) and one is from Germany (CAO/ARO/AIO 94). Unfortunately, low accrual resulted in early closure of both the NSABP R-03 and INT 0147 trials. The NSABP R-03 trial was designed to accrue 900 patients and accrued less than 300. In a preliminary report, the 123 patients in the preoperative arm had an improved 3-year survival (85% versus 78%) and decreased local failure (9% versus 5%) compared with the 130 patients in the postoperative arm (P = NS).[112]

The German trial completed the planned accrual of over 800 patients and randomized patients with uT3-4 and/or N+ rectal cancers less than 16 cm from the anal verge to conventional preoperative combined modality therapy (50.4 Gy in 28 fractions plus concurrent PVI 5-FU) versus postoperative combined modality therapy.[30] The PVI chemotherapy was delivered during weeks 1 and 5 of the radiation and the remaining four cycles of chemotherapy were bolus 5-FU/leucovorin. In order to help remove surgical bias, patients were stratified by surgeon. Compared with postoperative combined modality therapy, patients who received preoperative therapy had a significant decrease in local failure (6% vs 13%, P = .006) (see Table 48-4), acute toxicity (27% versus 40%, P = .001), chronic toxicity (14% versus 24%, P = .012), and, in those 194 patients judged by the surgeon pretreatment to require an APR, a significant increase in sphincter preservation (39% versus 20%, P = .004). With a median follow-up of 40 months there was no difference in 5-year survival (76% versus 74%) (see Table 48-5).

Given the improved local control, acute and long-term toxicity profile, and sphincter preservation reported in the German trial, patients with cT3 rectal cancer who require combined modality therapy should receive it preoperatively. In the German trial, 18% of patients who were clinically staged as uT3-4 and/or N+ preoperatively and underwent surgery without preoperative therapy had pT1-2N0 disease. Therefore, those patients would have been overtreated if they had received preoperative therapy. Although pretreatment MRI can help predict patients who may have positive circumferential margins,[33] neither MRI nor any other imaging modality or clinicopathologic factor can accurately identify patients with N+ disease.[34] Given that the INT pooled analysis[45] and the NCDB[46] suggest that some patients with node-negative disease may not require radiation, the development of more accurate imaging techniques and molecular markers to identify N+ disease are necessary.

Short-Course Preoperative Radiation Therapy Versus Conventional Preoperative Chemoradiation

Bujko and colleagues[113] from Warsaw preformed a randomized trial of two preoperative approaches. A total of 316 patients with cT3 rectal cancer were randomized to 5 Gy times 5 followed by surgery (median, 8 days) versus conventional preoperative combined modality therapy (50.4 Gy plus bolus 5-FU/leucovorin daily times 5, weeks 1 and 5) followed by surgery (median, 78 days). All tumors were above the anorectal ring, TME was performed for distal tumors, and there was no radiation quality control review. Local control and survival results were not reported.

Similar to the German CAO/ARO/AIO 94 trial, patients underwent a pretreatment clinical assessment by the operating surgeon. In the subset of patients who were thought to require an APR, sphincter preservation was achieved in 21% who received combined modality therapy and 26% in those who received short-course radiation. Although the pCR rate was 16% in patients who received combined modality therapy versus 1% for those who received the short course of radiation, this did not change the overall sphincter preservation rate (58% versus 61%, respectively). The authors emphasized that since the pCR rate was higher in the combined modality therapy arm, the absence of difference in sphincter preservation was likely related to a lack of the surgeon's commitment to the concept of sphincter preservation. Since modification of the surgical approach following preoperative therapy is contrary to traditional surgical oncologic principles, sphincter-preserving surgery in a patient who would normally require an APR requires a surgeon who is comfortable with this change. The German trial controlled for this bias since the randomization was stratified by surgeon.

Alternative Methods for Sphincter Preservation

Early localized tumors (3% to 5% of rectal cancers) include small, exophytic, mobile tumors without adverse pathologic factors (i.e., high grade, blood vessel invasion, lymphatic vessel invasion, colloid histology, or the penetration of tumor into or through the bowel wall) and are adequately treated with a variety of local therapies such as local excision or endocavitary radiation.

Endocavitary Radiation

Most investigators have used intracavitary irradiation alone[148-150] for early, noninvasive tumors. For more advanced tumors (cT2-3 and/or N+), it is generally combined with a temporary iridium-192 implant and/or external beam radiation.[59,151-153]

The technique of endocavitary radiation was introduced by Papillion and colleagues in Lyon, France. Prior to delivery, the anus is dilated and a 3-cm proctoscope is introduced. A low-energy x-ray unit is placed through the scope almost against the tumor. Generally, 50-kV x-rays, in doses of 30 Gy per treatment, are given using this "contact" approach. Three or four such treatments over 1 month are required. Bulky tumors may require additional irradiation with an iridium-192 implant or external beam to reach the deeper pararectal tissues. In an update of the Lyon experience expanded to 101 patients, the local failure rate was 15% and the 5-year survival was 81%.[156] In 22 patients who were stage T1 N0 by rectal ultrasound, none developed local failure.

Other institutions have reported similar results with endocavitary radiation alone. Using this technique, Hull and associates reported a 71% DFS rate in 126 patients.[154] With a median follow-up of 55 months, 10% local failure and 76% 5-year survival were reported in an initial analysis of Mayo Clinic experience. In a subsequent update, 29 patients had been treated with curative intent at Mayo Clinic with a total dose of up to 155 Gy in 1 to 5 fractions. Local control was 76% at 10 years; survival was 65% at 5 years and 42% at 10 years.[148] Maingon and colleagues treated 151 patients with this approach; the incidence of initial local control and ultimate local control by stage was T1, 78% and 87%; T2, 58% and 79%; and T3, 54% and 69%, respectively.[155]

Some institutions have chosen to combine endocavitary radiation with external beam radiation. At Washington University, patients received pelvic radiation (20 Gy in 5 fractions for those with cT1 disease and the remainder received 45 Gy in 25 fractions) followed 6 to 7 weeks later by two endocavitary treatments of 30 Gy each.[153] Results by stage were uT1, 100% DFS; uT2, 85% local control; uT3 (who were not optimal candidates for surgery) or tethered uT2, 56% local control (67% after salvage surgery). Aumock and associates also added external beam for cT2-3 tumors and reported local control rates of T1, 100%; mobile T2, 85%; and T3 or tethered T2, 56%.[152]

Most institutions do not have the 50-Kvp radiation machine required for this technique. Accordingly, there are limited centers that continue to treat patients with contact radiation.

Local Excision and Radiation Therapy

Local excision has been performed in combination with both preradiation and postradiation therapy. The advantage of performing a local excision prior to radiation is that pathologic details such as margins, depth of bowel wall penetration, and histologic features can be well characterized. Patients with pT1 tumors without adverse pathologic factors have a low enough incidence of local failure (5% to 10%) and positive nodes (<10%) that they do not require adjuvant therapy. However, once adverse pathologic factors are present (high grade, vascular invasion, or signet ring cells) or the tumor invades into or through the muscularis propria, the local failure rate is at least 17%, and the incidence of positive mesorectal and/or pelvic nodes is at least 10% to 15%.[157]

There are a variety of surgical approaches including transanal local excision, posterior proctotomy, and transsphincteric excision. Transanal endoscopy microsurgery (TEM) has emerged as another option for local treatment of rectal cancer.[158] Regardless of the technique the excision should be full thickness and nonfragmented and have negative margins.[159]

Local Excision Followed by Postoperative Therapy

A number of phase I/II trials have been reported. When the series are combined, the average crude local failure rate increases with T stage: pT1: 5%, pT2: 14%, and pT3:22% (Table 48-7).[160-170] However, in the series with more than 4-year follow-up (MGH,[164] Memorial Sloan-Kettering,[168] CALGB 8984,[232] Princess Margaret,[170] and RTOG 89-02[167]), the incidence of local failure for pT2 disease is 14% to 24%. Therefore, patients who are treated with local excision and postoperative adjuvant therapy require close follow-up beyond 5 years.

The few series that measure sphincter function after this combination therapy report favorable outcomes. All patients should receive 5-FU–based therapy concurrently with radiation. For patients with pT2-3 disease where the incidence of pelvic lymph nodes is at least 20%, an additional four cycles of adjuvant chemotherapy for a total of six cycles is recommended. Salvage of local failures is possible with most series reporting that at least half of the patients who undergo a salvage APR can be cured. pT3 tumors have a 25% local failure rate and are treated more effectively with radical surgery and preoperative or postoperative combined modality therapy.

Preoperative Therapy Followed by Local Excision

The experience with preoperative radiation plus 5-FU–based concomitant chemotherapy followed by local excision is more limited.[171-176] Most series are limited to highly selected patients with cT3 disease who are either medically inoperable or refuse radical surgery. For example, in the University of Florida series, only 11 of the 74 (15%) patients who had significant downstaging of their tumors were selected to undergo transanal excision of their residual rectal cancers.[171] Local failure rates range from 0% to 20% and 5-year survival ranges from 78% to 90%. Mohiuddin and associates treated 44 patients with tumors <3 cm from the dentate line; the local failure rate was 14% and the 5-year survival rate was 90%.[76]

Because most series limit this approach to those patients who responded to preoperative therapy, there is a need to identify prognostic factors to better define patients who are suitable for limited surgery. For example, tumor regression grade[177-179] may help predict the presence of positive nodes.

Functional Results after Local Excision and Adjuvant Therapy

Few series prospectively assess functional results after local excision and preoperative or postoperative therapy. The series from Memorial Sloan-Kettering[168] and Catholic University of the Sacred Heart, Rome,[165] report 94% and 100% good to excellent function, respectively. Using a different scale, investigators from Fox Chase Cancer Center[166] reported 82% good to excellent function, the University of Pennsylvania[163] reported 92% satisfactory function, and M. D. Anderson[162] reported that all patients were continent. In the preoperative setting sphincter function was reported good to excellent in 88% to 91%.[171,176]

Chemotherapy—Current with Radiation, Maintenance

There are limited data examining the use of chemotherapy in patients who undergo local excision and pre- or postoperative RT. In most series, 5-FU was delivered as a radiosensitizer rather than in the adjuvant setting. However, given the positive impact of chemotherapy on local control and survival in patients with resectable rectal cancer reported in the random-

Table 48-7 **Local Excision Plus Postoperative Therapy: Survival, Salvage, and Functional Results—Selected Series**

Series	No.	% T3	% 5-FU	Survival	Function	Local Failures Salvaged with APR
University of Florida[160]	45	2	4	88% cause specific	—	1 of 5
New England Deaconess[231]	48	10	54	94% crude	—	3 of 4
M.D. Anderson[161]	46	33	17	—	All continent	—
University of Pennsylvania[163]	16	32	0	94% 3-y actuarial 77% colostomy free	92% satisfactory*	2 of 2
Massachusetts General Hospital[164]	47	0	55	74% 5-y disease free	—	5 of 9
Catholic University[165]	21	0	0	81% 5-y actuarial	100% good to excellent*	1 of 2
Fox Chase[166]	21	19	10	77% 5-y actuarial	82% good to excellent*	3 of 4
CALGB[232]	51[†]	0	100	85% 6-y actuarial	—	4 of 7
MSKCC[168]	39	21	51	70% 5-y actuarial 87% colostomy free	94% good to excellent*	5 of 8
Vancouver[169]	23	9	0	81% 5-y disease free 77% cause specific	—	3 of 7
Princess Margaret[170] Hospital	73	11	0	67% 5-y actuarial 82% colostomy free	—	11 of 14

5-FU, 5-fluorouracil; APR, Abdominoperineal resection; CALGB, Cancer and Leukemia Group B; MSKCC, Memorial Sloan-Kettering Cancer Center.
*Memorial Sloan-Kettering Cancer Center Sphincter Function Scale.
†Analysis is limited to the 51 of 110 patients (all with T2 disease) who underwent a local excision and received postoperative radiation therapy plus chemotherapy.

ized postoperative rectal adjuvant trials,[180] all patients should be considered for two cycles of 5-FU–based therapy concurrently with radiation. For patients with pT2-3 disease where the incidence of pelvic lymph nodes is at least 20%, an additional four cycles of adjuvant chemotherapy for a total of six cycles is recommended.

LOCALLY ADVANCED DISEASE AND PALLIATION

Adenocarcinomas of the rectum are usually diagnosed as clinically resectable tumors. Less commonly they present with disease that is beyond the potentially curative surgical resection. In this setting it is more difficult to obtain the significant improvements in local control and survival that can be achieved for patients with resectable T3 rectal cancer with the use of combined modality therapy. The definition of resectability depends on the extent of the operation the surgeon is able to perform as well as the amount the patient is willing to undergo. Unresectable rectal cancer is a heterogeneous disease. It can range from a tethered or "marginally resectable" cancer to a fixed cancer with adherence to or direct invasion of adjacent organs or vital structures. Furthermore, both primary unresectable and locally recurrent rectal cancers are commonly analyzed together. The heterogeneity of the disease and absence of a uniform definition of resectability may explain some of the variation in results seen among the series.

The diagnostic work-up must evaluate the local spread and the presence and location of pelvic nodes and of metastases. The choice of one or more imaging studies such as CT scan,[181] MRI,[33] and PET[40,110] depends on the patient's presenting symptoms. Involvement of the sciatic notch indicated by symptoms or scans predicts a situation less likely to be helped by standard approaches of surgery followed or preceded by combined modality therapy. This has prognostic implications since patients with gross invasion of tumor into vital pelvic structures may be approached in a palliative rather than a curative fashion.

Approximately 10% of rectal cancers require extensive surgery such as a pelvic exenteration to obtain negative margins.[182] These include tumors invading the prostate, the base of bladder, or the uterus and vagina where the disease can be resected en bloc with negative margins. Midline posterior tumors adherent to or invading the distal sacrum may be resectable for cure with APR extended to include the sacrum. The 5-year survival rates range from 33% to 50%, with significant morbidity and mortality up to 6%.[183] Improvements in perioperative care, patient selection, and surgical techniques such as vascularized tissue flaps to facilitate the healing of pelvic and perineal wounds have improved the results.[184]

Extended surgery is still recommended even if there is a favorable response after preoperative therapy. Given the limitation of the total radiation dose that can be delivered to the bulky tumor in the pelvis[183] and the frequent problem of local recurrence, the surgeon should be aggressive since there is a risk of leaving microscopic residual tumor.[185]

With the exception of the uncommon "suture line only recurrence", patients with unresectable primary or locally recurrent disease should receive preoperative combined modality therapy as described above (45 to 50.4 Gy plus 5-FU–based chemotherapy). Although 50% to 90% will be able to undergo a resection with negative margins, depending on the degree of tumor fixation, 24% to 55% still develop a local recurrence.

Tethered cancers have the most favorable outcome of all T4 cancers. In a report from the MGH, the results of 28 patients with tethered rectal cancers treated with preoperative radiation were presented.[186] Although a complete resection with negative margins was possible in 93%, the local failure rate was 24%. Tobin and colleagues report a local failure rate of 14% and 5-year survival of 68% in 49 patients with tethered cancers treated with preoperative radiation.[187]

Intraoperative Radiation Therapy

The primary advantage of intraoperative radiation therapy (IORT) is that radiation can be delivered at the time of surgery to the site with the highest risk of local failure (the tumor bed) while decreasing the dose to the surrounding normal tissues. IORT can be delivered by two techniques: electron beam and brachytherapy. Brachytherapy is most commonly delivered by the high-dose rate (HDR) technique and the dose rate is similar to that used for electron beam IORT.[188-190] The results (and recommended dose) of IORT depend on whether the patient has primary unresectable or recurrent disease and on whether the margins of resection are negative or there is microscopic or gross residual disease. In general, series have used 10 to 20 Gy.

It is difficult to clearly separate treatment-related complications from disease-related complications in patients with unresectable primary and/or recurrent rectal cancers. The total incidence ranges from 15% to 50% in most series and is highest in patients with the most advanced disease (recurrent unresectable). Complications such as delayed healing, an increase in infection, fistula formation, and neuropathy may be the result of recurrent tumor, aggressive surgery, radiation, or a combination of these. In an IORT series from the Netherlands, 79 patients surveyed reported fatigue (44%), perineal pain (42%), sciatic pain (21%), walking difficulties (36%), and voiding dysfunction (42%).[191] In addition, functional impairment consisted of requiring help with basic activities (15%), sexual inactivity (56%), the loss of former lifestyle (44%), and the loss of professional occupation (40%).

The incidence of IORT related–neuropathy appears to increase with IORT doses of 15 to 20 Gy, and motor changes are seen primarily with 20 Gy.[66] While most neuropathy-related symptoms appear in the 6- to 9-month period following IORT, the University of Navarra reported peripheral neuropathy up to 5 years after IORT.[192]

The consequences of aggressive combined modality treatment approaches that include IORT must be weighed against the chance of cure if the patient is treated versus the disability, morbidity, and mortality eventually caused by uncontrolled tumor progression if the patient is not treated. Risk-benefit ratios must relate treatment-related morbidity and outcomes with tumor-related morbidity and outcomes in a careful discussion with the patient and family before treatment aims and goals are established (curative versus palliative intent).

Although sphincter preservation is a major goal for patients with primary resectable disease, this should be a lesser goal for patients with locally recurrent cancers. In view of the extensive surgery commonly required for patients with locally recurrent disease, although coloanal anastomosis or a very low anterior resection may be considered, patients may have a better functional outcome with a permanent colostomy.[193]

IORT techniques and results are described in more detail in Chapter 15.

Primary Unresectable Disease

Results of selected series are seen in Table 48-8. The largest experience and longest median follow-up of patients receiving preoperative therapy followed by IORT have been reported by the MGH.[194] Local failure in patients with negative margins decreased from 18% without IORT to 11% with IORT. For patients with positive margins, local failure decreased from 83% without IORT to 43% with IORT if there was gross residual disease, and to 32% with IORT if there was microscopic residual disease. For all patients in the series (with or without IORT), the 5-year DFS was 63% for patients with negative margins and 32% for patients with positive margins. These results underscore the importance of delivering preoperative therapy in order to help achieve negative margins. If negative margins cannot be obtained then microscopic residual disease is still preferable to gross residual disease. Reports from the Mayo Clinic[195] and Memorial Sloan-Kettering[196] revealed similar local failure rates in patients with negative margins (7% and 8%, respectively). Similar series from Munich,[197] Heidelberg,[180] and Eindhoven[198] have been reported. At the MGH, of the 95 patients with T4 disease who received preoperative irradiation and underwent complete resection, 40 patients had an IORT boost and 55 did not because it was not indicated secondary to a favorable response or it was not technically feasible.[199,200] Regardless of the response to preoperative therapy, higher local failure rates were seen in patients not receiving IORT (responders: 0% versus 16%, and nonresponders: 12% versus 27%). These data suggest that IORT should be delivered independent of the extent of tumor downstaging.

Locally Recurrent Disease

In general, patients with local recurrence have an unfavorable prognosis. The median survival ranges between 1 and 2 years.[201] Common symptoms include pain, hemorrhage, pelvic infection, and obstructive symptoms.

At the University of Wurzburg, sites of failure were analyzed in 155 patients.[202] The incidence of failure sites were similar for APR versus LAR: local plus nodal: 61% versus 66%, isolated lymph node: 4% versus 5%, internal iliac and presacral nodes: 47% versus 59%, and external iliac: 7% versus 2%. Local recurrence was most commonly seen in the presacral pelvis, and for patients who underwent an LAR, the anastomosis was involved in 93%.

Recurrences can be heterogeneous and the pattern of extension is more infiltrative within the operative bed compared with primary rectal cancer. Localized pelvic recurrences may be classified according to the tumor location within the pelvis. In a Mayo Clinic analysis by Suzuki and associates, 106 patients with subtotal resection for localized pelvic recurrence (no evidence of extrapelvic metastasis) were stratified during the surgical procedure according to the infiltration of the tumor to none (F0), one (F1), two (F2), or more than two pelvic sites (F3) (anterior, posterior, pelvic side wall [left, right]).[203] This classification system significantly correlated with survival. At the Catholic University of the Sacred Heart, Rome, 47 patients with locally recurrent, nonmetastatic rectal carcinoma were treated by preoperative chemoradiation + IORT and were classified by CT scan according to the Mayo Clinic system.[204] A further (F4) class was added when tumor infiltrated small bowel or bone. The classification system significantly predicted R0 resectability ($P = .01$) and survival ($P = .008$).

As with primary unresectable disease, patients should receive preoperative combined modality therapy if possible when considering normal tissue tolerance. However, in con-

Table 48-8 Primary Locally Advanced/Unresectable Rectal Cancer, External Beam ± Intraoperative Radiation (IORT)—Selected Series

Series	No.	Follow-up (mo)	Preoperative Treatment*	IORT	Local Failure Margins No.	Local Failure Margins Negative	No.	Positive	Total	Survival Margins Negative	Survival Margins Positive	Total
Massachusetts General Hospital[194]	145	41 median	45-50.4 Gy ± 5-FU ± 10-20 Gy IORT	Yes	45	11% 5 y	21 (micro) 7 (gross) 28 Total	32% 5 y 43% 5 y 35% 5 y	— — —	63% 5 y DSS	32% 5 y DSS	—
				No	66	18% 5 y	6 Total	83% 5 y	—	—	—	—
Mayo[195]	56	18 minimum	45-55 Gy ± 5-FU 10-20 Gy IORT	Yes	18	7% 5 y	19 (micro) 16 (gross)	14% 5-y 27% 5-y	16% 5-y	69% 5-y OS	(micro) 55% 5-y (gross) 21% 5-y	46% 5-y OS
Munich[197]	19	—	39.6 Gy BID + 5-FU 15 Gy HDR IORT	Yes	—	—	—	—	10% crude	—	—	—
Heidelberg[96]	40	18 median	41.4 Gy + 5-FU 10-18 Gy IORT	Yes	—	—	—	—	—	91% DFS	—	—
Memorial[196] Sloan-Kettering	18	18 median	50.4 Gy + 5-FU/LV 10-20 Gy HDR IORT	Yes	—	8% 2-y	—	62% 2-y	19% 2-y	77% 2-y DFS	38% 2-y DFS	69% 2-y
New England Deaconess[233] Hospital	27	24 median	50.4 Gy ± 5-FU 12.5-17 Gy IORT (orthovoltage)	Yes	—	—	—	—	27% crude	—	—	41% NED

BID, twice a day radiation; HDR IORT, high dose rate intraoperative radiation; NED, no evidence of disease; DSS, disease-specific survivial; DFS, disease-free survival; OS, overall survival.
*In most patients.

trast with primary disease, some patients in these series had prior external beam radiation and received either a limited dose or no additional external beam radiation.

The results of selected series are seen in Table 48-9. In the MGH series of 69 patients, the overall 5-year local control was 35% and was higher in those with negative margins (56%) versus positive margins (17%).[200] The overall 5-year survival was 27% and was higher in those with negative margins (40%) versus positive margins (14%). Similar results were reported in 74 patients treated at Memorial Sloan-Kettering.[189] The overall 5-year local control was 39% and was higher in patients with negative margins (43%) versus positive margins (26%). The overall 5-year survival was 23% and was higher with patients with negative margins (36%) versus positive margins (11%). In an IORT series of 123 colorectal cancer patients with local recurrence and no prior external radiation, the Mayo Clinic similarly reported lower 3-year local relapse rates in patients with microscopic versus gross residual disease after maximal resection (19% versus 32%, respectively). All patients received external beam radiation either alone ($N = 32$) or in conjunction with concurrent 5-FU ($N = 91$). However, the difference in local control by margin status did not translate into differences in 5-year survival. Patients with gross residual disease had a higher 5-year survival rate compared with other reported series (24% microscopic residual versus 18% gross residual).

Investigators at the M. D. Anderson and Oslo reported no benefit of IORT for patients with positive margins.[205] In a report from Olso, 107 patients with isolated pelvic recurrence received 46 to 50 Gy preoperatively.[206] Regardless of the volume of residual disease, there was no significant difference in local recurrence or survival whether or not they received IORT.

In summary, in contrast to patients who have negative or microscopically positive margins, it is less clear if patients with grossly positive margins benefit from aggressive therapy, in view of differing results by series. However, although the Oslo series reported no long-term survivors for patients with gross residual, U.S. IORT series report 10% to 18% 5-year survival for similar patients.

Reirradiation Followed by Surgery

The combination of adjuvant therapy and TME has appeared to significantly lower the incidence of local recurrence. However, there is a subset of patients who present with local only recurrence who have received previous pelvic radiation. In these patients, the recurrence is often not resectable with clear margins and reirradiation would be expected to be associated with a high risk of late toxicity. Few studies have analyzed the role of radiation retreatment in pelvic recurrence. Data from Mohiuddin and colleagues suggest that reirradiation with doses of 30 Gy, and if the small bowel can be excluded from the irradiation field, 40 Gy can be used for limited volumes.[207] A total of 103 patients with recurrent disease underwent reirradiation plus concurrent 5-FU–based chemotherapy. The initial radiation dose to the pelvis ranged from 30 to 74 Gy with a median dose of 50.4 Gy. Irradiation techniques consisted of two lateral fields with or without a posterior pelvic field to include recurrent tumor with a margin of 2 to 4 cm. Doses ranged from 15 to 49.2 Gy (median, 34.8 Gy). After reirradiation, 34 underwent surgical resection for residual disease. For the total group the median survival was 26 months and the 5-year actuarial survival was 19%. Patients who underwent resection had significantly higher median (44 versus 14 months) and 5-year survival rates (22% versus 15%, $P = .001$). Late complications were seen in 22 patients and were unrelated to radiation dose. These included 18 with persistent severe diarrhea, of whom 10 required long-term parenteral support, 15 with small bowel obstruction, 4 with fistula formation, and 2 with coloanal stricture.

A multicenter Italian trial of 59 patients with recurrent disease who had received less than 55 Gy were retreated preoperatively with concurrent 5-FU plus 30 Gy (1.2 Gy twice daily) to the GTV plus a 4-cm margin.[208] A boost was delivered, with the same fractionation schedule, to the GTV plus a 2-cm margin (10.8 Gy). Grade 3+ toxicity was 5% acute and 12% late. With a median follow-up of 36 months, local failure was 48%, median survival 42 months, and 5-year actuarial survival 39% (R0: 67% versus R1-2: 22%). Multivariate analysis confirmed the impact of longer disease-free interval on local control ($P = .016$) and DFS ($P = .002$). Patients who underwent an R0 resection had improved local control and DFS ($P = .016$).

Mayo Clinic investigators also have treated previously irradiated patients who develop local recurrence alone with aggressive approaches with curative intent (re-resection and IORT alone or in combination with additional pelvic radiation). In the initial group of 51 IORT patients who received prior radiation, 3-year local relapse rates after retreatment appeared to be higher than in the 123 IORT patients without prior radiation (55% versus 25%).[209] Survival was lower in the 51 patients who received prior radiation compared with the 123 who had not (median: 23 versus 28 months, 5-year: 12% versus 20%). At the Aachen 2002 ISIORT meeting, Haddock and colleagues presented results in 145 patients with recurrent rectal cancer who failed prior radiation and received IORT as a component of retreatment.[209] The 5-year overall survival was 18%. Improvements in long-term survival appeared to be related to more intensive treatment, including the more standard use of preoperative radiation with concurrent PVI 5-FU (25.2 to 30.6 Gy in 1.8-Gy fractions) and maintenance systemic chemotherapy.

Radiation Therapy Alone

Some investigators have advocated the use of radiation therapy alone.[151,210-212] A variety of techniques have been used including various combinations of external beam, brachytherapy, and intracavitary radiation.

Patients selected for radiation therapy alone are usually medically inoperable or have advanced local disease such that resection would compromise a vital pelvic structure. In most series, patients received pelvic RT followed by a boost with either external beam and/or brachytherapy. Brierley and associates from the Princess Margaret Hospital reported the results of external beam alone (40 to 60 Gy) in patients who refused surgery or had unresectable or medically inoperable disease.[213] The overall 5-year survival was 27% and was higher in more mobile tumors; mobile: 47%, partially fixed: 27%, and fixed: 4%. These data suggest that patients with mobile or partially fixed rectal cancers who are medically inoperable should be treated aggressively with pelvic RT as a component of their therapy.

Gerard and associates reported the combination of external beam, intracavitary, and brachytherapy in 63 patients with uT2-3 tumors.[212] For patients with uT3 disease, the 5-year local failure and survival rates were 20% and 35%, respectively.

Pelvic radiation offers effective palliation. In a subset of 80 patients with metastatic disease who received pelvic radiation, Crane and associates reported that 94% had complete resolution of pelvic symptoms and the 2-year pelvic symptom free control was 82%.[214] The Princess Margaret Hospital series

Table 48-9 Recurrent Rectal or Colorectal Cancer: The Role of Intraoperative Radiation (IORT)—Selected Series

Series	No.	Follow-up (mo)	Preoperative Treatment*	Local Failure Margin Status: No.	Negative	No.	Positive	Total	Survival Margin Status: Negative	Positive	Total
Mayo[234] (No prior RT)	123	—	50.4-54 Gy 7.5-20 Gy IORT	17	6% crude	40 (m) 65 (g)	19%, 3-y 32%, 3-y	25%, 3-y	44%, 3-y	(m) 24% 5-y (g) 18%, 5-y	20%, 5-y
Mayo[209] (Prior RT)	51	—	RT 37/51 25.2 Gy median	13	45%, 3-y	21 (m) 17 (g)	65%, 3-y 57%, 3-y	55%, 3-y	25%, 5-y	(m) 27%, 3-y (g) 21%, 3-y	12%, 5-y
Mayo (Prior RT)	145	—	25.5-30.6 Gy RT plus PVI 5FU	—	—	—	—	55%, 3-y	—	—	18%, 5-y
MDACC[235]	43[†]	26 mo median	45 Gy + 5-FU 10-20 GY IORT	—	—	—	—	36%	—	—	37% 5-y (DFS)
MSKCC[196]	46	18 mo median	(16) 50.4 Gy ± 5-FU/LV 10-20 Gy HDR IORT (25) 10-20 Gy IORT alone	—	18% 2-y	—	81%, 2-y	37%, 2-y	71%, 2-y DFS	0%, 2-y DFS	47%, 2-y DFS
MGH[200]	69	31 mo median	50.4 Gy ± 5-FU (49) 10-20 Gy IORT Some prior EBRT	25	44% 5-y	24	83%, 5-y (m + g)	65%, 5-y	40%, 5-y	14%, 5-y	27%, 5-y
French[236] Group	73	30 mo median	(30) 39 Gy ± 5-FU 10-15 Gy IORT (43) IORT alone	—	—	—	—	69%, 3-y 57% (R0)	—	—	31%, 3-y[‡]
Heidelberg[237]	31	28 mo median	41.4 Gy (22 preop) Mean 13.7 Gy IORT	14	22%, 4-y	9 (m) 8 (g)	39%, 4-y 40%, 4-y	29% crude	71%, 4-y DFS	29%, 4-y DFS	48%, 4-y (DFS) 58%, 4-y
New England Deaconess[233]	13	24 mo median	50.4 Gy ± 5-FU 12.5-17 Gy Orthovoltage IORT	—	—	—	—	73%	—	—	27%, NED
Catholic University[204]	47	80 mo median	45-47 Gy + 5-FU + MMC (11) 10-15 Gy IORT (31) Adjuvant CT	—	—	—	—	68%, 5-y (21%, 5-y, IORT)	—	—	22%, 5-y (41%, 5-y, IORT)
Eindhoven[198]	37	31 mo median	50.4 Gy (0-60 Gy) 10-17 Gy IORT	15	13% crude	8 (m) 14 (g)	13% crude 43% crude	40%, 3-y	74%, 3-y (R0 + R1)	(g) 35%, 3-y	58% 3-y
Oslo[206]	107	26 mo median	46-50 Gy RT (59) 12-18 Gy IORT	18	30% 5-y	29 (m) 12 (g)	65% 5-y Not eval	—	60% 5-y	(m) 25%, 5-y (g) 0%, 5-y	30% 5-y

*In most patients.
†Excluding 10 patients with multifocal or extrapelvic disease.
‡In 30 patients with IORT alone, no long-term survivors beyond 42 mo. vs 70% in patients with EBRT + IORT.
RT, external beam radiation; IORT, intraoperative radiation; HDR, high-dose rate; DFS, disease-free survival; m, microscopic; g, gross; NED, no evidence of disease; Mayo, Mayo Clinic; MDACC, M.D. Anderson Cancer Center; MSKCC, Memorial Sloan-Kettering Cancer Center; MGH, Massachusetts General Hospital; MMC, Mitomycin C; R0, resection margin negative; R1, resection margin microscopically positive; CT, chemotherapy.

reported similar palliative benefits.[213] In the subset of 84 patients who received more than 45 Gy, the following presenting symptoms were palliated within 6 to 8 weeks following the completion of radiation: pain: 89%, bleeding: 79%, neurologic: 52%, mass effect: 71%, discharge: 50%, urologic: 22%, and other: 42%.[230] In the Thomas Jefferson University series, complete plus partial symptomatic relief was achieved in the following categories: pain (65% + 28%), bleeding (100%), and mass effect (24% + 64%), respectively.[207] The duration of palliation was 8 to 10 months. In patients who are unable to receive radiation, laser or stents[215] offer some palliative benefit.

TECHNIQUES OF IRRADIATION

Patterns of Relapse That Define Radiation Portals

The design of pelvic RT fields is mainly based on the knowledge of local-regional failures after surgery. These occur as a result of residual disease in the soft-tissues of the pelvis as well as from residual nodal disease. For locally advanced disease, recurrences in the soft tissues may arise from tumor extension to the pelvic sidewall, the bladder, the prostate in men, the vagina in women, and the presacral space in all patients. This is especially true for tumors penetrating the mesorectal fascia or those with involved or close (<1 mm) circumferential margins. Incomplete mesorectal excision is also at higher risk to leave residual microscopic tumor cells behind.

The major lymphatic spread is in a cephalad direction contained within the perirectal fascia and along the mesenteric system that is commonly dissected by standard TME surgery. Outside the mesorectum is a space containing vessels, nerves, and lymphatics, which is not usually dissected. Series of Japanese surgeons who approached rectal cancer with lymph node dissection extended to the lateral space have shown that lesions at or below the peritoneal reflexion tend to spread laterally along the internal iliac and the obturator chains.[231] The external iliac nodes may only become at risk with anterior tumor extension and adjacent organ involvement. Lesions that extend to the anal canal or the lower third of the vagina can spread to the inguinal nodes.

The relative frequency and sites of pelvic failures were delineated by the early work of Gunderson and Sosin.[42] In this reoperative series of 75 patients (91% were initially treated with an APR), failure sites included soft tissue of the pelvis or the anastomotic site: 69%, pelvic lymph nodes: 42%, and the perineum: 25%. A more contemporary series of 269 patients by Hruby and colleagues confirmed that the majority of local failures occurred in the posterior central pelvis (47%) or at the anastomosis (21%), while anterior recurrences (11%) were mainly seen in T4 tumors. Perineal recurrences occurred in 16% of patients who underwent APR.[216] Figure 48-2 depicts sites and frequency of recurrences in a German series of 123 patients diagnosed with rectal cancer recurrences between 1998 and 2001.[217]

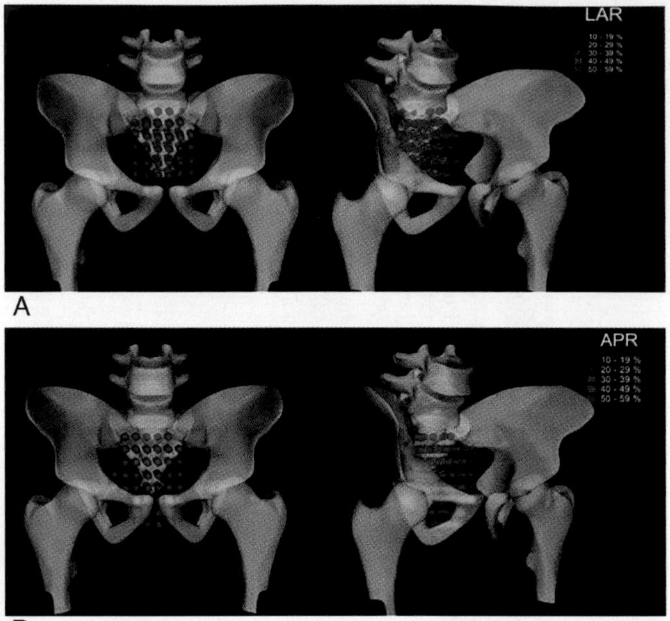

Figure 48-2 Sites of recurrences after low anterior resection (**A**) and abdominoperineal resection (APR) (**B**) in 123 patients with recurrent rectal cancer (areas involved in <10% excluded). Recurrent tumors are mainly situated in the posterior part of the bony pelvis. Note the higher percentage of recurrences in the lower part of the pelvis/perineum after APR. (From Hocht S, et al: Recurrent rectal cancer within the pelvis. Strahlenther Onkol 180:15-20, 2004. Reported by Urban and Vogel.)

Irradiation Fields

The whole pelvic radiation field should adequately cover the primary tumor/tumor bed as well as the primary nodes at risk. General guidelines for the design of pelvic RT fields are listed in Table 48-10. The intent of the boost is to treat the primary tumor and not to include clinically uninvolved nodes. Therefore, the exact size is determined by the size and location of the primary tumor. Whole pelvic and boost fields are usually treated with three-field (posteroanterior and lateral) or four-field (lateral and paired posterior obliques) techniques. A three-field technique allows more sparing of anterior pelvic structures. Field shaping by blocks is used to spare additional small intestine anteriorly and superiorly, the posterior muscle and soft tissue behind the sacrum, and inferior to the symphysis pubis. Specific examples of field arrangements for a variety of clinical presentations are seen in Figures 48-3 through 48-5.

Three-Dimensional Conformal Treatment Planning and Intensity-Modulated Radiation Therapy

Innovative techniques using three-dimensional (3-D) conformal treatment planning are being investigated. The most important contribution of 3-D treatment planning was the ability to plan and localize the target and normal tissues at all levels of the treatment volume, and to obtain dose volume histogram data. A randomized trial of conformal versus conventional RT in 266 evaluable patients with pelvic malignancies has been reported by Tait and associates. Patients were treated with a three-field technique with 6-MV photons and the most common dose was 64 Gy in 2-Gy fractions.[218] Although there was a decrease in normal tissue volumes in the radiation field with conformal versus conventional treatment (689 cm^3 versus 792 cm^3), there was no difference in the level of symptoms or in medication prescribed. Myerson and associates used a 3-D planned boost radiotherapy (0.9 Gy once or twice weekly to a total boost dose of 4.5 to 9 Gy) concurrently with pelvic irradiation (45 Gy/25 fractions).[219] Dose volume histogram information correlated with grade 3-4 toxicity, particularly with respect to small bowel complications. The authors concluded that every effort should be made to limit the volume of small

Table 48-10 General Guidelines for Pelvic Radiation Therapy

WHOLE PELVIC FIELD

AP/PA

Superior border: Sacral promontory (L5/S1 junction): the level of the attachment of the posterior peritoneum , above is little risk of soft tissue invasion by the primary tumor. Mesenteric lymphatics are adequately treated surgically. Para-aortic nodes are not treated since they are M1 disease.[79]

Lateral border: 1.5 cm lateral to the widest bony margin of the true pelvic walls to include possible lateral extension and the internal iliac chain.

Distal border: 3 to 5 cm distal to the tumor for patients receiving preoperative radiation (best determined by direct palpation, by an endoscopically placed clip, or by rectal contrast). For postoperative radiation, the distal field edge must include the perineum (as indicated by a radiopaque marker) if the surgery was an APR or 2-3 cm beyond the anastomosis for an anterior resection with reanastomosis. Note: bony anatomic landmarks such as the obturator foramina have no consistent relationship to the anal sphincter.

Laterals

Anterior border: T3 disease: include the rectum with a generous margin (determined by placing contrast in the rectum at simulation); the posterior margin of the symphysis pubis is the bony landmark to treat the internal iliac nodes, the posterior border of the vagina, or the prostate. T4 disease: 2-3 cm anterior to the anterior extent of the primary tumor; the anterior margin of symphysis pubis is a bony landmark to treat the external iliac nodes (preferably defined with CT based treatment planning). For anal canal involvement, the inguinal nodes may also be included. However, it is not clear that it is beneficial.[238]

Posterior border: 1.5 cm behind the anterior bony sacral margin.

BOOST FIELDS

Primary tumor/tumor bed + 3 cm margin

In general, field sizes measure 10 × 10 or 12 × 12 cm, corner blocks.

Oral contrast before simulation to exclude any small bowel within the boost volume.

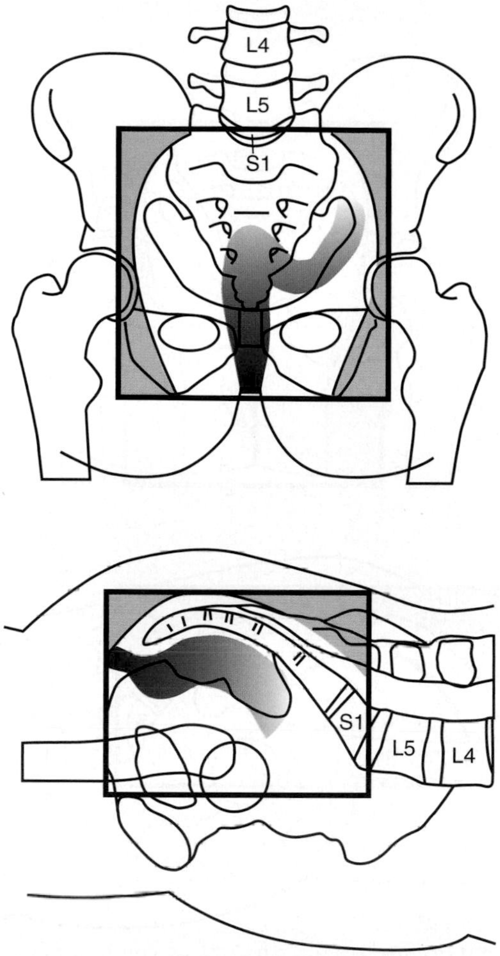

Figure 48-3 Treatment fields following an LAR for a T3 N1 M0 rectal cancer at 8 cm from the anal verge. In this example, the distal border is at the bottom of the obturator foramen and the perineum is blocked. Since the tumor was a T3, the anterior field is at the posterior margin of the symphysis pubis (to treat only the internal iliac nodes).

bowel receiving more than 40 Gy to less than 120 cm^3. Using a 3-D planning system, Koelbl and associates[220] found that in patients receiving postoperative radiation, the use of the prone position plus a belly board decreased the small bowel volume treated versus the supine position. Three-dimensional planned radiotherapy is desirable for patients who undergo reirradiation in order to limit dose to previously irradiated critical structures. Although not well studied to date, the use of intensity-modulated radiotherapy (IMRT) may further lower the dose to the critical structures while maintaining adequate doses in the planned target volume.[221,222]

Irradiation Dose

A meta-analysis of patients who received preoperative radiation with a variety of doses and fraction sizes concluded that biologically effective doses above 30 Gy, compared with less than 30 Gy, resulted in a statistically significant reduction in locoregional recurrences.[68] With conventional fractionation (1.8- to 2-Gy fractions, 5 days per week), the doses most commonly used for the whole pelvis fields for either pre- or postoperative irradiation are in the range of 45 to 50.4 Gy in 5 to 6 weeks. These doses are necessary to control for microscopic disease.[223] A boost of 5.4 Gy to the primary tumor or tumor bed may be delivered if the small bowel is excluded from the high dose field. However, it is not clear that higher doses improve local control. Higher preoperative doses to 60 Gy are associated with increased pCR rates; however, they may also significantly increase acute and long-term morbidity. The RTOG R-0012 phase II randomized trial compared BID preoperative chemoradiation up to 60 Gy (1.2 Gy to 45.6 Gy, with a boost of 9.6 to 14.4 Gy) with conventional fractionation (1.8 Gy to 45 Gy, with a boost of 5.4 to 9 Gy) plus 5-FU/irinotecan.[126] Both regimens resulted in a 28% pCR rate but were also associated with a greater than 40% rate of grade 3-4 acute toxicity.

In the postoperative setting, if there is incomplete resection (R1 or R2 resection), radiation doses of more than 60 Gy are required. External beam radiotherapy is limited in this situation by normal tissue tolerance, and results for patients with residual disease who received postoperative external RT are disappointing.[74,224] As previously discussed, IORT may help to overcome this problem by direct visualization and irradiation of the persistent tumor.

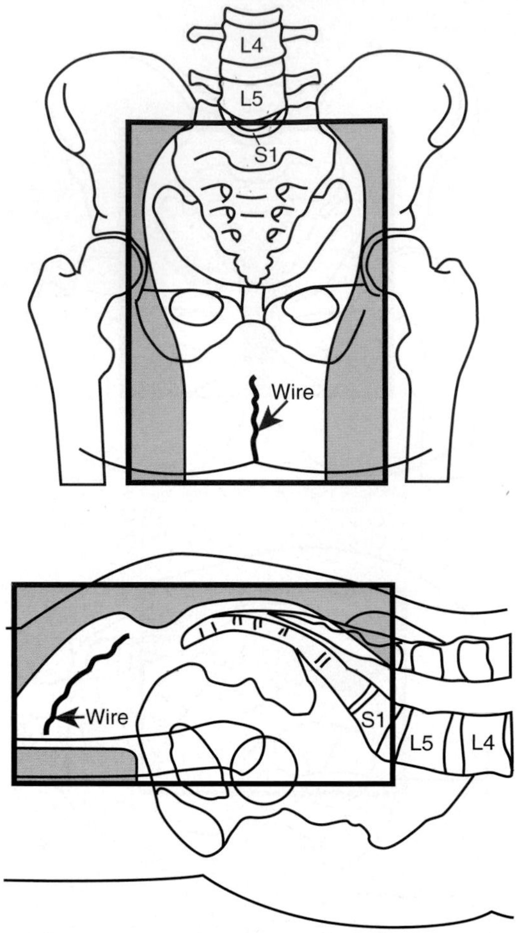

Figure 48-4 Treatment fields following an APR for a T3N1M0 rectal cancer 2 cm from the anal verge. In this example, the distal border is extended to include the perineal scar. Because the distal border is being extended only to include the scar, the remaining normal tissues can be blocked.

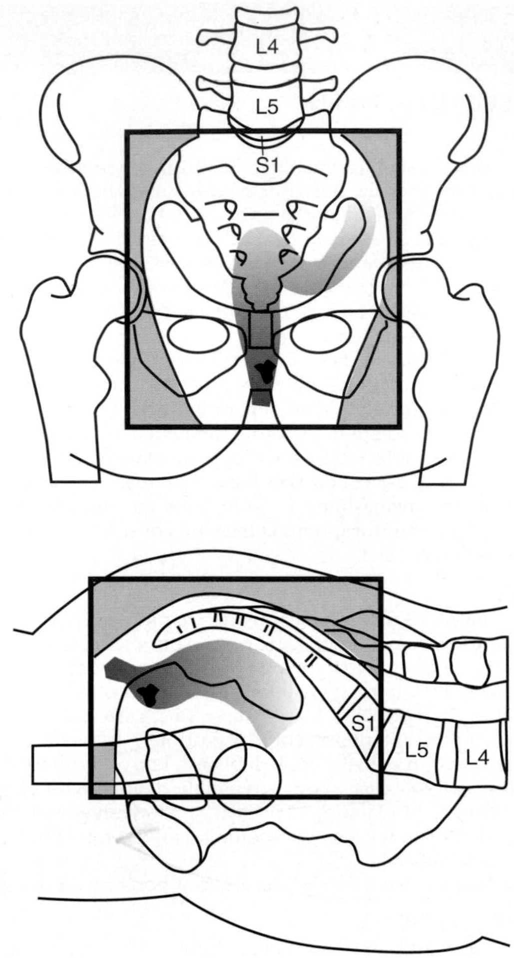

Figure 48-5 Treatment fields for preoperative radiation therapy for a low lying T3NxM0 (or following an LAR for a T3N1M0) rectal cancer. In this example the distal border is extended 3 cm beyond the primary tumor and the perineum is blocked. Because the tumor was a T3, the anterior field is at the posterior margin of the symphysis pubis (to treat only the internal iliac nodes).

Techniques to Reduce Acute and Chronic Toxicity

Complications of pelvic RT are a function of the volume of the radiation field, overall treatment time, fraction size, radiation energy, total dose, technique, and sequence of radiotherapy.[48] Acute side effects such as diarrhea and increased bowel frequency (small bowel), acute proctitis (large bowel), and dysuria are common during treatment.[225] These conditions are usually transient and resolve within a few weeks following the completion of radiation. The symptoms appear to be a function of the dose rate and fraction size rather than of the total dose. The mechanism is primarily the depletion of actively dividing cells in what is otherwise a stable cell renewal system. In the small bowel, loss of the mucosal cells results in malabsorption of various substances including fat, carbohydrate, protein, and bile salts. Examination during treatment frequently reveals an inflamed, edematous, and friable rectal mucosa. The bowel mucosa usually recovers completely in 1 to 3 months following radiation. Management usually involves the use of antispasmodic and/or anticholinergic medications. The use of concurrent chemotherapy, especially 5-FU, which has significant GI toxicity, will exacerbate the acute gastrointestinal effects.

Small bowel–related complications are directly proportional to the volume of small bowel in the radiation field.[226] In patients receiving combined radiation and chemotherapy, the volume of small bowel in the radiation field limits the ability to escalate the dose of 5-FU.[48]

Delayed complications occur less frequently but are more serious. The initial symptoms commonly occur 6 to 18 months following completion of radiation. Complications may include persistent diarrhea and increased bowel frequency, proctitis, strictures at the anastomotic site, small bowel obstruction, perineal/scrotal tenderness, delayed perineal wound healing, urinary incontinence, and bladder atrophy/bleeding. Injury to the vascular and supporting stromal tissues is the presumed pathophysiology.

The most common delayed severe complications are due to small bowel damage and include small bowel enteritis, adhesions, and small bowel obstruction requiring surgical intervention. The incidence of small bowel obstruction requiring surgery following postoperative pelvic radiation for rectal cancer is 4% to 12% in historical series. In the MGH series, the incidence of small bowel obstruction with postoperative RT was 6% compared with 5% with surgery alone.[49] It was 2% in the preoperative arm of the German CAO/ARO/AIO-94 trial.[30] Radiotherapeutic and surgical techniques, as well as general methods to decrease treatment-related toxicity, especially small bowel complications, are seen in Table 48-11.

Table 48-11 Techniques and Methods to Decrease Toxicity
RADIATION TECHNIQUE Multiple field techniques (PA:AP + laterals or preferably PA + laterals) use high-energy (preferably ≥15 MV) linear accelerators with computerized radiation dosimetry. Oral contrast to visualize the small bowel, rectal contrast, and a wire on the perineum help to guide field design. A 3-field rather than a 4-field technique will decrease the volume of small bowel in the pelvis that is carried to a higher radiation dose, male genitalia if they are in the treatment fields, and if there is a colostomy present. Shaped blocks and wedges should be used on the lateral fields. The perineal scar after APR should be included in the pelvic radiation fields since the use of a separate perineal field is associated with an increased risk of overlap. Treatment should be 5 days per week with all fields treated each day. Split course pelvic radiation is associated with increased chronic bowel complications.[239]
PHYSICAL MANEUVERS Prone position with abdominal wall compression and bladder distension and/or the use of immobilization molds or belly boards in the prone position generally decrease the volume of small bowel in the pelvis (though not consistently for all patients).[220] Some physical maneuvers such as a full bladder may be associated with patient discomfort leading to increased movement and daily set-up errors. The use of such techniques should be tailored to the individual patient.
SURGICAL MANEUVERS Placing clips in the high-risk areas intraoperatively or at the inferior aspect of the tumor in the preoperative setting helps to better define tumor volume or the inferior border of the fields. For patients treated postoperatively, especially after APR, the use of an absorbable dexon or vicryl mesh may temporarily remove the small bowel from the pelvis. Other techniques such as an inflatable pelvic small bowel displacement prosthesis[240,241] reconstruction of the pelvic floor, construction of an omental pedicle flap,[242] and retroversion of the uterus have had variable success.
SEQUENCING OF RADIOTHERAPY AND SURGERY Preoperative radiotherapy causes less acute and chronic toxicity compared with the postoperative treatment.[30,48] This is likely due to the fact that small bowel in an unviolated abdomen will be mobile and less likely to be within a pelvic radiation field and the irradiated volume does not require coverage of the perineum following an APR. In the German CAO/ARO/AIO-94 trial, grade 3-4 gastrointestinal toxicity was significantly reduced with the preoperative approach (acute: 12% versus 18%, $P = .04$, and long-term: 9% versus 15%, $P = .07$).[30] Strictures at the anastomotic site were also reduced (4% versus 12%, $P = .003$).
PHARMACOLOGIC APPROACHES AND RADIOPROTECTORS Randomized trials have investigated the use of sucralfate enemas to decrease acute radiation proctitis, olsalazine and mesalazine to decrease acute enteritis, and butyric acid to decrease chronic radiation proctitis.[243-246] All of these trials have been negative. The radioprotector WR-2721 did not reduce toxicity in early trials, but there is a suggestion of a benefit in a more recent study.[247] Rectal administered amifostine is well tolerated; however, its efficacy remains to be determined.[248]

TREATMENT ALGORITHMS, CONTROVERSIES, PROBLEMS, CHALLENGES, AND FUTURE POSSIBILITIES

Treatment Algorithms

The treatment of rectal cancer is multidisciplinary. It is important to develop treatment algorithms using a balanced approach with representation from all medical specialties including radiation, medical, and surgical oncology as well as radiology, gastroenterology, and pathology. Treatment algorithms developed by representatives of a single modality or institution may be biased.

Furthermore, treatment algorithms can be based on evidence, consensus, or both. While pure evidence based is the most rigorous, there are a variety of clinical settings where prospective trials do not specifically address a treatment controversy. Therefore, multidisciplinary panels that use evidence from both randomized trials as well as lower level sources, such as clinical experience, offer a more practical approach. The National Comprehensive Cancer Network (NCCN) uses this approach and their clinical practice guideline for rectal cancer is seen in Figure 48-6.[227]

Finally, two caveats: All treatment guideline recommendations should be interpreted with caution. Radiation oncology, as with other medical specialties, is both an art and a science. Therefore, these should serve as a guide rather than a "cookbook." Second, the ideal management for patients with rectal cancer is in a clinical trial and participation in these is encouraged.

Controversies and Future Directions

Significant progress has been made in the three conventional modalities used to treat rectal cancer: surgery, radiation, and chemotherapy. Identification of radial microscopic lymphatic spread within the mesorectum has led to the use of TME. With this type of surgery, local control rates appear to have been markedly increased (although not tested with standard resection in controlled phase III trials) and local failure rates above 15% to 20% are now no longer acceptable. Technical advances in radiotherapy, and improvements in the sequencing of radiotherapy, chemotherapy, and surgery will likely lead to further improvements. Moreover, novel cytotoxic chemotherapeutic agents, such as capecitabine, oxaliplatin, and irinotecan, as well as targeted therapies, such as bevacizumab and cetuximab, which have improved results of patients treated in the adjuvant and/or metastatic setting, are currently incorporated into combined modality programs. Clinicopathologic and molecular features and the development of more accurate preoperative imaging and staging methods will also play an important and integrative part in multimodality treatment of rectal cancer.

There are many controversies remaining. For example, should patients receive the short course (5 Gy times 5) or the long course (50.4 Gy) of radiation and is chemotherapy necessary with preoperative radiation and after surgery? Can we develop more accurate imaging techniques and/or molecular markers to identify patients with positive pelvic nodes to reduce the chance of overtreatment with preoperative therapy? Will more effective systemic agents both improve the results of combined modality therapy regimens and modify the need for pelvic radiation? These questions and others remain active areas of clinical investigation.

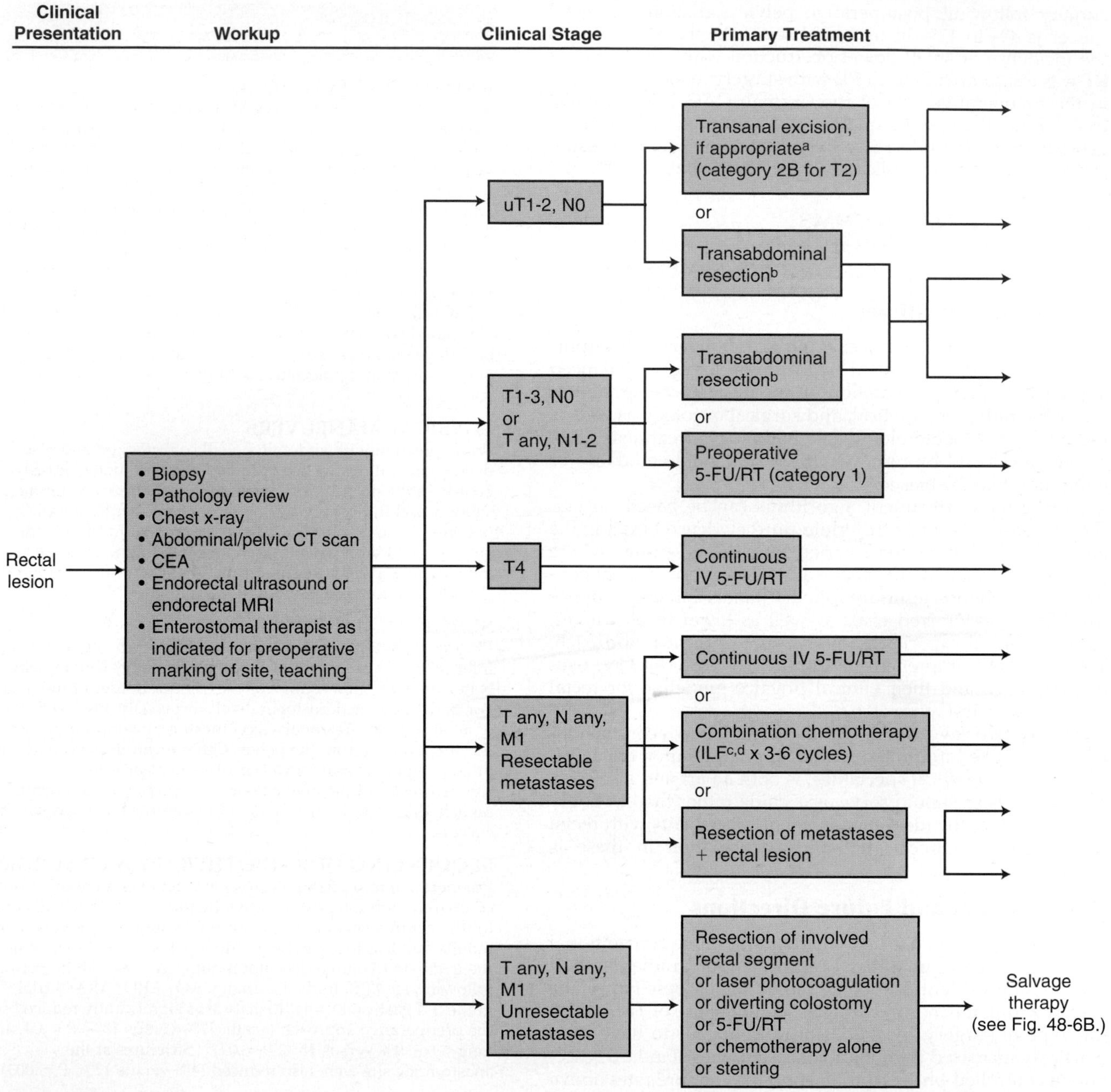

[a] Criteria for transanal excision:
- <30% circumference of bowel
- <3 cm in size
- margin clear (>3 mm)
- mobile, nonfixed
- within 8 cm of anal verge
- T1 or T2
- fragmented polyp with cancer, or indeterminate pathology (a full workup may be initiated if local excision reveals invasive cancer)
- no lymphovascular (LVI) or perineural invasion
- well to moderately differentiated
- Grade 1-2

[b] Abdominoperineal resection or low anterior resection or coloanal anastomosis using total mesorectal excision.

[c] A recent trial demonstrated an increased early 60-day mortality of bolus 5-FU/leucovorin/irinotecan. Careful monitoring of all regimens is required.

A

Figure 48-6 The National Comprehensive Cancer Network (NCCN) clinical practice guidelines for primary (**A**) and recurrent (**B**) rectal cancer. (From National Comprehensive Cancer Network: Rectal cancer—clinical practice guidelines in oncology. http://www.nccn.org/professional/physician_gLS/PDF/rectal.pdf)

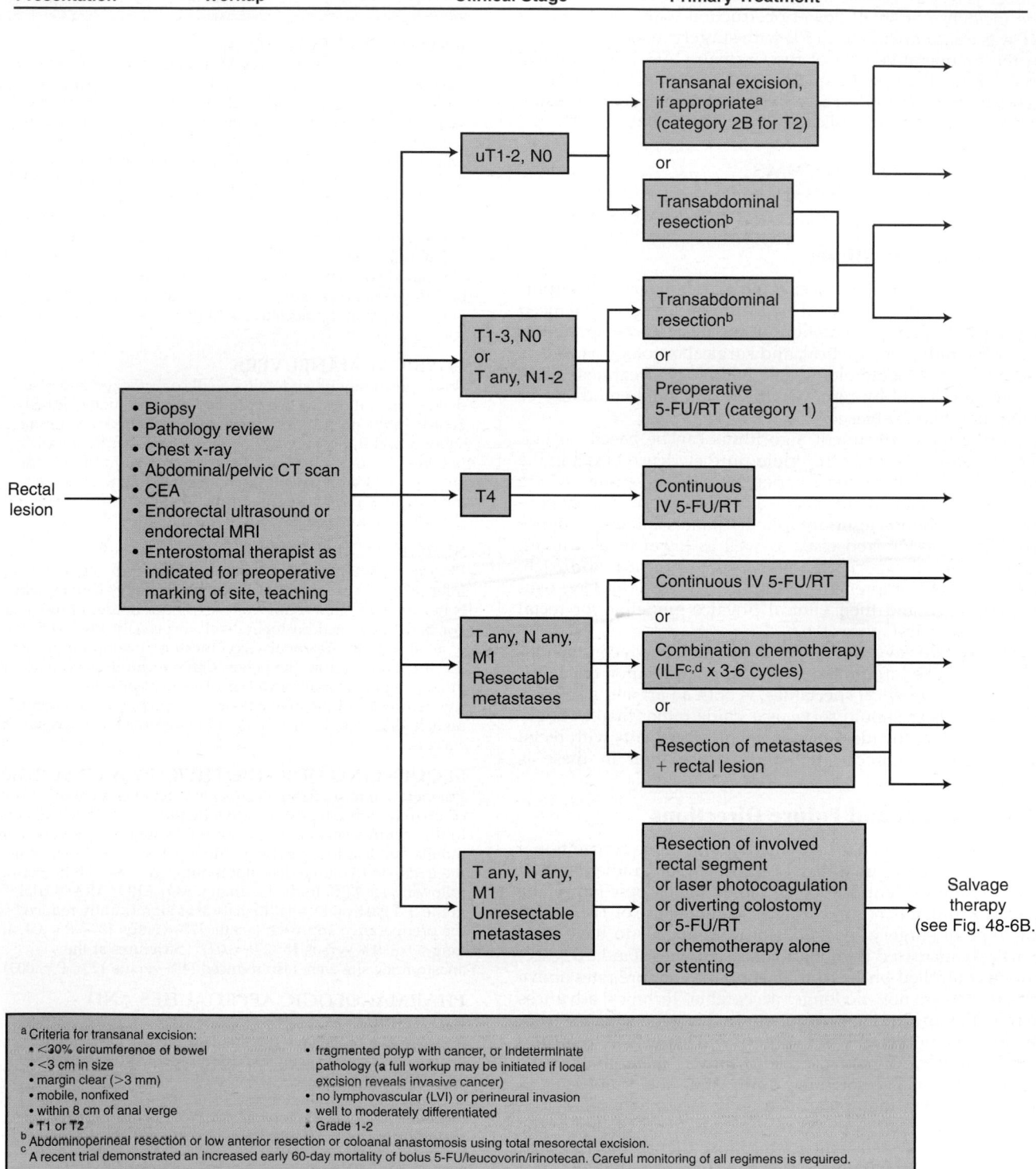

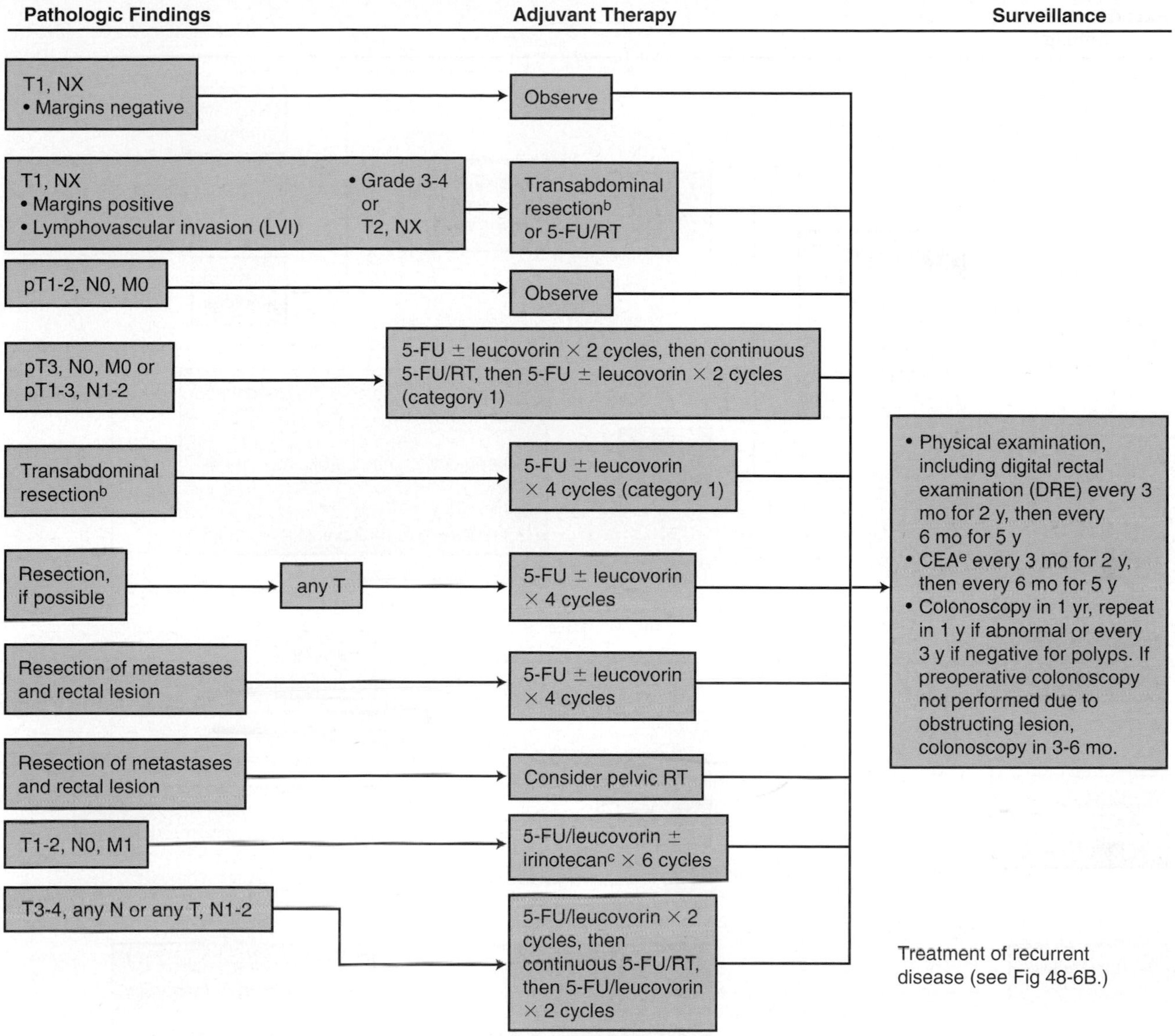

Rothenberg M, Meropol N, Poplin E, et al.: Mortality associated with irinotecan plus bolus fluorouracil/leucovorin: summary findings of an independent panel. J Clin Oncol 2001;19:3801-3807.

[d]ILF = 5-FU/leucovorin/irinotecan. Saltz L, Cox JV, Blanke C, et al.: Irinotecan plus fluorouracil and leucovorin for metastatic colorectal cancer. N Engl J Med 2000;343:905-914.

[e]If patient is a potential candidate for resection of isolated metastasis.

Disease Sites

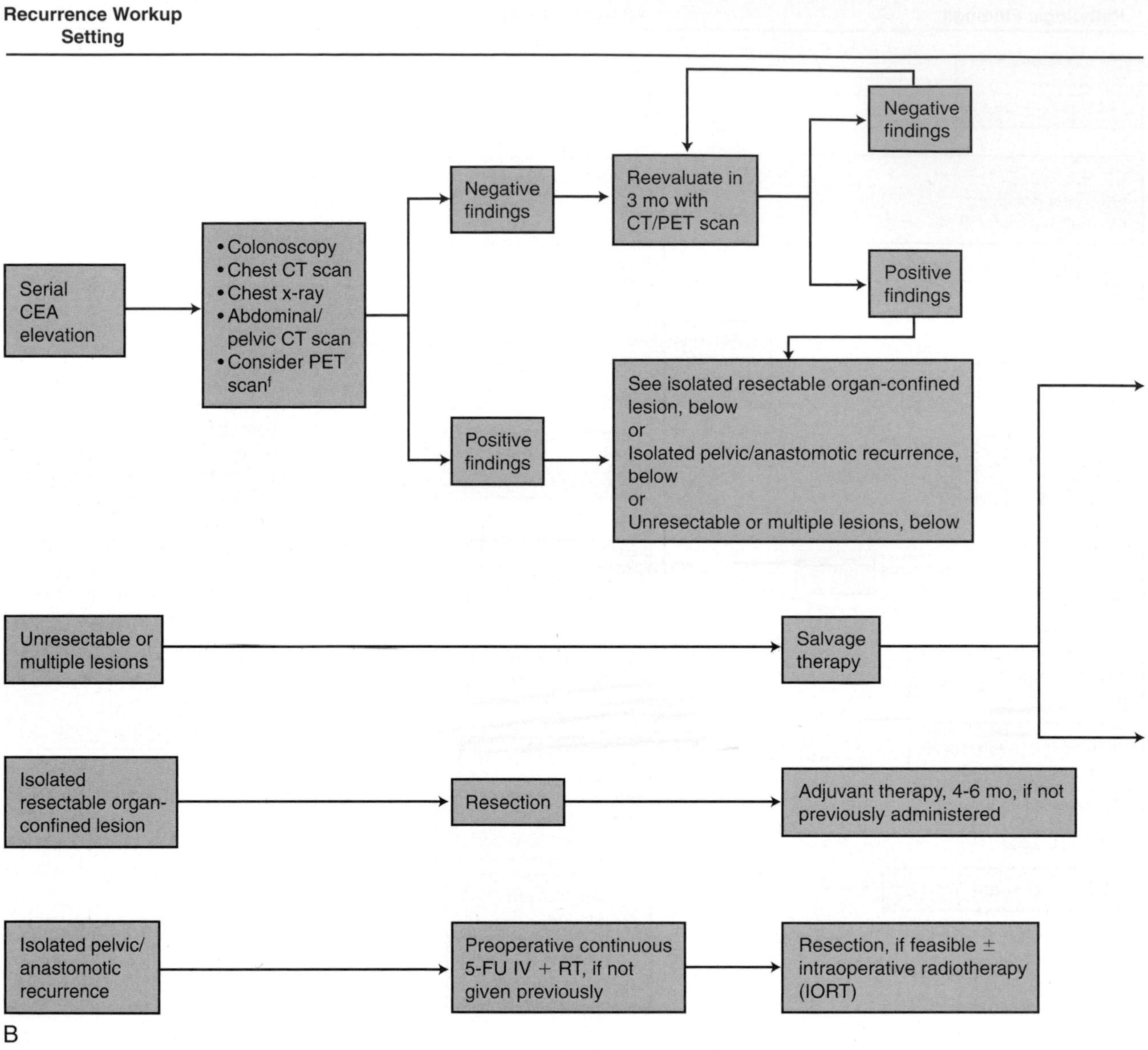

Figure 48-6—cont'd

Salvage Therapy[g,h]

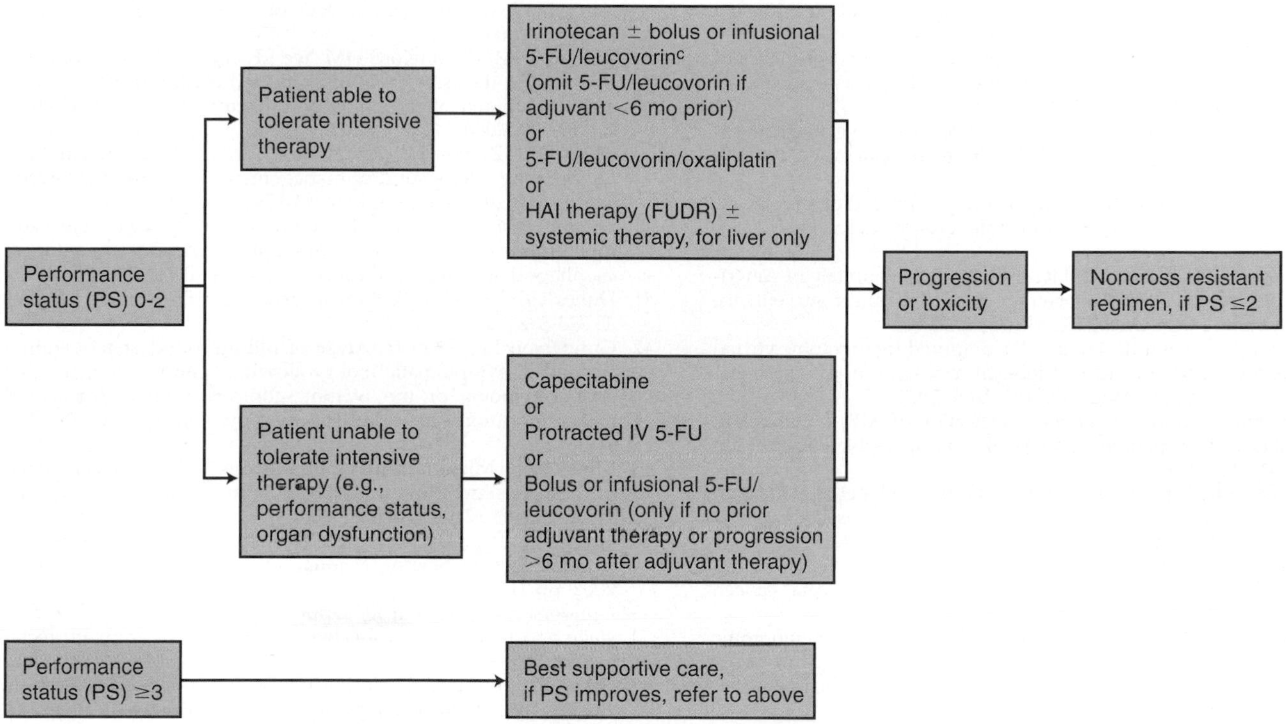

[f] When pelvic recurrence is suspected and salvage surgery is being considered.
[g] Combinations of 5-FU/leucovorin therapy with earlier irinotecan or oxaliplatin should be strongly considered in optimal treatment strategies. The exact sequence has not yet been defined.
[h] For chemotherapy references, review other sources.

REFERENCES

1. Leslie A, Carey FA, Pratt NR, et al: The colorectal adenoma-carcinoma sequence. Br J Surg 89:845-860, 2002.
2. Lynch HT, Watson P, Smyrk TC, et al: Colon cancer genetics. Cancer 70:1300-1312, 1992.
3. Whittemore AS, Wu-Williams AH, Lee M, et al: Diet, physical activity, and colorectal cancer among Chinese in North America and China. J Natl Cancer Inst 82:915-926, 1991.
4. Powell SM, Zilz N, Beazer-Barclay Y: APC mutations occur early during colorectal tumorigenesis. Nature 359:235-237, 1992.
5. Grady WM: Genomic instability and colon cancer. Cancer Metastasis Rev 23:11-27, 2004.
6. Gryfe R, Kim H, Hsieh ETK, et al: Tumor microsatellite instability and clinical outcome in young patients with colorectal cancer. New Engl J Med 342:69-77, 2000.
7. Watanabe T, Wu TT, Catalano PJ, et al: Molecular predictors of survival after adjuvant chemotherapy for colon cancer. New Engl J Med 344:1196-1206, 2001.
8. Lenz HJ, Danenberg KD, Leichman CG, et al: p53 and thymidylate synthase expression in untreated stage II colon cancer: associations with recurrence, survival, and site. Clin Cancer Res 4:1227-1234, 1998.
9. Garrity MM, Burgart LJ, Mahoney MR, et al: Prognostic value of proliferation, apoptosis, defective DNA mismatch repair, and p53 overexpression in patients with resected Dukes' B2 or C colon cancer: A North Central Cancer Treatment Group Study. J Clin Oncol 22:1572-1582, 2004.

10. Parkin DM, Pisani P, Ferlay J: Global cancer statistics. CA Cancer J Clin 49:33-64, 1999.
11. Jemal A, Siegal R, Ward E, et al: Cancer Statistics, 2006. CA Cancer J Clin 56:106-130, 2006.
12. Diep CB, Thorstensen L, Meling GI, et al: Genetic tumor markers with prognostic impact in Dukes' stages B and C colorectal cancer patients. J Clin Oncol 21:820-829, 2003.
13. Lashner BA, Provencher KS, Seidner DL: The effect of folic acid supplementation on the risk for cancer or dysplasia in ulcerative colitis. Gastroenterology 112:29-32, 1997.
14. Williams CS, Mann M, DuBois RN: The role of cyclooxygenases in inflammation, cancer, and development. Oncogene 18:7908-7916, 1999.
15. Winawer SJ, Fletcher RH, Miller L, et al: Colorectal cancer screening: clinical guidelines and rationale. Gastroenterology 112:594-642, 1997.
16. Benson AB III, Desch CE, Flynn PJ, et al: 2000 update of American Society of Clinical Oncology colorectal cancer surveillance guidelines. J Clin Oncol 18:3586-3588, 2000.
17. Pickhardt PJ, Choi JR, Hwang I: Computed tomographic virtual colonoscopy to screen for colorectal neoplasia in asymptomatic adults. New Engl J Med 349:2191-2200, 2003.
18. Traverso G, Shuber A, Levin B: Detection of APC mutations in fecal DNA from patients with colorectal tumors. New Engl J Med 346:311-320, 2002.
19. Compton C, Fenoglio-Preiser CM, Pettigrew N, et al: American Joint Committee on Cancer prognostic factors consensus conference. Colorectal Working Group. Cancer 88:1739-1757, 2000.
20. Brodsky JT, Richard GK, Cohen AM, et al: Variables correlated with the risk of lymph node metastasis in early rectal cancer. Cancer 69:322-326, 1992.
21. Meling GI, Rognum TO, Clausen OP: Serum carcinoembryonic antigen in relation to survival, DNA ploidy pattern, and recurrent disease in 406 colorectal carcinoma patients. Gastroenterology 27:1061-1068, 1992.
22. Minsky BD: Clinicopathologic impact of colloid in colorectal carcinoma. Dis Colon Rectum 33:714-719, 1990.
23. Chen JS, Hsieh PS, Tang R, et al: Clinical significance of signet ring cell carcinoma. Int J Colorectal Dis 19:102-107, 2004.
24. Bernick PE, Klimstra DS, Shia J, et al: Neuroendocrine carcinomas of the colon and rectum. Dis Colon Rectum 47:163-169, 2004.
25. Hatch KF, Blanchard DK, Hatch GF, et al: Tumors of the rectum and anal canal. World J Surg 24:437-443, 2000.
26. Grann A, Paty PB, Cohen AM, et al: Sphincter preservation of leiomyosarcoma of the rectum and anus with local excision and brachytherapy. Dis Colon Rectum 42:1296-1299, 1999.
27. Fan CW, Changchien CR, Wang JY, et al: Primary colorectal lymphoma. Dis Colon Rectum 43:1277-1282, 2000.
28. Gelas T, Peyrat P, Francois Y, et al: Primary squamous cell carcinoma of the rectum. Report of six cases and review of the literature. Dis Colon Rectum 45:1535-1540, 2002.
29. Quirke P, Durdey P, Dixon MF, et al: Local recurrence of rectal adenocarcinoma due to inadequate surgical resection. Histopathological study of lateral tumor spread and surgical excision. Lancet 1:996-999, 1986.
30. Sauer R, Becker H, Hohenberger P, et al: Preoperative chemoradiotherapy as compared with postoperative chemoradiotherapy for locally advanced rectal cancer. New Engl J Med 351:11-20, 2004.
31. Schaffzin DM, Wong WD: Endorectal ultrasound in the preoperative evaluation of rectal cancer. Clin Colorectal Cancer 4:124-132, 2004.
32. Hadfield MB, Nicholson AA, MacDonald AW, et al: Preoperative staging of rectal carcinoma by magnetic resonance imaging with a pelvic phased-array coil. Br J Surg 84:529-531, 1997.
33. Beets-Tan RGH, Beets GL: Rectal cancer: how accurate can imaging predict the T stage and the circumferential resection margin? Int J Colorectal Dis 18:385-391, 2003.
34. Kim JH, Beets GL, Kim MJ, et al: High-resolution MR imaging for nodal staging in rectal cancer: are there any criteria in addition to the size? Eur J Radiol 52:78-83, 2004.
35. Herrera L, Villarreal JR, Cert RT: Incidence of metastasis from rectal adenocarcinoma in small lymph nodes detected by a clearing technique. Dis Colon Rectum 35:783-788, 1992.
36. Harisinghani MG, Barentsz J, Hahn PF: Noninvasive detection of clinically occult lymph-node metastasis in prostate cancer. N Engl J Med 348:2491-2499, 2003.
37. Shami VM, Parmer KS, Waxman I: Clinical impact of endoscopic ultrasound and endoscopic ultrasound-guided fine-needle aspiration in the management of rectal carcinoma. Dis Colon Rectum 47:59-65, 2004.
38. Whiteford MH, Whiteford HM, Yee LF, et al: Usefulness of FDG-PET scan in the assessment of suspected metastatic or recurrent adenocarcinoma of the colon and rectum. Dis Colon Rectum 53:759-770, 2000.
39. Desai DC, Zervos EE, Arnold MW, et al: Positron emission tomography affects surgical management in recurrent colorectal cancer patients. Ann Surg Oncol 10:59-64, 2003.
40. Larson SM, Schoder H, Yeung H: Positron emission tomography/computerized tomography functional imaging of esophageal and colorectal cancer. Cancer J 10:243-250, 2004.
41. Dukes CE: The classification of cancer of the rectum. J Pathol 35:323-332, 1932.
42. Gunderson LL, Sosin H: Areas of failure found at reoperation (second or symptomatic look) following "curative surgery" for adenocarcinoma of the rectum: clinicopathologic correlation and implications for adjuvant therapy. Cancer 34:1278-1292, 1974.
43. Minsky BD, Mies C, Recht A, et al: Resectable adenocarcinoma of the rectosigmoid and rectum: 1. Patterns of failure and survival. Cancer 61:1408-1416, 1988.
44. Greene FL, Page DL, Fleming ID, et al (eds): Colon and Rectum. *In* AJCC Cancer Staging Manual, 6th ed. New York, Springer, 2002, pp 113-124.
45. Gunderson LL, Sargent D, Tepper JE, et al: Impact of T and N stage and treatment on survival and relapse in adjuvant rectal cancer: a pooled analysis. J Clin Oncol 22:1785-1796, 2004.
46. Green FL, Stewart AK, Norton HJ: New tumor-node-metastasis staging system for node-positive (stage III) rectal cancer: an analysis. J Clin Oncol 22:1778-1784, 2004.
47. Tepper JE, O'Connell MJ, Niedzwiecki D, et al: Impact of number of nodes retrieved on outcome in patients with rectal cancer. J Clin Oncol 19:157-163, 2001.
48. Minsky BD, Conti JA, Huang Y, et al: The relationship of acute gastrointestinal toxicity and the volume of irradiated small bowel in patients receiving combined modality therapy for rectal cancer. J Clin Oncol 13:1409-1416, 1995.
49. Willett CG, Tepper JE, Kaufman DS, et al: Adjuvant postoperative radiation therapy for rectal adenocarcinoma. Am J Clin Oncol 15:371-375, 1992.
50. Romsdahl MM, Withers HR: Radiotherapy combined with curative surgery: its use as therapy for carcinomas of the sigmoid colon and rectum. Arch Surg 113:446-453, 1978.
51. Balslev I, Pedersen M, Teglbjaerg PS, et al: Postoperative radiotherapy in Dukes' B and C carcinoma of the rectum and rectosigmoid: a randomized multicenter study. Cancer 58:22-28, 1986.
52. Gastrointestinal Tumor Study Group: Prolongation of the disease-free interval in surgically treated rectal carcinoma. N Engl J Med 312:1465-1472, 1985.
53. Arnaud JP, Nordlinger B, Bosset JF, et al: Radical surgery and postoperative radiotherapy as combined treatment in rectal cancer. Final results of a phase III study of the European Organization for Research and Treatment of Cancer. Br J Surg 84:352-357, 1997.
54. Medical Research Council Rectal Cancer Working Party: Randomized trial of surgery alone versus surgery followed by postoperative radiotherapy for mobile cancer of the rectum. Lancet 348:1610-1615, 1996.
55. Fisher B, Wolmark N, Rockette H, et al: Postoperative adjuvant chemotherapy or radiation therapy for rectal cancer: results from NSABP protocol R-01. J Natl Cancer Inst 80:21-29, 1988.
56. Krook JE, Moertel CG, Gunderson LL, et al: Effective surgical adjuvant therapy for high-risk rectal carcinoma. N Engl J Med 324:709-715, 1991.
57. Gastrointestinal Tumor Study Group: Adjuvant therapy of colon cancer: results of a prospectively randomized trial. N Engl J Med 310:737-743, 1984.

58. National Institutes of Health Consensus Conference.: Adjuvant therapy for patients with colon and rectal cancer. J Am Med Assoc 264:1444-1450, 1990.
59. Gerard JP, Chapet O, Nemoz C, et al: Improved sphincter preservation in low rectal cancer with high dose preoperative radiotherapy: the Lyon R96-02 randomized trial. J Clin Oncol 22: 2404-2409, 2004.
60. Wagman R, Minsky BD, Cohen AM, et al: Sphincter preservation with preoperative radiation therapy and coloanal anastomosis: long term follow-up. Int J Radiat Oncol Biol Phys 42:51-57, 1998.
61. Bonnel C, Pare YR, Pocard M, et al: Effects of preoperative radiotherapy for primary resectable adenocarcinoma on male sexual and urinary function. Dis Colon Rectum 45:934-939, 2002.
62. Dehni N, McNamara DA, Schlegel RD, et al: Clinical effects of preoperative radiation therapy on anorectal function after proctectomy and colonic J-pouch-anal anastomosis. Dis Colon Rectum 45:1635-1640, 2002.
63. Temple LKF, Wong WD, Minsky B: The impact of radiation on functional outcomes in patients with rectal cancer and sphincter preservation. Semin Radiat Oncol 13:469-477, 2003.
64. Nathanson DR, Espat NJ, Nash GM, et al: Evaluation of preoperative and postoperative radiotherapy on long-term functional results of straight coloanal anastomosis. Dis Colon Rectum 46:888-894, 2003.
65. Havenga K, Enker WE, McDermott K, et al: Male and female sexual and urinary function after total mesorectal excision with autonomic nerve preservation for carcinoma of the rectum. J Am Coll Surg 182:495-502, 1996.
66. Skibber JM, Hoff PM, Minsky BD: Cancer of the rectum. *In* DeVita VT, Hellman S, Rosenberg SA (eds): Cancer: Principles and Practice of Oncology 6th ed. Philadelphia, Lippincott, Williams and Wilkins, 2001, pp 1271-1318.
67. Camma C, Giunta M, Fiorica F, et al: Preoperative radiotherapy for resectable rectal cancer. A meta-analysis. J Am Med Assoc 284:1008-1015, 2000.
68. Colorectal Cancer Collaborative Group: Adjuvant radiotherapy for rectal cancer: a systematic overview of 22 randomised trials involving 8507 patients. Lancet 358:1291-1304, 2001.
69. Swedish Rectal Cancer Trial: Improved survival with preoperative radiotherapy in resectable rectal cancer. N Engl J Med 336:980-987, 1997.
70. Kapiteijn E, Marijnen CAM, Nagtegaal ID, et al: Preoperative radiotherapy combined with total mesorectal excision for resectable rectal cancer. New Engl J Med 345:638-646, 2001.
71. van de Velde CJH: Preoperative radiotherapy and TME-surgery for rectal cancer: detailed analysis in relation to quality control in a randomized trial. Proc ASCO 21:127a, 2002.
72. Marijnen CAM, Kapiteijn E, van de Velde CJH, et al: Acute side effects and complications after short-term preoperative radiotherapy combined with total mesorectal excision in primary rectal cancer: report of a multicenter randomized trial. J Clin Oncol 20:817-825, 2002.
73. van den Brink M, van den Hout WB, Stiggelbout AM, et al: Cost-utility analysis of preoperative radiotherapy in patients with rectal cancer undergoing total mesorectal excision: the Dutch Colorectal Cancer Group. J Clin Oncol 22:1-12, 2004.
74. Marijnen CAM, Nagtegaal ID, Kapiteijn E, et al: Radiotherapy does not compensate for positive resection margins in rectal cancer patients: report of a multicenter randomized trial. Int J Radiat Oncol Biol Phys 55:1311-1320, 2003.
75. Dzik-Jurask A, Domenig C, George M, et al: Diffusion MRI for prediction of response of rectal cancer to chemoradiation. Lancet 360:307-308, 2002.
76. Mohiuddin M, Derdel J, Marks G, et al: Results of adjuvant radiation therapy in cancer of the rectum: Thomas Jefferson University Hospital experience. Cancer 55:350-353, 1985.
77. Lusinchi A, Wibault P, Lasser P, et al: Abdominoperineal resection combined with pre and postoperative radiation therapy in the treatment of low-lying rectal carcinoma. Int J Radiat Oncol Biol Phys 37:59-65, 1997.
78. Sause WT, Pajak T, Noyes RD, et al: Evaluation of preoperative radiation therapy in operable colorectal cancer. Ann Surg 220:668-675, 1994.
79. Bosset JF, Horiot JC, Hamers HP, et al: Postoperative pelvic radiotherapy with or without elective irradiation of para-aortic nodes and liver in rectal cancer patients. A controlled clinical trial of the EORTC Radiotherapy Group. Radiother Oncol 61:7-13, 2001.
80. Lee JHL, Lee JH, Ahn JH, et al: Randomized trial of postoperative adjuvant therapy in stage II and III rectal cancer to define the optimal sequence of chemotherapy and radiotherapy: a preliminary report. J Clin Oncol 20:1751-1758, 2002.
81. O'Connell MJ, Martenson JA, Weiand HS, et al: Improving adjuvant therapy for rectal cancer by combining protracted infusion fluorouracil with radiation therapy after curative surgery. N Engl J Med 331:502-507, 1994.
82. Smalley SR, Benedetti J, Williamson S, et al: Intergroup 0144 A phase III rectal surgical adjuvant study of pelvic radiation (XRT) plus 5-FU based chemotherapy (bolus 5-FU before and after PVI + XRT versus PVI before, during, and after XRT versus biochemically modulated bolus 5-FU and XRT): mature outcome results and pelvic failure analysis. Int J Radiat Oncol Biol Phys 60:s137-s138, 2004.
83. Tepper JE, O'Connell MJ, Niedzwiecki D, et al: Adjuvant therapy in rectal cancer: analysis of stage, sex, and local control—final report of Intergroup 0114. J Clin Oncol 20:1744-1750, 2002.
84. Meyerhardt JA, Tepper JE, Niedzwiecki D, et al: Impact of body mass index on outcomes and treatment-related toxicity in patients with stage II and III rectal cancer: findings from Intergroup trial 0114. J Clin Oncol 22:648-657, 2004.
85. Meyerhardt JA, Tepper JE, Neidzwiecki D, et al: Impact of hospital procedure volume on surgical operation and long-term outcomes in high risk curatively resected rectal cancer: findings from the Intergroup 0114 study. J Clin Oncol 22:166-174, 2004.
86. Minsky BD, Cohen AM, Enker WE, et al: Combined modality therapy of rectal cancer: decreased acute toxicity with the preoperative approach. J Clin Oncol 10:1218-1224, 1992.
87. Chan AK, Wong A, Jenken DA, et al: Is postoperative adjuvant chemotherapy necessary in locally advanced rectal cancers after preoperative chemoradiation? Int J Radiat Oncol Biol Phys 60:s297, 2004.
88. Bosset JF, Calais G, Mineur L, et al: Does the addition of chemotherapy (CT) to preoperative radiotherapy (preop RT) increase the pathological response in patients with resected rectal cancer: report of the 22921 EORTC phase III trial. Proc ASCO 22:247, 2004.
89. Conroy T, Bonnetain F, Chapet O, et al: Preoperative (preop) radiotherapy (RT) + 5-FU/folinic acid (FA) in T3,4 rectal cancers: preliminary results of the FFCD 9203 randomized trial. Proc ASCO 22:227, 2004.
90. Willett CG, Badizadegan K, Ancukiewicz M, et al: Prognostic factors in stage T3N0 rectal cancer. Do all patients require postoperative pelvic irradiation and chemotherapy? Dis Colon Rectum 42:167-173, 1999.
91. Merchant NB, Guillem JG, Paty PB, et al: T3N0 rectal cancer: results following sharp mesorectal excision and no adjuvant therapy. J Gastrointest Surg 3:642-647, 1999.
92. Graf W, Dahlberg M, Osman MM, et al: Short-term preoperative radiotherapy results in down-staging of rectal cancer: a study of 1316 patients. Radiother Oncol 43:133-137, 1997.
93. Marijnen CAM, Nagtegaal ID, Kranenbarg EK, et al: No downstaging after short-term preoperative radiotherapy in rectal cancer patients. J Clin Oncol 19:1976-1984, 2001.
94. Francois Y, Nemoz CJ, Baulieux J, et al: Influence of the interval between preoperative radiation therapy and surgery on downstaging and on the rate of sphincter-sparing surgery for rectal cancer: the Lyon R90-01 randomized trial. J Clin Oncol 17:2396-2402, 1999.
95. Rouanet P, Saint Aubert B, Lemanski C, et al: Restorative and nonrestorative surgery for low rectal cancer after high dose radiation. Long term oncologic and functional results. Dis Colon Rectum 45:305-315, 2002.
96. Valentini V, Coco C, Cellini N, et al: Preoperative chemoradiation for extraperitoneal T3 rectal cancer: acute toxicity, tumor response and sphincter preservation. Int J Radiat Oncol Biol Phys 40:1067-1075, 1998.

97. Grann A, Feng C, Wong D, et al: Preoperative combined modality therapy for clinically resectable uT3 rectal adenocarcinoma. Int J Radiat Oncol Biol Phys 49:987-995, 2001.
98. Kuvshinoff B, Maghfoor I, Miedema B, et al: Distal margin requirements after preoperative chemoradiotherapy for distal rectal carcinomas: Are < 1 cm distal margins sufficient? Ann Surg Oncol 8:163-169, 2001.
99. Mehta VK, Cho C, Ford JM, et al: Phase II trial of preoperative three-dimensional conformal radiotherapy, protracted venous infusion 5-fluorouracil, and weekly CPT-11, followed by surgery for ultrasound-staged T3 rectal cancer. Int J Radiat Oncol Biol Phys 55:132-137, 2003.
100. Hyams DM, Mamounas EP, Petrelli N, et al: A clinical trial to evaluate the worth of preoperative multimodality therapy in patients with operable carcinoma of the rectum: a progress report of National Surgical Breast and Bowel Project Protocol R-03. Dis Colon Rectum 40:131-139, 1997.
101. Moore HG, Riedel E, Minsky BD, et al: Adequacy of 1-cm distal margin after restorative rectal cancer resection with sharp mesorectal excision and preoperative combined modality therapy. Ann Surg Oncol 10:80-85, 2003.
102. Grumann MM, Noack EM, Hoffman IA, et al: Comparison of quality of life in patients undergoing abdominoperineal extirpation or anterior resection for rectal cancer. Ann Surg 233:149-156, 2001.
103. Kollmorgen CF, Meagher AP, Pemberton JH, et al: The long term effect of adjuvant postoperative chemoradiotherapy for rectal cancer on bowel function. Ann Surg 220:676-682, 1994.
104. Valero G, Lujan JA, Hernandez Q, et al: Neoadjuvant radiation and chemotherapy in rectal cancer does not increase postoperative complications. Int J Colorectal Dis 18:495-499, 2003.
105. Habr-Gama A, de Souza PM, Ribeiro U Jr, et al: Low rectal cancer. Impact of radiation and chemotherapy on surgical treatment. Dis Colon Rectum 41:1087-1096, 1998.
106. Gavioli M, Bagni A, Piccagli I, et al: Usefulness of endorectal ultrasound after preoperative radiotherapy in rectal cancer. Dis Colon Rectum 43:1075-1083, 2000.
107. Barbaro B, Schulsinger A, Valentini V, et al: The accuracy of transrectal ultrasound in predicting the pathological stage of low-lying rectal cancer after preoperative chemoradiation therapy. Int J Radiat Oncol Biol Phys 43:1043-1047, 1999.
108. Hiotis SP, Weber SM, Cohen AM, et al: Assessing the predictive value of clinical complete response to neoadjuvant therapy for rectal cancer: an analysis of 488 patients. J Am Coll Surg 194:131-136, 2002.
109. Guillem JG, Moore HG, Akhurst T, et al: Sequential preoperative fluorodeoxyglucose-positron emission tomography assessment of response to preoperative chemoradiation: a means for determining long-term outcomes of rectal cancer. J Am Coll Surg 199:1-7, 2004.
110. Heriot AG, Hicks RJ, Drummond EGP, et al: Does positron emission tomography change management in primary rectal cancer? A prospective assessment. Dis Colon Rectum 47:451-458, 2004.
111. Pahlman L, Glimelius B: Pre- or postoperative radiotherapy in rectal and rectosigmoid carcinoma. Report from a randomized multicenter trial. Ann Surg 211:187-195, 1990.
112. Roh MS, Colangelo L, Wieand S, et al: Response to preoperative multimodality therapy predicts survival in patients with carcinoma of the rectum. Proc ASCO 22:247, 2004.
113. Bujko K, Nowacki MP, Nasierowska-Guttmejer A, et al: Sphincter preservation following preoperative radiotherapy for rectal cancer: report of a randomized trial comparing short-term radiotherapy versus conventionally fractionated radiochemotherapy. Radiother Oncol 72:15-24, 2004.
114. Cassidy J, Scheithauer W, McKendrick J, et al: Capecitabine (X) versus bolus 5-FU/Leucovorin (LV) as adjuvant therapy for colon cancer (the X-ACT study): efficacy results of a phase III trial. Proc ASCO 22:14, 2004.
115. Andre T, Boni C, Mounedji-Boudiaf L, et al: Oxaliplatin, fluorouracil, and leucovorin as adjuvant treatment for colon cancer. New Engl J Med 350:2343-2351, 2004.
116. Saltz LB, Cox JV, Blanke C, et al: Irinotecan plus fluorouracil and leucovorin for metastatic colorectal cancer. N Engl J Med 343:905-914, 2000.
117. Hurwitz HI, Fehrenbacher L, Novotny W, et al: Bevacizumab plus irinotecan, fluorouracil, and leucovorin for metastatic colorectal cancer. New Engl J Med 350:2335-2342, 2004.
118. Cunningham D, Humblet Y, Siena S, et al: Cetuximab monotherapy and cetuximab plus irinotecan in irinotecan-refractory metastatic colorectal cancer. New Engl J Med 351:337-345, 2004.
119. Fernandez-Martos C, Aparicio J, Bosch C, et al: Preoperative uracil, tegafur, and concomitant radiotherapy in operable rectal cancer: a phase II multicenter study with 3 years follow-up. J Clin Oncol 22:3016-3022, 2004.
120. Gambacorta MA, Valentini V, Morganti AG, et al: Chemoradiation with raltitrexed (Tomudex) in preoperative treatment of stage II-III resectable rectal cancer: a phase II study. Int J Radiat Oncol Biol Phys 60:130-138, 2004.
121. Ryan DP, Niedzwiecki D, Hollis D, et al: A phase I/II study of preoperative oxaliplatin (O), 5-fluorouracil, and external beam radiation therapy (XRT) in locally advanced rectal cancer: CALGB 89901. Proc ASCO 22:260, 2004.
122. Glynne-Jones R, Sebag-Montefiore D, McDonald A, et al: Preliminary phase II SOCRATES study results: capecitabine (CAP) combined with oxaliplatin (OX) and preoperative radiation (RT) in patients (pts) with locally advanced rectal cancer (LARC). Proc ASCO 22:264, 2004.
123. Rödel C, Grabenbauer GG, Papadopoulos T, et al: Phase I/II trial of capecitabine, oxaliplatin, and radiation for rectal cancer. J Clin Oncol 21:3098-3104, 2003.
124. Gerard JP, Chapet O, Nemoz C, et al: Preoperative concurrent chemoradiotherapy in locally advanced rectal cancer with high-dose radiation and oxaliplatin-containing regimen: the Lyon R0-04 phase II trial. J Clin Oncol 21:1119-1124, 2003.
125. Klautke G, Foitzik T, Ludwig K, et al: Intensified neoadjuvant chemoradiotherapy (CRT) with capecitabine and irinotecan in patients with locally advanced rectal cancer (LARC). Proc ASCO 22:293, 2004.
126. Mohiuddin M, Winter K, Mitchell E, et al: Results of RTOG-0012 randomized phase II study of neoadjuvant combined modality chemoradiation for distal rectal cancer. Int J Radiat Oncol Biol Phys 60:s138-s139, 2004.
127. Dupuis O, Vie G, Lledo G, et al: Capecitabine (X) chemoradiation (CRT) in the preoperative treatment of patients (pts) with rectal adenocarcinomas: a phase II GERCOR trial. Proc ASCO 22:255, 2004.
128. Ranson M, Hammond LA, Ferry D, et al: ZD1839, a selective oral epidermal growth factor receptor–tyrosine kinase inhibitor, is well tolerated and active in patients with solid, malignant tumors: results of a phase I trial. J Clin Oncol 20:2240-2250, 2002.
129. Willett CG, Boucher Y, di Tomaso E, et al: Direct evidence that VEGF-specific antibody bevacizumab has antivascular effects in human rectal cancer. Nature Med 10:145-147, 2004.
130. De Paoli A, Chiara S, Luppi G, et al: A phase II study of capecitabine (CAP) and preoperative radiation therapy (RT) in resectable, locally advanced rectal cancer (LARC). Proc ASCO 22:255, 2004.
131. Onaitis MW, Noone RB, Fields R, et al: Complete response to neoadjuvant chemoradiation for rectal cancer does not influence survival. Ann Surg Oncol 8:801-806, 2001.
132. Stein DE, Mahmoud NN, Anne PR, et al: Longer time interval between completion of neoadjuvant chemoradiation and surgical resection does not improve downstaging of rectal carcinoma. Dis Colon Rectum 46:448-453, 2003.
133. Janjan NA, Crane C, Feig BW, et al: Improved overall survival among responders to preoperative chemoradiation for locally advanced rectal cancer. Am J Clin Oncol 24:107-112, 2001.
134. Mohiuddin M, Hayne M, Regine WF, et al: Prognostic significance of postchemoradiation stage following preoperative chemotherapy and radiation for advanced/recurrent rectal cancers. Int J Radiat Oncol Biol Phys 48:1075-1080, 2000.
135. Read TE, Ogunbiyi OA, Fleshman JW, et al: Neoadjuvant external beam radiation and proctectomy for adenocarcinoma of the rectum. Dis Colon Rectum 44:1778-1790, 2001.
136. Garcia-Aguilar J, Hernandez de Anda E, Sirivongs P, et al: A pathologic complete response to preoperative chemoradiation is associated with lower local recurrence and improved survival in

rectal cancer patients treated by mesorectal excision. Dis Colon Rectum 46:298-304, 2003.
137. Ruo L, Tickoo S, Klimstra DS, et al: Long-term prognostic significance of extent of rectal cancer response to preoperative radiation and chemotherapy. Ann Surg 236:75-81, 2002.
138. Valentini V, Coco C, Picciocchi A, et al: Does downstaging predict improved outcome after preoperative chemoradiation for extraperitoneal locally advanced rectal cancer? A long term analysis of 165 patients. Int J Radiat Oncol Biol Phys 53:664-674, 2002.
139. Luna-Perez P, Segura J, Alvarado I, et al: Specific c-K-ras gene mutations as a tumor-response marker in locally advanced rectal cancer treated with preoperative chemoradiotherapy. Ann Surg Oncol 7:727-731, 2000.
140. Villafranca E, Okruzhnov Y, Dominguez MA, et al: Polymorphisms of the repeated sequences in the enhancer region of the thymidylate synthase gene promoter may predict downstaging after preoperative chemoradiation in rectal cancer. J Clin Oncol 19:1779-1786, 2001.
141. Esposito G, Pucciarelli S, Alaggio R, et al: p27kip1 expression is associated with tumor response to preoperative chemoradiotherapy in rectal cancer. Ann Surg Oncol 8:311-318, 2001.
142. Saw RPM, Morgan M, Koorey D, et al: p53, deleted in colorectal cancer gene, and thymidylate synthase as predictors of histopathologic response and survival in low, locally advanced rectal cancer treated with preoperative adjuvant therapy. Dis Colon Rectum 46:192-202, 2003.
143. Rödel C, Grabenbauer GG, Papadopoulos T, et al: Apoptosis as a cellular predictor for histopathologic response to neoadjuvant radiochemotherapy in patients with rectal cancer. Int J Radiat Oncol Biol Phys 52:294-303, 2002.
144. Giralt J, Eraso A, Armengol M, et al: Epidermal growth factor receptor is a predictor of tumor response in locally advanced rectal cancer patients treated with preoperative radiotherapy. Int J Radiat Oncol Biol Phys 54:1460-1465, 2002.
145. Giralt JL, Aranzazu E, Manuel D, et al: Prognostic significance of epidermal growth factor receptor (EGFR) in patients with rectal cancer treated with preoperative radiotherapy: a GICOR study. Int J Radiat Oncol Biol Phys 54:98, 2002.
146. Kandioler D, Zwrtek R, Ludwig C, et al: TP53 genotype but not p53 immunohistochemical result predicts response to preoperative short-term radiotherapy in rectal cancer. Ann Surg 235:493-498, 2002.
147. Adell G, Zhang H, Jansson A, et al: Decreased tumor cell proliferation as an indicator of the effect of preoperative radiotherapy of rectal cancer. Int J Radiat Oncol Biol Phys 50:659-663, 2001.
148. Lavertu S, Schild SE, Gunderson LL, et al: Endocavitary radiation therapy for rectal adenocarcinoma. 10 year results. Am J Clin Oncol 26:508-512, 2003.
149. Rauch P, Bey P, Peiffert D, et al: Factors affecting local control and survival after treatment of carcinoma of the rectum by endocavitary radiation: a retrospective study of 97 cases. Int J Radiat Oncol Biol Phys 49:117-124, 2001.
150. Gerard JP, Romestang P, Ardiet JM, et al: Endocavitary radiation therapy. Semin Radiat Oncol 8:13-23, 1998.
151. Coatmeur O, Truc G, Barillot I, et al: Treatment of T1-T2 rectal tumors by contact therapy and interstitial brachytherapy. Radiother Oncol 70:177-182, 2004.
152. Aumock A, Birnbaum EH, Fleshman JW, et al: Treatment of rectal adenocarcinoma with endocavitary and external beam radiotherapy: results for 199 patients with localized tumors. Int J Radiat Oncol Biol Phys 51:363-370, 2001.
153. Myerson RJ: Conservative alternatives to radical surgery for favorable rectal cancers. Ann Ital Chir 72:605-609, 2001.
154. Hull TL, Lavery IC, Saxton JP: Endocavitary irradiation. An option in select patients with rectal cancer. Dis Colon Rectum 37:1266-1270, 1994.
155. Maingon P, Guerif S, Darsouni R, et al: Conservative management of rectal adenocarcinoma by radiotherapy. Int J Radiat Oncol Biol Phys 40:1077-1085, 1998.
156. Gerard JP, Ayzac L, Coquard R, et al: Endocavitary irradiation for early rectal carcinomas T1 (T2). A series of 101 patients treated with the Papillon's technique. Int J Radiat Oncol Biol Phys 34:775-783, 1996.
157. Minsky BD, Mies C, Rich TA, et al: Lymphatic vessel invasion is an independent prognostic factor for survival in colorectal cancer. Int J Radiat Oncol Biol Phys 17:311-318, 1989.
158. Neary PC, Makin GB, White TJ, et al: Transanal endoscopic microsurgery: a viable operative alternative in selected patients with rectal lesions. Ann Surg Oncol 10:1106-1111, 2003.
159. Willett CG: Local excision followed by postoperative radiation therapy. Semin Radiat Oncol 8:24-29, 1998.
160. Mendenhall WM, Rout WR, Vauthey JN, et al: Conservative treatment of rectal adenocarcinoma with endocavitary irradiation or wide local excision and postoperative irradiation. J Clin Oncol 15:3241-3248, 1997.
161. Bleday R, Breen E, Jessup JM, et al: Prospective evaluation of local excision for small rectal cancers. Dis Colon Rectum 40:388-392, 1997.
162. Ota DM, Skibber J, Rich TA: M.D. Anderson Cancer Center experience with local excision and multimodality therapy for rectal cancer. Surg Oncol Clin N Am 1:147-152, 1992.
163. Rosenthal SA, Yeung RS, Weese JL, et al: Conservative management of extensive low-lying rectal carcinomas with transanal local excision and combined preoperative and postoperative radiation therapy: report of a phase I/II trial. Cancer 69:335-341, 1992.
164. Chakravarti A, Compton CC, Shellito PC, et al: Long-term follow-up of patients with rectal cancer managed by local excision with and without adjuvant irradiation. Ann Surg 230:49-54, 1999.
165. Valentini V, Morganti AG, De Santis M, et al: Local excision and external beam radiotherapy in early rectal cancer. Int J Radiat Oncol Biol Phys 35:759-764, 1996.
166. Fortunato L, Ahmad NR, Yeung RS, et al: Long-term follow-up of local excision and radiation therapy for invasive rectal cancer. Dis Colon Rectum 38:1193-1199, 1995.
167. Russell AH, Harris J, Rosenberg PJ, et al: Anal sphincter conservation for patients with adenocarcinoma of the distal rectum: long-term results of Radiation Therapy Oncology Group protocol 89-02. Int J Radiat Oncol Biol Phys 46:313-322, 2000.
168. Wagman RT, Minsky BD: Conservative management of rectal cancer with local excision and adjuvant therapy. Oncology 15:513-524, 2001.
169. Taylor RH, Hay JH, Larsson SN: Transanal local excision of selected low rectal cancers. Am J Surg 175:360-363, 1998.
170. Benson R, Wong CS, Cummings BJ, et al: Local excision and postoperative radiotherapy for distal rectal cancer. Int J Radiat Oncol Biol Phys 50:1309-1316, 2001.
171. Schell SR, Zlotecki RA, Mendenhall WM, et al: Transanal excision of locally advanced rectal cancers downstaged using neoadjuvant chemoradiotherapy. J Am Coll Surg 194:584-591, 2002.
172. Kim CJ, Yeatman TJ, Coppola D, et al: Local excision of T2 and T3 rectal cancers after downstaging chemoradiation. Ann Surg 234:352-358, 2001.
173. Lezoche E, Guerrieri M, Paganini AM, et al: Long-term results of patients with pT2 rectal cancer treated with radiotherapy and transanal endoscopic microsurgical excision. World J Surg 26:1170-1174, 2002.
174. Bonnen M, Crane C, Vauthey JN, et al: Long-term results using local excision after preoperative chemoradiation among selected T3 rectal cancer patients. Int J Radiat Oncol Biol Phys 60:1098-1105, 2004.
175. Ruo L, Guillem JG, Minsky BD, et al: Preoperative radiation with or without chemotherapy and full-thickness transanal excision for selected T2 and T3 distal rectal cancers. Int J Colorectal Dis 17:54-58, 2002.
176. Ahmad NR, Nagle DA: Preoperative radiation therapy followed by local excision. Semin Radiat Oncol 8:36-38, 1998.
177. Rödel C, Fietkau R, Raab R, et al: Tumor regression grading as a prognostic factor in patients with locally advanced rectal cancer treated with preoperative radiochemotherapy. Int J Radiat Oncol Biol Phys 60:s140, 2004.
178. Read TE, Andujar JE, Caushaj FP, et al: Neoadjuvant therapy for rectal cancer: histologic response of the primary tumor predicts nodal status. Dis Colon Rectum 47:825-831, 2004.
179. Vecchio FM, Valentini V, Minsky B, et al: The relationship of pathologic tumor regression grade (trg) and outcome after pre-

operative therapy in rectal cancer. Int J Radiat Oncol Biol Phys 2005 (in press).
180. Kallinowski F, Eble MJ, Buhr HJ, et al: Intraoperative radiotherapy for primary and recurrent rectal cancers. Eur J Surg Oncol 21:191-194, 1995.
181. Kim NK, Kim MJ, Yun SH, et al: Comparative study of transrectal ultrasonography, pelvic computerized tomography, and magnetic resonance imaging in preoperative staging of rectal cancer. Dis Colon Rectum 42:770-775, 1999.
182. Jimenez A, Shoup M, Cohen AM, et al: Contemporary outcomes of total pelvic exenteration in the treatment of colorectal carcinoma. Dis Colon Rectum 46:1619-1625, 2004.
183. Law WL, Chu KW, Choi HK: Total pelvic exenteration for locally advanced rectal cancer. J Am Coll Surg 190:78-83, 2004.
184. Goldberg JM, Piver MS, Hempling RE, et al: Improvements in pelvic exenteration: factors responsible for reducing morbidity and mortality. Ann Surg Oncol 5:399-406, 1998.
185. Reerink O, Verschueren RCJ, Szabo BG, et al: A favourable pathological stage after neoadjuvant radiochemotherapy in patients with initially irresectable rectal cancer correlates with a favorable prognosis. Eur J Cancer 39:192-195, 2003.
186. Willett CG, Shellito PC, Rodkey GV, et al: Preoperative irradiation for tethered rectal carcinoma. Radiother Oncol 21:141-142, 1991.
187. Tobin RL, Mohiuddin M, Marks G: Preoperative irradiation for cancer of the rectum with extrarectal fixation. Int J Radiat Oncol Biol Phys 21:1127-1132, 1991.
188. Strassmann G, Walter S, Kolotas C, et al: Reconstruction and navigation system for intraoperative brachytherapy using the flab technique for colorectal tumor bed irradiation. Int J Radiat Oncol Biol Phys 47:1323-1329, 2000.
189. Alekitar KM, Zelefsky MJ, Paty PB, et al: High dose rate intraoperative brachytherapy for recurrent colorectal cancer. Int J Radiat Oncol Biol Phys 48:219-226, 2000.
190. Nuyttens JJ, Kolkman-Deurloo IKK, Vermess M, et al: High dose intraoperative radiotherapy for close or positive margins in patients with locally advanced or recurrent rectal cancer. Int J Radiat Oncol Biol Phys 58:106-112, 2004.
191. Mannaerts GHH, Rutten HJT, Martijn H, et al: Effects on functional outcome after IORT-containing multimodality treatment for locally advanced primary and locally recurrent rectal cancer. Int J Radiat Oncol Biol Phys 54:1082-1088, 2002.
192. Azinovic I, Calvo FA, Puebla F, et al: Long-term normal tissue effects of intraoperative electron radiation therapy (IOERT): late sequelae, tumor recurrence, and second malignancies. Int J Radiat Oncol Biol Phys 49:597-604, 2001.
193. Shibata D, Guillem JG, Lanouette NM, et al: Functional and quality of life outcomes in patients with rectal cancer after combined modality therapy, intraoperative radiation therapy, and sphincter preservation. Dis Colon Rectum 43:752-758, 2000.
194. Nakfoor BM, Willett CG, Shellito PC, et al: The impact of 5-fluorouracil and intraoperative electron beam radiation therapy on the outcome of patients with locally advanced primary rectal and rectosigmoid cancer. Ann Surg 228:194-200, 1998.
195. Gunderson LL, Nelson H, Martenson JA, et al: Locally advanced primary colorectal cancer: intraoperative electron and external beam irradiation + 5-FU. Int J Radiat Oncol Biol Phys 37:601-614, 1997.
196. Harrison LB, Minsky BD, Enker WE, et al: High dose rate intraoperative radiation therapy (HDR-IORT) as part of the management strategy for locally advanced primary and recurrent rectal cancer. Int J Radiat Oncol Biol Phys 42:325-330, 1998.
197. Huber FT, Stepan R, Zimmermann F, et al: Locally advanced rectal cancer: resection and intraoperative radiotherapy using the flab method combined with preoperative or postoperative radiochemotherapy. Dis Colon Rectum 39:774-779, 1996.
198. Mannaerts GHH, Rutten HJT, Martijn H, et al: Comparison of intraoperative radiation therapy-containing multimodality treatment with historical treatment modalities for locally recurrent rectal cancer. Dis Colon Rectum 44:1749-1758, 2001.
199. Willett CG, Nakfoor BM, Daley W, et al: Pathologic downstaging does not guide the need for IORT in primary locally advanced rectal cancer. Front Radiat Ther Oncol 31:245-256, 1997.
200. Lindel K, Willett CG, Shellito PC, et al: Intraoperative radiation therapy for locally advanced recurrent rectal or rectosigmoid cancer. Radiother Oncol 58:83-87, 2001.
201. Gagliardi G, Hawley PR, Hershman MJ, et al: Prognostic factors in surgery for local recurrence of rectal cancer. Br J Surg 82:1401-1405, 1995.
202. Bagatzounis A, Kölbl O, Muller G, et al: The locoregional recurrence of rectal carcinoma. A computed tomographic analysis and a target volume concept for adjuvant radiotherapy. Strahlenther Onkol 173:68-75, 1997.
203. Suzuki K, Gunderson LL, Devine RM, et al: Intraoperative irradiation after palliative surgery for locally recurrent rectal cancer. Cancer 75:939-952, 1995.
204. Valentini V, Morganti AG, De Franco A, et al: Chemoradiation with or without intraoperative radiation therapy in patients with locally recurrent rectal carcinoma. Prognostic factors and long term outcome. Cancer 86:2612-2624, 1999.
205. Sanfilippo NJ, Crane CH, Skibber J, et al: T4 rectal cancer treated with preoperative chemoradiation to the posterior pelvis followed by multivisceral resection: patterns of failure and limitations of treatment. Int J Radiat Oncol Biol Phys 51:176-183, 2001.
206. Wiig JN, Tveit KM, Poulsen JP, et al: Preoperative irradiation and surgery for recurrent rectal cancer. Will intraoperative radiotherapy (IORT) be of additional benefit? Radiother Oncol 62:207-213, 2002.
207. Mohiuddin M, Marks G, Marks J: Long-term results of reirradiation for patients with recurrent rectal carcinoma. Cancer 95: 1144-1150, 2002.
208. Gambacorta MA, Valentini V, Mohiuddin M, et al: Preoperative hyperfractionated chemoradiation of locally recurrent rectal cancer in patients previously irradiated on the pelvis: a multicentric phase I-II trial. Int J Radiat Oncol Biol Phys 57:S385, 2003.
209. Haddock MG, Gunderson LL, Nelson H, et al: Intraoperative irradiation for locally recurrent coloredal cancer in previously irradiated patients. Int J Radiat Oncol Biol Phys 49:1267-1274, 2001.
210. Myerson RJ, Walz BJ, Kodner IJ, et al: Endocavitary radiation therapy for rectal cancer: Results with and without external beam. Endocurie Hypertherm Oncol 5:195-200, 1989.
211. Horiot JC, Roth SL, Calais G, et al: The Dijon clinical staging system for early rectal carcinomas amenable to intracavitary treatment techniques. Radiother Oncol 18:329-337, 1990.
212. Gerard JP, Chapet O, Ramaioli A, et al: Long-term control of T2-T3 rectal adenocarcinoma with radiotherapy alone. Int J Radiat Oncol Biol Phys 54:142-149, 2002.
213. Brierley JD, Cummings BJ, Wong CS, et al: Adenocarcinoma of the rectum treated by radical external radiation therapy. Int J Radiat Oncol Biol Phys 31:255-259, 1995.
214. Crane CH, Janjan NA, Abbruzzese JL, et al: Effective pelvic symptom control using initial chemoradiation without colostomy in metastatic rectal cancer. Int J Radiat Oncol Biol Phys 49:107-116, 2001.
215. Liberman H, Adams DR, Blatchford GJ, et al: Clinical use of the self-expanding metallic stent in the management of colorectal cancer. Am J Surg 180:407-412, 2001.
216. Hruby G, Barton M, Miles S: Sites of local recurrence after surgery, with or without chemotherapy, for rectal cancer: implications for radiotherapy field design. Int J Radiat Oncol Biol Phys 55:138-143, 2003.
217. Hocht S, Hammad R, Thiel H: A multicenter analysis of 123 patients with recurrent rectal cancer within the pelvis. Front Radiat Ther Oncol 38:41-51, 2004.
218. Tait DM, Nahum AE, Meyer LC, et al: Acute toxicity in pelvic radiotherapy: a randomised trial of conformal versus conventional treatment. Radiother Oncol 42:121-136, 1997.
219. Myerson RJ, Valentini V, Birnbaum EH, et al: A phase I/II trial of three-dimensionally planned concurrent boost radiotherapy and protracted venous infusion of 5-FU chemotherapy for locally advanced rectal carcinoma. Int J Radiat Oncol Biol Phys 50:1299-1308, 2001.
220. Koelbl O, Vordermark D, Flentje M: The relationship between belly board position and patient anatomy and its influence on dose-volume histogram of small bowel for postoperative radiotherapy of rectal cancer. Radiother Oncol 67:345-349, 2003.

221. Duthoy W, De Gersem W, Vergote K, et al: Clinical implementation of intensity-modulated arc therapy (IMAT) for rectal cancer. Int J Radiat Oncol Biol Phys 60:794-806, 2004.
222. Patel S, Vuong T, Ballivy O, et al: Phase II trial of pelvic intensity-modulated radiotherapy (IMRT) with concurrent chemotherapy for patients with rectal cancer. Int J Radiat Oncol Biol Phys 60:s424-s425, 2004.
223. Withers HR, Peters LJ, Taylor JM: Dose-response relationship for radiation therapy of subclinical disease. Int J Radiat Oncol Biol Phys 31:353-359, 1995.
224. De Neve W, Martijn H, Lybeert MM, et al: Incompletely resected rectum, rectosigmoid, or sigmoid carcinoma: results of postoperative radiotherapy and prognostic factors. Int J Radiat Oncol Biol Phys 21:1297-1302, 1991.
225. Miller RC, Sargent DJ, Martenson JA, et al: Acute diarrhea during adjuvant therapy for rectal cancer: a detailed analysis from a randomized Intergroup trial. Int J Radiat Oncol Biol Phys 54:409-413, 2002.
226. Gunderson LL, Russell AH, Llewellyn HJ, et al: Treatment planning for colorectal cancer: radiation and surgical techniques and value of small-bowel films. Int J Radiat Oncol Biol Phys 11:1379-1393, 1985.
227. National Comprehensive Cancer Network: Rectal cancer—clinical practice guidelines in oncology, vol. 2, 2006. http://www.nccn.org/professional/physicion_gLS/PDF/rectal.pdf
228. Kwok H, Bissett IP, Hill GL: Preoperative staging of rectal cancer. Int J Colorectal Dis 15:9-20, 2000.
229. Mitchell EP, Winter K, Mohiuddin M, et al: Randomized phase II trial of preoperative combined modality chemoradiation for distal rectal cancer. Proc ASCO 22:254, 2004.
230. Aschele C, Friso ML, Pucciarelli S, et al: A phase I-II study of weekly oxaliplatin (OXA), 5-fluorouracil (FU), continuous infusion (CI) and preoperative radiotherapy (RT) in locally advanced rectal cancer (LARC). Proc ASCO 21:132a, 2002.
231. Takahashi T, Ueno M, Azekura K: Lateral node dissection and total mesorectal excision for rectal cancer. Dis Colon Rectum 43:S59-S63, 2000.
232. Steele GD, Herndon JE, Bleday R, et al: Sphincter-sparing treatment for distal rectal adenocarcinoma. Ann Surg Oncol 6:433-441, 1999.
233. Kim HK, Jessup JM, Beard CJ, et al: Locally advanced rectal carcinoma: pelvic control and morbidity following preoperative radiation therapy, resection, and intraoperative radiation therapy. Int J Radiat Oncol Biol Phys 38:777-783, 1997.
234. Gunderson LL, Nelson H, Martenson J, et al: Intraoperative electron and external beam irradiation with or without 5-fluorouracil and maximun surgical resection for previously unirradiated locally recurrent colorectal cancer. Dis Colon Rectum 39:1379-1395, 1996.
235. Lowy AM, Rich TA, Skibber JM, et al: Preoperative infusional chemoradiation, selective intraoperative radiation, and resection for locally advanced pelvic recurrence of colorectal adenocarcinoma. Ann Surg 223:177-185, 1996.
236. Bussieres E, Gilly FN, Rouanet P, et al: Recurrences of rectal cancers: results of a multimodal approach with intraoperative radiation therapy. Int J Radiat Oncol Biol Phys 34:49-56, 1996.
237. Eble MJ, Lehnert T, Treiber M, et al: Moderate dose intraoperative and external beam radiotherapy for locally recurrent rectal carcinoma. Radiother Oncol 49:169-174, 1998.
238. Taylor N, Crane C, Skibber J, et al: Elective groin irradiation is not indicated for patients with adenocarcinoma of the rectum extending to the anal canal. Int J Radiat Oncol Biol Phys 51:741-747, 2001.
239. Sigmon WR, Randall ME, Olds WE, et al: Increased chronic bowel complications with split-course pelvic irradiation. Int J Radiat Oncol Biol Phys 28:349-353, 1993.
240. Hoffman JP, Sigurdson ER, Eisenberg BL: Use of saline-filled expanders to protect the small bowel from radiation. Oncology 12:51-54, 1998.
241. Tuech JJ, Chaudron V, Thoma V, et al: Prevention of radiation enteritis by intrapelvic breast prosthesis. Eur J Surg Oncol 30:900-904, 2004.
242. Chen JS, Chang Chien CR, Wang JY, et al: Pelvic peritoneal reconstruction to prevent radiation enteritis in rectal carcinoma. Dis Colon Rectum 35:897-903, 1992.
243. Talley NA, Chen F, King D, et al: Short-chain fatty acid in the treatment of radiation proctitis. A randomized, double-blind, placebo-controlled, cross-over pilot trial. Dis Colon Rectum 40:1046-1050, 1997.
244. O'Brien PC, Franklin CI, Poulsen M, et al: Acute symptoms, not rectally administered sucralfate, predict for late radiation proctitis: longer term follow-up of a phase III trial—Trans-Tasman Radiation Oncology Group. Int J Radiat Oncol Biol Phys 54:442-449, 2002.
245. Resbeut M, Marteau P, Cowen D, et al: A randomized double blind placebo controlled multicenter study of mesalazine for the prevention of acute radiation enteritis. Radiother Oncol 44:59, 1997.
246. Jahraus CD, Bettenhausen D, Sellitti M, et al: Randomized double-blind placebo controlled trial of balsalazide in the prevention of acute radiation enteritis as a consequence of pelvic radiotherapy. Int J Radiat Oncol Biol Phys 60:s253-s254, 2004.
247. Antonadou D, Athanassiou H, Sarris N, et al: Final results of a randomized phase III trial of chemoradiation treatment + amifostine in patients with colorectal cancer: Clinical Radiation Oncology Hellenic Group. Int J Radiat Oncol Biol Phys 60:s140-s141, 2004.
248. Ben-Joseph E, Han S, Tobi M, et al: A pilot study of topical intrarectal application of amifostine for prevention of late radiation rectal injury. Int J Radiat Oncol Biol Phys 53:1160-1164, 2002.
249. Borilis-Wassif S, Longenhorst BL, Hap WCJ: The contribution of preoperative radiotherapy in the management of borderline operability rectal cancer. *In* Jones SE, Lamon SE (eds): Adjuvant Therapy of Cancer II. New York, gune and stratton, 1974, pp 613-628.
250. Gerard A, Buyse M, Nordlinger B, et al: Preoperative radiotherapy as adjuvant treatment in rectal carcinoma. Ann Surg 108:606-614, 1988.
251. Treit KM, Guldrog I, Hagen S, et al: Randomized controlled trial of postoperative radiotherapy and short-tem time-scheduled 5-fluorouracil against surgery alone in the treatment of Dukes B and C rectal cancer. Am J Surg 84:1130-1135, 1997.
252. Wolmark N, Wieard JS, Hyams AM, et al: Randomized trial of postoperative adjuvant chemotherapy with or without radiotherapy for carcinoma of the rectum: National Surgical Adjuvant Breast and Bowel Protocol R-02. J Natl Cancer Inst 92:388-396, 2002.

CHAPTER 49

ANAL CARCINOMA

Michael G. Haddock and James A. Martenson

INCIDENCE

An estimated 4660 new cases of anal cancer will be diagnosed in the United States in 2006 (1910 in men and 2750 in women). The expected number of deaths is 660.

BIOLOGIC CHARACTERISTICS

Prognostic factors predictive for local control and survival are size and extent of the primary tumor and status of the regional lymph nodes.

STAGING EVALUATION

Staging should generally include a complete history and physical examination, anoscopy with biopsy, complete blood cell count, liver function tests, serum creatinine, chest radiograph, and computed tomography of the abdomen and pelvis.

Endoscopic ultrasound may be used to evaluate the depth of invasion.

PRIMARY THERAPY

Radiotherapy and concomitant chemotherapy are appropriate treatment for most patients with anal cancer. Five-year survival ranges from 65% to 80%.

Local control with anal preservation is achieved in more than 95% of patients with tumors less than 2 cm in size and in 60% to 75% of those with larger tumors.

ADJUVANT THERAPY

For those rare patients who are managed initially with abdominoperineal resection, adjuvant radiotherapy and chemotherapy are indicated in those with primary tumor extension beyond the anal sphincter or metastases to regional lymph nodes.

As many as 60% of patients with persistent or recurrent local disease after radiotherapy and chemotherapy may still be cured with abdominoperineal resection.

LOCALLY ADVANCED DISEASE

Radiotherapy and chemotherapy are effective in patients with large primary cancers with or without invasion of adjacent organs. Two thirds of patients with locally advanced primary tumors maintain a functional anus.

Patients with positive nodes have a 5-year survival of 50% to 60%.

PALLIATION

Palliative chemotherapy with 5-fluorouracil and mitomycin C in patients with metastatic disease is associated with a 50% response rate.

Brain and osseous metastases may be effectively palliated with hypofractionated radiotherapy.

Carcinoma of the anal canal accounts for about 1.5% of all malignancies of the digestive system in patients in the United States.[1] Despite the rarity of anal cancer, it is a model for successful oncology research, both in the laboratory and in the clinic. Epidemiologic observations about the increased incidence of anal cancer in some populations, along with advances in molecular biology that have allowed the identification of human papillomavirus (HPV) DNA in most anal tumors, have provided the initial clues to the mechanism of anal carcinogenesis. Retrospective studies have provided important information about the natural history and patterns of spread of anal cancer, as well as hypotheses to test in prospective trials. Prospective randomized trials have been completed successfully and have led to the adoption of a combination of radiotherapy and chemotherapy as the standard of care for patients with anal cancer. Yet, questions remain about the most effective and least toxic regimens of radiotherapy and chemotherapy.

This chapter focuses on the biology of anal cancer, the rationale for patient evaluation, treatment recommendations, and results of treatment. Radiotherapy techniques for patients with anal cancer will also be discussed.

ETIOLOGY AND EPIDEMIOLOGY

Anal cancer occurs much less frequently than other types of cancer of the digestive tract. It accounts for only 2% to 4% of all cancers of the anus or rectum.[2-5] In the United States, the annual incidence is 0.47 per 100,000 white men and 0.69 per 100,000 white women.[6] The annual incidence among African Americans is higher: 0.57 per 100,000 men and 0.78 per 100,000 women.[6] Overall, 87% of patients diagnosed with anal cancer are non-Hispanic whites, 5% are African American, and 3% are Hispanic.[7] The median age at diagnosis is 62 years.[7] Thus, the typical U.S. patient with anal cancer is a white woman in her seventh decade of life. An estimated 4660 new cases of anal cancer will be diagnosed in 2006 (1910 men, 2750 women), with an estimated 660 deaths (220 men, 440 women).[1]

Epidemiologic studies from Europe and the United States have reported an increased incidence of anal cancer in the past 30 to 40 years. Since 1960, the incidence of anal cancer in Connecticut has doubled in both men and women.[6] Between 1974 and 1985, the number of patients in Sweden diagnosed with anal cancer increased 4% per year, an increase similar to that reported for Swedish patients with malignant melanoma.[5] Similarly, the number of new cases of anal cancer in Denmark has doubled in men and tripled in women.[8]

The incidence of anal cancer is higher in urban than in rural populations, and increases in the incidence of anal cancer have been greater in urban than in rural populations.[5,6,8] In the United States, the increased incidence of anal cancer has been limited solely to densely populated regions. Young men account for a substantial proportion of this increase. In Denmark, the median age at diagnosis in men has decreased from 68 to 63 years, whereas in women, it has remained constant at 66 to 67 years.[8]

Association with Human Immunodeficiency Virus Infection

At least part of the increased incidence in young men can be explained by the observation that young homosexual men are at increased risk for the development of anal cancer, irrespective of their human immunodeficiency virus (HIV) status. Increased risk for anal cancer among never-married men, a surrogate marker for homosexuality,[6] has been noted in several epidemiologic studies.[9-12] In addition, men with anal cancer are more likely to never have married compared with control subjects who have stomach or colon cancer.[6,8] In most areas of the world, anal cancer is more common in women than in men of all age groups.[13,14] However, in areas with a relatively high proportion of homosexual men, anal cancer may be more common in men. In San Francisco, for example, the incidence of anal cancer in white men more than doubled from 0.53 per 100,000 in 1975 to 1.2 per 100,000 in 1989,[6] and in Los Angeles, anal cancer has become more common in men than in women under age 35.[9] A study of Danish homosexual men living in legally registered "marriage-like partnerships" identified an incidence of cancer double what was expected, which could be accounted for by HIV-related cancers, including Kaposi's sarcoma, non-Hodgkin's lymphoma, and anal cancer. The relative risk (RR) of anal cancer in this population was 31, and anal cancer appeared to be associated with a positive HIV status.[15]

The incidence of anal cancer is markedly increased in both men and women who have the acquired immunodeficiency syndrome (AIDS). The RR estimated from a linkage analysis of cancer registries and AIDS registries is 63, and it is higher for homosexual men (RR, 84) than for heterosexual men (RR, 38). The increased risk is also apparent during the 5-year period before an AIDS diagnosis. The absolute risk of anal cancer in AIDS patients is 1 per 1000.[16]

Risk Factors

The pathogenesis of anal cancer is multifactorial. A diagnosis of anal cancer represents the result of an interplay of multiple environmental and host factors. Patients with epidermoid anal cancer are more likely than control patients to have had a previous diagnosis of malignancy, including cancers of the vulva, vagina, or cervix and lymphoma or leukemia. Patients with anal cancer who are diagnosed before age 60 are at higher risk of subsequent development of malignancies of the respiratory system, bladder, vulva, vagina, and breast, but they are not at increased risk for subsequent development of colon or rectal cancers.[17] Overexpression of the *c-myc* oncogene has been implicated in the pathogenesis of both anal squamous cell neoplasia and breast cancer.[18,19] This finding, along with an observed pattern of second malignancies and prior malignancies in patients with anal cancer, suggests a multifactorial pathogenesis and common oncogenetic risk factors. These factors may include sexually transmitted viruses, environmental carcinogens such as cigarette smoke, immunosuppression, and genetic susceptibility.[17]

Anal cancer and cancers of the female genital tract share a common pathogenesis.[20] Embryologically, the anal and cervical canals are both derived from closely related anlagen.[21] Women patients with anal cancer are more likely than women with colon or stomach cancer to have had a prior diagnosis of cervical intraepithelial neoplasia.[20] An association between anal cancer and the number of lifetime sexual partners has been reported in women.[22] Case-control studies have also found an association between anal cancer and some sexually transmitted diseases.[13,22-24] This association, along with the increased incidence in young homosexual men, strongly suggests an etiologic factor for anal cancer associated with increased sexual activity.[6]

Among sexually transmittable infectious agents, HPV has been the most thoroughly studied potential causative agent. Although there are more than 60 types of HPV, those most commonly associated with benign genital condylomata acuminata are HPV 6 and HPV 11, whereas HPV 16, 18, 31, 33, and 35 are associated with malignancy or high-grade dysplasia.[25] Several investigators have also reported an association between genital warts and anal cancer in men and women.[23-27] The development of anal warts in both sexes has been linked with the practice of anal intercourse.[24]

The likelihood of finding HPV DNA in specimens of anal cancer varies according to patient demographics and laboratory technique. Patients with HPV-associated anal cancer are 10 years younger on average than are patients with reportedly HPV-negative cancers.[28] In addition, HPV-associated anal cancer has been reported more frequently in Europe and South America than in South Africa and India.[29] When in situ hybridization techniques are used to analyze biopsy specimens of anal cancer, the rate of HPV DNA detection ranges from 17% to 73%.[25,28] HPV DNA is more likely to be detected with polymerase chain reaction analysis. Studies comparing both techniques have found that polymerase chain reaction techniques detect HPV DNA in 78% to 85% of patients, whereas in situ hybridization techniques find HPV DNA in only 17% to 50% of the same patients.[25,30]

Exposure to HPV may be a risk factor even for patients in whom HPV DNA is not detected in the carcinoma specimen. Serum IgA antibodies to a peptide antigen from the E2 region of HPV 16 have been found in 89% of patients with anal cancer compared with only 24% of controls.[28] In another study, antibodies to HPV 16 capsids were elevated in 55% of patients with anal cancer compared with 3% of controls. Antibodies to HPV-capsid antigen were detected in an equal number of cancer specimens from patients whose HPV DNA was negative or positive (as assessed by in situ hybridization), which suggests that some presumed HPV-negative patients had been exposed to HPV.[31]

HPV infection and anal cytologic abnormalities are common in patients with HIV infection.[32] HIV-positive patients with HPV DNA found in anal biopsy specimens seem to have a high rate of cytologic abnormalities. In one study of 12 HIV-positive patients without AIDS, 11 patients (92%) with normal cytologic findings but with HPV DNA found in anal mucosa later had cytologic abnormalities at 17-month follow-up.[33] Many AIDS patients most likely die of opportunistic infections before anal cancer is manifested. Although the impact of effective antiretroviral therapy on the incidence of anal cancer is not yet clear,[34] further increases in the incidence of anal cancer may be observed in AIDS patients as survival time is prolonged.[32]

Although the true influence of HPV in anal carcinogenesis is uncertain, some laboratory findings point to the involvement of the HPV E6 and E7 proteins. These findings include the observation that the *E6* and *E7* oncogenes are consistently expressed in tumor cells but that normal E6 and E7 regulatory mechanisms are absent.[35] In addition, the E7 protein of HPV 16, in cooperation with the E6 protein, is able to transform mammalian cells in vitro while blocking *E6* and *E7* gene function, which results in reversal of the malignant phenotype.[35-37] Interactions of HPV oncoproteins with known tumor suppressor gene products have been reported. The E6 protein of HPV 16 and HPV 18 forms stable complexes with the p53 protein product of the *TP53* tumor suppressor gene.[38-40] The cellular p53–E6 protein complex results in a lack of appropriate G1 arrest and subsequent genomic instability. The E7 protein also forms complexes with the retinoblastoma gene product and with p107, p130, p33, cdk2, and cyclin A. E7 also activates the cyclin-A promoter and overrides two inhibitory functions that restrict the expression of cyclin A and cyclin E36.

Some evidence suggests that infectious agents other than HPV may contribute to anal carcinogenesis. Associations have been found between the development of anal cancer and a history of syphilis or gonorrhea in men[12,23] and between anal cancer and chlamydia and herpes simplex virus type 2 in both sexes.[22,24] In a study of patients in and around San Francisco, herpes simplex virus DNA was detected in 3 of 15 patients with invasive anal cancer and in 3 of 4 patients with high-grade intraepithelial neoplasia.[30] No Epstein-Barr virus or cytomegalovirus DNA was found in the tumor specimens of the 15 patients with anal cancer. Further studies are needed to determine whether these and other sexually transmitted agents are involved in anal oncogenesis or are merely surrogate markers for probable HPV infection.

Chronic immunosuppression is associated with an increased risk for anal malignancy. Renal transplant recipients have an increased incidence (as high as 100-fold) of carcinoma of the vulva or anus.[41,42] These cancers occur at an earlier age than they do in the general population.[41] Renal transplant patients also have an increased incidence of cutaneous neoplasia and viral warts. Those with a high susceptibility to cutaneous malignancy (four or more skin cancers) are more likely to have HPV DNA–associated skin cancer and are more likely to have an anogenital malignancy.[43] The increased incidence of anal malignancy in HIV-positive patients is most likely caused in part by chronic immunosuppression.

A number of authors have reported an association between anal cancer and cigarette smoking.[22,24,26,44] When compared with a control group of patients with colon cancer, both men and women smokers were found to have an increased risk of anal cancer.[24] In a population-based case-control study of patients with anogenital cancers in the Pacific Northwest, 60% of patients with newly diagnosed anal cancer were current smokers compared with 25% of the controls. The risk of anal cancer was positively correlated with both the number of cigarettes smoked per day and the number of years the patient had been a smoker.[44]

An association between anal cancer and benign anal conditions (e.g., hemorrhoids, anal fissure, or fistula) has been reported frequently,[14,45] and chronic irritation or inflammation of the anal tissue has been assumed to play a role in anal carcinogenesis.[26] In a Danish population-based study, patients with anal fissure, fistula, perianal abscess, or hemorrhoids were found to be at increased risk for anal cancer. However, the RR for invasive anal cancer was highest in the year immediately after a diagnosis of benign anal pathology, and it declined from a high of 12 the first year to 1.8 after 5 or more years, suggesting that a so-called benign anal condition is often a symptom rather than a cause of anal cancer.[46] Supporting evidence for this view is found in a study of patients treated for benign anal conditions at U.S. Veterans Affairs hospitals. The elevated RR for anal cancer in these patients was most pronounced in the first year after the benign pathologic condition was diagnosed, and it decreased rapidly thereafter until there was no increased risk of anal cancer between year 5 and year 22.[47]

PREVENTION AND EARLY DETECTION

Prevention of anal cancer should include educational efforts about the causal link of sexually transmitted HPV infection with malignancies of the anogenital tract. Recommendations of the 1996 National Institutes of Health Consensus Panel on cervical cancer prevention are also applicable to anal cancer and include encouragement to delay onset of sexual intercourse.[48] Barrier methods, such as condoms, do not prevent HPV transmission.[49] The panel also recommended development of an effective vaccine to prevent transmission of HPV, and a subsequent phase 3 clinical trial provided encouraging results in this regard.[50] Additional preventive efforts should be focused on the treatment of HPV infection, including the development of antiviral agents, targeting of E6 and E7 to block transforming activities, and vaccines to prevent progression of HPV infection.[48] Education is also required about the causal role of cigarette smoking in anal and other cancers.

Because of the rarity of anal cancer, efforts at early detection through widespread screening are not feasible. However, screening may be feasible in certain high-risk subsets. Anal intraepithelial neoplasia is a common finding in HPV-infected persons.[32,33] Analogous to the situation with cervical cancer, where cervical squamous intraepithelial lesions may progress to cervical carcinoma, high-grade squamous intraepithelial lesions (HSILs) may be a precursor to invasive anal cancer.[51-53] Anal cytologic smears have been used to diagnose HSILs in high-risk patients. Because the specificity of anal cytology for the detection of HSILs is low, anoscopy with biopsy is required to differentiate anal condylomata acuminata from HSILs.[51] However, the colposcopic criteria to distinguish low-grade squamous intraepithelial lesions (LSILs) from cervical HSILs have been used to distinguish LSILs from HSILs of the anus in homosexual and bisexual men.[54] This information may allow for a targeted biopsy of suspected HSILs, resulting in increased sensitivity for detection. One study of anal cytology in homosexual and bisexual men reported the sensitivity and specificity for detection of HSILs to be 69% and 59%, respectively, in HIV-positive men and 47% and 92%, respectively, in HIV-negative men.[53]

BIOLOGIC CHARACTERISTICS

Unlike most gastrointestinal tract malignancies, anal cancer is predominantly a locoregional disease, and distant metastasis is relatively rare. Most relapses after curative therapy are located in the pelvis, perineum, or inguinal regions.[55] Only 5% to 10% of patients will have cancer that has spread beyond the pelvis at diagnosis,[45,56,57] and 10% to 20% of patients will have disease relapse at distant sites after curative local therapy.[55,58,59] Although chemotherapy is considered a component of standard therapy for anal cancer, its addition has not decreased the number of patients with distant metastases.[57-59] As the number of metastatically involved regional nodes increases, so does the risk of distant metastasis.[60] The most common site of distant metastasis is the liver, followed, in variable order, by the lungs, extrapelvic lymph nodes, skin, or bones.[56,57,59,61-63]

Characteristics of anal cancer that have consistently been correlated with local control and survival are the size and extent of the primary tumor and the status of the inguinal and pelvic lymph nodes. The 5-year survival for patients with tumors 2 cm or more in diameter that are treated surgically is about 80% but declines to 55% to 65% when the tumor is 2 cm to 5 cm or to 40% to 55% when the tumor is more than 5 cm.[60,64] The depth of invasion and the size and extent of the primary tumor are prognostic for response to treatment, local control, and survival when patients are treated nonsurgically with radiotherapy and chemotherapy.[4,55,59,63,65-67]

The survival for patients with regional lymph node metastases who are treated primarily with surgical procedures with or without adjuvant therapy is about half that observed in similar patients without nodal metastases.[64,68] Similarly, 5-year survival rates after radiotherapy alone in patients with inguinal lymph node metastases range from 0% to 36% compared with 5-year survival rates of more than 50% in patients without lymph node involvement.[68-70] There is relatively little information in the medical literature about the prognostic significance of regional nodal metastases in patients who receive combined radiotherapy and chemotherapy. In a retrospective, recursive, partitioning analysis of patients treated at Princess Margaret Hospital, node-positive patients at 5-year follow-up were found to have a trend toward lower cause-specific survival (57% versus 81%; $P = .07$).[58] In the European Organization for Research and Treatment of Cancer (EORTC) randomized trial of radiotherapy alone versus radiotherapy and chemotherapy, regional nodal metastases were associated with significantly worse local control ($P = .004$) and survival ($P < .001$).[71] However, in node-positive patients, the number of involved nodes (≥1), their size (<2 cm or >2 cm), and the extent of involvement (N1 or N2 and N3) added no further prognostic information.[71]

Patient-related variables that have been evaluated as potential prognostic factors for local control and survival in patients with anal cancer include age, gender, race, and performance status. Age probably does not have independent prognostic significance for any end point. A retrospective Canadian study found that older patients were treated with less aggressive chemotherapy and were less likely to be offered salvage surgery for recurrence; thus, patients older than 65 years of age were found to be at higher risk for death from anal cancer.[72] Conflicting data exist about the impact of gender on prognosis. Several studies have reported no difference in outcome by gender in patients treated with radiotherapy or combined radiotherapy and surgery.[58,70,72,73] However, a trend toward higher survival in women has been reported in some surgical series[60,64] and, in the EORTC randomized trial, female sex was associated with better survival ($P = .12$) and local control ($P = .05$).[71] Lower survival in patients with anal cancer who received combined modality therapy has been reported in patients with lower performance status and in nonwhite patients.[74]

Several histopathologic variables have been evaluated as potential prognostic factors in patients with anal cancer. Histologic subtype (squamous cell versus cloacogenic), tumor cell morphology, extent of differentiation or keratinization, cell size, architecture, and pleomorphism are of no prognostic significance.[58,70,72,73,75] Extent of differentiation may be associated with tumor stage because patients with advanced-stage cancer tend to have tumors that are less differentiated.[60] The depth of invasion of the primary tumor has been reported to have prognostic significance in patients treated primarily with surgical resection.[75] DNA ploidy has also been associated with prognosis in surgically treated patients with DNA aneuploid tumors predictive of an inferior outcome.[75] In a Mayo Clinic study of surgically treated patients, those with aneuploid tumors had inferior survival compared with patients with DNA diploid or tetraploid tumors on univariate analysis. On multivariate analysis, however, DNA ploidy was not a significant predictive variable.[76]

There are currently no clinically useful tumor markers. Despite negative liver imaging, patients with elevated alkaline phosphatase or lactate dehydrogenase are at increased risk for subsequent liver metastases.[77] In one study, reduced expression of p21^{waf1}, a cyclin-dependent kinase inhibitor, was associated with shorter overall survival.[78] Preliminary information suggests that serum antibodies to HPV proteins may eventually be useful as prognostic markers. Elevated serum IgA antibodies to HPV 16 E2:9 peptide have been associated with lower survival independent of tumor size.[28] In another study, patients who died of anal cancer were found to have higher levels of IgG against HPV E7:5 peptide than did patients with anal cancer in complete remission or patients who died of other causes.[31]

PATHOLOGY AND PATHWAYS OF SPREAD

The World Health Organization (WHO) classification of malignant epithelial tumors of the anal canal includes squamous cell carcinoma, adenocarcinoma, small cell carcinoma, and undifferentiated carcinoma. Most cases of adenocarcinoma of the anus are actually distal rectal adenocarcinomas with extension into the anal canal. True primary anal canal adenocarcinoma is rare, as is small cell carcinoma of presumed neuroendocrine origin.[14,60] Subsets of squamous cell carcinoma in the WHO system include large-cell keratinizing, large-cell nonkeratinizing or transitional, and basaloid carcinoma.[79] Although basaloid carcinomas have historically been considered to be nonkeratinizing, most basaloid carcinomas exhibit keratinization and should be considered squamous cell carcinomas.[52]

Although most anal canal malignancies are squamous cell carcinomas or squamous cell variants, marked morphologic heterogeneity is characteristic.[52] Classification of epidermoid anal cancers on the basis of morphologic appearance has led to the use of several potentially confusing terms. These include transitional cell carcinoma, basaloid carcinoma, and mucoepidermoid carcinoma. These tumors all arise from the anal transition zone and are often grouped together as cloacogenic carcinoma. Mucoepidermoid carcinomas contain mucous microcysts and are histologically dissimilar to mucoepidermoid carcinomas of the salivary glands. The natural history is identical to that of squamous cell carcinoma of the anus without microcysts. Although sometimes considered to be distinct lesions in the medical literature, cloacogenic carcinoma, transitional cell carcinoma, basaloid carcinoma, and mucoepidermoid carcinoma are all subtypes of squamous cell carcinoma, because patients with these various tumor subtypes have similar clinical characteristics and the tumor subgroups do not differ in natural history or response to therapy.[14,45,55,80]

Primary anal melanoma is a rare tumor that accounts for only 1% of all anal cancers. Anal melanoma is similar to melanoma of the skin in that it rarely affects African Americans and is characterized by the distant spread of disease.[3,81] Outcome is poor after wide local excision or abdominoperineal resection, with just a 10% survival in most series at 5-year follow-up.[82]

Pathways of Tumor Spread

Anal cancer tumors spread by direct extension to surrounding tissues, lymphatic dissemination to pelvic and inguinal lymph nodes, or hematogenous spread to distant viscera.[83] At diagnosis, about half of all anal cancers have been found to invade the anal sphincter or surrounding soft tissue. Although Denonvilliers fascia is usually an effective barrier to prostatic invasion in men, direct extension to the rectovaginal septum is a common occurrence in women.[3]

The anal canal has several potential lymphatic drainage pathways. The superficial inguinal nodes are the primary drainage basin for that part of the anal canal distal to the dentate line.[84,85] Lymphatic drainage around the dentate line occurs to lymphatic plexuses of the rectal mucosa and along the pathway of the inferior and middle hemorrhoidal vessels to obturator and hypogastric lymph nodes. Lymphatic connections also join the anus to presacral, external iliac, and deep inguinal nodes.[86]

Metastatic involvement of pelvic lymph nodes has been reported in 25% to 35% of patients treated primarily with abdominoperineal resection.[45,60] Inguinal node metastases are found in about 10% of patients at diagnosis; the risk depends on the size and extent of the primary tumor.[55,56] The incidence of inguinal node metastases may be as high as 20% for tumors more than 4 cm in diameter and as high as 60% when there is direct invasion of adjacent pelvic organs.[56] Recurrence in undissected inguinal nodes has been reported in 13% of surgically managed patients with clinically negative inguinal lymph nodes.[60]

CLINICAL MANIFESTATIONS/PATIENT EVALUATION/STAGING

Rectal bleeding is the most common symptom of anal malignancy. Perineal pain, mass sensation at the anus, and a change in bowel habits are also frequently reported.[14,45,87-90] Many patients with symptoms of early anal cancer are diagnosed initially with a benign anal condition, such as hemorrhoids, anal fissures, or fistulas.[14,45]

Most patients with anal cancer are diagnosed at an early stage. A national survey of such patients found that 73% were diagnosed with stage 0 to II, whereas only 8% were diagnosed with stage IV.[7] The interval from the onset of symptoms to diagnosis may be quite prolonged, however, exceeding 1 month in 80% of patients and 6 months in 33%. A study of Norwegian patients with anal cancer found that nearly one third of them had a delay of more than 6 months from onset of symptoms to diagnosis.[90] This finding emphasizes the importance of a thorough digital rectal examination in patients with anal symptoms.[46,47,90]

Patient Evaluation

Evaluation of the patient with known or suspected anal cancer should begin with a thorough history and physical examination. The patient should be questioned about anal sphincter function and any history of risk factors (sexual or drug abuse) for HIV infection.

In addition to a complete general physical examination, a detailed examination should be conducted of the abdomen, inguinal region, anus, and rectum. The extent of circumferential involvement of the anal canal should be noted, and documentation should be made of the size, extent, and location of the primary tumor. The size, location, and mobility of palpable inguinal lymph nodes should be noted. Pararectal lymph nodes may be involved metastatically, but these are rarely palpable by digital rectal examination.[70]

Laboratory studies should include a complete blood cell count, measurement of serum creatinine, and liver function studies of bilirubin, alkaline phosphatase, lactate dehydrogenase, and glutamic-oxaloacetic transaminase. For patients with HIV risk factors, a determination of HIV status should be made before the initiation of therapy. Although concentrations of serum carcinoembryonic antigen (CEA) are elevated in 20% of patients with anal cancer, posttreatment CEA values have not been found to correlate with clinical outcomes and have not proved useful in patient management.[91] There are no other clinically useful tumor markers for anal cancer.

Radiographic evaluation should include chest radiographs and computed tomography (CT) of the abdomen and pelvis. The CT scan is generally inferior to the physical examination for the characterization of primary tumors, but it is useful for the evaluation of the liver and the perirectal, inguinal, pelvic, and para-aortic lymph nodes. Magnetic resonance imaging has not yet been proved more clinically useful than CT. The depth of invasion of the primary tumor may be evaluated with ultrasonography.[92]

Staging

Anal cancer should be staged according to the TNM staging system of the American Joint Committee on Cancer (AJCC) (Table 49-1).[93] Tumors are classified according to their maximum diameter and their invasion of adjacent structures, as determined by the physical examination and any imaging studies. In earlier editions of the staging system of the Union Internationale Contre le Cancer (International Union Against Cancer [UICC]),[70] primary tumors were classified not by size but rather according to the length and extent of their circumferential involvement with the anal canal. Tumors involving less than one third of the length and circumference of the anal canal were classified as T1, whereas those that involved more than one third of the length or circumference or that invaded the external sphincter were classified as T2. As in the current system, T3 tumors involved the rectum or perianal skin, and T4 tumors invaded adjacent structures.

The AJCC staging system for anal canal cancer is applicable to all carcinomas that arise from the anal canal. Cancers of the anal margin (distal to the anal verge) are staged as skin

Table 49-1 2002 TNM Staging System of the American Joint Committee on Cancer

Stage	T*	N†	M
0	Tis	N0	M0
I	T1	N0	M0
II	T2	N0	M0
	T3	N0	M0
IIIA	T1	N1	M0
	T2	N1	M0
	T3	N1	M0
	T4	N0	M0
IIIB	T4	N1	M0
	Any	N2	M0
	Any	N3	M0
IV	Any	Any	M1

*Tumor stages: Tis, carcinoma in situ; T1, tumor of 2 cm or less in greatest dimension; T2, tumor of more than 2 cm but 5 cm or less in greatest dimension; T3, tumor of more than 5 cm in greatest dimension; T4, tumor invades adjacent organs but not sphincter muscle alone.

†Nodal stages: N0, no regional lymph node metastases; N1, perirectal lymph node metastases; N2, unilateral internal iliac or unilateral inguinal lymph node metastases; N3, perirectal and inguinal or bilateral internal iliac or bilateral inguinal lymph node metastases.

From American Joint Committee on Cancer: Anal canal. *In* Greene FL, Page DL, Fleming ID, et al (eds): AJCC Cancer Staging Handbook, 6th ed. New York, Springer, 2002, pp 139-144.

cancers, but melanoma of the anal canal is excluded. For staging purposes, the regional lymph nodes in the AJCC system are the anorectal, perirectal, lateral sacral, internal iliac (hypogastric), and superficial and deep inguinal lymph nodes.[93]

PRIMARY THERAPY

Surgery Alone

Before the establishment in the 1980s of sphincter-sparing therapy as the standard of care for epidermoid anal cancer, most patients with anal cancer in North America were treated surgically with abdominoperineal resection. Reported 5-year survival after abdominoperineal resection for anal cancer ranged from 25% to 70% (average, 50%).[60,64,94] Locoregional recurrence developed in 25% to 35% of patients and distant metastasis in 10%.[60,64,94] Patients at highest risk for local recurrence (range, 36% to 48%) after abdominoperineal resection are those with extension of the primary tumor beyond the anal sphincter or metastases to inguinal or pelvic lymph nodes.[60] A component of locoregional disease is present in as many as 84% of patients with relapse after abdominoperineal resection.[60] When the inguinal lymph nodes are metastatically involved, the 5-year survival after primary surgical therapy is only 10% to 20%.[94] Although abdominoperineal resection is now rarely used initially, it is still useful for treatment of patients with local recurrence after conservative therapy and for management of complications after conservative therapy.[94]

Radiation Alone or Plus Chemotherapy

High-dose radiotherapy without surgical resection or other adjuvant therapy is an effective treatment for small T1 tumors without inguinal adenopathy. Table 49-2 summarizes the local control and survival results from retrospective series of radiotherapy alone for small anal cancers. For patients with anal cancers of 2 cm or less in diameter, 100% local control at 5 years after radiotherapy without chemotherapy has been reported in several small series of less than 10 patients each.[58,59,95] Local control rates at 5 years are lower (57% to 76%) in patients with 2- to 5-cm tumors.[58,59]

The only prospective randomized trial to compare radiotherapy alone with the combination of radiotherapy and chemotherapy in patients with node-negative anal cancers 5 cm or less in diameter (T1 to T2N0) was carried out by the UKCCCR (United Kingdom Coordinating Committee on Cancer Research) Anal Cancer Trial Working Party.[97] In this trial, 223 of 585 patients had T1 or T2N0 anal cancer and were randomized to receive 40 to 45 Gy of external beam radiotherapy to the pelvis, followed by a 15-Gy to 25-Gy boost with a perineal field or interstitial implant with or without two 4- or 5-day infusions of 5-fluorouracil (5-FU) and a single bolus injection of mitomycin C (MMC). Using local control as the end point, subset analysis showed a statistically significant advantage for combined modality therapy for patients with T1N0 or T2N0 anal cancer.[98]

Combined modality therapy with radiotherapy and chemotherapy is appropriate for most patients with anal cancer and has become the standard of care. Statistics from the U.S. National Cancer Data Base for 1988 and 1993 show that the use of chemotherapy has increased while the use of resection as the primary treatment has declined.[7]

The initial studies that led to the adoption of combined modality therapy with nonsurgical treatment were conducted at Wayne State University. Before scheduled surgical resection, 3000 cGy of radiation in 15 fractions was delivered to the true pelvis, medial inguinal nodes, and anal canal in conjunction with concomitant 5-FU 1000 mg/m^2 every 24 hours for 4 days as a continuous infusion and a single bolus injection of 15 mg/m^2 MMC. After five of the first six patients were found to have no residual tumor in the abdominoperineal resection specimen 4 to 6 weeks after the completion of radiotherapy, surgical resection was subsequently reserved for locally persistent or recurrent disease after radiotherapy and chemotherapy.[63] Overall, 86% (24 of 28) had a clinical complete response to radiotherapy and chemotherapy, and 7 (58%) of the 12 patients who had an abdominoperineal resection had a complete pathologic response.[99]

Table 49-3 summarizes the disease control and survival results with concomitant radiotherapy and chemotherapy from several series. Local failure after radiation doses of 45 to 60 Gy with concomitant chemotherapy occurred in 11% to 40% of patients, and 5-year actuarial survival rates were 65% to 80%.

Two randomized studies comparing radiotherapy alone with concomitant radiotherapy and 5-FU and MMC chemotherapy have been performed by the EORTC[71] and the UKCCCR Anal Cancer Trial Working Party.[97] For patient eligibility, the EORTC trial required a locally advanced primary tumor (T3 or T4) or involvement of regional lymph nodes, whereas the UKCCCR trial enrolled patients with any stage of disease, including distant metastases. Initial radiotherapy was

Table 49-2 5-Year Disease Control and Survival after Radiotherapy Alone for Early-Stage Anal Cancer

First Author/Reference	N	Total RT Dose, Gy	Tumor Size	Local Control, %	Overall Survival, %
Allal[59]	5	60-65*	≤2 cm	100	100
	37	60-65*	2-5 cm	76	63
Cummings[58]	6	45-55‡	≤2 cm	100	NR
	23	45-55‡	2-5 cm	57	NR
Martenson[95]	18	55-67	≤5 cm†	100	94
Schlienger[70]	63	60-65	T1-T2, UICC§	71	85
Doggett[56]	35	45-76	≤5 cm	77	92
Papillon[96]	63	45-50§	≤4 cm	87	76
Eschwege[69]	27	60-65	T1-T2, UICC‖	90	72

*Usually 40-Gy external beam, plus 20 to 25 Gy with interstitial implant.
†One patient with tumor >5 cm.
‡Overall 4-week treatment period.
§Equivalent to 30 Gy in 10 fractions, followed by 15 to 20 Gy with interstitial implant.
‖1979 UICC staging: T1, less than one-third length and circumference of anal canal; T2, more than one-third length or circumference of anal canal or infiltration of external sphincter.
NR, not reported; RT, radiotherapy; UICC, Union Internationale Contre le Cancer.

Table 49-3 Disease Control and Survival after Radiotherapy and Chemotherapy for Anal Cancer in Selected Series

First Author/ Reference	*N*	Median Follow-up, mo	Total RT Dose, Gy	Tumor Extent	Chemotherapy	Local Failure, No. (%)	Overall Survival, %
Rich[100]	39	54	45-66	T0-T4	5-FU*	13/39 (33)	74
Cummings[58]	66	24	48-50	T1-T4	5-FU	26/65 (40)	64
Hughes[101]	25	30	45-66	T0-T4	5-FU†	8/24 (33)	96 (2 y)
Martenson[74]	50	NR	50-53	T1-T4	5-FU, MMC	— (20)‡	58
Allal[59]	68	48	50-55§	T1-T4	5-FU, MMC	22/68 (32)	65
Doci[102]	56	49	54-56	T1-T3	5-FU, MMC	12/49 (24)	81
Tanum[61]	86	>36‖	50	T0-T4	5-FU, MMC	—	72
Cummings[58]	69	36 (min)	48-60	T1-T4	5-FU, MMC	10/69 (14)	76
Sischy[4]	26	32	40.8	<3 cm	5-FU, MMC	4/26 (15)	85 (3 y)
	50	—	40.8	≥3 cm	5-FU, MMC	18/50 (36)	68 (3 y)
Rich[100]	19	20	54-60	T2-T4	5-FU, CCDP	2/19 (11)	85 (3 y)
Doci[103]	35	37	54-58	T1-T3	5-FU, CDDP	4/35 (11)#	97, crude

*5-FU, 250-300 mg/m² per d, by infusion 5 d or 7 d weekly throughout radiotherapy.
†5-FU, 300 mg/m² per d throughout radiotherapy.
‡Kaplan-Meier estimate at 5 years.
§Usually 30 Gy external beam in 10 fractions plus 20 Gy with interstitial implant.
‖Investigators monitored for more than 3 y.
¶5-FU, 250 mg/m² per d, by infusion 5 d weekly throughout radiotherapy; CDDP, 4 mg/m² per d throughout radiotherapy.
#Crude.
CDDP, cisplatin; 5-FU, 5-fluorouracil; min, minimum; MMC, mitomycin C; NR, not reported; RT, radiotherapy.

Table 49-4 3-Year Disease Control and Survival in Randomized Studies Comparing Radiotherapy Alone with Radiation and Chemotherapy

Study	*N*	Median Follow-up, mo	Complete Response* %	Complete Response* *P* Value	Local Control† %	Local Control† *P* Value	Crude Distant Metastases, %	Overall Survival %	Overall Survival *P* Value
EORTC	103	42							
RT	52		54		55		21	64	
RT plus 5-FU, MMC	51		80	.02	69	.02	18	69	.17
UKCCCR	577	42							
RT	285		30		39		17	58	
RT plus 5-FU, MMC	292		39	.08	61	<.001	10	65	.25

*Assessment of complete response was 6 weeks after 45 Gy (before radiotherapy boost) in UKCCCR trial and 6 weeks after completion of 60 to 65 Gy in EORTC trial.
†Patients who had surgery to achieve local control at the completion of radiotherapy were considered locally controlled in the EORTC trial; in the UKCCCR trial, patients who had surgery at the completion of radiotherapy were considered local treatment failures, as were all patients who had surgery for treatment morbidity.
EORTC, European Organization for Research and Treatment of Cancer; 5-FU, 5-fluorouracil; MMC, mitomycin C; RT, radiotherapy; UKCCCR, United Kingdom Coordinating Committee on Cancer Research.

similar in both trials and consisted of 45 Gy to the pelvis over 4 to 5 weeks. In the EORTC trial, partial responders at 6 weeks after induction therapy were boosted with an additional 20 Gy and complete responders received 15 Gy. In the UKCCCR trial, a 15-Gy to 25-Gy boost was administered to patients with more than a 50% tumor response; patients with less than a 50% response had radical surgery. Chemotherapy in the EORTC trial consisted of 5-FU 750 mg/m² every 24 hours on day 1 to 5 and day 29 to 33 with a single 15-mg/m² dose of MMC on day 1. Chemotherapy in the UKCCCR trial consisted of 5-FU 1000 mg/m² every 24 hours on day 1 to 4 and day 29 to 32 or 750 mg/m² every 24 hours on day 1 to 5 and day 29 to 33, with a single MMC dose of 12 mg/m² given on the first day of radiotherapy.

Results of the EORTC[71] and UKCCCR[97] trials are summarized in Table 49-4. The complete response rate 6 weeks after boost radiotherapy was significantly improved with the addition of chemotherapy to radiotherapy (80% versus 54%; *P* = .02) in the EORTC trial. A nonstatistically significant trend toward a higher complete response rate was also reported in the UKCCCR trial. However, this end point was measured 6 weeks after the initiation of therapy compared with 6 weeks after the completion of all therapy in the EORTC trial. In both studies, local control was significantly improved with the addition of chemotherapy. Local control with radiotherapy alone was surprisingly low (39% at 3 years) in the UKCCCR study. The definition of local failure included tumor reduction of less than 50% 6 weeks after 45 Gy of radiation, surgery for morbidity, and failure to close a pretreatment colostomy for any reason. Conversely, EORTC investigators considered patients locally controlled even if they had to undergo surgery to achieve a complete response at the completion of radiotherapy. Neither study reported any significant impact of chemotherapy on the incidence of distant metastases or on survival, although absolute survival at 3 years slightly favored the chemoradiation arms numerically in both trials.

The EORTC and UKCCCR trials established combined modality therapy as the standard of care for patients with anal

Table 49-5 4-Year Disease Control, Survival, and Toxicity after Radiotherapy and 5-Fluorouracil with or without Mitomycin C: Results of RTOG/ECOG Randomized Trial 1289[104]

Treatment Arm	N	Total RT Dose, Gy	Negative Biopsy %	Negative Biopsy P Value	Local Control %	Local Control P Value	Colostomy Rate %	Colostomy Rate P Value	Colostomy-Free Survival %	Colostomy-Free Survival P Value	Disease-Free Survival %	Disease-Free Survival P Value	Overall Survival %	Overall Survival P Value	Grade 4-5 Toxicity %	Grade 4-5 Toxicity P Value
RT plus 5-FU	145	45-50.4	85		66		22		59		51		67		8	
RT plus 5-FU, MMC	146	45-50.4	92	.135	84	.0008	9	.002	71	.014	73	.003	76	.31	26	≤.001

ECOG, Eastern Cooperative Oncology Group; 5-FU, 5-fluorouracil; MMC, mitomycin C; RT, radiotherapy; RTOG, Radiation Therapy Oncology Group.

cancer. Further refinement in the understanding of optimal therapy is provided by the results of a phase 3 study conducted by the Radiation Therapy Oncology Group (RTOG) and the Eastern Cooperative Oncology Group (ECOG). In the RTOG/ECOG study (Table 49-5), patients were treated with radiotherapy (45 to 50.4 Gy in 25 to 28 fractions) and 5-FU and were randomized to receive or not receive MMC.[104] The addition of MMC was associated with fewer colostomies, higher local control, and better disease-free survival. The addition of MMC also significantly increased the risk of major toxicity. Survival was slightly higher in the MMC arm of the study, but the difference was not statistically significant. The chemotherapy regimen in this trial differed from that of the European trials because two doses of MMC 10 mg/m² were delivered on day 1 and day 29 instead of a single dose. Two of the four treatment-related deaths during the MMC arm were believed to be caused by a failure to follow protocol dose-reduction guidelines for the second MMC dose.

The biologic basis for improved outcome with the addition of chemotherapy to the treatment regimen is not known. However, the fact that several studies have reported no significant reduction in distant failure rates with chemotherapy suggests that the effect is predominantly locoregional, possibly because of an interaction with radiation.[58] For example, in the Princess Margaret Hospital experience, distant failure occurred in 18% of patients treated with radiotherapy alone, in 17% of those who received MMC and 5-FU, and in 10% of those receiving 5-FU alone.[58,105] Synergistic interactions between radiation and 5-FU or MMC and between 5-FU and MMC have been demonstrated in mammalian tumor cell lines in vitro.[106] Hypoxic mammalian tumor cells also have an increased sensitivity to MMC in vitro, although whether the hypoxia has any effect when anal cancer is treated with fractionated radiotherapy is not known.[107] Laboratory studies have also shown increased cytotoxicity associated with continuous infusion 5-FU compared with 5-FU delivery by intermittent bolus.[108]

It cannot be assumed that sequential therapy will duplicate the excellent results achieved with concomitant radiotherapy and chemotherapy. Complete pathologic response rates 6 weeks after 30 Gy of radiation, 5-FU, and MMC are in the range of 85% to 95%.[63,109-111] In contrast, only 45% of 42 patients who received sequential 5-FU and MMC, followed by radiotherapy, had a complete pathologic response.[88]

Anal function is preserved in 65% to 80% of patients after sphincter-sparing therapy.[58,59,73,101] The most common indication for abdominoperineal resection is recurrence, because 90% of patients for whom local control is achieved can be expected to maintain a functional anus.[58] Late treatment complications may result in the loss of anal function, and a colostomy may be required to manage complications in 2% to 10% of patients whose cancer is locally controlled.[56,58,59,70,73,95,103,112]

LOCALLY ADVANCED DISEASE AND PALLIATION

Tumor size appears to have a moderate impact on treatment outcome when anal cancer is treated with combined modality therapy. In the RTOG/ECOG study, 17% of patients with primary tumors 5 cm or more in diameter had positive biopsy findings 6 weeks after completion of therapy compared with 7% of those with a tumor less than 5 cm in diameter ($P = .02$). Preservation of anal function was also more likely in patients who had smaller tumors; 11% of patients with T1 or T2 cancer required a colostomy compared with 21% of those with T3 or T4 cancer.[104] Differences in local control have also been reported using tumor diameter cutoffs of less than 5 cm. In an earlier RTOG study, local control at 3 years was 84% among patients with tumors smaller than 3 cm and 62% among those with tumors 3 cm or larger.[4] Similarly, local control among patients treated at Princess Margaret Hospital was 94% for those with tumors of 2 cm or less and 72% for those with larger tumors. No difference in local control was reported between the subgroups of patients with tumors of 2 to 5 cm or with larger tumors (>5 cm), unless invasion of adjacent structures was discovered, in which case the local control rate was 62%.[58]

Preservation of anal function is possible in most patients with locally advanced disease. In the Princess Margaret Hospital experience, two thirds of patients with tumors that invaded adjacent structures maintained anal function after radiotherapy and chemotherapy, as did two thirds of the patients with tumors that involved more than 75% of the circumference of the anal canal.[58] Locally advanced disease is not an indication for abdominoperineal resection in patients who retain some measure of anal function at diagnosis.[58]

Node Involvement

Involvement of the inguinal lymph nodes at diagnosis is associated with a worse prognosis. In the EORTC randomized trial, patients with involved lymph nodes had inferior local control and inferior survival. However, the extent of nodal involvement did not add any prognostic information.[71] In a report from Princess Margaret Hospital, the 5-year cause-specific survival for clinically node-positive patients was 57% compared with 81% for node-negative patients ($P = .07$).

Combined modality therapy was effective in the treatment of patients with involved nodes. In such patients, control of cancer in metastatically involved lymph nodes was achieved 87% of the time.[58]

Radiotherapy without chemotherapy has been used for patients with metastatically involved inguinal lymph nodes, with control of nodal disease reported in 60% to 70% of patients.[56,73] However, survival is poor for these patients with radiotherapy alone (range, 0% to 36% at 5 years), and combined modality therapy with radiotherapy and chemotherapy is preferred.[68-70,73]

Salvage Therapy

Patients with local failure after radiotherapy and chemotherapy should be considered for abdominoperineal resection. Local control can be achieved with abdominoperineal resection in as many as 60% of these patients.[56,58,59,67,70,73] Ultimate local control is obtained in more than 90% of all patients with anal cancer, including patients who require surgery after radiotherapy for locally persistent or recurrent disease.[56,73]

Patients who have locally advanced recurrent disease that is not surgically resectable for cure may benefit from low-dose re-irradiation and chemotherapy followed by surgical resection of gross disease and intraoperative radiotherapy may result in successful salvage.

Palliation

Although anal cancer is predominantly a locoregional disease, 5% to 10% of patients will have disease beyond the pelvis at diagnosis and distant metastases will develop in 10% to 20% after locoregional therapy.[57-59] The most common site of distant metastases reported in most series is the liver; metastases to the lungs, lymph nodes, skin, bones, and brain have also been reported.[56,57,59,61-63] Palliative chemotherapy with 5-FU and MMC or cisplatin is associated with a 50% response rate and a median survival of 12 months.[57] Patients with brain metastases, symptomatic osseous metastases, or other localized symptomatic metastases should receive hypofractionated radiotherapy for palliation.

TECHNIQUES OF IRRADIATION

Field Design

Radiotherapy field design should be based on an understanding of the spread of anal cancer. Historical results in patients treated by abdominoperineal resection show that 35% to 46% had involvement of pelvic lymph nodes and that 13% to 16% had a recurrence in the inguinal lymph nodes.[60,64] Thus, pelvic and inguinal lymph nodes should be included in radiotherapy fields.

A portion of the inguinal lymph node chain is superficial to the femoral head and neck. It is important to use radiotherapy fields that decrease the radiation dose to these structures. Large anterior-posterior or posterior-anterior fields or four-field box techniques that include the inguinal lymph nodes deliver the full radiation dose to the femoral head and neck. Patients treated in this way may be at risk for radiation-induced fracture.[95] Radiotherapy techniques that treat the lateral inguinal lymph nodes only through anterior fields will minimize the dose to the femoral head and neck. One method is to treat the primary tumor, pelvic nodes, and inguinal nodes with an anterior photon field that encompasses all these structures. The posterior field is designed to treat only the primary tumor and the pelvic lymph nodes. Electron fields are used to supplement the dose to the lateral superficial inguinal nodes that are not included in the posterior photon field (Figs. 49-1 and 49-2). Another technique is to use CT-based simulation for optimal delineation of the inguinal lymph nodes and then to use this information to minimize the volume of the femur included within the radiotherapy field (Fig. 49-3).

Radiation Dose and Fractionation

The RTOG/ECOG randomized clinical trial has provided useful information about the most favorable combination of radiation dose and chemotherapy agents.[104] The best local control resulted from an aggressive regimen of radiotherapy and chemotherapy that consisted of 5-FU 1000 mg/m^2 per day on day 1 to 4 and day 29 to 32 of radiotherapy and of MMC 10 mg/m^2 on day 1 and day 29 of radiotherapy. The primary tumor, pelvic lymph nodes, and inguinal lymph nodes received a total dose of 36 Gy of radiation in 20 fractions, followed by a field reduction to include the primary tumor. An additional 9 Gy was administered in 5 fractions, for a total dose to the primary tumor of 45 Gy in 25 fractions. Patients who had residual tumor after 45 Gy received an additional dose of 5.4 Gy in 3 fractions, for a total cumulative primary tumor dose of 50.4 Gy in 28 fractions. The medial inguinal lymph nodes received 4500 cGy if clinically negative or 5040 cGy if clinically positive. This combination of radiotherapy and chemotherapy resulted in a 4-year local control rate of 84%, which was significantly better than the 4-year local control rate of 66% in patients randomized to receive an identical dose of radiotherapy and 5-FU without MMC ($P < .001$).

In the RTOG/ECOG study, 26% of the patients treated with radiotherapy, 5-FU, and MMC experienced life-threatening or fatal toxicity, including a 3% treatment-related death rate. This combination of a high rate of tumor control and significant toxicity indicates that a total radiation dose of 45 to 50.4 Gy, in conjunction with 5-FU and MMC, should result in a satisfactory therapeutic ratio. It is not yet known whether increasing the radiation dose to more than 50.4 Gy in conjunction with 5-FU and MMC chemotherapy will improve the therapeutic ratio. With both 5-FU and MMC, a higher radiation dose may produce an unacceptable risk of toxicity and is not recommended outside a controlled clinical trial. In an ongoing U.S. GI Intergroup clinical trial co-ordinated by RTOG, the recommended final boost dose is 55 to 59 Gy for patients with T3 to T4 disease, positive nodes, or T2 lesions with residual disease after 45 Gy.

The hypothesis that there will be fewer local failures when the radiation dose is increased to more than 50.4 Gy in combined modality therapy with both 5-FU and MMC has not been tested in prospective trials. Two retrospective series have contributed to the formation of this hypothesis. At the University of Texas M. D. Anderson Cancer Center, patients with anal cancer who were treated with radiotherapy and continuous infusion 5-FU 300 mg/m^2 during the entire radiotherapy course had better local control rates with radiation doses of 55 to 66 Gy (9 of 10) than with lower doses of 45 to 49 Gy (7 of 14).[101] Researchers at the University of Kansas evaluated treatment with or without chemotherapy and found local control rates of 92% for radiation doses of more than 55 Gy, 77% for 45 to 55 Gy, and 64% for 45 Gy or less.[113]

Radiotherapy without chemotherapy is appropriate for a few patients who are not candidates for combined modality therapy because of clinically significant comorbid illness or other reasons. A high rate of tumor control has been found in patients with small tumors treated with a radiation dose of 45 Gy in 25 fractions to the pelvis, inguinal lymph nodes, and primary tumor, followed by a boost dose to the primary tumor, for a total cumulative dose of 60 to 63 Gy in 33 to 35 fractions.[69,95]

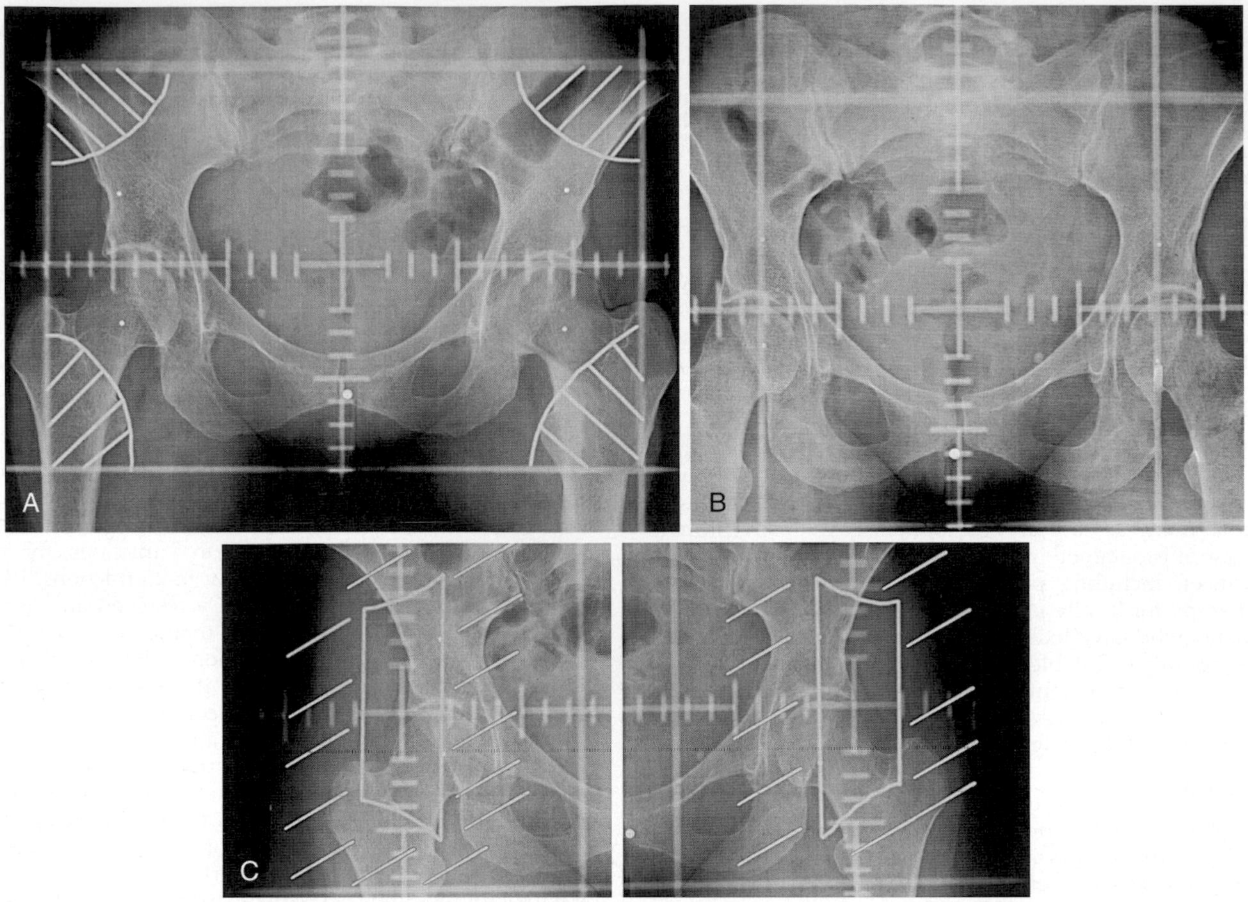

Figure 49-1 Anal cancer fields. **A**, Anterior photon field. **B**, Posterior photon field. **C**, Electron fields are used to give a supplementary radiation dose to lateral inguinal nodes not included in the posterior photon field. The medial border of each electron field is determined by placing radiopaque markers on the anterior abdominal wall at the lateral exit point of the posterior photon field (**B** and **C**) (From Martenson JA, Schild SE, Haddock MG: Disease sites. *In* Kahn FM, Potish RA [eds]: Treatment Planning in Radiation Oncology. Baltimore, Williams & Wilkins, 1998, p 321. By permission of the publisher.)

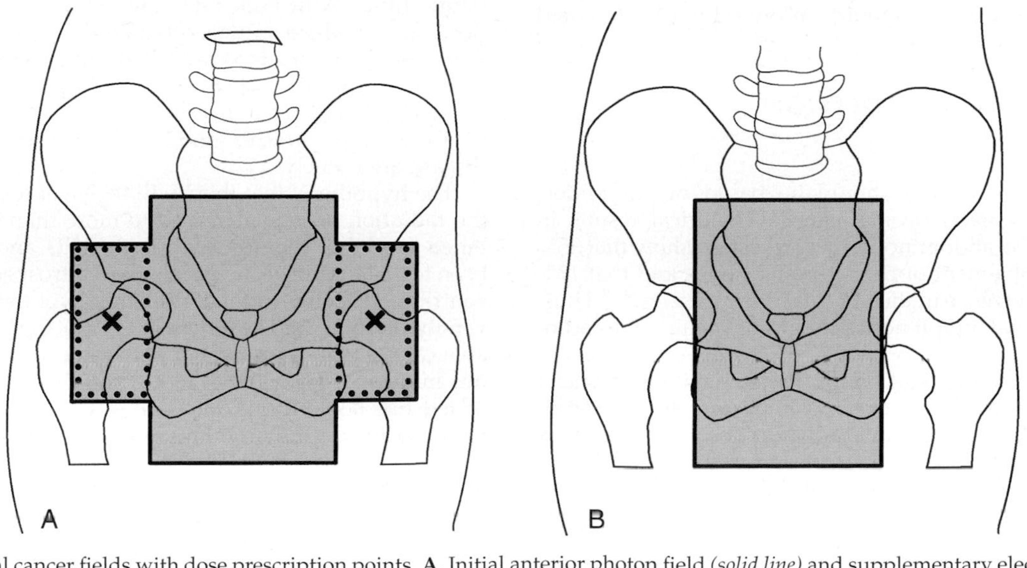

Figure 49-2 Anal cancer fields with dose prescription points. **A**, Initial anterior photon field *(solid line)* and supplementary electron fields *(dotted lines)*. **B**, Initial posterior photon field. A total dose of 36 Gy at 1.8 Gy/fraction is administered to the photon fields. The dose is specified on the central axis at the midplane of the patient. The electron fields provide daily supplementary irradiation during the first 20 treatments with the objective of giving 1.8 Gy each day at the depth of the inguinal nodes. This is done by calculating the daily dose from the anterior photon field at the depth of the inguinal nodes (point × in **A**). Typically, in a patient with inguinal lymph nodes at a depth of 3 cm (determined from imaging studies), the dose contribution to lateral inguinal nodes from the anterior photon field will be about 1.2 Gy per day (calculated separately for each individual patient). Thus, the daily dose to the supplementary electron fields would be 0.6 Gy per day, bringing the total daily dose to the inguinal nodes to 1.8 Gy from a combination of the anterior photon field and the supplementary electron field. After 36 Gy has been administered, an additional 9 to 14.4 Gy in 5 to 8 fractions is given to boost fields to a total cumulative dose to the tumor of 45 to 50.4 Gy. (From Martenson JA, Schild SE, Haddock MG: Anal carcinoma. *In* Kahn FM, Potish RA [eds]: Treatment Planning in Radiation Oncology. Baltimore; Williams & Wilkins, 1998, p 323. By permission of the publisher.)

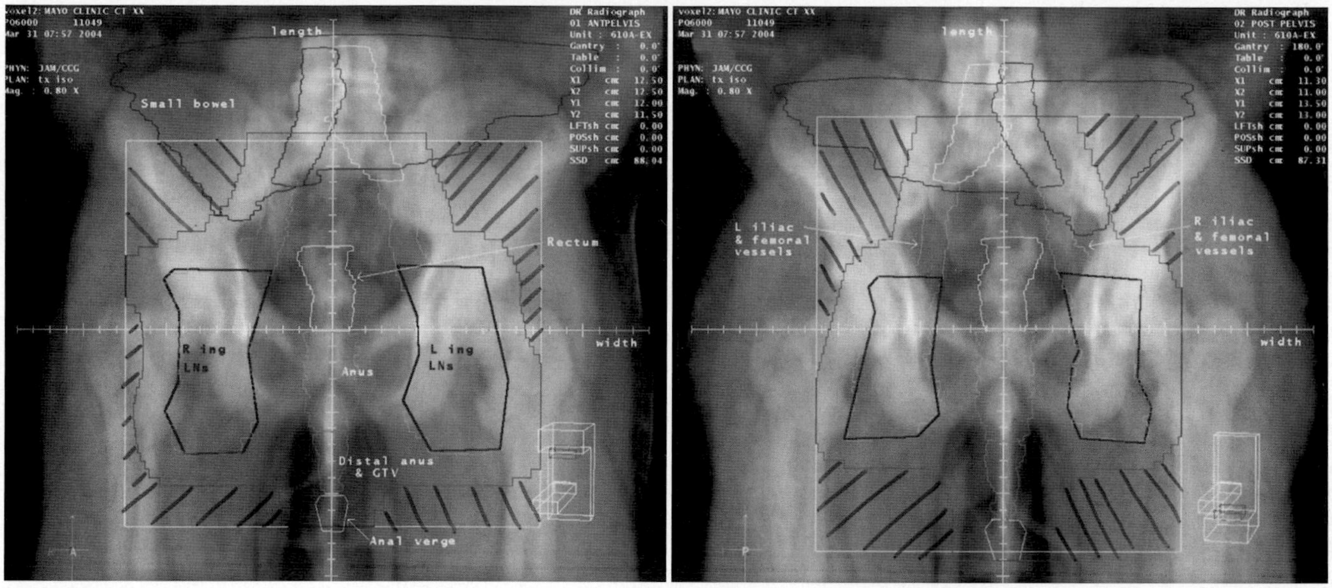

A B

Figure 49-3 Anterior (**A**) and posterior (**B**) radiation fields designed with computed tomographic simulation to allow optimal sparing of the femoral head and neck. GTV, gross tumor volume; ing, inguinal; L, left; LNs, lymph nodes; R, right.

Nearly all patients who receive concomitant radiotherapy and chemotherapy for anal cancer will have perineal skin reactions, and more than half will have confluent moist desquamation. The severity of such acute reactions is influenced by radiation fraction size. In a Princess Margaret Hospital study of 50 Gy in 20 fractions (2.5 Gy/fraction), the acute and late toxicities were considered unacceptably high.[58] Less severe toxicity was reported with the same fractionation schedule and a break in treatment or with a fractionation schedule of 48 Gy in 24 fractions.[58]

Overall, treatment time may affect the outcome of radiotherapy. In an RTOG pilot study evaluating 59.4 Gy with 5-FU and MMC that included a planned treatment break, 30% of patients required a colostomy by year 2 compared with only 7% in the RTOG/ECOG randomized trial, which did not use planned treatment breaks.[114,115]

Tumor Regression

Tumor regression may be slow after radiotherapy, with the time to complete regression ranging from 2 to 36 weeks (median, 12 weeks).[58] Most recurrences at the primary site manifest within 2 years of treatment.[58] When chemotherapy is not used, tumor regression may be even more prolonged. In a French study of 193 patients with anal cancer treated with radiotherapy alone, the mean time to a complete response was 3 months after the completion of therapy, and some patients required as long as 12 months for a complete response.[70]

Although routine biopsies have been required 4 to 6 weeks after the completion of therapy in several studies,[63,74,88] routine biopsies should not be performed on patients with regressing or clinically absent tumors. Treatment with 30 to 50 Gy and 5-FU and MMC is associated with negative biopsy findings in 85% to 90% of patients 4 to 6 weeks after completion of radiotherapy.[63,109,110] Because of accelerated repopulation in surviving clonogens, a low-dose radiation boost after a 6-week break is unlikely to provide any benefit. The purported benefit of additional therapy for 7 of 22 patients in the RTOG/ECOG study is more likely a result of continued slow tumor regression after initial therapy than the result of the addition of 9 Gy and cisplatin chemotherapy.

Treatment Tolerance

The acute toxicity associated with therapy for anal cancer may depend in part on radiation fraction size and schedule and how chemotherapy is used. Investigators at Princess Margaret Hospital reported a decrease from 75% to 40% in acute grade 3 toxicities when fraction size was reduced from 250 to 200 cGy or when a planned treatment break was used.[58] Acute toxicity is markedly higher when MMC is added to 5-FU and radiotherapy. In the RTOG/ECOG trial, 26% of patients who received 5-FU and MMC together experienced grade 4 or grade 5 toxicity (3% treatment-related deaths), compared with only 7% of patients receiving 5-FU (0.7% treatment-related deaths).[111]

For patients receiving both MMC and 5-FU, the most common life-threatening toxicity is bone marrow suppression resulting in neutropenic sepsis. In addition, essentially all patients will experience a perineal skin reaction.[4] In the RTOG/ECOG study, confluent moist desquamation was reported in 55% of patients treated with this combination.[115] Mild to moderate diarrhea may be experienced by two-thirds of patients, and nausea and vomiting by 25% and 15%, respectively.[4]

Late treatment-related complications are usually diagnosed within 2 years of treatment.[69] Asymptomatic or minimally symptomatic perineal fibrosis, telangiectasia, and minor intermittent bleeding from the anorectal region or bladder may be observed.[116] Severe late effects that affect social life or require surgical intervention have been reported in as many as 15% of patients.[58,61,69] These effects include anal incontinence, intestinal obstruction, chronic diarrhea, chronic pelvic pain, fistula, or bladder dysfunction.[61] Elderly women may be at increased risk for fractures of the femoral head and neck, especially if the radiotherapy fields encompass the entire femoral head and neck in both anterior and posterior treatment fields.[95] Late complications may necessitate colostomy for management in 2% to 10% of patients.[56,58,59,70,73,95]

Late complications of radiotherapy may be more likely when treatment is delivered with fraction sizes larger than 2 Gy.[58] Late complications are also more common in patients with locally advanced tumors; one series reported late effects in 23% of patients with T3 or T4 tumors compared with only 6% of patients with T1 or T2 tumors.[69]

Some investigators have reported that HIV-positive patients with anal cancer have reduced tolerance for combined radiotherapy and chemotherapy regimens.[117,118] Compared with HIV-negative patients, HIV-positive patients are more likely to require treatment breaks, hospitalization for acute reactions, and chemotherapy dose reductions.[117,119] In addition, survival of HIV patients is often limited; one report found a 29% 2-year survival for HIV-positive patients compared with 71% at 4 years for HIV-negative patients.[117] Although the best treatment strategy is unknown, low-dose radiation and chemotherapy in a small series of patients have been reported to result in satisfactory tolerance and response in HIV-positive patients and in patients with AIDS without major opportunistic infections.[119]

TREATMENT ALGORITHM AND FUTURE DIRECTIONS

Figure 49-4 is a diagnostic and treatment algorithm for patients with newly diagnosed anal cancer.

The optimum radiation dose and dose intensity in the combined modality setting are being investigated. Retrospective studies have indicated that prolongation of the overall treatment time leads to decreased local control.[112] An unexpectedly large number of patients requiring colostomies in a phase II RTOG study using a radiation dose of 59.4 Gy has been attributed to a planned treatment break in the protocol but may have been due, in part, to patient selection factors.[114] In a subsequent study with identical doses of radiotherapy and chemotherapy but no planned treatment break, the 1-year colostomy rate was reduced from 23% to 11%.[120]

Because locoregional failure continues to be an important problem, an escalation in the dose of radiation has been hypothesized to result in improved local control. The U.S. GI Intergroup protocol RTOG 9811 uses radiation doses as high as 59 Gy for patients with T3 or T4 lesions or for patients with T2 tumors who have residual cancer after receiving a total of 45 Gy. Results from RTOG 9811 may provide some indication as to whether an escalation in the radiation dose should be tested in a phase III clinical trial.

Although the addition of MMC to radiotherapy and 5-FU has been shown to improve local control and colostomy-free survival, the clinically significant acute toxicity associated with MMC suggests a need for equally effective but less toxic chemotherapy regimens. Cisplatin is currently being investigated as a potential substitute for MMC,[74] but whether it will result in equal efficacy or reduced toxicity has not been established; this regimen is not recommended outside clinical trials.[121]

The addition of chemotherapy to radiotherapy has resulted in improved local control of anal cancer without a significant reduction in distant metastases, which indicates a possible influence from the interaction of chemotherapy and radiotherapy. Alternative chemotherapy delivery schedules may enhance the interaction with radiotherapy. The combination of low-dose continuous-infusion 5-FU and cisplatin has been used in a series of 62 patients treated at M. D. Anderson Cancer Center, resulting in an overall 5-year survival of 90% and local control of 76% with acceptable acute and late toxicities.[122] No patient in the series required a treatment break for hematologic toxicity. Thus, this regimen is a good candidate for further testing in prospective clinical trials.

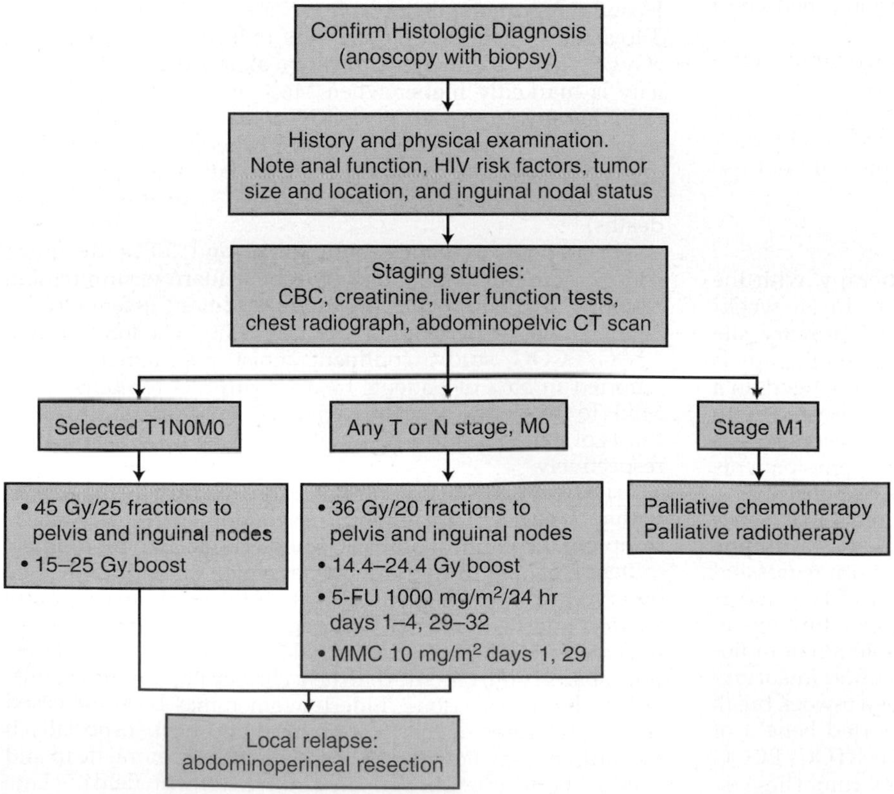

Figure 49-4 Diagnostic and treatment algorithm for patients with newly diagnosed anal cancer. CBC, complete blood cell count; CT, computed tomography; 5-FU, 5-fluorouracil; HIV, human immunodeficiency virus; MMC, mitomycin C.

Despite the rarity of anal cancer, major advances in the laboratory and clinic have led to an increased understanding of anal neoplasia that has improved treatment outcomes. As pathways leading to anal carcinogenesis are more fully described and the influences of HPV and other infectious agents are better defined, expanded research efforts focusing on prevention will be possible. However, further advances in the prevention and treatment of anal cancer will require continued commitment to prospective trials.

REFERENCES

1. Jemal A, Siegel R, Ward E, et al: Cancer statistics, 2006. CA Cancer J Clin 56:106-130, 2006.
2. McConnell EM: Squamous carcinoma of the anus: a review of 96 cases. Br J Surg 57:89-92, 1970.
3. Stearns MW Jr, Urmacher C, Sternberg SS, et al: Cancer of the anal canal. Curr Probl Cancer 4:1-44, 1980.
4. Sischy B, Doggett RL, Krall JM, et al: Definitive irradiation and chemotherapy for radiosensitization in management of anal carcinoma: interim report on Radiation Therapy Oncology Group study no. 8314. J Natl Cancer Inst 81:850-856, 1989.
5. Goldman S, Glimelius B, Nilsson B, et al: Incidence of anal epidermoid carcinoma in Sweden 1970-1984. Acta Chir Scand 155:191-197, 1989.
6. Melbye M, Rabkin C, Frisch M, et al: Changing patterns of anal cancer incidence in the United States, 1940-1989. Am J Epidemiol 139:772-780, 1994.
7. Myerson RJ, Karnell LH, Menck HR: The National Cancer Data Base report on carcinoma of the anus. Cancer 80:805-815, 1997.
8. Frisch M, Melbye M, Moller H: Trends in incidence of anal cancer in Denmark. BMJ 306:419-422, 1993.
9. Peters RK, Mack TM: Patterns of anal carcinoma by gender and marital status in Los Angeles County. Br J Cancer 48:629-636, 1983.
10. Biggar RJ, Burnett W, Mikl J, et al: Cancer among New York men at risk of acquired immunodeficiency syndrome. Int J Cancer 43:979-985, 1989.
11. Austin DF: Etiological clues from descriptive epidemiology: squamous carcinoma of the rectum or anus. Natl Cancer Inst Monogr 62:89-90, 1982.
12. Daling JR, Weiss NS, Klopfenstein LL, et al: Correlates of homosexual behavior and the incidence of anal cancer. JAMA 247:1988-1990, 1982.
13. Levi F, La Vecchia C, Randimbison L, et al: Patterns of large bowel cancer by subsite, age, sex and marital status. Tumori 77:246-251, 1991.
14. Beahrs OH, Wilson SM: Carcinoma of the anus. Ann Surg 184:422-428, 1976.
15. Frisch M, Smith E, Grulich A, et al: Cancer in a population-based cohort of men and women in registered homosexual partnerships. Am J Epidemiol 157:966-972, 2003.
16. Melbye M, Cote TR, Kessler L, et al, the AIDS Cancer Working Group: High incidence of anal cancer among AIDS patients. Lancet 343:636-639, 1994.
17. Frisch M, Olsen JH, Melbye M: Malignancies that occur before and after anal cancer: clues to their etiology. Am J Epidemiol 140:12-19, 1994.
18. Ogunbiyi OA, Scholefield JH, Rogers K, et al: *C-myc* oncogene expression in anal squamous neoplasia. J Clin Pathol 46:23-27, 1993.
19. Escot C, Theillet C, Lidereau R, et al: Genetic alteration of the *c-myc* protooncogene (MYC) in human primary breast carcinomas. Proc Natl Acad Sci U S A 83:4834-4838, 1986.
20. Melbye M, Sprogel P: Aetiological parallel between anal cancer and cervical cancer. Lancet 338:657-659, 1991.
21. Cabrera A, Tsukada Y, Pickren JW, et al: Development of lower genital carcinomas in patients with anal carcinoma: a more than casual relationship. Cancer 19:470-480, 1966.
22. Holmes F, Borek D, Owen-Kummer M, et al: Anal cancer in women. Gastroenterology 95:107-111, 1988.
23. Wexner SD, Milsom JW, Dailey TH: The demographics of anal cancers are changing: identification of a high-risk population. Dis Colon Rectum 30:942-946, 1987.
24. Daling JR, Weiss NS, Hislop TG, et al: Sexual practices, sexually transmitted diseases, and the incidence of anal cancer. N Engl J Med 317:973-977, 1987.
25. Zaki SR, Judd R, Coffield LM, et al: Human papillomavirus infection and anal carcinoma: retrospective analysis by in situ hybridization and the polymerase chain reaction. Am J Pathol 140:1345-1355, 1992.
26. Holly EA, Whittemore AS, Aston DA, et al: Anal cancer incidence: genital warts, anal fissure or fistula, hemorrhoids, and smoking. J Natl Cancer Inst 81:1726-1731, 1989.
27. Friis S, Kjaer SK, Frisch M, et al: Cervical intraepithelial neoplasia, anogenital cancer, and other cancer types in women after hospitalization for condylomata acuminata. J Infect Dis 175:743-748, 1997.
28. Heino P, Goldman S, Lagerstedt U, et al: Molecular and serological studies of human papillomavirus among patients with anal epidermoid carcinoma. Int J Cancer 53:377-381, 1993.
29. Scholefield JH, Kerr IB, Shepherd NA, et al: Human papillomavirus type 16 DNA in anal cancers from six different countries. Gut 32:674-676, 1991.
30. Palefsky JM, Holly EA, Gonzales J, et al: Detection of human papillomavirus DNA in anal intraepithelial neoplasia and anal cancer. Cancer Res 51:1014-1019, 1991.
31. Heino P, Eklund C, Fredriksson-Shanazarian V, et al: Association of serum immunoglobulin G antibodies against human papillomavirus type 16 capsids with anal epidermoid carcinoma. J Natl Cancer Inst 87:437-440, 1995.
32. Palefsky JM, Gonzales J, Greenblatt RM, et al: Anal intraepithelial neoplasia and anal papillomavirus infection among homosexual males with group IV HIV disease. JAMA 263:2911-2916, 1990.
33. Palefsky JM, Holly EA, Gonzales J, et al: Natural history of anal cytologic abnormalities and papillomavirus infection among homosexual men with group IV HIV disease. J Acquir Immune Defic Syndr 5:1258-1265, 1992.
34. Gates AE, Kaplan LD: AIDS malignancies in the era of highly active antiretroviral therapy. Oncology (Huntingt) 16:657-665, 2002.
35. Majewski S, Jablonska S: Human papillomavirus-associated tumors of the skin and mucosa. J Am Acad Dermatol 36:659-685, 1997.
36. Phelps WC, Yee CL, Munger K, et al: The human papillomavirus type 16 E7 gene encodes transactivation and transformation functions similar to those of adenovirus E1A. Cell 53:539-547, 1988.
37. zur Hausen H: Papillomavirus infections: a major cause of human cancers. Biochim Biophys Acta 1288:F55-F78, 1996.
38. Dyson N, Howley PM, Munger K, et al: The human papilloma virus-16 E7 oncoprotein is able to bind to the retinoblastoma gene product. Science 243:934-937, 1989.
39. Munger K, Werness BA, Dyson N, et al: Complex formation of human papillomavirus E7 proteins with the retinoblastoma tumor suppressor gene product. EMBO J 8:4099-4105, 1989.
40. Werness BA, Levine AJ, Howley PM: Association of human papillomavirus types 16 and 18 E6 proteins with p53. Science 248:76-79, 1990.
41. Penn I: Cancers of the anogenital region in renal transplant recipients: analysis of 65 cases. Cancer 58:611-616, 1986.
42. Blohme I, Brynger H: Malignant disease in renal transplant patients. Transplantation 39:23-25, 1985.
43. Arends MJ, Benton EC, McLaren KM, et al: Renal allograft recipients with high susceptibility to cutaneous malignancy have an increased prevalence of human papillomavirus DNA in skin tumours and a greater risk of anogenital malignancy. Br J Cancer 75:722-728, 1997.
44. Daling JR, Sherman KJ, Hislop TG, et al: Cigarette smoking and the risk of anogenital cancer. Am J Epidemiol 135:180-189, 1992.
45. Singh R, Nime F, Mittelman A: Malignant epithelial tumors of the anal canal. Cancer 48:411-415, 1981.
46. Frisch M, Olsen JH, Bautz A, et al: Benign anal lesions and the risk of anal cancer. N Engl J Med 331:300-302, 1994.

47. Lin AY, Gridley G, Tucker M: Benign anal lesions and anal cancer [letter]. N Engl J Med 332:190-191, 1995.
48. Consensus Development Conference: Cervical cancer. NIH Consensus Statement 14:1-38, 1996.
49. Winer RL, Lee SK, Hughes JP, et al: Genital human papillomavirus infection: incidence and risk factors in a cohort of female university students. Am J Epidemiol 157:218-226, 2003 (erratum in Am J Epidemiol 157:858, 2003).
50. Koutsky LA, Ault KA, Wheeler CM, et al: A controlled trial of a human papillomavirus type 16 vaccine. N Engl J Med 347: 1645-1651, 2002.
51. de Ruiter A, Carter P, Katz DR, et al: A comparison between cytology and histology to detect anal intraepithelial neoplasia. Genitourin Med 70:22-25, 1994.
52. Williams GR, Talbot IC: Anal carcinoma: a histological review. Histopathology 25:507-516, 1994.
53. Palefsky JM, Holly EA, Hogeboom CJ, et al: Anal cytology as a screening tool for anal squamous intraepithelial lesions. J Acquir Immune Defic Syndr Hum Retrovirol 14:415-422, 1997.
54. Jay N, Berry JM, Hogeboom CJ, et al: Colposcopic appearance of anal squamous intraepithelial lesions: relationship to histopathology. Dis Colon Rectum 40:919-928, 1997.
55. Salmon RJ, Zafrani B, Labib A, et al: Prognosis of cloacogenic and squamous cancers of the anal canal. Dis Colon Rectum 29: 336-340, 1986.
56. Doggett SW, Green JP, Cantril ST: Efficacy of radiation therapy alone for limited squamous cell carcinoma of the anal canal. Int J Radiat Oncol Biol Phys 15:1069-1072, 1988.
57. Tanum G: Treatment of relapsing anal carcinoma. Acta Oncol 32:33-35, 1993.
58. Cummings BJ, Keane TJ, O'Sullivan B, et al: Epidermoid anal cancer: treatment by radiation alone or by radiation and 5-fluorouracil with and without mitomycin C. Int J Radiat Oncol Biol Phys 21:1115-1125, 1991.
59. Allal A, Kurtz JM, Pipard G, et al: Chemoradiotherapy versus radiotherapy alone for anal cancer: a retrospective comparison. Int J Radiat Oncol Biol Phys 27:59-66, 1993.
60. Boman BM, Moertel CG, O'Connell MJ, et al: Carcinoma of the anal canal: a clinical and pathologic study of 188 cases. Cancer 54:114-125, 1984.
61. Tanum G, Tveit K, Karlsen KO, et al: Chemotherapy and radiation therapy for anal carcinoma: survival and late morbidity. Cancer 67:2462-2466, 1991.
62. Kuehn PG, Eisenberg H, Reed JF: Epidermoid carcinoma of the perianal skin and anal canal. Cancer 22:932-938, 1968.
63. Leichman L, Nigro N, Vaitkevicius VK, et al: Cancer of the anal canal: model for preoperative adjuvant combined modality therapy. Am J Med 78:211-215, 1985.
64. Frost DB, Richards PC, Montague ED, et al: Epidermoid cancer of the anorectum. Cancer 53:1285-1293, 1984.
65. Svensson C, Goldman S, Friberg B: Radiation treatment of epidermoid cancer of the anus. Int J Radiat Oncol Biol Phys 27:67-73, 1993.
66. Schlag PM, Hunerbein M: Anal cancer: multimodal therapy. World J Surg 19:282-286, 1995.
67. Longo WE, Vernava AM III, Wade TP, et al: Recurrent squamous cell carcinoma of the anal canal: predictors of initial treatment failure and results of salvage therapy. Ann Surg 220:40-49, 1994.
68. Dobrowsky W: Radiotherapy of epidermoid anal canal cancer. Br J Radiol 62:53-58, 1989.
69. Eschwege F, Lasser P, Chavy A, et al: Squamous cell carcinoma of the anal canal: treatment by external beam irradiation. Radiother Oncol 3:145-150, 1985.
70. Schlienger M, Krzisch C, Pene F, et al: Epidermoid carcinoma of the anal canal: treatment results and prognostic variables in a series of 242 cases. Int J Radiat Oncol Biol Phys 17:1141-1151, 1989.
71. Bartelink H, Roelofsen F, Eschwege F, et al: Concomitant radiotherapy and chemotherapy is superior to radiotherapy alone in the treatment of locally advanced anal cancer: results of a phase III randomized trial of the European Organization for Research and Treatment of Cancer Radiotherapy and Gastrointestinal Cooperative Groups. J Clin Oncol 15:2040-2049, 1997.
72. de Gara CJ, Basrur V, Figueredo A, et al: The influence of age on the management of anal cancer. Hepatogastroenterology 42:73-76, 1995.
73. Cantril ST, Green JP, Schall GL, et al: Primary radiation therapy in the treatment of anal carcinoma. Int J Radiat Oncol Biol Phys 9:1271-1278, 1983.
74. Martenson JA, Lipsitz SR, Lefkopoulou M, et al: Results of combined modality therapy for patients with anal cancer (E7283): an Eastern Cooperative Oncology Group study. Cancer 76:1731-1736, 1995.
75. Shepherd NA, Scholefield JH, Love SB, et al: Prognostic factors in anal squamous carcinoma: a multivariate analysis of clinical, pathological and flow cytometric parameters in 235 cases. Histopathology 16:545-555, 1990.
76. Scott NA, Beart RW Jr, Weiland LH, et al: Carcinoma of the anal canal and flow cytometric DNA analysis. Br J Cancer 60:56-58, 1989.
77. Tanum G, Hannisdal E, Stenwig B: Prognostic factors in anal carcinoma. Oncology 51:22-24, 1994.
78. Holm R, Skovlund E, Skomedal H, et al: Reduced expression of p21 WAF1 is an indicator of malignant behaviour in anal carcinomas. Histopathology 39:43-49, 2001.
79. Jass JR, Sobin LH: Histological Typing of Intestinal Tumors, 2nd ed. Berlin, Springer-Verlag, 1989, pp 41-47.
80. Dougherty BG, Evans HL: Carcinoma of the anal canal: a study of 79 cases. Am J Clin Pathol 83:159-164, 1985.
81. Quan SH: Anal cancers: squamous and melanoma. Cancer 70(Suppl 1):384-389, 1992.
82. Thibault C, Sagar P, Nivatvongs S, et al: Anorectal melanoma: an incurable disease? Dis Colon Rectum 40:661-668, 1997.
83. Cummings BJ: The place of radiation therapy in the treatment of carcinoma of the anal canal. Cancer Treat Rev 9:125-147, 1982.
84. Fenger C: Histology of the anal canal. Am J Surg Pathol 12:41-55, 1988.
85. Paradis P, Douglass HO Jr, Holyoke ED: The clinical implications of a staging system for carcinoma of the anus. Surg Gynecol Obstet 141:411-416, 1975.
86. Caplan I: The lymphatic vessels of the anal region: a study and investigation about 50 cases. Folia Angiol 24:260, 1976.
87. Salmon RJ, Fenton J, Asselain B, et al: Treatment of epidermoid anal canal cancer. Am J Surg 147:43-48, 1984.
88. Miller EJ, Quan SH, Thaler HT: Treatment of squamous cell carcinoma of the anal canal. Cancer 67:2038-2041, 1991.
89. Kuehn PG, Beckett R, Eisenberg H, et al: Epidermoid carcinoma of the perianal skin and anal canal: a review of 157 cases. N Engl J Med 270:614-617, 1964.
90. Tanum G, Tveit K, Karlsen KO: Diagnosis of anal carcinoma: doctor's finger still the best? Oncology 48:383-386, 1991.
91. Tanum G, Stenwig AE, Bormer OP, et al: Carcinoembryonic antigen in anal carcinoma. Acta Oncol 31:333-335, 1992.
92. Herzog U, Boss M, Spichtin HP: Endoanal ultrasonography in the follow-up of anal carcinoma. Surg Endosc 8:1186-1189, 1994.
93. American Joint Committee on Cancer: Anal canal. *In* Greene FL, Page DL, Fleming ID, et al (eds): AJCC Cancer Staging Handbook, 6th ed. New York, Springer-Verlag, 2002, pp 139-144.
94. Gordon PH: Squamous-cell carcinoma of the anal canal. Surg Clin North Am 68:1391-1399, 1988.
95. Martenson JA Jr, Gunderson LL: External radiation therapy without chemotherapy in the management of anal cancer. Cancer 71:1736-1740, 1993.
96. Papillon J, Montbarbon JF: Epidermoid carcinoma of the anal canal: a series of 276 cases. Dis Colon Rectum 30:324-333, 1987.
97. UKCCCR Anal Cancer Trial Working Party: Epidermoid anal cancer: results from the UKCCCR randomised trial of radiotherapy alone versus radiotherapy, 5-fluorouracil, and mitomycin. Lancet 348:1049-1054, 1996.
98. Bosset JF, Pavy JJ, Roelofsen F, et al: Combined radiotherapy and chemotherapy for anal cancer. Lancet 349:205-206, 1997.
99. Nigro ND, Seydel HG, Considine B, et al: Combined preoperative radiation and chemotherapy for squamous cell carcinoma of the anal canal. Cancer 51:1826-1829, 1983.
100. Rich TA, Ajani JA, Morrison WH, et al: Chemoradiation therapy for anal cancer: radiation plus continuous infusion of 5-

fluorouracil with or without cisplatin. Radiother Oncol 27:209-215, 1993.
101. Hughes LL, Rich TA, Delclos L, et al: Radiotherapy for anal cancer: experience from 1979-1987. Int J Radiat Oncol Biol Phys 17:1153-1160, 1989.
102. Doci R, Zucali R, Bombelli L, et al: Combined chemoradiation therapy for anal cancer: a report of 56 cases. Ann Surg 215:150-156, 1992.
103. Doci R, Zucali R, La Monica G, et al: Primary chemoradiation therapy with fluorouracil and cisplatin for cancer of the anus: results in 35 consecutive patients. J Clin Oncol 14:3121-3125, 1996.
104. Flam M, John M, Pajak TF, et al: Role of mitomycin in combination with fluorouracil and radiotherapy, and of salvage chemoradiation in the definitive nonsurgical treatment of epidermoid carcinoma of the anal canal: results of a phase III randomized intergroup study. J Clin Oncol 14:2527-2539, 1996.
105. Cummings BJ, Keane TJ, O'Sullivan B, et al: Mitomycin in anal canal carcinoma. Oncology 50 Suppl 1:63-69, 1993.
106. Dobrowsky W, Dobrowsky E, Rauth AM: Mode of interaction of 5-fluorouracil, radiation, and mitomycin C: in vitro studies. Int J Radiat Oncol Biol Phys 22:875-880, 1992.
107. Marshall RS, Rauth AM: Modification of the cytotoxic activity of mitomycin C by oxygen and ascorbic acid in Chinese hamster ovary cells and a repair-deficient mutant. Cancer Res 46:2709-2713, 1986.
108. Byfield JE, Calabro-Jones P, Klisak I, et al: Pharmacologic requirements for obtaining sensitization of human tumor cells in vitro to combined 5-fluorouracil or ftorafur and x rays. Int J Radiat Oncol Biol Phys 8:1923-1933, 1982.
109. Flam MS, John MJ, Mowry PA, et al: Definitive combined modality therapy of carcinoma of the anus: a report of 30 cases including results of salvage therapy in patients with residual disease. Dis Colon Rectum 30:495-502, 1987.
110. Tveit KM, Karlsen KO, Fossa SD, et al: Primary treatment of carcinoma of the anus by combined radiotherapy and chemotherapy. Scand J Gastroenterol 24:1243-1247, 1989.
111. Flam MS, John M, Pajak T, et al: Radiation (RT) and 5-fluorouracil (5FU) versus radiation, 5FU, and mitomycin-C (MMC) in the treatment of anal carcinoma: results of a phase III randomized RTOG/ECOG Intergroup trial [abstract]. Prog Proc Am Soc Clin Oncol 14:191, 1995.
112. Allal AS, Mermillod B, Roth AD, et al: The impact of treatment factors on local control in T2-T3 anal carcinomas treated by radiotherapy with or without chemotherapy. Cancer 79:2329-2335, 1997.
113. Nigh SS, Smalley SR, Elman AJ, et al: Conservative therapy for anal carcinoma: an analysis of prognostic factors [abstract]. Int J Radiat Oncol Biol Phys 21 Suppl 1:224, 1991.
114. John M, Pajak T, Flam M, et al: Dose escalation in chemoradiation for anal cancer: preliminary results of RTOG 92-08. Cancer J Sci Am 2:205, 1996.
115. John MJ, Pajak TJ, Flam MS, et al: Dose acceleration in chemoradiation (CRX) for anal cancer: preliminary results of RTOG 92-08. Int J Radiat Oncol Biol Phys 32 Suppl 1:157, 1995.
116. Cummings B, Keane T, Thomas G, et al: Results and toxicity of the treatment of anal canal carcinoma by radiation therapy or radiation therapy and chemotherapy. Cancer 54:2062-2068, 1984.
117. Holland JM, Swift PS: Tolerance of patients with human immunodeficiency virus and anal carcinoma to treatment with combined chemotherapy and radiation therapy. Radiology 193:251-254, 1994.
118. Chadha M, Rosenblatt EA, Malamud S, et al: Squamous-cell carcinoma of the anus in HIV-positive patients. Dis Colon Rectum 37:861-865, 1994.
119. Peddada AV, Smith DE, Rao AR, et al: Chemotherapy and low-dose radiotherapy in the treatment of HIV-infected patients with carcinoma of the anal canal. Int J Radiat Oncol Biol Phys 37:1101-1105, 1997.
120. John M, Pajak T, Kreig R, et al: Dose escalation without split-course chemoradiation for anal cancer: results of a phase II RTOG study [abstract]. Int J Radiat Oncol Biol Phys 39 Suppl:203, 1997.
121. Martenson JA, Lipsitz SR, Wagner H Jr, et al: Initial results of a phase II trial of high dose radiation therapy, 5-fluorouracil, and cisplatin for patients with anal cancer (E4292): an Eastern Cooperative Oncology Group study. Int J Radiat Oncol Biol Phys 35:745-749, 1996.
122. Paleologo FP, Goswitz MS, Skibber JM, et al: Results of radiation and concomitant continuous infusion 5-fluorouracil and cisplatin for anal cancer [abstract]. Int J Radiat Oncol Biol Phys 39 Suppl:135, 1997.

PART E

GENITOURINARY TUMORS

Overview

Anthony Zietman

Since the publication of the first edition of this textbook, the field of genitourinary oncology has changed dramatically. It is a field that is intensely multidisciplinary, and radiation oncologists, often substantially outnumbered in the multidisciplinary clinic, must be masters of the published data. Genitourinary oncology has become one of the areas in which practicing radiation oncologists are likely to spend a substantial proportion of their time and one that they cannot choose to ignore.

Developments in genitourinary oncology illustrate the best and some of the more problematic aspects of contemporary medicine. There is much research in areas of spectacular technologic advances, but too much has been widely adopted without sufficient and rigorous scientific evaluation. This overview provides highlights of the field that are reviewed in greater detail by the authors of the following chapters.

PROSTATE CANCER

Prostate cancer, along with breast and lung cancer, remains the bread and butter of the practicing radiation oncologist. Up to 40% of the referrals in some practices may be prostate cancer. This situation reflects the explosion in early case detection through the widespread use of the prostate-specific antigen (PSA) blood test and the successes of therapy. The incidence peaked in the early 1990s, a few years after the introduction of PSA, as the prevalence of the disease in the previously unscreened population was reduced. As predicted, the rate began to fall, but more recently, it has begun to rise again. The increase probably reflects the fact that sporadic early case detection has in time become an unofficial screening program, with more than 80% of American males having had their PSA tested. Detection rates far exceed the death rates, and many more men are being detected with prostate cancer than require treatment.[1] Because we cannot sort out the "tigers" from the "pussycats," radiation oncologists and urologists err on the side of caution and still treat most of those diagnosed with prostate cancer.[2] In the near future, it is likely that molecular markers will tell us who does not require treatment. At that time, our caseload will decline, and we can concentrate our energy and effective therapy on those who need it. However, which is the most effective therapy?

External irradiation has progressed substantially in recent years. The latest Patterns of Care Survey says that almost all radiation oncologists in the United States use three-dimensional (3D) conformal techniques.[3] The randomized trials show that conformal therapy reduces morbidity and that the increased radiation dose this allows gives higher cure rates. This is a superb example of practice changing on the basis of strong evidence. The introduction of intensity-modulated radiation and, in an increasing number of centers, proton beams will likely produce some dosimetric gains, but whether these will yield detectable clinical gains for the patient remains uncertain.

These substantial technical improvements have made external irradiation a much more lengthy and expensive process. As a result, alternative approaches have been proposed in an attempt to reduce the social and economic burden. One method is the use of hypofractionation, a previously heretical concept that has reappeared because of evidence suggesting that prostate cancer may have a low α/β ratio. This concept is being tested in randomized trials in the United States, Canada, and the United Kingdom. The other approach is the use of low and high dose rate (LDR, HDR) brachytherapy. Each approach has its proponents, and the early data look favorable for both. Some enthusiasm for brachytherapy has been industry rather than data driven, and it is the responsibility of radiation oncologists over the next decade to obtain and sift the data to determine whether either method offers real advantages and for which patients.

Patients with early prostate cancer have a disease that is so likely to be cured that quality-of-life issues become very important for the survivors. These topics are being reported using appropriate instruments at an increasing rate, and it is evident that the effects on quality of life will become one of the important ways that patients and physicians choose therapy in the years ahead.

For locally advanced disease, there have been tremendous efforts by the large U.S. and European cooperative groups to perform trials, answer questions, and determine standards of practice. The role of androgen therapy combined with external beam irradiation has become better defined. Results with radiation alone for low-risk disease are sufficiently good that these patients probably do not need androgen therapy (RTOG trial 94-08 is still awaited); intermediate-risk disease probably does, but only as a short neoadjuvant course[4,5]; and high-risk prostate cancer certainly needs it for years in a manner akin to breast cancer.[6] The role of pelvic lymph node irradiation in locally advanced disease is one that will not go away. RTOG 94-13 has suggested that there may be a small disease-specific survival advantage when it is given, and newer technology is being turned to treating the lymph nodes in a fashion less morbid than in the past.[7] Active trials are addressing the use of high-dose radiation in addition to androgen deprivation and the use of chemotherapy. The latter comes in the wake of recent randomized trials showing that chemotherapy can extend life in men with metastatic disease.

Prostate cancer now joins breast, testis, and lymphoma as an exemplary field of clinical research in which one trial builds on the shoulders of the next, and piece by piece, knowledge is built up to create a clearer picture of management. Prostate cancer also has become a model in its multidisciplinary approach. Through brachytherapy and combined-modality treatment, radiation oncologists, urologists, and medical oncologists have developed a new and productive spirit of cooperation.

BLADDER CANCER

Bladder cancer is an area in which substantial gains have been made. A growing body of supportive evidence has made the multimodality approach to bladder preservation a recognized alternative to the radical cystectomy.[8] The RTOG continues to refine technique in a series of trials optimizing radiation dose and chemotherapy. In the United Kingdom and northern Europe, there has been much work on better defining the treatment volume, and randomized trials are answering questions about nodal treatment and the value of whole- versus partial-bladder irradiation. There is interest in daily image guidance for this highly mobile tumor because the greatest morbidity of bladder cancer treatment is gastrointestinal rather than genitourinary. Any way to tighten volumes and reduce the volume of small bowel treated will be a step forward for these patients.

Several molecular markers and potential molecular targets have emerged in bladder cancer that are creating new avenues for clinical research. Future trial group research will be in the interaction of these agents with chemoradiation rather than in further adjustments in radiation dose or chemotherapy agents, which seem to have reached a plateau.

With all this progress, why is multimodality treatment with organ conservation not more popular with patients and urologists? The urologists have traditionally been the gatekeepers, and their belief that the bladder must be removed rapidly to maximize the chance for cure is strong, as is the belief that an irradiated bladder functions poorly and that superficial and invasive local failures are common and difficult to manage. The chapter on bladder cancer that follows summarizes the data that may be used by radiation and medical oncologists to argue for organ conservation as an alternative to immediate cystectomy for the willing patient.

TESTICULAR CANCER

Seminoma is one of the most radiation sensitive of all tumors, and radiation oncologists take particular pride in being able to promise a very high probability of cure. There are few cancers such as stage I-II seminoma, for which cure rates exceed 95%. For 40 years, adjuvant radiation therapy has been the principal player alongside orchiectomy, but more recently, there has been a stepwise retreat. Low-dose irradiation has a long-term legacy. Long ago, the mediastinal field was dropped because of concerns about cardiac toxicity and because improved chemotherapy offered a very effective salvage in cases in which it was needed. Recent concerns revolve around radiation-induced tumors.[9] Conformal techniques are now routinely used to spare some normal tissue, and, in a series of British and Canadian randomized trials, substantial reductions in target volume and dose have been tested.

Since the first edition of this book, the standard adjuvant treatment in Europe has shrunk from a full "dog-leg" field treated to 30 Gy down to a para-aortic field alone treated to only 20 Gy.[10] Trials are looking at single-agent carboplatin as an alternative to irradiation. In Canada, recognizing that most men with small tumors are disease free after orchiectomy, a policy of surveillance has become commonplace, with treatment deferred and given only to those who ultimately prove to have stage II disease. In Chapter 52, Warde documents these changes and the discussions that the contemporary radiation oncologist must have with any newly diagnosed patient. The recent story of irradiation in seminoma mirrors that of irradiation in Hodgkin's disease, for which the search for "how low can we go" has been driven by the success of the treatment.

PENILE CANCER

Penile carcinoma is another cancer for which organ conservation may be expected to be very popular. In Chapter 54, Crook and Mazeron demonstrate that penile cancer is not an ordinary skin cancer, but one with a high propensity for nodal spread. They also show that effective organ-sparing radiation treatment is possible. Treatment is technically challenging, and in the United States, where men are circumcised and the disease rare, there is little accumulated experience. However, treatment by brachytherapy or external beam irradiation follows simple first principles, and it is not beyond the reach of any skillful radiation oncologist.

RENAL CANCER, CANCER OF THE RENAL PELVIS, AND CANCER OF THE URETER

Renal cancer, cancer of the renal pelvis, and cancer of the ureter have traditionally been the preserve of the surgeon. There has been a tremendous stage shift in renal cancer with the routine discovery of small, incidental tumors on abdominal scans performed for other reasons. Development of the partial nephrectomy, laparoscopic nephrectomy, and percutaneous ultrasound ablation has provided effective therapy that cannot be matched by any medical or radiation therapy alternative.

Renal cell cancer is recognized to be relatively insensitive to radiation. Irradiation alone has a role to play in locally advanced or metastatic disease. It may be considered as an option after resection of disease with positive margins or after resection of an isolated local recurrence. Intraoperative irradiation may be used to deliver the high doses required without bowel toxicity. In metastatic disease, radiation therapy to a high dose has an important role in maintaining the quality of life of patients who may live many years.

Cancers of the renal pelvis and ureter are different from renal cell adenocarcinomas. Because they are transitional cell in origin, they behave more like bladder cancer and are more sensitive to irradiation and cisplatin-based chemotherapy, but organ-sparing approaches are not used. There is little gain in function or quality of life for preserving a kidney or ureter when another exists, and surgery is the mainstay of treatment. Chemoradiation may offer some assistance when the disease is locally advanced or has spread to nearby lymph nodes.

REFERENCES

1. Johansson JE, Andren O, Andersson SO, et al: Natural history of early, localized prostate cancer. JAMA 291:2713-2719, 2004.
2. Cooperberg MR, Lubeck DP, Meng MV, et al: The changing face of low-risk prostate cancer: trends in clinical presentation and primary management. J Clin Oncol 22:2141-2149, 2004.
3. Zelefsky MJ, Moughan J, Owen J, et al: Changing trends in national practice for external beam radiotherapy for clinically localized prostate cancer: 1999 Patterns of Care Survey for Prostate Cancer. Int J Radiat Oncol Biol Phys 59:1053-1062, 2004.
4. D'Amico AV, Manola J, Loffredo M, et al: Six month androgen suppression plus radiation therapy versus radiation therapy alone for patients with clinically localized prostate cancer. JAMA 292:821-827, 2004.

5. Hanks GE, Pajak TF, Porter A, et al: Phase III trial of long-term adjuvant androgen deprivation after neoadjuvant hormonal cytoreduction and radiotherapy in locally advanced carcinoma of the prostate. J Clin Oncol 21:3972-3978, 2003.
6. Bolla M, Colette L, Blank L, et al: Long-term results with immediate androgen suppression and external radiation in patients with locally advanced prostate cancer (an EORTC study); a phase III randomized trial. Lancet 360:103-106, 2002.
7. Roach M, DeSilvio M, Lawton C, et al: Phase III trial comparing whole pelvic versus prostate only radiotherapy and neoadjuvant versus adjuvant combined androgen suppression. J Clin Oncol 21:1904-1911, 2003.
8. Shipley WU, Kaufman DS, Thakral HK, et al: Long-term outcome of patients treated for muscle-invasive bladder cancer by trimodality therapy. Urology 60:62-68, 2002.
9. Travis LB, Curtis RE, Storm H, et al: Risk of second malignant neoplasms among long-term survivors of testicular cancer. J Natl Cancer Inst 89:1429-1439, 1997.
10. Jones WG, Fossa SD, Mead GM, et al: Randomized trial of 30 vs 20 Gy in the adjuvant treatment of stage I testicular seminoma: a report on Medical Research Council Trial TE18, European organization for the Research and Treatment of Cancer Trial 30942. J Clin Oncol 20:23:1200-1208, 2005.

CHAPTER 50

PROSTATE CANCER

Deborah A. Kuban, Louis Potters, Colleen A. Lawton, and Thomas M. Pisansky

INCIDENCE

An estimated 234,460 new cases of prostate cancer and 27,350 deaths will occur in 2006. These numbers have been relatively stable since 1994, when the level of prostate-specific antigen (PSA) began to be used as a screening tool that aided in diagnosing the backlog of existing cases in the population.

One in six American men will develop prostate cancer during his lifetime.

BIOLOGIC CHARACTERISTICS

PSA, clinical tumor stage, and tumor grade are predictive of extraprostatic tumor extension, lymphatic and hematogenous metastasis, and therefore therapeutic outcome. These factors may be combined to improve the accuracy of predicting disease-related survival.

STAGING

Tumor, node, and metastasis (TNM) classifications may be determined by clinical means or by pathologic examination of prostatectomy and lymphadenectomy specimens.

Digital rectal examination with or without ultrasound, Gleason score of the biopsy, and PSA level form the basis of the clinical staging workup. Bone scans and computed tomography or magnetic resonance imaging of the pelvis with or without the abdomen are selectively used for high-risk patients.

PRIMARY THERAPY

The selection of radiation therapy and radical prostatectomy as primary therapeutic modalities is based on life expectancy, comorbidities, tumor-related characteristics, and the patient's expectation with regard to quality-of-life issues.

In clinically localized disease, several years of observation are required to measure the impact of a particular treatment on the natural history of the disease. Radiation therapy provides outcomes for patients with organ-confined disease that compare favorably with expected survival durations.

Three-dimensional and intensity-modulated external beam radiation therapies allow treatment to conform to the target while minimizing exposure of nontarget (e.g., rectal and bladder) tissues.

Transperineal template ultrasound guidance provides a means for accurate radioactive source placement. Renewed interest in prostate brachytherapy resulted from this technical advantage, which has provided equivalent results for properly selected candidates.

ADJUVANT THERAPY

Risk factors for local tumor recurrence after postprostatectomy include tumor involvement of surgical margins, seminal vesicles, or pelvic lymph nodes. There is emerging evidence that adjuvant radiation therapy can improve local tumor control and disease-free survival.

LOCALLY ADVANCED DISEASE

External beam radiation therapy is the preferred primary treatment modality for locally advanced disease.

The addition of neoadjuvant androgen deprivation to radiation therapy improves local tumor control and progression-free survival rates.

Androgen deprivation as adjuvant therapy to external beam radiation therapy diminishes the risk for local tumor recurrence and metastatic disease relapse. Improved survival duration also may be observed, particularly for patients with high-grade tumors.

PALLIATION

External beam irradiation effectively relieves symptoms due to locally progressive disease or metastases.

Systemic radiation therapy (e.g., strontium 89, samarium 153) may increase the symptom-free interval in patients with osseous metastases, particularly when used in concert with localized external beam radiation therapy.

Prostate cancer is a significant health issue that provokes considerable discussion among various segments of the health care profession. The variable nature of the illness coupled with its prevalence in the elderly, who are subject to substantial medical comorbidity, and the dearth of outcomes-based evidence for medical decision-making fuels debate regarding the utility of early detection and the relative merits of therapeutic intervention. In this context, the radiation oncologist may engage in discussion with primary care physicians, urologists, and other health care professionals concerned with the welfare of patients with prostate cancer. A broad base of knowledge relevant to multispecialty interaction and detailed information regarding the "state of the (radiotherapeutic) art" is essential for productive dialog. The clinician should interpret the existing medical literature with a critical view and should strive to contribute to clinical research efforts that will ultimately improve the care of patients with this disease.

EPIDEMIOLOGY

The National Cancer Institute's Surveillance, Epidemiology, and End Results (SEER) Program estimated that 1,399,790 Americans would develop an invasive (other than cutaneous basal or squamous cell) cancer in 2006.[1] Among these Americans, an estimated 234,460 men with prostate cancer accounted for 33% of all newly diagnosed cancers. The annual age-adjusted incidence of prostate cancer dramatically increased over the past 2 decades.[2-4] For example, the age-adjusted annual incidence rate increased 6.4% per year between 1983 and 1989,[2] and there was a 66% overall increase between the periods of 1975 to 1979 and 1987 to 1991.[3] This change largely reflected the increased detection of localized, rather than regionally advanced or metastatic, prostate cancer cases.[2,5] Although the reason for this observation is not fully understood, it is at least in part due to the use of transurethral resection of the prostate[6] and to changes in the intensity of medical surveillance that occurred over time.[4,5] It appears that one in six American men will develop a clinically recognized invasive prostate cancer during his lifetime.[1] An estimated 27,350 men are expected to die of this disease in 2006.[1]

The incidence of incidental (or latent) prostate cancer observed at autopsy examination[7-9] and the incidence and prevalence of clinically manifest prostate cancer increase substantially with age.[1] Information from the SEER Program indicates that approximately 1.8% of American men between ages 40 and 59 years had a clinical diagnosis of prostate cancer, whereas 15% of men 60 to 79 years old would have prostate cancer by the time they attained this age. Although the prevalence of incidental carcinoma does not exhibit marked geographic variation, the regional disparity in the antemortem clinical expression of the disease and the cancer mortality rate of prostatic carcinoma is noteworthy.[7,10] North America, Australia, New Zealand, Western and Northern Europe, and the Caribbean have a much higher incidence of this disease than Asia and China.[10]

ETIOLOGY

Cohort and case-control studies are the two principal methods used to ascertain the cause of cancer.[11] Several reports describe various host-related and environmental factors that appear associated with prostate cancer (Table 50-1), but it is not yet understood which factors directly initiate or promote prostate carcinogenesis. Because this disease has shown age-related, racial/ethnic, and geographic variation,[1] it has been suggested that its development is primarily influenced by environmental agents and genetic factors. As discussed by several investigators,[12,13] long-term androgen exposure, which is required for normal prostatic development and for cancer growth and maintenance; advanced age[1]; race or ethnicity[14,15]; and familial history of prostate cancer[16,17] are viewed as the most likely risk factors. Other associations such as diet, especially fat intake, and body mass index are becoming more suspect.[18,19]

Hormonal Factors

Although several lines of investigation suggest the importance of hormones in the promotion of prostate cancer, their mechanism of action and interactions are not clearly understood. Animal studies indicate that chronic testosterone exposure markedly enhances the effects of carcinogens on prostatic tissues,[20] and the clinical expression of prostate cancer is rare in androgen-deprived men (e.g., eunuchs). Benign prostatic hypertrophy and prostate cancer simultaneously develop under androgen stimulation, and some reports suggest that men with benign hypertrophy are at increased risk for prostate cancer.[21,22] Various investigators report that men with prostate cancer have alterations in serum levels of androstenedione, dihydrotestosterone, sex hormone-binding globulin, or testosterone,[23-26] which can also vary according to race or ethnicity.[25,26]

Table 50-1 Potential Risk Factors for Prostate Cancer

Advanced age
Benign prostatic hyperplasia
Diet (e.g., fat intake)
Familial history of prostate cancer
Histologic precursors (e.g., prostatic intraepithelial neoplasia)
Hormonal factors (e.g., serum testosterone)
Occupational exposure (e.g., cadmium)
Race or ethnicity (e.g., black)
Sexual behavior (e.g., multiple partners)
Sexually transmitted disease (e.g., herpesvirus)
Tobacco use
Vasectomy

Age

Age may be the single most important factor associated with prostate cancer, as most elderly men have histologic evidence of cancer in the prostate gland,[8] and the rate of clinical detection is a direct function of age.[1] Although several causes may be invoked such as senescence of the immune system and prolonged exposure to carcinogens, an exact explanation for this association is lacking.

Hereditary Factors

Several investigators also observed familial clustering of prostate cancer and suggested that genetic constitution may increase susceptibility to the disease.[16,27-29] The characteristics of familial and hereditary prostate cancer are discussed by Carter and associates,[16] who describe an increased risk of the disease, a greater number of affected relatives, and an earlier age of onset with the familial type compared with the sporadic form. The hereditary type, considered a subset of the familial form, is characterized by autosomal dominant inheritance and may account for one in 10 cases.[16] The age-adjusted risk of developing prostate cancer in the setting of a familial predisposition is approximately twice that of the general population[16,27-29] but may be greater (i.e., 5- to 11-fold), depending on the number of affected first-degree relatives.[30] The increased risk associated with familial history is independent of age or of race or ethnicity.[28,29] It is uncertain whether a family history of breast or other cancers correlates with an excess risk for prostate cancer.[28,31]

Racial and Ethnic Variations

Prostate cancer incidence is characterized by marked racial/ethnic variation that is dependent on geographic factors.[1] For example, a 30- to 50-fold difference in the incidence of the disease is observed between black men and native Asians.[32] However, a complex interaction between race/ethnicity and environment exists. For example, the incidence of cancer in a particular racial/ethnic group (e.g., Japanese) tends to shift toward that of the population in the geographic area to which that group immigrates (e.g., the United States) as the group assimilates to its new environment and culture.[33] Certain racial or ethnic groups (e.g., blacks) present with more-advanced prostate cancer and appear to have a stage-adjusted outcome that is worse than for other members of their society (e.g., whites).[34,35] Racial variations of hormonal, dietary, genetic, and perhaps socioeconomic factors may account for such findings,[14,29,36] but definitive evidence in this regard is lacking, and further research is necessary to clarify the association between race/ethnicity and prostate cancer risk.

Dietary Factors

The role of dietary factors in prostate cancer pathogenesis is difficult to discern, because research in this area is confounded by complex interactions with other potential risk factors. These studies are often retrospective, and it is difficult to accurately document dietary patterns and isolate the effect of a particular nutrient that initiated carcinogenesis or promoted its clinical expression after a lengthy latency period. Nonetheless, there are striking racial/ethnicity and geographic variations in prostate cancer incidence that may have a dietary basis. In particular, a high-fat diet appears to correlate with prostate cancer incidence and mortality,[13,18,29,37,38] whereas ingestion of retinol,[39] certain carotenoids (e.g., lycopene),[13,40] phytoestrogens,[41] and vitamin D may be protective.[42] The influence of other vitamins (e.g., vitamin E) and minerals (e.g., zinc) is uncertain.[13] Whittemore and colleagues[29] studied the correlation of diet, physical activity, and body size with geographic and racial/ethnic factors. Prostate cancer risk was significantly and directly associated with total fat intake across all ethnic groups but was not related to body mass, physical activity patterns, or intake of micronutrients. Mills and colleagues made a similar observation that was not preserved when fruit and vegetable consumption was considered.[43]

Although studies have failed to consistently show that obesity is related to prostate cancer incidence, a study of more than 400,000 men begun by the American Cancer Society in 1982 (Cancer Prevention Study II) showed that men with higher body mass index (i.e., weight versus height) had an increased risk of prostate cancer death compared with men with a lower body mass index.[18,19] The mechanism through which obesity might cause prostate cancer or a higher mortality from prostate cancer is complex but is thought to be related to a state of hyperinsulinemia which leads to higher levels of insulin-like growth factor and available sex steroids (androgens).[44]

Other Lifestyle Factors

Research regarding other lifestyle factors such as tobacco use, alcohol consumption, physical activity level, body habitus, sexual behavior, and sexually transmitted diseases has provided mixed findings with regard to the importance of these factors in prostate cancer pathogenesis.[18-19,45-53] Although the results of these studies may be affected by the fact that several lifestyle factors may be simultaneously interacting and difficult to separate, nevertheless this research increasingly suggests that there may be an effect for at least some of these etiologic factors.

Environmental Exposure

A link between environmental or occupational exposure to carcinogens and development of prostate cancer has also been explored, but establishing a correlation and identifying causative agents have been difficult. For example, laborers in heavy industry, rubber manufacturers, and newspaper printers may have a somewhat higher incidence of prostate cancer,[54] but this association is weak, and its significance remains uncertain. Exposure to cadmium, as from cigarette smoke, nickel-cadmium batteries, or certain paints, has been implicated as a carcinogen, as cadmium workers have more aggressive prostate cancers and an increased cause-specific mortality.[55] Nonetheless, a clear association between these factors, environmental or occupational exposure, and prostate cancer is conjectural, and further study is required before firm conclusions can be formed.

Vasectomy

Some investigations suggest that vasectomy increases androgen levels[56] or produces an immunologic reaction[57] that might promote prostate carcinogenesis. Other studies indicate that vasectomy produces an approximately 1.6-fold increase in the risk of developing prostate cancer, which directly correlates with the interval from surgery.[53,58,59] However, DerSimonian and associates[60] concluded that these studies were inadequately designed and conducted, and John and colleagues[61] and Sidney and coworkers[62] could not confirm this association in large cohort studies. The National Institutes of Health determined that information regarding a putative association between vasectomy and prostate cancer was not convincing and that a causative relationship had not been established.[63] Vasectomy should not be considered a prostate cancer risk factor, and patient counseling and medical decision-making should not be altered on this basis.

Precancerous Lesions

Certain atypical epithelial lesions may be precursors of prostate cancer, and their presence in a prostatic biopsy may serve as a risk factor for this condition. These lesions are now classified into two categories: prostatic intraepithelial neoplasia (PIN) and atypical adenomatous hyperplasia.

Of the two categories, PIN represents the putative precancerous end of the morphologic continuum of cellular proliferation and is more strongly associated with prostate cancer.[64] PIN may appear hypoechoic by transrectal ultrasonography (TRUS), but biopsy is the definitive method with which to detect the condition. Two grades (low and high) are recognized, with high-grade PIN considered to be a precursor of invasive carcinoma.[64,65] Studies suggest that PIN predates prostate cancer by 10 years or more, with low-grade PIN first emerging in the third decade of life.[66] Although PIN is more common in the elderly, it may also be present at an early age. Sakr and colleagues[66] found PIN in 9% and 22% of men in their 20s and 30s, respectively, which appeared unrelated to race or ethnicity. Most foci of PIN in younger men were low-grade, with an increasing frequency of high-grade disease associated with advancing age. PIN is often found in proximity to carcinoma, and its presence warrants search for invasive carcinoma.[67] Davidson and associates[68] found that 35% of patients with PIN had prostate cancer identified on subsequent biopsy, which is consistent with the results of other studies.[69] Results such as these indicate that PIN is a likely and strong risk factor for prostate cancer that warrants close surveillance and follow-up (e.g., 6 month intervals for 2 years, and yearly intervals thereafter for life).[70,71]

PREVENTION AND EARLY DETECTION

Prostate cancer is an androgen-dependent tumor with a prolonged latency between initial malignant transformation and clinical expression, features well suited to disease prevention efforts.[7] Progression from tumor inception to invasive carcinoma often takes decades, allowing sufficient time for intervention.[9] Chemoprevention strategies that use high-risk target populations, particularly those with premalignant lesions (e.g., high-grade PIN), have the greatest potential to identify promising agents in a time-efficient manner.[72] The results of focused studies such as these can then be confirmed in large-scale trials applied to the general population. The ability to alter the hormonal environment of the host provides an excellent opportunity to interrupt the multistep process that results in clinical expression of the disease.[7] Advances in our understanding of the process of carcinogenesis and the availability of promising new chemopreventive agents, including those producing reversible androgen deprivation, have the potential to favorably affect the morbidity and mortality of prostate cancer in the foreseeable future.

Luteinizing hormone-releasing hormone analogues (e.g., goserelin, leuprolide) reduce luteinizing hormone and (secondarily) testosterone levels. The long-term use of these agents may cause anemia, atrophy of reproductive organs, diminished muscle mass, loss of libido, and vasomotor instability, which limits the utility of these agents for chemoprevention in the general population. Nonsteroidal antiandrogens (e.g., flutamide, bicalutamide) competitively bind to androgen receptors in target tissues. These agents are well tolerated in most patients, although adverse effects may include gastrointestinal disturbance, gynecomastia, and vasomotor instability. However, luteinizing hormone-releasing hormone (LHRH) analogues and nonsteroidal antiandrogens have not been introduced into the chemoprevention area, and their role in this setting is unknown.

Competitive inhibitors of 5α-reductase (e.g., finasteride) suppress intraprostatic dihydrotestosterone to castrate levels without a significant affect on libido, potency, or male musculature. The Prostate Cancer Prevention Trial was initiated to test the efficacy of finasteride as a chemoprevention agent.[73] This placebo-controlled phase III trial randomized 18,882 eligible men (≥55 years old, normal digital rectal examination [DRE] results, and prostate-specific antigen [PSA] levels <3 ng/mL) to finasteride (5 mg daily) or placebo for 7 years. As reported by Thompson and associates, there was a 25% reduction in the prevalence of prostate cancer over this 7-year period from 30.6% in the placebo group to 18.6% in the finasteride group.[73] However, more aggressive tumors (Gleason score of 7 to 10) were more common in patients who took finasteride: 37% of all tumors and 6.4% of all men on the finasteride arm versus 22% of all tumors and 5.1% of all men on the placebo arm. The advantage of preventing or delaying the appearance of prostate cancer must be weighed against the increased risk of high-grade disease.

Early Detection

Considerable controversy surrounds the use of early detection programs for prostate cancer. Some argue that early detection efforts are too costly and will lead to the recognition of an increased number of clinically insignificant tumors, as autopsy studies demonstrate a high prevalence of incidental tumors in older men.[9,10] There are concerns about the performance level of DRE, serum PSA, and TRUS in this setting, as well as the effects of lead-time and length-time bias in assessing the benefits of early detection. On the basis of indirect evidence, the American Cancer Society recommends that men older than 50 years of age with a life expectancy of at least 10 years undergo annual DRE and a serum PSA determination to identify prostate cancer at its earliest possible stage.[74] Annual screening is also endorsed for younger men (e.g., 45 years) at high risk, such as those with a strong family history (e.g., two or more affected first-degree relatives), and for black men. However, patients must be provided information about the risks and benefits of screening.[74] Because DRE and serum PSA measurements are considered fundamental components of early detection efforts, the results of these evaluations are often combined with TRUS findings when considering prostatic biopsy. Although DRE has high specificity for prostate cancer, it has a low sensitivity profile and is not considered an effective detection tool on its own.[75] The sensitivity of serum PSA, independent of other early detection methods, is difficult to determine, and its specificity is lower than DRE or TRUS.[76] Nonetheless, the positive predictive value (i.e., the likelihood a biopsy will demonstrate cancer) for an abnormal finding on DRE or TRUS, or both, is significantly enhanced by incorporating the findings of serum PSA testing.[76,77] The use of PSA may result in a diagnostic lead time of approximately 5 years[78] and in the detection of earlier-stage and lower-grade tumors.[77]

Economic Impact

The economic impact of screening strategies was evaluated by several investigators. Littrup and associates[79] used information from the American Cancer Society Prostate Cancer Detection Project to assess the economic impact of nine potential screening strategies. This benefit-cost analysis determined that a combination of DRE and PSA represented the least costly detection approach with the potential to decrease prostate cancer mortality. In a similar vein, Gustafsson and colleagues[80] evaluated the costs associated with six prostate cancer early detection strategies. Assessment with DRE and PSA, with TRUS for those with an elevated PSA value or abnormal DRE value, resulted in the highest (90%) cancer detection rate at a cost of $5530 per curable cancer case.

Benoit and Naslund[81] compared the cost of screening for prostate cancer and breast cancer. For the age range of 50 to 69 years, the cost of prostate cancer screening per cancer detected was $2372, compared with a cost of $10,975 for each detected cancer case in breast cancer screening programs. Unlike breast cancer screening, the effect of prostate cancer screening (particularly with the use of serum PSA) on mortality reduction has not been adequately evaluated, and additional study is essential to determine the worth of early detection programs for this condition. The Prostate, Lung, Colorectal, and Ovarian (PCLO) Cancer Screening Trial randomly assigned 38,350 men to the screening arm from 1993 through 2001, but it will be several years before the effect on mortality can be evaluated.[82]

Because serum PSA levels directly correlate with age in men without prostate cancer, several investigators sought to improve the diagnostic accuracy of PSA by defining the normal test range as a function of age and race (Table 50-2).[83-89] In particular, DeAntoni and coworkers[89] found that the mean PSA level was significantly different for successive decades of age, and there was increased variability in PSA values with advancing age. It was this age-related variability that largely accounted for the phenomenon of age-specific reference ranges. El-Galley and associates[88] studied the clinical impact of age-specific reference ranges in 2657 men who underwent prostatic biopsy. Analysis of the sensitivity, specificity, and positive predictive value profiles supported use of age-specific reference ranges because of increased detection sensitivity in younger men and increased specificity in older men. Receiver operating characteristic curve analysis was used to determine the optimal age-adjusted PSA cut-off points for DRE-negative patients, which are illustrated in Table 50-2.

Measuring PSA velocity (PSAV), defined as the change in serum PSA over time, is another method to account for prostatic changes that occur during the aging process. In men who develop prostate cancer, an exponential increase in PSA values begins approximately 5 years before the diagnosis is established,[90] and detecting a PSAV of 0.75 ng/mL/year or more appears to be a sensitive means to distinguish these men from those without prostatic disease or those with benign prostatic hypertrophy (BPH).[90-92] However, because of interassay variability, only a PSA change exceeding ±7.5% may be considered significant according to Kadmon and colleagues.[93]

Additional attempts to improve the screening accuracy of PSA measurements are based on the observation that serum

Table 50-2 **Upper Normal Age-Specific Limits for Prostate-Specific Antigen in Men without Prostate Cancer**

Study	No. of Patients	PROSTATE-SPECIFIC ANTIGEN LIMITS BY AGE GROUP* 40-49 Years	50-59 Years	60-69 Years	70-79 Years
Anderson et al[87]	1,716‡	1.5	2.5	4.5	7.5
Dalkin et al[83]	728‡	—	3.5	5.4	6.3
DeAntoni et al[89]	77,890‡	2.4	3.8	5.6	6.9
El-Galley et al[88]	2,657‡	—	3.5	5.0	7.0
Morgan et al[86]	1,693†	2.0	4.0	4.5	5.5
Oesterling et al[84]	471‡	2.5	3.5	4.5	6.5
Oesterling et al[85]	286‡	2.0	3.0	4.0	5.0

*Prostate-specific antigen values expressed in ng/mL.
†Black men only.
‡Japanese men only.

PSA level depends on cancer volume, tumor differentiation, and the amount of benign prostatic tissue.[94] To account for coexistent BPH, the concept of PSA density (PSAD) was introduced by Benson and colleagues.[95] PSAD is the total serum PSA value divided by the volume of the prostate gland, as determined by TRUS using the prolate ellipsoid formula (volume = length × width × height × 0.52). PSAD appears most useful for patients with a total serum PSA level in the range of 4 to 10 ng/mL, particularly when palpable prostatic abnormalities are absent. In this setting, it is believed a PSAD of 0.15 ng/mL/cm^3 or more best identifies men in whom prostatic biopsy should be considered.[96,97] In other investigations, diagnostic accuracy was not enhanced by the PSAD compared with using the upper normal PSA concentration, defined as 4.0 ng/mL, as a cutoff point for early detection.[98-100] Transition zone volume–adjusted PSA (PSAT) was introduced as an evolution in the PSAD concept for men with a serum PSA value in the indeterminate range (i.e., 4 to 10 ng/mL).[101] PSAT is calculated by dividing the serum PSA value by the TRUS-determined transition zone volume and is based on the rationale that BPH results exclusively from transition zone hyperplasia. Although preliminary results suggest PSAT may be more accurate than PSAD in predicting the presence of cancer,[101] confirmatory studies are necessary before this parameter is adopted.

Because the proportion of PSA complexed to α_1-antichymotrypsin is greater in patients with prostate cancer than in men with benign prostatic disease, the ratio of free-to-total (i.e., percent free) PSA will be lower in men with prostate cancer and may help discriminate between benign and malignant prostate conditions.[102-106] Although the free-to-total PSA ratio can be applied to any serum PSA level, performing a free PSA determination improves the specificity for prostate cancer detection when the total serum PSA range is approximately 3 ng/mL to 10 ng/mL.[104,107] To determine the optimal cutoff point that may warrant prostatic biopsy, various free-to-total PSA ratios were examined for their association with prostate cancer.[106,107] A multicenter clinical performance study demonstrated that a free-to-total PSA ratio of less than 7% was highly suspicious for cancer, whereas a free-to-total PSA ratio of above 25% was rarely associated with malignancy. In association with other study results, a diagnostic algorithm for the detection of early-stage prostate cancer based on the percent free PSA has been suggested.[107] However, larger population-based trials must be conducted and the utility of prostate cancer screening must be ascertained before widespread application can be recommended.[108]

PATHOLOGY AND PATHWAYS OF SPREAD

Anatomy

Prostatic anatomy is readily understood by using the urethra as a reference point. The verumontanum is a major anatomic landmark and protrudes from the posterior prostatic wall at the midpoint of the urethra and tapers distally to form the crista urethralis. Most prostatic ducts and the ejaculatory ducts empty into the urethra in this region, whereas the periurethral glands empty throughout the length of the urethra. Immediately proximal to the verumontanum is the müllerian remnant, the utricle, an approximate 0.5-cm length of epithelium-lined cul-de-sac. A circumferential sleeve of muscle surrounds the entire urethra and is composed of the proximal preprostatic smooth muscle sphincter, which prevents retrograde ejaculation, and a distal sphincter of striated and smooth muscle at the apex that is essential for urinary control.

The prostate is composed of three zones: peripheral, central, and transition. The peripheral zone includes approximately 70% of the prostatic volume and is the most common site of PIN and carcinoma. DRE often includes a description of the prostatic lobes based on palpation of the median furrow, which divides the peripheral zone into the right and left halves. The central zone is a cone-shaped area that includes the base of the prostate and encompasses the ejaculatory ducts; it represents approximately 25% of the volume of the prostate. The transition zone is the smallest component of the normal prostate, accounting for approximately 5% of the gland, but it usually enlarges as men age due to BPH and may grow to dwarf the remainder of the prostate. The central and peripheral zones are often referred to as the *nontransition zone*.

The prostatic capsule consists of an inner smooth muscle layer and an outer covering of collagen, with marked variability in the relative amount of each in different areas. At the apex, acinar elements are sparse, and the capsule is ill defined. As a result, the prostatic capsule cannot be regarded as a well-defined anatomic structure with constant features.

The nerve supply of the prostate is furnished by paired neurovascular bundles along the posterolateral edge of the prostate. Autonomic ganglia are clustered near the neurovascular bundles, and small nerve trunks arising at this site penetrate the capsule to form an extensive network within the gland.

The primary blood supply of the prostate is furnished by the internal iliac artery, and the venous drainage is directly into the prostatic plexus, which eventually empties into the internal iliac vein. This route may account for hematogenous metastases, most often in osseous sites.

The lymphatics of the prostate and the seminal vesicles were detailed through anatomic dissections described by Rouvière.[109] Lymphatic drainage of the prostate originates in an extensive intraprostatic network that coalesces to form a subcapsular system and henceforth coalesces into a periprostatic lymphatic network and the four pedicles of the collecting trunks: the external iliac, hypogastric (or internal iliac), and posterior and inferior pedicles that terminate in the external iliac (including the obturator), presacral, and hypogastric lymph nodes, respectively. The lymphatics of the seminal vesicle originate in the mucous and muscular networks and give rise to the superficial plexus, which culminates in the lymph nodes of the external iliac system.

Histologic Appearance

The prostatic epithelium consists of three main histologic types: secretory, basal, and neuroendocrine cells. Despite having the lowest proliferative activity of the epithelial elements, secretory cells produce PSA, prostatic acid phosphatase (PAP), acid mucin, and other secretory products. The basal cells form a flattened layer of cells surmounting the basement membrane at the periphery of the glands. These cells possess the highest proliferative activity of the prostatic epithelium and are thought to act as stem or "reserve" cells that repopulate the secretory cell layer.[110] Basal cells, selectively labeled with antibodies to high-molecular-weight keratin (e.g., 34βE12), are used to differentiate benign acinar processes from adenocarcinoma, which lacks a basal cell layer. Neuroendocrine cells are the least common epithelial cell type and are often not identified in routinely stained sections.

The seminal vesicles have a variable anatomic distribution, portions of which may occasionally be found within the prostatic capsule where they may be mistaken for prostatic nodularity or induration on examination. The cells of the epithelial component have large, irregular hyperchromatic nuclei with coarse chromatin and prominent nucleoli that often show nuclear abnormalities. When encountered in needle biopsies, such "pseudomalignant" cytologic atypia may lead to a mistaken diagnosis of prostatic adenocarcinoma. Cowper's glands consist of lobules of closely packed uniform acini and are noteworthy in that they may also be mistaken for prostatic carcinoma in biopsy specimens.

Pathology of Prostate Cancer

Prostatic Intraepithelial Neoplasia

PIN represents the putative precancerous end of the morphologic continuum of cellular proliferation within prostatic ducts, ductules, and acini.[64] The histologic diagnosis requires cytologic and architectural abnormalities, and lesions displaying some but not all such changes are considered atypical. PIN is designated as low grade or high grade, based on relative nuclear and nucleolar enlargement. The continuum culminating in high-grade PIN, and henceforth in early invasive cancer, is characterized by basal cell layer disruption, loss of markers of secretory differentiation, nuclear and nucleolar abnormalities, increased proliferative potential, and variations in DNA content (i.e., aneuploidy).[111-113] Virtually all measures of phenotype and nuclear abnormality by computer-based image analysis reveal similarities between PIN and invasive cancer, in contrast with normal and hyperplastic epithelium.[65] The recognition of PIN should serve as an indication for a thorough search for invasive cancer because of their close association.[64]

Histologic Appearance

Gross identification of prostate cancer may be difficult or impossible, and definitive diagnosis requires microscopic examination. In radical prostatectomy specimens, cancer is often multifocal, with a predilection for the peripheral zone. Tumor foci must be at least 5 mm in greatest dimension to be grossly apparent and appear yellow-white with a stony-hard consistency caused by stromal desmoplasia or inflammatory processes.

The minimal criteria necessary to establish a diagnosis of prostate cancer in biopsy material are described by Algaba and associates.[114] Approximately 99% of prostatic cancers are ductal or mucinous adenocarcinomas that have a microscopic appearance consisting of a proliferation of small acini with multiple patterns. Evaluation of small acinar proliferation of the prostate can be a diagnostic challenge, particularly when the suspicious focus is small.[115] Diagnosis relies on a combination of architectural and cytologic findings that may be enhanced by ancillary studies such as immunohistochemistry. Architectural features include irregular glandular contours that deviate from the smoothly rounded contours of normal prostatic glands. The fact that glands are usually regular in shape is useful, as malignancies often exhibit an irregular and haphazard arrangement. Noting variations in gland size can also be of value, and comparison with adjacent uninvolved prostatic glands may be useful. Cytologic features are also important for the diagnosis of cancer, because nuclear and nucleolar enlargements are seen in most suspected cancer cells.

The basal cell layer is critical to the diagnosis of adenocarcinoma, as an intact basal cell layer is present at the periphery of benign glands, whereas a basal cell layer is entirely lacking in carcinoma. However, small foci of adenocarcinoma clustered around larger glands, which have an intact basal cell layer, may occasionally compound diagnostic difficulty, and it may be useful to employ monoclonal antibodies against high-molecular-weight keratin (e.g., 34βE12) to evaluate the basal layer. Other ancillary histologic features that may aid in diagnosis include acidic mucin in the acinar lumen, eosinophilic crystalloids, and microvascular invasion. Inflammation should be identified when evaluating small glandular proliferation because reactive atypia may result or may be seen in the setting of prior radiation therapy, infarction, or other conditions. Granulomatous prostatitis is a vexing problem, and caution is warranted in the interpretation of biopsies with such a finding.[116]

Morphologic Variants

Several unusual morphologic variants (e.g., small cell tumors, ductal carcinoma, transitional cell carcinoma) of prostatic carcinoma have been identified but account for less than 10% of cases. These tumors are usually associated with typical acinar adenocarcinoma and rarely occur in pure form. It is important to recognize the special variants and to understand the criteria that distinguish them from benign mimics. Although data are limited, the clinical behavior and prognostic significance of the morphologic variants may differ from usual prostatic adenocarcinoma.[117]

Grading

The histologic pattern of prostate cancer correlates with disease outcome and therefore was used as a component of more than 30 grading systems proposed during this century. The Gleason system, based on a Veterans Administration study of more than 4000 patients, is the de facto standard in the United States and abroad (Fig. 50-1). The Gleason system

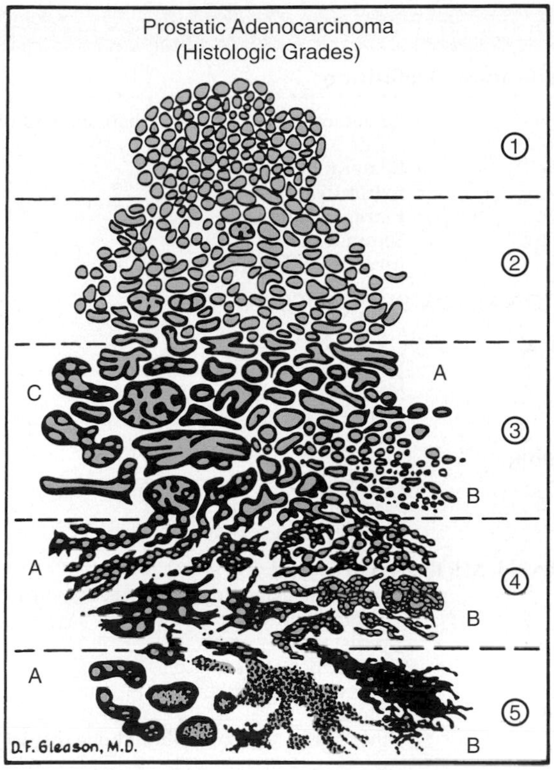

Figure 50-1 Standardized drawing for prostate cancer grading according to the Gleason system. (From Gleason DF: Histologic grading of prostatic carcinoma. *In* Bostwick DG [ed]: Pathology of the Prostate. New York, Churchill Livingstone, 1990, p 83.)

is based on the degree of glandular differentiation and an overall pattern of tumor growth at relatively low microscopic magnification (40 to 100 ×).[118] Five patterns of growth are recognized and numbered in order of increasing malignancy. Because of histologic variation in the tumor, two patterns are recorded for each case: a primary or predominant pattern (Gleason score of 1 to 5) and a secondary or lesser pattern (Gleason score of 1 to 5). The Gleason score is the sum of the primary and secondary patterns and ranges from 2 to 10. If only one pattern is present, the primary and secondary patterns receive the same designation. Gleason observed that more than 50% of prostate cancers contain two or more patterns,[119] and Aihara and colleagues[120] found an average of 2.7 different Gleason grades in a series of prostatectomy specimens. Interobserver and intraobserver variability has been reported with the Gleason and other grading systems, and Gleason found exact reproducibility of score in 50% of needle biopsies and ±1 score in 85% of cases.[119]

Although a correlation exists between the needle biopsy tumor grade and that found in the prostatectomy specimen, a higher grade (i.e., more poorly differentiated) is identified in approximately one third of cases, whereas downgrading is a less common observation.[118,121,122] Such grading errors are more common in biopsies with smaller amounts of tumor and lower tumor grades, which probably results from tissue sampling error, tumor heterogeneity, and undergrading of the needle biopsy. The correlation is strongest for the primary Gleason pattern, but the secondary pattern also provides useful predictive information, particularly when used to create the Gleason score.[118] Johnstone and coworkers[122] drew particular attention to the implications of biopsy undergrading with respect to estimates of prognosis and the potential limitations of using tumor grade to adjust for outcomes between different therapeutic modalities.

Pathologic Staging

The criteria for assigning pathologic classification and stage were developed by the American Joint Commission on Cancer (AJCC) and the Union Internationale Contre le Cancer (UICC) (Tables 50-3 and 50-4).[123,124] The sixth edition of the *AJCC Cancer Staging Manual* is now in use.[123] The details of handling, processing, and recording histologic findings of biopsy, radical prostatectomy, and nodal dissection tissue specimens are described in detail by the College of American Pathologists[125] and by Bostwick and associates.[126] Thorough examination of radical prostatectomy (RP) specimens is critical for tumor classification and should allow accurate determination of pathologic stage, Gleason score, tumor volume, and surgical margin status. Pathologic stage is assessed by determining the presence or absence of extraprostatic extension (EPE), seminal vesicle invasion (SVI), and lymph node involvement (LNI).

Extension of cancer beyond the edge or capsule of the prostate is diagnostic of EPE, which requires cancer in adipose tissue, perineural spaces of the neurovascular bundles, or anterior muscle. Difficulty is occasionally encountered in the presence of a dense desmoplastic response in extraprostatic tissue, particularly in cases treated by androgen deprivation. The neurovascular bundles are a path of least resistance and may be the earliest site of EPE. Although perineural invasion alone is not sufficient for EPE, there often are large nerve twigs within the prostate that may be mistaken for the neurovascular bundles. The anterior muscle is an uncommon site for EPE; this is observed only with large tumors involving the transition zone. Most patients (57% to 81%) with EPE have involved surgical margins,[127] which predicts a worse prognosis.

Positive surgical margins are defined as cancer cells touching the inked surface of the prostate. Care must be taken to avoid interpreting ink within tissue crevices created by postoperative handling of the specimen as margin positivity. The status of the surgical margin is not included in pathologic staging, and pathologists and clinical investigators should describe surgical margin status separately from EPE.

Seminal vesicle invasion is a pathologic finding associated with an increased risk for disease relapse[128,129] and occurs when a nontransition zone tumor extends into the region where vas deferens and seminal vesicle converge at the prostatic base.[130] Direct tumor growth from this location along the ejaculatory duct complex or through the prostatic capsule may result in seminal vesicle invasion. This mechanism accounts for the observations that tumor volume is often greatest at the prostatic end of the seminal vesicle in the vicinity of the vas deferens,[130] that involvement of both seminal vesicles is a common finding,[129] and that isolated deposits of prostate cancer remote from the ejaculatory duct complex are observed in only one eighth of seminal vesicle specimens involved with tumor.[129]

Postirradiation Histology

For approximately 18 to 24 months after external beam radiation therapy (EBRT), and perhaps longer for interstitial implantation, needle biopsy of the prostate in the absence of clinical disease progression is of limited value due to delayed and continuing tumor cell death.[131] After this period, needle biopsy is associated with a lower level of diagnostic error that is minimized by obtaining multiple specimens.[132-134] Histologic changes of prostatic radiation injury include acinar atrophy,

Table 50-3 American Joint Commission on Cancer TNM Staging Classification

Classification	Definition
PRIMARY TUMOR (T)	
Clinical	
TX	Primary tumor cannot be assessed
T0	No evidence of primary tumor
T1	Clinically inapparent tumor not palpable or visible by imaging
T1a	Tumor incidental histologic finding in 5% or less of tissue resected
T1b	Tumor incidental histologic finding in more than 5% of tissue resected
T1c	Tumor identified by needle biopsy (e.g., because of elevated prostate-specific antigen level)
T2	Tumor confined within the prostate*
T2a	Tumor involves one half of one lobe or less
T2b	Tumor involves more than one half of one lobe but not both lobes
T2c	Tumor involves both lobes
T3	Tumor extends through the prostatic capsule†
T3a	Extracapsular extension (unilateral or bilateral)
T3b	Tumor invades seminal vesicle(s)
T4	Tumor is fixed or invades adjacent structures other than the seminal vesicles: bladder neck, external sphincter, rectum, levator muscles, and/or pelvic wall
Pathologic (pT)	
pT2‡	Organ confined
pT2a	Unilateral involving one half of one lobe or less
pT2b	Unilateral involving more than one half of one lobe but not both lobes
pT2c	Bilateral disease
pT3	Extraprostatic extension
pT3a	Extraprostatic extension§
pT3b	Seminal vesicle invasion
pT4	Invasion of bladder, rectum
REGIONAL LYMPH NODES (N)	
Clinical	
NX	Regional lymph nodes cannot be assessed
N0	No regional lymph node metastasis
N1	Metastasis in regional lymph node or nodes
Pathologic	
pNX	Regional nodes not sampled
pN0	No positive regional nodes
pN1	Metastases in regional node(s)
DISTANT METASTASIS (M)¶	
MX	Distant metastasis cannot be assessed (not evaluated by any modality)
M0	No distant metastasis
M1	Distant metastasis
M1a	Nonregional lymph node(s)
M1b	Bone(s)
M1c	Other site(s) with or without bone disease

*Tumor found in one or both lobes by needle biopsy, but not palpable or reliably visible by imaging, is classified as T1c.
†Invasion into the prostatic apex or into (but not beyond) the prostatic capsule is classified as T2, not as T3.
‡There is no pathologic T1 classification.
§Positive surgical margin should be indicated by an R1 description (i.e., residual microscopic disease).
¶When more than one site of metastasis is present, the most advanced category (M1c) is used.
Reprinted from Brachytheraphy, vol.4: Crook J, Potters L, Stock R, et al: Critical organ dosimetry in permanent seed prostate brachytherapy: Defining the organs at risk. An American Brachytherapy Society Concensus Statement, pp 186-194. Copyright 2005, with permission from American Brachytherapy Society.

Table 50-4 American Joint Commission on Cancer Stage Grouping for Prostate Cancer

Stage	Tumor	Node	Metastasis	Grade
I	T1a	N0	M0	G1
II	T1a	N0	M0	G2, G3-4
	T1b	N0	M0	Any G
	T1c	N0	M0	Any G
	T1	N0	M0	Any G
	T2	N0	M0	Any G
III	T3	N0	M0	Any G
IV	T4	N0	M0	Any G
	Any T	N1	M0	Any G
	Any T	Any N	M1	Any G

Adapted from American Joint Committee on Cancer: Prostate. *In* Greene F, Page DL, Fleming ID, et al (eds): AJCC Cancer Staging Manual, 6th ed. Philadelphia, Springer, 2002, pp 337-345.

shrinkage and distortion, marked cytologic abnormalities of the epithelium, basal cell hyperplasia, stromal fibrosis, and a decreased ratio of acini to stroma.[131] Vascular sclerosis is also prominent and may involve small and large vessels. Although a definitive method to assess tumor viability after radiation therapy does not exist, PSA and PAP expression persists,[135] suggesting that tumor cells capable of protein production retain the potential for cell division and spread.[136,137] Keratin 34βE12 expression also persists and is often of value in separating treated adenocarcinoma from some of its mimics. Cancer grading after radiation therapy has yielded conflicting results; some observers found no difference in the pretherapy grade,[131] but others found an increased grade.[138] The consensus opinion is that grading should not be relied on after radiation therapy.

Effects of Androgen Deprivation

Androgen deprivation of normal, hyperplastic, and dysplastic epithelial cells causes acceleration of programmed cell death (i.e., apoptosis), with fragmentation of tumor DNA, emergence of apoptotic bodies, and inhibition of cell growth. There is reduced nuclear size, loss of nucleoli, chromatin condensation, nuclear pyknosis, and cytoplasmic vacuolation.[139-140] However, grading may be misleading and is to be avoided.[140] PSA, PAP, and keratin 34βE12 immunohistochemistry are useful in identifying carcinoma, as PSA and PAP are retained and 34βE12 remains negative. Expression of neuroendocrine differentiation markers (e.g., chromogranin, neuron-specific enolase), remains unaltered, whereas proliferative activity, as measured by proliferating cell nuclear antigen immunoreactivity, is reduced after androgen deprivation.[140]

BIOLOGIC CHARACTERISTICS

Molecular Biology

Oncogenesis probably occurs through the selection of several genetic changes, each modifying the expression or function of genes controlling cell growth or differentiation. Allelic loss is common in prostatic adenocarcinoma and appears to be more common in high-grade tumors. Chromosomes 8p, 10q, and 16q are typically involved,[141] and tumor suppressor genes appear to be present on chromosome 8p, which may play a role in carcinogenesis. Fluorescent in situ hybridization studies with centromere-specific probes for chromosomes 7, 8, 11, and 12 show that gains of chromosomes 7 and 8 are consistent numerical alterations and may be markers of tumor aggressiveness and prognosis.[142] Inactivation of *TP53*, a tumor suppressor gene on chromosome 17p, is present in as many as 25% of advanced prostate cancers but is rare in early disease, which suggests that it may play a role in tumor progression.[143] Another tumor suppressor gene, *DCC*, shows allelic deletion and loss of expression in 45% of cases, indicating that it is a common feature of prostate cancer. Loss of expression of the retinoblastoma gene on chromosome 13q is seen in a minority of prostate cancers, usually in advanced stages.[144] Activated oncogenes such as *RAS* and *ERBB2* (also called *HER2/NEU*) appear to be uncommon in early-stage prostate cancer.[145]

Predictive Factors

Pathologic End Points

The therapeutic efficacy of radiation therapy and radical prostatectomy depends on the accurate definition of grossly apparent tumor and on an appreciation for the nature of subclinical disease spread. Despite the clinical impression of a process confined to the prostate gland, occult tumor extension through the prostatic capsule or involvement of seminal vesicles or regional lymph nodes is common at the time of diagnosis. Compared with surgical-pathologic stage, the clinical staging of prostate cancer frequently underestimates disease extent, and many patients are upstaged after histologic examination of the radical prostatectomy and pelvic node dissection specimens.[146] Among patients thought to have intraprostatic disease by clinical assessment, various percentages of patients, depending on T stage, Gleason grade, and PSA level, will be found to have extracapsular extension, seminal vesicle or lymph node involvement at the time of prostatectomy (Table 50-5).[146]

Because these findings may have considerable importance for selection of an appropriate therapeutic strategy (e.g., radioactive seed implantation or radical prostatectomy versus EBRT), several investigators studied the association between readily available pretherapy factors and the pathologic end points of extraprostatic tumor extension, SVI, and pelvic LNI.

EXTRAPROSTATIC EXTENSION

EPE, the preferred term to describe tumor growth through the prostatic capsule into immediately surrounding tissues, is a pathologic feature that may portend an adverse disease outcome after radical prostatectomy,[147] and its presence may be important in patient selection for radical prostatectomy or radioactive seed implantation. Several pretherapy tumor-related factors are associated with EPE, and these include clinical tumor stage,[146] pretherapy serum PSA value,[146] prostatic biopsy tumor grade,[146] microvessel density (i.e., neovascularity),[148] and percent of biopsy containing cancer.[148] Although any of these factors may be individually used to estimate the likelihood for EPE, the accuracy of such estimates is enhanced by combining those factors that independently contribute to the predictive model.[146]

In the PSA era, Partin and coworkers[149] were among the first to use multivariate statistical analysis to identify pretherapy variables associated with EPE in patients who underwent radical prostatectomy and demonstrated that clinical tumor stage, Gleason score of the diagnostic biopsy, and serum PSA level independently correlate with this finding. The combination of these factors was used to develop probability estimates, which were displayed as a nomogram and later incorporated into clinical practice guidelines for patient management. Kattan and associates[150] conducted a separate validation study that confirmed that the nomogram discriminated well between men with organ-confined disease and those in whom the disease extended beyond the prostate gland. The updated Partin nomogram is shown in Table 50-5 and may be useful for predicting the probability of organ-confined status,[146] but any estimation should consider the confidence of the prediction, as indicated by the associated 95% confidence intervals, for the combination of factors relevant to the new patient under consideration.

SEMINAL VESICLE INVASION

SVI is a pathologic finding associated with an increased risk for disease relapse.[128,129,147] Although TRUS with needle biopsy of the seminal vesicles[151,152] or endorectal coil magnetic resonance imaging (MRI) by an experienced examiner[153] may identify SVI, conventional imaging techniques are not considered reliable methods for evaluating disease extent before therapeutic intervention.[154] Due to these limitations, several investigators correlated pretherapy tumor-related factors with SVI as a means to identify patients with a high likelihood for this condition.[129,146,152,155] These studies demonstrate that clinical tumor stage, tumor grade of the diagnostic biopsy specimen, percent cancer in the biopsy, and serum PSA level are associated with SVI in a statistically significant manner.

Although serum PSA level was the best single predictor, Partin and coworkers[149] observed that the clinical tumor stage and Gleason score contributed to SVI risk estimation, and they were among the first to combine these factors to develop nomograms for clinical use. Diaz and associates[156] used this information to create a prediction equation (i.e., percent probability of SVI = PSA + [Gleason score–6] × 10) to identify patient groups at high risk for SVI. However, Kattan and coworkers[150] applied the original SVI nomogram of Partin and colleagues[149] to an independent data set and concluded that the nomogram was suspect, particularly in the areas of high predicted probability, and ill suited to clinical application.

In response to Kattan and coworkers, Partin and colleagues performed a multi-institutional update in which new (and different) nomograms were developed and validated.[157] Although this provides useful information, patients were only assigned to the most advanced and mutually exclusive pathologic category based on the findings of the radical prostatectomy and PND specimens for the analysis. Although this may be appropriate for the surgical candidate, the risk of SVI may

Table 50-5 Clinical Staging Nomogram for Prostate Cancer

PSA Range (ng/ml)	Pathologic Stage	GLEASON SCORE* 2-4	5-6	3 + 4 = 7	4 + 3 = 7	8-10
CLINICAL STAGE T1C (NONPALPABLE. PSA ELEVATED)						
0-2.5	Organ confined	95% (89-99)	90 (88-93)	79 (74-85)	71 (62-79)	66 (54-76)
	Extraprostatic extension	5% (1-11)	9 (7-12)	17 (13-23)	25 (18-34)	28 (20-38)
	Seminal vesicle (+)	—	0 (0-1)	2 (1-5)	2 (1-5)	4 (1-10)
	Lymph node (+)	—	—	1 (0-2)	1 (0-4)	1 (0-4)
2.6-4.0	Organ confined	92 (82-98)	84 (81-86)	68 (62-74)	58 (48-67)	52 (41-63)
	Extraprostatic extension	8 (2-18)	15 (13-18)	27 (22-33)	37 (29-46)	40 (31-50)
	Seminal vesicle (+)	—	1 (0-1)	4 (2-7)	4 (1-7)	6 (3-12)
	Lymph node (+)	—	—	1 (0-2)	1 (0-3)	1 (0-4)
4.1-6.0	Organ confined	90 (78-98)	80 (78-83)	63 (58-68)	52 (43-60)	46 (36-56)
	Extraprostatic extension	10 (2-22)	19 (16-21)	32 (27-36)	42 (35-50)	45 (36-54)
	Seminal vesicle (+)	—	1 (0-1)	3 (2-5)	3 (1-6)	5 (3-9)
	Lymph node (+)	—	0 (0-1)	2 (1-3)	3 (1-5)	3 (1-6)
6.1-10.0	Organ confined	87 (73-97)	75 (72-77)	54 (49-59)	43 (35-51)	37 (28-46)
	Extraprostatic extension	13 (3-27)	23 (21-25)	36 (32-40)	47 (40-54)	48 (39-57)
	Seminal vesicle (+)	—	2 (2-3)	8 (6-11)	8 (4-12)	13 (8-19)
	Lymph node (+)	—	0 (0-1)	2 (1-3)	2 (1-4)	3 (1-5)
>10.0	Organ confined	80 (61-95)	62 (58-64)	37 (32-42)	27 (21-34)	22 (16-30)
	Extraprostatic extension	20 (5-39)	33 (30-36)	43 (38-48)	51 (44-59)	50 (42-59)
	Seminal vesicle (+)	—	4 (3-5)	12 (9-17)	11 (6-17)	17 (10-25)
	Lymph node (+)	—	2 (1-3)	8 (5-11)	10 (5-17)	11 (5-18)
CLINICAL STAGE T2A (PALPABLE < $^1/_2$ OF ONE LOBE)						
0-2.5	Organ confined	91 (79-98)	81 (77-85)	64 (56-71)	53 (43-63)	47 (35-59)
	Extraprostatic extension	9 (2-21)	17 (13-21)	29 (23-36)	40 (30-49)	42 (32-53)
	Seminal vesicle (+)	—	1 (0-2)	5 (1-9)	4 (1-9)	7 (2-16)
	Lymph node (+)	—	0 (0-1)	2 (0-5)	3 (0-8)	3 (0-9)
2.6-4.0	Organ confined	85 (69-96)	71 (66-75)	50 (43-57)	39 (30-48)	33 (24-44)
	Extraprostatic extension	15 (4-31)	27 (23-31)	41 (35-48)	52 (43-61)	53 (44-63)
	Seminal vesicle (+)	—	2 (1-3)	7 (3-12)	6 (2-12)	10 (4-18)
	Lymph node (+)	—	0 (0-1)	2 (0-4)	2 (0-6)	3 (0-8)
4.1-6.0	Organ confined	81 (63-95)	66 (62-70)	44 (39-50)	33 (25-41)	28 (20-37)
	Extraprostatic extension	19 (5-37)	32 (28-36)	46 (40-52)	56 (48-64)	58 (49-66)
	Seminal vesicle (+)	—	1 (1-2)	5 (3-8)	5 (2-8)	8 (4-13)
	Lymph node (+)	—	1 (0-2)	4 (2-7)	6 (3-11)	6 (2-12)
6.1-10.0	Organ confined	76 (56-94)	58 (54-61)	35 (30-40)	25 (19-32)	21 (15-28)
	Extraprostatic extension	24 (6-44)	37 (34-41)	49 (43-54)	58 (51-66)	57 (48-65)
	Seminal vesicle (+)	—	4 (3-5)	13 (9-18)	11 (6-17)	17 (11-26)
	Lymph node (+)	—	1 (0-2)	3 (2-6)	5 (2-8)	5 (2-10)
>10.0	Organ confined	65 (43-89)	42 (38-46)	20 (17-24)	14 (10-18)	11 (7-15)
	Extraprostatic extension	35 (11-57)	47 (43-52)	49 (43-55)	55 (46-64)	52 (41-62)
	Seminal vesicle (+)	—	6 (4-8)	16 (11-22)	13 (7-20)	19 (12-29)
	Lymph node (+)	—	4 (3-7)	14 (9-21)	18 (10-27)	17 (9-29)
CLINICAL STAGE T2B (PALPABLE, > $^1/_2$ OF ONE LOBE, NOT ON BOTH LOBES)						
0-2.5	Organ confined	88 (73-97)	75 (69-81)	54 (46-63)	43 (33-54)	37 (26-49)
	Extraprostatic extension	12 (3-27)	22 (17-28)	35 (28-43)	45 (35-56)	46 (35-58)
	Seminal vesicle (+)	—	2 (0-3)	6 (2-12)	5 (1-11)	9 (2-20)
	Lymph node (+)	—	1 (0-2)	4 (0-10)	6 (0-14)	6 (0-16)
2.6-4.0	Organ confined	80 (61-95)	63 (57-69)	41 (33-48)	30 (22-39)	25 (17-34)
	Extraprostatic extension	20 (5-39)	34 (28-40)	47 (40-55)	57 (47-67)	57 (46-68)
	Seminal vesicle (+)	—	2 (1-4)	9 (4-15)	7 (3-14)	12 (5-22)
	Lymph node (+)	—	1 (0-2)	3 (0-8)	4 (0-12)	5 (0-14)
4.1-6.0	Organ confined	75 (55-93)	57 (52-83)	35 (29-40)	25 (18-32)	21 (14-29)
	Extraprostatic extension	25 (7-45)	39 (33-44)	51 (44-57)	60 (50-68)	59 (49-69)
	Seminal vesicle (+)	—	2 (1-3)	7 (4-11)	5 (3-9)	9 (4-16)
	Lymph node (+)	—	2 (1-3)	7 (4-13)	10 (5-18)	10 (4-20)
6.1-10.0	Organ confined	69 (47-91)	49 (43-54)	26 (22-31)	19 (14-25)	15 (10-21)
	Extraprostatic extension	31 (9-53)	44 (39-49)	52 (46-58)	60 (52-68)	57 (48-67)
	Seminal vesicle (+)	—	5 (3-8)	16 (10-22)	13 (7-20)	19 (11-29)
	Lymph node (+)	—	2 (1-3)	6 (4-10)	8 (5-14)	8 (4-16)
>10.0	Organ confined	57 (35-86)	33 (28-38)	14 (11-17)	9 (6-13)	7 (4-10)
	Extraprostatic extension	43 (14-65)	52 (46-56)	47 (40-53)	50 (40-60)	46 (36-59)
	Seminal vesicle (+)	—	8 (5-11)	17 (12-24)	13 (8-21)	19 (12-29)
	Lymph node (+)	—	8 (5-12)	22 (15-30)	27 (16-39)	27 (14-40)

Table 50-5 Clinical Practice Guidelines for Prostate Cancer—cont'd

PSA Range (ng/ml)	Pathologic Stage	GLEASON SCORE* 2-4	5-6	3 + 4 = 7	4 + 3 = 7	8-10
CLINICAL STAGE T2C (PALPABLE, ON BOTH LOBES)						
0-2.5	Organ confined	86 (71-97)	73 (63-81)	51 (38-63)	39 (26-54)	34 (21-48)
	Extraprostatic extension	14 (3-29)	24 (17-33)	36 (26-48)	45 (32-59)	47 (33-61)
	Seminal vesicle (+)	—	1 (0-4)	5 (1-13)	5 (1-12)	8 (2-19)
	Lymph node (+)	—	1 (0-4)	6 (0-18)	9 (0-26)	10 (0-27)
2.6-4.0	Organ confined	78 (58-94)	61 (50-70)	38 (27-50)	27 (18-40)	23 (14-34)
	Extraprostatic extension	22 (6-24)	36 (27-45)	48 (37-59)	57 (44-70)	57 (44-70)
	Seminal vesicle (+)	—	2 (1-5)	8 (2-17)	6 (2-16)	10 (3-22)
	Lymph node (+)	—	1 (0-4)	5 (0-15)	7 (0-21)	8 (0-22)
4.1-6.0	Organ confined	73 (52-93)	55 (44-64)	31 (23-41)	21 (14-31)	18 (11-28)
	Extraprostatic extension	27 (7-48)	40 (32-50)	50 (40-60)	57 (43-68)	57 (43-70)
	Seminal vesicle (+)	—	2 (1-4)	8 (2-11)	4 (1-10)	7 (2-15)
	Lymph node (+)	—	3 (1-7)	12 (5-23)	16 (6-32)	16 (6-33)
6.1-10.0	Organ confined	67 (45-91)	46 (36-56)	24 (17-32)	16 (10-24)	13 (8-20)
	Extraprostatic extension	33 (9-55)	46 (37-55)	52 (42-61)	58 (46-69)	56 (43-69)
	Seminal vesicle (+)	—	5 (2-9)	13 (6-23)	11 (4-21)	16 (6-29)
	Lymph node (+)	—	3 (1-6)	10 (5-18)	13 (6-25)	13 (5-26)
>10.0	Organ confined	54 (32-85)	30 (21-38)	11 (7-17)	7 (4-12)	6 (3-10)
	Extraprostatic extension	46 (15-68)	51 (42-60)	42 (30-55)	43 (29-59)	41 (27-57)
	Seminal vesicle (+)	—	6 (2-12)	13 (6-24)	10 (3-20)	15 (5-28)
	Lymph node (+)	—	13 (6-22)	33 (18-49)	38 (20-58)	38 (20-59)

*The staging normogram is used to predict the probability (95% confidence interval) of each mutually exclusive pathologic stage from the preoperative clinical stage, biopsy Gleason score, and serum prostate-specific antigen (PSA) level (ng/mL). PSA, prostate-specific antigen. (From Partin AW, Mangold LA, Lamm DM, et al: Contemporary update of prostate cancer staging nomograms (Partin tables) for the new millennium. Urology 58: 845, 2001.)

be underestimated with this approach, and caution is necessary in using the revised nomogram for other purposes (e.g., radiation therapy target volume definition).

In contrast, Pisansky and associates[158] used a split-sample developmental and validation method based on a stepwise modeling process that identified clinical tumor stage (T1-2a, T2b-c, and T3a-b), diagnostic Gleason primary grade (1 to 2, 3, 4 to 5), and pretherapy serum PSA value as independent predictors. This methodology avoided the risk of constructing an overly optimistic model and allowed a reliable means to estimate the probability for SVI in the patient with newly diagnosed clinical T1-3b N0/X prostate cancer.

NODAL INVOLVEMENT

Clinical tumor stage, prostatic biopsy tumor grade, and serum PSA level are also associated with pelvic LNI, and a combination of these factors may be used to predict the probability of LNI in the patient with a new diagnosis of clinically localized prostate cancer.[146,152,159,160] Partin and colleagues[149] incorporated these factors in a LNI predictive nomogram, from which Roach and coworkers[161] derived a prediction equation (i.e., percent probability of LNI = $\frac{2}{3}$ PSA + [Gleason score −6] × 10). However, Kattan and associates[150] were not able to validate the LNI nomogram in a separate group of patients and suggested that the nomograms were not broadly applicable. As a result, Partin and colleagues[157] used a different mathematical method to analyze a larger and more diverse study population and later provided revised nomograms to estimate the probability of LNI.[146]

In addition to the nomogram model to predict LNI, other investigators have used probability plots that combine the independent predictors of clinical tumor stage, Gleason primary grade, and serum PSA level.[159] The split sample method was then used to validate these predictions, similar to the work related to the prediction of seminal vesicle involvement.[158] Although the nomogram is a handy tool for using pretherapy clinical characteristics to predict tumor extension which impacts therapeutic decision-making, Spevack and colleagues compared several predictive models to find that the split-sample developmental and validation method achieved the greatest accuracy.[162]

Clinical End Points

Factors predictive of clinical end points may be grouped according to whether they are patient related, are intrinsic to the neoplasm (i.e., tumor related), or are associated with treatment. It is essential to recognize that a factor may have importance only in certain patient subsets (e.g., those with clinically localized disease) but not in other settings (e.g., metastatic disease). Different end points may be considered (e.g., local tumor control, metastatic relapse, biochemical relapse [BCR], cause-specific or overall mortality), and a particular factor may have significance for some, but not other, end points. A potential prognostic factor is often evaluated by considering it alone (i.e., univariate analysis), but this approach may overestimate its importance due to an association or interaction with other factors. The most reliable method to control for this interaction is to use multivariate techniques, such as the Cox proportional hazards or logistic regression models,[163,164] particularly within the framework of carefully planned prospective studies that meet predetermined conditions. The statistical methodologies and issues common to prognostic factor studies in oncology are summarized by Simon and Altman,[165] and the special issue of evaluating a continuous variable (e.g., serum PSA level) is described by Altman and associates.[166] It is also possible to combine independent covariates to develop prognostic indices and groupings that have enhanced predictive accuracy for patient outcome.[209]

PATIENT-RELATED FACTORS

Age at diagnosis, comorbidity (i.e., the presence of coexistent medical conditions), race/ethnicity, performance status, and the presence of disease-related symptoms are important host-related prognostic factors. There is an implicit understanding that advanced age correlates with overall survival,[167,168] because it is considered an important comorbidity in long-term longitudinal studies.[169] However, age appears to affect disease-specific survival in expectant management (patients ≤60 years old fare better)[170,171] but not radiation therapy[172] or surgical[173] experiences. Although Pilepich and colleagues[174] found an association between age and postirradiation local tumor control and Leibel and coworkers[175] observed a higher rate of relapse in the younger (<60 years) patient, these findings were not confirmed in other series, including the end point of biochemical disease-free survival.[172,176-179]

Approximately one in eight American men with prostate cancer is a member of a racial minority population.[180] Although the stage at diagnosis varies between racial groups,[180] the effect of race on disease outcome is confounded by the influence of other prognostic variables. For example, when race was considered as a single factor, some reports suggested that African American patients with localized disease had a worse outcome than non-Hispanic whites.[35,180] However, racial variation in the use of surgical staging procedures, with its attendant impact on assignment of stage,[181] and consideration of additional disease-related characteristics suggest that outcome may be independent of racial background.[182,183] Nonetheless, Moul and associates[184] controlled for confounding factors in a series of patients who underwent radical prostatectomy at a single facility in an equal access (i.e., United States military) medical system. Although its cause could not be determined, the investigators observed that black race was associated with a higher likelihood for disease relapse after multivariate adjustment for certain tumor-related prognostic factors. Morton[14] postulated that racial variations in hormonal, nutritional, genetic, and socioeconomic factors may account for such findings, and more evidence in this regard is accruing.[185,186] There is evidence for differences in presentation and outcome for Hispanic men with localized prostate cancer,[187] but few to no reliable estimates exist for the Native American/Native Alaskan or Asian/Pacific Islander populations. Some evidence suggests biologic differences in patient subgroups.

The presence of coexistent medical ailments (e.g., ischemic heart disease) in the patient with prostate cancer is called a *comorbidity*. The prevalence and severity of comorbidity in a study population and the risk of death associated with the conditions may profoundly influence the results associated with a particular management strategy. Although not specifically designed for use in prostate cancer patients, several instruments are available to provide a semiquantitative measure of comorbidity. Albertsen and coworkers[188] aptly described three instruments (i.e., the Kaplan-Feinstein and Charlson indices and the index of coexistent disease) and applied each to a cohort of men with localized prostate cancer to assess the impact of comorbidity on patient survival. Although the index of coexistent disease had marginally better predictive value, each instrument was predictive of age-adjusted survival when corrected for the effect of Gleason score. The risk of death from causes other than prostate cancer (i.e., competing causes) strongly correlated with the severity of comorbidity, and a weak association with prostate cancer-related (i.e., cause-specific) mortality was also observed. The selection of a particular management approach based on overall health status has important implications in interpreting and comparing outcomes, because overall and, perhaps, cause-specific survival estimates will be influenced.[189] However, additional research is essential to quantify the confounding effect of comorbidity in the setting of prostate cancer outcomes reporting.

Tumor Stage

The anatomic extent of prostate cancer is an important tumor-related factor predictive of patient outcome and serves as a fundamental basis from which prognosis is established. Although different classification schemes have been used, studies consistently demonstrate the association of primary tumor stage with several end points in patients with localized disease. Cause-specific and overall survival rates are directly related to the extent of the primary tumor in radiation therapy[190,191] and expectant management[167,170] series. The probability of local tumor control[176] and the risk of clinical,[191,192] metastatic,[176,193] and biochemical relapse[172,178,179] are influenced in a similar manner. In patients treated solely with EBRT, Zagars and coworkers[194] determined that the AJCC system was a valid method for describing the primary tumor and provided a classification that was prognostically superior to the Whitmore-based system.[195] Despite the description of other prognostic factors (e.g., serum PSA level), the AJCC tumor stage remains an important predictor of relapse in patients treated with radiation therapy[172,176,179] and is a vital component of pretherapy disease evaluation.

Surgical Margins

The frequency of positive surgical margins has declined in the past decade, probably because of refinement in surgical technique and earlier cancer detection. Ohori and associates[196] found positive surgical margins in 24% of whole-mount radical prostatectomy specimens obtained before 1987. By modifying the surgical technique, a positive surgical margin rate of 8% was seen by 1993, despite similar tumor volume, grade, and pathologic stage of cancer. Positive margins are typically located at the apex (48%), rectal and lateral surfaces (24%), bladder neck (15%), and posterior pedicles (10%).[127] The significance of positive surgical margins in patients treated with radical prostatectomy is uncertain. Paulson and Robertson[197] found that patients with organ-confined cancer and positive surgical margins had a 60% probability of death from cancer, significantly greater than the 30% observed in patients without surgical margin involvement. In contrast, Ohori and coworkers[196] found that positive surgical margins had no effect on prognosis. Consensus regarding the prognostic significance of this finding is lacking and the need for adjuvant therapy is often debated.

Nodal Involvement

Tumor spread to regional lymph nodes is associated with a particularly poor outcome after radiotherapeutic or surgical management alone.[198-202] The prognostic significance of the number of involved nodes was identified in some[203,204] but not all reports.[199,205] Barzell and colleagues[206] were the first to quantify nodal cancer volume and evaluated its association with disease outcome. Schmid and associates[204] found that patients with micrometastasis (i.e., ≤5 mm in largest dimension) had significantly better progression-free and overall survivals compared with patients with more extensive nodal involvement. In contrast, Srignoli and colleagues[207] found no difference in the risk of subsequent distant metastasis. Cheng and coworkers[208] reported that the risk of distant metastasis in patients with regional nodal involvement was directly proportional to nodal cancer volume and that volume was the best predictor of 5-year metastasis-free survival. It may be that inconsistencies in the literature relate to differences in the study cohorts, treatment approach, duration of follow-up, or method of analysis used by various investigators. Extranodal extension of disease, as well as Gleason score of the primary tumor, may also be significant predictors of cancer-specific survival.[209]

Tumor Grade

Long-term case series of EBRT,[172,191,210] radical prostatectomy,[173,211] and expectant management[167,170] uniformly identify tumor grade as a strong predictor of disease relapse and mortality in clinically localized prostate cancer. Studies consistently demonstrate that patients with a poorly differentiated tumor (i.e., grade 4/5 or Gleason score ≥7) have an increased risk of metastatic disease progression, and reduced overall and disease-specific survival.[167,176,211] For the patient with clinical T1 or T2 disease, tumor grade has greater predictive value than does the distinction between T1 and T2 categories.[170,172,173,176] For example, Chodak and associates[170] observed a marked difference in 10-year disease-specific survival between patients with grade 1 or 2 prostate cancer (87%) and those with grade 3 tumors (34%) in an evaluation of expectant management. In the context of EBRT, Zagars and colleagues[191] performed perhaps the most detailed, long-term analysis of pretherapy prognostic factors in patients treated before the introduction of PSA. This study demonstrated that tumor grade was predictive of metastatic relapse and overall survival when controlling for other potential prognostic factors (e.g., tumor stage). The differences among 10-year survival rates for patients with grade 1 (64%), grade 2 or 3 (45%), and grade 4 (19%) tumors were highly significant. The association of tumor grade with metastatic relapse[172,176,192] and overall survival[176] is preserved when pretherapy serum PSA level is considered. Although tumor grade is also associated with disease-free survival and freedom from clinically evident disease relapse,[172,175,212,213] its impact on local tumor control after EBRT is less certain, because some reports found an association,[176,190] but others did not.[212] Recent investigations have focused on posttherapy serum PSA levels (i.e., biochemical relapse) as an end point by which to judge therapeutic efficacy. Multivariate analysis of pretherapy tumor-related factors for an association with biochemical relapse in radiation therapy[172,176,177,179] and surgical[173,211] series confirms the significance of tumor grade.

Prostate-Specific Antigen

An abundant literature attests to the importance of the pretherapy serum PSA level as an independent and highly significant predictor of therapeutic outcome.[172,176,177,214,215] In general the pretreatment PSA level is a measure of the amount of tumor present, although one must also consider the relative PSA contribution from the normal prostate tissue and the fact that some tumors, especially the poorly differentiated ones, may not produce PSA commensurate with the tumor burden. In assessment of postirradiation outcome, Landmann and Hunig[216] were the first to draw attention to this association, which was confirmed by the detailed statistical analysis of larger study populations.[172,177,192,193,217,218] The prognostic significance of PSA is not limited to patients treated with radiation therapy, as similar observations appear in surgical reports.[211,219,220]

Although pretherapy PSA is perhaps the strongest individual predictor of biochemical relapse,[176,214,221] the distinction between a "good" and a "bad" PSA is open to interpretation, because the effect of PSA on outcome increases in a continuous, rather than stepwise, fashion.[176,179] Outcome has also been shown to be related to radiation dose such that with higher radiation therapy doses patients with higher pretreatment PSA levels may have better outcome than would be expected with lower radiation therapy doses.[172,222,223] Accordingly, most investigators used a precedent established in the literature to select various PSA values to create categories for statistical analysis and presentation of outcome.[176,192,215] In particular, Zagars and colleagues used this method to emphasize the relationship between pretherapy PSA and clinical or biochemical relapse after radiation therapy.[176] In this series, there was a significant difference in the risk of relapse for pretherapy PSA categories of 4.0 or less, 4.1 to 10.0, 10.1 to 20.0, and more than 20 ng/mL, which was 16%, 34%, 51%, and 89% at 6-year follow-up, respectively. Pisansky and coworkers[179,221] presented outcomes in a similar manner but also constructed a model to display the relapse rate as a continuous function of PSA while accounting for the prognostic effect of clinical tumor stage and Gleason score (Fig. 50-2).

Although numerous studies relate pretherapy PSA level to biochemical relapse, reports using clinical end points are not as abundant.[176,192,224] Nonetheless, Crook and colleagues[224] affirmed that local tumor recurrence correlated with PSA in patients in whom serial postirradiation prostatic biopsies were performed. Zagars and associates[176] reported a similar finding in a study population in whom postirradiation prostatic biopsies were generally obtained to identify an otherwise unknown source for biochemical relapse. Studies with long enough follow-ups to document clinical disease relapse, local and distant, are now being reported and correlate clinical end points with pretreatment PSA levels.[172]

In an effort to improve the prognostic accuracy of pretherapy serum PSA, Zentner and associates[224] evaluated PSAD (i.e., the PSA value divided by prostatic volume) in patients treated with EBRT. Patients with a PSAD of 0.3 ng/mL/cm^3 or less had a 100% disease-free survival probability at 30 months, whereas the estimate for patients with PSAD of more than 0.3 ng/cm^3 was significantly worse (62%). Compared with other pretherapy tumor-related characteristics (e.g., serum PSA level, Gleason score), PSAD was the best predictor of disease outcome in this study.

In an attempt to confirm this, other investigators studied PSAD in concert with other pretherapy factors.[225-227] Although an association between PSAD and biochemical relapse was found,[225,227] this was a reflection of the interdependence of PSAD and the PSA level because multivariate analysis identified PSA level and Gleason score as independent covariates for this end point. PSAD does not appear to add significantly to the utility of serum PSA level as a predictor of outcome after EBRT, and it is not routinely used as a prognostic factor. As an extension of the PSAD concept, D'Amico and Propert[226]

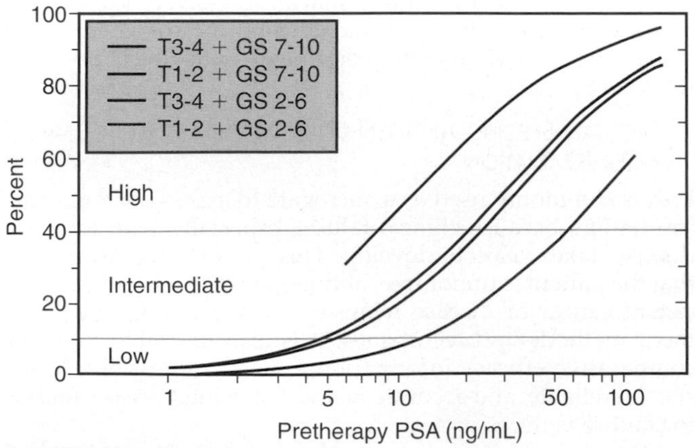

Figure 50-2 Probability of any relapse within 5 years of radiation therapy according to the combination of tumor stage and Gleason score as a function of the pretherapy prostate-specific antigen (PSA) level. (From Pisansky TM, Kahn MJ, Bostwick DG: An enhanced prognostic system for clinically localized carcinoma of the prostate. Cancer 79:2154, 1997.)

exploited the relationship between the contribution of normal epithelial cells to prostatic volume and the expression of PSA by normal and neoplastic cells (accounting for Gleason grade) to calculate the prostate cancer volume (V_{Ca}). Pretherapy V_{Ca} enhanced the predictive power of serum PSA level and Gleason score in identifying patients at increased risk for postirradiation biochemical relapse. Lankford and colleagues,[228] who preferred the term *PSA cancer volume*, confirmed this observation, which was particularly useful for patients with intermediate serum PSA values (i.e., 4 to 20 ng/mL).

The PSA doubling time (PSADT), which may reflect tumor proliferative activity (i.e., *aggressiveness*), uses regression analysis of serial serum PSA measurements over time to estimate prognosis.[229] Hanks and coworkers[230] used PSADT as a pretherapy predictive factor in patients treated with EBRT and found that a PSADT of less than 12 months adversely affected therapeutic outcome. Most investigation has focused on PSADT after therapy to predict the clinical outcome of patients with biochemical relapse after radiation therapy[212,229,231-233] or surgery.[234,235] In this setting, PSADT is related to pretherapy PSA level and tumor grade[212,218] and is associated with the anatomic location of tumor relapse.[212,218,234] Although there is considerable individual variation, a local tumor recurrence tends to correlate with a longer PSADT (median, 12 to 14 months), whereas a shorter PSADT (median, 4 to 6 months) is observed for metastatic relapse.[218,234] The posttherapy PSADT in patients treated with irradiation (median, 11 months)[218,236] is no different than that observed in surgical patients.[234,235]

After radiation therapy, residual prostatic epithelial cells may produce PSA under androgenic stimulation, and serum levels of PSA may be detected even in the absence of prostate cancer.[237] The postirradiation nadir PSA (nPSA) level is considered to be a predictive variable similar to pretherapy factors.[172,238,239] The nPSA correlates with pretherapy PSA level, tumor grade, and clinical tumor stage.[238,240] Nonetheless, nPSA is an independent predictor associated with biochemical or clinical relapse[218,238,240] and with local and metastatic tumor control.[224,239] As with pretherapy PSA, nPSA is associated with outcome in a continuous manner,[172,218] and an optimal cutoff point has not been established.[241] Although the nadir level can be used to predict the relative likelihood of failure after radiation, there is no absolute level which can determine success or failure after this therapy. Kuban and coworkers in a multi-institutional study of nearly 5000 patients treated by EBRT for prostate cancer demonstrated that progressively lower nadir levels were associated with incremental improvement in the disease-free survival rate correlated with the PSA level (PSA-DFS).[172]

Prostate-Specific Antigen Used to Assess Outcome after Irradiation

PSA is commonly used as a surrogate to assess outcome after irradiation, because clinical failure, especially with localized disease, takes years to develop. This can give the impression that the patient is tumor free, although PSA levels indicate persistent cancer or disease relapse.[192] In evaluating new treatment methods and techniques, it is also desirable to obtain comparative efficacy information as soon as possible. A consistent, reliable, and accurate method of using PSA as a marker for failure is necessary.

Over the past several years, it has become obvious that PSA failure definitions for surgery and radiation must use different criteria because of the inherent effect on the prostate by each of these modalities. The effect of various irradiation modalities, such as EBRT alone, brachytherapy alone, or the combination of EBRT and brachytherapy, on prostatic PSA production is also being studied. Because prostatectomy removes nearly all prostatic tissue, an absolute PSA level after surgery has been correlated with outcome. This level is very low, in the 0.1 to 0.4 ng/mL range, and is representative of the small amount of prostate typically left behind.[242,243] Although these levels have been correlated to postoperative relapse, further proof of progressive disease is evidenced by a rising PSA. For irradiated patients, a rising PSA is the criteria for relapse that must be used, because a very low target PSA value, especially soon after treatment is not very specific in predicting clinical failure.[244,245] This is because the prostate remains intact in irradiated patients and it takes a median of approximately 2 years for the PSA to reach the nadir, or lowest level.[246] Simultaneous with this gradual process, a PSA "bounce" can occur, mimicking failure because the bounce is a PSA rise but one derived from a benign cause, likely prostatitis.[247] The definition of PSA relapse after irradiation must take both factors into account to minimize false-positive failure reporting.

The American Society of Therapeutic Radiology and Oncology (ASTRO) held a Consensus Conference in 1996 for the purpose of devising a PSA-based failure definition after EBRT, which would standardize outcome reporting. The well-known ASTRO definition is characterized by 3 consecutive PSA rises with the time of failure backdated to half-way between the PSA nadir and the first PSA rise.[241] After several additional years of experience in the PSA era and more sophisticated statistical analysis, criticisms of the ASTRO definition were brought forward, and alternative definitions that were more sensitive and specific were advocated.[244,248]

A second Consensus Conference sponsored by ASTRO and the Radiation Therapy Oncology Group (RTOG) was held in 2005, at which several investigators presented analyses with more long-term follow-up than was available at the first conference.[249] A distinguished panel representing radiation and surgical specialties and clinical trials groups is formulating the latest consensus statement. The general feeling is that for at least 5 years after irradiation by EBRT or implantation, the PSA level cannot be expected to reach consistently low levels similar to surgically treated levels, and a threshold level for failure therefore must be relatively high; alternatively, failure must be based on a rising PSA, albeit perhaps with different criteria from those of the previous 3-year ASTRO definition. We have found that postirradiation PSA patterns of an intact prostate do not lend themselves to early outcome assessment, as we had previously enthusiastically hoped. It is difficult to make early outcome assessments for a tumor that characteristically relapses late after therapy.

Predictive Models

The use of multivariate statistical analysis to identify pretherapy predictive factors also provides the mathematical means to combine these variables to create prognostic indices and groupings that improve the accuracy of anatomically based systems (e.g., the AJCC system) to estimate therapeutic outcome. Hermanek and coworkers[250] and Burke and Henson[251] set forth the principles by which covariates may be combined to calculate the risk of relapse for the individual patient and to gather these relapse risks into prognostic groups. For patients with clinically localized prostate cancer, the serum PSA level, tumor grade, and tumor stage are relevant and readily available factors predictive of outcome. Several investigators used different combinations of these factors to display outcome after EBRT[176,178,179,226,252] or surgical resection.[211,253] A method often employed for constructing a prognostic group is to consolidate independent predictors into empirically derived subgroups that are further combined to define prognostic groupings. However, there are many different ways to combine prognostic variables (i.e., subgroups) to define a prognostic group, and a clear consensus regarding the optimal combination has not been established. For example, Fukunaga-Johnson and colleagues[178] used this method to divide their study population into *favorable* (i.e., tumor stage T1-2, Gleason score <7, and PSA ≤10 ng/mL) and *unfavorable* prognostic groups and reported an improved 5-year freedom from biochemical relapse (75% versus 33%) in the former group. However, Zagars and coworkers[176] arranged clinical tumor stage (T1-2 versus T3-4), Gleason score (2 to 6 versus 7 versus 8 to 10), and PSA (≤4 versus 4 to 10 versus 10 to 20 versus >20) characteristics in a different manner to describe 24 nonoverlapping categories. After inspection of the relapse risks (i.e., hazard indices) associated with these categories, certain categories were consolidated to define six prognostic groups with statistically different probabilities for clinical or biochemical relapse (Fig. 50-3), which for groups I, II, III, IV, V, and unfavorable were 6%, 30%, 40%, 46%, 57%, and 88% at 6 years, respectively.

Although empirically derived methods may aptly describe statistically distinct outcomes between patient subgroups within the study population from which they were obtained, this process does not necessarily provide a prediction for the as-yet-untreated patient with newly diagnosed prostate cancer. Schemes that compartmentalize a continuous factor (e.g., PSA) or do not adjust the relapse risk according to the interaction between prognostic factors may not render the optimal combination of variables by which to define prognostic groupings. Pisansky and coworkers[221] and Partin and associates[253] used cross-validation methods to develop predictive models that might be applied with greater confidence to the newly diagnosed prostate cancer patient. For patients treated with radiation therapy, Pisansky and colleagues[221] developed a risk score (R) defined as R = (1.07 × tumor stage risk) + (1.21 × Gleason score risk) + (1.2 × $\log_e$ PSA), in which tumor stage T1-2 indicates risk = 0, T3-4 indicates risk = 1, Gleason score of 2 to 6 indicates risk = 0, and Gleason score of

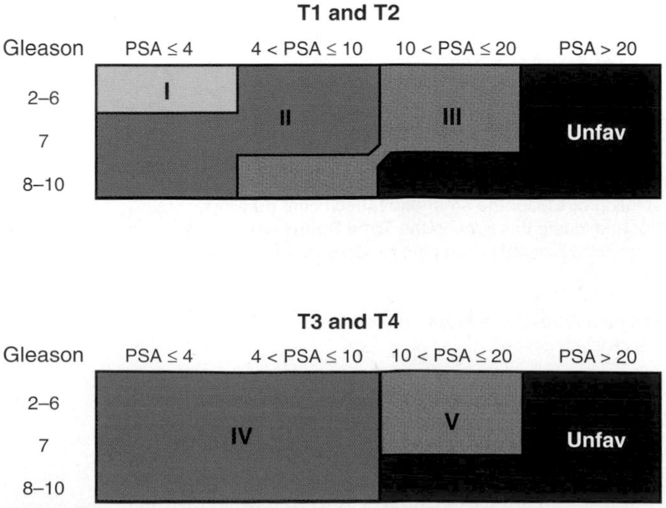

Figure 50-3 Prognostic groups are defined by tumor (T) stage, Gleason score, and prostate-specific antigen (PSA) level. Unfav, unfavorable. (From Zagars GK, Pollack A, von Eschenbach AC: Prognostic factors for clinically localized prostate carcinoma. Analysis of 938 patients irradiated in the prostate specific antigen era. Cancer 79:1370, 1997.)

7 to 10 indicates risk = 1. Patient groups considered to be at low (i.e., ≤10%), intermediate (i.e., similar to the entire study cohort), and high (i.e., ≥50%) risk for clinical or biochemical relapse were defined with receiver operator characteristic curve analysis as having risk scores of less than 3.1, 3.1 to 4.9, and more than 4.9, respectively. This prognostic grouping system was affirmed in the validation portion of this study, wherein the 5-year relapse-free risks for low- (92%), intermediate- (67%), and high-risk (24%) groups were nearly identical to those predicted by the model. These risk score prognostic groupings were highly predictive in an independent evaluation as well.[252]

Various predictive models have been advocated. The Partin tables are commonly used to combine prognostic factors to assess the chances of extraprostatic extension and seminal vesicle or lymph node involvement as these situations are associated with well-reported outcome estimates and can aid in determining the most advantageous treatment options.[146] Similarly, prognostic groupings representing low, intermediate, or high risk of relapse (risk groups) as suggested by D'Amico and associates and others have gained popularity because they are readily associated with outcome expectations.[254] Kattan and colleagues have developed nomograms for surgical and irradiation patients that directly use patient characteristics to generate a numeric percentage of risk for tumor relapse.[255,256] These systems rely on combining tumor stage, grade, pretreatment PSA level, and operative pathologic factors for surgical patients in predicting outcome after therapy (Fig. 50-4).

CLINICAL MANIFESTATIONS, PATIENT EVALUATION, AND STAGING

Clinical Symptoms and Signs

Because approximately three quarters of prostate cancers originate in the peripheral zone, patients with early-stage disease are often asymptomatic. However, the tumor may arise in the transition zone or may extend from a peripheral location to encroach on the prostatic urethra to produce obstructive symptoms. The resulting symptom complex, commonly referred to as prostatism, initially consists of urinary hesitancy, diminished force of stream, intermittency, and a sense of incomplete voiding. Thereafter, the bladder detrusor muscle may lose compliance, and irritative symptoms such as urgency, frequency, nocturia, dysuria, and incontinence may develop. Although acute urinary retention may ensue, it is no more likely to occur in the patient with prostate cancer than in the general population.[257,258] The constellation of obstructive symptoms now referred to as lower urinary tract symptoms is commonplace in the elderly male population[259] and is often associated with benign prostatic hypertrophy or other mechanical or functional disorders of the urinary bladder. Hematuria, which may result from tumor involvement of the prostatic urethra or bladder trigone, and hematospermia are uncommon signs of prostate cancer and should prompt further investigation to identify their causes.

Extraprostatic tumor spread is often asymptomatic and may not be apparent on physical or radiologic examination. However, extensive disease involvement of the periprostatic tissues may produce symptoms as a late manifestation of the disease process. Denonvilliers' fascia is usually an effective barrier to rectal involvement, but symptoms similar to those of a primary rectal cancer, such as hematochezia, constipation or intermittent diarrhea, reduced stool caliber, or abdominopelvic pain, may occur. Renal impairment as a result of prolonged bladder outlet obstruction or from tumor

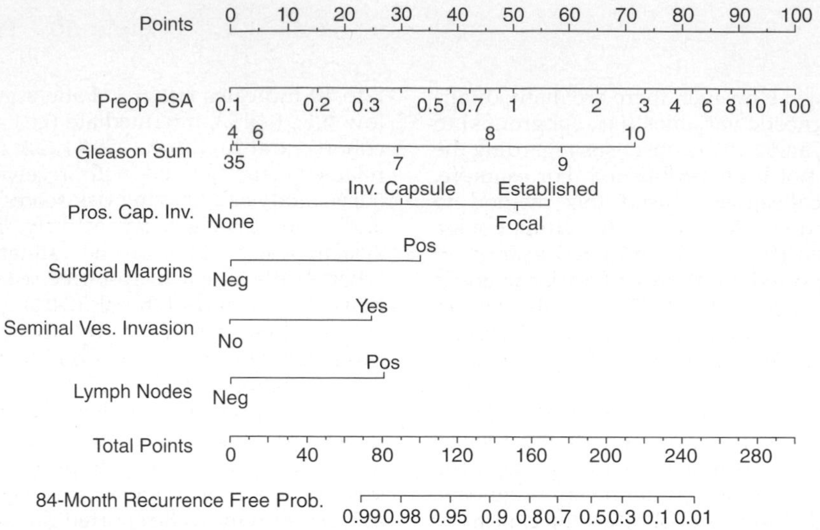

Instructions for Physician: Locate the patient's PSA on the **PSA** axis. Draw a line straight upward to the **Points** axis to determine how many points toward recurrence the patient receives for his PSA. Repeat this process for the other axis, each time drawing straight upward to the **Points** axis. Sum the points achieved for each predictor and locate this sum on the **Total Points axis**. Draw a line straight down to find the patient's probability of remaining recurrence free for 84 months assuming he does not die of another cause first.

Instruction to Patient: "Mr. X, if we had 100 men exactly like you, we would expect between <predicted percentage from nomogram – 10%> and <predicted percentage + 10%> to remain free of their disease at 7 years following radical prostatectomy, and recurrence after 7 years is very rare."

A

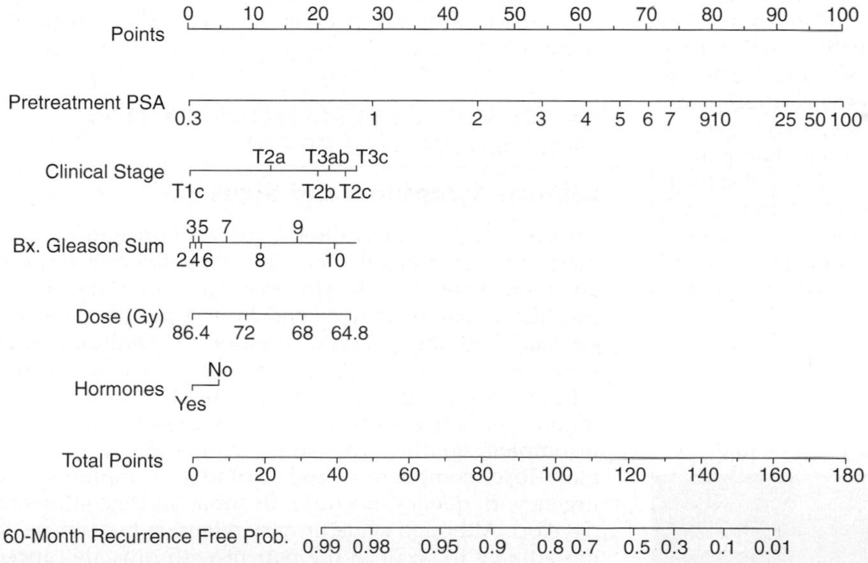

Instructions for Physician: Locate the patient's PSA on the **PSA** axis. Draw a line straight upward to the **Points** axis to determine how many points toward recurrence the patient receives for his PSA. Repeat this process for the other axes, each time drawing straight upward to the **Points** axis. Sum the points achieved for each predictor and locate this sum on the **Total Points** axis. Draw a line straight down to find the patients's probability of remaining recurrence free for 60 months assuming he does not die of another cause first.

Note: *This nomogram is not applicable to a man who is not otherwise a candidate for radiation therapy. You can use this only on a man who has already selected radiation therapy as treatment for his prostate cancer.*

Instruction to Patient: "Mr. X, if we had 100 men exactly like you, we would expect between <predicted percentage from nomogram – 10%> and <predicted percentage + 10%> to remain free of their disease at 5 years following conformal radiation therapy, and recurrence after 5 years is very rare."

B

Figure 50-4 **Top,** Postoperative nomogram based on 996 patients treated at The Methodist Hospital, Houston, Texas, for predicting tumor recurrence correlated with prostate-specific antigen (PSA) level after radical prostatectomy. Prognostic variables included pretreatment serum PSA level, specimen Gleason sum, prostatic capsular invasion, surgical margin status, seminal vesicle invasion, and lymph node status. For prostatic capsular invasion (Pros. Cap. Inv.), *none* refers to prostate cancer within the confines of the glandular prostate (group L0 in the original series) or in the prostatic stroma but beyond the limit of the normal acini (group L1); *invasion of the capsule* (Inv. Capsule) refers to group L2; *focal* refers to group L3F, and *established* refers to group L3E. Neg, negative; Pos, positive; Preop, preoperative; Prob, probability; Ves, vesicle. **Bottom,** Three-dimensional conformal radiation therapy nomogram based on 1042 patients treated at Memorial Sloan-Kettering Cancer Center for predicting PSA-correlated recurrence after radiation therapy.

involvement of the bladder trigone or periureteral tissues may cause symptoms or signs due to fluid retention or electrolyte imbalance. Invasion of the neurovascular bundles, urogenital diaphragm, and penile corporeal bodies may result in impotence, perineal pain, and priapism, respectively.

The pelvic, axial, and proximal regions of the appendicular skeleton are the most common sites of metastatic disease spread. Based on the distribution of uptake on radionuclide bone scan, the vertebral column (74%), ribs (70%), pelvis (60%), femora (44%), and shoulder girdle (41%) are the prevailing sites of involvement in patients with osseous metastases.[260] Although approximately one third to one half of those with bone metastases may be asymptomatic, pain in these areas is commonly described or may be elicited through examination of the skeletal system. The extent of osseous metastasis and the presence of symptoms[261] are associated with responsiveness to therapeutic intervention and survival duration. Pathologic fractures are uncommon but may affect the femora, humeri, and vertebral column. Extension of tumor into the epidural space or compression of nerve rootlets or peripheral nerves may cause neurologic deficits. Spinal cord compression is characterized by motor weakness, sensory changes, and bladder and bowel dysfunction. Its presence is considered an oncologic emergency that requires prompt recognition and treatment to avoid permanent disability.

Tumor involvement of pelvic or para-aortic lymph nodes is usually asymptomatic, and clinical signs, such as edema of the abdominal wall, genitalia, and lower extremities, are rarely apparent unless bulky nodal disease is present. Although metastases to other anatomic sites (e.g., adrenal glands, liver, lung, and skin) are described,[262] symptoms or signs due to functional compromise are uncommon. Paraneoplastic syndromes, including Cushing's syndrome, the syndrome of inappropriate antidiuretic hormone secretion and abnormalities of serum calcium levels, and hematologic manifestations (e.g., anemia, disseminated intravascular coagulation) may also be present in the patient with advanced metastatic disease.[263]

History and Physical Examination

A thorough history and physical examination are fundamental components of patient evaluation and may be instrumental in directing further diagnostic and staging procedures. In particular, detailed inquiry regarding urinary status, sexual function, and skeletal symptoms identifies the patient's baseline condition and may prompt further investigation and therapy. Assessment of comorbid illness may have relevance to therapeutic decision-making, and the family medical history may identify other family members at high risk for developing prostate cancer.

A complete physical examination is essential and may reveal metastatic disease or other clinically important conditions. Careful DRE of the prostate forms the cornerstone of the physical examination and is instrumental in tumor staging. The examination may be performed in the lithotomy, knee-chest, lateral prone (Sims'), or standing position with a well-lubricated, gloved index finger. The examiner should measure the craniocaudal and transverse dimensions of the gland and determine its overall consistency, sensitivity, and mobility, as well as the presence and size of any firm or elevated areas. Typically, an area of prostate cancer is quite hard, may or may not be raised above the surface of the gland, and is surrounded by compressible prostatic tissue. However, an area of prostatic induration is not pathognomonic of cancer, because the induration may result from prostatic calculi, infection, infarction, granulomatous prostatitis, or nodularity due to benign prostatic hyperplasia. Approximately 20% to 30% of patients with a prostatic abnormality that is suspected to be cancer have malignancy confirmed by biopsy.[77] The lateral rectal sulci and the urogenital diaphragm are also examined to determine whether extraprostatic tumor extension is present. Although the normal seminal vesicles are too soft to be palpated as discrete structures, firmness extending superior to the prostate gland suggests seminal vesicle involvement, and further investigation may be warranted.

Staging

Whitmore[264] is credited with developing the first widely accepted stage groupings for prostate cancer, and the general concepts set forth were later incorporated into the American Urological Association system.[195] Subsequently, the Organ Systems Coordinating Center of the National Cancer Institute initiated a process to align the Whitmore-based groupings and the TNM system. This and other efforts led to development of the AJCC TNM classification and stage groupings,[123] which were unified with the Union Internationale Contre le Cancer in 1987.[124] This system retains the general organizational scheme of prior systems and conforms to the TNM rules applied to tumors originating in other sites.

The TNM classifications and the stage groupings for prostate cancer are shown in Tables 50-3 and 50-4, respectively. Clinical staging involves primary tumor assessment with DRE, complete general examination to determine disease extent, serum PSA determination, and diagnostic imaging (including TRUS). The regional lymph nodes are defined as those confined to the true pelvis (i.e., those lying below the bifurcation of the common iliac arteries) and include the obturator, external and internal iliac, and sacral lymph node groups. All information available before definitive therapy may be used for clinical staging. Pathologic staging requires histologic examination of the prostatoseminalvesiculectomy and pelvic lymph node specimens; margin positivity should be specified.

Diagnostic Imaging

Ultrasonography

TRUS is an important tool in prostate cancer diagnosis and may be used to identify abnormalities of the prostate gland and seminal vesicles for staging purposes. TRUS is performed by inserting a 5- to 7.5-MHz transducer in the rectum and imaging the prostate in the axial and sagittal planes. Although the typical sonographic appearance of prostate cancer is an area of diminished echogenicity (hypoechoic) in the peripheral zone of the gland, between 14% and 29% of patients with prostate cancer have an isoechoic tumor that cannot be reliably distinguished from normal prostatic tissue.[76,265,266] Among prostate cancer screening participants with a hypoechoic finding on TRUS that prompts further evaluation, only 17% to 31% have a diagnosis of cancer established by needle biopsy of the prostate.[76,265,266]

Several investigations address the ability of TRUS to detect extraprostatic tumor extension, which may affect tumor stage, by correlating ultrasound observations with the findings from histologic examination of the prostatoseminalvesiculectomy specimen. In particular, the Radiology Diagnostic Oncology Group prospectively evaluated preoperative TRUS in 219 patients who underwent radical prostatectomy.[267] Among 85 patients considered to have disease confined to the prostate gland, 43 (51%) had extraprostatic tumor extension, whereas 50 of 134 patients (37%) with suspected extraprostatic disease did not have this confirmed by histologic examination.

Overall, the sensitivity and specificity of TRUS in identifying extraprostatic disease were 66% and 46%, respectively, and the test accuracy was only 58%. Based on these results, these investigators concluded that TRUS is not sufficiently accurate to assist in staging early-stage prostate cancer, mainly because of its limitations in identifying microscopic extraprostatic disease spread. Smith and associates[268] and Ohori and colleagues[269] found that TRUS is no more accurate than DRE in evaluating the local extent of disease, and inclusion of TRUS findings into tumor stage does not appear to influence radiotherapeutic outcome.[270]

Despite these limitations, tumor extension into the seminal vesicles may be appreciated by TRUS as echogenic abnormalities and by anterior displacement and enlargement of this structure. Terris and coworkers[151] demonstrated the feasibility of obtaining ultrasound-guided preoperative bilateral seminal vesicle biopsies. Among 73 prostate cancer patients suitable for prostatectomy, biopsy showed tumor involvement adjacent to seminal epithelium (i.e., a pathognomonic finding) in eight patients; all of these instances were confirmed after examination of the surgical specimen. Eleven of 133 negative preoperative seminal vesicle biopsies had involvement with cancer, resulting in a false-negative rate of 8%. Linzer and colleagues[271] also concluded that seminal vesicle biopsy accurately identifies extraprostatic tumor extension. Based on the estimated risk for occult seminal vesicle invasion,[146,156] consideration may be given to the selective use of ultrasound-guided seminal vesicle biopsy during the pretherapy staging process.

Computed Tomography

Computed tomography (CT) has little value in assessing intraprostatic anatomic changes due to the primary tumor, because the neoplasm usually has the same attenuation as the normal prostate gland. In the presence of EPE, the periprostatic fat planes may become indistinct, or there may be deformity of the bladder base, obliteration of the normal angle between the seminal vesicles and the posterior aspect of the bladder, or asymmetric enlargement of a seminal vesicle. However, caution must be exerted in interpreting these radiologic signs because they may be an artifact of biopsy or the plane between seminal vesicles and bladder may be obscured by rectal distention. EPE is often microscopic and cannot be detected with CT. This observation largely accounts for the low sensitivity of this procedure, which limits its utility in staging the primary tumor.[272]

A CT scan of the abdomen and pelvis is often obtained in the pretherapy staging of the patient with a new diagnosis of clinically localized prostate cancer. However, CT imaging can detect only abnormalities in lymph node size that may result from extensive tumor involvement. As a result, the diagnostic sensitivity of this procedure with respect to lymph node assessment is poor (≈ 25%),[272,273] and the routine use of this test is of little value in assignment of regional node stage for clinical practice or therapeutic research studies.[274] For example, Huncharek and Muscat[275] analyzed the CT results of 425 patients with newly diagnosed prostate cancer and found that only 12 patients (3%) had radiologic evidence of adenopathy. Because patients with adenopathy had higher serum PSA levels, these authors concluded that CT scanning was not indicated in the patient with a PSA value under 20 ng/mL, wherein fewer than 1% had adenopathy. Other investigators observed a similar association between serum PSA level and radiologic and histologic findings and concluded that CT imaging for nodal assessment should be reserved for patients with higher (>20 to 25 ng/mL) PSA values.[273,276] Particularly in high-risk patients fine-needle aspiration cytology may further enhance the specificity and accuracy of CT-based pelvic node evaluation.[253] In the patient in whom radiation therapy is the primary management approach, it appears prudent to perform the pelvic, with or without abdominal, CT scan in the treatment position to obtain diagnostic and treatment planning information at a single setting.[277]

Magnetic Resonance Imaging

In staging prostate cancer, high-resolution MRI requires equipment operating in the 1.5-T range to obtain the signal-to-noise ratio necessary to obtain thin section images in a small field of view. The T1- and T2-weighted spin-echo sequences are complementary and are used to optimize image resolution. The T1-weighted sequences provide high contrast between water density structures (e.g., prostate gland, seminal vesicles) and fat and are particularly useful for evaluating the periprostatic fat and veins, neurovascular bundles, perivesical tissues, and lymph nodes. The T2-weighted fast spin-echo (FASE) sequences demonstrate the internal zonal anatomy of the prostate and the architecture of the seminal vesicles. Although prostate cancer is typically a focal, peripheral region of decreased signal intensity surrounded by a normal (high-intensity) peripheral zone, nodules of benign prostatic hypertrophy, usually centrally located, may have similar signal characteristics.

Body-coil MRI for prostate cancer staging was prospectively evaluated in a multi-institutional trial conducted by the Radiology Diagnostic Oncology Group.[267] In this study, the findings of preoperative MRI were compared with step section histologic analysis of the prostate in 194 patients who underwent radical prostatectomy. MRI identified 60% of prostate cancers that measured 5 mm or more in size and had an overall tumor staging accuracy of 69%. Among 23 patients with tumor spread to pelvic lymph nodes, MRI identified nodal involvement in only 1 patient (sensitivity of 4%). Based on these observations, the Radiology Diagnostic Oncology Group concluded that body-coil MRI is not an accurate method for prostate cancer staging and has limited application to contemporary medical decision-making and patient care. Despite these reservations, technologic advances may allow for higher MRI resolution and improved staging accuracy. For example, MRI with FASE pulse sequence and a pelvic phased-array coil (multicoil)[278] may yield improved results compared with a conventional body coil. Recently, Harisinghani and colleagues have described the intravenous infusion of iron oxide lymphotropic superparamagnetic nanoparticles in normal saline to enhance MRI imaging of lymph nodes.[279] For lymph nodes which were considered normal by standard MRI criteria, the sensitivity of detecting tumor by this method was 96%. Further trials are in progress using this promising technology.

Endorectal surface-coil MRI of the prostate also has been studied by several investigators in an attempt to improve image quality and staging accuracy. The accuracy of endorectal MRI in staging the primary tumor (54% to 72%) appears comparable to that attained with conventional body-coil MRI.[153,154] Nonetheless, many false-negative readings are the result of microscopic perforation of the prostatic capsule, whereas the accuracy of detecting seminal vesicle invasion may be higher. Endorectal-coil MRI may be best applied in conjunction with the DRE, Gleason score, and pretherapy serum PSA findings in selected patients at high risk for tumor invasion of the seminal vesicles.

Magnetic resonance spectroscopy, which can noninvasively assess cellular metabolism, can be done in conjunction with MRI as a means to improve accuracy.[280]

Nuclear Medicine Imaging

BONE SCANS

Clinically apparent metastatic disease is limited to bone in 80% to 85% of patients with prostate cancer metastases and is observed in a pattern that correlates with the distribution of hematopoietic marrow in the adult. The high bone-to-soft-tissue ratio of uptake for technetium medronate conjugates provides a radiopharmaceutical agent well suited for use in bone scintigraphy, which is a highly sensitive method for detection of osteoblastic metastases. The scintigraphic appearance may range from a solitary focus of radionuclide uptake to the "superscan," in which the entire skeleton is uniformly affected. Recognition of the latter condition, distinguished by the lack of renal uptake and excretion of the radionuclide, is important because the scan may otherwise be interpreted as normal. Although the bone scan is a sensitive imaging tool, other conditions, such as arthritis, bone fracture, and Paget's disease, may also result in uptake of the radionuclide. In certain situations, standard bone radiography or tomography, CT, or MRI may be required to determine the nature of the findings seen on bone scan.

Since the advent of serum PSA testing, Chybowski and associates[281] were among the first to evaluate the utility of obtaining a routine bone scan in the pretherapy evaluation of the patient with newly diagnosed prostate cancer. These investigators conducted a retrospective evaluation of 521 randomly selected patients and correlated clinical tumor stage, tumor grade of the diagnostic biopsy specimen, acid phosphatase, PAP, and PSA serum levels with bone scan findings. In multivariate analysis, PSA, tumor stage, and acid phosphatase retained independent association with the results of the bone scan. The probability of a bone scan showing metastatic disease was most strongly associated with and was directly proportional to the serum PSA level, as illustrated in Figure 50-5. Analysis of the sensitivity and specificity profile of tumor stage and acid phosphatase showed that these tumor-related factors did not significantly enhance the predictive ability of PSA alone.

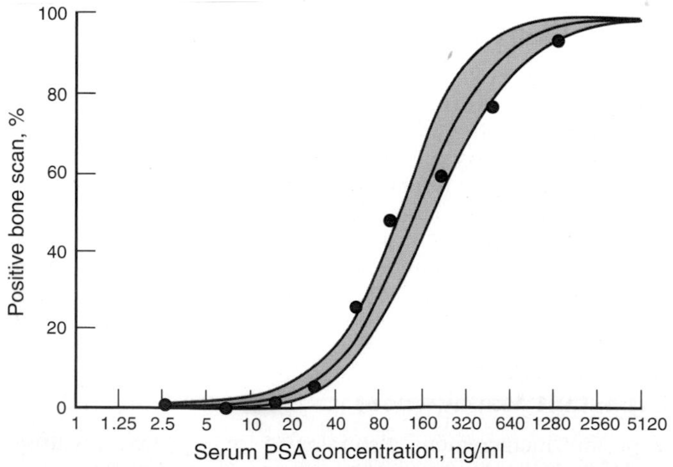

Figure 50-5 Results of bone scan findings as a function of pretherapy serum prostate-specific antigen (PSA) level; 95% confidence intervals are *shaded*. (From Chybowski FM, Larson Keller JJ, Bergstralh EJ, et al: Predicting radionuclide bone scan findings in patients with newly diagnosed, untreated prostate cancer: prostate-specific antigen is superior to all other clinical parameters. J Urol 145:313, 1991. Copyright 1991, with permission from American Urological Association.)

Because Chybowski and colleagues[281] showed that few patients (0.3%) with a pretherapy serum PSA level of 20 ng/mL or lower had a positive bone scan at disease presentation, Oesterling and coworkers[282] sought to confirm this finding in a successive study cohort. To this end, 852 consecutive patients with newly diagnosed untreated prostate cancer with a pretherapy serum PSA level of less than 20 ng/mL were evaluated. In this study, seven patients (0.8%) had scintigraphic evidence of bone metastases, and five of these patients were symptomatic in the area corresponding to the bone scan abnormality. The observed rates of false-negative bone scan results were 0.5% and 0.8% for patients with serum PSA levels of 10 ng/mL or less and less than 20 ng/mL, respectively. On the basis of these observations, the authors concluded that a bone scan was not routinely required in the staging evaluation of the patient without skeletal discomfort if the pretherapy serum PSA level was 10 ng/mL or less. This investigation confirmed the finding that serum PSA was most closely associated with the bone scan results and that neither clinical tumor stage nor tumor grade improved the predictive accuracy of PSA alone. Oesterling and colleagues[282] suggest that considerable economic savings could be realized if the use of a radionuclide bone scan were reserved for the symptomatic patient or for those with PSA levels above 10 ng/mL or (possibly) a high-grade tumor.

Radionuclide bone scintigraphy may also be of value in the posttherapy assessment of the patient with prostate cancer. The onset of skeletal symptoms, particularly in association with a rising serum PSA profile, should prompt radioscintigraphic investigation. However, posttherapy serum PSA monitoring is apt to identify tumor relapse before the occurrence of symptoms, as biochemical relapse may antedate development of bone scan abnormalities by several months. Freitas and coworkers[283] used receiver operating characteristic curve analysis to identify a serum PSA threshold level at which a posttherapy bone scan might be considered. This analysis indicated that few patients (1.5%) with a posttherapy PSA value of 8 ng/mL or less had a positive bone scan, whereas 38% of patients with a PSA level greater than this value had a bone scan indicative of osseous metastases. Although the optimal use of a bone scan in this setting has not been extensively investigated, this information may be of use in the posttherapy disease evaluation setting.

MONOCLONAL ANTIBODY IMAGING

Monoclonal antibody immunoconjugates have also been evaluated for nuclear medicine imaging purposes. Although radioimmunoscintigraphy with PSA- or PAP-directed monoclonal antibodies did not meet with great success, renewed interest in this area occurred with development of the murine monoclonal antibody CYT-356. This antibody is directed against the prostate-specific membrane antigen cytoplasmic epitope, which appears to predominate in prostatic tissues[284] and is enhanced after androgen deprivation.[285] The image performance of ^{111}In-labeled capromab pendetide (ProstaScint) has been assessed in the pretherapy evaluation of patients with clinically localized prostate cancer who are considered at high risk for disease spread to regional nodes and in the posttherapy setting when occult residual or recurrent disease is suspected. Before commercial availability, the manufacturer evaluated the test accuracy of ProstaScint with respect to pelvic nodal evaluation (68%) and in the setting of postprostatectomy biochemical relapse (63%). Subsequent evaluations suggest accuracy in the 70% range.[286,287] This imaging modality is usually used in special circumstances, such as in postprostatectomy patients with increasing PSA levels in whom it is important to differentiate between locoregional and distant disease, and not in routine pretreatment evaluation.

Laboratory Evaluation

Prostate-Specific Antigen

PSA is a serine protease produced by normal prostatic acinar and ductal epithelial cells and by neoplastic cells of prostatic origin.[287,288] It is detectable in the serum in a form immunologically identical to that purified from prostatic tissues and may be elevated in patients with benign (e.g., prostatic hypertrophy, prostatitis) or malignant disorders of the prostate gland.[287] Although PSA exists in several forms in the serum, the PSA-α_1-antichymotrypsin complex predominates,[289] whereas the free (noncomplexed) form of PSA is less abundant.[102,289]

The quantity of PSA in the serum is determined by commercially available immunoassays that use monoclonal antibodies to identify epitopes on the PSA molecule. The most frequently used assays in the United States are the IMx PSA assay and the Tandem-R and Tandem-E PSA assays. The Tandem assays use two murine monoclonal antibodies directed to separate epitopes on the PSA molecule, whereas the IMx PSA uses a monoclonal-polyclonal technique. The analytic characteristics of a single determination of the IMx and the mean of duplicates using the Tandem assays provide test results that correlate well.[290]

Serum PSA levels may exhibit interassay (run-to-run) and physiologic (i.e., intraindividual) variation that must be considered in interpreting serial determinations. Physiologic variation refers to the difference in PSA levels observed when a second sample is obtained from the same patient within a few weeks of the initial sample. For physiologic variation, the ratio difference variation is significantly greater than the interassay variation, is inversely related to the PSA level, and may be as high as 0.298 (95% confidence interval).[291] This means, for example, that a serum PSA of 4 ng/mL can increase to 5.2 ng/mL (4.0×0.298) and still remain in the range of physiologic variability.

The serum half-life of PSA is approximately 2.2 (±0.8) to 3.2 (±0.1) days,[292] which means that several weeks are required for serum levels to return to baseline after prostatic manipulation or for a nadir value to be reached after prostatectomy. Although digital examination of the prostate, prostatic massage, TRUS, ejaculation, and cystoscopy do not have a significant effect on the serum PSA level, prostate biopsy causes an immediate PSA elevation (median, 7.9 ng/mL) that requires several weeks to return to baseline.[293-295] Transurethral resection of the prostate (TURP) also causes PSA elevation (median, 5.9 ng/mL), with a median of 17 days required to arrive at the new baseline value.[295] Because the production and secretion of PSA are androgen dependent, androgen deprivation therapy often results in a striking reduction in the PSA level,[296] which should be considered in interpreting serum PSA values in this setting.

Pretherapy serum PSA is an important prognostic factor in predicting outcome after treatment for prostate cancer and should play an important role in consideration of treatment options. In general, the higher the PSA level, the more likely that the tumor is outside the capsule and into the seminal vesicles or lymph nodes, which has major impact on the choice of therapy.[172,176,255,256]

Acid Phosphatase

Although also produced in nonprostatic tissues, the glandular epithelium of the prostate is the dominant source of acid phosphatase in humans. The prostate-specific form of this enzyme (i.e., PAP) is distinct from other isoenzymatic forms and is influenced by hormonal factors, and its expression is altered in the androgen-deprived state. Several substrates (e.g., sodium thymolphthalein monophosphate) and biochemical assay methods were developed to measure the activity of acid phosphatase in the serum and in various tissue sources. Immunologic methods are available for serum quantification and immunohistochemical analysis of tissue specimens. Serum levels of PAP are affected by circadian rhythms, random diurnal fluctuation, prostatic massage, surgical manipulation of the prostate gland,[297] and the presence of benign prostatic hypertrophy.[298] Abnormally high serum acid phosphatase levels correlate with clinical tumor stage T3-4 disease, higher tumor grade, and pretherapy serum PSA.[191]

Since introduction of assays for serum PSA, controversy exists regarding the merit of acid phosphatase testing in patients with prostate cancer, and a striking decline in the use of serum PAP has occurred.[299] Several clinical observations support the assertion that serum PAP determinations add little to patient evaluation in before or after therapy. In patients with prostate cancer, serum PSA is at 2 to 10 times more likely to be elevated than is serum PAP,[218,299] and only 2% of patients with a normal serum PSA value will have an elevated serum PAP.[298] Fewer than 10% of patients treated for cure with radiation therapy have an elevated acid phosphatase level, whereas 80% to 90% have an abnormal (>4.0 ng/mL) PSA value.[217,218]

Although acid phosphatase levels eventually may be elevated in 67% to 81% of patients with established osseous metastatic disease,[298,300] only 20% of patients who develop a bone scan abnormality indicative of osseous metastases will have an antecedent rise in the serum acid phosphatase level.[300] Dupont and associates[301] demonstrated that serum PSA had greater sensitivity (87%), specificity (92%), and overall test accuracy (89%) compared with PAP for monitoring the disease status of patients treated with maximal androgen blockade for stage III-IV prostate cancer. Although there may be certain settings in which acid phosphatase determinations have clinical relevance, there appears to be little justification for the routine use of this serologic test for diagnosis, pretherapy evaluation, or posttherapy disease monitoring in the PSA era.

Staging Workup

The American College of Radiology (ACR)[302] and the National Comprehensive Cancer Network[303] have established guidelines for the pretherapy staging of patients with a recently established diagnosis of prostate cancer. The scheme proposed by the National Comprehensive Cancer Network is displayed in Figure 50-6,[303] and may be used for guidance. However, individual clinical circumstance may require departure from these guidelines, as independent medical judgment is necessary to meet needs unique to a particular situation.

PRIMARY THERAPY

Expectant Management

Expectant management, also referred to as watchful waiting or deferred therapy, is a policy wherein immediate therapeutic intervention is not pursued when a diagnosis of prostate cancer is established. With this approach, treatment is withheld until the time of disease progression or development of tumor-related symptoms. Intervention primarily relies on hormonal therapy to induce tumor regression and alleviate symptoms. This management strategy is used throughout the world and it is considered a satisfactory alternative to the use

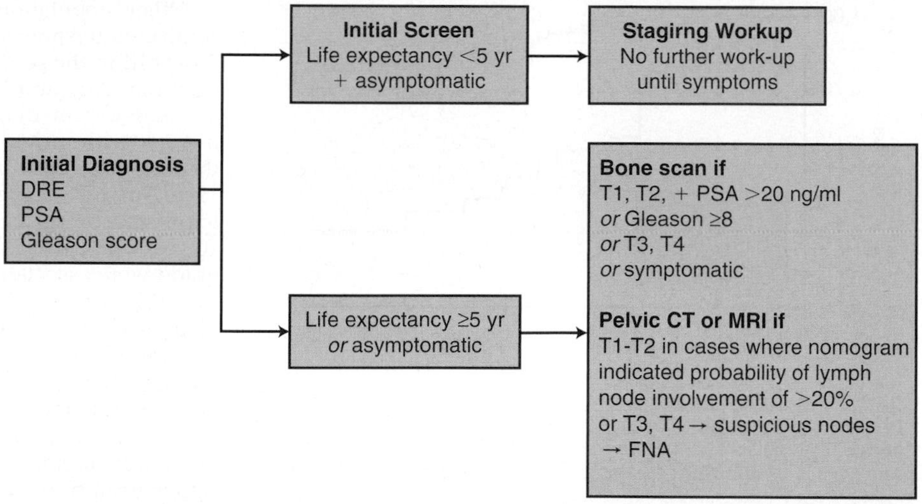

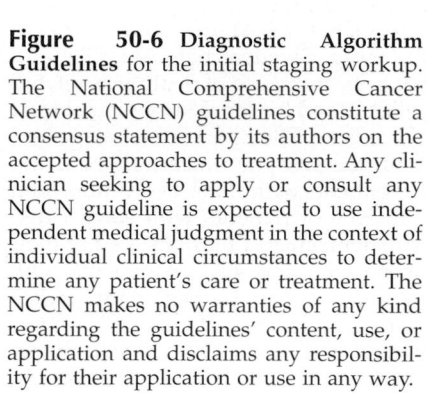

Figure 50-6 Diagnostic Algorithm Guidelines for the initial staging workup. The National Comprehensive Cancer Network (NCCN) guidelines constitute a consensus statement by its authors on the accepted approaches to treatment. Any clinician seeking to apply or consult any NCCN guideline is expected to use independent medical judgment in the context of individual clinical circumstances to determine any patient's care or treatment. The NCCN makes no warranties of any kind regarding the guidelines' content, use, or application and disclaims any responsibility for their application or use in any way.

of primary radiation therapy or radical prostatectomy by its proponents, especially in select patients.[170,304,305] In the United States, an evaluation of the National Cancer Data Base indicated that the proportion of men managed without definitive cancer-directed therapy for a new diagnosis of prostate cancer had declined during the past several years.[306] Nonetheless, approximately one in five American men did not receive immediate prostate cancer–directed therapy in the period from 1974 to 1990, and approximately one third of those with nonmetastatic disease did undergo expectant management.[307]

The rationale for expectant management is based on considerations related to the natural history of the condition, the age and comorbidity of the incident population, the perceived need (or lack thereof) for therapeutic intervention, and health-related quality-of-life issues. Incidental (or latent) prostate cancer is often found on autopsy examination of the prostate gland[8-10] and, although particularly common in the elderly,[9,10] is observed in as many as one third of men in their fourth and fifth decades.[8]

Incidental tumors bear some resemblance to their clinically apparent counterpart but are generally smaller, histologically well differentiated, and confined to the prostate gland. For example, Brawn and associates[308] performed autopsy examinations on 209 consecutive men without a diagnosis of prostate cancer. Among the 79 (38%) prostate glands that contained cancer, the median tumor volume was 0.24 cm^3 (range, .009 to 3.0 cm^3). All tumors were well (Gleason score of 2 to 4) or moderately (Gleason score of 5 to 7) differentiated, capsular penetration was present in only 13 cases (16%), and none of the tumors had spread to the pelvic or para-aortic lymph nodes. In contrast, Dugan and colleagues[309] examined 337 prostatectomy and pelvic lymph node dissection (PLND) specimens surgically removed for the treatment of clinically evident disease. In these patients, the median tumor volume was 6.7 cm^3 (range, 0.04 to 56.9 cm^3), and 40% had extraprostatic extension or nodal involvement, or both. Even among patients with PSA-detected, nonpalpable disease,[310] the tumor volume, Gleason score, and degree of EPE are not typical of incidental cancers found at autopsy.

Although the characteristics, and presumably the prognosis, of clinically apparent tumors differ from those seen at autopsy, several studies demonstrate that many localized prostate cancers have an indolent course that may support the use of expectant management for this condition. In particular, the prognosis appears quite favorable for the patient with a small-volume, low-grade tumor identified incidental to transurethral resection (stage T1a) for BPH.[311,312] However, the distinction between stage T1a and stage T1b is important, because the risk of disease progression and disease-specific mortality is highly dependent on tumor volume and grade.[312-314] Although various methods to further evaluate prognosis have been investigated (e.g., repeat resection, ultrasonography, postresection PSA level) in stage T1a disease, there is a low likelihood for disease progression in this condition,[311-314] and lifelong and attentive surveillance appears warranted for most patients.

For patients with more extensive nonmetastatic disease, several types of medical reports are cited in support of expectant management. These investigations include retrospective analyses of largely uncontrolled single-institution patient outcome experiences,[312,315-317] a meta-analysis of case records from select nonrandomized studies,[170] a few prospective or population-based studies,[167,304,314,318,319] and the results of two randomized clinical trials.[320,321]

The largest study of expectant management was performed by Chodak and coworkers,[170] who collected patient and disease characteristics from several nonrandomized institutional series and from a population-based study to evaluate the outcome of expectant management in patients with localized prostate cancer. These investigators identified 10 studies published during the preceding decade and obtained original data on 828 patients from six of these studies. In this meta-analysis, multivariate regression analysis identified tumor grade as the most significant factor associated with disease-specific survival. As shown in Figure 50-7, the 10-year disease-specific survival rate for a grade 1 or 2 tumor was significantly higher (87%) than for a grade 3 tumor (34%). For the U.S. and Swedish cohorts, the age-adjusted overall survival rate closely matched the expected survival of the general population from the same country. Nonetheless, patients with a grade 3 tumor had a substantially reduced rate of metastasis-free survival at 10 years (26%) than those with grade 1 (81%) or 2 (58%) tumors (Fig. 50-8). Based on these observations, the authors concluded that localized prostate cancer is a steadily progressive disorder but that observation with delayed hormonal therapy is a reasonable approach for some men with grade 1 or 2 disease.

Although single-institution series may include patients selected for expectant management on the basis of advanced

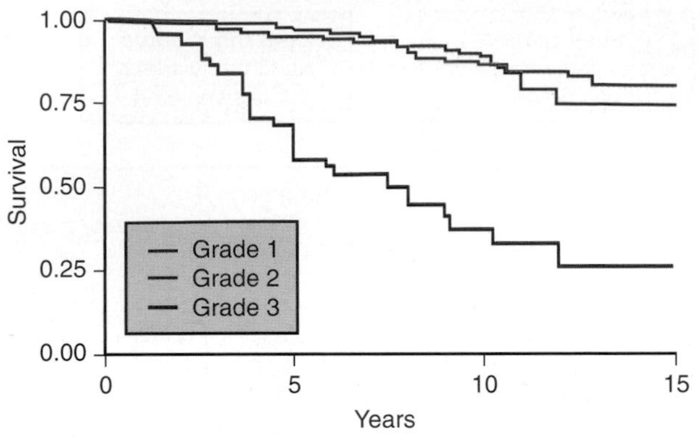

Figure 50-7 Disease-specific survival among untreated patients with localized prostate cancer according to tumor grade. (From Chodak GW, Thisted RA, Gerber GS, et al: Results of conservative management of clinically localized prostate cancer. N Engl J Med 330:242, 1994.)

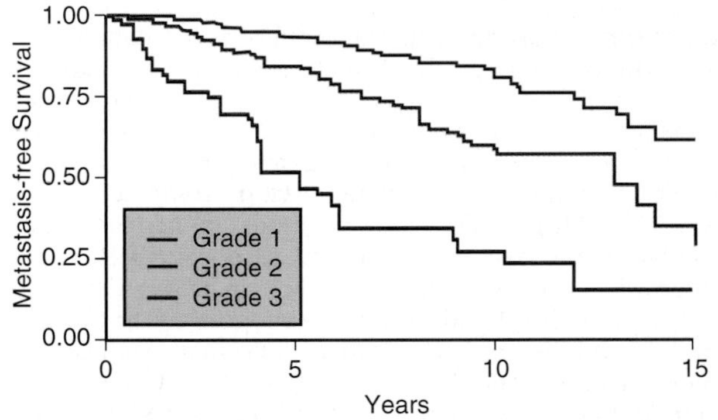

Figure 50-8 Metastasis-free survival times for untreated patients with localized prostate cancer according to tumor grade. (From Chodak GW, Thisted RA, Gerber GS, et al: Results of conservative management of clinically localized prostate cancer. N Engl J Med 330:242, 1994.)

age or life-limiting comorbidity, population-based studies are conducted to minimize this potential source of bias. In this regard, Johansson and colleagues[304] described a group of 300 consecutive patients diagnosed with stages T1-2 prostate cancer at the Örebro Medical Centre, a hospital serving a geographically well-defined population. Among these patients, 223 patients with predominantly low-grade tumors were treated with exogenous estrogen or orchiectomy if symptomatic tumor progression occurred. By the time of the last evaluation, extraprostatic tumor extension or metastatic disease had developed in 36% and 17%, respectively. Although the 15-year progression-free (45%) and overall survival (21%) rates were rather low, the high 15-year disease-specific survival (79%) appeared consistent with the results of several single-institution investigations.[317,319] In the latest update of this study, the prostate cancer mortality rate increased from 15 per 1000 person-years during the first 15 years to 44 per 1000 person-years beyond 15 years of follow-up.[304] Although most cancers had an indolent course during the first 10 to 15 years after diagnosis, follow-up from 15 to 20 years revealed a substantial decrease in progression-free survival (45% to 36%), survival without metastases (77% to 51%), and prostate cancer-specific survival (79% to 54%). These findings would tend to support early curative therapy for patients with an estimated life expectancy of more than 15 years.

Other population-based studies from Sweden have not confirmed the high 10 to 15 year disease-specific survival rate observed in the series from the Örebro Medical Centre.[304] For example, Aus and colleagues[322] identified all patients with an antemortem diagnosis of nonmetastatic prostate cancer treated with primary hormonal (63%) or deferred (36%) therapy who died in Goteborg, Sweden, between 1988 and 1990. Among 301 such patients, the cause of death was related to prostate cancer in 149 (50%), and for those surviving at least 10 years, 63% died of this disease. The initial tumor stage and grade were associated with the prostate cancer-related death rate. Whereas only 10% of patients with stage T1a tumors died of prostate cancer, 47% to 53% of patients with stage T1b-3 tumors and 70% of patients with stage T4 lesions died of their malignant disease. Between 43% and 48% of patients with grade 1 and grade 2 tumors and 60% of patients with grade 3 lesions died of prostate cancer. Of these patients, 58% underwent transurethral prostatic resection, 22% underwent an upper urinary tract procedure (e.g., pyelostomy) because of urinary obstruction, and 35% received palliative irradiation.[323] Norlén[324] had similar results in an evaluation of 44,300 patients with prostate cancer, representing 99% of all newly diagnosed cases reported to the Swedish Cancer Registry between 1960 and 1978. Survival rates were adjusted for mortality in the general population and were expressed as relative survival, which estimates the likelihood of dying of prostate cancer. Among patients with prostate cancer, the relative survival was 51%, 34%, and 17% after 5, 10, and 20 years of observation, respectively, representing an excess death rate of approximately 8% per year.

In the United States, Albertsen and associates[167] conducted a population-based, retrospective cohort analysis of men managed with immediate or delayed hormonal therapy for clinically localized prostate cancer. This study indicated that tumor grade and medical comorbidity were significant predictors of survival and suggested that life expectancy was not reduced in those with a low-grade (Gleason score of 2 to 4) tumor. However, for men with a Gleason score of 5, 6, 7 or 8 to 10, the ratios of other causes of death to prostate cancer death were 7 to 1, 2.5 to 1, 1 to 1, and 0.5 to 1, respectively. The risk of death from prostate cancer decreased with increasing age at diagnosis. The prostate cancer death rate did not increase after 15 years follow-up, as it did in the Swedish study reported by Johansson and colleagues.[304] This difference was attributed to differences in histologic tumor classification and accuracy in reporting cause of death. In the available no-treatment studies with long-term follow-up, PSA levels were not available, and tumors were more advanced at diagnosis than the current situation. The effect of lead time bias in PSA-screened patients will no doubt prove to be significant.

Another population-based study used the SEER program of the National Cancer Institute to determine whether therapeutic intervention affects the outcome of localized or regional prostate cancer.[171] Multivariate analysis of 104,577 patients demonstrated that radiation therapy and surgery resulted in improved disease-specific and overall survival compared with no treatment (Table 50-6). For example, patients treated with radiation therapy have a 34% reduction in the risk of prostate cancer-related death, a relative risk of 0.66, compared with patients in whom no treatment is given at diagnosis.

A randomized study from Sweden comparing radical prostatectomy to watchful waiting was reported.[321] Although the effect of treatment in relative terms was substantial, a decrease in disease-specific mortality of approximately 50% with 8.2 years median follow-up, in absolute terms, the impact was more modest. The disease-specific mortality decreased from 14.4% with watchful waiting to 8.6% with prostatec-

Table 50-6 Disease-Specific and Overall Survival for Localized or Regional Prostate Cancer

Treatment	No. of Patients	Disease-Specific Mortality (RR)*	Overall Mortality (RR)*	Median Survival (mo)
None	13,162	1.00	1.00	50
Radiation therapy	13,081	0.66	0.57	103
Surgery	63,908	0.62	0.75	73
Surgery and irradiation	16,949	0.81	0.67	93

*Relative risk (RR) is expressed relative to no treatment (RR = 1).
Adapted from Krongrad A, Lai H, Lamm SH, et al: Mortality in prostate cancer. J Urol 156:1084, 1996.

tomy.[321] Although after 5 years of follow-up, the overall mortality was similar (7.8% for prostatectomy patients versus 9.8% for the watchful waiting group), at 10 years' follow-up, there was a significant difference (P = .04) in favor of the treated patients (27% versus 32%), but the absolute difference remained only 5%. Because the men in this study were largely recruited before widespread PSA screening, the lead time introduced with earlier detection may erode the benefit of definitive treatment in contemporary populations, especially those with less than 10 to 15 years of life expectancy.

The U.S. based Prostate Cancer Intervention Versus Observation Trial (PIVOT), which was also designed to evaluate the relative efficacy of radical prostatectomy versus watchful waiting, continues to follow patients. Results will not be available until the next decade.[325,326]

In view of the observations previously discussed, a consensus regarding the relative merits of expectant management, prostatectomy, and radiation therapy is lacking. An exhaustive review of the literature performed by the Prostate Cancer Clinical Guidelines Panel,[327] convened by the American Urological Association and published in 1995, concluded that the available data on stage T2 prostate cancer were not adequate for a valid outcomes comparison of expectant management, radiation therapy, and radical prostatectomy. The Panel concluded that patients with newly diagnosed, clinically localized prostate cancer should be informed of all commonly accepted treatment options. The Panel identified a pressing need for randomized, prospective, controlled studies, particularly those investigating expectant management compared with early interventional therapies. Ten years later, these issues remain controversial and unresolved by the intervening randomized and retrospective studies that do not totally reflect the current situation.

Radiation Therapy

General Principles

Ionizing radiation has been used as curative therapy for clinically localized prostate cancer for nearly a century. Shortly after the discovery of radium, clinicians applied brachytherapy techniques to the management of this disease. Through the pioneering work of del Regato and Bagshaw, the modern era of megavoltage external beam radiation therapy (EBRT) emerged in the late 1960s, and soon thereafter EBRT was accepted as a standard therapeutic approach in men with clinically localized disease. Similarly, after the seminal work of Carlson[328] and Whitmore,[329] brachytherapy methods improved, and advances in imaging modalities, treatment planning software, and delivery methods allowed the application of brachytherapy to this condition. At present, the radiation oncologist has several radiotherapeutic options available to apply to the management of men with prostate cancer.

In clinically localized prostate cancer, several years of posttherapy observation are required to measure the impact of a particular treatment on the natural history of the disease. This presents a significant obstacle to timely assessment of newer therapeutic approaches. Although serum PSA held the hope of being an early surrogate end point to evaluate therapeutic efficacy, recent analyses seem to indicate that the most common PSA failure interval is 3 to 5 years after treatment and that approximately 15% of patients fail even after that. Although work is underway to try to determine prognostic PSA levels that indicate impending relapse at an earlier interval after treatment, it appears that this will remain a late relapsing disease in which early outcome assessment may be unreliable.[172,245,246,249] Due attention must be paid to the length of follow-up in reporting and reviewing outcome analyses.

Organ-Confined Disease

The literature contains few prospective, comparative clinical trials relevant to the treatment of patients with clinical stage T1-2 prostate cancer. Most reports were derived from single-institution observational case series in which a predetermined therapeutic approach and follow-up schedule were not established, and retrospective medical record review was used to assess efficacy and toxicity. Because the interpretation of observational case series presents certain problems,[330] statements about the utility of any treatment method, particularly compared with an alternative strategy, should be viewed with caution. In this context, the ensuing discussion emphasizes the experience from selected centers of urologic excellence and the Patterns of Care studies, as these sources present a relatively broad perspective on the results achieved across the spectrum of radiotherapeutic practice.

External Beam Radiation Therapy

Conventional EBRT refers to a treatment planning method wherein the prostate and other target tissues are identified by the anatomy of surrounding structures (e.g., bony landmarks and contrast-enhanced viscera). Although this approach appears crude compared with current technologic advances, the conventional method accounts for much of what is known about the long-term results of EBRT. Development of sophisticated imaging modalities, particularly CT, coupled with irradiation treatment planning computers, allowed for precise localization of the prostate gland and other target tissues with respect to the treatment beam. Accurate three-dimensional (3D) target volume definition was made possible, and individualized radiation therapy field definitions were devised to conform (i.e., conformal radiation therapy) to the shape of the target volumes. Without 3D dose calculation, this approach may be considered 2.5-dimensional conformal radiation therapy, whereas calculation of 3D dose distributions to further conform the high-dose target volume and the associated dose-volume histogram application to objectively evaluate beam coverage of the target and critical organs is designated *3D conformal radiation therapy* (3D-CRT).

Intensity-modulated radiation therapy (IMRT) is a technique that is similar to its predecessor, 3D-CRT, in that it uses multiple beam angles and CT-based computer planning to conform the dose to the prostate as closely as possible, thereby sparing the nearby normal structures. However, IMRT also takes this concept one step further. During each of the beam angles, usually 5 to 10, a part of the radiation field is blocked at a specified time to optimize treatment of the prostate but limit the dose to the critical structures (in this case, the bladder and rectum). This blocking is accomplished through small tungsten devices (leaves) contained within the head of the treatment machine which in total make up a multileaf collimator. Each treatment field can also be thought of as being divided into many small beamlets of radiation that can vary in intensity by dynamically blocking the opening delivering the radiation, allowing only a specified amount to reach the target. During each of the treatment fields, the collimator leaves move as directed by the individually designed computer treatment plan, and the desired amount of radiation is delivered in less than 1 minute per beam angle. Because multiple beams are consecutively cross-firing and converging at the treatment target, the dose is maximal at target and much reduced in the surrounding areas.

Simultaneous with advances in technology have been changes in outcome reporting and diagnostic imaging. Outcome reporting mainly uses PSA posttreatment to determine relapse but also uses PSA as a pretreatment factor to classify the disease burden and to categorize patients into prognostic risk groups. Because diagnostic imaging has improved markedly over the past several years, stage migration has also occurred. There is evidence that the year that treatment was delivered is an independent predictor of outcome in addition to all the other well-known prognostic factors, such as tumor stage, grade, dose, and technique.[331] Taken together, these circumstances have rendered pre-PSA era, conventional radiation therapy results obsolete. Because these are the studies with the longest follow-up, they can be used to gain perspective, although improved outcome is expected with more contemporary 3D-CRT and IMRT treatment techniques.

Results with Conventional External Beam Radiation Therapy. Representative long-term overall and disease-free survival estimates after conventional EBRT for clinically localized prostate cancer are summarized in Table 50-7.[191,192,332-336] Perhaps because patients were comparable with respect to age and tumor grade, similar overall survival probabilities of approximately 80%, 60%, and 35% at 5, 10, and 15 years, respectively, were reported. In most series, overall survival was associated with tumor grade and stage, and the experience of Zagars and associates[191] was particularly noteworthy in this regard. The most favorable subgroup of patients with T1-2 disease had low-grade disease and exhibited 15-year overall survival similar to that of an age-matched population without prostate cancer, whereas patients with a poorly differentiated tumor had a 20% likelihood for survival at 10 years. Most patients included in these series underwent clinical staging, and such patients fared worse than their counterparts who underwent staging lymphadenectomy and had histologically uninvolved regional nodes.[337] Nonetheless, the similarity of survival results attained at academic centers and the spectrum of practice types evaluated in the Patterns of Care study[334] suggested that a uniform expectation of survival outcome was achieved in this disease setting. As with overall survival, clinically determined (exclusive of PSA) disease-free survival probabilities for EBRT showed some similarities between series, and the disease-free survival in surgically staged, node-negative patients was higher than that of patients with clinical-radiologic node-negative or unknown nodal status.[337]

Because significant comorbid illness may reduce life expectancy, cause-specific survival may be a more appropriate end point to assess the efficacy of a particular treatment strategy. Cause-specific survival probabilities after conventional radiation therapy are summarized in Table 50-8.[192,332,333,335,336,338] In general, cause-specific survival is significantly higher than overall survival, which emphasizes the importance of comorbidity in assessment of therapeutic outcome. The importance of tumor grade as a predictor of cause-specific survival was particularly well demonstrated by

Table 50-7 Clinical Disease-Free and Overall Survival Rates after Conventional EBRT for Organ-Confined Disease

Study	Stage	No. of Patients	Disease-Free Survival (%) 5 y	10 y	15 y	Overall Survival (%) 5 y	10 y	15 y
Bagshaw et al[332]	T0*	96	≈ 85	≈ 75	≈ 75	~92	~72	≈ 43
	T1*	335	≈ 73	≈ 60	≈ 47	~81	~60	≈ 41
	T2*	242	≈ 62	≈ 39	≈ 26	~81	~53	≈ 29
Hanks et al[333]	T1-2†	104	85	67	—	87	63	—
Hanks et al[334]	T1	60	76	53	39	84	54	41
	T2	312	56	27	15	74	43	22
Hanks et al[434]	T1	116	74	52	—	85	63	—
	T2	415	53	34	—	75	46	—
Kuban et al[192]	T1	104	82	66	—	—	—	—
	T2a	72	79	57	—	—	—	—
	T2b-c	209	73	48	—	—	—	—
Lee and Sause[335]	T1-2†	20	89	70	64	85	60	40
Perez et al[336]	T1	41	≈ 78	—	—	79	67	—
	T2	185	≈ 67-75	≈ 46-53	—	80-82	63-70	—
Zagars et al[191]	T1	104	92	72	—	83	79	—
	T2	168	82	59	59	84	57	33

*Stanford staging system.
†Histologic pelvic node negative.
EBRT, external beam radiation therapy.

Table 50-8 **Cause-Specific Survival after Conventional EBRT for Organ-Confined Disease**

Study	Stage	No. of Patients	5 Years (%)	10 Years (%)	15 Years (%)
Bagshaw et al[332]	T0*	96	≈ 97	≈ 82	≈ 82
	T1*	335	≈ 88	≈ 77	≈ 65
	T2*	242	≈ 85	≈ 64	≈ 46
Hanks et al[333]	T1-2†	104	95	86	—
Lee and Sause[335]	T1-2†	20	100	82	75
Lu-Yao and Yao[338]	T1-2	16,869	—	74	—
Kuban et al[192]	T1	89	95	83	—
	T2a	60	97	93	—
	T2b-c	240	96	78	—
Perez et al[336]	T1	41	82	100	—
	T2	185	89-92	75-83	—

*Stanford staging system.
†Histologic pelvic node negative.
EBRT, external beam radiation therapy.

Table 50-9 **Clinically Determined Local Tumor Control after Conventional EBRT for Organ-Confined Disease**

Study	Stage	No. of Patients	5 Years (%)	10 Years (%)	15 Years (%)
Bagshaw et al[332]	T0*	96	≈ 95	≈ 90	≈ 85
	T1*	335	≈ 87	≈ 78	≈ 67
	T2*	242	≈ 82	≈ 61	≈ 48
Hanks et al[333]	T1-2	104	93	87	—
Hanks et al[334]	T1	60	96	96	83
	T2	312	83	71	65
Hanks et al[334]	T1	116	92	85	—
	T2	415	80	71	—
Kuban et al[341]	T1	101	≈ 96	≈ 92	≈ 62
	T2	281	≈ 87	≈ 66-75	≈ 50
Zagars et al[191]	T1	104	99	79	—
	T2	168	89	68	68

*Stanford staging system.
EBRT, external beam radiation therapy.

Kuban and colleagues[192] and Zietman and coworkers[236] wherein patients with a poorly differentiated tumor were at greater risk of prostate cancer-related mortality.

Although survival is a crucial and unequivocal end point, patient mortality (and, through inference, therapeutic efficacy) is strongly affected by underlying host- (e.g., age, comorbidity) and tumor-related (e.g., tumor grade) factors that may influence selection of a particular management approach. Complete and permanent eradication of the primary tumor (i.e., local tumor control) may be a more direct measure of radiotherapeutic efficacy. However, local tumor control is not consistently defined in the literature, and definitive evidence regarding the ability of EBRT to attain complete tumor ablation is elusive. Although most reports defined local tumor control as the absence of a progressively enlarging prostatic abnormality or of signs or symptoms suggesting local tumor recurrence (e.g., hematuria, urinary obstruction), there is considerable disparity between clinical assessment and the results of postirradiation prostatic biopsy,[339,340] and few investigations were constructed to address this issue. The likelihood for clinically determined, long-term local tumor control after EBRT is shown in Table 50-9.[191,332-334,341] These reports demonstrated that local tumor control is inversely related to tumor stage, in that patients with clinical stage T1 disease have a 10% to 15% greater local tumor control probability throughout follow-up. Although not consistently observed, there was the suggestion that poorly differentiated tumors were more likely to recur locally.[191,334] Patients remained at risk for local tumor recurrence for at least 15 years after conventional EBRT, which should urge caution in interpretation of reports with short-term follow-up. Results such as these suggest there is considerable room for improvement, especially in those patients with bilateral or poorly differentiated tumors. Strategies to improve local tumor control, which were subsequently applied, include dose escalation with conformal EBRT or IMRT, interstitial brachytherapy with or without EBRT, and the addition of androgen deprivation therapy.

Relatively few radiation therapy series evaluated regional nodal tumor relapse, but fewer than 3% of patients had this identified as a site of disease relapse.[191,341] However, the reported probability of regional nodal relapse was likely an underestimate, as serial radiologic imaging was not routinely performed during postirradiation patient follow-up. The mortality associated with regional nodal relapse has not been defined.

Median life expectancy after appearance of metastatic disease is approximately 2 to 3 years.[191,332] The likelihood of developing metastatic relapse after conventional EBRT for clinically localized prostate cancer is summarized in Table 50-10.[191,333,335,341] These data indicate that 5-year determinations underestimate the 10-year probability of metastases by one half to two thirds, which attests to the need for long-term disease monitoring. Heightened awareness may be of particular importance in the presence of local tumor recurrence, as

Table 50-10 **Distant Metastases after Conventional EBRT for Organ-Confined Disease**

Study	Stage	No. of Patients	5 Years (%)	10 Years (%)	15 Years (%)
Hanks et al[333]	T1-2	104	10	21	—
Kuban et al[341]	T1	101	≈ 12	≈ 23	—
	T2	281	≈ 16	≈ 81	≈ 31-46
Lee and Sause[335]	T1-2	20	11	30	30
Zagars et al[191]	T1	104	7	8	—
	T2	168	9	27	27

EBRT, external beam radiation therapy.

patients with this condition are at particularly high risk for subsequent metastatic relapse.[342-345] Whether tumor-related factors (e.g., tumor grade) that predispose to local recurrence place patients at risk for harboring subclinical metastases at presentation, or whether persistent disease at the primary site results in secondary tumor dissemination, is uncertain. However, Wheeler and colleagues[138] postulated that locally persistent tumor undergoes time-dependent dedifferentiation with emergence of a more virulent malignant type. Yorke and coworkers[346] proposed that more than half of metastases originate in association with local recurrence, and Coen and coworkers[347] reported a late wave of distant metastasis after local failure, suggesting that improved control of the primary tumor may enhance long-term survival.

Biochemical Relapse. More contemporary studies incorporate pretherapy and posttreatment serum PSA levels into outcome analyses to better define prognostic groups and disease-free status. Serial PSA measurements and the end point of PSA relapse-free survival have become the new benchmark for assessing treatment efficacy. Kuban and colleagues compared the clinical disease-free probability to that determined by PSA level for 385 stage T1-2 patients treated by conventional EBRT and found that clinical assessment alone may overestimate disease-free status by 10% to 20% at 5 years and by 20% to 40% at 10 years.[192] Because of serum stored before the PSA era, these authors were also able to group patients into pretreatment PSA prognostic categories which showed significant differences in outcome based on PSA level.

To study long-term outcome after EBRT in the PSA era, six institutions combined data and used the ASTRO PSA failure definition, defined by the Consensus conference in 1996, as the analysis end point.[348] Tumor stage, Gleason score, pretreatment PSA level, and PSA nadir after therapy were all established as important factors in outcome. Five years later, a follow-up study with data from nine institutions was completed and ultimately included 4839 patients with stage T1-2 prostate cancer treated from 1986 to 1995, with median of 6.3 years of follow-up.[172] Because of the treatment era, a conventional technique was used in earlier years and conformal therapy more recently. Doses were those common for the era as well. Sixteen percent of patients were treated to 60 to 65 Gy, 54% to 66 to 70 Gy, 19% to 70 to 72 Gy, 10% to 73 to 78 Gy, and 1% to levels above 78 Gy. Outcome analysis confirmed the prognostic factors established by the first study (i.e., tumor stage, Gleason score, pretreatment PSA, and posttreatment PSA nadir[348]) and established dose and year of treatment as independent prognostic variables.[172] PSA-related disease-free results for patients treated to at least 70 Gy are shown in Table 50-11, and Figure 50-9 demonstrates the relationship between nadir and eventual biochemical failure. Because of the long-term follow-up available for these patients, up to 14 years, this analysis also showed that of those patients who were disease free according to their PSA levels at 5 years, an additional 17% would develop PSA relapse by 10 years, pointing out the late relapsing nature of this disease. Clinical failure and survival analysis (Table 50-12) showed results more encouraging than those with PSA relapse as the end point.[349] In studying the relationship of PSA relapse to clinical relapse, this multi-institutional effort reported that 49% to 78% of patients were clinically disease-free at 5 years and 46% to 58% at 10 years after PSA failure, depending on risk group.[172] This further confirms the fact that clinical failure occurs late and that the use of posttreatment PSA improves accuracy when assessing the presence of disease.

Table 50-11 **Five- and 8-Year Disease-Free Survival Assessed by Prostate-Specific Antigen Level According to Prognostic Factor Category Treated to ≥70 Gy**

		Initial PSA (ng/mL)			
Stage	Gleason Score	*0-3.99* 5 y/8 y	*4-9.99* 5 y/8 y	*10-19.99* 5 y/8 y	*≥20* 5 y/8 y
T1b-c					
	2-4	100/—	75/75	70/70	36/24
	5-6	89/—	83/75	70/70	40/29
	7	100/100	63/59	53/47	17/—
	8-10	—/—	33/—	47/—	40/—
T2					
	2-4	93/84	80/74	78/69	16/16
	5-6	73/73	70/67	60/51	42/30
	7	68/54	64/57	53/45	12/—
	8-10	71/—	59/54	28/21	—/—

PSA, prostate-specific antigen.
From Kuban DA, Thames HD, Levy LB, et al: Long-term multi-institutional analysis of stage T1–T2 prostate cancer treated with radiotherapy in the PSA era. Int J Radiat Oncol Biol Phys 57(4):915-928, 2003.

Dose Escalation with Three-Dimensional Conformal Radiation Therapy, Intensity-Modulated Radiation Therapy, and Hypofractionation. With PSA outcome reports showing more room for improvement in treatment efficacy than was previously believed, effort was directed toward more conformal treatment techniques, 3D-CRT and IMRT to increase the prostate dose while avoiding adjacent nontarget tissues.

Single-institution studies have been reported for doses of 70 to 86 Gy according to pretreatment PSA category and risk group (Table 50-13).[222,223,350-353] Improvement in PSA-DFS has been demonstrated, and Hanks and colleagues showed that with long- term follow-up (8 to 12 years), there is a significant impact on the distant metastatic rate.[350] In patients with a pretreatment PSA level of 10 to 20 ng/mL, the 8-year PSA-DFS was 19% with a dose of less than 71.5 Gy, 31% with a dose of 71.5 to 75.5 Gy , and 84% with more than 75.5 Gy. Zelefsky

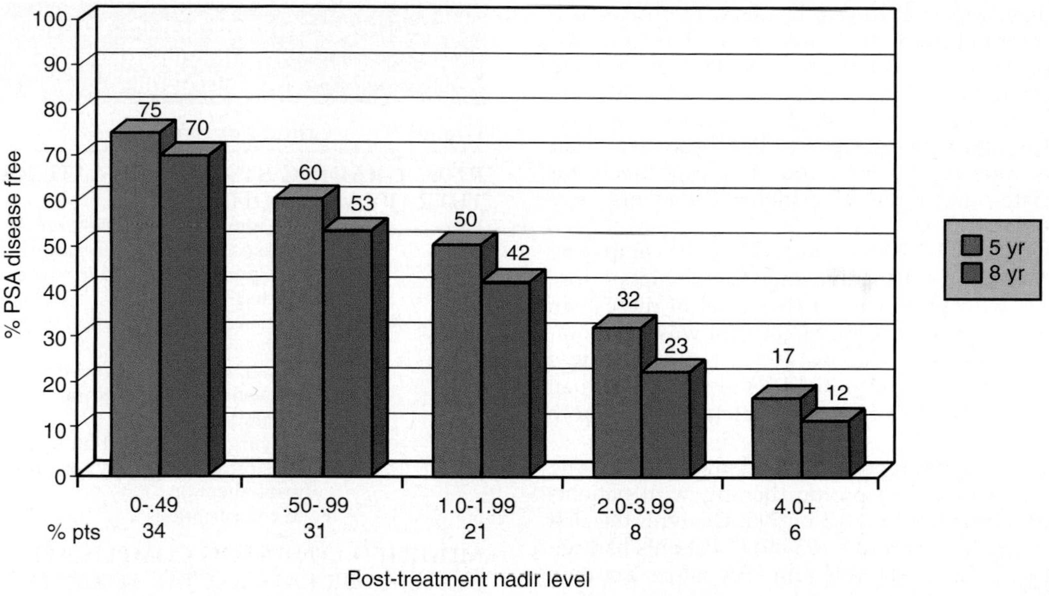

Figure 50-9 The likelihood for long-term local tumor control after external beam radiation therapy is shown as a percentage of all patients determined to be disease free by their prostate-specific antigen nadir level. The percentage of patients achieving each nadir level is given on the x-axis.

Table 50-12 Clinical Outcome for Patients with T1-2 Prostate Cancer

Risk Category	No. of Patients	OS (%) 5 Y	OS (%) 8 Y	LRF (%) 5 Y	LRF (%) 8 Y	MRF (%) 5 Y	MRF (%) 8 Y	CDF (%) 5 Y	CDF (%) 8 Y	CSS (%) 5 Y	CSS (%) 8 Y
All	4839	87	72	93	89	95	92	89	83	98	93
Low	1237	92	81	97	93	99	99	97	92	100	99
Intermediate	2191	86	72	94	90	96	94	91	84	99	95
High	1109	82	64	87	84	88	84	77	71	97	87

CDF, clinical disease-free survival; CSS, cause-specific survival; LRF, local recurrence-free survival; MRF, metastatic relapse-free survival; OS, overall survival; Y, years.

From Pisansky TM, Thames HD, Levy LB, et al: Clinical outcomes and prognostic factors in 4839 patients treated with external radiotherapy for stage T1-T2 prostate cancer [abstract 63]. Proceedings of the 46th annual ASTRO meeting. Int J Radiat Oncol Biol Phys 60:S167, 2004.

Table 50-13 Biochemical Relapse Rates with High Dose Conformal Radiation

Study	Dose (Gy)	No. of Patients	PSA (ng/mL)	PSA-DFS (%) 5 Y	PSA-DFS (%) 8 Y	PSA-DFS (%) 10 Y
Pollack et al[351]	72-75.9	235	<10 (Gl 2-6)	88	—	—
	72-75.9	45	<10 (Gl 7-10)	50	—	—
	72-75.9	97	<10-20	65	—	—
	≥76	129	10-20	79	—	—
	≥76	70	10-20	34	—	—
Zelefsky et al[352]	75.5	459*	Low risk	—	—	83
	75.5	—	Intermed risk	—	—	50
	75.5	—	High risk	—	—	42
Hanks et al[350]	>72	229	<10	—	69	—
	>75.5	—	10-20	—	84	—
	>75.5	—	>20	—	11	—

*All patients treated to 75.5 Gy. Total number of evaluable patients at all dose levels.

Gl, Gleason score; Gy, Gray; Intermed, intermediate; PSA, prostate-specific antigen; PSA-DFS, disease-free survival assessed by prostate-specific antigen level; Y, years.

and associates have reported 10-year results with dose escalation and 3D conformal irradiation.[352] For favorable-, intermediate-, and unfavorable-risk patients, the PSA-determined relapse-free rates for less than 70.2 Gy versus 75.6 Gy were 57% versus 83%, 42% versus 50%, and 24% versus 42%, respectively. Results from the same group with IMRT showed 3-year PSA relapse-free rates of 92%, 86%, and 81%, respectively, for low-, intermediate-, and high-risk patients.[353] Patients were treated to a dose of 81.0 or 86.4 Gy.

A randomized study by Pollack and colleagues comparing 70 Gy versus 78 Gy showed an advantage for the higher dose level for patients with pretreatment PSA level of more than 10 ng/mL. PSA-DFS at 6 years after treatment was 43% compared with 62%, a difference of almost 20%. No difference was demonstrated for patients with initial PSA levels of less than 10 ng/mL, with PSA-DFS of approximately 80% in both arms.[223]

Zietman and colleagues reported a randomized trial using a combination of photon and proton therapy, with patients randomized to treatment with 70.2 or 79.2 Gy, with the first 50.4 Gy given with photons (PROG 95-09).[354] Patients had relatively early stage (T1b-2b) disease with PSA values less than 15 ng/mL. This was also a positive study, with 5-year PSA-DFS rates of 65% and 60% for the low- and intermediate-risk, low-dose patients and PSA-DFS rates of 83% and 79% for their high-dose counterparts.

One way to increase dose and decrease treatment time is through hypofractionated radiation. Kupelian and coworkers have compared 70 Gy in 28 fractions (250 cGy/day) with IMRT to 78 Gy in 39 fractions (200 cGy/day) with 3D-CRT.[355] Although the median follow-up is short (21 months for the 70 Gy patients and 32 months for the 78 Gy patients), PSA disease-free outcome is similar (94% and 88%), and the late rectal complication rate is not greater for patients treated to the higher dose per day. Other similar studies are in progress in an attempt to decrease the number of fractions and shorten treatment time.

Complications. Complications that occur during or after EBRT can be grouped into four major categories: intestinal, urinary, sexual, and other. Intestinal toxicity occurring during radiation therapy manifests as an acute enteritis due to the effect of irradiation on the small and large intestine. The severity of this side effect is proportional to the volume of bowel included in the treatment fields but is usually well controlled with antidiarrheal medications and local steroidal type preparations for proctitis. After treatment, any such symptoms typically return to the baseline state within 2 to 4 weeks. However, long-term injury may occur in a small proportion of patients, and this may manifest as persistent diarrhea, tenesmus, rectal or anal strictures, or hematochezia; bowel ulceration, obstruction, or perforation is less common. The RTOG system for late (>90 days after completion of radiation therapy) morbidity is shown in Table 50-14 along with a more detailed Late Effects Normal Tissue (LENT) Task Force–RTOG modification used in some studies.

Most patients experience some degree of urinary toxicity during EBRT. The symptoms of cystitis/urethritis are characterized by urinary frequency, urgency, hesitancy, decreased force of stream, and dysuria. These symptoms are usually mild to moderate and resolve 2 to 4 weeks after treatment is completed. Significant long-term urinary sequelae are uncommon, but they may take the form of cystitis, hematuria, urethral stricture, or bladder contracture.

Although long-term rectal complications were typically acceptable for lower doses of radiation (<5% grade 2 for the dose range of 64 to 70 Gy), the use of higher EBRT doses with little alteration in radiation technique led to an alarming level of long-term complications.[222,356] Storey and colleagues, using data from the M. D. Anderson randomized dose response study with 3D-CRT, evaluated the amount of rectum which could be treated to a dose of 70 Gy while still keeping the rectal and bladder complication rates at a reasonable level.[357] This analysis showed that grade 2/3 rectal complications, which were mainly grade 2 (see Table 50-14), increased with 78 Gy compared with 70 Gy. According to the latest update, 26% of patients treated to 78 Gy developed complications compared with 12% treated to 70 Gy.[357] However, it was also shown that this complication rate could be minimized by decreasing the amount of rectum treated to the 70 Gy dose level. If less than 25% of the rectal volume was treated to more than 70 Gy, grade 2 or 3 complications occurred in 16% of patients compared with 46% of patients if more than 25% of the rectal volume was treated to this dose level. Additional work on this topic was done by Huang and associates at the same institution, defining additional parameters which serve to decrease the complication rate. It was found that the relative amount of rectum (as a percentage of the entire rectum) treated to lower dose levels such as 40 and 60 Gy and higher doses such as 75.6 and 80 Gy, as well as the absolute amount of treated rectum in cubic centimeters, were equally significant in predicting rectal complications.[358] Further study, using this same patient group, has shown that the correlation between rectal dose-volume histogram (DVH) and toxicity is a continuous function.[359] In patients treated with 3D-CRT, grade 3 rectal complications, still mainly rectal bleeding but more

Table 50-14 Grading System According to the Radiation Therapy Oncology Group Criteria

Grade	Criteria or Symptoms
RTOG GRADING SYSTEM FOR LATE RADIATION THERAPY MORBIDITY	
1	Minor symptoms requiring no treatment
2	Symptoms responding to simple outpatient management, lifestyle (performance status) not affected
3	Distressing symptoms altering patient's lifestyle (performance status)
	Hospitalization for diagnosis or minor surgical intervention (e.g., urethral dilatation) may be required
4	Major surgical intervention (e.g., laparotomy, colostomy, cystectomy) or prolonged hospitalization
5	Fatal complication
MODIFIED LENT-RTOG COMPLICATION GRADING SYSTEM FOR LATE RECTAL TOXICITY[358]	
1	Excess bowel movements twice baseline
	Slight rectal discharge or blood
2	>2 antidiarrheals/wk; ≤2 coagulations; occasional steroids or dilatation; intermittent pad use; regular non-narcotics or occasional narcotics
3	>2 antidiarrheals/d; >2 coagulations; ≥1 transfusion; prolonged daily steroid enemas; hyperbaric oxygen; regular dilation; daily pads; regular narcotics
4	Dysfunction requiring surgery; perforation; life-threatening bleeding
5	Fatal toxicity

LENT, Late Effects Normal Tissue Task Force; RTOG, Radiation Therapy Oncology Group.

severe, occur much less frequently (1% to 7% of treated patients).[356-360] Fortunately, the risk of grade 4 complications, those requiring a major surgical procedure, and grade 5 incidents, those causing the death of the patient, is practically zero and usually related to coexistent nonmalignant disease.[222,360]

IMRT consistently produces a very conformal dose distribution, decreasing the dose to surrounding organs. This has translated into the clinical benefit of decreased toxicity rates despite the delivery of significantly higher doses to the tumor. At the 81-Gy dose level with IMRT, grade 2 rectal toxicity rates of 3% are achievable, with grade 3 rates of just 1%.[353]

The correlation between DVH and bladder complication risk has not been as straightforward. With 3D-CRT, Pollack and colleagues did not see a difference in complication rates when increasing dose from the 70 Gy to the 78 Gy level.[223] In the RTOG dose escalation study, Michalski and coworkers saw a correlation between late bladder complications and the percent of bladder receiving radiation doses more than the defined reference doses of 60 and 65 Gy.[361] In general, the greater the percentage of bladder receiving higher doses, the higher the complication rate. However, there was no cut-off above which a complication was more expected as has been seen in rectal DVH analyses. Even more unexpectedly, a higher mean dose to the bladder was a predictor for a lower relative risk of bladder toxicity. An explanation for this might be that bladder complications occur late, as they did in the Massachusetts General Hospital proton boost dose escalation study, and the full incidence may not yet have been realized in later studies.[362] Alternatively, the lack of consistent correlation may be due to the relative proportion of bladder irradiated, which can change substantially as the treatment course proceeds. As irritative symptoms develop, the frequency of urination increases, which decreases bladder filling and therefore total bladder size. This has a direct effect on the percentage of bladder within the treatment field, which may differ substantially from that predicted by the initial treatment plan that is done with a desirably full bladder. Urinary toxicity data from Zelefsky and associates show an 11% incidence of grade 2 complications 3 years after IMRT with 81 Gy. Grade 3 complications, consisting of urethral strictures that required dilatation, occurred in less than 1% of patients at those dose levels.[353] There was little difference in the urinary complication rates for 3D-CRT and IMRT. This is likely explained by the fact that much of the toxicity is related to the urethra, which cannot be avoided with either technique.

Assessment of sexual function after EBRT is complex and may be fraught with difficulty. Potency typically begins to diminish one to 2 years after radiation and actuarial analysis appears similar to the natural aging process. Some patients have compromised potency due to concurrent illnesses such as diabetes or arteriosclerosis or as a result of certain medications taken for comorbid conditions. According to single-institution reports and meta-analyses, it appears that 50% to 60% of potent patients remain so after EBRT.[363] Other complications, including leg or genital edema and osteonecrosis, are rare with contemporary techniques. With more conformal radiation, complications appear to be very localized.

Of concern are the recent reports on second malignancies associated with radiation for prostate cancer. Although there is a long latency period (5 to 15 years), this is becoming a more significant consideration due to the younger age at diagnosis, presentation at earlier stages, improved treatment efficacy, and longer average life expectancy. Using SEER data from 1973-1993, Brenner and colleagues compared the risk of second malignancy in 51,584 irradiated men to 70,539 who had prostatectomy. There was a small but significant excess risk of solid tumors in men who underwent prostate radiation: 1 in 290 (all years), 1 in 125 for 5-year survivors, and 1 in 70 for 10-year survivors.[364] The most significant contributors to this increased risk were carcinomas of the bladder, rectum, lung and sarcomas within the treatment field. Using SEER data from 1973 to 1994, Baxter and colleagues[365] found a hazard ratio of 1.7 for the development of rectal cancers at the irradiated site that did not occur in the remainder of the colon. This 70% increased risk may appear more alarming than it actually is, because it translates into 1.4 more rectal cancers per 1000 irradiated men, the same approximate order of magnitude as the risk of having a first-degree relative with colorectal cancer or adding 10 years to a patient's age. Nevertheless, as potential candidates for radiation change, this should be considered.

BRACHYTHERAPY

Brachytherapy has involved the use of a variety of procedures and radioisotopes to treat prostate cancer for almost a century.[366,367] Contemporary overviews of the techniques and results achieved with this approach have been presented by Merrick and coworkers.[368]

The long-term results of interstitial brachytherapy as the sole means of prostate cancer treatment originated with the experience of Whitmore,[369] who developed a technique that required open laparotomy, prostatic mobilization, and retropubic insertion of trocars into the prostate with deposition of ^{125}I sources. However, this technique may result in irregular source placement and dose inhomogeneity,[370] which may account for the relatively high local tumor recurrence rate seen with this approach.[371] A retrospective analysis of 110 patients from the original retropubic Yale series with modern, 3D CT-based dosimetric parameters provides insight into the retropubic experience.[372] Several dosimetric parameters were evaluated to determine cutoff points that statistically separated these factors by local recurrence-free survival. When separated by favorable and unfavorable dosimetry parameters, there was a twofold increase in 10-year relapse-free survival. More importantly, a comparison of Yale's "inadequate" implants identified a group of patients with local control rates similar to other series from this era that have reported poor outcomes.

The experience with the open, free-hand approach suggests that optimal results could be achieved if accurate source placement was accomplished, if dose homogeneity and total dose were adequate, and if patients were appropriately selected.[373] Contemporaneous transperineal prostate brachytherapy relies on modern imaging procedures (e.g., ultrasonography, CT) to direct radioactive seed placement in an accurate and reproducible manner.

Patient Selection. The selection of patients for prostate brachytherapy is generally reserved for patients with clinically confined prostate cancer.[374] In this regard, the combination of pretreatment serum PSA, Gleason score, and clinical tumor stage may be useful for the selection of patients with a high probability of organ-confined disease (see Table 50-5).[146] The selection of brachytherapy as monotherapy versus brachytherapy as a boost with supplemental EBRT has primarily been based on pathologic risk factors. The American Brachytherapy Society (ABS) recommended monotherapy for patients with clinical stages T1-2a, a PSA value of 10 ng/mL or less, and a Gleason score of 6 or less, with the addition of supplemental EBRT for all patients with higher-risk features.[374] However, an increasing body of data indicates that supplemental EBRT may be omitted depending on implant quality and seed placement philosophy.[375]

Large prostate size is widely believed to be a relative contraindication to brachytherapy due to technical concerns and the perception that such patients are at higher risk for urinary morbidity. However, contrary to popular perception, several studies have reported that appropriately selected patients with a large prostate can be implanted with acceptable morbidity and with good dosimetry.[376,377] Pubic arch interference may represent a technical problem regardless of prostate size depending on the implantation technique used. With the preloaded needle technique, extended lithotomy position may be difficult to achieve during the planning phase, which may limit needle placement at the time of the implant. With intraoperative planning, patient positioning can be achieved at the time of implantation under anesthesia without pubic arch interference.

There appears to be a direct relationship between preimplantation International Prostate Symptom Scores (IPSS) and postimplantation urinary obstruction in men undergoing prostate brachytherapy, whether downsized with hormones or not (Fig. 50-10).[378] The use of prophylactic alpha-blockers may diminish the impact of a high initial IPSS score.[379] Nonetheless, patients with urinary symptoms should be informed of their risk of urinary retention after implantation.[380,381]

Patients who have been treated for benign prostatic hypertrophy with a TURP pose potential problems when treated with permanent prostate brachytherapy. A fresh TURP defect may lead to excessive morbidity and inadequate seed geometry.[382] In general, a preimplantation ultrasound is required for these patients to assess the TURP defect relative to the planned seed locations. Patients with a previous TURP may experience prolonged postimplantation dysuria and are at risk for urethral necrosis.[383] Current protocols for permanent prostate brachytherapy that place seeds peripherally in the prostate gland may not cause the high rates of urethral necrosis originally reported.[384]

Past TURP, prostate size, and history of inflammatory bowel disease, all relative contraindications in the past, need to be considered on an individual basis. Patients must also have a patent anus to allow for ultrasonography.

Isotope Selection. Radiobiologic data suggested that isotope dose-rate may be an important factor for treating prostate cancer as different grades of disease with different cell doubling times may have specific sensitivities to ^{125}I or ^{103}Pd.[385] Nonetheless, clinical data have been reported for ^{125}I and ^{103}Pd, regardless of tumor grade that does not indicate any difference in biochemical control.[386,387] The ABS does not recommend the use of one isotope over the other.[388]

Role of External Beam Irradiation. The reasons for combining EBRT and permanent prostate brachytherapy are based on the statistical risk of having extracapsular disease associated with Gleason score, PSA level, and stage.[146] A prostate implant provides a dose only to the prostate, with perhaps a 3- to 5-mm margin, and it may include just the base of the seminal vesicles.[389] The field effect of external radiation to encompass the seminal vesicles and a larger prostatic margin can potentially encompass the areas at risk for extracapsular disease not treated by the implant.

The clinical criteria recommended by the ABS for monotherapy include stage T1c and T2a, Gleason scores of 2 to 6 and a PSA level less than 10 ng/mL. Patients with stage T2b disease or a Gleason score of 8 to 10 or PSA level higher than 20 ng/mL are recommended to undergo EBRT and implantation.[374] Nonetheless, a review of the literature is not helpful to delineate whether there is a biochemical control difference between these approaches, as many centers do not stratify their patients accordingly (Table 50-15).[390] Detailed pathology studies indicate that the radial extent of extraprostatic cancer extension is almost always 5 mm or less, which is within the confines of a monotherapy brachytherapy dose distribution.[391] If the prostate gland is implanted with a generous periprostatic margin, supplemental EBRT may not improve the outcome in low-, intermediate-, or even high-risk cases.[376,388,390,392-394]

Results with brachytherapy alone or plus EBRT have been evaluated in several series. In an update of the Long Island experience, Potters and associates have shown little difference in PSA relapse-free survival (PSA-RFS) with combined external radiation and brachytherapy versus monotherapy brachytherapy,[375] provided that implantation dosimetry is acceptable. Likewise, Blasko and colleagues, have identified excellent 10-year BCR in all-risk patients undergoing monotherapy brachytherapy. In their study, 230 patients were treated with ^{103}Pd monotherapy, and they reported a 9-year PSA-RFS of 83%.[395] Forty percent of these patients presented with a Gleason score higher than 7, and 24% of the patients

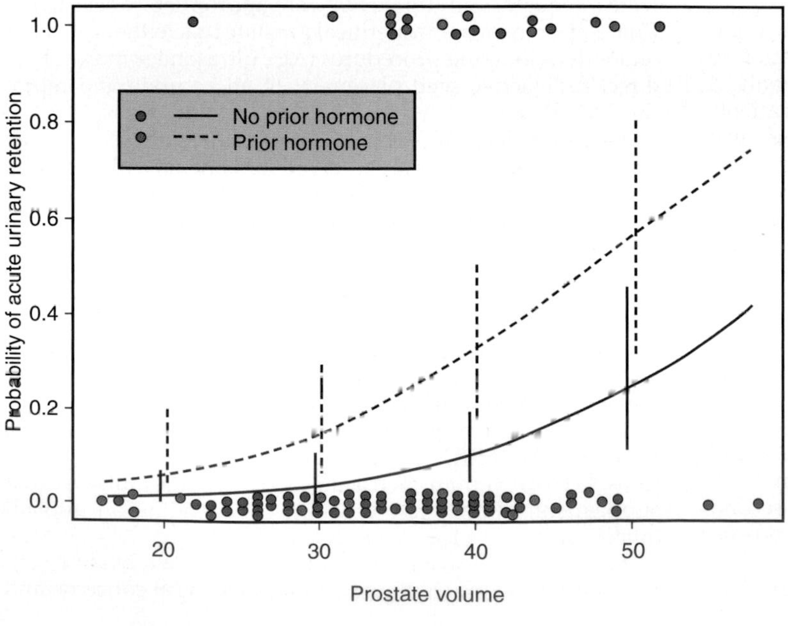

Figure 50-10 Risk of urinary retention according to prostate volume for patients treated with or without hormonal therapy. (From Crook J, McLean M, Catton C, et al: Factors influencing risk of acute urinary retention after TRUS-guided permanent prostate seed implantation. Int J Radiat Oncol Biol Phys 52:453, 2002.)

Table 50-15 **Review of the Literature on Permanent Prostate Brachytherapy Performed as Monotherapy or Combined with External Radiotherapy**

Study	No. of Patients	Median Follow-up (mo)	Biochemical Control	Definition	Comments
Ragde et al[418]		93		ASTRO†	High-risk patients treated with CMT; no analysis performed comparing groups
CMT	75		79%		
Monotherapy	144		66%		
Critz et al[393]					
CMT	689	48	88%	Nadir < 0.2 ng/mL	
Dattoli et al[392]					
CMT	73	36	79%	PSA < 1.0 ng/mL	All high-risk patients
Zelefsky et al[394]		48		ASTRO	CT-based ^{125}I implants; includes patients with clinical T3 disease
Monotherapy	248		71%		
Low risk*					
Monotherapy	112		88%		
Intermediate risk*					
Monotherapy	92		77%		
High risk*					
Monotherapy	22		38%		
Blasko et al[386]		58		ASTRO	
CMT	403		88%		
Monotherapy	231		79%		
Low risk*					
CMT	75		94%		
Monotherapy	279		79%		*P* = .06
Intermediate risk*					
CMT	104		85%		
Monotherapy	111		84%		*P* = .86
High risk*					
CMT	52		62%		
Monotherapy	11		54%		*P* = .53
Potters et al[390]		45		ASTRO (Kattan[413])	
CMT	314		81.5%		
Monotherapy	1162		82.1%		*P* = .54
Low risk* (matched)					
CMT	38		87.7%		
Monotherapy	40		93.4%		*P* = .54
Intermediate risk* (matched)					
CMT	174		84.8%		
Monotherapy	191		79.7%		*P* = .64
High risk* (matched)					
CMT	102		68.6%		
Monotherapy	84		60.5%		*P* = .49

ASTRO, American Society for Therapeutic Radiology and Oncology; CMT, combined-modality permanent prostate brachytherapy and external radiation therapy; PSA, prostate-specific antigen.

From Potters L, Fearn P, Kattan M: The role of external radiotherapy in patients treated with permanent prostate brachytherapy. Prostate Cancer Prostatic Dis 5:47-53, 2002.

†Three consecutive elevations with the failure date backdated to half-way between the PSA nadir and the first PSA elevation.

had a pretreatment PSA value of more than 20 ng/mL. These long-term results are as good as any series that routinely uses combined EBRT and permanent brachytherapy.[386,392,396]

Brachytherapy and Androgen-Ablative Therapy. With the development of real-time ultrasound permanent prostate brachytherapy in the mid 1980s, the role of combining neoadjuvant androgen deprivation (NAAD) and permanent prostate brachytherapy was to reduce the prostate size if it exceeded 60 g. This decreases the total isotope activity required and decreases pelvic arch interference.[397] Although this practice has continued, data suggest prostate size is less relevant to implantation quality than originally suspected.[377]

Although some prospective data indicate an improvement in disease-specific survival when combining NAAD and EBRT in patients with locally advanced and metastatic prostate cancer,[393] there are no prospective data to support the concept of NAAD as a radiosensitizer for early-stage prostate cancer.[398] Although Stock and coworkers initially reported on a potential role for combined permanent prostate brachytherapy and hormone therapy, they subsequently identified that any advantage of hormones is negated when postimplantation dosimetry is acceptable.[399] Likewise, in the 12-year Potters experience, the addition of hormonal therapy with prostate brachytherapy failed to significantly impact on biochemical freedom from relapse when including the impact of the postimplantation dosimetry.[400]

In patients with high-risk disease treated with EBRT and hormone therapy on the Radiation Therapy Oncology Group 9413 study, an improvement was observed when hormones and full pelvic external radiation were used with an EBRT prostate boost.[401] Future studies using permanent prostate brachytherapy may be worthwhile to incorporate a similar approach with adjuvant therapies. Nonetheless, a review of the literature does not appear to demonstrate any synergy based on current practices of combined use of hormones and permanent prostate brachytherapy.[390,402]

Postimplantation Dosimetry. Postimplantation analysis is an important process and needs to be performed on all patients undergoing permanent prostate brachytherapy (Table 50-16). Plain pelvic radiographs are insufficient because they do not accurately assess the spatial relationship of the prostate dose and surrounding tissues. CT-based dosimetry appears to be the best approach for postimplantation dosimetry.[403]

Postoperative CT-based dosimetric analysis provides detailed information regarding the coverage and uniformity of an implant, affords the ability to compare various intraoperative techniques, and provides a sound basis for future improvement. Although CT determination of prostate volume is widely accepted for EBRT planning, the use of CT for brachytherapy purposes is controversial. The accurate delineation of prostate contours on postimplantation CT may be difficult because of postoperative edema, degradation of the image due to implanted metallic seeds and a possible tendency to overestimate prostate volume from CT compared with transurethral ultrasound. However, a close correlation has been demonstrated for CT and ultrasound determined prostate volumes.[404]

Despite these recommendations, there are several problems with postimplantation CT studies that can limit permanent prostate brachytherapy dosimetry. The timing of the study is important as prostate edema may develop acutely after the traumatic insult associated with needle insertion.[405] Early CT scans after implantation may underestimate the prostate dose by up to 10% to 20%.[394] The reported edema half-life is approximately 10 to 14 days, and the best time to obtain this study may be 30 days after permanent prostate brachytherapy.[406] CT scans may by virtue of pixel size and the location of pelvic and periprostatic muscles overestimate the prostate size.[407] There is tremendous individual variability in drawing the prostate margin, which may over- or underestimate the delivered dose.[403] A difference of 1 to 2 mm can affect the prostate volume by as much as 30%. Each clinic needs to set up quality controls to ensure that prostate volumes are being appropriately drawn.

These problems aside, Stock and colleagues were able to define the D90 dose as the critical variable to assess permanent prostate brachytherapy. (The D90 represents the minimum dose to 90% of the prostate volume.)[408] Patients with a D90 dose greater than 140 Gy had a 4-year PSA-RFS of 92%, and those with a D90 dose less than 140 Gy had a 4-year PSA-RFS of 68% ($P = .04$). In the 12-year study, Potters and associates identified that the D90 (i.e., D90 dose reflecting the percent of the prescribed dose) was an independent predictor of biochemical freedom from relapse.[400]

Based on the unpredictable nature of prostatic edema during permanent prostate brachytherapy and its impact on dosimetry, dynamic real-time intraoperative treatment planning systems may ultimately improve the consistency of the D90 dose. Future studies with CT-ultrasound or CT-MRI spatial co-registration (fusion) may better define the prostate margin to determine the delivered dose. Studies on dose heterogeneity will better identify areas within the prostate based on dose that prove to be an independent predictor for toxicity or outcomes.

Standards have been suggested for postimplantation dosimetric analysis of implantation quality for the reporting of morbidity.[409] However, many diverse methods of defining the critical organs for morbidity, and of reporting the dose to these organs, are currently evident in the literature. This nonunifor-

Table 50-16 Recommendations for Postimplantation Dosimetric Analysis

All patients require post implant analysis
CT-based dosimetry is recommended (minimum)
Plain radiographs (to verify seed count)
Consistent post implant interval for performing dosimetry
Isodose displays for 50%, 80%, 90%, 100% and 200%
D90 dose from the dose volume histogram
Additional doses should be reported: D80, D100, V80, V90, V100, V150, V200*

URETHRAL DOSES

Anatomy
1. Contour a volume, not a point or line
2. Catheter or fusion with ultrasound to delineate the urethra.
3. Estimation is not accurate

Dosimetric parameters
1. Ur150: (volume in cc of urethra receiving 150% Rx dose)
2. UrD5 (in cGy)
3. UrD30 (in cGy)

RECTAL DOSES

Anatomy
1. Inner and outer wall contour on all CT slices where seeds are identified
2. Dose-percent parameters are too subjective.

Dosimetric Parameters:
1. R100: (volume of rectum in cc receiving 100% of recommended dose)
2. R150: (volume of rectum in cc receiving 150% of recommended dose)

ERECTILE RECOMMENDATIONS

1. Cannot make recommendations:
   Weight of evidence toward NVB dose
   No consensus on location and ability to contour the NVB on CT or ultrasound
2. Recommend study on NVB dosing and contouring
3. Could not support penile bulb dose measurements

CT, computed tomography; D80, D90, and D100, dose to the respective volume percent of the prostate (D90 represents the minimum dose to 90% of the prostate volume); NVB, neurovascular bundle. *V80, V90, V100, V150, and V200, volume of the prostate that received the respective dose percent.

From Crook J, Potters L, Stock R, et al: Critical organ dosimetry in permanent seed prostate brachytherapy: defining the organs at risk. An American Brachytherapy Society Consensus Statement. Brachytherapy 4:186-194, 2005.

mity of approach makes it difficult, if not impossible, to combine data from different centers to establish guidelines for minimizing toxicity.

An expert panel reached a consensus regarding dose parameters that should be tracked to normal tissues when performing prostate brachytherapy. It is hoped that collecting outcomes based on these parameters betters the understanding of normal tissue tolerances and side effects.[410] At this time, there are too little data to make any sound conclusions on any specific data-points that will predict the risk of complications. With the advent of real-time, dynamic implants, the role of postimplantation dosimetry assessment may become unnecessary.[411]

High Dose Rate Brachytherapy. An alternative to permanent prostate implants, high dose rate (HDR) remote afterloaded brachytherapy has been successfully used to treat prostate cancer where the preponderance of data using HDR for prostate cancer is in men with locally advanced disease. Generally, HDR treatments are combined with EBRT although rarely used as monotherapy. Modern HDR brachytherapy systems use computer planning programs and robotic delivery systems. During the treatment, a single, high-activity iridium 192 source is moved through the implantation catheters at 2.5- to 5-mm intervals. The programmable delivery system controls the amount of time the source stops at a particular location. This is also called the *dwell time*. By changing the combination of dwell times, an infinite variety of isovolume dose distributions can be generated. The brachytherapy treatment planning systems can optimize the dwell times based on their location in the implant using computer algorithms. This allows a more homogeneous dose within the implant volume and better coverage of the target volume. Recent advances in treatment planning may provide further refinement of dosimetry by using inverse planning algorithms.

Beside the dosimetric advantages, there are other practical advantages of HDR brachytherapy compared with traditional LDR brachytherapy. Because the HDR source has high activity (typically 10 curies), a treatment is delivered in a few minutes, similar to EBRT, and it is always carried out in the shielded controlled environment of the HDR treatment room. Between treatments, the patient does not need to be isolated and can stay in an unshielded room with other patients. There is no radiation exposure to hospital personnel or to the patient's family members. Because the HDR implant is a closed system, there is no risk of seed migration. The effect of postimplantation edema can be accounted for by performing dose calculation after implantation.

Outcome. Outcome is based specifically on the adopted definition of success or failure. During the retropubic era, the common definition of treatment failure was clinical relapse based on the digital rectal exam or the development of radiographic evidence of metastasis. In 1997, the American Society of Therapeutic Radiology and Oncology (ASTRO) convened a consensus panel that developed the current standard definition of biochemical failure.[412] Although this definition was specifically developed for patients undergoing EBRT, it has been employed in most series reporting outcomes after brachytherapy, despite its inherent deficiencies and problems.[413] The *time to failure* is defined as the midpoint between the PSA nadir and the first PSA rise. Unfortunately, until the ASTRO consensus definition was developed, the literature reporting outcomes from modern permanent prostate brachytherapy used various biochemical definitions, making comparative interpretations of the data difficult.

Five-year biochemical freedom from relapse after modern permanent brachytherapy is reported to be in the range of 75% to 100%, with 8- to 13-year results of 66% to 88%.[395,400,402,414,415] In the largest multi-institutional series of more than 3500 patients, Kattan and colleagues report a 5-year 79.8% biochemical freedom from relapse rate for those patients treated with monotherapy or EBRT and implant.[416] No patients treated with hormones were included in that study. Multivariate analysis from that series indicated that the pretreatment PSA value and the Gleason sum were highly significant factors predicting biochemical success (P = .0001 and .0003, respectively), but the addition of EBRT was significant (P = .0487).

Univariate and multivariate analysis from most studies of patients with clinically localized prostate cancer treated with permanent brachytherapy or EBRT concur that the pretreatment PSA values and Gleason sum are highly significant factors predicting biochemical success.[172,176,392] As a result, several methods for developing risk stratification schemes have been proposed, each of which appears to predict PSA-RFS (Fig. 50-11).[400]

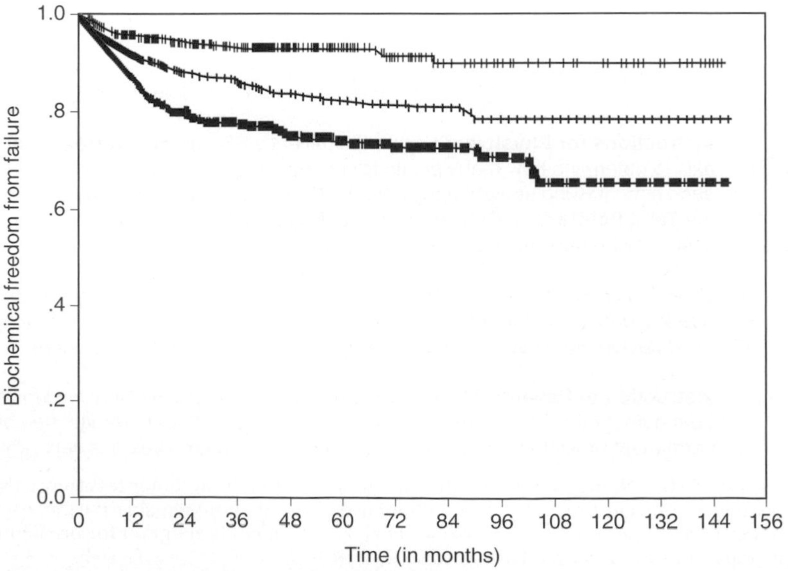

Figure 50-11 Biochemical freedom from failure at 12 years after permanent prostate brachytherapy. Patients were stratified by the following factors: pretreatment prostate-specific antigen (PSA) values < or ≥10 ng/mL, Gleason scores < or ≥7, and percent positive core-needle biopsy specimens < or ≥50%. Patients with three favorable factors were classified as low risk, and those with one adverse factor were classified as intermediate risk. Patients with two or more adverse factors were classified as high risk. (From Potters L, Morgenstern C, Calguaru E, et al: Twelve year outcomes following permanent prostate brachytherapy in patients with clinically localized prostate cancer. J Urol 173:1562, 2005.)

Although the concept of risk stratification is intuitive and simple to comprehend, recently developed nomogram analysis allows physicians to predict outcome better.[416] Although somewhat less intuitive, the nomogram approach assesses variables such as the pretreatment PSA value and Gleason sum in a continuous manner and independent of other factors to predict biochemical disease control (Fig 50-12). Use of additional pathology data such as percent positive core biopsy specimens has been identified to further enhance the ability to predict outcome.

Potters and coworkers examined information from brachytherapy patients identifying 26 independent variables.[417] This additional information predicted biochemical freedom from relapse better than that of the nomogram model. The concept of principle component analysis used in the Potters study to evaluate and compile multiple pathology variables can be used to construct a second-generation nomogram for patients considering brachytherapy.

Long-term biochemical freedom from relapse is reported for permanent prostate brachytherapy from several centers.[395,399,400,418,419] Although there are few data to correlate clinical outcomes with biochemical outcomes, several studies have compared treatment outcomes with surgery, EBRT, and prostate brachytherapy, with and without combination EBRT.[396,420] Treatment selection was not a significant factor to predict biochemical outcome except when EBRT doses were less than 72 Gy (Fig. 50-13).

Complications. Treatment-related morbidities after prostate brachytherapy may be acute, subacute, or chronic and affect most commonly the urinary, lower gastrointestinal, and sexual functions. Many factors have been shown to influence the likelihood of incurring complications, and may allow

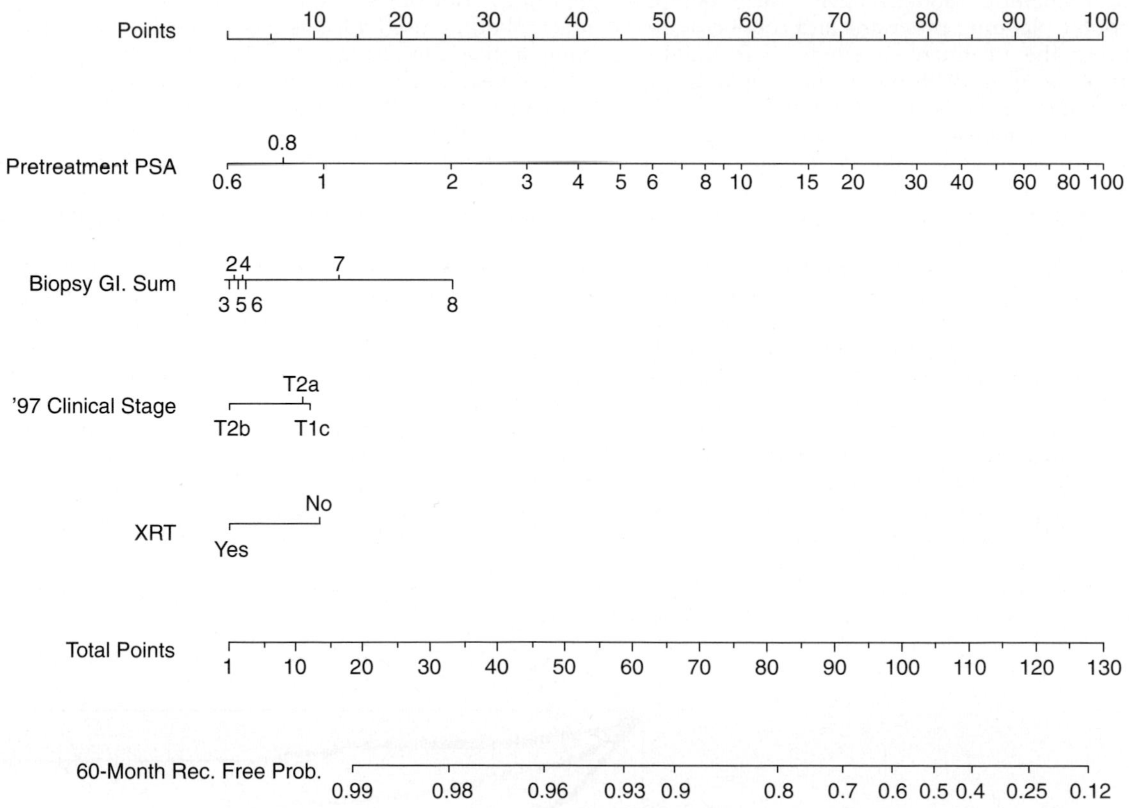

Instructions for Physician: Locate the patient's PSA on the **Pretreatment PSA** axis. Draw a line straight upward to the **Points** axis to determine how many points toward recurrence the patient receives for his PSA. Repeat this process for the other axes, each time drawing straight upward to the **Points** axis. Sum the points achieved for each predictor and locate this sum on the **Total Points** axis. Draw a line straight down to find the patient's probability of remaining recurrence free for 60 months assuming he does not die of another cause first.

Note: *This nomogram is not applicable to a man who is not otherwise a candidate for permanent prostate brachytherapy. You can use this only on a man who has already selected permanent prostate brachytherapy as treatment for his prostate cancer. You must decide upon use of adjuvant XRT prior to consulting this nomogram.*

Instruction to Patient: "Mr. X, if we had 100 men exactly like you, we would expect between <predicted percentage from nomogram – 30%> and <predicted percentage + 5%> to remain free of their disease at 5 years following permanent prostate brachytherapy, and recurrence after 5 years is very rare."

Figure 50-12 Nomogram for predicting 5-year freedom from tumor recurrence (Rec.) correlated with prostate-specific antigen (PSA) level after permanent prostate brachytherapy without neoadjuvant androgen-ablative therapy. Gl., Gleason score; Prob., probability; XRT, radiation therapy. (From Kattan MW, Potters L, Blasko JC, et al: Pretreatment nomogram for predicting freedom from recurrence after permanent prostate brachytherapy in prostate cancer. Urology 58:393, 2001.)

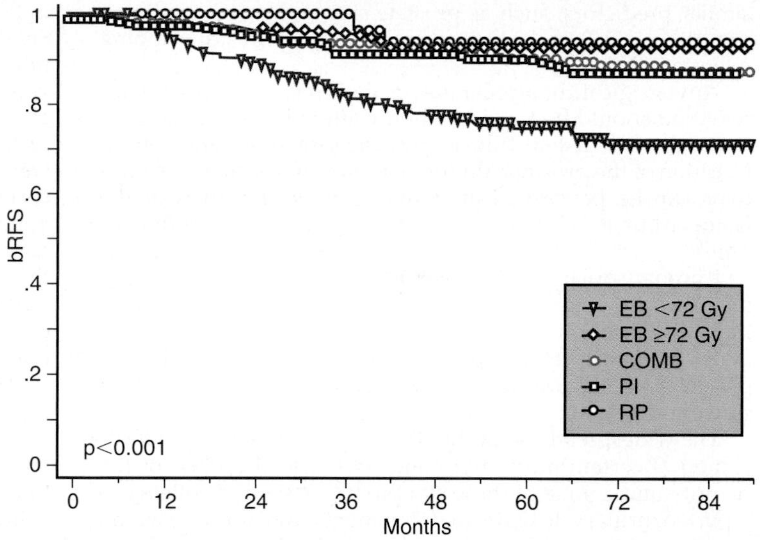

Figure 50-13 Biochemical freedom from recurrence for patients treated with permanent prostate brachytherapy (PI), external beam (EB) radiotherapy by dose (EB <72 Gy and EB ≥72 Gy), radical prostatectomy (RP), and combined methods (COMB). (From Kupelian PA, Potters L, Khuntia D, et al: Radical prostatectomy, external beam radiotherapy <72 Gy, external beam radiotherapy > or = 72 Gy, permanent seed implantation, or combined seeds/external beam radiotherapy for stage T1-T2 prostate cancer. Int J Radiat Oncol Biol Phys 58:25, 2004.)

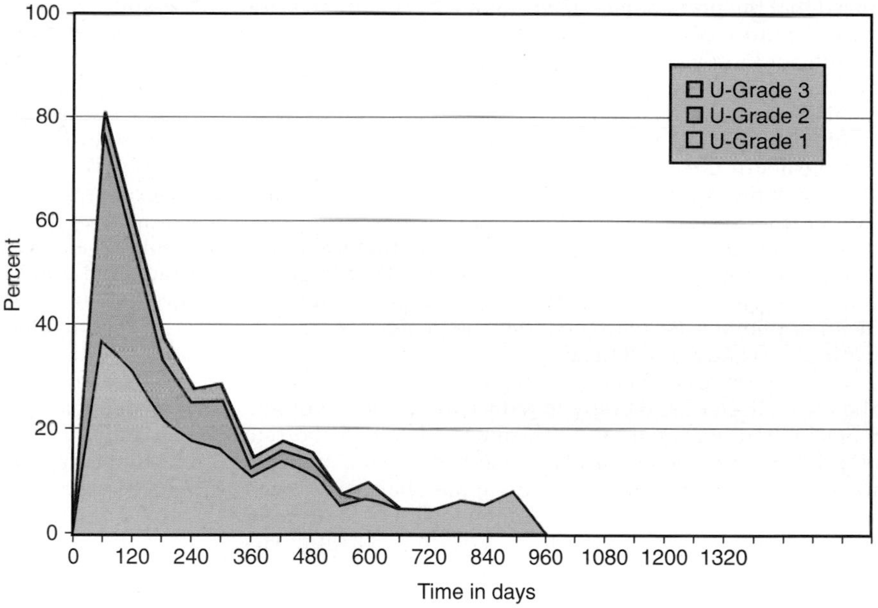

Figure 50-14 Cumulative reported urinary toxicity (i.e., frequency of urination or nocturia) for all patients using the modified Radiation Therapy Oncology Group (RTOG) toxicity scale. U-Grade 1 indicates dysuria, urgency, or bladder spasm requiring no or minimal medical intervention, such as phenazopyridine. U-Grade 2 indicates frequency with urgency and nocturia associated with early obstructive symptoms requiring other α-blocker–type therapy. U-Grade 3 indicates obstructive symptoms requiring an indwelling catheter or posttreatment transurethral resection of the prostate (TURP) for symptom relief. (From Gelblum DY, Potters L, Ashley R, et al: Urinary morbidity following ultrasound-guided transperineal prostate seed implantation. Int J Radiat Oncol Biol Phys 45:59, 1999.)

physicians to better select patients suitable for this approach.[380,409,421,422] These reports have also exposed the difficulties in evaluating morbidity due, in part, to the lack of standard assessment methods and potential biases. However, an updated consensus statement of the American Brachytherapy society has outlined standard data points from postimplantation dosimetry studies which may better allow the study of dose and normal tissue toxicity (see Table 50-16).[410]

Urinary Morbidity and Management. In the immediate postoperative period, patients will likely develop symptoms such as dysuria, frequency and hematuria (Fig. 50-14).[380] The inflammation in the prostate and adjacent tissues may result in weak stream or urinary retention.[422,423] Phenazopyridine is often helpful with dysuria, and alpha-blockers, such as tamsulosin, terazosin, and doxazosin, can be prescribed for irritative urinary symptoms such as frequency and weak stream. Hematuria generally improves spontaneously, but may cause urine retention requiring bladder irrigation. Patients who develop urinary retention may require catheter placement for an indefinite period of time. Local trauma to the prostate and seminal vesicles can result in hematospermia and orgasmalgia during the first few ejaculatory episodes, and may persist for several weeks.

Subacute urinary morbidity develops 1 to 2 weeks after the implant is placed and lasts for 6 to 12 weeks. Symptoms generally peak approximately 4 to 6 weeks after placement of ^{125}I or ^{103}Pd implants.[424] Although these symptoms usually resolve over time, many patients benefit from α-blocking agents. Locke and colleagues reported prospectively on urinary retention in 62 consecutive patients undergoing permanent prostate brachytherapy with or without EBRT.[425] At 1 week, the retention rate was 34%, and predictors for retention included prostate size larger than 36 g, and the preimplantation AUA symptom score was more than 10. The median duration of retention was 70 days (range, 0 to 469 days). Others have reported lower retention rates but observed that similar predictors, such as prostate size and preimplantation symptoms, affected the overall chance of developing retention.[378,380,422]

Any surgical manipulations of the prostate to correct for retention should be considered only after all medical options have been exhausted. Transurethral incision or a transurethral resection of the prostatic urethra for relief of obstructive symptoms can be performed after two to three half-lives of the isotope, but it is associated with up to a 26% incontinence rate.[426]

Chronic urinary morbidity can occur after 6 months and may include urinary frequency, incontinence, urethral strictures, and urethral necrosis.[427] Improvements in technique that avoid high periurethral radiation doses with peripheral seed placement have resulted in fewer severe long-term urinary side effects.[428,429]

The widespread use of the AUA score allows for standardization of certain morbidities and provides an outline of the severity and course of these symptoms. Desai and colleagues reported urinary toxicity in 117 patients and found a mean doubling of the baseline AUA score, peaking at 1 month after implantation and returning to baseline by about 24 months.[430] In a later study from the same institution, Terk and associates showed that the pretreatment IPSS was an independent factor to predict urinary retention in a multivariate analysis.[422] Gelblum and colleagues reported urinary toxicity using a modified RTOG scoring system from a large cohort of 693 patients undergoing permanent prostate brachytherapy with or without EBRT.[380] The IPSS scores 1 month after implantation were about three times that of the baseline scores. There was no significant difference in AUA scores between ^{125}I and ^{103}Pd implants at 60 and 120 days after the procedure.

There is much published on the urethral-sparing technique to help decrease acute urinary morbidity. Paradoxically, urinary toxicity is greatest in those with large prostates in which peripheral seed placement has the greatest impact on lowering the central prostatic dose.[431]

Another paradox associated with postimplantation toxicity is the use of hormonal therapy to reduce the prostate volume for brachytherapy. Crook and colleagues examined the rate and predictors of acute urinary retention in 150 patients undergoing implantation and multivariate analysis showed large prostate volume and prior hormone therapy to be independent predictors of urinary retention (see Fig. 50-10).[378] The explanation for this observation may be that cytoreduction of the prostate leaves mainly fibrous rather than glandular tissue, which does not allow the gland to accommodate to the acute reaction to implantation.

Lower Gastrointestinal Morbidity and Management. During the weeks after implantation, there may be changes in bowel habits in the form of diarrhea, constipation, tenesmus, or rectal pressure.[421,432,433] These symptoms generally respond to conservative management of symptoms.

Late injury includes proctitis, rectal ulceration, fistula formation, and incontinence.[433-435] The most common of these is proctitis, which often manifests as a painless bleeding that is usually self-limited. Bleeding from proctitis occurs late, about 1 to 2 years after implantation, and it may be exacerbated by constipation. Conservative management is recommended with stool softeners, local steroid creams, or foams. Aggressive measures such as biopsies and laser treatments may precipitate ulceration and fistula formation and should be avoided when possible.[434]

The incidence of proctitis has been reported to range from 1% to 12%.[436] Although the 12% proctitis rate reported by Wallner and coworkers represents the early experience with CT-based implants, subsequent refinements of the technique indicate that proctitis rates have decreased to 2% to 6%.[437,438] Snyder and associates, describing grade 2 proctitis after ^{125}I implantation, concluded that the incidence of proctitis was volume dependent for each dose studied.[439] The 5-year actuarial risk of grade 2 proctitis was 5% if 1.3 cc or less of the rectal volume received the prescription dose of 160 Gy, and it was 17% for more than 1.3 cc (P = .001). Others have tried to correlate the risk of proctitis relative to the delivered dose and volume of the rectum with less success.[433] Although there appears to be the suggestion of a dose-response relationship, the lack of conformity in the literature makes it difficult to recommend a specific dose to a certain volume of rectum. Intraoperative planning systems allow the operator to measure and limit the rectal dose during the case.[440]

The addition of EBRT to permanent prostate brachytherapy may be a risk factor for increased rectal toxicity. Zeitlin and coworkers reported a 2.3% fistula rate, raising concerns that combination therapy may be associated with more rectal injury.[441] This observation was also reported by Brandeis and colleagues in a study comparing quality-of-life indicators between implantation alone and implantation combined with external irradiation.[442] In that study, rectal intolerance was significantly higher in patients treated with combination therapy.

Sexual Function Morbidity and Management. Acute changes in sexual function after permanent prostate brachytherapy include pain with ejaculation and hematospermia. These symptoms generally dissipate over time and correlate with the acute prostatitis that the patient experiences. Erectile dysfunction (ED) after brachytherapy may be multifactorial, resulting from changes to the patient's neurologic, vascular, and psychological makeup. Zelefsky and coworkers identified a potential vascular mechanism for impotence after irradiation, and Merrick and colleagues examined and tried to correlate the radiation dose with the penile bulb as a mechanism for impotence.[443,444] Other confounding factors include comorbidities such as diabetes, hypertension, and smoking.

There are no prospective data looking at sexual potency after permanent prostate brachytherapy. However, retrospective data indicate a wide range of potency rates after brachytherapy, with as many as 80% to 85% of men younger than 60 years remaining potent when treated with an implant only, compared with 29% remaining potent after combination therapy with external irradiation, androgen deprivation, and implantation (Fig. 50-15).[445] The use of sildenafil to treat impotence showed a 62% response rate, with patients never having been treated with androgen deprivation responding more often.

In a study on 416 patients treated with implantation only, Stock and colleagues reported that preservation of potency was 79% at 3 years and 59% at 6 years.[446] In multivariate analysis, pretreatment potency and the implant dose were significant factors for erectile dysfunction after therapy.

High Dose Rate Brachytherapy Outcomes. The technique of HDR prostate brachytherapy has been in clinical practice since the 1980s.[447-449] Kovacs and coworkers reported one of the earliest experiences using HDR brachytherapy boost at University of Kiel.[450] Patients mostly had high-grade T2b-3 disease that was treated with a combination of split-course EBRT and two 15-Gy HDR treatments. The positive biopsy rate was 18% at 18 months after treatment. The result was updated at 10 years, and 78% of 171 patients remained free of disease at a median follow-up of 55 months. Mate and associates at Swedish Medical Center reported their experience with HDR brachytherapy.[451] This group used a more moderate hypofractionated schema with four HDR treatments of 3 to 4 Gy each combined with 45 to 50 Gy of EBRT. Pre-

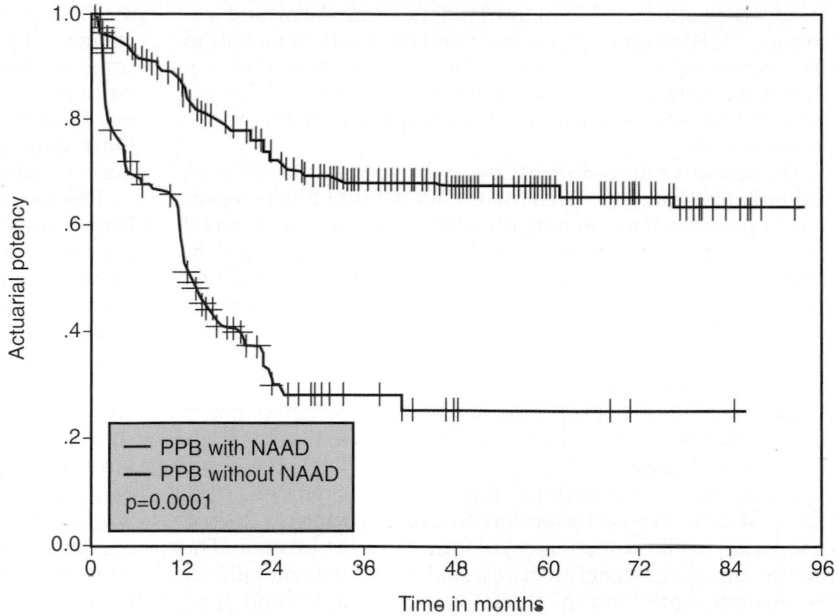

Figure 50-15 Actuarial potency of patients treated with or without neoadjuvant androgen ablation. NAAD, neoadjuvant androgen deprivation; PPB, permanent prostate brachytherapy. (From Potters L, Torre T, Fearn PA, et al: Potency after permanent prostate brachytherapy for localized prostate cancer. Int J Radiat Oncol Biol Phys 50:1235, 2001.)

treatment patient characteristics were stage T1b to T3c, mean initial PSA level of 12.9, and Gleason score of 3 to 9. The 5-year biochemical disease-free survival was 84%.

Martinez and colleagues at the William Beaumont Hospital reported the only on-going prospective dose escalation trial using increasingly larger fractions of HDR (5.5 to 6.5 Gy × 3 to 8.25 to 11.5 Gy × 2) combined with 46 Gy of EBRT.[449] The toxicity level using 9.5 Gy × 2 was acceptable. Patients with a PSA level of 10, T stage of T2b, and Gleason score of 7 were selected for this trial. Despite a high frequency of poor prognostic factors, the actuarial biochemical control rate was 89% at 2 years and 63% at 5 years.

The results from single-institutional clinical trials have shown that the technique of HDR brachytherapy for prostate cancer is feasible with minimal morbidity. However, the excellent results of single-institution studies must be validated in a multi-institutional setting and should be compared with other treatment techniques in prospective trials.

Postirradiation Prostate Biopsy

Although prostatic biopsy has been considered the gold standard for determining local tumor control after radiation therapy, these biopsies and their clinical significance may be difficult to interpret, as discussed in detail by Kuban and coworkers.[452] During the past few decades, a considerable range of postirradiation positive biopsy rates were reported (19% to 93%),[339,340,345,453] which likely reflected issues relevant to patient selection, interval from radiation therapy, biopsy extent, and therapeutic approach. The probability of obtaining a positive biopsy was related to pretherapy tumor stage, tumor grade, and postirradiation clinical examination findings. However, there are potential pitfalls in histologic interpretation of the postirradiation biopsy, and the distinction between radiation-induced epithelial atypia and residual neoplasm must be established to avoid erroneous histologic diagnosis.[131,454] Although ultrasound guidance and use of immunohistochemical stains (e.g., keratin 34βE12) may improve diagnostic accuracy,[454] most reports did not incorporate these aids.

Crook and colleagues[453,455] performed serial prostatic biopsies in a consecutive and unselected group of patients treated with EBRT. TRUS and prostatic biopsy were initially performed 12 months after radiation therapy and at 6-month intervals thereafter if the preceding biopsy result was positive or local tumor recurrence was suspected. These investigators concluded that complete postirradiation tumor clearance may require more than 2 years, that many patients (≥ one third) with an initially tumor-positive biopsy converted to negative on subsequent biopsy, that TRUS was no more predictive of biopsy result than clinical examination, and that patients with clinical local tumor recurrence had a higher nadir PSA level and required a longer time to achieve the nadir value.

Dugan and coworkers found that biopsy results correlated very well with PSA level after radiation,[133] and subsequent work on the predictive value of PSA nadir and rising PSA after therapy proved this to be a reliable, noninvasive means of establishing tumor recurrence. Because a rising trend in PSA may herald local failure and distant disease, situations that call for the documentation of local disease specifically, such as consideration of aggressive local therapy, still necessitate biopsy confirmation.

A few general conclusions about postirradiation prostatic biopsy may be made, Routine biopsy is justified only in a research setting; the tumor-positive biopsy rate is inversely related to the postirradiation interval and appears to plateau at about 3 years; tumor-positive biopsy results more than 2 or 3 years after radiation therapy are associated with reduced disease-free survival rates; and tumor-positive biopsy in an asymptomatic patient, particularly in the patient with normal DRE findings and a slowly rising PSA (doubling time at least 10 to 12 months), is not a mandate for intervention because the disease may take a slow, indolent course.[233,456]

Surgical Therapy

General Principles

The early history of radical prostatectomy can be traced to Hugh Hampton Young, who first performed the procedure through a perineal approach in 1904 at the Johns Hopkins Hospital. Although initially introduced for BPH some 40 years later, the retropubic technique was later modified for prostate cancer therapy. However, the procedure was accompanied by unacceptable morbidity (e.g., urinary incontinence, erectile dysfunction, and blood loss) until redefined by Walsh and colleagues,[457] Myers and coworkers,[458] and others. Refinements in the procedure gave the retropubic radical prostatectomy certain advantages over the perineal approach and set the stage for broader application and acceptance of this therapeutic modality.[459]

The operative procedure begins with a low midline incision and mobilization of the peritoneum. Bilateral PLND precedes radical prostatectomy in patients with sufficient risk of nodal involvement.[146] As described by Morgan and Lieber,[460] a standard or extended PLND may be performed, but the modified approach is more common in contemporaneous practice. Its margins of dissection are lateral, junction between external iliac artery and vein; inferior, femoral canal; posterior, obturator nerve and vasculature; and superior, bifurcation of the common iliac vessels. Frozen-section histologic examination is performed, and the procedure may be terminated in the presence of nodal disease.

Thereafter, the preprostatic adipose tissue is removed from the prostate to expose the endopelvic fascia, which is incised to separate the levator ani musculature from the prostate. The puboprostatic ligaments are transected to facilitate mobility of the prostatic apex, and the dorsal venous complex and anterior membranous urethra are transected in a manner to preserve the entire distal continence mechanism. The dissection continues by transecting the pillars of the prostate and the rectourethralis muscle, and a plane between the prostate and the anterior rectal wall is developed. If the nerve-sparing procedure is performed, the lateral pelvic fascia is incised, and the neurovascular bundles are allowed to fall away posterolaterally. After transecting and securing the pedicles to the prostate, Denonvilliers' fascia is incised to expose the vasa deferentia and seminal vesicles, and the vasa deferentia are transected. The seminal vesicles are dissected from the surrounding tissues, and the plane between prostate and bladder is developed until the longitudinal fibers of the bladder neck are identified. The bladder neck and proximal prostatic urethra are dissected from the prostatic parenchyma, the urethra is transected, and the prostate is removed. Attention is then turned to approximating the distal urethral stump and the proximal urethra at the bladder base to create the urethrourethral anastomosis. The bladder is brought down into the pelvis, the fascia is approximated in the midline, and the skin is closed.

Organ-Confined Disease

For patients with a life expectancy exceeding 10 years, radical prostatectomy is generally thought to be an appropriate option if disease is clinically confined to the prostate gland (i.e., stage I to II), although consideration is given to Gleason score and PSA level.[303] However, approximately one half (range, 41% to 64%) of patients thought to have organ-confined disease by clinical assessment have this confirmed by pathologic examination of the surgical specimen,[146,147,150] and one third of patients primarily treated with radical prostatectomy undergo additional cancer-directed therapy (i.e., radiation or androgen deprivation therapy) within 5 years.[461]

Disease outcome after radical prostatectomy is derived from retrospective analysis of study populations from single academic medical centers,[147,173,211,462-464] pooled analysis from selected centers,[465] or population-based cohorts[338,466] but is subject to the limitations of observational case series reports as described by Green and Byar.[330] The end points of metastasis-free, cause-specific, and overall survival likelihood from contemporary series of radical prostatectomy (with or without adjuvant or salvage therapy, or both) for patients with clinical stage I or II disease are displayed in Table 50-17. Recent reports indicate that biochemical and clinical failure rates are highly dependent on pretreatment prognostic factors such as tumor stage, Gleason score, and PSA level as well as surgical findings such as margin status, seminal vesicle and lymph node involvement.[462-464,467,468] As an example, the series reported by Han and associates is shown in Table 50-18.[463]

Although randomized trials comparing contemporary therapies for definitive treatment of prostate cancer have been nearly impossible to complete, available data suggest that irradiation (i.e., EBRT to current doses or a radioisotopic implant) and prostatectomy result in similar outcome for patients with equivalent prognostic factors.[396] Unfortunately, physician bias toward treatment options has been shown to be specialty related.[469,470] Many institutions have attempted to solve this problem through multidisciplinary clinics where patients have the benefit of obtaining consultation from multiple specialists.

Complications

Advances in surgical and anesthetic techniques and in postoperative care reduced intraoperative and postoperative complication rates. The anatomic approach to radical prostatectomy improved hemostasis and visualization during surgical dissection, which reduced the transfusion rate from 77% to approximately 16%.[471,472] Frank rectal injury is uncommon (≈ .5%),[471,472] and most patients do not require diverting colostomy, as primary closure of a small defect may suffice. Myocardial infarction (.7%), deep vein thrombosis (.8%), and pulmonary embolism (1%) are uncommon, and less than 1% of patients die in the perioperative period.[471,472]

Urinary incontinence is an often-cited complication of radical prostatectomy that typically improves during the first

Table 50-17 Radical Prostatectomy for Clinical Stage I-II Prostate Cancer

Study	Study Period	No. of Patients	BCR-Free (%)	Met-Free Survival (%)	CSS (%)	OS (%)	End Point
Amling et al[468]	1987-1993	2,782	60	—	—	—	10-y actuarial
Gerber et al[465]	1970-1993	2,758	—	70	85	—	10-y actuarial
Han et al[463]	1982-1999	2,494	79	82	—	—	15-y actuarial
Hull et al[464]	1983-1998	986	75	84	98	87	10-y actuarial
Kupelian et al[211]	1987-1993	423	58	91	—	94	5-y actuarial
Lu-Yao and Yao[338]	1983-1992	21,222	—	—	89	54-77*	10-y actuarial
Pound et al[462]	1982-1995	1,621	68	≈ 92	—	—	10-y actuarial
Trapasso et al[147]	1972-1992	725	47	—	94	86	10-y actuarial
Zincke et al[173]	1966-1991	3,170	52	82	90	75	10-y actuarial

*Outcome determined by histologic subgroup within specified range.
BCR, biochemical relapse; CSS, cause-specific survival; Met, metastasis; OS, overall survival.

Table 50-18 Actuarial 5-, 10- and 15-Year Relapse-Free Rates Following Anatomic Radical Retropubic Prostatectomy in Relation to Clinical Stage, Preoperative Prostate-Specific Antigen Level, and Gleason Score

Variable	Actuarial Percentage (95% CI) 5 Year	10 Year	15 Year
TNM			
T1a	100	100	100
T1b	90 (83-95)	85 (76-91)	75 (58-86)
T1c	91 (88-93)	76 (48-90)	76 (48-90)*
T2a	86 (83-88)	75 (71-79)	66 (59-72)
T2b	75 (70-79)	62 (56-68)	50 (41-58)
T2c	71 (61-79)	57 (45-68)	57 (45-68)
T3a	60 (45-72)	49 (34-63)	NA
Serum PSA (ng/mL)			
0-4.0	94 (92-96)	91 (87-93)	67 (34-86)
4.1-10.0	89 (86-91)	79 (74-83)	75 (69-80)
10.1-20.0	73 (68-78)	57 (48-64)	54 (44-63)*
>20.0	60 (49-69)	48 (36-59)	48 (36-59)*
Postoperative Gleason score			
2-4	100	100	100
5	98 (96-99)	94 (90-96)	86 (78-92)
6	95 (93-97)	88 (83-92)	73 (59-82)
7 (All)	73 (69-76)	54 (48-59)	48 (41-56)
7 (3 + 4)	81 (77-84)	60 (53-67)	59 (51-65)
7 (4 + 3)	53 (44-61)	33 (22-43)	33 (22-43)
8-10	44 (36-52)	29 (22-37)	15 (5-28)
Pathologic stage			
Organ confined	97 (95-98)	93 (90-95)	84 (77-90)
EPE+, GS < 7, SM−	97 (94-98)	93 (89-96)	84 (70-92)
EPE+, GS < 7, SM+	89 (80-94)	73 (61-82)	58 (41-71)
EPE+, GS ≥ 7, SM−	80 (75-85)	61 (52-68)	59 (50-67)
EPE+, GS ≥ 7, SM+	58 (49-66)	42 (32-52)	33 (23-44)
SV+, (LN−)	48 (38-58)	30 (19-41)	17 (5-35)
LN+	26 (19-35)	10 (5-18)	0

*Fourteen-year data.

CI, confidence interval; EPE, extraprostatic extension; GS, Gleason score; LN+, micrometastases to pelvic lymph nodes; NA, not available; PSA, prostate-specific antigen; SM, surgical margins; SV+, (LN−), involvement of seminal vesicles, negative lymph nodes; TNM, tumor-node-metastasis staging system; –, negative; +, positive.

From Han M, Partin AW, Pound CR, et al: Long-term biochemical disease-free and cancer-disease-free and cancer-specific survival following anatomic radical retropubic prostatectomy. Urol Clin North Am 28:555, 2001.

year. Although its precise cause is not fully understood, the remaining functional length of urethra and preservation of the muscular fibers about the bladder neck are probably critical factors. Depending on the severity of incontinence, it may be managed with protective pads, Cunningham clamp, transurethral collagen injection, or placement of an artificial genitourinary sphincter. Approximately one third (range, 6% to 63%) of patients experience a significant amount of postoperative urinary incontinence,[473-477] and most patients (97%) report some degree of voiding dysfunction.[478] The variation in incontinence rates may result from differences in patient characteristics (e.g., age), surgical technique, and the method through which information was obtained. Several reports suggest that physician-based assessments underestimate the presence and severity of incontinence,[473,478,479] as patients were hesitant to mention difficulties of this nature to their physician. Bladder neck or anastomotic stricture occurs in approximately 12% (range, 5% to 20%) of patients[473] and may require dilatation or incision to improve urinary flow.

Until recently, there was little awareness of bowel dysfunction as a possible postoperative complication. However, health-related quality-of-life instruments indicated that one third of patients had impaired bowel function (e.g., diarrhea, rectal urgency),[478] and one in five experienced fecal incontinence.[477] These difficulties often were not appreciated through physician inquiry and reporting[478] and were substantially greater than the expected incidence in a similar age group. Additional research is necessary to determine the cause of this problem so that modifications of surgical technique may be sought to reduce the risk of this complication.

Before introduction of the nerve-sparing procedure, erectile dysfunction was uniformly encountered. However, it was possible to preserve potency once the autonomic innervation of the corpora cavernosa was delineated and the nerve-sparing modification of the radical prostatectomy was made. Walsh and coworkers[474] reported that 68% of men retained potency, which was confirmed by Catalona and associates (59%).[480] Patient age, tumor stage, and excision or preservation of one or both neurovascular bundles correlated with the return of sexual function.[474] Nonetheless, population-based studies indicated that 21% (range, 11% to 27%) of patients were potent after radical prostatectomy,[473,475] and 97% of patients reported sexual dysfunction in a survey conducted by Litwin and colleagues.[478] As in other quality-of-life domains, physician-based assessment appeared to underestimate the incidence of impotence.[478]

Newer techniques such as laparoscopic prostatectomy and the robotic approach appear to be lesser surgical procedures with shorter hospital stays with the same or even lower rates of incontinence and impotence.[481,482]

Quality of Life

After the development of validated instruments, such as the UCLA Prostate Cancer Index and the Expanded Prostate Cancer Index Composite (EPIC), quality-of-life assessment has become an important component of posttreatment evaluation.[483,484] Litwin and colleagues[485] were among the first to evaluate quality of life in men treated for localized prostate cancer with an age-matched population. Since that time, investigators have generally found that bowel dysfunction is worse after EBRT than after radioisotopic implantation or prostatectomy.[486-488] This is typically evidenced by urgency, frequency, and bleeding. Urinary dysfunction, especially incontinence, is worse after prostatectomy, although irritative symptoms after implantation may be greater than after EBRT during the first 12 months.[487,488] Sexual function was similar for prostatectomy and EBRT, mainly because of the increasing dysfunction 2 to 5 years after irradiation, but better for implant recipients.[487,488] Age and comorbidities affected quality of life, as did the delivery of multiple therapies, especially hormonal therapy. Patient report surveys appear to give a more accurate assessment compared with physician- or chart-based reporting.[478,479]

LOCALLY ADVANCED DISEASE

Radiation Therapy

Locally advanced prostate cancer refers to clinical stage T3 or T4 disease and to bulky (e.g., tumor at least 25 cm^2 as determined by digital examination) T2 tumors.[489] Although there is limited information about the relative merits of various management approaches for this condition,[490,491] these patients generally are not managed with radical prostatectomy because

Table 50-19 Disease Outcome after External Beam Irradiation Alone for Locally Advanced Prostate Cancer*

Study	No. of Patients	Local Control (%) 5 y	Local Control (%) 10 y	Freedom from Relapse (%) 5 y	Freedom from Relapse (%) 10 y	Disease-Specific Survival (%) 5 y	Disease-Specific Survival (%) 10 y	Overall Survival (%) 5 y	Overall Survival (%) 10 y
Bagshaw et al[332]	446	75-80	60-75	30-45	15-30	35-70	25-50	35-65	15-35
Bolla et al[494]	198	77	—	48	—	—	—	62	—
Hanks et al[493]	269	72	65	47	38	—	—	58	38
Kuban et al[192]	≈ 445	—	—	47	29	75	50	—	—
Perez et al[190,336]	328/412	72	60	50†	33†	≈ 73	≈ 45	65	35
Pilepich et al[492]	523	78	—	≈ 40†	—	—	—	61-66	—
Pilepich et al[495]	468	71	—	44†	—	—	—	71	—
Zagars et al[191]	602	86	76	59	44	—	—	74	45

*Bulky T2, T3, or T4 disease.
†Disease-free survival.

the extent of disease often precludes complete surgical removal, and EBRT is generally considered the preferred treatment approach.

The clinical outcome after radiation therapy for these patients is modest (Table 50-19),[190-192,332,336,,492-495] and a substantial proportion of patients (half or more) develop clinically overt metastases by 10 years.[191] Incorporating posttherapy serum PSA monitoring into the assessment of disease status results in an outcome that is worse than previously recognized.[192,494,495] For example, Kuban and associates[192] used stored serum to evaluate the long-term PSA-based outcome of patients treated solely with EBRT and found a 13% decrement (47% versus 34%) at 5 years and an 18% decrement (29% versus 11%) at 10 years in comparing clinical to biochemical relapse-free estimates. In an effort to improve therapeutic outcome, clinical researchers have investigated dose escalation approaches with conformal and altered fractionation EBRT,[496-498] used neutron or proton beam therapy,[499-502] implanted radionuclide sources (e.g., ^{192}Ir) into the prostate,[503,504] or combined EBRT with androgen deprivation therapy[491,494,495,505-507] or hypoxic cell sensitizers.[508]

Specialized Techniques: Neutrons and Photon

Compared with photons, neutrons have a greater relative biologic effectiveness that results from higher linear energy transfer, lower dependence on oxygen enhancement (the effect of tumor hypoxia is reduced), diminished sublethal and potentially lethal damage repair, lesser variation in cell cycle–specific radiosensitivity, and direct (rather than free radical-mediated) DNA damage. However, neutron therapy has been the subject of only limited investigation in this setting.[499,500,502] The RTOG trial (study 7704) of mixed photon-neutron beam therapy versus proton irradiation alone showed improved local tumor control and disease-specific and overall survivals with the mixed beam.[499] As a further test of this approach, the Neutron Therapy Collaborative Working Group conducted a trial (study 8523) that randomized a larger study population to conventional photon irradiation or to neutron therapy.[500] This study demonstrated significantly improved local tumor control with neutrons, but an overall survival advantage was not apparent. Patients treated with neutron therapy had a significantly higher complication rate compared with those given photon RT. Nonetheless, work in this area continues in an attempt to capitalize on improved local tumor control and find the means to reduce treatment-related morbidity. Forman and coworkers[502] at Wayne State University achieved a negative posttherapy biopsy rate of 84% at 18 months and found that patient tolerance was satisfactory if the neutron dose level did not exceed 11 Gy.

Photons preferentially deposit energy at the end of their path (i.e., at the Bragg peak), which can be controlled to conform to an irregular 3D target volume. This results in a significant advantage in the dose distribution of photons compared with conventional proton-based radiation therapy, which potentially allows target dose escalation without increased normal tissue complications. Shipley and associates[501] randomly assigned patients with T3-4 disease to proton radiation therapy (67.2 Gy) or to photons (50.4 Gy) with a proton beam boost (25.2 Cobalt Gray Equivalent). The proton beam boost markedly enhanced local tumor control in patients with high-grade tumors. However, a difference in overall and disease-specific survivals was not observed, and gastrointestinal complications (e.g., rectal bleeding) were more common with the proton beam. In contrast, investigators at Loma Linda reported a low complication rate and excellent short-term local tumor control using photon (45 Gy) with proton boost (30 Cobalt Gray Equivalent) therapy.[509] Updates of the long-term results of this trial shows acceptable GI and GU toxicity levels.[510]

Given advances in photon beam dosimetry, including IMRT (see "Techniques of Irradiation") it is not known whether there is a true advantage to neutrons or protons over well-designed and dose-escalated photon radiation therapy.

High-dose brachytherapy combined with photon beam irradiation is another way to address locally advanced adenocarcinoma of the prostate with radiation therapy. (See brachytherapy section for details.)

Androgen Deprivation plus Irradiation

Androgen deprivation can induce apoptotic regression of androgen-responsive prostate tumors by reducing intracellular concentrations of dihydrotestosterone.[511] In the context of locally advanced prostate cancer; this may reduce the primary tumor volume (i.e., cytoreductive therapy), improve prospects for local tumor control, and extend the duration of survival free of metastatic disease. Pilepich and colleagues[174] used information from a prospective RTOG trial (study 75-06) to evaluate pretherapy factors for an association with disease outcome. Of particular relevance to cytoreductive therapy, multivariate analysis demonstrated that primary tumor size and concomitant or antecedent hormonal therapy correlated with local tumor control. This observation, along with the suggestion that addition of estrogen therapy to EBRT improved local tumor control,[512] prompted further study of hormonal cytoreduction in the setting of locally advanced prostate cancer. In preparation for a phase III trial, the RTOG (study 83-07) evaluated the efficacy and toxicity of megestrol and diethylstilbestrol (DES) in a phase II randomized study in which patients were assigned to either agent for 2 months before and during EBRT.[506] Both agents resulted in a high likelihood for clearance of the primary tumor (94% to 97%) and locoregional tumor control (93% to 94%) in conjunction with radiation therapy, but megestrol was associated with fewer side effects. However, in the advent of luteinizing hormone-releasing hormone (LHRH) agonists and nonsteroidal antiandrogen agents, the focus of the investigation in the RTOG (study 85-19) shifted to these agents, which were well tolerated and associated with a high rate of tumor clearance (100%).[507]

To determine the potential benefit of adding cytoreductive neoadjuvant androgen deprivation to conventional EBRT, the RTOG conducted a prospective comparative trial (study 86-10) that used goserelin (3.6 mg subcutaneously every 4 weeks for four doses) and oral flutamide (250 mg given three times daily) initiated 2 months before and continued during EBRT in patients with bulky (≥25 cm^2) T2-4 tumors.[489,512] After controlling for known prognostic variables, patients were randomized to irradiation alone, which consisted of 45 Gy to pelvic and lower para-aortic (if pelvic nodes were involved) nodes with a prostatic boost to 65 to 70 Gy, or to the combination of EBRT and neoadjuvant, cytoreductive androgen deprivation therapy. Updates of this trial, for which 456 patients were evaluable (226 who received neoadjuvant hormonal manipulation and 230 who received radiation alone), reveal a statistically significant improvement for the addition of hormone therapy at 5 and 8 years for local failure, distant metastasis, no evidence of disease (NED) survival, no biochemical evidence of disease (bNED) survival with a PSA level less than 1.5 ng/mL, and cause-specific survival.[512] At 8 years, the cause-specific survival rate was 69% for patients who received radiation alone and 77% for those who received irradiation plus the hormone therapy (P = .05).[512] Overall survival was not statistically improved (P = .10). Of interest is a subset analysis of centrally reviewed patients with Gleason scores of 2 to 6. This subset of patients did show a survival advantage at 8 years (70% versus 52%) in the irradiation plus hormone group versus irradiation alone (P = .015).[512] Severe treatment-related toxicity was not enhanced with goserelin and flutamide, and preservation of erectile function was similar between the two groups. Based on the findings from this study, Pilepich and associates concluded that in patients with locally advanced adenocarcinoma of the prostate Gleason score of 2 to 6, a short course of androgen ablation administered before and during EBRT is advised to improve local and distant outcomes as well as overall survival.[512]

During a similar time frame the question of androgen deprivation as an adjuvant to EBRT was evaluated by the RTOG and by the European Organization for Research and Treatment of Cancer (EORTC). The RTOG trial that evaluated androgen deprivation adjuvantly was study 85-31.[495,513] In this trial, there were 945 evaluable patients with nonbulky clinical T3, post prostatectomy pathologic T3, or node-positive prostate cancer assigned to irradiation alone or irradiation plus goserelin (3.6 mg SC, given every 4 weeks, beginning the last week of EBRT and continued indefinitely). EBRT consisted of 44 to 46 Gy to the pelvic and paraortic (in the presence of common iliac nodal disease) nodal regions with a prostatic boost to 65 to 70 Gy; post prostatectomy patients received 60 to 65 Gy to the prostatic fossa. The use of the adjuvant goserelin resulted in a statistically significant reduction in the risk of local tumor recurrence and distant metastasis as well as an improvement in overall survival, cause specific as well as bNED survival (Table 50-20).[513] The absolute survival difference estimated at 10 years was 53% versus 38% in favor of the goserelin adjuvant therapy.

Similarly, the EORTC conducted a trial which enrolled patients with locally advanced disease, i.e., T3-4 disease (367 patients) or those with high-grade tumors and localized disease, i.e., T1-2 (34 patients).[494,514] Patients were randomized to irradiation alone, with 50 Gy to the pelvic nodes and 70 Gy to the prostate and seminal vesicles at 2 Gy per fraction, or to irradiation plus androgen deprivation. Androgen deprivation consisted of goserelin (3.6 mg subcutaneously every 4 weeks) for 3 years beginning at the start of radiation therapy and patients were treated with 1 month of oral cyproterone acetate, (an antiandrogen) started 1 week before goserelin to inhibit the potential transient elevation of serum testosterone associated with LHRH agonist therapy. This trial, like the RTOG data, showed a survival advantage to the combined treatment over EBRT alone (Fig. 50-16). With a median follow-up of 66 months, overall survival was 62% for the irradiation-alone arm and 78% for the irradiation plus goserelin arm (P = .0002).[514] The 5-year cause-specific survival rate was 79% for the irradiation-alone arm and 94% for the irradiation plus goserelin arm, which was also statistically significant. The results of these two trials of adjuvant LHRH agonist therapy

Table 50-20 Results with the Use of Adjuvant Androgen Suppression

Assessment Measure	Study Arm	Estimated 5-Year Rate (%)	Estimated 10-Year Rate (%)	Significance
Local failure	I	15	23	$P < .001$
	II	30	39	
Distant metastases	I	15	25	$P < .001$
	II	29	39	
bNED PSA < 1.5 ng/mL	I	55	30	$P < .001$
	II	21	9	
Disease-specific mortality	I	9	17	$P < .0053$
	II	13	22	
Absolute survival	I	76	53	$P < .0043$
	II	71	38	

bNED, no biochemical evidence of disease; PSA, prostate-specific antigen.

Pilepich MV, Winter K, Lawton C, et al: Androgen suppression adjuvant to definitive radiotherapy in prostate carcinoma: long-term results of phase III RTOG 85-31. Int J Radiat Oncol Biol Phys 61:1285-1290, 2005.

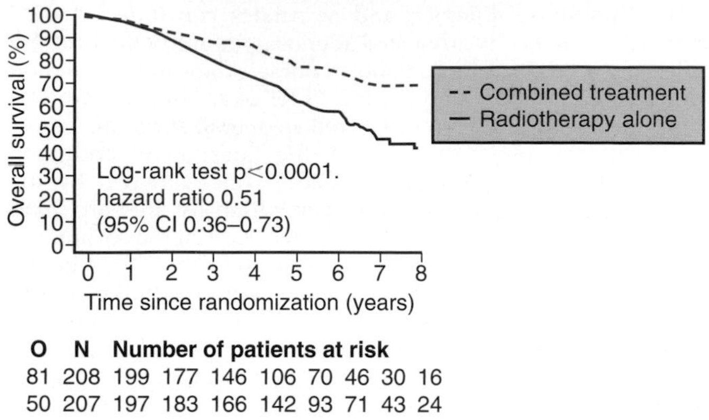

Figure 50-16 Kaplan-Meier estimates of overall survival by treatment group. N, number of patients; O, number of deaths. (From Bolla M, Collette L, Blank L, et al: Long-term results with immediate androgen suppression and external irradiation in patients with locally advanced prostate cancer [an EORTC study]: a phase III randomized trial. Lancet 360:103, 2002.)

and EBRT established the role for the adjuvant use of LHRH agonist in locally advanced prostate cancer.

Given the findings of RTOG 86-10, 85-31, and the EORTC trial discussed previously, questions remained about the timing and duration of hormonal manipulation, prompting the RTOG to investigate the duration of hormonal manipulation in protocol 92-02.[515] Included in the RTOG protocol 92-02 were patients with histologically confirmed adenocarcinoma of the prostate (clinical stage T2c-4) with no evidence of lymph node involvement in the common iliac or higher chains and pretreatment PSA levels less than 150 ng/mL. Patients were randomized to receive 2 months of neoadjuvant goserelin (3.6 mg SC, given every 4 weeks for a total of 4 months in arm I) along with flutamide (250 mg, given three times daily for a total of 4 months, 2 months neoadjuvantly and 2 months concurrently with irradiation). A radiation dose of 65 to 70 Gy was delivered to the prostate, and a dose of 45 to 50 Gy to the pelvic lymph nodes. Patients on arm II were randomized to receive the same neoadjuvant and concurrent hormonal manipulation, including goserelin and flutamide; they also received 24 months of goserelin (3.6 mg SC) every 4 weeks after cessation of irradiation. Of 1554 patients entered onto the study between June 1992 and April 1995, 779 received short-term androgen deprivation and radiation therapy, and 775 received long-term androgen deprivation with EBRT; 1514 patients were evaluable. With a median follow-up of 5.8 years, the long-term androgen deprivation radiation arm shows a statistically significant improvement in all efficacy end points except overall survival compared with the short-term androgen deprivation arm.[515] End points evaluated and showing statistically significant improvement to the addition of long-term hormonal manipulation included local progression, distant metastases, biochemical failure, and cause specific survival, as well as disease-free survival. In a subset of patients not part of the original study design, patients with tumors assigned Gleason scores of 8 to 10 had a statistically significant overall survival advantage of 81% versus 70.7% (P = .044). There was a small but significant increase in frequency of late gastrointestinal radiation injuries of grades 3, 4, and 5 associated with a long-term androgen-deprivation arm (2.6% versus 1.2% at 5 years; P = .037). Conclusions from this trial support the use of long-term androgen deprivation (a minimum of 2 years) after neoadjuvant and concurrent androgen deprivation and EBRT for locally advanced prostate cancer.[515]

With the question of the potential benefits of adding hormonal manipulation to EBRT largely answered, there remained the question of EBRT volumes. The issue regarding the treatment of pelvic lymph nodes was addressed by RTOG protocol 94-13, which accrued 1323 patients between April 1995 and June 1999.[516] Patients were randomly assigned to one of four arms: whole-pelvis EBRT plus neoadjuvant and concurrent hormonal manipulation, which included an LHRH agonist for a total of 4 months with goserelin (3.6 mg SC) or leuprolide (7.5 mg IM) with an antiandrogen (250 mg of flutamide PO, given three times daily for 4 months); prostate-only irradiation plus neoadjuvant and concurrent hormonal manipulation; whole-pelvis irradiation plus adjuvant hormonal manipulation; or prostate-only irradiation plus adjuvant hormonal manipulation. The hormonal manipulation in the adjuvant arm was the same 4-month course as in the neoadjuvant and concurrent arm. With a median follow-up of 59.5 months, 98% of the patients were considered eligible (n = 1292). Eligible patients included those with nonmetastatic prostate cancer, a PSA level less than 100 ng/mL, and an estimated risk of lymph node involvement of 15% as defined by the Roach formula (percent lymph node involvement = $\frac{2}{3}$ PSA + [GS − 6 × 10]). Progression-free survival was statistically impacted at 4 years by the use of whole-pelvis irradiation (54% versus 47%; P =.022). At 4 years, progression-free survival was not statistically different between the neoadjuvant and concurrent hormonal manipulation versus adjuvant hormonal manipulation arms (52% versus 49%; P = .56).[516] Conclusions of this study indicate that whole-pelvis irradiation plus neoadjuvant and concurrent hormonal manipulation improves progression-free survival compared with prostate-only irradiation and neoadjuvant plus concurrent or adjuvant hormonal manipulation. This study is the first prospective, randomized trial to suggest a benefit from whole-pelvis irradiation to address potential disease in the pelvic lymph nodes in patients with locally advanced prostate cancer.

Results of the RTOG and EORTC studies together provide appropriate justification to add immediate hormonal manipulation in the form of an LHRH agonist neoadjuvantly and adjuvantly to patients treated with irradiation for locally advanced adenocarcinoma of the prostate.[512-516]

Node-Positive Disease

Regional lymph node involvement (i.e., N1 disease) is an adverse prognostic factor for patients treated with radiation therapy or radical prostatectomy.[517,518] Several observational case series demonstrate that most patients with histologically confirmed pelvic lymph node-positive prostate cancer (pN+) experience disease relapse after radiation therapy alone.[200,201,517,519,520] For these patients, the most common site of relapse is metastatic (Table 50-21), which suggests that occult systemic metastases likely existed at the time of diagnosis. Prostate cancer–specific mortality, rather than comorbid illness, was the predominant cause of death, despite use of androgen deprivation at the time of clinical relapse.

The addition of adjuvant androgen deprivation to radiation therapy appears to improve disease outcome (see Table 50-21).[517,520-525] Particularly noteworthy in this regard was the national prostatic cancer project (study 1000) in which adjuvant systemic therapy (i.e., estramustine) significantly prolonged the likelihood of progression-free and overall survival compared with radiation therapy alone.[523] Likewise, subset analysis of pN+ disease patients entered on RTOG trial (85-31) who were assigned to irradiation with androgen deprivation

Table 50-21 **Outcome of Node-Positive Prostate Cancer after Radiation Therapy with or without Androgen Deprivation**

Study	No. of Patients	DFS (%)	CSS (%)	OS (%)	Metastasis (%)	End Point
RT ALONE						
Bagshaw et al[521]	60	—	—	20	—	10-y actuarial
Gervasi et al[517]	152	7*	43	32	83	10-y actuarial
Lawton et al[526]	23	55	—	63	—	5-y actuarial
Lawton et al[522]	345	≈ 72*	—	≈ 65	38	5-y actuarial
Schmidt et al[523]	118	<5	—	≈ 30	—	10-y actuarial
RT WITH ADT						
Cheng et al[524]	97	—	54	—	—	10-y actuarial
Lawton et al[522]	98	≈ 83*	—	≈ 73	27	5-y actuarial
Schmidt et al[523]	31	14	—	≈ 54	—	10-y actuarial
Whittington et al[525]	66	85	94	94	—	5-y actuarial

*Freedom from relapse.
ADT, androgen-deprivation therapy; CSS, cause-specific survival; DFS, disease-specific survival; OS, overall survival; RT, radiation therapy.

at disease progression versus those randomized to irradiation plus immediate androgen deprivation (goserelin) have shown (on multivariant analysis) that immediate hormonal manipulation has a statistically significant impact on all end points, including absolute survival, disease specific failure, metastatic failure, and biochemical control with a PSA level of less than 1.5 ng/mL.[522] The 5- and 9-year absolute survival rates were 72% and 62%, respectively, for all patients receiving immediate hormonal manipulation with irradiation, compared with 50% and 38% for patients receiving hormone therapy only at the time of relapse ($P = .030$).[522] Based on the data given earlier, contemporary practice guidelines rely on androgen deprivation and irradiation as the mainstay of treatment for patients with pN+ disease.[302,303,522,526]

Although local therapy (irradiation or surgery) may be beneficial,[522,527] definitive evidence for or against its use is lacking. When EBRT is administered, CT- or MR-based planning with complex conformal dosimetry is recommended to treat the pelvic lymphatics (45 to 50.4 Gy) with a boost to the site of nodal disease to a total dose of 50 to 55 Gy with at least similar doses to the seminal vesicles and doses above 70 Gy to the prostate. Prophylactic para-aortic irradiation is not beneficial.[492] For patients who are having local symptoms because of progressive disease in the prostate or regional area who were not treated with upfront local therapy and may be hormone refractory, a dose of at least 60 Gy at 2 Gy per fraction or more is required to significantly affect tumor size and symptoms.[528]

The optimal management strategy for node-positive patients remains controversial, and further research will help provide more information on the utility of radiation therapy in this setting. The RTOG conducted an open trial (96-08), which was a prospective trial randomizing patients with pelvic node-positive disease to androgen deprivation (orchiectomy or LHRH agonist and flutamide) or androgen deprivation plus radiation therapy, but this study closed prematurely due to inadequate patient accrual. Fortunately, the RTOG study 94-13 was successfully performed, and there appears to be a benefit to treating patients with high likelihood of lymph node involvement with whole-pelvis irradiation over prostate irradiation only.[516] In the face of the randomized data from the RTOG and the Messing trial,[527] for patients who have node-positive disease, local therapy in the form of EBRT versus surgery should be seriously considered in addition to hormonal manipulation.

Postoperative Radiation Therapy

Approximately one-third of men with prostate cancer undergo prostatectomy,[529] and approximately one-third to one-half of these patients develop recurrent disease 5 to 10 years later.[530-533] Postoperative curative EBRT is most commonly administered for three clinical situations: the presence of adverse risk factors after complete surgical resection (i.e., adjuvant therapy), subclinical disease suggested by a persistent or recurrent elevation of postoperative serum PSA level, or clinically apparent disease (i.e., positive DRE) suggesting tumor recurrence in the prostatic fossa. When strictly applied, the term *adjuvant* refers to treatment administered to reduce the risk of disease recurrence when all clinically detectable disease was removed by surgery, and this term should be reserved for patients with an undetectable postoperative PSA level. When a detectable PSA level persists after radical prostatectomy or occurs after a certain disease-free interval, the therapeutic goal changes to one of eradicating prostate cancer to render the patient free of all known disease, and treatment administered under this condition should be referred to as *salvage* therapy.

ADJUVANT EXTERNAL BEAM RADIATION THERAPY

Certain histologic findings of the radical prostatectomy and lymph node dissection specimen are associated with an increased risk of disease relapse and serve as possible indications for adjuvant EBRT. These risk factors include: higher Gleason score, tumor involvement of the surgical margins,[196,530,534] extension of the tumor through the prostatic capsule,[531-534] seminal vesicle,[149,533,534] and pelvic lymph node involvement.[527,530,533] Although the preoperative PSA level is also associated with disease relapse,[531-533] it typically has not been considered as a sole indication for adjuvant therapy. Several reports combined risk factors to predict the likelihood for postoperative failure,[255,532,535] and they may be referred to when considering adjuvant therapy. The rationale for adjuvant irradiation hinges on the premise that more than a million cancer cells may be present before PSA is detectable in the serum and that the greatest opportunity for eradicating the cancer exists when they are fewest in number, clinically occult, and remain localized.[536] There is also the suggestion that prostate cancer assumes a more aggressive phenotype with the passage of time,[537] and this indirectly suggests that earlier intervention may prevent delayed metastases.

Although uniform indications for adjuvant operative irradiation have not yet been adopted, suggested guidelines are available.[303,526] The National Comprehensive Cancer Network (NCCN) guidelines recommend 3D-CRT or IMRT or observation when there is a positive surgical margin.[303] The Patterns of Care 1996 Decision Trees and Management Guidelines advocate immediate postoperative irradiation for involved surgical margins or seminal vesicle invasion, but recognize that surveillance with serial PSA measurements is an appropriate alternative.[526] Adjuvant irradiation for patients with extraprostatic tumor extension, margin involvement or seminal vesicle invasion was supported by the results of a European Organization for Research and Treatment of Cancer (EORTC) clinical trial.[538]

Results

During the past decade, several observational series of adjuvant irradiation were added to the literature, and Table 50-22 summarizes the relevant reports with sufficient detail and follow-up duration.[539-545] Although its role is controversial, it is generally acknowledged that EBRT improves local tumor control compared with prostatectomy alone in patients at high risk for recurrence.[540-543,545] Clinically based local tumor control is observed in about 97% of patients with high-risk factors,[539-543,545] and actuarial estimates indicate that approximately 99% and 92% are free of local recurrence at 5 and 10 years, respectively. In contrast, the 5- and 10-year local control rates after radical prostatectomy alone in such patients are about 85% and 61%, respectively.[539-543,545] Overall clinical and biochemical relapse-free rates are also improved with adjuvant irradiation,[535,542,544-546] which generally reduces the risk of relapse by 43% to 88%.[535,541,542,545] Nonetheless, perhaps one fourth of patients with biochemical relapse only after adjuvant irradiation have persistent cancer in the prostatic fossa,[547] and this suggests that improved target definition, localization, or dose escalation may improve results.

The impact of adjuvant irradiation on metastasis-free, overall, and cause-specific survival is not clear, because inconsistent results are reported (see Table 50-22). This ambiguity may be due to difference in patient selection, time trends in disease presentation and therapeutic approach, inadequate patient numbers for statistical analysis, insufficient follow-up, and the confounding effect of subsequent androgen suppression. Nonetheless, a reduction in the risk of metastases and mortality due to prostate cancer was observed in some studies with longer follow-up.[540,541]

The ideal means to establish the role of adjuvant irradiation is through randomized clinical trials evaluating comparable and appropriately selected patient groups treated by prostatectomy with adjuvant irradiation or without it. The Southwest Oncology Group started a trial in 1988 that accrued three-quarters of its intended goal of 558 patients by 1996, but the results have not yet been published. However, early results from a similar but substantially larger trial conducted by the European Organization for Research and Treatment of Cancer (trial 22911) were reported.[538] One thousand five patients who had radical prostatectomy, were younger than 75 years, had a WHO performance status of 0 to 1, and had T0-T3 N0 M0 prostate cancer preoperatively were randomized to adjuvant irradiation versus observation within 4 months of surgery. Patients had pathologic risk factors of capsular invasion, positive surgical margins, or invasion of seminal vesicles after surgery.[538] The dose was 60 Gy using conventional radiation therapy delivered over 6 weeks. With a median follow-up of 5 years, the biochemical progression-free survival rate was 72.2% for patients who had adjuvant irradiation and 51.8% for those receiving surgery alone ($P < .0001$). Clinical progression-free survival was also improved from 74.8% to 83.3% at 5 years ($P = .004$). Further follow-up is needed to assess the impact on distant metastasis and overall survival, which currently are not statistically different.[538]

Complications

The morbidity of adjuvant irradiation is limited to the bladder, rectum, and erectile tissues, but side effects are generally mild and well tolerated.[540,543,544,548] The incidence of urinary incontinence is comparable to that which follows surgery alone,[543,544] and if attributed to radiation therapy is typically of a mild stress-induced nature.[543] Overall, significant genitourinary toxicity is observed in up to 5% to 10% of patients,[540,544] but it tends to respond well to a conservative or minimally invasive approach. The development of urethral strictures does not seem to be significantly affected by irradiation.[544] Most reports cite a 5% to 10% rate of mild or moderate radiation-induced proctopathy,[540,544] but the use of three-dimensional approaches and attention to rectal dose: volume parameters greatly diminishes this risk.[540,548] Formenti and colleagues reported that moderate doses of irradiation did not impair recovery of erectile function after nerve-sparing prostatectomy,[549] but this was not confirmed in another report.[550] Edema of the genitals or lower extremities (0% to 13%) is largely confined to patients

Table 50-22 Radical Prostatectomy with or without Adjuvant Radiation Therapy

	Local Control (%)		Disease-Free Survival (%)		Metastasis-Free Survival (%)		Survival (%)		
Study	RP	RP + RT	RP	RP + RT	RP	RP + RT	RP	RP + RT	End Point
Anscher et al[539]	60	92*	37	55	65	67	52	62	10-y actuarial
Cozzarini et al[540]	63	93*	31	69*	75	88*	80†	93*†	8-y actuarial
Hawkins et al[541]	87	98*	59	72*	—	NS*	≈ 92	≈ 92	5-y actuarial
	—	—	35	63*	—	NS*	84†	98*†	10-y actuarial
Leibovich et al[542]	≥84	100*	59	88*	≥84	100*	93	97	5-y actuarial
Petrovich et al[543]	—	—	66	70	—	—	91	91	5-y actuarial
	—	—	46	53	—	—	≈ 74	81	10-y actuarial
Schild et al[544]	83	100*	40	57*	≈ 92	≈ 92	92	≈92	5-y actuarial
Valcenti[545]	92‡	100‡	55	89*	100‡	100‡	100‡	100‡	5-y actuarial

*Statistically significant improvement with radiation therapy.
†Cause-specific survival.
‡Crude rate.
NS, specific value not stated; RP, radical prostatectomy; RT, radiation therapy.

in whom pelvic lymph node dissection is done and pelvic nodal irradiation is administered.[551,552]

Biochemical Relapse

Background

A detectable serum PSA level after prostatectomy is referred to as biochemical relapse or as biochemical failure, and it typically occurs months to years before there is clinical evidence of tumor recurrence.[213] Most surgical reports define biochemical relapse as equal to two PSA values that are at least 0.2 ng/mL. However, Amling and coworkers suggested that a PSA value equal to 0.04 ng/mL was a more appropriate threshold based on the likelihood of further PSA increases during the next 3 years,[219] and a Consensus Panel concluded that a level of 0.5 ng/mL provided more secure evidence to justify salvage therapy.[553] Low PSA levels may be due to residual benign prostatic glandular tissue, but PSA levels should not be 0.5 ng/mL. Although biochemical relapse often prompts a desire to identify the site of disease recurrence, physical examination, ultrasonography,[554,555] bone scintigraphy,[556,557] and CT[557] are often nonspecific or remain normal until the PSA level becomes markedly elevated.

Irregularities of the prostatic fossa may be apparent on clinical examination, but this finding does not strongly correlate with biopsy findings.[554,555] and it appears that prostatic fossa biopsy results do not influence the radiotherapeutic outcome.[558] A negative biopsy result does not exclude local recurrence as the source of biochemical relapse, and a positive biopsy result does significantly improve the prospects for radiotherapeutic success. A hypoechoic mass in the urethrovesicular anastomosis, bladder neck, or retrotrigone regions or disruption of the retroanastomotic fat plane are the ultrasonic features of local recurrence. Transrectal ultrasound is quite sensitive to these findings, but they are not highly specific for cancer and cannot be used to identify or exclude patients for radiotherapy.[555] CT of the pelvis and abdomen often demonstrates postoperative soft tissue effects that may be mistaken for tumor recurrence,[559] unless the PSA is markedly elevated.[557] Magnetic resonance imaging with an endorectal coil is a promising method to identify local recurrence after prostatectomy.[560] A neoplastic mass appears isointense on T1-weighted scans and hyperintense on T2-weighted scans, and it enhances with the addition of gadolinium. As additional information is gained with its use, these finding may help define the clinical target volume (CTV) and perhaps allow selective dose escalation. Bone scans are frequently normal in the asymptomatic patient, particularly so in those with a PSA level of less than 30 to 40 ng/mL and a PSA velocity of less than 0.5 ng/mL/month.[556,557] The optimal use of Prostascint imaging requires clarification, because its accuracy may be limited and its results are not associated with radiotherapeutic response.[561,562]

Partin and associates suggested that PSA velocity was associated with the site of disease relapse, such that patients with a PSA velocity of 0.75 ng/mL/year were more likely to have local tumor recurrence.[563] This group further evaluated PSA kinetics in association with other factors, and developed an algorithm to estimate the risk of metastasis after biochemical relapse.[213] The algorithm used all detectable PSA values within 2 years to calculate a PSA doubling time and combined it (10 months versus >10 months) with the interval to biochemical relapse (2 years versus >2 years after surgery) and the surgical Gleason score (5 to 7 versus 8 to 10). Patients with Gleason score of 5 to 7, an interval of 2 years, and a PSA doubling time of 10 months and those with a Gleason score of 8 to 10 and an interval of 2 years had a particularly high risk of metastatic relapse. Stephenson and colleagues found that patients with a shorter PSA doubling time were less likely to have PSA control after salvage radiation therapy.[564] However, salvage radiation therapy offered the possibility of biochemical control even for a substantial proportion of patients with a short PSA doubling time and high-grade cancer. It does not appear appropriate to use PSA kinetics alone to restrict the use of irradiation on an individual patient basis.

Several reports used multivariate analysis to identify factors that are associated with radiotherapeutic outcome. The surgical Gleason score,[561,564-568] PSA level immediately before irradiation,[561,564-566,569-572] and seminal vesicle invasion[564,565,573] are the factors most closely associated with biochemical control. Patients with a Gleason score of 8 to 10 tend to fare more poorly than those with lower-grade tumors.[561,564] Most investigators chose to evaluate the preirradiation PSA level by grouping various levels into distinct categories, and cutoff values from 1.0 ng/mL to 2.0 ng/mL often have been used.[561,564,566,569-571] However, Pisansky and coworkers concluded that there was a continuous risk of failure as the PSA level rose[565] and that each doubling of the PSA value increased the risk of biochemical relapse by approximately 40%. Most investigations support the conclusion that radiation therapy can be more effective if started earlier in the course of progressively rising serum PSA levels and that it is ill-advised to allow the PSA value to rise above 1.5 ng/mL.[553] Some reports suggest that the surgical margin status (involved margins),[564,573] postoperative PSA doubling time (>10 months),[564] and PSA levels during radiation therapy (stable or declining)[569] can favorably influence treatment results. The interval from surgery to biochemical relapse,[564,571,573] capsular perforation,[564,565] DNA ploidy,[565] neoadjuvant androgen suppression,[561,564,569,570] and radiation therapy dose level[564,565,568,573] have not been found to have prognostic significance.

Results

The outcome of patients selected to receive EBRT for biochemical relapse has been exclusively described through observational case series[561,564-575] as randomized clinical trial results are not presently available in this setting. The results presented in such reports (Table 50-23) should be considered tentative and any conclusions should be cautiously interpreted, because the series typically consist of small and heterogeneous study populations treated over an extended timeframe. It is likely that this variability accounts for the differences in outcome from one series to the next. In general, most patients received 64.8 Gy (series median) administered to the prostatic fossa without treatment of the regional lymphatics. With this approach, 75% (median) of patients had a significant biochemical response,[564-567,570-572] which indicates that incomplete surgical excision of the cancer is the source of biochemical relapse in most patients and that radiotherapy may be considered with intent to cure. Although more than 90% (median) of patients survive 5 years,[564-566,569] 45% (median) have biochemical control at this point.[564-570,574,575] Stephenson and associates demonstrated that prognostic factors can be combined to identify groups of patients likely to have more favorable radiotherapeutic outcomes (Fig. 50-17).[564] For example, patients with involved surgical margins, a PSA doubling time of more than 10 months, and a PSA level of 2.0 ng/mL before radiation therapy have an 80% likelihood of biochemical control at 4 years. Although the surgical findings and the PSA doubling time represent fixed and intrinsic determinants of prognosis, their impact on outcome is lessened when irradiation is given at lower PSA levels.[564-566,569-572]

Although observational series provide useful information, controlled clinical trials are necessary to define the optimal

Table 50-23 Contemporary Series of Salvage Radiotherapy for Biochemical Relapse after Prostatectomy

Study	No. of Patients	RT Median Dose (Gy)	Biochemical Response (%)*	BCR Free (%)	Overall Survival (%)	End Point
Anscher et al[574]	89	66.0	72	≈ 50	≤92	5-y actuarial
Catton et al[566]	43	60.0	≈ 60	≈ 18	88	5-y actuarial
Chawla et al[567]	54	64.8	76	35	—	5-y actuarial
Choo et al[575]	98	60.0	≈ 90	≈ 32	≈ 92	4-y actuarial
Do et al[570]	69	64.8	92	55	—	5-y actuarial
Katz et al[573]	115	66.6	—	46	≤95	4-y actuarial
Maier et al[569]	170	68.0	—	44	90	7-y actuarial
Perez et al[572]	92	≈ 62.5	79	20-75	—	4-y actuarial
Pisansky et al[565]	166	64.0	82	46	93	5-y actuarial
Song et al[561]	61	66.6	67	39	≤95	4-y actuarial
Stephenson et al[564]	501	64.8	67	40	≥82	5-y actuarial
Tsien et al[568]	57	64.8	—	35	—	5-y actuarial
Valicentl et al[571]	34	64.8	62	10-59	—	3-y actuarial

*Observed rate.
BCR, biochemical relapse; RT, radiation therapy.

Table 50-24 Contemporary Series of Salvage Radiotherapy for Clinically Apparent Local Recurrence after Prostatectomy

Study	No. of Patients	RT Median Dose (Gy)	Local Control (%)	BCR Free (%)	Overall Survival (%)	End Point
Cadeddu et al[580]	25	64.0*	—	14	—	5-y actuarial
Catton et al[566]	16	60.0	60	0	—	5-y actuarial
Choo et al[575]	44	63.0	97†	11	87	5-y actuarial
Koppie et al[558]	34	68.4*	—	39	—	3-y actuarial
Leventis et al[581]	15	66.0	—	18	—	5-y actuarial
Macdonald et al[582]	42	68.4	95†	27	78	5-y actuarial
Syndikus et al[550]	26	52.0*	54	—	—	10-y actuarial
Vander Kooy et al[579]	35	64.0	97†	56	97	8-y actuarial
Wiegel et al[578]	20	65.0	95†	68	51	5-y actuarial

*Mean. Mean daily fraction size was 2.76 Gy in Syndikus et al.[550]
†Observed (crude) rate.
BCR, biochemical relapse; RT, radiation therapy.

management approach for this clinical setting. The European Organization for Research and Treatment of Cancer (study 30943) is investigating the role of immediate versus delayed androgen deprivation in asymptomatic patients with biochemical relapse after prostatectomy or radiation therapy, or both, and the Radiation Therapy Oncology Group (study 9601) is testing the role of a nonsteroidal anti-androgen (i.e., bicalutamide) in association with prostatic fossa RT. Single-institution studies are emerging that suggest that adding hormonal therapy to radiation may be beneficial, especially in patients with higher PSA levels (>1.0 ng/mL).[576] Complications are similar to those reported for adjuvant irradiation. Although doses for biochemical relapse may be slightly higher, computed tomography–based treatment planning, using three dimensional conformal approaches, and the more recent use of intensity modulation has resulted in less treatment morbidity.[577]

Clinically Apparent Tumor Recurrence

Background

A thorough evaluation for metastatic disease should be performed before radiation therapy is contemplated, because many tumor-related characteristics that predispose to local recurrence are also associated with lymphatic and hematogenous dissemination. Transrectal ultrasonography or endorectal magnetic resonance imaging, radionuclide bone scintigraphy, CT of the pelvis ± abdomen, and renal function and serum PSA determinations are valuable supplements to the history and physical examination.

Results

Even though serum PSA is detectable with rare exception, salvage therapy is not initiated in some cases until tumor recurrence is evident on digital rectal examination or there is biopsy evidence of cancer in the prostatic fossa. The efficacy of salvage radiation therapy in this setting has been evaluated by relatively few investigators,[550,558,566,578-583] whose reports often include a heterogeneous and small study cohort. Table 50-24 displays the contemporary results of radiation therapy for this clinical condition. These observations suggest that clinically based local tumor control is achieved in about 85% of patients,[566,579,582,583] likelihood of biochemical disease-free[566,578-583] and overall survival[578,579,582,583] 5 years after irradiation is approximately 25% and 80%, respectively. These results suggest that irradiation may be of value in carefully selected patients with clinically apparent local tumor recurrence, and this approach appears to compare favorably with a primary androgen suppression management strategy.[584]

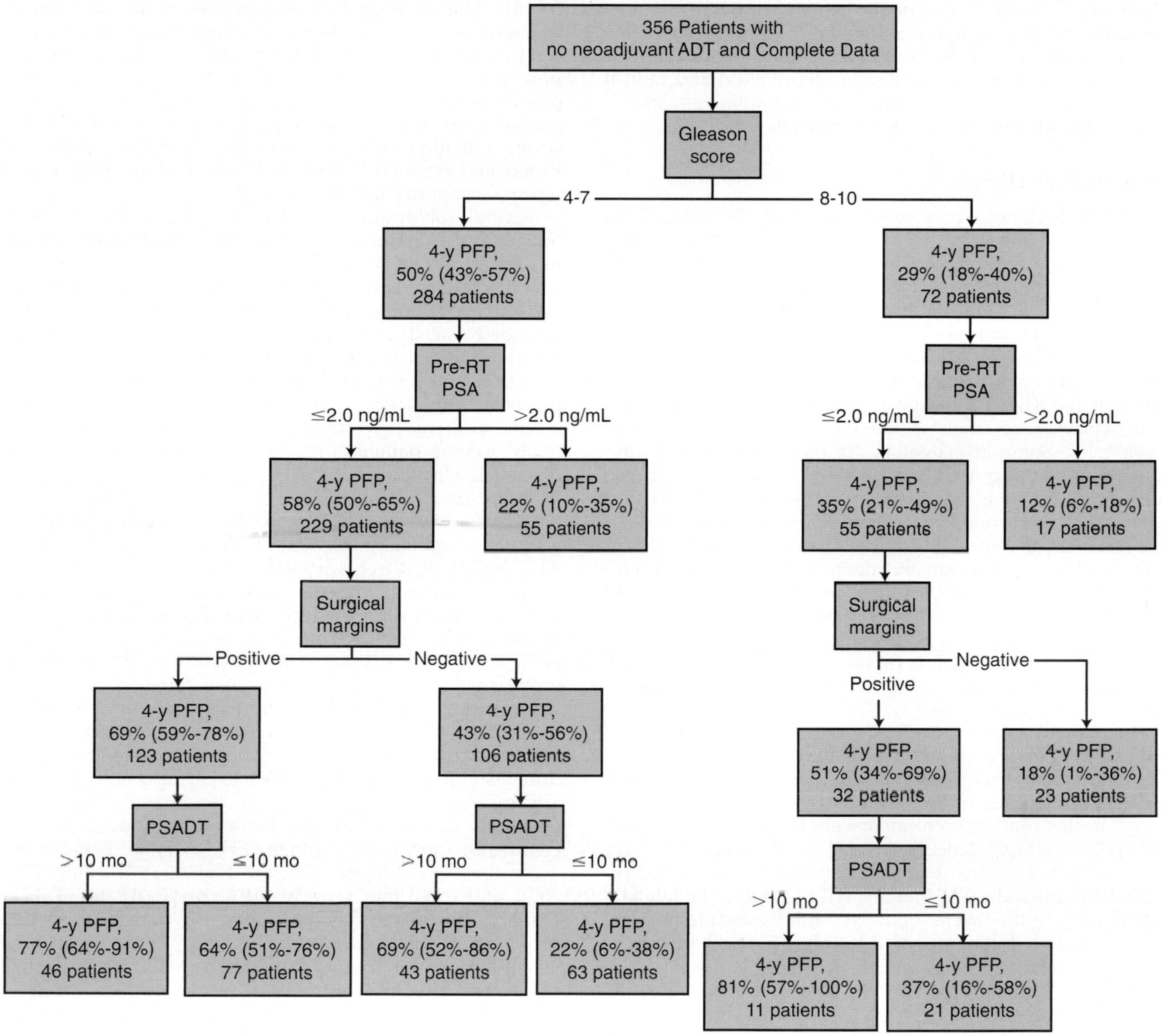

Figure 50-17 Four-year actuarial progression-free probability (PFP) after salvage radiotherapy. PFP is stratified by Gleason score, prostate-specific antigen (PSA) level before radiation therapy (RT), surgical margins, and PSA doubling time (PSADT). Patients receiving neoadjuvant androgen deprivation therapy (ADT) were excluded from this analysis. All values in parentheses are 95% confidence intervals. (From Stephenson AJ, Shariat SF, Zelefsky MJ, et al: Salvage radiotherapy for recurrent prostate cancer after radical prostatectomy. JAMA 291:1325, 2004.)

A shorter interval from prostatectomy to the detection of local recurrence, shorter PSA doubling time, pathologic tumor stage, Gleason score, and preirradiation PSA level are factors that appear to be associated with the efficacy of RT.[579,582] Given the benefit of hormonal manipulation in addition to irradiation in patients with locally advanced disease, physicians should consider hormonal manipulation in patients with clinically apparent postoperative tumor recurrence.[512-514]

Surgery

In general, radical prostatectomy is not recommended for patients with locally advanced (i.e. clinical stage T3) prostate cancer.[303] In a multi-institutional pooled analysis conducted by Gerber and coworkers,[585] 41% of patients with clinical stage T3 disease had histologic evidence of seminal vesicle invasion or pelvic LNI, and the 10-year cause-specific and overall survival probabilities were 57% and 32%, respectively. Although patients with well or moderately differentiated tumors had better outcome, these investigators concluded that further study was warranted to determine the optimal therapeutic approach for these patients. In contrast, Lerner and associates[586] reported better 10-year cause-specific (80%) and overall (70%) survival after radical prostatectomy with the selective use of adjuvant therapy and suggested that this approach should be considered for the patient with clinical stage T3 prostate cancer. It appears that further study is required before a clear consensus can be reached regarding the use of radical prostatectomy in this setting.

In an attempt to facilitate complete tumor resection, preoperative androgen deprivation has been given for approximately 3 months before radical prostatectomy for clinical stage

T3 disease,[587-594] but its therapeutic benefit is unknown and its role in this setting has not been defined.[590] Approximately one quarter (range, 14% to 59%) of patients have organ-confined disease after preoperative androgen deprivation and radical prostatectomy,[587,589-591] but surgical margin involvement[591,594] and therapeutic outcome do not appear altered.[589]

Node-Positive Disease

Several observational case series described the outcome of patients with node-positive disease (i.e., N1) after radical prostatectomy and pelvic node dissection.[198,199,205,207,523,530] Biochemical relapse is observed in nearly all such patients,[198,530,595,596] and the probability of survival free of clinical disease relapse at 10 years is compromised (≈ 15%)[199,207,523,597] by the development of metastatic disease.[199,207] Based on these observations, certain authors maintain that adjuvant androgen deprivation should be added to a management strategy that includes radical prostatectomy.[198,199,597] Some investigators are particularly strong proponents of this approach and consider immediate androgen deprivation the standard of care.[199] In this regard, Zincke and colleagues[199] performed a retrospective case series analysis and observed an improved 10-year disease-free likelihood for patients in whom adjuvant androgen deprivation was administered (76%) compared with those in whom it was withheld (24%). Although survival was not enhanced for all patients with N1 disease, the 10-year cause-specific survival probability for patients with a DNA diploid tumor was significantly better among those treated with adjuvant androgen deprivation (≈ 96% versus ≈ 70%).

For patients in whom radical prostatectomy is performed and positive pelvic lymph nodes are found, there is a prospective randomized trial performed by Messing and colleagues addressing the issue of the addition of hormonal manipulation.[527] In this trial, 98 men underwent radical prostatectomy and pelvic lymphadenectomy and were found to have nodal metastases. They were randomly assigned to receive immediate antiandrogen therapy with goserelin or bilateral orchiectomy, or they were followed until disease progression. With a median follow-up of 7.1 years, 7 of 47 men who received immediate antiandrogen treatment had died, compared with 18 of 51 men in the observation group who received surgery alone ($P = .02$) The cause of death was prostate cancer for 3 men in the immediate-treatment group and 16 men in the observation group ($P < .01$).[527] Based on this prospective, randomized data, patients who undergo radical prostatectomy and are found to have positive lymph nodes should undergo immediate androgen therapy. Whether they would benefit from additional radiation therapy remains unanswered.

Postirradiation Prostatectomy

As discussed by Corral and colleagues,[598] there is renewed interest in prostatectomy as a therapeutic option for select patients with biopsy-proven local tumor recurrence after radiation therapy. These authors recommend extensive preoperative evaluation to assess surgical feasibility and to exclude clinically overt metastatic disease. Cystoscopy, examination under anesthesia, CT or MRI of abdomen and pelvis, chest radiography, and radionuclide bone scintigraphy (with or without supplemental skeletal radiography or MRI) may be used to complement the history and clinical examination. The general health condition (i.e., comorbidity) and life expectancy of the patient and the patient's expectations should be considered in concert with the efficacy and morbidity of the procedure. The decision between prostatectomy and anterior exenterative surgery (e.g., cystoprostatectomy) requires careful preoperative and intraoperative evaluation. A cystoprostatectomy may be indicated in the presence of biopsy-proven bladder neck or seminal vesicle tumor invasion, incontinence from a noncompliant low-capacity bladder, severe radiation-induced cytopathy, or pelvic adhesions.[598] Pisters and Wajsman[599] provided a detailed description of the retropubic approach in this setting.

Several observational case series described disease outcome after surgical resection for postirradiation locally recurrent prostate cancer.[600-608] The most extensive experience was reported by Lerner and associates,[607] who demonstrated that salvage surgery (with or without androgen deprivation) provided encouraging tumor control and survival rates. Although resection was not feasible in 10 of the 132 patients (8%) in whom it was attempted, 60% successfully underwent prostatectomy, and cystoprostatectomy or total pelvic exenteration was performed in 29% and 4% of patients, respectively. Among patients in whom prostatectomy was accomplished, the likelihood of local tumor control was 92%, and the BCR-free survival and disease-specific survival estimates at 5 years were 65% and 89%, respectively. Rogers and coworkers[608] found similar outcomes (5-year disease-specific survival, 95%; 5-year BCR-free survival, 55%) in a case series of 40 patients. Although results with prostatectomy (with or without androgen deprivation) were favorable, patients who required cystoprostatectomy or total pelvic exenteration did not fare nearly as well.[603,607] Quality-of-life issues assume great importance when exenteration is considered.

Because radiation-induced fibrosis tends to obliterate the usual tissue planes used to establish surgical lines of resection, the increased technical difficulty and morbidity of the procedure result in a general reluctance to perform salvage surgery. The more common postoperative types and rates of complications described in the literature include urinary incontinence (mean, 32%; range, 15% to 79%), bladder neck contracture/anastomotic stricture (mean, 18%; range, 7% to 28%), and rectal injury (mean, 10%; range, 0% to 19%).[600-606] Urinary continence may be reestablished with an artificial sphincter,[602] and anastomotic stricture and rectal injury usually respond to minor interventions without resultant loss of organ integrity. Intraoperative blood loss may be increased[608] but generally is comparable to that encountered during prostatectomy as primary therapy.[585] Lerner and colleagues[607] observed a decreased need for blood transfusion and a reduced complication rate in patients treated with prostatectomy during more recent years, which highlights the importance of the anatomic approach and extent of surgical experience with this situation.

Postirradiation Cryosurgery

Another alternative to postradiation prostatectomy is cryosurgery, which is the killing of cells by the application of very cold temperatures. Cryosurgery was first used for prostate cancer in the 1960s and 1970s, but there was no transrectal ultrasound guidance or urethra warming so complications such as incontinence and urethral necrosis were common in addition to fistula formation. Given these problems the technology was abandoned until the late 1980s. Subsequently, transrectal ultrasound guidance and urethral warming were developed.[609-611] Currently there are no defined guidelines for urologists to appropriately select patients who have local failure after radiation for salvage cryosurgery. Optimally, patients would have locally recurrent disease without evidence of distant metastasis.[612] For patients whose PSA leve is more than 5 ng/mL, evaluation of the pelvic lymph nodes by CT, MRI, or pelvic lymph node dissection is reasonable, because salvage radical prostatectomy series report between 20% to 40% of patients as having metastatic disease to the pelvic lymph nodes in this setting.[612] The disease is best controlled with cryosurgery if it is confined to the prostate.

Several retrospective series have shown reasonable PSA control rates of 30% to 70% at 12 to 20 months with major complications in the 10% range in patients treated with cryosurgery after irradiation local failure.[613-616] Cryosurgery remains an option in these patients, although properly selecting candidates for this procedure remains a challenge.

METASTATIC DISEASE

Hormonal Therapy

In a particular prostatic tumor, three distinct cell populations may exist: androgen dependent, androgen sensitive, and androgen independent. Androgen-dependent cancer cells require a critical level of androgenic stimulation to maintain growth, whereas the growth rate of androgen-sensitive cells is decreased in the absence of androgenic stimulation. The clinical importance of this was established in the early 1940s by Huggins and colleagues,[617] who demonstrated the therapeutic benefit of androgen deprivation in the context of metastatic disease. The principles and efficacy of androgen deprivation therapy for patients with metastatic prostate cancer were well summarized by Griffiths and associates.[511]

Sex hormone production is regulated by the hypothalamic-pituitary axis. Gonadotropin-releasing hormone is synthesized by the hypothalamus and transported to the anterior lobe of the pituitary gland, where it controls the synthesis and secretion of the gonadotropic hormones, luteinizing hormone (LH) and follicle-stimulating hormone (FSH). The predominant means of controlling FSH and LH levels involves a closed-loop negative-feedback mechanism in which gonadal steroids have the capacity to inhibit FSH and LH secretion. The interaction of circulating LH with its receptor in the target cell results in production of circulating androgens through the following biosynthetic pathway:

$$\text{Cholesterol} \rightarrow \text{Pregnenolone}$$
$$\rightarrow 17\alpha\text{-Hydroxypregnenolone} \rightarrow \text{Dehydroepiandrosterone}$$
$$\rightarrow \text{Androstenediol} \rightarrow \text{Testosterone} \rightarrow \text{Dihydrotestosterone}$$

Under normal physiologic conditions, Leydig's cells account for 95% of testosterone production in adult men, with approximately 5% derived from adrenal androgen production (i.e., androstenedione) and its conversion in peripheral tissues to testosterone. After its diffusion into its target tissue, testosterone is converted to the more potent androgen α-dihydrotestosterone (DHT) by 5α-reductase. DHT forms an intracellular complex with the androgen receptor that targets specific DNA sequences. It is the androgen-responsive genes that determine the balance between cellular proliferation, cell death, and differentiation of the prostatic epithelial cell.

Several classes of androgen-deprivation agents are available for medical (versus surgical) castration and include estrogens (e.g., diethylstilbestrol, estramustine), progestational agents (e.g., cyproterone, medroxyprogesterone, megestrol), LHRH agonists (e.g., goserelin, leuprolide), and steroidal (e.g., cyproterone, medroxyprogesterone, megestrol) and nonsteroidal (e.g., bicalutamide, flutamide, nilutamide) antiandrogens. Although approximately 80% of patients with metastatic disease respond to androgen deprivation,[618] this response is often transient, such that only one fourth of patients remain alive after 5 years (median survival duration is about 2.5 years).[619,620]

Estrogenic therapy lowers LH concentration and thereby reduces serum testosterone levels. However, DES at 3 mg/day or more results in significant cardiovascular toxicity. Although lower doses (e.g., 1 mg/day) have fewer side effects, DES does not reliably reduce testosterone concentration to castrate levels. In addition to cardiovascular complications, estrogens may cause fluid retention, gynecomastia, and loss of libido and potency. Continuous administration of LHRH agonists causes inhibition of LH and FSH release and suppression of testosterone, which reaches castrate levels after 3 to 4 weeks. However, LHRH agonists initially produce a significant increase in testicular androgen production, known as the *flare reaction*, which can be inhibited with the administration of antiandrogens. The major side effects of the LHRH agonists include impotence, loss of libido, atrophy of the reproductive organs, and hot flashes. Antiandrogens competitively bind to androgen receptors at the target cell level. This class of agents blocks the effects of testicular and adrenal androgens. Antiandrogens are currently approved for use in combination therapy with an LHRH analogue to provide complete androgen blockade. Their use as a sole means of androgen deprivation has also been investigated.[621,622] At 150 mg per day, bicalutamide appeared to be equivalent to an LHRH agonist or castration in patients with locally advanced but nonmetastatic disease.[621] In patients with metastatic disease, bicalutamide as monotherapy showed a slight disadvantage (approximately 4 weeks less median survival) compared with medical or surgical castration.[622] Antiandrogens may offer a quality-of-life advantage over other androgen deprivation methods because they do not reduce serum testosterone and therefore do not have the marked inhibitory effect on libido and potency apparent with other agents. Gynecomastia can occur in as many as 70% of patients, and prophylactic breast radiation is therefore recommended.

The role of combined androgen blockade (i.e., LHRH agonist or orchiectomy and an antiandrogen) has been the subject of considerable investigation. Although Crawford and associates[619] and Janknegt and coworkers[623] demonstrated that progression-free and overall survivals were improved with the combination, the Prostate Cancer Trialists' Collaborative Group performed a systematic overview, or meta-analysis, of 22 clinical trials and concluded that survival duration was not enhanced with the combination.[620]

Chemotherapy

The utility of chemotherapy in the management of metastatic prostate cancer has not been thoroughly defined. This therapeutic option has been explored most in patients with hormone-resistant disease. Yagoda and Petrylak[624] reviewed 26 chemotherapy trials and found an overall 9% clinical tumor response rate. However, objective and reproducible methods for assessing therapeutic response were difficult to define. More recently, investigators have used serum PSA as an end point for assessing efficacy.

Although multiple combinations have been tested, docetaxel-based chemotherapy is now considered standard for hormone-refractory disease.[625,626] In a 1006-patient randomized trial, docetaxel plus prednisone showed a 2.4 month advantage in median survival compared with mitoxantrone plus prednisone.[625] A PSA response was seen in 45% of patients, and a pain response in 35% with this favored regimen. A meta-analysis of three randomized trials comparing docetaxel with mitoxantrone showed a reduction in death risk of 8% to 21% with docetaxel, which persisted 3 years after the start of therapy.[626] However, the absolute benefit remains quite small and is measured in months.

Studies exploring earlier use of chemotherapy, such as with hormone therapy before the disease is androgen independent, are in progress. Other promising strategies such as vaccines and molecular pathway inhibitors are under investigation. However, the most effective first-line therapy for metastatic prostate cancer is androgen deprivation.

Radiation Therapy

EBRT has an important role in the palliative care of patients with symptomatic metastatic disease. Painful osseous metastases are successfully palliated in more than 80% of patients.[627] Dose and fractionation schemes vary, but 30 Gy in 10 fractions is commonly used.[628] Although lower doses were initially thought to be equally effective, Blitzer found the duration of response was less for lower doses.[629] Patient longevity should be taken into account when considering fractionation schedules for palliative therapy. For patients with multiple sites of osseous pain, hemibody irradiation may provide pain relief. A single fraction or multiple treatments may be given.[630]

Systemic Radiotherapy

For the patient with multiple sites of painful osseous metastases, the administration of systemic radioisotopes may be considered. Strontium-89 is a calcium analogue that is absorbed by the newly forming bone. Approximately 80% of patients experience reduced pain with strontium-89, but only about 10% of patients become pain free.[631] Recent data suggests an improvement in quality of life for those patients who have a decrease in pain.[632] The major toxicity of this agent is myelosuppression, so adequate bone marrow reserve is required to safely use this form of radiation therapy. Other radionuclides, such as samarium 153 and rhenium 186, have somewhat less hematologic toxicity.[633]

A prospective, randomized trial by Sartor and coworkers showed samarium 153 to be safe and effective in the treatment of painful bony metastases in patients with hormone-refractory prostate cancer.[634] In this trial, 152 men with hormone-refractory prostate cancer and painful bony metastases were enrolled in a prospective, randomized, double-blind trial comparing radioactive samarium 153 and nonradioactive samarium 153. Twice as many patients (2:1) were randomized to the radioactive agent. The results of this trial demonstrated that 1 mCi/kg of samarium 153 is safe and effective for palliation of painful bony metastases in patients with hormone-refractory prostate cancer.[634]

Bisphosphonates

Another option for managing skeletal metastasis in metastatic prostate cancer is the use of bisphosphonates. Bisphosphonates have been shown in clinical trials to improve pain and analgesic scores in men with painful bony metastases,[635] but other trials have not corroborated these results.[636] A potential benefit of bisphosphonate therapy is in preventing osteoporosis caused by prolonged androgen deprivation use in patients with metastatic disease. Osteoporosis associated with androgen deprivation causes an increase in skeletal fractures[637] and potentially bisphosphonates could reduce such fractures. Although bisphosphonates have been shown to decrease skeletal-related events in a randomized clinical trial, optimal scheduling, timing, and duration of treatment still need to be evaluated.[636]

TECHNIQUES OF IRRADIATION

Primary Therapy

External Beam Radiation Therapy

Before starting EBRT, a comfortable and reproducible (supine or prone) position is established on a unit that reproduces the geometry of the treatment machine, and that allows radiologic imaging to define the appropriate treatment volume. According to current standards, this simulation process should incorporate the use of a patient immobilization device and is now typically done with CT imaging.[638] These immobilization devices reduce patient variations in daily patient position, thereby improving the accuracy of treatment delivery.[639,640] In the past, high-density contrast material was instilled into the bladder to help localize the position of the prostate, and contrast material or a radiopaque marker was used to delineate the rectum, but these treatment planning methods have largely been replaced by CT, which can provide more direct visualization of the target (e.g., prostate, seminal vesicles, pelvic nodes) and the adjacent normal tissues. A urethrogram can help in locating the urogenital diaphragm and therefore in locating the apex of the prostate. However, there is considerable debate about how advantageous this procedure is because of reported positional changes caused by the injected contrast material. It is used at some institutions in conjunction with CT planning.[641-644] Because bladder and rectal filling can cause positional changes in target organs and affect the amount of normal tissue irradiated, the amount of bladder and rectal distention should remain as consistent as possible throughout the course of therapy.[645,646] This is typically accomplished by simulating patients with a full bladder and an empty rectum.

Target Volumes

A fundamental consideration in EBRT planning is definition of treatment (i.e., target) volume, which consists of the primary tumor and its clinically or radiographically evident regional extensions (i.e., gross tumor volume), and tissues (e.g., seminal vesicle, lymph nodes) at risk of harboring subclinical tumor deposits (i.e., clinical target volume). The gross tumor volume (GTV) is the prostate gland and any extension of the primary tumor, as determined by clinical or radiologic examinations. The CTV includes GTV and regional sites to which the malignancy may spread but that are beyond the limits of clinical detection (i.e., subclinical disease). Determination of CTV is based on the risk of subclinical disease involvement that may be estimated by correlating pretherapy tumor-related factors with histologic findings of surgical specimens (see "Predictive Factors" and "Pathologic End Points"). Ideally, the decision to treat subclinical sites would also be based on sound clinical studies that attest to the value of such treatment. The planning target volume (PTV) is determined by adding margin to the CTV to account for internal target volume and patient motion, and the field margins are set to conform to the PTV with allowance for the radiation therapy beam dose build-up effect.

Movement of prostate, seminal vesicles, and surrounding tissues (e.g., bladder, rectum) throughout the course of EBRT is a well-recognized phenomenon that is a function of bladder and rectal distention and has particular relevance to the design and dosimetric consequences of a tightly conformed beam arrangement.[645-650] The degree of prostatic motion as demonstrated in several studies can be summarized as follows. Mean right-to-left (RL) motion is generally 1 mm or less with a standard deviation of 4 mm or less; mean anteroposterior (AP) motion is 1.5 mm or less, but the standard deviation is 5 to 6 mm; and the mean motion along the superoinferior (SI) axis is approximately 2 to 3 mm, with a standard deviation of approximately 5 mm.[638] Seminal vesicle motion can be greater and more inconsistent than that of the prostate, and it is more difficult to correct because of a greater degree of deformation from bladder and rectal filling.[651] Little and colleagues, in a study evaluating correction for prostate motion by port films versus B-mode acquisition and targeting (BAT) ultrasound, found that margins that covered the prostate with a 95% confidence level without BAT were 5.3, 10.4, and 10.4 mm in the RL, SI, and AP directions, respectively.[650] The study by Chandra and associates showed that the prostate would be outside the planning target volume approximately one third of the time when using a 5-mm margin without BAT ultrasound to correct for interfractional prostate movement.[648] Studies have compared BAT ultrasound to other methods of prostate localization such as CT and fiducial markers with port films.[648] Results tend to vary by approximately 5 to 7 mm, such that margins of this magnitude are still necessary even when using a method for prostate localization more accurate than port films.

The regional lymphatic tissues may be considered part of the CTV in certain situations, and several observational case series suggested that elective nodal irradiation (ENI) contributed a therapeutic benefit for certain patient subsets.[521,652-654] The RTOG conducted a prospective, randomized trial that evaluated ENI in patients with stage T1b-2 (study 7706) prostate cancer.[655] Patients who had no evidence of nodal involvement by lymphangiography, CT imaging, or lymphadenectomy were assigned to pelvic nodal plus prostatic irradiation or to prostatic irradiation alone. Although ENI did not improve clinical outcome, the study design may not have been sufficient to exclude a therapeutic benefit.[274] Preliminary results of a subsequent trial, RTOG 94-13, show a higher biochemical disease-free survival rate in patients with a risk of lymph node involvement greater than 15%, provided that hormonal therapy was given neoadjuvantly.[516] Some think it is appropriate to use models that estimate the risk of pelvic nodal involvement [146,160] when defining target volume and considering ENI when the risk of LNI reaches or exceeds 15%.[516] Whether to irradiate pelvic lymph nodes remains a controversial issue. For the patient with clinical stage T3 or pelvic node-positive prostate cancer, ENI of the para-aortic nodes does not appear justified.[492]

The goal of ENI of the pelvis is to include the obturator, internal and external iliac lymph nodes. This is often accomplished with a four-field beam arrangement that consists of AP, posteroanterior (PA), and opposed lateral fields (Fig. 50-18). In the past, field margins were typically established through their relationship with certain bony landmarks as follows: superior, the L5-S1 interspace; inferior, bottom of ischial tuberosities; lateral, 2 cm lateral to pelvic inlet; anterior, approximately 1 cm anterior to anterior projection of pubic symphysis; and posterior, the S3-4 interspace. The nodal sites can be contoured using CT scan planning and pelvic fields designed accordingly.[656] Complex blocking to shield portions of the small intestine and rectum is recommended.[657] Alternatively, IMRT can be used. A dose of 45 to 50.4 Gy is recommended[303,526,657] and is often administered in 1.8-Gy once-daily fractions.

The seminal vesicles may also be a site of subclinical tumor extension in patients with clinically localized prostate cancer. The likelihood of SVI may be estimated from predictive models.[146,156,158] Ultrasound-guided biopsy[151] or endorectal-coil MRI[153] may be used in the pretherapy evaluation. However, the role of elective irradiation of the seminal vesicles is controversial,[658,659] and strict indications for its use have not been firmly established. Nonetheless, the seminal vesicles may be included in the CTV if the risk of SVI is 15% or greater,[156] as was suggested for ENI.[160,516] A dose of 50 to 55 Gy was recommended in this setting, whereas 55 to 65 Gy may be given in the presence of established tumor involvement.[526] Exclusion of the seminal vesicles in patients with a low likelihood of SVI may reduce the volume of, and radiation therapy dose to, nontarget normal tissues (e.g., rectum).[156,658] Because the extent of SVI is generally within 1 cm of the junction of the

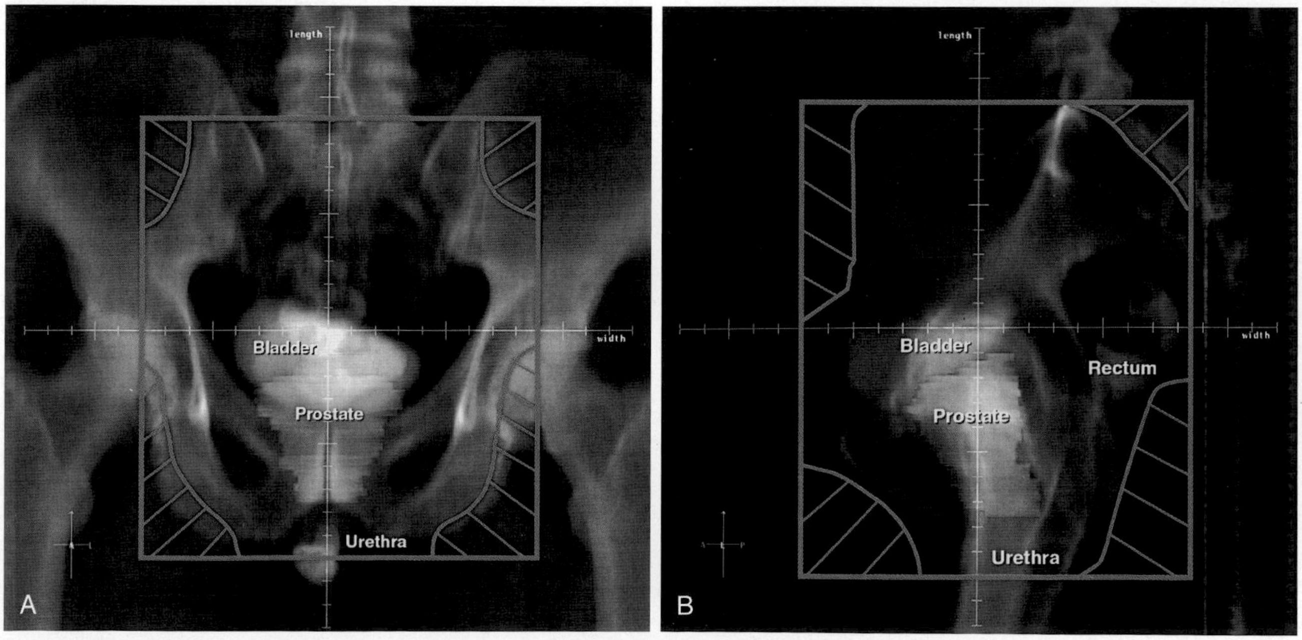

Figure 50-18 Anteroposterior (**A**) and lateral (**B**) views of CT-generated, digitally reconstructed simulation radiographs of a typical four-field arrangement for elective pelvic nodal radiation therapy.

seminal vesicles with the prostatic base,[130] it is not certain whether inclusion of the entire seminal vesicle within the high-dose target volume is routinely required. Although further study is necessary, D'Amico and coworkers[659] concluded that satisfactory outcome could be achieved with irradiation directed solely to the prostate in patients with clinical stage T1-2a disease, a Gleason score of 6 or lower, and a PSA value of 10 ng/mL or less.

IMAGE-BASED TREATMENT PLANNING AND DELIVERY

To accurately delineate target (e.g., prostate) and nontarget (e.g., rectum and bladder) structures, radiologic imaging-based treatment planning should be performed to define target volumes. Although MRI may be used,[660,661] images are typically obtained from a CT scan that reproduces treatment conditions. After GTV is determined, internal (e.g., isocenter) and external (i.e., fiducial) fixed points are established, a margin is added to account for subclinical disease extension,[161,645] and the CTV is defined as part of the prescription procedure. Thereafter, variation in the shape, size, and position of the CTV in relation to the internal fixed point and the position of the patient and radiation therapy beam in relation to external fixed points are accounted for as the internal motion and set-up margins to establish the PTV; these margins are typically in the range of 0.5 cm to 1.0 cm. Roach and associates[161] advocated nonuniform margins, because of the direction and various amounts of prostatic internal motion and the different tolerances of the surrounding (e.g., fibroadipose versus rectal) tissues. With this scheme, the margins added to GTV were defined as anterior and inferior: 2.0 cm; superior and lateral: 1.5 cm; and posterior: 0.5 to 0.75 cm by Roach and colleagues.[161] Techniques for prostate localization before each treatment fraction are now available, such that margins have been decreased substantially to increase dose and limit normal tissue complications. These techniques include BAT ultrasound, fiducial markers with port films, and CT scan.[647-651]

Various EBRT beam arrangements may be used. The latest include six-field (right and left anterior oblique, right and left posterior oblique, opposed lateral) techniques and six- to eight-beam IMRT techniques (Fig. 50-19).[193,662,663]

Sophisticated treatment-planning computers also allow display of DVHs to determine the radiation dose to target (i.e., prostate) and nontarget (e.g., bladder, rectum) tissues, and "idealized" treatment plans may be derived through analysis of DVHs and computerized beam optimization. Studies have provided DVH parameters that serve as treatment planning guidelines for limiting rectal toxicity (Table 50-25).[358,664]

Table 50-25 Dose-Volume Histogram Parameters for Limiting Rectal Complications*

Dose (Gy)	Rectum (%)	Rectal Volume (cc)
30	82†	—
60	40	—
70	26	—
75.6	15.8	3.8
78	5.1	1.4

*Significant cutpoints: $P < .05$.

†Data from Tucker SL, Dong L, Cheung R, et al: Comparison of rectal dose-wall histogram versus dose-volume histogram for modeling the incidence of late rectal bleeding after radiotherapy. Int J Radiat Oncol Biol Phys 60:1589-1601, 2004.

Data from Huang EH, Pollack A, Levy L, et al: Late rectal toxicity: dose volume effects of conformal radiotherapy for prostate cancer. Int J Radiat Oncol Biol Phys 58:1513-1519, 2004.

Brachytherapy

Several techniques for permanent seed brachytherapy have been developed based on prostate imaging. The CT-based method, initially used by Wallner and colleagues, was associated with high rectal and urinary complications, and has largely been discontinued as it does not offer direct intraoperative visualization.[665]

Most permanent prostate brachytherapy incorporates real-time ultrasonography to visualize the prostate (Fig. 50-20). The probe is placed on a fixed stepping device that allows its independent movement relative to the transperineal template. With or without the addition of fluoroscopy, the use of a bi-plane ultrasound probe allows prostate visualization in sagittal and axial mode for accurate prostate imaging. Others are using real-time MRI techniques to perform permanent prostate brachytherapy.[666] Most centers use real-time ultrasonography imaging with various techniques. The Seattle technique employs the use of a preplan based on serial axial transrectal ultrasonography performed in lithotomy position in advance of the implant.[382] Based on an approved plan, needles are loaded with I-125 or Pd-103 and spacers, and used in the operating room to correspond with the plan. Needle placement follows the plan with deposition of each successive needle's seeds. Use of fluoroscopy may assist to assure that the needles are positioned against a zero plane as a reference position. Several vendor-specific products have been developed to mimic this process with seed links or strands. An advantage of this approach is that it allows for multiple plans to be developed in advance of the case and that needle placement in the operating room is generally easy and can be performed in a timely manner. The disadvantage of this process is that it remains difficult to achieve the exact position of the prostate relative to the preplan and that there is no ability to compensate for discrepancies during the case, except to add additional sources at the discretion of the physician.

An alternative technique, originally developed at Mount Sinai, uses an interstitial gun to place each seed individually.[667] The interstitial gun can be used with a preplan but is more commonly used for a real-time implant, where needle positions can be adjusted as needed. Likewise, use of the interstitial applicator is operator dependent and requires a higher degree of dexterity and ultrasound skills.

There are no studies that have directly compared these techniques. However, it is generally understood that implantation quality is similar between the real-time and preplanned techniques.[402]

With advances in software treatment planning systems, Potters and coworkers have reported on a dynamic intraoperative technique that achieves dose conformality based on set parameters for minimum and maximum prostate dose with inverse planning.[440] Using treatment planning software in the operating room, seed location can be determined on actual needle placement, and then followed by dynamic assessment of the dosimetry during the case. Final intraoperative dosimetry appears to correlate to the CT-based dosimetry, with the advantage of using 8% less isotope activity per case (Fig. 50-21). Others are using techniques such as the integration of intraoperative computerization and seed planning to allow greater flexibility during the procedure and to achieve good implantation quality with fewer seeds.[667-669]

HIGH DOSE RATE PROSTATE BRACHYTHERAPY

Generally reserved for patients with locally advanced patients, HDR brachytherapy (HDR-BT) offers a boost treat-

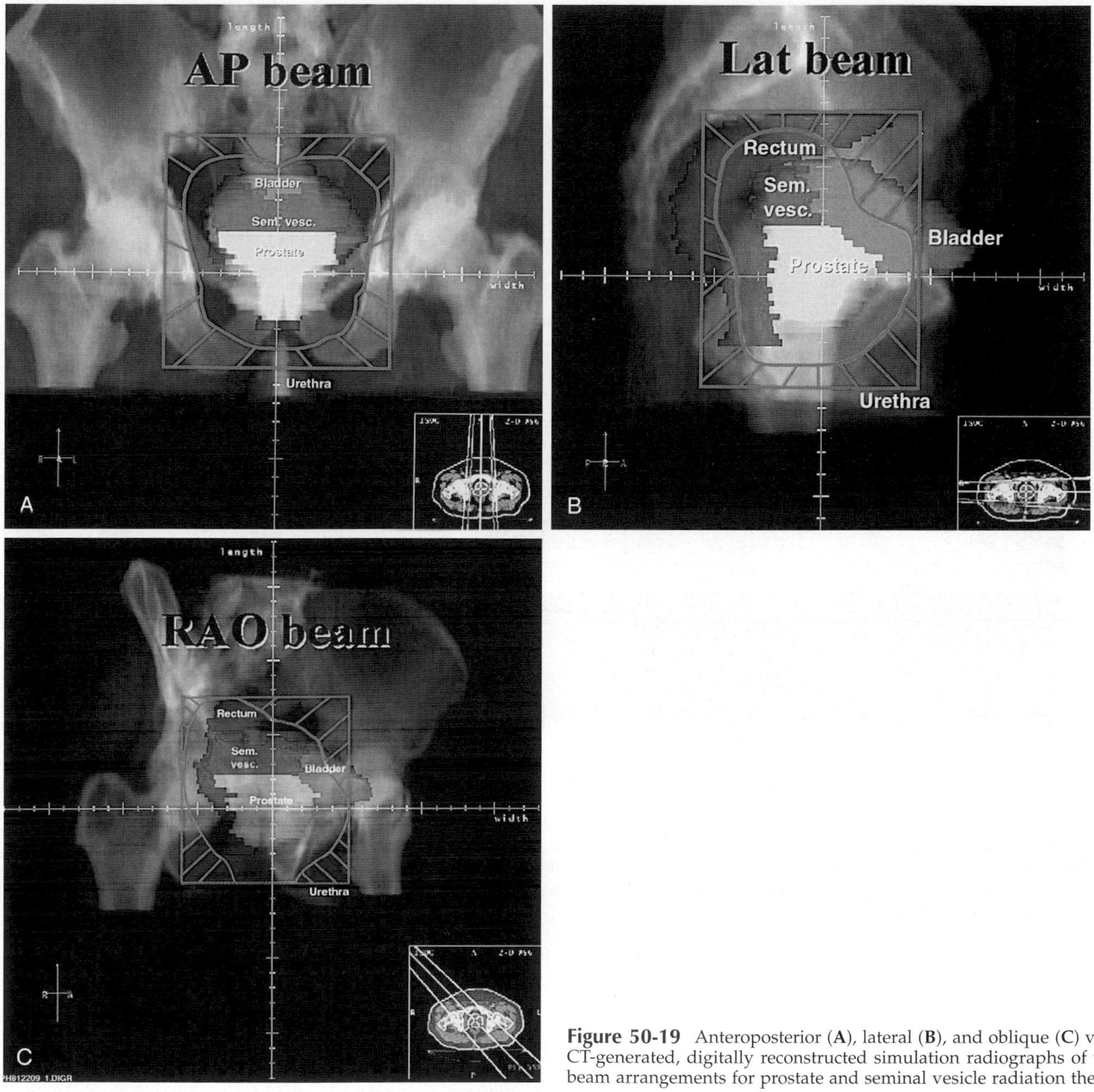

Figure 50-19 Anteroposterior (**A**), lateral (**B**), and oblique (**C**) views of CT-generated, digitally reconstructed simulation radiographs of various beam arrangements for prostate and seminal vesicle radiation therapy.

ment option to EBRT. By placing HDR afterloading needles directly into the prostate gland under real-time ultrasound guidance, a steep dose gradient between the prostate and adjacent normal tissues can be generated that is unaffected by organ motion and edema or treatment setup uncertainties. The ability to control the amount of time the single radioactive source dwells at each position along the length of each brachytherapy catheter further enhances the conformity of the dose. Data from several groups performing HDR-BT in patients with locally advanced disease suggest similar tumor control as 3D-conformal EBRT with the added advantages of reduced treatment times, less acute toxicity, and no additional technologic requirements to account and correct for treatment setup uncertainties and organ motion.[670-673] The issues that remain unresolved with this technique (as with other methods of dose escalation) revolve around the amount of additional dose required to provide optimal tumor control, the role of androgen deprivation in the management of patients with locally advanced disease, and whether the regional lymphatics should be irradiated. Real-time, conformal techniques control for dose to normal tissues while boosting the prostate, usually in 3 fractions, and better eliminate problems associated with catheter movement between fractions, when performed as a single needle implant.[674]

Postoperative Therapy

Adjuvant Irradiation

Adjuvant irradiation typically begins 2 to 4 months after surgery, when maximal urinary control is established and there is complete wound healing without urinary extravasation or anastomotic stricture. Evidence-based recommenda-

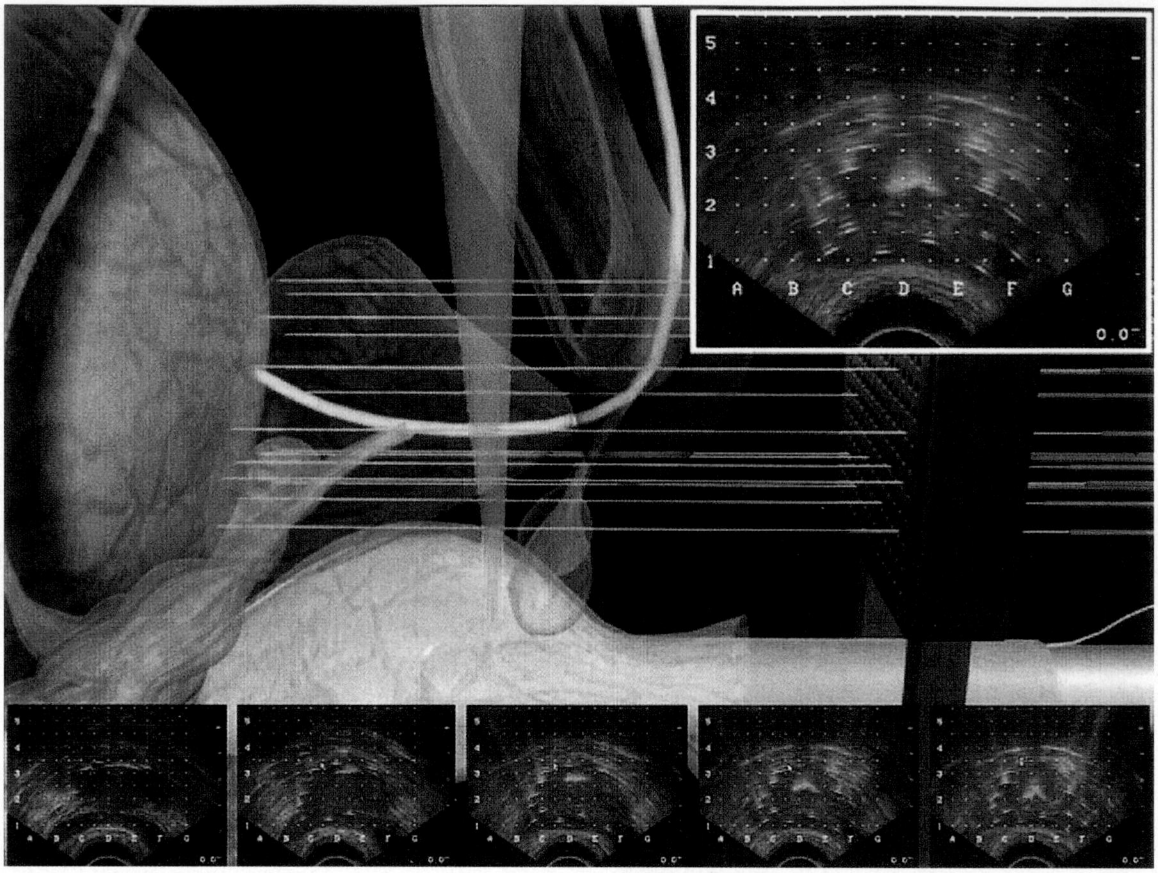

Figure 50-20 Axial-view image of permanent prostate brachytherapy. (Courtesy of Louis Potters, MD, Memorial Sloan-Kettering Cancer Center at Mercy Medical Center, Rockville Center, NY.)

tions for preirradiation evaluation are not available, but it is prudent to obtain a serum PSA level.

Although pelvic nodal irradiation was sometimes used in early reports, more recent series and clinical trials defined the prostatic fossa as the target,[538,543,545] which is optimally identified with CT scan. Definition of the clinical target volume (CTV) can be aided by use of bladder, rectal, and urethral contrast instilled at simulation, and by combining preoperative radiologic imaging information and the details of the operative procedure and pathologic examination (e.g., prostatic dimensions, sites of extraprostatic tumor extension, and margin involvement). A preoperative CT may be valuable for determining the positions of the prostate and seminal vesicles in relation to bony landmarks. The preoperative location of the prostate ± seminal vesicles with their surrounding fibroadipose and fascial tissues is considered the CTV,[628] which is customized to individual patient-specific circumstances (Fig. 50-22). In the presence of seminal vesicle invasion, tumor extent is generally within 2 cm of the junction of the seminal vesicle with the prostatic base.[675] and this observation may be considered when designing the field and prescribing dose. The vesicourethral anastomosis can be quite low in the pelvis, and a CT urethrogram can aid in defining this structure.

The planning target volume (PTV) encompasses the CTV with margins to account for daily set-up variation and internal target movement. Although ideal margins have not been defined, the addition of 5 to 15 mm to the CTV is appropriate.[676] The field margins are then set by considering the field edge/dose buildup characteristics of the treatment equipment. Customized complex blocking material, multileaf collimation, or intensity-modulation should be used to conform the dose to the PTV.

There is limited information about the dose-volume characteristics of the normal critical structure and the risk of side effects,[548] so the ideal planning constraints are not sufficiently defined. Cozzarini and associates contoured from the anal verge to the rectosigmoid junction as a solid organ and found that the dose-volume histogram correlated with the risk of late intermittent or more severe hematochezia.[548] This risk was about 7% by 3 years if the rectal volume that received 50 Gy (i.e., V50) was less than 63%, V55 for less than 57%, or V60 for less than 50%, whereas it was approximately three times greater if these parameters were exceeded. Although a dose-volume relationship for erectile dysfunction has not been reported with postoperative radiation therapy, there is an association in the context of primary irradiation. Erectile dysfunction is more common when the mean dose to the penile bulb exceeds 52.5 Gy,[677] or when 60% of the penile bulb (i.e., D60) receives more than 42 Gy.[678] Studies of conformal primary irradiation do not demonstrate a clear relationship between bladder dose-volume parameters and complications, but a literature review suggested that a 5% to 10% rate of moderate to severe complications exists when the whole bladder dose does not surpass 50 Gy, or the V55-65 is 33% to 50% and the V65-75 is less than 20%.[679]

The American College of Radiology Appropriateness Criteria and the Patterns of Care Consensus Committee recommend treatment of the prostatic fossa to 59.4 to 66.6 Gy,[526,680] and this is consistent with reports in the literature. For the

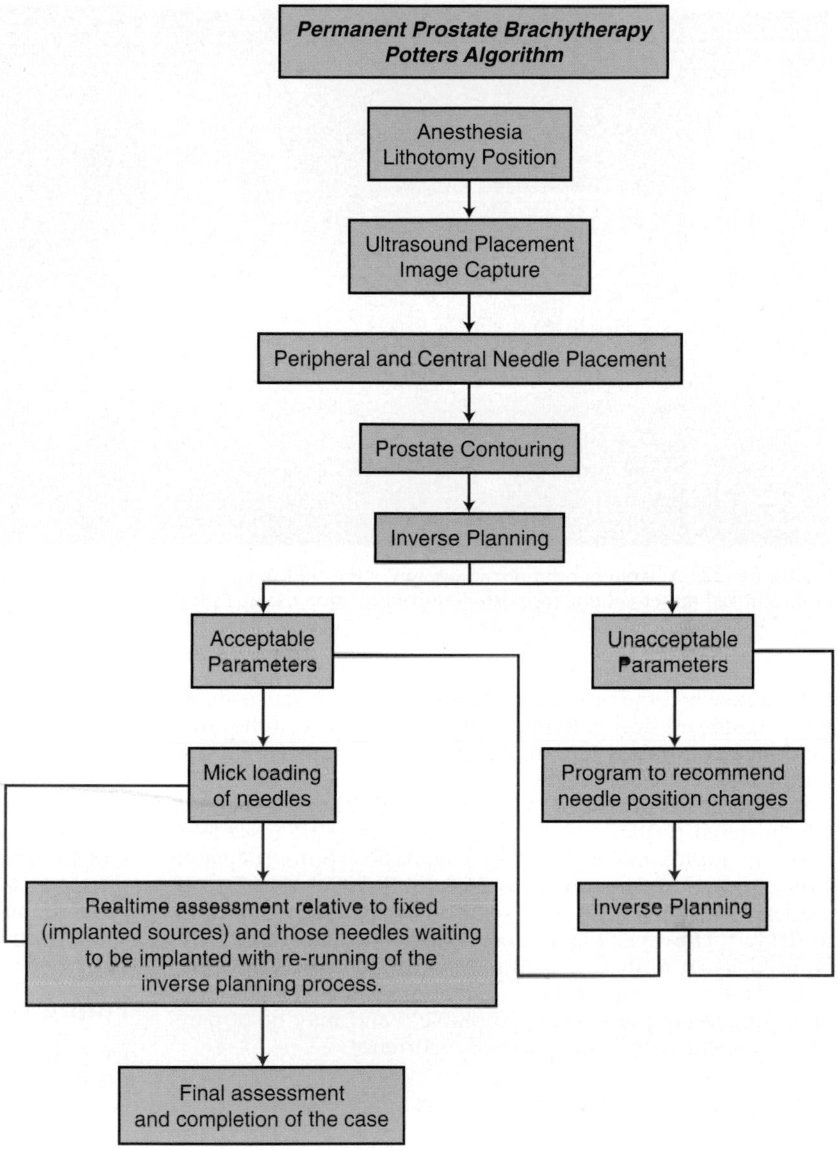

Figure 50-21 Dynamic prostate implant algorithm using treatment planning systems that employ inverse planning techniques. (Reprinted from Brachytherapy, vol. 2 [3]: Potters L, Calguaru E, Thornton B, et al: Toward a dynamic real-time intraoperative permanent prostate brachytherapy methodology, pp 172-180. Copyright 2003, with permission from American Brachytherapy Society.)

patient with regional lymph node involvement, androgen deprivation therapy should be considered.[527] The role of adjuvant radiotherapy is uncertain in this setting.

Biochemical Relapse

The principles of EBRT target volume definition are similar to those used in the adjuvant setting (previously discussed), as the prostatic fossa only was treated in most reports and this is typically considered the CTV (see Fig. 50-22) when the initial surgery showed no evidence for pelvic nodal involvement.[526] The CTV is determined by CT-based planning with complex blocking, which is aided by use of bladder and urethral contrast, and by considering preoperative, operative, and pathology information. Connolly and colleagues documented the sites of sonographically apparent local tumor recurrence, which was at the anastomosis (69%), bladder neck (17%), or retrotrigone (14%),[555] and this information may also be instrumental in designing the CTV. The PTV encompasses the CTV with margins to account for daily set-up variation and internal target movement. Although ideal margins have not been defined, the addition of 5 to 15 mm to the CTV is appropriate.[676]

The optimal dose has not been defined, but 64.0 to 64.8 Gy given in 32 to 36 fractions is typical in the literature. Somewhat higher doses, up to 70 Gy, may be considered if a favorable dose-volume relationship can be achieved in the surrounding organs at risk. Dose-volume constraints for the bladder and rectum are similar to those described for adjuvant therapy.

Clinical Local Recurrence

The focus and intensity of EBRT changes when a prostatic fossa mass is present. More extensive radiologic evaluation and fusion (that is, overlaying and merging the digital magnetic resonance and computed tomographic images) of complementary imaging modalities may provide optimal identification of the complete extent of the mass. It may also be possible to use the surgical clips placed during prostatectomy or insert gold markers into the mass to allow precise localization of the tumor at each daily treatment session, as is

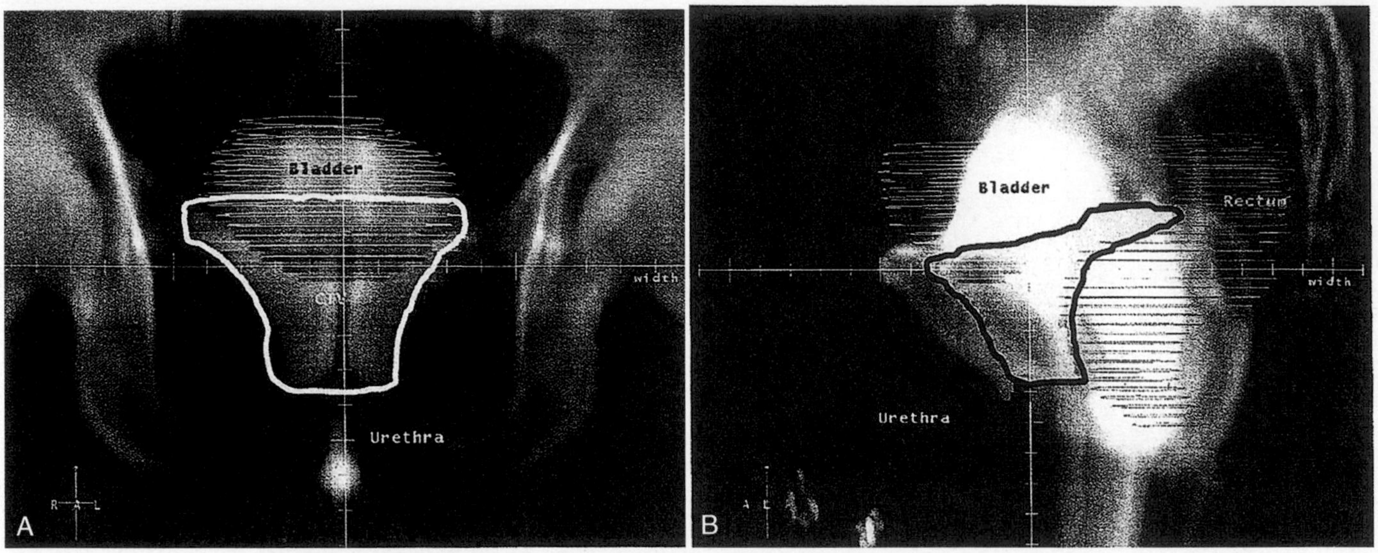

Figure 50-22 **A,** Anteroposterior radiograph of the clinical target volume for postoperative radiation therapy planning. **B,** Lateral radiograph of the clinical target volume for postoperative radiation therapy planning.

now done when the prostate is in situ.[681] IMRT may also allow for a significant dose differential in the targeted volume, and this can be exploited to administer a higher dose within the tumor than in the remaining prostatic fossa.

For the series described in Table 50-24, EBRT was generally administered to the local recurrence and prostatic fossa to a dose of approximately 65 Gy. The ACR Appropriateness Criteria advocate treatment to 66.6 to 70.2 Gy over 7 to 8 weeks,[680] and the PCS Consensus Committee recommends 65 to 70 Gy.[526] However, higher doses may be necessary and may be used when normal structure dose-volume constraints are considered with three-dimensional approaches. The addition of androgen suppression is acceptable[526] and may be of particular benefit with a bulky tumor recurrence.

TREATMENT ALGORITHM AND FUTURE DIRECTIONS

Practice guideline development methods were set forth by the Agency for Healthcare Policy and Research. Multidisciplinary efforts of this nature are centered on analysis of existing scientific outcome and technology assessment studies in an environment of consensus building. Clinical practice guidelines so derived are meant to apply to most, but not all, patients with the specified condition. It is essential that patient evaluation and the management decisions are made in light of all circumstances of an individual case. In this context, the ACR,[302,657,680] the National Comprehensive Cancer Network (NCCN),[303] the Patterns of Care Study Consensus Committee,[526] and the Preferred Oncology Network of America[682] provided management pathways relevant to pretherapy evaluation, radiotherapeutic care, posttherapy surveillance, and salvage therapy for patients with prostate cancer. Application of these guidelines will not necessarily ensure optimal outcome, so the clinician must exercise independent medical judgment to determine an individual patient's best care program. Likewise, as new studies are reported and more current information emerges, this must drive diagnostic and treatment decisions because formal guidelines are only updated periodically. There has been a rapidly advancing technologic revolution in diagnostic imaging and radiation treatment derived from computer-driven applications that can quickly make adopted guidelines and recommendations obsolete.

The latest NCCN recommendations are presented in Figure 50-23.[303] The recent trend has been toward evidence-based medicine tailored as much as possible for the individual patient. This is especially pertinent in cancer care, in which prospectively randomized and retrospective studies often provide generalized information for a disease that can have significantly diverse variables in selected populations and individuals.

Future Directions

Despite an abundant medical literature, nearly all facets of prostate cancer are under active investigation. The variable natural history of a condition with a high autopsy incidence[7,8] calls for an improved understanding of the role of early detection and the factors that initiate and promote clinical expression of the disorder.[683] Once the diagnosis is established, appropriate combinations of host- and tumor-related characteristics are necessary to establish reliable prognostic indices and groupings to identify suitable patient groups for management strategies that befit the risk for and nature of tumor progression.[250,251] Use of artificial neural networks[684] may allow departure from an anatomic-based and compartmentalized (i.e., bin) stage grouping system to a model that incorporates a broad spectrum (e.g., anatomic, histologic, serologic, molecular) of reproducible predictors into a unified system that may improve prognostic accuracy. Identification of intermediate and surrogate end points for clinical outcomes (e.g., PSA relapse) may allow enrollment of patient groups apt to benefit from a particular intervention while the statistical efficiency of the trial is enhanced and the required number of participants and trial duration are reduced.[685] Future research efforts may uncover therapeutic advances more rapidly than previously possible.

During the next few years, advances in radiation oncology are apt to occur along several fronts, many of which were discussed in the foregoing sections in concert with its pertinent subject matter (see "Locally Advanced Disease"). Some of these areas include evaluation of new methods; modalities

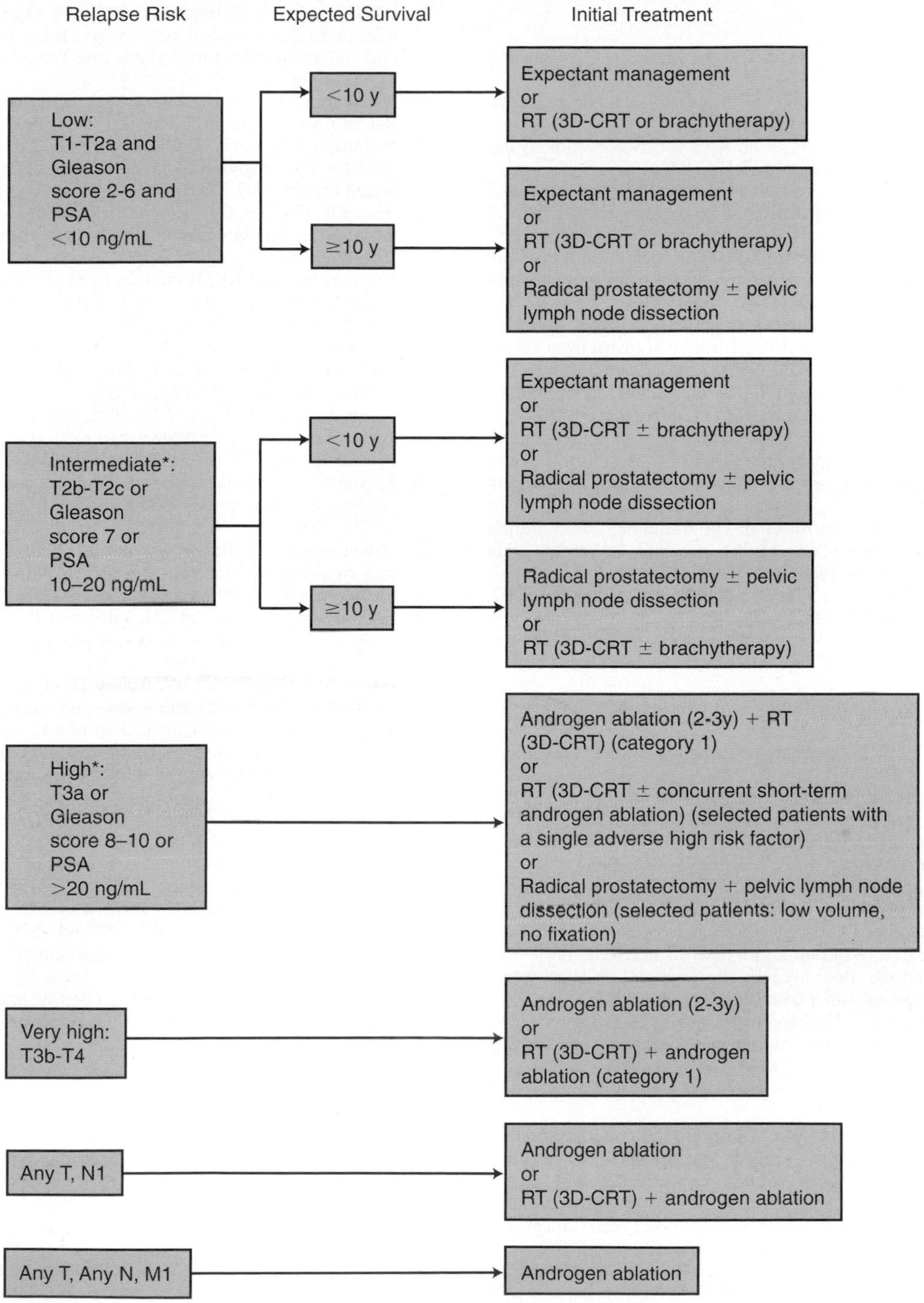

*Patients with multiple adverse factors may be shifted into the next higher risk group.

Figure 50-23 Prostate cancer treatment algorithm: Clinical practice guidelines by the National Comprehensive Cancer Network: prostate cancer version 1:2004. 3D-CRT, three-dimensional conformal radiation therapy; PSA, prostate-specific antigen; RT, radiation therapy. (From National Comprehensive Cancer Network: Prostate cancer NCCN clinical practice guidelines for oncology. J NCCN 2:224, 2004.)

and technologies such as IMRT, proton therapy, and image-guided therapy in general; better application and delivery in prostate brachytherapy; dose-response and toxicity relationships for escalated dose levels; hormonal, chemotherapeutic, and molecular therapy interactions with radiation; better treatment for relapse after irradiation; and economic and quality-of-life assessments. In these and other areas, hypotheses derived from the observational case series will yield to the scientific method as embodied in the prospective clinical trial, which will serve as the avenue through which undisputed improvements in the care of patients with prostate cancer will become a reality.

REFERENCES

1. Jemal A, Siegal R, Ward E, et al: Cancer statistics. CA Cancer J Clin 56:106-130, 2006.
2. Lu-Yao GL, Greenberg ER: Changes in prostate cancer incidence and treatment in USA. Lancet 343:251, 1994.
3. Devesa SS, Blot WJ, Stone BJ, et al: Recent cancer trends in the United States. J Natl Cancer Inst 87:175, 1995.
4. Potosky AL, Miller BA, Albertsen PC, et al: The role of increasing detection in the rising incidence of prostate cancer. JAMA 273:548, 1995.
5. Jacobsen SJ, Katusic SK, Bergstralh EJ, et al: Incidence of prostate cancer diagnosis in the eras before and after serum prostate-specific antigen testing. JAMA 274:1445, 1995.
6. Potosky AL, Kessler L, Gridley G, et al: Rise in prostatic cancer incidence associated with increased use of transurethral resection. J Natl Cancer Inst 82:1624, 1990.
7. Breslow N, Chan CW, Dhom G, et al: Latent carcinoma of prostate of autopsy in seven areas. Int J Cancer 20:680, 1977.
8. Stemmermann GN, Nomura AM, Chyou PH, et al: A prospective comparison of prostate cancer at autopsy and as a clinical event: the Hawaii Japanese experience. Cancer Epidemiol Biomarkers Prev 1:189, 1992.
9. Sakr WA, Haas GP, Cassin BF, et al: The frequency of carcinoma and intraepithelial neoplasia of the prostate in young male patients. J Urol 150:379, 1993.
10. Parkin DM, Bray F, Ferlay J, et al: Global cancer statistics, 2002. CA Cancer J Clin 55:74, 2005.
11. Begg CB: Methodological issues in studies of the treatment, diagnosis, and etiology of prostate cancer. Semin Oncol 21:569, 1994.
12. Haas GP, Sakr WA: Epidemiology of prostate cancer. CA Cancer J Clin 47:273, 1997.
13. Pienta KJ, Esper PS: Risk factors for prostate cancer. Ann Intern Med 118:793, 1993.
14. Morton RA: Racial differences in adenocarcinoma of the prostate in North American men. Urology 44:637, 1994.
15. Smith DS, Bullock AD, Catalona WJ, et al: Racial differences in a prostate cancer screening study. J Urol 156:1366, 1996.
16. Carter BS, Bova GS, Beaty TH, et al: Hereditary prostate cancer: epidemiologic and clinical features. J Urol 150:797, 1993.
17. Gronberg H, Damber L, Damber JE: Studies of genetic factors in prostate cancer in a twin population. J Urol 152:1484, 1994.
18. Neugut AI, Chen AC, Petrylak DP: The "skinny" on obesity and prostate cancer prognosis. J Clin Oncol 22:395, 2004.
19. Calle EE, Rodriquez C, Walker-Thurmond K, et al: Overweight, obesity, and mortality from cancer in a prospectively studied cohort of U.S. adults. N Engl J Med 348:1625, 2003.
20. Isaacs JT: Hormonal balance and the risk of prostatic cancer. J Cell Biochem Suppl 16H:107, 1992.
21. Armenian HK, Lilienfeld AM, Diamond EL, et al: Relation between benign prostatic hyperplasia and cancer of the prostate: a prospective and retrospective study. Lancet 2:115, 1974.
22. Greenwald P, Kirmss V, Polan AK, et al: Cancer of the prostate among men with benign prostatic hyperplasia. J Natl Cancer Inst 53:335, 1974.
23. Barrett-Connor E, Garland C, McPhillips JB, et al: A prospective, population-based study of androstenedione, estrogens, and prostatic cancer. Cancer Res 50:169, 1990.
24. Nomura A, Heilbrun LK, Stemmermann GN, et al: Prediagnostic serum hormones and the risk of prostate cancer. Cancer Res 48:3515, 1988.
25. Ross R, Bernstein L, Judd H, et al: Serum testosterone levels in healthy young black and white men. J Natl Cancer Inst 76:45, 1986.
26. Ross RK, Bernstein L, Lobo RA, et al: 5-Alpha-reductase activity and risk of prostate cancer among Japanese and U.S. white and black males. Lancet 339:887, 1992.
27. Aprikian AG, Bazinet M, Plante M, et al: Family history and the risk of prostatic carcinoma in a high-risk group of urological patients. J Urol 154:404, 1995.
28. Hayes RB, Liff JM, Pottern LM, et al: Prostate cancer risk in U.S. blacks and whites with a family history of cancer. Int J Cancer 60:361, 1995.
29. Whittemore AS, Kolonel LN, Wu AH, et al: Prostate cancer in relation to diet, physical activity, and body size in blacks, whites, and Asians in the United States and Canada. J Natl Cancer Inst 87:652, 1995.
30. Steinberg GD, Carter BS, Beaty TH, et al: Family history and the risk of prostate cancer. Prostate 17:337, 1990.
31. Tulinius H, Egilsson V, Olafsdottir GH, et al: Risk of prostate, ovarian, and endometrial cancer among relatives of women with breast cancer. BMJ 305:855, 1992.
32. Ross RK, Coetzee GA, Reichardt J, et al: Does the racial-ethnic variation in prostate cancer risk have a hormonal basis? Cancer 75:1778, 1995.
33. Shimizu H, Ross RK, Bernstein L, et al: Cancers of the prostate and breast among Japanese and white immigrants in Los Angeles County. Br J Cancer 63:963, 1991.
34. Natarajan N, Murphy GP, Mettlin C: Prostate cancer in blacks: an update from the American College of Surgeons' Patterns of Care studies. J Surg Oncol 40:232, 1989.
35. Pienta KJ, Demers R, Hoff M, et al: Effect of age and race on the survival of men with prostate cancer in the metropolitan Detroit tri-county area 1973 to 1987. Urology 45:93, 1995.
36. Baquet CR, Horm JW, Gibbs T, et al: Socioeconomic factors and cancer incidence among blacks and whites. J Natl Cancer Inst 83:551, 1991.
37. Armstrong B, Doll R: Environmental factors and cancer incidence and mortality in different countries, with special reference to dietary practices. Int J Cancer 15:617, 1975.
38. Le Marchand L, Kolonel LN, Wilkens LR, et al: Animal fat consumption and prostate cancer: a prospective study in Hawaii. Epidemiology 5:276, 1994.
39. Hsing AW, Comstock GW, Abbey H, et al: Serologic precursors of cancer. Retinol, carotenoids, and tocopherol and risk of prostate cancer. J Natl Cancer Inst 82:941, 1990.
40. Giovannucci E, Ascherio A, Rimm EB, et al: Intake of carotenoids and retinol in relation to risk of prostate cancer. J Natl Cancer Inst 87:1767, 1995.
41. Stephens FO: Phytoestrogens and prostate cancer. Possible preventive role. Med J Aust 167:138, 1997.
42. Hanchette CL, Schwartz GG: Geographic patterns of prostate cancer mortality: evidence for a protective effect of ultraviolet radiation. Cancer 70:2861, 1992.
43. Mills PK, Beeson WL, Phillips RL, et al: Cohort study of diet, lifestyle, and prostate cancer in Adventist men. Cancer 64:598, 1989.
44. Calle EE, Kaaks R: Overweight, obesity, and cancer: epidemiological evidence and proposed mechanisms. Nat Rev Can 8:579, 2004.
45. Checkoway H, DiFerdinando G, Hulka BS, et al: Medical, lifestyle, and occupational risk factors for prostate cancer. Prostate 10:79, 1987.
46. van der Gulden JW, Verbeek AL, Kolk JJ: Smoking and drinking habits in relation to prostate cancer. Br J Urol 73:382, 1994.
47. Cerhan JR, Torner JC, Lynch CF, et al: Association of smoking, body mass, and physical activity with risk of prostate cancer in the Iowa 65+ Rural Health study (United States). Cancer Causes Control 8:229, 1997.
48. Thune I, Lund E: Physical activity and the risk of prostate and testicular cancer: a cohort study of 53,000 Norwegian men. Cancer Causes Control 5:549, 1994.
49. Moyad MA, Carroll PR: Lifestyle recommendations to prevent prostate cancer. Part I. Time to redirect our attention? Urol Clin North Am 31:289, 2004.
50. Pierotti B, Altieri A, Talamini R, et al: Lifetime physical activity and prostate cancer risk. Int J Cancer 114:639, 2005.
51. Cuzick J: Human papillomavirus infection of the prostate. Cancer Surveys 23:91, 1995.
52. Ross RK, Deapen DM, Casagrande JT, et al: A cohort study of mortality from cancer of the prostate in Catholic priests. Br J Cancer 43:233, 1981.
53. Honda GD, Bernstein L, Ross RK, et al: Vasectomy, cigarette smoking, and age at first sexual intercourse as risk factors for prostate cancer in middle-aged men. Br J Cancer 57:326, 1988.
54. van der Gulden JW, Kolk JJ, Verbeek AL: Prostate cancer and work environment. J Occup Med 34:402, 1992.

55. Elghany NA, Schumacher MC, Slattery ML, et al: Occupation, cadmium exposure, and prostate cancer. Epidemiology 1:107, 1990.
56. Ross RK, Paganini-Hill A, Henderson BE: The etiology of prostate cancer. What does the epidemiology suggest? Prostate 4:333, 1983.
57. Anderson DJ, Alexander NJ, Fulgham DL, et al: Immunity to tumor-associated antigens in vasectomized men. J Natl Cancer Inst 69:551, 1982.
58. Giovannucci E, Ascherio A, Rimm EB, et al: A prospective cohort study of vasectomy and prostate cancer in U.S. men. JAMA 269:873, 1993.
59. Giovannucci E, Tosteson TD, Speizer FE, et al: A retrospective cohort study of vasectomy and prostate cancer in U.S. men. JAMA 269:878, 1993.
60. DerSimonian R, Clemens J, Spirtas R, et al: Vasectomy and prostate cancer risk. Methodological review of the evidence. J Clin Epidemiol 46:163, 1993.
61. John EM, Whittemore AS, Wu AH, et al: Vasectomy and prostate cancer—results from a multiethnic case-control study. J Natl Cancer Inst 87:662, 1995.
62. Sidney S, Quesenberry CP Jr, Sadler MC, et al: Vasectomy and the risk of prostate cancer in a cohort of multiphasic health-checkup examinees. Second report. Cancer Causes Control 2:113, 1991.
63. Healy B: From the National Institutes of Health. JAMA 269:2620, 1993.
64. Bostwick DG: High grade prostatic intraepithelial neoplasia. The most likely precursor of prostate cancer. Cancer 75:1823, 1995.
65. Bostwick DG, Pacelli A, Lopez-Beltran A: Molecular biology of prostatic intraepithelial neoplasia. Prostate 29:117, 1996.
66. Sakr WA, Grignon DJ, Haas GP, et al: Age and racial distribution of prostatic intraepithelial neoplasia. Eur Urol 30:138, 1996.
67. Qian J, Wollan P, Bostwick DG: The extent and multicentricity of high-grade prostatic intraepithelial neoplasia in clinically localized prostatic adenocarcinoma. Hum Pathol 28:143, 1997.
68. Davidson D, Bostwick DG, Qian JQ, et al: Prostatic intraepithelial neoplasia is a risk factor for adenocarcinoma. Predictive accuracy in needle biopsies. J Urol 154:1295, 1995.
69. Abdel-Khalek M, El-Baz M, Ibrahiem el-H, et al: Predictors of prostate cancer on extended biopsy in patients with high-grade prostatic intraepithelial neoplasia: a multivariate analysis model. BJU Int 94:528, 2004.
70. Shepherd D, Keetch DW, Humphrey PA, et al: Repeat biopsy strategy in men with isolated prostatic intraepithelial neoplasia on prostate needle biopsy. J Urol 156:460, 1996.
71. Ashida S, Nakagawa H, Katagiri T, et al: Molecular features of the transition from prostatic intraepithelial neoplasia (PIN) to prostate cancer; genome-wide gene expression profiles of prostate cancers and PINs. Cancer Res 64:5963, 2004.
72. Bostwick DG: Target populations and strategies for chemoprevention trials of prostate cancer. J Cell Biochem Suppl 19:191, 1994.
73. Thompson IM, Goodman PJ, Tangen CM, et al: The influence of finasteride on the development of prostate cancer. N Engl J Med 349:215, 2003.
74. von Eschenbach A, Ho R, Murphy GP, et al: American Cancer Society guideline for the early detection of prostate cancer: update 1997. CA Cancer J Clin 47:261,1997.
75. Gerber GS, Thompson IM, Thisted R, et al: Disease-specific survival following routine prostate cancer screening by digital rectal examination. JAMA 269:61, 1993.
76. Mettlin C, Murphy GP, Babaian RJ, et al: The results of a five-year early prostate cancer detection intervention. Cancer 77:150, 1996.
77. Catalona WJ, Richie JP, Ahmann FR, et al: Comparison of digital rectal examination and serum prostate specific antigen in the early detection of prostate cancer: results of a multicenter clinical trial of 6,630 men. J Urol 151:1283, 1994.
78. Gann PH, Hennekens CH, Stampfer MJ: A prospective evaluation of plasma prostate-specific antigen for detection of prostatic cancer. JAMA 273:289, 1995.
79. Littrup PJ, Goodman AC, Mettlin CJ: The benefit and cost of prostate cancer early detection. CA Cancer J Clin 43:134, 1993.
80. Gustafsson O, Carlsson P, Norming et al: Cost-effectiveness analysis in early detection of prostate cancer: an evaluation of six screening strategies in a randomly selected population of 2,400 men. Prostate 26:299, 1995.
81. Benoit RM, Naslund MJ: An economic rationale for prostate cancer screening. Urology 44:795, 1994.
82. Andriole GL, Levin DL, Crawford ED, et al: Prostate cancer screening in the Prostate, Lung, Colorectal and Ovarian (PLCO) cancer screening trial: findings from the initial screening round of a randomized trial. J Natl Cancer Inst 97:433, 2005.
83. Dalkin BL, Ahmann FR, Kopp JB: Prostate specific antigen levels in men older than 50 years without clinical evidence of prostatic carcinoma. J Urol 150:1837, 1993.
84. Oesterling JE, Jacobsen SJ, Chute CG, et al: Serum prostate-specific antigen in a community-based population of healthy men. Establishment of age-specific reference ranges. JAMA 270:860, 1993.
85. Oesterling JE, Kumamoto Y, Tsukamoto T, et al: Serum prostate-specific antigen in a community-based population of healthy Japanese men: lower values than for similarly aged white men. Br J Urol 75:347, 1995.
86. Morgan TO, Jacobsen SJ, McCarthy WF, et al: Age-specific reference ranges for serum prostate-specific antigen in black men. N Engl J Med 335:304, 1996.
87. Anderson JR, Strickland D, Corbin D, et al: Age-specific reference ranges for serum prostate-specific antigen. Urology 46:54, 1995.
88. El-Galley RE, Petros JA, Sanders WH, et al: Normal range prostate-specific antigen versus age-specific prostate-specific antigen in screening prostate adenocarcinoma. Urology 46:200, 1995.
89. DeAntoni EP, Crawford ED, Oesterling JE, et al: Age- and race-specific reference ranges for prostate-specific antigen from a large community-based study. Urology 48:234, 1996.
90. Carter HB, Pearson JD, Metter J, et al: Longitudinal evaluation of prostate-specific antigen levels in men with and without prostate disease. JAMA 267:2215, 1992.
91. Smith DS, Catalona WJ: Rate of change in serum prostate specific antigen levels as a method for prostate cancer detection. J Urol 152:1163, 1994.
92. Carter HB, Pearson JD, Waclawiw Z, et al: Prostate-specific antigen variability in men without prostate cancer: effect of sampling interval on prostate-specific antigen velocity. Urology 45:591, 1995.
93. Kadmon P, Weinberg AD, Williams RH, et al: Pitfalls in interpreting prostate specific antigen velocity. J Urol 155:1655, 1996.
94. Partin AW, Carter HB, Chan DW, et al: Prostate specific antigen in the staging of localized prostate cancer: influence of tumor differentiation, tumor volume and benign hyperplasia. J Urol 143:747, 1990.
95. Benson MC, Whang IS, Olsson CA, et al: The use of prostate specific antigen density to enhance the predictive value of intermediate levels of serum prostate specific antigen. J Urol 147:817, 1992.
96. Bazinet M, Meshref AW, Trudel C, et al: Prospective evaluation of prostate-specific antigen density and systematic biopsies for early detection of prostatic carcinoma. Urology 43:44, 1994.
97. Meshref AW, Bazinet M, Trudel C, et al: Role of prostate-specific antigen density after applying age-specific prostate-specific antigen reference ranges. Urology 45:972, 1995.
98. Brawer MK, Aramburu EAG, Chen GL, et al: The inability of prostate specific antigen index to enhance the predictive value of prostate specific antigen in the diagnosis of prostatic carcinoma. J Urol 150:369, 1993.
99. Catalona WJ, Richie JP, deKernion JB, et al: Comparison of prostate specific antigen concentration versus prostate specific antigen density in the early detection of prostate cancer-receiver operating characteristic curves. J Urol 152:2031, 1994.
100. Mettlin C, Littrup PJ, Kane RA, et al: Relative sensitivity and specificity of serum prostate specific antigen (PSA) level compared with age-referenced PSA, PSA density and PSA change-data from the American Cancer Society National Prostate Cancer Detection Project. Cancer 74:1615, 1994.
101. Kalish J, Cooner WH, Graham SD Jr: Serum PSA adjusted for volume of transition zone (PSAT) is more accurate than PSA

adjusted for total gland volume (PSAD) in detecting adenocarcinoma of the prostate. Urology 43:601, 1994.
102. Stenman UH, Leinonen J, Alfthan H, et al: A complex between prostate-specific antigen and alpha 1-antichymotrypsin is the major form of prostate-specific antigen in serum of patients with prostatic cancer: assay of the complex improves clinical sensitivity for cancer. Cancer Res 51:222, 1991.
103. Catalona WJ, Smith DS, Wolfert RL, et al: Evaluation of percentage of free serum prostate-specific antigen to improve specificity of prostate cancer screening. JAMA 274:1214, 1995.
104. Luderer AA, Chen YT, Soriano TF, et al: Measurement of the proportion of free to total prostate-specific antigen improves diagnostic performance of prostate-specific antigen in the diagnostic gray zone of total prostate-specific antigen. Urology 46:187, 1995.
105. Oesterling JE, Jacobsen SJ, Klee GG, et al: Free, complexed and total serum prostate specific antigen: the establishment of appropriate reference ranges for their concentrations and ratios. J Urol 154:1090, 1995.
106. Thiel RP, Oesterling JE, Wojno KJ, et al: Multicenter comparison of the diagnostic performance of free prostate-specific antigen. Urology 48:45, 1996.
107. Vashi AR, Oesterling JE: Percent free prostate-specific antigen. Entering a new era in the detection of prostate cancer. Mayo Clin Proc 72:337, 1997.
108. Gohagan JK, Prorok PC, Kramer BS, et al: The Prostate, Lung, Colorectal, and Ovarian Cancer Screening Trial of the National Cancer Institute. Cancer 75:1869, 1995.
109. Rouvière H: Anatomy of the Human Lymphatic System. Ann Arbor, MI, Edwards Brothers, 1938.
110. Bonkhoff H, Stein U, Remberger K: The proliferative function of basal cells in the normal and hyperplastic human prostate. Prostate 24:114, 1994.
111. Bostwick DG, Brawer MK: Prostatic intra-epithelial neoplasia and early invasion in prostate cancer. Cancer 59:788, 1987.
112. Petein M, Michel P, van Velthoven R, et al: Morphonuclear relationship between prostatic intraepithelial neoplasia and cancers as assessed by digital cell image analysis. Am J Clin Pathol 96:628, 1991.
113. Qian JQ, Bostwick DG, Takahashi S, et al: Chromosomal anomalies in prostatic intraepithelial neoplasia and carcinoma detected by fluorescence in situ hybridization. Cancer Res 55:5408, 1995.
114. Algaba F, Epstein JI, Aldape HC, et al: Assessment of prostate carcinoma in core needle biopsy—definition of minimal criteria for the diagnosis of cancer in biopsy material. Cancer 78:376, 1996.
115. Iczkowski KA, MacLennan GT, Bostwick DG: Atypical small acinar proliferation suspicious for malignancy in prostate needle biopsies: clinical significance in 33 cases. Am J Surg Pathol 21:1489, 1997.
116. Oppenheimer JR, Kahane H, Epstein JI: Granulomatous prostatitis on needle biopsy. Arch Pathol Lab Med 121:724, 1997.
117. Bostwick DG, Dundore PA: Biopsy Pathology of the Prostate. London, Chapman & Hall, 1997.
118. Gleason DF: Histologic grading of prostatic carcinoma. *In* Bostwick DG (ed): Pathology of the Prostate. New York, Churchill Livingstone, 1990, p 83.
119. Gleason DF: Histologic grading of prostate cancer: a perspective. Hum Pathol 23:273, 1992.
120. Aihara M, Wheeler TM, Ohori M, et al: Heterogeneity of prostate cancer in radical prostatectomy specimens. Urology 43:60, 1994.
121. Spires SE, Cibull ML, Wood DP Jr, et al: Gleason histologic grading in prostatic carcinoma. Correlation of 18-gauge core biopsy with prostatectomy. Arch Pathol Lab Med 118:705, 1994.
122. Johnstone PA, Riffenburgh R, Saunders EL, et al: Grading inaccuracies in diagnostic biopsies revealing prostatic adenocarcinoma: implications for definitive radiation therapy. Int J Radiat Oncol Biol Phys 32:479, 1995.
123. American Joint Committee on Cancer: Prostate. *In* Greene F, Page DL, Fleming ID, et al (eds): AJCC Cancer Staging Manual, 6th ed. Philadelphia, Springer, 2002, pp 337-345.
124. International Union Against Cancer: Prostate. *In* Sobin LH, Wittekind C (eds): TNM Classification of Malignant Tumours, 5th ed. New York, Wiley-Liss, 1997, p 170.
125. Henson DE, Hutter RVP, Farrow GM, et al: Practice protocol for the examination of specimens removed from patients with carcinoma of the prostate gland-a publication of the Cancer Committee, College of American Pathologists. Arch Pathol Lab Med 118:779, 1994.
126. Bostwick DG, Myers RP, Oesterling JE: Staging of prostate cancer. Semin Surg Oncol 10:60, 1994.
127. Blute ML, Bostwick DG, Seay TM, et al: Pathologic classification of prostate carcinoma: the impact of margin status. Cancer 82:902, 1998.
128. Epstein JI, Pizov G, Walsh PC: Correlation of pathologic findings with progression after radical retropubic prostatectomy. Cancer 71:3582, 1993.
129. Ohori M, Scardino PT, Lapin SL, et al: The mechanisms and prognostic significance of seminal vesicle involvement by prostate cancer. Am J Surg Pathol 17:1252, 1993.
130. Villers AA, McNeal JE, Redwine EA, et al: Pathogenesis and biological significance of seminal vesicle invasion in prostatic adenocarcinoma. J Urol 143:1183, 1990.
131. Bostwick DG, Egbert BM, Fajardo LF: Radiation injury of the normal and neoplastic prostate. Am J Surg Pathol 6:541, 1982.
132. Brawer MK, Bostwick DG: Interpretation of postirradiation prostate biopsies. *In* Bostwick DG (ed): Pathology of the Prostate. New York, Churchill Livingstone, 1990, p 193.
133. Dugan TC, Shipley WU, Young RH, et al: Biopsy after external beam radiation therapy for adenocarcinoma of the prostate: correlation with original histological grade and current prostate specific antigen levels. J Urol 146:1313, 1991.
134. Siders DB, Lee F: Histologic changes of irradiated prostatic carcinoma diagnosed by transrectal ultrasound. Hum Pathol 23:344, 1992.
135. Mahan DE, Bruce AW, Manley PN, et al: Immunohistochemical evaluation of prostatic carcinoma before and after radiotherapy. J Urol 124:488, 1980.
136. Crook J, Robertson S, Esche B: Proliferative cell nuclear antigen in postradiotherapy prostate biopsies. Int J Radiat Oncol Biol Phys 30:303, 1994.
137. Ljung G, Egevad L, Norberg M, et al: Assessment of proliferation indicators in residual prostatic adenocarcinoma cells after radical external beam radiotherapy. Prostate 29:303, 1996.
138. Wheeler JA, Zagars GK, Ayala AG: Dedifferentiation of locally recurrent prostate cancer after radiation therapy: evidence for tumor progression. Cancer 71:3783, 1993.
139. Murphy WM, Soloway MS, Barrows GH: Pathologic changes associated with androgen deprivation therapy for prostate cancer. Cancer 68:821, 1991.
140. Armas OA, Aprikian AG, Melamed J, et al: Clinical and pathobiological effects of neoadjuvant total androgen ablation therapy on clinically localized prostatic adenocarcinoma. Am J Surg Pathol 18:979, 1994.
141. Cher ML, Bova GS, Moore DH, et al: Genetic alterations in untreated metastases and androgen-independent prostate cancer detected by comparative genomic hybridization and allelotyping. Cancer Res 56:3091, 1996.
142. Jenkins RB, Qian J, Lee HK, et al: A molecular cytogenetic analysis of 7q3l in prostate cancer. Cancer Res 58:759, 1998.
143. Ljung G, Egevad L, Norberg M, et al: Expression of p21 and mutant p53 gene products in residual prostatic tumor cells after radical radiotherapy. Prostate 32:99, 1997.
144. Theodorescu D, Broder SR, Boyd JC, et al: P53, bcl-2 and retinoblastoma proteins as long-term prognostic markers in localized carcinoma of the prostate. J Urol 158:131, 1997.
145. Moyret-Lalle C, Marcals C, Jacquemler J, et al: Ras, p53 and HPV status in benign and malignant prostate tumors. Int J Cancer 64:124, 1995.
146. Partin AW, Mangold LA, Lamm DM, et al: Contemporary update of prostate cancer staging nomograms (Partin tables) for the new millennium. Urology 58:843, 2001.
147. Trapasso JG, deKernion JB, Smith RB, et al: The incidence and significance of detectable levels of serum prostate specific antigen after radical prostatectomy. J Urol 152:1821, 1994.
148. Bostwick DG, Wheeler TM, Blute M, et al: Optimized microvessel density analysis improves prediction of cancer stage from prostate needle biopsies. Urology 48:47, 1996.

149. Partin AW, Yoo J, Carter HB, et al: The use of prostate specific antigen, clinical stage and Gleason score to predict pathological stage in men with localized prostate cancer. J Urol 150:110, 1993.
150. Kattan MW, Stapleton AM, Wheeler TM, et al: Evaluation of a nomogram used to predict the pathologic stage of clinically localized prostate carcinoma. Cancer 79:528, 1997.
151. Terris NM, McNeal JE, Freiha FS, Stamey TA: Efficacy of transrectal ultrasound-guided seminal vesicle biopsies in the detection of seminal vesicle invasion by prostate cancer. J Urol 149:1035, 1993.
152. Stone NN, Stock RG, Unger P: Indications for seminal vesicle biopsy and laparoscopic pelvic lymph node dissection in men with localized carcinoma of the prostate. J Urol 154:1392, 1995.
153. Chelsky MJ, Schnall MD, Seidmon EJ, et al: Use of endorectal surface coil magnetic resonance imaging for local staging of prostate cancer. J Urol 150:391, 1993.
154. Tempany CM, Zhou X, Zerhouni EA, et al: Staging of prostate cancer-results of Radiology Diagnostic Oncology Group project comparison of three MR imaging techniques. Radiology 192:47, 1994.
155. Bostwick DG, Qian J, Bergstralh E, et al: Prediction of capsular perforation and seminal vesicle invasion in prostate cancer. J Urol 155:1361, 1996.
156. Diaz A, Roach M, Marquez C, et al: Indications for and the significance of seminal vesicle irradiation during 3D conformal radiotherapy for localized prostate cancer. Int J Radiat Oncol Biol Phys 30:323, 1994.
157. Partin AW, Kattan MW, Subong ENP, et al: Combination of prostate-specific antigen, clinical stage, and Gleason score to predict pathological stage of localized prostate cancer: a multi-institutional update. JAMA 277:1445, 1997.
158. Pisansky TM, Blute ML, Suman VJ, et al: Correlation of pretherapy prostate cancer characteristics with seminal vesicle invasion in radical prostatectomy specimens. Int J Radiat Oncol Biol Phys 36:585, 1996.
159. Pisansky TM, Zincke H, Suman VJ, et al: Correlation of pretherapy prostate cancer characteristics with histologic findings from pelvic lymphadenectomy specimens. Int J Radiat Oncol Biol Phys 34:33, 1996.
160. Roach M, Marquez C, Yuo HS, et al: Predicting the risk of lymph node involvement using the pre-treatment prostate specific antigen and Gleason score in men with clinically localized prostate cancer. Int J Radiat Oncol Biol Phys 28:33, 1994.
161. Roach M, Pickett B, Rosenthal SA, et al: Defining treatment margins for six field conformal irradiation of localized prostate cancer. Int J Radiat Oncol Biol Phys 28:267, 1994.
162. Spevack L, Killion LT, West JC, et al: Predicting the patient at low risk for lymph node metastasis with localized prostate cancer: an analysis of four statistical models. Int J Radiat Oncol Biol Phys 34:543, 1996.
163. Cox DR: Regression models and life tables. J R Stat Soc 34:187, 1972.
164. Hosmer D, Lemeshow S: Applied Logistic Regression. New York, John Wiley & Sons, 1989.
165. Simon R, Altman DG: Statistical aspects of prognostic factor studies in oncology. Br J Cancer 69:979, 1997.
166. Altman DG, Lausen B, Sauerbrei W, et al: Dangers of using "optimal" cutpoints in the evaluation of prognostic factors. J Natl Cancer Inst 86:829, 1994.
167. Albertsen PC, Hanley JA, Fine J: 20-Year outcomes following conservative management of clinically localized prostate cancer. JAMA 293:2095, 2005.
168. Borre M, Nerstrom B, Overgaard J: The natural history of prostate carcinoma based on a Danish population treated with no intent to cure. Cancer 80:917, 1997.
169. Charlson ME, Pompei P, Ales KL, et al: A new method of classifying prognostic comorbidity in longitudinal studies: development and validation. J Chronic Dis 40:373, 1987.
170. Chodak GW, Thisted RA, Gerber GS, et al: results of conservative management of clinically localized prostate cancer. N Engl J Med 330:242, 1994.
171. Krongrad A, Lai H, Lamm SH, et al: Mortality in prostate cancer. J Urol 156:1084, 1996.
172. Kuban DA, Thames HD, Levy LB, et al: Long-term multi-institutional analysis of stage T1-T2 prostate cancer treated with radiotherapy in the PSA era. Int J Radiat Oncol Biol Phys 57:915, 2003.
173. Zincke H, Oesterling JE, Blute ML, et al: Long-term (15 years) results after radical prostatectomy for clinically localized (stage T2c or lower) prostate cancer. J Urol 152:1850, 1994.
174. Pilepich MV, Krall JM, Sause WT, et al: Prognostic factors in carcinoma of the prostate-analysis of RTOG study 75-06. Int J Radiat Oncol Biol Phys 13:339, 1987.
175. Leibel SA, Hanks GE, Kramer S: Patterns of Care outcome studies: results of the national practice in adenocarcinoma of the prostate. Int J Radiat Oncol Biol Phys 10:401, 1984.
176. Zagars GK, Pollack A, von Eschenbach AC: Prognostic factors for clinically localized prostate carcinoma: analysis of 938 patients irradiated in the prostate specific antigen era. Cancer 79:1370, 1997.
177. Zietman AL, Coen JJ, Shipley WU, et al: Radical radiation therapy in the management of prostatic adenocarcinoma: the initial prostate specific antigen value as a predictor of treatment outcome. J Urol 151:640,1994.
178. Fukunaga-Johnson N, Sandler HM, McLaughlin PW, et al: results of 3D conformal radiotherapy in the treatment of localized prostate cancer. Int J Radiat Oncol Biol Phys 38:311, 1997.
179. Pisansky TM, Kahn MJ, Rasp GM, et al: A multiple prognostic index predictive of disease outcome following irradiation for clinically localized prostatic carcinoma. Cancer 79:337, 1997.
180. Mettlin CJ, Murphy G: The National Cancer Data Base report on prostate cancer. Cancer 74:1640, 1994.
181. Harlan L, Brawley O, Pommerenke F, et al: Geographic, age, and racial variation in the treatment of local/regional carcinoma of the prostate. J Clin Oncol 13:93, 1995.
182. Roach M III, Krall J, Keller JW, et al: The prognostic significance of race and survival from prostate cancer based on patients irradiated on Radiation Therapy Oncology Group protocols (1976-1985). Int J Radiat Oncol Biol Phys 24:441, 1992.
183. Brawn PN, Johnson EH, Kuhl DL, et al: Stage at presentation and survival of white and black patients with prostate carcinoma. Cancer 71:2569, 1993.
184. Moul JW, Douglas TH, McCarthy WF, et al: Black race is an adverse prognostic factor for prostate cancer recurrence following radical prostatectomy in an equal access health care setting. J Urol 155:1667, 1996.
185. Richardson JT, Webster JD, Fields NJ: Uncovering myths and transforming realities among low-SES African-American men: implications for reducing prostate cancer disparities. J Natl Med Assoc 96:1295, 2004.
186. Abdelrahaman E, Raghavan S, Baker L, et al: Racial difference in circulating sex hormone-binding globulin levels in prepubertal boys. Metabolism 54:91, 2005.
187. Rosser CJ, Kuban DA, Levy LB, et al: Clinical features and treatment outcome of Hispanic men with prostate cancer following external beam radiotherapy. J Urol 170:1856, 2003.
188. Albertsen PC, Fryback DG, Storer BE, et al: The impact of comorbidity on life expectancy among men with localized prostate cancer. J Urol 156:127, 1996.
189. Fowler JE Jr, Terrell FL, Renfroe DL: Co-morbidities and survival of men with localized prostate cancer treated with surgery or radiation therapy. J Urol 156:1714, 1996.
190. Perez CA, Lee HK, Georgiou A, et al: Technical and tumor-related factors affecting outcome of definitive irradiation for localized carcinoma of the prostate. Int J Radiat Oncol Biol Phys 26:581,1993.
191. Zagars GK, von Eschenbach AC, Ayala AG: Prognostic factors in prostate cancer: analysis of 874 patients treated with radiation therapy. Cancer 72:1709, 1993.
192. Kuban DA, Elmahdi AM, Schellhammer PF: Prostate-specific antigen for pretreatment prediction and posttreatment evaluation of outcome after definitive irradiation for prostate cancer. Int J Radiat Oncol Biol Phys 32:307, 1995.
193. Leibel SA, Zelefsky MJ, Kutcher GJ, et al: The biological basis and clinical application of three-dimensional conformal external beam radiation therapy in carcinoma of the prostate. Semin Oncol 21:580, 1994.

194. Zagars GK, Geara FB, Pollack A, et al: The T classification of clinically localized prostate cancer: an appraisal based on disease outcome after radiation therapy. Cancer 73:1904, 1994.
195. Catalona WJ, Whitmore WF Jr: New staging systems for prostate cancer. J Urol 142:1302, 1989.
196. Ohori M, Wheeler TM, Kattan MW, et al: Prognostic significance of positive surgical margins in radical prostatectomy specimens. J Urol 154:1818, 1995.
197. Paulson DF, Robertson CN: Positive margins. Is adjunctive radiation therapy indicated? Acta Oncol 30:263, 1991.
198. deKernion JB, Neuwirth H, Stein A, et al: Prognosis of patients with stage D1 prostate carcinoma following radical prostatectomy with and without early endocrine therapy. J Urol 144:700, 1990.
199. Zincke H, Bergstralh EJ, Larson-Keller JJ, et al: Stage DI prostate cancer treated by radical prostatectomy and adjuvant hormonal treatment: evidence for favorable survival in patients with DNA diploid tumors. Cancer 70:311, 1992.
200. Leibel SA, Fuks Z, Zelefsky MJ, et al: The effects of local and regional treatment on the metastatic outcome in prostatic carcinoma with pelvic lymph node involvement. Int J Radiat Oncol Biol Phys 28:7, 1994.
201. Lawton CA, Winter K, Byhardt R, et al: Androgen suppression plus radiation versus radiation alone for patients with D1 (pN+) adenocarcinoma of the prostate (results based on a national prospective randomized trial, RTOG 85-31). Int J Radiat Oncol Biol Phys 38:931, 1997.
202. Hanks GE, Buzydlowski J, Sause WT, et al: Ten-year outcomes for pathologic node-positive patients treated in RTOG 75-06. Int J Radiat Oncol Biol Phys 40:765, 1998.
203. Smith JA Jr, Middleton RG: Implications of volume of nodal metastasis in patients with adenocarcinoma of the prostate. J Urol 133:617, 1985.
204. Schmid HP, Mihatsch MJ, Hering F, et al: Impact of minimal lymph node metastasis on long-term prognosis after radical prostatectomy. Eur Urol 31:11, 1997.
205. Steinberg GD, Epstein JI, Piantadosi S, et al: Management of stage D1 adenocarcinoma of the prostate: the Johns Hopkins experience 1974 to 1987. J Urol 144:1425, 1990.
206. Barzell W, Bean MA, Hilaris BS, et al: Prostatic adenocarcinoma: relationship of grade and local extent to the pattern of metastases. J Urol 118:278, 1977.
207. Srignoli AR, Walsh PC, Steinberg GD, et al: Prognostic factors in men with stage D1 prostate cancer—identification of patients less likely to have prolonged survival after radical prostatectomy. J Urol 152:1077, 1994.
208. Cheng L, Bergstralh EJ, Cheville JC: Cancer volume of lymph node metastasis predicts progression in prostate cancer. Am J Surg Pathol 22:1491, 1998.
209. Griebling TL, Ozkutlu D, See WA, et al: Prognostic implications of extracapsular extension of lymph node metastasis in prostate cancer. Mod Pathol 10:804, 1997.
210. Swanson GP, Cupps RE, Utz DC, et al: Definitive therapy for prostate carcinoma—Mayo Clinic results at 15 years after treatment. Br J Radiol 67:877, 1994.
211. Kupelian PA, Katcher J, Levin HS, et al: Stage T1-2 prostate cancer: a multivariate analysis of factors affecting biochemical and clinical failures after radical prostatectomy. Int J Radiat Oncol Biol Phys 37:1043, 1997.
212. Lee WR, Hanks GE, Hanlon A: Increasing prostate-specific antigen profile following definitive radiation therapy for localized prostate cancer: clinical observations. J Clin Oncol 15:230, 1997.
213. Pound Cr, Partin AW, Eisenberger MA, et al: Natural history of progression after PSA elevation following radical prostatectomy. JAMA 281:1591, 1999.
214. Kuban DA, El-Mahdi AM, Schellhammer PF: PSA for outcome prediction and posttreatment evaluation following radiation for prostate cancer: do we know how to use it? Semin Radiat Oncol 8:72, 1998.
215. Martinez AA, Gonzalez JA, Chung AK, et al: A comparison of external beam radiation therapy versus radical prostatectomy for patients with low risk prostate carcinoma diagnosed, staged, and treated at a single institution. Cancer 88:425, 2000.
216. Landmann C, Hunig R: Prostatic-specific antigen as an indicator of response to radiotherapy in prostate cancer. Int J Radiat Oncol Biol Phys 17:1073, 1989.
217. Lee WR, Hanks GE, Schultheiss TE, et al: Localized prostate cancer treated by external-beam radiotherapy alone: serum prostate-specific antigen-driven outcome analysis. J Clin Oncol 13:464, 1995.
218. Zagars GK, Pollack A, Kavadi VS, et al: Prostate-specific antigen and radiation therapy for clinically localized prostate cancer. Int J Radiat Oncol Biol Phys 32:293, 1995.
219. Amling CL, Bergstralh EJ, Blute ML, et al: Defining prostate specific antigen progression after radical prostatectomy: what is the most appropriate cut point? J Urol 165:1146, 2001.
220. Gretzer MB, Trock BJ, Han M, et al: A critical analysis of the interpretation of biochemical failure in surgically treated patients using the American Society for Therapeutic Radiation and Oncology Criteria. J Urol 168:1419, 2002.
221. Pisansky TM, Kahn MJ, Bostwick DG: An enhanced prognostic system for clinically localized carcinoma of the prostate. Cancer 79:2154, 1997.
222. Zelefsky MJ, Fuks Z, Hunt M, et al: High dose radiation delivered by intensity modulated conformal radiotherapy improves the outcome of localized prostate cancer. J Urol 166:876, 2001.
223. Pollack A, Zagars GK, Starkschall G, et al: Prostate cancer radiation dose response: results of the M. D. Anderson phase III randomized trials. Int J Radiat Oncol Biol Phys 53:1097, 2002.
224. Zentner PG, Pao LK, Benson MC, et al: Prostate-specific antigen density: a new prognostic indicator for prostate cancer. Int J Radiat Oncol Biol Phys 27:47, 1993.
225. Corn BW, Hanks GE, Lee WR, et al: Prostate specific antigen density is not an independent predictor of response for prostate cancer treated by conformal radiotherapy. J Urol 153:1855, 1995.
226. D'Amico AV, Propert KJ: Prostate cancer volume adds significantly to prostate-specific antigen in the prediction of early biochemical failure after external beam radiation therapy. Int J Radiat Oncol Biol Phys 35:273, 1996.
227. Pollack A, Lankford S, Zagars GK, et al: Prostate specific antigen density as a prognostic factor for patients with prostate carcinoma treated with radiotherapy. Cancer 77:1515, 1996.
228. Lankford SP, Pollack A, Zagars GK: Prostate-specific antigen cancer volume: a significant prognostic factor in prostate cancer patients at intermediate risk of failing radiotherapy. Int J Radiat Oncol Biol Phys 38:327, 1997.
229. Pollack A, Zagars GK, Kavadi VS: Prostate specific antigen doubling time and disease relapse after radiotherapy for prostate cancer. Cancer 74:670, 1994.
230. Hanks GE, Hanlon AL, Lee WR, et al: Pretreatment prostate-specific antigen doubling times: clinical utility of this predictor of prostate cancer behavior. Int J Radiat Oncol Biol Phys 34:549, 1996.
231. Zagars GK, Pollack A: Kinetics of serum prostate-specific antigen after external beam radiation for clinically localized prostate cancer. Radiother Oncol 44:213, 1997.
232. D'Amico AV, Moul JW, Carroll PR, et al: Surrogate end point for prostate cancer-specific mortality after radical prostatectomy or radiation therapy. J Natl Cancer I 95:1376, 2003.
233. Kuban DA, Thames H, Horwitz E, et al: Predicting outcome after PSA failure in prostate cancer patients treated by radiation. Who needs salvage therapy? Int J Radiat Oncol Biol Phys 60(Suppl): S167, 2004.
234. Swindle PW, Kattan MW, Scardino PT: Markers and meaning of primary treatment failure. Urol Clin North Am 30:377, 2003.
235. Moul JW: Variables in predicting survival based on treating "PSA-only" relapse. Urol Oncol 21:292, 2003.
236. Zietman AL, Coen JJ, Dallow KC, et al: The treatment of prostate cancer by conventional radiation therapy: an analysis of long-term outcome. Int J Radiat Oncol Biol Phys 32:287, 1995.
237. Willett CG, Zietman AL, Shipley WU, et al: The effect of pelvic radiation therapy on serum levels of prostate specific antigen. J Urol 151:1579, 1994.
238. Zietman AL, Tibbs MK, Dallow KC, et al: Use of PSA nadir to predict subsequent biochemical outcome following external beam radiation therapy for T1-2 adenocarcinoma of the prostate. Radiother Oncol 40:159, 1996.

239. Hanlon AL, Diratzouian H, Hanks GE: Post-treatment prostate-antigen nadir highly predictive of distant failure and death from prostate cancer. Int J Radiat Oncol Biol Phys 53:297, 2002.
240. Kavadi VS, Zagars GK, Pollack A: Serum prostate-specific antigen after radiation therapy for clinically localized prostate cancer-prognostic implications. lnt J Radiat Oncol Biol Phys 30:279, 1994.
241. Consensus statement. Guidelines for PSA following radiation therapy. American Society for Therapeutic Radiology and Oncology Consensus Panel. Int J Radiat Oncol Biol Phys 37:1035, 1997.
242. Partin AW, Pound CR, Clemens JQ, el al: Serum PSA after anatomic radiation prostatectomy: the Johns Hopkins experience after 10 years. Urol Clin North Am 20:713, 1993.
243. Fowler JE Jr, Brooks J, Pandey P, et al: Variable histology of anastomotic biopsies with detectable prostate specific antigen after radical prostatectomy. J Urol 153:1011, 1995.
244. Thames H, Kuban D, Levy L, et al: Comparison of alternative biochemical failure definitions based on clinical outcome in 4839 prostate cancer patients treated by external beam radiotherapy between 1986 and 1995. Int J Radiat Oncol Biol Phys 57:929, 2003.
245. Kuban D, Thames H, Levy L, et al: Failure definition-dependent differences in outcome following radiation for localized prostate cancer: can one size fit all? Int J Radiat Biol Phys 61:409, 2005.
246. Kuban DA, Thames HD, Levy LB: PSA after radiation for prostate cancer. Oncology (Williston Park) 18:595, 2004.
247. Horwitz EM, Levy LB, Kuban DA, et al: The biochemical and clinical significance of the post-treatment PSA bounce for prostate cancer treated with external beam radiation therapy alone: a multi-institutional pooled analysis. Int J Radiat Oncol Biol Phys 60(Suppl):S235, 2004.
248. Kestin LL, Vicini FA, Martinez AA: Practical application of biochemical failure definitions: what to do and when to do it. Int J Radiat Oncol Biol Phys 53:304, 2002.
249. Roach M, Thames H, Schellkamver S, et al: A revised consensus definition for biochemical failure following radiotherapy with curative intent for clinically localized prostate cancer. Int J Radiat Oncol Biol Phys (In press).
250. Hermanek P, Hutter RV, Sobin LH: Prognostic grouping: the next step in tumor classification. J Cancer Res Clin Oncol 116:513, 1990.
251. Burke HB, Henson DE: The American Joint Committee on Cancer criteria for prognostic factors and for an enhanced prognostic system. Cancer 72:3131, 1993.
252. Movsas B, Hanlon AL, Teshima T, et al: Analyzing predictive models following definitive radiotherapy for prostate carcinoma. Cancer 80:1093, 1997.
253. Partin AW, Piantadosi S, Sanda MG, et al: Selection of men at high risk for disease recurrence for experimental adjuvant therapy following radical prostatectomy. Urology 45:831, 1995.
254. D'Amico AV, Whittington R, Malkowicz SB, et al: Predicting prostate specific antigen outcome preoperatively in the prostate specific antigen era. J Urol 166:2185, 2001.
255. Kattan MW, Wheeler TM, Scardino PT: Postoperative nomogram for disease recurrence after radical prostatectomy for prostate cancer. J Clin Oncol 17:1499, 1999.
256. Kattan MW, Zelefsky MJ, Kupelian PA, et al: Pretreatment nomogram for predicting the outcome of three-dimensional conformal radiotherapy in prostate cancer. J Clin Oncol 18:3352, 2000.
257. Moul JW, Davis R, Vaccaro JA, et al: Acute urinary retention associated with prostatic carcinoma. J Urol 141:1375, 1989.
258. Chute CG, Panser LA, Girman CJ, et al: The prevalence of prostatism: a population-based survey of urinary symptoms. J Urol 150:85, 1993.
259. Kuritzky L: Role of primary care clinicians in the diagnosis and treatment of LUTS and BPH. Urology 6(Suppl 9):S53, 2004.
260. Grayhack JT, Grayhack JJ: Clinical dilemmas and problems in assessing prostatic metastasis to bone: the scientific challenge. Adv Exp Med Biol 324:1, 1992.
261. Chodak GW, Vogelzang NJ, Caplan RJ, et al: Independent prognostic factors in patients with metastatic (stage D2) prostate cancer. The Zoladex Study Group. JAMA 265:618, 1991.
262. Saitoh H, Hida M, Shimbo T, et al: Metastatic patterns of prostatic cancer: correlation between sites and number of organs involved. Cancer 54:3078, 1984.
263. Matzkin H, Braf Z: Paraneoplastic syndromes associated with prostatic carcinoma. J Urol 138:1129, 1987.
264. Whitmore WF Jr: Hormone therapy in prostatic cancer. Am J Med 697:613, 1956.
265. Brawer MK, Chetner MP, Beatie J, et al: Screening for prostatic carcinoma with prostate specific antigen. J Urol 147:841,1992.
266. Flanigan RC, Catalona WJ, Richie JP, et al: Accuracy of digital rectal examination and transrectal ultrasonography in localizing prostate cancer. J Urol 152:1506, 1994.
267. Rifkin MD, Zerhouni EA, Gatsonis CA, et al: Comparison of magnetic resonance imaging and ultrasonography in staging early prostate cancer: results of a multi-institutional cooperative trial. N Engl J Med 323:621, 1990.
268. Smith JA, Scardino PT, Resnick MI, et al: Transrectal ultrasound versus digital rectal examination for the staging of carcinoma of the prostate: results of a prospective, multi-institutional trial. J Urol 157:902, 1997.
269. Ohori M, Egawa S, Shinohara K, et al: Detection of microscopic extracapsular extension prior to radical prostatectomy for clinically localized prostate cancer. Br J Urol 74:72, 1994.
270. Pinover WH, Hanlon A, Lee WR, et al: Prostate carcinoma patients upstaged by imaging and treated with irradiation: an outcome-based analysis. Cancer 77:1334, 1996.
271. Linzer DG, Stock RG, Stone NN, et al: Seminal vesicle biopsy. Accuracy and implications for staging of prostate cancer. Urology 48:757, 1996.
272. Engeler CE, Wasserman NF, Zhang G: Preoperative assessment of prostatic carcinoma by computerized tomography: weaknesses and new perspectives. Urology 40:346, 1992.
273. Flanigan RC, McKay TC, Olson M, et al: Limited efficacy of preoperative computed tomographic scanning for the evaluation of lymph node metastasis in patients before radical prostatectomy. Urology 48:428, 1996.
274. Hanks GE, Krall JM, Pilepich MV, et al: Comparison of pathologic and clinical evaluation of lymph nodes in prostate cancer: implications of RTOG data for patient management and trial design and stratification. Int J Radiat Oncol Biol Phys 23:293, 1992.
275. Huncharek M, Muscat J: Serum prostate-specific antigen as a predictor of staging abdominal/pelvic computed tomography in newly diagnosed prostate cancer. Abdominal Imaging 21:364, 1996.
276. Levran Z, Gonzalez JA, Diokno AC, et al: Are pelvic computed tomography, bone scan and pelvic lymphadenectomy necessary in the staging of prostatic cancer? Br J Urol 75:778, 1995.
277. Van Poppel H, Ameye F, Oyen R, et al: Accuracy of combined computerized tomography and fine needle aspiration cytology in lymph node staging of localized prostatic carcinoma. J Urol 151:1310, 1994.
278. Kier R Wain S, Troiano R, et al: Fast spin-echo MR images of the pelvis obtained with a phased-array coil: value in localizing and staging prostatic carcinoma. AJR Am J Roentgenol 150:391, 1993.
279. Harisinghani MG, Barentsz J, Hahn PF, et al: Noninvasive detection of clinically occult lymph-node metastases in prostate cancer. N Engl J Med 348:2491, 2003.
280. Roach M, Kurhanewicz J, Carroll P: Spectroscopy in prostate cancer: hope or hype? Oncology (Williston Park) 11:1399, 2001.
281. Chybowski FM, Larson Keller JJ, Bergstralh EJ, et al: Predicting radionuclide bone scan findings in patients with newly diagnosed, untreated prostate cancer: prostate specific antigen is superior to all other clinical parameters. J Urol 145:313, 1991.
282. Oesterling JE, Martin SK, Bergstralh EJ, et al: The use of prostate-specific antigen in staging patients with newly diagnosed prostate cancer. JAMA 269:57, 1993.
283. Freitas JE, Gilvydas R, Ferry JD, et al: The clinical utility of prostate-specific antigen and bone scintigraphy in prostate cancer follow-up. J Nucl Med 32:1387, 1991.
284. Silver DA, Pellicer I, Fair WR, et al: Prostate-specific membrane antigen expression in normal and malignant human tissues. Clin Cancer Res 3:81, 1997.
285. Wright GL Jr, Grob BM, Haley C, et al: Upregulation of prostate-specific membrane antigen after androgen-deprivation therapy. Urology 48:326, 1996.
286. Babaian RJ, Sayer J, Podoloff DA, et al: Radioimmunoscintigraphy of pelvic lymph nodes with ^{111}indium-labeled monoclonal antibody CYT-356. J Urol 152:1952, 1994.

287. Purohit RS, Shinohara K, Meng MV, et al: Imaging clinically localized prostate cancer. Urol Clin North Am 30:279, 2003.
288. Nadji M, Tabei SZ, Castro A, et al: Prostate-specific antigen: an immunohistologic marker for prostate neoplasms. Cancer 48:1229, 1981.
289. Lilja H, Christensson A, Dahlen U, et al: Prostate-specific antigen in serum occurs predominantly in complex with alpha 1-antichymotrypsin. Clin Chem 37:1618, 1991.
290. Oesterling JE, Moyad MA, Wright GL, et al: An analytical comparison of the three most commonly used prostate-specific antigen assays: Tandem-R, Tandem-E, and IMx. Urology 46:524, 1995.
291. Komatsu K, Wehner N, Prestigiacomo AF, et al: Physiologic (intraindividual) variation of serum prostate-specific antigen in 814 men from a screening population. Urology 47:343, 1996.
292. Stamey TA, Yang N, Hay AR, et al: Prostate-specific antigen as a marker for adenocarcinoma of the prostate. N Engl J Med 317:909, 1987.
293. Yuan JJ, Coplen DE, Petros JA, et al: Effects of rectal examination, prostatic massage, ultrasonography and needle biopsy on serum prostate specific antigen levels. J Urol 147:810, 1992.
294. Glenski WJ, Klee GG, Bergstralh EJ, et al: Prostate-specific antigen: establishment of the reference range for the clinically normal prostate gland and the effect of digital rectal examination, ejaculation, and time on serum concentrations. Prostate 21:99, 1992.
295. Oesterling JE, Rice DC, Glenski WJ, et al: Effect of cystoscopy, prostate biopsy, and transurethral resection of prostate on serum prostate-specific antigen concentration. Urology 42:276, 1993.
296. Guess HA, Heyse JF, Gormley GJ, et al: Effect of finasteride on serum PSA concentration in men with benign prostatic hyperplasia: results from the North American phase III clinical trial. Urol Clin North Am 20:627, 1993.
297. Rubenstein M, Guinan PD, McKiel CF, et al: Review of acid phosphatase in the diagnosis and prognosis of prostatic cancer. Clin Physiol Biochem 6:241, 1988.
298. Bogdanowicz JFAT, Bentvelsen FM, Oosterom R, et al: Evaluation of prostate-specific antigen and prostatic acid phosphatase in untreated prostatic carcinoma and benign prostatic hyperplasia. Scand J Urol Nephrol 138:97, 1991.
299. Jones GT, Mettlin C, Murphy GP, et al: Patterns of care for carcinoma of the prostate gland: results of a national survey of 1984 and 1990. J Am Coll Surg 180:545, 1995.
300. Merrick MV, Ding CL, Chisholm GD, et al: Prognostic significance of alkaline and acid phosphatase and skeletal scintigraphy in carcinoma of the prostate. Br J Urol 57:715, 1985.
301. Dupont A, Cusan L, Gomez JL, et al: Prostate specific antigen and prostatic acid phosphatase for monitoring therapy of carcinoma of the prostate. J Urol 146:1064, 1991.
302. Forman JD, Lee WR, Roach M III, et al: Staging Evaluation for Patients with Adenocarcinoma of the Prostate. ACR Appropriateness Criteria. Radiology 215(Suppl):1373, 2000.
303. National Comprehensive Cancer Network: Prostate cancer NCCN clinical practice guidelines for oncology. J NCCN 2:224, 2004.
304. Johansson JE, Andren O, Anderson SO, et al: Natural history of early, localized prostate cancer. JAMA 291:2713, 2004.
305. Wilt TJ: Prostate carcinoma practice patterns: what do they tell us about the diagnosis, treatment, and outcomes of patients with prostate carcinoma? Cancer 88:1277, 2000.
306. Mettlin CJ, Murphy GP, Ho R, et al: The National Cancer Data Base report on longitudinal observations on prostate cancer. Cancer 77:2162, 1996.
307. Mettlin CJ, Murphy GP, Cunningham MP, et al: The National Cancer Data Base report on race, age, and region variations in prostate cancer treatment. Cancer 80:1261, 1997.
308. Brawn PN, Kuhl D, Speights VO, et al: The incidence of unsuspected metastases from clinically benign prostate glands with latent prostate carcinoma. Arch Pathol Lab Med 119:731, 1995.
309. Dugan JA, Bostwick DG, Myers RP, et al: The definition and preoperative prediction of clinically insignificant prostate cancer. JAMA 275:288, 1996.
310. Epstein JI, Walsh PC, Carmichael M, et al: Pathologic and clinical findings to predict tumor extent of nonpalpable (stage T1c) prostate cancer. JAMA 271:368, 1994.
311. Epstein JI, Paull G, Eggleston JC, et al: Prognosis of untreated stage Al prostatic carcinoma: a study of 94 cases with extended followup. J Urol 136:837, 1986.
312. Lowe BA, Listrom MB: Incidental carcinoma of the prostate: an analysis of the predictors of progression. J Urol 140:1340, 1988.
313. Zhang G, Wasserman NF, Sidi AA, et al: Long-term follow-up results after expectant management of stage A1 prostatic cancer. J Urol 146:99, 1991.
314. Haapiainen R, Rannikko S, Makinen J, et al: To carcinoma of the prostate: influence of tumor extent and histologic grade on prognosis of untreated patients. Eur Urol 12:16, 1986.
315. Moskovitz B, Nitecki S, Levin D: Cancer of the prostate: is there a need for aggressive treatment? Urol Int 42:49, 1987.
316. Stenzl A, Studer UE: Outcome of patients with untreated cancer of the prostate. Eur Urol 24:1, 1993.
317. Warner J, Whitmore WF: Expectant management of clinically localized prostatic cancer. J Urol 152:1761, 1994.
318. Adolfsson J, Oksanen H, Salo JO, et al: Localized prostate cancer and 30 years of follow-up in a population-based setting. Prostate Cancer Prostatic Dis 3:37, 2000.
319. George NJR: Natural history of localised prostatic cancer managed by conservative therapy alone. Lancet 1:494, 1988.
320. Graversen PH, Nielsen KT, Gasser TC, et al: Radical prostatectomy versus expectant primary treatment in stages I and II prostatic cancer: a fifteen-year follow-up. Urology 36:493, 1990.
321. Bill-Axelson A, Holmberg L, Ruutu M, et al: Radical prostatectomy versus watchful waiting in early prostate cancer. N Engl J Med 352:1977, 2005.
322. Aus G, Hugosson J, Norlen L: Long-term survival and mortality in prostate cancer treated with noncurative intent. J Urol 154:460, 1995.
323. Aus G, Hugosson J, Norlen L: Need for hospital care and palliative treatment for prostate cancer treated with noncurative intent. J Urol 154:466, 1995.
324. Norlén BJ: Survival and mortality in prostatic cancer: a study based on the Swedish Cancer Registry. Acta Oncol 30:141, 1991.
325. Wilt TJ, Brawer MK: The Prostate Cancer Intervention Versus Observation Trial—a randomized trial comparing radical prostatectomy versus expectant management for the treatment of clinically localized prostate cancer. J Urol 152:1910, 1994.
326. Wilt TJ, Brawer MK: The Prostate Cancer Intervention versus Observation Trial (PIVOT). Oncology (Williston Park) 11:1133, 1997.
327. Middleton RG, Thompson IM, Austenfeld MS, et al: Prostate cancer clinical guidelines panel summary report on the management of clinically localized prostate cancer. J Urol 154:2144, 1995.
328. Eastham JA, Kattan MW, Groshen S, et al: Fifteen-year survival and recurrence rates after radiotherapy for localized prostate cancer. J Clin Oncol 15:3214, 1997.
329. Zelefsky MJ, Whitmore WF Jr: Long-term results of retropubic permanent 125 iodine implantation of the prostate for clinically localized prostatic cancer. J Urol 158:23, 1997.
330. Green SB, Byar DP: Using observational data from registries to compare treatments: the fallacy of omnimetrics. Stat Med 3:361, 1984.
331. Kupelian P, Kuban D, Thames H, et al: Improved biochemical relapse-free survival with increased external radiation doses in patients with localized prostate cancer the combined experience of nine institutions in patients treated in 1994 and 1995. Int J Radiat Oncol Biol Phys 61:415, 2005.
332. Bagshaw MA, Kaplan ID, Cox RS: Radiation therapy for localized disease. Cancer 71:939, 1993.
333. Hanks GE, Asbell S, Krall JM, et al: Outcome for lymph node dissection negative T-1b, T2 (A-2, B) prostate cancer treated with external beam radiation therapy in RTOG 77-06. Int J Radiat Oncol Biol Phys 21:1099, 1991.
334. Hanks GE, Krall JM, Hanlon AL, et al: Patterns of Care and RTOG studies in prostate cancer: Long-term survival, hazard rate observations, and possibilities of cure. Int J Radiat Oncol Biol Phys 28:39, 1994.

335. Lee RJ, Sause WT: Surgically staged patients with prostatic carcinoma treated with definitive radiotherapy: fifteen-year results. Urology 43:640, 1994.
336. Perez CA, Pilepich MV, Garcia D, et al: Definitive radiation therapy in carcinoma of the prostate localized to the pelvis: experience at the Mallinckrodt Institute of Radiology. NCI Monogr 7:85, 1988.
337. Asbell SO, Martz KL, Pilepich MV, et al: Impact of surgical staging in evaluating the radiotherapeutic outcome in RTOG phase III study for A_2 and B prostate carcinoma. Int J Radiat Oncol Biol Phys 17:945, 1989.
338. Lu-Yao GL, Yao SL: Population-based study of long-term survival in patients with clinically localised prostate cancer. Lancet 349:906, 1997.
339. Scardino PT, Wheeler TM: Local control of prostate cancer with radiotherapy: frequency and prognostic significance of positive results of post-irradiation prostate biopsy. NCI Monogr 7:95, 1988.
340. Prestidge BR, Kaplan I, Cox RS, et al: The clinical significance of a positive post-irradiation prostatic biopsy without metastases. Int J Radiat Oncol Biol Phys 24:403, 1992.
341. Kuban DA, El-Mahdi AM, Schellhammer PF: Potential benefit of improved local tumor control in patients with prostate carcinoma. Cancer 75:2373, 1995.
342. Kuban DA, El-Mahdi AM, Schellhammer PF: Effect of local tumor control on distant metastasis and survival in prostatic adenocarcinoma. Urology 30:420, 1987.
343. Fuks Z, Leibel SA, Wallner KE, et al: The effect of local control on metastatic dissemination in carcinoma of the prostate: long-term results in patients treated with ^{125}I implantation. Int J Radiat Oncol Biol Phys 21:537, 1991.
344. Zagars GK, von Eschenbach AC, Ayala AG, et al: The influence of local control on metastatic dissemination of prostate cancer treated by external beam megavoltage radiation therapy. Cancer 68:2370, 1991.
345. Kuban DA, El-Mahdi AM, Schellhammer P: The significance of post-irradiation prostate biopsy with long-term follow-up. Int J Radiat Oncol Biol Phys 24:409, 1992.
346. Yorke ED, Fuks Z, Norton L, et al: Modeling the development of metastases from primary and locally recurrent tumors: comparison with a clinical database for prostatic cancer. Cancer Res 53:2987, 1993.
347. Coen JJ, Zietman AL, Thakral H, et al: Radical radiation for localized prostate cancer: local persistence of disease results in a late wave of metastases. J Clin Oncol 20:3199, 2002.
348. Shipley WU, Thames HD, Sandler HM, et al: Radiation therapy for clinically localized prostate cancer: a multi-institutional pooled analysis. JAMA 281:1598, 1999.
349. Pisansky TM, Thames HD, Levy LB, et al: Clinical outcomes and prognostic factors in 4839 patients treated with external radiotherapy for stage T1-T2 prostate cancer [abstract 63]. Proceedings of the 46th annual ASTRO meeting. Int J Radiat Oncol Biol Phys 60:S167, 2004.
350. Hanks GE, Hanlon AL, Epstein B, et al: Dose response in prostate cancer with 8-12 years follow-up. Int J Radiat Oncol Biol Phys 54:427, 2002.
351. Pollack A, Hanlon AL, Horwitz EM, et al: Prostate cancer radiotherapy dose response: an update of the Fox Chase experience. J Urol 171:1132, 2004.
352. Zelefsky M, Fuks Z, Chan H, et al: Ten-year results of dose escalation with 3-dimensional conformal radiotherapy for patients with clinically localized prostate cancer. 60:S149, 2004.
353. Zelefsky MJ, Fuks Z, Hunt M, et al: High-dose intensity modulated radiation therapy for prostate cancer: early toxicity and biochemical outcome in 722 patients. Int J Radiat Oncol Biol Phys 53:1111, 2002.
354. Zietman AL, DeSilvo M, Slater JD, et al: A randomized trial comparing conventional dose (70.2 GYE) and high dose (79.2 GYE) conformal radiation in early stage adenocarcinoma of the prostate: results of an interim analysis of PROG 95-09 JAMA 294:1233, 2005.
355. Kupelian PA, Reddy CA, Carlson TP, et al: Preliminary observations on biochemical relapse-free survival rates after short-course intensity-modulated radiotherapy (70 Gy at 2.5 Gy/fraction) for localized prostate cancer. Int J Radiat Oncol Biol Phys 53:904, 2002.
356. Chism DB, Horwitz EM, Hanlon AL, et al: Late morbidity profiles in prostate cancer patients treated to 79-84 Gy by a simple four-field coplanar beam. Int J Radiat Oncol Biol Phys 55:71, 2003.
357. Storey MR, Pollac A, Levy L, et al: Complications from radiotherapy dose escalation in prostate cancer: preliminary results of a randomized trial. Int J Radiat Oncol Biol Phys 48:635, 2000.
358. Huang EH, Pollack A, Levy L, et al: Late rectal toxicity: dose volume effects of conformal radiotherapy for prostate cancer. Int J Radiat Oncol Biol Phys 58:1513, 2004.
359. Cheung R, Tucker LS, Ye JS, et al: Characterization of rectal normal tissue complication probability after high-dose external beam radiotherapy for prostate cancer. Int J Radiat Oncol Biol Phys 57:S151, 2003.
360. Michalski J, Winter K, Purdy JA, et al: Toxicity following 3D radiation therapy for prostate cancer on RTOG 9406 dose level V. Int J Radiat Oncol Biol Phys 57:S151, 2003.
361. Michalski HM, Purdy JA, Winter K, et al: Preliminary report of toxicity following 3D radiation therapy for prostate cancer on 3DOG/RTOG 9406 dose levels I and II. Int Radiat Oncol Biol Phys 56:192, 2003.
362. Gardner BG, Zietman AL, Shipley WU, et al: Late normal tissue sequelae in the second decade after high dose radiation therapy with combined photons and conformal photons for locally advanced prostate cancer. J Urol 167:123, 2002.
363. Robinson JW, Moritz S, Fung T: Meta-analysis of rates of erectile function after treatment of localized prostate carcinoma. Int J Radiat Oncol Biol Phys 54:1063, 2002.
364. Brenner DJ, Curtis RE, Hall EJ, et al: Second malignancies in prostate carcinoma patients after radiotherapy compared with surgery. Cancer 88:398, 2000.
365. Baxter NN, Tepper JE, Durham SB, et al: Increased risk of rectal cancer after prostate radiation: a population-based study. Gastroenterology 128:819, 2005.
366. Pasteau O: Traitment du cancer de la prostate par le radium. Rev Mal Nutr 363, 1911.
367. Young HH: The use of radium in cancer of the prostate and bladder. JAMA 68:1174, 1917.
368. Merrick GS, Wallner KE, Butler WM: Permanent interstitial brachytherapy for the management of carcinoma of the prostate gland. J Urol 169:1643, 2003.
369. Whitmore WF Jr, Batata M, Hilaris B: Prostatic irradiation: iodine-125 implantation. Proceedings of the 23rd Clinical Conference on Cancer. Houston, TX, MD Anderson Hospital and Tumor Institute, 1978, p 195.
370. Whitmore WF Jr, Hilaris B, Batata M, et al: Interstitial radiation: short-term palliation or curative therapy? Urology 25:24, 1985.
371. Grossman HB, Batata M, Hilaris B, et al: ^{125}I implantation for carcinoma of prostate: further follow-up of first 100 cases. Urology 20:591, 1982.
372. Peschel RE, Fogel TD, Kacinski BM, et al: Iodine-125 implants for carcinoma of the prostate. Int J Radiat Oncol Biol Phys 11:1777, 1985.
373. Blasko JC, Ragde H, Luse RW, et al: Should brachytherapy be considered a therapeutic option in localized prostate cancer? Urol Clin North Am 23:633, 1996.
374. Nag S, Beyer D, Friedland J, et al: American Brachytherapy Society (ABS) recommendation for transperineal permanent brachytherapy of prostate cancer. Int J Radiat Oncol Biol Phys 44:789, 1999.
375. Potters L, Huang D, Calugaru E, et al: Importance of implant dosimetry for patients undergoing prostate brachytherapy. Urology 62:1072, 2003.
376. Merrick GS, Butler WM, Dorsey AT, et al: Effect of prostate size and isotope selection on dosimetric quality following permanent seed implantation. Tech Urol 7:233, 2001.
377. Stone NN, Stock RG: Prostate brachytherapy in patients with prostate volumes >/= 50 cm (3): dosimetric analysis of implant quality. Int J Radiat Oncol Biol Phys 46:1199, 2000.
378. Crook J, McLean M, Catton C, et al: Factors influencing risk of acute urinary retention after TRUS-guided permanent prostate seed implantation. Int J Radiat Oncol Biol Phys 52:453, 2002.

379. Merrick GS, Butler WM, Wallner KE, et al: Prophylactic versus therapeutic alpha-blockers after permanent prostate brachytherapy. Urology 60:650, 2002.
380. Gelblum DY, Potters L, Ashley R, et al: Urinary morbidity following ultrasound-guided transperineal prostate seed implantation. Int J Radiat Oncol Biol Phys 45:59, 1999.
381. Landis D, Wallner K, Locke J, et al: Late urinary function after prostate brachytherapy. Brachytherapy 1:21, 2002.
382. Blasko JC, Ragde H, Grimm PD: Transperineal ultrasound-guided implantation of the prostate morbidity and complications. Scand J Urol Nephrol Suppl 137:113, 1991.
383. Wallner K, Lee H, Wasserman S, et al: Low risk of urinary incontinence following prostate brachytherapy in patients with a prior transurethral prostate resection. Int J Radiat Oncol Biol Phys 37:565, 1997.
384. Stone NN, Stock RG: Dynamic cystography can replace cystoscopy following prostate seed implantation. Tech Urol 6:112, 2000.
385. Cha CM, Potters L, Ashley R, et al: Isotope selection for patients undergoing prostate brachytherapy. Int J Radiat Oncol Biol Phys 45:391, 1999.
386. Blasko JC, Grimm PD, Sylvester JE, et al: The role of external beam radiotherapy with I-125/Pd-103 brachytherapy for prostate carcinoma. Radiother Oncol 57:273, 2000.
387. Dicker AP, Lin CC, Leeper DB, et al: Isotope selection for permanent prostate implants? An evaluation of ^{103}Pd versus ^{125}I based on radiobiological effectiveness and dosimetry. Semin Urol Oncol 18:152, 2000.
388. Nag S, Bice WS, DeWyngaert JK, et al: The American Brachytherapy Society recommendations for transperineal permanent brachytherapy of prostate cancer. Int J Radiat Oncol Biol Phys 44:789, 1999.
389. Han B, Wallner K, Aggarwal S, et al: Treatment margins for prostate brachytherapy. Semin Urol Oncol 18:137, 2000.
390. Potters L, Fearn P, Kattan M: The role of external radiotherapy in patients treated with permanent prostate brachytherapy. Prostate Cancer Prostatic Dis 5:47, 2002.
391. Davis BJ, Haddock MG, Wilson TM, et al: Treatment of extraprostatic cancer in clinically organ-confined prostate cancer by permanent interstitial brachytherapy: is extraprostatic seed placement necessary? Tech Urol 6:70, 2000.
392. Dattoli M, Wallner K, True L, et al: Long-term outcomes after treatment with external beam radiation therapy and palladium 103 for patients with higher risk prostate carcinoma: influence of prostatic acid phosphatase. Cancer 97:979, 2003.
393. Critz FA, Williams WH, Levinson AK, et al: Simultaneous irradiation for prostate cancer: intermediate results with molern techniques J Urol 164:738, 2000.
394. Zelefsby MJ, Hollister T, Raben A, et al: Five-year biochemical outcome and toxicity with transperineal CT-planned permanent I-125 prostate implantation for patients with localized prostate cancer. Int J Radiat Oncol Biol Phys 47:1261, 2000.
395. Blasko JC, Grimm PD, Sylvester JE, et al: Palladium-103 brachytherapy for prostate carcinoma. Int Radiat Oncol Biol Phys 46:839, 2000.
396. Kupelian PA, Potters L, Khuntia D, et al: Radical prostatectomy, external beam radiotherapy <72 Gy, external beam radiotherapy > or = 72 Gy, permanent seed implantation, or combined seeds/external beam radiotherapy for stage T1-T2 prostate cancer. Int J Radiat Oncol Biol Phys 58:25, 2004.
397. Wallner K, Ellis W, Russell K, et al: Use of TRUS to predict pubic arch interference of prostate brachytherapy. Int J Radiat Oncol Biol Phys 43:583, 1999.
398. Potters L, Torre T, Ashley R, et al: Examining the role of neoadjuvant androgen deprivation in patients undergoing prostate brachytherapy. J Clin Oncol 18:1187, 2000.
399. Stock RG, Cahlon O, Cesaretti JA, et al: Combined modality treatment in the management of high-risk prostate cancer. Int J Radiat Oncol Biol Phys 59:1352, 2004.
400. Potters L, Morgenstern C, Calugaru E, et al: Twelve year outcomes following permanent prostate brachytherapy in patients with clinically localized prostate cancer. J Urol 173:1562, 2005.
401. Roach M III, DeSilvio M, Lawton C, et al: Phase III trial comparing whole-pelvic versus prostate-only radiotherapy and neoadjuvant versus adjuvant combined androgen suppression: Radiation Therapy Oncology Group 9412. J Clin Oncol 21:1901, 2003.
402. Merick GS, Wallner KE, Butler WM: Permanent interstitial brachytherapy for the management of carcinoma of the prostate gland. J Urol 169:1643, 2003.
403. Prestidge BR, Bice WS, Kiefer EJ, et al: Timing of computed tomography-based postimplant assessment following permanent transperineal prostate brachytherapy in the United States. Int J Radiat Oncol Biol Phys 40:1111, 1998.
404. Badiozamani KR, Wallner K, Cavanagh W, et al: Comparability of CT-based and TRUS-based prostate volumes. Int J Radiat Oncol Biol Phys 43:375, 1999.
405. Waterman FM, Dicker AP: Impact of postimplant edema on V(100) and D(90) in prostate brachytherapy: can implant quality be predicted on day 0? Int J Radiat Oncol Biol Phys 53:610, 2002.
406. Yue N, Dicker AP, Nath R, et al: The impact of edema on planning ^{125}I and ^{103}Pd prostate implants. Med Phys 26:763, 1999.
407. Roy JN, Wallner KE, Harrington PJ, et al: A CT-based evaluation method for permanent implants: application to prostate. Int J Radiat Oncol Biol Phys 26:163, 1993.
408. Stock RG, Stone NN, Tabert A, et al: A dose-response study for I-125 prostate implants. Int J Radiat Oncol Biol Phys 41:101, 1998.
409. Nag S, Ellis RJ, Merrick GS, et al: American Brachytherapy Society recommendation for reporting morbidity after prostate brachytherapy. Int J Radiat Oncol Biol Phys 54:462, 2002.
410. Crook J, Potters L, Stock R, et al: Critical organ dosimetry in permanent seed prostate brachytherapy: defining the organs at risk. An American Brachytherapy Society consensus statement. Brachytherapy 4:186, 2005.
411. Beyer DC, Shapiro RH, Puente F: Real-time optimized intraoperative dosimetry for prostate brachytherapy: a pilot study. Int J Radiat Oncol Biol Phys 48:1583, 2000.
412. American Society for Therapeutic Radiology and Oncology Consensus Panel: Consensus statement: guidelines for PSA following radiation therapy. Int J Radiat Oncol Biol Phys 37:1035, 1997.
413. Kattan MW, Fearn PA, Leibel S, et al: The definition of biochemical failure in patients treated with definitive radiotherapy. Int J Radiat Oncol Biol Phys 48:1469, 2000.
414. Grimm PD, Blasko JC, Sylvester JE, et al: 10-Year biochemical (prostate-specific antigen) control of prostate cancer with ^{125}I brachytherapy. Int J Radiat Oncol Biol Phys 51:31, 2001.
415. Ragde H, Grado GL, Nadir BS: Brachytherapy for clinically localized prostate cancer: thirteen-year disease free survival of 769 consecutive prostate cancer patients treated with permanent implants alone. Arch Esp Urol 54:739, 2001.
416. Kattan MW, Potters L, Blasko JC, et al: A pretreatment nomogram for predicting freedom from recurrence after permanent prostate brachytherapy in prostate cancer. Urology 58:393-399, 2001.
417. Potters L, Purrazzella R, Brustein S, et al: A comprehensive and novel predictive modeling technique using detailed pathology factors in men with localized prostate carcinoma. Cancer 95:1451, 2002.
418. Ragde H, Korb LJ, Elgamal AA, et al: Modern prostate brachytherapy: prostate specific antigen results in 219 patients with up to 12 years of observed follow-up. Cancer 89:135, 2000.
419. Sylvester JE, Blasko JC, Grimm PD, et al: Ten-year biochemical relapse-free survival after external beam radiation and brachytherapy for localized prostate cancer: the Seattle experience. Int J Radiat Oncol Biol Phys 57:944, 2003.
420. Potters L, Klein EA, Kattan MW, et al: Monotherapy for stage T1-T2 prostate cancer radical prostatectomy, external beam radiotherapy, or permanent seed implantation. Radiother Oncol 71:29, 2004.
421. Galblum DY, Potters L, Ashley R, et al: Rectal complications associated with transperineal interstitial brachytherapy for prostate cancer. Int Radiat Oncol Biol Phys 48:119, 2000.
422. Terk MD, Stock RG, Stone NN: Identification of patients at increased risk for prolonged urinary retention following radioactive seed implantation of the prostate [see comments]. J Urol 160:1379, 1998.

423. Crook J: Morbidity after brachytherapy for prostate adenocarcinoma. Mayo Clin Proc 79:945, 2004.
424. Wallner K, Merrick G, True L, et al: I-125 versus Pd-103 for low-risk prostate cancer: morbidity outcomes from a prospective randomized multicenter trial. Cancer J 8:67, 2002.
425. Locke J, Ellis W, Wallner K, et al: Risk factors for acute urinary retention requiring temporary intermittent catheterization after prostate brachytherapy: a prospective study. Int J Radiat Oncol Biol Phys 52:712, 2002.
426. Hu K, Wallner K: Urinary incontinence in patients who have a TURP/TUIP following prostate brachytherapy. Int J Radiat Oncol Biol Phys 40:783, 1998.
427. Stone NN, Stock RG: Complications following permanent prostate brachytherapy. Eur Urol 41:427, 2002.
428. Gray G, Wallner K, Roof J, et al: Cystourethroscopic findings before and after prostate brachytherapy. Tech Urol 6:109, 2000.
429. Merick GS, Wallner KE, Butler WM: Minimizing prostate brachytherapy-related morbidity. Urology 62:786, 2003.
430. Desai J, Stock RG, Stone NN, et al: Acute urinary morbidity following I-125 interstitial implantation of the prostate gland. Radiat Oncol Investig 6:135, 1998.
431. Merrick GS, Butler WM, Tollenaar BG, et al: The dosimetry of prostate brachytherapy-induced urethral strictures. Int J Radiat Oncol Biol Phys 52:461, 2002.
432. Merrick GS, Butler WM, Dorsey AT, et al: Rectal function following prostate brachytherapy. Int J Radiat Oncol Biol Phys 48:667, 2000.
433. Waterman FM, Dicker AP: Probability of late rectal morbidity in ^{125}I prostate brachytherapy. Int J Radiat Oncol Phys 55:342, 2003.
434. Han B, Wallner KE: Dosimetric and radiographic correlates to prostate brachytherapy-related rectal complications. Int J Cancer 96:372, 2001.
435. Merrick GS, Butler WM, Wallner KE, et al: Late rectal function after prostate brachytherapy. Int J Radiat Oncol Biol Phys 57:42, 2003.
436. Merrick GS, Butler WM: Rectal function following permanent prostate brachytherapy. W V Med J 100:18, 2004.
437. Hu K, Wallner K: Clinical course of rectal bleeding following I-125 prostate brachytherapy. Int J Radiat Oncol Biol Phys 41:263, 1998.
438. Merick GS, Wallner KE, Butler WM: Morbidity after brachytherapy for prostate adenocarcinoma. Mayo Clin Proc 79:945, 2004.
439. Snyder KM, Stock RG, Hong SM, et al: Defining the risk of developing grade 2 proctitis following ^{125}I prostate brachytherapy using a rectal dose-volume histogram analysis. Int J Radiat Oncol Biol Phys 50:335, 2001.
440. Potters L, Calguaru E, Thornton B, et al: Toward a dynamic real-time intraoperative permanent prostate brachytherapy methodology. Brachytherapy 2:172, 2003.
441. Zeitlin SI, Sherman J, Raboy A, et al: High dose combination radiotherapy for the treatment of localized prostate cancer. J Urol 160:91, 1998.
442. Brandeis JM, Litwin MS, Burnison CM, et al: Quality of life outcomes after brachytherapy for early stage prostrate cancer. J Urol 163:851, 2000.
443. Merrick GS, Wallner K, Butler WM, et al: A comparison of radiation dose to the bulb of the penis in men with and without prostate brachytherapy-induced erectile dysfunction. Int J Radiat Oncol Biol Phys 50:597, 2001.
444. Zelesky MJ, McKee AB, Lee H, et al: Efficacy of oral sildenafil in patients with erectile dysfunction after radiotherapy for carcinoma of the prostate. Urology 53:775, 1999.
445. Potters L, Torre T, Fearn PA, et al: Potency after permanent prostate brachytherapy for localized prostate cancer. Int J Radiat Oncol Biol Phys 50:1235, 2001.
446. Stock RG, Kao J, Stone NN: Penile erectile function after permanent radioactive seed implantation for treatment of prostate cancer. J Urol 165:436, 2001.
447. Kestin LL, Martinez AA, Stromberg JS, et al: Matched-pair analysis of conformal high-dose brachytherapy boost versus external-beam radiation therapy alone for locally advanced prostate cancer. J Clin Oncol 18:2869, 2000.
448. Martinez A, Gonzalez J, Stromberg J, et al: Conformal prostate brachytherapy: initial experience of a phase I/II dose-escalating trial. Int J Radiat Oncol Biol Phys 33:1019, 1995.
449. Martinez AA, Kestin LL, Stromberg JS, et al: Interim report of image-guided conformal high-dose-rate brachytherapy for patients with unfavorable prostate cancer: the William Beaumont phase II dose-escalating trial. Int J Radiat Oncol Biol Phys 47:343, 2000.
450. Kovacs G, Wirth B, Bertermann H, et al: Prostate preservation by combined external beam and HDR brachytherapy at nodal negative prostate cancer patients—an intermediate analysis after ten years' experience. Int J Radiat Oncol Biol Phys 36(Suppl):198, 1996.
451. Mate TP, Gottesman JE, Hatton J, et al: High-dose-rate afterloading ^{192}iridium prostate brachytherapy: feasibility report. Int J Radiat Oncol Biol Phys 41:525, 1998.
452. Kuban DA, El-Mahdi AM, Schellhammer PF: Prognostic significance of post-irradiation prostate biopsies. Oncology 7:29, 1993.
453. Crook JM, Perry GA, Robertson S, et al: Routine prostate biopsies following radiotherapy for prostate cancer: results for 226 patients. Urology 45:624, 1995.
454. Brawer MK, Nagle RB, Pitts W, et al: Keratin immunoreactivity as an aid to the diagnosis of persistent adenocarcinoma in irradiated human prostates. Cancer 63:454, 1989.
455. Crook J, Robertson S, Collins G, et al: Clinical relevance of transrectal ultrasound, biopsy, and serum prostate-specific antigen following external beam radiotherapy for carcinoma of the prostate. Int J Radiat Oncol Biol Phys 27:31, 1993.
456. Albertsen PC, Hanley JA, Penson DF, et al: Validation of increasing prostate specific antigen as a predictor of prostate cancer death after treatment of localized prostate cancer with surgery or radiation. J Urol 171:2221, 2004.
457. Walsh PC: Radical prostatectomy—a procedure in evolution. Semin Oncol 21:662, 1994.
458. Myers RP, Goellner JR, Cahill DR: Prostate shape, external striated urethral sphincter and radical prostatectomy: the apical dissection. J Urol 138:543, 1987.
459. Lu-Yao GL, McLerran D, Wasson J, et al: An assessment of radical prostatectomy: time trends, geographic variation, and outcomes. JAMA 269:2633, 1993.
460. Morgan WR, Lieber MM: Pelvic lymphadenectomy. *In* Crawford ED, Das S (eds): Current Genitourinary Cancer Surgery. Philadelphia, Lea & Febiger, 1990, p 162.
461. Lu-Yao GL, Potosky AL, Albertsen PC, et al: Follow-up prostate cancer treatments after radical prostatectomy: a population-based study. J Natl Cancer Inst 88:166, 1996.
462. Pound CR, Partin AW, Epstein JI, et al: Prostate-specific antigen after anatomic radical retropubic prostatectomy: patterns of recurrence and cancer control. Urol Clin North Am 24:395, 1997.
463. Han M, Partin AW, Pound CR, et al: Long-term biochemical disease-free and cancer-disease-free and cancer-specific survival following anatomic radical retropubic prostatectomy. Urol Clin North Am 28:555, 2001.
464. Hull GW, Rabbani F, Abbas F, et al: Cancer control with radical prostatectomy alone in 1,000 consecutive patients. J Urol 167:528, 2002.
465. Gerber GS, Thisted RA, Scardino PT, et al: Results of radical prostatectomy in men with clinically localized prostate cancer. JAMA 276:615, 1996.
466. Murphy GP, Mettlin C, Menck H, et al: National patterns of prostate cancer treatment by radical prostatectomy—results of a survey by the American College of Surgeons Commission on Cancer. J Urol 152:1817, 1994.
467. Iselin CE, Robertson JE, Paulson DF: Radical perineal prostatectomy: oncological outcome during a 20-year period. J Urol 161:163, 1999.
468. Amling CL, Blute ML, Bergstralh EJ, et al: Long-term hazard of progression after radical prostatectomy for clinically localized prostate cancer: continued risk of biochemical failure after 5 years. J Urol 164:101, 2000.
469. Wilt TJ: Uncertainty in prostate cancer care: the physician's role in clearing the confusion. JAMA 283:3258, 2000.
470. Fowler FJ, McNaughton Collins M, Albertsen PC, et al: Comparison of recommendations by urologists and radiation oncologists

for treatment of clinically localized prostate cancer. JAMA 283:3217, 2000.
471. Andriole GL, Smith DS, Rao G, et al: Early complications of contemporary anatomical radical retropubic prostatectomy. J Urol 152:1858, 1994.
472. Zincke H, Bergstralh EJ, Blute ML, et al: Radical prostatectomy for clinically localized prostate cancer-long-term results of 1,143 patients from a single institution. J Clin Oncol 12:2254, 1994.
473. Fowler FJ Jr, Barry MJ, Lu-Yao G, et al: Patient-reported complications and follow-up treatment after radical prostatectomy. The national Medicare experience: 1988-1990 (updated June 1993). Urology 42:622, 1993.
474. Walsh PC, Partin AW, Epstein JI: Cancer control and quality of life following anatomical radical retropubic prostatectomy-results at 10 years. J Urol 152:1831, 1994.
475. Fowler FJ, Barry MJ, Lu-Yao G, et al: Effect of radical prostatectomy for prostate cancer on patient quality of life: results from a Medicare survey. Urology 45:1007, 1995.
476. Jonler M, Madsen FA, Rhodes PR, et al: A prospective study of quantification of urinary incontinence and quality of life in patients undergoing radical retropubic prostatectomy. Urology 48:433, 1996.
477. Bishoff JT, Motley G, Optenberg SA, et al: Incidence of fecal and urinary incontinence following radical perineal and retropubic prostatectomy in a national population. J Urol 160:454, 1998.
478. Litwin MS, Lubeck DP, Henning JM, et al: Differences in urologist and patient assessments of health related quality of life in men with prostate cancer: results of the CaPSURE database. J Urol 159:1988, 1998.
479. Wei JT, Montie JE: Comparison of patients' and physicians' rating of urinary incontinence following radical prostatectomy. Semin Urol Oncol 18:76, 2000.
480. Catalona WJ, Basler JW: Return of erections and urinary continence following nerve sparing radical retropubic prostatectomy. J Urol 150:905, 1993.
481. Omar AM, Townell N: Laparoscopic radical prostatectomy: a review of the literature and comparison with open techniques. Prostate Cancer Prostatic Dis 7:295, 2004.
482. Smith JA: Robotically assisted laparoscopic prostatectomy: an assessment of its contemporary role in the surgical management of localized prostate cancer. Am J Surg 188(Suppl):63S, 2004.
483. Litwin MS, Hays RD, Fink A, et al: The UCLA Prostate Cancer Index: development, reliability, and validity of a health-related quality of life measure. Med Care 36:1002, 1998.
484. Wei JT, Dunn RL, Litwin MS, et al: Development and validation of the expanded prostate cancer index composite (EPIC) for comprehensive assessment of health-related quality of life in men with prostate cancer. Urology 56:899, 2000.
485. Litwin MS, Hays RD, Fink A, et al: Quality-of-life outcomes in men for localized prostate cancer. JAMA 273:129,1995.
486. Litwin MS, Sadetsky N, Pasta DJ, et al: Bowel function and bother after treatment for early stage prostate cancer: a longitudinal quality of life analysis from CaPSURE. J Urol 172:515, 2004.
487. Davis JW, Kuban DA, Lynch DF, et al: Quality of life after treatment for localized prostate cancer: differences based on treatment modality. J Urol 166:947, 2001.
488. Potosky AL, Davis WW, Hoffman RM, et al: Five-year outcomes after prostatectomy or radiotherapy for prostate cancer: the prostate cancer outcomes study. J Natl Cancer Inst 95:1358, 2004.
489. Pilepich MV, Krall JM, Al-Sarraf M, et al: Androgen deprivation with radiation therapy compared with radiation therapy alone for locally advanced prostatic carcinoma: a randomized comparative trial of the Radiation Therapy Oncology Group. Urology 45:616, 1995.
490. Paulson DF, Hodge GB, Hinshaw W: Radiation therapy versus delayed androgen deprivation for stage C carcinoma of the prostate. J Urol 131:901, 1984.
491. Aro J, Haapiainen R, Kajanti M, et al: Comparison of endocrine and radiation therapy in locally advanced prostatic cancer. Eur Urol 15:182, 1988.
492. Pilepich MV, Krall JM, Johnson RJ, et al: Extended field (periaortic) irradiation in carcinoma of the prostate—analysis of RTOG 75-06. Int J Radiat Oncol Biol Phys 12:345, 1986.
493. Hanks GE, Diamond JJ, Krall JM, et al: A ten-year follow-up of 682 patients treated for prostate cancer with radiation therapy in the United States. Int J Radiat Oncol Biol Phys 13:499, 1987.
494. Bolla M, Gonzalez D, Warde P, et al: Improved survival in patients with locally advanced prostate cancer treated with radiotherapy and goserelin. N Engl J Med 337:295, 1997.
495. Pilepich MV, Caplan R, Byhardt RW, et al: Phase III trial of androgen suppression using goserelin in unfavorable-prognosis carcinoma of the prostate treated with definitive radiotherapy. Report of Radiation Therapy Oncology Group protocol 85-31. J Clin Oncol 15:1013, 1997.
496. Sandler HM, Perez-Tamayo C, Ten Haken RK, et al: Dose escalation for stage C (T3) prostate cancer: minimal rectal toxicity observed using conformal therapy. Radiother Oncol 23:53, 1992.
497. Leibel SA, Heimann R, Kutcher GJ, et al: Three-dimensional conformal radiation therapy in locally advanced carcinoma of the prostate: preliminary results of a phase I dose-escalation study. Int J Radiat Oncol Biol Phys 28:55,1994.
498. Forman JD, Duclos M, Shamsa F, et al: Hyperfractionated conformal radiotherapy in locally advanced prostate cancer: results of a dose escalation study. Int J Radiat Oncol Biol Phys 34:655, 1996.
499. Laramore GE, Krall JM, Thomas FJ, et al: Fast neutron radiotherapy for locally advanced prostate cancer. Final report of a Radiation Therapy Oncology Group randomized clinical trial. Am J Clin Oncol 16:164, 1993.
500. Russell KJ, Caplan RJ, Laramore GE, et al: Photon versus fast neutron external beam radiotherapy in the treatment of locally advanced prostate cancer: results of a randomized prospective trial. Int J Radiat Oncol Biol Phys 28:47, 1994.
501. Shipley WU, Verhey LJ, Munzenrider JE, et al: Advanced prostate cancer. The results of a randomized comparative trial of high dose irradiation boosting with conformal photons compared with conventional dose irradiation using photons alone. Int J Radiat Oncol Biol Phys 32:3, 1995.
502. Forman JD, Duclos M, Sharma R, et al: Conformal mixed neutron and photon irradiation in localized and locally advanced prostate cancer: preliminary estimates of the therapeutic ratio. Int J Radiat Oncol Biol Phys 35:259, 1996.
503. Stromberg J, Martinez A, Benson R, et al: Improved local control and survival for surgically staged patients with locally advanced prostate cancer treated with up-front low dose rate iridium-192 prostate implantation and external beam irradiation. Int J Radiat Oncol Biol Phys 28:67, 1994.
504. Stromberg J, Martinez A, Gonzalez J, et al: Ultrasound-guided high dose rate conformal brachytherapy boost in prostate cancer: treatment description and preliminary results of a phase I/II clinical trial. Int J Radiat Oncol Biol Phys 33:161, 1995.
505. Zagars GK, Johnson DE, von Eschenbach AC, et al: Adjuvant estrogen following radiation therapy for stage C adenocarcinoma of the prostate: long-term results of a prospective randomized trial. Int J Radiat Oncol Biol Phys 14:1085, 1988.
506. Pilepich MV, Krall JM, John MJ, et al: Hormonal cytoreduction in locally advanced carcinoma of the prostate treated with definitive radiotherapy: preliminary results of RTOG 83-07. Int J Radiat Oncol Biol Phys 16:813, 1989.
507. Pilepich MV, John MJ, Krall JM, et al: Phase II Radiation Therapy Oncology Group study of hormonal cytoreduction with flutamide and Zoladex in locally advanced carcinoma of the prostate treated with definitive radiotherapy. Am J Clin Oncol 13:461, 1990.
508. Lawton CA, Coleman CN, Buzydlowski JW, et al: Results of a phase II trial of external beam radiation with etanidazole (SR 2508) for the treatment of locally advanced prostate cancer (RTOG protocol 90-20). Int J Radiat Oncol Biol Phys 36:673, 1996.
509. Yonemoto LT, Slater JD, Rossi CJ Jr, et al: Combined proton and photon conformal radiation therapy for locally advanced carcinoma of the prostate: preliminary results of a phase I/II study. Int J Radiat Oncol Biol Phys 37:21, 1997.
510. Gardner BG, Zietman AL, Shipley WU, et al: Late normal tissue sequelae in the second decade after high dose radiation therapy with combined photons and conformal protons for locally advanced prostate cancer. J Urol 167:123, 2002.

511. Griffiths K, Eaton CL, Harper ME, et al: Hormonal treatment of advanced disease—some newer aspects. Semin Oncol 21:672, 1994.
512. Pilepich MV, Winter K, John MJ, et al: Phase III Radiation Therapy Oncology Group (RTOG) trial 86-10 of androgen deprivation adjuvant to definitive radiotherapy in locally advanced carcinoma of the prostate. Int J Radiat Oncol Biol Phys 50:1243, 2001.
513. Pilepich MV, Winter K, Lawton C, et al: Androgen suppression adjuvant to definitive radiotherapy in prostate carcinoma: long-term results of phase III RTOG 85-31. Int J Radiat Oncol Biol Phys 61:1285-1290, 2005.
514. Bolla M, Collette L, Blank L, et al: Long-term results with immediate androgen suppression and external irradiation in patients with locally advanced prostate cancer (an EORTC study) a phase III randomized trial. Lancet 360:103, 2002.
515. Hanks GE, Pajak T, Potter A, et al: Phase III trial of long-term adjuvant androgen deprivation after neoadjuvant hormonal cytoreduction and radiotherapy in locally advanced carcinoma of the prostate: the Radiation Therapy Oncology Group Protocol 92-02. J Clin Oncol 21:3972, 2003.
516. Roach M III, DeSilvio M, Lawton C, et al: Phase III trial comparing whole-pelvic vs prostate only radiotherapy and neoadjuvant vs. adjuvant combined androgen suppression: Radiation Therapy Oncology Group 94-13. J Clin Oncol 21:1904, 2003.
517. Gervasi LA, Provet J, Al-Askari S, et al: Prognostic significance of lymph nodal metastases in prostate cancer. J Urol 142:332,1989.
518. Johnson DE, von Eschenbach AC, Prout G Jr, et al: Roles of lymphangiography and pelvic lymphadenectomy in staging prostate cancer. Nodal involvement as a prognostic indicator in patients with prostatic carcinoma. J Urol 124:226, 1980.
519. Paulson DF, Cline WA, Koefoot RB, et al: Extended field radiation therapy versus delayed hormonal therapy in node positive prostatic adenocarcinoma. J Urol 127:935, 1982.
520. Lawton CA, Cox JD, Glisch C, et al: Is long-term survival possible with external beam irradiation for stage D1 adenocarcinoma of the prostate? Cancer 69:2761, 1992.
521. Bagshaw MA: Radiotherapeutic treatment of prostatic carcinoma with pelvic node involvement. Urol Clin North Am 11:297, 1984.
522. Lawton CA, Winter K, Grignon D, et al: Androgen suppression plus radiation vs radiation alone for patients with D1 (pN+) adenocarcinoma of the prostate: updated results based on a national prospective randomized trial, RTOG 85-31 [erratum in J Clin Oncol 23:8921, 2005]. J Clin Oncol 23:800, 2005.
523. Schmidt JD, Gibbons RP, Murphy GP, et al: Evaluation of adjuvant estramustine phosphate, cyclophosphamide, and observation only for node-positive patients following radical prostatectomy and definitive irradiation. Prostate 28:51, 1996.
524. Cheng CWS, Bergstralh EJ, Zincke H: Stage D1 prostate cancer. A nonrandomized comparison of conservative treatment options versus radical prostatectomy. Cancer 71:996, 1993.
525. Whittington R, Malkowicz SB, Machtay M, et al: The use of combined radiation therapy and hormonal therapy in the management of lymph node-positive prostate cancer. Int J Radiat Oncol Biol Phys 39:673, 1997.
526. Coia LR, Minsky BD, John M, et al: 1996 decision trees and management guidelines. Semin Radiat Oncol 7:163, 1997.
527. Messing EM, Manola J, Sarosdy M, et al: Immediate hormonal therapy combined with observation after radical prostatectomy and pelvic lymphadenectomy in men with node-positive prostate cancer. N Engl J Med 341:1781, 1999.
528. Lankford SP, Pollack A, Zagars GK: Radiotherapy for regionally localized hormone refractory prostate cancer. Int J Radiat Oncol Biol Phys 33:907, 1995.
529. Cooperberg MR, Broering JM, Litwin MS, et al: The contemporary management of prostate cancer in the United States: lessons from the Cancer of the Prostate Strategic Urologic Research Endeavor (CaPSURE), a national disease registry. J Urol 17:1499, 2004.
530. Amling CL, Blute ML, Bergstralh EJ, et al: Long-term hazard of progression after radical prostatectomy for clinically localized prostate cancer: continued risk of biochemical failure after 5 years. J Urol 164:101, 2000.
531. Moul JW, Connelly RR, Lubeck DP, et al: Predicting risk of prostate specific antigen recurrence after radical prostatectomy with the Center for Prostate Disease Research and Cancer of the Prostate Strategic Urologic Research Endeavor databases. J Urol 166:1322, 2001.
532. Han M, Partin AW, Zahurak M, et al: Biochemical (prostate specific antigen) recurrence probability following radical prostatectomy for clinically localized prostate cancer. J Urol 169:517, 2003.
533. Roehl KA, Han M, Ramos CG, et al: Cancer progression and survival rates following anatomical radical retropubic prostatectomy for clinically localized prostate cancer. J Urol 172:910, 2004.
534. Kupelian P, Katcher J, Levin H, et al: Correlation of clinical and pathologic factors with rising prostate-specific antigen profiles after radical prostatectomy alone for clinically localized prostate cancer. Urology 48:249, 1996.
535. Blute ML, Bergstralh EJ, Iocca A, et al: Use of Gleason score, prostate specific antigen, seminal vesicle and margin status to predict biochemical failure after radical prostatectomy. J Urol 165:119, 2000.
536. Anscher MS: Adjuvant radiotherapy following radical prostatectomy is more effective and less toxic than salvage radiotherapy for a rising prostate specific antigen. Int J Can 20:91, 2001.
537. Connolly JA, Presti JC Jr, Cher ML, et al: Accelerated tumor proliferation rates in locally recurrent prostate cancer after radical prostatectomy. J Urol 158:515, 1997.
538. Bolla M, Van Poppel H, Van Cangh P, et al: Post operative radiotherapy (P-XRT) after radical prostatectomy (PX) improves progression-free survival (PFS) in pT3N0 prostate cancer (PC) (EORTC 22911). Int J Radiat Oncol Biol Phys 60(Suppl):S186, 2004.
539. Anscher MS, Robertson CN, Prosnitz LR: Adjuvant radiotherapy for pathologic stage T3/4 adenocarcinoma of the prostate: ten-year update. Int J Radiat Oncol Biol Phys 33:37, 1995.
540. Cozzarini C, Bolognesi A, Ceresoli GL, et al: Role of postoperative radiotherapy after pelvic lymphadenectomy and radical retropubic prostatectomy: a single institute experience of 415 patients. Int J Radiat Oncol Biol Phys 59:674, 2004.
541. Hawkins CA, Bergstralh EJ, Lieber MM, et al: Influence of DNA ploidy and adjuvant treatment on progression and survival in patients with pathologic stage T3 (PT3) prostate cancer after radical retropubic prostatectomy. Urology 46:356, 1995.
542. Leibovich BC, Engen DE, Patterson DE, et al: Benefit of adjuvant radiation therapy for localized prostate cancer with a positive surgical margin. J Urol 163:1178, 2000.
543. Petrovich Z, Lieskovsky G, Langholz B, et al: Nonrandomized comparison of surgery with and without adjuvant pelvic irradiation for patients with pT3N0 adenocarcinoma of the prostate. Am J Clin Oncol 24:537, 2001.
544. Schild SE, Wong WW, Grado GL, et al: The results of radical retropubic prostatectomy and adjuvant therapy for pathologic stage C prostate cancer. Int J Radiat Oncol Biol Phys 34:535, 1996.
545. Valcenti RK, Gomella LG, Ismail M, et al: The efficacy of early adjuvant radiation therapy for pT3N0 prostate cancer: a matched-pair analysis. Int J Radiat Oncol Biol Phys 45:53, 1999.
546. Schild SE, Pisansky TM: The role of radiotherapy after radical prostatectomy. Urol Clin North Am 28:629, 2001.
547. Ligtner DJ, Lange PH, Reddy PK, et al: Prostate specific antigen and local recurrence after radical prostatectomy. J Urol 144:921, 1990.
548. Cozzarini C, Fiorino C, Ceresoli GL, et al: Significant correlation between rectal DVH and late bleeding in patients treated after radical prostatectomy with conformal or conventional radiotherapy (66.6-70.2 Gy). Int J Radiat Oncol Biol Phys 55:668, 2003.
549. Formenti SC, Lieskovsky G, Simoneau AR, et al: Impact of moderate dose of postoperative radiation on urinary continence and potency in patients with prostate cancer treated with nerve sparing prostatectomy. J Urol 155:616, 1996.
550. Syndikus I, Pickles T, Kostashuk E, et al: Postoperative radiotherapy for stage pT3 carcinoma of the prostate: improved local control. J Urol 155:1983, 1996.
551. Eisbruch A, Perez CA, Roessler EH, et al: Adjuvant irradiation after prostatectomy for carcinoma of the prostate with positive surgical margins. Cancer 73:384, 1994.
552. Wiegel T, Bressel M, Carl UM: Adjuvant radiotherapy following radical prostatectomy: results of 56 patients. Eur J Cancer 31A:5, 1995.

553. Cox JD, Gallagher MJ, Hammond EH, et al: Consensus statements on radiation therapy of prostate cancer: guidelines for prostate re-biopsy after radiation and for radiation therapy with rising prostate-specific antigen levels after radical prostatectomy. J Clin Oncol 17:1155, 1999.
554. Fowler JE, Brooks J, Pandey P, et al: Variable histology of anastomotic biopsies with detectable prostate specific antigen after radical prostatectomy. J Urol 153:1011, 1995.
555. Connolly JA, Shinohara K, Presti JC, et al: Local recurrence after radical prostatectomy: characteristics in sizes, location, and relationship to prostate-specific antigen and surgical margins. Urology 47:225, 1996.
556. Cher ML, Bianco FJ, Lam JS, et al: Limited role of radionuclide bone scintigraphy in patients with prostate specific antigen elevations after radical prostatectomy. J Urol 160:1387, 1998.
557. Kane CJ, Amling CL, Johnstone PA, et al: Limited value of bone scintigraphy and computed tomography in assessing biochemical failure after radical prostatectomy. Urology 61:607, 2003.
558. Koppie TM, Grossfeld GD, Nudell DM, et al: Is anastomotic biopsy necessary before radiotherapy after radical prostatectomy? J Urol 166:111, 2001.
559. Summers RM, Korobkin M, Quint Le, et al: Pelvic CT findings after radical prostatectomy. J Comput Tomogr 17:767, 1993.
560. Sella T, Schwartz LH, Swindle PW, et al: Suspected local recurrence after radical prostatectomy: endorectal coil MR Imaging. Radiology 231:379, 2004.
561. Song DY, Thompson TL, Ramakrishnan V, et al: Salvage radiotherapy for rising or persistent PSA after radical prostatectomy. Urology 60:281, 2002.
562. Thomas CT, Bradshaw PT, Pollock BH, et al: Indium-111-capromab pendetide radioimmunoscintigraphy and prognosis for durable biochemical response to salvage radiation therapy in men after failed prostatectomy. J Clin Oncol 21:1715, 2003.
563. Partin AW, Pearson JD, Landis PK, et al: Evaluation of serum prostate-specific antigen velocity after radical prostatectomy to distinguish local recurrence from distant metastases. Urology 43:649, 1994.
564. Stephenson AJ, Shariat SF, Zelefsky MJ, et al: Salvage radiotherapy for recurrent prostate cancer after radical prostatectomy. JAMA 291:1325, 2004.
565. Pisansky TM, Kozelsky TF, Myers RP, et al: Radiotherapy for isolated serum prostate specific antigen elevation after prostatectomy for prostate cancer. J Urol 163:845, 2000.
566. Catton C, Gospodarowicz M, Warde P, et al: Adjuvant and salvage radiation therapy after radical prostatectomy for adenocarcinoma of the prostate. Radiother Oncol 59:51, 2001.
567. Chawla AS, Thakral HK, Zeitman AL, et al: Salvage radiotherapy after radical prostatectomy for prostate adenocarcinoma: analysis of efficacy and prognostic factors. Urology 59:726, 2002.
568. Tsien C, Griffith KA, Sandler HM, et al: Long-term results of three-dimensional conformal adjuvant and salvage radiotherapy after radical prostatectomy. Urology 62:93, 2003.
569. Maier J, Forman J, Tekyi-Mensah S, et al: Salvage radiation for a rising PSA following radical prostatectomy. Urology 22:50, 2004.
570. Do T, Parker RG, Do C, et al: Salvage radiotherapy for biochemical and clinical failures following radical prostatectomy. Cancer J Sci Am 4:324, 1998.
571. Valicenti RK, Gomella LG, Ismail M, et al: Effect of higher radiation dose on biochemical control after radical prostatectomy for pT2N0 prostate cancer. Int J Radiat Oncol Biol Phys 42:501, 1998.
572. Perez CA, Michalski JM, Baglan K, et al: Radiation therapy for increasing prostate-specific antigen levels after radical prostatectomy. Clin Prostate Cancer 1:235, 2003.
573. Katz MS, Zelefsky MJ, Venkatraman ES, et al: Predictors of biochemical outcome with salvage conformal radiotherapy after radical prostatectomy for prostate cancer. J Clin Oncol 21:483, 2003.
574. Anscher MS, Clough R, Dodge R: Radiotherapy for a rising prostate-specific antigen after radical prostatectomy: the first 10 years. Int J Radiat Oncol Biol Phys 48:369, 2000.
575. Choo R, Hruby G, Hong J, et al: (In)-efficacy of salvage radiotherapy for rising PSA or clinically isolated local recurrence after radical prostatectomy. Int J Radiat Oncol Biol Phys 53:269, 2002.
576. King CR, Presti JC Jr, Gill H, et al: Radiotherapy after radical prostatectomy: does transient androgen suppression improve outcomes? Int J Radiat Oncol Biol Phys 59:341, 2004.
577. Teh BS, Mai WY, Augspurger ME, et al: Intensity modulated radiation therapy (IMRT) following prostatectomy: more favorable acute genitourinary toxicity profile compared to primary IMRT for prostate cancer. Int J Radiat Oncol Biol Phys 49:465, 2001.
578. Wiegel T, Bressel M, Arps H, et al: Radiotherapy of local recurrence following radical prostatectomy. Strahlenther Onkol 168:333, 1992.
579. Vander Kooy MJ, Pisansky TM, Cha SS, et al: Irradiation for locally recurrent carcinoma of the prostate following radical prostatectomy. Urology 49:65, 1997.
580. Cadeddu JA, Partin AW, Deweese TL, et al: Long-term results of radiation therapy for prostate cancer recurrence following radical prostatectomy. J Urol 159:173, 1998.
581. Leventis AK, Shariat SF, Kattan MW, et al: Prediction of response to salvage radiation therapy in patients with prostate cancer recurrence after radical prostatectomy. J Clin Oncol 19:1030, 2001.
582. Macdonald OK, Schild SE, Vora SE, et al: Salvage radiotherapy for palpable, locally recurrent prostate cancer after radical prostatectomy. Int J Radiat Oncol Biol Phys 58:1530, 2004.
583. Choo R, Morton G, Danjoux C, et al: Limited efficacy of salvage radiotherapy for biopsy confirmed or clinically palpable local recurrence of prostate carcinoma after surgery. Radiother Oncol 74:163, 2005.
584. Anscher MS, Prosnitz LR: Radiotherapy vs. hormonal therapy for the management of locally recurrent prostate cancer following radical prostatectomy. Int J Radiat Oncol Biol Phys 17:953, 1989.
585. Gerber GS, Thisted RA, Chodak GW, et al: results of radical prostatectomy in men with locally advanced prostate cancer: multi-institutional pooled analysis. Eur Urol 32:385, 1997.
586. Lerner SE, Blute ML, Zincke H: Extended experience with radical prostatectomy for clinical stage T3 prostate cancer. Outcome and contemporary morbidity. J Urol 154:1447, 1995.
587. Narayan P, Lowe BA, Carroll PR, et al: Neoadjuvant hormonal therapy and radical prostatectomy for clinical stage C carcinoma of the prostate. Br J Urol 73:544, 1994.
588. Smit WG, Helle PA, van Putten WL, et al: Late radiation damage in prostate cancer patients treated by high dose external radiotherapy in relation to rectal dose. Int J Radiat Oncol Biol Phys 18:23, 1990.
589. Gomella LG, Liberman SN, Mulholland SG, et al: Induction androgen deprivation plus prostatectomy for stage T3 disease. Failure to achieve prostate-specific antigen-based freedom from disease status in a phase II trial. Urology 47:870, 1996.
590. Garnick MB, Fair WR: First International Conference on Neoadjuvant Hormonal Therapy of Prostate Cancer. Overview consensus statement. Urology 49:1, 1997.
591. Van Poppel H, Deridder D, Elgamal AA, et al: Neoadjuvant hormonal therapy before radical prostatectomy decreases the number of positive surgical margins in stage T2 prostate cancer: Interim results of a prospective randomized trial. J Urol 154:429, 1995.
592. Gleave ME, Goldenberg SL, Jones EC, et al: Biochemical and pathological effects of 8 months of neoadjuvant androgen withdrawal therapy before radical prostatectomy in patients with clinically confined prostate cancer. J Urol 155:213, 1996.
593. Labrie F, Cusan L, Gomez JL, et al: Neoadjuvant hormonal therapy. The Canadian experience. Urology 40:56, 1997.
594. Witjes WP, Schulman CC, Debruyne FM: Preliminary results of a prospective randomized study comparing radical prostatectomy versus radical prostatectomy associated with neoadjuvant hormonal combination therapy in T2-3 N0 M0 prostatic carcinoma. The European Study Group on Neoadjuvant Treatment of Prostate Cancer. Urology 49:65, 1997.
595. Ghavamian R, Bergstralh EJ, Blute ML, et al: Radical retropubic prostatectomy plus orchiectomy versus orchiectomy alone for pTxN+ prostate cancer: a matched comparison. J Urol 161:1223, 1999.
596. Palapattu GS, Allaf ME, Trock BJ, et al: Prostate specific antigen progression in men with lymph node metastases following

radical prostatectomy: results of long-term followup. J Urol 172:1860, 2004.

597. Myers RP, Larson-Keller JJ, Bergstralh EJ, et al: Hormonal treatment at time of radical retropubic prostatectomy for stage D1 prostate cancer: results of long-term follow-up. J Urol 147:910, 1992.
598. Corral DA, Pisters LL, von Eschenbach AC: Treatment options for localized recurrence of prostate cancer following radiation therapy. Urol Clin North Am 23:677, 1996.
599. Pisters LL, Wajsman Z: Salvage surgery following full-dose radiation therapy for prostate cancer. *In* Bland KI, Karakousis CP, Copeland EM (eds): Atlas of Surgical Oncology. Philadelphia, WB Saunders, 1995, p 605.
600. Neerhut GJ, Wheeler T, Cantini M, et al: Salvage radical prostatectomy for radiorecurrent adenocarcinoma of the prostate. J Urol 140:544, 1988.
601. Thompson IM, Rounder JB, Spence CR, et al: Salvage radical prostatectomy for adenocarcinoma of the prostate. Cancer 61:1464, 1988.
602. Link P, Freiha FS: Radical prostatectomy after definitive radiation therapy for prostate cancer. Urology 37:189, 1991.
603. Mout JW, Paulson DF: The role of radical surgery in the management of radiation recurrent and large volume prostate cancer. Cancer 68:1265, 1991.
604. Ahlering TE, Lieskovsky G, Skinner DG: Salvage surgery plus androgen deprivation for radioresistant prostatic adenocarcinoma. J Urol 147:900, 1992.
605. Stein A, Smith RB, deKernion JB: Salvage radical prostatectomy after failure of curative radiotherapy for adenocarcinoma of prostate. Urology 40:197, 1992.
606. Pontes JE, Montie J, Klein E, et al: Salvage surgery for radiation failure in prostate cancer. Cancer 71:976, 1993.
607. Lerner SE, Blute ML, Zincke H: Critical evaluation of salvage surgery for radio-recurrent resistant prostate cancer. J Urol 154:1103, 1995.
608. Rogers E, Ohori M, Kassabian VS, et al: Salvage radical prostatectomy—outcome measured by serum prostate specific antigen levels. J Urol 153:104, 1995.
609. Onik G, Cobb C, Cohen J, et al: US characteristics of frozen prostate. Radiology 168:529, 1988.
610. Cohen JK, Miller RJ: Thermo protection of urethra during cryosurgery of prostate. Cryobiology 31:313, 1994.
611. Cohen JK, Miller RJ, Shuman BA: Urethral warming catheter for use during cryoablation of the prostate. Urology 45:861, 1995.
612. Lam JS, Belldergun AS: Salvage cryosurgery of the prostate after radiation failure. Rev Urol 6(Suppl):S27, 2004.
613. Pisters LL, von Eschenbach AC, Scott SM, et al: The efficacy and complications of salvage cryotherapy of the prostate. J Urol 157:921, 1997.
614. Ghafar Ma, Johnson CS, De La Taille A, et al: Salvage cryotherapy using an argon base system for locally recurrent prostate cancer after radiation therapy: the Columbia experience. J Urol 166:1333, 2001.
615. Han KR, Belldegrun AS: Third-generation cryosurgery for primary and recurrent prostate cancer. BJU Int 93:14, 2004.
616. Chen JL, Pautler SE, Mouraviev V, et al: Results of salvage and cryoablation of the prostate after radiation: identifying predictors of treatment failure and complications. J Urol 165:1937, 2001.
617. Huggins C, Stevens RE, Hodges CV: Studies on prostate cancer. II. The effects of castration on advanced carcinoma of the prostate gland. Arch Surg 43:209, 1941.
618. Vogelzang NJ, Chodak GW, Soloway MS, et al: Goserelin versus orchiectomy in the treatment of advanced prostate cancer: final results of a randomized trial. Zoladex Prostate Study Group. Urology 46:220, 1995.
619. Crawford ED, Blumenstein BA, Goodman PJ, et al: Leuprolide with and without flutainide in advanced prostate cancer. Cancer 66:1039, 1990.
620. Prostate Cancer Trialists' Collaborative Group: Maximum androgen blockade in advanced prostate cancer: an overview of the randomized trials. Lancet 355:1491, 2000.
621. Iversen P, Tyrrell CJ, Kaisary AV, et al: Casodex (bicalutamide) 150-mg monotherapy compared with castration in patients with previously untreated nonmetastic prostate cancer: results from two multicenter randomized trials at a median follow-up of 4 years. Urology 51:389, 1998.
622. Tyrrell CJ, Kaisary AV, Iversen P, et al: A randomized comparison of Casodex (bicalutamide) 150 mg monotherapy versus castration in the treatment of metastatic and locally advanced prostate cancer. Eur Urol 33:447, 1998.
623. Janknegt RA, Abbou CC, Bartoletti R, et al: Orchiectomy and nilutamide or placebo as treatment of metastatic prostatic cancer in a multinational double-blind randomized trial. J Urol 149:77, 1993.
624. Yagoda A, Petrylak D: Cytotoxic chemotherapy for advanced hormone-resistant prostate cancer. Cancer 71:1098, 1993.
625. Eisenberger MA, De Witt R, Berry W, et al: A multicenter phase III comparison of docetaxel (D) + prednisone (P) and mitoxantrone (MTZ) + P in patients with hormone-refractory prostate cancer (HRPC). J Clin Oncol 22(Suppl):4, 2004.
626. Smith DC, Chay CH, Dunn RL, et al: Phase II trial of paclitaxel, estramustine, etoposide, and carboplatin in the treatment of hormone-refractory prostate cancer. Cancer 98:269, 2003.
627. Tong D, Gillick L, Hendrickson FR: The palliation of symptomatic osseous metastases. Final results of the study by the Radiation Therapy Oncology Group. Cancer 50:893, 1982.
628. Coia LR, Hanks GE, Martz K, et al: Practice patterns of palliative care for the United States 1984-1985. Int J Radiat Oncol Biol Phys 14:1261, 1988.
629. Blitzer PH: Reanalysis of the RTOG study of the palliation of symptomatic osseous metastasis. Cancer 55:1468, 1985.
630. Wilkins W, Keen CW: Hemi-body radiotherapy in the management of metastatic carcinoma. Clin Radiol 38:267, 1987.
631. Robinson RG, Preston DF, Schiefelbein M, et al: Strontium-89 therapy for the palliation of pain due to osseous metastases. JAMA 274:420, 1995.
632. Turner SL, Gruenewald S, Spry N, et al: Less pain does equal better quality of life following strontium-89 therapy for metastatic prostate cancer. Br J Cancer 84:297, 2001.
633. Kim SI, Chen DC, Muggia FM: A new look at radionuclide therapy in metastatic disease of bone. Anticancer Res 8:681, 1988.
634. Sartor O, Reid RH, Hoskin PJ, et al: Samarium-153-Lexidroam complex for treatment of painful bone metastases in hormone-refractory prostate cancer. Urology 63:940, 2004.
635. Smith MR: Bisphosphonates to prevent bony skeletal complications in men with metastatic prostate cancer. J Urol 170(Pt 2):S55, 2003.
636. Heindenreich A: Bisphosphonates in the management of metastatic prostate cancer. Oncology 65(Suppl 1):5, 2003.
637. Shahinian VB, Kuo YF, Freeman JL, et al: Risk of fracture after androgen deprivation for prostate cancer. N Engl J Med 352:154, 2005.
638. Valicenti RK, Waterman FM, Croce RJ, et al: Efficient CT simulation of the four-field technique for conformal radiotherapy of prostate carcinoma. Int J Radiat Oncol Biol Phys 37:953, 1997.
639. Rosenthal SA, Roach M III, Goldsmith BJ, et al: Immobilization improves the reproducibility of patient positioning during six-field conformal radiation therapy for prostate carcinoma. Int J Radiat Oncol Biol Phys 27:921, 1993.
640. Hunt MA, Schultheiss TE, Desobry GE, et al: An evaluation of setup uncertainties for patients treated to pelvic sites. Int J Radiat Oncol Biol Phys 32:227, 1995.
641. Sharma R, Duclos M, Chuba PJ, et al: Enhancement of prostate tumor volume definition with intravesical contrast: a three-dimensional dosimetric evaluation. Int J Radiat Oncol Biol Phys 38:575, 1997.
642. Schild SE, Buskirk SJ, Robinow JS: Prostate cancer: Retrograde urethrography to improve treatment planning for radiation therapy. Radiology 181:885, 1991.
643. Roach M III, Pickett B, Holland J, et al: The role of the urethrogram during simulation for localized prostate cancer. Int J Radiat Oncol Biol Phys 25:299, 1993.
644. Cox JA, Zagoria RJ, Raben M: Prostate cancer-comparison of retrograde urethrography and computed tomography in radiotherapy planning. Int J Radiat Oncol Biol Phys 29:1119, 1994.
645. Ten Haken RK, Forman JD, Heimburger DK, et al: Treatment planning issues related to prostate movement in response to dif-

ferential filling of the rectum and bladder. Int J Radiat Oncol Biol Phys 20:1317, 1991.
646. Balter JM, Sandler HM, Lam K, et al: Measurement of prostate movement over the course of routine radiotherapy using implanted markers. Int J Radiat Oncol Biol Phys 31:113, 1995.
647. Lattanzi J, McNeeley S, Donnelly S: Ultrasound-based stereotactic guidance in prostate cancer—quantification of organ motion and set-up errors in external beam radiation therapy. Comput Aided Surg 5:289, 2000.
648. Chandra A, Doug L, Huang E: Experience of ultrasound-based daily prostate localization. Int J Radiat Oncol Biol Phys 56:436, 2003.
649. Langen KM, Pouliot J, Anezinos C: Evaluation of ultrasound-based prostate localization for image-guided radiotherapy. Int J Radiat Oncol Biol Phys 57:535, 2003.
650. Little DJ, Dong L, Levy LB: Use of portal images and BAT ultrasonography to measure set up error and organ motion for prostate IMRT: implications for treatment margins. Int J Radiat Oncol Biol Phys 56:1218, 2003.
651. Kuban DA, Dong L, Cheung R, et al: Ultrasound based localization. Semin Radiat Oncol 15:180, 2005.
652. McGowan DG: The value of extended field radiation therapy in carcinoma of the prostate. Int J Radiat Oncol Biol Phys 7:1333, 1981.
653. Polysongsang S, Aron BS, Shehata WM, et al: Comparison of whole pelvis versus small-field radiation therapy for carcinoma of prostate. Urology 27:10, 1986.
654. Perez CA, Michalski J, Brown KC, et al: Nonrandomized evaluation of pelvic lymph node irradiation in localized carcinoma of the prostate. Int J Radiat Oncol Biol Phys 36:573, 1996.
655. Asbell SO, Krall JM, Pilepich W, et al: Elective pelvic irradiation in stage A2, B carcinoma of the prostate: analysis of RTOG 77-06. Int J Radiat Oncol Biol Phys 15:1307, 1988.
656. Forman JD, Lee Y, Roberson P, et al: Advantages of CT and beam's eye view display to confirm the accuracy of pelvic lymph node irradiation in carcinoma of the prostate. Radiology 186:889, 1993.
657. Pollack A, Paryani SB, Hussey D, et al: Locally advanced (high-risk) prostate cancer. American College of Radiology. ACR Appropriateness Criteria. Radiology 215(Suppl):1401, 2000.
658. Katcher J, Kupelian PA, Zippe C, et al: Indications for excluding the seminal vesicles when treating clinically localized prostatic adenocarcinoma with radiotherapy alone. Int J Radiat Oncol Biol Phys 37:871, 1997.
659. D'Amico AV, Whittington R, Kaplan I, et al: Equivalent 5-year bNED in select prostate cancer patients managed with surgery or radiation therapy despite exclusion of the seminal vesicles from the CTV. Int J Radiat Oncol Biol Phys 39:335, 1997.
660. Roach M, Faillace-Akazawa P, Malfatti C, et al: Prostate volumes defined by magnetic resonance imaging and computerized tomographic scans for three-dimensional conformal radiotherapy. Int J Radiat Oncol Biol Phys 35:1011, 1996.
661. Kagawa K, Lee WR, Schultheiss TE, et al: Initial clinical assessment of CT-MRI image fusion software in localization of the prostate for 3D conformal radiation therapy. Int J Radiat Oncol Biol Phys 38:319, 1997.
662. Pickett B, Roach M, Verhey L, et al: The value of nonuniform margins for six-field conformal irradiation of localized prostate cancer. Int J Radiat Oncol Biol Phys 32:211, 1995.
663. Kuban DA, Dong L: High-dose intensity modulated radiation therapy for prostate cancer. Curr Urol Rep 5:197, 2004.
664. Tucker SL, Dong L, Cheung R, et al: Comparison of rectal dose-wall histogram versus dose-volume histogram for modeling the incidence of late rectal bleeding after radiotherapy. Int J Radiat Oncol Biol Phys 60:1589, 2004.
665. Wallner K, Chiu-Tsao ST, Roy J, et al: An improved method for computerized tomography-planned transperineal ^{125}iodine prostate implants. J Urol 146:90, 1991.
666. D'Amico A, Cormack R, Kumar S, et al: Real-time magnetic resonance imaging-guided brachytherapy in the treatment of selected patients with clinically localized prostate cancer. J Endourol 14:367, 2000.
667. Stone NN, Hong S, Lo YC, et al: Comparison of intraoperative dosimetric implant representation with postimplant dosimetry in patients receiving prostate brachytherapy. Brachytherapy 2:17, 2003.
668. Todor DA, Zaider M, Cohen GN, et al: Intraoperative dynamic dosimetry for prostate implants. Phys Med Biol 48:1153, 2003.
669. Woolsey J, Bissonette E, Schneider BF, et al: Prospective outcomes associated with migration from preoperative to intraoperative planned brachytherapy: a single center report. J Urol 172(Pt 2):2528, 2004.
670. Bezou AR, Monsour P, Buhler C, et al: High dose rate after loading 192 iridium prostate brachytherapy. J La State Med Soc 154:37, 2002.
671. Galalae RM, Kovacs G, Schultze J, et al: Long-term outcome after elective irradiation of the pelvic lymphatics and local dose escalation using high-dose rate brachytherapy for locally advanced prostate cancer. Int J Radiat Oncol Biol Phys 52:81, 2002.
672. Vicini F, Vargas C, Gustafson G, et al: High dose rate brachytherapy in the treatment of prostate cancer. World J Urol 21:220, 2003.
673. Vicini FA, Vargas C, Edmundson G, et al: The role of high-dose rate brachytherapy in locally advanced prostate cancer. Semin Radiat Oncol 13:98, 2003.
674. Martinez AJ, Gonzalez J, Spencer W, et al: Conformed high dose rate brachytherapy improves biochemical control and cause specific survival in patients with prostate cancer and poor prognostic factors. J Urol 169:974, 2003.
675. Kestin L, Goldstein N, Vicini F, et al: Treatment of prostate cancer with radiotherapy: should the entire seminal vesicles be included in the clinical target volume? Int J Radiat Oncol Biol Phys 54:686, 2002.
676. Kruse JJ, Herman MG, Hagness CR, et al: Daily monitoring of patient setup variation and prostatic fossa tissue motion with an electronic portal imaging device. Int J Radiat Oncol Biol Phys 51(Suppl):387, 2001.
677. Roach M, Winter K, Michalski JM, et al: Penile bulb dose and impotence after three-dimensional conformal radiotherapy for prostate cancer on RTOG 9406: finding from a prospective, multi-institutional, phase I/II dose-escalation study. Int J Radiat Oncol Biol Phys 60:1351, 2004.
678. Wernicke AG, Valicenti R, DiEva K, et al: Radiation dose delivered to the proximal penis as a predictor of the risk of erectile dysfunction after three-dimensional conformal radiotherapy for localized prostate cancer. Int J Radiat Oncol Biol Phys 60:1357, 2004.
679. Marks LB, Carroll PR, Dugan TC, et al: The response of the urinary bladder, urethra, and ureter to radiation and chemotherapy. Int J Radiat Oncol Biol Phys 31:1257, 1995.
680. Perez CA, Beyer DC, Blasko JC, et al: Postradical prostatectomy irradiation in carcinoma of the prostate. American College of Radiology. ACR Appropriateness Criteria. Radiology 215(Suppl): 1419, 2000.
681. Herman MG, Pisansky TM, Kruse JJ, et al: Technical aspects of daily online positioning of the prostate for three-dimensional conformal radiotherapy using an electronic portal-imaging device. Int J Radiat Oncol Biol Phys 57:1131, 2003.
682. Ahlering T, Parker R, Kumar S, et al: Practice guidelines for prostate cancer. Cancer J Sci Am 2:S77, 1996.
683. Partin AW, Carter BB, Epstein JI, et al: The biology of prostate cancer: new and future directions in predicting tumor behavior. Monogr Pathol 34:198, 1992.
684. Burke HB: Artificial neural networks for cancer research: outcome prediction. Semin Surg Oncol 10:73, 1994.
685. Burke HB: Increasing the power of surrogate endpoint biomarkers: the aggregation of predictive factors. J Cell Biochem 19(Suppl):278, 1994.

CHAPTER 51

BLADDER CANCER

Anthony L. Zietman and William U. Shipley

INCIDENCE

The American Cancer Society estimates that in 2006 there will be 61,420 new cases of carcinoma of the bladder, of which approximately one third will have muscle invasive disease. And 13,060 will likely die from bladder cancer. Transitional cell cancer has strong etiologic connections with smoking. The less common squamous cell cancer is more closely associated with chronic inflammation such as *Schistosoma* infection or indwelling catheter.

BIOLOGIC CHARACTERISTICS

The most important predictors of progression from superficial to the muscle-invasive stage are high grade, penetration of the lamina propria, and the presence of carcinoma in situ. Once muscle invasion has occurred, the strongest predictors of metastasis and death are bulk of tumor and depth of invasion.

EGFR and *Her-2* are commonly overexpressed and abnormalities of *p53* expression commonly seen. Their prognostic and predictive significance remains uncertain.

STAGING EVALUATION

Painless hematuria is the most common presentation. Urine cytology commonly indicates cancer, but cystoscopy and transurethral resection are necessary for definitive assessment of the primary tumor.

MRI may define penetration of the bladder wall and either MRI or CT scan can evaluate abdominopelvic lymph nodes. The upper tracts must also be evaluated with CT or retrograde ureteroscopy as synchronous tumors are common. Chest radiography and bone scan are usually obtained when cancer deeply invades the muscle.

PRIMARY THERAPY

Superficial tumors are managed by transurethral resection of bladder tumor alone in the case of low-grade lesions and together with intravesical BCG for high grade, lamina propria invasion, or carcinoma in situ. Over 10 years, as many as 50% of the latter group will progress to muscle invasion.

Radical cystectomy is the US standard for the management of muscle-invading cancers. There is 90% control within the pelvis but 50% ultimately die of distant metastasis. Radical radiation alone provides only 30% to 40% local control, though the use of salvage cystectomy keeps cure rates close to those of primary cystectomy. When limited surgery (transurethral resection of bladder tumor) is combined with radiation and cisplatin-based chemotherapy, over 70% of patients keep their native bladders, and cure rates are comparable to published cystectomy series. Quality-of-life studies show high levels of satisfaction with the retained bladder.

ADJUVANT THERAPY

Neoadjuvant chemotherapy downstages the primary tumor over 50% of the time but only adds 5% to 10% to the chance for cure. Adjuvant chemotherapy is commonly used but has proven utility only in the case of node positive disease.

Adjuvant radiation may be given after cystectomy for locally advanced disease but the morbidity is high and the benefits unclear.

LOCALLY ADVANCED DISEASE AND PALLIATION

When there is hydronephrosis, extension into adjacent organs or nodal spread, the likelihood of cure is small. Cystectomy or radiation may be used for palliation of voiding symptoms or bleeding but the mainstay of care is combination chemotherapy. Bladder cancer is a chemoresponsive disease and cisplatin-based regimens give responses in over 60% of cases and are often quite durable. Second-line treatment with taxotere and gemcitabine is also very active.

Radiation therapy is effective in palliating painful bone metastases and in alleviating symptoms from brain metastases.

More than 80% of bladder cancer patients present with early disease that has not yet invaded the detrusor smooth muscle. In the absence of muscle invasion, endoscopic transurethral resection (TUR) with or without intravesical therapy is the therapy of choice. The radiation oncologist plays only a limited and occasional role. For muscle-invading disease, the most appropriate treatment algorithm remains controversial. Although radical cystectomy has long been the standard treatment in the United States, organ-preserving regimens using radiation with concurrent chemotherapy are comparably effective alternatives in a subset of patients.

In this chapter, we separately discuss the treatment of superficial and locally advanced (muscle-invading) disease. Special emphasis is placed on the development of combined-modality therapy in muscle-invading bladder cancer with and without bladder preservation.

ETIOLOGY AND EPIDEMIOLOGY

Bladder cancer is the fourth most common cancer among men and the eighth most common cancer among women. It is estimated that there will be 61,420 new cases and 13,060 bladder cancer deaths in 2006.[1,2] There is little or no association between socioeconomic status and bladder cancer.[3]

Internationally, incidence rates of bladder cancer vary Almost 10-fold. Highest rates occur in western Europe and North America; relatively low rates are found in Eastern Europe and several areas of Asia (China, India, Philippines).[4,5]

Cancer of the bladder occurs primarily in older white men. The incidence rate among black men is about 50% of that among whites. The male-female ratio is at least 3:1, approaching 4:1 in whites. Two thirds of cases occur among persons aged 65 and older.

From the period 1969 to 1971 to the period 1988 to 1990, incidence rates increased 31% to 37% among whites and 15% to 21% among blacks. Mortality rates declined 18% to 24% during this period of increasing incidence. Incidence of locally advanced and metastatic bladder cancer remained virtually constant.[6]

RISK FACTORS

Cigarette smoking and occupational exposures are the major risk factors for bladder cancer. Cigarette smoking accounts for an estimated 48% of bladder cancer diagnosed in men and 32% among women in the United States. Occupational exposure among white men accounts for 25% of bladder cancer diagnoses in men and 11% in women. Emerging evidence also suggests that chlorinated organic compounds formed as a byproduct of drinking water chlorination may account for 10% to 15% of cases. Infection with *Schistosoma haematobium* is a well-documented risk factor and an important cause of bladder cancer in developing countries.

Cigarette smoking increases the risk of bladder cancer two- to three-fold. Risk estimates for moderate to heavy smokers range from 2 to 5 compared with nonsmokers.[7-9] Some studies indicate a reduction in risk within the first 2 to 4 years after cessation of smoking, but no further decrease in risk with increased time since quitting.[10,11] Other studies, however, suggested a decline of risk comparable to that of nonsmokers.[12,13]

In the 1950s, occupational exposures to aromatic amines in the British dyestuff and rubber industries were found to be associated with bladder cancer.[14,15] The mean time from start of exposure to death was 25 years, with the greatest risk for workers who started before age 25. Workers in the leather industry are at increased risk for bladder cancer, but the carcinogen has not yet been identified.[16,17] The increased risk for painters seems to be due to many known carcinogens in paint such as benzidine, polychlorinated biphenyls, formaldehyde, asbestos, and solvents such as benzene, dioxane, and methylene chloride.[18] Drivers of trucks, buses, or taxicabs are suspected to have an increased exposure to exhaust emissions containing polycyclic aromatic hydrocarbons (PAHs) and nitro-PAHs.[19]

It was first recognized in the 1970s that chlorination of drinking water generates a wide array of halogenated organic compounds. A number of epidemiologic studies investigated the possible association between exposure to these compounds and cancer. A 1992 meta-analysis of these studies found a significant association between exposure to chlorination byproducts and bladder cancer.[20] Several studies published subsequently supported this conclusion.[21,22]

Aromatic amines are detoxified by *N*-acetylation. The *N*-acetyltransferase enzyme in the liver is polymorphic, displaying a slow and a rapid acetylator phenotype. The allele that confers a slow acetylator phenotype is assumed to be associated with an increased risk of bladder cancer (relative risk, 1.1 to 1.9).[23,24]

There are several other well-documented risk factors. Exposure to *S. haematobium* infection is associated with a predominantly increased risk of squamous cell carcinoma of the bladder.[25] Heavy consumption of phenacetin-containing analgesics was linked to cancer of the renal pelvis, ureter, and bladder.[26] Cyclophosphamide, an alkylating agent, and pelvic radiation have also been linked to the risk of bladder cancer.[27,28]

PREVENTION AND EARLY DETECTION

Primary prevention involves identification and avoidance of cancer-causing factors.[29] In public health terms, avoidance of cigarette smoking is the most effective means available for the prevention of bladder cancer.

Secondary prevention involves screening individuals at high risk for a particular cancer with the goal of early detection and treatment. Cytologic evaluation of the urine may be a satisfactory screening test, with a sensitivity of approximately 75% (higher for high-grade lesions than for low-grade lesions: 50% to 80% versus 20%), a specificity between 95% and 99.9%, and low cost and risk. However, the prevalence of preclinical bladder cancer is probably too low in the general population for large-scale screening programs to be rewarding. Testing for asymptomatic hematuria does not appear to be a useful method for screening. A single test has a low sensitivity. Repeat testing at short intervals, such as weeks, has been advocated but yields unacceptably high rates of false-positive results.[30,31]

Chemoprevention involves the administration of a natural or synthetic agent to healthy people or patients with precancerous conditions who are at high risk for bladder cancer to prevent or retard the development or progression of cancer. The vitamin A analogue, 13-*cis*-retinoic acid, as well as high-dose multivitamins, polyamine synthesis inhibitors, and oltipraz are currently under investigation as potential chemopreventive agents,[32] but nothing definitive exists at present.

PATHOLOGY AND PATHWAYS OF SPREAD

In the United States, over 90% of cancers arising in the bladder are transitional cell carcinoma (TCC). Less common pathologies are adenocarcinoma, squamous cell carcinoma (SCC), and small cell carcinoma, accounting approximately 6%, 2%, and for less than 1% of bladder tumors, respectively. In Egypt, SCC accounts for 70% of all bladder cancers.

Macroscopically, papillary growth is more frequent than solid tumors (approximately 80% versus 20%). Solid tumors are more likely than papillary tumors to be high grade and invasive into the muscularis propria layer.

Although the collective term "superficial cancer" is still commonly used, it is a category that comprises several classes of transitional cell cancers with different rates of recurrence, different rates of progression to muscle invasion, and quite different treatments. The tumors that arise in the epithelium and develop in an exophytic pattern are known as Ta tumors. They are usually low grade (I or II) and considered to be relatively benign lesions that closely resemble the normal urothelium. Although they have more than the normal seven layers of urothelium, they show normal nuclear polarity in more than 95% of tumors and no or only slight pleomorphism. When progression deeper into the lamina propria occurs, the tumor is described as T1 and carries a higher risk of progression and even of metastasis.

Grade is an important predictor of relapse and progression for all categories of superficial disease. Pathologic grades I to III (low, intermediate, or high) are based on the number of mitoses, presence of nuclear abnormalities, and cellular atypia. High-grade tumors show loss of polarization of the nuclei and moderate to prominent pleomorphism. Muscle-invasive disease, however, is usually high grade, and depth of invasion is the more important prognostic factor for outcome.

Carcinoma in situ (Tcis) is defined as noninvasive, high-grade, flat cancer confined to the epithelium, which can be localized or diffuse, and it may occur in association with either superficial or muscle-invasive TCC. Tcis can also occur without a concurrent exophytic tumor. Endoscopically, Tcis presents as a friable red area indistinguishable from inflammation and spreads laterally, displacing normal epithelium. Urine cytology is positive in 90% of patients with Tcis because of a loss in the cohesiveness of cells.

Squamous cell cancers are associated with chronic inflammation or infection with *Schistosoma* and tend to grow as large masses with a high degree of necrosis. In North America they are more commonly associated with chronic bladder irritation or stasis such as a lifelong indwelling catheter. The North American variant has the distinction of higher metastatic propensity.

Transitional cell cancer is often multifocal both in place and in time (polychronotropism). This is a striking characteristic of this disease but the etiology is uncertain. Two of the most commonly held explanatory theories are a genetic field defect with multiple new tumors spontaneously arising or alternatively the local reimplantation of tumor cells ("local metastasis"). Evidence strongly suggests that tumor reimplantation or submucosal migration is the predominant mechanism. Multifocal tumors as well as upper tract and lower tract lesions arising in one individual demonstrate clonality.[33]

External and internal iliac chains as well as perivesical lymph nodes are first-echelon lymph nodes. Common iliac, para-aortic, and paracaval lymph nodes are considered second-echelon lymph nodes.

Bladder cancer can also spread by direct extension or hematogenous metastases. Direct extension can be to the pelvic side wall, anterior pelvis and symphysis pubis, rectum, or sigmoid colon. Hematogenous metastatic spread is most frequently seen to the lung and bone. Peritoneal metastases are another route of spread.

MOLECULAR BIOLOGY

Newly discovered cellular mechanisms and their associated proteins have become the subject of intense interest. This is partly for what they tell us about the biology of a tumor but also because of their potential role as prognostic markers and/or therapeutic targets. It has long been recognized that invasive bladder tumors are extremely heterogeneous in nature despite almost always being of high-grade transitional cell morphology. The search to understand the heterogeneity and use it to therapeutic advantage is only just beginning. At the moment the best prognostic indicators we have in bladder cancer are clinical: tumor size, uni- or multi-focality, and the presence or absence of either hydronephrosis or lymph node involvement (vide infra). No molecular marker yet comes close to improving upon these clinical markers but it is anticipated that they will in the next decade.

Apoptosis and Cell Cycle Receptors

These receptors provide malignant cells with an evolutionary selective advantage. These include cellular immortalization, escape from G1 checkpoint control, loss of DNA damage checkpoints (G2/M), loss of normal DNA repair mechanisms, loss of apoptotic response, and the development of invasive capabilities.[34-37] The *pRb* and *p53* pathways, which involve several common molecules, provide G1 checkpoint control and regulate the response to DNA damage. Although the Rb gene itself is only mutated in a few specific cancers, it is thought that abnormalities of its function are far more common; transitional cell bladder cancer is one of these. Disruption of its function is required to overcome the restraint it imposes on cell-cycle progression. The proapoptotic tumor suppressor gene eliminates cells with abnormalities in their Rb pathways and thus tumors commonly have abnormalities at *p16* and *p14ARF* and abnormalities at these loci may also be required to overcome the checkpoints that protect the cell from aberrant stimuli. *P53* abnormalities, which may be easily detected by nuclear immunohistochemistry, appear to be related to the progression of bladder cancer and to outcome following treatment. In an analysis of cystectomy patients at the University of Southern California, patients who had mutant *p53* had a significantly increased risk of death from disease compared with those patients bearing tumors with wild-type *p53*.[35,37,38] New cooperative group trials are under way, testing the role of 3 cycles of combination chemotherapy in patients with negative nodes but mutated *p53*. Work from the RTOG on patients who were treated with chemotherapy and radiation has not, however, shown any clear association between either *p16* or *p53* and outcome.[39] Clearly, the implication of the expression of these markers will vary according to the treatment planned.

In other centers other genes regulating apoptotic function have been studied retrospectively.[40-42] In examining a large database containing bladder cancer of different stages all treated by a variety of methods, it did seem that those who had *Bax* or *CD40L* tumors lived longer. *Bcl-2* positivity appeared to predict worse survival. The caveat, however, is that these were not prospective studies balanced for other prognostic variables.

Workers from Germany have suggested that one does not have to analyze the molecular pathways relating to apoptosis to predict response; a measure of the baseline spontaneous apoptotic rate of the tumor may be easier and quite sufficient. The inability to undergo spontaneous apoptosis whether due to overexpression of *bcl-2* or surviving predicts local failure after irradiation and chemotherapy.[43]

The RAS family of transforming genes is often overexpressed in bladder cancer. Their presence may be related to the original development of the tumor. In a mouse model farnesyl-transferase inhibitors that inhibit the post-translational modifications of *H-ras* worked synergistically with radiation in reducing tumor recurrence.[44]

Growth Factor Receptors

The epidermal growth factor (*EGFR*) family of receptor tyrosine kinases is known to initiate a complex program of signal transduction events that modulate cell survival, invasion, migration, proliferation, and differentiation. This family has four known members, of which *erb-1* (*EGFR*) and *erb-2* (*Her-2*) are the best characterized. The role of these receptors has been studied extensively in recent years in a variety of malignancies and there is evidence that increased activity through this pathway is common. The FDA has recently approved the use of ZD1839, an inhibitor of *EGFR1*, for lung cancer patients and of trastuzumab, a monoclonal antibody against *EGFR2* or *Her-2*, for appropriate breast cancer patients. In breast cancer, overexpression of *Her-2* is associated with poor prognosis, and the activity of trastuzumab unequivocally correlates with overexpression of *Her-2*.

Both *EGFR* and *Her-2* are commonly overexpressed in urothelial tumors. Numerous studies have investigated expression of *Her-2* in bladder cancer using immunohistochemistry, and have found overexpression in 40% to 80% of tumors.[39,45-48] There are, however, conflicting data on the relationship between the expression of these receptors with response to treatment and clinical outcome. A recent RTOG study pointed to a more *favorable* prognosis in those who overexpress *EGFR* but a lower complete response rate in patients with TCC who overexpress *Her-2*.[39] These patients had all been treated with chemotherapy and radiation and it may be that *EGFR* has a more direct involvement in improving the response of TCC to these agents than it does other tumors. It will be crucial to elucidate this relationship clearly as a growth factor receptor may be either a favorable or an unfavorable marker depending upon the proposed therapy. The RTOG data would suggest that targeting the *Her-2* pathway may be more profitable than *EGFR* in the initial therapy of muscle-invasive bladder cancer. There is certainly experimental evidence that *Her-2* has an antiapoptotic effect and that tumor radiosensitization can result from targeting this mechanism.[49]

Hypoxia

It is well recognized to be strongly associated with both radiation and chemotherapy resistance. It results in the upregulation of genes that facilitate anerobic metabolism and promote tumor vascularization. One such hypoxia-inducible factor is carbonic anhydrase IX (CA IX). It appears to be useful as a surrogate marker of hypoxia within bladder tumors. Several studies have showed the majority of bladder tumor expressing this marker though it appears, strangely, to be more strongly expressed in superficial than invasive tumors. Evidence on its role as a prognostic marker has been conflicting.[50,51]

CLINICAL PRESENTATION, PATIENT EVALUATION, AND STAGING

Clinical Presentation

Painless, episodic, hematuria is the most frequent presenting manifestation of bladder cancer (80%). It may be associated with irritative symptoms but is often painless and episodic. Hematuria is typically present through urination. Seventeen percent of patients present with severe bleeding and clot formation, and 20% present with dysuria. Some asymptomatic patients proved to have bladder cancer are found to have microscopic hematuria or, less frequently, pyuria. Bladder tumors can cause strangury (pain on straining to urinate), urinary retention, ureteral obstruction, sepsis, and rarely life-threatening hematuria. Regional pelvic disease may cause flank pain because of nerve invasion, edema, and ureteral obstruction. The signs and symptoms of bone, liver, pulmonary, and central nervous system metastases may be present if disease has disseminated.

Work-up of a Patient with Hematuria or Suspected Bladder Tumor

Patient work-up should include voided urine analysis, urinary cytology, intravenous pyelogram or CT urogram, and cystoscopy with biopsy of suspicious lesions. If the disease is classified as T1 or greater, the work-up must include abdominopelvic CT scan or MRI, bone scan, and chest radiograph. For those with muscle-invading disease a bone scan is also necessary.

Endoscopy

The endoscopic evaluation forms the mainstay of diagnosis and staging. Initially, an outpatient cystoscopy with biopsy is performed, and urine is obtained for cytology. Cystoscopy provides direct visualization of the bladder and facilitates biopsy of the bladder. Number, size, shape, and location of tumors as well as appearance of the surrounding mucosa, urethra, and urethral orifice are documented. Size (<2 cm, >5 cm), shape (papillary or flat), and associated Tcis lesions are of predictive importance. Using an illustrative bladder map, the location, number, size, and characteristics (papillary versus sessile) of the bladder tumor as well as presence or absence of CIS should be noted. If the pathology is positive for bladder cancer, a subsequent cystoscopy with TUR of the bladder tumor (TURBT), which is generally performed using epidural anesthesia, is scheduled.

Transurethral Resection of Bladder Tumor and Bladder Biopsy

Cold cup biopsies of all suspicious areas, the mucosa surrounding the area, any exophytic lesions, and the prostatic urethra as well as random biopsies of all four quadrants are obtained. All material is collected. When diffuse CIS is present, the prostatic urethra contains neoplastic cells in up to 25% of cases. For evaluation of muscle invasion, sufficient resection to provide adequate pathologic staging has to be done. An attempt is usually made to resect the bladder tumor as completely as is safely possible.

Bimanual Examination

Bimanual examination before and after complete TUR is performed, and the size and mobility of any palpable mass are evaluated. A residual palpable mass suggests muscle invasion. Most invasive bladder cancers are located near the trigone or posterior bladder wall and cannot be reliably palpated. This procedure alone leads to understaging in up to 50% of patients.

Urinary Cytology

Urine cytology should be used to complement the findings of cystoscopy. It is extremely valuable for the diagnosis of high-grade TCC, especially CIS that might be difficult for the endoscopist to visualize. The presence of high-grade TCC in the cytology specimen in patients with low-grade papillary TCC suggests either unrecognized CIS or less commonly high-grade disease in the upper urinary tracts.[52,53] For the diagnosis of low-grade papillary tumors, cytology is not sensitive because grade 1 TCC appears to be identical to normal urethral cells.

Cytology has been regarded as the gold standard for noninvasive screening of urine for bladder cancer. It has a sensitivity of 40% to 60% with specificity in excess of 90%. Nuclear matrix protein (NMP22), fibrin/fibrinogen degradation products (FDP), urinary bladder cancer antigen (BTA) and basic fetoprotein have all been compared to cytology in bladder cancer screening studies. Other methods utilized include fluorescence in situ hybridization (FISH), microsatellite analysis of free DNA, and telomerase reverse transcriptase determination. Unfortunately, all of these tests have a sensitivity which ranges only from 40% to 75% with a specificity of 50% to 90%.[54,55] Cytology is illustrative of the problems of noninvasive screening. Poorly differentiated tumors have a 20% false-negative detection rate whereas well-differentiated tumors have up to an 80% false-negative detection rate. Most of the other noninvasive screening tests have similar levels of false-positive and false-negative rates but have the benefit of lack of subjectivity by the person reading the test.[55]

Imaging

Although fewer than 60% of bladder cancers are seen on intravenous urography, this imaging modality provides valuable information about the status of the upper urinary tract.[56] Ureteral obstruction or a nonfunctioning kidney predicts muscle-invasive disease in 90% of cases.[57] Concomitant or subsequent upper urinary tract tumors are found in 2% to 5% of patients.

Evaluation of a patient with potential muscle-invading bladder cancer should include CT scan of the abdomen and pelvis. Although it is not very sensitive in reliably describing the depth of invasion or lymph node involvement, it can be helpful in the planning for subsequent treatment. Gadolinium-enhanced MRI imaging may prove useful in distinguishing superficial from invasive disease and in distinguishing intravesical from extravesical tumor.[58-61] Lymphangiography using iron nanoparticles and MRI might be particularly useful in detecting early nodal metastases.[62] All bladder-specific imaging should ideally be performed before TURBT, because of postsurgical edema.

Patients with Ta or low-grade T1 tumors do not require extensive metastatic work-up. However, those with muscle-invading tumors have a 50% risk of occult metastatic disease and should have chest imaging and a bone scan.

STAGING

The basis for the major staging systems is the classic clinicopathologic study by Jewett and Strong,[63] which correlates the probability of regional lymph node and distant metastases with the depth of invasion of the primary bladder tumor. The TNM (tumor, node, metastasis) system of 2002 is shown in Table 51-1 and Figure 51-1.[64] However, in clinical practice, the correlation between depth of invasion, based on cystoscopic evaluation, and the final cystectomy specimen is only 50% to 60%. The accuracy of the determination of degree of muscle infiltration is, therefore, modest at best. The clinical staging system as proposed by Union Internationale Contre Cancer was often more practical. Cancer without residual induration after TURBT was staged as T2 and cancer with palpable residual induration, T3. The most important determination of treatment outcome seems to be whether the tumor is organ confined (T3a) or non–organ confined (T3b). Stage T3b also includes tumors that extend to the perivesical fat. When comparing outcome for different treatment modalities, it is very important to consider whether the disease was staged clinically or whether a cystectomy specimen was available for a thorough pathologic staging.

Table 51-1 AJCC 2002 TNM Bladder Cancer Staging

PRIMARY TUMOR (T)	
Tis	Carcinoma in situ
Ta	Noninvasive papillary tumor
T1	Tumor invades the lamina propria, but not beyond
T2	Tumors invading the muscularis propria
pT2a	Tumor invades superficial muscle (inner half)
pT2b	Tumor invades deep muscle (outer half)
T3	Tumors invade perivesical tissue
pT3a	Microscopically
pT3b	Macroscopically (extravesical mass)
T4	Tumor invades any of the following: prostate, uterus, vagina, pelvic or abdominal wall.
T4a	Tumors invade prostate, uterus, vagina.
T4b	Tumor invades pelvic or abdominal wall.
REGIONAL LYMPH NODES (N)	
NX	Regional lymph nodes cannot be assessed
N0	No regional lymph node metastasis
N1	Metastasis in a single lymph node, ≤2 cm in greatest dimension
N2	Metastasis in a single lymph node >2 cm but <5 cm in greatest dimension; or multiple lymph nodes, none >5 cm in greatest dimension
DISTANT METASTASIS (M)	
MX	Distant metastasis cannot be assessed
M0	No distant metastasis
M1	Distant metastasis

American Joint Committee on Cancer: Bladder. In Greene FL, Page DL, Fleming ID, et al. (eds). AJCC Cancer Staging Manual, 6th ed. New York, Springer, 2002.

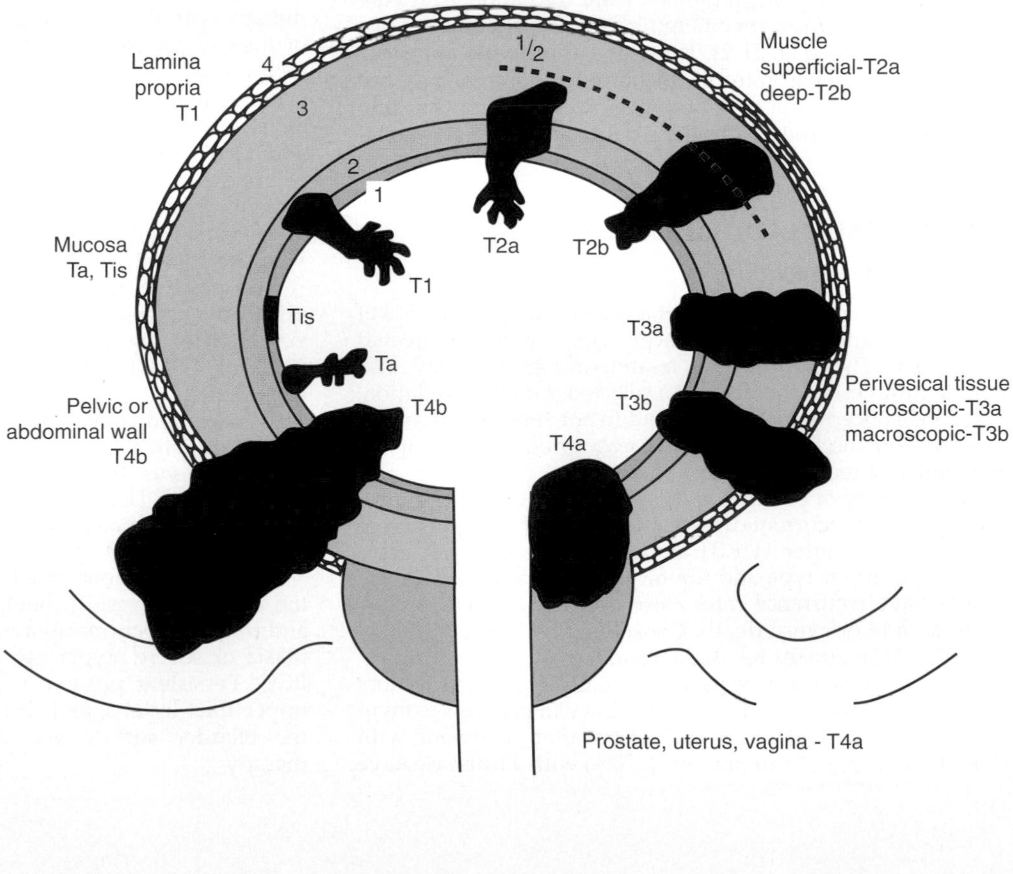

Figure 51-1 Staging of bladder tumors.

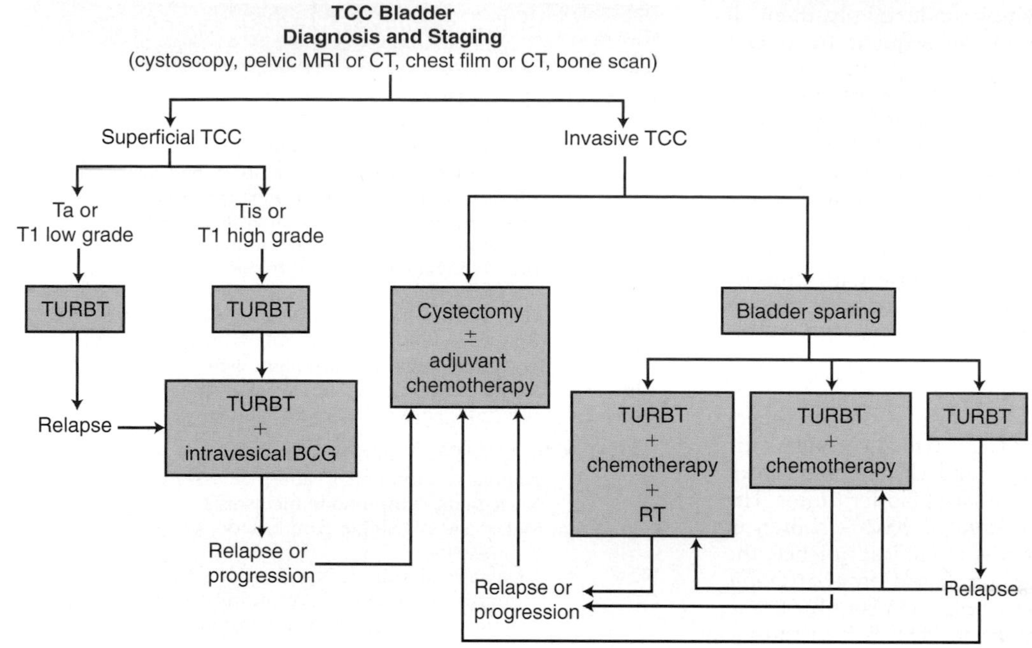

Figure 51-2 Diagnostic and treatment algorithm.

PRIMARY THERAPY

The presence or absence of muscle invasion is the key factor in determining the appropriate treatment option for bladder cancer. In the absence of muscle invasion, endoscopic TUR with or without intravesical therapy is the therapy of choice.

The most appropriate treatment algorithm for muscle-invading disease remains controversial. Although radical cystectomy has long been the standard treatment in the United States, organ-preserving regimens using radiation with concurrent chemotherapy are emerging as viable alternatives in a subset of patients (Fig. 51-2). These two approaches appear to have similar survival rates in uncontrolled comparisons, but strong physician and patient preferences have so far prevented a randomized, controlled trial comparing these treatment options.

SUPERFICIAL BLADDER CANCER

Transurethral Resection

Patients with superficial TCC, who account for 70% to 75% of all newly diagnosed bladder cancer cases, are initially treated by TURBT. The appropriate treatment regimen may also include intravesical therapy for a selected patient population. Decisions concerning the use of adjuvant therapy are based primarily on the probability of disease progression, not the probability of recurrence.

The majority of patients with superficial TCC will eventually experience recurrent disease after TURBT.[65] Progression to invasive disease after TURBT alone, however, is closely associated with tumor type and tumor grade.[66,67] Although Ta, G1 tumors have recurrence rates close to 100% at 5 years, they rarely invade or cause death. Consequently, TUR alone may be sufficient treatment for these tumors.

The risk of progression is substantially higher for tumors of higher grade or stage. Ta, G2-3 disease will progress to invasive TCC in 20% of cases at 5 years after treatment with TURBT alone. Nearly all patients (>70%) with T1 disease have high-grade tumors, and approximately 50% experience invasive disease at 5 years. In patients with T1 disease with CIS in the pathologic specimen, the rate of progression rises to 80% at 5 years.[68]

Intravesical Therapy

Bacille Calmette-Guérin: Intravesical therapy involves the instillation of a therapeutic agent into the bladder. Bacille Calmette-Guérin (BCG) is currently the most effective intravesical agent for treatment of superficial TCC of the bladder. Intravesical therapy with BCG has been shown effective in reducing rates of disease progression, improving survival, and decreasing recurrence.

Several randomized, controlled trials compared TURBT alone with TURBT with BCG.[69-72] For patients with Ta, G2-3 and T1 disease, adjuvant therapy with BCG reduces the rate of progression to 5% to 15% at 5 years. Nonetheless, 50% of patients with T1/CIS will experience muscle-invading cancer at 10 years. Progression rates among patients who respond to BCG are 1% at 1 year, 5% at 3 years, and 15% at 5 years.

The positive impact on progression translates into a survival advantage. With long-term follow-up, adjuvant intravesical BCG improved survival rates to 88% compared with 63% with TURBT alone and reduced the cystectomy rates from 42% to 20%.[73]

Besides reducing progression and improving survival, BCG treatment also delays tumor recurrence in approximately 50% of patients. In the six published randomized, controlled trials in which TUR with BCG was compared with TUR alone, recurrence rates ranged from 20% to 42% with intravesical therapy versus 42% to 100% without.

Several conditions other than those just outlined call for the use of intravesical therapy with BCG. These include CIS and frequent recurrence of low-grade disease. Urothelial dysplasia or severe atypia can be treated prophylactically with BCG. Persistent positive urine cytology without associated upper tract lesions, and disease involving more than 40% of the bladder surface are also indications for intravesical therapy.

Intravesical therapy is the first-line treatment for diffuse CIS. The average complete response rate of CIS to BCG is greater than 70% for more than 1 year.[74] It prevents subsequent disease in 60% of cases for up to 5 years and in 40% of cases for up to 10 years. Particularly in CIS of the prostatic urethra, BCG has spared many patients cystectomy. TUR is recommended to stage the disease and to open the bladder neck to allow BCG to bathe the prostatic urethra. Low-grade superficial disease with frequent recurrence is also considered an indication for intravesical therapy.

One consequence of controlling the bladder component of disease in a patient with TCC is an increase in the frequency of extravesical relapse. Relapses can develop anywhere transitional epithelium is found: renal pelvis, ureters, and urethra. The risk for upper tract tumor is 20% at 5 years, 25% at 10 years, and 33% at 15 years. Prostatic urethra and duct involvement at 5 years is 10% to 15% and at 10 years, 20%. If a complete resection of tumors of the urethra cannot be obtained, patients are managed with cystectomy. Patients with a positive cytology and no obvious bladder tumor need careful monitoring of the upper tracts. Ureteroscopic resection and instillation of BCG through the renal pelvis is possible.

Although BCG is the treatment of choice for intravesical therapy, a variety of other agents have been investigated. Intravesical chemotherapy such as thiopeta, doxorubicin, and mitomycin decreases short-term tumor recurrence rates but not disease progression or survival rates.[74] Relapsed superficial disease may also be treated with intravesical interferon, which in some provides a second remission and may stave off the time to a cystectomy.

Role of Radiation in High-Risk Superficial Bladder Cancer

It is well recognized that TURBT may clinically understage tumors as superficial when they have already invaded into the muscle wall (approximately 20% to 30%). Radiation therefore has an advantage in that it can reach tumor deposits too deep for instillation therapy. There have been no randomized trials comparing radiotherapy to current intravesical treatment options. The Dutch South Eastern Bladder Cancer Group has, however, recently presented data in 121 patients with T1G3 cancers.[75] External radiotherapy with 50 Gy was one treatment option and 17 patients received this. Though the numbers are limited it appeared to be as effective as intravesical BCG or mitomycin. Good results have also been achieved at the University of Rotterdam with interstitial implants.[76] In this selective but prospective series, patients with single T1 tumors less than 5 cm in diameter underwent TURBT and subsequent local irradiation of the tumor area in the bladder wall by an interstitial radium implant. The definitive local control rate was 82% and the 10-year survival rate 76%. Recently, another group in the Netherlands has published their results using a combination of transurethral resection, external beam radiotherapy (3 to 4 × 3.5 Gy), and interstitial radiotherapy (mean implant dose of 55 Gy) in patients with solitary T1G3 and T2 tumors.[77] The local control rate was 70% in the whole patient population. The 5-year disease-specific survival rate was 80% for stage T1 and 60% for T2a.

A large series of high-risk T1 cancers treated with either TURBT plus RT/RCT comes from the University of Erlangen.[159] In this series only 15% progressed to muscle-invasive disease after 5 years, which compares favorably to most studies of TURBT and instillation therapy. More than 80% of those alive at 5 years preserved their bladder. These results certainly suggest that radiation may have a role to play in those with high grade or recurrent T1 lesions and may be attempted ahead of cystectomy on a protocol or in place of cystectomy in those who are medically inoperable.

MUSCLE-INVADING BLADDER CANCER (T2-4)

Muscle-invading tumors constitute 20% to 25% of all newly diagnosed bladder cancers. The most appropriate treatment algorithm for muscle-invading disease remains controversial. Although radical cystectomy has been the standard treatment for two decades, organ-preserving regimens using predominantly multiple-modality therapy, consisting of TUR followed by irradiation with concurrent chemotherapy, are emerging as viable alternatives in a subset of patients. Refining the treatment choice by maximizing quality of life without compromising survival is the ultimate goal.

Radical Cystectomy

Surgical Methods

During radical cystectomy in male patients, bladder, prostate, seminal vesicle, proximal vas deferens, and proximal urethra, with a margin of adipose tissue and peritoneum, are resected en bloc. In females, the procedure involves an anterior pelvic exenteration to remove the bladder, urethra, uterus, fallopian tubes, ovaries, anterior vaginal wall, and surrounding fascia en bloc. Before cystectomy, grossly abnormal lymph nodes are sampled. In case of metastases, cystectomy is aborted unless urinary diversion is required to relieve symptoms. Urinary diversion is usually accomplished through an ileal conduit opening onto the anterior abdominal wall through a urostoma.

Incontinent urinary tract reconstruction: In the early 1950s, Bricker and colleagues developed what was to become the most common type of diversion after cystectomy, the ileal conduit diversion. Urine drains directly from the ureters through a segment of ileum to the skin surface, where it is collected by an external collection appliance.

Continent urinary tract reconstruction: Techniques for performing continent urinary diversions have been developed over the past 15 years. The two most important approaches are formation of a continent urinary reservoir made of bowel, which drains to a stoma that can be catheterized, and creation of an orthotopic neobladder, in which a newly formed urinary reservoir made out of bowel is anastomosed to the urethra.

Cutaneous urinary reservoir: The two main options are reservoirs made from colon and small bowel (Indiana pouch) or entirely from small bowel (Kock pouch).[78,79] The Indiana pouch consists of approximately 25 cm of right colon, often including some distal ileum which is brought to the abdominal wall. It relies on the ileocecal valve for continence. Patients catheterize the pouch on average four to six times per day.

The Kock pouch is a cutaneous continent urinary reservoir constructed from 60 cm of ileum, with an afferent antireflux nipple valve for the ureteral intestinal anastomosis and an efferent nipple valve for the catheterizable stoma. Major complication rates of around 20% are reported. Incontinence, difficulty with catheterization, loss of antireflux features of the nipple valve, and urinary leaks are the major problems with these diversions.

Orthotopic diversion: A neobladder is constructed from ileum, ileocolon, or sigmoid colon and anastomosed to the native urethra as opposed to the abdominal wall. This permits the patient to void in a relatively normal fashion per urethram.

The Mainz pouch (neobladder) consists of an ileocecal segment, which is detubularized and anastomosed to the urethra.[80] The Hautmann pouch consists of a W-shaped ileoneobladder, in which 60 cm of ileum is configured into a sphere.[81]

Orthotopic bladders are contraindicated when the tumor involves the urethra. Orthotopic neobladders are becoming increasingly common in patients undergoing cystectomy but have been predominantly used in men. They are less common in women because of the technical difficulties maintaining continence and the risk of urethral recurrence given the shorter length of the female urethra.[82] It remains true, however, that in 2004 the majority of patients still did not receive a continent reservoir because of intercurrent disease, impaired renal function, surgery time, dilated ureters, or bowel disease.

Morbidity of Cystectomy

Operative mortality from cystectomy in modern series ranges from 1% to 2%, with postoperative complication rates ranging from 15% to 32%.[83,84] These included hemorrhage, rectal injury, deep venous thrombosis, pulmonary embolus, pelvic abscess, sepsis, wound infection, and small-bowel obstruction. The need for urinary diversion and loss of sexual function in patients undergoing radical cystectomy are the most serious side effects and may impair quality of life dramatically. In women, loss of sexual function occurs secondary to subtotal vaginectomy and in men secondary to prostatectomy with loss of vascular supply or nerves serving penile erection. Newer nerve-sparing techniques for men allow up to 40% to 70% of selected patients to regain their erectile potency.[85]

When feasible, continent urinary diversions achieve 82% continence rates with early complication rates of 15% to 20% and mild hypochloremic acidosis in 50% of the patients. Intestinal obstruction, acute pyelonephritis, ureteral obstruction, stomal stenosis, intestinal fistula, and ureteroileal urinary leakage are also reported. Ten percent of patients experience ureteral-intestinal strictures, reservoir dysfunction requiring augmentation of the pouch, and dysfunction of the stoma. Overall, 10% to 15% of patients require reoperation.

Cancer Outcome after Cystectomy

Two large recent series provide the best data on outcome after radical cystectomy. The University of Southern California recently reported on 633 patients undergoing radical cystectomy with pathologic stages pT2-T4a with an actuarial overall survival rate at 5 years of 48% and at 10 years of 32%.[86] The series from the Memorial Sloan-Kettering Cancer Center showed that in 184 patients with tumors of pT2-4, the 5-year overall survival rate was 36%. The actuarial 5-year survival rate for all the 269 patients with pathologic stages ranging from pT0-pT4 was 45%.[87]

T category is a significant independent predictor of survival and local control. By clinical stage, 5-year survival rates were 56% for T1, 50% for T2, and 23% for T3a-b. Five-year local relapse rates by pathologic stage ranged from 6% for pT2 disease to 51% for pT3b.

The presence or absence plus the extent of lymph node disease is also a significant determinant of survival. The estimated probability of 5-year survival of patients with nodal metastases is 29%; with one to five nodes positive 35%, and with six or more nodes positive 17%.[88] The incidence of positive lymph nodes varies according to pathologic tumor stage. In cystectomy series, it ranged from 0% to 6% for superficial disease, 18% to 22% for muscle-invasive disease (pT2, 6% to 20%; pT3a, 30% to 31%), 30% to 64% for disease invading the perivesical fat (pT3b), and 45% to 59% for disease invading adjacent organs (pT4).[89-91]

Although the disease is locally controlled, many patients will ultimately develop disease metastases (5-year distant disease rate for T3-4, 40% to 50%; T2, 30%). Median time to diagnosis of distant metastases is approximately 18 months. The most common sites for distant metastases are bone, lung, and liver.

Radiation as an Adjunct to Cystectomy

Preoperative Radiation Therapy

The recognition that moderate-dose radiation (20 to 50 Gy) may reduce the volume of gross disease and eradicate microscopic TCC led to its frequent use before cystectomy in the 1970s. In nonrandomized studies, these doses were found to reduce the frequency of metastases in the lymphadenectomy specimens by approximately 50%.[92] By the 1980s, improvements in the technique of radical cystectomy, together with the introduction of more extensive therapeutic lymphadenectomies, made many question the need for radiation.[93] It has been argued that radiation delays the time to definitive surgery, increases its morbidity, and may compromise the surgeon's ability to perform continent urinary diversions. Furthermore, the question was addressed by an intergroup trial reported in 1997.[94] 140 patients with invasive or recurrent superficial bladder cancers were randomized to receive cystectomy either with or without preoperative radiation (20 Gy in 5 fractions). There was no significant survival advantage to either group at 5 years. The trial was small, the doses low, and the predominant pattern of failure distant, all factors that would make it practically impossible to detect any advantage to radiation. Parsons and Million[95] did, however, demonstrate an apparent survival advantage for patients with clinical T3 tumors who received preoperative radiation.

Cole and colleagues reported on 133 patients with T3b disease treated at the M. D. Anderson Cancer Center.[96] This retrospective review documented that when pelvic wall recurrence occurs following modern radical cystectomy, it is usually only in patients who had clinical stage T3b or T4 tumors. They report a 28% incidence of pelvic recurrence in stage T3b patients treated by radical cystectomy, with or without multidrug chemotherapy. However, when stage T3b patients were treated with preoperative radiation therapy (which this institution used extensively prior to 1980), the pelvic recurrence rate was only 10%. Before 1983, all patients underwent 50-Gy preoperative irradiation, followed 4 weeks later by cystectomy. Actuarial 5-year pelvic control was 91%. After 1983, radiation was discontinued, and subsequent pelvic control rates have fallen to 73% despite improvements in surgical technique, staging, and the addition of systemic chemotherapy. A survival decrement (52% to 42%) was also seen. The extent to which patient-selection factors contributed to this observed difference is unknown. Others have reported lower rates of pelvic recurrence using cystectomy alone for this subset of patients, and it therefore remains uncertain whether these findings are widely applicable.[93]

The morbidity of preoperative irradiation is small. Whitmore reported comparable rates of wound healing and perioperative mortality for patients who received and those who did not receive irradiation before cystectomy.[92] There is limited experience in the creation of continent urinary diversions after preoperative irradiation, although Housset and colleagues report that it is possible after the delivery of 44 Gy.[97]

Transitional cell cancers of the bladder have a high propensity to autotransplantation. Iatrogenic wound seeding after cystotomy was commonly reported by those who performed partial cystectomies or bladder brachytherapy. Low-dose preoperative radiation (8.5 to 20 Gy) profoundly reduced the incidence of this problem.[98] Low dose radiation is still occasionally given in the United States prior to a partial cystectomy. The partial cystectomy is, however, not commonly performed because it is limited to small, unifocal tumors of the dome, an unusual location.

Postoperative Radiation Therapy

When the cystectomy specimen shows extensive extravesical disease and positive surgical margins, the risk for pelvic recurrence is high. Postoperative radiation therapy has been evaluated in only one randomized study. The National Cancer Institute of Egypt reported on 236 patients with T3-4 tumors (68% squamous cell) who received either no adjuvant therapy or postoperative radiation.[99] The incidence of pelvic recurrence was significantly reduced in the latter group (50% versus 10%). Whether this finding is as applicable to transitional as to squamous cell tumors remains an unanswered question. Today, patients with such extensive disease commonly receive adjuvant chemotherapy, although the ability of this modality to prevent local recurrence has been called into question by Cole and colleagues.[96] Radiation rarely cures patients with pelvic wall recurrences following radical cystectomy.[100] Perhaps some could be cured if given adjuvant radiotherapy.

The morbidity of postoperative irradiation is high because of the large volumes of small bowel that occupy the pelvis after cystectomy if the urologist does not use pelvic reconstruction techniques to displace small bowel loops from the tumor bed (omental pedicle flap, mesh, other). Two series reported a greater than 30% incidence of small-bowel obstruction when 50 Gy was delivered using conventional fractionation.[101] If radiation is envisaged as an accompaniment to cystectomy for advanced disease, it appears to be safer if delivered preoperatively. If this was not done then the radiation volumes should be kept small, limited to the floor of the pelvis, and with a dose of no more than 45 Gy.

A final postoperative pathology demonstrating positive pelvic lymph nodes is not an indication for pelvic radiation as a single adjuvant. There is a high likelihood of occult micrometastatic disease (>80%) and thus a far greater need for adjuvant chemotherapy. If positive margins exist in addition to positive lymph nodes then again the primary need is for the systemic treatment. Radiation can be given to the bladder bed in addition to the chemotherapy in a younger patient when the pathologic indications are strong but it must be recognized that the risks are high and the benefits likely small.

Salvage Radiation Therapy

Attempts to salvage patients with TCC of the bladder at the time of symptomatic or gross pelvic recurrence after radical cystectomy with RT or with combined chemotherapy and RT are usually unsuccessful. Some palliation can be achieved.[100] In some centers consideration is given to preoperative chemoradiation followed by attempted resection of the pelvic mass and intraoperative radiation. There is no large published experience looking at this approach.

BLADDER PRESERVATION

Conservative Surgery

Partial Cystectomy

Surgical resection by partial cystectomy requires that the lesion is solitary and is located in a region of the bladder that allows for complete excision with a 2-cm tumor-free margin (e.g., the bladder dome). The portion of the bladder to be resected should be small enough to allow adequate bladder capacity. Contraindications include association with CIS in other sites of the bladder and bladder neck or trigone tumors in which ureteral reimplantation would be required to achieve an adequate margin. Given these constraints, only 6% to 19% of patients with primary, muscle-invading bladder cancer are potential candidates.[102] Even for this select group of patients, local recurrence rates range from 38% to 78%; one half of the recurrences appear in the first year and two thirds by 2 years.

Transurethral Resection of Bladder Tumor

Clinical complete response rates (assessed cystoscopically with repeat biopsy 3 weeks after initial TURBT) after TURBT for T2 and T3 cancers overall are in the 10% to 20% range.[103,104] Five-year survival in 85 patients with grades 1 and 2 T2 cancers was an unacceptable 27%.[105] A few studies have reported 5-year survival rates as high as 78%, but these results included only those patients who had no residual disease or no invasive disease on repeat biopsy and urine cytology. Although potentially effective in a small proportion of favorable T2 tumors, TURBT is usually not sufficient as monotherapy in muscle-invading bladder cancer.

Radical External Beam Radiation

In the past, EBRT was widely used as a single modality for T2-4 bladder cancers, particularly in Europe. In the United States, however, the use of radiation was frequently limited to patients whose tumor characteristics made them poor candidates for surgical monotherapy.

The total radiation dose used in modern series (Table 51-2) varied from 55 to 65 Gy, with 1.8 Gy to 2 Gy/fraction in North America, and from 50 to 55 Gy at 2.5 to 2.75 Gy/fraction in the United Kingdom.[106-119] Most patients were treated with one fraction per day five times a week. Patient response was evaluated by cystoscopic examination and biopsy 3 to 6 months after completion of RT. Patients with residual tumor and no known metastatic disease underwent salvage surgery (range of salvage cystectomy rate, 13% to 24%) if they were suitable surgical candidates. Those unfit received palliative measures.

The 5-year local control ranged from 31% to 45% for the entire patient population and from 49% to 79% for the subgroup of patients with complete response. Factors reported as having a significant favorable effect on local control[119] with RT include

- Early clinical stage (T2 and T3a)
- Absence of ureteral obstruction
- Complete response
- Visibly complete TURBT
- Absence of coexisting CIS
- Small tumor size (<5-cm maximum diameter)
- Solitary tumors
- Tumor configuration (papillary versus sessile)
- Hemoglobin level (>10 mg/dl)

Tumor eradication may range from as high as 66% for those with solitary T2 tumors to as low as 9% for those with multiple tumors and hydronephrosis. The 5-year overall survival in these reports ranged from 25% to 46%. Stage-specific 5-year survival rates ranged from 49% to 71% for T2 to 37% for T3b.

The success of any bladder conserving strategy rests upon the ability to rapidly recognize local recurrence and treat promptly with salvage surgery. Salvage cystectomy can be undertaken safely without increased morbidity after a

Table 51-2 External Beam Radiotherapy Alone for Muscle-Invasive Bladder Cancer

Study	No.	5-Y Survival by T Category (%) T2	T3 (T3a/T3b)	T4	Overall
Duncan, 1986[106]	963	40	26	12	30
Blandy, 1988[107]	614	27	38	9	—
Jenkins, 1988*[108]	182	46	35	—	40
Gospodarowicz, 1991*[111]	355	50	(38/28)	—	46
Jansson, 1991*[112]	319	31	16	6	28
Davidson, 1990*[117]	709	49	28	2	25
Greven, 1990[109]	116	59	10	0	—
Smaaland, 1991[110]	146	26	10†	—	—
Fossa, 1993[113]	308	38‡	14§	—	24
Pollack, 1994[114]	135	42	20	0	26
Moonen, 1998[115]	379	25	17	—	22
Borgaonkar, 2002*[118]	163	48	26	—	45

*Cause-specific survival.
†T3/T4.
‡T2/T3a.
§T3b/T4.

Table 51-3 Treatment Outcome for Brachytherapy in Combination with External Beam

Series	Local Control (5 y)	Overall Survival (5 y)	Disease-Specific Survival (5 y)	Survival with Preserved Bladder (5 y)
Moonen[125]	84%	86%	—	90%
Wijnmaalen[126]	88%	48%	69%	—
Van der Steen[77]	70%	—	T1 80%	—
			T2 60%	—
Mazeron[128]	77%	72%	73%	95%
Rozan[129]	—	67%	83%	96.1%
Pernot[129a]	73%	71%	77%	—

All series employed combinations of EBRT and brachytherapy. Usually preoperative EBRT dose of <15 Gy to reduce the risk of tumor seeding. The series of Moonen gave 30 Gy and those of Van der Steen and Wijnmaalen gave 40 Gy to tumors of stage T2b or higher.

complete course of RT or chemoradiation regimens.[120] After radiation, an ileal conduit, rather than a neobladder, is the more likely method of urinary diversion. A Kock pouch urinary diversion may also be performed safely in patients who received prior RT to the pelvis.[121]

Interstitial Brachytherapy

This was developed as a technique in the early part of the 20th century but has progressively declined in popularity and is mainly performed in specialist centers in France and the Netherlands. The early technique involved the implantation of permanent radon seeds or temporary radium or cobalt needles.[122,123] Although effective, there were substantial problems with radiation safety and significant morbidity from urinary leakage. Hospital stays were protracted. As alternative techniques employing external radiation became available, and as the morbidity and mortality of the cystectomy declined, so these became preferred approaches. Over the last two decades, however, afterloading techniques and computer planning mean that some centers are again looking at this as an option for selected patients. Appropriate candidates for brachytherapy are those with a solitary TCC with a diameter of <5 cm, stage T1 (with high grade) to T3a (muscle invasion but no extension through wall).

Early experience made clear that TCC is a tumor that may be surgically seeded either into the wound or to the peritoneal cavity. Van der Werf-Messing demonstrated the value of small doses of preoperative radiation to prevent iatrogenic scar implantation.[124] In those centers using brachytherapy, low doses of external radiation are given preoperatively with fractionation schemes that fit the convenience and ideology of the center. These range from 1 × 8.5 Gy or 3 × 3.5 Gy to 15 × 2 Gy. Historically, wound implants occurred in 10% to 20% and are now rarely seen.

Five-year local control rates for selected patients do appear excellent, varying between 70% and 90% with correspondingly high rates of bladder preservation[125-129] (Table 51-3). The most serious acute morbidity is fistula with wound leakage. This is most strongly predicted by tumor size, active length of radioactive sources, and use of a partial cystectomy. Serious late toxicity is rarely reported because the treated bladder volumes are relatively small. A study reported by Pos does, however, raise the possibility that there is more late morbidity using fractionated HDR than continuous LDR.[130]

COMBINED-MODALITY THERAPY

Chemotherapy as monotherapy achieves a clinical complete response in only 25% to 37% of patients.[131-137] This is more frequently reported in lower stage disease, small tumors (<5 cm), and papillary tumors.[131,133-135] Two-year survival rate with chemotherapy alone is approximately 30% (cT3-4). Even in responders, chemotherapy alone spares the bladder in only 15% to 20% of patients. Chemotherapy is therefore rarely used alone for localized disease and almost invariably in combination with other therapies.

Chemotherapy and Conservative Surgery

Chemotherapy has been used with TURBT in an attempt to spare the bladder. In a highly selected patient population, 5-year local control rates of up to 48% have been reported. Complete response rates after chemotherapy and TURBT range from 45% to 48%.[111,138-142] These findings suggest that the addition of TURBT to MVAC (methotrexate, vinblastine, doxorubicin [Adriamycin], and cisplatin) confers a considerable local control advantage over either alone. In a highly selected patient population, chemotherapy followed by partial cystectomy in conjunction with pelvic lymphadenectomy has been used in an attempt to spare the bladder.[143] Patients should meet the following criteria to be considered for such treatment:

- Complete or major response to chemotherapy
- Solitary lesion in the dome or the anterior wall of the bladder
- No history of prior invasive bladder cancer
- No CIS
- A good bladder capacity.

Although 5-year survival is high at close to 50%, less than half of these patients preserve their bladders.

Chemotherapy and Radical Local Therapy

Neoadjuvant Chemotherapy Before Definitive Local Therapy

Chemotherapy before definitive local therapy has been well tested in invasive bladder cancer. The results of the major randomized controlled trials are shown in Table 51-4.[144-153,166]

Many of the earlier trials comparing neoadjuvant chemotherapy and definitive local therapy alone used single-drug chemotherapy regimens. None of these studies detected a survival difference. The survival rates among both treatment arms were almost identical. The Spanish trial using neoadjuvant cisplatin reported a significant prolongation of disease-free interval with chemotherapy (mean time to progression, 13 months versus 30 months, $P = .03$).[146] It is important to note that in these trials the definitive treatment of the primary bladder cancer was delayed for 3 months during the administration of chemotherapy, but ultimate survival was not reduced.

A number of more recent trials[145,148-153,182] used cisplatin-based multidrug chemotherapy regimens. These studies, unfortunately, do not provide a clear and consistent indication of the efficacy of neoadjuvant cisplatin-based chemotherapy. The Nordic 1 Cooperative Bladder Cancer Study Group randomized T1G3-T4a bladder cancer patients to two cycles of neoadjuvant cisplatin and doxorubicin or to no chemotherapy. Patients in both arms received preoperative irradiation (20 Gy in 5 fractions) and cystectomy as definitive local treatment. A significant survival advantage was seen in the chemotherapy arm for the subgroup of patients with cT3-4a disease (5-year survival 52% versus 37%, $P = .03$), but not for the entire patient population.

The RTOG 89-03 trial evaluated two cycles of neoadjuvant MCV (methotrexate, cisplatin, and vinblastine) chemotherapy before concurrent cisplatin and definitive radiation. Neoadjuvant chemotherapy did not confer any detectable survival advantage. Rates of distant metastases, local metastases, and complete responses were similar in the two arms.[148]

The MRC-EORTC trial randomized 975 patients to three cycles of neoadjuvant MCV versus no chemotherapy.[149] Definitive local treatment was cystectomy, radical RT, or preoperative RT followed by immediate cystectomy as determined by physician or patient preference. Final analysis, with a median follow-up of 7.4 years, reported a small but significant survival gain for chemotherapy. At 8 years, the survival for the chemotherapy patients was 43% compared with 37% in the control arm ($p = .048$).

M-VAC, the most aggressive regimen, has been tested in an intergroup trial led by SWOG.[182] The results, after slow accrual and very long follow-up, achieved borderline significance ($p = .06$) with a 25% reduction in the risk of death through the addition of M-VAC. An almost identical study by the Italian GUONE group showed no significant difference.[153] Debate continues as to the relevance of these conflicting findings, especially when set against the morbidity of chemotherapy.

Although neoadjuvant chemotherapy seems to improve survival only marginally, it certainly has a significant impact in terms of tumor downstaging. Major responses (defined as transition from invasive disease to T0, CIS, Ta, or T1) occurred in approximately 40% of patients. Complete clinical response, as evaluated by repeat cystoscopy and biopsy after chemotherapy, ranges from 25% to 37%.

Table 51-4 Randomized Phase III Trials of Neoadjuvant Chemotherapy

Study Group	Neoadjuvant Arm	Standard Arm	Patients	Survival
Cisplatin Trials				
Aust/UK[144]	DDP/RT	RT	255	No difference
Canada/NCI[166]	DDP/RT or preoperative RT + Cyst	RT or preoperative RT + Cyst	99	No difference
Spain (CUETO)[39]	DDP/Cyst	Cyst	121	No difference
Combination Chemotherapy				
EORTC/MRC[149]	MCV/RT or Cyst	RT or Cyst	976	5.5% difference in favor of CMV
RTOG[148]	MCV/RT + C	RT + C	126	No benefit
SWOG Intergroup[182]	M-VAC/Cyst	Cyst	298	Benefit with M-VAC
Italy (GUONE)[153]	M-VAC/Cyst	Cyst	206	No difference
Italy (GISTV)[147]	M-VEC/Cyst	Cyst	171	No difference
Genoa[150]	DDP/5-FU/RT/Cyst	Cyst	104	No difference
Nordic 1[145]	ADM/DDP/RT/Cyst	RT/Cyst	311	No difference, 15% benefit with ADM + DDP in T3-T4a
Nordic 2[151]	MTX/DDP/Cyst	Cyst	317	No difference
Abol-Enein[152]	CarboMV/Cyst	Cyst	194	Benefit with CarboMV

ADM, doxorubicin; Carbo, carboplatin; Cyst, cystectomy; DDP or C, cisplatin; E, epirubicin; MTX, methotrexate; RT, radiation therapy; V, vinblastine.

Response to neoadjuvant therapy certainly seems to predict survival. Survival rates at 5 years range from 62% to 75% among responders versus 20% to 26% among nonresponders in several of the trials.

Adjuvant Chemotherapy after Definitive Local Therapy

Five randomized, controlled trials provide information on the value of adjuvant chemotherapy after radical primary therapy (Table 51-5).[154-157] All of these studies used three to four cycles of platinum-based multiagent chemotherapy. As with neoadjuvant therapy the results have been conflicting.

In three studies, a significant progression-free survival benefit at 3 and 5 years was observed when patients were randomized to adjuvant chemotherapy compared with observation. However, overall survival was not significantly different. Patients in the observation group were treated with chemotherapy at relapse except in the study reported by Stöckle and colleagues.[152] The failure to provide salvage chemotherapy in this study may explain the low survival rates in the observation arm (5-year crude survival, 17%). The progression-free survival benefit does not translate into an overall survival benefit if patients receive salvage chemotherapy. In other words, observation with salvage chemotherapy might be just as effective as adjuvant chemotherapy in terms of survival.

Trimodality Therapy Using Limited Resection, Chemotherapy, and Irradiation in Bladder Preservation

The rationale for combining chemotherapy with RT is twofold.

1. Certain cytotoxic agents, in particular cisplatin and 5-FU, are capable of sensitizing tumor tissue to radiation, thus increasing cell kill in a synergistic fashion.
2. Patients with muscle-invading TCC harbor occult metastases in approximately 50% of cases, which makes a case for the addition of systemic chemotherapy in an attempt to control occult distant disease.

Trimodality therapy consisting of TUR with concurrent chemoradiation may, therefore, increase the efficacy of bladder-sparing protocols. The evolution of approach over the past 2 decades is shown in Figure 51-3.

Many phase II trials have combined chemotherapy and RT in different sequences in patients with invasive bladder cancer. Although a variety of different drugs and radiation doses have been used, it is apparent that the highest clinical complete response rate (T0) was achieved in patients who received concurrent chemotherapy and RT compared with sequential regimens.[158-163] Table 51-6 shows results from several modern series of multimodality bladder preservation therapy.[97,148,159,164]

One of the clearest indications of the potential of multimodality therapy for bladder preservation can be found in a study from the University of Paris.[158] In this study, TURBT followed by concomitant cisplatin, 5-FU, and accelerated RT was initially used as a precystectomy regimen. The first 18 patients who had no residual tumor on cystoscopy and repeat biopsy (clinical complete response) underwent radical cystectomy as planned. None of these patients had any evidence of malignancy in the cystectomy specimens, a 100% pathologic complete response rate. Previous studies using TUR and chemotherapy found residual tumor in as many as 50% of the cystectomy specimens in clinical complete responders.

After this striking evidence of tumor eradication, the University of Paris investigators changed their protocol to one of selective bladder preservation. In 1988, they converted to induction chemoradiation, restaging with cystoscopy, and repeat biopsy of the tumor site 4 to 6 weeks after completion of the chemoradiation. Subsequent consolidation chemoradiation was only selectively given to patients who did not have

Table 51-5 Randomized, Controlled Trials of Adjuvant Chemotherapy

Series	Stage	Treatment	5-y Disease-Free Survival (%)	5-y Overall Survival (%)	Significance
Skinner, 1991[154]	pT3-4	Cyst + 4 × CAP	52	49	Sign. for N+
	Nx	Cyst	38	43	—
Stöckle, 1992[155]	pT3b-4 52—	Cyst + 3 × MVAC	52	—	Sign.
	N+	Cyst	14	—	—
Studer[156]	pTa-4	Cyst + 3 × Cis	—	57	Neg
	N+	Cyst	—	54	—
Freiha, 1996[157]	pT3b-4	Cyst + 4 × CMF	50	55	Sign
	Nx	Cyst	22	35	—

Cyst, cystectomy; Cis, cisplatin; CMF, cisplatin, methotrexate, 5-fluorouracil; MVAC, methotrexate, vinblastine, adriamycin, cisplatin; CAP, cyclophosphamide, adriamycin, cisplatin; Sign, significant; neg, negative; N+, node positive.

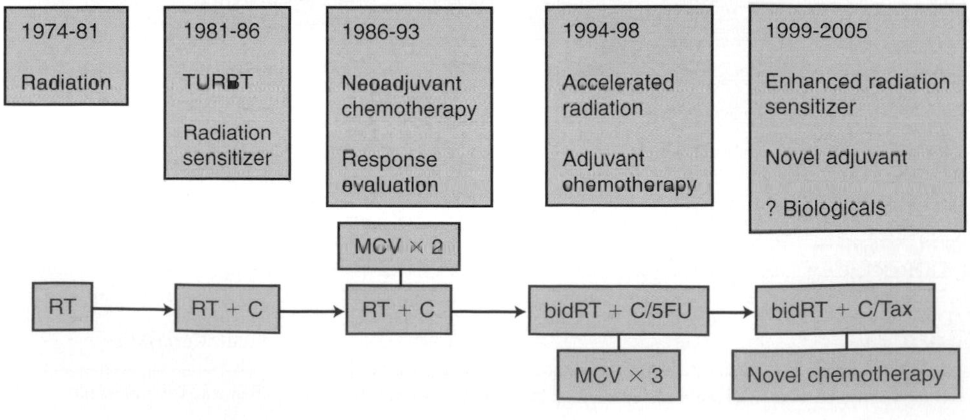

Figure 51-3 Bladder Conservation: Evolution of multimodality approach. RT, radiation; C, cisplatin; M, methotrexate; V, vinblastine; Tax, taxotere.

Table 51-6 **Results of Multimodality Treatment for Muscle-Invading Bladder Cancer**

Series	Multimodality Therapy Used	No.	5-y Overall Survival (%)	5-y Disease-Free Survival (%)
RTOG 8802, 1996	TURBT, MCV, external beam radiation + cisplatin	91	51%	44% (4 y)
RTOG 8903, 1998[148]	TURBT ± MCV, external beam radiation + cisplatin	123	49%	38%
University of Paris, 1997[97]	TURBT, 5-FU, external beam radiation + cisplatin	120	63%	NA
Erlangen, 2002[159]	TURBT, external beam radiation, cisplatin, carboplatin, or cisplatin and 5-FU	415	50%	42%
Massachusetts General Hospital, 2002[164]	TURBT ± MCV, external beam radiation + cisplatin	190	54%	45%

5-FU, 5-fluorouracil; MCV, methotrexate, cisplatin, vinblastine; TURBT, transurethral resection of bladder tumor.

any evidence of disease at restaging (complete response). In cases of persistent disease, patients underwent immediate cystectomy. The 5-year survival rate for all patients who entered the protocol was 63%.

At the University of Erlangen in Germany, a prospective bladder preservation study was started in 1982. The first 106 consecutive patients, however, were treated only with TURBT followed by radiation to 50.2 to 56 Gy at 2 Gy daily. A multimodality approach was initiated in 1985 when chemotherapy (cisplatin or carboplatin) was added concurrently with the radiation regimen in 139 subsequent patients.[159] This protocol differed in two aspects from the University of Paris study. All recruited patients underwent the entire course of chemoradiation. Restaging TURBT was performed at 6 to 8 weeks, only after completion of the entire protocol. In addition, only patients with invasive persistent disease or poorly differentiated residual superficial tumors underwent cystectomy. Patients with well-differentiated superficial disease (Ta, CIS) were treated further conservatively with TUR and intravesical chemo- or immunotherapy. Overall survival for the 245 patients was 47% at 5 years and 26% after 10 years.

When the outcomes of the two patient groups who received and did not receive concurrent chemotherapy were compared, concomitant chemotherapy was found to improve complete response rates but did not significantly impact distant metastasis rates or survival. Five-year survival rates were 52% with chemotherapy and 50% without chemotherapy, respectively. The subgroup of patients who either had persistent invasive tumor (nonresponders) at first restaging or needed a cystectomy for early invasive recurrences within 9 months after completion of the treatment had dismal survival rates (5-year overall survival, 16%) because of early systemic spread. Patients who needed salvage cystectomy later than 9 months after completion of the treatment achieved a 5-year survival rate comparable to that of the entire group.

In June 1986, MGH implemented a selective bladder preservation protocol for patients with muscle-invading bladder cancer. To improve on earlier results in terms of both local and distant control, two cycles of neoadjuvant MCV chemotherapy were added before the chemoradiation regimen. MCV was chosen because three- or four-drug (e.g., MVAC) chemotherapy has been shown to be more effective than single-agent cisplatin in metastatic bladder cancer. Five-year overall survival was 52%, and 42% of patients survived 5 years and conserved their bladders.

From 1989 through 1994, the RTOG assessed long-term efficacy of neoadjuvant MCV chemotherapy in 126 patients with muscle-invading bladder cancer before a selective bladder preservation (combined-modality therapy with selection for consolidation by either cystectomy or consolidation chemoradiation based on initial response) by a randomized trial (RTOG 89-03).[148] Patients were randomized to neoadjuvant MCV or no neoadjuvant chemotherapy. Only 62% of the patients in the MCV arm (arm 1) were able to complete the protocol compared with 82% in arm 2. No differences in the complete response rate (60% in arm 1 and 55% in arm 2), actuarial 5-year survival (arm 1, 50%; arm 2, 50%), 5-year survival with preserved bladder (32% in arm 1 and 32% in arm 2), and distant metastases (35% in arm 1 and 43% in arm 2) were observed. Treatment-related morbidity, however, was significantly higher in the neoadjuvant chemotherapy arm (4% of patients in arm 2 and 14% of patients in arm 1 died of treatment-related causes). In summary, two cycles of MCV neoadjuvant chemotherapy did not significantly improve the rate of complete response to induction chemoradiation, the rate of distant metastases, or overall survival. An unexpectedly high protocol deviation rate of 38% was observed as a result of toxicity in the MCV arm.

The RTOG protocol 97-06 demonstrated the safety and feasibility of induction chemoradiation involving accelerated hyperfractionation for the tumor with a standard dose schedule for the pelvis.[167] Outpatient cisplatin is included as radiation sensitizer. Adjuvant MCV chemotherapy (methotrexate, 30 mg/m^2; vinblastine, 3 mg/m^2; cisplatin, 70 mg/m^2) is to be given after consolidation chemoradiation or radical cystectomy as an outpatient regimen and is repeated every 28 days for three cycles. The rationale for this protocol was to reduce the duration of the induction treatment to 12 days, thereby decreasing the delay between onset of consolidation chemoradiation or cystectomy for those patients in whom induction therapy fails.

Another original way to combine chemotherapy and radiation has been employed by Eapen and colleagues. This group has combined conventionally fractionated external radiation with intra-arterial cisplatin. Their durable complete response rates are as high as any in the literature. The principal problem they have faced is a high level of sacral neuropathy, which, in recent years, they have reduced through reducing the dose of infused cisplatin.[168]

The primary goal of bladder-preserving therapy, as with any therapy for muscle-invading TCC of the bladder, is patient survival. Bladder preservation in the interest of quality of life can only be considered a secondary objective.

The *overall survival* of the *modern bladder preservation series* at 5 years ranges from 45% to 52%; 54% to 67% of surviving patients have a tumor-free, normally functioning bladder. Overall survival with this approach has not been compared in a randomized fashion with modern radical cystectomy (Table 51-7). Selection bias of more favorable patients in the cystectomy studies makes a nonrandomized comparison very difficult. Surgical patients are generally younger, with a better performance status. Surgery allows for a more accurate

Table 51-7 Muscle-Invasive Bladder Cancer: Survival Outcomes in Contemporary Series

Series	Stages	No.	Overall Survival 5 y	10 y
Cystectomy				
USC, 2001[86]	pT2-pT4a	633	48%	32%
MSKCC, 2001[87]	pT2-pT4a	181	36%	27%
SWOG/ECOG/CALGB,*† 2002[182]	cT2-cT4a	307	50%	34%
Selective Bladder Preservation				
University of Erlangen,* 2002[159]	cT2-cT4a	326	45%	29%
MGH,* 2002[164]	cT2-cT4a	190	54%	36%
RTOG,* 1998[148]	cT2-cT4a	123	49%	—

*These series include all patients by their intention-to-treat.
†50% of patients were randomly assigned to receive 3 cycles of neoadjuvant M-VAC.

pathologic staging and identification of only surgically identifiable metastatic disease, which leads to a discontinuation of approximately 15% of cystectomies. Results reported by clinical stage are better for comparison with bladder-conserving strategies, but, unfortunately, most cystectomy studies do not provide data on the initial clinical staging. It is, therefore, very challenging to compare these two approaches in a meaningful manner in a nonrandomized fashion. Martinez-Pineiro and associates did, however, report their cystectomy series by clinical stage.[146] The 5-year survival rate was 41% (48% for clinical stage T2); this is similar to that of the bladder preservation strategy (5-year survival ranges from 45% to 52%), in which all patients who initiated their therapy are reported, not only those whose tumor response was satisfactory to complete the organ preservation program. It is important to remember that the appropriate strategy for bladder preservation therapy includes cystectomy for nonresponders. Any comparison of cystectomy protocols with bladder preservation protocols must include these nonresponders to avoid being biased by patient selection.

Prognostic Factors in Chemoradiation

Complete Response

Clinical complete response (or T0 response), evaluated by cystoscopy with tumor site biopsy with or without cytology 2 to 8 weeks after completion of the induction chemoradiation, ranged from 70% to 80%. The complete response rate was significantly higher in patients in whom a macroscopically *visible complete resection* could be achieved compared with patients with residual macroscopic disease after TURBT (92% versus 60%, $P < .001$).[97] Patients with *clinical stage* T2-3a achieved significantly more frequent complete responses than those with T3b-4 disease (83% versus 58%, $P < .001$, University of Paris T2, 81% versus MGH T3-4, 64%). Patients who presented with *hydronephrosis* achieved a 66% complete response versus 83% in patients who had no hydronephrosis at presentation (University of Paris, $P < .05$; MGH, 52% versus 77%). The Erlangen group has shown that those with Tcis disease in the bladder in addition to the invasive tumor are less likely to have a durable response and more likely to require cystectomy.

Chemoradiation added significant improvement to the clinical complete response rates compared with the "early" complete response after the induction chemotherapy alone. After two cycles of MCV, the complete response rate for patients with T2 disease was 62% and with T3 or T4 disease, 41%. After adding a course of concurrent chemoradiation, the complete response rate increased to 81% and 64%, respectively (MGH). Factors predicting for a complete response also predict local control and, ultimately, bladder preservation.

Survival

Clinical complete responders generally have significantly higher 5-year survival rates than nonresponders. The amount of residual tumor after TURBT is also a prognostic factor for survival as for local control. The same is true for those with T2 clinical stage compared with T3-4 and those presenting without hydronephrosis. Overall, visibly completely resected T2-3a tumors had the best prognosis.

The 5-year distant metastasis rate for all patients entered in the protocols ranged from 34% to 40%. In the MGH series, the 5-year distant metastasis rate in the T0 responder group was only 20%. Patients who did not respond rapidly ($T > 0$) and underwent immediate cystectomy had a 50% distant metastasis rate at 5 years. However, it was similar to the 5-year rate of initial T0 responders who subsequently underwent salvage cystectomy for local failure (5-year distant metastasis rate, 54%).

Follow-up after Chemoradiation

All patients with bladder cancer (either superficial or invasive) treated with bladder-preserving therapies must be willing to return for regular, thorough clinical examinations, cystoscopy, and urine cytology follow-up so that transurethral surgery, intravesical chemotherapy, or cystectomy can be implemented at the earliest opportunity if necessary. The optimal timing of cystoscopy after RT is unclear but is usually first done at 3 months.[110] At the MGH our protocol mandates 3 monthly cystoscopy and urine cytology for the first 2 years, then 6 monthly until 5 years, and annual thereafter.

Managing Recurrent Disease in the Bladder

Of patients who have complete responses, 80% to 89% remained free from invasive recurrence in the bladder at 5 years, and 60% remained free from any noninvasive or invasive occurrence. Of patients whose invasive recurrence was cured, 20% to 30% subsequently experienced superficial TCC. Eighty-four percent of patients who experienced superficial recurrences (Ta or CIS) at MGH have been maintained in remission by TUR and intravesical drug therapy with 15 to 49 months of follow-up. Patients with hydronephrosis were significantly less likely to achieve local control compared with those without hydronephrosis at presentation (66% versus 83%, $P < .05$, MGH).

Invasive recurrences are generally managed with cystectomy. Superficial tumors may be managed by TURBT and intravesical therapy.[169,170] In selected series, salvage cystectomy results in a 40% to 50% survival rate at 5 years and locoregional control rates of 60%.

Conclusions Regarding Combined Chemoradiation and TURBT

The *ideal candidate for bladder preservation* meets the following criteria:

1. Primary T2-3a tumors that are unifocal
2. Tumor size less than 5 cm in maximum diameter
3. No presence of ureteral obstruction
4. Good capacity of the bladder
5. Visibly complete TURBT

Quality-of-Life Studies

Radical cystectomy causes changes in many areas of quality of life, including urinary, sexual, and social function, daily living activities and satisfaction with body image.[171-175] Sexual function has been particularly emphasized because of the high prevalence of erectile dysfunction. Researchers have, over the last decade, concentrated on the relative merits of continent and noncontinent diversions. Available data have been mixed with some groups, surprisingly, reporting few differences between the quality of life of those with an ileal conduit and those with continent diversions. Until recently, little comparative data have been available on those who have neobladders. Hart and colleagues have compared outcome in cystectomy patients who have either ileal conduits, cutaneous Koch pouches, or urethral Koch pouches.[175] Of 1074 patients undergoing cystectomy for bladder cancer at the University of Southern California, 368 were eligible for study because they were alive, spoke English, and had no major health issues that could affect global quality of life. Of these, 61% completed self-reporting questionnaires. Regardless of the type of urinary diversion, the majority of patients reported good overall quality of life, little emotional distress, and few problems with social, physical, or functional activities. Problems with their diversions and with sexual function were the most commonly reported. After controlling for age, no significant differences were seen among urinary diversion subgroups in any quality-of-life area. It might be anticipated that those receiving the urethral Koch diversions would be the most satisfied and the explanation why this is not so is unclear. It may be that the subgroups were too small to detect differences but perhaps it is more likely that each group adapts in time to the specific difficulties presented by that type of diversion.

Zietman and coworkers have performed a study on patients receiving TURBT, chemotherapy, and radiation in the treatment of their bladder cancer at the Massachusetts General Hospital.[176] Of 221 patients with clinical T2-4a cancer of the bladder treated at the Massachusetts General Hospital from 1986 to 2000, 71 were alive with their native bladders and disease free in 2001. These patients were asked to undergo a urodynamic study (UDS) and to complete a quality-of-life questionnaire. Sixty-nine percent participated in some component of this study, with a median time from trimodality therapy of 6.3 years. This log follow-up is sufficient to capture the majority of late radiation effects. Seventy-five percent of patients had normally functioning bladders by UDS. Reduced bladder compliance, a recognized complication of radiation, was seen in 22% but in only one third of these was it reflected in distressing symptoms. Two of twelve women showed bladder hypersensitivity, involuntary detrusor contractions, and incontinence. The questionnaire showed that bladder symptoms were uncommon, especially among men, with the exception of control problems. These were reported by 19%, with 11% wearing pads (all women). Distress from urinary symptoms was half as common as their prevalence. Bowel symptoms occurred in 22%, with 14% recording any level of distress. The majority of men retained sexual function. Global health–related quality of life was high. The great majority of patients treated by trimodality therapy therefore retain good bladder function. It was concluded that there is a small but detectable level of lasting bowel dysfunction and distress and that this might be judged the additional price that these patients have had to pay to retain their bladders.

A prospective multicenter study from France has recently been presented.[177] It tracks voiding symptoms and quality of life in 53 patients from before their trimodality treatment. Thirty-three retained their bladders, and these were interviewed 6, 12, and 24 months later. Levels of urinary symptoms were very high but only 5% reported any EORTC grade 3 symptoms. It was also notable that most patients experienced improvement of symptoms over the two years after treatment, presumably because of the eradication of a symptomatic tumor.

Two recent cross-sectional questionnaire studies, one from Sweden and one from Italy, have compared the outcome following radiation with the outcome following cystectomy.[178,179] The questionnaire results for urinary function following radiation were very similar to those recorded in the MGH study. Over 74% of patients reported good urinary function. Both studies compared bowel function in irradiated patients with that seen in patients undergoing cystectomy. In both the bowel symptoms were greater for those receiving radiation than for those receiving cystectomy (10 versus 3% and 32 versus 24%, respectively) but in neither was this statistically significant.

In the assessment of sexual function, most women in the MGH study preferred not to answer the questions and no data was therefore available for them. Almost all men, however, did. In contrast to patients who have been irradiated for prostate cancer, the majority of male bladder-sparing patients reported adequate erectile function (full or sufficient for intercourse), and only 8% reported dissatisfaction with their sex lives. These are in line with those obtained in the Swedish and Italian series in which 38% and 25% of men retained useful erections as compared with 13% and 8% of cystectomized controls. The MGH series allowing the use of sildenafil probably contributed to the better outcome.

LOCALLY ADVANCED DISEASE AND PALLIATION

When bladder cancer has invaded adjacent organs or spread to the pelvic lymph nodes cure is rare, as the primary tumors are usually bulky and distant metastases usually present, even if subclinical. In this situation if the voiding symptoms are not too severe and the renal function allows, it is common to give combination chemotherapy and reassess after several cycles. If the patients have had a good response they may receive consolidation chemoradiation delivered with "curative" intent. If renal function is poor, patients may be given non–platinum-based regimens such as taxol either before or with the radiation. If voiding symptoms are severe or there is bilateral hydronephrosis, they may be better served by percutaneous urinary drainage and then cystectomy with urinary diversion.

For patients with locally advanced T4 primary tumors or locally recurrent cancer, there is a rationale for combining resection with intraoperative radiation therapy (IORT) but experience is limited. Resection and IORT would preferably be preceded by several cycles of multiagent chemotherapy, then pelvic radiation (45 to 50.4 Gy in 1.8-Gy fractions) plus concurrent weekly cisplatin (see prior section). Trials have been published from our colleagues in Lyon, France, and Pamplona, Spain, demonstrating the potential value of pursuing such approaches in other centers with IORT capabilities.[180-182]

If the patient is unfit for cystectomy then radiation may be given to the bladder for palliation. Duchesne and colleagues reported an MRC trial in the UK in which 500 patients were randomized to two palliative fractionation schedules: 35 Gy in 10 fractions and 21 Gy in 3 fractions (given weekly). When assessed at 3 months, 68% had had some symptomatic improvement but there was no difference between the arms.[183] There was no evidence for a difference in toxicity justifying the use of this very hypofractionated regimen for the palliation of patients at the end of their lives.

Metastatic bladder cancer is very responsive to platinum-based chemotherapy. MVAC or MCV are the usual choices as first line drugs but taxotere and gemcitabine are showing equivalence. It is remarkable that, unlike most other solid tumors, complete responses are not unusual and durable responses do occur.

Radiation is often used in the palliation of bone and brain metastases. Palliative radiation may also relieve the IVC or lymphatic obstruction that can occur when there is heavy involvement of the para-aortic nodes.

TECHNIQUE OF IRRADIATION

External Beam

In almost all work on bladder cancer published to date radiation therapy has been delivered by conventional 2-D radiotherapy. Although 3-D techniques are now readily available there is uncertainty as to how best to employ them when treating an organ as mobile as the bladder. In the future "4-D" techniques which employ daily imaging and real time tracking of the bladder will likely become routine.

The 2-D technique is well established and it is worth discussing the advantages and pitfalls in detail. At the MGH the following technique has been used on- and off-protocol through the 1990s. Though we are currently changing technique and testing new doses and fraction sizes this remains the approach that we recommend off-protocol. The standard protocol for radical RT as well as combined-modality therapy uses a four-field isocentric technique, which consists of shaped anterior, posterior, right, and left lateral fields for the initial or induction treatment field. This is followed by a boost or consolidation field.

Simulation

All simulations begin with the insertion of a Foley catheter into the patient shortly after they have voided. The post-void urine residual is measured and this volume is replaced by an equal volume of bladder contrast plus 25 additional mL of contrast and 15 mL of air. The contrast defines the inner walls of the bladder as they are positioned shortly after voiding. The air aids visualization of the anterior bladder on a lateral simulation film. The amount of contrast should not be less than the postvoid residual because this amount of urine will be present in the bladder during treatment. The postvoid residual is determined at catheterization for the introduction of contrast. If the postvoid residual exceeds 25 mL, additional contrast is added so that the total amount of contrast equals the postvoid residual. Treatments are given with the bladder empty as this makes tumor localization far more predictable. The patient is then immobilized in a supine position and the simulation must proceed rapidly to avoid confusion due to changes in bladder size from subsequent bladder filling. The simulation may either be formed using APPA and lateral radiographs or it may be performed in a CT simulator.

TARGET VOLUMES

During the first phase of treatment the bladder is treated along with a margin of 2 cm. If using a radiographic rather than a CT simulation, the contrast only lines the inner wall of the bladder and another 5 to 10 mm must be added to account for wall thickness, depending upon the degree of bladder filling. In men the entire prostate is also covered in this first phase as there may be occult stromal invasion or extension into the prostatic urethra. In women the proximal 2 cm of urethra are also considered target. Care must be taken to avoid the inferior border of the field glancing the vulva as this greatly limits tolerance. The internal and external iliac lymph nodes of the pelvis are also covered for this phase of therapy. The top border of the field usually lies only at the level of the bifurcation of the common iliac vessels and does not include the entire pelvis. This is because a significant number of irradiated patients will subsequently require salvage cystectomy with urinary diversion. It is therefore prudent to limit the amount of radiation to bowel that may subsequently be needed for this purpose. Another good reason to limit the bowel volume is that quality of life studies have shown that the most troublesome consequences of irradiation for bladder cancer relate to the small bowel irradiation rather than the bladder irradiation.[176,179]

During the boost phase of treatment we, at the MGH, treat the tumor alone with a 1.5-cm margin rather than the entire bladder. Defining the tumor may be difficult but we employ a combination of a bladder map drawn by the urologist at the time of TURBT, and CT and MR information from the staging work-up. CT scan after TURBT often overestimates the tumor residuum because of edema in the bladder wall. Using these sources of information it is usually possible to exclude approximately one third of the bladder from the boost volume (Fig. 51-4). While this may not seem like much, it does mean that less than the entire volume is treated to full dose, a factor that may contribute to the good functional results seen after use of this technique.

FIELDS

The first phase treats the pelvic lymph nodes and bladder using a 4-field arrangement. The second phase boosts the

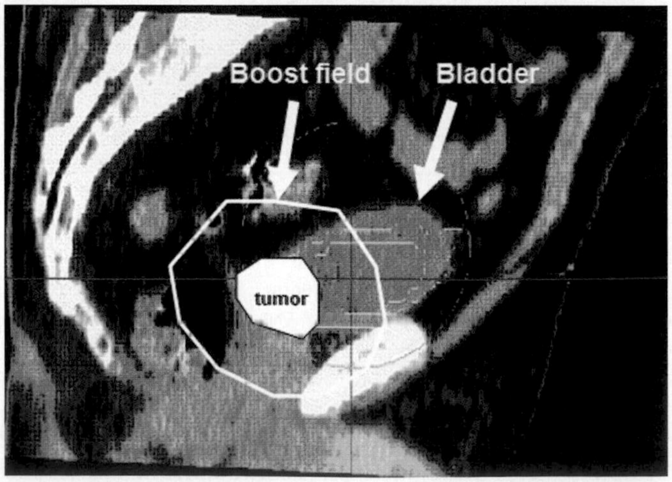

Figure 51-4 Sagittal CT image showing how a lateral boost may be given to a tumor to spare the anterior bladder.

bladder tumor alone. As most tumors are on the bladder trigone or on the postero-lateral walls it is easiest to boost with opposed lateral fields. If this is anticipated the 4-field box used in the first phase has to be weighted more heavily toward the AP and PA to save femoral head tolerance and allow the lateral boost. For the planning of the parallel-opposed lateral fields, 50 mL of dilute barium is introduced via the rectal catheter for localization of the rectum.

Patients are treated with empty bladders to achieve a reproducible target and to minimize volume irradiated. Many patients with bladder cancer have significant postvoid residual volume so artificial emptying of the bladder by catheterization may give a false impression of the shape and size of the target volume at simulation. Introducing proportionally more contrast during simulation may give a more accurate volume.

Total Dose

At the MGH we have traditionally given doses in the order of 65 Gy together with chemotherapy and an aggressive TURBT. 45 Gy is given in the first phase to the larger field covering the entire bladder and the low pelvic lymph nodes. The tumor is then boosted to the full dose. Fractions of 1.8 Gy are used throughout. Invasive local recurrence is limited to only 15% to 18% of all complete responders, implying that this is an adequate dose for permanent control in the vast majority of those who respond to radiation.

Treatment Break to Evaluate Response

At the MGH we have routinely built a 3-week break into the treatment program following the delivery of 39 to 42 Gy followed by repeat cystoscopy (see Fig. 51-3). Patients are selected to continue and complete radiation (the consolidation) on the basis of their response at this point. Those who have had complete responses or in whom the tumor residuum is less than T1 by stage (Ta or Tis) continue. The others are recommended to undergo a cystectomy. This can thus be performed before the patient has had full dose radiation, an easier proposition for the surgeon. It also means that a patient responding poorly can be identified early and recommended surgery promptly rather than waiting for an entire course of radiation to be completed, by which time progression may have occurred that could threaten the efficacy of salvage. Concerns have been expressed on radiobiological grounds that split course treatment compromises efficacy.[184,185] There is also the worry that those who have not been complete responders after 40 Gy might yet become complete responders after 65 Gy and thus some may be recommended an unnecessary cystectomy. This concern, however, probably affects only a tiny minority of patients.

Controversial Issues in External Radiation Technique

Nodal Treatment

Lymph node involvement is common in this disease and is seen in approximately 25% of those coming to a radical cystectomy.[86] The number of lymph nodes involved is well established as a prognostic indicator which surgeons use to determine the extent of their lymph node dissection and the need for adjuvant chemotherapy. This information is, however, unavailable to radiation oncologists. More interesting for them is the knowledge that some patients with positive lymph nodes may be cured by a lymphadenectomy, a situation different from prostate cancer and more akin to breast or head and neck cancers. The thoroughness of a lymph node dissection (<10 nodes removed) also correlates with outcome independent of nodal status.[186,187] Thus, radiation to the pelvis might confer a survival advantage though it comes at the price of additional morbidity. Centers that do irradiate the bladder alone do not report either an increased pelvic failure rate or reduced survival, although direct comparisons are difficult and randomized data are not available.[188] It may be that either chemotherapy does the job of the nodal irradiation or that nodal disease extends beyond the confines of the current pelvic template. Surgeons are now starting to explore extended lymphadenectomies to the level of the inferior mesenteric artery; randomized trials are planned.[44,189]

Partial Bladder Treatment

Estimates of bladder tolerance have been made which suggest that up to 80 Gy could be given if one third of the bladder is spared, whereas 65 Gy is the limit for whole bladder treatment.[190,191] In addition the low rate of development of new invasive tumors elsewhere in the bladder after brachytherapy (5% to 7%) suggests that localized partial bladder radiation is a reasonable strategy.[125] Careful selection is, however, necessary, with such approaches being limited to smaller tumors (<5 cm), unifocal tumors, and those without extensive Tis tumor elsewhere in the bladder. A randomized trial in the United Kingdom has shown that partial bladder irradiation does allow for the delivery of a higher dose to the tumor than whole bladder radiation without an increase in morbidity.[192] It did not, however, show either improvements in local control or survival. 149 patients were randomized to receive whole bladder conformal RT to 52.5 Gy in 20 fractions or partial bladder conformal radiation to either 57.5 Gy in 20 fractions or 55 Gy in 16 fractions. The 5-year local control rates for these 3 regimens were 58%, 59%, and 38%, respectively, without any significant differences between arms.

Treatment Margins

At the MGH in expanding the CTV to the PTV we have adopted isotropic 2-cm margins around either the bladder (first phase of treatment) or tumor (boost) in all three dimensions. This is to account for set-up errors and organ motion. Several studies employing serial CT scans have shown that margins less than this may be inadequate. Turner and coworkers demonstrated that bladder wall movement of >1.5 cm occurs at least once during a course of treatment in over 60% of patients.[193] Several others have reported that the GTV moves outside the PTV on at least one occasion in at least 20%.[194,195] Our own analysis showed that these variations are highly patient dependent and occurred even when strict instructions were given regarding bladder and rectal filling.[196] The greatest degree of bladder wall positional change occurred in the cranial direction, with the least variation in the anteroinferior direction, limited by the pubic symphysis. In light of this information it is clear that organ motion is the dominant source of error and that the magnitude of the error depends upon the region of the bladder. The solutions are clear though difficult to achieve. Graham and colleagues have recommended anisotropic margin widths of 1.6 cm anterior and posterior, 1.4 cm laterally, 3 cm superior, and 1.4 cm inferior.[197] The problem is that these margins incorporate much normal tissue. Daily image-guided therapy will be the only way to reduce these margins significantly. Daily CT or cone-beam therapy, which could delineate the bladder, may be practicable in the near future. There is also interest in the use of fiducial markers that could be placed by the urologist at the time of TURBT in the bladder wall around the tumor crater (Fig. 51-5). Roof and associates have shown that if the daily treatment is centered on the bladder centroid rather than referenced to bony anatomy, margins of <1.5 cm could be feasible.[196] None of these studies accounts for the fact that the bladder not only changes in size but also in shape; it is

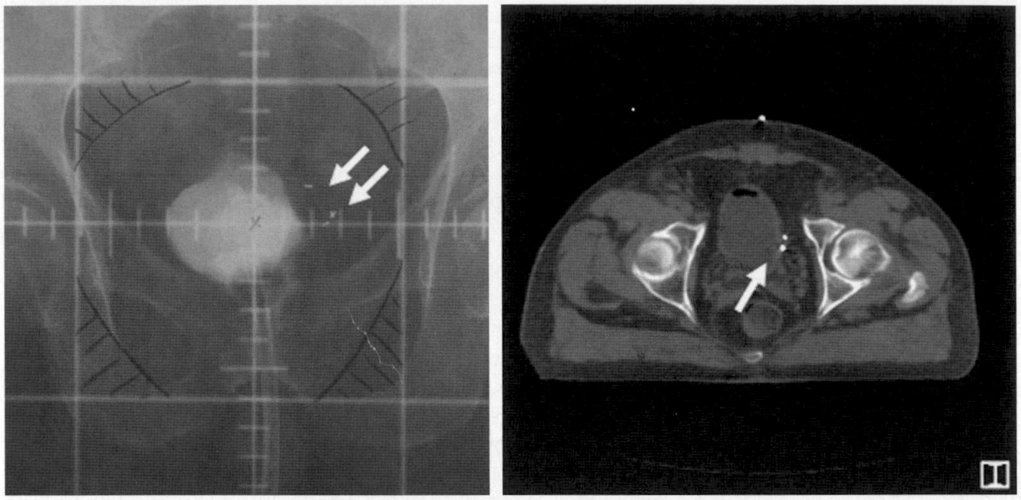

Figure 51-5 Fiducial markers placed adjacent to bladder tumor at time of transurethral resection. Note distances from outer wall of bladder to contrast on cystogram, a point that must be appreciated on drawing target volumes.

deformable. This will likely set a limit on our ability to shrink margins in the near future.

Radiation Dose

There is evidence for a dose response curve in bladder cancer, with most studies showing that doses of <62 Gy (at 1.8 to 2 Gy/fraction) predict poor outcome.[198-200] Most of these studies, however, have employed radiation alone and the curve is likely to be greatly modified by effective debulking of the tumor or by radiation sensitization with chemotherapy. Increasing dose may result in increased complete response rates but may add to the morbidity and may also be limited by the rapid proliferative index and short doubling time of these tumors.[201] Interest recently has therefore concentrated on dose intensification using accelerated regimes rather than an increase in total dose.. Acceleration may be achieved through hypofractionation but this is better limited to the palliative setting, or through the use of conventional 2 Gy fractionation given twice a day.[202] The Royal Marsden Hospital has reported on 85 patients with twice-daily fractions of 1.8 to 2.0 Gy 5 days a week to doses between 57.6 Gy and 64 Gy in 32 fractions over 26 days. Of 70 patients who had cystoscopic reevaluation 3 to 6 months after RT, 80% were found to be complete responders (i.e., cystoscopy and biopsy negative for tumor 3 to 6 months later).[203] Plataniotis and colleagues reported a total response rate of 67% when a twice-daily fractionation was used during the last week (fifth week) of RT.[204]

Unfortunately, acceleration with fraction sizes of 2 Gy seems to increase acute toxicity. The RTOG has therefore explored acceleration with hyperfractionation and recent protocols have employed fraction sizes of 1.2 to 1.8 Gy with a concomitant boost technique. No comparative studies have yet been performed but morbidity appears low.[167]

Hyperfractionation has also been used to increase the total tumor dose. A randomized trial of 168 patients with T2-4 tumors, unsuited for cystectomy, compared hyperfractionated EBRT (1 Gy three times a day to a total dose of 84 Gy) with conventional fractionation (2.0 Gy every day to 64 Gy).[205,206] Hyperfractionation achieved superior results with respect to survival at 5 years (27% versus 18%), local control (12% versus 7%), and clinical complete response rates (59% versus 36%) with an increase in late toxicity. Both study arms were treated by a split-course of RT with a 2-week gap after the first 3 weeks, the effect of which is unknown. The benefit of the hyperfractionated schedule persisted over a 10-year follow-up period, both for local control and survival. It should be noted, however, that patients in the conventional fractionation arm did poorly compared with those receiving similar treatment in other studies largely because patients unfit for cystectomy were entered in this study.

Future improvements in the complete response rate may also come without any need to escalate radiation dose: from better selection of patients; better radiation sensitization; or a more aggressive TURBT. Others have argued that doses of 65 Gy at 1.8 to 2 Gy/fraction may actually be more than is needed, especially for those who have had visibly complete transurethral resections. The Erlangen group has delivered doses tailored to the estimated residuum following resection. These doses are in the range of 50 to 59 Gy (1.8 to 2 Gy/fraction) depending upon whether disease to be treated is microscopic or gross in volume.[207]

Brachytherapy

Shortly after completion of the preoperative radiation (<2 weeks) a suprapubic cystotomy is performed to ascertain the true dimensions of the tumor and to confirm that it is indeed unifocal. There are regional differences in the type of surgery performed on the primary tumor. In France a partial cystectomy is preferred. In the Netherlands, citing concerns about the risk of fistula, this is only performed for lesions on the dome or in a diverticulum. The target area is determined by the surgery and is either the bladder scar after partial cystectomy or the macroscopic tumor plus a 1.5- to 2.0-cm margin. It may be marked by fiducials at this point. Narrow afterloading tubes are then inserted into the target area parallel and halfway through the bladder wall. In the case of a partial cystectomy two tubes one on either side of the scar are sufficient. If a partial cystectomy is not perfomed then 3 to 5 tubes in a single plane will encompass most lesions. The tubes are then brought out to the anterior abdominal wall and a suprapubic catheter inserted for drainage. The tubes are removed without anesthesia after the completion of radiation; the urinary catheter is removed 2 weeks later.

Radiation planning may be performed using stereo-shifted radiographs but it is now preferable to use CT. Doses given vary greatly in the literature according to the additional external beam given and whether or not high or low dose rate brachytherapy is planned. If less than 10 to 15 Gy is given preoperatively, then 30 to 60 Gy are given using low-dose rate. The lower doses are given to those who have had partial cystectomies or complete resections. In the Netherlands 30 Gy external beam is either supplemented with 40 Gy LDR or 10 × 3.2 Gy HDR (2 fractions per day with a 6-hour interval).

SUMMARY, TREATMENT ALGORITHM, CHALLENGES, AND FUTURE POSSIBILITIES

Selective bladder preservation is based on the response of the tumor to induction combined-modality therapy, which includes a TUR of as much of the primary bladder tumor as is judged safely possible combined with concurrent chemotherapy and RT; early cystectomy is recommended for patients whose tumors are not responding to combined-modality therapy to maximize the possibility of cure (Fig. 51-6). In appropriately selected patients, bladder-preserving treatment with chemoradiation therapy offers a chance for long-term cure and survival comparable to cystectomy while affording a 60% to 70% chance of maintaining a normally functioning bladder (see Fig. 51-2, Table 51-6, and Table 51-7). This approach is not suitable for patients with tumors obstructing a ureter. Between 20% and 30% of patients cured of muscle-invading bladder cancer will subsequently acquire a new superficial tumor, but these superficial tumors have generally responded well to the usual intravesical drug therapy. These patients require close urologic surveillance, as do any patients with superficial bladder cancer treated conservatively. Bladder-preserving treatment usually results in a normally functioning bladder without incontinence or hematuria for stage T2 and T3a patients. However, T3b-4 patients experience local control less frequently using these techniques.

No data exist, however, to suggest that patients with more advanced disease are in any way disadvantaged by preoperative chemoradiation as an attempt at bladder conservation. Although many urologists have found merit in a selective bladder-sparing approach to muscle-invading transitional cell bladder cancer, many more will need to become convinced if there is to be a significant change in treatment practices for bladder cancer across the country. As studies addressing the possibility of organ preservation continue to demonstrate positive results, it is hoped that more patients will become informed about and be offered selective bladder-sparing approaches as an alternative to radical cystectomy.

The immediate therapeutic challenges for radiation oncologists include:

- More effective radiographic tumor definition and tracking during radiation therapy. This may allow tighter margins, higher dose delivery, and higher rates of bladder preservation.
- More effective radiation sensitization. Gemcitabine is currently under evaluation in several centers.

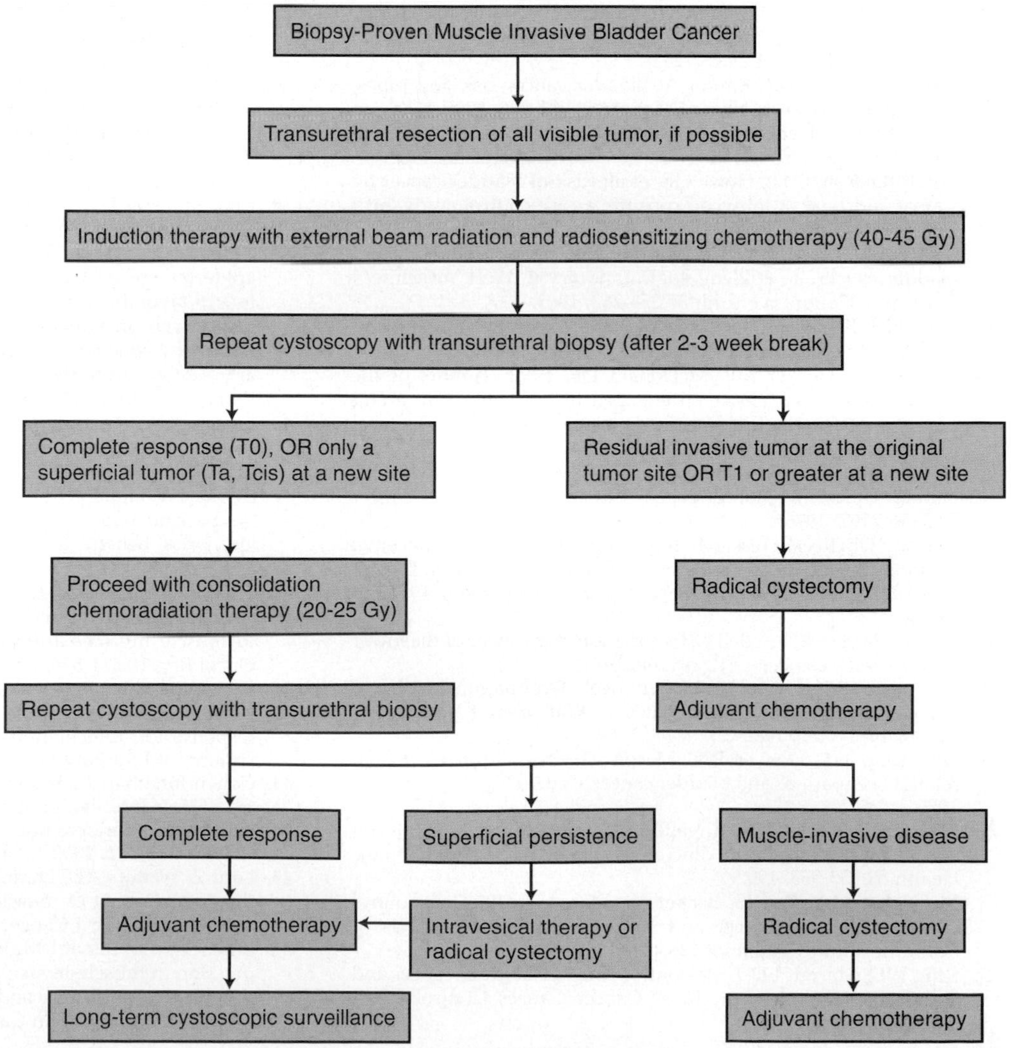

Figure 51-6 Treatment algorithm for the trimodality management of invasive bladder cancer.

- More effective evaluation of pelvic lymph nodes using, perhaps, iron nanoparticle MR lymphangiography, and more effective treatment of pelvic lymph nodes with either extended lymphadenectomy or radiation delivered using IMRT.
- Integrating rational biologic strategies into primary therapy. The RTOG will soon explore the combination of radiation, taxotere, and herceptin.

REFERENCES

1. Jemal A, Siegal R, Ward E, et al: Cancer statistics, 2006. CA Cancer J Clin 56:106-130, 2006.
2. Vaidya A, Soloway MS, Hawke C, et al: De novo muscle invasive bladder cancer: is there a change in trend? J Urol 165:47-50; discussion 50, 2001.
3. Rubben H, Lutzeyer W, Wallace DMA: The epidemiology and aetiology of bladder cancer. *In* Zingg EJ, Wallace DMA (eds): Bladder Cancer. New York, Springer-Verlag, 1985, pp 1-21.
4. Parkin DM, Muir CS, Whelan SL, et al: Cancer Incidence in Five Continents, 1992, vol VI (IARC Publ. No. 120). Lyon, International Agency for Research on Cancer, 1992.
5. Parkin DM, Pisani P, Ferlay J: Global cancer statistics. CA Cancer J Clin 49:33-64, 1999.
6. Cohen SM, Johansson SL: Epidemiology and etiology of bladder cancer. Urol Clin North Am 19:421-428, 1992.
7. Nomura A, Kolonel LN, Yoshizawa CN: Smoking, alcohol, occupation and hair dye use in cancer of the lower urinary tract. Am J Epidemiol 130:1159-1163, 1989.
8. Schifflers E, Jamart J, Renard V: Tobacco and occupational risk factors in bladder cancer: a case-control study in southern Belgium. Int J Cancer 39:287-292.
9. Hartge P, Hoover R, Kantor A: Bladder cancer risk and pipes, cigars and smokeless tobacco. Cancer 55:901-906, 1985.
10. Augustine A, Hebert JR, Kabat GC, et al: Bladder cancer in relation to cigarette smoking. Cancer Res 48:4405-4408, 1988.
11. Burch JD, Rohan TE, Howe GR, et al: Risk of bladder cancer by source and type of tobacco exposure: a case-control study. Int J Cancer 44:622-628, 1989.
12. Cartwright RA, Adib R, Appleyard I, et al: Cigarette smoking and bladder cancer: an epidemiological inquiry in West Yorkshire. J Epidemiol Commun Health 37:256-263, 1983.
13. D'Avanzo B, Negri E, La Vecchia C, et al: Cigarette smoking and bladder cancer. Eur J Cancer 26:714-718, 1990.
14. Case RAM, Hosker ME, McDonald DB, et al: Tumors of the urinary bladder in workmen engaged in the manufacture and use of certain dyestuff intermediates in the British chemical industry. Br J Indust Med 11:75-104, 1954.
15. Schulte PA, Ringen K, Hemstreet GP, et al: Risk factors for bladder cancer in a cohort exposed to aromatic amines. Cancer 58:2156-2162, 1986.
16. Clayson DB: Recent research into occupational bladder cancer. *In* Connolly JG (ed): Carcinoma of the Bladder. Progress in Cancer Research and Therapy, vol 18. New York, Raven Press, 1981, pp 13-24.
17. Cole P, Hoover R, Friedell G: Occupation and cancer of the lower urinary tract. Cancer 29:1250-1260, 1972.
18. Silverman DT, Levin LI, Hoover RN: Occupational risks of bladder cancer in the United States: I. White men. J Natl Cancer Inst 81:1472-1480, 1989.
19. Silverman DT, Hoover RN, Mason TJ, et al: Motor exhaust-related occupations and bladder cancer. Cancer Res 46:2113-2116, 1986.
20. Morris RD, Audet AM, Angellllo IF, et al: Chlorination, chlorination by-products, and cancer: a meta-analysis. Am J Public Health 82:955-963, 1992.
21. McGeehin MA, Reif JS, Becher JC, Mangione EJ: Case-control study of bladder cancer and water disinfection methods in Colorado. Am J Epidemiol 138:492-501, 1993.
22. King WD, Marrett LD: Case-control study of bladder cancer and water chlorination by-products. Cancer Causes Control 7:596-604, 1996.
23. Evans DAP: Acetylation. *In* Ethnic Differences in Reactions to Drugs and Menobiotics. New York, Alan R Liss, 1989, pp 209-242.
24. Evans DAP: Survey of the human acetylator polymorphism in spontaneous disorders. J Med Genet 21:243-253, 1984.
25. Bhagwandeen SB: Schistosomiasis and carcinoma of the bladder in Zambia. S Afr Med J 50:1616-1620, 1976.
26. McCredie M, Stewart JH, Ford JM, et al: Phenacetin-containing analgesics and cancer of the bladder or renal pelvis in women. Br J Urol 55:220-224, 1983.
27. Levine LA, Richie JP: Urological complications of cyclophosphamide. J Urol 141:1063-1069, 1989.
28. Travis LB, Curtis RE, Glimelius B, et al: Bladder and kidney cancer following cyclophosphamide therapy for non-Hodgkin's lymphoma. J Natl Cancer Inst 87:524-530, 1995.
29. Johnson DE, Boileau MA: Bladder cancer overview. *In* Johnson DE, Boileau MA (eds): Genitourinary Tumors: Fundamental Principles and Surgical Techniques. New York, Grune & Stratton, 1982, pp 399-447.
30. Messing EM, Young TB, Hunt VB, et al: The significance of asymptomatic microhematuria in men 50 or more years old: findings of a home screening study using dipsticks. J Urol 137:919-922, 1987.
31. Messing EM, Young TB, Hunt VB, et al: Urinary tract cancers found by home screening with hematuria dipsticks in healthy men over 50 years of age. Cancer 64:2361-2367, 1989.
32. Joseph JV, Messing EM: Chemoprevention of bladder and prostate cancer. Cancer Control 4:136-141, 1997.
33. Sidransky D, Frost P, Eschenbach AV, et al: Clonal origin of bladder cancer. N Engl J Med 326:737-740, 1992.
34. Knowles MA: What we could do now: molecular pathology of bladder cancer. Mol Pathol. 54:215-221, 2001.
35. Pollack A, Wu CS, Czerniak B: Abnormal bcl-2 and pRb expression are independent correlates of radiation response in muscle-invasive bladder cancer. Clin Cancer Res 3:1823-1829, 1997.
36. Cote RJ, Chatterjee SJ: Molecular determinants of outcome in bladder cancer. Cancer J Sci Am 5:1-15, 1999.
37. Esrig D, Elmajian D, Groshen S, et al: Accumulation of nuclear p53 and tumor progression in bladder cancer. N Eng J Med 331:1259-1264, 1994.
38. Cote RJ, Esrig D, Groshen S, et al: p53 and treatment of bladder cancer. Nature 385:285-292, 1997.
39. Chakravarti A, Winter K, Wu CL, et al: Expression of the epidermal growth factor receptor (EGFR) and Her-2 are predictors of favorable outcome and reduced complete response rates respectively in patients with muscle-invading bladder cancers treated by concurrent radiation and cisplatin-based chemotherapy: a report from the Radiation Therapy Oncology Group. Int J Radiat Oncol Biol Phys 62:318-327, 2005.
40. Hussain SA, Ganesan R, Hiller L, et al: BAX and CD40L are predictors of survival in transitional cell carcinoma of the bladder. Br J Cancer 88:586-592, 2003.
41. Cooke PW, James ND, Ganesan R, et al: BCL2 expression identifies patients with advanced bladder cancer treated by radiotherapy who benefit from neoadjuvant chemotherapy. BJU Int 85:829-835, 2000.
42. Hussain SA, Ganesan R, Hiller L, et al: BCL2 expression predicts survival in patients receiving synchronous chemoradiotherapy in muscle invasive transitional cell carcinoma of the bladder. Oncol Rep 10:571-576, 2003.
43. Rödel C, Grabenbauer GG, Rödel F: Apoptosis, p53, bcl-2, and Ki-67 in invasive bladder carcinoma: possible predictors for response to radiochemotherapy and successful bladder preservation. Int J Radiat Oncol Biol Phys 46:1213-1221, 2000.
44. Cohen-Jonathan E, Muschel RJ, Gillies McKenna W: Farnesyltransferase inhibitors potentiate the antitumor effect of radiation on a human tumor xenograft expressing activated HRAS. Radiat Res 154:125-132, 2000.
45. Latif Z, Watters AD, Dunn I, et al: HER2/neu overexpression in the development of muscle-invasive transitional cell carcinoma of the bladder. Br J Cancer 89:1305-1309, 2003.
46. Jimenez RE, Hussain M, Bianco FJ Jr, et al: Her-2/neu overexpression in muscle-invasive urothelial carcinoma of the bladder: prognostic significance and comparative analysis in primary and metastatic tumors. Clin Cancer Res 7:2440-2447, 2001.

47. Chow NH, Chan SH, Tzai TS, et al: Expression profiles of ErbB family receptors and prognosis in primary transitional cell carcinoma of the urinary bladder. Clin Cancer Res 7:1957-1962, 2001.
48. Underwood M, Bartlett J, Reeves J, et al: C-erbB-2 gene amplification: a molecular marker in recurrent bladder tumors? Cancer Res 55:2422-2430, 1995.
49. Bellmunt J, Hussain M, Dinney CP: Novel approaches with targeted therapies in bladder cancer. Therapy of bladder cancer by blockade of the epidermal growth factor receptor family. Crit Rev Oncol Hematol 46:85-104, 2003.
50. Turner KJ, Crew JP, Wykoff CC, et al: The hypoxia-inducible genes VEGF and CA9 are differentially regulated in superficial versus invasive bladder cancer. Br J Cancer 86:1276-1282, 2002.
51. Hoskin PJ, Sibtain A, Daley FM, Wilson GD: GLUT1 and CA IX as intrinsic markers of hypoxia in bladder cancer: relationship with vascularity and proliferation as predictors of outcome of ARCON. Br J Cancer 89:1290-1297, 2003.
52. Harving N, Wolf H, Melsen F: Positive urine cytology after tumor resection: an indicator for concomitant carcinoma in situ. J Urol 140:495-497, 1988.
53. Koss L, Dietch D, Ramanathan R, et al: Diagnostic value of cytology of voided urine. Acta Cytol 29:810-816, 1985.
54. Lin C, Young D, Kirley SD, et al: Detection of tumor cells in bladder washings by a monoclonal antibody to human bladder tumor-associated antigen. J Urol 140:672-677, 1988.
55. Boman H, Hedelin H., Holmang H: Four bladder tumor markers have a disappointingly low sensitivity for small size and low grade recurrence. J Urol 167:80-83, 2002.
56. Hillman B, Silvert M, Cook G, et al: Recognition of bladder tumors by excretory urography. Radiology 138:319-323, 1981.
57. Hatch TR, Berry JM: The value of excretory radiography in staging bladder cancer. J Urol 135:49, 1986.
58. Voges G, Tauschke E, Stöckle M, et al: Computerized tomography: an unreliable method for accurate staging of bladder tumors in patients who are candidates for radical cystectomy. J Urol 142:972-974, 1989.
59. Nishimura K, Hida S, Nishio Y, et al: The validity of magnetic resonance imaging (MRI) in the staging of bladder cancer: Comparison with computed tomography (CT) and transurethral ultrasonography (US). Jpn J Clin Oncol 18:217-226, 1988.
60. Neuerburg J, Bohndorf K, Sohn M, et al: Urinary bladder neoplasms: Evaluation with contrast-enhanced MR imaging. Radiology 172:739-743, 1989.
61. Mallampati GK, Siegelman ES: MR imaging of the bladder. Magn Res Imaging Clin N Am 12:545-555, 2004.
62. Deserno WM, Harisinghani MG, Taupitz MJ, et al: Urinary bladder cancer: preoperative nodal staging with ferumoxtran-10-enhanced MR imaging. Radiology 233:449-456, 2004.
63. Jewett H, Strong G: Infiltrating carcinoma of the bladder: relation of depth of penetration of the bladder wall to incidence of local extension and metastases. J Urol 55:366-372, 1946.
64. American Joint Committee on Cancer: Bladder. *In* Greene FL, Page DL, Fleming ID, et al (eds): AJCC Cancer Staging Manual, 6th ed. New York, Springer, 2002.
65. Heney NH, Ahmad S, Flanagan MJ, et al: Superficial bladder cancer: progression and recurrence. J Urol 130:1083-1086, 1983.
66. Fitzpatrick JM, West AB, Butler MR, et al: Superficial bladder tumors (stage, pTa, grades 1 and 2): the importance of recurrence pattern following initial resection. J Urol 135:920-922, 1986.
67. Malmstrom PU, Busch C, Norlen BJ: Recurrence, progression and survival in bladder cancer: a retrospective analysis of 232 patients with greater or equal to 5-year follow-up. Scand J Urol Nephrol 21:185-195, 1987.
68. Lamm DL: Carcinoma in situ. Urol Clin North Am 19:499-508, 1992.
69. Herr HW, Pinsky CM, Whitmore WF, et al: Experience with intravesical bacillus Calmette-Guérin therapy of superficial bladder tumors. Urology 25:119-123, 1985.
70. Pagano F, Bassi P, Milani C, et al: A low dose bacillus Calmette-Guérin regimen in superficial bladder cancer therapy: is it effective? J Urol 146:32-35, 1991.
71. Melekos MD, Chionis H, Panatzakos A, et al: Intravesical bacillus Calmette-Guérin immunoprophylaxis of superficial bladder cancer: results of a controlled prospective trial with modified treatment schedule. J Urol 149:744-748, 1993.
72. Shahin O, Thalmann GN, Rentsch C, et al: A retrospective analysis of 153 patients treated with or without intravesical bacillus Calmette-Guerin for primary state T1 grade 3 bladder cancer: recurrence, progression and survival. J Urol 169:96-100, 2003.
73. Davis JW, Sheth SI, Doviak MJ, et al: Superficial bladder carcinoma treated with bacillus Calmette-Guérin: progression-free and disease specific survival with minimum 10-year followup. J Urol 167(2 Pt 1):494-500, 2002.
74. Lamm DL: Long-term results of intravesical therapy for superficial bladder cancer. Urol Clin North Am 19:573-580, 1992.
75. Mulders PF, Hoekstra WJ, Heybrock RP: Prognosis and treatment of T1G3 bladder tumours. A prognostic factor analysis of 121 patients. Dutch South Eastern Bladder Cancer Study Group. Eur J Cancer 30:914-917, 2001.
76. Van der Werf-Messing B, Hop WJC: Carcinoma of the urinary bladder (T1N0M0) treated either by radium implant or transurethral resection only. Int J Radiat Oncol Biol Phys 7:299-303, 2001.
77. Van der Steen-Banasik EM, Visser AG, Reinders JG: Saving bladders with brachytherapy: implantation technique and results. Int J Radiat Oncol Biol Phys 53:622-629, 2002.
78. Rowland RG, Mitchell ME, Bihrle R: The cecoileal continent urinary reservoir. World J Urol 3:185-190, 1985.
79. Kock NG: Continent ileostomy. Prog Surg 12:180, 1973.
80. Thuroff JW, Alken P, Riemiller H, et al: The Mainz pouch for augmentation or substitution of the bladder and continent diversion. Semin Urol 5:69, 1987.
81. Hautmann RE, Egshart G, Frohenberg D, et al: The ileal neobladder. J Urol 139:39-42, 1988.
82. Ghoneim MA: Orthotopic bladder substitution in women following cystectomy for bladder cancer. Urol Clin North Am 24:225-239, 1997.
83. Frazier HA, Robertson JE, Paulson DF: Complications of radical cystectomy and urinary diversion: a retrospective review of 675 cases in 2 decades. J Urol 148:1401-1405, 1992.
84. Chang SS, Cookson MS, Baumgartner RG, et al: Analysis of early complications after radical cystectomy: results of a collaborative care pathway. J Urol 167:2012-2016, 2002.
85. Schlegel PN, Walsh PC: Neuroanatomical approach to radical cystoprostatectomy with preservation of sexual function. J Urol 138:1402-1406, 1987.
86. Stein JP, Lieskoversusky G, Cote R, et al: Radical cystectomy in the treatment of invasive bladder cancer: long-term results in 1,054 patients. J Clin Oncol 19:666-675, 2001.
87. Dalbagni G, Genega E, Hashibe M: Cystectomy for bladder cancer: a contemporary series. J Urol 165:1111-1116, 2001.
88. Lerner SP, Skinner DG, Lieskoversusky G, et al: The rationale for en bloc pelvic lymph node dissection for bladder cancer patients with nodal metastases: Long-term results. J Urol 149:758-765, 1993.
89. Herr HW, Bochner BH, Dalbagni G, et al: Impact of the number of lymph nodes retrieved on outcome in patients with muscle invasive bladder cancer. J Urol 167:1295-1298, 2002
90. Poulsen AL, Horn T, Steven K: Radical cystectomy: extending the limits of pelvic lymph node dissection improves survival for patients with bladder cancer confined to the bladder wall. J Urol 160:2015-2019; discussion 2020, 1998.
91. Konety BR, Joslyn SA, O'Donnell MA: Extent of pelvic lymphadenectomy and its impact on outcome in patients diagnosed with bladder cancer: analysis of data from the Surveillance, Epidemiology and End Results Program data base. J Urol 169:946-950, 2003.
92. Whitmore W: Integrated irradiation and cystectomy for bladder cancer. Br J Urol 52:1-9, 1980.
93. Skinner D, Lieskoversusky G: Contemporary cystectomy with pelvic node dissection compared to preoperative radiation plus cystectomy in management of invasive bladder cancer. J Urol 131:1069-1072, 1984.
94. Smith JA, Crawford ED, Paradelo JC, et al: Treatment of advanced bladder cancer with combined preoperative irradiation and radical cystectomy versus radical cystectomy alone: a phase III intergroup study. J Urol 157:805-807, 1997.

95. Parsons J, Million R: Planned preoperative irradiation in the management of clinical stage B2-C (T3) bladder carcinoma. Int J Radiat Oncol Biol Phys 14:797-810, 1988.
96. Cole C, Pollack A, Zagars G, et al: Local control of muscle-invasive bladder cancer: preoperative radiotherapy and cystectomy versus cystectomy alone. Int J Radiat Oncol Biol Phys 32:331-340, 1995..
97. Houssett M, Maulard C, Chretien Y, et al: Combined radiation and chemotherapy for invasive transitional-cell carcinoma of the bladder: a prospective study. J Clin Oncol 11:2150-2157, 1993.
98. van der Werf-Messing B: Carcinoma of the bladder treated by suprapubic radium implants. The value of additional external irradiation. Eur J Cancer 5:277, 1969.
99. Zaghloul M, Awaad H, Akoush H, et al: Post-operative radiotherapy of carcinoma in bilharzial bladder: improved disease free survival through improving local control. Int J Radiat Oncol Biol Phys 23:511-517, 1992.
100. Fromenti SC: Management of patients with pelvic recurrence following radical cystectomy. *In* Petrovich Z, Baert L (eds): Carcinoma of the urinary bladder innovation in management. Berlin: Springer-Verlag, 1998, pp 249-258.
101. Reisinger SA, Mohuiddin M, Mulholland SG: Combined pre- and post-operative adjuvant radiation therapy for bladder cancer—a ten-year experience. Int J Radiat Oncol Biol Phys 24:463-468, 1992.
102. Sweeny P, Kursh ED, Resnick MI: Partial cystectomy. Urol Clin North Am 19:10701-10711, 1992.
103. Herr HW: Conservative management of muscle-infiltrating bladder cancer: Prospective experience. J Urol 138:1162-1163, 1987.
104. Henry K, Miller J, Mori M, et al: Comparison of transurethral resection to radical therapies for stage B bladder tumors. J Urol 140:964-967, 1988.
105. Barnes RW, Dick AL, Hadley HL, et al: Survival following transurethral resection of bladder carcinoma. Cancer Res 37:2895-2898, 1977.
106. Duncan W, Quilty PM: The results of a series of 963 patients with transitional cell carcinoma of the urinary bladder primarily treated by radical megavoltage x-ray therapy. Radiother Oncol 7:299-310, 1986.
107. Blandy JP, Jenkins BJ, Fowler CG, et al: Radical radiotherapy and salvage cystectomy for T2/3 cancer of the bladder. Progr Clin Biol Res 260:447-451, 1988.
108. Jenkins BJ, Caulfield MJ, Fowler CG, et al: Reappraisal of the role of radical radiotherapy and salvage cystectomy in the treatment of invasive (T2/T3) bladder cancer. Br J Urol 62:342-346, 1988.
109. Greven KM, Solin LJ, Hanks GE: Prognostic factors in patients with bladder carcinoma treated with definitive irradiation. Cancer 65:908-912, 1990.
110. Smaaland R, Akslen L, Tonder B, et al: Radical radiation treatment of invasive and locally advanced bladder cancer in elderly patients. Br J Urol 67:61-69, 1991.
111. Gospodarowicz MK, Rider WD, Keen CW, et al: Bladder cancer: long term follow-up results of patients treated with radical radiation. Clin Oncol 3:155-161, 1991.
112. Jahnson S, Pedersen J, Westman G: Bladder carcinoma—a 20-year review of radical irradiation therapy. Radiother Oncol 22:111-117, 1991.
113. Fossa SD, Waehre H, Aass N, et al: Bladder cancer definitive radiation therapy of muscle-invasive bladder cancer. A retrospective analysis of 317 patients. Cancer 72:3036-3043, 1993.
114. Pollack A, Zagars GK, Swanson DA: Muscle-invasive bladder cancer treated with external beam radiotherapy: prognostic factors. Int J Radiat Oncol Biol Phys 30:267-277, 1994.
115. Moonen L, Voet H, Nijs R, et al: Muscle-invasive bladder cancer treated with external beam radiotherapy: pretreatment prognostic factors and the predictive value of cystoscpic re-evaluation during treatment. Radiother Oncol 49:149-155, 1998.
116. Quilty PM, Duncan W, Chisholm GD, et al: Results of surgery following radical radiotherapy for invasive bladder cancer. Br J Urol 58:396-405, 1986.
117. Davidson SE, Symonds RP, Snee MP, et al: Assessment of factors influencing the outcome of radiotherapy for bladder cancer. Br J Urol 66:288-293, 1990.
118. Borgaonkar S, Jain A, Bollina P, et al: Radical radiotherapy and salvage cystectomy as the primary management of transitional cell carcinoma of the bladder. Results following the introduction of a CT planning technique. Clin Oncol 14:141-147, 2002.
119. Mameghan H, Fisher R, Mameghan J, Brook S: Analysis of failure following definitive radiotherapy for invasive transitional cell carcinoma of the bladder. Int J Radiat Oncol Biol Phys 31:247-254, 1995.
120. Sell A, Jakobsen A, Nerstrom B: Treatment of advanced bladder cancer category T2, T3 and T4a. A randomized multicenter study of preoperative irradiation and cystectomy versus radical irradiation and early salvage cystectomy for residual tumor. Scand J Urol Nephrol Suppl 138:893-901, 1991.
121. Ahlering TE, Kanellos A, Boyd SD, et al: A comparative study of perioperative complications with Kock pouch urinary diversion in highly irradiated versus nonirradiated patients. J Urol 139:1202-1204, 1988.
122. Barringer BS: Twenty-five years of radon treatment of cancer of the bladder. JAMA 135:616-618; 1947.
123. Herger C, Sauer HR: Radium treatment of cancer of the bladder. Report of 267 cases. AJR 47:909-915, 1942.
124. van der Werf-Messing B: Carcinoma of the bladder treated by suprapubic radium implants. The value of additional external irradiation. Eur J Cancer 5:277, 1969.
125. Moonen LM, Horenblas S, van der Voet JC, et al: Bladder conservation in selected T1G3 and muscle-invasive T2-T3a bladder carcinoma using combination therapy of surgery and iridium-192 implantation. Br J Urol 74:322-327, 1994.
126. Wijnmaalen A, Helle PA, Koper PC, et al: Muscle invasive bladder cancer treated by transurethral resection, followed by external beam radiation and interstitial iridium-192. Int J Radiat Oncol Biol Phys 39:1043-1052, 1997.
127. Van der Steen-Banasik EM, Visser AG, Reinders JG, et al: Saving bladders with brachytherapy: implantation technique and results. Int J Radiat Oncol Biol Phys 53:622-629, 2002.
128. Mazeron JJ, Crook J, Chopin D, et al: Conservative treatment of bladder carcinoma by partial cystectomy and interstitial iridium 192. Int J Radiat Oncol Biol Phys 15:1323-1330, 1988.
129. Rozan R, Albuisson E, Donnarieix D, et al: Interstitial iridium-192 for bladder cancer (a multicentric survey: 205 patients). Int J Radiat Oncol Biol Phys 24:469-477, 1992.
129a. Pernot M, Hubert J, Guillemin F, et al: Combined surgery and brachytherapy in the treatment of some cancers of the bladder (partial cystectomy and interstitial iridium-192). Radiother Oncol 38:115-120, 1996.
130. Pos FJ, Horenblas S, Lebesque J, et al: LDR is superior to HDR brachytherapy for bladder cancer. Int J Radiat Oncol Biol Phys 59:696-705, 2004.
130a. Rintala E, Hannisdal E, Fossa SD, et al: Neoadjuvant chemotherapy in bladder cancer: a randomized study. Scand J Nephrol 27:355-362, 1993.
131. Roberts JT, Fossa SP, Richards SB, et al: Results of Medical Research Council phase II study of low dose cisplatin and methotrexate in the primary treatment of locally advanced (T3 and T4) transitional cell carcinoma of the bladder. Br J Urol 68:162-168, 1991.
132. Farah R, Chodak GW, Vogelzang NI, et al: Curative radiotherapy following chemotherapy for invasive bladder carcinoma (a preliminary report). Int J Radiat Oncol Biol Phys 20:413-417, 1991.
133. Herr HW, Whitmore WF, Morse MJ, et al: Neoadjuvant chemotherapy in invasive bladder cancer: the evolving role of surgery. J Urol 144:1083 1088, 1990.
134. Sternberg C, Arena M, Calabresi F, et al: Neo-adjuvant M-VAC (methotrexate, vinblastine, Adriamycin, and cisplatin) for muscle infiltrating transitional cell carcinoma of the urothelium. Cancer 72:1975-1982, 1993.
135. Splinter TAW, Pavone-Macaluso M, Jacqmin D, et al: European Organization for Research and Treatment of Cancer-Genitourinary Group phase 2 study of chemotherapy in stage T3-4N0-XM0 transitional cell carcinoma of the bladder. J Urol 148:1793-1796, 1992.
136. Dreicer R, Messing EM, Loehrer PJ, Trump DL: Perioperative methotrexate, vinblastine, doxorubicin, and cisplatin (M-VAC) for poor risk transitional cell carcinoma of the bladder: an

Eastern Cooperative Oncology Group Pilot Study. J Urol 144:1123-1127, 1990.
137. Angulo J, Sanchez-Chapado M, Lopez JI, Flores N: Primary cisplatin, methotrexate and vinblastine aiming at bladder preservation in invasive bladder cancer: Multivariate analysis on prognostic factors. J Urol 155:1897-1902, 1996.
138. Scher H, Herr H, Sternberg C, et al: Neo-adjuvant chemotherapy for invasive bladder cancer. Experience with the M-VAC regimen. Br J Urol 64:250-256, 1989.
139. Prout GR, Shipley WU, Kaufman D, et al: Preliminary results in invasive bladder cancer with transurethral resection, neoadjuvant chemotherapy and combined pelvic irradiation plus cisplatin chemotherapy. J Urol 144:1128-1134, 1990.
140. Parsons JT, Million RR: Bladder cancer. *In* Perez CA, Brady LW (eds): Principles and Practice of Radiation Oncology. Philadelphia, JB Lippincott, 1991, pp 1036-1058.
141. Farah R, Chodak GW, Vogelzang NJ, et al: Therapy for invasive bladder carcinoma (a preliminary report). Int J Radiat Oncol Biol Phys 20:413-417, 1991.
142. Hall RR: Bladder preserving treatment: the role of transurethral surgery alone and with combined modality therapy for muscle-invading bladder cancer. *In* Vogelzang NJ, Scardino PT, Shipley WU, Coffey DS (eds): Comprehensive Textbook of Genitourinary Oncology. Baltimore, Williams & Wilkins, 1995, pp 509-513.
143. Herr HE, Scher HI: Neoadjuvant chemotherapy and partial cystectomy for invasive bladder cancer. J Clin Oncol 12:975-980, 1994.
144. Wallace DMA, Radhavan D, Kelly KA, et al: Neo-adjuvant (preemptive) cisplatin therapy in invasive transitional cell carcinoma of the bladder. Br J Urol 67:608-615, 1991.
145. Malmstrom Per-Uno, Rintala E, Members of the Nordic Cooperative Bladder Cancer Study Group: Five-year follow-up of a prospective trial of radical cystectomy and neoadjuvant chemotherapy: Nordic Cystectomy Trial 1. J Urol 115:1903, 1996.
146. Martinez-Pineiro JA, Martin MG, Arocena M, et al: Neoadjuvant cisplatin chemotherapy before radical cystectomy in invasive transitional cell carcinoma of the bladder: a prospective randomized phase III trial. J Urol 153:964-973, 1995.
147. GISTV (Italian Bladder Cancer Study Group): Neoadjuvant treatment for locally advanced bladder cancer: a randomized prospective clinical trial. J Chemother 8:345-346, 1996.
148. Shipley WU, Winter KA, Lee R, et al: Initial results of RTOG 89-03: a phase III trial of neoadjuvant chemotherapy in patients with invasive bladder cancer treated with selective bladder preservation by combined radiation therapy and chemotherapy [Abstract 41]. Int J Radiat Oncol Biol Phys 39:155, 1997.
149. Hall RR: Updated results of a randomised controlled trial of neoadjuvant cisplatin (C), methotrexate (M) and vinblastine (V) chemotherapy for muscle-invasive bladder cancer. Proc Ann Meet Am Soc Clin Oncol 21:178a, 2002.
150. Orsatti M, Curotto A, Canobbio L: Alternating chemo-radiotherapy in bladder cancer: a conservative approach. Int J Radiat Oncol Biol Phys 33:173-178, 1995
151. Sherif A, Rintala E, Mestad O, et al: Neoadjuvant cisplatin-methotrexate chemotherapy of invasive bladder cancer—Nordic cystectomy trial 2. Scand J Urol Nephrol 36:419-425, 2002.
152. Abol-Enein H, El Makresh M, El Baz M, Ghoneim M: Neoadjuvant chemotherapy in treatment of invasive transitional bladder cancer: a controlled, prospective randomised study. Br J Urol 80(suppl 2):49, 1997.
153. Bassi P, Pagano F, Pappagallo G: Neo-adjuvant M-VAC of invasive bladder cancer: The G.U.O.N.E. multicenter phase III trial. Eur Urol 33(Suppl 1):142, 1998.
154. Skinner DG, Daniels JR, Russell C, et al: The role of adjuvant chemotherapy following cystectomy for invasive bladder cancer: a prospective comparative trial. J Urol 145:459-467, 1991.
155. Stöckle M, Meyenburg W, Wellek S, et al: Fortgeschrittenes Blasenkarzinom (Stadien pT3b, pT4a, pN1, pN2). Verbesserte Überlebensraten nach radikaler Zystektomie durch 3 adjuvante Zyklen M-VAC/M-VEC-Erste Ergebnisse einer kontrollierten Studie. Akt Urol 22:201, 1991.
156. Studer UE, Bacchi M, Biedermann C, et al: Adjuvant cisplatin chemotherapy following cystectomy for bladder cancer: results of a prospective randomized trial. J Urol 152:81-84, 1994.
157. Freiha F, Reese J, Torti FM: A randomized trial of radical cystectomy versus radical cystectomy plus cisplatin, vinblastine and methotrexate chemotherapy for muscle invasive bladder cancer. J Urol 155:496, 1996.
158. Housset M, Maulard C, Chretien YC, et al: Combined radiation and chemotherapy for invasive transitional-cell carcinoma of the bladder: a prospective study. J Clin Oncol 11:2150-2157, 1993.
159. Rodel C, Grabenbauer GG, Kuhn R, et al: Invasive bladder cancer: organ preservation by radiochemotherapy. Front Radiat Ther Oncol 36:118-130, 2002.
160. Vogelzang NJ, Moormeier JA, Awan AM, et al: Methotrexate, vinblastine, doxorubicin and cisplatin followed by radiotherapy or surgery for muscle invasive bladder cancer: the University of Chicago experience. J Urol 149:753-757, 1993.
161. Cervak J, Cufer T, Kragelj B: Sequential transurethral surgery, multiple drug chemotherapy, and radiation therapy for invasive bladder carcinoma: Initial report. Int J Radiat Oncol Biol Phys 25:777-782, 1993.
162. Coppin C, Gospodarowicz M, James K, et al: Improved local control of invasive bladder cancer by concurrent cisplatin and preoperative or definitive radiation. J Clin Oncol 14:2901-2907, 1996.
163. Russell K, Boileau M, Higano C, et al: Combined 5-fluorouracil and irradiation for transitional cell carcinoma of the urinary bladder. Int J Radiat Oncol Biol Phys 19:693-699, 1990.
164. Shipley WU, Kaufman DS, Thakral HK, et al: Long-term outcome of patients treated for muscle-invasive bladder cancer by trimodality therapy. Urology 60:62-68, 2002.
165. Tester W, Caplan R, Heaney J, et al: Neoadjuvant combined modality program with selective organ preservation for invasive bladder cancer: results of RTOG phase II trial 88-02. J Clin Oncol 14:119-126, 1996.
166. Housset M, Dufour B, Maulard-Durdux C, et al: Concomitant fluorouracil (5-FU)-cisplatin (CDDP) and bifractionated split course radiation therapy (BSCRT) for invasive bladder cancer. Proc ASCO 16:319a, 1997.
167. Hagan MP, Winter KA, Kaufman DS, et al: RTOG 97-06: initial report of a phase I-II trial of selective bladder conservation using TURBT, twice-daily accelerated irradiation sensitised with cisplatin, and adjuvant MCV combination chemotherapy. Int J Radiat Oncol Biol Phys 57:665-672, 2003.
168. Eapen L, Stewart D, Collins J, Peterson R: Effective bladder sparing therapy with intra-arterial cisplatin and radiotherapy for localized bladder cancer. J Urol 172:1276-1280, 2004.
169. Pisters LL, Tykochinsky G, Wajsman Z: Intravesical bacillus Calmette-Guérin or mitomycin C in the treatment of carcinoma in situ of the bladder following prior pelvic radiation therapy. J Urol 146:1514-1517, 1991.
170. Zietman AL, Grocela J, Zehr E, et al: Selective bladder conservation using trans-urethral resection, chemotherapy, and radiation: the risk and consequences of superficial recurrences within the retained bladder. Urology 58:380-385, 2001.
171. Boyd SD, Feinberg SM, Skinner DG, et al: Quality of life survey of urinary diversion patients: comparison of ileal conduits versus continent Koch urinary reservoirs. J. Urol 138:1386, 1987.
172. Mansson A, Johnson G, Mansson W: Quality of life after cystectomy: comparison between patients with conduit and those with caecal reservoir urinary diversion. Br J Urol 62:240, 1988.
173. Raleigh ED, Berry M, Monite JE: A comparison of adjustments to urinary diversions: a pilot study. J Wound Ostomy Continence Nurs 22:58, 1995.
174. Bjerre BD, Johansen C, Steven K: Health related quality of life after cystectomy: bladder substitution compared with ileal conduit diversion. A questionnaire survey. Brit J Urol 75:200, 1995.
174. Hart S, Skinner EC, Meyerowitz BE, et al: Quality of life after radical cystectomy for bladder cancer in patients with an ileal conduit, or cutaneous or urethral Kock pouch. J Urol 162:77-81, 1999.
176. Zietman AL, Sacco D, Skowronski U, et al: Organ-conservation in invasive bladder cancer treated by trans-urethral resection, chemotherapy, and radiation: results of a urodynamic and quality of life study on long-term survivors. J Urol 2003.

177. Chauvet B, Lagrange JL, Geoffrois L, et al: Quality of life assessment after concurrent chemoradiation for invasive bladder cancer: preliminary results of a French multicentric prospective study. Int J Radiat Oncol Biol Phys 57(Suppl 2):177, abstract 88, 2003.
178. Caffo O, Fellin G, Graffer U, Luciani L: Assessment of quality of life after cystectomy or conservative therapy for patients with infiltrating bladder carcinoma. Cancer 78:1089-1097, 1996.
179. Henningsohn L, Wijkstrom H, Dickman PW, et al: Distressful symptoms after radical radiotherapy for urinary bladder cancer. Radiother Oncol 60:215-225, 2002.
180. Gerard JP, Hulewicz G, Saleh M, et al: Pilot study of IORT for bladder carcinoma. Front Radiat Ther Oncol 31:250-252, 1997.
181. Calvo FA, Aristu J, Abuchaibe O, et al: Intraoperative and external preoperative radiotherapy in invasive bladder cancer: effect of neoadjuvant chemotherapy in tumor downstaging. Am J Clin Oncol 16:61-66, 1993.
182. Calvo FC, Zincke H, Gunderson LL, et al: Genitourinary IORT. *In* Gunderson LL, Willett CG, Harrison LB, Calvo FC (eds): Intraoperative Irradiation: Techniques and Results. Totowa, NJ, Humana Press, 1999, pp 421-436.
183. Duchesne GM, Bolger JJ, Griffiths GO, et al: A randomized trial of hypofractionated schedules of palliative radiotherapy in the management of bladder carcinoma: results of medical research council trial BA09. Int J Radiat Oncol Biol Phys 47:379-388, 2000.
184. Maciejewski B, Majewski S: Dose fractionation and tumour repopulation in radiotherapy for bladder cancer. Radiother Oncol 21:163-170, 1991.
185. Moonen L, van der Voet H, de Nijs R, et al: Muscle-invasive bladder cancer treated with external beam radiation: influence of total dose, overall treatment time, and treatment interruption on local control. Int J Radiat Oncol Biol Phys 42:525-530, 1998.
186. Grossman HB, Natale RB, Tangen CM, et al: Neoadjuvant chemotherapy plus cystectomy compared with cystectomy alone for locally advanced bladder cancer. N Engl J Med 349:859-866, 2003.
187. Herr HW, Faulkner JR, Grossman MB, et al: Surgical factors influence bladder cancer outcomes: a co-operative group report. J Clin Oncol 22:2781-2789, 2004.
188. Sengelov L, von der Masse H: Radiotherapy in bladder cancer. Radiother Oncol 52:1-14, 1999.
189. Leissner J, Ghoneim MA, Abol-Enein H, et al: Extended radical lymphadenectomy in patients with urothelial bladder cancer: results of a prospective multicenter study. J Urol 171:139-144, 2004.
190. Emani B, Lyman J, Brown A, et al: Tolerance of normal tissue to therapeutic irradiation. Int J Radiat Oncol Biol Phys 21:109-122, 1991
191. Marks LB, Carroll PR, Dugan TC, Anscher MS: The response of the urinary bladder, urethra and ureter to radiation and chemotherapy. Int J Radiat Oncol Biol Phys 31:1257-1280, 1995.
192. Cowan RA, McBain CA, Ryder WDRR, et al: Radiotherapy for muscle invasive carcinoma of the bladder: results of a randomised trial comparing whole bladder with dose-escalated partial bladder irradiation. Int J Radiat Oncol Biol Phys 59:197-207, 2004.
193. Turner SL, Swindell R, Bowl N: Bladder movement during radiation therapy for bladder cancer: implications for treatment planning. Int J Radiat Oncol Biol Phys 39:355-360, 1997.
194. Harris SJ, Buchanan RB: An audit and evaluation of bladder movements during radical radiotherapy. Clin Oncol 10:262-264, 1998.
195. Sur RK, Clinkard J, Jones WG, et al: Changes in target volume during radiotherapy treatment of invasive bladder carcinoma. Clin Oncol 5:30-33, 1993.
196. Roof KS, Mazal A, Sarkar S, et al: Three-dimensional CT based analysis of inter-fraction bladder motion during radiotherapeutic treatment of bladder cancer. [Submitted for publication.]
197. Graham J, Gee A, Hilton S, et al: Geometric uncertainties in radiotherapy of the prostate and bladder. *In* Geometric Uncertainties in Radiotherapy. London, British Institute of Radiology, 2003.
198. Shipley WU, Rose MA: Bladder cancer: the selection of patients for treatment by full-dose irradiation. Cancer 55:2278-2284, 1985.
199. Morrison R: The results of treatment of cancer of the bladder—a clinical contribution to radiobiology. Clin Radiol 26:67-75, 1975.
200. Maciejewski B, Majewski S: Dose fractionation and tumour repopulation in radiotherapy for bladder cancer. Radiother Oncol 21:163-170, 1991.
201. Wilson GD, McNally NJ, Dische S, et al: Cell proliferation in human tumours measured by in-vivo labelling with bromodeoxyuridine. Br J Radiol 61:419-422, 1988.
202. Cole DJ, Durrant KR, Roberts JT, et al: A pilot study of accelerated fractionation in the radiotherapy of invasive carcinoma of the bladder. Br J Radiol. 65:792-798, 1992.
203. Horwich A, Pendlebury S, Dearnaley DP: Organ conservation in bladder cancer. Eur J Cancer 31(Suppl 5):208, 1995.
204. Plataniotis G, Michalopoulos E, Kouvaris J, et al: A feasibility study of partially accelerated radiotherapy for invasive bladder cancer. Radiother Oncol 33:84-87, 1994.
205. Edsmyr F, Andersson L, Espostl PL, et al: Irradiation therapy with multiple small fractions per day in urinary bladder cancer. Radiother Oncol 4:197, 1985.
206. Naslund I, Nilsson B, Littbrand B: Hyper-fractionated radiotherapy of bladder cancer: a 10 year follow up of a randomized clinical trial. Acta Oncol 33:397-402, 1994.
207. Sauer R, Birkenhake S, Kühn R: Efficacy of radiochemotherapy with platin derivates compared to radiotherapy alone in organsparing treatment of bladder cancer. Int J Radiat Biol Phys 40:121-127, 1998.

CHAPTER 52

TESTICULAR CANCER

Padraig R. Warde, Jeremy F. G. Sturgeon, and Mary K. Gospodarowicz

INCIDENCE

Testicular cancer accounts for 1% of all male malignancies.

There were 48,500 new cases and 8900 deaths worldwide in 2002, and 8250 new cases and 370 deaths projected in the United States in 2006.

It is the most common malignancy in men aged 15 to 35 years.

BIOLOGIC CHARACTERISTICS

Isochromosome 12p is present in more than 80% of cases.

STAGING EVALUATION

Evaluation includes history and physical examination, serum tumor markers (alpha-fetoprotein [AFP], β-human chorionic gonadotropin [β-hCG], lactate dehydrogenase [LDH]), complete blood cell count, creatinine, chest radiograph, computed tomography (CT) scan of abdomen and pelvis, and CT scan of thorax (omit in seminoma if CT scan of abdomen is normal).

PRIMARY AND ADJUVANT THERAPY

Radical inguinal orchidectomy is performed.

SEMINOMA

Stage I—Surveillance: 15% relapse *or* adjuvant retroperitoneal radiation therapy, 5% relapse; 5-year survival ~100%. Adjuvant chemotherapy remains experimental.

Stage II—≤5 cm nodes, radiation therapy 10% relapse; >5 cm nodes, chemotherapy 5% relapse; 5-year survival ~97%.

Stage III—Chemotherapy, no visceral metastases (except pulmonary); 5-year survival 86%; visceral metastases 5-year survival 72%.

NONSEMINOMA

Stage I—Surveillance, 30% relapse *or* retroperitoneal lymphadenectomy *or* adjuvant chemotherapy in high-risk patients; 5-year survival ~100%.

Stage II—≤5 cm nodes, chemotherapy or RPLD, >5 cm nodes, chemotherapy, 5-year survival ~95%.

Stage III—Chemotherapy: Good prognosis group (60% of cases); testis/retroperitoneal primary, no visceral metastases (except pulmonary), AFP < 1000, βHCG < 5000, LDH < 1.5 ULN; 5-year survival ~86%.

Intermediate prognosis group (26% of cases); testis/retroperitoneal primary, no visceral metastases (except pulmonary), and AFP, 1,000–10,000, or βHCG 5,000–50,000 or LDH 1.5–10 ULN; 5-year survival ~79%.

Poor prognosis group (14% of cases); mediastinal primary or nonpulmonary visceral metastases or any of AFP > 10,000, βHCG > 50,000, LDH > 10 ULN; 5-year survival ~48%.

Testicular tumors are uncommon but constitute an important group of malignancies in young men. Worldwide it is estimated that there were more than 48,500 new cases and 8900 deaths from disease in 2002.[1] The vast majority are primary germ cell tumors (GCTs). The incidence of GCTs has doubled in the past 30 years and while most patients present with early-stage and highly curable disease, the continued rise in incidence of these tumors presents a major challenge. The identification of prognostic factors in patients with both early and advanced disease has helped to refine management strategies for these patients. The management of patients with testicular tumors is significantly affected by histology and disease extent. In this chapter we will discuss the management principles for patients with primary GCTs of the testis, extragonadal germ cell malignancies, and other rare testicular tumors.

ETIOLOGY AND EPIDEMIOLOGY

Testicular cancer accounts for 1% to 2% of all cancers in men in most white populations across the world.[2] Germ cell testicular tumors are the most common solid malignancies in males between 20 and 35 years of age and it is estimated that in 2006 there will be 8250 new cases and 370 deaths from testicular cancer in the United States.[3] The cumulative lifetime risk of developing a GCT for an American white male is 0.2%.[4] Between 1973 and 1998 the incidence of testicular GCTs rose 44% in the United States with the major rise occurring in seminoma rather than nonseminoma.[5]

The age distribution of testicular cancer is similar in all white populations. There is a small peak in early childhood around 2 years of age, with rates then remaining low until 15 years of age. There is a second peak in young adults around 25 to 40 years of age and the rate then declines with a small peak again between 65 and 75 years of age. Testicular cancers occurring in childhood and in the young adult years are usually GCTs while those occurring after age 65 are principally non–germ cell malignancies, mainly lymphomas. Nonseminomatous tumors are more common in childhood and in the 15-to-30 age group; seminomas are seen on average one decade later (25 to 40 years).

There is considerable geographic and ethnic variation in the incidence of testicular tumors, with the highest incidence being reported from Denmark (8.4 per 100,000 per year) and Switzerland (6.2 to 8.8 per 100,000 per year).[2] The incidence of testicular cancer is lower in nonwhites compared with whites. In the United States, white males (5.6 per 100,000 per year) are five to six times more likely to develop testicular cancers than African Americans (1.04 per 100,000 per year); low incidence rates are seen in other ethnic groups, such as Americans of Chinese and Japanese descent.[5] A high incidence of testicular cancer is seen in some nonwhite populations such as the Maoris in New Zealand and Native Americans.[2]

While major variations in risk in genetically similar populations and the rapidly rising incidence suggest a significant contribution of environmental factors in the etiology of germ cell testicular tumors, the only well-established risk factors are a history of testicular maldescent, presence of a contralateral testis tumor, a family history of testis cancer, and gonadal dysgenesis. Men with a history of cryptorchidism have approximately a five fold increased chance of developing a testicular cancer.[6] Orchiopexy prior to puberty appears to lower the risk of developing a subsequent tumor, and may help preserve Leydig cell function and enhance fertility.[7,8] While most testicular cancers in men with a history of maldescent occur on the ipsilateral side, approximately 5% to 20% of tumors develop in the contralateral testicle.[9] The mechanism by which cryptorchidism increases the risk of developing GCTs is unknown but the effects of maldescent on the testis (increased temperature, increased risk of trauma if inguinal) have been suggested as possible factors. However, the increase in incidence of tumor in the contralateral testicle suggests that both maldescent and testicular cancer may be the result of the same prenatal etiologic process. Other genitourinary abnormalities associated with testicular cancers include hydrocele and hypospadias.[10,11]

Prior testicular cancer is a major risk factor for the development of a contralateral malignancy. In a large population-based follow-up study of 2850 patients with unilateral testicular cancer, the cumulative risk (at 25 years after diagnosis of the primary tumor) of developing a contralateral malignancy was 5.2% and was greater in nonseminoma (8.4% at 25 years) than in seminoma (3.6% at 25 years).[12]

Other factors linked to the development of testicular cancer include mumps orchitis, history of testicular trauma, immunosuppression following organ transplant, and human immunodeficiency virus (HIV) infection.[6,13] There is no evidence to suggest a causal relationship between testicular trauma and the development of a tumor, and the likely explanation is that testicular trauma leads to examination of the testes. Because of the age distribution of testicular cancer, exposure must occur early in life if there is an environmental contribution in the etiology of these tumors. Prenatal factors linked to the later development of testicular cancers include threatened miscarriage, excessive maternal nausea, and delivery by cesarean section.[6,14] To explain these associations, it has been suggested that exposure of the germinal epithelium in utero to an elevated level of free unbound maternal estrogen could give rise to subsequent cryptorchidism and an elevated risk of developing a testicular tumor. However, the prenatal estrogen theory remains unproved.[6]

PREVENTION AND EARLY DETECTION

The identification of carcinoma in situ (CIS) or testicular intraepithelial neoplasia (TIN) as a precursor of testicular GCTs has raised the possibility that the development of invasive testicular cancer could be prevented by treating CIS. In adults, CIS is found adjacent to GCTs in virtually 100% of cases and it is thought that, with the exception of spermatocytic seminoma, it precedes the development of all invasive tumors.[15] The natural history of testicular CIS is unknown, but the Danish experience suggests that all cases of adult CIS will ultimately progress to invasive cancer.[16]

The management of patients with testicular CIS is controversial. Orchidectomy has been suggested for unilateral disease, and low dose irradiation (15 to 20 Gy) has been recommended in bilateral cases, or when a previous orchidectomy has been performed.[17] The optimal dose of radiotherapy is unknown; however, doses of 16 Gy or lower are likely not effective and should not be used.[18] The goal of radiation therapy (RT) in this setting is to eradicate CIS and prevent development of invasive cancer while preserving sufficient Leydig cell function to obviate the need for lifelong androgen replacement therapy. At present, the methods of androgen replacement therapy are less than satisfactory, and many patients suffer problems with sexual dysfunction and mood swings.[19]

The diagnosis of testicular CIS can only be made by testicular biopsy. Because the incidence of CIS in the general population is low (at most 0.7%), screening biopsies are not recommended at present. However, they should be considered in high-risk patients including those with presumed extragonadal germ cell cancer, intersex individuals, and patients with contralateral GCTs.[16]

Testicular self-examination has been advocated by many for the early detection of invasive tumors but its usefulness is unproved. There is no evidence to indicate that a screening program would be of benefit; however, there is a need for education about the early signs and symptoms of testicular cancer to reduce delay at presentation. The optimal follow-up of patients with unilateral testicular GCTs and those with cryptorchidism, both of whom have an approximately 2% to 5% chance of developing a testicular cancer, is unclear, but a yearly testicular ultrasound from age 15 would seem reasonable. These patients also have an increased risk of CIS (3% to 5%) and in some centers in Europe are considered for testicular biopsy.[16]

BIOLOGIC CHARACTERISTICS/ MOLECULAR BIOLOGY

Germ cell tumors have a distinctive capacity for totipotential differentiation as demonstrated by the frequent finding of combinations of choriocarcinoma, embryonal carcinoma, and seminoma in a single tumor. They also can retain their ability to differentiate as displayed by the not infrequent identification of mature teratoma in residual posttreatment retroperitoneal masses. Cytogenetic analysis of GCTs has shown that chromosome numbers are more homogeneous in seminomas than in nonseminomas.[20,21] Triploid and tetraploid chromosomal patterns are common in seminomas, and hyperdiploid to hypertriploid counts are common in nonseminomas. A characteristic chromosome anomaly in GCTs of all histologic types is the presence of an isochromosome of the short arm of chromosome 12.[22] This isochromosome consists essentially of two chromosome 12 short arms.[21] It is present in more than 80% of cases, and GCTs without a 12p isochromosome have extra copies of 12p segments incorporated into other chromosomes. The 12p isochromosome is also found in testicular CIS.[22] Isochromosome copies tend to be more numerous in nonseminomas than in seminomas.

It is not known how these chromosomal changes contribute to the development of the neoplastic phenotype. However, the frequent finding of the 12p isochromosome in both CIS and invasive tumors indicates that it plays a role in the biology of these tumors. The possibility of amplification of normal or modified genes such as DAD-R on the 12p isochromosome is currently being investigated.[22] Proto-oncogenes present on the short arm of chromosome 12 could be activated by point mutations, deletions, or translocations to become oncogenes, which could then act in a dominant manner.[23] The *K-ras* gene is located on the short arm of chromosome 12, and amplification or enhanced expression of this gene has been reported to occur in testicular tumors and derived cell lines. Other candidate genes being studied include the *c-kit* oncogene, the *SCF* gene, the *c-mos* oncogene, and the *CCND2* gene. In addition to chromosome 12, 17q is overrepresented in 50% of cases of GCT and this area contains a number of genes of interest including GRB7 and plakoglobin.[22]

The study of the genetics and molecular biology of GCTs has enhanced our understanding of these tumors. To date, however, cytogenetics has had little impact in the clinic, with the possible exception of the use of various markers for the identification of nontesticular germ cell cancers located elsewhere in the body.[24-26]

PATHOLOGY AND PATHWAYS OF SPREAD

Pathology

Testicular cancers arise from intratesticular and paratesticular cells (Table 52-1). The vast majority are of germ cell origin and three major classification schemes have been in use worldwide (Table 52-2).[27-29] The Dixon and Moore classification as modified by Mostofi has been adopted by the World Health Organisation (WHO) and is the classification scheme most widely used in North America.[30]

Table 52-1 Histologic Classification of Testicular Neoplasms

Germ Cell Tumors (Demonstrating One or More of the Following Components)
Seminoma
Embryonal carcinoma
Teratoma
Choriocarcinoma
Yolk sac tumor (endodermal sinus tumor: embryonal adenocarcinoma of the prepubertal testis)
Sex Cord-Stromal (Gonadal Stromal) Tumors
Leydig cell tumor
Sertoli cell tumor
Granulosa cell tumor (adult and juvenile types)
Both Germ Cell and Gonadal Stromal Elements
Gonadoblastoma
Adnexal and Paratesticular Tumors
Mesothelioma
Soft tissue origin (e.g., sarcomas)
Adnexal (e.g., adenocarcinoma) of the rete testis
Miscellaneous Neoplasms
Carcinoid
Lymphoma
Cyst
Metastatic Neoplasms

For clinical purposes, GCTs are classified into two major groups: seminomas and nonseminomas (NSGCTs), although patients with pure seminoma may recur with pure NSGCT and vice versa. Approximately 60% of GCTs are pure seminoma, 30% are NSGCT, and 10% are mixed tumors (both seminoma and NSGCT elements present).[5] Patients with mixed tumors are clinically considered to have a NSGCT, the only exception being the presence of syncytiotrophoblastic cells in cases of seminoma.

Carcinoma In Situ

Intratubular germ cell neoplasia, or CIS, is felt to precede the development of all cases of seminoma and NSGCTs in adults (with the exception of spermatocytic seminoma).[31] On light microscopy, CIS cells closely resemble seminoma cells and in most cases are found within the seminiferous tubules. Cytologically, there is no difference between the CIS cells that develop into seminomas and NSGCT. In the general population the incidence of CIS is very low (0.2%), but it is somewhat higher in men with impaired fertility (0.5%) and in patients with cryptorchid testes (2% to 4%).[16]

Seminomas

Seminoma, the most common type of testicular GCT, is most commonly seen in the fourth decade of life. On gross examination the tumors are usually well demarcated from the residual testicular tissue and rarely have foci of necrosis or hemorrhage. On microscopic examination the classic or typical seminoma type is made up of large cells with abundant cytoplasm divided by connective tissue septa into sheets or cords.[32] These cells typically have round, hyperchromatic or vesicular nuclei with prominent nucleoli. Frequently, there is a lymphocytic infiltrate, and macrophages, plasma cells, and multinucleated giant cells are often present. Syncytiotrophoblasts are present in 15% to 20% of cases and their presence does not appear to alter prognosis.

On immunohistochemistry, virtually all seminomas express placental leukocyte alkaline phosphatase (PLAP) and do not express low-molecular-weight keratins, blood group antigens, or vimentin. Several histologic variants of seminoma have been identified, including anaplastic seminoma and spermatocytic seminoma. Anaplastic seminoma is diagnosed when there are three or more mitoses seen per high power field.[32] Spermatocytic seminoma is a rare subtype mainly seen in older men and is not associated with CIS or bilateral disease.[31] Also, these tumors do not stain for PLAP on immunohistochemistry and rarely, if ever, metastasize. An

Table 52-2 Three Classifications of Germ Cell Tumor

Dixon and Moore (1953)[29]	WHO Classification[30]	Pugh, 1976[27]
Group I	Seminoma	Seminoma
Seminoma	Spermatocytic seminoma	Spermatocytic seminoma
Spermatocytic seminoma	Embryonal carcinoma, adult-type	Malignant teratoma, undifferentiated
Group II	Teratoma	Teratoma, differentiated
Embryonal carcinoma	Mature	Malignant teratoma, intermediate
Group III	Immature	Yolk sac tumor; orchioblastoma
Teratoma, pure	Teratoma with malignant areas other than seminoma, embryonal carcinoma, or choriocarcinoma	
Group IV	Embryonal carcinoma and teratoma (teratocarcinoma)	
Teratoma with carcinoma or sarcoma	Infantile embryonal carcinoma	
Group V	Polyembryoma	
Teratoma with embryonal carcinoma or choriocarcinoma		
Embryonal carcinoma, adult-type		

Disease Sites

atypical variant of seminoma with some features similar to NSGCT on immunohistochemistry, while morphologically appearing like classic seminoma, has been reported.[33] Usually, there is little or no lymphocytic infiltrate and the tumor cells have less cytoplasm than classic seminoma cells. In terms of prognosis, this atypical variant appears to have the same prognosis as the classical type.

Nonseminomatous Germ Cell Tumors

Nonseminomatous tumors constitute 40% of germ cell testicular cancers and occur most commonly in the third decade of life. In the WHO classification system, NSGCTs include embryonal carcinoma, teratoma (mature, immature, or with malignant differentiation), choriocarcinoma, yolk sac tumor, and mixed GCTs. Most tumors are mixed with two or more cell types present. While some tumors have a component of seminoma, the association of seminoma within a histologically confirmed NSGCT has no major impact on the clinical outcome.[34] However, patients with combined tumors present at an age (median age, 33 years) intermediate between those with seminoma (median age, 36 years) and those with nonseminoma (median age, 27 years).[34] On gross examination there is usually a soft and irregular mass poorly demarcated from the surrounding testicular tissue, and a considerable amount of necrosis and hemorrhage is often present. Immunohistochemical studies usually demonstrate cytoplasmic expression of low-molecular-weight keratins in embryonal carcinomas, and yolk sac elements, low-molecular-weight keratin, and/or vimentin expression in mature teratomas.

Teratomas are tumors composed of cells derived from two or more of the germ cell layers (ectoderm, mesoderm, or endoderm). When one of the component tissues in either type of teratoma exhibits the histologic appearance of another malignancy, such as sarcoma or carcinoma, the term 'teratoma with malignant transformation' is used. Choriocarcinomas are tumors composed of both multinucleated syncytiotrophoblasts and mononuclear cytotrophoblast cells. Pure choriocarcinoma is very rare and usually manifests with widespread metastases and very high levels of β-human chorionic gonadotropin (β-hCG), and has a poor prognosis. Elements of choriocarcinoma are found in up to 10% of NSGCTs and do not appear to affect prognosis. Yolk sac tumor, also known as endodermal sinus tumor, is composed of cells that usually produce alpha-fetoprotein (AFP) and resemble those seen in the yolk sac in an embryo. Pure yolk sac tumors are rare but are the most common variant of childhood GCT. Elements of yolk sac tumor are found in up to 50% of NSGCTs.

Pathways of Spread

Local or direct extension of tumor into epididymis, through tunica vaginalis, into spermatic cord (T3) and rarely into scrotum (T4) can occur, but the prognostic impact of such spread is small. For patients with GCT, lymphatic spread is the most common route of metastasis. The lymphatic drainage of the testis is directly to the para-aortic lymph nodes. There are minor differences in the distribution of metastases from left or right testis tumors. The left testicular vein drains to the left renal vein and the lymphatic drainage is primarily to the lymph nodes in the para-aortic area, directly below the left renal hilum. On the right side, the testicular vein drains directly to the inferior vena cava below the level of the renal vein and, therefore, paracaval and interaortocaval nodes are the first ones to be involved in right-sided tumors. The distribution of retroperitoneal lymph node metastases in NSGCT is shown in Figure 52-1.[35] Contralateral nodal involvement occurs in approximately 15% of cases and is rarely found in the absence of ipsilateral involvement. Supradiaphragmatic spread can occur through the thoracic duct, and while left supraclavicular nodal disease is infrequent at presentation, it is often seen at the time of relapse.

Pelvic and inguinal lymph node involvement is rare (<3%). Factors predisposing to inguinal lymph node involvement include prior unrelated scrotal or inguinal surgery, scrotal orchidectomy with incision of the tunica albuginea, tumor invasion of the tunica vaginalis or lower third of the epididymis, and cryptorchid testis.[36,37] Disruption of lymphatic vessels in the spermatic cord during inguinal surgery has been shown to induce anastomoses between the testicular lymphatic vessels and the regional lymphatics destined for inguinal or pelvic lymph nodes. In an occasional patient, a connection with the contralateral inguinal lymph nodes may be established, but this is very uncommon. In a small propor-

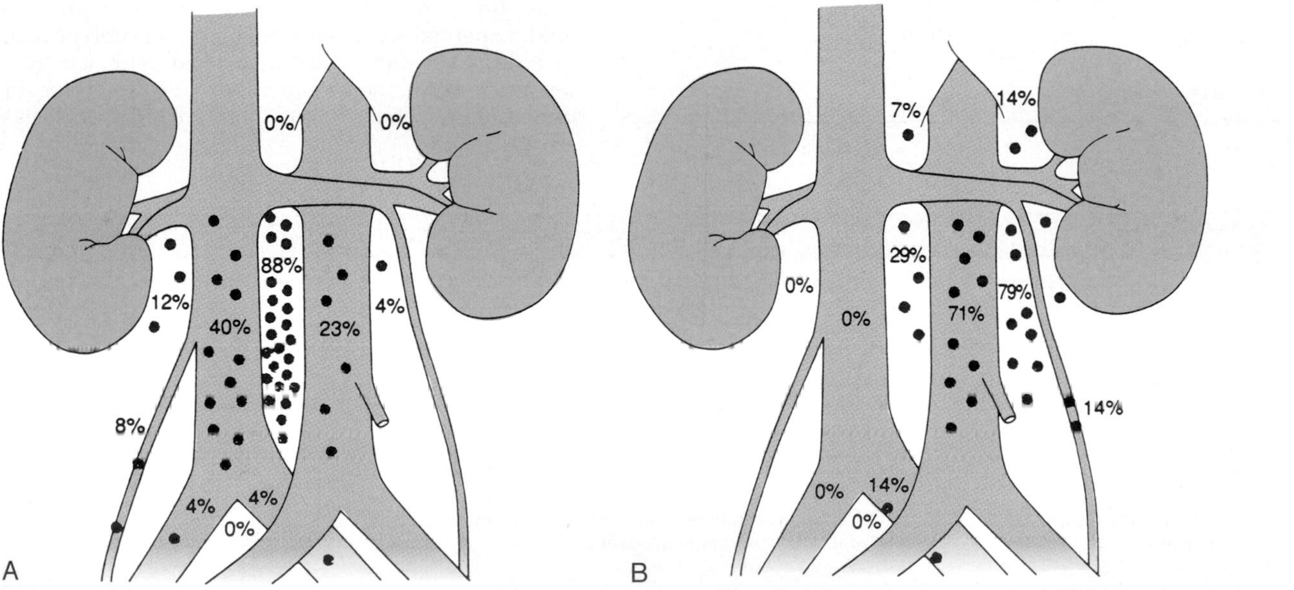

Figure 52-1 Distribution of retroperitoneal lymph node metastases in early stage nonseminoma germ cell tumor. **A,** Right testis primary tumor. **B,** Left testis primary tumor.

tion of patients with inguinal relapse, no predisposing factors may be apparent.[37]

In patients with NSGCTs, hematogenous spread occurs early in the course of the disease. The pulmonary parenchyma is the commonest site of hematogenous spread but liver, bone, brain, kidney, and gastrointestinal metastases are also seen. In a review of over 5000 patients with metastatic GCT, pulmonary metastases were present in 44% of cases, liver metastases were present in 6% of cases, with all other areas of hematogenous spread present in 1% or less of patients.[38] Mediastinal and neck node involvement were present in 11% to 12% of cases.

CLINICAL MANIFESTATIONS, PATIENT EVALUATION, AND STAGING

Clinical Manifestations

Patients with testis tumors most commonly present with a painless testicular mass. Up to 45% of patients have testicular pain, with signs and symptoms suggestive of acute epididymitis in up to 25% of cases. Much less common presenting features include those related to the presence of metastases, for example, back pain, dyspnea, and gynecomastia (from human chorionic gonadotropin [hCG] producing malignancies). The differential diagnosis of a testicular mass (in addition to tumor) includes torsion, hydrocele, varicocele, spermatocele, and epididymitis. A small percentage of tumors are associated with a hydrocele so the presence of transillumination on examination does not rule out a diagnosis of malignancy.

Patient Evaluation

In patients who present with no evidence of metastasis a diagnostic and therapeutic radical orchidectomy is usually performed after a solid mass is detected on physical examination or by ultrasonography. Serum tumor markers, including AFP, β-hCG, and LDH, should be obtained preoperatively to allow monitoring of decay with treatment (Fig. 52-2). Staging investigations are performed after the histologic diagnosis is confirmed, with the exception of patients with poor performance status and metastatic disease, for whom systemic therapy may be instituted based on a clinical diagnosis supported by unequivocal elevation of AFP and β-hCG. In these cases, the histologic diagnosis can often be obtained via needle biopsy.

Staging investigations include CT thorax, abdomen, and pelvis, and tumor markers, preferably both preoperatively and postoperatively. Since CT of the thorax is of little value in patients with seminoma and no evidence of retroperitoneal lymph node involvement, chest x-ray can be substituted in this setting. In stage II and III seminoma, especially in patients with bulky retroperitoneal disease, a bone scan should be performed. Abnormal serum marker levels should be monitored to document decay according to the expected half-lives. Patients with extensive metastatic disease, nonpulmonary visceral metastases (NPVM), or very high tumor marker levels are at risk for brain metastases, and a CT of the brain should be performed in these patients.[39] Baseline pulmonary and renal functions are assessed in patients who require chemotherapy.

Tumor Markers

Measurements of AFP, β-hCG, and LDH are essential in the diagnosis and management of patients with GCTs.[40] The hCG is a glycoprotein with a molecular weight of 45,000, composed of two subunits, of which the α subunit is identical to that of LH, FSH, and TSH, and a distinct β subunit. hCG is normally produced by the placenta. As well as occurring in nonseminomatous GCTs, about 15% of patients with seminoma have elevated β-hCG levels. Low levels of β-hCG may be found in other neoplasms, including prostate, bladder, and renal tumors. The use of marijuana derivatives also may lead to elevated levels. Some cross-reactivity with LH does occur, and in cases where an elevated hCG level is thought to be due to this, consideration should be given to having levels remeasured after treatment with testosterone.[41] The half-life of β-hCG in human serum is approximately 22 hours.

AFP is the major serum protein of fetal life. It is a glycoprotein with a molecular weight of 70,000. In addition to NSGCTs, it may be elevated in hepatocellular carcinomas, cirrhosis, hepatitis, and pregnancy. The half-life of AFP is approximately 5 days. AFP is not found in pure seminoma; its elevation in this setting implies the presence of nonseminomatous tumor elements. Liver disease should be considered in the differential diagnosis in patients whose disease appears to be responding, and in whom AFP fails to fall appropriately or is found to be increasing.

One or both of these markers are elevated in 85% of patients with NSGCTs. Experience with surveillance of patients with

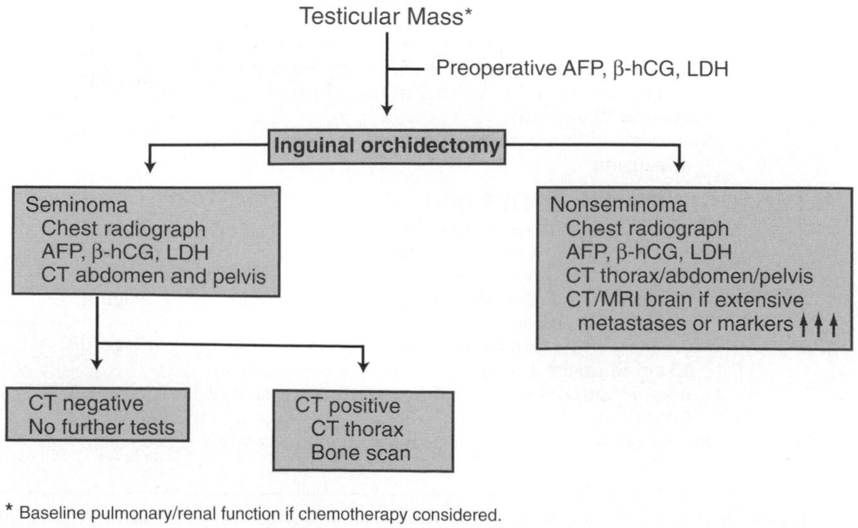

Figure 52-2 **Diagnostic algorithm** for a patient with a testicular mass. AFP, alpha-fetoprotein; β-hCG, β-human chorionic gonadotropin; LDH, lactate dehydrogenase.

early-stage disease has shown that normal markers do not exclude the presence of occult disease.[42]

LDH is a tumor marker and an independent prognostic factor in patients with GCTs. It is elevated in up to 60% of patients with nonseminomas, and also in a high proportion of patients with advanced seminoma.[38,43]

Both AFP and β-hCG are useful evidence of malignancy when measured before orchidectomy. The rate of decline after orchidectomy indicates the likelihood of residual tumor. Determination of tumor marker levels is used to assess response to treatment, predict the likelihood of achieving complete remission, and in regular follow-up to indicate recurrence, often in the absence of symptoms, physical findings, or abnormal imaging.

Placental alkaline phosphatase (PLAP) is an isoenzyme of alkaline phosphatase and is normally expressed by placental syncytiotrophoblasts. It is also expressed by testis tissue and has been investigated as a tumor marker in seminoma. While PLAP is often elevated in patients with seminoma, it has proved to be of little value in clinical management.[44]

Staging

The 2002 UICC TNM classification (Table 52-3), which combines anatomic and nonanatomic prognostic factors, is the recommended staging system.[45] In stage I disease one of the most important determinants of outcome is the presence of vascular invasion in the primary tumor, and this differentiates a pT1 tumor from a pT2 tumor.[46] Tumors with invasion of the spermatic cord are staged as pT3 cancers and the rare tumors with scrotal invasion are classified as pT4 lesions. In stage II disease, the extent of retroperitoneal adenopathy and serum tumor marker level determines treatment and outcome. Patients with retroperitoneal lymph nodes less than 5 cm in diameter (N1-2 disease) are often successfully treated with regional therapy, either retroperitoneal lymph node dissection

Table 52-3 Staging of Testis Tumors: American Joint Committee on Cancer

The extent of primary tumor is classified after radical orchidectomy.

PRIMARY TUMOR

pTX	Primary tumor cannot be assessed. (If no radical orchidectomy has been performed, Tx is used.)
pT0	No evidence of primary tumor (e.g., histologic scar in testis)
pTis	Intratubular germ cell neoplasia (carcinoma in situ)
pT1	Tumor limited to the testis and epididymis without vascular/lymphatic invasion. Tumor may invade into the tunica albuginea but not the tunica vaginalis.
pT2	Tumor limited to the testis and epididymis with vascular/lymphatic invasion, or tumor extending through the tunica albuginea with involvement of the tunica vaginalis.
pT3	Tumor invades the spermatic cord with or without vascular/lymphatic invasion.
pT4	Tumor invades the scrotum with or without vascular/lymphatic invasion.

REGIONAL LYMPH NODES (N), CLINICAL

NX	Regional lymph nodes cannot be assessed.
N0	No regional lymph node metastasis
N1	Metastasis with a lymph node mass ≤2 cm in greatest dimension; or multiple lymph nodes, none >2 cm in greatest dimension.
N2	Metastasis with a lymph node mass >2 cm but not >5 cm in greatest dimension; or multiple lymph nodes, any one mass >2 cm but not >5 cm in greatest dimension.
N3	Metastasis with a lymph node mass >5 cm in greatest dimension

PATHOLOGIC LYMPH NODES (pN)

pNX	Regional lymph nodes cannot be assessed.
pN0	No regional lymph node metastasis
pN1	Metastasis with a lymph node mass ≤2 cm in greatest dimension and ≤5 nodes positive, none >2 cm in greatest dimension.
pN2	Metastasis with a lymph node mass >2 cm but not >5 cm in greatest dimension; or >5 nodes positive, none >5 cm; or evidence of extranodal extension of tumor.
pN3	Metastasis with a lymph node mass >5 cm in greatest dimension

DISTANT METASTASIS (M)

MX	Distant metastasis cannot be assessed.
M0	No distant metastasis
M1	Distant metastasis
M1a	Nonregional nodal or pulmonary metastasis
M1b	Nonpulmonary visceral metastasis

SERUM TUMOR MARKERS (S)

SX	Marker studies not available or not performed
S0	Marker study levels within normal limits
S1	LDH <1.5 × N and hCG (mIU/ml) <5000 and AFP (ng/ml) <1000
S2	LDH 1.5-10 × N or hCG (mIU/ml) 5000-50,000 or AFP (ng/ml) 1000-10,000
S3	LDH >10 × N or hCG (mIU/ml) >50,000 or AFP (ng/ml) >10,000
N	Indicates the upper limit of normal for the LDH assay

Stage Grouping

Stage 0	pTis	N0	M0	S0
Stage I	pT1-4	N0	M0	SX
Stage IA	pT1	N0	M0	S0
Stage 1B	pT2	N0	M0	S0
	pT3	N0	M0	S0
	pT4	N0	M0	S0
Stage IS	Any T	N0	M0	S1-3
Stage II	Any T	N1-3	M0	SX
Stage IIA	Any T	N1	M0	S0
	Any T	N1	M0	S1
Stage IIB	Any T	N2	M0	S0
	Any T	N2	M0	S1
Stage IIC	Any T	N3	M0	S0
	Any T	N3	M0	S1
Stage III	Any T	Any N	M1	SX
Stage IIIA	Any T	Any N	M1a	S0
	Any T	Any N	M1a	S1
Stage IIIB	Any T	N1-3	M0	S2
	Any T	Any N	M1a	S2
Stage IIIC	Any T	N1-3	M0	S3
	Any T	Any N	M1a	S3
	Any T	Any N	M1B	Any S

Greene FL, Page DL, Fleming ID, et al, eds. AJCC Cancer Staging Manual, 6th ed. New York, Springer-Verlag, 2002.

(RPLD) in NSGCTs, or external beam radiation therapy in seminomas; however, those with nodal disease greater than 5 cm in diameter have a high risk of distant failure following regional therapy and are usually treated with systemic chemotherapy.

With the use of cisplatin-based chemotherapy, the survival of patients with metastatic testis tumors is excellent.[40] However, a minority of patients still succumb to testis cancer in spite of treatment. Adverse prognostic factors associated with a lower cure rate have been identified and a number of prognostic classifications of low risk or good prognosis groups have been published.[47,48]

In 1991, the International Germ Cell Cancer Collaborative Group (IGCCCG) of investigators from the United Kingdom, United States, and Europe set out to study prognostic factors and outcome in over 5000 adult patients with GCTs treated between 1975 and 1990 with cisplatin-based chemotherapy.[38] (See section on primary therapy.) Adverse prognostic factors identified included the presence of an extragonadal primary tumor (liver, bone, brain), or other NPVMs (kidney, skin, gastrointestinal). Elevation of all three tumor markers had a clear effect on survival. The information obtained by the IGCCCG has been used to construct the revised 2002 TNM staging classification for testis tumors[45] and three distinct subgroups (good prognosis, intermediate prognosis, and poor prognosis) were identified. This classification system has recently been validated by van Dijk and associates using Cox regression and recursive partitioning in a cohort of 3048 NSGCT patients.[43] They were able to subdivide the poor prognosis group of the IGCCCG into three subgroups with clearly distinct outcomes and this may be helpful in evaluating treatment results in the future.

PRIMARY THERAPY

The initial management involves a radical inguinal orchidectomy in almost all cases. Postorchidectomy management is based on the histology and extent of disease. The management policies for both seminomas and nonseminomatous tumors have evolved separately but currently are quite similar, with the exception of the use of RT in early-stage seminoma. Sperm testing and banking should be considered before treatment with chemotherapy, RPLD, and RT.

Surgery

Initial management involves a radical inguinal orchidectomy to allow high division of the spermatic cord. Orchidectomy is both diagnostic and therapeutic by providing adequate tissue to ascertain the diagnosis and offering cure in a high proportion (60% to 90%) of patients with stage I disease.[49,50] Although not recommended, a scrotal approach does not appear to compromise the outcome, and no additional therapy is required following scrotal violation, provided that the scrotal cavity has not been grossly contaminated by tumor. In patients with life-threatening metastatic disease and a clear cut diagnosis of germ cell malignancy, initial management should be with chemotherapy, and surgery should be postponed until completion of systemic treatment.[51] The role of orchidectomy as essential for local control has been questioned in patients with metachronous or synchronous bilateral tumors.[52]

Seminoma

The majority of patients (70% to 80%) with seminoma present with clinical stage I disease; 15% to 20% have infradiaphragmatic lymph node involvement on radiologic investigation (stage II disease), and less than 5% present with distant disease. Treatment options in patients with stage I seminoma include RT, surveillance, and adjuvant chemotherapy. While adjuvant retroperitoneal RT was the standard of care for the past 50 to 60 years, it is now accepted that a policy of surveillance provides the optimal outcomes, minimizing the burden of treatment while maintaining the cure rate at 100%.[53-55] Adjuvant radiation therapy remains a viable treatment option, with low rates of acute and late toxicity, for those unable to follow a surveillance protocol. The acute morbidity of the relatively low dose RT used in this setting is minimal; however, impaired spermatogenesis and increased rates of gastrointestinal symptoms, cardiac disease, and peptic ulceration on long-term follow-up have been reported.[56-59] There has also been increasing concern regarding the possible induction of second malignancies by RT.[56,60,61]

In stage II disease, retroperitoneal RT is usually recommended for patients with nonbulky tumor (stage IIA-B), while chemotherapy is the treatment of choice for patients with more advanced disease. In certain rare instances RPLD can be considered. In stage III disease chemotherapy is the treatment of choice.[61,62]

Management of Patients with Stage I Disease

SURVEILLANCE

The data on seminoma surveillance is now mature and relapse rates have consistently been reported to be approximately 15% in unselected populations of patients with stage I disease. The results of prospective nonrandomized studies of surveillance are shown in Table 52-4.[53,63-69] The two largest reported series are from the Rigshospitalet in Copenhagen and the Princess Margaret Hospital (PMH) in Toronto.[68,69] In the Rigshospitalet series of 394 patients, the crude relapse rate was 17% with a median follow-up of 60 months. In the PMH series of 345 patients, with a median follow-up of 9.4 years, the actuarial 5-year relapse-free rate was 85%. The other studies with adequate follow-up (>36 months) have reported similar relapse

Table 52-4 Results of Surveillance in Stage I Seminoma

Series	No. of Patients	Follow-up Median (mo)	Relapse No. (%)	CSS (%)
Allhoff (Hanover)[63-69,71]	33	—	3 (9)	100
Charig (Oxford)	15	31	5 (33)	100
Germa Lluch (Barcelona)	45	34	5 (11)	100
Horwich (Royal Marsden Hospital)	103	62	17 (16.5)	100
Oliver (Royal London Hospital)	67	61	16 (24)	97
Ramakrishnan (Royal Hallamshire Hospital)	72	44	13 (18)	100
Daugaard (Copenhagen)	394	60	69 (17.5)	100
Warde (Princess Margaret Hospital)	345	100	55 (16)	99.7

CSS, cause-specific survival.

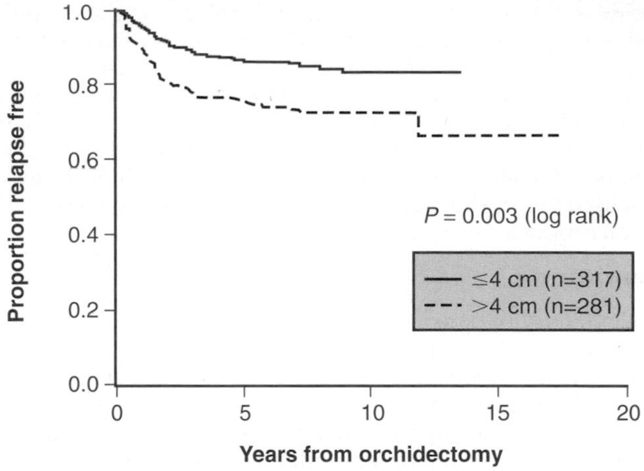

Figure 52-3 Relapse-free rate based on primary tumor size. (From Warde P, Specht L, Horwich A, et al: Prognostic factors for relapse in stage I seminoma managed by surveillance: a pooled analysis. J Clin Oncol 20:4448-4452, 2002. Copyright © American Society of Clinical Oncology.)

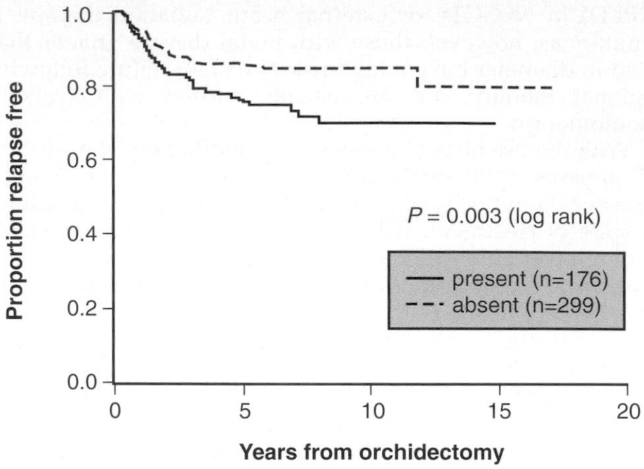

Figure 52-4 Relapse-free rate based on rete testis invasion. (From Warde P, Specht L, Horwich A, et al: Prognostic factors for relapse in stage I seminoma managed by surveillance: a pooled analysis. J Clin Oncol 20:4448-4452, 2002. Copyright © American Society of Clinical Oncology.)

rates. The predominant site of relapse in all studies was in the para-aortic lymph nodes—41 of 49 (82%) of relapses in the Danish Testicular Cancer Study Group (DATECA) study and 47 of 55 (85%) in the PMH series.[54] The median time to relapse ranged from 12 to 18 months, but late relapses (>4 years) have also been reported.[70]

Prognostic factors for relapse have been examined in a number of the surveillance studies.[54,71-73] In the PMH series on multivariate analysis, age and tumor size were predictive of relapse while small vessel invasion (SVI) approached statistical significance.[72] In the Danish Testicular Study Group (DATECA) report, tumor size was the only significant predictive factor for relapse on multivariate analysis.[54] In the Royal Marsden Hospital series of 103 patients managed with surveillance, the only significant factor predicting for relapse was the presence of lymphatic and/or vascular invasion (9% versus 17% relapse rate).[53]

To more accurately determine prognostic factors for relapse in patients with stage I testicular seminoma managed by surveillance a pooled analysis of 4 large surveillance series using individual patient data was performed.[73] Data on 638 patients was obtained from 4 centers—Royal Marsden Hospital, Danish Testicular Cancer Study Group, Princess Margaret Hospital and the Royal London Hospital. On multivariate analysis tumor size and rete testis invasion predicted for relapse. The effect of tumor size on relapse rate is shown in Figure 52-3, rete testis invasion in Figure 52-4, and both adverse prognostic factors present in Figure 52-5. The hazard ratio for relapse with a tumor size greater than 4 cm was 2.0 (95% confidence interval [CI], 1.3 to 3.2) relative to baseline (tumor size < 4 cm and no rete testis invasion). The hazard ratio for rete testis involvement was 1.7 (95% CI, 1.1 to 2.6) and with both adverse prognostic factors present the hazard ratio for relapse was 3.4 (95% CI, 2.0 to 6.1).

At relapse, most patients have been treated with retroperitoneal RT. The incidence of second relapse after RT was 12.5% in the PMH series and 11% in the DATECA series. The likelihood of detecting progression in the retroperitoneal lymph nodes early (nodes < 5 cm) and therefore suitable for RT, depends on the frequency of follow-up CT scans of the abdomen and pelvis. The current PMH follow-up policy is shown in Table 52-5. One of the concerns regarding the routine

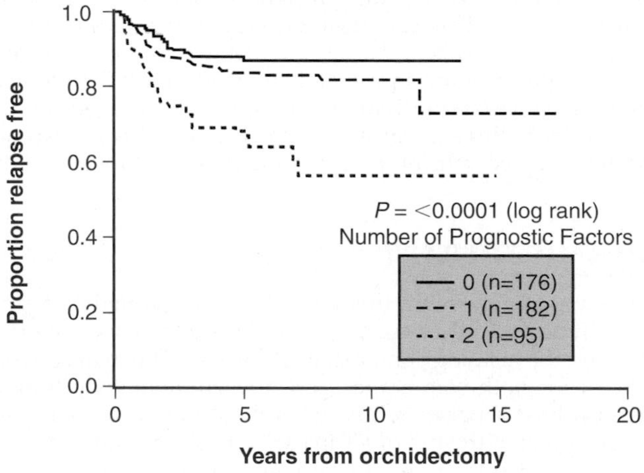

Figure 52-5 Relapse-free rate based on effect of both tumor size >4 cm and rete testis invasion. (From Warde P, Specht L, Horwich A, et al: Prognostic factors for relapse in stage I seminoma managed by surveillance: a pooled analysis. J Clin Oncol 20:4448-4452, 2002. Copyright © American Society of Clinical Oncology.)

use of surveillance is the potential for an increased use of chemotherapy, which involves a more prolonged and toxic treatment. In the 1981-1999 PMH experience, a similar percentage of patients managed with surveillance (5.1%) and adjuvant RT (3.5%) required chemotherapy as part of their management. This concern is difficult to address because, in some centers, chemotherapy was used electively at relapse, and some patients have contraindications to RT.

Radiation Therapy

The overall survival rate in most series in the modern era ranges between 92% and 99% at 5 to 10 years with cause-specific survival approaching 100%. Most deaths are due to intercurrent illness but concern exists that premature death may be occurring from radiation-induced cancers or cardiac disease.[56,59] In large single or multi-institutional series in the modern era, the relapse rate has varied from 0.5% to 5% (Table 52-6).[69,74-78] In-field relapse is rare and when suspected, biopsy

Table 52-5 **Follow-up Protocol for Stage I Seminoma**

	Month 4	Month 6	Month 8	Month 12
Years 1-2	Markers CXR CT Ab/Pel*		Markers CXR CT Ab/Pel*	Markers CXR CT Ab/Pel*
Years 3-5		CXR CT Ab/Pel*		CXR CT Ab/Pel*
Years 6,7		CT Ab/Pel*		CXR CT Ab/Pel*
Years 8-10				CXR CT Ab/Pel*

CXR, chest x-ray; CT, computed tomography; Ab/Pel, abdomen/pelvis .
*CT abdomen and pelvis done only if on surveillance.

Table 52-6 **Results of Retroperitoneal Radiation Therapy in Stage I Seminoma**

Author[74-78,80]	Years of Study	No. Patients	% Relapse	CSS (%)
Bayens	1975-1985	132	4.5	99
Coleman	1980-1995	144	4.2	100
Fossa	1989-1993	242	3.7	100
Hultenschmidt	1978-1992	188	1	100
Santoni	1970-1999	487	4.3	99.4
Warde	1981-1989	282	5	100

CSS, cause-specific survival.

should be performed to rule out nonseminomatous disease. The commonest sites of relapse following adjuvant radiation therapy are the mediastinum, lungs, and left supraclavicular fossa. A small proportion of patients, usually with predisposing factors, relapse in the inguinal nodes. Uncommon sites of isolated metastases such as brain and tonsil have been noted in case reports.[39,79] For supradiaphragmatic relapse, chemotherapy is the treatment of choice and gives close to 100% cure. Inguinal relapse can often be treated successfully with RT to the involved area.[80]

Most relapses occur within 2 years of RT. In the PMH series of 282 patients treated between 1981 and 1999, the median time to relapse was 18 months with the latest relapse occurring at 6 years. Follow-up efforts should therefore concentrate on the 2 years after RT, and the current PMH follow-up policy is shown in Figure 52-6. This is similar to the policy used for patients on surveillance except that a CT abdomen and pelvis is also done at all visits.

With such excellent results the prognostic factors for relapse are difficult to establish. One of the potential factors predicting relapse is the presence of anaplastic histology. In the PMH experience, 8 of 55 patients with anaplastic seminoma relapsed compared to 2 of 116 patients with classic seminoma (14.5% versus 1.7%).[80] The WHO criteria for the diagnosis of anaplastic seminoma (3 or more mitoses per high power field) are not uniformly used, and other series indicate that the prognosis for patients with anaplastic seminoma is similar to that for patients with classic seminoma.[81] Other factors reported to be associated with higher risk of relapse include tumor invasion of the tunica albuginea, lymphovas-

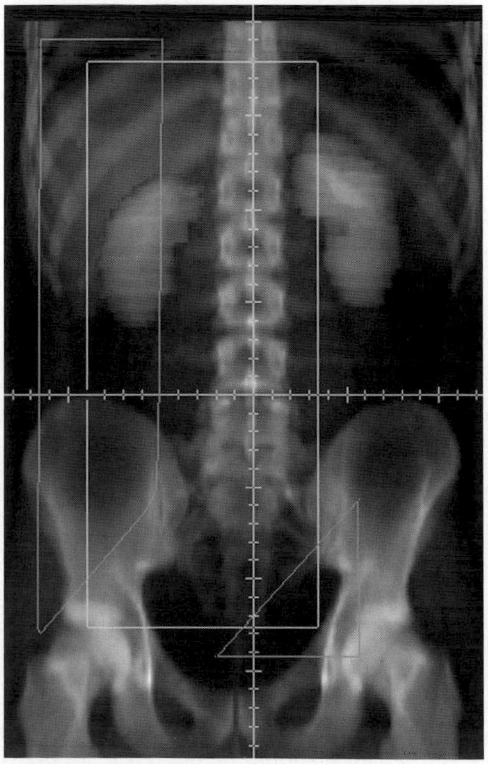

Figure 52-6 Radiation fields stage I.

cular invasion, invasion of epididymis, raised preoperative hCG level, and spermatic cord involvement.[74,80]

SURGERY

Retroperitoneal lymph node dissection is another often forgotten treatment option available in seminoma. It is an alternative approach available for patients unwilling to comply with surveillance or those unable to be treated with RT, such as those with inflammatory bowel disease or those previously treated with retroperitoneal RT. RPLD may also be appropriate in patients with concurrent or previous malignancy for whom histologic examination of lymph nodes is essential to plan treatment.

CHEMOTHERAPY

Adjuvant chemotherapy using carboplatin has been investigated as an alternative strategy to radiation therapy or surveillance in stage I seminoma. The use of one to two courses of carboplatin as adjuvant therapy after orchidectomy was initially reported by Oliver and colleagues, who treated 78 patients (53 patients had two courses; 25 patients had one course).[82] With a median follow-up of 44 months, only one patient had relapsed.

The Medical Research Council (MRC) UK has conducted a randomized phase III study of 1447 patients comparing adjuvant RT and a single course of carboplatin.[83] The relapse rate in both arms of the study was similar at 3 years (3.4% RT versus 4.6% carboplatin) with most of the relapses in the carboplatin arm occurring in the retroperitoneal lymph nodes. One benefit of adjuvant carboplatin noted in this setting was a reduction in the incidence of second primary testicular GCTs. This data would suggest that if single agent carboplatin is used then continued surveillance of the retroperitoneal lymph nodes is required.

Data from other single institution series indicate that if adjuvant carboplatin is given in this setting then two courses of treatment are necessary.[84,85] Even with two cycles of carboplatin a small but significant percentage of patients recur in the retroperitoneum and the usefulness of this approach is questionable.[84,85] In addition, the long-term toxicity of this strategy is unknown and, except in highly select cases, such as patients with coincidental inflammatory bowel disease, it should only be used in a study setting.

OVERVIEW OF MANAGEMENT OF STAGE I SEMINOMA

Almost 100% of patients with stage I testicular seminoma are cured regardless of the choice of postorchidectomy management. One of the most attractive features of surveillance is the ability to limit treatment to orchidectomy alone. Surveillance must not compromise survival, and it is reassuring to find only one disease-related death in the two largest surveillance series.[68,69] Surveillance requires a commitment to close and prolonged follow-up from both patients and clinicians; patient compliance with follow-up is essential, as failure to detect relapse at an early stage may compromise survival. However, failure to attend for follow-up may also compromise the outcome for patients treated with RT. While isolated occurrences of second nontesticular tumor following treatment of seminoma with RT have been reported for decades, there is now convincing data from long-term studies indicating that patients with seminoma treated with RT have an increased risk of developing a second malignancy, and this factor must be considered when deciding on postorchidectomy management.[61,62]

While physicians may view one management approach as preferable, surveillance should be offered to all patients with stage I seminoma and individual patients' preferences must be considered.[86] These preferences may be based on many socioeconomic factors as well as the side effects associated with both approaches. Also, the identification of prognostic factors for occult disease will allow patients and clinicians to choose management based on a more accurate assessment of an individual patient's risk of relapse.

Management of Patients with Stage II Seminoma

Approximately 15% to 20% of patients have radiologically involved para-aortic lymph nodes and are classified as having stage II disease. Patients are divided into three groups depending on the transverse diameter of the largest retroperitoneal lymph node mass: ≤2 cm (stage IIA), 2.1 to 5 cm (stage IIB), and >5 cm (stage IIC).[87,88] Approximately 70% of stage II patients have small bulk retroperitoneal disease at presentation with lymph nodes that are less than 5 cm. The definition of the substages of stage II seminoma has varied over time and the literature has to be interpreted cautiously. The number of patients with stage II disease is too small to mount phase III studies of management, and treatment decisions must be based on data from single institutions where patients have been treated in a uniform fashion.

The most important prognostic factor in stage II seminoma is the bulk of retroperitoneal disease, usually defined by the transverse diameter of the largest lymph node mass visible on CT scan. This was the only prognostic factor for relapse in a consecutive series of 95 patients with stage II seminoma treated with radiotherapy at the PMH between 1981 and 1999.[89] The 5-year relapse-free rate in 79 patients with nodal disease of less than 5 cm (IIA/B) was 91% compared to 44% in 16 patients with bulkier disease (IIC). Relapse occurred most commonly in mediastinal or supraclavicular lymph nodes, lung, or bone. Thirteen patients were treated with chemotherapy at relapse, and nine were free of disease at last follow-up. Two patients had salvage RT in the early 1980s (they would now be treated with salvage chemotherapy) and one was free of disease on follow-up. These five patients plus one additional patient who refused salvage treatment died of progressive seminoma. Thirty one patients (23 stage IIC) received initial chemotherapy for stage II disease with two relapses, one of whom was salvaged by second line chemotherapy. These results are similar to other series in the literature (Table 52-7) and support the continued use of primary radiotherapy in stage II patients with small bulk disease.[74,89-92] However, in patients with bulky retroperitoneal disease, the high failure rate following radiotherapy and the fact that not all patients with relapse were salvaged mandates the use of primary chemotherapy instead of radiation therapy.

Staging should not be the only parameter used to decide on treatment of retroperitoneal disease in patients with stage II seminoma. Tumor bulk, location of disease relative to normal tissue, as well as anatomic variants must also be considered. Patients with nodal disease extending 10 cm from L1-L5 in the retroperitoneum with a maximum transverse diameter of 4 cm are classified as having IIB disease and these patients with bulky disease should be treated with chemotherapy. Lymph node masses that are situated laterally may necessitate irradiating a large volume of one or both kidneys or the liver in order to adequately encompass the tumor. The same situation may arise in cases of abnormal anatomy, such as with horseshoe or pelvic kidney. These patients are better treated with chemotherapy because of an unacceptably high risk of radiation toxicity. Patients in whom radiotherapy and chemotherapy are contraindicated or the diagnosis is uncertain should be considered for retroperitoneal lymph node dissection.

The use of combination carboplatin and RT in stage IIA/B seminoma has been suggested by Patterson and associates.[93]

Table 52-7 Results of Retroperitoneal RT in Stage II A/B Seminoma

Author (Year of Publication)[74,89-92]	Years of Study	No. Patients	No. Relapse (%)	CSS (%)
Bayens (1992)	1975-1985	29	7 (24)	93
Chung (2004)	1981-1999	79	7 (8.8)	97.5
Classen (2004)	1991-1994	87	4 (4.6)	100
Vallis (1995)	1974-1989	48	3 (6)	98
Zagars (2001)	1984-1999	37	5 (13.5)	100

CSS, cause-specific survival.

He and his colleagues described a series of 30 patients treated with one course of carboplatin 4 to 6 weeks prior to RT. They reported a 5-year relapse survival rate of 96.9% compared with 80.7% in a historical cohort (largely treated in the 1980s) managed with radiation alone. The major problems with this report include the possibility of stage migration improving the results in the combined therapy group as well as a low control rate with RT alone, by modern standards. This approach cannot be accepted as routine practice without further data.

The commonest sites of relapse following radiotherapy in stage II patients with small bulk lymph node metastases are mediastinal or supraclavicular nodes, lung, and bone. Most relapsing patients are cured with chemotherapy, which emphasizes the importance of regular follow-up with clinical examination and chest x-ray after radiation. CT imaging of the abdomen and pelvis is not necessary after complete resolution of abdominal disease. In the PMH series, two of the seven patients who relapsed after RT had bone metastases, and both presented with spinal cord compression as the first sign of relapse. Therefore, all patients with unexplained back pain should have a bone scan to exclude metastases, and those with new-onset neurologic deficits require urgent imaging of the spine with MRI.

Residual Retroperitoneal Mass

The presence of a residual retroperitoneal mass after treatment of stage II seminoma is common and the management of these patients remains controversial. In contrast to NSGCTs, it is uncommon to find residual teratoma at RPLD and stable persistent masses often represent fibrosis or necrosis and only a minority contain active tumor. In addition, surgery may be technically difficult in patients with seminoma and is associated with higher morbidity compared with surgery in patients with NSGCTs.[94] The possibility of a nonseminomatous component to explain a residual mass needs to be kept in mind even in patients whose primary tumors show pure seminoma. Therapeutic options for patients with residual masses after treatment include observation, surgical removal or, very rarely after primary chemotherapy, RT can be considered. Positron emission tomography (PET) scanning has been reported to be of little value in this setting by some authors but others have reported it is a clinically useful predictor of tumor especially if the mass is greater than 3 cm in diameter.[95,96]

The most extensive experience in the management of residual masses in seminoma has been reported by the MSKCC group, where 55 of 104 patients with a residual retroperitoneal mass underwent surgical exploration or multiple biopsies.[97] Thirty-two patients (58%) had a formal RPLD and 23 (42%) had multiple intraoperative biopsies performed, as the residual mass was deemed unresectable. No patient with a preoperative mass less than 3 cm in diameter had residual tumor, whereas 30% of those with a mass greater than 3 cm had viable disease on pathologic examination. Given this high proportion of persistent malignancy, Memorial Sloan-Kettering Cancer Center (MSKCC) investigators have recommended resection or biopsy of masses of 3 cm or larger. In contrast, Culine and Droz have suggested that as long as the retroperitoneal mass continues to decrease in size after treatment, then continued observation is a reasonable strategy.[98] Similar results have been reported by other centers.[89,99] It seems clear that patients with a residual mass of 3cm or less can safely be observed. For patients with bulkier disease, up front surgery or observation can be instituted with therapy reserved for masses that increase in size. In all patients with residual masses after treatment, periodic CT examinations are mandatory and treatment is indicated for disease that increases in size on follow-up.

The use of RT in patients with a postchemotherapy residual mass has been shown to be of little benefit.[99,100] Horwich and associates have reported on the outcome in 29 patients with residual mass after cisplatin-based combination chemotherapy (15 treated with adjuvant RT and 14 managed by observation alone) and there was no evidence that risk of relapse was influenced by the use of adjuvant RT.[99] The MRC Testicular Tumor Working Party published a retrospective pooled analysis assessing the role of RT for postchemotherapy residual mass among men with seminoma.[100] Among the 123 patients with a residual abdominal mass 56% received adjuvant radiotherapy. There was no significant difference in outcome among patients who did or did not receive RT. Given these data routine RT is not indicated for a post-chemotherapy residual mass.

Management of Patients with Stage III Seminoma

This is an uncommon presentation (less than 5%). Seminoma has been shown to be exceptionally chemosensitive and the use of cisplatin-based regimens has changed the outcome of patients with metastatic disease. Mencel and colleagues have reported the MSKCC results in 140 patients with bulky stage II, stage III, and extragonadal tumors treated from 1979 to 1992.[101] One hundred and thirty patients (93%) achieved a favorable response (complete response [CR] or partial response [PR] with negative serum tumor markers). One hundred and twenty five patients (88%) were alive and 120 (86%) progression free at the time of the analysis (median follow-up 43 months). Fifty-five of 60 patients (92%) treated with four courses of cisplatin and etoposide were progression free. Based on this (and other) analyses, four courses of etoposide and cisplatin is the currently accepted standard management approach.[102]

Nonseminoma

The major advances in the treatment of nonseminomatous tumors of the testis occurred in the 1970s. Tumor markers (AFP, β-hCG, LDH) were used to measure response to treatment and to detect disease relapse. New drugs with clinical efficacy were identified with the introduction of cisplatin, bleomycin, and vinblastine. Before these drugs were available, nonseminomatous tumors were treated with a wide range of chemotherapeutic agents, and there were occasional reports of long-term remissions with the use of single-agent mithramycin and actinomycin D.[103] The modern era in treating advanced disease began at the M.D. Anderson Hospital with the use of continuous infusions of bleomycin and vinblastine,[104] the vincristine + actinomycin D + bleomycin (VAB) regimens from MSKCC,[105] and later the cisplatin + vinblastine + bleomycin (CVB) regimen from Indiana University.[106] With these regimens, complete responses to treatment were frequent and cures were apparent in patients with metastatic disease.

Stage I Disease

Current treatment strategies for these patients include either a modified bilateral RPLD or a policy of surveillance in which chemotherapy and surgery are reserved for patients with evidence of disease progression. The clinical factors associated with a high risk of occult nodal disease on RPLD, and therefore the factors that predict for disease progression on surveillance, include the presence of vascular invasion in the primary tumor, the presence of embryonal carcinoma, and the size of the primary tumor (Table 52-8).[107-109] In the MRC UK study of 259 patients managed by orchidectomy, four factors (presence of embryonal carcinoma, absence of yolk sac elements, and invasion of blood vessels or lymphatics) were identified on multivariate analysis as predictive of relapse.[46] When three or four adverse features were present in the primary tumor the risk of relapse was 58%, with two features present the risk of relapse was 24%, and with one or no adverse factors the probability of relapse was only 9%.

On surveillance protocols, tumor markers, chest radiographs, and physical examination are performed every two months, with CT of the abdomen and pelvis every four months. Published studies of surveillance have shown a 30% risk of disease progression (Table 52-9).[46,50,68,107,109-115] Up to 95% of patients will progress within 12 months of diagnosis; progression more than 24 months from diagnosis is extremely rare. Approximately 60% of patients progress in the retroperitoneal lymph nodes, with or without other evidence of disease (see Table 52-8). The other common presentations of disease progression are lung metastases or tumor marker elevation alone. At the time of progression patients are usually treated with chemotherapy, although RPLD is used in selected cases with small retroperitoneal lymph nodes. Most patients are cured at relapse and the cause-specific survival in most series is greater than 95% (see Table 52-8).

RPLD is a recognized alternative to surveillance in clinical stage I disease. Surgical techniques have undergone considerable modification in the last 20 years. In this setting a modified unilateral infrahilar RPLD is now performed, with nerve-sparing techniques to preserve ejaculation. The technique used has evolved from the bilateral RPLD, which included the renal suprahilar nodes. Usually, a midline transperitoneal approach is employed. For right-sided tumors the interaortocaval nodes and paracaval nodes are removed with preservation of the left sympathetic chain, and for left-sided tumors the para-aortic and interaortocaval nodes are removed and the right autonomic chain is preserved. If significant lymphadenopathy is discovered at the time of surgery, a more extensive surgical resection is performed. The relapse rate following surgery is approximately 10% for patients with pathologic stage I disease if there is no SVI in the primary tumor, versus 19.4% if SVI is present. As with relapses on surveillance, most patients who relapse after RPLD are cured with subsequent chemotherapy.[116] Pulmonary metastases are the most common site of relapse.

In some centers patients with clinical stage I NSGCT at high risk of relapse on surveillance are offered immediate adjuvant chemotherapy.[117,118] The MRC UK showed that two courses of adjuvant bleomycin + etoposide + cisplatin (BEP) chemotherapy achieve a 98% to 99% relapse-free rate in the high-risk

Table 52-8 Features Associated with High Risk of Relapse on Surveillance for Clinical Stage I Nonseminomatous Germ Cell Tumor

Vascular invasion[107-109,221]
Lymphatic invasion[107]
Absence of yolk sac elements[107]
Presence of embryonal carcinoma[107]
Absence of AFP preoperatively[108]
T category[108,110]
Percentage of teratoma in specimen

Table 52-9 Prospective Trials of Surveillance in Stage I Nonseminoma

Study	No. of Patients	Progression (%)	Deaths from Disease	Retroperitoneal Progression (%)
Daugaard et al (Copenhagen)[68]	301	29	0	—
Freedman et al (MRC)[107]	259	32	3	55
Freiha et al (Stanford)[112]	23	13	—	67
Jacobsen et al (Denmark)[109]	83	28	—	65
Peckham and Brada (RMH)[113]	132	27	1	60
Nicolai and Pizzocaro (Milan)[222]	85	29	3	66
Raghavan et al (Australia)[114]	49	28	2	38
Read et al (MRC)[46]	396	25	5	61
Sogani et al (MSKCC)[223]	102	25	3	72
Sharir et al (PMH)[50]	170	75	1	65
Thompson et al (New Zealand)[115]	36	33	1 (? + 1)	33
Wishnow et al (M. D. Anderson Cancer Center)[111]	82	29	—	—

MRC, Medical Research Council; MSKCC, Memorial Sloan-Kettering Cancer Center; PMH, Princess Margaret Hospital; RMH, Royal Marsden Hospital.

Table 52-10 Prognostic Factors for Relapse in Metastatic Germ Cell Tumors

Center	Histology	AFP	hCG	LDH	Liver/Lung/Brain	Extragonadal Primary Site	Lung Metastases
MSKCC	Yes	No	Yes	Yes	One site each in model	Yes	One site in model
Indiana	No	No	No	No	Yes	No	≥3 cm or >5/Luisa field
MRC (UK)	Yes	100	>1000	No	Yes	≥5-cm mediastinal mass	≥20 lung metastases

AFP, alpha-fetoprotein; hCG, human chorionic gonadotropin; LDH, lactate dehydrogenase; MSKCC, Memorial Sloan-Kettering Cancer Center; MRC, Medical Research Council.

Adapted from Paulson D (ed): Staging and substaging of metastatic germ cell tumors using prognostic factors. Probl Urol 8:76-86, 1994.

group, and this finding has been supported by other studies.[119] In this setting it should be recognized that at least 50% of the patients who receive chemotherapy do not require treatment, and the toxicity is significant. To reduce treatment-related toxicity, one study has tested a single cycle of adjuvant BEP. Forty two patients with stage I nonseminomatous GCTs received bleomycin 20 mg/m^2, etoposide 120 mg/m^2, and cisplatin 40 mg/m^2 daily for 3 days.[120] One patient relapsed and died in remission from treatment-related toxicity.

Surveillance was introduced as a way of preventing patients with true stage I disease from having unnecessary surgery, but now the morbidity previously associated with retroperitoneal lymphadenectomy has been reduced by nerve-sparing procedures to preserve ejaculatory function.[121,122] Ironically, as some centers routinely give chemotherapy to patients with clinical stage I who are judged to be at high risk of progression, an increasing number of patients may be exposed to chemotherapy who do not, in fact, require any further treatment.

Clinical Stage II

Treatment options for patients with clinical stage II NSGCT include RPLD, chemotherapy, or a combination of both.[123,124] Patients with retroperitoneal nodes greater than 5 cm in diameter have been shown to have a high relapse rate following RPLD and therefore are usually approached with chemotherapy. The outcome is excellent and will be discussed further in the section on management of stage III disease. In North America patients with solitary nodal masses less than 3 cm in size are most commonly treated with RPLD. A modified bilateral infrahilar lymphadenectomy is the current standard management in this setting. Patients with retroperitoneal disease between 3 and 5 cm in size may be treated with initial surgery or primary chemotherapy. Published data suggest that 8% to 44% of patients will relapse following RPLD if fewer than 6 lymph nodes are involved, with no node greater than 2 cm in diameter.[123-128] For this group of patients close monitoring, with chemotherapy reserved for relapse, is the recommended approach for compliant patients. Almost all patients who relapse can be salvaged with chemotherapy.

For noncompliant patients with pathologic stage II disease and for patients with more than 6 nodes involved, or with any node greater than 2 cm in diameter, adjuvant chemotherapy should be considered. A number of trials using two to four cycles of chemotherapy have been reported. Williams and associates reported the results of a randomized trial of 195 patients with N1-3 nodal disease who received two cycles of PVB or two cycles of VAB-4 or observation with standard treatment at relapse.[125] Equivalent survival was shown in this study with observation and two cycles of adjuvant chemotherapy. A more recent study of 50 patients treated with two cycles of adjuvant etoposide and cisplatin has shown no relapses with a median follow-up of 35 months, suggesting that bleomycin can be omitted in this group of patients.[129]

Table 52-11 Tumor Markers Risk Groups

Markers	AFP (mg/mL)	hCG(mg/mL)	LDH (× N)
Good	<1000	<1000	<1.5 × N
Intermediate	<1000	1000-10,000	1.5-10 × N
Poor	>10,000	>10,000	>10 × N

AFP, alpha-fetoprotein; hCG, human chorionic gonadotropin; LDH, lactate dehydrogenase; N, upper limit of normal.

Stage III

Although the cure of many patients with metastatic nonseminomatous testis tumors is one of the most remarkable advances in cancer therapy in the last 20 years, difficulty in comparing published results from different centers arose because of a lack of common agreement on those prognostic factors that predict a favorable or unfavorable outcome. Table 52-10 shows the prognostic factors used to classify patients into treatment groups in three major centers (MRC UK, Indiana University, and MSKCC).[130] These different prognostic groupings have made comparison of trial results impossible. Stage migration and other similar factors could have accounted for observed differences, rather than different treatment protocols.

In order to promote greater uniformity in assigning patients to risk groups and interpreting results from different treatment centers, the IGCCCG analyzed data from 5168 patients with nonseminomatous tumors.[38] Independent prognostic variables identified by the IGCCCG included

- Tumor markers, divided into three risk groups (Table 52-11)
- The presence of mediastinal primary disease (MED1°)
- The presence or absence of NPVM, for example, liver, gastrointestinal tract

Based on the results of multivariate analysis, the IGCCCG recommended three prognostic groups for nonseminomatous tumors and two prognostic groups for seminoma. For NSGCTs the good prognosis group included patients with a testis/retroperitoneal primary, no NPVM, and an AFP level of less than 1000 ng/ml, βhCG of less than 1000 ng/mL (or less than 5000 IU/mL), and LDH less than 1.5 times the normal value (Table 52-12). The intermediate prognosis group included patients with a testis or retroperitoneal primary, no NPVM, and marker levels of AFP more than 1000 ng/mL but less than 10,000 ng/mL, or β-hCG of more than 1000 ng/mL but less than 10,000 ng/mL (or < 50,000 IU/mL), or LDH more than 1.5 times but less than 10 times the normal value. The poor prognosis group included patients with a mediastinal primary, or NPVM, or an AFP level of more than 10,000 ng/mL, or β-hCG of more than 10,000 ng/ml (or

Table 52-12 **Prognostic Groups in Advanced Nonseminomatous Germ Cell Tumors**

Variable	Markers	MED 1°	NPVM	Patients (%)	3-y PFS	3-y Overall Survival
Good (all of)	Good	No	No	56	90	92
Intermediate	Intermediate	No	No	28	78	81
Poor (any of)	Poor	Yes	Yes	16	45	50

MED1°, mediastinal primary disease; NPVM, nonpulmonary visceral metastases; PFS, progression-free survival.

< 50,000 IU/mL), or LDH of more than 10 times the normal value. With these criteria, the 5-year survival for the good prognosis group was 92%; for the intermediate group, 80%; and for the poor prognosis group, 48%. For seminoma, only two prognostic groups were identified: a good prognosis group without NPVM with a 5-year survival of 86%, and an intermediate prognosis group with NPVM with a 5-year survival of 72%. The value of this prognostic classification was further validated in the analysis of survival from the MRC UK/The European Organization for Research on Treatment of Cancer (EORTC) database of NSGCTs treated between 1990 and 1993, and by analysis of data from the Eastern Cooperative Oncology Group/Southwest Oncology Group/Cancer and Leukemia Group B (ECOG/SWOG/CALGB).[38] The IGCCCG classification system has recently been updated by van Dijk and colleagues using Cox regression and recursive partitioning in a cohort of 3048 NSGCT patients.[43] They were able to subdivide the poor prognosis group of the IGCCCG into three subgroups with clearly distinct outcomes and this may be helpful in evaluating treatment results in the future.

TREATMENT

Chemotherapy has evolved since the recognition of the efficacy of cisplatin, bleomycin, and vinblastine–containing regimens. More recently, ifosfamide, etoposide, paclitaxel, gemcitabine, and irinotecan have been found to be effective drugs. By the end of the 1970s, most patients with metastatic disease received treatment with either the PVB regimen or the VAB-6 regimen. It was also recognized that maintenance chemotherapy was unnecessary for patients achieving complete clinical remission.[131,132]

The next step forward came with publication of a comparison of the PVB regimen with the BEP regimen in which vinblastine was replaced by etoposide.[133] Complete remission and 2-year survival rates were similar overall, but BEP was considered more effective in poor-prognosis, advanced disease. Importantly, there was a significant reduction in neuromuscular toxicity using BEP. A number of subsequent trials have examined the optimum number of causes of treatment, the need for bleomycin, and the replacement of cisplatin with carboplatin.

The Southeastern Cancer Study Group (SECSG) carried out a randomized trial comparing four courses of BEP to three courses of BEP for patients with favorable-prognosis tumors, and concluded that in this group, three courses of BEP were preferable because of reduced toxicity with no decrease in disease-free status.[134] An EORTC/MRC trial randomized 800 patients to receive three courses of BEP or three courses of BEP plus one course of etoposide + cisplatin (EP). The progression-free survival was equivalent in each group, but there was an improvement in the quality of life and a decrease in toxicity with three cycles of BEP.

The MSKCC group compared four cycles of EP with three cycles of VAB-6 in a randomized trial of 164 patients with good-prognosis GCTs, and found similar complete remission rates, and relapse-free and event-free survivals, with less toxicity in the EP arm.[135] The question of whether or not bleomycin is essential to the treatment regimen remains controversial. An ECOG trial comparing three cycles of EP to three cycles of BEP in 178 patients with minimal or moderate stage disease found increased toxicity and inferior failure-free and overall survival in the EP arm, leading to a recommendation that bleomycin continue to be used in this patient group.[136] Culine and associates reported in 1999 on 209 patients randomized to receive three cycles of BEP or four cycles of EP. Although there was no difference in overall survival and the toxicities were equivalent, an updated report at ASCO in 2003 showed that with a mean follow-up of 51 months, the overall survival did not differ significantly between patients in the two groups. However, they noted a non–statistically significant trend towards an inferior event-free survival in the group who did not receive bleomycin, and they now recommend that bleomycin be included in the treatment regimen.[137]

A randomized trial at MSKCC compared four cycles of EP with four cycles of EC (etoposide and carboplatin) in 270 patients with good-risk disease.[138] Although CR rates were comparable, event-free and relapse-free survivals were less favorable for those treated with EC. The authors recommended restricting carboplatin to investigational status in GCTs and the routine use of cisplatin-based regimens. Horwich reported in 1997 for the MRC and EORTC a study of 598 patients randomized to receive four courses of BEP or four courses of bleomycin, etoposide and carboplatin.[139] The 3-year survival rate was superior in the BEP group (97% versus 90%, $P = .003$). These results confirmed the inferior status of carboplatin compared to cisplatin.

At the present time, the standard of care for patients with good-risk disease is to treat with three courses of BEP or four courses of EP.[134] Some experts recognize a favorable subgroup which may be treated with EP alone, such as patients with positive markers only. Complete remission rates of 90% to 98% would be expected in this patient group.

Patients with intermediate and poor-risk disease have durable CR rates of 28% to 79% with current treatment regimens. The standard of primary chemotherapy for such patients today would be to give four courses of BEP, or treat with a similar cisplatin-based regimen (Table 52-13). About 25% to 30% of patients who present with poor-risk disease will fail to achieve CR or will relapse from CR following first-line chemotherapy. For these patients further attempts at curative therapy have included the use of other active agents in conventional dosage or high-dose chemotherapy followed by autologous stem cell transplant.[140-142]

A frequently used second-line regimen includes vinblastine, ifosfamide, and cisplatin. Motzer has reported a trial in which patients received paclitaxel, ifosfamide, and cisplatin as second-line therapy.[143] Thirty patients were treated at first relapse, and achieved a 77% CR rate. Seventy-three percent of patients had durable responses with a median follow-up of 33 months. At the present time these two regimens have not been compared to each other in a randomized trial. More recently, gemcitabine and irinotecan have been shown to be effective

Table 52-13 Chemotherapy Regimens in Use

BEP*	
Bleomycin	30 units IV weekly on days 2, 9, 16
Etoposide	100 mg/m^2 IV daily × 5
Cisplatin	20 mg/m^2 IV daily × 5
EP†	
Etoposide	100 mg/m^2 IV daily × 5
Cisplatin	20 mg/m^2 IV daily × 5
VIP‡	
Etoposide	75 mg/m^2 IV daily × 5 days
Ifosfamide	1.2 g/m^2 IV daily × 5 days, with mesna
Cisplatin	20 mg/m^2 IV daily × 5 days

*Cycles repeated every 21 days.
†Cycles repeated every 21 days.
‡Cycles repeated every 21-28 days.

drugs for second-line therapy, but no precise statement can be made from the trials reported on whether they are preferable as second-line therapy to the other two regimens previously described.[144,145]

High-dose chemotherapy combined with autologous stem cell or bone marrow transplantation may be employed as salvage therapy for relapse after first-line therapy, or as part of first-line therapy if the marker decline is slower than predicted. Predictors for poor outcome with such treatment include progressive disease before high-dose chemotherapy is started, mediastinal nonseminomatous primary tumors, patients who are refractory to conventional doses of cisplatin, and hCG levels above 1000 U/L before high-dose treatment is started. Motzer[146] has reported on 37 platinum-resistant patients treated with paclitaxel, ifosfamide, high-dose carboplatin, and etoposide followed by stem cell transplant. Fifty-seven percent of these patients achieved CR with 41% being disease free for a median follow-up of 30 months. Similar results have been published by other groups.

Rosti and colleagues presented data in 2002 from the European group for blood and marrow transplantation.[147] This was the first randomized trial utilizing high-dose chemotherapy with stem cell support as salvage therapy for patients who responded incompletely to first-line platinum therapy, or who relapsed after treatment. Two hundred and eighty patients were randomized. One group received chemotherapy with four cycles of a combination including vinblastine, etoposide, ifosfamide, and cisplatin. The second group received three cycles of the same chemotherapy followed by one course of high-dose carboplatin and stem cell transplantation. Forty one percent of patients in the conventional treatment arm achieved CR compared to 44% in the group receiving stem cell transplant. At 3 years, the curves for overall and disease-free survival were not significantly different in either arm. There were nine treatment-related deaths in the stem cell arm and two in the standard chemotherapy arm.

Patients who present with bulky retroperitoneal disease commonly have residual disease seen on CT scan after induction chemotherapy. Remission rates in GCTs usually refer to the response following induction chemotherapy and subsequent surgery, if this is required to resect residual tumor masses. Less frequently, residual mediastinal or pulmonary metastases may be seen in the lungs following treatment. It is recommended that residual disease be resected and that in the abdomen an RPLD be performed.[148-150] Approximately 85% to 90% of patients will have necrosis or teratoma, mature or immature, in the pathology specimens, and 5% to 10% of patients with normal tumor markers will have active cancer. In the latter group, two additional cycles of platinum-based chemotherapy are often recommended.

Treatment Complications

Radiation Therapy

With the low dose RT used in seminoma acute complications are minor in most patients.[78,151,152] Mild nausea and vomiting are common, and a small proportion of patients require regular antiemetics and are unable to complete daily tasks while receiving RT. Diarrhea develops in a minority of patients. Severe late radiation complications are rare and usually, no severe complications are expected unless the patient has an underlying medical problem or a technical error occurs. An increased incidence of peptic ulceration in patients treated with 30 to 45 Gy has been reported.[57]

Late Gonadal Toxicity

Testicular germinal epithelium is exquisitely sensitive to ionizing radiation. Although the contralateral testis is not located directly in the radiation field, scatter dose can be significant and may cause profound depression of spermatogenesis and compromise future fertility. A radiation dose between 20 and 50 cGy may produce temporary aspermia, and doses greater than 50 cGy may preclude recovery of spermatogenesis.[153] The use of scrotal shielding reduces the scattered radiation dose to the testis, but cannot assure protection of spermatogenesis in all patients. In men who recover spermatogenesis after RT for seminoma, there is no evidence of an increased incidence of genetic abnormalities among offspring.[154] Limiting RT target volume to the para-aortic and common iliac area does not eliminate concerns regarding RT-induced fertility issues. In the MRC randomized trial of para-aortic radiation alone versus para-aortics and pelvis the median time to a normal posttreatment sperm count was 13 months in those patients treated to the para-aortics alone.[155] This was significantly better than the patients treated to the para-aortic and pelvic lymph nodes (20 months). However, at 3 years of follow-up there was no significant difference in sperm counts between the 2 groups. Testicular shielding should be used in all patients who wish to retain fertility after treatment.[156]

Cardiovascular Toxicity

Mediastinal irradiation has resulted in an increased risk of heart disease.[157,158] In the Patterns of Care study, Hanks and associates found an increased incidence of cardiac disease in patients treated with mediastinal RT compared with those treated with infradiaphragmatic RT alone.[159] The true incidence of cardiac disease following mediastinal RT is not known, and patients and physicians should be made aware of this risk. Recent data from M.D. Anderson and the Royal Marsden Hospital suggest that long term survivors of testicular seminoma treated with postorchiectomy RT are at significant excess risk of death as a result of cardiac disease.[56,59] However, the relevance of this data to the modern practice of radiotherapy has been questioned.[160]

Second Malignancy

In discussing second malignancies after treatment of testicular cancer a distinction must be made between second GCTs of the testis, which reflect a common risk factor for this disease, and unrelated malignancies, which may be treatment induced. An increased risk of second cancers has been documented in a number of studies, and since this increased risk is expressed more than 10 to 15 years following RT, it is often not apparent in series with shorter follow-up.[161,162] Zagars and colleagues have reported an increased cancer-specific standardized mortality ratio (SMR) in 453 long-term survivors of

RT for testicular seminoma.[56] The cancer-specific SMR was 1.91 (99% CI, 1.14 to 2.98) and this increased mortality was detected only after 15 years of follow-up. The largest study of second cancers in long-term survivors of testicular cancer was conducted by Travis and associates at the National Cancer Institute Cancer Epidemiology Division.[61] Over 28,000 patients with testis cancer, including over 15,000 with seminoma from 16 population-based registries worldwide, were evaluated. Overall, 1406 second cancers, excluding contralateral testis tumors, occurred against 981 expected (observed/expected [O/E] = 1.43). The actuarial risk of developing a second nontesticular malignancy increased over time from diagnosis of testicular cancer and was 18.2% at 25 years. Secondary leukemia was linked with RT and chemotherapy, while an excess of the stomach, bladder, and possibly pancreas tumors was associated with prior RT.[61,62] Limitation of the radiotherapy field to the infradiaphragmatic region appears to result in a lower risk of second malignancy than more extensive fields and it is likely that limiting the treatment volume to the para-aortic area alone would decrease the risk further.[61]

Psychological Toxicity

The majority of patients do not have any serious psychological sequelae from their diagnosis or treatment, and some patients report an improved outlook on life compared to their premorbid state and to that of control groups.[163,164] Some patients, however, do experience severe psychological symptoms in the areas of sexual activity, infertility, distress, and social upheaval.[165,166] Appropriate social support should be offered to patients with testis tumors. Although this is a highly curable disease, it is still a life-threatening condition in young patients with a concomitant threat of infertility and impaired sexual function as a result of the disease or its treatment.[167]

Chemotherapy Complications

The complications of chemotherapy in testicular GCTs are related to the drugs employed.[168] Nausea and vomiting occur with all the drugs used, but are controlled effectively in most patients with 5-HT_3 antagonists and steroids. Myelosuppression is frequent. Febrile neutropenia is seen in about 10% to 15% of patients receiving EP and such patients may benefit from hematopoietic growth factors. Nephrotoxicity, primarily a reduction in the glomerular filtration rate, occurs with the use of cisplatin and ifosfamide.[169] Renal tubule function is normal in most patients, but hypomagnesemia is seen in patients after repeated use of cisplatin. Raynaud's phenomenon has been reported in 23% to 49% of patients, although resolution of symptoms is common.[170] Chronic peripheral neuropathy (often asymptomatic) is well recognized after treatment with cisplatin, vinblastine, and etoposide. Pulmonary toxicity is seen with the use of bleomycin and is dose related.[171] Impaired fertility, which may precede the use of chemotherapy, may also continue after its use. Although chemotherapy also produces infertility, recovery of sperm counts has been observed in the majority of patients.[172] In the study of second cancers in long-term survivors of testicular cancer conducted by Travis and colleagues,[61] an increased risk of secondary leukemia was associated with prior treatment with chemotherapy.

Other Testicular Tumors

Leydig Cell Tumors

Leydig or interstitial cell tumors account for approximately 2% of all testicular tumors.[173] Twenty-five percent occur in children and can manifest with signs of prepubertal virilization. Seventy-five percent occur in adults, usually with a painless testicular mass. Most Leydig cell tumors are benign and there are no definite histologic criteria for malignancy.[174-177] The regional lymph nodes are the commonest site of metastatic disease but lung, bone, and liver metastases have also been reported.

The initial management is similar to GCTs with a radical inguinal orchidectomy followed by staging assessment with chest x-ray (CXR) and CT abdomen and pelvis. Urinary and serum steroids should also be assessed. Retroperitoneal lymph node dissection can be considered in selected cases.[177] There is no role for adjunctive or definitive RT or chemotherapy.

Sertoli Tumors

Sertoli cell tumors account for less than 1% of all testicular tumors.[178] They have been classified into three subtypes: classic, large cell calcifying, and sclerosing.[179] Most present with a painless testicular mass and initial management is with a radical inguinal orchidectomy. Both precocious puberty and feminization have been reported associated with Sertoli cell tumors in children. Most Sertoli cell tumors are benign and orchidectomy is nearly always curative.

Extragonadal Germ Cell Tumors

Extragonadal germ cell tumors (EGCTs) have a similar histology to testicular GCTs but are found in other parts of the body, in the absence of a testicular mass. They account for 1% to 5% of all GCTs, and like testicular GCTs tend to occur in young men, although the median age of presentation is 5 to 10 years older than with testicular GCTs.[40] Of adult EGCTs, 10% occur in women, usually as ovarian dysgerminomas, and these will be discussed elsewhere (see Chapter 58). In infants, EGCTs are more common than testicular primary tumors (usually sacrococcygeal teratomas).[180]

Overall, patients with EGCTs (especially NSGCTs) have a worse prognosis than patients with testicular primaries.[181] Cytogenetic analysis of tumor tissue shows a similar pattern to that found in testicular tumors, with isochromosome 12(p) present in 70% to 80% of cases.[182,183] An increased incidence of EGCTs is seen in Klinefelter's syndrome.[184] A number of patients present with poorly differentiated carcinomas (predominantly in midline locations) with a similar cytogenetic pattern to those with typical EGCTs, and do respond to cisplatin-based chemotherapy regimens.[185]

EGCTs most commonly arise in three midline sites in the mediastinum, the pineal and suprasellar regions, and the sacrococcyx (usually in infants). There have been rare case reports of tumors arising in the orbit, prostate, vagina, and liver. Tumors arising in the retroperitoneum are usually thought to be associated with an occult testicular primary lesion. Mediastinal GCTs usually occur in the anterior superior region of the mediastinum adjacent to the thymus. Patients may present with cough, dyspnea, and chest pain, and tumor marker levels are frequently abnormal. Local invasion or metastatic disease to the lungs, liver, or bone is common. Biopsy should always be performed since treatment is dependent on the histologic subtype. For mature teratomatous tumors surgery is advised, whereas for NSGCTs or seminomas the preferred approach is cisplatin-based chemotherapy. Surgical resection is recommended for residual mass after chemotherapy. However, the precise role of locoregional therapy after primary chemotherapy is unclear.

The results of an international analysis of 635 consecutive patients with EGCTs treated in 11 European and U.S. centers have recently been reported.[181] Patients with pure seminomatous histology had a long-term cure rate of 89%, irrespective of site of primary (retroperitoneum or mediastinum).

However, in patients with nonseminomatous tumors mediastinal primary was an adverse feature with only 45% of these patients alive at 5 years compared with 63% of patients with retroperitoneal presentations.[181] Prognostic variables for response and outcome have been identified and four prognostic risk groups have been identified based on histology; presence of liver, lung, or CNS metastases; elevation of β-hCG; and number of metastatic sites involved with disease.[186] The best prognostic group has an 89% 5-year survival rate and encompasses all patients with seminoma. The other groups all have nonseminomatous histology and 5-year survivals of 69%, 55%, and 17%, respectively. The excellent treatment results with chemotherapy alone of mediastinal seminomatous tumors would suggest that there is no routine role for RT in their management. Platinum-based chemotherapy regimen is recommended and a 5-year survival of 73% has been reported with the use of cisplatin + vincristine + methotrexate + bleomycin + actinomycin D + cyclophosphamide + etoposide (POMB/ACE) chemotherapy.[187]

Special Treatment Situations

Germ Cell Tumors in Patients with a Horseshoe Kidney

Horseshoe kidney occurs in approximately 1 in 400 of the general population.[188] There is an association between renal fusion abnormalities and cryptorchidism, which in turn is associated with an increased incidence of testicular neoplasms. The association of horseshoe kidney and testicular tumors may occur more commonly, as it represents another abnormality in the development of the urogenital ridge.[189] Because of this anomaly, variation in the normal pathways of lymphatic spread may be expected.

There are two main problems in the management of GCTs associated with horseshoe or pelvic kidney. The first is related to the technical problem of delivery of RT in patients with seminoma. In a number of cases of horseshoe kidney, a large part of the renal parenchyma directly overlies the regional lymph nodes and lies within the standard radiation volume. The delivery of a standard radiation dose would be associated with an unacceptable risk of radiation nephritis. The second problem is related to the possible abnormalities in lymphatic drainage of the testis and, therefore, the possibility of relapse when the standard radiation fields are used. Unusual patterns of relapse have been observed in patients managed by surveillance, confirming concerns regarding abnormal lymphatic pathways.[190] For these reasons, in patients with seminoma and NSGCTs, postorchidectomy surveillance in stage I and chemotherapy in stage II have usually been recommended. However, an RPLD is another option for patients unwilling to follow the surveillance program. Reports in the literature suggest that RPLD is both safe and effective in the selected cases where it was performed.[190-192] However, horseshoe kidney poses special technical problems during RPLD for testicular tumors due to anomalous renal and intra-abdominal vascular patterns and helical CT angiography is useful for meticulous surgical planning and the safe performance of surgery in this setting.[193]

Testicular Tumors Developing in Immunosuppressed Patients

It is well established that the risks of developing Kaposi's sarcoma and non-Hodgkin's lymphoma are markedly increased in patients with HIV infection.[194] Although there was initially some controversy about whether these patients have an increased risk of developing testicular neoplasms, it is now clear that HIV-infected men have an increased incidence of testicular cancer.[195,196] Organ transplant patients also have an increased incidence of testicular tumors.[196] The clinical course of immunosuppressed patients with testicular tumors is similar to that of nonimmunosuppressed patients, and these patients should be offered standard oncologic therapy. Both chemotherapy and RT reduce the CD4 count even when antiretroviral therapy is used; therefore, wherever possible, surveillance should be used in patients with stage I disease.[13] Caution must be exercised as benign retroperitoneal adenopathy related to AIDS may be mistaken for metastasis from a testicular primary tumor. For those receiving chemotherapy, consideration should be given to concomitant prophylaxis for opportunistic infection. The majority can be cured of their tumor and the outcome of patients with HIV-related GCTs is similar to non-HIV patients.[197] In transplant patients requiring retroperitoneal RT, the kidney or pancreatic allograft should be shielded wherever possible. If this cannot be safely achieved, then RPLD or chemotherapy should be used instead. Posttransplant patients appear to tolerate platinum-based chemotherapy without any problems.[198,199]

Bilateral Testicular Germ Cell Tumors or Tumors Arising in a Single Testicle

Patients with testis cancer in one testicle are significantly more likely to develop a testis tumor in the contralateral testicle with rates of metachronous or synchronous development of second testis cancers of 1% to 5% reported in various studies.[200,201] Bilateral orchidectomy is still recommended as standard management resulting in infertility, lifelong dependency on androgen substitution, and possible psychological morbidity due to castration at a young age.[202] Recommendations for assessing patients prior to initiation of androgen replacement and ongoing monitoring have recently been published and include serum PSA testing on a regular basis.[203] In order to preserve endogenous hormonal function, organ sparing surgery, followed by low dose RT to the remaining testis to eradicate residual CIS where present , may be a viable therapeutic approach with a high likelihood of cure in a highly select group of patients.[204] Patients with large tumors (greater than 20 mm) or clinical evidence of metastatic disease should not be considered for this approach. The largest series reported to date is by Heidenreich and associates who reported on 73 patients with bilateral tumors (52 metachronous, 17 synchronous, and 4 GCTs in a solitary testicle).[202] Fifty-six patients had adjuvant irradiation to the remaining testis and 17 did not. Overall, there were three systemic relapses and four local failures (all in patients who did not receive RT). With a median follow-up of 7.5 years, 72 patients (98.6%) are alive and free of disease; 85% have normal exogenous serum testosterone levels and do not need hormone replacement therapy. The recent European Consensus on the diagnosis and treatment of testis cancer has emphasized the need for organ sparing approaches to be conducted only in centers with experience in this area.[51]

Central Nervous System Metastases

Approximately 2% to 3% of patients with metastatic GCTs will present clinically with brain metastases and up to 40% of patients who die of progressive disease will have brain metastases at autopsy. Patients who present at time of diagnosis with brain metastases can achieve approximately 50% 5-year cause-specific survival with aggressive treatment.[205] The optimal local therapy in patients with resectable disease is unclear but in those with unresectable disease RT to a dose of 40 to 45 Gy should be given to gross disease, preferably using a stereotactic approach. The role of total brain irradiation is unclear but if given, the dose should not exceed 40 Gy. Patients presenting with late relapse with CNS metastases should be treated aggressively as long-term disease-free survival is possible.[206] Patients who develop brain metastases during systemic chemotherapy have a very poor prognosis and should likely receive palliative RT only.[206]

Spermatocytic Seminoma

Spermatocytic seminoma is a rare testicular tumor and accounts for only 1% to 2% of all seminomas. It usually occurs at age 50 to 60 years but is seen in younger patients.[207] It is distinct in its histologic characteristics with usually three different cell sizes, spherical nuclei, lack of cytoplasmic glycogen and sparse or absent lymphocytic infiltrate when compared to classic seminoma.[31] Unlike classic seminoma, it does not appear to arise from CIS and it occurs solely in the testis and has no ovarian equivalent. All patients presented as stage I and there is only one case in the literature that has been confirmed as developing subsequent metastatic disease.[208] In the past it has been treated in a similar fashion to seminoma with adjuvant RT to the para-aortic and pelvic nodes; however, the likelihood of benefit from this approach is low and all patients should be placed on surveillance.[209]

TECHNIQUES AND DOSE OF IRRADIATION

Stage I Seminoma

Radiation Fields

The traditional management of stage I seminoma patients after orchiectomy has consisted of RT to the para-aortic and pelvic (retroperitoneal) lymph nodes. The most frequently used field arrangement is parallel-opposed anteroposterior fields, and patients are treated with 10- to 18-MeV linear accelerator photons. The clinical target volume includes the para-aortic lymph nodes and ipsilateral pelvic lymph nodes and is defined with the help of the information obtained from CT scan of the abdomen and pelvis to avoid irradiation of renal parenchyma. With left-sided tumors the left renal hilum is included in the field by shaping the left lateral border of the RT portal. This classic plan was called "hockey stick" in North America and "dogleg" in the United Kingdom and Europe. Usually, the radiation fields extended from the top of the T11 vertebral body (or T10) to the inguinal ligament. With this technique the penis is moved out of the field and, in addition, the contralateral testis is placed in a scrotal shield to protect fertility and hormonal function. Verification, simulator and port fields are routine. The inguinal lymph nodes are not routinely treated with this technique and in patients with risk factors for inguinal lymph node involvement, these can be treated either by extending the radiation field inferiorly or by adding a direct anterior field. In general, scrotal radiation is avoided even in patients with scrotal violation. The only instance where scrotal radiation may be recommended is in patients with very extensive local disease, incomplete surgery, and gross scrotal contamination prior to surgery.

The low incidence of pelvic lymph node involvement in stage I seminoma has led to the investigation of adjuvant RT directed to the para-aortic lymph nodes alone. The advantages of such an approach include decreased scatter to the remaining testicle and a reduction in the integral radiation dose the patient receives, presumably decreasing the risk of second malignancy.[210,211] Reports from phase II trials and retrospective single institutional experiences have shown excellent results with few pelvic failures.[81,90,212]

The MRC Testicular Study Group in the United Kingdom has conducted a prospective randomized trial of the traditional para-aortic and pelvic radiation versus para-aortic irradiation alone.[155] The results of this study of 478 patients showed a 96% relapse-free survival for patients treated with para-aortic RT alone versus 96.6% relapse-free survival for those treated to the para-aortic and pelvic lymph nodes. Sperm counts after treatment were significantly higher in the para-aortic alone group and there was some decrease in incidence of diarrhea in the patients treated to the para-aortic and pelvic lymph nodes. However, the 33% incidence of diarrhea in these patients likely reflects the use of a high dose per fraction (200 cGy/day) in this study compared with the 125 cGy/day used in many other studies. All patients who received para-aortic and pelvic RT relapsed in supradiaphragmatic sites, but four patients in the para-aortic alone group failed with disease in the pelvis. This trial showed that reduced RT volume gives excellent results, but, when used, a small risk of pelvic failure remains. Therefore, if this treatment approach is adopted, regular surveillance with CT of the pelvic lymph nodes must be performed to ensure that when pelvic relapse occurs it is detected early. Data from the Christie Hospital in Manchester where no routine evaluation of the pelvic nodes is carried out after para-aortic radiation alone has shown that the median size of the pelvic lymph nodes at time of detection of relapse was 5 cm (range, 2.5 to 9 cm).[81] The advantage of para-aortic RT alone is therefore not clear, particularly in comparison to surveillance.

A compromise between traditional RT fields and para-aortic RT alone may be to irradiate the para-aortic and ipsilateral common iliac lymph nodes by positioning the inferior border of the radiation fields at midpelvis as is currently done at PMH (see Fig. 52-6).[213] This encompasses the lymph nodes that are typically removed at lymphadenectomy in patients with nonseminomatous tumors and also covers the vast majority of pelvic nodal relapses in patients treated with para-aortic RT alone.[90,121] This approach may reduce the risk of second malignancy by reducing the integral dose of RT and has the potential to reduce the scatter dose to the remaining testis and preserve fertility without the requirement for ongoing pelvic surveillance.[214]

Radiation Dose

The minimum dose of radiation required to control occult seminomatous tumor has not been defined. At PMH in Toronto, a dose of 25 Gy prescribed at midline and delivered in 20 daily fractions of 1.25 Gy has been used for over 25 years with no in-field recurrences observed. While it is apparent from our experience that a dose greater than 25 Gy is unnecessary, the question of whether a lesser dose would be sufficient has not been answered. Results from the MRC TE18 trial comparing 20 Gy in 10 fractions to 30 Gy in 15 fractions to the para-aortic lymph nodes alone show equivalent relapse rates in both arms with a median follow-up of 61 months.[215] However, in a single institution study of 53 patients, 1 patient (of any expected 8 with micrometastatic nodal disease based on surveillance data) relapsed in-field[216] when treated with 20 Gy in 10 fractions to the para-aortic and iliac lymph nodes. Further follow-up is clearly necessary before this schedule can be adopted. Radiation doses of less than 20 Gy have been associated with in-field failures reported in the literature.[216-218] The results of a hypofractionated approach using 20 Gy in 8 fractions over 1.5 weeks in 431 patients (para-aortic RT only) has been reported by Logue and colleagues.[81] No in-field recurrences were observed and the overall relapse rate was 3.5% with a median follow-up of 62 months. Forty-six percent of

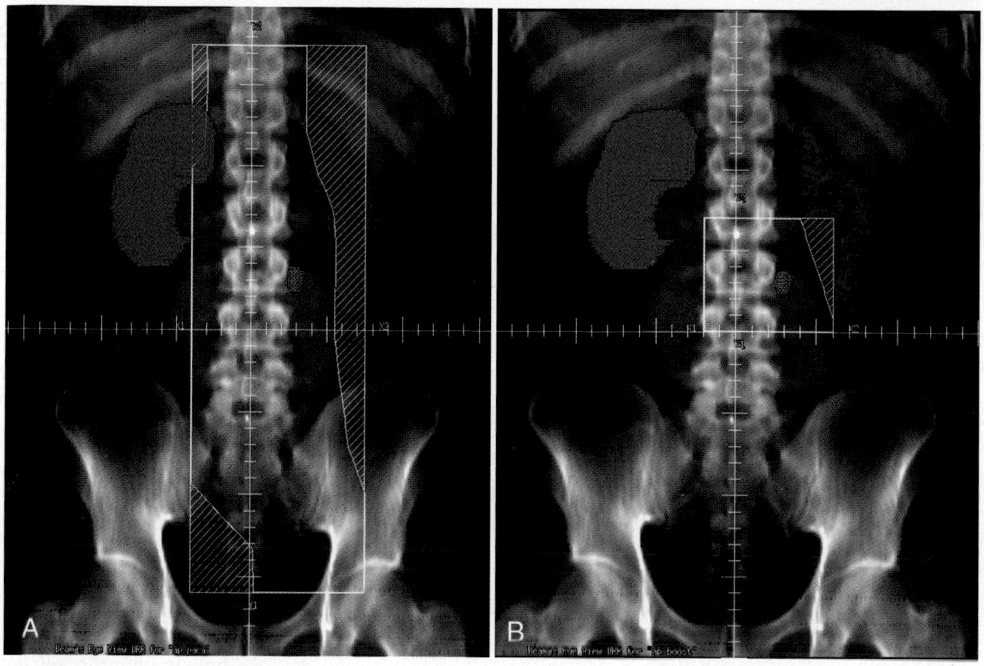

Figure 52-7 Radiation fields stage II. **A,** Extended field. **B,** Boost field.

patients developed nausea during treatment with 12% of patients reporting episodes of vomiting. With 1.25 Gy/day as given at PMH, little acute toxicity is observed.[80] However, patients may be willing to trade off a more severe acute toxicity for the convenience of a shorter treatment regimen.

Stage II Seminoma

The technique of radiation in stage II seminoma is similar to that used in stage I disease. The penis is always positioned out of the field and the contralateral testis is placed in a scrotal shield. The treatment volume includes the gross tumor as well as the para-aortic and ipsilateral common and external iliac lymph nodes (Fig. 52-7A). The radiation dose is typically 25 Gy in 20 daily fractions plus a boost of a further 10 Gy in 5 to 8 fractions to the gross lymphadenopathy (see Fig. 52-7B). At PMH, this boost is given concurrently with the large-field treatment. A CT scan with the patient in treatment position is used to ensure that the gross tumor is adequately encompassed by the radiation fields and that the minimal possible volume of kidney and liver are irradiated. The contralateral iliac lymph nodes may also be treated in cases where lymphadenopathy in the low para-aortic area is deemed to increase the risk of these nodes being involved by tumor. However, this is probably of most concern in patients with bulky retroperitoneal lymphadenopathy who are better treated with primary chemotherapy as discussed previously. Adjuvant radiation of supraclavicular lymph nodes in patients with stage II disease has been recommended by some although it is not justified on a routine basis in view of the low risk of isolated supraclavicular recurrence (2/79 patients with IIA/B disease in the PMH series).[92,219] The ease with which supraclavicular lymph nodes can be followed clinically, the availability of effective salvage chemotherapy for these cases, and the possibility of compromising bone marrow reserve for subsequent chemotherapy should it be necessary, as well as the potential for radiation-induced cardiac toxicity, must be considered.

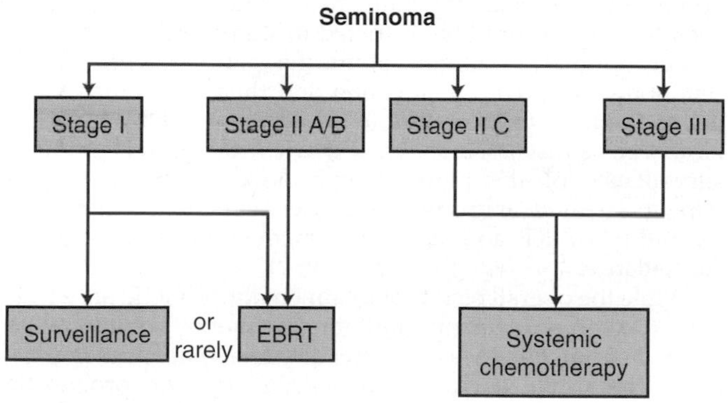

Figure 52-8 **Treatment algorithm for testicular seminoma** based on TNM stage groupings.

ALGORITHMS, CONCLUSIONS, AND FUTURE POSSIBILITIES

The recommended treatment algorithms for seminomas and nonseminomas based on TNM stage groupings are outlined in Figures 52-8 and 52-9. Despite the major advances in treatment over the past 20 years, there are ongoing controversies regarding the optimal management of GCTs. In seminoma the major area of controversy is the optimal management of stage I disease. The available data from surveillance and adjuvant RT series suggest that almost 100% of patients with stage I testicular seminoma are cured whichever approach is chosen as postorchidectomy management. However, there are increasingly persuasive data that adjuvant RT in this setting is associated with a small but definite risk of second malignancy. In addition, long-term data from surveillance series have documented the safety of this approach. In a compliant patient surveillance should be considered the management option of choice. It is disturbing to note that a considerable proportion of urologists and radiation oncologists do not discuss the

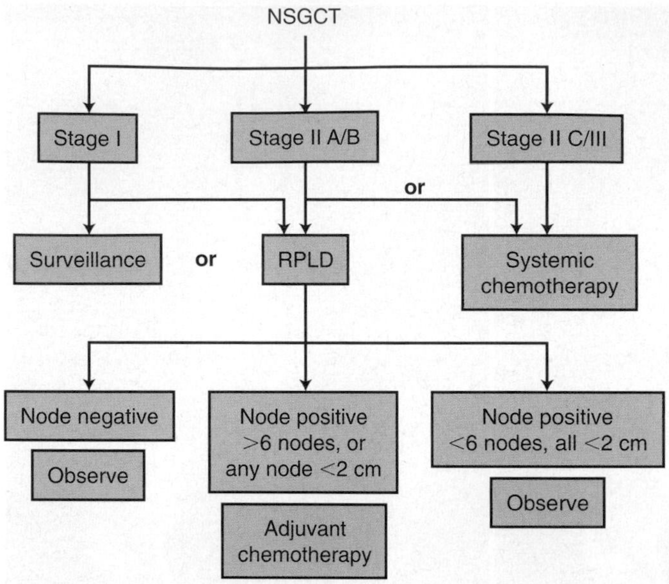

Figure 52-9 Treatment algorithm for testicular nonseminomatous germ cell tumors (NSGCTs) based on clinical TNM stage groupings.

option of surveillance with their patients.[86,220] Adjuvant chemotherapy should be restricted to study settings.

The optimal RT target volume for patients with stage I seminoma is under investigation and there is an increasing interest in limiting treatment to the para-aortic lymph nodes. However, as discussed above, if pelvic irradiation is omitted, surveillance of the pelvic lymph nodes is required and patients treated with this approach experience both the morbidity of RT and have the ongoing inconvenience of surveillance.

While the overall results of treatment for NSGCTs are excellent, further refinements and improvements remain to be made. In stage I disease, it is necessary to define optimal treatment, individualized for each patient based on prognostic factors, and with patient participation in the decision making. For good-risk metastatic disease, randomized trials are needed to identify subgroups of patients who may be safely treated with fewer courses of chemotherapy or with treatment that omits bleomycin. In advanced or poor-risk disease, clinical trials are needed to further evaluate favorable reports from high-dose regimens with stem cell support, and to identify subgroups of patients most likely to benefit from this aggressive approach. Finally, new drugs with similar clinical efficacy but less toxicity would be a welcome addition in the treatment of these neoplasms.

ACKNOWLEDGMENT

The authors would like to thank Mrs. Eleni Sachinidis for her help in manuscript preparation.

REFERENCES

1. http://www-dep.iarc.fr/globocan/GLOBOframe.htm.
2. Huyghe E, Matsuda T, Thonneau P: Increasing incidence of testicular cancer worldwide: a review. J Urol 170:5-11, 2003.
3. Jemal A, Siegel R, Ward E, et al: Cancer Statistics, 2006. CA Cancer J Clin 56:106-130, 2006.
4. Parkin D, Muir C, Whelan S, et al: Cancer incidence in five continents. Comparability and quality of data. Vol 120: Lyon, France, IARC Scientific Publications, 1992.
5. McGlynn KA, Devesa SS, Sigurdson AJ, et al: Trends in the incidence of testicular germ cell tumors in the United States. Cancer 97:63-70, 2003.
6. Dieckmann KP, Pichlmeier U: Clinical epidemiology of testicular germ cell tumors. World J Urol 22:2-14, 2004.
7. Lee PA, Coughlin MT: The single testis: paternity after presentation as unilateral cryptorchidism. J Urol 168:1680-1682; discussion 1682-1683, 2002.
8. Herrinton LJ, Zhao W, Husson G: Management of cryptorchism and risk of testicular cancer. Am J Epidemiol 157:602-605, 2003.
9. Strader CH, Weiss NS, Daling JR, et al: Cryptorchism, orchiopexy, and the risk of testicular cancer. Am J Epidemiol 127:1013-1018, 1988.
10. Tollerud D, Blattner W, Fraser M, et al: Familial testicular cancer and urogenital developmental anomalies. Cancer 55:1849-1854, 1985.
11. Prener A, Engholm G, Jensen OM: Genital anomalies and risk for testicular cancer in Danish men. Epidemiology 7:14-19, 1996.
12. Osterlind A, Berthelsen JG, Abildgaard N, et al: Risk of bilateral testicular germ cell cancer in Denmark: 1960-1984. J Natl Cancer Inst 83:1391-1395, 1991.
13. Powles T, Bower M, Daugaard G, et al: Multicenter study of human immunodeficiency virus-related germ cell tumors. J Clin Oncol 21:1922-1927, 2003.
14. Buetow SA: Epidemiology of testicular cancer. Epidemiol Rev 17:433-449, 1995.
15. Grigor KM, Rorth M: Should the contralateral testis be biopsied? Round table discussion. Eur Urol 23:129-135, 1993.
16. Rorth M, Rajpert-De Meyts E, Andersson L, et al: Carcinoma in situ in the testis. Scand J Urol Nephrol Suppl 166-186, 2000.
17. Giwercman A, Skakkebaek NE: Carcinoma in situ of the testis: biology, screening and management. Eur Urol 2:19-21, 1993.
18. Classen J, Dieckmann K, Bamberg M, et al: Radiotherapy with 16 Gy may fail to eradicate testicular intraepithelial neoplasia: preliminary communication of a dose-reduction trial of the German Testicular Cancer Study Group. Br J Cancer 88:828-831, 2003.
19. Fossa SD, Opjordsmoen S, Haug E: Androgen replacement and quality of life in patients treated for bilateral testicular cancer. Eur J Cancer 35:1220-1225, 1999.
20. Sandberg AA, Meloni AM, Suijkerbuijk RF: Reviews of chromosome studies in urological tumors. III. Cytogenetics and genes in testicular tumors. J Urol 155:1531-1556, 1996.
21. Atkin N, Baker M: High chromosome numbers of testicular germ cell tumors. Cancer Genet Cytogenet 88:90, 1995.
22. Oosterhuis JW, Looijenga LH: Current views on the pathogenesis of testicular germ cell tumors and perspectives for future research: highlights of the 5th Copenhagen Workshop on Carcinoma in situ and Cancer of the Testis. APMIS 111:280-289, 2003.
23. Shuin T, Misaki H, Kubota Y, et al: Differential expression of protooncogenes in human germ cell tumors of the testis. Cancer 73:1721-1727, 1994.
24. Motzer RJ, Amsterdam A, Prieto V, et al: Teratoma with malignant transformation: diverse malignant histologies arising in men with germ cell tumors. J Urol 159:133-138, 1998.
25. Ilson DH, Motzer RJ, Rodriguez E, et al: Genetic analysis in the diagnosis of neoplasms of unknown primary tumor site. Semin Oncol 20:229-237, 1993.
26. Donadio AC, Motzer RJ, Bajorin DF, et al: Chemotherapy for teratoma with malignant transformation. J Clin Oncol 21:4285-4291, 2003.
27. Pugh R: Pathology of Testis. Oxford, Blackwell, 1976.
28. Mostofi F, Price EJ: Tumors of the male genital system. *In* Hartmann W, Cowan W, eds. Atlas of Tumor Pathology, 6th ed. Washington, DC, Armed Forces Institute of Pathology, 1973, p 85.
29. Dixon F, Moore R: Tumors of the male sex organs. *In* Atlas of Tumor Pathology. Washington, DC, Armed Forces Institute of Pathology, 1953, pp 31-32.

30. Ebele J, Sauter G, Epstein J, et al, eds: Pathology and Genetics of Tumors of the Urinary System and Male Genital Organs. Lyon, France, IARC Press, 2004.
31. Grigor KM: A new classification of germ cell tumors of the testis. Eur Urol 23:93-100; discussion 101-103, 1993.
32. Ulbright TM: Germ cell neoplasms of the testis. Am J Surg Pathol 17:1075-1091, 1993.
33. Tickoo SK, Hutchinson B, Bacik J, et al: Testicular seminoma: a clinicopathologic and immunohistochemical study of 105 cases with special reference to seminomas with atypical features. Int J Surg Pathol 10:23-32, 2002.
34. Thomas R, Dearnaley D, Nicholls J, et al: An analysis of surveillance for stage I combined teratoma–seminoma of the testis. Br J Cancer 74:59-62, 1996.
35. Donohue J, Zachary J, Maynard B: Distribution of nodal metastases in nonseminomatous testis cancer. J Urol 128:315-320, 1982.
36. Mason MD, Featherstone T, Olliff J, et al: Inguinal and iliac lymph node involvement in germ cell tumors of the testis: implications for radiological investigation and for therapy. Clin Oncol 3:147-150, 1991.
37. Klein FA, Whitmore W, Sogani PC, et al: Inguinal lymph node metastases from germ cell testicular tumors. J Urol 131:497-500, 1984.
38. International Germ Cell Cancer Collaborative Group: International Germ Cell Consensus Classification: a prognostic factor-based staging system for metastatic germ cell cancers. J Clin Oncol 15:594-603, 1997.
39. Raina V, Singh SP, Kamble N, et al: Brain metastasis as the site of relapse in germ cell tumor of testis. Cancer 72:2182-2185, 1993.
40. Bosl G, Motzer R: Testicular germ-cell cancer. N Engl J Med 337:242-253, 1997.
41. Catalona W, Vaitukaitis J, Fair W: Falsely positive specific human chorionic gonadotropin assays in patients with testicular tumors: conversion to negative with testosterone administration. J Urol 122:126-128, 1979.
42. Sturgeon JF, Jewett MA, Alison RE, et al: Surveillance after orchidectomy for patients with clinical stage I nonseminomatous testis tumors. J Clin Oncol 10:564-568, 1992.
43. Van Dijk MR, Steyerberg EW, Stenning SP, et al: Identifying subgroups among poor prognosis patients with nonseminomatous germ cell cancer by tree modelling: a validation study. Ann Oncol 15:1400-1405, 2004.
44. Nielsen OS, Munro AJ, Duncan W, et al: Is placental alkaline phosphatase (PLAP) a useful marker for seminoma? Eur J Cancer 26:1049-1054, 1990.
45. Sobin LH, Wittekind C: UICC TNM Classification of Malignant Tumors, 6th ed. New York, John Wiley & Sons, 2002.
46. Read G, Stenning S, Cullen M, et al: Medical Research Council prospective study of surveillance for stage I testicular teratoma. Medical Research Council Testicular Tumors Working Party. J Clin Oncol 10:1762-1768, 1992.
47. Bajorin D, Katz A, Chan E: Comparison of criteria for assigning germ cell tumor patients to "good risk" and "poor risk" studies. J Clin Oncol 6:786-792, 1988.
48. Hitchins RN, Newlands ES, Smith D, et al: Long-term outcome in patients with germ cell tumors treated with POMB/ACE chemotherapy: comparison of commonly used classification systems of good and poor prognosis. Br J Cancer 59:1989, 1989.
49. Fleshner N, Warde P: Controversies in the management of testicular seminoma. Semin Urol Oncol 20:227-233, 2002.
50. Sharir S, Jewett M, Sturgeon J, et al: Progression detection of stage I nonseminomatous testis cancer on surveillance: implication for the followup protocol. J Urol 161:472-476, 1999.
51. Schmoll HJ, Souchon R, Krege S, et al: European consensus on diagnosis and treatment of germ cell cancer: a report of the European Germ Cell Cancer Consensus Group (EGCCCG). Ann Oncol 15:1377-1399, 2004.
52. Weissbach L: Organ preserving surgery of malignant germ cell tumors. J Urol 153:90-93, 1995.
53. Horwich A: Surveillance for stage I seminoma of the testis. *In*: Horwich A, ed. Testicular Cancer. Investigation and Management. London: Chapman and Hall Medical, 1991, pp. 109-116.
54. Von der Maase H, Specht L, Jacobsen GK, et al: Surveillance following orchidectomy for stage I seminoma of the testis. Eur J Cancer 14:1931-1934, 1993.
55. Warde P, Gospodarowicz M, Panzarella T, et al: Results of adjuvant radiation therapy and surveillance in stage I seminoma. Br J Urol 80, A1144:291, 1997.
56. Zagars GK, Ballo MT, Lee AK, et al: Mortality after cure of testicular seminoma. J Clin Oncol 22:640-647, 2004.
57. Hamilton CR, Horwich A, Bliss JM, et al: Gastrointestinal morbidity of adjuvant radiotherapy in stage I malignant teratoma of the testis. Radiother Oncol 10:85-90, 1987.
58. Fossa SD, Moynihan C, Serbouti S: Patients' and doctors' perception of long-term morbidity in patients with testicular cancer clinical stage I. A descriptive pilot study. Supp Care Cancer 4:118-128, 1996.
59. Huddart RA, Norman A, Shahidi M, et al: Cardiovascular disease as a long-term complication of treatment for testicular cancer. J Clin Oncol 21:1513-1523, 2003.
60. Travis L, Andersson M, Holowaty E, et al: Risk of leukemia following radiotherapy and chemotherapy for testicular cancer. J Clin Oncol 18:308a, 1999.
61. Travis LB, Curtis RE, Storm H, et al: Risk of second malignant neoplasms among long-term survivors of testicular cancer. J Natl Cancer Inst 89:1429-1439, 1997.
62. Travis LB, Andersson M, Gospodarowicz M, et al: Treatment-associated leukemia following testicular cancer. J Natl Cancer Inst 92:1165-1171, 2000.
63. Allhoff EP, Liedke S, de Riese W, et al: Stage I seminoma of the testis. Adjuvant radiotherapy or surveillance? Br J Urol 68:190-194, 1991.
64. Charig MJ, Hindley AC, Lloyd K, et al: 'Watch policy' in patients with suspected stage I testicular seminoma: CT as a sole staging and surveillance technique. Clin Radiol 42:40-41, 1990.
65. Germa Lluch JR, Climent MA, Villavicencio H, et al: Treatment of stage I testicular tumors. Br J Urol 71:473-477, 1993.
66. Oliver R, Lore S, Ong J: Alternatives to radiotherapy in the management of seminoma. Br J Urol 65:61-67, 1990.
67. Ramakrishnan S, Champion AE, Dorreen MS, et al: Stage I seminoma of the testis: is post-orchidectomy surveillance a safe alternative to routine postoperative radiotherapy? Clin Oncol 4:284-286, 1992.
68. Daugaard G, Petersen PM, Rorth M: Surveillance in stage I testicular cancer. APMIS 111:76-83; discussion 83-75, 2003.
69. Warde P, Gospodarowicz M, Panzarella T, et al: Surveillance is an appropriate management strategy in patients with stage I seminoma. Int J Radiat Oncol Biol Phys 54:61, 2002.
70. Chung P, Parker C, Panzarella T, et al: Surveillance in stage I testicular seminoma—risk of late relapse. Can J Urol 9:1637-1640, 2002.
71. Horwich A, Alsanjari N, A'Hern R, et al: Surveillance following orchidectomy for stage I testicular seminoma. Br J Cancer 65:775-778, 1992.
72. Warde P, Specht L, Masse H, et al: Prognostic factors for relapse in stage I seminoma managed by surveillance. J Urol 161:158, 1999.
73. Warde P, Specht L, Horwich A, et al: Prognostic factors for relapse in stage I seminoma managed by surveillance: a pooled analysis. J Clin Oncol 20:4448-4452, 2002.
74. Bayens YC, Helle PA, Van PW, et al: Orchidectomy followed by radiotherapy in 176 stage I and II testicular seminoma patients: benefits of a 10-year follow-up study. Radiother Oncol 25:97-102, 1992.
75. Coleman JM, Coleman RE, Turner AR, et al: The management and clinical course of testicular seminoma: 15 years' experience at a single institution. Clin Oncol (R Coll Radiol) 10:237-241, 1998.
76. Fossa SD, Horwich A, Russell JM, et al: Optimal planning target volume for stage I testicular seminoma: a Medical Research Council randomized trial. J Clin Oncol 17:1146-1154, 1999.
77. Hultenschmidt B, Budach V, Genters K, et al: Results of radiotherapy for 230 patients with stage I-II seminomas. Strahlenther Onkol 172:186-192, 1996.
78. Santoni R, Barbera F, Bertoni F, et al: Stage I seminoma of the testis: a bi-institutional retrospective analysis of patients treated with radiation therapy only. BJU Int 92:47-52; discussion 52, 2003.

79. Rathmell AJ, Mapstone NP, Jones WG: Testicular seminoma metastasizing to palatine tonsil. Clin Oncol 5:185-186, 1993.
80. Warde P, Gospodarowicz MK, Panzarella T, et al: Stage I testicular seminoma: results of adjuvant irradiation and surveillance. J Clin Oncol 13:2255-2262, 1995.
81. Logue JP, Harris MA, Liversusey JE, et al: Short course para-aortic radiation for stage I seminoma of the testis. Int J Radiat Oncol Biol Phys 57:1304-1309, 2003.
82. Oliver RT, Edmonds PM, Ong JY, et al: Pilot studies of 2 and 1 course carboplatin as adjuvant for stage I seminoma: should it be tested in a randomized trial against radiotherapy? Int J Radiat Oncol Biol Phys 29:3-8, 1994.
83. Oliver R, Mason M, von der Maase H, et al: A randomised comparison of single agent carboplatin with radiotherapy in the adjuvant treatment of stage I seminoma of the testis, following orchidectomy: MRC TE19/EORTC 30982. J Clin Oncol 22:386s, 2004.
84. Steiner H, Holtl L, Wirtenberger W, et al: Long-term experience with carboplatin monotherapy for clinical stage I seminoma: a retrospective single-center study. Urology 60:324-328, 2002.
85. Aparicio J, Garcia del Muro X, Maroto P, et al: Multicenter study evaluating a dual policy of postorchiectomy surveillance and selective adjuvant single-agent carboplatin for patients with clinical stage I seminoma. Ann Oncol 14:867-872, 2003.
86. Choo R, Sandler H, Warde P, et al: Survey of radiation oncologists: practice patterns of the management of stage I seminoma of testis in Canada and a selected group in the United States. Can J Urol 9:1479-1485, 2002.
87. Sobin LH, Wittekind CL, eds: International Union Against Cancer (UICC): TNM Classification of Malignant Tumors, 6th ed. New York, John Wiley & Sons, 2002.
88. Greene FL, Page DL, Fleming ID, et al, eds: AJCC Cancer Staging Manual, 6th ed. New York, Springer-Verlag, 2002.
89. Chung PW, Gospodarowicz MK, Panzarella T, et al: Stage II testicular seminoma: patterns of recurrence and outcome of treatment. Eur Urol 45:754-759; discussion 759-760, 2004.
90. Classen J, Schmidberger H, Meisner C, et al: Para-aortic irradiation for stage I testicular seminoma: results of a prospective study in 675 patients. A trial of the German Testicular Cancer Study Group (GTCSG). Br J Cancer 90:2305-2311, 2004.
91. Vallis KA, Howard GC, Duncan W, et al: Radiotherapy for stages I and II testicular seminoma: results and morbidity in 238 patients. Br J Radiol 68:400-405, 1995.
92. Zagars GK, Pollack A: Radiotherapy for stage II testicular seminoma. Int J Radiat Oncol Biol Phys 51:643-649, 2001.
93. Patterson H, Norman AR, Mitra SS, et al: Combination carboplatin and radiotherapy in the management of stage II testicular seminoma: comparison with radiotherapy treatment alone. Radiother Oncol 59:5-11, 2001.
94. Mosharafa AA, Foster RS, Leibovich BC, et al: Is post-chemotherapy resection of seminomatous elements associated with higher acute morbidity? J Urol 169:2126-2128, 2003.
95. De Santis M, Pont J: The role of positron emission tomography in germ cell cancer. World J Urol 22:41-46, 2004.
96. Ganjoo KN, Chan RJ, Sharma M, et al: Positron emission tomography scans in the evaluation of postchemotherapy residual masses in patients with seminoma. J Clin Oncol 17:3457-3460, 1999.
97. Herr HW, Sheinfeld J, Puc HS, et al: Surgery for a post-chemotherapy residual mass in seminoma. J Urol 157:860-862, 1997.
98. Culine S, Droz JP: Optimal management of residual mass after chemotherapy in advanced seminoma: there is time for everything. J Clin Oncol 14:2884-2885, 1996.
99. Horwich A, Paluchowska B, Norman A, et al: Residual mass following chemotherapy of seminoma. Ann Oncol 8:37-40, 1997.
100. Duchesne GM, Stenning SP, Aass N, et al: Radiotherapy after chemotherapy for metastatic seminoma—a diminishing role. Eur J Cancer 33:829-835, 1997.
101. Mencel PJ, Motzer RJ, Mazumdar M, et al: Advanced seminoma: treatment results, survival, and prognostic factors in 142 patients. J Clin Oncol 12:120-126, 1994.
102. Gholam D, Fizazi K, Terrier-Lacombe MJ, et al: Advanced seminoma—treatment results and prognostic factors for survival after first-line, cisplatin-based chemotherapy and for patients with recurrent disease: a single-institution experience in 145 patients. Cancer 98:745-752, 2003.
103. Kennedy B: Mithramycin therapy in advanced testicular neoplasms. Cancer 26:755-766, 1970.
104. Samuels M, Johnson E, Holoye P: Continuous infusion bleomycin therapy with vinblastine in stage III testicular neoplasms. Cancer Chemother Rep 59:563-570, 1975.
105. Vugrin D, Herr H, Whitmore WJ, et al: VAB-6 combination chemotherapy in disseminated cancer of the testis. Ann Intern Med 95:59-61, 1981.
106. Einhorn L, Donohue J: Cis-diammine dichloroplatinum, vinblastine + bleomycin combination chemotherapy in disseminated testicular cancer. Ann Intern Med 87:293-298, 1977.
107. Freedman LS, Parkinson MC, Jones WG, et al: Histopathology in the prediction of relapse of patients with stage I testicular teratoma treated by orchidectomy alone. Lancet 2:294-298, 1987.
108. Klepp O, Olsson AM, Henrikson H, et al: Prognostic factors in clinical stage I nonseminomatous germ cell tumors of the testis: multivariate analysis of a prospective multicenter study. Swedish-Norwegian Testicular Cancer Group. J Clin Oncol 8:509-518, 1990.
109. Jacobsen GK, Rorth M, Osterlind K, et al: Histopathological features in stage I non-seminomatous testicular germ cell tumors correlated to relapse. Danish Testicular Cancer Study Group. APMIS 98:377-382, 1990.
110. Nicolai N, Pizzocaro G: A surveillance study of clinical stage I nonseminomatous germ cell tumors of the testis: 10-year followup. J Urol 154:1045-1049, 1995.
111. Wishnow KI, Johnson DE, Swanson DA, et al: Identifying patients with low-risk clinical stage I nonseminomatous testicular tumors who should be treated by surveillance. Urology 34:339-343, 1989.
112. Freiha F, Torti F: Orchiectomy only for clinical stage I nonseminomatous germ cell testis tumors: comparison with pathologic stage I disease. Urology 34:347-348, 1989.
113. Peckham MJ, Brada M: Surveillance following orchidectomy for stage I testicular cancer. Int J Androl 10:247-254, 1987.
114. Raghavan D, Colls B, Levi J, et al: Surveillance for stage I nonseminomatous germ cell tumors of the testis: the optimal protocol has not yet been defined. Br J Urol 61:522-526, 1988.
115. Thompson PI, Nixon J, Harvey VJ: Disease relapse in patients with stage I nonseminomatous germ cell tumor of the testis on active surveillance. J Clin Oncol 6:1597-1603, 1988.
116. Sesterhenn IA, Weiss RB, Mostofi FK, et al: Prognosis and other clinical correlates of pathologic review in stage I and II testicular carcinoma: a report from the Testicular Cancer Intergroup Study. J Clin Oncol 10:69-78, 1992.
117. Pont J, Albrecht W, Postner G, et al: Adjuvant chemotherapy for high-risk clinical stage I nonseminomatous testicular germ cell cancer: long-term results of a prospective trial. J Clin Oncol 14:441-448, 1996.
118. Oliver R, Raja M, Ong J, et al: Pilot study to evaluate impact of a policy of adjuvant chemotherapy for high risk stage 1 malignant teratoma on overall relapse rate of stage 1 cancer patients. J Urol 148:1453-1455, 1992.
119. Cullen MH, Stenning SP, Parkinson MC, et al: Short-course adjuvant chemotherapy in high-risk stage I nonseminomatous germ cell tumors of the testis: a Medical Research Council report. J Clin Oncol 14:1106-1113, 1996.
120. Schefer H, Mattmann S, Borner M, et al: Single course adjuvant bleomycin, etoposide and cisplatin (BEP) for high risk stage I non-seminomatous germ cell tumors (NSGCT). Am Soc Clin Oncol 19:340a, 2000.
121. Donohue J, Thornhill J, Foster R, et al: Retroperitoneal lymphadenectomy for clinical stage A testis cancer (1965-1989): modifications of technique and impact on ejaculation. J Urol 149:237-243, 1993.
122. Jewett M: Nerve-sparing technique for retroperitoneal lymphadenectomy in testis cancer. Urol Clin North Am 17:449-459, 1990.
123. Vogelzang NJ, Fraley EE, Lange PH, et al: Stage II nonseminomatous testicular cancer: a 10-year experience. J Clin Oncol 1:171-178, 1983.

124. Richie JP, Kantoff PW: Is adjuvant chemotherapy necessary for patients with stage B1 testicular cancer? J Clin Oncol 9:1393, 1991.
125. Williams SD, Stablein DM, Einhorn LH, et al: Immediate adjuvant chemotherapy versus observation with treatment at relapse in pathological stage II testicular cancer. N Engl J Med 317:1433-1438, 1987.
126. Skinner DG, Scardino PT: Relevance of biochemical tumor markers and lymphadenectomy in management of nonseminomatous testis tumors: current perspective. J Urol 123:378-382, 1980.
127. Hartlapp JH, Weissbach L, Bussar-Maatz R: Adjuvant chemotherapy in nonseminomatous testicular tumor stage II. Int J Androl 10:277-284, 1987.
128. Pizzocaro G, Piva L, Salvioni R, et al: Adjuvant chemotherapy in resected stage II nonseminomatous germ cell tumors of the testis. In which cases is it necessary? Eur Urol 10:151-158, 1984.
129. Motzer R, Sheinfeld J, Mazumdar M, et al: Etoposide and cisplatin adjuvant therapy for patients with pathologic stage II germ cell tumors. J Clin Oncol 13:2700-2704, 1995.
130. Paulson D (ed): Staging and substaging of metastatic germ cell tumors using prognostic factors. Problems in Urology. Vol 8. Philadelphia, Lippincott, 1994, pp 76-86.
131. Sturgeon J, Alison R, Comisarow R, et al: Advanced nonseminomatous testicular tumors: maintenance chemotherapy is unnecessary. Proc AACR 21:610:153, 1980.
132. Einhorn L, Williams S, Troner M, et al: The role of maintenance therapy in disseminated testicular cancer. N Engl J Med 305:727-731, 1981.
133. Williams S, Birch R, Einhorn L, et al: Treatment of disseminated germ-cell tumors with cisplatin, bleomycin, and either vinblastine or etoposide. N Engl J Med 316:1435-1440, 1987.
134. Einhorn L, Williams S, Loehrer P, et al: Evaluation of optimal duration of chemotherapy in favorable-prognosis disseminated germ cell tumors: a Southeastern Cancer Study Group protocol. J Clin Oncol 7:387-391, 1989.
135. Bosl G, Geller N, Bajorin D, et al: A randomized trial of etoposide + cisplatin versus vinblastine + bleomycin + cisplatin + cyclophosphamide + dactinomycin in patients with good-prognosis germ cell tumors. J Clin Oncol 6:1231-1238, 1988.
136. Loehrer P Sr, Johnson D, Elson P, et al: Importance of bleomycin in favorable-prognosis disseminated germ cell tumors: an Eastern Cooperative Oncology Group trial. J Clin Oncol 13:470-476, 1995.
137. Culine S, Kerbrat P, Bouzy J, et al: The optimal chemotherapy regimen for good-risk metastatic non-seminomatous germ cell tumors (MNSGCT) is 3 cycles of bleomycin, etoposide and cisplatin: Mature results of a randomized trial. Am Soc Clin Oncol 22:382, 2003.
138. Bajorin D, Sarosdy M, Pfister D, et al: Randomized trial of etoposide and cisplatin versus etoposide and carboplatin in patients with good-risk germ cell tumors: a multiinstitutional study. J Clin Oncol 11:598-606, 1993.
139. Horwich A, Sleijfer DT, Fossa SD, et al: Randomized trial of bleomycin, etoposide, and cisplatin compared with bleomycin, etoposide, and carboplatin in good-prognosis metastatic nonseminomatous germ cell cancer: a Multiinstitutional Medical Research Council/European Organization for Research and Treatment of Cancer Trial. J Clin Oncol 15:1844-1852, 1997.
140. Motzer R, Bajorin D, Bosl G: "Poor-risk" germ cell tumors: current progress and future directions. Semin Oncol 19:206-214, 1992.
141. Nichols C, Williams S, Lehrer P, et al: Randomized study of cisplatin dose intensity in poor-risk germ cell tumors: a Southeastern Cancer Study Group and Southwest Oncology Group protocol. J Clin Oncol 9:1163-1172, 1991.
142. Ozols R, Ihde D, Linehan W, et al: A randomized trial of standard chemotherapy v a high-dose chemotherapy regimen in the treatment of poor prognosis nonseminomatous germ-cell tumors. J Clin Oncol 6:1031-1040, 1988.
143. Motzer RJ, Sheinfeld J, Mazumdar M, et al: Paclitaxel, ifosfamide, and cisplatin second-line therapy for patients with relapsed testicular germ cell cancer. J Clin Oncol 18:2413-2418, 2000.
144. Bokemeyer C, Gerl A, Schoffski P, et al: Gemcitabine in patients with relapsed or cisplatin-refractory testicular cancer. J Clin Oncol 17:512-516, 1999.
145. Kollmannsberger C, Rick O, Derigs HG, et al: Activity of oxaliplatin in patients with relapsed or cisplatin-refractory germ cell cancer: a study of the German Testicular Cancer Study Group. J Clin Oncol 20:2031-2037, 2002.
146. Motzer RJ, Mazumdar M, Sheinfeld J, et al: Sequential dose-intensive paclitaxel, ifosfamide, carboplatin, and etoposide salvage therapy for germ cell tumor patients. J Clin Oncol 18:1173-1180, 2000.
147. Rosti G, Pico J-L, Wandt H, et al: High-dose chemotherapy (HDC) in the salvage treatment of patients failing first-line platinum chemotherapy for advanced germ cell tumors (GCT): first results of a prospective randomised trial of the European Group for Blood and Marrow Transplantation (EBMT): IT-94 study. ASCO Annual Meeting 2002.
148. Einhorn L, Williams S, Mandelbaum I, et al: Surgical resection in disseminated testicular cancer following chemotherapeutic cytoreduction. Cancer 48:904-908, 1981.
149. Fox E, Weathers T, Williams S, et al: Outcome analysis for patients with persistent nonteratomatous germ cell tumor in postchemotherapy retroperitoneal lymph node dissections. J Clin Oncol 11:1294-1299, 1993.
150. Toner G, Panicek D, Heelan R, et al: Adjunctive surgery after chemotherapy for nonseminomatous germ cell tumors: recommendations for patient selection. J Clin Oncol 8:1683-1694, 1990.
151. Malas S, Sur RK, Levin V, et al: Toxicity in patients with testicular seminoma treated with radiotherapy. Different dose levels and treatment fields. Acta Oncol 35:201-206, 1996.
152. Yeoh E, Horowitz M, Russo A, et al: The effects of abdominal irradiation for seminoma of the testis on gastrointestinal function. J Gastroenterol Hepatol 10:125-130, 1995.
153. Fossa SD, Abyholm T, Normann N, et al: Post-treatment fertility in patients with testicular cancer. III. Influence of radiotherapy in seminoma patients. Br J Urol 58:315-319, 1986.
154. Senturia YD, Peckham CS, Peckham MJ: Children fathered by men treated for testicular cancer. Lancet 2:766-769, 1985.
155. Fossa S, Horwich A, Russell J, et al: Radiotherapy of seminoma stage I: optimal field size. A Medical Research Council (UK) study. *In* Jones W, Appleyard I, Harnden P, et al, eds: Germ Cell Tumors IV. The Proceedings of the Fourth Germ Cell Tumor Conference. Leeds, November 1997. London, John Libbey & Company Ltd., 1998, pp. 121-129.
156. Bieri S, Rouzaud M, Miralbell R: Seminoma of the testis: is scrotal shielding necessary when radiotherapy is limited to the para-aortic nodes? Radiother Oncol 50:349-353, 1999.
157. Stewart JR, Fajardo LF: Radiation induced heart disease: an update. Progr Cardiovasc Dis 28:173-194, 1984.
158. Corn BW, Trock BJ, Goodman RL: Irradiation-related ischemic heart disease. J Clin Oncol 8:741-750, 1990.
159. Hanks GE, Peters T, Owen J: Seminoma of the testis: long-term beneficial and deleterious results of radiation. Int J Radiat Oncol Biol Phys 24:913-919, 1992.
160. Horwich A: Radiotherapy in stage I seminoma of the testis. J Clin Oncol 22:585-588, 2004.
161. Moller H, Mellemgaard A, Jacobsen GK, et al: Incidence of second primary cancer following testicular cancer. Eur J Cancer 5:672-676, 1993.
162. van Leeuwen F, Stiggelbout AM, van den Belt-Dusebout AW, et al: Second cancer risk following testicular cancer: a follow-up study of 1,909 patients. J Clin Oncol 11:415-424, 1993.
163. Fossa SD, Aass N, Kaalhus O: Testicular cancer in young Norwegians. J Surg Oncol 39:43-63, 1988.
164. Kaasa S, Aass N, Mastekaasa A, et al: Psychosocial well-being in testicular cancer patients. Eur J Cancer 27:1091-1095, 1991.
165. Jonker-Pool G, Van de Wiel HB, Hoekstra HJ, et al: Sexual functioning after treatment for testicular cancer—review and meta-analysis of 36 empirical studies between 1975-2000. Arch Sex Behav 30:55-74, 2001.
166. Jonker-Pool G, Hoekstra HJ, van Imhoff GW, et al: Male sexuality after cancer treatment—needs for information and support: testicular cancer compared to malignant lymphoma. Patient Educ Couns 52:143-150, 2004.

167. Barrass BJ, Jones R, Graham JD, et al: Practical management issues in bilateral testicular cancer. BJU Int 93:1183-1187, 2004.
168. Boyer M, Raghavan D: Toxicity of treatment of germ cell tumors. Semin Oncol 19:128-142, 1992.
169. Prestayko A, D'Aoust J, Issell B, et al: Cisplatin (cis-diamminedichloroplatinum II). Cancer Treat Rev 6:17-39, 1979.
170. Vogelzang N, Bosl G, Johnson K, et al: Raynaud's phenomenon: a common toxicity after combination chemotherapy for testicular cancer. Ann Intern Med 95:288-292, 1981.
171. Comis R: Detecting bleomycin pulmonary toxicity: a continued conundrum. J Clin Oncol 8:765-767, 1990.
172. Aass N, Fossa S, Theodorsen L, et al: Prediction of long-term gonadal toxicity after standard treatment for testicular cancer. Eur J Cancer 27:1087-1091, 1991.
173. Papatsoris AG, Triantafyllidis A, Gekas A, et al: Leydig cell tumor of the testis. New cases and review of the current literature. Tumori 90:422-423, 2004.
174. Thrasher J, Frazier H: Non-germ cell testicular tumors. Probl Urol 8:167, 1994.
175. Mostofi F, Sobin L: International Histological Classification of Tumors of Testes. Geneva, World Health Organization, 1977.
176. Grem J, Robins H, Wilson K, et al: Metastatic Leydig cell tumor of the testis: report of three cases and review of the literature. Cancer 58:2116-2119, 1986.
177. Kim I, Young R, Scully R: Leydig cell tumors of the testis: a clinicopathological analysis of 40 cases and review of the literature. Am J Surg Pathol 9:177-192, 1985.
178. Peterson RO: Testis. *In* Urologic Pathology. Philadelphia, JB Lippincott, 1992, pp 487-491.
179. Giglio M, Medica M, De Rose AF, et al: Testicular Sertoli cell tumors and relative sub-types. Analysis of clinical and prognostic features. Urol Int 70:205-210, 2003.
180. Mann J, Pearson D: Results of the United Kingdom Children's Cancer Study Group's malignant germ cell tumor studies. Cancer 63:1657, 1989.
181. Bokemeyer C, Nichols CR, Droz JP, et al: Extragonadal germ cell tumors of the mediastinum and retroperitoneum: results from an international analysis. J Clin Oncol 20:1864-1873, 2002.
182. Chaganti R, Rodriguez E, Mathew S: Origin of adult male mediastinal germ-cell tumors. Lancet 343:1130, 1994.
183. Chaganti RS, Houldsworth J: Genetics and biology of adult human male germ cell tumors. Cancer Res 60:1475-1482, 2000.
184. Nichols C, Heerema N: Klinefelter's syndrome associated with mediastinal germ cell neoplasms. J Clin Oncol 5:1290, 1987.
185. Motzer RJ, Rodriguez E, Reuter VE, et al: Genetic analysis as an aid in diagnosis for patients with midline carcinomas of uncertain histologies. J Natl Cancer Inst 83:341-346, 1991.
186. Hartmann JT, Nichols CR, Droz JP, et al: Prognostic variables for response and outcome in patients with extragonadal germ-cell tumors. Ann Oncol 13:1017-1028, 2002.
187. Bower M, Brock C, Holden L, et al: POMB/ACE chemotherapy for mediastinal germ cell tumors. Eur J Cancer 33:838-842, 1997.
188. Bauer SB, Perlmutter AD, Retik AB: Anomalies of the upper urinary tract. *In* Walsh PC, Retik AB, Stamey TA, et al, eds.: Campell's Urology, 6th ed. Philadelphia, WB Saunders, 1992, pp 1357-1442.
189. Li FP, Fraumeni JF: Testicular cancers in children: epidemiologic characteristics. J Natl Cancer Inst 48:1575-1582, 1972.
190. Elyan SA, Reed DH, Ostrowski MJ, et al: Problems in the management of testicular seminoma associated with a horseshoe kidney. Clin Oncol 2:163-167, 1990.
191. Sogani PC, Whitmore W Jr: Retroperitoneal lymphadenectomy for germ cell tumor of testis in association with horseshoe kidney. Urology 18:446-452, 1981.
192. Key DW, Moyad R, Grossman HB: Seminoma associated with crossed fused renal ectopia. J Urol 143:1015-1016, 1990.
193. Evans CP, Tunuguntla HS, Saffarian AR, et al: Does retroperitoneal lymphadenectomy for testicular germ cell tumor require a different approach in the presence of horseshoe kidney? J Urol 169:503-506, 2003.
194. Tirelli U, Bernardi D, Spina M, et al: AIDS-related tumors: integrating antiviral and anticancer therapy. Crit Rev Oncol Hematol 41:299-315, 2002.
195. Powles T, Nelson M, Bower M: HIV-related testicular cancer. Int J STD AIDS 14:24-27, 2003.
196. Leibovitch I, Baniel J, Rowland RG, et al: Malignant testicular neoplasms in immunosuppressed patients. J Urol 155:1938-1942, 1996.
197. Powles T, Bower M, Shamash J, et al: Outcome of patients with HIV-related germ cell tumors: a case-control study. Br J Cancer 90:1526-1530, 2004.
198. Dahl O, Vagstad G, Iversen B: Cisplatin-based chemotherapy in a renal transplant recipient with metastatic germ cell testicular cancer. Acta Oncol 35:759-761, 1996.
199. Lindley C, Gordon T, Tremont S: Cisplatin-based chemotherapy in a renal transplant recipient. Cancer 68:1113, 1991.
200. Bokemeyer C, Schmoll HJ, Schoffski P, et al: Bilateral testicular tumors: prevalence and clinical implications. Eur J Cancer 6:874-876, 1993.
201. Osterlind A, Berthelsen JG, Abildgaard N, et al: Incidence of bilateral testicular germ cell cancer in Denmark, 1960-84: preliminary findings. Int J Androl 10:203-208, 1987.
202. Heidenreich A, Weissbach L, Holtl W, et al: Organ sparing surgery for malignant germ cell tumor of the testis. J Urol 166:2161-2165, 2001.
203. Rhoden EL, Morgentaler A: Risks of testosterone-replacement therapy and recommendations for monitoring. N Engl J Med 350:482-492, 2004.
204. Yossepowitch O, Baniel J: Role of organ-sparing surgery in germ cell tumors of the testis. Urology 63:421-427, 2004.
205. Fossa SD, Bokemeyer C, Gerl A, et al: Treatment outcome of patients with brain metastases from malignant germ cell tumors. Cancer 85:988-997, 1999.
206. Bokemeyer C, Nowak P, Haupt A, et al: Treatment of brain metastases in patients with testicular cancer. J Clin Oncol 15:1449-1454, 1997.
207. Pendlebury S, Horwich A, Dearnaley DP, et al: Spermatocytic seminoma: a clinicopathological review of ten patients. Clin Oncol 8:316-318, 1996.
208. Matoska J, Ondrus D, Hornak M: Metastatic spermatocytic seminoma. A case report with light microscopic, ultrastructural, and immunohistochemical findings. Cancer 62:1197-1201, 1988.
209. Chung PW, Bayley AJ, Sweet J, et al: Spermatocytic seminoma: a review. Eur Urol 45:495-498, 2004.
210. Fraass BA, Kinsella TJ, Harrington FS, et al: Peripheral dose to the testes: the design and clinical use of a practical and effective gonadal shield. Int J Radiat Oncol Biol Phys 11:609-615, 1985.
211. Jacobsen KD, Olsen DR, Fossa K, et al: External beam abdominal radiotherapy in patients with seminoma stage I: field type, testicular dose, and spermatogenesis. Int J Radiat Oncol Biol Phys 38:95-102, 1997.
212. Melchior D, Hammer P, Fimmers R, et al: Long term results and morbidity of para-aortic compared with para-aortic and iliac adjuvant radiation in clinical stage I seminoma. Anticancer Res 21:2989-2993, 2001.
213. Thomas GM: Is "optimal" radiation for stage I seminoma yet defined? J Clin Oncol 17:3004-3005, 1999.
214. Schmidberger H, Bamberg M, Meisner C, et al: Radiotherapy in stage IIA and IIB testicular seminoma with reduced portals: a prospective multicenter study. Int J Radiat Oncol Biol Phys 39:321-326, 1997.
215. Jones WG, Fossa SD, Mead GM, et al: Randomized trial of 30 versus 20 Gy in the adjuvant treatment of stage I testicular seminoma: a report on Medical Research Council Trial TE18, European Organisation for the Research and Treatment of Cancer Trial 30942 (ISRCTN18525328). J Clin Oncol 23:1200-1208, 2005.
216. Gurkaynak M, Akyol F, Zorlu F, et al: Stage I testicular seminoma: para-aortic and iliac irradiation with reduced dose after orchiectomy. Urol Int 71:385-388, 2003.
217. Dosoretz DE, Shipley WU, Blitzer PH, et al: Megavoltage irradiation for pure testicular seminoma: results and patterns of failure. Cancer 48:2184-2190, 1981.
218. Lester SG, Morphis J, Hornback NB: Testicular seminoma: analysis of treatment results and failures. Int J Radiat Oncol Biol Phys 12:353-358, 1986.

219. Chung PW, Warde PR, Panzarella T, et al: Appropriate radiation volume for stage IIA/B testicular seminoma. Int J Radiat Oncol Biol Phys 56:746-748, 2003.
220. Bagnell S, Choo R, Klotz LH, et al: Practice patterns of Canadian urologists in the management of stage I testicular seminoma. Can J Urol 11:2194-2199, 2004.
221. Sturgeon JFG: The status of surveillance in the management of stage 1 nonseminomatous testis tumors. Probl Urol 8:111-117, 1994.
222. Nicolai N, Pizzocaro G: A surveillance study of clinical stage I nonseminomatous germ cell tumors of the testis: 10-year followup. J Urol 154:1045-1049, 1995.
223. Sogani PC, Perrotti M, Herr HW, et al: Clinical stage I testis cancer: long-term outcome of patients on surveillance. J Urol 159:855-858, 1998.

CHAPTER 53

KIDNEY AND URETERAL CARCINOMA

Steven J. Buskirk, William W. Wong, Michael G. Haddock,
Alexander S. Parker, Winston W. Tan, and Michael J. Wehle

INCIDENCE

The American Cancer Society estimated that there were 38,890 new cases of carcinoma of the kidney and renal pelvis and 12,840 deaths, as well as 2430 new cases of ureter cancer and 770 deaths in 2006.

BIOLOGIC CHARACTERISTICS

Historically, factors predicting outcomes for patients with cancer of the kidney have included tumor stage, nuclear and Fuhrman grades, tumor size, extension through the renal capsule, nodal involvement, renal vein involvement, histologic pattern, and presence of necrosis. Several independent groups have combined individual prognostic factors into multivariate scoring algorithms that possess a higher degree of ability for predicting outcome. Molecular markers are not widely used to predict outcome.

For renal pelvis or ureter cancer, the most important prognostic factors for survival are stage (i.e., reflects local extent of disease and regional lymph node involvement) and histologic grade of the tumor.

STAGING EVALUATION

Evaluation of the patient with kidney cancer should include a history and physical examination, complete blood cell count, liver chemistries, urinalysis, chest radiograph, intravenous pyelography, computed tomography of the abdomen and pelvis, and bone scan.

Magnetic resonance angiography may be used in some cases for preoperative mapping of the vasculature.

Evaluation of the patient with renal pelvis or ureter cancer should include a history and physical examination, complete blood cell count, liver chemistries, urinalysis, urine cytology, chest radiograph, intravenous pyelography, and computed tomography of the abdomen and pelvis. Cystoscopy and ureteroscopy are needed to rule out synchronous lesions in the remainder of the urothelial tract.

PRIMARY THERAPY

Surgical resection (i.e., partial or radical nephrectomy) is the primary treatment for renal cell carcinoma. The 5-year survival rate is about 90% for patients with tumor confined to the kidney, about 60% if it has spread only to nearby tissues, and about 9% if it has spread to distant sites.

Nephroureterectomy with resection of a bladder cuff at the ureterovesical junction is standard therapy for resectable tumors of the renal pelvis and ureter. Survival rates are 60% to 80% or more for minimally invasive disease, 20% to 30% for deeply invasive disease, and 10% to 15% for cases involving the regional lymphatics. More conservative nephron-sparing surgery is an option for patients with small, solitary, low-grade, and low-stage disease.

ADJUVANT THERAPY

Adjuvant therapy for renal cancer is selectively indicated on the basis of failure patterns and survival results with surgery alone. Patients who undergo a gross total resection of tumor have a low risk for local failure and moderate risk for distant metastases.

There is no proven adjuvant role for radiation therapy, chemotherapy, immunotherapy, or molecularly targeted treatment as part of the primary management for patients with localized renal cancer.

Patients with renal pelvis and ureteral carcinomas that are high grade or locally advanced or have lymph node involvement are at significant risk for distant metastases and locoregional relapse. Adjuvant radiation therapy decreases local failure rates and may be given with or without concomitant and adjuvant chemotherapy.

LOCALLY ADVANCED DISEASE

For renal cancer, a combined treatment consisting of preoperative external beam irradiation and cytoreductive surgical resection with or without intraoperative irradiation has the greatest potential for local control of disease.

For patients who have locally advanced or unresectable renal pelvis and ureteral carcinoma at presentation, combined radiation therapy and chemotherapy or radiation therapy alone can palliate local symptoms. If there is adequate downstaging of disease, resection may be feasible and lead to long-term, disease-free survival for some patients.

PALLIATION

Nephrectomy can be used to alleviate local symptoms of renal cancer. Radiation therapy is effective in palliating painful bone metastases and in alleviating the symptoms of brain metastases. Systemic treatment with chemotherapy, hormone therapy, immunotherapy, and molecularly targeted treatment provides response rates of up to 20%, but these methods have not affected survival.

For metastatic renal pelvis and ureter cancer, objective response rates of 50% to 70% are achieved with systemic chemotherapy regimens. Radiation therapy provides palliation of local symptoms in most patients and improves their quality of life.

INTRODUCTION

Kidney

Renal cell carcinoma (RCC), also called hypernephroma or Growitz's tumor, was first reported by Konig in 1826.[1] In 1883, Growitz observed that the fatty content of RCC was similar to that of adrenal cells. He therefore postulated that these tumors arose from adrenal rests within the kidney.[2] In 1894, Birch-Hirschfel first used the term *hypernephroid* to describe these tumors. This description led to the commonly used term *hypernephroma*.[1]

RCC has diverse clinical manifestations, and surgery continues to be the primary treatment modality. RCC appears to be more resistant to radiation therapy and chemotherapy than most epithelial tumors.[1] Immunomodulation and molecularly targeted treatment may have a potential role in the systemic treatment of this disease.[3,4]

Renal Pelvis and Ureter

Primary cancers of the renal pelvis and ureter are uncommon. Most published reports are retrospective studies with relatively small numbers of patients. Surgery is the primary treatment for these patients. Standard surgery includes a nephroureterectomy with removal of the bladder cuff. In selected patients, more conservative surgery provides acceptable results. However, for patients with adverse prognostic factors such as high-grade tumor or advanced-stage disease, the prognosis remains poor. Chemotherapy and radiation therapy as adjuvant or primary treatment for selected patients may improve treatment outcome, and their roles need to be better defined.

ETIOLOGY AND EPIDEMIOLOGY

Kidney

Etiology

A number of risk factors have been implicated in the development of RCC. Given the paucity of data from cohort studies focusing on RCC, most of the information regarding these risk factors has come from case-control investigations. The only widely accepted risk factors for RCC are cigarette smoking and obesity.[5,6] Each of these factors is believed to increase the risk of developing RCC by approximately twofold. There is also some evidence to support hypertension as a third major risk factor; however, the effects of hypertension on RCC development are difficult to disentangle from its well-known association with smoking and obesity.[5] Population-attributable risk estimates suggest that roughly one half of all cases of RCC diagnosed in the United States can be attributed to smoking, obesity, or hypertension.[7] Other factors shown to increase the risk for RCC include a positive family history,[8] phenacetin use,[9] diets high in red meat,[10] a history of urinary tract infections,[11] reproductive factors related to exposure to high levels of endogenous estrogen,[12,13] exposure to Thoratrast,[14] and a variety of occupational exposures, including organic solvents, petroleum products, heavy metals, and asbestos.[15] Conversely, factors such as diets high in fruits and vegetables,[10] moderate alcohol intake,[16] and physical activity[13] are associated with a decreased risk for RCC. The role of these factors in protecting against the development of RCC remains unclear and will require independent confirmation in future studies.

Epidemiology

Kidney cancer accounts for approximately 3% of new cancer cases and 3% of cancer deaths in the United States each year. More than 90% of kidney cancers among adults are classified as RCC.[17] In 2006, the American Cancer Society estimated that approximately 38,890 new cases of RCC would be diagnosed in the United States and approximately 12,840 deaths would be attributed to RCC.[17,18] According to data from the National Cancer Institute's Surveillance, Epidemiology, and End Results (SEER) program, the overall incidence of RCC in the United States has increased at a rate of 2% per year since the early 1970s.[19] Moreover, it has been suggested that early detection of subclinical tumors by increased abdominal imaging cannot fully explain the rising incidence of RCC.[19,20]

RCC is typically diagnosed in the seventh decade of life (median age at diagnosis is 65 years), but it has been observed in children as young as 6 months.[1] Incidence rates for RCC are higher among men (15.7 per 100,000) than women (7.8 per 100,000) but very similar between whites and blacks.[18] Globally, the incidence of RCC is highest in developed countries and shows considerable variability worldwide. The highest rates are reported in North America and Scandinavia, and the lowest rates are reported in Asia and South America.[21]

Renal Pelvis and Ureter

Etiology

Patients with carcinomas of the renal pelvis and ureter have a 30% to 50% risk of developing metachronous or synchronous bladder cancer, whereas the risk of developing upper urinary tract malignancy after treatment of superficial bladder cancer is up to 9.8% in one report.[22] The same risk factors and environmental agents that cause bladder cancers appear to play significant roles in the development of upper urinary tract cancers.

There is a strong association between cigarette smoking and the development of renal and ureter carcinomas. Population-based case-control studies have demonstrated a significant increase in risk of these cancers in smokers.[23-26] Smokers have 2.6- to 7.2-fold increased risk, and the relative risk is proportional to the amount of cigarettes consumed. It is estimated that 40% to 70% of these cancers can be attributed to cigarette smoking.

Other etiologic agents have been implicated. Habitual use of analgesics that contain phenacetin has been implicated as a cause of renal pelvis and ureter cancers.[27-29] Capillarosclerosis is a pathognomonic change seen in patients with long-standing abuse of compound analgesics.[29] The histologic grade of renal pelvic tumors has been shown to increase in a dose-dependent fashion with phenacetin consumption.[30] Ingestion of Chinese herbs containing *Aristolochia fangchi*, which is used for weight reduction, results in a nephropathy characterized by progressive renal fibrosis and increased risk of developing urothelial cancers.[31,32] There is a 57- to 100-fold increase in the incidence of renal pelvis and ureter cancers in Balkan countries affected by an endemic nephropathy.[33,34] The renal pathology is an interstitial nephritis. The cause of the endemic nephropathy is postulated to be related to high concentrations of radon and minerals in the drinking water in the area. In a Swedish population-based cohort study, patients with a history of kidney or ureteral stones have a 2.5-fold increase in the risk of renal and ureter cancers, suggesting that chronic irritation and infection may play a role.[35] Occupational exposure to organic chemicals has been associated with a higher risk of developing upper urinary tract urothelial cancers for workers in the chemical, petrochemical, or plastics industries.[23] There are reports of kindreds with familial urothelial cancers of the upper urinary tract.[36,37] Families with Lynch syndrome II also have an increased risk of these malignancies.[38]

Epidemiology

Based on data from the SEER program, the age-adjusted annual incidence of renal pelvic and ureter cancers is 0.73 to 1.15 cases per 100,000 person-years.[39] These cancers represent about 5% to 7% of all urinary tract tumors.[40] The incidence increases with age, with the peak age at diagnosis in the sixth and seventh decades of life. There is a male predominance of cases, and the incidence of upper urinary tract urothelial cancers has increased in recent years.[41]

PREVENTION AND EARLY DETECTION

Kidney

Cessation of cigarette smoking is the most effective method of preventing RCC. Investigators using data from a large case-control investigation in Iowa reported that the risk of RCC development decreases steadily from the point of smoking cessation. Moreover, 15 years from the point of cessation, the risk of developing RCC returns to that of someone who never smoked cigarettes.[42] It is unclear whether reductions in weight translate to a reduction in risk for RCC because inquiries into this matter have only recently been initiated. Similarly, there is some indication that daily moderate alcohol consumption and physical activity reduce the risk of RCC development[13,16]; but further confirmatory investigations are required. Avoiding phenacetin-containing analgesics and exposure to heavy metals and asbestos may help to prevent the disease.[3]

Because the tumor usually remains clinically occult for many years, RCC is a challenging diagnosis. Over the past 3 decades, the percentage of patients presenting with the classic triad of flank pain, hematuria, and a palpable mass has dropped to less than 10%. Between 25% and 39% of patients with RCC are asymptomatic at the time of diagnosis.[43]

Early detection of RCC has been dramatically enhanced by the increased use of imaging modalities, including computed tomography (CT) and ultrasonography.[44] Tumors are being discovered at earlier stages in the disease process, which should ultimately translate to improved probability of surgical cure and better patient outcomes.[3]

Renal Pelvis and Ureter

The risk of renal and ureter cancers is significantly reduced in smokers by smoking cessation, with the reduction in risk correlating with the time of quitting cigarette smoking.[25] A case-control study in Japan suggests frequent intake of green and yellow vegetables can also decrease the risk of urothelial cancers.[45] There is no known intervention that can prevent future development of metachronous lesions of the urothelial tract after a primary tumor has been diagnosed.

The role of routine urine cytology as a screening test is unclear, even in the population at increased risk of developing these cancers (e.g., heavy smokers, workers in petrochemical industries). For patients with a history of bladder cancer, screening of the upper urinary tract is often advocated. However, the use of screening intravenous pyelogram (IVP) is controversial in this setting.[46] Urine cytology should be done on a regular basis for these patients.

PATHOLOGY AND PATHWAYS OF SPREAD

Kidney

Pathology

In 1997, an international consensus conference on RCC sponsored by the Union Internationale Contre le Cancer (UICC) and the American Joint Committee on Cancer (AJCC) outlined recommendations for the classification of RCC.[47] The UICC/AJCC adopted the classification system originally proposed at the Heidelberg conference in 1996.[48] The participants at both conferences proposed that RCC be categorized as clear cell, papillary, chromophobe, or collecting duct RCC subtypes. RCC that does not fall into one of these four groups is classified as RCC, not otherwise specified. Granular cell RCC was considered an ambiguous term not specific to a single subtype because it encompassed oncocytoma (i.e., benign kidney tumor) and chromophobe and clear cell RCCs. The UICC/AJCC and Heidelberg classification no longer includes the granular cell RCC subtype. This classification system recognizes that RCC consists of several histologic subtypes with distinct morphologic and genetic characteristics. Previous reports have demonstrated significant differences in patient outcome by histologic subtype using the UICC/AJCC and Heidelberg classification.[49-51] Patients with clear cell RCC have a worse prognosis compared with patients with papillary and chromophobe RCC, although there does not appear to be a statistically significant difference in outcome between patients with papillary and chromophobe RCC.[52] Features predictive of outcome, particularly histologic tumor necrosis, have been shown to differ by subtype.[50,52,53]

Pathways of Spread

RCC may spread by local extension through the renal capsule into the perinephric fat or the adrenal gland[54] or by direct extension through the renal vein to the inferior vena cava (occasionally reaching the right atrium).[3] Lymphatic drainage is to the renal hilar, para-aortic, and paracaval lymph nodes.[54] RCC may also spread by bloodborne metastasis to the lung[3] or by retrograde venous drainage to the ovary or testis.[54]

Renal Pelvis and Ureter

Pathology

The most common type of renal pelvis and ureter cancers is transitional cell carcinoma.[55,56] Squamous cell carcinoma accounts for 5% to 8% of the cases.[57] Other cell types such as adenocarcinomas or sarcomas are uncommon.

Pathways of Spread

Synchronous or metasynchronous involvement of multiple areas of the urothelial epithelium by transitional cell carcinoma is common in patients with renal pelvis and ureter cancers. This finding provides support for the theory that the entire urothelial epithelium is affected by carcinogens, resulting in a field defect.[56,58] As the tumor progresses, it invades the surrounding tissues with direct extension through the ureteral wall into periureteral tissues or to adjacent renal parenchyma and extrarenal tissues. Lymph node metastasis is the most common site of metastasis in cancer of the upper urinary tract.[55,59] Nodal metastasis usually occurs near or superior to the primary tumor site, involving the periaortic or pericaval lymph nodes and the renal hilar nodes. In patients with high-grade or high-stage disease, the risk of lymph node metastasis is as high as 60%, whereas the risk is 0% to 10% for patients with low-grade or low-stage disease.[60,61] The finding of lymph vessel invasion in the tumor is predictive of regional lymph node metastasis.[62] Lymph node metastasis is a good predictor for the development of distant metastasis.[55,63] Patients with high-grade or advanced-stage disease are also at significant risk of developing distant metastasis.

The most common sites of distant failure are lung, liver, and bone.

BIOLOGIC CHARACTERISTICS AND MOLECULAR BIOLOGY

Kidney

Similar to cancers of the breast, prostate, and colon, RCC occurs in familial and sporadic forms. Much of our understanding of the genetic basis and underlying biology of RCC has come from investigations of the hereditary forms of this tumor, with the hope that identifying the genes for the hereditary forms of renal carcinoma might lead to the genes for the common forms of sporadic RCC. Several hereditary syndromes are associated with the development of RCC, including von Hippel-Lindau (VHL) syndrome, tuberous sclerosis, hereditary papillary renal carcinoma (HPRC), Britt Hogg-Dubé (BHD) syndrome, and hereditary renal carcinoma.[64] VHL syndrome, an autosomal dominant disorder affecting 1 in 40,000 individuals, is caused by a mutation of the *VHL* tumor suppressor gene located on chromosome 3p. Silencing of the *VHL* gene by somatic mutation or hypermethylation is thought to play a role in 50% to 60% of sporadic clear cell RCC.[65] Tuberous sclerosis is an autosomal dominant disorder affecting 1 in 10,000 individuals, and it results from mutations of the *TSC1* gene on chromosome 9q or the *TSC2* gene on chromosome 6p.[66] Hereditary papillary renal carcinoma is also an autosomal dominant disorder. Patients develop bilateral, multifocal lesions with associated germline mutations of the *MET* proto-oncogene located on chromosome 7q.[67] BHD is a dominantly inherited predisposition to benign fibrofolliculomas and other skin and soft tissue tumors, including RCC. The gene for BHD *(FLCN)* has been mapped to chromosome 17p12-q11.2.[68]

The past decade has seen the emergence of high-throughput gene expression profiling as a means of improving our understanding of the genetic basis of cancer,[69] including RCC.[70-72] A number of novel candidate genes in addition to *VHL* have been implicated in the initiation, development, and progression of RCC. Specific genes that have been shown to have a role in renal carcinogenesis include the *FHIT* and *RASSF1* tumor suppressor genes,[73,74] several forms of *TGFBR* for the transforming growth factor-β receptor,[75] forms of *HIF* for hypoxia-inducible factors,[76] *PTEN*,[77] *VEGF* for vascular endothelial growth factor,[78] and forms for carbonic anhydrases.[79] Other genes that have been investigated but for which the data suggest little involvement in RCC include those for E-cadherin, *TP53*,[80,81] *BCL2*, retinoblastoma *(RB1)*, *MYC*,[82] and *ERBB2*.[83]

Renal Pelvis and Ureter

The available data show that the karyotypic abnormalities in these tumors are similar to those in bladder cancers. Loss of the entire chromosome or partial loss of the short arm of chromosome 9 is a common finding, suggesting that it may be an early pathogenetically important event in tumorigeneis.[84,85] Overexpression of TP53, cyclin E, and cyclin A is seen in many tumors and is associated with a worse prognosis.[86-88] Tumors in patients with hereditary nonpolyposis colorectal cancer syndrome are characterized by mutations in a number of DNA mismatch repair genes that are detectable as microsatellite instability.[89]

CLINICAL MANIFESTATIONS, PATIENT EVALUATION, AND STAGING

Kidney

Clinical Manifestations

Patients with RCC have multiple presenting signs and symptoms that are usually caused by local extension or metastatic disease.[44] Because of these multiple symptoms, RCC has been called the *internist's tumor*.[3] Symptoms resulting from local tumor extension include hematuria, abdominal pain, and a flank mass.[44] However, the simultaneous presentation of this classic triad occurs in only about 10% of cases.[3,44] Symptoms caused by metastatic disease include fever, weight loss, and night sweats.[44] Two percent of male patients present with a varicocele, usually left sided, as a result of impaired drainage of the testicular vein.[90] Paraneoplastic syndromes occur in about 30% of patients with RCC. Symptoms include hypertension, hypercalcemia, pyrexia, and hepatic dysfunction.[91,92]

Patient Evaluation

During the past 20 years, the widespread use of CT, magnetic resonance imaging (MRI), and ultrasonography to evaluate the upper abdomen has significantly increased the incidental finding of RCC.[93,94] Between 25% and 40% of diagnoses are made after the incidental detection of a renal mass.[93-95] These tumors usually are smaller and are therefore more likely to be associated with surgical cure.[94-96]

After RCC has been diagnosed, patients should undergo further evaluation and staging (Table 53-1), including a history and physical examination, complete blood cell count, serum chemistries, urinalysis, chest radiograph, IVP, CT, and a bone scan. CT can predict tumor extent preoperatively in 90% of cases.[97] MRI with gadolinium is superior to CT in determining inferior vena cava tumor extent.[98] Magnetic resonance angiography can be used to evaluate vasculature preoperatively, especially when nephron-sparing surgery (NSS) is being considered for patients with bilateral cancers.

Staging

Two staging systems are used to define disease extent in RCC. Historically, Robson's modification of the Flocks and Kadesky system was used.[99] More recently, the American Joint

Table 53-1 Patient Evaluation for Kidney and Ureteral Carcinoma

COMPLETE HISTORY AND PHYSICAL EXAMINATION
Laboratory tests
Complete blood cell count
Serum chemistries
Urinalysis

RADIOLOGIC STUDIES
Chest radiograph
Chest computed tomography (optional)
Intravenous pyelography
Computed tomography of the abdomen and pelvis
Bone scan

SELECTED ADDITIONAL STUDIES
Ultrasonography (kidney)
Magnetic resonance imaging with intravenous gadolinium of the abdomen (kidney)
Magnetic resonance angiography (kidney)

Committee on Cancer Staging and End Results Reporting Classification has been used (Table 53-2).[100] This system appears to be superior to the Robson system because it delineates more clearly local tumor extent and quantifies lymph node involvement.[44]

Renal Pelvis and Ureter

Clinical Manifestations

About 75% to 80% of patients present with gross or microscopic hematuria, and 35% to 45% have flank pain.[55,58,101] The pain may mimic that of ureteral calculus. Urinary symptoms such as frequency and dysuria are reported in 25% to 50% of patients. A palpable mass may be found in up to 10% of patients, and it is usually a hydronephrotic kidney. Constitutional symptoms such as malaise and weight loss are frequently seen in patients with extensive disease or metastases.

Patient Evaluation

Patients are evaluated with urine cytology, IVP, and ureteroscopy. Cytology of voided urine detects 35% to 59% of upper urinary tract transitional carcinomas and is more useful for detecting higher-grade cancers.[102] The positive yield is improved with urine specimens obtained by ureteral catheterization or by washings of the upper urinary tract. The positive predictive value of renal pelvis washing for high-grade cancer is 93%, but it is only 43% for low-grade cancer.[103,104] IVP findings for these tumors include a radiolucent filling defect or obstructive hydronephrosis. Ureteroscopy or percutaneous nephroscopy is performed if exfoliative cytology or IVP has suspicious findings. Ureteroscopic biopsy provides the tissue diagnosis of upper tract urothelial cancer in up to 89% of cases.[105]

After the diagnosis has been made, additional studies should be performed to evaluate the stage of disease. These studies include a complete blood cell count, chemistries, and a chest radiograph or chest CT. CT of the abdomen and pelvis is useful to demonstrate the local extent of disease and intra-abdominal metastasis, although it is not a sensitive or specific test for nodal staging.[106]

Staging

The current tumor-node-metastasis (TNM) staging system is listed in Table 53-2.[100] Another staging system that is often used is the Jewett-Strong classification, which was originally used for bladder cancer: stage 0, limited to the mucosa; stage A, submucosal infiltration; stage B, invasion into but not through the muscle wall; stage C, invasion through the wall; stage D, lymphatic or distant metastasis.[55,107] Tumor grade has a strong association with disease stage (Table 53-3). Stage and tumor grade are important prognostic factors for survival.[59,101,107-109] Table 53-4 illustrates the impact of stage and grade on overall survival.

Table 53-2 **2002 American Joint Committee on Cancer Staging Classification System for Kidney and Ureteral Carcinoma**

Stage	Description
PRIMARY TUMOR (T)	
TX	Primary tumor cannot be assessed
T0	No evidence of primary tumor
KIDNEY	
T1	Tumor 7 cm or less in greatest dimension, limited to the kidney
T1a	Tumor 4 cm or less in greatest dimension, limited to the kidney
T1b	Tumor more than 4 cm but not more than 7 cm in greatest dimension, limited to the kidney
T2	Tumor more than 7 cm in greatest dimension, limited to the kidney
T3	Tumor extends into major veins or invades adrenal gland or perinephric tissues but not beyond Gerota's fascia
T3a	Tumor invades adrenal gland or perinephric tissue but not beyond Gerota's fascia
T3b	Tumor grossly extends into renal vein(s) or its segmental muscle containing branches, or invades the wall of the vena cava below the diaphragm
T3c	Tumor grossly extends into the vena cava above the diaphragm
T4	Tumor invades beyond Gerota's fascia
URETERAL-RENAL PELVIS	
Ta	Papillary noninvasive carcinoma
Tis	Carcinoma in situ
T1	Tumor invades subepithelial connective tissue
T2	Tumor invades muscularis
T3	Renal pelvis only: tumor invades beyond muscularis into peripelvic fat or renal parenchyma
T3	Ureter only: tumor invades beyond muscularis into periureteric fat
T4	Tumor invades adjacent organs or through kidney into perinephric fat
REGIONAL LYMPH NODE (N)*	
NX	Regional lymph nodes cannot be assessed
N0	No regional lymph node metastasis
N1	Metastasis in a single regional lymph node (ureteral-pelvis: 2 cm or less in greatest dimension)
N2	Metastasis in a single lymph node, more than 2 cm but not more than 5 cm in greatest dimension; or multiple lymph nodes, none more than 5 cm in greatest dimension
N3	Metastasis in a lymph node more than 5 cm in greatest dimension
DISTANT METASTASIS (M)	
MX	Distant metastasis cannot be assessed
M0	No distant metastasis
M1	Distant metastasis
STAGE GROUPINGS, RENAL AND URETERAL	
0a	Ta N0 M0
0is	Tis N0 M0
I	T1 N0 M0
II	T2 N0 M0
III	T3 N0 M0
IV	T4 N0 M0
	Any T N1-3 M0
	Any T Any N M1

*Laterality does not affect the N classification.

From Greene F, Page DL, Fleming ID, et al (eds): AJCC Cancer Staging Manual, 6th ed. Philadelphia, Springer, 2002.

PRIMARY THERAPY

Kidney

Surgery

Surgical resection is the only possible curative treatment for RCC. In 1883, Growitz[110] performed the first successful nephrectomy as treatment for RCC. Mortensen reported the first radical nephrectomy in 1948, although simple nephrectomy remained the primary surgical treatment until the early 1960s.[3,111] Robson described removing the kidney with its perirenal fat, regional lymph nodes, and ipsilateral adrenal gland.[112] Because of the concern about potential tumor exten-

Table 53-3 Correlation between Tumor Grade and Stage of Disease for Renal Pelvis and Ureter Cancer

	Stage (%) Rubenstein et al[107]				Stage (%) Heney et al[108]					Stage (%) Corrado et al[109]				
Grade	*A*	*B*	*C*	*D*	*0*	*A*	*B*	*C*	*D*	*0*	*A*	*B*	*C*	*D*
I	77	23	0	0	100	0	0	0	0	50	50	0	0	0
II	47	33	7	13	23	42	19	4	12	2	64	13	13	8
III	13	13	41	33	4	8	17	33	38	0	28	16	24	32
IV	8	33	50	8	—	—	—	—	—	0	0	13	25	62

Table 53-4 Renal Pelvic and Ureteral Carcinoma: Five-Year Survival Rates Categorized by Stage and Grade

	Survival by Stage (%)					Survival by Grade (%)			
Study	*N*	*I or A*	*II or B*	*III or C*	*IV or D*	*1*	*2*	*3*	*4*
Ozsahin et al[59]	138	45	61	15	16	67	52	16	—
Bloom et al[101]	54	62	25	33	0	83	52	18	13
Rubenstein et al[107]	70	72	64	33	0	90	56	40	11
Heney et al[108]	60	95	82	29	0	100	81	29	—
Corrado et al[109]	92	83	72	51	16	83	75	52	0

Table 53-5 Survival Rates after Radical Nephrectomy for Renal Cell Carcinoma

			Survival by Stage (%)			
Study	No. of Patients	Length of Survival (y)	*I*	*II*	*III*	*IV*
Robson et al[99] (1969)	88	5	66	64	42	11
		10	60	67	38	0
Skinner et al[113] (1971)	309	5	65	47	51	8
		10	56	20	37	7
McNichols et al[114] (1981)	506	5	67	51	34	14
		10	56	28	20	3
Selli et al[115] (1983)	115	5	93	63	80	13
Golimbu et al[116] (1986)	326	5	88	67	40	2
		10	66	35	15	—
Dinney et al[117] (1992)	314	5	73	68	51	20

sion through the renal capsule into the perinephric fat or to the ipsilateral adrenal gland, radical nephrectomy eventually became the standard surgical treatment.[44] Survival results for treatment with standard open radical nephrectomy are delineated in Table 53-5.[99,113-117]

Upper pole cancers may necessitate adrenal gland removal with nephrectomy, depending on the size, pathologic type, and extent of invasion of the renal tumor, but this is rarely indicated for middle or lower pole cancers. Preoperative CT has demonstrated 99.6% specificity and a 94.4% negative predictive value for adrenal gland involvement.[118,119] In a review of 511 radical nephrectomies with adrenal gland removal, the incidence of renal cancer involvement with the adrenal was 5.7%. In examining the specimens by stage, T1-2 tumors had an incidence of adrenal involvement of 0.6%.[118]

Radical nephrectomy often includes resection of hilar lymph nodes and occasionally includes regional lymph node dissection.[44] Although regional lymph node dissection provides additional prognostic information, it has not been proved to prolong survival.[44] The Mayo Clinic reviewed 955 patients who underwent a lymph node dissection as part of a radical nephrectomy. Multivariate analysis demonstrated that high-grade tumor, presence of sarcomatoid features, tumor size greater than or equal to 10 cm, stage T3, and histologic tissue necrosis were significant predictors of lymph node–positive disease. The investigators concluded that these high-risk factors could be considered in deciding which patients might benefit from an extensive lymph node dissection during the radical nephrectomy.[120]

The risk of local failure after radical nephrectomy is approximately 5% for patients who have had a gross total resection of all tumor.[121] Prognostic factors having a significant impact on local failure include disease-positive surgical margins and positive lymph nodes.[121]

The risk of distant metastasis after gross resection of all tumor is approximately 26%.[121] Lymph node involvement, pathologic tumor type, and renal vein involvement significantly affect the incidence of distant metastases.[121]

Partial nephrectomy (NSS) has been performed to treat small tumors. The initial indications for this surgery are presence of bilateral tumors or a cancer involving an anatomic or functional solitary kidney.[44] Because of the low incidence (<6%) of local recurrence in patients who underwent partial nephrectomy for these significant indications, this procedure has been extended to include patients with small tumors (<4 cm).[122] The incidence of local recurrence in these "electively" treated patients is 3% or less.[122] Recent data from several institutions suggest larger tumors (7 cm) can also be considered for NSS.[123,124] The trend to perform NSS is fostered by the fact that patients undergoing NSS had a decreased cumulative incidence of chronic renal insufficiency compared with patients who underwent radical nephrectomy.[125,126]

Laparoscopic radical nephrectomy has become a popular surgical approach for patients with renal carcinoma. Data indicate that pure and hand-assisted laparoscopic radical nephrectomy compares with the standard open approach in oncologic control.[127-129] Both laparoscopic approaches have demonstrated advantages regarding blood loss, length of hospital stay, pain medication use, cosmesis, and patient recovery compared with the standard open approach of radical nephrectomy.[127,128] The rationale for and uses of laparoscopic partial nephrectomy continue to expand. With the increase in detection of small incidental renal masses, the development of minimally invasive procedures as a surgical therapy has emerged.

Radiofrequency heating, cryosurgical freezing, and other techniques to obliterate suspicious small renal lesions have been reported in clinical trials.[130,131] These techniques have been employed through open, laparoscopic, and percutaneous approaches.[130-132] Larger clinical trials and longer follow-up periods will be necessary to determine the role of minimally invasive techniques in surgical management of renal carcinoma.

Adjuvant Irradiation

The use of neoadjuvant or postoperative irradiation in the management of locally advanced primary RCC is controversial. Preoperative irradiation reduces the size of renal tumors and causes fibrosis, with thickening of the tumor capsule and sclerosis of small blood vessels.[133] In a retrospective review, Riches and colleagues reported apparent survival advantages of patients treated with preoperative irradiation versus surgery alone (49% versus 30% 5-year survival rates).[134]

Two prospective clinical trials evaluating the role of neoadjuvant irradiation have been conducted (Table 53-6).[135,136] Van der Werf-Messing reported a series of 126 evaluable patients from 1965 to 1972 randomized to undergo nephrectomy alone versus low-dose preoperative radiation therapy (30 Gy in 15 fractions for 3 weeks) followed by immediate nephrectomy.[135] There was no significant survival difference between the two groups by overall P stage. However, in patients with stage P3 lesions (i.e., tumor infiltrating intrarenal or extrarenal veins or lymph vessels), complete resection of tumor was more frequent in the group treated with radiation therapy. Survival in patients with stage P2 (i.e., extension beyond kidney) or P3 lesions was better when complete resection was performed.[135]

Juusela and associates also conducted a prospective, randomized study of preoperative irradiation followed by nephrectomy (38 patients) versus nephrectomy alone (44 patients).[136] Patients treated with preoperative irradiation received 2.2 Gy per day to a total dose of 33 Gy. Patients treated with preoperative irradiation had a 47% 5-year survival compared with 63% for patients treated with nephrectomy alone.[136]

The role of postoperative irradiation has also been evaluated retrospectively and prospectively (Table 53-7).[137-141] In a nonrandomized comparison of surgery with or without postoperative irradiation, Rafla found an overall survival advantage at 5 years in 94 patients undergoing postoperative irradiation versus 96 patients treated by nephrectomy alone (overall 5-year survival rate of 56% versus 37%).[137] These data were confirmed in an expanded updated analysis by Rafla.

Table 53-6 Preoperative Irradiation for Renal Cell Carcinoma

Study	Type of Study	No. of Patients	Treatment	Total Radiation Dose (Gy)/Fx	5-Year Survival Rate (%)
Riches et al[134] (1951)	R	685	N	NS	30
		131	RT + N		49
Van der Werf-Messing et al[135] (1973)	P	85	N	30/15	50
		89	RT + N		45
Juusela et al[136] (1977)	P	44	N	33/15	63
		38	RT + N		47

Fx, fractions; N, nephrectomy; NS, not stated; P, prospective; R, retrospective; RT, radiation therapy.

Table 53-7 Postoperative Irradiation for Renal Cell Carcinoma

Study	Type of Study	No. of Patients	Treatment	Total Radiation Dose (Gy)/Fx	5-Year Survival Rate (%)
Rafla[137] (1970)	R	96	N	NS	37
		94	N + RT		56
Finney[138] (1973)	P	49	N	55/25	51
		51	N + RT		45
Kjaer et al[139] (1987)	P	33	N	50/20	62
		32	N + RT		38
Stein et al[140] (1992)	R	63	N	46/23	40
		56	N + RT		50
Kao et al[141] (1994)	R	12	N	45/25	62*
		12	N + RT		75*

*Disease-free survival.
Fx, fractions; N, nephrectomy; NS, not stated; P, prospective; R, retrospective; RT, radiation therapy.

The 5-year survival rate was 38% (40 of 105) for patients who received postoperative irradiation versus 18% (24 of 135) for those undergoing nephrectomy alone.[142]

In a pseudorandomized trial of 100 patients (i.e., randomization by odd versus even date of birth), Finney found that incidence of distant metastases, local recurrence, and crude survival were not affected by the addition of postoperative radiation therapy (55 Gy in 25 fractions in 5 weeks).[138] These results are difficult to interpret because randomization was not blinded or stratified on the basis of risk factors.

A prospective, randomized study of postoperative radiation therapy involving a small number of patients was conducted by the Copenhagen Renal Cancer Study Group. Patients were randomized to nephrectomy alone (33 patients) versus nephrectomy and postoperative radiation therapy (32 patients).[139] Postoperative irradiation consisted of 50 Gy in 20 fractions. The 5-year survival was 62% for nephrectomy alone versus 38% for nephrectomy and postoperative radiation therapy.[139] Forty-four percent of the patients treated with radiation therapy had significant complications involving the stomach, duodenum, or liver.[139] These complications contributed to the death of the patients in 19% of the patients who received postoperative irradiation.

Three retrospective studies evaluated the role of postoperative radiation therapy in patients at high risk for local recurrence after surgery.[140,141,143] Patients received doses of 45 to 46 Gy with 1.8- to 2-Gy fractions using multiple treatment fields and CT-based planning. Local recurrence was decreased significantly, and one major treatment complication (i.e., radiation-induced liver disease) occurred. Survival and disease-free survival were not significantly improved with postoperative radiation.

Adjuvant Chemotherapy, Immunotherapy, and Molecularly Targeted Treatment

Adjuvant therapy is given to patients at high risk for disease relapse after curative surgery with the intention of preventing disease relapse systemically. Three separate clinical trials evaluating adjuvant interferon-α after nephrectomy failed to demonstrate a survival benefit.[144-146] The Cytokine Working Group had conducted a high-dose intravenous bolus interleukin-2 (IL-2) trial versus observation in postnephrectomy patients, and it did not show any survival benefit.[147] A different approach was studied by Jocham and colleagues, using autologous tumor cell vaccine; 558 patients with resected pT2-3b pN0-3 M0 RCC were randomly assigned to vaccine or to observation. At 4.5 years, the progression-free survival rate was 77% with the vaccine and 68% with observation. These results are very interesting, but long-term follow-up of these patients will determine its effect on overall survival.[148]

Summary of Treatment

Radical nephrectomy continues to be the first line of therapy for apparent localized renal carcinoma. Less invasive techniques, such as laparoscopic radical nephrectomy, play a larger role in the surgical management of renal carcinoma. NSS is considered with increased frequency for patients with small and medium-sized tumors. The role of postoperative irradiation in the management of RCC is not established. Because the risk of local failure is only 5% in patients treated with gross total resection of tumor during radical nephrectomy,[121] routine use of postoperative radiation therapy is not indicated. However, the risk of local failure is higher in patients with positive margins and with lymph node involvement. Patients with these pathologic features at surgery may be candidates for future clinical trials. There is no evidence that adjuvant immunotherapy or molecularly targeted treatment in patients with resected RCC is beneficial.

Renal Pelvis and Ureter

Surgery

Surgery is the mainstay of treatment for patients with cancers of the renal pelvis or ureter. Nephroureterectomy with removal of the bladder cuff is the standard surgery. Locoregional failure develops in 9% to 15% of patients with low-grade, low-stage disease and in 30% to 50% of patients with high-grade or high-stage disease.[149,150] Ureteral stump recurrence has been reported in 16% to 64% of patients if the stump is left in place.[55,101,149,150] Laparoscopic nephroureterectomy has equal anticancer effectiveness, decreases need for postoperative analgesia, shortens recovery time, and reduces the duration of hospital stay.[151,152] More conservative NSS or partial ureterectomy, many of which can be done endoscopically, is an acceptable option in selected patients.[153-156] These include patients with low-grade and low-stage disease, small lesion size (<1 to 1.5 cm), absence of multifocal disease, solitary kidney, bilateral disease, or major medical comorbidities.

Primary Radiation Therapy

Reports on the use of radiation therapy alone for cancers of the renal pelvis or ureter have been limited to case reports or small numbers of patients, and primary irradiation is not considered to be a standard treatment.[157,158] Some patients with gross residual disease after surgery or who have recurrent disease are treated with external beam radiation therapy (EBRT). Batata and colleagues reported long-term disease control in one of eight patients who received EBRT for gross residual disease after surgery.[55] In a study by Cozad and coworkers, 2 of 11 patients were disease free after receiving 45 and 50.4 Gy, respectively, for gross residual disease postoperatively.[149] Brady and associates reported that 2 of 6 patients with locally recurrent or gross residual disease were disease free at 36 months and 84 months after receiving 50 and 60 Gy, respectively.[158]

Combined chemotherapy and radiation therapy has been used in the management of TCC of the bladder to achieve organ preservation.[159,160] Such approach appears reasonable as the primary treatment in selected patients with TCC of the upper urinary tract if surgery is not an option. Studies evaluating combined chemotherapy and irradiation are warranted.

Adjuvant Irradiation

Despite aggressive surgery, local recurrence of disease frequently occurs. Many studies reported local recurrence rates up to 45%. The risk of local relapse correlates with the stage of disease and tumor grade. The pattern of failure for these cancers is demonstrated nicely in a study by Cozad and colleagues.[149] Five-year local control rate was 90% for grade 1 and 2 tumors and 41% for grade 3 and 4 tumors for patients who were treated with surgery alone. For stage I and II disease, the 5-year local control rate was 83%, compared with 52% for stage III disease. About one half of all the local relapses manifested initially as an isolated site of recurrence, and the other half manifested as combined local and distant recurrence. Distant metastasis occurred in 19% in patients with stage I or II disease and in 53% of those with stage III disease. Most distant relapses in stage III disease manifested as the initial site of failure. In another report by Johansson and coworkers,

10 of 23 patients had local recurrence after surgery, but 4 of these 10 patients had no further tumor spread.[56] In patients with high-grade or high-stage disease, the risk of lymph node metastasis is up to 60%, whereas the risk is 0% to 10% for patients with low-grade or low-stage disease.[62,63] These data suggest that although patients who have high-grade or high-stage disease have substantial risks for distant and local recurrence of disease, many of them have locoregional failure as the only initial site of failure. Adjuvant irradiation would improve locoregional control in these selected patients. They should also be considered for adjuvant chemotherapy to reduce the risk of distant metastasis.

Few studies have evaluated the role of adjuvant irradiation in the management of renal pelvis and ureter carcinomas.[55,158,160-162] Several series suggest that adjuvant irradiation has a significant impact on the local control of disease in high-risk patients, although the number of patients included is small. In a study by Cozad and associates, 26 patients with T3-4N0/+ disease had radical surgery, 9 of whom received adjuvant irradiation to a median dose of 50 Gy.[161] Local failure occurred in 9 of 17 without and 1 of 9 with adjuvant irradiation (*P* = .07). The effect of adjuvant irradiation was seen only in high-grade tumors, because no local relapse developed in patients with low-grade disease, regardless of whether adjuvant therapy was given. Metastasis developed in 4 of 9 and 8 of 17 with and without radiation therapy, respectively. The 5-year actuarial survival rate was 44% with and 24% without adjuvant irradiation (*P* = .23). In a study by Brookland and Richter, adjuvant irradiation was given to 11 of 23 patients who had tumor grade 3 or 4 or pathologic stage C or D disease.[162] The median dose was 50 Gy to the ureteropelvic bed, with or without inclusion of the para-aortic nodes. For the nonirrradiated group, the median survival was 26 months, and the local relapse rate was 45%, compared with 35 months and 11%, respectively, for those who received adjuvant irradiation.

The impact of adjuvant irradiation on overall survival of these high-risk patients has not been well demonstrated, partly because of the small number of patients in the published studies. Some investigators have questioned the routine use of adjuvant irradiation.[63] To improve survival, the significant risk of distant metastasis in these patients has to be addressed. Studies incorporating chemotherapy are needed to demonstrate the benefits of adjuvant therapy on overall survival.[163]

LOCALLY ADVANCED DISEASE

Kidney

Large RCCs rarely invade adjacent organs at presentation. Instead, they displace and compress adjacent tissues.[44] However, if the tumor directly invades contiguous tissues such as the liver, duodenum, large intestine, and perinephric muscle, initial surgical resection may not be successful. In a prospective study of 126 evaluable patients randomized to nephrectomy alone or to preoperative EBRT (30 Gy in 3 weeks) followed by immediate nephrectomy, van der Werf-Messing observed that complete resection in patients with tumor infiltrating intrarenal or extrarenal veins or lymph vessels was more common in the preoperative irradiation group.[135] This significant increase of complete resection in patients with locally advanced disease who received preoperative radiation produced a considerably higher survival at 18 months compared with that for patients treated with surgery alone. However, at 5 years, there was no significant difference in survival.[135]

Intraoperative Irradiation

MAYO CLINIC RESULTS

In addition to neoadjuvant EBRT, an intraoperative irradiation supplement with electrons (IOERT) or high dose rate brachytherapy (HDR-IORT) may be considered as an additive component of treatment in patients with locally advanced primary or recurrent disease. Frydenberg and colleagues described two patients with locally advanced RCC and six patients with locally recurrent RCC treated with preoperative EBRT (45 to 50 Gy) followed by resection and IOERT at Mayo Clinic.[164] The two patients with primary locally advanced disease were alive without evidence of disease at 15 and 50 months from initiation of EBRT.[164] Of the six patients with locally recurrent disease, two were alive with no evidence of disease at 29 and 42 months. The locoregional control rate was 87.5%.[164]

The Mayo Clinic IOERT series was updated to include 14 patients with locally advanced primary (n = 2) or recurrent (n = 12) renal cancers (Table 53-8).[165] Preoperative EBRT was given in 11 of the 14 patients (dose of 44 Gy in 8 fractions). The IOERT dose was 10 to 20 Gy in 12 of 14 patients (dose of

Table 53-8 Locally Advanced and Recurrent Renal Cell Carcinoma: Survival, Disease Status, and Patterns of Failure after External Beam plus Intraoperative Electron Irradiation at the Mayo Clinic

Disease Category	No. of Patients	Status	Survival (mo)	Failure Patterns
Primary RCC	2 total			
	1	Alive NED	56	—
	1	Dead NED	31	Liver, lungs
Recurrent RCC	8 total			
	2	Alive NED	37, 55	—
	2	Alive WD	21.5, 44	Local failure, lymph nodes, bone
	2	Dead NED	10.5, 19	
	2	Dead WD	16, 19	Regional failure, lung, CNS
Recurrent TCC-SCC	3 total			
	1	Dead NED	28.5	Central failure, liver
	2	Dead WD	5, 12	
Wilms' tumor	1	Dead WD	8	Lymph nodes, liver

CNS, central nervous system; NED, no evidence of disease; RCC, renal cell carcinoma; SCC, squamous cell cancer; TCC, transitional cell cancer; WD, with disease.

25 Gy given to 2 patients who received high-dose EBRT before referral to Mayo Clinic with disease progression).

In the RCC group of patients, 5 of 10 patients were alive. Three (30%) of 10 were free of disease at 37, 55, and 56 months from initiation of treatments, and 2 others died free of disease at 10.5 and 19 months (5 of 10, or 50%, relapse free). Two patients were alive with disease at 22 and 44 months, and three died of disease at 16, 19, and 31 months. Of the four patients with other cell types, one died free of disease at 28.5 months, and three died of disease at 5, 8, and 12 months. Local or central relapse occurred in only one patient in each category. The distant metastasis rate was high at 57% (8 of 14 patients).[165]

In the latest update of the Mayo Clinic series, IOERT had been used as a supplement to EBRT and resection in 49 patients with genitourinary malignancies, including 28 patients with renal cancer (8 with bladder, 7 with prostate, 2 with ureter, and 4 with miscellaneous cancers).[166] Survival was best for patients with primary or recurrent renal cancer (5 year, 37% versus 16%; $P = .05$), for patients with gross total resection preceding IOERT (5 year, 41% versus 0%; $P < .0001$), and for primary versus recurrent disease (5 year, 48% versus 25%; $P = .019$). For the 28 patients with renal primaries, disease control was as follows: 90% (5 year) for local control, 88% (5 year, within IOERT field) for central control, and 28% (3 year) for distant control.

Pamplona Series

The University Clinic of Navarra in Pamplona used IOERT as a component of treatment for 11 patients with locally advanced primary ($n = 8$) or locally recurrent ($n = 3$) lesions.[165,167] Patients received IOERT after maximal surgical resection, and 7 of the 11 received postoperative EBRT (30 to 45 Gy). Gross residual disease remained in four patients; the remaining seven had close or micropositive margins. Histologic examination revealed RCC in 10 patients and transitional cell carcinoma in 1. The IOERT dose ranged from 10 to 20 Gy (10 Gy for two patients; 15 Gy for eight patients; 20 Gy for one patient).

In an early analysis[167] (follow-up time of 2 to 33 months; median, 8 months), distant metastases occurred in three patients (three in lung; two in liver), and local relapse occurred in one of the three (microresidual disease, IOERT dose of 20 Gy and no EBRT). In an analysis update,[165] 3 of 11 patients were free of disease at 3 or more years, similar to the results of the Mayo Clinic series.

Heidelberg Results

Elbe and others reported a University of Heidelberg series of 11 patients with renal cancer in whom IOERT was given as a component of treatment (3 with primary disease; 8 with locally recurrent disease).[168] Patients had maximal resection, IOERT (12 to 20 Gy), and postoperative EBRT (40 Gy in 2-Gy fractions, 5 days per week). With mean follow-up of 24 months, no local relapses occurred. Distant metastases, however, occurred in 5 of 11 patients, or 45% (lung in 3; bone in 2). Overall and disease-free survival rates at 3 years were 47% and 34%, respectively.

Renal Pelvis and Ureter

For patients with locally advanced or unresectable disease, the overall prognosis is poor. Treatment decision has to be individualized. The performance status and medical comorbidities of these patients are major considerations in deciding the aggressiveness of treatment. Radiation therapy, with or without chemotherapy, has been shown to achieve long-term disease control in some patients who have gross residual or locally recurrent disease.[55,149,158] In a study by Cozad and colleagues, 19 patients had gross residual disease after surgery, 11 of which received postoperative irradiation.[149] The median survival of the irradiated group was 11 months, versus 4 months for those receiving no radiation. Two patients who were treated with 45 Gy to 50.4 Gy of EBRT were free of disease at 21 and 28 months. For these patients, the role of combined-modality therapy incorporating chemotherapy and radiation therapy should be further studied. In selected patients, preoperative irradiation with or without chemotherapy may downstage the disease. If there is adequate tumor shrinkage, surgical resection with or without intraoperative irradiation to the tumor bed may become possible.

METASTATIC DISEASE AND PALLIATION

Kidney

In patients with demonstrated widespread metastatic disease at initial diagnosis, nephrectomy is not justified if the intent is to induce a spontaneous regression; the incidence of such a regression is less than 1%, compared with the high morbidity and mortality rates associated with nephrectomy.[3,169] A palliative nephrectomy can be considered in patients suffering from repeated hemorrhages, tumor pain, or significant paraneoplastic syndromes.[44]

Solitary Metastases: Role of Surgery or Irradiation

The role of nephrectomy has been evaluated in patients who present with solitary metastatic disease. Of 158 patients who presented to the Mayo Clinic between 1970 and 1980 with documented metastatic disease and no prior treatment at diagnosis, 56 patients (35%) had a solitary metastasis.[170] The survival rates at 2 and 3 years for patients with solitary metastasis were 29.1% and 19%, respectively, compared with 6.8% and 4.3% for patients with multiple lesions.[170] Nephrectomy was performed on 67.6% of patients who presented with multiple metastases and 83.9% of patients with solitary metastasis. Nephrectomy markedly influenced survival only in patients with solitary metastasis, low-grade primary tumor, and weight loss of less than 10%.[170]

Treatment of the solitary metastatic site has been evaluated in patients with synchronous or metachronous solitary metastasis.[171,172] Of 18 patients who presented with a solitary metastasis at diagnosis, the only patients who survived longer than 2 years were 4 (22%) who underwent surgical treatment of the primary and metastatic sites.[171]

Patients with metachronous solitary metastasis have a more favorable outlook. Of 26 patients treated with surgery or radiation therapy at the Mayo Clinic, 18 (69%) lived more than 2 years, and the 5-year survival rate from the time of nephrectomy was 50%.[171] Six (23%) of the 26 patients lived more than 5 years after removal of the solitary metastatic lesion.[171]

Kjaer evaluated 25 patients with RCC and solitary metastasis.[172] Twelve patients had a focus in the bone, and the remaining 13 patients had metastasis in soft tissue, including the lungs, thyroid, flank, and epididymis. Radiation therapy was used primarily to treat the bone lesions. The 13 patients with soft tissue metastasis were treated with surgery (7 patients) and radiation therapy (6 patients). The median survival of this select group of patients was 4.3 years. The 5- and 10-year survival rates were 36% and 16%, respectively. Females had 5- and 10-year survival rates of 76% and 38%, respectively, versus 18% and 12% for males. This difference was determined to be statistically significant ($P = .05$).[172]

Two clinical trials have shown that debulking nephrectomy may enhance the effect of immunotherapy. The Southwest Oncology Group (SWOG) randomized 246 patients to initial nephrectomy followed by interferon versus interferon alone.[173] The median survival of the nephrectomy group was significantly improved by 3 months in the subset of patients with an Eastern Cooperative Oncology Group (ECOG) performance status of 0 to 1. The European Organization for Research and Treatment of Cancer (EORTC) conducted a trial similar to the SWOG trial that enrolled 83 patients. Patients undergoing nephrectomy experienced a 10-month median survival benefit.[174] Based on these debulking nephrectomy trials, patients with a good initial performance status who subsequently receive interferon immunotherapy appear to experience an improved survival. There have been no prospective trials evaluating debulking nephrectomy followed by IL-2.

Bone Metastases

Metastases to the bone (solitary or multiple) may occur in 25% to 50% of patients with RCC.[175] Althausen and associates evaluated 38 patients with osseous metastases from RCC.[175] Patients were treated with resection with or without allograft implantation, radiation therapy alone, or a combination of treatments. The survival for the entire group was 90% at 6 months, 84% at 1 year, 55% at 5 years, and 39% at 10 years. Age, gender, and presence of a pathologic fracture had no influence on survival. Presentation without metastasis, long disease-free interval between nephrectomy and first metastases, appendicular skeletal location, and solitary metastases were correlated with longer survival.[175] The study authors concluded that patients who have an appendicular (preferably solitary) metastasis and who have a long duration from diagnosis of disease to metastasis should be treated with complex orthopedic surgical procedures if necessary.[175] Postoperative radiation therapy should be considered in selected cases.

The results of radiation therapy alone in the treatment of bone metastases have been evaluated.[176,177] Halperin and Harisiadis evaluated the results of 36 sites irradiated for bone pain.[176] The pain responded in 77% of the treated sites, and most sites received a time-dose fractionation (TDF) equivalent dose ranging from 45 to 85. No relation was observed between the TDF equivalent dose given and the probability of response.[176] Twenty-four (86%) of the 28 sites were partially or completely free of pain for the remainder of the patients' lives.[176]

Onufrey and Mohiuddin evaluated the effectiveness of radiation therapy to alleviate bone pain.[177] Eighty-six bone sites were treated with TDF values ranging from less than 40 to 80 or more. Twenty-six of 39 patients (67%) who received a TDF of more than 70 experienced significant relief of symptoms compared with 14 of 47 patients (30%) who received a TDF of less than 70. There was no difference in response in the peripheral versus the axial skeleton.[177]

Wilson and coworkers reported partial and symptomatic response rates to palliative reduction of 67% and 73%, respectively. They were not able to establish a dose-response relationship based on the biologic effective dose (BED).[178]

Brain Metastases

Brain metastases are diagnosed in approximately 10% of patients with metastatic RCC.[179] Wronski and others evaluated the results of whole-brain radiation therapy in a retrospective study of 119 patients treated at M. D. Anderson Cancer Center.[179] The median radiation dose was 30 Gy (range, 18 to 56 Gy). The overall median survival from the time of diagnosis of the brain metastases was 4.4 months.[179] Seventy patients (58.8%) had multiple brain tumors, with a survival of 3.0 months compared with 4.4 months for patients with a single brain metastasis ($P = .043$). The cause of death was determined to be neurologic in 90 (76%) of the 119 patients. Patients with brain metastases diagnosed synchronously with the renal primary (24 patients) had a median survival of 3.4 months, compared with 3.2 months for the 95 patients diagnosed metachronously. Multivariate analysis revealed favorable prognostic factors to be a single brain metastasis, lack of distant metastases at diagnosis, and tumor diameter less than 2 cm.[179]

Because patients with brain metastases from RCC treated with whole-brain radiation alone have a poor survival and a high probability of a neurologic death, more aggressive treatments have been evaluated in selected patients with favorable prognostic features. Patients who could undergo surgical resection of brain metastases from RCC had a 12-month median survival.[180] Stereotactic radiosurgery in conjunction with whole-brain radiation therapy produced a local control rate of more than 80% in nine lesions in patients with brain metastases from RCC.[181]

Radiosurgery alone or in combination with whole-brain radiation therapy for renal cell brain metastasis has been evaluated by several institutions. These retrospective studies have reported local tumor control rates of 88% to 96%.[182-185] Brown and associates reported that the addition of whole-brain irradiation to radiosurgery improved local control and decreased distant brain failure rates.[183] These studies also demonstrated that the Radiation Therapy Oncology Group recursive partitioning analysis (RPA) class strongly influenced the survival of these patients.[182,186]

Soft Tissue Masses

Halperin and Harisiadis found that 9 (64%) of 14 "tumor masses" responded to various doses of radiation.[176] The doses ranged from a TDF equivalent of 45 to more than 100. No definite dose response was apparent. Radiation therapy can be effective in palliating symptoms of pain and bleeding in patients with massive RCC.

Chemotherapy, Immunotherapy, and Molecularly Targeted Treatment

Treatment options for patients with metastatic RCC include hormonal therapy, chemotherapy, immunotherapy, and molecularly targeted treatment. Hormonal therapy has been studied in RCC, with responses to progestins, androgen, or antiestrogens between 0% and 10%. Hormonal therapy is not effective for RCC. Multiple chemotherapy regimens have been tested in patients with RCC and a response rate of 5.6% was obtained.[187] One regimen worth mentioning is the gemcitabine and continuous 5-fluorouracil (5-FU) combination, which in the second-line setting in a phase II study produced a response rate of 17%.[188] RCC is not a chemotherapy-sensitive disease. In certain subsets of renal cancer (non–clear cell type), the responses to chemotherapy appear to be better. In non–clear cell RCC, responses of more than 10% to 15% have been reported with carboplatin plus paclitaxel, cisplatin plus gemcitabine, and doxorubicin plus gemcitabine (for collecting duct or sarcomatoid histology).[189]

Immunotherapy for Renal Cell Carcinoma

RCC is an immunologically responsive disease. Spontaneous remissions have been reported because of this phenomenon in 0.5% of patients. In an attempt to reproduce this accentuated response, the efficacy of IL-2 or interferon had been studied in RCC. The overall response rate of alfa interferon is 15%, with a delay in time to progression of 4 months. There are no long-term remissions.[190] IL-2 has been used since the mid-1980s for metastatic RCC. Objective responses of 14% to 19% have been reported, with 7% of patients having long-term remission, including survival of 10 years or more.[191] Intravenous bolus IL-2 treatment is associated with significant toxicity, including renal failure, congestive heart failure, respiratory failure from capillary leak syndrome, coma, liver failure, and arrhythmias.[192] Other important considerations include the fact that patients have to be admitted in a monitored unit, staff must be familiar with the administration of the drug, patients have to be otherwise healthy to be eligible for this treatment, and most oncologists have not been trained to administer it. During past years, modified doses of IL-2 have been given by subcutaneous or inhalation routes instead of being administered intravenously. Most of the regimens have been able to produce responses of 10% to 19%.

Yang and colleagues compared high-dose intravenous and low-dose intravenous bolus of subcutaneous IL-2. They found higher responses with high-dose bolus IL-2 (21%) compared with low-dose bolus intravenous IL-2 (13%) and subcutaneous IL-2 (10%). Significantly superior complete response durability and survival were found in the patients that received high-dose bolus intravenous IL-2.[193] Atzpodien and coworkers showed that subcutaneous IL-2, interferon, and 5-FU could improve 3-year survival rates for patients with metastatic RCC compared with a non–IL-2 regimen (25 versus 16 months).[194] IL-2 is still the standard regimen for metastatic RCC. Based on the premise that decreasing the tumor burden would enhance the effect of immunotherapy, two trials were conducted and showed that nephrectomy in patients with metastatic RCC in combination with interferon-α in patients with good functional status (ECOG 0-1) could improve survival by 7 months.[173,174]

Molecularly Targeted Treatment

A randomized trial of bevacizumab, a vascular endothelial growth factor (VEGF) antibody, resulted in a significant prolongation of progression survival of 2.3 months in patients with metastatic RCC.[195] This study opened the door for further trials using molecularly targeted treatments for this disease. Several drugs, including tyrosine kinase inhibitors, rafkinase inhibitors, and epidermal growth factor inhibitors, have been tested, with responses in phase II studies of 20% or more.[196] It is hoped that less toxic drugs can be developed to produce long-term remissions in RCC and even cure. With better understanding of the biology of the disease, clinical investigators are combining multiple molecularly targeted treatments, moving them closer to achieving these goals.[196]

Renal Pelvis and Ureter

Systemic chemotherapy should be considered for patients presenting with metastatic disease.[197-199] In patients who have symptomatic metastases, EBRT can provide palliation of local symptoms and improve the quality of life. Most painful metastases respond to 20 to 40 Gy of irradiation, using fraction size of 2 to 4 Gy. For patients with poor performance status and very short life expectancy, a single treatment of 8 Gy may provide short-term palliation of painful bone metastasis.

TECHNIQUES OF IRRADIATION

Kidney

Preoperative irradiation treatment volumes for patients with locally advanced disease should encompass the primary tumor, renal hilar lymph nodes, para-aortic lymph nodes, and vascular extent of tumor (Fig. 53-1). Anteroposterior and posteroanterior (AP-PA) fields with high-energy photons should be used initially. To spare dose-limiting organs, including the liver, small intestine, and spinal cord, three-dimensional conformal field combinations of AP-PA, laterals, or obliques should be considered. Intensity-modulated radiation therapy (IMRT) can also be used to minimize the dose to normal tissues. Total doses of 45 to 50.4 Gy in 1.8-Gy fractions using multiple fields or IMRT should be given preoperatively, followed by surgery in 4 to 6 weeks. If possible, an IORT supplement should be considered if residual disease or narrow margins exist after maximal surgical resection. At the Mayo Clinic, doses of 10 to 20 Gy are usually delivered with IOERT; the dose depends on margin status and the amount of EBRT delivered preoperatively or planned postoperatively.[164]

Postoperative radiation should be considered for patients at high risk for local recurrence after surgery. Pathologic features predictive of local recurrence include positive lymph nodes and positive surgical margins.[121] The target volume should include the tumor bed, regional lymph nodes (hilar and para-aortic lymph nodes), and vascular extent of tumor. If feasible, the scar should be included in the target volume because scar recurrences have occasionally happened.[140] Total radiation doses of 45 to 50.4 Gy should be delivered with 1.8- to 2-Gy fractions using multiple-field techniques. Small-volume fields can be used to boost areas of residual disease to a total of 55 to 60 Gy. IMRT can be used to treat the target volume and minimize the dose to the normal tissues (i.e., liver, small bowel, stomach, opposite kidney, and spinal cord).

Patients in whom a local recurrence has developed in the tumor bed or regional nodes after radical nephrectomy should be considered for aggressive treatment.[164] This treatment includes preoperative three-dimensional (3D) or IMRT external beam irradiation to the recurrent tumor volume, postoperative tumor bed, and renal hilar and para-aortic lymph nodes. A total dose of 45 Gy in 25 fractions should be delivered using multiple treatment fields. Maximal surgical debulking with consideration of IORT should occur within 4 to 6 weeks of completion of EBRT.

Treatment-Related Toxicity

CT-aided radiation therapy treatment planning (3D or IMRT) is essential to reduce the risk of treatment-related toxicity. The Copenhagen Renal Study Group randomized 32 patients to receive postoperative irradiation after surgery.[139] Twenty-seven of the 32 patients randomized completed the course of postoperative radiation therapy to a dose of 50 Gy in 20 fractions. Significant complications to the stomach, duodenum, or liver occurred in 12 of the 27 patients within 1 to 44 months (median, 5 months) after completion of radiation therapy. Postirradiation complications contributed to the death of 5 (19%) of the 27 patients. The increased fraction size of 2.5 Gy may have partially contributed to the high complication rate.

Renal Pelvis and Ureter

The radiation treatment field should include the primary tumor bed with an adequate margin plus the regional lymph nodes adjacent to the primary tumor bed. For renal pelvis and upper ureteral lesions, nodal metastasis most commonly occurs near or superior to the primary tumor site, involving the periaortic or pericaval lymph nodes and the renal hilar nodes. The superior and inferior extent of the periaortic or pericaval nodal chain to be included in the treatment field is not well described in the literature. A minimum of 4 to 5 cm is reasonable, although a bigger margin may be justified in

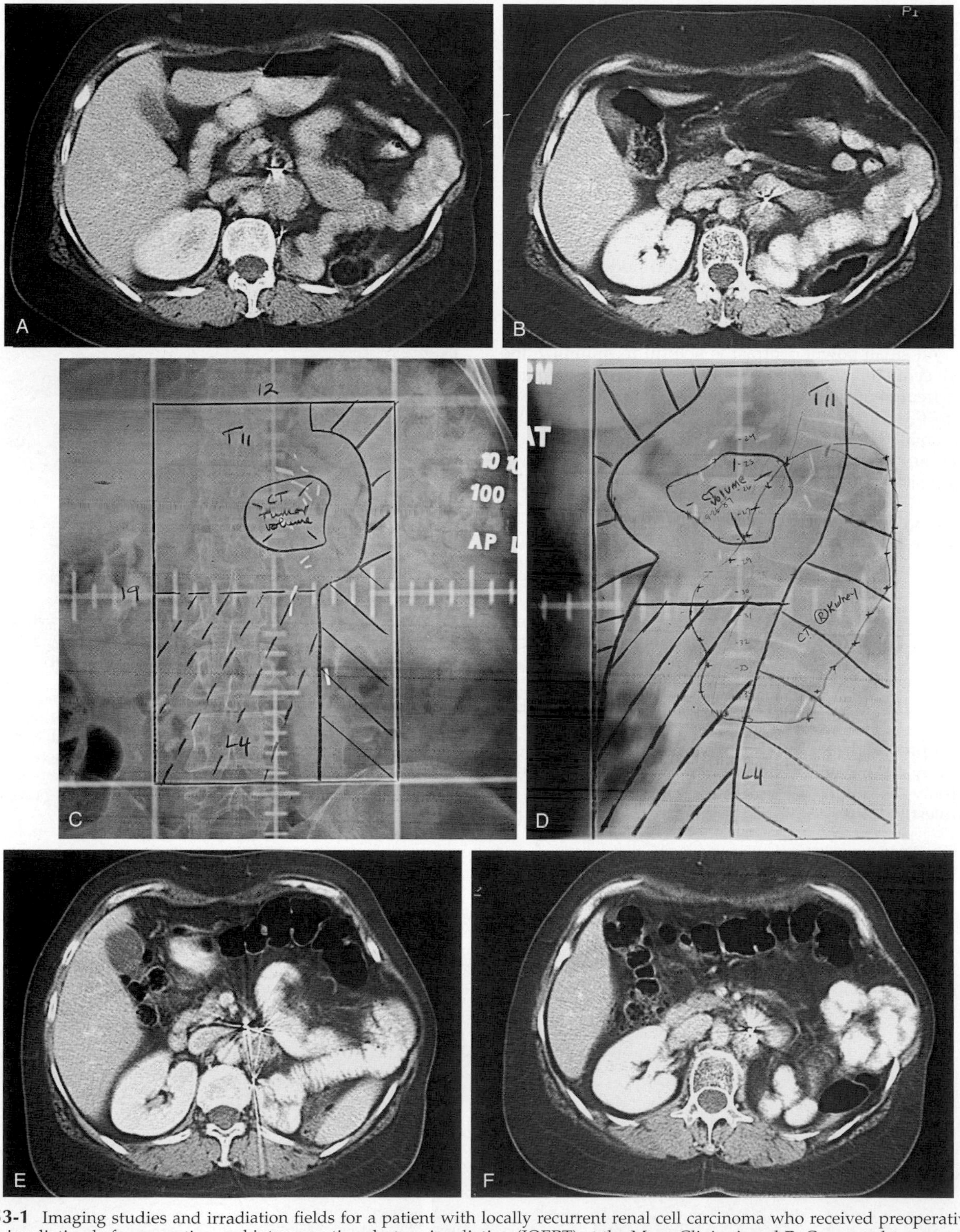

Figure 53-1 Imaging studies and irradiation fields for a patient with locally recurrent renal cell carcinoma who received preoperative external beam irradiation before resection and intraoperative electron irradiation (IOERT) at the Mayo Clinic. **A** and **B,** Computed tomography (CT) before irradiation demonstrates bulky para-aortic adenopathy and lack of a fat plane adjacent to the aorta. **C** and **D,** Irradiation fields encompass the recurrent tumor and para-aortic lymph nodes using a multifield technique of anteroposterior-posteroanterior (AP-PA) (**C**) plus paired laterals (**D**) to deliver 45 Gy in 25 fractions to large fields from T11 through L4 *(solid lines)*. The right kidney was excluded from AP-PA fields (**C**), except for the upper medial components (>75% excluded). Because approximately 50% of the right kidney was within the lateral fields (**D**), the lateral dose contribution was limited to less than 18 Gy. The spinal cord was excluded from the lateral fields. After 45 Gy, the field was altered to block from isocenter inferiorly *(dashed lines)*. **E** and **F,** Posttreatment CT of the abdomen 4 weeks after 50.4 Gy given in 28 fractions over 5 weeks and 2.5 months after the pretreatment scan. Notice shrinkage of the mass with the improved fat planes relative to the aorta. An IOERT dose of 12.5 Gy was given after a marginal gross total resection. (**A, B, E,** and **F,** From Calvo FA, Zincke H, Gunderson LL, et al: Genitourinary IORT. *In* Gunderson LL, Willett CG, Harrison JB, Calvo F [eds]: Intraoperative Irradiation: Techniques and Results. Totowa, NJ, Humana Press, 1999.)

patients with extensive nodal involvement. The initial treatment field should be treated to 45 to 50.4 Gy in 1.8 Gy per fraction. Areas of gross disease may be boosted to 54 to 60 Gy by small-volume fields, using techniques to minimize the small bowel in the treatment field. The dose to the contralateral functioning kidney should not exceed 18 Gy. The volume of irradiated liver (for patients with left-sided lesions) and stomach (for patients with right-sided lesions) can be reduced with AP/PA fields. Lateral fields may be used to deliver part of the treatment to keep the dose to the spinal cord within tolerance. Representative fields for a local recurrence of renal pelvis cancer are shown in Figure 53-2.

For lower ureteral lesions, pelvic lymph nodes should be included in the treatment field. The posterior location of the ureter allows the use of a four-field or three-field (PA and opposed laterals) technique. The use of a prone treatment position and small bowel contrast is helpful to minimize the amount of small bowel in the treatment field. A representative radiation treatment field for a lower ureter cancer is shown in Figure 53-3. Some centers have advocated the use of IMRT to spare small bowel during pelvic irradiation.[200,201] Boost volumes can be treated by multiple field arrangement, depending on the clinical situation.

TREATMENT ALGORITHM, CONCLUSIONS, AND FUTURE POSSIBILITIES

Kidney

RCC continues to be an intriguing medical problem. Some progress has been made in identifying the environmental, occupational, hormonal, cellular, and genetic factors associated with disease development. Significant progress has also been made in the early detection of these tumors through the expanded use of abdominal ultrasonography, CT, and MRI.[3,44] This has improved the probability of surgical cure with radical nephrectomy and has led to the development of partial nephrectomy as definitive treatment of selected tumors. Future investigations should be directed to prevent local and distant recurrence after surgical resection and to control locally advanced and metastatic disease.

Figure 53-4 presents an algorithm for the current Mayo Clinic philosophy on evaluation and management of RCC. Patients with a tumor 4 cm in diameter or smaller, a solitary

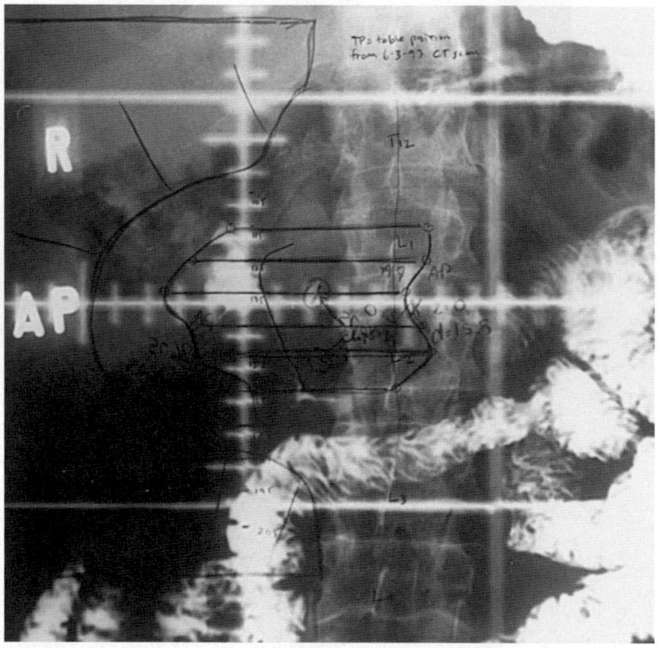

Figure 53-2 Irradiation fields for a locally recurrent renal pelvis transitional cell carcinoma. Original location of the primary tumor is identified by clips. Current size of the gross, unresectable (due to invasion of the inferior vena cava and other vascular structures) tumor is identified by computed tomography–based reconstruction. Periaortic lymph nodes are included within the anteroposterior-posteroanterior field.

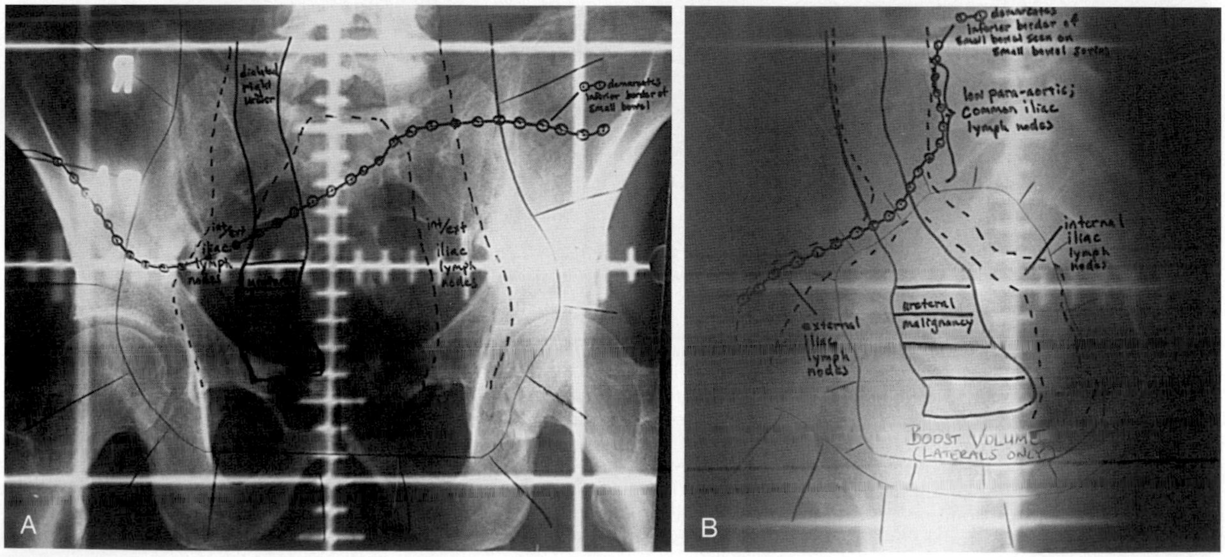

Figure 53-3 **A** and **B**, Radiation therapy fields for a low transitional cell carcinoma being managed by primary radiation therapy because of severe medical comorbidity preventing surgery. A beam's eye view reconstruction of the lower ureteral tumor, bladder, and draining pelvic lymph nodes is superimposed on the simulation films. Initial blocking for the tumor nodal fields is shown with final boost volumes to the primary lesion plus several centimeters of margin based on location of the small bowel identified by small-bowel series.

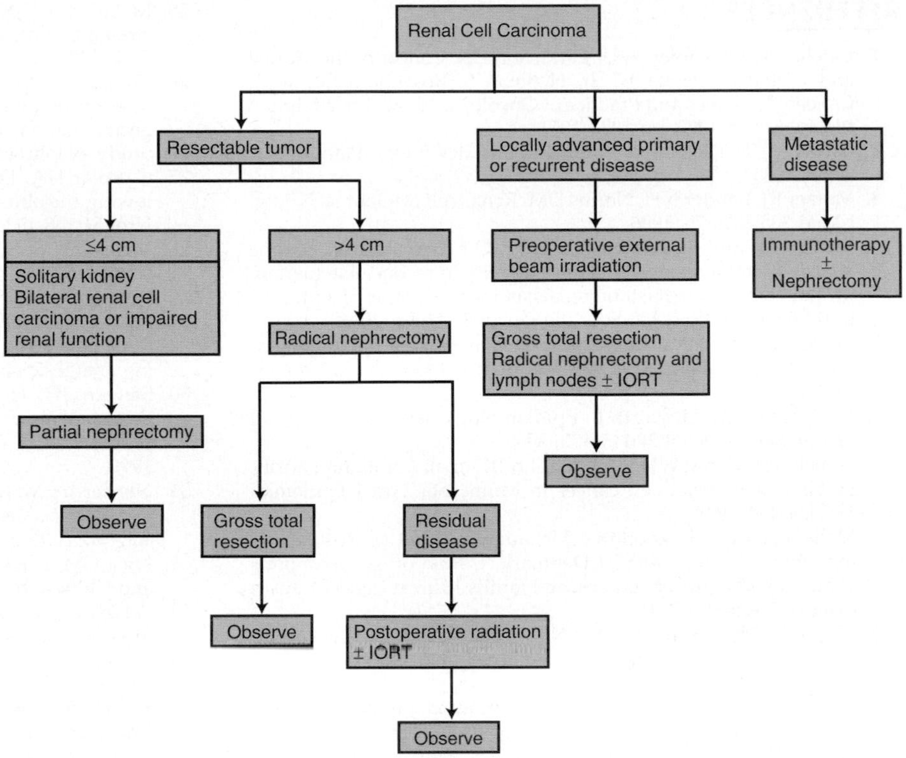

Figure 53-4 Algorithm for the evaluation and management of renal cell carcinoma. IORT, intraoperative irradiation.

kidney, bilateral RCCs, or impaired renal function may be candidates for partial nephrectomy. Patients with tumors larger than 4 cm and a normally functioning opposite kidney should be treated with radical nephrectomy. If gross total resection with negative margins is accomplished, the patient should be monitored. If positive surgical margins or lymph node involvement is present at radical nephrectomy, consideration should be given to postoperative EBRT.[140,141]

If locally advanced or locally recurrent disease is present, patients should receive preoperative EBRT to the tumor, regional lymph nodes, and vascular extent of tumor. Maximal resection, preferably combined with IORT to narrow or positive margins, should be planned for 4 to 6 weeks after completion of EBRT.[164]

Potential Clinical Trials

Patients who present with metastatic disease should be considered for participation in clinical trials using immunotherapy, molecularly targeted treatment, or other systemic treatments. Palliative nephrectomy should be considered only for patients with solitary metastasis, low-grade primary tumor, and weight loss of less than 10%.[170]

Future clinical trials should evaluate local and systemic treatment modalities. Patients who have undergone radical nephrectomy with gross total resection of tumor and who have negative surgical margins, negative lymph nodes, and no renal vein involvement have a favorable prognosis, and observation is appropriate.

Patients who have positive surgical margins or positive lymph nodes are at increased risk for local failure (with or without abdominal seeding). These patients could be entered into a prospective trial randomizing them to observation versus postoperative irradiation (with or without concomitant systemic therapy). The use of CT-based three-dimensional treatment planning (3D and IMRT) and conventional fractionation of 1.8 to 2 Gy per day to a total of 45 to 50 Gy should have a low risk of treatment-related complications and may improve local control and survival. If surgical reconstruction has been used to displace small intestine or stomach, areas of residual disease marked by surgical clips can be safely boosted to 60 to 65 Gy with 3D techniques, prone positioning, and false tabletop techniques.

Patients who have positive lymph nodes and renal vein involvement are at increased risk for distant metastases. Future trials should evaluate the use of adjuvant systemic treatment for these patients. Molecular target therapy may have potential value in the adjuvant setting in the future.

Patients with locally advanced disease appear to benefit from aggressive treatment, including preoperative radiation therapy, surgical debulking, and IORT. Future trials should evaluate the use of radiation sensitizers and systemic agents to improve local control and reduce distant spread of disease.

Renal Pelvis and Ureter

The management of early-stage and low-grade cancer is surgical. The standard surgery is nephroureterectomy. However, many patients are candidates for ureteroscopic NSS or partial ureterectomy, reserving nephroureterectomy for recurrence. For patients with locally advanced disease, the risks of locoregional and distant failure are substantial despite radical surgery. Studies are urgently needed to better define the roles of combined-modality treatment with newer chemotherapy regimens and radiation therapy as adjuvant or primary treatments. The use of IMRT may reduce the side effects of EBRT and deserves further validation. Development of therapeutic agents that target molecular pathways necessary for malignant cell growth or dissemination, as seen in lung cancer and colon cancer, could add to the treatment options for these cancers. Because these are relatively uncommon cancers, clinical trials involving multiple centers and cooperative groups should be encouraged to increase the number of patients participating in studies.

REFERENCES

1. Linehan WM, Shipley WU, Parkinson DR: Cancer of the kidney and ureter. *In* Devita VT Jr, Hellman S, Rosenberg RA (eds): Cancer: Principles and Practice of Oncology, 4th ed. Philadelphia: JB Lippincott; 1993, pp 1023-1051.
2. Growitz VP: Die sogenannten Lipome der Niere. Pathol Anat 93:39, 1883.
3. Motzer RJ, Bander NH, Nanus DM: Renal-cell carcinoma. N Engl J Med 335:865-875, 1996.
4. Motzer RJ, Rini BI, Michaelson D: SUO 11248, a novel tyrosine kinase inhibitor shows antitumor activity in second-line therapy for patients with metastatic renal carcinoma: results of a phase 2 trial [abstract]. Proc Am Soc Clin Oncol 22:4500a, 2004.
5. Mellemgaard A: Human Renal-Cell Carcinoma—Epidemiological and Mechanistic Aspects. Lyon, France, IARC Press, 1999, pp 69-80.
6. McLaughlin JK, Lipworth L: Epidemiologic aspects of renal cell cancer. Semin Oncol 27:115-123, 2000.
7. Benichou J, Chow WH, McLaughlin JK, et al: Population attributable risk of renal cell cancer in Minnesota. Am J Epidemiol 148:424-430, 1998.
8. Mellemgaard A, Engholm G, McLaughlin JK, et al: Risk factors for renal cell carcinoma in Denmark. I. Role of socioeconomic status, tobacco use, beverages, and family history. Cancer Causes Control 5:105-113, 1994.
9. McCredie M, Stewart JH, Day NE: Different roles for phenacetin and paracetamol in cancer of the kidney and renal pelvis. Int J Cancer 53:245-249, 1993.
10. Wolk A, Gridley G, Niwa S, et al: International renal cell cancer study. VII. Role of diet. Int J Cancer 65:67-73, 1996.
11. Parker AS, Cerhan JR, Lynch CF, et al: History of urinary tract infection and risk of renal cell carcinoma. Am J Epidemiol 159:42-48, 2004.
12. Chow WH, McLaughlin JK, Mandel JS, et al: Reproductive factors and the risk of renal cell cancer among women. Int J Cancer 60:321-324, 1995.
13. Nicodemus KK, Sweeney C, Folsom AR: Evaluation of dietary, medical and lifestyle risk factors for incident kidney cancer in postmenopausal women. Int J Cancer 108:115-121, 2004.
14. Kauzlaric D, Barmeir E, Luscieti P, et al: Renal carcinoma after retrograde pyelography with Thorotrast. AJR Am J Roentgenol 148:897-898, 1987.
15. Mandel JS, McLaughlin JK, Schlehofer B, et al: International renal-cell cancer study. IV. Occupation. Int J Cancer 61:601-605, 1995.
16. Parker AS, Cerhan JR, Lynch CF, et al: Gender, alcohol consumption, and renal cell carcinoma. Am J Epidemiol 155:455-462, 2002.
17. Eble JN, Sauter G, Epstein JI, et al: World health organization classification of tumors: pathology and genetics of tumors of the urinary system and male genital organs. Lyon, France, IARC Press, 2004, p 12.
18. Jemal A, Tiwari RC, Murray T, et al: Cancer statistics, 2004. CA Cancer J Clin 54:8-29, 2004.
19. Chow WH, Devesa SS, Warren JL, et al: Rising incidence of renal cell cancer in the United States. JAMA 281:1628-1631, 1999.
20. Pantuck AJ, Zisman A, Belldegrun AS: The changing natural history of renal cell carcinoma. J Urol 166:1611-1623, 2001.
21. Parkin DM, Pisani P, Ferlay J: Estimates of the worldwide incidence of eighteen major cancers in 1985. Int J Cancer 54:594-606, 1993.
22. Hurle R, Losa A, Manzetti A, et al: Upper urinary tract tumors developing after treatment of superficial bladder cancer: 7-year follow-up of 591 consecutive patients. Urology 53:1144-1148, 1999.
23. Jensen OM, Knudsen JB, McLaughlin JK, et al: The Copenhagen case-control study of renal pelvis and ureter cancer: role of smoking and occupational exposures. Int J Cancer 41:557-561, 1988.
24. Ross RK, Paganini-Hill A, Landolph J, et al: Analgesics, cigarette smoking, and other risk factors for cancer of the renal pelvis and ureter. Cancer Res 49:1045-1048, 1989.
25. McLaughlin JK, Silverman DT, Hsing AW, et al: Cigarette smoking and cancers of the renal pelvis and ureter. Cancer Res 52:254-257, 1992.
26. Pommer W, Bronder E, Klimpel A, et al: Urothelial cancer at different tumour sites: role of smoking and habitual intake of analgesics and laxatives. Results of the Berlin Urothelial Cancer Study. Nephrol Dial Transplant 14:2892-2897, 1999.
27. Gaakeer HA, De Ruiter HJ: Carcinoma of the renal pelvis following the abuse of phenacetin-containing analgesic drugs. Br J Urol 51:188-192, 1979.
28. McCredie M, Stewart JH, Carter JJ, et al: Phenacetin and papillary necrosis: independent risk factors for renal pelvic cancer. Kidney Int 30:81-84, 1986.
29. Palvio DH, Andersen JC, Falk E: Transitional cell tumors of the renal pelvis and ureter associated with capillarosclerosis indicating analgesic abuse. Cancer 59:972-976, 1987.
30. Stewart JH, Hobbs JB, McCredie MR: Morphologic evidence that analgesic-induced kidney pathology contributes to the progression of tumors of the renal pelvis. Cancer 86:1576-1582, 1999.
31. Nortier JL, Martinez MC, Schmeiser HH, et al: Urothelial carcinoma associated with the use of a Chinese herb *(Aristolochia fangchi)*. N Engl J Med 342:1686-1692, 2000.
32. Lord GM, Cook T, Arlt VM, et al: Urothelial malignant disease and Chinese herbal nephropathy. Lancet 358:1515-1516, 2001.
33. Petkovic SD: Epidemiology and treatment of renal pelvic and ureteral tumors. J Urol 114:858-865, 1975.
34. Cukuranovic R, Ignjatovic M, Stefanovic V: Urinary tract tumors and Balkan nephropathy in the South Morava River Basin. Kidney Int Suppl 34:S80-S84, 1991.
35. Chow WH, Lindblad P, Gridley G, et al: Risk of urinary tract cancers following kidney or ureter stones. J Natl Cancer Inst 89:1453-1457, 1997.
36. Frischer Z, Waltzer WC, Gonder MJ: Bilateral transitional cell carcinoma of the renal pelvis in the cancer family syndrome. J Urol 134:1197-1198, 1985.
37. Orphali SL, Shols GW, Hagewood J, et al: Familial transitional cell carcinoma of renal pelvis and upper ureter. Urology 27:394-396, 1986.
38. Lynch HT, Ens JA, Lynch JF: The Lynch syndrome II and urological malignancies. J Urol 143:24-28, 1990.
39. Munoz JJ, Ellison LM: Upper tract urothelial neoplasms: incidence and survival during the last 2 decades. J Urol 164:1523-1525, 2000.
40. Kirkali Z, Tuzel E: Transitional cell carcinoma of the ureter and renal pelvis. Crit Rev Oncol Hematol 47:155-169, 2003.
41. Mellemgaard A, Carstensen B, Norgaard N, et al: Trends in the incidence of cancer of the kidney, pelvis, ureter and bladder in Denmark 1943-88. Scand J Urol Nephrol 27:327-332, 1993.
42. Parker AS, Cerhan JR, Janney CA, et al: Smoking cessation and renal cell carcinoma. Ann Epidemiol 13:245-251, 2003.
43. Curti BD: Renal cell carcinoma. JAMA 292:97-100, 2004.
44. Sokoloff MH, deKernion JB, Figlin RA, et al: Current management of renal cell carcinoma. CA Cancer J Clin 46:284-302, 1996.
45. Wakai K, Hirose K, Takezaki T, et al: Foods and beverages in relation to urothelial cancer: case-control study in Japan. Int J Urol 11:11-19, 2004.
46. Hastie KJ, Hamdy FC, Collins MC, et al: Upper tract tumours following cystectomy for bladder cancer. Is routine intravenous urography worthwhile? Br J Urol 67:29-31, 1991.
47. Storkel S, Eble JN, Adlakha K, et al: Classification of renal cell carcinoma: Workgroup No. 1. Union Internationale Contre le Cancer (UICC) and the American Joint Committee on Cancer (AJCC). Cancer 80:987-989, 1997.
48. Kovacs G, Akhtar M, Beckwith BJ, et al: The Heidelberg classification of renal cell tumours. J Pathol 183:131-133, 1997.
49. Ljungberg B, Alamdari FI, Stenling R, et al: Prognostic significance of the Heidelberg classification of renal cell carcinoma. Eur Urol 36:565-569, 1999.
50. Moch H, Gasser T, Amin MB, et al: Prognostic utility of the recently recommended histologic classification and revised TNM staging system of renal cell carcinoma: a Swiss experience with 588 tumors. Cancer 89:604-614, 2000.

51. Amin MB, Tamboli P, Javidan J, et al: Prognostic impact of histologic subtyping of adult renal epithelial neoplasms: an experience of 405 cases. Am J Surg Pathol 26:281-291, 2002.
52. Cheville JC, Lohse CM, Zincke H, et al: Comparisons of outcome and prognostic features among histologic subtypes of renal cell carcinoma. Am J Surg Pathol 27:612-624, 2003.
53. Delahunt B, Eble JN: Papillary renal cell carcinoma: a clinicopathologic and immunohistochemical study of 105 tumors. Mod Pathol 10:537-544, 1997.
54. Lai PP: Kidney, renal pelvis, and ureter. *In* Perez CA, Brady LW (eds): Principles and Practice of Radiation Oncology, 2nd ed. Philadelphia, JB Lippincott, 1992, pp 1025-1035.
55. Batata MA, Whitmore WF, Hilaris BS, et al: Primary carcinoma of the ureter: a prognostic study. Cancer 35:1626-1632, 1975.
56. Johansson S, Angervall L, Bengtsson U, et al: A clinicopathologic and prognostic study of epithelial tumors of the renal pelvis. Cancer 37:1376-1383, 1976.
57. Li MK, Cheung WL: Squamous cell carcinoma of the renal pelvis. J Urol 138:269-271, 1987.
58. Abeshouse BS: Primary benign and malignant tumors of the ureter. Am J Surg 91:237, 1956.
59. Ozsahin M, Zouhair A, Villa S, et al: Prognostic factors in urothelial renal pelvis and ureter tumours: a multicentre Rare Cancer Network study. Eur J Cancer 35:738-743, 1999.
60. Charbit L, Gendreau MC, Mee S, et al: Tumors of the upper urinary tract: 10 years of experience. J Urol 146:1243-1246, 1991.
61. Miyao N, Masumori N, Takahashi A, et al: Lymph node metastasis in patients with carcinomas of the renal pelvis and ureter. Eur Urol 33:180-185, 1998.
62. Miyake H, Hara I, Gohji K, et al: The significance of lymphadenectomy in transitional cell carcinoma of the upper urinary tract. Br J Urol 82:494-498, 1998.
63. Maulard-Durdux C, Dufour B, Hennequin C, et al: Postoperative radiation therapy in 26 patients with invasive transitional cell carcinoma of the upper urinary tract: no impact on survival? J Urol 155:115-117, 1996.
64. Linehan WM, Walther MM, Zbar B: The genetic basis of cancer of the kidney. J Urol 170:2163-2172, 2003.
65. Gnarra JR, Tory K, Weng Y, et al: Mutations of the VHL tumour suppressor gene in renal carcinoma. Nat Genet 7:85-90, 1994.
66. van Slegtenhorst M, de Hoogt R, Hermans C, et al: Identification of the tuberous sclerosis gene TSC1 on chromosome 9q34. Science 277:805-808, 1997.
67. Iliopoulos O, Eng C: Genetic and clinical aspects of familial renal neoplasms. Semin Oncol 27:138-149, 2000.
68. Khoo SK, Bradley M, Wong FK, et al: Birt-Hogg-Dube syndrome: mapping of a novel hereditary neoplasia gene to chromosome 17p12-q11.2. Oncogene 20:5239-5242, 2001.
69. Kim AS: Clinical impact of gene expression profiling on oncology diagnosis, prognosis, and treatment. Comb Chem High Throughput Screen 7:183-206, 2004.
70. Gieseg MA, Cody T, Man MZ, et al: Expression profiling of human renal carcinomas with functional taxonomic analysis. BMC Bioinformatics 3:26, 2002.
71. Boer JM, Huber WK, Sultmann H, et al: Identification and classification of differentially expressed genes in renal cell carcinoma by expression profiling on a global human 31,500-element cDNA array. Genome Res 11:1861-1870, 2001.
72. Takahashi M, Rhodes DR, Furge KA, et al: Gene expression profiling of clear cell renal cell carcinoma: gene identification and prognostic classification. Proc Natl Acad Sci U S A 98:9754-9759, 2001.
73. Martinez A, Fullwood P, Kondo K, et al: Role of chromosome 3p12-p21 tumour suppressor genes in clear cell renal cell carcinoma: analysis of VHL dependent and VHL independent pathways of tumorigenesis. Mol Pathol 53:137-144, 2000.
74. Morrissey C, Martinez A, Zatyka M, et al: Epigenetic inactivation of the RASSF1A 3p21.3 tumor suppressor gene in both clear cell and papillary renal cell carcinoma. Cancer Res 61:7277-7281, 2001.
75. Copland JA, Luxon BA, Ajani L, et al: Genomic profiling identifies alterations in TGFbeta signaling through loss of TGFbeta receptor expression in human renal cell carcinogenesis and progression. Oncogene 22:8053-8062, 2003.
76. Turner KJ, Moore JW, Jones A, et al: Expression of hypoxia-inducible factors in human renal cancer: relationship to angiogenesis and to the von Hippel-Lindau gene mutation. Cancer Res 62:2957-2961, 2002.
77. Shin Lee J, Seok Kim H, Bok Kim Y, et al: Expression of PTEN in renal cell carcinoma and its relation to tumor behavior and growth. J Surg Oncol 84:166-172, 2003.
78. Igarashi H, Esumi M, Ishida H, et al: Vascular endothelial growth factor overexpression is correlated with von Hippel-Lindau tumor suppressor gene inactivation in patients with sporadic renal cell carcinoma. Cancer 95:47-53, 2002.
79. Ashida S, Nishimori I, Tanimura M, et al: Effects of von Hippel-Lindau gene mutation and methylation status on expression of transmembrane carbonic anhydrases in renal cell carcinoma. J Cancer Res Clin Oncol 128:561-568, 2002.
80. Kuczyk MA, Serth J, Bokemeyer C, et al: Detection of p53 gene alteration in renal-cell cancer by micropreparation techniques of tumor specimens. Int J Cancer 64:399-406, 1995.
81. Papadopoulos I, Rudolph P, Weichert-Jacobsen K: Value of p53 expression, cellular proliferation, and DNA content as prognostic indicators in renal cell carcinoma. Eur Urol 32:110-117, 1997.
82. Shimazui T, Oosterwijk E, Debruyne FM, et al: Molecular prognostic factor in renal cell carcinoma. Semin Urol Oncol 14:250-255, 1996.
83. Rasmuson T, Grankvist K, Ljungberg B: Soluble ectodomain of c-erbB-2 oncoprotein in relation to tumour stage and grade in human renal cell carcinoma. Br J Cancer 75:1674-1677, 1997.
84. Fadl-Elmula I, Gorunova L, Mandahl N, et al: Cytogenetic analysis of upper urinary tract transitional cell carcinomas. Cancer Genet Cytogenet 115:123-127, 1999.
85. Rigola MA, Fuster C, Casadevall C, et al: Comparative genomic hybridization analysis of transitional cell carcinomas of the renal pelvis. Cancer Genet Cytogenet 127:59-63, 2001.
86. Rey A, Lara PC, Redondo E, et al: Overexpression of p53 in transitional cell carcinoma of the renal pelvis and ureter. Relation to tumor proliferation and survival. Cancer 79:2178-2185, 1997.
87. Furihata M, Ohtsuki Y, Sonobe H, et al: Prognostic significance of cyclin E and p53 protein overexpression in carcinoma of the renal pelvis and ureter. Br J Cancer 77:783-788, 1998.
88. Furihata M, Ohtsuki Y, Sonobe H, et al: Cyclin A overexpression in carcinoma of the renal pelvis and ureter including dysplasia: immunohistochemical findings in relation to prognosis. Clin Cancer Res 3:1399-1404, 1997.
89. Blaszyk H, Wang L, Dietmaier W, et al: Upper tract urothelial carcinoma: a clinicopathologic study including microsatellite instability analysis. Mod Pathol 15:790-797, 2002.
90. Ritchie AW, Chisholm GD: The natural history of renal carcinoma. Semin Oncol 10:390-400, 1983.
91. Sufrin G, Chasan S, Golio A, et al: Paraneoplastic and serologic syndromes of renal adenocarcinoma. Semin Urol 7:158-171, 1989.
92. Chisholm GD: Nephrogenic ridge tumors and their syndromes. Ann N Y Acad Sci 230:403-423, 1974.
93. Porena M, Vespasiani G, Rosi P, et al: Incidentally detected renal cell carcinoma: role of ultrasonography. J Clin Ultrasound 20:395-400, 1992.
94. Konnak JW, Grossman HB: Renal cell carcinoma as an incidental finding. J Urol 134:1094-1096, 1985.
95. Thompson IM, Peek M: Improvement in survival of patients with renal cell carcinoma—the role of the serendipitously detected tumor. J Urol 140:487-490, 1988.
96. Smith SJ, Bosniak MA, Megibow AJ, et al: Renal cell carcinoma: earlier discovery and increased detection. Radiology 170:699-703, 1989.
97. Johnson CD, Dunnick NR, Cohan RH, et al: Renal adenocarcinoma: CT staging of 100 tumors. AJR Am J Roentgenol 148:59-63, 1987.
98. Semelka RC, Shoenut JP, Magro CM, et al: Renal cancer staging: comparison of contrast-enhanced CT and gadolinium-enhanced fat-suppressed spin-echo and gradient-echo MR imaging. J Magn Reson Imaging 3:597-602, 1993.
99. Robson CJ, Churchill BM, Anderson W: The results of radical nephrectomy for renal cell carcinoma. J Urol 101:297-301, 1969.
100. Greene F, Page DL, Fleming ID, et al (eds): AJCC Cancer Staging Manual, 6th ed. Philadelphia, Springer, 2002.

101. Bloom NA, Vidone RA, Lytton B: Primary carcinoma of the ureter: a report of 102 new cases. J Urol 103:590-598, 1970.
102. Chow NH, Tzai TS, Cheng HL, et al: Urinary cytodiagnosis: can it have a different prognostic implication than a diagnostic test? Urol Int 53:18-23, 1994.
103. Zincke H, Aguilo JJ, Farrow GM, et al: Significance of urinary cytology in the early detection of transitional cell cancer of the upper urinary tract. J Urol 116:781-783, 1976.
104. Witte D, Truong LD, Ramzy I: Transitional cell carcinoma of the renal pelvis the diagnostic role of pelvic washings. Am J Clin Pathol 117:444-450, 2002.
105. Guarnizo E, Pavlovich CP, Seiba M, et al: Ureteroscopic biopsy of upper tract urothelial carcinoma: improved diagnostic accuracy and histopathological considerations using a multi-biopsy approach. J Urol 163:52-55, 2000.
106. Badalament RA, Bennett WF, Bova JG, et al: Computed tomography of primary transitional cell carcinoma of upper urinary tracts. Urology 40:71-75, 1992.
107. Rubenstein MA, Walz BJ, Bucy JG: Transitional cell carcinoma of the kidney 25-year experience. J Urol 119:594-597, 1978.
108. Heney NM, Nocks BN, Daly JJ, et al: Prognostic factors in carcinoma of the ureter. J Urol 125:632-636, 1981.
109. Corrado F, Ferri C, Mannini D, et al: Transitional cell carcinoma of the upper urinary tract: evaluation of prognostic factors by histopathology and flow cytometric analysis. J Urol 145:1159-1163, 1991.
110. Gilbert JB: Diagnosis and treatment of malignant renal tumors. J Urol 39:223, 1937.
111. Mortensen RA: Transthoracic nephrectomy. J Urol 60:855, 1948.
112. Robson CJ: Radical nephrectomy for renal cell carcinoma. J Urol 89:37-42, 1963.
113. Skinner DG, Colvin RB, Vermillion CD, et al: Diagnosis and management of renal cell carcinoma: a clinical and pathologic study of 309 cases. Cancer 28:1165-1177, 1971.
114. McNichols DW, Segura JW, DeWeerd JH: Renal cell carcinoma: long-term survival and late recurrence. J Urol 126:17-23, 1981.
115. Selli C, Hinshaw WM, Woodard BH, et al: Stratification of risk factors in renal cell carcinoma. Cancer 52:899-903, 1983.
116. Golimbu M, Joshi P, Sperber A, et al: Renal cell carcinoma: survival and prognostic factors. Urology 27:291-301, 1986.
117. Dinney CP, Awad SA, Gajewski JB, et al: Analysis of imaging modalities, staging systems, and prognostic indicators for renal cell carcinoma. Urology 39:122-129, 1992.
118. Tsui KH, Shvarts O, Barbaric Z, et al: Is adrenalectomy a necessary component of radical nephrectomy? UCLA experience with 511 radical nephrectomies. J Urol 163:437-441, 2000.
119. Paul R, Mordhorst J, Busch R, et al: Adrenal sparing surgery during radical nephrectomy in patients with renal cell cancer: a new algorithm. J Urol 166:59-62, 2001.
120. Blute ML, Leibovich BC, Cheville JC, et al: A protocol for performing extended lymph node dissection using primary tumor pathological features for patients treated with radical nephrectomy for clear cell renal cell carcinoma. J Urol 172:465-469, 2004.
121. Rabinovitch RA, Zelefsky MJ, Gaynor JJ, et al: Patterns of failure following surgical resection of renal cell carcinoma: implications for adjuvant local and systemic therapy. J Clin Oncol 12:206-212, 1994.
122. Lerner SE, Hawkins CA, Blute ML, et al: Disease outcome in patients with low stage renal cell carcinoma treated with nephron sparing or radical surgery. J Urol 155:1868-1873, 1996.
123. Patard JJ, Shvarts O, Lam JS, et al: Safety and efficacy of partial nephrectomy for all T1 tumors based on an international multicenter experience. J Urol 171:2181-2185, quiz 2435, 2004.
124. Lam JS, Shvarts O, Alemozaffard M: Nephro-sparing surgery as the new gold standard for T1 renal cell carcinoma: results of a contemporary UCLA series [abstract 1774]. J Urol 171(Suppl 4):471, 2004.
125. Lau WK, Blute ML, Weaver AL, et al: Matched comparison of radical nephrectomy vs nephron-sparing surgery in patients with unilateral renal cell carcinoma and a normal contralateral kidney. Mayo Clin Proc 75:1236-1242, 2000.
126. McKiernan J, Simmons R, Katz J, et al: Natural history of chronic renal insufficiency after partial and radical nephrectomy. Urology 59:816-820, 2002.
127. Ono Y, Kinukawa T, Hattori R, et al: Laparoscopic radical nephrectomy for renal cell carcinoma: a five-year experience. Urology 53:280-286, 1999.
128. Portis AJ, Yan Y, Landman J, et al: Long-term followup after laparoscopic radical nephrectomy. J Urol 167:1257-1262, 2002.
129. Stifelman M, Taneja C, Cohen M: Hand assisted laparoscopic nephrectomy: a multi-institutional study evaluation oncological control [abstract]. J Urol 167:668, 2002.
130. Harmon J, Parulkar B, Doble A: Critical assessment of cancer recurrence following renal cryoablation: a multi-center review [abstract 175]. J Urol 171(Suppl 4):469, 2004.
131. Shingleton B, Sewell P: Percutaneous renal tumor cryoablation: results in the first 90 patients [abstract 1751]. J Urol 171(Suppl 4):463, 2004.
132. Savage SJ, Gill IS: Renal tumor ablation: energy-based technologies. World J Urol 18:283-288, 2000.
133. Malkin RB: Regression of renal carcinoma following radiation therapy. J Urol 114:782-783, 1975.
134. Riches EW, Griffiths IH, Thackray AC: New growths of the kidney and ureter. Br J Urol 23:297, 1951.
135. van der Werf-Messing B: Proceedings: carcinoma of the kidney. Cancer 32:1056-1061, 1973.
136. Juusela H, Malmio K, Alfthan O, et al: Preoperative irradiation in the treatment of renal adenocarcinoma. Scand J Urol Nephrol 11:277-281, 1977.
137. Rafla S: Renal cell carcinoma: natural history and results of treatment. Cancer 25:26-40, 1970.
138. Finney R: The value of radiotherapy in the treatment of hypernephroma—a clinical trial. Br J Urol 45:258-269, 1973.
139. Kjaer M, Iversen P, Hvidt V, et al: A randomized trial of postoperative radiotherapy versus observation in stage II and III renal adenocarcinoma. A study by the Copenhagen Renal Cancer Study Group. Scand J Urol Nephrol 21:285-289, 1987.
140. Stein M, Kuten A, Halpern J, et al: The value of postoperative irradiation in renal cell cancer. Radiother Oncol 24:41-44, 1992.
141. Kao GD, Malkowicz SB, Whittington R, et al: Locally advanced renal cell carcinoma: low complication rate and efficacy of postnephrectomy radiation therapy planned with CT. Radiology 193:725-730, 1994.
142. Rafla S: The role of adjuvant radiotherapy in the management of renal cell carcinoma. *In* Javadpour N (ed): Cancer of the Kidney. New York, Thieme-Stratton, 1984, pp 93-107.
143. Gez E, Libes M, Bar-Deroma R, et al: Postoperative irradiation in localized renal cell carcinoma: the Rambam Medical Center experience. Tumori 88:500-502, 2002.
144. Messing EM, Manola J, Wilding G, et al: Phase III study of interferon alfa-NL as adjuvant treatment for resectable renal cell carcinoma: an Eastern Cooperative Oncology Group/Intergroup trial. J Clin Oncol 21:1214-1222, 2003.
145. Pizzocaro G, Piva L, Colavita M, et al: Interferon adjuvant to radical nephrectomy in Robson stages II and III renal cell carcinoma: a multicentric randomized study. J Clin Oncol 19:425-431, 2001.
146. Porzsolt F: Adjuvant therapy of renal cell cancer with interferon alpha-2a [abstract]. Proc Am Soc Clin Oncol 11:202a, 1992.
147. Clark JI, Atkins MB, Urba WJ, et al: Adjuvant high-dose bolus interleukin-2 for patients with high-risk renal cell carcinoma: a Cytokine Working Group randomized trial. J Clin Oncol 21:3133-3140, 2003.
148. Jocham D, Richter A, Hoffmann L, et al: Adjuvant autologous renal tumour cell vaccine and risk of tumour progression in patients with renal-cell carcinoma after radical nephrectomy: phase III, randomised controlled trial. Lancet 363:594-599, 2004.
149. Cozad SC, Smalley SR, Austenfeld M, et al: Transitional cell carcinoma of the renal pelvis or ureter: patterns of failure. Urology 46:796-800, 1995.
150. Zincke H, Neves RJ: Feasibility of conservative surgery for transitional cell cancer of the upper urinary tract. Urol Clin North Am 11:717-724, 1984.
151. McDougall EM, Clayman RV, Elashry O: Laparoscopic nephroureterectomy for upper tract transitional cell cancer: the Washington University experience. J Urol 154:975-979, discussion 979-980, 1995.

152. Klingler HC, Lodde M, Pycha A, et al: Modified laparoscopic nephroureterectomy for treatment of upper urinary tract transitional cell cancer is not associated with an increased risk of tumour recurrence. Eur Urol 44:442-447, 2003.
153. Wallace DM, Wallace DM, Whitfield HN, et al: The late results of conservative surgery for upper tract urothelial carcinomas. Br J Urol 53:537-541, 1981.
154. Leitenberger A, Beyer A, Altwein JE: Organ-sparing treatment for ureteral carcinoma? Eur Urol 29:272-278, 1996.
155. Pohar KS, Sheinfeld J: When is partial ureterectomy acceptable for transitional-cell carcinoma of the ureter? J Endourol 15:405-408, discussion 409, 2001.
156. Elliott DS, Segura JW, Lightner D, et al: Is nephroureterectomy necessary in all cases of upper tract transitional cell carcinoma? Long-term results of conservative endourologic management of upper tract transitional cell carcinoma in individuals with a normal contralateral kidney. Urology 58:174-178, 2001.
157. Lieber MM, Lupu AN: High grade invasive ureteral transitional cell carcinoma with a congenital solitary kidney: long-term survival after ureterectomy and radiation therapy. J Urol 120:368-369, 1978.
158. Brady LW, Gislason GJ, Faust DS, et al: Radiation therapy: a valuable adjunct in the management of carcinoma of the ureter. JAMA 206:2871-2874, 1968.
159. Zietman AL, Grocela J, Zehr E, et al: Selective bladder conservation using transurethral resection, chemotherapy, and radiation: management and consequences of Ta, T1, and Tis recurrence within the retained bladder. Urology 58:380-385, 2001.
160. Tester W, Caplan R, Heaney J, et al: Neoadjuvant combined modality program with selective organ preservation for invasive bladder cancer: results of Radiation Therapy Oncology Group phase II trial 8802. J Clin Oncol 14:119-126, 1996.
161. Cozad SC, Smalley SR, Austenfeld M, et al: Adjuvant radiotherapy in high stage transitional cell carcinoma of the renal pelvis and ureter. Int J Radiat Oncol Biol Phys 24:743-745, 1992.
162. Brookland RK, Richter MP: The postoperative irradiation of transitional cell carcinoma of the renal pelvis and ureter. J Urol 133:952-955, 1985.
163. Bamias A, Deliveliotis C, Fountzilas G, et al: Adjuvant chemotherapy with paclitaxel and carboplatin in patients with advanced carcinoma of the upper urinary tract: a study by the Hellenic Cooperative Oncology Group. J Clin Oncol 22:2150-2154, 2004.
164. Frydenberg M, Gunderson L, Hahn G, et al: Preoperative external beam radiotherapy followed by cytoreductive surgery and intraoperative radiotherapy for locally advanced primary or recurrent renal malignancies. J Urol 152:15-21, 1994.
165. Calvo F, Zincke H, Gunderson LL: Genitourinary IORT. In Gunderson LL, Willet CG, Harrison JB, Calvo F (eds): Intraoperative Irradiation—Techniques and Results. Totowa, NJ, Humana Press, 1999, pp 421-436.
166. Haddock MG, Miller RC, Zincke H, et al: Intraoperative electron irradiation (IOERT) for locally advanced genitourinary malignancies. 3rd International ISIORT Meeting, Aachen, Germany. ISIORT abstract 5.1, 2002.
167. Santos M, Ucar A, Ramos H, et al: [Intraoperative radiotherapy in locally advanced carcinoma of the kidney: initial experience]. Actas Urol Esp 13:36-40, 1989.
168. Eble MJ, Stahler G, Wannenmacher M: IORT for locally advanced or recurrent renal cell carcinoma. Front Radiat Ther Oncol 31:253-255, 1997.
169. McCaffrey JA, Motzer RJ: What is the role of nephrectomy in patients with metastatic renal cell carcinoma? Semin Oncol 23:19, 1996.
170. Neves RJ, Zincke H, Taylor WF: Metastatic renal cell cancer and radical nephrectomy: identification of prognostic factors and patient survival. J Urol 139:1173-1176, 1988.
171. O'Dea MJ, Zincke H, Utz DC, et al: The treatment of renal cell carcinoma with solitary metastasis. J Urol 120:540-542, 1978.
172. Kjaer M: The treatment and prognosis of patients with renal adenocarcinoma with solitary metastasis: 10 year survival results. Int J Radiat Oncol Biol Phys 13:619-621, 1987.
173. Flanigan RC, Salmon SE, Blumenstein BA, et al: Nephrectomy followed by interferon alfa-2b compared with interferon alfa-2b alone for metastatic renal-cell cancer. N Engl J Med 345:1655-1659, 2001.
174. Mickisch GH, Garin A, van Poppel H, et al: Radical nephrectomy plus interferon-alfa-based immunotherapy compared with interferon alfa alone in metastatic renal-cell carcinoma: a randomised trial. Lancet 358:966-970, 2001.
175. Althausen P, Althausen A, Jennings LC, et al: Prognostic factors and surgical treatment of osseous metastases secondary to renal cell carcinoma. Cancer 80:1103-1109, 1997.
176. Halperin EC, Harisiadis L: The role of radiation therapy in the management of metastatic renal cell carcinoma. Cancer 51:614-617, 1983.
177. Onufrey V, Mohiuddin M: Radiation therapy in the treatment of metastatic renal cell carcinoma. Int J Radiat Oncol Biol Phys 11:2007-2009, 1985.
178. Wilson D, Hiller L, Gray L, et al: The effect of biological effective dose on time to symptom progression in metastatic renal cell carcinoma. Clin Oncol (R Coll Radiol) 15:400-407, 2003.
179. Wronski M, Maor MH, Davis BJ, et al: External radiation of brain metastases from renal carcinoma: a retrospective study of 119 patients from the M. D. Anderson Cancer Center. Int J Radiat Oncol Biol Phys 37:753-759, 1997.
180. Wronski M, Arbit E, Russo P, et al: Surgical resection of brain metastases from renal cell carcinoma in 50 patients. Urology 47:187-193, 1996.
181. Fuller BG, Kaplan ID, Adler J, et al: Stereotaxic radiosurgery for brain metastases: the importance of adjuvant whole brain irradiation. Int J Radiat Oncol Biol Phys 23:413-418, 1992.
182. Sheehan JP, Sun MH, Kondziolka D, et al: Radiosurgery in patients with renal cell carcinoma metastasis to the brain: long-term outcomes and prognostic factors influencing survival and local tumor control. J Neurosurg 98:342-349, 2003.
183. Brown PD, Brown CA, Pollock BE, et al: Stereotactic radiosurgery for patients with "radioresistant" brain metastases. Neurosurgery 51:656-665, discussion 665-657, 2002.
184. Amendola BE, Wolf AL, Coy SR, et al: Brain metastases in renal cell carcinoma: management with gamma knife radiosurgery. Cancer J 6:372-376, 2000.
185. Payne BR, Prasad D, Szeifert G, et al: Gamma surgery for intracranial metastases from renal cell carcinoma. J Neurosurg 92:760-765, 2000.
186. Hernandez L, Zamorano L, Sloan A, et al: Gamma knife radiosurgery for renal cell carcinoma brain metastases. J Neurosurg 97:489-493, 2002.
187. Yagoda A, Petrylak D, Thompson S: Cytotoxic chemotherapy for advanced renal cell carcinoma. Urol Clin North Am 20:303-321, 1993.
188. Rini BI, Vogelzang NJ, Dumas MC, et al: Phase II trial of weekly intravenous gemcitabine with continuous infusion fluorouracil in patients with metastatic renal cell cancer. J Clin Oncol 18:2419-2426, 2000.
189. Milowsky MI, Rosmarin A, Tickoo SK, et al: Active chemotherapy for collecting duct carcinoma of the kidney: a case report and review of the literature. Cancer 94:111-116, 2002.
190. Motzer RJ, Bacik J, Murphy BA, et al: Interferon-alfa as a comparative treatment for clinical trials of new therapies against advanced renal cell carcinoma. J Clin Oncol 20:289-296, 2002.
191. Fyfe G, Fisher RI, Rosenberg SA, et al: Results of treatment of 255 patients with metastatic renal cell carcinoma who received high-dose recombinant interleukin-2 therapy. J Clin Oncol 13:688-696, 1995.
192. Fisher RI, Rosenberg SA, Fyfe G: Long-term survival update for high-dose recombinant interleukin-2 in patients with renal cell carcinoma. Cancer J Sci Am 6(Suppl 1):S55-S57, 2000.
193. Yang JC, Sherry RM, Steinberg SM, et al: Randomized study of high-dose and low-dose interleukin-2 in patients with metastatic renal cancer. J Clin Oncol 21:3127-3132, 2003.
194. Atzpodien J, Kirchner H, Jonas U, et al: Interleukin-2- and interferon alfa-2a-based immunochemotherapy in advanced renal cell carcinoma: a prospectively randomized trial of the German Cooperative Renal Carcinoma Chemoimmunotherapy Group (DGCIN). J Clin Oncol 22:1188-1194, 2004.
195. Yang JC, Haworth L, Sherry RM, et al: A randomized trial of bevacizumab, an anti-vascular endothelial growth factor anti-

body, for metastatic renal cancer. N Engl J Med 349:427-434, 2003.
196. Hainsworth JD, Sosman JA, Spigel R: Phase II trial of bevacizumab and erlotinib in patients with metastatic renal carcinoma [abstract]. Proc Am Soc Clin Oncol 22:4502a, 2004.
197. Burch PA, Richardson RL, Cha SS, et al: Phase II study of paclitaxel and cisplatin for advanced urothelial cancer. J Urol 164:1538-1542, 2000.
198. Lerner SE, Blute ML, Richardson RL, et al: Platinum-based chemotherapy for advanced transitional cell carcinoma of the upper urinary tract. Mayo Clin Proc 71:945-950, 1996.
199. Moore MJ, Winquist EW, Murray N, et al: Gemcitabine plus cisplatin, an active regimen in advanced urothelial cancer: a phase II trial of the National Cancer Institute of Canada Clinical Trials Group. J Clin Oncol 17:2876-2881, 1999.
200. Mundt AJ, Lujan AE, Rotmensch J, et al: Intensity-modulated whole pelvic radiotherapy in women with gynecologic malignancies. Int J Radiat Oncol Biol Phys 52:1330-1337, 2002.
201. Heron DE, Gerszten K, Selvaraj RN, et al: Conventional 3D conformal versus intensity-modulated radiotherapy for the adjuvant treatment of gynecologic malignancies: a comparative dosimetric study of dose-volume histograms small star, filled. Gynecol Oncol 91:39-45, 2003.

CHAPTER 54

PENILE CANCER

Juanita Crook and Jean-Jacques Mazeron

INCIDENCE

Penile cancer occurs in approximately 1 of 100,000 North Americans and Europeans (0.4% to 0.6% of all male cancers), but it represents as much as 10% of male malignancies in parts of Asia, Africa, and South America.

BIOLOGIC CHARACTERISTICS

Human papillomavirus types 16 and 18 are detected in 40% to 45% of penile cancers. Moderate or poor differentiation, invasion of the corpora, and the presence of tumor emboli in lymphovascular channels predict regional spread.

STAGING EVALUATION

Circumcision is recommended for full evaluation of the primary tumor. Magnetic resonance may supplement palpation in the determination of invasion of the corpora. Computed tomography for staging lacks sufficient sensitivity for evaluation of lymph nodes. For adverse pathology (grade, invasion of corpora, or lymphovascular spaces) bilateral staging and superficial inguinal lymph node dissection are recommended.

PRIMARY THERAPY

Penile conservation is recommended for T1-2 tumors up to 4 cm in diameter and for selected T3 tumors.

Laser surgery for T1s and T1 tumors yields satisfactory local control and cosmesis.

Interstitial brachytherapy for stage T1-2 tumors allows penile preservation in 70% to 85% of patients. The most common sequelae of treatment are urethral stenosis (12% to 45%) and soft tissue necrosis (8% to 25%).

For external beam radiation therapy, penile preservation rates are 50% to 65%.

ADJUVANT THERAPY

Adjuvant external beam radiation therapy is recommended after lymph node dissection for patients with multiple positive groin nodes or extracapsular disease.

LOCALLY ADVANCED DISEASE

Locally advanced penile cancer is a highly lethal malignancy that requires a multimodality approach, beginning with total or partial penectomy and lymph node dissection, followed by systemic chemotherapy with or without pelvic and inguinal irradiation.

PALLIATION

Unresectable nodes are rarely controlled by radiation therapy, but palliation may be possible with irradiation. A combined approach with systemic chemotherapy is warranted if the patient's general condition permits.

The penis is divided into three portions: the root, the body (or shaft), and the glans. The root is embedded in the superficial perineum. The shaft consists of the erectile bodies composed of two corpora cavernosa, the corpus spongiosum, and the overlying skin. The glans constitutes the distal part of the corpus spongiosum and is covered by a skin fold known as the prepuce. The arbitrary limit between glans and body is the coronal sulcus.

Early-stage, well-differentiated cancers of the penis can be effectively managed with local therapy, and attention should be paid to preservation of penile function and morphology. Primary surgical management is effective but can be associated with considerable psychosexual morbidity. Even partial penectomy can have a profound effect on sexual health and self-image.[1,2] Suicide or attempted suicide after partial penectomy has been reported.[3-5] External or interstitial radiation therapy is an organ-sparing alternative that preserves penile morphology and function without compromising disease control or survival in selected patients. Unfortunately, many urologists do not routinely offer this penis-conserving option.[6] Quality of life and sexual health after surgery is rarely studied or reported. Sexuality and expectations should be discussed when deciding on primary management. Advanced or poorly differentiated tumors require a multimodality approach.

ETIOLOGY AND EPIDEMIOLOGY

Carcinoma of the penis is rare, with an estimated incidence of 1 case per 100,000 men in North America and Europe, where it accounts for 0.4% to 0.6% of cancers.[7] Higher incidences are seen in parts of Asia, Africa, and South America, where it represents up to 10% of malignancies in male patients.[7,8] The peak incidence is in the sixth decade in developed countries but earlier where the incidence is higher.[9]

Case-control studies have identified important risk factors (OR > 10) to be phimosis, chronic inflammatory conditions such as lichen sclerosis, treatment with psoralen and ultraviolet A photochemotherapy (PUVA), smoking (dose-dependent association), and a history of genital condylomas (threefold to fivefold increase in risk). Neonatal circumcision is associated with a threefold decrease in risk of penile carcinoma, although in some series, up to 20% of patients had been circumcised neonatally.[10] Human papillomavirus (HPV) types 16 and 18 have been identified in about 50% of invasive penile cancers.[10,11]

PREVENTION AND EARLY DETECTION

Infant circumcision is highly effective in prevention of this disease, but it is no longer recommended on these grounds alone.[12] The emphasis is instead on education, the promotion of good hygiene for the normally retractile foreskin, and surgical correction of phimosis. Men should be made aware of the association between certain HPV subtypes, venereal warts, and cancer, as well as the premalignant nature of conditions such as lichen sclerosis, which may precede the diagnosis of cancer by many years.

BIOLOGIC CHARACTERISTICS AND MOLECULAR BIOLOGY

The overall incidence of HPV in penile carcinoma is 40% to 45%, as detected by polymerase chain reaction (PCR) amplification of DNA.[9,13] HPV-16[13] and HPV-18[14] are the most frequent subtypes detected. The frequency of HPV detection depends on the histopathologic subtype of penile cancer. HPV association is seen in 80% to 100% of basaloid and warty penile cancers but in only approximately 35% of verrucous or squamous cell carcinomas.[9] The difference in prevalence of HPV in these two groups suggests different pathogenesis. HPV presence in a tumor does not appear to confer a worse prognosis.[13]

In one series, *p53* positivity was found in 41% of 82 cases of invasive penile cancer. In multivariate analysis, *p53* positivity and lymphatic embolization were predictive of lymph node metastases.[15]

PATHOLOGY AND PATHWAYS OF SPREAD

Premalignant lesions are associated with invasive cancers in 20% to 30% of cases. Intraepithelial neoplasias such as bowenoid papulosis, Bowen's disease, and erythroplasia of Queryat[16] are precursor lesions of warty and basaloid penile cancers. Lichen sclerosis (balanitis xerotica obliterans) is associated with non-HPV variants of penile carcinoma.[17,18] Condylomas, Buschke-Löwenstein disease, Kaposi's sarcoma, and leukoplakia are also associated with penile cancer.

The primary tumor most frequently occurs on the glans (48%) or prepuce (25%), with the glans and prepuce involved in 9%, the coronal sulcus in 6%, and the shaft in only 2%.[8] Squamous cell carcinomas represent 95% of invasive cancers of the penis. Most are low-grade tumors. Other histopathologic primary tumor types are malignant melanoma, transitional cell carcinoma, basal cell carcinoma, and sarcoma.[8]

The lymphatics of the prepuce and the skin of the shaft drain into the superficial inguinal nodes located above the fascia lata. The glans and the deep penile structure drain into the superficial or deep inguinal nodes. Lymphatics thereafter drain into those that accompany the femoral vessels and extend to the external iliac, common iliac, and para-aortic regions. The sentinel nodes are located above and medial to the junction of the inferior epigastric and saphenous veins.

CLINICAL MANIFESTATIONS, PATIENT EVALUATION, AND STAGING

General Approach

Because of the rarity of carcinoma of the penis, many series span several decades. Three different staging systems are encountered in a review of the literature of the past 2 decades (Table 54-1).[19-21]

Clinical staging of carcinoma of the penis is very subjective, and it may be difficult to distinguish T1 (i.e., invasion of subepithelial connective tissue) from T2 (i.e., invasion of corpus spongiosum or cavernosum). For this reason, techniques that treat less than the full thickness of the penis must be restricted to very carefully selected cases. Magnetic resonance imaging (MRI) may be helpful in cases that are difficult to stage clinically, with a positive predictive value for invasion of the corpora cavernosa of 75% (6 of 8 patients).[22] When combined with artificial erection, MRI-guided staging showed good agreement with ultimate pathologic stage.[23]

Any patient who presents with phimosis and chronic discharge, bleeding, balanitis, or swelling in the region of the coronal sulcus or glans under an unretractable foreskin should have a dorsal slit of the foreskin to allow inspection of the glans and should preferably have a full circumcision. Any suspicious lesions should be biopsied (Fig. 54-1).

Table 54-1 Staging Systems for Carcinoma of the Penis

Stage	Description
JACKSON STAGING SYSTEM*	
1	Tumor limited to the glans or prepuce
2	Tumor extending into the shaft or corpora but without node involvement
3	Tumor confined to the shaft but with malignant but operable lymph nodes
4	Invasion beyond the shaft with inoperable lymph nodes or distant metastases
TNM STAGING OF THE UICC, 1978†	
Tis	Carcinoma in situ
T1	Tumor ≤ 2 cm
T2	Tumor > 2 cm and ≤ 5 cm
T3	Tumor > 5 cm or deep invasion including urethra
T4	Tumor invades adjacent structures
N1	Metastases in unilateral inguinal lymph nodes
N2	Metastases in bilateral inguinal lymph nodes
N3	Fixed inguinal lymph nodes
TNM STAGING OF THE UICC, 1987-2002‡	
T1	Tumor in subepithelial connective tissue
T2	Tumor in corpus spongiosum/cavernosum
T3	Tumor in urethra/prostate
T4	Tumor in other adjacent structures
N1	Tumor in one superficial inguinal lymph node
N2	Tumor in multiple/bilateral superficial inguinal lymph nodes
N3	Tumor in deep inguinal or pelvic lymph nodes

UICC, International Union Against Cancer (Union Internationale Contre le Cancer).
*From Jackson S: The treatment of carcinoma of the penis. Br J Surg 53:33-35, 1966.
†From Harmer M: Penis (ICD-0187). *In* TNM Classification of Malignant Tumours, 3rd ed. Berlin, Springer-Verlag, 1978, pp 126-128.
‡From Hermanek PS, Sobin LH. Penis (ICD-0187). *In* Hermanek PS, Sobin LH (eds): TNM Classification of Malignant Tumours, 4th ed. Berlin, Springer-Verlag, 1987, 130-132.

Lymph Node Assessment: The N0 Patient

Management of the patient with clinically negative groins remains controversial. Although the gold standard treatment for invasive penile cancer remains amputation and bilateral groin dissection,[8,15] most radiotherapy series advocate a "wait and see" policy, with no systematic staging investigations such as computed tomography (CT) scans or fine-needle aspiration.[5,24-27] Because only about 20% of clinically negative nodes have micrometastases,[5,24-27] staging lymph node dissection is not warranted for all patients. Only 50% of clinically suspicious nodes are histologically positive.[28] Inguinal node dissection may be complicated in one third of cases by infec-

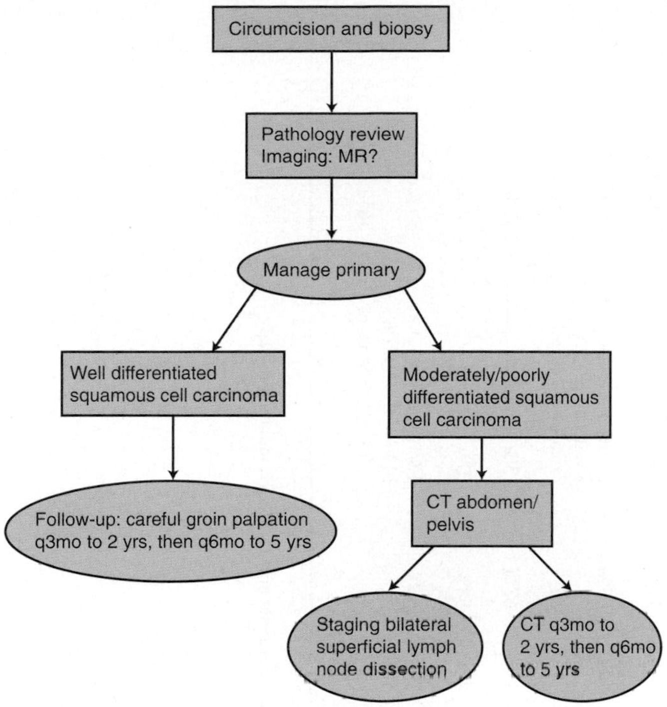

Figure 54-1 Diagnostic algorithm for a clinically node-negative patient. CT, computed tomography; MR, magnetic resonance.

tion, skin flap necrosis, deep vein thrombosis, or severe leg edema.[29-31]

Nodal status is, however, the strongest predictive factor for overall survival.[5,32,33] Lymph node dissection may be curative for men with microscopic regional spread. Several surgical series have identified that *therapeutic* node dissection confers an inferior survival compared with *prophylactic* node dissection.[34] McDougal found a 5-year survival after inguinal node dissection of 92% for clinically N0 patients, compared with 33% for those with clinically involved nodes.[35] Modified inguinal lymphadenectomy, sparing the saphenous vein and limiting the dissection laterally, distally, and proximally, may reduce morbidity.[29]

Histopathologic factors help to identify patients at high risk for microscopic regional spread. Grade is predictive for regional failure, which occurs with 30% of well-differentiated and 81% of moderately to poorly differentiated tumors.[30] T stage, vascular invasion, and the presence of more than 50% poorly differentiated cancer in the primary tumor are also predictive for nodal relapse.[32] McDougal reported that tumor grade and the presence of corporeal invasion (T stage) were strong predictors of nodal relapse. Patients with clinically negative nodes but with poorly differentiated cancers or invasion of the corpora had a 78% rate of node positivity after inguinal dissection, compared with 4% for moderately or well-differentiated tumors and no invasion of the corpora.[35]

The difficulty with applying this information to decision-making in radiotherapy is that the primary tumor is not available for complete histopathologic examination. Invasion of the corpora may be underappreciated clinically. However, an additional prognostic factor for regional spread is the presence of tumor emboli in venous or lymphatic channels.[36] If, on examination of the biopsy, tumor emboli are present in lymphovascular spaces or the tumor shows moderate or poor differentiation, assessment of regional lymph nodes is warranted by bilateral modified inguinal node dissection. The specificity and sensitivity of CT are not sufficiently reliable,[37] and fine-needle aspiration is only applicable to nodes that are enlarged or suspected of containing disease.

Dynamic sentinel node mapping using a gamma probe after intradermal injection of technetium 99m around the primary tumor is promising in the detection of early lymph node involvement.[37] Reports indicate a false-negative rate of 11% to 22%,[37-39] but this procedure has yet to be accepted as an alternative to modified inguinal node dissection.

PRIMARY THERAPY

Surgery

Circumcision is the first step in all cases. Small tumors that are limited to the prepuce can be treated by circumcision alone. Penis-conserving surgical techniques such as laser or Mohs' surgery may be suitable for selected tumors. Mohs' surgery[40] for carcinoma in situ or very superficial tumors involves excision of tissue in successive layers with complete microscopic scanning of each horizontally cut layer to identify any tumor outgrowths that may extend beyond the visible or palpable lesion. Successive layers are removed until margins are histologically clear.

Laser surgery using carbon dioxide or neodymium: yttrium-aluminum-garnet (Nd:YAG) lasers has been reported to provide a superior functional and cosmetic result compared with standard surgical techniques for selected premalignant and malignant lesions.[41-43] Most tumors appropriate for this modality are carcinoma in situ or T1, although the occasional T2 tumor is included in reported series. Windahl reported a 19% local recurrence rate for 67 patients; 50% of failures could be retreated with laser. Extended, careful follow-up is required because only 57% of local recurrences occurred within the first 2 years, 30% between 6 and 10 years, and 15% after 10 years.[42] Whether these late failures represent true local recurrences or new primary tumors is unknown.

Selected cases, especially those involving only skin, can be treated by wide excision, but local wedge excision is associated with a high recurrence rate. Total or partial penectomy is indicated for larger or more invasive tumors. An adequate resection margin of 1 to 2 cm and tumor-free margins on frozen section should be obtained. Partial penectomy may be possible when the tumor involves the glans or the distal shaft, and the penile remnant will allow the patient to direct the urinary stream. Total amputation is indicated for larger or proximal tumors and requires a perineal urethrostomy.

Irradiation

Radical radiotherapy in the form of brachytherapy or external beam radiation therapy (EBRT) is effective in achieving local control in a high percentage of patients. Except for Rozan's collaborative report from France,[24] the number of patients in each series in Table 54-2 is relatively small. Often, series span several decades, during which time treatment techniques and dose prescriptions evolve. Staging systems have also undergone significant modifications (see Table 54-1).

Interstitial brachytherapy yields a 5-year local tumor control rate of 70% to 86%, with penile preservation rates at 5 years ranging from 72% to 83%. For EBRT, local control rates are less favorable, 41% to 70% at 5 years. The increased need for surgical salvage decreases penile preservation rates to 36%

Table 54-2 Comparative Results from Radiotherapy Series

Study	No. of Patients	RT Type	Dose (Gy)	Months of Follow-up (range)	5-Year Local Control by RT	5-Year CSS*	Complications	Penile Preservation
Chaudhery et al[61] (1999)	23	BT	50 LDR	21 (4-117)	70% (8 y)	—	No necrosis 2/23 with stenosis	70% (8 y)
Crook et al[46] (2004)	49	BT	60 @ 65 cGy/h	33 (4-140)	85.3%	90%	16% necrosis 12% stenosis	85%, 5-y actuarial rate
Delannes et al[27] (1992)	51	BT	50-65 @ 60 cGy/h	65 (12-144)	86% crude	85%	23% necrosis 45% stenosis	75%
Kiltie et al[26] (2000)	31	BT	64 @ 47 cGy/h	61.5	81%	85.4%	8% necrosis 44% stenosis	75%
Mazeron et al[25] (1984)	50	BT	60-70 LDR	36-96	78% crude	—	3/50 necrosis 19% stenosis	74%
Rozan et al[24] (1995)	184	BT	59 @ 50 cGy/h	139	86%	88%	21% necrosis 45% stenosis	78%
Soria et al[5] (1996)	102	BT	61-70 over 5-7 d	111	77%	72%	Not stated	72% (6 y)
Gotsadze et al[62] (2000)	155	Ext	40-60 @ 2 Gy/Fx	4 decades' experience	65%	86%	1 with necrosis 5 with stenosis	65%
McLean et al[53] (1993)	26	Ext	35/10 Fx to 60/25 Fx	116 (84-168)	61.5%	69%	7/26 unspecified	66% crude
Neave et al[54] (1993)	24	Mold	56/84 h (12 h/d)	36-mo minimum	69.7%	67%	13% stenosis	55%
	20	Ext	50-55/20-22 Fx	36-mo minimum	69.7%	58%	10% stenosis	60%
Sarin et al[4] (1997)	59	Ext	60/30 Fx	62 (2-264)	55%	66%	3% necrosis 14% with stenosis	50% crude
Zouhair et al[44] (2001)	23	Ext	45-74/25-37 Fx	12 (5-139)	41%	—	2/23 with stenosis	36%

*Corrected for intercurrent deaths.
BT, brachytherapy; CSS, cause-specific survival; Ext, external beam; Fx, fractions; LC, local control; LDR, low dose rate (actual dose rate not stated); RT, radiation therapy.

Table 54-3 Type of Salvage Surgery for Local Recurrence or Necrosis after External Beam Radiation Therapy or Brachytherapy

Study	Type of Irradiation	Local Excision	Partial Penectomy	Total Penectomy
Chaudhery et al[61]	BT	—	4	—
Crook et al[46]	BT	—	5	2
Delannes et al[27]	BT	—	4	3
Kiltie et al[26]	BT	—	2	3
Rozan et al[24]	BT	3	16	12
Zouhair et al[44]	RT	1	6	7

BT, brachytherapy; RT, external beam radiation.

to 66%. Careful extended follow-up is recommended because local failures can occur several years after treatment. Mazeron reported that of the 11 local failures in a brachytherapy series of 50 patients, only 36% occurred in the first 2 years; 45% occurred between years 2 and 5, and 18% occurred between years 5 and 8.[25] This late recurrence pattern is strikingly similar to that seen after penile-conserving therapy using a laser.[42]

Surgery for Salvage

Surgery for salvage is successful in more than 80% of failures.[24,44] Local excision is rarely appropriate as surgical salvage, with procedures equally divided between total and partial penectomy (Table 54-3).[24,26,27,44] The choice depends on penile length and the proportion of the shaft irradiated by the primary treatment. The localized nature of brachytherapy should result in less radical salvage operations, but this is not apparent in the literature.

Patient Selection for Radiation Therapy

Several prognostic factors have been identified for penile preservation. For EBRT, a total dose of less than 60 Gy, a protracted treatment time of more than 45 days, and a daily fraction size of less than 2 Gy are all associated with an increased risk of local failure.[4,44]

For brachytherapy, the volume of tumor and depth of invasion are predictive of local control.[5,25,26,45] The ideal tumor for brachytherapy should be less than 4 cm in its maximum diameter,[5,25,26,45] with less than 1 cm of invasion.[5,25] Local failure rates of 60% for tumors larger than 4 cm in diameter have been reported, compared with 14% for those smaller than 4 cm. Use of more than six brachytherapy needles and tumor volumes greater than 8 cc are also associated with an increased risk of failure.[5,22,23] Mazeron reported an 11% local failure rate for T1 (<2 cm), 22% for T2 (2 to 5 cm), and 29% for T3 disease.[25]

Histopathology does not appear to be a factor in local control. Most penile cancers are well-differentiated squamous cell carcinomas. A more favorable outcome for verrucous cancers has been reported, but most series do not specify this pathology subtype. Moderate to poor differentiation influences overall survival and the risk of nodal involvement[45,46] but does not preclude a penile-conserving approach.

LOCALLY ADVANCED DISEASE AND PALLIATION

Although a penile-sparing approach is occasionally warranted for a T3 tumor in a younger patient, most locally advanced tumors require partial or total penectomy with a perineal urostomy and bilateral groin dissection.

Node-Positive Disease

Involved nodes should be resected if possible. As in squamous cancers of other sites that drain to the inguinal regions, patients with pathologic findings of multiple positive nodes or extracapsular spread should be offered postoperative radiotherapy.[46,47] If dissection of deep pelvic nodes is negative, treatment can be limited to the involved groin. A direct anterior electron field of suitable energy to deliver a dose of 45 to 50 Gy over 5 weeks to the depth of the nodes is appropriate.[48] If the status of the pelvic nodes is unknown, they should be included in the treatment volume.

Unresectable nodes are rarely controlled by radiotherapy but can be palliated. A combined approach with systemic chemotherapy may be warranted if the patient's general condition permits an aggressive approach. Reports using combination chemotherapy (5-fluorouracil [5-FU] and mitomycin C[49] or various cisplatin-based regimens) indicate limited success.[50] Intra-arterial chemotherapy for locally advanced or recurrent penile cancer using cisplatin, methotrexate, and bleomycin (CMB)[51] or CMB plus 5-FU and mitomycin C[51] has shown promise. The Southwest Oncology Group has reported a trial using CMB in locally advanced or metastatic penile cancer in 40 men, with a response rate of 32.5%.[52] Surgery or irradiation, or both, can be used after a response to chemotherapy.

TECHNIQUES OF IRRADIATION

External Beam Radiation

External radiotherapy has several advantages in that it is widely available, delivers a reliably homogeneous dose, and does not require the specific expertise of brachytherapy. Well-localized carcinoma in situ (Tis) may be treated effectively using 125- to 250-kV orthovoltage beams or 13-MeV electrons with suitable bolus, using fractionation schemes commonly employed for skin cancer such as 35 Gy given in 10 fractions over 2 weeks.[53] However, for most penile cancers, irradiation to the full thickness of the penis with a full dose to the skin surface is required. Fraction sizes less than 2 Gy may be suboptimal,[4] and fraction sizes larger than 2 Gy may be associated with increased long-term sequelae.[54] Doses range from 60 Gy given in 25 fractions over 5 weeks to 74 Gy given in 37 fractions over 7.5 weeks, avoiding interruptions due to acute reactions (e.g., edema, pain, desquamation).[4] An easily reproducible setup over the 6-week period that is comfortable for the patient despite increasing local reaction and easily verified by technologists is essential.

Wax Block

A 10 × 10 cm to 10 × 15 cm wax block can be constructed in two halves with a central cylindrical chamber.[44,53] The patient is positioned supine on the treatment couch, and the penis is supported in a vertical position, encased in the wax block. Tissue-equivalent material must be placed in the distal portion of the cylindrical chamber to maintain full dose to the glans. Parallel-opposed beams of cobalt 60 or 4- to 6-MV photons treat the entire length of the penis (Fig. 54-2).

This technique may become increasingly uncomfortable for the patient as treatment progresses. Penile swelling may require modification of the wax block. Verification of penile position within the wax is impossible, but catheterization throughout the 6 weeks of treatment may prevent the penis from "slumping" inside the wax.

Perspex Block

A Perspex block is a good alternative to the wax block technique, providing full buildup to the skin surface and allowing treatment by parallel-opposed beams.[4] Preconstructed blocks in a range of sizes of the central cylindrical chamber can be sterilized for reuse. Penile swelling can be accommodated easily by choosing the next larger size, and penile position within the transparent block can be easily verified visually (Fig. 54-3).

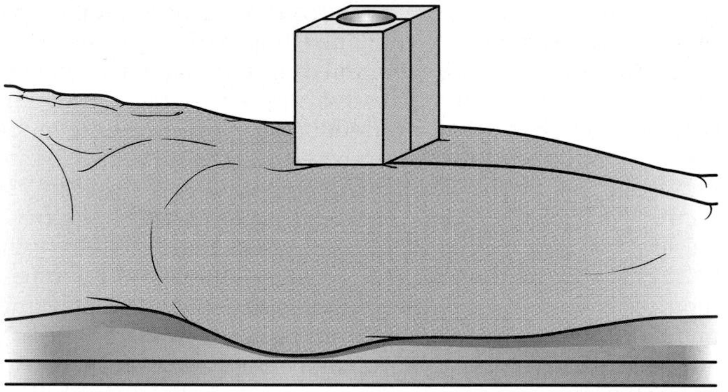

Figure 54-2 Wax block technique. A wax block with a central cylindrical chamber for the penis provides a full buildup of dose to the skin surface for parallel-opposed megavoltage beams.

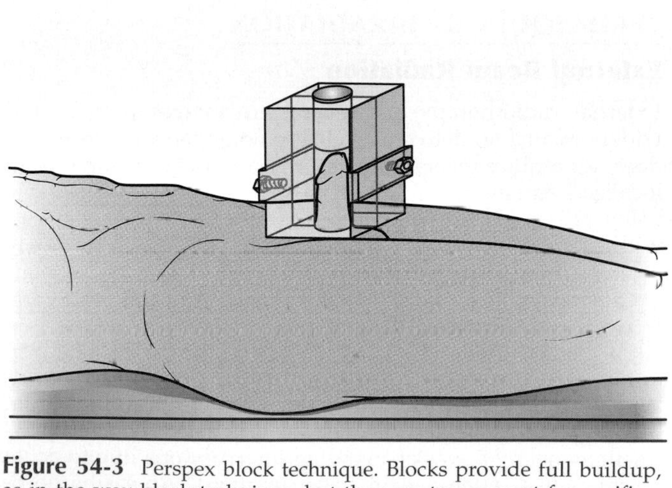

Figure 54-3 Perspex block technique. Blocks provide full buildup, as in the wax block technique, but they are transparent for verification of penile position. The blocks are bivalved and can be made in a range of sizes to accommodate penile swelling as treatment progresses.

Water Bath

A water bath can also be used in place of wax or Perspex to provide full dose to the penile surface.[55,56] The patient is positioned prone on the treatment couch, the upper and lower portions of his body supported on Styrofoam slabs, with the water bath positioned to contain the suspended penis (Fig. 54-4). Visual inspection of correct positioning is easy, and the setup results in the least discomfort for the patient. Beam arrangement and fractionation are the same as for a wax or Perspex block.

Brachytherapy

The penis is well suited to brachytherapy. For centers with appropriate expertise, surface molds or interstitial techniques can be used with good effect. Circumcision should be performed before brachytherapy to ensure complete exposure of the tumor and prevent subsequent phimosis or annular fibrosis of the foreskin.

Molds

Unlike interstitial brachytherapy, a mold is not invasive and does not require anesthesia.[54] The acute reaction develops after the treatment is finished. A surface dose of 55 to 60 Gy is prescribed, with a central axis dose of 46 to 50 Gy over 84 hours (12 h/day).[57] Techniques using a Perspex tube[54] or silicon monomer[58] have been described.

Interstitial Brachytherapy

There is broad experience with interstitial brachytherapy for T1 or T2 penile carcinoma, with reports from many European countries and from Canada. Circumcision should always precede penile brachytherapy. Implants are usually placed under general anesthesia. The Paris system of dosimetry[59] is applicable to manually afterloaded implants and remote afterloading pulse dose rate (PDR) systems, although for the latter, some optimization can be introduced.

Penile brachytherapy is generally performed as a volume implant delivering full-thickness irradiation, although well-selected, very superficial tumors may be treated with a single-plane implant. For volume implants, two or three parallel planes of sources are inserted, with two or three needles in each plane. Equal intersource and interplane spacing ranges from 12 to 18 mm. The distribution, spacing, and total number of needles depend on tumor size. Planes are usually oriented with the needles passing from the dorsal to the ventral surface of the glands, but a left-right orientation may be acceptable depending on tumor location. Visual verification of coverage can be readily accomplished. Care must be taken to adhere to the rules of the Paris system[59] and to be aware of the relation-

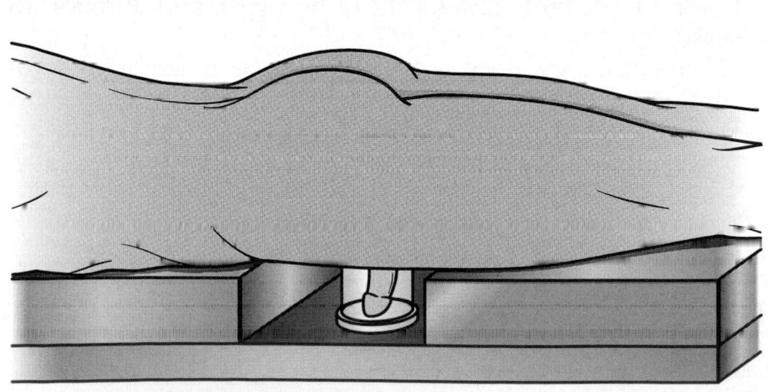

Figure 54-4 Water bath technique. The patient lies prone on the Styrofoam slabs such that the penis is suspended in the water bath. The overflow tray catches the run-off water. Transparent sides on the water bath permit a visual check of penile position.

ship of the treated volume to the needles such that placement ensures that the entire tumor and desired margin are within the high-dose volume (Fig. 54-5).

Needle placement requires 30 to 45 minutes in the operating room. Catheterization aids in identification of the urethra so as to avoid transfixing it with implant needles. The 19.5-gauge needles are appropriate for manually afterloaded ^{192}Ir wire, and 17.5-gauge needles are compatible with a PDR remote afterloader. The needles are stabilized through the duration of the implantation with predrilled Plexiglas templates. The prescribed dose is generally 60 Gy at a dose rate of 50 to 60 cGy per hour over 100 to 120 hours (4 to 5 days). No dose rate correction is required for PDR (hourly fractions) compared with continuous LDR. A Styrofoam collar positioned around the base of the penis proximal to the needles supports the penis, distances the implant from the testicles, and minimizes unnecessary irradiation of adjacent tissue. A thin sheet of lead can be inserted into the Styrofoam collar to decrease transmitted dose to the testicles if subsequent fertility is an issue.

The brachytherapy needles are generally well tolerated. The patient remains catheterized and in bed for the duration of the implant, although with PDR, the source cables can be disconnected from the needles to allow the patient to mobilize for brief periods between fractions. Sufficient analgesia is usually provided by acetaminophen, with or without codeine. Leg exercises and prophylactic subcutaneous heparin (5000 U every 12 hours) are recommended. Removal of the needles occurs at the bedside after premedication with a narcotic analgesic.

Tolerance: Acute and Chronic Reactions

Toxicity: Acute Reaction

The acute reaction after brachytherapy is limited to the implant site. Moist desquamation peaks in 2 to 3 weeks but may take 2 to 3 months to heal completely. Local hygiene is important, including frequent soaks in baking soda and water. Sterile distal urethritis is common, but urethral adhesions, causing a divided or deviated urinary stream, should be

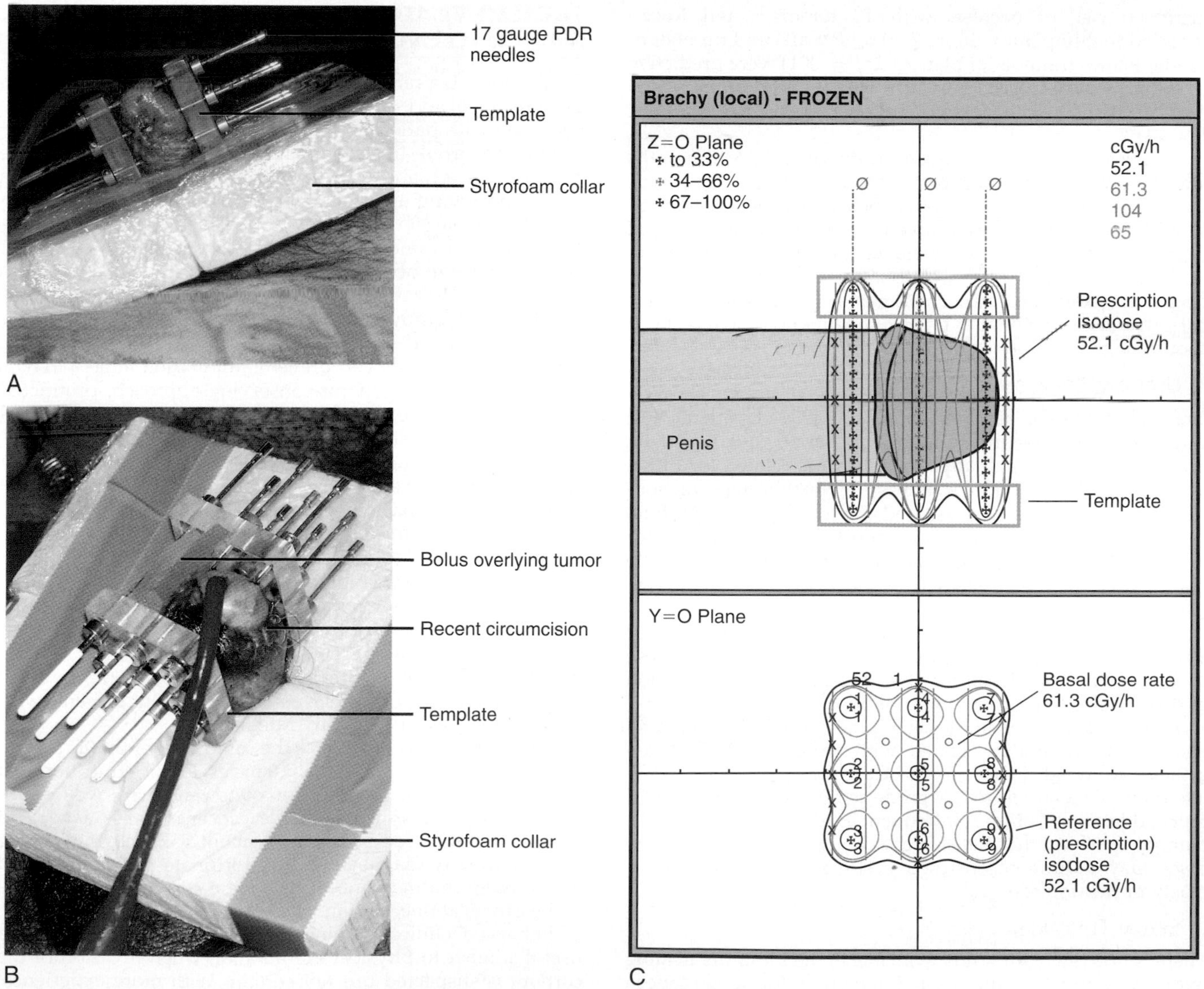

Figure 54-5 Interstitial brachytherapy according to the Paris system of dosimetry. **A,** A six-needle, two-plane implant. **B,** A nine-needle, three-plane implant. **C,** Dose distribution for **B.** According to the Paris system,[59] dose rate minima in the central plane (61.3 cGy/h in this case) are the basal dose rate. The prescription isodose is 85% of the basal dose rate (52.1 cGy/h in this case).

separated by passing an 18-Fr Foley catheter a few centimeters into the distal urethra. Intercourse can be resumed as soon as the patient is comfortable, but because the healing epithelium is fragile, additional water-based lubricant is recommended.

The acute reaction to EBRT peaks during treatment and may involve edema of the penile shaft and more extensive desquamation. Management is similar to that for brachytherapy patients.

Late Reactions

The two most common and significant late complications of radiotherapy for penile cancer are soft tissue necrosis and urethral stenosis. Either can occur with EBRT or brachytherapy (see Table 54-2).

Soft Tissue Necrosis

Soft tissue necrosis is reported in 0% to 23% of patients and is more common after brachytherapy than after external radiation. Necrosis is the most common reason for amputation of a tumor-free penis. The risk of necrosis or fibrosis increases with increasing dose over 60 Gy.[19] Mazeron has reported an increased risk of necrosis with T3 tumors,[25] and Rozan reported that implant volume (>30 cc; $P = .01$) and number of needle planes (number of planes >2; $P = .001$) were predictive of subsequent necrosis.[24] Similarly, Crook found an increased risk of necrosis with a larger number of needles ($n = 49$; $P = .04$).[46]

The peak time for soft tissue ulceration is 7 to 18 months after brachytherapy, but it can occur much later.[27] Causative factors include trauma and cold exposure. Areas of ulceration should be treated conservatively, with attention to good hygiene, antibiotics, and steroid creams. Biopsy should be avoided unless there is suspicion of concomitant tumor. A deeper or painful area of necrosis may respond well to hyperbaric oxygen treatment.[46] If such treatment is available, it should be tried before resorting to amputation.

Urethral Stenosis

Urethral stenosis is reported in 10% to 45% of patients and tends to occur later in the follow-up period, but it usually occurs before 3 years. It appears to be dose related for EBRT, as seen in 30% of Duncan's series,[60] in which a hypofractionated treatment regimen was used (50 to 57.5 Gy in 16 fractions). For brachytherapy, Rozan reported that the only factor predictive of urethral stenosis was the number of needle planes used in the implant ($P = 0.001$ for more than two planes).[24]

When a three-plane implant is indicated because of tumor size or morphology, needles of the central plane will be close to the urethra. A PDR remote afterloader allows optimization of dwell times to limit the urethral dose.

Urethral adhesions in the acute phase should be separated and the distal urethra dilated with an 18- to 20-Fr Foley catheter to avoid development of a chronic problem. Many late urethral stenoses are low grade and can be managed with repeat dilatations, often at infrequent intervals. Patients can be taught to perform this themselves as required, although severe cases may require reconstructive surgery such as urethroplasty or meatoplasty.

Sexual Function

There is no systematic study available in the literature dealing with sexual function after radiation therapy for penile cancer. The impact on sexual function is often not assessed.[4,5,24] Crook found that in a series of 49 men treated with brachytherapy, 22 of 27 who were potent at baseline reported satisfactory potency at last follow-up.[46] Delannes observed that apart from one patient who developed painful erections due to sclerosis, "sexual function did not appear to be altered by the implant."[27] Sarin provided details for only 14 of the 59 patients, commenting that 12 were normal and 2 had minor impairment.[4] Mazeron stated that for noninfiltrating or moderately infiltrating tumors less than 4 cm in diameter, "sexual function remained the same as before treatment."[25]

Thermoluminescent dosimeter measurements for pulse dose rate penile brachytherapy after incorporation of a layer of 2 mm of lead into the Styrofoam collar around the penis indicate a total dose to the anterior testicle of 53 to 58 cGy and 26 cGy to the posterior testicle during a 60 Gy treatment course.[46] No data are available on postbrachytherapy sperm counts.

Other Sequelae

Mottled hypopigmentation or hyperpigmentation, telangiectasia, and mild to moderate focal fibrosis may occur. Some atrophy of the glans in areas of deep tumor infiltration is common.

TREATMENT ALGORITHM, CONTROVERSIES, AND CHALLENGES

Penile cancer is a rare but psychologically devastating disease. The functional and sexual implications of treatment should be discussed with patients.

Our preferred treatment algorithm is shown in Figure 54-6. For T1s, T1, and T2 tumors less than 4 cm in diameter, a penile-conserving approach as primary management is warranted. Laser surgery can provide satisfactory cosmesis, function, and local tumor control, especially for T1s or small T1 lesions, with the option of re-treating local recurrences with further laser. The radiotherapeutic treatment of choice is interstitial brachytherapy and results in penile preservation in 70% to 85% of cases. If brachytherapy expertise is not available, external radiotherapy can prevent amputation in 50% to 60% of patients. With any penis-conserving approach, protracted follow-up is necessary because surgical salvage of local failures can be curative.

Observation of regional nodes is acceptable for low-risk T1 and T2 tumors that are well differentiated with no evidence of lymphovascular space invasion. Moderately or poorly differentiated tumors and all T3 tumors should have surgical staging of regional lymph nodes.

Squamous cell carcinoma of the penis remains a clinical challenge. Although it is highly curable in its early stages, the challenge is to minimize the psychosexual morbidity of treatment through less aggressive surgical approaches or alternatives to surgery such as brachytherapy without compromising cure. When diagnosis is delayed and the patient presents with advanced disease, the fatality rate is high.

Rare tumors do not achieve the same level of public awareness as the more common malignancies. Public education and support groups for breast or prostate cancer are well established and successful. For penile cancer, there is a need to educate the public and physicians about risk factors, warning signs, and early diagnosis. It is unfortunate that men should ever present with advanced disease on such a readily visible and easily examined organ.

Enhanced clinical staging with MRI may prove to be a useful adjunct to physical examination when invasion of the corpora is suspected but not certain. With more experience, dynamic sentinel node mapping may spare patients with high-risk disease (T3 or moderately or poorly differentiated) the morbidity of a staging superficial inguinal node dissection.

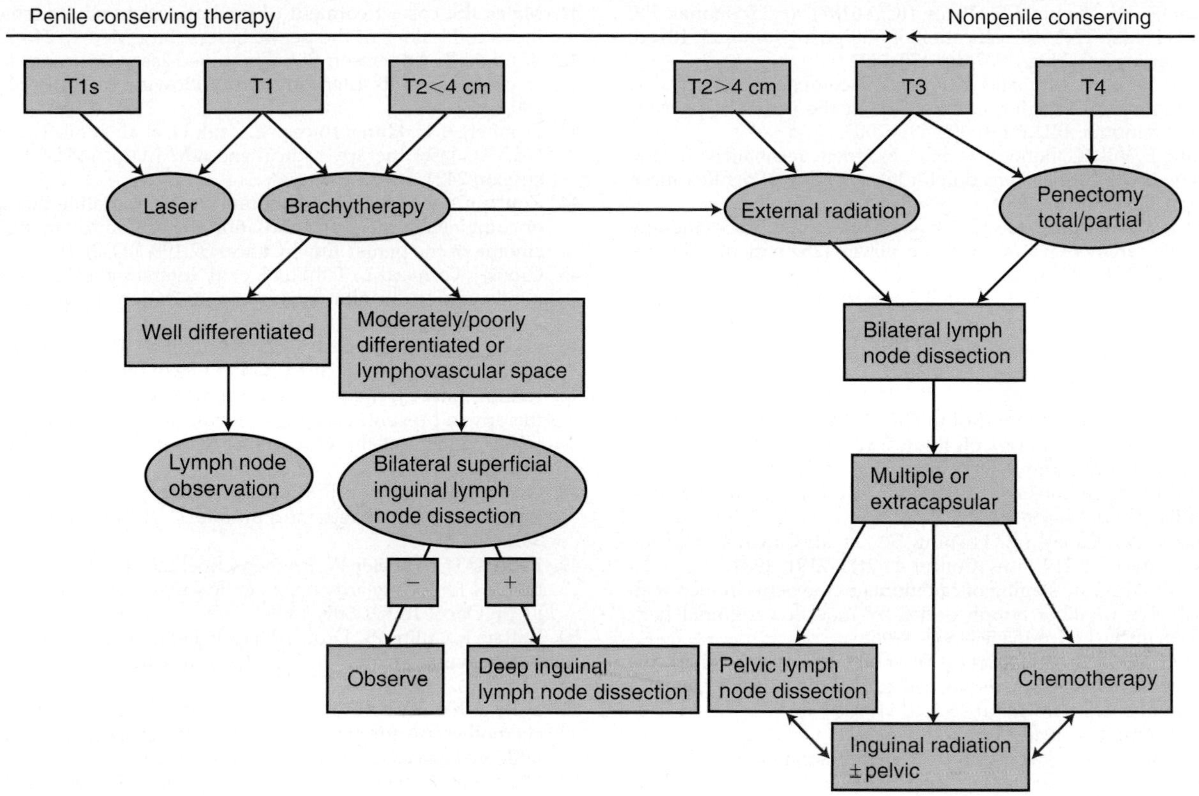

Figure 54-6 Algorithm for the treatment of penile cancer. External radiation is a reasonable option for T1 and small T2 tumors if brachytherapy is not available.

Cooperative group trials are required to determine the most effective aggressive multimodality approach for the patient with advanced disease.

REFERENCES

1. Opjordsmoen S, Fossa SD: Quality of life in patients treated for penile cancer: a follow-up study. Br J Urol 74:652-657, 1994.
2. Opjordsmoen S, Waehre H, Aass N, Fossa SD: Sexuality in patients treated for penile cancer: patients' experience and doctors' judgment. Br J Urol 73:554-560, 1994.
3. Hanash KA, Furlow WL, Utz DC, Harrison EG Jr: Carcinoma of the penis: a clinicopathologic study. J Urol 104:291-297, 1970.
4. Sarin R, Norman AR, Steel GG, Horwich A: Treatment results and prognostic factors in 101 men treated for squamous carcinoma of the penis. Int J Radiat Oncol Biol Phys 38:713-722, 1997.
5. Soria JC, Fizazi K, Piron D, et al: Squamous cell carcinoma of the penis: multivariate analysis of prognostic factors and natural history in monocentric study with a conservative policy. Ann Oncol 8:1089-1098, 1997.
6. Harden SV, Tan LT: Treatment of localized carcinoma of the penis: a survey of current practice in the UK. Clin Oncol (R Coll Radiol) 13:284-287, quiz 288, 2001.
7. Rippentrop JM, Joslyn SA, Konety BR: Squamous cell carcinoma of the penis: evaluation of data from the surveillance, epidemiology, and end results program. Cancer 101:1357-1363, 2004.
8. Stancik I, Holtl W: Penile cancer: review of the recent literature. Curr Opin Urol 13:467-472, 2003.
9. Rubin MA, Kleter B, Zhou M, et al: Detection and typing of human papillomavirus DNA in penile carcinoma: evidence for multiple independent pathways of penile carcinogenesis. Am J Pathol 159:1211-1218, 2001.
10. Dillner J, von Krogh G, Horenblas S, Meijer CJ: Etiology of squamous cell carcinoma of the penis. Scand J Urol Nephrol Suppl 205:189-193, 2000.
11. McCance DJ, Kalache A, Ashdown K, et al: Human papillomavirus types 16 and 18 in carcinomas of the penis from Brazil. Int J Cancer 37:55-59, 1986.
12. Lerman SE, Liao JC: Neonatal circumcision. Pediatr Clin North Am 48:1539-1557, 2001.
13. Bezerra AL, Lopes A, Santiago G, et al: Human papillomavirus as a prognostic factor in carcinoma of the penis: analysis of 82 patients treated with amputation and bilateral lymphadenectomy. Cancer 91:2315-2321, 2001.
14. Picconi MA, Eijan AM, Distefano AL, et al: Human papillomavirus (HPV) DNA in penile carcinomas in Argentina: analysis of primary tumors and lymph nodes. J Med Virol 61:65-69, 2000.
15. Lopes A, Bezerra AL, Pinto CA, et al: P53 as a new prognostic factor for lymph node metastasis in penile carcinoma: analysis of 82 patients treated with amputation and bilateral lymphadenectomy. J Urol 168:81-86, 2002.
16. Gross G, Pfister H: Role of human papillomavirus in penile cancer, penile intraepithelial squamous cell neoplasias and in genital warts. Med Microbiol Immunol (Berl) 193:35-44, 2004.
17. Perceau G, Derancourt C, Clavel C, et al: Lichen sclerosus is frequently present in penile squamous cell carcinomas but is not always associated with oncogenic human papillomavirus. Br J Dermatol 148:934-938, 2003.
18. Velazquez EF, Cubilla AL: Lichen sclerosus in 68 patients with squamous cell carcinoma of the penis: frequent atypias and correlation with special carcinoma variants suggests a precancerous role. Am J Surg Pathol 27:1448-1453, 2003.
19. Jackson S: The treatment of carcinoma of the penis. Br J Surg 53:33-35, 1966.
20. Harmer M: Penis (ICD-0187). *In* TNM Classification of Malignant Tumours, 3rd ed. Berlin, Springer-Verlag, 1978, pp 126-128.

21. Hermanek PS, Sobin LH. Penis (ICD-0187). *In* Hermanek PS, Sobin LH (eds): TNM Classification of Malignant Tumours, 4th ed. Berlin, Springer-Verlag, 1987, pp 130-132.
22. Lont AP, Besnard AP, Gallee MP, et al: A comparison of physical examination and imaging in determining the extent of primary penile carcinoma. BJU Int 91:493-495, 2003.
23. Scardino E, Villa G, Bonomo G, et al: Magnetic resonance imaging combined with artificial erection for local staging of penile cancer. Urology 63:1158-1162, 2004.
24. Rozan R, Albuisson E, Giraud B, et al: Interstitial brachytherapy for penile carcinoma: a multicentric survey (259 patients). Radiother Oncol 36:83-93, 1995.
25. Mazeron JJ, Langlois D, Lobo PA, et al: Interstitial radiation therapy for carcinoma of the penis using iridium 192 wires: the Henri Mondor experience (1970-1979). Int J Radiat Oncol Biol Phys 10:1891-1895, 1984.
26. Kiltie AE, Elwell C, Close HJ, Ash DV: Iridium-192 implantation for node-negative carcinoma of the penis: the Cookridge Hospital experience. Clin Oncol (R Coll Radiol) 12:25-31, 2000.
27. Delannes M, Malavaud B, Douchez J, et al: Iridium-192 interstitial therapy for squamous cell carcinoma of the penis. Int J Radiat Oncol Biol Phys 24:479-483, 1992.
28. Narayana AS, Olney LE, Loening SA, et al: Carcinoma of the penis: analysis of 219 cases. Cancer 49:2185-2191, 1982.
29. Parra RO: Accurate staging of carcinoma of the penis in men with nonpalpable inguinal lymph nodes by modified inguinal lymphadenectomy. J Urol 155:560-563, 1996.
30. Theodorescu D, Russo P, Zhang ZF, et al: Outcomes of initial surveillance of invasive squamous cell carcinoma of the penis and negative nodes. J Urol 155:1626-1631, 1996.
31. Bevan-Thomas R, Slaton JW, Pettaway CA: Contemporary morbidity from lymphadenectomy for penile squamous cell carcinoma: the M. D. Anderson Cancer Center Experience. J Urol 167:1638-1642, 2002.
32. Slaton JW, Morgenstern N, Levy DA, et al: Tumor stage, vascular invasion and the percentage of poorly differentiated cancer: independent prognosticators for inguinal lymph node metastasis in penile squamous cancer. J Urol 165:1138-1142, 2001.
33. Horenblas S, van Tinteren H: Squamous cell carcinoma of the penis. IV. Prognostic factors of survival: analysis of tumor, nodes and metastasis classification system. J Urol 151:1239-1243, 1994.
34. Ornellas AA, Seixas AL, Marota A, et al: Surgical treatment of invasive squamous cell carcinoma of the penis: retrospective analysis of 350 cases. J Urol 151:1244-1249, 1994.
35. McDougal WS: Carcinoma of the penis: improved survival by early regional lymphadenectomy based on the histological grade and depth of invasion of the primary lesion. J Urol 154:1364-1366, 1995.
36. Lopes A, Hidalgo GS, Kowalski LP, et al: Prognostic factors in carcinoma of the penis: multivariate analysis of 145 patients treated with amputation and lymphadenectomy. J Urol 156:1637-1642, 1996.
37. Horenblas S, van Tinteren H, Delemarre JF, et al: Squamous cell carcinoma of the penis. II. Treatment of the primary tumor. J Urol 147:1533-1538, 1992.
38. Tanis PJ, Lont AP, Meinhardt W, et al: Dynamic sentinel node biopsy for penile cancer: reliability of a staging technique. J Urol 168:76-80, 2002.
39. Valdes Olmos RA, Tanis PJ, Hoefnagel CA, et al: Penile lymphoscintigraphy for sentinel node identification. Eur J Nucl Med 28:581-585, 2001.
40. Mohs FE, Snow SN, Larson PO: Mohs micrographic surgery for penile tumors. Urol Clin North Am 19:291-304, 1992.
41. Malek RS: Laser treatment of premalignant and malignant squamous cell lesions of the penis. Lasers Surg Med 12:246-253, 1992.
42. Windahl T, Andersson SO: Combined laser treatment for penile carcinoma: results after long-term followup. J Urol 169:2118-2121, 2003.
43. Frimberger D, Hungerhuber E, Zaak D, et al: Penile carcinoma. Is Nd:YAG laser therapy radical enough? J Urol 168:2418-2421, discussion 2421, 2002.
44. Zouhair A, Coucke PA, Jeanneret W, et al: Radiation therapy alone or combined surgery and radiation therapy in squamous-cell carcinoma of the penis? Eur J Cancer 37:198-203, 2001.
45. Crook J, Grimard L, Tsihlias J, et al: Interstitial brachytherapy for penile cancer: an alternative to amputation. J Urol 167:506-511, 2002.
46. Crook JM, Jezioranski J, Grimard L, et al: Penile brachytherapy results for 49 patients. Int J Radiat Oncol Biol Phys 62:460, 2005.
47. Katz A, Eifel PJ, Jhingran A, Levenback CF: The role of radiation therapy in preventing regional recurrences of invasive squamous cell carcinoma of the vulva. Int J Radiat Oncol Biol Phys 57:409-418, 2003.
48. Gerbaulet A, Lambin P: Radiation therapy of cancer of the penis. Indications, advantages, and pitfalls. Urol Clin North Am 19:325-332, 1992.
49. Pedrick TJ, Wheeler W, Riemenschneider H: Combined modality therapy for locally advanced penile squamous cell carcinoma. Am J Clin Oncol 16:501-505, 1993.
50. Kattan J, Culine S, Droz JP, et al: Penile cancer chemotherapy: twelve years' experience at Institut Gustave-Roussy. Urology 42:559-562, 1993.
51. Huang XY, Kubota Y, Nakada T, et al: Intra-arterial infusion chemotherapy for penile carcinoma with deep inguinal lymph node metastasis. Urol Int 62:245-248, 1999.
52. Haas GP, Blumenstein BA, Gagliano RG, et al: Cisplatin, methotrexate and bleomycin for the treatment of carcinoma of the penis: a Southwest Oncology Group study. J Urol 161:1823-1825, 1999.
53. McLean M, Akl AM, Warde P, et al: The results of primary radiation therapy in the management of squamous cell carcinoma of the penis. Int J Radiat Oncol Biol Phys 25:623-628, 1993.
54. Neave F, Neal AJ, Hoskin PJ, Hope-Stone HF: Carcinoma of the penis: a retrospective review of treatment with iridium mould and external beam irradiation. Clin Oncol (R Coll Radiol) 5:207-210, 1993.
55. Sagerman RH, Yu WS, Chung CT, et al: External-beam irradiation of carcinoma of the penis. Radiology 152:183-185, 1984.
56. Vujovic Olga GJB, Davis Stewart: Carcinoma of the penis: a treatment technique with external beam radiation. Ann R Coll Physicians Surg Can 34:495-497, 2001.
57. el-Demiry MI, Oliver RT, Hope-Stone HF, et al: Reappraisal of the role of radiotherapy and surgery in the management of carcinoma of the penis. Br J Urol 56:724-728, 1984.
58. Akimoto T, Mitsuhashi N, Takahashi I, et al: Brachytherapy for penile cancer using silicon mold. Oncology 54:23-27, 1997.
59. Pierquin B, Chassagne D, Wilson F: Modern Brachytherapy. New York, Masson, 1987.
60. Duncan W, Jackson SM: The treatment of early cancer of the penis with megavoltage x-rays. Clin Radiol 23:246-248, 1972.
61. Chaudhary AJ, Ghosh S, Bhalavat RL, et al: Interstitial brachytherapy in carcinoma of the penis. Strahlenther Onkol 175:17-20, 1999.
62. Gotsadze D, Matveev B, Zak B, Mamaladze V: Is conservative organ-sparing treatment of penile carcinoma justified? Eur Urol 38:306-312, 2000.

PART F

GYNECOLOGIC TUMORS

Overview

Gillian M. Thomas

This overview provides an introduction to the chapters on specific gynecologic tumors that follow, including discussions of cancer of the cervix, uterine corpus, ovary, vulva, and vagina. It highlights important clinical issues, areas of controversy, and areas of progress for each tumor site. The etiologic and epidemiologic differences among these tumors are addressed in the relevant chapters.

CERVICAL CANCER

The incidence of invasive cervical cancer continues to decline in the developed world, particularly in areas and countries where effective population-wide screening programs have been implemented.[1] Nevertheless, the number of patients who develop cervical cancer and who die of this disease is steadily rising in the developing world. Relatively wealthy nations can afford to implement strategies that have improved outcomes in cervical cancer, such as the use of concurrent chemotherapy and irradiation in locally advanced disease, but few patients in the developing world have access to these improvements. Few can access even basic radiation treatment or surgery.[2]

With human papillomavirus (HPV) infection recognized as the cause of cervical cancer, studies are emerging on the utility of preventive vaccines based on the most common causative agents, HPV-16 and HPV-18.[3,4] The proof of principle has been established that these vaccines can prevent HPV infection.[5,6,7] Over the next decade, it is hoped that vaccines to prevent the development of cervical cancer may be available to young females worldwide. Nevertheless, even with widespread population-based use of vaccines, the slow progression of preinvasive to invasive cervical cancer implies that at least another decade of treatment of established invasive disease will be necessary.

The International Federation of Gynecology and Oncology (FIGO) staging classification for cervical cancer has remained unchanged over many years and is in need of revision.[8] The internationally used staging system fails to take into account the predictive importance of nodal involvement; it does not officially incorporate modern radiologic methods of staging, including computed tomography (CT), magnetic resonance imaging (MRI), and positron emission tomography (PET), that are being used increasingly for pretreatment evaluation but that are largely unavailable in the developing world.

PET[9] appears to hold the most promise in accuracy for predicting nodal and other involvement in the pelvis and at extrapelvic sites. Before the recognition of the utility of PET scans for staging patients with cervical cancer, there was no noninvasive, relatively accurate means of identifying potentially curable extrapelvic disease in the para-aortic node-bearing regions. It is anticipated that PET, where available, will become a standard pretreatment investigation; it can more accurately delineate the extent of nodal disease and therefore influence therapy. The identification of incurable disseminated disease may spare some patients radical treatment with chemotherapy and irradiation, whereas for others, it may direct effective treatment to previously unrecognized sites of disease. It may also guide radiation dose escalation to sites of bulky disease using intensity-modulated radiation therapy (IMRT).[10]

In the management of locally advanced disease (stage IB2-IVA), concurrent chemotherapy with radiation has become a standard of treatment. Positive results from five clinical trials supported incremental benefit from the addition of concurrent chemotherapy to irradiation in adjuvant and definitive settings. The 1999 National Cancer Institute (NCI) alert about this benefit led to rapid uptake and implementation of the evidence. Two analyses in the United States and Canada have shown that approximately 70% of patients with invasive disease receive concurrent chemotherapy with definitive irradiation.[11,12] However, there has been little progress on determining whether particular patient subsets may have a differential benefit from the addition of concurrent chemotherapy. Some subset analyses of the phase III trials suggest that benefits in patients with smaller bulk disease (i.e., those with stage IB2 and small IIB) may be greater than for those with IIIB disease.[13,14] No progress has been made in identifying possibly more effective regimens than cisplatin-based chemotherapy. After the NCI alert was issued, a subsequent randomized trial of the Gynecologic Oncology Group (GOG) was abandoned when a planned interim analysis suggested that a peripheral constant infusion of concurrent 5-fluorouracil (5-FU) during external beam irradiation did not improve outcomes over those obtained with the commonly used regimen of weekly concurrent cisplatin.[15]

Research is assessing more "targeted" therapies for locally advanced disease. The presence of hypoxia in most cervical cancers, its association with poorer treatment outcomes, and its stimulation of the angiogenic and proliferative pathways present a rational target for focused treatment interventions.[16] The next study of the GOG will compare concurrent weekly cisplatin and irradiation with weekly cisplatin and irradiation plus tirapazamine; the target is hypoxic tumor cells. Tirapazamine is a logical drug to examine because it is a specifically cytotoxic to hypoxic cells and is significantly more active in this capacity than mitomycin C; it is also synergistic when used with platinum and with irradiation. Phase I/II studies of inhibitors of the pathways of angiogenesis such as antibodies to vascular endothelial growth factor (VEGF) and tyrosine kinase inhibitors are being conducted, and these agents will undoubtedly be incorporated into the next generation of phase III trials of treatment of advanced disease.

Significant controversy remains about the optimal primary treatment for stage IB/IIA cervical cancer: surgery or chemoradiation. The results of primary surgery followed by concurrent chemotherapy and irradiation appear comparable to those of concurrent chemoradiation alone, although no study directly comparing these treatment approaches using three modalities versus two has been completed. Although neoadjuvant chemotherapy before surgery is widely used in some countries of the world,[17] the data on the efficacy of this strategy remain inconclusive. One study suggested benefits of neoadjuvant chemotherapy before surgery compared with irradiation alone, but the results in both study arms were markedly inferior to those achieved with irradiation alone in most other large series.[18] The European Organization for Research and Treatment of Cancer (EORTC) is conducting a randomized clinical trial comparing neoadjuvant chemotherapy before surgery with definitive concurrent chemoradiation in patients with stage IB2 and IIB cervical cancers.

Technical aspects of planning radiation therapy in cervical cancer are changing rapidly. CT planning has been adopted widely to more accurately delineate the location and gross extent of the primary tumor and pelvic lymph nodes for external beam irradiation planning.[19] Functional imaging with PET and MRI may also improve tumor delineation. Various observational studies are examining the role of IMRT for pelvic irradiation in cervical cancer, particularly the impact on complication rates. No studies have compared pelvic control or survival rates with the use of IMRT versus conventional external beam irradiation planning.[20] The use of IMRT is still considered experimental. Significant innovations are occurring in the area of image-guided brachytherapy planning.[21] Conformal dosing for brachytherapy planning is limited by the accuracy of the CT and MR diagnostic images used to delineate gross tumor volume.

ENDOMETRIAL CANCER

Prognostic factors in endometrial carcinoma are extensively reviewed in Chapter 56. Numerous studies have confirmed the importance of stage, histologic type, grade, depth of myometrial invasion, patient age, and the presence of lymphovascular space invasions.[22-24] The FIGO system staging contains three grades, but suggestions have been made for binary grading systems.[25] Scholten has demonstrated that FIGO grade 2 tumors do not have a significantly different outcome compared with grade 1; a two-tiered grading system would overcome the limited clinical value and poor reproducibility of the intermediate grade.[26] It is hoped that these data will influence the FIGO staging system sufficiently to incorporate a binary grading system, which has better prognostic power, is more reproducible, and will have more clinical utility.

Controversy continues about the role of surgical staging in clinical stage I-II disease. Although the FIGO classification system requires surgical staging, the probability of finding occult extrauterine disease in most patients with clinical stage I disease, particularly for grade 1-2 tumors, is extremely small, and staging for most clinical stage I patients is therefore irrelevant, adding morbidity without significantly influencing treatment or survival. Because the incidence of extrauterine disease may rise to 40% to 50% for those with grade 3 tumors or outer half invasion of the myometrium,[27] it is not unreasonable to consider surgical staging in these patients to direct further therapy, be it to the pelvis or to extrapelvic sites.

There is no consistency in surgical staging practices within the United States, Europe, or the rest of the world. Some oncologists stage all patients, regardless of the potential yield of performing reoperation, even patients who have had bilateral salpingo-oophorectomy and hysterectomy for low-risk disease. Others stage none, and some stage only the patients deemed at high risk for extrauterine disease by virtue of pathologic factors of the primary uterine tumor, including tumor grade and depth of myometrial invasion.

Intimately associated with controversies around staging is the use of adjuvant postoperative irradiation in stage I endometrial cancer. Two studies[23,28] have shown no overall survival benefit for the use of adjuvant external beam irradiation for patients with clinical stage I disease, although pelvic recurrence is decreased. The salvage rate for patients with isolated vaginal vault recurrence after surgery alone is high, accounting for the discrepancy between prevention of pelvic recurrence and the lack of ultimate impact on survival.[23,29] Many argue that adjuvant irradiation could be withheld from most patients with clinical stage I disease, with therapy delivered only for overt recurrence confined to the vaginal vault or pelvis. Notwithstanding the psychological impact of clinical recurrence for patients, it is doubtful that the prevention of pelvic recurrence leads to significant survival gains for most patients given the results of the randomized studies.

The observational study by Creutzberg of the subset of patients with stage IC, grade 3 tumors treated with surgery plus adjuvant external beam pelvic irradiation in a dose of 46 Gy demonstrated a pelvic relapse rate of 13% and a distant relapse rate of 31%, both significantly higher than for other patients with stage I disease treated with adjuvant postoperative external beam irradiation.[27] Because of the high risk of relapse, many favor pelvic irradiation at least for patients with grade 3 tumors with deep myometrial invasion if surgical staging has not been performed. Although some argue that adjuvant irradiation is unnecessary for patients with surgically proven negative nodes, Keys identified a group with a significantly high risk for relapse by virtue of combinations of tumor grade, depth, lymphovascular space involvement, and patient age despite having negative nodes.[24] The high rate of distant metastases[27] will undoubtedly lead to future studies of systemic therapies for those with grade 3 tumors penetrating the outer half of the myometrium.

Controversy exists about the use of adjuvant vault brachytherapy alone for patients with proven negative lymph nodes. No data exist to confirm or refute the use of adjuvant vault brachytherapy versus observation and treatment at the time of relapse in those with proven negative nodes. Given the low relapse rates for most clinical stage I disease, except for those identified by Keys and Creutzberg as high risk, and given our lack of understanding of factors predicting vaginal vault relapse alone, an argument can be made against the probable cost effectiveness of the former strategy.

Optimal treatment for patients with stage III endometrial cancer remains undefined. The GOG conducted a randomized trial of patients with stage III or IV disease and up to 2 cm of residual cancer that confirmed a small survival benefit for the use of chemotherapy (Adriamycin [doxorubicin] and cisplatin) compared with the use of pelvic and whole-abdomen irradiation.[30] Unfortunately, this study included the diversity of patients within the stage III category: those with a very good prognosis (i.e., adnexal disease only or positive cytology only)[31-33] and those with a poor prognosis (i.e., disease in multiple sites including lymph nodes, unfavorable (nonendometrioid) cell type, and gross residual disease up to 2 cm in diameter). Although some have accepted this study as confirmation that chemotherapy alone should be used for all stage

III/IV patients, others feel that subsets of stage III patients (including IIIA) who have good outcomes with surgery and irradiation alone should be spared the toxicity of doxorubicin- and platinum-containing chemotherapy. Similarly for those with nodal involvement only within stage IIIC, adjuvant irradiation without chemotherapy provides very good results.[34,35] Some evidence suggests that pelvic control with chemotherapy alone in stage III patients is poor (3-year actuarial pelvic failure rate of 47%, 31% for pelvic failures as the first or only site of relapse) and that pelvic or pelvic and para-aortic irradiation should be integrated with systemic therapy in patients with stage III disease.[36]

The optimal integration of irradiation and chemotherapy for stage III disease, however, has not been defined. The randomized trials attesting to efficacy of chemotherapy have used taxol, doxorubicin, and cisplatin or doxorubicin plus cisplatin.[37] Despite these findings, physicians typically use a regimen combining carboplatin and taxol as chemotherapy for adjuvant or definitive treatment of advanced endometrial cancer, arguing the toxicity of the latter regimen is less that than of the doxorubicin-containing combinations and that phase II data support its efficacy.

VULVAR AND VAGINAL CANCER

The rarity of vulvar and vaginal cancers, with their diversity of disease extent and location within the relevant organs, makes them difficult to study in a systematic, rigorous fashion. Locally advanced vaginal cancers are most commonly treated with concurrent chemotherapy and irradiation, extrapolating expected improved results from the many solid tumor sites in which the use of concurrent therapy has improved results over the use of definitive irradiation alone. Vaginal cancer remains rare, hindering the needed accrual to perform randomized trials to confirm or refute the hypothesis of additional benefits from concurrent chemotherapy. More conformal external beam radiation techniques may offer advantages for the residual primary disease after whole-pelvis irradiation, particularly for those in whom brachytherapy cannot encompass the tumor residuum.

Vulvar cancer treatments should integrate the unique and individual benefits of surgery, irradiation, and chemotherapy.[38] Progress in defining optimal management for all stages and extents of vulvar cancer is usually based on the results of careful observational studies in which consistent management policies have been employed. Recognition of the efficacy of modest-dose irradiation (47.6 Gy) in combination with chemotherapy in the preoperative management of locally advanced vulvar cancer[39,40] has led to a marked decrease in extirpative or exenterative surgery in advanced disease. Current studies explore the efficacy of increased doses of radiation (57.6 Gy with chemotherapy in the current preoperative GOG study); a planned study in the Netherlands will examine the results of definitive chemoradiation using doses of 62 to 64 Gy with concurrent chemotherapy without planned surgery (Van der Zee A: Personal communication, 2005). It is anticipated that these two studies will establish important points on the radiation dose-control curve when chemotherapy is added to radiotherapy for the management of locally advanced vulvar disease.

Controversy remains about the optimal treatment of inguinal regions in vulvar cancer. Because the metachronous development of nodal recurrence in vulvar cancer almost inevitably leads to the patient's death, initial management decisions with respect to the inguinal nodes are critical. Sentinel node studies in early disease will establish the accuracy of this procedure and may lead to a decline in the morbidity of complete inguinofemoral node dissection in those with negative sentinel nodes (Van de Zee A: Personal communication, 2005).[41] Management of the patient with positive nodes on sentinel node study consists of completing the inguinal node dissection. For those with positive nodes, adjuvant postoperative radiation therapy is usually administered. Proposed international studies originating in the Netherlands include treating patients with positive sentinel nodes with definitive nodal irradiation without inguinal node dissection. Controversy also exists about whether there is a role for definitive irradiation or chemoradiation instead of groin node dissection in patients with clinically negative nodes with early disease or in those with advanced primary disease in the vulva where definitive chemoradiation is planned.

OVARIAN CANCER

Many pieces of evidence suggest that patients with ovarian cancer are best managed by physicians with expertise in the area, particularly gynecologic oncologists who can perform adequately the necessary staging and debulking procedures that appear to contribute to overall patient survival. The challenges in the management of patients with ovarian cancer remain focused on the fact that 75% of patients present with advanced disease because of the lack of an effective screening strategy.[42] Definitive whole-abdomen irradiation has been largely abandoned, even for patients with cure rates approaching 70%.[43-46] Chemotherapy using carboplatin and paclitaxel has become the standard of management for most patients with ovarian cancer.[47] Studies have confirmed that surgically staged patients with stage I disease may not benefit from adjuvant chemotherapy.[48] The challenge in advanced disease has been to identify systemic agents other than the standard one that may further improve the overall 5-year survival rate of 52%, which was achieved in the 1990s. Various doublet and triplet combinations of antineoplastic drugs showing activity in ovarian cancer have been examined, but major gains have not been achieved.

Three multicenter, randomized trials in small-volume, residual advanced epithelial ovarian cancer have been reported. The results suggest that intraperitoneal chemotherapy provides a survival and progression-free survival advantage compared with intravenous regimens.[49-51] Although it has been suggested that intraperitoneal chemotherapy become the standard of care in ovarian cancer based on these results, some suggest that the results using intraperitoneal paclitaxel and cisplatin have not been compared with what is considered the standard intravenous regimen of paclitaxel and cisplatin in comparable doses. In the most recent trial of the GOG,[51] significant toxicities were related specifically to the chemotherapy and to peritoneal catheter complications. Many physicians are not prepared to adopt the regimen used in the randomized trial despite the improvement in overall survival from 49.7 months to 65.6 months ($P = .017$) and the prolongation in the median progression-free survival from 18.3 months to 24 months ($P = .027$). At present, there seems to be variable uptake and implementation of intraperitoneal chemotherapy in advanced ovarian cancer. It appears that many centers and physicians are adopting different dosing schedules and drugs for intraperitoneal chemotherapy. A number of groups are conducting randomized phase II trials in an attempt to define less toxic intraperitoneal regimens that may be more easily used in routine clinical practice.

Future research efforts to improve therapy for advanced ovarian cancer will focus on the integration of biologic agents, including antibodies to VEGF and tyrosine kinase inhibitors.

The palliative benefit of localized radiation treatment for masses that can be encompassed, even if they are chemotherapy resistant, should not be ignored.[50-53] Response rates to palliative irradiation are substantial and usually exceed those to second- and third-line chemotherapy.

REFERENCES

1. Ferlay J, Bray F, Pisani P, Parkin DM: Globocan 2000. Cancer Incidence, Mortality and Prevalence Worldwide. Lyon, IARC Press, 2001.
2. Tatsuzaki H, Levin CV: Quantitative status of resources for radiation therapy in Asia and Pacific region. Radiother Oncol 60:81-89, 2001.
3. Boshart M, Gissmann L, Ikenberg H, et al: A new type of papillomavirus DNA, its presence in genital cancer biopsies and in cell lines divided from cervical cancer. EMBO J 3:1151-1157, 1984.
4. Dunst M, Gissmann L, Ikenberg H, et al: A papillomavirus DNA from a cervical carcinoma and its prevalence in cancer biopsy specimens from different geographic regions. Proc Natl Acad Sci U S A 80:3812-3815, 1983.
5. Koutsky LA, Adult KA, Wheeler CM, et al: A controlled trial of a human papillomavirus type 16 vaccine. N Engl J Med 347:1645-1651, 2002.
6. Tjalma WAA, Arbyn M, Paavonen J, et al: Prophylactic human papillomavirus vaccines: the beginning of the end of cervical cancer. Int J Gynecol Cancer 14:751-761, 2004.
7. Bell MC, Alvarez RD: Chemoprevention and vaccines: a review of the nonsurgical options for the treatment of cervical dysplasia. Int J Gynecol Cancer 15:4-12, 2005.
8. International Federation of Gynecology and Obstetrics (FIGO): Staging announcement. FIGO staging of gynecologic cancers; cervical and vulva. Intl J Gynecol Cancer 5:319, 1995.
9. Grigsby PW, Siegel BA, Dehdashti F, et al: Posttherapy [18F] fluorodeoxyglucose positron emission tomography in carcinoma of the cervix; response and outcome. J Clin Oncol 22:2167-2171, 2004.
10. Mundt AJ, Mell LK, Roeske JC: Preliminary analysis of chronic gastrointestinal toxicity in gynecology patients treated with intensity-modulated whole pelvic radiation therapy. Int J Radiat Oncol Biol Phys 56;1354-1360, 2003.
11. Eifel PJ, Moughan J, Erickson B, et al: Patterns of radiotherapy practice for patients with carcinoma of the uterine cervix: a patterns of care study. Int J Radiat Oncol Biol Phys 60:1144-1153, 2004.
12. Barbera L, Paszat L, Thomas G, et al: The rapid uptake of concurrent chemotherapy for cervix cancer patients treated with curative radiation. Int J Radiat Oncol Biol Phys 64:1389-1394, 2006.
13. Eifel PJ, Winter K, Morris M, et al: Pelvic irradiation with concurrent chemotherapy versus pelvic and para-aortic irradiation for high-risk cervical cancer: an update of Radiation Therapy Oncology Group trial (RTOG) 90-01. J Clin Oncol 22:972-980, 2004.
14. Thomas G, Dembo A, Ackerman I, et al: A randomized trial of standard versus partially hyperfractionated radiation with or without concurrent 5-fluorouracil in locally advanced cervical cancer. Gynecol Oncol 69:137-145, 1998.
15. Lanciano R, Calkins A, Bundy BN, et al: A randomized comparison of weekly cisplatin or protracted venous infusion in combination with pelvic radiation in advanced cervix cancer. J Clin Oncol 23:8289-8295, 2005.
16. Coleman N, Mitchell J, Camphausen K: Tumor hypoxia: chicken, egg, or a piece of the farm? J Clin Oncol 20:610-615, 2001.
17. Sardi JE, Giaroli A, Sananes C, et al: Long-term follow-up of the first randomized trial using neoadjuvant chemotherapy in stage Ib squamous carcinoma of the cervix: the final results. Gynecol Oncol 67:61-9, 1997.
18. Benedetti-Panici P, Greggi S, Colombo A, et al: Neoadjuvant chemotherapy and radical surgery versus exclusive radiotherapy in locally advanced squamous cell cervical cancer: results from the Italian multicenter randomized study. J Clin Oncol 20:179-88, 2002.
19. Kim RY, McGinnis S, Spencer SA, et al: Conventional four-field pelvic radiotherapy technique with computed tomography treatment planning in cancer of the cervix: potential geographic miss and its impact on pelvic control. Int J Radiat Oncol Biol Phys 31:109-112, 1994.
20. Portalance L, Chao KSC, Grigsby PW, et al: Intensity-modulated radiation therapy (IMRT) reduces bowel, rectum, and bladder doses in patients with cervical cancer receiving pelvic and para-aortic radiation. Int J Radiat Oncol Biol Phys 51:261-266, 2001.
21. Nag S, Cardenes H, Chang S, et al: Proposed guidelines for image-based intracavitary brachytherapy for cervical carcinoma: report from Image-Guided Brachytherapy Working Group. Int Radiat Oncol Biol Phys 60:1160-1172, 2004.
22. Aalders J, Abeler V, Kolstad P, et al: Postoperative external irradiation and prognostic parameters in stage I endometrial carcinoma: clinical and histopathological study of 540 patients. Obstet Gynecol 56:419-427, 1980.
23. Creutzberg CL, van Putten WL, Koper PC, et al: Surgery and postoperative radiotherapy versus surgery alone for patients with stage-1 endometrial carcinoma: multicentre randomized trial. Postoperative Radiation Therapy in Endometrial Carcinoma (PORTEC) Study Group [see comments]. Lancet 355:1404-1411, 2000.
24. Keys HM, Roberts JA, Brunetto VL, et al: A phase III trial of surgery with or without adjunctive external pelvic radiation therapy in intermediate risk endometrial adenocarcinoma: A Gynecologic Oncology Group Study. Gynecol Oncol 92:744-751, 2004.
25. Lax SF, Kurman RJ, Pizer ES, et al: A binary architectural grading system for uterine endometrioid carcinoma has superior reproducibility compared with FIGO grading and identifies subsets of advance-stage tumors with favorable and unfavorable prognosis. Am J Surg Pathol 24:1201-1208, 2000.
26. Scholten AN, Creutzberg CL, Noordijk EM, et al: Long-term outcome in endometrial carcinoma favors a two instead of a three-tiered grading system. Int J Radiat Oncol Biol Phys 52:1067-1074, 2002.
27. Creutzberg CL, van Putten WL, Warlam-Rodenhuis CC, et al: Outcome of high-risk stage IC, grade 3, compared with stage I endometrial carcinoma patients: the postoperative radiation therapy in endometrial carcinoma trial. J Clin Oncol 22:1234-1241, 2004.
28. Aalders J, Abeler V, Kolstad P, et al: Postoperative external irradiation and prognostic parameters in stage I endometrial carcinoma: clinical and histopathologic study of 540 patients. Obstet Gynecol 56:419-427, 1980.
29. Creutzberg CL, van Putten WLJ, Koper PC, et al: Survival after relapse in patients with endometrial cancer: results from a randomized trial. Gynecol Oncol 89:201-209, 2003.
30. Randall ME, Brunetto VL, Muss H: Whole abdominal radiotherapy versus combination doxorubicin-cisplatin chemotherapy in advanced endometrial carcinoma: a randomized phase III trial of the Gynecologic Oncology Group [abstract 3]. Proc Am Soc Clin Oncol 22:2, 2003.
31. Mackillop WJ, Pringle JF: Stage III endometrial carcinoma. A review of 90 cases. Cancer 56:2519-2523, 1985.
32. Mariani A, Webb MJ, Keeney GL, et al: Stage III endometrioid corpus cancer includes distinct subgroups. Gynecol Oncol 87:112-117, 2002.
33. Mariani A, Webb MJ, Keeney GL, et al: Assessment of prognostic factors in stage IIIA endometrial cancer. Gynecol Oncol 86:38-44, 2002.
34. Mundt AJ, Murphy KT, Rotmensch J, et al: Surgery and postoperative radiation therapy in FIGO stage IIIIC endometrial carcinoma. Int J Radiat Oncol Biol Phys 50:1154-1160, 2001.
35. Nelson G, Randall M, Sutton G, et al: FIGO stage IIIC endometrial carcinoma with metastases confined to pelvic nodes: analysis of treatment outcomes, prognostic variables, and failure patterns following adjuvant radiation therapy. Gynecol Oncol 75:211-214, 1999.
36. Mundt AJ, McBride R, Rotmensch J, et al: Significant pelvic recurrence in high-risk pathologic stage I-IV endometrial carcinoma patients after adjuvant chemotherapy alone: implications for adjuvant radiation therapy. Int J Radiat Oncol Biol Phys 50:1145-1153, 2001.
37. Fleming GF, Brunetto VL, Cella D, et al: Phase III trial of doxorubicin plus cisplatin with or without paclitaxel plus filgrastim in

advanced endometrial carcinoma: a Gynecologic Oncology Group Study. J Clin Oncol 22:2159-2166, 2004.
38. Thomas GM, Dembo AJ, Bryson SCP, et al: Changing concepts in the management of vulvar cancer. Gynecol Oncol 42:9-21, 1991.
39. Moore DH, Thomas GM, Montana S, et al: Preoperative chemoradiation for advanced vulvar cancer: a phase II study of the Gynecologic Oncology Group. Int J Radiat Oncol Biol Phys 42:79-85, 1998.
40. Montana GS, Thomas GM, Moore DH, et al: Preoperative chemoradiation for carcinoma of the vulva with N2/N3 nodes: a gynecologic oncology group study. Int J Radiat Oncol Biol Phys 48:1007-1013, 2000.
41. Levenback C, Coleman RL, Burke TW, et al: Lymphatic mapping and sentinel node identification in patients with cervix cancer undergoing radical hysterectomy and pelvic lymphadenectomy. J Clin Oncol 20:688-693, 2002.
42. Hogg R, Friedlander M: Biology of epithelial ovarian cancer. Implications for screening women at high genetic risk. J Clin Oncol 22:1315-1327, 2004.
43. Dembo AJ, Davy M, Stenwig AE, et al: Prognostic factors in patients with stage I epithelial ovarian cancer. Obstet Gynecol 75:263-27390.
44. Lederman JA, Dembo AJ, Sturgeon JFG, et al: Outcome of patients with unfavorable optimally cytoreduced ovarian cancer treated with chemotherapy and whole abdominal radiation. Gynecol Oncol 41:30-35, 1991.
45. Dembo AJ, Bush RS: Choice of postoperative therapy based on prognostic factors. Int J Radiat Oncol Biol Phys 8:893-897, 1982.
46. Dembo AJ: Abdominopelvic radiotherapy in ovarian cancer: a 10-year experience. Cancer 55:2285-2290, 1985.
47. Ozols RF, Bundy BN, Greer BE, et al: Phase III trial of carboplatin and paclitaxel compared with cisplatin and paclitaxel in patients with optimally resected stage III ovarian cancer: a Gynecologic Oncology Group study. J Clin Oncol 21:3194-3200, 2003.
48. Trimbos JB, Parmar M, Vergote I, et al: International Collaborative Ovarian Neoplasm Trial 1 and Adjuvant Chemotherapy in Ovarian Neoplasm Trial: two parallel randomized phase III trials of adjuvant chemotherapy in patients with early stage ovarian carcinoma. J Natl Cancer Inst 95:105-112, 2003.
49. Alberts DS, Lui PY, Hannigan EV, et al: Intraperitoneal cisplatin plus intravenous cyclophosphamide versus intravenous cisplatin plus intravenous cyclophosphamide for stage III ovarian cancer. N Engl J Med 335:1950-1955, 1996.
50. Markman M, Bundy BN, Alberts DS, et al: Phase III trial of standard-dose intravenous cisplatin plus paclitaxel versus moderately high-dose carboplatin followed by intravenous paclitaxel and intraperitoneal cisplatin in small-volume stage III ovarian carcinoma: an intergroup study of the Gynecologic Oncology Group, Southwestern Oncology Group, and Eastern Cooperative Oncology Group. J Clin Oncol 19:1001-1007, 2001.
51. Armstrong DK, Bundy B, Wenzel L, et al: Intraperitoneal cisplatin and paclitaxel in ovarian cancer. N Engl J Med 354:34-43, 2006.
52. Corn BW, Lanciano RM, Boente M, et al: Recurrent ovarian cancer: effective radiotherapeutic palliation after chemotherapy failure. Cancer 74:2979-2983, 1994.
53. Davidson SA, Rubin SC, Mychalczak B, et al: Limited-field radiotherapy as salvage treatment of localized persistent or recurrent epithelial ovarian cancer. Gynecol Oncol 51:349-354, 1993.
54. Fujiwara K, Suzuki S, Yoden E, et al: Local radiation therapy for localized relapse or refractory ovarian cancer patients with or without symptoms after chemotherapy. Int J Gynecol Cancer 12:250-256, 2002.
55. Corn BW, Greven KM, Randall ME, et al: The efficacy of cranial irradiation in ovarian cancer metastatic to the brain: analysis of 32 cases. Obstet Gynecol 86:955-959, 1995.

CHAPTER 55

CERVICAL CANCER

Wui-Jin Koh and David H. Moore

INCIDENCE

The expected incidence is 9710 cases in 2006 (invasive), accounting for 2% of cancer deaths (3700 in 2006) in U.S. women.

It is still the leading cause of cancer death in women of medically underserved countries.

Successful screening programs correlate with a low incidence of invasive disease.

BIOLOGY

Histology is 80% to 90% squamous, with increasing frequency of adenocarcinoma. In 93% of patients, there is an association with human papilloma virus infection.

Prognostic factors are stage, tumor size, lymph node metastasis, hemoglobin level, and other factors.

STAGING EVALUATION

International Federation of Gynecology and Obstetrics (FIGO) staging includes physical examination, chest radiography, and intravenous pyelography and, in selected cases, cystoscopy, proctoscopy or barium enema, and bone films.

It may be useful (but does not influence FIGO stage) to include computed tomography, magnetic resonance imaging, lymphangiogram, positron emission tomography, and lymph node sampling.

PRIMARY THERAPY

See Table 55-1.

Table 55-1 **Primary Therapy**

Stage	Primary Therapy	5-yr Survival (%)
0/select IA1	Cone biopsy; simple hysterectomy; brachytherapy	>98
IA2	Radical hysterectomy + pelvic node dissection (PND); irradiation (RT)	≥95
IB1/small IIA	Radical hysterectomy + PND; RT	~90
IB2/IIA	Chemoradiation (ChemoRT)	80-85
IIB	ChemoRT	70-75
III	ChemoRT	~50
IVA	ChemoRT; selective exenteration	15-25
IVB	Chemotherapy; palliative RT	~0

Primary therapy (PT) and survival are related to disease extent at the time of initial diagnosis and staging evaluation.

ADJUVANT THERAPY

Radiation therapy with or/without cisplatin-based chemotherapy after hysterectomy is for patients with high-risk features.

Adjuvant hysterectomy after radiation therapy is not routinely recommended but may benefit patients with poor vaginal anatomy or persistent cervical disease.

Neoadjuvant chemotherapy has no benefit prior to radiation therapy for locally advanced disease but possible benefit prior to radical hysterectomy for stage IB2 disease.

Concurrent chemotherapy and radiation therapy have resulted in five positive phase III trials for survival.

PALLIATION

Cisplatin in combination with paclitaxel or topotecan chemotherapy is given but is rarely, if ever, curative.

Radiation therapy often provides excellent short-term relief of pain and bleeding.

The incidence of and mortality from invasive cervical cancer have steadily declined in the United States over the past five decades, in part because of the successful implementation of screening programs that detect many cancers at a preinvasive stage. Unfortunately, cytologic screening programs have failed to penetrate many medically underserved communities, and invasive cervical cancer continues to be a major public health problem internationally. In the United States, 60% of women with newly diagnosed invasive cervical cancer have not had a Papanicolaou (Pap) smear in at least 5 years.[1]

During the past decade, much has been learned about the etiology and biology of this disease. Epidemiologic studies have long demonstrated that cervical cancers occur in a pattern that suggests that they stem from a sexually transmitted agent. We now know that nearly all cervical cancers contain human papillomavirus (HPV) DNA. Recent studies of the epidemiology and molecular biology of these cancers have provided compelling evidence of a causal relationship between HPV and cervical carcinoma.

Even invasive cervical cancers are highly curable if they are detected at an early stage. Radiation and surgery yield comparable cure rates of 80% to 90% for patients with early-stage disease. Radiation therapy plus concurrent chemotherapy, which is the treatment of choice for patients with locally advanced disease, is curative in over 70% of patients with FIGO stage II disease and in about 50% of patients with FIGO stage III disease.

EPIDEMIOLOGY AND ETIOLOGY

In the United States, cervical cancer is responsible for about 2% of the cancer deaths in women, with about 9710 new cases of invasive disease and 3700 deaths in 2006.[2] Worldwide, invasive cervical cancer is the third most common malignancy in women (after breast and colorectal) and accounts for nearly 371,000 cases and 190,000 deaths per year.[3] Incidence rates range from as low as 3 to 4 per 100,000 in Israel to more than 80 per 100,000 in Recife, Brazil.[4] Presumably, this wide range reflects a variation in epidemiologic risk factors that is compounded by the lack of adequate screening programs in poor communities. The relatively high international mortality rates may also reflect the greater number of women who present with advanced disease when screening programs and patient education are inadequate.

Risk factors for the development of carcinoma of the cervix and its intraepithelial precursors follow a pattern typical of sexually transmitted diseases. These include first coitus at a young age, multiple sexual partners, history of other sexually transmitted diseases, and high parity.[5] Weaker associations have been suggested with cigarette smoking and the use of oral contraceptives. In contrast, the risk of developing cervical cancer is low in women who are nulliparous or virginal. Among women with only one lifetime sexual partner, past and current high-risk sexual behavior by the male partner have a substantial role in the development of cervical carcinogenesis.[6] Conversely, male circumcision is associated with a reduced prevalence of penile HPV infection and a reduced risk of cervical cancer in their current sexual partners.[7]

Until recently, the reasons for these associations were only the subject of speculation. However, today, the epidemiologic findings, combined with the results of molecular studies (discussed in detail later), are generally thought to be sufficient to identify human HPV infection acquired through sexual intercourse as an etiologic agent in the development of most cervical cancers.[8,9]

Although the epidemiology of cervical adenocarcinoma is somewhat less well understood, studies also reveal the presence of HPV DNA in most cases.[10] It is interesting that in the United States, the incidence of adenocarcinoma appears to have increased in opposition to the steady decrease in the rate of invasive squamous carcinoma. This may reflect, in part, differences in the effectiveness of cytologic screening in detecting adenocarcinoma at a preinvasive stage.[11] Some investigators have implicated oral contraceptives as a possible risk factor for adenocarcinoma, but this remains controversial.[12]

Clear cell carcinoma, a rare form of cervical and vaginal adenocarcinomas, has been clearly linked with prenatal exposure to diethylstilbestrol (DES), a drug that was used to prevent miscarriages in the 1940s and 1950s.[13] Prenatal DES exposure arrests development of the transformation zone in the upper third of the vagina, which accounts for the location of these lesions. The average age at which cancer in DES-exposed patients was diagnosed was 19 years, much younger than the average age of patients with newly diagnosed squamous carcinoma or non–DES-related adenocarcinoma. New diagnoses of DES-related clear cell carcinoma have declined now that the youngest cohort of DES-exposed patients has passed the age of peak incidence.

PREVENTION AND EARLY DETECTION

Although there have been significant changes in the fields of radiation and gynecologic oncology, the dramatic decrease in cervical cancer mortality from the 1940s to the 1980s is primarily due to the success of mass screening programs.[14,15] The cervix is an ideal target for cancer screening because of its accessibility, the long average time interval from the initial DNA insult to the development of invasive cancer, and the high cure rate with appropriate treatment of preinvasive and early invasive lesions.

Squamous cell carcinomas originate at the squamocolumnar junction (transformation zone) of the cervix. Invasive lesions are frequently associated with adjacent carcinoma in situ (CIS).

Longitudinal studies suggest a long average time to progression from CIS to invasive disease. Peterson[16] described 127 patients with CIS who were followed for at least 3 years. At the end of 10 years, invasive carcinoma had developed in about 30%. Koss and colleagues[17] observed a spontaneous regression rate of 25% in 67 patients with untreated CIS who were observed for 3 years. In a later analysis of this series, the authors reported that invasive lesions had developed in 40% of the original 67 patients.[18] In another longitudinal study of patients with untreated CIS, Kottmeier[19] observed progression to invasive carcinoma in 71% and 80% of patients followed for 12 and 30 years, respectively.

Longitudinal studies have also demonstrated a relatively long time between the diagnosis of dysplasia and the development of CIS. One large prospective study reported mean times for progression to CIS development of 58, 38, and 12 months for patients with mild, intermediate, or severe dysplasia, respectively.[20] These results are consistent with the finding that the mean age of women diagnosed with cervical intraepithelial neoplasia (CIN) is about 16 years younger than that of women diagnosed with invasive carcinoma.[21]

Although a number of classifications have been used, the Bethesda system is currently the most widely accepted method of categorizing cervical cytologic specimens in the United States.[22] The relationship between this system and earlier classification systems is outlined in Table 55-2.

Table 55-2 Relationship of the Bethesda System to Previous Classifications

Normal Limits	Benign Cellular Changes	Epithelial Cell Abnormalities				
	Infection Reactive repair	ASCUS AGUS	LGSIL HPV Mild dysplasia CIN1	HGSIL Moderate dysplasia CIN2	Severe dysplasia CIS, CIN3	Invasive carcinoma
I	II		III		IV	V
			The Papanicolaou Classification			

BETHESDA SYSTEM TERMINOLOGY

ASCUS, atypical squamous cells of unknown significance
AGUS, atypical glandular cells of unknown significance
LGSIL, low-grade squamous intraepithelial lesion
HGSIL, high-grade squamous cell intraepithelial lesion
HPV, human papillomavirus

CIS, carcinoma in situ; CIN, cervical intraepithelial neoplasia.
Adapted from Shingleton HM, Patrick RL, Johnston WW, et al: The current status of the Papanicolaou smear. CA Cancer J Clin 45:305-320, 1995.

There is some controversy concerning the ideal frequency of cytologic screening, but the American College of Obstetrics and Gynecology and the American Cancer Society have recommended that annual screening commence approximately 3 years after the onset of vaginal intercourse and should begin no later than 21 years of age.[23] After initiation of screening, cervical screening should be performed annually with conventional cervical cytology smears or every 2 years using liquid-based cytology. At or after age 30, women who have had three consecutive technically satisfactory and normal/negative cytology results may be screened every 2 to 3 years (unless they have a history of in utero DES exposure, are HIV positive, or are immunocompromised). As compared with annual screening, mathematical modeling predicts the excess risk of cervical cancer with less frequent screening intervals to be approximately 3 in 100,000.[24]

Despite the proved efficacy of cytologic screening, many women remain unscreened. Fifty percent of the women with newly diagnosed invasive cervical cancer have never had a Pap smear, and another 10% have not had a Pap smear in 5 years.[9] Women who tend to be underscreened in the United States fall into groups of postmenopausal, uninsured, ethnic minority, and, especially, elderly black and poor in rural areas. In the United States, about 25% of the cervical cancer cases and 41% of the deaths occur in women who are aged 65 years or older. In addition, nearly 50% of women older than 60 years have not had a Pap smear in 3 years, even though many have seen a physician for other medical needs.

PATHOLOGY AND PATHWAYS OF SPREAD

Eighty percent to 90% of cervical cancers are squamous. Squamous cell neoplasms are frequently subcategorized as either large cell keratinizing, large cell nonkeratinizing, or small cell carcinomas.[25,26] The latter should not be confused with anaplastic small cell carcinomas, which have histologic features that resemble small cell neuroendocrine neoplasms of the lung and tend to have a particularly aggressive clinical course.[27,28]

The frequency of primary cervical adenocarcinoma is about 10% to 20% but appears to have been increasing recently, particularly in younger women.[29,30] Cervical adenocarcinomas can originate high in the endocervical canal and can be missed with standard cytologic screening collection methods. The perceived increased frequency of cervical adenocarcinomas may be attributed to a decreased incidence of squamous cell carcinomas in the screened population without a concomitant decreased incidence of cervical adenocarcinomas. Whether conventional screening methods are insensitive to the detection of adenocarcinoma precursor lesions or whether such precursor lesions progress more quickly to invasive disease has not been determined. Nonetheless, women who participate in a cytologic screening program and develop cervical adenocarcinoma are more likely to have early-stage disease than an unscreened cohort. Most cervical adenocarcinomas are mucinous with features suggestive of endocervical glandular epithelium; about 20% demonstrate other müllerian neoplastic patterns.

The cervix is richly supplied with lymphatics organized into three anastomosing plexuses that drain the mucosal, muscularis, and serosal layers.[31] The most important lymphatic collecting trunks exit laterally from the uterine isthmus in three groups[31,32]: the upper branches originate in the anterior and lateral cervix and follow the uterine artery, the middle branches drain to the deeper hypogastric (obturator) nodes, and the lowest branches drain posteriorly to the inferior and superior gluteal, common iliac, presacral, and subaortic lymph nodes.

The incidences of pelvic lymph node involvement for patients with FIGO stages IB, IIB, and IIIB cervical cancer are approximately 15%, 30%, and 50%, respectively.[33-36] The incidence of periaortic lymph node metastasis also increases with tumor stage; about 5%, 20%, and 30% of patients with FIGO stage IB, IIB, and IIIB disease, respectively, have para-aortic lymph node metastasis at diagnosis.[33,37] For each stage, the risk of lymph node involvement is correlated with tumor size.[38,39]

Hematogenous metastases are rarely detectable at diagnosis, and recurrent pelvic disease is seen in about two thirds of patients who relapse after treatment. However, distant metastases are also a common feature of disease relapse. In a study of disease relapse patterns from the Mallinckrodt Institute of Radiology, Fagundes and associates[40] reported 10-year actuarial rates for distant metastasis of 16%, 31%, 26%, and 39% for patients treated with radiation for FIGO stages IB, IIA, IIB, and III disease, respectively. The most common site of extrapelvic metastasis was the lungs, followed by the para-aortic lymph nodes. Although the lumbar spine has been reported to be a relatively frequent site of skeletal metastasis, studies that include computed tomography (CT) scanning suggest that patients who appear to have had metastases isolated to the lumbar spine may actually have had direct tumor extension from para-aortic disease.[41]

Prognostic Factors

With the exception of distant hematogeneous metastases, the presence of retroperitoneal nodal involvement represents the most significant negative prognostic factor in patients with cervical cancer.[34,42] However, the evaluation of other prognostic factors is to a great degree predicated on whether patients have early-stage tumors that are managed surgically or more advanced cancers that require definitive radiotherapy or chemoradiotherapy. The availability of a hysterectomy specimen for full pathologic review allows finer assessment of intratumoral risk factors when cancer remains confined to the cervix, factors that may be superseded in larger tumors with clear extracervical extension.

In a prospective surgicopathologic evaluation of 645 patients with clinical stage IB disease who underwent radical hysterectomy and pelvic lymphadenectomy, independent prognostic factors for disease-free survival included pelvic nodal metastases, clinical tumor size (within stage IB classification), capillary-lymphatic space invasion, and depth of tumor infiltration into the cervical stroma.[34]

In more advanced lesions, a multivariate analysis of 642 patients entered into three Gynecologic Oncology Group (GOG) prospective clinical trials of definitive radiotherapy demonstrated that the presence of positive para-aortic nodes was the single most important independent predictor for relapse and survival, overwhelming all other risk factors. The next two most important prognostic factors, pelvic nodal involvement and tumor size, retained significance only in the absence of para-aortic metastases. Other weaker prognostic variables included clinical stage, patient age, and performance status. In this analysis of more advanced tumors, cell type, histologic grade, and pretreatment hematocrit were not significant prognostic factors when the preceding variables were accounted for.[42]

MOLECULAR BIOLOGY

HPV is a small, double-stranded DNA virus that belongs to the papovavirus group. To date, more than 80 different strains of HPV have been isolated using polymerase chain reaction analysis.[43] HPV infection occurs in the basal cell layer of the epithelium, which becomes a continuous reservoir of HPV DNA as the viral genome replicates itself in the dividing cells. As the epithelial cells mature, viral DNA replication continues in the absence of basal cell division, increasing the HPV DNA copy number per cell.[44] Microscopically, this process is associated with koilocytosis, a finding that is considered pathognomonic of HPV infection.[45]

Of the many strains that have been characterized, HPV-16 and HPV-18 have been most commonly associated with squamous cell carcinoma and adenocarcinoma, respectively.[46,47] HPV-31, HPV-33, and HPV-35 have also been associated with malignancy, whereas HPV-6 and HPV-11 are usually associated with benign viral condyloma or mild dysplastic epithelial changes such as CIN-1.[46,48-53]

Initially, HPV carcinogenesis was postulated to have been mediated through oncogenes *E6* and *E7*. Transgenic mouse experiments provide some of the strongest in vivo evidence linking *E6* and *E7* expression to the development of cervical cancer.[54,55] Figure 55-1 outlines the mechanisms by which HPV influences oncogenic activity. The E6 protein of HPV oncogenes binds with the E6-associated protein (E6-AP) to the p53 protein, which results in the degradation of p53. The p53 protein is an important negative regulator of cell growth. Thus, by binding and degrading the p53 protein, E6 proteins contribute to the pathogenesis of cancer by removing the critical and protective function of p53.[56] The E6 proteins of oncogenes from an HPV strain most likely involved in carcinogenesis, such as oncogenes for HPV-16 and HPV-18, bind p53 more efficiently than oncogenes from HPV strains not involved in carcinogenesis, which possibly explains the differences in oncogenicity of these strains.[57] By itself, *E6* is not capable of inducing transformation, but it has been shown to induce immortalization of primary human keratinocytes in conjunction with *E7*, whose protein binds to and functionally inactivates the gene product of the retinoblastoma (*rb*) tumor-suppressor gene. This binding results in the uncontrolled release of active transcription factors (E2F) and unregulated progression through the cell cycle. Biologic differences between low-risk and high-risk HPV viruses include observations that the latter are capable of inducing chromosome abnormalities in normal keratinocytes and are more likely to interfere with cell cycle regulatory proteins and checkpoints.[58]

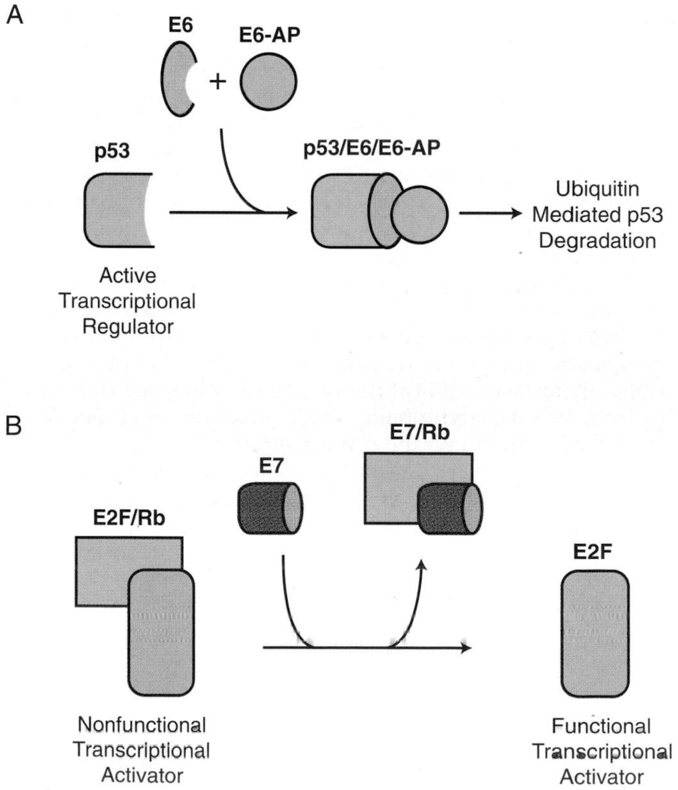

Figure 55-1 Biologic consequences of viral oncoprotein interactions with cellular tumor suppressors. **A,** Schematic representation of mechanism by which *E6* is hypothesized to inactivate p53 protein through ubiquitin-mediated degradation of p53. **B,** Role of *E7* in altering activity of the cellular transcription factor E2F via its capacity to bind Rb protein.

The evidence implicating HPV in the pathogenesis of cervical cancer includes (1) multiple epidemiologic studies demonstrating that HPV infection is the most important risk factor for the development of squamous intraepithelial lesions and cervical carcinomas, (2) detection of HPV DNA in more than 90% of cervical cancers and their precursor lesions, (3) evidence of HPV transcriptional activity in neoplastic tissues, and (4) evidence that HPV oncogenes can mediate malignant transformation in transgenic mice.[54,55] The precise rate of development for both low- and high-grade squamous intraepithelial lesions in women infected with HPV is unknown; however, it is evident that an HPV-associated cervical carcinoma ultimately develops in a very small proportion of HPV-infected women,[9] a finding that has prompted researchers to look for other cofactors in cervical carcinogenesis.

Longitudinal studies have demonstrated that the incidence of HPV infections among cytologically normal sexually active young women is high.[59] Many women infected with HPV eliminate the infection and are at low or no risk for developing cervical neoplasia. The median duration of most new HPV infections is less than 1 year.[59] More than one third of women remain consistently or intermittently positive for HPV DNA and many of these women will subsequently test positive for an HPV type that is different from the original HPV type.[60] The transient nature of HPV infections in younger women substantiates the common observation that low-grade cervical neoplasia frequently regresses to normal.[61]

Theoretically, other factors may interact with HPV to attenuate the body's immune response, promote persistent HPV infection, upregulate *E6/E7* expression, or enhance the genetic damage caused by HPV oncogene expression. Possible factors currently under investigation include smoking, oral contraceptive use, and infection with the human immunodeficiency virus (HIV).[62] Several case-control studies have linked smoking behavior to an increased risk of cervical neoplasia.[63,64] Carcinogens found in cigarette smoke are concentrated in cervical mucus,[65] and women who smoke have decreased numbers of antigen-presenting cells in cervical epithelium.[66] Thus, smoking may increase the risk for cervical cancer via changes in local immunity. Immunosuppression has long been recognized as a risk factor for the development of cervical carcinoma.[67] A positive link between oral contraceptive use and cervical cancer, however, is still uncertain.[68]

Marked advances in molecular biology in the 1990s resulted in an understanding of HPV function, recognition of HPV oncogene expression in cervical tissue, and delineation of the pathogenesis of cervical cancer. Although other cofactors may be involved and are under investigation, the acquisition and persistence of HPV infection are critical to the development of cervical neoplasia.

Koutsky and colleagues reported results from a prospective, double-blind placebo-controlled study of a monovalent HPV 16 virus–like vaccine. With median duration of follow-up of 17 months, the incidence of persistent HPV 16 infection was 3.8 per 100 woman-years at risk in the placebo group versus 0 per 100 woman-years in the vaccine group.[69] A number of other HPV-directed vaccines are in development as potential chemopreventive agents and offer hope for the future prevention of invasive cervical cancer and its precursors.[70,71] Prospects for the primary prevention of cervical neoplasia, particularly in areas of the world where screening is unavailable, are exciting.

CLINICAL MANIFESTATIONS, PATIENT EVALUATION, AND STAGING

Preinvasive and minimally invasive cervical cancers are usually detected by routine cytologic screening. Most patients with more advanced disease present with some form of abnormal vaginal bleeding—postcoital, menstrual, intermenstrual, or postmenopausal—that may be associated with a clear or foul-smelling discharge. Extreme pelvic tenderness, particularly if associated with fever, should be fully evaluated to rule out complicating pelvic inflammatory disease. The triad of sciatic pain, leg edema, and hydronephrosis is almost always associated with extension of disease into the pelvic side wall and indicative of unresectable disease. Bladder and rectal symptoms also suggest locally advanced pelvic disease and the need for evaluation of the urinary and gastrointestinal tracts.

Staging and Patient Evaluation

The current clinical staging system for cervical cancer by the International Federation of Gynecology and Oncology (FIGO) is detailed in Table 55-3.[72] This staging system has been criticized for its failure to consider important prognostic variables such as tumor size and lymph node involvement.[73] FIGO partially recognized the prognostic importance of tumor size by subdividing tumors confined to the cervix (FIGO stage IB) into those measuring ≤4 cm (FIGO stage IB1) and >4 cm (stage IB2) in diameter.[72] FIGO stage IA was redefined to separate very early lesions that invade ≤3 mm into the cervical stroma, measure ≤7 mm in diameter, and have a negligible risk of regional metastasis from slightly larger lesions that have been reported to involve lymph nodes in up to 5% of cases[74] (FIGO stage IA2). FIGO stage IA1 is now close, but not equivalent, to the Society of Gynecologic Oncologists' (SGO) long-standing definition for microinvasion. This definition, still widely used in the United States, defines microinvasion as ≤3-mm invasion into cervical stroma without infiltration of lymph-vascular spaces.

According to FIGO, only the results of palpation, inspection, colposcopy, endocervical curettage, hysteroscopy, cytoscopy, proctoscopy, intravenous urography, and plain films of the lungs and skeleton can be used to influence stage assignment. Suspected bladder or rectal involvement should be confirmed by biopsy. FIGO clearly indicates that the results of other imaging studies, such as lymphangiography, CT, and magnetic resonance imaging (MRI), and the findings of operative procedures, including laparoscopy or open lymphadenectomy, cannot be used to change the stage assignation. However, if CT is obtained, the urographic findings may be used to rule out hydronephrosis. The results of these other tests are of prognostic value and often influence treatment decisions, but institutions that publish reports on cervical cancer must adhere strictly to FIGO's rules for staging to minimize confusion and to enable comparisons among studies. Adherence to FIGO's staging guidelines avoids inconsistencies that arise when stage assignments are based on information gained from methods that are not universally available or routinely used.

Surgical staging of the pelvic and para-aortic lymph nodes has been used to obtain prognostic information, to identify patients who would benefit from extended-field irradiation, and to debulk grossly enlarged lymph nodes. Early reports of

Table 55-3 International Federation of Gynecology and Obstetrics Staging of Carcinoma of the Cervix[72]

Stage 0	Carcinoma in situ, intraepithelial carcinoma; *cases of stage 0 should not be included in any therapeutic statistics for invasive carcinoma.*
Stage I	The carcinoma is strictly confined to the cervix (*extension to the corpus should be disregarded*).
Stage IA	Invasive cancer identified only microscopically. All gross lesions, even with superficial invasion, are stage 1B cancers. Invasion is limited to measured stromal invasion with a maximum depth of 5 mm and no wider than 7 mm. (*The depth of invasion should not be more than 5 mm taken from the base of the epithelium, either surface or glandular, from which it originates. Vascular space involvement, either venous or lymphatic, should not alter the staging.*)
Stage IA1	Measured invasion of stroma no greater than 3 mm in depth and no wider than 7 mm.
Stage IA2	Measured invasion of stroma greater than 3 mm and no greater than 5 mm in depth and no wider than 7 mm.
Stage IB	Clinical lesions confined to the cervix or preclinical lesions greater than IA.
Stage IB1	Clinical lesions no greater than 4 cm in size.
Stage IB2	Clinical lesions greater than 4 cm in size.
Stage II	The carcinoma extends beyond the cervix, but has not extended onto the pelvic wall; the carcinoma involves the vagina, but not as far as the lower third.
Stage IIA	No obvious parametrial involvement.
Stage IIB	Obvious parametrial involvement.
Stage III	The carcinoma has extended onto the pelvic wall; on rectal examination there is no cancer-free space between the tumor and the pelvic wall; the tumor involves the lower third of the vagina; all cases with a hydronephrosis or nonfunctioning kidney should be included, unless they are known to be due to another cause. No extension onto the pelvic wall, but involvement of the lower third of the vagina.
Stage IIIA	Extension onto the lower third of the vagina.
Stage IIIB	Extension onto the pelvic wall or hydronephrosis or nonfunctioning kidney.
Stage IV	The carcinoma has extended beyond the true pelvis or has clinically involved the mucosa of the bladder or rectum.
Stage IVA	Spread of the growth to adjacent organs.
Stage IVB	Spread to distant organs.

high complication rates in patients treated with radiation following transperitoneal lymphadenectomy discouraged the use of this procedure,[75,76] but more recent studies have documented a significantly lower incidence of major complications if the operation is performed with a retroperitoneal approach.[77] Laparoscopic biopsy of pelvic and aortic lymph nodes is a means of cervical cancer surgical staging that is less invasive, with shorter times to recuperation and less potential for adhesions that can increase the potential for treatment-related bowel toxicity. Several investigators have demonstrated the feasibility of laparoscopic surgical staging.[78,79] Using a variety of surgical approaches, Goff and colleagues[80] reported that pretreatment surgical staging resulted in modifications in planned radiation therapy in 43% of patients. The value of pretreatment surgical debulking of tumor-involved lymph nodes is unproven, and although the information gained from surgical staging may be valuable in selected patients, its routine use should probably be limited to investigational settings.[81]

Other studies used to assess the extent of lymph node involvement include CT, MRI, lymphangiography, and PET. In a prospective study, the Gynecologic Oncology Group (GOG) compared the accuracy of CT and lymphangiography in assessing para-aortic lymph node involvement.[37] The sensitivities of CT versus lymphangiography were 34% and 79%, respectively, and the specificities were 73% and 96%, respectively. However, it should be noted that the technical and interpretive methodologies of CT used thresholds that are no longer acceptable today. Lymphangiography also facilitates the design of radiation fields. Unfortunately, although lymphangiography was determined to be a very good imaging technique for assessing the status of the para-aortic lymph nodes,[9] it is no longer available in many medical communities.

MRI of the pelvis is a relatively new modality that has been increasingly utilized to evaluate local tumor extent.[82] MRI provides better definition of the extent of disease in the cervix than CT does and may be particularly useful in assessing disease in patients for whom surgery is being considered for primary treatment.[83] Pelvic MRI can also be helpful in designing radiation portals, particularly in defining the borders of lateral fields.[84]

Positron emission tomography (PET) has been compared to CT for assessing lymph node status prior to planned radiation therapy. Grigsby and associates[85] compared PET to CT in a retrospective study of 101 consecutive patients with newly diagnosed cervical carcinoma. CT demonstrated enlarged pelvic lymph nodes in 20%, and aortic lymph nodes in 7% of patients. PET demonstrated abnormal uptake in pelvic lymph nodes in 67%, and aortic lymph nodes in 21% of patients. Surgical staging was not routinely performed to verify the accuracy of imaging findings. A multivariate analysis showed that positive aortic lymph nodes detected by PET imaging was the most important prognostic factor for progression-free survival. Yen and colleagues[86] conducted a prospective evaluation of PET versus MRI and/or CT staging of patients with newly diagnosed (35%) or recurrent (65%) cervical cancer. Verification of lesions identified on imaging was obtained via surgical biopsy or clinical follow-up. Although its diagnostic accuracy was similar for local lesions, PET was superior to both MRI and CT in identifying metastatic lesions. As of January 2005, the Centers for Medicare and Medicaid Services (CMS) has approved the use of PET scanning in the evaluation of newly diagnosed, locally advanced cervical cancer as an adjunct to conventional anatomic imaging. A suggested approach in the work-up of newly diagnosed cervical cancer is shown in Figure 55-2.

PRIMARY THERAPY

Because patients with cervical cancer usually present with disease that is clinically confined to the pelvis, locoregional disease control is the primary challenge for physicians. Treatment with carefully tailored surgery or radiation therapy has produced impressive cure rates in patients with early-stage disease.

It should be recalled that in cervical cancer, progression-free survival rates are closely tracked by overall survival rates, reflecting the limited options for salvage in patients with locally recurrent or metastatic disease. This is unlike the situations with some other malignancies such as prostate and breast cancers or lymphomas, where indolent tumor biology or the availability of multiple salvage options can lead to wide variances between the above two outcome measures. It also highlights the importance of achieving ultimate tumor control, and hence cure, with up-front definitive therapy in cervical cancer.

Primary surgery is typically reserved for physiologically fit patients with tumors clinically confined to the cervix, or those with minimal contiguous vaginal extension (stages I and selected IIA). Current guidelines generally advise that where possible, patients should be treated with either definitive surgery or definitive radiotherapy, thereby avoiding the potential increased toxicity with the use of both modalities in a single patient. Recognizing that most patients with pathologic extracervical spread (e.g., positive lymph nodes, parametrial invasion), or with multiple adverse primary tumor characteristics identified after surgery will be offered adjuvant radiation, or chemoradiation, most surgeons now further limit radical hysterectomy to patients with smaller lesions, often those less than 4 cm in maximal diameter.

Radical radiation therapy is effective for patients with local-regional confined cervical cancer of any stage. Treatment must be carefully tailored to the patient and to the extent of disease but usually consists of a combination of external-beam irradiation and brachytherapy. Overall, historically reported 5-year survival rates of patients treated with *radiation alone* are approximately 75% to 85% for FIGO stage IB, 65% to 70% for FIGO stage II, 30% to 40% for FIGO stage III, and 10% to 15% for FIGO stage IVA disease.[87-92] Within stage subsets, cure rates are strongly correlated with the size of the primary tumor and the extent of regional involvement.[38,91-93]

Treatment Variables Associated with Radiotherapy in Management of Cervical Cancer

The delivery of optimal radiotherapy for patients with cervical cancer requires careful consideration and integration of several critical treatment decisions. These include the role of concurrent chemotherapy with radiation, the use and timing of brachytherapy in combination with external-beam therapy, the total dose and overall duration of radiotherapy, and the volume of elective nodal coverage. These treatment variables clearly need to be judiciously balanced against tumor risk factors and overall patient performance status.

Chemoradiation

Although radiation therapy is the single most effective modality for treatment of local-regional disease not amenable to surgical sterilization, the cure rates for patients with bulky central or regionally metastatic disease treated with radiation alone left room for improvement. As radiation doses typically used already approached conventionally accepted adjacent normal

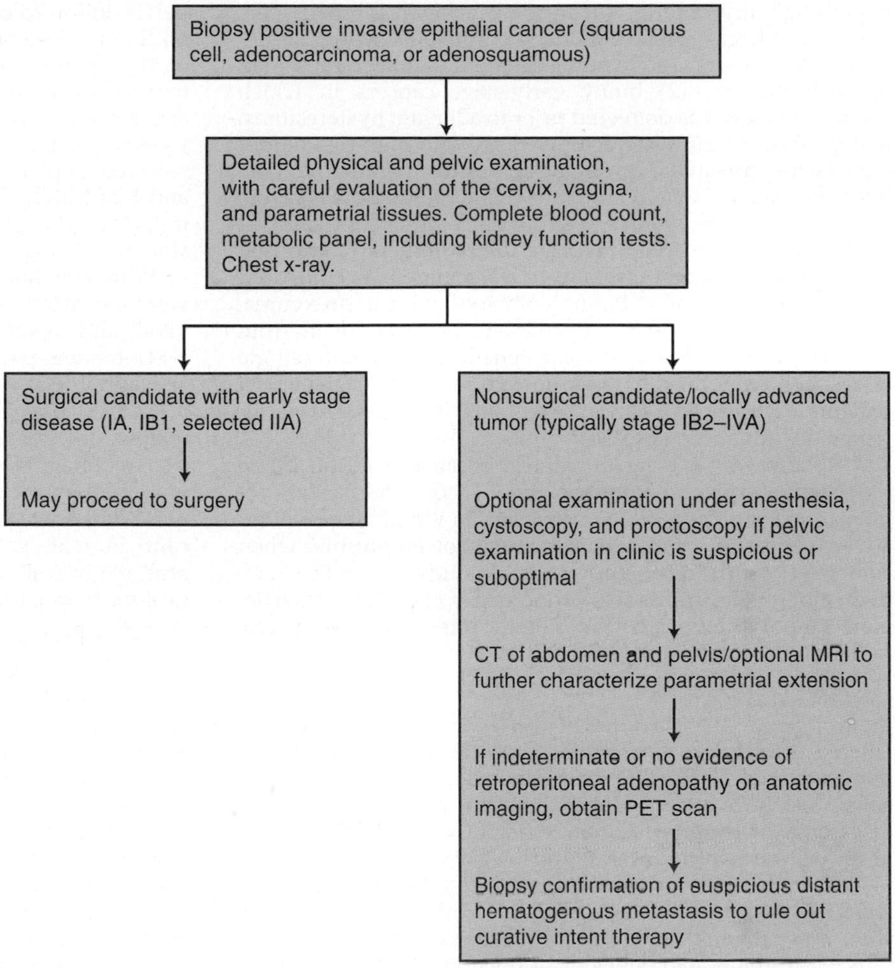

Figure 55-2 Diagnostic algorithm for cervical cancer.

tissue tolerance limits, many trials have been conducted over the past three decades to evaluate the potential benefit of adding systemic agents to primary radiotherapy.

Initial efforts to identify a drug providing radiosensitization focused on the potential role of hydroxyurea with radiotherapy. In an early phase III trial, the GOG compared primary radiation combined with hydroxyurea versus placebo in patients with pelvic-confined FIGO stage IIIB or IVA cervical squamous cell cancers. This study (GOG protocol 4) showed a statistically significant improvement in complete tumor response, progression-free survival, and overall survival favoring the hydroxyurea arm. This study has been criticized because only 104 out of a total 190 randomized patients were eligible and evaluable for outcome analysis, and the survival in patients treated with radiotherapy alone was lower than what might have been expected based on other large institutional-based reports.[94] Other studies that purported to show a benefit to hydroxyurea combined with radiation were conducted at the Roswell Park Memorial Cancer Institute; however, these reports were hampered by small sample sizes, patient overlap, and duplicate reporting.[95] While the GOG, based on the results of GOG protocol 4, selected the combination of concurrent hydroxyurea and radiation as the control arm for further studies in patients with locally advanced cervical cancer, the regimen did not gain widespread acceptance within the oncologic community. Furthermore, a recent meta-analysis has concluded that there was no evidence to support the use of hydroxyurea combined with radiotherapy in the treatment of cervical cancer.[96]

Subsequently, in postulating that tumor hypoxia represented a significant cause of treatment failure following radiotherapy in patients with bulky cervical cancer, investigators attempted to enhance outcome by studying the impact of first-generation nitroimadazole hypoxic-cell radiosentizers. However, multi-institutional phase III trials consistently showed no improvement in outcome with the use of misonidazole or pimonidazole combined with radiotherapy, when compared to the control arms of radiotherapy with or without hydroxyurea.[97-101] The preceding reports formed the basis for the conclusion, in the 1996 National Institutes of Health Consensus Statement on Cervical Cancer, that there was "no proven benefit to combining chemotherapy with radiation" in locally advanced cervical cancer.[102]

Most recently, there has been a profound shift in the paradigm of radiotherapy in the management of cervical cancer. In February 1999, the National Cancer Institute (NCI) issued a clinical announcement stating that "strong consideration should be given to the incorporation of concurrent cisplatin-based chemotherapy with radiation therapy in women who require radiation therapy for treatment of cervical cancer."[103] This recommendation was based on the results of five phase III randomized clinical trials, conducted in North America under the aegis of the National Cancer Institute–sponsored Clinical Trials Cooperative Groups. The five studies had different eligibility criteria, but in total included a broad spectrum of clinical presentations: (1) patients with locally advanced tumors for whom chemoradiation represented primary therapy, (2) bulky early-stage cancers in which chemoradiation was delivered prior to adjuvant hysterectomy, and (3) postradical hysterectomy cases with high-risk pathologic factors (positive lymph nodes, positive parametria, positive margins) for whom adjuvant chemoradiation was given. In each of the five studies, a statistically significant survival advantage was observed favoring the radiotherapy arm that included a concurrent cisplatin-based regimen, as compared to radiation alone or radiation combined with hydroxyurea, with a dramatic 30% to 50% decrease in the risk of death from cervical cancer.[104-108] The outcome benefit represents the single largest contemporary therapeutic gain in the management of patients with cervical cancer, especially in those with local-regionally advanced disease.

Cisplatin was a drug of interest because it is the single most active systemic cytotoxic agent in cervical cancer, demonstrated radiosensitizing properties in vitro,[109] had limited adverse effects on hematopoiesis, and showed promise when combined with radiotherapy in pilot studies.[110-112] The relatively nonmyelosuppressive properties of cisplatin are particularly important when considering the impact of whole pelvic radiation on bone marrow function.

GOG Protocol 85/SWOG 8695

From 1986 to 1990, a total of 368 evaluable patients were entered into this two-arm joint GOG/SWOG phase III randomized trial.[104] Eligible cases included locally advanced squamous cell cancer, adenocarcinoma, or adenosquamous carcinoma of the uterine cervix (FIGO stage IIB-IVA), with negative para-aortic nodes and negative intra-abdominal metastases based on surgical staging. Radiotherapy guidelines were identical in both arms. Patients with stage IIB tumors were prescribed 40.8-Gy external-beam radiotherapy (EBRT) directed to the whole pelvis in 24 fractions (1.7 Gy/fraction), followed by low-dose-rate (LDR) brachytherapy in one or two applications for an additional dose of 40 Gy to point A, or a cumulative point A dose of 80.8 Gy. Further limited supplemental parametrial external radiation was permitted to bring the point B dose to 55 Gy (combining both EBRT and brachytherapy contributions). Patients with stage III or IVA tumors received 51 Gy EBRT in 30 fractions to the whole pelvis, followed by intracavitary brachytherapy delivering an additional dose of 30 Gy to point A (cumulative point A dose of 81 Gy), plus an optional parametrial boost to bring point B to a total dose of 60 Gy. Patients randomized to the control arm received hydroxyurea orally at a dose of 80 mg/kg twice weekly during EBRT. Patients on the experimental arm received cisplatin and 5-fluorouracil (5-FU) during weeks 1 and 5 of EBRT. Cisplatin was given as a slow IV bolus at 50 mg/m^2 on days 1 and 29, and 5-FU delivered as a 4-day infusion of 1000 mg/m^2/24 h on days 2 to 5 and 30 to 33 of EBRT.

With a median at-risk follow-up interval of 8.7 years, there were statistically significant improvements in disease-free survival and overall survival rates favoring the cisplatin/5-FU–treated patients (5-year survival rate of 62% in the cisplatin/5-FU arm versus 50% in the hydroxyurea arm; $p = 0.018$) (Fig. 55-3). Analysis of patterns of first sites of relapse did not identify significant differences between the two treatment groups. The cisplatin/5-FU arm was associated with a lower incidence of severe or life-threatening leukopenia. While there was a slight increase (not statistically significant) in acute gastrointestinal toxicity in the cisplatin/5-FU arm, the overall late complication rates at 3 years were identical for both patient cohorts.[104]

GOG Protocol 120

While awaiting the maturation of data from GOG 85/SWOG 8695, the GOG conducted another phase III randomized trial of concurrent chemoradiotherapy in patients with locally advanced cervical cancer.[105] Eligibility criteria for GOG 120 were similar to those in the previously described GOG 85, and included patients with locally advanced (FIGO stage IIB-IVA) cervical cancer with negative para-aortic nodal and intraperitoneal metastases following surgical staging. Radiation guidelines in this study were identical to those in GOG85/SWOG 8695, and were held constant across all three study arms. Given that the results from GOG85/SWOG 8695 were not yet known, the control arm remained hydroxyurea concurrent with radiation, with the drug given at 3 g/m^2 twice weekly during EBRT. The two experimental arms each contained cisplatin, but with different schedules. In one arm, patients received cisplatin at 50 mg/m^2, followed by infusional 5-FU at 1000 mg/m^2/d for 4 days, starting on days 1 and 29 of EBRT (similar to GOG 85/SWOG 8695), *and* hydroxyurea at 2 g/m^2 twice weekly throughout EBRT. In the other

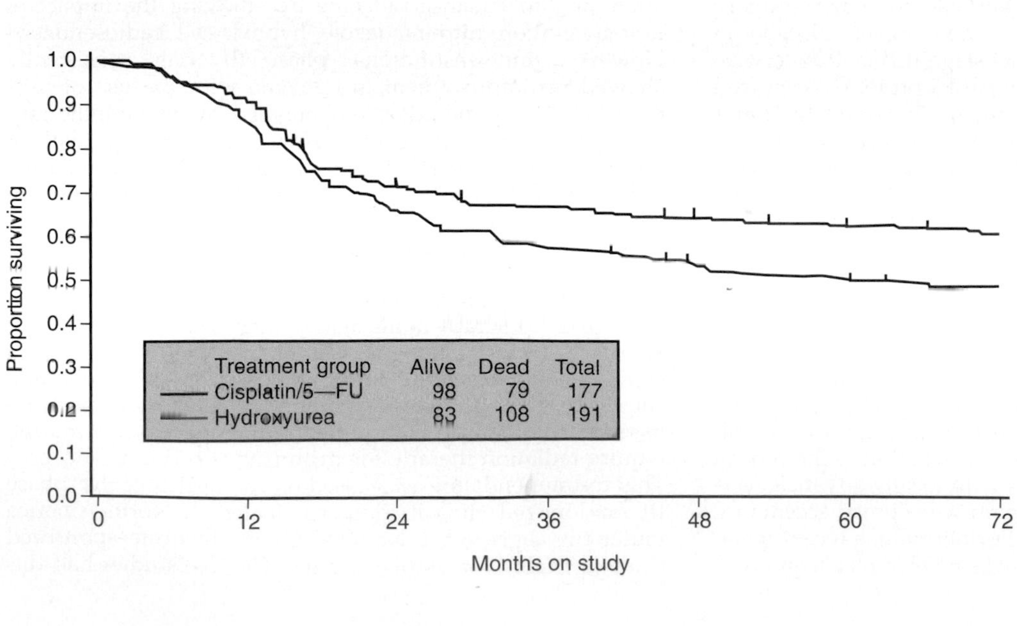

Figure 55-3 Overall survival by treatment arm in GOG 85 ($p = 0.018$). (From Whitney CS, Sause W, Bundy BN, et al: Randomized comparison of fluorouracil plus cisplatin versus hydroxyurea as an adjunct to radiation therapy in stages IIB-IVA carcinoma of the cervix with negative para-aortic lymph nodes. A Gynecologic Oncology Group and Southwest Oncology Group Study. J Clin Oncol 17:1344, Fig. 2, 1999. Reprinted with permission from the American Society of Clinical Oncology.)

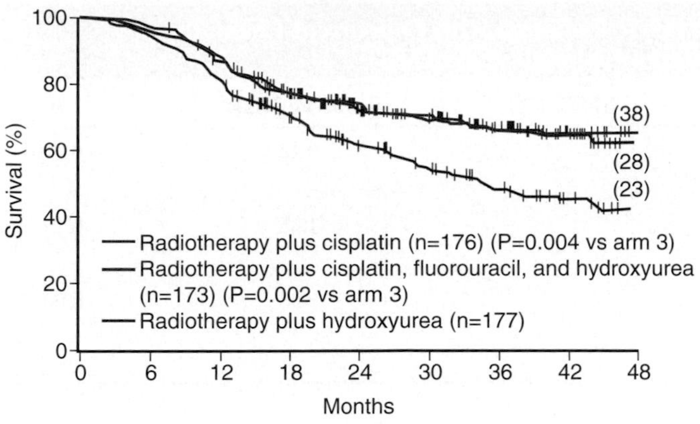

Figure 55-4 Overall survival by treatment arm in GOG 120 ($p < 0.005$ for both cisplatin-containing arms compared to the hydroxyurea control group). (From Rose PG, Bundy BN, Watkins EB, et al: Concurrent cisplatin-based chemoradiation improves progression-free and overall survival in advanced cervical cancer: results of a randomized Gynecologic Oncology Group study. New Engl J Med 340:1144-1153, 1999.Copyright © 1999 Massachusetts Medical Society. All rights reserved.)

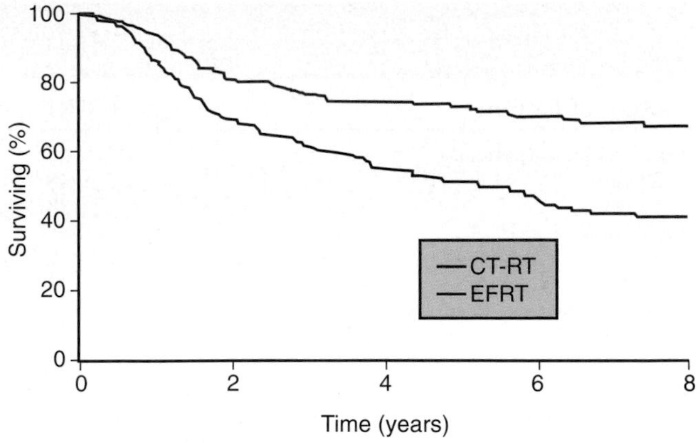

Figure 55-5 Updated overall survival by treatment arm in RTOG 90-01, comparing concurrent chemoradiation (CT-RT) with extended-field radiotherapy alone (EFRT) ($p < 0.0001$). (From Eifel PJ, Winter K, Morris M, et al: Pelvic irradiation with concurrent chemotherapy versus pelvic and para-aortic irradiation for high-risk cervical cancer: an update of Radiation Therapy Oncology Group trial (RTOG) 90-01. J Clin Oncol 22:876, Fig. 1, 2004. Reprinted with permission from the American Society of Clinical Oncology.)

cisplatin treatment group, patients received cisplatin as the sole chemotherapy agent at 40 mg/m^2 weekly during EBRT.

A total of 526 analyzable patients were entered into this trial from 1992 to 1997. With a median at-risk follow-up interval of 35 months, there was a significant improvement in progression-free and overall survival rates favoring both cisplatin-containing arms over the arm with radiotherapy and hydroxyurea alone. Actuarial 3-year overall survival rates were 65% for both cisplatin-containing arms, versus 47% for the hydroxyurea alone group ($p < 0.005$ for both cisplatin-containing arms compared to the hydroyurea cohort) (Fig. 55-4). Patients in both cisplatin-treated groups had a significantly lower frequency of pelvic relapse (19% to 20%) compared to the patients receiving hydroxyurea alone (30%). There was also a slight reduction in distant failures favoring the cisplatin-treated patients, but this did not reach statistical significance. Although both cisplatin-containing arms had essentially identical progression-free and overall survival rates, treatment with cisplatin alone resulted in significantly less acute toxicity than with the three-drug regimen, and hence it was selected as the preferred regimen from this study.[105]

RTOG Protocol 90-01

From 1990 to 1997, the RTOG conducted a phase III randomized trial comparing radiation alone to concurrent chemoradiation.[106] Eligible patients included women with FIGO stage IIB-IVA locally advanced epithelial cervical cancers, as well as those with earlier stage IB/IIA tumors if the primary lesion size was 5 cm or larger or if there were biopsy-proved pelvic nodal metastases. Patients with known extrapelvic disease, as evaluated by bipedal lymphagiography or retroperitoneal surgical staging, were ineligible. Based on an earlier RTOG study that indicated a benefit to prophylactic para-aortic nodal irradiation in patients with stage IB2-IIB cancers,[113] the control arm of radiation alone included contiguous extended field coverage to the L1-2 vertebral interspace. The pelvis and para-aortic nodes were prescribed a dose of 45 Gy in 25 fractions, supplemented by LDR intracavitary brachytherapy to boost the point A cumulative dose to at least 85 Gy. Institutions were allowed to initiate brachytherapy earlier, at an EBRT dose of 20 to 30 Gy, provided that the final point A dose specification was adhered to and that further external-beam pelvic radiation be delivered with a midline block. In the experimental arm, patients were selected to receive pelvic radiation only, with the superior field edge defined at the L4-5 vertebral interspace. With the exception of eliminating prophylactic para-aortic coverage, radiation parameters for the experimental arm were similar to the control group's. Concurrent with their radiotherapy, patients randomized to the experimental group received 3 cycles of cisplatin/5-FU chemotherapy (cisplatin 75 mg/m^2, 5-FU 1000 mg/m^2/d for 4 d) administered at 3-week intervals, with the third cycle often given at the time of brachytherapy insertion.

A total of 388 analyzable patients were included. At a median at-risk follow-up interval of 43 months, preceding the NCI clinical announcement, there was a statistically significant advantage for disease-free and overall survival rates favoring the chemoradiation arm. The actuarial 5-year overall survival rate was 73% in patients treated with chemotherapy and radiation, compared to 58% in patients treated with extended field radiation alone ($p = 0.004$).[106]

The results of RTOG 90-01 have been recently updated, with a median at-risk follow-up duration of 6.6 years.[114] The significant outcome benefit of concurrent chemotherapy and radiation over radiation alone has been maintained, with 8-year overall survival rates of 67% and 41%, respectively ($p < 0.0001$) (Fig. 55-5). The advantage of chemoradiation was noted regardless of FIGO stage (IB and II versus III and IVA), pelvic nodal involvement, or the method of pretherapy nodal evaluation (lymphangiography versus retroperitoneal nodal staging). The rate of cumulative overall grade 3 or higher late complications was similar in both treatment groups (14% at 5 years). Analysis of patterns of failure noted a significant reduction in local-regional and distant metastases (excluding para-aortics) relapse rates favoring the patients treated with radiation and cisplatin/5-FU. Although there was a slightly higher para-aortic failure rate in patients receiving chemoradiation compared to extended field radiation alone, this did not reach statistical significance.

The patterns of failure recorded in RTOG 90-01 (Table 55-4) may allow the hypothesis that concurrent chemotherapy

Table 55-4 **Patterns of Failure in RTOG 90-01, Comparing Pelvic Radiation with Concurrent Chemotherapy (CT-RT) versus Extended Field Radiotherapy without Chemotherapy (EFRT)[114]**

Pattern of Failure	CT-RT (%)	EFRT (%)	Relative Risk*	*p*
Local-regional (pelvic)			0.42	<0.0001
5 years	18	34		
8 years	18	35		
Para-aortic			1.65	0.15
5 years	7	4		
8 years	9	4		
Distant metastases (excluding para-aortics)			0.48	0.0013
5 years	18	31		
8 years	20	35		

*A value less than 1.0 indicates an advantage in favor of CT-RT.

not only provides local-regional radiosensitization but also addresses pre-existing micrometastases, although it should be recognized that the risk of distant metastases is closely linked to the incidence of pelvic failure.[40] At the very least, this trial indicates that for patients at some risk of para-aortic nodal metastases, albeit without grossly identifiable disease, chemoradiation with radiation limited only to the pelvis achieves better outcomes than extended-field radiation alone without chemotherapy.

GOG Protocol 123

From 1992 to 1997, the GOG conducted a phase III randomized trial comparing preoperative treatment with radiation versus radiation and concurrent cisplatin in patients presenting with an earlier tumor stage than those included in the preceding three described studies.[107] Eligible patients were those with stage IB2 cervical cancers (≥4 cm tumor diameter), with no evidence of retroperitoneal adenopathy on radiologic (CT or lymphangiography) or surgical assessment. Radiotherapy specifications were identical in both treatment arms. The pelvis was prescribed a dose of 45 Gy in 25 fractions with EBRT, followed by LDR intracavitary brachytherapy to boost the cumulative point A dose to 75 Gy. In the experimental arm, patients received weekly cisplatin at a dose of 40 mg/m^2 (with a maximal dose of 70 mg/wk), for up to 6 doses. The final dose of cisplatin could be given during brachytherapy insertion. Based on the interim results of a previous GOG trial that evaluated the role of adjuvant hysterectomy in centrally bulky tumors (GOG 71), all patients in this study underwent extrafascial hysterectomy following either radiation alone or radiation plus concurrent cisplatin.

A total of 369 patients were evaluated, with a median at-risk follow-up interval of 36 months. Patients who received concurrent cisplatin had a significantly higher incidence of pathologic complete response in the hysterectomy specimen, as well as improved pelvic control, progression-free survival, and overall survival rates compared to those treated without chemotherapy. The 3-year overall survival rates were 83% and 74% in the chemoradiation and radiation arms, respectively ($p = 0.008$) (Fig. 55-6). Although there was an increase in acute toxicities in the patients treated with cisplatin and radiation, these reactions were predominantly of transient hematologic perturbations, and severe late toxicities were infrequent and equally divided between the two groups.[107]

Intergroup Protocol 0107 (SWOG 8797/GOG 109/RTOG 91-12)

The last of the five phase III trials that formed the basis for the 1999 NIH clinical announcement investigated the role of chemoradiation as an adjunct to primary surgery for clinically early stage disease, but in whom postoperative high-risk pathologic features are discovered.[108] Eligible patients for this intergroup study consisted of patients with stage IA2, IB, or IIA carcinoma of the cervix who were initially treated with radical hysterectomy and pelvic lymphadenectomy and who were found to have positive pelvic lymph nodes, positive margins, and/or positive parametrial infiltration on microscopic evaluation. Taken together, these high-risk factors have the unifying theme of pathologically identified extracervical/extrauterine disease extension. In this two-arm trial, patients were randomized to pelvic radiation alone (EBRT to 49.3 Gy in 29 fractions, without brachytherapy), or to the same radiation combined with chemotherapy. Chemotherapy consisted of cisplatin (70 mg/m^2) and 5-FU (1000 mg/m^2/d for 4 d) given for four cycles beginning on days 1, 22, 43, and 64 of therapy. Two of the chemotherapy cycles were delivered concurrently with pelvic radiation, followed by two additional cycles after completion of EBRT.

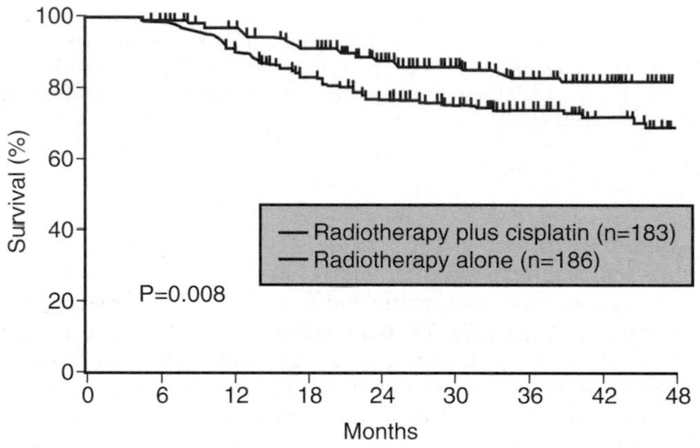

Figure 55-6 Overall survival by treatment arm in GOG 123 ($p = 0.008$). (From Keys HW, Bundy BN, Stehman FB, et al: A comparison of weekly cisplatin during radiation therapy versus irradiation alone, each followed by adjuvant hysterectomy in bulky stage IB cervical carcinoma: A randomized trial of the Gynecologic Oncology Group. N Engl J Med 340:1154-1161, 1999. Copyright © Massachusetts Medical Society. All rights reserved.)

A total of 243 eligible patients were entered into the trial from 1991 to 1996. With a median at-risk follow-up time of 42 months, patients receiving combined adjuvant chemoradiation had a statistically significant improvement in progression-free and overall survival rates compared to those

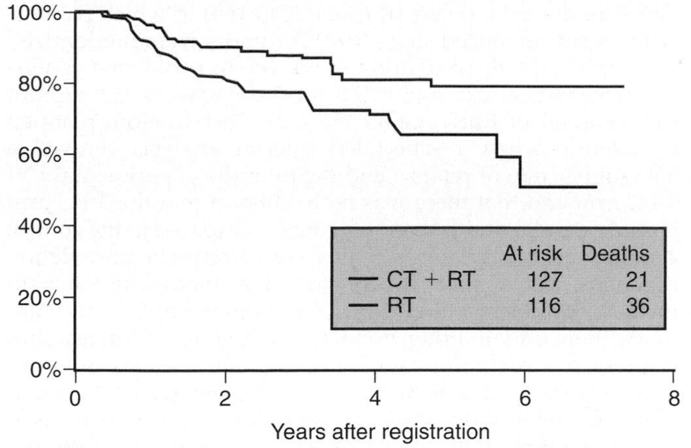

Figure 55-7 Overall survival, by treatment arm, in Intergroup protocol 0107, comparing postoperative chemoradiation (CT+RT) to radiation alone (RT) ($p = 0.007$). (From Peters WA, Liu PY, Barrett RJ II, et al: Concurrent chemotherapy and pelvic radiation therapy compared with pelvic radiation therapy alone as adjunctive therapy after radical surgery in high-risk, early-stage carcinoma of the cervix. J Clin Oncol 18:1609, Fig. 2, 2000. Reprinted with permission from the American Society of Clinical Oncology.)

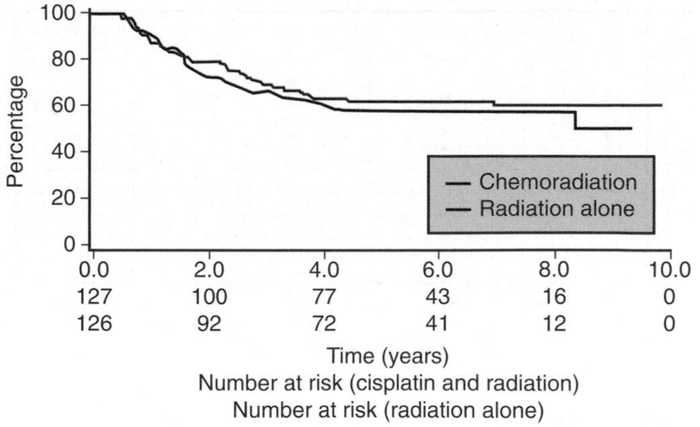

Figure 55-8 Overall survival by treatment arm (chemoradiation; radiation alone) in the NCIC study ($p = 0.53$). (From Pearcey R, Brundage M, Drouin P, et al. Phase III trial comparing radical radiotherapy with and without cisplatin chemotherapy in patients with advanced squamous cell cancer of the cervix. J Clin Oncol 20:970, Fig. 3, 2002. Reprinted with permission from the American Society of Clinical Oncology.)

undergoing radiation alone. The estimated 4-year overall survival rates were 81% and 71% for the chemoradiation and radiation only arms, respectively ($p = 0.007$) (Fig. 55-7). The outcome benefit for adjuvant chemoradiotherapy appeared to arise from reduction in both pelvic and distant failures, although comparisons of relapse patterns between treatment arms did not reach statistical significance. There was an increase in acute toxicities in the combined modality arm, but these were mostly limited to transient, and manageable hematologic and gastrointestinal effects.

National Cancer Institute of Canada Trial

In contrast to the consistent therapeutic benefits seen for combining cisplatin-based chemotherapy with radiation in the preceding five phase III trials, the National Cancer Institute of Canada (NCIC) published the results of another randomized study that questioned the role of concurrent chemoradiation in locally advanced cervical cancers.[115] Eligible patients included those with stage IIB-IVA squamous cell cancers, or earlier stage disease (IB/IIA) if the primary tumor was at least 5 cm in diameter or if there were histologically positive pelvic nodal involvement. Radiation specifications, which were identical in both treatment arms, prescribed a dose of 45 Gy in 25 fractions to the pelvis with EBRT. This was followed by intracavitary brachytherapy using various allowable dose rates, but each calibrated to provide an LDR biologically equivalent dose of 35 Gy to point A (total cumulative point A dose of 80 Gy in conventional equivalents). Careful quality control was maintained to complete all radiation therapy within 7 weeks. Patients randomized to receive chemotherapy were given weekly cisplatin at a dose of 40 mg/m^2 for a total of 5 administrations concurrently with EBRT.

Between 1991 and 1996, 253 eligible patients were entered into the trial. With a median at-risk follow-up duration of 82 months, there were no observable differences in progression-free or overall survival between the two treatment arms[115] (Fig. 55-8).

Various reasons for the lack of a demonstrable effect of cisplatin concurrent with radiation in the NCIC study have been promulgated by the authors and others.[116] These include the lack of surgical staging, a relatively small sample size, the confounding factor of treatment-related anemia in the chemotherapy arm, and the omission of 5-FU (which may be synergistic with cisplatin) from the chemotherapy regimen. Perhaps most provocative is the suggestion that concurrent cisplatin-containing chemotherapy exhibits its greatest benefit primarily in patients with suboptimal and prolonged overall radiation therapy durations. In contrast to the studies reported by Whitney[104] and Rose,[105] where the median duration of the treatment course was 64 and 62 days, respectively, the timing for completion of radiation in the NCIC study was carefully controlled, with a median duration of 51 days.[115] However, the potential reduced impact of concurrent cisplatin with optimum radiation schedules have been refuted by others.[116] Nonetheless, the NCIC authors conclude that despite their negative trial, "... the balance of evidence favors the use of combined-modality treatment for the types of patients studied in this trial. The best results are certainly achieved by careful attention to RT details, including dose and overall delivery time, the use of brachytherapy whenever possible, and probably the addition of concurrent cisplatin chemotherapy to RT."[115]

Synopsis Regarding Platinum-Based Chemotherapy Concurrent with Radiation

In an overview, Rose and Bundy summated the collective results of the six North American randomized trials (including the NCIC study) and showed a cumulative and statistically significant 36% reduction in the risk of death favoring combined cisplatin-based chemotherapy and radiotherapy over radiotherapy alone or combined with hydroxyurea and suggested that the negative results of the NCIC study might simply be a product of statistical variation[116] (Fig. 55-9). Furthermore, a formalized meta-analysis of all known randomized trials of concurrent chemoradiation in cervical cancer showed a statistically significant improvement in overall survival for combined modality therapy, especially for those patients receiving cisplatin.[117]

There remains ongoing debate as to what represents the current standard cisplatin-containing regimen to use when combined with radiotherapy. The GOG has selected weekly cisplatin at 40 mg/m^2 (maximum 70 mg weekly dose) for up to 6 cycles, concurrent with EBRT, as its standard for chemora-

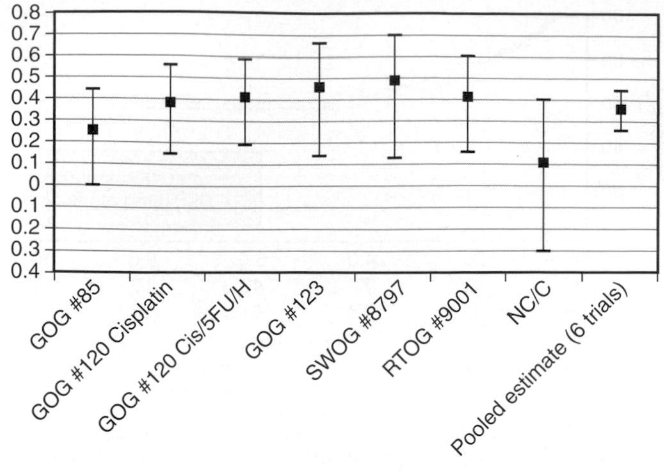

Figure 55-9 Reduction in the risk (1 – relative risk) of death from six chemoradiation clinical trials in cervical cancer, with 95% confidence intervals. A value above 0 represents a benefit for cisplatin-containing chemoradiation. Cis, cisplatin; 5-FU, fluorouracil; SWOG, Southwest Oncology Group (Intergroup Protocol 0107); H, hydroxyurea. (From Rose PG, Bundy BN: Chemoradiation for locally advanced cervical cancer: does it help? J Clin Oncol 20:891, Fig. 1, 2002. Reprinted with permission from the American Society of Clinical Oncology.)

diation of cervical cancer. Others believe that 5-FU should not be omitted and thus combine cisplatin at 50 to 75 mg/m^2 with 5-FU at 1000 $mg/m^2/d$ for 4 days, given on a 3-week cycle. It is clear that hydroxyurea is no longer a drug of interest in the context of chemoradiation for cervical cancer. Taken in total, the overall data provide compelling support for the use of chemoradiation in all cervical cancer patients, except perhaps for those with the earliest presentations of disease.

It should be emphasized, however, that radiotherapy remains the single most effective modality in the management of patients with locally advanced cervical cancer, where surgical extirpation of tumor is infeasible or incomplete. Even in the absence of chemotherapy, radiotherapy alone is able to cure many patients with bulky cervical tumors. Some patients present with hydronephrosis and renal dysfunction or other medical cormobidities that preclude the use of cisplatin. The use of concurrent carboplatin, which avoids nephrotoxicity, has been suggested by some as an alternative to cisplatin, but its comparative efficacy remains unproven.[118] Ultimately, the selection of concurrent cisplatin-based chemotherapy requires sound medical judgement, balancing the potential improvement in tumor control with patient physiology, disease presentation, and the increased toxicities (notably hematologic, metabolic, and gastrointestinal) associated with the addition of chemotherapy.

Noncisplatin Chemoradiation Regimens

Although there is general acknowledgement of the efficacy of cisplatin in combination with radiotherapy, various investigators have evaluated other noncisplatin chemoradiation regimens, primarily infusion 5-FU. Thomas and colleagues reported a four-arm randomized trial evaluating the impact of infusional 5-FU as a single chemotherapeutic agent, given at 1000 $mg/m^2/d$ for 4 days during the first and last week of EBRT. Both the radiation alone and chemoradiation cohorts were further divided into standard versus partially hyperfractionated radiation schedules. There was no overall benefit seen for the addition of 5-FU to radiotherapy in this study of patients with locally advanced cervical cancer.[119] The GOG conducted a phase III trial (GOG 165) in which patients with locally advanced stage IIB-IVA tumors were randomized to weekly cisplatin at 40 $mg/m^2/wk$ versus protracted venous infusion 5-FU at 225 $mg/m^2/d$ for 5 days/week throughout the duration of EBRT. GOG 165 was closed before planned completion when a scheduled interim analysis showed a 35% higher rate of relapse and death in the experimental PVI 5-FU arm and that there was no likelihood that the 5-FU arm would ever show improved outcomes compared to the control arm of weekly cisplatin.[119a] Other concurrent chemoradiation regimens tested that appear to have therapeutic benefit include epirubicin[120] and 5-FU plus mitomycin-C.[121] In summary, there remain other nonplatinum agents of interest, but at present, a platinum-containing regimen remains the standard of care in combination with radiotherapy in the treatment of patients with cervical cancer. While 5-FU may be used in combination with cisplatin, current evidence does not support the use of 5-FU alone in chemoradiation algorithms.

Neoadjuvant Chemotherapy

Although concurrent cisplatin-based chemoradiation has become the widely accepted standard of care, caution is raised regarding the use of strategies employing neoadjuvant chemotherapy before radiotherapy. Multiple randomized trials, most with small patient numbers, have failed to identify an effective strategy of neoadjuvant chemotherapy followed by definitive radiotherapy. A systematic review and individual patient data meta-analysis showed no benefit, and indeed, an overall trend to detriment, for patients receiving neoadjuvant chemotherapy (predominantly cisplatin-based) before radical radiation.[122] In two of the randomized trials, it was reported that the neoadjuvant chemotherapy approach, although associated with a reasonable initial response, ultimately resulted in statistically significant inferior pelvic control and overall survival compared to patients treated with definitive radiotherapy alone.[123,124]

A plausible explanation for the lack of benefit seen with chemotherapy preceding radiation is that although responses can be seen with systemic cytotoxics alone, the remaining clonogens undergo accelerated repopulation, thereby offsetting the efficacy of radiotherapy.[125] Questions remain regarding potential benefit of initial chemotherapy in surgical candidates or where the dose and intercycle interval of systemic agents are optimized, but the use of neoadjuvant chemotherapy strategies should be considered only in the context of carefully designed clinical trials. Unless more effective cytotoxic agents are identified, there is no current reason to consider neoadjuvant chemotherapy followed by definitive radiotherapy in patients with localized, curable cervical cancer.

Brachytherapy Plus External-Beam Radiation Therapy

The importance of brachytherapy in the curative treatment of intact cervical cancer is indisputable. Clinicians have sometimes been inclined to de-emphasize the use of brachytherapy in patients with FIGO stage III disease, arguing that disease at the pelvic wall is beyond the reach of traditional intracavitary therapy. However, reports from the Patterns of Care Study[126] and from M.D. Anderson Cancer Center (MDACC)[93] have demonstrated significantly better survival rates for patients treated with a combination of external-beam and intracavitary radiation. In the MDACC report of 1007 patients treated with radiation for FIGO stage IIIB disease, the disease-specific survival rate was 43% for patients who had intracavitary irradiation versus 21% for those treated with external-beam radiation (EBRT) alone. Patients treated during periods when policies emphasized the use of brachytherapy had significantly better survival rates. Patients who received higher doses of EBRT (and concomitantly lower doses of intracavitary radiation) to the central pelvis had poorer survival rates. The rate of major complications was also correlated with the proportion of central pelvic treatment given with EBRT, and this correlation suggested that the therapeutic ratio narrows when the dose of external-beam radiation given to the whole pelvis exceeds 45 Gy.[93] Nonetheless, a careful balance between external-beam and brachytherapy components of therapy, accounting for tumor volume, anatomic presentation, and disease regression rate, represents the hallmark of proper cervical cancer radiotherapy planning.

Radiation Dose and Duration

In general, a cumulative dose of at least 85 Gy to point A is considered desirable for patients undergoing primary radiotherapy for locally bulky cervical cancer (stage IB2-IVA), with a dose of at least 45 Gy to all volumes at risk for microscopic tumor spread. These dose levels represent current protocol standards for large cooperative groups such as the GOG and the RTOG. Smaller and earlier tumors (stage IA-IB1), may be treated to somewhat lower overall doses of 75 to 80 Gy. The relative contributions of EBRT and brachytherapy to the overall dose vary according to institutional preferences. Many centers favor initiating external whole pelvic radiation to a dose of 40 to 45 Gy before proceeding with brachtherapy. Gross parametrial or pelvic nodal disease can then be boosted with limited external fields, blocking critical central pelvic structures, to a cumulative dose of 55 to 65 Gy (combining external-beam and brachytherapy components), depending on disease volume and the ability to avoid adjacent normal tissues. Other institutions prefer to emphasize and initiate brachytherapy earlier, at external whole pelvic doses of 20 to 30 Gy, especially for patients with earlier stage and smaller volume disease. External beam radiation is then continued to the pelvis, with or without midline blocking. Although recommendations have been made to try to limit the rectal and bladder reference points to maximal summated doses of 70 Gy and 75 Gy, respectively, it is recognized that the most important consideration is to deliver adequate tumoricidal doses, even if the normal tissue dose recommendations are somewhat exceeded. On the other hand, a total point A dose of 85 to 90 Gy for intact bulky cervical cancer probably represents a reasonable limit, based on integral doses to surrounding normal pelvic structures, and there is no evidence that significant further radiation dose escalation will result in therapeutic gain. For adjuvant radiotherapy following primary surgery, where there is no gross tumor residual, an external-beam dose of 45 to 50 Gy to the pelvis is considered sufficient and tolerable.

These preceding dose discussions are based on conventional external fractionation of 1.8 to 2.0 Gy daily and LDR brachytherapy. The use of altered fractionation, or in particular high-dose-rate (HDR) brachytherapy, necessitates a different system of reference doses and is discussed in greater detail later.

The adverse impact of treatment duration protraction in cervical cancer has been evaluated by several investigators. There is general consensus that prolonging a course of radical radiotherapy beyond approximately 7 weeks is associated with a 0.5% to 1% decrease in pelvic control per extra day.[127-131] Although debate remains about whether an increase in treatment duration adversely affects outcome or is simply a reflection of unfavorable tumor or patient characteristics, there is compelling radiobiologic demonstration of accelerated tumor repopulation that mitigates the efficacy of radiotherapy.[125] In contrast, there is no evidence that prolongation of treatment duration results in a reduction of late normal tissue sequalae.[132] Thus, it is now considered prudent to complete a course of definitive radiotherapy for cervical cancer within 7 to 8 weeks by eliminating all elective treatment breaks, delivering external-beam parametrial boosts between, or interdigitated with, brachytherapy insertions, and actively supporting patients through acute toxicities so as to avoid radiation interruptions.

Role of Extended-Field Irradiation

The prognosis of patients with cervical carcinoma is inversely related to the extent of regional involvement. However, because hematogeneous metastasis is usually a late event in the course of this disease, patients with lymph node metastases often can be cured with regional irradiation if pelvic disease can be controlled. Even patients with documented para-aortic lymph node metastases have a 20% to 50% 5-year survival rate, depending on the extent of pelvic disease.[33,133-136]

Two groups have explored the use of prophylactic extended-field irradiation in patients who do not have overt para-aortic metastases. The Radiation Therapy Oncology Group (RTOG) randomized patients who had bulky FIGO stages IB-IIA or FIGO stage IIB disease to receive either standard pelvic irradiation or extended-field irradiation (including the pelvic and para-aortic nodes) combined with brachytherapy.[113] Patients with known para-aortic lymph node metastases were excluded from the study, but no consistent method of lymph node evaluation was specified in the protocol. Results demonstrated a significantly better overall survival rate for patients treated with extended-field irradiation (67% versus 55% at 5 years, $p = 0.02$). However, this survival advantage for extended field radiation has raised questions because the study paradoxically did not show a significant increase in progression-free survival.[113]

A second trial from the European Oncology and Radiation Therapy Consortium (EORTC)[137] randomized patients who had more advanced pelvic disease (bulky FIGO stage IIB, FIGO stage III, or biopsy-proved pelvic lymph node metastases) but required a lymphangiogram to assess the regional lymph nodes. In this study, the disease-free survival rates of patients in the two treatment arms were not significantly different at 4 years although the rate of relapse in para-aortic lymph nodes was higher in patients who had not received radiation to this site. Overall survival rates were not reported. The more accurate and consistent pretreatment nodal evaluation and the relatively high rate of pelvic disease recurrence in the EORTC study may have reduced the margin for improvement and obscured any advantage derived from extended-field irradiation.

Although the role of prophylactic para-aortic nodal irradiation remains to be fully defined, the results of RTOG 90-01 clearly indicate that concurrent chemotherapy with pelvic radiation leads to significant outcome benefits over extended field radiation without chemotherapy.[114] Underlying the question of prophylactic para-aortic radiation is the assumption that the para-aortic nodes represent isolated occult extrapelvic disease in some patients for whom sterilization by radiotherapy would translate to cure (assuming achievable pelvic control). The results of RTOG 90-01, which showed significant reductions in both pelvic and distant relapse with chemoradiation, suggest that the use of concurrent chemotherapy to some degree addresses subclinical metastases beyond the volume of irradiation. Unanswered is the question of whether prophylactic extended-field radiation in addition to systemic chemotherapy would provide additional therapeutic gain.

At present, it is the practice pattern at the University of Washington to include prophylactic para-aortic nodal irradiation to 45 Gy, concurrent with chemotherapy (to the level of the renal vessels, or at the L1-2 vertebral interspace), for patients with the highest potential risk of para-aortic disease—those with common iliac adenopathy, or with extensive pelvic lymphadenopathy by radiologic imaging who do not undergo surgical staging. Whereas the efficacy of such an approach has not been proven, the use of concurrent cisplatin-based chemotherapy with extended field radiation has been shown to be tolerable in several phase II trials.[138,139]

Impact of Anemia and Tumor Hypoxia on Radiotherapy Outcome: Potential as Therapeutic Targets

The adverse association of anemia on outcome following primary radiotherapy for cervical cancer has been well documented in many previous clinical reviews.[140,141] Whether this association reflects cause and effect or whether anemia is simply a surrogate for larger and more refractory tumors is still being debated. Potential mechanisms for a negative impact of anemia on cervical cancer radiotherapy outcomes may be linked to tumor hypoxia and consequent radioresistance, as well as induction of angiogenesis, increased tumor aggressiveness, and enhanced metastatic potential.

A large Canadian multicenter retrospective analysis provided intriguing evidence that anemia is an independent negative prognostic factor in cervical cancer. The study found that it was the average hemoglobin (Hgb) level *during* radiotherapy rather than *before* therapy that was more predictive of poor outcome. The adverse impact of anemia during radiotherapy was second only to tumor stage in prognostic significance on multivariate analysis. The magnitude of the increment in survival for nonanemic compared with anemic patients exceeded the gain achieved with concurrent chemoradiation strategies. The most provocative suggestion of the Canadian study was that correction of anemia (by transfusion, to a Hgb level ≥12 g/dl) abrogated the adverse impact of preexisting anemia.[142] These findings have been echoed by another recent single-institution retrospective report from Austria, although a different threshold Hgb level (≤11 g/dl) for anemia was used.[143] Despite the potential prognostic and therapeutic implications of anemia in cervical cancer, only one small prospective randomized trial directly addressing this issue has been completed, in the 1970s. This study indicated improved pelvic control for irradiated patients whose Hgb level was corrected by transfusion, but the analysis was hampered by limited patient numbers and lack of stratification.[144]

In an attempt to provide definitive answers, the GOG conducted a prospective phase III trial (GOG protocol 0191) in which patients with locally advanced cervical cancer undergoing primary chemoradiation (radiotherapy with concurrent weekly cisplatin at a dose of 40 mg/m^2) were randomized to Hgb maintenance at a level of 10 g/dl versus aggressive intervention to raise Hgb levels to 12 to 13 g/dl (by transfusion and erythropoietin). However, due to concerns about an increased incidence of thromboembolic events, this trial was prematurely closed.

As standard of practice, radiation oncologists attempt to maintain patient hemoglobin levels at generally 10 g/dl during treatment for cervical cancer. Although the impact of maintaining this hemoglobin level on tumor control is unclear (recognizing that the studies discussed above had noted optimal outcome at hemoglobin levels of 12 g/dl), it is recognized that lower hemoglobin levels adversely affect patient quality of life and may affect their ability to tolerate aggressive chemoradiation. Besides the use of transfusion and/or erythropoietic factors, every effort should be made to minimize cervical trauma and blood loss during a patient's evaluation and treatment. Local hemostatic agents (Monsel's solution) and vaginal packing should minimize blood loss after necessary biopsies and examinations. When local hemostatic measures fail to control bleeding, radiotherapeutic hemostasis may be achieved with transvaginal orthovoltage irradiation or with prompt initiation of external-beam irradiation, possibly using 2 or 3 days of hyperfractionated pelvic irradiation. In patients with curable cancers, use of a hyperfractionated EBRT approach (for example, 1.5 to 1.8 Gy/fraction twice daily for 2 to 3 days) achieves the same likelihood of hemostasis as larger daily fractions, while preserving normal tissue tolerance and ultimate treatment planning flexibility. Although some authors have recommended emergency intracavitary therapy to control bleeding, this approach is more likely to compromise subsequent curative treatment.

Tumor hypoxia, as measured by oxygen electrodes, has been identified in many cervical cancers and is a predictor of poor outcome.[145,146] Although there may be a link, the relationship between host status (anemia and hemoglobin level) and tumor milieu (hypoxia) remains ambiguous. To exploit hypoxia as a potential therapeutic target, the GOG has opened a randomized phase III trial (GOG 219) that will investigate the efficacy of a new-generation bioreductive drug—tirapazamine, added to the present standard of concurrent cisplatin and radiation for locally advanced cervical cancer. In addition to its radiosensitizing effects, tirapazamine has generated significant interest because it is itself a potent and selective hypoxic cell cytotoxin and is also potentially synergistic with cisplatin.[147,148]

Recent studies have identified significant modulations of gene expression in hypoxic tumors that may be associated with tumor aggressiveness and progression, including hypoxia-inducible factor 1, p53, VEGF, platelet-derived endothelial cell growth factor, nitric oxide synthase, and matrix metalloproteinases.[149] These biomolecular markers provide potential new targets for future therapeutic investigations.

Primary Therapy By Disease Stage

Preinvasive Disease

Preinvasive lesions are usually treated with local ablative procedures (cryosurgery or laser ablation) or excisional procedures (loop excision or cervical conization). Hysterectomy is an appropriate treatment option for women with high-grade cervical dysplasia who no longer desire fertility preservation. Ablative treatment is contraindicated if the entire transformation zone has not been well visualized, if there is a marked discrepancy between Pap smear results and colposcopy findings, or if colposcopy evaluation with biopsies leaves unresolved the presence of invasive disease. In these situations, conization should be performed to exclude the presence of invasion.

Microinvasive Disease (FIGO Stage IA)

Early microinvasive (FIGO stage IA1 or SGO stage IA) disease is conventionally treated with a simple (type I) abdominal or vaginal hysterectomy after the depth of invasion has been confirmed by cone biopsy. However, for selected patients who wish to maintain fertility and who agree to close follow-up, therapeutic conization of the cervix may be adequate treatment.

Although early microinvasive carcinomas of the cervix (SGO stage IA or FIGO stage IA1) are usually treated with hysterectomy, patients with medical contraindications to surgery can be treated very effectively with brachytherapy alone, for which 10-year progression-free survival rates of 98% to 100% have been reported.[150-152] Treatment usually consists of one or two LDR intracavitary insertions that deliver 65 to 75 Gy exposure to point A, 6500 to 7500 mg-h of exposure, and a maximal vaginal surface dose of 100 to 120 Gy, depending on the extent of microinvasive disease, size of the cervix, and normal tissue anatomy.[150,153,154]

The risk of regional spread from more deeply invasive FIGO stage IA2 carcinomas is about 5%. Surgical treatment, therefore, usually includes a radical hysterectomy combined with a pelvic lymph node dissection. Attempts to treat stage IA2 cervical cancer with conservative surgery have yielded poor results.[155] The use of irradiation for stage IA2 tumors usually warrants treatment with a combination of external-beam and intracavitary radiation, in which 40 to 45 Gy of pelvic EBRT (often with midline blocking), is combined with intracavitary brachytherapy to deliver a cumulative point A dose of at least 75 to 80 Gy. Five-year survival with either surgical or radiation treatment is at least 95%.

Recognizing the outstanding cure rates with radiotherapy alone in stage IA cervical cancer, combined with the fact that radiation is typically used in lieu of primary surgery in such early stage patients who have significant medical comorbidities, the use of concurrent chemoradiation for these cases is not routinely justifiable. Furthermore, clinical trials to evaluate the role of chemoradiation in this patient population, who have an excellent oncologic prognosis, would not be feasible statistically.

FIGO Stages IB, IIA

Primary surgical management is probably best suited to physiologically fit patients with small FIGO stage IB or IIA cervical cancers without clinical evidence of regional metastasis. Depending on the size of the cervical tumor, surgeons may vary somewhat the extent of their resection of the paracervical tissues and uterosacral ligaments (Fig. 55-10). The risk of major complications, particularly bladder and rectal dysfunction or ureter injury, is proportional to the extent of surgical resection and may therefore be greater when radical hysterectomy is used to treat larger tumors. The ovaries of premenopausal women are usually not removed, which provides an advantage for radical surgery over irradiation in young women with relatively small tumors. Massive obesity and other medical problems that increase the risk of a major pelvic surgical procedure are usually considered relative contraindications to a primary surgical approach.

Reported results of treatment with radical hysterectomy versus those of radiation therapy for FIGO stage IB cervical carcinomas are comparable, with 80% to 90% of patients surviving after 5 years. However, because surgeons tend to select young patients who have relatively small tumors for surgical treatment and to refer patients who have large tumors or evidence of regional spread for irradiation, the compared findings may be misleading.

For patients with FIGO stages IB and IIA disease, treatment results are strongly correlated with tumor size, which thus influences appropriate selection of primary therapy. Most FIGO stage IB1 tumors can be treated effectively with radical hysterectomy or combined external-beam and intracavitary radiation; both have cure rates of 85% to 90%.[38,156] In a report of the only randomized trial comparing radical surgery (with or without postoperative irradiation) with irradiation alone,

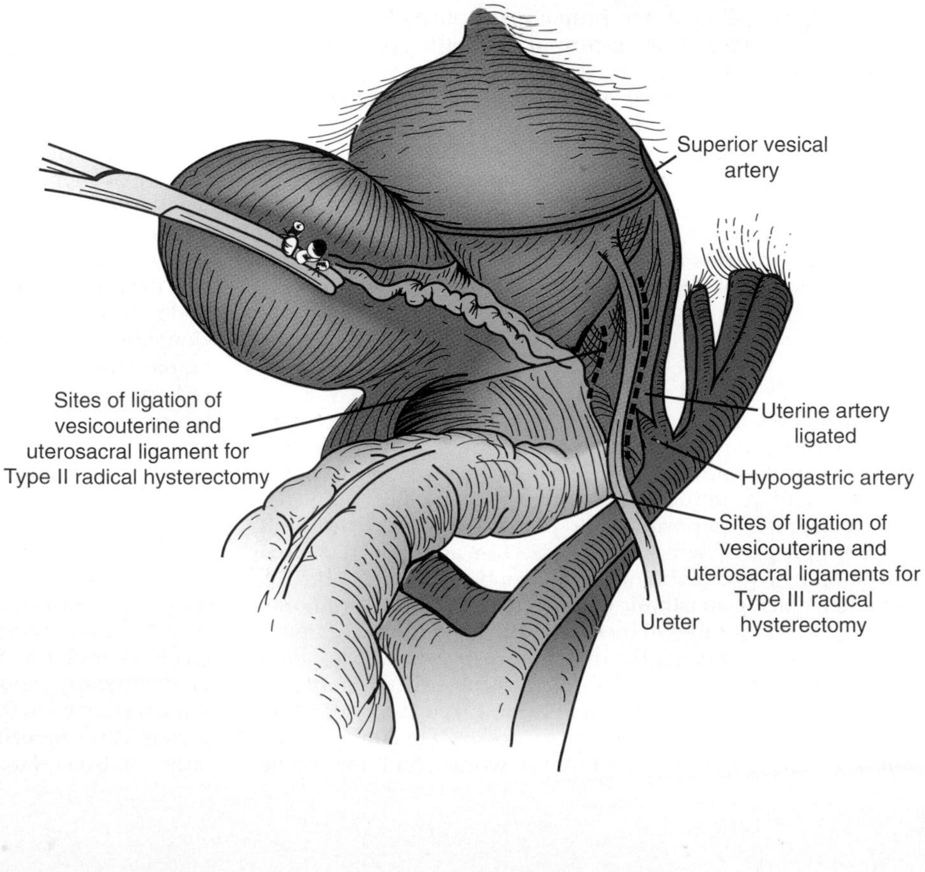

Figure 55-10 Sites of ligation of the vesicouterine and uterosacral ligaments for a type II or type III radical hysterectomy. (From Berek JS, Hacker NF: Practical Gynecologic Oncology. Baltimore, Williams & Wilkins, 1994, p 256.)

Landoni and colleagues[157] reported a 5-year actuarial survival rate of 87% for patients with FIGO stage IB-IIA tumors 4 cm or less in diameter treated with primary surgery compared with 90% for patients treated with definitive irradiation. Morbidity was somewhat greater in patients initially treated with surgery, particularly for those who also received postoperative pelvic irradiation for parametrial or lymph node involvement, positive tumor margins, or deep invasion into stroma. In the same study, the 5-year survival rate of patients with bulky FIGO stages IB2 and IIA tumors larger than 4 cm was similar for both treatments (70% for patients treated with surgery and 72% for patients treated with radiation). However, 84% of patients with the larger lesions had the aforementioned high-risk features and received postoperative pelvic irradiation. As a result, morbidity was again greater in surgically treated patients. The combined dose of external and LDR intracavitary radiation used to treat patients in this study (median cumulative dose to point A was 76 Gy) was lower than that recommended by some investigators.

Although some authors recommend radical surgical treatment for patients with FIGO stage IB2 carcinomas, the risk of pelvic recurrence is high for most of these patients unless they also receive postoperative irradiation. To avoid exposing these patients to the combined risks of a radical hysterectomy and irradiation, radiation therapy with concurrent chemotherapy is often preferred as the primary treatment. For the same reason, other findings that have been associated with an increased risk of pelvic lymph node metastasis and pelvic recurrence (extensive lymphovascular space invasion, deep stromal penetration) are considered by some clinicians to be contraindications to surgery as primary disease management. Unfortunately, the presence or absence of these factors cannot be reliably determined with conventional clinical staging. A recent cohort analysis suggested that elevated preoperative squamous cell carcinoma (SCC) antigen levels predicted an increased likelihood of postoperative radiation therapy and cancer relapse.[158] Although intriguing, these observations should be validated with further studies.

In patients selected for primary radiotherapy for stage IB/IIA tumors, the use of concurrent chemotherapy should be based on tumor size and/or the presence of retroperitoneal lymphadenopathy. In small volume disease (IB1), with no clinical evidence of pelvic nodal disease, radiation alone provides excellent tumor control and cure rates. Similar to patients with stage IA tumors, many of these cases are referred for radiation based on medical conditions that render primary surgery less desirable. However, with increased tumor size (i.e., stage IB2) or the presence of pelvic nodal metastases, present evidence indicates the benefit of concurrent cisplatin-based chemotherapy to radiation.

Fertility-Preserving Surgery

Approximately 10% to 15% of cervical cancers will occur in women during reproductive years, and some of these patients are hesitant to undergo radical pelvic surgery or radiation therapy with resulting permanent loss of fertility. Dargent and colleagues[159] reported their pioneering experience with laparoscopic pelvic lymph node dissection and radical vaginal trachelectomy (for highly selected, nonbulky stage I and IIA patients), placing an isthmic cerclage around the lower uterine segment that is sutured to the vaginal cuff. A number of investigators have subsequently reported their experiences with fertility-preserving surgery for early-stage (predominantly IA2 and IB tumors no larger than 2 cm) cervical cancer using both vaginal and abdominal approaches.[160-162] In 2003, Bernardini and colleagues[163] reported that 80 women had undergone radical trachelectomy at their institution. There were 39 women who subsequently attempted pregnancy, resulting in a total of 22 pregnancies among 18 patients. The rate of cancer relapse following these procedures appears to be comparable to that of women undergoing radical hysterectomy. The rate of relapse is higher for larger tumors (>2 cm) and in the presence of lymphovascular space invasion.

Postoperative Irradiation

Postoperative irradiation is most commonly recommended in two clinical situations: (1) when pathologic findings in specimens resected during radical hysterectomy suggest a significant risk of pelvic disease recurrence without adjuvant treatment and (2) when findings in specimens resected during simple hysterectomy show clinically unsuspected invasive cervical cancer.

Most clinicians recommend postoperative pelvic irradiation when histologic examination of a specimen resected during radical hysterectomy reveals multiple or bulky positive lymph nodes, parametrial involvement, or positive tumor margins. Historically, the use of adjuvant radiotherapy in these patients led to an improvement in pelvic control but without clear evidence of survival benefit.[164,165] Tumor features that are associated with a high risk of local recurrence, especially nodal metastases, also tend to be predictors of distant metastasis, decreasing the effect of local control on survival. In addition, a number of factors may reduce the efficacy of postoperative irradiation.[166] Higher doses of radiation may be required to sterilize microscopic disease in a disturbed operative site. Furthermore, clinicians' fears of causing major complications in patients who have had an extensive transperitoneal pelvic surgical procedure often limit the radiation dose that can be administered safely.[167-170] However, present evidence, based on the results of Intergroup Protocol 0107 (discussed earlier), clearly show an outcome advantage, including overall survival benefit, for concurrent chemoradiation in such patients, who may be collectively defined as having pathologic evidence of extracervical disease following radical hysterectomy for clinically early stage disease.[108] In the absence of any gross tumor residual, a dose of 50 Gy to the whole pelvis is typically prescribed as adjuvant treatment. Although some clinicians also add vaginal brachytherapy boost, the added therapeutic benefit of this is unclear, and it should be remembered that the results of Intergroup Protocol 0107 were achieved without the use of intravaginal brachytherapy.

More controversial indications for postoperative irradiation may include findings of a single microscopically positive node, bulky primary disease, deep stromal penetration, invasion into lymph-vascular space, or high-grade adenocarcinoma. The GOG conducted a trial (GOG 92) of postoperative radiotherapy versus observation alone following radical hysterectomy in stage IB cervical cancer with risk factors limited to the primary tumor (without extracervical spread or nodal metastases).[171] Eligible patients were those modeled to have an approximately 3-year risk of failure of 30% following surgery alone, based on varying permutations of tumor size, lymphovascular space involvement, and depth of cervical stromal invasion. A total of 277 eligible patients were entered into the study between 1988 and 1995. Patients randomized to postoperative radiotherapy (no concurrent chemotherapy) received 50.4 Gy whole pelvic radiation, without vaginal brachytherapy boost. There was a statistically significant improvement in the relapse-free survival at 2 years (88% versus 79%) favoring the irradiation arm over observation-only controls. However, no formal comparative survival analysis was reported. There was also a higher incidence of severe toxicity in the radiation cohort (6%) compared with the surgery-only cohort (2.1%).[171] At present, the use of adjuvant radiotherapy following radical hysterectomy for patients with risk factors confined to the cervix should be based on careful consideration of patient physiology, surgicopathologic findings, and multidisciplinary consultation between the patient, surgeon, and radiation oncologist.

An NCI consensus conference concluded that "primary therapy should avoid the routine use of both radical surgery and radiation therapy."[9] If clinical evaluation reveals risk factors that would require pelvic irradiation after radical hysterectomy, radiotherapy should be considered the primary treatment of choice. Although improvements in imaging technology allow better determination of nodal disease and may eventually permit evaluation of more subtle intratumoral risk features such as depth of stromal invasion and lymphvascular space involvement, the only tumor parameter that can be routinely evaluated before hysterectomy is tumor size. It is clear that the larger the cervical lesion, the more likely the indications for postoperative radiotherapy following radical hysterectomy. For this reason, many clinicians avoid primary surgery in patients with tumor diameters greater than 4 cm (stage IB2), because 50% to 80% of such cases undergo recommended postoperative radiation.[157,172,173]

Although it is standard practice to screen women for cervical cancer before a hysterectomy is performed for any reason, unsuspected invasive cancer is occasionally discovered in the resected specimen from a simple hysterectomy performed for benign disease or CIN. If cancer invasion is >3 mm or if there is extensive invasion into lymph-vascular space, then there is a significant risk of paracervical or pelvic lymph node involvement, and postoperative pelvic irradiation is indicated. With this treatment, the prognosis is still very good, with a 5-year survival rate of approximately 80% if the tumor appears to have been confined to the cervix and if surgical margins are negative.[174] Patients who have gross residual disease after hysterectomy may still be curable but have a 5-year survival rate of only about 30%. Given the poor prognosis of patients with gross residual disease after "cut-through" hysterectomy, it would seem reasonable to consider concurrent chemoradiation for this subset of cases.

ADJUNCTIVE SURGERY

In a retrospective study of cases from the University of Texas MDACC, Durrance and associates[175] suggested that the rate of central disease recurrence after radiation therapy of bulky (≥6 cm) endocervical cancers may be reduced when irradiation is combined with an extrafascial hysterectomy. Authors of a subsequent report[176] emphasized that acceptable complication rates could be achieved only if the dose of radiation was reduced and if surgery was limited to a simple (type I) extrafascial hysterectomy performed with careful, sharp dissection. After these reports, the use of combined treatment increased, and some clinicians began using adjunctive hysterectomy to treat patients with smaller endocervical tumors (<6 cm in diameter) and tumors with an exophytic morphology.

Although combined treatment is routinely used by many practitioners, there is still no evidence that it improves survival rates over treatment with radiation alone. In 1992, Thoms and colleagues[177] reexamined the experience of the MDACC and concluded that biases that led to the selection of patients with more favorable disease for combined treatment made it impossible to compare meaningfully the relative efficacy of the two approaches. Mendenhall and colleagues[178] compared the outcome of patients treated before or after treatment policy changed at the University of Florida to include planned adjuvant hysterectomy. No difference in outcome was seen between patients treated before or after the change in policy.

The GOG conducted a phase III trial (GOG 71) in patients with stage IB2 cervical cancer randomized to receive radiation therapy alone versus radiation therapy followed by extrafascial hysterectomy (this trial, which did not involve chemotherapy, preceded the GOG 123 trial discussed earlier in the chemoradiation section). Although adjuvant hysterectomy following primary radiotherapy appeared to reduce the rate of local recurrence, there was no improvement in overall survival.[179]

Based on the preceding discussion there are no clear data to support the routine role of adjuvant hysterectomy after primary irradiation for bulky but cervix-confined tumors, particularly after optimal doses of radiation have been delivered. However, it may be selectively applied in patients with poor tumor response to radiotherapy or in those whose tumor and pelvic anatomy precluded good brachytherapy geometry.

LOCOREGIONALLY ADVANCED DISEASE (STAGES IIB-IVA) AND PALLIATION

The treatment of choice for most patients with locoregionally advanced disease (IIB-IVA) is definitive radiation therapy with concurrent cisplatin-based chemotherapy. Radiation consists of a combination of external-beam irradiation and brachytherapy. Most authorities today consider optimal radiotherapy as a cumulative point A dose of 85 to 90 Gy (in conventional equivalents), with all treatment completed within 8 weeks. The 5-year survival rates of patients treated with chemoradiation now approach 70% to 80% for stage IIB, 50% to 60% for stage IIIB, and perhaps 15% to 25% for stage IVA disease.[104-106,114] With aggressive treatment, even patients with massive, locoregionally advanced tumors have a realistic chance of being cured.

Salvage Therapy for Recurrent Disease

Following primary management for cervical cancer, a small percentage of patients will present with isolated local-regional failure for whom radical salvage therapy may be contemplated. Patient selection, careful "restaging," and individualization of therapy are essential.[180] The most important determinant of therapy options is whether a patient has received prior pelvic radiotherapy.

Patients who experience local recurrence after initial surgery alone may be salvaged by radical radiotherapy, using customized combinations of external-beam radiation and intracavitary or interstitial brachytherapy. Salvage radiotherapy is particularly effective for small central failures limited to the vagina or paravaginal tissues, with a 5-year survival rate of 69% reported in one series.[181] In the adverse setting of tumor recurrence, the use of chemotherapy concurrent with radiation (as extrapolated from the primary management of locally advanced disease) may provide added therapeutic benefit.[182]

There are limited reports of radical reirradiation for patients who relapse following prior pelvic radiotherapy.[183,184] However, radical surgery forms the primary cornerstone of salvage for isolated pelvic recurrences in previously irradiated patients. In most cases, the only potentially curative option is pelvic exenteration. For highly selected patients with central recurrences, in whom pelvic exenteration is successfully completed, 5-year survival rates approximating 50% may be achieved.[185-187]

Proximity or fixation of recurrent tumor to the pelvic side wall is an adverse prognostic finding, leading some previous investigators to suggest that attempted surgical salvage be abandoned with intraoperatively detected side wall involvement. However, several institutions have incorporated intraoperative radiation therapy (IORT) directed to the involved pelvic side wall for incompletely resected tumor or insecure margins following pelvic exenteration, allowing for tumor control and long-term survival in these patients who were previously considered incurable.[188,189] (see Chapter 15 with regard to techniques and results for multiple disease sites, including cervical cancer).

Advanced Disease, Palliation

The prognosis is extremely poor for patients with recurrent or metastatic cervical cancer that is not amenable to surgery or radiation with curative intent. Systemic chemotherapy is a therapeutic option, although no trials to date have compared chemotherapy to best supportive care in this setting.

Cisplatin has long been considered the most active single chemotherapy agent for the treatment of cervical carcinoma.[190] Compared to cisplatin 50 mg/m^2 administered as a short infusion, phase III studies have not confirmed an advantage with either higher doses or alternative infusion schedules.[191,192] Furthermore, a phase II study conducted by the GOG resulted in inferior response rates with the platinum analogues carboplatin and iproplatin.[193] Subsequent phase II studies have identified a number of drugs with single-agent activity against cervical carcinoma including mitolactol, ifosfamide, paclitaxel, topotecan, gemcitabine, and vinorelbine (Table 55-5).

In an attempt to improve therapeutic efficacy, a number of phase III trials have investigated the use of drug combinations with cisplatin. Compared to cisplatin alone, Omura and colleagues[200] showed a higher objective response rate and progression-free survival with cisplatin plus ifosfamide; however, there was no improvement in overall survival, and toxicity with combination chemotherapy therapy was significantly increased. Awaiting maturation of these data, the GOG conducted another phase III trial demonstrating no advantage with the addition of bleomycin to the cisplatin plus ifosfamide combination.[201] More recently, the GOG compared single-agent cisplatin to a combination of cisplatin plus paclitaxel with quality of life assessments included among outcomes measures. The combination of cisplatin plus paclitaxel resulted in a higher objective response rate, longer progression-free survival, and higher toxicity—without an apparent decrement in patient reported quality of life.[202]

Long and associates presented results of a prospective randomized trial comparing cisplatin versus cisplatin plus topotecan, which, for the first time, demonstrated an improvement in overall survival with the combination regimen.[203] Although some cisplatin-based combinations have yielded statistically superior results, the benefits of salvage chemotherapy remain modest, at best (Table 55-6). A new GOG trial (protocol 204) will directly compare four cisplatin-containing regimens: cisplatin plus paclitaxel versus topotecan versus gemcitabine versus vinorelbine. Although the results of this trial will not be available for several years, it is clear from existing clinical trials data that single-agent cisplatin is no longer appropriate treatment for recurrent or metastatic cervical carcinoma for patients who have previously received cisplatin concurrent with primary radiation therapy.

Radiation therapy can also play an important role in the palliation of patients with incurable advanced disease. Hypofractionated pelvic irradiation usually controls bleeding and frequently provides prompt relief of pelvic pain. A variety of fractionation schemes have been used. The RTOG reported the results of a phase I/II study in which patients with advanced pelvic malignancies were given up to three fractions of 10 Gy at 1-month intervals with misonidazole.[204] The overall objective response rate was 57%, but the rate of grade 3 and 4

Table 55-5 Phase II Chemotherapy Trials in Metastatic or Recurrent Squamous Cell Carcinoma of the Cervix

Drug Dose and Schedule	Reference	Patients	Partial Response Rate	Complete Response Rate
Mitolactol 180 mg/m^2 PO daily × 10 d, q4wk	Stehman, 1989[194]	55	2%	27%
Ifosfamide 1.5 g/m^2/d × 5 d, q3wk (with MESNA)	Sutton, 1993[195]	51	4%	12%
Paclitaxel 170 mg/m^2 over 24 h, q3wk	McGuire, 1996[196]	30	3%	14%
Topotecan 1.5 mg/m^2/d × 5 d, q4wk	Bookman, 2000[197]	40	3%	10%
Gemcitabine 800 mg/m^2/wk × 3 wk, q4wk	Schilder, 2000[198]	27	0%	8%
Vinorelbine 30 mg/m^2 weekly	Morris, 1998[199]	35	3%	15%

Table 55-6 Phase III Trials of Cisplatin and Cisplatin-Containing Regimens in Advanced, Recurrent, or Metastatic Cervical Carcinoma

Reference	Regimen	No. of Patients	OR	CR	PFS (mo)	OS (mo)
Omura, 1997	P	140	19%	6%	3.2	8.0
	P + IFX	151	31%	13%	4.6	8.3
Bloss, 2002	P + IFX	146	32%	NS	4.6	8.5
	P + IFX + B	141	32%	NS	5.1	8.4
Moore, 2004	P	134	19%	6%	3.0	8.9
	P + T	130	36%	15%	4.9	9.9
Long, 2004	P	145	13%	NS	2.9	7.0
	P + Topo	148	26%	NS	4.6	9.2

B, bleomycin; CR, complete response rate; IFX, ifosfamide plus MESNA; OR, objective response rate; OS, overall survival; PFS, progression-free survival; P, cisplatin; T, paclitaxel; Topo, topotecan; NB, not stated.

toxicities was high (45%). Studies of the MDACC experience with this method have demonstrated a symptomatic response rate of approximately 75% with two fractions of 10 Gy but have also revealed an unacceptable rate of major complications when a third fraction of 10 Gy was given.[205,206]

In a second RTOG study, accelerated split-course irradiation was used as palliative treatment for patients with advanced pelvic malignancies. Patients received up to three courses of 14.8 Gy given in 3.7-Gy fractions twice daily over 2 days.[207] A 3- to 6-week rest interval was given between courses. Patients who completed the three courses of radiation had an overall response rate of about 60%, with complete relief of pain achieved in 50% of patients.

Other fractionation schemes, such as 30 Gy in 10 fractions, have been used successfully. Prolonged fractionation is rarely indicated for palliation of patients with extraregional metastases from cervical cancer because the median life expectancy for these patients is very short. Above all, these patients benefit from close monitoring of their symptoms; prompt, aggressive treatment with analgesic drugs; and sensitive, supportive care. Anesthetic or neuroablative treatments may be helpful in selected cases, and prompt referral to a multidisciplinary pain service is warranted for patients with intractable pain.

TECHNIQUES OF IRRADIATION

External-Beam Irradiation

In the radical radiation treatment of carcinoma of the cervix, EBRT is used to treat central disease and to sterilize known or suspected regional metastases. For patients with bulky central disease, a course of EBRT to the pelvis usually causes significant tumor regression, potentially improving the dose distribution of subsequent intracavitary radiation by shrinking endocervical disease to bring it within the high-dose range of intracavitary therapy or by reducing exophytic tumor that would have caused undesirable caudad displacement of intracavitary vaginal applicators. For these reasons, patients who have locally advanced disease usually begin treatment with external-beam radiation.

However, the proportion of treatment given with external-beam or intracavitary radiation must be balanced carefully. Because of the relatively large volume of bladder, rectum, and small bowel included in external pelvic fields, the dose of intracavitary therapy that can be safely given is seriously compromised when a high dose (>45 to 50 Gy) of whole pelvic EBRT is delivered. Some radiation oncologists prefer to begin intracavitary irradiation as early as possible, even in patients with initial bulky disease, shielding central normal structures with a midline block on anteroposterior-posteroanterior (AP-PA) fields after 20 to 30 Gy. In the past, use of a 3- to 4-cm-diameter midline block was considered standard. A review of urinary tract complications in patients treated with radiation for FIGO stage I cervical cancers at MDACC demonstrated a significantly higher rate of ureteral stenosis when parametrial irradiation was combined with relatively high doses of intracavitary therapy, presumably because the relatively narrow standard central blocks failed to protect the ureters from radiation.[208] For this reason, customized blocks are preferred when a high dose of parametrial boost irradiation is given.

To optimize the match between external-beam and intracavitary irradiation, Perez[154] developed an elaborate central gradient step-wedge block designed to compensate for the lateral dose gradient from intracavitary treatment. For this method, one of several standard gradient blocks is matched to the patient's intracavitary distribution and used to shield central structures on AP-PA fields. Perez has been able to deliver very high paracentral radiation doses by using intracavitary therapy to give most of the central treatment. However, the gradient blocks can only be matched to the dose distribution calculated in a single plane (usually in the center mid-coronal plane of the implant). Theoretically, anterior and posterior structures (such as the uterosacral ligaments) may be underdosed with this method, although the survival rates reported by Perez and associates have generally been excellent.[154]

Alternatively, a somewhat higher dose of radiation (35 to 45 Gy) may be given to the whole pelvis before intracavitary irradiation. Although this approach somewhat reduces the total paracentral dose that can be delivered via brachytherapy, it may be advantageous to deliver a more homogeneous dose sufficient to eradicate microscopic disease to the entire pelvis, particularly for locally advanced tumors. Additional focal external treatment can be delivered to persistent disease involving the pelvic wall or lymph nodes after the first intracavitary treatment. The medial edge of such boost fields is usually placed at about the 50 cGy/h isodose margin of the intracavitary dose distribution or about 0.5 cm from the lateral surface of the vaginal applicator.

In all cases, care must be taken to include all areas at risk for disease in the pelvis. High-energy (≥15 MV) anterior and posterior opposed fields treat the entire pelvic contents with low morbidity as long as the total pelvic dose does not exceed 40 to 45 Gy. The inferior border is usually placed at the mid or lower pubis and at least 3-4 cm below the lowest extent of cervical or vaginal disease, and lateral borders should be placed about 1.5 cm lateral to the bony margins of the true pelvis. Typical illustrated guidelines for design of pelvic external-beam fields are shown in Figure 55-11. Many clinicians prefer to treat with four fields (anterior, posterior, and two laterals), sparing some small bowel anterior to the iliac nodes. However, because all the major pelvic lymph node groups and pelvic supporting structures can be involved in patients with locally advanced cervical cancer, careless shielding of lateral fields can cause the tumor to be undertreated. Lateral fields that include a posterior border at S2-3 (previously considered standard by some practitioners) frequently shield gross tumor in patients with locally advanced disease. Some have advocated the use of CT or MRI to guide planning of lateral fields (Fig. 55-12).[84] Although this can be helpful, such studies may still underestimate the extent of microscopic spread in the pelvis.

Historically, field borders that define the volume of EBRT have been based on empirically derived bony anatomic landmarks. These bony landmarks, which are still widely promulgated in textbooks and radiotherapy protocol guidelines, represent the careful attempts of past clinical investigators to match skeletal anatomy, which can be readily appreciated radiographically, with potential soft tissue tumor extent, nodal drainage, and pathways of regional spread. While broadly useful, the routine use of these "standardized fields" has been questioned as lacking in individual case coverage, based on intraoperative measurements,[209] MRI,[84] CT,[210] and lymphangiography.[211]

Recent advances in imaging technology and radiation treatment planning have allowed more precise delineation of soft tissue anatomy, independent of skeletal structures. The use of CT-based treatment planning is widespread, and many centers are increasing incorporating MRI and PET data in designing radiation fields. Although these imaging technologies provide clear improvement in our abilities to define gross tumor extent, they also underscore several critical issues

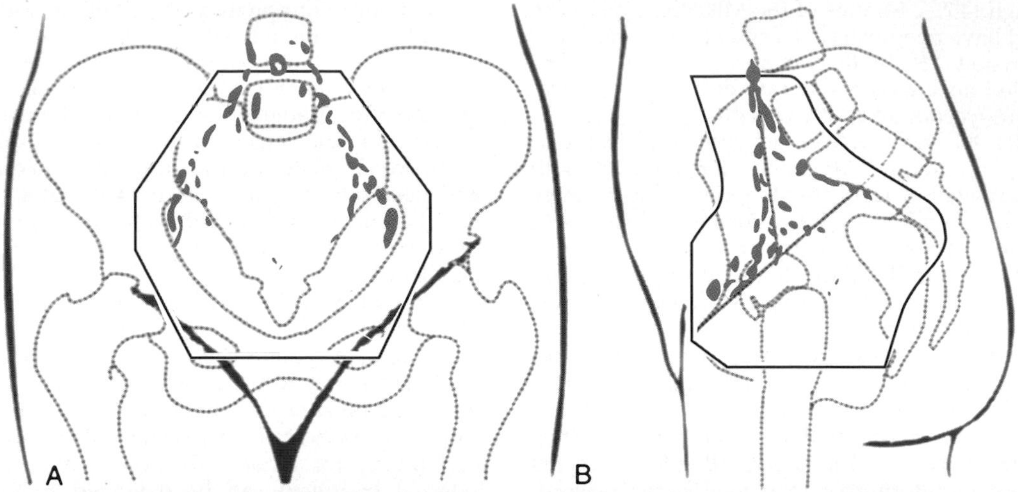

Figure 55-11 Typical anteroposterior-posteroanterior **(A)** and lateral **(B)** fields for treatment of carcinoma of the cervix. On the lateral view, external iliac nodes are typically centered about a plane between S1-2 and the tip of the pubis and common iliac nodes along a plane from the anterior aspect of L4 to the bisector of the external iliac plane. Care must be taken to design fields that cover regional lymph nodes and the primary tumor with margin.

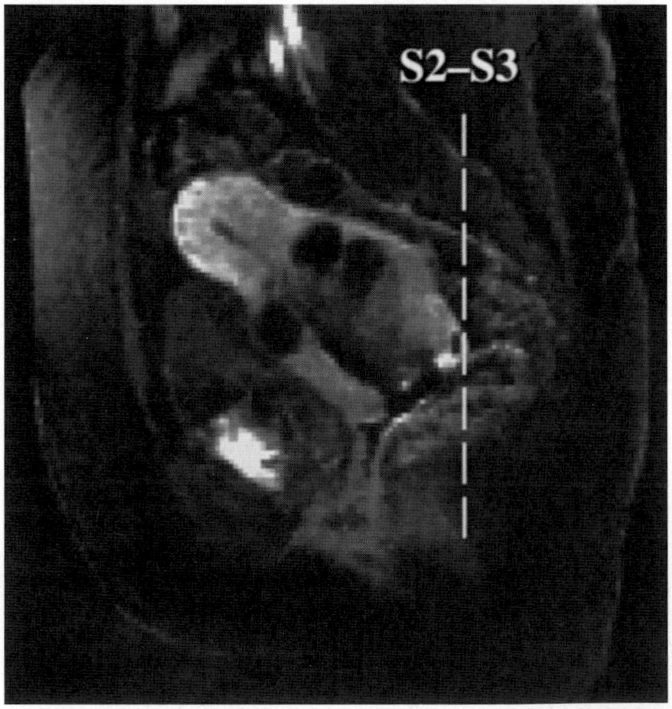

Figure 55-12 Sagittal MRI of a patient with a bulky stage IB2 adenocarcinoma. MRI demonstrated a normal uterine fundus and a bulky endocervical tumor, clarifying the site of origin of this lesion. The study also illustrates the risk of using a "standard" posterior margin for lateral fields because the posterior extent of gross disease extends posterior to the S2-3 interspace.

that need to be addressed. To take full advantage of these imaging modalities, radiation oncologists must have adequate training and formalized experience in interpreting radiologic studies. Findings from a detailed pelvic examination must be carefully incorporated into the treatment plan, because there are areas of potential tumor extension, such as in the vagina and medial parametria, that may not be well-imaged. Finally, there needs to be a clear awareness of the potential pathways of regional and nodal spread from cervical cancer, as it is not possible to image microscopic disease, and lack of such recognition may lead to inadequate coverage of the volume at risk.

Examples of EBRT ports for patients with cervical cancer based on contemporary CT simulation are shown in Figures 55-13 and 55-14. An example of a composite external-beam dosimetry plan is illustrated in Figure 55-15. Although CT-based treatment planning and field design allow customization based on individual patient findings, it should be noted that the general similarity of these fields to the traditional "standardized" bony anatomy–based fields serve as a testament to the clinical acumen and observational skills of previous clinicians who did not have access to the imaging modalities of today.

Intensity-modulated radiation therapy (IMRT) represents an exciting new technology in radiotherapy delivery that combines high-resolution imaging, advances in computer treatment software and linear accelerator collimation capabilities, inverse planning, and radiation beam flux modulation to produce highly conformal dose distributions unachievable using conventional approaches. It has been most widely used in head and neck and prostate cancers, simultaneously allowing sparing of surrounding normal structures and dose intensification to the tumor target volume. Dosimetric evaluation of its use in gynecologic cancers suggests IMRT may significantly reduce unwanted radiation exposure to adjacent bowel and bladder while preserving tumor coverage.[212] Early clinical experience at the University of Chicago has demonstrated a reduction in acute gastrointestinal toxicity for gynecologic cancer patients undergoing pelvic IMRT compared with contemporaneous historical controls treated with traditional standard techniques.[213] Recent analysis has also indicated a decrease in acute hematologic suppression, favoring patients treated with IMRT, especially in those who also received chemotherapy.[214] Although there is excitement about the potential eventual application of IMRT to cervical cancer radiotherapy, serious questions remain about target definitions, treatment standardization, intrapatient and interpatient reproducibility, and time-intensive requirements for treatment planning and delivery. At this time, the use of IMRT in cervical cancer should be considered experimental and should be

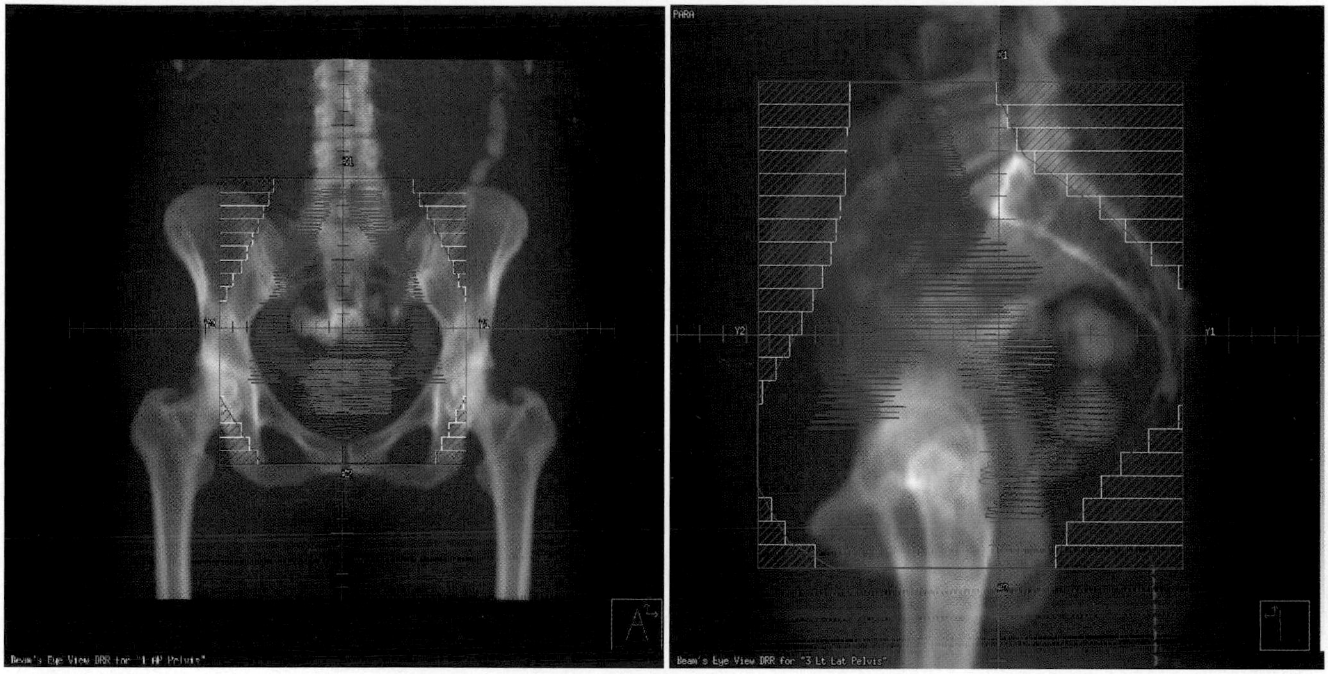

A B

Figure 55-13 Anterior **(A)** and left lateral **(B)** digitally reconstructed radiographs (DRRs) of external-beam pelvic fields for a patient with stage IIIB cervical cancer with bilateral parametrial extension and left pelvic side wall involvement but without nodal metastases on radiologic imaging. (Objects selectively illustrated: *pink*, cervical tumor gross tumor volume; *green*, fundus; *brown*, rectum; *blue*, pelvic vessels as surrogates for nodal basins, including internal iliacs, external iliacs, and common iliacs. Other objects such as bladder and small bowel can be alternately turned on or off on the computer screen to facilitate visualization.)

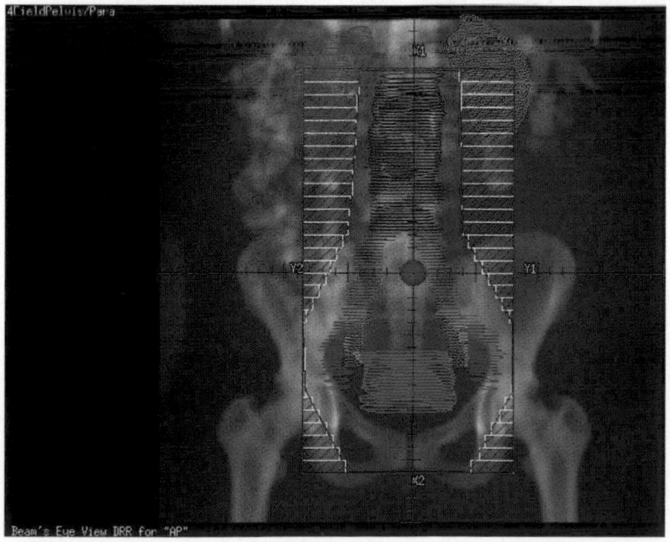

Figure 55-14 Anterior digital reconstructed radiograph of an extended pelvic and para-aortic external-beam field in a different patient with stage IIIB cervical cancer and multiple pelvic and low para-aortic lymph node metastases. Objects selected on this image included the cervical tumor gross tumor volume (*pink*), the areas of gross nodal involvement as determined by CT/PET imaging (*yellow*), the associated pelvic and para-aortic nodal basins, and bilateral kidneys.

undertaken only in the context of a rigorously conducted clinical trial.

External-beam irradiation tends to cause some retraction of the vaginal apex. Because the vaginal capacity may limit the size of vaginal applicators, small tumors in women who have a narrow (usually postmenopausal) vagina may be more effectively treated by administering intracavitary irradiation before external-beam therapy or early in the course of treatment.

Brachytherapy

Encapsulated radium sources were first used to treat cervical cancers shortly after Marie Curie's discovery more than a century ago. The origin of cervical cancers at the mouth of a hollow, relatively radioresistant organ made the disease ideal for intracavitary treatment. With careful placement of sources in the uterus and vagina, clinicians are able to capitalize on the inverse square law, delivering a high dose of radiation to cervical tumor with much lower radiation exposure to critical normal tissues such as the bladder and rectum.

Empirical evidence, in vitro studies of the effect of dose rate on tumor cell kill and late normal tissue effects, available technology and radiation protection considerations led to the initial use of sources that delivered ionizing radiation at relatively low dose rates over time. Although LDR intracavitary brachytherapy has traditionally been used for most patients with cervical cancer treated in the United States, HDR brachytherapy has been widely used in other countries, especially in those where inpatient facilities for brachytherapy were limited. Over the past decade, comparison data from several randomized trials,[215-218] reviews,[219] and large single-

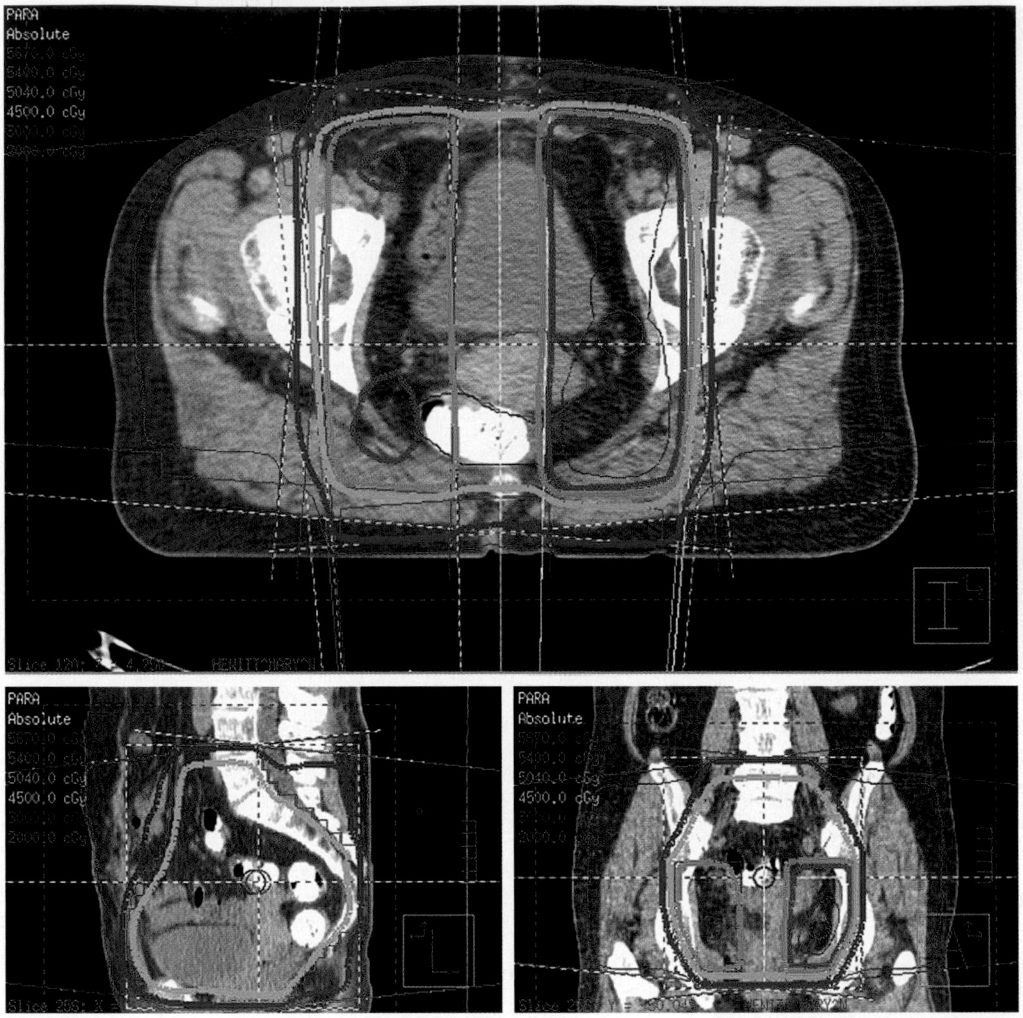

Figure 55-15 External beam dosimetry planning (for patient shown in Fig. 55-13). The prescribed dose was 45 Gy to the whole pelvis, with parametrial boosts to 50.4 Gy to the right and 54 Gy to the left (patient had bulkier disease on the left, with extension to the pelvic side wall). Central dose in this patient was supplemented by intracavitary brachytherapy.

institutional retrospective experiences[220,221] have led to an increasing acceptance of the efficacy and tolerability of HDR brachytherapy for cervical cancer in the United States. Large clinical cooperative trials groups such as the GOG and RTOG now accept that when performed appropriately and within clearly specified guidelines of dosing and fractionation, HDR and LDR intracavitary cervical brachytherapy are therapeutically similar. Faced with issues related to LDR-associated personnel exposure, source regulation and storage, and source replacement, many centers have turned to outpatient-based HDR brachytherapy for cervical cancer. In a patterns of care survey, 16.4% of patients who underwent brachytherapy for cervical cancer between 1996 and 1999 had at least part of their therapy delivered using HDR[222]—undoubtedly, the use of HDR brachytherapy has since increased substantially.

Low-Dose-Rate Intracavitary Therapy

Until the early 1980s, most intracavitary therapy was delivered using radioactive radium (^{226}Ra). Although the long half-life (1620 years) was an advantage, the possibility that radon gas, one of the daughter products of ^{226}Ra, could escape from encapsulated sources was a potential radiation protection problem. For this reason cesium 137 (^{137}Cs), an artificially produced isotope of similar average energy, gradually began to replace ^{226}Ra in most practices. Because the half-life of ^{137}Cs is only about 30 years, the sources must be replaced periodically. It is also important to remember that most of the published long-term results of radiation therapy for carcinoma of the cervix are based on patients treated with linear sources of ^{226}Ra, which were usually 22 mm long. Commercially available cesium sources are usually shorter (≤17 to 20 mm). Standard loadings designed for radium will produce higher dose rates to critical structures if short cesium sources are used without spacers.

Many intracavitary applicator systems have been used to position sources in the uterus and vagina. All include a central uterine tandem; the major differences are in the design of the vaginal source holders. In the United States, most radiation oncologists use some variation of the Fletcher-Suit-Delclos applicator system that was first developed at MDACC. The most characteristic feature of this system is the pair of cylindrical vaginal colpostats that are placed against the cervix on either side of the tandem. These holders position the axis of the vaginal sources approximately perpendicular to the uterine tandem (Fig. 55-16). This positioning is designed to take advantage of the anisotropy of the sources, and, combined with the anterior and posterior tungsten shields incorporated in the design, to reduce the volume of bladder and rectum exposed to high doses of radiation. For patients with a narrow vagina, unshielded mini-ovoids and Lucite cylinders of various sizes can be used to position the intravaginal sources. Another applicator system used successfully by a

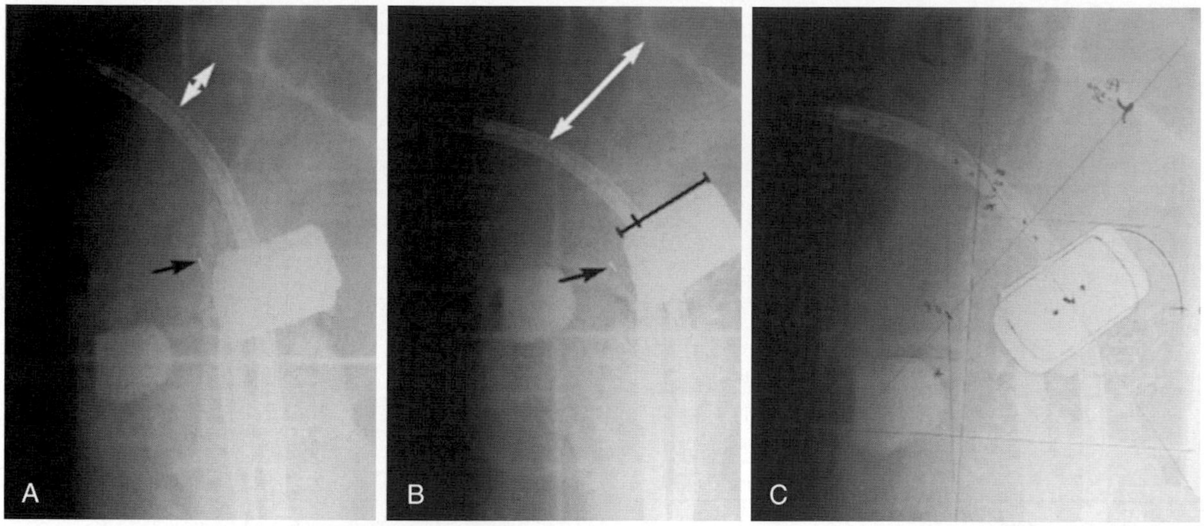

Figure 55-16 Lateral views of Fletcher-Suit-Delclos intracavitary placements in a young woman with an FIGO IB2 endocervical tumor. **A,** This patient had a very pliable vagina, and aggressive packing pushed the uterus and the system high in the pelvis against the sacrum, potentially trapping bowel between the intracavitary system and the sacrum. **B,** The system was repacked, using a suture slipped through the cervix to provide countertraction during packing. This kept the system lower in the pelvis, but the ovoids were allowed to fall posteriorly. This position can lead to overdosage of the rectum, particularly cephalad to the ovoids. **C,** A second repacking resulted in a good placement with acceptable positioning of the system midway between the sacrum and bladder. Ovoids are bisected by the tandem and are close to the cervical marker seeds; posterior packing protects the rectum. It is rare to need two adjustments of an intracavitary system, but the significant improvement achieved with this effort should improve the therapeutic ratio for this patient and underscores the importance of intraoperative radiographs in cervical cancer brachytherapy.

number of groups, including Memorial Sloan-Kettering Hospital, is the Henschke applicator. With this system, the vaginal sources are positioned parallel to the axis of the intrauterine tandem.

Today, all these systems are afterloading, meaning that the sources are inserted after the applicators have been placed and secured and accurate positioning has been confirmed; this minimizes personnel's exposure to the radiation. Radiation exposure from LDR implants can be further reduced to negligible levels with computerized remote afterloading equipment that removes the cesium sources automatically when visitors or personnel enter the room.

Successful intracavitary therapy requires experience, skill, some imagination, and a willingness to persist until an optimal placement has been achieved.[223] Radiation sources must be positioned in the uterus and vagina in a way that avoids underdosing areas in the cervix and paracervical tissues, with a sensitivity to the limits of mucosal tolerance. Every tumor presents a somewhat different challenge because of the wide variations in tumors and patient anatomy encountered clinically. A thorough discussion of the methods that can be used to address these variations is beyond the scope of this chapter, but some basic principles apply to most common clinical situations.

Although there has been considerable debate regarding the "optimal" intracavitary brachytherapy system, and there is no doubt that brachytherapy requires technical skill and attention to detail, it is also apparent that *whether* intracavitary brachytherapy is used is more important than *how* it is placed. In the United States, most radiation oncologists are familiar with some variation of the Fletcher-Suit-Delclos applicator system, but other systems are also used. A recent dosimetric evaluation of the Fletcher-Suit-Delclos applicator system compared to the Henschke shielded applicator suggested that the latter system provided dose-distribution advantage.[224] Other large institutions in North America have successfully used linear intrauterine sources alone, without colpostats, provided that the tandem sources extended to 1 cm below the cervix or the inferior-most extent of vaginal disease.[119] What is clear is that the introduction of radioactive sources into the endocervical and endometrial canal permits a central tumor dose intensification that is unachievable by any external-beam technique, regardless of the nuances of source placement (Fig. 55-17). It is this very high radiation dose, placed in direct juxtaposition to tumor, within a radiotolerant organ, that allows for control of even large cervical cancers.

In most cases, the highest sources in the tandem should extend superiorly at least 6 cm above the external os or, if the uterus is small, as high as possible in the uterine cavity. A relatively long line of sources will provide better lateral dose penetration and coverage of high endocervical tumor. However, except in unusual circumstances, the benefit of source loadings that extend more than 8 cm above the external os is probably outweighed by the additional radiation exposure to the small bowel and sigmoid. A tandem of 6.5 to 8 cm will accommodate 35 to 40 mgRaEq of cesium distributed in three linear sources spaced with their centers 22 to 25 mm apart. Typical loadings (cephalad to caudad) of LDR linear cesium sources would be 15-15-10 for relatively large tumors that still expand the endocervix at the time of intracavitary placement, or 15-10-10 for smaller tumors. The caudad source in the tandem should not protrude more than a couple of millimeters below the superior surface of the colpostats to avoid a hot spot in the adjacent bladder and rectum. Similar distributions can be achieved with remote afterloading units by distributing 5 mgRaEq point sources along the length of the tandem.

The choice of vaginal applicator is determined by the vaginal capacity and by the distribution of any vaginal disease. Vaginal cylinders are usually reserved for patients who have a very narrow vagina or significant vaginal mucosal disease. In general, when colpostats are used, their medial sur-

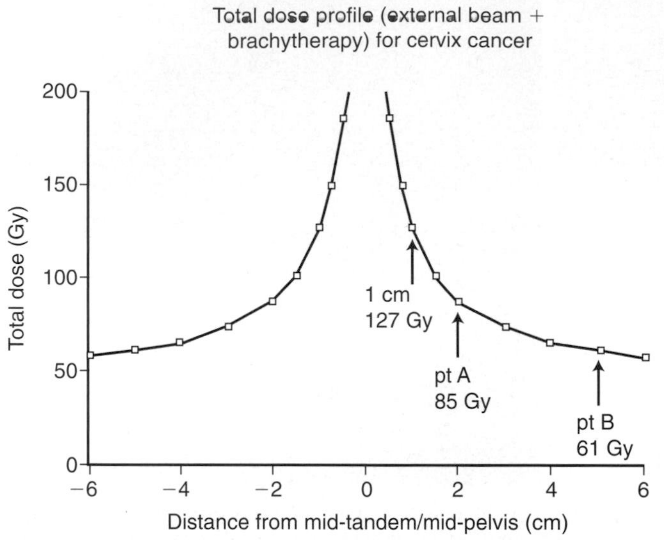

Figure 55-17 Illustration of the central dose escalation achieved when combining intracavitary brachytherapy with external-beam radiation. Although the diagram is idealized, it is based on current GOG guidelines for radiation dosing in locally advanced cervical cancer: 45 Gy to the whole pelvis, intracavitary brachytherapy to an LDR equivalent dose of 85 Gy to point (pt) A, and additional external-beam parametrial boost of 4.5 to 9 Gy with central structures shielded. The *x*-axis represents distance from the centrally placed tandem toward each pelvic side wall, along the transaxial plane encompassing bilateral pt As.

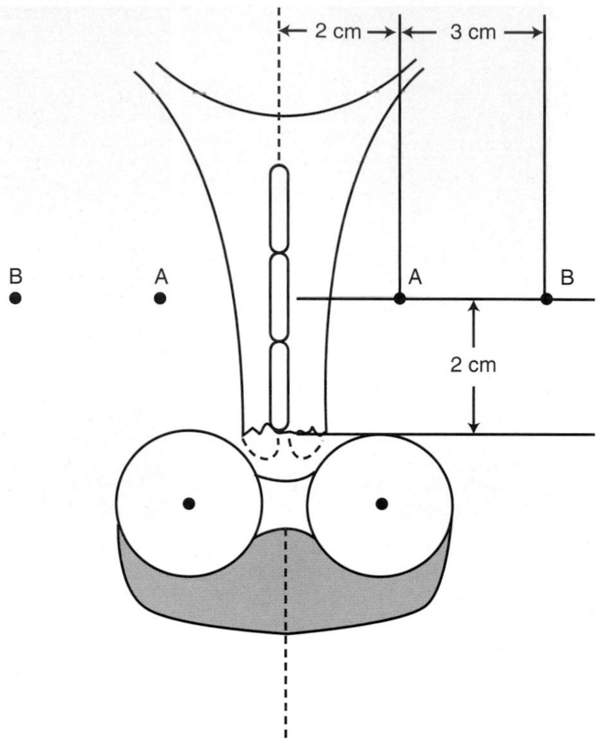

Figure 55-18 Location of point A and point B using the method recommended in ICRU 38. (From International Commission on Radiation Units and Measurement, Bethesda. 38:1-23, 1985.)

faces should be separated by ≤1 cm to avoid a central cold spot. Instead, to maximize the dose deliverable from intravaginal sources, the vagina should be fitted with the largest ovoids that can be placed snugly against the cervix. The anterior and posterior lips of the cervix should always be marked with radiopaque seeds (see Fig. 55-16) so the relationship between the cervix and vaginal applicators can be verified on intraoperative films. Significant caudad displacement of the colpostats will dramatically reduce the dose to cervical tumor and lead to increased vaginal stenosis. The colpostats should be centered over the cervical portion; unless the anterior or posterior lip is disproportionately involved, the colpostats should be bisected by the tandem on the lateral view. Very posterior displacement of the colpostats usually result in an underdosage to anterior disease and an unacceptable overdosage to the rectum, particularly to the portion of the rectum that is superior to the colpostat. The standard loadings for Fletcher-Suit-Delclos ovoids are 10 or 15 mgRaEq for 2 cm (small), 15 or 20 mgRaEq for 2.5 cm (medium), 20 or, rarely, 25 mgRaEq for 3 cm (large), and 5 to 10 mgRaEq for mini-ovoids. These loadings will result in a dose rate at the lateral vaginal surface of approximately 75 to 110 cGy/h. The higher activity sources are used when the placement is excellent or when the patient has bulky central disease. The lower activities tend to be used for patients with small tumors, for suboptimal (but acceptable) positioning, and to keep the total vaginal surface dose beneath the cumulative maximum of 120 to 140 Gy.

Once the appropriate equipment has been chosen, the system must be packed in place. Although the procedure can be performed under intravenous sedation with monitored anesthesia care, general or regional anesthesia may be preferred, unless the patient is at increased risk for anesthetic complications, because it permits a good examination of the pelvis and provides maximal relaxation of the perineal musculature during placement and packing of the intracavitary applicator.

The system should be packed in place with lubricated gauze, preferably a type that contains a radiopaque thread, while the vagina is retracted by an assistant. Packing should be carefully placed anteriorly and posteriorly, displacing the rectum and bladder away from the system. Care should be taken not to force the cervix away from the colpostats during the packing. Gradual withdrawal of the retractors during the procedure permits placement of additional packing in the space occupied by the retractors. With firm packing, the risk of displacement during a 48- to 72-hour placement is minimal. However, when vaginal cylinders are used instead of packing or when a remote afterloading device is used, a stitch should be placed in the labia and secured to the system to prevent displacement. The accuracy of the applicator position should be confirmed while the patient is still under sedation by anteroposterior and lateral x-rays. If the placement is unsatisfactory, the system should be repositioned and repacked (see Fig. 55–16).

Dose Specification

Several methods have been used to specify the radiation dose delivered by an intracavitary system. Today, most clinicians describe treatment using one of several variations of the Manchester system. With this approach, the dose and dose rate are specified to a paracentral point (point A) and to a point near the pelvic wall (point B) (Fig. 55-18). Point A is usually placed 2 cm lateral and superior to the external cervical os along the axis of the intrauterine tandem, although a number of methods have been used to identify the position of this reference point. Because point A lies in a region of steep dose gradient, relatively small variations in its position can result in substantial differences in the calculated dose rate. For this reason the use of point A or similar reference points was criticized by the International Commission on Radiation Units and Measurements in its 1985 report on intracavitary dose and volume specification.[225] The Commission recommended a system, used in some parts of Europe, in which the volume of tissue treated to a certain dose (usually 60 Gy) and the reference air kerma (in μGy at 1 m) are specified. At MDACC, a somewhat similar system is used, with additional emphasis on the vaginal surface dose, substituting mgRaEqHrs for reference air kerma as a means of limiting pelvic integral dose and relying on a set of empirically derived rules concerning the position and activity of the radiation sources. When point A is used as a reference point for dosing and reporting, attention must also be given to the three-dimensional isodose distributions surrounding the entire implant.

In fact, the Manchester system was originally meant to be applied in the context of relatively standard intracavitary source arrangements and loadings. Unexpected results can occur when a standard dose is delivered to point A from a system that is poorly positioned or has very unusual source arrangements. For this reason, the use of point A to specify the dose from interstitial implants is probably particularly dangerous.

A well-placed LDR system loaded according to the preceding recommendations will produce a dose rate at point A of approximately 45 to 55 cGy/h. Somewhat higher activity loadings have been recommended and used successfully. However, higher activity sources will result in higher dose rates and may have a somewhat greater biologic effect. Dose rates > 65 cGy/h to point A should be used with caution. In a prospective randomized study, Haie-Meder and colleagues reported an increased rate of major complications when the dose rate to point A was increased from 40 to 80 cGy/h.[226]

Patients who have bulky central disease and favorable anatomy can usually be treated to 85 to 90 Gy to point A (40 to 45 Gy with external-beam and 40 to 50 Gy with brachytherapy) with an acceptably low risk of late complications. Higher doses of central external-beam treatment tend to compromise the total paracentral dose that can be delivered. Somewhat lower doses (75 to 85 Gy) are usually recommended for smaller (IA-IB1) tumors. However, adjustments to these doses and to the distribution of sources in the intracavitary applicators may be needed, taking into account the position of the system in relation to other pelvic structures and the distribution of tumor as determined by physical examination and imaging studies.

LDR brachytherapy has been used successfully in combination with external-beam irradiation since the 1950s to treat thousands of patients and to achieve high local control and cure rates with a low risk of complications. The radiobiologic advantages of delivering brachytherapy at LDR has been emphasized by many, and a number of clinicians continue to express skepticism about the comparability of HDR, particularly in the treatment of patients with unfavorable anatomy, for whom the dose to critical normal tissues may be similar to the paracentral dose.[227] On the other hand, increased acceptance of, experience with, and training in HDR brachytherapy techniques have led many to adopt outpatient-based HDR brachytherapy as the approach of choice. Whether using LDR or HDR, the importance of attention to anatomic detail, an understanding of normal tissue tolerance, an appreciation of radiobiologic principles, and an adherence to guidelines for loading and fractionation cannot be overemphasized.

High-Dose-Rate Brachytherapy

Computerized remote afterloading technology has now made it possible to deliver intracavitary radiation at very high doses in minutes instead of hours or days. Worldwide use of HDR brachytherapy as an alternative to LDR brachytherapy has increased rapidly in recent years. Because HDR treatment is always delivered with remote afterloading equipment, radiation exposure to personnel is eliminated. Patients do not have to be hospitalized for treatment, providing a possible economic advantage, and the delivery of treatment in several short fractions may permit greater control over the position of sources during treatment. The most important concern has been that treatment with large HDR fractions reduces the opportunity for recovery of sublethal normal tissue injury and therefore may narrow the therapeutic ratio between tumor control and complications. Other possible disadvantages include the labor intensity of the process and the opportunity for an irreversible error that is not discovered during a very short duration of exposure.

Investigators have been reporting their experiences with HDR brachytherapy for more than 20 years, describing thousands of patients with cervical cancer who were treated with this approach. The authors of numerous retrospective studies have demonstrated that HDR treatment is feasible, effective, and safe.[219] In addition, there have been four randomized trials of HDR versus LDR brachytherapy (Table 55-7).[215-218] While each study had flaws, the data would suggest, in total, that HDR brachytherapy, within carefully applied dosing and fractionation guidelines, provides therapeutic equivalency to traditional LDR approaches.

Depending on the size of the radiation fractions used to deliver HDR brachytherapy, the biologic effect (particularly to normal tissues) of a nominal dose of radiation will be significantly greater when it is given with HDR as compared with LDR brachytherapy. To select an HDR schedule that may be comparable with LDR treatment, it is helpful to consider the fractionation and dose-rate effects, and specifically, applications of the linear quadratic (LQ) model used to describe these effects.

The LQ model has been used to describe a biologically effective dose, given as

$$\text{BED} = \text{total dose}[1 + \text{dose per fraction}/(\alpha/\beta)]$$

where α/β describes the varying influence of fraction size on radiation effects in different tumors and normal tissues.

HDR fractionation schedules reported in the literature vary markedly, with insertion numbers and point A dose fraction sizes ranging from 2 to 7 and 3 to 14 Gy, respectively.[219] However, applications of the LQ model support the use of at least 5 fractions. Assuming an α/β ratio of 3 for late damage to normal tissues, Stitt and coworkers[228] used the LQ model to predict how a dose of HDR brachytherapy would have to be divided so its effect on normal tissue was comparable to that of 70 Gy of LDR brachytherapy. According to their model, 5 or 6 fractions are sufficient if the dose to critical normal tissues is 80% or less of the dose to the paracentral reference point. However, if the anatomy is somewhat less favorable and the normal tissue dose is 90% of the tumor dose, more fractions are required.

The use of the LQ equation allows one to calculate and approximate the biologic equivalency of HDR to traditional LDR-based dosing. Typically, an α/β ratio of 10 is used for tumor and acute responding tissues, and a ratio of 3 is used for late responding normal tissues. Using the LQ equation, tumor doses of 80 to 85 Gy to point A in LDR equivalent would result in BEDs of 96 to 102 Gy_{10}. Conservatively accounting for late responding normal tissue tolerances, an LDR equivalent doses of 70 Gy to the rectum and 75 Gy to the bladder correspond to 120 Gy_3 and 125 Gy_3, respectively.

Table 55-7 Randomized Trials of High (HDR)-Versus Low-Dose-Rate (LDR) Brachytherapy in Cervical Cancer

Series (Reference)	No. of Patients	Survival	Severe Late Toxicity	Comments
Patel[215]	Group I—early stage LDR: n = 36 HDR: n = 34 Group II—bulky/ advanced tumor LDR: n = 210 HDR: n = 202	Group I—5-y OS LDR—72% HDR—82% Group II LDR—55% HDR 54%	Group I LDR—GI 3% HDR—GI 0% Group II LDR—GI 2% HDR—GI 1%	Equivalent outcomes for HDR and LDR in local control, survival, and late toxicity. No severe late GU toxicity noted.
Teshima[216]	LDR: n = 171 HDR: n = 259	LDR—5-y CSS St I /II/III 93%/78%/47% HDR St I/II/III 85%/73%/53%	LDR—4% HDR—10%	Unbalanced randomization—includes older patients specifically referred for HDR. Equivalent local control and CSS. Higher late toxicity with HDR, but still considered within acceptable levels.
Hareyama[217]	Stage II LDR: n = 26 HDR: n = 22 Stage III LDR: n = 45 HDR: n = 39	Stage II—5-y DSS LDR—87% HDR—69% Stage III LDR—60% HDR—51%	Stage II/III LDR—13% HDR—10%	No significant differences in DSS and complication rates
Lertsanguansinchai[218]	LDR: n = 109 HDR: n = 112	3 y RFS LDR—70% HDR—70%	LDR—3% HDR—7%	Comparable local control, RFS, and complication rates

CSS, cause-specific survival; DSS, disease-specific survival; OS, overall survival; RFS = relapse-free survival.

There is emerging evidence that small volumes of the rectum and bladder can tolerate a total of 130 to 140 Gy$_3$. Ogino and associates[229] did not observe any grade 4 to 5 rectal complications with a dose equivalent of less than 147 Gy$_3$ to the rectum. Grade 3 to 4 rectal toxicity was reported in less than 5% of patients with a BED of less than 119 Gy$_3$ and in less than 10% with a BED of less than 146 Gy$_3$. Their current fractionation schedules are designed to keep the BED for late-responding tissues to less than 119 Gy$_3$ for early stage disease and to less than 147 Gy$_3$ for locally advanced cancers, allowing a tailoring of dose to disease extent.

A detailed analysis of 24 reported series of HDR brachytherapy failed to identify a dose-response relationship for either tumor control or late tissue complications.[230] Although this does not refute the importance of radiobiologic considerations and calculations in the implementation of HDR brachytherapy, it underscores the complexity of patient- and treatment-related variables involved in the radiotherapeutic management of cervical cancer and the difficulty in reducing HDR dosing issues to a simple mathematical formula.

At present, a consensus HDR scheme for cervical cancer adopted by the GOG consists of 5 fractions of 6 Gy per insertion to point A, for a nominal total HDR dose of 30 Gy. Based on the LQ model, this dose has been calculated to be the biologic equivalent of 40 Gy LDR to point A. When combined with a dose of 45 Gy external-beam radiation to the pelvis, this results in a cumulative dose of 85 Gy to point A in conventional equivalents, which is the current standard for radiation prescription in GOG trials of locally advanced cervical cancer. To preserve biologic equivalency dosing to late reacting normal tissues, the GOG has recommended that the ICRU rectal dose point receive no more than 4.1 Gy (68% of point A dose), and the bladder dose point no more than 4.6 Gy (77% of point A dose) per insertion. The increased flexibility in dose shaping with HDR brachytherapy may be useful in optimizing tumor to normal tissue dose ratios. Although the LQ model is a useful tool for comparing fractionation schemes, no mathematical formula can take the place of clinical judgment and observation.

As with LDR brachytherapy, the timing of HDR insertions depends on the stage and volume of disease and its response to external-beam irradiation. For small cervical cancers, brachytherapy may be initiated during the first 2 weeks of radiation; for more advanced lesions, brachytherapy is performed near or at the end of external-beam irradiation, which provides time for bulky tumors to regress. However, the addition of multiple HDR fractions at the end of pelvic irradiation should not be allowed to protract treatment excessively. If most or all of external radiation is to be given before brachytherapy, two, or even three, HDR fractions are given per week, if necessary, to avoid exceeding a total treatment time of 8 weeks. On days in which HDR brachytherapy is performed, external-beam radiotherapy must not be given.

The literature describes a wide range of sedation methods (none to spinal or general anesthesia) used during the administration of HDR brachytherapy. Most commonly, conscious sedation is used. This involves administration of intravenous midazolam and fentanyl by a trained nurse. To accommodate conscious sedation in the radiation oncology clinic, the patient must at least be continuously monitored by pulse oximetry and blood pressures. The physician and nurse must be certified in conscious sedation procedures, be up to date on cardiopulmonary resuscitation measures, and have ready access to a resuscitation cart. In a review of 124 patients with cervical cancer treated at the University of Wisconsin with HDR brachytherapy, the median doses of midazolam and fentanyl given during each procedure were 8 mg (2 to 40 mg) and 200 μg (50 to 600 μg), respectively.[231] At the University of Washington, the first HDR insertion in each patient is done under transabdominal ultrasound guidance to facilitate placement of the intrauterine tandem. If the anatomy for insertion of the tandem is particularly difficult, an intrauterine Smit sleeve is placed at the first implant to facilitate subsequent applications.

At present, most HDR loading schemes attempt to recapitulate the familiar and symmetrical "pear-shaped" dose distribution typically used in LDR brachytherapy. This isodose distribution can be obtained by designating a series of dose points surrounding the tandem and colpostat and letting the dosimetry program calculate source dwell times in each source location to create the desired dose distribution. Alternatively, the physician may specify the relative weight of each selected dwell position in the brachytherapy apparatus, somewhat analogous to the loading of individual sources in an LDR system. Most HDR practitioners use tandem and ovoids that are based on the LDR Fletcher-Suit-Delclos applicator. However, others favor a tandem and ring system that has the advantage of having fixed geometry and potentially simplified dosimetric planning (Fig. 55-19). A further advantage of HDR brachytherapy that has yet to be fully exploited is the greater degree of dose optimization that can be achieved compared to LDR approaches. Nascent efforts in image-guided brachytherapy may eventually lead to a shift from the present central symmetry toward a more asymmetrical dose distribution biased toward residual tumor volume.

Although HDR brachytherapy has had a shorter history than that of LDR brachytherapy, the cumulative experience to date is not trivial. Results indicate that HDR has provided effective treatment for many patients with cervical cancer over the past 3 decades, and is an acceptable alternative to LDR for intracavitary radiation implants. As with LDR, practitioners of HDR must be well trained and sufficiently experienced in the system of brachytherapy they ultimately choose to use.

Interstitial Brachytherapy

Interstitial brachytherapy has long been used to treat patients with vaginal disease recurrence after hysterectomy and to increase the dose of radiation delivered to the distal vagina in the rare patient who presents with extensive vaginal disease. However, several groups have advocated a broader role for interstitial irradiation by reporting on the use of large interstitial implants, usually guided by a perineal template, for patients with a variety of clinical presentations, including poor anatomy, bulky disease, or extensive involvement in the parametrium or pelvic wall. Initial reports of this technique were enthusiastic and high local control rates were reported.[232-234] Unfortunately, despite having more than 20 years of clinical experience, there have been few reports of long-term outcome in patients with primary cervical carcinoma treated with this technique. A 1995 report[235] of the combined experiences of Stanford and the Joint Center for Radiation Therapy at Harvard was disappointing, with 3-year disease-free survival rates of only 36% and 18% for patients with FIGO stages IIB and IIIB disease, respectively, and high rates of major complications. A review of 1992-1994 practice patterns from the Patterns of Care Study indicates that less than 6% of patients in the United States are treated with interstitial brachytherapy. Comparisons across series are rendered difficult by patient selection and the inherent case individualization in technique and dosimetry.

For selected patients with very difficult clinical presentations, this may, however, be a useful technique. Full understanding of its efficacy awaits further reports of mature clinical experiences, but its use should probably be limited to selected institutions with sufficient experience in using an interstitial approach. Because of the variability of interstitial approaches, the use of interstitial brachytherapy is currently not permitted in phase III randomized trials of radiation or chemoradiation in cervical cancer.

Normal Tissue Effects of Radiation

An appreciation of the tolerance of normal tissues to radiation is needed to determine optimal treatment doses. Experience suggests that the upper one third of the vaginal mucosa can tolerate radiation doses as high as 120 to 140 Gy, whereas the lower two thirds usually should not receive more than 80 to 85 Gy. Most institutions do not exceed 75 to 80 Gy (combined external-beam and LDR intracavitary dose) to the International Commission on Radiological Units and Measurements (ICRU) bladder reference point and 70 to 75 Gy to the ICRU rectal point.[153,236] However, these reference doses should be used only as general guidelines. Several studies of CT-based dosimetry have demonstrated that small volumes of rectum and bladder routinely receive much higher doses than those calculated from orthogonal films.[237] Also, concern about reference dose limits should always be balanced against the need to deliver a tumoricidal dose to the cancer.

Historical reports of severe late normal complications, usually defined as injury to the bladder, rectum, or small bowel requiring hospitalization or surgical intervention, typically range from 5% to 10% using crude estimates, but they may be higher using actuarial calculations.[238,239] Complications are related to the presenting stage and volume of disease, as well as to the dose delivered to the individual normal tissues. The severe complications occur in the first 3 to 5 years after completion of radiation, but there remains a small but continuous added risk thereafter.[239] Smoking during radiotherapy has been associated with a significantly higher risk of late complications.[240] Most reports of late morbidity have focused on severe GI and GU toxicities—only recently have rigorous efforts been made to monitor for less severe sequalae that, while not requiring surgery or extensive medical care, still have an impact on patients' quality of life. The recent use of concurrent chemoradiation has been clearly shown to increase acute toxicities, especially with respect to hematologic and gastrointestinal function, compared to radiation alone, but there does not appear to be a coincident increase in late morbidity.[241]

Radiobiology principles would predict an unacceptable complication rate for patients treated with curative HDR brachytherapy if the rectum and bladder receive the same dose as point A. However, with careful retraction and packing, the doses to these tissues can usually be substantially reduced, and studies generally have not demonstrated an increased complication rate when the dose of HDR is adequately fractioned.[215,219] As with LDR brachytherapy, careful technique and the expertise of the brachytherapist may be as important as any other factor. These parameters are very difficult to evaluate. Studies have suggested that the complication rates from HDR treatment of cervical cancer tend to decrease with increasing institutional experience.[242-244]

TREATMENT ALGORITHM, CONCLUSIONS, AND FUTURE POSSIBILITIES

Although cytologic screening programs have made it possible to prevent most invasive cervical cancers, and recent molecular biologic discoveries have raised hopes for a future vaccine against the sexually transmitted virus that appears to induce malignant transformation, cervical cancer remains a major public health problem worldwide.

Both radical hysterectomy and radiation therapy achieve high cure rates for patients with stage IB1 disease (Fig. 55-20). The rates of major toxicity from the two treatments are similar, but the types of side effects differ. Surgery tends to be the preferred treatment for young women with small squamous car-

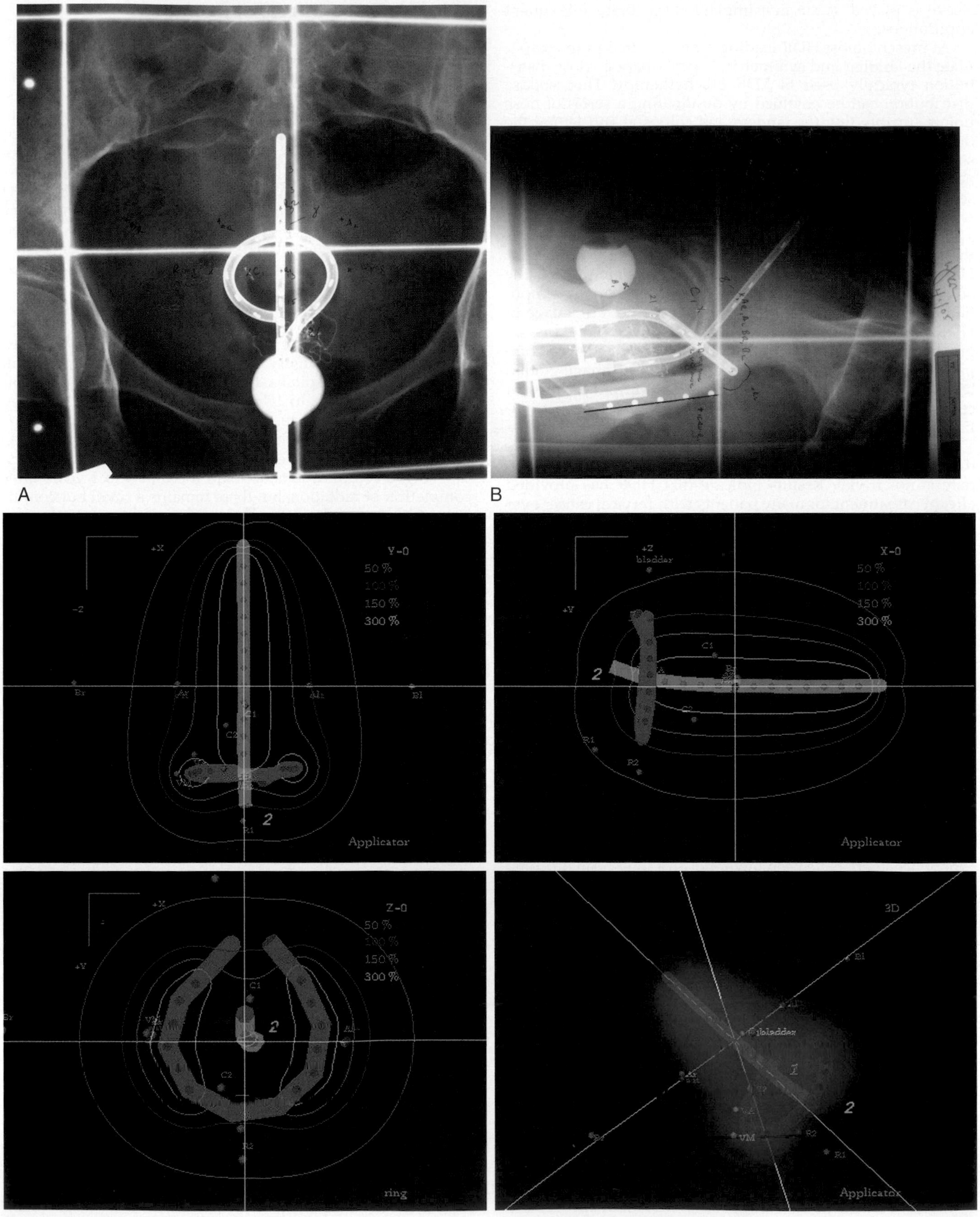

Figure 55-19 Anterior **(A)** and lateral **(B)** radiographs of an intracavitary tandem and ring insertion for HDR afterloading brachytherapy. The source dwell positions selected for "loading" include those in the intrauterine tandem, as well as the lateral positions in the ring corresponding to the lateral vaginal fornices, thereby mimicking the dosimetry distribution of tandem and ovoids **(C)**. Computerized brachytherapy dosimetry allows visualization of dose in the traditional planes of calculation (coronal, sagittal, and transverse) but also permit three-dimensional representation of dose distribution that may be exploited to conform better to unusual tumor geometries.

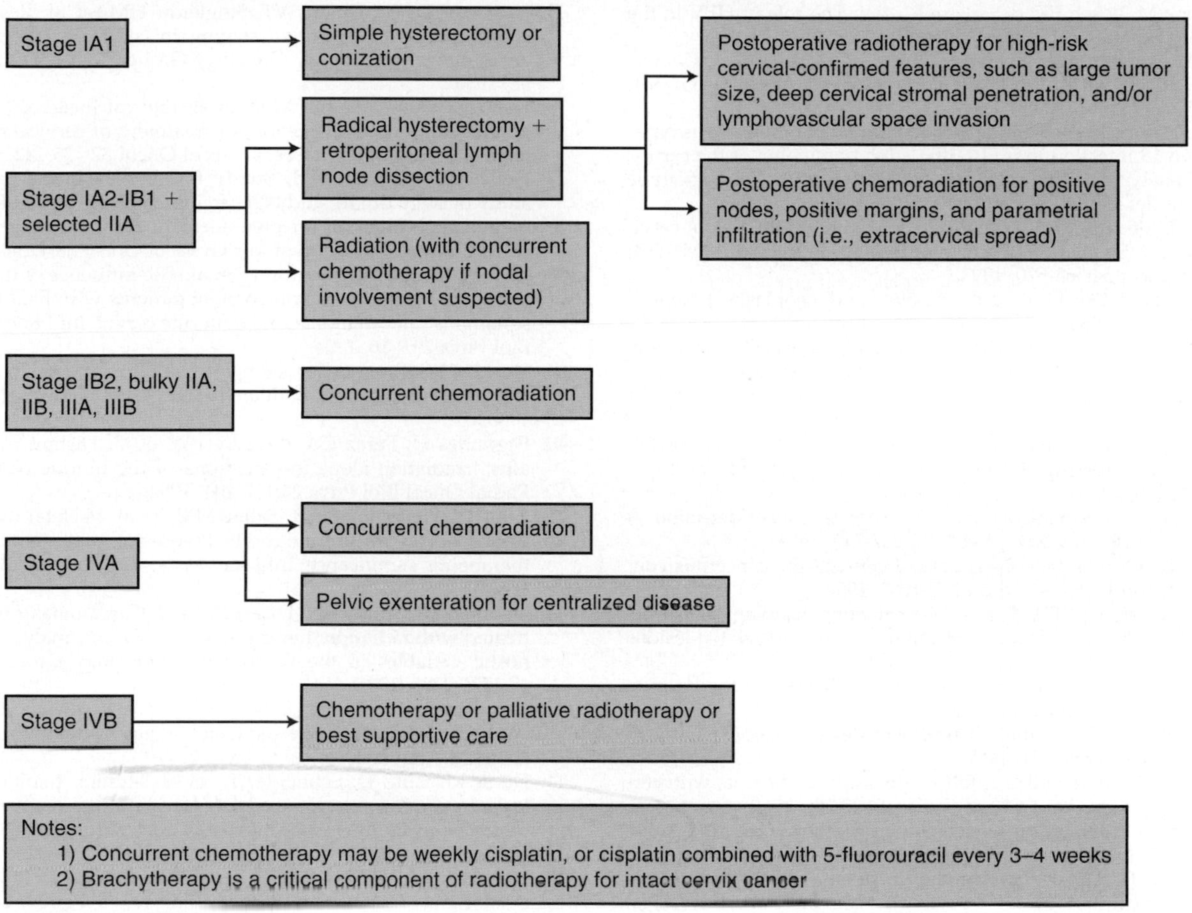

Figure 55-20 Treatment algorithm for cervical cancer.

cinomas to avoid radiation-related ovarian failure and to minimize the risk of sexual dysfunction.

Aggressive radiation therapy, including a combination of external-beam irradiation and brachytherapy, concurrent with cisplatin-based chemotherapy, is now the primary treatment of choice in the management of bulky and locoregionally advanced disease (see Fig. 55-20). Radiation remains the most active single modality for the treatment of cervical cancer not amenable to surgical resection or sterilization. Improvements in radiotherapy targeting and delivery will be realized by advances in imaging modalities, including PET, careful conformal radiation treatment planning, and appropriate incorporation of brachytherapy.

Adjuvant hysterectomy has not been shown to improve the outcome of patients treated with radiation therapy for stage IB2 disease if adequate doses of radiation therapy are delivered. Radical radiation therapy or chemoradiation is also preferred over a combination of radical hysterectomy and postoperative radiation therapy because the increased cost and complications of combined treatment are not justified by any significant improvement in local control or survival. Although treatment is successful in most primary cervical cancer cases, pelvic disease recurrence continues to be an important problem, particularly for patients who present with extensive local-regional disease. Recent studies have emphasized the influence of radiation dose, volume, fractionation, and treatment time on locoregional control and survival for patients with locally advanced disease.

The present focus on improving outcomes in bulky and local-regionally advanced cervical cancer is on the addition of promising systemic agents to the current standard of cisplatin and radiotherapy. Compounds of interest include tirapazamine, paclitaxel, topotecan, and anti-EGFR and antiangiogenic agents. Finally, there remains the need to identify new drugs, including nonplatinum regimens, that have efficacy for patients with advanced, recurrent, or metastatic disease not amenable to definitive surgery or radiotherapy.

REFERENCES

1. Makuc DM, Freid VM, Kleinman JC: National trends in the use of preventive health care by women. Am J Public Health 79:21-26, 1989.
2. Jemal A, Siegal R, Ward E, et al: Cancer Statistics, 2006. CA Cancer J Clin 56:106-130, 2006.
3. Parkin DM, Pisani P, Ferlay J: Global cancer statistics. CA Cancer J Clin 49:33-64, 1999.
4. Whelan SL, Parkin DM, Masuyer E: Patterns of cancer in five continents. Lyons, International Agency for Research on Cancer, 1990.
5. Cannistra SA, Niloff JM: Cancer of the uterine cervix. N Engl J Med 334:1030-1038, 1996.
6. Agarwal SS, Sehgal A, Sardana S, et al: Role of male behavior in cervical carcinogenesis among women with one lifetime sexual partner. Cancer 72:1666-1669, 1993.
7. Castellsague X, Bosch FX, Munoz N, et al: Male circumcision, penile human papillomavirus infection, and cervical cancer in female partners. N Engl J Med 346:1105-1112, 2002.

8. Munoz M, Bosch FX, deSanjose S, et al: The role of HPV in the etiology of cervical cancer. Mutat Res 305:293-301, 1994.
9. National Institutes of Health Consensus Development Conference Statement on Cervical Cancer. Gynecol Oncol 66:351-361, 1997.
10. Tenti P, Romagnoli S, Silini E, et al: Human papillomavirus types 16 and 18 infection in infiltrating adenocarcinoma of the cervix: PCR analysis of 138 cases and correlation with histologic type and grade. Am J Clin Pathol 106:52-56, 1996.
11. Sigurdsson K: Effect of organized screening on the risk of cervical cancer. Evaluation of screening activity in Iceland, 1964-1991. Int J Cancer 54:563-570, 1993.
12. Stubblefield PG: Oral contraceptives and neoplasia. J Reprod Med 29:524, 1984.
13. Herbst AL, Cole P, Norusis MJ: Epidemiologic aspects and factors related to survival in 384 registry cases of clear cell adenocarcinoma of the vagina and cervix. Am J Obstet Gynecol 135:876-886, 1979.
14. Devessa SS, Silverman DT, Young JLJ, et al: Cancer and mortality trends among whites in the United States. J Natl Cancer Inst 79:701-770, 1987.
15. Koss LG: The Papanicolaou test for cervical cancer detection: A triumph and a tragedy. JAMA 261:737-743, 1989.
16. Peterson O: Spontaneous course of cervical pre-cancerous conditions. Am J Obstet Gynecol 72:1063, 1956.
17. Koss LG, Stewart FW, Foote FW, et al: Some histological aspects of behavior of epidermoid carcinoma in situ and related lesions of the uterine cervix. Cancer 16:1160, 1963.
18. Clemmesen J, Poulsen H: Report of the Ministry of the Interior, Document 3. Copenhagen, 1971.
19. Kottmeier HL: Evolution et traitment des epitheliomas. Rev Fr Gynecol Obstet 56:821, 1961.
20. Richart RM, Barron BA: A follow-up study of patients with cervical dysplasia. Am J Obstet Gynecol 105:386, 1969.
21. Walton RJ: Cervical cancer screening programs. Can Med Assoc J 127:953, 1982.
22. Solomon D, Davey D, Kurman R, et al: The 2001 Bethesda System: terminology for reporting results of cervical cytology. JAMA 287:2114-2119, 2001.
23. Saslow D, Runowicz CD, Solomon D, et al: American Cancer Society guideline for the early detection of cervical neoplasia and cancer. CA Cancer J Clin 52:342-362, 2002.
24. Sawaya GF, McConnell KJ, Kulasingam SL, et al: Risk of cervical cancer associated with extending the interval between cervical-cancer screenings. N Engl J Med 349:1501-1509, 2003.
25. Robert ME, Fu YS: Squamous cell carcinoma of the uterine cervix: A review with emphasis on prognostic factors and unusual variants. Semin Diagn Pathol 7:173, 1990.
26. Wentz WB, Reagan JW: Survival in cervical cancer with respect to cell type. Cancer 12:384-388, 1959.
27. Sheets EE, Berman ML, Hrountas CK, et al: Surgically treated, early-stage neuroendocrine small-cell cervical carcinoma. Obstet Gynecol 71:10-14, 1988.
28. Silva EG, Kott M, Ordonez NG: Endocrine carcinoma intermediate cell type of the uterine cervix. Cancer 54:1705, 1984.
29. Parazzini F, LaVecchia C: Epidemiology of adenocarcinoma of the cervix. Gynecol Oncol 39:40, 1990.
30. Peters RK, Chao A, Mack TM, et al: Increased frequency of adenocarcinoma of the uterine cervix in young women in Los Angeles County. J Natl Cancer Inst 1986:423, 1986.
31. Plentl AA, Friedman EA: Lymphatics of the cervix uteri. *In* Lymphatic System of Female Genitalia. Philadelphia, WB Saunders, 1971, pp 75-115.
32. Netter FH: The CIBA Collection of Medical Illustrations, Vol 2: Reproductive System. Summit, NJ, CIBA Pharmaceutical Products, 1988.
33. Berman ML, Keys H, Creasman W, et al: Survival and patterns of recurrence in cervical cancer metastatic to periaortic lymph nodes (a Gynecologic Oncology Group study). Gynecol Oncol 19:8-16, 1984.
34. Delgado G, Bundy BN, Fowler WC, et al: A prospective surgical pathological study of Stage I squamous carcinoma of the cervix: A Gynecologic Oncology Group study. Gynecol Oncol 36:314-320, 1989.
35. Lagasse LD, Creasman WT, Singleton HM, et al: Results and complications of operative staging in cervical cancer: Experiences of the Gynecologic Oncology Group. Gynecol Oncol 9:90-98, 1980.
36. Lee Y-N, Wang KL, Lin M-H, et al: Radical hysterectomy with pelvic lymph node dissection for treatment of cervical cancer: A clinical review of 954 cases. Gynecol Oncol 32:135-142, 1989.
37. Heller PB, Malfetano JH, Bundy BN, et al: Clinical-pathologic study of stage IIB, III, and IVA carcinoma of the cervix: Extended diagnostic evaluation for para-aortic node metastasis—a Gynecologic Oncology Group study. Gynecol Oncol 38:425-430, 1990.
38. Eifel PJ, Morris M, Wharton JT, et al: The influence of tumor size and morphology on the outcome of patients with FIGO stage IB squamous cell carcinoma of the uterine cervix. Int J Radiat Oncol Biol Phys 29:9-16, 1994.
39. Hoskins WJ: Prognostic factors for risk of recurrence in Stages Ib and IIa cervical cancer. Baillière's Clin Obstet Gynecol 2:817-828, 1988.
40. Fagundes H, Perez CA, Grigsby PW, et al: Distant metastases after irradiation alone in carcinoma of the uterine cervix. Int J Radiat Oncol Biol Phys 24:197-204, 1992.
41. Kim RY, Weppelmann B, Salter MM, et al: Skeletal metastases from cancer of the uterine cervix: Frequency, patterns, and radiotherapeutic significance. Int J Radiat Oncol Biol Phys 13:705-708, 1987
42. Stehman FB, Bundy BN, Disaia PJ, et al: Carcinoma of the cervix treated with radiation therapy. I. A multivariate analysis of prognostic variables in the Gynecologic Oncology Group. Cancer 67:2776-2785, 1991.
43. Los Alamos National Laboratory HPV sequence database: Available at http://www.stdgen.lanl.gov/stdgen-virus/hpv/; accessed August 2006.
44. Durst M, Glitz D, Schneider A, et al: Human papillomavirus type 16 gene expression and DNA replication in cervical neoplasia analysis by *in situ* hybridization. Virology 189:132-140, 1992.
45. Ferenczy A, Winkler B: Cervical intraepithelial neoplasia and condyloma. *In* Kurman R (ed): Blaustein's Pathology of the Female Genital Tract. New York, Springer-Verlag, 1987, pp 117-217.
46. Boshart M, Gissmann L, Ikenberg H, et al: A new type of papillomavirus DNA, its presence in genital cancer biopsies and in cell lines derived from cervical cancer. EMBO J 3:1151-1157, 1984.
47. Durst M, Gissman L, Ikenberg H, et al: A papillomavirus DNA from a cervical carcinoma and its prevalence in cancer biopsy specimens from different geographic regions. Proc Natl Acad Sci U S A 80:3812-3815, 1983.
48. Crum CP, Levine RU: Human papillomavirus infection and cervical neoplasia: New perspectives. Int J Gynecol Pathol 3:376-388, 1984.
49. Crum CP, Ikenberg H, Richart RM, et al: Human papillomavirus type 16 and early cervical neoplasia. N Engl J Med 310:880-883, 1984.
50. Crum CP, Mitao M, Levine RU, et al: Cervical papillomaviruses segregate within morphologically distinct precancerous lesions. J Virol 54:675-681, 1985.
51. Koutsky LA, Holmes KK, Critchow CW, et al: A cohort study of the risk of cervical intraepithelial neoplasia grade 2 or 3 in relation to papillomavirus infection. N Engl J Med 327:1272-1278, 1992.
52. Reid R, Crum CP, Herschmann BR, et al: Genital warts and cervical cancer. III. Subclinical papillomaviral infection and cervical neoplasia are linked by a spectrum of continuous morphologic and biologic change. Cancer 53:943-953, 1984.
53. Willett GD, Kurman RJ, Reid R, et al: Correlation of the histologic appearance of intraepithelial neoplasia of the cervix with human papillomavirus types: Emphasis on low grade lesions including so-called flat condyloma. Int J Gynecol Pathol 8:18-25, 1989.
54. Arbeit JM, Munger K, Howley PM, et al: Neuroepithelial carcinomas in mice transgenic with human papillomavirus type 16 E6/E7 ORFs. Am J Pathol 142:1187-1197, 1993.
55. Lambert PF, Pan H, Pitot HC, et al: Epidermal cancer associated with expression of human papillomavirus type 16 E6 and E7

oncogenes in the skin of transgenic mice. Proc Natl Acad Sci U S A 90:356-364, 1993.
56. Griep AE, Lanbert PF: Role of papillomavirus oncogenes in human cervical cancer: Transgenic animal studies. Proc Soc Exp Biol Med 206:24-34, 1994.
57. Werness BA, Levine AJ, Howley PM: Association of human papillomavirus types 16 and 18 E6 proteins with p53. Science 248:76-79, 1990.
58. Southern SA, Herrington CS: Disruption of cell cycle control by human papillomaviruses with special reference to cervical carcinoma. Int J Gynecol Oncol 10:263-274, 2000.
59. Ho GYF, Bierman R, Beardsley L, Chang CJ, Burk RD: Natural history of cervicovaginal papillomavirus infection in young women. N Engl J Med 338;423-438, 1998.
60. Moscicki AB, Palefsky J, Smith G, Siboshski S, Schoolnik G. Variability of human papillomavirus DNA testing in a longitudinal cohort of young women. Obstet Gynecol 82:578-585, 1993.
61. Nasiell K, Roger V, Nasiell M: Behavior of mild cervical dysplasia during long-term follow-up. Obstet Gynecol 67:665-669, 1986.
62. Vernon SD, Hart CE, Reeves WC, et al: The HIV-1 tat protein enhances E2-dependent human papillomavirus 16 transcription. Virus Res 27:133-145, 1993.
63. Slattery ML, Robison LM, Schuman KL, et al: Cigarette smoking and exposure to passive smoke are risk factors for cervical cancer. JAMA 261:1593-1598, 1989.
64. Sierra-Torres CH, Tyring SK, Au WW: Risk contribution of sexual behavior and cigarette smoking to cervical neoplasia. Int J Gynecol Cancer 13:617-625, 2003.
65. Hellberg D, Nilsson S, Haley NJ, et al: Smoking and cervical intraepithelial neoplasia: nicotine and cotinine in serum and cervical mucus in smokers and nonsmokers. Am J Obstet Gynecol 158:910-913, 1988.
66. Barton SE, Maddox PH, Jenkins D, et al: Effect of cigarette smoking on cervical epithelial immunity: a mechanism for neoplastic change? Lancet 2:652-654, 1988.
67. Halpert R, Fruchter RG, Sedlis A, et al: Human papillomavirus and lower genital neoplasia in renal transplant patients. Obstet Gynecol 68:251-258, 1986.
68. Piper JM. Review: oral contraceptives and cervical cancer. Gynecol Oncol 22:1-14, 1985.
69. Koutsky LA, Ault KA, Wheeler CM, et al: A controlled trial of a human papillomavirus type 16 vaccine. N Engl J Med 347:1645-1651, 2002.
70. Tjalma WAA, Arbyn M, Paavonen J, et al: Prophylactic human papillomavirus vaccines: the beginning of the end of cervical cancer. Int J Gynecol Cancer 14:751-761, 2004.
71. Bell MC, Alvarez RD: Chemoprevention and vaccines: a review of the nonsurgical options for the treatment of cervical dysplasia. Int J Gynecol Cancer 15:4-12, 2005.
72. International Federation of Gynecology and Obstetrics: Staging announcement. FIGO staging of gynecologic cancers: cervical and vulva. Int J Gynecol Cancer 5:319-324, 1995.
73. Eifel PJ: Problems with the clinical staging of carcinoma of the cervix. Semin Radiat Oncol 4:1-8, 1994.
74. Fu YS, Berek JS: Minimal cervical cancer: Definition and histology. *In* Grundmann E, Beck L (eds): Minimal Neoplasia-Diagnosis and Therapy. Recent Results in Cancer Research. Berlin, Springer-Verlag, 1988, pp 47-56.
75. Piver MS, Barlow JJ: High dose irradiation to biopsy confirmed aortic node metastases from carcinoma of the uterine cervix. Cancer 39:1243-1246, 1977.
76. Wharton JT, Jones HWI, Day T, et al: Preirradiation celiotomy and extended field irradiation for invasive carcinoma of the cervix. Obstet Gynecol 49:333-338, 1977.
77. Weiser EB, Bundy BN, Hoskins WJ, et al: Extraperitoneal versus transperitoneal selective para-aortic lymphadenectomy in the pretreatment surgical staging of advanced cervical carcinoma (a Gynecologic Oncology Group study). Gynecol Oncol 33:283-289, 1989.
78. Querleau D, LeBlanc E, Castelain B: Laparoscopic pelvic lymphadenectomy in the staging of early carcinoma of the cervix. Am J Obstet Gynecol 164:579-581, 1991.
79. Benedetti-Panici P, Maneschi F, Cutillo G, et al: Laparoscopic abdominal staging in locally advanced cervical cancer. Int J Gynecol Cancer 9:194-197, 1999.
80. Goff BA, Muntz HG, Paley PJ, et al: Impact of surgical staging in women with locally advanced cervical cancer. Gynecol Oncol 74:436-442, 1999.
81. Moore DH, Stehman FB: What is the appropriate management of early stage cervical cancer (International Federation of Gynecology and Obstetrics Stages I and IIA), surgical assessment of lymph nodes, and role of therapeutic resection of lymph nodes involved with cancer? Monogr Natl Cancer Inst 21:43-46, 1996.
82. Russell AH, Shingleton HM, Jones WB, et al: Diagnostic assessments in patients with invasive cancer of the cervix: A national pattern of care study of the American College of Surgeons. Gynecol Oncol 63:159-165, 1996.
83. Hricak H, Powell CB, Yu KK, et al: Invasive cervical carcinoma: Role of MR imaging in pretreatment work-up-cost minimization and diagnostic efficacy analysis. Radiology 198:403-409, 1996.
84. Russell AH, Walter JP, Anderson MW, et al: Sagittal magnetic resonance imaging in the design of lateral radiation treatment portals for patients with locally advanced squamous cancer of the cervix. Int J Radiat Oncol Biol Phys 23:449-455, 1992.
85. Grigsby PW, Siegel BA, Dehdashti F: Lymph node staging by positron emission tomography in patients with carcinoma of the cervix. J Clin Oncol 19:3745-3749, 2001.
86. Yen TC, Ng KK, Ma SY, et al: Value of dual-phase 2-fluoro-2-deoxy-D-glucose positron emission tomography in cervical cancer. J Clin Oncol 21:3651-3658, 2003.
87. Barillot I, Horiot JC, Pigneux J, et al: Carcinoma of the intact uterine cervix treated with radiotherapy alone: A French Cooperative Study: Update and multivariate analysis of prognostic factors. Int J Radiat Oncol Biol Phys 38:969-978, 1997.
88. Lanciano RM, Won M, Coia L, et al: Pretreatment and treatment factors associated with improved outcome in squamous cell carcinoma of the uterine cervix: A final report of the 1973 and 1978 Patterns of Care Studies. Int J Radiat Oncol Biol Phys 20:667-676, 1991.
89. Perez CA, Camel HM, Kuske RR, et al: Radiation therapy alone in the treatment of carcinoma of the uterine cervix: A 20-year experience. Gynecol Oncol 23:127-140, 1986.
90. Horiot JC, Pigneux J, Pourquier H, et al: Radiotherapy alone in carcinoma of the intact uterine cervix according to G. H. Fletcher guidelines: A French cooperative study of 1383 cases. Int J Radiat Oncol Biol Phys 14:605-611, 1988.
91. Lowrey GC, Mendenhall WM, Million RR: Stage IB or IIA-B carcinoma of the intact uterine cervix treated with irradiation: A multivariate analysis. Int J Radiat Oncol Biol Phys 24:205-210, 1992.
92. Perez CA, Grigsby PW, Nene SM, et al: Effect of tumor size on the prognosis of carcinoma of the uterine cervix treated with irradiation alone. Cancer 69:2796-2806, 1992.
93. Logsdon MD, Eifel PJ: FIGO IIIB squamous cell carcinoma of the cervix: an analysis of prognostic factors emphasizing the balance between external-beam and intracavitary radiation therapy. Int J Radiat Oncol Biol Phys 43:763-775, 1999.
94. Hreshchyshyn MM, Aron BS, Boronow RC, et al: Hydroxyurea or placebo combined with radiation to treat stages IIIB and IV cervical cancer confined to the pelvis. Int J Radiat Oncol Biol Phys 5:317-322, 1979.
95. Stehman FB: Experience with hydroxyurea as a radiosensitizer in carcinoma of the cervix. Sem Oncol 19(suppl 9):48-52, 1992.
96. Symonds P, Kirwan J, Williams C, et al: Concomitant hydroxyurea plus radiotherapy versus radiotherapy for carcinoma of the uterine cervix (review). Cochrane Database Syst Rev 1:CD003918, 2004.
97. Overgaard J, Bentzen SM, Kolstad P, et al: Misonidazole combined with radiotherapy in the treatment of carcinoma of the uterine cervix. Int J Radiat Oncol Biol Phys 16:1069-1072, 1989.
98. Stehman FB, Bundy BN, Thomas G, et al: Hydroxyurea versus misonidazole with radiation in cervical carcinoma: long-term follow-up of a gynecology oncology group trial. J Clin Oncol 11:1523-1528, 1993.
99. Dische S, Chassagne D, Hope-Stone HF, et al: A trial of Ro 03-8799 (pimonidazole) in carcinoma of the uterine cervix: an

interim report from the Medical Research Council Working Party on advanced carcinoma of the cervix. Radiother Oncol 26:93-103, 1993.
100. Grigsby PW, Winter K, Wasserman TH, et al: Irradiation with or without misonidazole for patient with stages IIIB and IVA carcinoma of the cervix: final results of RTOG 80-05. Int J Radiat Oncol Biol Phys 44:513-517, 1999.
101. Chan P, Milosevic M, Fyles A, et al: A phase III randomized study of misonidazole plus radiation versus radiation alone for cervix cancer. Radiother Oncol 70:295-299, 2004.
102. National Institutes of Health:: Cervical Cancer. Consens Statement 14:1-38, 1996.
103. National Cancer Institute: Clinical Announcement—Concurrent chemoradiation for cervical cancer. National Institutes of Health Bethesda, MD, February 1999.
104. Whitney CW, Sause W, Bundy BN, et al: Randomized comparison of fluorouracil plus cisplatin versus hydroxyurea as an adjunct to radiation therapy in stages IIB-IVA carcinoma of the cervix with negative para-aortic lymph nodes. A Gynecologic Oncology Group and Southwest Oncology Group Study. J Clin Oncol 17:1339-1348, 1999.
105. Rose PG, Bundy BN, Watkins EB, et al: Concurrent cisplatin-based chemoradiation improves progression-free and overall survival in advanced cervical cancer: Results of a randomized Gynecologic Oncology Group study. N Engl J Med 340:1144-1153, 1999.
106. Morris M, Eifel PJ, Lu J, et al: Pelvic radiation with concurrent chemotherapy versus pelvic and para-aortic radiation for high-risk cervical cancer: A randomized Radiation Therapy Oncology Group clinical trial. N Engl J Med 340:1137-1143, 1999.
107. Keys HM, Bundy BN, Stehman FB, et al: A comparison of weekly cisplatin during radiation therapy versus irradiation alone, each followed by adjuvant hysterectomy in bulky stage IB cervical carcinoma: A randomized trial of the Gynecologic Oncology Group. N Engl J Med 340:1154-1161, 1999.
108. Peters WA, Liu PY, Barrett RJ, et al: Concurrent chemotherapy and pelvic radiation therapy compared with pelvic radiation therapy alone as adjunctive therapy after radical surgery in high-risk, early-stage carcinoma of the cervix. J Clin Oncol 18:1606-1713, 2000.
109. Dewil L: Combined treatment of radiation and cis-diaminedichloroplatinum (II): A review of experimental and clinical data. Int J Radiat Oncol Biol Phys 13:403-426, 1987.
110. Malfetano J, Keys H, Kredentser D, et al: Weekly cisplatin and radical radiation therapy for advanced, recurrent and poor prognosis cervical carcinoma. Cancer 71:3703-3706, 1993.
111. Potish RA, Twiggs LB, Adcock LL, et al: Effect of cis-platinum on tolerance to radiation therapy in advanced cervical cancer. Am J Clin Oncol 9:387-391, 1986.
112. Runowicz CD, Wadler S, Rodriguez-Rodriguez L, et al: Concomitant cisplatin and radiotherapy in locally advanced cervical carcinoma. Gynecol Oncol 34:387-391, 1989.
113. Rotman M, Pajak M, Choi K, et al: Prophylactic extended-field irradiation of para-aortic lymph nodes in stages IIB and bulky IB and IIA cervical carcinomas. Ten-year treatment results of RTOG 79-20. JAMA 274:387-393, 1995.
114. Eifel PJ, Winter K, Morris M, et al: Pelvic irradiation with concurrent chemotherapy versus pelvic and para-aortic irradiation for high-risk cervical cancer: an update of Radiation Therapy Oncology Group trial (RTOG) 90-01. J Clin Oncol 22:972-880, 2004.
115. Pearcey R, Brundage M, Drouin P, et al: Phase III trial comparing radical radiotherapy with and without cisplatin chemotherapy in patients with advanced squamous cell cancer of the cervix. J Clin Oncol 20:966-972, 2002.
116. Rose PG, Bundy BN: Chemoradiation for locally advanced cervical cancer: does it help? J Clin Oncol 20:891-893, 2002.
117. Green JA, Kirwan JM, Terney JF, et al: Survival and recurrence after concomitant chemotherapy and radiotherapy for cancer of the uterine cervix: a systematic review and meta-analysis. Lancet 358:781-786, 2001.
118. Higgins RV, Naumann WR, Hall JB, Ha-ake M: Concurrent carboplatin with pelvic radiation therapy in the primary treatment of cervical cancer. Gynecol Oncol 89:499-503, 2003.
119. Thomas G, Dembo A, Ackerman I, et al: A randomized trial of standard versus partially hyperfractionated radiation with or without concurrent 5-fluorouracil in locally advanced cervical cancer. Gynecol Oncol 69:137-145, 1998.
119a. Lanciano R, Calkins A, Bundy BN, et al: Randomized comparison of weekly cisplatin or protracted venous infusion of fluorouracil in combination with pelvic radiation in advanced cervix cancer: a Gynecologic Oncology Group study. J Clin Oncol 23:8289-8295, 2005.
120. Wong LC, Ngan HYS, Cheung ANY et al: Chemoradiation and adjuvant chemotherapy in cervical cancer. J Clin Oncol 17:2055-2060, 1999.
121. Lorvidhaya V, Chitapanarux I, Sangruchi S, et al: Concurrent Mitomycin-C, 5-Fluorouracil, and radiotherapy in the treatment of locally advanced carcinoma of the cervix: a randomized trial. Int J Radiat Oncol Biol Phys 55:1226-1232, 2003.
122. Neoadjuvant Chemotherapy for Cervical Cancer Meta-analysis Collaboration: Neoadjuvant chemotherapy for locally advanced cervical cancer: a systematic review and meta-analysis of individual patient data from 21 randomized trials. Eur J Cancer 39:2470-2486, 2003.
123. Souhami L, Gil R, Allan S, et al: A randomized trial of chemotherapy followed by pelvic radiation therapy in Stage IIIB carcinoma of the cervix. Int J Radiat Oncol Biol Phys 9:970-997, 1991.
124. Tattersall MHN, Lorvidhaya V, Vootiprux V, et al: Randomized trial of epirubicin and cisplatin chemotherapy followed by pelvic radiation in locally advanced cervical cancer. J Clin Oncol 13:444-451, 1995.
125. Withers HR, Taylor JMG, Maciejewski B: The hazard of accelerated tumor clonogen repopulation during radiotherapy. Acto Oncologica 27:131-146, 1988.
126. Lanciano RM, Martz K, Coia LR, et al: Tumor and treatment factors improving outcome in stage III-B cervix cancer. Int J Radiat Oncol Biol Phys 20:95-100, 1991.
127. Fyles A, Keane TJ, Barton M, Simm J: The effect of treatment duration in the local control of cervix cancer. Radiother Oncol 25:273-279, 1992.
128. Lanciano RM, Pajak TF, Martz K, Hanks GE: The influence of treatment time on outcome for squamous cell cancer of the uterine cervix treated with radiation: a Patterns-of-Care study. Int J Radiat Oncol Biol Phys 25:391-397, 1993.
129. Girinsky T, Rey A, Roche B, et al: Overall treatment time in advanced cervical carcinomas: a critical parameter in treatment outcome. Int J Radiat Oncol Biol Phys 27:1051-1056, 1993.
130. Perez CA, Grigsby PW, Castro-Vita H, Lockett MA: Carcinoma of the uterine cervix. I. Impact of prolongation of overall treatment time and timing of brachytherapy on outcome of radiation therapy. Int J Radiat Oncol Biol Phys 32:1275-1288, 1995.
131. Petereit DG, Sarkaria JN, Chappell R, et al: The adverse effect of treatment prolongation in cervical carcinoma. Int J Radiat Oncol Biol Phys 32:1301-1307, 1995.
132. Perez CA, Grigsby PW, Castro-Vita H, Lockett MA: Carcinoma of the uterine cervix. II. Lack of impact of prolongation of overall treatment time on morbidity of radiation therapy. Int J Radiat Oncol Biol Phys 34:3-11, 1996.
133. Cunningham M, Dunton C, Corn B, et al: Extended-field radiation therapy in early-stage cervical carcinoma: Survival and complications. Gynecol Oncol 43:51-54, 1991.
134. Rubin SC, Brookland R, Mikuta JJ, et al: Para-aortic nodal metastases in early cervical carcinoma: Long-term survival following extended-field radiotherapy. Gynecol Oncol 18:213-217, 1984.
135. Komaki R, Mattingly RF, Hoffman RG, et al: Irradiation of para-aortic lymph node metastases from carcinoma of the cervix or endometrium: Preliminary results. Radiology 147:245-248, 1983.
136. Rotman M, Aziz H, Eifel PJ: Irradiation of pelvic and para-aortic nodes in carcinoma of the cervix. Semin Radiat Oncol 4:23-29, 1994.
137. Haie C, Pejovic MH, Gerbaulet A, et al: Is prophylactic para-aortic irradiation worthwhile in the treatment of advanced cervical carcinoma? Results of a controlled clinical trial of the EORTC radiotherapy group. Radiother Oncol 11:101-112, 1988.
138. Varia MA, Bundy BN, Deppe G, et al: Cervical carcinoma metastatic to para-aortic nodes: extended field radiation therapy with concomitant 5-fluorouracil and cisplatin chemotherapy: a

Gynecologic Oncology Group study. Int J Radiat Oncol Biol Phys 42:1015-1023, 1998.
139. Malfetano JH, Keys H, Cunningham MJ, et al: Extended field radiation and cisplatin for stage IIB and IIIB cervical cancer. Gynecol Oncol 67:203-207, 1997.
140. Bush R: The significance of anemia in clinical radiation therapy. Int J Radiat Oncol Biol Phys 12:2047-2050, 1986.
141. Girinski T, Pejovic-Lenfant M, Bourhis J, et al: Prognostic value of hemoglobin concentrations and blood transfusions in advanced carcinoma of the cervix treated by radiation therapy: Results of a retrospective study of 386 patients. Int J Radiat Oncol Biol Phys 16:37-42, 1989.
142. Grogan M, Thomas GM, Melamed I, et al: The importance of hemoglobin levels during radiotherapy for carcinoma of the cervix. Cancer 86:1528-1536, 1999
143. Kapp KS, Poschauko J, Geyer E, et al: Evaluation of the effect of routine packed red blood cell transfusion in anemic cervix cancer patients treated with radical radiotherapy. Int J Radiat Oncol Biol Phys 54:58-66, 2002.
144. Bush RS, Jenkin RDT, Allt WEC, et al: Definitive evidence for hypoxic cells influencing cure in cancer therapy. Br J Cancer 37:302-306, 1978 (suppl 3).
145. Hockel M, Schlenger K, Aral B, et al: Association between tumor hypoxia and malignant progression in advanced cancer of the uterine cervix. Cancer Res 56:4509-4515, 1996.
146. Fyles AW, Milosevic M, Wong R, et al: Oxygenation predicts radiation response and survival in patients with cervix cancer. Radiother Oncol 48:149-156, 1998.
147. Dorie MJ, Brown JM: Tumor-specific, schedule-dependent interaction between tirapazamine (SR 4233) and cisplatin. Cancer Res 53:4633-4636, 1993.
148. Gatzemeier U, Rodriguez, G, Treat J, et al: Tirapazamine-cisplatin: the synergy. Br J Cancer 77(suppl 4):15-17, 1998.
149. Dachs GU, Tozer GM. Hypoxia modulated gene expression: angiogenesis, metastasis, and therapeutic exploitation. Eur J Cancer 36:1649-1660, 2000.
150. Grigsby PW, Perez CA: Radiotherapy alone for medically inoperable carcinoma of the cervix: Stage IA and carcinoma in situ. Int J Radiat Oncol Biol Phys 21:375-378, 1991.
151. Kolstad P: Follow-up study of 232 patients with stage Ia1 and 411 patients with stage Ia2 squamous cell carcinoma of the cervix (microinvasive carcinoma). Gynecol Oncol 33:265-272, 1989.
152. Hamberger AD, Fletcher GH, Wharton JT: Results of treatment of early Stage I carcinoma of the uterine cervix with intracavitary radium alone. Cancer 41:980-985, 1978.
153. Fletcher GH: Textbook of Radiotherapy. Philadelphia, Lea & Febiger, 1980.
154. Perez CA: Uterine cervix. *In* Perez CA, Brady LW (eds): Principles and Practice of Radiation Oncology, 2nd ed. Philadelphia, JB Lippincott, 1992.
155. Burghardt E, Pickel H: Local spread and lymph node involvement in cervical cancer. Obstet Gynecol 52:138-145, 1978.
156. Alvarez RD, Potter ME, Soong SJ, et al: Rationale for using pathologic tumor dimensions and nodal status to subclassify surgically treated stage IB cervical cancer patients. Gynecol Oncol 43:108-112, 1991.
157. Landoni F, Maneo A, Colombo A, et al: Randomised study of radical surgery versus radiotherapy for stage Ib-IIa cervical cancer. Lancet 350:535-540, 1997.
158. Reesink-Peters N, van der Velden J, ten Hoor KA, et al: Preoperative serum squamous cell carcinoma antigen levels in clinical decision making for patients with early-stage cervical cancer. J Clin Oncol 23:1455-1462, 2005.
159. Dargent D, Brun JL, Roy M, Remy I: Pregnancies following radical trachelectomy for invasive cervical cancer [abstract]. Gynecol Oncol 52:105, 1994.
160. Roy M, Plante M: Pregnancies after radical vaginal trachelectomy for early-stage cervical cancer. Am J Obstet Gynecol 179:1491-1496, 1998.
161. Covens A, Shaw P, Murphy J, et al: Is radical trachelectomy a safe alternative to radical hysterectomy for patients with stage IA-B carcinoma of the cervix? Cancer 86:2273-2279, 1999.
162. Rodriguez M, Guimares O, Rose PG: Radical abdominal trachelectomy and pelvic lymphadenectomy with uterine conservation and subsequent pregnancy in the treatment of early invasive cervical cancer. Am J Obstet Gynecol 185;370-374, 2001.
163. Bernardini M, Barrett J, Seaward G, Covens A: Pregnancy outcomes in patients with radical trachelectomy. Am J Obstet Gynecol 189:1378-1382, 2003.
164. Thomas GM, Dembo AJ: Is there a role for adjuvant pelvic radiotherapy after radical hysterectomy in early stage cervical cancer? Int J Gynecol Cancer 1:1-8, 1991.
165. Koh WJ, Panwala K, Greer B: Adjuvant therapy for high-risk, early stage cervical cancer. Sem Radiat Oncol 10:51-60, 2000.
166. Stock RG, Chen ASJ, Karasek K: Patterns of spread in node-positive cervical cancer: the relationship between local control and distant metastases. Cancer J Sci Am 2:256-262, 1996.
167. Bandy LC, Clarke-Pearson DL, Soper JT, et al: Long-term effects on bladder function following radical hysterectomy with and without postoperative radiation. Gynecol Oncol 26:160-168, 1987.
168. Barter JF, Soong SJ, Shingleton HM, et al: Complications of combined radical hysterectomy-postoperative radiation therapy in women with early stage cervical cancer. Gynecol Oncol 32:292-296, 1989.
169. Montz FJ, Holschneider CH, Solh S, et al: Small bowel obstruction following radical hysterectomy: risk factors, incidence and operative findings. Gynecol Oncol 53:114-120, 1994.
170. Remy JC, Fruchter RG, Choi K, et al: Complications of combined radical hysterectomy and pelvic radiation. Gynecol Oncol 24:317-326, 1986.
171. Sedlis A, Bundy BN, Rotman MZ, et al: A randomized trial of pelvic radiation therapy versus no further therapy in selected patients with stage IB carcinoma of the cervix after radical hysterectomy and pelvic lymphadenectomy: a Gynecologic Oncology Group study. Gynecol Oncol 73:177-183, 1999.
172. Finan MA, DeCesare S, Fiorica JV, et al: Radical hysterectomy for stage IB1 versus IB2 carcinoma of the cervix: does the new staging system predict morbidity and survival? Gynecol Oncol 62:139-147, 1996.
173. Rutledge TL, Kamelle SA, Tillmanns TD, et al: A comparison of stages IB1 and IB2 cervical cancers treated with radical hysterectomy. Is size the real difference? Gynecol Oncol 95:70-76, 2004.
174. Roman LD, Morris M, Mitchell MF, et al: Prognostic factors for patients undergoing simple hysterectomy in the presence of invasive cancer of the cervix. Gynecol Oncol 50:179-184, 1993.
175. Durrance FY, Fletcher GH, Rutledge FN: Analysis of central recurrent disease in stages I and II squamous cell carcinomas of the cervix on intact uterus. Am J Roentgenol 106:831-838, 1969.
176. O'Quinn AG, Fletcher GH, Wharton JT: Guidelines for conservative hysterectomy after irradiation. Gynecol Oncol 9:68-79, 1980.
177. Thoms WW, Eifel PJ, Smith TL, et al: Bulky endocervical carcinomas: A 23-year experience. Int J Radiat Oncol Biol Phys 23:491-499, 1992.
178. Mendenhall WM, McCarty PJ, Morgan LS, et al: Stage IB-IIA-B carcinoma of the intact uterine cervix greater than or equal to 6 cm in diameter: Is adjuvant extrafascial hysterectomy beneficial? Int J Radiat Oncol Biol Phys 21:899-904, 1991.
179. Keys HM, Bundy BN, Stehman FB, et al: Radiation therapy with and without extrafascial hysterectomy for bulky stage IB cervical carcinoma: a randomized trial of the Gynecologic Oncology Group. Gynecol Oncol 89:343-353, 2003.
180. Koh WJ, Paley PJ, Comsia ND, Greer B: Radical management of recurrent cervical cancer. *In* Eifel PJ, Levenback C (eds): Cancer of the Female Lower Genital Tract—American Cancer Society Atlas of Clinical Oncology. London, BC Decker, 2001, pp 169-182.
181. Ijaz T, Eifel PJ, Burke T, Oswold MJ: Radiation therapy of pelvic recurrence after radical hysterectomy for cervical carcinoma. Gynecol Oncol 70:241-246, 1998.
182. Thomas GM, Dembo AJ, Myhr T, et al: Long-term results of concurrent radiation and chemotherapy for carcinoma of the cervix recurrent after surgery. Int J Gynecol Cancer 3:193-198, 1993.
183. Russell AH, Koh WJ, Markette K, et al: Radical reirradiation for recurrent or second primary carcinoma of the female reproductive tract. Gynecol Oncol 27:226-232, 1987.

184. Randall ME, Evans L, Greven KM, et al: Interstitial reirradiation for recurrent gynecologic malignancies: results and analysis of prognostic factors. Gynecol Oncol 48:23-31, 1993.
185. Morley GW, Hopkins MP, Lindenauer SM, Roberts JA: Pelvic exenteration, University of Michigan: 100 patients at 5 years. Obstet Gynecol 74:934-943, 1989.
186. Shingleton HM, Soong SJ, Gelder MS, et al: Clinical and histopathologic factors predicting recurrence and survival after pelvic exenteration for cancer of the cervix. Obstet Gynecol 73:1027-1034, 1989.
187. Stanhope CR, Webb MJ, Prodratz KC: Pelvic exenteration for recurrent cervical cancer. Clin Obstet Gynecol 33:897-909, 1990.
188. Stelzer KJ, Koh WK, Greer BE, et al: The use of intraoperative radiation therapy in radical salvage for recurrent cervical cancer: outcome and toxicity. Am J Obstet Gynecol 172:1881-1888, 1995.
189. Garton GR, Gunderson LL, Webb MJ, et al: Intraoperative radiation therapy in gynecologic cancer: update of the experience at a single institution. Int J Radiat Oncol Biol Phys 37:839-843, 1997.
190. Thigpen JT, Singleton H, Homesley H, et al: cis-Platinum in treatment of advanced or recurrent squamous cell carcinoma of the cervix: a phase II trial of the Gynecologic Oncology Group. Cancer 48:899-903, 1981.
191. Bonomi P, Blessing JA, Stehman FB, et al: Randomized trial of three cisplatin dose schedules in squamous-cell carcinoma of the cervix: a Gynecologic Oncology Group study. J Clin Oncol 3:1079-1085, 1985.
192. Thigpen JT, Blessing JA, DiSaia PJ, et al: A randomized comparison of rapid versus prolonged (24 hr) infusion of cisplatin in therapy of squamous cell carcinoma of the uterine cervix: a Gynecologic Oncology Group study. Gynecol Oncol 32:198-202, 1989.
193. McGuire WP, Arseneau JC, Blessing JA, et al: A randomized comparative trial of carboplatin and iproplatin in advanced squamous carcinoma of the uterine cervix: a Gynecologic Oncology Group study. J Clin Oncol 7:1462-1468, 1989.
194. Stehman FB, Blessing JA, McGehee R, Barrett RJ: A phase II evaluation of mitolactol in patients with advanced squamous cell carcinoma of the cervix: a Gynecologic Oncology Group study. J Clin Oncol 7:1892-1895, 1989.
195. Sutton GP, Blessing JA, McGuire WP, et al: Phase II trial of ifosfamide and mesna in patients with advanced or recurrent squamous carcinoma of the cervix who had never received chemotherapy: a Gynecologic Oncology Group study. Am J Obstet Gynecol 168:805-807, 1993.
196. McGuire WP, Blessing JA, Moore DH, et al: Paclitaxel has moderate activity in squamous cervix cancer: a Gynecologic Oncology Group study. J Clin Oncol 14:792-795, 1996.
197. Bookman MA, Blessing JA, Hanjani P, et al: Topotecan in squamous cell carcinoma of the cervix: a phase II study of the Gynecologic Oncology Group. Gynecol Oncol 77:446-449, 2000.
198. Schilder RJ, Blessing JA, Morgan M, et al: Evaluation of gemcitabine in patients with squamous cell carcinoma of the cervix: a phase II study of the Gynecologic Oncology Group. Gynecol Oncol 76:204-207, 2000.
199. Morris M, Brader KR, Levenback C, et al: Phase II study of vinorelbine in advanced and recurrent squamous cell carcinoma of the cervix. J Clin Oncol 16:1094-1098, 1998.
200. Omura GA, Blessing JA, Vaccarello L, et al: A randomized trial of cisplatin versus cisplatin plus mitolactol versus cisplatin plus ifosfamide in advanced squamous carcinoma of the cervix: a Gynecologic Oncology Group study. J Clin Oncol 15:165-171, 1997.
201. Bloss JD, Blessing JA, Behrens BC, et al: Randomized trial of cisplatin and ifosfamide with or without bleomycin in squamous carcinoma of the cervix: a Gynecologic Oncology Group study. J Clin Oncol 20:1832-1837, 2002.
202. Moore DH, Blessing JA, McQuellon RP, et al: Phase III study of cisplatin with or without paclitaxel in stage IVB, recurrent, or persistent squamous cell carcinoma of the cervix: a Gynecologic Oncology Group trial. J Clin Oncol 22:3113-9, 2004.
203. Long HJ, Bundy BN, Grendys EC, et al: Randomized phase III trial of cisplatin with or without topotecan in carcinoma of the uterine cervix: a Gynecologic Oncology Group study. J Clin Oncol 23:4626-4633, 2005.
204. Spanos WJ, Wasserman T, Meoz R, et al: Palliation of advanced pelvic malignant disease with large fraction pelvic radiation and misonidazole: Final report of RTOG phase I/II study. Int J Radiat Oncol Biol Phys 13:1479-1482, 1987.
205. Adelson MD, Wharton JT, Delclos L, et al: Palliative radiotherapy for ovarian cancer. Int J Radiat Oncol Biol Phys 13:17-21, 1987.
206. Boulware RJ, Caderao JB, Delclos L, et al: Whole pelvis megavoltage irradiation with single doses of 1000 rad to palliate advanced gynecologic cancers. Int J Radiat Oncol Biol Phys 5:333-338, 1979.
207. Spanos WJ, Perez CA, Marcus S, et al: Effect of rest interval on tumor and normal tissue response-a report of phase III study of accelerated split course palliative radiation for advanced pelvic malignancies (RTOG-8502). Int J Radiat Oncol Biol Phys 25:399-403, 1993.
208. McIntyre JF, Eifel PJ, Levenback C, et al: Ureteral stricture as a late complication of radiotherapy for stage IB carcinoma of the uterine cervix. Cancer 75:836-843, 1995.
209. Greer BE, Koh WJ, Figge DC, et al: Gynecologic radiotherapy fields defined by intraoperative measurements. Gynecol Oncol 38:421-424, 1990.
210. Kim RY, RY, McGinnis S, Spencer SA, et al: Conventional four-field pelvic radiotherapy technique without computed tomography-treatment planning in cancer of the cervix: potential geographic miss and its impact on pelvic control. Int J Radiat Oncol Biol Phys 31:109-112, 1994.
211. Bonin SR, Lanciano RM, Corn BW, et al: Bony landmarks are not an adequate substitute for lymphangiography in defining pelvic node location for the treatment of cervical cancer with radiotherapy. Int J Radiat Oncol Biol Phys 34:167-172, 1996.
212. Portalance L, Chao KSC, Grigsby PW, et al: Intensity-modulated radiation therapy (IMRT) reduces small bowel, rectum, and bladder doses in patients with cervical cancer receiving pelvic and para-aortic radiation. Int J Radiat Oncol Biol Phys 51:261-266, 2001.
213. Mundt AJ, Lujan AE, Rotmensch J, et al: Intensity-modulated whole pelvic radiotherapy in women with gynecologic malignancies. Int J Radiat Oncol Biol Phys 52:1330-1337, 2002
214. Brixey CJ, Roeske JC, Lujan AE, et al: Impact of intensity-modulated radiotherapy on acute hematologic toxicity in women with gynecologic malignancies. Int J Radiat Oncol Biol Phys 54:1388-1396, 2002.
215. Patel FD, Sharma SC, Negi PS et al: Low dose rate versus high dose rate brachytherapy in the treatment of carcinoma of the uterine cervix: a clinical trial. Int J Radiat Oncol Biol Phys 28:335-341, 1994.
216. Teshima T, Inoue T, Ikeda T, et al: High-dose rate and low-dose rate intracavitary therapy for carcinoma of the uterine cervix. Final results of Osaka University Hospital. Cancer 72:2409-2414, 1993.
217. Hareyama M, Sakata K, Oouchi A, et al: High-dose-rate versus low-dose-rate intracavitary therapy for carcinoma of the uterine cervix: a randomized trial. Cancer 94:117-124, 2002.
218. Lertsanguansinchai P, Lertbutsayanukul C, Shotelersuk K, et al: Phase III randomized trial comparing LDR and HDR brachytherapy in treatment of cervical cancer. Int J Radiat Oncol Biol Phys 59:1424-1431, 2004.
219. Orton CG, Seyedsadr M, Somnay A: Comparison of high and low dose rate remote afterloading for cervix cancer and the importance of fractionation. Int J Radiat Oncol Biol Phys 21:1425-1426, 1991.
220. Petereit DG, Sarkaria JN, Petter DM, Schink JC: High-dose-rate versus low-dose-rate brachytherapy in the treatment of cervical cancer; analysis of tumor recurrence—the University of Wisconsin experience. Int J Radiat Oncol Biol Phys 45:1267-1274, 1999.
221. Arai T, Nakano T, Morita S, et al: High dose rate remote afterloading intracavitary radiation therapy for cancer of the uterine cervix. Cancer 69:175-180, 1992.
222. Eifel PJ, Moughan J, Erickson B, et al: Patterns of radiotherapy practice for patients with carcinoma of the uterine cervix: a pat-

terns of care study. Int J Radiat Oncol Biol Phys 60:1144-1153, 2004.

223. Katz A, Eifel PJ: Quantification of intracavitary brachytherapy parameters and correlation with outcome in patients with carcinoma of the cervix. Int J Radiat Oncol Biol Phys 48:1417-1425, 2000.
224. Thirion P, Kelly C, Salib O, et al: A randomized comparison of two brachytherapy devices for the treatment of uterine cervical carcinoma. Radiother Oncol 74:247-250, 2005.
225. International Commission on Radiation Units and Measurements: Dose and Volume Specification for Reporting Intracavitary Therapy in Gynecology. Vol 38. Bethesda, MD, International Commission on Radiation Units and Measurements, 1985, pp 1-23.
226. Haie-Meder C, Kramar A, Lambin P, et al: Analysis of complications in a prospective randomized trial comparing two brachytherapy low dose rates in cervical carcinoma. Int J Radiat Oncol Biol Phys 29:1195-1197, 1994.
227. Scalliet P, Gerbaulet A, Dubray B: HDR versus LDR gynecological brachytherapy revisited. Radiother Oncol 28:118-126, 1993.
228. Stitt JA, Fowler JF, Thomadsen BR, et al: High dose rate intracavitary brachytherapy for carcinoma of the cervix: The Madison system: I. Clinical and radiobiological considerations. Int J Radiat Oncol Biol Phys 24:383-386, 1992.
229. Ogino I, Kitamura T, Okamoto N, et al: Late rectal complication following high dose rate intracavitary brachytherapy in cancer of the cervix. Int J Radiat Oncol Biol Phys 31:725-734, 1995.
230. Petereit DG, Pearcey R: Literature analysis of high dose rate brachytherapy fractionation schedules in the treatment of cervical cancer: is there an optimal fractionation schedule? Int J Radiat Oncol Biol Phys 43:359-366, 1999.
231. Brandt K, Petereit DG, Sarkaria J, et al: Conscious sedation in outpatient GYN HDR brachytherapy. Proceedings, First Annual Multidisciplinary Radiation Oncology Conference. Philadelphia, 1996.
232. Aristizabal SA, Woolfitt B, Valencia A, et al: Interstitial parametrial implants in carcinoma of the cervix stage II-B. Int J Radiat Oncol Biol Phys 13:445-450, 1987.
233. Martinez A, Edmundson GK, Cox RS, et al: Combination of external-beam irradiation and multiple-site perineal applicator (MUPIT) for treatment of locally advanced or recurrent prostatic, anorectal, and gynecologic malignancies. Int J Radiat Oncol Biol Phys 11:391-398, 1985.
234. Syed AMN, Puthwala AA, Neblett D, et al: Transperineal interstitial-intracavitary "Syed-Neblett" applicator in the treatment of carcinoma of the uterine cervix. Endocuriether Hyperther Oncol 2:1-13, 1986.
235. Hughes-Davies L, Silver B, Kapp D: Parametrial interstitial brachytherapy for advanced or recurrent pelvic malignancy: The Harvard/Stanford experience. Gynecol Oncol 58:24-27, 1995.
236. Eifel PJ, Morris M, Delclos L, et al: Radiation therapy for cervical carcinoma. *In* Dilts PV Jr, Sciarra JJ (eds): Gynecology and Obstetrics. Philadelphia, JB Lippincott, 1993, pp 1-25.
237. Schoeppel SJ, LaVigne M, Martel MK, et al: Three-dimensional treatment planning of intracavitary gynecologic implants: analysis of ten cases and implications for dose specification. Int J Radiat Oncol Biol Phys 28:277-283, 1993.
238. Perez CA, Grigsby PW, Lockett MA, Chao KS, Williamson J: Radiation therapy morbidity in carcinoma of the uterine cervix: dosimetric and clinical correlation. Int J Radiat Oncol Biol Phys 44:855-866, 1999.
239. Eifel PJ, Levenback C, Wharton JT, Oswald MJ: Time course and incidence of late complications in patients treated with radiation therapy for FIGO stage IB carcinoma of the uterine cervix. Int J Radiat Oncol Biol Phys 32:1289-1300, 1995.
240. Eifel PJ, Jhingran A, Bodurka DC, Levenback C, Thames H: Correlation of smoking history and other patient characteristics with major complications of pelvic radiation therapy for cervical cancer. J Clin Oncol 20:3651-3657, 2002.
241. Kirwan JM, Symonds P, Green JA, et al: A systematic review of acute and late toxicity of concomitant chemoradiation for cervical cancer. Radiother Oncol 68:217-226, 2003.
242. Rotte K: Comparison of HDR afterloading and classical techniques for radiation therapy of cancer of the cervix uteri. Acta Select Brachyther (Suppl) 2:42-46, 1991.
243. Kataoka M, Kawamura M, Nishiyama Y, et al: Results of the combination of external-beam and high dose rate intracavitary irradiation for patients with cervical carcinoma. Gynecol Oncol 44:48-52, 1992.
244. Utley J, von Essen C, Horn R, et al: High-dose-rate afterloading brachytherapy in carcinoma of the uterine cervix. Int J Radiat Oncol Biol Phys 10:2259-2263, 1984.

CHAPTER 56

ENDOMETRIAL CANCER

Carien L. Creutzberg

INCIDENCE

Endometrial cancer is the most common gynecologic malignancy, and it is the fourth most common cancer in women, with an incidence rate in the United States of 25 cases per 100,000 women.

The estimated incidence for U.S. women in 2006 was 41,200 cases. The mortality rate was 4 deaths per 100,000 women, with an estimated 7350 deaths in 2006.

BIOLOGIC CHARACTERISTICS

Two types of endometrial carcinoma have been distinguished: type I, which is associated with estrogen and has a favorable prognosis, and type 2, which is unrelated to estrogen, is more often non-endometrioid, and has an inferior outcome.

More than 75% of endometrial cancers are endometrioid carcinomas, and 20% to 25% are non-endometrioid cancers, including 5% to 10% serous carcinomas, 1% to 5% clear cell carcinomas, and 1% to 3% mucinous carcinomas. Up to 5% are other uterine cancers, including uterine sarcomas (i.e., carcinosarcoma, leiomyosarcoma, and endometrial stroma sarcoma).

Risk factors include tumor stage, histologic cell type, tumor grade, depth of myometrial invasion, lymph node metastases, lymphovascular invasion, and the patient's age.

STAGING EVALUATION

Evaluation should include the patient's history and physical examination, including vaginal inspection and bimanual pelvic examination, endometrial biopsy, chest radiograph, complete blood cell count, and chemistries. The International Federation of Gynecology and Obstetrics (FIGO) staging is based on the surgical and pathology findings.

Computed tomography or magnetic resonance imaging of the abdomen and pelvis is indicated for locally advanced disease and medically inoperable patients.

PRIMARY THERAPY AND RESULTS

Abdominal hysterectomy with bisalpingo-oophorectomy is the primary therapy.

The role of lymphadenectomy remains a subject of controversy. It is used primarily for staging purposes and to tailor adjuvant therapy. It may have therapeutic value for grade 3 cancers, unfavorable histologic types, and advanced disease; however, no survival benefit was seen in a phase III trial.

The 5-year survival rate is 80% to 90% for patients with stage I endometrial carcinoma, 60% to 80% for stage II, and 30% to 80% for stage III disease because of the diverse extent of and prognosis for tumors classified as stage III.

Primary radiation therapy for medically inoperable patients provides 5-year survival rates of 50% to 85% and local control rates of 70% to 90% for stage I disease.

ADJUVANT THERAPY

Radiation therapy can significantly improve local control and disease-free survival for patients with stage I disease, but it confers no overall survival advantage. For intermediate-risk disease, the indication for radiation therapy is tailored to prognostic factors. Patients with grade 3 tumors, outer 50% myometrial invasion, advanced age, or lymphovascular space invasion should be considered for adjuvant pelvic irradiation. Brachytherapy alone may be considered for stage IC, grade 1 or 2 disease, preferably within the scope of clinical trials.

Adjuvant therapy is not indicated for treating low-risk disease (i.e., stage IA-B, grade 1-2 endometrioid carcinoma).

Pelvic irradiation is indicated for high-risk and locally advanced disease. Adjuvant chemotherapy, concurrent chemoradiation, or sequential irradiation and chemotherapy should be considered; however, these patients should be enrolled in clinical trials.

LOCALLY ADVANCED DISEASE

Patients with locally advanced pelvic disease should have optimal debulking surgery followed by radiation therapy. These patients should be considered for clinical trials of chemotherapy or concurrent chemoradiation.

Gross residual disease should be considered for palliative treatment.

PALLIATION

Metastatic disease or nonresectable local disease can be treated with chemotherapy or hormonal therapy.

Palliative irradiation should be offered to symptomatic patients because it provides excellent relief of symptoms such as blood loss, vaginal discharge, pain and edema caused by local disease or lymphadenopathy, and symptoms from distant metastases, such as pain caused by bone involvement or symptomatic brain metastases.

Endometrial carcinoma is the most frequent gynecologic malignancy diagnosed in the United States and European countries, and it is the fourth most common cancer in women. Because most patients present with early-stage disease, their prognosis is usually favorable. The relative 5-year survival rate is 84% for all patients. Patients with uterus-confined disease have a 5-year relative survival rate of 96%, compared with 67% for those with regional involvement.[1]

Even after the publication of three randomized trials, controversies in the management of stage I endometrial carcinoma remain. The optimal extent of surgery, especially the role of pelvic and para-aortic lymphadenectomy, is one of these issues. The indications for pelvic irradiation and the use of brachytherapy are also a source of dispute. Trials investigating these issues are being conducted.

Despite the favorable outcome for most patients, there remain patients with advanced disease or poor histologic subtypes who have poor prognoses. The optimal treatment for these patients is the challenge for the next decade of research, including studies of extended surgery and appropriate adjuvant therapies, such as radiation therapy with concurrent and adjuvant chemotherapy. Clinical and basic research continues to investigate the biology, especially of non-endometrioid cancers, and searches for new molecular markers and targeted therapies, including biologic agents.

EPIDEMIOLOGY AND ETIOLOGY

Epidemiology

The incidence of endometrial cancer in the United States is 25 cases per 100,000 women, and it has remained stable since 1995.[1] The U.S. incidence is among the highest in the world. European countries report incidence rates ranging from 15 to 20 cases per 100,000 women.[2] The American Cancer Society estimates that a total of 41,200 new cancers of the uterus will be diagnosed in 2006.[1] This represents 6% of the estimated 668,470 new female malignancies, and it is the most common gynecologic malignancy and the fourth most common cancer in women. The mortality rate for uterine cancer in the United States is 4 deaths per 100,000, and the estimate for 2006 was 7350 deaths, which was 2.5% of all cancer deaths among women and 25% of all deaths from gynecologic malignancies. The mortality rates decreased from 5.3 to 4.1 deaths per 100,000 women between 1973 and 1995; however, the mortality rate has remained stable since 1995.[1]

Uterine cancer is typically a cancer of postmenopausal women between 55 and 85 years old, with peak incidence rates exceeding 95 per 100,000 women 65 to 80 years old.[1] Less than 5% of the patients are younger than 40 years. Uterine sarcomas also manifest primarily in the postmenopausal population. Leiomyosarcomas occur at an earlier age than carcinosarcomas.[3]

Etiology

The cause of endometrial carcinoma is related to exposure of the endometrium to unopposed estrogens. Many studies have documented the association of endometrial cancer with increased exogenous or endogenous estrogen exposure.[4] Early menarche, late menopause, obesity, nulliparity, infertility, and estrogen-producing ovarian tumors are classically associated with the development of endometrial cancer. In obese women, elevated estrogen levels due to increased peripheral conversion of androstenedione may be the underlying mechanism for the increased risk. Endometrial cancer has also been associated with conditions such as hypertension and diabetes, but it is not clear whether these are true independent risk factors or related to obesity.[5] Unopposed exogenous estrogen levels have strong association with the risk of endometrial cancer.[6] The use of tamoxifen for the prevention or treatment of breast cancer has been documented to statistically increase the risk of subsequent endometrial cancer.[7-10] Despite its antiestrogen effects on breast tissue, tamoxifen has some weak estrogenic effects on other organs of the body, including the uterus, which accounts for this risk.

Patients who have endometrial biopsies confirming complex hyperplasia with atypia have a 30% to 40% risk of subsequent development of endometrial cancer. Hyperplasia with atypia is considered a premalignant phase of endometrioid carcinoma and has a similar origin.[11]

An increased risk associated with a family history of endometrial cancer has been observed, especially in women younger than 50 years, but less than 1% of all endometrial cancers were attributable to familial and potentially genetic factors.[12-14] Familial clustering of ovarian and endometrial cancers specific to the endometrioid morphology has been reported.[15,16] The risk of developing other malignancies, especially of the colon and breast, is increased after the diagnosis of endometrial carcinoma.[15,17] Women with mutations in the *MLH1* or *MSH2* genes, which are responsible for hereditary nonpolyposis colorectal cancer (HNPCC) syndrome, are at increased risk for developing endometrial cancer.[18,19] HNPCC, or Lynch syndrome, is classified based on the presence or absence of tumors other than colorectal cancers. Lynch syndrome II patients have a high risk of endometrial cancer, second only to that of colorectal cancers.[20,21] Women with Lynch syndrome II have a 20% risk of developing endometrial cancer before 50 years of age, which increases to 60% by 60 years.

PREVENTION AND DETECTION

No measures to prevent endometrial cancer other than avoiding unopposed estrogen use have been identified. Prophylactic hysterectomy is recommended in patients with known hyperplasia with atypia[11,22,23] and prophylactic hysterectomy and oophorectomy in Lynch syndrome II gene carriers, for whom the risk of concurrent or subsequent endometrial cancer is substantial.[20,21] Chemoprevention using Depo-Provera (depomedroxyprogesterone acetate) or oral contraceptives is being studied among HNPCC mutation carriers in the M.D. Anderson Cancer Center.

Screening for endometrial cancer has not been performed in the general population. The early symptoms and favorable prognosis of this disease preclude efficacy of population screening.[24] Vaginal ultrasound studies alone have not been found effective for screening purposes.[25] Prompt analysis of every patient with postmenopausal or abnormal vaginal bleeding with vaginal ultrasound studies and endometrial biopsy is indicated.

Screening of patients using tamoxifen has been suggested. However, the characteristic hyperplastic aspect of the endometrium at ultrasound studies leads to high false-positive rates and frequent invasive diagnostic procedures in asymptomatic tamoxifen users.[26,27] In a prospective ultrasound screening study of 247 tamoxifen users, it was shown that of 52 asymptomatic patients with a thickened endometrium, most had an atrophic endometrium, and only 1 had cancer, whereas in 2 of 20 patients with vaginal bleeding, endometrial cancer was diagnosed.[27] The study authors concluded that routine ultrasound screening is not indicated in asymptomatic women using tamoxifen but that all women with abnormal bleeding should be evaluated.

Studies evaluating intensive screening programs of HNPCC gene carriers not electing prophylactic surgery are ongoing (GOG, M.D. Anderson). Because transvaginal ultrasound alone has not been found effective, serial ultrasound studies are used in conjunction with annual endometrial biopsy.

PATHOLOGY AND PATTERNS OF SPREAD

Pathology

Almost all uterine epithelial cancers are adenocarcinomas. The World Health Organization (WHO) has described several subtypes (Table 56-1). The most common type of endometrial adenocarcinoma is the endometrioid type, which accounts for 75% of cases.[28,29] Other histologic types, also referred to as

Table 56-1 World Health Organization Histologic Classification of Epithelial Tumors of the Uterus

Endometrioid adenocarcinoma
Villoglandular
Secretory
Ciliated cell
Variant with squamous differentiation
Mucinous adenocarcinoma
Serous adenocarcinoma
Clear cell adenocarcinoma
Mixed cell adenocarcinoma
Squamous cell carcinoma
Transitional cell carcinoma
Small cell carcinoma
Undifferentiated carcinoma

Table 56-2 World Health Organization Histologic Classification of Mesenchymal and Mixed Tumors of the Uterus

MESENCHYMAL TUMORS
Smooth muscle tumors
Leiomyoma, not otherwise specified
Smooth muscle tumor of uncertain malignant potential
Leiomyosarcoma
Epithelioid variant
Myxoid variant
Endometrial stromal and related tumors
Endometrial stromal nodule
Endometrial stromal sarcoma, low grade
Undifferentiated endometrial sarcoma
Miscellaneous mesenchymal tumors
Mixed endometrial stromal and smooth muscle tumor
Adenomatoid tumor
Perivascular epithelioid cell tumor
Other mesenchymal tumors (benign and malignant)
MIXED EPITHELIAL AND MESENCHYMAL TUMORS
Adenofibroma
Adenomyoma
Atypical polypoid adenomyoma
Adenosarcoma
Carcinosarcoma (malignant mixed müllerian tumor)
Carcinofibroma

non-endometrioid endometrial carcinomas (NEECs), include serous (5% to 10%), mucinous (1% to 3%), and clear cell carcinomas (1% to 5%). Uterine mesenchymal and mixed tumors, usually called the uterine sarcomas, include leiomyosarcoma, endometrial stromal sarcoma, and carcinosarcoma (or malignant mixed müllerian tumor [MMMT]). The WHO classification of mesenchymal and mixed tumors of the uterus is summarized in Table 56-2. Carcinosarcoma is the most common type of uterine sarcoma (45%), followed by leiomyosarcoma (40%) and endometrial stromal sarcoma (10% to 15%). Carcinosarcomas are composed of malignant epithelial and stromal components, and because of this biphasic appearance, their origin has long been debated. Based on molecular genetic analysis, the current opinion is that these cancers should be considered metaplastic carcinomas. Clinical data support this view that carcinosarcomas should be considered high-risk carcinomas.[28,30,31]

Non-endometrioid histologic types have a poorer prognosis. Serous and clear cell carcinomas are uniformly identified in this category. Serous adenocarcinoma has also been called uterine papillary serous carcinoma (UPSC). It is histologically similar to its ovarian counterpart. UPSC was first described in 1982 and was found to have a higher rate of failure within the abdomen, as in ovarian cancer.[32,33] This entity can be confused with the papillary villoglandular subtype of endometrioid adenocarcinoma, which carries a significantly more favorable prognosis. Serous carcinoma is frequently diagnosed at a higher stage than endometrioid adenocarcinomas. Clear cell carcinoma has been reported to have the same poor prognosis, with more advanced disease at diagnosis.[34,35] Serous and clear cell carcinomas have been shown to have outcomes similar to grade 3 endometrioid carcinoma.[36,37]

Adenosquamous cell carcinoma has been suggested by some investigators to be another poor histologic subtype,[34,35] but others think the prognosis of these patients is no different from that for the typical endometrioid adenocarcinoma.[38,39] Zaino[38] evaluated a large population of patients who were part of a Gynecologic Oncology Group (GOG) study and found a parallel between the glandular grade and the degree of differentiation in the squamous component. It was subsequently suggested that the name of this histologic subtype should reflect the lack of importance of this feature by calling it adenocarcinoma with squamous differentiation.

Endometrial hyperplasia frequently precedes endometrial carcinoma. Endometrial hyperplasia is considered a precursor of endometrioid carcinoma, and endometrial intraepithelial carcinoma has been associated with the development of non-endometrioid carcinoma. The International Society of Gynecological Pathologists has identified two architectural forms of endometrial hyperplasia, simple and complex. Endometrial hyperplasia displaying marked architectural abnormalities is designated *complex hyperplasia*, whereas lesions with a lesser degree of architectural abnormalities are designated *simple hyperplasia*. Atypical nuclear changes can be associated with the simple or complex types and are regarded separately from hyperplasia that is not displaying atypia. Progression of simple hyperplasia to endometrioid carcinoma is rare (<2%), whereas progression to carcinoma occurs in 30% to 40% of the patients with simple and complex hyperplasia with atypia.[11,22,23,40,41] The risk of subsequent endometrial cancer warrants hysterectomy in patients with hyperplasia displaying atypia.

Not all endometrial cancers arise in a setting of atypical hyperplasia. Non-endometrioid cancers, especially serous carcinomas, are related to endometrial intraepithelial carcinoma, which appears to represent malignant transformation of atrophic endometrium. It is found in the adjacent endometrium of up to 90% of serous carcinomas.[42]

Patterns of Spread

Endometrial cancer remains confined to the uterine body for a long time. The initial spread occurs by local extension along the endometrial surface. Subsequent growth continues in the radial and longitudinal directions. Longitudinal growth results in involvement of the lower uterine segment and the cervix, initially involving the endocervical glands and later spreading by cervical stromal invasion. The tumor can also extend along the cornua to the fallopian tubes. Radial growth results in myometrial invasion, initially superficially and later penetrating to the subserosa and the serosa. Two patterns of myometrial invasion have been described: an expansive growth pattern with pushing borders and an infiltrating growth pattern with cancer cells and nests penetrating the myometrium haphazardly.[43,44] The infiltrating growth pattern is associated with frequent lymphovascular space invasion and early lymphatic spread. After the tumor breaches the serosa, transperitoneal dissemination can occur, with a pattern resembling that of ovarian cancer. Occasionally, after extensive penetration of the myometrium or the cervix, direct invasion of the bladder or the rectum may occur, or the tumor may involve the pelvic soft tissues and continue to reach the pelvic sidewall. Peritoneal seeding can result from growth through the serosa or from transtubal spillage of tumor cells into the peritoneal cavity.

The more extensive the direct invasion, the higher the risk of lymph node metastasis.[45,46] The endometrium has few lymphatics, but after the tumor penetrates the myometrium and especially when it reaches the lymphatic-rich subserosa, spread by lymphatic invasion is common. Lymphatics from the uterine fundus can drain directly to the para-aortic lymph nodes. Typically, the internal and external iliac lymph node groups are the first echelon of spread. Sentinel node detection studies[47-49] have shown the sentinel nodes to be located in the obturator, external iliac, and para-aortic regions. Lymphatic spread is also believed to be responsible for involvement of the vagina and for isolated adnexal involvement.

Overall, about 11% of patients with clinical stage I and occult stage II endometrial carcinoma and 5% to 7% of patients with tumors confined to the uterus have pelvic or para-aortic lymph node involvement.[45,50] The extent of myometrial penetration correlates strongly with the histologic grade of the tumor, and the depth of invasion and tumor grade correlate with the risk of lymphatic involvement. The risk of intra-abdominal dissemination is higher in patients with non-endometrioid carcinoma. Abdominal involvement of endometrioid carcinoma is associated with other risk factors, such as lymph node involvement, adnexal involvement, and lymphovascular space invasion.

Hematogenous spread is uncommon in endometrial cancer, occurring mainly with high-grade tumors, unfavorable histologies, or advanced stages. The most common metastatic sites include the lungs, liver, and bones. Distant nodal metastases (i.e., supraclavicular or inguinal) result from extensive lymphatic involvement or from hematogenous spread.

Table 56-3 Predominant Features of Type I and II Endometrial Cancer

Characteristic	Type I	Type II
CLINICOPATHOLOGIC FEATURES		
Estrogen relation	Yes	No
Precursor lesion	Hyperplasia	Intraepithelial carcinoma
Age	Younger	Older
Histologic type	Endometrioid	Non-endometrioid
Grade	1 or 2	3
Stage	Stage 1	More advanced
Prognosis	Good	Poor
GENETIC FEATURES		
Ploidy	Diploid	Aneuploid
TP53 mutation	10-20% (late event)	60-90% (early event)
PTEN inactivation	35-50%	5-10%
HER2 overexpression	10-15%	20-25% (serous: 60%)
EGFR overexpression	10-30%	60-80%
KRAS mutation	15-30%	0-5%
Microsatellite instability	20-30%	0-5%

BIOLOGIC CHARACTERISTICS AND PROGNOSTIC FACTORS

Biologic Features

Two different types of endometrial carcinoma have been described.[51] Type I tumors are estrogen related, are often preceded by hyperplasia, and are typically low-grade endometrioid carcinomas. They usually develop in an estrogen-rich environment (e.g., obesity, premenopausal and perimenopausal phases), and they have a good prognosis. Type II tumors are unrelated to estrogen and develop in atrophic endometrium, presumably preceded by endometrial intraepithelial carcinoma, and they are more often serous and clear cell carcinomas. Patients with type II tumors are older postmenopausal patients; have high-grade, deeply invasive tumors; and have an unfavorable prognosis.[28,51] A summary of the differences between these two groups is shown in Table 56-3. The genetic abnormalities involved in the carcinogenesis of endometrial cancer are different for type I and II carcinomas.

Modern biologic techniques have provided new insights in the genetics and molecular biology of cancers. Mutations in three types of genes are considered to be the cause of most cancers: oncogenes, tumor suppressor genes, and mismatch repair genes. The protein products of oncogenes such as *KRAS* and *ERBB2* (previously designated *HER2/NEU* and now often designated *HER2*) participate in growth pathways in normal cells. A mutation in an oncogene can induce unrestrained proliferation. Loss or inactivation of tumor suppressor genes such as *TP53* and *PTEN* may promote uncontrolled growth by losing the normal cellular response to DNA damage, i.e., cell cycle arrest or apoptosis. Mismatch repair genes such as *MLH1* and *MSH2* are responsible for detecting and correcting DNA damage. A marker for defects in mismatch repair genes is microsatellite instability.

Specific molecular alterations have been found in type I and II endometrial cancers. In type II cancers, *TP53* mutations have been found in up to 90% of cases (invasive and intraepithelial carcinomas), suggesting it to be an early event in carcinogenesis. HER2 protein overexpression due to a mutation in the *ERBB2* gene has been identified in a significant proportion (up to 80%) of serous carcinomas. The HER2 gene product, similar to the epidermal growth factor receptor, is a transmembrane receptor protein that plays an important role in the ERBB signaling network that is responsible for regulating cell growth and differentiation. HER2 overexpression is associated with aggressive biologic behavior and poor survival. Targeted therapy using trastuzumab (Herceptin), a monoclonal antibody to HER2, may be an attractive therapeutic strategy for serous cancers.[52,53] Epidermal growth factor receptor (EGFR) overexpression occurs in 60% to 80% of type II cancers, and it correlates with advanced-stage disease and poor prognosis.[54] Targeted therapy with EGFR tyrosine kinase inhibitors such as erlotinib or cetuximab is being investigated.[55]

No specific abnormalities have been associated with type I cancers in general, which suggests that type I is a heterogeneous group of tumors with different combinations of abnormalities. *TP53* mutations have been found in 10% to 20% of type I cancers, are associated with grade 3 tumors, and may be related to dedifferentiation. Mutant TP53 protein expression has been associated with advanced stage and other adverse factors, such as poor differentiation, deep invasion, and poor survival.[56] More general markers of genetic damage such as DNA aneuploidy have consistently been associated with an inferior outcome.[57-59]

Table 56-4 Prognostic Value of Genetic Abnormalities

Genetic Abnormality	Prognostic Value
Aneuploidy	Decreased survival*
TP53 mutation	Decreased survival
PTEN inactivation	Conflicting data
HER2 overexpression	Decreased survival
EGFR overexpression	Decreased survival
KRAS mutation	Conflicting data
Microsatellite instability	No prognostic significance

*Remains significant prognostic factor in multivariate analysis.

As listed in Table 56-4, some molecular abnormalities such as *PTEN* and *KRAS* mutations, which are considered early events in the development of endometrioid carcinomas, are associated with a favorable prognosis, whereas others predict an unfavorable outcome. In most multivariate analyses, however, the prognostic significance of these molecular markers is lost in the presence of the traditional major prognostic factors: stage, grade, depth of invasion, and histologic subtype. The molecular markers have no defined role in guiding clinical management, and their major promise seems to be the identification of specific targets for therapy.

Prognostic Factors

Numerous studies have identified the major prognostic factors in endometrial carcinoma. Comprehensive retrospective analyses and prospective, randomized studies have established the major prognostic factors for survival and relapse to be stage, patient age, histologic cell type, tumor grade, depth of myometrial invasion, and presence of lymphvascular space invasion.[46,60,61] Randomized trials have confirmed the prognostic value of these factors.[62-64] Among stage I patients, grade has been found to be a major factor, with grade 3 tumors associated with a threefold to fivefold increased risk of relapse and cancer death.[65,66] In most studies, grade 2 tumors do not have significantly different outcomes compared with grade 1, and two-tiered grading systems have been proposed to overcome the limited clinical value and poor reproducibility of the intermediate grade.[43,67] The binary grading system proposed by Lax[43] is based on the proportion of solid growth, the pattern of myometrial invasion, and the presence of tumor cell necrosis. In a comparative analysis of the prognostic significance and the interobserver variability of these grading systems in a series of 800 stage I endometrial cancers, the reproducibility of the binary system was not found to be greater than that of the International Federation of Gynecology and Obstetrics (FIGO) grading system, but the prognostic power of the systems was equally strong. A simple two-tiered system, dividing tumors into low or high risk based on the proportion of solid growth (<50% versus >50%), was shown to have superior prognostic power and greater reproducibility.[68] Alternatively, the FIGO grading system may be used as a binary system by dividing tumors into grades 1 and 2 versus grade 3. Such a binary FIGO system has been shown to have strong prognostic significance, and it has the additional advantages of being highly reproducible and familiar to practicing pathologists worldwide.[68,69]

In most studies, depth of myometrial invasion had less strong prognostic value than tumor grade. Deep invasion, particularly into the outer third of the myometrial wall, has been associated with increased risk of relapse and inferior outcome.[60] A diffusely infiltrating pattern of myometrial invasion, as opposed to an expansive growth pattern with pushing borders, has been suggested to be a stronger adverse prognostic factor than the depth of invasion.[66,70] Because the effluent lymphatics and capillaries are mainly located in the subserosa, the tumor-free distance from the serosa may prove to be the strongest prognostic factor. In a multivariate analysis of 153 patients, tumor-free distance was found to be a highly significant predictor of relapse and death from disease, stronger than depth of invasion, and to have greater reproducibility.[71]

Lymphovascular space invasion has been found to be a major prognostic factor that significantly and independently increases the risk of relapse, especially distant relapse.[64,65,72] In an analysis of 609 stage I-III endometrial cancer patients, those with lymphovascular space invasion (LVSI) were found to have a 5-year relapse rate of 39%, in contrast to 19% for patients without LVSI ($P < .0001$). Even in otherwise low-risk stage I disease, the presence of LVSI significantly increased the risk of relapse (28% with versus 14% without LVSI). In stage I patients with high-risk features, those with LVSI had a 43% relapse rate.[72]

CLINICAL MANIFESTATIONS/PATIENT EVALUATION/STAGING

Clinical Manifestations

Abnormal uterine bleeding is the most common presenting sign of patients with endometrial cancer. Because blood loss is an early sign of endometrial proliferation, 75% of patients present with early-stage disease. However, only about 15% to 20% of the patients with postmenopausal bleeding are found to have endometrial cancer. Another, rather nonspecific symptom is profuse, watery discharge. In premenopausal or perimenopausal patients, the presenting symptom may be irregular blood loss or menorrhagia. It is unusual for screening cervical cytology to be the method of diagnosis, but malignant endometrial cells occasionally are found in routine Pap smears. Pain is usually absent unless there is pyometra. Patients with more advanced stages of endometrial cancer can present with abdominal symptoms, gastrointestinal symptoms, back pain, or lymphedema.

Patient Evaluation

Patient evaluation for confirmed or suspected malignancy includes a medical history and physical examination, including vaginal inspection and bimanual pelvic examination. Medical history should include the presence of risk factors associated with endometrial cancer, such as obesity, hypertension, diabetes mellitus, estrogen or tamoxifen use, nulliparity, and a family history, especially of colon, endometrial, breast, or ovarian cancer.

Most endometrial carcinoma patients have early-stage disease and do not have significant abnormalities on pelvic examination. However, a complete pelvic examination should be performed to exclude gross cervical extension, vaginal metastases, and adnexal pathology.

Outpatient procedures, such as transvaginal ultrasonography and endometrial biopsy or aspiration curettage, establish the diagnosis in more than 90% of patients suspected to have endometrial cancer. Various endometrial biopsy tools are available, such as small Novak curette, Pipelle instrument, or Vabra aspirator, that permit the procedure to be performed without general anesthesia. If these procedures are not conclusive, a formal dilation and fractional curettage (D&C) should be carried out, with or without hysteroscopy. Hysteroscopy allows direct visual assessment of the endocervix

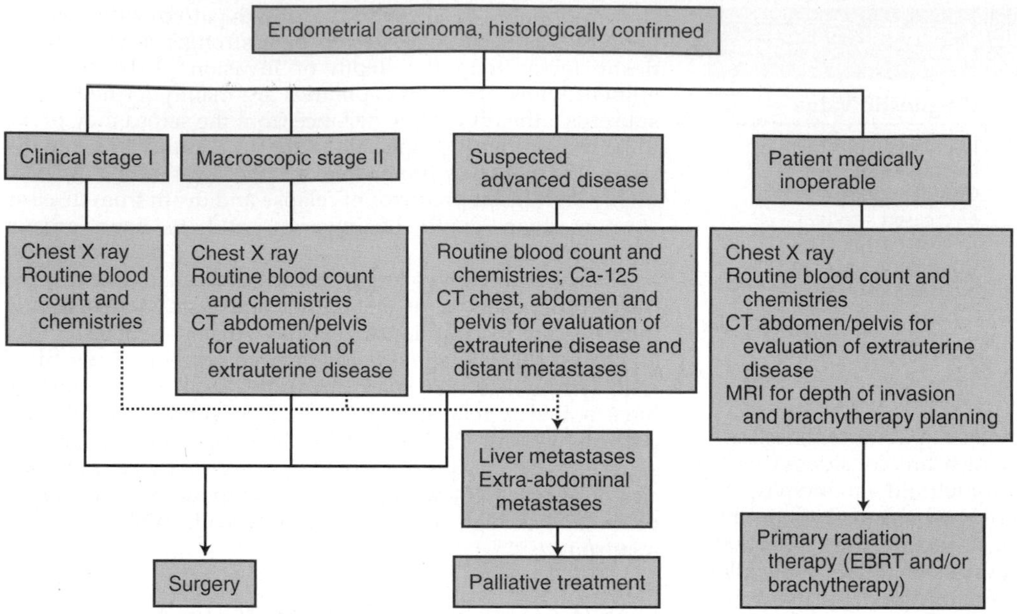

Figure 56-1 Diagnostic algorithm for patients with endometrial carcinoma.

and the endometrial cavity and can be useful in guiding biopsy of any visible abnormality in symptomatic patients when other procedures have been nondiagnostic. Figure 56-1 presents an algorithm for patient workup and evaluation.

Staging

After a diagnosis of malignancy is established, the preoperative evaluation and staging workup are done. Definitive staging according to the 1988 FIGO system is based on the surgical and pathology findings (Table 56-5). The previous nonsurgical FIGO staging system (1971) continues to be used for patients not undergoing surgery. The patient's general evaluation should include standard blood tests and a chest radiograph. Endometrial carcinoma patients are often elderly and frail and may have a number of concurrent medical problems that influence selection of the appropriate treatment. Computed tomography (CT) and magnetic resonance imaging (MRI) are not routinely performed for patients with clinical stage I disease who will be undergoing surgery, but imaging should be done if locally advanced disease is suspected. The major limitations of CT are its unreliability in assessing myometrial invasion, especially if less than one third to one half of the myometrial thickness or in atrophic uteri, and the failure to detect minor parametrial, lymph nodal, or local extrauterine invasion.[73] The greatest value of CT may be staging of clinical stage III or IV patients and medically inoperable patients, for whom CT is useful for evaluating the size and extent of the tumor, for excluding extrauterine disease, and for planning of radiation therapy. MRI using intravenous contrast is superior to CT in determining myometrial invasion and diagnosing stage II disease.[74]

Although the 1988 FIGO staging system requires a pelvic lymphadenectomy, the role of lymphadenectomy and the optimal extent of lymphadenectomy (e.g., lymph node sampling, selective or complete lymphadenectomy, pelvic or aortic lymphadenectomy) are subjects of controversy, as is the question of whether lymphadenectomy is a purely diagnostic and prognostic procedure or therapeutic benefit can be obtained. Completeness of the surgical staging procedure can upstage patients otherwise considered stage I, and the problems of stage migration and patient selection preclude definitive conclusions on the value of lymphadenectomy in the absence of randomized data. The approach to these surgical staging issues varies among gynecologists and gynecologic oncologists and among different countries. The variability in staging of patients clearly affects the distribution of stages in endometrial cancer patients.

Table 56-5 Federation of Gynecology and Obstetrics (FIGO) Surgical Staging System for Endometrial Carcinoma, 1988

Stage and Grade		Description
IA	(G1,2,3)	Tumor limited to endometrium
IB	(G1,2,3)	Invasion limited to <50% of the myometrium
IC	(G1,2,3)	Invasion of >50% of the myometrium
IIA	(G1,2,3)	Endocervical glandular involvement only
IIB	(G1,2,3)	Cervical stromal invasion
IIIA	(G1,2,3)	Tumor invades serosa and/or adnexa and/or positive peritoneal cytology
IIIB	(G1,2,3)	Vaginal metastases
IIIC	(G1,2,3)	Metastases to pelvic and/or para-aortic lymph nodes
IVA	(G1,2,3)	Tumor invasion to bladder and/or bowel mucosa
IVB	(G1,2,3)	Distant metastases including intra-abdominal and/or inguinal lymph nodes
FIGO HISTOLOGIC GRADING		
G1		<5% nonsquamous or nonmorular solid growth pattern
G2		5-50% of a nonsquamous or nonmorular solid growth pattern
G3		>50% of a nonsquamous or nonmorular solid growth pattern

PRIMARY THERAPY

Surgery

Surgery is the mainstay of treatment of endometrial carcinoma. Surgical evaluation should start with exploration and collection of ascites or peritoneal lavage fluid for cytologic evaluation. Thorough examination and palpation of the pelvic and abdominal organs and lymph node regions should be carried out, and any suspicious sites should be biopsied. After initial assessment, the standard surgical procedure is a total abdominal hysterectomy with bilateral salpingo-oophorectomy (TAH-BSO). In situations with gross cervical involvement (macroscopic stage II disease), a radical hysterectomy should be considered. Literature data support the use of radical hysterectomy in macroscopic stage II disease, although a survival advantage over TAH-BSO and pelvic radiation therapy has not been proved.[75,76]

The standard surgical approach is laparotomy through a midline incision, which allows full exposure of the abdomen, pelvic areas, and lymphatic sites. However, laparoscopic techniques for staging and treatment have been developed, and a number of institutions have evaluated laparoscopic staging and laparoscopic-assisted vaginal hysterectomy, especially for early-stage disease.[77-79] The advantages of laparoscopy are the shorter hospitalization and recovery time and decrease of surgical morbidity. Disadvantages are the increased length of the operation and the learning curve involved with laparoscopic techniques. Increased risks of malignant cells in the peritoneal cytology specimen[80] and vaginal cuff recurrence or port site metastases[81] have been reported. The importance of early occlusion of the fallopian tubes and uterine artery and avoidance of intrauterine manipulators to prevent such peritoneal spread and vaginal cuff recurrence has been stressed.[77,81-83] First results from retrospective studies and a small, single-center randomized trial have shown the overall and relapse-free survival rates to be similar to laparotomy, with fewer complications and earlier recovery.[77,78] Laparotomy remains preferable to laparoscopy in very obese patients and in patients with intra-abdominal adhesions.

The GOG is conducting a randomized study comparing conventional laparotomy with laparoscopic surgery and vaginal hysterectomy. Patients with clinical stages I or IIA and all grades of disease are included. End points of the study are surgical complications, morbidity and mortality, length of hospital stay, quality of life, and the incidence of disease relapse. The target number of patients for this study is 2550 during an accrual period of 10 years.

The role of pelvic and para-aortic lymphadenectomy or lymph node sampling has been widely debated. Determination of nodal involvement has prognostic implications, and in patients with nodal involvement, it directs further therapy. The potential therapeutic implications of lymphadenectomy are directly related to the a priori risk of nodal disease in the population studied. Prospective and retrospective studies of lymphadenectomy in patients with clinical stage I or II endometrial carcinoma without extrauterine spread identified at surgery have shown the rates of pelvic and aortic nodal involvement to be 7% to 9% and 2% to 3%, respectively.[45,50,84,85] The risk of lymph node involvement varies with the major risk factors, as was demonstrated in the landmark GOG surgical pathologic staging study (Table 56-6).[45,46] Some of these features can be identified at the time of hysterectomy and used to evaluate the indication for lymph node dissection. The addition of lymphadenectomy, especially if pelvic and aortic lymphadenectomies are performed, prolongs operation time and has side effects such as leg edema (5%), lymphocysts (symptomatic in 5% to 7%), increased rates of deep vein thrombosis (2%) and small bowel obstruction (up to 5%), and increased blood loss and higher transfusion rates (5% to 10%).[85-87] Studies suggesting a survival advantage were small, single-center retrospective analyses, flawed by patient selection and stage migration.[86-88] The larger National Cancer Institute and Duke University analyses reported a survival benefit with multiple-site lymphadenectomy for grade 3 cancers, whereas no benefit was found for grade 1 or 2 disease.[84,85] Lymphadenectomy should therefore be considered for patients with grade 3 disease, cervical involvement, and high-risk histologies.[50,84,85] It has been shown that if pelvic lymphadenectomy is performed, a minimum of 11 nodes should be removed from multiple sites.[84,85,88] Because only retrospective analyses have been published, it cannot be ruled out that the survival benefit was caused by elimination of patients from earlier-stage categories (i.e., stage migration) and by exclusion of patients at increased surgical risk due to advanced age or concurrent morbidities (i.e., selection bias). The first multicenter randomized trial on lymphadenectomy, the UK Medical Research Council ASTEC study, accrued 1408 women (704 randomized to TAH-BSO and 704 to TAH-BSO plus lymphadenectomy). Preliminary results did not show a survival benefit for lymphadenectomy (H. Kitchener, oral presentation, ESGO, September 2005). Definitive published results are expected by late 2006.

Sentinel node detection may be an alternative way to identify patients requiring more intensive therapy. In breast cancer, it has been shown that removal and meticulous analysis of

Table 56-6 Risk Factors for Lymph Node Metastases

Risk Level	Lymph Node Metastasis: Pelvic Nodes (%)	Lymph Node Metastasis: Aortic Nodes (%)
ALL CLINICAL STAGE I		
Low risk		
Grade 1, endometrium only, no intraperitoneal disease	0	0
Moderate risk		
No intraperitoneal disease		
Inner-middle invasion or grade 2 or 3	3	2
Both factors	6	2
High risk		
Deep invasion	18	15
Intraperitoneal disease	33	8
Both	61	30
NO GROSS EXTRAUTERINE DISEASE		
Low risk		
No invasion or grade 1 with invasion	<5	<2
Moderate risk		
All other	5-10	<5
High risk		
Grade 3, outer 33% invasion	>10	>10

*Excluding serous or clear cell histology.

Data from Creasman WT, Morrow CP, Bundy BN, et al: Surgical pathologic spread patterns of endometrial cancer. A Gynecologic Oncology Group Study. Cancer 60:2035-2041, 1987.

sentinel nodes with serial sectioning and immunohistochemistry more adequately identifies occult nodal involvement while sparing most patients the risks and added toxicities of more extensive procedures. First results from sentinel node studies in endometrial carcinoma have shown that the combined use of radiocolloid labeling and patent blue dye results in a sentinel node detection rate of 82% to 94%, with identification of two or three sentinel nodes per patient.[47-49] The sentinel nodes were located in the obturator, external iliac, or para-aortic regions. In the study by Barranger,[48] macrometastases were identified in three sentinel nodes from two patients with routine staining, and immunohistochemical analysis identified six additional micrometastatic sentinel nodes in three other patients and one sentinel node containing isolated tumor cells. No false-negative sentinel nodes were found. Additional larger studies are needed to further explore this concept and develop reliable sentinel node detection procedures.

Primary Radiation Therapy: Indications and Results

The approximately 3% of patients who have severe medical conditions that render them medically inoperable can be offered primary radiation therapy for their endometrial cancer. Substantial local control and disease-specific survival rates have been reported, although these patients have a high mortality rate because of their coexisting medical conditions. Patients at low risk for extrauterine spread may be treated with intrauterine brachytherapy alone. External beam radiation therapy (EBRT) to the pelvis is based on the risk of extrauterine disease, and it is usually employed in cases with grade 3 disease, larger uterine volume, or cervical involvement. Primary radiation therapy (i.e., radical or definitive radiation) refers to treatment done with curative intent. Because of their coexisting illnesses, some patients are not candidates for primary irradiation, but they should be offered palliative radiation therapy.

Several studies have demonstrated the efficacy of primary radiation therapy for clinical stage I disease. Using uterine brachytherapy with or without EBRT, 5-year uterine control rates of 70% to 90% and disease-free survival rates ranging from 50% to 80% have been reported.[89-96] Grade 3 tumors had significantly lower pelvic control and survival rates than grade 1 or 2 disease. Studies that included stage II patients reported 5-year pelvic control rates of 40% to 60% and disease-specific survival rates of about 50% to 60%.[91,95,96]

Surgical Results: Early-Stage Disease

Many retrospective studies have reported invariably good outcomes for stage IA and IB grade 1 and 2 endometrioid carcinoma treated with TAH-BSO alone, with a 5-year relapse-free survival rate of 95% and 5-year vaginal relapse rates of 2% to 5%.[97-100] Several investigators stressed that lymphadenectomy is not indicated in these low-risk patients.[99,100] In some studies, vaginal brachytherapy was used.[100] The addition of brachytherapy to TAH-BSO may reduce vaginal relapse rates from between 2% and 5% to between 0% and 2% but without a survival difference and at the cost of (albeit minimal) morbidity. Effective salvage treatment is available for the occasional patient with vaginal relapse.

Adjuvant Therapy: Stages I and II

Three prospective, randomized trials have been published that evaluated the role of postoperative pelvic irradiation in intermediate-risk endometrial carcinoma,[62-64] and they are summarized in Table 56-7. The Norwegian trial, published in 1980, included 540 women with clinical stage I endometrial carcinoma. After hysterectomy and postoperative vaginal brachytherapy (60 Gy to the mucosal surface), patients were randomly assigned to additional pelvic irradiation (40 Gy in 2-Gy fractions, with a midline block after 20 Gy) or observation. Although additional pelvic irradiation reduced vaginal and pelvic relapse rates (2% at 5 years versus 7% in the control group), more distant metastases were found in the pelvic irradiation group (10% versus 5%), and survival was not improved (89% versus 91% at 5 years).[101] The subgroup with grade 3 tumors with deep (>50%) myometrial invasion showed improved local control and survival after pelvic irradiation (18% versus 27% cancer-related deaths); however, there were too few patients in this category to reach significance.

In the Postoperative Radiation Therapy in Endometrial Carcinoma (PORTEC) trial, 715 patients with stage I endometrial carcinoma, grade 1 or 2 with deep (>50%) myometrial invasion or grade 2 or 3 with superficial (<50%) invasion were randomized after TAH-BSO to receive pelvic radiation therapy (46 Gy in 2-Gy fractions) or no further treatment.[63] The 10-year locoregional relapse rates were 5% in the radiation therapy group and 14% in the control group ($P < .0001$). There was no significant survival difference between the treatment arms, with 10-year overall survival rates of 66% (irradiation) and 73% (controls; $P = .09$). Endometrial cancer–related death

Table 56-7 Comparison of the Randomized Trials of Adjuvant Radiation Therapy for Stage I Endometrial Carcinoma

Trial	No. of Eligible Patients	Surgery	Randomization	Locoregional Recurrence	Survival	Severe Complications
Norwegian[62] 1968-1974	540 Stage I	TAH-BSO	BT vs BT plus pelvic RT	7% vs 2% at 5 y $P < .01$	89% vs 91% at 5 y P = NS	NA
PORTEC[63] 1990-1997	714 Stage IB, G 2-3 Stage IC, G 1-2	TAH-BSO	NAT vs pelvic RT	14% vs 4% at 5 y $P < .001$	85% vs 81% at 5 y $P = .31$	3% GI at 5 y (actuarial)
GOG-99[64] 1987-1995	392 Stage IB, IC Stage II (occult)	TAH-BSO and lymphadenectomy	NAT vs pelvic RT	12% vs 3% at 2 y $P < .01$	86% vs92% at 4 y $P = .56$	8% GI at 2 y (crude)

TAH-BSO, total abdominal hysterectomy with bilateral salpingo-oophorectomy; BT, brachytherapy; G, grade; GI: gastrointestinal; NA: not available; NAT: no additional treatment; RT: radiation therapy.

rates were 10% in the radiation therapy group and 8% in the control group (P = .47). The patients younger than 60 years (both arms) had a 5-year locoregional relapse rate of 3%, compared with 9% and 10% for patients 60 to 70 years old and those older than 70 years, respectively. Patients with grade 2 tumors with superficial invasion had a 5-year locoregional relapse rate of 5%. Risk criteria for relapse were grade 3, age older than 60 years, and outer 50% invasion.

The 5-year survival rate after any relapse was 13% in the radiation therapy group and 48% in the control group (P < .001). After vaginal relapse, 5-year actuarial survival rates were 38% in the radiation therapy group and 70% in the control group, which shows the high salvage rates of vaginal relapse in patients not previously irradiated. Most (87%) of the 39 patients with isolated vaginal relapse could be treated with curative intent, usually with pelvic irradiation and brachytherapy and with surgery in some. A complete remission was obtained in 89%, and 77% remained in complete remission after further follow-up.[102] In contrast, only 4 of 10 patients who were treated for pelvic relapse reached a complete remission, and the outcome after pelvic and distant relapse was poor, with only 6% and 11% of patients, respectively, surviving 5 years.

The GOG-99 trial included 392 evaluable patients with stage IB, IC, or IIA endometrial carcinoma of any histologic grade, who were randomized after TAH-BSO and lymphadenectomy to receive pelvic irradiation (50.4 Gy in 1.8-Gy fractions) or no additional treatment (NAT).[64] A high-intermediate risk (HIR) group was defined based on the prognostic factors of age, histologic grade, myometrial invasion, and the presence of lymphovascular space invasion. The HIR group (33% of the study population) had a 2-year incidence of relapse in the NAT arm of 27%, in contrast to 6% for the low-intermediate risk (LIR) group (67% of patients). Radiation therapy resulted in similar hazard reductions for the HIR and LIR subgroups (58% and 54%), but in absolute terms, the differences were greater for HIR patients, with a reduction of 4-year cumulative relapse from 27% (NAT) to 13% (irradiation). There was even a slight, although nonsignificant survival benefit: 4-year overall survival was 86% for NAT and 92% for radiation therapy. The 2-year estimated vaginal and pelvic failure rate was 12% in the NAT group and 3% in the radiation therapy group, for a 58% hazard reduction by irradiation. These results are strikingly similar to those obtained in the PORTEC study without lymphadenectomy. However, the 4-year crude rate of severe complications in GOG-99 was 13% for patients who had received irradiation, compared with a 5-year actuarial rate of 3% in the PORTEC trial, which underlines the increased risk of toxicity when combining extended surgery with pelvic radiation therapy.

Conclusions that can be drawn from these randomized trials of pelvic radiation therapy in stage I endometrial carcinoma are that pelvic irradiation provides a highly significant improvement of local control but offers no survival advantage. A large proportion of endometrial cancer patients has a very favorable prognosis, and these patients should be observed after TAH-BSO. Radiation therapy is a very effective salvage treatment for vaginal relapse in patients not previously irradiated. The data suggest that the use of postoperative radiation therapy should be limited to the group of patients at sufficiently high risk for locoregional relapse (≥15%) to warrant the risk of treatment-associated morbidity to maximize initial local control and relapse-free survival. In the PORTEC study, patients with two of the three major risk factors (grade 3, age 60 or older, and outer 50% myometrial invasion) were found to have an increased risk of locoregional relapse and to have the highest absolute benefit from pelvic irradiation. The 10-year locoregional relapse rates in this "high-risk" category were 4.6% in the radiation therapy group and 23.1% in the control group. In the GOG-99 trial, similar high risk criteria were identified, with reduction of isolated 4-year local relapse in the HIR group from 13% to 5%. The risk criteria as defined in the PORTEC and GOG-99 trials and the risk reduction with radiation therapy in the high-risk groups are listed in Table 56-8.

Because most relapses occur in the vagina, the use of vaginal brachytherapy alone has been advocated, especially after extensive surgical staging. Data from mostly retrospective studies that used vaginal brachytherapy alone for stage I endometrial cancer have shown the 5-year risk of vaginal relapse to be 0% to 7%.[50,62,103-111] Pelvic and distant failure rates, however, remain similar to those of patients treated with

Table 56-8 Comparison of the Risk Groups in the PORTEC and GOG-99 Trials and Risk Reduction with Radiation Therapy

Risk Levels	Risk Groups: *PORTEC*[63]	*GOG-99*[64]
Risk factors		
Age	<60 vs >60	<50 vs <70 vs >70
Grade	Grade 1-2 vs 3	Grade 1 vs 2-3
Deep invasion	<50% vs >50%	<66% vs >66%
Lymphovascular space invasion	—	Absent vs present
High-risk group	At least 2 of the 3 factors	Any age and 3 factors Age ≥ 50 and 2 factors Age ≥ 70 and 1 factor
Results for the high-risk group	10-year locoregional relapse RT: 5% NAT: 23% Rel. risk: 0.22 With GOG high-risk criteria RT: 8% NAT: 22% Rel. risk: 0.36	4-year relapse (any) RT: 13% NAT: 27% Rel. risk: 0.48 4-year isolated local relapse RT: 5% NAT: 13% Rel. risk: 0.38

GOG, Gynecologic Oncology Group; PORTEC, Postoperative Radiation Therapy in Endometrial Carcinoma; NAT, no additional treatment; rel. risk, relapse with RT compared with NAT; RT, radiation therapy.

surgery alone, which is the reason that most studies included only or mainly low-risk patients (i.e., grade 1 to 2 disease with no or superficial invasion).

Vaginal control and complication rates for high dose rate (HDR) vaginal brachytherapy are comparable to those of low dose rate (LDR) therapy.[108] Petereit and Pearcey[112] reviewed the results of HDR brachytherapy for stage I endometrial cancer patients and concluded that local control rates of 98% and higher were obtained with modest doses (e.g., 35 Gy HDR therapy to the surface or 21 Gy to a 5-mm depth in three fractions). The use of higher doses did not further increase local control, but complication rates were higher. Several HDR studies using surgical staging included patients with high-risk stage I or stage II disease and reported vaginal control rates of 98% to 100%.[109,110,113,114] Pelvic and distant relapses were found mainly in the high-risk stage I or II patients; the 5-year disease-free survival (DFS) rates were 90% to 95% and 74%, respectively.

These data suggest that even for patients with high-risk features, vaginal brachytherapy may be used instead of EBRT to maximize local control with fewer side effects and better quality of life. The phase III PORTEC-2 trial is randomly assigning patients with stage I-IIA endometrial carcinoma with risk features (i.e., age of at least 60 years, grade 1 or 2 tumors with outer 50% invasion or grade 3 with inner 50% invasion) to EBRT or vaginal brachytherapy. In addition to evaluation and comparison of relapse, survival, and complication rates, the PORTEC-2 trial includes prospective quality-of-life evaluation to assess the short-term and long-term impact of these treatment modalities on quality of life.

Stage IC, Grade 3 Disease

Stage IC, grade 3 endometrial carcinoma should be regarded separately, because this subgroup of patients is at increased risk for pelvic relapse and distant metastases and has lower survival rates.[65,115,116] Straughn and colleagues[116] analyzed the outcome of 220 stage IC endometrial cancer patients who had surgical staging, including pelvic and para-aortic lymphadenectomy, comparing 99 (45%) patients treated with radiation therapy (pelvic irradiation [20%] and brachytherapy alone [25%]; selection criteria not specified) with 121 (55%) who did not receive radiation therapy. The 5-year DFS rates were significantly lower for the observation group (75% versus 93%), but overall survival rates were similar (90% versus 92%). Among the 47 patients with stage IC, grade 3 cancers, 5-year DFS rates were 90% after radiation therapy and 59% for the observation group.

During the inclusion period of the PORTEC trial, 99 evaluable patients with grade 3 tumors with deep myometrial invasion were registered and received radiation therapy. The 5-year actuarial vaginal and pelvic relapse rate was 13% in the IC grade 3 group, significantly higher than for other stage I patients, who had excellent pelvic control (97% to 99%) after pelvic irradiation. The 5-year rates of distant metastases were increased in both subgroups with grade 3 tumors: 20% for grade 3 with less than 50% invasion and 31% for grade 3 with more than 50% invasion, compared with 3% to 8% for grade 1 and 2 disease. Overall survival at 5 years was 58% for those with stage IC, grade 3 disease; 74% for those with stage IB, grade 3 disease; and 83% to 86% for those with stage IB, grade 2 or stage IC, grade 1 and 2 disease ($P < .001$).[65] In multivariate analyses, grade 3 was the most important adverse prognostic factor, with hazard ratios for any relapse and for endometrial carcinoma–related death of 5.4 ($P = .0001$) and 5.5 ($P = .0004$), respectively.

Whether surgical staging has been performed or not, pelvic irradiation is generally recommended for grade 3 tumors with deep myometrial invasion.[115,117-120] In view of the increased risk of distant relapse and cancer-related death, adjuvant chemotherapy is being investigated by several groups (see "Adjuvant Chemotherapy").

Stage II Disease

Stage II endometrial carcinoma includes patients with minimal microscopic involvement of the cervix (often called *stage II occult*) and those with macroscopic cervical involvement, even though these two groups have different prognoses. Cervical involvement has been associated with a poorer prognosis due to the increased risk of lymphovascular space involvement and pelvic lymph node metastases.[61] Patients with minimal extension to the endocervix, especially stage IIA, have outcomes identical to those of patients with stage I disease, and treatment should be the same as for stage I. Patients with stage IIB disease have a less favorable outcome.[121]

Patients with occult stage II disease have already undergone TAH-BSO. Pelvic irradiation with vaginal cuff boost is usually recommended for stage IIB occult disease treated with TAH-BSO because cervical involvement increases the risk of parametrial lymphatic disease.[122] For stage I disease, the addition of vaginal irradiation does not significantly add to local control when pelvic EBRT is used, but it does increase toxicity.[123-125] Although not extensively evaluated, this also may apply to occult stage II disease,[125] but because a vaginal cuff is usually not taken at TAH-BSO, most investigators continue to recommend a cuff boost for stage IIB occult disease. Reported adverse prognostic factors among patients with stage II disease are stage IIB, grade 3, lymphovascular space invasion, and advanced age.[121,126]

Patients with macroscopic stage II disease should be considered for radical hysterectomy, with adjuvant pelvic irradiation depending on the surgical findings (e.g., parametrial or vaginal extension, lymph node involvement, surgical margin involvement). Retrospective studies have shown that radical hysterectomy alone for macroscopic stage II endometrial cancer has local control and survival rates similar to those obtained with TAH-BSO plus pelvic irradiation.[75,76,122,127-129] Some studies reported improved survival after radical hysterectomy compared with TAH-BSO alone, but the selection criteria for radical hysterectomy and for radiation therapy were unclear and might have influenced the results.[76,127,128] Pelvic irradiation improved local control for patients treated with TAH-BSO.[126,127] Table 56-9 presents an overview of the results for stage II disease.

Patients with macroscopic stage II tumors with bulky cervical extension, precluding radical hysterectomy with adequate margins, should be treated with preoperative pelvic irradiation, followed by hysterectomy if feasible. In case of insufficient tumor regression after pelvic irradiation, intrauterine brachytherapy should be added. Depending on the regression and clinical situation after brachytherapy, completion hysterectomy should again be considered.

Unfavorable Histologic Types

Serous and clear cell cancers, approximately 10% and 5% of endometrial carcinomas, respectively, have been identified as histologic types with an inferior prognosis due to aggressive growth and spread patterns with frequent diffuse intra-abdominal dissemination. These histologic types often manifest with advanced disease (46% stage II-IV, compared with 21% for all endometrial cancers). Different treatment approaches (e.g., extended surgery, surgery with whole-abdomen irradiation [WAI], surgery with adjuvant chemotherapy) have

Table 56-9 **Outcome for Patients with Stage II Endometrial Carcinoma**

Study	No. of Patients	Stage	Treatment	5-Year Survival Rate	5-Year Relapse Rate
Ayhan et al[75] (2004)	48	II	21 RH alone 22 SH + EBRT 5 SH + VBT	OS: 86% SH: 83% RH: 90%	17%
Sartori et al[76] (2001)	203	IIA: 111 IIB: 92	135 SH 68 RH IIA: 66 EBRT IIB: 67 EBRT	IIA: 86% IIB: 74% SH: 79% RH: 94%	14% RT: 11% No RT: 19%
Mariani et al[127] (2001)	82	II, III II: 57	22 SH 35 RH 38 EBRT	DRS: 73% SH: 68% RH: 76% St III: 47%	RH and RT both produce fewer relapses
Jobsen et al[121] (2001)	42	II occult IIA: 21 IIB: 21	SH + EBRT	DFS: IIA: 95% IIB: 74%	21% IIB: 33%
Eltabbakh and Moore[122] (1999)	48	II	11 RH alone 20 SH + EBRT + VBT 13 SH + EBRT 4 SH + VBT	OS: 92% IIA: 93% IIB: 91% No diff RH vs SH + RT	6.3%
Leminen et al[129] (1995)	112	Clinical II 55 surg I 35 surg II 21 surg III	All preoperative RT 45 SH 55 RH 57 EBRT	DFS: 72% No diff SH vs RH	24%

DFS: disease-free survival; diff, difference between; DRS: disease-related survival; EBRT: external beam radiation therapy; OS: overall survival; RH: radical hysterectomy; RT: radiation therapy; SH: simple hysterectomy (i.e., total abdominal hysterectomy with bilateral salpingo-oophorectomy); surg, surgery; VBT: vaginal brachytherapy.

been suggested. Several studies have shown that serous and clear cell carcinomas have similar relapse and survival rates compared with grade 3 endometrioid carcinomas.[36,37] In an analysis of 5694 surgically staged endometrial cancer patients in the 25th annual report of FIGO, 3996 were stage I. Serous and clear cell cancers represented 5.2% of stage I cancers, and grade 3 carcinomas accounted for 8.1%. There were more stage I cancers among serous and clear cell cancers than among grade 3 carcinomas (54% and 49% versus 42%). Five-year survival rates were 72% and 81%, respectively, for serous and clear cell cancers, compared with 76% for grade 3 disease. Postoperative radiation therapy improved survival by about 8% for these histologic types (76% versus 68% for grade 3; 74% versus 66% for serous cancers; and 83% versus 77% for clear cell carcinoma), but these differences were not significant.[37] Results from an analysis of 68 stage I and II serous cancers showed adjuvant treatment with chemotherapy or radiation therapy, or both, to significantly improve survival.[130]

Conclusions from these analyses are that serous and clear cell cancers should be treated as grade 3 carcinomas. Adjuvant treatment using radiation therapy with concurrent or sequential chemotherapy should be considered, preferably within clinical trials (discussed later).

Adjuvant Hormonal Therapy

Adjuvant hormonal therapy for endometrial cancer has been extensively studied in view of the high incidence of progesterone receptor positivity and the 18% to 34% response rates to progesterone therapy seen in metastatic grade 1 or 2 disease. However, a meta-analysis of six randomized trials with a total of 3544 patients did not show a survival benefit for adjuvant progesterone treatment.[131] A randomized trial enrolling 1148 patients showed a higher intercurrent death rate in the progesterone group due to an increased risk of thromboembolic disease.[132] Among the 461 high-risk patients, a tendency toward fewer cancer-related deaths in the progesterone group was observed, but overall survival was unchanged. The COSA-NZ-UK trial showed a decrease in the rate of relapse with 3 years of adjuvant progestins, but it did not make a difference in disease-specific survival.[133]

Adjuvant Chemotherapy

Two randomized trials evaluated the efficacy of chemotherapy in the adjuvant setting. The first trial, using single-agent doxorubicin, did not show any benefit.[134] The results of GOG 122, a randomized trial comparing WAI with combination doxorubicin-cisplatin chemotherapy in advanced endometrial carcinoma (i.e., stages III-IV; up to 2 cm residual disease after surgery allowed) showed combination chemotherapy to improve progression-free and overall survival rates, with a predicted difference in disease-free survival of 15% at 5 years (50% versus 35%) and an overall 5-year survival rate difference of 11% (53% versus 42%).[135] However, relapses remained common (55%), occurring predominantly in the pelvis and abdomen in both arms, and adverse effects were substantial, especially in the doxorubicin-cisplatin arm. Because residual disease was allowed, this trial did not study true adjuvant treatment for microscopic disease, and it can be debated whether the radiation dose used would be appropriate for macroscopic residual disease. Further results of this and other trials are awaited to assess the impact of chemotherapy on overall survival and the cost in terms of added morbidity or even mortality in this elderly patient group. Increased pelvic relapse rates have been reported when using adjuvant chemotherapy alone in patients with high-risk or advanced-stage endometrial carcinoma.[136] Of the 67% who relapsed, 40% had pelvic relapse, and 56% had distant relapse. The 3-year pelvic failure rate was 47%, and in 31%, the pelvis was the first or only site of relapse.

Because these data support the use of pelvic irradiation in high-risk patients undergoing adjuvant chemotherapy, future trials should explore the optimal sequencing of therapy and the use of concurrent radiation therapy and chemotherapy. Initial pilot studies have indicated combined therapy to be tolerable.[137,138] A phase II trial of concurrent radiation therapy and cisplatin (two courses) followed by four courses of cisplatin and paclitaxel after irradiation for high-risk or advanced-stage endometrial carcinoma (66% stage III) showed a 98% treatment completion rate and expected, but still significant toxicity (chronic grade 3 and 4 toxicity in 16% and 2%, respectively). The 2-year disease-free and overall survival rates were 83% and 90%, respectively, but longer follow-up is needed to assess the outcome.[139] A phase III RTOG trial, randomizing between pelvic irradiation and pelvic irradiation with chemotherapy, has been started.

Results of studies of adjuvant chemotherapy in the high-risk histologic types (mainly serous carcinoma) have been disappointing. One study indicated a 2-year progression-free survival of only 22.5% for serous carcinoma after adjuvant cisplatin, doxorubicin, and cyclophosphamide (PAC) chemotherapy.[140] An analysis of stage I cases suggested even worse outcome with adjuvant chemotherapy compared with surgery alone.[141] Because many serous carcinomas are ERBB2 positive, trastuzumab appears to be a promising agent, and trials of adjuvant trastuzumab have been started.[52,142]

LOCALLY ADVANCED DISEASE AND PALLIATION

Locally Advanced Disease: Stages III and IV

Since the use of the FIGO 1988 staging system, the stage III category has included a patient group with a wide variation in tumor volume and extension and with a wide range of survival rates. Stage IIIA disease varies from the isolated finding of malignant cells in the peritoneal cytologic specimen to extensive macroscopic involvement of the pelvic tissues and ovaries. Because stage IIIB disease is rare (<1% of all endometrial carcinomas), outcome data are scarce. Nicklin[143] reported inferior outcome for clinical stage IIIB disease compared with stage IIIC, but survival was not different from stage IIIC or IV disease. Treatment should be individualized, and depending on the degree of vaginal extension, it may involve radical surgery or primary radiation therapy. Stage IIIC varies from microscopic involvement of a single pelvic node to extensive macroscopic disease involving the pelvic and para-aortic nodes. To best assess treatment, stage III disease must be evaluated as several different entities rather than as a single stage or disease entity. Table 56-10 outlines some of the experience with locally advanced disease.

Stage IIIA Disease

Patients with stage IIIA disease are those with uterine serosal involvement, positive peritoneal cytology, or adnexal involvement, and they have a poorer outcome than patients with stage I or II disease.[119,144-146] Positive peritoneal cytology has been associated with an increased risk of intra-abdominal spread. However, positive cytology is most frequently seen in patients with other high-risk factors, such as high-grade, deep myometrial invasion or vascular space invasion, and cytologic status has been demonstrated to lose its prognostic significance in the absence of other adverse factors.[147-149] Several studies have demonstrated that if positive peritoneal cytology is the only adverse factor (cytologic stage IIIA), the outcome is identical to stage I disease, and treatment should be based on the primary tumor factors, similar to stage I.[145,147-149] Use of extended-field radiation therapy (EFRT) or WAI would only add unnecessary toxicity. Care should be taken when interpreting an isolated finding of positive peritoneal cytology in patients with otherwise favorable disease, because increased risk of malignant cytology has been reported for patients with previous hysteroscopies.[150,151]

For patients with other risk factors, different issues apply. Patients with microscopic stage III disease have a better outcome than those with gross clinical stage III disease.[146,152] Patients with stage IIIA disease due to involvement of the serosa have a better DFS (42% versus 20%) than patients with multiple extrauterine disease sites.[144] The number of extrauterine disease sites correlates with probability of relapse. Patients with one, two and three or more extrauterine sites had 5-year DFS rates of 68%, 56%, and 0%, respectively.[153] In a large series of 126 patients with stage III disease, ovarian or tubal involvement had a better outcome (60% 5-year survival) than pelvic peritoneal or parametrial involvement (44%). Local control and survival were improved with surgical resection.[146]

Most stage III endometrial carcinoma patients have adjuvant pelvic irradiation.[146,154,155] In view of the high rate of abdominal relapse, the use of WAI has been supported, and several studies have demonstrated favorable results with WAI.[156,157] However, because of the toxicity and limited efficacy of WAI, adjuvant chemotherapy has been studied in locally advanced disease. The initial results of GOG 122, a randomized trial comparing WAI with doxorubicin-cisplatin chemotherapy in advanced (stages III-IV) endometrial carcinoma, have shown combination chemotherapy to improve progression-free and overall survival rates compared with WAI.[135] However, relapses remained common (55%), occurring predominantly in the pelvis and abdomen in both arms, and adverse effects were substantial. Current studies are focusing on the combined use of chemotherapy and pelvic irradiation.[139]

Stage IIIC Disease

Patients with stage IIIC disease without intraperitoneal involvement have a more favorable outcome compared with patients with abdominal disease. If the disease is limited to the pelvic and para-aortic nodes, EFRT is potentially curative, especially if only microscopic para-aortic disease is found.[155,158] Women with only pelvic node metastases have a better outcome than those with metastases in pelvic and para-aortic nodes, and disease-free survival rates up to 80% have been reported.[158-160] The risk of microscopic para-aortic disease increases with clinical stage. Microscopic para-aortic nodal metastases were diagnosed in 10%, 22%, and 71% of patients with clinical stage I (with risk factors of grade 3 tumors or deep invasion, or both), stage II, and stage III disease, respectively.[161] A retrospective analysis reported a 27% 5-year disease-free survival rate for 11 patients with microscopic para-aortic nodal disease treated with EFRT, but none of 8 patients treated with pelvic radiation therapy combined with progestins survived.[162] Complete removal of macroscopic or microscopic para-aortic nodal disease followed by EFRT resulted in 5-year survival rates of 46% and 53% among 50 and 17 patients, respectively, whereas patients with residual macroscopic nodal disease or omission of para-aortic field radiation had significantly decreased survival rates (13% to 18%).[161,163,164] The combination of extended surgery and EFRT has, however, a substantial complication rate, with reported intestinal obstruction rates of 12% to 27%.[161,162] EFRT therefore should be reserved for patients with suspected or proven para-aortic lymph node involvement; however, it has been

Table 56-10 **Outcome For Patients with Stage III Endometrial Carcinoma**

Study	No. of Patients	Stage	Treatment	5-Year Survival Rate
Tebeu et al[148] (2004)	53	IIIA	TAH-BSO; EBRT	Cytologic IIIA: CSS 91% Histologic IIIA: CSS 50% RT: CSS 60%; No RT: CSS 20%
Randall et al[135] (2006)	388	III-IV	TAH-BSO; LND; randomization between WAR and AP chemo	5-y DFS: WAI 38% 5-y OS: WAI 42%
Bristow et al[164] (2003)	41	IIIC Pelvic: 21 PAO: 20	TAH-BSO; LND; EBRT; 17 EFRT; 15 chemo	CSS median 30 mo No residual disease: 37 mo Residual nodal disease: 9 mo
Ayhan et al[160] (2002)	68	IIIA 26 IIIC 42	TAH-BSO; LND; full staging	All: DFS 58%. OS 64% IIIA: DFS 60%, OS 68% IIIC: DFS 68%, OS 62%
Mariani et al[145] (2002)	51	IIIC	TAH-BSO + LND; EBRT	Nodes only: CSS 72%, RFS: 68% Nodes + other sites: CSS 33%, RFS 25%
Ashman et al[144] (2001)	39	IIIA 19 IIIB/C 8 IV 12	TAH-BSO; LND; 26 EBRT; 13 chemo	DFS: 29% Serosa only: 42%
Mundt et al[158] (2001)	30	IIIC	TAH-BSO; staging + LND; 20 EBRT; 10 EFRT; 5 chemo; 7 hormones	DFS: 34% CSS: 56%
Nelson et al[159] (1999)	17	IIIC pelvic	TAH-BSO; LND; 13 EBRT; 4 WAR	DFS: 81% OS: 72%
Schorge et al[155] (1996)	86	III	TAH-BSO; LND; EBRT; some chemo or hormones	OS: 54% DFS: 44% IIIC: RT increased DFS
Greven et al[153] (1993)	105	III	TAH-BSO; 60 LND; EBRT or EFRT	DFS: 64%
Gibbons et al[156] (1991)	17	III	TAH-BSO or resection; WAR	DFS: 58% OS: 68%
Greven et al[146] (1989)	74	III	TAH-BSO or debulking; EBRT	OS: 54%
Grigsby et al[154] (1987)	30	III	TAH-BSO or resection; EBRT	DFS: 56%
Potish et al[157] (1985)	27	IIIA	TAH-BSO; WAR	OS: 71% Adnexa or cytology: 90% Beyond adnexa: 0% relapse free
Aalders et al[152] (1984)	67	III	TAH-BSO or debulking; EBRT	OS: 40%

AP: doxorubicin plus cisplatin chemotherapy; chemo, chemotherapy; CSS: cause-specific survival; DFS: disease-free survival; EBRT: external beam pelvic radiation therapy; EFRT: extended-field radiotherapy; LND: lymph node dissection; OS: overall survival; PAO: para-aortic; RFS: relapse-free survival; TAH-BSO: total abdominal hysterectomy and bilateral salpingo-oophorectomy; WAI: whole abdominal irradiation.

suggested that EFRT should be used for patients with positive pelvic nodes in combination with other adverse factors such as grade 3 disease.[158] Trials of additional chemotherapy are being conducted.

Stage IV Disease

Patients with stage IV disease have a poor prognosis with reported median survival rates of 12 to 15 months. Retrospective analyses have shown that maximal cytoreduction is the most important prognostic factor, with median survival rates of 18 to 30 months for optimal (<2 cm) cytoreduction, in contrast to 3 to 7 months without debulking.[165-167] However, if debulking did not result in optimal cytoreduction, survival was severely impaired due to a 37% rate for major postoperative complications and 13% rate for mortality.[167] In an analysis of 45 stage III-IV patients treated after surgery (usually TAH-BSO) with chemotherapy (four courses of cisplatin, epirubicin, and cyclophosphamide) and radiation therapy, 9-year progression-free and overall survival rates of 30% and 53%, respectively, were reported.[168]

Patients with bulky stage III or IV disease should be considered for clinical trials to find the optimal combination and sequencing of (extensive) surgery, chemotherapy, and radiation therapy. Because many patients are elderly and have concurrent morbidities, such trials should include quality-of-life analysis. Outside the scope of clinical trials, treatment for these patients is highly individualized, depending on the extent of the disease and the patient's condition.

Radiation Therapy for Recurrent Disease

Management of locoregional recurrent disease requires consideration of factors such as prior surgical and radiation therapy, extent and location of the relapse, the presence of distant metastases, and the performance status of the patient.

Factors determining the prognosis after treatment for relapse are the size and stage of the recurrence, the initial histology and grade, the recurrence-free interval, and the initial treatment.[169-174]

Reported local control rates after radical treatment for isolated vaginal relapse in previously unirradiated patients range from 80% to 90% for patients with recurrences confined to the mucosa to 60% to 80% for those with more advanced disease. Five-year overall survival rates are 40% to 70%.[102,169,172,175-178] For patients previously treated with pelvic irradiation, survival rates after vaginal relapse of 10% to 30% have been reported. In the PORTEC trial, the 5-year actuarial survival rate after vaginal relapse was 38% in the radiation therapy group and 70% in the control group.

Curative treatment for isolated vaginal recurrence in patients not previously irradiated consists of pelvic irradiation and vaginal brachytherapy. The use of a brachytherapy boost is essential.[176] Distal vaginal recurrence in the suburethral region or more extensive vaginal recurrence requires careful individualized brachytherapy planning to encompass the target volume with vaginal cylinder or interstitial brachytherapy, or both.[179]

Pelvic and distant relapses generally have a poor prognosis. Complete remission rates of treatment for pelvic relapse range from less than 5% for patients who had previous pelvic irradiation and those with sidewall disease to 5% to 30% for patients not previously irradiated.[180]

Radiation therapy is effective in palliation of bleeding, vaginal discharge, pain, and obstructive symptoms. Selected patients with pelvic relapse may be candidates for a curative approach with extended surgery with or without preoperative chemoradiation or intraoperative irradiation, or both. Patients with isolated distant metastasis such as a single lung nodule may have long symptom-free periods after local resection.

The frequency of follow-up examinations and their value in detecting asymptomatic recurrences have been subject of discussion.[181-184] It has been argued that 50% to 75% of women with relapsed disease were symptomatic and that regular follow-up is not cost effective because patients after relapse can only occasionally be salvaged. However, patients with early-stage disease treated with surgery alone should be followed closely, especially during the first 3 years, to diagnose vaginal relapse at an early, usually asymptomatic stage, because salvage rates are high. Regular evaluations, including visual inspection of the vagina and bimanual rectovaginal examinations taking Pap smears or biopsies only if abnormalities are found, are sufficient to diagnose vaginal recurrence. Because distant relapse can only occasionally be treated with a view to a long symptom-free interval, it cannot be recommended to actively screen for distant metastases outside the scope of clinical trials.

Radiation Therapy for Palliation

Radiation therapy has an important role in palliation of symptoms from locally advanced, recurrent, or metastatic endometrial cancer. Vaginal bleeding, vaginal discharge, or pain from advanced or recurrent disease or lymphedema from enlarged pelvic lymph nodes can be successfully palliated with a short course of fractionated EBRT using 3- to 4-Gy fractions to a dose of 20 to 30 Gy over 1 to 2 weeks. Other sites of symptomatic metastases, such as brain metastases or distant lymph node disease, are uncommon but can also be effectively palliated with similar radiation doses. Rapid and effective palliation of pain from bone metastases can be obtained using a single 8-Gy dose.[185]

Systemic Therapy for Recurrent or Metastatic Disease

Hormonal Therapy

Progestational agents are the standard hormonal therapy for advanced or metastatic grade 1 or 2 disease, especially for progesterone receptor–positive tumors. Reported response rates range from 15% to 34%, with a median response duration of several months. For progesterone receptor– and estrogen receptor–positive tumors response rates up to 77% have been observed, in contrast to 9% for receptor-negative tumors.[186,187] For relatively asymptomatic patients with unknown receptor status and grade 1 or 2 disease, progestins should be considered. Grade 3 disease is unlikely to respond to hormonal therapy (<10%). High-dose therapy (800 mg/day of megestrol acetate or 1000 mg/day of medroxyprogesterone acetate [MPA]) was not found to be more effective than standard doses (160 mg/day of megestrol or 200 mg/day of MPA).[186,188] For patients with disease progression after a response to progestins, tamoxifen and aromatase inhibitors may be considered.

Chemotherapy

Symptomatic patients with recurrent or metastatic disease, especially grade 3 or receptor-negative tumors, should be considered for chemotherapy. Because most patients with advanced disease are elderly women, their performance status and concurrent diseases may preclude the use of multiagent chemotherapy, and this should be kept in mind when counseling these patients. Cisplatin, doxorubicin, cyclophosphamide, ifosfamide, and paclitaxel are the most active agents for endometrial carcinoma, and multiagent chemotherapy has been shown to be more effective than single-agent therapy. Platinum- or paclitaxel-containing multiagent therapy provides response rates of 30% to 75%, with median remission duration of 6 to 12 months.[189-192] Adriamycin (doxorubicin) plus cisplatin therapy (AP regimen) has been shown to be as effective as the traditional combination of these agents with cyclophosphamide (CAP regimen), with a better toxicity profile.[189] Doxorubicin plus paclitaxel was not found to be superior to doxorubicin plus cisplatin in terms of response (40% and 43%), survival, or toxicity.[193] A randomized GOG trial comparing AP therapy with doxorubicin, cisplatin and paclitaxel with filgrastim support (TAP regimen) showed an improved response rate (57% versus 34%) and somewhat longer survival (58% versus 50% 1-year survival) for TAP, but at the cost of significant paclitaxel neurotoxicity.[192] Carboplatin and paclitaxel therapy, which is the standard for ovarian cancer and is used commonly in the community, has less toxicity than AP or TAP, and it may be equally effective.[142,194] A GOG trial is comparing carboplatin and paclitaxel with TAP.

Optimally, all patients with advanced or metastatic disease should be enrolled in randomized studies to evaluate the appropriate treatment. Molecular targeted therapies, such as cetuximab or erlotinib for tumors showing significant EGFR receptor activity and trastuzumab for tumors with strong (3+ by immunohisochemisty assay) HER2 expression are being explored and may prove to be effective and less toxic alternatives for subsets of patients.

TREATMENT OF UTERINE SARCOMAS

Uterine sarcomas are rare, and management is therefore variable because data from randomized studies are lacking. Most patients present with vaginal bleeding, much like patients with adenocarcinomas, but the tumor is typically larger before this occurs. Uterine sarcoma may also be an unexpected diagnosis in a uterus resected for presumed symptomatic leiomyoma.[195] Other patients can present with local discomfort from uterine enlargement.

Uterine sarcomas comprise three distinct types with different characteristics and different outcomes: carcinosarcomas (or malignant mixed müllerian tumors [MMMT]), 45%; leiomyosarcomas, 40%; and endometrial stromal sarcomas, 15%. Uterine sarcomas, especially leiomyosarcomas, have a higher metastatic rate without preceding lymph node involvement compared with the adenocarcinomas. The lungs are the most common sites of metastatic disease. Because of the high rate of metastases especially to the lung, initial evaluation should include CT of the chest.

Because patterns of failure are different for the different sarcoma types, treatment should be tailored to the specific sarcoma type. Treatment of uterine sarcomas is primarily focused on the initial surgery. Hysterectomy is the mainstay of treatment.

Endometrial stromal sarcomas (ESS), formerly called low-grade ESS, are composed of cells that resemble normal proliferation phase endometrial stroma and are almost all estrogen and progesterone receptor positive. ESS are usually diagnosed at stage I (90%) and should be treated with TAH-BSO alone. Hormone-replacement therapy should not be prescribed in view of their hormone sensitivity. Chemotherapy and radiation therapy should not be used. In case of pelvic or abdominal recurrent disease, debulking surgery should be employed, followed by hormonal therapy (i.e., progestins such as MPA). Aromatase inhibitors, gonadotropin-releasing hormone agonists, and selective estrogen-receptor modulators (SERMs) are used as second- and third-line hormonal therapy. Because of the indolent growth pattern of ESS, patients with advanced or recurrent disease usually have a long survival and may have second or third debulking surgery and several lines of hormonal therapies. For the rare hormone receptor–negative recurrence, chemotherapy with doxorubicin and ifosfamide may be considered.

Undifferentiated uterine sarcoma, formerly called high-grade ESS, should be treated with more extensive surgery. Carcinosarcomas and undifferentiated uterine sarcomas warrant lymph node evaluation, and most current authors favor full surgical staging, including TAH-BSO, peritoneal cytology, full pelvic lymph node dissection, and omentectomy. Clinical data support the view that carcinosarcomas should be considered high-risk carcinomas and should be treated accordingly.[196] In leiomyosarcoma, the risk of lymph node involvement is very low, and lymphadenectomy is therefore not considered indicated.

Retrospective studies of adjuvant radiation therapy have shown improved pelvic control, especially for carcinosarcomas, but no survival benefit.[196-200] The European Organization for Research and Treatment of Cancer (EORTC) completed a prospective, randomized trial (55874) of pelvic irradiation versus no further therapy in 224 patients with uterine sarcomas stage I and II (any types). Radiation therapy provided a significant reduction of pelvic recurrence, with 5-year pelvic recurrence rates of 18% with irradiation versus 36% for the control group (P = .0012). However, survival was not improved (5-year survival rates of 58% and 56%, P = .92). This trial showed the need to separate the different sarcoma types. Carcinosarcomas were found to benefit from pelvic irradiation in terms of pelvic control, but survival was not improved. Leiomyosarcomas had no apparent benefit from irradiation because they were most likely to relapse at distant sites. There were too few endometrial stromal sarcomas included to allow specific comments (Reed N: personal communication, 2005).

In carcinosarcoma, the risk of relapse and patterns of relapse seem to be related to the epithelial component, and molecular genetic and clinical data support the current opinion that carcinosarcomas should be treated as high-risk carcinomas. Based on the data summarized earlier, pelvic radiation therapy is indicated for patients with risk factors similar to those with carcinomas (e.g., high mitotic count, deep myometrial invasion, age older than 60 years, cervical involvement) and for cases with residual microscopic or macroscopic pelvic disease. For patients with leiomyosarcoma or undifferentiated uterine sarcoma, pelvic irradiation can be considered for microscopic or macroscopic residual disease, preferably within clinical trials evaluating radiation therapy with concurrent or sequential chemotherapy.

Adjuvant chemotherapy has been investigated in uterine sarcomas in view of their increased risk of distant metastases. Most trials included only carcinosarcomas. A randomized study evaluating doxorubicin showed no benefit.[201] Studies of chemotherapy for advanced or recurrent disease showed only 18% response to paclitaxel monotherapy,[202] but combination therapy with cisplatin, doxorubicin, and ifosfamide was found to be more effective, with an overall-response rate of 56%, albeit with considerable toxicity.[203] First reports of other platinum-based regimens such as carboplatin and paclitaxel[204] or cisplatin and epirubicin followed by radiation therapy[205] suggest a better toxicity profile and equal efficacy.

Further trials investigating platinum-based regimens with sequential radiation therapy are being conducted to determine optimal treatment of patients with uterine sarcomas.[205,206]

TECHNIQUES OF IRRADIATION

External Beam Pelvic Irradiation

Most patients receive pelvic radiation therapy in the postoperative setting. The clinical target volume for pelvic irradiation consists of the site of the uterus and cervix, the parametrial tissues, the proximal half of the vagina, and the pelvic lymph nodes (i.e., internal and external iliac and the lower common iliac lymph node regions). The planning target volume is derived by adding an appropriate margin around the clinical target to allow for the beam penumbra, geometric uncertainties, and variability in daily patient setup. The main organs at risk for complications are the rectosigmoid, small bowel, and the bladder. Most acute and late complications are of the gastrointestinal tract, and it is essential to reduce the volume of small bowel within the treatment fields as much as possible. A four-field box technique is usually employed, which has a smaller volume of small bowel in the high-dose region compared with anterior and posterior parallel-opposed ports. The patient should be instructed to keep the bladder filled during treatment. The prone treatment position reduces the volume of small bowel within the pelvis, and special belly board devices have been designed that are more effective in pushing the small bowel out of the treatment fields and that ensure reproducible positioning by acting as an positioning device.[207] The use of a belly board device has been shown to be more effective in the postoperative setting than for primary treatment. In thin patients with firm abdominal walls, there may be less benefit, but there is still some advantage to this position. High-energy photons from a linear accelerator are preferred to ensure a homogeneous dose distribution.

The use of a vaginal marker such as a catheter or a gauze with radiopaque contrast helps ensure the vagina is covered in the treatment volume with adequate margins. However, the marker should not distend the vagina to preclude the irradiation of a larger volume of the rectum. Rectal contrast may be used to opacify its contour if conventional simulation is used. Most radiation therapy departments are using CT simulation and three-dimensional CT planning, and multileaf collimators are used in all fields to shield organs at risk and reduce the treated volume. The use of CT planning has the clear advantage of delineating the actual nodal sites, instead of using standard field borders, which risk insufficiently or too generously encompassing the lymphatic chains. The classic field extends from the L4-5 or L5-S1 interspace to the mid-obturator foramen; laterally 2 cm from the widest plane of the true pelvis; ventrally to the pubic symphysis; and dorsally to S3 (Fig. 56-2 A to C).

A total dose of 45 to 46 Gy is usually prescribed in the postoperative setting, with daily fractions of 1.8 to 2.0 Gy for 5 fractions per week. For cases with involved margins or residual macroscopic disease, the target dose is 50.4 Gy with a boost dose to the areas of involvement using CT planning to a cumulative dose of 60 to 70 Gy, depending on the situation. Ideally, these risk areas should be marked with clips during surgery and an omentoplasty should be used to move the small bowel out of the high-dose area.[208]

Extended Field Irradiation

Patients undergoing treatment to the pelvic and para-aortic regions are usually treated in the supine position to ensure a dorsal position of the kidneys. CT-directed planning ensures adequate sparing of the kidneys when using a four-field technique, usually with more weight from the anterior and posterior fields. The superior field border is usually placed at the T12-L1 junction, but it may be individualized according to the level of detected or suspected lymph node involvement. Three-dimensional conformal planning using multiple fields has been shown to significantly reduce the volume of small bowel in the high-dose region compared with anterior and posterior parallel-opposed fields (Fig. 56-2 D and E).[209]

Doses used for pelvic and para-aortic treatment are typically 45 to 50.4 Gy with standard 1.8-Gy fractions. For macroscopic involved lymph nodes a boost dose may be used. Technical aspects of WAI are outlined in Chapter 58.

Intensity-Modulated Radiation Therapy

In view of the additional toxicities when combining surgery, EBRT, and chemotherapy in high-risk endometrial cancer patients, several groups have been investigating the use of intensity-modulated radiation therapy (IMRT) to reduce the dose to critical organs surrounding the target tissues. Pelvic irradiation results in the irradiation of large volumes of the small bowel and rectum, and it may lead to gastrointestinal toxicity in a significant proportion of the patients.

IMRT uses multiple beams of various intensities that conform the high-dose region to the shape of the target tissues in three dimensions, minimizing the dose to the surrounding organs. Treatment planning studies[210-212] have shown that a substantial reduction of the doses to the small bowel, rectum, and the pelvic bone marrow can be realized (Fig. 56-3). The volume of small bowel irradiated to the prescription dose is reduced by a factor of 2, compared with a CT-based, conventional, three-dimensional, four-field box technique.[210,212] First results of clinical studies have shown a modest reduction of acute gastrointestinal toxicity in patients treated with pelvic IMRT[210] and of acute hematologic toxicity in gynecologic cancer patients receiving pelvic IMRT combined with chemotherapy.[213] In an analysis of 36 gynecologic cancer patients treated with pelvic irradiation with or without chemotherapy or brachytherapy (or both), IMRT also resulted in a significant reduction of patients experiencing chronic gastrointestinal toxicity (11% mild symptoms compared with 50% in a historical series of patients receiving pelvic irradiation) and less severe gastrointestinal complications (0% versus 3%).[214] Especially for the increasing number of high-risk endometrial carcinoma patients treated with surgery, radiation therapy, and chemotherapy, IMRT may be an essential tool in reducing the chronic toxicities of multimodality treatment.

Complications of Pelvic Irradiation

Side effects of radiation therapy for gynecologic malignancies have been well documented. Complication rates are dose and volume dependent and are higher for the combination of pelvic EBRT and vaginal brachytherapy (VBT) than for EBRT or VBT alone.[97,119,123,124,215] Complication rates after EBRT are also increased if a full lymphadenectomy is added to the hysterectomy.[215-219] Other treatment-related factors associated with the risk of complications are treatment volume, daily fractionation, radiation therapy technique, and the (historical) use of one field per day.[217,220,221] Patient-related risk factors are prior abdominal surgery, young age, low weight, and concurrent diabetes, hypertension, inflammatory bowel disease, or other pelvic inflammatory conditions, although literature data show conflicting results regarding several of these factors. The most significant complications are obstruction of the small bowel, chronic diarrhea, proctitis, fistula formation, vaginal stenosis, and insufficiency fractures of bone. The use of EBRT is associated with the risk of small bowel complications.[219] The addition of VBT to EBRT especially increases the incidence of vaginal and rectal side effects, such as fibrosis, stenosis, ulcers, and fistula.[123,124,215,216] Reported rates of severe complications after TAH-BSO plus EBRT range from 2% to 6%; after surgery followed by EBRT and VBT, from 4% to 13%; after VBT alone, from 0% to 7% (dose dependent); and after EBRT and surgery, including lymphadenectomy, from 7% to 18%.

The rates of mild to moderate complications are less well established. Acute side effects of EBRT, such as diarrhea, urgency, abdominal cramps, and urinary frequency are usually not reported if they do not cause an interruption or discontinuation of treatment.[222] Mild late side effects (including increased bowel movements, episodes of diarrhea, abdominal cramps, frequent urination, and minor incontinence) are underreported.[223,224]

In the PORTEC trial, 63% of the patients were treated during radiation therapy with medication or dietary measures, or both, for mild, acute symptoms. Discontinuation of irradiation due to acute symptoms occurred in 2% of cases. The 5-year actuarial rates of any late complication were 26% in the radiation therapy group and 4% in the control group ($P < .0001$).[225] Most complications (67%) were mild (grade 1), and almost 50% of symptoms resolved in the course of 2 to 3 years. Gastrointestinal symptoms were the predominant side effects, with a 5-year actuarial rate of (mostly mild) gastrointestinal complications in the radiation therapy group of 20%. The 5-year actuarial rates of severe (grade 3 or 4) late complications were 3% in the radiation therapy group and 0% in the control group. No severe late genitourinary or vaginal complications occurred.

The presence of acute treatment-related symptoms was the most important risk factor for late complications ($P = .001$). The association between acute and late treatment complications has become a topic of interest and research.[226-229] The fact that a subset of patients with acute toxicity have no symptom-free interval between acute and late complications supports

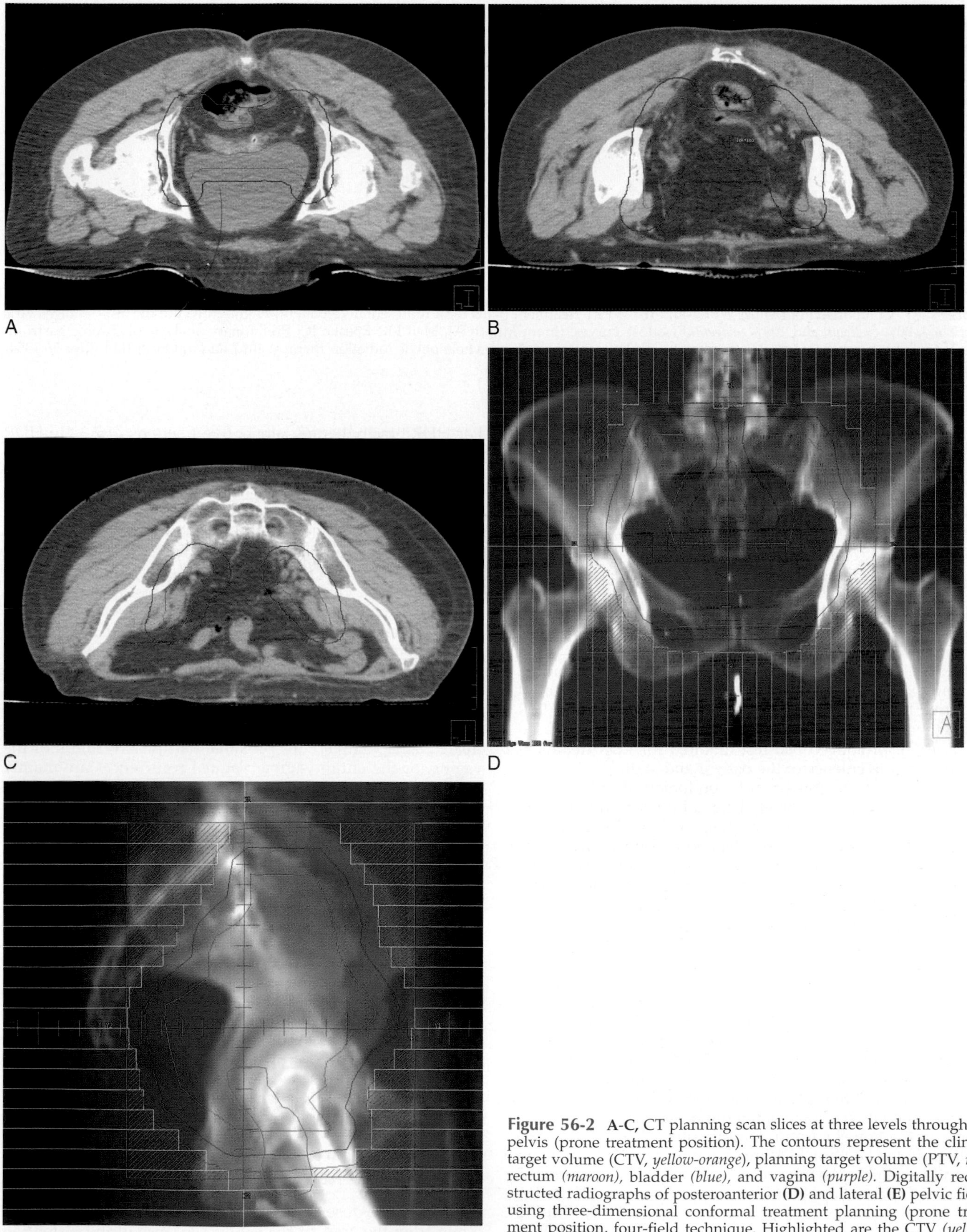

Figure 56-2 **A-C,** CT planning scan slices at three levels through the pelvis (prone treatment position). The contours represent the clinical target volume (CTV, *yellow-orange*), planning target volume (PTV, *red*), rectum *(maroon)*, bladder *(blue)*, and vagina *(purple)*. Digitally reconstructed radiographs of posteroanterior **(D)** and lateral **(E)** pelvic fields using three-dimensional conformal treatment planning (prone treatment position, four-field technique. Highlighted are the CTV *(yellow-orange)* and PTV *(red)*.

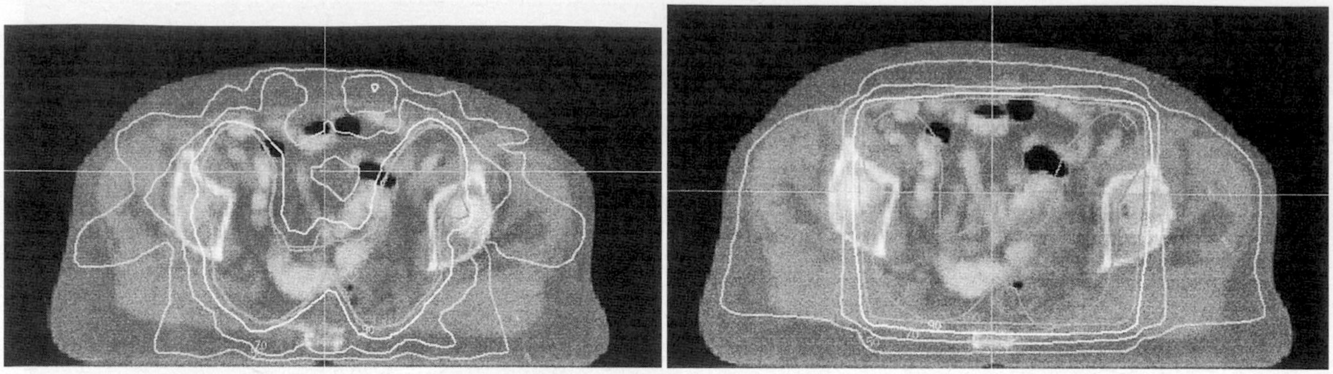

Figure 56-3 Comparison of **(A)** IM-WPRT and **(B)** WPRT treatment plans for a representative patient. Highlighted are the 50% *(orange)*, 70% *(light blue)*, 90% *(yellow)*, and 100% *(magenta)* isodose curves. (From Mundt AJ, Mell LK, Roeske JC: Preliminary analysis of chronic gastrointestinal toxicity in gynecology patients treated with intensity-modulated whole pelvic radiation therapy. Int J Radiat Oncol Biol Phys 56:1354-1360, 2003. Reproduced with permission.)

the theory that late injury occurs as a consequence of persisting acute injury of the intestinal mucosa.[226] Pelvic irradiation is associated with short-term and long-term effects on gastrointestinal function, most notably increased frequency of bowel actions, less bile acid absorption, and faster intestinal transit.[224] Most of these changes improve with time, but some long-term effects persist.

Brachytherapy Techniques

LDR and HDR brachytherapy techniques are available with a variety of manual and remote afterloading applicators for intracavitary and interstitial brachytherapy. LDR is being replaced in most centers by pulsed dose rate (PDR) techniques simulating LDR treatment, but with the convenience of modern HDR machines. Iridium 192 is used for PDR and HDR brachytherapy. HDR may be preferred in view of the increased morbidity of prolonged bed rest required for LDR treatment and for the convenience of the patient and staff.

In primary treatment of endometrial carcinoma, brachytherapy has traditionally been administered with LDR techniques such as Heyman packing or Simon capsules or with a single intrauterine tube, depending on the size of the uterus. The technical aspects of intracavitary placement of a single tube are similar to those for cervical carcinoma, but different dose specification points have been used (e.g., point *My* for myometrium, 2 cm laterally and caudally to the tip of the most advanced applicator, or the *A-line*, 2 cm laterally from the tip). A small uterus can be treated with a single tube, using a stepping source and increasing the dwell times at the fundus to obtain a pear-shaped isodose distribution (i.e., inverted pear). However, an individualized approach is preferable, with dose specification at the serosa at the site of the tumor. An MRI or CT scan is used, ideally with the intrauterine tubes in place, to determine the depth of tumor invasion and the myometrial width in relation to the tubes. CT or MRI planning ensures adequate coverage of the tumor while avoiding overdosing in the bowel surrounding the uterus. Specific uterine applicators for HDR or PDR intracavitary brachytherapy are currently available. An intermediate-size uterus can be treated with a two-channel applicator (one applicator in each uterine cornu), which results in a pear-shaped isodose distribution at the fundus. For treatment of a large uterus with a tumor deeply infiltrating the myometrium, Heyman packing using Norman-Simon applicators is preferred. The American Brachytherapy Society has published treatment guidelines.[230]

For HDR brachytherapy alone, five fractions of 7.3-Gy HDR prescribed at 2 cm from the midpoint of the uterine sources are recommended. If used in conjunction with EBRT, 2 fractions of 8.5 Gy to 4 fractions of 5.2 Gy are suggested. CT or MRI planning is recommended to individualize treatment prescription to the thickness of the uterine wall.

Vaginal Brachytherapy

In patients with vaginal recurrence, the most common site is the upper vagina, and vaginal cuff brachytherapy has long been used to decrease the risk of vaginal cuff recurrence after hysterectomy. Since the mid-1990s, HDR fractionated vaginal cuff brachytherapy alone has been increasingly used as adjuvant therapy after hysterectomy in selected patients. There are institutional variations in the target volume for vaginal brachytherapy, especially the length of the vagina to be treated—the vaginal cuff, proximal half or two thirds of the vagina, or the entire vagina. Vaginal recurrences are mainly located in the vaginal vault and upper vagina, with a ratio of proximal to distal recurrences of 4:1.[50] It is recommended to treat only the upper half of the vagina, because this is associated with lower complication rates (i.e., vaginal stenosis and fistula) than treating the entire length of the vagina. Although most radiation oncologists use vaginal cylinders treating the upper half to two thirds of the vagina, others claim that vaginal colpostats have the advantage of providing a better dose distribution around the vaginal vault with lower doses to the bladder and rectum.[107]

Convenient, moderate-dose fractionation schedules of vaginal brachytherapy provide very high vaginal control rates (>95%) and very low morbidity rates.[112] The use of higher doses increases the risk of side effects and does not further increase the vaginal control rates. Based on these data, optimal LDR and HDR dose schedules seem to be those that give an equivalent of 45 to 50 Gy to the mucosal surface of the upper half of the vagina. Typical examples are LDR 30 Gy, specified at a 5-mm depth at a dose rate of 60 to 65 cGy per hour and given in one session of 2 to 3 days, or HDR 21 Gy, specified at a 5-mm depth and given in 3 fractions of 7 Gy each 1 week apart.

Usually, the dose is specified at 5 mm from the surface and 5 mm from the apex of the vagina. Because of the distention of the vagina after placement of the vaginal cylinder, it has been argued that the wall becomes less than 5 mm thick and that the reference isodose should be chosen at a 3-, 4-, or 5-

mm depth, depending on a clinical estimation of the mucosal thickness. By individualizing the depth and avoiding applicators with small diameters, the rate of vaginal side effects was significantly reduced (17% and 1% for grade 1 and 2, compared with 26% and 8%), without a difference in vaginal control.[231] In individual cases, the target depth can be adjusted according to the clinical situation. For example, in case of a thick scar at the cuff the dose can be specified at 10 mm from the apex and 5 mm along the wall.

Vaginal brachytherapy can be performed as an outpatient procedure, especially when a vaginal cylinder is used, for which no sedation or anesthesia is needed. If vaginal colpostats are used with vaginal gauze packing, intravenous sedation or general or regional anesthesia is commonly used. Most U.S. centers use fentanyl and midazolam intravenously for sedation. With the patient in the lithotomy position, an indwelling bladder catheter is inserted in the bladder, and the balloon is filled with radiopaque contrast material to visualize the bladder base on applicator placement radiographs. Two radiopaque metal seed markers may be inserted submucosally in the vaginal cuff to assess applicator position on radiographs. The colpostats are positioned in the upper vagina against the cuff. Vaginal packing is used to secure the colpostats in place and to displace the bladder base and anterior

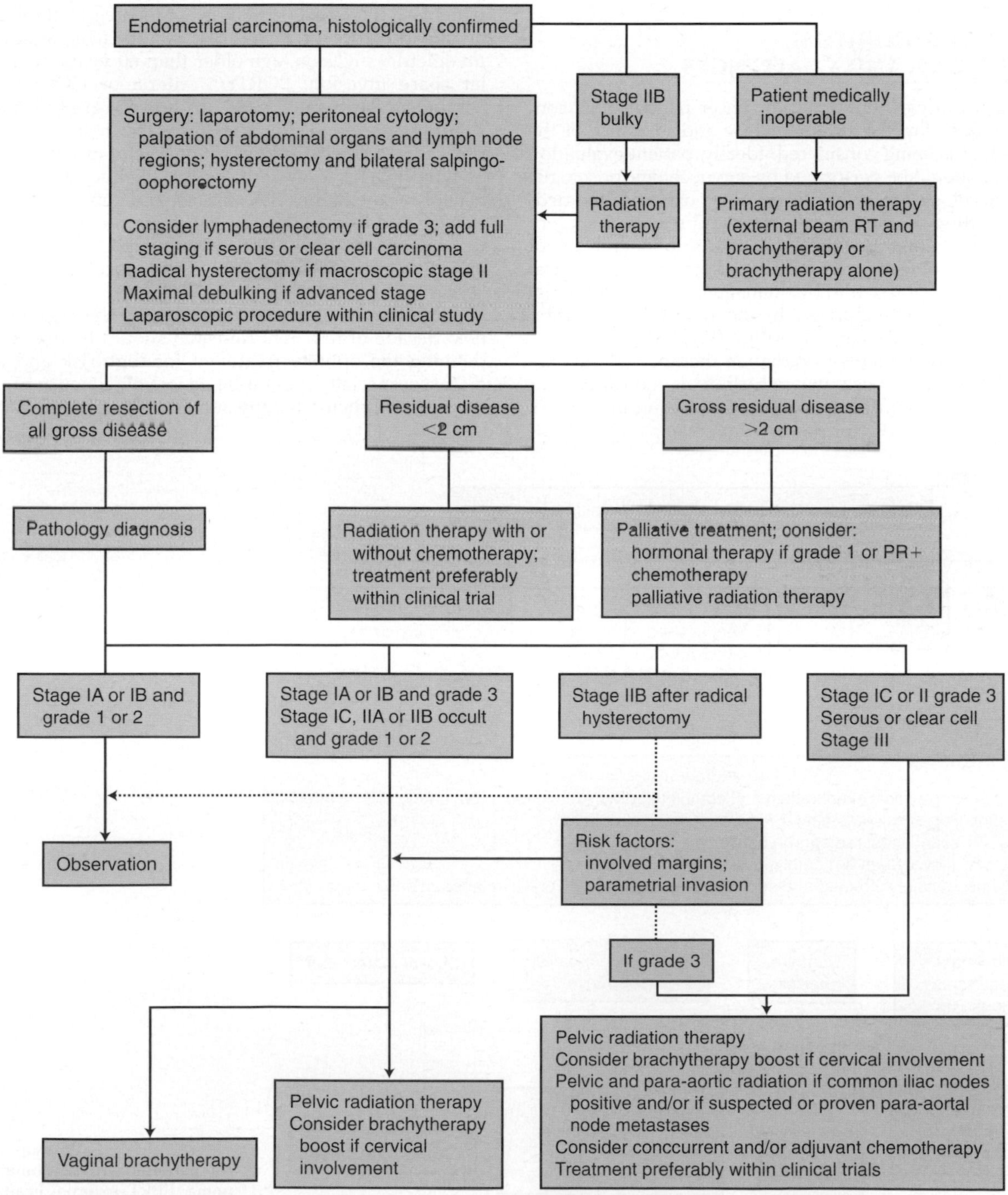

Figure 56-4 Treatment algorithm for patients with endometrial carcinoma. PR, palliative radiation; RT, radiation therapy.

rectum away. When a vaginal cylinder is used, the largest diameter that smoothly fits the vagina should be chosen, because with smaller diameters, the volume of the vaginal mucosa receiving more than 150% of the dose is increased. The applicator is held in place by an external immobilization device. Orthogonal radiographs are obtained to verify the appropriate placement of the applicator in relation to the vaginal cuff markers and for dosimetric calculations. A small amount of rectal contrast agent is injected before the lateral radiograph is filmed. After the appropriate quality assurance checks, the HDR treatment is administered, which takes less than 10 minutes, depending on the dose and the source activity. Applicators and catheters are then removed, and the patient is discharged.

TREATMENT ALGORITHM, CONCLUSIONS, AND CHALLENGES

The treatment of each endometrial cancer patient must consider the risk factors for tumor relapse and tolerance of the treatment that is being considered. Ideally, patient evaluation and surgery should be performed by a gynecologic oncologist or by a gynecologist with specific oncology expertise and dedication. Deciding on the indication for and extent of surgery and adjuvant therapy requires a multidisciplinary team of gynecologic oncologists, radiation oncologists, and medical oncologists. The approach to the management of endometrial cancer patients is summarized in the treatment algorithm (Fig. 56-4) and the follow-up algorithm (Fig. 56-5).

The main developments in radiation therapy for endometrial carcinoma have been the reduction of indications for pelvic irradiation, shifting the role of irradiation in low-risk disease toward treatment reserved for patients with vaginal or pelvic relapse, the increasing use of vaginal brachytherapy alone for intermediate-risk disease, and the use of adjuvant chemotherapy and radiation therapy for high-risk and advanced disease. Radiation therapy techniques have been developed that reduce the risk of acute and late complications, especially in conjunction with extended surgery or chemotherapy.

The role of pelvic irradiation in treating intermediate-risk endometrial carcinoma has been established with the results of randomized trials. Pelvic irradiation provides a highly significant improvement of local control, but it does not increase overall survival and does not reduce the risk of distant metastases. The use of pelvic irradiation should be limited to patients at increased (>15%) risk of locoregional relapse based on the presence of major risk factors (e.g., grade 3, deep myometrial invasion, age older than 60 years, lymphovascular space invasion; PORTEC criteria or GOG-HIR criteria having similar results). Stage IA and IB, grade 1 and 2 cases should be observed after TAH-BSO. The inclusion of such low-risk cases in clinical studies of the role of radiation therapy or of lymphadenectomy reduces the likelihood of observing a benefit for the higher-risk subsets, and subjects these patients to increased risks of toxicity. Radiation therapy is a very effective salvage treatment for vaginal relapse in patients not previously irradiated, with 80% to 90% local control rates and 5-year survival rates of 50% to 70%.

High-risk endometrial carcinoma is the challenge for the next decade of research. Research should be directed toward defining the optimal treatment for high-risk and advanced disease, especially the combined use of (concurrent) radiation therapy and chemotherapy and the role of lymphadenectomy.

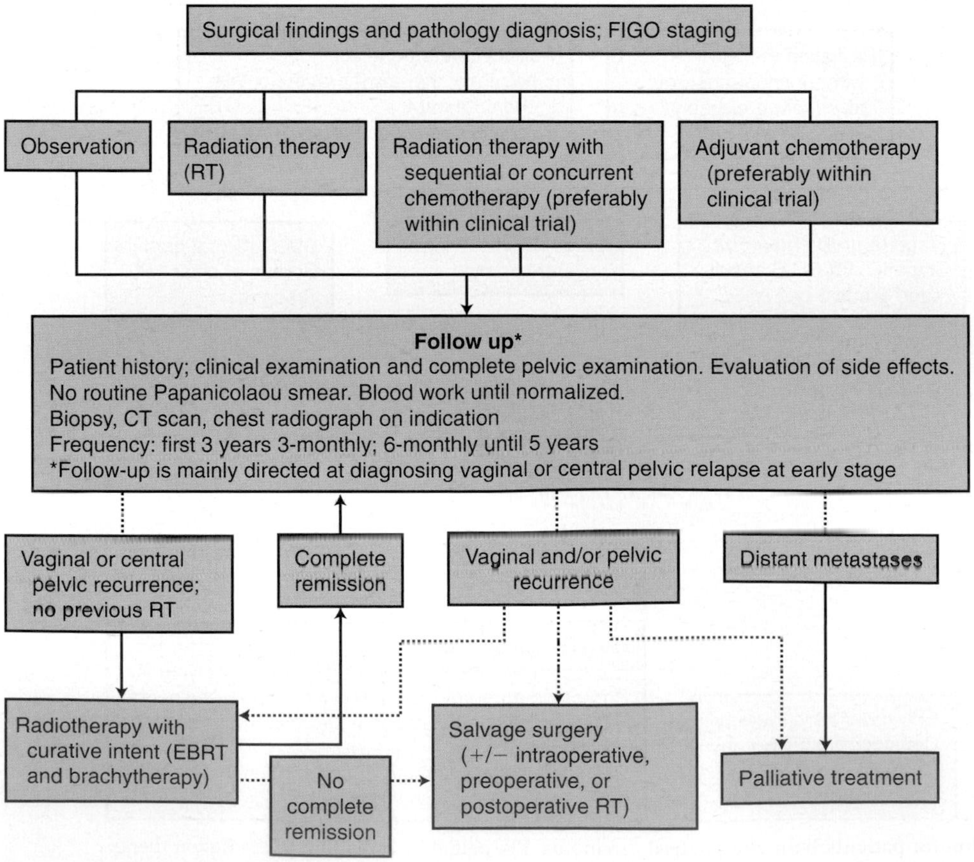

Figure 56-5 Follow-up algorithm for patients with endometrial carcinoma. EBRT, external beam radiation therapy.

Targeted therapies may prove to be effective, especially in the treatment of serous carcinoma. Newer radiation therapy techniques that reduce the risk of complications should be further developed, especially in conjunction with multimodality treatment. For patients with locally advanced disease in whom trimodality treatment (i.e., surgery, irradiation, and chemotherapy) is indicated, laparoscopic staging followed by preoperative concurrent chemoradiation, restaging, and surgical resection alone or plus intraoperative radiation therapy and adjuvant chemotherapy should be evaluated.

Quality-of-life and cost-effectiveness analyses will become essential because patients with high-risk and advanced-stage disease are typically elderly and have concurrent medical illnesses. The approach to these patients needs to balance the benefit of more aggressive adjuvant therapies with the cumulative toxicities. The ultimate goal of treatment for endometrial cancer patients remains the maximization of event-free and complication-free survival.

REFERENCES

1. Jemal A, Siegel R, Ward E, et al: Cancer statistics, 2006. CA Cancer J Clin 56:106-130, 2006.
2. Visser O, Coebergh JWW, Scouten LJ, Van Dijck JAAM: Incidence of cancer in the Netherlands 2000. Utrecht, Netherlands Cancer Registry, 2004.
3. Harlow BL, Weiss NS, Lofton S: The epidemiology of sarcomas of the uterus. J Natl Cancer Inst 76:399-402, 1986.
4. Gambrell RD Jr, Bagnell CA, Greenblatt RB: Role of estrogens and progesterone in the etiology and prevention of endometrial cancer: review. Am J Obstet Gynecol 146:696-707, 1983.
5. Purdie DM, Green AC: Epidemiology of endometrial cancer. Best Pract Res Clin Obstet Gynaecol 15:341-354, 2001.
6. Shapiro S, Kelly JP, Rosenberg L, et al: Risk of localized and widespread endometrial cancer in relation to recent and discontinued use of conjugated estrogens. N Engl J Med 313:969-972, 1985.
7. Fisher B, Costantino JP, Redmond CK, et al: Endometrial cancer in tamoxifen-treated breast cancer patients: findings from the National Surgical Adjuvant Breast and Bowel Project (NSABP) B-14. J Natl Cancer Inst 86:527-537, 1994.
8. Magriples U, Naftolin F, Schwartz PE, et al: High-grade endometrial carcinoma in tamoxifen-treated breast cancer patients. J Clin Oncol 11:485-490, 1993.
9. van Leeuwen FE, Benraadt J, Coebergh JW, et al: Risk of endometrial cancer after tamoxifen treatment of breast cancer. Lancet 343:448-452, 1994.
10. Bergman L, Beelen ML, Gallee MP, et al: Risk and prognosis of endometrial cancer after tamoxifen for breast cancer. Comprehensive Cancer Centres' ALERT Group. Assessment of Liver and Endometrial Cancer Risk following Tamoxifen. Lancet 356:881-887, 2000.
11. Kurman RJ, Kaminski PF, Norris HJ: The behavior of endometrial hyperplasia. A long-term study of "untreated" hyperplasia in 170 patients. Cancer 56:403-412, 1985.
12. Parslov M, Lidegaard O, Klintorp S, et al: Risk factors among young women with endometrial cancer: a Danish case-control study. Am J Obstet Gynecol 182:23-29, 2000.
13. Parazzini F, La Vecchia C, Moroni S, et al: Family history and the risk of endometrial cancer. Int J Cancer 59:460-462, 1994.
14. Olson JE, Sellers TA, Anderson KE, et al: Does a family history of cancer increase the risk for postmenopausal endometrial carcinoma? A prospective cohort study and a nested case-control family study of older women. Cancer 85:2444-2449, 1999.
15. Hemminki K, Aaltonen L, Li X: Subsequent primary malignancies after endometrial carcinoma and ovarian carcinoma. Cancer 97:2432-2439, 2003.
16. Hemminki K, Granstrom C: Familial clustering of ovarian and endometrial cancers. Eur J Cancer 40:90-95, 2004.
17. Re A, Taylor TH, DiSaia PJ, Anton-Culver H: Risk for breast and colorectal cancers subsequent to cancer of the endometrium in a population-based case series. Gynecol Oncol 66:255-257, 1997.
18. Aarnio M, Sankila R, Pukkala E, et al: Cancer risk in mutation carriers of DNA-mismatch-repair genes. Int J Cancer 81:214-218, 1999.
19. Wijnen J, de Leeuw W, Vasen H, et al: Familial endometrial cancer in female carriers of MSH6 germline mutations. Nat Genet 23:142-144, 1999.
20. Lynch HT, Smyrk TC, Watson P, et al: Genetics, natural history, tumor spectrum, and pathology of hereditary nonpolyposis colorectal cancer: an updated review. Gastroenterology 104:1535-1549, 1993.
21. Vasen HF, Wijnen JT, Menko FH, et al: Cancer risk in families with hereditary nonpolyposis colorectal cancer diagnosed by mutation analysis. Gastroenterology 110:1020-1027, 1996.
22. Lindahl B, Willen R: Spontaneous endometrial hyperplasia: a prospective, 5 year follow-up of 246 patients after abrasio only, including 380 patients followed-up for 2 years. Anticancer Res 14:2141-2146, 1994.
23. Janicek MF, Rosenshein NB: Invasive endometrial cancer in uteri resected for atypical endometrial hyperplasia. Gynecol Oncol 52:373-378, 1994.
24. Gerber B, Krause A, Muller H, et al: Ultrasonographic detection of asymptomatic endometrial cancer in postmenopausal patients offers no prognostic advantage over symptomatic disease discovered by uterine bleeding. Eur J Cancer 37:64-71, 2001.
25. Dove-Edwin I, Boks D, Goff S, et al: The outcome of endometrial carcinoma surveillance by ultrasound scan in women at risk of hereditary nonpolyposis colorectal carcinoma and familial colorectal carcinoma. Cancer 94:1708-1712, 2002.
26. Mourits MJ, Van der Zee AG, Willemse PH, et al: Discrepancy between ultrasonography and hysteroscopy and histology of endometrium in postmenopausal breast cancer patients using tamoxifen. Gynecol Oncol 73:21-26, 1999.
27. Gerber B, Krause A, Muller H, et al: Effects of adjuvant tamoxifen on the endometrium in postmenopausal women with breast cancer: a prospective long-term study using transvaginal ultrasound. J Clin Oncol 18:3464-3470, 2000.
28. Kurman RJ (ed): Blaustein's Pathology of the Female Genital Tract: Endometrial Carcinoma (ed 4). New York, Springer-Verlag, 1994, pp 439-486.
29. Christopherson WM, Connelly PJ, Alberhasky RC: Carcinoma of the endometrium. V. An analysis of prognosticators in patients with favorable subtypes and stage I disease. Cancer 51:1705-1709, 1983.
30. Abeln EC, Smit VT, Wessels JW, et al: Molecular genetic evidence for the conversion hypothesis of the origin of malignant mixed mullerian tumours. J Pathol 183:424-431, 1997.
31. Bitterman P, Chun B, Kurman RJ: The significance of epithelial differentiation in mixed mesodermal tumors of the uterus: a clinicopathologic and immunohistochemical study. Am J Surg Pathol 14:317-328, 1990.
32. Hendrickson M, Ross J, Eifel P, et al: Uterine papillary serous carcinoma: a highly malignant form of endometrial adenocarcinoma. Am J Surg Pathol 6:93-108, 1982.
33. Eifel PJ, Ross J, Hendrickson M, et al: Adenocarcinoma of the endometrium. Analysis of 256 cases with disease limited to the uterine corpus: treatment comparisons. Cancer 52:1026-1031, 1983.
34. Wilson TO, Podratz KC, Gaffey TA, et al: Evaluation of unfavorable histologic subtypes in endometrial adenocarcinoma. Am J Obstet Gynecol 162:418-423, 1990.
35. Fanning J, Evans MC, Peters AJ, et al: Endometrial adenocarcinoma histologic subtypes: clinical and pathologic profile. Gynecol Oncol 32:288-291, 1989.
36. Alektiar KM, McKee A, Lin O, et al: Is there a difference in outcome between stage I-II endometrial cancer of papillary serous/clear cell and endometrioid FIGO grade 3 cancer? Int J Radiat Oncol Biol Phys 54:79-85, 2002.
37. Creasman WT, Kohler MF, Odicino F, et al: Prognosis of papillary serous, clear cell, and grade 3 stage I carcinoma of the endometrium. Gynecol Oncol 95:593-596, 2004.
38. Zaino RJ, Kurman R, Herbold D, et al: The significance of squamous differentiation in endometrial carcinoma. Data from a Gynecologic Oncology Group study. Cancer 68:2293-2302, 1991.

39. Abeler VM, Kjorstad KE: Endometrial adenocarcinoma with squamous cell differentiation. Cancer 69:488-495, 1992.
40. Baloglu H, Cannizzaro LA, Jones J, et al: Atypical endometrial hyperplasia shares genomic abnormalities with endometrioid carcinoma by comparative genomic hybridization. Hum Pathol 32:615-622, 2001.
41. Hunter JE, Tritz DE, Howell MG, et al: The prognostic and therapeutic implications of cytologic atypia in patients with endometrial hyperplasia. Gynecol Oncol 55:66-71, 1994.
42. Ambros RA, Sherman ME, Zahn CM, et al: Endometrial intraepithelial carcinoma: a distinctive lesion specifically associated with tumors displaying serous differentiation. Hum Pathol 26: 1260-1267, 1995.
43. Lax SF, Kurman RJ, Pizer ES, et al: A binary architectural grading system for uterine endometrial endometrioid carcinoma has superior reproducibility compared with FIGO grading and identifies subsets of advance-stage tumors with favorable and unfavorable prognosis. Am J Surg Pathol 24:1201-1208, 2000.
44. Mittal KR, Barwick KW: Diffusely infiltrating adenocarcinoma of the endometrium: a subtype with poor prognosis. Am J Surg Pathol 12:754-758, 1988.
45. Creasman WT, Morrow CP, Bundy BN, et al: Surgical pathologic spread patterns of endometrial cancer. A Gynecologic Oncology Group study. Cancer 60:2035-2041, 1987.
46. Morrow CP, Bundy BN, Kurman RJ, et al: Relationship between surgical-pathological risk factors and outcome in clinical stage I and II carcinoma of the endometrium: a Gynecologic Oncology Group study. Gynecol Oncol 40:55-65, 1991.
47. Niikura H, Okamura C, Utsunomiya H, et al: Sentinel lymph node detection in patients with endometrial cancer. Gynecol Oncol 92:669-674, 2004.
48. Barranger E, Cortez A, Grahek D, et al: Laparoscopic sentinel node procedure using a combination of patent blue and radiocolloid in women with endometrial cancer. Ann Surg Oncol 11:344-349, 2004.
49. Burke TW, Levenback C, Tornos C, et al: Intraabdominal lymphatic mapping to direct selective pelvic and paraaortic lymphadenectomy in women with high-risk endometrial cancer: results of a pilot study. Gynecol Oncol 62:169-173, 1996.
50. COSA-NZ-UK Endometrial Cancer Study Group: Pelvic lymphadenectomy in high risk endometrial cancer. Int J Gynecol Cancer 6:102-107, 1996.
51. Bokhman JV: Two pathogenetic types of endometrial carcinoma. Gynecol Oncol 15:10-17, 1983.
52. Santin AD, Bellone S, Gokden M, et al: Overexpression of HER-2/neu in uterine serous papillary cancer. Clin Cancer Res 8:1271-1279, 2002.
53. Santin AD: HER2/neu overexpression: has the Achilles' heel of uterine serous papillary carcinoma been exposed? Gynecol Oncol 88:263-265, 2003.
54. Khalifa MA, Mannel RS, Haraway SD, et al: Expression of EGFR, HER-2/neu, P53, and PCNA in endometrioid, serous papillary, and clear cell endometrial adenocarcinomas. Gynecol Oncol 53:84-92, 1994.
55. Jasas KV, Fyles A, Elit L, et al: Phase II study of erlotinib (OSI 774) in women with recurrent or metastatic endometrial cancer: NCIC CTG IND-148. 2004 ASCO annual meetings proceedings. J Clin Oncol 22:5019, 2005.
56. Jeon YT, Kang S, Kang DH, et al: Cyclooxygenase-2 and p53 expressions in endometrial cancer. Cancer Epidemiol Biomarkers Prev 13:1538-1542, 2004.
57. Mariani A, Sebo TJ, Katzmann JA, et al: Pretreatment assessment of prognostic indicators in endometrial cancer. Am J Obstet Gynecol 182:1535-1544, 2000.
58. Baak JPA, Snijders W, van Diermen B, et al: Prospective multicenter validation confirms the prognostic superiority of the endometrial carcinoma prognostic index in International Federation of Gynecology and Obstetrics stage 1 and 2 endometrial carcinoma. J Clin Oncol 21:4214-4221, 2003.
59. Lukes AS, Kohler MF, Pieper CF, et al: Multivariable analysis of DNA ploidy, p53, and HER-2/neu as prognostic factors in endometrial cancer. Cancer 73:2380-2385, 1994.
60. Zaino RJ, Kurman RJ, Diana KL, et al: Pathologic models to predict outcome for women with endometrial adenocarcinoma: the importance of the distinction between surgical stage and clinical stage—a Gynecologic Oncology Group study [published erratum appears in Cancer 79:422, 1997]. Cancer 77:1115-1121, 1996.
61. Greven KM, Corn BW, Case D, et al: Which prognostic factors influence the outcome of patients with surgically staged endometrial cancer treated with adjuvant radiation? Int J Radiat Oncol Biol Phys 39:413-418, 1997.
62. Aalders J, Abeler V, Kolstad P, et al: Postoperative external irradiation and prognostic parameters in stage I endometrial carcinoma: clinical and histopathologic study of 540 patients. Obstet Gynecol 56:419-427, 1980.
63. Creutzberg CL, van Putten WL, Koper PC, et al: Surgery and postoperative radiotherapy versus surgery alone for patients with stage-1 endometrial carcinoma: multicentre randomised trial. PORTEC Study Group. Post Operative Radiation Therapy in Endometrial Carcinoma [see comments]. Lancet 355:1404-1411, 2000.
64. Keys HM, Roberts JA, Brunetto VL, et al: A phase III trial of surgery with or without adjunctive external pelvic radiation therapy in intermediate risk endometrial adenocarcinoma: a Gynecologic Oncology Group study. Gynecol Oncol 92:744-751, 2004.
65. Creutzberg CL, van Putten WL, Warlam-Rodenhuis CC, et al: Outcome of high-risk stage IC, grade 3, compared with stage I endometrial carcinoma patients: the Postoperative Radiation Therapy in Endometrial Carcinoma Trial. J Clin Oncol 22:1234-1241, 2004.
66. Scholten AN, Creutzberg CL, Noordijk EM, et al: Long-term outcome in endometrial carcinoma favors a two- instead of a three-tiered grading system. Int J Radiat Oncol Biol Phys 52:1067-1074, 2002.
67. Taylor RR, Zeller J, Lieberman RW, et al: An analysis of two versus three grades for endometrial carcinoma [see comments]. Gynecol Oncol 74:3-6, 1999.
68. Scholten AN, Smit VTHB, Beerman H, et al: Prognostic significance and interobserver variability of histologic grading systems for endometrial carcinoma. Cancer 100:764-772, 2004.
69. Alkushi A, Abdul-Rahman ZH, Lim P, et al: Description of a novel system for grading of endometrial carcinoma and comparison with existing grading systems. Am J Surg Pathol 29:295-304, 2005.
70. Suzuki C, Matsumoto T, Sonoue H, et al: Prognostic significance of the infiltrative pattern invasion in endometrioid adenocarcinoma of the endometrium. Pathol Int 53:495-500, 2003.
71. Lindauer J, Fowler JM, Manolitsas TP, et al: Is there a prognostic difference between depth of myometrial invasion and the tumor-free distance from the uterine serosa in endometrial cancer? Gynecol Oncol 91:547-551, 2003.
72. Briet JM, Hollema H, Reesink N, et al: Lymphvascular space involvement: an independent prognostic factor in endometrial cancer. Gynecol Oncol 96:799-804, 2005.
73. Dore R, Moro G, D'Andrea F, et al: CT evaluation of myometrium invasion in endometrial carcinoma. J Comput Assist Tomogr 11:282-289, 1987.
74. Manfredi R, Mirk P, Maresca G, et al: Local-regional staging of endometrial carcinoma: role of MR imaging in surgical planning. Radiology 231:372-378, 2004.
75. Ayhan A, Taskiran C, Celik C, et al: The long-term survival of women with surgical stage II endometrioid type endometrial cancer. Gynecol Oncol 93:9-13, 2004.
76. Sartori E, Gadducci A, Landoni F, et al: Clinical behavior of 203 stage II endometrial cancer cases: the impact of primary surgical approach and of adjuvant radiation therapy. Int J Gynecol Cancer 11:430-437, 2001.
77. Malur S, Possover M, Michels W, et al: Laparoscopic-assisted vaginal versus abdominal surgery in patients with endometrial cancer—a prospective randomized trial. Gynecol Oncol 80:239-244, 2001.
78. Eltabbakh GH, Shamonki MI, Moody JM, et al: Laparoscopy as the primary modality for the treatment of women with endometrial carcinoma. Cancer 91:378-387, 2001.
79. Gemignani ML, Curtin JP, Zelmanovich J, et al: Laparoscopic-assisted vaginal hysterectomy for endometrial cancer: clinical outcomes and hospital charges. Gynecol Oncol 73:5-11, 1999.

80. Sonoda Y, Zerbe M, Smith A, et al: High incidence of positive peritoneal cytology in low-risk endometrial cancer treated by laparoscopically assisted vaginal hysterectomy. Gynecol Oncol 80:378-382, 2001.
81. Chu CS, Randall TC, Bandera CA, et al: Vaginal cuff recurrence of endometrial cancer treated by laparoscopic-assisted vaginal hysterectomy. Gynecol Oncol 88:62-65, 2003.
82. Schneider A: Vaginal cuff recurrence of endometrial cancer treated by laparoscopic-assisted vaginal hysterectomy. Gynecol Oncol 94:861-2004.
83. Holub Z: Vaginal cuff recurrence of endometrial cancer treated by laparoscopic-assisted vaginal hysterectomy. Gynecol Oncol 90:495-497, 2003.
84. Trimble EL, Kosary C, Park RC: Lymph node sampling and survival in endometrial cancer. Gynecol Oncol 71:340-343, 1998.
85. Cragun JM, Havrilesky LJ, Calingaert B, et al: Retrospective analysis of selective lymphadenectomy in apparent early-stage endometrial cancer. J Clin Oncol 23:3668-3675, 2005.
86. Mohan DS, Samuels MA, Selim MA, et al: Long-term outcomes of therapeutic pelvic lymphadenectomy for stage I endometrial adenocarcinoma. Gynecol Oncol 70:165-171, 1998.
87. Fanning J, Nanavati PJ, Hilgers RD: Surgical staging and high dose rate brachytherapy for endometrial cancer: limiting external radiotherapy to node-positive tumors. Obstet Gynecol 87:1041-1044, 1996.
88. Kilgore LC, Partridge EE, Alvarez RD, et al: Adenocarcinoma of the endometrium: survival comparisons of patients with and without pelvic node sampling. Gynecol Oncol 56:29-33, 1995.
89. Nguyen TV, Petereit DG: High-dose-rate brachytherapy for medically inoperable stage I endometrial cancer. Gynecol Oncol 71:196-203, 1998.
90. Fishman DA, Roberts KB, Chambers JT, et al: Radiation therapy as exclusive treatment for medically inoperable patients with stage I and II endometrioid carcinoma with endometrium. Gynecol Oncol 61:189-196, 1996.
91. Rouanet P, Dubois JB, Gely S, et al: Exclusive radiation therapy in endometrial carcinoma. Int J Radiat Oncol Biol Phys 26:223-228, 1993.
92. Lehoczky O, Bosze P, Ungar L, et al: Stage I endometrial carcinoma: treatment of nonoperable patients with intracavitary radiation therapy alone. Gynecol Oncol 43:211-216, 1991.
93. Kucera H, Knocke TH, Kucera E, et al: Treatment of endometrial carcinoma with high-dose-rate brachytherapy alone in medically inoperable stage I patients. Acta Obstet Gynecol Scand 77:1008-1012, 1998.
94. Grigsby PW, Kuske RR, Perez CA, et al: Medically inoperable stage I adenocarcinoma of the endometrium treated with radiotherapy alone. Int J Radiat Oncol Biol Phys 13:483-488, 1987.
95. Varia M, Rosenman J, Halle J, et al: Primary radiation therapy for medically inoperable patients with endometrial carcinoma—stages I-II. Int J Radiat Oncol Biol Phys 13:11-15, 1987.
96. Knocke TH, Kucera H, Weidinger B, et al: Primary treatment of endometrial carcinoma with high-dose-rate brachytherapy: results of 12 years of experience with 280 patients. Int J Radiat Oncol Biol Phys 37:359-365, 1997.
97. Carey MS, O'Connell GJ, Johanson CR, et al: Good outcome associated with a standardized treatment protocol using selective postoperative radiation in patients with clinical stage I adenocarcinoma of the endometrium [see comments]. Gynecol Oncol 57:138-144, 1995.
98. Poulsen HK, Jacobsen M, Bertelsen K, et al: Adjuvant radiation therapy is not necessary in the management of endometrial carcinoma stage I, low-risk cases. Int J Gynecol Cancer 6:38-43, 1996.
99. Mariani A, Webb MJ, Keeney GL, et al: Low-risk corpus cancer: Is lymphadenectomy or radiotherapy necessary? Am J Obstet Gynecol 182:1506-1516, 2000.
100. Alektiar KM, McKee A, Venkatraman E, et al: Intravaginal high-dose-rate brachytherapy for Stage IB (FIGO Grade 1, 2) endometrial cancer. Int J Radiat Oncol Biol Phys 53:707-713, 2002.
101. Aalders J, Abeler V, Kolstad P, et al: Postoperative external irradiation and prognostic parameters in stage I endometrial carcinoma: clinical and histopathologic study of 540 patients. Obstet Gynecol 56:419-427, 1980.
102. Creutzberg CL, van Putten WLJ, Koper PC, et al: Survival after relapse in patients with endometrial cancer: results from a randomized trial. Gynecol Oncol 89:201-209, 2003.
103. Bond WH: Early uterine body carcinoma: has post-operative vaginal irradiation any value? Clin Radiol 36:619-623, 1985.
104. Eltabbakh GH, Piver MS, Hempling RE, et al: Excellent long-term survival and absence of vaginal recurrences in 332 patients with low-risk stage I endometrial adenocarcinoma treated with hysterectomy and vaginal brachytherapy without formal staging lymph node sampling: report of a prospective trial. Int J Radiat Oncol Biol Phys 38:373-380, 1997.
105. Rose PG, Tak WK, Fitzgerald TJ, et al: Brachytherapy for early endometrial carcinoma: a comparative study with long-term follow-up. Int J Gynecol Cancer 9:105-109, 1999.
106. Elliott P, Green D, Coates A, et al: The efficacy of postoperative vaginal irradiation in preventing vaginal recurrence in endometrial cancer. Int J Gynecol Cancer 4:84-93, 1994.
107. Petereit DG, Tannehill SP, Grosen EA, et al: Outpatient vaginal cuff brachytherapy for endometrial cancer. Int J Gynecol Cancer 9:456-462, 1999.
108. Pearcey RG, Petereit DG: Post-operative high dose rate brachytherapy in patients with low to intermediate risk endometrial cancer. Radiother Oncol 56:17-22, 2000.
109. Chadha M, Nanavati PJ, Liu P, et al: Patterns of failure in endometrial carcinoma stage IB grade 3 and IC patients treated with postoperative vaginal vault brachytherapy. Gynecol Oncol 75:103-107, 1999.
110. Weiss E, Hirnle P, Arnold-Bofinger H, et al: Adjuvant vaginal high-dose-rate afterloading alone in endometrial carcinoma: patterns of relapse and side effects following low-dose therapy. Gynecol Oncol 71:72-76, 1998.
111. Anderson JM, Stea B, Hallum AV, et al: High-dose-rate postoperative vaginal cuff irradiation alone for stage IB and IC endometrial cancer. Int J Radiat Oncol Biol Phys 46:417-425, 2000.
112. Petereit DG, Pearcey R: Literature analysis of high dose rate brachytherapy fractionation schedules in the treatment of cervical cancer: is there an optimal fractionation schedule? Int J Radiat Oncol Biol Phys 43:359-366, 1999.
113. Anderson JM, Stea B, Hallum AV, et al: High-dose-rate postoperative vaginal cuff irradiation alone for stage IB and IC endometrial cancer. Int J Radiat Oncol Biol Phys 46:417-425, 2000.
114. Rittenberg PV, Lotocki RJ, Heywood MS, et al: High-risk surgical stage 1 endometrial cancer: outcomes with vault brachytherapy alone. Gynecol Oncol 89:288-294, 2003.
115. Greven KM, Randall M, Fanning J, et al: Patterns of failure in patients with stage I, grade 3 carcinoma of the endometrium. Int J Radiat Oncol Biol Phys 19:529-534, 1990.
116. Straughn JM, Huh WK, Orr JW, et al: Stage IC adenocarcinoma of the endometrium: survival comparisons of surgically staged patients with and without adjuvant radiation therapy. Gynecol Oncol 89:295-300, 2003.
117. Naumann RW, Higgins RV, Hall JB: The use of adjuvant radiation therapy by members of the Society of Gynecologic Oncologists. Gynecol Oncol 75:4-9, 1999.
118. Koh WJ, Tran AB, Douglas JG, et al: Radiation therapy in endometrial cancer. Best Pract Res Clin Obstet Gynaecol 15:417-432, 2001.
119. Greven KM, Corn BW: Endometrial cancer. Curr Probl Cancer 21:65-127, 1997.
120. Jereczek-Fossa BA: Postoperative irradiation in endometrial cancer: still a matter of controversy. Cancer Treat Rev 27:19-33, 2001.
121. Jobsen JJ, Schutter EM, Meerwaldt JH, et al: Treatment results in women with clinical stage I and pathologic stage II endometrial carcinoma. Int J Gynecol Cancer 11:49-53, 2001.
122. Eltabbakh GH, Moore AD: Survival of women with surgical stage II endometrial cancer. Gynecol Oncol 74:80-85, 1999.
123. Irwin C, Levin W, Fyles A, et al: The role of adjuvant radiotherapy in carcinoma of the endometrium—results in 550 patients with pathologic stage I disease. Gynecol Oncol 70:247-254, 1998.
124. Randall ME, Wilder J, Greven K, et al: Role of intracavitary cuff boost after adjuvant external irradiation in early endometrial carcinoma. Int J Radiat Oncol Biol Phys 19:49-54, 1990.

125. Greven KM, D'Agostino RB Jr, Lanciano RM, et al: Is there a role for a brachytherapy vaginal cuff boost in the adjuvant management of patients with uterine-confined endometrial cancer? Int J Radiat Oncol Biol Phys 42:101-104, 1998.
126. Pitson G, Colgan T, Levin W, et al: Stage II endometrial carcinoma: prognostic factors and risk classification in 170 patients. Int J Radiat Oncol Biol Phys 53:862-867, 2002.
127. Mariani A, Webb MJ, Keeney GL, et al: Role of wide/radical hysterectomy and pelvic lymph node dissection in endometrial cancer with cervical involvement. Gynecol Oncol 83:72-80, 2001.
128. Cornelison TL, Trimble EL, Kosary CL: SEER data, corpus uteri cancer: treatment trends versus survival for FIGO stage II, 1988-1994. Gynecol Oncol 74:350-355, 1999.
129. Leminen A, Forss M, Lehtovirta P: Endometrial adenocarcinoma with clinical evidence of cervical involvement: accuracy of diagnostic procedures, clinical course, and prognostic factors. Acta Obstet Gynecol Scand 74:61-66, 1995.
130. Hamilton CA, Liou WS, Osann KN, et al: Impact of adjuvant therapy on survival of patients with early-stage uterine papillary serous carcinoma. Int J Radiat Oncol Biol Phys 63:839-844, 2005.
131. Martin-Hirsch PL, Lilford RJ, Jarvis GJ: Adjuvant progestagen therapy for the treatment of endometrial cancer: review and meta-analyses of published randomised controlled trials. Eur J Obstet Gynecol Reprod Biol 65:201-207, 1996.
132. Vergote I, Kjorstad K, Abeler V, et al: A randomized trial of adjuvant progestagen in early endometrial cancer. Cancer 64:1011-1016, 1989.
133. COSA-NZ-UK Endometrial Cancer Study Groups: Adjuvant medroxyprogesterone acetate in high-risk endometrial cancer. Int J Gynecol Cancer 8:387-391, 1998.
134. Morrow CP, Bundy BN, Homesley HD, et al: Doxorubicin as an adjuvant following surgery and radiation therapy in patients with high-risk endometrial carcinoma, stage I and occult stage II: a Gynecologic Oncology Group Study. Gynecol Oncol 36:166-171, 1990.
135. Randall ME, Filliaci VL, Muss H, et al: Randomized phase III trial of whole-abdominal irradiation versus doxorubicin and cisplatin chemotherapy in advanced endometrial carcinoma: a Gynecologic Oncologic Group Study. J Clin Oncol 24:36-44, 2006.
136. Mundt AJ, McBride R, Rotmensch J, et al: Significant pelvic recurrence in high-risk pathologic stage I-IV endometrial carcinoma patients after adjuvant chemotherapy alone: implications for adjuvant radiation therapy. Int J Radiat Oncol Biol Phys 50:1145-1153, 2001.
137. Frigerio L, Mangili G, Aletti G, et al: Concomitant radiotherapy and paclitaxel for high-risk endometrial cancer: first feasibility study. Gynecol Oncol 81:53-57, 2001.
138. Reisinger SA, Asbury R, Liao SY, et al: A phase I study of weekly cisplatin and whole abdominal radiation for the treatment of stage III and IV endometrial carcinoma: a Gynecologic Oncology Group pilot study. Gynecol Oncol 63:299-303, 1996.
139. Greven K, Winter K, Underhill K, et al: Preliminary analysis of RTOG 9708: Adjuvant postoperative radiotherapy combined with cisplatin/paclitaxel chemotherapy after surgery for patients with high-risk endometrial cancer. Int J Radiat Oncol Biol Phys 59:168-173, 2004.
140. Burke TW, Gershenson DM, Morris M, et al: Postoperative adjuvant cisplatin, doxorubicin, and cyclophosphamide (PAC) chemotherapy in women with high-risk endometrial carcinoma. Gynecol Oncol 55:47-50, 1994.
141. Elit L, Kwon J, Bentley J, et al: Optimal management for surgically Stage 1 serous cancer of the uterus. Gynecol Oncol 92:240-246, 2004.
142. Santin AD, Bellone S, O'Brien TJ, et al: Current treatment options for endometrial cancer. Expert Rev Anticancer Ther 4:679-689, 2004.
143. Nicklin JL, Petersen RW: Stage 3B adenocarcinoma of the endometrium: a clinicopathologic study. Gynecol Oncol 78:203-207, 2000.
144. Ashman JB, Connell PP, Yamada D, et al: Outcome of endometrial carcinoma patients with involvement of the uterine serosa. Gynecol Oncol 82:338-343, 2001.
145. Mariani A, Webb MJ, Keeney GL, et al: Assessment of prognostic factors in stage IIIA endometrial cancer. Gynecol Oncol 86:38-44, 2002.
146. Greven KM, Curran WJ Jr, Whittington R, et al: Analysis of failure patterns in stage III endometrial carcinoma and therapeutic implications. Int J Radiat Oncol Biol Phys 17:35-39, 1989.
147. Kadar N, Homesley HD, Malfetano JH: Positive peritoneal cytology is an adverse factor in endometrial carcinoma only if there is other evidence of extrauterine disease. Gynecol Oncol 46:145-149, 1992.
148. Tebeu PM, Popowski Y, Verkooijen HM, et al: Positive peritoneal cytology in early-stage endometrial cancer does not influence prognosis. Br J Cancer 91:720-724, 2004.
149. Kasamatsu T, Onda T, Katsumata N, et al: Prognostic significance of positive peritoneal cytology in endometrial carcinoma confined to the uterus. Br J Cancer 88:245-250, 2003.
150. Obermair A, Geramou M, Gucer F, et al: Does hysteroscopy facilitate tumor cell dissemination? Incidence of peritoneal cytology from patients with early stage endometrial carcinoma following dilatation and curettage (D & C) versus hysteroscopy and D & C. Cancer 88:139-143, 2000.
151. Revel A, Tsafrir A, Anteby SO, et al: Does hysteroscopy produce intraperitoneal spread of endometrial cancer cells? Obstet Gynecol Surv 59:280-284, 2004.
152. Aalders JG, Abeler V, Kolstad P: Clinical (stage III) as compared to subclinical intrapelvic extrauterine tumor spread in endometrial carcinoma: a clinical and histopathological study of 175 patients. Gynecol Oncol 17:64-74, 1984.
153. Greven KM, Lanciano RM, Corn B, et al: Pathologic stage III endometrial carcinoma: prognostic factors and patterns of recurrence. Cancer 71:3697-3702, 1993.
154. Grigsby PW, Perez CA, Kuske RR, et al: Results of therapy, analysis of failures, and prognostic factors for clinical and pathologic stage III adenocarcinoma of the endometrium. Gynecol Oncol 27:44-57, 1987.
155. Schorge JO, Molpus KL, Goodman A, et al: The effect of postsurgical therapy on stage III endometrial carcinoma. Gynecol Oncol 63:34-39, 1996.
156. Gibbons S, Martinez A, Schray M, et al: Adjuvant whole abdominopelvic irradiation for high risk endometrial carcinoma. Int J Radiat Oncol Biol Phys 21:1019-1025, 1991.
157. Potish RA, Twiggs LB, Adcock LL, et al: Role of whole abdominal radiation therapy in the management of endometrial cancer: prognostic importance of factors indicating peritoneal metastases. Gynecol Oncol 21:80-86, 1985.
158. Mundt AJ, Murphy KT, Rotmensch J, et al: Surgery and postoperative radiation therapy in FIGO stage IIIC endometrial carcinoma. Int J Radiat Oncol Biol Phys 50:1154-1160, 2001.
159. Nelson G, Randall M, Sutton G, et al: FIGO stage IIIC endometrial carcinoma with metastases confined to pelvic lymph nodes: analysis of treatment outcomes, prognostic variables, and failure patterns following adjuvant radiation therapy. Gynecol Oncol 75:211-214, 1999.
160. Ayhan A, Taskiran C, Celik C, et al: Surgical stage III endometrial cancer: analysis of treatment outcomes, prognostic factors and failure patterns. Eur J Gynaecol Oncol 23:553-556, 2002.
161. Rose PG, Cha SD, Tak WK, et al: Radiation therapy for surgically proven paraaortic node metastasis in endometrial carcinoma. Int J Radiat Oncol Biol Phys 24:229-233, 1992.
162. Hicks ML, Piver MS, Puretz JL, et al: Survival in patients with paraaortic lymph-node metastases from endometrial adenocarcinoma clinically limited to the uterus. Int J Radiat Oncol Biol Phys 26:607-611, 1993.
163. Corn BW, Lanciano RM, Greven KM, et al: Endometrial cancer with paraaortic adenopathy—patterns of failure and opportunities for cure. Int J Radiat Oncol Biol Phys 24:223-227, 1992.
164. Bristow RE, Zahurak ML, Alexander CJ, et al: FIGO stage IIIC endometrial carcinoma: Resection of macroscopic nodal disease and other determinants of survival. Int J Gynecol Cancer 13:664-672, 2003.
165. Chi DS, Welshinger M, Venkatraman ES, et al: The role of surgical cytoreduction in stage IV endometrial carcinoma. Gynecol Oncol 67:56-60, 1997.

166. Cook AM, Lodge N, Blake P: Stage IV endometrial carcinoma: a 10 year review of patients. Br J Radiol 72:485-488, 1999.
167. Lambrou NC, Gomez-Marin O, Mirhashemi R, et al: Optimal surgical cytoreduction in patients with stage III and stage IV endometrial carcinoma: a study of morbidity and survival. Gynecol Oncol 93:653-658, 2004.
168. Bruzzone M, Miglietta L, Franzone P, et al: Combined treatment with chemotherapy and radiotherapy in high-risk FIGO stage III-IV endometrial cancer patients. Gynecol Oncol 93:345-352, 2004.
169. Wylie J, Irwin C, Pintilie M, et al: Results of radical radiotherapy for recurrent endometrial cancer. Gynecol Oncol 77:66-72, 2000.
170. Jereczek-Fossa B, Badzio A, Jassem J: Recurrent endometrial cancer after surgery alone: results of salvage radiotherapy. Int J Radiat Oncol Biol Phys 48:405-413, 2000.
171. Curran WJ Jr, Whittington R, Peters AJ, et al: Vaginal recurrences of endometrial carcinoma: the prognostic value of staging by a primary vaginal carcinoma system. Int J Radiat Oncol Biol Phys 15:803-808, 1988.
172. Sears JD, Greven KM, Hoen HM, et al: Prognostic factors and treatment outcome for patients with locally recurrent endometrial cancer. Cancer 74:1303-1308, 1994.
173. Podczaski E, Kaminski P, Gurski K, et al: Detection and patterns of treatment failure in 300 consecutive cases of "early" endometrial cancer after primary surgery. Gynecol Oncol 47:323-327, 1992.
174. Poulsen MG, Roberts SJ: Prognostic variables in endometrial carcinoma. Int J Radiat Oncol Biol Phys 13:1043-1052, 1987.
175. Ackerman I, Malone S, Thomas G, et al: Endometrial carcinoma—relative effectiveness of adjuvant irradiation vs therapy reserved for relapse [see comments]. Gynecol Oncol 60:177-183, 1996.
176. Hoekstra CJ, Koper PC, van Putten WL: Recurrent endometrial adenocarcinoma after surgery alone: prognostic factors and treatment. Radiother Oncol 27:164-166, 1993.
177. Pai HH, Souhami L, Clark BG, et al: Isolated vaginal recurrences in endometrial carcinoma: treatment results using high-dose-rate intracavitary brachytherapy and external beam radiotherapy. Gynecol Oncol 66:300-307, 1997.
178. Hart KB, Han I, Shamsa F, et al: Radiation therapy for endometrial cancer in patients treated for postoperative recurrence. Int J Radiat Oncol Biol Phys 41:7-11, 1998.
179. Nag S, Yacoub S, Copeland LJ, et al: Interstitial brachytherapy for salvage treatment of vaginal recurrences in previously unirradiated endometrial cancer patients. Int J Radiat Oncol Biol Phys 54:1153-1159, 2002.
180. Burke TW, Heller PB, Woodward JE, et al: Treatment failure in endometrial carcinoma. Obstet Gynecol 75:96-101, 1990.
181. Burke TW: How should we monitor women treated for endometrial carcinoma? Gynecol Oncol 65:377-378, 1997.
182. Berchuck A, Anspach C, Evans AC, et al: Postsurgical surveillance of patients with FIGO stage I/II endometrial adenocarcinoma. Gynecol Oncol 59:20-24, 1995.
183. Reddoch JM, Burke TW, Morris M, et al: Surveillance for recurrent endometrial carcinoma: development of a follow-up scheme. Gynecol Oncol 59:221-225, 1995.
184. Shumsky AG, Brasher PM, Stuart GC, et al: Risk-specific follow-up for endometrial carcinoma patients. Gynecol Oncol 65:379-382, 1997.
185. Van den Hout WB, van der Linden YM, Steenland E, et al: Single- versus multiple-fraction radiotherapy in patients with painful bone metastases: cost-utility analysis based on a randomized trial. J Natl Cancer Inst 95:222-229, 2003.
186. Thigpen JT, Brady MF, Alvarez RD, et al: Oral medroxyprogesterone acetate in the treatment of advanced or recurrent endometrial carcinoma: a dose-response study by the Gynecologic Oncology Group. J Clin Oncol 17:1736-1744, 1999.
187. Moore TD, Phillips PH, Nerenstone SR, et al: Systemic treatment of advanced and recurrent endometrial carcinoma: current status and future directions. J Clin Oncol 9:1071-1088, 1991.
188. Lentz SS, Brady MF, Major FJ, et al: High-dose megestrol acetate in advanced or recurrent endometrial carcinoma: a Gynecologic Oncology Group study. J Clin Oncol 14:357-361, 1996.
189. Thigpen JT, Brady MF, Homesley HD, et al: Phase III trial of doxorubicin with or without cisplatin in advanced endometrial carcinoma: a gynecologic oncology group study. J Clin Oncol 22:3902-3908, 2004.
190. Aapro MS, Van Wijk FH, Bolis G, et al: Doxorubicin versus doxorubicin and cisplatin in endometrial carcinoma: definitive results of a randomised study (55872) by the EORTC Gynaecological Cancer Group. Ann Oncol 14:441-448, 2003.
191. Dimopoulos MA, Papadimitriou CA, Georgoulias V, et al: Paclitaxel and cisplatin in advanced or recurrent carcinoma of the endometrium: long-term results of a phase II multicenter study. Gynecol Oncol 78:52-57, 2000.
192. Fleming GF, Brunetto VL, Cella D, et al: Phase III trial of doxorubicin plus cisplatin with or without paclitaxel plus filgrastim in advanced endometrial carcinoma: a Gynecologic Oncology Group study. J Clin Oncol 22:2159-2166, 2004.
193. Fleming GF, Filiaci VL, Bentley RC, et al: Phase III randomized trial of doxorubicin + cisplatin versus doxorubicin + 24-h paclitaxel + filgrastim in endometrial carcinoma: a Gynecologic Oncology Group study. Ann Oncol 15:1173-1178, 2004.
194. Hoskins PJ, Swenerton KD, Pike JA, et al: Paclitaxel and carboplatin, alone or with irradiation, in advanced or recurrent endometrial cancer: a phase II study. J Clin Oncol 19:4048-4053, 2001.
195. Sagae S, Yamashita K, Ishioka S, et al: Preoperative diagnosis and treatment results in 106 patients with uterine sarcoma in Hokkaido, Japan. Oncology 67:33-39, 2004.
196. Gerszten K, Faul C, Kounelis S, et al: The impact of adjuvant radiotherapy on carcinosarcoma of the uterus. Gynecol Oncol 68:8-13, 1998.
197. Salazar OM, Bonfiglio TA, Patten SF, et al: Uterine sarcomas: analysis of failures with special emphasis on the use of adjuvant radiation therapy. Cancer 42:1161-1170, 1978.
198. Perez CA, Askin F, Baglan RJ, et al: Effects of irradiation on mixed mullerian tumors of the uterus. Cancer 43:1274-1284, 1979.
199. Livi L, Andreopoulou E, Shah N, et al: Treatment of uterine sarcoma at the Royal Marsden Hospital from 1974 to 1998. Clin Oncol (R Coll Radiol) 16:261-268, 2004.
200. Le T: Adjuvant pelvic radiotherapy for uterine carcinosarcoma in a high risk population. Eur J Surg Oncol 27:282-285, 2001.
201. Omura GA, Blessing JA, Major F, et al: A randomized clinical trial of adjuvant adriamycin in uterine sarcomas: a Gynecologic Oncology Group study. J Clin Oncol 3:1240-1245, 1985.
202. Curtin JP, Blessing JA, Soper JT, et al: Paclitaxel in the treatment of carcinosarcoma of the uterus: a Gynecologic Oncology Group study. Gynecol Oncol 83:268-270, 2001.
203. van Rijswijk RE, Vermorken JB, Reed N, et al: Cisplatin, doxorubicin and ifosfamide in carcinosarcoma of the female genital tract. A phase II study of the European Organization for Research and Treatment of Cancer Gynaecological Cancer Group (EORTC 55923). Eur J Cancer 39:481-487, 2003.
204. Toyoshima M, Akahira J, Matsunaga G, et al: Clinical experience with combination paclitaxel and carboplatin therapy for advanced or recurrent carcinosarcoma of the uterus. Gynecol Oncol 94:774-778, 2004.
205. Manolitsas TP, Wain GV, Williams KE, et al: Multimodality therapy for patients with clinical stage I and II malignant mixed mullerian tumors of the uterus. Cancer 91:1437-1443, 2001.
206. Pautier P, Rey A, Haie-Meder C, et al: Adjuvant chemotherapy with cisplatin, ifosfamide, and doxorubicin followed by radiotherapy in localized uterine sarcomas: results of a case-control study with radiotherapy alone. Int J Gynecol Cancer 14:1112-1117, 2004.
207. Olofsen-Van Acht M, van den BH, Quint S, et al: Reduction of irradiated small bowel volume and accurate patient positioning by use of a bellyboard device in pelvic radiotherapy of gynecological cancer patients. Radiother Oncol 59:87-93, 2001.
208. Logmans A, van Lent M, van Geel AN, et al: The pedicled omentoplasty, a simple and effective surgical technique to acquire a safe pelvic radiation field; theoretical and practical aspects. Radiother Oncol 33:269-271, 1994.
209. Olofsen-van Acht MJ, Quint S, Seven M, et al: Three-dimensional treatment planning for postoperative radiotherapy in patients with node-positive cervical cancer: comparison between a conventional and a conformal technique. Strahlenther Onkol 175:462-469, 1999.

210. Mundt AJ, Lujan AE, Rotmensch J, et al: Intensity-modulated whole pelvic radiotherapy in women with gynecologic malignancies. Int J Radiat Oncol Biol Phys 52:1330-1337, 2002.
211. Lujan AE, Mundt AJ, Yamada SD, et al: Intensity-modulated radiotherapy as a means of reducing dose to bone marrow in gynecologic patients receiving whole pelvic radiotherapy. Int J Radiat Oncol Biol Phys 57:516-521, 2003.
212. Heron DE, Gerszten K, Selvaraj RN, et al: Conventional 3D conformal versus intensity-modulated radiotherapy for the adjuvant treatment of gynecologic malignancies: a comparative dosimetric study of dose-volume histograms. Gynecol Oncol 91:39-45, 2003.
213. Brixey CJ, Roeske JC, Lujan AE, et al: Impact of intensity-modulated radiotherapy on acute hematologic toxicity in women with gynecologic malignancies. Int J Radiat Oncol Biol Phys 54:1388-1396, 2002.
214. Mundt AJ, Mell LK, Roeske JC: Preliminary analysis of chronic gastrointestinal toxicity in gynecology patients treated with intensity-modulated whole pelvic radiation therapy. Int J Radiat Oncol Biol Phys 56:1354-1360, 2003.
215. MacLeod C, Fowler A, Duval P, et al: Adjuvant high-dose rate brachytherapy with or without external beam radiotherapy post-hysterectomy for endometrial cancer. Int J Gynecol Cancer 9:247-255, 1999.
216. Greven KM, Lanciano RM, Herbert SH, et al: Analysis of complications in patients with endometrial carcinoma receiving adjuvant irradiation. Int J Radiat Oncol Biol Phys 21:919-923, 1991.
217. Corn BW, Lanciano RM, Greven KM, et al: Impact of improved irradiation technique, age, and lymph node sampling on the severe complication rate of surgically staged endometrial cancer patients: a multivariate analysis. J Clin Oncol 12:510-515, 1994.
218. Lewandowski G, Torrisi J, Potkul RK, et al: Hysterectomy with extended surgical staging and radiotherapy versus hysterectomy alone and radiotherapy in stage I endometrial cancer: a comparison of complication rates. Gynecol Oncol 36:401-404, 1990.
219. Potish RA, Dusenbery KE: Enteric morbidity of postoperative pelvic external beam and brachytherapy for uterine cancer. Int J Radiat Oncol Biol Phys 18:1005-1010, 1990.
220. Letschert JG, Lebesque JV, Aleman BM, et al: The volume effect in radiation-related late small bowel complications: results of a clinical study of the EORTC Radiotherapy Cooperative Group in patients treated for rectal carcinoma. Radiother Oncol 32:116-123, 1994.
221. Jereczek-Fossa B, Jassem J, Nowak R, et al: Late complications after postoperative radiotherapy in endometrial cancer: analysis of 317 consecutive cases with application of linear- quadratic model. Int J Radiat Oncol Biol Phys 41:329-338, 1998.
222. Jereczek-Fossa BA, Badzio A, Jassem J: Factors determining acute normal tissue reactions during postoperative radiotherapy in endometrial cancer: analysis of 317 consecutive cases. Radiother Oncol 68:33-39, 2003.
223. Pedersen D, Bentzen SM, Overgaard J: Reporting radiotherapeutic complications in patients with uterine cervical cancer: the importance of latency and classification system. Radiother Oncol 28:134-141, 1993.
224. Yeoh E, Horowitz M, Russo A, et al: Effect of pelvic irradiation on gastrointestinal function: a prospective longitudinal study. Am J Med 95:397-406, 1993.
225. Creutzberg CL, van Putten WL, Koper PC, et al: The morbidity of treatment for patients with Stage I endometrial cancer: results from a randomized trial. Int J Radiat Oncol Biol Phys 51:1246-1255, 2001.
226. Wang CJ, Leung SW, Chen HC, et al: The correlation of acute toxicity and late rectal injury in radiotherapy for cervical carcinoma: evidence suggestive of consequential late effect (CQLE). Int J Radiat Oncol Biol Phys 40:85-91, 1998.
227. Schultheiss TE, Lee WR, Hunt MA, et al: Late GI and GU complications in the treatment of prostate cancer. Int J Radiat Oncol Biol Phys 37:3-11, 1997.
228. Bourne RG, Kearsley JH, Grove WD, et al: The relationship between early and late gastrointestinal complications of radiation therapy for carcinoma of the cervix. Int J Radiat Oncol Biol Phys 9:1445-1450, 1983.
229. Weiss E, Hirnle P, Arnold-Bofinger H, et al: Therapeutic outcome and relation of acute and late side effects in the adjuvant radiotherapy of endometrial carcinoma stage I and II. Radiother Oncol 53:37-44, 1999.
230. Nag S, Erickson B, Parikh S, et al: The American Brachytherapy Society recommendations for high-dose-rate brachytherapy for carcinoma of the endometrium. Int J Radiat Oncol Biol Phys 48:779-790, 2000.
231. Onsrud M, Strickert T, Marthinsen AB: Late reactions after postoperative high-dose-rate intravaginal brachytherapy for endometrial cancer: a comparison of standardized and individualized target volumes. Int J Radiat Oncol Biol Phys 49:749-755, 2001.

CHAPTER 57

VULVAR AND VAGINAL CARCINOMA

Anthony H. Russell

VULVAR CARCINOMA

INCIDENCE

Vulvar carcinoma accounts for 3% to 5% of all gynecologic malignancies.

It constitutes 1% to 2% of cancers in women.

BIOLOGY

Approximately 80% to 90% of primary vulvar tumors are squamous cell carcinomas.

Carcinomas of the vestibular glands (Bartholin's glands) often are adenocarcinomas or adenocystic carcinomas, but 30% to 50% have squamous histology.

Melanoma, basal cell carcinoma, Merkel cell tumor, sarcoma, Paget's disease, and metastatic lesions constitute rare histologic types of vulvar malignancy.

ETIOLOGY

Young patients with vulvar carcinoma more commonly smoke and have a higher incidence of human papillomavirus (HPV) infection; these factors are commonly associated with vulvar intraepithelial neoplasia.

In elderly patients, HPV infection is unusual, and concurrent vulvar intraepithelial neoplasia is uncommon.

Invasive vulvar cancer is often seen arising in a background of lichen sclerosus and squamous hyperplasia in older patients, although only approximately 4% of patients with these associated lesions develop clinically apparent neoplasia.

RISK FACTORS

International Federation of Gynecology and Obstetrics (FIGO) stage, primary tumor size, depth of invasion, presence of capillary-lymphatic space involvement, and width of surgical margins correlate with primary recurrence risk. Number and size of lymph node metastases and extracapsular extension in metastatic adenopathy correlate with risk of regional recurrence and distant dissemination.

STAGING EVALUATION

Evaluation includes the patient's history, a physical examination, and the pathologic status of lymph nodes.

Regional imaging assessments may include computed tomography, positron emission tomography, magnetic resonance imaging, and ultrasonography. Imaging findings may aid in selecting therapy, but they do not affect assignment of stage.

PRIMARY THERAPY

For primary disease, initial treatment is based on clinical evaluation of the disease extent, and adjuvant therapy in patients treated with primary surgery is based on the presence or absence of pathologic risk factors. Except when surgery would compromise the anatomy or function of midline structures, radical local excision is standard therapy for primary disease of limited volume and extent.

For locally advanced primary lesions or lesions invading or encroaching on functionally important midline structures (e.g., clitoris, urethra, anorectum, ischial rami), initial chemoradiation, possibly followed by conservative excision, is preferred to extirpative surgery.

Treatment of regional lymph nodes consists of unilateral or bilateral inguinal node dissection, depending on extent and location of the primary tumor (lateralized versus midline) and involvement of nodes. In rare patients with primary cancers of limited size (<2 cm) and depth of invasion (<1 mm), groin dissection may be omitted.

Although groin dissection remains the standard of care, elective irradiation of groins that are negative for disease (based on clinical and imaging assessment) may replace groin node dissection in selected patients undergoing initial chemoradiation because of the extent of the primary lesion.

For patients with fixed or ulcerating groin lymph nodes, concurrent chemoradiation, alone or followed by limited groin dissection, may provide regional control.

ADJUVANT THERAPY

For the primary tumor, adjuvant local vulvar and tumor bed irradiation may be administered for certain risk factors, including involved or close surgical margins (<8 mm) or capillary lymphatic space involvement and deep invasion (>5 mm).

For one macroscopic node metastasis, two or more microscopically involved nodes, or extracapsular extension, unilateral or bilateral irradiation to the groin and pelvic lymph nodes is given after surgical resection of inguinofemoral nodes.

PALLIATION

Radiation therapy often provides relief of pain or bleeding.

Chemotherapy alone is generally ineffective.

Vulvar carcinoma is an uncommon disease, accounting for only 3% to 5% of all gynecologic cancers. Diversity in the location and clinical extent of disease at presentation, ranging from in situ or small-volume invasive primary disease to neglected extensive tumors that may locally extend to involve the vagina, urethra, or anus, suggests the wisdom of individualized treatment. The presence or absence of metastatic spread to inguinal lymph nodes adds to the heterogeneity of the patient population at the time of diagnosis. The range of patient age at diagnosis, the existence of medical comorbidities, and the diversity of patients' concerns regarding function and cosmesis further complicate treatment decisions. Appreciation of the broad clinical spectrum of patients afflicted with vulvar cancer has resulted in major changes in disease management in the past 20 years.

Historically, radical vulvectomy and bilateral inguinal node dissection was the standard approach for most patients, regardless of disease extent.[1-4] Most large series from which survival data are available are from the era when vulvar cancer was preferentially treated with surgery alone. Data compiled from seven large series in the literature suggest that the overall survival rate for operable patients is approximately 70%.[5-11] Corrected 5-year survival results from the compiled series for International Federation of Gynecology and Obstetrics (FIGO) stages I, II, III, and IV are 90%, 77%, 51%, and 18%, respectively.

Because of the chronic, often debilitating physical and psychological sequelae of radical vulvectomy in long-term survivors, questions arose regarding the need for radical vulvectomy in patients with limited disease at diagnosis. Unsatisfactory rates of locoregional control in patients with advanced disease stimulated exploration of novel combinations of therapies. Increasing awareness of the sensitivity of squamous vulvar cancer to radiation further suggested management changes. Although optimal therapy for many situations remains to be defined, avenues of change include conservative surgery for selected patients with early disease and multimodality therapy (i.e., chemoradiation alone or integrated with less extensive surgery) for the patients with locally advanced disease for whom ultraradical surgery produced inadequate local control and survival results in decades past. Definitive irradiation or chemoradiation is increasingly accepted as alternative therapy for patients with disease that would require partial or total exenteration if treated by initial surgery. Preoperative or postoperative adjuvant irradiation or chemoradiation are commonly used to complement conservative surgery in patients with adverse clinical or histopathologic features.

Mature published results remain sparse for patients treated on the basis of the newer concepts of integrated multimodality management tailored to the site and extent of disease. Valuable information continues to accumulate from a number of phase I/II study reports, all of which support the concept of integrated therapy. Selecting the order in which therapies are employed, defining the intensity and scope of radiation and the extent of surgery when these complementary modalities are used sequentially, and optimizing the choice and schedule of chemotherapy when combined with radiation are issues that require further study.

ETIOLOGY AND EPIDEMIOLOGY

No universal cause for vulvar cancer has been identified. The cause is likely multifactorial, and some risk factors have been identified. Many patients with vulvar carcinoma have had previous malignant or premalignant lesions of the genital tract.[12-14] Between 2% and 5% of vulvar intraepithelial neoplasia-3 (VIN-3) lesions (i.e., severe dysplasia or carcinoma in situ) will progress to invasive carcinoma.[15] The risk factors for progression to invasive cancer are poorly understood but do include advanced age. One study observed that the relative risk for vulvar or vaginal carcinoma after treatment for cervical carcinoma was 2.9%, regardless of whether the patient received irradiation for treatment of the cervical cancer. Compromised immune status, whether iatrogenic in the setting of organ transplantation, congenital, or acquired based on human immunodeficiency virus (HIV) infection, leads to an increased risk of cancers in the lower genital tract, including the vulva and vagina. Improvement in immune function with antiretroviral therapy may decrease the risk in HIV-infected patients.[16-25]

The human papillomavirus (HPV) has been implicated as a cause of vulvar cancer. Brinton and colleagues established a relative risk of vulvar cancer of 14.6% when there is a history of condylomata acuminata.[26] HPV has been detected widely in sexually active women. The type of HPV is related to the risk of benign or malignant tumors of the vulva. In patients with condylomata acuminata, the detected HPV is usually type 6 or 11, whereas for vulvar in situ neoplasia or vulvar carcinoma, HPV-16 and HPV-18 are more common.[27,28] Invasive vulvar cancer and condyloma may be present synchronously in the same patient, delaying diagnosis of malignancy in some patients. Multiple studies have investigated the presence of HPV in vulvar carcinoma. It is reported to be present in 0% to 80% of examined tumors and may be detected in primary tumors and nodal metastases.[29,30] Smoking is an additional risk factor for vulvar carcinoma, and the combination of smoking with a history of genital warts results in a strong increase in the relative risk for vulvar cancer.[13,26] It is probable that smoking and HPV infection have a synergistic effect on the genesis of vulvar cancer, with smoking functioning as a promoter.[31,32]

Data are conflicting about the etiologic role of vulvar dystrophies (i.e., lichen sclerosus or squamous cell hyperplasia) in the cause of vulvar cancer. These epithelial alterations may be seen in approximately one half of patients with vulvar cancer.[33-35] Patients with vulvar cancer and associated lichen sclerosus are on average significantly older than patients with newly diagnosed lichen sclerosus with or without squamous hyperplasia.[36] However, less than 5% of these epithelial alterations will progress to invasive vulvar malignancy.

There are two broadly different groups of vulvar cancer patients. The first consists of younger patients who more frequently smoke and are at higher risk for HPV infection and whose invasive cancers are commonly associated with VIN. The second, more common group consists of elderly patients whose disease may be unrelated to smoking or HPV infection and in whom concurrent VIN is unusual, but lichen sclerosus and squamous hyperplasia are common associated findings.[37]

Investigators have examined a number of molecular and genetic parameters in an effort to define prognostic factors in patients with invasive cancer and to identify patients with lichen sclerosus, squamous hyperplasia, or VIN who are at highest risk for development of invasive malignancy.[38-45] However, molecular markers have not yet entered routine clinical practice.

PREVENTION AND EARLY DETECTION

Because most vulvar malignancies arise from cutaneous surfaces readily accessible to examination visibly and palpably, invasive lesions should be diagnosed when small and easily treated. Unfortunately, most advanced vulvar cancers are a result of the patient's delay or neglect or the physician's failure to diagnose. Some elderly patients may be mentally impaired. Inappropriate modesty, anxiety, or frank denial may lead a patient to ignore or minimize symptoms of pruritus, oozing, bleeding, and pain. There is little justification for failure of a physician to perform a thorough examination when patients have such symptoms.

No known measures to prevent invasive vulvar cancer exist, except for the appropriate treatment of VIN when it is detected. BecauseVIN-3 may be associated with an occult invasive lesion in as many as 20% of patients, care must be taken when employing treatment techniques that do not include full-thickness histologic evaluation.[46] Excisional techniques, provided that there is minimal loss of functionality and cosmesis, may be preferable to ablative techniques without histologic material for study. Wedge biopsy or excisional biopsy of smaller lesions is suggested for most vulvar abnormalities, performed if necessary under colposcopic guidance. Even if vulvar lesions appear to have a warty appearance and are believed to be benign, confluent warts should undergo biopsy to exclude an underlying diagnosis of squamous cell carcinoma. Whether treatment of lichen sclerosus and squamous hyperplasia reduces the risk of subsequent development of invasive cancer remains unknown.

A history of smoking tobacco is associated with VIN and invasive vulvar malignancy. Patients who smoke should be encouraged to quit, because the statistical risk of anogenital malignancy associated with former smoking is substantially less than that associated with current smoking, and it diminishes with increasing time since cessation of smoking.[31] Women with vulvar or vaginal cancer appear to have a fourfold increased risk of subsequently developing a second primary cancer of the lung.[47]

Because of the risk for multifocal disease throughout the lower genital tract and anus, it is appropriate to perform colposcopy of the cervix, vagina, and vulva and digital rectal examination or anoscopy to identify possible synchronous lesions at other sites.

PATHOLOGY AND PATHWAYS OF SPREAD

Pathology

Squamous cell cancer is the most common malignant lesion of the vulva and constitutes 80% to 90% of vulvar tumors. Variants of squamous cell cancer include cancers with discontiguous, infiltrative borders permeating lymphatic spaces with a so-called spray pattern of local invasion[48-50] and verrucous cancers (Fig. 57-1).[51-55]

Poorly differentiated cancers with a trabecular growth pattern manifesting finger-like projections and an infiltrative border with discontiguous islands and nests of malignant cells may spread to regional nodes, even when small, and frequently recur beyond the margins of local excision within dermal lymphatic channels. Recognition of this pattern of growth should prompt consideration of adjuvant postoperative radiation therapy.

Verrucous cancers may clinically manifest a warty appearance resembling a cauliflower, with exuberant hyperkeratosis seen microscopically. Broad, bulbous borders characterize these tumors, which rarely metastasize to regional nodes. Morphologic and biologic studies on 10 cases of verrucous carcinoma of the vulva support the theory that verrucous cancers constitute a discrete clinicopathologic subset of vulvar cancer.[56] Treatment is radical local excision. Despite a tendency to recur locally, the role of irradiation as adjuvant treatment for this variant remains controversial because of anecdotal reports of clinical radioresistance.

Much less common tumors found in the vulva include malignant melanoma, basal cell carcinoma, Merkel cell tumors, transitional cell carcinomas, adenocystic carcinoma, vulvar Paget's disease, and a variety of sarcomas. Tumors metastasizing from other sites may manifest in the vulva.[57]

Melanomas constitute less than 10% of primary tumors, but they are the second most common malignancy of the vulva. Even tertiary referral centers see only one or two such patients annually. Melanomas may arise de novo or from preexisting junctional or compound nevi. Rare, amelanotic vulvar melanomas may occur. Diagnostic assessments, staging, and treatment broadly parallel the treatment of cutaneous melanoma arising at other sites. Prognosis correlates with depth of invasion using the classifications of Clark, Breslow, and Chung and with the presence or absence of spread to regional nodes.[58-60] Locoregional therapy is primarily surgical.

Primary malignant tumors of the vulva may arise in Bartholin's gland, and many of these are variants of adenocarcinomas. Adenocystic carcinomas rarely disseminate to regional nodes, and they may have an indolent natural history with late local and hematogenous relapse.[61] Tumors in the Bartholin's gland areas may also be squamous cell neoplasms, and they are thought to arise in distal ductal squamous epithelium.

Bartholin's tumors tend to be deeply infiltrative and solid, often with the overlying skin remaining intact. This clinical presentation may be confused with benign cysts or infection, causing delayed diagnosis and difficulty in accomplishing surgical clearance with wide, negative margins. Outcomes data from nonrandomized patients with Bartholin's tumors suggest that those with more locally extensive primary tumors administered postoperative adjuvant irradiation are less likely to manifest local failure than more favorable patients treated with surgery as monotherapy.[61]

The International Society for the Study of Vulvar Disease recommended abandoning the term "microinvasion" when

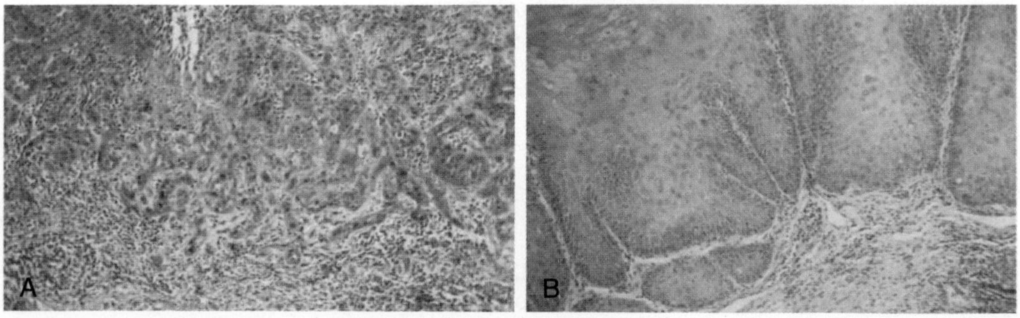

Figure 57-1 Variants of squamous cell cancer of the vulva. **A,** Infiltrative pattern of growth with discontinuous satellites of malignant cells, sometimes called a *spray pattern* of growth. **B,** Verrucous cancer with a bulbous, pushing front of invasion into the surrounding stroma. (Photomicrographs courtesy of Dr. Richard Oi, Department of Pathology, University of California at Davis.)

Table 57-1 Incidence of Groin Node Metastasis Correlated with Depth of Invasion for Primary Tumors 2 cm or Smaller

Depth of Invasion (mm)	Number of Patients	Number of Positive Nodes	Incidence (%)
≤1	120	0	0
1.1-2	121	8	6.6
2.1-3	97	8	8.2
3.1-4	50	11	22.0
4.1-5	40	10	25.0
>5	32	12	37.5

Data from references 49, 50, 72, 78, 80, 82.

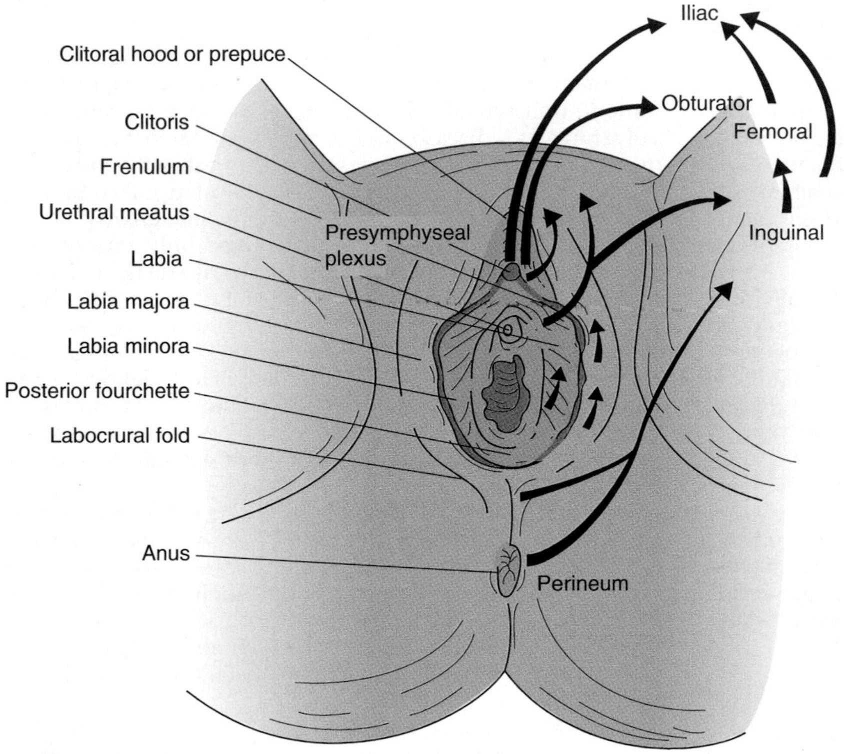

Figure 57-2 Lymphatic drainage of the vulva and perineum. *Arrows* indicate the flow patterns. (Adapted from Russell AH: Cancer of the vulva. *In* Leibel SA, Phillips TL [eds]: Textbook of Radiation Oncology, 2nd ed. Philadelphia, WB Saunders, 2004, p 1179.)

applied to carcinoma of the vulva and proposed the use of stage IA, a substage of FIGO stage I that incorporates criteria for tumor size and depth. The depth of invasion is defined as the distance from the epithelial stromal junction of the most superficial adjacent dermal papillae to the deepest point of invasion. Stage IA is defined as a solitary squamous cell cancer of the vulva measuring less than 2 cm in diameter, with clinically negative nodes and a depth of invasion that is 1 mm or less.[62,63] This definition encompasses the previous understanding of microinvasion, because the risk of nodal involvement with invasion less than 1 mm is close to 0% (Table 57-1). In addition to tumor stage and depth, other pathologic features of the primary tumor should be assessed, including presence or absence of vascular space invasion, tumor grade, and tumor growth pattern.[64]

Pathways of Spread

Vulvar cancer spreads by direct extension to adjacent structures, including the vagina, urethra, perineum, anus, and ischial rami. Tumor may spread by embolization through the lymphatics to the regional nodes. Permeation of lymphatics is uncommon but may account for the occasional patient with recurrence in the skin bridge conserved when vulvar cancer is treated surgically employing separate incisions for the primary and the regional node dissection. This is rare in the absence of extensive groin node metastases.[65]

The lymphatics of the vulva (Fig. 57-2) consist of a network that covers the entire labia minora, fourchette, prepuce, and distal vagina below the hymenal membrane.[55] Lymphatics coalesce anteriorly, forming larger trunks, which run lateral to the clitoris to the mons veneris, acquiring tributaries from the lymphatics of the labia majora, which run in a parallel fashion anteriorly from the perineal body. At the mons veneris, the vulvar lymphatic trunks diverge laterally to the inguinal nodes. Study of the localization of dye or radiolabeled tracer in regional lymph nodes after focal injection of discrete sites in the vulva and on the perineum reveals that the lymphatic drainage of the perineum, clitoris, and anterior labia minora is bilateral, whereas the lymph flow from well-lateralized sites (>2 cm from midline structures) in the vulva is predominantly to the ipsilateral groin.[66,67]

The vulvar lymphatics run through the vulva and do not traverse the labiocrural fold. Perineal lymphatics course lateral to the labiocrural fold through the superficial tissues of the upper medial thigh. In the radiation treatment of patients with advanced vulvar cancer that extends to the perineal skin, these lateral channels should be taken into consideration. Advanced vulvar cancer extending up the vagina proximal to the hymenal ring may spread through vaginal lymphatics directly to pelvic nodes.

From the superficial inguinal nodes, secondary lymphatic drainage occurs through the cribriform fascia to the femoral nodes, with subsequent tertiary flow under the inguinal ligaments to the external iliac nodes. However, metastases have been reported to the femoral lymph nodes without involvement of the superficial inguinal lymph nodes, especially from carcinomas of the clitoris and Bartholin's gland.[67,68] A Gynecologic Oncology Group (GOG) study also found an unexpectedly high incidence of ipsilateral groin recurrences secondary to presumed involvement of lymph nodes deep to the cribriform fascia despite negative superficial nodes.[69] Levenback has further supported these data by lymphatic mapping studies.[70] Actuarial risk of groin recurrence at 5 years was 16% (19 of 119) among vulvar cancer patients treated with groin node dissection alone at M.D. Anderson Cancer Center, of whom 111 had superficial inguinal node dissections. Of these patients, 117 had groin specimens histopathologically negative for metastases.[71]

The frequency of lymph node metastases to the inguinofemoral nodes is related to the lesion size and depth of stromal invasion.[72] For lesions less than 1 cm in diameter, the incidence is approximately 5%. For lesions exceeding 4 cm, the rate of inguinofemoral lymph node metastases is 30% to 50%.[73,74] The incidence of groin node metastasis is correlated with depth of invasion of the primary in clinical stage I (T1) vulvar cancer in Table 57-1. The depth of invasion is defined as the distance from the epithelial stromal junction of the most superficial adjacent dermal papillae to the deepest point of invasion. The incidence of occult nodal involvement in clinically nonsuspicious groin nodes treated by complete lymphadenectomy is cross-tabulated by primary tumor size and T category in Table 57-2.[75]

Metastases to the contralateral groin in the absence of ipsilateral groin metastases may be seen in up to 15% of patients with very advanced primaries.[76] Metastases to contralateral groin nodes in the setting of uninvolved ipsilateral groins have been reported in patients with Bartholin's gland primaries[77] and tumors of the anterior labia minora.[78] In the absence of spread to ipsilateral nodes, discrete (2 cm in diameter or less), well-lateralized primary cancers limited to the vulva and not approaching midline structures (T1) spread to contralateral groin nodes in less than 1% of patients undergoing bilateral lympahadenectomy.[72,73,78-82] However, 5 patients (2.6%) of 192 pooled patients with T1 lateralized cancers managed with negative ipsilateral groin dissection have manifested contralateral groin recurrence.[69,82-87] A theoretical explanation for this discrepancy is the possibility that dissection of negative groin nodes may be therapeutic in a small number of patients in whom routine sectioning of groin nodes may fail to detect minute micrometastases because of undersampling.

The overall incidence of metastases to the pelvic lymph nodes is 5%. Lymphadenectomy can detect metastatic involvement in pelvic nodes in 15% to 28% of patients with metastases to inguinal nodes.[5,10,11,74,76,88-92] However, pelvic node metastasis is uncommon in the absence of three or more positive inguinofemoral lymph nodes and rare in the context of occult involvement of a single groin node.

Hematogenous spread, usually to lung and bone, is uncommon in the absence of inguinofemoral lymph node involvement and usually occurs late in the course of the disease. Most patients die of uncontrolled locoregional disease. However, in patients with three or more positive lymph nodes, the ultimate risk of hematogenous spread is 66%. In contrast, patients with fewer than three positive lymph nodes have only a 4% risk of hematogenous spread.[93,94]

BIOLOGY AND PROGNOSTIC FACTORS

In multivariate analysis the presence or absence of lymph node involvement remains the single most important prognostic factor in outcomes of treatment for vulvar cancer.[95] For those with negative lymph nodes, the average 5-year survival from nine large literature series is 91% (range, 83% to 100%).[5,10,11,76,88,89,96-98] For those with involved lymph nodes treated with curative intent, the average 5-year survival rate

Table 57-2 Probability of Clinically Occult Metastasis to Inguinofemoral Lymph Nodes Correlated with Primary Tumor Category and Size in Operable Vulvar Cancer

Tumor Category and Size	N0* *n* (%)†	N1* *n* (%)†	Total *N* (%)
T CATEGORY			
T1	13/84 (15.5)	3/21 (14.3)	16/105 (15.2)
T2	17/56 (30.4)	4/14 (28.5)	21/70 (30)
T3	11/38 (28.9)	1/11 (9.1)	12/49 (24.4)
T4	0/1	0/0	0/1
Total	41/179 (22.9)	8/46 (17.4)	49/225 (21.7)
CLINICAL TUMOR SIZE (cm)			
0-1.0	3/39 (7.7)	0/4	3/43 (7)
1.1-2.0	11/46 (23.9)	3/17 (17.6)	14/63 (22.2)
2.1-3.0	13/42 (31)	1/10 (10)	14/52 (26.9)
3.1-5.0	12/33 (36.4)	2/8 (25)	14/41 (34.1)
>5.0	1/10 (10)	2/5 (40)	3/15 (20)
Total‡	40/170 (23.5)	8/44 (18.2)	48/214 (22.4)

*N0, no palpable inguinal nodes; N1, nodes palpable, not suspicious.
†Staging from International Federation of Gynecology and Oncology (FIGO), 1969.
‡Clinical tumor measurements not available for all patients.
Adapted from Gonzalez Bosquet J, Kinney WK, Russell AH, et al: Risk of occult inguinofemoral lymph node metastasis from squamous carcinoma of the vulva. Int J Radiat Oncol Biol Phys 57:419-424, 2003.

Table 57-3 **Width of Surgical Margin and Risk of Local Recurrence**

Study	Margin <8 mm	Margin ≥8 mm
Heaps et al[64]	21/44 (48%)	0/91
Faul et al[109]	18/31(58%)	NA
De Hullu et al[108]*	9/40 (23%)	0/39

*Surgical margins of ≤ 8 mm versus > 8 mm.
NA. not available.

Table 57-4 **Clinical Assessment of Inguinofemoral Nodes by Palpation**

Clinical Assessment	Histologically Negative	Histologically Positive
Clinically negative (n = 451 patients)	363 (80.5%)	88 (19.5%)
Clinically positive (n = 243 patients)	53 (21.8%)	190 (78.2%)

Data pooled from six institutions.[4,10,11,89,92,113]

is 52% (range, 38% to 61%).[5,8,10,11,88,96,99] Ninety-five percent of relapses after primary surgical treatment occur in the vulva, perineum, or groins.[72,100-105] The extent of lymphatic involvement is prognostic and includes type of nodal spread (unilateral or bilateral), volume of tumor in the involved nodes, extracapsular penetration number of positive nodes, and level of metastatic disease in the nodal chain.[8,30,96,106,107]

Because of the dominant negative impact of inguinal node metastasis, some investigators examine only primary tumor-related characteristics in relation to their correlation with nodal involvement rather than their impact on risk of recurrence of disease at the primary site. A number of primary tumor-related characteristics, identified on multivariate analysis, predict for vulvar relapse regardless of nodal involvement, among them tumor size and depth of invasion.[11] The latter correlates with locoregional recurrence and with the risk of nodal metastasis. Because most relapses after primary surgical treatment occur in the vulva or groin, to improve outcomes, it is necessary to understand factors predictive of overall survival and those predictive of local recurrence and nodal relapse. Although risk probably increases continuously with depth, two data sets suggested that a sharply defined classification into low-risk versus high-risk groups may occur depending on tumor depth (first series, low risk <5 mm and high risk ≥5 mm; second series, low risk <9 mm, high risk ≥9 mm).[73,103] Heaps and colleagues identified stage, width of surgical margin, depth of invasion, tumor thickness, growth pattern (infiltrative rather than pushing), and presence of vascular space invasion as factors predictive of local recurrence after primary surgery.[64]

Three publications (Table 57-3) have reported a clear association between risk of vulvar recurrence and adequacy of surgical resection margins. When microscopic margins are 8 mm or less in formalin-fixed tissue, local recurrence has been observed in 48 (43%) of 115 patients.[64,108,109] Allowing for shrinkage artifact, this correlates with a margin of at least 1.0 cm in unfixed tissue. A minimal clinical free space of 1 cm of uninvolved normal tissue provides a practical guideline for identifying patients who are highly likely to be advised to undergo postoperative local irradiation for inadequate margins if treated by initial surgery. Under such circumstances, preoperative irradiation or chemoradiation may be preferable to secure better margins and to reduce the scope of subsequent conservative surgery.

CLINICAL MANIFESTATIONS, PATIENT EVALUATION, AND STAGING

Clinical Features and Evaluation

The virus-related cause of vulvar cancer, its association with preinvasive or invasive cancers in other parts of the lower genital tract, and its histologic features suggest that vulvar cancer is sometimes one manifestation of a multifocal disease, or *field cancerization*.[44,110] However, at the time of diagnosis, only about 5% of vulvar cancers are multifocal. Patients usually present with a vulvar mass or ulcer, often after a long history of pruritus or vulvar discomfort. Depending on the location and size of the lesion within the vulva, the patient may also complain of dysuria, difficulty with defecation, bleeding, or discharge. Rarely, patients may present with advanced inguinal node involvement, occasionally with ulcerating masses in the groins or with lower extremity lymphedema resulting from obstruction.

The diagnosis of vulvar cancer requires biopsy. For lesions smaller than 1 cm, a definitive excisional biopsy, including surrounding skin, underlying dermis, and connective tissue, may be preferable to obtain surgical margins of at least 1 cm grossly in all dimensions around the lesion. For larger lesions, a wedge biopsy should be performed. When vulvar dystrophy is present and the vulva is difficult to assess visually, colposcopy of the vulva should be performed with appropriately directed biopsies of abnormal areas to assess disease extent. The remainder of the lower genital tract and anus should be examined, if necessary with a colposcope and anoscopy, to identify the possible presence of synchronous preinvasive or invasive cancers.

Clinical evaluation of the groin nodes is inaccurate in approximately 20% of cases. Iversen reported that up to 36% of palpably normal groins in patients with vulvar cancer may harbor occult metastases.[111] Based on pooled surgical data on 694 patients from six institutions, 19.5% of patients with clinically negative groin nodes will have histologically proven groin metastasis. Assessment by palpation may be compromised by the depth at which groin nodes lie beneath overlying skin. The average depth may be 6 cm, and it is frequently greater in obese patients.[112] Conversely, 21.8% of patients with clinically positive groins are found to have negative nodes if surgically dissected, presumably because of the confounding presence of inflammatory or reactive adenopathy (Table 57-4).[4,10,11,89,92,113]

Staging

In 1988, FIGO introduced a surgical staging system for vulvar cancer that has since undergone several revisions. The American Joint Committee on Cancer (AJCC), International Union Against Cancer (UICC), and FIGO (AJCC/UICC/FIGO) tumor-node-metastasis (TNM) categories and stage groupings of 2002 are provided in Table 57-5. Staging systems are intended to standardize reporting of treatment efficacy, allowing comparison of the outcomes of treatment from different institutions and comparison of results employing different treatment strategies. Ideally, stage should not be employed to determine therapy. Unfortunately, the current clinical-pathologic system defines stage for many patients based on information derived after surgical treatment. Because of the

Table 57-5 FIGO/AJCC/UICC 2002 TNM Classification and Stage Grouping

PRIMARY TUMOR (T)

TX	Primary tumor cannot be assessed
T0	No evidence of primary tumor
Tis	Carcinoma in situ (preinvasive carcinoma)
T1	Tumor confined to the vulva and perineum 2 cm or less in greatest dimension
T1a	Tumor confined to the vulva or vulva and perineum, 2 cm or less in greatest dimension, and with stromal invasion no greater than 1 mm*
T1b	Tumor confined to the vulva or vulva and perineum, 2 cm or less in greatest dimension, and with stromal invasion greater than 1 mm
T2	Tumor confined to the vulva and perineum, more than 2 cm in greatest dimension
T3	Tumor of any size with contiguous spread to the lower urethra and/or vagina or anus
T4	Tumor of any size invading the upper urethra, bladder mucosa, or rectal mucosa, or tumor fixed to the pubic bone

REGIONAL LYMPH NODES (N)†

NX	Regional lymph nodes cannot be assessed
N0	No nodal metastases
N1	Unilateral regional lymph node metastasis
N2	Bilateral regional lymph node metastasis

DISTANT METASTASIS (M)

MX	Distant metastasis cannot be assessed
M0	No evidence of distant metastasis
M1	Distant metastasis (including pelvic lymph node metastasis)

FIGO/AJCC/UICC STAGE GROUPING

0	Tis N0 M0
IA	T1a N0 M0
IB	T1b N0 M0
II	T2 N0 M0
III	T3 N0 M0
	T1-3 N1 M0
IVA	T1-3 N2 M0
	T4 Any N M0
IVB	Any T Any N M1

*Depth of invasion is defined as the measurement of the tumor from the epithelial-stromal junction of the adjacent most superficial dermal papilla to the deepest point of invasion.

†Assessment of inguinofemoral nodes is histologic.

AJCC, American Joint Commission on Cancer; FIGO, International Federation of Gynecology and Oncology; TNM, tumor-node-metastisis; UICC, International Union Against Cancer.

understandable desire to confirm nodal status by histology, the staging system appears to implicitly endorse initial surgical management of the groin nodes when this may not be prudent in all clinical circumstances.

Considerable heterogeneity of prognosis exists within the stages as currently defined. Staging systems lump patients together who may overall have similar prognoses but whose tumors have different biologic behavior, require different treatments, and can be expected to have different patterns of relapse. For example, a T3 N0 M0 cancer is categorized as stage III, as is a T1 N1 M0 cancer. In isolation, the FIGO stage formalism does not function well as an aid to clinical treatment decisions.

To fully comply with FIGO staging requirements, histologic confirmation of groin node status should be obtained. Assignment of FIGO or AJCC stage may not be necessary or feasible in all patients, however, to develop a rational plan for treatment. A patient with a well-lateralized T1b lesion with clinically negative groin nodes may not require histologic confirmation of the status of the contralateral groin nodes if surgical therapy confirms the ipsilateral nodes to be histologically uninvolved. Similarly, for a patient with a locally advanced primary tumor requiring preoperative chemoradiation in an effort to avoid compromise of functionally important midline structures, it may be medically sensible to electively include the groin nodes in the irradiated volume, provided that they appear grossly uninvolved by physical examination and diagnostic imaging. Without subsequent groin dissection and without sampling of groin nodes before treatment, such patients are reported to have a very low probability of groin failure if treatment is carried out with appropriate technique.[114,115] Strictly speaking, they are "unstaged" or may be categorized as NX. Comprehensive pretreatment evaluation of disease extent may be less important when institutional treatment policy is to carry out initial surgery in all medically operable and technically resectable patients, even in the presence of limited node metastasis.

If the detection of nodal disease pretreatment will affect the selection, sequencing, or intensity of treatment modalities, the diagnostic algorithm illustrated in Figure 57-3 may help to guide therapy. There exists no consensus standard for the pretreatment evaluation of disease extent. Positron emission tomography (PET) or computed tomography (CT) may not be available in many locations, and lack of reimbursement may prove an additional obstacle even when the technology is available for other indications. Experience with sentinel node identification is not universal, and its use remains controversial. The diagnostic algorithm in Figure 57-3 may not be applicable in all venues.

Confirmation of node status is usually accomplished by surgical exploration of the inguinal nodes. The most common surgical practice is to obtain histologic examination of the ipsilateral superficial inguinal lymph nodes for lateralized lesions of the vulva and of bilateral superficial nodes for lesions considered to be midline. Although there is no widely accepted definition of midline, a minimum of 1 cm of clinically involved tissue separating the border of the tumor from a structure that has bilateral lymphatic drainage should be mandatory before considering omission of contralateral node assessment, and many clinicians recommend 2 cm.

Because lymphatic drainage from the anterior labia minora may be bilateral,[66,116] bilateral groin assessment should be considered for lesions arising in these areas even if otherwise apparently lateralized, because contralateral groin metastases with negative ipsilateral groin nodes have been described with primary tumors in this location.[78] Possibly because precise tumor extent may be more difficult to appreciate on physical examination, contralateral groin node metastases with negative ipsilateral groin nodes have similarly been reported in patients with primary cancers of Bartholin's gland, suggesting consideration of bilateral histologic groin assessment in such patients.[77]

Sentinel nodes may be identified for selective excisional biopsy by injection of dye at the primary site and by lym-

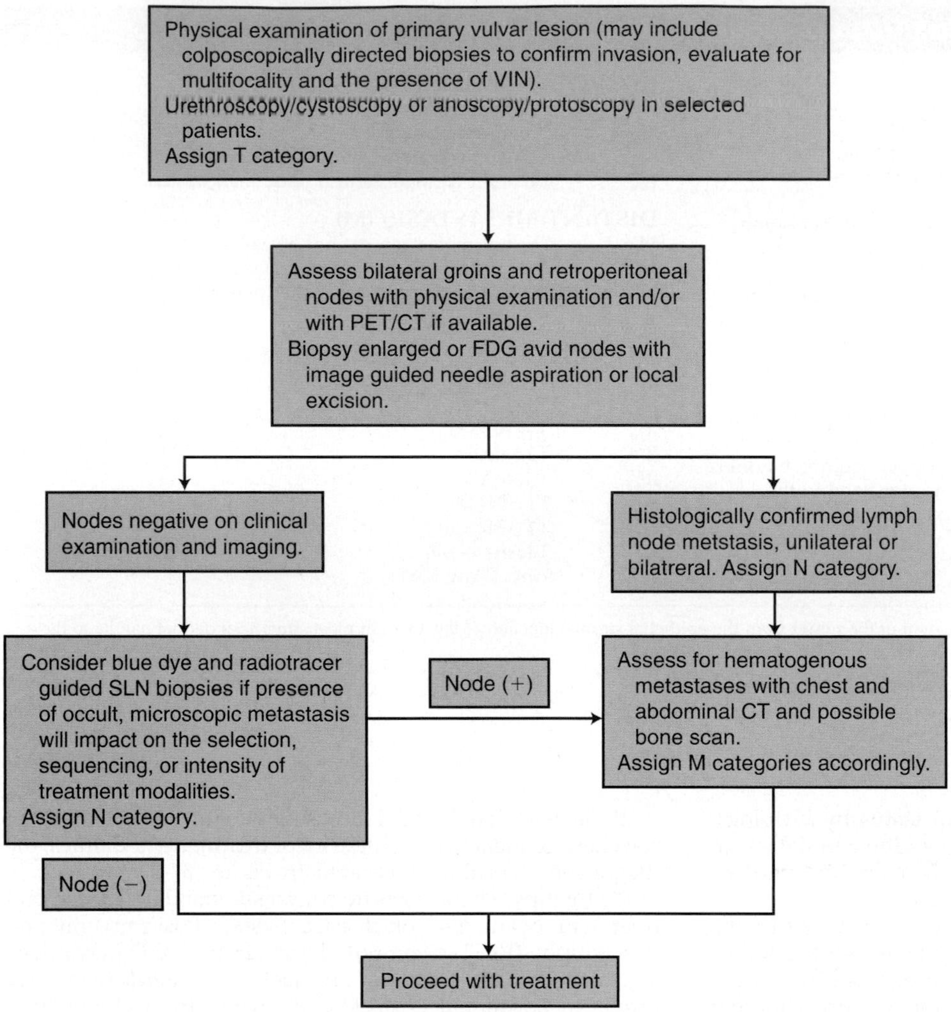
Physical examination of primary vulvar lesion (may include colposcopically directed biopsies to confirm invasion, evaluate for multifocality and the presence of VIN).
Urethroscopy/cystoscopy or anoscopy/protoscopy in selected patients.
Assign T category.
Assess bilateral groins and retroperitoneal nodes with physical examination and/or with PET/CT if available.
Biopsy enlarged or FDG avid nodes with image guided needle aspiration or local excision.
Nodes negative on clinical examination and imaging.
Histologically confirmed lymph node metstasis, unilateral or bilatreral. Assign N category.
Consider blue dye and radiotracer guided SLN biopsies if presence of occult, microscopic metastasis will impact on the selection, sequencing, or intensity of treatment modalities.
Assign N category.
Node (+)
Assess for hematogenous metastases with chest and abdominal CT and possible bone scan.
Assign M categories accordingly.
Node (−)
Proceed with treatment

Figure 57-3 Diagnostic algorithm for vulvar cancer. CT, computed tomography; FDG-PET, ^{18}F-fluorodeoxyglucose positron emission tomography; M, metastasis; N, node; SLN, sentinel lymph node; T, tumor; VIN, vulvar intraepithelial neoplasia.

phoscintography.[70,117-123] It is unclear whether use of a blue dye alone is sufficient to identify sentinel nodes. Reported results appear to be better when a radioactive tracer is employed alone or in combination with blue dye.

Pathologic ultrastaging of groin nodes has been proposed to increase the sensitivity of sentinel node excisional biopsy in the detection of microscopic groin node metastases.[122,124] Ultrastaging may include thin step-sectioning of retrieved nodes with or without immunohistochemical staining.[125] The prognostic and therapeutic implications of lymph node metastasis identified only by ultrastaging remain undefined but are the subject of ongoing investigation. These techniques have not yet entered routine clinical practice.

When nodal disease is advanced and initial surgery to the groin area is not planned, histologic confirmation of metastatic contamination may be obtained by fine-needle aspiration.

Noninvasive imaging, including CT, PET, magnetic resonance imaging (MRI), and ultrasonography may assist in assessing lymph node status, particularly in larger or obese patients, in whom femoral nodes may be many centimeters below the skin and well beyond a depth where node palpation is feasible.[126-129] Metabolic imaging may detect metastases in the absence of gross nodal enlargement. Spatial imaging may identify nodes accessible for image-guided fine-needle aspiration. Although clinically useful in some patients, the results of imaging assessment, unless confirmed histologically, do not alter assignment of FIGO stage. Accurate measurement of the depth of femoral nodes below the anterior skin surface at the level of the femoral artery as it passes under the inguinal ligament is critical in the design and implementation of radiation-based therapy of undissected groins, as well as in the context of adjuvant irradiation of the groins after superficial or total inguinal lymph node dissection.[112,130]

PRIMARY THERAPY

The treatment of patients with vulvar cancer has been in a state of evolution for the past 3 decades. Previously, en bloc radical vulvectomy with bilateral groin dissection with or without bilateral pelvic node dissection was the treatment of choice for all patients with vulvar cancer.[2,4,88] Although extirpative surgery improved cancer outcomes compared with results obtained during previous eras, it is associated with substantial acute and chronic postoperative morbidity as well as major psychological sequelae. Leg lymphedema after radical groin and pelvic node dissection may be temporary or permanent and disabling.[88,131] Pelvic relaxation, organ prolapse, and urinary incontinence can develop in some patients, particularly when removal of the distal urethra or a portion of the lower vagina is required to achieve surgical clearance. Vaginal introital stenosis can occur, and the absence of the vulva and venereal fat can have the functional equivalence of shortening effective vaginal depth and removing a protective cushion from the pubic arch. These changes may contribute to dyspareunia in many patients. Clitorectomy profoundly diminishes the capacity for arousal and climax. The psychosexual consequences of vulvectomy are frequently devastating.[132-134]

The clinical extent of vulvar cancer at the time of diagnosis may be decreasing, possibly because of more enlightened attitudes regarding the pathogenesis of the disease and improved access to health care. Among operable patients undergoing radical groin dissection, the frequency of lymph node metastasis has fallen from approximately 50% in reports from the 1940s and 1950s[1,135] to approximately 30% in surgical literature from the 1970s and 1980s.[8,89,96-98] Because preinvasive disease or unifocal disease of minimal volume and depth of invasion is being diagnosed in younger, sexually active patients, modifications in the surgical approach to vulvar cancer have been provoked by concerns about the chronic morbidities of ablative surgery in patients with disease of limited extent.

Refined understanding of pathologic predictive factors, patterns of failure after standard radical surgery, and efficacy and tolerability of radical radiation in vulvar cancer has led to progressive change from the recommendation for radical surgery in all patients. The focus of vulvar cancer management has moved toward decreasing the morbidity and mortality of radical vulvectomy in patients with early-stage, prognostically favorable tumors and toward improving results without increasing morbidity in patients with advanced, poor-prognosis disease by using integrated multimodality therapy that includes irradiation, chemotherapy, and surgery.[3] The diversity of the disease and the afflicted patients requires tailoring the nature and extent of treatment to the location and severity of the cancer, cognizant of the activity, efficacy, and toxicity of each available treatment modality used alone or in combination.

Decisions regarding management of the primary tumor in the vulva are made on the basis of primary tumor volume and anatomic extent (i.e., direct involvement or impingement on functionally important midline structures). The impact of biopsy and definitive surgery on anatomic function and cosmesis must be evaluated.

Decisions regarding management of the groin nodes are directed by whether histologically confirmed node metastases are present, their extent, and the size, location, and depth of invasion of the vulvar primary.

Surgical Trends

Radical surgery for vulvar cancer has moved away from the classic radical vulvectomy with en bloc bilateral inguinal lymph node dissection toward less extensive vulvar surgery, particularly in patients with early-stage lesions. This includes separate ipsilateral or bilateral groin incisions with preservation of the skin bridge, less radical inguinal node surgery, and omission of pelvic node removal.[73,80,136] The definition of radical vulvar surgery has changed with the realization that the therapeutic effect of radical surgery is limited by the closest resection margin rather than by achievement of total organ ablation (i.e., vulvectomy).[64,108,109]

In patients with limited disease and clinically tumor-negative groin nodes, use of separate incisions for the primary and groins is associated with decreased morbidity without compromise of survival.[137] In patients with occult groin node metastases, use of triple incisions has no significant impact on disease-specific and overall survival compared with en bloc resection. However, when corrected for other prognostic variables in a multivariate analysis, the type of surgical treatment (i.e., triple incision versus en bloc) was an independent predictor for vulvar recurrence but not for inguinal or pelvic relapse.[138] The lack of impact on disease-specific survival and overall survival may be attributed to high salvage rates for isolated vulvar recurrence reported in some clinical series,[102,139] although the 2-year actuarial survival rate after vulvar recurrence has been reported to be as low as 25%, and uncontrolled local recurrence was a contributing cause of death in 15 of 16 patients dying of cancer in one series.[109]

If the tumor is removed widely, the terms *radical local excision*, *radical wide local excision*, *radical wide excision*, or *wide local excision* are used. Although there is some uncertainty about the optimal extent of surgical margin after wide local excision, data from two clinical series reveal high local control rates for cases in which the surgical margin was greater than 8 mm in the fixed state postoperatively (see Table 57-3).[64,108] This suggests that tumor margins of at least 1 cm in all dimensions in the nonfixed state are desirable to achieve high local control rates. Many clinicians endorse a margin of 2 cm. Implicit is the understanding that radical local excision should include dissection below the lesion down to the deep perineal fascia. Although radical local excision is widely accepted in the treatment of small lesions, there is a growing trend to extend its use to lesions larger than 2 cm.[72,79,91,136]

Successful management of the inguinal nodes is essential because 90% of patients who experience relapse in regional lymph nodes after primary therapy will ultimately die of cancer.[91,102,104,105,140-142] Patients whose primary lesion in the vulva invades to a depth less than 1 mm and is smaller than 2 cm have a minimal risk of groin node metastasis and do not require treatment of the inguinal region (see Table 57-1). In every patient with a primary tumor larger or more deeply invasive, treatment should include, as a minimum, the ipsilateral groin.

The move toward more conservative, tailored surgical management has led to changes in the extent of groin dissection and the use of unilateral groin dissection for selected patients. The standard radical bilateral inguinofemoral lymph node dissection, including superficial and deep nodes, results in a 50% incidence of wound breakdown, a 30% incidence of groin complications (e.g., breakdown, lymphangitis, lymphocyst), and a 10% to 15% incidence of extremity lymphedema.[11,88,131,143] The surgical morbidity associated with limited, superficial groin dissections is generally acknowledged to be less than that associated with superficial and deep dissections.[136] The rationale for limiting the extent or depth of groin dissection relates to the observed orderly sequence of metastatic progression in the groin nodal chain. Metastases in the deep femoral nodes without involvement of the superficial nodes are uncommon.[136] However, the actuarial risk of groin recurrence at 5 years was 16% among vulvar cancer patients treated with superficial groin node dissection alone at M.D. Anderson Cancer Center.[71] Results may be improved by extending the superficial groin dissection to remove the medial portion of the cribriform fascia and underlying femoral nodes en bloc with the superficial inguinal fat pad.[144] Identification of sentinel nodes by injection of blue dye and lymphoscintigraphy may further reduce the risk of groin failure by identifying patients with direct lymphatic pathways to deep nodes.[70,117-123]

For lateralized lesions, the ipsilateral superficial groin nodes are believed to be the sentinel nodes for predicting possible further lymphatic involvement. If the superficial ipsilateral nodes are involved with tumor, surgery will generally proceed to complete the deep groin node dissection. For patients undergoing postoperative irradiation to the groin after superficial and deep groin node dissection, the risk of subsequent lymphedema is substantial.[68,145] However, whether groin irradiation or chemoradiation can prudently substitute for completion of the groin dissection under these circumstances remains speculative.

For patients with lateralized lesions and no involvement of the ipsilateral nodes, the incidence of contralateral groin node involvement is extremely low,[66,73] and routine dissection of the contralateral nodes is omitted. Bilateral superficial dissections are recommended for patients whose tumors involve or are within 1 cm of midline structures or involve the anterior labia minora.

When nodal disease is fixed or ulcerating, the local tumor burden is large and unlikely to be controlled by surgery or irradiation alone. In such patients, combined therapy with chemoradiation and surgery may offer the best chances of local control.[146]

Radiation Therapy

Radiation therapy for vulvar cancer was pioneered in Europe in the early 20th century in an era when surgical options for advanced vulvar cancer were limited. As radical surgery became more feasible and surgical results improved because of improvements in anesthesia, postoperative nutritional support, blood transfusion, antibiotics, and refinements in reconstructive surgery and wound care that evolved in response to the carnage of two world wars, primary radiation therapy fell into disrepute. Because of perceptions that vulvar cancer was resistant to radiation therapy and because of the acute desquamation accompanying radical irradiation of the vulva and the severe late effects of radiation on the vulva in long-term survivors, the use of radiation was largely restricted to palliative cases and patients with anatomic extent of disease or medical comorbidities precluding operative intervention.[147-151] With focused hindsight, radiation therapy equipment and techniques were primitive compared with modern technology, and radiation fractionation and total dose were often naïve with respect to late effects. The perception that radiation was a poor second choice as a curative modality stemmed in part from the low survival rates reported in early series for patients selected for radiation therapy who were unsuitable for primary surgery because of poor general medical condition or very advanced tumors, or both. Despite these concerns, a number of pieces of information emerged to support the radiocurability of vulvar cancer and the use of irradiation alone or as adjuvant therapy before or after more conservative surgical resection.

In Frischbier and Thomsen's report, the 5-year survival rate for 33 patients treated with irradiation for stages III or IV disease was 39%.[148] Backstrom provided valuable dose-control data in a series of 19 inoperable patients with T4 disease.[147] Six patients remained disease free after radiation therapy, and local control correlated with the radiation dose delivered.

Prempree demonstrated that interstitial brachytherapy, alone or combined with teletherapy, could be successfully employed as salvage therapy in patients with local or regional recurrence of vulvar cancer. Results were particularly favorable (6 of 6 patients salvaged) for small recurrences at the vaginal introitus.[142]

In an effort to prevent regional recurrence after initial surgery, the GOG conducted a randomized trial that compared pelvic lymphadenectomy with radiation therapy (45 to 50 Gy) administered to the bilateral groins and pelvis (excluding the tumor bed and residual vulva) in 114 surgically treated patients who were found to have groin node metastasis.[90] Metastases were detected in pelvic nodes in 15 (28%) of 53 patients undergoing pelvic lymphadenectomy, 9 of whom expired within 1 year. Overall survival at 2 years was 68% in patients treated with radiation and 54% in patients treated surgically. Survival benefit was limited to patients with macroscopic groin metastasis or two or more groin nodes contaminated (63% for radiation therapy versus 37% for surgery). The beneficial effect of radiation therapy can be attributed predominantly to a reduction in groin failures in the irradiated patients, who had a 5% incidence of groin relapse compared with a 24% incidence in patients treated surgically. A 9% incidence of vulvar cancer recurrence was observed across both treatment arms.

Data from two other studies suggest that macroscopic involvement of a single node and extracapsular invasion confer a risk of inguinal recurrence after surgery that is as high as in those with multiple lymph node involvement. It is suggested that such patients may also benefit from postoperative groin and pelvic nodal irradiation.[107,152]

The target volume for adjuvant postoperative radiation therapy depends on the indications for adjuvant therapy. For patients with disease-negative groin nodes but adverse histopathologic factors discerned on study of the excised primary, focal irradiation targeted at inadequate margins, residual vulva, and adjacent perineal skin is appropriate. For patients with unilateral node metastases in whom the contralateral groin has been dissected, it may not always be necessary to include the contralateral groin and pelvic nodes, which were treated in the GOG study of adjuvant irradiation.[90]

Many patients with node involvement also have indications to treat the primary tumor bed and residual vulva. However, whether to routinely include the tumor bed and residual vulva in all patients undergoing adjuvant postoperative radiation therapy because of node metastasis remains an issue of controversy. Dusenbery reported 27 patients with squamous cell carcinoma of the vulva and 1 to 15 (average, 4) histologically involved inguinal lymph nodes who were treated after radical vulvectomy and bilateral lymphadenectomy (25 patients), radical vulvectomy and unilateral lymphadenectomy (1 patient), or hemivulvectomy and bilateral lymphadenectomy (1 patient). Postoperative irradiation was directed at the bilateral groin and pelvic nodes (19 patients), unilateral groin and pelvic nodes (6 patients), or unilateral groin only (1 patient). Twenty-six patients had the midline blocked. Actuarial 5-year overall survival and disease-free survival estimates were 40% and 35%. Relapses developed in 63% (17 of 27) of the patients at a median of 9 months from surgery (range, 3 months to 6 years). Central recurrences (i.e., under the midline block) were present in 13 of these 17 patients (representing 50% of the patients treated with the midline blocked), occurring as central disease only (8 patients), central and regional disease (4 patients), or central and distant disease (1 patient), leading the study authors to conclude that the target volume for adjuvant postoperative radiation for patients with node metastases should include the tumor bed.[153]

Of the 114 node-positive patients in the GOG trial of adjuvant groin and pelvis radiation, 44 developed relapse. Eleven patients (9.7% of 114 patients, 25% of 44 patients with recurrence) developed relapse at the unirradiated vulva or tumor bed.[90] Because follow-up was short in the GOG study, this may represent an underestimate of the true risk of local recurrence in such patients. Conversely, some late local recurrences may represent true second primary cancers in conserved vulvar tissue that is predisposed to malignant transformation. This would seem to be the case when second lesions develop in residual contralateral vulva after wide local excision of initially well-lateralized lesions. Whether adjuvant irradiation can reduce the risk of such second primary cancers is unknown. Whether to include the residual vulva or tumor bed in the target volume for adjuvant postoperative radiation in node-positive patients remains controversial. Assessment of risk factors associated with the primary tumor may assist in making this determination.

Whether adjuvant local radiation can overcome the negative prognostic impact of close or positive margins, capillary lymphatic space involvement, and depth of invasion is unproved. However, strongly suggestive evidence regarding margins is provided by the outcomes observational study of Faul.[109] Sixty-two patients with invasive vulvar carcinoma and positive or close (<8 mm) margins of excision were retrospectively studied. Thirty-one patients were treated with adjuvant radiation therapy to the vulva, and 31 patients were observed after surgery. Local recurrences were diagnosed in 58% of observed patients and 16% of patients treated with adjuvant radiation therapy. Adjuvant irradiation significantly reduced local recurrence rates in the close-margin and positive-margin groups. On multivariate analysis, adjuvant irradiation and margins of excision were significant prognostic predictors for local control. The positive-margin observed group had a significantly poorer actuarial 5-year survival than the other groups ($P = .0016$), and adjuvant irradiation significantly improved survival for this group. The 2-year actuarial survival rate after developing local recurrence was only 25%, lower than is often reported for salvage therapy. Local recurrence was a significant predictor for death from vulvar carcinoma (risk ratio = 3.54).

Preoperative Irradiation

In the 1960s, Boronow pioneered the use of preoperative radiation therapy followed by more conservative surgery in patients with locally advanced or recurrent vulvovaginal cancers as an alternative to pelvic exenteration. Updating his experience with a total of 48 treated cases (37 primary cases and 11 cases of recurrent disease), he reported a 72% 5-year survival rate for all 48 cases treated. One patient required a total pelvic exenteration for local failure, and one had a posterior exenteration for local failure. One bladder and one rectum were lost to permanent diversion because of radiation injury. Five of 96 viscera (48 urinary bladders and 48 rectums) were lost, and 91 (94.8%) were retained.[154]

Three small series totaling 26 patients treated with 30 to 55 Gy preoperatively reported histologically negative surgical specimens from 13 patients (50%). Only microscopic residual disease was found in additional patients.[155-157]

Preoperative Chemoradiation

Several single-institution studies reported encouraging results employing preoperative chemoradiation before conservative resection in locally advanced or locally recurrent vulvar cancer.[158,159] These reports, along with reported treatment successes using chemoradiation for anal and esophageal cancer patients, provided much of the foundation for protocol work commencing in 1989 by the GOG.

GOG protocol 101 used preoperative chemoradiation consisting of 47.6 Gy in once- or twice-daily fractions of 1.7 Gy synchronously with two courses of infusional 5-fluorouracil (5-FU) and cisplatin as initial therapy for 73 patients with extensive squamous cell cancer of the vulva (FIGO stages III and IV), followed by surgical excision of residual primary tumor plus bilateral inguinofemoral lymph node dissection.[160] The dose-fractionation schedule for chemoradiation employed in GOG protocol 101 is schematically depicted in Figure 57-4. The planned 1.5- to 2.5-week treatment interruption was intended to mitigate the severity of acute radiation dermatitis that can progress to confluent moist desquamation and to permit hematologic recovery. Twice-daily radiation was employed to optimize the radiation-drug synergism. Seven patients did not undergo a post-treatment surgical procedure: deteriorating medical condition (2 patients); other medical condition (1 patient); unresectable residual tumor (2 patients); patient refusal (2 patients).

After chemoradiotherapy, 33 (46.5%) of 71 patients had no visible vulvar cancer at the time of planned surgery, and 38 (53.5%) of 71 had gross residual cancer at the time of operation. Five of the 38 had positive resection margins and underwent further radiation therapy to the vulva (3 patients), wide local excision and vaginectomy necessitating colostomy (1 patient), or no further therapy (1 patient). Only 2 (2.8%) of 71 had residual unresectable disease. In only three patients was it not possible to preserve urinary or gastrointestinal continence. The study authors concluded that preoperative chemoradiotherapy was feasible and that it might reduce the need for more radical surgery, including primary pelvic exenteration.

In parallel with the study of preoperative chemoradiation for patients with locally advanced primary vulvar cancer, the GOG studied patients presenting with advanced disease in the inguinofemoral nodes, 1969 nodal classification N2/N3, including some patients with matted, fixed, or ulcerated groin nodes not judged resectable by initial surgery. The identical preoperative chemoradiation schedule was employed to treat 46 patients. Three patients died during treatment, and one refused to complete the therapy. Four patients who completed chemoradiation did not undergo planned surgery; two patients died of non–cancer-related causes, and two patients had unresectable disease. After preoperative chemoradiation, the disease in the lymph nodes was judged resectable in 38 of 40 patients. Two patients who completed chemoradiation did not undergo surgery because of pulmonary metastasis. One underwent radical vulvectomy and unilateral node dissection, and the other had only radical vulvectomy. The operative lymph node specimen was histologically negative in 15 of 37 patients. Nineteen patients developed recurrent or metastatic disease, or both. Local control of the disease in the lymph nodes was achieved in 36 of 37, and in the primary area, local control was achieved in 29 of 38 of the patients. Two patients died of treatment-related complications. The investigators concluded that resectability and local control of advanced nodal disease could be obtained with a high probability after preoperative chemoradiation in patients with carcinoma of the vulva with extensive groin adenopathy.[146]

Acute toxicity associated with the preoperative chemoradiation program employed by the GOG might be reduced by pragmatic reductions in the intensity of chemotherapy administered. Hematologic tolerance to the GOG regimen may be improved in elderly patients by reducing the daily 5-FU dose to 750 to 800 mg/m^2 or shortening the duration of infusion to 72 hours from 96 hours. Because cisplatin appears to potentiate radiation response at 40 mg/m^2 in patients with cervical cancer, reduction in the dose of cisplatin from 50 to 40 mg/m^2 may also improve tolerance in frail patients without sacrificing therapeutic efficacy. Hematologic tolerance may be improved by reversing the order of the third and fourth treatment weeks, such that the second cycle of chemotherapy is administered during the last week of treatment (days 29 to 33). Responses tend to be rapid and frequently may be discerned before embarking on the second half of the chemoradiation program. The duration of treatment interruption can usually be limited to 11 rest days (including weekends) by treating with 10 instead of 9 fractions of twice-daily radiation during the weeks of chemotherapy treatment and 4 fractions during the nonchemotherapy weeks, completing the preoperative regimen of 47.6 Gy with 2 cycles of chemotherapy in 5 elapsed weeks. These minor modifications of the GOG regimen are

Cycle #1

	MON.—FRi.		MON.—FRi.
Day	1 2 3 4 5	6 7	8 9 10 11 12
Radiation	R R R R R	0 0	R R R R R
1.7 Gy/Fx	R R R R		
5-FU	F F F F		
1000 mg/m2/24 hrs			
Cisplatin	P		
50 mg/m2			

1 1/2—2 1/2 Week Planned Rest

Cycle #2

	MON.—FRi.		MON.—FRi.
Day	1 2 3 4 5	6 7	8 9 10 11 12
Radiation	R R R R R	0 0	R R R R R
1.7 Gy/Fx	R R R R		
5-FU	F F F F		
1000 mg/m2/24 hrs			
Cisplatin	P		
50 mg/m2			

Figure 57-4 Gynecologic Oncology Group (GOG) protocol 101 for treating advanced vulvar cancer with preoperative chemoradiation. Patients who are judged to have unresectable disease after completion of 47.6 Gy preoperative chemoradiation receive an addition 20 Gy in fractions (Fx) of 1.7 to 2.0 Gy, with a reduced treatment volume encompassing gross residual disease, or they may receive an additional radiation dose by brachytherapy. A third cycle of chemotherapy is recommended if teletherapy is employed. 0, a day without radiation treatment; F, 5-fluorouracil given by continuous intravenous infusion (1000 $mg/m^2/24$ h for 96 h on days 1 to 4 of each cycle); P, short infusion of cisplatin (50 mg/m^2 on day 1 of each cycle); R, a fraction of external radiation encompassing the primary site and regional extensions; a 4-hour minimum intertreatment interval is mandatory, but 6 hours or more are suggested when feasible. (Adapted from Moore DH, Thomas GM, Montana GS, et al: Preoperative chemoradiation for advanced vulvar cancer: a phase II study of the Gynecologic Oncology Group. Int J Radiat Oncol Biol Phys 42:79-85, 1998.)

routinely employed to treat elderly patients with extensive disease at Massachusetts General Hospital (MGH) (Fig. 57-5). The initial radiation treatment volume at MGH electively encompasses the groin nodes bilaterally in all patients, regardless of whether groin node metastases have been histologically verified. Evaluation for potential surgical resection of residual disease is carried out 2 weeks after completion of 47.6 Gy. If resection can be carried out without compromising functionally important midline structures, this is considered preferred management at MGH to avoid the chronic sequelae of high-dose radiation on the vulva and perineum.

In patients with initially negative groin nodes (i.e., palpably and by diagnostic imaging assessment, with or without biopsy), electively irradiated groin nodes are not routinely dissected. In patients with initial gross groin node metastases, residual palpable nodes may be removed surgically, independent of the decision regarding surgical intervention for the vulvar primary. For patients with residual, unresectable node metastases, limited volume boost radiation is used to carry nodes to 61.2 to 64.6 Gy with twice-daily fractions of 1.7 Gy concurrently with a third cycle of infusional chemotherapy. Similarly, reduced volume boost treatment is administered to gross residual primary disease that has not become resectable by conservative excision.

In some patients, a complete clinical response may be seen after moderate-dose preoperative chemoradiation. In the GOG study of preoperative chemoradiation for patients with locally advanced primary tumors, preoperative chemoradiation resulted in a complete clinical response in 34 of 71 patients evaluable for therapeutic efficacy (48%) and a pathologic complete response in 70% (22 of 31) of the 34 complete responders undergoing surgery.[160]

Possible options for further management of patients with a clinical complete response to preoperative chemoradiation include generous biopsy to confirm pathologic complete response, conservative surgery to remove palpable scar tissue and the tumor bed, and a modest dose of radiation for purpose of consolidation (8.5 to 9 Gy in 5 fractions over 1 week).

Primary Irradiation or Chemoradiation

Treatment of Primary Lesions

Whether irradiation in higher dose than employed preoperatively, alone or combined with concurrent chemotherapy, can replace radical surgery as treatment for vulvar cancer is unknown. Reports of radiation therapy using contemporary techniques and dose-fractionation schedules used as monotherapy after biopsy are uncommon. Because of probable selection biases in choosing patients for such treatment, it is impossible to meaningfully compare outcomes to alternative treatment strategies. It can be concluded that some patients enjoy locoregional control and prolonged disease-free survival when managed in this fashion.[161,162]

Increasingly, the trend is to employ chemoradiation (i.e., irradiation and synchronous radiopotentiating chemotherapy) as definitive therapy for patients with disease judged

Cycle #1

	MON.—FRi.		MON.—FRi.
Days	1 2 3 4 5	6 7	8 9 10 11 12
Radiation* 1.7 Gy/Fx	R R R R R R R R R R	0 0	R R R R 0
5-FU	F F F F		
Cisplatin 40-50 mg/m² day 2	P		

5-FU: 750-1000 mg/m²/24 hr × 96 hr days 1-5 generally commencing after first fraction of radiation on day 1 and discontinued between first and second radiation fractions day 5.

— 11 planned rest days (12-21)—

Cycle #2

	MON.—FRi.		MON.—FRi.
Days	22 23 24 25 26	27 28	29 30 31 32 33
Radiation* 1.7 Gy/Fx	0 R R R R	0 0	R R R R R R R R R R
5-FU			F F F F
Cisplatin 40-50 mg/m² day 30			P

5-FU: 750-1000 mg/m²/24 hr × 96 hr days 29-33 generally commencing after first fraction of radiation on day 29 and discontinued between first and second radiation fraction day 33. 72-hour infusion may be employed if hematologic suppression is severe wth 96-hour infusion days 1-5.

Cycle #3

	MON.—FRi.
Days	50 51 52 53 54
Boost Volume Radiation (B) 1.7 Gy/Fx 8-10 fractions	B B B B B B B B B B
5-FU	F F F F
Cisplatin 40-50 mg/m2 day 51	P

5-FU: 750-1000 mg/m²/24 hr × 72-96 hr generally commencing after first fraction of radiation on day 50 and discontinued between the first and second radiation fractions day 54. 72-hour infusion may be employed if hematologic suppression is severe with 96-hour infusion days 1-5 or days 29-33.

Figure 57-5 Modified Gynecologic Oncology Group (GOG) regimen as employed at Massachusetts General Hospital. The initial radiation volume *(asterisk)* includes the primary tumor, regional extensions, and bilateral groins. Patients judged to have unresectable disease 2 weeks after completion of 47.6 Gy receive 13.6 to 17 Gy in 8 to 10 twice-daily fractions (Fx) of 1.7 Gy to a reduced treatment volume (B) encompassing gross residual primary disease and gross unresectable regional nodes. A third cycle of concurrent chemotherapy (72 to 96 hours) is administered on days 50 to 54. Resectable groin metastases may be removed surgically in lieu of boost radiation. The cumulative dose to unresected gross disease is 61.2 to 64.6 Gy over the 8 elapsed weeks. Rarely, reduced boost volumes are treated with brachytherapy. 0, a day without radiation treatment; F, 5-fluorouracil given by continuous intravenous infusion (750 to 1000 mg/m²/24 h for 96 h commencing after the first fraction of radiation on days 1, 29, and 50); P, short infusion of cisplatin (40 to 50 mg/m² on days 2, 30, and 51); R, a fraction of external radiation encompassing the primary and regional nodes; a 4-hour minimum intertreatment interval is mandatory, but 6 hours or more are suggested when feasible.

too extensive for functionally conservative surgery. Reports of response rates for initial chemoradiation used preoperatively or as definitive therapy are tabulated in Table 57-6.[115,158-161,163-177] Unfortunately, the small numbers of patients selected for this approach, the variable selection criteria, the drugs employed, the radiation doses used, and the duration of follow-up are so diverse as to defy identification of an optimal regimen. However, as experience continues to accumulate and observational data become more mature, it seems probable that definitive chemoradiation will emerge as a viable treatment plan for patients with unresectable, extensive disease or who are inoperable because of comorbidities.

Treatment of Inguinal Nodes

It is unclear whether primary radiation or chemoradiation can replace primary surgery as definitive therapy for the inguinal

Table 57-6 Results of Chemoradiation for Previously Untreated Locally Advanced Vulvar Cancer

Study	Year	No of Patients	RT Dose (Gy)	Chemotherapy Agents*	Response (%)†
Kalra et al[176]	1981	1	30	5-FU/Mit-C	100 R
Iversen[175]	1982	9	15-40	Bleomycin	22 R
Levin et al[158]	1986	6	18-60.5	5-FU/Mit-C	100 R
Evans et al[174]	1988	4	20-65	5-FU/Mit-C	100 R
Thomas et al[159]	1989	9	44-60	5-FU/Mit-C	67 CR
Carson et al[164]	1990	6	45-50	5-FU/Mit-C/CDDP	67 CR, 17 PR
Whitaker et al[177]	1990	9	45-50	5-FU/Mit-C	44 CR, 56 PR
Berek et al[163]	1991	12	46.5-54	5-FU/CDDP	67 CR, 25 PR
Russell et al[166]	1992	18	47-56	5-FU/Mit-C/CDDP	89 CR, 44 PCR
Koh et al[165]	1993	17	34-70.4	5-FU/Mit-C/CDDP	53 CR, 35 PR
Sheistroen and Trope C[167]	1993	20	30-45	Bleomycin	25 CR, 50 PR
Sebag-Montefiore et al[169]	1994	37	45-50	5-FU/Mit-C	47 CR, 34 PR
Wahlen et al[115]	1995	19	43.2-70	5-FU/Mit-C	53 CR, 37 PR
Eifel et al[168]	1995	11	40-50	5-FU/CDDP	91R, 27 PCR
Lupi et al[173]	1996	24	54-60	5-FU/Mit-C	42 CR, 54 PR, 33 PCR
Landoni et al[172]	1996	41	54	5-FU/Mit-C	24 PCR ,56 PR
Cunningham et al[171]	1997	14	50-65	5-FU/CDDP	64 CR, 28 PR
Moore et al[160]	1998	73	40.9-47.8	5-FU/CDDP	47 CR, 30 PCR
Akl et al[170]	2000	12	30-36	5-FU/Mit-C	100 CR
Han et al[161]	2000	10	40-62	5-FU/Mit-C/CDDP	80 CR, 20 PR

*Some patients within individual series received 5-FU alone or in combination with cisplatin or mitomycin C.

†Response (R), partial response (PR), complete response (CR), and pathologic complete response (PCR) percentages are calculated based on the initial number of patients treated, not on the number of patients completing treatment or on the number undergoing repeat biopsy or surgery.

5-FU, 5-fluorouracil; CDDP, cisplatin; CR, clinical complete locoregional response; Mit-C, mitomycin C; PCR, pathologic complete response based on repeat biopsy or surgical excision; PR, partial clinical locoregional response; R, clinical locoregional response; RT, radiation therapy.

Data from references 115, 158-161, 163-177.

regions. Experience with radiation as primary treatment of the inguinal region is evolving but incomplete.

A randomized study conducted by the GOG compared primary inguinal dissection with primary groin irradiation to control the inguinal-femoral nodes in conjunction with radical vulvectomy in patients with squamous cell cancer of the vulva and clinically nonsuspicious groins.[178] This study was terminated before completion of accrual when interim monitoring revealed an excess of nodal relapse and death among patients treated with nodal irradiation. Radiation therapy consisted of 50 Gy in daily fractions of 2-Gy administered to a depth of 3 cm below the anterior skin surface. On the groin dissection arm, 5 (20.0%) of 25 patients had positive groin nodes. Those node-positive patients received postoperative irradiation. There were five groin relapses (18.5%) among the 27 patients randomized to receive groin irradiation, and none among patients treated with initial groin dissection. Initial groin dissection patients had significantly better progression-free interval (P = .03) and survival (P = .04).

Although resistance of the inguinal nodes to irradiation is one possible reason for the unacceptable groin failures in patients treated without groin dissection, a subsequent analysis of that study indicated that the groin irradiation technique employed was inadequate.[112] The irradiation technique was based on the assumption that the inguinal lymph nodes lay 3 to 4 cm below the surface, and a substantial percentage of treatment was delivered using electrons of energy appropriate to that depth. Koh's study illustrated that the median depth of lymph nodes in the groin was 6 cm from the surface but could be as deep as 17 cm in large patients. Kalidas[130] obtained measurements of the inguinal node depths of 31 patients with cervical, vaginal, or vulvar malignancies from their planning CT scans. Twenty-four of 81 superficial inguinal node depth measurements were greater than 3 cm, and all of 84 deep inguinal (femoral) node measurements were beyond the 3-cm range.[130] The irradiation technique used in the GOG study almost certainly resulted in significant underdose of the nodal bed. In planning radiation-based therapy to the groins, there can be no substitute for direct measurement of groin node depth by CT or other means. Depth of the deep femoral lymphatics is usually specified as the depth of the femoral artery as it passes beneath the inguinal ligament.

A review of primarily observational studies[71,154,178-184] indicates that the risk of groin node failure after irradiation in the patient with clinically disease-negative groin nodes is approximately 10% (Table 57-7). These studies did not always report the expected incidence of nodal disease in the patients irradiated, so the efficacy of irradiation is uncertain. However, approximately 15% to 25% of patients with clinically nonsuspicious groin nodes are expected to have subclinical metastases if elective nodal dissection is performed (see Table 57-2).

Two of the articles provide indirect evidence that irradiation without surgery can eradicate microscopic disease in clinically negative groin nodes in some patients. Frankendal and associates[179] performed radical vulvectomy without inguinal node dissection in 29 patients with clinically disease-negative groin nodes. Twelve patients received elective inguinal nodal irradiation; the radiation dose ranged from 30 to 60 Gy given over 15 to 55 days. There were no nodal recurrences. Seventeen patients received no radiation therapy, and three experienced inguinal failure. Manavi reported 135 patients who underwent simple vulvectomy for T1 cancers without groin dissection.[183] Sixty-five patients underwent elective groin irradiation. On average, those patients had less favorable primary tumors than the 70 patients who had no treatment to their groins. There were three groin recurrences (4.6%) in the irradiated patients and seven groin recurrences (10%) in the unirradiated patients.

Two observational studies totaling 36 patients reported the outcome for patients treated for locally advanced vulvar cancer with chemoradiation that included elective treatment

Table 57-7 Results of Elective Groin Irradiation or Chemoradiation in Patients with Vulvar Cancer and Clinically Negative Inguinofemoral Lymph Nodes

Study	No. of Patients	Groin Failure*	Failure Rate (%)
RADIATION ALONE			
Frankendal et al[179]	12	0	0
Simonsen et al[181]	65	11	16.9
Boronow et al[154]	13	0	0
Perez et al[180]	39	2	5.1
Lee et al[182]	16	3	18.8
Petereit et al[184]	23	2	8.7
Stehman et al[178]	27	5	18.5
Manavi et al[183]	65	3	4.6
Katz et al[71]	29	3	11
Total	289	29	10
CHEMORADIATION			
Leiserowitz et al[114]	19	0	0
Wahlen et al[115]	17	0	0
Total	36	0	0

*Patients had International Federation of Gynecology and Oncology (FIGO) 1969 N0-1 negative groin nodes determined by clinical evaluation.

of undissected groin nodes.[114,115] There were no groin relapses (see Table 57-7).

Treatment Approaches

The initial management decision for vulvar cancer is based on clinical features, including the extent of the primary, presence or absence of detectable node metastases, and the age, comorbidities, and preferences of the patient. The need for adjunctive therapies is determined by histopathologic findings. Management of the nodes and the primary tumor is based on the merits of each entity. Because there are no precise definitions of what constitutes favorable or early disease versus locally advanced disease, clinical definitions are provided to outline the principles that guide therapeutic choices.

Early, Favorable Low-Risk Disease

A practical definition of early, favorable disease (i.e., low risk) is disease that can be expected to be curatively managed by surgery alone. The extent and location of the primary tumor are amenable to radical excision without sacrificing the function of the urethra, the anorectum, the clitoris, and the vagina. Generally, this category includes patients without palpable or imaging evidence of inguinal node metastasis. For low-risk cancers that are unifocal and well-lateralized, wide local excision of the primary lesion in the vulva is recommended for most patients. The reported results from observational studies of wide local excision for T1 or T2 tumors suggest an average survival rate of approximately 90%. The criteria proposed for the selection of patients for such conservative surgical resection vary but generally include patients with tumors less than 2 cm in diameter and depth of invasion less than 5 mm.[69,73,83,136,185]

The role and indications for postoperative adjuvant vulvar irradiation are ill defined. Although data have clearly demonstrated that surgical margins less than 8 mm, increasing depth of invasion, presence of capillary lymphatic space involvement, and increasing size of primary cancer portend increased risk for vulvar recurrence after excision of any extent, it is still unclear to what extent postoperative adjuvant irradiation can overcome these risks.

Although wider excision may for some patients eliminate the risk of close margins, it may not be feasible or advisable for midline or deep margins and cannot overcome other risk factors. One retrospective series of 62 patients with positive or close (<8 mm) margins showed on multivariate analysis that adjuvant irradiation significantly reduced local recurrence rates and significantly improved survival rates for the positive margin group.[109] The role of adjuvant irradiation after wide local excision of vulvar cancer was being explored in a GOG randomized clinical trial, but the trial had to be abandoned because of lack of accrual.

Standard management of the inguinal regions for all patients with invasive disease of greater than 1 mm depth is groin dissection. Postoperative radiation therapy to the inguinal and pelvic nodes is recommended for patients with involvement of two or more nodes and for those with a single node with macroscopic metastasis or extranodal extension. In patients with diagnostic imaging that shows no evidence of pelvic adenopathy, the superior border of the treatment volume extends no more cephalad than the middle of the sacroiliac joints to limit acute and chronic enteric morbidity. The randomized study from which these recommendations are largely drawn gave prophylactic adjuvant irradiation to both groins, even when involvement was unilateral only.[90] The contribution of adjuvant irradiation to the contralateral negative groin is uncertain and may be unnecessary. Two issues remain controversial. Whether residual vulva and tumor bed should routinely be included in the treatment volume when groins and pelvic nodes require irradiation remains unclear, although histopathologic features associated with the primary may suggest that this is prudent in selected patients, if not all. Whether concurrent chemotherapy should be administered with purely adjuvant treatment to further enhance the regional efficacy of radiation is also the substance of conjecture and debate. Hypothetically, the increase in acute toxicity could be offset by improved regional control, possibly with a reduced dose of radiation that might translate into diminished late radiation effects. This hypothesis remains untested. A treatment algorithm for management of patients with early, lateralized disease is found in Figure 57-6.

Management of Small Primary Tumors Encroaching on Midline Structures

Although surgical excision remains the historical standard treatment for patients with small, midline primary tumors, it is not unreasonable to consider treating a primary midline lesion, regardless of size, with a localized field of primary irra-

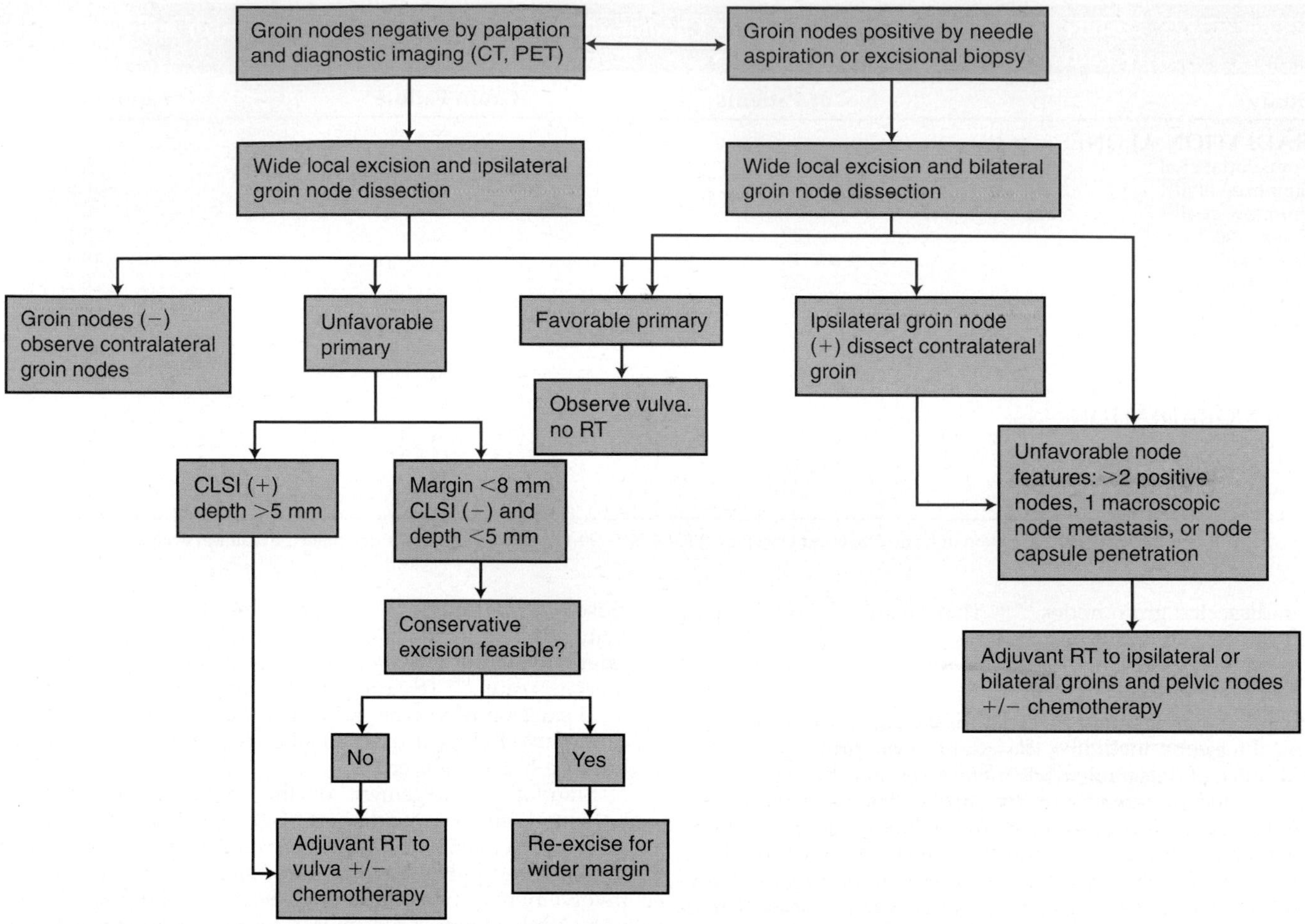

Figure 57-6 **Treatment algorithm for limited vulvar cancer** CLSI, capillary lymphatic space involvement; CT, computed tomography, PET, positron emission tomography; RT, radiation therapy.

diation or chemoirradiation if surgical excision would result in predictable loss of cosmesis or function. Although these patients can be cured with surgery as monotherapy, the functional and cosmetic impairments can be psychologically devastating. For many patients, clinical shrinkage after modest-dose (45 to 54 Gy) irradiation or chemoradiation can permit conservative excision of residual tumor with excellent preservation of function and cosmesis. (Fig. 57-7) This recommendation remains controversial, not because of a lack of efficacy for radiation (which has been valuable in more locally advanced disease), but because no systematic studies of subsequent sexual function and morbidity have been performed. Anecdotally, clitoral function can be preserved in some sexually active patients after 45 Gy combined with 5-FU–based chemotherapy supplemented by clitoris-sparing local excision. Such patients are sexually active and orgasmic before treatment, are sexually active and orgasmic 12 or more months after completion of treatment, and subjectively report intact sensation and vascular engorgement and erectile clitoral function. Whether this is also feasible after higher doses of radiation alone is unknown.

LOCALLY ADVANCED DISEASE AND PALLIATION

Patients may be considered to have locally advanced disease if the location and extent of the primary lesion in the vulva is such that radical excision would require functional compromise or sacrifice of functionally important midline structures. Patients with clinically involved groin nodes, particularly nodular, ulcerating, or fixed, are also considered to have locally advanced disease. These patients are predictably inadequately treated by surgery as monotherapy, and combined-modality therapy (i.e., chemoradiation or chemoradiation coordinated with conservative surgery) should be considered by multidisciplinary consultation before initiation of any therapeutic intervention.

Historically, adequate surgical clearance of large primary tumors that involve the anus, rectum, rectovaginal septum, or proximal urethra usually included radical vulvectomy plus some type of pelvic exenteration. Five-year survival rates with primary surgery for advanced disease range up to 50%.[7] The physical and psychological morbidities from such surgical procedures are high.

In a landmark study, Boronow and colleagues explored the use of preoperative radiation in locally advanced disease with the intent to reduce the scope of subsequent surgery.[154] Thirty-seven patients with locally advanced vulvar cancer were treated with variable doses of radiation (median, 48 Gy) followed by surgery. The 5-year survival rate was 75.6%. Approximately 40% of patients had no residual disease in the operative specimen after preoperative irradiation.[154]

Subsequently, multiple investigators reported favorable results with preoperative chemoradiation in patients with

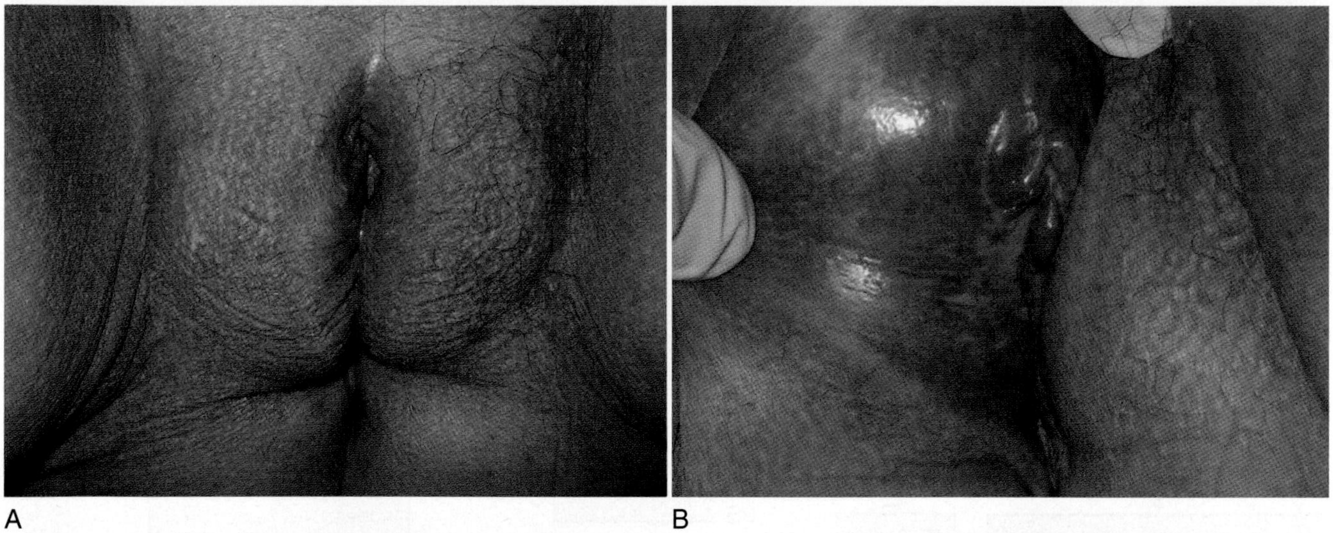

Figure 57-7 Clinical results after combined-modality therapy for a small, T2N0, anterior right labia minora primary tumor invading the clitoris. The images were obtained at a follow-up examination 18 months after treatment that consisted of 45 Gy given in 25 fractions to a volume encompassing the primary and electively including the groin nodes bilaterally with two courses of concurrent infusional 5-fluorouracil and bolus cisplatin. Conservative excision of residual tissue spared the clitoris and most of the vulva. Images were obtained with the labia apposed (**A**) and with the right labium majorum retracted, revealing the excision scar (**B**).

locally advanced disease. Patients were treated with chemoradiation preoperatively if shrinkage permitted non-exenterative surgery (see Table 57-6).

A GOG study evaluated concurrent 5-FU and cisplatin in conjunction with a modest radiation dose (47.6 Gy) as preoperative therapy for patients with clinical stage III or IV squamous cell cancer of the vulva.[160] After completing preoperative chemoirradiation, 33 (46.5%) of 71 patients had no visible vulvar cancer at the time of planned surgery, and only 2 (2.8%) of 71 had residual disease judged unresectable. In three patients, urinary or gastrointestinal continence could not be preserved. Because of this study and the single-institution phase II studies, there is a growing acceptance by gynecologic oncologists that concurrent chemotherapy and irradiation constitutes the treatment of choice for primary management of patients with locally advanced disease.

Randomized trials for vulvar cancer have not been performed to test whether concurrent chemotherapy confers additional benefit to radiation alone. The drugs currently used include 5-FU, alone or in combination with cisplatin or mitomycin C (see Table 57-6). Results with bleomycin have been unsatisfactory because of gross tumor persistence or a high local relapse rate after initial favorable response.[167,175] The GOG is evaluating weekly cisplatin as a radiation potentiator in the treatment of advanced vulvar cancer. Information from prospective, controlled trials of chemoradiation (i.e., radiation alone compared with radiation with concurrent 5-FU and mitomycin C) for cancers of the anal canal suggests that the addition of chemotherapy is useful and may permit some reduction in the total radiation dose necessary to eradicate disease.[186,187] An algorithm for the management of patients with locally advanced primary cancer, with or without locally extensive groin metastases, is provided in Figure 57-8.

Management of Patients with Advanced Nodal Disease

When groin nodes are ulcerating or fixed, initial treatment of the inguinal regions consists of primary irradiation or chemoradiation. Because it is unclear whether chemoradiation in tolerable doses can eradicate bulky nodal disease, if there is substantial regression of nodal disease, it is reasonable to subsequently operate to remove any residual adenopathy.

Patients with bulky involved nodes that are initially resectable may undergo initial surgical removal of the bulky nodes followed by postoperative radiation or initial irradiation or chemoradiation followed by operative removal of any residuum. The optimal sequencing of therapies remains controversial because surgery can delay initiation of irradiation, and preoperative irradiation may compromise wound healing. Commonly, patients with bulky inguinal nodes also have locally advanced primary tumors, in which case initial irradiation or chemoradiation is the logical sequence choice. If there is clinical uncertainty about whether all gross adenopathy can be removed from the groins, imaging with ultrasound, CT, or MRI may aid in elucidating the spatial relationships among blood vessels, nerves, bone, and metastatic adenopathy. These imaging modalities may be particularly useful in defining disease extent in large patients in whom the femoral nodes lie deeper than can be realistically assessed by clinical palpation.

Regardless of the sequencing of therapies, groin surgery should be limited to removal of gross adenopathy rather than an en bloc removal of all lymphatic tissue. It should be accomplished through the smallest feasible incision to accomplish this objective. The intent of such surgery is to reduce groin cancer volume to a microscopic or occult burden that can be controlled by modest doses of fractionated radiation. Conversely, a radiation dose administered before or after surgical cytoreduction should be restricted to an effective dose for controlling microscopic or occult disease. By limiting the extent of groin dissection in anticipation of subsequent irradiation and by limiting the radiation dose in anticipation of surgical removal of residual, bulky disease, some acute complications (e.g., wound dehiscence, infection) and late sequelae (e.g., lymphedema, femoral fracture) can be reduced or avoided.

Locally Recurrent or Metastatic Cancer

The outcome for patients who experience relapse of vulvar cancer after primary therapy markedly depends on the site of

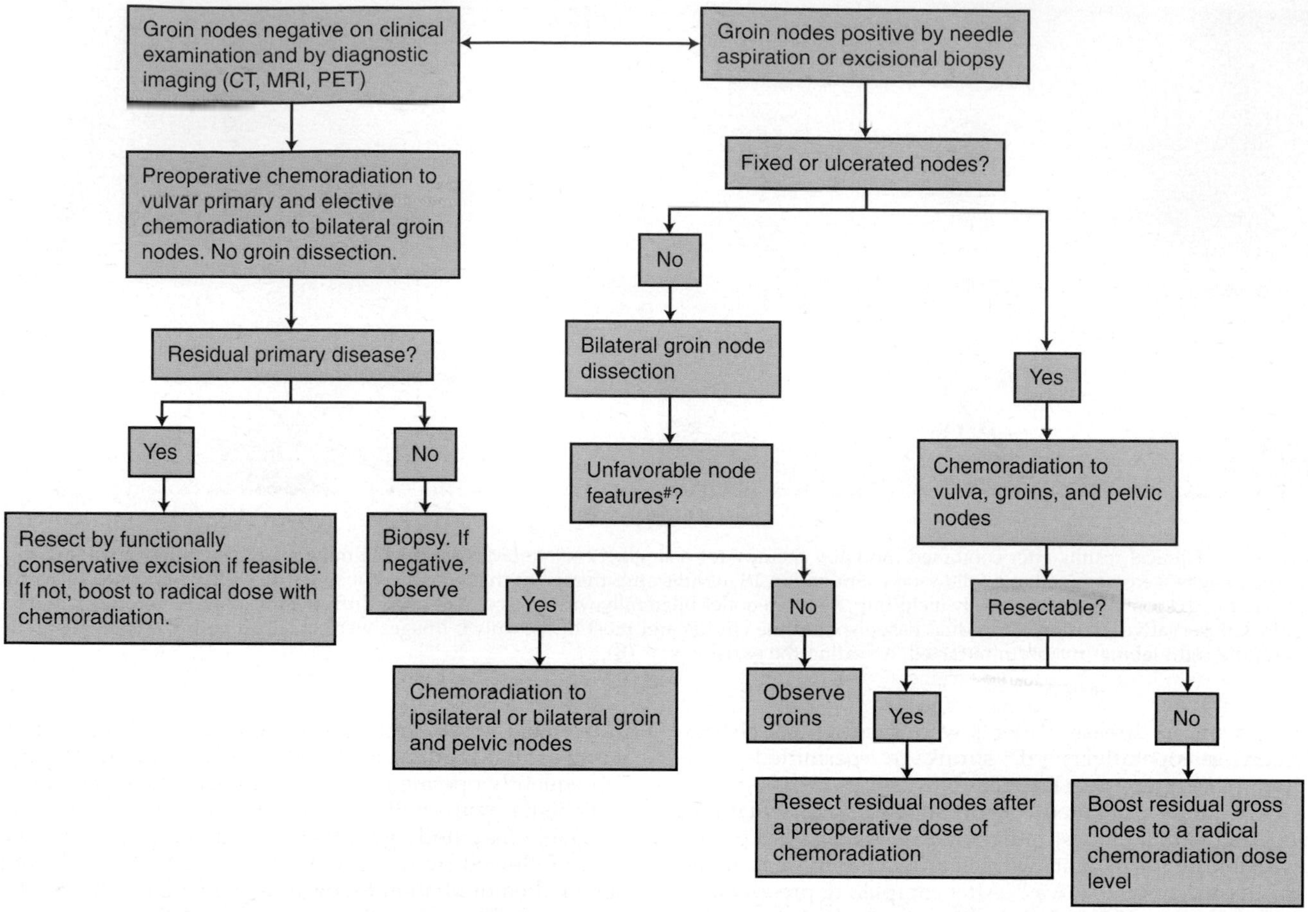

Figure 57-8 Treatment algorithm for an extensive vulvar primary tumor. An extensive primary lesion is one that encroaches on or invades functionally important midline structures (e.g., clitoris, urethra, anorectum) and can not be surgically resected without potential compromise to the functional integrity of those structures. Unfavorable node features include more than two positive nodes, one macroscopic node metastasis, or metastatic spread through node capsule. CT, computed tomography, MRI, magnetic resonance imaging; PET, positron emission tomography.

relapse. For those with distant metastases, chemotherapy with agents active against squamous cell cancer is often offered, but response rates and durations are generally poor.[102,188-197]

Agents (e.g., 5-FU, cisplatin, mitomycin C) that may be useful when given concurrently with irradiation may have limited efficacy when given alone. Inferential evidence for this statement includes patients with regionally extensive vulvar cancer treated with irradiation and synchronous cytotoxic chemotherapy who manifest prompt and marked response within the irradiated volume while simultaneously developing overt metastatic disease outside the irradiated volume. This finding may, however, be an indication of inadequate dose levels of chemotherapy necessary to result in a systemic treatment effect rather than evidence of chemoresistance.

Inguinal recurrences may be amenable to management with irradiation or chemoradiation to provide local control. Few patients survive long term.[102,104,105,141,142]

Local vulvar recurrence appears to be related to the previously described risk factors and particularly to inadequate surgical resections with margins less than 8 mm pathologically. Several reports suggested that up to 75% of patients with vulvar recurrence of cancer may be cured, usually when treated with surgical re-excision.[104,198] Boronow and colleagues reported a 5-year survival rate of 63% with modest-dose irradiation.[154] However, Faul and associates reported only a 25% 2-year actuarial survival rate after vulvar recurrence.[109] Radiation therapy or chemoradiation for local recurrence is an option, particularly when the lesion is not amenable to repeat resection without predictably inadequate surgical margins or compromise of functionally important midline structures.[159,166]

Because vulvar neoplasia is often a field defect, second tumors may develop but are often labeled vulvar recurrences. New primary cancers often develop in sites remote from the initial tumor. It is important, if possible, to differentiate a new occurrence of cancer from a recurrence because the latter would attribute a treatment failure to the original treatment modalities used and lead to an underestimate of the efficacy of the original therapy.

TECHNIQUES OF IRRADIATION

Groin and Nodal Irradiation

The GOG study that established the usefulness of postoperative adjuvant groin irradiation used external beam radiation bilaterally to the inguinal and femoral dissection beds and pelvic nodes, even when node involvement was unilateral.[90] This study forms the basis on which most radiation oncologists use postoperative adjuvant nodal irradiation, and the specific radiation volumes and doses in the study—45 to 50 Gy in 1.8- to 2.0-Gy fractions—are often those prescribed. These doses are sufficient to offer a high probability of control of microscopic disease. The technique used was an anterior and posterior (AP) parallel-opposed pair of fields. The inferior border of the volume recommended is usually determined clinically using a margin lying parallel and 6 to 8 cm inferior to the inguinal skin crease or ligament. The GOG study used a superior border at the L5-S1 interspace, although the value of extending the field to this level superiorly is uncertain. The observed survival gains appear to be related to improved control of the inguinal regions and not to improved control of the pelvic nodes. Involved nodes located high in the pelvis or in the common iliac region connote a high probability of extrapelvic failure. In the interest of reducing bowel morbidity, it seems sensible to limit the superior border in a comparable fashion to that used in some institutions for carcinoma of the anal canal (1 or 2 cm above the inferior sacroiliac joint), unless there is radiographic evidence of higher pelvic nodal involvement.

The patient is usually treated in the supine position with the feet apart or in the frog-leg position to minimize skin reaction in the medial thigh and to allow appropriate blocking of the vulvar tissue centrally. The lymphadenectomy scar usually lies within the limits normally used for the lateral margins of the volume. The necessity for specifically encompassing the inguinal lymphadenectomy scar is unclear because the incidence of scar recurrence is unknown. The medial two thirds of distance between the origin and insertion of the inguinal ligament (i.e., between the pubic tubercle and the anteroinferior iliac spine) should be included unless surgical clips indicate more lateral nodal involvement. For patients receiving nodal irradiation only, with no indications for vulvar irradiation, a midline AP block is used to exclude residual vulva and central pelvis from the radiation field. It is important to confirm clinically that the lateral borders of the block do not encroach on the medial aspects of the inguinal node bed and obturator nodes, resulting in underdosage. Generally, the width of the midline block should be no greater than the distance between the pubic tubercles. It is intended only to reduce dose to midline structures (distal urethra, vagina, and anorectum) and residual vulva. Use of the midline block has been associated with a high risk of local recurrence in the shielded midline.[153] It should be used only if risk factors for local recurrence are minimal. Generally, the radiation fields for inguinal and pelvic nodal irradiation exclusive of the vulva resemble the inverted Y used in lymphoma therapy with appropriate modifications of the lateral extent to encompass the groins as described (Fig. 57-9).

For patients with clinically and radiographically negative groin nodes in whom elective nodal irradiation or chemoradiation is to be used without subsequent surgical dissection, the techniques and volume of radiation are similar to those described for adjuvant therapy. Generally, this can be done when preoperative irradiation or chemoradiation is needed for a locally advanced vulvar primary. The inguinofemoral nodal depth should be confirmed by CT, magnetic resonance imaging (MRI), or ultrasonography because the delivery of an adequate dose is critically dependent on establishing the appropriate depth and location for dose prescription and calculation. The dose given must be substantially increased for patients with fixed or ulcerating lymph nodes. Although the optimal dose is not defined, a dose of 64.6 Gy, usually in combination with several cycles of concurrent chemotherapy, may be necessary to provide the highest probability of locoregional control while remaining within the tolerance of adjacent normal tissues.

A recognized complication of groin irradiation is femoral neck fracture.[71,199] This is a particular risk in older patients who may have some degree of osteoporosis and who are vulnerable to falls and fractures in the absence of radiation. Equally weighted parallel-opposed photon fields are inappropriate if

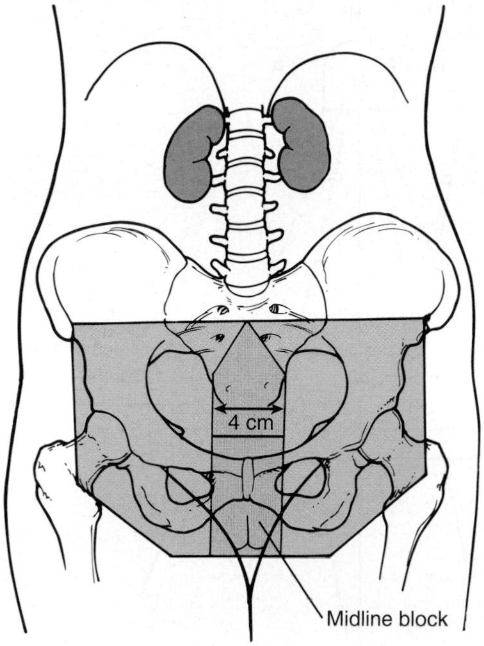

Figure 57-9 The radiation fields for groin and pelvic nodal irradiation exclusive of the vulva resemble the inverted Y used in lymphoma therapy with appropriate modifications to encompass the lateral groins.

the dose prescribed will exceed 45 Gy. Techniques for minimizing femoral neck dose include partial central transmission block technique in which dose to the deep groin nodes is prescribed through a large anterior photon field employing low-energy photons of 4 to 6 MV. Dose to deeper pelvic nodes and the vulva is calculated and supplemented by a smaller, opposed posterior pelvic field using photons of higher energy. A central partial transmission block is placed over the anterior field corresponding to the narrower posterior field that attenuates the contribution of the anterior field to the deep pelvic nodes and vulva, allowing better dose homogeneity. If inguinal nodes are superficial, dose may be further supplemented by administering a portion of the treatment with high-energy electrons. When abutting photon fields or photon and electron fields to encompass nodal tissue overlying the femoral necks, there is considerable potential for "hot" and "cold" spots. Hot spots may injure the femoral arteries and the femurs, and cold spots hazard disease recurrence within the clinical target volume. Moving the field abutments once or twice during a course of treatment can diminish these hazards. Technical alternatives include the use of intensity-modulated radiation therapy (IMRT) or proton beam.

Called a *modified segmental boost technique*, the use of right and left anterior oblique, partially beam-split photon fields to supplement the groin node dose is a technique suitable for any department with an isocentric linear accelerator with appropriate beam energies (Fig. 57-10).[200] With this technique, the oblique fields are angled so the medial border of each anterior oblique field corresponds to the beam divergence of the lateral border of the posterior field, minimizing the potential for hot and cold spots. The tumor dose must be brought to the skin surface if there is evidence of cutaneous involvement. Bolus material may be required.

Axial dose profiles employing various techniques are depicted in Figure 57-11. The magnitudes of hot spots at the boundaries of treatment fields are shown.

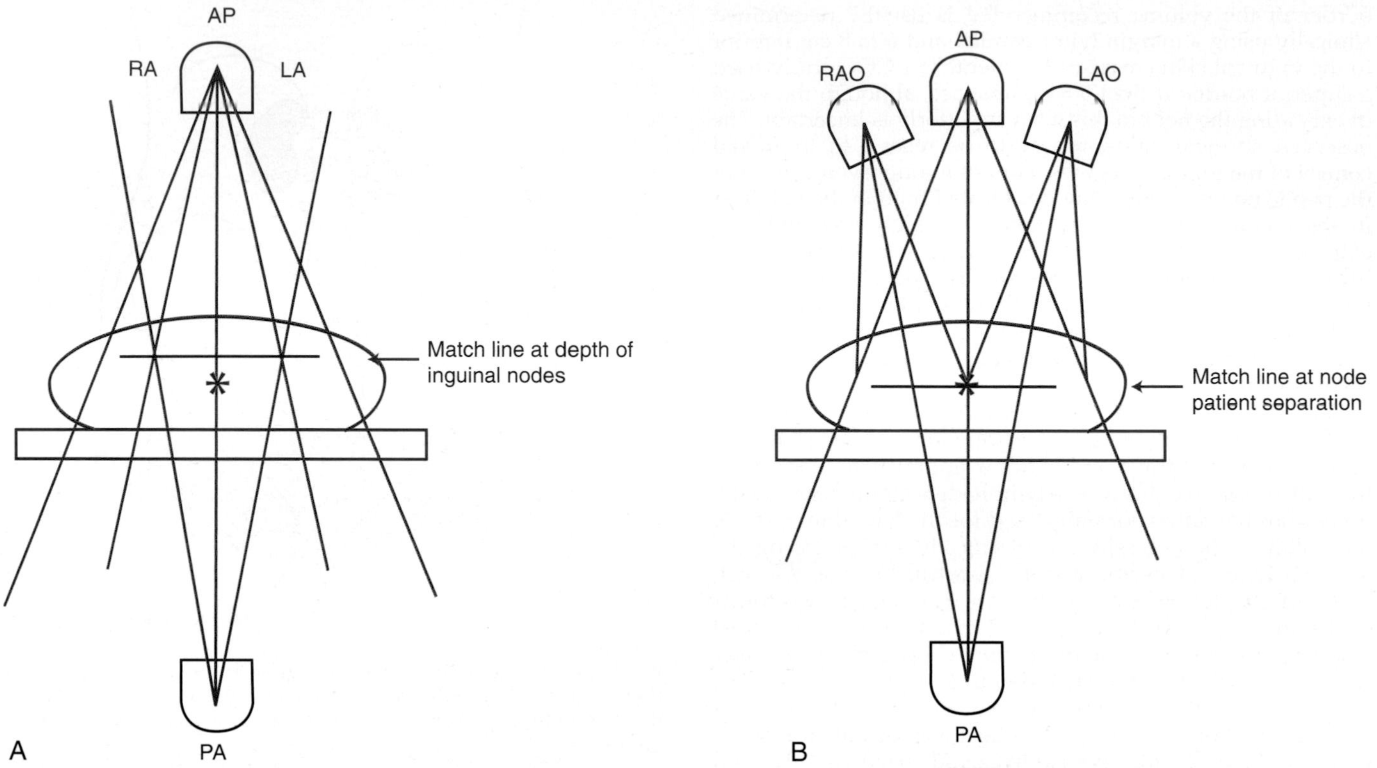

Figure 57-10 Treatment technique for irradiation of the pelvis and inguinal nodes. Beam arrangements for two techniques: segmental boost technique (**A**) and modified segmental boost technique (**B**). AP, anteroposterior; LA, left anterior; LAO, left anterior oblique; PA, posteroanterior; RA, right anterior; RAO, right anterior oblique. (Data from Moran M, Lund MW, Ahmad M, et al: Improved treatment of pelvis and inguinal nodes using modified segmental boost technique: dosimetric evaluation. Int J Radiat Oncol Biol Phys 59:1523-1530, 2004.)

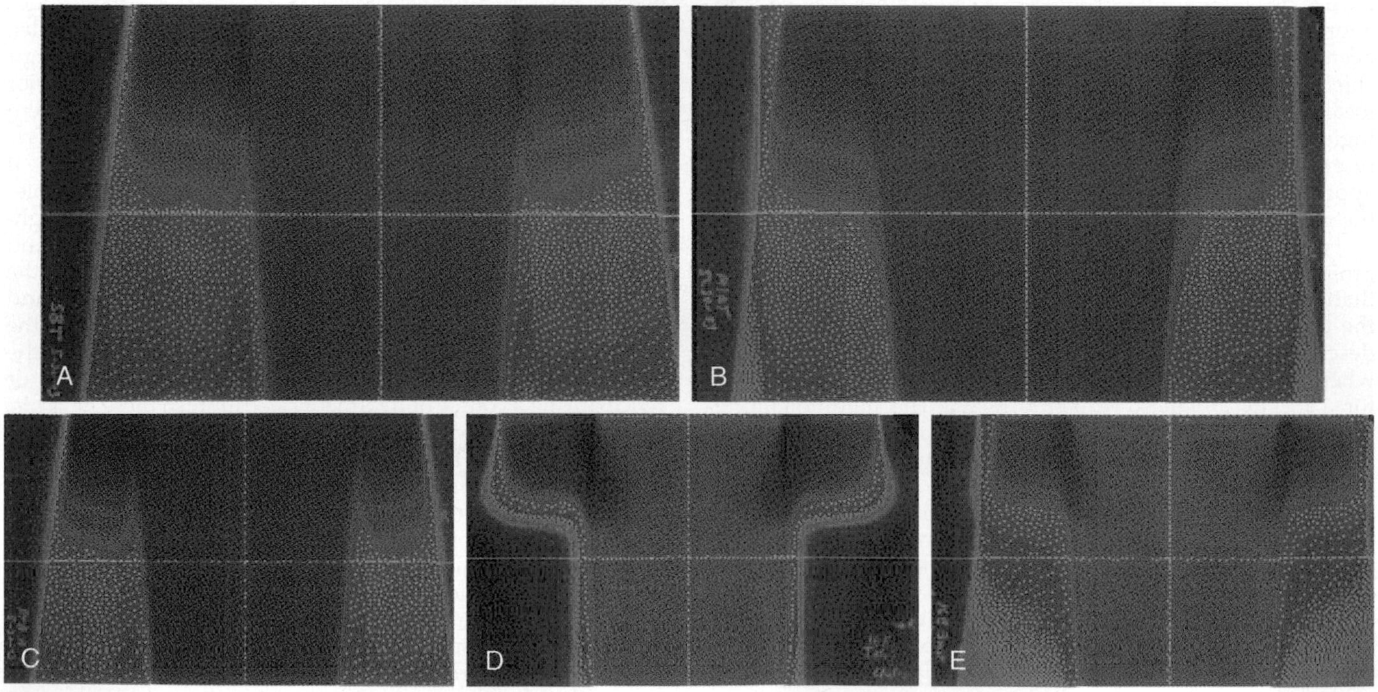

Figure 57-11 Comparative dose profiles for various techniques employed to treat the pelvis and groin nodes. Color rendering of axial dose distribution generated from vertical film irradiation in a plastic-water (PW) phantom using five different techniques for treating pelvis and inguinal nodes. High-dose areas are visible in field overlap regions. **A,** Segmental boost technique. **B,** Modified segmental boost technique. **C,** Partial transmission block technique. **D,** Photon with electron tag technique. **E,** Photon with electron boost technique. (Data from Moran M, Lund MW, Ahmad M, et al: Improved treatment of pelvis and inguinal nodes using modified segmental boost technique: dosimetric evaluation. Int J Radiat Oncol Biol Phys 59:1523-1530, 2004.)

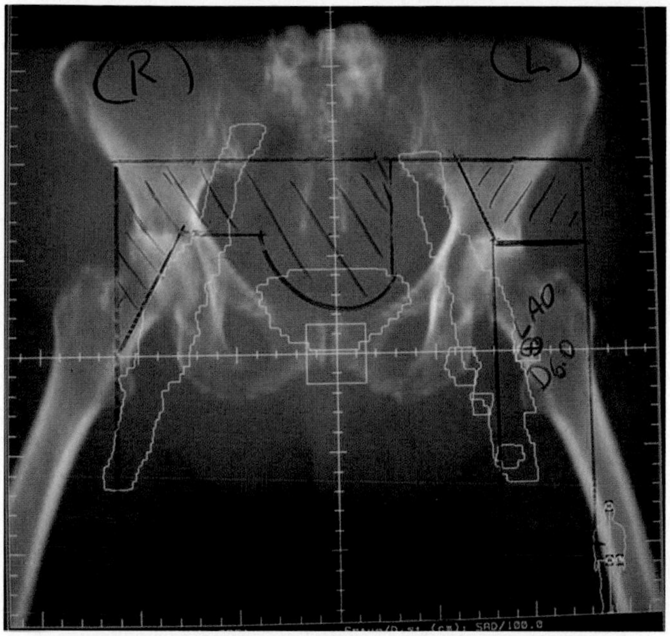

Figure 57-12 Simulation digitally reconstructed radiograph for treatment of a patient with a lateralized T3N1 squamous carcinoma of the left labium majorum and minorum with metastases in two medial left groin nodes based on fused positron emission tomography/computed tomography (PET/CT). The volume encompasses the clinically negative contralateral groin nodes medial to the femoral vessels, which have been reconstructed from CT images. On the involved side, the treatment volume is extended cephalad to encompass the obturator and caudal external iliac nodes while shielding central pelvic soft tissues. The left lateral groin has a portion of the treatment delivered by an anterior oblique field using modified segmental boost technique, with the medial beam border corresponding to the left lateral border of the posterior field.

Selection of target volumes, choice of treatment technique, and prescription of radiation dose and fractionation should be individualized based on tumor factors, patient comorbidities, availability of equipment, and sophistication of medical dosimetry support. An example of individualization of target volume, portal design, and technique is depicted in Figure 57-12.

Adjuvant Irradiation of the Vulva

When adjuvant irradiation to the vulva is indicated because of risk of local recurrence, an appositional perineal portal may be used with the patient in dorsal lithotomy position. Just as surgical concepts are changing to limit radical excision to the site of the primary cancer rather than extirpation of the entire vulva, radiation volumes are also being modified. A localized field of radiation may be used to encompass the vulvar scar with an appropriate margin. This allows maximal sparing of uninvolved vulvar tissues from acute and late radiation reactions. When therapy is adjuvant, irradiation alone employing doses of 45 to 54 Gy is recommended. The role of chemoradiation in the adjuvant setting is not established. The beam energy should be tailored to the estimated depth or thickness of the original lesion from the vulvar surface, with appropriate use of bolus to deliver the prescribed tumor dose to the skin of the vulva. An electron beam or low-energy photon beam is employed. If the target volume in the vulva is localized and can be encompassed using a perineal vulvar port, even if there is also an indication to treat the regional nodes, the use of separate fields to the groin region and vulva may spare a significant volume of the vulva from radiation effects. Care must be exercised to establish the location of the exit beam from the perineal port and ensure safety with respect to possible overlap with the nodal irradiation volumes. Alternatively, anterior and posterior photon fields may be employed when insecure margins are treated with less than precise definition of where the at-risk tissue lies.

Definitive Vulvar Irradiation

When definitive irradiation is selected for primary management of a small or early midline vulvar primary, a technique may be used similar to that described for adjuvant treatment (i.e., perineal portal tailored to the depth and thickness and size of the lesion). Most vulvar cancers appear to be extremely responsive, and rapid, visible response to irradiation is often apparent after a tumor dose of 30 to 36 Gy in fractions of 1.8 to 2.0 Gy.

Because available dose-control data for vulvar cancer are scant and seldom correlated with the volume of disease treated and because it is unproved whether the addition of concurrent chemotherapy can modify the total dose required to sterilize disease, dosage guidelines are imprecise. In general, concurrent 5-FU or 5-FU plus cisplatin with or without mitomycin C is recommended for definitive treatment. For small vulvar tumors (<4 cm), total doses of 54 to 61.6 Gy at 1.8 to 2 Gy per fraction with concurrent chemotherapy may be adequate. For larger or inoperable tumors, the entire vulva may need to be irradiated using an AP-PA parallel-opposed pair of fields. Tumor doses should be escalated to 64 to 72 Gy if no surgery is contemplated. Total dose depends on the fractionation employed, the elapsed time to complete treatment, whether concurrent chemotherapy is employed, and if so, how much.

Because most patients are thicker in the low pelvis where central axis dose is frequently calculated when parallel-opposed fields are treated, dose per fraction may be significantly higher at the vulva due to reduced tissue attenuation of the beams. This depends significantly on beam energies. Compensators may be employed to minimize the impact of this effect. Thermoluminescent dosimeters placed on the tumor and in the cleft between the labia are a simple mechanism to confirm actual absorbed dose at the vulva. This permits tailoring of compensatory measures should the dose inhomogeneity be excessive, which is sometimes the case in large patients.

Although planned split-course irradiation is to be avoided because of the concern for increased tumor proliferation with protracted overall treatment times, most patients require a short rest to allow epithelial regeneration before completing a planned definitive course of chemoradiation to the vulva. Use of twice-daily fractionation schemes is a tactic to compensate for treatment interruption and to keep overall elapsed time to complete therapy reasonable while maximizing radiation-drug synergism.

Some oncologists have used interstitial radiation implants, particularly for boosting bulky disease or boosting the involved vagina.[201,202] No randomized data are available to evaluate the relative benefits and toxicities of interstitial versus external boost irradiation. A potential pitfall of interstitial techniques is difficulty in achieving dose homogeneity, and late effects may be increased because of the inevitable hot spots in tissues in direct contact with interstitial sources.

Radiation Treatment Sequelae

When vulvar irradiation is used as an adjuvant treatment to wide local excision or as definitive treatment, the 100% tumor dose usually needs to be delivered to the skin and mucosal surfaces of the distal vagina. Even when doses of 45 to 50 Gy are given in the adjuvant setting, it is expected that all patients will experience moist desquamation. This may vary from patchy, moist desquamation to confluent, moist desquamation over the treatment volume. Generally, this reaction heals in the 2 or 3 weeks after completion of radiation therapy. The reaction is usually managed with symptomatic measures, including frequent sitz baths, exposure to air, application of topical ointments such as those used to treat superficial burns, and pain medication. In some situations, particularly for elderly, frail patients, hospitalization for skin care may be required. Depending on the volume treated, acute effects may include urethritis, cystitis, and proctitis. Diarrhea is unusual unless a full pelvic volume is irradiated.

The late effects of radiation may include skin changes of atrophy or telangiectasis, which in small volumes are not usually functionally distressing. Some patients may experience more extensive skin atrophy and dense subcutaneous fibrosis. The development of mucosal or perineal ulcers is rare. Late effects on the vulva appear to be minimized by limiting the radiation fraction size to 1.6 to 1.8 Gy. When the radiation volume has included the anus and lower rectum, radiation bowel injury may occur, with rectal bleeding, fibrosis, or stricture.

Irradiation of the node-bearing areas may result in similar acute effects if full doses are required at the skin. Acute effects may vary from erythema to moist desquamation, particularly in intertriginous areas and along skin folds.

The contribution of radiation therapy to the problem of leg edema induced by groin surgery is unknown. One series suggested that after concurrent chemotherapy and radiation, 4 of 14 surviving patients treated for advanced primary or recurrent disease experienced leg edema. In two patients, the edema was minimal and did not require treatment. Two patients did require treatment with compression and diuretics. Both had an inguinal lymphadenectomy before chemoradiation.[166]

Radiation therapy to the groins may induce femoral neck fracture.[71,199] The risk of hip fracture may not correlate well with the dose delivered to the hips and may be more common in frail, elderly women with osteoporosis.[203] Fractures through the ischial rami may occasionally be seen in patients carried to higher radiation dose for unresectable primary disease. Rarely, groin radiation may induce hemodynamically significant femoral artery stenosis.

Acute complications from chemoradiation can be severe. Reviewing 5-FU plus mitomycin C or mitomycin C alone used as concurrent radiopotentiators in the treatment of 17 patients with vulvar cancer, Mulayim observed grade 4 neutropenia in six patients (35%) using the 1998 Standard Toxicity Criteria.[204] Three patients experienced life-threatening neutropenic sepsis after their second cycle of chemotherapy. In four patients, the second cycle of chemotherapy was cancelled because of the severity of the acute reactions after the first cycle. Severe enterocolitis was a direct contributing cause of death of two patients. Skin toxicity necessitated treatment interruption for nine patients at a median dose of 32.4 Gy (range, 16.2 to 48 Gy). Nine patients (53%) required more than 9 weeks to complete chemoradiation. Eleven (65%) of 17 patients were older than 70 years.[204] With the benefit of hindsight and better understanding of pharmacokinetics in elderly women, chemotherapy dose reduction may have been appropriate from the outset of treatment in some of these patients.[205] Mitomycin C has been associated with significant bowel toxicity in other irradiation-chemotherapy contexts,[206] and cisplatin is more likely to be used as a second drug in conjunction with 5-FU.

Treatment interruption necessitated by severe acute radiation dermatitis can delay treatment longer than a planned, elective interruption, as was required in GOG protocol 101 and as is practiced routinely at MGH after 23.8 Gy. Despite a second 2-week break in this schedule after 47.6 Gy and before reduced-volume boost therapy, almost all patients are able to complete a radical course of chemoradiation within 8 weeks consisting of 64.6 Gy given in 38 fractions with three cycles of concurrent 5-FU and cisplatin chemotherapy. Thirty of the radiation fractions are administered twice daily during the weeks of chemotherapy infusion to compensate for treatment interruption and to maximize radiation-drug synergism.

CHALLENGES, CONTROVERSIES, AND FUTURE POSSIBILITIES

Because of the diversity of clinical presentations, the relative rarity of the disease, and the availability of multiple effective treatment strategies, the systematic exploration of treatment options in phase III clinical trials is difficult. For many questions, observational studies of outcomes after standardized therapy may be the best information available to guide future therapeutic choices. Several important questions must be addressed:

1. For resectable primary cancers involving the clitoris, lower urethra, or vaginal introitus, will primary surgery, primary irradiation, or chemoirradiation provide the best therapeutic ratio? Of particular relevance to this question would be a prospective comparison of local cancer control and of psychosexual and physical quality of life.
2. What is the optimal fractionation and dose of radiation to small-volume and large-volume (nonresectable) vulvar cancers to obtain local control with acceptable morbidity?
3. In advanced vulvar cancer, when irradiation or chemoirradiation is selected for initial therapy, is it better to try to increase the radiation dose sufficiently to eradicate disease, or is there less morbidity with a lower radiation dose combined with planned surgical removal of residual disease?
4. Does concurrent chemotherapy allow the use of a decreased radiation dose with decreased late radiation sequelae?
5. Does chemotherapy improve local control compared with the same radiation dose alone?
6. If chemotherapy is useful, what agents should be used: 5-FU, cisplatin, or mitomycin C or combinations of these drugs?
7. Can appropriately planned irradiation or chemoirradiation be used instead of inguinal node dissection for patients with clinically and radiographically negative groin nodes?
8. In what circumstances is adjuvant nodal irradiation indicated? Is it beneficial for patients with involvement of one macroscopic node or extranodal extension in addition to those with involvement of two or more nodes? Might patients with only one positive node benefit?
9. Will concomitant chemotherapy with adjuvant irradiation result in better control and survival than irradiation alone?
10. When adjuvant groin and pelvic nodal irradiation is used, is it necessary to treat bilaterally if positive nodes are only unilateral?
11. Should primary concurrent chemotherapy and radiation replace the use of wide local excision for small lesions that involve midline structures?

An understanding of the answers to these questions will come from carefully documented reporting from centers where sufficient numbers of patients are treated in a uniform fashion and where techniques and doses of radiation and the use of concomitant chemotherapy are carefully documented with respect to the site and extent of disease treated.

MELANOMA OF THE VULVA

Malignant melanomas of the vulva are rare and constitute about 10% of all vulvar malignancies. Even large, tertiary cancer referral centers treat only one or two patients annually.[60,207,208] Malignant melanoma occurs predominantly in postmenopausal white women, with a peak incidence between the sixth and seventh decades. These lesions may arise de novo or from preexisting junctional or compound nevi.

Three basic histologic types exist. Superficial spreading melanoma is most common and tends to remain superficial in its early course; lentigo malignant melanoma is a "flat freckle" that has a tendency to remain superficial; and nodular melanoma is the most aggressive variety, carries the worst prognosis, and tends to invade deeply early.[207] Prognosis and staging are based on measurements of tumor depth of penetration as described by the melanoma staging systems of Clark, Breslow, and Chung.[58-60] The FIGO staging system for vulva is not usefully applied to melanoma.

Treatment

The main method of vulvar melanoma management is surgery. Just as in the management of vulvar squamous cell carcinomas, surgery has tended to become more conservative. Surgical management is being individualized to take into account identification of the depth of tumor invasion and the tumor size and location. Wide local excision of vulvar melanoma is used increasingly. Reduction in the scope of surgery does not appear to have compromised survival, although only limited observational studies have been reported.[209,210] For level I or II lesions (superficial), the risk of nodal spread is rare, and wide local excision is adequate therapy. For deeper lesions, radical vulvectomy with en bloc bilateral inguinofemoral lymphadenectomy has been the historical standard of care. PET and sentinel node groin biopsies may be tools to aid in tailoring the extent of regional surgery. Systemic adjuvant therapies for vulvar melanoma parallel adjuvant strategies for cutaneous melanomas arising at other primary sites.

Inguinal node dissection is recommended for patients with tumor invasion greater than 1 mm. Nodal involvement is unlikely for melanomas whose depth of invasion is less.[58] The prognosis of patients with positive pelvic lymph nodes is so poor that pelvic lymphadenectomy is not recommended for management.

Common sites of relapse include the groin, perineum, and vaginal urethral margin, which often predate the clinical appearance of hematogenous metastases.[60,207,211-213] However, patients who die of melanoma usually have widespread metastases to parenchymal organs.

Radiation therapy has no established role in the routine management of vulvar melanomas, although anecdotal information suggests that melanoma arising in this location may be more radiosensitive than melanoma from other cutaneous sites.[214] Given the high locoregional recurrence rate after what has often been extensive and sometimes mutilating surgery, prospective investigation of adjuvant regional irradiation or chemoradiation, administered preoperatively or postoperatively, appears warranted (see Chapter 39). Radiation may be used for palliation of symptomatic recurrent disease and for patients with initially unresectable disease or those declining exenterative surgery.

Prognosis

Although an overall 5-year survival rate as high as 50% has been reported,[213] most series record 5-year survival rates between 15% and 30%, except for patients with stage I disease.[208] Patients with nodal spread are not commonly cured.[60] The overall 5-year survival rate with negative and positive nodes is 38% and 13%, respectively.[215]

As with melanoma arising at other sites, the spectrum of biologic virulence is broad. Recurrences and metastases 10 years or longer after initial treatment are not uncommon.[60,207,211,212]

VERRUCOUS CARCINOMA

Verrucous carcinoma of the vulva represents a variant of squamous cell carcinoma. These lesions were originally described as occurring in the oral cavity but have also been described involving the vagina, cervix, and vulva. Lesions grossly resemble cauliflower. Usually large and pearly gray to white, this cancer characteristically invades with a sharply circumscribed pushing margin. Clinically, these tumors are usually slow growing. Because metastases to regional lymph nodes are rare, radical local excision is the standard treatment.[51-54] If there are suspicious groin nodes, fine-needle aspiration or excisional biopsy should be carried out. Usually, nodes are enlarged because of inflammatory hypertrophy, but if they do contain metastases, groin node dissections are indicated.

Verrucous carcinoma has a reputation of being radioresistant, and reports of favorable outcomes after radiation are uncommon. Surgery remains the treatment of choice whenever feasible, with the use of irradiation limited to circumstances in which potentially curative surgery cannot be performed.

VAGINAL CARCINOMA

INCIDENCE

Carcinoma of the vagina accounts for 1% to 3% of all gynecologic malignancies.

BIOLOGIC CHARACTERISTICS

Most (80%) lesions are squamous cell carcinoma. The second most common type is melanoma. Sarcomas and lymphomas may be primary in the vagina. Adenocarcinomas are commonly metastatic from other primary sites (e.g., uterus, colon, ovary, kidney, breast), with the exception of primary clear cell cancers. True primary adenocarcinomas of the vagina are rare.

Seventy percent of patients are 60 years old or older.

STAGING EVALUATION

Cancer extending to the external cervical os or on to the vulva is considered a cervical or vulvar primary in the International Federation of Gynecology and Oncology (FIGO) formalism and staged accordingly, even if the epicenter of the cancer is in the vagina.

FIGO staging includes clinical assessment of the pelvis, chest radiograph, and renal evaluation. Depending on the clinical situation, CT, MRI, and PET may be used to assess local and nodal extent of disease, but findings do not alter the FIGO stage. Cystoscopy and proctoscopy may be appropriate when primary disease is extensive and involves the anterior vagina or rectovaginal septum.

Patients with vaginal adenocarcinoma should be assessed for potential primaries arising in other organs.

Patients with melanoma require systemic evaluation.

PRIMARY THERAPY

Patients with vaginal intraepithelial neoplasia (VAIN) may be treated with local excision, laser ablation, topical 5-fluorouracil, or irradiation.

Primary therapy for invasive disease consists of external and intracavitary or interstitial irradiation, except in selected early cases that may be treated surgically with local excision or with brachytherapy alone.

Radical surgery, which may entail partial or total pelvic exenteration, is generally reserved for isolated pelvic recurrence after irradiation and for patients with fistulas at diagnosis.

RESULTS

Five-year actuarial cancer-free survival for patients treated with irradiation alone approaches 100% for stage 0, 85% for stage I, and 75% for stage II disease.

Of patients with stage III disease, approximately 30% to 50% will be cured. Long-term cancer-free survival for rare patients with stage IVA disease is anecdotal, and the rate is usually less than 20%.

Patients who experience relapse usually do so within 2 years. Most patients have locoregional persistence or recurrence as a component of the pattern of failure. Distant failure alone without antecedent locoregional failure occurs in less than 30% of relapsing patients.

ADJUVANT THERAPY

Concurrent chemotherapy with irradiation has had favorable results for a small number of patients, paralleling similar treatment for anal, cervical, and vulvar cancers. Randomized, controlled trials comparing chemoradiation to irradiation alone have not been performed.

SALVAGE

Radical surgery, usually exenterative, may be appropriate for persistent or locally recurrent disease, but the likelihood of salvage is low.

PALLIATION

Individualized irradiation may be effective to reduce local symptoms.

Chemotherapy is generally ineffective for disseminated disease.

Primary invasive cancer of the vagina is rare. According to the FIGO staging formalism, a cancer of the vagina that involves the cervical os or the vulva must be classified as arising from that structure, even if the tumor epicenter appears to be in the vagina. Only if involvement of these adjacent organs can be excluded can an invasive cancer of the vagina be classified as primary. Because of the infrequency with which the disease occurs, standardized therapeutic approaches have not evolved, and few centers have extensive experience with these tumors.

Approximately 80% of vaginal malignancies are squamous cell cancers.[216] The following discussion refers to squamous cell disease of the vagina except when otherwise stated.

ETIOLOGY AND EPIDEMIOLOGY

Approximately 70% of primary vaginal malignancies are detected in women 60 years old or older. Approximately 60% occur in patients older than 70 years.[216,217]

In a population-based case-control study of 156 women with vaginal intraepithelial neoplasia (VAIN) or invasive vaginal cancer, the number of lifetime sexual partners (>5), early onset of intercourse (age <17), and current smoking were identified as lifestyle risk factors. Antibodies to HPV-16 were much more common in VAIN and cancer patients than controls, and HPV DNA was detected in 80% of patients with in situ disease and 60% of patients with invasive disease.[218] Approximately 30% of patients had a history of treatment for a prior anogenital in situ or invasive malignancy, most commonly of the cervix. Early hysterectomy appears to be a risk factor in some studies, but only if done for malignant or premalignant disease.[218,219]

The criteria for considering a vaginal squamous cell carcinoma as primary include vaginal location not involving the external cervical os or vulva and a specified length of time from a previous diagnosis of cervical or vulvar cancer. There is no uniformly accepted interval, although 5 years from a previous invasive cancer seems sensible.

Immunosuppression (e.g., among organ transplant recipients) predisposes to lower genital tract intraepithelial neoplasia, including VAIN, although a higher incidence of invasive vaginal cancer has not been demonstrated. Previous ionizing radiation for prior malignancy may also predispose to VAIN or vaginal cancer, usually after a latent period of many years,[220] suggesting that the radiation may be a contributing factor in some patients. Given the similarly increased incidence of vaginal cancer after surgical treatment of cervical malignancy, multiple factors may contribute.

The natural history of VAIN is not well understood, and the potential for VAIN to progress to invasive squamous cell malignancy is not known with precision. In most VAIN series, there is a clinically significant incidence of subsequent invasive vaginal cancer. The congruence of risk factors for VAIN and invasive disease[218] and the younger average age of VAIN patients compared with patients with invasive disease give credence to the theory that VAIN is a precursor lesion in some or all patients with invasive disease.

Aho and colleagues identified 23 patients with VAIN followed for at least 3 years without treatment.[221] The mean age was 41 years. One half of the VAIN lesions were multifocal, and one half were associated with cervical intraepithelial neoplasia (CIN) or vulvar dysplasia. The spontaneous regression rate of VAIN was high (78%), including four of five VAIN-3 patients, but two cases (9%) progressed to invasive cancer. Three studies have shown that only 2% to 5% of patients with VAIN treated with various methods progress to having invasive vaginal carcinoma.[220-222]

The normal vagina does not contain glandular elements, and primary adenocarcinomas of the vagina are therefore rare. Most commonly, adenocarcinomas involving the vagina are metastases from other organs. Common primary sites include the uterine corpus, ovaries, kidneys, breast, colon, and rectum.[223] Therapy for such patients is largely determined by the primary site of origin. Direct extension from primary adenocarcinomas in the cervix, Bartholin's glands, or paraurethral Skene's glands may involve the vagina, but it should be clinically apparent on physical examination.

The clear cell variant of vaginal adenocarcinoma (CCAC) has been linked to in utero exposure to the synthetic estrogen diethylstilbestrol (DES) that was used in the late 1940s, 1950s, and 1960s to support high-risk pregnancies and to prevent threatened spontaneous abortion.[224] Use continued despite minimal evidence of efficacy until the drug was banned for use in pregnancy in 1975. Vaginal adenosis, morphologically identical to rare cases of vaginal adenosis in women born before the DES era, has been detected in approximately one third of patients with in utero DES exposure. Three patterns of adenosis have been described: mucinous, resembling endocervical glands; tubo-endometrial;, and embryonic.[225,226] Clear cell cancer of the vagina is associated with vaginal adenosis in as many as 95% of cases, most commonly the tubo-endometrial morphology, implicating adenosis as the cell line of origin.[227,228] The Registry for Research on Hormonal Transplacental Carcinogenesis accessioned more than 580 cases of clear cell carcinoma of the vagina and cervix. In utero exposure to synthetic estrogens accounted for approximately two thirds of reported cases, leaving a significant number of cases unexplained.

Work by Herbst and coworkers suggested that the age distribution for clear cell adenocarcinoma of the vagina had two separate peaks.[229,230] The first peak contained women with a mean age of 26 years, and the second peak contained women with a mean age of 71 years. The first peak contained all DES daughters, and the second peak contained women born well before 1950 and therefore not exposed to DES. However, even when the DES daughters were excluded, a bimodal pattern was observed. The age range of DES-related clear cell adenocarcinoma is 7 to 42 years. The actual risk of DES-exposed women for developing CCAC is estimated at only 1 in 1000, with the highest risk for women exposed before 12 weeks' gestation.[231]

PREVENTION AND EARLY DETECTION

There is no consensus regarding the utility of vaginal vault screening after hysterectomy. Although early detection clearly benefits the woman in whom vaginal cancer is destined to develop, based on the low frequency of the disease and the limited apparent effectiveness of vaginal cytology to make the diagnosis, "there is insufficient evidence to recommend routine vaginal smear screening in women after total hysterectomy for benign disease."[232,233]

The utility of vault screening cytology among women who have undergone hysterectomy for invasive or preinvasive disease has not been adequately studied to prove effectiveness, although in the absence of evidence, such screening would seem prudent given the multicentric nature of lower genital tract neoplasia and its association with invasive disease. Patients whose vaginal cancer manifests with abnormal cytology are more likely to have early disease and the most favorable outcomes.

Physicians should be encouraged to continue Papanicolaou smear screening in this higher-risk population well into their older years, because approximately 70% of vaginal cancers are diagnosed in women older than 60 years. Careful inspection by palpation and direct visualization of the entire length of the vagina is necessary. This usually necessitates rotation of the vaginal speculum to avoid obscuring lesions under the speculum blades.

Histologic and cytologic criteria for VAIN and invasive vaginal cancer parallel those for cervical lesions. In postmenopausal women or women with a history vaginal irradiation, distinguishing dysplasia from inflammatory or postirradiation changes can be difficult, because atrophy and radiation effects can mimic the features seen in neoplasia. Topical estrogen therapy before sampling of the vagina can minimize atrophic and inflammatory changes and may facilitate more accurate assessment of specimens.

PATHOLOGY AND PATHWAYS OF SPREAD

Eighty percent of vaginal lesions are squamous cell carcinoma. The second most common histologic type is melanoma. Sarcomas and lymphomas may be primary neoplasms in the vagina. Adenocarcinomas are commonly metastatic from other primary sites (e.g. uterus, colon, ovary, kidney, breast), with the exception of primary clear cell cancers. True primary adenocarcinomas of the vagina are rare.

Most vaginal cancers involve the upper two thirds of the vagina, where direct extension can involve the parametrium, paracolpos, bladder, or rectum. Lymphatic drainage of the proximal third to half of the vagina parallels that of the cervix: by the obturator nodes to the hypogastric, external iliac, and common iliac nodes. Lesions of the lower one third of the vagina may follow vulvar lymphatic drainage patterns to the inguinal-femoral nodes and subsequently to the pelvic nodes. Lesions infiltrating the rectovaginal septum may spread to pararectal and presacral nodes. Interconnections between lymphatic channels exist, and the pattern of lymphatic metastasis from primary vaginal cancer is not reliably predictable based on location of the primary within the vagina.

Table 57-8 **Vaginal Cancer: Staging Systems**

Disease Site	AJCC TNM	FIGO	Definition
Primary tumor	TX		Primary tumor cannot be assessed
	T0		No evidence of primary tumor
	Tis	0	Carcinoma in situ
	T1	I	Tumor confined to the vagina
	T2	II	Tumor invades paravaginal tissues but not to the pelvic wall
	T3	III	Tumor extends to the pelvic wall
	T4	IVA	Tumor invades mucosa* of the bladder or rectum and/or extends beyond the true pelvis
		IVB	Distant metastasis
Regional lymph nodes	NX		Regional lymph nodes cannot be assessed
	N0		No regional lymph node metastasis
Upper two thirds of vagina	N1		Pelvic node metastasis
Lower one third of vagina	N1		Unilateral inguinal node metastasis
	N2		Bilateral inguinal node metastases
Distant metastasis	MX		Presence of distant metastasis cannot be assessed
	M0		No distant metastasis
	M1		Distant metastasis

*Presence of bullous edema is not sufficient evidence to classify as T4 or FIGO IVA.
AJCC, American Joint Committee on Cancer; FIGO, International Federation of Gynecology and Oncology; TNM, tumor-node-metastasis system.

Hematogenous dissemination is rare at diagnosis. It is more common patients with far advanced, neglected lesions.

CLINICAL MANIFESTATIONS, PATIENT EVALUATION, AND STAGING

Presenting symptoms of early disease include bleeding (including contact bleeding), discharge, pruritus, and dyspareunia. Pain and alterations of urinary bladder or anorectal function are associated with locally advanced disease.

Staging includes careful clinical examination of the vagina and pelvis, possibly under anesthesia, with careful examination of the cervix and vulva to exclude involvement of those sites. Cystoscopy and proctosigmoidoscopy may be necessary in women with locally advanced disease or with bladder or bowel symptoms. Assessment of the pelvic and groin nodes by CT, MRI, or PET is advisable to plan treatment in most cases of invasive disease, although results do not affect assignment of FIGO clinical stage. MRI may supplement physical examination in assessing primary disease extent and determining teletherapy and interstitial brachytherapy target volumes for radiation-based therapy.

Patients are staged using the AJCC TNM formalism or, more commonly, the FIGO formalism (Table 57-8). A modification of the FIGO staging system proposed by Perez and colleagues in 1973 divides stage II into stage IIa, which includes patients with paravaginal infiltration without parametrial invasion, and stage IIB, which includes patients with parametrial infiltration that does not extend to the pelvic sidewall.[234] This distinction is recognized as prognostically important by some radiation oncologists but has not been incorporated into FIGO staging.

PRIMARY THERAPY

Vaginal Intraepithelial Neoplasia

VAIN is commonly detected by cytologic screening and is best localized by colposcopy and iodine staining, with careful attention being paid to the vaginal vault angles, which are commonly distorted by previous hysterectomy. VAIN may be multifocal in the vagina in up to 60% of patients.[235] The high frequency of apical involvement facilitates detection by colposcopy. For low-grade lesions, there appears to be a significant spontaneous regression rate.

Treatments with surgical excision, laser vaporization, and intravaginal topical 5-FU have proved partially effective.[220,222,236] Local excision, when feasible without functional compromise, is the treatment associated with the lowest risk of recurrence, but it is limited in applicability because the disease is frequently multifocal. Recurrence after laser vaporization has been reported for 38% of cases, and recurrence after topical vaginal 5-FU has been reported for 59%.[235]

For selected cases, intracavitary brachytherapy may be appropriate.[222,237-239] Often, irradiation is reserved for patients relapsing after conservative therapies with less potential for late morbidity. Control of VAIN by intracavitary brachytherapy alone approaches 100%. Prospective data are not available regarding alterations in vaginal depth and diameter, elasticity, sexual function, and quality of life after vaginal brachytherapy.

Invasive Cancer

Primary vaginal malignancies are rare. Single-institution treatment outcome reports retrospectively analyze limited numbers of patients often spanning multiple decades, during which diagnostic techniques and management philosophies have evolved. Because of the correlation of prognosis with stage and tumor size and the fact that treatments feasible for earlier-stage, smaller primaries without nodal spread may be quite different from management strategies for patients with more extensive disease, it is difficult to compare outcomes reflecting different therapeutic techniques and modalities. Without compelling prospective data, treatment inevitably represents some measure of extrapolation from general principles of oncologic management tailored on the basis of tumor location and extent and the constraining comorbidities of an individual patient.

Rationale and General Principles

Radical irradiation constitutes the treatment of choice for most patients with vaginal cancer. Primary surgery is appropriate in the earliest of invasive lesions when curative or potentially curative resection can be achieved without exenteration or

Table 57-9 Range of Surgical Treatments Used According to FIGO Stage

FIGO Stage	Surgical Treatment
I	Partial or total vaginectomy Radical hysterectomy/vaginectomy ± pelvic ± para-aortic node dissection; inguinal node dissection for lower third of vagina
II	Partial or total vaginectomy + parametrectomy + paracolpectomy + pelvic ± para-aortic node dissection
III	Radical hysterectomy/vaginectomy + parametrectomy + pelvic/inguinal node ± para-aortic node dissection
IV	Exenterative surgery, usually total with formation of urinary and bowel bypass

FIGO, International Federation of Gynecology and Oncology.
From Tjalma WA, Monaghan JM, de Barros Lopes A, et al: The role of surgery in invasive squamous carcinoma of the vagina. Gynecol Oncol 81:360-365, 2001.

functionally morbid surgery. Primary surgery may be appropriate for rare patients who present with primary disease-related fistulas that require surgery for restoration of continence. The magnitude of surgical intervention may be quite variable, as reported from a single institution with a strong surgical bias (Table 57-9).[240]

Primary surgery may be used in patients previously irradiated for other malignancies because further radical irradiation is rarely an option. Given the intimate proximity of bowel and bladder to the vagina, exenterative surgery is usually necessary to achieve clear margins and to promote postoperative healing.

Surgical cancer control in selected stage I and II patients can be quite good. Tjalma and colleagues[240] reported surgical results for 37 patients (26 stage I, 6 stage II, 2 stage III, and 3 stage IV) employing the surgical procedures detailed in Table 57-9. Seven patients required postoperative irradiation for incomplete excision or node metastasis. The 5- and 10-year survival rates were 92% and 74% for patients managed with surgery alone, and the 5-year survival rate was 71% for patients undergoing combined-modality therapy. Eighteen patients in the series reported by Tjalma and associates were managed with primary radiation therapy (1 stage I, 6 stage II, 4 stage III, and 7 stage IV), with 44% alive at 5 years and 35% alive at 10 years. However, nonrandomized data reflecting strong selection biases do not permit comparison of the relative efficacy of treatment modalities employed nor of the morbidities experienced by cancer survivors. Total pelvic exenteration was employed to treat two patients with stage I disease and 1 patient with stage III disease in this series. Anterior exenteration was employed to treat two patients with stage II disease. Five (14%) of 37 patients in this surgical series were treated with exenterative procedures who may have been amenable to organ-conserving therapy with radiation-based treatment, with surgery reserved for salvage of patients with persistent or recurrent disease. Three additional patients with stage IV disease had exenterative procedures.[240]

No widely accepted standardized treatment technique has been developed for radiation treatment of vaginal cancer. Generally, brachytherapy may be employed alone or in conjunction with teletherapy (external beam radiation), depending on the local and regional extent of disease. Teletherapy alone is employed for patients with locally extensive or bulky disease. Brachytherapy may include intravaginal sources or interstitial needle implants done freehand or with custom templates. Custom molds or partially shielded intravaginal cylinders can be used to selectively administer higher-dose radiation to only a portion of the length and diameter of the vagina. Patients with early-stage disease usually receive a higher proportion of their dose from brachytherapy, whereas those with more advanced pelvic disease receive a greater component of their radiation dose from teletherapy.

The principles of irradiation include treating the draining regional lymph nodes when there is a risk of nodal involvement. Because lesions of the lower third of the vagina have the potential to metastasize to inguinal lymph nodes, it is usual to electively include the medial inguinal lymph nodes in the radiation volume for distal primaries. Usually, no attempt is made to extend the volume to include the entire inguinal region because relapse in nodes lateral to the femoral vessels is rare. However, when groin nodes are involved at diagnosis, the entire inguinofemoral group of nodes may be irradiated employing techniques similar to those employed for groin irradiation in patients with primary vulvar cancers.

Usually, 40 to 50 Gy is delivered using external beam irradiation to the whole pelvis, and intracavitary or interstitial irradiation is used to bring the primary tumor dose up to between 70 and 85 Gy. When scrutinizing the radiation therapy literature, care must be employed to understand whether brachytherapy dose (and therefore cumulative dose) is specified at the vaginal mucosa or at a depth in tissue below the vaginal mucosa. Because of the rapid fall-off in dose from intracavitary sources, brachytherapy dose at 5 mm depth may be 75% or less of the vaginal mucosal dose, accounting for at least some of the width of the spectrum of cited radiation doses employed in patients treated for cure. When irradiation is employed as monotherapy, cumulative dose to all portions of the gross tumor volume should not be less than 70 Gy when conventional low dose rate brachytherapy techniques are used.

Results

Series from single institutions often span multiple decades, during which diagnostic assessments of tumor extent have changed and treatment strategies and techniques have not remained static. Some series pool patients with squamous cell carcinoma and patients with nonsquamous histologies, and they include patients with noninvasive lesions and patients with prior treatment for other primary pelvic cancers. Outcomes analyses are challenging to interpret. In their series of 301 patients, Chyle and associates found that histologic type (non-CCAC versus squamous cell carcinoma) was a strong adverse prognostic factor.[241] Similarly, melanoma of the vagina is associated with a grim prognosis, and it should not be pooled with squamous cell cancers in analyzing treatment efficacy and survival.[211,242,243]

Mature outcomes from an unusually large series spanning 30 years at the M.D. Anderson Cancer Center are reported in Table 57-10. This series consisted exclusively of previously untreated patients with primary invasive cancer of the vagina treated wholly or predominantly with irradiation.[244]

For squamous cell cancer, tumor stage is generally found to be the most important prognostic variable for local control and survival after treatment with irradiation. Tumor size (smaller or larger than 4 cm) and histologic grade may be influential.[241,245] Neither of these factors is reflected in FIGO staging.

Treatment techniques (e.g., brachytherapy alone, teletherapy alone, combinations of external beam and intracavitary or interstitial brachytherapy) and total radiation dose appropriately vary with stage, disease distribution, and tumor size.

Table 57-10 Results of Radical Radiation Therapy for 193 Previously Untreated Patients with Invasive Squamous Cell Carcinoma of the Vagina, 1970-2000

FIGO Stage	No. of Patients	Pelvic Disease Control (%) at 5 Years	Disease-Specific Survival (%) at 5 Years
I*	50	86	85
II	97	84	78
III	39	69	NS
IVA	7	86	NS
III + IVA†	46	71	58

*Eighteen patients had gross excision of their primary tumors before irradiation, of which 10 were stage I.

†Five percent of patients with stages III + IVA received neoadjuvant chemotherapy, and 17% received concurrent radiation therapy and cisplatin-based chemotherapy regimens.

FIGO, International Federation of Gynecology and Oncology; NS, percentage not stated.

From Frank SJ, Jhingran A, Levenback C, Eifel PJ: Definitive radiation therapy for squamous cell carcinoma of the vagina. Int J Radiat Oncol Biol Phys 62:138-147, 2005.

Therefore, it is difficult to make any statement regarding comparative efficacy of radiotherapeutic modalities or techniques.

According to numerous analyses, almost all failures occur within the first 5 years.[241,244-248] It is not feasible to distinguish potential second primary cancer in the vagina from possible marginal recurrence. Rare late failures in the vagina may reflect an underlying field defect rather than inadequate initial therapy. Because virtually the entire vagina is usually treated by teletherapy in many patients, late vaginal failures outside the irradiated volume are uncommon.

Relapse is more likely to be pelvic than systemic. In a series from M.D. Anderson Cancer Center, 21 (68%) of 31 patients with stage I or II disease who relapsed had failure in the vagina or pelvis as all or a component of their relapse pattern, whereas 10 (32%) of 31 failed distantly only. Among patients with stage III or IV disease, 15 (83%) of 18 who relapsed had pelvic or vaginal recurrence as all or a component of their pattern of initial relapse. Three (17%) of 18 patients who relapsed had distant metastases only.[244] Rare relapse in inguinal nodes is seen in patients whose primary initially involved the distal one third of the vagina and in whom the inguinal nodes were not included in the treatment volume or were grossly contaminated with metastatic disease at the time of diagnosis.[244,249]

Except for isolated vaginal recurrence in patients with VAIN or stage I disease, salvage therapy is usually ineffective. Surgical salvage implies partial or total exenteration in virtually all previously irradiated patients.

LOCALLY ADVANCED DISEASE AND PALLIATION

Because combined-modality treatment with concurrent chemotherapy demonstrates improved outcomes for patients with squamous cell cancers of the cervix, anus, and other sites, it is not unreasonable to extrapolate the use of synchronous treatment with irradiation and chemotherapy to similar patients with locally advanced vaginal cancer. Because of the rarity of this disease, very limited numbers of patients have been reported using this approach.[245,250] It is unlikely that a prospective comparison of chemoradiation and irradiation alone will be feasible.

Analogous to the evolution of chemoradiation in the treatment of cancer of the vulva, chemoradiation for vaginal cancer may become more widespread and popular based on the clinical impression of usefulness rather than on the basis of prospective, randomized data. Although anal canal cancers are amenable to cure with high-dose irradiation alone,[251] better local cancer control is achieved with chemoradiation.[186,187] Long-term complications are generally lower and functional results more satisfactory because of the use of lower total doses of radiation using fewer conventional fractions rather than reduced dose per fraction. Reduction in total radiation dose from 65 to 70 Gy to approximately 54 Gy has reduced the need for diverting colostomy or abdominoperineal resection for radiation-related complications in cured patients.

Concurrent chemotherapy with irradiation appears to significantly enhance radiation effects on cancer and cycling epithelial cells, but it does not appear to proportionately increase late effects in normal tissues. Late complications in patients treated for cervical cancer with chemoradiation are not dramatically different from those seen in patients treated with irradiation alone using comparable radiation dose and fractionation regimens.[252-254] Part of the clinical cost of chemoradiation is increased acute toxicity. The compensatory benefit may be in reduced late complications if the total radiation dose is reduced, analogous to the situation in treatment of anal canal cancers. Most publications reporting treatment outcomes for patients with vaginal cancer report late bowel and urinary bladder complications. Few comment on vaginal depth, diameter, or elasticity; sexual function; and quality of life. No prospective evaluation of the impact of radical irradiation administered to the vagina has been undertaken. A potential benefit from integrating concurrent chemotherapy and accepting radiation dose reduction may be in improved long-term vaginal function, with reduced risk of atrophy and stenosis. Such potential benefit is largely hypothetical. If accumulating experience suggests that chemoradiation improves local control in patients with stages III or IVA vaginal cancers, extrapolation to patients with earlier disease may be warranted in the interests of preserving normal tissue integrity.

TECHNIQUES OF IRRADIATION

Brachytherapy

Brachytherapy as monotherapy is appropriate for patients with VAIN and selected patients with small volume, minimally invasive disease confined to the vaginal wall. This approach can be used if the entire tumor volume can be encompassed without delivering an unacceptable dose to the vaginal mucosal surface. Precise selection criteria have not been universally agreed on, and some patients treated with brachytherapy alone have relapses in pelvic sites remote from the vagina, presumably caused by lymphatic spread.

Generally, brachytherapy is used to supplement teletherapy dose given to a large volume encompassing the primary disease, potential subclinical extensions of the primary cancer, and lymph node volumes at risk. After 45 to 50 Gy of conventionally fractionated teletherapy, brachytherapy is employed to boost the cumulative dose (i.e., external beam plus low dose rate brachytherapy dose) to 70 to 80 Gy when irradiation is employed as the sole modality of therapy.

Intravaginal irradiation is usually accomplished using some form of vaginal cylinder. The largest possible diameter cylinder is used to improve the ratio of dose to the tumor surface to dose at maximal tumor depth. Because of the rapid fall-off in dose with distance from intravaginal sources, it is usually inappropriate to use intracavitary brachytherapy to treat primary cancers that are more than 5 mm thick at the completion of teletherapy.

When conventional low dose rate intravaginal brachytherapy is employed, the labia are usually sutured closed, sealing the vagina shut and securing the implant in place. When high dose rate brachytherapy delivers treatment over a few minutes, fixation of the cylinder to a locking base plate ensures rigid immobility of the system. In addition to the convenience of outpatient treatment, the short treatment times of fractionated high dose rate brachytherapy secured with rigid external fixation makes it feasible to employ partial shielding of the vaginal circumference with reproducible treatment of smaller lengths of the vaginal tube. This may contribute to improvement in functional outcomes. Daily high dose rate treatments may employ fractions of 2 Gy at depth to a cumulative brachytherapy dose of 20 to 26 Gy to supplement the external beam dose of 45 to 50 Gy.

For disease involving the upper vagina or vaginal fornices, an intrauterine tandem may be placed to function as an anchor for vaginal cylinders or spacers while ensuring adequate dose at the proximal end of the vagina. Individual, custom vaginal molds have been used to treat vaginal cancer.[255]

For cancers more than 5 mm thick, deep paravaginal invasion, or parametrial extension, brachytherapy boosts may be delivered using isotopes such as iridium 192 in interstitial implants. Interstitial implants may be performed freehand or through a template sutured to the perineum.[256,257] In patients with cancers involving a vaginal fornix or extending into the parametrium, intersitial needles commonly penetrate into the peritoneal cavity. Under these circumstances, needle placement may be safer with simultaneous laparoscopy to reduce risk of perforation of abdominal viscera. Similarly, in patients who have undergone prior hysterectomy, laparoscopy, or minilaparotomy, it may be helpful to avoid perforation of loops of bowel that may be adherent to the vaginal apex and pelvic floor.

External Beam Irradiation

External beam irradiation is similar to that given for carcinoma of the cervix, except that the full length of the vagina usually is included in the initial teletherapy volume. Rare exceptions may include patients with unifocal disease less than 2 cm long that is confined to the vaginal fornices or the very distal vagina. Parallel-opposed anterior and posterior pelvic portals rather than a four-field box technique may be employed for slender patients and when medial inguinal nodes are included for patients with involvement of the caudal third of the vagina. For larger patients, a four-field technique may be used in an effort to reduce total dose and dose per fraction to the bladder dome and anterior small bowel. Medial groin nodes may be treated with this technique by expanding the anteroinferior portion of the lateral fields, provided that the dose to the proximal femurs is kept to less than 45 Gy by excluding these structures to the maximal extent feasible on the anterior and posterior fields. Rarely, when inguinal nodes are involved at the time of diagnosis, techniques that are used to encompass the entire inguinofemoral node volumes in patients with cancer of the vulva may be successfully deployed for vaginal cancer patients.

The initial target volume may be influenced by the results of diagnostic imaging studies, and larger volumes may be appropriate for patients with pelvic nodal metastases. Conventionally, the superior extent of the teletherapy volume has been at the L5-S1 interspace. Use of this landmark ensures coverage of retroperitoneal nodes caudal to the bifurcations of the common iliac arteries in almost all patients and includes the distal common iliac nodes in many patients.[258,259] Analysis of sites of relapse in one clinical series suggested that this volume may be excessive for most patients, contributing to avoidable acute and delayed toxicities of treatment.[249] Because initial failures predominantly occur in the vagina, paracolpos, and parametria, expanded volumes to electively encompass secondary nodal volumes may not be routinely advisable. In patients with negative imaging assessment of regional nodes, a superior border 1 to 2 cm cephalad to the inferior margin of the sacroiliac joints may be sufficient.

The target volume for initial teletherapy treatment remains controversial. In patients with documented node metastases, extension of the treatment volume to encompass the next echelon of clinically uninvolved nodes seems prudent at present. As imaging technology evolves, future improvements in sensitivity may make treatment of smaller teletherapy volumes more secure.

For patients with bulky disease, including patients with gross lymph node metastasis, boost therapy by intracavitary or interstitial brachytherapy techniques may not be feasible. Under such circumstances, tailored volume reductions based on clinical findings and results from diagnostic imaging studies often permit treatment by external beam techniques alone. Tailored volumes may be treated to a cumulative dose between 65 and 70 Gy using teletherapy alone. Rarely can a higher dose be achieved with teletherapy without substantial risk of late radiation complications in vulnerable normal tissues (e.g., urethra, bladder, rectum) adjacent to the gross target volume. Administration of concurrent radiopotentiating chemotherapy may be a means to derive maximal potential benefit from a reduced radiation dose that can be delivered using external treatment alone.

Complications of Treatment

Acute effects in patients undergoing teletherapy as all or a major component of their treatment may include radiation urethritis or cystitis with frequency, urgency, and dysuria. Oral anticholinergic and antispasmodic medications may be beneficial for patients in whom these symptoms are more than a temporary irritant, as well as a urinary tract analgesic such as phenazopyridine hydrochloride (Pyridium).

Depending on the volume of small bowel unavoidably included in the irradiated volume, most patients experience some degree of erratic bowel function that usually includes more frequent and often unformed bowel movements that may progress to watery diarrhea. Dietary modification and medications such as loperamide hydrochloride or atropine with diphenoxylate hydrochloride (Imodium, Lomotil) may be beneficial.

Acute effects on the anorectum may cause tenesmus and small-volume blood loss. Topical medications such as those employed for the treatment of hemorrhoids can be beneficial to some patients and may be applied directly to the anal area externally or to the anorectum by suppository.

Vaginal effects may include serous discharge and pruritus. Oral antihistamines and topical vaginal moisturizing agents may provide some symptomatic relief.

Acute radiation dermatitis may progress to moist desquamation on the vulva and portions of the perineum when the primary lesion involves the distal vagina. Soaks, air exposure, and topical balms and creams that may or may not include antibiotics such as 1% silver sulfadiazine cream are soothing for many patients. Occlusive dressings may be temporarily required for severe cases. Therapy generally parallels skin treatment for thermal burns.

Because of the paucity of large data sets reporting treatment outcomes and the variability in the equipment, techniques, and doses of radiation employed over several decades to address different stages and extent of disease, it is difficult to predict the risk of serious late complications for an individual patient.

Complications of treatment have been reviewed in various publications. In a historical series, Dancuart and colleagues treated a group of patients between 1955 and 1982. Reported late effects included vaginal fibrosis (10%) and cystitis, proctitis, or vaginal necrosis (12%). A further 5% of patients experienced rectal or sigmoid stenosis, hemorrhage, or multiple fistulas.[246] Over a similar period, in which patients were treated with radical irradiation from 1953 to 1991, Perez and associates[247] reported late complications in 205 patients from an initial population of 212 patients with VAIN (20 patients) or invasive carcinomas of the vagina (192 patients). Twenty-five major local complications (12% crude rate) attributable all or in part to radiation injury were observed, including six rectovaginal fistulas, three vesicovaginal fistulas, four bladder neck contractures or urethral strictures, two rectal strictures, two cases of proctitis, and one instance each of rectal ulcer, vaginal necrosis, small bowel obstruction, cystitis, leg edema, neuritis, severe vaginal stenosis, and diverticulitis. Tewari and colleagues[257] reported the complications in a series of 71 patients treated between 1976 and 1997 with interstitial brachytherapy alone (10 patients) or in combination with teletherapy (61 patients) to a cumulative dose of 80 Gy. Nine patients had major complications, including four necroses, four fistulas, and one small bowel obstruction, for a crude rate of 13%.

Chyle and others at M.D. Anderson Cancer Center found that transperitoneal staging pelvic lymphadenectomy before radiation therapy contributed significantly to complications of therapy.[241] Because this technique has largely been abandoned in the treatment of cervical cancer patients for this reason, it seems sensible to do so for patients with vaginal cancer.

In a subsequent retrospective series from M.D. Anderson Cancer Center, 193 patients with invasive squamous cell cancers of the vagina treated between 1970 and 2000 were analyzed employing the formalism of the National Cancer Institute Common Terminology Criteria for Adverse Events.[244] The cumulative rate of grade 3 or 4 complications was 10% at 5 years and 17% at 10 years. Twenty patients had a total of 25 major complications, 19 of which involved the gastrointestinal tract, including proctitis requiring transfusion (7 patients), fistulas (5 patients), small bowel obstruction (4 patients), and large bowel obstruction, rectal ulceration, and fecal incontinence (1 patient each). Eight of 11 patients with major rectal complications had primary tumors involving the posterior vaginal wall. Genitourinary complications included vesicovaginal fistulas (2 patients), hemorrhagic cystitis (3 patients), and urethral stricture (1 patient). All major urinary tract complications were seen in patients with primary cancers involving the anterior wall of the vagina. With univariate analysis, the incidence of complications correlated with primary tumor stage and smoking history. Current smokers had a 25% incidence of complications, compared with 18% in former smokers who quit 6 months or longer before irradiation and 5% in patients who had never smoked.[244]

Vaginal stenosis is probably the complication that occurs with greatest frequency, but it is almost certainly underreported. The average age of this population, many of whom may not regularly experience vaginal intercourse, probably increases the likelihood of significant stenosis and decreases the rate at which this is reported as a functionally limiting complication. The morbidity of vaginal stenosis may be limited to difficulty and discomfort with subsequent vaginal examinations in patients who are not active sexually. Stenosis may also compromise early diagnosis and subsequent salvage of local relapse and prevent surveillance of the cervix in patients who have not had prior hysterectomy. Anecdotally, severe radiation vaginitis progressing to fusion of the upper vagina can restore urinary continence in some patients with vesicovaginal fistulas at the time of diagnosis.

Vaginal stenosis can be prevented with variable success with the use of vaginal dilators. Topical intravaginal estrogen on a chronic basis is the most effective treatment for vaginal mucosal atrophy in the irradiated patient and should be used in addition to systemic hormone replacement in younger patients in whom radiation has ablated ovarian function. Because some intravaginal estrogen is absorbed systemically, the precise balance of oral or transdermal hormone replacement with vaginal estrogen administration varies from patient to patient.

TREATMENT ALGORITHM AND FUTURE POSSIBILITIES

A diagnostic and treatment algorithm for invasive cancer of the vagina is depicted in Figure 57-13. Confirmation of invasive disease should be obtained by biopsy. In selected patients in whom excisional biopsy can be accomplished without functional compromise, wide local excision may be diagnostic and therapeutic. Critical in planning therapy is definition of disease extent. Careful physical examination, possibly including colposcopy, cystourethroscopy, anoscopy, and proctoscopy, can aid in the evaluation of primary disease extent and in screening for synchronous primaries of the cervix, vulva, and anus. Although the value of PET has not been established specifically for vaginal cancer, its use to assess regional node metastasis and distant metastasis seems a logical extrapolation from the use of PET in patients with cervical cancer. Fused PET/CT is preferred to PET alone because of improved spatial resolution and ability to distinguish pelvic lymph node involvement from nonspecific ^{18}F-fluorodeoxyglucose activity in bowel. MRI is superior to CT in distinguishing soft tissue tumor extensions within the pelvis. Effective use of MRI requires gadolinium contrast administration and selection of the correct pulse sequences optimized for visualization of pelvic soft tissues. Findings may be helpful in planning radiation dose distributions, particularly for brachytherapy techniques and in the design of reduced boost volumes for teletherapy. None of these imaging technologies alters assignment of FIGO clinical stage. However, imaging results may affect selection, sequencing, and intensity of treatment modalities.

Patients with small-volume primary tumors confined to the vaginal wall that do not encroach on functionally important midline structures (e.g., urethra, bladder, rectum) may be treated with primary surgical excision if the surgery will not compromise sexual function. This depends on the diameter of

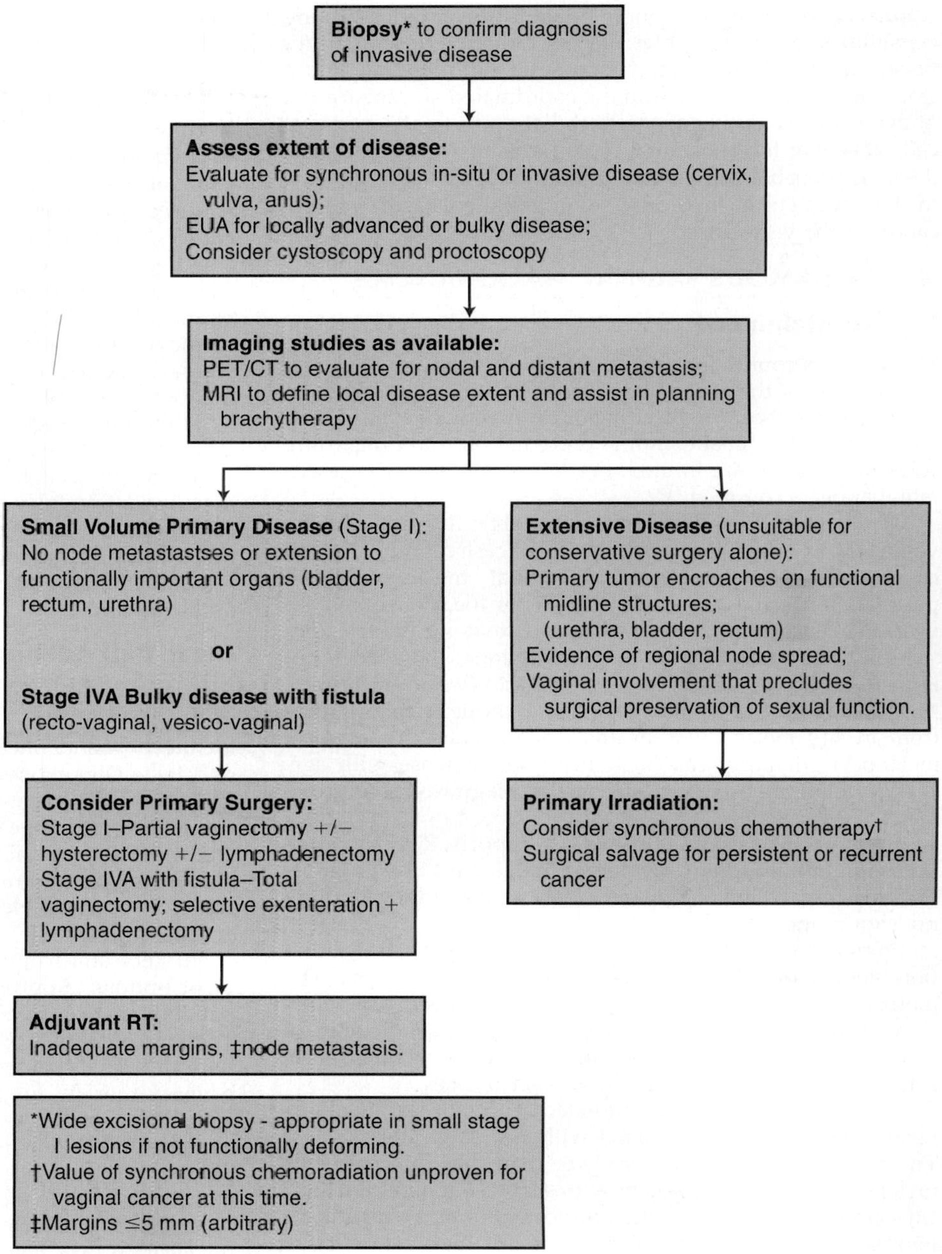

Figure 57-13 Diagnostic and therapeutic algorithm for invasive squamous cell cancer of the vagina. An *asterisk* indicates wide excisional biopsy that is appropriate for small stage I lesions if it is not functionally deforming; a *dagger* indicates that the value of synchronous chemotherapy (chemoradiation) is unproved for vaginal cancer; and the *double dagger* indicates margins of less than 5 mm (arbitrary measure). CT, computed tomography; EUA, examination under anesthesia; MRI, magnetic resonance imaging; PET, positron emission tomography.

the patient's vagina, which is usually related to her reproductive history (e.g., vaginal parity) and location within the vagina. Rarely are patients with more extensive disease suitable for initial surgery. An exception is patients with stage IVA bulky central disease and fistula formation (i.e., vesicovaginal or rectovaginal fistulas) in whom total vaginectomy with selective or total exenteration may be necessary initial treatment for hygienic reasons. However, fistula formation is not the inevitable consequence of radiotherapeutic management of patients with stage IVA disease. Anecdotally, some patients presenting with small vesicovaginal fistulas have urinary continence restored if the vaginal walls fuse after radical radiation therapy, effectively sealing the fistula. If that is the intent, use of a vaginal dilator after irradiation is counterproductive.

Use of chemotherapy synchronously with irradiation is not of established value in patients with primary vaginal cancer. Employment of chemoradiation represents a logical extrapolation from the treatment of patients with primary cancers of the anus, cervix, and vulva. It is reasonable to consider in patients for whom conventional techniques do not have a high probability of success, primarily patients with stage III or IVA disease. The value of synchronous chemotherapy as a tactic by which the radiation dose may be reduced while yielding equivalent or better tumor control and improved late normal tissue function remains largely theoretical.

Because of the rarity of vaginal cancer, prospective, randomized clinical trials are unlikely in the context of decentralized cancer care. Progress in improving local and regional control may come from refined understanding of dose-control probabilities for volume of disease and optimization of dose delivery to more precisely defined tumor volumes. Application of increasingly sophisticated spatial and metabolic imaging modalities to the initial assessment of patients with vaginal cancer, along with more powerful treatment planning capabilities rendering tighter, elegant radiation dose distributions, should improve the therapeutic ratio. Extrapolating from the benefits reaped from the coordinated administration of cytotoxic chemotherapy with radiation to treat squamous cell cancers of the anogenital region arising at adjacent sites, it seems probable that chemoradiation will play a larger role in the treatment of medically suitable patients with vaginal cancer in the years ahead.

NONSQUAMOUS VAGINAL MALIGNANCIES

Vaginal Melanoma

Melanoma accounts for approximately 3% of vaginal malignancies and is the second most common histologic type of primary vaginal cancer. Bleeding or protrusion of a mass from the vagina is the most common presentation. Data regarding stage distribution are limited, but advanced stage at presentation appears common.[242]

Of all melanomas in women, less than 1% arise in the vagina. Most of the literature consists of case reports or small case series. The incidence of vaginal melanoma from population-based data is 0.026 to 0.030 per 100,000 women per year, and consistent with the assumption that ultraviolet exposure is not a causal factor in these lesions, there does not appear to be an effect of race or latitude on incidence. Melanomas arising in the vagina are thought to originate from in situ melanocytes in areas of melanosis or atypical melanocytic hyperplasia. Incidence does increase with age. The population-based median age at diagnosis is approximately 70 years.[243]

In a meta-analysis of published case reports, Reid and associates found only tumor size larger than 3 cm to be prognostic for survival. Patient age and tumor stage and location are not significant.

Primary treatment includes radical surgery, radical radiation therapy, or combinations of irradiation and surgery. The modality of treatment does not appreciably affect survival.[242]

Most relapses are local or regional. Of metastatic sites of relapse, the lung, usually concomitant with pelvic recurrence, is the most common site among published cases.

Overall survival is poor, estimated at 15% or less, and survival seems limited to patients with low-stage disease.[242,243] The rate of survival is much lower than that for cutaneous melanomas, but it is consistent with survival at other mucosal sites and the generally large tumor volume at diagnosis. Because inadequate surgical margins are highly predictive of relapse and because salvage after relapse is unlikely, patients treated with primary surgery must have a definitive first procedure, frequently entailing partial or total pelvic exenteration.

Given the very poor survival and the high morbidity of such procedures, thorough preoperative assessment for disease spread beyond the boundaries of surgical resection should be undertaken in each patient for whom such surgery is contemplated. Investigations may include whole-body CT, PET, and possibly MRI of the brain. Surgical therapy must also be individualized in the context of patient comorbidities and the patient's willingness to undergo procedures that imply profound changes in quality of life in exchange for a slender prospect of cure.

Although melanomas have traditionally been considered radioresistant, among the few long-term survivors reported are some patients who have been treated with irradiation. Local irradiation may provide palliation and growth restraint in patients with proven metastatic deposits for whom exenterative surgery may not be appropriate. Adjuvant systemic therapy and treatment of disseminated melanoma parallels the treatment of melanoma arising at other sites.

Sarcomas

Vaginal sarcomas make up 3% of primary vaginal malignancies. Of the 68 cases of vaginal sarcoma reported by Peters and colleagues,[260] leiomyosarcomas accounted for 68%. Other reported sarcomas include endometrial stromal sarcoma, malignant mixed müllerian tumor, and rhabdomyosarcoma.[261]

Surgical resection is the treatment of choice. The benefit of chemotherapy or radiation therapy is not established in the treatment of adult vaginal sarcomas, but irradiation may be employed preoperatively or postoperatively for inadequate surgical margins or regional spread, analogous to the treatment of extremity and truncal sarcomas.

Embryonal rhabdomyosarcoma (i.e., sarcoma botryoides) is a highly malignant sarcoma that occurs in children up to 6 years old (mean age, 1.8 years). This sarcoma generally manifests as soft nodules that fill and protrude from the vagina or as abnormal bleeding. The prognosis for patients with this malignancy has improved dramatically with the use of multimodality therapy, including surgery, polyagent chemotherapy, and irradiation.[262]

Clear Cell Adenocarcinoma of the Vagina

Prognostic factors for all CCACs of the vagina include stage at diagnosis, tumor size, and grade of the lesion, including architecture and nuclear grade, and they appear to pertain equally to DES-exposed and DES-unexposed patients. Among DES-exposed patients, very young age is also a poor prognostic factor. It appears from the Netherlands Registry that DES-exposed vaginal CCAC cases are diagnosed after shorter durations of symptoms.[263] Possibly because of early occurrence of abnormal bleeding, most cases are stage I or stage II at diagnosis.

Surgery and irradiation have been used as primary treatment options. Approximately one half of all vaginal CCAC patients in the U.S. Registry for Research on Hormonal Transplacental Carcinogenesis were treated initially with radical surgery alone.[264] Radical irradiation is offered as primary therapy for patients with locally advanced disease and those who are not surgical candidates or decline radical surgery. Irradiation may be given as adjuvant therapy for patients at high risk for pelvic relapse. Irradiation may be used alone or in combination with surgical resection to treat locally recurrent disease. Optimal treatment of recurrent disease is not clear; in 1979, Herbst and coworkers reported a 5-year survival rate after pelvic relapse of 40%.[265]

Most relapses are local or locoregional, although the incidence of distant relapse in CCAC is higher than in squamous vaginal cancers. In the study of Waggoner and colleagues, 9% of all DES-exposed CCAC patients presented with lung or distant nodal metastases.[264] Among DES-unexposed patients, the rate of distant disease was 24%. Although most relapses occur within 3 years of treatment, later relapses, including 12 cases of relapse more than 8 years after diagnosis, have been reported.[266]

REFERENCES

1. Green TH Jr, Ulfelder H, Meigs JV: Epidermoid carcinoma of the vulva: an analysis of 238 cases. Parts I and II. Am J Obstet Gynecol 73:834-840, 1958.
2. Taussig FJ: Cancer of the vulva: an analysis of 155 cases. Am J Obstet Gynecol 40:764-770, 1940.
3. Thomas GM, Dembo AJ, Bryson SC, et al: Changing concepts in the management of vulvar cancer. Gynecol Oncol 42:9-21, 1991.

4. Way S: Carcinoma of the vulva. Am J Obstet Gynecol 79:692-697, 1960.
5. Benedet JL, Turko M, Fairey RN, Boyes DA: Squamous carcinoma of the vulva: results of treatment 1938 to 1976. Am J Obstet Gynecol 134:201-207, 1979.
6. Boutselis JG: Radical vulvectomy for invasive squamous cell carcinoma of the vulva. Obstet Gynecol 39:827-836, 1972.
7. Cavanagh D, Shepherd JH: The place of pelvic exenteration in the primary management of advanced carcinoma of the vulva. Gynecol Oncol 13:318-322, 1982.
8. Hacker NF, Berek JS, Lagasse LD, et al: Management of regional lymph nodes and their prognostic influence in vulvar cancer. Obstet Gynecol 61:408-412, 1983.
9. Japaze H, Garcia-Bunuel R, Woodruff JD: Primary vulvar neoplasia: a review of in situ and invasive carcinoma 1935-1972. Obstet Gynecol 49:404-411, 1977.
10. Morley GW: Infiltrative carcinoma of the vulva: results of surgical treatment. Am J Obstet Gynecol 124:874-888, 1976.
11. Rutledge F, Smith JP, Franklin EW: Carcinoma of the vulva. Am J Obstet Gynecol 106:1117-1130, 1970.
12. Choo YC, Morley GW: Multiple primary neoplasms of the anogenital region. Obstet Gynecol 56:365-369, 1980.
13. Mabuchi K, Bross DS, Kessler II: Epidemiology of cancer of the vulva. A case-control study. Cancer 55:1843-1848, 1985.
14. Merrill JA, Ross NL: Cancer of the vulva. Cancer 14:13-20, 1961.
15. Buscema J, Woodruff JD, Parmley TH, Genadry R: Carcinoma in situ of the vulva. Obstet Gynecol 55:225-230, 1980.
16. Abercrombie PD, Korn AP: Vulvar intraepithelial neoplasia in women with HIV. AIDS Patient Care STDS 12:251-254, 1998.
17. Caterson RJ, Furber J, Murray J, et al: Carcinoma of the vulva in two young renal allograft recipients. Transplant Proc 16:559-561, 1984.
18. Halpert R, Fruchter RG, Sedlis A, et al: Human papillomavirus and lower genital neoplasia in renal transplant patients. Obstet Gynecol 68:251-258., 1986
19. Korn AP, Abercrombie PD, Foster A: Vulvar intraepithelial neoplasia in women infected with human immunodeficiency virus-1. Gynecol Oncol 61:384-386, 1996.
20. Kuhn L, Sun XW, Wright TC Jr: Human immunodeficiency virus infection and female lower genital tract malignancy. Curr Opin Obstet Gynecol 11:35-39, 1999.
21. Wright TC, Koulos JP, Liu P, Sun XW: Invasive vulvar carcinoma in two women infected with human immunodeficiency virus. Gynecol Oncol 60:500-503, 1996.
22. Porreco R, Penn I, Droegemueller W, et al: Gynecologic malignancies in immunosuppressed organ homograft recipients. Obstet Gynecol 45:359-364, 1975.
23. Giaquinto C, Del Mistro A, De Rossi A, et al: Vulvar carcinoma in a 12-year-old girl with vertically acquired human immunodeficiency virus infection. Pediatrics 106:E57, 2000.
24. Massad LS, Silverberg MJ, Springer G, et al: Effect of antiretroviral therapy on the incidence of genital warts and vulvar neoplasia among women with the human immunodeficiency virus. Am J Obstet Gynecol 190:1241-1248, 2004.
25. Adami J, Gabel H, Lindelof B, et al: Cancer risk following organ transplantation: a nationwide cohort study in Sweden. Br J Cancer 89:1221-1227, 2003.
26. Brinton LA, Nasca PC, Mallin K, et al: Case-control study of cancer of the vulva. Obstet Gynecol 75:859-866, 1990.
27. Buscema J, Naghashfar Z, Sawada E, et al: The predominance of human papillomavirus type 16 in vulvar neoplasia. Obstet Gynecol 71:601-606, 1988.
28. Gissmann L, Schwarz E: Persistence and expression of human papillomavirus DNA in genital cancer. Ciba Found Symp 120:190-207, 1986.
29. Ansink AC, Heintz AP: Epidemiology and etiology of squamous cell carcinoma of the vulva. Eur J Obstet Gynecol Reprod Biol 48:111-115, 1993.
30. Pinto AP, Schlecht NF, Pintos J, et al: Prognostic significance of lymph node variables and human papillomavirus DNA in invasive vulvar carcinoma. Gynecol Oncol 92:856-865, 2004.
31. Daling JR, Sherman KJ, Hislop TG, et al: Cigarette smoking and the risk of anogenital cancer. Am J Epidemiol 135:180-189, 1992.
32. zur Hausen H: Human genital cancer: synergism between two virus infections or synergism between a virus infection and initiating events? Lancet 2:1370-1372, 1982.
33. Buscema J, Stern J, Woodruff JD: The significance of the histologic alterations adjacent to invasive vulvar carcinoma. Am J Obstet Gynecol 137:902-909, 1980.
34. Zaino RJ, Hussein Zadeh N, Nahhas W, Mortel R: Epithelial alterations in proximity to invasive squamous carcinoma of the vulva. Int J Gynecol Pathol 1:173-184, 1982.
35. Rouzier R, Morice P, Carnot F, et al: Prognostic significance of epithelial disorders adjacent to invasive vulvar carcinomas. Gynecol Oncol 81:414-419, 2001.
36. Jones RW, Sadler L, Grant S, et al: Clinically identifying women with vulvar lichen sclerosus at increased risk of squamous cell carcinoma: a case-control study. J Reprod Med 49:808-811, 2004.
37. Crum CP, McLachlin CM, Tate JE, Mutter GL: Pathobiology of vulvar squamous neoplasia. Curr Opin Obstet Gynecol 9:63-69, 1997.
38. Lerma E, Matias-Guiu X, Lee SJ, Prat J: Squamous cell carcinoma of the vulva: study of ploidy, HPV, p53, and pRb. Int J Gynecol Pathol 18:191-197, 1999.
39. Rolfe KJ, MacLean AB, Crow JC, et al: TP53 mutations in vulval lichen sclerosus adjacent to squamous cell carcinoma of the vulva. Br J Cancer 89:2249-2253, 2003.
40. Bamberger ES, Perrett CW: Angiogenesis in benign, pre-malignant and malignant vulvar lesions. Anticancer Res 22:3853-3865, 2002.
41. Johnson GA, Mannel R, Khalifa M, et al: Epidermal growth factor receptor in vulvar malignancies and its relationship to metastasis and patient survival. Gynecol Oncol 65:425-429, 1997.
42. Kagie MJ, Kenter GG, Tollenaar RA, et al: P53 protein overexpression, a frequent observation in squamous cell carcinoma of the vulva and in various synchronous vulvar epithelia, has no value as a prognostic parameter. Int J Gynecol Pathol 16:124-130, 1997.
43. Gordinier ME, Steinhoff MM, Hogan JW, et al: S-phase fraction, p53, and HER-2/neu status as predictors of nodal metastasis in early vulvar cancer. Gynecol Oncol 67:200-202, 1997.
44. Braakhuis BJ, Tabor MP, Kummer JA, et al: A genetic explanation of Slaughter's concept of field cancerization: evidence and clinical implications. Cancer Res 63:1727-1730, 2003.
45. Scheistroen M, Trope C, Petersen EO, Nesland JM: P53 protein expression in squamous cell carcinoma of the vulva. Cancer 85:1133-1138, 1999.
46. Husseinzadeh N, Recinto C: Frequency of invasive cancer in surgically excised vulvar lesions with intraepithelial neoplasia (VIN 3). Gynecol Oncol 73:119-120, 1999.
47. Frisch M, Melbye M: Risk of lung cancer in pre- and postmenopausal women with anogenital malignancies. Int J Cancer 62:508-511, 1995.
48. Crissman JD, Azoury RS: Microinvasive carcinoma of the vulva. A report of two cases with regional lymph node metastasis. Diagn Gynecol Obstet 3:75-80, 1981.
49. Wilkinson EJ, Rico MJ, Pierson KK: Microinvasive carcinoma of the vulva. Int J Gynecol Pathol 1:29-39, 1982.
50. Kneale BLG, Elliott PM, McDonald IA: Microinvasive carcinoma of the vulva: clinical features and management. *In* Coppleson M (ed): Gynecologic Oncology. Edinburgh, Churchill Livingstone, 1981, p 320.
51. Foye G, Marsh MR, Minkowitz S: Verrucous carcinoma of the vulva. Obstet Gynecol 34:484-488, 1969.
52. Gallousis S: Verrucous carcinoma. Report of three vulvar cases and review of the literature. Obstet Gynecol 40:502-507, 1972.
53. Japaze H, Van Dinh T, Woodruff JD: Verrucous carcinoma of the vulva: study of 24 cases. Obstet Gynecol 60:462-466, 1982.
54. Lucas WE, Benirschke K, Lebherz TB: Verrucous carcinoma of the female genital tract. Am J Obstet Gynecol 119:435-440, 1974.
55. Russell AH: Cancer of the vulva. *In* Leibel SA, Phillips TL (eds): Textbook of Radiation Oncology. Philadelphia, WB Saunders, 2004, p 1674.
56. Gualco M, Vonin S, Foglia G, et al: Morphologic and biologic studies on ten cases of verrucous carcinoma of the vulva supporting the theory of a discrete clinico-pathologic entity. Int J Gynecol Cancer 13:317-24, 2003.

57. Neto AG, Deavers MT, Silva EG, Malpica A: Metastatic tumors of the vulva: a clinicopathologic study of 66 cases. Am J Surg Pathol 27:799-804, 2003.
58. Breslow A: Thickness, cross-sectional areas and depth of invasion in the prognosis of cutaneous melanoma. Ann Surg 172:902-908, 1970.
59. Clark WH Jr, From L, Bernardino EA, Mihm MC: The histogenesis and biologic behavior of primary human malignant melanomas of the skin. Cancer Res 29:705-727, 1969.
60. Chung AF, Woodruff JM, Lewis JL Jr: Malignant melanoma of the vulva: a report of 44 cases. Obstet Gynecol 45:638-646, 1975.
61. Copeland LJ, Sneige N, Gershenson DM, et al: Adenoid cystic carcinoma of Bartholin gland. Obstet Gynecol 67:115-120, 1986.
62. Kneale BL: Carcinoma of the vulva then and now. The 1987 ISSVD presidential address. J Reprod Med 33:496-499, 1988.
63. Kneale BL, Fortune DW: Pathology of the vulva. Curr Opin Obstet Gynecol 3:548-52, 1991.
64. Heaps JM, Fu YS, Montz FJ, et al: Surgical-pathologic variables predictive of local recurrence in squamous cell carcinoma of the vulva. Gynecol Oncol 38:309-314, 1990.
65. Hacker NF, Leuchter RS, Berek JS, et al: Radical vulvectomy and bilateral inguinal lymphadenectomy through separate groin incisions. Obstet Gynecol 58:574-579, 1981.
66. Iversen T, Aas M: Lymph drainage from the vulva. Gynecol Oncol 16:179-189, 1983.
67. Chu J, Tamimi HK, Figge DC: Femoral node metastases with negative superficial inguinal nodes in early vulvar cancer. Am J Obstet Gynecol 140:337-339, 1981.
68. Burke TW, Levenback C, Coleman RL, et al: Surgical therapy of T1 and T2 vulvar carcinoma: further experience with radical wide excision and selective inguinal lymphadenectomy. Gynecol Oncol 57:215-220, 1995.
69. Stehman FB, Bundy BN, Dvoretsky PM, Creasman WT: Early stage I carcinoma of the vulva treated with ipsilateral superficial inguinal lymphadenectomy and modified radical hemivulvectomy: a prospective study of the Gynecologic Oncology Group. Obstet Gynecol 79:490-497, 1992.
70. Levenback C, Burke TW, Morris M, et al: Potential applications of intraoperative lymphatic mapping in vulvar cancer. Gynecol Oncol 59:216-220, 1995.
71. Katz A, Eifel PJ, Jhingran A, Levenback CH: The role of radiation therapy in preventing regional recurrences of invasive squamous cell carcinoma of the vulva. Int J Radiat Oncol Biol Phys 57:409-418, 2003.
72. Hacker NF, Berek JS, Lagasse LD, et al: Individualization of treatment for stage I squamous cell vulvar carcinoma. Obstet Gynecol 63:155-162, 1984.
73. Wharton JT, Gallager S, Rutledge FN: Microinvasive carcinoma of the vulva. Am J Obstet Gynecol 118:159-162, 1974.
74. Boyce J, Fruchter RG, Boyce J, et al: Prognostic factors in carcinoma of the vulva. Gynecol Oncol 20:364-377, 1985.
75. Gonzalez Bosquet J, Kinney WK, Russell AH, et al: Risk of occult inguinofemoral lymph node metastasis from squamous carcinoma of the vulva. Int J Radiat Oncol Biol Phys 57:419-424, 2003.
76. Krupp PJ, Bohm JW: Lymph gland metastases in invasive squamous cell cancer of the vulva. Am J Obstet Gynecol 130:943-952, 1978.
77. Mazouni C, Morice P, Duvillard P, et al: Contralateral groin recurrence in patients with stage I Bartholin's gland squamous cell carcinoma and negative ipsilateral nodes: report on two cases and implications for lymphadenectomy. Gynecol Oncol 94:843-845, 2004.
78. Magrina JF, Webb MJ, Gaffey TA, Symmonds RE: Stage I squamous cell cancer of the vulva. Am J Obstet Gynecol 134:453-459, 1979.
79. Iversen T, Abeler V, Aalders J: Individualized treatment of stage I carcinoma of the vulva. Obstet Gynecol 57:85-89, 1981.
80. Parker RT, Duncan I, Rampone J, Creasman WL: Operative management of early invasive epidermoid carcinoma of the vulva. Am J Obstet Gynecol 123:349-355, 1975.
81. Buscema J, Stern JL, Woodruff JD: Early invasive carcinoma of the vulva. Am J Obstet Gynecol 140:563-569, 1981.
82. Hoffman JS, Kumar NB, Morley GW: Microinvasive squamous carcinoma of the vulva: search for a definition. Obstet Gynecol 61:615-618, 1983.
83. Burke TW, Stringer CA, Gershenson DM, et al: Radical wide excision and selective inguinal node dissection for squamous cell carcinoma of the vulva. Gynecol Oncol 38:328-332, 1990.
84. Lin JY, DuBeshter B, Angel C, Dvoretsky PM: Morbidity and recurrence with modifications of radical vulvectomy and groin dissection. Gynecol Oncol 47:80-86, 1992.
85. Andrews SJ, Williams BT, DePriest PD, et al: Therapeutic implications of lymph nodal spread in lateral T1 and T2 squamous cell carcinoma of the vulva. Gynecol Oncol 55:41-46, 1994.
86. Tham KF, Shepherd JH, Lowe DG, et al: Early vulval cancer: the place of conservative management. Eur J Surg Oncol 19:361-367, 1993.
87. Farias-Eisner R, Cirisano FD, Grouse D, et al: Conservative and individualized surgery for early squamous carcinoma of the vulva: the treatment of choice for stage I and II (T1-2N0-1M0) disease. Gynecol Oncol 53:55-58, 1994.
88. Green TH Jr: Carcinoma of the vulva: a reassessment. Obstet Gynecol 52:462-469, 1978.
89. Iversen T, Aalders JG, Christensen A, Kolstad P: Squamous cell carcinoma of the vulva: a review of 424 patients 1956-1974. Gynecol Oncol 9:271-279, 1980.
90. Homesley HD, Bundy BN, Sedlis A, Adcock L: Radiation therapy versus pelvic node resection for carcinoma of the vulva with positive groin nodes. Obstet Gynecol 68:733-740, 1986.
91. Dean RE, Taylor ES, Weisbrod DM, Martin JW: The treatment of premalignant and malignant lesions of the vulva. Am J Obstet Gynecol 119:59-68, 1974.
92. Morris JM: A formula for selective lymphadenectomy. Its application to cancer of the vulva. Obstet Gynecol 50:152-158, 1977.
93. Hacker NF: Current treatment of small vulvar cancers. Oncology (Williston Park) 4:21-25, discussion 26, 28, 33, 1990.
94. Homesley HD, Bundy BN, Sedlis A, et al: Assessment of current International Federation of Gynecology and Obstetrics staging of vulvar carcinoma relative to prognostic factors for survival (a Gynecologic Oncology Group study). Am J Obstet Gynecol 164:997-1003, discussion 1003-1004, 1991.
95. Franklin EW 3rd, Rutledge FD: Prognostic factors in epidermoid carcinoma of the vulva. Obstet Gynecol 37:892-901, 1971.
96. Curry SL, Wharton JT, Rutledge F: Positive lymph nodes in vulvar squamous carcinoma. Gynecol Oncol 9:63-67, 1980.
97. Monaghan JM, Hammond IG: Pelvic node dissection in the treatment of vulval carcinoma—is it necessary? Br J Obstet Gynaecol 91:270-274, 1984.
98. Podratz KC, Symmonds RE, Taylor WF, Williams TJ: Carcinoma of the vulva: analysis of treatment and survival. Obstet Gynecol 61:63-74, 1983.
99. Cavanagh D, Roberts WS, Bryson SC, et al: Changing trends in the surgical treatment of invasive carcinoma of the vulva. Surg Gynecol Obstet 162:164-168, 1986.
100. Cavanagh D, Fiorica JV, Hoffman MS, et al: Invasive carcinoma of the vulva. Changing trends in surgical management. Am J Obstet Gynecol 163:1007-1015, 1990.
101. Malfetano J, Piver MS, Tsukada Y: Stage III and IV squamous cell carcinoma of the vulva. Gynecol Oncol 23:192-198, 1986.
102. Podratz KC, Symmonds RE, Taylor W: Carcinoma of the vulva: analysis of treatment failures. Am J Obstet Gynecol 143:340-351, 1982.
103. Bryson SC, Dembo AJ, Colgan TJ, et al: Invasive squamous cell carcinoma of the vulva: defining low and high risk groups for recurrence. Int J Gynecol Cancer 1:25-31, 1991.
104. Piura B, Masotina A, Murdoch J, et al: Recurrent squamous cell carcinoma of the vulva: a study of 73 cases. Gynecol Oncol 48:189-195, 1993.
105. Tilmans AS, Sutton GP, Look KY, et al: Recurrent squamous carcinoma of the vulva. Am J Obstet Gynecol 167:1383-1389, 1992.
106. van der Velden J, van Lindert AC, Lammes FB, et al: Extracapsular growth of lymph node metastases in squamous cell carcinoma of the vulva. The impact on recurrence and survival. Cancer 75:2885-2890, 1995.
107. Origoni M, Sideri M, Garsia S, et al: Prognostic value of pathological patterns of lymph node positivity in squamous cell

carcinoma of the vulva stage III and IVA FIGO. Gynecol Oncol 45:313-316, 1992.
108. De Hullu JA, Hollema H, Lolkema S, et al: Vulvar carcinoma. The price of less radical surgery. Cancer 95:2331-2338, 2002.
109. Faul CM, Mirmow D, Huang Q, et al: Adjuvant radiation for vulvar carcinoma: improved local control. Int J Radiat Oncol Biol Phys 38:381-389, 1997.
110. Slaughter DP, Southwick HW, Smejkal W: Field cancerization in oral stratified squamous epithelium: clinical implications of multicentric origin. Cancer 6:963-968, 1953.
111. Iversen T: The value of groin palpation in epidermoid carcinoma of the vulva. Gynecol Oncol 12:291-295, 1981.
112. Koh WJ, Chiu M, Seltzer KJ, et al: Femoral vessel depth and the implications for groin node radiation. Int J Radiat Oncol Biol Phys 27:969-974, 1993.
113. Goplerud DR, Keettel WC: Carcinoma of the vulva: a review of 156 cases from the University of Iowa Hospitals. Am J Obstet Gynecol 100:550-553, 1968.
114. Leiserowitz GS, Russell AH, Kinney WK, et al: Prophylactic chemoradiation of inguinofemoral lymph nodes in patients with locally extensive vulvar cancer. Gynecol Oncol 66:509-514, 1997.
115. Wahlen SA, Slater JD, Wagner RJ, et al: Concurrent radiation therapy and chemotherapy in the treatment of primary squamous cell carcinoma of the vulva. Cancer 75:2289-2294, 1995.
116. Parry-Jones E: Lymphatics of the vulva. J Obstet Gynecol Br Emp 70:751-765, 1963.
117. De Cicco C, Sideri M, Bartolomei M, et al: Sentinel node biopsy in early vulvar cancer. Br J Cancer 82:295-299, 2000.
118. Ansink AC, de Hullu JA, van der Zee AG: Further data on the usefulness of sentinel lymph node identification and ultrastaging in vulvar squamous cell carcinoma. Gynecol Oncol 88:29-34, 2003. (Gynecol Oncol 90:688-689, 2003; author reply 689-690.)
119. Ansink AC, Sie-Go DM, van der Velden J, et al: Identification of sentinel lymph nodes in vulvar carcinoma patients with the aid of a patent blue V injection: a multicenter study. Cancer 86:652-656, 1999.
120. de Hullu JA, Hollema H, Piers DA, et al: Sentinel lymph node procedure is highly accurate in squamous cell carcinoma of the vulva. J Clin Oncol 18:2811-2816, 2000.
121. Rodier JF, Janser JC, Routiot T, et al: Sentinel node biopsy in vulvar malignancies: a preliminary feasibility study. Oncol Rep 6:1249-1252, 1999.
122. Terada KY, Shimizu DM, Wong JH: Sentinel node dissection and ultrastaging in squamous cell cancer of the vulva. Gynecol Oncol 76:40-44, 2000.
123. Decesare SL, Fiorica JV, Roberts WS, et al: A pilot study utilizing intraoperative lymphoscintigraphy for identification of the sentinel lymph nodes in vulvar cancer. Gynecol Oncol 66:425-428, 1997.
124. Puig-Tintore LM, Ordi J, Vidal-Sicart S, et al: Further data on the usefulness of sentinel lymph node identification and ultrastaging in vulvar squamous cell carcinoma. Gynecol Oncol 88:29-34, 2003.
125. Moore RG, Granai CO, Gajewski W, et al: Pathologic evaluation of inguinal sentinel lymph nodes in vulvar cancer patients: a comparison of immunohistochemical staining versus ultrastaging with hematoxylin and eosin staining. Gynecol Oncol 91:378-382, 2003.
126. Cohn DE, Dehdashti F, Gibb RK, et al: Prospective evaluation of positron emission tomography for the detection of groin node metastases from vulvar cancer. Gynecol Oncol 85:179-184, 2002.
127. Hall TB, Barton DP, Trott PA, et al: The role of ultrasound-guided cytology of groin lymph nodes in the management of squamous cell carcinoma of the vulva: 5-year experience in 44 patients. Clin Radiol 58:367-371, 2003.
128. Sohaib SA, Moskovic ED: Imaging in vulval cancer. Best Pract Res Clin Obstet Gynaecol 17:543-556, 2003.
129. Sohaib SA, Richard PS, Ind T, et al: MR imaging of carcinoma of the vulva. AJR Am J Roentgenol 178:373-377, 2002.
130. Kalidas H: Influence of inguinal node anatomy on radiation therapy techniques. Med Dosim 20:295-300, 1995.
131. McKelvey JL, Adcock LL: Cancer of the vulva. Obstet Gynecol 26:455-466, 1965.
132. Andersen BL, Hacker NF: Psychosexual adjustment after vulvar surgery. Obstet Gynecol 62:457-462, 1983.
133. Green MS, Naumann RW, Elliot M, et al: Sexual dysfunction following vulvectomy. Gynecol Oncol 77:73-77, 2000.
134. Stellman RE, Goodwin JM, Robinson J, et al: Psychological effects of vulvectomy. Psychosomatics 25:779-783, 1984.
135. Way S: The anatomy of the lymphatic drainage of the vulva and its furtherance on the radical operation for carcinoma. Ann R Coll Surg Engl 3:187-197, 1948.
136. DiSaia PJ, Creasman WT, Rich WM: An alternate approach to early cancer of the vulva. Am J Obstet Gynecol 133:825-832, 1979.
137. Ansink A, van der Velden J: Surgical interventions for early squamous cell carcinoma of the vulva. Cochrane Database Syst Rev (2):CD002036, 2000.
138. van der Velden J, Schilthuis MS, Hyde SE, et al: Squamous cell cancer of the vulva with occult lymph node metastases in the groin: the impact of surgical technique on recurrence pattern and survival. Int J Gynecol Cancer 14:633-638, 2004.
139. Maggino T, Landoni F, Sartori E, et al: Patterns of recurrence in patients with squamous cell carcinoma of the vulva: a multicenter CTF study. Cancer 89:116-122, 2000.
140. Lingard D, Free K, Wright RG, Battistutta D: Invasive squamous cell carcinoma of the vulva: behaviour and results in the light of changing management regimens. A review of clinicohistological features predictive of regional lymph node involvement and local recurrence. Aust N Z J Obstet Gynaecol 32:137-145, 1992.
141. Krupp PJ, Lee FY, Bohm JW, et al: Prognostic parameters and clinical staging criteria in the epidermoid carcinoma of the vulva. Obstet Gynecol 46:84-88, 1975.
142. Prempree T, Amornmarn R: Radiation treatment of recurrent carcinoma of the vulva. Cancer 54:1943-1949, 1984.
143. Figge DC, Gaudenz R: Invasive carcinoma of the vulva. Am J Obstet Gynecol 119:382-395, 1974.
144. DiSaia PJ: What is the proper extent of an inguinal lymphadenectomy for early vulvar cancer? Gynecol Oncol 90:687-688, author reply 689-690, 2003.
145. Gould N, Kamelle S, Tillmanns T, et al: Predictors of complications after inguinal lymphadenectomy. Gynecol Oncol 82:329-332, 2001.
146. Montana GS, Thomas GM, Moore DH, et al: Preoperative chemoradiation for carcinoma of the vulva with N2/N3 nodes: a gynecologic oncology group study. Int J Radiat Oncol Biol Phys 48:1007-1013, 2000.
147. Backstrom A, Edsmyr F, Wicklund H: Radiotherapy of carcinoma of the vulva. Acta Obstet Gynecol Scand 51:109-115, 1972.
148. Frischbier HJ, Thomsen K: Treatment of cancer of the vulva with high energy electrons. Am J Obstet Gynecol 111:431-435, 1971.
149. Helgason NM, Hass AC, Latourette HB: Radiation therapy in carcinoma of the vulva: a review of 53 patients. Cancer 30:997-1000, 1972.
150. Kuipers T: Carcinoma of the vulva. Radiol Clin (Basel) 44:475-483, 1975.
151. Tod MD: Radium implantation in treatment of carcinoma of the vulva. Br J Radiol 22:508-512, 1949.
152. Ansink AC, van Tinteren H, Aartsen EJ, Heintz AP: Outcome, complications and follow-up in surgically treated squamous cell carcinoma of the vulva 1956-1982. Eur J Obstet Gynecol Reprod Biol 42:137-143, 1991.
153. Dusenbery KE, Carlson JW, LaPorte RM, et al: Radical vulvectomy with postoperative irradiation for vulvar cancer: therapeutic implications of a central block. Int J Radiat Oncol Biol Phys 29:989-998, 1994.
154. Boronow RC, Hickman BT, Reagan MT, et al: Combined therapy as an alternative to exenteration for locally advanced vulvovaginal cancer. II. Results, complications, and dosimetric and surgical considerations. Am J Clin Oncol 10:171-181, 1987.
155. Acosta AA, Given FT, Frazier AB, et al: Preoperative radiation therapy in the management of squamous cell carcinoma of the vulva: preliminary report. Am J Obstet Gynecol 132:198-206, 1978.
156. Hacker NF, Berek JS, Julliard GJ, Lagasse LD: Preoperative radiation therapy for locally advanced vulvar cancer. Cancer 54:2056-2061, 1984.

157. Jafar K, Magalotti F, Magalotti M: Radiation therapy in carcinoma of the vulva. Cancer 47:686-691, 1981.
158. Levin W, Goldberg G, Altaras M, et al: The use of concomitant chemotherapy and radiotherapy prior to surgery in advanced stage carcinoma of the vulva. Gynecol Oncol 25:20-25, 1986.
159. Thomas G, Dembo A, DePetrillo A, et al: Concurrent radiation and chemotherapy in vulvar carcinoma. Gynecol Oncol 34:263-267, 1989.
160. Moore DH, Thomas GM, Montana GS, et al: Preoperative chemoradiation for advanced vulvar cancer: a phase II study of the Gynecologic Oncology Group. Int J Radiat Oncol Biol Phys 42:79-85, 1998.
161. Han SC, Kim DH, Higgins SA, et al: Chemoradiation as primary or adjuvant treatment for locally advanced carcinoma of the vulva. Int J Radiat Oncol Biol Phys 47:1235-1244, 2000.
162. Perez CA, Grigsby PW, Chao C, et al: Irradiation in carcinoma of the vulva: factors affecting outcome. Int J Radiat Oncol Biol Phys 42:335-344, 1998.
163. Berek JS, Heaps JM, Fu YS, et al: Concurrent cisplatin and 5-fluorouracil chemotherapy and radiation therapy for advanced-stage squamous carcinoma of the vulva. Gynecol Oncol 42:197-201, 1991.
164. Carson LF, Twiggs LB, Adcock LL, et al: Multimodality therapy for advanced and recurrent vulvar squamous cell carcinoma. A pilot project. J Reprod Med 35:1029-1032, 1990.
165. Koh WJ, Wallace HJ 3rd, Greer BE, et al: Combined radiotherapy and chemotherapy in the management of local-regionally advanced vulvar cancer. Int J Radiat Oncol Biol Phys 26:809-816, 1993.
166. Russell AH, Mesic JB, Scudder SA, et al: Synchronous radiation and cytotoxic chemotherapy for locally advanced or recurrent squamous cancer of the vulva. Gynecol Oncol 47:14-20, 1992.
167. Scheistroen M, Trope C: Combined bleomycin and irradiation in preoperative treatment of advanced squamous cell carcinoma of the vulva. Acta Oncol 32:657-661, 1993.
168. Eifel PJ, Morris M, Burke TW, et al: Prolonged continuous infusion cisplatin and 5-fluorouracil with radiation for locally advanced carcinoma of the vulva. Gynecol Oncol 59:51-56, 1995.
169. Sebag-Montefiore DJ, McLean C, Arnott SJ, et al: Treatment of advanced carcinoma of the vulva with chemoradiotherapy—can exenterative surgery be avoided? Int J Gynecol Cancer 4:150-155, 1994.
170. Akl A, Akl M, Boike G, et al: Preliminary results of chemoradiation as a primary treatment for vulvar carcinoma. Int J Radiat Oncol Biol Phys 48:415-420, 2000.
171. Cunningham MJ, Goyer RP, Gibbons SK, et al: Primary radiation, cisplatin, and 5-fluorouracil for advanced squamous carcinoma of the vulva. Gynecol Oncol 66:258-261, 1997.
172. Landoni F, Maneo A, Zanetta G, et al: Concurrent preoperative chemotherapy with 5-fluorouracil and mitomycin C and radiotherapy (FUMIR) followed by limited surgery in locally advanced and recurrent vulvar carcinoma. Gynecol Oncol 61:321-327, 1996.
173. Lupi G, Raspagliesi F, Zucali R, et al: Combined preoperative chemoradiotherapy followed by radical surgery in locally advanced vulvar carcinoma. A pilot study. Cancer 77:1472-1478, 1996.
174. Evans LS, Kersch CR, Constable WC, Taylor PT: Concomitant 5-fluorouracil, mitomycin-C, and radiotherapy for advanced gynecologic malignancies. Int J Radiat Oncol Biol Phys 15:901-906, 1988.
175. Iversen T: Irradiation and bleomycin in the treatment of inoperable vulval carcinoma. Acta Obstet Gynecol Scand 61:195-197, 1982.
176. Kalra JK, Grossman AM, Krumholz BA, et al: Preoperative chemoradiotherapy for carcinoma of the vulva. Gynecol Oncol 12(Pt 1):256-260, 1981.
177. Whitaker SJ, Kirkbride P, Arnott SJ, et al: A pilot study of chemoradiotherapy in advanced carcinoma of the vulva. Br J Obstet Gynaecol 97:436-442, 1990.
178. Stehman FB, Bundy BN, Thomas G, et al: Groin dissection versus groin radiation in carcinoma of the vulva: a Gynecologic Oncology Group study. Int J Radiat Oncol Biol Phys 24:389-396, 1992.
179. Frankendal B, Larsson LG, Westling P: Carcinoma of the vulva. Results of an individualized treatment schedule. Acta Radiol Ther Phys Biol 12:165-174, 1973.
180. Perez CA, Grigsby PW, Galakatos A, et al: Radiation therapy in management of carcinoma of the vulva with emphasis on conservation therapy. Cancer 71:3707-3716, 1993.
181. Simonsen E, Nordberg UB, Johnsson JE, et al: Radiation therapy and surgery in the treatment of regional lymph nodes in squamous cell carcinoma of the vulva. Acta Radiol Oncol 23:433-442, 1984.
182. Lee WR, McCollough WM, Mendenhall WM, et al: Elective inguinal lymph node irradiation for pelvic carcinomas. The University of Florida experience. Cancer 72:2058-2065, 1993.
183. Manavi M, Berger A, Kucera E, et al: Does T1, N0-1 vulvar cancer treated by vulvectomy but not lymphadenectomy need inguinofemoral radiation? Int J Radiat Oncol Biol Phys 38:749-753, 1997.
184. Petereit DG, Mehta MP, Buchler DA, Kinsella TJ: Inguinofemoral radiation of N0,N1 vulvar cancer may be equivalent to lymphadenectomy if proper radiation technique is used. Int J Radiat Oncol Biol Phys 27:963-967, 1993.
185. Berman ML, Soper JT, Creasman WT, et al: Conservative surgical management of superficially invasive stage I vulvar carcinoma. Gynecol Oncol 35:352-357, 1989.
186. UK Coordinating Committee on Cancer Research: Epidermoid anal cancer: results from the UKCCCR randomised trial of radiotherapy alone versus radiotherapy, 5-fluorouracil, and mitomycin. UKCCCR Anal Cancer Trial Working Party. Lancet 348:1049-1054, 1996.
187. Bartelink H, Roelofsen F, Eschwege F, et al: Concomitant radiotherapy and chemotherapy is superior to radiotherapy alone in the treatment of locally advanced anal cancer: results of a phase III randomized trial of the European Organization for Research and Treatment of Cancer Radiotherapy and Gastrointestinal Cooperative Groups. J Clin Oncol 15:2040-2049, 1997.
188. Belinson JL, Stewart JA, Richard AL, McClure M: Bleomycin, vincristine, mitomycin-C, and cisplatin in the management of gynecological squamous cell carcinomas. Gynecol Oncol 20:387-393, 1985.
189. Benedetti-Panici P, Greggi S, Scambia G, et al: Cisplatin (P), bleomycin (B), and methotrexate (M) preoperative chemotherapy in locally advanced vulvar carcinoma. Gynecol Oncol 50:49-53, 1993.
190. Deppe G, Bruckner HW, Cohen CJ: Adriamycin treatment of advanced vulvar carcinoma. Obstet Gynecol 50(Suppl):13s-14s, 1977.
191. Deppe G, Cohen CJ, Bruckner HW: Chemotherapy of squamous cell carcinoma of the vulva: a review. Gynecol Oncol 7:345-348, 1979.
192. Durrant KR, Mangioni C, Lacave AJ, et al: Bleomycin, methotrexate, and CCNU in advanced inoperable squamous cell carcinoma of the vulva: a phase II study of the EORTC Gynaecological Cancer Cooperative Group (GCCG). Gynecol Oncol 37:359-362, 1990.
193. Huang GS, Juretzka M, Ciaravino G, et al: Liposomal doxorubicin for treatment of metastatic chemorefractory vulvar adenocarcinoma. Gynecol Oncol 87:313-318, 2002.
194. Shimizu Y, Hasumi K, Masubuchi K: Effective chemotherapy consisting of bleomycin, vincristine, mitomycin C, and cisplatin (BOMP) for a patient with inoperable vulvar cancer. Gynecol Oncol 36:423-427, 1990.
195. Srivannaboon S, Boonyanit S, Vatananusara C, Sophak P: A clinical trial of bleomycin on carcinoma of the vulva: a preliminary report. J Med Assoc Thai 56:101-108, 1973.
196. Wagenaar HC, Colombo N, Vergote I, et al: Bleomycin, methotrexate, and CCNU in locally advanced or recurrent, inoperable, squamous-cell carcinoma of the vulva: an EORTC Gynaecological Cancer Cooperative Group Study. European Organization for Research and Treatment of Cancer. Gynecol Oncol 81:348-354, 2001.
197. Thigpen JT, Blessing JA, Homesley HD, Lewis GC Jr: Phase II trials of cisplatin and piperazinedione in advanced or recurrent squamous cell carcinoma of the vulva: a Gynecologic Oncology Group Study. Gynecol Oncol 23:358-363, 1986.

198. Hopkins MP, Reid GC, Morley GW: The surgical management of recurrent squamous cell carcinoma of the vulva. Obstet Gynecol 75:1001-1005, 1990.
199. Grigsby PW, Roberts HL, Perez CA: Femoral neck fracture following groin irradiation. Int J Radiat Oncol Biol Phys 32:63-67, 1995.
200. Moran M, Lund MW, Ahmad M, et al: Improved treatment of pelvis and inguinal nodes using modified segmental boost technique: dosimetric evaluation. Int J Radiat Oncol Biol Phys 59:1523-1530, 2004.
201. Carlino G, Parisi S, Montemaggi P, Pastore G: Interstitial radiotherapy with Ir192 in vulvar cancer. Eur J Gynaecol Oncol 5:183-185, 1984.
202. Pao WM, Perez CA, Kuske RR, et al: Radiation therapy and conservation surgery for primary and recurrent carcinoma of the vulva: report of 40 patients and a review of the literature. Int J Radiat Oncol Biol Phys 14:1123-1132, 1988.
203. Guarischi A, Keane TJ, Elhakim T: Metastatic inguinal nodes from an unknown primary neoplasm: a review of 56 cases. Cancer 59:572-577, 1987.
204. Mulayim N, Foste-Silver D, Schwartz PE, Higgins S: Chemoradiation with 5-fluorouracil and mitomycin C in the treatment of vulvar squamous cell carcinoma. Gynecol Oncol 93:659-666, 2004.
205. Tebbutt NC, Norman AR, Cunningham D, et al: Analysis of the time course and prognostic factors determining toxicity due to infused fluorouracil. Br J Cancer 88:1510-1515, 2003.
206. Thomas G, Dembo A, Fyles A, et al: Concurrent chemoradiation in advanced cervical cancer. Gynecol Oncol 38:446-451, 1990.
207. Podratz KC, Gaffey TA, Symmonds RE, et al: Melanoma of the vulva: an update. Gynecol Oncol 16:153-168, 1983.
208. Verschraegen CF, Benjapibal M, Supakarapongkul W, et al: Vulvar melanoma at the M. D. Anderson Cancer Center: 25 years later. Int J Gynecol Cancer 11:359-364, 2001.
209. Davidson T, Kissin M, Westbury G: Vulvo-vaginal melanoma—should radical surgery be abandoned? Br J Obstet Gynaecol 94:473-476, 1987.
210. Trimble EL, Lewis JL Jr, Williams LL, et al: Management of vulvar melanoma. Gynecol Oncol 45:254-258, 1992.
211. Brand E, Fu YS, Lagasse LD, Berek JS: Vulvovaginal melanoma: report of seven cases and literature review. Gynecol Oncol 33:54-60, 1989.
212. Fenn ME, Abell MR: Melanomas of vulva and vagina. Obstet Gynecol 41:902-911, 1973.
213. Morrow CP, Rutledge FN: Melanoma of the vulva. Obstet Gynecol 39:745-752, 1972.
214. Cascinelli N, Di Re F, Lupi G, Balzarini GP: Malignant melanoma of the vulva. Tumori 56:345-352, 1970.
215. Phillips GL, Bundy BN, Okagaki T, et al: Malignant melanoma of the vulva treated by radical hemivulvectomy. A prospective study of the Gynecologic Oncology Group. Cancer 73:2626-2632, 1994.
216. Creasman WT, Phillips JL, Menck HR: The National Cancer Data Base report on cancer of the vagina. Cancer 83:1033-1040, 1988.
217. Beller U, Maisonneuve P, Benedet JL, et al: Carcinoma of the vagina. Int J Gynaecol Obstet 83(Suppl 1):27-39, 2003.
218. Daling JR, Madeleine MM, Schwartz SM, et al: A population-based study of squamous cell vaginal cancer: HPV and cofactors. Gynecol Oncol 84:263-270, 2002.
219. Herman JM, Homesley HD, Dignan MB: Is hysterectomy a risk factor for vaginal cancer? JAMA 256:601-603, 1986.
220. Lenehan PM, Meffe F, Lickrish GM: Vaginal intraepithelial neoplasia: biologic aspects and management. Obstet Gynecol 68:333-337, 1986.
221. Aho M, Vesterinen E, Meyer B, et al: Natural history of vaginal intraepithelial neoplasia. Cancer 68:195-197, 1991.
222. Benedet JL, Murphy KJ, Fairey RN, Boyes DA: Primary invasive carcinoma of the vagina. Obstet Gynecol 62:715-719, 1983.
223. Mazur MT, Hsueh S, Gersell DJ: Metastases to the female genital tract: analysis of 325 cases. Cancer 53:1978-1984, 1984.
224. Herbst AL, Scully RE: Adenocarcinoma of the vagina in adolescence: a report of 7 cases including 6 clear-cell carcinomas (so-called mesonephromas). Cancer 25:745-757, 1970.
225. Robboy SJ, Hill EC, Sandberg EC, Czernobilsky B: Vaginal adenosis in women born prior to the diethylstilbestrol era. Hum Pathol 17:488-492, 1986.
226. Robboy SJ, Scully RE, Herbst AL: Pathology of vaginal and cervical abnormalities associated with prenatal exposure to diethylstilbestrol (DES). J Reprod Med 15:13-18, 1975.
227. Robboy SJ, Welch WR, Young RH, et al: Topographic relation of cervical ectropion and vaginal adenosis to clear cell adenocarcinoma. Obstet Gynecol 60:546-551, 1982.
228. Robboy SJ, Young RH, Welch WR, et al: Atypical vaginal adenosis and cervical ectropion. Association with clear cell adenocarcinoma in diethylstilbestrol-exposed offspring. Cancer 54:869-875, 1984.
229. Herbst AL: Diethylstilbestrol and adenocarcinoma of the vagina. Am J Obstet Gynecol 181:1576-1578, discussion 1579, 1999.
230. Herbst AL, Ulfelder H, Poskanzer DC, Longo LD: Adenocarcinoma of the vagina. Association of maternal stilbestrol therapy with tumor appearance in young women. 1971. Am J Obstet Gynecol 181:1574-1575, 1999.
231. Melnick S, Cole P, Anderson D, Herbst A: Rates and risks of diethylstilbestrol-related clear-cell adenocarcinoma of the vagina and cervix. An update. N Engl J Med 316:514-516, 1987.
232. Fetters MD, Fischer G, Reed BD: Effectiveness of vaginal Papanicolaou smear screening after total hysterectomy for benign disease. JAMA 275:940-947, 1996.
233. Pearce KF, Haefner HK, Sarwar HF, Nolan TE: Cytopathological findings on vaginal Papanicolaou smears after hysterectomy for benign gynecologic disease. N Engl J Med 335:1559-1562, 1996.
234. Perez CA, Arneson AN, Galakatos A, Samanth HK: Malignant tumors of the vagina. Cancer 31:36-44, 1973.
235. Dodge JA, Eltabbakh GH, Mount SL, et al: Clinical features and risk of recurrence among patients with vaginal intraepithelial neoplasia. Gynecol Oncol 83:363-369, 2001.
236. Petrilli ES, Townsend DE, Morrow CP, Nakao CY: Vaginal intraepithelial neoplasia: biologic aspects and treatment with topical 5-fluorouracil and the carbon dioxide laser. Am J Obstet Gynecol 138:321-328, 1980.
237. Mock U, Kucera H, Fellner C, et al: High-dose-rate (HDR) brachytherapy with or without external beam radiotherapy in the treatment of primary vaginal carcinoma: long-term results and side effects. Int J Radiat Oncol Biol Phys 56:950-957, 2003.
238. Perez CA, Grigsby PW, Garipagaoglu M, et al: Factors affecting long-term outcome of irradiation in carcinoma of the vagina. Int J Radiat Oncol Biol Phys 44:37-45, 1999.
239. Teruya Y, Sakumoto K, Moromizato H, et al: High dose-rate intracavitary brachytherapy for carcinoma in situ of the vagina occurring after hysterectomy: a rational prescription of radiation dose. Am J Obstet Gynecol 187:360-364, 2002.
240. Tjalma WA, Monaghan JM, de Barros Lopes A, et al: The role of surgery in invasive squamous carcinoma of the vagina. Gynecol Oncol 81:360-365, 2001.
241. Chyle V, Zagard GK, Wheeler JA, et al: Definitive radiotherapy for carcinoma of the vagina: outcome and prognostic factors. Int J Radiat Oncol Biol Phys 35:891-905, 1996.
242. Reid GC, Schmidt RW, Roberts JA, et al: Primary melanoma of the vagina: a clinicopathologic analysis. Obstet Gynecol 74:190-199, 1989.
243. Weinstock MA: Malignant melanoma of the vulva and vagina in the United States: patterns of incidence and population-based estimates of survival. Am J Obstet Gynecol 171:1225-1230, 1994.
244. Frank SJ, Jhingran A, Levenback C, Eifel PJ: Definitive radiation therapy for squamous cell carcinoma of the vagina. Int J Radiat Oncol Biol Phys 62:138-147, 2005.
245. Kirkbride P, Fyles A, Rawlings GA, et al: Carcinoma of the vagina—experience at the Princess Margaret Hospital (1974-1989). Gynecol Oncol 56:435-443, 1995.
246. Dancuart F, Delclos L, Wharton JT, Silva EG: Primary squamous cell carcinoma of the vagina treated by radiotherapy: a failures analysis—the M. D. Anderson Hospital experience 1955-1982. Int J Radiat Oncol Biol Phys 14:745-749, 1988.
247. Perez CA, Camel HM, Galakatos AE, et al: Definitive irradiation in carcinoma of the vagina: long-term evaluation of results. Int J Radiat Oncol Biol Phys 15:1283-1290, 1988.

248. Chau PM, Green AE: Radiotherapeutic management of malignant tumors of the vagina. Prog Clin Cancer 10:728-750, 1965.
249. Yeh AM, Marcus RB Jr, Amdur RJ, et al: Patterns of failure in squamous cell carcinoma of the vagina treated with definitive radiotherapy alone: what is the appropriate treatment volume? Int J Cancer 96(Suppl):109-116, 2001.
250. Dalrymple JL, Russell AH, Lee SW, et al: Chemoradiation for primary invasive squamous carcinoma of the vagina. Int J Gynecol Cancer 14:110-117, 2004.
251. Deniaud-Alexandre E, Touboul E, Tiret E, et al: Results of definitive irradiation in a series of 305 epidermoid carcinomas of the anal canal. Int J Radiat Oncol Biol Phys 56:1259-1273, 2003.
252. Eifel PJ, Winter K, Morris M, et al: Pelvic irradiation with concurrent chemotherapy versus pelvic and para-aortic irradiation for high-risk cervical cancer: an update of radiation therapy oncology group trial (RTOG) 90-01. J Clin Oncol 22:872-880, 2004.
253. Lukka H, Hirte H, Fyles A, et al: Concurrent cisplatin-based chemotherapy plus radiotherapy for cervical cancer—a meta-analysis. Clin Oncol (R Coll Radiol) 14:203-212, 2002.
254. Peters WA 3rd, Liu PY, Barrett RJ 2nd, et al: Concurrent chemotherapy and pelvic radiation therapy compared with pelvic radiation therapy alone as adjuvant therapy after radical surgery in high-risk early-stage cancer of the cervix. J Clin Oncol 18:1606-1613, 2000.
255. Bertoni F, Bertoni G, Bignardi M: Vaginal molds for intracavitary curietherapy: a new method of preparation. Int J Radiat Oncol Biol Phys 9:1579-1582, 1983.
256. Gupta AK, Vicini FA, Frazier AJ, et al: Iridium-192 transperineal interstitial brachytherapy for locally advanced or recurrent gynecological malignancies. Int J Radiat Oncol Biol Phys 43:1055-1060, 1999.
257. Tewari KS, Cappuccini F, Puthawala AA, et al: Primary invasive carcinoma of the vagina: treatment with interstitial brachytherapy. Cancer 91:758-770, 2001.
258. Greer BE, Koh WJ, Figge DC, et al: Gynecologic radiotherapy fields defined by intraoperative measurements. Gynecol Oncol 38:421-424, 1990.
259. McAlpine J, Schlaerth JB, Lim P, et al: Radiation fields in gynecologic oncology: correlation of soft tissue (surgical) to radiologic landmarks. Gynecol Oncol 92:25-30, 2004.
260. Peters WA 3rd, Kumar NB, Morley GW, et al: Primary sarcoma of the adult vagina: a clinicopathologic study. Obstet Gynecol 65:699-704, 1985.
261. Curtin JP, Saigo P, Slucher B, et al: Soft-tissue sarcoma of the vagina and vulva: a clinicopathologic study. Obstet Gynecol 86:269-272, 1995.
262. Andrassy RJ, Hays DM, Raney RB, et al: Conservative surgical management of vaginal and vulvar pediatric rhabdomyosarcoma: a report from the Intergroup Rhabdomyosarcoma Study III. J Pediatr Surg 30:1034-1036, discussion 1036-1037, 1995.
263. Hanselaar A, van Loosbroek M, Schuurbiers O, et al: Clear cell adenocarcinoma of the vagina and cervix. An update of the central Netherlands registry showing twin age incidence peaks. Cancer 79:2229-2236, 1997.
264. Waggoner SE, Mittendorf R, Biney N, et al: Influence of in utero diethylstilbestrol exposure on the prognosis and biologic behavior of vaginal clear-cell adenocarcinoma. Gynecol Oncol 55:238-244, 1994.
265. Herbst AL, Norusis MJ, Rosenow PJ, et al: An analysis of 346 cases of clear cell adenocarcinoma of the vagina and cervix with emphasis on recurrence and survival. Gynecol Oncol 7:111-122, 1979.
266. Fishman DA, Williams S, Small W Jr, et al: Late recurrences of vaginal clear cell adenocarcinoma. Gynecol Oncol 62:128-132, 1996.

CHAPTER 58

OVARIAN CANCER

Higinia Cardenes and Jeanne Schilder

INCIDENCE AND ETIOLOGY

Epithelial ovarian cancer (EOC) accounts for 4% of all cancer diagnosis and 5% of all cancer deaths in the United States (U.S.). An estimated 20,180 women will be diagnosed with ovarian cancer in the U.S. in 2006 and 15,310 will die of the disease.

Epidemiologic studies have identified hormonal, environmental, and genetic factors in ovarian carcinogenesis.

PREVENTION AND EARLY DETECTION

Women at increased risk for EOC are best identified by an adequate family history and genetic testing.

Available data indicate that the optimal management of women with familial ovarian cancer syndrome with *BRCA1/2* mutations is prophylactic bilateral oophorectomy.

BIOLOGIC CHARACTERISTICS

Common epithelial tumors account for 60% of all ovarian tumors and 80% to 90% of EOCs.

FIGO stage, histologic subtype and grade, surgical staging, and extent of residual disease after debulking surgery are the most significant prognostic factors.

STAGING EVALUATION

Approximately 70% of patients have advanced EOC (stage III-IV) at diagnosis.

Diagnosis and evaluation of the extent of ovarian cancer require a thorough evaluation, including an adequate history and physical examination, computed tomography (CT) or radiography, and laboratory studies, to elucidate potential sites of disease.

Surgery is crucial in the diagnosis, accurate staging, and optimal cytoreduction of EOC.

PRIMARY THERAPY

The *goal of surgery* is to establish the diagnosis, determine the extent of the disease, and obtain optimal cytoreduction. Unilateral salpingo-oophorectomy may be considered for a patient with stage IA disease who desires to preserve fertility after comprehensive surgical staging confirms no evidence of extraovarian disease.

Recommendations regarding management of patients with incompletely staged EOC remain controversial. Patients with stage IA-B, grade 1 EOC should undergo complete surgical staging, because no adjuvant therapy is required if the stage is confirmed. Patients with EOC more advanced than stage IA-B, grade 1 can be offered second-look laparotomy to complete surgical staging or adjuvant chemotherapy (e.g., six cycles of cisplatin-based chemotherapy). If residual disease is suspected, complete surgical staging and debulking is recommended in all cases.

ADJUVANT THERAPY

Completely staged low-risk patients (i.e., stages IA-IB, grade 1, and perhaps grade 2 disease) do not require adjuvant therapy because 5-year survival rate after complete surgical staging is greater than 90%.

Patients with more advanced stages I-II or poorly differentiated (or aneuploid) tumors require adjuvant therapy because the 5-year survival is 70% to 80%, with a relapse rate of 25% to 40%.

The best adjuvant therapy for the intermediate- and high-risk groups remains to be defined, although the trend, based on the results of two European trials (ACTION and ICON), is to treat them with *systemic chemotherapy* (i.e., cisplatin or carboplatin and paclitaxel) for a total of three to six cycles.

The *role of radiation therapy* (intraperitoneal radioactive phosphorus 32 [^{32}P] or whole-abdomen irradiation [WAI]) has been limited since the introduction of cisplatin and taxane chemotherapy.

ADVANCED DISEASE

Adjuvant chemotherapy is recommended for all patients with advanced-stage EOC after appropriate cytoreductive surgery. The preferred regimen is a combination of carboplatin and paclitaxel for a total of six cycles.

Long-term survival for patients with advanced disease ranges from 60% for stage IIIA to 30% for stage IIIC and less than 20% for stage IV. More than 70% of patients experience disease relapse, with a median time to progression of less than 2 years. Maintenance and consolidation chemotherapy (systemic and intraperitoneal) have not improved survival.

Selection of second-line chemotherapy at relapse depends on whether the patient is sensitive or resistant to initial platinum-containing adjuvant chemotherapy. No standard chemotherapy regimen is considered to be the treatment of choice for recurrent EOC.

The *role of secondary surgery* for advanced-stage EOC remains controversial. For patients with optimally cytoreduced disease at diagnosis, in the absence of randomized data demonstrating a survival benefit, there is no defined role for second-look laparotomy (SLL) after definitive primary therapy. If optimal cytoreduction is not performed initially, SLL appears to confer a benefit in terms of overall survival and disease-free survival based on a European randomized trial.

Secondary cytoreductive surgery at the time of relapse is of limited value in light of data indicating prolonged survival with the currently available salvage chemotherapy.

RADIATION THERAPY (RT)

The results of sequential WAI for consolidation and salvage have been disappointing, probably because of inadequate patient selection.

Results of a prospective, randomized trial suggest that WAI may be an option for consolidation RT in selected subgroups of patients with complete pathologic response after adjuvant chemotherapy, but there is no benefit for consolidation WAI in patients with residual disease.

Patients with chemotherapy-refractory EOC may have prolonged survival after salvage RT, particularly those with minimal residual or relapsed disease limited to the pelvis. The relapse-free survival rates at 3 to 4 years have been between 30% and 50% in selected series.

Randomized data have failed to show benefit for consolidation therapy using intraperitoneal ^{32}P in terms of tumor relapse and survival.

PALLIATION

Surgery is usually is limited to debulking of large masses to improve patients' symptoms and quality of life and to relieve intestinal obstruction.

Several chemotherapy agents are available for second- and third-line treatment of recurrent or metastatic EOC. The response rates range from 14% to 30%, and the duration of response usually is on the order of 6 months or less.

Radiation therapy may improve local abdominopelvic symptoms in 50% to 70% of patients. Irradiation also offers good palliation in patients with brain metastasis, and the effect usually is maintained until death for about 70% of patients.

Patients who progress after several chemotherapy and irradiation regimens without evidence of clinical benefit should be carefully evaluated for potential clinical trials or the best supportive care.

Epithelial ovarian cancer (EOC) is the leading cause of death among women with gynecologic malignancies, and it is the fifth most common cancer in women in the United States.[1] Ovarian cancer is overall the fourth most common cause of cancer death in females, behind lung, breast, and colorectal cancer. On the basis of distinct clinical and pathologic features, EOC can be separated into three major entities: epithelial carcinomas (>90%), germ cell tumors, and sex cord-stromal carcinomas.

Unfortunately, only one third of patients with epithelial EOC present with stage I or II, whereas more than 70% of the patients with EOC have stage III or IV at the time of diagnosis. With the introduction of platinum compounds in the late 1970s and the introduction of paclitaxel in the early 1990s, response rates to chemotherapy increased significantly.[2] After almost 15 years of experience with these drugs, there has been only a moderate improvement in the overall 5-year survival (37% in 1970s versus 52% in 1990s), primarily due to more adequate surgical cytoreduction and the introduction of cisplatin-based adjuvant therapy.[1,3] However, although response to initial therapy is expected, most patients eventually develop progressive disease or relapse and die of their disease.

In the past two decades, major efforts have been directed toward increased understanding of potential risk factors involved in ovarian carcinogenesis, including genetic risk; surgical procedures have been refined and therapeutics strategies extensively evaluated in an attempt to improve outcome among women with EOC.

EPIDEMIOLOGY AND ETIOLOGY

Epidemiology

It has been estimated that 20,180 new cases of ovarian cancer will be diagnosed and 15,310 deaths are expected in the United States in 2006, representing 4% of all cancer diagnosis and 5% of all female cancer deaths.[1] Incidence rates, which have remained relatively stable over the past 20 years, are higher in white compared with black women. Black women in the United States have a lower incidence ($10.3/10^5$ women) compared with white women ($13–15/10^5$),[4] but both have similar stage distribution and stage-specific 5-year survival rates.[1,3] The cumulative probabilities of developing or dying from EOC among U.S. women are 1.4% and 0.7%, respectively, by age 80.[5] Most EOC is diagnosed in postmenopausal women, with a median age at diagnosis of 63 years. The incidence of EOC rises with increasing age and peaks in the eighth decade, after which the rate plateaus.[1] Data from the Surveillance, Epidemiology and End Results (SEER) Program of the National Cancer Institute (NCI) indicate that EOC is infrequent in women younger than 40 years old. The age-specific incidence increases from $15/10^5$ in the 40 to 44 age group to a peak rate of $57/10^5$ in the 70 to 74 age group.[4]

Overall, there has been little change in EOC mortality in the last quarter century.[1] During the same period, some authors have found an increasing EOC mortality rate in women older than 65 years compared with younger women. Estimated 5-year survival of 66% and 33% for women younger and older than 65 years, respectively, have been reported by Harlan and colleagues.[6] Similarly, women older than 65 years with advanced EOC have a worse prognosis than younger patients (13% and 45% 5-year survival, respectively).[6] Although the mortality rate has not changed significantly, there has been an improvement in 5-year relative survival rates among whites and blacks, from 37% and 41% in 1974 to 1976 to 40% and 42% for the period of 1983 to 1985 and 52% in 1992 to 1999, respectively, by race and year of diagnosis.[1]

Etiology

Although the molecular events leading to the development of EOC are unknown, several epidemiologic studies have identified hormonal, environmental, and genetic factors as playing an important role in ovarian carcinogenesis. The pathogenetic mechanisms explaining the link between these risk factors and the development of EOC have not been determined. A history of pregnancy with an age at first birth of 25 years or younger, multiple births, tubal ligation, history of breast feeding, and the use of oral contraception appear to reduce the risk for developing EOC by 30% to 60%.[7] Conversely, nulliparity or age at first birth of older than 35 years confers an increased risk. In the World Health Organization (WHO) study, the relative risk of EOC in women who had used oral contraceptives was 0.75,[8] and it was further decreased with longer duration of use. However, EOC risk appears to be increased among women who have undergone infertility treatment, particularly for borderline tumors.[9] Postmenopausal estrogen replacement therapy may also increase the risk for EOC, although conflicting findings have been published. From the published data, it seems that the prolonged use of unopposed estrogens versus combined estrogen-progestin therapy may be associated with increased risk for EOC.[10,11] Additionally, the increased risk for EOC in patients with history of breast cancer and vice versa, provides further evidence of the influence of hormonal factors in the etiology of EOC.[12]

A positive family history is the single most important risk factor for the development of EOC. It is clinically useful to separate genetic risk into familial and hereditary EOC. Women with a single family member affected by EOC have a 4% to 5% risk, whereas those with two affected family members have a 7% risk for developing EOC. In contrast, women with hereditary EOC syndrome, defined as having at least two first-degree relatives with EOC, have a lifetime probability as high as 25% to 50% of developing the disease. However, fewer than 10% of cases can be classified as hereditary EOC.

EOC is more common in industrialized countries. Multiple other possible risk factors have been explored. Although there are some reports indicating a relationship between obesity and risk for EOC, the role of a particular diet, consumption of coffee and smoking, and industrial exposure to carcinogens or to diagnostic and therapeutic radiation has not been clearly established. There are some conflicting reports regarding the association of the use of talc powder and the development of EOC.

PREVENTION AND EARLY DETECTION

Screening

Survival of patients with EOC is primarily influenced by the stage of the disease at diagnosis. Unfortunately, only one fourth of women with epithelial EOC present with localized disease, and despite the good prognosis associated with early-stage disease, overall 5-year survival in women with EOC is less than 35%, in large part because of the presence of advanced disease at the time of diagnosis in 75% of patients. Therefore, there is significant interest in evaluating potential screening methods that would allow the diagnosis of EOC in an earlier phase of development and therefore with potentially more curable stages of the disease.

By definition, a good screening test should be accurate, simple, inexpensive, and safe, and, more importantly, it should result in a decrease in disease-specific mortality. Currently, there is no reliable, cost-effective screening test for EOC that satisfies these criteria. This is probably related partially to the fact that neither the natural history nor the etiology of this disease is clearly understood, unlike cervical cancer. There is no direct evidence for a premalignant lesion in EOC; no experimental data exist to suggest that a benign ovarian cyst can progress to a borderline tumor that can lead to an invasive carcinoma.

A number of screening strategies have been investigated, in particular pelvic examination, transvaginal sonography, CA 125 (cancer antigen derived from the coelomic epithelium), or a combination of any of them. However, these are not sufficiently accurate for general screening and are limited by their sensitivity and specificity. Hogg and Friedlander,[13] after a thorough review of the literature, demonstrated the lack of conclusive data supporting a reduction in mortality rate with the use of screening for EOC either in the general population or among genetically high-risk groups.

None of the North American expert groups recommends routine screening for EOC. The National Cancer Institute has made the following recommendation: "There is insufficient evidence to establish that screening for ovarian cancer with serum markers such as CA 125 levels, transvaginal ultrasound, or pelvic examinations would result in a decrease in the mortality from ovarian cancer (levels of evidence 4, 5)." There is good evidence that screening for ovarian cancer with the tests mentioned would result in more diagnostic laparoscopies and laparotomies than new ovarian cancers found, and unnecessary oophorectomies may also result.[14] Screening procedures, such as CA-125 testing and ultrasonography, were recommended only for women with a presumed hereditary cancer syndrome. The U.S. Preventive Service Task Force, the American College of Physicians, the American College of Obstetricians and Gynecologists, and the Canadian Task Force on the Periodic Health Examination all recommend against routine screening for EOC in asymptomatic women, despite pressure from patient-advocacy groups.

Several large ovarian-cancer screening trials are currently in progress. The National Cancer Institute's Prostate, Lung, Colon, Ovarian Cancer (PLCO) trial compares screening with annual CA-125 measurement, transvaginal ultrasound, and pelvic examination to usual medical care in 76,000 women aged 60 through 74, with the participants in the study followed for 10 years.[15] A European multicentric study headquartered at St. Bartholomew's Hospital in London will evaluate 120,000 postmenopausal women randomized to receive no screening or screening with transvaginal ultrasound followed by color flow Doppler examinations in women with abnormal transvaginal ultrasounds. Serial CA 125 levels will be used to determine which participants should proceed to color flow Doppler examination.

Studies are also in progress to identify more sensitive tumor markers. Macrophage colony-stimulating factor (M-CSF) has been detected in epithelial ovarian tumors and in 70% of the serum or ascites of patients with diagnosed carcinoma.[16] Similarly, OVX-1 is a newly developed antibody that may also complement CA-125.[17] A panel of CA-125, M-CSF, and OVX-1 was shown to identify early-stage EOC with extremely high sensitivity and moderate specificity in preliminary studies.[18] It is hoped that in the near future, genomics and proteomics technology may be proved effective tools for EOC screening.

Currently, the only method available to identify women who are at increased risk for EOC is by an adequate family history and genetic testing. The American Society of Clinical Oncology (ASCO) has made a recommendation for genetic testing to be performed in patients with personal or family history that is suggestive of a genetic cancer susceptibility condition, if the test can be adequately interpreted and if the results will aid in diagnosis or influence the medical or surgical management of the patient or family members who are at hereditary risk for cancer.

The optimal management strategy for a woman with an inherited susceptibility to EOC but no overt cancer is unclear. Although close surveillance and screening with transvaginal sonography and CA-125 levels are frequently used in women who are at high risk for hereditary EOC, there is no clear evidence of its utility in decreasing mortality.[19] The National Institutes of Health Consensus Development Panel on Ovarian Cancer[14] and the American College of Obstetricians and Gynecologists[20] have recommended that prophylactic bilateral oophorectomies (PBO) should be strongly considered in women with hereditary EOC who are older than 35 years or who do not intend to bear any more children. However, the Cancer Genetics Consortium reviewed the same information and concluded that the evidence is insufficient to recommend for or against it.[21] Prophylactic bilateral oophorectomy does not completely eliminate the risk for developing primary peritoneal carcinomatosis in women with hereditary risks for EOC. On the other hand, patients with *BRCA1* and *BRCA2* mutations are obviously at risk for both breast and EOC, and the recommendations regarding prophylactic surgery to the breasts and ovaries are very challenging for patients when both risks are considered together.

The currently available data seem to indicate that currently the optimal management for women with familial ovarian cancer syndromes with *BRCA 1/2* mutations is a PBO, because this approach has been shown to reduce mortality among these high-risk patients.[22] However, women should be counseled that they may be at some risk for the development of peritoneal serous papillary carcinomatosis, even in the presence of histologically normal ovaries.[23] Oral contraceptives have also been shown to decrease the incidence of EOC among this high-risk population.[24] A multicenter prospective evaluation of the role of PBO in high-risk individuals is in progress, conducted by the Gynecologic Oncology Group (GOG #199) titled "Prospective Screening Study of Risk Reducing Salpingo-Oophorectomy (RRSO) and Longitudinal CA 125 Screening in Participants at Increased Genetic Risk of Ovarian Cancer." Eligible women will be older than 30, and have at least one intact ovary, documented deleterious *BRCA 1 / 2* mutation, or a first- or second-degree relative with the mutation, as well as women with family history of at least two ovarian and/or breast cancers among first- or second-degree relatives, or women with breast cancer diagnosed prior to menopause (or equals 50 years of age if menopause unknown).

BIOLOGIC CHARACTERISTICS/ MOLECULAR BIOLOGY

The two most relevant clinical syndromes associated with hereditary EOC have been identified. The hereditary breast-ovarian cancer syndrome (HBEOC) is the most common of these and accounts for 85% to 90% of all hereditary ovarian cancer cases currently identified.[25] Most of these tumors are associated with mutations of the *BRCA1* locus (17q21). A second breast-ovarian cancer susceptibility gene, *BRCA2*, has been localized to chromosome 13q12.[26] The lifetime risk for EOC for a woman with a *BRCA1* mutation is approximately 30% to 60%, although some estimates are as high as 85%,[27] whereas for patients with *BRCA2* mutations, estimates are 10% to 20%.[28] Female carriers of *BRCA1* mutations also have a risk for fallopian tube carcinoma that is 50 to 120 times that of the general population as well as marked increase in the risk for peritoneal cancer.[29] Hereditary EOC is also a component of the hereditary nonpolyposis colorectal cancer syndrome (HNPCC),[30] an autosomal dominant disorder associated with defects in the genes responsible for DNA mismatch repair, also known as Lynch syndrome II.[31] This syndrome includes a high predisposition to site-specific colorectal cancer as well as an increased risk for several other cancers, including endometrial, ovarian, gastric, and upper urinary tract. The cumulative risk for EOC by age 70 among persons with mutations in one of the mismatch repair genes is approximately 12%.[32] Most EOCs associated with germline mutations of *BRCA1* are serous adenocarcinomas, with an average age at diagnosis of 48 years. *BRCA1*-associated cancer may have a more favorable outcome than sporadic EOC,[33] probably related to a higher cisplatin sensitivity of these tumors. A large, prospective study is currently in progress by the GOG to compare the clinical course of sporadic EOC with that associated with *BRCA1* and *BRCA2* mutations.

A statistically significant reduction in ovarian and breast cancer risk after oophorectomy when compared to the control cohort has been reported by Rebbeck and colleagues.[34] Oral contraceptives may reduce the risk for EOC in women with *BRCA1* or *BRCA2* gene mutations.[35]

Other genetic abnormalities reported in ovarian cancer include mutations in the *p53* gene, altered *c-myc*, *H-ras*, and *K-ras*, and overexpression of epidermal growth factor receptor (EGFR) as the most frequent findings. The prognostic significant of these abnormalities is still unclear.

Prognostic Factors

The most significant prognostic factors in EOC include Federation of Gynecology and Obstetrics (FIGO) stage, histologic subtype and grade, and, in early-stage tumor, excrescences on the ovarian surface, intraoperative rupture of the capsule, bilaterality, and the presence of dense ovarian adhesions. Surgical prognostic factors include the presence of a large-volume malignant ascites, and volume of residual disease after cytoreductive surgery.[36] Tumor stage remains the most important prognostic variable. GOG data have shown that comprehensively assessed stage IA patients with well- or moderately differentiated tumors have a greater than 90% 5-year survival rate, whereas patients with unfavorable prognosis early-stage EOC have a 5-year survival rate of approximately 80%.[36] Patients with stage III disease have a 5-year survival rate of approximately 15% to 20% that is dependent in large part on the volume of disease present in the upper abdomen,[37] whereas patients with stage IV disease have less than a 5% 5-year survival. Tumor size, bilaterality, and cytologically negative ascites have no prognostic significance in advanced disease.

Volume of residual disease after cytoreductive surgery has a significant impact on survival; patients who have been optimally debulked have a 22-month improvement in median survival compared to those undergoing suboptimal cytoreductive surgery.[37] It is hard to determine how much of this is related directly to the natural history of the disease, i.e., tumor "aggressiveness," and how much incremental benefit accrues from surgical debulking. Although no prospective data exist to prove a benefit of "maximal surgical effort," theories surrounding tumor growth as well as nonrandomized studies support this practice. Griffiths[38] reported results of 102 patients with stage II and III disease treated with melphalan following primary debulking surgery. Median survival was 39 months in those with no gross residual disease, 29 months with residual tumor less than 0.5 cm, 18 months if residual disease was between 0.6 and 1.5 cm, and 11 months when it was greater than 1.5 cm.[38] Total volume of residual disease measured in cubic centimeters has not been found to differ from the volume of the single largest residual mass.[39] Prognosis is often measured in terms of "optimal" versus "suboptimal" debulking. The GOG study reported by Hoskins and colleagues[37] showed a significant progression-free and survival advantage in patients with stage III disease that was cytoreduced to 1 cm or less,[37] but optimal is no overt residuum —that is, presumed "microscopic only." This study also demonstrated that optimal cytoreduction in those patients who present with large-volume disease does not confer the same prognosis as that for patients initially found to have small-volume disease.[37] Additionally, they have shown that the number of residual lesions remaining after cytoreductive surgery as well as the site of disease in the abdomen and degree of omental involvement may be predictors of the extent and aggressiveness of the disease.[37,39] More recently, Chi and colleagues[40] found a significant 5-year survival advantage for patients without residual disease (50%), compared to those with residual disease of 1 to 2 cm (28%) and those with greater than 2 cm (21%). Despite variations in this definition of optimal debulking, the GOG currently defines optimal debulking as residual disease of less than 1 cm.

The true prognostic impact of histologic subtype and grade in patients with EOC remains to be determined. It seems to be particularly important in patients with early-stage EOC, as indicated earlier.[36,41,42] Cell type has less prognostic significance than grade. In advanced-stage patients, mucinous and clear-cell histologies have been shown to have an adverse prognostic significance.[37,42]

Serum CA-125 levels generally reflect the volume of disease and, therefore, in multivariate analysis, preoperative levels have not been found to be an independent prognostic factor for survival.[43] However, postoperative CA-125 levels appear to have greater prognostic significance, independent of the amount of residual disease, primarily in determining the probability of a patient achieving a complete remission after adjuvant chemotherapy.[44]

A number of biologic factors with prognostic significance have been identified. Some investigators have found aneuploidy to be a significant prognostic factor in their selection of high-risk early-stage EOC patients for adjuvant therapy.[45] In the GOG, aneuploidy has not been included as a criterion for risk in early-stage disease. Molecular factors with potential prognostic significance in EOC include abnormalities in oncogene products (HER-2-neu, p20),[46] suppressor gene products (p53, p16, pRB), and markers of proliferation (DNA index, S-fraction, KI-67 index, proliferating cell nuclear antigen). There have been a number of reports regarding measures of drug sensitivity (PgP, BAX) or drug resistance (MDR1), DNA repair, and serum cytokine levels (interleukin-6). Additionally, there are contradictory reports regarding the prognostic significance of EGFR,[46] cyclooxygenase (COX)-2 expression,[47] genes associated with tumor invasion, and metastases (microvessel density and presence of vascular endothelial growth factor [VEGF]).[48] However, most of these factors have been identified in retrospective studies and have significant shortcomings, owing to their subjectivity, lack of reproducibility, and low prognostic power. Currently, none of these markers is routinely used to select therapy for patients with EOC or to accurately predict outcome.

PATHOLOGY AND PATHWAYS OF SPREAD

Pathogenesis

The common epithelial tumors are by far the most frequent, accounting for 60% of all ovarian tumors and for 80% to 90% of EOC. The remaining tumors arise from germ or stromal cells. The exact cell of origin of EOC is not known, nor has a premalignant precursor lesion of the ovary been identified. The EOC arises from the embryologic derivatives of the surface epithelium, or serosa, of the ovary. During embryogenesis, the coelomic cavity forms with a mesothelial lining of cells of mesodermal origin, and the gonadal ridge is covered by serosal epithelium. Müllerian ducts, which give rise to the fallopian tubes, uterus, and vagina, are the result of invagination of the mesothelial lining. As the ovary develops, the surface epithelium extends into the ovarian stroma to form inclusion glands and cysts. Therefore, when the epithelium becomes malignant, it can exhibit a variety of müllerian-type cell differentiations: serous carcinomas can resemble the fallopian tube; mucinous tumors resemble the endocervix; endometrioid carcinomas, the endometrium, and clear cell tumors—glycogen-rich cells—can resemble endometrial glands in pregnancy. Germ cell tumors are derived from primordial germ cells which undergo defective meiosis. The intraovarian matrix that supports the germ cells and is covered by the surface epithelium consists of cells originating from the sex cords and mesenchyma of the embryonic gonad, from which derive the sex cord–stromal tumors.

Histologic Classification of Common Epithelial Tumors

Table 58-1 shows the classification of common epithelial tumors developed by the WHO, FIGO, the International Society of Gynecologic Pathologists, and the Society of Gynecologic Oncologists (SGO).[49] This classification is based on cell type, location of the tumor, and degree of malignancy, including benign epithelial tumors and tumors of low malignant potential to invasive carcinomas.

Patients with tumors of *low malignant potential* ("borderline tumor") (LMP) are generally younger than the ones with frankly malignant tumors, and have an excellent prognosis. LMP represent approximately 10% of ovarian neoplasms and include a heterogeneous group of lesions defined histologically by atypical epithelial proliferation without apparent stromal invasion. The differentiation between LMP and carcinomas is primarily made on the architectural basis of invasion, pushing borders versus destructive invasion, respectively, rather than on a cytologic basis. The presence of foci of microinvasion up to 3 mm in the stroma, often with associated desmoplastic reaction, does not seem to alter the excellent prognosis of LMP tumors.

The *invasive epithelial carcinomas* are uncommon in women younger than age 35 years, and generally present as solid or mixed masses with areas of necrosis and hemorrhage, often with extensive intraperitoneal disease. These tumors are characterized by histologic type and grade.

Serous tumors account for almost half of all common EOC, of which approximately one third are malignant. Mucinous tumors represent one third of common EOC, of which only approximately 5% are malignant; the great majority are benign. Endometrioid tumors represent only 8% of EOC, and most of them are malignant. Clear-cell tumors are very uncommon (3%) and often associated with endometriosis; most of them are malignant. Other histologic types are very uncommon.

Pathways of Spread

EOC arises from the surface epithelium of the ovary, and early in the natural history of the disease it is characterized by cystic growths within epithelial inclusion cysts within the stroma of the ovary. Subsequently, the tumor penetrates through the capsule, causing exfoliation of malignant cells throughout the peritoneal cavity. The normal circulation of the peritoneal fluid up the right paracolic gutter, along the intestinal mesentery, to the undersurface of the right hemidiaphragm and omentum, facilitates the widespread dissemination and implantation of tumor cells throughout the peritoneal cavity. Papillary serous tumors have a much greater incidence of extraovarian spread than do mucinous tumors, which tend to remain confined to the ovary and often become very large (18–20 cm). There can also be direct extension of the tumor from the ovary to involve the peritoneal surfaces of the bladder, rectosigmoid, and pelvic peritoneum.

A second pattern of spread is via the retroperitoneal lymphatics that drain the ovary. Lymphatic drainage occurs following the ovarian blood supply in the infundibulopelvic ligament to lymph nodes around the aorta and vena cava to the level of the renal vessels, as well as lymphatics through the broad ligament and parametrial channels to the pelvic wall nodal regions (external iliac, obturator, and hypogastric).

Table 58-1 WHO Classification of Tumors of the Ovary

COMMON EPITHELIAL TUMORS
Serous
- Adenocarcinoma
- Surface papillary adenocarcinoma
- Adenocarcinofibroma (malignant adenofibroma)

Mucinous
- Adenocarcinoma
- Adenenocarcinofibroma (malignant adenofibroma)
- Mucinous cystic tumor with mural nodules
- Mucinous cystic tumor with pseudomyxoma peritonei

Endometrioid (including variants with squamous differentiation)
- Adenocarcinoma NOS
- Adenocarcinofibroma (malignant adenofibroma)
- Malignant müllerian mixed tumor (carcinosarcoma)
- Adenosarcoma
- Endometrioid stromal sarcoma
- Undifferentiated ovarian sarcoma

Clear cell (mesonephroid)
- Adenocarcinoma
- Adenocarcinofibroma (malignant adenofibroma)

Transitional cell tumors
Squamous cell tumors
Mixed epithelial tumors (specific components)
Undifferentiated and unclassified tumors

SEX CORD—STROMAL TUMORS

Granulosa-stromal cell tumors
- Granulosa cell tumor group
- Thecoma-fibroma group
- Fibroma
- Cellular fibroma
- Fibrosarcoma
- Stromal tumor with minor sex-cord elements
- Sclerosing stromal tumor
- Signet-ring stromal tumor
- Unclassified (fibrothecoma)

Sertoli-stromal cell tumors
- Sertoli-Leydig cell tumor group (androblastoma)
- Sertoli cell tumor
- Stromal-Leydig cell tumor

Sex cord-stromal tumors of mixed or unclassified cell types
- Sex-cord tumor with annular tubules
- Gynandroblastoma (specify components)
- Sex cord-stromal tumor, unclassified

Steroid cell tumors
- Leydig cell tumor group
- Steroid cell tumor, NOS

GERM CELL TUMORS

Primitive germ cell tumors
- Dysgerminoma
- Yolk sac tumor
- Embryonal carcinoma
- Polyembryoma
- Nongestational choriocarcinoma
- Mixed germ cell tumor (specify components)

Byphasic or triphasic teratoma
- Immature teratoma
- Mature teratoma

Monodermal teratoma and somatic type tumors associated with dermoid cysts
- Thyroid tumor group: Struma ovarii: benign or malignant
- Carcinoid group
- Neuroectodermal tumor group
- Carcinoma group
- Melanocytic group
- Sarcoma group
- Sebaceous tumor group
- Pituitary type tumor group
- Retinal anlage tumor group
- Others

NOS, not otherwise specified.
From Tavassoli FA, Devilee P (eds), for the International Agency for Research on Cancer (IARC): WHO Classification of Tumors: Pathology and Genetics of Tumors of the Breast and Female Genital Organs. Lyon, IARC Press, 2003, p 114.

More rarely, spread may occur along the round ligament, resulting in involvement of inguinal lymph nodes. Lymph node metastasis is correlated with the stage of the disease. Approximately 10% to 15% of patients with ovarian cancer that appears to be confined to the ovaries have metastases to para-aortic lymph nodes, whereas nodal metastases occur in most cases of advanced EOC.[50] Many patients whose tumors appear confined to the pelvis have occult metastatic disease in the pelvic or retroperitoneal nodes or in the upper abdomen.

Young and colleagues[41] published the results of a cooperative national study in which 100 patients with a diagnosis of "early" (stage Ia-IIb) EOC referred to the Ovarian Cancer Study Group underwent systematic restaging. Almost one third of the patients (31%) believed to have stage I or II disease at the time of the initial surgery were upstaged following a second, surgical staging procedure, and 77% of the upstaged patients were found to have stage III disease. Sites of unsuspected disease were most likely to be peritoneal washings/ascites fluid, periaortic nodes, pelvic peritoneum and other pelvic tissues, omentum, and diaphragm. Tables 58-2 and 58-3 illustrate the results of restaging laparotomy in early EOC.[41]

Table 58-2 Results of Restaging Laparotomy in "Early"-Stage (Ia-IIb) Epithelial Ovarian Cancer

Initial Stage	Patients (*N*)	Upstaged (%)
IA	37	16
IB	10	30
IC	2	0
IIA	4	100
IIB	38	39
IIC	9	33
Total	100	31/100 = 31

Upstaged to Stage III: 31/31.
From Young RC, Decker DG, Wharton JT, et al: Staging laparotomy in early ovarian cancer. JAMA 250:3072-3076, 1983.

Table 58-3 Sites of Disease in 31 Upstaged Patients

Site	Biopsies, Positive/Total	Percentage (%)	Total Upstaged (%)
Washings	14/31	45	45
Periaortic nodes	9/20	45	29
Pelvic tissue	9/19	47	29
Omentum	8/24	33	26
Diaphragm	7/24	29	23
Other abdominal tissue	6/19	32	19
Cul-de-sac peritoneum	5/19	26	16

Reprinted with permission from Young RC, Decker DG, Wharton JT, et al: Staging laparotomy in early ovarian cancer. JAMA, 250:3072-3076, 1983.

Hematogenous dissemination at the time of diagnosis can occur, but is uncommon. Only 2% to 3% of patients are found to have parenchymal involvement of the liver or lungs.

CLINICAL MANIFESTATIONS, DIAGNOSIS, AND STAGING

Clinical Manifestations

Approximately 70% of patients with EOC have stage III or IV disease at diagnosis, whereas 70% of patients with germ cell ovarian malignancies present with stage I disease. Possible explanations for this difference in stage distribution are, first, that, unlike EOC, ovarian germ cell malignancies tend to stretch and twist the infundibulopelvic ligament, causing severe pain while the disease is still confined to the ovary and, second, the lack of intraperitoneal spread common in EOC.

Functioning ovarian tumors of the sex cord-stromal type may present with symptoms suggestive of excessive endogenous estrogen or androgen production. Young girls with granulosa cell tumors generally present with precocious puberty, whereas women in the reproductive years often complain about amenorrhea, and postmenopausal women may present with painless postmenopausal bleeding. Sertoli-Leydig cell tumors may present with symptoms of virilization.

Generally, patients with EOC report a history of several months of vague and ill-defined symptoms such as abdominal discomfort and bloating, nausea, anorexia, or early satiety, owing to the presence of malignant ascites or large intra-abdominal masses. Other common symptoms include irregular vaginal bleeding, and gastrointestinal and/or urinary tract symptoms. Unfortunately, these symptoms are nonspecific and occur relatively commonly in the general population without the diagnosis of ovarian cancer.

Diagnosis

The diagnosis of early-stage EOC is made when an asymptomatic adnexal mass is noted at the time of a routine pelvic examination. However, it is important to recognize that the majority of these palpable adnexal masses are not malignant (5% in premenopausal patients and 30%–60% in postmenopausal patients are malignant). Patients presenting with nonspecific abdominal discomfort require a prompt and careful pelvic examination. The presence of a large, solid, irregular fixed mass on pelvic examination or presence of palpable upper abdominal mass and ascites are highly suggestive of an ovarian malignancy.

There is not a reliable noninvasive method to determine the malignant potential of an ovarian mass. Endovaginal ultrasound allows identifying characteristics of pelvic masses that characterizes them as highly suggestive to be benign or highly suggestive to be malignant. Morphology indices, based on tumor volume and wall structure, have been developed to indicate the likelihood of pelvic masses being malignant. Sonographic findings suggestive of malignancy in patients with a pelvic mass include a solid component, often nodular or papillary; thick septations; presence of ascites and presence of peritoneal masses; enlarged lymph nodes; or matted loops of bowel.[51] Initial hopes that color flow Doppler and Doppler techniques evaluating resistance index (RI) and pulsatility index (PI) of adnexal masses have proved to be disappointing. The suspicion of ovarian malignancy in a patient with a pelvic mass and ascites is usually high enough to warrant operative intervention. A pelvic mass in the absence of ascites or the presence of liver metastases, however, may raise the suspicion of a metastatic process such as colon cancer or other gastrointestinal malignancies. Whether or not to proceed with operative intervention, the type of procedure to be performed, and the type of surgeon (gynecologic oncologist vs. general surgeon or surgical oncologist) may vary depending on the differential diagnosis, and, therefore, preoperative evaluation is indicated.

Among other possible preoperative tests, a serum CA-125 measurement may help distinguish a gynecologic etiology from other pathologic processes such as primary gastrointestinal malignancies. Eighty percent of women with advanced ovarian cancer have elevation of CA-125. The incidence of elevated CA-125 is highest in women with serous histology and lowest in those with mucinous tumors. However CA-125 is not specific for EOC. There are a number of gynecologic and nongynecologic conditions associated with elevated CA-125, including endometrial cancer and certain pancreatic, lung, and colon cancers as well as benign conditions such as endometriosis, inflammatory bowel disease, uterine leiomyoma, menstruation, and pregnancy, although levels are rarely greater than 100 to 200 U/mL.[52] CA-125 is most clinically useful in monitoring response in patients receiving therapy for pathologically confirmed EOC.

Enlarged ovaries are relatively common in premenopausal women and frequently are due to either functioning ovarian cysts, such as endometriomas or corpus luteum cysts, or to benign ovarian cysts. Adnexal masses that are mobile, purely cystic, unilateral, less than 8 to 10 cm in diameter, and have smooth internal and external contours by ultrasound are highly unlikely to be malignant and can be followed for a period of 2 months. Surgical exploration is indicated if there is no resolution within this period of time. However, women who have solid, fixed, irregularly shaped or larger masses should undergo exploratory surgery. Rising values of serial CA-125 assays obtained during the observation period are an indication that a malignancy may be present. The role of laparoscopic staging is still undefined, and the evidence supports the management of all malignant ovarian lesions via laparotomy and adequate surgical staging, although many are not so managed at present.

In postmenopausal patients, the threshold for surgical intervention is lower than in premenopausal women, given the lower prevalence of nonmalignant conditions that could produce an elevated CA-125 when compared with premenopausal women. Cysts less than 3 cm do not need to be removed if they appear to be unilocular and are associated with a normal level of CA-125 and normal transvaginal ultrasound (morphology index) or color Doppler flow studies. Postmenopausal women with complex asymptomatic pelvic masses or simple cysts in association with elevated serum CA-125 levels (>65 U/mL) should undergo prompt surgery, because these are more likely to indicate ovarian cancer.

When a germ cell tumor is suspected, because of the presence of a solid adnexal mass in a premenarchal or adolescent patient, measurement of serum alpha-fetoprotein (AFP) and human chorionic gonadotropin (β-hCG) are helpful in establishing a preoperative diagnosis of an endodermal sinus tumor, embryonal carcinoma, choriocarcinoma, or mixed germ cell tumor. However, most young women with these diseases are not recognized preoperatively, with the diagnosis being discovered incidentally on final pathology reports, after laparoscopic oophorectomy or cystectomy. Levels of AFP and β-hCG are very useful in serially monitoring the presence of residual disease and the effectiveness of therapy.

Routine blood work and chest radiograph should be part of the overall preoperative evaluation of a patient with suspected ovarian cancer before surgical staging. Computed tomography (CT) scan and magnetic resonance imaging (MRI) are not helpful in establishing the diagnosis in a patient with a definite pelvic mass for which surgery is usually indicated. These tests allow assessment of retroperitoneal lymph nodes, identification of intraperitoneal and mesenteric implants, and presence of visceral metastasis. A barium enema or Hypaque enema can be very helpful in determining whether there is compromise of the sigmoid colon lumen in women with obstructive symptoms. Positron emission tomography (PET) imaging has not been shown to be useful in the differential diagnosis of ovarian neoplasms.

For patients with advanced disease, the preoperative diagnosis of malignancy is usually apparent. However, gastrointestinal malignancies such as stomach, pancreatic, and colon cancers can mimic advanced EOC; similarly, breast, stomach, colon, and other malignancies can metastasize to the ovaries, making the primary diagnosis difficult. History and physical examination, as well as judicious use of diagnostic studies, such as upper and lower endoscopies, CT scan, barium enema, and serum tumor markers (CA-125, carcinoembryonic antigen [CEA], and CA 19-9) can help clarify the diagnosis preoperatively. A thorough preoperative evaluation would potentially influence a decision regarding neoadjuvant chemotherapy in those patients who are found to have extensive unresectable or metastatic disease. Patients with family history of ovarian or breast cancer should also be considered for consultation by clinical cancer genetics.

Staging

Surgery is crucial in diagnosis, accurate staging, and optimal cytoreduction as it contributes to improve outcome in the management of EOC. Ovarian cancer is surgically staged according to the 2002 revised FIGO and American Joint Committee on Cancer (AJCC) staging system (Table 58-4).[53] Our understanding of the natural history and patterns of spread of EOC constitutes the basis and rationale for the specific recommendations regarding surgical staging (Table 58-5).[41]

Patients with apparent early-stage disease require adequate surgical staging with thorough evaluation of all areas at risk to properly evaluate the extent of the disease and to guide appropriate subsequent treatment recommendations. The goal of surgery in patients with advanced disease is optimal cytoreduction. A recent report from the NCI-SEER database indicates that only about 10% of the U.S. women with apparent early-stage EOC undergo appropriate surgical staging and recommends postoperative therapy.[54] A gynecologic oncologist should be consulted to perform the surgical procedure if

Table 58-4 FIGO staging for Primary Carcinoma of the Ovary*

Stage I:	Growth limited to the ovaries.
Stage IA	Growth limited to one ovary; no ascites containing malignant cells. No tumor on the external surface; capsule intact.
Stage IB	Growth limited to both ovaries; no ascites containing malignant cells. No tumor on the external surfaces; capsules intact.
Stage IC*	Tumor either stage IA or IB but with tumor on the surface of one or both ovaries; or with capsules ruptured; or with ascites present containing malignant cells or with positive peritoneal washings.
Stage II	Growth involving one or both ovaries with pelvic extension.
Stage IIA	Extension and/or metastasis to the uterus and/or tubes.
Stage IIB	Extension to other pelvic tissues.
Stage IIC†	Tumor either stage IIA or IIB but with tumor on the surface of one or both ovaries; or with capsules ruptured; or with ascites present containing malignant cells or with positive peritoneal washings.
Stage III	Tumor involving one or both ovaries with peritoneal implants outside the pelvis and/or retroperitoneal or inguinal nodes. Superficial liver metastasis equals stage III. Tumor is limited to the true pelvis but with histologically proven malignant extension to small bowel or omentum.
Stage IIIA	Tumor grossly limited to the true pelvis with negative nodes but with histologically confirmed microscopic seeding of abdominal peritoneal surfaces.
Stage IIIB	Tumor of one or both ovaries with histologically confirmed implants of the abdominal peritoneal surfaces, none exceeding 2 cm in diameter. Nodes negative.
Stage IIIC	Abdominal implants >2 cm in diameter and/or positive retroperitoneal or inguinal nodes.
Stage IV	Growth involving one or both ovaries with distant metastasis. If pleural effusion is present, there must be positive cytologic test results to allot a case to stage IV. Parenchymal liver metastasis equals stage IV.

*These categories are based on findings at clinical examination or surgical exploration.

†To evaluate the impact on prognosis of the different criteria for allotting cases to stage IC-IIC, it would be of value to know if rupture of the capsule was (a) spontaneous or (b) caused by the surgeon, and if the source of malignant cells detected was (a) peritoneal washings or (b) ascites.

From American Joint Committee on Cancer (AJCC). AJCC Cancer Staging Manual, Sixth Edition. Published by Springer-Verlag, New York, Inc., Eds. Greene FL, Page DI, Flemming ID et al, 2002; 257-287.

Table 58-5 Diagnostic Algorithm and Comprehensive Surgical Staging for Early EOC

History and physical examination
Labs—CBC, blood chemistries, preoperative CA-125
Imaging—chest radiograph (posteroanterior and lateral), CT abdomen and pelvis
Comprehensive surgical staging:
Examination under anesthesia
Appropriate surgical incision
Cytologic evaluation: ascites or peritoneal washings
Pelvic cul-de-sac
Bilateral paracolic gutters
Left hemi-diaphragm
Inspection of serosal surfaces: biopsies of adhesions or suspicious findings
Stomach
Small bowel: Ileocecal junction to ligament of Treitz
Large bowel: Ileocecal junction to rectum
Peritoneal surfaces and mesentery
Solid organs: kidneys, liver, spleen, gallbladder, pancreas
Total abdominal hysterectomy*
Unilateral or bilateral salpingo-oophorectomy*
Infracolic omentectomy
Appendectomy*
Pelvic and aortic lymph-node biopsies
Peritoneal biopsies
Pelvic cul-de-sac
Bladder
Bilateral sidewalls
Bilateral paracolic gutters
Diaphragm

*Tailor to individual.

an ovarian malignancy is diagnosed or suspected preoperatively, or incidentally found intraoperatively. Survival data suggest that those patients operated on by gynecologic oncologists have an improved progression-free and overall survival, at least in part because of more appropriate surgical staging and more aggressive cytoreductive surgery performed before initiating subsequent treatment.[54,55] Patients with previous diagnosis of malignancy are often referred to a gynecologic oncologist after "incomplete" staging. Identical work-up procedures are recommended in this situation, in addition to a careful pathology review.

Proper surgical staging should be accomplished as outlined in Table 58-5. A vertical abdominal incision should be used, except perhaps in the young, when ovarian preservation may be considered, to allow adequate access to the upper abdomen. Information gained from examination under anesthesia can help establish the proper incision, and it should be performed in all cases. On entering the peritoneal cavity, aspiration of ascites if present or peritoneal washings from the pelvis, should be obtained and sent for cytology. In the absence of ascites, washings prove positive for malignancy in 10% to 36% of apparent stage IA patients.[56] Adhesions should be lysed and samples sent for microscopic evaluation. If intraperitoneal carcinomatosis is not present, the affected adnexa should be removed intact, paying special attention to avoid, if possible, rupture and spillage of malignant cells. Frozen section should be obtained to confirm the diagnosis.

If cancer diagnosis is established, in postmenopausal women or women in whom fertility is no longer desired, bilateral salpingo-oophorectomy and total abdominal hysterectomy should be performed, primarily because the serosal surface of the uterus is a large peritoneal surface for implantation of malignant cells. Field effects may be present whereby the epithelium of the fallopian tubes or uterus are involved with premalignant or malignant processes that may not be grossly recognized at the time of surgery. Preservation of the uterus and normal-appearing contralateral ovary could be an option in a woman of reproductive age with either a borderline malignant tumor or an invasive epithelial cancer that is grossly confined to one ovary. A frozen section assessment of any abnormality involving the contralateral ovary helps guide the surgeon in determining whether to remove that ovary.[57]

Subsequently, surgical staging should be carried out in the absence of gross upper abdominal disease, including careful inspection of all the peritoneal surfaces and viscera (all intestinal serosal surfaces, mesentery, paracolic gutters, undersurfaces of both hemidiaphragms, gallbladder, and liver). Any suspicious areas in the abdominal cavity should be biopsied. If there is no evidence of gross disease, samples of pelvic peritoneum from the area of the ipsilateral infundibulopelvic and round ligaments, the pouch of Douglas, both gutters, right hemidiaphragm, bladder peritoneum, and bowel mesentery are obtained. A complete infracolic omentectomy should be performed. Any enlarged pelvic or retroperitoneal lymph nodes are removed, regardless of their locations. Although the true incidence of lymph node metastases is not known, several series have reported pelvic lymph node involvement of 0 to 22% and aortic lymph node involvement of 9% to 25%, with an overall incidence among all studies of 21%.[50] Approximately 10% to 15% of patients with ovarian cancer apparently confined to the ovaries will have metastasis to the periaortic nodes.[41,50] Metastases to contralateral lymph nodes have been reported by Flanagan and colleagues,[58] indicating the necessity of bilateral lymph node assessment in all patients. If bulky residual disease (greater than 1 cm) is present in the abdomen, there is no role for para-aortic lymphadenectomy, given the lack of benefit in survival.[59] Appendectomy should be performed in patients with mucinous tumors, because 8% of these patients will have involvement of the appendix. However, routine appendectomy in early EOC is controversial but it should be performed in patients with grade 3 or mucinous tumors.

An incomplete surgical staging, because of unsuspected ovarian malignancy at the time of the initial surgery or inappropriate procedure, often results in understaging of EOC. Young and colleagues[41] found that in almost one third of the patients (31%) believed to have stage I or II disease at the time of the initial surgery were upstaged following a second staging surgical procedure, and 77% of the upstaged patients were found to have stage III disease (see Tables 58-2 and 58-3). Women with incompletely staged EOC represent a clinical dilemma. The simplest and best approach is to proceed with a properly performed staging laparotomy by a gynecologic oncologist with maximum cytoreduction. However, if this is not possible, an alternative is to clinically stage the patient and evaluate extent of potential residual disease by CT scan and CA-125 levels. If the histology demonstrates an LMP, additional surgical intervention is not recommended; close clinical observation is the best approach. If CT, CA-125 levels, or a review of the operative report suggests evidence of residual disease, potential options include upfront complete surgical staging with maximum debulking followed by adjuvant chemotherapy or neoadjuvant chemotherapy followed by subsequent surgical reassessment and interval cytoreduction, a concept tested by the European Organization for Research and Treatment of Cancer (EORTC).[60,61]

The National Comprehensive Cancer Network (NCCN)[62] offered recommendations regarding the treatment of patients with incompletely staged EOC. Complete surgical staging should be performed in all patients with suspected stage IA-B, grade 1 tumors, because if the stage is confirmed, no further therapy is indicated. If potentially resectable residual disease is suspected, a complete surgical staging and debulking are recommended for all stages. For patients with stages higher than IA-B, grade 1, if no residual disease is suspected, chemotherapy for six cycles is recommended if no further surgery is to be performed; complete surgical staging with debulking is an option for all patients with stage IA-B, grade 1-3, or stage IC tumors. Tumor reductive surgery should be conducted for patients with stage II-IV disease with suspected potentially resectable residual disease (to be offered to patients with stage IV disease on an individual basis, particularly in the case of large intra-abdominal masses or bowel obstruction).

PRIMARY THERAPY

Early-Stage Epithelial Ovarian Cancer

Primary Surgery

Adequate surgical staging allows definition of the appropriate candidates for adjuvant therapy. Unilateral salpingo-oophorectomy may be considered only if a thorough surgical staging has confirmed no evidence of extraovarian spread of the disease, in a patient with stage IA, who strongly desires preservation of fertility. In a series of 118 women with stage I EOC, biopsy of the contralateral ovary proved malignancy in only 2.5% when the ovary appeared normal; on the other hand, under these circumstances, biopsy of the contralateral normal ovary, in a patient wishing to retain fertility, might actually compromise her ability to conceive secondary to tubo-ovarian adhesions.[63] A dilation and curettage should be performed if hysterectomy is not performed, particularly in patients with endometrioid histology, which carries a 20% risk for a synchronous endometrial primary malignancy.

Adjuvant Therapy

The role of adjuvant treatment in patients with early EOC after comprehensive surgical staging is still controversial. GOG data[36] have established that patients with stages IA and IB, well and moderately differentiated tumors (diploid tumors), are at low risk for relapse after comprehensive surgical staging. A GOG study[64] randomized patients in the favorable prognosis category to receive no treatment or oral intermittent melphalan. With a median follow-up of more than 6 years, the 5-year disease-free and overall survival rates for untreated patients and those receiving melphalan were 91% and 94%, and 98% and 96%, respectively, a nonstatistically significant difference. This group of patients can be spared the acute and chronic toxicities of chemotherapy.

In contrast, patients with poorly differentiated (and grade 1 aneuploid tumors?)[45] or more advanced stages I or II (rupture of the capsule, dense adhesions, clear-cell histology, extraovarian spread, or positive peritoneal washings) have poorer outcomes (70%-80% 5-year survival rate among the treated patients, 25%-40% relapse rate). For these "high-risk" early EOC patients, the majority of gynecologic oncologists would advise adjuvant therapy, although the optimum treatment remains an area of controversy. There has been significant controversy regarding the role of immediate therapy versus delaying treatment until disease progression. A consensus has not been established about the prognostic significance of some clinicopathologic features, such as positive peritoneal cytology, presence of ascites, and dense adhesions.[65] Clinicopathologic factors currently used by the GOG to define unfavorable-prognosis early-stage disease include FIGO stage II and IC, clear-cell histology, and poorly differentiated tumors.

The benefit of adjuvant chemotherapy for all patients with early-stage EOC has been questioned. No improvement in either overall survival or relapse-free survival (RFS) was shown in patients undergoing comprehensive surgical staging, in the retrospective subset analysis in the Adjuvant Chemotherapy in Ovarian Neoplasm (ACTION) trial, suggesting that platinum-based adjuvant chemotherapy benefits primarily patients who are incompletely staged.[66]

Adjuvant Radiation Therapy

Historically, intraperitoneal (IP) radiocolloids and whole-abdomen irradiation (WAI) with/without pelvic irradiation have been used in the management of EOC. Despite its long history in the treatment of EOC and its proven curative role in patients with microscopic or minimal residual disease, the proper role of radiotherapy (RT) in the management of this disease is controversial and not clearly established. Similarly, the potential roles of RT in the consolidative treatment and as salvage therapy following chemotherapy failure remain controversial.

Intraperitoneal Radioactive Chromic Phosphate Suspension (^{32}P)

Radioactive phosphorus 32 (^{32}P) seems to be the most attractive radiocolloid for IP administration because it is a pure β emitter that avoids the hazard of γ radiation. ^{32}P has a half-life of 14.3 days, average tissue penetration of 1.4 to 3.0 mm, and a maximum and average β energies of 1.71 MeV and 0.69 MeV, respectively. Chromic ^{32}P is a blue-green, chemically inert colloidal form of ^{32}P used for intracavitary instillation. Unfortunately, the precise distribution and dose delivered by ^{32}P to the peritoneal surface is unknown and often unpredictable. The IP isotope distribution should be tested prior to instillation with radioactive technetium sulfur colloid (^{99m}Tc) or after radiocolloid administration with scintigraphic imaging of Bremsstrahlung photons.

The best available data supporting that 10 to 15 mCi of ^{32}P delivers superficial but therapeutic dosages to the peritoneal surfaces are from Currie and colleagues.[67] There appears to be predominantly an abdominal distribution with much smaller systemic absorption. The majority of the ^{32}P is either absorbed by the peritoneal surface, by the macrophages lining the peritoneal cavity, or phagocytized by free-floating macrophages. The rest of the ^{32}P is carried by the abdominal current to the right hemidiaphragm where it passes through the diaphragmatic lymphatics and enters the mediastinal lymphatics. It then passes to the right subclavian vein via the right thoracic trunk and enters the general circulation where it is rapidly cleared by the liver and deposited to a lesser extent in other tissues (spleen and bone marrow). Pelvic and para-aortic lymph nodes receive relatively low nontherapeutic doses. Several studies using imaging techniques confirm that the distribution of chromic ^{32}P is dynamic for the first 6 to 24 hours but thereafter is fixed. Boye and colleagues[68] reported that the estimated peritoneal surface dose from 10 mCi of ^{32}P is approximately 30 Gy, although the uptake and distribution of ^{32}P in the peritoneal cavity often shows significant inhomogeneity. They noted an increase in measurable levels of ^{32}P in the blood for 7 days, following which it declined; the estimated maximum dose to the peripheral blood even at its peak was 1.2 cGy. The dose to the bone marrow was higher by 2-5 times, but the maximum dose was still very low, in the order of 6 cGy.

RANDOMIZED TRIALS USING INTRAPERITONEAL ^{32}P

Table 58-6 shows the results of randomized trials using IP ^{32}P in the adjuvant setting for early-stage EOC. Young and colleagues[36] reported in 1990 the results of a GOG trial in which 141 eligible patients with FIGO stage IC and II, or poorly differentiated tumors FIGO stage IA or IB after comprehensive surgical staging, were randomized between ^{32}P at the time of surgery, or melphalan. The outcomes for the two treatment groups, with a median follow-up of more than 6 years, were similar with respect to 5-year disease-free survival (DFS) (80% in both groups) and overall survival (81% with melphalan versus 78% with ^{32}P; P = .48). Seven percent of the patients could not receive the prescribed ^{32}P because of catheter difficulties, and 6% subsequently required surgery for bowel obstruction. However, although there was no observation arm, the GOG concluded that the added cost, inconvenience, and risk for alkylating agent induced leukemia were not justified, and ^{32}P was chosen as the control arm for the next GOG trial. However, the observed survival could be attributed to favorable tumor characteristics rather than to the therapy employed (17% of the patients entered had grade I or borderline tumors and, therefore, were at low risk for relapse).[36]

The second major GOG trial[69] in early EOC included a similar high-risk/unfavorable group of early-stage patients, randomized to receive either IP ^{32}P or cyclophosphamide plus cisplatin (CP). Of the 229 patients included in the analysis, 110 received ^{32}P, and 119 received CP chemotherapy. Percentage relapse-free at 10 years were 72% for CP and 65% for ^{32}P groups. After adjusting for stage and histologic grade, the estimated relapse rate was 29% less for CP than for ^{32}P, and the death rate was 17% lower for patients receiving CP (difference not significant). Combining the two arms, the 10-year cumulative incidence of relapse for all stage I patients was 27% compared with 44% for stage II patients (P = .01). Survival at 5 years was 83% for CP and 76% for ^{32}P. Eight patients randomized to ^{32}P were unable to receive the treatment, and two patients had small-bowel perforations during catheter insertion. Although there were no statistically significant differences between the two arms, the better progression-free interval for CP and the problems with adequate distribution and late toxicities associated with ^{32}P made the platinum-based combination the preferred standard treatment for patients with early-stage, high-risk EOC.[69] The recently closed GOG trial (GOG 157) has omitted ^{32}P and randomizes patients with stage IC and II and poor prognosis IA and IB early EOC, after complete surgical staging, to receive three versus six cycles of carboplatin and paclitaxel. The end points for this investigation will be DFS, overall survival, and comparative toxicity.

The NCI of Canada Clinical Trials Group[70] randomized 257 eligible patients with high-risk stage I, stage IIA, and completely resected stages IIB or III, to IP ^{32}P (10-15 mCi), oral melphalan, or WAI by moving strip technique (2250 cGy/20 fractions) and pelvic radiation (2250 cGy if prior WAI; 4500 cGy if prior ^{32}P or melphalan). Comprehensive surgical staging was not mandatory. No difference in actuarial 5-year survival was observed between the arms, with a median follow-up of 8 years (66%, 61%, and 62% 5-year survival for ^{32}P, melphalan, and WAI, respectively). The ^{32}P plus pelvic RT arm was closed prematurely because of the high incidence of bowel complications.

In the Norwegian Radium Hospital study,[71] adjuvant IP-^{32}P was compared with six cycles of cisplatin in a group of 347 patients with stages I-III EOC without residual tumor following primary surgical debulking. Patients with extensive adhesions randomized to ^{32}P were treated with WAI (17%). The median follow-up was 62 months. No difference in actuarial survival or DFS was seen between the two treatment groups. The estimated 5-year crude and DFS in the group randomized to receive ^{32}P were 83% and 81%, respectively. For the patients randomized to receive cisplatin, the estimated 5-year crude and DFS were 81% and 75%, respectively. Late bowel obstruction requiring surgery occurred more often in the group treated with ^{32}P (4%) or WAI (11%) compared with the cisplatin group (1%). The authors recommended that cisplatin be

Table 58-6 Early-Stage Ovarian Cancer. Intraperitoneal-^{32}P Prospective Randomized Trials

Study	High-Risk	Patients (*N*)	Study Design	5-year DFS (%)	5-year Survival (%)
GOG (Young, 1990)	IA,IB,G3 IC-II OpD	141	P-32 vs melphalan	80 80	78 81
GOG (Young, 2003)	IA,IB,G3 IC-II OpD	229	P-32 vs CTX + CDDP	65* 72*	76 83
NCI Canada (Klaassen, 1988)	IA,IB,G3 IC-III, OpD	257	Pelvic RT + P-32 vs pelvic RT + melphalan vs pelvic RT + WAI	— — —	66 61 62
Norwegian Radium Hospital (Vergote, 1992)	I-III OpD	347	CDDP vs P-32	75† 81†	81 83
GICOG (Bolis, 1995)	IC	176	CDDP vs P-32	81 66	83 79

*10-year DFS.

†5-year DFS rates in patients with stage I by treatment subgroups: 86%, 95%, and 83% for ^{32}P, WAI, and cisplatin, respectively.

From Young RC, Walton LA, Ellenberg SS, et al: Adjuvant therapy in stage I and stage II epithelial ovarian cancer: results of two prospective randomized trials. N Engl J Med 322:1021-1027, 1990; Young RC, Brady MF, Nieberg RM, et al: Adjuvant treatment for early ovarian cancer: a randomized Phase III trial of intraperitoneal ^{32}P or intravenous cyclophosphamide and cisplatin—a Gynecology Oncology Group (GOG) study. J Clin Oncol 21:4350-4355, 2003; Klaasen D, Shelley W, Starreveld A, et al: Early stage ovarian cancer: a randomized clinical trial comparing whole abdominal radiotherapy, melphalan, and intraperitoneal chromic phosphate: a National Cancer Institute of Canada Clinical Trials Group report. J Clin Oncol 6:1254-1263, 1988; Vergote IB, Vergote-DeVos LN, Abeler VN, et al: Randomized trial comparing cisplatin with radioactive phosphorus or whole abdomen irradiation as adjuvant treatment of ovarian cancer. Cancer 69:741-749, 1992; Bolis G, Colombo N, Pecorelli S, et al: Adjuvant treatment for early epithelial ovarian cancer: results of two randomized clinical trials comparing cisplatin to no further therapy or chromic phosphate. Ann Oncol 9:887-893, 1995.

used as standard adjuvant treatment for subsequent controlled studies, although this group had inferior median survival, median time to relapse, and a greater percentage of patients relapsing.

In 1993, the same authors[72] reported 313 patients with EOC who received IP ^{32}P as primary adjuvant treatment (245 patients), consolidating therapy after negative second-look laparotomy (SLL) (59 patients) or after positive SLL with minimal residuum (9 patients). The actuarial 5-year crude survival was 81% in the group treated adjuvantly and 79% in the group treated after SLL. However, the morbidity rate was substantial: two patients died of treatment complications attributed to ^{32}P, and small bowel obstruction without tumor relapse occurred in 22 (7%) patients (13 treated surgically and 9 medically). The authors concluded that without an untreated observation group, it was unclear if adjuvant ^{32}P conferred a survival advantage.

The Italian study by the Gruppo Italiano Collaborativo Oncologica Ginecologica (GICOG) performed two multicenter randomized clinical trials.[73] After surgical staging, eligible patients in Study 1 (83 eligible patients, stages IA and IB, grades 2 and 3) were randomized to either cisplatin or no further treatment (control). Patients in Study 2 (176 eligible patients, stage IC, any grade) were randomized to cisplatin or IP ^{32}P. The 5-year DFS in Study 1 was 83% for cisplatin and 64% for the control group ($P = .09$), but no difference in overall survival could be detected (5-year survival 87% and 81% for the cisplatin and control groups, respectively). When the control group patients were treated with cisplatin at relapse, they had the same 5-year survival as the immediate cisplatin group. In Study 2, the 5-year DFS was 81% for the cisplatin group and 66% for the ^{32}P group ($P = .008$). Again, there was no difference in overall survival (5-year survival 83% and 79% for the cisplatin and ^{32}P groups, respectively). These two studies also demonstrated that the cisplatin-treated patients had a poorer outcome at relapse than the non–cisplatin-treated patients. In both trials, the difference in relapse pattern was primarily due to a reduction in relapses in the pelvis only. The fact that there was no difference in the overall survival in any of the two trials may be due to a) the limited impact of this adjuvant therapy, b) the relatively low doses of cisplatin, c) the impact of salvage treatment at the time of relapse, or d) simply that the power of the study was too low. One possible explanation for failure to demonstrate a therapeutic benefit for ^{32}P is the relatively low radiation dose delivered to sites of possible tumor involvement.[74]

Because the previously mentioned studies for high-risk groups lack a control group, the optimal adjuvant therapy for this group of patients with intermediate prognosis (stage I, G2-3; stage II no residuum, any grade; stage II, 2-cm residuum, G1-2) remains subject to question. The trend in the United States, and probably around the world, is to treat patients with high-risk stage I and II EOC with systemic chemotherapy, primarily platinum/taxane combinations.

Whole-Abdomen Irradiation

Theoretical and practical advantages of the WAI over ^{32}P are mainly a more homogeneous dose distribution, better coverage of the pelvic and periaortic lymph nodes, and the ability to treat all the peritoneal surfaces without limitations due to the presence of postoperative adhesions. However, WAI is associated with a higher incidence of acute and late toxicity primary related to dose-limiting organs including the liver, kidneys, and small bowel.

The use of external beam RT in the treatment of EOC began to decline significantly following the publication of the M.D. Anderson randomized trial in 1975.[75] This trial included 108 evaluable patients with stage I-II EOC, randomized to single-agent melphalan versus WAI with pelvic boost. The overall actuarial 2-year survivals were 85% and 90%, and 55% and 58%, for WAI and melphalan, respectively. However, this study has been criticized for not irradiating the diaphragm adequately, low RT doses to the liver and kidney areas, imbalance in stage distribution between the two arms (significant preponderance of more advanced stages IIB versus I-IIA in the radiotherapy arm), and short follow-up.

Only in the past decade has a clear appreciation emerged of the risk factors within FIGO stages. In 1977, early-stage disease was subdivided into high-risk (all stage II, all stage IC, and stages IA and IB with high-grade tumors) and low-risk groups (all other types). Dembo and colleagues[76] and Lederman and colleagues[77] defined several risk groups to select those patients most suitable for primary postoperative adjuvant RT. All patients were optimally debulked with no macroscopic residual disease in the upper abdomen and up to 2-cm residual disease in the pelvis, because the latter site can be safely boosted. Dembo and Bush[78,79] recommended adjuvant WAI for the patients in the intermediate risk group (stage I-II, grades 2-3, and stage III grade 1, with less than 2-cm residual disease). This group has an approximately 70% 5-year freedom from relapse (FFR) following RT. Patients in the high-risk group, including stage III grade 2-3 and stage II grade 3 with small residuum, have only a 20% 5-year FFR following RT, and were subsequently treated in Toronto with combined chemotherapy and radiation.

Randomized Trials of Whole-Abdomen Irradiation in Stage I and II Disease

Table 58-7 shows the results of randomized trials of WAI as adjuvant therapy in the management of early-stage EOC. In 1979, Dembo and associates[80] published results of a randomized trial between postoperative WAI and pelvic RT alone or followed by chlorambucil. The study included 147 patients with stage I-III EOC with minimal (<2 cm) or no residual disease demonstrating a 10-year survival advantage of 64% versus 40%, in favor of WAI ($P = .0007$). No survival benefit was seen for patients with gross (>2 cm) residual disease. Therefore, it appears that WAI, when administered to appropriate volumes with adequate techniques in patients with minimal residual-disease EOC, results in treatment outcomes comparing favorably with those obtained by modern chemotherapy regimens.[81] Subsequently, Fyles and colleagues[82] reported the results of a randomized study to determine whether an increased dose of WAI (27.5 Gy) resulted in improved disease control and survival when compared with standard WAI dose (22.5 Gy). A pelvic boost of 22.5 Gy was used in both arms. One hundred and twenty-five patients with early-stage EOC, optimally debulked, intermediate-risk, were entered in the study. No difference was found between both arms in terms of 5-year survival (83% and 72% in the low-dose and high-dose arms, respectively), patterns of relapse, hematologic toxicity, or late complications.[82]

Three other randomized trials have been reported comparing WAI with chemotherapy, although only one study involved cisplatin-based chemotherapy.[70,83,84] None of these trials demonstrated a significant difference between the WAI and chemotherapy arms. Sell and colleagues[83] randomized patients between WAI versus pelvic RT plus cyclophosphamide, observing 4-year overall survivals of 63% for WAI versus 55% for pelvic RT plus cyclophosphamide (not statistically significant). In 1985, the Northwest Oncologic Cooperative Group of Italy[84] initiated a prospective randomized trial in high-risk group, early-stage disease (stage IA-IB, grade 3; stage IC and stage II). Patients were randomized between

Table 58-7 **Early-Stage Ovarian Cancer: WAI—Randomized Studies**

Study	Patient Population (Stage)	Patients (N)	Study Design	Outcome
NCI Canada Klaassen, 1988	I-III	107 106	Randomized: WAI vs Pelvic RT + melphalan	62%—5 y RFS 61%—5 y RFS
Dembo, 1979	I-III OpD	76 71	Randomized: WAI vs Pelvic RT ± chlorambucil	64%—10 y RFS* 40%—10 y RFS*
Smith, 1975	I	14 28	Randomized: WAI vs melphalan	85%—2 y RFS 90%—2 y RFS
Smith, 1975	II	37 29	Randomized: WAI vs melphalan	55%—2 y RFS 58%—2 y RFS
Sell, 1990	I	60 58	Randomized: WAI vs pelvic RT + CTX	63%—4 y survival 55%—4 y survival
Chiara, 1994	I-II	44 25	Randomized: CDDP + CTX vs WAI	73%—5 y survival 68%—5 y survival

Differences not statistically significant except for Dembo's series* ($P = .0007$)

CDDP, cisplatin; CTX, cyclophosphamide; OpD, optimally debulked; RFS, relapse-free survival; RT, radiotherapy; WAI, whole abdomen irradiation.

From Klaasen D, Shelley W, Starreveld A, et al: Early stage ovarian cancer: a randomized clinical trial comparing whole abdominal radiotherapy, melphalan, and intraperitoneal chromic phosphate: a National Cancer Institute of Canada Clinical Trials Group report. J Clin Oncol 6:1254-1263, 1988; Smith JP, Rutledge FN, Delclos L: Postoperative treatment of early cancer of the ovary: a random trial between postoperative irradiation and chemotherapy. J Natl Cancer Inst 42:149-153, 1975; Dembo AJ, Bush RS, Beale FA, et al: Ovarian carcinoma: Improved survival following abdominopelvic irradiation in patients with a complete pelvic operation. Am J Obstet Gynecol 134:793-800, 1979; Sell A, Bertelsen K, Andersen JE, et al: Randomized study of whole abdomen irradiation versus pelvic irradiation plus cyclophosphamide in treatment of early ovarian cancer. Gynecol Oncol 37:367-373, 1990; Chiara S, Pierfranco C, Franzone P: High-risk early-stage ovarian cancer: Randomized trial comparing cisplatin plus cyclophosphamide versus whole abdominal radiotherapy. Am J Clin Oncol 17:72-76, 1994.

cisplatin plus cyclophosphamide and WAI. When the data were analyzed according to treatment received rather than treatment assigned, no significant differences could be detected in terms of RFS or overall survival between the patients receiving chemotherapy versus WAI (73% vs 60% and 73% vs 68%, respectively).[84]

In 1986 the GOG activated a randomized protocol to compare WAI versus platinum-based chemotherapy. This trial asked a crucial question, namely, which therapy given adjuvantly produced better survival and DFS, but was closed because patient accrual was inadequate. Therefore, the question remains unanswered.

In terms of the role of pelvic RT, two randomized trials conducted by the GOG and Princess Margaret Hospital compared pelvic RT to observation, in stage I, grades 2-3, EOC. They failed to demonstrate a decreased relapse rate.[64,85,86]

The 2004 NCCN clinical practice guidelines[62] have made the following recommendations regarding adjuvant therapy for early-stage EOC: (1) Patients with stage IA or IB grade 1 tumors do not require adjuvant therapy, and observation alone is recommended because survival is greater than 90%. (2) Some disagreement continues regarding stage IA or IB grade 2 tumors. If residual disease is suspected or observation is considered, a complete surgical staging is recommended for all patients. If no residual disease is suspected, surgical staging is an option, or alternatively, patients may be treated with six cycles of chemotherapy. (3) For patients with grade 3 tumors or higher stages of the disease, systemic chemotherapy is indicated after appropriate surgery.

Adjuvant Chemotherapy

Approximately 20% to 30% of women with early-stage EOC eventually die from their disease. Because early-stage EOC appears relatively infrequently, few randomized trials have been conducted in this group. Table 58-8 shows the results of several randomized trials of observation versus cisplatin-based chemotherapy in early-stage EOC. The most discussed studies are the small U.S. trial of observation versus melphalan,[36] an Italian study[73] of observation versus cisplatin, and a Scandinavian study[45] of observation versus carboplatin. The randomized trial conducted by the Gruppo Italiano Collaborativo Oncologica Ginecologica[73] demonstrated improved DFS with adjuvant cisplatin, but there was no difference in terms of overall survival. The other two trials did not reveal any difference between the observation and the chemotherapy arms. The lack of demonstrated benefit may be related to lack of power to demonstrate a survival advantage in this patient population with relatively long-term survival, the efficacy of cisplatin at the time of disease relapse, or both.

The EORTC-ACTION[66] trial and the International Collaborative Ovarian Neoplasm (ICON1)[87] are the two largest randomized trials conducted in early-stage EOC comparing platinum-based adjuvant chemotherapy with observation following surgery. A total of 448 patients were accrued in the ACTION trial, and 477 patients in the ICON1 trial. Although both trials had similar randomization, there were significant differences between them in terms of patient inclusion criteria. The ACTION trial[66] recruited patients with stages IA-IB, grade 2-3, all grades IC and IIA, and all I-IIA clear-cell histologies. The ICON1[87] included all patients with early stages, grades, and histologic cell types, and those where the responsible clinician had uncertainty regarding the benefit from adjuvant therapy. The ACTION trial had more strict guidelines for surgery, requiring comprehensive surgical staging, in addition to tumor typing and grading. However, in ICON1, surgery consisted of hysterectomy and bilateral salpingo-oophorectomy without a requirement for surgical staging. Chemotherapy in the intervention arm of the ACTION trial consisted of at least four cycles of a platinum-containing regimen; patients in the control arm who suffered a relapse were to receive the same regimen. In ICON1, chemotherapy with CAP (cyclophosphamide, doxorubicin, and cisplatin) or single-agent carboplatin was recommended, although other

Table 58-8 **Randomized Trials of No Adjuvant Therapy Versus Cisplatin-Based Chemotherapy in Early-Stage Ovarian Cancer**

Study	High-Risk	Patients (*N*)	Median Follow-Up (mo)	Study Design	5-year DFS (%)	5-year Survival (%)
GOG Young, 1990[36]	IA, IB Grade 1-2 Optimal staging	81	>72	Melphalan vs observation	98 91 NS	98 94 NS
GICOG Bolis, 1995[73]	IA, IB Grade 2-3 Optimal staging	83	76	Cisplatin vs observation	83 64 NS	87 81 NS
Trope, 2000[45]	I, grade 2-3 Grade I aneuploid or clear cell Suboptimal staging	162	46	Carboplatin vs observation	70 71 NS	86 85 NS
ICON1, 2003[87]	I-II MD uncertain if pt would benefit from Tx No surgical staging	477	51	Platinum-based vs observation	73 62 *P* = .01	79 70 *P* = .03
ACTION Trimbos, 2003[66]	IA, IB Grade 2-3 IC-IIA all grades; clear cell Optimal staging in 1/3 pts	448	59	Platinum-based vs observation	76 68 *P* = .02	85 78 *P* = .10

From Young RC, Walton LA, Ellenberg SS, et al: Adjuvant therapy in stage I and stage II epithelial ovarian cancer: results of two prospective randomized trials. N Engl J Med 322:1021-1027, 1990; Trope CG, Kaern J, Hogberg T, et al: Randomized study on adjuvant chemotherapy in stage I ovarian cancer with evaluation of DNA ploidy as prognostic instrument. Ann Oncol 11:281-288, 2000; Bolis G, Colombo N, Pecorelli S, et al: Adjuvant treatment for early epithelial ovarian cancer: results of two randomized clinical trials comparing cisplatin to no further therapy or chromic phosphate. Ann Oncol 9:887-893, 1995; Trimbos JB, Vergote I, Bolis G, et al: Impact of adjuvant chemotherapy and surgical staging in early-stage ovarian carcinoma: European Organization for Research and Treatment of Cancer—Adjuvant Chemotherapy in Ovarian Neoplasm Trial (EORTC-ACTION). J Natl Cancer Inst 95:113-125, 2003; Colombo N, Guthrie D, Chiari S, et al: International Collaborative Ovarian Neoplasm Trial 1: a randomized trial of adjuvant chemotherapy in women with early stage ovarian cancer. J Natl Cancer Inst 95:125-132, 2003.

platinum-based regimens were allowed. The primary end point in both trials was survival; clinical relapse was a secondary end point. The trials have been combined for analysis.[88] A total of 925 patients were randomized between the two trials. After a median follow-up of more than 4 years, the 5 year overall survival was 82% in the chemotherapy arm and 74% in the observation arm ($P = .008$). RFS at 5 years was also better in the adjuvant chemotherapy arm, 76%, when compared with the observation arm, 65% ($P = .001$).[88] In the ACTION trial, completeness of surgical staging was an independent prognostic factor. When this trial was analyzed separately, there was no benefit in overall survival or DFS associated with the use of adjuvant chemotherapy, whereas in the suboptimally staged patients cisplatin-based chemotherapy improved the outcome.[66] This has been interpreted to suggest that adjuvant chemotherapy is beneficial in incompletely staged patients with potential occult residual disease. Conflicting interpretations of these trials have led to a lack of consensus on the need and indication for adjuvant therapy in early-stage EOC. Estimates of risk for relapse in early disease are not clear, although most agree that carefully staged patients with grade 1 stage IA disease do not require adjuvant therapy.

Molecular markers, including gene expression profiles, are needed to better identify the group of patients with unfavorable prognosis who may benefit from adjuvant therapy. The ongoing EORTC trial randomizes nonoptimally staged patients, without overt evidence of extraovarian disease to restaging followed by observation versus adjuvant chemotherapy without restaging.

The preliminary results of the most recent GOG randomized trial (GOG 157),[89] in which 321 evaluable patients with stage IA-IB, grade 3, and stage IC-II completely resected EOC (70% stage I) were randomized to receive three versus six courses of paclitaxel and carboplatin, has been published in abstract form. The risk for relapse was 33% lower among women receiving six cycles, and survival was improved by 5%, but the differences were not statistically significant. Hematologic toxicity and neurotoxicity were substantially greater than in the group receiving six cycles of chemotherapy. The GOG is currently investigating the use of carboplatin and paclitaxel (three cycles), with or without maintenance paclitaxel (40 mg/m^2/week) for 24 weeks in patients with completely resected stage IC and IIA-C EOC and stage IA-B poorly differentiated or clear-cell tumors.

The 2004 NCCN guidelines[62] recommend the combination of carboplatin (AUC 5-7.5) and paclitaxel 175 mg/m^2 over 3 hours, for three to six cycles every 3 weeks.[90] Alternative regimens include cisplatin and paclitaxel, or carboplatin and docetaxel. New biologic agents, in particular the antiangiogenesis agents, appear of promise in EOC and hopefully will be investigated in the near future in patients with early stage disease.

ADVANCED-STAGE EPITHELIAL OVARIAN CANCER

Role of Surgery

Primary Cytoreductive Surgery

Although surgery represents the cornerstone of the initial management, it is insufficient even if complete tumor resection is performed. Additional therapy is almost always indicated. The management of patients with advanced EOC requires surgical staging with maximal (optimal) cytoreduction, if possible, leaving no or minimal residual tumor. The GOG currently defines optimal cytoreduction as leaving no residual disease greater than 1 cm in maximum tumor diameter.[37] Unfortunately, this definition does not accurately assess the "volume" of residual disease because numerous lesions of less than 1 cm in maximum diameter may be present. Potential benefits of aggressive debulking with presumed reduction in clonogenic cell number include improved survival because chemotherapy may be more effective in eradicating disease residuum. Improvement of disease-related symptoms, primarily abdominal pain, distension, and early satiety may contribute to better quality of life.

Retrospective evidence supports the advantages of cytoreductive surgery. Relapse-free interval and median survival are inversely related to the size of the largest residual mass at the completion of the debulking surgery, prior to initiation of chemotherapy (see Biology/Prognostic Factors sections).[37-40] A meta-analysis of 6885 patients found that maximum cytoreduction was one of the most important prognostic factors for survival in patients with advanced EOC, such that each 10% increase in maximal cytoreduction was associated with a 5.5% increase in median survival time.[91] Surgery should be performed by a board-certified gynecologic oncologist who is more likely to adequately stage patients, achieve optimal cytoreduction, and render a higher proportion of long-term surviving patients.[91] Although EOC typically does not invade into the muscularis and mucosa of the intestine, metastatic implants in the bowel mesentery or serosa can cause obstruction and resection may be indicated. In addition to the rectosigmoid, the most frequent sites of bowel resection are the terminal ileum, cecum, and transverse colon. Appendectomy should be performed if gross involvement with tumor is present or in patients with mucinous tumors.

Retroperitoneal lymph node metastasis could be identified in up to 70% of patients with advanced EOC. In patients with enlarged pelvic or para-aortic nodes, removal is mandatory in an effort to obtain maximal cytoreduction. However, the role of systemic lymphadenectomy in patients with nonpalpable enlarged nodes with advanced metastatic disease is debated.[92]

The magnitude of incremental benefit from debulking surgery in various circumstances remains unclear, because patients with tumors that can be optimally debulked may have biologically more favorable disease. The therapeutic value of cytoreductive surgery seems to be more evident for patients in whom it can be performed without excessive morbidity. However, there are no data to confirm or refute therapeutic benefit when extensive surgery, such as splenectomy, extensive bowel resection with diverting colostomy, partial hepatectomy, and/or diaphragmatic resection, is required. Associated morbidities and impact on quality of life have not been clearly evaluated.

Secondary Surgery

The term secondary surgery is a broad definition that includes (1) SLL or comprehensive surgical-staging procedure in patients clinically free of disease after completion of primary therapy; (2) secondary cytoreductive surgery or surgical debulking of relapse after clinical remission following initial therapy; and (3) interval cytoreductive surgery, which is surgical debulking after a limited course of neoadjuvant chemotherapy (Table 58-9).[92]

1. *Second look laparotomy (SLL):* The potential value of SLL is in accurate definition of extent of residual disease following chemotherapy. Current imaging modalities and CA-125 serum levels are inaccurate in assessing small volume disease at the completion of the primary treatment. SLL was initially used to establish the response to chemotherapy, particularly in patients with an apparent clinically complete response. In assessing the efficacy of new chemotherapy regimens used in clinical trials, a complete response was initially thought to be a surrogate for survival. There was a theory that early identification of potential resistant disease and resection thereof could alter the course of the disease. Although SLL may provide prognostic information,[93] it is not used routinely, given the lack of proven benefit, potential surgical morbidity, subsequent impact on patient's quality of life, lack of effective consolidation regimens for those shown to be free of disease, and no available curative second-line chemotherapy regimens for those patients with residuum.

SLL demonstrates residual disease in 30% to 50% of patients with clinically complete response. The proportion with residuum seems to be directly related to the initial stage of the disease.[92,93] The survival benefit of the SLL or SLL with interval debulking was evaluated in a trial of the GOG.[94] More than 800 patients with advanced, optimally debulked stage III EOC were randomized to receive six cycles of paclitaxel plus either cisplatin or carboplatin. At the time of the initial randomization, women were given the option to undergo (393) or not (399) SLL, after completion of chemotherapy. Women with negative SLL were followed without further therapy, whereas those with residual disease underwent maximal debulking followed by additional chemotherapy.[94] Median progression-free and overall survivals were 19.4 and 48.7 months for patients randomized to cisplatin and paclitaxel compared with 20.7 and 57.4 months for the patients

Table 58-9 Surgical Procedures for Ovarian Carcinoma

Surgical Staging	Initial extirpation of gynecologic organs, assessment of peritoneal surfaces, omentum, and lymph nodes to determine stage in apparent early-stage disease
Debulking	Initial extirpation of gynecologic organs and bulky tumor with the goal of cytoreduction. Residual disease of less than 1 cm is considered optimal debulking; residual disease of greater than 1 cm is suboptimal debulking
Interval Debulking	Secondary debulking procedure, usually performed following 3-6 cycles of chemotherapy and usually reserved for individuals who underwent initial suboptimal debulking. Because disease is usually encountered, additional chemotherapy usually follows.
Second-Look Laparotomy	Evaluation of peritoneal surfaces and lymph nodes in an asymptomatic patient following adjuvant chemotherapy to facilitate recommendations for surveillance versus additional salvage therapy.
Palliative Surgery	Operating on a patient with complications from treatment or known disease when the procedure can improve quality of life. Examples include repair of a fistula, or diversion of bowel secondary to obstruction.

receiving carboplatin and paclitaxel, respectively.[87] The study showed that women selecting SLL were more likely than those in the no SLL group to have gross residual disease at the time of the initial surgery (69% vs. 60%, respectively). Although women with negative SLL had a significantly better DFS and overall survival than those with residual disease, the performance of an SLL itself was not associated with improved outcome when compared with those patients who elected observation after completion of the initial adjuvant chemotherapy. The authors concluded that SLL did not appear to identify those women for whom further chemotherapy was associated with a better survival.[94] Despite the initial enthusiasm in the early 1980s, in the absence of data from randomized trials demonstrating a survival benefit, there is little place for SLL after primary therapy, and it should be reserved for patients on clinical trials.

2. *Secondary* and 3. *Interval cytoreductive surgery:* Women in whom initial optimal cytoreductive surgery cannot be achieved may be treated with three to six cycles of neoadjuvant or induction chemotherapy, followed by an attempt at maximal cytoreduction, in those experiencing a good response. One potential advantage of this approach is the avoidance of an aggressive surgery in women with potentially chemoresistant disease, who would have a poor outcome regardless of the treatment.

There have been two large randomized trials evaluating the outcome after interval cytoreduction, with conflicting results. A survival benefit for neoadjuvant chemotherapy was suggested in the EORTC trial published by van der Burg and coworkers.[60] In this trial, 319 patients with residual disease >1 cm in diameter after primary surgery were randomized to continue chemotherapy or undergo interval cytoreduction, after having received three cycles of cisplatin and cyclophosphamide without progression of disease. Cytoreduction was associated with longer DFS and a significant 6-month prolongation in median survival (26 months for those who underwent interval cytoreduction vs. 20 months for those who did not, $P = .04$). This study has been much debated and even criticized because of the imperfections in its design, in particular the fact that maximum cytoreduction up front was not required (no indication of the extent of attempted cytoreduction at diagnosis). This could explain the benefit of interval cytoreduction. The mature results of the study have just been announced verifying the continued superiority in survival in the cohort treated with interval cytoreduction compared to those who received chemotherapy alone.[61] The GOG conducted a similar trial in which 550 patients with advanced EOC suboptimally debulked, but with an initial attempt to obtain maximum cytoreduction, were randomized to receive three cycles of paclitaxel and cisplatin followed by interval cytoreductive surgery versus continued chemotherapy, if there was no evidence of progressive disease. There was not improvement in either the median time to progression or death (10.5 months in the secondary-surgery group vs. 10.7 months in the chemotherapy-alone group) or survival (34 months for the interval-cytoreductive surgery and chemotherapy-alone groups).[95]

Available evidence suggests that neoadjuvant chemotherapy followed by later cytoreduction does not provide superior outcome over that achieved by aggressive initial surgical debulking followed by taxane-based chemotherapy, although it may spare some initial surgical morbidity. The EORTC is investigating the role of neoadjuvant chemotherapy in a randomized, phase III study comparing upfront debulking surgery versus neoadjuvant chemotherapy in patients with stage IIIC or IV epithelial ovarian cancer (EORTC 55971).

Secondary cytoreductive surgery at the time of disease relapse requires the expertise of a well-trained gynecologic oncologist. Its benefit, however, is unclear, given the lack of prospective, randomized trials evaluating its role. Munkarah and Coleman[96] recently performed an extensive analysis of the published data on secondary cytoreduction in recurrent EOC. The authors recognized that evaluation of the impact of secondary cytoreduction on survival was limited by 1) interinvestigator differences in defining optimal cytoreduction, 2) heterogeneity of patients included, and 3) lack of information on postoperative therapy and its potential impact. From their review of the literature, it seems that patients without evidence of gross residual disease after secondary cytoreduction at the time of the recurrence have prolonged survival in the range of 44 to 60 months. However, current data on the use of salvage chemotherapy without surgery for recurrent EOC may be associated with median survival of approximately 35 months. They concluded that "the available data suggest a benefit for secondary surgical cytoreduction in recurrent ovarian cancer. This needs to be considered in the light of recent data reporting prolonged survival with the use of combination salvage chemotherapy without surgery."

Although the available literature does not provide information regarding which patients may benefit from secondary cytoreduction, it seems that patients who had complete or optimal resection at the primary surgery or a disease-free interval of more than 6 to 12 months and in whom an optimal debulking of all recurrent disease is possible are most likely to benefit. However, factors that predict optimal resectability in this group of patients have not been defined. Currently, there are two ongoing large prospective trials conducted by the EORTC and GOG, which may provide additional information regarding the optimal management of patients with recurrent EOC after an initial complete remission.

Role of Chemotherapy

First Line—Adjuvant Chemotherapy

Patients with advanced-stage EOC (stages III and IV) are rarely if ever cured with surgery alone. Current standard therapies for women with advanced EOC have developed as a consequence of data from randomized trials. Historically, patients were treated with alkylating agents, resulting in 40% to 50% clinical response rates, with 15% to 20% of patients experiencing complete responses. In the early 1980s, the standard of care for advanced EOC was the combination of cyclophosphamide and doxorubicin (AC) as established by the GOG.[97] Chemotherapy for EOC has evolved significantly since that time, with the introduction of platinum compounds and the taxanes. GOG 47 demonstrated the superiority of CAP over AC, with improvement in the complete response rate (51% vs. 26%) and progression-free survival (PFS) (13 months vs. 8 months).[98] As a result, CAP became standard therapy in the 1980s in the United States. A subsequent GOG trial failed to reveal a survival advantage to the inclusion of doxorubicin.[99] Two meta-analyses did demonstrate a modest survival benefit,[100,101] but because of the additional toxicity of doxorubicin, the combination of cyclophosphamide and cisplatin was widely accepted as first-line therapy in advanced EOC in the early 1990s.

By the early 1990s, the new taxane class of compounds was available for clinical trials. Paclitaxel was the first drug to be evaluated demonstrating significant activity as a single agent in "platinum-refractory" patients.

Two phase III studies of paclitaxel in combination with cisplatin as a first-line therapy resulted in the standard front-line treatment being changed from cisplatin/cyclophosphamide to cisplatin/paclitaxel. GOG 111[2] evaluated 386 patients with suboptimal stage III or IV disease. Patients were randomized to paclitaxel and cisplatin versus cyclophosphamide and cisplatin. The cisplatin–paclitaxel regimen was found to be superior with a 5- month median PFS advantage (18 vs. 13 months, $P < .001$), a 14-month median survival advantage (38 vs. 24 months, $P < .001$), and an increased clinical complete response rate (54% vs. 32%).[2] These results were subsequently confirmed by a European-Canadian trial, including patients with stages IIB-IV. Similar chemotherapy regimens were compared.[102] In this trial, cisplatin was combined with paclitaxel administered as a 3-hour infusion (24-hour infusion in the GOG trial). Despite differences in design, a significant advantage was again noted in clinical response rate, median PFS, and median survival among the women receiving paclitaxel.[102]

Since the establishment of a platinum and taxane as standard first-line therapy, little progress has been achieved in overall survival. More than 70% of patients still experience disease relapse, with a median to progression of less than 2 years. There remains a need for more effective therapy. Different dosing schedules and platinum and taxane compounds have been examined. Several studies and a meta-analysis have demonstrated that outcomes using cisplatin and carboplatin are equivalent, although a detailed review of these trials is out of the scope of this chapter. In a GOG study, 792 patients with optimally debulked stage III EOC were randomized to receive cisplatin–paclitaxel versus carboplatin–paclitaxel.[90] No difference was shown in median progression-free and overall survival between the two regimens, but the toxicities of both regimens differ substantially. The advantages of carboplatin over cisplatin include more convenient infusion time and lower incidence of gastrointestinal toxicity and peripheral neuropathy. Although carboplatin results in greater bone marrow toxicity, this is reversible with very little long-term toxicity. Whereas the efficacy of the two platinum analogs is comparable, quality of life issues have resulted in carboplatin replacing cisplatin as the standard treatment in combination with paclitaxel.

A recently completed intergroup study compared the standard carboplatin and paclitaxel to two triplets (paclitaxel+ gemcitabine+carboplatin and carboplatin+ doxil+paclitaxel) and two sequential doublets (topotecan+carboplatin → paclitaxel+carboplatin and gemcitabine+carboplatin → paclitaxel+carboplatin). The study was designed to evaluate the potential benefit from the addition of agents known to be active in the recurrent setting, to determine their role as first-line therapy. Maturation of the data is pending.

The lack of progress made through multiple trials evaluating various standard antineoplastic regimens has led to research evaluating more biologically targeted therapies based on the genetic variations of ovarian tumors. These abnormalities include overexpression of *p53* and *p27*, and mutations in cyclin E, HER2/neu, platelet-derived growth factor (PDGF), transforming growth factor-β (TGF-β), VEGF, and Bcl-2. Specific agents designed to target these abnormalities include angiogenesis inhibitors, metalloproteinase inhibitors, anti-HER-2/*neu*, farnesyltransferase inhibitors, and tyrosine kinase inhibitors. The multiple molecular pathways underlying primary tumor progression and metastases are complex. Nevertheless, interventions at a molecular level, tailored to the individual patient and tumor characteristics, as well as agents to reverse drug resistance, and the potential for gene therapy, may hold promise in the future for improved treatment strategies.

Maintenance and Consolidation Chemotherapy

Unfortunately, only about 20% of women enjoy long-term PFS with modern carboplatin/taxane-based chemotherapy. High relapse rates have resulted in a number of trials investigating the role of maintenance or consolidation chemotherapy to improve survival. These include use of continuation or maintenance chemotherapy beyond the standard six cycles and high-dose strategies (IP chemotherapy alone or with intravenous therapy and high-dose chemotherapy with stem cell support). None of these strategies has been shown to improve survival, except a small benefit with prolonged administration of paclitaxel. Maintenance therapy cannot be considered a standard of care.

Second Line—Salvage Chemotherapy

Despite 50% improvement in survival with current regimens, the 5-year survival remains dismal for patients with stage III-IV disease, ranging from almost 60% for stage IIIA disease to around 30% for stage IIIC and less than 20% for those patients with stage IV at presentation. Relapse is expected in at least 75% of patients who initially achieve a complete clinical response. The selection of salvage therapy is generally based on whether women are sensitive or resistant to initial platinum-based chemotherapy. Patients who respond to initial platinum-based therapy and have a significant relapse-free interval (>6 months) have a higher probability of responding again to platinum-based therapy at the time of relapse. These patients are called *platinum sensitive*. The optimal retreatment regimen for them is not clear, although generally a platinum (cisplatin or carboplatin) plus paclitaxel alone or in combination is often recommended. The duration of previous response is highly predictive of response rate and median survival after salvage chemotherapy. Those patients with a treatment-free interval between 5 to 12 months following initial therapy have a response rate of 25% to 30% compared with almost 60% response rate for those with treatment-free interval longer than 24 months. For patients with platinum-resistant disease (defined as progression during platinum therapy, stable disease or relapse <6 months from the initial platinum-based therapy), numerous single agents have shown some activity, including paclitaxel (if not part of the initial regimen), etoposide, liposomal doxorubicin, and topotecan. Response rates range between 20% and 35%. Less-active agents with response rates between 10% and 20% include gemcitabine, navelbine, and ifosfamide. Unfortunately, the duration of response to these "second-line" agents is generally short, on the order of 3 to 6 months. Sequential administration of these agents can result in palliation of symptoms.

The current NCCN clinical guidelines[62] state "no single chemotherapy agent should be considered the treatment of choice for recurrent EOC." They also say "in vitro chemosensitivity testing to choose a chemotherapy regimen for recurrent disease could not be recommended, because of the lack of demonstrable efficacy for such an approach."

Role of Radiation Therapy

The value of combined modality therapy (sequential chemotherapy and radiation) and salvage RT after failure following chemotherapy remains undefined. These strategies have been used in a wide variety of circumstances and usually in uncontrolled observational studies. Toxicity may be severe when multiple chemotherapy regimens and/or surgical procedures have been used before RT. Comparisons to other potential consolidation or salvage treatments are lacking.

Whole-Abdomen Irradiation as Initial Therapy in Patients with Limited Residual Disease

The National Institutes of Health (NIH) consensus conference in 1994[103] indicated "the role of RT in advanced epithelial EOC is controversial. Long-term RFSs have been demonstrated for stages II and III after optimal debulking and postoperative RT, but no prospective trials of WAI compared with CT have been performed." They also recommended, "WAI should be reevaluated and newer RT techniques evaluated in the treatment of optimally debulked stage II and III disease."

Dembo[78,79,104] reported 5-year survival rates of 58% and 42% in EOC patients with stage II and III, respectively, optimally debulked (<2 cm residuum) and treated with WAI. Goldberg and Peschel[105] reviewed the Yale experience with adjuvant WAI in 74 EOC patients with stage I-III and none or limited (<2 cm) residual disease. The actuarial survival and DFS at 10 years were 77% and 79%, respectively. Weiser and colleagues[106] reported on 68 stage II-III patients treated with WAI after cytoreductive surgery at Walter Reed Army Medical Center. Patients with no residual disease had a 10-year actuarial survival of 59% and a median survival in excess of 10 years. Those with less than 2 cm residual disease had a 10-year survival of 42% and a median survival of 6 years. Seventeen percent of the patients experienced late severe toxicity, probably as a result of the higher doses delivered to the entire abdomen when compared with other series (40 Gy in 20 fractions), without liver shielding. Fuller and colleagues[107] published the results of postoperative WAI in 106 patients with stage I-III EOC. Those patients who had stages I-IIIA with no postoperative residual disease, or <.5 cm abdominal and/or <2 cm pelvic residual disease had a 10-year RFS of 71% with WAI, compared with 40% when subtotal abdominopelvic techniques were used.

Advanced-Stage Ovarian Cancer: Consolidation and Salvage Radiation Therapy

Planned sequential combined-modality therapy (SCMT) has utilized RT after chemotherapy. With SCMT, many have a spectrum of residual disease from none pathologically detected at SLL through to gross residual disease variously treated with or without further surgical resection.

Although consolidation treatment may be justified since even 33% to 50% of patients with negative SLL would experience clinical disease relapse, its value remains controversial. After the work of Dembo and colleagues[108] in 1979, which showed that WAI was an effective adjuvant treatment for patients with early EOC with minimal residual disease, it was believed than in advanced EOC in which surgery and chemotherapy have successfully reduced bulky stage II or III disease, WAI might prolong survival.[109]

A phase II trial was conducted at the Princess Margaret Hospital[77] of six cycles of cyclophosphamide, doxorubicin, and cisplatin followed by WAI in patients with stage III, high-grade histology or macroscopic residual disease in the pelvis. The results were compared to a matched control group with similar prognostic features receiving WAI alone. The median survival was extended from 2.4 to 5.7 years, and 43% of the patients receiving combined therapy were free of relapse at 5 years compared to 22% treated with WAI alone ($P = .03$).

Planned SCMT theoretically may be of benefit to some patients, particularly those with microscopic or no residual abdominal disease or those with minimal residual disease confined to an area that could receive an RT dose higher than what can be delivered to the whole abdomen. An observational study[110] suggested prolonged survival after planned sequential therapy in those with grade 1-2 disease or minimal residuum (2 cm) prior to and after chemotherapy.

Lambert and colleagues[111] from the North Thames Ovary Group Study, reported in 1993 the results of a randomized trial in patients with advanced EOC (stages IIB-IV, <2 cm residual disease at SLL) designed to determine whether consolidation therapy with WAI after chemotherapy improved survival and DFS compared with the continued chemotherapy. A total of 254 patients were entered in the study. This consisted of 5 monthly courses of 400 mg/m^2 of carboplatin. One hundred seventeen patients with residual disease <2 cm at SLL or laparoscopy, were then randomized to receive consolidation therapy, either 5 further courses of carboplatin at the same dosage or WAI. There was no statistical difference in either survival or DFS between arms (less than 30% 5-year survival and DFS).

Bruzzone and colleagues[112] conducted a randomized trial of platinum-based chemotherapy versus RT (WAI 30.2 Gy, pelvis 43.2 Gy) in 41 patients with stage III-IV ovarian cancer with pathologic complete response or minimal residual disease at SLL, after primary aggressive surgery and three courses of platinum-based chemotherapy. With a median follow-up of 22 months, disease progression was observed in 55% and 28.5% of the patients randomized to RT and chemotherapy, respectively. The authors admitted that the two arms were not well balanced (no residual disease at SLL in 71% and 50% of the chemotherapy and RT patients, respectively). Similar results have been reported by Lawton and colleagues.[113]

Hoskins and colleagues[114] reported a series of EOC patients with stages I-II grade 3 or stage III any grade tumors, receiving either six cycles of chemotherapy alone or the same platinum-based chemotherapy with WAI between the third and fourth cycle. Five-year survivals were 78% and 64%, favoring the group receiving RT.

Thomas and Dembo[115,116] reported disappointing results in a review of 28 trials of sequential WAI (both for consolidation and salvage) after chemotherapy in advanced EOC. A strong association was found between tumor residuum before WAI and survival (76% for those patients with no residuum compared with 49% and 17% for patients with microscopic or less than 5-mm residuum and macroscopic gross residual disease, respectively). The study author indicated that "if therapy is to be successfully completed with minimal morbidity, WAI should be limited to = 2500 cGy, initial chemotherapy to six courses and surgery to initial debulking and SLL."[116]

Pickel and colleagues[117] evaluated the effect of consolidation RT after carboplatin-based chemotherapy, in patients with advanced optimally debulked EOC. Sixty four of 94 patients with EOC (stages IC-IV), without evidence of gross residual disease after six courses of carboplatin, epirubicin, and prednimustine, were randomized to receive consolidation WAI versus no further therapy. The RFS and overall survival rates of patients who received adjuvant chemoradiotherapy were significantly higher than those of patients who received adjuvant chemotherapy only (68% vs. 56% and 49% vs. 26%, 2- and 5-year RFS, respectively; 87% vs. 61% and 59% vs. 33%, 2- and 5-year overall survival, respectively).

Whelan and colleagues[118] reviewed the records of 105 patients with advanced EOC treated with cisplatin combination chemotherapy followed by WAI at the Princess Margaret Hospital, in order to assess morbidity of this approach and identify those factors predictive of toxicity. Nine of the 105 patients (8.6%) required surgery for bowel obstruction that was not due to recurrent disease, three had a bowel obstruction treated conservatively, and a further five underwent surgery for obstruction secondary to recurrent tumor. The presence of both a dose of WAI over 2250 cGy, as well as a SLL prior to RT, was associated with an increased risk for serious bowel complications.

Sorbe and colleagues[119] recently published the results of a randomized trial conducted by the Swedish-Norwegian Ovarian Cancer Study Group. A total of 742 patients with stage III EOC were entered in the study to evaluate the role of consolidation RT. Patients underwent primary cytoreductive surgery followed by four cycles of induction chemotherapy (cisplatin + doxorubicin or epirubicin). Patients with no evidence of disease and complete or partial clinical response underwent SLL. Patients with complete surgical but not pathologic response were further randomized to WAI versus additional six cycles of chemotherapy, whereas patients with complete pathologic response were randomized to WAI, additional six cycles of chemotherapy, or observation. Despite the fact that 742 patients were enrolled in the study, only 172 patients (23%) were randomized to consolidative treatment. In the subgroup with complete surgical and pathologic response, the 5-year PFS was significantly better in the RT group (56%) than in the chemotherapy group (36%) and the observation group (35%). The relapse rate was lower in the RT group (65%), when compared with chemotherapy (71%) or the control group (74%). No differences were noted between both therapies in the subgroup with microscopic residual disease. Toxicity was worse in the RT group with 10% severe late intestinal complications.[119] Although the trial suffers from the lack of statistical power, the significant improvement in PFS with consolidative WAI warrants further investigation.

It seems intuitive to assume that if WAI as sole postoperative adjuvant treatment is only effective in those with presumed microscopic disease, then it is unlikely to be effective in the consolidation setting in those with macroscopic residuum after chemotherapy. Although the optimum intensity and duration of chemotherapy given prior to surgical reassessment and consolidation WAI remains unclear, it seems that the ability to deliver potentially tumoricidal doses of RT to the abdomen is compromised in patients heavily pretreated with myelotoxic chemotherapy. Another potential advantage of limiting the amount of chemotherapy is the emergence of cisplatin-radiation cross-resistance. Louie and colleagues[120] demonstrated the emergence of radiation resistance simultaneously with cisplatin resistance during chronic cisplatin exposure. In a human ovarian cancer cell line, Britten and colleagues[121] demonstrated a threefold reduction in radiation sensitivity in cells that had developed cisplatin resistance compared to the cisplatin-naïve parent cell line. Because some data suggest a substantial cross-resistance between cisplatin and radiation,[122] it is possible that prolonged exposure to cisplatin renders residual tumor cells less radiosensitive.

Salvage Irradiation after Chemotherapy with/without SLL

Favorable experiences with salvage RT in chemotherapy-refractory EOC continue to be reported, although the published studies offer widely differing experiences with regard to response rates, duration of response, and toxicity. Eifel and colleagues[123] published the M.D. Anderson experience in 37 patients with EOC and positive SLL after platinum-based chemotherapy, or recurrent disease after initial complete response to chemotherapy, who received hyperfractionated WAI with split. Their results were disappointing, with 3-year RFS of 10% and 14% for patients with grade II and III EOC, respectively, and microscopic residual disease. Twelve patients with gross residual disease had rapid relapse (median time to relapse of 4.9 months) and all died from their disease. However, Reddy and colleagues[124] reported a 4-year actuarial survival and RFS rates of 23% and 22%, respectively, in 44 patients receiving salvage WAI after they had failed one or more chemotherapy regimens. Patients with microscopic residual disease prior to WAI had a 4-year survival and RFS of 37% and 42%, respectively. The results were more impressive in patients with disease limited to the pelvis (RFS of 56% compared with 0% when the upper abdomen was involved). Eight patients (18%) developed bowel complications, five of which needed surgical intervention. Similar results have been reported by Fein and colleagues[125] and Cmelak and Kapp[126] with encouraging results in selected patients with chemotherapy-refractory EOC, who had been debulked to small amounts of residual disease (<1 cm). In these patients, salvage WAI can be delivered with acceptable toxicity with long-term survival of approximately 35%. Probably those patients with chemotherapy-refractory disease, who have failed several previous chemotherapy regimens, with disease limited to the pelvis, are the ones who could potentially benefit the most from salvage pelvic irradiation. Given the potential toxicity of salvage radiotherapy after extensive chemotherapy, it is important to limit the volume of irradiation to the area of gross disease by using three-dimensional conformal radiotherapy.

Consolidation/Salvage IP ^{32}P Therapy after Chemotherapy with/without SLL

^{32}P has been considered by several authors as possible adjuvant therapy for patients with negative or microscopic residual disease at SLL, after cisplatin-based chemotherapy. In the Duke experience,[127] patients with only microscopic residual or resected macroscopic residual disease had a median DFS of 24 months and a 3- and 4-year DFS of 36% and 27%, respectively. Vergote and colleagues[72] in 1993 reported on 68 patients who received ^{32}P as consolidation therapy after SLL (59 patients with no residual disease and 9 patients with microscopic or gross residual disease). Fifty patients without residual tumor after primary surgery and negative SLL were included in a prospective randomized trial to receive either the isotope or no treatment (only 12% of the patients had stage III disease). The estimated 5-year crude and DFS rates were 79% and 66%, respectively. No difference was observed in survival between those patients receiving adjuvant ^{32}P (245 patients) and the ones treated with ^{32}P after SLL. ^{32}P was associated with a considerable number of bowel complications. In Spanos and colleagues' observational series,[128] a significant reduction in complications from 21% to 4.1% was noted in patients who received ^{32}P within 12 hours of surgery compared with longer time after surgery; the 5-year survival following SLL was 75% for negative, 48% for microscopic, and 32% for gross residual disease.

Rogers and colleagues[129] reported their results in 51 patients with stages I-III disease, who were found to have no evidence of disease at SLL and received 15 mCi of IP ^{32}P. They compared the results with a group of 35 patients who were otherwise eligible for ^{32}P, who did not receive it primarily due to other treatment protocols, peritoneal adhesions, or the recommendation that no further therapy be given following a negative SLL. Patients in both groups were comparable with regard to stage, histology, grade, median age, residual disease following initial surgery, and chemotherapy regimen. Although this was not a randomized study, the 5-year actuarial DFS rate from the date of the SLL was 86% for those receiving ^{32}P and 67% for those not receiving ^{32}P (P = .05). The corresponding 5-year overall survival rates were 90% and 78%, again favoring treatment with ^{32}P. Late adverse effects were similar in both groups. It seems that with adequate technique of administration and patient selection of those least likely to have adhesions, ^{32}P can be delivered safely with minimal long-term toxicity.

In 1996, the GOG completed a prospective, randomized trial comparing ^{32}P with no additional therapy for stage III ovarian cancer patients after negative SLL.[130] Two hundred and two patients were included in the study. There was no difference in tumor relapse rate or survival between both groups. Despite a complete pathologic remission at SLL after initial surgery and platinum-based regimen, 60% of the patients had tumor relapse within 5 years of a negative SLL.[130]

Patillo and colleagues[131] studied the in vitro enhancement of ^{32}P cytotoxicity by cisplatin in cultured human ovarian adenocarcinoma (CHOA) cell lines and conducted a limited observational study combining fractionated low-dose IP ^{32}P instillations (5 mCi, 8 administrations) with up to eight monthly cycles of cisplatin or carboplatin, in 30 patients with advanced disease. Complete and partial response rates were 47% and 40%, respectively. Three-year survival was 63%, with a mean survival time of 17 months. Based on their laboratory and clinical data, the authors concluded that cisplatin enhances the tumor cell–killing effect of ^{32}P with a supra-additive effect. These conclusions have not been further tested in a controlled clinical trial.

Palliative Therapy in Ovarian Cancer

Palliative Surgery

In the majority of patients, the disease eventually progresses within the abdominal cavity, and may be potentially amenable to cytoreductive surgery, although the benefit is unclear. Because early relapses are often associated with a very poor prognosis, the role of additional surgery is generally limited. Although successful palliation can be achieved surgically in a selected subset of women, the identification of those who might benefit remains a challenge.

The role of surgery in the palliative setting in EOC involves primarily 1) debulking large masses in an attempt to improve patients' symptoms and quality of life and 2) an attempt to relieve intestinal obstruction generally related to a mechanical obstruction from recurrent masses. Careful preoperative evaluation is indicated before any surgical intervention, including assessment of the patient's performance and nutritional status and history of previous RT. Imaging studies may help to delineate the number and location of obstructions as well as the extent of intra-abdominal disease, to guide the surgical decision-making process. Patients with recurrent disease and short life expectancy are unlikely to benefit from exploration. In patients in whom surgery may be indicated the procedure to be performed needs to be carefully evaluated. Successful surgical palliation can be achieved in up to 70% of patients in the absence of large abdominopelvic masses, large volume of ascites, multiple obstructive sites, and severe weight loss.[132] For those who are not candidates for surgical palliation, adequate analgesia and hydration are the most important factors; percutaneous gastrotomy or endoscopic stent placement may be indicated for palliation in some circumstances. It is important to exercise good judgment and expertise to maximize outcome for these patients with short life expectancy to improve their quality of life.

Palliative Radiotherapy

Patients with grossly recurrent and metastatic ovarian cancer following chemotherapy often have significant symptoms that are unresponsive to further systemic therapy. Symptoms may be due to recurrent disease in the pelvis, causing pain and/or bleeding; but relapses in the brain, chest, groin, and other areas may require palliation as well. Even after demonstrated chemotherapy resistance, recurrent disease may respond to palliative irradiation. Corn and colleagues[133] reported an overall symptomatic response rate of 79% with complete palliative response in 51% in 33 patients receiving palliative RT. Symptoms remained palliated until death in 90%. Davidson and colleagues[134] found limited-field RT in patients with localized persistent/recurrent disease to be well tolerated, with limited acute or late morbidity, even in patients heavily pretreated with systemic and intraperitoneal chemotherapy. Fujiwara and colleagues[135] reported symptomatic relief in 50% of patients undergoing RT for localized relapsed or refractory EOC, with improved survival in those patients treated before the development of symptoms or in those with limited nodal disease only.

With increasingly effective systemic therapy, some authors have reported an increasing incidence of brain metastases, presumably due to prolonged survival time and the CNS acting as a "sanctuary site" from systemic chemotherapy. Although the median survival of patients with brain metastasis is only 4 to 6 months when treated with whole-brain RT, certain subsets appear to enjoy longer survival. Corn and colleagues[136] published a series of 32 patients who received RT for symptomatic cerebral metastases, finding clinical response in 23 patients, maintained until death in 71%.

TECHNIQUES OF IRRADIATION

WAI—Technique

Surgical staging information, as well as analysis of patterns of failure, suggests that to be effective the RT volume must include all peritoneal surfaces. The ability of WAI to alter failure patterns by decreasing upper-abdominal relapse compared to no or smaller volume RT has been clearly demonstrated.[70,78,107,137] Dembo and associates[78,108] emphasized the necessity of covering the diaphragm with adequate margin during all phases of normal respiration. This requires that liver shielding be limited or absent. Appropriate kidney localization and blocking should be undertaken to keep total doses within tolerance. Although few are willing to accept a role for definitive RT in EOC or to consider exploration of concurrent chemotherapy and WAI, if there is a role in the future, modern, three-dimensional planning techniques should be employed. CT simulation and possibly intensity-modulated RT[138] may more precisely shield the liver and kidneys (Figs. 58-1 and 58-2). Boost doses should be directed at areas of risk rather than routinely to the pelvis. Although most old RT series describe the routine administration of the pelvic boost, this is not universally true.[139,140]

In definitive primary treatment of selected subsets of patients with early disease, the moving strip technique for WAI has been replaced by the open field technique (AP/PA). Dembo and coworkers[141] showed the therapeutic equivalence of these techniques in a prospective, randomized trial. WAI doses of 22.5 to 25 Gy (at 130 to 150 cGy/fraction) over 4 weeks appear to be associated with a favorable long-term toxicity profile while maintaining considerable therapeutic efficacy in appropriately selected patients. Periaortic and pelvic boost may be recommended in patients without complete lymph node sampling or in the presence of completely debulked retroperitoneal lymphadenopathy (median dose, 45 Gy). Additional conformal pelvic boost may be given to those patients who are at high risk for pelvic recurrence (to sites of macroscopic (<1 to 2 cm) residual disease, defined intraoperatively or radiographically). Theoretically, three-dimensional conformal therapy, using multiple-beam arrangement with limited margins, may potentially decrease long-term toxicity

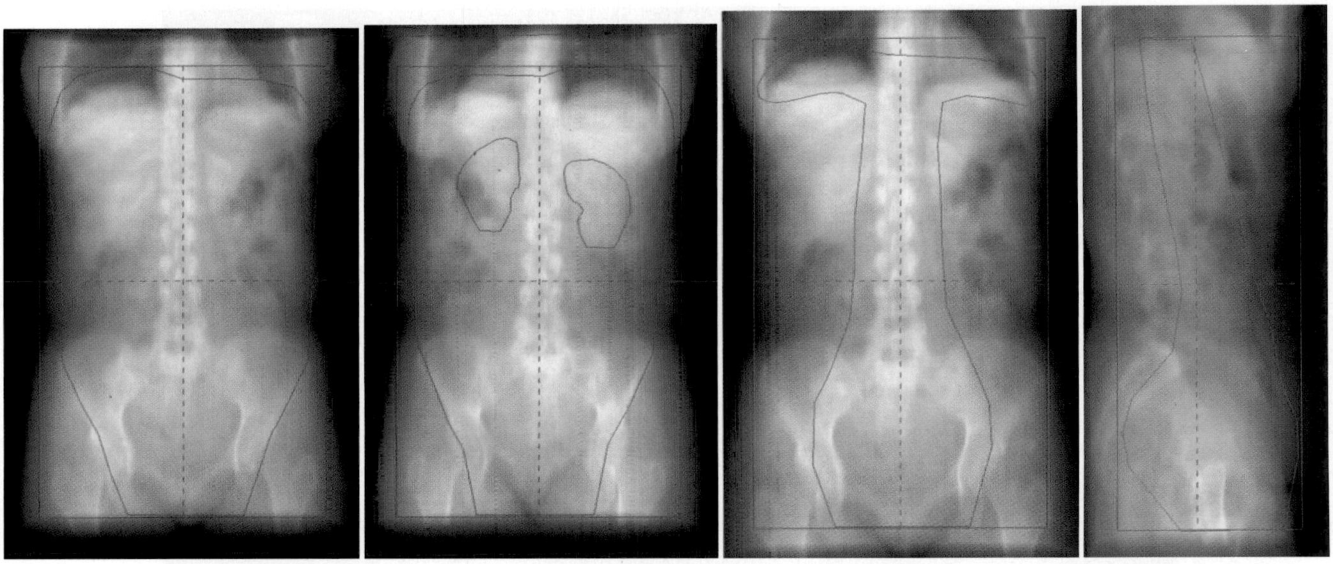

Figure 58-1 **A,** Anteroposterior, whole-abdomen radiation field. **B,** Posteroanterior, whole-abdomen radiation field. **C,** Anteroposterior, periaortic field boost. **D,** Lateral, periaortic field boost.

while boosting sites such as the diaphragm or nodes, although its therapeutic efficacy is unproven.

Older, limited studies have explored changed fractionation schemes for WAI such as hyperfractionation.[125,139] Such approaches are unlikely to be adopted because they are unlikely to be therapeutically superior to once-per-day regimens and are difficult to utilize secondary to patient convenience issues.

A basic criticism of WAI has been whether the limited RT doses tolerated by the whole abdomen (22–30 Gy) can be effective in sterilizing disease, because they are considerably below doses conventionally used to control microscopic disease in epithelial malignancies. Fletcher[142] suggested that approximately 50 Gy is required to sterilize microscopic disease in the majority (assuming 10^8-10^9 residual clonogenic cells). More recently, theoretical bases for this observation have been challenged by Marks[143] and by Withers and Suwinski.[144] The model proposed by Withers and Suwinski assumes that not all patients with microscopic residuum have as large as 10^8 or 10^9 clonogenic cells, and there may be an equal distribution of patients with 1 to 10 logs. Therefore, it appears that radiation in dose levels within limits of whole abdominal tolerance should be able to sterilize disease in some patients with more limited deposits of ovarian cancer and fewer clonogenic cells.

WAI—Toxicity

The initiation of WAI generally results in rather immediate toxicity. Fyles and colleagues[145] reported the WAI toxicity in 598 patients. Acute complications included nausea and vomiting in 61% (severe 10%), diarrhea in 68% (severe 10%)—before the era of effective antiemetic therapy (5-HT_3 inhibitors)—leukopenia, and thrombocytopenia (11% each). Treatment interruptions occurred in 23%, and 10% of the patients did not complete the treatment. Late complications included chronic diarrhea (14%), transient hepatic enzyme elevation (44%), and symptomatic basal pneumonitis (4%). Severe late bowel complications were infrequent, with 25 (4%) patients developing bowel obstruction, 16 requiring surgery. In multivariate analysis, the moving-strip technique was associated with a significantly higher risk for chronic complications compared with the open technique. Whelan and colleagues[118] reported the toxicity of WAI after cisplatin-containing chemotherapy in 105 patients from Princess Margaret Hospital. They found that both an abdominal dose greater than 22.5 Gy and the use of SLL increased the risk for severe bowel complications. Although the gastrointestinal side effects can generally be managed, the associated myelosuppression (neutropenia and thrombocytopenia) can result in a deleterious protraction of treatment. Efforts to ameliorate neutropenia with growth factors (e.g., granulocyte colony-stimulating factor) have not been successful in limiting treatment breaks as thrombocytopenia becomes dose-limiting.[146]

TREATMENT ALGORITHM, CONTROVERSIES, AND FUTURE DIRECTIONS

Treatment Algorithm

EOC continues to be one of the leading causes of cancer-related death in women. In the past decade, intense clinical research and significant resources have resulted in defining the current standard of care for the majority of patients with this disease (Fig. 58-3).

Controversies and Future Directions

A number of questions remain unanswered. Some of the current areas of controversy in the management of patients with EOC include:

1. Who should be screened for EOC and how? Who should undergo genetic testing? What is the appropriate management of patients at high risk for EOC? What is the role of prophylactic bilateral salpingo-oophorectomy in reducing the risk of EOC and its impact in overall survival and quality of life?
2. What is the role of molecular markers and gene expression signature in determining prognosis and selecting appropriate therapy in EOC?

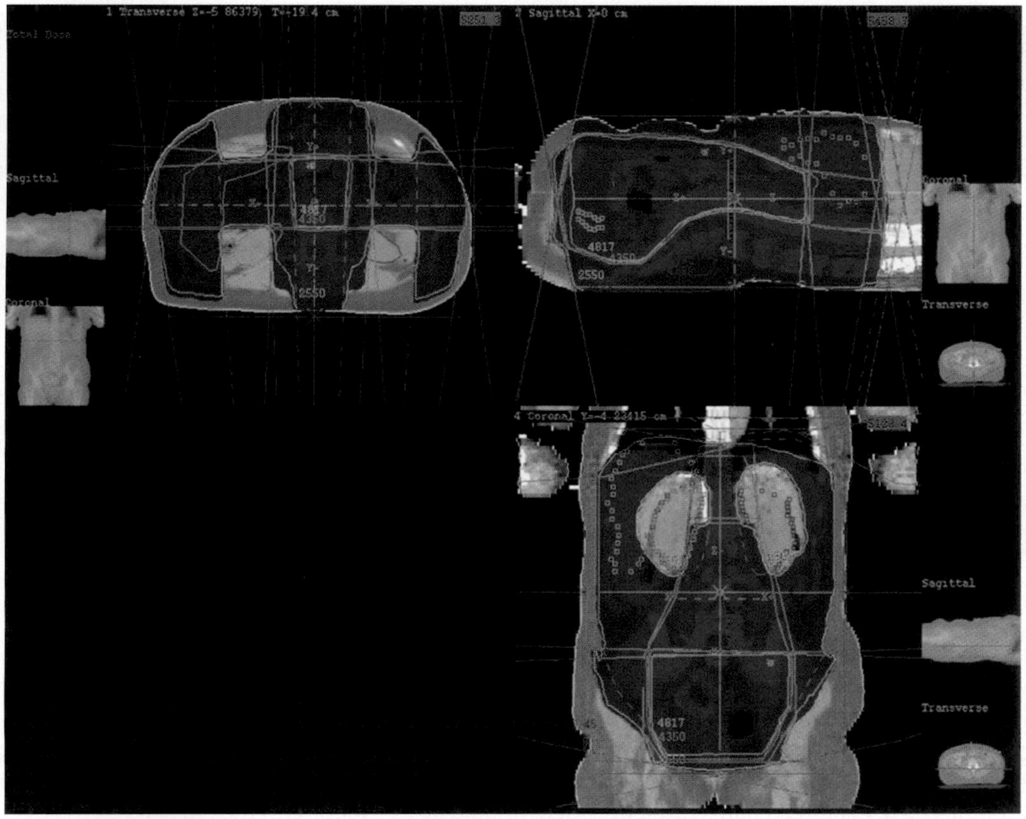

A

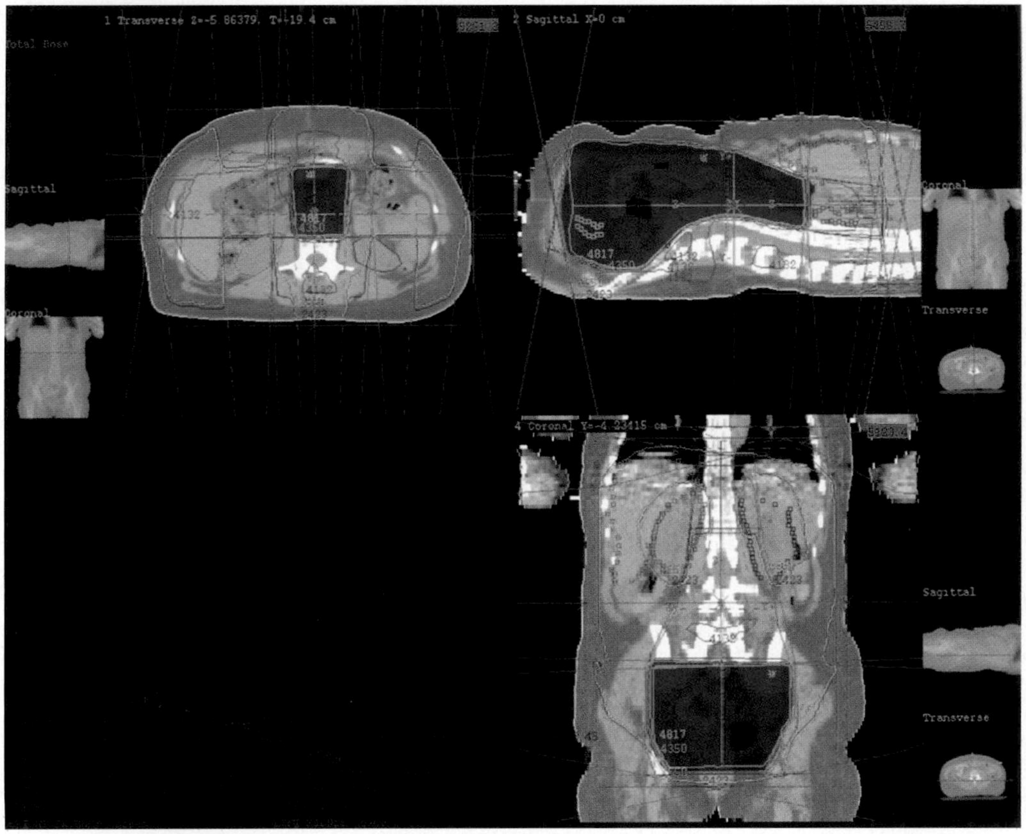

B

Figure 58-2 Isodose clouds for whole-abdomen irradiation. **A,** Periaortic boost. **B,** Pelvic boost.

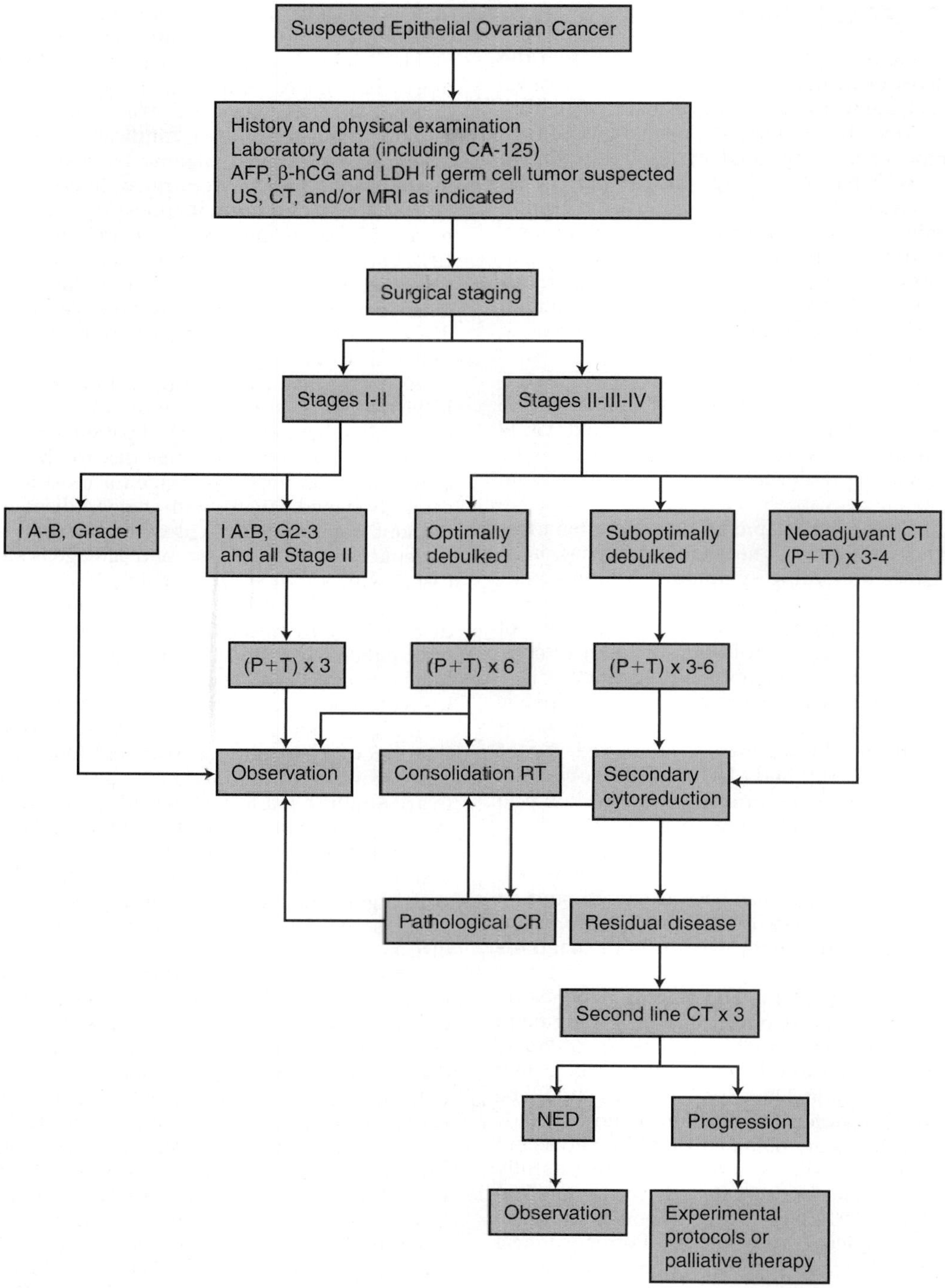

Figure 58-3 Treatment algorithm for epithelial ovarian cancer. AFP, alpha-fetoprotein; β-hCG, beta-human chorionic gonadotropin, CR, complete response; CT, chemotherapy; EOC, epithelial ovarian cancer; LDH, lactate dehydrogenase; MRI, magnetic resonance imaging; NED, no evidence of disease; P+T, platinum plus taxane chemotherapy; RT, radiation therapy; US, ultrasonography.

3. What is the role of adjuvant chemotherapy for early-stage, high-risk EOC, selection of more effective chemotherapy agents, and duration of therapy?
4. What is the optimal chemotherapy combination in patients with advanced EOC after optimal surgery? Is there a role for interval debulking surgery in advanced EOC?
5. What is the role of maintenance/consolidation therapy in EOC? Is there still a role for consolidation WAI or IP ^{32}P in EOC?
6. What is the best chemotherapy combination for patients with recurrent disease (platinum-sensitive versus platinum-refractory)?
7. What is the role of molecular targeted therapy in EOC? Is there a role for a combination of chemotherapy and biologic therapy in first-line maintenance salvage therapy in EOC?
8. Is there a role for chemosensitizing radiotherapy in combination with taxanes or other agents in early, advanced EOC (GOG 99-15)?

OVARIAN GERM CELL TUMORS

Germ cell tumors (GCTs) of the ovary are derived from the germ cell derivatives of ovarian tissue. The WHO classifies these tumors as belonging to one of three main categories, including benign (mostly dermoids), malignant tumors arising from components of dermoid cysts, and primitive malignant GCTs (see Table 58-1).[49] Age distribution varies among these three groups. Dermoid cysts are usually seen in the second and third decades, but can span all age groups. Malignant tumors arising in dermoid cysts are usually squamous, and are most often encountered in the same age range as women affected by EOC. The most distinct age distribution is that of primitive GCTs, which nearly always occur in young women, with a median of 16 to 20 years. Dysgerminomas account for approximately 50% of all malignant GCTs, followed in frequency by yolk sac tumors and immature teratomas, which account for 20% each, with mixed GCTs making up the remaining 10%. The other types are extremely rare. Germ cell tumors represent less than 5% of all ovarian malignancies.

Most malignant GCTs exhibit rapid growth and often manifest with signs and symptoms of an abdominal mass or an acute abdomen. Other presenting symptoms include abnormal uterine bleeding, precocious puberty, and fever. Differential diagnoses can include appendicitis or complications of pregnancy. Because of the age distribution of these tumors, they can occur concurrently with a normal pregnancy.

Evaluation of a young woman presenting with a pelvic mass should include diagnostic studies to rule out appendicitis and pregnancy. If an adnexal mass is identified, tumor markers including β-hCG, AFP, and LDH should be obtained. Characteristic tumor markers of various GCTs are shown in Table 58-10. CA-125 is often elevated in patients with an adnexal mass, but is nonspecific, and does not help delineate the histology of GCTs. Once an adnexal mass is identified, other intra-abdominal pathology has been excluded, and an attempt has been made to classify the mass with tumor markers, surgical evaluation is indicated for both diagnosis and treatment.

The extent of surgical debulking and staging depends on intraoperative findings. GCTs are often quite large, ranging in size in one series from 7 to 40 cm. This requires an adequate vertical midline incision followed by evaluation of the extent of disease. Ascites is present in 20% of patients; this should be evacuated and sent for cytologic evaluation. If no ascites is present, cytologic washings are obtained from the pelvis and bilateral paracolic gutters. Both ovaries should be carefully inspected. Bilaterality ranges from 5% for yolk sac tumors and immature teratomas to 10% with dysgerminomas. Surgical staging should be completed as per EOC. Retroperitoneal lymph nodes are palpated, and suspicious nodes are excised.

Table 58-10 Tumor Markers for Germ Cell Tumors

Histology	β-hCG	AFP	LDH
Dysgerminoma	+/−	−	+
Yolk sac tumor	−	+	−
Immature teratoma	−	+/−	−
Mixed GCT	+/−	+/−	+/−
Choriocarcinoma	+	−	−
Embryonal carcinoma	+	+/−	−
Polyembryoma	+	+/−	−

AFP, alpha-fetoprotein; β-hCG, beta-human chorionic gonadotropin; GCT, germ cell tumor; LDH, lactate dehydrogenase.

If no suspicious nodes are present, the bilateral pelvic and para-aortic lymph nodes are sampled; a complete lymphadenectomy has not been shown to be indicated. Disease is most often grossly confined to one ovary; 60% to 70% of patients will have stage I disease. In these cases, unilateral salpingo-oophorectomy is indicated; if no extraovarian disease is appreciated, staging biopsies and retroperitoneal lymphadenectomy are performed. In cases of pure dysgerminoma, biopsy of a normal-appearing contralateral ovary can be considered, as microscopic involvement can be as high as 10%. Otherwise, ovarian biopsy is not indicated. Fortunately, preservation of the uterus and contralateral ovary and maintenance of fertility are usually possible. If grossly metastatic disease is present, debulking is performed in a similar fashion to that described for EOC.

Adjuvant therapy for dysgerminomas is stage-dependent. If the patient is unstaged, she can be offered a staging operation versus chemotherapy. Most patients with dysgerminomas are diagnosed with early-stage disease. Because preservation of fertility is an important issue for most of these women, all carefully staged patients with stage IA disease can be observed without compromising cure, because only 15% to 25% of patients experience relapse, and salvage is successful in these cases, with survival approaching 100%.[147] Patients who are unstaged and decline staging operation, and those with disease more advanced than stage IA require adjuvant therapy with either radiation or chemotherapy. Similarly, any histologic evidence of other germ cell elements increases the risk for recurrence, and requires adjuvant therapy.

Dysgerminomas are exquisitely sensitive to RT, which was the preferred modality of treatment following surgery in the past. However, infertility resulting from radiation-induced ovarian failure led to a search for less toxic regimens in this young population. Until the demonstration that metastatic dysgerminomas could be cured with cisplatin-based chemotherapy, most patients with stage I disease and all patients with higher-stage disease were treated with RT. Virtually all patients with early-stage tumors were cured of their disease.

The evolution of chemotherapy for GCTs has been based on the successful treatment of similar histology testicular GCTs. Initially, patients with advanced ovarian GCTs were treated with surgical debulking followed by vincristine, dactinomycin, and cyclophosphamide chemotherapy (VAC), with cure rates of approximately 50%.[148] Because of very high cure rates achieved even in advanced testicular GCT using cisplatin, vinblastine, and bleomycin, the GOG evaluated a similar regimen in ovarian GCTs, and noted a 70% 4-year survival.[149] Etoposide reduced toxicity and improved cure rates in testicular GCTs. Using three to four cycles of bleomycin, etoposide, and cisplatin (BEP) led to its adoption as the standard regimen for ovarian GCTs with a 79% to 83% PFS.[150,151] Patients who have no evidence of disease after surgical staging followed by three cycles of BEP can expect a 96% to 100% PFS.[152-154]

Nondysgerminomatous tumors are treated similarly to dysgerminomas, with a few notable exceptions. This group of tumors differs from dysgerminomas in their radioresistance, and in the past, they had a grim prognosis. However, they respond to chemotherapy, with results of VAC and BEP mirroring the results seen with dysgerminomas. Most nondysgerminomatous GCTs of the ovary are treated with surgery followed by combination chemotherapy. The current standard therapy for nondysgerminomatous tumors is similar to that for the dysgerminomas: three cycles of BEP when complete surgical resection has been accomplished, and four cycles when residual disease remains.

The most important prognostic feature in nondysgerminomatous tumors, and that which is used to dictate therapy, is the grade of the lesion. Careful pathologic review of the specimen is imperative, as the presence of other germ cell elements requires adjuvant therapy, even in those with stage IA grade 1 disease, similar to patients with stage IA dysgerminomas, as mentioned earlier. However, the notable exception is patients with adequately confirmed stage IA, grade 1 immature teratoma, for whom adjuvant chemotherapy is not necessary.[147,154–156] Even patients with stage IA, grade 2 and 3 disease have such a high relapse rate that postoperative chemotherapy is indicated.[147,151–153]

Endodermal sinus (yolk sac) tumors, derived from the primitive yolk sac, are the third most frequent GCT of the ovary. These tumors secrete AFP, which can be used as a marker for response to therapy and recurrence. Most patients present with early-stage disease, but all patients, regardless of stage and extent of initial surgery (generally unilateral oophorectomy or salpingo-oophorectomy) are treated with platinum-based chemotherapy.[153]

Embryonal carcinoma and nongestational choriocarcinoma of the ovary are both extremely rare. Embryonal carcinomas can secrete both AFP and β-hCG, whereas pure choriocarcinomas secrete only β-hCG. The recommended treatment approach involves surgery, generally unilateral oophorectomy or salpingo-oophorectomy, followed by combination chemotherapy using the BEP regimen.[153] Prognosis for mixed GCTs is related to the relative amount of the most aggressive malignant component. The most frequent combination consists of elements of endodermal sinus tumor and dysgerminoma. Mixed GCTs may secrete any combination of markers, depending on the histologic components of the tumor.

The prognosis for ovarian GCTs is excellent, and fertility-sparing surgery is possible in most cases, even with advanced disease. Future directions include improving prognosis in advanced disease through evaluation of new chemotherapeutic regimens, and reducing toxicity while maintaining the excellent prognosis of those with early-stage disease.

OVARIAN SEX CORD-STROMAL TUMORS

Ovarian sex cord-stromal tumors (SCSTs) arise from the mesenchymal and connective tissue elements of the ovary, and constitute 7% of all ovarian malignancies. Unlike the extremes in age distribution of the malignancies discussed earlier, older populations affected with EOC and younger populations affected with GCTs, SCSTs are relatively evenly distributed from the second to the eighth decades. A hallmark of this class of tumors is their ability to secrete hormones, in particular estrogen and testosterone. Presenting signs are often related to the effects of these hormones. Evaluation of precocious puberty or frank virilization may identify a pelvic mass, which in the presence of elevated testosterone or estrogen levels, is highly suggestive of a SCST. Patients with an estrogen-secreting ovarian tumor can present with endometrial carcinoma and an adnexal mass. Subclassification of these tumors is listed in Table 58-1.

The most common SCST is the adult granulosa cell tumor, which accounts for 70% of all malignant SCSTs and 95% of all granulosa cell tumors. The extreme rarity of the other tumors in this category makes them difficult to study.

Abnormalities of menstruation ranging from menometrorrhagia and oligomenorrhea to amenorrhea can occur in premenstrual women, whereas postmenopausal bleeding may be the presenting complaint in older patients. Additional signs of hyperestrogenemia include breast tenderness and endometrial hyperplasia or carcinoma. Increasing abdominal girth and abdominal discomfort may be signs of associated ascites, torsion, or mass effect. Granulosa cell tumors are often suspected on the basis of the gross appearance, including a multicystic mass interspersed with a hemorrhagic, friable stromal component. Hemorrhage into these cystic spaces can result in acute abdominal pain and anemia, which is another common presentation. Adult granulosa cell tumors may be suspected, but are rarely diagnosed preoperatively.

Management includes exploratory laparotomy for a pelvic mass; when granulosa cell tumor is diagnosed, staging is similar to that for EOC. A fertility-sparing procedure can be accomplished by unilateral oophorectomy in a patient desiring to maintain her reproductive capability, as long as the contralateral ovary appears normal, and there is no evidence of endometrial carcinoma. If metastatic disease is present, or if the patient is postmenopausal, hysterectomy and bilateral salpingo-oophorectomy are performed.

Recommendations for additional treatment with chemotherapy or RT depend on disease extent. Adjuvant chemotherapy is not recommended for stage I disease. Rather, chemotherapy is recommended following maximal surgical debulking of stage II-IV disease, although its contribution to improved survival is unproven. Patients with stage IC disease may be offered chemotherapy on an individualized basis. Although these tumors may respond to RT it is usually not recommended, as adjuvant therapy is of no proven value. Two retrospective series have found similar outcomes in stage I patients treated with adjuvant RT. Savage and colleagues[157] found 10-year DFS rates of 77% in those treated with adjuvant RT versus 78% in those treated with surgery alone. A role for primary treatment was noted, however, in eight patients who could not undergo primary surgical debulking, or had residual disease. This population showed a 50% response rate, which lasted between 16 months and 5 years. The M.D. Anderson Cancer Center reported a series of 34 patients with granulosa cell tumor, 14 of whom had measurable disease. In this group of 14, six demonstrated a complete response, and three had durable responses.[158] Although adjuvant therapy does not appear to be warranted, some patients have success with primary treatment or treatment of residual disease.

The standard therapy for patients with stage II-IV granulosa cell tumor is a platinum-containing chemotherapy regimen, although controlled trials have not been conducted because of its rarity. Therefore, results are difficult to interpret. Between 1991 and 1997, the GOG evaluated 57 patients with stage II-IV incompletely resected or recurrent histologically confirmed SCSTs.[159] These included 48 granulosa cell tumors, seven Sertoli-Leydig tumors, one malignant thecoma, and one unclassified. All patients were treated with four cycles of BEP. Eleven of 16 patients with primary disease and 21 of 41 with recurrent disease experienced PFS, with a median of 3 years.[159] Other regimens with some activity include combination cisplatin, doxorubicin, and cyclophosphamide,[160] single agent paclitaxel (in patients who have failed platinum-based chemotherapy),[160] and combination platinum/paclitaxel.[161] Rationale exists for the use of hormonal regimens as well with success, demonstrated in patients with recurrent or persistent granulosa cell tumors, treated with medroxyprogesterone or leuprolide acetate.[162,163]

Granulosa cell tumors are notorious for late relapse, even after years apparently disease-free. Disease relapse has been noted up to 20 years following the initial diagnosis and often consists of isolated intrapelvic or abdominal masses. Further surgical resections or RT may control disease for protracted periods of years. A reliable marker for relapse is yet to be elucidated. Often, patients will have an elevation in certain proteins derived from granulosa cells, including inhibin, müllerian-inhibiting substance, and follicle-regulating protein, heralding recurrent disease. None of these has been proved to be entirely reliable, but inhibin levels are frequently followed on an annual to semi-annual basis following surgical resection and/or adjuvant therapy. It is not clear that earlier intervention at the first sign of tumor relapse improves symptom-free overall survival. Future directions include determining improved noninvasive methods to detect relapse of disease, and finding active agents in the treatment of these rare tumors.

REFERENCES

1. Jemal A, Siegel R, Ward E, et al: Cancer Statistics, 2006. CA Cancer J Clin 56:106-130, 2006.
2. McGuire WP, Hoskins WJ, Brady MF, et al: Cyclophosphamide and cisplatin compared with paclitaxel and cisplatin in patients with stage III and stage IV ovarian cancer. N Engl J Med 334:1-6, 1996.
3. Landis SH, Murray T, Bolden S, Wingo PA: Cancer statistics. CA Cancer J Clin 49:8, 1999.
4. Yancik R, Ries LG, Yates JW: Ovarian cancer in the elderly: an analysis of surveillance, epidemiology and end results program data. Am J Obstet Gynecol 154:639, 1986.
5. Ries LAG, Eisner M, Kosary CL, et al (eds): SEER Cancer Statistics Review: 1973-1999. Bethesda, MD: National Cancer Institute, 2002.
6. Harlan LC, Clegg LX, Trimble EL: Trends in surgery and chemotherapy for women diagnosed with ovarian cancer in the United States. J Clin Oncol 21:3488-3494, 2003.
7. Daly M, Obrams GI: Epidemiology and risk assessment for ovarian cancer. Semin Oncol 25:255-264, 1998.
8. Anonymous: Epithelial ovarian cancer and combined oral contraceptives. The WHO Collaborative Study of Neoplasia and Steroid Contraceptives. Int J Epidemiol 18:538-545, 1989.
9. Rossing MA, Daling JR, Weiss NS, et al: Ovarian tumors in a cohort of infertile women. N Engl J Med 331:771-776, 1994.
10. Lacey JV, Mink PJ, Lubin JH, et al: Menopausal hormone replacement therapy and risk of ovarian cancer. JAMA 288:334, 2002.
11. Anderson GL, Judd HL, Kaunitz AM, et al: Effects of estrogen plus progestin on gynecologic cancers and associated diagnostic procedures. JAMA 290:1739-1748, 2003.
12. Risch HA: Hormonal etiology of epithelial ovarian cancer, with a hypothesis concerning the role of androgens and progesterone. J Natl Cancer Inst 90:1774-1786, 1998.
13. Hogg R, Friedlander M: Biology of epithelial ovarian cancer. Implications for screening women at high genetic risk. J Clin Oncol 22:1315-1327, 2004.
14. NIH Consensus Development Panel on Ovarian Cancer: Ovarian cancer: screening, treatment and follow-up. JAMA 273:491, 1995.
15. Kramer BS, Gohagan J, Prorok PC, Smart C: A National Cancer Institute sponsored screening trial for prostatic, lung, colorectal, and ovarian cancers. Cancer 71:589, 1993.
16. Ramakrishnan S, Xu FJ, Brandt SJ, et al: Elevated levels of macrophage colony stimulating factor (M-CSF) in serum and ascites from patients with epithelial ovarian cancer. Gynecol Oncol 21:40, 1990.
17. Xu FJ, Yu YH, Daly L, et al: OVX1 radioimmunoassay complements CA-125 for predicting the presence of residual ovarian carcinomas at second-look surgical surveillance procedures. J Clin Oncol 11:1506, 1993.
18. Woolas RP, Xu FJ, Jacobs IJ, et al: Elevation of multiple serum markers in patients with stage I ovarian cancer. J Natl Cancer Inst 85:1748, 1993.
19. Boyd J, Rubin SC: Hereditary ovarian cancer: molecular genetics and clinical implications. Gynecol Oncol 64:196, 1997.
20. American College of Obstetricians and Gynecologists Committee on Quality Assessment: ACOQ criteria set for prophylactic bilateral oophorectomy to prevent epithelial carcinoma. Int J Gynecol Obstet 52:101, 1996.
21. Burke W, Daly M, Garber J, et al: Recommendations for follow-up care of individuals with an inherited predisposition to cancer. II. BRCA1 and BRCA2. Cancer Genetics Studies Consortium. JAMA 277:997, 1997.
22. Olopade OI, Artioli G: Efficacy of risk-reducing salpingo-oophorectomy in women with BRCA 1 and BRCA 2 mutations. Breast J 10(Suppl 1):S5-S9, 2004.
23. Karlan BY, Baldwin RL, Lopez-Luevanos ES, et al: Peritoneal serous papillary carcinoma, a phenotypic variant of familial ovarian cancer: implications for ovarian cancer screening. Am J Obstet Gynecol 180:917, 1999.
24. Narod SA, Sun P, Risch HA: Hereditary Ovarian Cancer Clinical Study Group. Ovarian cancer, oral contraceptives, and BRCA mutations. N Engl J Med 345: 1706-1707, 2001.
25. Boyd J: Molecular genetics of hereditary ovarian cancer. Oncology 12:399, 1998.
26. Wooster R, Neuhausen SL, Mangion J, et al: A strong candidate for the breast and ovarian cancer susceptibility gene BRCA2. Science 266:66, 1994.
27. Frank TS: Testing for hereditary risk of ovarian cancer. Cancer Control 6:327-334, 1999.
28. Ford D, Easton DF: The genetics of breast and ovarian cancer. Br J Cancer 72:805, 1995.
29. Brose MS, Rebbeck TR, Calzone KA, et al: Cancer risk estimates for BRCA1 mutation carriers identified in a risk evaluation program. J Natl Cancer Inst 94:1365-1372, 2002.
30. Bewtra C, Watson P, Conway T, et al: Hereditary ovarian cancer: a clinicopathologic study. Int J Gynecol Pathol 11:180, 1992.
31. Lynch HT, Kimberling W, Albano WA, et al: Hereditary non-polyposis colorectal cancer (Lynch syndrome I and II). I. Clinical description of resource. Cancer 56:934, 1985.
32. Aarnio M, Sankila R, Pukkala E, et al: Cancer risk in mutation carriers of DNA-mismatch repair genes. Int J Cancer 81:214-218, 1999.
33. Rubin SC, Benjamin I, Behbakht K, et al: Clinical and pathological features of ovarian cancer in women with germ-line mutations of BRCA1. N Engl J Med 335:1413, 1996.
34. Rebbeck TR, Levin AM, Eisen A, et al: Breast cancer risk after bilateral prophylactic oophorectomy in BRCA1 mutation carriers. J Natl Cancer Inst 91:1475, 1999.
35. Narod SA, Risch H, Moslehi R, et al: Oral contraceptives and the risk of hereditary ovarian cancer. N Engl J Med 339:424, 1998.
36. Young RC, Walton LA, Ellenberg SS, et al: Adjuvant therapy in stage I and stage II epithelial ovarian cancer: results of two prospective randomized trials. N Engl J Med 322:1021-1027, 1990.
37. Hoskins WJ, Bundy BN, Thigpen JT, Omura GA: The influence of cytoreductive surgery on recurrence-free interval and survival in small volume stage III epithelial ovarian cancer: a Gynecologic Oncology Group study. Gynecol Oncol 47:159-166, 1992.
38. Griffiths CT: Surgical resection of tumor bulk in the primary treatment of ovarian cancer. Natl Cancer Inst Monogr 42:101-105, 1975.
39. Redman JR, Petroni GR, Saigo PE, et al: Prognostic factors in advanced ovarian carcinoma. J Clin Oncol 4:515-523, 1986.
40. Chi DS, Leon LF, Venkatraman ES, et al: Identification of prognostic factors in advanced epithelial ovarian carcinoma. Gynecol Oncol 82:532-537, 2001.
41. Young RC, Decker DG, Wharton JT, et al: Staging laparotomy in early ovarian cancer. JAMA 250:3072-3076, 1983.
42. Omura GA, Brody MF, Homesley HD, et al: Long-term follow-up and prognostic factor analysis in advanced ovarian carcinomas: the Gynecologic Oncology Group experience. J Clin Oncol 9:1138, 1991.
43. Makar APH, Kristensen GB, Kaern J, et al: Prognostic value of pre- and postoperative serum CA-125 levels in ovarian cancer: new aspects and multivariate analysis. Obstet Gynecol 79:1002-1010, 1992.
44. Fayers PM, Rustin G, Wood R, et al: The prognostic value of serum CA-125 in patients with advanced ovarian carcinoma: an analysis of 573 patients by the Medical Research Council Working Party on gynecological cancer. Int J Gynecol Cancer 3:285-292, 1993.
45. Trope CG, Kaern J, Hogberg T, et al: Randomized study on adjuvant chemotherapy in stage I ovarian cancer with evaluation of

DNA ploidy as prognostic instrument. Ann Oncol 11:281-288, 2000.
46. Skirnisdottir I, Sorbe B, Seidal T: The growth factor receptors HER-2/neu and EGFR, their relationship and their effects on the prognosis in early stage (FIGO I-II) epithelial ovarian carcinoma. Int J Gynecol Cancer 11:119-129, 2001.
47. Denkert C, Kobel M, Pest S, et al: Expression of cyclo-oxygenase 2 is an independent prognostic factor in human ovarian carcinoma. Am J Pathol 160: 893-903, 2002.
48. Raspollini MR, Amunni G, Villanuchi A, et al: Prognostic significance of microvessel density and vascular endothelial growth factor expression in advanced ovarian serous carcinoma. Int J Gynecol Cancer 14:815-823, 2004.
49. Tavassoli FA, Devilee P (eds), for the International Agency for Research on Cancer (IARC): WHO Classification of Tumors: Pathology and Genetics of Tumors of the Breast and Female Genital Organs. Lyon, IARC Press, 2003, p 114.
50. Piver MS, Barlow JJ, Lele SB: Incidence of subclinical metastasis in stage I and stage II ovarian carcinoma. Obstet Gynecol 52:100, 1978.
51. Herrmann UJ: Sonographic patterns of ovarian tumors. Clin Obstet Gynecol 36:375, 1993.
52. Chen D, Schwartz PE, Li X, Yang Z: Evaluation of CA125 levels in differentiating malignant from benign tumors in patients with pelvic masses. Obstet Gynecol 72:23, 1988.
53. Greene FL, Page DI, Flemming ID, et al: American Joint Committee on Cancer (AJCC): AJCC Cancer Staging Manual, ed 6. New York, Springer-Verlag, 2002, pp 257-287.
54. Munoz KA, Harlan LC, Trimble EL: Patterns of care for women with ovarian cancer in the United States. J Clin Oncol 15:3408-3415, 1997.
55. Elit L, Bondy SJ, Paszat L, et al: Outcomes in surgery for ovarian cancer. Gynecol Oncol 87:260, 2002.
56. Keettel WC, Pixley EE, Buchsbaum HJ: Experience with peritoneal cytology in the management of gynecologic malignancies. Am J Obstet Gynecol 120:174, 1974.
57. Schilder JM, Thompson AM, DePriest PD, et al: Outcome of reproductive age women with stage IA or IC invasive epithelial ovarian cancer treated with fertility-sparing therapy. Gynecol Oncol 87:1-7, 2002.
58. Flanagan CW, Mannel RS, Walker JL, Johnson GA: Incidence and location of para-aortic lymph node metastases in gynecologic malignancies. J Am Coll Surg 181:72, 1995.
59. Scarabelli C, Gallo A, Zarrelli A, et al: Systematic pelvic and para-aortic lymphadenectomy during cytoreductive surgery in advanced ovarian cancer: potential benefit on survival. Gynecol Oncol 56:328, 1995.
60. van der Burg MEL, van Lent M, Buyse M, et al: The effect of debulking surgery after induction chemotherapy on the prognosis in advanced epithelial ovarian cancer. N Engl J Med 332:629-634, 1995.
61. van der Burg MEL, Coens C, van Lent M, et al: After 10 years follow-up interval debulking surgery remains a significant prognostic factor for survival and progression-free survival for advanced ovarian cancer: The EORTC Gynecological Cancer Group Study. Abstract # 008. Int J Gynecol Cancer 14:Suppl 1, 2004.
62. Morgan RJ, Alvarez RD, Armstrong DK, et al: Ovarian cancer. Clinical Practice Guidelines. National Comprehensive Cancer Network (NCCN). JNCCN 2:526-547, 2004.
63. Benjamin I, Morgan MA, Rubin SC: Occult bilateral involvement in stage I epithelial ovarian cancer. Gynecol Oncol 72:288, 1999.
64. Hreshchyshyn MM, Park RC, Blessing JA: The role of adjuvant therapy in stage I ovarian cancer. Am J Obstet Gynecol 138:139-145, 1980.
65. Vergote I, DeBravanter J, Fyles A, et al: Prognostic importance of degree of differentiation and cyst rupture in stage I invasive epithelial ovarian carcinoma. Lancet 357:176-182, 2001.
66. Trimbos JB, Vergote I, Bolis G, et al: Impact of adjuvant chemotherapy and surgical staging in early-stage ovarian carcinoma: European Organization for Research and Treatment of Cancer—Adjuvant Chemotherapy in Ovarian Neoplasm Trial (EORTC-ACTION). J Natl Cancer Inst 95:113-125, 2003.
67. Currie JL, Bagne F, Harrix C, et al: Radioactive chromic phosphate suspension: studies on distribution, dose absorption, and effective therapeutic radiation in phantoms, dogs and patients. Gynecol Oncol 12:193-218, 1981.
68. Boye E, Lindergaad MW, Paus E, et al: Whole-body distribution of radioactivity after intraperitoneal administration of ^{32}P colloids. Br J Radiol 57:395-402, 1984.
69. Young RC, Brady MF, Nieberg RM, et al: Adjuvant treatment for early ovarian cancer: a randomized Phase III trial of intraperitoneal ^{32}P or intravenous cyclophosphamide and cisplatin—a Gynecology Oncology Group (GOG) study. J Clin Oncol 21:4350-4355, 2003.
70. Klaasen D, Shelley W, Starreveld A, et al: Early stage ovarian cancer: a randomized clinical trial comparing whole abdominal radiotherapy, melphalan, and intraperitoneal chromic phosphate: a National Cancer Institute of Canada Clinical Trials Group report. J Clin Oncol 6:1254-1263, 1988.
71. Vergote IB, Vergote-DeVos LN, Abeler VN, et al: Randomized trial comparing cisplatin with radioactive phosphorus or whole abdomen irradiation as adjuvant treatment of ovarian cancer. Cancer 69:741-749, 1992.
72. Vergote IB, Winderen M, De Vos LN, Trope CG: Intraperitoneal radioactive phosphorus therapy in ovarian carcinoma. Analysis of 313 patients treated primarily or at second-look laparotomy. Cancer 71:2250-2260, 1993.
73. Bolis G, Colombo N, Pecorelli S, et al: Adjuvant treatment for early epithelial ovarian cancer: results of two randomized clinical trials comparing cisplatin to no further therapy or chromic phosphate. Ann Oncol 9:887-893, 1995.
74. Ott RJ, Flower MA, Jones A, McCready VR: The measurement of radiation doses from ^{32}P chromic phosphate therapy of the peritoneum using SPECT. Eur J Nucl Med 11:305-308, 1985.
75. Smith JP, Rutledge FN, Delclos L: Postoperative treatment of early cancer of the ovary: a random trial between postoperative irradiation and chemotherapy. J Natl Cancer Inst 42:149-153, 1975.
76. Dembo AJ, Davy M, Stenwig AE, et al: Prognostic factors in patients with stage I epithelial ovarian cancer. Obstet Gynecol 75:263, 1990.
77. Lederman JA, Dembo AJ, Sturgeon JFG, et al: Outcome of patients with unfavorable optimally cytoreduced ovarian cancer treated with chemotherapy and whole abdominal radiation. Gynecol Oncol 41:30-35, 1991.
78. Dembo AJ, Bush RS: Choice of postoperative therapy based on prognostic factors. Int J Radiat Oncol Biol Phys 8:893-897, 1982.
79. Dembo AJ: Abdominopelvic radiotherapy in ovarian cancer: a 10-year experience. Cancer 55:2285-2290, 1985.
80. Dembo AJ, Bush RS, Beale FA, et al: Ovarian carcinoma: improved survival following abdominopelvic irradiation in patients with a complete pelvic operation. Am J Obstet Gynecol 134:793-800, 1979.
81. Carey M, Dembo AJ, Simm JE, et al: Testing the validity of a prognostic classification in patients with surgically optimal ovarian carcinoma: a 15-year review. Int J Gynecol Cancer 3:24-35, 1993.
82. Fyles AW, Thomas GM, Pintilie M, et al: A randomized study of two doses of abdominopelvic radiation therapy for patients with optimally debulked stage I, II and III ovarian cancer. Int J Radiat Oncol Biol Phys 41:543-549, 1998.
83. Sell A, Bertelsen K, Andersen JE, et al: Randomized study of whole abdomen irradiation versus pelvic irradiation plus cyclophosphamide in treatment of early ovarian cancer. Gynecol Oncol 37:367-373, 1990.
84. Chiara S, Pierfranco C, Franzone P: High-risk early-stage ovarian cancer: randomized trial comparing cisplatin plus cyclophosphamide versus whole abdominal radiotherapy. Am J Clin Oncol 17:72-76, 1994.
85. Bush RS, Allt WEC, Beale FA: Treatment of carcinoma of the ovary: operation, irradiation and chemotherapy. Am J Obstet Gynecol 127:692-704, 1977.
86. Dembo AJ, Bush RS, Beale FA, et al: The Princess Margaret Hospital study on ovarian cancer: stage I, II and asymptomatic III presentations. Cancer Treat Rep 63:249-254, 1979.
87. Colombo N, Guthrie D, Chiari S, et al: International Collaborative Ovarian Neoplasm Trial 1: a randomized trial of adjuvant

chemotherapy in women with early stage ovarian cancer. J Natl Cancer Inst 95:125-132, 2003.
88. Trimbos JB, Parmar M, Vergote I, et al: International Collaborative Ovarian Neoplasm Trial 1 and Adjuvant Chemotherapy in Ovarian Neoplasm Trial: Two parallel randomized phase III trials of adjuvant chemotherapy in patients with early stage ovarian carcinoma. J Natl Cancer Inst 95:105-112, 2003.
89. Young R, Rose G, Lage J, et al: A randomized phase III trial of three versus six cycles of carboplatin and paclitaxel as adjuvant treatment in early stage ovarian epithelial carcinoma. A Gynecologic Oncology Group Study. 34th Annual Meeting of the Society of Gynecologic Oncologists (Abst #1001), 2003.
90. Ozols RF, Bundy BN, Greer BE, et al: Phase III trial of carboplatin and paclitaxel compared with cisplatin and paclitaxel in patients with optimally resected stage III ovarian cancer: a Gynecologic Oncology Group study. J Clin Oncol 21:3194-3200, 2003.
91. Bristow RE, Tomacruz RS, Armstrong DK, et al: Survival effect of maximal cytoreductive surgery for advanced ovarian carcinoma during the platinum era: a meta-analysis. J Clin Oncol 20:1248-1259, 2002.
92. Greer BE, Swensen RE, Gray HJ, et al: Surgery for ovarian cancer: rationale and guidelines. JNCCN 1:561-568, 2004.
93. Van der Berg ME: More than 20 years second-look surgery in advanced epithelial ovarian cancer: What did we learn? Ann Oncol 8:627, 1997.
94. Greer BE, Bundy BN, Ozols RF, et al: Implications of second look laparotomy (SLL) in the context of Gynecologic Oncology Group (GOG) Protocol 158: a non-randomized comparison using an explanatory analysis (Abstract 1). Gynecol Oncol 88:156-157, 2003.
95. Rose P, Nerenstone S, Brady M, et al: Secondary surgical cytoreduction for advanced ovarian carcinoma: a Gynecologic Oncology Group (GOG) study. N Engl J Med 351:2489-2497, 2004.
96. Munkarah AR, Coleman RL: Critical evaluation of secondary cytoreduction in recurrent ovarian cancer. Gynecol Oncol 95:273-280, 2004.
97. Omura GA, Morrow CP, Blessing JA, et al: A randomized comparison of melphalan versus melphalan plus hexamethylmelamine versus adriamycin plus cyclophosphamide in ovarian carcinoma. Cancer 51:783, 1983.
98. Omura GA, Blessing JA, Ehrlich CE, et al: A randomized trial of cyclophosphamide and doxorubicin with or without cisplatin in advanced ovarian carcinoma. A GOG study. Cancer 57:1725, 1986.
99. Omura GA, Bundy BN, Berek JS, et al: Randomized trial of cyclophosphamide plus cisplatin with or without doxorubicin in ovarian carcinoma. A GOG study. J Clin Oncol 7:457, 1989.
100. West RJ, Zweig SF: Meta-analysis of chemotherapy regimens for ovarian carcinoma: a reassessment of cisplatin, cyclophosphamide and doxorubicin versus cisplatin and cyclophosphamide. Eur J Gynaecol Oncol 18:343, 1997.
101. Fanning J, Bennett TZ, Hilgers RD: Meta-analysis of cisplatin, doxorubicin and cyclophosphamide versus cisplatin and cyclophosphamide chemotherapy for ovarian carcinoma. Obstet Gynecol 80:954, 1992.
102. Piccart MJ, Bertelsen K, James K, et al: Randomized intergroup trial of cisplatin-paclitaxel versus cisplatin-cyclophosphamide in women with advanced epithelial ovarian cancer. Three years results. J Natl Cancer Inst 92:699-708, 2000.
103. National Institutes of Health Consensus Development Conference Statement: Ovarian cancer: screening, treatment and follow-up. Gynecol Oncol 5S:S4-S14, 1994.
104. Dembo AJ: Radiotherapeutic management of ovarian cancer. Semin Oncol 11:238-250, 1984.
105. Goldberg N, Peschel RE: Postoperative abdominopelvic radiation therapy for ovarian cancer. Int J Radiat Oncol Biol Phys 14:425-429, 1988.
106. Weiser EB, Burke TW, Heller PB, et al: Determinants of survival of patients with epithelial ovarian carcinoma following whole abdominal irradiation (WAR). Gynecol Oncol 30:201-208, 1988.
107. Fuller DB, Sause WT, Plenk HP, Menlove RL: Analysis of postoperative radiation therapy in stage I through III epithelial ovarian carcinoma. J Clin Oncol 5:897-905, 1987.
108. Dembo AJ, Bush RS, Beale FA, et al: Ovarian carcinoma: improved survival following abdominopelvic irradiation in patients with a complete pelvic operation. Am J Obstet Gynecol 134:793-800, 1979.
109. Fuks Z, Rizel S, Anteby S: The multimodal approach to the treatment of stage III ovarian carcinoma. Int J Radiat Oncol Biol Phys 8:903-908, 1982.
110. Schray MF, Martinez A, Howes AE, et al: Advanced epithelial ovarian cancer: salvage abdominal irradiation for patients with recurrent or persistent disease after combination chemotherapy. J Clin Oncol 6:1433-1439, 1988.
111. Lambert HE, Rustin GJS, Gregory WM, Nelstrop AE: A randomized trial comparing single-agent carboplatin with carboplatin followed by radiotherapy for advanced ovarian cancer: a North Thames Ovary Group Study. J Clin Oncol 11:440-448, 1993.
112. Bruzzone M, Repetto L, Chiara S, et al: Chemotherapy versus radiotherapy in the management of ovarian cancer patients with pathological complete response or minimal residual disease at second-look. Gynecol Oncol 38:392-395, 1990.
113. Lawton F, Luesley D, Blackledge G, et al: A randomized trial comparing whole abdominal radiotherapy with chemotherapy following cisplatinum cytoreduction in epithelial ovarian cancer. West Midlands Ovarian Cancer Group Trial II. Clin Oncol 2:4-9, 1990.
114. Hoskins PJ, Swenerton KD, Wong F, et al: Platinum plus cyclophosphamide plus radiotherapy is superior to platinum alone in "high risk" epithelial ovarian cancer (residual negative and either stage I or II, grade 3, or stage III, any grade). Int J Gynecol Cancer 5:134-142, 1995.
115. Thomas GM, Dembo AJ: Integrating radiation therapy into the management of ovarian cancer. Cancer 71:1710-1718, 1993.
116. Thomas GM: Is there a role for consolidation or salvage radiotherapy after chemotherapy in advanced epithelial ovarian cancer? Gynecol Oncol 51:97-103, 1993.
117. Pickel H, Lahousen M, Petru E, et al: Consolidation radiotherapy after carboplatin-based chemotherapy in radically operated advanced ovarian cancer. Gynecol Oncol 72:215-219, 1999.
118. Whelan TJ, Dembo AJ, Bush RS, et al: Complications of whole abdominal and pelvic radiotherapy following chemotherapy for advanced ovarian cancer. Int J Radiat Oncol Biol Phys 22:853-858, 1992.
119. Sorbe B, on behalf of the Swedish-Norwegian Ovarian Cancer Study Group: Consolidation treatment of advanced (FIGO stage III) ovarian carcinoma in complete surgical remission after induction chemotherapy: a randomized, controlled, clinical trial comparing whole abdominal radiotherapy, chemotherapy and no further treatment. Int J Gynecol Cancer 13:278-286, 2003.
120. Louie KG, Behrens BC, Kinsella TJ, et al: Radiation survival parameters of anti-neoplastic drug-sensitive and resistant human ovarian cancer cell lines and their modification by buthionine sulfoxime. Cancer Res 45:2110-2115, 1985.
121. Britten RA, Peacock J, Warenious HM: Collateral resistance to photon and neutron irradiation is associated with acquired cisplatin resistance in human ovarian tumor cells. Radiother Oncol 23:170-175, 1992.
122. Schwartz JL, Rotmensch J, Beckett MA, et al: X-Ray and cis-diammine dichloroplatinum cross-resistance in human tumor cell lines. Cancer Res 48:5133-5135, 1988.
123. Eifel PJ, Gershenson DM, Delclos L, et al: Twice-daily, split-course abdominopelvic radiation therapy after chemotherapy and positive second-look laparotomy for epithelial ovarian carcinoma. Int J Radiat Oncol Biol Phys 21:1013-1018, 1991.
124. Reddy S, Lee M-S, Yordan E, et al: Salvage whole abdomen radiation therapy: its role in ovarian cancer. Int J Radiat Oncol Biol Phys 27:879-884, 1993.
125. Fein DA, Morgan LS, Marcus RB, et al: Stage III ovarian carcinoma: an analysis of treatment results and complications following hyperfractionated abdominopelvic irradiation for salvage. Int J Radiat Oncol Biol Phys 29:169-176, 1994.
126. Cmelak AJ, Kapp DS: Long-term survival with whole abdominopelvic irradiation in platinum-refractory persistent or recurrent ovarian cancer. Gynecol Oncol 65:453-460, 1997.
127. Soper JT, Wilkinson RH Jr, Bandy LC, et al: Intraperitoneal chromic phosphate (^{32}P) as salvage therapy for persistent carci-

noma of the ovary after surgical restaging. Am J Obstet Gynecol 156:1153-1158, 1987.
128. Spanos WJ, Day T, Jose B, et al: Use of ^{32}P in stage III epithelial carcinoma of the ovary. Gynecol Oncol 54:35-39, 1994.
129. Rogers L, Varia M, Halle J, et al: ^{32}P following negative second-look laparotomy for epithelial ovarian cancer. Gynecol Oncol 50:141-146, 1993.
130. Varia MA, Stehman FB, Bundy BN, et al: Intraperitoneal radioactive phosphorus (^{32}P) versus observation after negative second-look laparotomy for stage III ovarian carcinoma: a randomized trial of the Gynecologic Oncology Group. J Clin Oncol 21:2849-2855, 2003.
131. Patillo RA, Collier BD, Abdel-Dayem H, et al: Phosphorus-32-chromic phosphate for ovarian cancer: I. Fractionated low-dose intraperitoneal treatments in conjunction with platinum analog chemotherapy. J Nucl Med 36:29-36, 1995.
132. Pothuri B, Vaidya A, Aghajanian C, et al: Palliative surgery for bowel obstruction in recurrent ovarian cancer: an updated series. Gynecol Oncol 89:309-313, 2003.
133. Corn BW, Lanciano RM, Boente M, et al: Recurrent ovarian cancer: effective radiotherapeutic palliation after chemotherapy failure. Cancer 74:2979-2983, 1994.
134. Davidson SA, Rubin SC, Mychalczak B, et al: Limited-field radiotherapy as salvage treatment of localized persistent or recurrent epithelial ovarian cancer. Gynecol Oncol 51:349-354, 1993.
135. Fujiwara K, Suzuki S, Yoden E, et al: Local radiation therapy for localized relapsed or refractory ovarian cancer patients with or without symptoms after chemotherapy. Int J Gynecol Cancer 12: 250-256, 2002.
136. Corn BW, Greven KM, Randall ME, et al: The efficacy of cranial irradiation in ovarian cancer metastatic to the brain: analysis of 32 cases. Obstet Gynecol 86:955-959, 1995.
137. Martinez A, Schray MF, Howes AE, Bagshaw MA: Post-operative radiation therapy for epithelial ovarian cancer: the curative role based on 24-year experience. J Clin Oncol 3:901-911, 1985.
138. Hong L, Alektiar K, Chui C, et al: IMRT of large fields: whole abdomen irradiation. Int J Radiat Oncol Biol Phys 54:278-289, 2002.
139. Randall ME, Barrett RJ, Spirtos NM, et al: Chemotherapy, early surgical reassessment and hyperfractionated abdominal radiotherapy in stage III ovarian cancer: results of a Gynecologic Oncology Group study. Int J Radiat Oncol Biol Phys 34:139-147, 1996.
140. Kuten A, Stein M, Steiner M, et al: Whole abdominal irradiation following chemotherapy in advanced ovarian carcinoma. Int J Radiat Oncol Biol Phys 14:273-279, 1988.
141. Dembo AJ, Bush RS, Beale FA, et al: A randomized clinical trial of moving strip versus open field whole abdominal irradiation in patients with invasive epithelial cancer of the ovary. Int J Rad Oncol Biol Phys 9:97, 1983.
142. Fletcher GH: Textbook of Radiotherapy, 3rd ed. Philadelphia, Lea & Febiger, 1980.
143. Marks LB: A standard dose of radiation for "microscopic disease" is not appropriate. Cancer 66:2498-2502, 1990.
144. Withers HR, Suwinski R: Radiation dose response for subclinical metastases. Semin Radiat Oncol 8:224-228, 1998.
145. Fyles AW, Dembo AJ, Bush RS, et al: Analysis of complications in patients treated with abdominopelvic radiation therapy for ovarian carcinoma. Int J Radiat Oncol Biol Phys 22:847-851, 1992.
146. Fyles AW, Manchul L, Levin W, et al: Effect of filgrastim (G-CSF) during chemotherapy and abdomino-pelvic radiation therapy in patients with ovarian carcinoma. Int J Radiat Oncol Biol Phys 41:843-847, 1998.
147. Williams SD: Ovarian germ cell tumors: an update. Semin Oncol 25:407-413, 1998.
148. Slayton RE, Park RC, Silverberg SG, et al: Vincristine, dactinomycin, and cyclophosphamide in the treatment of malignant germ cell tumors of the ovary: a Gynecologic Oncology Group study (a final report). Cancer 56:243, 1985.
149. Williams SD, Blessing JA, Moore DH, et al: Cisplatin, vinblastine, and bleomycin in advanced and recurrent ovarian germ-cell tumors. Ann Intern Med 111:22, 1989.
150. Mayordomo JI, Paz-Ares L, Rivera F, et al: Ovarian and extragonadal malignant germ-cell tumors in females: a single-institution experience with 43 patients. Ann Oncol 5:225, 1994.
151. Gershenson DM, Morris M, Cangir A, et al: Treatment of malignant germ cell tumors of the ovary with bleomycin, etoposide, and cisplatin. J Clin Oncol 8:715, 1990.
152. Gershenson DM: Update on malignant ovarian germ cell tumors. Cancer Suppl 71:1581-1590, 1993.
153. Williams S, Blessing JA, Liao S, et al: Adjuvant therapy of ovarian germ cell tumors with cisplatin, etoposide, and bleomycin: a trial of the Gynecologic Oncology Group. J Clin Oncol 12:701-706, 1994.
154. Marina NM, Cushing B, Giller R, et al: Complete surgical excision is effective treatment for children with immature teratomas with or without malignant elements: a Pediatric Oncology Group/Children's Cancer Group intergroup study. J Clin Oncol 17:2137-2143, 1999.
155. Dark CG, Bower M, Newlands ES, et al: Surveillance policy for stage I ovarian germ cell tumors. J Clin Oncol 15:620-624, 1997.
156. Bonazzi C, Peccatori F, Columbo N, et al: Pure ovarian immature teratoma, a unique and curable disease: 10 years' experience of 32 prospectively treated patients. Obstet Gynecol 84:598-604, 1994.
157. Savage P, Constenela D, Fisher C, et al: Granulosa cell tumours of the ovary: demographics, survival and the management of advanced disease. Clin Oncol 10:242-245, 1998.
158. Wolf JK, Mullen J, Eifel PJ, et al: Radiation treatment of advanced or recurrent granulose cell tumor of the ovary. Gynecol Oncol 73:35-41, 1999.
159. Homesley HD, Bundy GN, Hurteau JA: Bleomycin, etoposide, and cisplatin combination therapy of ovarian granulose cell tumors and other stromal malignancies: a Gynecologic Oncology Group Study. Gynecol Oncol 72:131-137, 1999.
160. Gershenson DM, Copeland LJ, Kavanagh JJ, et al: Treatment of metastatic stromal tumors of the ovary with cisplatin, doxorubicin, and cyclophosphamide. Obstet Gynecol 70:765-769, 1987.
161. Tresukosol D, Kudelka AP, Edwards CL, et al: Recurrent ovarian granulosa cell tumor: a case report of a dramatic response to Taxol. Int J Gynecol Cancer 5:156-159, 1995.
162. Malik ST, Slevin ML: Medroxyprogesterone acetate (MPA) in advanced granulose cell tumours of the ovary—a new therapeutic approach? Br J Cancer 63:410-411, 1991.
163. Fishman A, Kudelka AP, Tresukosol D, et al: Leuprolide acetate for treating refractory or persistent ovarian granulose cell tumor. J Reprod Med 41:393-396, 1996.

PART G

BREAST CANCER

Overview

Jay R. Harris

INCIDENCE AND MORTALITY

Breast cancer is the most frequently diagnosed cancer in U.S. women and the second most frequent cause of cancer mortality. An estimated 211,240 new patients were diagnosed in 2005, and 40,410 women died of breast cancer.

Incidence rates have continued to rise over the past 10 years of full records, but the mortality rate has decreased. The incidence rates are lower for black American women than for white American women, but the mortality rates are higher.

ETIOLOGY

The causes of breast cancer are largely unknown. It is a disease resulting from a complex series of genetic and epigenetic events that result in the dysfunction of several cellular and microenvironmental processes.

Genetic mutations, in which specific nucleotide base pairs of a gene are altered or lost, are common in breast cancers. Most genetic mutations in breast cancer are somatic, developing during the lifetime of the cell rather than occurring as an inherited condition.

Germline mutations in tumor suppressor genes are estimated to play a role in 5% to 10% of all breast cancers. The most common of these inherited mutations are mutations in *BRCA1* or *BRCA2*.

SCREENING

Meta-analysis of mammographic screening trials demonstrates a 20% to 35% reduction in breast cancer mortality in women between the ages of 50 and 69 years and a slightly lower reduction in women between the ages of 40 and 49 years.

Screening with breast magnetic resonance imaging has not been established, but it appears to be useful in young women at high risk for the disease, such as those with a *BRCA1/2* mutation.

NATURAL HISTORY

Breast cancer is a heterogeneous disease with a predisposition for systemic involvement, and it commonly has a long natural history.

The major regional drainage site for the breast is the axilla. The likelihood of axillary nodal involvement is directly related to the size of the primary tumor. Even small tumors (less than 1 cm) are associated with a 20% risk of axillary involvement. Histologic involvement of axillary nodes has a high correlation with prognosis.

PROGNOSTIC AND PREDICTIVE FACTORS

The prognosis of an individual patient based on the standard prognostic factors can be estimated using AdjuvantOnline.

Several gene-based approaches have been and are being developed. One is a reverse transcriptase–polymerase chain reaction assay of 21 prospectively selected genes that can quantify the likelihood of distant recurrence in tamoxifen-treated patients with node-negative, estrogen receptor–positive breast cancer and has also been a predictive factor for the use of chemotherapy in these patients.

TREATMENT

Adjuvant systemic treatment in addition to local treatment has demonstrated significant improvements in survival for treated patients compared with controls and is largely responsible for the recent decrease in the mortality rate.

Systemic therapy can be hormonal therapy, which is useful only for patients with estrogen receptor–positive or progesterone receptor–positive breast cancer, or chemotherapy.

Additional biologic therapies, such as trastuzumab (Herceptin) a humanized immunoglobulin directed against the Erbb2 (Her2/neu) receptor, are useful.

Radiation therapy plays an important role in the management of the disease as part of primary treatment and for palliation.

Breast cancer is a major public health problem throughout most of the world. As part of primary treatment and for palliation, radiation therapy plays an important role in the management of the disease. This chapter summarizes the anatomy, incidence, risk factors, screening, natural history, and the general treatment approaches to breast cancer. For a more detailed description, please refer to a general text on this topic.[1]

ANATOMY

The mammary gland, situated on the anterior chest wall, is composed of glandular tissue with a dense fibrous stroma. The glandular tissue consists of lobules that group together into 15 to 25 lobes arranged approximately in a spoke-like pattern. Multiple major and minor ducts connect the milk-secreting lobular units to the nipple. Small milk ducts course throughout the breast, converging into larger collecting ducts that open into the lactiferous sinus at the base of the nipple. Most cancers form initially in the terminal duct lobular units of the breast. Glandular tissue is more abundant in the upper outer portion of the breast; as a result, half of all breast cancers occur in this area. The chest wall includes ribs, intercostal muscles, and serratus anterior muscle, but not the pectoral muscles. The breast lymphatics drain by way of three major routes: axillary, transpectoral, and internal mammary. Intramammary lymph nodes are coded as axillary lymph nodes for staging purposes. Supraclavicular lymph nodes are classified as regional lymph nodes for staging purposes. Metastasis to any other lymph node, including cervical or contralateral internal mammary lymph nodes, is classified as a distant metastasis. The regional lymph nodes are as follows:

1. Axillary (ipsilateral): interpectoral (Rotter's) nodes and lymph nodes along the axillary vein and its tributaries that may be (but are not required to be) divided into the following levels:
   a. Level I (low-axilla): lymph nodes lateral to the lateral border of the pectoralis minor muscle.
   b. Level II (mid-axilla): lymph nodes between the medial and lateral borders of the pectoralis minor muscle and the interpectoral (Rotter's) lymph nodes.
   c. Level III (apical axilla): lymph nodes medial to the medial margin of the pectoralis minor muscle, including those designated as apical.
2. Internal mammary (ipsilateral): lymph nodes in the intercostal spaces along the edge of the sternum in the endothoracic fascia.
3. Supraclavicular: lymph nodes in the supraclavicular fossa, a triangle defined by the omohyoid muscle and tendon (lateral and superior border), the internal jugular vein (medial border), and the clavicle and subclavian vein (lower border).

TRENDS IN INCIDENCE AND MORTALITY

The following information is provided by the American Cancer Society.[2] The incidence and mortality rates for white and black females in the United States from 1975 to 2001 is shown in Figure G-1. Breast cancer is the most frequently diagnosed cancer in U.S. women and the second most frequent cause of cancer mortality. An estimated 211,240 new patients were diagnosed in 2005, and 40,410 women died from breast cancer. In addition to invasive breast cancer, 58,490 new cases of in situ breast cancer are expected to be diagnosed among women during 2005. Of these, 85% will be ductal carcinoma in situ. Breast cancer incidence rates increased rapidly in the 1980s due to increased use of mammographic screening and have increased gradually since then. Breast cancer incidence

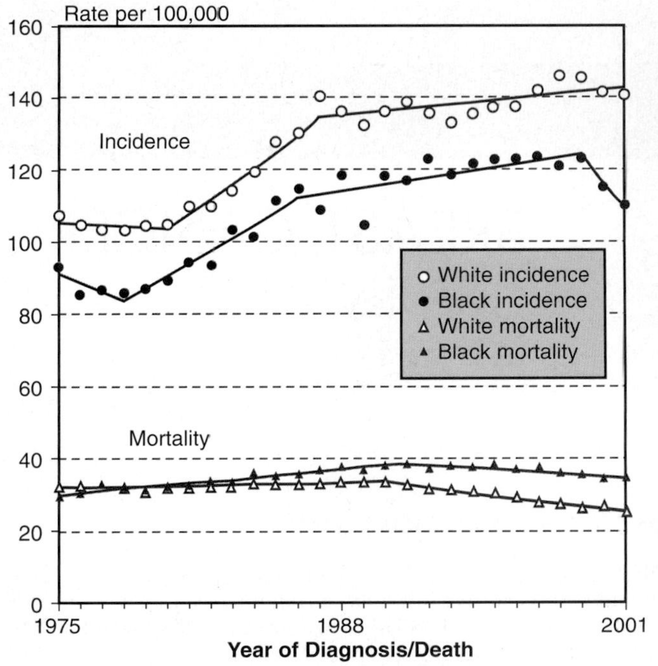

Figure G-1 Breast cancer incidence and mortality for white and black women between 1975 and 2001. Rates are age-adjusted to the 2000 U.S. standard million population by 5-year age groups. Regression lines were calculated using the Joinpoint Regression Program Version 2.7, September 2003, from the National Cancer Institute. (From Ries LAG, Eisner MP, Kosary CL, et al [eds]: SEER Cancer Statistics Review, 1975-2001. Bethesda, MD, National Cancer Institute, 2004, http://seer.cancer.gov/csr/1975_2001/)

rates vary by race and are highest for white Americans and lowest for Native Americans and Alaska natives, with African American, Asian American, and Hispanic or Latin American rates intermediate in decreasing incidence. The mortality rates for breast cancer declined by 2.3% per year from 1990 to 2001 for all women, with larger decreases for women younger than 50 years. However, the mortality rate for African Americans is considerably higher than that for white Americans. Internationally, the United States has the 18th highest mortality rate of 50 countries (19.0 per 100,000, age adjusted) with Denmark the highest (27.8) and China the lowest (5.5).

The incidence rate increases steeply with age until the late 40s, then increases less steeply for the rest of the life span. The lifetime risk (0 to 110 years) of developing breast cancer is 13.4%. The risk of being diagnosed with breast cancer over different age intervals (incorporating age-specific incidence rates for primary breast cancer while adjusting for other causes of death) is shown in Table G-1. According to the National Cancer Institute, the risk between the ages of 30 and 39 is 0.44% (1 of 227), the risk between the ages of 40 and 49 is 1.49% (1 of 67), that between the ages of 50 and 59 is 2.79% (1 of 36), and that between the ages of 60 and 69 is 3.83% (1 of 26).[3] This approach is particularly useful when advising women about their individual risk of developing breast cancer.

RISK FACTORS FOR BREAST CANCER

There are several well-established risk factors for breast cancer, but these do not account for the major international differences or allow for practical preventive measures. Genetic

Table G-1 **Risk of Being Diagnosed with Breast Cancer in 10, 20, and 30 Years and in the Remaining Lifetime***

Current Age	+10 years	+20 years	+30 Years	Eventually
0	0.00	0.00	0.05	13.39
10	0.00	0.05	0.49	13.54
20	0.05	0.49	1.95	13.57
30	0.44	1.91	4.57	13.59
40	1.49	4.18	7.64	13.31
50	2.79	6.36	9.77	12.21
60	3.83	7.49	9.63	10.11

*Given cancer-free status at the current age, lifetime risk (%) of being diagnosed with cancer was determined according to 12 Surveillance, Epidemiology, and End Results (SEER) areas; the lifetime risk of dying of cancer was 2.98% (determined for U.S. totals, 1999-2001).

factors are responsible for only a small percentage of cases. Environmental factors have been speculated to have major roles because incidence rates vary greatly between countries, and rates among migrants moving from low- and high-risk countries converge to the rate of the destination country. However, the environmental factors responsible for this variation are unknown.

The risk factors with strongest association with breast cancer are breast cancer in a mother or sister, high blood estrogens for postmenopausal women, and high blood IGF-1 levels for premenopausal women. Risk factors with a moderate strength of association are age at first birth greater than 34 years, a family history of breast cancer in a first-degree relative, estrogen plus progesterone replacement for more than 5 years, high blood prolactin levels, and a diagnosis of benign breast disease. Other risk factors are obesity for postmenopausal women, height greater than 5 feet 7 inches, alcohol use of more than 1 drink/day, late age at menopause, none or only one child, and exposure to ionizing radiation.[4]

GENETIC AND FAMILIAL FACTORS

A family history may be due to chance, nongenetic risk factors shared by relatives, or the inheritance of a specific germline mutation from the mother or father. Between 5% and 10% of all breast cancers are directly attributable to inherited factors. This rate is higher in women diagnosed at the age of 45 or younger. Inherited breast cancer may be distinguished clinically from sporadic breast cancer by a younger age of onset, a higher prevalence of bilateral breast cancer, and the presence of associated tumors in family members.

The major genes responsible for an inherited susceptibility to breast cancer are *BRCA1* and *BRCA2*. Inherited mutations are much more common in Ashkenazi Jews than in the general population. Other genetic syndromes are seen with inherited mutations in *Tp53* (Li-Fraumeni), *PTEN* (Cowden), ATM (Ataxia-telangiectasia), *CHEK2* and *MSH2/MLH1* (Muir-Toree). The risk of breast cancer in women with an inherited mutation in *BRCA1/2* is 40% to 85% by age 70 and the risk of ovarian cancer is 25% to 65% for *BRCA1* and 15% to 25% for *BRCA2* by age 70.[5] Carriers diagnosed with breast cancer have about a 40% risk of an opposite breast cancer in the next 10 years.[6,7] Histopathologically, *BRCA1*-associated cancers typically are high grade with pushing borders and are estrogen and progesterone negative and Her-2/neu negative ("triple negative"), whereas *BRCA2*-associated cancers do not have a characteristic pattern.[8] More than 100 distinct mutations in *BRCA1/2* have been characterized in high-risk families. It is not known whether all mutations carry the same risk.

Radiation oncologists need to consider the likelihood of an inherited mutation when patients are seen in consultation or in follow-up. The key to this assessment is a careful family history of breast and/or ovarian cancer, including age at diagnosis. An inherited mutation should be considered in any woman diagnosed with breast cancer before the age of 40, any woman of Ashkenazi descent diagnosed with breast cancer before the age of 50, any woman of Ashkenazi descent diagnosed at any age with a close relative with ovarian cancer, and any woman diagnosed before age 50 with multiple first- and second-degree relatives with breast or especially with ovarian cancer. Various models are now available to guide clinicians in estimating the likelihood of an inherited mutation, based on cancer and family history and ethnic background.[9] Several of these models can be run through the CancerGene software package available at www.utsouthwestern.edu/cancergene.[10] Any patient with an estimated probability of a *BRCA1/2* mutation of 10% or greater should be referred to a breast cancer medical geneticist or a genetic counselor.

In women with a *BRCA1/2* mutation, but without a diagnosis of breast cancer, the three main management options currently available include close surveillance, prophylactic mastectomy and/or prophylactic oophorectomy, and chemoprevention. Prophylactic mastectomy has a proven record of substantially reducing breast cancer risk.[11] Similarly, prophylactic oophorectomy substantially reduces the risk of ovarian cancer and also reduces the risk of breast cancer by about 50% in premenopausal women.[12] For high-risk women who choose close surveillance, annual mammography and twice-yearly physical examinations are typically performed. It has been demonstrated that the breast MRI is more effective than mammography in early detection among women with *BRCA* mutations.[13] Tamoxifen appears to reduce breast risk, and various chemoprevention trials are available.

Management of women with a diagnosis of breast cancer and an inherited mutation in *BRCA1/2* is discussed in Chapter 60. Such patients can elect breast-conserving therapy, but need to be apprised that their risk of subsequent additional breast cancers is very high.

MAMMOGRAPHIC SCREENING

Mammographic screening, which allows breast cancer to be detected earlier than by physical examination, is an important strategy in the reduction of breast cancer mortality. The objective of this approach is to institute treatment before metastases develop, averting death from the disease. Mammography and physical examination are the main methods used for early detection.

The most recent meta-analysis of mammographic screening trials demonstrates a 20% to 35% reduction in breast cancer mortality in women between the ages of 50 and 69 years and a slightly lower reduction in women between the ages of 40 and 49.[14] All major medical organizations in the United States recommend screening mammography for women 40 years old or older. There is still uncertainty about the optimal frequency of screening and whether it is useful in women older than 70 years.

NATURAL HISTORY OF BREAST CANCER

Breast cancer is a heterogeneous disease with a predisposition for systemic involvement and it commonly has a long natural history. There is debate as to whether breast cancer is a systemic disease at its inception or whether it spreads at some point in its clinical evolution.[15] The major argument against breast cancer being a strictly systemic disease is the significant reduction in breast cancer mortality that results from early detection using screening mammography.

The natural history of untreated breast cancer has been documented in a series of 250 patients from Middlesex Hospital in England between 1805 and 1933.[16] The median survival time from the onset of symptoms was 2.7 years. Eighteen percent of the patients survived 5 years, and 4% survived 10 years, indicating that survival can be lengthy even if the disease is untreated.

Brinkley and Haybittle[17] reported the survival of a group of 704 patients with breast cancer from Cambridge, England, who were treated between 1947 and 1950. The minimum period of follow-up for survivors was 31 years. Survival curves for these patients with breast cancer at no time became parallel with those for the normal population. Even after 25 years, the number of deaths from breast cancer was 15 times higher than expected in a normal population. Similarly, other studies have indicated a persistent excess risk of mortality after treatment for breast cancer.[18,19] Nevertheless, a considerable proportion of patients treated for breast cancer will live their normal life expectancy, free of further evidence of the disease. This is especially true for those with breast cancer 2 cm or smaller and without axillary lymph node involvement.[15,20]

Most invasive breast cancers are epithelial neoplasms; invasive ductal carcinoma accounts for approximately 85% of breast cancers. Invasive lobular carcinoma comprises 5% to 10% of breast cancers and has an overall prognosis similar to the invasive ductal type. Several special types of breast carcinoma are much less common than the invasive ductal and lobular kinds and generally have a more favorable prognosis. These include mucinous, classic medullary, papillary, tubular, and adenoid cystic carcinoma. Patients with node-negative disease with special tumor types measuring 3 cm or less in diameter have a relatively good prognosis, equivalent to that of patients with node-negative disease with infiltrating ductal or lobular carcinoma measuring 1 cm or less in diameter.[21]

The primary site of breast cancer usually is described by its location according to quadrant in the breast. In one series of 696 cases, 48% were located in the upper outer quadrant, 15% in the upper inner quadrant, 11% in the lower outer quadrant, 6% in the lower inner quadrant, and 17% in the central region.[22] An additional 3% were called diffuse because of multicentric or massive involvement of the breast. In one large series of node-negative patients, women with medial tumors did slightly worse than women with lateral tumors (recurrence rates, 18% versus 14%, $P < 0.005$).[23] This observation is likely related to preferential involvement of internal mammary nodes (IMNs) with medial tumors. IMN involvement is uncommon (about 10%) when axillary nodes are negative, but is more common (30%) when axillary nodes are positive. Recurrence in the IMN chain is very uncommon.

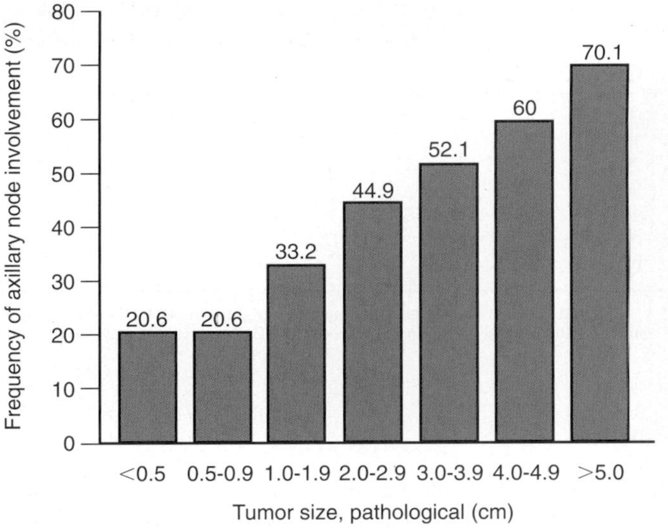

Figure G-2 Frequency of axillary node involvement related to tumor size. (Adapted from Carter CL, Allen C, Henson DE: Relation of tumor size, lymph node status, and survival in 27,740 breast cancer cases. Cancer 63:181-187, 1989.)

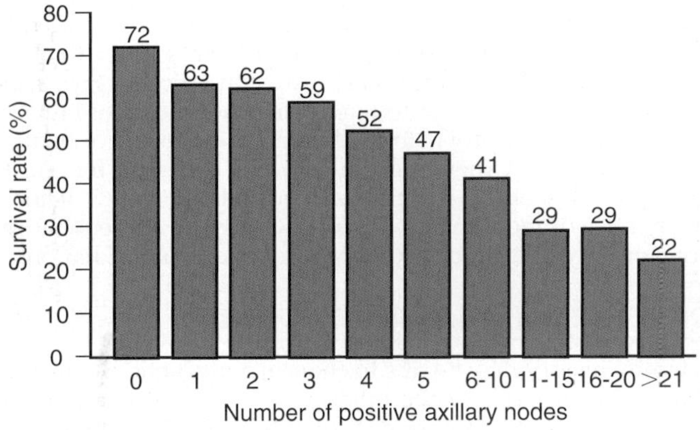

Figure G-3 Five-year results related to the number of pathologically positive axillary nodes. (Adapted from Nemoto T, Vana J, Bedwani RN, et al: Management of survival of female breast cancer: results of a national survey by the American College of Surgeons. Cancer 45:2917-2924, 1980.)

The major regional drainage site for the breast is the axilla. The likelihood of axillary nodal involvement is directly related to the size of the primary tumor.[24,25] In one large survey of patients, small tumors (<1 cm) were associated with a 20% risk of axillary involvement (Fig. G-2).[25] Patients with microinvasive breast cancer (i.e., ductal carcinoma in situ with foci of invasion) are the only subgroup in whom the risk of axillary nodal involvement is consistently reported to be 3% or less. Histologic involvement of axillary nodes has a high correlation with prognosis. This is illustrated in Figure G-3, which demonstrates that prognosis progressively declined with increasing numbers of positive nodes.[24]

STAGING

The sixth edition of the AJCC TNM staging system is provided in Tables G-2 and G-3.[26] It represents a significant change from the fifth edition published in 1997. Among the reasons cited for the major revision were the increased diagnosis of breast cancer at a very early stage based on the widespread use of screening mammography; the increasing use of sentinel node procedure instead of axillary node dissection, accompanied by an increased use of more detailed sectioning of nodes and of immunochemical and molecular techniques for the detection of metastatic tumor deposits; and increased knowledge about the prognostic significance of the location and extent of nodal involvement in the axillary, internal mammary, and supraclavicular lymph node areas.[27] An editorial on the new staging system praised the advances in the revision, but pointed out that the new staging system is complicated and difficult to use.[28] There is a clear need to develop new reliable markers of biologic aggressiveness of breast cancer to better account for the large inhomogeneity seen within stage. It should be noted that stage reclassification using the new staging system results in significant changes in outcome by stage.[29]

This staging system for carcinoma of the breast applies to infiltrating (including microinvasive) and in situ carcinomas. Microscopic confirmation of the diagnosis is mandatory, and the histologic type and grade of carcinoma should be recorded. The evaluation of patients for metastatic disease before primary treatment includes clinical staging, a careful history and physical examination, appropriate breast imaging and liver function tests. In patients at high risk, bone and body CT scans are also performed. The use of PET scans for the detection of metastases is being evaluated. For breast cancer, there is clinical staging (based on physical examination, imaging and the pathology used to establish the diagnosis) and pathologic staging (which also includes the pathology of the definitive surgical procedure). If surgery occurs after the patient has received neoadjuvant systemic or radiation therapy, the prefix "y" should be used with the TNM classification. Of note in the staging system, "isolated tumor cells" (ITCs) are defined as single cells or small clusters of cells not greater than 0.2 mm in largest dimension, usually with no histologic evidence of malignant activity (such as proliferation or stromal reaction) and are classified as pN0. Micrometastases are defined as tumor deposits greater than 0.2 mm but not greater than 2.0 mm in largest dimension that may have histologic evidence of malignant activity (such as proliferation or stromal reaction).

SURGICAL TREATMENT OF BREAST CANCER

The "modified radical mastectomy" combines total resection of the breast with an axillary dissection with preservation of both pectoral muscles. This procedure is the most common operative treatment for patients with invasive breast cancer in the United States. In recent years, sentinel node biopsy has become increasingly used. If the sentinel node is negative, the patient can be spared the morbidity of an axillary dissection.[30]

Conservative approaches to breast surgery include quadrantectomy, wide excision, and local excision. Quadrantectomy is a resection of the tumor, along with the involved quadrant of the breast, including the overlying skin. A wide excision involves resection of the tumor with 1 to 2 cm of adjacent breast tissue, designed to provide clear margins of resection. A local excision is a simple excision of the tumor, without regard to the microscopic margins of resection.

PROGNOSTIC AND PREDICTIVE FACTORS

A prognostic factor is defined as a biologic or clinical measurement associated with disease-free or overall survival, which can be used to estimate the prognosis of the patient. A predictive factor is any measurement associated with response or lack of response to a particular therapy, which can be used to guide the use of that particular therapy in an individual patient.

The role of prognostic factors in optimizing treatment for patients with breast cancer has changed with the trend toward the widespread use of adjuvant systemic therapy. The most established prognostic factor in primary breast cancer is the number of positive axillary nodes. Other important factors are histologic type and grade and tumor size. Other possible prognostic factors are lymphatic and/or vascular invasion and measures of proliferation. Estrogen and progesterone receptor status, although a good predictive factor for response to hormonal therapy, is a relatively weak prognostic factor. *HER2* gene amplification and HER2 protein overexpression are predictive factors for the use of Herceptin and have prognostic value. A wide range of prognostic and predictive factors has been evaluated, but they are beyond the scope of this chapter.

It is possible to estimate on-line the prognosis of an individual patient based on the standard prognostic factors. One such on-line service, which has been validated, is Adjuvant-Online (www.adjuvantonline.com).[31]

Several gene-based approaches have been developed.[32] One of these is a multigene test developed by NSABP investigators.[33] The test employs a reverse transcriptase–polymerase chain reaction (RT-PCR) assay of 21 prospectively selected genes in paraffin-embedded tumor tissue to quantify the likelihood of distant recurrence in tamoxifen-treated patients with node-negative, estrogen receptor-positive breast cancer. The test has been validated and is commercially available. The test has recently been shown to also be a predictive factor for the use of chemotherapy in these patients.[34] Another approach has been using microarray analysis to identify gene-expression profiles or signatures associated with a poor prognosis or a good prognosis. One group developed a 70-gene prognosis profile, which is being validated in Europe.[35]

ADJUVANT SYSTEMIC THERAPY

The use of adjuvant systemic therapy is based on the theory that occult metastases (or micrometastases) are commonly present at the time of presentation. Evidence for this theory arises from the fact that many patients manifest metastatic involvement over time, and improvements in local control have been shown to provide only a small decrease in subsequent distant metastases.

Adjuvant treatment in addition to local treatment has demonstrated significant improvements in survival for treated patients compared with controls. An Overview or meta-analysis of 194 prospective randomized clinical trials involving over 45,000 women with early breast cancer has been conducted.[36] The Overview was organized on the premise that small, but clinically important, improvements in outcome often require very large trials or a combination of many trials. The information provided below (unless otherwise specified) is from the recently published results of the 2000 Overview.[36] All of the comparisons provided below for the Overview results are statistically significant.

Hormonal Therapy

The development of hormonal therapy for breast cancer has arguably been the first successful "targeted" therapy for

Table G-2 TNM Staging System for Breast Cancer

PRIMARY TUMOR (T)

TX	Primary tumor cannot be assessed
T0	No evidence of primary tumor
Tis	Carcinoma in situ
Tis (DCIS)	Ductal carcinoma in situ
Tis (LCIS)	Lobular carcinoma in situ
Tis (Paget's)	Paget's disease of the nipple with no tumor
T1	Tumor of 2 cm or less in greatest dimension
T1mic	Microinvasion of 0.1 cm but not more than 0.5 cm in greatest dimension
T1a	Tumor more than 0.1 cm but not more than 0.5 cm in greatest dimension
T1b	Tumor more than 0.5 cm but not more than 1 cm in greatest dimension
T1c	Tumor more than 1 cm but not more than 2 cm in greatest dimension
T2	Tumor more than 2 cm but not more than 5 cm in greatest dimension
T3	Tumor more than 5 cm in greatest dimension
T4	Tumor of any size with direct extension to (a) chest wall or (b) skin only as described below
T4a	Extension to chest wall, not including pectoralis muscle
T4b	Edema (including peau d'orange) or ulceration of the skin of the breast, or satellite skin nodules confined to the same breast
T4c	Features of T4a and T4b
T4d	Inflammatory carcinoma

REGIONAL LYMPH NODES (N)

Clinical Staging

NX	Regional lymph nodes cannot be assessed (e.g., previously removed)
N0	No regional lymph node metastasis
N1	Metastasis to movable ipsilateral axillary lymph node(s)
N2	Metastases in ipsilateral axillary lymph nodes fixed or matted, or in clinically apparent* ipsilateral internal mammary nodes in the *absence* of clinically evident axillary lymph node metastasis
N2a	Metastasis in ipsilateral axillary lymph nodes fixed to one another (matted) or to other structures
N2b	Metastasis only in clinically apparent* ipsilateral internal mammary nodes and in the *absence* of clinically evident axillary lymph node metastasis
N3	Metastasis in ipsilateral infraclavicular lymph node(s) with or without axillary lymph node involvement, or in clinically apparent* ipsilateral internal mammary lymph node(s) and in the *presence* of clinically evident axillary lymph node metastasis; or metastasis in ipsilateral supraclavicular lymph node(s) with or without axillary or internal mammary involvement
N3a	Metastasis in ipsilateral infraclavicular lymph node(s)
N3b	Metastasis in ipsilateral internal mammary lymph node(s) and axillary lymph node(s)
N3c	Metastasis in ipsilateral supraclavicular lymph node(s)

Pathologic Staging (pN)

pNX	Regional lymph nodes cannot be assessed (e.g., previously removed or not removed for pathologic study)
pN0	No regional lymph node metastasis histologically, no additional examination for isolated tumor cells (ITC)
pN1	Metastasis in 1 to 3 axillary lymph nodes and/or in internal mammary nodes with microscopic disease detected by sentinel lymph node dissection but not clinically apparent†
pN1mi	Micrometastasis greater than 0.2 mm, none greater than 2.0 mm
pN1a	Metastasis in 1 to 3 axillary lymph nodes
pN1b	Metastasis in internal mammary nodes with microscopic disease detected by sentinel lymph node dissection but not clinically apparent†
pN1c	Metastasis in 1 to 3 axillary lymph nodes and in internal mammary lymph nodes with microscopic disease detected by sentinel lymph node dissection but not clinically apparent.† (If associated with more than 3 positive axillary lymph nodes, the internal mammary nodes are classified as pN3b to reflect increased tumor burden.)
pN2	Metastasis in 4 to 9 axillary lymph nodes or in clinically apparent* internal mammary lymph nodes in the *absence* of axillary lymph node metastasis
pN2a	Metastasis in 4 to 9 axillary lymph nodes (at least one tumor deposit greater than 2.0 mm)
pN2b	Metastasis in clinically apparent* internal mammary lymph nodes in the *absence* of axillary lymph node metastasis
pN3	Metastasis in 10 or more axillary lymph nodes, or in infraclavicular lymph nodes, or in clinically apparent* ipsilateral internal mammary lymph nodes in the *presence* of 1 or more positive axillary lymph nodes; or in more than 3 axillary lymph nodes with clinically negative microscopic metastasis in internal mammary lymph nodes; or in ipsilateral supraclavicular lymph nodes
pN3a	Metastasis in 10 or more axillary lymph nodes (at least one tumor deposit greater than 2.0 mm) or metastasis to the infraclavicular lymph nodes
pN3b	Metastasis in clinically apparent* ipsilateral internal mammary lymph nodes in the *presence* of 1 or more positive axillary lymph nodes; or in more than 3 axillary lymph nodes and in internal mammary lymph nodes with microscopic disease detected by sentinel lymph node dissection but not clinically apparent†
pN3c	Metastasis in ipsilateral supraclavicular lymph nodes

DISTANT METASTASIS (M)

MX	Distant metastasis cannot be assessed
M0	No distant metastasis
M1	Distant metastasis

*Clinically apparent is defined as detected by imaging studies (excluding lymphoscintigraphy) or by clinical examination or as grossly visible pathologically.

†Not clinically apparent is defined as not detected by imaging studies (excluding lymphoscintigraphy) or by clinical examination.

From Greene FL, Page DL, Fleming ID, et al (eds), for the American Joint Committee on Cancer: AJCC Cancer Staging Manual, 6th ed. New York, Springer-Verlag, 2002.

Table G-3 Stage Grouping

Stage 0*	Tis	N0	M0
Stage I	T1†	N0	M0
Stage IIA	T0	N1	M0
	T1†	N1	M0
	T2	N0	M0
Stage IIB	T2	N1	M0
	T3	N0	M0
Stage IIIA	T0	N2	M0
	T1*	N2	M0
	T2	N2	M0
	T3	N1	M0
	T3	N2	M0
Stage IIIB	T4	N0	M0
	T4	N1	M0
	T4	N2	M0
Stage IIIC	Any T	N3	M0
Stage IV	Any T	Any N	M1

*A stage designation may be changed if postsurgical imaging studies reveal the presence of distant metastases, provided that the studies are carried out within 4 months of diagnosis in the absence of disease progression and provided that the patient has not received neoadjuvant therapy.

†T1 includes T1mic.

From Greene FL, Page DL, Fleming ID, et al (eds), for the American Joint Committee on Cancer: AJCC Cancer Staging Manual, 6th ed. New York, Springer-Verlag, 2002.

cancer. The mainstay of hormonal therapy for breast cancer has been tamoxifen. The benefit of Tamoxifen, an anti-estrogen taken orally (20 mg per day), has been shown to be restricted to patients with ER-positive tumors. Tamoxifen for 5 years results in a 41% proportional reduction in breast cancer recurrence and a 33% proportional reduction in breast cancer mortality. The benefit of tamoxifen is similar in all patient age groups with and without the use of adjuvant chemotherapy. The 15-year recurrence rate for a group of patients (30% of whom are node positive and 20% of whom have unknown ER) is 45% in controls and 33% with about 5 years of tamoxifen. The 15-year breast cancer mortality rate for the same group of patients is 35% in controls and 26% with about 5 years of tamoxifen. Tamoxifen also reduces the risk of contralateral breast cancer by about 40%. These beneficial effects of tamoxifen outweigh the slightly higher risk of endometrial cancer and thromboembolic events associated with this drug in most patients.

The oldest form of adjuvant hormonal therapy is ovarian ablation. More recently, the option of ovarian suppression has been developed. This therapy is only appropriate for premenopausal patients. The 15-year recurrence rate for a group of patients aged less than 50 (61% of whom are node positive and 47% of whom have unknown ER) is 52% in controls and 47% with ovarian ablation/suppression. The 15-year breast cancer mortality rate for the same group of patients is 44% in controls and 40% with ovarian ablation/suppression.

The newest form of adjuvant hormonal therapy is the use of aromatase inhibitors, which have shown comparable or superior effectiveness as tamoxifen as front-line adjuvant therapy[37] and have substantial effectiveness after 2 to 3 years[38] or 5 years[39] of tamoxifen.

Adjuvant Chemotherapy

The Overview results demonstrate that the use of polychemotherapy is clearly superior to the use of single agents. Polychemotherapy has been shown to result in a long-term benefit in disease-free survival and overall survival for patients with breast cancer. (In the Overview, about one half of the trials used CMF-based regimens, and about one third used anthracycline-based regimens.) Optimal results are achieved with 4 to 6 months of adjuvant chemotherapy. The magnitude of the benefit is related to patient age, with greater benefit in premenopausal women compared with postmenopausal patients. For patients aged less than 50 years, the 15-year recurrence rate is 54% in controls and 41% with polychemotherapy for an absolute benefit of 13%. For patients between the ages of 50 and 69 years, the 15-year recurrence rate is 58% in controls and 53% with polychemotherapy for an absolute benefit of 5%. For patients aged less than 50 years, the 15-year breast cancer mortality rate is 42% in controls and 32% with polychemotherapy for an absolute benefit of 10%. For patients between the ages of 50 and 69 years, the 15-year recurrence rate is 50% in controls and 47% with polychemotherapy for an absolute benefit of 3%. Anthracycline-based regimens show a moderate, but statistically significant advantage over CMF-based regimens. Later advances in the use of polychemotherapy include the addition of taxanes to anthracycline-based regimens[40] and the use of every-2-week administration compared with every-three-week administration ("dose dense").[41] The use of escalating doses of chemotherapy, even with bone marrow rescue, has not shown benefit over conventional doses.

Adjuvant Biologic Therapy

A number of newer biologic or targeted approaches have been developed and are in various phases of evaluation. This includes tyrosine kinase inhibitors, angiogenesis inhibitors, and immunotherapy. The most developed of these is traztuzumab (Herceptin), a humanized immunoglobulin directed against the Her-2/neu receptor. Traztuzumab is used for Her-2/neu-positive metastatic and locally advanced breast cancer and has been established as an adjuvant therapy in operable Her-2-positive disease.[42]

Preoperative or Neoadjuvant Systemic Therapy

Preoperative systemic therapy is routinely performed in locally advanced breast cancer. It is also used in patients with a large operable breast cancer to facilitate breast-conserving therapy. In early-stage breast cancer, preoperative systemic therapy has not been shown to improve survival compared with conventional adjuvant systemic therapy, but it does allow assessment of response. This assessment may help individualize systemic therapy, and it provides an earlier end point than survival, which may hasten the pace of progress in clinical breast cancer research.

Selecting Adjuvant Systemic Therapy for the Individual Patient

The guidelines for selecting adjuvant systemic therapy for the individual patient are complex and evolving. It begins with an assessment of the risk of systemic recurrence in the absence of systemic therapy (see "Prognostic and Predictive Factors"). The approach to the individual patient is based on whether the patient has hormonally responsive breast cancer (estrogen receptor-positive and/or progesterone-receptor positive) or not. Other considerations are the patient's age, menopausal status, and general health status. The anticipated benefits of the various systemic therapies can also be estimated on AdjuvantOnline (www.adjuvantonline.com).[31] The benefits and risks of these therapies are discussed with the patient. Given the magnitude of the benefit from these adjuvant systemic therapies and the lack of curative treatment of a systemic recurrence, systemic therapy is generally used, except for patients with very early-stage breast cancer.

ASSESSING CONTRIBUTIONS OF LOCAL AND SYSTEMIC THERAPY

There has been substantial progress in treating breast cancer.[43] Most of this progress has come from advances in adjuvant systemic therapy, particularly for hormone-responsive breast cancer. The substantial decrease in breast cancer mortality is primarily due to these advances in systemic therapy. Radiation therapy, however, has also played an important role. Some of the earliest randomized trials in all of clinical medicine, conducted in the 1950s, tested the use of radiation therapy in patients with invasive breast cancer treated with mastectomy.[44] Subsequently, beginning in the 1960s, trials of breast-conserving surgery combined with radiation therapy compared with mastectomy were started.[45,46] Over time, considerable information has been accumulated on the use of radiation therapy in patients with invasive breast cancer after mastectomy and after breast-conserving surgery. The success of breast-conserving therapy has been an important quality-of-life advance in the management of the disease.

There are a couple of major themes in reviewing these trials. One is the important issue of assessing the value of radiation therapy separately when used in the absence of or when used in conjunction with adjuvant systemic therapy. Given the demonstrated value of adjuvant systemic therapy in improving relapse-free and overall survival, systemic therapy is now typically used in patients with invasive breast cancer. In the absence of systemic therapy, radiation therapy reduces local recurrence after mastectomy or breast-conserving surgery by about 70%.[47] Theoretically, the use of adjuvant systemic therapy by itself may lower the chance of local recurrence, lessening the need for irradiation. Systemic therapy could also interact with radiation therapy to make it more, or possibly less, effective, and could provide spatial complementarity (i.e., radiation therapy for local and systemic therapy for systemic disease) to improve survival when both are used. Serendipitously, these systemic therapies, hormonal therapy more than chemotherapy, interact with radiation therapy to substantially improve local tumor control.[48] More important is the finding that irradiation used with systemic therapy decreases distant metastases and improves survival.[49,50] In prior trials, such as NSABP Trial B-04,[51] where systemic therapy was not used, radiation therapy was found not to influence survival. The more recent trials suggest that when systemic therapy is effective at controlling micrometastatic disease, it is important to obtain local tumor control. Eventually, it is anticipated that systemic therapy will advance in its effectiveness so that no local therapy is needed; however, up to now, the use of systemic therapy has increased the role of local therapy. Of note in the Danish postmastectomy trials testing radiation therapy in patients treated with adjuvant systemic therapy, there was about a 30% rate of local recurrence in the absence of radiation therapy, and irradiation resulted in a 10% absolute improvement in survival.[52,53] If the benefit of radiation therapy is proportional, as is seen with most therapies in breast cancer, and acts through its reduction in local recurrence, it would suggest that patients with a 15% rate of local recurrence would have a 5% absolute improvement in survival. Unfortunately, given the failure to accrue to the large, randomized trial of postmastectomy radiation therapy for patients with one to three positive nodes treated with adjuvant systemic therapy (a group with an anticipated local recurrence rate of about 15%), this extrapolation remains conjectural. The recent meta-analysis of radiation therapy and extent of surgery clearly demonstrates that reduction in 5-year local recurrence leads to an improvement in 15-year survival.[56]

Another major theme is the need to balance the benefits of radiation therapy against its costs, complications and inconvenience. One of the most serious complications seen with radiation therapy for breast cancer, particularly for left-sided cancers, is increased late cardiac mortality.[44] Early techniques of breast cancer irradiation, especially those that intended to treat the internal mammary nodes, resulted in substantial doses of radiation to the heart. It is fortunate that improved irradiation techniques, especially with the use of CT-based simulation, allow for exclusion of the entire heart in the high-dose areas.[54] Efforts are continuing to identify patients who do not require radiation therapy, and these efforts are ongoing. There are no "predictive factors" for radiation therapy; the benefit from irradiation in reducing local recurrence is proportionally similar in all subgroups. The emphasis has been on identifying prognostic factors in cases for which the risk of local recurrence without radiation therapy is sufficiently low, such that radiation therapy is not justified.

REFERENCES

1. Harris J, Lippman ME, Morrow M, Osborne CK (eds): Diseases of the Breast, 3rd ed. Philadelphia, Lippincott Williams & Wilkins, 2004.
2. American Cancer Society: Cancer Facts and Figures 2005. Atlanta, American Cancer Society, 2005.
3. National Cancer Institute: Breast cancer rates. Available at www.cis.nci.nih.gov/fact.
4. Willett W, Rockhill B, Hankinson SE, et al: Non-genetic factors in the causation of breast cancer. *In* Harris J, Lippman ME, Morrow M, Osborne CK (eds): Diseases of the Breast, 3rd ed. Philadelphia, Lippincott Williams & Wilkins, 2004, pp 223-276.
5. Isaacs C, Peshkin BN, Schwartz M: Evaluation and management of women with a strong family history. *In* Harris J, Lippman ME, Morrow M, Osborne CK (eds): Diseases of the Breast, 3rd ed. Philadelphia, Lippincott Williams & Wilkins, 2004, pp 315-345.
6. Metcalfe K, Lynch HT, Ghadirian P, et al: Contralateral breast cancer in BRCA1 and BRCA2 mutation carriers. J Clin Oncol 22:2328-2335, 2004.
7. Pierce LJ, Strawderman M, Narod SA, et al: Effect of radiotherapy after breast-conserving treatment in women with breast cancer and germline BRCA1/2 mutations. J Clin Oncol 18:3360-3369, 2000.
8. Eerola H, Heikkila P, Tamminen A, et al: Histopathological features of breast tumours in BRCA1, BRCA2 and mutation-negative breast cancer families. Breast Cancer Res 7:R93-R100, 2005.
9. Domchek SM, Eisen A, Calzone K, et al: Application of breast cancer risk prediction models in clinical practice. J Clin Oncol 21:593-601, 2003.
10. CancerGene software: Available at: www.utsouthwestern.edu/cancergene.
11. Rebbeck TR, Friebel T, Lynch HT, et al: Bilateral prophylactic mastectomy reduces breast cancer risk in BRCA1 and BRCA2 mutation carriers: the PROSE Study Group. J Clin Oncol 22:1055-1062, 2004.
12. Rebbeck TR, Lynch HT, Neuhausen SL, et al: Prophylactic oophorectomy in carriers of BRCA1 or BRCA2 mutations. N Engl J Med 346:1616-1622, 2002.
13. Kriege M, Brekelmans CT, Boetes C, et al: Efficacy of MRI and mammography for breast-cancer screening in women with a familial or genetic predisposition. N Engl J Med 351:427-437, 2004.
14. Elmore JG, Armstrong K, Lehman CD, Fletcher SW: Screening for breast cancer. JAMA 293:1245-1256, 2005.
15. Hellman S: Karnofsky Memorial Lecture. Natural history of small breast cancers. J Clin Oncol 12:2229-2234, 1994.
16. Bloom HJ, Richardson WW, Harries EJ: Natural history of untreated breast cancer (1805-1933). Comparison of untreated and

treated cases according to histological grade of malignancy. Br Med J 5299:213-221, 1962.
17. Brinkley D, Haybittle JL: Long-term survival of women with breast cancer. Lancet 1:1118, 1984.
18. Rutqvist LE, Wallgren A: Long-term survival of 458 young breast cancer patients. Cancer 55:658-665, 1985.
19. Hibberd AD, Horwood LJ, Wells JE: Long term prognosis of women with breast cancer in New Zealand: study of survival to 30 years. Br Med J 286:1777-1779, 1983.
20. Rosen PR, Groshen S, Saigo PE, et al: A long-term follow-up study of survival in stage I (T1N0M0) and stage II (T1N1M0) breast carcinoma. J Clin Oncol 7:355-366, 1989.
21. Rosen PP, Groshen S, Kinne DW, Norton L: Factors influencing prognosis in node-negative breast carcinoma: analysis of 767 T1N0M0/T2N0M0 patients with long-term follow-up. J Clin Oncol 11:2090-2100, 1993.
22. Spratt J, Donegan W: Cancer of the Breast. Philadelphia, WB Saunders, 1971.
23. Nemoto T, Natarajan N, Bedwani R, et al: Breast cancer in the medial half. Results of 1978 National Survey of the American College of Surgeons. Cancer 51:1333-1338, 1983.
24. Nemoto T, Vana J, Bedwani RN, et al: Management and survival of female breast cancer: results of a national survey by the American College of Surgeons. Cancer 45:2917-2924, 1980.
25. Carter CL, Allen C, Henson DE: Relation of tumor size, lymph node status, and survival in 24,740 breast cancer cases. Cancer 63:181-187, 1989.
26. Greene FL, Page DL, Fleming ID, et al (eds), for the American Joint Committee on Cancer: AJCC Cancer Staging Manual, 6th ed. New York, Springer-Verlag, 2002.
27. Singletary SE, Allred C, Ashley P, et al: Revision of the American Joint Committee on Cancer staging system for breast cancer. J Clin Oncol 20:3628-3636, 2002.
28. Bunnell CA, Winer EP: Lumping versus splitting: the splitters take this round. J Clin Oncol 20:3576-3577, 2002.
29. Woodward WA, Strom EA, Tucker SL, et al: Changes in the 2003 American Joint Committee on Cancer staging for breast cancer dramatically affect stage-specific survival. J Clin Oncol 21:3244-3248, 2003.
30. Grube BJ, Giuliano AE: The current role of sentinel node biopsy in the treatment of breast cancer. Adv Surg 38:121-166, 2004.
31. AdjuvantOnline: Available at: www.adjuvantonline.com.
32. Van't Veer LJ, Paik S, Hayes DF: Gene expression profiling of breast cancer: a new tumor marker. J Clin Oncol 23:1631-1635, 2005.
33. Paik S, Shak S, Tang G, et al: A multigene assay to predict recurrence of tamoxifen-treated, node-negative breast cancer. N Engl J Med 351:2817-2826, 2004.
34. Paik S, Shak S, Tang G, et al: Expression of the 21 genes in the recurrence score assay and prediction of clinical benefit from tamoxifen in NSABP study B-14 and chemotherapy in NSABP study B-20. Paper presented at the San Antonio Breast Cancer Conference, 2004, San Antonio, TX.
35. van de Vijver MJ, He YD, van't Veer LJ, et al: A gene-expression signature as a predictor of survival in breast cancer. N Engl J Med 347:1999-2009, 2002.
36. Early Breast Cancer Trialists' Collaborative Group(EBCTCG): Chemotherapy and hormonal therapy for early breast cancer: effects on recurrence and 15-year survival in an overview of the randomized trials. Lancet 365:1687-1717, 2005.
37. Howell A, Cuzick J, Baum M, et al: Results of the ATAC (Arimidex, tamoxifen, alone or in combination) trial after completion of 5 years' adjuvant treatment for breast cancer. Lancet 365:60-62, 2005.
38. Coombes RC, Hall E, Gibson LJ, et al: A randomized trial of exemestane after two to three years of tamoxifen therapy in postmenopausal women with primary breast cancer. N Engl J Med 350:1081-1092, 2004.
39. Goss PE, Ingle JN, Martino S, et al: A randomized trial of letrozole in postmenopausal women after five years of tamoxifen therapy for early-stage breast cancer. N Engl J Med 349:1793-1802, 2003.
40. Henderson IC, Berry DA, Demetri GD, et al: Improved outcomes from adding sequential Paclitaxel but not from escalating Doxorubicin dose in an adjuvant chemotherapy regimen for patients with node-positive primary breast cancer. J Clin Oncol 21:976-983, 2003.
41. Citron ML, Berry DA, Cirrincione C, et al: Randomized trial of dose-dense versus conventionally scheduled and sequential versus concurrent combination chemotherapy as postoperative adjuvant treatment of node-positive primary breast cancer: first report of Intergroup Trial C9741/Cancer and Leukemia Group B Trial 9741. J Clin Oncol 21:1431-1439, 2003.
42. Romond EH, Perez EA, Bryant J, et al: Trastuzumab plus adjuvant chemotherapy for operable HER2-positive breast cancer. N Engl J Med 353:1673-1684, 2005.
43. Harris JR: Radiation therapy for invasive breast cancer: not just for local control. J Clin Oncol 23:1607-1608, 2005.
44. Jones JM, Ribeiro GG: Mortality patterns over 34 years of breast cancer patients in a clinical trial of post-operative radiotherapy. Clin Radiol 40:204-208, 1989.
45. Fisher B, Bauer M, Margolese R, et al: Five-year results of a randomized clinical trial comparing total mastectomy and segmental mastectomy with or without radiation in the treatment of breast cancer. N Engl J Med 312:665-673, 1985.
46. Veronesi U, Saccozzi R, Del Vecchio M, et al: Comparing radical mastectomy with quadrantectomy, axillary dissection, and radiotherapy in patients with small cancers of the breast. N Engl J Med 305:6-11, 1981.
47. Early Breast Cancer Trialists' Collaborative Group: Favourable and unfavourable effects on long-term survival of radiotherapy for early breast cancer: an overview of the randomised trials. Lancet 355:1757-1770, 2000.
48. Morrow M, Harris JR: Local management of invasive breast cancer. In Harris JR, Lippman ME, Morrow M, Osborne CK (eds): Diseases of the Breast. Philadelphia, Lippincott Williams and Wilkins, 2004, pp 718-744.
49. Whelan T, Julian J, Wright J, et al: Does locoregional radiation therapy improve survival in breast cancer? A meta-analysis. J Clin Oncol 18:1220-1229, 2000.
50. Vinh-Hung V, Verschraegen C: Breast-conserving surgery with or without radiotherapy: pooled-analysis for risks of ipsilateral breast tumor recurrence and mortality. J Natl Cancer Inst 96:115-121, 2004.
51. Fisher B, Redmond C, Fisher ER, et al: Ten-year results of a randomized clinical trial comparing radical mastectomy and total mastectomy with or without radiation. N Engl J Med 312:674-681, 1985.
52. Overgaard M, Hansen PS, Overgaard J, et al: Postoperative radiotherapy in high-risk premenopausal women with breast cancer who receive adjuvant chemotherapy. Danish Breast Cancer Cooperative Group 82b Trial. N Engl J Med 337:949-955, 1997.
53. Overgaard M, Jensen MB, Overgaard J, et al: Postoperative radiotherapy in high-risk postmenopausal breast-cancer patients given adjuvant tamoxifen. Danish Breast Cancer Cooperative Group DBCG 82c randomised trial. Lancet 353:1641-1648, 1999.
54. Hurkmans CW, Cho BC, Damen E, et al: Reduction of cardiac and lung complication probabilities after breast irradiation using conformal radiotherapy with or without intensity modulation. Radiother Oncol 62:163-171, 2002.
55. Piccart-Gebhart MJ, Procter M, Leyland-Jones B, et al: Trastuzumab after adjuvant chemotherapy in HER2-positive breast cancer. N Engl J Med 353:1659-1672, 2005.
56. Clarke M, Collins R, Darby S, et al: Effects of radiotherapy and of differences in the extent of surgery for early breast cancer on local recurrence and 15-year survival: an overview of the randomised trials. Lancet 366:2087-2106, 2005.

CHAPTER 59

NONINVASIVE BREAST CANCER

Douglas W. Arthur and Frank A. Vicini

INCIDENCE

Noninvasive breast disease accounts for 22% of all breast cancer.

Lobular carcinoma in situ (LCIS) represents less than 15% of noninvasive disease, Paget's disease accounts for .5% to 5%, and ductal carcinoma in situ (DCIS) constitutes 85%.

BIOLOGIC AND PATHOLOGIC CHARACTERISTICS

Noninfiltrating lobular proliferation (LCIS) is characterized by loose, discohesive cells filling the acinar space. It is frequently estrogen and progesterone receptor positive, lacks E-cadherin gene *(CDH1)* expression, and rarely has overexpression of ERBB2 (i.e., HER2 or HER2/NEU) or TP53 proteins.

The presence of Paget's cells in the epidermis indicates an underlying malignancy in more than 95% of cases.

The noninfiltrating clonal proliferative process of DCIS is confined to the ductal lumens of the breast, and it is a precursor to invasive disease. The estrogen receptor is present in 70% of DCIS lesions, but the rate of expression is high (90%) in low-grade lesions and is significantly lower (25%) in high-grade lesions. About 50% of all DCIS lesions overexpress the product of the proto-oncogene *HER2*, and 25% overexpress the *TP53* tumor suppressor gene.

STAGING EVALUATION

For most noninvasive breast disease, staging entails bilateral mammograms and excision with pathologic evaluation to include lesion size, histology, estrogen and progesterone receptor status, and margin status.

For LCIS, pathologic evaluation is limited to identification and estrogen and progesterone receptor status.

PRIMARY TREATMENT

Standard management for LCIS is observation. Because the risk for in-breast failure is less than 15% at 12 years, the diagnosis of LCIS usually has minimal survival impact. Alternative treatment approaches for high-risk disease include tamoxifen and bilateral mastectomy.

Treatment for Paget's disease is breast-conservation therapy. Excision with negative margins followed by whole-breast irradiation produces in-breast disease-control rates of 87% to 95%. An alternative treatment approach for high-risk disease (i.e., diffuse disease with positive margins despite re-excision) is mastectomy.

Treatment for DCIS is breast-conservation therapy. Excision with negative margins followed by whole-breast irradiation produces in-breast disease-control rates of 85% to 95%. An alternative treatment approach for low-risk disease (i.e., size <1 cm, grade 1, and negative margins of >1 cm) is to consider excision only. The alternative approach to high-risk disease (i.e., diffuse disease and positive margins despite re-excision) is mastectomy.

Noninvasive breast cancer is composed of three distinct histologic entities: lobular carcinoma in situ (LCIS), Paget's disease, and ductal carcinoma in situ (DCIS). As a result of the increase in the quality and use of mammography, these three histologies comprise a larger percentage of all breast cancer cases seen today. Historically, mastectomy was common, but with a better understanding of the natural history of these noninvasive disease processes, investigation has led to breast-conserving treatment options. Controversy regarding the optimal treatment approach continues to exist, and treatment recommendations range from observation to breast-conserving therapy to mastectomy. To appropriately formulate a patient's treatment options, it is important to understand the distinguishing pathologic appearances, biologic characteristics, and natural history of these three noninvasive breast disease entities.

LOBULAR CARCINOMA IN SITU

LCIS was first described as a pathologic entity by Foote and Stewart in 1941.[1] Microscopically, LCIS appears as a noninfiltrating process of lobular proliferation. LCIS has been reported to manifest with multicentric breast involvement in up to 90% of mastectomy specimens, with bilateral involvement documented in 35% to 59%.[2-5] Histologically, LCIS is characterized by loose, discohesive epithelial cells filling the acinar space.[2-5] The degree of lobular involvement ranges from a simple filling of the ductal lumens to exhibiting moderate to overt distention with extension into the adjacent extralobular ducts.[6] As a result of this spectrum of appearances, the lines of histologic delineation can become blurred between atypical ductal hyperplasia, LCIS, and when ductal extension is seen, DCIS. This may introduce a source of complexity when comparing publications from varying institutions.[3-5,7] As guidance, further description has stated that the process must result in the distention and distortion of more than one half of the acini in a lobular unit to be labeled as LCIS, distinguishing it from atypical ductal hyperplasia.[3] The use of molecular markers has been suggested for distinguishing LCIS in problematic cases.[4] LCIS cells are frequently estrogen receptor positive, and rarely is ERBB2 overexpressed or TP53 protein accumulated.[4,8-10] Loss of E-cadherin gene *(CDH1)* expression is documented in more than 95% of LCIS.[10-13] The *CDH1* product is a calcium-dependent cellular adhesion molecule that is responsible for epithelial organization, and the absence of this adhesion molecule in LCIS may explain its discohesive morphology.[10-13] Conclusions regarding the application of these tests require further clinical study.

Publications on biopsy results report LCIS incidence rates to be 0.5% to 3.6%, and cases of LCIS represent less than 15% of all noninvasive lesions recorded.[5,14,15] Some reports indicate a continued increase in the incidence of LCIS between 1978 and 1998, possibly as a result of the increased use of mammographic screening and consequent biopsies during this period.[16] Because there are no clinical or mammographic indicators, LCIS without additional histologic findings is typically an incidental finding when biopsy is performed for alternative reasons.[1-4,14] Although mammographically detected calcifications corresponding with LCIS have been reported, the calcifications are more commonly unassociated and manifest in the adjacent tissue.[17-19] DCIS and invasive disease are frequently identified (22% to 27%) in the subsequent lumpectomies performed when LCIS is the sole histologic entity seen on core biopsy.[20-22] Criteria identifying patients for whom observation only is sufficient after core biopsy showing LCIS have not been clearly established.

Management considerations for LCIS depend on whether it is associated with a diagnosis of DCIS or infiltrative disease or is the sole histologic entity encountered. Only 5% to 12% of early-stage breast cancers have an associated component of LCIS.[23-25] The effect that the presence of LCIS has on the outcome of breast-conservation management of early-stage breast cancer has only recently been evaluated, and the conflicting data are based on limited numbers. The accepted treatment approach is to manage the breast according to the dominant histology present (i.e., DCIS or invasive) and disregard the presence of LCIS. Additional surgery is not pursued to obtain LCIS-clear margins. Moran and Haffty reported their experience with breast conservation for early-stage breast cancer, comparing 51 patients with LCIS with 1045 patients without LCIS.[23] They found no statistically significant difference between the two groups regarding 10-year overall survival, distant disease-free survival, or ipsilateral breast tumor recurrence (IBTR)-free survival. Abner and associates reported similar findings for their cohort of early-stage breast cancer patients, with a median follow-up of 161 months.[24] They reported a local recurrence rate of 13% for the 119 patients with LCIS and 12% for the 1062 patients without LCIS. The risks for contralateral disease and distant failure were not affected by the presence or extent of LCIS. In contrast, Sasson and coworkers reported a comparable cohort of patients, 65 of whom had associated LCIS and 1274 of whom did not.[25] Fifteen percent of patients with LCIS developed an IBTR, compared with 5% of patients without LCIS. The cumulative incidence estimated the 10-year IBTR rate to be 29% and 6%, respectively. Analysis found age less than 50 years, tumor size less than 2 cm, associated invasive ductal carcinoma, disease-negative axillary nodes, and absence of systemic therapy to be associated with an increased risk of IBTR. The need for the addition of tamoxifen or a more aggressive treatment approach in this group of high-risk patients is uncertain, and further study is necessary.

If LCIS is the sole histologic diagnosis, treatment recommendations range from conservative to extreme (Fig. 59-1). When first described as a pathologic entity, the significance of LCIS was unknown, and mastectomy was consistently pursued.[1] Knowledge of frequent contralateral involvement extended treatment recommendations to random contralateral biopsy and bilateral mastectomy.[1,2] However, observational studies after lumpectomy only have led to a better understanding of the natural history of this disease, and a more conservative approach is now commonly practiced.[5,7,14,15] Although reports using E-cadherin and loss of heterozygosity (LOH) studies suggest LCIS may be a precursor to invasive disease, historically, LCIS has been considered a marker for an increased risk of developing invasive disease that is 9 to 12 times that of the normal population, and this risk requires long-term follow-up exceeding 20 years.[3,12,16,21] A range of ipsilateral and contralateral breast failure rates are reported. This variation reflects differences in the length of follow-up, the definitions used for histologic classification (i.e., atypical lobular hyperplasia versus lobular carcinoma in situ), and the extent of excision used in these observational studies.[26,27] In a 12-year follow-up report on a 182-patient cohort treated with lumpectomy only for LCIS, the National Surgical Adjuvant Breast and Bowel Project (NSABP) found a 14.4% IBTR rate and a 7.8% contralateral breast tumor recurrence (CBTR) rate.[27] Of the IBTRs, 9 (34.6%, 5% of the total cohort) were invasive malignancies and 17 (65.4%, 9% of the total cohort) were noninvasive malignancies. Although the frequency of CBTR was less than IBTR, the frequency of invasive CBTR (5.6% of total cohort) was similar to invasive IBTR (5% of total cohort). All of the IBTRs were documented to be at the site of the index lesion except for one, characterized as pure LCIS, which was found at a remote site. This report continues to support the indolent nature of LCIS and a conservative management approach.

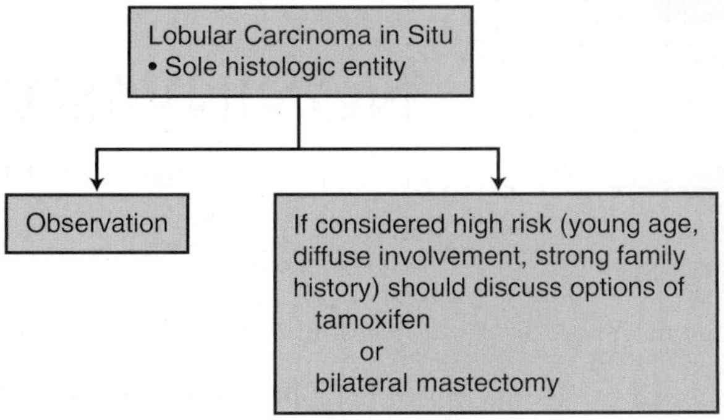

Figure 59-1 Treatment algorithm for lobular carcinoma in situ.

The impact of subsequent development of invasive disease on mortality was estimated in earlier publications to be 5% to 7%.[7,14] However, with contemporary use of close mammographic and clinical follow-up leading to early detection of subclinical abnormalities, it is reasonable to expect this mortality risk to be reduced. This reduction is reflected in the lower mortality risk (1%) reported by the NSABP.[27]

Close observation with regular physical examinations and mammographic surveillance is the accepted management approach.[5,7,14,15,26,27] There is no role for radiation therapy in the management of LCIS. Knowing that this is a bilateral breast disease process means that a unilateral treatment approach (i.e., ipsilateral mastectomy) is inadequate. Bilateral prophylactic mastectomy is thought to be excessive in all cases, except for patients believed to be at higher risk (e.g., young, diffuse process, with a significant family history). A less radical approach is the use of tamoxifen. Tamoxifen has been studied in the prevention of malignancy. Although the long-term risks versus benefits are not yet available, at 5 years, the risk of subsequent disease development was reduced with the use of tamoxifen by 56%.[28]

PAGET'S DISEASE

The clinical presentation of crusting, bleeding, and ulceration of the nipple was first described in 1856, but it was not until 1874 that the association with an underlying breast carcinoma was recognized by Sir James Paget.[29,30] Paget's disease of the nipple is characterized histologically by the presence of unique, clearly identifiable Paget's cells that are described as large, round to oval cells that contain hyperchromatic nuclei and prominent nucleoli. Mitoses are frequently seen. These Paget's cells occur singly or in clusters, and they are scattered throughout the epidermis.[31-33]

The fact that Paget's disease is associated with an underlying malignancy in more than 95% of cases has generated discussion regarding the origin of these malignant cells. The epidermotropic theory appears to be the prevailing opinion with the belief that the disease originates from the underlying in situ or invasive disease. This is supported by histologic evidence of intraepithelial extension, immunohistochemical studies, and evidence suggesting that the epidermal keratinocytes release a motility factor, heregulin-α, that results in the chemotaxis of Paget's cells that migrate to the overlying nipple epidermis.[31,34,35]

Reported in 0.5% to 5% of breast cancer patients, Paget's disease is an uncommon diagnosis.[31,36-40] The disease is most commonly unilateral, but reports of bilaterality and male Paget's disease can be found.[41-45] Women describe itching and burning of the nipple and areola, and crusting is often described. There is a slow progression toward an eczematoid appearance that can extend to the skin. If neglected, bleeding, pain, and ulceration can occur.[37,46] Alternatively, Paget's disease may be asymptomatic and manifest as a pathologic finding after surgical removal.[39] The differential diagnosis includes superficially spreading melanoma, pagetoid squamous cell carcinoma in situ, and clear cells of Toker.[32,33] A palpable mass is detected in about 50% of patients at diagnosis. If there is a palpable mass, more than 90% of cases will be invasive carcinoma. If no palpable mass is detected, 66% to 86% will have an underlying DCIS. These adjacent, underlying malignancies are usually located centrally; however, the location of these malignancies has also been reported to be elsewhere in the breast.[31,37,40]

Mammographic findings range from thickening of the nipple-areolar complex to parenchymal changes associated with an underlying malignancy. Although mammographic findings are frequent in the presence of a palpable mass, normal mammograms are reported in as many as 50% of cases.[37,47]

The appropriate management of Paget's disease remains unsettled, but in accordance with physician and patient preference, attempts have been made to investigate the role of breast-conserving therapy. After mastectomy was initially shown to be effective, transition to breast-conserving treatment has been cautious because of the inability to accumulate a significant number of uniform patients similarly treated.[36,41,48] The cause stems from the infrequent occurrence of this disease entity, the range of disease presentation (i.e., nipple involvement with or without an underlying mass and association with invasive versus noninvasive disease), and the variable extent of surgical resection. Limited series have described results with various forms of treatment including limited surgical resection alone, radiation therapy alone, and limited resection followed by irradiation (Table 59-1). Conservative surgery alone for Paget's disease has not been successful, and local recurrence rates of 25% to 40% have been reported, reflecting the experience seen with local excision only with early-stage invasive breast cancer.[49,54-58] Polgar and associates reported a database review of 33 women with Paget's disease who were treated with cone excision alone.[49] The clinicopathologic characteristics for this group of patients was comparable to other reports, with 91% presenting without a palpable mass and 91% with associated underlying DCIS. The median follow-up was 6 years, with a total of 11 (33.3%) failures and a 5-year actuarial local failure rate of 28.4%.

A report described the successful use of irradiation alone in a small series of 19 patients with Paget's disease of the nipple without an underlying palpable mass.[50] In this series, 16 of 19 remained locally controlled, with a median follow-up of 5 years and 3 months. However, this approach has not been adopted because of the limited experience and because of the unknown extent and character of the underlying disease, leading to questions in field design and total dose prescription.

The combination of limited surgical resection and postoperative irradiation appears to be the most successful breast-conservation approach. Two collaborative studies have shown the successful use of breast-conserving therapy in Paget's disease of the nipple. The European Organization for Research and Treatment of Cancer (EORTC) study 10873 was a multi-institutional registration study, for which Bijker and colleagues reported a 5-year local recurrence rate of 5.2%.[51] In this study, complete excision with tumor-free margins of the nipple-areolar complex and underlying breast tissue was followed by whole-breast radiation therapy to 50 Gy. The median follow-up was 6.4 years, and most patients were found to have an underlying DCIS without a palpable mass. The second study, updated by Marshall and coworkers, was a seven-institution collaborative review of 36 patients with Paget's disease without a palpable mass or mammographic density.[52,53] Median follow-up was 9.4 years, and all patients had at least 12 months of follow-up. The extent of surgical resection varied. Patients underwent complete (69%) or partial (25%) excision of the nipple-areolar complex and underlying breast tissue, with 6% reported as biopsy only. The final margin status was documented as negative in 56%, positive in 6%, and unknown in 39% of patients. All received whole-breast irradiation (median dose, 50 Gy), and most received an additional boost dose to the tumor bed. Actuarial rates of local in-breast failure as the only site of first recurrence were 9% at 5 years, 13% at 10 years, and 13% at 15 years. Two additional patients

Table 59-1 Breast Conservation in the Treatment of Paget's Disease

Study	No. of Patients	Median Follow-up	Treatment Approach	Palpable Mass *Yes*	*No*	DCIS Only *With*	*Without*	Local Control (5-Year Actuarial)
Polgar et al[49]	33	6 y	Only cone excision	91	9	91	9	71.6
Stockdale et al[50]	19	5.25 y	RT alone	0	19	—	—	84.2 (crude)
Bijker et al[51]	61	6.4 y	Cone excision + RT	3	97	93	7	94.8
Marshall et al[52,53]	36	9.4 y	Excision* + RT	0	100	75	25†	91 (5 y)‡ 87 (10 y)‡ 87 (15 y)‡

*Final margin status: 56% negative, 6% positive, and 39% unknown.
†Six percent were DCIS and invasive, 3% were invasive only, and for 16%, there was no underlying pathology.
‡Breast was only site of failure.
DCIS, ductal carcinoma in situ; RT, radiation therapy.

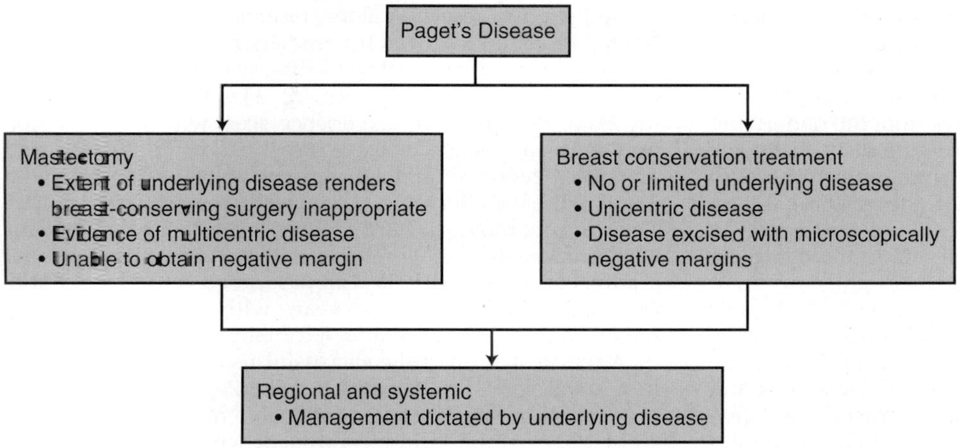

Figure 59-2 Treatment algorithm for Paget's disease.

had disease recurrence in the treated breast simultaneously with regional and distant metastasis at the extended time intervals of 69 and 122 months. Despite the variation of clinical, pathologic, and treatment factors, statistical evaluation did not identify any factors that significantly predicted for risk of local recurrence.

On presentation, the workup and evaluation should include bilateral breast examination, mammography, and biopsy to confirm the diagnosis of Paget's disease and fully evaluate the extent of underlying malignancy. An individual's prognosis does not depend on the diagnosis of Paget's disease, but on the associated underlying malignancy. Local treatment decisions and risk management for systemic and regional nodal disease should be based on the underlying disease (Fig. 59-2). Because breast-conserving therapy, which includes lumpectomy and standard whole-breast irradiation, has been proved effective for early-stage infiltrating duct carcinoma and DCIS, it appears that Paget's disease can be approached with the same conservative surgical methods. Standard principles governing patient selection, surgical resection, and irradiation should be applied. Proper patient selection includes patients without evidence of multicentric disease and limited underlying disease extent. In the limited published experiences, most cases have been associated with underlying noninvasive disease; however, to include cases with underlying invasive disease is thought to be appropriate for breast-conserving surgery. Complete surgical resection of the disease process (i.e., nipple-areolar complex excision in conjunction with any underlying disease) with a negative microscopic surgical margin is followed by standard whole-breast irradiation.

DUCTAL CARCINOMA IN SITU

Epidemiology

DCIS is represented by a heterogeneous spectrum of histologic appearances that all arise within and are confined to the ductal lumens of the breast. This clonal proliferation does not breach the epithelial basement membrane, and there is no evidence of invasion into the adjacent breast stroma.[59] DCIS lacks the ability to metastasize; the rarely reported axillary nodal metastasis or distant metastasis has been attributed to the probable presence of an undetected component of invasive carcinoma.[59-63]

Before 1980, the incidence of DCIS was low, representing only 1.4% of all breast biopsies and 5% of all breast malignancies.[64-69] With the increased use of mammography and as pathologists began to recognize DCIS as its own pathologic entity, the incidence of DCIS has dramatically increased.[70-74] The incidence of DCIS increased from 4800 cases reported in 1983 to more than 50,000 cases reported in 2003, and this represents a 10-fold increase in only 20 years.[59,75,76] Of the estimated 215,990 new breast cancers diagnosed in 2004, 59,390 were noninvasive, of which 85% were DCIS.[77] With this increase, there has been a corresponding change in the presentation of DCIS lesions from predominantly palpable to more than 90% nonpalpable.[75,76] Studies have shown that the rate of screen-detected DCIS increases with age, whereas DCIS accounts for a progressively smaller percentage of the total cancers detected (i.e., invasive plus DCIS).[78,79] The rate of DCIS detection has been shown to increase from 0.56 per 1000 mammograms among women 40 to 49 years old to 1.07 per 1000 mammograms among women 70 to 84 years old.[79]

Associated risk factors for the development of DCIS compare with risk factors for invasive disease. They include older age, benign breast disease, family history, and reproductive factors, including nulliparity or older age at pregnancy.[59,80-82]

Prevention and Early Detection

Although successful treatment options are in use, improved outcomes can be realized through prevention of DCIS development and the early detection of new lesions. The role of tamoxifen in the prevention of disease development has been studied by the NSABP in a protocol that randomized patients at high risk for the development of breast cancer to tamoxifen or placebo.[28] Patients eligible included those who were 60 years of age or older, had a history of LCIS, or were between the ages of 35 and 59 years, with a 5-year predicted risk for breast cancer of at least 1.66%. The predicted risk for breast cancer was determined using the Gail model that incorporates combinations of risk factors to estimate the probability of occurrence of breast cancer over time. These variables include age, number of first-degree relatives with breast cancer, nulliparity or age at first live birth, number of breast biopsies, pathologic diagnosis of atypical hyperplasia, and age at menarche. The 5-year follow-up data reveal that for noninvasive breast cancer, tamoxifen use was associated with a 50% reduction in risk. Through 69 months, the cumulative incidence of noninvasive breast cancer among the placebo group was 15.9 per 1000 women, compared with 7.7 per 1000 women in the tamoxifen group. The average annual rate of noninvasive breast cancer per 1000 women was 2.68 in the placebo group and 1.35 in the tamoxifen group, yielding a relative risk of 0.50 (95% CI, 0.33 to 0.77).[28]

Mammography plays an essential role in the early detection of noninvasive lesions, providing an opportunity for intervention early in the course of disease development. The distinctive mammographic feature of DCIS is the presence of microcalcifications, which has been reported in 84% to 98% of cases.[83-86] Between 72% and 76% of the DCIS lesions appear as microcalcifications as the sole mammographic finding and an additional 12% as microcalcifications in combination with other mammographic abnormalities.[84-86] Approximately 10% manifest as noncalcified irregularities described as a circumscribed nodule or a poorly defined mass, or they are represented by asymmetry or architectural distortion.[87,88]

Beyond detection, several attempts have been made to correlate the mammographic appearance of the lesion to the histologic type, grade, and extent of disease. Linear branching microcalcifications have been associated with high-grade DCIS or comedo necrosis. Heterogeneous granular calcification is commonly associated with moderately differentiated DCIS, and fine granular microcalcifications are typically associated with low-grade, noncomedo DCIS.[79,85,86] Although there is a degree of correlation between appearance and histology, there is considerable overlap, which limits the use of this information in clinical decision-making. Whether this represents a loose correlation of mammographic appearance with histologic type or the lack of consensus on histologic classification is unknown. Microcalcifications are not always present throughout the histologic abnormality, and the estimated mammographic size and extent of disease therefore frequently underestimates the true pathologic extent of the disease process. Although the mammographic extent can be used to guide the extent of surgical excision, caution should be exercised because the size is typically underestimated by 1 to 2 cm.[89,90] In patients presenting with nipple discharge and a negative mammographic evaluation, galactography may be helpful in distinguishing the presence of a papilloma from an underlying DCIS.[91]

Investigations into the use of ultrasound, digital mammography, and magnetic resonance imaging (MRI) have not suggested a prominent role in the radiographic evaluation of DCIS. Mammography has been a reliable and cost-effective screening tool, but improvements in the assessment of disease extent within the breast would improve surgical guidance and have a potential impact on treatment decisions before surgical intervention. MRI, a more sensitive modality, has the potential to refine clinical decision-making and surgical planning in selected cases, although further investigation is needed. In a study of 51 patients who had undergone prior surgery for DCIS, the sensitivity of MRI for detection of residual disease and multicentricity remained impressive at 96% and 86%, respectively. The investigators concluded that a negative MRI finding after surgical excision was superior to a mammogram in the detection of residual DCIS, occult invasive cancer, and multicentricity, and the presence of these forms of residual disease could be ruled out with a negative MRI.[92]

Biologic Characteristics and Molecular Markers

DCIS is a precursor lesion to invasive ductal carcinoma and exists along an evolutionary continuum that starts with benign breast tissue and ends with invasive breast cancer.[93] This concept has been verified in several ways. For years, pathologists have recognized and documented confirmation of a histologic progression from benign breast cells to invasive breast cancer and have found that this histologic evidence was more commonly present when an invasive lesion was discovered. The evolutionary concept is further supported by the acknowledged association between the presence of DCIS and the subsequent increased risk of developing an invasive breast cancer.[59,94,95] In some series, a 10-fold risk of developing an invasive lesion has been reported. The presence of shared identical genetic abnormalities between DCIS and synchronous invasive breast cancer demonstrates a clonal relationship of biologic progression.[59,94-96] The biologic evolution from benign breast cells to invasive breast cancer occurs through highly diverse genetic mechanisms. Knowledge of these mechanisms may allow us to alter the pathways and prevent progression, and they are the subjects of investigation.

Documented genetic and molecular differences can differentiate DCIS from normal breast tissue. Genetic alterations have been evaluated with an analysis of LOH that has demonstrated gain or loss of multiple loci.[94-98] LOH is not seen in normal breast tissue, but it occurs with increasing frequency that correlates with histologic progression from benign to malignant. In hyperplasias from noncancerous breasts, LOH is rarely documented; it is more common (42% to 50%) in atypical ductal hyperplasia. Among specimens harvested from cancerous breasts, 77% of noncomedo and 80% of comedo DCIS lesions share LOH with the synchronous invasive lesion in at least one locus.[96] Molecular markers have a heterogeneous distribution of expression.[59] The estrogen receptor is present in 70% of DCIS lesions, but the rate of expression is 90% in low-grade lesions and is 25% in high-grade lesions. This trend is reversed for the rate of overexpression of the *ERBB2 (HER2)* proto-oncogene and the *TP53* tumor suppression gene. About 50% of all DCIS overexpress *HER2*, and 25% overexpress *TP53*. However, both molecular markers are identified in less than 20% of low-grade lesions but in two thirds of the high-grade lesions.

Pathology and Pathways of Spread

The primary goal of pathologic assessment is to differentiate DCIS from invasive cancer, because the presence of invasive disease alters the focus of treatment from breast only to include treatment that may also need to address a risk of regional and distant metastasis. Once identified, pathologic classification of DCIS follows in an attempt to predict clinical outcome and direct treatment management. Historically, an architectural classification system has been used dividing patients into the five classic subtypes: comedo, solid, cribriform, papillary, and micropapillary.[99-101] Less common subtypes include apocrine, neuroendocrine, signet-cell cystic, hypersecretory carcinoma, and clinging DCIS.[62] The difficulty with an architectural classification method is that there can be a mixture of architectural subtypes identified within the same lesion, and the reproducibility of classification is unreliable because pathologists apply various criteria.[63,90,102-104] The value of an architectural classification system is questionable because the architectural subtypes do not correlate well with clinical behavior.[105] Although this was not an issue when mastectomy was routinely used, the ability to predict clinical behavior has become important because breast-conservative approaches are more commonly applied.

In an attempt to better predict clinical behavior, several classification systems have been proposed.[91,106-109] These are based on nuclear grade of the tumor cells and presence of comedo necrosis with and without architectural features. These characteristics appear to correlate with the risk of local recurrence.[81] In 1997, an international consensus conference was convened to discuss several pathologic aspects concerning DCIS with the goal of reaching a consensus.[110] The committee stated that a DCIS classification system should reflect its biology and predict the probability of local recurrence, risk of mastectomy, probability of subsequent invasive cancer, and breast cancer–specific mortality. It was recognized that several classification systems have been proposed, and although a specific system was not endorsed, the group recommended that four features be routinely described: nuclear grade, necrosis, polarization, and architectural pattern. They also recommended that several additional features be documented in the pathology report. These features include margin status, size, description of microcalcification location in relation to the DCIS lesion, and correlation of the tissue specimen with the specimen radiographic and mammographic findings.

Stereoscopic, three-dimensional analysis of DCIS within the mammary glandular tree has led to a better understanding of the distribution and growth pattern of this disease entity. In a study by Ohtake and associates, the extension of intraductal carcinoma was mapped out through a process of three-dimensional reconstruction, and an interesting pattern of ductal spread was observed.[111] The investigators described ductal anastomoses that established a connection between the ductal-lobular units, providing a pathway for widespread intraductal extension. They described three directional patterns of spread: central type of extension, described as the continuous extension from the primary lesion centrally toward the nipple; peripheral type of extension, defined as the continuous extension in peripheral and lateral directions; and a mixed type. The most common type of extension was central (68%). In a study by Faverly and colleagues, the growth pattern of DCIS was described and its impact on surgical margin discussed.[112] They documented unicentric and multicentric growth patterns, defined as one area versus two distinct areas separated by more than 4 cm, respectively.

They also described two patterns of extension along the duct: continuous and discontinuous or multifocal. The continuous form extended along the ducts without gaps, and 90% of poorly differentiated DCIS showed a continuous growth pattern. The discontinuous or multifocal form was defined as two or more areas of DCIS separated by less than 4 cm. Seventy percent of well-differentiated DCIS had a discontinuous growth pattern, with 63% of foci separated by a gap of less than 5 mm, 83% with foci separated by less than 10 mm, and only 8% with gaps of more than 10 mm. Because less than 10% of lesions exhibiting a discontinuous growth pattern demonstrated a gap of more than 1 cm, the study authors concluded that a 1-cm clear margin of normal tissue would result in complete surgical removal of the lesion in 90% of cases.

Primary Therapy

Patient evaluation focuses on bilateral mammography, with which the presence of additional breast malignancies can be excluded and the extent of the DCIS process defined. After it is determined that DCIS is the only disease entity requiring treatment, the primary focus becomes local management of the breast. In concert with the spectrum of clinical presentations encountered with DCIS, there are several treatment approaches. They range from the treatment of the whole breast to the treatment of a partial-breast target. On the one end of this spectrum, when multicentric disease or a diffuse DCIS process is documented, a mastectomy is considered to be the standard of care. If a focal area of DCIS is confronted, breast-conservative approaches are favored. Supported with phase III trial data, the use of standard breast-conserving therapy with lumpectomy and standard whole-breast irradiation is most commonly recommended, and newer partial-breast treatment techniques (with and without irradiation) are being offered with increased frequency.

All presentations of DCIS can be successfully managed with total mastectomy. This is supported by the reports from mastectomy series showing disease control rates that approach 100% and cancer-specific mortality rates of less than 4%.[65,113-118] However, it is recognized that the availability of mammographic screening has shifted the most common presentation of DCIS from one of a palpable mass with advanced involvement to one of early stage and limited extent, for which a total mastectomy intuitively appears to be excessive. To promote mastectomy in the management of noninvasive disease would be in opposition to the increasing use of breast-conserving therapy for invasive disease. Although a phase III trial comparing total mastectomy to breast-conserving therapy for DCIS has never been done, the psychological benefits of preserving the breast and the acceptable rates of local control achieved with breast-conserving therapy support the use of total mastectomy only when necessary. Total mastectomy is most commonly reserved for patients presenting with multicentric or diffuse disease, patients for whom the use of radiation therapy is contraindicated, when an unacceptable cosmetic result is anticipated after appropriate surgical excision, or for salvage in the event of in-breast recurrence after standard breast-conserving therapy.[119]

Breast-conservation treatment is composed of an initial surgical excision of the primary lesion with a negative surgical margin followed by whole-breast irradiation delivered with standard, accepted techniques, such as those used for early-stage invasive breast cancer. Literature supporting this approach is found as retrospective series and prospective phase III trials comparing lumpectomy only to lumpectomy followed by whole-breast irradiation.

Retrospective analysis of lumpectomy and whole-breast irradiation has reported a 5-year cause-specific survival rate that approaches 100% and local control rates that range from 85% to 95%.[120-132] Prospective, randomized trials have been completed evaluating the role of postoperative irradiation and tamoxifen in the management of DCIS with breast-conserving therapy (Tables 59-2 and 59-3). The NSABP initiated the first trial, protocol B-17, designed to evaluate the role of postoperative irradiation.[133,136-138] All 814 evaluable patients enrolled were initially diagnosed with DCIS, and they underwent lumpectomy and achieved clear surgical margins (i.e., inked specimen margins histologically tumor free). Patients were subsequently randomized to receive postoperative whole-breast irradiation or no irradiation. Randomization was stratified using age (≤49 or >49), tumor type (i.e., DCIS or DCIS plus LCIS), and method of detection (i.e., mammographic or clinical, or both) and whether an axillary dissection was performed. Eighty-three percent of patients presented with nonpalpable tumors and pathologic assessment documented no gross tumor in 54.1%. The radiation therapy guidelines used consisted of whole-breast tangential fields treated to 50 Gy as in previous NSABP studies; boost to the surgical bed was not included. In a study with a 12-year follow-up, the rate of in-breast tumor recurrence with lumpectomy only was 31.7%, compared with 15.7% when irradiation was delivered ($P < .000005$). Most in-breast failures were close to the site of lumpectomy. The time to recurrence ranged from 2 to 123 months, with a median time of 36 months. Nine pathologic features (i.e., comedo necrosis, histologic type, margin status, lymphoid infiltrate, nuclear grade, focality, cancerization, stroma, and tumor size) were evaluated for their ability to predict for in-breast recurrence, and only comedo necrosis was a significant predictor for recurrence. The average annual hazard rates for IBTR were lower for all nine pathologic characteristics when radiation therapy was added.

In 1996, the EORTC completed its randomized phase III trial 10853.[134,139] This trial evaluated the role of radiation therapy after complete local excision of DCIS. Five hundred

Table 59-2 Randomized Clinical Trials Evaluating the Role of Postoperative Radiation Therapy in the Management of Ductal Carcinoma In Situ

Trial	No. of Patients	Follow-up	LOCAL RECURRENCE (CUMULATIVE %) Histology of Recurrence	L	L + XRT	P Value	OVERALL SURVIVAL (%) L	L + XRT	P Value
NSABP B-17[133]	818	12 y actuarial	DCIS	14.6	8.0	.001			
			Invasive	16.8	7.7	.00001	86	87	.80
			DCIS + invasive	31.7	15.7	<.000005			
EORTC 10853[134]	1002	4.25 y median	DCIS	8.0	5.0	.06			
			Invasive	8.0	4.0	.04	99	99	.94
			DCIS + invasive	16.0	9.0	.005			
UKCCCR[135]	1030	4.38 y median	DCIS	6.0	3.0	.01			
			Invasive	7.0	3.0	.0004	—	—	—
			DCIS + invasive	14.0	6.0	<.0001			

DCIS, ductal carcinoma in situ; EORTC, European Organization for Research and Treatment of Cancer; L, lumpectomy; L+XRT, lumpectomy and postoperative radiation therapy; NSABP, National Surgical Adjuvant Bowel and Breast Project; UKCCCR, United Kingdom Coordinating Committee on Cancer Research.

Table 59-3 Randomized Clinical Trials Evaluating the Role of Tamoxifen in the Management of Ductal Carcinoma In Situ

Trial	No. of Patients	Follow-up	LOCAL RECURRENCE (CUMULATIVE %) Histology of Recurrence	−Tam	+Tam	P Value	OVERALL SURVIVAL (%) −Tam	+Tam	P Value
NSABP B-17[133]	1798	7 y actuarial	DCIS	5.8	5.0	.48			
			Invasive	5.3	2.6	.01	3.2	1.8	.16
			DCIS + invasive	11.1	7.7	.02	4.9	2.3	.01
UKCCCR[135]	1576	4.38 y median	DCIS	10.0	7.0	.08			
			Invasive	4.0	8.0	.23	2.0	1.0	.30
			DCIS + invasive	15.0	13.0	.42	6.0	7.0	.59

DCIS, ductal carcinoma in situ; NSABP, National Surgical Adjuvant Bowel and Breast Project; −Tam, without tamoxifen; +Tam, with tamoxifen; UKCCCR, United Kingdom Coordinating Committee on Cancer Research.

patients were treated and followed in the excision-only group, and 502 received excision plus irradiation. All patients had histologically confirmed tumor-free margins, defined as no DCIS at the inked margin, and the prescribed radiation therapy consisted of whole-breast tangential fields treated to 50 Gy in 25 fractions. A boost dose was not advised, and only 5% received a boost to the surgical bed. For the patients enrolled, 21% of tumors were palpable, 72% were nonpalpable, and 7% of patients presented with nipple discharge only. At a follow-up interval of 4.25 years, the investigators reported a 16% in-breast failure rate with excision only and a 9% in-breast failure rate with excision plus irradiation. The local recurrence-free interval was significantly longer ($P = .005$) in the irradiation arm compared with the no-irradiation arm. Risk factors for recurrence were evaluated, and it was found that even with the addition of irradiation, local recurrence rates ranging between 15% and 20% were seen in the worst subgroups (i.e., high nuclear grade, presence of necrosis, clinically detected lesions, involved or unknown margin status, and age younger than 40 years).

The United Kingdom Coordinating Committee on Cancer Research (UKCCCR) DCIS Working Group conducted a randomized trial investigating the role of adjuvant irradiation.[135] Within a more complex 2 × 2 factorial protocol design, the aim was to compare excision alone, excision plus tamoxifen, excision plus irradiation, and excision plus irradiation and tamoxifen. Tamoxifen was prescribed at 20 mg/day, and radiation therapy was delivered through whole-breast tangential fields to a total dose of 50 Gy. Boost was not recommended. A total of 1030 patients were enrolled. When reported with a 52.6-month follow-up, the crude incidence of local recurrence was documented in 14% of the 508 patients who were treated with excision only and reduced to 6% when the excision was followed by radiation therapy (522 patients). The addition of tamoxifen offered minimal benefit toward overall ipsilateral local control rates when added to irradiation; however, it did appear to reduce the ipsilateral recurrence rate of DCIS in the absence of irradiation.[135]

In a trial asking a similar question about the role of tamoxifen and building on the results from B-17, the NSABP initiated a trial to determine whether the addition of tamoxifen to lumpectomy and postoperative irradiation would be more effective than lumpectomy and postoperative irradiation alone.[133,140] Women with DCIS or DCIS and LCIS were eligible. They included women with one or more masses or calcification clusters if all were excised. Women with microscopically positive margins for DCIS or LCIS were also included, representing 15% of each treatment arm. All of the 1804 women underwent excision and were randomized to whole-breast irradiation and placebo ($n = 902$) or whole-breast irradiation followed by tamoxifen ($n = 902$). Patients were stratified according to age (≤49 years or >49 years), tumor type (i.e., DCIS or DCIS and LCIS), and method of detection (i.e., mammography or clinical examination, or both). Eighty percent of patients presented with nonpalpable lesions that were measured as 1 cm or less. Postoperative irradiation was delivered with standard tangential fields to a total dose of 50 Gy. The placebo or tamoxifen (10 mg, twice daily) was continued for

5 years. At 7 years of follow-up, the in-breast failure rate after lumpectomy, radiation therapy, and placebo was 11.1%, and the rate was reduced to 7.7% when tamoxifen was added to lumpectomy and irradiation ($P = .02$). The contralateral breast occurrence rate was also reduced with the addition of tamoxifen, decreasing from 4.9% to 2.3% ($P = .01$).

Risk factor assessment has been performed with the goal of determining which patients are ideal for breast-conserving therapy, identifying patients better treated with mastectomy, and establishing which patients can be successfully managed with lumpectomy only. Single-institution studies and randomized studies have identified factors that predict for an increased risk of recurrence.[125,127,138-145] Tumor size, comedo necrosis, nuclear grade, young age, and margin status have been identified as factors associated with a higher risk of in-breast recurrence. Most series report higher local recurrence rates for younger women less than 40, 45, or 50 years old. It is therefore appropriate to take age into consideration when determining appropriateness for breast-conserving therapy and when presenting options to the patient.[141,145] Whether this increased risk of local failure could be offset with an increase in the boost dose or a wider resection margin is uncertain. However, the addition of radiation therapy reduces the risk of recurrence in all cases, and it is only when diffuse disease, signified by mammographic appearance or the inability to achieve clear surgical margins, is encountered that a mastectomy is the preferred method of surgical management.

In the absence of high-risk factors, the question is whether a less comprehensive treatment approach (i.e., wide excision only or lumpectomy and accelerated partial-breast irradiation) is sufficient. Although failure pattern data and retrospective analysis confirm these more directed treatment approaches to be valid, they lack confirmation in an appropriately designed clinical trial.[75,133,136,137,143,146] The Radiation Therapy Oncology Group (RTOG) is conducting a prospective, randomized trial evaluating the need for radiation therapy in low-risk DCIS. After lumpectomy with 3-mm clear margins of resection, patients are stratified according to age (<50 versus ≥50), tumor size (≤1 cm versus >1 to 2.5 cm), margin status (negative re-excision versus 3 to 9 mm versus ≥10 mm), grade, and the use of tamoxifen (at the discretion of the managing physician). After stratification, patients are randomized to whole-breast irradiation or observation. The NSABP and RTOG jointly launched a phase III accelerated partial-breast irradiation trial in 2005 that randomized patients to standard whole-breast irradiation after lumpectomy or to accelerated partial-breast irradiation to determine whether in-breast control rates were comparable. Because the in-breast failure patterns for DCIS suggest that treatment directed to the primary lesion plus a 2-cm margin should achieve local control rates that are equal to whole-breast treatment approaches, patients with pure DCIS or DCIS and LCIS were eligible for stratified randomization.

In summary, DCIS is a noninvasive malignancy that is managed successfully with treatment directed toward the breast only (Fig. 59-3). Treatment approaches addressing the

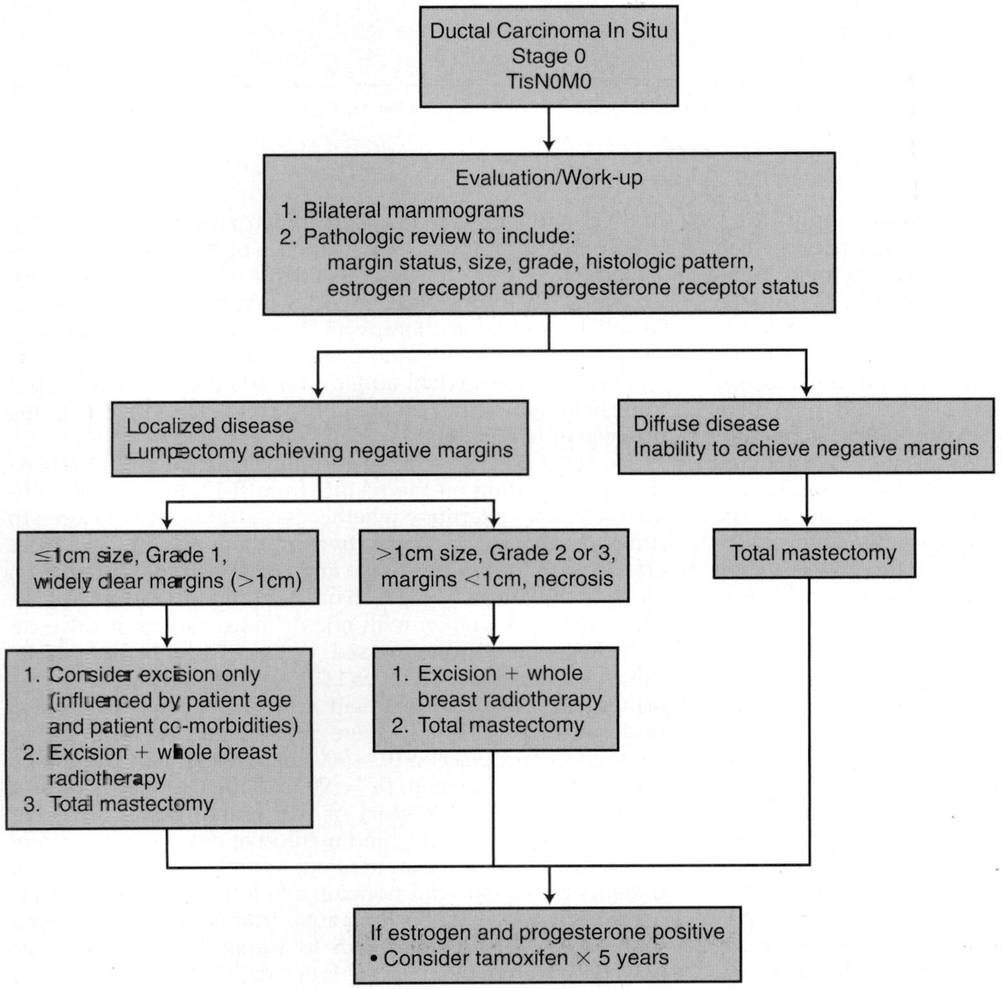

Figure 59-3 Management decision tree for ductal carcinoma in situ.

whole breast are considered the standard of care, although partial-breast treatment (i.e., wide excision only versus lumpectomy plus partial-breast irradiation) is being evaluated. Although mastectomy can always be considered a treatment option, breast-conserving therapy is the preferred treatment approach. When considering a patient for standard breast-conserving therapy, it is important to first ensure that clinical and mammographic information confirms it to be a unicentric lesion. When surgical excision of the lesion is performed, negative pathologic margins should be established and an acceptable cosmetic result achieved. Postoperative irradiation should be delivered with whole-breast tangential fields to a homogeneous dose of 46 to 50 Gy given in 1.8 to 2.0 Gy per fraction. The surgical bed is then given an appropriately designed electron boost that covers the surgical bed plus margin (2 cm) to a total cumulative dose of 60 to 66 Gy.

REFERENCES

1. Foote FW, Stewart FW: Lobular carcinoma in situ—a rare form of mammary cancer. Am J Pathol 17:491-495, 1941.
2. Rosen PP, Lieberman PH, Braun DW, et al: Lobular carcinoma in situ of the breast. Am J Surg Pathol 2:225-251, 1978.
3. Page DL, Kidd TE, Dupont WE, et al: Lobular neoplasia of the breast: higher risk for subsequent invasive cancer predicted by more extensive disease. Hum Pathol 22:1232-1239, 1991.
4. Schnitt SJ, Morrow M: Lobular carcinoma in situ: current concepts and controversies. Semin Diagn Pathol 16:209-223, 1999.
5. Wheeler JE, Enterline HT, Roseman JM, et al: Lobular carcinoma in situ of the breast—long term follow-up. Cancer 34:554-563, 1974.
6. Tavassoli FA: Lobular neoplasia. *In* Tavassoli FA (ed): Pathology of the Breast, 2nd ed. New York, Elsevier, 1999, pp 373-400.
7. Frykberg ER, Bland KI: In situ breast carcinoma. Adv Surg 26:29-72, 1993.
8. Albonico G, Querzoli P, Ferretti S, et al: Biological profile of in situ breast cancer investigated by immunohistochemical technique. Cancer Detect Prev 22:313-318, 1998.
9. Bur ME, Zimarowski MJ, Schmitt SJ, et al: Estrogen receptor immunohistochemistry in carcinoma in situ of the breast. Cancer 69:1174-1181, 1992.
10. Acs G, Lawton TJ, Rebbeck TR, et al: Differential expression of E-cadherin in lobular and ductal neoplasms of the breast and its biologic and diagnostic implications. Am J Clin Pathol 115:85-98, 2001.
11. Jacobs TW, Pliss N, Kouria G: Carcinoma in situ of the breast with indeterminate features. Am J Surg Pathol 25:229-236, 2001.
12. Vos CB, Cleton-Jansen AM, Verx G, et al: E-cadherin inactivation in lobular carcinoma in situ of the breast: an early event in tumorigenesis. Br J Cancer 76:1131-1133, 1997.
13. Goldstein NS, Kestin LL, Vicini FA: Clinicopathologic implications of E-cadherin reactivity in patients with lobular carcinoma in situ of the breast. Cancer 92:738-747, 2001.
14. Andersen JA: Lobular carcinoma in situ of the breast—an approach to rational treatment. Cancer 39:2597-2602, 1977.
15. Haagensen CD, Bodian C, Haagensen DE: Lobular neoplasia (lobular carcinoma in situ). Breast Carcinoma: Risk and Detection. Philadelphia, WB Saunders, 1981, pp 238-292.
16. Li CI, Anderson BO, Daling JR, et al: Changing incidence of lobular carcinoma in situ of the breast. Breast Cancer Res Treat 75:259-268, 2002.
17. Georgian-Smith D, Lawton TJ: Calcifications of lobular carcinoma in situ of the breast: radiologic-pathologic correlation. AJR Am J Roentgenol 176:1255-1259, 2001.
18. Sapino A, Frigerio A, Peterse JL, et al: Mammographically detected in situ lobular carcinomas of the breast. Virchows Arch 436:421-430, 2000.
19. Sonnenfeld MR, Frenna TH, Weidner N, et al: Lobular carcinoma in situ: mammographic-pathologic correlation of results of needle-directed biopsy. Radiology 181:363-367, 1991.
20. Liberman L, Sama M, Susnik B, et al: Lobular carcinoma in situ at percutaneous breast biopsy: surgical biopsy findings. AJR Am J Roentgenol 173:219-299, 1999.
21. Cohen MA: Cancer upgrades at excisional biopsy after diagnosis of atypical lobular hyperplasia or lobular carcinoma in situ at core-needle biopsy: some reasons why. Radiology 231:617-621, 2004.
22. Foster MC, Helvie MA, Gregory NE, et al: Lobular carcinoma in situ or atypical lobular hyperplasia at core-needle biopsy: is excisional biopsy necessary? Radiology 231:813-819, 2004.
23. Moran M, Haffty B: Lobular carcinoma in situ as a component of breast cancer: the long-term outcome in patients treated with breast-conservation therapy. Int J Radiat Oncol Biol Phys 40:353-358, 1998.
24. Abner AL, Connolly JL, Recht A, et al: The relationship between the presence and extent of lobular carcinoma in situ and the risk of local recurrence for patients with infiltrating carcinoma of the breast treated with conservative surgery and radiation therapy. Cancer 88:1072-1077, 2000.
25. Sasson AR, Fowble B, Hanlon AL, et al: Lobular carcinoma in situ increases the risk of local recurrence in selected patients with stages I and II breast carcinoma treated with conservative surgery and radiation. Cancer 91:1862-1869, 2001.
26. Fisher ER, Costantino J, Fisher B, et al: Pathologic findings from the National Surgical Adjuvant Breast Project (NSABP) protocol B-17—five-year observations concerning lobular carcinoma in situ. Cancer 78:1403-1416, 1996.
27. Fisher ER, Land SR, Fisher B, et al: Pathologic findings from the National Surgical Adjuvant Breast and Bowel Project—twelve-year observations concerning lobular carcinoma in situ. Cancer 100:238-244, 2004.
28. Fisher B, Costantino J, Wickerham DL, et al: Tamoxifen for prevention of breast cancer: report of the national surgical adjuvant breast and bowel project P-1 study. J Natl Cancer Inst 90:1371-1388, 1998.
29. Velpeau S: A Treatise on Diseases of the Breast and Mammary Region. London, Sydenham Society, 1856.
30. Paget J: On the disease of the mammary areola preceding cancer of the mammary gland. St Bartholomew Hosp Rep 10:87-89, 1874.
31. Jamali FR, Ricci A, Deckers PJ: Paget's disease of the nipple-areola complex. Surg Clin North Am 76:365-381, 1996.
32. Kohler S, Rouse RV, Smoller BR: The differential diagnosis of pagetoid cells in the epidermis. Mod Pathol 11:79-92, 1998.
33. Lloyd J, Flanagan AM: Mammary and extramammary Paget's disease. J Clin Pathol 53:742-749, 2000.
34. Muir R: The pathogenesis of Paget's disease of the nipple. Br J Surg 30:451-471, 1935.
35. Schelfhout VR, Coene ED, Delaey B, et al: Pathogenesis of Paget's disease: epidermal heregulin-α, motility factor, and the HER receptor family. J Natl Cancer Inst 92:622-628, 2000.
36. Ashikari R, Park K, Huvos AG, et al: Paget's disease of the breast. Cancer 26:680-685, 1970.
37. Sakorafas GH, Blanchard K, Sarr MG, et al: Paget's disease of the breast. Cancer Treat Rev 27:9-18, 2001.
38. Nance FC, DeLoach DH, Welsh RA, et al: Paget's disease of the breast. Ann Surg 171:864-872, 1970.
39. Inwang ER, Fentiman IS: Paget's disease of the nipple. Br J Hosp Med 44:392-395, 1990.
40. Chaudary MA, Millis RR, Lane B, et al: Paget's disease of the nipple: a ten year review including clinical, pathological, and immunohistochemical findings. Breast Cancer Res Treat 8:139-146, 1986.
41. Paone JF, Baker RR: Pathogenesis and treatment of Paget's disease of the breast. Cancer 48:825-829, 1981.
42. Markpoulos CH, Gogas H, Sampalis F, et al: Bilateral Paget's disease of the breast. Eur J Gynaecol Oncol 18:495-496, 1997.
43. Fernandes F, Costa M, Bernando M: Bilateral Paget's disease of the breast: a case report. Eur J Surg Oncol 16:172-174, 1990.
44. Desai DC, Brennan EJ, Carp NZ: Paget's disease of the male breast. Am Surg 62:1068-1072, 1996.
45. Hayes R, Cummings B, Miller RAW, et al: Male Paget's disease of the breast. J Cutan Med Surg 4:208-212, 2000.

46. Ward KA, Burton JL: Dermatological diseases of the breast in young women. Clin Dermatol 15:45-52, 1997.
47. Ikeda DM, Helvie MA, Frank TS, et al: Paget disease of the nipple: radiologic-pathologic correlation. Radiology 189:89-94, 1993.
48. Yim JH, Wick MR, Philpott GW, et al: Underlying pathology in mammary Paget's disease. Ann Surg Oncol 4:287-292, 1997.
49. Polgar C, Orosz Z, Kovacs T, et al: Breast-conserving therapy for Paget disease of the nipple. Cancer 94:904-905, 2002.
50. Stockdale AD, Brierly JD, White WF, et al: Radiotherapy for Paget's disease of the nipple: a conservative alternative. Lancet 2:664-666, 1989.
51. Bijker N, Rutgers EJT, Duchateau L, et al: Breast-conserving therapy for Paget disease of the nipple. Cancer 91:472-477, 2001.
52. Pierce LJ, Haffty BG, Solin LJ, et al: The conservative management of Paget's disease of the breast with radiotherapy. Cancer 80:1065-1072, 1997.
53. Marshall JK, Griffith KA, Haffty BG, et al: Conservative management of Paget disease of the breast with radiotherapy. Cancer 97:2142-2149, 2003.
54. Lagios MD, Westdahl PR, Marye RR, et al: Paget's disease of the nipple. Cancer 54:545-551, 1984.
55. Dixon AR, Galea RR: Pathogenesis and treatment of Paget's disease of the breast. Cancer 48:835, 1981.
56. Fischer B, Anderson S, Bryant J, et al: Twenty-year follow-up of a randomized trial comparing total mastectomy, lumpectomy, and lumpectomy plus irradiation for the treatment of invasive breast cancer. N Engl J Med 347:1233-1241, 2002.
57. Veronesi U, Cascinelli N, Mariani L, et al: Twenty-year follow-up of randomized study comparing breast-conserving surgery with radical (Halstead) mastectomy for early breast cancer. N Engl J Med 347:1227-1232, 2002.
58. Fourquet A, Campana F, Vielh P, et al: Paget's disease of the nipple without detectable breast tumor: conservative management with radiation therapy. Int J Radiat Oncol Biol Phys 13:1463-1465, 1987.
59. Burstein HJ, Polyak K, Wong JS, et al: Ductal carcinoma in situ of the breast. N Engl J Med 350:1430-1441, 2004.
60. Page DL, Anderson TJ: Diagnostic Histopathology of the Breast. Edinburgh, Churchill Livingstone, 1987.
61. Page DL, Dupont WD, Rogers LW, et al: Continued local recurrence of carcinoma 15-25 years after a diagnosis of low grade ductal carcinoma in situ of the breast treated only by biopsy. Cancer 76:1197-1200, 1995.
62. Lagios MD: Ductal carcinoma in situ: controversies in diagnosis, biology, and treatment. Breast J 1:68-78, 1995.
63. Lennington WJ, Jensen RA, Dalton LW, et al: Ductal carcinoma in situ of the breast. Cancer 73:118-124, 1994.
64. Anderson JA, Schiodt T: On the concept of carcinoma in situ of the breast. Pathol Res Pract 166:407-414, 1980.
65. Ashikari R, Huvos AG, Snyder RE: Prospective study of non-infiltrating carcinoma of the breast. Cancer 39:435-439, 1977.
66. Blichert-Toft M, Graversen HP, Andersen JA, et al: In situ breast carcinomas: a population-based study on frequency, growth pattern, and clinical aspects. World J Surg 12:845-851, 1988.
67. Rosen PP, Braun DW, Kinne DE: The clinical significance of pre-invasive breast carcinoma. Cancer 46:919-925, 1980.
68. Rosner D, Bedwani RN, Vana J, et al: Noninvasive breast carcinoma: results of a national survey by the American College of Surgeons. Ann Surg 192:139-147, 1980.
69. Wilson RE, Donegan WL, Mettlin C, et al: The 1982 national survey of carcinoma of the breast in the United States by the American College of Surgeons. Surg Gynecol Obstet 159:309-318, 1984.
70. Lenhard RE: Cancer statistics: a measure of progress. CA Cancer J Clin 46:3-7, 1996.
71. Schnitt SJ, Silen W, Sadowsky NL, et al: Ductal carcinoma in situ (intraductal carcinoma) of the breast. N Engl J Med 318:898-903, 1988.
72. Seidman H, Gelb SK, Silverberg E, et al: Survival experience in the breast cancer detection demonstration project. CA Cancer J Clin 37:258-290, 1987.
73. Simon MS, Lemanne D, Schwartz AG, et al: Recent trends in the incidence of in situ and invasive breast cancer in the Detroit Metropolitan area (1975-1988). Cancer 71:769-774, 1993.
74. Simon MS, Schwartz AG, Martino S, et al: Trends in the diagnosis of in situ breast cancer in the Detroit Metropolitan area, 1973 to 1987. Cancer 69:466-469, 1992.
75. Silverstein MJ: An argument against routine use of radiotherapy for ductal carcinoma in situ. Oncology 17:1511-1533, 2003.
76. Ernster VL, Barclay J, Kerlikowske K, et al: Incidence of and treatment for ductal carcinoma in situ of the breast. JAMA 275:913-918, 1996.
77. Jemal A, Tiwari RC, Murray T, et al: Cancer statistics, 2004. CA Cancer J Clin 54:8-29, 2004.
78. Kopans DB: Detection of ductal carcinoma in situ in women undergoing screening mammography. J Natl Cancer Inst 95:487, 2003.
79. Ernster VL, Ballard-Barbash R, Barlow WE, et al: Detection of ductal carcinoma in situ in women undergoing screening mammography. J Natl Cancer Inst 94:1546-1554, 2002.
80. Trentham-Dietz A, Newcomb PA, Storer BE, et al: Risk factors for carcinoma in situ of the breast. Cancer Epidemiol Biomarkers Prev 9:697-703, 2000.
81. Kerlikowske K, Molinaro A, Cha I: Characteristics associated with recurrence among women with ductal carcinoma in situ treated by lumpectomy. J Natl Cancer Inst 95:1692-1702, 2003.
82. Kerlikowske K, Barclay J, Grady D, et al: Comparison of risk factors for ductal carcinoma in situ and invasive breast cancer. J Natl Cancer Inst 89:76-82, 1997.
83. Dershaw DD: Breast imaging and the conservative treatment of breast cancer. Radiol Clin North Am 40:501-516, 2002.
84. Stomper PC, Connolly JL: Ductal carcinoma in situ of the breast: correlation between mammographic calcification and tumor subtype. AJR Am J Roentgenol 159:483-485, 1992.
85. Tabar L, Fagerberg CJG, Gad A, et al: Reduction in mortality from breast cancer after mass screening with mammography. Lancet 1:829-832, 1985.
86. Tabar L, Gad A, Parsons WC, et al: Mammographic appearances of in situ carcinomas. *In* Silverstein MJ (ed): Ductal Carcinoma In Situ of the Breast, 2nd ed. Philadelphia, Lippincott Williams & Wilkins, 2002, pp 87-104.
87. Sakorafas GH, Farley DR: Optimal management of ductal carcinoma in situ of the breast. Surg Oncol 12:221-240, 2003.
88. Winchester DP, Jeske JM, Goldschmidt RA: The diagnosis and management of ductal carcinoma in-situ of the breast. CA Cancer J Clin 50:184-200, 2000.
89. Holland R, Hendriks J, Verbeek A, et al: Extent, distribution and mammographic/histological correlations of breast ductal carcinoma in situ. Lancet 335:519-522, 1990.
90. Satake H, Shimamoto K, Sawaki A, et al: Role of ultrasonography in the detection of intraductal spread of breast cancer: correlation with pathologic findings, mammography and MR imaging. Eur Radiol 10:1726-1732, 2000.
91. Patchefsky AS, Schwartz GF, Finkelstein SD, et al: Heterogeneity of intraductal carcinoma of the breast. Cancer 63:731-741, 1989.
92. Hwang ES, Kinkel K, Esserman LJ, et al: Magnetic resonance imaging in patients diagnosed with ductal carcinoma-in-situ: value in the diagnosis of residual disease, occult invasion, and multicentricity. Ann Surg Oncol 10:381-388, 2003.
93. Allred DC, Mohsin SK, Fuqua SAW: Histological and biological evolution of human premalignant breast disease. Endocr Relat Cancer 8:47-61, 2001.
94. Radford DM, Phillips NHJ, Fair KL, et al: Allelic loss and the progression of breast cancer. Cancer Res 55:5180-5183, 1995.
95. Stratton MR, Collins N, Lakhani SR, et al: Loss of heterozygosity in ductal carcinoma in situ of the breast. J Pathol 175:195-201, 1995.
96. O'Connell P, Pekkel V, Fuqua SA, et al: Analysis of loss of heterozygosity in 399 premalignant breast lesions at 15 genetic loci. J Natl Cancer Inst 90:697-703, 1998.
97. Aubele MM, Cummings MC, Mattis AE, et al: Accumulation of chromosomal imbalances from intraductal proliferative lesions to adjacent in situ and invasive ductal breast cancer. Diagn Mol Pathol 9:14-19, 2000.

98. Farabegoli F, Champeme MH, Bieche I, et al: Genetic pathways in the evolution of breast ductal carcinoma in situ. J Pathol 196:280-286, 2002.
99. Page DL, Anderson TJ: Diagnostic Histopathology of the Breast. Edinburgh, Churchill Livingstone, 1987.
100. Page DL, Rogers LW: Combined histologic and cytologic criteria for the diagnosis of mammary atypical ductal hyperplasia. Hum Pathol 23:1095-1097, 1992.
101. Rosen PP: Rosen's Breast Pathology. New York, Lippincott-Raven, 1997, pp 237-245.
102. Quinn CM, Ostrowski JL: Cytological and architectural heterogeneity in ductal carcinoma in situ of the breast. J Clin Pathol 50:596-599, 1997.
103. Schnitt SJ, Connolly JL, Tavassoli FA, et al: Interobserver variability in the diagnosis of ductal proliferative breast lesions using standardized criteria. Am J Surg Pathol 16:1133-1143, 1992.
104. Elston CW, Sloane JP, Amendoeira J, et al: Causes of inconsistency in diagnosing and classifying intraductal proliferations of the breast. European Commission Working Group on Breast Screening Pathology. Eur J Cancer 36:1769-1772, 2000.
105. Bavde S, A'Hern RP, Ward AM, et al: Prediction of local recurrence of ductal carcinoma in situ of the breast using five histological classifications: a comparative study with long follow-up. Hum Pathol 29:915-923, 1998.
106. Silverstein MJ: Current management of noninvasive (in situ) breast cancer. Adv Surg 34:17-41, 2000.
107. Lagios MD: Ductal carcinoma in situ: pathology and treatment. Surg Clin North Am 70:853-871, 1990.
108. Silverstein MJ, Poller DN, Waisman JR, et al: Prognostic classification of breast ductal carcinoma in-situ. Lancet 345:1154-1157, 1995.
109. Holland R, Peterse JL, Millis RR, et al: Ductal carcinoma in situ: a proposal for a new classification. Semin Diagn Pathol 11:167-180, 1994.
110. The Consensus Conference Committee: Consensus conference on the classification of ductal carcinoma in situ. Cancer 80:1798-1802, 1997.
111. Ohtake T, Abe R, Kimijima I, et al: Intraductal extension of primary invasive breast carcinoma treated by breast-conservation surgery. Cancer 76:32-45, 1995.
112. Faverly DRG, Burgers L, Bult P, et al: Three dimensional imaging of mammary ductal carcinoma in situ: clinical implications. Semin Diagn Pathol 11:193-198, 1994.
113. Sunshine JA, Moseley MS, Fletcher WS, et al: Breast carcinoma in situ: a retrospective review of 112 cases with a minimum 10-year follow-up. Am J Surg 150:44-51, 1985.
114. Farrow JH: Current concepts in the detection and the treatment of the earliest of the early breast cancers. Cancer 25:468-477, 1970.
115. Silverstein MJ, Cohlan BF, Gierson ED, et al: Duct carcinoma in situ: 228 cases without microinvasion. Eur J Cancer 28:630-634, 1992.
116. Kinne DW, Petrek JA, Osborne MP, et al: Breast carcinoma in situ. Arch Surg 124:33-36, 1989.
117. Schuh ME, Nemoto T, Penetrante R, et al: Intraductal carcinoma. Analysis of presentation, pathologic findings, and outcome of disease. Arch Surg 121:1303-1307, 1986.
118. Arnesson LG, Smeds S, Fagerberg G, et al: Follow-up of two treatment modalities for ductal carcinoma in situ of the breast. Br J Surg 76:672-675, 1989.
119. Solin L, Fourquet A, Vicini FA, et al: Salvage treatment for local recurrence after breast-conserving surgery and radiation as initial treatment for mammographically detected ductal carcinoma in situ of the breast. Cancer 91:1090-1097, 2001.
120. McCormick B, Rosen PP, Kinne D, et al: Duct carcinoma in situ of the breast: an analysis of local control after conservative surgery and radiotherapy. Int J Radiat Oncol Biol Phys 21:289-292, 1991.
121. Haffty BG, Peschel RE, Papadopoulus D, et al: Radiation therapy for ductal carcinoma in situ of the breast. Conn Med 54:482-484, 1990.
122. Kurtz JM, Jacquemier J, Torhorst J, et al: Conservation therapy for breast cancers other than infiltrating ductal carcinoma. Cancer 63:1630-1635, 1989.
123. Ray GR, Adelson J, Hayhurst E, et al: Ductal carcinoma in situ of the breast: results of treatment by conservative surgery and definitive irradiation. Int J Radiat Oncol Biol Phys 19:843-850, 1990.
124. Solin LJ, Fowble BL, Schulz DJ, et al: Definitive irradiation for intraductal carcinoma of the breast. Int J Radiat Oncol Biol Phys 19:843-850, 1990.
125. Van Zee KJ, Liberman L, Samli B, et al: Long term follow-up of women with ductal carcinoma in situ treated with breast conserving surgery: the effect of age. Cancer 86:1757-1767, 1999.
126. Hiramatsu H, Bornstein BA, Recht A, et al: Local recurrence after conservative surgery and radiation therapy for ductal carcinoma in situ. Possible importance of family history. Cancer J Sci Am 1:55-61, 1995.
127. Sneige N, McNeese MD, Atkinson EN, et al: Ductal carcinoma in situ treated with lumpectomy and irradiation: histological analysis of 49 specimens with emphasis on risk factors and long term results. Hum Pathol 26:642-649, 1995.
128. Fourquet A, Zafrani B, Campana F, et al: Breast conserving treatment of ductal carcinoma in situ. Semin Radiat Oncol 2:116-124, 1992.
129. Solin LJ, Recht A, Fourquet A, et al: Ten-year results of breast conserving surgery and definitive irradiation for intraductal carcinoma (ductal carcinoma in situ) of the breast. Cancer 68:2337-2344, 1991.
130. Solin LJ, Kurtz J, Fourquet A, et al: Fifteen-year results of breast conserving surgery and definitive breast irradiation for the treatment of ductal carcinoma in situ (intraductal carcinoma of the breast). J Clin Oncol 14:754-763, 1996.
131. Amichetti M, Caffo O, Richetti A, et al: Ten-year results of treatment of ductal carcinoma in situ (DCIS) of the breast with conservative surgery and radiotherapy. Eur J Cancer 33:1559-1565, 1997.
132. Mirza NQ, Vlastos G, Meric F, et al: Ductal carcinoma-in situ: long-term results of breast conserving therapy. Ann Surg Oncol 7:656-664, 2000.
133. Fisher B, Land S, Mamounas E, et al: Prevention of invasive breast cancer in women with ductal carcinoma in situ: an update of the National Surgical Adjuvant Breast and Bowel Project Experience. Semin Oncol 28:400-418, 2001.
134. Julien JP, Bijker N, Fentimen IS, et al: Radiotherapy in breast-conserving treatment for ductal carcinoma in situ: first results of the EORTC randomized phase III trial 10853. EORTC Breast Cancer Cooperative Group and EORTC Radiotherapy Group. Lancet 355:528-533, 2000.
135. Houghton J, George WD, Cuzick J, et al: Radiotherapy and tamoxifen in women with completely excised ductal carcinoma in situ of the breast in the UK, Australia, and New Zealand: randomized controlled trial. Lancet 362:95-102, 2003.
136. Fisher B, Costantino J, Redmond C, et al: Lumpectomy compared with lumpectomy and radiation therapy for the treatment of intraductal breast cancer. N Engl J Med 328:1581-1586, 1993.
137. Fisher B, Dignam J, Wolmark N, et al: Lumpectomy and radiation therapy for the treatment of intraductal breast cancer: findings from National Surgical Breast and Bowel Project B-17. J Clin Oncol 16:441-452, 1998.
138. Fisher ER, Costantino JP, Fisher B, et al: Pathologic findings from the National Surgical Breast and Bowel Project (NSABP) protocol B-17: intraductal carcinoma (ductal carcinoma in situ). Cancer 75:1310-1319, 1995.
139. Bijker N, Peterse JL, Duchateau L, et al: Risk factors for recurrence and metastasis after breast-conserving therapy for ductal carcinoma-in-situ: analysis of European Organization for Research and Treatment of Cancer Trial 10853. J Clin Oncol 19:2263-2271, 2001.
140. Fisher B, Dignam J, Wolmark N, et al: Tamoxifen in treatment of intraductal breast cancer: National Surgical Breast and Bowel Project B-24 randomised controlled trial. Lancet 353:1993-2000, 1999.
141. Fowble B: Overview of conservative surgery and radiation therapy in ductal carcinoma in situ. *In* Silverstein MJ, Recht A, Lagios MD (eds): Ductal Carcinoma In Situ of the Breast, 2nd ed. Philadelphia, Lippincott Williams & Wilkins, 2002, pp 287-302.

142. Eusebi V, Feudale E, Foschini MP, et al: Long-term follow-up of in situ carcinoma of the breast. Semin Diagn Pathol 11:223-235, 1994.
143. Silverstein MJ, Lagios MD, Groshen S, et al: The influence of margin width on local control of ductal carcinoma in situ of the breast. N Engl J Med 340:1455-1461, 1999.
144. Ottensen GL, Graversen HP, Blichert-Toft M, et al: Ductal carcinoma in situ of the female breast: short-term results of a prospective nationwide study. The Danish Breast Cancer Cooperative Group. Am J Surg Pathol 16:1183-1196, 1992.
145. Vicini FA, Kestin LL, Goldstein NS, et al: Impact of young age on outcome in patients with ductal carcinoma in situ treated with breast conserving therapy. J Clin Oncol 18:296-306, 2000.
146. Kuske RR: Should all ductal carcinoma in situ patients receive radiation therapy and is partial breast irradiation an option? *In* Silverstein MJ, Recht A, Lagios MD (eds): Ductal Carcinoma In Situ of the Breast, 2nd ed. Philadelphia, Lippincott Williams & Wilkins, 2002, pp 287-302.

CHAPTER 60

BREAST CANCER: STAGES T1 AND T2

Abram Recht

PATIENT SELECTION

Most patients with stage I or II invasive breast cancer are candidates for breast-conserving therapy.

For a few patients, treatment with conservative surgery plus radiation therapy is absolutely or relatively contraindicated due to concerns about toxicity. For some, the anticipated cosmetic results of conservative surgery and irradiation may be so poor that mastectomy with immediate reconstruction is a more appealing alternative.

Probably relatively few patients have a low risk of local recurrence when conservative surgery is used without irradiation. Physicians treating patients in such a manner, whether on a formalized study or not, must adequately inform them of the uncertainties and potential dangers of this approach.

Proper pretreatment evaluation is a critical aspect of deciding on the most appropriate treatment approach. Careful physical examination should be performed. All patients should have mammograms before biopsy and, in selected patients, after biopsy to ensure the completeness of resection. Specimen radiography should be performed routinely, including for patients who present with a nonpalpable mass without microcalcifications.

Careful evaluation of the tumor specimen is mandatory, especially with regard to the margins of resection. The edges of the specimen should be inked or otherwise evaluated or marked before the specimen is sectioned. It is critical for the pathologist to know how far tumor extends beyond the edges of any grossly apparent mass and whether calcifications are associated with the tumor or benign tissue, or both. A detailed description of the size of the invasive component, histologic type, presence of an extensive intraductal component or lymphovascular invasion, grade, and other features of the lesion should be recorded.

TREATMENT

The exact size of microscopically "adequate" negative margins for patients being considered for breast-conserving therapy (with or without irradiation) cannot be defined. Microscopically uninvolved margins are preferred, but selected patients with involved margins have excellent local control.

The dose-response curve for local control and complications has not been adequately studied. Most patients with uninvolved margins have excellent local control and cosmetic results when given whole-breast doses of 50 Gy in 2-Gy fractions or its biologic equivalent, with or without a boost dose to the tumor bed. Patients younger than 50 years or those with certain histologic findings may benefit most from the addition of a boost dose.

Three-dimensional compensation using physical devices or intensity-modulated radiation therapy improves the homogeneity of dose distribution within the breast, but its ultimate clinical value is uncertain.

Accelerated partial-breast irradiation may allow patients to undergo breast-conserving therapy more quickly and with less risk of long-term complications than with conventional treatment with whole-breast irradiation. However, few long-term results from studies of partial-breast irradiation are available, and there are substantial uncertainties regarding most aspects of selecting patients for and performing partial-breast irradiation.

The value of irradiation directed at regional lymph nodes is uncertain. There is no consensus on when and which regional nodes should be irradiated.

The timing of surgery, irradiation, and systemic therapy with regard to each other may affect treatment results, but many details of how to best combine these modalities are unknown.

Concurrent administration of chemotherapy and irradiation generally increases the risks of complications and is probably not needed for most patients.

Tamoxifen may be given before, during, or after radiation therapy without apparent deleterious effects on local control rates.

FOLLOW-UP

Follow-up should focus on detecting potentially curable recurrences and new primary tumors in the ipsilateral and contralateral breasts.

The optimal follow-up schedule and testing regimen is unknown, but many oncologists prefer to perform biannual or annual physical examinations and annual mammograms indefinitely.

SALVAGE THERAPY

Mastectomy ordinarily is the treatment of choice for patients with a local recurrence who have received prior radiation therapy.

For patients not previously irradiated, if on careful clinical, radiologic, and pathologic evaluation the lesion appears limited and no evidence of multicentric disease is found, consideration may be given to management with further breast-conserving therapy, rather than mastectomy.

The value of further adjuvant systemic therapy for patients with invasive tumors at recurrence is unknown.

Table 60-1 Randomized Trials Comparing Mastectomy with Breast-Conserving Therapy

Trial	Study Period	No. of Patients	Follow-up (y)*	Time Point (y)	Distant Failure† M	Distant Failure† BCT	Overall Survival† M	Overall Survival† BCT
WHO[362]	1972-1979	179	22 (mean)	—	.7 (.04-1.2)‡		.7 (.5-1.1)‡	
Milan I[363]	1973-1980	701	20	20	24%§	23%§	41%	42%
NSABP B-06[364¶]	1976-1984	1406	20.7 (mean)	20	51%	54%	47%	46%
US NCI[365]	1979-1989	279	18.4	20	33%¶	40%¶	58%	53%
EORTC 10801[366]	1980-1986	903	13.4	10	34%	39%	66%	65%
Denmark 82TM[367]	1983-1989	859	3.3	6	34%¶	30%¶	79%	82%
Combined EORTC/ Danish trials[368]	—	1772	9.8	10	32%	34%	67%	67%

*The length of follow-up is a median value unless otherwise stated.
†Rates given are actuarial values at time point indicated unless otherwise stated.
‡Odds ratio for comparing BCT with mastectomy, with the 95% confidence interval given parenthetically; exact rates were not given.
§Crude rate.
¶For the NSABP B-06 trial, comparison included only lumpectomy patients receiving radiotherapy.
¶Total relapse rate; the distant metastasis rate was not given separately.
BCT, breast-conserving therapy (includes radiation therapy); EORTC, European Organization for Research and Treatment of Cancer; M, mastectomy; NSABP, National Surgical Adjuvant Bowel and Breast Project; US NCI, United States National Cancer Institute; WHO, World Health Organization.

Approximately 70% to 80% of patients with stage I or II invasive breast cancers are potential candidates on technical grounds for treatment with breast-conserving therapy.[1,2] This approach has been one of the great success stories of modern radiation oncology.

Since 1970, six major randomized trials have compared mastectomy to breast-conserving therapy performed using modern radiation therapy techniques (Table 60-1). There were no significant differences in disease-free or overall survival between the two arms. A meta-analysis of these and other trials reached the same conclusions.[3]

Nonetheless, many questions remain regarding optimal patient selection and management, the choice of radiation therapy techniques and doses, and the integration of irradiation with systemic therapy. This chapter concentrates on the selection and treatment of patients with early-stage invasive cancer with breast-conserving surgery with or without irradiation. Other sources discuss this topic in much greater depth than is possible here.[4-7] Chapter 59 discusses the management of patients with ductal carcinoma in situ (DCIS), those with locally advanced breast cancer, and the use of radiation therapy in patients with early or more advanced disease treated with mastectomy.

PRETREATMENT IMAGING AND PATHOLOGIC EVALUATION

Preoperative Imaging

Mammography should always be performed before treatment,[8] but it does not always accurately delineate the pathologic extent of disease.[9] The roles of other modalities in evaluating patients for breast-conserving therapy, such as ultrasound[10,11] and magnetic resonance imaging (MRI),[12,13] are not fully defined. One problem in interpreting their clinical significance is that only a few studies of these other modalities enrolled consecutive patients, rather than selected ones.[11,14,15] Although these studies may show lesions not detected by mammography, they also have a significant number of false-positive and false-negative results. Such studies may be most useful for patients with radiologically dense breast tissue.[16]

Intraoperative and Postoperative Imaging

Conventional single-view specimen radiographs are not very accurate in assessing the completeness of excision.[17] The value of routine postoperative mammograms is uncertain in patients with negative margins. In a series from Philadelphia, their use made no difference to the recurrence rate for patients with DCIS.[18] Studies differ on whether having residual calcifications found on postoperative mammograms increases the risk of local failure.[19-21] Postoperative MRI also seems to have limited accuracy in assessing the presence or amount of residual disease.[22]

Pathologic Evaluation

The College of American Pathologists[23] has promulgated minimum standards for handling, pathologic evaluation, and reporting of findings for breast specimens. The most common approach is for the surgeon to remove a single specimen, which the pathologist later rolls in India ink and sequentially sections ("bread-loafs") perpendicular to its long axis. Marking different edges of the specimen with different colors of ink may allow more directed re-excision to be performed, if needed. Some pathologists prefer to "shave" each face of a specimen (especially for large resections); the margin is considered involved when any tumor is seen in one of the shaved margin slides. The clinical implications may be quite different for these two approaches.[24] Some surgeons take cavity specimens, which are additional pieces of tissue at each edge of the excision cavity, in addition to the main specimen.[25] It is not clear whether this approach yields improved results compared with removal of a single specimen.

SURGICAL TECHNIQUES

Breast-Conserving Surgery

It is beyond the scope of this chapter to discuss the technical aspects of surgery in detail; such information may be found elsewhere.[4-7] There is enormous variability from surgeon to surgeon and institution to institution in the performance of breast-conserving surgery. The only randomized study of the effect of different widths of resection for patients with invasive breast cancer is the Milan II trial.[26,27] In one arm, a very wide excision (i.e., quadrantectomy) was performed, and in the other arm, a narrow excision (i.e., tumorectomy) was used. The local failure rate in the tumorectomy group was 17% (57 of 345), compared with 6% (21 of 360) in the quadrantectomy group. However, the techniques of irradiation were not the same in the two arms. No difference was seen in recurrence rates between patients treated with tumorectomy or quadrantectomy and the same radiation therapy technique in a study from Rome.[28]

Axillary Dissection

Most surgeons follow the practice of Berg[29] by dividing the axilla into three anatomic levels: level I, the nodes lying laterally and inferiorly to the border of the pectoralis minor muscle; level II, those lying under the pectoralis minor; and level III (also called the infraclavicular nodes), those lying medially and superiorly to the border of the pectoralis minor. Removal of level I nodes alone is likely to find evidence of metastasis in most patients with axillary involvement, with almost all remaining node-positive patients being identified if level II nodes are also removed.[30]

Two randomized trials have compared axillary failure rates, survival rates, and morbidity after limited dissection (i.e., removal of level I and II nodes only) with complete dissection (i.e., removal of levels I, II, and III).[31,32] There were no differences in disease-free or overall survival rates between the arms, but limited dissection caused less morbidity.

Axillary failures are rare in patients treated with a level I-II dissection with negative or positive nodes.[30] Failure rates are higher in patients treated with inadequate surgery or in patients with eight or more positive nodes.[33]

Sentinel Node Biopsy

The rationale, techniques, and results with sentinel node biopsy (SNB) are described in the sources previously cited and in other reviews.[34,35] In brief, a radionuclide tracer or a vital dye is injected in the breast, with the surgeon then finding the axillary nodes that take it up. This approach allows removal of a much more limited amount of tissue than does conventional axillary dissection, with accordingly lower morbidity.[36] The false-negative rate for SNB is 0% to 12% in different studies. Randomized trials comparing SNB with conventional level I-II axillary dissection have been or are being conducted by a number of cooperative groups in North America and Europe; results are not yet available. Although the risk of axillary failure in patients with negative SNB results appears very low, the need for completion dissection or specific axillary irradiation in patients with involved sentinel nodes is controversial. Several trials in Europe and North America are examining this issue.

BREAST-CONSERVING SURGERY WITH RADIATION THERAPY

To rationally choose between breast-conserving surgery plus irradiation and mastectomy, patients and physicians must compare their relative effectiveness in the individual situation, estimate the risk of complications, and then evaluate what choice best fits their needs. This requires an assessment of how patient, clinical, and pathologic factors affect these outcomes. The risk of local failure and complications in relation to these factors may also be modulated by treatment parameters, particularly the use of systemic therapy.

Patient Factors

Pregnancy

Unless terminated, pregnancy is an absolute contraindication to radiation therapy because of the possible teratogenic and carcinogenic effects on the fetus, which can occur even at low doses because of scattered radiation resulting from tangential-field irradiation of the breast.[37]

Prior Treatment with Radiation Therapy

Most physicians have recommended mastectomy for individuals previously treated to the thorax with irradiation for another malignancy due to concerns about long-term toxicities (especially soft tissue and cardiac effects) from further irradiation. However, there were no unusual acute or chronic sequelae among 12 women treated with breast-conserving therapy, including radiation therapy, at the University of Pittsburgh 10 to 29 years after receiving irradiation for treatment of Hodgkin's disease or non-Hodgkin's lymphoma.[38] One of two such patients treated at Stanford University developed severe soft tissue necrosis in the lateral breast and chest wall.[39]

Rheumatologic Disorders

Only three studies have performed a formal comparison of the risk of complications of patients with rheumatologic diseases with those of a matched, normal population.[40-42] Their results are consistent with each other, although the numbers of patients with any one diagnosis vary and are generally quite small. For example, a case-control study from Yale University, found no increased risk of acute or long-term complications except for patients with scleroderma.[41] Although the data are very limited, I feel patients with lupus, rheumatoid arthritis, and similar illnesses can be safely treated with breast-conserving surgery and irradiation, whereas radiation therapy should be avoided in those with scleroderma, mixed connective tissue disorder, or CREST syndrome, a form of systemic sclerosis characterized by *c*alcinosis, *R*aynaud's phenomenon, loss of *e*sophageal muscle control, *s*clerodactyly, and *t*elangiectasia.

Breast Size

In older studies, women with very large breasts generally had a greater risk of significant retraction and fibrosis than patients with smaller breasts. However, such patients seem likely to have much better cosmetic results when treated using higher-energy photons[43] or intensity-modulated radiation therapy (IMRT); the use of a lateral decubitus or prone position may also be helpful. The risk of acute skin reactions can also be reduced by the use of 1.8-Gy daily fractions. Although such patients can be technically challenging to treat, they should not be denied radiation therapy solely on that basis.

Patient Age

In most series, patients younger than 35 to 40 years at diagnosis had a substantially higher risk of breast recurrence after breast-conserving therapy than older patients.[44] However, few studies have examined the interaction of age with other factors, especially the tumor-free margin width. For example, a study from Fox Chase Cancer Center in Philadelphia found that the 5-year actuarial local failure rate was only 3% among 38 patients 35 years old or younger whose tumor did not contain an extensive intraductal component and who had tumor-free margins wider than 2 mm.[45] The rate was 13% among 10 patients with close or positive margins. In a series from Tufts–New England Medical Center, Boston, for patients with close margins (≤2 mm), the 12-year actuarial failure rate for 28 patients 45 years old or younger was 19%, compared with 5% for 71 older patients.[46] There were no differences between local failure rates for these age cohorts when the margins were wider. Systemic therapy also substantially improves local control rates for young patients after breast-conserving therapy.[44] The limited evidence available does not show a superior outcome with mastectomy compared with breast conservation.[47] Young age at diagnosis should not be a contraindication to breast-conserving therapy.

Although some physicians have been reluctant to refer older patients for radiation therapy after breast-conserving surgery, older patients tolerate irradiation extremely well and have excellent local control rates.[48,49] Older patients appear to have lower risks of local failure after breast-conserving surgery alone than younger patients, but patients generally should not undergo different local treatment solely because of their age.

Genetic Factors

A family history of breast cancer by itself does not increase the risk of local failure in most series.[50,51] Some studies found that mutations of the *BRCA1* or *BRCA2* genes had no effect on local failure rates after breast-conserving therapy,[52-57] but in other series, patients with mutations had substantially higher rates.[58-60] Patients with mutations have a substantially higher risk of contralateral breast cancer development than patients without mutations (e.g., 25% in mutation carriers versus 4% in noncarriers in one series at 10 years[55]). The risks of ipsilateral local failure[55] and contralateral new primary development[55,61] in mutation carriers seem to be substantially reduced by the use of tamoxifen or oophorectomy. There is no evidence whether long-term breast-cancer-specific survival rates are superior when patients with such mutations are treated by mastectomy rather than breast-conserving therapy.

Individuals likely to be heterozygous for the *ATM* gene (ataxia telangiectasia mutated) or *BRCA1* or *BRCA2* gene do not seem at markedly higher risk of developing irradiation-related toxicities than normal individuals.[55,62,63] However, one preliminary study suggested that patients having two *ATM* mutations may be more sensitive than normal individuals.[64]

Indirect evidence suggests that irradiation does not increase the risk of contralateral breast cancers in patients with *ATM* mutations.[65,66] There are no data on this issue for patients with *BRCA1* and *BRCA2* mutations. A positive family history or finding of an abnormal breast-cancer linked gene should not be considered a contraindication to breast-conserving surgery.

Clinical Factors

Means of Detection

The risk of local recurrence appears to be the same for patients with palpable and nonpalpable cancers.[67] Patients who present with nipple discharge do not have higher local failure rates than other patients when resection margins are not involved.[68]

Tumor Size and Location

Tumor size does not influence recurrence rates after breast-conserving surgery and irradiation.[45] However, it is difficult to achieve acceptable cosmetic results while obtaining negative margins in most patients with tumors larger than 4 to 5 cm. For such patients, neoadjuvant chemotherapy may sometimes allow the use of breast-conserving therapy.[69,70]

Patients with lesions in the subareolar or periareolar area that do not directly extend to the nipple or areola have high local control rates after wide excision with negative margins and without nipple-areolar resection.[71,72] Even when nipple-areolar resection must be performed, the appearance and texture of the remaining breast is at least as good as that after reconstruction procedures, and sensation in the remaining breast mound is preserved.

Bilateral Breast Cancers

Patients with bilateral breast cancer (synchronous or metachronous) can be treated successfully with breast-conserving therapy without an increased risk of complications.[73,74]

Multiple Ipsilateral Primary Cancers

Patients are found to have two nonadjacent primaries in the same breast on radiologic evaluation. In a consecutive series of 200 patients in Edinburgh with palpable masses, 6 patients (3%) had two or more lesions in the breast on mammography.[75] In a study of 225 selected patients with a single biopsy-proven invasive cancer or DCIS who then were imaged with MRI at the Hospital of the University of Pennsylvania in Philadelphia, 17 patients (8%) were found to have suspicious lesions in a separate quadrant from the index lesion; however, only 8 had lesions that were found to be malignant on biopsy (4% of the entire population).[76] Such multiple primaries are also rare in histopathologic studies. In a study of 183 mastectomy specimens performed in Tokushima, Japan, only 3 patients (2%) had multiple lesions without any demonstrable continuity between them.[77]

A substantial number of patients who are initially thought to have multiple independent lesions may have a single primary tumor with wide but unappreciated spread within the breast. Several studies that have taken care to exclude such individuals have found local failure rates in patients with multiple ipsilateral primaries undergoing irradiation after excisions with negative resection margins to be similar to those of patients with single lesions.[74,78-80] Performing breast-conserving surgery appears reasonable in such individuals.

Pathologic Factors

Margin Status

Margin status appears to be the single most important prognostic factor for the risk of local recurrence after breast-conserving therapy that includes irradiation. Definitions of margin status vary between investigators, but most appear to define a *positive* or *involved margin* as the presence of invasive cancer or DCIS in an inked surface when a bread-loafing technique is used to process the specimen or the finding of tumor anywhere in a shaved-margin specimen.

There is general agreement that patients with involved or positive margins should usually undergo further surgery before starting radiation therapy. However, some studies have shown a low risk of failure for patients with positive margins. In a study from Fox Chase Cancer Center, none of 42 patients with positive margins had a local recurrence by 5 years.[81] Similarly, in a study from Tufts–New England Medical Center, the 5-year local failure rate was 5% for 80 patients with positive margins who did not receive tamoxifen, with no local failures occurring among 25 patients who did.[82]

The amount of disease at the margins may be important in determining the risk of local recurrence. In a study from the Joint Center for Radiation Therapy (JCRT) with a median follow-up time of 127 months, the crude 8-year local failure rate was 14% for 122 patients with focal margin involvement (i.e., DCIS and invasive cancer across all examined slides that could be encompassed by three or fewer low-power microscopic fields); however, for 66 patients with extensive margin involvement, the rate was 27%.[83] The 45 patients with focally positive margins who received systemic therapy had a 7% local recurrence rate, compared with 18% for the 77 patients who did not receive systemic therapy. In a study from Marseille, France, with a median follow-up of 72 months, the risk of local failure was 14% (10 of 70) for patients with a single positive margin, compared with 36% (17 of 47) for patients with multiple involved margins.[84] Similarly, in a study from Thomas Jefferson University Hospital in Philadelphia, in which shaved margins were used to evaluate patients, the 5-year rate of local failure was 9% for the 59 patients with a single positive margin, compared with 23% for 27 patients with two or more positive margins.[85] However, by 10 years, the rates of failure had substantially increased in both groups (26% and 37%, respectively).

There is little evidence on how the exact tumor-free margin width affects the risk of local recurrence. Different investigators have arbitrarily distinguished between *negative* and *close* margins (usually defined as less than 1 mm or less than 2 mm between the tumor and the inked surface). In several studies with a median follow-up of 5 years or longer, wider margins were associated with lower failure rates.[86-88] However, only three published studies have subdivided results for patients according to relatively narrow margin-width intervals in a way that allows this division to be critically evaluated (Table 60-2). Although patients with very wide margins (>5 to 10 mm) might be expected to have much lower risks of failure than patients with narrower margins, such an effect was not consistently observed.

Only one study (from William Beaumont Hospital near Detroit) has studied how the volume of disease near uninvolved margins affects the risk of local recurrence.[89] With a median follow-up time of 103 months, the 5-year actuarial Kaplan-Meier local failure rates increased only slightly with increasing tumor burden in the tissue within 2.1 mm of the inked margin (1%, 3%, and 6% in the three subgroups they defined, respectively); however, by 12 years, the differences were much larger (rates of 6%, 18%, and 24%, respectively).

Randomized trials have demonstrated that chemotherapy and tamoxifen substantially reduce failure rates in patients with uninvolved margins treated with breast-conserving surgery and radiation therapy.[90-93] However, there are few data on how the tumor-free margin width affects this interaction. In a retrospective study of patients with estrogen receptor protein-positive invasive cancers treated with irradiation and tamoxifen (without chemotherapy) at Fox Chase Cancer Center, the 5-year actuarial rate of local failure among patients with negative microscopic margins (>2 mm wide) was 5% for 205 patients not receiving tamoxifen and 4% for 107 patients who did.[81] For patients with close margins, the respective rates were 11% (32 patients) and 0% (18 patients), a difference that was not statistically significant.

Other Histologic Features

Infiltrating ductal cancers are described as having an *extensive intraductal component* (EIC) when two features are simultaneously present: intraductal carcinoma constituting a prominent portion of the area of the primary mass (in an earlier definition, 25% or more) and intraductal carcinoma clearly extending beyond the infiltrating margin of the tumor or present in sections of grossly normal adjacent breast tissue.[94] Predominantly noninvasive tumors, with only focal areas of invasion, are also included in this category. Some investigators have used other definitions, most of which probably describe the same entity. Tumors with an EIC extend more widely through the breast than others.[95] It is much more difficult to obtain uninvolved resection margins when an EIC is present than when it is absent, and the volume of residual disease may be greater.

In past studies from the JCRT and other institutions in which microscopic margins were not examined, the presence of EIC was a major risk factor for local failure. However, its impact is uncertain when margin status is accounted for. The presence of an EIC had no impact in a study from the JCRT,[83] but in a series of patients with margins wider than 2 mm treated in Philadelphia, the presence of an EIC increased the 10-year Kaplan-Meier actuarial local failure rate from 6% to 16%.[86] The presence of an EIC was also an independent risk factor for local recurrence in patients 55 years old or younger in a later analysis of their experience.[45]

Patients with infiltrating lobular carcinomas or tumors with mixed ductal and lobular features appear to have comparable recurrence rates to patients with infiltrating ductal carcinomas.[96-98] Experience with other histologic subtypes is

Table 60-2 Tumor-Free Margin Width and the Risk of Local Failure after Breast-Conserving Therapy with Radiation Therapy

Characteristic	JCRT[83]	Tufts-NEMC[46]	William Beaumont[89]
Median follow-up (mo)	127	121	103
Measure	8-y crude	12-y KM	12-y KM
Margin width (mm)			
Involved	22% (166)*	17% (105)	17% (105)
.1-1	7% (94)	—	14% (94)
1.1-2	6% (33)	—	18% (45)
.1-2	7% (127)	9% (99)	—
2.1-3	—	—	15% (59)
3.1-5	—	—	13% (43)
2.1-5	4% (47)	5% (84)	—
>5 (NOS)	12% (56)	0 (69)	—
5.1-10	—	—	13% (90)
>10 (NOS)	—	—	5% (52)
No tumor on re-excision	8% (101)	6% (137)	2% (160)

*The number of patients in a subgroup is given in parentheses.

JCRT, Joint Center for Radiation Therapy, Boston; KM, Kaplan-Meier estimator; NOS, not otherwise specified; Tufts-NEMC, Tufts–New England Medical Center, Boston; William Beaumont, William Beaumont Hospital, Detroit.

Adapted from Recht A: Lessons of studies of breast-conserving therapy with and without whole-breast irradiation for patient selection for partial-breast irradiation. Semin Radiat Oncol 15:123-132, 2005.

much more limited, but results appear similar to those with more common tumors.[96,99-101]

Atypical hyperplasia and other benign proliferative diseases do not appear to affect the risk of local failure.[102] Studies conflict on whether the presence of lobular carcinoma in situ does[103] or does not[104] increase local failure rates.

Conclusions about Breast-Conserving Therapy with Irradiation

Most individuals with early-stage breast cancer are candidates for breast-conserving surgery and irradiation. For a few patients, radiation therapy is absolutely or relatively contraindicated because of concerns about toxicity. If the margins of the initial excision are microscopically involved or equivocal, re-excision should be done. In most patients, a cosmetically and pathologically satisfactory re-excision can be performed. For some individuals, the anticipated cosmetic results may be so poor because of the need for very extensive resection or small breast size that mastectomy with immediate reconstruction may be a more appealing alternative. If the margins of the re-excision specimen are still involved microscopically, the patient should understand that she may have a substantial risk for local recurrence, although the risk for some may be reduced by systemic therapy. Some patients are willing to accept the possible increased risk of local recurrence and systemic failure to avoid mastectomy. Treatment decisions must be guided by the values of the affected individual.

BREAST-CONSERVING SURGERY WITHOUT RADIATION THERAPY

Results for Relatively Unselected Patients

Radiation therapy is time consuming and expensive, and it may cause complications. Some have argued that local failure is of only cosmetic or psychological importance, rather than affecting the ultimate chance of cure.

Table 60-3 summarizes the largest randomized studies comparing outcome with breast-conserving surgery alone with conservative surgery with radiation therapy for relatively unselected patients. These trials had fairly broad entry criteria, and they required only very small microscopically tumor-free margins for entry (in the Scottish trial, only grossly tumor-free margins[105]). Local failure rates were much higher for patients treated with breast-conserving surgery alone. In a meta-analysis of 15 published trials enrolling 9422 patients, the relative risk of ipsilateral breast tumor recurrence after conservative surgery alone was increased threefold, and for 13 trials with a total of 8206 patients for whom data were available, there was an excess mortality rate of 8.6%.[106]

Results for Highly Selected Patient Subgroups

Several investigators have tried to identify patient subgroups with a low risk of local recurrence after conservative surgery alone, particularly when tamoxifen is used.[107] Results for such studies with approximately 5-year median follow-up or longer are listed in Table 60-4.

The benefits of radiation therapy in such patients may be quite limited. For example, in the Uppsala-Örebro (Sweden) trial, the 10-year risk of local failure was 11% for patients older than 55 years whose tumors did not have any comedo or lobular features, compared with 6% in the irradiated arm.[108] In the British Association of Surgical Oncology (BASO) II trial, which included patients with tumors 2 cm or smaller of histologic grade 1 with pathologically uninvolved axillary nodes, the local failure rate was reduced from only 2% (8 of 411) to .5% (2 of 396) by the addition of irradiation to tamoxifen.[109]

Elderly patients may have relatively low risks of local failure after treatment with breast-conserving surgery alone, especially if tamoxifen is used. In the Milan III trial, the risk of local failure was the same in unirradiated patients (1 of 23) and irradiated patients (1 of 25) older than 65 years, with an unreported number of patients receiving tamoxifen or chemotherapy.[110] An American Intergroup trial (Cancer and Leukemia Group B trial 9343) for patients 70 years old or older

Table 60-3 Randomized Trials Comparing Breast-Conserving Surgery Alone with Breast-Conserving Surgery and Irradiation for Relatively Unselected Patients with Early-Stage Invasive Breast Cancer, with a Median Follow-Up Time Longer than Five Years

Trial	Period	No. of Patients	Follow-up (mo)	Time Point (y)	Local Failure (%)* CS Alone	Local Failure (%)* CS + RT	Distant Failure or Breast Cancer Death (%)* CS Alone	Distant Failure or Breast Cancer Death (%)* CS + RT	Death, All Causes (%)* CS Alone	Death, All Causes (%)* CS + RT
NSABP B-06[364]	1976-1984	1137	248 (mean)	20	39	14	42†	35†	53	50
Uppsala-Örebro[108]	1981-1988	381	103 (CS alone)/ 109 (CS + RT)	10	24	9	20‡	10‡	22	22
Ontario[359]	1984-1989	799	91	Crude	35	11	30‡	23‡	24	21
Milan III[110]	1987-1989	567	109	10	15	3	16†§	12†§	23	18
Scotland[105]	1985-1991	585	68	Crude	24	6	20†	13†	.98¶	
St. George/ Royal Marsden[368]	1981-1990	391	82 (mean)	Crude	35	12	¶	¶	¶	¶

*Rates given are actuarial at the time point indicated unless otherwise stated.
†Breast cancer deaths.
‡Distant failure.
§Crude rate.
¶Hazard ratio for comparison of CS + RT with CS alone; actual rates were not reported.
¶Unknown or not reported.
CS, breast-conserving surgery; CS + RT, breast-conserving surgery and radiation therapy; NSABP, National Surgical Adjuvant Bowel and Breast Project.

Table 60-4 Local Failure Rates for Highly Selected Patient Subgroups Treated with Conservative Surgery without Radiotherapy with Median Follow-Up of Approximately Five Years or Longer

Study	Period	Age	Nodes	Max. Size	Subgroup Features	Margins	Tamoxifen Used	Follow-up (mo)*	No. of Patients	LF†
Milan III[110]	1987-1989	≥66	pN0/1	2.5	NA	Neg	Optional (TAM or CT)	109	23	4%
Women's College Hospital[369]	1977-1986	≥65	pN0	NA	ER^+, $LVPI^-$, no comedo DCIS	Neg	None	109	34	9%
Uppsala-Örebro[108]	1981-1998	≥56	pN0	2	No comedo or lobular features	Neg	None	103	84	11% (10 y)
NSABP B-21[93]	1991-1998	Any	pN0	1	ER^+	Neg	All	89	197	10%
GBSG V[113]	1991-1998	45-75	pN0	2	HG 1-2, EIC^-, LVI^-, ER+, or PRP^+	Neg	All	71	80	3%
Ontario-British Columbia Trial[112]	1992-2000	≥51	pN0 or cN0	5	≤1 cm, ER^+ or PR^+	Neg	All	67	139	3% (5 y)
Boston-Providence[370]	1978-2003	≥51	cN0	1.5	HG 1-2	≥10 mm (gross)	Some	61	80	6%
Vienna[371]	1983-1994	≥61	pN0	4	ER^+	Neg	Some	60	83	1%
CALGB 9343[111]	1994-1999	≥70	pN0 or cN0	2	ER^+	Neg	All	60	319	4%
BASO II[109]	1992-2000	≤69	pN0	2	HG 1	Neg	All	54	411	2%

*Follow-up length is given as the median time.

†Crude local failure rates are given, unless a time is given in parentheses, in which case the results are actuarial.

CALGB, Cancer and Acute Leukemia Group B; cN0, clinically uninvolved axillary lymph nodes; CT, chemotherapy; EIC^-, no extensive intraductal component; ER^+, positive for the estrogen-receptor protein; GBSG V, German Breast Cancer Study Group Trial V; HG, histologic grade; LF, local failure rate (crude unless otherwise specified); LVI^-, lymphovascular invasion; $LVPI^-$, no lymphovascular or perineural invasion; NA, not available or unknown; Neg, disease-negative margins, not otherwise defined in the study; NG, nuclear grade; NSABP, National Surgical Adjuvant Breast and Bowel Project; pN0, pathologically uninvolved axillary lymph nodes; PR^+, positive for the progesterone-receptor protein.

From Recht A: Lessons of studies of breast-conserving therapy with and without whole-breast irradiation for patient selection for partial-breast irradiation. Semin Radiat Oncol 15:123-132, 2005.

found, with a median follow-up time of 60 months, that the risk of locoregional failure was 4% for patients treated with conservative surgery plus tamoxifen, compared with 1% for patients also receiving radiation therapy.[111] In a trial conducted in Ontario and British Columbia in which the median patient age was 68 years and the median follow-up time was 5.6 years, the 5-year actuarial local failure rates for unirradiated patients 60 years old or older with hormone receptor–positive tumors 1 cm or smaller was 1%.[112]

Routine use of hormonal therapy may be needed to achieve low failure rates in patients treated without irradiation, even in highly selected populations. In the German Breast Cancer Study Group (GBSG) V trial, with a median follow-up time of 5.9 years, the rate of local failure in patients treated with breast-conserving surgery without tamoxifen or irradiation was 29% (23 of 79 patients), compared with 3% (2 of 80) for patients treated with conservative surgery plus tamoxifen.[113] Failure rates in the patients receiving breast-conserving surgery plus irradiation were 5% for 94 patients not receiving tamoxifen and 3% for 94 patients who did. In the BASO II trial, with a median follow-up time of 54 months, the risk of local failure in patients receiving neither tamoxifen nor irradiation was 9% (15 of 174); for patients receiving tamoxifen but not irradiation, the rate was 2% (8 of 411).[109]

Conclusions about Breast-Conserving Surgery without Irradiation

Randomized trials that included relatively unselected patients found that treatment with breast-conserving surgery alone resulted in a high local failure rate compared with initial treatment with conservative surgery and irradiation, which reduced overall survival rates. However, some patient subgroups have an acceptably low risk of local failure after treatment with conservative surgery alone, especially when hormonal therapy is used. Even these patients may prefer to reduce the risks of local failure further by being irradiated.[114,115] The risk of ipsilateral breast tumor recurrence may increase with further follow-up (e.g., in the Ontario-British Columbia trial, from 7.7% at 5 years to 17.6% at 8 years for the arm randomized to tamoxifen without irradiation[112]). The decision to omit radiation therapy should be made by the patient and her physicians together, not unilaterally.

TIMING OF POSTOPERATIVE RADIATION THERAPY AND SYSTEMIC THERAPY IN RELATION TO SURGERY AND EACH OTHER

Interval Between Breast Surgery and the Start of Radiation Therapy

The interval between surgery and irradiation may influence the risk of local failure because of tumor proliferation occurring during this time. Local failure rates do not seem to be affected by exactly when radiation therapy is started up to 4 months after the last breast surgery.[116-120] However, prolonging the interval between surgery and irradiation beyond 4 months may increase failure rates for patients with narrow, although uninvolved, margins. In the upfront-outback trial performed at the JCRT and affiliated institutions from 1984 to 1992, patients with clinical stage I or II breast carcinoma were randomized after breast-conserving surgery and axillary dissection to receive four cycles of chemotherapy at 3-week intervals before or after irradiation.[121,122] With a median follow-up time of 135 months, the risk of local failure for patients receiving irradiation first was 11%, compared with 16% for patients receiving chemotherapy first.[122] However, local failure rates were similar in the irradiation-first (13%) and chemotherapy-first arms (6%) for the 123 patients with margins greater than 1 mm in width, but for the 47 patients with close margins, the respective failure rates in the two arms were 4% and 32%. The risks of local failure among the 51 patients with positive margins in the two arms were 20% and 23%, respectively.

Similarly, in a study from Rush-Presbyterian Hospital in Chicago, 48 patients with margin widths of 2 mm or more had a low risk of local failure whether the interval between surgery and irradiation was shorter than 120 days (no patient had recurrent disease) or longer (5% failure rate).[123] However, when margins were close, positive, or unknown (37 patients), the risk of local recurrence was substantially lower in the early-irradiation group (6%) compared with the delayed-irradiation group (24%). Unfortunately, the actual tumor-free margin width has not been reported in other studies examining the role of the interval between surgery and irradiation.

Three additional randomized trials have examined the effect of prolonged delays on starting radiation therapy. A consortium of the French national cancer centers conducted a trial from 1994 to 1999, in which 638 eligible patients with one to seven positive axillary nodes treated with breast-conserving therapy or mastectomy were randomized to receive irradiation concurrently with the first cycles of a regimen combining mitoxantrone, 5-fluorouracil, and cyclophosphamide (FNC regimen) or irradiation after completion of epirubicin, 5-fluorouracil, and cyclophosphamide (FEC regimen).[124] With a median follow-up of 41 months, there was no difference in locoregional control between the arms. However, the actual rates of failure have not been reported, nor have results been separately given for the mastectomy and lumpectomy patients. A similar trial was conducted from 1996 to 2000 at the Institut Curie in Paris and collaborating institutions for patients treated with lumpectomy.[125] Patients received irradiation concurrently with the first three cycles of FNC or began irradiation 3 to 5 weeks after six cycles of FNC given every 3 weeks. Forty-four percent of the 706 accrued patients had disease-negative axillary nodes. The microscopic margin width was wider than 1 mm in 86% of patients. With a median follow-up time of 37 months, the locoregional failure rates in the concurrent and sequential arms were 3.5% and 4.3%, respectively.

The Sequencing of Chemotherapy and Radiotherapy in Adjuvant Breast Cancer/OlmeSartan and Calcium Antagonists Randomized (SECRAB/OSCAR) trial, conducted from 1998 to 2004 in the United Kingdom, compared results of a sandwich approach (i.e., two cycles of cyclophosphamide, methotrexate, and 5-fluorouracil [CMF regimen], then irradiation, followed by further CMF) with six cycles of CMF followed by irradiation in 2250 patients. Patients could receive anthracycline-based chemotherapy before starting the protocol. No results are available yet from this trial.

Interval Between Surgery and the Start of Chemotherapy

Some studies suggest that certain patient subgroups may have higher distant failure rates when chemotherapy is delayed too long after surgery. In the JCRT retrospective experience, for patients aged 50 years or younger at diagnosis with one to three positive axillary nodes, treated with the CMF regimen without doxorubicin, the actuarial 5-year freedom from distant failure was 84% for 83 patients beginning chemotherapy within 8 weeks of axillary dissection, compared with 78%

for 37 patients beginning chemotherapy more than 8 weeks after dissection.[116] This difference was not statistically significant. In the JCRT upfront-outback trial,[121,122] the crude rate of distant or regional nodal failure (as a first site of failure) was 47% for patients with four or more positive nodes in the irradiation-first arm, compared with 31% for patients in the chemotherapy-first arm. In contrast, the respective rates for patients with one to three positive nodes were 27% and 28%. However, the opposite relationship between nodal status and the surgery-to-chemotherapy approach was found in a nonrandomized series from the University of Arizona.[126] In a study from the M.D. Anderson Cancer Center in Houston, Texas, when chemotherapy began made no difference in outcome for early-stage patients with one to three or with four or more positive nodes.[127] The optimal timing of chemotherapy with regard to surgery remains uncertain.

Concurrent versus Sequential Administration of Chemotherapy and Radiation Therapy and Local Control

Concurrent administration of chemotherapy and irradiation (i.e., within a few hours to two days of each other) does not by itself appear to improve local control rates for most patients when the interval between surgery and irradiation is not thereby affected. In the JCRT retrospective experience, the incidence of local recurrence was the same whether patients received irradiation before chemotherapy, sequential "sandwich" chemoradiation (in which some cycles were given before and some cycles after radiation therapy), or concurrent chemoradiation with or without preceding chemotherapy cycles.[116] However, specific patient subgroups may benefit from concurrent chemoradiation programs. A pilot study of a concurrent CMF regimen and irradiation conducted at the JCRT found that with a median follow-up time of 94 months, the crude 5-year local failure rate was the same for patients (1 [4%] of 25) with positive margins as for patients (1 [6%] of 16) with close margins (≤1 mm) or those (3 [4%] of 70) with more widely negative margins.[128]

There are few studies about the impact of interruptions in chemotherapy regimens on their effectiveness. In the randomized International Breast Cancer Study Group trial VI, 5-year disease-free and overall survival rates were identical whether patients received a total of six cycles of CMF given over 6 months or over 12 months.[129] Similarly, in the retrospective JCRT experience, distant failure rates were almost identical in patients with one to three positive nodes who received sandwich therapy or concurrent chemoradiation (18%).[116]

Tamoxifen and Radiation Therapy

Several randomized trials found that giving tamoxifen concurrently with irradiation (and for prolonged periods after irradiation) reduced the risk of local failure after breast-conserving therapy by one half to two thirds.[91,93,130] Nonrandomized studies have found no difference in local failure rates between patients receiving tamoxifen concurrently with or only after irradiation.[131,132]

Conclusions about the Timing of Therapy

There is little consensus regarding the optimal combination of systemic therapy with conservative surgery and irradiation for patients with early-stage breast cancer.[133,134] Available data on this subject are often contradictory. I think patients should use chemotherapy and irradiation sequentially, rather than concurrently, because of the increased risk of toxicity with concurrent regimens (discussed later) without clear evidence of advantages in tumor control. Radiation therapy can be safely started 2 to 3 weeks after completing chemotherapy. Most American centers give all the planned chemotherapy before irradiation, which may not be optimal for all patients, particularly those with uninvolved but close margins (≤1 mm wide). In such patients, it seems prudent to start radiation therapy within approximately 4 months of the last breast surgery before chemotherapy or after a short chemotherapy regimen or by using a sandwich approach. This requires close communication among the surgeon, medical oncologist, and radiation oncologist. For selected patients with positive margins, the toxicities of concurrent chemoradiation may be justified in an attempt to achieve low local failure rates.

WHEN TO USE NODAL IRRADIATION

Axillary Irradiation

Radiation therapy is highly effective in preventing axillary recurrence in patients with clinically uninvolved (N0) nodes, with failure rates of 1% to 3%, very similar to those achieved with axillary dissection.[135] Axillary failure rates and overall survival rates were very similar in the NSABP B-04 trial[136] and a trial conducted at the Institut Curie in Paris comparing these approaches.[137] Axillary failure is more common (3% to 30%) in patients with clinically suspicious (N1) axillary disease when treated with irradiation than with axillary dissection. These patients should undergo a level I-II dissection.

The lower portions of the axilla (levels I and at least part, but not always all, of level II) and sentinel nodes are ordinarily included in the same fields used to treat the breast.[138,139] Several studies in selected patients with clinically uninvolved axillary nodes treated with irradiation directed to the breast alone have had axillary failure rates of 0% to 10%.[111,112,140-143] In an Italian trial directly comparing axillary irradiation and breast irradiation for patients older than 45 years with tumors of 1.2 cm or smaller, with a median follow-up time of 42 months, there were no differences in the overall survival rates or risk of metastases at 5 years and only minimal differences in the risk of axillary recurrence (.5% and 1% in the two arms, respectively).[144]

Axillary failure is rare in patients found to have positive nodes on conventional dissection, and full axillary irradiation is not usually indicated. Axillary irradiation may be an important alternative to complete dissection in patients who are found to have positive nodes on limited axillary surgery, such as SNB or axillary sampling.[145-147] However, it is not clear whether full axillary irradiation or further axillary surgery is superior in particular situations. Randomized trials are testing these different approaches.

Supraclavicular Nodal Irradiation

In most series, supraclavicular recurrences occur in only a few percent of patients when the axillary nodes are pathologically negative or only one to three nodes are positive.[33,148] Supraclavicular nodal failures are much more common in patients with four or more pathologically positive axillary nodes.[33,149,150] Data from the JCRT suggested that lymphatic vessel invasion in the primary tumor may increase the risk of supraclavicular failure in patients with negative or one to three positive axillary nodes, but the number of patients in these subgroups was small.[148] A study from Taiwan of 2658 consecutive patients found that high grade, having four or more positive nodes, and having positive nodes at axillary level II or III were associated with statistically significant increased risks of supraclavicular failure on multivariate analysis.[151] However, this analysis included patients who did or did not have nodal irradiation. The incidence of supraclavicular failure can be reduced to 1% or less for patients receiving doses of 45 to 50 Gy in 1.8- to 2-Gy fractions.[152]

Internal Mammary Nodal Irradiation

Internal mammary node (IMN) metastases occur in 1% to 10% of patients with pathologically negative axillary nodes, with most studies demonstrating incidences of less than 5%.[153,154] Reported rates are 20% to 50% for patients with positive dissections. Tumor size and the number of involved nodes likely influence this risk. For example, in a study from Nice, France, the incidence of IMN involvement in patients with positive axillary nodes with T1-2 tumors was 26% (12 of 45), compared with 47% (8 of 17) for patients with T3 lesions and positive axillary nodes.[155] In a study conducted in Kanazawa, Japan, the risk of involvement of IMNs was 17% (5 of 30) for patients with one to three positive axillary nodes, compared with 43% (10 of 23) for patients with four or more positive axillary nodes.[156] In a series from Chicago, the respective rates in these groups were 30% (21 of 71) and 56% (44 of 78).[154] The location of the primary tumor in the breast appears to have only a minor impact on the risk of IMN involvement when tumor size and nodal status are taken into account.

Most studies report a rate of 1% or less for clinical IMN recurrences in patients. Retrospective studies have differed on whether patients benefit from IMN irradiation.[157-159] However, large, randomized trials have not shown improved outcome after specific IMN treatment with surgery or irradiation.[160-163] A trial of IMN and supraclavicular nodal irradiation conducted by the European Organization for Research and Treatment of Cancer (EORTC) from 1996 to 2004 accrued more than 4000 patients; results are pending. The National Cancer Institute of Canada began a similar protocol in 2000 for patients undergoing breast-conserving therapy, with an accrual goal of 1822 patients.

Conclusions about When to Use Nodal Irradiation

Axillary or supraclavicular irradiation need not routinely be given after removal of level I-II nodes when the nodes are negative or only one to three nodes are positive. Insufficient data are available to justify firm recommendations regarding axillary and supraclavicular irradiation for patients with four or more positive nodes. The benefits of such treatment, if any, are likely to be small. A supraclavicular field is adequate for treating most such individuals. Treating a full axillary field may be useful for patients with very extensive nodal involvement or a more limited dissection, but because of the risks of arm edema, only a supraclavicular field should be treated in patients who have had a dissection that included level III nodes. IMN irradiation results in treating larger volumes of lung or heart than treating just the breast. Given its uncertain value and its potential risks, such treatment is never mandatory in my view.

PATIENT POSITIONING AND IMMOBILIZATION, SIMULATION, TARGET VOLUMES, AND RADIATION TREATMENT TECHNIQUES

Patient Position and Immobilization

Although patients are ordinarily treated in the supine position, the lateral decubitus[164] and prone positions[165] may be useful in the treatment of patients with very large breasts. Numerous immobilization techniques with specialized breast boards, custom foam cradles, and other methods have been used. Regardless of the immobilization technique employed, the uncertainty of patient position in daily treatment by well-trained radiation therapists due to set-up errors and patient movement is rarely more than 5 mm.[166-168]

Respiration causes modest movement of the breast during treatment. In one study, respiratory excursions resulted in the medial field border moving an average of 6 mm anteriorly and 3 mm posteriorly, compared with the computed tomography (CT) simulation images obtained during free breathing; the corresponding movements of the lateral field border were an average of 4 mm anteriorly and 2 mm posteriorly.[169] Respiratory gating or breath-hold techniques have been described, and by treating patients in moderate or deep inspiration, these methods may reduce the amount of heart treated, often quite substantially, compared with free breathing.[167,169,170] However, such techniques may increase the dose given to the contralateral breast for patients receiving nodal irradiation and the volume of lung irradiated to doses above 20 Gy for patients treated to the breast alone compared with tangential fields. Not all patients are able to cooperate with this approach.[171] The effects of set-up and respiratory motions on the cumulative dose distribution within the breast as a whole or at the excision cavity are small,[166,169,172] but there may be a substantial effect of respiration on the doses given to the IMNs.[169]

There is no fully satisfactory way to immobilize the breast itself. Netting is useful in treating large-breasted women to improve the reproducibility of setup and to move the breast tissue medially to limit the amount of normal tissue treated. Other devices, such as a plastic ring to help hold the breast in place[173] or cellulose acetate[174] or plastic immobilization casts, have been used for this purpose, but they tend to increase the skin dose.

Simulation

Many detailed descriptions of fluoroscopically based simulation and treatment techniques are available.[175-179] CT-based simulation techniques have been used to aid conventional treatment planning or to replace it entirely. CT simulation enables reconstruction of the true dose distribution in three dimensions within the entire treated volume by allowing corrections for lung inhomogeneity and changes in contour at multiple levels, as well as measurements of the irradiated volumes of lung and heart. However, there is substantial interphysician variation in delineating the breast tissue on CT.[180] Care must be taken to include the entire tumor bed in the tangential fields with adequate margin to account for respiration and normalization; having surgical clips in place may be helpful, particularly when CT-guided simulation is not performed.[181]

Regional lymph nodes cannot be directly seen on planning CT, unless pathologically enlarged. Because of the variable position of the IMNs,[182] techniques employing radionuclide lymphoscintigraphy or CT are preferred to minimize the volumes of normal heart and lung in the treatment fields while ensuring adequate coverage.[183,184] The IMNs may lie medial or lateral to the vessels, which are usually visible at the sternal-pleural junction. The subclavian and axillary vessels typically are used as surrogates for the position of the axillary nodes, and the sternocleidomastoid, pectoralis minor and major, and anterior scalene muscles and the clavicle are used to define the boundaries of the infraclavicular and supraclavicular nodal regions.[185] Changes in arm position have little effect on the positions of the IMNs and medial supraclavicular nodes, but there may be substantial changes in the position of the axillary nodes.[186] It is best to maintain the same arm position between simulation and treatment.

Whole-Breast Irradiation

The field borders of standard tangential fields are designed to include nearly the entire volume of the breast with adequate margin for daily set-up error and to achieve full dose to the breast tissue (Table 60-5). Blocking or gantry rotation should be used to make the posterior field edges coplanar to reduce exposure to the heart, lung, and contralateral breast (Fig. 60-1).

In patients with large breasts or medial-to-lateral separations (more than 22 to 24 cm), it may be preferable to use high-energy photons (≥10 MV) to keep the maximum inhomogeneity less than 110%. Skin failures are rare, regardless of treatment energy,[43] and a bolus or beam-spoiler does not need to be used routinely for such patients. For patients 45 years old or younger, it is desirable to reduce the risk of radiation carcinogenesis by reducing the dose to the contralateral breast by not using wedges for the medial field.[187]

Matchline and Nodal Irradiation Techniques

When the supraclavicular or supraclavicular and axillary regions need to be irradiated, it is generally necessary to use fields separate from the tangential fields used to treat the breast, because breast tangential fields cover only a portion of these areas.[138,188,189] Techniques using modified tangential fields that include the axillary nodes have been described elsewhere.[190] As a result, problems of achieving an adequate geometric match arise. Many techniques are available that use field geometry and blocking with templated blocks or multileaf collimators to avoid hot spots due to field overlap or underdosing due to fields being too far apart (Figs. 60-2 and 60-3).[175-179] Situations calling for doses above 45 to 50 Gy to be given to the axilla require the use of an en face or posterior boost field or opposed anteroposterior fields to avoid excessive fibrosis in the pectoralis muscle.

Treatment of IMNs with a photon hockey-stick field should be discouraged (Fig. 60-4). Such a technique results in a mismatch between the nodal field and the tangential fields in the lateral plane between them, resulting in overdosage or underdosage. Photon fields that directly irradiate the heart in this manner also appear to increase the risk of late cardiac deaths.[3] Although this problem may be limited by the use of electron or mixed-beam direct internal mammary fields,[183,184] the problem of achieving adequate field junctions with the tangential fields remains. The commonly used "partially wide tangent" technique included only the IMNs in the third interspace and above (which are the ones most likely to be involved) to reduce the irradiated volumes of lung and

Table 60-5 Field Borders and Blocks

TANGENTS

Inferior: 1 cm margin inferior to the inframammary fold

Superior: The margin of the breast is determined by palpation and will be given a 1-cm margin. When a three-field technique is used, the placement of the matchline depends on the location of the primary tumor and the breast tissue. Ordinarily, the matchline is at the second intercostal space or the second rib (radiographically, usually at the inferior edge of the sternoclavicular junction).

Lateral: Include all breast tissue with a 1-cm margin. This usually places this border at the posterior to midaxillary line.

Medial: This point is at the midline in most patients. When the internal mammary nodes are to be included, the medial border is best determined with the aid of lymphoscintigraphy or computed tomography; otherwise, the medial border is arbitrarily placed 3 cm across the midline. When the contralateral breast has been previously treated or when both breasts are to be treated simultaneously, care should be taken to ensure that treatment fields do not overlap. A gap of .5 cm on the skin between the medial borders of the two pairs of fields is adequate.

Anterior: A 2-cm margin of light is given above the highest point of the breast.

Posterior: The deep edges of the tangents should be coincident. The medial and lateral borders determine their exact position.

Blocks: When a three-field technique is used, a block is drawn along the hanging wire that defines the matchline at the superior border with the en face supraclavicular-axillary field.

BOOST

Include the breast tissue from approximately the skin surface to the anterior chest wall, with 1 to 2 cm around the excision cavity as the planning target volume.

SUPRACLAVICULAR-AXILLARY FIELD

Borders: This field is angled approximately 10 degrees from the vertical toward the medial side to avoid treating the cervical spinal cord.

Inferior: Determined by the matchline with the tangential fields. With the Joint Center for Radiation Therapy technique, the central-axis plane is located here.

Superior: Radiologically, this is usually the superiormost portion of the first rib. Except in unusual situations, it is preferable not to clear skin ("flash") in the supraclavicular region.

Lateral: Usually, two thirds of the medial-to-lateral distance through the humeral head. In some patients with extensive axillary disease, it may be necessary to clear skin laterally.

Medial: Set up to the center of the suprasternal notch (midline), and then angle the gantry.

Blocks: The inferior border is defined by a block through the central axis. In most patients, the lateral third of the humeral head should be blocked. In some patients with very extensive axillary disease, this may not be possible.

SUPRACLAVICULAR FIELD

The borders are the same as for the full axillary-supraclavicular field, except the lateral field border is at the coracoid process.

EN FACE AXILLARY BOOST

The couch, gantry, and collimator are angled to direct the beam from the axilla toward the supraclavicular nodes by aiming toward the suprasternal notch. The isocenter is placed at a point 3- to 4-cm lateral to the head of the clavicle in the supraclavicular fossa. The field size varies with the patient's body size but is usually on the order of 6 × 8 cm. The anterior border is set to run posteriorly to the anterior edge of the pectoralis major muscle, as determined visually and by palpation. The other borders are determined by the desired volume of treatment.

POSTERIOR AXILLARY BOOST

Inferior: Block the field to match the superior border of the tangential fields.

Superior: It is parallel to the clavicle.

Medial: It is 2 cm into the lung tissue medial to the chest wall.

Lateral: It is at the middle of the humeral head.

EN FACE INTERNAL MAMMARY FIELD

Use CT simulation to plan the depth and width.

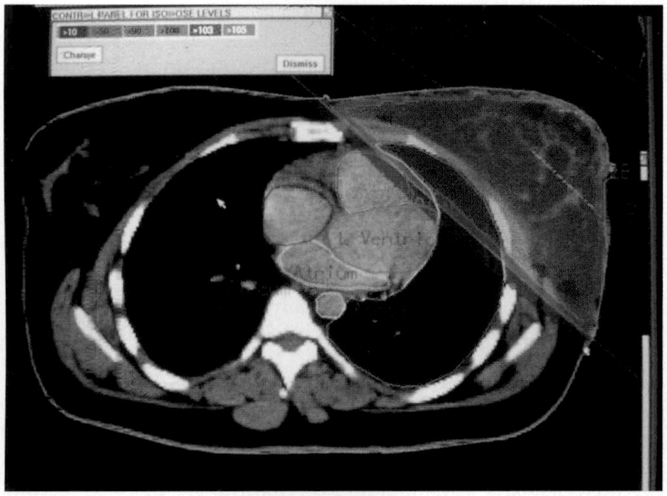

Figure 60-1 Color wash rendition of the dose distribution for typical whole-breast tangential fields, superimposed on a transverse CT image. Notice the relationships of the field borders to the cardiac chambers and the left anterior descending coronary artery (LAD). Color code: dark blue, dose more than 10% to 50% of the prescribed dose; light blue, more than 50% to 90%; green, more than 90% to 100%; yellow, more than 100% to 103%; orange, more than 103% to 105%; red, more than 105%.

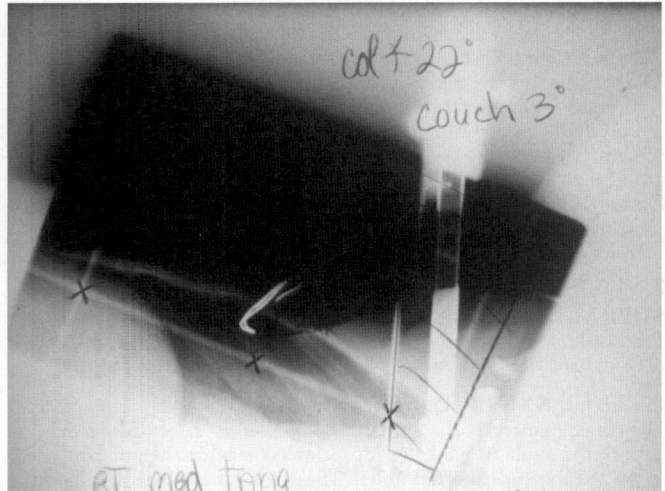

Figure 60-2 Example of a block placed at the superior end of tangential fields (toward the right side in this simulator radiograph) to achieve a geometrically acceptable match with the supraclavicular or supraclavicular-axillary field. In this example, the patient is being treated after mastectomy.

heart.[191] However, such blocks may increase the risk of local failure for patients with inferiorly located tumors.[192] Field border recommendations for nodal fields are provided in Table 60-5.

Breast Boosts

Local control and cosmetic results are similar with interstitial implantation (Fig. 60-5), photons, or electrons.[193,194] The preoperative description of the lesion, mammograms, and the operative report can help to define the location of the tumor

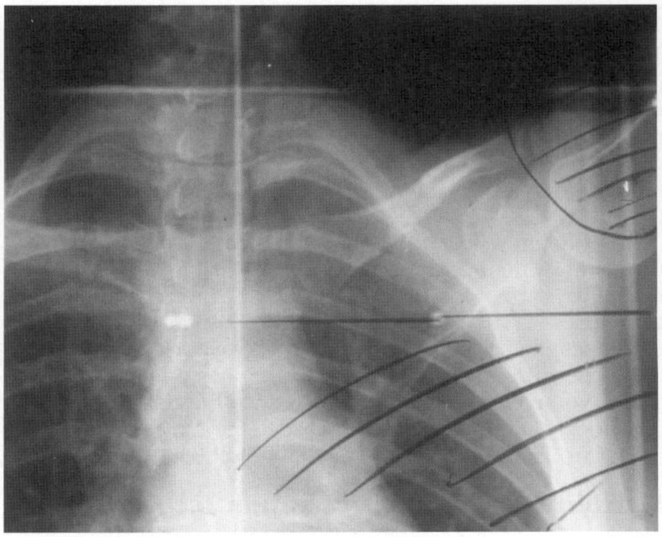

Figure 60-3 Simulator radiograph of a supraclavicular-axillary field. Notice the block at the central axis plane inferiorly (which serves to match with the tangential fields) and the block over a portion of the humeral head. A cervical spine block was not used in this case.

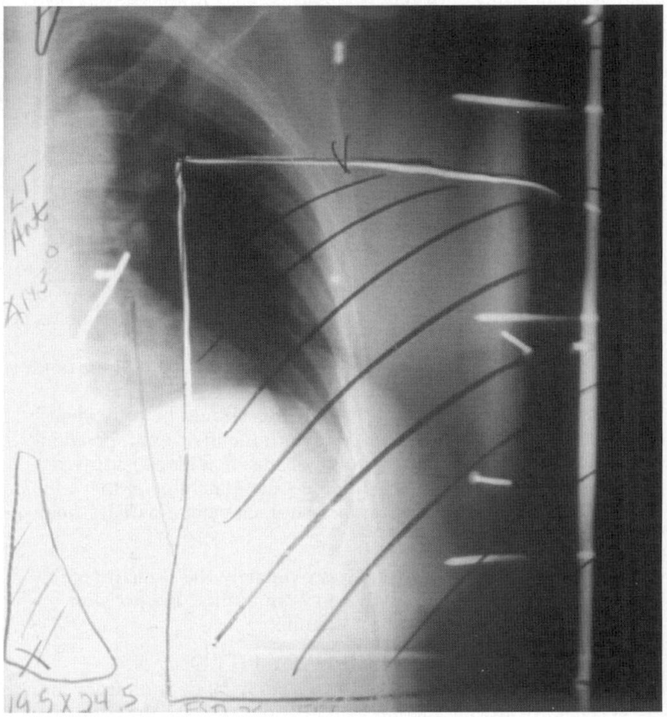

Figure 60-4 Simulator radiograph of a hockey-stick field. The wire medially represents the limits of the patient's breast tissue. The right-angled wire more laterally represents the limits of the tangential field borders, and a block has been indicated to try to avoid overlap. Notice the large volume of the heart that is irradiated.

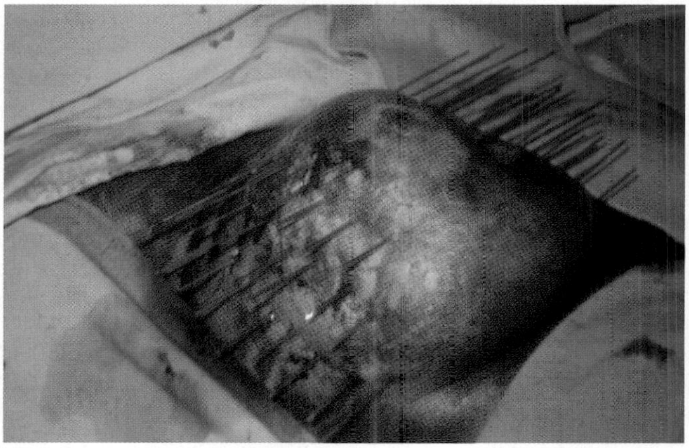

Figure 60-5 Placement of stainless steel needles through the breast for interstitial implant boost. Plastic tubes are inserted through the needles, which are then removed. Metal buttons are then placed over the ends. After the radioactive material is inserted, the ends are crimped to hold the implant securely in place when the patient returns to her room. In this example, the ends of the tubes have not yet been trimmed.

bed. However, because the position of the breast in the treatment position is often substantially different from the position used in these other procedures (especially mammography), such information must be used cautiously. Palpation may reveal a tissue defect, although in many patients the breast tissue is reapproximated after resection. Similarly, the surgical scar is not always a reliable guide to the area of excision.[181,195] Ultrasound is very useful in determining the thickness of the breast tissue when clinical boost planning is performed.[196]

Radiologic techniques of locating and planning the boost volume rely on the placement of surgical clips with subsequent fluoroscopic simulation,[197] ultrasound delineation of the excision cavity,[198,199] or CT to localize the clips and cavity.[200,201] However, the clinical value of more accurate localization of the tumor bed is not clear in patients receiving whole-breast irradiation. In a study from Philadelphia, the availability of surgical clips for planning the boost did not reduce the local failure rate.[202]

It is not certain what the margins around the tumor bed should be for the boost planning target volume. In most institutions, 1- to 2-cm margins are used. Small inaccuracies in the size of the boost volume seem unlikely to have a major impact on the risk of recurrence.

RADIATION THERAPY DOSE AND SCHEDULE PARAMETERS

Whole-Breast Fractionation

Conventions for prescribing doses to tangential breast treatment fields vary substantially from one institution to another.[203,204] Almost all look solely at the dose distribution in the central axis plane, and dose distributions in more caudal or cephalic planes are usually substantially different from those in the central axis plane unless some form of three-dimensional compensation is used. Failure to correct for the effect of lung inhomogeneity on dose distribution from tangential fields further increases the artificiality of the concept of *prescribed dose*.[205,206] Few studies examine the impact of interfraction[166,167] and intrafraction motion (e.g., due to respiration[169]) on the actual dose delivered. Fortunately, these effects appear to be small. Differences in prescribing conventions for boost fields are even more substantial. The following data on dose-response relationships must be interpreted with caution.

Most centers in the United States and Western Europe give whole-breast doses of 45 to 50 Gy in 1.8- to 2-Gy daily fractions. Schemes using larger fractions frequently have been used in Canada and the United Kingdom with excellent results (e.g., 40 Gy in 15 or 16 fractions).[207,208]

Only a few randomized clinical trials have compared different fractionation schemes. In a trial conducted at the Royal Marsden and Cheltenham General Hospitals in England from 1986 to 1998, 1410 patients were randomized to receive 50 Gy in 25 fractions or 42.9 Gy or 39 Gy given in 13 fractions delivered over 5 weeks (alternating between two fractions and three fractions in successive weeks).[209] Elective boost treatment (14 Gy in 7 fractions) was the same in all three arms. There was no difference in tumor control between the study arms. Cosmetic outcome in the 39-Gy arm was superior to that of the patients receiving 50 Gy, which was superior to that of patients receiving 42.9 Gy.[210]

A trial conducted from 1993 to 1996 in Ontario, Canada, included 1234 women with pathologically clear resection margins and negative axillary lymph nodes. Patients were randomly assigned to receive whole-breast irradiation of 42.5 Gy in 16 fractions over 22 days or 50 Gy in 25 fractions over 35 days.[211] A boost was not given. With a median follow-up of 69 months, the 5-year rate of local recurrence of invasive cancer in each of the two arms was 3%. Seventy-seven percent of patients in each arm had excellent or good global cosmetic outcome at 3 and 5 years.

The largest fractionation study is the START trial, conducted in the United Kingdom between 1999 and 2002.[212,213] It included two subtrials. In trial A (2236 patients), a control arm of 50 Gy in 25 fractions was compared with 41.6 Gy in 13 fractions or 39 Gy in 13 fractions given over 5 weeks. Trial B (2215 patients) compared 50 Gy in 25 fractions to 40 Gy in 15 fractions over 3 weeks. Results of this study are not yet available.

Even more hypofractionated schemes have been tried.[214-216] A randomized study at the Hôpital Necker (Paris) compared giving 45 Gy in 25 fractions delivered in 5 weeks with 23 Gy delivered as 5 Gy on days 1 and 3 and 6.5 Gy on days 15 and 17.[214] With a minimum follow-up of 4 years, the locoregional recurrence rates in patients undergoing tumorectomy were 7% (4 of 56) in the conventional fractionation arm and 4% (2 of 45) in the hypofractionation arm. The incidence of fibrosis and telangiectasias appeared greater in the hypofractionated group, although the severity of these was not described. The FAST trial, begun in the United Kingdom, randomly allocates patients 50 years old or older with cancers 3 cm or smaller and negative axillary nodes to one of five different schedules: a control arm of 50 Gy in 2-Gy fractions over 35 days (5 fractions per week); 30 Gy in 6-Gy fractions given over 35 days (1 fraction weekly); 28.5 Gy in 5.7-Gy fractions given over 35 days; 30 Gy in 6-Gy fractions over 15 days (2 or 3 fractions per week); or 28.5 Gy in 5.7-Gy fractions in 15 days.[217] No boost is used. The primary end point is change in breast appearance at 2 years, and the study has an accrual goal of 1500 patients.

Preliminary data from one pilot study of hyperfractionated radiation therapy (48 Gy whole-breast dose followed by a boost of 9.6 Gy, delivered twice daily in 1.6-Gy fractions) showed it to be well tolerated acutely.[218] However, no long-term data are available yet on this approach.

Total Dose to the Primary Tumor Site

Several retrospective studies have found that doses of approximately 50 Gy given in 2-Gy fractions or its biologic equivalent resulted in excellent local control rates in patients with uninvolved resection margins, with no improvement in local control when higher doses were used.[211,219,220] However, the impact of histology and age was not analyzed in these studies. None of these randomized or retrospective studies has examined the effect of the exact tumor-free margin width on the dose-response curve.

Four randomized trials have compared whole-breast irradiation alone with whole-breast irradiation plus a boost for patients with uninvolved margins.[221-225] All trials showed a lower risk of local failure for patients receiving higher doses, but the absolute differences were only 2% to 3% for the overall populations. In the EORTC trial, the boost reduced the local failure rate from 20% to 10% for patients younger than 40 years, but little benefit was seen in older patients, especially those older than 60 years.[224] However, in this trial, margin status was defined only in relation to the invasive component of the tumor, ignoring DCIS, which severely limits the applicability of these results.

Giving doses above 50 Gy to the tumor bed may be of greater benefit for patients whose specimen resection margins are positive or not evaluated.[226] However, doses above 60 Gy probably yield little added benefit. In the EORTC randomized trial, for patients with involved margins, the rate of local failure at 5 years was 8% for those receiving a total dose of 76 Gy, compared with 10% for those receiving a dose of 60 Gy.[227]

Nodal Irradiation Doses

Axillary and supraclavicular nodes are commonly prescribed by giving treatment to an anterior field at a fixed depth (typically 5 cm and 3 cm, respectively). However, the position of the nodes varies substantially, and such fixed-point dosing may not give adequate coverage.[228] Whether clinical results would be improved by individualized dose prescriptions is not clear.

Doses of 45 to 50 Gy result in a very low incidence of nodal failure in patients with clinically uninvolved nodes.[30,152] There is little evidence regarding the nature of the dose-response relationship for suspiciously enlarged nodes.

Conclusions about Dose and Schedule Parameters

Whole-breast and nodal doses of approximately 50 Gy in 25 fractions or its biologic equivalent seem effective at controlling microscopic residual disease in most patients. It is not clear whether larger fraction sizes may increase complication rates in some patient subsets (discussed later). A boost dose to the excision cavity and its environs increases the local control rate very modestly for patient populations as a whole. Based on age, histology, margin status, and other factors, it is not certain which patient subgroups may be most likely to benefit from a boost. When given, the total dose to the primary tumor site should be approximately 60 to 65 Gy.

INNOVATIVE IRRADIATION TECHNIQUES

Three-Dimensional Compensation and Intensity-Modulated Radiation Therapy

Several investigators have reported using three-dimensional physical compensators[174,229] or IMRT to treat the entire breast,[230,231] with or without simultaneous boost treatment of the excision site[232,233] and with or without treating regional lymph nodes.[234-236] Dose delivery is substantially more homogeneous than with conventional wedged techniques (Fig. 60-6).

The only completed randomized trial comparing traditional and three-dimensionally compensated approaches was conducted from 1997 to 2000 at the Royal Marsden Hospital in the United Kingdom, in which 306 moderate- or large-breasted patients were treated with standard two-dimensional or three-dimensional techniques (i.e., physical compensation or static-field IMRT).[237] At 2 years, a change in the appearance of the breast was apparent in 52% (60 of 116) evaluable patients treated with the conventional technique, compared with 36% (42 of 117) of those treated with three-dimensional techniques.

The true value of such approaches is not clear. Most patients treated with conventional approaches already have low local failure rates, excellent cosmetic results, and few complications. Simple maneuvers, such as use of high-energy photons and reduced fraction sizes, may be able to achieve many of the same results. The dose to the contralateral breast and lung may be increased, at least with certain IMRT techniques.[235] The Royal Marsden Hospital and similar trials being conducted in Cambridge, England, and in Canada may help delineate the proper place of three-dimensional compensation and IMRT in breast irradiation.

Accelerated Partial-Breast Irradiation

Traditionally, the entire breast has been treated in all patients, but because of the characteristics of localized breast cancers, it is possible that treatment of only a more limited volume surrounding the tumor would be equally effective. Occult synchronous primary cancers are rare in patients with clinically unicentric cancers. Most residual tumor cells remaining after lumpectomy are located within a few centimeters of the excision cavity.[95] Two thirds or more of local recurrences are at or near the site of the primary tumor, whether radiation therapy is used or not.[238-241]

Accelerated partial-breast irradiation (APBI) may be defined as any scheme that delivers radiation to the tumor site and limited surrounding tissue over a short overall time (e.g., 1 week). In principle, this approach can avoid the complications associated with whole-breast irradiation and allow treatment to be completed more quickly.[240] Among the approaches used are low dose rate interstitial implantation; high-dose brachytherapy using implantation or a balloon catheter[242]; single-fraction intraoperative irradiation using 50-kV photons[243] or high-energy electrons[244]; and three-dimensional conformal external beam irradiation.[245-247]

Several studies of APBI using interstitial implantation with median follow-up times of 5 years or longer have found local failure rates of 1% to 9%.[248-250] The only randomized trial completed that compared APBI with conventional whole-breast irradiation was conducted from 1982 to 1987 in Manchester, England, which randomly allocated 708 evaluable patients to receive irradiation to the entire breast and regional lymph nodes or treatment to the affected quadrant without whole-breast or nodal irradiation.[251] Microscopic margin status was not examined. With a median follow-up of 65 months, the incidences of breast recurrence in the two arms were 7% (26 of 355) and 14% (51 of 353) by 7 years, respectively. The actuarial 7-year breast recurrence rates in the whole-breast arm and in the limited-field group were similar for patients with infiltrating ductal carcinomas (11% and 15%, respectively); however, for patients with infiltrating lobular tumors, the respective recurrence rates were 8% and 34%. Other trials have

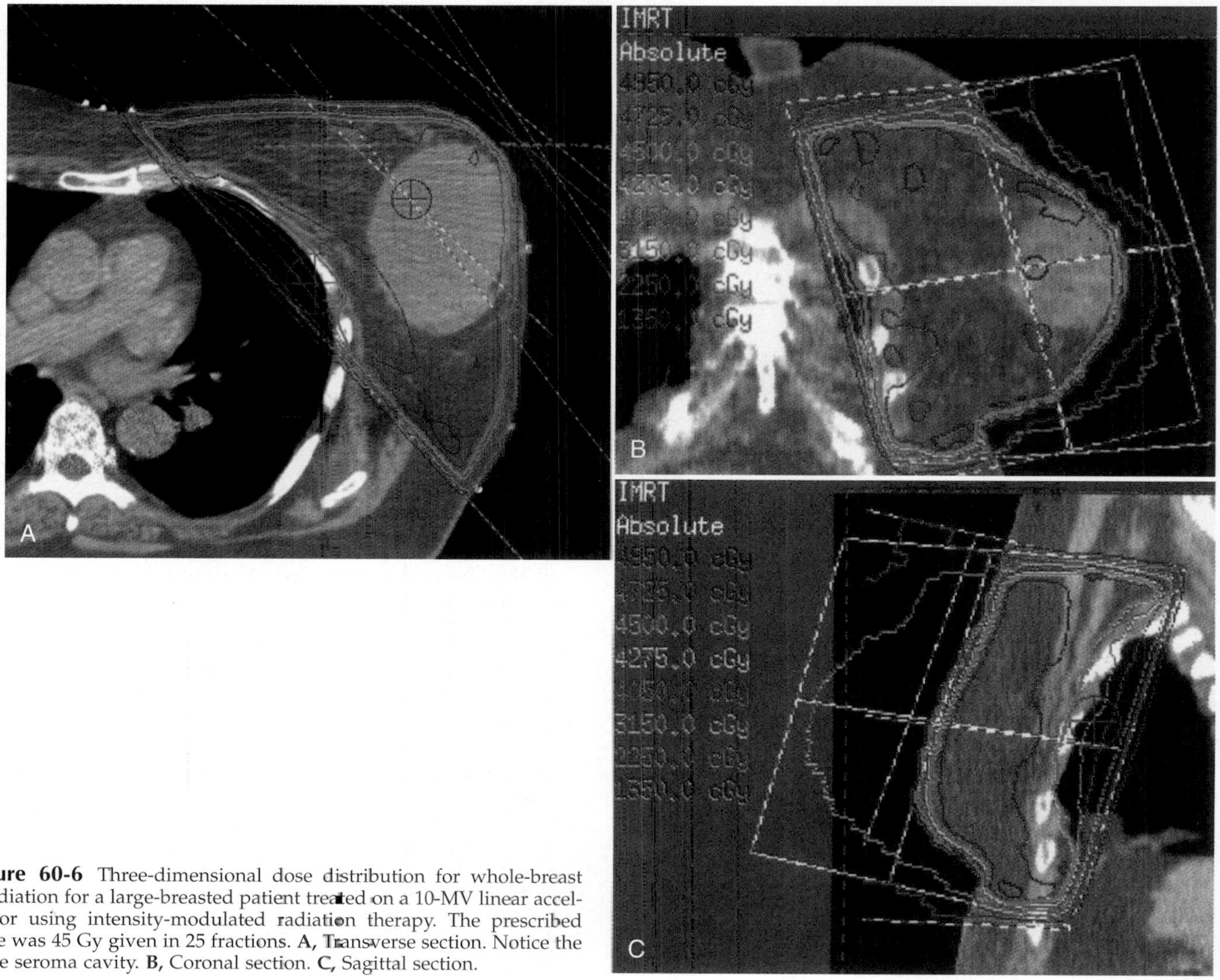

Figure 60-6 Three-dimensional dose distribution for whole-breast irradiation for a large-breasted patient treated on a 10-MV linear accelerator using intensity-modulated radiation therapy. The prescribed dose was 45 Gy given in 25 fractions. **A,** Transverse section. Notice the large seroma cavity. **B,** Coronal section. **C,** Sagittal section.

been completed or are being conducted by investigators in Europe and North America.

APBI is a promising approach, but much work remains to refine patient selection, treatment techniques, and doses. Patients must be fully informed about the limited data on the results of APBI and its possible risks compared with whole-breast irradiation.

ACUTE AND CHRONIC COMPLICATIONS AND COSMETIC RESULTS

Acute Reactions and Their Management

Patients should be seen at least weekly during treatment. The most common problem requiring attention is skin reactions. Skin care recommendations vary greatly from center to center and have rarely been subjected to comparative testing. Two randomized trials found that washing with soap and water reduces the severity of skin reactions, compared with not washing at all or using water alone.[252,253] Several trials have shown no differences in reactions between patients using different skin care products when compared with each other or when no products were applied.[254-257] One double-blind trial suggested that a cream including hyaluronic acid (which serves to retain moisture in the underlying dermis) was more effective in preventing severe skin reactions than one containing only the base of polyethylene glycol, glycerol, and sorbitol.[258] Another trial found that applying a potent steroid cream from the beginning of treatment decreased the intensity of the acute skin reaction.[259] However, there were no data on whether this cream caused any long-term changes in the skin. One commonly held view is that applying skin-care products before radiation treatment increases the skin dose given, but measurements have shown this effect is minimal.[260] Patients may apply such products whenever and as often as needed.

About 10% to 15% of patients treated with radiation therapy alone or sequential chemotherapy and irradiation develop moist desquamation during or shortly after completion of radiation therapy[121]; the rate may be 50% or higher for patients receiving concurrent chemoradiation (Fig. 60-7).[133] Most patients who have only limited areas of moist desquamation (especially in the inframammary fold) can continue radiation therapy without interruption. In some cases, it may be desirable to temporarily switch from tangential fields to the boost field, rather than giving a complete treatment break. When treatment must be interrupted due to skin reaction, the patient should be seen at least twice weekly to resume

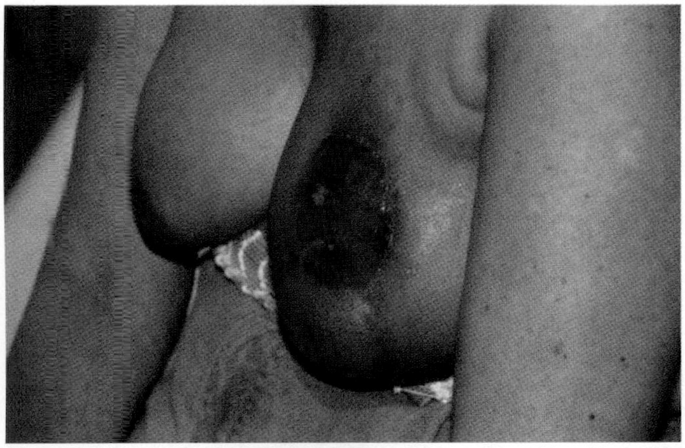

Figure 60-7 Moist desquamation occurred in the electron boost field after completion of radiation therapy. Such reactions are uncomfortable but rarely become infected.

radiation therapy at the earliest opportunity. Treatment breaks of more than 1 week are rarely necessary. Re-epithelialization need not be complete for treatment to begin. Skin care commonly used in this setting includes chlorhexidine gluconate or other antibacterial soaps to cleanse the area, alleviating discomfort with mild analgesics if needed, and using nonadherent dressings to absorb drainage and maintain moisturization. However, in a randomized trial performed in Scotland, patients with moist desquamation took longer to heal when a hydrogel dressing was used than when a dry dressing was applied.[257]

Myelosuppression of clinical significance in patients receiving irradiation alone is extremely unusual, and their blood counts do not need to be routinely checked except for patients who receive concurrent chemotherapy and irradiation. Treatment breaks generally need not be given for myelosuppression, unless signs and symptoms of infection are also present, because the volume of marrow irradiated is small and rarely interferes with recovery. Hematologic and other acute toxicities appear to be slightly greater in patients treated with chemotherapy after irradiation than with chemotherapy given before irradiation.[121] For patients receiving concurrent chemotherapy, special attention should be given to signs of infection (local or systemic) or radiation pneumonitis. However, the incidence of these problems is low.[128]

Postoperative cellulitis or abscess should be dealt with before radiation therapy is started if possible. When noticed after radiation therapy has started, antibiotics or surgical consultation, or both, should be initiated promptly. It is probably not necessary to interrupt radiation therapy unless abscess drainage is required. If the treatment is interrupted for more than 2 weeks, I consider increasing the total dose to the primary tumor site, although there are no data on the value of doing this.

Radiation pneumonitis occurring during treatment is very unusual, although concurrent use of chemotherapy may increase this risk.[133] Because radiation pneumonitis is a diagnosis of exclusion (discussed later), a prompt evaluation should be undertaken to exclude other causes of cough, dyspnea, and fever. If symptoms are severe, however, it may be necessary to stop radiation therapy until a complete evaluation can be performed.

Fatigue is a nearly universal complaint. A prospective study performed in Munich, Germany, did not find any factors correlated with the development or severity of fatigue.[261] Fatigue is generally mild and resolves within 2 months after completion of radiation therapy.

Subacute and Chronic Complications

Skin, Soft Tissue, and Bone

Patients may develop a skin reaction, *radiation recall*, when chemotherapy (particularly doxorubicin) is given after irradiation. However, this is rare when chemotherapy begins more than 2 weeks after the completion of radiation therapy.[133]

Breast abscesses or cellulitis probably develop in 5% to 10% of patients at any time after surgery.[262,263] Cellulitis may be more frequent in patients with hematomas or seromas requiring drainage, large volumes of resected breast tissue, or arm edema.[264,265] Sometimes, cellulitis or abscess mimics an inflammatory-type recurrence,[262,266] although the presence of pain, possible systemic symptoms of infection, and the time course of development usually make the distinction clear.

Rarely, patients develop patches of white or yellowish, well-circumscribed sclerosis and induration weeks to years after irradiation. This phenomenon has been called *post-irradiation morphea* or *circumscribed scleroderma*.[267] Sometimes, the patches may be preceded by the development of erythema, and they may be surrounded by a more highly pigmented, bruiselike area.

Radiation therapy may cause various histologic changes of fibrosis and atrophy,[268] which rarely result in clinical symptoms. The most common parenchymal change clinically is fibrosis. The fibrosis is generally mild, but when it is severe, the cosmetic results of treatment can be impaired.

Some individuals develop fat necrosis, which typically causes a painless mass located superficially in the breast, accompanied by retraction or dimpling of the overlying skin.[269] The skin may be thickened clinically and radiologically. Fat necrosis is firm and relatively circumscribed on palpation. Mammography usually reveals a spiculated, often poorly defined mass that may contain punctate or large, irregular calcifications. Attachment to the skin, dimpling, and thickening of the skin are often evident. Cystic degeneration may develop in the center of such a lesion, resulting in a cavity that contains oily fluid or necrotic fat. Calcification frequently develops in the cyst wall. Fat necrosis may mimic a carcinoma radiologically. Although fat necrosis is usually associated with pain, biopsy is required to be certain of the diagnosis.

After irradiation, patients commonly notice intermittent, transient breast pain, which can be sharp and shooting or dull and aching and can last a few seconds, minutes, or rarely longer. In a randomized trial in which patients were allocated to receive radiation therapy or not after breast-conserving surgery, patients treated with irradiation had more breast discomfort initially, but with further follow-up, the degree of discomfort became equal in both groups.[270] Pain is generally mild, although it can be severe in a few individuals. Some patients with severe pain or fibrosis have responded to treatment with pentoxifylline, alone or in combination with vitamin E.[271,272]

Soft tissue necrosis is rare. In the JCRT experience, most patients were treated with a boost, but only three patients (.2%) developed tissue necrosis requiring surgical resection.[273] All three were treated in ways not used today. One of these patients suffered osteoradionecrosis of the medial sternum after a total dose of 60 Gy in 24 fractions, and in two cases, necrosis was associated with use of an interstitial implant, with a total dose of 67 Gy in each case.

The incidence of rib fractures is related to the energy of the treatment machine and the total breast dose given.[273] With modern methods, the incidence of rib fractures should be less than 1%.[274]

Arm Edema and Shoulder and Arm Function

Axillary dissection may result in substantial morbidity. Arm edema may cause psychological and functional morbidity, and it may predispose patients to cellulitis. The most feared complication of arm edema is the development of lymphangiosarcoma, or Stewart-Treves syndrome, which is rare.[275]

The risk of developing symptomatic arm edema is only a few percent when sentinel node biopsy, level I-II axillary dissection, or irradiation alone is employed.[36,276] However, the risk is substantially increased after a complete axillary dissection.[31] The risk of arm edema is increased further when full axillary irradiation is given to patients who have had a complete dissection, although not when patients have undergone a more limited dissection.[277-279] In contrast, the risk of arm edema was only 3% in a series of 82 node-positive patients who had a level I-II or complete dissection who were treated with a supraclavicular field.[280]

The management of lymphedema is controversial, partly because few randomized trials have compared different approaches. For example, a trial conducted in Edmonton, Canada, found that manual lymphatic massage (widely used in treating arm edema) had no benefits in addition to compression bandaging, except perhaps in patients with mild lymphedema.[281]

The most common neurologic complication due to axillary dissection is the *intercostobrachial nerve syndrome*, which is characterized by paresthesias of the upper arm, shoulder, and axilla and occasionally of the more anterior portion of the chest wall. The pain may be dull, aching, or burning in character. It is usually constant but may become better with rest. Treatment tends to be ineffective, although some patients respond to nerve blocks or topical measures.[282,283] This syndrome may be permanent for the most severely affected individuals. Motor injury resulting from axillary dissection should be unusual, because the thoracodorsal, long thoracic, and pectoral nerves can be exposed and protected. Nonetheless, many patients experience decreased muscle strength and range of motion after a complete axillary dissection.[284,285] In some, these problems may persist for a year or longer. Early physical therapy may help reduce this problem.[286]

Axillary irradiation may also cause changes in shoulder mobility and arm functioning. There is a very broad range of reported incidence of these problems.[287] Such changes are rare in patients treated with doses of 50 Gy or less in 1.8- to 2.0-Gy fractions.

Brachial Plexopathy

Brachial plexopathy must be distinguished from neuropathies caused by axillary dissection or recurrence. In the JCRT experience, the radiation dose and the use of chemotherapy affected this risk.[273] When the axillary dose was 50 Gy or lower, the incidence of plexopathy was .4% (3 of 724) when no chemotherapy was given and 3.4% (10 of 267) when chemotherapy was employed. When the axillary dose was more than 50 Gy, the incidence of plexopathy was 3% (2 of 63) when chemotherapy was not used, compared with 8% (5 of 63) when chemotherapy was given. Four of the 20 affected patients had severe or permanent injuries. In other series, the risk of developing brachial plexopathy appears to be substantial only when doses above 50 Gy or large fraction sizes are used.[30] There is no satisfactory treatment for brachial plexopathy.

Pulmonary Effects

Radiographic pulmonary changes, such as infiltrates and localized interstitial fibrosis, are common in patients treated with radiation therapy.[288] These usually stabilize by 12 months after treatment, although some may resolve after that and some continue to progress for as long as 5 years.

Clinical radiation pneumonitis is much less common than radiologic changes. It is characterized by a chronic cough, fever, and nonspecific infiltrate on the chest radiograph.[288] It usually appears 4 to 9 months after completion of radiation therapy. Rarely, irradiation appears to precipitate a more generalized syndrome (i.e., bronchiolitis obliterans organizing pneumonia).[289]

Radiation pneumonitis is rare in patients treated with irradiation to the breast alone, whether chemotherapy is given or not.[290-292] When chemotherapy is given, the sequencing of chemotherapy and irradiation, the drugs used, and the volume of treated lung may be important in determining this effect. For example, in the JCRT experience, the incidence of symptomatic radiation pneumonitis was 8% for patients treated concurrently with a CMF regimen and irradiation, compared with 1% in those treated sequentially.[290] However, at the University of Pennsylvania, only 2% of patients treated with concurrent chemoradiation without methotrexate developed symptomatic pneumonitis.[293] There are also conflicting data regarding the risk of clinical pneumonitis in patients treated with irradiation and concurrent or sequential paclitaxel.[133]

Two studies found that tamoxifen increased the risk of radiologic pulmonary fibrosis after irradiation.[294,295] However, in a series from Fox Chase Cancer Center, tamoxifen did not affect the risk of clinical radiation pneumonitis.[81]

Cardiac Complications

Radiation therapy may cause acute or chronic damage to the heart.[296] Acute and subacute complications such as pericarditis and cardiac failure have been reported infrequently.[273] Long-term increased cardiac mortality has been found in meta-analyses[3] and registry-based studies[297,298] that included predominantly patients treated with outmoded techniques of irradiation. However, several studies using modern irradiation techniques (which expose less of the heart, even when the IMNs are deliberately included) and daily fraction sizes of 1.8 to 2 Gy have not shown any increased risk of cardiac morbidity and mortality at median follow-up times of 10 to 20 years.[299-302]

Most studies have not shown an increased risk of anthracycline cardiac toxicity in irradiated patients, but the number of patients at risk in these studies and their follow-up evaluations are limited.[133,274] Although an initial study of patients treated with concurrent doxorubicin and irradiation in Milan found an increased risk of congestive heart failure in patients who received left-sided irradiation,[303] an update reported that breast irradiation did not impact on the risk of systolic dysfunction.[304] Similar studies from Rotterdam and France also found that irradiation did not increase the risk of cardiac dysfunction.[305,306] There is little information about long-term cardiac toxicities in patients treated with irradiation and taxanes, anthracycline-taxane combinations, or new biologic agents such as trastuzumab.

Carcinogenesis

The effect of radiation therapy on the risk of developing new contralateral primary cancers appears small. In a study using data from the Connecticut Tumor Registry, only patients 45 years old or younger at exposure had an increased risk of developing a contralateral breast cancer, compared with unexposed patients; the relative risk was 1.21 at a dose of 1 Gy, which is probably the minimum achievable with standard

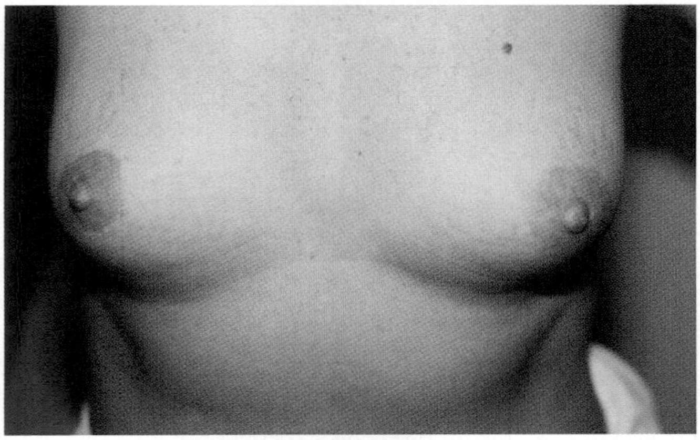

Figure 60-8 The left breast was irradiated 19 months earlier, and the cosmetic result is excellent.

current techniques.[307] In an analysis of the Surveillance, Epidemiology, and End Results (SEER) database, an increased risk was seen also for patients older than 55 years, but (confusingly) not for patients between the ages of 45 and 55 years.[308] Treatment techniques can minimize but cannot eliminate this risk.[187]

Most cancers developing within the radiation therapy fields are soft tissue sarcomas or angiosarcomas. They tend to occur 8 to 10 years or longer after treatment, but they may appear as soon as 1.5 to 2 years.[309] The reported incidence of soft tissue sarcomas is 9 to 14 cases per 100,000 patient-years of observation.[310-312] In a series from the Institut Gustav-Roussy near Paris, the 10-year actuarial incidence was .2%, the 20-year incidence was .43%, and the 30-year incidence was .78%.[311] The incidence of angiosarcomas in patients treated with breast-conserving therapy is not clear, with estimates of 5 to 13 cases per 10,000 treated patients.[309,313,314]

Other solid tumors, such as lung and esophageal cancers, may also be increased in incidence in areas within or adjacent to the radiation therapy fields. In one study, postmastectomy irradiation was associated with an estimated excess of seven or eight lung cancer cases per 10,000 women who survived more than 10 years from diagnosis.[315] Such cancers are almost entirely limited to patients who had been or are smokers.[316,317] Later studies found no increase in the risk of lung cancer after the use of irradiation as part of breast-conserving therapy, perhaps in part due to the smaller volume of lung treated.[318,319]

Radiation-induced leukemia appears rare in patients not receiving chemotherapy.[274] Results of studies suggest that irradiation increases the risk of leukemia by .3% to .5% in patients who receive anthracycline-based standard-dose chemotherapy.[320,321]

Cosmetic Results

Most patients have acceptable cosmetic results, with little or no change in the size, shape, or texture of the breast compared with its pretreatment characteristics (Fig. 60-8).[193] Patients tend to have more favorable views of cosmetic outcome than do physicians.[322,323] Cosmetic results tend to decline for the first 3 years after treatment but then remain stable.

Cosmetic outcome appears to have improved over time because of changes in surgical and irradiation techniques (Fig. 60-9). However, cosmetic results in different series are difficult to compare because there is no standard for describing results. Schemes for objectively measuring changes in breast size, shape, fibrosis, or contour have been described,[324,325] but they

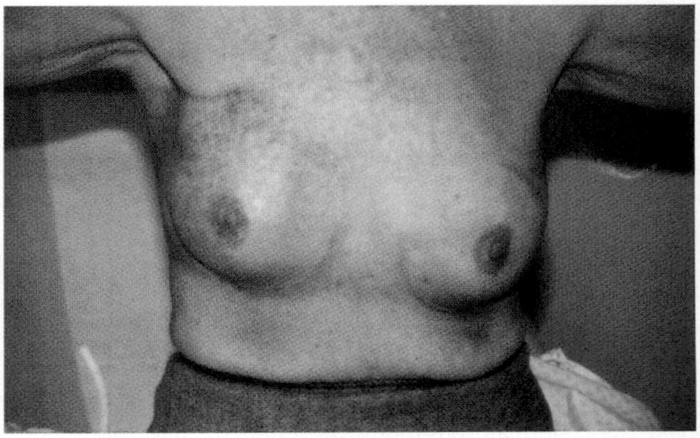

Figure 60-9 This patient was treated for right breast cancer in 1974 and left breast cancer in 1991. The photograph was taken 2 years after the last treatment. The right side was treated using a 4-MV linear accelerator to a dose of 46.8 Gy to the breast and regional nodes, followed by an electron boost. The left side was treated on a 6-MV accelerator, giving 45 Gy to the breast only, followed by an electron boost. On the right, she has substantial fibrosis and retraction of the breast superiorly, a hyperpigmented and fibrotic ridge superiorly due to match-line overlap between the tangential and supraclavicular-axillary fields, and substantial telangiectasias in the electron-boost field. In contrast, the cosmetic result on the left is good, with an easily visible surgical scar in the upper outer quadrant but few other changes. At follow-up in February 1997, telangiectasias had begun to appear in the left-sided electron boost field (not shown).

are not widely used. One reason is that they may not capture skin changes and other significant sequelae.

Surgery appears the most important factor responsible for cosmetic outcome.[193,326] Greater breast size has been associated with increased retraction after breast-conserving therapy using irradiation (Fig. 60-10).[327-329] However, this problem can be at least partially overcome by the use of higher photon energies[43] and use of the prone or lateral decubitus position. Doses to the entire breast much above 50 Gy in 2-Gy fractions seem to worsen results,[330] as does the use of large fraction sizes when doses above 45 Gy are given.[331] Giving a breast boost worsens results modestly, although in the EORTC trial the cosmetic results obtained with implantation and external beam boosts were comparable.[326] The use of a hockey-stick field or other techniques resulting in imperfectly matched field edges can cause substantial fibrosis and skin changes at areas of overlap (see Fig. 60-10).

Cosmetic results appear to be similar whether chemotherapy is given before or after radiation therapy.[121] However, the cosmetic results in patients receiving methotrexate (as part of the CMF regimen) or doxorubicin concurrently with irradiation tend to be inferior to sequential regimens, although not all oncologists agree on this point.[133] There are no data on how the taxanes affect cosmesis in irradiated patients. Overall cosmetic results were unaffected by tamoxifen in two studies.[81,82] In a study from the University of Pennsylvania, complication rates and cosmetic results were very similar whether tamoxifen was given concurrently or sequentially with irradiation, although breast edema was slightly more common in the former group (79% versus 65%).[332]

PATIENT FOLLOW-UP

Goals and Scheduling of Follow-Up Visits and Testing

The major goal of surveillance after breast-conserving therapy is to detect and treat ipsilateral local recurrences and new

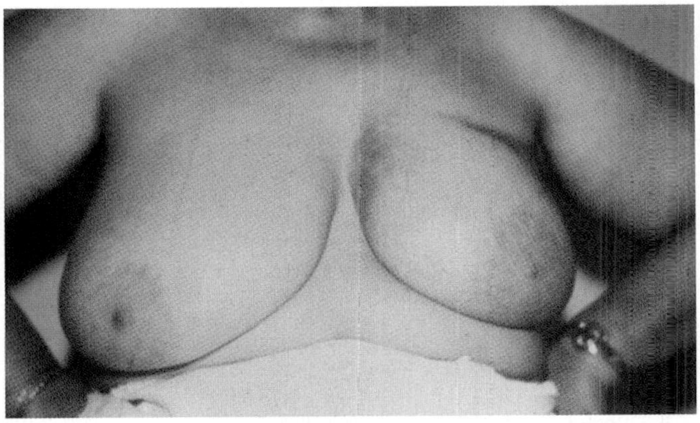

Figure 60-10 A poor cosmetic result in a patient with large breasts was caused by excessive fibrosis and retraction. The hyperpigmented and fibrotic ridges seen at the medial and superior borders of the left breast resulted from overlap between a hockey-stick field and breast tangential fields.

ipsilateral or contralateral primary tumors before they can metastasize. A secondary goal is to allow the use of a second breast-conserving approach for selected individuals.

The optimal intervals between office visits and mammograms are unknown. Some physicians recommend unilateral films every 6 months for as long as several years after treatment, although there are no data supporting this approach. A study performed at the Netherlands Cancer Institute in Amsterdam found no difference in rates of discovery of impalpable contralateral breast cancers or tumor stage whether mammograms were performed annually or every 2 years.[333] The value of other breast imaging modalities such as MRI in follow-up is uncertain.[334] Routine use of bone scans, chest radiographs, blood tests, and other studies used to detect distant metastases in asymptomatic patients is not warranted.[335] In my practice, patients have an interval history and physical examination performed by one of their treating physicians every 3 to 4 months for the first several years and then at least every 6 to 12 months indefinitely, with bilateral mammograms performed approximately 6 months after completing radiation therapy and then yearly.

Local Recurrence

The location of tumor recurrence in the treated breast changes with time. In the first 5 to 10 years, most relapses are in or near the original tumor bed, but with increasing follow-up, more are seen in other quadrants of the breast.[336-340] This suggests that two processes are reflected in the observed incidence of ipsilateral breast recurrence: regrowth of tumor cells left after the initial therapy and the development of new primary tumors unrelated to the original one.

Roughly one third to one half of local recurrences are detected solely by follow-up mammography, with the rest divided almost equally between those found on physical examination without any suspicious radiologic signs and those detected by examination and mammography. The physical and radiologic characteristics of the recurrence differ from those of the original presentation in a substantial proportion of patients.[341] Patients presenting with radiologically occult primaries should be followed with mammography and physical examination.

Physical examination after treatment usually reveals only mild thickening without a mass effect. However, surgery or irradiation may cause masslike regions of fibrosis that may occasionally be difficult to distinguish from a local recurrence. Recurrences may be especially difficult to detect for patients with infiltrating lobular carcinomas, which often produce only minimal thickening or retraction at the biopsy site without a mass. Rarely, the only sign of recurrence may be diffuse breast retraction. Recurrence in the nipple alone, manifesting as Paget's disease, has been reported but seems to be rare. Although some changes on examination that occur more than 1 to 2 years after the completion of radiation therapy may have benign causes (e.g., fat necrosis), they should be viewed as suspicious for recurrence.

Changes on mammogram usually stabilize within 4 to 12 months after treatment, but the radiologic appearance may take 2 to 3 years to reach its final state. There can be substantial overlap between benign and malignant lesions in radiologic appearance and on palpation. Suspicious microcalcifications that develop after treatment may be benign or malignant, although those that develop in a quadrant different from the initial tumor have a high likelihood of being malignant.[342] Benign and malignant radiologic changes may coexist. Recurrences of infiltrating lobular carcinomas are particularly likely to be radiographically occult.

Differential Diagnosis

The most common benign cause of suspected recurrence is probably fat necrosis. Biopsy is often required to confirm the clinical impression. Sarcomas are fortunately rare in this patient population but must be kept in mind, particularly for patients at longer intervals from treatment.

Further Evaluation of Possible Local Recurrence

Ultrasound may sometimes be helpful in differentiating benign and malignant lesions. Significant early contrast enhancement with gadolinium is seen on MRI in most patients with suspicious findings in whom biopsy reveals recurrent cancer, but the effect is rare with benign findings.[343] However, it is unclear what the role of these modalities should be, because highly accurate, minimally invasive biopsy techniques are readily available.

Fine-needle aspiration cytology and image-guided core biopsy are likely to be sufficient to establish the presence or absence of recurrence for most patients. However, they must be used cautiously. It is sometimes difficult to distinguish between radiation-induced cellular atypia and malignancy, even on open biopsies,[268] and consultation with an expert pathologist is prudent in such a situation. A negative result should not stop further pursuit of a suspicious or equivocal lesion.

SALVAGE OF LOCOREGIONAL FAILURE

Between 5% and 10% of patients with a recurrence in the treated breast present with concurrent distant metastases at the time of discovery of the breast recurrence.[344] A similar proportion of patients has locally extensive recurrence that precludes surgery or has concomitant inoperable regional nodal recurrences.

The 5-year relapse-free survival rates for patients with an isolated operable breast relapse treated with mastectomy are approximately 60% to 75%. Overall or cause-specific survival rates are 80% to 85%.[344] The ultimate risk of distant relapse after local failure after initial treatment with conservative surgery alone appears similar to that of patients failing locally after treatment with breast-conserving surgery and irradiation.[345]

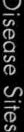

The most important variable affecting subsequent outcome of patients undergoing mastectomy may be the histology of the recurrence. Patients with noninvasive recurrences have very low rates of distant or regional nodal failure, whereas patients with invasive cancers have failure rates of 30% to

50%.[346-349] Patients with recurrences in the skin alone or with an inflammatory-type picture have a very poor prognosis, more similar to patients with extensive and rapid chest wall recurrence after mastectomy than to patients with breast parenchymal failures.[350] Tumor size greater than 2 cm at recurrence and diffuse involvement of the breast or dermal lymphatic involvement also are poor prognostic signs. In most series, the longer the time to failure after initial therapy, the better the prognosis. Variables for which there is not agreement on prognostic importance include the clinical size of the original primary tumor, the original clinical stage, original axillary nodal status, axillary involvement at recurrence, the location of the tumor with regard to the original lesion, and the means of detection of the recurrence (when other factors are accounted for).

The incidence of chest wall recurrence after salvage mastectomy is 10% or less, although most such patients have progressive local disease despite further treatment. It is rare that axillary exploration finds nodal tissue in patients who have had prior dissection, and repeat dissection does not seem warranted in the absence of suspicious adenopathy. Postoperative complications after mastectomy are rare. However, reconstructions using purely autologous tissue[351,352] appear much better tolerated by irradiated tissues than do reconstructions using prostheses.[353]

Some studies have tried using further conservative surgery in patients with a local failure after breast-conserving surgery and irradiation. Second local failure rates have been 20% to 30%.[354,355] Some groups have added further irradiation after excision. Their results appear comparable to those of patients treated with salvage conservative surgery alone, although the risk of serious complications appears low.[356,357] Patients initially treated with salvage lumpectomy may not ultimately achieve the same local control as if they had initially been treated with salvage mastectomy.[358] However, there has been little analysis of factors correlating with outcome after such treatment.

After local relapse, breast-conserving therapy has been performed in 30% to 70% of patients initially treated with breast-conserving surgery alone.[108,110,359,360] Such patients should probably also receive radiation therapy. In a series from Women's College Hospital, Toronto, the 5-year actuarial second local recurrence rate was 69% for patients treated with further conservative surgery alone and 11% for 14 patients treated with breast-conserving surgery and irradiation.[361]

The role of adjuvant chemotherapy or hormonal therapy after breast recurrence is unclear.[349] Some individuals with chest wall fixation may respond sufficiently to chemotherapy or hormonal therapy to allow mastectomy. However, systemic therapy alone cannot prevent local progression for long.

CONCLUSIONS

Breast-conserving therapy provides highly satisfactory cosmetic results without compromise of local tumor control or survival for most patients with early-stage breast cancer. Cooperation among the surgeon, radiologist, pathologist, medical oncologist, and radiation oncologist is critical in achieving this goal.

REFERENCES

1. Morrow M, Strom EA, Bassett LW, et al: Standard for breast conservation therapy in the management of invasive breast carcinoma. CA Cancer J Clin 52:277, 2002.
2. Tyldesley S, Foroudi F, Barbera L, et al: The appropriate rate of breast conserving surgery: an evidence-based estimate. Clin Oncol 15:144, 2003.
3. Early Breast Cancer Trialists' Collaborative Group: Favourable and unfavourable effects on long-term survival of radiotherapy for early breast cancer: an overview of the randomised trials. Lancet 355:1757, 2000.
4. Bonadonna G, Hortobagyi GN, Gianni AM: Textbook of Breast Cancer. A Clinical Guide to Therapy, 2nd ed. London, Martin Dunitz, 2001.
5. Donegan WL, Spratt JS: Cancer of the Breast, 5th ed. Philadelphia, WB Saunders, 2002.
6. Bland KI, Copeland EM III: The Breast: Comprehensive Management of Benign and Malignant Disorders, 3rd ed. St. Louis, WB Saunders, 2004.
7. Harris JR, Lippman ME, Morrow M, et al: Diseases of the Breast, 3rd ed. Philadelphia, Lippincott Williams & Wilkins, 2004.
8. Berg WA: Imaging the local extent of disease. Semin Breast Dis 4:153, 2001.
9. Holland R, Hendriks JHCL: Microcalcifications associated with ductal carcinoma in situ: mammographic-pathologic correlation. Semin Diagn Pathol 11:181, 1994.
10. Golshan M, Fung BB, Wolfman J, et al: The effect of ipsilateral whole breast ultrasonography on the surgical management of breast carcinoma. Am J Surg 186:391, 2003.
11. Hata T, Takahashi H, Watanabe K, et al: Magnetic resonance imaging for preoperative evaluation of breast cancer: a comparative study with mammography and ultrasonography. J Am Coll Surg 198:190, 2004.
12. International Breast Cancer Consensus Conference: Image-detected breast cancer: state of the art diagnosis and treatment. J Am Coll Surg 193:297, 2001.
13. Orel SG, Schnall MD: MR imaging of the breast for the detection, diagnosis, and staging of breast cancer. Radiology 220:13, 2001.
14. Fischer U, Kopka L, Grabbe E: Breast carcinoma: effect of preoperative contrast-enhanced MR imaging on the therapeutic approach. Radiology 213:881, 1999.
15. Schelfout K, Van Goethem M, Kersschot E, et al: Contrast-enhanced MR imaging of breast lesions and effect on treatment. Eur J Surg Oncol 30:501, 2004.
16. Sardanelli F, Giuseppetti GM, Panizza P, et al: Sensitivity of MRI versus mammography for detecting foci of multifocal, multicentric breast cancer in fatty and dense breasts using the whole-breast pathologic examination as a gold standard. AJR Am J Roentgenol 183:1149, 2004.
17. Lee CH, Carter D: Detecting residual tumor after excisional biopsy of impalpable breast carcinoma: efficacy of comparing preoperative mammograms with radiographs of the biopsy specimen. AJR Am J Roentgenol 164:81, 1995.
18. Fowble B, Hanlon AL, Fein DA, et al: Results of conservative surgery and radiation for mammographically detected ductal carcinoma in situ (DCIS). Int J Radiat Oncol Biol Phys 38:949, 1997.
19. McCormick B, Rosen PP, Kinne D, et al: Duct carcinoma in situ of the breast: an analysis of local control after conservation surgery and radiotherapy. Int J Radiat Oncol Biol Phys 21:289, 1991.
20. Sneige N, McNeese MD, Atkinson EN, et al: Ductal carcinoma in situ treated with lumpectomy and irradiation: histopathological analysis of 49 specimens with emphasis on risk factors and long term results. Hum Pathol 26:642, 1995.
21. Aref A, Youssef E, Washington T, et al: The value of postlumpectomy mammogram in the management of breast cancer patients presenting with suspicious microcalcifications. Cancer J Sci Am 6:25, 2000.
22. Lee JM, Orel SG, Czerniecki BJ, et al: MRI before reexcision surgery in patients with breast cancer. AJR Am J Roentgenol 182:473, 2004.
23. Henson DE, Oberman HA, Hutter RV: Practice protocol for the examination of specimens removed from patients with cancer of the breast: a publication of the Cancer Committee, College of American Pathologists. Arch Pathol Lab Med 121:27, 1997.
24. Guidi AJ, Connolly JL, Harris JR, et al: The relationship between shaved margin and inked margin status in breast excision specimens. Cancer 79:1568, 1997.
25. Macmillan RD, Purushotham AD, Mallon E, et al: Tumour bed positivity predicts outcome after breast-conserving surgery. Br J Surg 84:1559, 1997.

26. Veronesi U, Luini A, Galimberti V, et al: Conservation approaches for the management of stage I/II carcinoma of the breast: Milan Cancer Institute trials. World J Surg 18:70, 1994.
27. Salvadori B: Local recurrences after breast-conserving treatment: an open problem. Semin Surg Oncol 12:46, 1996.
28. Arcangeli G, Micheli A, D'Angelo L, et al: A comparison between tumorectomy (TART) and quadrantectomy (QUART) followed by radiotherapy in early stage breast cancer [abstract]. Radiother Oncol 40(Suppl 1):S77, 1996.
29. Berg JW: The significance of axillary node levels in the study of breast cancer. Cancer 8:776, 1955.
30. Recht A, Houlihan MJ: Axillary lymph nodes and breast cancer: a review. Cancer 76:1491, 1995.
31. Semiglazov VF, Krivorotko PV, Petrovskyi SG, et al: Prognostic significance of the number of axillary lymph nodes removed in patients with breast cancer T1-3N0, T1-2N1M0 [abstract]. Eur J Surg Oncol 30:137, 2004.
32. Tominaga T, Takashima S, Danno M: Randomized clinical trial comparing level II and level III axillary node dissection in addition to mastectomy for breast cancer. Br J Surg 91:38, 2004.
33. Recht A, Gray R, Davidson NE, et al: Locoregional failure ten years after mastectomy and adjuvant chemotherapy with or without tamoxifen without irradiation: experience of the Eastern Cooperative Oncology Group. J Clin Oncol 17:1689, 1999.
34. Posther KE, Wilke LG, Giuliano AE: Sentinel lymph node dissection and the current status of American trials on breast lymphatic mapping. Semin Oncol 31:426, 2004.
35. Jakub JW, Cox CE, Pippas AW, et al: Controversial topics in breast lymphatic mapping. Semin Oncol 31:324, 2004.
36. Rietman JS, Dijkstra PU, Geertzen JH, et al: Short-term morbidity of the upper limb after sentinel lymph node biopsy or axillary lymph node dissection for stage I or II breast carcinoma. Cancer 98:690, 2003.
37. Mazonakis M, Varveris H, Damilakis J, et al: Radiation dose to conceptus resulting from tangential breast irradiation. Int J Radiat Oncol Biol Phys 55:386, 2003.
38. Deutsch M, Gerszten K, Bloomer WD, et al: Lumpectomy and breast irradiation for breast cancer arising after previous radiotherapy for Hodgkin's disease or lymphoma. Am J Clin Oncol 24:33, 2001.
39. Wolden SL, Hancock SL, Carlson RW, et al: Management of breast cancer after Hodgkin's disease. J Clin Oncol 18:765, 2000.
40. Ross JG, Hussey DH, Mayr NA, et al: Acute and late reactions to radiation therapy in patients with collagen vascular diseases. Cancer 71:3744, 1993.
41. Chen A, Obedian E, Haffty BG: Breast-conserving therapy in the setting of collagen vascular disease. Cancer J Sci Am 7:480, 2001.
42. Phan C, Mindrum M, Silverman C, et al: Matched-control retrospective study of the acute and late complications in patients with collagen vascular diseases treated with radiation therapy. Cancer J 9:461, 2003.
43. Monson JM, Chin L, Nixon A, et al: Is machine energy (4-8 MV) associated with outcome for stage I-II breast cancer patients? Int J Radiat Oncol Biol Phys 37:1095, 1997.
44. Zhou P, Recht A: Young age and outcome for women with early-stage invasive breast cancer. Cancer 101:1264, 2004.
45. Freedman GM, Hanlon AL, Fowble BL, et al: Recursive partitioning identifies patients at high and low risk for ipsilateral tumor recurrence after breast-conserving surgery and radiation. J Clin Oncol 20:4015, 2002.
46. Neuschatz AC, DiPetrillo T, Safaii H, et al: Long-term follow-up of a prospective policy of margin-directed radiation dose escalation in breast-conserving therapy. Cancer 97:30, 2003.
47. Kroman N, Holtveg H, Wohlfahrt J, et al: Effect of breast-conserving therapy versus radical mastectomy on prognosis for young women with breast carcinoma. Cancer 100:688, 2004.
48. Solin LJ, Schultz DJ, Fowble BL: Ten-year results of the treatment of early-stage breast carcinoma in elderly women using breast-conserving surgery and definitive breast irradiation. Int J Radiat Oncol Biol Phys 33:45, 1995.
49. Vlastos G, Mirza NQ, Meric F, et al: Breast conservation therapy as a treatment option for the elderly: the M.D. Anderson experience. Cancer 92:1092, 2001.
50. Chabner E, Gelman R, Nixon AJ, et al: Family history and treatment outcome in young women after breast-conserving surgery and radiation therapy for early-stage breast cancer. J Clin Oncol 16:2045, 1998.
51. Vlastos G, Mirza NQ, Meric F, et al: Breast-conservation therapy in early-stage breast cancer patients with a positive family history. Ann Surg Oncol 9:912, 2002.
52. Verhoog LC, Brekelmans CTM, Seynaeve C, et al: Survival and tumour characteristics of breast-cancer patients with germline mutations of *BRCA1*. Lancet 351:316, 1998.
53. Chappuis PO, Kapusta L, Bégin LR, et al: Germline BRCA1/2 mutations and $p27^{Kip1}$ protein levels independently predict outcome after breast cancer. J Clin Oncol 18:4045, 2000.
54. Delaloge S, Kloos I, Ariane D, et al: Young age is the major predictor of local relapse among conservatively treated BRCA1-, BRCA2-, or non-BRCA-linked hereditary breast cancer (BC) [abstract 41]. Proc Am Soc Clin Oncol 22:11, 2003.
55. Pierce L, Levin A, Rebbeck T, et al: Ten-year outcome of breast-conserving surgery (BCS) and radiotherapy (RT) in women with breast cancer (BC) and germline BRCA 1/2 mutations: results from an international collaboration [abstract 5]. Breast Cancer Res Treat 82:S7, 2003.
56. Kirova YM, Stoppa-Lyonnet D, Savignoni A, et al: Risk of breast recurrence in relation to BRCA1/2 mutation status following breast-conserving surgery and radiotherapy [abstract 329]. EJC Suppl 2:150, 2004.
57. Robson ME, Chappuis PO, Satagopan J, et al: A combined analysis of outcome following breast cancer: differences in survival based on BRCA1/BRCA2 mutation status and administration of adjuvant treatment. Breast Cancer Res 6:R8, 2004.
58. Robson M, Levin D, Federici M, et al: Breast conservation therapy for invasive breast cancer in Ashkenazi women with BRCA gene founder mutations. J Natl Cancer Inst 91:2112, 1999.
59. Haffty BG, Harrold E, Khan AJ, et al: Outcome of conservatively managed early-onset breast cancer by BRCA1/2 status. Lancet 359:1471, 2002.
60. El-Tamer M, Russo D, Troxel A, et al: Survival and recurrence after breast cancer in BRCA1/2 mutation carriers. Ann Surg Oncol 11:157, 2004.
61. Metcalfe K, Lynch HT, Ghadirian P, et al: Contralateral breast cancer in BRCA1 and BRCA2 mutation carriers. J Clin Oncol 22:2328, 2004.
62. Chenevix-Trench G, Spurdle AB, Gatei M, et al: Dominant negative ATM mutations in breast cancer families. J Natl Cancer Inst 94:205, 2002.
63. Bremer M, Klopper K, Yamini P, et al: Clinical radiosensitivity in breast cancer patients carrying pathogenic ATM gene mutations: no observation of increased radiation-induced acute or late effects. Radiother Oncol 69:155, 2003.
64. Iannuzzi CM, Atencio DP, Green S, et al: ATM mutations in female breast cancer patients predict for an increase in radiation-induced late effects. Int J Radiat Oncol Biol Phys 52:606, 2002.
65. Shafman TD, Levitz S, Nixon AJ, et al: Prevalence of germline truncating mutations in ATM in women with a second breast cancer after radiation therapy for a contralateral tumor. Genes Chromosomes Cancer 27:124, 2000.
66. Geoffroy-Perez B, Janin N, Ossian K, et al: Variation in breast cancer risk of heterozygotes for ataxia-telangiectasia according to environmental factors. Int J Cancer 99:619, 2002.
67. Taylor ME, Perez CA, Halverson KJ, et al: Mammographic presentation and local failure analysis in patients with stage I and II breast cancer treated with conservation therapy [abstract]. Int J Radiat Oncol Biol Phys 36(Suppl 1):279, 1996.
68. Cabioglu N, Krishnamurthy S, Kuerer HM, et al: Feasibility of breast-conserving surgery for patients with breast carcinoma associated with nipple discharge. Cancer 101:508, 2004.
69. Veronesi U, Bonadonna G, Zurrida S, et al: Conservation therapy after primary chemotherapy in large carcinomas of the breast. Ann Surg 222:612, 1995.
70. Fisher ER, Wang J, Bryant J, et al: Pathobiology of preoperative chemotherapy: findings from the National Surgical Adjuvant Breast and Bowel Protocol (NSABP) B-18. Cancer 95:681, 2002.
71. Bussières E, Guyon F, Thomas L, et al: Conservation treatment in subareolar breast cancers. Eur J Surg Oncol 22:267, 1996.
72. Gajdos C, Tartter PI, Bleiweiss IJ: Subareolar breast cancers. Am J Surg 180:167, 2000.

73. Gollamudi SV, Gelman RS, Peiro G, et al: Breast-conserving therapy for stage I-II synchronous bilateral breast cancer. Cancer 79:1362, 1997.
74. Heaton KM, Peoples GE, Singletary SE, et al: Feasibility of breast conservation therapy in metachronous or synchronous bilateral breast cancer. Ann Surg Oncol 6:102, 1999.
75. Dixon JM, Chetty U: Mammography in the management of patients with small breast cancers. Br J Surg 78:218, 1991.
76. Bedrosian I, Schlencker J, Spitz FR, et al: Magnetic resonance imaging-guided biopsy of mammographically and clinically occult breast lesions. Ann Surg Oncol 9:457, 2002.
77. Morimoto T, Okazaki K, Komaki K, et al: Cancerous residue in breast-conserving surgery. J Surg Oncol 52:71, 1993.
78. Hartsell WF, Recine DC, Griem KG, et al: Should multicentric disease be an absolute contraindication to the use of breast-conserving therapy? Int J Radiat Oncol Biol Phys 30:49, 1994.
79. Cho LC, Senzer N, Peters GN: Conservative surgery and radiation therapy for macroscopically multiple ipsilateral invasive breast cancers. Am J Surg 183:650, 2002.
80. Kaplan J, Giron G, Tartter PI, et al: Breast conservation in patients with multiple ipsilateral synchronous cancers. J Am Coll Surg 197:726, 2003.
81. Fowble B, Fein DA, Hanlon AL, et al: The impact of tamoxifen on breast recurrence, cosmesis, complications, and survival in estrogen receptor-positive early-stage breast cancer. Int J Radiat Oncol Biol Phys 35:669, 1996.
82. Wazer DE, Morr J, Erban JK, et al: The effects of postirradiation treatment with tamoxifen on local control and cosmetic outcome in the conservatively treated breast. Cancer 80:732, 1997.
83. Park C, Mitsumori M, Nixon A, et al: Outcome at 8 years following breast-conserving surgery and radiation therapy for invasive breast cancer: influence of margin status and systemic therapy on local recurrences. J Clin Oncol 18:1668, 2000.
84. Cowen D, Houvenaeghel G, Bardou V, et al: Local and distant failures after limited surgery with positive margins and radiotherapy for node-negative breast cancer. Int J Radiat Oncol Biol Phys 47:305, 2000.
85. DiBiase SJ, Komarnicky LT, Schwartz GF, et al: The number of positive margins influences the outcome of women treated with breast preservation for early stage breast carcinoma. Cancer 82:2212, 1998.
86. Freedman G, Fowble B, Hanlon A, et al: Patients with early stage invasive cancer with close or positive margins treated with conservative surgery and radiation have an increased risk of breast recurrence that is delayed by adjuvant systemic therapy. Int J Radiat Oncol Biol Phys 44:1005, 1999.
87. Smitt MC, Nowels K, Carlson RW, et al: Predictors of reexcision findings and recurrence after breast conservation. Int J Radiat Oncol Biol Phys 57:979, 2003.
88. Santiago RJ, Wu L, Harris E, et al: Fifteen-year results of breast-conserving surgery and definitive irradiation for stage I and II breast carcinoma: the University of Pennsylvania experience. Int J Radiat Oncol Biol Phys 58:233, 2004.
89. Goldstein NS, Kestin L, Vicini F: Factors associated with ipsilateral breast failure and distant metastases in patients with invasive breast carcinoma treated with breast-conserving therapy. A clinicopathologic study of 607 neoplasms from 583 patients. Am J Clin Pathol 120:500, 2003.
90. Fisher B, Dignam J, Mamounas EP, et al: Sequential methotrexate and fluorouracil for the treatment of node-negative breast cancer patients with estrogen receptor-negative tumors: eight-year results from the National Surgical Adjuvant Breast and Bowel Protocol (NSABP) B-13 and first report of findings from NSABP B-19 comparing methotrexate and fluorouracil with conventional cyclophosphamide, methotrexate, and fluorouracil. J Clin Oncol 14:1982, 1996.
91. Fisher B, Dignam J, Bryant J, et al: Five versus more than five years of tamoxifen therapy for breast cancer patients with negative lymph nodes and estrogen receptor-positive tumors. J Natl Cancer Inst 88:1529, 1996.
92. Dalberg K, Johansson H, Johansson U, et al: A randomized trial of long term adjuvant tamoxifen plus postoperative radiation therapy versus radiation therapy alone for patients with early stage breast carcinoma treated with breast-conserving surgery. Cancer 82:2204, 1998.
93. Fisher B, Bryant J, Dignam JJ, et al: Tamoxifen, radiation therapy, or both for prevention of ipsilateral breast tumor recurrence after lumpectomy in women with invasive breast cancers of one centimeter or less. J Clin Oncol 20:4141, 2002.
94. Schnitt SJ, Connolly JL: Processing and evaluation of breast excision specimens: a clinically oriented approach. Am J Clin Pathol 98:125, 1992.
95. Holland R, Connolly JL, Gelman R, et al: The presence of an extensive intraductal component following a limited excision correlates with prominent residual disease in the remainder of the breast. J Clin Oncol 8:113, 1990.
96. Weiss MC, Fowble BL, Solin LJ, et al: Outcome of conservative therapy for invasive breast cancer by histologic subtype. Int J Radiat Oncol Biol Phys 23:941, 1992.
97. Warneke J, Berger R, Johnson C, et al: Lumpectomy and radiation treatment for invasive lobular carcinoma of the breast. Am J Surg 172:496, 1996.
98. Peiró G, Bornstein BA, Connolly JL, et al: The influence of infiltrating lobular carcinoma on the outcome of patients treated with breast-conserving surgery and radiation therapy. Breast Cancer Res Treat 59:49, 2000.
99. Kurtz JM, Jacquemier J, Torhorst J, et al: Conservation therapy for breast cancers other than infiltrating ductal carcinoma. Cancer 63:1630, 1989.
100. Thurman SA, Schnitt SJ, Connolly JL, et al: Outcome after breast-conserving therapy for patients with stage I or II mucinous, medullary, or tubular breast carcinoma. Int J Radiat Oncol Biol Phys 59:152, 2004.
101. Millar BA, Kerba M, Youngson B, et al: The potential role of breast conservation surgery and adjuvant breast radiation for adenoid cystic carcinoma of the breast. Breast Cancer Res Treat 87:225, 2004.
102. Fowble B, Hanlon AL, Patchefsky A, et al: The presence of proliferative breast disease with atypia does not significantly influence outcome in early-stage invasive breast cancer treated with conservative surgery and radiation. Int J Radiat Oncol Biol Phys 42:105, 1998.
103. Sasson AR, Fowble B, Hanlon AL, et al: Lobular carcinoma in situ increases the risk of local recurrence in selected patients with stages I and II breast carcinoma treated with conservative surgery and radiation. Cancer 91:1862, 2001.
104. Abner A, Connolly JL, Recht A, et al: The relationship between the presence and extent of lobular carcinoma in situ and the risk of local recurrence in patients with infiltrating cancer of the breast treated with conservative surgery and radiation therapy. Cancer 88:1072, 2000.
105. Forrest AP, Stewart HJ, Everington D, et al: Randomized controlled trial of conservation therapy for breast cancer: 6-year analysis of the Scottish trial. Lancet 348:708, 1996.
106. Vinh-Hung V, Verschraegen C: Breast-conserving surgery with or without radiotherapy: pooled-analysis for risks of ipsilateral breast tumor recurrence and mortality. J Natl Cancer Inst 96:115, 2004.
107. Recht A: Lessons of studies of breast-conserving therapy with and without whole-breast irradiation for patient selection for partial-breast irradiation. Semin Radiat Oncol 15:123, 2005.
108. Liljegren G, Holmberg L, Bergh J, et al: 10-Year results after sector resection with or without postoperative radiotherapy for stage I breast cancer: a randomized trial. J Clin Oncol 17:2326, 1999.
109. Blamey R, Chetti U, George D, et al: Update of the BASO II trial of primary treatment of tumours of excellent prognosis [abstract 360]. EJC Suppl 2:161, 2004.
110. Veronesi U, Marubini E, Mariani L, et al: Radiotherapy after breast-conserving surgery in small breast carcinoma: long-term results of a randomized trial. Ann Oncol 12:997, 2001.
111. Hughes KS, Schnaper LA, Berry D, et al: Lumpectomy plus tamoxifen with or without irradiation in women 70 years of age or older with early breast cancer. N Engl J Med 351:971, 2004.
112. Fyles AW, McCready DR, Manchul LA, et al: Tamoxifen with or without breast irradiation in women 50 years of age or older with early breast cancer. N Engl J Med 351:963, 2004.
113. Winzer K-J, Sauer R, Sauerbrei W, et al: Radiation therapy after breast-conserving surgery: first results of a randomised clinical trial in patients with low risk of recurrence. Eur J Cancer 40:998, 2004.

114. Palda VA, Llewellyn-Thomas HA, Mackenzie RG, et al: Breast cancer patients' attitudes about rationing postlumpectomy radiation therapy: applicability of trade-off methods to policy-making. J Clin Oncol 15:3192, 1997.
115. Hayman JA, Fairclough DL, Harris JR, et al: Patient preferences concerning the trade-off between the risks and benefits of routine radiation therapy after conservative surgery for early-stage breast cancer. J Clin Oncol 15:1252, 1997.
116. Recht A, Come SE, Gelman RS, et al: Integration of conservative surgery, radiotherapy, and chemotherapy for the treatment of early-stage node-positive breast cancer: sequencing, timing, and outcome. J Clin Oncol 9:1662, 1991.
117. Nixon AJ, Recht A, Neuberg D, et al: The relation between the surgery-radiotherapy interval and treatment outcome in patients treated with breast-conserving surgery and radiotherapy without systemic therapy. Int J Radiat Oncol Biol Phys 30:17, 1994.
118. Froud PJ, Mates D, Jackson JS, et al: Effect of time interval between breast-conserving surgery and radiation therapy on ipsilateral breast recurrence. Int J Radiat Oncol Biol Phys 46:363, 2000.
119. Hébert-Croteau N, Freeman CR, Latreille J, et al: Delay in adjuvant radiation treatment and outcomes of breast cancer—a review. Breast Cancer Res Treat 74:77, 2002.
120. Huang J, Barbera L, Brouwers M, et al: Does delay in starting treatment affect the outcomes of radiotherapy? A systematic review. J Clin Oncol 21:555, 2003.
121. Recht A, Come SE, Henderson IC, et al: The sequencing of chemotherapy and radiation therapy after conservative surgery for early-stage breast cancer. N Engl J Med 334:1356, 1996.
122. Bellon JR, Come SE, Gelman RS, et al: The sequencing of chemotherapy and radiation therapy in early stage breast cancer: updated results of a randomized trial. J Clin Oncol 23:1934, 2005.
123. Hartsell WF, Recine DC, Griem KL, et al: Delaying the initiation of intact breast irradiation for patients with lymph node positive breast cancer increases the risk of local recurrence. Cancer 76:2497, 1995.
124. Rouëssé J, Cvitkovic F, De Lalande B, et al: Concomitant or sequential chemo-radiotherapy (CRT) in operable breast cancer. Final results of a French multicentric phase III study [abstract 649]. Breast Cancer Res Treat 76:S160, 2002.
125. Calais G, Serin D, Fourquet A, et al: Randomized study comparing adjuvant radiotherapy (RT) with concomitant chemotherapy (CT) versus sequential treatment after conservative surgery for patients with stages I and II breast carcinoma [abstract 95]. Int J Radiat Oncol Biol Phys 54(Suppl):57, 2002.
126. Dalton WS, Brooks RJ, Jones SE, et al: Breast cancer adjuvant therapy trials at the Arizona Cancer Center using adriamycin and cyclophosphamide. *In* Salmon ES (ed): Adjuvant Therapy of Cancer V. Orlando, Grune & Stratton, 1987, pp 263-269.
127. Buzdar AU, Smith TL, Powell KC, et al: Effect of timing of initiation of adjuvant chemotherapy on disease-free survival in breast cancer. Breast Cancer Res Treat 2:163, 1982.
128. Bellon JR, Shulman LN, Come SE, et al: A prospective study of concurrent cyclophosphamide/methotrexate/5-fluorouracil and reduced-dose radiotherapy in patients with early-stage breast carcinoma. Cancer 100:1358, 2004.
129. International Breast Cancer Study Group: Duration and reintroduction of adjuvant chemotherapy for node-positive premenopausal breast cancer patients. J Clin Oncol 14:1885, 1996.
130. Rutqvist LE, Cedermark B, Glas U, et al: Randomized trial of adjuvant tamoxifen in node negative postmenopausal breast cancer. Acta Oncol 31:265, 1992.
131. Ahn PH, Vu HT, Lannin D, et al: Sequence of radiotherapy with tamoxifen in conservatively managed breast cancer does not affect local relapse rates. J Clin Oncol 23:17, 2005.
132. Pierce LJ, Hutchins LF, Green SR, et al: Sequencing of tamoxifen and radiotherapy after breast-conserving surgery in early-stage breast cancer. J Clin Oncol 23:24, 2005.
133. Recht A: Integration of systemic therapy and radiation therapy for patients with early-stage breast cancer treated with conservative surgery. Clin Breast Cancer 4:104, 2003.
134. Recht A: Tamoxifen and radiotherapy for women with early-stage breast cancer. Breast Dis Yearbook Q 15:238, 2004.
135. Recht A: Should irradiation replace dissection for patients with breast cancer with clinically negative axillary lymph nodes? [Guest editorial]. J Surg Oncol 72:184, 1999.
136. Fisher B, Jeong JH, Anderson S, et al: Twenty-five-year follow-up of a randomized trial comparing radical mastectomy, total mastectomy, and total mastectomy followed by irradiation. N Engl J Med 347:567, 2002.
137. Louis-Sylvestre C, Clough K, Asselain B, et al: Axillary treatment in conservative management of operable breast cancer: dissection or radiotherapy? Results of a randomized study with 15 years of follow-up. J Clin Oncol 22:97, 2004.
138. Goodman RL, Grann A, Saracco P, et al: The relationship between radiation fields and regional lymph nodes in carcinoma of the breast. Int J Radiat Oncol Biol Phys 51:99, 2001.
139. Chung MA, DiPetrillo T, Hernandez S, et al: Treatment of the axilla by tangential breast radiotherapy in women with invasive breast cancer. Am J Surg 184:401, 2002.
140. Halverson KJ, Taylor ME, Perez CA, et al: Regional nodal management and patterns of failure following conservative surgery and radiation therapy for stage I and II breast cancer. Int J Radiat Oncol Biol Phys 26:593, 1993.
141. Wong JS, Recht A, Beard CJ, et al: Treatment outcome after tangential radiation therapy without axillary dissection in patients with early-stage breast cancer and clinically negative axillary nodes. Int J Radiat Oncol Biol Phys 39:915, 1997.
142. McKinna F, Gothard L, Ashley S, et al: Selective avoidance of lymphatic radiotherapy in the conservative management of women with early breast cancer. Radiother Oncol 52:219, 1999.
143. Fujimoto N, Amemiya A, Kondo M, et al: Treatment of breast carcinoma in patients with clinically negative axillary lymph nodes using radiotherapy versus axillary dissection. Cancer 101:2155, 2004.
144. Zurrida S, Orecchia R, Galimberti V, et al: Axillary radiotherapy instead of axillary dissection: a randomized trial. Ann Surg Oncol 9:156, 2002.
145. Fodor J, Tóth J, Major T, et al: Incidence and time of occurrence of regional recurrence in stage I-II breast cancer: value of adjuvant irradiation. Int J Radiat Oncol Biol Phys 44:281, 1999.
146. Chetty U, Jack W, Prescott RJ, et al: Management of the axilla in operable breast cancer treated by breast conservation: a randomized clinical trial. Br J Surg 87:163, 2000.
147. Galper S, Recht A, Silver B, et al: Is radiation alone adequate treatment to the axilla for patients with limited axillary surgery? Implications for treatment after a positive sentinal node biopsy. Int J Radiat Oncol Biol Phys 48:125, 2000.
148. Galper S, Recht A, Silver B, et al: Factors associated with regional nodal failure in patients with early-stage breast cancer with 0-3 positive axillary nodes following tangential irradiation alone. Int J Radiat Oncol Biol Phys 45:1157, 1999.
149. Ewers S-B, Attewell R, Baldetorp B, et al: Flow cytometry analysis and prediction of loco-regional recurrences after mastectomy in breast carcinoma. Acta Oncol 31:733, 1992.
150. Kuske RR, Hayden D, Bischoff R, et al: The impact of extracapsular axillary nodal extension (ECE) with and without irradiation on patterns of failure and survival from breast cancer [abstract]. Int J Radiat Oncol Biol Phys 36(Suppl 1):277, 1996.
151. Chen SC, Chen MF, Hwang TL, et al: Prediction of supraclavicular lymph node metastasis in breast carcinoma. Int J Radiat Oncol Biol Phys 52:614, 2002.
152. Recht A, Pierce SM, Abner A, et al: Regional nodal failure after conservative surgery and radiotherapy for early-stage breast carcinoma. J Clin Oncol 9:988, 1991.
153. Veronesi U, Cascinelli N, Greco M, et al: Prognosis of breast cancer patients after mastectomy and dissection of internal mammary nodes. Ann Surg 202:702, 1985.
154. Sugg SL, Ferguson DJ, Posner MC, et al: Should internal mammary nodes be sampled in the sentinal lymph node era? Ann Surg Oncol 7:188, 2001.
155. Abbès M, Pagin G, Guillaume B, et al: À propos de 195 curages mammaires internes pour cancer du sein. Lyon Chir 79:99, 1983.
156. Noguchi M, Taniya T, Koyasaki N, et al: A multivariate analysis of en bloc extended radical mastectomy versus conventional radical mastectomy in operable breast cancer. Int Surg 77:48, 1992.

157. Arriagada R, Le MG, Mouriesse H, et al: Long-term effect of internal mammary chain treatment. Results of a multivariate analysis of 1195 patients with operable breast cancer and positive axillary nodes. Radiother Oncol 11:213, 1988.
158. Obedian E, Haffty BG: Internal mammary nodal irradiation in conservatively managed breast cancer patients: is there a benefit? Int J Radiat Oncol Biol Phys 44:997, 1999.
159. Fowble B, Hanlon A, Freedman G, et al: Internal mammary node irradiation neither decreases distant metastases nor improves survival in stage I and II breast cancer. Int J Radiat Oncol Biol Phys 47:883, 2000.
160. Lacour J, Bucalossi P, Cacers E, et al: Radical mastectomy versus radical mastectomy plus internal mammary dissection: five-year results of an international cooperative study. Cancer 37:206, 1976.
161. Lacour J, Lê MG, Hill C, et al: Is it useful to remove internal mammary nodes in operable breast cancer? Eur J Surg Oncol 13:309, 1987.
162. Veronesi U, Marubini E, Mariani L, et al: The dissection of internal mammary nodes does not improve the survival of breast cancer patients. 30-year results of a randomized trial. Eur J Cancer 35:1320, 1999.
163. Romestaing P, Ecochard R, Hennequin C, et al: The role of internal mammary chain irradiation on survival after mastectomy for breast cancer—results of a phase III SFRO trial [abstract]. Radiother Oncol 56(Suppl 1):S85, 2000.
164. Fourquet A, Campana F, Rosenwald J-C, et al: Breast irradiation in the lateral decubitus position: technique of the Institut Curie. Radiother Oncol 22:261, 1991.
165. Griem KL, Fetherston P, Kuznetsova M, et al: Three-dimensional photon dosimetry: a comparison of treatment of the intact breast in the supine and prone position. Int J Radiat Oncol Biol Phys 57:891, 2003.
166. Hector CL, Webb S, Evans PM: The dosimetric consequences of inter-fractional patient movement on conventional and intensity-modulated breast radiotherapy treatments. Radiother Oncol 54:57, 2000.
167. Remouchamps VM, Letts N, Yan D, et al: Three-dimensional evaluation of intra- and interfraction immobilization of lung and chest wall using active breathing control: a reproducibility study with breast cancer patients. Int J Radiat Oncol Biol Phys 57:968, 2003.
168. Baroni G, Garibaldi C, Scabini M, et al: Dosimetric effects within target and organs at risk of interfractional patient mispositioning in left breast cancer radiotherapy. Int J Radiat Oncol Biol Phys 59:861, 2004.
169. Frazier RC, Vicini FA, Sharpe MB, et al: Impact of breathing motion on whole breast radiotherapy: a dosimetric analysis using active breathing control. Int J Radiat Oncol Biol Phys 58:1041, 2004.
170. Pedersen AN, Korreman S, Nyström H, et al: Breathing adapted radiotherapy of breast cancer: reduction of cardiac and pulmonary doses using voluntary inspiration breath-hold. Radiother Oncol 72:53, 2004.
171. Remouchamps VM, Letts N, Vicini FA, et al: Initial clinical experience with moderate deep-inspiration breath hold using an active breathing control device in the treatment of patients with left-sided breast cancer using external beam radiation therapy. Int J Radiat Oncol Biol Phys 56:704, 2003.
172. Das IJ, Cheng C-W, Fosmire H, et al: Tolerances in setup and dosimetric errors in the radiation treatment of breast cancer. Int J Radiat Oncol Biol Phys 26:883, 1993.
173. Bentel GC, Marks LB, Whiddon CS, et al: Acute and late morbidity of using a breast positioning ring in women with large/pendulous breasts. Radiother Oncol 50:277, 1999.
174. Valdagni R, Ciocca M, Busana L, et al: Beam modifying devices in the treatment of early breast cancer: 3-D stepped compensating technique. Radiother Oncol 23:192, 1992.
175. Siddon RL, Buck BA, Harris JR, et al: Three-field technique for breast irradiation using tangential field corner blocks. Int J Radiat Oncol Biol Phys 9:583, 1983.
176. Klein EF, Taylor M, Michaletz-Lorenz M, et al: A mono-isocentric technique for breast and regional nodal therapy using dual asymmetric jaws. Int J Radiat Oncol Biol Phys 28:753, 1994.
177. Galvin JM, Powlis W, Fowble B, et al: A new technique for positioning tangential fields. Int J Radiat Oncol Biol Phys 26:877, 1993.
178. Rosenow UF, Valentine ES, Davis LW: A technique for treating local breast cancer using a single set-up point and asymmetric collimation. Int J Radiat Oncol Biol Phys 19:183, 1990.
179. Lu XQ, Sullivan S, Eggleston T, et al: A three-field breast treatment technique with precise geometric matching using multileaf collimator-equipped linear accelerators. Int J Radiat Oncol Biol Phys 55:1420, 2003.
180. Hurkmans CW, Borger JH, Pieters BR, et al: Variability in target volume delineation on CT scans of the breast. Int J Radiat Oncol Biol Phys 50:1366, 2001.
181. Krawczyk JJ, Engel B: The importance of surgical clips for adequate tangential beam planning in breast conserving surgery and irradiation. Int J Radiat Oncol Biol Phys 43:347, 1999.
182. Bentel G, Marks LB, Hardenbergh P, et al: Variability of the location of internal mammary vessels and glandular breast tissue in breast cancer patients undergoing routine CT-based treatment planning. Int J Radiat Oncol Biol Phys 44:1017, 1999.
183. Arthur DW, Arnfield MR, Warwicke LA, et al: Internal mammary node coverage: an investigation of presently accepted techniques. Int J Radiat Oncol Biol Phys 48:139, 2000.
184. Krueger EA, Schipper MJ, Koelling T, et al: Cardiac chamber and coronary artery doses associated with postmastectomy radiotherapy techniques to the chest wall and regional nodes. Int J Radiat Oncol Biol Phys 60:1195, 2004.
185. Madu CN, Quint DJ, Normolle DP, et al: Definition of the supraclavicular and infraclavicular nodes: implications for three-dimensional CT-based conformal radiation therapy. Radiology 221:333, 2001.
186. Dijkema IM, Hofman P, Raaijmakers CP, et al: Loco-regional conformal radiotherapy of the breast: delineation of the regional lymph node clinical target volumes in treatment position. Radiother Oncol 71:287, 2004.
187. Kelly CA, Wang X-Y, Chu JCH, et al: Dose to the contralateral breast: a comparison of four primary breast irradiation techniques. Int J Radiat Oncol Biol Phys 34:727, 1996.
188. Aristei C, Chionne F, Marsella AR, et al: Evaluation of level I and II axillary nodes included in the standard breast tangential fields and calculation of the administered dose: results of a prospective study. Int J Radiat Oncol Biol Phys 51:69, 2001.
189. McCormick B, Botnick M, Hunt M, et al: Are the axillary lymph nodes treated by standard tangent breast fields? J Surg Oncol 81:12, 2002.
190. Takeda A, Shigematsu N, Ikeda T, et al: Evaluation of novel modified tangential irradiation technique for breast cancer patients using dose-volume histograms. Int J Radiat Oncol Biol Phys 58:1280, 2004.
191. Marks LB, Hebert ME, Bentel G, et al: To treat or not to treat the internal mammary nodes: a possible compromise. Int J Radiat Oncol Biol Phys 29:903, 1994.
192. Raj KA, Hardenbergh P, Hollis D, et al: Local recurrence under the heart block in patients with left-sided breast cancer. Int J Radiat Oncol Biol Phys 60(Suppl 1):S403, 2004.
193. De la Rochefordière A, Abner A, Silver B, et al: Are cosmetic results following conservative surgery and radiotherapy for early breast cancer dependent on technique? Int J Radiat Oncol Biol Phys 23:925, 1992.
194. Poortmans P, Bartelink H, Horiot JC, et al: The influence of the boost technique on local control in breast conserving treatment in the EORTC "boost versus no boost" randomised trial. Radiother Oncol 72:25, 2004.
195. Machtay M, Lanciano R, Hoffman J, et al: Inaccuracies in using the lumpectomy scar for planning electron boosts in primary breast carcinoma. Int J Radiat Oncol Biol Phys 30:43, 1994.
196. Gillian D, Hendry JA, Yarnold JR: The use of ultrasound to measure breast thickness to select electron energies for breast boost radiotherapy. Radiother Oncol 32:265, 1994.
197. Bedwinek J: Breast conserving surgery and irradiation: the importance of demarcating the excision cavity with surgical clips. Int J Radiat Oncol Biol Phys 26:675, 1993.
198. Leonard C, Harlow CL, Coffin C, et al: Use of ultrasound to guide radiation boost planning following lumpectomy for carcinoma of the breast. Int J Radiat Oncol Biol Phys 27:1193, 1993.

199. Ringash J, Whelan T, Elliott E, et al: Accuracy of ultrasound in localization of breast boost field. Radiother Oncol 72:61, 2004.
200. Regine WF, Ayyangar KM, Komarnicky LT, et al: Computer-CT planning of the electron boost in definitive breast irradiation. Int J Radiat Oncol Biol Phys 20:121, 1991.
201. Smitt MC, Birdwell RL, Goffinet DR: Breast electron boost planning: comparison of CT and US. Radiology 219:203, 2001.
202. Fein DA, Fowble BA, Hanlon AL, et al: Does the placement of surgical clips within the excision cavity influence local control for patients treated with breast-conserving surgery and irradiation? Int J Radiat Oncol Biol Phys 34:1009, 1996.
203. Das IJ, Cheng C-W, Fein DA, et al: Patterns of dose variability in radiation prescription of breast cancer. Radiother Oncol 44:83, 1997.
204. Kantorowitz DA: The impact of dose-specification policies upon nominal radiation dose received by breast tissue in the conservation treatment of breast cancer. Int J Radiat Oncol Biol Phys 47:841, 2000.
205. Solin LJ, Chu JCH, Sontag MR, et al: Three-dimensional photon treatment planning of the intact breast. Int J Radiat Oncol Biol Phys 21:193, 1991.
206. Buchholz TA, Gurgoze E, Bice WS, et al: Dosimetric analysis of intact breast irradiation in off-axis planes. Int J Radiat Oncol Biol Phys 39:261, 1997.
207. Olivotto IA, Weir LM, Kim-Sing C, et al: Late cosmetic results of short fractionation for breast conservation. Radiother Oncol 41:7, 1996.
208. Magee B, Stewart AL, Swindell R: Outcome of radiotherapy after breast conserving surgery in screen detected breast cancers. Clin Oncol 11:40, 1999.
209. Owen JR, Ashton A, Regan J, et al: Fractionation sensitivity of breast cancer. Results of a randomised trial [abstract 19]. EJC Suppl 1:S9, 2003.
210. Yarnold JR, Owen JR, Ashton A, et al: Fractionation sensitivity of change in breast appearance after radiotherapy for early breast cancer: long-term results of a randomised trial [abstract 77]. Radiother Oncol 64(Suppl 1):S25, 2002.
211. Whelan T, MacKenzie R, Julian J, et al: Randomized trial of breast irradiation schedules after lumpectomy for women with lymph node-negative breast cancer. J Natl Cancer Inst 94:1143, 2002.
212. START Trial Management Group: Standardization of breast radiotherapy (START) trial. Clin Oncol 11:145, 1999.
213. Yarnold JR: Altered fractionation schemes [abstract 32]. EJC Suppl 2:65, 2004.
214. Baillet F, Housset M, Maylin C, et al: The use of a specific hypofractionated radiation therapy regimen versus classical fractionation in the treatment of breast cancer: a randomized study of 230 patients. Int J Radiat Oncol Biol Phys 19:1131, 1990.
215. Maher M, Campana F, Mosseri V, et al: Breast cancer in elderly women: a retrospective analysis of combined treatment with tamoxifen and once-weekly irradiation. Int J Radiat Oncol Biol Phys 31:783, 1995.
216. Koukourakis MI, Giatromanolaki A, Kouroussis C, et al: Hypofractionated and accelerated radiotherapy with cytoprotection (HypoARC): a short, safe, and effective postoperative regimen for high-risk breast cancer patients. Int J Radiat Oncol Biol Phys 52:144, 2002.
217. Yarnold J, Bloomfield D, LeVay J, et al: Prospective randomised trial testing 5.7 Gy and 6.0 Gy fractions of whole-breast radiotherapy in women with early breast cancer ("fast" trial) [abstract P3.02]. Clin Oncol 16:S30, 2004.
218. Schomberg PJ, Shanahan TG, Ingle JN, et al: Accelerated hyperfractionation radiation therapy after lumpectomy and axillary lymph node dissection in patients with stage I or II breast cancer: pilot study. Radiology 202:565, 1997.
219. Pezner RD, Wagman LD, Ben-Ezra J, et al: Breast conservation therapy: local tumor control in patients with pathologically clear margins who receive 5000 cGy breast irradiation without local boost. Breast Cancer Res Treat 32:261, 1994.
220. Smitt MC, Nowels KW, Zdeblick MJ, et al: The importance of the lumpectomy surgical margin status in long term results of breast conservation. Cancer 76:259, 1995.
221. Romestaing P, Lehingue Y, Carrie C, et al: Role of a 10-Gy boost in the conservative treatment of early breast cancer: results of a randomized clinical trial in Lyon, France. J Clin Oncol 15:963, 1997.
222. Romestaing P, Lehingue Y, Delauney C, et al: Role of a 10-Gy boost in the conservation treatment of early breast cancer: results of a randomized clinical trial in Lyon, France [abstract 1]. Int J Radiat Oncol Biol Phys 51(Suppl 1):3, 2001.
223. Tessier E, Héry M, Ramaioli A, et al: Boost in conservative treatment: 6 years results of randomized trial [abstract 345]. Breast Cancer Res Treat 50:287, 1998.
224. Bartelink H, Horiot JC, Poortmans P, et al: Recurrence rates after treatment of breast cancer with standard radiotherapy with or without additional radiation. N Engl J Med 345:1378, 2001.
225. Polgár C, Fodor J, Orosz Z, et al: Electron and high-dose-rate brachytherapy boost in the conservative treatment of stage I-II breast cancer: first results of the randomized Budapest boost trial. Strahlenther Onkol 178:615, 2002.
226. Wazer DE, Schmidt-Ullrich RK, Ruthazer R, et al: Factors determining outcome for breast-conserving irradiation with margin-directed dose escalation to the tumor bed. Int J Radiat Oncol Biol Phys 40:851, 1998.
227. Jones HA, Antonini N, Hart G, et al: Significance of margins of excision on breast cancer recurrence (on behalf of the EORTC Radiotherapy, Breast Cancer Groups) [abstract 316]. EJC Suppl 2:147, 2004.
228. Bentel GC, Marks LB, Hardenbergh PH, et al: Variability of the depth of supraclavicular and axillary lymph nodes in patients with breast cancer: is a posterior axillary boost field necessary? Int J Radiat Oncol Biol Phys 47:755, 2000.
229. Evans PM, Donovan EM, Fenton N, et al: Practical implementation of compensators in breast radiotherapy. Radiother Oncol 49:255, 1998.
230. Chang SX, Deschesne KM, Cullip TJ, et al: A comparison of different intensity modulation treatment techniques for tangential breast irradiation. Int J Radiat Oncol Biol Phys 45:1305, 1999.
231. Vicini FA, Sharpe M, Kestin L, et al: Optimizing breast cancer treatment efficacy with intensity-modulated radiotherapy. Int J Radiat Oncol Biol Phys 54:1336, 2002.
232. Lo YC, Yasuda G, Fitzgerald TJ, et al: Intensity modulation for breast treatment using static multi-leaf collimators. Int J Radiat Oncol Biol Phys 46:187, 2000.
233. Guerrero M, Li XA, Earl MA, et al: Simultaneous integrated boost for breast cancer using IMRT: a radiobiological and treatment planning study. Int J Radiat Oncol Biol Phys 59:1513, 2004.
234. Cho BC, Hurkmans CW, Damen EM, et al: Intensity modulated versus non-intensity modulated radiotherapy in the treatment of the left breast and upper internal mammary lymph node chain: a comparative planning study. Radiother Oncol 62:127, 2002.
235. Krueger EA, Fraass BA, McShan DL, et al: Potential gains for irradiation of chest wall and regional nodes with intensity modulated radiotherapy. Int J Radiat Oncol Biol Phys 56:1023, 2003.
236. Lomax AJ, Cella L, Weber D, et al: Potential role of intensity-modulated photons and protons in the treatment of the breast and regional nodes. Int J Radiat Oncol Biol Phys 55:785, 2003.
237. Yarnold JR, Donovan E, Bleackley N, et al: Randomised trial of standard 2D radiotherapy (RT) versus 3D intensity modulated radiotherapy (IMRT) in patients prescribed breast radiotherapy [abstract 47]. Radiother Oncol 64(Suppl 1):S15, 2002.
238. Arthur D: Accelerated partial breast irradiation: a change in treatment paradigm for early breast cancer. J Surg Oncol 84:185, 2003.
239. Vicini FA, Kestin L, Chen P, et al: Limited-field radiation therapy in the management of early-stage breast cancer. J Natl Cancer Inst 95:1205, 2003.
240. Kuerer HM, Julian TB, Strom EA, et al: Accelerated partial breast irradiation after conservative surgery for breast cancer. Ann Surg 239:338, 2004.
241. Vaidya JS, Tobias JS, Baum M, et al: Intraoperative radiotherapy for breast cancer. Lancet Oncol 5:165, 2004.
242. Keisch M, Vicini F, Kuske RR, et al: Initial clinical experience with the MammoSite breast brachytherapy applicator in women with early-stage breast cancer treated with breast-conserving therapy. Int J Radiat Oncol Biol Phys 55:289, 2003.
243. Vaidya JS, Baum M, Tobias JS, et al: Targeted intra-operative radiotherapy (Targit): an innovative method of treatment for early breast cancer. Ann Oncol 12:1075, 2001.

244. Veronesi U, Gatti G, Luini A, et al: Full-dose intraoperative radiotherapy with electrons during breast-conserving surgery. Arch Surg 138:1253, 2003.
245. Formenti SC, Rosenstein B, Skinner KA, et al: T1 stage breast cancer: adjuvant hypofractionated conformal radiation therapy to tumor bed in selected postmenopausal breast cancer patients—pilot feasibility study. Radiology 222:171, 2002.
246. Baglan KL, Sharpe MB, Jaffray D, et al: Accelerated partial breast irradiation using 3D-conformal radiation therapy (3D-CRT). Int J Radiat Oncol Biol Phys 55:302, 2003.
247. Taghian A, Doppke K, Recht A, et al: Accelerated partial-breast irradiation (APBI) using 3D conformal external beam radiotherapy (3D-CRT) for patients with early-stage breast cancer: preliminary results of an ongoing phase I trial [abstract]. Int J Radiat Oncol Biol Phys 60(Suppl 1):S274, 2004.
248. King TA, Bolton JS, Kuske RR, et al: Long-term results of wide-field brachytherapy as the sole method of radiation therapy after segmental mastectomy for Tis,1,2 breast cancer. Am J Surg 180:299, 2000.
249. Benitez PR, Chen PY, Vicini FA, et al: Partial breast irradiation in breast conserving therapy by way of interstitial brachytherapy. Am J Surg 188:355, 2004.
250. Polgár C, Major T, Fodor J, et al: High-dose-rate brachytherapy alone versus whole breast radiotherapy with or without tumor bed boost after breast-conserving surgery: seven-year results of a comparative study. Int J Radiat Oncol Biol Phys 60:1173, 2004.
251. Ribeiro GG, Magee B, Swindell R, et al: The Christie Hospital breast conservation trial: an update at 8 years from inception. Clin Oncol 5:278, 1993.
252. Campbell IR, Illingworth MH: Can patients wash during radiotherapy to the breast or chest wall? A randomized controlled trial. Clin Oncol 4:78, 1992.
253. Roy I, Fortin A, Larochelle M: The impact of skin washing with water and soap during breast irradiation: a randomized study. Radiother Oncol 58:333, 2001.
254. Williams MS, Burk M, Loprinzi CL, et al: Phase III double-blind evaluation of an aloe vera gel as a prophylactic agent for radiation-induced skin toxicity. Int J Radiat Oncol Biol Phys 36:345, 1996.
255. Olsen DL, Raub W Jr, Bradley C, et al: The effect of aloe vera gel/mild soap versus mild soap alone in preventing skin reactions in patients undergoing radiation therapy. Oncol Nurs Forum 28:543, 2001.
256. Heggie S, Bryant GP, Tripcony L, et al: A phase III study on the efficacy of topical aloe vera gel on irradiated breast tissue. Cancer Nurs 25:442, 2002.
257. Wells M, Raab G, MacBride S, et al: Prevention and management of radiation skin reactions: a randomised controlled trial of skin care approaches in patients with breast, head and neck, and anorectal cancer [abstract 688]. EJC Suppl 1:S207, 2003.
258. Liguori V, Guillemin C, Pesce GF, et al: Double-blind, randomized clinical study comparing hyaluronic acid cream to placebo in patients treated with radiotherapy. Radiother Oncol 42:155, 1997.
259. Böstrom A, Lindman H, Swartling C, et al: Potent corticosteroid cream (mometasone furoate) significantly reduces acute radiation dermatitis: results from a double-blind, randomized study. Radiother Oncol 59:257, 2001.
260. Burch SE, Parker SA, Vann AM, et al: Measurement of 6-MV x-ray surface dose when topical agents are applied prior to external beam irradiation. Int J Radiat Oncol Biol Phys 38:447, 1997.
261. Geinitz H, Zimmermann FB, Stoll P, et al: Fatigue, serum cytokine levels, and blood cell counts during radiotherapy of patients with breast cancer. Int J Radiat Oncol Biol Phys 51:691, 2001.
262. Keidan RD, Hoffman JP, Weese JL, et al: Delayed breast abscesses after lumpectomy and radiation therapy. Ann Surg 56:440, 1990.
263. Mertz KR, Baddour LM, Bell JL, et al: Breast cellulitis following breast conservation therapy: a novel complication of medical progress. Clin Infect Dis 26:481, 1998.
264. Bowers GJ, Prestidge B, Getz JB, et al: Infectious complications in irradiated breasts following conservative breast therapy. The Breast J 1:295, 1995.
265. Brewer VH, Hahn KA, Rohrbach BW, et al: Risk factor analysis for breast cellulitis complicating breast conservation therapy. Clin Infect Dis 31:654, 2000.
266. Staren ED, Klepek S, Smith AP, et al: The dilemma of breast cellulitis after breast conservation therapy. Arch Surg 131:651, 1996.
267. Schaffer JV, Carroll C, Dvoretsky I, et al: Postirradiation morphea of the breast: presentation of two cases and review of the literature. Dermatology 200:67, 2000.
268. Schnitt SJ, Connolly JL, Harris JR, et al: Radiation-induced changes in the breast. Hum Pathol 15:545, 1984.
269. Boyages J, Bilous M, Barraclough B, et al: Fat necrosis of the breast following lumpectomy and radiation therapy for early breast cancer. Radiother Oncol 13:69, 1988.
270. Rayan G, Dawson LA, Bezjak A, et al: Prospective comparison of breast pain in patients participating in a randomized trial of breast-conserving surgery and tamoxifen with or without radiotherapy. Int J Radiat Oncol Biol Phys 55:154, 2003.
271. Delanian S, Porcher R, Balla-Mekias S, et al: Randomized, placebo-controlled trial of combined pentoxifylline and tocopherol for regression of superficial radiation-induced fibrosis. J Clin Oncol 21:2545, 2003.
272. Okunieff P, Augustine E, Hicks JE, et al: Pentoxifylline in the treatment of radiation-induced fibrosis. J Clin Oncol 22:2207, 2004.
273. Pierce SM, Recht A, Lingos T, et al: Long-term radiation complications following conservative surgery (CS) and radiation therapy (RT) in patients with early stage breast cancer. Int J Radiat Oncol Biol Phys 23:915, 1992.
274. Shapiro CL, Recht A: Side effects of adjuvant therapy for breast cancer. N Engl J Med 344:1997, 2001.
275. Petrek JA: Post-treatment sarcomas. *In* Harris JR, Hellman S, Henderson IC, et al (eds): Breast Diseases, 2nd ed. Philadelphia, JB Lippincott, 1991, pp 834-839.
276. Cabanes PA, Salmon RJ, Vilcoq JR, et al: Value of axillary dissection in addition to lumpectomy and radiotherapy in early breast cancer. Lancet 339:1245, 1992.
277. Larson D, Weinstein M, Goldberg I, et al: Edema of the arm as a function of the extent of axillary surgery in patients with stage I-II carcinoma of the breast treated with primary radiotherapy. Int J Radiat Oncol Biol Phys 12:1575, 1986.
278. Delouche G, Bachelot F, Premont M, et al: Conservation treatment of early breast cancer: long term results and complications. Int J Radiat Oncol Biol Phys 13:29, 1987.
279. Pierquin B, Huart J, Raynal M, et al: Conservative treatment for breast cancer: long-term results (15 years). Radiother Oncol 20:16, 1991.
280. Pierce LJ, Oberman HA, Strawderman MH, et al: Microscopic extracapsular extension in the axilla: is this an indication for axillary radiotherapy? Int J Radiat Oncol Biol Phys 33:253, 1995.
281. McNeely ML, Magee DJ, Lees AW, et al: The addition of manual lymph drainage to compression therapy for breast cancer related lymphedema: a randomized controlled trial. Breast Cancer Res Treat 86:95, 2004.
282. Vecht CJ, Van de Brand HJ, Wajer OJM: Post-axillary dissection pain in breast cancer due to a lesion of the intercostobrachial nerve. Pain 38:171, 1989.
283. Watson CPN, Evans RJ, Watt VR: The post-mastectomy pain syndrome and the effect of topical capsaicin. Pain 38:177, 1989.
284. Gerber L, Lampert M, Wood C, et al: Comparison of pain, motion, and edema after modified radical mastectomy vs. local excision with axillary dissection and radiation. Breast Cancer Res Treat 21:139, 1992.
285. Lin PP, Allison DC, Wainstock J, et al: Impact of axillary lymph node dissection on the therapy of breast cancer patients. J Clin Oncol 11:1536, 1993.
286. Gutman H, Kersz T, Barzilai T, et al: Achievements of physical therapy in patients after modified radical mastectomy compared with quadrantectomy, axillary dissection, and radiation for carcinoma of the breast. Arch Surg 125:389, 1990.
287. Rietman JS, Dijkstra PU, Hoekstra HJ, et al: Late morbidity after treatment of breast cancer in relation to daily activities and quality of life: a systematic review. Eur J Surg Oncol 29:229, 2003.
288. Marks LB: The pulmonary effects of thoracic irradiation. Oncology (Huntingt) 8:89, 1994.
289. Takigawa N, Segawa Y, Saeki T, et al: Bronchiolitis obliterans organizing pneumonia syndrome in breast-conserving therapy

for early breast cancer: radiation-induced lung toxicity. Int J Radiat Oncol Biol Phys 48:751, 2000.

290. Lingos TI, Recht A, Vicini F, et al: Radiation pneumonitis in breast cancer patients treated with conservative surgery and radiation therapy. Int J Radiat Oncol Biol Phys 21:355, 1991.
291. Lind PA, Wennberg B, Gagliardi G, et al: Pulmonary complications following different radiotherapy techniques for breast cancer, and the association to irradiated lung volume and dose. Breast Cancer Res Treat 68:199, 2001.
292. Lind PA, Marks LB, Hardenbergh PH, et al: Technical factors associated with radiation pneumonitis after local +/− regional radiation therapy for breast cancer. Int J Radiat Oncol Biol Phys 52:137, 2002.
293. Overmoyer B, Fowble B, Solin L, et al: The long term results of conservative surgery and radiation with concurrent chemotherapy for early stage breast cancer [abstract]. Proc Am Soc Clin Oncol 11:90, 1992.
294. Bentzen SM, Skoczylas JZ, Overgaard M, et al: Radiotherapy-related lung fibrosis enhanced by tamoxifen. J Natl Cancer Inst 88:918, 1996.
295. Koc M, Polat P, Suma S: Effects of tamoxifen on pulmonary fibrosis after cobalt-60 radiotherapy in breast cancer patients. Radiother Oncol 64:171, 2002.
296. Theodoulou M, Seidman AD: Cardiac effects of adjuvant therapy for early breast cancer. Semin Oncol 30:730, 2003.
297. Rutqvist LE, Johansson H: Mortality by laterality of the primary tumor among 55,000 breast cancer patients from the Swedish Cancer Registry. Br J Cancer 61:866, 1990.
298. Paszat LF, Mackillop WJ, Groome PA, et al: Mortality from myocardial infarction after adjuvant radiotherapy for breast cancer in the Surveillance, Epidemiology, and End-Results cancer registries. J Clin Oncol 16:2625, 1998.
299. Gyenes G, Rutqvist LE, Liedberg A, et al: Long-term cardiac morbidity and mortality in a randomized trial of pre- and post-operative radiation therapy versus surgery alone in primary breast cancer. Radiother Oncol 48:185, 1998.
300. Nixon AJ, Manola J, Gelman R, et al: No long-term increase in cardiac-related mortality after breast-conserving surgery and radiation therapy using modern techniques. J Clin Oncol 16:1374, 1998.
301. Rutqvist LE, Liedberg A, Hammar N, et al: Myocardial infarction among women with early-stage breast cancer treated with conservative surgery and breast irradiation. Int J Radiat Oncol Biol Phys 40:359, 1998.
302. Højris I, Overgaard M, Christensen JJ, et al: Morbidity and mortality of ischemic heart disease in high-risk breast-cancer patients after adjuvant postmastectomy systemic treatment with or without radiotherapy: analysis of DBCG 82b and 82c randomized trials. Lancet 354:1425, 1999.
303. Valagussa P, Zambetti M, Biasi S, et al: Cardiac effects following adjuvant chemotherapy and breast irradiation in operable breast cancer. Ann Oncol 5:209, 1994.
304. Zambetti M, Moliterni A, Materazzo C, et al: Long-term cardiac sequelae in operable breast cancer patients given adjuvant chemotherapy with or without doxorubicin and breast irradiation. J Clin Oncol 19:37, 2001.
305. Meinardi MT, van Veldhuisen DJ, Gietema JA, et al: Prospective evaluation of early cardiac damage induced by epirubicin-containing adjuvant chemotherapy and locoregional radiotherapy in breast cancer patients. J Clin Oncol 19:2746, 2001.
306. Bonneterre J, Roche H, Kerbrat P, et al: Long-term cardiac follow-up in relapse-free patients after six courses of fluorouracil, epirubicin, and cyclophosphamide, with either 50 or 100 mg of epirubicin, as adjuvant therapy for node-positive breast cancer: French adjuvant study group. J Clin Oncol 22:3070, 2004.
307. Boice JD, Harvey EB, Blettner M, et al: Cancer in the contralateral breast after radiotherapy for breast cancer. N Engl J Med 326:781, 1992.
308. Gao X, Fisher SG, Emami B: Risk of second primary cancer in the contralateral breast in women treated for early-stage breast cancer: a population-based study. Int J Radiat Oncol Biol Phys 56:1038, 2003.
309. Monroe AT, Feigenberg SJ, Mendenhall NP: Angiosarcoma after breast-conserving therapy. Cancer 97:1832, 2003.
310. Kurtz JM, Amalric R, Brandone H, et al: Contralateral breast cancer and other second malignancies in patients treated by breast-conserving therapy with radiation. Int J Radiat Oncol Biol Phys 15:277, 1988.
311. Taghian A, de Vathaire F, Terrier P, et al: Long-term risk of sarcoma following radiation treatment for breast cancer. Int J Radiat Oncol Biol Phys 21:361, 1991.
312. Huang J, Mackillop WJ: Increased risk of soft tissue sarcoma after radiotherapy in women with breast carcinoma. Cancer 92:172, 2001.
313. Strobbe LJA, Peterse HL, van Tinteren H, et al: Angiosarcoma of the breast after conservation therapy for invasive cancer, the incidence and outcome. An unforeseen sequela. Breast Cancer Res Treat 47:101, 1998.
314. Marchal C, Weber B, de Lafontan B, et al: Nine breast angiosarcomas after conservative treatment for breast carcinoma: a survey from French comprehensive cancer centers. Int J Radiat Oncol Biol Phys 44:113, 1999.
315. Inskip PD, Stovall M, Flannery FT: Lung cancer risk and radiation dose among women treated for breast cancer. J Natl Cancer Inst 86:983, 1994.
316. Neugut AI, Murray T, Santos J, et al: Increased risk of lung cancer after breast cancer radiation therapy in cigarette smokers. Cancer 73:1615, 1994.
317. Ford MB, Sigurdson AJ, Petrulis ES, et al: Effects of smoking and radiotherapy on lung carcinoma in breast carcinoma survivors. Cancer 98:1457, 2003.
318. Zablotska LB, Neugut AI: Lung carcinoma after radiation therapy in women treated with lumpectomy or mastectomy for primary breast carcinoma. Cancer 97:1404, 2003.
319. Deutsch M, Land SR, Begovic M, et al: The incidence of lung carcinoma after surgery for breast carcinoma with and without postoperative radiotherapy. Results of National Surgical Adjuvant Breast and Bowel Project (NSABP) clinical trials B-04 and B-06. Cancer 98:1362, 2003.
320. Crump M, Tu D, Shepherd L, et al: Risk of acute leukemia following epirubicin-based adjuvant chemotherapy: a report from the National Cancer Institute of Canada Clinical Trials Group. J Clin Oncol 21:3066, 2003.
321. Smith RE, Bryant J, DeCillis A, et al: Acute myeloid leukemia and myelodysplastic syndrome after doxorubicin-cyclophosphamide adjuvant therapy for operable breast cancer: the National Surgical Adjuvant Breast and Bowel Project experience. J Clin Oncol 21:1195, 2003.
322. Kaija H, Rauni S, Jorma I, et al: Consistency of patient- and doctor-assessed cosmetic outcome after conservative treatment of breast cancer. Breast Cancer Res Treat 45:225, 1997.
323. Hoeller U, Kuhlmey A, Bajrovic A, et al: Cosmesis from the patient's and the doctor's view. Int J Radiat Oncol Biol Phys 57:345, 2003.
324. Vrieling C, Collette L, Bartelink E, et al: Validation of the methods of cosmetic assessment after breast-conserving therapy in the EORTC "boost versus no boost" trial. Int J Radiat Oncol Biol Phys 45:667, 1999.
325. Marinus J, Niel CG, de Bie RA, et al: Measuring radiation fibrosis: the interobserver reliability of two methods of determining the degree of radiation fibrosis. Int J Radiat Oncol Biol Phys 47:1209, 2000.
326. Vrieling C, Collette L, Fourquet A, et al: The influence of patient, tumor and treatment factors on the cosmetic results after breast-conserving therapy in the EORTC "boost vs. no boost" trial. Radiother Oncol 55:219, 2000.
327. Pezner RD, Patterson MP, Lipsett JA, et al: Factors affecting cosmetic outcome in breast-conserving cancer treatment—objective quantitative assessment. Breast Cancer Res Treat 20:85, 1991.
328. Gray JR, McCormick B, Cox L, et al: Primary breast irradiation in large-breasted or heavy women: analysis of cosmetic outcome. Int J Radiat Oncol Biol Phys 21:347, 1991.
329. Moody AM, Mayles WPM, Bliss JM, et al: The influence of breast size on late radiation effects and association with radiation dose inhomogeneity. Radiother Oncol 33:106, 1994.
330. Taylor ME, Perez CA, Halverson KJ, et al: Factors influencing cosmetic results after conservation therapy for breast cancer. Int J Radiat Oncol Biol Phys 31:753, 1995.

331. Van Limbergen E, Rijnders A, van der Scheuren E, et al: Cosmetic evaluation of breast conserving treatment for mammary cancer. 2. A quantitative analysis of the influence of radiation dose, fractionation schedules and surgical treatment techniques on cosmetic results. Radiother Oncol 16:253, 1989.
332. Christensen VJ, Harris E, Hwang W-T, et al: The impact of concurrent versus sequential tamoxifen and radiation therapy in breast cancer patients undergoing breast conservation therapy [abstract 40]. Proc Am Soc Clin Oncol 22:11, 2003.
333. Kaas R, Hart AA, Besnard AP, et al: Impact of mammographic interval on stage and survival after the diagnosis of contralateral breast cancer. Br J Surg 88:123, 2001.
334. Morakkabati N, Leutner CC, Schmiedel A, et al: Breast MR imaging during or soon after radiation therapy. Radiology 229:893, 2003.
335. Smith TJ, Davidson NE, Schapira DV, et al: American Society of Clinical Oncology 1998 update of recommended breast cancer surveillance guidelines. J Clin Oncol 17:1080, 1999.
336. Fourquet A, Campana F, Zafrani B, et al: Prognostic factors of breast recurrence in the conservative management of early breast cancer: a 25-year follow-up. Int J Radiat Oncol Biol Phys 17:719, 1989.
337. Kurtz JM, Amalric R, Brandone H, et al: Local recurrence after breast-conserving surgery and radiotherapy: frequency, time course, and prognosis. Cancer 63:1912, 1989.
338. Veronesi W, Salvadori B, Luini A: Conservative treatment of early breast cancer. Long-term results of 1232 cases treated with quadrantectomy, axillary dissection, and radiotherapy. Ann Surg 211:250, 1990.
339. Vicini FA, Recht A, Abner A, et al: Recurrence in the breast following conservative surgery and radiation therapy for early-stage breast cancer. J Natl Cancer Inst Monogr 11:33, 1992.
340. Krauss DJ, Kestin LL, Mitchell C, et al: Changes in temporal patterns of local failure after breast-conserving therapy and their prognostic implications. Int J Radiat Oncol Biol Phys 60:731, 2004.
341. Chen C, Orel SG, Harris EE, et al: Relation between the method of detection of initial breast carcinoma and the method of detection of subsequent ipsilateral local recurrence and contralateral breast carcinoma. Cancer 98:1596, 2003.
342. Solin LJ, Fowble BL, Troupin RH, et al: Biopsy results of new calcifications in the postirradiated breast. Cancer 63:1956, 1989.
343. Belli P, Costantini M, Romani M, et al: Magnetic resonance imaging in breast cancer recurrence. Breast Cancer Res Treat 73:223, 2002.
344. Lannin DR, Haffty BG: End results of salvage therapy after failure of breast-conservation surgery. Oncology (Huntingt) 18:272, 2004.
345. Fredriksson I, Liljegren G, Arnesson LG, et al: Local recurrence in the breast after conservative surgery—a study of prognosis and prognostic factors in 391 women. Eur J Cancer 38:1860, 2002.
346. Voogd AC, van Tienhoven G, Peterse HL, et al: Local recurrence after breast conservation therapy for early stage breast cancer: detection, treatment, and outcome in 266 patients. Cancer 85:437, 1999.
347. McBain CA, Young EA, Swindell R, et al: Local recurrence of breast cancer following surgery and radiotherapy: incidence and outcome. Clin Oncol 15:25, 2003.
348. Vicini FA, Kestin L, Huang R, et al: Does local recurrence affect the rate of distant metastases and survival in patients with early-stage breast carcinoma treated with breast-conserving therapy? Cancer 97:910, 2003.
349. Galper S, Blood E, Gelman R, et al: Prognosis following local recurrence after conservative surgery and radiation for early-stage breast cancer. Int J Radiat Oncol Biol Phys 61:348, 2005.
350. Gage I, Schnitt SJ, Recht A, et al: Skin recurrences after breast-conserving therapy for early stage breast cancer. J Clin Oncol 16:480, 1998.
351. Williams JK, Bostwick J, Bried JT, et al: TRAM flap breast reconstruction after radiation treatment. Ann Surg 221:756, 1995.
352. Kroll SS, Schusterman MA, Reece GP, et al: Breast reconstruction with myocutaneous flaps in previously irradiated patients. Plast Reconstr Surg 93:460, 1994.
353. Spear SL, Onyewu C: Staged breast reconstruction with saline-filled implants in the irradiated breast: recent trends and therapeutic implications. Plast Reconstr Surg 105:930, 2000.
354. Dalberg K, Mattsson A, Sandelin K, et al: Outcome of treatment for ipsilateral breast tumor recurrence in early-stage breast cancer. Breast Cancer Res Treat 49:69, 1998.
355. Salvadori B, Marubini E, Miceli R, et al: Reoperation for locally recurrent breast cancer in patients previously treated with conservative surgery. Br J Surg 86:84, 1999.
356. Deutsch M: Repeat high-dose external beam irradiation after lumpectomy for in-breast tumor recurrences after previous lumpectomy and breast irradiation. Int J Radiat Oncol Biol Phys 53:687, 2002.
357. Resch A, Fellner C, Mock U, et al: Locally recurrent breast cancer: pulse dose rate brachytherapy for repeat irradiation following lumpectomy—a second chance to preserve the breast. Radiology 225:713, 2002.
358. Dalberg K, Liedberg A, Johansson U, et al: Uncontrolled local disease after salvage treatment for ipsilateral breast tumour recurrence. Eur J Surg Oncol 29:143, 2003.
359. Clark RM, Whelan T, Levine M, et al: Randomized clinical trial of breast irradiation following lumpectomy and axillary dissection for node-negative breast cancer: an update. J Natl Cancer Inst 88:1659, 1996.
360. Malmström P, Holmberg L, Anderson H, et al: Breast conservation surgery, with and without radiotherapy, in women with lymph node-negative breast cancer: a randomised clinical trial in a population with access to public mammography screening. Eur J Cancer 39:1690, 2003.
361. McCready DR, Chapman J-A, Wall JL, et al: Characteristics of local recurrences following lumpectomy for breast cancer. Cancer Invest 12:568, 1994.
362. Arriagada R, Lê MG, Guinebretiere JM, et al: Late local recurrences in a randomised trial comparing conservative treatment with total mastectomy in early breast cancer patients. Ann Oncol 14:1617, 2003.
363. Veronesi U, Cascinelli N, Mariani L, et al: Twenty-year follow-up of a randomised study comparing breast-conserving surgery with radical mastectomy for early breast cancer. N Engl J Med 347:1227, 2002.
364. Fisher B, Anderson S, Bryant J, et al: Twenty-year follow-up of a randomized trial comparing total mastectomy, lumpectomy, and lumpectomy plus irradiation for the treatment of invasive breast cancer. N Engl J Med 347:1233, 2002.
365. Poggi MM, Danforth DN, Sciuto LC, et al: Eighteen-year results in the treatment of early breast carcinoma with mastectomy versus breast conservation therapy: The National Cancer Institute Randomized Trial. Cancer 98:697, 2003.
366. Van Dongen JA, Voogd AC, Fentiman IS, et al: Long-term results of a randomized trial comparing breast-conserving therapy with mastectomy: European Organization for Research and Treatment of Cancer 10801 trial. J Natl Cancer Inst 92:1143, 2000.
367. Blichert-Toft M, Rose C, Andersen JA, et al: A Danish randomized trial comparing breast conservation with mastectomy in mammary carcinoma. J Natl Cancer Inst Monogr 11:19, 1992.
368. Renton SC, Gazet J-C, Ford HT, et al: The importance of the resection margin in conservative surgery for breast cancer. Eur J Surg Oncol 22:17, 1996.
369. McCready DR, Chapman JA, Hanna WM, et al: Factors associated with local breast cancer recurrence after lumpectomy alone: postmenopausal patients. Ann Surg Oncol 7:562, 2000.
370. Lee SH, Chung MA, Chelmow D, Cady B: Avoidance of adjuvant radiotherapy in selected patients with invasive breast cancer. Ann Surg Oncol 11:316, 2004.
371. Gruenberger T, Gorlitzer M, Mittlboeck M, et al: Adjuvant radiotherapy has no benefit after primary breast cancer treatment in selected postmenopausal patients (Abstr.). Eur J Cancer 34 (suppl. 1):S31, 1998.

CHAPTER 61

BREAST CANCER: STAGES T3 AND T4

Locally Advanced and Inflammatory Breast Cancer and Postmastectomy Radiation Therapy

Thomas A. Buchholz, Massimo Cristofanilli, and Eric A. Strom

INCIDENCE

Although the overall incidence of breast cancer has increased since 1980, the percentage of cancers diagnosed as T3 or T4 primary disease has consistently declined. Reasons for this decline include the increasing use of screening mammography and the public campaign aimed at promoting women's health through education and self-awareness.

BIOLOGIC CHARACTERISTICS

T3 or T4 primary disease usually occurs because of lack of screening to detect the lesion at an earlier stage, a delay in treating an apparent lesion due to misdiagnosis, or aggressive tumor biology with rapid disease growth.

Advanced breast cancer represents a diverse spectrum of biologic characteristics. As with early-stage disease, most T3 or T4 breast tumors are of the infiltrating ductal subtype.

Patients who are diagnosed with locally advanced breast cancer shortly after the first sign or symptom of the disease commonly have a tumor with high nuclear grade, high proliferative indices, estrogen and progesterone receptor–negative disease, and amplification of the *ERBB2 (HER2/NEU)* oncogene.

Patients who present long after symptoms first appear are more likely to have tumors with a lower nuclear grade, lower proliferative indices, and estrogen and progesterone receptor–positive disease.

Inflammatory breast cancer is a subgroup of advanced breast cancer that is commonly associated with a clinical history of rapid disease growth, a high propensity for metastatic spread, and a tendency to invade the dermal lymphatics.

STAGING EVALUATION

Patients with advanced primary tumors warrant comprehensive staging to exclude the presence of metastatic disease and to delineate the extent of locoregional disease.

All patients should provide a history and undergo physical examination. Evaluation should include diagnostic mammography, serum chemistry studies, chest radiography, bone scan, and imaging of the liver.

Although less commonly used, pretreatment ultrasonography of the breast and lymphatics can be clinically valuable in assessing the extent of locoregional disease.

THERAPY

Locally advanced breast cancer requires multimodality treatment that includes multiagent chemotherapy, surgery, and radiation therapy.

Neoadjuvant chemotherapy plays an important role in helping patients with initially unresectable disease become operative candidates, and it may allow carefully selected patients to undergo breast-conserving surgery.

After chemotherapy and surgery, all patients with locally advanced breast cancer should receive irradiation to the breast or chest wall and the draining lymphatics.

All patients with hormonally responsive disease should also receive adjuvant tamoxifen or an aromatase inhibitor, or both.

OUTCOMES

Outcomes of patients with stage III breast cancer have significantly improved over the past 2 decades. With anthracycline chemotherapy, surgery, radiation therapy, and hormonal treatments, approximately two thirds of patients with stage IIB or IIIA disease and one third of patients with stage IIIB disease survive 10 years without disease recurrence. These outcome data may be underestimations because they do not incorporate the added survival benefits of taxanes, other new chemotherapeutics, aromatase inhibitors, and improvements in radiation therapy and surgery.

Long-term locoregional recurrence rates after surgery and radiation therapy for patients with advanced disease range from 10% to 25%, depending on the particular features of the disease.

Locally advanced breast cancer remains a therapeutic challenge for oncology specialists. Patients who present with large primary tumors or extensive regional disease usually are at high risk for distant and locoregional disease recurrence. These patients benefit from aggressive systemic and locoregional treatment approaches. The administration of these treatments requires careful coordination among all disciplines involved in oncology. Previous data have indicated that the degree to which this coordination exists and the experience of the treating center can affect the treatment outcome. In a study of breast cancer patients in California, those treated at large teaching hospitals had significantly better survival rates than those treated at small community or health maintenance organization hospitals.[1] Multidisciplinary care is of particular importance for patients with advanced disease because the optimal sequencing of various therapies is less straightforward than for patients with early-stage breast cancer.

Locally advanced breast cancer was once considered a fatal disease. Before the routine use of chemotherapy, most patients developed distant metastases and died.[2-4] In the past, locoregional treatments—mastectomy alone, radiation therapy alone, or combined surgery and irradiation—were attempted to prevent uncontrolled locoregional disease progression. With such strategies, the outcome of patients was poor.[2-4] Fortunately, the current outlook for patients with locally advanced breast cancer is much more optimistic. Although distant metastases remain a persistent problem, long-term disease-free survival rates have significantly improved with systemic treatments.[5] This improvement in metastatic disease control has also heightened the importance of achieving locoregional control. Arguably, the success of chemotherapy in eradicating micrometastatic disease has allowed the advances achieved in surgery and radiation therapy to also contribute to improved patient survival. Because of the improvements in locoregional and systemic treatments, combined-modality therapy has become the standard of care for all patients with stage IIB and III breast cancer.

The term *locally advanced breast cancer* represents a heterogeneous category of biologically diverse diseases. The term itself most commonly refers to patients with stage III breast cancer, but this definition is not universally accepted. In addition to the ambiguity of the term *locally advanced breast cancer*, the disease within this category is itself heterogeneous. At one end of the spectrum, stage III breast cancer includes biologically aggressive and rapidly proliferating inflammatory breast cancer. At the other end of the spectrum, stage III breast cancer can also represent estrogen receptor–positive indolent disease that has over many years grown to a considerable size but failed to metastasize. These diverse disease characteristics should be considered when making treatment decisions and predicting outcomes.

ETIOLOGY

Breast cancer is a disease resulting from a complex series of genetic and epigenetic events that result in the dysfunction of several cellular and microenvironmental processes. Genetic mutations, in which specific nucleotide base pairs of a gene are altered or lost, are common in breast cancers, particularly in cases of locally advanced disease. Most genetic mutations in breast cancer are somatic, meaning they developed during the lifetime of the cell rather than occurring as an inherited condition. A mutation in the *TP53* gene is one example of a common somatic mutation seen in locally advanced breast cancer.[6] This mutation results in a loss of the critical tumor suppressor functions of the normal *TP53* gene, including cell cycle arrest or induction of apoptosis after injury to cellular DNA.

Germline mutations in tumor suppressor genes can also play a role in the development of some locally advanced breast cancers. The most common of these inherited mutations are mutations in *BRCA1* or *BRCA2*. The *BRCA1* mutations are particularly relevant to locally advanced breast cancer because they are associated with a biologically aggressive phenotype that is characterized by a higher nuclear grade, estrogen receptor–negative disease, and a higher proliferative index.[7,8]

Many locally advanced breast cancers also have abnormalities in growth-promoting proto-oncogenes. The best-characterized proto-oncogene abnormality is the overexpression of ERBB2 (also designated HER2 and formerly called HER2/NEU), a cell surface receptor with an internal tyrosine kinase domain that activates a variety of downstream signaling pathways. HER2 protein overexpression has been associated with an increased proliferative capacity, enhancement of the metastatic potential, and increased rate of tumorigenesis.[9,10]

Environmental and epigenetic factors also play important roles in breast cancer development and disease progression. Radiation exposure, alcohol consumption, and a variety of estrogenic conditions are known to be associated with breast cancer development.[11-13] Data suggest that the microenvironment of the breast is a critical element of breast cancer formation and progression. For example, the proliferation of vasculature in the microenvironment (i.e., angiogenesis) is of critical importance to tumor progression.

EPIDEMIOLOGY

The incidence of locally advanced breast cancer is decreasing in the United States, despite the fact that the overall incidence of breast cancer is increasing. The American Cancer Society estimated that between 1980 and 1987 the incidence of breast cancer increased at a rate of 4% per year; since that time, the incidence has continued to increase at a rate of 0.4% per year.[14,15] The 4% annual increase between 1980 and 1987 in part reflected an increase in mammography screening during this period, and the more gradual subsequent increases have resulted from more women moving into the higher-risk age groups and more women having risk factors such as delayed child birth, nulliparity, and postmenopausal use of estrogen and progesterone.

Despite the annual increase in breast cancer incidence, the proportion of breast cancers that are diagnosed as locally advanced disease and the incidence of locally advanced disease have both decreased. The incidence rates for tumors 3.0 cm or larger decreased 27% between 1980 and 1987, and in more recent years, the rates of larger tumors have continued to decline by 1.9% annually.[14,15] In the year 2000, it was estimated that only 6% of breast cancers were larger than 5.0 cm at the time of diagnosis. Given this trend, it was reasonable to estimate that 12,000 patients would be diagnosed with T3 or T4 breast cancer in 2004.

There are two major reasons for the decline in the incidence of locally advanced breast cancer. First, mammographic screening has shifted the extent of disease at diagnosis toward earlier disease stages. Second, public education and women's health initiatives have prompted women to seek out medical care at the first sign of a breast mass and have helped educate the medical community about appropriate standards for evaluating a breast mass.

There are still subgroups of patients for whom locally advanced breast cancer remains an epidemiologic problem. For example, black women in the United States are more often diagnosed with locally advanced disease than white women.[14,15] This finding was first noticed during the 1980s and continues to be true today. There are many possible reasons for the higher incidence of locally advanced breast cancer in African Americans, including decreased access to medical care, less use of screening mammography, and biologic differences in the cancer. Specifically, breast cancers in black women tend to be of higher grade and more often lack estrogen receptors compared with those in white women in the United States.[16,17]

BIOLOGIC CHARACTERISTICS AND MOLECULAR BIOLOGY

Locally advanced breast cancer can result from rapid disease growth with early spread to the lymphatics or from a delay in treatment. A thorough patient history and physical examination combined with an assessment of the tumor's biologic features can help to distinguish these two categories. Typically, rapid disease growth occurs in the setting of high-grade tumors that have high proliferative indices, high rates of estrogen receptor-negative disease, and high rates of HER2 overexpression. Advanced primary tumors in patients who present for treatment many years after first appreciating a breast abnormality are more commonly of lower grade and are estrogen receptor positive.

Advances in genomics and molecular biology have permitted a more comprehensive assessment of the genetic heterogeneity of breast cancers. For example, DNA microarray technology permits investigators to measure the expression of a tumor's entire genome rather than focusing on one or two genes of interest. In doing so, breast cancers can be classified in various general categories based on their genetic expression patterns. Perou and colleagues first described this classification, and a number of groups have subsequently reproduced these results.[18,19] These categories predict the biologic aggressiveness of the disease.[19] Microarray studies have demonstrated that the expression patterns of breast cancers are strongly influenced by the estrogen receptor gene. The newer classifications of the biologic spectrum of breast cancer based on genomic categories include two classes of predominantly estrogen receptor–negative tumors with basal-like gene expression patterns (i.e., one is *HER2* positive, and the other is *HER2* negative). The basal-like expression pattern is associated with a poor prognosis and biologically aggressive phenotype. Three other major classes include estrogen receptor–positive tumors with luminal expression patterns, which usually carry a better prognosis than basal-like breast cancers. These molecular classifications are further delineated in Figure 61-1.[19]

Inflammatory breast cancer, which is a subcategory of locally advanced disease, has unique biologic traits. The diagnosis of inflammatory carcinoma is made on the basis of the clinical history and physical examination findings. The clinical history should describe breast erythema, warmth, and heaviness that have a relatively rapid onset and progression. Physical examination may reveal brawny edema of the breast, which may or may not be associated with a breast mass. It is important to distinguish inflammatory breast cancers from neglected breast primaries that slowly progress over many months to up to a year. Neglected locally advanced cancers can cause secondary inflammatory changes in the breast that mimic those of inflammatory breast cancer.

Most commonly, inflammatory breast cancer is characterized by high histologic grade, a high percentage of cells in the S phase, aneuploidy, absent estrogen receptor expression, and high expression of TP53 and epidermal growth factor.[20] Most investigators have found that HER2 is not more commonly overexpressed in inflammatory breast cancer than in nonin-

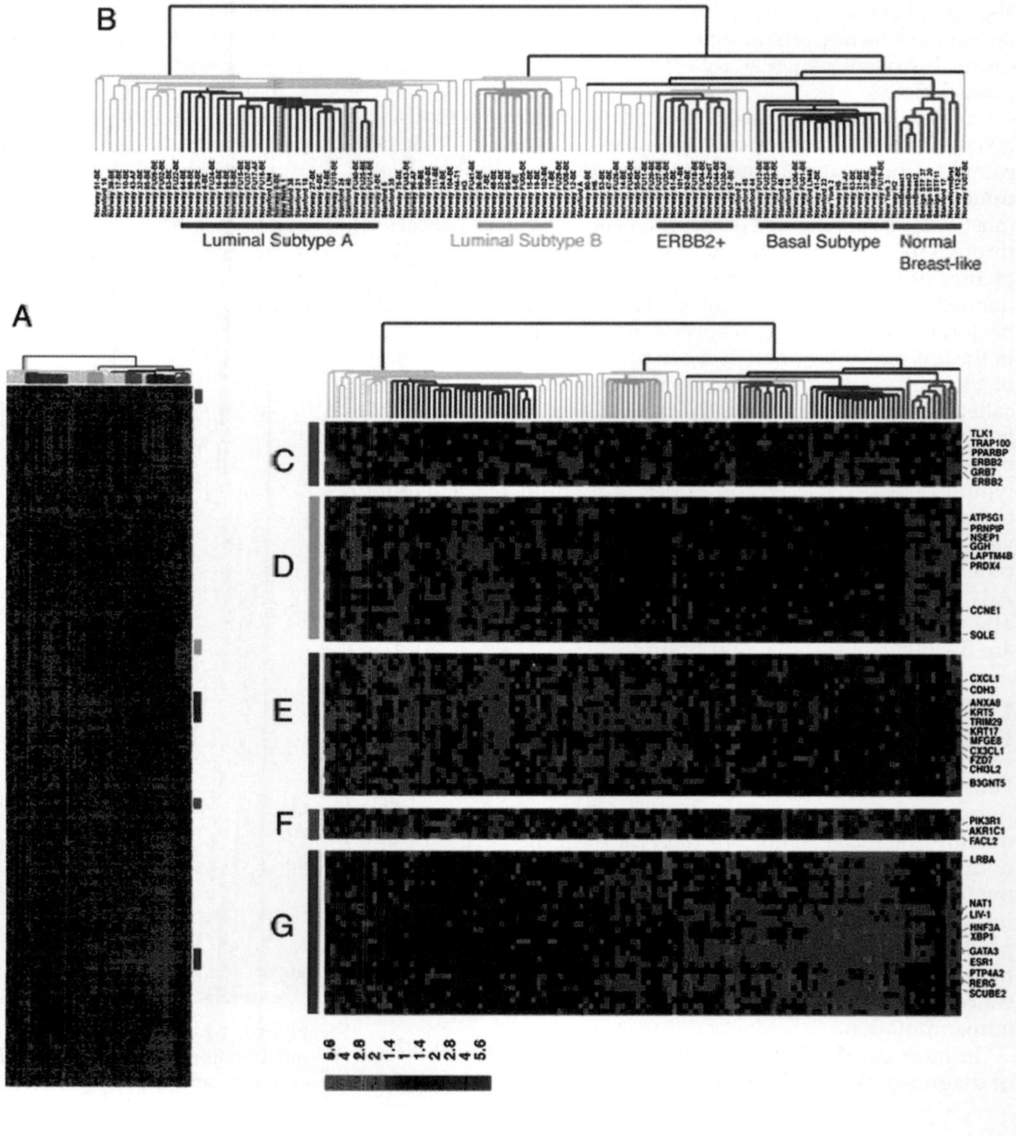

Figure 61-1 Global gene expression patterns of breast carcinomas show how they can cluster according to distinctive basal and luminal subtypes. These gene expression patterns have been found to correlate with estrogen receptor status and clinical outcome. The horizontal axes represent the individual tumors statistically segregated into groups based on the degree of similarity in gene expression patterns. The horizontal axis and corresponding *green* and *red matrix* reflect the expression of an individual gene within each of the tumors.

flammatory advanced disease.[20,21] However, later work suggests that many of these tumors overexpress RhoC GTPase and have loss of expression of the tumor suppressor gene *WIPS3*. If confirmed and validated, these markers may prove to be useful for diagnosis and may offer therapeutic targets.[22,23]

One of the pathologic hallmarks of inflammatory breast cancer is invasion into the dermal lymphatics and erythema of the skin, which may in part be representative of tumor angiogenesis. Alpaugh and associates established the first transplantable human inflammatory breast cancer xenograft, and unlike other breast cancer xenografts that grow as isolated subcutaneous nodules, this xenograft grows exclusively within the lymphatics and blood vessels and causes striking erythema of the overlying skin.[24,25] Shirakawa and coworkers found inflammatory breast cancer xenografts to have a particular pattern of neovascular growth, in which blood vessels within cancer tissue did not have a lining of endothelial cells.[25-27] These data help to provide insights into how the tumor lymphatics and vasculature may be therapeutic targets in inflammatory breast cancer.

PATHOLOGY AND PATHWAYS OF SPREAD

As in early-stage disease, most locally advanced breast cancers are infiltrating ductal carcinomas. Lobular cancers are more difficult to detect with mammography, and this histology can also manifest as locally advanced disease. However, it is unusual for locally advanced disease to have favorable breast cancer histologies such as tubular, medullary, and mucinous characteristics.

As primary breast cancers grow, they have the potential to invade nearby structures, including the skin, the nipple-areola complex, the pectoralis major muscle, and the chest wall. As tumors grow, their potential for dissemination increases. The most common route of spread for primary breast cancers is through the lymphatic channels of the breast. Most breast lymphatics drain directly to levels I or II of the axilla, which are defined anatomically as being inferolateral to and beneath the pectoralis minor muscle, respectively. After disease is present in the low axilla lymphatics, it can progress to involve level III of the axilla (i.e., superomedial to the pectoralis minor, also called the infraclavicular lymph nodes) and the supraclavicular lymph nodes. Tumors arising in the inner, lower, or central breast can also drain directly into the internal mammary lymph nodes. These lymph nodes are within the ipsilateral thorax and in proximity to the internal mammary artery and vein. Internal mammary lymph node disease is most commonly limited to the first three intercostal interspaces. Advanced primary tumors also may spread hematogenously. The most common sites of distant metastases in breast cancer are the bone, liver, lung, and brain.

CLINICAL MANIFESTATIONS, PATIENT EVALUATIONS, AND STAGING

Patients with locally advanced breast cancer commonly present after detecting a breast mass on self-examination. Frequently, there is a significant interval from the period of first noticing the breast abnormality to the time of presentation for medical care. During this interval, the breast mass usually increases in size. After a long delay before seeking treatment, patients can present with a bleeding or ulcerative mass that occupies most of the breast. Over time, some breast cancers can involute the breast, giving the appearance of an autoamputation.

In most cases, regional adenopathy is evident at the time of diagnosis of T3 or T4 primary breast cancers. Pain, limited range of motion, edema, and weakness or numbness of the arm is possible in patients with advanced axillary and supraclavicular adenopathy.

Patients with inflammatory breast cancers most frequently describe a rapid onset of breast erythema and increasing breast size or heaviness. Often, these changes progress over days or weeks and are frequently initially misdiagnosed as breast cellulitis. Figure 61-2 shows the presenting appearance of the breast in a patient with inflammatory breast cancer. The history of presenting signs and symptoms is the critical determinant in classifying a breast cancer as inflammatory.

All patients presenting with locally advanced disease require a comprehensive initial history and physical examination. While obtaining the history, it is critical to establish the time course of presenting signs and symptoms, because these elements are necessary to differentiate inflammatory breast cancer from other T4 tumors. In addition to breast symptoms, the history should include questions concerning changes in general health and questions specifically relating to symptoms possibly due to metastases (e.g., bone pain, change in neurologic status).

The initial physical examination is of critical importance in patients with locally advanced breast cancer. Unlike patients with early-stage disease, most patients with T3 or T4 tumors are treated with neoadjuvant chemotherapy. This treatment significantly shrinks the tumor in most patients, and the pretreatment extent of disease is critical for determination of subsequent locoregional therapies. The breast examination should document breast asymmetry, mass size and whether the mass is freely mobile, skin erythema or edema, and skin or nipple retraction. Mobility of the primary mass should be tested with the pectoralis major muscle contracted and relaxed to distinguish chest wall invasion from invasion into the pectoralis muscle. Skin edema is best assessed with the patient in the supine position. Edema of the skin causes thickening, which makes the hair follicle more prominent, resulting in the classic peau d'orange appearance. This can best be appreciated by gently pinching the affected skin between the thumb and first finger. Figure 61-3 shows a patient who presented with T4

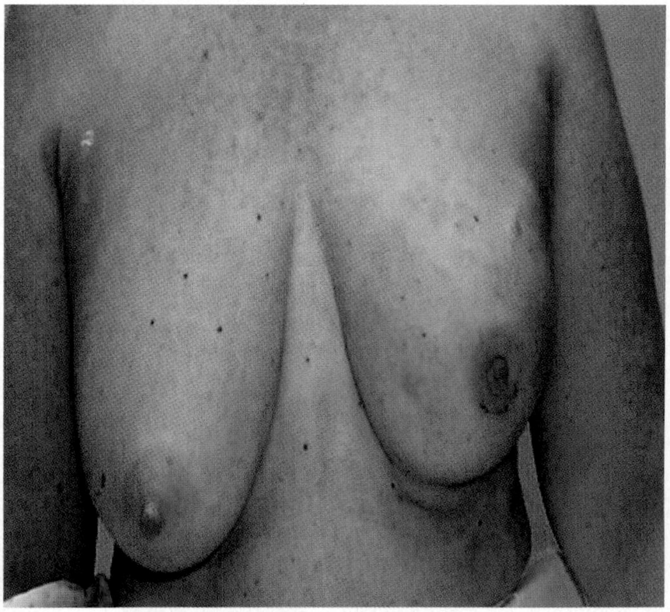

Figure 61-2 Photograph of a patient who presented with T4d inflammatory breast cancer of the left breast. The breast has central erythema and edema in the nipple-areola region.

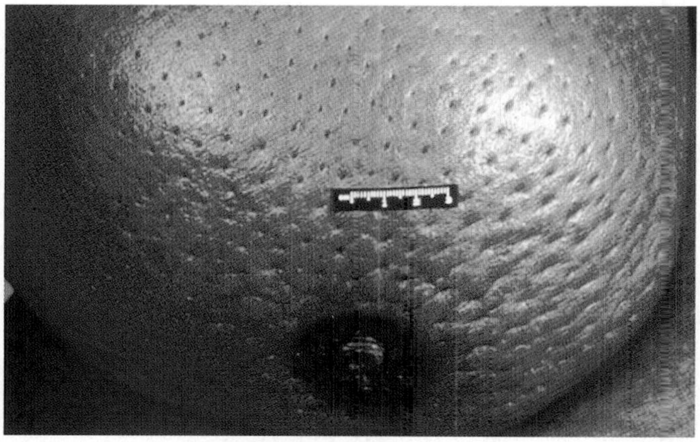

Figure 61-3 Photograph of a patient with a T4 breast cancer who presented with the classic peau d'orange pattern due to edema of the skin.

primary disease and was found to have peau d'orange on initial examination. The axilla and supraclavicular fossa should be examined with the patient upright, and regional adenopathy should be described and include the size, consistency, and mobility of axillary, infraclavicular, and supraclavicular lymph nodes. The internal mammary lymph nodes are infrequently palpable, even when involved with disease. Despite this, the parasternal area should be examined for asymmetric prominence with the patient supine.

After completion of an examination, the primary tumor and nodal basin should be assigned a clinical T and N stage. The American Joint Commission on Cancer (AJCC) 2003 clinical and pathologic staging system is provided in the breast cancer overview chapter.

All patients with advanced disease should be staged using bilateral diagnostic mammography, basic serum chemistry tests and blood cell counts, a chest radiograph, computed tomography (CT) of the upper abdomen, and a bone scan. Patients with T4 disease should have pretreatment photographs taken of the sites of dermal involvement. At our institution, we routinely use ultrasonography to assess the extent of disease in the regional lymph nodes. This is particularly useful in patients treated with neoadjuvant chemotherapy. Ultrasonography can frequently detect unsuspected regional disease in the infraclavicular fossa and supraclavicular fossa. Involved lymph nodes can appear to be enlarged or have abnormal hilar architecture on ultrasonography. We routinely perform fine-needle aspiration to assess the presence of disease in lymphatic locations in which it was not detected by clinical examination. Magnetic resonance imaging (MRI) and positron emission tomography (PET) continue to be investigated and are not considered to be the standard of care. However, as refinements of these modalities improve their positive predictive value, they will likely play important roles in the staging evaluation. Serum tumor markers such as carcinoembryonic antigen (CEA), CA 15.3, and CA 27-29 are used by some practitioners but are not recommended as the standard of care.[28]

TREATMENT OVERVIEW

Patients with stage III disease are optimally treated with a combined-modality approach. The incorporation of systemic treatments into the management of locally advanced disease, along with improvements in surgical and radiation therapies, has significantly improved the outcomes of patients with advanced disease. For example, early studies in which patients with advanced disease were treated with mastectomy or radiation therapy, or both, reported 5-year survival rates of only 25% to 45%.[2-4] In contrast, later data have shown that patients with advanced-stage disease, when treated with a combination of surgery, radiation therapy, and chemotherapy, have 5-year survival rates approaching 80% for patients with stage IIIA disease and 45% for patients with stage IIIB disease.[5]

Combined-modality treatments are best administered with input from a coordinated multidisciplinary team of surgeons, medical oncologists, and radiation oncologists. For patients with advanced operable breast cancer, mastectomy followed by adjuvant chemotherapy and radiation therapy is an appropriate therapeutic approach. Equally appropriate is the use of chemotherapy as the first therapeutic intervention (i.e., neoadjuvant chemotherapy). For patients who are not optimal surgical candidates at the time of diagnosis because of T4 primary tumors or advanced lymph node disease, neoadjuvant chemotherapy is considered to be the standard of care.

Treating patients with advanced primary tumors with chemotherapy before surgery has several potential advantages. One advantage is that it gives selected patients with T3 or T4 tumors the option of being treated with breast-preservation surgery. Numerous studies have indicated that neoadjuvant chemotherapy achieves a substantial reduction in the size of the primary tumor and nodal metastases in more than 80% of cases, which often permits a breast-conserving surgery that achieves an acceptable aesthetic outcome.[29-32] A second advantage is that neoadjuvant chemotherapy allows physicians to assess the primary tumor's response to a particular chemotherapy regimen. For the minority of patients whose disease does not respond or progresses, this assessment enables a change to a different regimen, allowing for the most effective chemotherapy to be given as early as possible and avoiding the unnecessary toxicity from an ineffective therapy. A third advantage of neoadjuvant chemotherapy is that it permits clinical trials that test new systemic treatments to be conducted and reported in a much more expeditious fashion. Data from multiple clinical trials have indicated that pathologic complete remission (pCR) (i.e., no residual cancer in the breast or lymph nodes after neoadjuvant chemotherapy) is associated with an excellent long-term prognosis.[29,33,34] Data from our institution indicated that the 5-year survival rate of patients with relatively advanced breast cancer was 89% in those in whom a pCR was achieved, compared with 64% for patients in whom a pCR was not achieved ($P < .01$).[34] Because higher pCR rates correlate with excellent long-term survival rates, phase III clinical trials have been designed using pCR as the primary end point. For example, we conducted a phase III randomized trial that indicated that 12 cycles of weekly paclitaxel had much greater activity than paclitaxel administered in the traditional method of 4 cycles given every 3 weeks.[35] Our trial found that the 12-week schedule followed by four cycles of 5-fluorouracil, doxorubicin, and cyclophosphamide (FAC regimen) resulted in twice the pCR rate of the every-3-week schedule of paclitaxel followed by four cycles of FAC. It would likely take 5 to 10 years of follow-up for an adjuvant chemotherapy trial to show this improved activity.

One desired advantage of neoadjuvant chemotherapy that has not been realized is the hope that earlier administration of chemotherapy would increase the probability of eradicating preexisting micrometastatic disease. Unfortunately, the two largest trials that compared neoadjuvant and adjuvant chemotherapy found that sequencing chemotherapy before surgery provided no overall survival advantage. Specifically, the National Surgical Adjuvant Breast and Bowel Project (NSABP) B-18 protocol randomized 1523 patients with early-stage, operable breast cancer to receive four cycles of doxorubicin plus cyclophosphamide (AC regimen) before or after surgical treatment. After 9 years, the overall survival and disease-free survival rates were almost identical between the two groups ($P = .80$ and $P = .50$, respectively).[29] A second large, randomized, prospective trial conducted by the European Organization for Research and Treatment of Cancer (EORTC) also demonstrated equivalent rates of survival and distant metastases between preoperative and postoperative chemotherapy treatment with four cycles of fluorouracil, epirubicin, and cyclophosphamide (FEC regimen).[32]

The increasing use of neoadjuvant chemotherapy has raised many questions concerning the surgical and radiotherapeutic management of patients with locally advanced breast cancer. Accordingly, it is best to have surgeons, radiation oncologists, and medical oncologists participate in decisions regarding treatment sequencing and provide the necessary multidisciplinary coordination to address the added complexity that neoadjuvant chemotherapy brings to the treatment of patients with locally advanced breast cancer.

LOCOREGIONAL TREATMENT OF PATIENTS WITH ADVANCED PRIMARY DISEASE

Breast Conservation after Neoadjuvant Chemotherapy

Historically, all patients with advanced primary breast cancers underwent mastectomy and postmastectomy radiation therapy as the preferred locoregional treatment. However, the high response rates associated with neoadjuvant chemotherapy have allowed for breast conservation in selected patients with advanced disease. The NSABP and EORTC trials comparing neoadjuvant chemotherapy with adjuvant chemotherapy in patients with stage II or III breast cancer found that rates of breast conservation were higher in the neoadjuvant chemotherapy arms.[29,30] This increase directly resulted from a greater percentage of patients with T3 disease being offered breast conservation after first responding to chemotherapy. One concern about using chemotherapy before breast-conserving surgery is that many advanced breast cancers do not shrink concentrically to a solitary nidus in response to neoadjuvant chemotherapy. In such cases, a surgery directed at the primary core may leave a high burden of microscopic disease around the tumor bed site, which may be associated with higher rates of breast cancer recurrence.

Some clinical data indicate that patients with advanced tumors who have been treated with breast-conservation surgery after neoadjuvant chemotherapy have higher rates of breast cancer recurrence. For example, in the NSABP B-18 trial, the cancer recurrence rate in patients with large primary tumors in whom a response to neoadjuvant chemotherapy allowed breast-conservation surgery was twice that in patients with smaller tumors who were treated with surgery first (15.7% versus 7.6%).[29]

Other series have also shown relatively high breast cancer recurrence rates in patients who receive neoadjuvant chemotherapy.[36,37] From these data, it is clear that breast-conservation procedures after neoadjuvant chemotherapy are more complex, that multidisciplinary coordination is important, and that proper patient selection for breast-conservation procedures is critical.

Investigators at the University of Texas M.D. Anderson Cancer Center published the results of one of the largest studies investigating breast conservation after neoadjuvant chemotherapy.[38] In this study, 340 carefully selected patients were treated with breast-conservation therapy after showing a favorable response to chemotherapy. Patient selection criteria for a breast-conserving approach included no postoperative residual malignant calcifications, no residual T4 breast skin abnormalities, negative surgical margins, no multicentric disease, and a willingness and ability to undergo surgery and radiation therapy. With such criteria, the outcome was favorable, with 5- and 10-year local recurrence rates of 5% and 10%, respectively, despite the fact that 72% of patients in the study had clinical stage IIB or III disease.

The authors of this series also identified the following four factors associated with breast cancer recurrence and locoregional recurrence: clinical N2 or N3 disease, lymphovascular space invasion, a multifocal pattern of residual disease (defined as noncontiguous foci of disease interspersed among fibrosis, necrosis, granulomas, and giant cells within the resected specimen), and residual disease greater than 2 cm in diameter.[38] Eighty-four percent of patients had just one of these factors or none of the factors, and this group had a 4% breast cancer recurrence rate at 10 years.[39] In contrast, the 4% of patients with three of these factors had a 45% breast cancer recurrence rate. Having a T3 or T4 tumor did not correlate with breast cancer recurrence in most cases in which the primary tumor responded to a solitary nidus or no residual disease was found in the breast after chemotherapy. However, the breast cancer recurrence rate was 20% in patients with T3 or T4 tumors that broke up and left a multifocal pattern of residual disease.[38] Improvements in breast imaging, such as the use of MRI, may prove to be of value in detecting this pattern of residual disease before a surgical intervention.

Patients with stage III breast cancer are at risk for locoregional recurrence even after mastectomy is performed. Patients with advanced disease are at significant risk for distant metastases, which is an additional incentive to avoid removing the entire breast when breast-conserving surgery can be done with acceptable recurrence rates.

Mastectomy and Postmastectomy Radiation Therapy

A modified radical mastectomy (i.e., resection of the breast with a level I-II axillary lymph node dissection) remains the most common locoregional treatment for patients with locally advanced breast cancer. This treatment is highly effective in achieving excellent rates of long-term locoregional control for many patients with invasive breast cancer, and postmastectomy radiation therapy benefits a cohort of patients who maintain clinically relevant rates of local regional recurrence despite undergoing a modified radical mastectomy. However, a significant controversy remains concerning the indications for postmastectomy radiation therapy, despite the fact that combinations of mastectomy, radiation therapy, and systemic treatments have been used in the treatment of breast cancer for more than 30 years.

More than 25 randomized, prospective clinical trials have evaluated the benefits of radiation therapy after mastectomy for patients with breast cancer. However, some of these trials date back more than 50 years, and it is not surprising that there is considerable heterogeneity in the surgical and radiation therapy treatments used in these trials. Despite the variability in trial design and treatments, a number of groups have performed meta-analyses of the data from these studies. In 1987, Cuzick and colleagues published the first meta-analysis of data from postmastectomy radiation therapy trials and reported that radiation use was associated with a poorer overall survival rate.[40] In a subsequent analysis, Cuzick and associates reported that postmastectomy radiation therapy decreased the breast cancer death rate but increased the non–breast cancer death rate,[41] which resulted in equivalent overall survival rates between the two groups.

The Early Breast Cancer Trialists' Collaborative Group (EBCTCG) performed a comprehensive meta-analysis of trials investigating postmastectomy radiation therapy.[42] This group analyzed the actual data from more than 15,000 patients and demonstrated two positive findings. The first was that postmastectomy radiation therapy reduced isolated locoregional recurrence rates. For patients with lymph node–positive disease, the 10-year isolated locoregional recurrence rate was 9% in the radiation therapy group and 24% in the no-irradiation group. This benefit was seen in the trials that included a standard modified radical mastectomy and the trials that allowed mastectomy with axillary sampling. The second benefit was that by reducing locoregional recurrences, postmastectomy radiation therapy significantly improved breast cancer–specific survival (20-year rates of 53.4% versus 48.6% for patients not treated with radiation therapy; $P = .0001$).[42] Unfortunately, in the meta-analysis, the improvement in breast cancer deaths was offset by an increase in non–breast cancer deaths ($P = .0003$). In further analysis of this end point, the study authors found that cardiovascular deaths were significantly higher in the patients treated with radiation therapy, whereas deaths due to pulmonary toxicity or treatment-related cancers were not statistically different in the two groups. It is conceivable that postmastectomy radiation therapy could improve overall survival rates if new techniques that selectively avoid treating the heart and vasculature were used.

It is important to recognize limitations of meta-analyses when considering the relevancy of these data to modern breast cancer patients. Many of the trials included patients at low risk for locoregional recurrence, and many used unconventional radiation doses, fractionation patterns, and radiation field designs. To minimize these confounding effects, Van de Steene and coworkers conducted a similar meta-analysis but excluded trials that began before 1970, trials with small sample sizes, trials with relatively poor survival rates, and trials that used radiation fractionation schedules that are no longer standard practice.[43] When these less than optimal studies were excluded, postmastectomy radiation therapy significantly improved overall survival, with an odds reduction for death of 12.4%. Whelan and associates performed a meta-analysis of the published postmastectomy radiation trials that included systemic therapy in both treatment arms. In this analysis, the addition of radiation after mastectomy was also shown to reduce the risk of any recurrence (odds ratio of 0.69) and mortality (odds ratio of 0.83).[44]

The 10-year data from three randomized trials investigating postmastectomy radiation therapy provided new insights into the potential benefits of radiation therapy. These studies differed from previous trials in that they used relatively more modern radiation treatment techniques and included systemic therapy for all patients. Table 61-1 displays the results from these trials. The Danish Breast Cancer Cooperative Group (DBCCG) 82b trial randomized 1708 premenopausal women with stage II or III breast cancer to receive mastectomy followed by nine cycles of a CMF regimen (i.e., cyclophosphamide, methotrexate, and 5-fluorouracil) or mastectomy, radiation therapy, and eight cycles of CMF chemotherapy.[45] Patients randomized to receive radiation therapy had a lower 10-year rate of locoregional recurrence and a higher 10-year overall survival rate. A smaller trial, conducted in Vancouver, British Columbia, randomized 318 premenopausal women with lymph node–positive disease to receive mastectomy and CMF chemotherapy with or without postmastectomy radiation therapy.[46] Patients who underwent radiation therapy had lower 20-year rates of locoregional recurrence and similar improvement in the 20-year overall survival rate. The third trial, the DBCCG 82c study, randomized more than 1300 postmenopausal women to receive mastectomy and tamoxifen or mastectomy, tamoxifen, and radiation therapy.[47] Similar benefits were again found.

Taken together, these three studies demonstrate that by reducing locoregional recurrence, postmastectomy radiation therapy can improve overall survival. These trials differed from many of their predecessors in that all patients were treated with systemic therapy. In theory, the addition of systemic treatments lowers the competing risk of distant metastases, thereby making the achievement of locoregional control more important. The Danish studies also found that with more modern radiation therapy techniques, cardiac toxicity from irradiation could be avoided. In the combined 82b and 82c trial populations, there were equivalent rates of heart disease–related hospital admissions and cardiac deaths in the patients treated with radiation therapy compared with those in the no-irradiation arm.[48]

The latest phase III clinical trials indicated that radiation therapy improved the overall survival rates of breast cancer patients who had a 25% to 30% risk of locoregional recurrence after mastectomy and chemotherapy. It is clear from a number of studies that patients with more than four positive lymph nodes or T3 or T4 primary disease have this degree of risk.[49-52] It is also generally accepted that women with stage T1 N0 or T2 N0 disease have a low risk for recurrence after mastectomy and therefore are not expected to benefit from radiation therapy. What is less clear is whether postmastectomy radiation therapy is indicated for patients with stage II breast cancer with one to three positive lymph nodes. In part, this

Table 61-1 Ten-Year Locoregional Recurrence and Overall Survival Rates in Randomized Trials Investigating Irradiation after Mastectomy and Systemic Treatments

Trial	No. of Patients	Treatment Arm	Locoregional Recurrence (%)	Overall Recurrence Survival (%)
Danish 82b[45]	1708	Irradiation	9	54
		No irradiation	32	45
Vancouver[46]	318	Irradiation	13	54
		No irradiation	33	46
Danish 82c[47]	1375	Irradiation	8	45
		No irradiation	35	36

controversy arose because in the 82b trial, 63% of the patients had one to three positive lymph nodes.[45] The difficulty in interpreting these data, however, is that many patients in this trial did not undergo a formal level I-II axillary dissection. The median number of axillary lymph nodes resected in the trial was only 7, with 76% of the patients having fewer than 10 lymph nodes removed and 15% having 3 or fewer lymph nodes removed.[45] Accordingly, some of the patients reported to have three or fewer positive lymph nodes likely would have had four or more positive lymph nodes if a more extensive surgical procedure had been performed. Correspondingly, their risk of a chest wall or supraclavicular recurrence would be higher than that usually estimated for patients with one to three positive nodes. Failure to remove these additional involved axillary lymph nodes would predispose patients to axillary recurrence, which could be avoided by a more complete axillary dissection. An earlier publication of the Danish 82b trial reported that 45% of all locoregional recurrences were found in the axilla.[53]

In an effort to further define the locoregional recurrence risk, a number of groups have evaluated the outcomes of women with stage II breast cancer with one to three positive lymph nodes who were treated with mastectomy that included a level I-II axillary dissection, systemic treatment, and no irradiation. These data and those for patients with more advanced disease are summarized in Table 61-2.[49-52] In general, these data suggest that the 10-year locoregional recurrence risk for patients with one to three positive lymph nodes is approximately 12%, which is almost three times lower than the locoregional recurrence rate in the no-irradiation arm of the Danish trials. Correspondingly, the expected benefit gained from the addition of postmastectomy radiation therapy would be expected to be much less. Woodward and colleagues found that the use of postmastectomy irradiation reduced locoregional recurrence in patients with stage II disease and one to three positive lymph nodes from 13% to 3%.[54] Whether this degree of benefit is clinically meaningful with respect to patients' survival is unknown. Another important consideration is that locoregional recurrences after mastectomy can develop after 10 years of follow-up. The 10-year data presented in Table 61-2 therefore may be underestimations of the true percentage of patients with persistent locoregional disease after surgery and chemotherapy. Specifically, in the 20-year update of the Vancouver randomized trial, approximately 20% of the total number of locoregional recurrences in the group randomized to not receive postmastectomy irradiation developed after 10 years of follow-up.[46]

Some series have identified subgroups of patients with stage II breast cancer and one to three positive lymph nodes that have higher risks of locoregional recurrence.[49,51,52,55,56] Factors that identify these subgroups include young age, the presence of extracapsular extension greater than 2 mm, tumor size larger than 4 cm, positive or close (2 mm) surgical margins, lymphovascular space invasion, invasion of the skin, nipple, or pectoralis muscle, fewer than 10 lymph nodes resected, and a 20% or higher rate of lymph node involvement. It is important to recognize that these factors were identified in retrospective subset analyses and have yet to be validated.

The American Society for Therapeutic Radiology and Oncology (ASTRO) and the American Society of Clinical Oncology (ASCO) have published consensus statements recommending postmastectomy radiation therapy for women with four or more positive lymph nodes or advanced primary disease. Both statements recommended that an additional trial be performed to further clarify the benefit of postmastectomy radiation therapy for women with stage II disease and one to three positive lymph nodes.[57,58] Unfortunately, an Intergroup trial designed to determine the benefits of postmastectomy radiation therapy for these patients closed because of poor accrual.

Postmastectomy Radiation Therapy after Neoadjuvant Chemotherapy

The use of neoadjuvant chemotherapy has significantly increased, particularly for patients with advanced primary tumors. One of the most important questions raised by this increased use concerns the indications for postmastectomy radiation therapy. In patients treated with mastectomy first, the decision to administer radiation therapy is made on the basis of the pathologic extent of disease. This is because pathologic quantification of disease is much more precise than clinical and radiographic examinations. The ASTRO and ASCO consensus statements regarding postmastectomy radiation therapy have recommended that treatments be based in large part on the pathologic determination of disease extent in lymph nodes.[57,58] Neoadjuvant chemotherapy changes the extent of pathologic disease in 80% to 90% of cases, and it is unclear how the posttreatment pathologic information should guide decisions regarding radiation treatments. One study compared how the pathologic extent of disease correlated with locoregional recurrence after mastectomy for patients treated with surgery first or chemotherapy first.[59] Not surprisingly, this study found that the locoregional recurrence rate associated with a particular pathologic extent of disease was higher in patients treated with chemotherapy first than in patients treated with surgery first. These data imply that patients treated with neoadjuvant chemotherapy have a risk of locoregional recurrence that is affected by the pretreatment clinical stage and the extent of pathologically residual disease after chemotherapy.

Table 61-2 Ten-Year Locoregional Recurrence Rates in Clinical Trials That Treated with Mastectomy and Systemic Treatments without Irradiation

Study	No. of Patients	Systemic Therapy	Locoregional Recurrence Rate: *Patients with 1-3 PLN*	Locoregional Recurrence Rate: *Patients with >3 PLN*
Recht et al[50]	2016	CMF	13%	29%
Katz et al[49]	1031	Doxorubicin based	10%	21%
Wallgren et al[51]	5352	Varied	14% 19% to 27%*	24% 24% to 34%*
Taghian et al[52]	5758	Varied	13%*	24% to 32%

*Higher rates were associated with high-grade disease and lymphovascular space invasion.
CMF, cyclophosphamide, methotrexate, and 5-fluorouracil; PLN, positive lymph nodes.

Few studies have investigated the efficacy of radiation therapy in patients treated with neoadjuvant chemotherapy and mastectomy and reported how clinical and pathologic factors are associated with locoregional recurrence in patients who do not receive irradiation. Two questions concerning postmastectomy radiation therapy are unique to patients treated with neoadjuvant chemotherapy. Do patients with advanced clinical stage disease who achieve an excellent response to neoadjuvant chemotherapy continue to have a clinically relevant risk of locoregional recurrence? Do patients with clinical stage II disease who have no lymph node involvement or one to three positive lymph nodes after neoadjuvant chemotherapy and surgery have a higher rate of locoregional recurrence than those who are treated with surgery first and are found to have stage II disease with one to three positive lymph nodes?

Only one published study has evaluated the efficacy of postmastectomy radiation therapy in patients treated with neoadjuvant chemotherapy. This study compared the outcomes of 579 patients who received neoadjuvant chemotherapy, mastectomy, and radiation therapy with those of 136 patients who were treated with neoadjuvant chemotherapy and mastectomy alone.[60] All of the patients included in this study were treated on prospective trials at the M.D. Anderson Cancer Center, but radiation therapy was not a randomized variable in any of these trials. There were significant imbalances in the prognostic factors between the two groups, with patients being referred for radiation therapy having more extensive disease. Despite the imbalances in T and N clinical stages, the locoregional recurrence rate was significantly lower in the patients treated with postmastectomy radiation therapy than in those treated with neoadjuvant chemotherapy and mastectomy alone (10-year locoregional recurrence rates were 8% and 22%, respectively; $P = .001$). As indicated in Table 61-3, treatment with radiation therapy was associated with better overall and cause-specific survival rates for selected groups of patients with high-risk disease. A multivariate analysis for the end point of cause-specific survival showed that treatment with radiation therapy was independently associated with a better outcome, and the hazard ratio for patients who did not receive radiation therapy was 2.03 (95% CI, 1.41 to 2.92; $P < .0001$). The hazard ratio for not receiving radiation therapy for the end point of locoregional recurrence was 4.7 (95% CI, 2.7 to 8.1; $P < .0001$).

The same study also addressed the two aforementioned clinically important questions. The data indicated that patients with locally advanced clinical disease who had favorable responses to chemotherapy and were treated with mastectomy still benefited from the addition of radiation therapy.[60] For patients with stage III disease who achieved a pCR, the locoregional recurrence rate for those treated with radiation therapy was 3%, compared with 33% for those who did not receive radiation therapy ($P = .006$). Using a broader definition of favorable response as having less than 5 cm of disease and fewer than four positive lymph nodes, similar benefits were observed. For those with stage III disease who achieved a favorable response using these criteria, the locoregional recurrence rates were 9% for those receiving radiation therapy and 20% for those not receiving radiation therapy.

A second publication from this group specifically attempted to address the question of which patients treated with neoadjuvant chemotherapy for clinical stage II breast cancer should receive radiation therapy. The study authors examined 132 such patients who had not received radiation therapy and found that the small number of patients with clinical T3N0 disease and those with four or more positive lymph nodes had high rates of locoregional recurrence.[61] However, the 42 patients with clinical stage II disease who had one to three positive lymph nodes after neoadjuvant chemotherapy had a relatively low rate of locoregional recurrence (5-year rate of 8%). More data are needed to better define the risk in these patients, and similar data should be forthcoming from the patients treated with mastectomy on the NSABP B-18 trial.

On the basis of these data, it is reasonable to recommend postmastectomy radiation therapy for all patients with clinical T3 or T4 tumors or clinical stage III disease regardless of their response to the chemotherapy regimen. In terms of clinical stage I or II breast cancer, postmastectomy radiation therapy should be recommended for patients with four or more positive lymph nodes after chemotherapy and for the unusual patient in whom the disease progresses and the primary tumor exceeds 5 cm in diameter. Additional studies are needed to quantify the locoregional recurrence risk in patients who present with T1 or T2 disease and have one to three positive lymph nodes after neoadjuvant chemotherapy.

TECHNIQUES OF IRRADIATION

Because radiation treatment plays a critical role in the management of locally advanced breast cancer, the design of treatment fields is important. For patients with stage III disease, the initial target volume should include the breast, chest wall, and draining lymphatics. At a minimum, the undissected axillary apex and the supraclavicular fossa lymph nodes should be included. At our institution, we also include the internal mammary lymph nodes as a therapeutic target. One rationale for including these structures is that the internal mammary

Table 61-3 Ten-Year Locoregional Recurrence and Overall Survival Rates for Selected Subgroups of Patients in the M.D. Anderson Cancer Center Series Investigating the Efficacy of Postmastectomy Irradiation after Neoadjuvant Chemotherapy

Subgroup	Treatment	Locoregional Recurrence (%)	Cause-Specific Survival (%)
T4 disease	Irradiation	15	45
	No irradiation	46	24
N2 or N3 disease	Irradiation	12	49
	No irradiation	40	27
Stage IIIB or IIIC	Irradiation	15	44
	No irradiation	51	22

Adapted from Huang EH, Tucker SL, Strom EA, et al: Radiation treatment improves local-regional control and cause-specific survival for selected patients with locally advanced breast cancer treated with neoadjuvant chemotherapy and mastectomy. J Clin Oncol 22:4691-4699, 2004.

lymph nodes frequently contain disease in patients with locally advanced disease, particularly those with medial or central tumors.

A variety of techniques can be adopted to include these targets in the radiation field. Initially, patients should be immobilized with their ipsilateral arm abducted (90 to 120 degrees) and externally rotated. In assessing arm position, it is important to have the soft tissues of the arm cranial to the junction of the tangent and supraclavicular fossa field. Skin folds within the supraclavicular fossa should be avoided if possible. After positioning and immobilization, the patients are placed on a 10- to 15-degree angle board to flatten the slope of the chest wall in the region of the sternum.

At our institution, we use a CT simulator that is specially equipped with a large bore to accommodate the patient's arm position. Radiopaque wires are placed on the surgical scar and around the borders of the breast and the treatment field. The interface border between the chest wall–breast field and the supraclavicular fields is typically placed at the bottom of the clavicular head. A scout view of the patient is obtained to assess patient position. After optimal patient positioning is confirmed, CT images are acquired and the appropriate isocenters are determined and marked along with appropriate set-up points. Areas of interest are then contoured on the CT slices. Typically, we contour the tumor bed (for cases of breast conservation) and the internal mammary artery and vein in the upper three interspaces. Regions of adenopathy are also contoured.

For patients treated with breast-conservation surgery, the breast is typically treated with medial and lateral tangent photon fields. These fields are created with matched nondivergent deep and cranial borders. A nondivergent cranial border is created through rotation of the couch. The nondivergent deep border is typically achieved by over-rotating the gantry or a half-beam block. The collimators are rotated to match the chest wall slope, and any volume that extends into the supraclavicular field is blocked. For patients with advanced disease and tumor locations in the central or medial breast, we attempt to include the contoured internal mammary structures by widening the deep border in the upper half of the field (often called *deep tangents* or *half-wide tangents*). CT simulation allows physicians to assess a variety of gantry angles for these tangents and pick the optimal angle that minimizes lung volume while avoiding irradiation of the contralateral breast. Figure 61-4 shows an example of a deep tangent field that includes the upper internal mammary lymph nodes in the field. A supraclavicular-axillary apex field is matched to the tangents with a nondivergent half-beam block. The gantry of this field is rotated 15 degrees to be off the spinal cord. For patients with advanced disease, we typically place the border lateral to the humeral head to cover the anterior soft tissues of the breast, chest wall, and axilla. Figure 61-5 shows an example of such a field. We use a posterior axillary boost only when there is gross disease present in the midaxilla or in instances where the axillary dissection was omitted or inadequate.

For patients treated after mastectomy, we target the chest wall and draining lymphatics with a four-field technique. The supraclavicular-axillary apex field is identical to that described previously. The lateral chest wall is treated with an opposed tangent technique similar to that used for a breast. The medial chest wall and internal mammary lymph nodes are treated with a medial electron field (that includes the contoured internal mammary vessels) that is angled 15 degrees. This field is matched to the tangents on the skin. Figure 61-6 shows examples of such fields. One advantage of this tech-

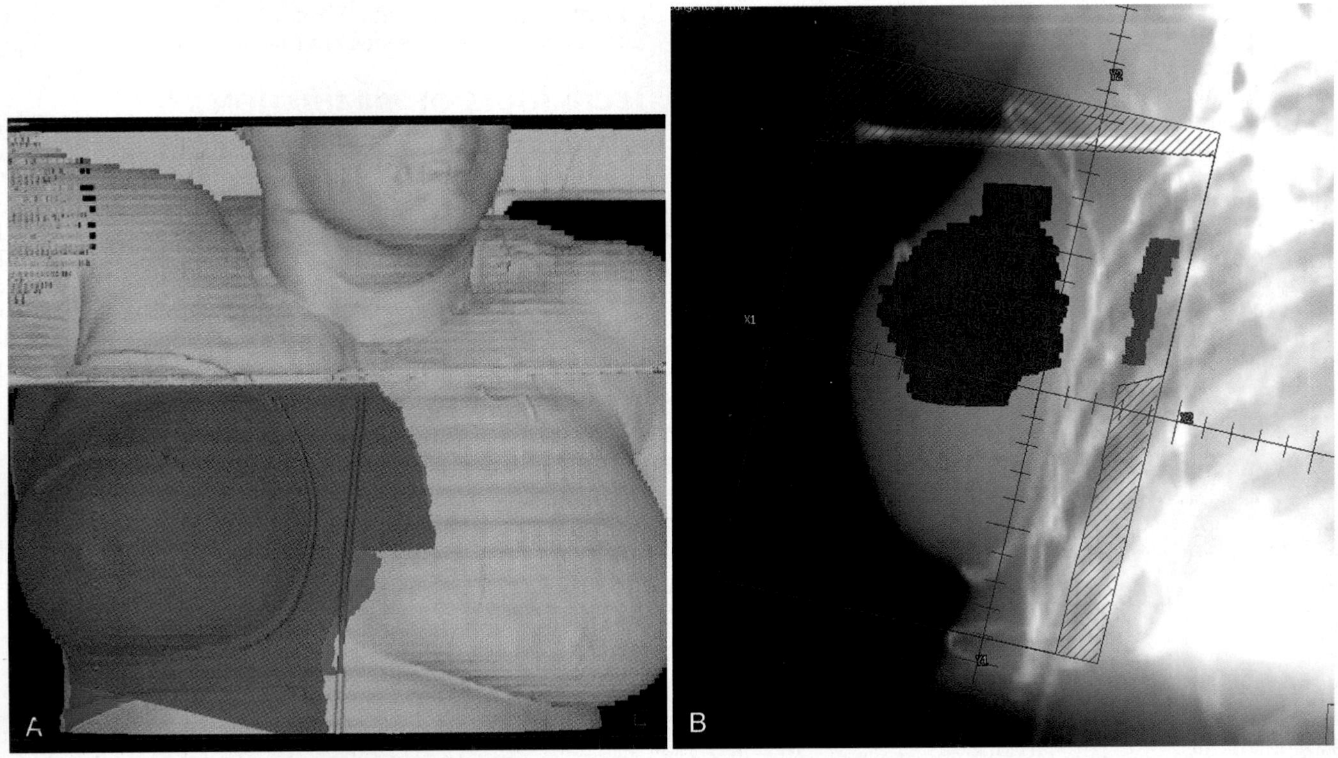

Figure 61-4 An example of deep tangent fields used to treat the breast and first three interspaces of the internal mammary lymph node chain. **A,** Skin surface rendering of the treatment fields as projected on the reconstructed images from the treatment planning study. **B,** Beam's eye view reconstructed radiograph of the medial tangent beam. The tumor bed *(red)* and the internal mammary lymph node region *(yellow)*, as defined by the internal mammary vessels, were contoured on consecutive CT axial images before determining the orientation of the field.

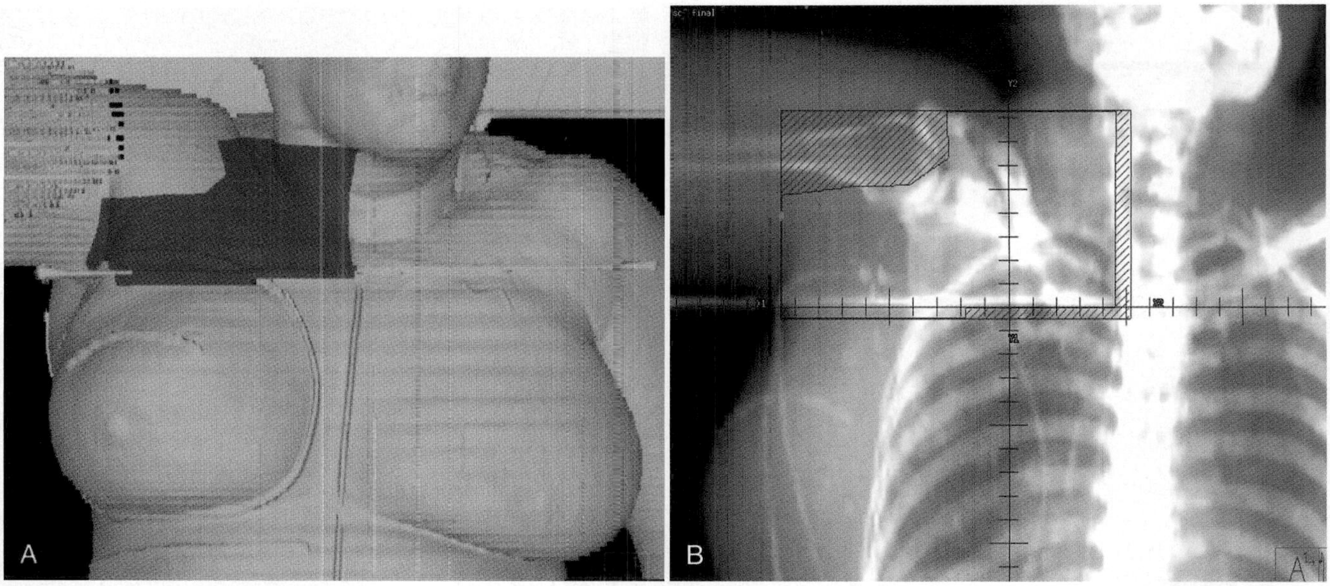

Figure 61-5 Example of a field used to treat the supraclavicular and axillary apex lymph nodes and the superolateral breast and chest wall. In this case, the tumor bed was high in the breast and approached the junction of this field with those shown in Figure 61-4. A 5-mm overlap of the field was purposefully designed in this region. **A,** Skin surface rendering of the treatment fields as projected on the reconstructed images from the CT treatment planning study. **B,** Beam's eye view reconstructed radiograph of the field.

nique is that it provides relatively broad circumferential coverage of the chest wall, something that is important, particularly for patients with T4 tumors. The technique enables avoidance of heart irradiation.

We treat our initial targets to a total dose of 50 Gy in 25 fractions over 5 weeks. For patients treated with mastectomy, we use a 3- to 5-mm bolus over the chest wall every other day for 2 weeks and then as needed to ensure that a brisk radiation dermatitis develops. However, this dermatitis should not lead to a treatment interruption. For patients with T4 tumors involving the skin, we slightly overlap the junctions of the matched fields. After completing a course of treatment to 50 Gy, we treat the chest wall with a generous boost of electron fields (5 to 10 cm beyond the mastectomy scar and covering the tumor bed location of the original primary) for an additional 10 Gy in 5 fractions over 1 week. We treat all sites of unresected but initially involved adenopathy in the internal mammary, infraclavicular, and supraclavicular regions with a radiation boost. If ultrasonography has shown a resolution of disease in these areas down to 1 cm or less, we treat this region with an additional boost of 10 Gy. If more than 1 cm of disease exists, we increase the boost treatment to 16 Gy. We treat patients with inflammatory cancer with an accelerated radiation schedule, based on a retrospective study that suggested that this schedule improved the outcome over comparison to a historical data set.[62] The initial target volumes are treated to 51 Gy in 1.5-Gy fractions given twice daily for 17 treatment days. Subsequently, the boost fields are treated with an additional 15 Gy in 1.5-Gy twice-daily fractions over 5 treatment days. We have found that this fractionation schedule is associated with an improved rate of locoregional control and has an acceptable toxicity profile.

Treatment plans showing radiation dose in multiple off-axis slices should be used to determine optimal beam parameters. For patients treated with breast-conservation surgery, a forward-planned field-in-field technique is used to achieve optimal three-dimensional dose homogeneity. CT treatment planning with heterogeneity correction factors is also used for patients treated with mastectomy. Electron energies for the medial chest wall–internal mammary lymph node fields ensure that the 90% isodose curve covers the contoured volume and avoids irradiation of the heart. The supraclavicular dosimetry should be checked to verify that the 90% isodose curve fully covers the undissected level III axilla.

SYSTEMIC TREATMENT

Systemic treatments benefit patients with advanced disease. In general, these patients have a relatively high risk for metastatic disease. Unless medically contraindicated, all patients with advanced breast cancer should be treated with chemotherapy, and all patients with tumors that are positive for estrogen receptors or progesterone receptors, or both, should also be treated with hormonal therapy.

Several regimens are considered appropriate standard treatment for patients with locally advanced disease. The most widely adopted regimens include combinations of an anthracycline and a taxane (i.e., paclitaxel or docetaxel). In part, this recommendation is based on an Intergroup trial that randomized patients who had been treated with four cycles of the AC regimen (doxorubicin and cyclophosphamide) to receive four cycles of paclitaxel or no additional chemotherapy. This study found a disease-free survival benefit for those treated with paclitaxel.[63] These data are supported by a similar study conducted by the NSABP (the B22 trial), which also found that patients who received four cycles of AC plus four cycles of paclitaxel had higher disease-free survival rates than those who received four cycles of AC alone.[64] Another trial from the M.D. Anderson Cancer Center comparing four cycles of FAC and four cycles of paclitaxel with eight cycles of FAC found a similar trend toward an improved outcome for patients treated with taxanes.[65] The NSABP B27 trial demonstrated that the sequence of neoadjuvant AC-docetaxel (given over eight cycles) was associated with a higher pCR rate compared with standard AC given over four cycles.[66] A small trial from

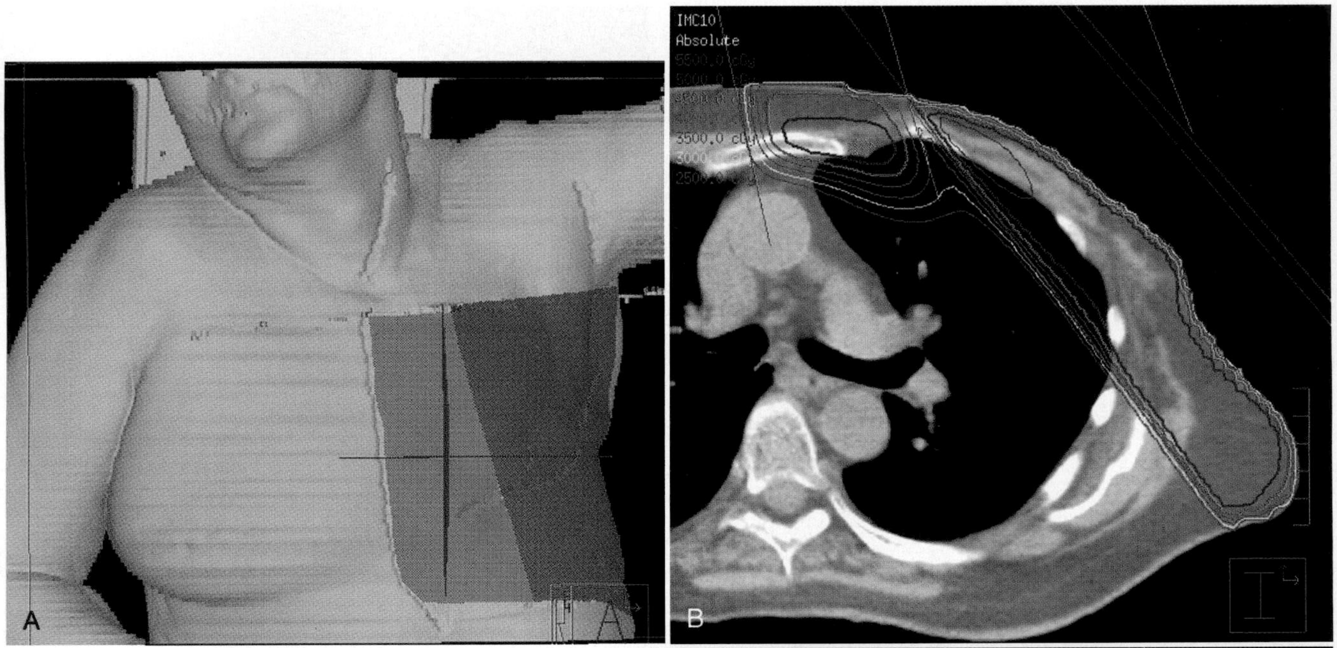

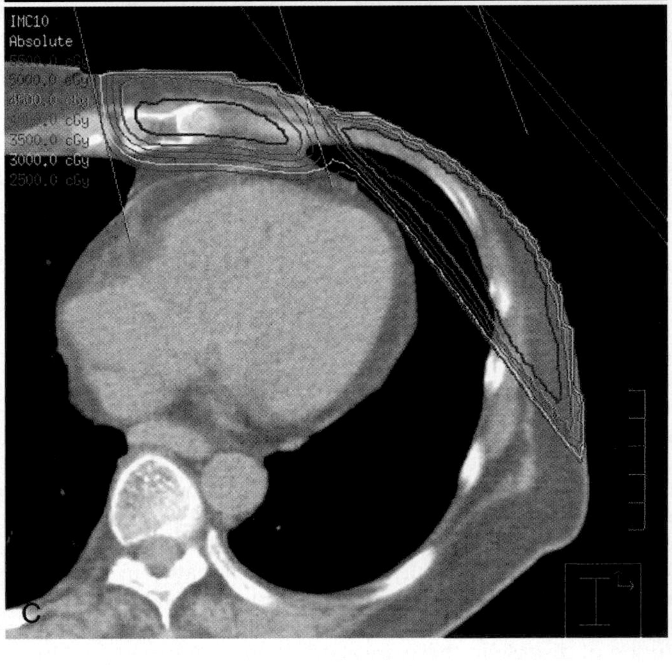

Figure 61-6 Example of three-field technique used to treat the internal mammary lymph nodes and chest wall while sparing the radiation dose to the heart. The three fields consist of a medial electron field that includes the chest wall and internal mammary lymph node chain. CT treatment planning is used to determine the appropriate electron energy such that the contoured internal mammary lymph node region in the upper three interspaces is covered by the 90% isodose curve. The field is angled 15 degrees off vertical. The lateral chest wall is treated with medial and lateral photon tangent fields. **A,** Skin surface rendering of the treatment fields as projected on the reconstructed images from the CT treatment planning study. **B,** Axial CT slice demarcating the three treatment fields and the resulting radiation dose distribution, including how the dose is able to cover the upper internal mammary region as depicted by the *yellow contour*. **C,** Axial CT slice in a region of the heart, showing how this technique allows for dose shaping around the cardiac structures.

Aberdeen randomized patients who had responded to neoadjuvant anthracycline chemotherapy to continue this treatment alone or to cross over to a taxane.[67] Despite selecting for patients whose disease responded to an anthracycline, the study showed that patients who crossed over to a taxane had a significantly higher rate of pCR.

Subsequent chemotherapy trials have investigated how to optimally combine taxane and anthracycline chemotherapy. In an Intergroup trial, it was found that giving four cycles of AC followed by four cycles of paclitaxel in a dose-dense fashion improved disease-free survival compared with the usual 3-week dosing schedule of the same chemotherapy.[68] A similar finding was observed in a randomized trial conducted at the M.D. Anderson Cancer Center. In this study, which compared different dose schedules of paclitaxel as neoadjuvant treatment, the pCR rate was 29% for patients treated with 12 weekly cycles of paclitaxel followed by four cycles of FAC, compared with a 14% pCR rate for the dosing schedule adopted from their previous trials (four cycles of paclitaxel given every 3 weeks, followed by four cycles of FAC).[35] The Breast Cancer International Research Group conducted a trial that randomized patients with lymph node-positive breast cancer to receive six cycles of a TAC regimen (i.e., docetaxel, doxorubicin, and cyclophosphamide) or six cycles of FAC and found a disease-free survival rate improvement in the TAC arm.[69] Taken together, these data suggest that any of the following chemotherapy regimens can be considered acceptable for patients with lymph node-positive breast cancer: dose-dense scheduling of AC plus paclitaxel, weekly paclitaxel plus FAC, or TAC.

In addition to chemotherapy, hormonal therapy is indicated for all patients with estrogen or progesterone receptor-positive disease. Premenopausal women who continue to have ovarian function after chemotherapy should receive tamoxifen as the preferred therapy. For postmenopausal women, the use of an aromatase inhibitor is equally appropriate. There are a number of options for postmenopausal patients, including anastrozole for 5 years, initial tamoxifen for 2 to 3 years followed by exemestane, or tamoxifen for 5 years followed by 5 years of letrozole.[70-72]

The use of trastuzumab for patients with *HER2*-positive breast cancer remains an area of continued research. An important study from M.D. Anderson randomized patients to four cycles of neoadjuvant paclitaxel and four cycles of FEC with or without concurrent trastuzumab. The pCR for patients treated with concurrent trastuzumab was a remarkable 65%, compared with a 26% rate of pCR for patients treated with chemotherapy alone ($P = .016$).[73] In addition to this neoadjuvant trial, several cooperative group trials are investigating the addition of trastuzumab to chemotherapy in the adjuvant setting.

OUTCOMES

The routine use of chemotherapy and hormonal therapy has significantly improved the outcomes for patients with stage III breast cancer. Before the use of systemic treatments, very few patients survived 10 years after surgery or radiation therapy, or both.[2-4] In comparison, 67% of patients with stage IIB or IIIA disease and 33% of patients with stage IIIB/C disease survive 10 years if treated with anthracycline chemotherapy, surgery, radiation therapy, and hormonal treatments.[5] Patients currently diagnosed with locally advanced disease are likely to have even better long-term survival rates than these statistics indicate because the data were obtained before the incorporation of taxanes, other new chemotherapeutics, aromatase inhibitors, and improvements in radiation therapy and surgery.

Multimodality treatment has also been able to improve long-term locoregional recurrence rates. For patients treated with chemotherapy, appropriate surgery, and radiation therapy, the locoregional recurrence rates are predicted to be less than 15%.[60]

The subgroup of patients with locally advanced breast cancer that responds poorly to initial neoadjuvant chemotherapy remains a therapeutic challenge. Patients with a significant volume of residual primary disease or with four or more positive lymph nodes after neoadjuvant chemotherapy have a poor prognosis, with a disease-free survival rate of only 25% and a locoregional recurrence rate as high as 25%.[60] New therapeutic approaches are needed for this cohort.

INFLAMMATORY BREAST CANCER

Inflammatory breast cancer is a unique and aggressive subgroup of locally advanced breast cancer manifested by rapid disease onset and the clinical findings of skin erythema, edema (peau d'orange), and breast induration, warmth, and asymmetric enlargement. Typically, there is extensive lymphovascular invasion by tumor emboli that involves the superficial dermal plexus of vessels in the papillary and high reticular dermis.[74]

Inflammatory breast cancer makes up only 1% to 6% of primary breast cancers.[75] Data from the Surveillance, Epidemiology, and End Results (SEER) database indicate that the incidence of inflammatory breast cancer increased from 0.3 to 0.7 cases per 100,000 person-years from between 1975 and 1977 to between 1990 and 1992. This increase was much larger than that observed for noninflammatory forms of breast cancer during the same period.[76] This study also found that inflammatory breast cancer was associated with a statistically significant lower overall survival rate ($P = .0001$) than that of noninflammatory breast cancers.

No randomized, prospective clinical trials have specifically evaluated treatments in patients with inflammatory breast cancer. M.D. Anderson has one of the largest single-institution experiences in the treatment of inflammatory breast cancer. In this institution, six prospective inflammatory breast cancer trials were conducted between 1974 and 2001, and 242 patients were treated on these trials. The resulting data suggest that aggressive trimodality treatment and the incorporation of taxanes into the chemotherapy regimen have had a favorable impact on the outcomes of patients, because there has been a significant improvement in the 3-year overall survival rate (71% versus 53%; $P = .12$) and the progression-free survival rate (46% versus 39%; $P = .19$).[77]

The current standard of care for patients with inflammatory breast cancer is initial neoadjuvant chemotherapy followed by mastectomy, if feasible, and postmastectomy radiation therapy. At our institution, we have used an accelerated radiation schedule, giving patients twice-daily treatments (1.5 Gy twice daily to a total dose of 51 Gy to the chest wall and draining lymphatics, followed by a boost to the chest wall of an additional 15 Gy). In a retrospective analysis, this twice-daily schedule to a total dose of 66 Gy was associated with a locoregional recurrence rate of 16%, which was much lower than the 42% rate during the era when treatment was given to 60 Gy or when once-daily irradiation schedules were used.[62]

Patients who do not respond favorably to neoadjuvant chemotherapy have a very poor prognosis. They may require locoregional therapy with preoperative radiation therapy or definitive radiation therapy alone.

TREATMENT ALGORITHMS AND NEW THERAPEUTIC APPROACHES

Figures 61-7 and 61-8 show treatment algorithms for patients with locally advanced breast cancer and patients with inflammatory breast cancer, respectively.

The current era is arguably the most exciting in the history of breast cancer therapeutics. During the 1990s, the U.S. Food and Drug Administration approved twice the number of drugs for breast cancer treatment than it had during the 1980s.[78] More exciting is the move from developing additional nonselective cytotoxic chemotherapies toward the development of new biologic therapies designed against tumor-specific genetic targets. The clearest example of such a strategy has been the successful use of trastuzumab for patients with tumors that overexpress the HER2 receptor. Incorporation of this targeted therapy has significantly improved the outcomes of patients with metastatic disease, has shown initial promise as a neoadjuvant treatment, and is under active investigation as a component of adjuvant therapies.

In addition to the HER2 receptor, therapies have been developed against a number of other biologic targets, including other growth-promoting receptors, the tumor vasculature, and products of other oncogenes. Many of these new therapeutics have shown significant promise in preclinical studies and have moved into phase I and phase II trials in human breast cancer patients.

Advances in molecular biology have also led to improvements in understanding patients' prognoses and the likelihood of their disease responding to a particular treatment.

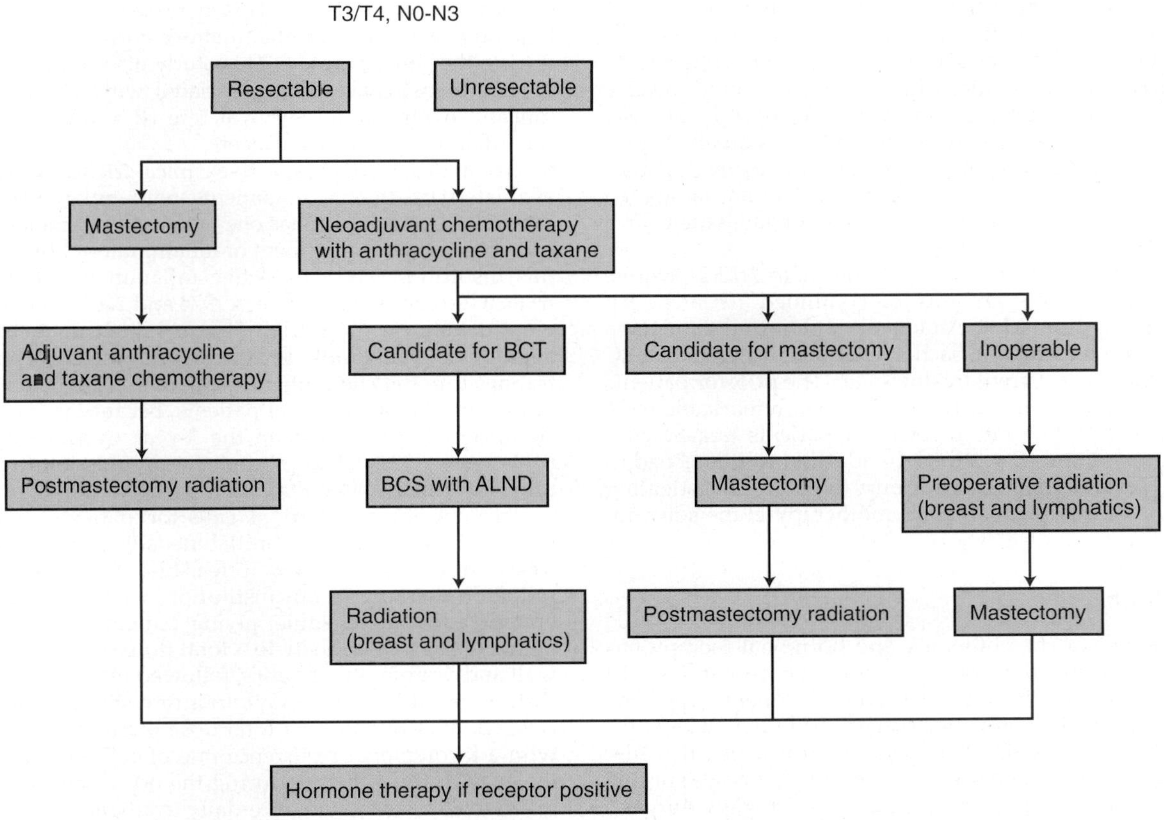

Figure 61-7 Treatment algorithm for locally advanced, noninflammatory breast cancer. ALND, axillary lymph node dissection; BCT, breast-conserving therapy; BCS, breast-conserving surgery.

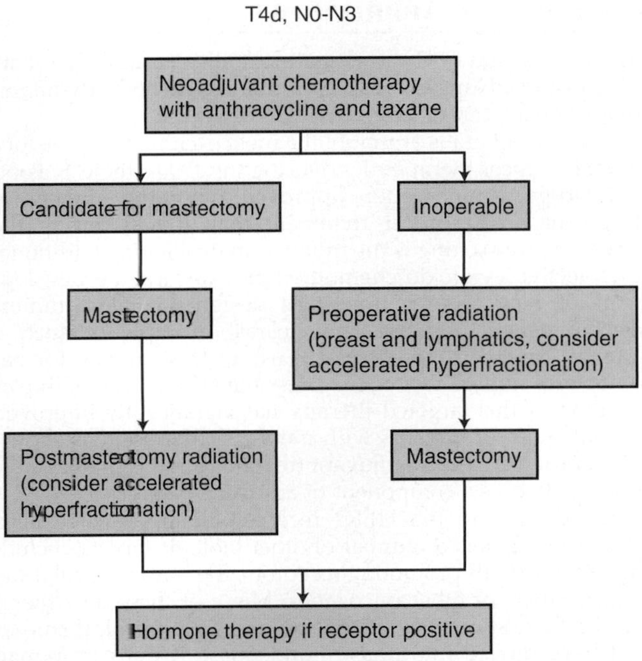

Figure 61-8 Treatment algorithm for inflammatory breast cancer.

Historically, new molecular markers have been studied in breast cancer as a single gene product. DNA microarray analyses permit rapid assessment of the expression pattern of the entire genome of a tumor. By comparing the expression pattern with clinical outcome, investigators have been able to identify gene sets that predict the development of distant metastases, which may lead to more selective use of available therapeutics.[79,80] We have identified an expression profile of a set of genes that correlated with the probability of achieving a pCR after paclitaxel plus FAC chemotherapy.[81] Such insights eventually may allow therapies to be selected for an individual patient based on the genetic characteristics of that patient's disease, rather than offering uniform treatments to entire classes of breast cancer patients.

CONCLUSIONS

Significant advances in public education and increasing use of mammography screening have led to fewer breast cancer patients found to have locally advanced disease at the time of diagnosis. The cure rate for breast cancer remains strongly influenced by the initial disease stage, and this important fact is a major contributor to the finding that the annual death rate from breast cancer is decreasing. Several exciting advances in therapy for breast cancer have incrementally added survival benefits for patients with locally advanced disease. The future of breast cancer treatment looks very promising as new molecular targets are identified and new tumor-selective therapeutics are developed.

REFERENCES

1. Lee-Feldstein A, Anton-Culver H, Feldstein PJ: Treatment differences and other prognostic factors related to breast cancer survival. JAMA 271:1163-1168, 1994.
2. Haagensen CD, Stout AP: Carcinoma of the breast: criteria of inoperability. Ann Surg 118:859-870, 1943.
3. Fracchia AA, Evans JF, Eisenberg BC: Stage III carcinoma of the breast—a detailed analysis. Ann Surg 192:705, 1980.
4. Haagensen CD, Cooley E: Radical mastectomy for mammary carcinoma. Ann Surg 170:884, 1969.
5. Hortobagyi GN, Singletary SE, Buchholz TA: Locally advanced breast cancer. *In* Singletary SE, Robb GL, Hortobagyi GN (eds): Advanced Therapy of Breast Disease, 2nd ed. Hamilton, Ontario, BC Decker, 2004, pp 498-508.
6. Hollstein M, Sidransky D, Vogelstein B, et al: P53 mutations in human cancer. Science 253:49-53, 1991.
7. Gretarsdottir S, Thorlacius S, Valgardsdottir R, et al: BRCA2 and p53 mutations in primary breast cancer in relation to genetic instability. Cancer 58:859-862, 1998.
8. Greenblatt MS, Chappuis PO, Bond JP, et al: TP53 mutations in breast cancer associated with BRCA1 or BRCA2 germ-line mutations. Cancer Res 61:4092-4097, 2001.
9. Slamon DJ, Godolphin W, Jones LA, et al: Studies of the HER2/neu proto-oncogene in human breast and ovarian cancer. Science 244:707-712, 1989.
10. Slamon DJ, Clark GM, Wong SG, et al: Human breast cancer: correlation of relapse and survival with amplification of the HER-2/neu oncogene. Science 235:177-182, 1987.
11. Tokunaga M, Land CE, Tokuoka S, et al: Incidence of female breast cancer among atomic bomb survivors, 1950-1985. Radiat Res 138:209-233, 1994.
12. Smith-Warner SA, Spiegelman D, Yaun S, et al: Alcohol and breast cancer in women: a pooled analysis of cohort studies. JAMA 279:535-540, 1998.
13. Chlebowski RT, Hendrix SL, Langer RD, et al: Influence of estrogen plus progestin on breast cancer and mammography in healthy postmenopausal women: the Women's Health Initiative Randomized Trial. JAMA 289:3243-3253, 2003.
14. Breast Cancer Facts and Figures 2003-2004. Atlanta, GA, American Cancer Society, 2003, pp 1-25.
15. Cancer Facts & Figures 2004. Atlanta, GA: American Cancer Society, 2004, pp. 1-58.
16. Li CI, Malone KE, Daling JR: Differences in breast cancer hormone receptor status and histology by race and ethnicity among women 50 years of age and older. Cancer Epidemiol Biomarkers Prev 11:601-607, 2002.
17. Elledge RM, Clark GH, Chamness GC, et al: Tumor biologic factors and breast cancer prognosis among white, Hispanic, and black women in the United States. J Natl Cancer Inst 86:705-712, 1994.
18. Perou CM, Sorlie T, Eisen MB, et al: Molecular portraits of human breast tumours. Nature 406:747-752, 2000.
19. Sorlie T, Perou CM, Tibshirani R, et al: Gene expression patterns of breast carcinomas distinguish tumor subclasses with clinical implications. Proc Natl Acad Sci U S A 98:10869-10874, 2001.
20. Guerin M, Gabillot M, Mathieu M, et al: Structure and expression of c-erB-2 and EGF receptor genes in inflammatory and non-inflammatory breast cancer: prognostic significance. Int J Cancer 43:201-208, 1989.
21. Pro B, Cristofanilli M, Buzdar AU, et al: The evaluation of p53, HER-2/neu, and serial MDR protein expression as possible markers of chemoresistance and their use as prognostic markers in inflammatory breast cancer [abstract]. Proc Am Soc Clin Oncol 17:553a, 1998.
22. Kleer CG, Zhang Y, Pan Q, et al: WISP3 and RhoC guanosine triphosphatase cooperate in the development of inflammatory breast cancer. Breast Cancer Res 6:R110-R115, 2004.
23. van Golen KL, Davies S, Wu ZF, et al: A novel putative low-affinity insulin-like growth factor-binding protein, LIBC (lost in inflammatory breast cancer), and RhoC GTPase correlate with the inflammatory breast cancer phenotype. Clin Cancer Res 5:2511-2519, 1999.
24. Alpaugh ML, Tomlison JS, Shao ZM, et al: A novel human xenograft model of inflammatory breast cancer. Cancer Res 59:5079-5084, 1999.
25. Shirakawa K, Tsuda H, Heike Y, et al: Absence of endothelial cells, central necrosis, and fibrosis are associated with aggressive inflammatory breast cancer. Cancer Res 61:445-451, 2001.
26. Shirakawa K, Kobayashi H, Heike Y, et al: Hemodynamics in vasculogenic mimicry and angiogenesis in inflammatory breast cancer. Cancer Res 62:560-566, 2002.
27. Shirakawa K, Shibuya M, Heike Y, et al: Tumor-infiltrating endothelial cells and endothelial precursor cells in inflammatory breast cancer. Int J Cancer 99:344-351, 2002.
28. Boccardo F, Bruzzi P, Cionini L, et al: Appropriateness of the use of clinical and radiologic examinations and laboratory tests in the follow-up of surgically-treated breast cancer patients. Results of the Working Group on the Clinical Aspects of Follow-up. Ann Oncol 6(Suppl 2):57-59, 1995.
29. Fisher B, Brown A, Mamounas E, et al: Effect of preoperative chemotherapy on local-regional disease in women with operable breast cancer: findings from National Surgical Adjuvant Breast and Bowel Project B-18. J Clin Oncol 15:2483-2493, 1997.
30. Fisher ER, Wang J, Bryant J, et al: Pathobiology of preoperative chemotherapy: findings from the National Surgical Adjuvant Breast and Bowel (NSABP) protocol B-18. Cancer 95:681-695, 2002.
31. Wolmark N, Wang J, Mamounas E, et al: Preoperative chemotherapy in patients with operable breast cancer: nine-year results from National Surgical Adjuvant Breast and Bowel (NSABP) protocol B-18. Cancer 30:96-102, 2001.
32. van der Hage JA, Cornelis JH, van de Velde CJ, et al: Preoperative chemotherapy in primary operable breast cancer: results from the European Organization for Research and Treatment of Cancer trial 10902. J Clin Oncol 19:4224-4237, 2001.
33. Buzdar AU, Singletary SE, Booser DJ, et al: Combined modality treatment of stage III and inflammatory breast cancer. M.D. Anderson Cancer Center experience. Surg Oncol Clin North Am 4:715-734, 1995.
34. Kuerer HM, Newman LA, Smith TL, et al: Clinical course of breast cancer patients with complete pathologic primary tumor and axillary lymph node response to doxorubicin-based neoadjuvant chemotherapy. J Clin Oncol 17:460-469, 1999.
35. Green MC, Buzdar AU, Smith T, et al: Weekly paclitaxel improves pathological complete remission in operable breast cancer compared with paclitaxel once every 3 weeks. J Clin Oncol 23:5983-5992, 2005.
36. Mauriac L, MacGrogan G, Avril A, et al: Neoadjuvant chemotherapy for operable breast carcinoma larger than 3 cm: a unicentre randomized trial with a 124-month median follow-up. Ann Oncol 10:47-52, 1999.
37. Rouizer R, Extra JM, Carton M, et al: Primary chemotherapy for operable breast cancer: incidence and prognostic significance of ipsilateral breast tumor recurrence after breast-conserving surgery. J Clin Oncol 19:3828-3835, 2001.
38. Chen AM, Meric-Bernstam F, Hunt KK, et al: Breast-conserving therapy after neoadjuvant chemotherapy: the M.D. Anderson Cancer Center experience. J Clin Oncol 22:2303-2312, 2004.
39. Chen AM, Meric-Bernstam F, Hunt KK, et al: Breast conservation after neoadjuvant chemotherapy: a prognostic index for clinical decision-making. Cancer 103:689-695, 2005.
40. Cuzick J, Stewart H, Peto R, et al: Overview of randomized trials of postoperative adjuvant radiotherapy in breast cancer. Cancer Treat Rep 71:15-29, 1987.
41. Cuzick J, Stewart H, Rutqvist L, et al: Cause-specific mortality in long-term survivors of breast cancer who participated in trials of radiotherapy. J Clin Oncol 12:447-453, 1994.
42. Early Breast Cancer Trialists' Collaborative Group: Favourable and unfavourable effects on long-term survival of radiotherapy for early breast cancer: an overview of the randomised trials. Lancet 355:1757-1770, 2000.
43. Van de Steene J, Soete G, Storme G: Adjuvant radiotherapy for breast cancer significantly improves overall survival: the missing link. Radiother Oncol 55:263-272, 2000.
44. Whelan TJ, Julian J, Wright J, et al: Does locoregional radiation therapy improve survival in breast cancer? A meta-analysis. J Clin Oncol 18:1220-1229, 2000.

45. Overgaard M, Hansen PS, Overgaard J, et al: Postoperative radiotherapy in high-risk premenopausal women with breast cancer who receive adjuvant chemotherapy. N Engl J Med 337:949-955, 1997.
46. Ragaz J, Olivotto IA, Spinelli JJ, et al: Locoregional radiation therapy in patients with high-risk breast cancer receiving adjuvant chemotherapy: 20-year results of the British Columbia randomized trial. J Natl Cancer Inst 97:116-126, 2005.
47. Overgaard M, Jensen MB, Overgaard J, et al: Randomized trial evaluating postoperative radiotherapy in high risk postmenopausal breast cancer patients given adjuvant tamoxifen: results from the DBCG 82c trial. Lancet 353:1641-1648, 1999.
48. Hojris I, Overgaard M, Christensen JJ, et al: Morbidity and mortality of ischaemic heart disease in high-risk breast cancer patients after adjuvant postmastectomy systemic treatment with or without radiotherapy: analysis of DBCG 82b and 82c randomised trials. Lancet 354:1425-1430, 1999.
49. Katz A, Strom EA, Buchholz TA, et al: Loco-regional recurrence patterns following mastectomy and doxorubicin-based chemotherapy: implications for postoperative irradiation. J Clin Oncol 18:2817-2827, 2000.
50. Recht A, Gray R, Davidson NE, et al: Locoregional failure ten years after mastectomy and adjuvant chemotherapy with or without tamoxifen without irradiation: experience of the Eastern Cooperative Oncology Group. J Clin Oncol 17:1689-1700, 1999.
51. Wallgren A, Bonetti M, Gelber RD, et al: Risk factors for locoregional recurrence among breast cancer patients: results from International Breast Cancer Study Group trials I through VII. J Clin Oncol 21:1205-1213, 2003.
52. Taghian A, Jeong JH, Mamounas E, et al: Patterns of locoregional failure in patients with operable breast cancer treated by mastectomy and adjuvant chemotherapy with or without tamoxifen and without radiotherapy: results from five National Surgical Adjuvant Breast and Bowel Project randomized clinical trials. J Clin Oncol 22:4247-4254, 2004.
53. Overgaard M, Christensen JJ, Johansen H, et al: Evaluation of radiotherapy in high-risk breast cancer patients: report from the Danish Breast Cancer Cooperative Group (DBCG 82) Trial. Int J Radiat Oncol Biol Phys 19:1121-1124, 1990.
54. Woodward W, Strom EA, Tucker SL, et al: Locoregional recurrence after doxorubicin-based chemotherapy and postmastectomy radiation: implications for patients with early stage disease and predictors for recurrence after radiation. Int J Radiat Oncol Biol Phys 57:336-344, 2003.
55. Katz A, Buchholz TA, Strom EA, et al: Recursive partitioning analysis of locoregional recurrence following mastectomy and doxorubicin-based chemotherapy: implications for postoperative irradiation. Int J Radiat Oncol Biol Phys 50:397-403, 2001.
56. Katz A, Strom EA, Buchholz TA, et al: The influence of pathologic tumor characteristics on locoregional recurrence rates following mastectomy. Int J Radiat Oncol Biol Phys 50:735-742, 2001.
57. Harris JR, Halpin-Murphy P, McNeese M, et al: Consensus statement on postmastectomy radiation therapy. Int J Radiat Oncol Biol Phys 44:989-990, 1999.
58. Recht A, Edge SB, Solin LJ, et al: Postmastectomy radiotherapy: clinical practice guidelines of the American Society of Clinical Oncology. J Clin Oncol 19:1539-1569, 2001.
59. Buchholz TA, Katz A, Strom EA, et al: Pathologic tumor size and lymph node status predict for different rates of locoregional recurrence after mastectomy for breast cancer patients treated with neoadjuvant versus adjuvant chemotherapy. Int J Radiat Oncol Biol Phys 53:880-888, 2002.
60. Huang EH, Tucker SL, Strom EA, et al: Radiation treatment improves local-regional control and cause-specific survival for selected patients with locally advanced breast cancer treated with neoadjuvant chemotherapy and mastectomy. J Clin Oncol 22: 4691-4699, 2004.
61. Garg A, Strom EA, McNeese MD, et al: T3 disease at presentation or pathologic involvement of four or more lymph nodes predict for local-regional recurrence in stage II breast cancer treated with neoadjuvant chemotherapy and mastectomy without radiation. Int J Radiat Oncol Biol Phys 59:138-145, 2004.
62. Liao Z, Strom EA, Buzdar AU, et al: Locoregional irradiation for inflammatory breast cancer: effectiveness of dose escalation in decreasing recurrence. Int J Radiat Oncol Biol Phys 47:1191-2000, 2000.
63. Henderson IC, Berry DA, Demetri GD, et al: Improved outcomes from adding sequential paclitaxel but not from escalating doxorubicin dose in an adjuvant chemotherapy regimen for patients with node-positive primary breast cancer. J Clin Oncol 21:976-983, 2003.
64. Mamounas EP, Bryant J, Lembersky B, et al: Paclitaxel after doxorubicin plus cyclophosphamide as adjuvant chemotherapy for node-positive breast cancer: results from N5ABP B-28. J Clin Oncol 23:3686-3696, 2005.
65. Buzdar AU, Singletary SE, Theriault RL, et al: Prospective evaluation of paclitaxel versus combination chemotherapy with fluorouracil, doxorubicin, and cyclophosphamide as neoadjuvant therapy in patients with operable breast cancer. J Clin Oncol 17:3412-3417, 1999.
66. Bear HD, Anderson S, Brown A, et al: The effect on tumor response of adding sequential preoperative docetaxel to preoperative doxorubicin and cyclophosphamide: preliminary results from National Surgical Adjuvant Breast and Bowel Project protocol B-27. J Clin Oncol 21:4165-4174, 2003.
67. Hutcheon AW, Heys SD, Sarker TK, et al: Neoadjuvant docetaxel in locally advanced breast cancer. Breast Cancer Res Treat 79:S19-S24, 2003.
68. Citron ML, Berry DA, Cirrincione C, et al: Randomized trial of dose-dense versus conventionally scheduled and sequential versus concurrent combination chemotherapy as postoperative adjuvant treatment of node-positive primary breast cancer: first report of Intergroup trial C9741/Cancer and Leukemia Group B trial 9741. J Clin Oncol 21:1431-1439, 2003.
69. Martin M, Peienkowski T, Mackey JR, et al: TAC improves disease free survival and overall survival over FAC in node positive early breast cancer patients, BCIRG 001: 55 months follow-up [abstract]. Breast Cancer Res Treat 82:A43, 2003.
70. Baum M, Buzdar AU, Cuzick J, et al: Anastrozole alone or in combination with tamoxifen versus tamoxifen alone for adjuvant treatment of postmenopausal women with early breast cancer: first results of the ATAC randomised trial. Lancet 359:2131-2139, 2002.
71. Coombes RC, Hall E, Gibson LJ, et al: Intergroup exemestane study. A randomized trial of exemestane after two to three years of tamoxifen therapy in postmenopausal women with primary breast cancer. N Engl J Med 350:1081-1092, 2004.
72. Goss PE, Ingle JN, Martino S, et al: A randomized trial of letrozole in postmenopausal women after five years of tamoxifen therapy for early-stage breast cancer. N Engl J Med 349:1793-1802, 2003.
73. Buzdar AU, Ibrahim N, Francis D, et al: Significantly higher pathological complete remission rate following neoadjuvant therapy with trastuzumab, paclitaxel and anthracycline-containing chemotherapy: results of a randomized trial in HER2-positive operable breast cancer. J Clin Oncol 23:3676-3685, 2005.
74. Haagensen C: Diseases of the Breast, 2nd ed. Philadelphia, WB Saunders, 1971, pp 576-584.
75. Levine P, Steinhorn S, Ries L, et al: Inflammatory breast cancer. The experience of the Surveillance Epidemiology and End Results (SEER) Program. J Natl Cancer Inst 74:291-297, 1985.
76. Chang S, Parker SL, Pham T, et al: Inflammatory breast carcinoma incidence and survival. The Surveillance Epidemiology and End Results (SEER) Program of the National Cancer Institute, 1975-1992. Cancer 82:2366-2372, 1998.
77. Cristofanilli M, Buzdar AU, Hortobagyi GN: Update on the management of inflammatory breast cancer. Oncologist 8:141-148, 2003.
78. Giordano SH, Buzdar AU, Smith TL, et al: Is breast cancer survival improving? Cancer 100:44-52, 2004.
79. van't Veer LJ, Dai H, van de Vijver MJ, et al: Gene expression profiling predicts clinical outcome of breast cancer. Nature 415:530-536, 2002.
80. van de Vijver MJ, He YD, van't Veer LJ, et al: A gene-expression signature as a predictor of survival in breast cancer. N Engl J Med 347:1999-2009, 2002.
81. Ayers M, Symmans WF, Stec J, et al: Gene expression profiles predict complete pathologic response to neoadjuvant paclitaxel and fluorouracil, doxorubicin, and cyclophosphamide chemotherapy in breast cancer. J Clin Oncol 22:2284-2293, 2004.

PART H

SARCOMA AND BENIGN DISEASE

CHAPTER 62

SOFT TISSUE SARCOMA

Brian O'Sullivan, Peter Chung, Colleen Euler, and Charles Catton

EPIDEMIOLOGY/PATHOLOGY

Soft tissue sarcomas (STSs) are derived from mesenchymal tissue and contribute to approximately 1% of adult cancers in the United States or almost 9000 new cases annually; approximately 5000 are male and 4000 are female patients. Although all age groups are affected, the median onset of STS is generally from 50 to 55 years of age. Just more than half originate in the limbs (extremities) and torso (truncal), whereas the retroperitoneum or visceral tissues (approximately 35%) and the head and neck (10%) consist of the remainder. The most common pathologic classification scheme for STS is based on histogenesis, wherein tumors are named according to the normal tissues that they most resemble. Numerous subtypes are recognized, the most common being the liposarcoma and malignant fibrous histiocytoma subtypes. Attempts are underway to classify according to distinct molecular characteristics that recognize distinct behavioral and functional characteristics.

BIOLOGIC CHARACTERISTICS

Major prognostic factors are tumor size, pathologic grade, and depth of involvement of the tumor as it relates to the superficial investing fascia that separates the subcutaneous compartment of the body from the deeper *muscular* tissues. These characteristics combined with the presence of nodal involvement and distant metastases make up the tumor, node, metastasis (TNM) stage classification. Lymph-node involvement is a grave characteristic in STS, but it is also rarely encountered other than for certain histologic subtypes. The predominant pattern of relapse is to the lungs for most STS, but intra-abdominal lesions will generally relapse within the abdomen, including the liver. Gastrointestinal stromal tumors (GISTs) are rare STSs that predominantly arise in the stomach or small intestine. These represent the first solid tumor with a consistent favorable response to molecular targeted therapy governed by the presence of a specific point mutation in the *KIT* receptor tyrosine kinase that reliably predicts response to imatinib (Gleevec). Other sarcomas also have extensive cytogenic abnormalities that can aid in their differential diagnosis and may ultimately provide therapeutic targets.

STAGING EVALUATION

In addition to diagnostic interventions, clinical examination should heed particular attention to lesion size and mobility and the relationship to the investing fascia deep to the subcutaneous fat (i.e., superficial versus deep) and adjacent neurovascular structures or bone. All soft tissue masses deep to the investing fascia should be considered sarcoma until proved otherwise. Before embarking on treatment, histologic confirmation of the diagnosis is necessary; and prebiopsy cross-sectional imaging with computed tomography (CT) or magnetic resonance imaging (MRI) is necessary to avoid compromising the outcome of local treatment by contaminating tissues that were uninvolved initially. For metastatic staging CT of the chest is required, excepting very low-grade lesions or small lesions where a plain chest radiograph may be sufficient. If the underlying diagnosis is rhabdomyosarcoma (RMS), a bone marrow biopsy is necessary as well as cerebrospinal fluid analysis in parameningeal lesions.

PRIMARY THERAPY

In general the approach is confined to surgery with or without local radiotherapy (RT). The latter may include external beam approaches delivered preoperatively, postoperatively, or using brachytherapy. Chemotherapy remains controversial and is generally restricted to established chemoresponsive lesions and in some high-risk cases. The 5-year survival of patients with STS overall can be expected to be approximately 60%; but this depends on the site of the primary lesion in addition to the known prognostic factors. Vigilance in the detection of both local and metastatic relapse is warranted, because a proportion of patients may be successfully salvaged by additional intensive treatment with surgery and adjuvant approaches.

PALLIATION

It is sometimes difficult to separate the objectives of long-term disease control from symptom relief, because the same treatment approaches may be warranted for both goals. Palliative management usually ends with a decision whether chemotherapy should be used in the patient for whom no other options remain. A complete and durable response to systemic chemotherapy is uncommon and generally seen only in certain histologic subtypes, such as liposarcoma and synovial sarcoma. Single-agent doxorubicin is preferred over doxorubicin-based combination chemotherapy based on the available evidence. RT has its usual indications in the management of symptoms of bone metastases but surgery can have an important role in the relief of obstruction or for mechanical problems including fracture.

Soft tissue sarcomas (STS) are rare malignancies derived from mesenchymal tissue and contribute approximately 1% of adult cancers in the United States or almost 9000 new cases annually; approximately 5000 patients are male and 4000 are female.[1] No obvious association with ethnicity seems present. The disease is characterized by heterogeneity in anatomical site, histologic tumor subtype, and the risk of metastatic progression. Although all age groups are affected, the median onset of STS is generally from 50 to 55 years of age. Slightly more than half originate in the limbs (extremities) and torso (truncal), and the retroperitoneum or visceral tissues (approximately 35%) and the head and neck (10%) make up the remainder. Because of different conventions in attribution of certain sarcomas to the abdomen and thorax, there has been a spurious increase in incidence in these sites recently. The only gender relationship concerns a putative link to lower risk of synovial sarcoma in females potentially related to its hallmark translocation[2] (see Pathologic Features and Natural History).

The anatomic location, size, depth (with respect to the superficial fascia), and pathologic characteristics dictate the natural history and treatment of STS. The pathologic classification is still determined by light microscopy enhanced by ultrastructure and immunohistochemical characteristics. For certain sarcomas, however, evaluation for the presence of specific molecular signatures is becoming routine in the diagnostic assessment. The overall 5-year survival remains approximately 50% to 60% for all stages and sites combined. Lesions of the extremity and superficial trunk (torso) are usually controlled at the local site; and death results from lung metastases, manifesting almost entirely within 2 to 3 years of initial diagnosis. In contrast, retroperitoneal lesions commonly exhibit inexorable continued attrition from continued local recurrence at the primary site many years following initial treatment. Lesions in the head and neck provide an intermediate situation where local disease seems more difficult to control than in the extremity. In addition, unusual patterns of disease relapse are not infrequent among several histologies including rhabdomyosarcoma (RMS), liposarcoma, epithelioid sarcoma, and others.

ETIOLOGY AND EPIDEMIOLOGY

Environmental Etiologic Factors

A perplexing issue about STS is that in most cases there is no evident, clearly defined etiologic factor. Notwithstanding this, multiple factors have been identified that either predispose or are associated with the development of STS. Several possible risk factors must be further assessed in STS such as herbicide exposure and constitutional and hormonal factors during childhood, puberty, and adulthood. STS was identified recently in a group of nondefining-AIDS neoplasms linked to various concurrent viral infections in the HIV-infected host, including children.[3,4] No clear demographic features have been identified in normal populations, but one Italian study questioned whether body weight contributed to increased risk.[5]

The factor with perhaps the greatest notoriety is radiation resulting from accidental, therapeutic, or diagnostic exposure. The resulting risk of cancer has been enshrined in the collective oncology consciousness from as early as 1922.[6] However, certain conditions in themselves are associated with intrinsic host predisposition to radiation-induced neoplasia, most notably retinoblastoma. Although rare in the cancer incidence statistics, children are an obvious concern because of the available latent period that can span many decades.

Although the risk associations with RT are well appreciated, the molecular mechanisms and real antecedent cause of these lesions are poorly understood. Germline mutations in tumor suppressor genes and accumulated damage to DNA repair genes may lead to neoplasia; but it remains unknown if most individuals have a genetic defect that underpinned the development of the first cancer, for which RT was administered, and in turn led to the induction of the irradiation-induced cancer.[7] If this is the case, there may be subgroups of individuals at considerably greater risk, whereas others have relatively low risk.[7] One hypothesis is that incomplete damage in normal tissues results in mutagenic responses and disorganized reparative proliferation that can eventually trigger tumor induction.[8] This may provide a basis for the observation that RT-induced sarcomas commonly originate on the perimeter of the previous RT target volume and nor necessarily in the high-dose region.

RT use in the primary management of breast cancer remains a problem from the standpoint of sarcoma induction. Karlsson and colleagues studied all 122,991 women with breast cancer in Sweden from 1958 to 1992 and found 116 STSs[9] (40 angiosarcomas and 76 other). Breast cancer also may have additional risk, because lymphedema following the treatment of breast cancer is independently associated with the development of lymphangiosarcoma.[10] In this setting the lymphangiosarcoma generally develops beyond the immediate irradiated volume in addition to the area that was targeted.[11]

Trauma is a controversial factor. Often, a minor episode of injury may draw attention to a preexisting mass, or awkward malignant masses may be more prone to trauma and consequent injury. Pukkala studied cancer incidences in world-class athletes in Finland.[12] Smoking-related cancers were less frequent, whereas the incidence of other cancers was not reduced. The authors speculated whether injuries during active sport may predispose to sarcoma; and in turn there has been concern that operative trauma, including arthroplasty surgery, may increase STS risk. However, Scandinavian studies on more than 100,000 patients who had undergone total hip or knee arthroplasty showed no increased risk of sarcoma; and there was no sarcoma case presenting at the site of operation.[13,14] Desmoid tumors are commonly seen in the anterior abdominal wall following pregnancy, but the biologic and traumatic basis for this is unclear.[15]

Several chemical carcinogens, including thorotrast, vinyl chloride, and arsenic, are established in the causation of hepatic angiosarcomas. Workers exposed to phenoxyherbicides, chlorophenols, and dioxins had higher mortality rates from cancer compared to controls; and the increase was highest for STS.[16-18] There have been conflicting reports about occupational exposure to phenoxyacetic acids detectable in chlorophenols (frequent in wood preservatives) and certain herbicides.[19-22]

Molecular Pathogenetic Mechanisms

Two major types of genetic alterations appear to play a role in the development of STS. Specific genetic-alteration tumors make up one broad group that include simple karyotypes, such as fusion genes caused by reciprocal translocations (Table 62-1), and specific point mutations such as *KIT* mutations in gastrointestinal stromal tumors. The second broad sarcoma distinction involves complex unbalanced karyotypes and nonspecific genetic alterations, representing numerous genetic losses and gains.[23]

Table 62-1 Cytogenetic Abnormalities and Fusion Genes in Soft Tissue Sarcoma

Histologic Subtype	Usual Translocations	Genes Involved
Alveolar sarcoma of soft parts	t(X;17) (p11;q15)	*ASPL/TFE3*
Chondrosarcomas extraskeletal myxoid	t(9;22) (q22;q12)	*NR4/A3*
Clear cell sarcoma	t(12;22) (q13;q12)	*ETV6/NTRK3*
Dermatofibrosarcoma protuberans	t(17;22) (q22;q13)	*PDGF-B*
Desmoplastic small round cell tumor	t(11;22) (p13;q12)	*EWS/WT1*
Fibrous histiocytoma (angiomatoid)	t(12;16) (q13;p11)	*TLS/ATF1*
Liposarcoma (myxoid)	t(12;16) (q13;p11)	*TLS/CHOP*
	t(12;22) (q13;p12)	*CHOP/EWS*
RMS (alveolar)	t(2;13) (q35;q14)	*PAX3/FKHR*
	t(1;13) (p36;14)	*PAX7/FKHR*
Synovial sarcoma	t(X;18) (p11;q11)	*SYT/SSX1* or *SSX2*

RMS, rhabdomyosarcoma.

Simple Karyotypic Sarcomas with Specific Genetic Alterations

Fusion gene–related sarcomas may account for approximately 30% of sarcomas. Many of the resulting fusion genes arising from the specific genetic alterations derived from chromosomal translocations have already been identified (see Table 62-1).[24,25] They frequently include fusions involving the *EWS* family members, *TLS* and *TAF2N*, now designated *TAF15*, or the *EWS* gene. Fusion genes provide specific diagnostic markers but also encode chimeric proteins that are important regulators of the biology and pathogenesis of these sarcomas by governing the transcription of multiple downstream genes and pathways.[25]

Complex Karyotypic Sarcomas without Specific Genetic Alterations

Karyotypically complex lesions, exemplified by malignant fibrous histiocytoma (MFH) (a changing diagnostic entity discussed later), leiomyosarcoma, nonmyxoid-type liposarcoma, angiosarcoma, and fibrosarcoma appear to be differentiated from sarcomas with simple genetic alterations by the prevalence of inactivation of the *p53*, now designated *TP53*, pathway. This appears to be a common early event in the abrogation of *TP53* checkpoint function, which ultimately leads to the progression of these lesions. This may explain why these lesions cannot be readily characterized into distinct clinical stereotypes compared to their STS counterparts with more specific genetic alterations.[23]

Genetic Conditions Associated with Sarcomas

Given the genetic knowledge described earlier, it is not surprising that STS is associated with several genetic conditions. Patients with neurofibromatosis have a 5% to 10% lifetime risk of developing a malignant neurofibrosarcoma arising in a neurofibroma[26-29] most commonly in the central nervous system (CNS). These patients frequently present the additional diagnostic dilemma of distinguishing between potential metastases or other benign neurofibromas found on staging investigations. A significant risk of STS is found in individuals with somatic mutations in the *TP53* tumor suppressor gene (Li-Fraumeni syndrome, characterized by a familial cluster of sarcoma [12%], breast cancer [25%], leukemia, adrenal carcinoma, brain tumors [12%], lung cancer, skin cancer, and pancreatic cancer).[30,31]

Long-term survivors of retinoblastoma with the associated *Rb* gene abnormality often develop tumors later in life, with a risk approximating 10% to 15%.[32,33] For hereditary retinoblastoma the cumulative incidence of a second cancer at 50 years after diagnosis is 50% compared to only 5% for nonhereditary retinoblastoma.[34] Wong and colleagues showed that the relative risk of STS increases with doses beginning at 5 Gy rising 10.7-fold at dose levels exceeding 60 Gy.[34]

Gardner's syndrome, a subset of familial adenomatous polyposis, is associated with the development of intra-abdominal desmoids.[35]

PREVENTION AND EARLY DETECTION

General Screening

General screening for sarcoma in the population at large is problematic given its rarity. Patients at increased risk for sarcoma require a more detailed clinical evaluation at a lower threshold of intervention than might be used in general practice. Deep lesions always require investigation, especially if there is a history of growth; any superficial or deep abnormality of skin or soft tissues in patients with a history of prior RT requires careful evaluation. Predisposing genetic tendencies should be considered.

Implications for Prevention

Unfortunately, in the clinical management context, the etiology of an individual sarcoma has only limited significance because it generally does not affect therapeutic decision-making beyond the fact that patients who have sarcomas arising in a previously irradiated field cannot easily receive further RT, and there may be limitations in surgery as well.

BIOLOGIC CHARACTERISTICS/MOLECULAR BIOLOGY

As already mentioned, sarcomas have extensive cytogenic abnormalities that may aid in their differential diagnosis and may ultimately provide therapeutic targets. Unfortunately, molecular prognostication and prediction of treatment response are proving more elusive than originally anticipated. For example, the presence of the translocation t(X;18) (p11;q11) has been used to confirm the diagnosis of synovial cell sarcoma for patients with poorly differentiated lesions that cannot be otherwise characterized. Irrespective of their histologic appearance, almost all synovial sarcomas contain the t(X;18) (*SYT-SSX*) translocation involving the *SSX1* gene (associated with monophasic histology) or *SSX2* gene (associated with biphasic histology) gene, two closely related genes from chromosome Xp11, and the *SYT* gene from chromosome 18q11. The result is the formation of a chimeric gene, which is thought to function by encoding a transcription-activating protein. It was suggested that the transcripts of these fusion genes had specific prognostic significance (n = 45),[36-38] but results have been contradictory.[39]

Additional biologic prognostic information has been studied and includes mutations in p53 and *MDM2*, Ki-67 status, altered expressions of the retinoblastoma gene product (pRb) in high-grade sarcomas with uncertain conclusions.[23,40,41] Also, tissue hypoxia appears associated with the development of distant metastases independently from depth, size, and grade.[42]

PATHOLOGY AND PATHWAYS OF SPREAD

Pathology

Classical Pathology Classification

Although originating from the mesoderm and, in some lesions from ectoderm, a beguiling feature of the legacy of the nomenclature of sarcoma pathology is the traditional view of histologic subtypes originating from similar appearing normal tissue counterparts. The most common classification scheme for STS is still based on histogenesis, as outlined in the World Health Organization (WHO) classification (Table 62-2).[43] However, as the degree of histologic differentiation becomes less apparent, the determination of a putative cellular origin becomes increasingly difficult.

This view of pathogenesis and histogenesis is now being contested. Although some benign lesions (especially lipomas) may resemble mature differentiated normal tissue, many STSs arise in tissues that do not typically possess the putative normal tissues mentioned. For example, synovial sarcomas are only rarely found in synovial tissues. Because the necessary genetic information is contained in all diploid cells, a more plausible explanation may be that a given set of genes may program differentiation in any mesenchymal cell, thereby giving origin to almost any mesenchymal neoplasm.[43] It seems unlikely that there is a single precursor primitive mesenchymal stem cell for each STS.

Classification by Functional Genomics

With advances in molecular characterization of STS, and the emerging dissatisfaction with traditional methods of classification, it is not unexpected that recent proposals have explored gene expression profiling of STS to attempt to identify a genomic-based classification scheme.[44-46] For example, Segal and colleagues examined RNA sarcoma samples and found that synovial sarcomas, round cell/myxoid liposarcomas (MLSs), clear-cell sarcomas, and gastrointestinal stromal tumors displayed distinct and homogeneous gene expression profiles. In a separate study, Nielsen observed that *KIT* appeared to be one of the prominent discriminator genes for MFH.[45] There may be a genomic basis for diagnosis, with both high sensitivity and specificity, and gene-expression profiling may be useful in classification; further research may ultimately lead to enhancement of *classical* methods of defining subtypes of STS.[44-46]

Grading of Sarcoma

Despite the fact that histologic grade continues to be the most powerful independent prognostic factor, there is no agreement about which grading system should be used. Two of the best known are the French Federation of Cancer Centers Sarcoma Group[47] and U.S. National Cancer Institute (NCI) systems.[48] Both classify using degrees of necrosis and mitotic rate; but the American system considers histologic type or subtype, location, cellularity, and nuclear pleomorphism, whereas the French system relies more on differentiation. Recent views suggest that the French method may be prognostically more useful.[23,49] The situation is further complicated by the existence of a two-grade system (e.g., high versus low grade), and the four-grade system of the International Union Against Cancer (UICC) and the American Joint Committee on Cancer (AJCC). The TNM stage classification (see the following text) uses a two-tiered grade classification (low versus high). Because different grading systems are used, a simple formula to *translate* three- and four-tiered grading systems into a two-tiered system is provided for TNM. In the most commonly employed three-tiered classification, grade 1 is considered *low grade* and grades 2 and 3 *high grade.* In the less common four-tiered systems, grades 1 and 2 are considered low grade and grades 3 and 4 high grade.[50,51]

PATHOLOGIC FEATURES AND NATURAL HISTORY

Selected Pathologic Subtypes

Malignant Fibrous Histiocytoma

A recent development in the histologic deliberations about STS concerns MFH, long regarded the prototypical STS and the most common soft tissue malignancy of the past two decades. MFH is now becoming a diagnosis of exclusion and potentially synonymous with undifferentiated pleomorphic sarcoma.[52] Recent evidence suggests that MFH is a more general diagnosis that can be subtyped by immunohistochemical and ultrastructural means in most patients.[53] The most common subclassifications are myxofibrosarcoma and leiomyosarcoma. Recent evaluations have shown profound changes to the classification of previously diagnosed cases with more than 50% of cases undergoing significant modification. Daugaard studied a series of cases where the number of MFHs was reduced from 72 to 2; 22 cases were renamed myxofibrosarcomas and 20 (7%) were found not to be sarcomas.[54]

Angiosarcoma

Angiosarcoma is no longer included in the TNM stage classification because its natural history is inconsistent with the general behavior of STS.[50,51] Particularly unique is the propensity of superficial angiosarcoma to occur in the head and neck region in approximately 50% of cases and to demonstrate a radial growth pattern within the dermis of the scalp and facial tissues, often in an older and typically male patient. Lesions appear at considerable distance between separate ulcerated nodules and exhibit a characteristic patchy macularis of purplish hue. Involvement of the eyelid and periorbital tissues is particularly troublesome. This sinister growth pattern makes it difficult to control, in part because of difficulty determining the optimal extent of surgical and RT margins from gross tumor. The disease has an ominous natural history, and local recurrence beyond the treatment areas is frequent.[55,56] Regional node metastases (10%-20% rates) are also more frequent than in most STS subtypes and distant metastasis is common.

Another rare variant is one complicating the treatment of breast carcinoma with superficial angiosarcoma appearing extensively within the confines of the previously irradiated volume and a tendency to develop disease in the opposite breast. A further interesting predisposition in angiosarcoma is its tendency to arise in cardiac tissues where it represents one of the most common pathologic subtypes of a rare presentation of STS.

Table 62-2 Histologic Classification of Soft Tissue Sarcoma

FIBROUS TUMORS
- Fibromatoses
  - Superficial fibromatoses
    - Palmar and plantar (Dupuytren's contracture fibromatoses)
    - Penile (Peyronie's fibromatosis)
    - Knuckle pads
  - Deep fibromatoses
    - Abdominal fibromatosis (abdominal desmoid)
    - Extra-abdominal fibromatosis (extra-abdominal desmoid)
    - Intra-abdominal fibromatosis (intra-abdominal desmoid)
    - Mesenteric fibromatosis (including Gardner's syndrome)
    - Infantile (desmoid-type) fibromatosis
- Fibrosarcoma
  - Adult fibrosarcoma
  - Inflammatory fibrosarcoma

FIBROHISTIOCYTIC TUMORS
- Dermatofibrosarcoma protuberans (including pigmented form, Bednar tumor)
- Malignant fibrous histiocytoma
  - Storiform-pleomorphic
  - Myxoid (myxofibrosarcoma)
  - Giant cell (malignant giant cell tumor of soft parts)
  - Inflammatory

LIPOMATOUS TUMORS
- Atypical lipoma
- Liposarcoma
  - Well-differentiated liposarcoma
  - Lipoma-like liposarcoma
  - Sclerosing liposarcoma
  - Inflammatory liposarcoma
  - Dedifferentiated liposarcoma
  - Myxoid/round cell liposarcoma
  - Pleomorphic liposarcoma

SMOOTH MUSCLE SARCOMAS
- Leiomyosarcoma
- Epithelioid leiomyosarcoma

SKELETAL MUSCLE SARCOMAS
- RMS
  - Embryonal RMS
  - Botryoid RMS
  - Spindle cell RMS
  - Alveolar RMS
  - Pleomorphic RMS
  - RMS with ganglionic differentiation (ectomesenchyme)

MALIGNANT TUMORS OF BLOOD AND LYMPH VESSELS
- Epithelioid hemangioendothelioma
- Angiosarcoma and lymphangiosarcoma
- Kaposi's sarcoma

MALIGNANT PERIVASCULAR TUMORS
- Malignant glomus (glomangiosarcoma) tumor
- Malignant hemangiopericytoma

MALIGNANT SYNOVIAL TUMORS
- Malignant giant cell tumor of tendon sheath

MALIGNANT NEURAL TUMORS
- MPNST (neurofibrosarcoma)
  - Malignant Triton tumor (MPNST with RMS)
  - Glandular MPNST
  - Epithelioid MPNST
  - Malignant granular cell tumor
- Primitive neuroectodermal tumor
  - Neuroblastoma
  - Ganglioneuroblastoma
  - Neuroepithelioma (peripheral neuroectodermal tumor)

PARAGANGLIONIC TUMORS
- Malignant paraganglioma

EXTRASKELETAL CARTILAGINOUS AND OSSEOUS TUMORS
- Extraskeletal chondrosarcoma
- Myxoid chondrosarcoma
- Mesenchymal chondrosarcoma
- Extraskeletal osteosarcoma

PLURIPOTENTIAL MALIGNANT MESENCHYMAL TUMORS
- Malignant mesenchymoma
- Alveolar soft part sarcoma
- Epithelioid sarcoma
- Malignant extrarenal rhabdoid tumor
- Desmoplastic small cell tumor
- Ewing's sarcoma (extraskeletal)
- Clear cell sarcoma (melanoma of soft parts)
- Gastrointestinal stromal tumors
- Synovial sarcoma
  - Biphasic synovial sarcoma
  - Monophasic synovial sarcoma

Benign lesions other than fibromatosis and atypical lipoma are not included in the present tabulation.
MPNST, malignant peripheral nerve sheath tumor; RMS, rhabdomyosarcoma.
Modified from: Fletcher CDM, Unni K, Mertens K (eds): World Health Organization Classification of Tumours: Pathology and Genetics of Tumours of Soft Tissue and Bone. Lyon, France, IARC Press (International Agency for Research on Cancer) publishers, 2002.[43]

Rhabdomyosarcoma

RMS is especially important because it is the fifth most common cancer in childhood[57] but is also represented in the adult where the outcome is significantly less favorable.[58] One feature concerns the *spindle cell rhabdomyosarcoma* that is only rarely described in the adult compared to children and carries a relatively favorable prognosis. In the adult, it appears to have a predilection for the head and neck and may be unusually aggressive compared to childhood.[59,60] RMS is generally subdivided into embryonal (approximately 70% of cases), alveolar (approximately 20%), and pleomorphic subtypes according to histologic pattern and molecular alterations.[61,62] Both embryonal and alveolar RMS have been studied extensively for cytogenetic and molecular genetic alterations. No consistent findings have been observed in the embryonal variant; in contrast, the majority of alveolar subtypes possess the t(2;13) aberration (see Table 62-1). Both translocations may be associated with different clinical phenotypes.[63] The translocations and the gene fusion products are characteristic, and the *PAX3* gene family involved in the disease fingerprint may have a role in muscle development.[64]

RMS is also one of the sarcomas associated with a risk of lymph node metastasis. Irrespective of age the alveolar and embryonal subtypes manifest high rates of response to chemotherapy and RT. The initial evaluation of RMS is similar to regular STS but should include bone marrow examination. In addition, the CSF should be sampled in parameningeal

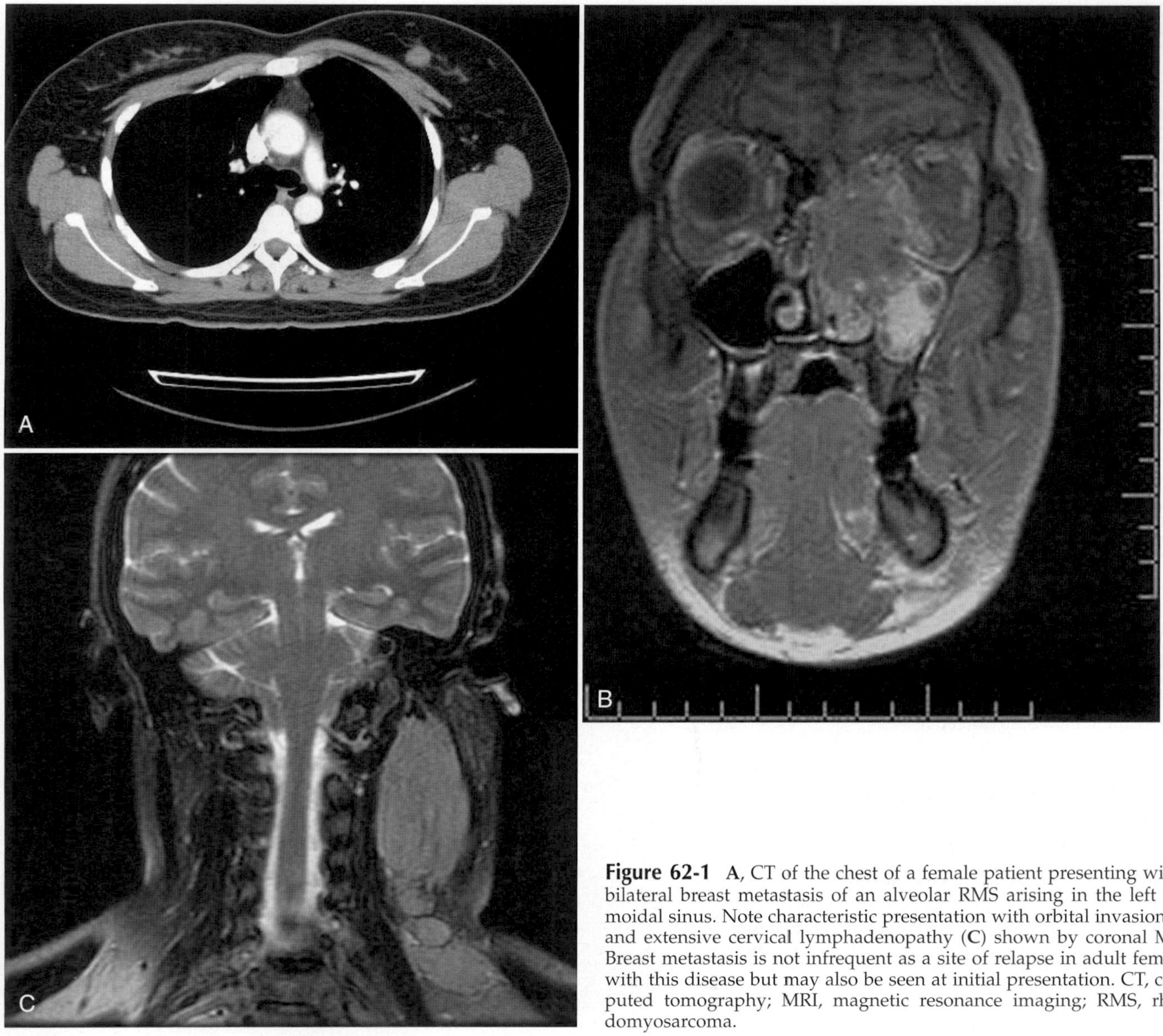

Figure 62-1 **A**, CT of the chest of a female patient presenting with a bilateral breast metastasis of an alveolar RMS arising in the left ethmoidal sinus. Note characteristic presentation with orbital invasion (**B**) and extensive cervical lymphadenopathy (**C**) shown by coronal MRI. Breast metastasis is not infrequent as a site of relapse in adult females with this disease but may also be seen at initial presentation. CT, computed tomography; MRI, magnetic resonance imaging; RMS, rhabdomyosarcoma.

lesions. Rarely but distinctly, these lesions tend to develop synchronous or metachronous metastases in one or both breasts (Fig. 62-1).

Liposarcoma

Liposarcoma is the second most commonly encountered STS subtype and MLS is the most common variant.[65] Classical MLS has a t(12:16) translocation resulting in the *TLS-CHOP* fusion shared with the more aggressive round cell variant and not seen in predominantly myxoid well-differentiated liposarcoma.[66] It also has an unusual pattern of recurrence that includes a predilection for soft tissue metastases.[67-70]

Apparent multifocal presentation or recurrence at two or more anatomically separate soft tissue sites (with predilection for the retroperitoneum and mediastinum) (Fig. 62-2) and bone metastases are a striking yet unpredictable feature of MLS and contrasts with other STS. Surgery and RT may result in relatively long disease-free intervals (e.g., many years). Uncertainty had existed about whether such multifocal lesions represent an unusual pattern of metastasis or multiple separate primary tumors until Antonescu and colleagues showed that all cases of multifocal MLS bore the identical molecular lineage of the parent primary tumor.[71]

More favorable survival in a large cohort of liposarcoma patients compared with other histologic subtypes was recently reported in a series exceeding 1000 cases. The observation was independent of other prognostic factors including grade, depth, and tumor size.[72] MLS also appears to manifest an unusually sensitive response to RT[73] (Fig. 62-3) that may explain the propensity for unexpectedly favorable local control following adjuvant RT.[74]

Dermatofibrosarcoma Protuberans

Dermatofibrosarcoma protuberans (DFSP) is a superficial tumor that often manifests as deceptive dermal, raised purple/red lesion(s) in the lower neck, upper chest, and shoulder girdle regions. DFSPs arise from the dermis and exhibit a characteristic slow but persistent growth over many years. Hallmark immunohistochemical staining for the *CD34* gene suggests evidence of neural differentiation. Although

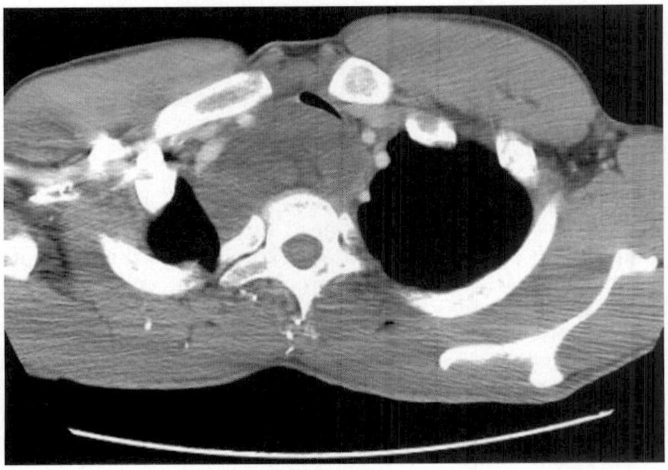

Figure 62-2 CT showing isolated mediastinal relapse with tracheal obstruction occurring in a patient who had presented 7 years previously with a MLS in the popliteal fossa similar to the lesion shown in Figure 62-8. The initial limb lesion was treated with preoperative RT and maintained local control. This patient underwent airway management, preoperative RT, and surgical resection and was disease free with 15 months of follow-up. Isolated soft-tissue relapse in this fashion is a hallmark of the behavior of MLS and may result in long-term remission or salvage of such lesions. CT, computed tomography; MLS, myxoid liposarcoma; RT, radiation therapy.

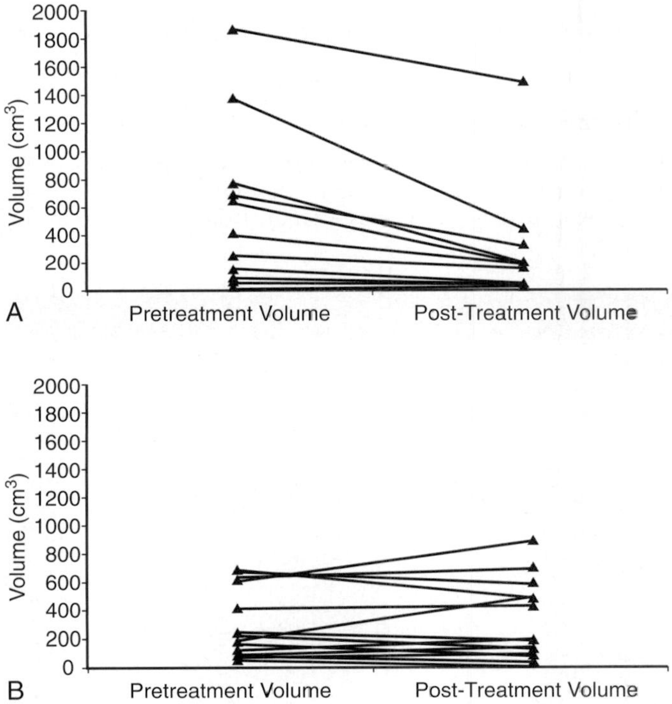

Figure 62-3 Pretreatment and post-treatment three-dimensional tumor volumes obtained in an identical manner for (**A**) MLS (experimental group) and (**B**) malignant fibrous histiocytoma (control group) treated with preoperative RT (50 Gy in 25 fractions) at the Princess Margaret Hospital. These results provide the first objective data to support the idea that MLS tumors show a statistically significant reduction in size when treated with RT and that this response is greater than that of MFH tumors given the same RT. MFH, malignant fibrous histiocytoma; MLS, myxoid liposarcoma; RT, radiation therapy. (Adapted from Pitson G, Robinson P, Wilke D, et al: Radiation response: An additional unique signature of myxoid liposarcoma. Int J Radiat Oncol Biol Phys 60:522-526, 2004.)

borderline to low grade in histologic appearance, it has a propensity for local recurrence after simple excision. Its indolence renders it exempt from the TNM stage classification system.[50,51] Chromosomal translocation and gene fusion products have also been observed (see Table 62-1). Specifically, platelet-derived growth factor beta (PDGFB) is increased locally, resulting in autocrine or paracrine tumor growth. Of importance, imatinib (Gleevec) is an inhibitor of the PDGF receptor tyrosine kinase. Recent data have shown response to imatinib in DFSP predicted by the presence of the t(17;22) translocation.[75] In general, however, the typical cases fare extremely well with surgery alone or supplemented with adjuvant RT,[76-78] and these should remain the conventional management approaches at this time for curable disease.

Synovial Sarcoma

Synovial sarcoma often exhibits a biphasic cellular pattern consisting of a stroma of fibroblast spindle- and epithelial-like cells in a glandular pattern on light microscopy and immunohistochemistry. Typically occurring in the para-articular areas of the tendon sheaths and joints of young adults, at least 50% of the cases are in the lower limbs (especially the knee), and most of the remainder are seen in the upper limbs.[79] Calcification may be apparent. It may also be encountered in regions without apparent relationship to synovial structures.[80] Local treatment follows the general principles of STS treatment. This histologic subtype exhibits more favorable responses to chemotherapy than most other histologies.[81] The disease also has a reputation for higher risk of lymph node metastasis (<2% to 14%).[82,83] As noted earlier, in synovial sarcoma the t(x;18) translocation can almost invariably be detected with the demonstration of a fusion between the *SSX1* and *SYT* genes.

Gastrointestinal Stromal Tumors

Gastrointestinal stromal tumors (GISTs) are rare soft tissue sarcomas that represent the first solid tumor with a consistent favorable response to molecular targeted therapy. These tumors predominantly arise in the stomach or small intestine but can also develop from omentum and retroperitoneum. Metastases occur predominantly within the peritoneal cavity and to the liver. GISTs harbor so-called gain-of-function mutations in the *c-KIT* or *platelet-derived growth factor receptor A* (*PDGFRA*) genes in 85% and 5% of cases, respectively.[84,85] Through these mutations the receptors are constitutively activated. The advent of the tyrosine kinase inhibitor imatinib was a major breakthrough in the management of advanced GIST lesions because the response rates were dramatic and effective treatment options had not previously been available.[86,87] Patients whose tumors contained exon 11 *KIT* mutations are more likely to respond to imatinib than those whose tumors have an exon 9 *KIT* mutation or those with no detectable kinase mutation.[88]

Clear Cell Sarcoma (Malignant Melanoma of Soft Parts)

For many years this unusual tumor has also been termed *malignant melanoma of soft parts*, or *clear cell sarcoma of tendons and aponeuroses*. Like melanoma it has a predilection to develop lymph node metastases but in contrast presents as a deep soft tissue mass rather than a cutaneous lesion. Clear cell sarcoma has a distinct chromosomal translocation, t(12;22) (q13;q13) involving *EWS* and *ATF1* genes. Because of the presence of intracellular melanin and immunoreactivity for *S100* and HMB45, it has been suggested that this entity is better considered a subtype of melanoma and not a STS. Recent analysis by genomic profiling and cluster analysis appears to confirm this view.[89]

Pathways of Spread

Local Disease

Most STSs tend to spread in a longitudinal direction within the muscle groups where they originate, typically an extremity. As they extend, lesions invade muscle, and contiguous structures may envelop major neurovascular structures. The extending border comprises an outer perimeter of edematous tissue intermixed with a reactive zone of neovascularity with interspersed tumor satellites and pseudopodia. This surrounding area is generally termed the *pseudocapsule,* and may encourage erroneous interpretation of anatomic disease containment and enucleation. Such operations, frequently termed *shell outs,* almost invariably mean that residual diseases remain. STS generally respect barriers to tumor spread in the axial plane of the extremity such as bone, interosseous membrane, major fascial planes, and this feature should be exploited in planning tissue preserving approaches to management. Thus the margins of RT should be wide in the cephalocaudal direction, but in the cross-section there may be much greater security in defining nontarget structures. For nonextremity lesions, the direction of sarcoma growth is also along the involved musculature, but care must be taken to ensure that the fascial planes are appropriately recognized and encompassed in surgical or radiation target volumes.[90]

A complete description of all the body's anatomic planes and fascial compartments is beyond the scope of this chapter. Nonetheless, they guide the principles used to manage these lesions. The importance of the osteofascial compartments of the extremities is that, from an anatomic standpoint, they operate as functional units and are protected from each others' risks of tumor contamination in the absence of inappropriate violation of the subdividing fascial septae. The latter may occur with misplaced surgical intrusion, including inappropriate placement of drain or biopsy tracts.[91]

The fascial structures are also important because they guard tumors arising superficial to the fascia investing the muscles of the region from the deeper structures. Tumors arising in subcutaneous tissues are staged differently to those arising deep to the fascia. In the event that the fascia has been disrupted, as is often the case following an *unplanned* sarcoma resection with positive margins, it may provide a route for deep contamination by tumor.

Regional Lymph Node Involvement

In STS, there is generally no need for any specific regional lymph node treatment. Important exceptions to this generalization include epithelioid sarcoma, clear cell sarcoma, angiosarcoma, and RMS (Table 62-3).[82,83] Generally, lymph node involvement has been associated with an adverse prognosis[50,51] rivaling that of distant metastasis. However, recent data suggest that isolated lymph node metastasis may not be as deleterious a factor.[92,93]

Distant Metastasis

Most sarcomas present with localized disease and overt metastasis is present in only 10% of cases at diagnosis. Typically the patient is asymptomatic, and staging investigations are required to demonstrate metastases. The predominant risk is to the lungs. Spread to bone may be seen following lung metastases but is seen with the greatest regularity in MLS where it may be the first site of relapse. MLS also has the unusual characteristic of developing isolated soft tissue metastases. In patients with retroperitoneal sarcoma (RPS) and intra-abdominal visceral sarcomas, the liver is a more common site of first metastasis.

CLINICAL MANIFESTATIONS/PATIENT EVALUATION/STAGING

Clinical Manifestations

The presenting feature of extremity and superficial torso STS is most often with a painless mass. Evidence of pain or other symptoms usually indicates origin from or invasion of

Table 62-3 Histologic Type of Sarcomas and Lymph Node Metastasis*

Histologic Subtype	MAZERON 1987 SERIES[82] *n*	(%)	FONG 1993 SERIES[83] *n*	(%)
Alveolar soft part	3/24	12.5	0/13	0
Angiosarcoma	—	—	5/37	13.5
Chondrosarcoma	—	—	1/46	2.2
Clear cell sarcoma	11/40	27.5	—	—
Epithelioid sarcoma	14/70	20.0	2/12	16.7
Fibrosarcoma	54/215	4.4	0/162	0
Hemangiopericytoma	—	—	0/21	0
Leiomyosarcoma	21/524	4.0	9/328	2.7
Liposarcoma	16/504	3.2	3/403	0.7
Lymphangiosarcoma	—	—	1/4	25.0
Malignant fibrous histiocytoma	84/823	10.2	8/316	2.6
Neurofibrosarcoma (MPNST)	3/476	0.6	2/96	2.1
Osteosarcoma	—	—	0/11	0
RMS (embryonal)	—	—	12/88	13.6
RMS (other)	201/1354	14.8	1/35	2.9
Synovial sarcoma	117/851	13.7	2/145	1.4
Undifferentiated spindle cell	—	0	0/42	—
Vascular	43/376	11.4	—	—
Other	—	—	0/27	0
Total	567/5257	10.8	47/1772	2.6

*Number (*n*) of nodal metastases/all sarcoma patients in two studies and proportion (%) of all lesions.
MPNST, malignant peripheral nerve sheath tumor; RMS, rhabdomyosarcoma.
Data from Mazeron and Suit summarizing literature studies[82] and Fong, et al. from a single institution.[83]

neurovascular structures. Erythema and warmth may be evident depending on the vascular and tissue response. Some patients will present with large, slow-growing lesions that may restrict joint motion, and larger tumors may ulcerate skin or invade adjacent compartments and bone leading to fracture.

In general, superficial (or subcutaneous) lesions are smaller than those deep to fascia or in the retroperitoneum. Growth rate appears to be an important determinant of the clinical course. Low-grade sarcoma (especially low-grade liposarcoma) may grow at an imperceptible rate without symptoms, and the lesion may be enormous at presentation. This is especially the case for massive low-grade liposarcomas of the retroperitoneum. Otherwise, patients with intra-abdominal sarcoma commonly present with nonspecific abdominal pain or a palpable mass of prodigious size before symptoms such as anorexia and chronic subacute intestinal obstruction with subsequent weight loss appear. Uterine sarcoma often presents with a pelvic mass preceded by menorrhagia.

Head and neck sarcomas may originate within the upper aerodigestive tract and present symptoms of nasal obstruction, cranial nerve dysfunction, proptosis, and associated mass effect in sensitive locations; the latter may include pain or pharynx and airway compromise depending on the location and size of lesions. Sarcomas also arise in the subcutaneous tissues of the scalp, facial tissues, or neck, or may present with a superficial mass.

Patient evaluation

Initial Assessment

The overall initial evaluation of an STS patient is summarized in the diagnostic algorithm shown in Figure 62-4. All soft tissue masses deep to the investing fascia should be considered sarcoma until proved otherwise. The type of biopsy, or a prior inappropriate excision, may jeopardize the form and outcome of local treatment by contaminating tissues that were uninvolved initially. Before embarking on treatment, histologic confirmation of the diagnosis is necessary. To minimize the risk of undesirable outcome, prebiopsy cross-sectional imaging is necessary to avoid compromising the planning of management.

In addition to the diagnostic interventions, assessment should include a thorough clinical assessment including history and clinical examination. Particular attention should be given to the relationship of the investing fascia deep to the subcutaneous fat (i.e., whether superficial versus deep) and adjacent neurovascular structures or bone, and lesion size and mobility.

Both computed tomography (CT) scan and magnetic resonance imaging (MRI) are used widely to evaluate the primary local disease. CT provides better bony detail than MRI and has the advantage of exhibiting calcification characteristic of certain histologies (e.g., synovial sarcoma). However, MRI provides pluridirectional images and superior contrast resolution and is likely the best instrument for tumor definition. It is also essential to evaluate peritumoral edema, which is less apparent with CT. Low signal intensity on T1-weighted images and a high signal on T2-weighted images are typical and can be readily separated from normal soft tissue structures, but they cannot distinguish subtypes of STS and benign from malignant lesions. In general a prominent anatomic area (e.g., a joint) should be included in the field of view to permit adequate localization for treatment planning.

A *blinded* study by the Radiation Diagnostic Oncology Group that compared MRI and CT in patients with malignant

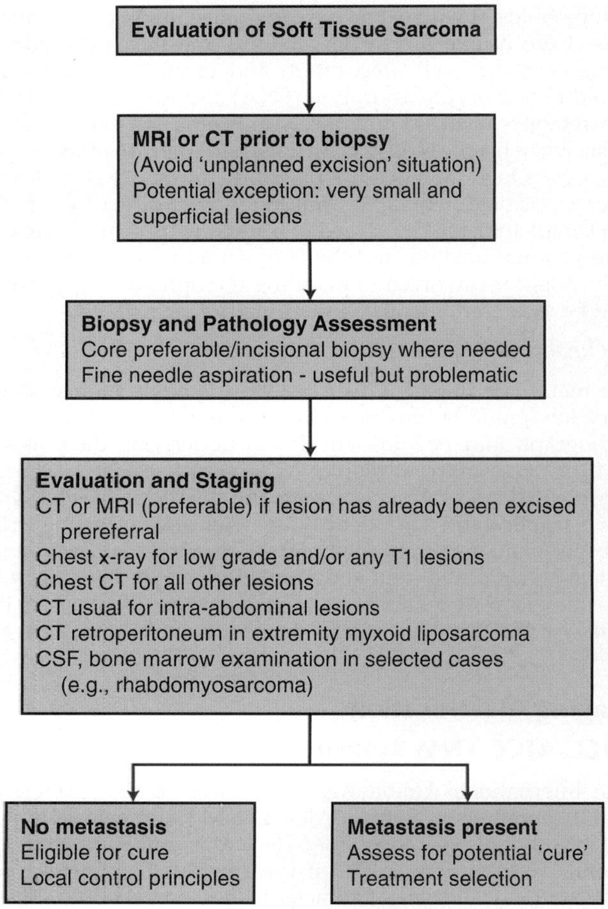

Figure 62-4 Diagnostic algorithm for the initial evaluation of a STS patient. All soft tissue masses deep to the investing fascia should be considered sarcoma until proved otherwise. Emphasis is needed on the type of biopsy and pathological assessment. Most patients require CT or MRI for the local disease assessment, and most patients require CT to exclude metastatic disease. CSF analysis for tumor cytology is indicated in parameningeal RMS. CSF, cerebrospinal fluid; MLS, myxoid liposarcoma; MRI, magnetic resonance imaging; RMS, rhabdomyosarcoma; RT, radiation therapy; STS, soft tissue sarcoma.

bone and soft tissue tumors showed no specific advantage of MRI over CT.[94] Although the diagnostic evaluation may be equally served by both modalities, the treatment planning requirements (for both surgery and RT) frequently require additional information including advantages through MRI/CT image-fusion techniques. Positron emission tomography (PET) scan has the putative advantage over MRI in quantifying biological tumor activity, and evidence suggests it may have prognostic value in identifying tumors of higher grade. It may also demonstrate prediction of better outcome in patients who respond to induction regimens.[95,96] The value of ^{18}F-fluorodeoxyglucose positron emission tomography (FDG-PET) in the detection as well as grading and response to therapy of soft tissue and bone sarcoma has been assessed in a systematic review and meta-analysis of 29 clinical studies; and the authors concluded that there is no indication for its use in the standard treatment of sarcomas.[97]

Establishing the Diagnosis

Fine-needle aspiration biopsy (FNAB) as a primary diagnostic tool is controversial and should only be used where a cytopathologist with extensive experience in sarcoma is available. Core needle biopsy under local anesthesia provides a more consistent cell preparation and tissue specimen compared to fine-needle aspiration (FNA) and is recommended.[23] Open biopsy of STS is only rarely indicated but yields a diagnosis when needle biopsy is unsuccessful (approximately 10% of cases). Open incisional biopsy of deep tumors is preferred over excisional biopsy to minimize the difficulty of the *unplanned* excision.[98-100] Needle tracts are potential sites of tumor contamination, and the surgeon and radiation oncologist should be involved in planning the optimal biopsy route and be aware of potential contamination.

Exclusion of Metastasis

For metastatic staging, CT of the chest is required, except for very low-grade lesions or small lesions where a plain chest radiograph may be sufficient. If the underlying diagnosis is RMS, a bone marrow biopsy is necessary as well as cerebrospinal fluid analysis in parameningeal lesions. PET may have applicability in identifying metastases in high-risk subsets (e.g., recurrent high-grade tumors). For retroperitoneal, visceral, and intra-abdominal lesions, the site of metastasis that is most common (i.e., the liver) should be evaluated with the modality that is used for evaluation of the primary lesion.

Staging Classifications

UICC/AJCC TNM System

The International Union Against Cancer (UICC)/American Joint Committee on Cancer (AJCC) TNM staging system[50,51] is the most widely employed for STSs and is unusual within the overall TNM system in that it incorporates histologic grade with anatomical disease characteristics. Generally, the system is based on an ascending hierarchy of risk depending on whether a lesion is deemed to have no adverse features for relapse or one, two, or three factors present represented by size partitioned at the 5-cm break point, grade (high versus low), and lesion depth as *a* (superficial tumor arising outside the investing fascia) or *b* (a deep tumor that arises beneath the fascia or invades the fascia) (Table 62-4). All STS subtypes are included excepting visceral sarcomas, where an international system is lacking, and dermatofibrosarcoma protuberans, because it is considered to have only borderline malignant potential; finally, angiosarcoma is no longer included because of the differences in natural history from other sarcomas.

Table 62-4 International Union Against Cancer (UICC) and American Joint Committee on Cancer (AJCC) TNM Classification (6th ed) of Soft Tissue Sarcomas[50,51]

PRIMARY TUMOR	
TX	Primary tumor cannot be assessed.
T0	No evidence of primary tumor.
T1	Tumor ≤5 cm in greatest dimension.
	T1a superficial tumor*
	T2b deep tumor*
T2	Tumor ≥5 cm in greatest dimension.
	T2a superficial tumor*
	T2b deep tumor*
REGIONAL LYMPH NODES	
NX	Regional lymph nodes cannot be assessed.
N0	No regional lymph node metastasis.
N1	Regional lymph node metastasis.
DISTANT METASTASIS	
MX	Distant metastasis cannot be assessed.
M0	No distant metastasis.
MI	Distant metastasis.

STAGE GROUPING				
Stage I	G1-2	T1a, 1b, 2a, 2b	N0	M0
Stage II	G3-4	T1a, 1b, 2a	N0	M0
Stage III	G3-4	T2b	N0	M0
Stage IV	Any G	Any T	N1	M0
	Any G	Any T	N0	M1

**Note:* Superficial tumor is located exclusively above the superficial fascia without invasion of the fascia; deep tumor is located either exclusively beneath the superficial fascia, superficial to the fascia with invasion of or through the fascia, or both superficial yet beneath the fascia.

G, grade; M, distant metastasis; N, regional lymph nodes; T, primary tumor; X, category cannot be assessed.

Rhabdomyosarcoma

Two separate classifications of disease extent exist for RMS. The original description of disease extent had been by a postoperative surgical classification developed by the North American Intergroup Rhabdomyosarcoma Study Group (IRSG). Currently, such lesions will frequently be treated with induction protocols well in advance of surgery. Therefore reliance on a surgical staging system is problematic. The International Society of Pediatric Oncology (SIOP) employs a TNM presurgical staging system more in keeping with contemporary TNM staging and both systems.

Retroperitoneum Proposed Staging

Retroperitoneal sarcomas are currently classified by the TNM system. However, a classification system has been developed based on grade, completeness of resection, and distant metastases.[101] For class 1 (low grade/grossly complete resection/no metastases) the 5-year overall survival was 68% to 89%. For class 2 (high grade/grossly complete resection/no metastases) the 5-year overall survival was 46%-40%. For class 3 (incomplete resection/no metastases) the 5-year overall survival was 24% to 26%; and for class 4 (distant metastases) it was 0% to 17%. Validation is required before it can be considered for general use.

PRIMARY THERAPY OF SOFT TISSUE SARCOMA

Results of Treatment (General Issues)

The expected 5-year survival of patients with STS overall is approximately 60%.[102] The benchmark for local control in extremity sarcomas is approximately 90% in Table 62-5. There has been little progress in reducing the risk of metastases. The overall approach to the local management of nonmetastatic extremity, head and neck, and superficial trunk, including the body wall, STS is summarized in Figure 62-5. In general the approach is confined to surgery with or without RT; and we recommend chemotherapy in selected cases including chemoresponsive lesions and in some high-risk cases, but the evidence for the latter is less substantial.

Evidence about Local Management (Randomized Trials)

The origins of contemporary extremity STS management can be traced to the landmark trial at the NCI where patients with high-grade sarcoma of the extremities were randomized to receive amputation versus a limb-sparing operation followed by adjuvant RT (see Table 62-5).[103] In addition to the

Table 62-5 Phase III Randomized Controlled Trials in the Local Management of Soft Tissue Sarcoma

Centers & Authors	Study Period	Site	Trial Schema	*N*	Local Control or Response	Comments
Feldkirch, Austria	1978-1988	Multiple	60 Gy alone	66	30.5%	64% had equally balanced gross disease.
Rhomberg, et al.[126]			60 Gy + razoxane	64	64%	Toxicity equivalent; lower EBRT dose in RPS.
NCI	1975-1982	Extrem	Amputation	16	100%	Small trial with imbalance.
Rosenberg, et al.[103]			Surg & EBRT	27	4%	No survival difference.
NCI	Not given	RPS	IORT & postop RT	15	60%	Small trial; significant toxicity.
Sindelar, et al.[212]			Postop EBRT	20	20%	No survival difference.
MSKCC high grade[104]	1982-1992	Extrem	Surg	63	70%	No survival difference.
Pisters, et al.[104]		Trunk	Surg & BRT	56	91%	
NCI high grade	1983-1991	Extrem	Surg	44	80%	No survival difference.
Yang, et al.[105]			Surg & postop EBRT	47	100%	Concurrent chemotherapy administered.
MSKCC low grade	1982-1992	Extrem	Surg	23	74%	Subset of main MSKCC trial.
Pisters, et al.[104]		Trunk	Surg & BRT	22	64%	Poor control in low grade with BRT.
NCI low grade	1983-1991	Extrem	Surg	24	67%	Subset of main trial.
Yang, et al.[105]			Surg & postop EBRT	26	96%	Equal control with EBRT for low grade.
CSG/NCIC CTG	1994-1997	Extrem	Preop EBRT	94	93%	No survival difference.
O'Sullivan, et al.[106,121]			Postop EBRT	96	92%	Wound complications with preop; late fibrosis with postop. Abstract results: full manuscript pending.
UCLA	1984-1988	Extrem	Concurrent RT & IV Dox	52	92%	Chemotherapy trial with local control endpoint.
Eilber, et al.[153]			Concurrent RT & IA Dox	44	93%	Published in abstract form.
IGR	2000-2003	Extrem	ILP-melphalan (with 0.5 mg TNF-α)	25	68% Resp	Outcome was imaging response assessment.
Bonvalot, et al.[157]			ILP-melphalan (with 1 mg TNF-α)	25	56% Resp	No dose effect detected for the objective tumor response.
			ILP-melphalan (with 2 mg TNF-α)	25	72% Resp	Systemic toxicity was significantly correlated with higher TNF-αdoses.
			ILP-melphalan (3 mg upper limit + 4 mg (lower limit) TNF-α	25	64% Resp	
EORTC	1997-2004	Extrem Nonextrem	EIA chemotherapy alone	127	Too early	Early progressive disease within 3 months: 9%; survival
Lindner, et al.[213]			EIA chemotherapy & RHT	127	Too early	Early progressive disease within 3 months: 12%. Abstract results: full manuscript pending.

BRT, brachytherapy; CSG/NCIC CTG, Canadian Sarcoma Group/National Cancer Institute of Canada Clinical Trials Group; EBRT, external beam radiation therapy; EIA, etoposide, ifosfamide, doxorubicin; EORTC, European Organization for Research and Treatment of Cancer; Extrem, extremity; IGR: Institut Gustave Roussy; ILP, isolated limb perfusion; MSKCC, Memorial Sloan-Kettering Cancer Center; NCI, U.S. National Cancer Institute; Nonextrem, nonextremity; Postop, postoperative; Preop, preoperative; Resp, response; RHT, regional hyperthermia; RPS, retroperitoneal sarcoma; Surg, conservative surgery; TNF-α, tumor necrosis factor-α.

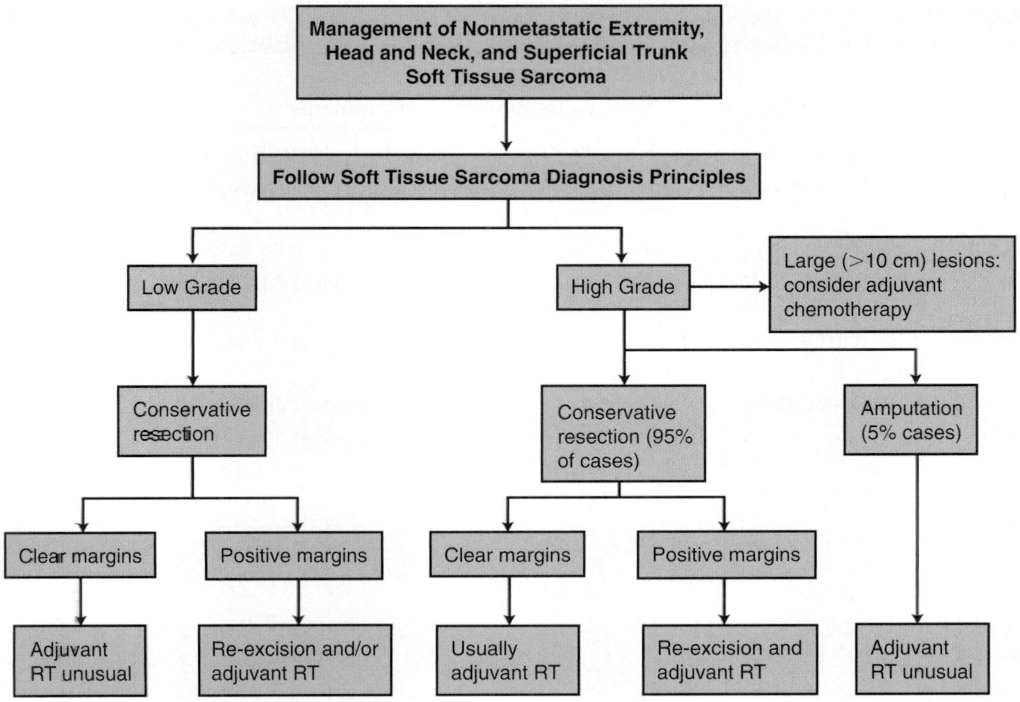

Figure 62-5 The focus of this schema predominantly addresses the local treatment of these lesions and recognizes that systemic chemotherapy is controversial. In unfavorable presentations in a fit patient, chemotherapy may be considered although in general this is an institution-specific preference. Of note, the predominant approach involves tissue preservation with conservative surgery and adjuvant RT. Selected patients may be treated with surgery alone and rare patients (5% of cases) require amputation. RT, radiation therapy.

amputation versus limb sparing NCI trial, there have been a number of others addressing several important controversies (see Table 62-5). Notably, two trials compared conservative surgery alone to similar surgery with adjuvant RT (one addressing brachytherapy and the second postoperative external beam radiation therapy [EBRT]).[104,105] Another trial addressed preoperative versus postoperative EBRT in extremity STS.[106]

Philosophy of Local Management

Surgery is the mainstay of the management of STS and was formerly used alone, albeit often in the form of an amputation. Better understanding of the fascial containment and routes of spread have led to tissue preservation in most patients. Inappropriate violation of fascia should not take place, because tumors usually involve either the superficial or the deep compartment, but rarely both. If the deep compartment is involved or has been contaminated, re-excision, RT, or frequently both may be required. RT needs to generously include the deep compartment together with the original subcutaneous tissue site if it was involved or contaminated.

For most superficial STS (the *a* subcategory in the TNM), the clinician's preoccupation should be with margins of resection above the fascia. The deep margin can be safely secured by either resecting the lesion en bloc with the investing fascia, which acts as a *wide* deep resection margin; or giving RT after a negative but narrow margin excision in which the fascia remains intact. In this latter situation, the clinical target volume (CTV) only needs to encompass the superficial tumor region with the underlying fascia but not widely within the deeper muscle compartment. Generally, we recommend that RT is not indicated in the presence of adequate resection margins, irrespective of pathologic features including grade, because the principle of anatomic containment and tissue protection should govern the use and indications for the local treatment modalities.

Surgical Management Issues

Extent of Surgery and Causes of Different Resection Margins

Of more importance than the description of the type of surgery is the actual extent of viable residual disease remaining after surgery. This is not a precise variable but is best represented by expert pathologic assessment of the surgical *resection margin.* Characterization of the margin guides the need for adjuvant RT for those tumors with insufficient normal tissue surrounding the tumor to reliably prevent local recurrence. Having positive margins nearly doubles the risk of local recurrence and increases the risk of distant recurrence and disease-related death.[107]

We have shown that positive resection margins may have different causes. Patients with microscopically positive margin low-grade liposarcomas have a low risk of local failure, as do patients where a positive margin is anticipated before surgery to preserve critical structures; and RT is able to sterilize the minimal residual disease. However, two categories of positive surgical margins are associated with a higher risk of local recurrence: patients who present after prereferral unplanned excision and have a positive margin on subsequent re-excision, and those with unanticipated positive margins occurring during primary sarcoma resection.[108] The policy in STS surgery should be to achieve negative surgical margins, and this is best accomplished by performing surgery at an experienced referral center. In this setting it appears that a small isolated positive resection margin, planned from the outset by the multidisciplinary team with the intention of sparing a critical anatomic structure (e.g., at a major nerve, vessel, or bone) has a favorable outcome (local recurrence 3.6%) compared with an *unplanned excision* margin-positive situation (local recurrence 31.6%).[108] RT must obviously be used in both circumstances. Although recent data indicate that the unplanned surgery (without re-excision) situation can often be managed successfully with immediate RT,[109] we remain concerned that substantial contamination means that subsequent RT will be less successful. In addition, the burden of residual disease is often underestimated.[108]

Surgery Alone in the Treatment of Soft Tissue Sarcoma

Conservation Approaches

Most deep sarcomas present with disease expanding out of a single muscle unit or may have undergone a *contaminating* biopsy prior to referral and therefore need RT combined with surgery.[110] There is undoubtedly a subgroup of patients who do not need RT.[111-114] The problem with these data are that they are retrospective and emanate from large centers with experience in sarcoma management, and case selection is present. The challenge remains in how to select those cases that can be managed by single modality approach versus those who also require RT.

Amputation

The polar opposite circumstance where RT is usually omitted is when amputation is performed. There rarely is a need to deliver RT following amputation when there has been unsatisfactory clearance of at-risk tissues, especially in very proximally positioned extremity lesions.

Even in a milieu where limb preservation with adjuvant RT is a preferred policy, there always remains a group of patients who are better treated with amputation.[115] At Memorial Sloan-Kettering Cancer Center (MSKCC), from 1968 to 1990 the amputation rate fell from 50% to less than 5%[116] and at the Princess Margaret Hospital (PMH) amputation was never popular and only used in 7 of 226 patients with extremity STS treated between 1980 and 1988,[117] strong evidence that the indications for this approach should be rare.[118] Amputation should only be performed: (1) where it is impossible to achieve adequate surgical clearance, because the lesion involves major neurovascular structures or multiple compartments (Fig. 62-6); (2) potential major RT complication would result from dose and volume considerations; and (3) some lower extremity distal lesions where a below-knee amputation prosthesis may be more serviceable than a limb damaged by extensive surgery and radiation.[119]

Radiation Therapy Management Issues

Rationale for Adjuvant Radiation Therapy

Adjuvant RT is generally used to permit more conservative tissue resections and therefore less-extensive operations than usual. External-beam photons delivered preoperatively or postoperatively, or brachytherapy are the usual modes of administration. Strander and associates, in a systematic overview involving 4579 patients,[120] employed data from five randomized trials, six prospective studies, 25 retrospective studies, and three additional articles. Adjuvant RT improved the local control rate in combination with conservative surgery in the treatment of STS of extremities and trunk in patients with negative, marginal, or minimal microscopic positive surgical margins. A local control rate of 90% is expected. Improvement is obtained with RT following intralesional surgery, but the local control rate is less satisfactory. For STS in other anatomic sites, such as retroperitoneum, head and neck, breast, and uterus, they concluded that the benefit in local control with adjuvant RT was less compelling.[120]

Details of the Randomized Trials of Adjuvant Radiation Therapy

As mentioned earlier, adjuvant RT with conservative surgical resection has been evaluated in two randomized clinical trials.[104,105] Yang and colleagues at the NCI randomized high-grade extremity lesions following limb-sparing surgery to receive adjuvant RT or no further treatment following the surgery. Concurrent chemotherapy was also used depending on grade. The local control for those receiving RT was 99% compared to 70% in the control group ($P = 0.0001$).[105] The results were similar for high- and low-grade tumors. Adjuvant

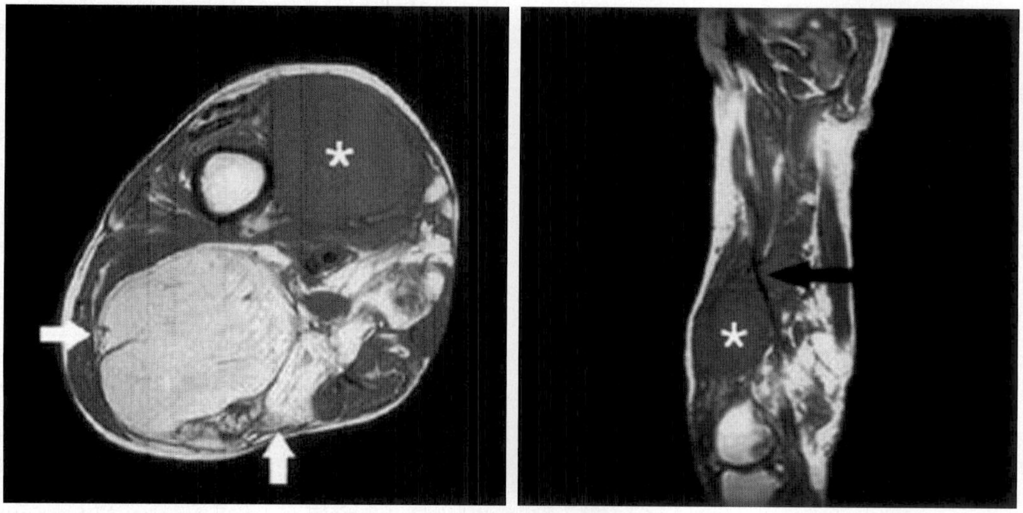

A B

Figure 62-6 (**A**) An axial T1-weighted (TR, 800 msec; TE, 10 msec) image of a complex dedifferentiated liposarcoma of the right thigh necessitating above-knee amputation because of multicompartmental and composite soft-tissue involvement. A large multilobulated mass encases the sciatic nerve and femoral neurovascular bundle. The posterior component of the mass was predominantly composed of fat signal (*white arrows*) and involved the posterior compartment of the thigh. The more anterior and higher-grade component (*) lay predominantly within the vastus medialis muscle and was of intermediate signal. (**B**) A corresponding sagittal view demonstrates encasement of the femoral neurovascular bundle (*black arrow*) by the dedifferentiated component of the tumor (*). TE, time to echo signal; TR, time to repetition signal. (Adapted from Ghert MA, Abudu A, Driver N, et al: The indications for and the prognostic significance of amputation as the primary surgical procedure for localized soft tissue sarcoma of the extremity. Ann Surg Oncol 12:10-17, 2005. With Rind permission of Springer and Business Media.)

RT, using brachytherapy, was also evaluated in a randomized trial at MSKCC with a similar effect in high-grade lesions.[104] No improvement in local control was evident in the low-grade tumors (see Table 62-5), attributed to more slowly cycling cells that are thereby excluded from the radiosensitive phases of the cycle during brachytherapy.[104]

Scheduling: Preoperative versus Postoperative Radiation Therapy

The two most common methods of RT delivery are preoperative or postoperative external beam. A Canadian randomized trial compared preoperative and postoperative RT in extremity STS.[106,121] Wound complications were twice as common with preoperative RT as with postoperative RT (35% versus 17%), but the increased risk was almost entirely confined to patients with sarcomas of the lower extremity.[106] RT toxicity rates in the Canadian trial after 2 years differed between the two arms of the study with a tendency to manifest greater fibrosis in the postoperative arm of the study.[122] This analysis strongly suggested that field size was predictive of greater joint stiffness and fibrosis and may also contribute to limb edema. Patients with late treatment responses such as fibrosis, joint stiffness, or limb edema had significantly lower limb function scores at later time points.[122]

With 3.3 years median follow-up, the initial report of the Canadian trial showed identical local control between the two arms of the trial and identified an early improvement in overall survival ($P = 0.0481$) in the preoperative RT arm,[106] which was not substantiated with 5-year results.[121] The 5-year results for preoperative versus postoperative respectively were local control: 93% versus 92%; metastatic-relapse free: 67% versus 69%; recurrence-free survival: 58% versus 59%; overall survival: 73% versus 67% ($P = 0.48$); and cause-specific survival: 78% versus 73% ($P = 0.64$). Only resection margins were significant for local control. Tumor size and grade were the only significant factors for metastatic relapse, overall survival, and cause-specific survival. Grade was the only consistent predictor of recurrence-free survival.[121]

Radiation Therapy Alone in Soft Tissue Sarcoma

Although every effort should be made to attempt resection, there are patients for whom definitive radiation may be considered because of unresectability, or medical comorbidity, or both, or to achieve palliation where surgery is considered inappropriate. Tepper and colleagues treated 51 patients with definitive photon beam irradiation to a total dose of 64 to 66 Gy. The 5-year local control and survival rates were 33% and 25%, respectively. Local control was better for tumors less than 5 cm (87.5%) than in tumors 5 to 10 cm (53%) or greater than 10 cm (30%).[123] More recently, Kepka and colleagues updated this series, which now contains 112 patients who underwent RT for gross disease. Local control at 5 years was 51%, 45%, and 9% for tumors less than 5 cm, 5 to 10 cm, and greater than 10 cm, respectively (Fig. 62-7A). Patients who received doses of less than 63 Gy had inferior 5-year outcomes compared to those receiving higher doses including local control, 22% versus 60% (Fig. 62-7B); disease-free survival, 10% versus 36%; and overall survival rates, 14% versus 52%.[124] Kepka and colleagues also noted a rise in complications at doses of 68 Gy or more, which appears to provide a therapeutic window.[124]

Potentially, higher doses of RT with concurrent dose-intensified chemotherapy regimens, possibly delivered with conformal RT volumes to further protect normal tissues, provide an opportunity to enhance local control in this setting. Preliminary data using concurrent ifosfamide-based protocol exist and may provide an opportunity to address unresectable disease.[125] Rhomberg and colleagues used the radiation sensitizer razoxane.[126] Among 82 patients with gross disease, RT combined with razoxane demonstrated an increased response rate compared to photon irradiation alone (74% versus 49%) with improved local control (64% versus 30%; $P < 0.05$). Acute skin reactions were enhanced in the *sensitizer* arm, but late toxicity was not increased.[126]

Radiation Therapy Modality

EBRT and brachytherapy represent the two common methods of RT for STS, but randomized data comparing these modalities directly are unavailable.

EXTERNAL BEAM

EBRT may include photons or particle beam (electrons, protons, pions, or neutrons) but in practice is generally confined to photon treatments.[105,106,121]

An alternative approach is the use of intraoperative radiation therapy (IORT) delivered with electron beam. The major interest for IORT has been in retroperitoneal sarcoma where the proximity to bowel limits RT delivery and surgical margins are often compromised because of anatomical constraints. Some reports also describe IORT for extremity sarcomas,[127] but formal clinical trials have not compared the relative merits of this approach. Its use may be governed as much by its availability at a given center as by any special advantage that it may confer.

BRACHYTHERAPY

Brachytherapy has several advantages over EBRT including its prompt initiation following surgery when clonogen numbers are at a minimum; and is more easily administered with chemotherapy when this is part of the treatment approach because the skin is relatively protected; and the shorter overall treatment time (typically 4 to 6 days versus 5 to 6.5 weeks for EBRT) is operationally attractive and acceptable to patients. However, brachytherapy results, when not administered in centers with high referral populations of patients treated with brachytherapy, may fall short of those expected with EBRT. There is also the lack of efficacy for low-grade tumors noted earlier, a feature not apparent with EBRT.[105] Brachytherapy may not provide optimal results when the anatomy of the lesion is unsuited for ideal implant geometry.

The American Brachytherapy Society (ABS) has also recommended that brachytherapy should not be used as a sole treatment modality in several situations: (1) if the CTV cannot be adequately encompassed in the implant geometry, (2) where the proximity of critical anatomy is anticipated to prevent administration of meaningful dose, (3) where the resection margins are positive, and (4) if there is skin involvement.[128] In such situations, use of EBRT alone or with brachytherapy may be used. Thus an alternative approach is a combination of EBRT with a brachytherapy boost. There is greater security from the comprehensive coverage typical of EBRT and additional radiobiologic and dosimetric advantages of perioperative brachytherapy. This has resulted in high control rates comparable to full-dose external-beam RT. Typical approaches could employ 45 Gy with EBRT followed by 20 Gy delivered using brachytherapy realizing local control rates of approximately 90%.[129-131] This approach is particularly useful when satisfactory geometry is achievable and the tumor is located in sites where external irradiation as a sole modality has a relatively high probability of producing major toxicity.

One circumstance where brachytherapy is particularly useful is when surgery alone results in resection margins being

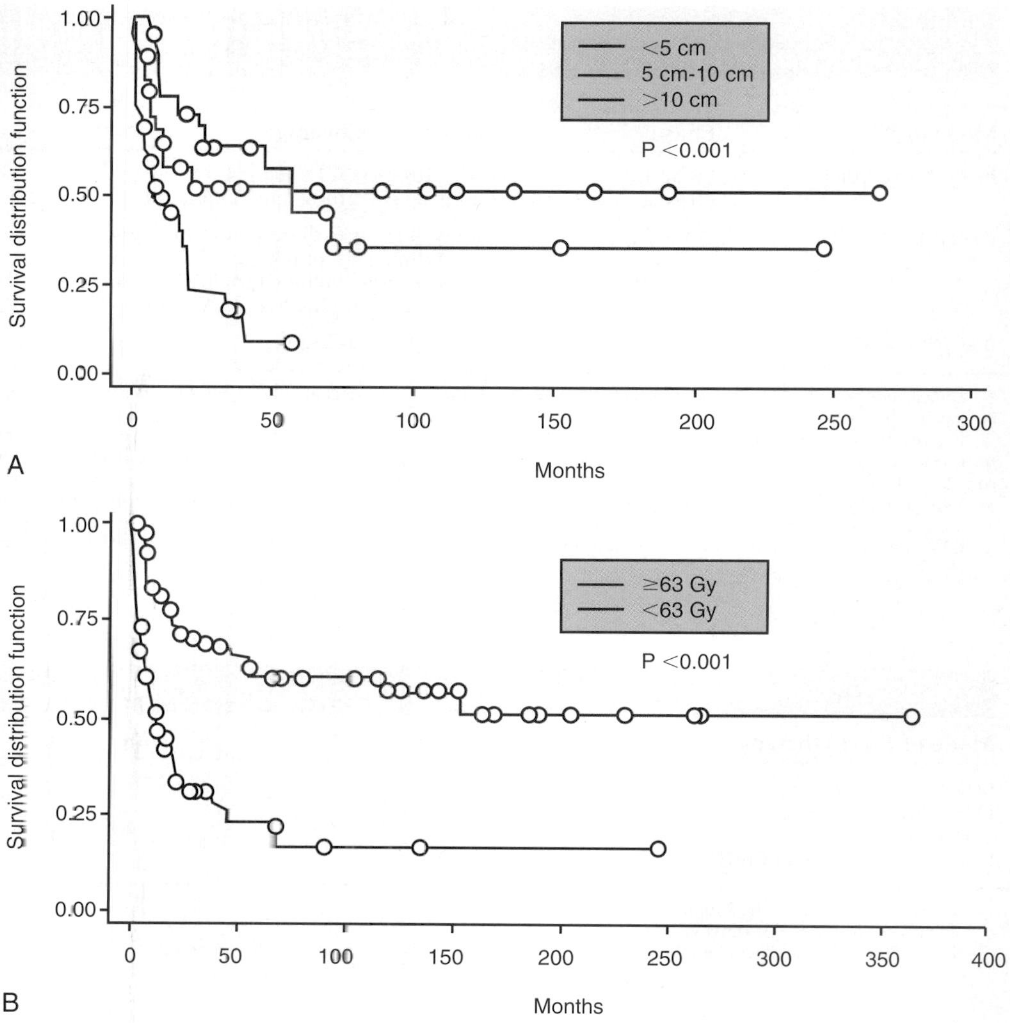

Figure 62-7 (**A**) Local control according to tumor size of unresected STS in a single institution using definitive RT, an uncommon approach in the management. (**B**) Local control by total radiation dose partitioned at the 63 Gy level. RT, radiation therapy; STS, soft tissue sarcoma. (From Kepka L, Delaney TF, Suit HD, Goldberg SI: Results of radiation therapy for unresected soft-tissue sarcomas. Int J Radiat Oncol Biol Phys 63:852-859, 2005.)

too close. In this situation, brachytherapy allows early delivery of radiation to a reduced and select volume of tissue precisely mapped by the intraoperative findings. If the surgical and pathologic findings are satisfactory, the unused brachytherapy catheters can be removed.

The technical delivery aspects of brachytherapy remain varied and have been defined in an experiential manner and without clinical trials at this time. Various options are available that include low-dose rate (LDR) monotherapy, LDR combined with EBRT, fractionated high-dose rate (HDR), and intraoperative HDR.

Radiation Therapy Dose

External Beam Dose Fractionation

EBRT prescriptions for postoperative RT depend on the tumor grade and involvement of the surgical margin but typically employ 60 and 66 Gy for low- and high-grade tumors respectively, with a *shrinking field* technique following 50 Gy at 1.8 to 2 Gy per fraction (Table 62-6). Not infrequently, doses may need to be limited to 45 to 50 Gy in certain anatomic areas containing critical structures (e.g., head and neck, intra-abdominal sites, etc.) to minimize morbidity. In these situations the preoperative approach probably has an advantage.

Sparing of late effects may be expected with smaller fraction size in altered fractionation protocols and may be important when critical structures are irradiated. However, an improvement in therapeutic gain remains unproven.

Alternative EBRT strategies have also used modified dose fractionation approaches in combination with chemotherapy. Thus far it is unclear what additional advantages these approaches may provide, and they have not been widely adopted despite being originally reported two decades previously.[132,133]

Our interpretation of Kepka and colleagues' results[124] is that unresected disease treated with the goal of long-term control should receive at least 70 Gy in 35 fractions or equivalent when this is anatomically feasible, bearing in mind adjacent normal tissues that may demand dose modification. Doses may also need to be higher when employing smaller dose per fraction strategies to ameliorate late-responding tissue effects. In this situation, the therapeutic ratio may be further enhanced by the addition of systemic treatments to augment the RT response.[126]

Brachytherapy Dose

The optimal adjuvant doses for postoperative brachytherapy remain undefined.[128] Doses will vary depending on the dose rate and whether it is being used as a sole modality or in conjunction with EBRT (Table 62-7). The prescription point for the implant may also vary but is generally recommended at an

Table 62-6 Dose-Volume Guidelines for Adjuvant Radiotherapy of Extremity Soft Tissue Sarcoma Based on Two Randomized Controlled Trials[104,106]

Mode of RT	Treatment Phase	Volumetric Coverage	Dose
Preoperative EBRT	Phase 1	GTV plus 4-cm CTV margin	50 Gy in 25 fractions
	Phase 2	Original GTV plus 2-cm CTV margin	If required (if positive margins)*
Postoperative EBRT	Phase 1	Limits of surgical dissection including scars and drain sites plus 4-cm CTV margin	50 Gy in 25 fractions
	Phase 2	*High-risk* target volume (original GTV and surgical scar) plus 1-cm CTV margin	16 Gy in 8 fractions
Brachytherapy	Course	*Surgical bed* plus 2 cm†	45 Gy in 4-6 days

Dimensions provided refer to longitudinal coverage. Axial dimensions are generally 2-cm CTV coverage or coverage of the adjacent barrier to tumor incursion (e.g., a fascial plane) if closer.

External beam fractionation doses outlined are within normal accepted premises for 2 Gy per fraction as used in the Canadian trial. Alternative dose fractionation regimens may use 1.8 Gy per fraction to 50.4 Gy (phase 1) and other equivalent regimens and corresponding higher doses for phase 1 and 2 combined. Total doses and fractionation may not be modified for altered fraction or when administering concurrent chemotherapy.

*Not generally required, but administered in approximately 15% of cases in the Canadian trial that compared preoperative versus postoperative EBRT.

†*Surgical bed* for brachytherapy is the GTV plus 2-cm longitudinal margin; dose recommendations are for low-dose rate treatments.

CTV, clinical target volume; EBRT, external beam radiation therapy; GTV, gross tumor volume; RT, radiation therapy.

Table 62-7 Guidelines for Adjuvant Doses for Postoperative LDR and HDR Brachytherapy for Soft Tissue Sarcoma

Mode of Brachytherapy	Total Dose	Time	Dose Rate
LDR monotherapy	45-50 Gy	4-6 d	~0.45 Gy/h
LDR with EBRT	15-25 Gy	2-3 d	~0.45 Gy/h
Fractionated HDR	32-50 Gy	4-7 d	bid; q6h (activity 3-10 Ci)
Fractionated HDR with EBRT*	12-18 Gy	3 d	bid; q6h (activity 3-10 Ci)

Information derived from citations or recommendations in references 128 and 134.

*Published experience existing with this technique is limited.

d, day; EBRT, external beam radiation therapy; h, hour; HDR, high-dose rate; LDR, low-dose rate.

isodose line 5 to 10 mm from the plane of the implant. There is general agreement about the dose for LDR as monotherapy (see Table 62-7), and doses of 45 to 50 Gy at approximately 0.45 Gy/hour seem acceptable with the skin dose not exceeding 20 to 25 Gy where large areas of skin are treated.[128,134] Where LDR brachytherapy is used with external beam (typically 45 to 50 Gy), doses of 15 to 25 Gy are generally administered over 2 to 3 days.[128] Fractionated HDR is more problematic, in part because it is a new technique with little clinical experience in a rare disease; in addition there are radiobiologic issues governing serious late toxicity. For example, caution should be exercised when placing catheters in contact with neurovascular structures, and the dose per fraction should probably be curtailed. Generally, doses of approximately 36 Gy in 10 fractions using a 6-hour interfraction interval have been suggested, but some authors have used higher doses.[134] Guided by the more abundant breast cancer experience, a dose of 32 to 34 Gy in twice-daily fractions of 3.4 to 4 Gy over 4 to 5 days[135-137] seems useful and safe; but even here there have reports of fat necrosis.[137]

An additional comment concerns the use of intraoperative HDR, a novel and rarely used approach, which has been reported for the treatment of retroperitoneal sarcoma. Doses of 10 to 15 Gy as single treatment prescribed at 0.5 cm were used to supplement EBRT doses of 45 to 50 Gy, depending on surgical margins.[138] The large single doses required make this a problematic approach in the vicinity of the vulnerable anatomy of the retroperitoneum.

Factors Influencing Choice of Radiation Therapy Dose

Ongoing problems of fibrosis that appear to be volume related were discussed previously.[122] In addition we have noted a fracture rate that appears dose related (doses of 60 Gy or greater to bone) in a series of 363 patients with lower extremity sarcomas treated with EBRT and surgery, but without chemotherapy, and followed for a median of 50 months.[139] A total of 27 postradiation fractures were identified (6.3%). Seventeen of these patients had received postoperative radiation (with 15 patients receiving 66 Gy and 2 receiving 60 Gy), and 3 had received preoperative radiation with a postoperative boost (total dose, 66 Gy). Twenty patients had received 60 to 66 Gy (fracture rate 20 of 192, or 10%) and 3 had received 50 Gy (fracture rate 3 of 172, or 2%). The results also demonstrate that female gender confers a higher risk of fracture, and others have shown that chemotherapy aggravates the risk.[140-142]

Because of these dose-related issues, it may be more useful to tailor the external beam (or brachytherapy) strategy to the needs of the anatomic setting and the volume of tissue that needs to be irradiated, especially if there is need to encompass vulnerable normal tissue structures. Such modifications may include combining moderate dose levels of both brachytherapy and EBRT, choosing preoperative versus postoperative external beam approaches to reduce risks of fracture or peripheral nerve injury, or using techniques such as intensity modulated RT.[143]

Radiation Target Volume

The existence of a zone of uncertain size and location that may contain subclinical disease in proximity to the presenting site of the primary tumor presents a frequent dilemma. The size and extent of the putative *risk zone* depends on a number of factors, such as the amount of disturbance of tissue planes and barriers to tumor incursion that may already have taken place, including scars and drain sites. Such areas will need to be included with an appropriate margin. In the preoperative setting, the gross tumor volume (GTV) is typically represented by the radiologically defined tumor but the acceptable volume margin remains problematic, depending on the nature of the prior biopsy, the anatomic containment of the lesion, and the imaging characteristics of the lesion. The latter feature concerns the imaging changes evident on MRI beyond the overt tumor evident on clinical examination or even CT scanning and how this information should impact on treatment planning.

The local growth characteristics of STSs have suggested that tumor cells may be located in the surrounding soft tissues at some distance from the main tumor mass.[144,145] The original observation led to the development of the concept of a *reactive zone* surrounding the lesion, situated between the tumor margin and pseudocapsule and more remote normal tissues. The reactive zone was described as consisting of a granulation tissue-like proliferation with characteristics including edema and neovascularity and, in addition, might contain satellite tumor cells.[145] MRI has documented high T2-weighted signal changes surrounding STSs. These radiographic abnormalities are thought to be because of increased water content and have, therefore, been labeled *peritumoral edema*. However, it is unclear whether these MRI findings are actually the result of tissue edema and correspond to the reactive zone noted earlier or also contain tumor cells.[146]

Recently we reported a small series (n = 15) of patients where satellite tumor cells can be identified histologically in the tissues surrounding a STS and whether their presence correlates with increased T2-weighted signal intensity on MRI (Fig. 62-8). Sarcoma cells were identified histologically in the tissues beyond the tumor in 10 of 15 cases. In six cases tumor cells were located within 1 cm of the tumor margin, and in four cases malignant cells were found at a distance greater than 1 cm and up to a maximum of 4 cm. The location of tumor cells beyond the margin did not correlate with tumor size or the location or extent of peritumoral changes.[147]

In the discussion that follows, recommended dose-volume guidelines for both external beam and brachytherapy are summarized (see Table 62-6) based on what was used in the two randomized controlled trials and bearing in mind anatomic and imaging characteristics of the lesions and normal tissues.

External Beam Volumes

Within the framework of uncertainty noted previously, our policy has been to use a 4-cm CTV margin (approximating a 5-cm field margin after the PTV and penumbra are considered) beyond any imaging abnormalities, including *peritumoral edema,* or areas of surgical disruption irrespective of grade or size of the tumor. However, practice is variable and there have been no randomized trials in this area. Our policy reflects the practice undertaken in a randomized trial that provided very acceptable 5-year local control rates (see Table 62-5).[106,121]

A postoperative RT trial is being initiated by the United Kingdom National Cancer Research Network (NCRN) that will compare a 5-cm longitudinal and 3-cm axial margin (standard arm) versus smaller margins (likely 1.5-cm longitudinal and 2-cm axial) from the surgical bed. Patients in both arms of the study will receive 66 Gy over 6.5 weeks with a volume reduction after 25 fractions (50 Gy) in the standard arm to the same volume as used from the outset in the experimental arm. Limb function is to be assessed using the Toronto Extremity Salvage Score (TESS)[148] (Written personal communication, Martin Robinson: http://pfsearch.ukcrn.org.uk/StudyDetail.aspx?TopicID=1@StudyID=1472).

Brachytherapy Volumes

The ABS recommends at least 2- to 5-cm longitudinal margin beyond the CTV, and at least 1 cm beyond the lateral edge of the CTV (Fig. 62-9).[128] These are based on general agreement by experts, but there is no consensus on the exact size of the margin beyond the tumor bed. The CTV may be difficult to define but in general is represented by the volume of tissue considered at risk for microscopic extension of tumor and includes the tumor bed visualized on radiographic studies and under direct inspection intraoperatively.[128] The brachytherapy protocol at MSKCC uses margins of 2 cm around the surgical bed.[149,150]

Other Local Management Approaches

Combined Preoperative Chemotherapy and Radiation Therapy

Enhancing the local effect of RT with concurrent chemotherapy while also promptly addressing the distant metastasis risk

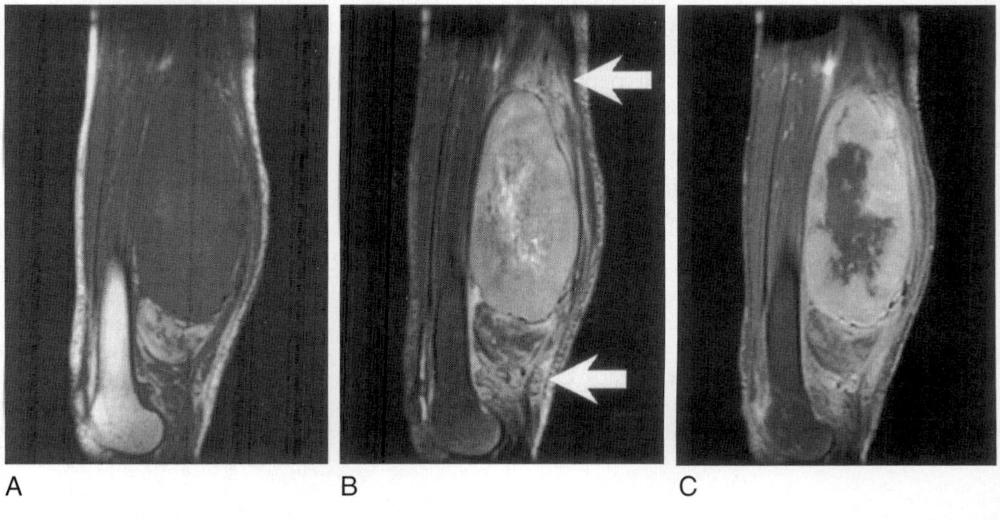

Figure 62-8 (**A**) Sagittal T1-weighted and (**B**) fat-suppressed fast spin-echo T2-weighted, and (**C**) contrast-enhanced fat suppressed T1-weighted MRI scans of a liposarcoma of the posterior thigh. Peritumoral increased T2-weighted signal intensity (*arrows*) seen both proximally and distally to tumor periphery on T2-weighted image (**B**), with mild corresponding enhancement on postcontrast-enhanced T1-weighted image (**C**). MRI, magnetic resonance imaging. (Adapted from White LM, Wunder JS, Bell RS, et al: Histologic assessment of peritumoral edema in soft tissue sarcoma. Int J Radiat Oncol Biol Phys 61:1439-1445, 2005.)

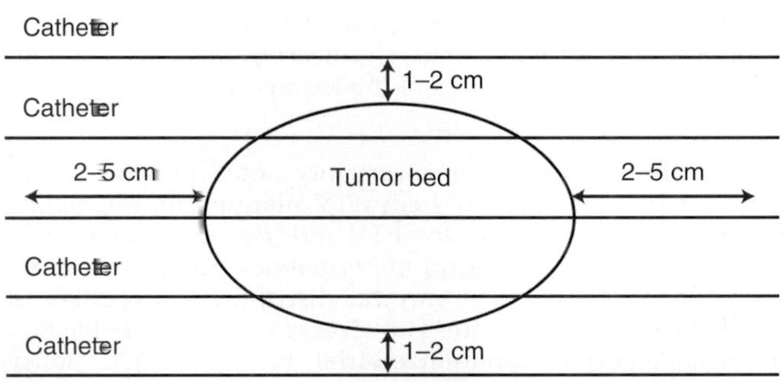

Figure 62-9 American Brachytherapy Guidelines for catheter positioning for STS. Catheters are placed 1-2 cm beyond the lateral edge of the CTV and 2-5 cm beyond the CTV in the longitudinal direction. CTV, clinical target volume; STS, soft tissue sarcoma. (From Nag S, Shasha D, Janjan N, et al: The American Brachytherapy Society recommendations for brachytherapy of soft tissue sarcomas. Int J Radiat Oncol Biol Phys 49:1033-1043, 2001.)

prior to the surgery is an attractive concept. Strategies include the use of perfusion techniques (see the following text) as well as a sequential intravenous chemotherapy and radiation strategy in patients with localized, high-grade, large (>8 cm) extremity STS described by DeLaney and colleagues.[151] The protocol involved three courses of doxorubicin, ifosfamide, mesna, and dacarbazine (MAID) interdigitated with two 22-Gy courses of radiation (11 fractions each) for a total preoperative radiation dose of 44 Gy. This was followed by surgical resection. An additional 16 Gy (8 fractions) boost dose was delivered if the surgical margins were microscopically positive. The outcomes of 48 patients treated with this regimen appeared superior to those of a matched cohort of historical controls. The 5-year overall survival rates were 87% versus 58% ($P = 0.0003$) for the MAID versus control patient cohorts with the difference linked to an improvement in the distant metastases rate with 5-year freedom from distant metastasis rate of 75% versus 44% ($P = 0.0016$); and the local control was similar in both groups. Febrile neutropenia occurred in 25% of patients receiving the chemotherapy and radiation sequential therapy; 14 (29%) of the patients treated with MAID also experienced wound complications. Late fatal myelodysplasia was seen in one patient who received chemotherapy.

Intra-arterial Chemotherapy

Two unusual and distinct approaches involving limb perfusion have been used in the management of STS. The first is intra-arterial chemotherapy with doxorubicin or other agents. This infusional approach is conceptually attractive because it provides high doses of chemotherapy directly into the affected limb, but it has not been shown to confer benefit compared to intravenous chemotherapy. A further modification of the approach is to combine it with RT, an approach that has been advocated for decades at University of California, Los Angeles (UCLA). A feature of their protocol is the use of higher dose per fraction (3.5 Gy per fraction). The total dose has varied over eras with doses of 17.5 Gy, 28 Gy, and the original protocol of 35 Gy preceded by a three-day infusion of intra-arterial doxorubicin. In the first of two randomized trials, post-RT chemotherapy was of no additional benefit compared to no further chemotherapy.[152] In the second trial ($n = 99$), the intra-arterial approach with 28 Gy was compared to an intravenous approach, and they were found not to be different.[153]

Isolated Limb Perfusion

Isolated lymph perfusion (ILP) is a very different approach and has been popularized in Europe. It was likely developed predominantly as a means of addressing the more prevalent local control problem of limb threat from satellitosis and in-transit metastases complicating malignant melanoma. The essential requirement is limb arterial and venous access to isolate the limb from the remainder of the body through an extracorporeal circulation system. A heart-lung machine is used to reoxygenate the blood recirculating from the limb. The blood in the extracorporeal circuit is also often warmed to 39°C to 40°C to enhance the effect of chemotherapy.[154] After isolation of the extremity, a chemotherapeutic agent is perfused into the limb. Several have been used, the most effective or popular of which is melphalan with tumor necrosis factor-α (TNF-α) at a highly lethal dose under normal circumstances.[155] TNF-α was initially approved in Europe after a multicenter trial in patients with locally advanced STSs, deemed unresectable by an independent review committee; the response rate to isolated limb perfusion with TNFα plus melphalan was 76%, and the limb was saved in 71% of patients.[155] Both components of the regimen (melphalan and TNF-α) appear important and omission of TNF-α has resulted in a decrease in the tissue dose of melphalan, probably from its effects on the tumor vasculature. Recent efforts, including a randomized trial (see Table 62-5) have focused on attempts to reduce the dose of TNF to try to reduce toxicity.[156,157] Other authors recently reported results using doxorubicin instead of melphalan and higher temperature (42°C).[158]

The major component of the selection for the ILP approach hinges on the decision that patients would otherwise require amputation or marked loss of function if treated in conventional ways. Following this, patients who develop resectable disease usually undergo surgery. The response rates for multiple STS and melanoma appear very similar: overall response of 95% and 96% for both diseases and complete response of 69% (in melanoma) and 61% (in multiple primary STS).[154] Grunhagen and associates have also reported efficacy of this treatment for locally advanced extremity desmoid tumors in a small study of 11 patients. Amputation was avoided in all cases, and the authors suggest ILP should be considered when resection without important functional sacrifice may be deemed improbable.[159]

Adjuvant Chemotherapy in Soft Tissue Sarcoma

Background

The use of chemotherapy in the adjuvant setting to combat microscopic metastatic disease remains controversial. The standard of care for nearly all pediatric sarcomas involves chemotherapy. It has proven benefit in patients with osteogenic sarcoma, Ewing's sarcoma, and RMS. If chemotherapy is going to be adopted and have the same impact as radiation and surgery in the management of STS, more effective drugs must be identified that clearly indicate efficacy in this disease.

Meta-analysis of Randomized Trials

The results from 14 randomized trials performed over three decades were comprehensively combined from 1568 patients in a landmark meta-analysis that used individual patient data.[160] This study addressed the role of doxorubicin-based adjuvant chemotherapy in STS. In the meta-analysis, the figures for distant relapse-free interval and overall recurrence-free survival were significantly in favor of the use of adjuvant chemotherapy. However, and most important, the difference in overall survival, the ultimate aim of adjuvant chemotherapy, was not significantly different between the chemotherapy and the control groups ($P = 0.12$).

Only three trials in the meta-analysis had a relatively large sample size.[161-163] The inclusion of cases with minimal or only small risk of metastatic failure may dilute the power of the studies to detect an effect that may exist only for patients at substantial risk of metastasis.

Studies Since the Meta-Analysis

Since the publication of the meta-analysis, an important study was reported from Italy. The inclusion criteria for this trial were appropriately restricted to very adverse tumors (large high-grade lesions) and a very intensive cytotoxic regimen (five cycles of 4'-epidoxorubicin 60 mg/m^2 days 1 and 2 and ifosfamide 1.8 g/m^2 days 1 through 5, with hydration, mesna, and granulocyte colony-stimulating factor) compared to no systemic treatment.[164] The disease-free and overall survival rates were statistically improved at preliminary analysis. However, by the time of publication, the metastatic rate in both arms was virtually identical (44% and 45%); and it can be expected that the ultimate survival rate will also be the same.[164] Unfortunately, this raises the question of whether the potential value of aggressive chemotherapy may largely be in delaying the manifestation of distant metastasis but not in their prevention.

Recent Analyses of Multicenter Data

Recently, several attempts have been made to pool data from large established cancer centers in the United States. One such study included all patients treated or not treated with adjuvant or neoadjuvant chemotherapy at M. D. Anderson Cancer Center (MDACC), Houston, and MSKCC but showed no statistical difference in overall survival for patients treated with chemotherapy versus no adjuvant chemotherapy.[165] In contrast, combined nonrandomized data from UCLA and MSKCC showed that adjuvant chemotherapy may be useful for some STS subsets, including myxoid and round cell liposarcoma.[166] Moreover, data from the MSKCC and Dana Farber Cancer Institute databases have suggested a significant improvement in disease-specific survival in patients with high-grade extremity STSs greater than 10 cm.[167] In interpreting such data, it is important to recognize biases that may exist, and it is clear that randomized trials should continue.

Influence of Chemotherapy on Local Control

The largest trial in the meta-analysis (that of the European Organization for Research and Treatment of Cancer [EORTC]) compared the outcome of adjuvant cyclophosphamide, vincristine, doxorubicin, and dacarbazine (CYVADIC) chemotherapy compared to control in 468 patients. The relapse-free survival was significantly better after CYVADIC (56% versus 43% for controls; $P = 0.007$) and local recurrence was significantly reduced by CYVADIC (17% versus 31%; $P = 0.01$).[162] The favorable result in this subset analysis was confined to head, neck, and trunk tumors. In contrast, distant metastases rates were similar in both arms as were overall survival rates (63% versus 56%; $P = 0.64$). Thus adjuvant chemotherapy may improve local control in high risk groups of STS, where local control has traditionally not been as satisfactory.

Summary of Evidence about Adjuvant Chemotherapy

For the high-risk patients, those presenting with large, high-grade, and deep lesions (stage III disease), a benefit to adjuvant chemotherapy appears to be small, if present at all. For this reason we tend to individualize treatment for a given clinical setting. Younger patients with relatively chemotherapy-sensitive subtypes such as myxoid and round cell liposarcoma and synovial sarcoma may experience benefit; and it has also been our policy to advise chemotherapy in patients presenting with lymph-node involvement, and in adverse presentations of head and neck or torso sarcoma when surgery and RT delivery are compromised.

SEPARATE MANAGEMENT ISSUES

Intra-Abdominal Soft Tissue Sarcoma

Retroperitoneal Sarcomas

Soft-tissue sarcomas of the retroperitoneum (RPS) represent 10% to 15% of all STSs and their treatment results have recently been reviewed comprehensively.[168] Liposarcoma (30% to 60%) and leiomyosarcoma (20% to 30%) are the most common, although all sarcoma histologies may appear. In most reports median tumor size at diagnosis is greater than 10 cm in diameter, and tumors of less than 5 cm are uncommon because symptoms develop late and are often nonspecific.[169] The management of a suspected RPS is summarized in Figure 62-10, and the mainstay of treatment is complete surgical resection. The main adjuvant approach is RT, but the benefits are uncertain with this approach. Current chemotherapy strategies have not shown an improvement in outcome.

SURGERY FOR RETROPERITONEAL SARCOMA

The optimal primary treatment of RPS is en-bloc excision of the tumor with adjacent involved viscera and a margin of uninvolved tissue. However, local disease extension with involvement of vital viscera and vascular structures makes this difficult to achieve. Published treatment results for RPS since 1994 are shown in Table 62-8. Grossly complete resection rates have improved to 80% to 90% in more recent reports. The five-year local control rates are only 40% to 60%, and unlike extremity sarcomas, local relapse continues out to 10 years. Overall 5-year survival for RPS is 50% to 60%, and most deaths are caused by local rather than systemic relapses.

ADJUVANT RADIATION THERAPY

The high risk of local failure following surgery has made neoadjuvant and adjuvant therapy an attractive option for RPS, but their role remains controversial. Postoperative RT for RPS is compromised by presence of adhesed bowel in the tumor bed, the presence of adjacent radiosensitive vital structures that limit the radiation dose, and a poorly defined treatment volume. The limited data available for postoperative RT for RPS shows that it may delay local relapse but not prevent it.[170]

RT given with the tumor in situ has the advantages of treating a well-defined and undisturbed tumor volume where the tumor also acts as a tissue-expander to displace small bowel and other radiosensitive viscera from the radiation field. Reports of preoperative EBRT for RPS demonstrate that it is associated with minimal acute[171] and late[172] toxicity and no increase in wound healing complications.[171] This attractive option for combining RT with surgery for RPS is currently the subject of an American College of Surgical Oncologists (ACOSOG) randomized trial comparing preoperative RT and en-bloc surgical excision to surgery alone for primary RPS.

Three-dimensional conformal RT and intensity-modulated radiation therapy (IMRT) are particularly well suited for preoperative RT of RPS (Fig. 62-11). A CTV margin of 1.5 to 2.0 cm around the GTV is optimal but may need to be reduced to protect vital radiosensitive viscera. A dose of 45 to 50.4 Gy

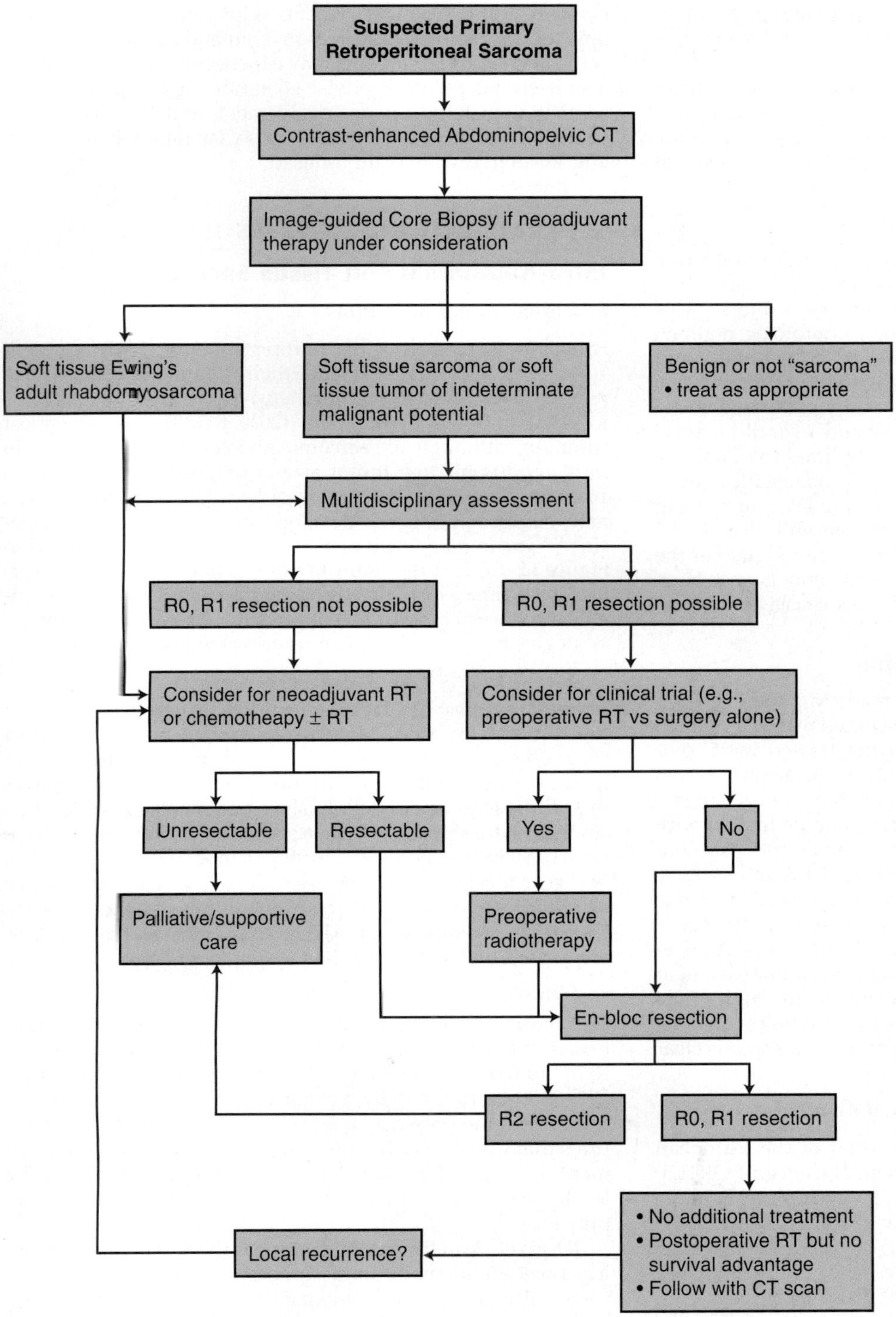

Figure 62-10 Treatment and diagnostic algorithm for a suspected retroperitoneal STS. These lesions are often low-grade liposarcomas and resemble mature fat, presenting difficulties for the pathologist in ascertaining a pathology diagnosis of sarcoma even when multiple image-guided biopsies are attempted. The clinician may need to determine the appropriate choice of treatment even when the diagnosis is clinically highly suspicious, but biopsy sampling artifact may make confirmation of pathological diagnosis improbable without definitive resection. The place of induction approaches, especially preoperative RT, needs to be considered on an individual basis in such cases. CT, computerized tomography; R0, microscopically clear resection; R1, microscopically positive but grossly clear resection; R2, resection with macroscopic gross residual disease; RT, radiation therapy.

in 1.8 to 2-Gy fractions may be given to large CTV volumes with acceptable acute and late toxicity.

For postoperative RT, the identification of an appropriate treatment volume is problematic and is best accomplished when preoperative cross-sectional tumor imaging is available.

Intraoperative radiotherapy (IORT) provides the opportunity to directly target areas identified to be at high risk at the time of surgery with a single fraction of radiation and may be used alone or in combination with EB therapy. The Massachusetts General Hospital experience with intraoperative electron boost following preoperative external beam therapy (40-50 Gy) for RPS reported an improved local control and overall survival (83% and 74%, respectively) in a selected subgroup of 16 patients who underwent complete excision and who received 10 to 20 Gy IORT compared to no IORT (30% and 61%, respectively). Complications in four patients included hydronephrosis, neuropathy, and ureteroarterial fistula.[172] Petersen and colleagues at the Mayo Clinic also reported improved local control, using a similar treatment approach.[173] These studies were not randomized, and potentially more favorable lesions may have been chosen for IORT.

Table 62-8 Treatment Outcome for Retroperitoneal Sarcoma[a]

Author/year (Reference No.)	Complete Resection Rate[b] n	(%)	Overall Survival[c] 5 y (%)	10 y (%)	Local Control after Complete Resection[d] (%)
Gronchi, et al., 2004[214]	167	88	54	27	46
Hassan, et al.,[e] 2004[215]	97	78	45	29	43
Ferrario, et al., 2003[216]	130	95	60	48	43 at 5 y[e] 34 at 10 y[e]
Jones, et al.,[f] 2002[171]	55	84	78 at 2 y	NA	NA
Stoeckle, et al., 2001[217]	165	65	46	NA	42
Van Dalen, et al., 2001[218]	142	54	NA	NA	42
Petersen, et al.,[g] 2002[173]	87	83	47	NA	59[h]
Herman, et al., 1999[219]	70	73	53[i]	40[i]	NA
Lewis, et al.,[j] 1998[169]	500	62	54[e]	35[e]	59[e]
Jenkins, et al, 1996[220]	119	49	20	NA	NA
Kilkenny, et al., 1996[221]	63	78	48[i]	37[i]	NA
Singer, et al., 1995[222]	83	NA	60	50	NA
Catton, et al., 1994[170]	104	43	36	14	50 at 5 y 18 at 10 y
Gieschen, et al., 2001[172]	37	78	50	NA	72

[a]Series of 50 or more patients published in English since 1994. All series are retrospective except for Jones, et al.[171]; Petersen, et al.[173]; Lewis, et al.[169]; and Jenkins, et al.[220] Where the same center has published sequential series that includes patients also included in a previous series, only the most recent qualifying publication is quoted.

[b]The proportion of patients with retroperitoneal sarcoma undergoing surgical exploration at that center who had a grossly complete resection, irrespective of the microscopic margin status. The denominator used to calculate this proportion does not always correspond to *n*, the number of patients included in the series.

[c]Actuarial survival, irrespective of resection status.

[d]Locoregional control rate in patients undergoing complete resection, with or without the use of adjuvant radiation therapy or chemotherapy. Unless otherwise indicated, figure quoted is actuarial and at 5 y postresection.

[e]Limited to patients with primary tumors.

[f]All patients received preoperative RT.

[g]All patients received intraoperative RT with EBRT.

[h]Includes cases irradiated for gross residual tumor.

[i]Survival quoted for completely resected patients only.

[j]Complete resection rate is quoted for patients with primary or recurrent disease excluding those with distant metastases ($n = 397$); survival rates quoted are disease specific survival in all patients with primary disease ($n = 278$); local control rate quoted is for patients with primary disease undergoing either complete ($n = 185$) or partial ($n = 62$) resection.

EBRT, external beam radiation therapy; NA, not available; RT, radiation therapy; y, year.

In a series of 32 patients treated with HDR brachytherapy with or without postoperative EBRT for RPS, Alektiar and colleagues reported a 5-year actuarial local control rate of 62% (74% for primary presentation). Complications included bowel obstruction (18%), fistula (9%), neuropathy (6%), hydronephrosis (3%), and wound complication (3%).[138]

Primary Gastrointestinal Sarcomas and Gastrointestinal Stromal Tumors

Primary gastrointestinal sarcomas are uncommon and make up approximately 0.1% to 3% of all gastrointestinal neoplasms[174] and 14% of all sarcomas.[175] MSKCC reported on 239 patients with GIST and 322 with leiomyosarcoma arising within the abdomen.[175] The 5-year, disease-specific survival was 28% and 29% for GIST and leiomyosarcoma, respectively. Complete gross excision was achieved for 49% of cases. Favorable factors for overall Disease Specific Survival (DSS) with liposarcoma and GIST were primary presentation, tumor size less than 5 cm, and complete excision. Local recurrence was a component of initial recurrence in 36% of GIST and 40% of leiomyosarcoma, and pulmonary metastases constituted 30% of first recurrences for liposarcoma but only 5% of GIST. Hepatic metastases accounted for 50% of first recurrences for GIST but only 20% for leiomyosarcoma.

The predominantly intra-abdominal location and the predilection for failure from peritoneal seeding and hematogenous metastases limit the role of adjunctive RT for gastrointestinal sarcomas. Specific circumstances may arise where the tumor had infiltrated, such as pelvic or retroperitoneal wall structures; and adjunctive RT may be considered for these cases to improve local control following marginal resection. GIST is now recognized as a distinct entity. A randomized phase II trial of two doses of imatinib mesylate in patients with unresectable, metastatic, or recurrent GIST demonstrated a partial response in 68%, and stable disease in 20% of 147 heavily pretreated patients, with modest associated toxicity.[176] Follow-up is too short to determine if imatinib mesylate can be curative; and patients who respond should be considered for complete resection of any residual, because subsequent acquired resistance to the drug has been identified. The role of imatinib mesylate as a postoperative adjuvant for resectable disease is the subject of two ongoing randomized trials.

Soft Tissue Sarcomas of the Thorax (Chest Wall, Thoracic Cavity, and Breast)

Chest-Wall, Mediastinum, and Intrathoracic Lesions

Sarcomas of the thorax are uncommon. The treatment of choice is wide surgical resection where possible, and where it cannot be accomplished the outcomes are extremely unfavorable. The role of adjuvant local and systemic therapy follows the same principles as for other STS, especially in the case of chest-wall lesions (see Fig. 62-5). For chest-wall sarcoma, the overall 5-year survival is reported to be 50% to 66%, with local control exceeding 70% and metastatic rate of 40%.[177-180] In

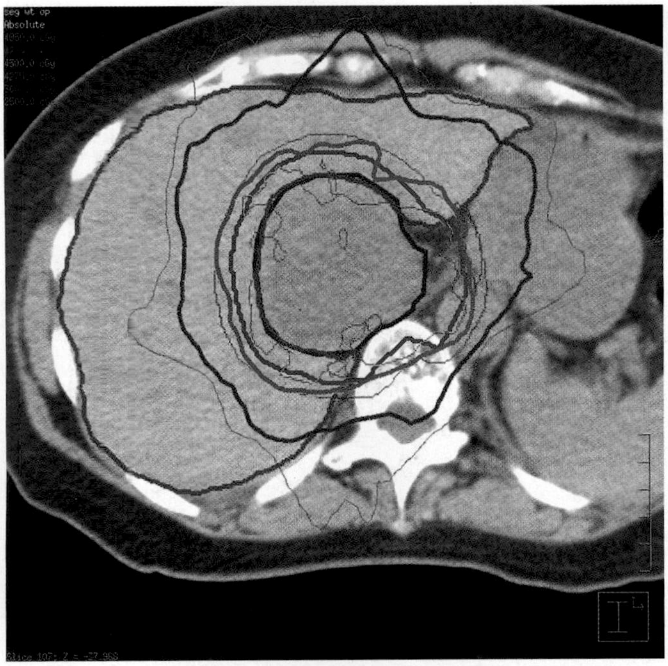

Figure 62-11 Preoperative IMRT treatment plan for a patient with a retroperitoneal leiomyosarcoma arising behind the inferior vena cava and displacing the liver. The GTV is shown in *red* and is virtually surrounded by the sensitive liver structure (delineated in *green*). The prescribed dose is 45 Gy to the CTV minimum. The 30-Gy isodose line is well conformed to the CTV and offers maximal protection to the uninvolved liver. CTV, clinical target volume; GTV, gross tumor volume; IMRT, intensity-modulated radiation therapy.

lung sarcomas overall 5-year survival was 49%. Patients who did not undergo resection died within 19 months of diagnosis.[181] Mediastinal sarcomas fare poorly, with 5-year overall survival rates of 32%, and patients with high-grade tumors had a reduction in survival compared to low-grade tumors (27% versus 66%).[182] Cardiac sarcomas should also be managed with surgery, but this is often not feasible and some authors have advocated heart transplantation as definitive treatment.[183,184]

Breast Sarcomas

Primary breast sarcomas are comprised of phyllodes and nonphyllodes tumors. Although distinction is made on histologic basis, the natural history may be similar. The incidence of malignant phyllodes tumors is 2.1 per million women.[185] Primary nonphyllodes sarcomas of the breast have an incidence of approximately 17 per million women.[186]

PHYLLODES TUMORS OF THE BREAST

Phyllodes tumors are composed of both epithelial elements and connective tissue stroma. The stroma determines malignancy where marked cellular pleomorphism, nuclear atypia, increased mitotic activity, and overgrowth of the stroma signify malignancy. In contrast to epithelial breast cancer, it is relatively unusual to have enlarged axillary nodes, and when these do occur they are often reactive because of necrotic or infected tumor.[187,188]

The treatment of choice is surgical excision with a wide margin. Breast conservation surgery has been practiced particularly if lesion to breast size ratio allows excision with reasonable cosmesis. In malignant tumors and also where lesions are large or the surgical margins close, or both, RT has been added to surgical treatment. However, breast conservation without RT has also been reported to provide local control.[189] The routine use of chemotherapy is not established.[189,190] Both benign and malignant phyllodes tumors may recur locally and metastasize (seen in 25%).[190] Local recurrence has been reported as high as 40%[191] but has averaged about 15%.[189,192-195] Disease-free survival at 5 years for patients with malignant tumors has been reported at 66%.[189]

NONPHYLLODES BREAST SARCOMA

Surgical treatment is indicated to widely excise the tumor using breast-conserving surgery if possible but may require mastectomy. Axillary node dissection is not indicated because of the rare occurrence of axillary metastases.[196,197] The use of adjuvant RT is based on tumor size, grade, and margins; but its use in the breast is not as well defined as for extremity sarcoma. Angiosarcoma may have a worse prognosis compared to other STSs with poor local control, a tendency to develop bilateral involvement, and low survival rates.[197,198] Overall survival has been reported to be 60% to 70% at 5 years[197,199,200] with local control reported in 55% to 75% of cases.[196,197,201]

Head and Neck Soft Tissue Sarcoma

Head and neck STSs only make up approximately 10% of STS, and patients frequently succumb from local disease failure without metastases. Underlying this behavior pattern is the anatomic proximity to nonexpendable local or, in the interest of sparing tissue, a tendency to compromise the extent of local tissues resected or irradiated. This is particularly the case for lesions in the proximity of the spinal cord, brain stem, and optic apparatus. Some uniquely aggressive sarcomas are represented more commonly in the head and neck, such as angiosarcoma of the scalp and facial regions and parameningeal RMS. In the case of the latter diseases, there is a high risk of lymph node metastases and distant disease.

The overall approach to the management of head and neck STS have recently been described in detail.[202,203] Other than the exceptions noted earlier, these lesions behave similarly to STS elsewhere; and similar principles can be applied (see Fig. 62-5).[203] RT is an effective local adjuvant to surgery capable of elevating the local control rate from 52% with surgery alone to 90%.[204] Data from the Princess Margaret Hospital showed that patients with clear margins treated without adjuvant RT had a control rate of 74% compared to 70% in positive-margin patients who received adjuvant RT.[117] Because they usually do not present with great size, tumor size is relatively less important in prognosis, but outcome remains linked to tumor grade and to the ability to obtain a satisfactory resection. In general the results of local management have not been satisfactory (overall local control rates of approximately 60%-70%) and similar survival rates (60%-70%). As with other sarcomas, the role of chemotherapy in ameliorating the risk of distant metastasis remains unproven; however, there are exploratory data that suggest that chemotherapy may have a beneficial influence on reducing local failure rates.[162]

Management of Lymph Node Metastasis

Elective treatment of nodal regions is unusual apart from certain high-risk histologic subtypes. However, in the presence of overt regional lymph-node disease, patients generally would be treated with surgery and radiation if they are being considered for curative management. The presence of lymph-node metastasis is a grave prognostic factor with outcome similar to other stage IV disease. Selected patients undergoing radical lymphadenectomy for isolated lymph-node metastasis had 46% 5-year survival in a series reported from MSKCC.[83] Behranwala and colleagues from the Royal Marsden reported that the 5-year survival of isolated lymph-node metastasis was 24% (95% CI, 12.6%-37.1%) compared to 0% with lymph-node metastasis and distant disease. At the Princess Margaret Hospital, patients who presented with isolated nodal metastases had a 4-year survival of 71%, which was significantly better than patients with synchronous lymphatic and systemic metastases.[93]

Princess Margaret Hospital's policy is to offer surgery for lymph-node metastases and frequently add chemotherapy, but this is not the usual practice in patients without lymph node involvement.[93] RT is also added for patients where there is risk of recurrence within the surgically dissected tissues because of extracapsular nodal spread (especially when the resection margins are narrow), or when nodes are very large or multiple, or both. In general the lymph-node pathway will follow the vascular structures in the involved nodal basin (Fig. 62-12). It is customary to provide at least a microscopic dose of EBRT into the next echelon of apparently uninvolved nodal tissues, and the targeting and technical delivery for such lesions may be complex (Fig. 62-13).

Aggressive Fibromatosis

Also termed *extra-abdominal desmoid tumors,* aggressive fibromatosis is a benign neoplasm capable of local infiltration and destruction. The disease can infiltrate by a pattern of sinuous fibrotic stranding into the soft tissues, along fascial planes, and for a considerable distance from the main tumor mass. Wide surgical excision is the treatment of choice, but recurrence is frequent. At the MDACC surgery alone resulted in a 10-year local recurrence rate of approximately 33%, despite negative margins. If resection margins were positive following surgery alone, the 10-year recurrence rate exceeded 50% but was reduced to 31% in margin-positive cases that received RT (P = 0.007). Overall, patients treated with combined surgery and RT experienced a 10-year actuarial local relapse rate of 25%. In addition, in patients treated with RT for gross disease, the 10-year actuarial relapse rate was 24%, making this a viable option for such patients. Similar outcomes were noted by Nuyttens and colleagues in a comparative review of 22 articles; they reported that both RT alone (local control 78%) and RT and surgery (local control 78%) were superior to surgery alone (local control 61%).[205] Because positive surgical margins are frequent, we usually advise adjuvant RT depending on lesion location and consideration of salvage options for any subsequent recurrence. Adjuvant EBRT can be delivered either preoperatively or postoperatively. Although postoperative RT is usually employed, the Princess Margaret Hospital has reported the efficacy of preoperative RT in a group of 58 patients. With median follow-up of 69 months, there were 11 local recurrences (19%).[206] Hormonal manipulations, EBRT, and chemotherapy can be used for symptomatic unresectable disease; but a trial of surveillance to evaluate the presence or pace of progression, or both, may also be considered.

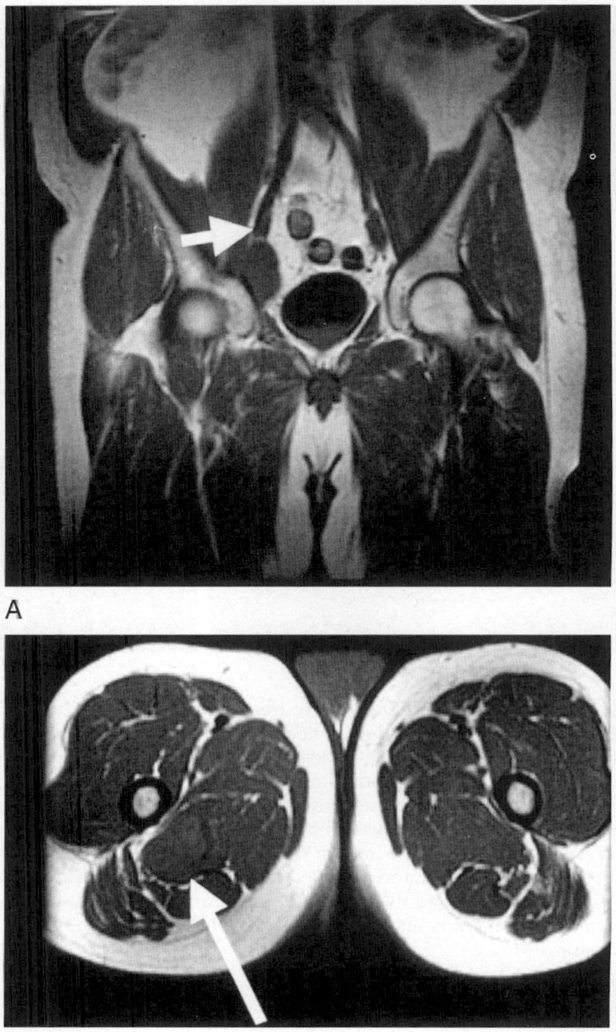

A

B

Figure 62-12 **(A)** Coronal MRI view of a young male patient shows an external iliac lymph node mass located adjacent to the right common iliac artery (*arrow*). **(B)** The primary tumor (*arrow*) was subclinical and identified in the posterior thigh compartment in adductor magnus and close to the sciatic nerve. Because of the complexity of the target, preoperative RT was chosen to include both the primary tumor and the femoral, external iliac, and common iliac lymph node regions (see Fig. 62-13). RT, radiation therapy. (Adapted from O'Sullivan B, Wunder J, Pisters PW: Target description for RT of soft tissue sarcoma. *In* Gregoire V, Scalliet P, Ang KK [eds]: Clinical Target Volumes in Conformal Radiotherapy and Intensity Modulated Radiotherapy. Heidelberg, Germany, Springer; 2003. pp. 205-227. With permission of Springer and Business Media.)

SALVAGE TREATMENT AND PALLIATION

Salvage

Salvage treatment of patients with STS needs to be considered because selected patients may enjoy long disease-free outcomes following intervention for recurrence, either locally or distant (regional nodal and lung). Salvage of other metastasis is unlikely, but soft tissue lesions may also be associated with subsequent long disease-free survival, especially in selected cases of MLS. The border between salvage treatment and aggressive palliation is blurred and should be individualized.

Local Recurrence

An outline for the evaluation and management of locally recurrent STS must consider the dual goals of tumor control and normal tissue protection in a manner that is even more complicated than the treatment of primary disease (Fig. 62-14).

In patients with STS not previously treated with RT or chemotherapy, combined-modality therapy should be used, especially because these can generally be administered safely. The potential for adjuvant chemotherapy to enhance local control may mean it could have a role in local salvage because

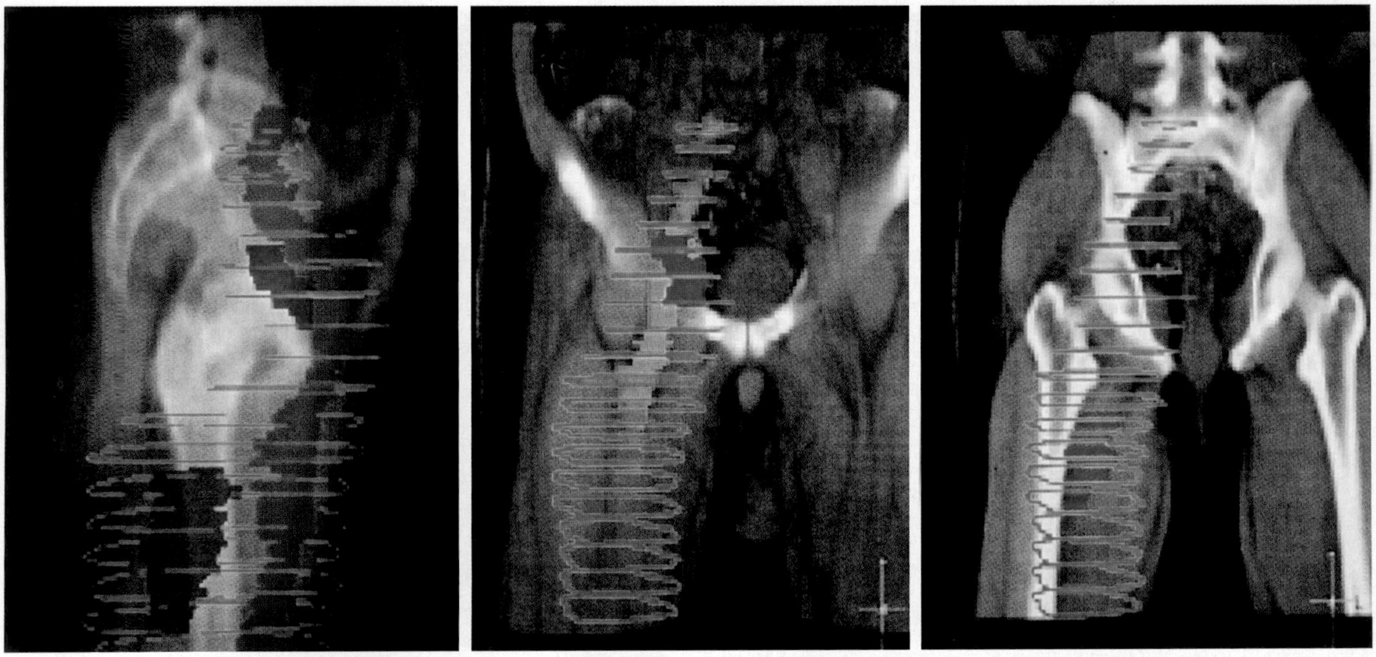

Figure 62-13 The CTV delineation to treat the patient described in Figure 62-12 with preoperative RT that included the primary tumor in the thigh and the local draining lymph node areas following induction chemotherapy. The sagittal view (**A**) shows the GTV for the primary (*red*), the solitary external iliac lymph node (*dark blue*), and the CTV (*pale blue* wire frame) for concurrent preoperative RT of the primary and the lymphatic areas. The CTV for the nodal region encompasses both the vascular structures (*yellow*) and the GTV for the macroscopic lymph node. The CTV also extends to include the common iliac region in the upper part of the figure. The coronal projections of the same targets used in **A** are represented in the different positional planes: vascular target (*yellow*) and the lymph node GTV (*dark blue*) in **B;** primary GTV (*red*) in **C.** This patient has remained disease-free for 6 years following treatment with 50 Gy in 25 fractions administered preoperatively, followed by resection of both the primary tumor and involved lymph nodes. CTV, clinical target volume; GTV, gross tumor volume; RT, radiation therapy. (From O'Sullivan B, Wunder J, Pisters PW: Target description for radiotherapy of STS. *In* Gregoire V, Scalliet P, Ang KK [eds], Clinical Target Volumes in Conformal Radiotherapy and Intensity Modulated Radiotherapy. Heidelberg, Germany, Springer; 2003. pp. 205-227. With permission of Springer and Business Media.)

it is improbable that it was used initially. Preoperative or postoperative RT can be used with the same caveats relating to the volume and dose issues previously discussed for the management of primary disease.

For previously irradiated lesions, greater individualization is needed and the possibility may also exist that the lesion may be an irradiation-induced sarcoma. Prior irradiated lesions would generally undergo tumor bed implantation with brachytherapy catheters in conjunction with a wide local excision where possible. Brachytherapy should be administered with the same guidelines and restrictions as described earlier for primary disease. When EBRT is indicated, preoperative RT probably has an advantage because of the smaller doses and volumes involved.

Local Recurrence with Metastasis

Concurrent metastases are occasionally identified with local relapse. Patients who recur with multiple symptomatic metastases after a short disease-free interval are best managed with palliative approaches. Aggressive surgical palliation is rarely indicated in this situation, but local excision of a small or superficial recurrence may delay or prevent local complications. The occasional patient presenting with local recurrence and limited systemic disease may benefit from aggressive treatment, especially after a long disease-free interval. This should include local salvage according to the principles outlined previously and consideration of metastasectomy (Fig. 62-15).

Metastatic Disease

In selected cases, pulmonary metastasectomy is potentially curative, although distant disease at other sites is unlikely to be cured, excepting soft tissue metastasis in liposarcoma (see Fig. 62-15). Treatment of metastatic bone disease is likely always palliative. Although, once more and rarely, MLS can exhibit an unusually indolent course. For first-time pulmonary metastasectomy the five-year survival rates range from 15% to 35% and from 12% to 52% for subsequent pulmonary resections.[207] The most adverse features for outcome of pulmonary metastasectomy were incomplete resection, tumor doubling time exceeding 40 days, more than four metastatic lesions, and disease-free interval shorter than 12 months. A retrospective study of 255 STS patients at the EORTC also showed 5-year disease-free and overall survival figures of 35% and 38%.[208] The International Registry of Lung Metastases reported 5206 patients with pulmonary metastases resection, 2173 of whom had bone or STS. Patients with single metastases and long disease-free intervals were recognized as having better outcome.[209]

Palliative Treatment

General Approach Including Surgery

Palliative management is complicated and usually ends with a decision about whether chemotherapy should be used in the patient for whom no other options remain. It is some-

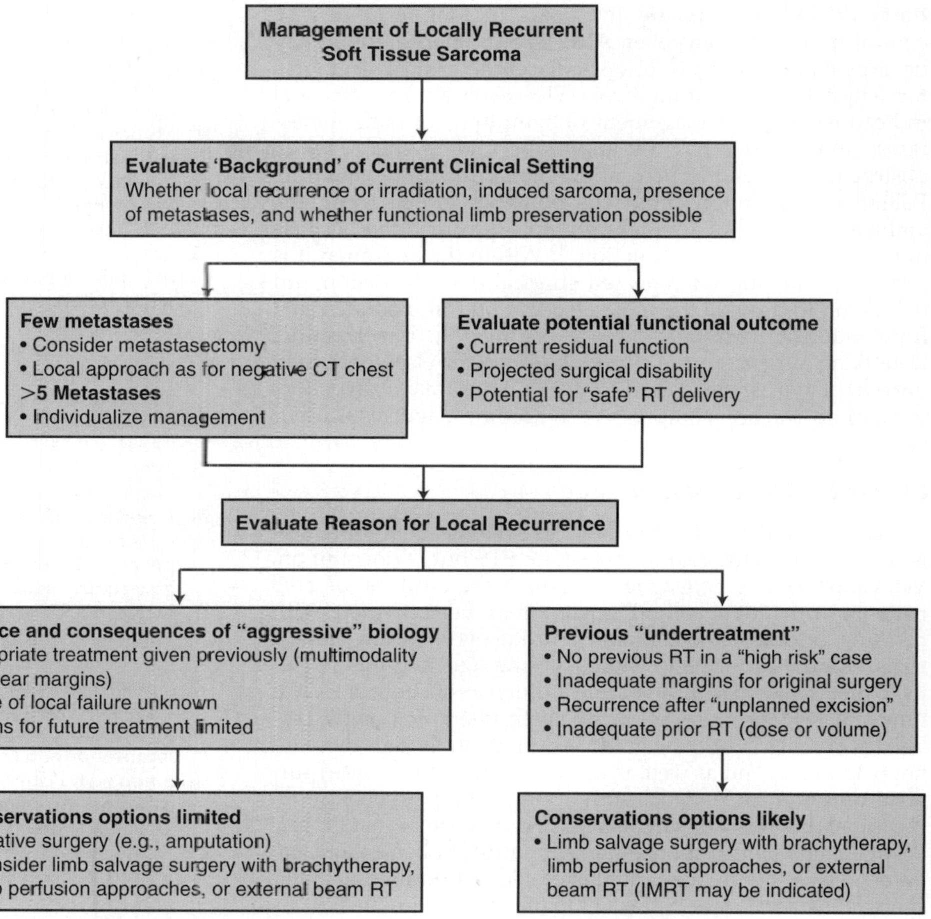

Figure 62-14 Management algorithm for the treatment of locally recurrent STS.

These lesions are complex to manage and the clinician must consider various elements that include the potential that the lesion may be an irradiation-induced sarcoma, appreciating the reasons underlying the recurrence, the impact of concurrent metastases on decision-making, and the options for protecting functioning tissue at the site of the recurrence. EBRT, external beam radiation therapy; IMRT, intensity-modulated radiation therapy; RT, radiation therapy.

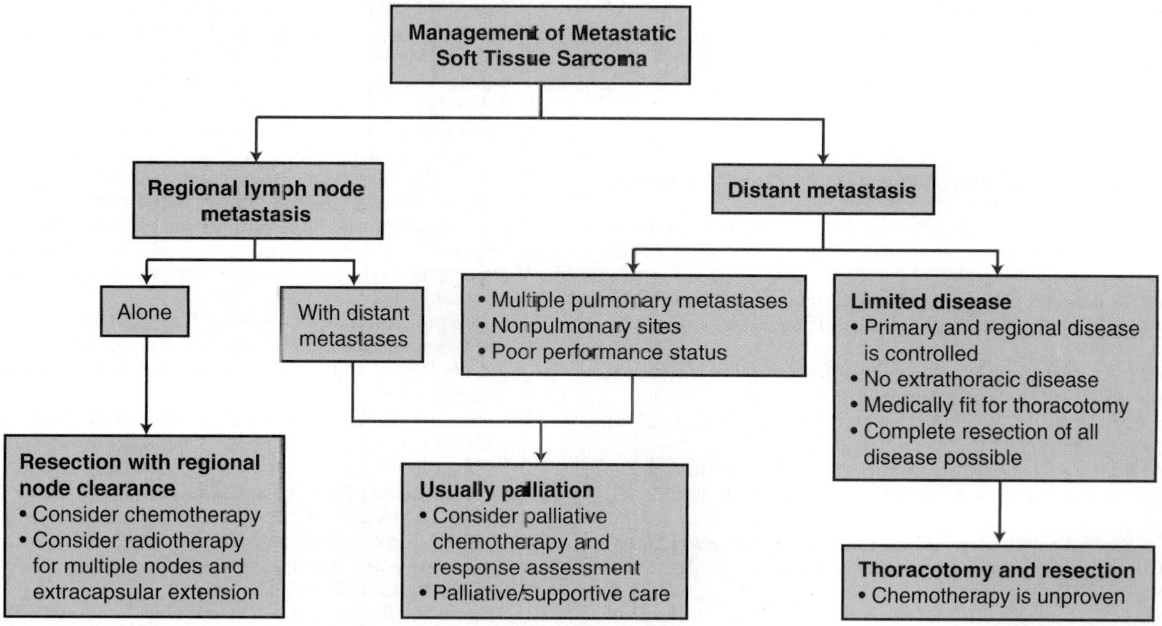

Figure 62-15 Management algorithm for the treatment of metastatic STS.

Patients with these lesions have potentially salvageable disease that requires careful selection prior to initiating intensive treatment approaches.

times difficult to separate the goals of long-term disease control from symptom relief. Also, in STS relapse, there may be large malignant mass lesions adjacent to critical structures for which RT has a limited role. However, RT has its usual indications in the management of symptoms of bone metastases, and surgery has an important role in the relief of obstruction or for mechanical problems including fracture. Palliative amputations hold the potential for restoring the ambulatory status of a patient previously bedridden because of extreme pain and dysfunction.[210] Within the abdomen it is relatively common for repeated surgical decompression and debulking to provide the most effective and immediate relief from indolent metastatic disease confined to this location. Debulking surgery in the chest, abdomen, or elsewhere may prevent or at least delay morbidity from intestinal obstruction, ureteral obstruction compressive syndromes, and respiratory embarrassment.[210]

Chemotherapy for Metastases

A complete and durable response to systemic chemotherapy is certainly a useful goal in metastatic STS but is uncommon. Van Glabbeke and colleagues described the outcome of 2185 patients with advanced STSs who had been treated with first-line anthracycline-containing protocols in seven clinical trials.[81] Good performance status, young age, and absence of liver metastases had a favorable influence on both survival time and response rate following chemotherapy. Longer survival is expected with low grade lesions even though these do not tend to respond as well. In addition, there is increased survival duration for patients with a long time period between the initial diagnosis of sarcoma and occurrence of metastases, despite equivalent response rates. In addition better survival is associated with certain histologies: liposarcoma and synovial sarcoma fare better compared to malignant fibrous histiocytoma. Another issue is whether single agent or combination chemotherapy should be used in incurable locally advanced or metastatic STS. Bramwell and colleagues performed a meta-analysis on data on 2281 participants from eight RCTs from reports of single-agent doxorubicin versus doxorubicin-based combination chemotherapy and concluded that single-agent doxorubicin was the optimal therapy.[211] Median survival ranged from 7.7 to 12.0 months with single agent doxorubicin and ranged from 7.3 to 12.7 months with combination chemotherapy.

REFERENCES

1. Jemal A, Tiwari RC, Murray T, et al: Cancer statistics, 2004. CA Cancer J Clin 54:8-29, 2004.
2. Bu X, Bernstein L, Brynes RK: Reduced risk of synovial sarcoma in females: X-chromosome inactivation? Br J Cancer 87:28-30, 2002.
3. Wistuba II, Behrens C, Gazdar AF: Pathogenesis of non-AIDS-defining cancers: A review. AIDS Patient Care STDS 13:415-426, 1999.
4. Olsson H: An updated review of the epidemiology of soft tissue sarcoma. Acta Orthop Scand Suppl 75:16-20, 2004.
5. Tavani A, Soler M, La Vecchia C, et al: Body weight and risk of soft-tissue sarcoma. Br J Cancer 81:890-892, 1999.
6. Beck A: Zur frage des Rontgensarkoms, zugleich ein Beitrag zur pathogenese des Sarkoms. Muench med Wochenschr 69:623-625, 1922.
7. Spiro IJ, Suit HD: Radiation-induced bone and soft tissue sarcomas: Clinical aspects and molecular biology. Cancer Treat Res 91:143-155, 1997.
8. Sheppard DG, Libshitz HI: Post-radiation sarcomas: A review of the clinical and imaging features in 63 cases. Clin Radiol 56:22-29, 2001.
9. Karlsson P, Holmberg E, Samuelsson A, et al: Soft tissue sarcoma after treatment for breast cancer—a Swedish population-based study. Eur J Cancer 34:2068-2075, 1998.
10. Stewart F, Treves N: Lymphangiosarcoma in post-mastectomy lymphedema. Cancer 1:64-81, 1943.
11. Muller R, Hajdu S, Brennan M: Lymphangiosarcoma associated with chronic filarial lymphedema. Cancer 59:179-183, 1987.
12. Pukkala E, Kaprio J, Koskenvuo M, et al: Cancer incidence among Finnish world class male athletes. Int J Sports Med 21:216-220, 2000.
13. Paavolainen P, Pukkala E, Pulkkinen P, Visuri T: Cancer incidence in Finnish hip replacement patients from 1980 to 1995: A nationwide cohort study involving 31,651 patients. J Arthroplasty 14:272-280, 1999.
14. Visuri T, Pukkula E, Pulkkinen P, Paavolainen P: Decreased cancer risk in patients who have been operated on with total hip and knee arthroplasty for primary osteoarthrosis: A meta-analysis of 6 Nordic cohorts with 73,000 patients. Acta Orthop Scand 74:351-360, 2003.
15. Fong Y, Rosen P, Brennan M: Multifocal desmoids. Surgery 114:902-906, 1993.
16. Kogevinas M, Kauppinen T, Winkelmann R, et al: Soft tissue sarcoma and non-Hodgkin's lymphoma in workers exposed to phenoxy herbicides, chlorophenols, and dioxins: Two nested case-control studies. Epidemiology 6:396-402, 1995.
17. Lynge E: Cancer incidence in Danish phenoxy herbicide workers, 1947-1993. Environ Health Perspect 106 Suppl 2:683-688, 1998.
18. Hardell L, Erikson M, Degerman A: Meta-analysis of four Swedish case-control studies on exposure to pesticides as risk factors for soft tissue sarcoma including the relation to tumour localization and histopathologic type. Int J Oncol 6:847-851, 1995.
19. Smith AH, Pearce NE, Fisher DO, et al: Soft tissue sarcoma and exposure to phenoxyherbicides and chlorophenols in New Zealand. J Natl Cancer Inst 73:1111-1117, 1984.
20. Balarajan R, Acheson ED: Soft tissue sarcomas in agriculture and forestry workers. J Epidemiol Community Health 38:113-116, 1984.
21. Hoar SK, Blair A, Holmes FF, et al: Agricultural herbicide use and risk of lymphoma and soft-tissue sarcoma. JAMA 256:1141-1147, 1986.
22. Hoppin JA, Tolbert PE, Flanders WD, et al: Occupational risk factors for sarcoma subtypes. Epidemiology 10:300-306, 1999.
23. Borden EC, Baker LH, Bell RS, et al: Soft tissue sarcomas of adults: State of the translational science. Clin Cancer Res 9:1941-1956, 2003.
24. Tomescu O, Barr FG: Chromosomal translocations in sarcomas: Prospects for therapy. Trends Mol Med 7:554-559, 2001.
25. Ladanyi M, Bridge JA: Contribution of molecular genetic data to the classification of sarcomas. Hum Pathol 31:532-538, 2000.
26. Zoller ME, Rembeck B, Oden A, et al: Malignant and benign tumors in patients with neurofibromatosis type 1 in a defined Swedish population. Cancer 79:2125-2131, 1997.
27. Doorn PF, Molenaar WM, Buter J, Hoekstra HJ: Malignant peripheral nerve sheath tumors in patients with and without neurofibromatosis. Eur J Surg Oncol 21:78-82, 1995.
28. Angelov L, Davis A, O'Sullivan B, et al: Neurogenic sarcomas: Experience at the University of Toronto. Neurosurgery 43:56-64; discussion 64-55, 1998.
29. Feldkamp MM, Lau N, Provias JP, et al: Acute presentation of a neurogenic sarcoma in a patient with neurofibromatosis type 1: A pathological and molecular explanation. Case report. J Neurosurg 84:867-873, 1996.
30. Kleihues P, Schauble B, zur Hausen A, et al: Tumors associated with p53 germline mutations: A synopsis of 91 families. Am J Pathol 150:1-13, 1997.
31. Li FP, Fraumeni JF, Jr: Prospective study of a family cancer syndrome. JAMA 247:2692-2694, 1982.
32. Moll AC, Imhof SM, Bouter LM, Tan KE: Second primary tumors in patients with retinoblastoma. A review of the literature. Ophthalmic Genet 18:27-34, 1997.
33. Abramson DH, Melson MR, Dunkel IJ, Frank CM: Third (fourth and fifth) nonocular tumors in survivors of retinoblastoma. Ophthalmology 108:1868-1876, 2001.

34. Wong FL, Boice JD, Jr, Abramson DH, et al: Cancer incidence after retinoblastoma. Radiation dose and sarcoma risk. JAMA 278:1262-1267, 1997.
35. Posner MC, Shiu MH, Newsome JL, et al: The desmoid tumor. Not a benign disease. Arch Surg 124:191-196, 1989.
36. Kawai A, Woodruff J, Healey JH, et al: SYT-SSX gene fusion as a determinant of morphology and prognosis in synovial sarcoma. N Engl J Med 338:153-160, 1998.
37. Ladanyi M, Antonescu CR, Leung DH, et al: Impact of SYT-SSX fusion type on the clinical behavior of synovial sarcoma: A multi-institutional retrospective study of 243 patients. Cancer Res 62:135-140, 2002.
38. Nilsson G, Skytting B, Xie Y, Bet al: The SYT-SSX1 variant of synovial sarcoma is associated with a high rate of tumor cell proliferation and poor clinical outcome. Cancer Res 59:3180-3184, 1999.
39. Guillou L, Benhattar J, Bonichon F, et al: Histologic grade, but not SYT-SSX fusion type, is an important prognostic factor in patients with synovial sarcoma: A multicenter, retrospective analysis. J Clin Oncol 22:4040-4050, 2004.
40. Brennan MF, Singer SS, Maki R, et al (eds): Principles and Practice of Oncology. Philadelphia, Lippincott Williams and Wilkins; 2005, pp. 1581-1637.
41. O'Sullivan B, Pisters PW: Staging and prognostic factor evaluation in soft tissue sarcoma. Surg Oncol Clin N Am 12:333-353, 2003.
42. Maseide K, Kandel RA, Bell RS, et al: Carbonic anhydrase IX as a marker for poor prognosis in soft tissue sarcoma. Clin Cancer Res 10:4464-4471, 2004.
43. Fletcher CDM, Unni K, Mertens K (eds): World Health Organization Classification of Tumours: Pathology and Genetics of Tumours of Soft Tissue and Bone. Lyon, France, IARC Press (International Agency for Research on Cancer); 2002.
44. Segal NH, Pavlidis P, Antonescu CR, et al: Classification and subtype prediction of adult soft tissue sarcoma by functional genomics. Am J Pathol 163:691-700, 2003.
45. Nielsen TO, West RB, Linn SC, et al: Molecular characterisation of soft tissue tumours: A gene expression study. Lancet 359:1301-1307, 2002.
46. Baird K, Davis S, Antonescu CR, et al: Gene expression profiling of human sarcomas: Insights into sarcoma biology. Cancer Res 65:9226-9235, 2005.
47. Trojani M, Contesso G, Coindre JM, et al: Soft-tissue sarcomas of adults; study of pathological prognostic variables and definition of a histopathological grading system. Int J Cancer 33:37-42, 1984.
48. Costa J, Wesley RA, Glatstein E, Rosenberg SA. The grading of soft tissue sarcomas. Results of a clinicohistopathologic correlation in a series of 163 cases. Cancer 53:530-541, 1984.
49. Guillou L, Coindre JM, Bonichon F, et al: Comparative study of the National Cancer Institute and French Federation of Cancer Centers Sarcoma Group grading systems in a population of 410 adult patients with soft tissue sarcoma. J Clin Oncol 15:350-362, 1997.
50. Sobin L, Wittekind C: TNM Classification of Malignant Tumours, 6th ed. New York, Wiley-Liss, 2002.
51. Greene FL, Page D, Norrow M, et al: AJCC Cancer Staging Manual, 6th ed. New York, Springer; 2002.
52. Fletcher CDM: Pleomorphic malignant fibrous histiocytomas: fact or fiction? A reappraisal based on 159 tumors diagnosed as pleomorphic sarcoma. Am J Surg Pathol 16:213-228, 1992.
53. Fletcher CD, Gustafson P, Rydholm A, et al: Clinicopathologic re-evaluation of 100 malignant fibrous histiocytomas: prognostic relevance of subclassification. J Clin Oncol 19:3045-3050, 2001.
54. Daugaard S: Current soft-tissue sarcoma classifications. Eur J Cancer 40:543-548, 2004.
55. Mark RJ, Tran LM, Sercarz J, et al: Angiosarcoma of the head and neck. The UCLA experience 1955 through 1990. Arch Otolaryngol Head Neck Surg 119:973-978, 1993.
56. Holden CA, Spittle MF, Jones EW: Angiosarcoma of the face and scalp, prognosis and treatment. Cancer 59:1046-1057, 1987.
57. Ruymann FB, Grovas AC: Progress in the diagnosis and treatment of rhabdomyosarcoma and related soft tissue sarcomas. Cancer Invest 18:223-241, 2000.
58. La Quaglia MP, Heller G, Ghavimi F, et al: The effect of age at diagnosis on outcome in rhabdomyosarcoma. Cancer 73:109-117, 1994.
59. Rubin BP, Hasserjian RP, Singer S, et al: Spindle cell rhabdomyosarcoma (so-called) in adults: Report of two cases with emphasis on differential diagnosis. Am J Surg Pathol 22:459-464, 1998.
60. Nascimento AF, Fletcher CD: Spindle cell rhabdomyosarcoma in adults. Am J Surg Pathol 29:1106-1113, 2005.
61. Frascella E, Toffolatti L, Rosolen A: Normal and rearranged PAX3 expression in human rhabdomyosarcoma. Cancer Genet Cytogenet 102:104-109, 1998.
62. Barr FG, Chatten J, D'Cruz CM, et al: Molecular assays for chromosomal translocations in the diagnosis of pediatric soft tissue sarcomas. JAMA 273:553-557, 1995.
63. Kelly KM, Womer RB, Sorensen PH, et al: Common and variant gene fusions predict distinct clinical phenotypes in rhabdomyosarcoma. J Clin Oncol 15:1831-1836, 1997.
64. Goulding M, Lumsden A, Paquette AJ: Regulation of PAX3 expression in the dermomyotome and its role in muscle development. Development 120:957-971, 1994.
65. Enzinger F, Weiss S: Soft Tissue Tumors. St. Louis, Mosby, 1995.
66. Antonescu CR, Elahi A, Humphrey M, et al: Specificity of TLS-CHOP rearrangement for classic myxoid/round cell liposarcoma: Absence in predominantly myxoid well-differentiated liposarcomas. J Mol Diagn 2:132-138, 2000.
67. Cheng EY, Springfield DS, Mankin HJ: Frequent incidence of extrapulmonary sites of initial metastasis in patients with liposarcoma. Cancer 75:1120-1127, 1995.
68. Spillane AJ, Fisher C, Thomas JM: Myxoid liposarcoma—The frequency and the natural history of nonpulmonary soft tissue metastases. Ann Surg Oncol 6:389-394, 1999.
69. Pearlstone DB, Pisters PW, Bold RJ, et al: Patterns of recurrence in extremity liposarcoma: Implications for staging and follow-up. Cancer 85:85-92, 1999.
70. Estourgie SH, Nielsen GP, Ott MJ: Metastatic patterns of extremity myxoid liposarcoma and their outcome. J Surg Oncol 80:89-93, 2002.
71. Antonescu CR, Elahi A, Healey JH, et al: Monoclonality of multifocal myxoid liposarcoma: Confirmation by analysis of TLS-CHOP or EWS-CHOP rearrangements. Clin Cancer Research 6:2788-2793, 2000.
72. Weitz J, Antonescu CR, Brennan MF: Localized extremity soft tissue sarcoma: Improved knowledge with unchanged survival over time. J Clin Oncol 21:2719-2725, 2003.
73. Pitson G, Robinson P, Wilke D, et al: Radiation response: An additional unique signature of myxoid liposarcoma. Int J Radiat Oncol Biol Phys 60:522-526, 2004.
74. Hatano H, Ogose A, Hotta T, et al: Treatment of myxoid liposarcoma by marginal or intralesional resection combined with radiotherapy. Anticancer Res 23:3045-3049, 2003.
75. McArthur GA, Demetri GD, van Oosterom A, et al: Molecular and clinical analysis of locally advanced dermatofibrosarcoma protuberans treated with imatinib: Imatinib Target Exploration Consortium Study B2225. J Clin Oncol 23:866-873; 2005.
76. Ballo MT, Zagars GK, Pisters P, Pollack A: The role of radiation therapy in the management of dermatofibrosarcoma protuberans. Int J Radiat Oncol Biol Phys 40:823-827, 1998.
77. Suit H, Spiro I, Mankin HJ, et al: Radiation in management of patients with dermatofibrosarcoma protuberans. J Clin Oncol 14:2365-2369, 1996.
78. Sun LM, Wang CJ, Huang CC, et al: Dermatofibrosarcoma protuberans: Treatment results of 35 cases. Radiother Oncol 57:175-181, 2000.
79. Spillane AJ, A'Hern R, Judson IR, et al: Synovial sarcoma: A clinicopathologic, staging, and prognostic assessment. J Clin Oncol 18:3794-3803, 2000.
80. Essary LR, Vargas SO, Fletcher CD: Primary pleuropulmonary synovial sarcoma: Reappraisal of a recently described anatomic subset. Cancer 94:459-469, 2002.
81. Van Glabbeke M, van Oosterom AT, Oosterhuis JW, et al: Prognostic factors for the outcome of chemotherapy in advanced soft tissue sarcoma: An analysis of 2,185 patients treated with anthracycline-containing first-line regimens—A European Organiza-

tion for Research and Treatment of Cancer Soft Tissue and Bone Sarcoma Group Study. J Clin Oncol 17:150-157, 1999.
82. Mazeron JJ, Suit HD: Lymph nodes as sites of metastases from sarcomas of soft tissue. Cancer 60:1800-1808, 1987.
83. Fong Y, Coit DG, Woodruff JM, Brennan MF: Lymph node metastasis from soft tissue sarcoma in adults. Analysis of data from a prospective database of 1772 sarcoma patients. Ann Surg 217:72-77, 1993.
84. Hirota S, Isozaki K, Moriyama Y, et al: Gain-of-function mutations of C-KIT in human gastrointestinal stromal tumors. Science 279:577-580, 1998.
85. Heinrich MC, Corless CL, Duensing A, et al: PDGFRA activating mutations in gastrointestinal stromal tumors. Science 299:708-710, 2003.
86. Joensuu H, Roberts PJ, Sarlomo-Rikala M, et al: Effect of the tyrosine kinase inhibitor STI571 in a patient with a metastatic gastrointestinal stromal tumor. N Engl J Med 344:1052-1056, 2001.
87. Joensuu H, Fletcher C, Dimitrijevic S, et al: Management of malignant gastrointestinal stromal tumours. Lancet Oncol 3:655-664, 2002.
88. Heinrich MC, Corless CL, Demetri GD, et al: Kinase mutations and imatinib response in patients with metastatic gastrointestinal stromal tumor. J Clin Oncol 21:4342-4349, 2003.
89. Segal NH, Pavlidis P, Noble WS, et al: Classification of clear-cell sarcoma as a subtype of melanoma by genomic profiling. J Clin Oncol 21:1775-1781, 2003.
90. O'Sullivan B, Wunder J, Pisters PW: Target description for radiotherapy of soft tissue sarcoma. *In* Gregoire V, Scalliet P, Ang KK (eds): Clinical Target Volumes in Conformal Radiotherapy and Intensity Modulated Radiotherapy. Heidelberg, Germany, Springer; 2003. pp 205-227.
91. Mankin HJ, Mankin CJ, Simon MA: The hazards of the biopsy, revisited. J Bone Joint Surg Am 78:656-663, 1996.
92. Behranwala KA, A'Hern R, Omar AM, Thomas JM: Prognosis of lymph node metastasis in soft tissue sarcoma. Ann Surg Oncol 11:714-719, 2004.
93. Riad S, Griffin AM, Liberman B, et al: Lymph node metastasis in soft tissue sarcoma in an extremity. Clin Orthop Relat Res 426:129-134, 2004.
94. Panicek DM, Gatsonis C, Rosenthal DI, et al: CT and MR imaging in the local staging of primary malignant musculoskeletal neoplasms: Report of the Radiology Diagnostic Oncology Group. Radiology 202:237-246, 1997.
95. Jones DN, McGowage GB, Sostman HT, et al: Monitoring of neoadjuvant therapy response of soft tissue and musculoskeletal sarcoma using fluorine-18 FDG PET. J Nucl Med 37:1438-1444, 1996.
96. Dimitrakopoulou-Strauss A, Strauss LG, Scharzbach M, et al: Dynamic PET 18F-FDG studies in patients with primary and recurrent soft tissue sarcoma: Impact on diagnosis and correlation with grading. J Nucl Med 42:713-720, 2001.
97. Bastiaannet E, Groen H, Jager PL, et al: The value of FDG-PET in the detection, grading and response to therapy of soft tissue and bone sarcomas; a systematic review and meta-analysis. Cancer Treat Rev 30:83-101, 2004.
98. Noria S, Davis A, Kandel R, et al: Residual disease following unplanned excision of soft tissue sarcoma of an extremity. J Bone Joint Surg Am 78:650-655, 1996.
99. Davis AM, Kandel RA, Wunder JS, et al: The impact of residual disease on local recurrence in patients treated by initial unplanned resection for soft tissue sarcoma of the extremity. J Surg Oncol 66:81-87, 1997.
100. Siebenrock KA, Hertel R, Ganz R: Unexpected resection of soft-tissue sarcoma. More mutilating surgery, higher local recurrence rates, and obscure prognosis as consequences of improper surgery. Arch Orthop Trauma Surg 120:65-69, 2000.
101. van Dalen T, Hennipman A, Van Coevorden F, et al: Evaluation of a clinically applicable post-surgical classification system for primary retroperitoneal soft-tissue sarcoma. Ann Surg Oncol 11:483-490, 2004.
102. Pollock R, Karnell L, Menck H, Winchester D: The National Cancer Data Base report on soft tissue sarcoma. Cancer 78:2247-2257, 1996.
103. Rosenberg SA, Tepper J, Glatstein E, et al: The treatment of soft-tissue sarcomas of the extremities: Prospective randomized evaluations of (1) limb-sparing surgery plus radiation therapy compared with amputation and (2) the role of adjuvant chemotherapy. Ann Surg 196:305-315, 1982.
104. Pisters PW, Harrison LB, Leung DH, et al: Long-term results of a prospective randomized trial of adjuvant brachytherapy in soft tissue sarcoma. J Clin Oncol 14:859-868, 1996.
105. Yang JC, Chang AE, Baker AR, et al: Randomized prospective study of the benefit of adjuvant radiation therapy in the treatment of soft tissue sarcomas of the extremity. J Clin Oncol 16:197-203, 1998.
106. O'Sullivan B, Davis AM, Turcotte R, et al: Preoperative versus postoperative radiotherapy in soft-tissue sarcoma of the limbs: A randomised trial. Lancet 359:2235-2241, 2002.
107. Stojadinovic A, Leung DH, Hoos A, et al: Analysis of the prognostic significance of microscopic margins in 2,084 localized primary adult soft tissue sarcomas. Ann Surg 235:424-434, 2002.
108. Gerrand CH, Wunder JS, Kandel RA, et al: Classification of positive margins after resection of soft-tissue sarcoma of the limb predicts the risk of local recurrence. J Bone Joint Surg Br 83-B: 1149-1155, 2001.
109. Kepka L, Suit HD, Goldberg SI, et al: Results of radiation therapy performed after unplanned surgery (without re-excision) for soft tissue sarcomas. J Surg Oncol 92:39-45, 2005.
110. Stotter A, Fallowfield M, Mott A, et al: Role of compartmental resection for soft tissue sarcoma of the limb and limb girdle. Br J Surg 77:88-92, 1990.
111. Karakousis C, Emrich L, Rao U, Khalil M: Limb salvage in soft tissue sarcomas with selective combination of modalities. Eur J Surg Oncol 17:71-80, 1991.
112. Geer RJ, Woodruff J, Casper ES, Brennan MF: Management of small soft-tissue sarcoma of the extremity in adults. Arch Surg 127:1285-1289, 1992.
113. Baldini EH, Goldberg J, Jenner C, et al: Long-term outcomes after function-sparing surgery without radiotherapy for soft tissue sarcoma of the extremities and trunk. J Clin Oncol 17:3252-3259, 1999.
114. Rydholm A, Gustafson P, Rooser B, et al: Limb-sparing surgery without radiotherapy based on anatomic location of soft tissue sarcoma. J Clin Oncol 9:1757-1765, 1991.
115. Mann GN: Less is (usually) more: When is amputation appropriate for treatment of extremity soft tissue sarcoma? Ann Surg Oncol 12:1-2, 2005.
116. Williard WC, Collin C, Casper ES, et al: The changing role of amputation for soft tissue sarcoma of the extremity in adults. Surg Gynecol Obst 175:389-396, 1992.
117. Le Vay J, O'Sullivan B, Catton C, et al: Outcome and prognostic factors in soft tissue sarcoma in the adult. Int J Radiat Oncol Biol Phys 27:1091-1099, 1993.
118. Ghert MA, Abudu A, Driver N, et al: The indications for and the prognostic significance of amputation as the primary surgical procedure for localized soft tissue sarcoma of the extremity. Ann Surg Oncol 12:10-17, 2005.
119. Colterjohn NR, Davis AM, O'Sullivan B, et al: Functional outcome in limb-salvage surgery for soft tissue tumours of the foot and ankle. Sarcoma 1:67-74, 1997.
120. Strander H, Turesson I, Cavallin-Stahl E: A systematic overview of radiation therapy effects in soft tissue sarcomas. Acta Oncol 42:516-531, 2003.
121. O'Sullivan B, Davis A, Turcotte R, et al: Five year results of a randomized phase III trial of pre-operative vs post-operative radiotherapy in extremity soft issue sarcoma. ASCO Annual Meeting Proceedings (Abstract 9007). J Clin Oncol 22:14S, 2004.
122. Davis AM, O'Sullivan B, Turcotte R, et al: Late radiation morbidity following randomization to preoperative versus postoperative radiotherapy in extremity soft tissue sarcoma. Radiother Oncol 75:48-53, 2005.
123. Tepper JE, Suit HD: Radiation therapy alone for sarcoma of soft tissue. Cancer 56:475-479, 1985.
124. Kepka L, Delaney TF, Suit HD, Goldberg SI: Results of radiation therapy for unresected soft-tissue sarcomas. Int J Radiat Oncol Biol Phys 63:852-859, 2005.

125. Cormier JN, Patel SR, Herzog CE, et al: Concurrent ifosfamide-based chemotherapy and irradiation. Analysis of treatment-related toxicity in 43 patients with sarcoma. Cancer 92:1550-1555, 2001.
126. Rhomberg W, Hassenstein EO, Gefeller D: Radiotherapy vs. radiotherapy and razoxane in the treatment of soft tissue sarcomas: final results of a randomized study. Int J Radiat Oncol Biol Phys 36:1077-1084, 1996.
127. Dubois JB, Debrigode C, Hay M, et al: Intra-operative radiotherapy in soft tissue sarcomas. Radiother Oncol 34:160-163, 1995.
128. Nag S, Shasha D, Janjan N, et al: The American Brachytherapy Society recommendations for brachytherapy of soft tissue sarcomas. Int J Radiat Oncol Biol Phys 49:1033-1043, 2001.
129. Delannes M, Thomas L, Martel P, et al: Low-dose-rate intraoperative brachytherapy combined with external beam irradiation in the conservative treatment of soft tissue sarcoma. Int J Radiat Oncol Biol Phys 47:165-169, 2000.
130. O'Connor MI, Pritchard DJ, Gunderson LL: Integration of limb-sparing surgery, brachytherapy, and external-beam irradiation in the treatment of soft-tissue sarcomas. Clin Orthop Relat Res 289:73-80; 1993.
131. Rosenblatt E, Meushar N, Bar-Deroma R, et al: Interstitial brachytherapy in soft tissue sarcomas: the Rambam experience. Isr Med Assoc J 5:547-551, 2003.
132. Abbatucci JS, Boulier N, de Ranieri J, et al: Radiotherapy as an integrated part of the treatment of soft tissue sarcomas. Radiother Oncol 2:115-121, 1984.
133. Eilber FR, Guiliano AE, Huth J, et al: High-grade soft-tissue sarcomas of the extremity: UCLA experience with limb salvage. Prog Clin Biol Res 201:59-74, 1985.
134. Ballo MT, Lee AK: Current results of brachytherapy for soft tissue sarcoma. Curr Opin Oncol 15:313-318, 2003.
135. Arthur DW, Koo D, Zwicker RD, et al: Partial breast brachytherapy after lumpectomy: Low-dose-rate and high-dose-rate experience. Int J Radiat Oncol Biol Phys 56:681-689, 2003.
136. Ott OJ, Potter R, Hammer J, et al: Accelerated partial breast irradiation with iridium-192 multicatheter PDR/HDR brachytherapy. Preliminary results of the German-Austrian multicenter trial. Strahlenther Onkol 180:642-649, 2004.
137. Wazer DE, Berle L, Graham R, et al: Preliminary results of a phase I/II study of HDR brachytherapy alone for T1/T2 breast cancer. Int J Radiat Oncol Biol Phys 53:889-897, 2002.
138. Alektiar KM, Hu K, Anderson L, et al: High-dose-rate intraoperative radiation therapy (HDR-IORT) for retroperitoneal sarcomas. Int J Radiat Oncol Biol Phys 47:157-163, 2000.
139. Holt GE, Griffin AM, Pintilie M, et al: Fractures following radiotherapy and limb-salvage surgery for lower extremity soft-tissue sarcomas. A comparison of high-dose and low-dose radiotherapy. J Bone Joint Surg Am 87:315-319, 2005.
140. Lin PP, Schupak KD, Boland PJ, et al: Pathologic femoral fracture after periosteal excision and radiation for the treatment of soft tissue sarcoma. Cancer 82:2356-2365, 1998.
141. Alektiar KM, Zelefsky MJ, Brennan MF: Morbidity of adjuvant brachytherapy in soft tissue sarcoma of the extremity and superficial trunk. Int J Radiat Oncol Biol Phys 47:1273-1279, 2000.
142. Helmstedter CS, Goebel M, Zlotecki R, Scarborough MT: Pathologic fractures after surgery and radiation for soft tissue tumors. Clin Orthop Relat Res 389:165-172; 2001.
143. O'Sullivan B, Ward I, Haycocks T, Sharpe M: Techniques to modulate radiotherapy toxicity and outcome in soft tissue sarcoma. Curr Treat Options Oncol 4:453-464, 2003.
144. Simon MA, Enneking WF: The management of soft-tissue sarcomas of the extremities. J Bone Joint Surg Am 58:317-327, 1976.
145. Enneking WF, Spanier SS, Malawer MM: The effect of the Anatomic setting on the results of surgical procedures for soft parts sarcoma of the thigh. Cancer 47:1005-1022, 1981.
146. Panicek DM, Schwartz LH: Soft tissue edema around musculoskeletal sarcomas at magnetic resonance imaging. Sarcoma 1:189-191, 1997.
147. White LM, Wunder JS, Bell RS, et al: Histologic assessment of peritumoral edema in soft tissue sarcoma. Int J Radiat Oncol Biol Phys 61:1439-1445, 2005.
148. Davis AM, Wright JG, Williams JI, et al: Development of a measure of physical function for patients with bone and soft tissue sarcoma. Qual Life Res 5:508-516, 1996.
149. Alektiar KM, Leung D, Zelefsky MJ, Brennan MF: Adjuvant radiation for stage II-B soft tissue sarcoma of the extremity. J Clin Oncol 20:1643-1650, 2002.
150. Harrison LB, Franzese F, Gaynor JJ, Brennan MF: Long-term results of a prospective randomized trial of adjuvant brachytherapy in the management of completely resected soft tissue sarcomas of the extremity and superficial trunk. Int J Radiat Oncol Biol Phys 27:259-265, 1993.
151. DeLaney TF, Spiro IJ, Suit HD, et al: Neoadjuvant chemotherapy and radiotherapy for large extremity soft-tissue sarcomas. Int J Radiat Oncol Biol Phys 56:1117-1127, 2003.
152. Eilber FR, Giuliano AE, Huth JF, Morton DL: A randomized prospective trial using postoperative adjuvant chemotherapy (Adriamycin) in high-grade extremity soft-tissue sarcoma. Am J Clin Oncol 11:39-45, 1988.
153. Eilber FR, Giuliano AE, Huth JF, Other AN: Intravenous (IV) vs. intraarterial (IA) Adriamycin, 2800r radiation and surgical excision for extremity soft tissue sarcomas: A randomized prospective trial (Abstract 1194). Proceedings of the American Society of Clinical Oncology 9:309, 1990.
154. Grunhagen DJ, Brunstein F, Graveland WJ, et al: Isolated limb perfusion with tumor necrosis factor and melphalan prevents amputation in patients with multiple sarcomas in arm or leg. Ann Surg Oncol 12:473-479, 2005.
155. Eggermont AM, de Wilt JH, ten Hagen TL: Current uses of isolated limb perfusion in the clinic and a model system for new strategies. Lancet Oncol 4:429-437, 2003.
156. Grunhagen DJ, de Wilt JH, van Geel AN, et al: TNF dose reduction in isolated limb perfusion. Eur J Surg Oncol 31:1011-1019, 2005.
157. Bonvalot S, Laplanche A, Lejeune F, et al: Limb salvage with isolated perfusion for soft tissue sarcoma: could less TNF-alpha be better? Ann Oncol 16:1061-1068, 2005.
158. Rossi CR, Mocellin S, Pilati P, et al: Hyperthermic isolated perfusion with low-dose tumor necrosis factor alpha and doxorubicin for the treatment of limb-threatening soft tissue sarcomas. Ann Surg Oncol 12:398-405, 2005.
159. Grunhagen DJ, de Wilt JH, Verhoef C, et al: TNF-based isolated limb perfusion in unresectable extremity desmoid tumours. Eur J Surg Oncol 31:912-916, 2005.
160. Sarcoma Meta-analysis Collaboration: Adjuvant chemotherapy for localised resectable soft-tissue sarcoma of adults: meta-analysis of individual data. Lancet 350:1647-1654, 1997.
161. Alvegard TA, Sigurdsson H, Mouridsen H, et al: Adjuvant chemotherapy with doxorubicin in high-grade soft tissue sarcoma: A randomized trial of the Scandinavian Sarcoma Group. J Clin Oncol 7:1504-1513, 1989.
162. Bramwell V, Rouesse J, Steward W, et al: Adjuvant CYVADIC chemotherapy for adult soft tissue sarcoma—Reduced local recurrence but no improvement in survival: A study of the European Organization for Research and Treatment of Cancer Soft Tissue and Bone Sarcoma Group. J Clin Oncol 12:1137-1149, 1994
163. Omura GA, Blessing JA, Major F: Randomised trial of adjuvant adriamycin in uterine sarcomas: A Gynecologic Oncology Group study. J Clin Oncol 3:1240-1245, 1985.
164. Frustaci S, Gherlinzoni F, De Paoli A, et al: Adjuvant chemotherapy for adult soft tissue sarcomas of the extremities and girdles: Results of the Italian randomized cooperative trial. J Clin Oncol 19:1238-1247, 2001.
165. Cormier JN, Huang X, Xing Y, et al: Cohort analysis of patients with localized, high-risk, extremity soft tissue sarcoma treated at two cancer centers: Chemotherapy-associated outcomes. J Clin Oncol 22:4567-4574, 2004.
166. Eilber FC, Eilber FR, Eckardt J, et al: The impact of chemotherapy on the survival of patients with high-grade primary extremity liposarcoma. Ann Surg 240:686-695; discussion 695-687, 2004.
167. Grobmyer SR, Maki RG, Demetri GD, et al: Neo-adjuvant chemotherapy for primary high-grade extremity soft tissue sarcoma. Ann Oncol 15:1667-1672, 2004.

168. Mendenhall WM, Zlotecki RA, Hochwald SN, et al: Retroperitoneal soft tissue sarcoma. Cancer 104:669-675, 2005.
169. Lewis JJ, Leung D, Woodruff JM, Brennan MF: Retroperitoneal soft-tissue sarcoma: analysis of 500 patients treated and followed at a single institution. Ann Surg 228:355-365, 1998.
170. Catton C, O'Sullivan B, Kotwell C, et al: Outcome and prognosis in retroperitoneal soft tissue sarcoma. Int J Radiat Oncol Biol Phys 29:1005-1010, 1994.
171. Jones JJ, Catton CN, O'Sullivan B, et al: Initial results of a trial of preoperative external-beam radiation therapy and postoperative brachytherapy for retroperitoneal sarcoma. Ann Surg Oncol 9:346-354, 2002.
172. Gieschen HL, Spiro IJ, Suit HD, et al: Long-term results of intraoperative electron beam radiotherapy for primary and recurrent retroperitoneal soft tissue sarcoma. Int J Radiat Oncol Biol Phys 50:127-131, 2001.
173. Petersen IA, Haddock MG, Donohue JH, et al: Use of intraoperative electron beam radiotherapy in the management of retroperitoneal soft tissue sarcomas. Int J Radiat Oncol Biol Phys 52:469-475, 2002.
174. Crosby JA, Catton CN, Davis A, et al: Malignant gastrointestinal stromal tumors of the small intestine: A review of 50 cases from a prospective database. Ann Surg Oncol 8:50-59, 2001.
175. Clary BM, DeMatteo RP, Lewis JJ, et al: Gastrointestinal stromal tumors and leiomyosarcoma of the abdomen and retroperitoneum: A clinical comparison. Ann Surg Oncol 8:290-299, 2001.
176. Demetri GD, von Mehren M, Blanke CD, et al: Efficacy and safety of imatinib mesylate in advanced gastrointestinal stromal tumors. N Engl J Med 347:472-480, 2002.
177. Gordon MS, Hajdu SI, Bains MS, Burt ME: Soft tissue sarcomas of the chest wall. Results of surgical resection. J Thorac Cardiovasc Surg 101:843-854, 1991.
178. Graeber GM, Snyder RJ, Fleming AW, et al: Initial and long-term results in the management of primary chest wall neoplasms. Ann Thorac Surg 34:664-673, 1982.
179. Greager JA, Patel MK, Briele HA, et al: Soft tissue sarcomas of the adult thoracic wall. Cancer 59:370-373, 1987.
180. Perry RR, Venzon D, Roth JA, Pass HI: Survival after surgical resection for high-grade chest wall sarcomas. Ann Thorac Surg 49:363-368; discussion 368-369, 1990.
181. Petrov DB, Vlassov VI, Kalaydjiev GT, et al: Primary pulmonary sarcomas and carcinosarcomas—Postoperative results and comparative survival analysis. Eur J Cardiothorac Surg 23:461-466, 2003.
182. Burt M, Ihde JK, Hajdu SI, et al: Primary sarcomas of the mediastinum: Results of therapy. J Thorac Cardiovasc Surg 115:671-680, 1998.
183. Michler RE, Goldstein DJ: Treatment of cardiac tumors by orthotopic cardiac transplantation. Semin Oncol 24:534-539, 1997.
184. Uberfuhr P, Meiser B, Fuchs A, et al: Heart transplantation: An approach to treating primary cardiac sarcoma? J Heart Lung Transplant 21:1135-1139, 2002.
185. Bernstein L, Deapen D, Ross RK: The descriptive epidemiology of malignant cystosarcoma phyllodes tumors of the breast. Cancer 71:3020-3024, 1993.
186. Moore MP, Kinne DW: Breast sarcoma. Surg Clin North Am 76:383-392, 1996.
187. Mangi AA, Smith BL, Gadd MA, et al: Surgical management of phyllodes tumors. Arch Surg 134:487-492; discussion 492-483, 1999.
188. Rowell MD, Perry RR, Hsiu JG, Barranco SC: Phyllodes tumors. Am J Surg 165:376-379, 1993.
189. Reinfuss M, Mitus J, Duda K, et al: The treatment and prognosis of patients with phyllodes tumor of the breast: An analysis of 170 cases. Cancer 77:910-916, 1996.
190. Kapiris I, Nasiri N, A'Hern R, et al: Outcome and predictive factors of local recurrence and distant metastases following primary surgical treatment of high-grade malignant phyllodes tumours of the breast. Eur J Surg Oncol 27:723-730, 2001.
191. Hines JR, Murad TM, Beal JM: Prognostic indicators in cystosarcoma phylloides. Am J Surg 153:276-280, 1987.
192. Cohn-Cedermark G, Rutqvist LE, Rosendahl I, Silfversward C: Prognostic factors in cystosarcoma phyllodes. A clinicopathologic study of 77 patients. Cancer 68:2017-2022, 1991.
193. Salvadori B, Cusumano F, Del Bo R, et al: Surgical treatment of phyllodes tumors of the breast. Cancer 63:2532-2536, 1989.
194. Chua CL, Thomas A, Ng BK: Cystosarcoma phyllodes: A review of surgical options. Surgery 105:141-147, 1989.
195. Zurrida S, Bartoli C, Galimberti V, et al: Which therapy for unexpected phyllode tumour of the breast? Eur J Cancer 28:654-657, 1992.
196. Barrow BJ, Janjan NA, Gutman H, et al: Role of radiotherapy in sarcoma of the breast—A retrospective review of the M.D. Anderson experience. Radiother Oncol 52:173-178, 1999.
197. Zelek L, Llombart-Cussac A, Terrier P, et al: Prognostic factors in primary breast sarcomas: A series of patients with long-term follow-up. J Clin Oncol 21:2583-2588, 2003.
198. Donnell RM, Rosen PP, Lieberman PH, et al: Angiosarcoma and other vascular tumors of the breast. Am J Surg Pathol 5:629-642, 1981.
199. Pollard SG, Marks PV, Temple LN, Thompson HH: Breast sarcoma. A clinicopathologic review of 25 cases. Cancer 66:941-944, 1990.
200. Adem C, Reynolds C, Ingle JN, Nascimento AG: Primary breast sarcoma: Clinicopathologic series from the Mayo Clinic and review of the literature. Br J Cancer 91:237-241, 2004.
201. Callery CD, Rosen PP, Kinne DW: Sarcoma of the breast. A study of 32 patients with reappraisal of classification and therapy. Ann Surg 201:527-532, 1985.
202. Sturgis EM, Potter BO: Sarcomas of the head and neck region. Curr Opin Oncol 15:239-252, 2003.
203. O'Sullivan B, Audet N, Catton C, Gullane P: Soft tissue and bone sarcomas of the head and neck. *In* Harrison LB, Sessions RB, Hong WK (eds): Head and Neck Cancer: A Multidisciplinary Approach, 2nd ed. Philadelphia, Lippincott Williams & Wilkins; 2004. pp 786-823.
204. Tran LM, Mark R, Meier R, et al: Sarcomas of the head and neck. Prognostic factors and treatment strategies. Cancer 70:169-177, 1992.
205. Nuyttens JJ, Rust PF, Thomas CR Jr, Turrisi AT III: Surgery versus radiation therapy for patients with aggressive fibromatosis or desmoid tumors: A comparative review of 22 articles. Cancer 88:1517-1523, 2000.
206. O'Dea FJ, Wunder J, Bell RS, et al: Preoperative radiotherapy is effective in the treatment of fibromatosis. Clin Orthop Relat Res 19-24, 2003.
207. Frost DB: Pulmonary metastasectomy for soft tissue sarcomas: Is it justified? J Surg Oncol 59:110-115, 1995.
208. van Geel AN, Pastorino U, Jauch KW, et al: Surgical treatment of lung metastases: The European Organization for Research and Treatment of Cancer-Soft Tissue and Bone Sarcoma Group study of 255 patients. Cancer 77:675-682, 1996.
209. Friedel G, Pastorino U, Buyse M, et al: Resection of lung metastases: Long-term results and prognostic analysis based on 5206 cases—The International Registry of Lung Metastases. Zentralbl Chir 124:96-103, 1999.
210. Sheldon DG, James TA, Kraybill WG: Palliative surgery of soft tissue sarcoma. Surg Oncol Clin N Am 13:531-541, ix, 2004.
211. Bramwell VH, Anderson D, Charette ML: Doxorubicin-based chemotherapy for the palliative treatment of adult patients with locally advanced or metastatic soft tissue sarcoma. Cochrane Database Syst Rev CD003293, 2003.
212. Sindelar WF, Kinsella TJ, Chen PW, et al: Intraoperative radiotherapy in retroperitoneal sarcomas. Final results of a prospective, randomized, clinical trial. Arch Surg 128:402-410, 1993.
213. Lindner LH, Schlemmer M, Hohenberger P, et al: Risk assessment of early progression among 213 pts with high-risk soft tissue sarcomas (HR-STS) treated with neoadjuvant chemotherapy +/- regional hyperthermia: EORTC 62961 + ESHO-RHT95. Intergroup Phase III Study. ASCO Annual Meeting Proceedings (Abstract 9020). J Clin Oncol 23:16S, 2005.
214. Gronchi A, Casali PG, Fiore M, et al: Retroperitoneal soft tissue sarcomas: patterns of recurrence in 167 patients treated at a single institution. Cancer 100:2448-2455, 2004.
215. Hassan I, Park SZ, Donohue JH, et al: Operative management of primary retroperitoneal sarcomas: a reappraisal of an institutional experience. Ann Surg 239:244-250, 2004.

216. Ferrario T, Karakousis CP: Retroperitoneal sarcomas: Grade and survival. Arch Surg 138:248-251, 2003.
217. Stoeckle E, Coindre JM, Bonvalot S, et al: French Federation of Cancer Centers Sarcoma Group. Prognostic factors in retroperitoneal sarcoma: A multivariate analysis of a series of 165 patients of the French Cancer Center Federation Sarcoma Group. Cancer 92:359-368, 2001.
218. van Dalen T, Hoekstra HJ, van Geel AN, et al: Dutch Soft Tissue Sarcoma Group. Locoregional recurrence of retroperitoneal soft tissue sarcoma: Second chance of cure for selected patients. Eur J Surg Oncol 27:564-568, 2001.
219. Herman K, Gruchala A, Niezabitowski A, et al: Prognostic factors in retroperitoneal sarcomas: Ploidy of DNA as a predictor of clinical outcome. J Surg Oncol 71:32-35, 1999.
220. Jenkins MP, Alvaranga JC, Thomas JM: The management of retroperitoneal soft tissue sarcomas. Eur J Cancer 32A:622-626, 1996.
221. Kilkenny JW, Bland KI, Copeland EM: Retroperitoneal sarcoma: The University of Florida experience. J Am Coll Surg 182:329-339, 1996.
222. Singer S, Corson JM, Demetri GD, et al: Prognostic factors predictive of survival for truncal and retroperitoneal soft-tissue sarcoma. Ann Surg 221:185-195, 1995.

CHAPTER 63

NONMALIGNANT DISEASES

Michael Heinrich Seegenschmiedt

DEFINITION AND CLASSIFICATION OF NONMALIGNANT DISEASES

Many nonmalignant or "benign" diseases can be successfully treated with ionizing radiation. Its use for painful musculoskeletal diseases has a long tradition in Europe.[1] Sokoloff[2] reported positive results in radiotherapy of painful "rheumatoid diseases" as early as 1898. The traditional classification of benign diseases amenable to radiotherapy as inflammatory, degenerative, hyperproliferative, functional, and other types of disorders is currently outdated. Worldwide, irradia-tion of nonmalignant diseases has become more important recently, although indications and treatment concepts have changed considerably, and there are clear differences between countries owing to clinical traditions and differences in organization and training.[3–6]

Indications for the Implementation of Radiotherapy

Nonmalignant diseases have several features that may justify the use of radiotherapy. They can grow invasively and aggressively without forming metastases. Desmoids can be cosmetically disfiguring and functionally disturbing. Keloids or endocrine orbitopathies may be life-threatening. Refractory hepatic hemangioma (Kasabach-Merritt Syndrome) or juvenile angiofibroma in facial regions of children or adolescents may require radiotherapy. There may be an indication for radiation therapy when nonmalignant diseases have a lasting effect on quality of life by causing pain or other serious symptoms, or if other methods are not available, have failed, or may induce more side-effects. Overall, radiotherapy is rarely the first option for treatment of most nonmalignant diseases.

The application of radiotherapy in most nonmalignant diseases is classified as an elective measure, and, therefore, a particularly thorough informed consent has to be conducted. Particular attention should focus on the risk for long-term consequences, such as the triggering of secondary malignancies or leukemia.

Long-Term Risk for Tumor Induction

Considering international data about the emergence of tumors and leukemias after whole-body exposure to ionizing radiation (UNSCEAR, BEIR), the risk for tumor induction can be calculated on a gender- and age-related basis, according to Jansen and associates.[7] The average lifetime risk for exposure to radiation is lower in men (9.5%) than in women (11.5%). Table 63-1 summarizes the age- and gender-specific risk for tumor induction.[7]

Principles of Irradiation of Nonmalignant Diseases

The principles of irradiation of nonmalignant diseases can be summarized in 10 statements (Table 63-2).

RADIOBIOLOGIC ASPECTS

The radiobiologic mechanisms, which are known from tumor therapy, and the identified proliferating target cells are only partially applicable to nonmalignant diseases. Other radiation-sensitive target cells, and cellular and functional mechanisms should be considered as target points for ionizing radiation. However, radiotherapy is probably not working via one particular mechanism but rather through a complex interaction of different effects.

Reactions in Connective Tissue

Several *mechanisms* are triggered by ionizing radiation in connective tissues. Following any trauma or acute or chronic inflammation, several cell systems regulate the repair process where fibroblasts play a central role, particularly during the *reparative phase*, which is characterized by high cell production and stimulation of specific growth factors. Furthermore, ionizing radiation also has a pivotal influence on cellular differentiation.[8,9]

For some hyperproliferative events, *fibroblast overreaction* is responsible for the disease process—for example, during the early stage of Dupuytren's contracture, during the early phase of Peyronie's disease, in keloids, and in the progression of aggressive fibromatosis. The increased fibroblast production can be influenced by ionizing radiation, which influences differentiation and suppresses cell proliferation.

Reactions in the Vascular System

The *endothelial cells* of the capillaries and the larger arterial and venous blood vessels are the origin of various cytokine-mediated cellular reactions and possess a high proliferative potential. Amongst others, intercellular adhesion molecule 1 (ICAM-1), a mediator of the leukocyte-endothelial interaction, is induced by low radiation doses.[10,11] Similarly, selectins mediate the penetration of mononuclear blood cells into the interstitial tissue.[11] Endothelial prostaglandin release is also modulated by ionizing radiation.[12] Cellular and membrane functions can be modified when exposed to radiation.

Large single or total doses may cause endothelial damage, leading to sclerosis and obliteration of small blood vessels. Higher fractionated doses or single doses are used for cerebral arteriovenous malformations (AVMs) or symptomatic vertebral hemangiomas, and lower single and total doses are applied to reduce inflammatory processes such as endocrine orbitopathy, pseudotumor orbitae, furuncles, and sweat-gland abscesses.

Reactions in Painful Processes

Degenerative processes in hypotrophic tissues such as tendons, ligaments, and joints can cause pain by chronic inflammation and trigger various forms of functional impairment of the musculoskeletal system. Radiation does not influence the degenerative process, but may reduce the inflammation and, as a consequence, improve function of affected joints and limbs and achieve pain relief.

Table 63-1 Tumor Induction Depending on Age and Gender. Relative Life-Time Risk

Age Group (yr)	Men (%/Sv)	Women (%/Sv)
≤10	25-26	32-33
11–20	15	19
21–30	13-14	17
31–40	7	8
41–50	5	6
51–60	4.5	5
61–70	3.5	4.5
71–80	2.5	3.0
>80	1.0	1.5

From Jansen JTM, Broerse J, Zoetelief J, et al: Assessment of carcinogenic risk in the treatment of benign disease of knee and shoulder joint. *In* Seegenschmiedt MH, Makoski H-B: Kolloquium Radioonkologie/Strahlentherapie, Radiotherapie bei gutartigen Erkrankungen, vol 15. Altenberge: Diplodocus-Verlag, 2001, pp. 13-15.

Table 63-3 Mechanisms of Action and Dose Concepts

Mechanisms of Action	Single Dose (Gy)	Total Dose (Gy)
Cellular gene and protein expression, e.g., eczemas	<2.0	<2
Inhibition of inflammation in lymphocytes, e.g., in pseudotumor orbitae	0.3-1.0	2-6
Inhibition of fibroblast proliferation, e.g., in keloids	1.5-3.0	8-12
Inhibition of proliferation in benign tumors, e.g., in desmoids	1.8-3.0	45-60

Table 63-2 Principles of Irradiation of Nonmalignant Diseases

1. Estimate the *natural course of disease* without therapy.
2. Consider potential consequences of non-treatment of the patient.
3. Review data about *alternative therapies* and their therapeutic results.
4. Conduct a *risk-benefit analysis* compared with other possible measures.
5. Prove that the indication is justified if *conventional therapies* have failed, if risks and consequences of other therapies are greater, and if nontreatment would have more dramatic consequences than irradiation for the patient.
6. Consider the individual *potential long-term radiogenic risks.*
7. Inform *each patient* about all relevant details of radiotherapy: target volume, dose concept (single and total dose), duration of single session and whole irradiation series, relevant radiogenic risks, and side effects.
8. Obtain *written consent* from the patient following *thorough patient education.*
9. Ensure *long-term aftercare* to document result.
10. Request a competent *second opinion* in case of doubt and if the provided patient's data or treatment decisions are uncertain.

Data from Seegenschmiedt MH, Katalinic A, Makoski H, et al: Radiation therapy for benign diseases: patterns of care study in Germany. Int J Radiat Oncol Biol Phys 47:195-202, 2000; Micke O, Seegenschmiedt MH: The German Working Group guidelines for radiation therapy of benign diseases: a multicenter approach in Germany. Int J Radiat Oncol Biol Phys 52:496-513, 2002.

Mechanism of Action

To know individual target cells and potential pathogenic mechanisms of the various nonmalignant diseases also means to coordinate the radiation therapy concepts accordingly and consistently. The dose concepts applied in nonmalignant diseases differ greatly from each other due to other potential mechanisms of action (Table 63-3).

NONMALIGNANT DISORDERS OF THE HEAD AND NECK

Nonmalignant tumors of the central nervous system (CNS) can lead to severe, life-threatening symptoms due to local expansion and pressure on neighboring structures. Depending on growth rate, the surrounding tissue can adapt and delay clinical diagnosis. Percutaneous radiotherapy with single or fractionated stereotactic radiotherapy as well as brachytherapy presents a great advantage for some benign diseases of the brain and the head and neck region.

Pituitary adenoma and meningioma are important benign diseases treated with radiation therapy. These are covered fully in Chapters 25 and 26.

Craniopharyngioma

Definition and Clinical Features

Craniopharyngiomas are rare dysontogenetic midline tumors originating from Rathke's pocket or the ductus craniopharyngicus. They make up 6% to 10% of CNS tumors in children and appear mostly between ages 5 and 15. They are located near the sella, with a close connection to pituitary gland, hypothalamus, chiasma opticum, and visual nerves. Intrasellar tumors are rare; some are also located suprasellarly or intrasellarly. Main symptoms are visual impairment or loss of vision, visual field impairment (bitemporal hemianopia), and endocrine dysfunctions such as dwarfism, fat tissue disturbance, or adrenal cortex insufficiency. Signs of intracranial pressure can appear as well. Diagnosis is made from skull radiographs (sella expansion), CT (typical calcifications), and MRI (cystic or mixed solid and cystic tumor components).[13,14]

Nonradiotherapeutic Treatment

Primary therapy consists of complete resection, which is equivalent to permanent cure. Due to relatively high postoperative aftereffects, such as visual impairment (20%) and panhypopituitarism (in up to 95%) following radical neurosurgical procedure,[15,16] less radical surgery with adjuvant three-dimensional (3D), conformal RT is the preferred method. Ten-year control rates after complete tumor resection are 60% to 93%.[16,17]

Radiotherapeutic Options

In primary inoperable tumors or after subtotal resection, percutaneous RT is indicated because otherwise the progression rate after 2 to 3 years amounts to 70% to 90%.[18] After subtotal resection alone, the recurrence rate is 30%, which, with postoperative RT, reaches a control rate of 80% to 95% after 5 to 20 years.[18–20] Long-term control rate after primary RT or after subtotal resection or cyst punctuation with adjuvant radiotherapy (RT), respectively, with 50 to 54 Gy total dose (1.8–2 Gy/fx) is comparable with complete resection.[21,22]

Stereotactic RT provides less stress on normal tissue. Due to the proximity to the chiasm and the visual nerves, fractionated stereotactic RT (FSRT) is preferred to single-dose irradiation. Using FSRT, a local 10-year control rate of 100% was reached in Heidelberg. According to MRI, four of 26 patients reached complete and 14 partial remission; eight had a stable MRI finding. In five patients, visual improvement was reached. The hypophyseal hormonal situation deteriorated in seven patients. There were no radionecroses, secondary malignancies, or visual deteriorations.[23] Another option is the local application of radionuclides in the craniopharyngiomal cysts, which can bring tumor growth to a halt.

After conformal RT, the rate of visual deterioration is up to 10%. Severe side effects such as radionecroses, cognitive changes, and secondary malignancies occur with an incidence of less than 2%.[14]

Acoustic Neuromas (Schwannomas)

Definition and Clinical Features

Acoustic neuromas are benign neuroectodermal tumors originating from the Schwann cells at the 4th cranial nerve. They make up 5% of primary brain tumors. Their incidence is 1 in 100,000, and 5% of patients are affected by neurofibromatosis type II. The growth in the cerebellopontine angle exerts pressure on the *N. vestibularis* and the *N. cochlearis*, causing hearing impairment, tinnitus, and vertigo. Further growth leads to facial paresis (cranial nerve [CN] VII), trigeminal neuropathy (CN V), and brainstem symptoms. Diagnosis is made via high-resolution CT and MRI. Therefore, it is possible to distinguish intrameatal from extrameatal tumors; further classification is done depending on tumor location and size (Table 63-4).[24]

Nonradiotherapeutic Treatment

Complete tumor resection is standard therapy. Because of the option of radiosurgery, particularly the large tumors (>25 mm) are surgically resected today. Therefore, the anatomic and functional conservation of CN VII and CN VIII is problematic. Nerve injury can be avoided intraoperatively by electrophysiologic monitoring. If transection cannot be avoided, function can be maintained in more than 90% of cases through reconstruction or anastomosis to CN XI. Hearing is maintained in only 40% of cases, depending on tumor size. In addition, approximately 10% of patients develop fistulas postoperatively, 6% pareses of the caudal cranial nerves, 2% hydrocephalus, 1% meningitis, and 1% hemiparesis. Postoperative mortality is approximately 1%.[25–27]

Table 63-4 Classification of Acoustic Neuromas

Tos Classification	Extrameatal Part of the Tumor (mm)
0	Only intrameatal
1	1-10
2	11-25
3	26-40
4	>40

From Tos M, Thomsen J: Proposal of classification of tumor size in acoustic neuroma surgery. *In* Tos M, Thomsen J (eds): Proceedings of the First International Conference on Acoustic Neuroma. Amsterdam, Kugler, 1992.

Radiotherapeutic Options

Stereotactic single-dose irradiation (SRT; radiosurgery) with gamma knife or modified linear accelerator is the preferred therapy because of the dose localization. Besides the direct damage of proliferating benign tumor cells, the effect is due to the reaction of the associated tumor vessels, which develop vessel occlusions just as do angiomas.[28,29] Further growth is inhibited; in 40% to 70% of cases, there is even tumor remission in the long-run. There is an indication for SRT in progressive and symptomatic *primary or recurrent acoustic neuromas* up to a size of 25 mm. With larger tumors, radiation exposure of the cranial nerves and the brainstem increases as well as the side-effect rate. The aim of therapy is not only the disappearance of tumor and symptoms but also the prevention of tumor progression and the maintenance of the remaining ability to hear.

Tolerance doses for *N. vestibulocochlearis*, *N. facialis*, and *N. trigeminus* are known[30] and depend on the length of nerves that are irradiated, tumor diameter, and dose at the tumor edge. Due to refined SRT techniques, complications to the facial and trigeminal nerves are seen only rarely today, but because the *N. vestibulocochlearis* goes right through the tumor, it cannot always be fully protected. Protection is only possible through dose reduction and/or fractionated RT.

With single doses of 12 to 14 Gy at the tumor edge (depending on reference isodose 15–25 Gy centrally), local control rates of up to 95% can be reached.[31–37] Radiogenic side effects occur very rarely. Stereotactic RT planning is done with high-resolution CT and MRI with suitable software for image fusion. With a modified linear accelerator, multiple stationary fields or rotational techniques are used. To decrease the side effects, some centers use FSRT. Typical RT doses are 5 × 5/10 × 3/25 × 2 and 30 × 1.8 Gy.[34,38–43] Recently, there has been a trend in favor of FSRT.

In a comparison between SRT, surgery, and monitoring alone, a current overview from Japan with more than 7000 patients shows that under monitoring, 50% of tumors showed progression within 3 years, as detected by MRI, and 20% of those cases needed to undergo surgery. With SRT, up to 8% have recurrences after 3 years and only 5% have to have surgery. After primary surgery, 2% have recurrences and in 3% of cases, surgery leads to functional impairment (*Yamakami et al., 2003*). Recent studies consider SRT to be as effective as surgery but with fewer side effects.[44,45]

Arteriovenous Malformation

Definition and Clinical Features

Intracranial AVM are rare vascular abnormalities consisting of widened arteries with connections to the normal capillary bed; this enables oxygenated blood to enter directly into the venous system. About 80% of AVM are located supratentorially. Incidence of AVM is unknown. Its prevalence is below 0.01% (about 18:100,000) in the Western Hemisphere. Most AVM are discovered at the age of 20 to 40 years. AVM can extend to aneurysms and rupture (2%–5% per year).[46] Neurologic symptoms (headaches, hemorrhage, cramp attacks) to the point of sudden death through bleeding characterize the clinical course. Diagnosis is made with special imaging techniques (angiography, MRI).

Untreated AVM have a bleeding risk of 2% to 4% per year, which increases after a rupture Large AVM with deep arterial feeders or those located at the basal ganglia or thalamus (9%)

have an increased bleeding risk.[47] Lethality after the first bleed is up to 30%; 10% to 20% of survivors have long-term neurologic defects. Spontaneous regression is very rare.

For therapy planning, precise knowledge about size, location, arterial feeders, and venous drainage of the nidus is required

The aim of therapy is the prevention of bleeding by complete obliteration of the nidus; if possible, the improvement of neurologic malfunctions; and at the same time, the prevention of therapy-induced side effects. For this purpose, the options of minimally invasive endoscopic surgery, endovascular embolization, and single-dose stereotaxy (radiosurgery) are available.

Nonradiotherapeutic Treatment

The therapy of choice is the elective *complete excision* of the AVM vessel abnormality. Particularly with small AVM in superficial, noneloquent regions of the brain, *microsurgery* reaches high cure rates. Larger AVM are treated initially with embolization before surgery or radiosurgery. Only in special cases is surgery performed under emergency conditions to remove life-threatening brain hemorrhages.

Radiotherapeutic Options

AVM are irradiated with SRT with a linear accelerator or gamma knife.[48,49] Fractionated RT with total doses of up to 60 Gy produced inadequate results.[50–53] Depending on the size and location of the AVM, a singe dose of 15 to 25 Gy is required in the periphery of the nidus. If the therapy is successful, complete obliteration of the nidus will occur within a few years. However, the bleeding risk continues to exist during the interval between SRT and complete obliteration. The obliteration rate after SRT is 65% to 95% (Table 63-5).

The side effects of SRT are mostly chronic and follow the time course of AVM obliteration: focal radionecroses or leukencephalopathies occur 9 to 36 months after SRT,[54–56] but they may also appear after several weeks.[57] The risk correlates strongly with the irradiated brain volume and the total dose[58–60]: the brain volume irradiated with >10 Gy is an important predictive factor.[61,62]

Chordomas

Definition and Clinical Features

Chordomas are rare, slowly growing, midline tumors originating from embryonal notochord rests in the region of the skull base and clivus (35%), the vertebral column (15%), or the sacral or tail bone region (50%). They have to be distinguished immunohistochemically from *low-grade chondrosarcomas*, which have a more favorable prognosis. Typical neurologic symptoms and magnetic resonance tomography lead to diagnosis.

Nonradiotherapeutic Treatment

Complete tumor resection is the therapy of choice. Large tumor rests, evidence of tumor necrosis, and female gender are unfavorable prognostic factors.[75] Due to the proximity to critical brain structures, complete removal near the base of skull is only rarely possible so that recurrences occur in more than 50% of operated cases.

Radiotherapeutic Options

The most important indication for high-dose RT is in case of inoperability and after incomplete resection. There is a clear dose–effect relation with significantly improved local control when total doses of >65 Gy are given.[76] Such high doses are difficult to administer without complications when conventional photon therapy is used, and, therefore, protons and heavy ions are often used for base of skull lesions.

Using fractionated photon therapy and total doses of up to 60 Gy, 5-year control rates of 17% to 33% have been reached. Higher total doses can be given when FSRT is used, but the clinical experiences with this method are limited. In Heidelberg, 37 patients received a median total dose of 66.6 Gy. The local control rate after 5 years was 50%.[77] Radiosurgical techniques are possible with smaller tumors and when there is sufficient distance to visual nerves, chiasma, and brainstem. The selected patient collective thus reached local control rates of 67%.[78]

With protons, total doses of 65 to 80 Gy equivalent are given. At the Massachusetts General Hospital, a total of 519 patients were treated with a total dose of 66 to 83 Gy equivalent resulting in local control rates of 73% after 5 years.[79,80] Other centers combine photon and proton therapy.

For chordomas of the sacrum, surgical resection is the primary therapy, but local recurrences can occur. Therefore, a number of centers have used preoperative radiation therapy in the management of these tumors.

Glomus Tumor/Chemodectoma

Definition and Clinical Features

The glomus tumors (synonyms: chemodectomas; nonchromaffin paragangliomas) are rare benign tumors that can occur in multiple anatomic locations:

1. Paragangliomas at the carotid glomus—along the carotid, mostly near the bifurcation

Table 63-5 Obliteration Rate and Radiogenic Side Effects after Radiosurgery

Study (chronologically)	*n*	Obliteration (%)	Moderate Side Effects (%)	Severe Side Effects (%)
Steiner et al.[49]	247	81	8	1
Colombo et al.[63]	153	80	6	2
Engenhart et al.[48]	212	72	4	4
Deruty et al.[64,65]	115	82	10	Not stated
Flickinger et al.[67]	1255	72	5	3
Miyawaki et al.[68]	73	64	13	5
Wolbers et al.[69]	29	71	Not stated	0
Chang et al.[70]	254	79	3	2
Schlienger et al.[71]	169	64	4	1
Pollock et al.[72]	144	76	10	<1
Shin et al.[73]	100	95 (5 years)	Not stated	4
Friedman et al.[74]	269	53	4	1

2. Jugular paraganglioma—location near the skull base in the region of the jugular bulb
3. Paraganglioma of the tympanic glomus—located in the region of the tympanum
4. Other paragangliomas—at the larynx; near the aorta; pulmonary; orbital cavity.

About 50% of tumors are located near the skull base in the jugular fossa. The age peak is 45 years. The tumors are usually unilateral; only 10% to 20% are bilateral or multiple.[81] They grow slowly, are rarely endocrinally active, and degenerate into malignant forms in 5% to 10%; they can also infiltrate bone, vessels, the middle ear, and cranial nerves. Main symptoms are headaches, CN failure (CN V–XII), dysphagia, pulsatile tinnitus, vertigo, and hypacusis. Without therapy, there is the risk for CN injury; the swelling can increase to a life-threatening size. Diagnosis is made clinically and with high-resolution CT and MRI .

Nonradiotherapeutic Treatment

Although glomus tumors grow slowly, they can cause severe problems, and, therefore, they must be treated. In the carotid region, primary tumor resection after previous embolization is the therapy of choice. At the skull base or at the tympanum, neurosurgical interventions are more risky; therefore, fractionated RT is often favored. In the case of incomplete surgery, the patient should initially be observed, and further treatment should only be started if the tumor grows.

Radiotherapeutic Options

Depending on the size and location of the lesions, the indication for RT may be either *primary irradiation* in case of functional or other inoperability (mostly jugular paragangliomas) or *additive irradiation* for R1-2 resection or *irradiation of recurrence* if there is progression after surgery. Conventional fractionated 3D-conformal RT with 45 to 55 Gy is the norm. The CTV is restricted to the tumor region with safety margin, to cover microscopic extensions.

Two overviews show that RT of paragangliomas produces control rates as good as or even better than surgery. Even in large, diffusely growing or multiple tumors, RT produces a local control rate of 88% to 93%.[82,83] Kim and associates[82] noticed a recurrence rate of 22% with doses of less than 40 Gy, whereas recurrences occurred in only 1.4% with doses of more than 40 Gy. Frequently, tumor rests are detectable on imaging for several years. Therapeutic success is usually assessed in terms of the regression of CN failures and the lack of tumor progression. A dose of 45 to 50 Gy does not complicate surgery that might become necessary later.

During the past decade, stereotactic single-dose RT and gamma knife have been used for the treatment of paragangliomas. Although the observation time after surgery is short, the results are very favorable.

Irradiation of paragangliomas of the carotid glomus can acutely cause pharyngeal mucositis and chronically may lead to skin fibrosis and dryness of the pharyngeal mucosa on the irradiated side. Irradiation of jugular or tympanic paragangliomas can lead to acute skin reactions in the external acoustic canal; tube ventilation dysfunction, reduced sound conduction, and salivary retention may occur in the middle ear. Long-term sequelae are rare.[83]

Juvenile Nasopharyngeal Fibroma

Definition and Clinical Features

Juvenile nasopharyngeal fibromas (JNF; synonym: angiofibromas) are very rare benign, strongly vascularized tumors in the head and neck region, affecting mainly male juveniles. JNF develop in the sphenoethmoidal suture and can spread from the epipharynx and the main nasal cavity via the sphenopalatine foramen and into the pterygopalatine fossa. After bony destruction, there is spread into the paranasal sinuses, the infratemporal fossa, the orbital space, and the middle cranial fossa.

Intracranial spread occurs in about 25% of cases. Typical symptoms are epistaxis and impaired nose breathing; depending on the spread, facial swelling as well as orbital (e.g., blindness) and intracranial symptoms (e.g., CN failure) may occur. A biopsy can cause massive bleeding so that histologic confirmation of diagnosis is often not performed. The presence of hormone receptors shows the influence of androgynous hormones. Spontaneous remission after puberty is possible but therapy can hardly be delayed when the symptoms increase and when complications are threatening.[84]

Nonradiotherapeutic Treatment

In JNF, the main emphasis is placed on surgery combined with embolization to decrease the size of the tumor. Small tumors that are restricted to the posterior nasal cavity and the nasopharynx can be completely removed after embolization. Equally, JNF with lateral spread are indications for surgery. Through surgery, most JNF without intracranial spread have local control rates of up to 100% with minimal toxicity.[85,86]

Radiotherapeutic Options

Radiotherapy is a very effective treatment for JNF. In advanced stages, complete resection is often not possible. Especially tumors with intracranial spread (stage IV) should receive primary irradiation. Other indications for 3D-conformal RT are tumor rests, inoperability, or recurrences after initial surgery. With modern CT-based treatment planning, high control rates are achieved in advanced JNF as well. FSRT is often recommended.[87]

Total doses of 30 to 55 Gy (1.8–2 Gy per fraction) are said to be effective,[88] but for large tumors, doses of 40 to 46 Gy are currently recommended.[89] With conventional fractionated RT, control rates of 80% to 100% can be reached. JNF often require several months after RT to remit[90]; sometimes, complete remission, as detected by imaging techniques, does not occur even after years, although there is no further growth.

Radiation side effects include mucositis, xerostomia and caries, dysfunction of the pituitary gland, CN failure, temporal-lobe necrosis, osteoradionecrosis, growth impairment of the facial skull, cataract, glaucoma, and atrophic rhinitis, but these can be limited through careful RT planning and highly conformal RT. Radiation-induced tumors occur in up to 4% of cases and particularly in young patients; this has to be weighed against the risk for sudden death or severe morbidity after surgery.

NONMALIGNANT DISORDERS OF THE EYE AND ORBIT

Pterygium

Definition and Clinical Features

Pterygium is a wig-shaped fibrovascular proliferating tissue originating at the lens epithelium at the border between conjunctiva and cornea. It normally extends from the medial (nasal) corner of the eye to the cornea and beyond. The highest incidence occurs in hot, dusty, dry, and sun-exposed regions ("desert belts"); here, even people in their 20s and 30s are affected.[91,92] Typical symptoms are foreign body feeling and tearing, sometimes motility problems. Affection of the cornea can cause impaired vision.

Nonradiotherapeutic Treatment

Therapy is indicated if vision is threatened by the pterygium growing toward the pupil and if esthetics are subjectively affected. *Complete surgical excision* is the therapy of choice; there are several alternatives: open-wound defect ("bare sclera technique"), primary conjunctival occlusion, rotation flap, keratoplasties, or free transplant. The local control rate is 50% to 70%.[91] In case of recurrence, additional treatments are indicated postoperatively. In those cases, *local cytostatics* (e.g., mitomycin C) are administered, which may lead to severe local complications such as scleral ulceration, secondary glaucoma, corneal edema, corneal perforation, iritis, or cataracts.[93–95]

Radiotherapeutic Options

Radiotherapy in case of recurrence is indicated after local resection of the pterygium; some centers also report success with primary and/or preoperative RT of the pterygium.[96] Besides rare orthovoltage therapy,[97] brachytherapy with beta radiators and eye applicators is usually employed. Normally, radionuclide strontium-90, a fission product of uranium-235 (half-life period 28 years), which decays to yttrium-90 (half-life period 64 days) is used. Strontium-90 radiation has a maximum energy of .546 MeV; for yttrium-90 it reaches 2.27 MeV.[98] The eye applicators have an effective diameter of 8 to 12 mm. The affected lesion is either generously covered by the applicator for a certain time or very large lesions are treated with a circular motion toward the corneal limbus.[99]

Most clinical studies have used postoperative RT for recurrence prophylaxis. Van den Brenk[100] observed only 1.4% recurrences in 1300 treated pterygia (1064 patients); irradiation was carried out once a week (days 0, 7, and 14 postoperatively). Paryani and others[99] achieved a recurrence rate of only 1.7% in 825 eyes with 6 × 10 Gy (1× / week). Wilder and associates[91] report more than 11% recurrences in 244 eyes after 3 × 8 Gy (1×/week). In comparison to placebo irradiation, a Dutch double-blind randomized study with 1 × 25 Gy showed significantly lower recurrence rates.[101]

Radiogenic consequences such as severe scleromalacia and corneal ulcerations occur in up to 4% to 5% of cases after application of higher total doses and after single-dose RT with 1 × 20 to 22 Gy.[102,103]

Choroidal Hemangioma

Definition and Clinical Features

Choroid membrane hemangiomas are slowly growing benign tumors originating from the vessels of the choroid. They can also occur in congenital Sturge-Weber syndrome. The *diffuse* (at ages 5–10) and the *local type* (at ages 30–50) can be distinguished.[104] Symptoms are determined by the size and location of the tumor: if the hemangioma is located close to the papilla or macula, "fuzzy or blurred vision," metamorphopsia, and secondary retinal detachment are observed; in case of direct macular involvement, chronic glaucoma frequently develops. Sometimes there is complete loss of vision. Hemangiomas appear ophthalmoscopically as red-orange swelling and concomitant clinical phenomena (glaucoma, retinal detachment etc.). Further diagnostic procedures are ultrasound, fluorescence angiography, CT, MRI, and scintigraphy (phosphorus-32).[105]

Nonradiotherapeutic Treatment

Indication for therapy depends on the progression of the lesion and the severity of symptoms (in case of visual impairment, retinal detachment, or secondary glaucoma). Small lesions outside the central vision are treated with photodynamic therapy, photocoagulation, or transpapillary thermotherapy[106,107] (e.g., to prevent retinal detachment). Lesions near the macula or papilla are not coagulated because there is a risk for central scotoma; the same holds for incomplete retinal detachment and for the diffuse type (Sturge-Weber syndrome). Overall, ophthalmologists currently favor *photodynamic therapy.*

Radiotherapeutic Options

Irradiation can be done with photons, protons, or brachytherapy. It is indicated in case of no response to photocoagulation and particularly in case of critical proximity to the macula or papilla because invasive measures threaten vision.[108] After successful irradiation, the retina reattaches partially or, perhaps, completely; the lesion becomes flatter, eye and vision are maintained, and visual acuity is often improved. Reductions of visual acuity affect almost exclusively eyes with existing location-dependent maculopathy. The earlier RT starts, the better the long-term results.[109,110] Schilling and associates[111] irradiated 36 localized and 15 diffuse hemangiomas with 10 × 2 Gy; after 5 years, 23 (64%) eyes of the localized type achieved complete retinal reattachment; visual acuity was stable in 50% and improved in 50%; favorable results were also achieved for the diffuse type. In advanced cases, irradiation of the hemangioma cannot conserve visual acuity but it can often maintain the eye as a whole.

RT is conventionally fractionated with 18 to 20 Gy (local type) or 30 Gy (diffuse type) (1.8–2 Gy per fraction). In case of unilateral location, a lateral stationary field that tilts slightly backward is used to protect the other eye and the chiasm. In bilateral disease, opposing lateral fields with lens protection are used.

Brachytherapy is carried out in localized hemangiomas with eye plaques; iodine-125 seeds are preferred. Doses from the apex to the base of the lesion vary between 30 and 240 Gy. Results are excellent in the sense of a permanent resorption of the subretinal edema, complete retinal attachment, and maintenance of vision.[110,113–115]

Potential radiogenic side effects are retinopathy and papillopathy with doses of greater than 30 Gy. In spite of lens-protecting RT techniques, cataracts occasionally develop as well.

Age-related Macular Degeneration

Definition and Clinical Features

Macular degeneration is age-dependent (AMD) and thus appears with increasing frequency from the age of 40 onward. The incidence for 75- to 80-year-olds is 1.2%. Prevalence rises from 20% in 65- to 74-year-olds to 35% in 75- to 84-year-olds. When one eye is affected, the risk for the other eye is 7% to 12% per year. An important risk factor is nicotine abuse, especially for neovascular forms.

The disease frequently results in loss of vision.[116] In terms of progression, it is possible to distinguish *early* and *late forms*—topographically there are *foveal, extrafoveal, and subfoveal forms;* at the final stage, there are *dry* (geographic) and *wet* (neovascular) *forms.*[117] The *classic form* is well demarcated in contrast to the *occult form.* Dry forms with drusen, small atrophies, and slight loss of visual acuity appear most frequently (80%). Approximately 20% develop wet (exudative) forms with effects ranging from visual impairment to blindness; in 90% there is choroidal neovascularization (CNV) with edema (exudation) and bleeding. Without successful therapy, there is the risk for complete loss of vision.

Nonradiotherapeutic Treatment

Due to type, location, and size of CNV, *laser coagulation* is only suitable for a few lesions; in the long run, visual impairment frequently reappears, corresponding to the natural disease progress. The rare "classic" extrafoveal CNV is treated with *photocoagulation*. In subfoveal CNV, irreversible damage and loss of central vision are impending. In this case, *antiangiogenic substances* and transpapillary thermotherapy are employed: *photodynamic therapy* with intravenous verteporfin leads to selective photochemical vessel wall damage[118]; in classic CNV, this treatment can delay or prevent visual loss.[119] Initially, 3 to 4 therapies are required because new leaks often appear due to CNV. Improvement of visual acuity in wet AMD is rare; in contrast, cases of classic (nonoccult) CNV benefit frequently.

Radiotherapeutic Options

In principle, photons, protons, and brachytherapy can be used for irradiation. So far, there are no systematic studies with homogeneous collectives and identical criteria for selection and evaluation. Comparisons with natural cause of disease or control groups (Macular Photocoagulation Study Group) are rather misleading. *Photon therapy* from a linear accelerator is done with mask fixation via lateral stationary fields in semifield technique. The unaffected eye is spared through posterior gantry inclination by 10°[120]; anterior angled fields (1 cm diameter) with lens protection[121] or rotational techniques[122] are also possible.

Results of Radiotherapy

The era of radiotherapy triggered an Irish dose-finding study; after 1 year of RT, visual acuity was stable or improved in 63%; membranes degenerated in 77%. The control group showed loss of vision in all cases except for one, and the membranes increased in all cases; in the long run and on average, visual acuity decreased by less than 1 line after RT and by 3.5 lines in the control group.[123] Retrospectively, total doses of 5 to 36 Gy produced positive effects; studies with negative results were outnumbered. Overall, the therapeutic tolerance for antiangiogenic effects is small, and with increasing total doses, which might cause regression of neovascular membranes, the risk for radiogenic retinopathy increases as well.[122,124–236]

The German RAD study compared placebo irradiation with 8×2 Gy RT; visual acuity was identical.[130] A Swiss study compared 1 Gy (control), 8 Gy, or 16 Gy total dose; after 12 or 18 months, respectively, the corrected visual acuity with 8 or 16 Gy total dose was significantly better than with 1 Gy; patients with classic CNV or initial visual acuity of more than 20/100 had a greater benefit; otherwise, there was no difference in reading ability or size of the CNV between the groups.[120] A German group compared 5×2 and 18×2 Gy with a control group; in classic CNV, the higher dose stabilized visual acuity more frequently than the low dose or control; there was no difference in occult CNV. The study was discontinued because 25% of cases irradiated with 36 Gy developed retinopathy (without consequences to visual acuity).[135] In single-dose RT with 7.5 Gy, there was a significant improvement in visual acuity compared with the control group (78% vs 38%).[125]

Overall, the value of radiotherapy in AMD is not adequately defined. In primarily occult CNV, visual acuity appears to remain stable for a certain length of time. Therefore, clinical radiotherapy should be evaluated.[137]

Endocrine Orbitopathy

Definition and Clinical Features

Endocrine orbitopathy (EO, Grave's disease) is an inflammatory fibrosing disease of the eye socket that is often associated with hyperthyroidism and toxic struma (autoimmune thyropathy; morbus Basedow). On rare occasions, it appears also as Hashimoto's thyroiditis, myxedema without previous thyrotoxicosis, or even without thyroid disease. It is considered an *autoimmune disease* where autoantibodies against thyroid-stimulating hormone (TSH) receptors are formed in the eye musculature, triggering inflammatory and fibrosing tissue reactions in the eye muscles and orbital adipose tissue.[138] During the late stage, there is fibrosis and scarring of the orbital tissue. However, the symptoms are often only moderate and not progressive so that no therapy is required.

Typical *symptoms* are tears, photophobia, feeling of pressure, and pain. Other signs are periorbital edema, proptosis, eye muscle pareses, corneal irritation, and visual nerve impairment to the point of blindness. Diagnosis is obtained clinically with imaging and thyroid diagnostics (antibody determination). Histologic backup through biopsy is only required in exceptional cases.

Nonradiotherapeutic Treatment

Treatment of EO focuses on the *intensity of symptoms*. Spontaneous remission is always possible. Reaching *euthyrosis* in cases of underlying thyroid disease is the most important precondition for any further therapy because it can influence the symptoms in the eye. In cases of mild progression of EO, *local-topical therapy* alone is recommended. In more severe progression, the use of *glucocorticoids* and possibly other medication, such as cyclosporin-A, is indicated. *Operative measures* on the eyelids and eye muscles are usually done in stable primary disease (at least 6 months) and when diplopia has not recurred. On rare occasions, surgery is performed to resect orbital fatty tissue in severe exophthalmos with cosmetic impairment; there may even be short-term or emergency surgery to achieve decompression of the visual nerves—for example, through removal of one or several bony walls of the eye socket.[139]

Radiotherapeutic Options

Ionizing radiation has effects on the cellular reactions mediated by T lymphocytes during the early stage and on fibroblasts during the late stage of EO.

RT of both orbits can be effective in extensive inflammatory EO.[140] Due to the possibility of spontaneous remission and the effectiveness of other measures, it is only indicated in progressive and recidivating cases. Data obtained in a prospective, randomized study at the University of Utrecht speak against the early use of RT; there was no effect on EO for early disease, but good effectiveness for more advanced disease.[141] A prospective, randomized study investigated the effectiveness of orbital RT combined with corticosteroids against corticosteroids alone; in this case, the combination was superior to monotherapy.[142] Another double-blind study compared RT with high-dose corticosteroid therapy and showed that RT alone was more effective.[143]

For bilateral disease, both orbits are irradiated via lateral opposing fields with 6 to 10 MV photons. "Half-beam technique"and fields with 10-degree posterior angled fields are used to minimize the dose to the lens and eye posterior chamber. The size of the effective radiation fields reaches 5×5 cm^2 to 6×7 cm^2. The posterior border of the field covers the ring of Zinn at the superior orbital fissure and thus the entire length of the eye muscles. The posterior part of the lateral counterfields is blocked by lead absorbers; the central beam or the anterior border of the field respectively is located 5 to 6 mm behind the iris/pupil; the posterior border of the field covers the ring of Zinn at the superior orbital fissure.

Dose concepts: The doses used are generally 2.0 Gy per fraction to 2.4–30 Gy total dose; There are no controlled stage-related dose escalation studies so far. Frequently, pretherapeutic corticosteroids are administered during RT. However, the dose reduction of corticosteroids should not take place during RT.

Clinical Results of Radiotherapy

Many patients show "good" to "very good" clinical responses after percutaneous RT. After clinical response to an effective RT dose, recurrences occur only very rarely.

Petersen and associates[144] carried out the largest clinical study so far by collecting long-term results at Stanford of a total of 311 patients from 1968 to 1988. The patients had all been irradiated with 20 or 30 Gy via lateral counterfields. The best responses were observed in the categories "soft tissue" (II), "cornea" (V), and "loss of vision" (VI), but the condition of more than 50% of patients with "proptosis" (III) and "eye muscle involvement" (IV) also improved after RT. In addition, several prognostic factors were established (e.g., age, gender, concurrent thyrostatic therapy, functional status of thyroid). Approximately 30% of patients required surgical correction of the eye muscles or eyelids after RT, which is by no means a negative statement against the effectiveness of RT! Subjectively and objectively, the final success was "good" or "very good" in more than 80% of operated patients.

In individual cases, irradiation may even replace eye surgery or corticosteroids when there is a relevant contraindication.[145]

Side Effects of Radiotherapy

Low-dose RT has almost no side effects. Large clinical studies showed no severe acute or chronic side effects, such as cataract or retinopathy.[144,146]

Reactive Lymphoid Hyperplasia/ Pseudotumor Orbitae

Definition and Clinical Features

Lymphoid diseases of the orbit are rare and have a broad range, including pseudotumor orbitae (PO) and malignant lymphomas.[147] There are three possible causes: (1) an infectious process, for example, in transmitted sinusitis; (2) an autoimmune process; (3) a fibroproliferative process. Experience shows that corticosteroids or immune suppressants can cause remission.

In differential diagnosis, other causes of orbital space requirement such as granulomatous diseases (e.g., sarcoidosis, Wegener's granulomatosis), local infections, or autoimmune diseases have to be excluded. Frequently, the acute onset of symptoms, unilateral disease, and impaired eye motility point to pseudotumor. On imaging, the infiltrates appear in retrobulbar adipose tissue (up to 80%), enlarged eye muscles (up to 60%), thickening of the optic nerve (up to 40%), and proptosis (up to 70%).

Clinical diagnosis and diagnostic imaging can hardly differentiate between benign and malignant changes, and, therefore, biopsy is essential.[148]

Nonradiotherapeutic Treatment

Surgical excision can be used in accessible lesions, but recurrences are frequent.[149] Corticosteroids are the most important component of medical therapy, but up to 50% do not respond adequately.[150] Some patients have to discontinue medication because of side effects. According to Lambo and coworkers,[148] adequate radiotherapy achieves complete remission in 70% to 100% of cases; without therapy, visual acuity can deteriorate seriously and permanently; there is no correlation between duration of progression and irreversible loss of visual acuity. The potential for malignant transformation of orbital pseudotumors is unclear.

Radiotherapeutic Options

Radiotherapy has response rates of 70% to 100%.[147,151–153] Recommended doses vary between 0.5 and 3.0 Gy per fraction and 20 and 35 Gy total dose. Careful treatment planning helps to keep radiation side effects low.

Initially, a treatment attempt with a low dose of 2 × 0.5 Gy per week up to 5 Gy total dose (first series) can be used. In acute or chronic inflammation, gradual dose increase can initiate an early response on the one hand[154]; in case of nonresponse after 4 weeks, irradiation is changed to daily fractionation with 1.5 to 2 Gy single dose and up to 30 to 40 Gy total dose (second series). In the United States, most patients are treated with initial doses of approximately 30 Gy at standard fractionation.

Irradiation Technique

After CT planning, patients are treated via anterior and lateral fields with 1:3 weighting and wedged filters for dose homogenization while the patient's eyes are open. In bilateral disease, parallel opposing lateral fields with half-block technique[149] or two anterior electron fields are used.

Radiogenic Side Effects

Hardly any severe complications are observed. With higher doses, there may be dry-eye syndrome and cataract formation.

NONMALIGNANT DISEASES OF JOINTS AND TENDONS

General Aspects

Dose Concepts

It has been known since the beginning of the 20th century that low doses of ionizing radiation have an analgesic and anti-inflammatory effect.[155]

Nonradiotherapeutic Treatment

Numerous conservative measures, such as oral, local, or systemic application of medication, are the mainstay of management. Radiation therapy is rarely used in the United States for primary management of these diseases, but its use is more common in other countries.

In Germany, guidelines and dose concepts for radiotherapy of nonmalignant diseases were developed during the past 10 years where dose per fraction of 0.5 Gy to total doses of 6 Gy can be used. Conditions that have been treated include bursitis, tendonitis, subacromial syndrome (rotator cuff syndrome), tennis elbow (epicondylopathia humeri), calcaneodynia (heel spur), and degenerative joints with cartilaginous destruction (osteoarthritis).

NONMALIGNANT DISEASES OF CONNECTIVE TISSUE AND SKIN

Desmoid (Aggressive Fibromatosis)

Definition and Clinical Features

A desmoid is a benign growth of connective tissue originating in the deep muscular-aponeurotic structures in the region of muscle fascias, aponeuroses, tendons, and scar tissue. The incidence of new cases is two to four per 1 million inhabitants per year. Women are usually affected twice as frequently as men are (1:1.5–2.5). Desmoids occur most frequently during the third and fourth decades of life, but children can be affected as well.

Desmoids are differentiated into extra-abdominal (≈70%) and intra-abdominal (≈10%) desmoids and those located in the abdominal wall (≈20%). Extra-abdominal forms tend to recur, intra-abdominal forms are associated with the autosomal dominantly inherited Gardner syndrome. Histologically, desmoids are similar to highly differentiated (G1) fibrosarcomas. Mitotic activity is low, and cellular atypias are rare. Locally infiltrating growth has earned the name of "aggressive fibromatosis" for this disease. Local recurrences after resection alone are quite common.[156–158] Pretherapeutic diagnostics are made with magnetic resonance tomography to estimate the size and infiltration into other organs as well as incision biopsy to distinguish benign from malignant lesions.

Nonradiotherapeutic Treatment

Desmoids can regress spontaneously or they can grow to huge size, but they rarely cause death.[159] Surgery with a safety margin of 2 to 5 cm is considered the "gold standard." After R0 resection, no therapy is usually required; however, in the case of initial R1 resection, one can wait to see if recurrences appear. Good long-term control can be achieved by resection alone, but up to 50% local recurrences require surgical and other measures subsequently.[160] Tamoxifen and progesterone can exert growth inhibitory effects.[161] Nonsteroidal antirheumatics, vitamin C,[162,163] and alkylating substances (vincristine, methotrexate) have been tested.

Radiotherapeutic Options

Radiotherapy is indicated in cases of local inoperability, after R2 resection and in R1 resection if repeated surgery has already been performed for recurrence.[158,164,165] Radiotherapy is often used adjuvantly or primarily as the only measure. Adjuvant radiotherapy significantly reduces recurrence rates compared to surgery alone: with total doses of greater than 50 Gy, recurrence rate decreases from 60% to 80% to 10% to 30%. With normal fractionation and single doses of 1.8 to 2.0 Gy, a total dose of 50 to 55 Gy is recommended postoperatively; for inoperable or recurring desmoids, the recommended total dose is 60 to 65 Gy. After primary radiotherapy, the local control rate does not differ a lot from that after adjuvant irradiation.[158,165–176]

Results of Radiotherapy

In most studies, tumor size has no prognostic influence on local control.[170] According to a meta-analysis (698 cases in 13 studies),[164] the local control rate after R0 resection and radiotherapy was improved by 17% compared with surgery alone; for macroscopic (R2) and microscopic tumor rests (R1), patients treated with adjuvant radiotherapy had even better results.

In 2001 to 2002, the patterns of care study on the use of radiotherapy for treatment of desmoids was carried out in Germany; 345 patients were subjected to evaluation.[177] The desmoids were distributed in the extremities (81.2%; $n = 280$), the trunk (13.9%; $n = 48$), and the head and neck region (4.9%; $n = 17$). A total of 204 patients (59%) were irradiated primarily for recrudescing or nonresectable desmoids, 141 (40.8%) postoperatively in high-risk situations (marginal or unclear resection), unclear R-state ($n = 44$), R1 resection ($n = 49$), or R2 resection ($n = 28$). Most patients were intensively pretreated, on average with 2 (1–5) operations.

The median time of observation after therapy was 43 (4–306) months. A total of 67 recurrences (19%) occurred after RT. The long-term local control rate was 81.4% after primary radiotherapy of nonresectable desmoids and 79.6% after postoperative irradiation of resected desmoids. A precise topographic analysis of recurrences was possible in 124 patients or 22 recurrences (18%); 12 (54%) of the recurrences were located within and 10 (46%) outside the target volume or at the edge of the field.

Peyronie's Disease

Definition and Clinical Features

Peyronie's disease is a chronic and mostly progressive inflammation and connective tissue excrescence of the tunica albuginea in the cavernous bodies of the penis. It usually affects men at the age of 40 to 60 years. Its cause is unknown. Strands of scar lead to the typical bending of the penis, which may cause severe pain during erection. Spontaneous remission is described only very rarely.

Nonradiotherapeutic Treatment

There is no simple and successful standard treatment. Vitamin E, para-aminobenzoate, and steroids are said to have a favorable influence during the early phase. There are also local therapeutic attempts with ultrasound or shock waves as well as with corticoid, procaine, and hyaluronic acid injections. Resection and plastic surgery, for example, after Nesbit,[178] is associated with complications and is only carried out in advanced stages. After radical resection, inflatable implants are used to maintain erection ability. Ionizing radiation can delay further induration and lead to softening of lumps and strands, thus causing pain, bending, and functional problems of the penis.

Radiotherapeutic Options

Radiotherapy can be used during the early stages but in the later stages, there are hardly any radiosensitive fibroblasts and inflammatory cells left. Therapy is carried out with gonadal protection (lead apron or capsule), and the glans penis is spared. The nonerect penis is pulled forward manually by the patient and is irradiated via a dorsal stationary field with orthovoltage or electrons up to 6 MeV with 5 to 10 mm bolus.

Conventional fractionation is 20 Gy in 2 Gy fractions, but it is possible to use hypofractionation with 2 to 4 Gy single dose two to three times per week up to a total dose of 12 to 15 Gy.

Results of Radiotherapy

Within 12 to 24 months, radiotherapy leads to an improvement of symptoms in two thirds of all early-stage patients. Local pain and associated clinical symptoms decrease in up to 75%. Angulation (25%-30%) and dysfunction of the penis (30%-50%) show less response because these symptoms often indicate that the disease is already in a more advanced stage.[179–190]

Dupuytren's Contracture (Morbus Dupuytren) and Morbus Lederhose

Morbus Dupuytren (MD) (Dupuytren's contracture) and morbus Lederhose (ML) are two spontaneous connective tissue diseases in which the palmar or plantar aponeurosis is affected. Two thirds of patients show bilateral involvement. The disease is more common in the hands (MD) than in the feet (ML). It mostly appears from the age of 40 years onwards. Depending on geographic region and racial factors, its prevalence is up to 1% to 3%. Subcutaneous lumps with skin fixation appear; later, there are strands that may reach as far as the periosteum. With increasing connective tissue hardening, flexion contractures develop in the metacarpophalangeal or proximal interphalangeal joints, and grabbing (MD) or walking (ML) is impaired. Mostly, the 4th/5th phalanges of the hand (MD) or the 1st/2nd toes of the foot (ML) are affected. The extent of the extension deficit determines clinical staging in MD.

Nonradiotherapeutic Treatment

Spontaneous regression is initially possible. Without any further therapy, more than 50% of people affected show disease progression after 5 years. Surgery is indicated if there is functional impairment. Prophylactic use of radiotherapy during the early stages is feasible.

Radiotherapeutic Options

Radiotherapy can be considered during the early stages of disease. The target cells are the strongly proliferating radiosensitive fibroblasts and inflammatory cells. The aim of therapy is to avoid further progression.

Normal fractionation is 2 Gy per fraction to 20 Gy total dose or 3 to 4 Gy per fraction to a total dose of 12 to 15 Gy.

Results of Radiotherapy

Many studies showed a very good response to radiotherapy in the form of stabilized disease (70%–80%). However, only a small number of early-stage patients experience degeneration of lumps and strands (20%–30%). Only a few studies have controlled long-term observation for more than 2 years.[191,192]

Keloids and Hypertrophic Scars

Definition and Clinical Features

Keloids are excessive tissue excrescences in the region of scars, and they may occur in case of skin injury from surgery, burns, chemical burns, inflammation (e.g., acne), or even spontaneously. They differ from hypertrophic scars due to their infiltrating character, causing local pain and inflammation reactions or even triggering long-term progression; hypertrophic scars only show thickening without surrounding reaction, and they can flatten spontaneously.

Keloids appear mostly in the upper body and in regions with high skin tension—for example, above the sternum, at the earlobes, and in the joint regions. The cause of disease is still unknown, but there is a genetic and race-specific predisposition.

Nonradiotherapeutic Treatment

Besides surgical excision of hyperplastic tissue with cosmetic disfigurement and functional disruptions, it is possible to use a conservative procedure with pressure and silicon bandages, steroids, plant extracts, or steroid injections for smaller lesions. In more than 50% of cases, there is local recurrence after excision of keloids alone.

Radiotherapeutic Options

Indications for irradiation are either demonstrated recurrences postoperatively or a high recurrence risk (e.g., marginal resection borders, wider spread, unfavorable location). Fibroblasts, mesenchymal cells, and inflammatory cells are the target cells. Prophylactic irradiation immediately after excision of the recurrence is most effective. Recurrence rate after postoperative irradiation is 20% to 25%.

Irradiation is initiated 24 hours after surgery at the latest. Conventional radiography (70–150 kV), electrons (<6 MeV), and brachytherapy with iridium-192 implants[193,194] or with strontium-90 dermaplate[195] are used. The target volume is limited to the scar plus 1-cm safety margin. The recommended dose is 12 to 20 Gy, typically with 3 Gy fractions.[196] Single-dose irradiation with 7.5 to 10 Gy is effective.[197,198]

Other Diseases of Connective Tissue and Skin/Cutaneous Appendages

Acute and chronic inflammatory changes of the skin (furuncle, carbuncle), the nailbed (panaritium, paronychia) and at the sweat glands of the armpit and groin (hidradenitis suppurativa) can lead to chronic and therapy-refractive inflammations that are painful and that can seriously impair those affected by disease. If all local measures are exhausted, if there is a confirmed antibiotic resistance, and if further surgical measures are rejected in those cases, "inflammation irradiation" can be used with single doses of 0.5 to 1.0 Gy daily up to 10 Gy.

Gynecomastia: Recently, there has been an increased interest in the use of radiotherapy of the male mammary gland for gynecomastia prophylaxis or therapeutic irradiation in painful gynecomastia for patients undergoing hormone therapy in prostate carcinoma. Bilateral radiotherapy of the mammillary region is done with 8 to 12 MeV electrons. Usually, 4 to 5 × 3 Gy up to a total dose of 12 to 15 Gy are used. This treatment can prevent pain or growth of the mammary gland in 70% of male patients.[199] Radiotherapy cannot reverse gynecomastia.

Plantar warts can be painful and functionally as well as cosmetically very disturbing. In older studies, control rates of more than 80% were achieved with conventional orthovolt technique (1 × 10 Gy or 5 × 3 Gy). The warts fell off without consequences after several weeks.[200]

NONMALIGNANT DISORDERS OF BONY TISSUES

Aneurysmal Bone Cysts

Definition and Clinical Features

Aneurysmal bone cysts are benign, vascular cystic lesions in the metaphase of bones, which can cause functional impairment, pathologic fractures, and damage of neighboring structures. They can infiltrate the surrounding soft tissue. In spite of their nonmalignant character, cysts can lead to bone destruction and thus lead to serious problems, which is why treatment is recommended once a cyst has been diagnosed, particularly if the vertebral column is affected.[201]

Nonradiotherapeutic Measures

Therapy is primarily surgical (resection or curettage) as long as this does not lead to a considerable functional impairment. Following curettage, recurrence occurs in up to 60% of patients.[202] After complete resection, there is normally no recurrence.[201]

Radiotherapeutic Possibilities

Radiotherapy can be used in patients with cysts that cannot be treated by surgery or if curettage is difficult due to the size or location of cysts. Cyst progression or repeated recurrences are also indications for radiotherapy. Because more than 50% of patients are 10 to 19 years old, radiation doses should be kept as low as possible. Nobler and associates[203] report one recurrence in a total of 11 patients who were irradiated with doses from 12 to 31.6 Gy. A dosage of 10 to 20 Gy for 1 to 2 weeks seems to be adequate to control aneurysmal bone cysts reliably.

Pigmented Villonodular Synovitis

Definition and Clinical Features

Pigmented villonodular synovitis is a rare proliferative disease affecting the synovia of joints and the tendon sheaths.[204] There are two types of disease: the strictly localized and the diffuse involvement of synovial membranes.[205] In the majority of cases, the lesion is restricted to one joint and can spread to muscles, tendons, and skin.

Nonradiotherapeutic Measures

Surgical excision normally consists of synovectomy, which is rarely complete, particularly in the large joints like the knee.[206] Therefore, recurrences occur with a frequency of up to 45%.[207]

Radiotherapeutic Possibilities

O´Sullivan and coworkers[205] report on 14 patients who were irradiated with 30-50 Gy in 15 to 35 fractions. The patients had different risk factors: microscopic residual (7), macroscopic tumor (7), tumor >10 cm (5), tumor 5 to 10 cm (7), recurrences (8), skin infiltration with ulceration (2). During an average observation period of 69 months (13–250 months), one patient had a persisting finding 8 months after radiotherapy with 30 Gy in 15 fractions. All but two patients had tumor control. On the basis of this experience from the Princess Margaret Hospital, irradiation with a total dose of 40 Gy in 20 fractions can be recommended.

Vertebral Hemangiomas

Definition and Clinical Features

Vertebral hemangiomas are benign lesions that can lead to a resorption of the affected bone.[208–210] Normally, only one vertebral body is affected. Hemangiomas are usually diagnosed by their radiologic picture of rarefaction with vertical, dense trabeculas of a honeycomb pattern. Most lesions require no therapy. In most cases, symptoms occur during the fourth or fifth decade of life.[211–215] Women are affected more frequently than men.[216] Spread of the tumor into the extradural space, hemorrhage, or rare compression fractures can lead to bone-marrow compression.

Nonradiotherapeutic Measures

Surgical relief can become necessary, but it is difficult owing to the danger of hemorrhage.[212,217–220] In most cases, only partial resection is possible, and postoperative irradiation can be considered.[208,209]

Radiotherapeutic Possibilities

Rades and associates[221] analyzed data from 339 patients with symptomatic vertebral hemangiomas from publications of the past 50 years. Two-hundred-twenty-two patients had to be excluded, either because surgery was part of the treatment (n = 98) or because the data were incomplete (n = 124). Of the remaining 117 patients, 54 patients received 36 to 44 Gy (group A), and 62 patients 20 to 34 Gy (group B). After a median observation period of 36 months (6–312 months), 39% of group A and 82% of group B patients had complete pain relief. They recommend a total dose of 40 Gy.

Heterotopic Ossifications

Definition and Clinical Features

Heterotopic ossifications (HO) appear following trauma or surgery (total hip replacement) of the hip in 10% to 80% of cases and with varying degrees of severity. HO consist of real bone and are located in the periarticular soft tissue.[222] Ten percent develop extensive HO, causing pain and functional impairment. Patients with HO frequently complain of pain only a few days after surgery. Radiologically, calcified structures with blurred contours are detected 3 to 6 weeks postoperatively.

Etiology of HO is only partially known. It is assumed that the pluripotent mesenchymal cells, which are present ubiquitously in periarticular soft tissue, develop into osteoblastic stem cells under certain conditions.[223]

For all patients with an indication for a hip replacement, there should be an individual estimation of the risk of HO before carrying out surgery. Patients who already have ipsilateral or contralateral HO carry the greatest risk. After second surgery, 90% to 100% of those patients redevelop HO.[224–227] Patients with moderate or severe osteophytes at the femoral head and socket also have a high risk for HO, with an incidence of more than 50%.[224,228,229] After acetabular fractures, HO appear in 90% of hips. Fifty percent of those patients develop HO with clinical pathology.[230,231] Ankylosing spondylitis and the (rare) idiopathic hyperostosis of the skeleton are other influencing factors.

Diagnosis and Classification

Extensive ossifications lead to mobility impairment of the hip joint and cause pain. If HO is suspected, radiographs of the hip should be taken. Discrete changes in the radiograph can be seen at 2 weeks after surgery at the earliest. The literature provides a multitude of staging approaches. The most frequent one is the classification of HO according to Brooker and colleagues[222] (Fig. 63-1). To keep it simple, HO grades III and IV, according to Brooker and colleagues, are designated as severe or clinically relevant, although there may not be any pain or mobility impairment.

Nonradiotherapeutic Treatment

SURGERY

Clinically relevant (i.e., usually ankylosing) HO that have appeared after surgery should be removed to mobilize the joint and to remove pain. Complete removal of HO is not essential if this is difficult and burdened with a higher risk. Most authors consider it necessary to wait for maturation of the forming ectopic bone and to reoperate only after 6 months to 1.5 years.

MEDICINAL THERAPY

Although ethane hydroxydiphosphates (EHDPs) have been used as prophylaxis, the treatment results are not convincing.[232–234]

In contrast, some studies show that indomethacin, a prostaglandin synthesis inhibitor, is also effective in patients with high risk.[235–240]

Like indomethacin, ibuprofen inhibits prostaglandin synthesis. After treatment with indomethacin and ibuprofen, the

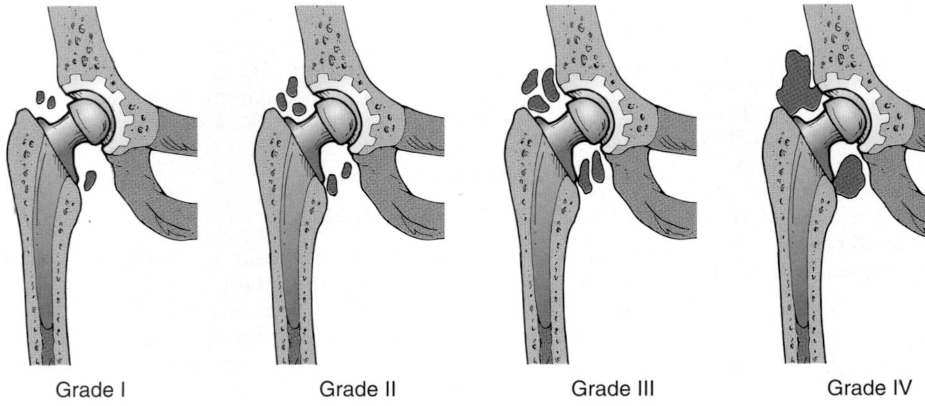

Figure 63-1 Staging of heterotrophic ossifications. **Grade I**. Bone islands within soft tissue around hip. **Grade II.** Exophytes of pelvis or proximal femur end with a minimum distance of 1 cm. **Grade III.** Exophytes of pelvis or proximal femur end with a distance of <1 cm. **Grade IV.** Bony ankylosis between proximal femur and pelvis.

(From Brooker AF, Bowerman JW, Robinson RA, Riley LH: Ectopic ossification following total hip replacement. J Bone Joint Surg 55:A1629–1632, 1973.)

incidence of HO was significantly lower than in the placebo group[228,241]; this was not the case after EHDP treatment.[232,242]

Radiotherapeutic Options

Radiotherapy for prophylaxis of HO has been employed since the late 1970s and has proved to be effective.[243] The initial dose was 20 Gy in 10 fractions.[243–248] Multiple dose schedules have been used.

In three randomized studies, 10 Gy were compared with 20 Gy,[246] or with 17.5 Gy in 5 fractions,[249] and 8 Gy in 1 fraction with 10 Gy.[250] There was no significant difference between the effectiveness of high and low doses. Severe ossifications occurred in 7% of patients with low and 5% of patients with high irradiation doses. No difference could be observed between fractionated and single-dose irradiation.

Various authors pointed out that radiotherapy should be started no later than day 4 after surgery.[223,226,243,246–249,251]

Preoperative radiation treatment with 7 to 8 Gy in one fraction was used successfully in high-risk patients.[253] There was no significant difference in clinically relevant HO compared to patients who were irradiated postoperatively.

Irradiation is tolerated well. Neither fractionated irradiation nor high single doses leads to an increased frequency of wound-healing disturbances. So far, none of the patients developed a malignant tumor within the irradiation field. Because radiation-induced tumors appear very rarely and only after latencies of 10 to 30 years, this risk is irrelevant for most patients because the median age of patients is 65.

Radiotherapeutic Procedure

The irradiation field contains the typical localizations of periarticular ossifications, where the cranial field border is located approximately 3 cm above the acetabulum, and the irradiation field includes about two thirds of the implant shaft. Normally, the field size is 14 × 14 cm.

The effect of radiotherapy on the ingrowth of bone and fixation of noncemented implants was investigated in rabbits[254] and dogs.[253] After irradiation with 10 Gy (in 5 or 4 fractions), the fixation was significantly decreased within 2 to 6 weeks.[254,255] Sumner and associates[256] were also able to show that irradiation initially decreases the grade of fixation during the early postoperative phase, but, after 4 weeks, the implants in irradiated and nonirradiated bone had the same strength.

In clinical application, the protection of hip prosthesis with absorbers as recommended by Jasty and coworkers[257] and the use of smaller blocks restricted to acetabular and femoral parts of the prosthesis can lead to ossifications underneath the block. Inadequate irradiation fields led to HO in 13 of 18 hips (76%) after irradiation with 7 Gy.[258] An open irradiation field covers the entire periarticular risk region more completely.

Nonfixation of cementless implants was not observed after 6 Gy in one fraction,[259] after 7 Gy in one fraction,[252] or 17.5 Gy in 5 fractions.[249,251,260] Due to those animal experimental and clinical studies, there appears to be no objection to irradiating hips with noncemented TEP without absorber.

REFERENCES

1. Von Pannewitz G: Degenerative Erkrankungen. *In* Zuppinger A, Ruckensteiner E (Hrsg): Handbuch der medizinischen Radiologie. Berlin-Heidelberg-New York, Springer, 1970, pp 96-98.
2. Sokoloff N: Röntgenstrahlen gegen Gelenkrheumatismus. Fortschr Röntgenstr 1:209-213, 1898.
3. Leer JWH, van Houtte P, Davelaar J: Indications and treatment schedules for irradiation of benign diseases: a survey. Radiother Oncol 48:249-257, 1998.
4. Order EO, Donaldson SS (eds): Radiation Therapy of Benign Diseases, 2nd ed. Berlin, Heidelberg, New York, Springer, 1998.
5. Seegenschmiedt MH, Katalinic A, Makoski H, et al: Radiation therapy for benign diseases: patterns of care study in Germany. Int J Radiat Oncol Biol Phys 47:195-202, 2000.
6. Seegenschmiedt MH, Micke O, Willich N: Radiation therapy for nonmalignant diseases in Germany—current concepts and future perspectives. Strahlenther Onkol 180:718-730, 2004.
7. Jansen JTM, Broerse J, Zoetelief J, et al: Assessment of carcinogenic risk in the treatment of benign disease of knee and shoulder joint. *In* Seegenschmiedt MH, Makoski H-B: Kolloquium Radioonkologie/Strahlentherapie, Radiotherapie bei gutartigen Erkrankungen, vol 15. Altenberge, Diplodocus-Verlag, 2001, pp 13-15.
8. Rodemann HP, Bamberg M: Cellular basis of radiation-induced fibrosis. Radiother Oncol 35:83-90, 1995.
9. Von Wangenheim KH, Petersen HP, Schwenke K: A major component of radiation action: interference with intracellular control of differentiation. Int J Radiat Biol 68:369-388, 1995.
10. Behrends U, Peter RU, Hintermeier-Knabe R, et al: Ionizing radiation induces human intercellular adhesion molecule 1 in vitro. J Invest Dermatol 103:726-730, 1994.
11. Deleted in print.
12. Hopewell JW, Robbins MEC, Van den Aardweg GJMJ, et al: The modulation of radiation-induced damage to pig skin by essential fat acids. Br J Cancer 58:1-7, 1993.
13. Sanford RA, Muhlbauer MS: Craniopharyngioma in children. Neurol Clin 9:453-465, 1991.
14. Sanford RA: Craniopharyngioma: results of survey of the American Society of Pediatric Neurosurgery. Pediatr Neurosurg 21(Suppl 1):39-43, 1994.
15. DeVile CJ, Grant DB, Hayward RD, et al: Growth and endocrine sequelae of craniopharyngioma. Arch Dis Child 75:108-114, 1996.

16. Hoffmann HJ, DeSilva M, Humphreys RP, et al: Aggressive surgical management of cranio-pharyngiomas in children. J Neurosurg 76:47-52, 1992.
17. Tomita T, McLone D: Radical resection of childhood craniopharyngiomas. Pediatr Neurosurg 19:6-14, 1993.
18. Sung DI, Chang CH, Harisiadis L, et al: Treatment results of craniopharyngiomas. Cancer 47:847-852, 1981.
19. Rajan B, Ashley S, Gorman C, et al: Craniopharyngioma: long-term results following limited surgery and radiotherapy. Radiother Oncol 26:1-10, 1993.
20. Bloom HJ, Glees J, Bell J: The treatment and long-term prognosis of children with intracranial tumors: a study of 610 cases, 1950-1981. Int J Radiat Oncol Biol Phys 18:723-745, 1990.
21. Becker G, Kortmann RD, Skaley M, et al: The role of radiotherapy in the treatment of craniopharyngioma: indications, results, side effects. Front Radiat Ther Oncol 33:100-113, 1999.
22. Habrand JL, Ganry O, Couanet D, et al: The role of radiation therapy in the management of craniopharyngioma: a 25-year experience and review of the literature. Int J Radiat Oncol Biol Phys 44:255-263, 1999.
23. Schulz-Ertner D, Frank C, Herfarth KK, et al: Fractionated stereotactic radiotherapy for craniopharyngiomas. Int J Radiat Oncol Biol Phys 54:1114-1120, 2002.
24. Tos M, Thomsen J: Proposal of classification of tumor size in acoustic neuroma surgery. *In* Tos M, Thomsen J (eds): Proceedings of the First International Conference on Acoustic Neuroma. Amsterdam, Kugler, 1992.
25. Samii M, Matthies C: Management of 1000 vestibular schwannomas (acoustic neuromas): surgical management and results with an emphasis on complications and how to avoid them. Neurosurgery 40:11-21, 1997.
26. Samii M, Matthies C: Management of 1000 vestibular schwannomas (acoustic neuromas): hearing function in 1000 tumor resections. Neurosurgery 40:248-260, 1997.
27. Samii M, Matthies C: Management of 1000 vestibular schwannomas (acoustic neuromas): the facial nerve preservation and restitution of function. Neurosurgery 40:684-694, 1997.
28. Linskey ME, Martinez AJ, Kondziolka D, et al: The radiobiology of human acoustic schwannoma xenografts after stereotactic radiosurgery evaluated in the subrenal capsule of athymic mice. J Neurosurg 78:645-653, 1993.
29. Seo Y, Fukuoka S, Nakagawara J, et al: Effect of gamma knife radiosurgery on acoustic neurinomas. Stereotact Funct Neurosurg 66(Suppl 1):93-102, 1996.
30. Flickinger JC, Kondziolka D, Lunsford L: Dose and diameter relationships for facial, trigeminal, and acoustic neuropathies following acoustic neuroma radiosurgery. Radiother Oncol 41:215-219, 1996.
31. Flickinger JC, Kondziolka D, Niranjan A, Lunsford LD: Results of acoustic neuroma radiosurgery: an analysis of 5 years' experience using current methods. J Neurosurg 94:1-6, 2001.
32. Foote KD, Friedman WA, Buatti JM, et al: Analysis of risk factors associated with radiosurgery for vestibular schwannoma. J Neurosurg 95:440-449, 2001.
33. Iwai Y, Yamanaka K, Shiotani M, Uyama T: Radiosurgery for acoustic neuromas: results of low-dose treatment. Neurosurgery 53:282-287, 2003.
34. Meijer OW, Vandertop WP, Baayen JC, Slotman BJ: Single-fraction vs. fractionated linac-based stereotactic radiosurgery for vestibular schwannoma: a single-institution study. Int J Radiat Oncol Biol Phys 56:1390-1396, 2003.
35. Niranjan A, Lunsford LD, Flickinger JC, et al: Dose reduction improves hearing preservation rates after intracanalicular acoustic tumor radiosurgery. Neurosurgery 45:753-762, 1999.
36. Petit JH, Hudes RS, Chen TT, et al: Reduced-dose radiosurgery for vestibular schwannomas. Neurosurgery 49:1299-1306, 2001.
37. Rowe JG, Radatz MW, Walton L, et al: Gamma knife stereotactic radiosurgery for unilateral acoustic tumors. J Neurol Neurosurg Psychiatry 74:1536-1542, 2003.
38. Andrews DW, Suarez O, Goldmann HW, et al: Stereotactic radiosurgery and fractionated stereotactic radiotherapy for the treatment of acoustic schwannomas: comparative observations of 125 patients treated at one institution. Int J Radiat Oncol Biol Phys 50:1265-1278, 2001.
39. Fuss M, Debus J, Lohr F, et al: Conventionally fractionated stereotactic radiotherapy (FSRT) for acoustic neuromas. Int J Radiat Oncol Biol Phys 48:1381-1387, 2000.
40. Sakamoto T, Shirato H, Takeichi N, et al: Annual rate of hearing loss falls after fractionated stereotactic irradiation for vestibular schwannoma. Radiother Oncol 60:45-48, 2001.
41. Sawamura Y, Shirato H, Sakamoto T, et al: Management of vestibular schwannoma by fractionated stereotactic radiotherapy and associated cerebrospinal fluid malabsorption. J Neurosurg 99:685-692, 2003.
42. Shirato H, Sakamoto T, Takeichi N, et al: Fractionated stereotactic radiotherapy for vestibular schwannoma (VS): a comparison between cystic-type and solid-type VS. Int J Radiat Oncol Biol Phys 48:1395-1401, 2000.
43. Williams JA: Fractionated stereotactic radiotherapy for acoustic neuromas. Int J Radiat Oncol Biol Phys 54:500-504, 2002.
44. Karpinos M, Teh BS, Zeck O, et al: Treatment of acoustic neuroma: stereotactic radiosurgery vs. microsurgery. Int J Radiat Oncol Biol Phys 54:1410-1421, 2002.
45. Regis J, Pellet W, Delsanti C, et al: Functional outcome after gamma knife surgery or micro-surgery for vestibular schwannomas. J Neurosurg 97:1091-1100, 2002.
46. Graf CJ, Perret GE, Torner JC: Bleeding from cerebral arteriovenous malformations as part of their natural history. J Neurosurg 58:331-337, 1983.
47. Stefani MA, Porter PJ, terBrugge KG, et al: Large and deep brain arteriovenous malformations are associated with risk of future hemorrhage. Stroke 33:1220-1224, 2002.
48. Engenhart R, Wowra B, Debus J, et al: The role of high-dose, single-fraction irradiation in small and large intracranial AVMs. Int J Radiat Oncol Biol Phys 30:521-529, 1994.
49. Steiner L, Lindquist C, Adler JR, et al: Clinical outcome of radiosurgery for cerebral arteriovenous malformations. J Neurosurg 77:1-8, 1992.
50. Lindquist C, Steiner L, Blomgren H, et al: Stereotactic radiation therapy of intracranial arteriovenous malformations. Acta Radiol 368(Suppl):610-613, 1986.
51. Laing RW, Childs J, Brada M: Failure of conventionally fractionated radiotherapy to decrease the risk of hemorrhage in inoperable AVMs. Neurosurgery 30:872-875, 1992.
52. Poulsen MG: Arteriovenous malformation—a summary of 6 cases treated with radiation therapy. Int J Radiat Oncol Biol Phys 13:1553-1557, 1987.
53. Wilms M, Kocher M, Makoski H-B, et al: Langzeitergebnisse der semistereotaktischen konventionell fraktionierten Strahlenbehandlung arterio-venöser Malformationen des Gehirns. Strahlenther Onkol 179(Suppl):69, 2003.
54. Fajardo LF: Morphology of radiation effects on normal tissue. *In* Perez CA, Brady LW (eds): Principles and Practice of Radiation Oncology, 2nd ed. Philadelphia, Lippincott, 1992, pp 114-123.
55. van der Kogel AJ: Central nervous system radiation injury in small animal models. *In* Gutin PH, Leibel SA, Sheline GE (eds): Radiation Injury to the Nervous System. Raven Press Ltd., New York, 1991.
56. Nakata H, Yoshimine T, Murasawa A, et al: Early blood-brain barrier disruption after high-dose single-fraction irradiation in rats. Acta Neurochir (Wien) 136:82-86, 1995.
57. Kocher M, Voges J, Mueller R-P, et al: Linac radiosurgery for patients with a limited number of brain metastases. J Radiosurg 1:9-15, 1998.
58. Flickinger JC, Schell MC, Larson DA: Estimation of complications for linear accelerator radio-surgery with the integrated logistic formula. Int J Radiat Oncol Biol Phys 19:143-148, 1990.
59. Flickinger JC, Kondziolka D, Maitz AH, et al: Analysis of neurological sequelae from radio-surgery of AVMs: how location affects outcome. Int J Radiat Oncol Biol Phys 40:273-278, 1998.
60. Flickinger JC, Kondziolka D, Maitz AH, et al: An analysis of the dose-response for arteriovenous malformation radiosurgery and other factors affecting obliteration. Radiother Oncol 63:347-354, 2002.
61. Voges J, Treuer H, Sturm V, et al: Risk analysis of linear accelerator radiosurgery. Int J Radiat Oncol Biol Phys 36:1055-1063, 1996.

62. Voges J, Treuer H, Lehrke R, et al. Risk analysis of LINAC radiosurgery in patients with arteriovenous malformation (AVM). Acta Neurochir (Wien) 68(Suppl):118-123, 1997.
63. Colombo F, Pozza F, Chierego G, et al: Linear accelerator radiosurgery of cerebral arteriovenous malformations: an update. Neurosurgery 34:14-21, 1994.
64. Deruty R, Pelissou-Guyotat I, Amat D, et al: Complications after multidisciplinary treatment of cerebral arteriovenous malformations. Acta Neurochir (Wien) 138:119-131, 1996.
65. Deruty R, Pelissou-Guyotat I, Morel C, et al: Reflections on the management of cerebral arteriovenous malformations. Surg Neurol 50:245-255, 1998.
66. Fleetwood IG, Marcellus ML, Levy RP, et al: Deep arteriovenous malformations of the basal ganglia and thalamus: natural history. J Neurosurg 98:747-750, 2003.
67. Flickinger JC, Pollock BE, Kondziolka D, et al: A dose-response analysis of arteriovenous malformation obliteration after radiosurgery. Int J Radiat Oncol Biol Phys 36:873-879, 1996.
68. Miyawaki L, Dowd C, Wara W, et al: Five year results of linac radiosurgery for arteriovenous malformations: outcome for large avms. Int J Radiat Oncol Biol Phys 44:1089-1106, 1999.
69. Wolbers JG, Mol HC, Kralendonk JH, et al: Stereotactic radiosurgery with adjusted linear accelerator for cerebral arteriovenous malformations: preliminary results in the Netherlands. Ned Tijdschr Geneeskd 143:1215-1221, 1999.
70. Chang JH, Chang JW, Park YG, Chung S: Factors related to complete occlusion of arteriovenous malformations after gamma knife radiosurgery. J Neurosurg 93(Suppl 3):96-101, 2000.
71. Schlienger M, Atlan D, et al: Linac radiosurgery for cerebral arteriovenous malformations: results in 169 patients. Int J Radiat Oncol Biol Phys 46:1135-1142, 2000.
72. Pollock BE, Kline RW, Stafford SL: The rationale and technique of staged-volume arteriovenous malformation radiosurgery. Int J Radiat Oncol Biol Phys 48:817-824, 2000.
73. *Ibid.*
74. Friedman WA, Bova FJ, Bollampally S, et al: Analysis of factors predictive of success or complications in arteriovenous malformation radiosurgery. Neurosurgery 52:296-308, 2003.
75. Rich TA, Schiller A, Suit HD, et al: Clinical and pathologic review of 48 cases of chordoma. Cancer 56:182-187, 1985.
76. Romero J, Cardenes H, la Torre A, et al: Chordoma: results of radiation therapy in eighteen patients. Radiother Oncol 29:27-32, 1993.
77. Debus J, Schulz-Ertner D, Schad L, et al: Stereotactic fractionated radiotherapy for chordomas and chondrosarcomas of the skull base. Int J Radiat Oncol Biol Phys 47:591-596, 2000.
78. Muthukumar N, Kondziolka D, Lunsford LD, et al: Stereotactic radiosurgery for chordoma and chondrosarcoma: further experience. Int J Radiat Oncol Biol Phys 41:387-392, 1998.
79. Austin-Seymour M, Munzenrider J, Goitein M, et al: Fractionated proton radiation therapy for chordomas and low grade chondrosarcomas of the base of skull. J Neurosurg 70:13-17, 1989.
80. Munzenrider JE, Liebsch NJ: Proton therapy for tumors of the skull base. Strahlenther Onkol 175(Suppl II):57-63, 1999.
81. Million RR, Cassisi NJ, Mancuso AA, Stringer SP: Chemodectomas (glomus body tumors). *In* Million RR, Cassisi NJ (eds.): Management of Head and Neck Cancer. A Multidisciplinary Approach, 2nd ed. Philadelphia, Lippincott, 1994, pp 765-783.
82. Kim JA, Elkon D, Lim ML, Constable WC: Optimum dose of radiotherapy for chemodectomas in the middle ear. Int J Radiat Oncol Biol Phys 6:815ff, 1980.
83. Springate SC, Weichselbaum RR: Radiation or surgery for chemodectomas of the temporal bone: a review of local control and complications. Head Neck 12:303ff, 1990.
84. Spector JG: Management of juvenile angiofibromata. Laryngoscope 98:1016-1026, 1998.
85. Antonelli AR, Cappiello J, Donajo CA, et al: Diagnosis, staging and treatment of juvenile nasopharyngeal angiofibroma. Laryngoscope 97:1319-1325, 1997.
86. Waldman SR, Levine HL, Astor F, et al: Surgical experience with nasopharyngeal angiofibroma. Arch Otolaryngol 107:677-682, 1981.
87. Kuppersmith RB, Teh BS, Donovan DT, et al: The use of intensity modulated radiotherapy for the treatment of extensive and recurrent juvenile angiofibroma. Int J Pediatr Otorhinolaryngol 52:261-268, 2000.
88. Million RR, Cassisi NJ, Mancuso AA, Stringer SP: Juvenile angiofibroma. *In* Million RR, Cassisi NJ (eds.): Management of Head and Neck Cancer. A Multidisciplinary Approach, 2nd ed. Philadelphia, Lippincott, 1994, pp 627-641.
89. McGahan RA, Durrance FY, Parke RB Jr, et al: The treatment of advanced juvenile nasopharyngeal angiofibroma. Int J Radiat Oncol Biol Phys 17:1067-1072, 1989.
90. Reddy KA, Mendenhall WM, Amdur RJ, et al: Long-term results of radiation therapy for juvenile nasopharyngeal angiofibroma. Am J Otolaryngol 22:172-175, 2001.
91. Wilder RB, Buatti JM, Kittelson JM, et al: Pterygium treated with excision and post-operative beta-irradiation. Int J Radiat Oncol Biol Phys 23:533-537, 1992.
92. Monteiro-Grillo I, Gaspar L, Monteiro-Grillo M, et al: Postoperative irradiation of primary or recurrent pterygium: results and sequelae. Int J Radiation Oncol Biol Phys 48:865-869, 2000.
93. Chen PO, Ariyasu RG, Kaza V, et al: A randomized trial comparing mitomycin C and conjunctival autograft after excision of primary pterygium. Am J Ophthalmol 12:151-160, 1995.
94. Mahar PS, Nwokora GE: Role of mitomycin C in pterygium surgery. Br J Ophthalmol 77:433-435, 1993.
95. Rubinfield RS, Pfister RR, Stein RM, et al: Serious complication of topical mitomycin C after pterygium surgery. Ophthalmology 99:1647-1654, 1992.
96. Pajic B, Pallas A, Aebersold D, Greiner RH: Prospective study about course of primary pterygia after exclusive treatment with Sr-/Y-90 irradiation. Strahlenther Oncol, in press.
97. Willner J, Flentje M, Lieb W, et al: Soft X-ray therapy of recurrent pterygium-an alternative to Sr-90 eye applicators. Strahlenther Oncol 177:404-409, 2001.
98. Jaakkola A, Heikkonen J, Tommula P, et al: Strontium plaque irradiation of subfoveal neovascular membranes image-related macular degeneration. Graefes Arch Clin Exp Ophthalmol 236:24-30, 1998.
99. Paryani SB, Scott WP, Wells JW Jr, et al: Management of pterygium with surgery and radiation therapy. The North Florida Pterygium Study Group. Int J Radiat Oncol Biol Phys 28:101-103, 1994.
100. Van den Brenk HA: Results of prophylactic postoperative irradiation on 1300 cases of pterygium. Am J Radiol 103:723-733, 1968.
101. Mourits MP, Lombardo SH, van der Sluijs FA, Fenton S: Reliability of exophthalmos measurement and the exophthalmometry value in a healthy Dutch population and in Graves' patients. Orbit 23:161-168, 2004.
102. Aswad M, Baum J: Optimal time for postoperative irradiation of pterygia. Ophthalmology 94:1450-1451, 1987.
103. MacKenzie FS, Hirst LW, Kynaston B, Bain C: Recurrence rate and complications after beta irradiation for ptergyia. Ophthalmology 98:1776-1780, 1991.
104. Witschel H, Font RL: Hemangioma of the choroid: a clinicopathologic study of 71 cases and a review of the literature. Surv Ophthalmol 20:415-431, 1976.
105. Shields JA, Shields CL: Atlas of Orbital Tumors. Lippincott, Williams & Wilkins, Philadelphia, 1999.
106. Mashayekhi A, Shields CL: Circumscribed choroidal hemangioma. Curr Opin Ophthalmol 14:142-149, 2003.
107. Shields CL, Honavar SC, Shields JA, et al: Circumscribed choroidal hemangioma. Clinical manifestations and factors predictive of visual outcome in 200 consecutive cases. Ophthalmology 108:2237-2248, 2001.
108. Shields JA, Shields CL, Materin MA, et al: Changing concepts in management of circumscribed choroidal hemangioma. The 2003 J. Howard Stokes Lecture (Part 1). Ophthalmol Surg Lasers 35:383-393, 2004.
109. Madreperla SA: Choroidal hemangioma treated with photodynamic therapy using verteporfin. Arch Ophthalmol 119:1606-1610, 2001.
110. Augsburger JJ, Freire J, Brady LW: Radiation therapy for choroidal and retinal hemangiomas. *In* Wiegel T, Bornfeld N, Foerster MH, Hinkelbein W (eds): Radiotherapy of Ocular Disease, vol 30. Basel, Karger, 1997, pp 265-280.

111. Schilling H, Sauerwein W, Lommatzsch A, et al: Long-term results after low dose ocular irradiation for choroidal hemangiomas. Br J Ophthalmol 81:267-273, 1997.
112. No reference.
113. Kreusel KM, Bornfeld N, Lommatzsch A, et al: Ruthenium-106 brachytherapy for peripheral retinal capillary hemangioma. Ophthalmology 105:1386-1392, 1998.
114. Madreperla SA: Choroidal hemangioma treated with photodynamic therapy using verteporfin. Arch Ophthalmol 119:1606-1610, 2001.
115. Zografos L, Bercher L, Chamot L, et al: Cobalt-60 treatment of choroidal hemangiomas. Am J Ophthalmol 121:190-199, 1996.
116. Pauleikhoff D, Holz FG: Die altersabhängige Makuladegeneration. Ophthalmologe 93:299-315, 1996.
117. International ARM Epidemiological Study Group: An international classification system for ARM. Surv Ophthalmol 39:367-374, 1995.
118. Miller JW, Walsh AW, Kramer M, et al: Photodynamic therapy of experimental choroidal neo-vascularisation using lipoprotein-delivered benzoporphyrin. Arch Ophthalmol 113:810-818, 1995.
119. Treatment of Age-related Macular Degeneration with Photodynamic Therapy (TAP) Study Group: Photodynamic therapy of subfoveal choroidal neovascularisation in age-related macular degeneration with verteporfin. One-year results of two randomised clinical trials-TAP report I. Arch Ophthalmol 117:1329-1345, 1999.
120. Valmaggia C, Ries G, Ballinari P: Radiotherapy for subfoveal choroidal neovascularization in age-related macular degeneration: a randomized clinical trial. Am J Ophthalmol 133:521-529, 2002.
121. Bergink GJ, Deutman AF, Van den Broek JFCM, et al: Radiation therapy for subfoveal choroidal neovascular membranes in age-related macular degeneration. Graefes Arch Clin Exp Ophthalmol 232:591-598, 1994.
122. Mauget-Faysse M, Chiquet C, Milea D, et al: Long term results of radiotherapy for subfoveal choroidal neovascularisation in age related macular degeneration. Br J Ophthalmol 83:923-928, 1999.
123. Hart PM, Chakravarthy U, MacKenzie G, et al: Teletherapy for subfoveal choroidal neovascularisation of age related macular degeneration: Results of follow up in a non-randomised study. Br J Ophthalmol 80:1046-1050, 1996.
124. Bergink GJ, Hoyng CB, Van der Maazen RWM, et al: A randomized controlled clinical trial on the efficacy of radiation therapy in the control of subfoveal choroidal neovascularization in age-related macular degeneration: radiation versus observation. Graefes Arch Clin Exp Ophthalmol 236:321-325, 1998.
125. Char DH, Irvine AI, Posner MD, et al: Randomized trial of radiation for age-related macular degeneration. Am J Ophthalmol 127:574-578, 1999.
126. Hoeller U, Fuisting B, Schwartz R, et al: Results of radiotherapy of subfoveal neovascularization with 16 and 20 Gy. Eye 19:1151-1156, 2005.
127. Hollick EJ, Goble RR, Knowles PJ, et al: Radiotherapy treatment of age-related subfoveal neovascular membranes in patients with good vision. Eye 10:609-616, 1996.
128. Pöstgens H, Bodanowitz S, Kroll P: Low dose radiation therapy for age-related macular degeneration. Graefes Arch Clin Exp Ophthalmol 235:656-661, 1997.
129. Prettenhofer M, Haas A, Mayer R, Oechs A, et al: The photon therapy of subfoveal choroidal neovascularisation in age-dependent macular degeneration—the result of a prospective study in 40 patients. Strahlenther Onkol 174:613-617, 1998.
130. RAD (The Radiation Therapy for Age-related Macular Degeneration Study): A prospective, randomized, double-masked trial on radiation therapy for neovascular age-related degeneration. Ophthalmology 106:2239-2247, 1999.
131. Sasai K, Murara R, Mandai M, et al: Radiation therapy for ocular choroidal neovascularization (phase I/II study): preliminary report. Int J Radiat Oncol Biol Phys 39:173-178, 1997.
132. Spaide RF, Guyer DR, McCormick B, et al: External beam radiation therapy for choroidal neo-vascularisation. Ophthalmology 105:24-30, 1998.
133. Stalmans P, Leys A, Van Limbergen E: External beam radiotherapy (20 Gy, 2 fractions) fails to control the growth of choroidal neovascularization in age-related macular degeneration: a review of 111 cases. Retina 17:481-492, 1997.
134. Staar S, Krott R, Mueller R-P, et al: External beam radiotherapy for subretinal neovascularisation in age-related macular degeneration. Is this treatment efficient? Int J Radiat Oncol Biol Phys 45:467-473, 1999.
135. Thölen A, Meister A, Bernasconi PP, et al: Radiotherapie von subretinalen Neovaskularisations-membranen bei altersabhängiger Makuladegeneration. Ophthalmologe 95:691-698, 1998.
136. Yonemoto LT, Slater JD, Blacharski PB, et al: Dose response in the treatment of subfoveal choroidal neovascularization in age-related macular degeneration: results of a phase I/II dose escalation study using proton radiotherapy. J Radiosurg 3:47-54, 2000.
137. Fine SL, Maguire MG: It is not time to abandon radiotherapy for neovascular age-related macular degeneration. Arch Ophthalmol 119:275-276, 2001.
138. Bahn RS, Dutton CM, Naff N, et al: Thyrotropin receptor expression in Graves' orbital adipose/connective tissues: potential autoantigen in Graves' ophthalmopathy. J Clin Endocrinol Metab 83:998-1002, 1998.
139. Mourits M, Koornneef L, Wiersinga WM, et al: Orbital decompression for Graves' ophthalmopathy by inferomedial plus lateral and by coronal approach. Ophthalmology 97:636-641, 1990.
140. Kahaly G, Förster G, Pitz S, et al: Aktuelle interdisziplinäre Diagnostik und Therapie der endokrinen Orbitopathie. Dtsch Med Wochenschr 122:27-32, 1997.
141. Deleted in print.
142. Bartalena L, Marcocci C, Chiovato L, et al: Orbital cobalt irradiation combined with systemic corticosteroids for Graves' ophthalmopathy: comparison with systemic corticosteroids alone. J Clin Endocrinol Metab 56:1139-1144, 1983.
143. Prummel MF, Mourits MP, Blank L, et al: Randomized double-blind trial of prednisone versus radiotherapy. In: Graves' Ophthalmopathy. Lancet 342:949-954, 1993.
144. Petersen IA, Donaldson SS, McDougall IR, Kriss JP: Prognostic factors in the radiotherapy of Graves' ophthalmopathy. Int J Radiat Oncol Biol Phys 19:259-264, 1990.
145. Burch HB, Wartofsky L: Graves' ophthalmopathy: current concepts regarding pathogenesis and management. Endocr Rev 146:747-793, 1993.
146. Donaldson SS, Bagshaw MA, Kriss JP: Supervoltage orbital radiotherapy for Graves' ophthalmopathy. J Clin Endocrinol Metab 37:276-285, 1973.
147. Austin-Seymour MM, Donaldson SS, Egbert PR, et al: Radiotherapy of lymphoid diseases of the orbit. Int J Radiat Oncol Biol Phys 11:371-379, 1985.
148. Lambo MJ, Brady LW, Shields CL: Lymphoid tumors of the orbit. *In* Alberti WE, Sagerman RH (eds): Radiotherapy of Intraocular and Orbital Tumors. Berlin, Springer (1. Auflage): 1993, pp 205-216.
149. Donaldson SS, McDougall IR, Kriss JP: Graves' Disease. *In* Alberti WE, Sagerman RH (eds.): Radiotherapy of intraocular and orbital tumors. Berlin, Springer (1 Auflage), 1993, pp 191-197.
150. Leone C, Lloyd T: Treatment protocol for orbital inflammatory disease. Ophthalmology 92:1325-1331, 1985.
151. Barthold HJ, Harvey A, Markoe AM, et al: Treatment of orbital pseudotumors and lymphoma. Am J Clin Oncol 9:527-532, 1986.
152. Fritzpatrick PI, Macko SL: Lymphoreticular tumors of orbit. Int J Radiat Oncol Biol Phys 10: 333-340, 1984.
153. Lanciano R, Fowble B, Sergott R, et al: The results of radiotherapy for orbital pseudotumor. Int J Radiat Oncol Biol Phys 18:407-411, 1989.
154. Notter M: Strahlentherapie bei pseudotumor orbitae. *In* Seegenschmiedt MH, Makoski HB (eds): Radiotherapie gutartiger Erkrankungen, Symposium 5.-6. März 2000 Altenberge, Germany, Diplodocus Verlag, 2000, pp 123-136.
155. Gocht H: Therapeutische Verwendung der Röntgenstrahlen. Fortschr Röntgenstr 1:14, 1897.
156. Atahan I, Lale F, Akyol F, et al: Radiotherapy in the management of aggressive fibromatosis. Br J Radiol 62:854-856, 1989.

157. Goy BW, Lee SP, Eilber F, et al: The role of adjuvant radiotherapy in the treatment of resectable desmoid tumors. Int J Radiat Oncol Biol Phys 39:659-665, 1997.
158. Hoffmann W, Weidmann B, Schmidberger H, et al: Klinik und Therapie der aggressiven Fibromatose (Desmoide). Strahlenther Onkol 169:235-241, 1993.
159. Posner MC, Shiu MH, Newsome JL: The desmoid tumor—not a benign disease. Arch Surg 124:191-196, 1989.
160. Suit HD, Spiro I: Radiation treatment of benign mesenchymal disease. Semin Radiat Oncol 9:171-178, 1999.
161. Wilcken N, Tattersall MH: Endocrine therapy for desmoid tumors. Cancer 68:1384-1388, 1991.
162. *Ibid.*
163. Wadell WR, Gerner RE: Indomethacin and ascorbate inhibit desmoid tumors. J Surg Oncol 15:85-90, 1980.
164. Kirschner MJ, Sauer R: Die Rolle der Radiotherapie bei der Behandlung von Desmoidtumoren. Strahlenther Onkol 169:77-82, 1993.
165. Kamath SS, Parsons JT, Marcus RB: Radiotherapy for local control of aggressive fibromatosis. Int J Radiat Oncol Biol Phys 36:325-328, 1996.
166. Assad WA, Nori D, Hilaris BS, et al: Role of brachytherapy in the management of desmoid tumors. Int J Radiat Oncol Biol Phys 12:901-906, 1986.
167. Bataini JP, Belloir C, Mazabraud A, et al: Desmoid tumors in adults: the role of radiotherapy in their management. Am J Surg 155:754-760, 1988.
168. Ballo MT, Zagars GK, Pollack A: Desmoid tumor: Prognostic factors and outcome after surgery, radiation therapy or combined surgery and radiation therapy. J Clin Oncol 17:158-167, 1999.
169. Enzinger FM, Shiraki M: Musculo-aponeurotic fibromatosis of the shoulder girdle (extra-abdominal desmoid). Cancer 20:1131-1140, 1967.
170. Kiel KD: Radiation therapy in the treatment of aggressive fibromatoses (desmoid tumors). Cancer 54:2051-2055, 1984.
171. Kinzbrunner B, Ritter S, Domingo J: Remission of rapidly growing desmoid tumors after tamoxifen. Cancer 52:2201-2204, 1983.
172. Klein WA, Miller HH, Anderson M: The use of indomethacin, sulindac and tamoxifen for the treatment of desmoid tumors associated with familial polyposis. Cancer 60:2863-2868, 1987.
173. Leibel SA, Wara WM, Hill D, et al: Desmoid tumors: local control and patterns of relapse following radiation therapy. Int J Radiat Oncol Biol Phys 9:1167-1171, 1983.
174. Leithner A, Schnack B, Katterschafka T, et al: Treatment of extra-abdominal desmoid tumors with interferon-alpha with or without tretinoin. J Surg Oncol 73:21-25, 2000.
175. Suit HD: Radiation dose and response of desmoid tumors. Int J Radiat Oncol Biol Phys 9:225-227, 1990.
176. Walther E, Hünig R, Zalad S: Behandlung der aggressiven Fibromatose. Orthopädie 17:193-200, 1998.
177. Seegenschmiedt MH, Micke O, Willich N, GCG-BD: Radiation Therapy for Nonmalignant Diseases in Germany: Current Concepts and Future Perspectives. Verlag, Germany, 2004.
178. Nesbit RM: Congenital curvature of the phallus. Report of three cases with description of corrective operation. J Urol 93:230-232, 1950.
179. Feder BH: Peyronie's disease. J Am Geriatr Soc 19:947- 951, 1971.
180. Helvie WW, Ochsner SF: Radiation therapy in Peyronie's disease. South Med J 65:1192-1196, 1972.
181. Martin CL: Long time study of patients with Peyronie's disease treated with irradiation. AJR Am J Roentgenol 114:492-495, 1972.
182. Wagenknecht LV, Meyer WH, Kiskemann A: Wertigkeit verschiedener Therapieverfahren bei Induratio penis plastica. Urol Int 37:335-348, 1982.
183. Pambor M, Schmidt W, Wiesner M, Jahr U: Induratio penis plastica-Ergebnisse nach kombinierter Behandlung mit Röntgenbestrahlung und Tokopherol. Z Klin Med 40:1425-1427, 1985.
184. Weisser GW, Schmidt B, Hübener KH, et al: Die Strahlenbehandlung der Induratio penis plastica. Strahlenther Onkol 163:23-28, 1987.
185. Mira JG, Chahbazian CM, del Regato JA: The value of radiotherapy for Peyronie's disease: presentation of 56 new case studies and review of the literature. Int J Radiat Oncol Biol Phys 6:161-166, 1989.
186. Viljoen IM, Goedhals L, Doman MJ: Peyronie's disease: a perspective on the disease and the long-term results of radiotherapy. S Afr Med J 83:19-20, 1993.
187. Rodrigues CI, Hian Njo, Karim AB: Results of radiotherapy and vitamin E in the treatment of Peyronie's disease. Int J Radiat Oncol Biol Phys 31:571-576, 1995.
188. Williams JL, Thomas CG: The natural history of Peyronie's disease. J Urol 103:75-76, 1970.
189. Bruns F, Kardels B, Schäfer U, et al: Strahlentherapie bei Induratio penis plastica. Röntgenpraxis 52:33-37, 1999.
190. Incrocci L, Wijnmaalen A, Slob AK, et al: Low-dose radiotherapy in 179 patients with Peyronie's disease: treatment outcome and current sexual function. Int J Radiat Oncol Biol Phys 47:1353-1356, 2000.
191. Keilholz L, Seegenschmiedt MH, Sauer R: Radiotherapy in early stage Dupuytren's contracture: initial and long-term results. Int J Radiat Oncol Biol Phys 36:891-897, 1996.
192. Adamietz B, Keilholz L, Grünert J, Sauer R: Die Radiotherapie des Morbus Dupuytren im Frühstadium. Langzeitresuktate nach einer medianen Nachbeobachtungszeit von 10 Jahren. Strahlenther Onkol 177:604-610, 2001.
193. Escarmant P, Zimmermann S, Amar A, et al: The treatment of 783 keloid scars by Iridium 192 interstitial irradiation after surgical excision. Int J Radiat Oncol Biol Phys 26:245-251, 1993.
194. Guix B, Henriquez I, Andres A, et al: Treatment of keloids by high-dose-rate brachytherapy: a seven-year-study. Int J Radiat Oncol Biol Phys 50:167-172, 2001.
195. Prott FJ, Micke O, Wagner W, et al: Narbenkeloidprophylaxe durch Bestrahlung mit Strontium-90. MTA 12:425-428, 1997.
196. Micke O, Seegenschmiedt MH: The German Working Group guidelines for radiation therapy of benign diseases: a multicenter approach in Germany. Int J Radiat Oncol Biol Phys 52:496-513, 2002.
197. Lo TCM, Seckel BR, Salzman FA, Wright KA: Single-dose electron beam irradiation in treatment and prevention of keloids and hypertrophic scars. Radiother Oncol 19:267-272, 1990.
198. Janssen de Limpens MP: Comparison of the treatment of keloids and hypertrophic scars. Eur J Plast Surg 9:18-21, 1986.
199. Metzger H, Junker A, Voss AC: Die Bestrahlung der Brustdrüsen als Prophylaxe der östrogen-induzierten Gynäkomastie beim Prostatakarzinom. Strahlenther Onkol 156:102-104, 1980.
200. Chou JL, Easley JD, Feldmeier JJ: Effective radiotherapy in palliating mammalgia associated with gynecomastia after DES therapy. Int J Radiat Oncol Biol Phys 15:749-751, 1988.
201. Clough JR, Price CGH: Aneurysmal bone cyst: pathogenesis and long term results of treatment. Clin Orthop 97:52-63, 1973.
202. Marcove RC, Sheth DS, Takemoto S, et al: The treatment of aneurysmal bone cyst. Clin Orthop 311:157, 1995.
203. Nobler MP, Higinbotham ML, Phillips RF: The cure of aneurysmal bone cyst. Irradiation superior to surgery in analysis of 33 cases. Radiology 90:1185, 1968.
204. Goldman AB, DiCarlo EF: Pigmented villonodular synovitis. Diagnosis and differential diagnosis. Radiol Clin North Am 266:1327-1347, 1988.
205. O'Sullivan B, Cummings B, Catton C, et al: Outcome following radiation treatment for high-risk pigmented villonodular synovitis. Int J Radiat Oncol Biol Phys 32:777-786, 1995.
206. Wiss DA: Recurrent villonodular synovitis of the knee. Successful treatment with yttrium-90. Clin Orthop Rel Res 169:139-144, 1982.
207. Granowitz SP, D´Antonio J, Mankin HL: The pathogenesis and long-term end results of pigmented villonodular synovitis. Clin Orthop 114:335-351, 1976.
208. Unni KK, Ivins JC, Beabout JW, et al: Hemangioma, hemangiopericytoma and hemangioendothelioma (angiosarcoma) of bone. Cancer 27:1403-1414, 1971.
209. McAllister VL, Kendall BE, Bull JWD: Symptomatic vertebral hemangiomas. Brain 98:71-80, 1975.
210. Raco A, Ciappetta P, Artico M, et al: Vertebral hemangiomas with cord compression: the role of embolization in five cases. Surg Neurol 34:164-168, 1990.

211. Laredo JD, Reizine D, Bard M, et al: Vertebral hemangiomas. Radiologic evaluation. Radiology 161:183-189, 1986.
212. No reference.
213. Bremnes RM, Hauge HN, Sagsveen R: Radiotherapy in the treatment of symptomatic vertebral hemangiomas: technical case report. Neurosurgery 39:1054-1058, 1996.
214. Doppman JL, Oldfield EH, Heiss JD: Symptomatic vertebral hemangiomas: treatment by means of direct intralesional injection of ethanol. Radiology 214:341-348, 2000.
215. Kleinert H: Über die Telekobalttherapie der Wirbelhämangiome. Strahlenther Onkol 134:504-510, 1967.
216. Winkler C, Dornfeld S, Baumann M, et al: Effizienz der Strahlentherapie bei Wirbelhämangiomen. Strahlenther Onkol 172:681-684, 1996.
217. Pastushyn AI, Slinko EI, Mirzoyeva GM: Vertebral hemangiomas: diagnosis, management, natural history and clinicopathological correlates in 86 patients. Surg Neurol 50:535-547, 1998.
218. Padovani R, Acciarri N, Giulioni M, et al: Cavernous angiomas of the spinal district: surgical treatment of 11 patients. Eur Spine J 6:298-303, 1997.
219. Fox MW, Onofrio BM: The natural history and management of symptomatic and asymptomatic vertebral hemangiomas. J Neurosurg 78:36-45, 1993.
220. Harrison MJ, Eisenberg MB, Ullman JS, et al: Symptomatic cavernous malformations affecting the spine and spinal cord. Neurosurgery 37:195-205, 1995.
221. Rades D, Bajrovic A, Alberti A, Rudat V: Is there a dose-effect relationship for the treatment of symptomatic vertebral hemangioma? Int J Radiat Oncol Biol Phys 55:178-181, 2002.
222. Brooker AF, Bowerman JW, Robinson RA, Riley LH: Ectopic ossification following total hip replacement. J Bone Joint Surg 55:A1629-A1632, 1973.
223. Ayers DC, Pellegrini VD, Evarts CM: Prevention of heterotopic ossification in high-risk patients of radiation therapy. Clin Orthop 263:87-93, 1991.
224. De Lee J, Ferrari A, Charnley J: Ectopic bone formation following low friction arthroplasty of the hip. Clin Orthop 121:53, 1976.
225. Ritter MA, Vaughan RB: Ectopic ossifications after total hip arthroplasty: predisposing factors, frequency and effect on results. J Bone Joint Surg 59:A 345-351, 1977.
226. Ayers DC, Evarts CM, Parkinson JR: The prevention of heterotopic ossification in high-risk patients by low-dose radiation therapy after total hip arthroplasty. J Bone Joint Surg 68:A1423-A1430, 1986.
227. Pedersen NW, Kristensen SS, Schmidt SA, et al: Factors associated with heterotopic bone formation following total hip replacement. Arch Orthop Trauma Surg 108:92-95, 1989.
228. Schmidt SA, Kjaersgaard-Andersen P, Pedersen NW, et al: The use of indomethacin to prevent the formation of heterotopic bone after total hip replacement. J Bone Joint Surg 70:A834-A838, 1988.
229. Goel A, Sharp DJ: Heterotopic bone formation after hip replacement. J Bone Joint Surg 73:B255-257, 1991.
230. Bosse MJ, Poka A, Reinert CM, et al: Heterotopic bone formation as a complication of acetabular fractures. J Bone Joint Surg 70:A1231-A1237, 1988.
231. Slawson RG, Poka A, Bathon H, et al: The role of postoperative radiation in the prevention of heterotrophic ossification in patients with posttraumatic acetabular fracture. Int J Radiat Oncol Biol Phys 17:669-672, 1989.
232. Bijvoet OLM, Nollen AJG, Sloof TJJH, Feith R: Effect of diphosphonate on para-articular ossification after total hip replacement. Acta Orthop Scand 45:926-934, 1974.
233. Garland DE, Betzabe A, Kenneth GV, Vogt JC: Diphosphonate treatment for heterotopic ossification in spinal cord injury patients. Clin Orthop 176:197-200, 1983.
234. Thomas BJ, Amstutz HC: Results of administration of diphosphonate for prevention of heterotopic ossification after total hip arthroplasty. J Bone Joint Surg 67:A400-A403, 1985.
235. Almasbakk K, Roysiand P: Does indomethacin prevent postoperative ectopic ossification in total hip replacement? Acta Orthop Scand 48:556, 1977.
236. Kjaersgaard-Andersen P, Schmidt SA: Indomethacin for the prevention of ectopic ossification after hip arthroplasty. Acta Orthop Scand 57:12-14, 1986.
237. Ritter MA, Sieber JM: Prophylactic indomethacin for the prevention of heterotopic bone formation following total hip arthroplasty. Clin Orthop 196:217-225, 1985.
238. Cella JP, Salvati EA, Sculco TP: Indomethacin for the prevention of heterotopic ossification following total hip arthroplasty. J Arthroplasty 3:229-234, 1988.
239. Sodemann B, Persson PE, Nilsson OS: Prevention of heterotopic ossification by non-steroid anti-inflammatory drugs after total hip arthroplasty. Clin Orthop 237:158-237, 1988.
240. McLaren AC: Prophylaxis with indomethacin for heterotopic bone. J Bone Joint Surg 72:A245-A247, 1990.
241. Elmstedt E, Lindholm TS, Nilsson OS, Tornkvist H: Effect of ibuprofen on heterotopic ossification after hip replacement. Acta Orthop Scand 56:25-27, 1985.
242. Finerman GA, Stover S: Ossification following hip replacement or spinal cord injury: Two clinical studies with EHDP. Met Bone Dis Relat Res 3:337-342, 1981.
243. Coventry MB, Scanlon PW: The use of radiation to discourage ectopic bone. A nine-year study in surgery about the hip. J Bone Joint Surg 63:A201-A208, 1981.
244. Van der Werf GJIM, van Hasselt NGM, Tonino AJ: Radiotherapy in the prevention of recurrence of paraarticular ossification in total hip prosthesis. Arch Orthop Trauma Surg 104:85-88, 1985.
245. McLennan I, Keys HM, Evarts CM, Rubin P: Usefulness of postoperative hip irradiation in the prevention of bone formation in a high risk group of patients. Int J Radiat Oncol Biol Phys 10:49-53, 1984.
246. Anthony P, Keys H, McCollister-Evarts C, et al: Prevention of heterotopic bone formation with early postoperative irradiation in high risk patients undergoing total hip arthroplasty: comparison of 10 Gy versus 20 Gy schedules. Int Radiat Oncol Biol Phys 13:365-369, 1987.
247. Sylvester JE, Greenberg P, Selch MT, et al: The use of postoperative irradiation for the prevention of heterotopic bone formation after total hip replacement. Int J Radiat Oncol Biol Phys 14:471-476, 1988.
248. Blount LH, Thomas BJ, Tran L, et al: Postoperative irradiation for prevention of heterotopic bone: analysis of different dose schedules and shielding considerations. Int J Radiat Oncol Biol Phys 19:577-581, 1990.
249. Seegenschmiedt MH, Goldmann AR, Wölfel R, et al: Prevention of heterotopic ossification (HO) after total hip replacement: randomized high versus low dose radiotherapy. Radiother Oncol 26:271-274, 1993.
250. Konski A, Pellegrini V, Poulter C, et al: Randomized trial comparing single dose versus fractionated irradiation for prevention of heterotopic bone. Int J Radiat Oncol Biol Phys 18:1139-1142, 1990.
251. Seegenschmiedt MH, Goldmann AR, Martus P, et al: Prophylactic radiation therapy for prevention of heterotopic ossification after hip arthroplasty: results in 141 high-risk hips. Radiology 188:257-264, 1993.
252. Alberti W, Quack G, Krischke W, et al: Verhinderung ektoper Ossifikationen nach Totalendoprothese des Hüftgelenks durch Strahlentherapie. Dtsch Med Wochenschr 120:983-989, 1995.
253. Gregoritch S, Chadha M, Pellegrini V, et al: Preoperative irradiation for prevention of heterotopic ossification following prosthetic total hip replacement. Preliminary results. Int J Radiat Oncol Biol Phys 27(Suppl 1):157-158, 1993.
254. Konski A, Weiss C, Rosier R, et al: The use of postoperative irradiation for prevention of heterotopic bone after total hip replacement with biological fixation (porous coated) prosthesis: an animal model. Int J Radiat Oncol Biol Phys 18:861-865, 1990.
255. Wise MW 3d, Robertson ID, Lachiewicz PF, et al: The effect of radiation therapy on the fixation strength of an experimental porous-coated implant in dogs. Clin Orthop 261:276-280, 1990.
256. Summer DR, Turner TM, Pierson RH, et al: Effects of radiation on fixation of non-cemented porous-coated implants in a canire model. Bone Joint Surg Am 72:1527-1533, 1990.

257. Jasty M, Schutzer S, Tepper J, et al: Radiation-blocking shields to localize periarticular radiation precisely for prevention of heterotopic bone formation around uncemented total hip arthroplasties. Clin Orthop 257:138-145, 1990.
258. De Flitch DJ, Stryker JA: Postoperative hip irradiation in prevention of heterotopic ossification: causes of treatment failure. Radiology 188:265-270, 1993.
259. Hedley AK, Leon PM, Douglas HH: The prevention of heterotopic bone formation following total hip arthroplasty using 600 rad in a single dose. Arthroplasty 4:319-325, 1989.
260. Sauer R, Seegenschmiedt MH, Goldmann A, et al: Prophylaxe periartikulärer Verknöcherungen nach endoprothetischen Hüftgelenksersatz durch postoperative Bestrahlung. Strahlenther Onkol 16:889-899, 1992.

PART I

CHILDHOOD CANCERS

Overview

Larry Kun

Approximately 9000 children and adolescents present with newly diagnosed cancer in the United States each year (Table I-1).[1,2] Most pediatric cancers manifest as readily identifiable syndromes that link presenting features with the disease entity and with molecular and genetic characteristics. Approximately two thirds of children in North America are treated on clinical protocols, reflecting the major pediatric clinical cooperative group (the Children's Oncology Group [COG]), one of the pediatric-specific consortia (New Approaches to Neuroblastoma Therapy Study [NANTS] and the Pediatric Brain Tumor Consortium [PBTC]), independent studies at a few major institutions, and collaborative trials. With contemporary therapies, long-term disease control—*cure*—is achieved in 70% to 80% of children and adolescents. Survivors of childhood cancer often have physical and functional limitations that prevent them from achieving their full potential and compromise their quality of life.[2-14] Current strategies and clinical investigations seek to maintain or improve disease control for the more favorable disease types and presentations; equally, studies aim toward reducing the therapies most associated with long-term morbidity and mortality. For children with disease presentations less likely to be controlled, clinical trials incorporate further intensification of therapy and possibly introduce newer biologic or molecularly targeted agents.[15,16]

Radiation therapy is a major component of therapy for most children presenting with cancer. Between 10 and 20 years ago, radiation therapy was most frequently used as "preventive central nervous system therapy" in acute lymphoblastic leukemia (ALL) (the most common type of cancer occurring in children), but contemporary therapeutic approaches focus more on the pediatric solid tumors and stem cell transplantation.[12,17-24] A decade ago, clinical research on the role of radiation therapy was almost entirely focused on reducing indications and dose; the current focus is more on optimizing the risk-benefit ratio and defining the irradiation parameters for selective use.

Radiation therapy has an expanding role in treating many pediatric brain tumors (the second most common group of cancers occurring in children) and sarcomas (soft tissue and bone neoplasms), as well as neuroblastoma and pediatric Hodgkin's disease.[19-22,25-30] Data from St. Jude Children's Research Hospital show the proportion of newly diagnosed children with all forms of cancer receiving irradiation has increased over the past decade (from approximately 40% to almost 60%), even with the elimination of preventive cranial irradiation in institutional protocols. The mean age of children undergoing irradiation has decreased from 11.4 to 9.6 years. Greater use of radiation therapy reflects the improvements in dose conformality and the ability to limit radiation exposure to critical normal structures, fully recognizing the increased vulnerability of young children and growing adolescents to radiation-related normal-tissue effects while acknowledging the critical goal of achieving local tumor control. In most settings, the defensive position of the radiation oncologist has been replaced by the required knowledge base in pediatric oncology and the details of radiation oncology at a time when a relative plateau has been reached in the efficacy of conventional cytotoxic chemotherapy and expectations are more limited for high-dose chemotherapy in treating most pediatric solid tumors.[22,23,29,31-36]

The introduction of three-dimensional treatment planning and the use of sophisticated treatment delivery techniques have had enormous impact on the risk-benefit ratio in pediatric radiation oncology. Current approaches essentially demand use of three-dimensional conformal (3D-CRT) or intensity-modulated radiation therapy (IMRT) in most settings.[23,25,37-39] Interest in newer physical modalities (e.g., proton beam, potentially charged carbon particles) is keen because further sparing of normal tissues is objectively more critical in the pediatric setting than in most adult cancer presentations. Early data are available for rhabdomyosarcoma, other soft tissue sarcomas, and several central nervous system (CNS) tumor histiotypes (e.g., ependymomas, low-grade gliomas, craniopharyngiomas), suggesting realization of the goals of maintaining or enhancing local tumor control while diminishing some of the most common radiation dose-limiting normal tissue effects.[28,37,38,40-43]

The newer molecularly targeted therapies are of interest in combination with radiation therapy. Several classes of drugs under investigation for anticancer effect in childhood cancers show radiosensitizing potential in preclinical studies, such as the platelet-derived growth factor (PDGF) inhibitors, farnesyl transferase inhibitors (FTIs), and histone deacetylase inhibitors (HDACs), which are in phase I and II trials in conjunction with local irradiation for treating pediatric brain and solid tumors.[15,16,44,45]

Stem cell transplantation (i.e., high-dose chemotherapy with allogeneic bone marrow transplantation or hematopoietic rescue with autologous marrow or peripheral stem cells) has been relatively successful in selected leukemias (i.e., ALL and acute myelogenous leukemia [AML] in children) and solid tumors (e.g., neuroblastoma). Total-body irradiation (TBI) is a relatively standard component of the conditioning regimen for most allogeneic transplantations, particularly at a time when the use of haploidentical or matched, unrelated donors requires the more effective immune suppression achievable with TBI.[24,46,47]

Whether for locoregional tumor control or as a systemic agent, the use of ionizing radiation demands a balance between its documented efficacy in the more common tumors

Table I-1 Common Neoplasms Occurring in Children and Adolescents

Disease Type	Proportion of Childhood Cancers	Role for Radiation Therapy
Acute leukemias	*24%*	
Acute lymphoblastic leukemia (ALL)	18%	1. Limited benefit from preventive cranial irradiation (high-risk T-cell leukemia, <5% ALL cases) 2. Therapeutic CNS RT for CNS relapse 3. TBI in BMT for recurrent or high-risk ALL
Acute myeloid leukemia (AML)	4%	1. TBI in BMT
CNS tumors	*18%*	
Glial tumors	12%	1. Local RT for many low-grade tumors, often at progression 2. Local RT for all high-grade tumors
Ependymomas	1%	1. Local RT for virtually all tumors
Craniopharyngiomas	1%	1. Local RT for incompletely resected, progressive, or recurrent tumors
Medulloblastomas and other embryonal CNS tumors	3%	1. Systematic craniospinal irradiation + local boost for children ≥3 years old 2. Local RT for children <3 years old (investigational)
Malignant lymphomas	*15%*	
Hodgkin's disease	9%	1. Local (involved field) in combined-modality therapy 2. TBI in transplantation settings for recurrent disease
Malignant lymphoid tumors	6%	1. Limited local or TBI (BMT) indications
Neuroblastoma	5%	1. Locoregional RT for regionally advanced disease 2. Palliative RT (bone, soft tissue) 3. TBI in high-dose therapy or stem cell rescue regimens (investigational)
Wilms' tumor	4%	1. Locoregional RT in advanced disease or for unfavorable histology 2. Visceral RT in metastatic disease
Retinoblastoma	4%	1. Ocular RT in consolidative settings or for progressive or recurrent disease
Soft tissue sarcomas	*7%*	
Rhabdomyosarcomas	4%	1. Locoregional RT for most presentations (intermediate, advanced, or alveolar histology)
Other soft tissue	3%	1. Locoregional RT based on histology, site, size, and age
Bone sarcomas	*6%*	
Osteosarcoma	3%	1. Limited postoperative use in central sites
Ewing's sarcoma	2%	1. Local RT for "nondispensable" primary site 2. Local postoperative RT after marginal resection 3. Visceral and bone RT in metastatic disease
Hepatic tumors	1%	1. Limited postoperative or palliative RT
Germ cell tumors	5%	1. Limited locoregional RT

BMT, bone marrow transplantation; CNS, central nervous system; RT, radiation therapy; TBI, total-body irradiation.

Adapted from SEER Cancer Statistics: http://seer.cancer.gov; Gurney JG, Davis S, Severson RK, et al: Trends in cancer incidence among children in the U.S. Cancer 78:532-541, 1996; Smith M, Hare ML: An overview of progress in childhood cancer survival. J Pediatr Oncol Nurs 21:160-164, 2004.

in children and its potential long-term toxicities. Radiation-related late effects are often more pronounced in children than in adults, especially in somatic changes (i.e., growth and development of musculoskeletal tissues) and functional effects (i.e., neurocognitive, auditory, and endocrine).[3-9,13,48,49] Infants and young children tend to be particularly vulnerable to the effects of radiation and certain chemotherapeutic agents (e.g., alkylating agents, cisplatin, doxorubicin).[3,50-53] Alterations in bone growth, muscle development, and intermediate-size arteries tend to be more prevalent in younger patients than in adolescents or adults. Threshold radiation levels are recognized for epiphyseal growth, but even low-dose exposures can be correlated with changes in height and bone development (i.e., contour and integrity). Similarly, muscular underdevelopment is noted even with radiation doses less than 15 Gy.[13,54] It is not clear whether visceral tolerances are significantly lower in this age group, although the frequent use of combined-modality therapy introduces added concerns regarding radiation tolerance for the heart, lungs, liver, and kidneys.[53,55-60] Intermediate-size vessels, particularly at the circle of Willis, show reduced caliber and flow in a notably high proportion of children younger than 1 to 3 years, whereas major vascular effects are otherwise uncommon at the dose levels used in most pediatric instances.[61-63] A high proportion of children evidence hypothyroidism after even low-dose exposures of the neck; manifestations of reduced testosterone levels after low-dose irradiation are also more common after irradiation in childhood or adolescence.[7,49,64,65]

Neurocognitive effects of CNS irradiation have been well described and correlated directly with radiation dose and volume, as well as indirectly with patient age. Concerns regarding limited life potential attendant to diminished learning and IQ have driven much of the recent protocol-based attempts to limit radiation use, volume, and dose in treating children with CNS tumors.[3,66-69] Data from the use of narrow targets to rather high doses have shown preservation of intellectual function in children as young as 12 months of age with ependymomas.[25] Prospective measurements of learning disabilities are key to further assessing the impact of sophisticated radiation therapy in localized brain tumors. Evidence indicates that specific interventions (e.g., pharmacologic, cognitive rehabilitation) can ameliorate some of the learning problems that precede measurable cognitive decline.[70,71]

In considering pediatric radiation therapy, the physician must always address the issue of secondary carcinogenesis, an overall risk that approximates 5% to 10% over 3 decades of follow-up.[6,72,73] The long survival intervals of successfully treated children and the added risk of secondary cancers in some of the growing or developing tissues (e.g., the pubescent and adolescent breast) require exquisite balance in including irradiation and in selecting techniques that to some degree limit volume exposure potentially associated with added carcinogenic phenomena.[74-78] Unanticipated interactions of chemotherapy and irradiation have also been associated with increased carcinogenesis; at St. Jude, the long-term incidence of secondary brain tumors in patients with treated ALL increased from between less than 1% and 3% to 20% in a single protocol, with the latter figure uniquely associated with concurrent cranial irradiation and high-dose antimetabolite chemotherapy (6-MP).[79,80,88]

It is important to be cognizant of settings associated with relatively increased risk of radiation-induced carcinogenesis. Several of the pediatric cancer syndromes are associated with constitutional genetic effects that uniquely increase the risks of radiation carcinogenesis. These include the Li-Fraumeni syndrome and ataxia-telangiectasia, both with associated *TP53* abnormalities (seen in children with sarcomas and multiple cancers); Gorlin's syndrome, associated with *PTCH* mutations in the sonic hedgehog pathway (seen in a subset of children with medulloblastoma); and hereditary forms of retinoblastoma with deletions of the retinoblastoma gene on chromosome 13.[81-87]

The following chapters outline the biology, clinical features, and outcome of the more common pediatric cancers, summarizing the current and evolving roles of radiation therapy in the multidisciplinary approach to childhood cancer.

REFERENCES

1. Gurney JG, Davis S, Severson RK, et al: Trends in cancer incidence among children in the U.S. Cancer 78:532-541, 1996.
2. Smith M, Hare ML: An overview of progress in childhood cancer survival. J Pediatr Oncol Nurs 21:160-164, 2004.
3. Mulhern RK, Merchant TE, Gajjar A, et al: Late neurocognitive sequelae in survivors of brain tumours in childhood. Lancet Oncol 5:399-408, 2004.
4. Adams MJ, Lipsitz SR, Colan SD, et al: Cardiovascular status in long-term survivors of Hodgkin's disease treated with chest radiotherapy. J Clin Oncol 22:3139-3148, 2004.
5. Barr RD, Sala A: Quality-adjusted survival: a rigorous assessment of cure after cancer during childhood and adolescence. Pediatr Blood Cancer 44:201-204, 2005.
6. Mertens AC, Yasui Y, Neglia JP, et al: Late mortality experience in five-year survivors of childhood and adolescent cancer: the Childhood Cancer Survivor Study. J Clin Oncol 19:3163-3172, 2001.
7. Constine LS, Woolf PD, Cann D, et al: Hypothalamic-pituitary dysfunction after radiation for brain tumors. N Engl J Med 328:87-94, 1993.
8. Stovall M, Donaldson SS, Weathers RE, et al: Genetic effects of radiotherapy for childhood cancer: gonadal dose reconstruction. Int J Radiat Oncol Biol Phys 60:542-552, 2004.
9. Sklar CA, Robison LL, Nesbit ME, et al: Effects of radiation on testicular function in long-term survivors of childhood acute lymphoblastic leukemia: a report from the Children's Cancer Study Group. J Clin Oncol 8:1981-1987, 1990.
10. Tucker MA, D'Angio GJ, Boice JD Jr, et al: Bone sarcomas linked to radiotherapy and chemotherapy in children. N Engl J Med 317:588-593, 1987.
11. Bhatia S, Yasui Y, Robison LL, et al: High risk of subsequent neoplasms continues with extended follow-up of childhood Hodgkin's disease: report from the Late Effects Study Group. J Clin Oncol 21:4386-4394, 2003.
12. Pui CH, Cheng C, Leung W, et al: Extended follow-up of long-term survivors of childhood acute lymphoblastic leukemia. N Engl J Med 349:640-649, 2003.
13. Paulino AC: Late effects of radiotherapy for pediatric extremity sarcomas. Int J Radiat Oncol Biol Phys 60:265-274, 2004.
14. Hudson MM, Poquette CA, Lee J, et al: Increased mortality after successful treatment for Hodgkin's disease. J Clin Oncol 16:3592-3600, 1998.
15. Jones HA, Hahn SM, Bernhard E, McKenna WG: Ras inhibitors and radiation therapy. Semin Radiat Oncol 11:328-337, 2001.
16. Geyer JR, Boyett J, Douglas J, et al: Phase I trial of ZD1839 (Iressa™) and radiation in pediatric patients newly diagnosed with brain stem tumors or incompletely resected supratentorial malignant gliomas. Int J Radiat Oncol Biol Phys 60(S1):S251, 2004.
17. Pui CH: Toward optimal central nervous system-directed treatment in childhood acute lymphoblastic leukemia. J Clin Oncol 21:179-181, 2003.
18. Clarke M, Gaynon P, Hann I, et al: CNS-directed therapy for childhood acute lymphoblastic leukemia: Childhood ALL Collaborative Group overview of 43 randomized trials. J Clin Oncol 21:1798-1809, 2003.
19. Haas-Kogan DA, Swift PS, Selch M, et al: Impact of radiotherapy for high-risk neuroblastoma: a Children's Cancer Group Study. Int J Radiat Oncol Biol Phys 56:28-39, 2003.
20. Schuck A, Ahrens S, Paulussen M, et al: Local therapy in localized Ewing tumors: results of 1058 patients treated in the CESS 81, CESS 86, and EICESS 92 trials. Int J Radiat Oncol Biol Phys 55:168-177, 2003.
21. Wolden SL, Anderson JR, Crist WM, et al: Indications for radiotherapy and chemotherapy after complete resection in rhabdomyosarcoma: a report from the Intergroup rhabdomyosarcoma studies I to III. J Clin Oncol 17:3468-3475, 1999.
22. Wolden SL, Gollamudi SV, Kushner BH, et al: Local control with multimodality therapy for stage 4 neuroblastoma. Int J Radiat Oncol Biol Phys 46:969-974, 2000.
23. Wolden SL, La TH, LaQuaglia MP, et al: Long-term results of three-dimensional conformal radiation therapy for patients with rhabdomyosarcoma. Cancer 97:179-185, 2003.
24. Davies SM, Ramsay NK, Klein JP, et al: Comparison of preparative regimens in transplants for children with acute lymphoblastic leukemia. J Clin Oncol 18:340-347, 2000.
25. Merchant TE, Mulhern RK, Krasin MJ, et al: Preliminary results from a phase II trial of conformal radiation therapy and evaluation of radiation-related CNS effects for pediatric patients with localized ependymoma. J Clin Oncol 22:3156-3162, 2004.
26. Wolden SL: Radiation therapy for non-rhabdomyosarcoma soft tissue sarcomas in adolescents and young adults. J Pediatr Hematol Oncol 27:212-214, 2005.
27. Fouladi M, Wallace D, Langston JW, et al: Survival and functional outcome of children with hypothalamic/chiasmatic tumors. Cancer 97:1084-1092, 2003.
28. Marcus KJ, Goumnerova L, Billett AL, et al: Stereotactic radiotherapy for localized low-grade gliomas in children: final results of a prospective trial. Int J Radiat Oncol Biol Phys 61:374-379, 2005.
29. Dorffel W, Luders H, Ruhl U, et al: Preliminary results of the multicenter trial GPOH-HD 95 for the treatment of Hodgkin's disease in children and adolescents: analysis and outlook. Klin Padiatr 215:139-145, 2003.
30. Ruhl U, Albrecht MR, Lueders H, et al: The German multinational GPOH-HD 95 trial: treatment results and analysis of failures in pediatric Hodgkin's disease using combination chemotherapy with and without radiation. Int J Radiat Oncol Biol Phys 60:S131, 2004.
31. Tekautz TM, Fuller CE, Blaney S, et al: Atypical teratoid/rhabdoid tumors (ATRT): improved survival in children 3 years of age and older with radiation therapy and high-dose alkylator-based chemotherapy. J Clin Oncol 23:1491-1499, 2005.

32. Blaney SM, Boyett J, Friedman H, et al: Phase I clinical trial of mafosfamide in infants and children aged 3 years or younger with newly diagnosed embryonal tumors: a Pediatric Brain Tumor Consortium study (PBTC-001). J Clin Oncol 23:525-531, 2005.
33. Duffner PK, Krischer JP, Sanford RA, et al: Prognostic factors in infants and very young children with intracranial ependymomas. Pediatr Neurosurg 28:215-222, 1998.
34. Wharam MD, Hanfelt JJ, Tefft MC, et al: Radiation therapy for rhabdomyosarcoma: local failure risk for clinical group III patients on Intergroup Rhabdomyosarcoma Study II. Int J Radiat Oncol Biol Phys 38:797-804, 1997.
35. Michalski JM, Meza J, Breneman JC, et al: Influence of radiation therapy parameters on outcome in children treated with radiation therapy for localized parameningeal rhabdomyosarcoma in Intergroup Rhabdomyosarcoma Study Group trials II through IV. Int J Radiat Oncol Biol Phys 59:1027-1038, 2004.
36. Nachman JB, Sposto R, Herzog P, et al: Randomized comparison of low-dose involved-field radiotherapy and no radiotherapy for children with Hodgkin's disease who achieve a complete response to chemotherapy. J Clin Oncol 20:3765-3771, 2002.
37. Wolden SL, Dunkel IJ, Souweidane MM, et al: Patterns of failure using a conformal radiation therapy tumor bed boost for medulloblastoma. J Clin Oncol 21:3079-3083, 2003.
38. Saran FH, Baumert BG, Khoo VS, et al: Stereotactically guided conformal radiotherapy for progressive low-grade gliomas of childhood. Int J Radiat Oncol Biol Phys 53:43-51, 2002.
39. Krasin MJ, Crawford BT, Zhu Y, et al: Intensity-modulated radiation therapy for children with intraocular retinoblastoma: potential sparing of the bony orbit. Clin Oncol (R Coll Radiol) 6:215-222, 2004.
40. Merchant TE, Gould CJ, Xiong X, et al: Early neuro-otologic effects of three-dimensional irradiation in children with primary brain tumors. Int J Radiat Oncol Biol Phys 58:1194-1207, 2004.
41. Yock T, Schneider R, Friedmann A, et al: Proton radiotherapy for orbital rhabdomyosarcoma: clinical outcome and a dosimetric comparison with photons. Int J Radiat Oncol Biol Phys 63:1161-1168, 2005.
42. Hug EB, Muenter MW, Archambeau JO, et al: Conformal proton radiation therapy for pediatric low-grade astrocytomas. Strahlenther Onkol 178:10-17, 2002.
43. Merchant TE, Zhu Y, Thompson SJ, et al: Preliminary results from a phase II trial of conformal radiation therapy for pediatric patients with localised low-grade astrocytoma and ependymoma. Int J Radiat Oncol Biol Phys 52:325-332, 2002.
44. Valerie K, Dritschilo A, McKenna G, et al: Novel molecular targets for tumor radiosensitization: Molecular Radiation Biology and Oncology Workshop: translation of molecular mechanisms into clinical radiotherapy. Int J Cancer 90:51-58, 2000.
45. Delmas C, Heliez C, Cohen-Jonathan E, et al: Farnesyltransferase inhibitor, R115777, reverses the resistance of human glioma cell lines to ionizing radiation. Int J Cancer 100:43-48, 2002.
46. Litzow MR, Perez WS, Klein JP, et al: Comparison of outcome following allogeneic bone marrow transplantation with cyclophosphamide-total body irradiation versus busulphan-cyclophosphamide conditioning regimens for acute myelogenous leukaemia in first remission. Br J Haematol 119:1115-1124, 2002.
47. Woolfrey AE, Anasetti C, Storer B, et al: Factors associated with outcome after unrelated marrow transplantation for treatment of acute lymphoblastic leukemia in children. Blood 99:2002-2008, 2002.
48. Williams GB, Kun LE, Thompson JW, et al: Hearing loss as a late complication of radiotherapy in children with brain tumors. Ann Otol Rhinol Laryngol 114:328-331, 2005.
49. Gurney JG, Kadan-Lottick NS, Packer RJ, et al: Endocrine and cardiovascular late effects among adult survivors of childhood brain tumors: Childhood Cancer Survivor Study. Cancer 97:663-673, 2003.
50. Kenney LB, Yasui Y, Inskip PD, et al: Breast cancer after childhood cancer: a report from the Childhood Cancer Survivor Study. Ann Intern Med 141:590-597, 2004.
51. Pein F, Sakiroglu O, Dahan M, et al: Cardiac abnormalities 15 years and more after adriamycin therapy in 229 childhood survivors of a solid tumour at the Institut Gustave Roussy. Br J Cancer 91:37-44, 2004.
52. Lipshultz SE, Rifai N, Dalton VM, et al: The effect of dexrazoxane on myocardial injury in doxorubicin-treated children with acute lymphoblastic leukemia. N Engl J Med 351:145-153, 2004.
53. Green DM, Grigoriev YA, Nan B, et al: Congestive heart failure after treatment for Wilms' tumor: a report from the National Wilms' Tumor Study Group. J Clin Oncol 19:1926-1934, 2001.
54. Thomas PR, Griffith KD, Fineberg BB, et al: Late effects of treatment for Wilms' tumor. Int J Radiat Oncol Biol Phys 9:651-657, 1983.
55. van der Pal HJ, van Dalen EC, Kremer LC, et al: Risk of morbidity and mortality from cardiovascular disease following radiotherapy for childhood cancer: a systematic review. Cancer Treat Rev 31:173-185, 2005.
56. Jakacki RI, Goldwein JW, Larsen RL, et al: Cardiac dysfunction following spinal irradiation during childhood. J Clin Oncol 11:1033-1038, 1993.
57. Mertens AC, Yasui Y, Liu Y, et al: Pulmonary complications in survivors of childhood and adolescent cancer. A report from the Childhood Cancer Survivor Study. Cancer 95:2431-2441, 2002.
58. Ritchey ML, Green DM, Thomas PR, et al: Renal failure in Wilms' tumor patients: a report from the National Wilms' Tumor Study Group. Med Pediatr Oncol 26:75-80, 1996.
59. Irwin C, Fyles A, Wong CS, et al: Late renal function following whole abdominal irradiation. Radiother Oncol 38:257-261, 1996.
60. Tefft M, Mitus A, Das L, et al: Irradiation of the liver in children: review of experience in the acute and chronic phases, and in the intact normal and partially resected. AJR Am J Roentgenol 108:365-385, 1990.
61. Rajakulasingam K, Cerullo LJ, Raimondi AJ: Childhood moyamoya syndrome. Postradiation pathogenesis. Childs Brain 5:467-475, 1979.
62. Rudoltz MS, Regine WF, Langston JW, et al: Multiple causes of cerebrovascular events in children with tumors of the parasellar region. J Neurooncol 37:251-261, 1998.
63. Grill J, Couanet D, Cappelli C, et al: Radiation-induced cerebral vasculopathy in children with neurofibromatosis and optic pathway glioma. Ann Neurol 45:393-396, 1999.
64. Hancock SL, McDougall IR, Constine LS: Thyroid abnormalities after therapeutic external radiation. Int J Radiat Oncol Biol Phys 31:1165-1170, 1995.
65. Shalet SM, Brennan BM: Puberty in children with cancer. Horm Res 57(Suppl 2):39-42, 2002.
66. Grill J, Renaux VK, Bulteau C, et al: Long-term intellectual outcome in children with posterior fossa tumors according to radiation doses and volumes. Int J Radiat Oncol Biol Phys 45:137-145, 1999.
67. Walter AW, Mulhern RK, Gajjar A, et al: Survival and neurodevelopmental outcome of young children with medulloblastoma at St Jude Children's Research Hospital. J Clin Oncol 17:3720-3728, 1999.
68. Ris MD, Packer R, Goldwein J, et al: Intellectual outcome after reduced-dose radiation therapy plus adjuvant chemotherapy for medulloblastoma: a Children's Cancer Group study. J Clin Oncol 19:3470-3476, 2001.
69. Palmer SL, Gajjar A, Reddick WE, et al: Predicting intellectual outcome among children treated with 35-40 Gy craniospinal irradiation for medulloblastoma. Neuropsychology 17:548-555, 2003.
70. Butler RW, Mulhern RK: Neurocognitive interventions for children and adolescents surviving cancer. J Pediatr Psychol 30:65-78, 2005.
71. Mulhern RK, Khan RB, Kaplan S, et al: Short-term efficacy of methylphenidate: a randomized, double-blind, placebo-controlled trial among survivors of childhood cancer. J Clin Oncol 22:4795-4803, 2004.
72. Gold DG, Neglia JP, Dusenbery KE: Second neoplasms after megavoltage radiation for pediatric tumors. Cancer 97:2588-2596, 2003.
73. Hawkins MM: Second primary tumors following radiotherapy for childhood cancer. Int J Radiat Oncol Biol Phys 19:1297-1301, 1990.
74. Sankila R, Garwicz S, Olsen JH, et al: Risk of subsequent malignant neoplasms among 1,641 Hodgkin's disease patients diagnosed in childhood and adolescence: a population-based cohort study in the five Nordic countries. Association of the Nordic

Cancer Registries and the Nordic Society of Pediatric Hematology and Oncology. J Clin Oncol 14:1442-1446, 1996.
75. Neglia JP, Meadows AT, Robison LL, et al: Second neoplasms after acute lymphoblastic leukemia in childhood. N Engl J Med 325:1330-1336, 1991.
76. Guibout C, Adjadj E, Rubino C, et al: Malignant breast tumors after radiotherapy for a first cancer during childhood. J Clin Oncol 23:197-204, 2005.
77. Hancock SL, Tucker MA, Hoppe RT: Breast cancer after treatment of Hodgkin's disease. J Natl Cancer Inst 85:25-31, 1993.
78. Bhatia S, Robison LL, Oberlin O, et al: Breast cancer and other second neoplasms after childhood Hodgkin's disease. N Engl J Med 334:745-751, 1996.
79. Relling MV, Rubnitz JE, Rivera GK, et al: High incidence of secondary brain tumours after radiotherapy and antimetabolites. Lancet 354:34-39, 1999.
80. Edick MJ, Cheng C, Yang W, et al: Lymphoid gene expression as a predictor of risk of secondary brain tumors. Genes Chromosomes Cancer 42:107-116, 2005.
81. Melean G, Sestini R, Ammannati F, Papi L: Genetic insights into familial tumors of the nervous system. Am J Med Genet C Semin Med Genet 129:74-84, 2004.
82. Lynch HT, Shaw TG, Lynch JF: Inherited predisposition to cancer: a historical overview. Am J Med Genet C Semin Med Genet 129:5-22, 2004.
83. Swift M, Sholman L, Perry M, Chase C: Malignant neoplasms in the families of patients with ataxia-telangiectasia. Cancer Res 36:209-215, 1976.
84. Romer J, Curran T: Targeting medulloblastoma: small-molecule inhibitors of the Sonic Hedgehog pathway as potential cancer therapeutics. Cancer Res 65:4975-4978, 2005.
85. Wetmore C, Eberhart DE, Curran T: The normal patched allele is expressed in medulloblastomas from mice with heterozygous germ-line mutation of patched. Cancer Res 60:2239-2246, 2000.
86. Fletcher O, Easton D, Anderson K, et al: Lifetime risks of common cancers among retinoblastoma survivors. J Natl Cancer Inst 96:357-363, 2004.
87. Moll AC, Imhof SM, Schouten-Van Meeteren AY, et al: Second primary tumors in hereditary retinoblastoma: a register-based study, 1945-1997: is there an age effect on radiation-related risk? Ophthalmology 108:1109-1114, 2001.
88. Walter AW, Hancock ML, Pui CH, et al: Secondary brain tumors in children treated for acute lymphoblastic leukemia at St. Jude Children's Research Hospital. J Clin Oncol 16:3761-3767, 1998.

CHAPTER 64

CENTRAL NERVOUS SYSTEM TUMORS IN CHILDREN

Thomas E. Merchant

INCIDENCE AND OVERALL SURVIVAL

Annual incidence of 3 cases per 100,000 population ages 0 to 19 years.

There are 3000 cases annually in United States, including all brain and spinal cord tumors.

The 5-year overall survival has increased from 60% (1975-1984) to 65% (1985-1994) to 68% (1995-2004).

ETIOLOGY

Parental employment in agricultural, electrical, or motor-vehicle–related occupations and textile industry. Prenatal diagnostic and postnatal exposure to ionizing radiation; prenatal exposure to *N*-nitrosamines and *N*-nitrosamides, insecticides, herbicides, and agricultural and nonagricultural fungicides. Parental exposures to polycyclic aromatic hydrocarbons including chemical, petrochemical, and paint exposures. Family history of malignant brain tumor.

Genetic syndromes including neurofibromatosis, Li-Fraumeni syndrome, Gorlin's syndrome, Turcot's syndrome, and ataxia telangiectasia.

Biologic features include mutations of *p53* (predominantly glioma in young patients), loss of 22q (ependymoma), and alterations in the tumor suppressor *NF1* and *NF2* genes on chromosomes 17q and 22q, respectively.

HISTOLOGIC SUBTYPES

- Astrocytic tumors
  - Pilocytic astrocytoma (World Health Organization [WHO] grade I)
  - Pleomorphic xanthoastrocytoma (WHO grade I)
  - Astrocytoma (WHO grade II)
  - Anaplastic astrocytoma (WHO grade III)
  - Glioblastoma multiforme (WHO grade IV)
  - Oligodendroglial tumors
  - Oligodendroglioma (WHO grade II)
  - Anaplastic oligodendroglioma (WHO grade III)
- Ependymoma
  - Ependymoma (cellular, papillary, clear cell)
  - Anaplastic ependymoma
  - Myxopapillary ependymoma
- Mixed glioma
- Tumors of uncertain origin
  - Astroblastoma
- Choroid plexus tumors
  - Choroid plexus papilloma
  - Choroid plexus carcinoma
- Neuronal and glial-neuronal tumors
  - Ganglioglioma
  - Central neurocytoma
  - Dysembryoplastic neuroepithelial tumor
- Embryonal tumors
  - Primitive neuroectodermal tumors
    - Infratentorial primitive neuroectodermal tumor (PNET) including medulloblastoma
    - Supratentorial PNET including pineoblastoma
  - Atypical teratoid rhabdoid tumor
- Craniopharyngioma
- Meningioma
- Germ cell tumors
  - Germinoma
  - Nongerminomatous germ cell tumors
    - Embryonal carcinoma
    - Yolk sac tumor
    - Choriocarcinoma
    - Teratoma
    - Mixed germ cell tumors

EVALUATION

History and physical examination (all patients)

Magnetic resonance imaging (MRI) of the brain and spine (all patients, but spinal imaging may be omitted for localized astrocytoma)

Computed tomography (CT) for craniopharyngioma and germ cell tumors

Lumbar cerebrospinal fluid (CSF) cytology for embryonal tumors, germ cell tumors, ependymoma

Alpha-fetoprotein and ß-human chorionic gonadotropin for germ cell tumors

THERAPY

- Surgery
  - No biopsy—certain optic pathway gliomas and germ cell tumors
  - Biopsy—accessible optic pathway gliomas and germ cell tumors
  - Subtotal resection—limited or decompressive surgery to alleviate symptoms including low-grade glioma, craniopharyngioma, germ cell tumor, myxopapillary ependymoma
  - Gross-total resection—maximal resection compatible with acceptable neurologic outcome, for patients with embryonal tumor, high-grade glioma, ependymoma, certain low-grade glioma, and primary spinal cord tumor
  - Ventriculostomy and/or CSF shunting—symptomatic or persistent hydrocephalus with or without biopsy or attempted resection
- Radiation therapy
  - Craniospinal irradiation—required for cases of neuraxis dissemination or tumors with high propensity to neuraxis dissemination including embryonal tumors and germ cell tumors (governed by the age of the patient, generally older than 3 years)
  - Focal irradiation—low- and high-grade glioma, ependymoma, craniopharyngioma, meningioma, localized spinal cord tumors, pituitary tumors, and germinoma treated with combined modality therapy
- Chemotherapy
- Radiation therapy delayed or avoided—embryonal tumors (age < 36 months), low-grade glioma (typically young patients with age limits undefined)
- Combined modality therapy—embryonal tumors, germ cell tumors, high-grade glioma, brainstem glioma

CURRENT TRENDS

Radiation therapy continues to play an important role in the treatment of pediatric central nervous system (CNS) tumors.

Reducing late effects through reductions in radiation dose and volume are important issues.

The acceptable age for irradiation has been lowered from 36 to 12 months in clinical trials for patients with embryonal tumors and ependymoma.

The acceptable age for irradiation for patients with low-grade astrocytoma remains undefined.

Disease-control and functional outcomes for children with CNS tumors continues to improve.

The central role radiation therapy currently plays in treating pediatric brain tumors could not have been predicted a decade ago. Radiation therapy avoidance was at its peak then and was the central theme of clinical trial designs in pediatric neuro-oncology. The resurgence of radiation therapy as a frontline treatment and its application in very young children has resulted from a number of simultaneous developments.

Investigators recognized that treatment regimens omitting or delaying irradiation had inferior disease control. This difference was demonstrated in successive prospective trials for embryonal tumors in children younger than 3 years and by comparing disease control between younger and older patients. Patients treated on regimens without radiation therapy experienced acute and long-term side effects that would have otherwise been attributed to radiation therapy, and prospective research showed a high incidence of morbidity in newly diagnosed patients. Newer radiation methods also came about at a time when the need for a "new agent" was greatest—when chemotherapy dose intensification showed no benefit over conventional dose regimens. The advent of magnetic resonance imaging (MRI) and its increasing availability during the past 2 decades has directly impacted the diagnosis, staging, neurosurgery, chemotherapy response evaluation, radiation therapy planning, and surveillance of these patients. Image-guided neurosurgical navigation came of age, including widespread use of the operative microscope, improving the rate of tumor resection and the ability of radiation therapy to eradicate local tumors. Investigators initiated studies to systematically reduce radiation dose and volume with or without adjuvant chemotherapy. The most important development having an impact on radiation therapy was the advent of three-dimensional radiation therapy planning. The dosimetry advantages were obvious and understood by the larger neuro-oncology community. Although limited data have been generated from single institution studies, the first clinical trials implementing conformal treatment technology are currently underway.

This is a pivotal time for radiation therapy in the treatment of children with brain tumors. Despite the increasing availability of advanced treatment technology, children should be treated on clinical trials designed to improve tumor control, to objectively study CNS effects, and to build a consensus for treatment guidelines. Even though the impact of pediatric CNS tumors on public health is small—there are fewer than 3000 cases diagnosed annually in the United States—these patients provoke tremendous emotion and represent 20% of all childhood malignancies.[1] Most children with brain tumors require radiation therapy during the course of their management. Broadly subdivided into the more common gliomas (1648 cases/year), embryonal tumors (484 cases/year), ependymomas (200 cases/year), germ cell tumors (131 cases/year), craniopharyngiomas (100 cases/year), and pituitary tumors (92 cases/year), these tumors require special care and remain a leading cause of cancer death in children.

EMBRYONAL CNS TUMORS

Embryonal tumors of the CNS are the most common malignant brain tumors in children. They are characterized by their infiltrative nature, aggressive patterns of growth, propensity for dissemination, and common need for intensive combined modality therapy. These tumors are found throughout the CNS and are further classified according to histologic and molecular features into two groups: primitive neuroectodermal tumor (PNET) and atypical teratoid/rhabdoid tumor (ATRT). PNET includes two distinct entities, medulloblastoma (Fig. 64-1) and pineoblastoma (Fig. 64-2), named for their site of origin in the posterior fossa and pineal region, respectively. Regarding classification, the radiation oncologist should be aware of the aggressive histologic variant of medulloblastoma (large cell anaplastic medulloblastoma) that is more prone to cerebrospinal fluid (CSF) dissemination.[2,3] They should also know that the pathologist is now able to more consistently identify genetic abnormalities such as monosomy 22 or deletion of 22q11 and alterations in the *INI1* gene characteristic of ATRT.[4] ATRTs unknowingly were considered the same as other PNETs but are now known to carry a worse prognosis.

Medulloblastoma and supratentorial PNET are commonly diagnosed in young children. The relatively large number of patients and the cooperative spirit among neurosurgeons, pediatric oncologists, and radiation oncologists have led to considerable understanding and progress in the treatment of these tumors. Patients are risk classified for treatment based on the most important prognostic factors for tumor control: extent of disease, extent of resection, and age at the time of irradiation (the most important prognostic factor for functional outcome). The treatment for patients with embryonal tumors of the CNS is remarkably similar regardless of subtype or tumor location and consists of surgery, postoperative radiation therapy, and chemotherapy. The requirement of craniospinal irradiation, regardless of extent of disease, is the element that distinguishes the treatment of these tumors. Approximately one third of patients present with neuraxis dissemination at the time of diagnosis as determined by MRI of the brain and spine (Fig. 64-3) and CSF cytology.[5] Because the negative predictive value of these staging procedures remains relatively low, and the most common mode of failure remains distant, craniospinal irradiation (CSI) is a mainstay in the treatment of these tumors.[6]

The side effects attributed to radiation therapy are a primary concern for patients with medulloblastoma. The concern is greatest for patients with average-risk disease, for whom long-term disease control is likely and the side effects of therapy have a lasting impact. The treatment of this tumor is technically demanding and consists of CSI that has also included boost treatment of the anatomic posterior fossa. Until recently, the standard of care for an average-risk patient was postoperative CSI to 36 Gy and a boost treatment to 54 Gy

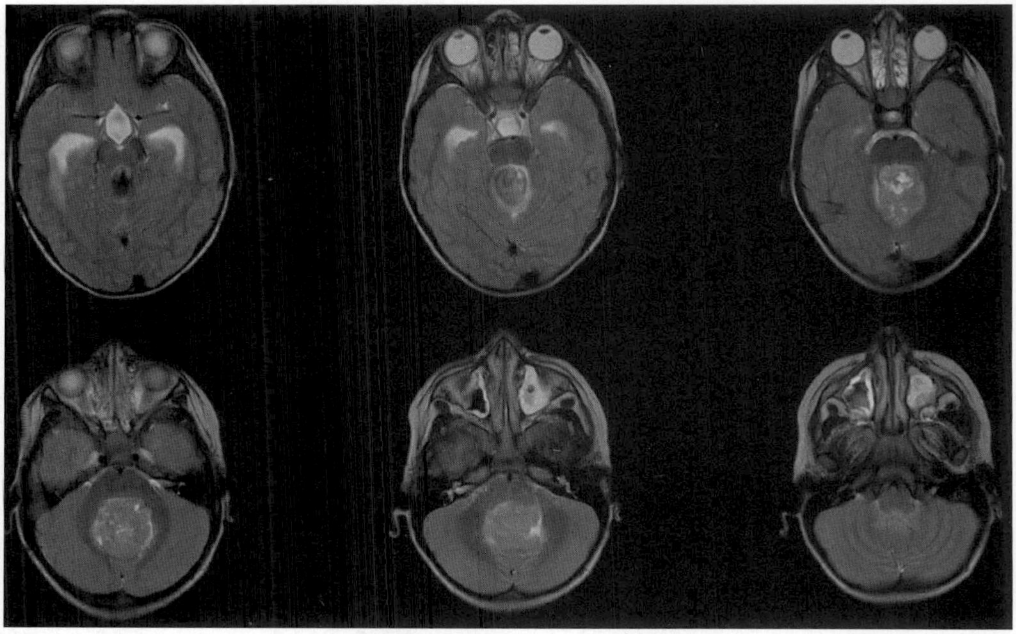

Figure 64-1 A IVth ventricular tumor (medulloblastoma) on T2-weighted MRI. Dilated temporal horns result from obstructive hydrocephalus.

using conventional fractionation of 1.8 Gy/day. In a cooperative group trial, CSI dose was lowered to 23.4 Gy for average-risk patients in a randomized comparison with 36 Gy CSI. This trial showed an increased risk of relapse in patients receiving the reduced CSI dose.[7] Multiagent chemotherapy combined with reduced-dose CSI was found to be equivalent to standard-dose CSI and now has been adopted as a treatment standard for average-risk patients.[8] Cognitive impairment continues to be a significant problem with an IQ loss of 4.3 points per year reported from a recent single arm trial of low-dose (23.4 Gy) CSI and chemotherapy.[9]

The most recent Children's Oncology Group (COG) study sought to define the best chemotherapy regimen (lomustine [CCNU], cisplatin, vincristine vs cyclophosphamide, cisplatin, vincristine) to accompany low-dose CSI and the standard posterior fossa boost. No differences were observed in disease control (3-year event-free survival > 83% in both arms); however, patients treated with the cyclophosphamide-containing regimen appeared to have more severe toxicity (18% vs 25%).[10] Attention has now turned to combining the two chemotherapy regimens and randomizing patients between 18 Gy and 23.4 Gy CSI, followed by a second randomization between conventional boost treatment and treatment of less than the entire posterior fossa. This is an ambitious four-arm randomized trial developed for pediatric patients between the ages of 3 and 8 years. For those older than 8 years, the CSI dose will remain 23.4 Gy, and the trial will also include a randomized comparison of conventional posterior fossa boost and boost treatment of the tumor bed using a 1.5-cm clinical target volume margin.

Reducing the CSI dose does little to reduce the volume that receives the highest doses because the boost dose is prescribed to the entire posterior fossa. Reducing the boost volume for average-risk patients from the entire posterior fossa to the tumor bed with a limited margin is recognized as critical to the goal of reducing the normal tissue volume that receives the highest doses (Fig. 64-4).

Treatment of less than the entire posterior fossa after 23.4 Gy CSI using focal radiation delivery techniques appears to be as effective as treatment of the entire posterior fossa based on recent trial results from St. Jude Children's Research Hospital and participating centers involving 84 patients. In this prospective trial, the cumulative incidence of posterior fossa failure was only 6.3% at 3 years.[11] Treatment for these patients included postoperative CSI to 23.4 Gy, conformal posterior fossa boost to 36 Gy, and focal treatment of the tumor bed with a 2-cm margin. Chemotherapy was administered after radiation therapy. Patients in this study experienced a dose reduction to the anatomic posterior fossa of approximately 13%. The risks associated with reducing the CSI dose and limiting the boost treatment to the postoperative tumor bed with a limited margin must be balanced against the observed effects of radiation therapy on cognition, neurologic function, and growth and development.

Hyperfractionation for reducing toxicity is currently being tested in Europe.[12] Pursuit of different strategies in the United States and abroad may someday provide the basis for a worldwide trial for patients with medulloblastoma.

Current cooperative group trials for very young children (younger than 3 years) with medulloblastoma highlight the importance of radiation therapy in the treatment of these tumors. The current COG protocol for children younger than 3 years with localized medulloblastoma includes 20 weeks of combination chemotherapy followed by a second surgery, when indicated, and sequential irradiation of the posterior fossa and primary site before 20 additional weeks of maintenance chemotherapy.[13] CSI has been omitted for these patients, and the doses to the posterior fossa (18-23.4 Gy) and primary site (45-54 Gy) are prescribed based on patient age, response, and risk status. A similar strategy was used in the Pediatric Brain Tumor Consortium (PBTC) protocol for similar patients with one exception: Intrathecal chemotherapy (mafosfamide) was given during the first 20 weeks of chemotherapy as a substitute for CSI.[14] Both protocols included radiation therapy after 20 weeks based on results from prior trials that showed a median time to progression of approximately 24 weeks.[15,16] The targeting guidelines used in these studies are largely empirical—investigators attempt to minimize the dose to normal tissues while maintaining an acceptable rate of local tumor control.

Fear of cognitive deficits is the driving force in the design of current treatment trials for this young patient population.

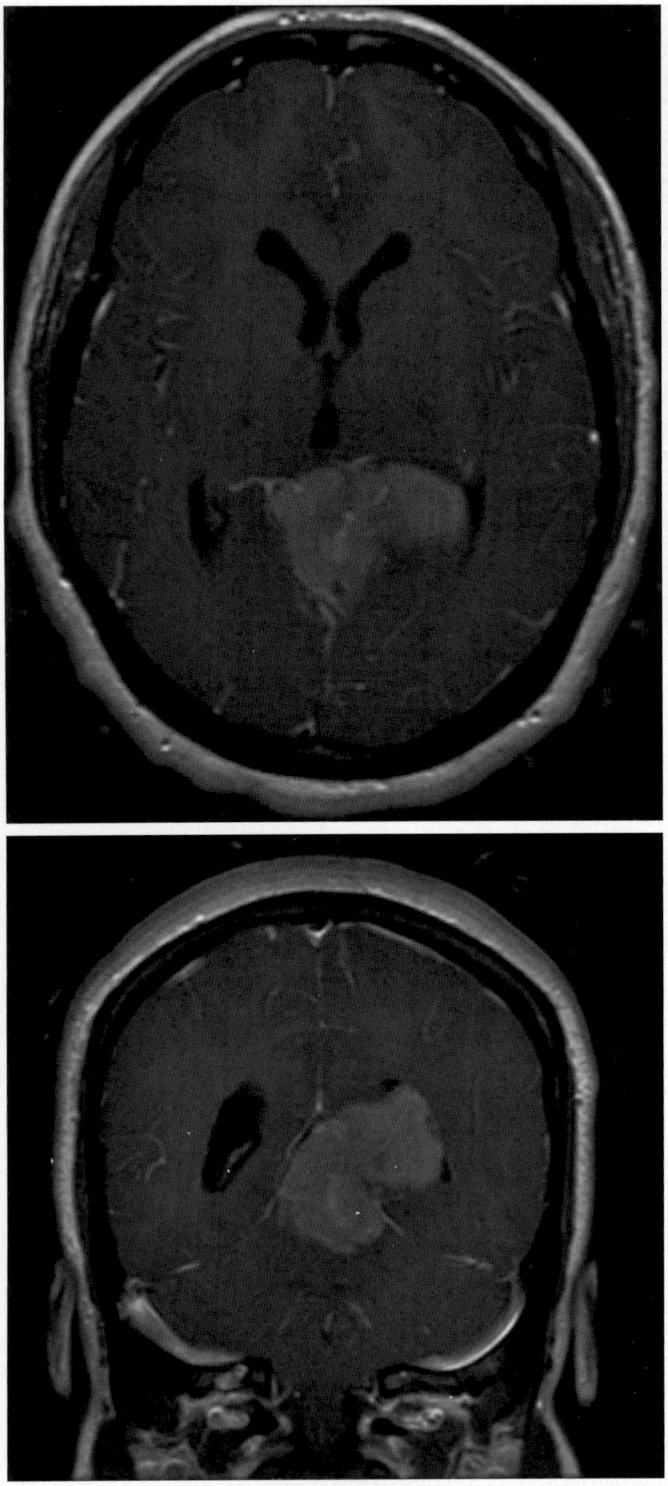

Figure 64-2 Pineal region tumor (pineoblastoma) on axial (*upper*) and coronal (*lower*) postcontrast T1-weighted MRI.

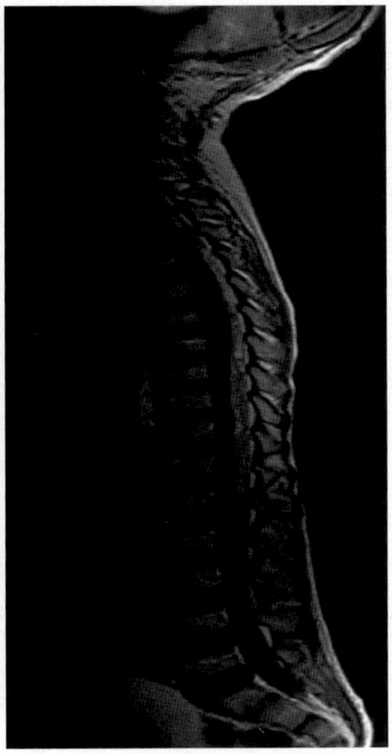

Figure 64-3 Sagittal postcontrast T1-weighted MRI demonstrating metastatic medulloblastoma filling the spinal subarachnoid space.

For very young children with medulloblastoma, a persistent decline in cognitive function has been observed by Walter and colleagues.[17] The decline is not surprising given the median cranial dose of 35.2 Gy for patients with a median age of 2.6 years and the additive effects of the tumor, surgery, and chemotherapy. Because a significant decline has also been observed for older children with medulloblastoma treated with lower craniospinal doses,[9] CSI for the youngest children no longer appears to be a reasonable treatment option. Data concerning the effectiveness of yet lower CSI doses are extremely limited.[18] These findings form the basis of the current COG and PBTC trials for very young children. CSI has been omitted with the hope that the side effects of treatment will be reduced enough to provide for a meaningful quality of life among long-term survivors.

EPENDYMOMA

Ependymoma is the third most common CNS tumor in children, affecting approximately 200 individuals younger than 19 years annually in the United States.[1] It shares many of the clinical characteristics of more common gliomas, embryonal tumors, and less common germ cell tumors. Ependymoma may occur anywhere within the CNS and has the highest prevalence within the posterior fossa arising from the floor or roof of the IVth ventricle or cerebellopontine angle where it is known to invade the brainstem or envelop cranial nerves or vascular structures. Ependymoma also arises within the parenchyma of the cerebral hemispheres in older patients and, rarely, in the spinal cord. The interval from the onset of symptoms to diagnosis may be influenced by the young age at the time of diagnosis, the perceived slow growth rate of this tumor, and the remitting signs and symptoms of increased intracranial pressure resulting from obstructive hydrocephalus.

Ependymoma is most commonly diagnosed in children who are younger than 4 years of age. For the past 2 decades, progress in the treatment of this tumor has been slowed by concerns about late effects. Recent advances in neuroimaging, surgery, and radiation therapy have moved the field of neuro-oncology forward in the treatment of this tumor resulting in more acceptable outcomes and providing new disease control benchmarks. Investigators treating these patients with

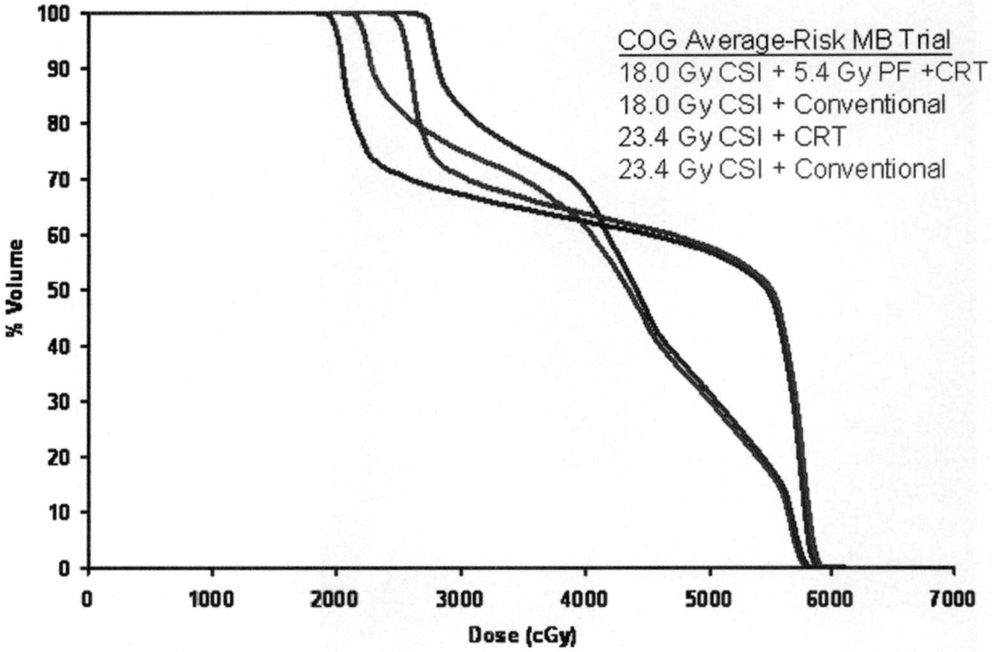

Figure 64-4 Left-temporal lobe cumulative dose-volume histogram simulated for a typical average-risk medulloblastoma (MB) patient treated according to the four arms of the current medulloblastoma study of the Children's Oncology Group (COG). The trial includes randomization of CSI (craniospinal irradiation) dose (18 Gy vs 23.4 Gy) and randomization of primary site boost volume (conventional posterior fossa volume [PF] vs conformal radiation therapy of tumor/tumor bed + 1.5 cm clinical target volume margin) to 55.8 Gy. CRT, conformal radiation therapy.

contemporary surgery and radiation therapy have been able to increase the 3-year event-free survival from approximately 55% to 62% to 75% with remarkably limited treatment-related effects.[19,20]

The standard of care for a child with *localized* ependymoma is to attempt gross-total resection, perform a second surgery for potentially resectable residual tumor, and proceed with postoperative radiation therapy directed at the primary site using a 10-mm, anatomically-confined, clinical target volume surrounding the residual tumor or tumor bed, or both, as defined on postoperative neuroimaging. The recommended total dose is 59.4 Gy using conventional fractionation, because these tumors are prone to recur locally. Conventions regarding organs at risk apply; for patients with tumors arising in the lower aspect of the posterior fossa, avoidance of the spinal cord should be considered after 54 Gy. Special considerations for patients with posterior fossa tumors may apply to very young children (generally younger than 18 months) with no evidence of a residual tumor, or patients who have signs and symptoms of severe brainstem injury after resection (postoperative seizure, hypertension, and ischemic changes on neuroimaging) who are at increased risk for necrosis. Although data support the irradiation of children with ependymoma under the age of 3 years, the current trial of the COG seeks to form a national consensus and supports the enrollment of children as young as 12 months for postoperative irradiation (see *www.clinicaltrials.gov* NLM Identifier NCT00027846).

The prognosis for a patient with ependymoma is determined by tumor grade and extent of resection.[21-23] Patients with overtly anaplastic tumors have inferior disease control compared to those with differentiated tumors; however, the assignment of tumor grade can be difficult for those cases where focal anaplasia occurs in the setting of a largely differentiated tumor. All patients should be treated with curative intent regardless of tumor grade. Extent of resection is an unequivocal prognostic factor: patients with substantial residual tumor have the worst prognosis. Because patients with varying amounts of residual tumor have achieved long-term survival after radiation therapy and modern surgical resection has altered the definition of near-total and subtotal resection, the volume of residual tumor differentiating between patients with good and poor prognosis remains unknown. Radiation oncologists contribute to the care of a child with ependymoma when they emphasize the need for resection of residual tumor before the initiation of radiation therapy (Fig. 64-5).

HIGH-GRADE ASTROCYTOMA

Although astrocytoma is the most common brain tumor in adults and children, major differences exist in the relative proportion of the various tumor subtypes and their management and outcomes. Tumors such as glioblastoma multiforme (GBM), anaplastic astrocytoma, anaplastic oligodendroglioma, malignant pleomorphic xanthoastrocytoma, and other malignant glial-neuronal tumors are uncommon in children, representing fewer than 10% of pediatric brain tumors, and are rarely seen in children younger than 4 years. Resection compatible with acceptable neurologic outcome followed by postoperative radiation therapy to dose levels approaching 59.4 Gy, using generous clinical target volume margins surrounding the residual tumor, tumor bed, and suspicious abnormality on neuroimaging, are standard. Concurrent or postirradiation chemotherapy using conventional or investigational agents is routinely administered for patients with glioblastoma and anaplastic astrocytoma and on an individual basis for the other tumor types. For targeting purposes, the radiation oncologist should be aware that children with high-grade brain tumors may present with extensive changes throughout the brain that represent tumor extension along white matter tracts (Fig. 64-6), that neuraxis dissemination is not uncommon and should be ruled out before irradiation, and that treatment volumes for these patients may appear to be relatively large but should not be compromised because of the patient's age despite the myth that children with high-grade brain tumors stand a better chance of survival than their adult counterparts.

One irreproducible study showed a benefit for chemotherapy.[24] This study included a randomization of 58 patients with

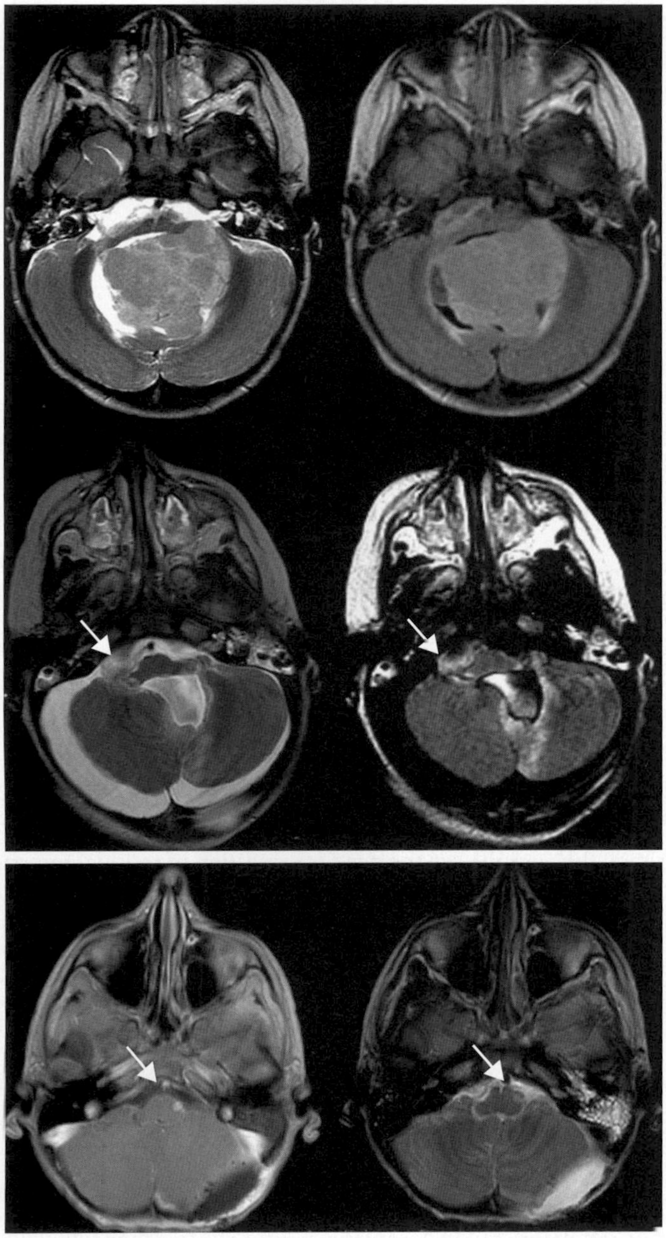

Figure 64-5 Ependymoma of the IVth ventricle with preoperative extension through the left foramen of Luschka to cerebellopontine angle on T2-weighted (*upper left*) and fluid-attenuated inversion recovery (*upper right*). MRI and postoperative residual tumor (*arrows*) anterolateral to brainstem is described as subtotal resection (*center*). Separate case of ependymoma showing postoperative residual tumor (*arrow*) is described as near-total resection.

high-grade astrocytoma to local irradiation versus local irradiation plus weekly vincristine followed by 12 months of carmustine, vincristine, and prednisone. The reported 5-year progression-free survival (PFS) rate was 18% versus 46% favoring the use of chemotherapy, and patients with GBM (n = 40) had a 5-year PFS of 6% versus 42% favoring the use of chemotherapy. A larger study with 172 patients randomized between local irradiation versus local irradiation plus pre- and postirradiation 8-in-1 chemotherapy (vincristine, carmustine, procarbazine, cytarabine, hydroxyurea, cisplatin, dacarbazine, and methylprednisolone) showed no difference between the two arms with a 5-year PFS of 26% and 33%, respectively.[25] This study was illustrative for the lack of concordance between institutional and expert pathology review. Thirty percent of patients in this study did not have high-grade glioma, and the survival estimates were in fact lower than originally reported.[26]

LOW-GRADE ASTROCYTOMA

Low-grade astrocytomas are found throughout the nervous system in children, yet are clustered predominantly in subsites of the cerebellum (cerebellum, cerebellar peduncles, and dorsally exophytic brainstem glioma) or diencephalon including the optic chiasm, optic pathways, hypothalamus, and thalami (Fig. 64-7). Slow-growing tumors located in these critical links of the nervous and endocrine systems result in presenting signs and symptoms that differ markedly from the other types of pediatric tumors, which are prone to obstruction of CSF pathways. Loss of vision, dysdiadochokinesia, dysmetria, ataxia, tremor, endocrinopathies including precocious puberty, and cognitive dysfunction are a few of the insidious signs and symptoms that are often overlooked in the developing child and lead to well-established deficits.

Few inroads have been made in radiation therapy for pediatric low-grade astrocytoma in recent years, mainly because most who would be candidates for radiation therapy are younger children with optic pathway tumors. However, advances in surgery have resulted in successful primary resection of most cerebellar and peripheral cerebral lesions with long-term disease control exceeding 90% when measured at 5 years. In the setting of residual tumor after initial resection and in the absence of persistent symptoms, most children should follow a course of observation with second surgery at the time of progression contingent on the associated risks. In a landmark study conducted from 1991 to 1996, which enrolled 726 patients with the intention of observation after surgery, the PFS at 5 years was 92% for patients after gross-total resection, 53% with near-total resection, and 61% with subtotal resection. More than 75% of patients had juvenile pilocytic astrocytoma, and PFS was lowest in midline (59%) and hypothalamic-chiasmatic tumors (50%) compared to tumors of the cerebellar hemisphere (89%), cerebellar vermis (84%), and cerebral hemisphere (89%).[27] Without information regarding the ability of follow-up surgery to render these individuals disease free or symptom free, disease-free or asymptomatic these individuals, a large proportion of patients remain candidates for adjuvant therapy including external beam radiation therapy.

Newly diagnosed patients with optic pathway tumors present a formidable challenge to the entire oncology team, and many radiation oncologists avoid rendering opinions. Radiation therapy is the most effective treatment for optic pathway tumors, combining noninvasive therapy with durable tumor control in the majority of patients and an excellent track record in stabilizing and, in rare cases, reversing symptoms. Surgery may have a role to play when decompression of chiasm or nerves may be safely accomplished or when neuroimaging suggests that the tumor is localized and extrinsic to critical structures. Resection should be avoided or curtailed when disability is certain and the treatment plan calls for radiation therapy regardless of outcome.

In some centers, chemotherapy is recommended regardless of patient age; in these settings, the patient is seldom seen by the radiation oncologist. Chemotherapy has a track record of success in delaying radiation therapy for patients with pediatric low-grade astrocytoma but cannot be considered curative; the majority of patients will eventually require radiation therapy.[28,29] Among the important observations

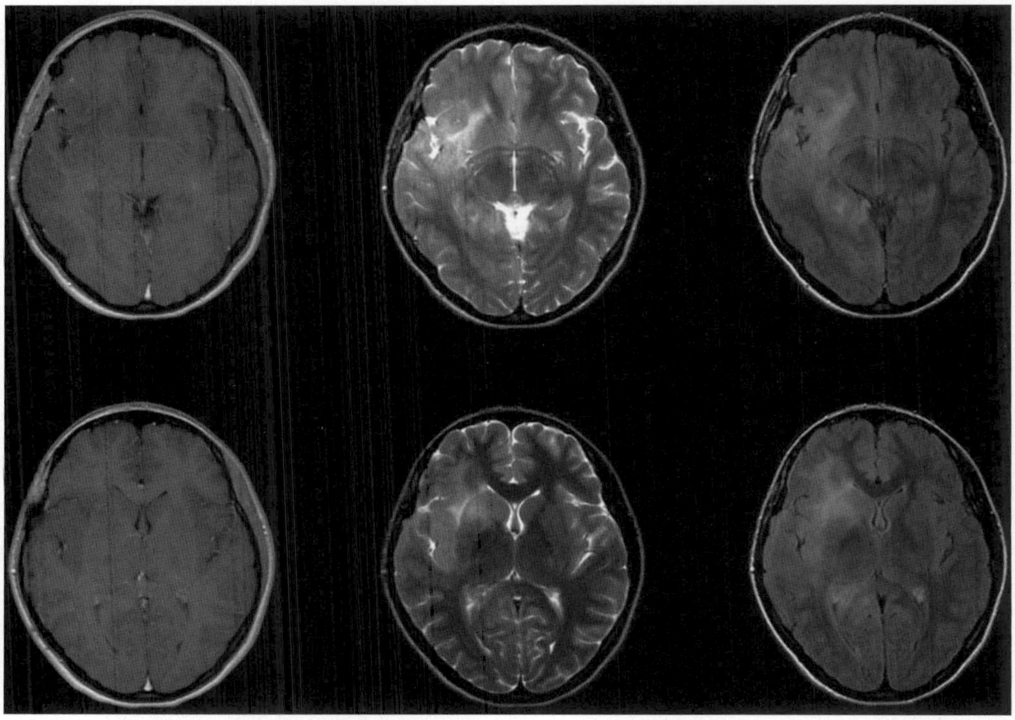

Figure 64-6 Anaplastic astrocytoma involving the right hemisphere with extension to the contralateral hemisphere via the corpus callosum. Postcontrast T1-weighted MRI (*left upper and lower*) does not demonstrate diffuse hemispheric and transcallosal involvement observed on T2-weighted (*center upper and lower*) and fluid-attenuated inversion recovery (*right upper and lower*) MRI.

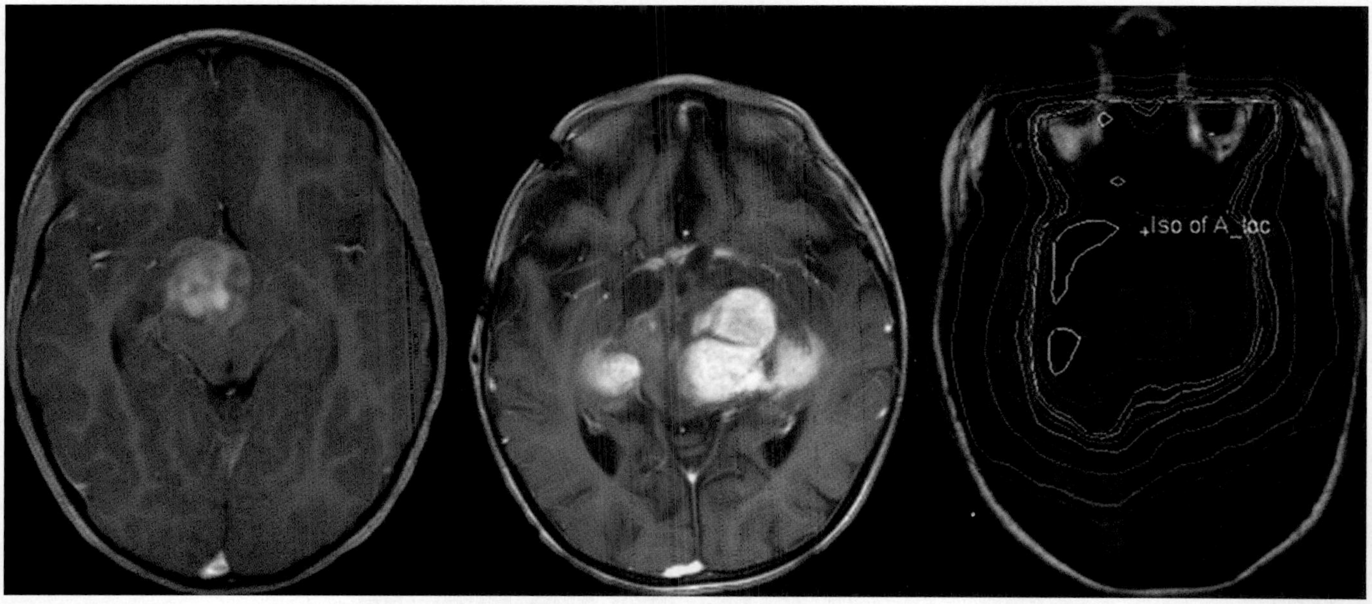

Figure 64-7 Three different cases of optic pathway glioma. Localized hypothalamic-chiasmatic (*left*), diffuse optic pathway tumor (*center*), and typical large treatment volume for an optic pathway tumor with involvement of bilateral optic nerves, optic chiasm, and bilateral optic tracts (*right*) are shown.

about chemotherapy to remember are that most patients receive first-line chemotherapy for 16 to 18 months and that patients who progress do so at a median time of approximately 36 months. Patients who progress often receive second-line chemotherapy, and the radiation therapy avoidance rate is approximately 50% when measured at 5 years. Given the natural history of these tumors, plus experience gained from observing patients after a primary surgical approach that resected only a portion of the tumor, it is plausible that a certain proportion of these tumors might have stabilized or waxed or waned in terms of progression. A number of the patients included in the reported series include children with neurofibromatosis type 1 (NF1)—15% of patients with NF1 have optic pathway glioma. These patients are often diagnosed through screening procedures at an early age and have tumors that are prone to spontaneous progression and regression. Radiation therapy has the best PFS rates when comparing irradiated, chemotherapy-treated, and observation patients.[30]

In the future, several points regarding the management of these patients will need to be clarified. What is the appropriate age for radiation therapy? (The recommended age currently ranges from 5 to 15 years depending on the treatment center.) Are alkylating agents appropriate as first-line therapy? Is second-line chemotherapy appropriate in a patient who has progressed on chemotherapy or after chemotherapy and observation? Is it appropriate to observe an ophthalmologically unreliable patient who has completed chemotherapy with a presenting history of visual deficit when the next treatment will be instituted only at the time of further visual change? For a given patient's age, what interval of delay is clinically significant? Along the same lines, is the risk of hearing loss from the combination of chemotherapy and radiation therapy worth the interval of time in a patient with compromised vision? And finally, what are the true risks of vasculopathy (Fig. 64-8), endocrinopathy, cognitive decline, and malignancy induction in patients with low-grade astrocytoma treated with radiation therapy? The aforementioned side effects of radiation therapy are the cornerstones of radiation therapy avoidance, yet solid data have not been objectively derived and functional outcome data have been lacking from most chemotherapy series. One should ask the question: Do these tumors respond more quickly to radiation therapy or chemotherapy? Although most would consider radiation therapy in this regard, there are no data to support this perception.

Although single fraction irradiation (radiosurgery) has been used to treat well-defined areas of residual tumors, targeting guidelines have not been developed for external beam radiation therapy. Prospective data suggest that a clinical target volume margin of 10 mm or even smaller may be appropriate for these tumors, although additional follow-up is required and the advantages of small volume irradiation, in terms of side effect reduction, have not been proved. Most children with low-grade astrocytoma have World Health Organization (WHO) grade 1 tumors, and conventionally fractionated radiation therapy to 54 Gy is recommended. Patients with disseminated low-grade astrocytoma should be approached with curative intent using craniospinal irradiation. Although dissemination is rare at presentation, the natural history of hypothalamic low-grade astrocytoma suggests a pattern of failure that is distant. Spinal imaging might be considered in the evaluation of these patients, especially those with hypothalamic tumors that have a relatively higher propensity to disseminate.

BRAINSTEM GLIOMA

Brainstem glioma in our definition refers to the diffuse intrinsic tumors most often involving the pons. These tumors have a characteristic appearance on MRI and do not require biopsy. Their outcome is uniformly fatal despite excellent responses to radiation therapy and corticosteroids. After years of attempting to escalate dose, alter fractionation, and sensitize tumors to the effects of irradiation, investigators have now turned to more targeted therapies in conjunction with conventionally fractionated radiation therapy to approximately 54 to 55.8 Gy (Fig. 64-9).

CENTRAL NERVOUS SYSTEM GERM CELL TUMORS

CNS germ cell tumors are rare among brain tumors affecting adults and children. Based on data from the Central Brain Tumor Registry of the United States, fewer than 93 are expected to be diagnosed annually in the United States in boys younger than 19 years, and the number of tumors diagnosed in girls is expected to be less than 38.[1] These numbers demonstrate the male preponderance of this disease.

Progress in the treatment of CNS germ cell tumors has been slowed by the number of patients for protocol enrollment, the diversity of tumor histiotypes, the multitude of clinical presentations, the range of disease extent at diagnosis, the presence or absence of tumor markers, and the variable radiographic characteristics. The approach to the treatment of these tumors can be decided by histology into two groups, germinomatous and nongerminomatous germ cell tumors, with little overlap. Germinoma, analogous to seminoma in the extra-CNS setting, is highly sensitive to all forms of therapy, making decisions regarding management difficult, with a major emphasis on side effects of treatment instead of disease control. Nongerminomatous germ cell tumors, in

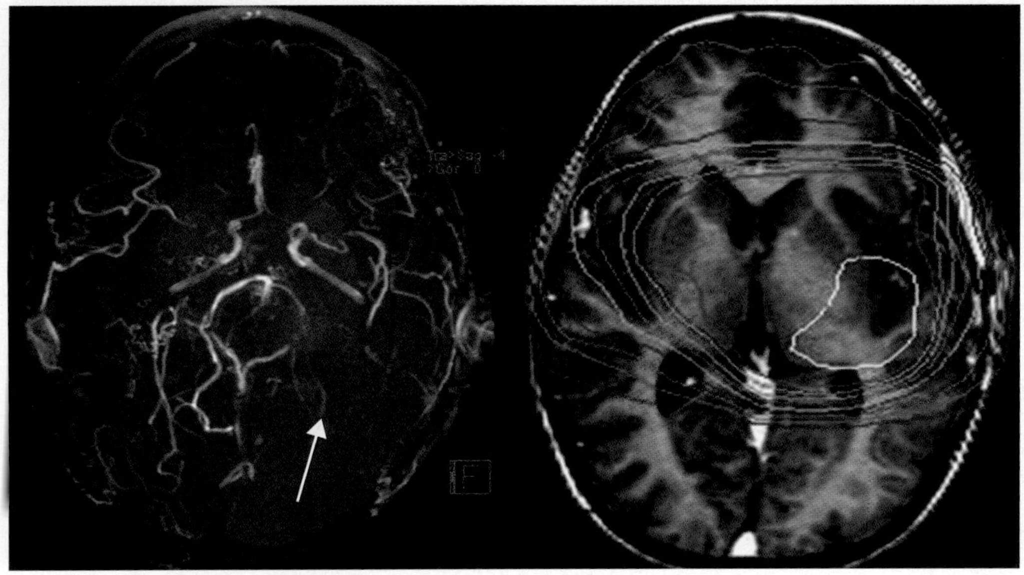

Figure 64-8 Posterior cerebral vasculopathy 4 years after focal irradiation of an optic pathway tumor. Magnetic resonance angiogram (*left*) shows loss of vascularity (*arrow*) corresponding to treatment dosimetry (*right*).

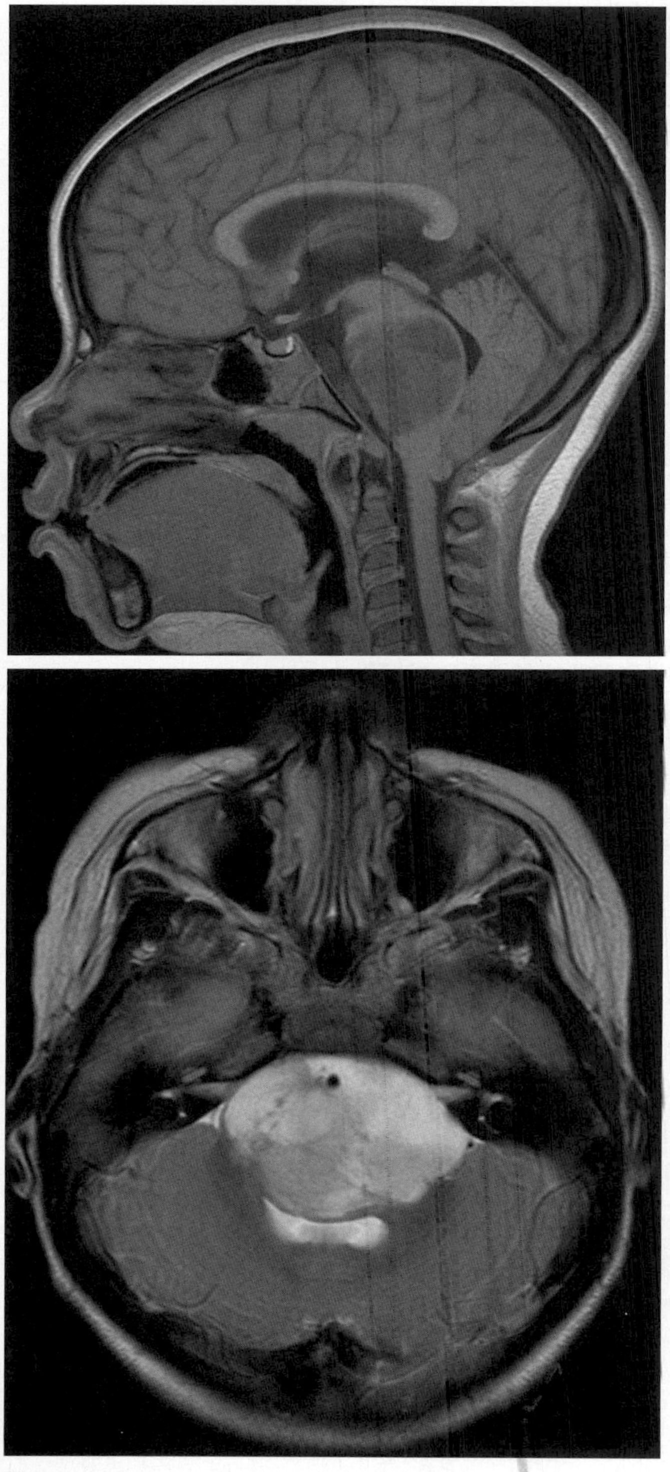

Figure 64-9 Brainstem glioma on T1-sagittal (*upper*) and T2-axial (*lower*) weighted MRI.

contradistinction to their extra-CNS analogs, are less sensitive to all forms of therapy.

The importance of staging cannot be overemphasized in the management of these patients. Poor staging affects classification for outcomes analysis, response evaluation, radiation dose, and volume prescriptions as well as the cure of these patients. A high-quality spinal MRI is required along with adequate CSF sampling. The negative predictive value of a single lumbar CSF cytologic analysis remains unclear and should be considered an important secondary objective in any major study. Serum and CSF alpha-fetoprotein and β-human chorionic gonadotropin (ß-hCG) are important for diagnostic and staging purposes, including response evaluation and making decisions regarding the use of surgery and radiation therapy; however, each institution and cooperative group has its own criteria for cutoff values and risk classification, and ratios of serum-to-CSF values and the normal values in the CSF have not been established. Standardization in the use of serum and CSF markers is required as well as the assays used for their measurement. In addition, markers such as carcinoembryonic antigen (CEA); placental alkaline phosphatase; lactate dehydrogenase (LDH); and the soluble form of c-kit, a transmembrane tyrosine kinase receptor, should be investigated.[31]

The diagnosis of germinoma requires a biopsy. Although its radiographic appearance and location may be characteristic, because of the absence of markers and the differences in management between germinoma and other tumor types, a tissue diagnosis should be established. Histopathology in the setting of elevated markers is not necessary; however, when the markers are negative and ß-hCG is low but elevated, or when there is any question concerning the diagnosis, we favor biopsy when it can be performed with a low risk of side effects. Although most biopsies are extremely small and provide limited detail regarding tumor heterogeneity, tissue can be invaluable after a poor or mixed response to therapy.

Based on the curability of extra-CNS germ cell tumors with multiagent chemotherapy, it was logical for investigators to consider chemotherapy alone as a treatment option. This option was pursued for a number of years because of concerns about the effects of radiation therapy. There have been two approaches with chemotherapy: chemotherapy alone and chemotherapy as a component of a combined modality approach involving the use of reduced-dose and volume irradiation. There have been two successive trials attempting to treat patients with chemotherapy alone.[32,33] These trials differed in the types of agents used as well as their intensity and sequencing. Our impression from the first trial is that the event-free survival was short, the progression rate was high, and there were a noticeable number of toxic deaths. Our impression from the second trial was that outcomes were similarly poor and toxicity remained high. The key finding from these trials is that there is a subset of patients that may be effectively treated without irradiation and that salvage with radiation therapy, at least for the patients with germinoma, may be feasible. It is important to find a way to determine which patients might be candidates to avoid irradiation and to consider this treatment approach only for the youngest patients. Toxic deaths using chemotherapy alone have made a bad impression; however, such studies were carried out at centers that might not have been equipped to handle this type of patient and treatment intensity.

There are too many combined modality approaches for CNS germ cell tumors to list them all, and hopefully the current and proposed studies through the COG are the best of prior experiences. The aim of the current nongerminomatous germ cell tumor study is to assess the ability of neoadjuvant chemotherapy, with or without preirradiation surgery, to reduce or eliminate measurable disease before radiation therapy (Fig. 64-10). Patients receive alternating combinations of carboplatin/etoposide and ifosfamide/etoposide every 3 weeks for 18 weeks (induction) followed by response assessment. Patients with progressive disease are taken off protocol; those with a complete response proceed to craniospinal irradiation that includes neuraxis irradiation to 36 Gy and a focal

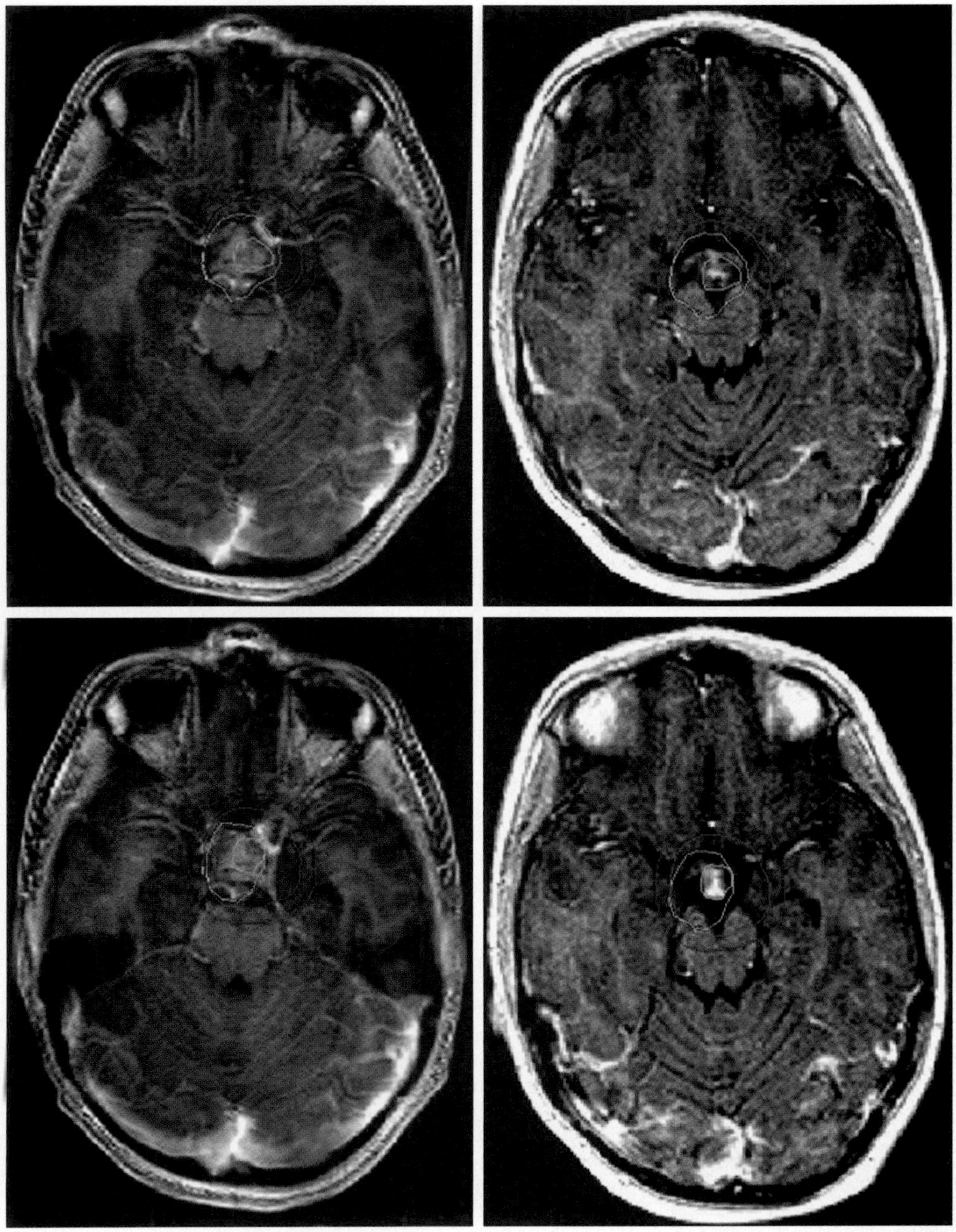

Figure 64-10 Prechemotherapy (*left column*) and postchemotherapy (*right column*) T1-weighted MRIs of a central nervous system germ cell tumor at two anatomic levels, superior (*upper*) and inferior (*lower*), showing the effect of the chemotherapy response on the targeted volume. Prechemotherapy gross tumor volume (*yellow*), postchemotherapy gross tumor volume (*blue*), clinical target volume (10 mm) (*magenta*), and planning target volume (5 mm) (*red*) are shown.

boost to 54 Gy using a 1-cm clinical target volume margin based on assessment of pre- and postinduction neuroimaging. Those with less than a complete response (CR) have the option of surgical resection. Patients with more than 65% reduction in their volume of disease (partial response [PR]) after induction chemotherapy or induction chemotherapy and preirradiation surgery, will proceed to craniospinal irradiation if their markers have normalized. Those with stable disease or less than PR and abnormal markers receive consolidative chemotherapy using thiotepa/etoposide and peripheral stem cell rescue before radiation therapy. The combined CR and PR rates are expected to be more than 70% for this study group and will hopefully translate into improved outcomes.

The upcoming COG study for CNS germinoma is ambitious for it proposes to randomize patients between "standard" radiation therapy and combined modality therapy consisting of two cycles of carboplatin and etoposide (induction) followed by radiation therapy (complete responders) or further chemotherapy and radiation therapy based on response assessment, mainly those with minimal residual disease, partial responses or stable disease. As proposed, there are at least eight possible treatment groups combining the different possible stages of disease, responses, and randomization arms.

Standard radiation therapy for patients with localized disease is considered ventricular irradiation to 24 Gy followed by focal irradiation with 21 Gy, for a total primary site dose of 45 Gy. Standard radiation therapy for patients with disseminated disease is considered craniospinal irradiation to 24 Gy followed by focal irradiation with 21 Gy, for a total primary site dose of 45 Gy. The lack of consensus with regard to treatment volumes, the noticeable risk of failure outside the irradiated volume in many series, and the adequacy of staging procedures have made decisions about radiation therapy treatment guidelines controversial.[34] Patients treated in the combined modality arm of the COG CNS germinoma study will receive response- and risk-adapted radiation therapy to include focal irradiation to 30 Gy for patients with localized disease in CR after induction; focal irradiation to 40.5 Gy for patients in PR after induction and CR or minimal residual disease after two additional cycles of cisplatin and cyclophosphamide. Variations to the proposed regimen are included for those with neuraxis dissemination at diagnosis. They will receive combined-modality treatment with craniospinal irradiation to 24 Gy, except for those patients who have a CR to induction for whom 21 Gy will be administered.

This study hopes to answer a number of important questions, including the ability of chemotherapy to treat microscopic residual disease, the ability of chemotherapy to reduce the dose of irradiation, the ability to predict outcome based on response to chemotherapy, the adequacy of ventricular irradiation, and the ability to differentiate the neurocognitive outcomes between patients who receive radiation therapy alone or a combined modality approach.

CRANIOPHARYNGIOMA

Craniopharyngioma represents one of the most difficult brain tumors treated by the radiation oncologist because of concerns about postirradiation morbidity and the technical and medical aspects of the treatment. Radical surgery is appropriate for patients with tumors that may be completely resected without damaging the anterior hypothalamus and affecting personality and quality of life. For other patients limited surgery followed by conformal fractionated external beam radiation therapy is recommended. The limited surgery approach includes surgical decompression of the cystic or solid components of the tumor to alleviate symptoms, restore vision, improve CSF flow, and reduce the volume of irradiation. The use of radiosurgery and intracystic isotopes should be reserved for recurrence. Radiosurgery is useful for treating small solid residual tumors. Intracystic isotopes have some usefulness in treating cystic components measuring more than 2 to 3 cm in diameter. Neither is effective for treating both cystic and solid components. Further, concerns have been raised about irradiation of the optic nerves, chiasm, and proximal optic pathways.

Combined modality therapy (limited surgery and radiation therapy) was first proposed by colleagues at the St. George's and Royal Marsden Hospitals more than 50 years ago where long-term survivors were found to have functional outcomes, whereas those treated with primary surgery seldom reached any level of independence and productivity. The Royal Marsden results for limited surgery and radiation therapy remain the standard to which others compare for disease control, reporting 10- and 20-year PFSs of 83% and 79%, respectively.[35]

Because there are fewer than 100 pediatric patients diagnosed with craniopharyngioma in the United States each year, the experience of any given institution in the treatment of these patients is limited.

In most centers the radiation oncologist is one of the last to see these patients, who are referred only after numerous attempts at resection because radiation therapy avoidance has taken such a high priority in management.

One of the questions often asked concerns the consequences of delaying radiation therapy. One advantage of delaying is that when progression occurs, and if there are no further sequelae, nothing has been lost and the patient proceeds with treatment with no difference in disease control. The negative side is that when a patient requires additional surgery at the time of progression and radiation therapy is going to be administered regardless, the patient may postoperatively return to a poor functional state; radiation therapy in this setting can be very difficult. If surgery is done again, the arachnoid layer is often adherent to the brain and there is scarring and bleeding, and the postoperative course is difficult.

In some reports, the type of imaging, extent of resection, and preirradiation progression are prognostic factors; however, there are no recent prospective series. When the tumor recurs after treatment, there are a number of options ranging from surgery followed by aspiration and observation to radiosurgery, intracystic isotopes including P32 and Y90 (in Europe), and intracystic bleomycin.

The debate between surgery and radiation therapy centers on the side effects of each treatment. Surgical morbidity tends to be acute and permanent. Radiation-related side effects may be early and transient or late and permanent. These patients experience a wide range of side effects that include neurologic, endocrine, and cognitive function. They are at risk for vasculopathy, necrosis, and second tumors. The indication for radiation therapy includes any patient whose tumor cannot be completely resected without resulting in significant damage to the hypothalamus. External beam radiation therapy is recommended to the entire solid and cystic tumor using a limited clinical target volume margin, generally less than 10 mm, and doses of 54 Gy or more. Royal Marsden investigators used 1.67 Gy to approximately 50.1 Gy.

Although we have not developed age criteria for the treatment of these patients, we understand that young patients with these centrally located tumors are at risk for late sequelae. In certain patients in whom the cyst has been resected and there remains only a small solid residual tumor, we might be inclined to just observe if the patient is very young (<5 years). Patients in whom cystic progression is likely should receive radiation therapy because accelerated cyst formation in response to radiation therapy is relatively frequent. Treatment of these tumors should not be urgent. The time to response is approximately 9 months. Considerations should be given to imaging studies during radiation therapy when there is a chance that cystic enlargement might occur. There are numerous absolute and relative contraindications to radiation therapy. Listed in order are active cysts, young age, uncontrolled diabetes mellitus, vasculopathy and stroke, significant preirradiation morbidity including visual or other neurologic deficits, prior intracystic isotopes or radiosurgery with radiation-related effects including decreased vision and necrosis, possible iatrogenic seeding after surgery, poorly defined tumor volumes, and extremely active cysts, as mentioned.

Craniopharyngioma is amenable to the spectrum of focal irradiation delivery methods. The major debate over the two treatments involves side effects, many of which are similar but many of which are also different. Prominent side effects of radiation therapy include effects on neurologic, endocrine, and cognitive function. In addition, vasculopathy (affecting the circle of Willis and its branches into the basal ganglia) and the risk of second tumors are concerns (anaplastic astrocytoma and glioblastoma multiforme). Patients who receive radiation therapy regardless of preirradiation status are likely to develop panhypopituitarism. Diabetes insipidus is not common. Patients may develop metabolic syndromes in part because of the combined effects of surgery and poorly treated endocrine deficiencies. Patients develop short- and long-term side effects from radiation including changes in appetite, nausea and vomiting, headache, and the effects of increased cyst formation.

CHOROID PLEXUS TUMORS

Choroid plexus papilloma is treated with surgery and observation. Choroid plexus carcinomas, because of their vascular nature, are often treated with pre-resection chemotherapy and postoperative focal irradiation when localized and the residual micro- or macroscopic tumor is known to remain at the primary site. Craniospinal irradiation has fallen from favor because of the young age at presentation and through the effectiveness of chemotherapy, but remains an option.

SPINAL CORD TUMORS

Spinal cord tumors are exceedingly rare and require special consideration.[36,37] The most common presentation is a localized low-grade astrocytoma involving the cervicothoracic spinal cord. Other locations and tumor types include myxopapillary ependymoma, generally involving the cauda equina or conus medullaris; localized ependymoma; and a variety of high-grade neoplasms including anaplastic astrocytoma, GBM, and PNET.

Neuraxis imaging should be carried out in the absence of an inflammatory or paramagnetic artifact from surgery. This is especially true for high-grade tumors and myxopapillary ependymoma where metastatic spread occurs with a relatively high frequency. In the latter case, craniospinal irradiation may be given with curative intent when dissemination is documented early in the course of planning. Irradiation of the spinal cord–bearing tumor should not be undertaken unless the patient has been evaluated and even explored by an expert neurosurgeon. Because uncomplicated gross-total resection makes irradiation of ependymal and low-grade spinal cord tumors unnecessary, every effort should be made to consider resection. As most practicing radiation oncologists fear spinal cord injury and resist irradiation of the spinal cord to dose levels of more than 45 Gy, treatment should be left to those who will consider curative dose levels, generally 54 Gy and higher. Finally, care must be taken to ensure that the rostral and caudal extent of these tumors are encompassed with an appropriate margin despite the relative large volume in a small individual. Homogeneity of dose and minimizing dose to normal tissues is requisite in the treatment of these patients (Fig. 64-11).

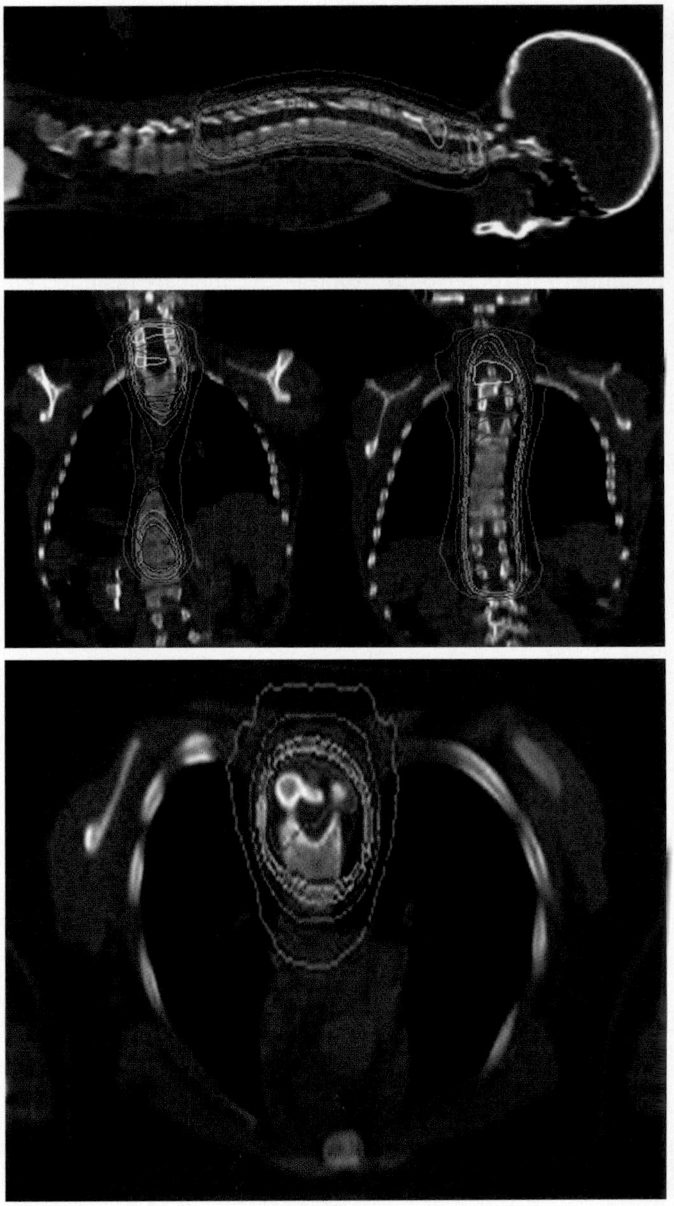

Figure 64-11 Sagittal (*upper*), coronal (*middle*), and axial (*lower*) treatment dosimetry for a low-grade spinal cord astrocytoma treated with surgery and chemotherapy before eventual progression and 54 Gy radiation therapy.

NORMAL TISSUE TOLERANCES AND SIDE EFFECTS

Long-term side effects are central to decisions about the use of radiation therapy in children with CNS tumors. Despite their significance, the data are limited, often leaving the radiation oncologist unprepared to accurately estimate the long-term effects of treatment.[38]

Radiation therapy for pediatric CNS tumors may affect neurologic, endocrine, and cognitive functions and lead to somatic effects, parenchymal or vascular damage, and secondary neoplasms (Fig. 64-12). The risk associated with side effects is unequivocally governed by the age of the patient, time after treatment, location of the primary site, and the prescribed dose and volume. As the dose and volume of irradiation have been systematically reduced for specific patient groups, additional factors have been found to be significant including the effects of surgery, chemotherapy, and the premorbidity from the tumor. Any or all of the aforementioned side effects may be present before the initiation of radiation therapy. The focus of discussion should be the combination of possible effects and the long-term prospects for disease control and independent functional outcome. Long-term predictions about the quality of survivorship are difficult to make because of the tremendous differences in current treatment compared to the treatment administered to those for whom long-term data are available. Long-term survivors of brain tumor are more likely to have diminished social function.[39]

The cognitive effects of radiation therapy include effects on global intelligence, learning, memory, attention, and behavior. The adverse cognitive effects of radiation therapy in children with brain tumors are generally known only for children who have received whole-brain irradiation as a component of their treatment to dose levels of 18, 24, and 36 Gy. These doses are representative of those customarily used in the treatment of acute lymphoblastic leukemia (ALL) and medulloblastoma.

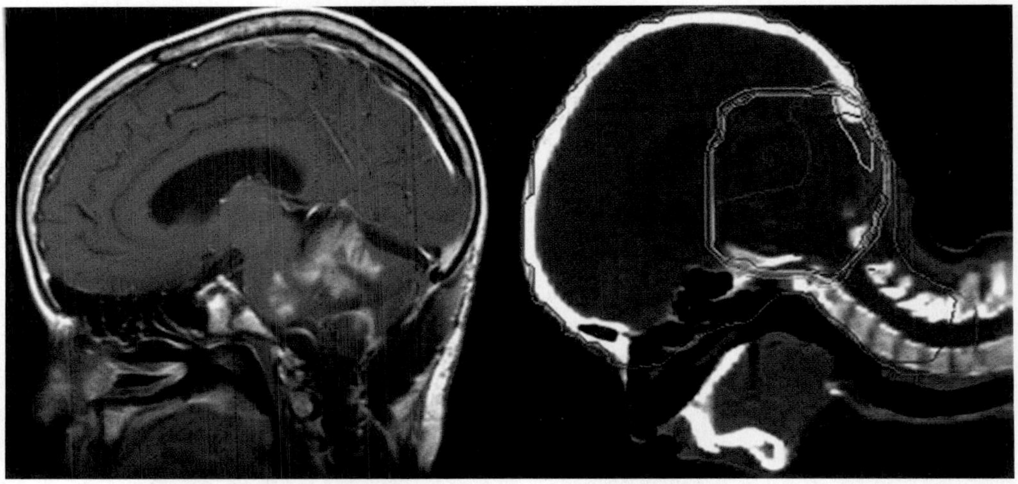

Figure 64-12 Example of radiation-induced secondary brain tumor (glioblastoma multiforme) after treatment for medulloblastoma.

Fewer data are available showing the effects of partial brain irradiation in patients with other tumor types.[40,41] Most studies show a relationship between discrete doses and age at treatment.[42] Age and dose-related decline in IQ was first demonstrated in children who received 36 Gy. These patients had IQ scores approximately 8.2 points lower than those who received 24 Gy, and 12.3 points lower than those who received 18 Gy.[43] At least one study found no difference in effect on IQ between doses of 18 and 24 Gy among children older than 6 years, but doses greater than 24 Gy adversely affected IQ.[40] Young age at the time of irradiation is the most important prognostic factor regardless of dose. Volume of irradiation is an important prognostic factor for functional outcome.[41] Children treated with partial brain irradiation were more likely to have an IQ greater than 90 points at 5 years (60%) compared to those who received craniospinal irradiation. Additional data that describe the effects of focal irradiation to more limited volumes are needed. The use of focal radiation techniques in the treatment of children with brain tumors, especially those who do not require craniospinal irradiation, presents a unique opportunity to study the cognitive effects of radiation dose to more limited volumes. The combined advantages of newer treatment methods and more limited volume guidelines have been demonstrated in children with ependymoma. Among 88 patients with localized ependymoma who received radiation therapy using a 1-cm clinical target volume margin, there was no decline in IQ, memory, and academic achievement including 48 children younger than 3 years old at the time of irradiation.[20] These same patients have contributed to separate reports correlating the effects of hydrocephalus and treatment dosimetry on outcome.[44,45] Similar encouraging findings have been demonstrated for a variety of patients in the assessment of attention, impulsivity, and reaction time.[46]

Irradiation of the hypothalamic-pituitary axis (HPA) leads to endocrine deficiencies. The incidence and time to onset of clinically significant endocrinopathies depend on the total dose to the HPA, time after irradiation, and the direct (tumor invasion or mass effect) and indirect (hydrocephalus) effects of the tumor. Residents have long been taught that the pituitary is the organ at risk in the intracranial portion of the endocrine system and that panhypopituitarism is a foregone conclusion after irradiation of the sellar or suprasellar region. More recent data show the importance of the hypothalamus and the intrinsic and differential sensitivity of the hypothalamic nuclei.[47] Among hormone deficiencies observed after radiation therapy, growth hormone deficiency is most common followed by adrenocorticotropin, gonadotropin secretion abnormality, and, less common, hypothyroidism (central). Growth hormone deficiency has been observed after doses as low as 10 Gy and as early as 6 to 12 months after radiation therapy at higher doses.[48] Although recent attention has been focused on the contribution of radiation therapy to hypothalamic obesity, other deficiencies, such as diabetes insipidus and hyperprolactinemia, are attributed to local tumoral effects and often surgery when it affects the structural integrity of the HPA. Supporting what radiation oncologists often suspected, provocative endocrine testing before the administration of radiation therapy has revealed a surprising level of preexisting endocrine deficiencies.[48] Hydrocephalus has been implicated in at least one series as the provoking factor.[44] These experiences illustrate the importance of prospective baseline and serial testing for side effects and the presence of transient or permanent effects as a result of the effects of tumor, surgery, and chemotherapy.

Hearing loss is a potential complication of radiation therapy in children. Radiation may affect the conducting system of the ear. The best example is serous otitis media resulting from mucociliary dysfunction during and after radiation therapy. Soft tissue infections of the ear should be treated aggressively, and instrumentation of the external auditory canal should be undertaken cautiously. Sensorineural hearing loss may occur as a result of damage to the cochlea or other parts of the auditory system. Because the doses administered are below the threshold for obvious neurologic impairment of hearing, effects of radiation on the cochlea are more common and usually noted months or years after treatment. The incidence and time course resulting from radiation are unknown. Most children also receive ototoxic chemotherapy and are therefore at risk for the combined effects of both treatments.[49,50]

Dental complications are uncommon but may occur in brain tumor patients who receive craniospinal irradiation when the salivary glands are subtended by the irradiated volume. Other long-term somatic complications include permanent hair loss, wound healing problems, softening of the bone and ligaments of the spine, and spinal growth impairment. Patients with optic pathway glioma, and to a lesser extent craniopharyngioma, appear to have a higher incidence of vasculopathy in general, a higher incidence after radiation therapy, and an acceleration of preexisting abnormalities. As more children become long-term survivors and neuroimaging improves, subclinical abnormalities on follow-up imaging are seen with increasing frequency including microangiopathy with calcifications, lacunar infarcts, and transient or permanent enhancing or T2-signal abnormalities most often but not always in the region that receives the highest dose. Some changes are more apparent in patients who receive chemotherapy or those known to have suffered ischemia at the time of surgery. Second tumors are an unfortunate complication of radiation therapy for CNS tumors. They tend to occur years after treatment, usually when the patient is considered cured. Contoured examples of organs at risk are given in Figures 64-13 and 64-14.

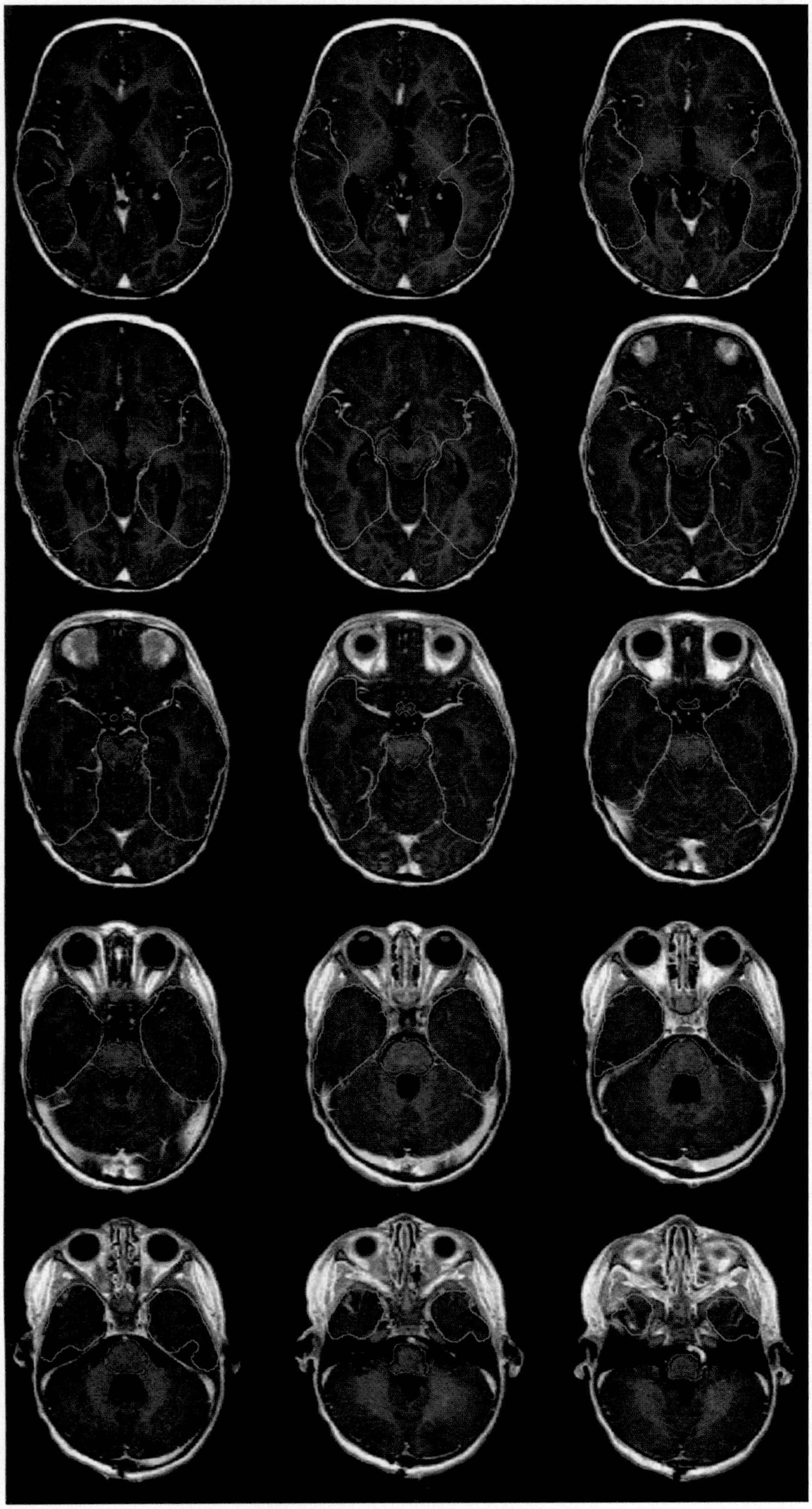

Figure 64-13 Panel of T1-weighted MRIs showing important organs at risk for pediatric brain tumor patients. Contoured structures serve as an approximate guide to the definition of the brainstem (*orange*), temporal lobes (*light blue*), optic chiasm (*yellow*), pituitary gland (*red*), and hypothalamus (*magenta*). Upper aspect of the temporal lobes terminate at the atria of the lateral ventricles. Aspect of the temporal lobes posteromedial to the lateral ventricles is not included.

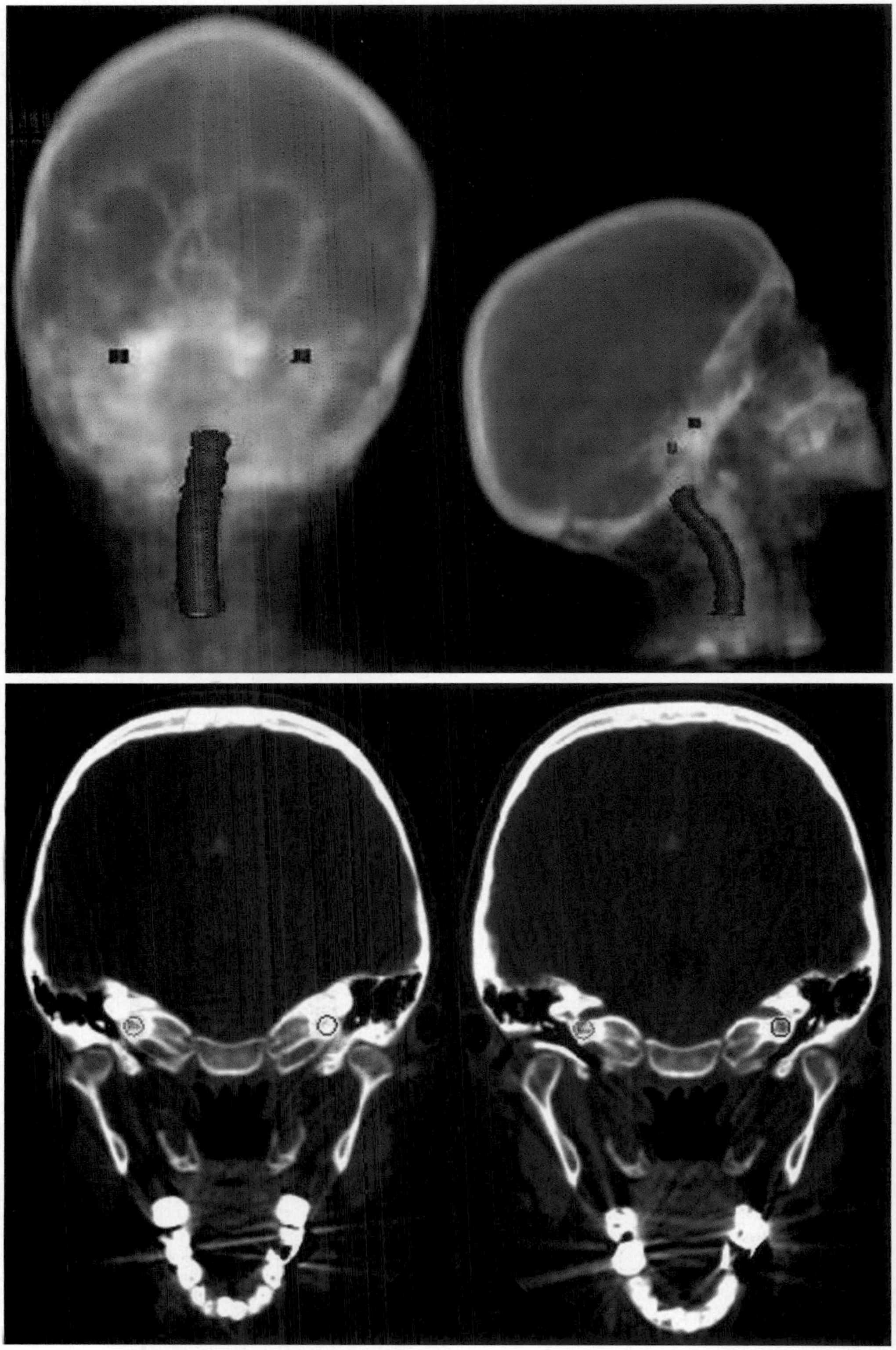

Figure 64-14 Anterior and lateral digitally reconstructed radiographs (*upper*) showing left (*green*) and right (*red*) cochleae and spinal cord (*yellow*). Spinal cord volume definition begins inferior to the foramen magnum. Cochleae are contoured on two axial CT images (*lower*) and are represented as a circular structure in the temporal bone.

SUPPORTIVE CARE

Supportive care for children with brain tumors is required throughout the course of radiation therapy. Short-term side effects may occur including nausea, vomiting, fatigue, loss of appetite, headache, and recurrence of neurologic symptoms present at the time of diagnosis. Treatment with antiemetics regardless of symptoms may be appropriate because many children are not able to articulate their feelings of nausea and reversal of appetite suppression may be difficult once established. First-line medications should include Zofran (ondansetron) or a similar $5HT_3$ (5-hydroxytryptamine type 3); second-line medications include Phenergan (promethazine) and Reglan (metoclopramide); and third-line medications include the use of corticosteroids, which should be reserved for patients with intractable nausea, vomiting, and neurologic symptoms including headache. Persistent nausea over several months occurs in patients whose tumors arose along the dorsum of the brainstem.

Children are less likely to be placed on prophylactic antiseizure medication after surgery and require corticosteroids during radiation therapy. It is therefore important to determine the true need for antiseizure medications and to encourage and monitor steroid tapering. Patients treated with steroids need to be monitored for oral candidiasis and the need for gastrointestinal prophylaxis. For some patients, the need for CSF shunting may not be apparent in the perioperative period and should therefore be monitored carefully.

Sedation and anesthesia have become imperative in treating young children with brain tumors. The demand has increased owing to the requirements of focal radiation delivery protocols and the need to reduce the set-up margin component of the planning target volume. At most centers, most children younger than 6 to 7 years require radiation therapy. Sedation or anesthesia is generally safe and does not appear to add to the acute effects of treatment; the use of sedation on a repeated basis does not appear to be as effective as anesthesia.

REFERENCES

1. CBTRUS 2002: Statistical report: primary brain tumors in the United States, 1995-1999: Central Brain Tumor Registry of the United States, 2002.
2. Eberhart CG, Kepner JL, Goldthwaite PT, et al: Histopathologic grading of medulloblastomas: a Pediatric Oncology Group study. Cancer 94:552-560, 2002.
3. Giangaspero F, Rigobello L, Badiali M, et al: Large-cell medulloblastomas. A distinct variant with highly aggressive behavior. Am J Surg Pathol 16:687-693, 1992.
4. Packer RJ, Biegel JA, Blaney S, et al: Atypical teratoid/rhabdoid tumor of the central nervous system: report on workshop. J Pediatr Hematol Oncol 24:337-342, 2002.
5. Merchant TE, Wang MH, Haida T, et al: Medulloblastoma: long-term results for patients treated with definitive radiation therapy during the computed tomography era. Int J Radiat Oncol Biol Phys 36:29-35, 1996.
6. Straathof CS, de Bruin HG, Dippel DW, et al: The diagnostic accuracy of magnetic resonance imaging and cerebrospinal fluid cytology in leptomeningeal metastasis. J Neurol 246:810-814, 1999.
7. Thomas PR, Deutsch M, Kepner JL, et al: Low-stage medulloblastoma: final analysis of trial comparing standard-dose with reduced-dose neuraxis irradiation. J Clin Oncol 18:3004-3011, 2000.
8. Packer RJ, Goldwein J, Nicholson HS, et al: Treatment of children with medulloblastomas with reduced-dose craniospinal radiation therapy and adjuvant chemotherapy: a Children's Cancer Group study. J Clin Oncol 17:2127-2136, 1999.
9. Ris MD, Packer R, Goldwein J, et al: Intellectual outcome after reduced-dose radiation therapy plus adjuvant chemotherapy for medulloblastoma: a Children's Cancer Group study. J Clin Oncol 19:3470-3476, 2001.
10. Packer R, Gajjar A, Vezina G, et al: Preliminary report of A9961: a phase III randomized study of craniospinal radiation therapy (CSRT) followed by one of two adjuvant chemotherapy regimens (CCNU, CPDD, VCR or CPM, CPDD, VCR) in children with newly diagnosed average-risk medulloblastoma (MB) [abstract]. The 11th International Symposium on Pediatric Neuro-Oncology, Boston, 2004. Available online at http://home.comcast.net/~turne038/abstracts.htm [abstract Ther 61].
11. Merchant TE, Kun LE, Krasin MJ, et al: A multi-institution prospective trial of reduced-dose craniospinal irradiation (23.4 Gy) followed by conformal posterior fossa (36 Gy) and primary site irradiation (55.8 Gy) and dose-intensive chemotherapy for average-risk medulloblastoma. Int J Radiat Oncol Biol Phys 57:S194-S195, 2003.
12. Carrie C, Muracciole X, Gomez F, et al: Conformal radiotherapy, reduced boost volume, hyperfractionated radiotherapy and online quality control in standard-risk medulloblastoma without chemotherapy: results of the French M-SFOP 98 protocol. Int J Radiat Oncol Biol Phys 57:S195, 2003.
13. Merchant TE, Pritchard DL, Vargo JA, Sontag MR: Radiation therapy for the treatment of childhood medulloblastoma: the rationale for current techniques, strategies, and dose-volume considerations. Electromedica 69:69-71, 2001.
14. Blaney SM, Boyett J, Friedman H, et al: Phase I clinical trial of mafosfamide in infants and children aged 3 years or younger with newly diagnosed embryonal tumors: a Pediatric Brain Tumor Consortium Study (PBTC-001). J Clin Oncol 23:525-531, 2005.
15. Duffner PK, Horowitz ME, Krischer JP, et al: Postoperative chemotherapy and delayed radiation in children less than three years of age with malignant brain tumors. N Engl J Med 328:1725-1731, 1993.
16. Geyer JR, Zeltzer PM, Boyett JM, et al: Survival of infants with primitive neuroectodermal tumors or malignant ependymomas of the CNS treated with eight drugs in 1 day: a report from the Children's Cancer Group. J Clin Oncol 12:1607-1615, 1994.
17. Walter AW, Mulhern RK, Gajjar A, et al: Survival and neurodevelopmental outcome of young children with medulloblastoma at St. Jude Children's Research Hospital. J Clin Oncol 17:3720-3728, 1999.
18. Goldwein JW, Radcliffe J, Johnson J, et al: Updated results of a pilot study of low dose craniospinal irradiation plus chemotherapy for children under five with cerebellar primitive neuroectodermal tumors (medulloblastoma). Int J Radiat Oncol Biol Phys 34:899-904, 1996.
19. Garvin J, Sposto R, Stanley P, et al: Childhood ependymoma: improved survival for patients with incompletely resected tumors with the use of pre-irradiation chemotherapy [abstract]. 11th International Symposium on Pediatric Neuro-Oncology, Boston, 2004. Available online at http://home.comcast.net/~turne038/abstracts.htm [abstract Ther 29].
20. Merchant TE, Mulhern RK, Krasin MJ, et al: Preliminary results from a phase II trial of conformal radiation therapy and the evaluation of radiation-related CNS effects for pediatric patients with localized ependymoma. J Clin Oncol 22(15):3156-3162, 2004.
21. Merchant TE, Jenkins JJ, Burger PC, et al: Influence of tumor grade on time to progression after irradiation for localized ependymoma in children. Int J Radiat Oncol Biol Phys 53:52-57, 2002.
22. Pollack IF, Gerszten PC, Martinez AJ, et al: Intracranial ependymomas of childhood: long-term outcome and prognostic factors. Neurosurgery 37:655-666; discussion 666-667, 1995.
23. Sutton LN, Goldwein J, Perilongo G, et al: Prognostic factors in childhood ependymomas. Pediatr Neurosurg 16:57-65, 1990.
24. Sposto R, Ertel IJ, Jenkin RD, et al: The effectiveness of chemotherapy for treatment of high grade astrocytoma in children: results of a randomized trial. A report from the Children's Cancer Study Group. J Neurooncol 7:165-177, 1989.
25. Finlay JL, Boyett JM, Yates AJ, et al: Randomized phase III trial in childhood high-grade astrocytoma comparing vincristine, lomustine, and prednisone with the eight-drugs-in-1-day regimen. Children's Cancer Group. J Clin Oncol 13:112-123, 1995.
26. Pollack IF, Boyett JM, Yates AJ, et al: The influence of central review on outcome associations in childhood malignant gliomas: results from the CCG-945 experience. Neuro-oncol 5:197-207, 2003.
27. Wisoff JH, Sanford RA, Holmes E, et al: Impact of surgical resection on low grade gliomas of childhood: a report from the CCG9891/POG9130 low grade astrocytoma study. Proceedings of the 39th American Society of Clinical Oncology meeting, 100 (abstr 401), Chicago, 2003.
28. Packer RJ, Lange B, Ater J, et al: Carboplatin and vincristine for recurrent and newly diagnosed low-grade gliomas of childhood. J Clin Oncol 11:850-856, 1993.
29. Laithier V, Grill J, Le Deley MC, et al: Progression-free survival in children with optic pathway tumors: dependence on age and the quality of the response to chemotherapy—results of the first

French prospective study for the French Society of Pediatric Oncology. J Clin Oncol 21:4572-4578, 2003.
30. Fouladi M, Wallace D, Langston JW, et al: Survival and functional outcome of children with hypothalamic/chiasmatic tumors. Cancer 97:1084-1092, 2003.
31. Takeshima H, Kuratsu J: A review of soluble c-kit (s-kit) as a novel tumor marker and possible molecular target for the treatment of CNS germinoma. Surg Neurol 60:321-324; discussion 324-325, 2003.
32. Balmaceda C, Heller G, Rosenblum M, et al: Chemotherapy without irradiation—a novel approach for newly diagnosed CNS germ cell tumors: results of an international cooperative trial. The First International Central Nervous System Germ Cell Tumor Study. J Clin Oncol 14:2908-2915, 1996.
33. Kellie SJ, Boyce H, Dunkel IJ, et al: Primary chemotherapy for intracranial nongerminomatous germ cell tumors: results of the second international CNS germ cell study group protocol. J Clin Oncol 22:846-853, 2004.
34. Shirato H, Aoyama H, Ikeda J, et al: Impact of margin for target volume in low-dose involved field radiotherapy after induction chemotherapy for intracranial germinoma. Int J Radiat Oncol Biol Phys 60:214-217, 2004.
35. Rajan B, Ashley S, Gorman C, et al: Craniopharyngioma—long-term results following limited surgery and radiotherapy. Radiother Oncol 26:1-10, 1993.
36. Merchant TE, Nguyen D, Thompson SJ, et al: High-grade pediatric spinal cord tumors. Pediatr Neurosurg 30:1-5, 1999.
37. Merchant TE, Kiehna EN, Thompson SJ, et al: Pediatric low-grade and ependymal spinal cord tumors. Pediatr Neurosurg 32:30-36, 2000.
38. Gajjar A, Vezina G, Langston J, et al: Results of central imaging review for patients enrolled on average risk medulloblastoma (MB) protocol A9961 [abstract]. The 11th International Symposium on Pediatric Neuro-Oncology, Boston, 2004. Available online at http://home.comcast.net/~turne038/abstracts.htm [abstract Imag 3].
39. Zebrack BJ, Gurney JG, Oeffinger K, et al: Psychological outcomes in long-term survivors of childhood brain cancer: a report from the childhood cancer survivor study. J Clin Oncol 22:999-1006, 2004.
40. Fuss M, Poljanc K, Hug EB: Full scale IQ (FSIQ) changes in children treated with whole brain and partial brain irradiation. A review and analysis. Strahlenther Onkol 176:573-581, 2000.
41. Hoppe-Hirsch E, Brunet L, Laroussinie F, et al: Intellectual outcome in children with malignant tumors of the posterior fossa: influence of the field of irradiation and quality of surgery. Childs Nerv Syst 11:340-345, 1995.
42. Mulhern RK, Hancock J, Fairclough D, et al: Neuropsychological status of children treated for brain tumors: critical review and integrative analysis. Med Pediatr Oncol 20:181-191, 1992.
43. Silber JH, Radcliffe J, Peckham V, et al: Whole-brain irradiation and decline in intelligence: the influence of dose and age on IQ score. J Clin Oncol 10:1390-1396, 1992.
44. Merchant TE, Lee H, Zhu J, et al: The effects of hydrocephalus on IQ before and after focal irradiation of children with localized infratentorial ependymoma. J Neurosurg 101(2 Suppl):159-168, 2004.
45. Merchant TE, Kiehna EN, Li C, et al: The effect of radiation dosimetry on IQ after conformal radiation therapy in pediatric patients with localized ependymoma [abstract]. The 11th International Symposium on Pediatric Neuro-Oncology, Boston, 2004. Available online at http://home.comcast.net/~turne038/abstracts.htm [abstract LE22].
46. Merchant TE, Kiehna EN, Miles MA, et al: Acute effects of irradiation on cognition: changes in attention on a computerized continuous performance test during radiotherapy in pediatric patients with localized primary brain tumors. Int J Radiat Oncol Biol Phys 53:1271-1278, 2002.
47. Robinson IC, Fairhall KM, Hendry JH, et al: Differential radiosensitivity of hypothalamo-pituitary function in the young adult rat. J Endocrinol 169:519-526, 2001.
48. Merchant TE, Goloubeva O, Pritchard DL, et al: Radiation dose-volume effects on growth hormone secretion. Int J Radiat Oncol Biol Phys 52:1264-1270, 2002.
49. Merchant TE, Gould CJ, Xiong X, et al: Early neuro-otologic effects of three-dimensional irradiation in children with primary brain tumors. Int J Radiat Oncol Biol Phys 58:1194-1207, 2004.
50. Landier W, Merchant TE. Adverse effects of cancer treatment on hearing. *In* Schwartz C, Hobbie W, Constine L, Ruccione K (eds): Survivors of Childhood Cancer: Assessment and Management, 2nd ed. New York, Springer-Verlag (under contract).

CHAPTER 65

PEDIATRIC SOFT TISSUE SARCOMAS

Laurie E. Blach and Alberto S. Pappo

INCIDENCE

Soft tissue sarcomas (STSs) account for approximately 7% of all childhood cancers.

Of all STSs, 40% are rhabdomyosarcoma (RMS).

Approximately 4.3 cases of RMS (1 million children) occur per year.

BIOLOGIC CHARACTERISTICS

Embryonal RMS: loss of heterozygosity chromosome 11p

Alveolar RMS: chromosomal translocation t(2;13) involving the *PAX* gene

Nonrhabdomyosarcoma soft tissue sarcoma (NRSTS): familial cancer syndromes, genetic abnormalities, and chromosomal translocations

STAGING EVALUATION

RMS: IRS clinical grouping system; TNM pretreatment staging classification based on location of primary disease, presence of nodal and distant metastases

NRSTS: American Joint Committee on Cancer (AJCC) staging system using grade, size, nodal and distant metastases, and IRS system

PRIMARY THERAPY

RMS: VAC (vincristine, actinomycin D, cyclophosphamide)-based chemotherapy
- Surgery and radiation therapy for primary disease
- 5-year survival 70% to 95%

NRSTS: surgical resection ± adjuvant radiation therapy
- ± neoadjuvant or adjuvant chemotherapy
- 5-year survival 70% to 90%

LOCALLY ADVANCED DISEASE

RMS: aggressive chemotherapy
- Radiation therapy to primary and metastatic disease
- 5-year survival 20% to 35%
- Favorable subset (embryonal histology and <10 years of age) 5-year survival 50%

NRSTS: surgery, chemotherapy, and radiotherapy
- 5-year survival
- <10% metastatic disease
- 10% to 30% unresectable disease

Rhabdomyosarcoma (RMS) is the most common soft tissue sarcoma (STS) of childhood.[1] Most children with RMS in North America are treated on clinical protocols developed by the Intergroup Rhabdomyosarcoma Study Group (IRSG), now known as the Soft Tissue Sarcoma Committee of the Children's Oncology Group (COG). This combined effort has tripled the survival rate of patients with RMS since 1972. Radiotherapy (RT) plays a major role in the treatment of RMS and is the main focus of this chapter.

The nonrhabdomyosarcoma soft tissue sarcomas (NRSTSs) of childhood are a heterogeneous group of neoplasms that have been poorly studied in pediatrics. Only three prospective studies that included fewer than 200 patients have been conducted in North America to date.[2,3] Given the paucity of literature in pediatrics, most of these children (excluding those with infantile fibrosarcoma) have been treated in a similar fashion to adults. However, it is unclear whether results of treatment from one age group can be transferred to another.

ETIOLOGY AND EPIDEMIOLOGY

Soft tissue sarcomas account for approximately 7% of all childhood cancers, and approximately 40% of these are RMS.[4,5] The age-adjusted incidence rate of RMS for patients younger than 20 years of age is 4.3 per million children.[4] RMS is more frequent in boys and men,[1] and black females are less commonly affected than white females.[1] There is a bimodal age distribution, with a peak incidence occurring in the 2- to 6-year age group and a small peak during adolescence.[1] The typical age of presentation varies with histology and location of the primary site (Table 65-1). RMS is associated with congenital anomalies, particularly of the genitourinary system. Other organ systems with associated anomalies include the central nervous system (CNS) and gastrointestinal, cardiovascular, and respiratory systems. Autopsies confirm anomalies in up to 32% of patients.[6]

The specific cause of these tumors in most cases is unknown. However, an increased incidence of STSs has been reported in a variety of syndromes including Li-Fraumeni, neurofibromatosis, Costello, and Beckwith-Wiedemann syndromes.[7-10] Prior radiation exposure may induce chromosomal abnormalities and result in the development of these malignancies.[11] Immunosuppression may increase the risk of developing certain types of NRSTS.[12] Development of RMS has been associated with maternal and paternal use of marijuana and cocaine and exposure to radiographs or chemicals in utero.[13,14] However, a direct causative link between these agents and RMS has not been established.

PATHOLOGY AND PATHWAYS OF SPREAD

RMS is one of the small round cell malignant tumors of childhood.[13] The different histologic subtypes of RMS and their relative frequency are listed in Table 65-1. Embryonal RMS is the most common histologic subtype, consisting of spindle-shaped rhabdomyoblasts, small round cells with hyperchromatic nuclei on a background of myxoid stroma.[15] The alveolar subtype has tumors arranged in cords with pseudolining cleft-like spaces similar to alveoli.[15] Botryoides, a subset of embryonal RMS, presents grossly with grapelike clusters and histologically as a layer of small round cells surrounding a polypoid tumor.[15] Originally, extraosseous Ewing's sarcoma

Table 65-1 Rhabdomyosarcoma (RMS) Histology, Frequency, Outcome, and Sites[16,17]

Histology	Frequency (%)	Outcome (5-y OS) (%)	Age (y)	Sites
Favorable				
Embryonal	60-70	70-80	3-12	GU, H&N, orbit
Botryoid	5-10	85-95	0-3	Mucosal sites
Unfavorable		50-60	6-21	Extremity, trunk
Alveolar	20-30			
Undifferentiated sarcoma	<5			

GU, genitourinary; H&N, head and neck; OS, overall survival; y, year.

Table 65-2 Rhabdomyosarcoma (RMS) Prognosis by Primary Site[16,17]

	Outcome (5-y Survival) (%)
Favorable sites	80-90 Orbit Nonparameningeal H&N GU: nonbladder/nonprostate Biliary tract
Unfavorable sites	50-70 Parameningeal H&N Bladder/prostate Other (trunk, retroperitoneum, extremity, etc.)

GU, genitourinary; H&N, head and neck; y, year.

was considered a subset of RMS but is now included in the Ewing's sarcoma family of tumors and treated accordingly.

The specific pathologic subtypes of RMS are prognostic and associated with outcome (see Table 65-1).[16,17] Children with embryonal pathology have a better clinical outcome than those with alveolar histology. Botryoid histology is associated with an excellent survival. Certain histologies are also associated with occurrence in particular primary sites (see Table 65-1). Alveolar histology and undifferentiated lesions often occur in the extremity and truncal regions. Botryoid tumors occur in the genitourinary region, biliary tract, nasopharynx, and external auditory canal.[13]

RMS occurs most frequently in the head and neck (H&N) region followed by the genitourinary and extremity regions. The location of the primary site impacts outcome (Tables 65-2 and 65-3).[16,17] RMS of the orbit, nonparameningeal H&N sites, and paratesticular primary sites are associated with an excellent clinical outcome. Those of the extremities and truncal areas do less well.

Metastatic disease is present in approximately 20% of patients at diagnosis. The most common metastatic site is the lung, followed by the bone marrow and bone. Lymph node spread is unusual but is commonly seen with paratesticular primaries (especially those older than 10 years of age) and extremity RMS.[18-20]

NRSTS pathologic subtypes are similar to those in adults and can occur anywhere in the body.[21,22] Although controversial, they are believed to derive from multipotential mesenchymal cells.[22] Infantile fibrosarcoma and infantile hemangiopericytoma are two unique types of NRSTS seen during the first 2 years of life, which are exceptions to those discussed previously. They are highly chemosensitive tumors, and attempts to do radical surgical resections in these patients should be avoided.[23,24]

The natural history of NRSTS depends on histologic grade, invasiveness, and size. Factors associated with an increased risk of local recurrence include site, use of radiotherapy or positive margins, and clinical group.[25] Factors associated with an increased risk of distant metastases include tumor size (>5 cm), invasiveness, and tumor grade.[25] Low-grade tumors tend to recur locally but rarely metastasize. High-grade sarcomas recur locally and distantly. Twenty percent of children present with distant metastases at diagnosis. The most common site of metastases is to the lung. Lymph node metastases are rare in pediatric patients; but in adults a high incidence has been reported in patients with epithelioid sarcoma and angiosarcoma.

BIOLOGIC CHARACTERISTICS AND MOLECULAR BIOLOGY

Embryonal RMS is associated with the loss of heterozygosity at chromosome 11p, which is the location of insulin-like growth factor II (IGF-II).[26] Alveolar RMS has the associated chromosomal translocation t(2;13)(q35;q14) involving the *PAX3* gene.[27,28] Rarely, a translocation takes place at chromosome 1p36 involving the *PAX7* gene.[29] Amplification of certain proto-oncogenes and DNA ploidy have been identified as possible prognostic indicators.[30]

NRSTSs are associated with familial cancer syndromes such as Li-Fraumeni syndrome and neurofibromatosis.[10,31] Abnormalities of chromosome 17 or mutated p53 have been detected in many NRSTSs.[32] A variety of chromosomal translocations that result in specific fusion genes that can be detected by the use of reverse transcription–polymerase chain reaction (RT-PCR) have been described in NRSTS. Some examples include the translocations seen in synovial sarcoma t(X;18) (fusion of *SYT* and *SSX*), myxoid liposarcoma t(12;16) (fusion of *TLS* and *CHOP*), clear cell sarcoma t(12;22) (fusion of *FUS* and *DDIT3*), and congenital fibrosarcoma t(12;15) (fusion of *ETV6* and *NTRK3*).[32,33]

CLINICAL MANIFESTATIONS

The most common presenting symptom of an STS is a painless mass. Local symptoms occur because of local extension of the tumor into the neurovascular structures, bone, or other surrounding organs. The growth of these tumors may result in a disturbance of function that can lead to the presenting complaint. Specific presenting symptoms are site specific (see Table 65-3).

Table 65-3 **Rhabdomyosarcoma (RMS) Presenting Symptoms, Workup, and Outcome by Primary Site**[16,17]

Primary Site	Presenting Symptoms	Workup	Outcome (5-y Survival) (%)
Orbit	Eyelid swelling Globe displacement	MRI brain/orbits	95
Parameningeal H&N	Headache	Cranial nerve exam	70-75
Nonparameningeal H&N	Cranial nerve abnormalities Mass	MRI brain/primary CT neck	80-85
Paratesticular	Unilateral painless scrotal mass	ABD/pelvic CT LN evaluation and LN dissection for ≤10 y	80
Vagina/vulva	Genital mass Genital discharge	Ultrasound EUA	90
Bladder/prostate	Bladder outlet obstruction	Ultrasound, EUA MRI pelvis	70-75
Extremity	Mass	LN evaluation Angiography MRI primary	60-70

ABD, abdomen; CT, computed tomography; EUA, examination under anesthesia; H&N, head and neck; LN, lymph node; MRI, magnetic resonance imaging; y, year.

Table 65-4 **Workup for Pediatric Soft Tissue Sarcoma**

History and physical exam
Measurement of lesion
CBC
Blood work
Urinalysis
CXR
CT and MRI of primary, or both
CT chest
Bone scan
Bone marrow biopsy*
LN evaluation*

*Bone marrow biopsy and LN evaluation not needed for nonrhabdomyosarcoma.
CBC, complete blood (cell) count; CT, computed tomography; CXR, chest radiograph; LN, lymph node; MRI, magnetic resonance imaging.

Table 65-5 **International Rhabdomyosarcoma Study (IRS) Clinical Grouping Classification**

Clinical group I	Completely resected localized disease Confined to muscle of origin Involvement outside of muscle of origin (contiguously)
Clinical group II	Microscopic residual disease and regional nodal involvement Microscopic residual disease (after gross resection, N0) Regional nodal involvement (without microscopic residual disease) Regional nodal involvement (with microscopic residual disease)
Clinical group III	Gross residual disease After biopsy After gross major resection (>50% of disease)
Clinical group IV	Distant metastasis*

*Liver, lung, bones, bone marrow, distant muscle, positive CSF cytology, pleural or abdominal fluids, peritoneal or pleural implants.
CSF, cerebrospinal fluid; N0, Not clinically involved.

PATIENT EVALUATION

A complete history and physical examination is performed with particular attention to the presenting local signs and symptoms of the primary site. Evidence of symptomatic metastasis is evaluated. The diagnostic evaluation is directed by the location of the primary site and is obtained to determine extent of disease, size, invasiveness, and the presence or absence of lymph node metastasis. This is defined by a combination of plain film radiograph, computed tomography (CT) scan, and magnetic resonance imaging (MRI) of the primary lesion. Additional evaluation is performed based on the location of the primary disease (see Table 65-3). Standard evaluation of RMS for evidence of metastasis includes a chest CT, bone scan, bone marrow biopsy, and clinical lymph node evaluation (Table 65-4). Pathologic examination of lymph nodes is not routinely recommended except for extremity RMS, paratesticular RMS for boys (10 years of age or older),[18,19] and clinically suspicious lymph nodes. For NRSTS the evaluation is similar, but it does not include a bone marrow biopsy or lymph node evaluation.

A biopsy should be performed after complete evaluation of the primary lesion. The same principles for surgical biopsy of adult STS apply including careful placement of the biopsy site to avoid an increase in the extent of surgery, avoiding hematoma development and contamination of uninvolved areas and vital structures. The placement of the biopsy should not interfere with the ability to perform an organ-sparing procedure and spare a strip of skin outside of the radiation port.

STAGING

The initial RMS staging system was a clinical group classification based on the extent of residual disease after surgical resection (Table 65-5). This system proved to be prognostic of outcome. A tumor, node, metastasis (TNM)-based pretreatment staging system was developed later (Table 65-6) and has been proved to be predictive of outcome.[34] Currently, both the TNM pretreatment staging system and the clinical group classification are used for treatment recommendations and

Disease Sites

Table 65-6 Tumor, Node, Metastasis (TMN) Pretreatment Staging Classification

Stage	Site	Tumor Invasiveness	Tumor Size	Nodal Status	Metastasis
1	Favorable	T1/T2	A/B	N0/N1/NX	M0
2	Unfavorable	T1/T2	A	N0/NX	M0
3	Unfavorable	T1/T2	A	N1	M0
			B	N0/N1/NX	M0
4	Any site	T1/T2	A/B	N0/NX	M1

A, ≤5 cm in diameter; B, >5 cm in diameter; M0, no distant metastasis; M1, distant metastasis; N0, not clinically involved; N1, clinically involved by tumor; NX, clinical status unknown; T1, confined to site of origin; T2, extension and fixation to surrounding tissue; TMN, tumor, node, metastasis.

Table 65-7 International Rhabdomyosarcoma Study (IRS)-V Risk Categories[39]

Risk	Failure-Free Survival (%)	Survival (%)
LOW	80-90	90-95
Embryonal/botryoid RMS		
Stage 1, clinical groups I, II, III		
Stage 2, clinical groups I, II		
Stage 3, clinical groups I, II		
INTERMEDIATE		
Embryonal/botryoid	60-80	70-85
Stage 2, clinical group III		
Stage 3, clinical group III		
Alveolar RMS	50-55	55-60
Clinical groups I-III		
Embryonal RMS, <10 y		
Clinical group IV		
HIGH	<25	25-35
Clinical group IV		
(Embryonal RMS >10 y)		

RMS, rhabdomyosarcoma.

Table 65-8 International Rhabdomyosarcoma Study (IRS) I-IV Results[16,35-38]

IRS	Failure-Free Survival (5 y)	Overall Survival (5 y)
I	51%	55%
II	55%	63%
III	65%	71%
IV*	77%	86%

*3-y results.
y, year.

patient stratification. In IRS-V, patients are stratified into risk groups (Table 65-7), and treatment recommendation is tailored specifically for each group. NRSTS is staged according to IRS and TNM from the International Union Against Cancer (UICC).[25]

PRIMARY THERAPY

Historically, the outcome for children with RMS was poor, with fewer than 20% surviving 5 years. Since the 1970s there has been a dramatic improvement in the survival rate of children with this disease. Recent studies show an approximate 5-year survival of 75% (Table 65-8).[35] This significant progress is caused, in part, by the role of the IRSG and the thousands of children who enrolled in the IRS studies over the past few decades. Children with RMS should be treated under the care of a pediatric oncology team and enrolled in RMS protocols when possible.

The first IRS-I trial (1972-1978) used a combined modality approach that included chemotherapy, radiotherapy, and surgery. Results revealed a significant improvement in outcome with this approach (5-year survival 55%).[36]

IRS-II (1978-1984) intended to intensify treatment for children who did poorly, while minimizing toxicity without diminishing the good outcome for those who did well. Overall outcomes were improved compared to IRS-I (see Table 65-8).[16,36] The results of the first two studies confirmed that certain histologic subtypes and primary locations were prognostic (see Tables 65-1 and 65-2).[16,36]

In IRS-III (1984-1991), the children were randomized to a treatment regimen based on clinical group, histology, and primary site (see Table 65-6). Overall, outcomes were improved compared with the prior IRS studies (see Table 65-8). However, there was no difference in outcome between the different randomized groups.[37] The addition of doxorubicin to the standard VAC (vincristine, actinomycin D, and cyclophosphamide) did not improve the outcome of patients with advanced-stage disease in three consecutive IRSG trials.[16,36,37]

IRS-IV, which spanned from 1991 to 1997, used the TNM pretreatment staging system (see Table 65-6) to separate patients into risk groups based on primary site of disease, disease extent, and presence or absence of nodal and distant metastatic disease. The use of different chemotherapy combinations in stages 1 through 3 was evaluated and compared with standard VAC chemotherapy.[38] Results showed no significant difference in outcome between the different arms. In patients with stage IV disease, an "up-front window" was used to investigate new combinations of agents followed by standard VAC chemotherapy. Patients with stage 1, clinical group (CG) II N1 and III; stage 2, CG II; and stage 3, CG I and II benefited most from the therapy that was delivered in IRS-IV.[38]

Currently, for IRS-V, children are separated into low-, intermediate-, and high-risk categories based on prognostic factors from IRS-III data (see Table 65-7).[39] Low-risk patients are defined as those with primary tumors at favorable sites, completely resected or microscopic residual, or orbit and eyelid primaries with gross residual disease and tumors less than 5 cm at unfavorable sites but completely resected. Intermediate-risk patients are all other patients with local or regional tumors.[38] High-risk patients are those with metastatic disease or undifferentiated sarcoma, excluding children younger than 10 years of age with embryonal histology (see Table 65-7). The IRS-V schema is shown in Figure 65-1.

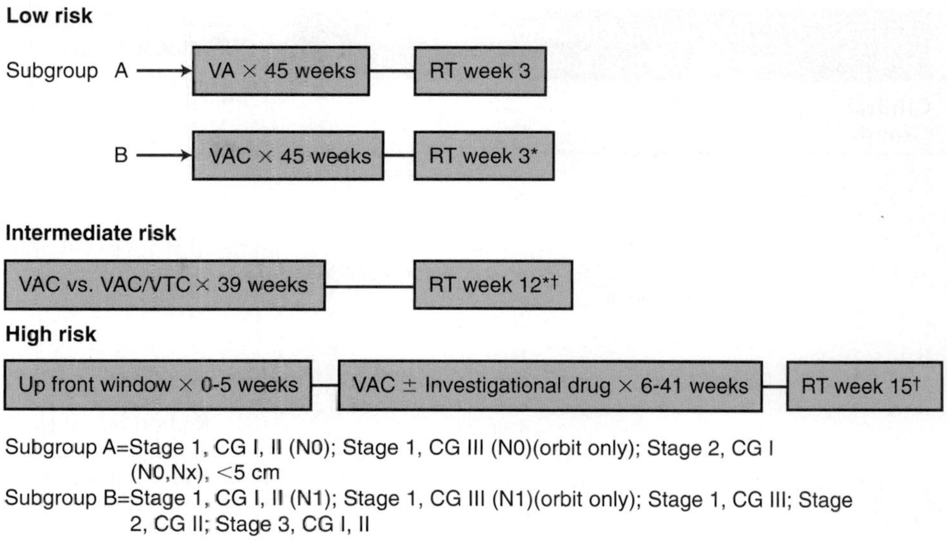

Figure 65-1 Intergroup Rhabdomyosarcoma Study Group V Treatment Schema.

*Week 12 if low-risk uterus, vagina, vulva, or superficial special parameningeal site, or if intermediate clinical group III, to allow for possible second-look surgery. †Unless emergency or parameningeal site with extracranial extension, RT given day 0. V, vincristine; A, actinomycin D; C, cyclophosphamide; T, topotecan; RT, radiotherapy; CG, clinical group.

Table 65-9 Alveolar Rhabdomyosarcoma (RMS) and Undifferentiated Sarcoma[40]

	Failure-Free Survival (10 y)			Overall Survival (10 y)		
	XRT	No XRT	p value	XRT	No XRT	p value
IRS I, II	73%	44%	.03	82%	52%	.02
IRS III	95%	69%	.01	95%	86%	.23

IRS, International Rhabdomyosarcoma Study; XRT, external radiation therapy; y, year.

The goals of treatment continue to improve results in patients who do less well and minimize toxicity in those with good outcomes. Organ preservation continues to be important. Subgroups of patients within each category continue to be defined, and treatment recommendations are tailored to each group.

LOCAL TREATMENT FOR RMS

Before the IRSG studies, radical surgery was the mainstay of therapy for RMS. Radiotherapy is now considered an integral part of the treatment of RMS and is used in most patients. Radiotherapy has allowed an increase in organ preservation and limb-sparing treatment. Certain primary sites require special consideration regarding local therapy.

Recommendations for local therapy have been modified through the years based on IRS results. In the first IRS study, the addition of radiotherapy to patients with completely resected tumors (CG I) did not improve the outcome.[36] Therefore radiotherapy was not recommended for completely resected disease (CG I) in the first three IRS studies. Results of this approach showed that children with alveolar RMS and undifferentiated sarcoma had a significantly worse failure-free survival (FFS) and overall survival (OS) when radiotherapy was omitted (Table 65-9).[40] Radiotherapy is now recommended for all children with alveolar RMS and undifferentiated sarcoma, even for completely resected disease (CG I).[40]

In IRS-IV children with CG III (gross residual disease) were randomized between 5040 cGy with conventional fractionation or 5940 cGy given with hyperfractionation. Hyperfractionation did not improve outcome in IRS-IV and is therefore no longer used for RMS.[41]

IRS-V is investigating the use of lower radiotherapy doses in patients with low-risk disease and has incorporated second-look surgery after induction chemotherapy with dose-adjusted radiotherapy recommendations based on findings and results of second-look surgery for certain subsets (Table 65-10).

Radiotherapy Techniques

Children with RMS should be treated on or according to the most recent available protocols in institutions familiar with treating pediatric malignancies. The current protocols outline radiotherapy guidelines in exquisite detail. The general guidelines for radiotherapy delivery are outlined in Table 65-10 and Table 65-11. However, exceptions exist to most of these basic rules. Details of some of these exceptions are discussed for individual primary sites in the following text.

The RMS treatment volume is described in general as the prechemotherapy volume with a 2-cm margin. More specifically, the gross tumor volume (GTV) is defined as the preoperative visible and palpable disease defined by physical examination, operative findings, and imaging evaluation. The clinical target volume (CTV) is defined as the GTV + 1.5 cm, modified to take into account barriers to tumor spread. The CTV includes the draining lymph node chain if the nodes are involved with a tumor, either clinically or pathologically. The planning target volume (PTV) is defined as the CTV plus a margin to account for setup error and intrinsic motion. The GTV is usually not changed by surgical resection or response to chemotherapy except under certain circumstances as defined in the protocol. For patients with primary sites in the H&N as well as vulva and uterus CG III disease, who do not

Table 65-10 International Rhabdomyosarcoma Study (IRS)-V Radiotherapy (RT) Doses

Clinical Group	Risk	Dose
I	Low	No radiation therapy
	Intermediate	3600 cGy
	High	No radiation therapy (embryonal) 3600 cGy-alveolar RMS
	After second-look surgery*	3600 cGy
II	Low	3600 cGy
	Intermediate	N0-3600 cGy N1-4140 cGy
	High	4140 cGy
	After second-look surgery*	4140 cGy
III	Low	3600 cGy (orbit) 4500 cGy (nonorbit)
	Intermediate	4140 cGy (CR biopsy negative) 5040 cGy
	High	5040 cGy
	After second-look surgery*	5040 cGy

*If low-risk uterus, vagina, vulva, superficial special parameningeal site or if immediate risk, clinical group III, patient may be a candidate for second-look surgery. Radiation therapy given based on clinical group after second-look surgery.

CR, complete response; N0, Not clinically involved; N1, clinically involved by tumor; RMS, rhabdomyosarcoma.

Table 65-11 Radiotherapy Volume

GTV	Extent of primary disease at diagnosis*
CTV	GTV + 1.5-cm margin
PTV	CTV + margin for motion

*The GTV is changed by chemotherapy response and surgery in selected circumstances.

CTV, clinical target volume; GTV, gross tumor volume; PTV, planning target volume.

undergo a second look operation, a total dose of 5040 cGy is given with a second CTV and PTV defined for a cone down at 3600 cGy if there is a radiographic response to induction chemotherapy. The boost volume is defined at the CTV of the original GTV at diagnosis + 0.5 cm margin.

Radiotherapy doses to the primary disease range from 3600 cGy to 5040 cGy and are based on risk category, clinical group, TMN stage, and status after second-look surgery (see Table 65-10). For stage 4 disease, the primary is treated with radiotherapy to 5040 cGy with conventional fractionation. Metastatic disease sites are treated with doses dependent on tolerance of surrounding normal structures.

Timing of radiotherapy delivery is outlined in Table 65-12. Radiotherapy is begun at week 12 except for patients with low-risk disease (stage 1 CG II, III; stage 2, 3 CG II), in which radiotherapy is given at week 3. However, patients with low risk CG III disease of the vulva, uterus, biliary tumors, and special nonparameningeal H&N will have radiotherapy delayed to week 12 to allow for possible second-look surgery. Patients with metastatic disease receive radiotherapy at week 15. In patients with high-risk parameningeal disease, defined as those with intracranial extension, and those with emergent situations, radiotherapy starts at day 0.

Table 65-12 Timing of Radiotherapy

Low-risk disease	Week 3*
Intermediate-risk disease	Week 12
Metastatic disease	Week 15

*Exceptions: low-risk clinical group III disease of vulva, vagina, and special nonparameningeal H&N primary sites, week 12 (to allow second-look surgery)

H&N, head and neck.

Radiotherapy treatment delivery techniques are evolving from traditional 2-dimensional (2D) approaches to highly conformal 3D techniques, use of intensity-modulated radiotherapy (IMRT), proton beam therapy and brachytherapy. The potential benefit of these approaches to improve treatment delivery and minimize toxicity is quite promising.

Individual Sites

Parameningeal Sites

Children with parameningeal RMS had a poor outcome (3-year disease-free survival of 33%) in the first IRS studies secondary to meningeal relapse.[42-45] In IRS-II, craniospinal radiation therapy and later whole-brain radiotherapy were recommended to decrease the local failure rate. This resulted in an improved outcome (3-year relapse-free survival of 57%).[43] The treatment volume was then progressively reduced. In IRS-IV the recommended margin on gross residual disease was decreased to 2 cm without obvious compromise.[46] Recent reviews confirm that whole-brain radiotherapy is unnecessary.[44] The initial failures were probably because of inadequate dose and tumor coverage in the pre-CT era.[43] Using current complex treatment planning techniques with CT and MRI may further improve target definition, improve dose delivery, and reduce dose to surrounding normal tissue structures, thereby improving outcomes and minimizing toxicity.[44,45] Analysis of IRS II-IV studies combined revealed a 5-year OS of 73%.[44] Histology, primary site, and meningeal involvement continue to be prognostic.[45] The availability of neuroimaging is associated with an increase in identification of meningeal impingement.[44]

Local therapy by radiotherapy continues to be standard. Figure 65-2 illustrates a 3D plan and isodose distribution for a patient with parameningeal RMS. Patients with meningeal impingement (cranial nerve palsy or cranial base bone erosion with or without intracranial extension) start radiotherapy on day 0, but the volume of radiation treatment is not extended.[45] Initiation of radiotherapy within 2 weeks of diagnosis for children with meningeal impingement within was associated with a lower rate of local failure.[44]

Orbit

RMS of the orbit is a favorable primary site (stage I) and results have been excellent. IRS III confirmed that only two chemotherapy agents (vincristine and actinomycin) were needed rather than three.[37] Surgery is usually limited to biopsy only. Therefore most patients have CG III disease (gross residual disease) and receive radiotherapy. There was a superior outcome in patients treated on IRS-IV (100%) compared with IRS-III (83%), possibly because of more intensive treatment, higher radiation therapy dose, and improved compliance with radiation therapy guidelines.[47]

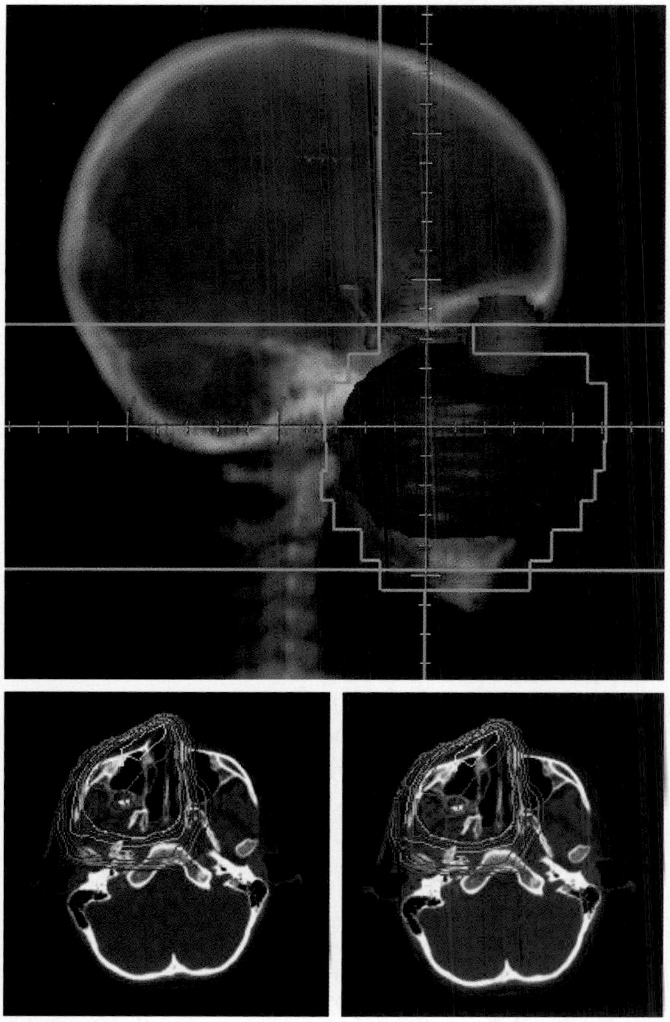

Figure 65-2 3D plan and isodose distribution for RMS of parameningeal rhabdomyosarcoma.

The radiotherapy treatment volume is gross tumor volume with a 2-cm margin. However, the CTV does not extend outside of the bony orbit, providing there is no bony erosion of the orbit. Treatment approaches can include an angled anterior field or a wedged pair. Figure 65-3 illustrates a treatment plan for orbital RMS. Patients should be treated with mask immobilization and their eye open to avoid a bolusing effect. Attempts should be made to shield the lens, cornea, lacrimal gland, pituitary, hypothalamus, and optic chiasm without skimping on the recommended margin. Most common sequelae include cataract formation, decreased visual acuity, hypoplastic orbit, ptosis, and dry eye.[48] Serious complications are rare.

Four international collaborative groups compared their data at an international workshop: IRSG, Sarcoma Committee; International Society of Paediatric Oncology (SIOP); German Collaborative Soft Tissue Sarcoma Group (CWS); and Italian Cooperative Soft Tissue Sarcoma Group (ICG). The overall 10-year EFS and OS were 77% and 87%, respectively.[48] The use of radiotherapy differed between the groups (93% in IRSG, 76% in ICG, 70% in CWS, and only 37% in SIOP). Use of radiotherapy positively impacted EFS (82% versus 53% radiotherapy versus 0% radiotherapy), and there was a statistically significant difference on EFS by treatment group (IRS 86%, CWS 70%, ICG 64%, SIOP 58%); but there was no difference in OS (88%-85%).[48] Histology and age younger than 3 years were negative prognostic factors.[47] The side effects of radiotherapy must be weighed against the improvement in EFS and the need for additional combined therapy (and its potential side effects) in those who relapse. Currently, IRS-V is investigating the use of lower radiotherapy doses, which may potentially reduce radiotherapy–related toxicity (see Table 65-7). IMRT or proton beam therapy may prove to further reduce radiotherapy toxicity.

Special Pelvic Sites

Before the use of combined modality therapy, pelvic exenteration was used to treat patients with tumors in the bladder and prostate. The use of delayed local therapies using a primary chemotherapy approach in an attempt to decrease the use of radiotherapy or radical surgeries was tested in IRS-II. Local treatment was reserved for patients with residual or progressive disease. This resulted in a poor bladder preservation

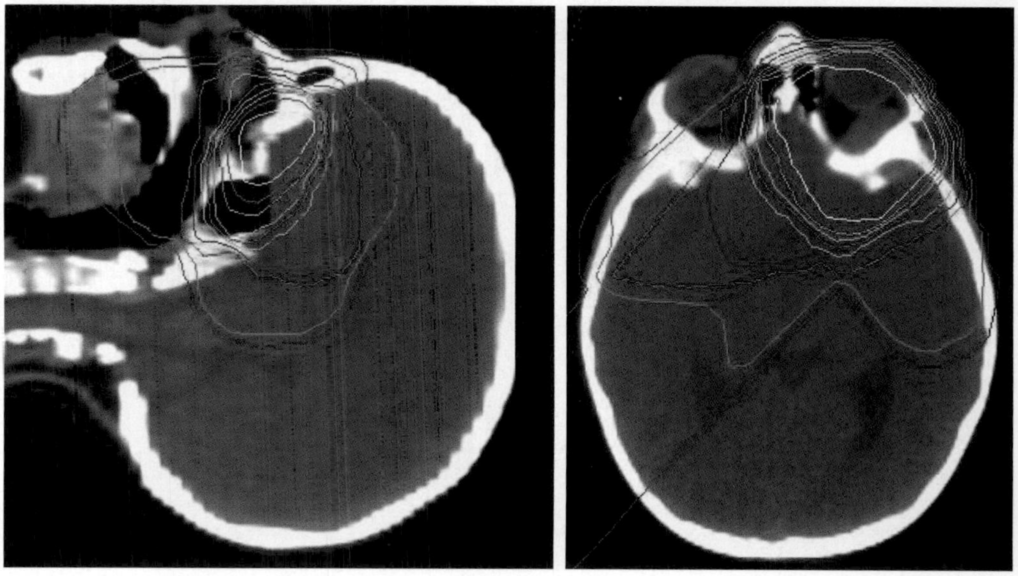

Figure 65-3 3D isodose distribution for an orbital rhabdomyosarcoma.

rate (22%) and an inferior 3-year disease-free survival (52% versus 70%).[49] Therefore in IRS-III, local treatment with radiotherapy was instituted and surgical resection was used for gross residual disease after chemotherapy and radiotherapy. This approach resulted in improved organ preservation (60%) and disease-free survival (73%).[50] In IRS-IV, children with nonmetastatic bladder and prostate RMS had an 82% survival, with bladder function preserved in 55% of event-free survivors after 6 years.[51] Radiotherapy was used for the majority of patients, and most received second-look operations after radiotherapy.

Patients with vulvar and vaginal tumors did well with the chemotherapy-based approach used in IRS-II.[49] Therefore children with these tumors are recommended to undergo biopsy, chemotherapy, and limited surgical resection, with radiotherapy reserved for residual disease. Results of this approach revealed that children ages 1 to 9 years have a 98% 5-year survival, whereas children outside of this age range did less well in the first two IRS studies (5-year survival 67%).[52] There was a significant improvement in outcome with IRS III/IV therapy for these children (90%).[51]

The overall cure rate for RMS of the genital tract has steadily improved with an increased rate of organ preservation.[52] However, some have questioned the use of radiotherapy for pelvic tumors, claiming that radiotherapy leads to poor functional outcomes, second primary malignancies, and abnormal growth and development of pelvic organs.[53,54] SIOP recommends initial chemotherapy with radiotherapy reserved for those who do not achieve a complete response, have residual tumor after initial chemotherapy, or recur locally.[55] In IRS-V the use of radiotherapy is tailored to the patient based on histology, response to treatment, surgical procedure, findings at second surgery, and location of disease. It appears that there is a high salvage rate for children who recur locally, particularly if they have not had radiotherapy as part of their treatment.[52,56] However, radiotherapy should be used up front if indicated to avoid a local recurrence, a decrease in event-free survival, and the need for a second course of combined modality therapy.[52,56]

In IRS-V, to select children for radiotherapy, the timing of local control and radiotherapy is delayed until week 12 (week 28 for node-negative vaginal tumors) to allow for second-look surgery. Reduced dose radiotherapy and further local treatment recommendations are then determined by findings at that time (see Table 65-7). The goal remains to minimize toxicity while maintaining excellent overall results.

The optimal radiation therapy approach to treatment of the pelvic region must be individualized. The GTV is defined as the preoperative tumor volume excluding the intraabdominal or intrapelvic tumor that was debulked. However, all areas of preoperative involvement of the peritoneum or mesentery and the site of origin will be included in the GTV. Figure 65-4 illustrates a treatment plan of RMS of the pelvis. Traditionally, simple anterior and posterior fields have been used, because they have the added benefit of sparing the femoral epiphysis and proximal femur. However, highly conformal treatment planning and delivery techniques including IMRT, proton beam therapy, and brachytherapy may help spare the surrounding normal and critical structures, while potentially minimizing toxicity. Toxicity of radiotherapy includes nonfunctioning bladder, bladder dysfunction, dribbling, enuresis, incontinence, hydronephrosis, urethral stricture,[51] vaginal stenosis, bony hypoplasia, scoliosis, infertility, hormonal dysfunction, musculoskeletal abnormalities, and rectal and bowel injury.

Extremities

Patients with extremity RMSs tend to have alveolar histology and therefore a poorer outcome. Radiotherapy is used for all patients with alveolar histology, regardless of extent of resection (see Table 65-9).[40] The same principles apply to the treatment of these lesions as in other STSs of the extremities. Wide local excision followed by radiotherapy for microscopic or gross residual disease is the general approach. Regional nodal evaluation is recommended, and regional radiotherapy is given if the results are positive. The use of chemotherapy and radiotherapy may be appropriate before resection if initial surgery would preclude organ preservation. Radiotherapy is delivered to the original tumor volume with a 2-cm margin. Special attention must be paid to the tumor location, immobilization, and complex treatment planning with the use of wedges, compensators, or bolus as indicated. Inclusion of all

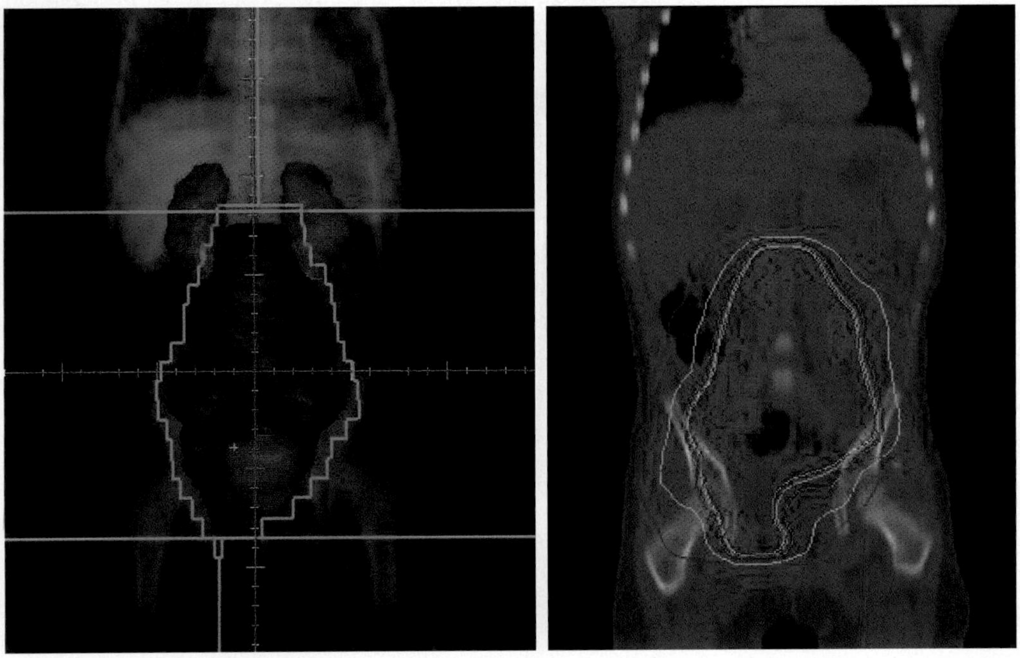

Figure 65-4 3D simulation film and isodose distribution for rhabdomyosarcoma of the pelvis.

scars and drain sites is recommended. Attempts must be made to spare a strip of skin, portion of joints, and adjacent and opposite epiphysis. The use of brachytherapy should be considered to minimize normal tissue toxicity and decreased growth and development.

Paratesticular Sites

For RMS of the paratesticular region, the recommended surgical treatment is radical inguinal orchiectomy with high ligation of the spermatic cord. Ipsilateral retroperitoneal lymph node dissection (RPLND) is now indicated for all patients older than 10 years of age.[19] In IRS-IV there was a reduction in the rate of positive retroperitoneal lymph nodes from 24% to 8% and a decrease in failure-free survival secondary to an increase in local and regional relapse.[57] This is believed to be caused by an underestimation of nodal involvement by CT staging evaluation. Therefore the role of CT scans in place of an RPLND has undergone re-evaluation.[57] As part of staging evaluation, an ipsilateral RPLND is now considered standard for boys older than 10 years of age.[19] Lymph node sampling is performed for children younger than 10 years of age only if there are positive or concerning findings on CT. Retroperitoneal lymph node irradiation is indicated for positive lymph nodes. Violation of the scrotum from transscrotal biopsy renders the patient with CG II disease and then requires radiotherapy to the hemiscrotum. Resection of violated scrotal tissue should be performed and possible hemiscrotectomy considered. The survival of children with paratesticular RMS is greater than 80% at 5 years of age.

Relapse

Analysis of the first three IRS protocols revealed that the median survival from first recurrence was 0.8 years with 17% surviving 5 years.[56] Tumor histology, initial stage or group, and location of recurrence has been determined to be prognostic.[56] There is a subset with improved outcomes (50% at 5 years) that has been identified. A treatment protocol for relapsed RMS is being developed by COG using a risk-based approach.

LOCAL TREATMENT: NONRHABDOMYOSARCOMA

The primary treatment of NRSTS is surgical resection. Studies at the National Cancer Institute and Massachusetts General Hospital confirmed the equivalence of a limb-sparing approach with wide local excision and radiotherapy to an amputation.[58,59] In children, however, there are concerns regarding the use of radiotherapy, including abnormal bone growth and development and the induction of second malignancies. Therefore radiotherapy is used less often than in adults.

The recommendations for radiotherapy in pediatric NRSTS are not clear-cut. Radiotherapy appears to be unnecessary for small low-grade tumors amenable to wide local excision. Large unresectable low-grade malignancies, recurrent low-grade lesions, and those in difficult locations to achieve clean margins may need adjuvant radiotherapy. Based on results of the Pediatric Oncology Group (POG) study No. 8653, radiation therapy appears unnecessary for children who undergo radical resection of a high-grade NRSTS.[60] Adjuvant radiation is recommended for high-grade tumors that are unresectable, marginally resected, or with close and positive margins.[60] Preoperative radiotherapy should be considered in patients who might be converted to an organ-sparing procedure or in whom a gross total resection would result in significant functional morbidity.

The current recommended dose to the tumor bed is approximately 5000 to 6000 cGy in conventional fractionation with a shrinking field technique.[60] Brachytherapy should be considered adjuvant local treatment. A new study proposed by COG will better define the role and dose of radiotherapy in these patients.

Chemotherapy

There are no clear-cut guidelines regarding the use of chemotherapy in NRSTS. A randomized study (POG No. 8653) investigating patients with localized disease did not demonstrate a benefit of adjuvant chemotherapy for localized disease.[2] Chemotherapy is not routinely recommended for localized, resectable NRSTS.[2,25] A POG study is currently investigating the use of chemotherapy for unresectable or metastatic NRSTS.

TOXICITY

Radiotherapy-induced toxicity depends on the location of the radiotherapy treatment. The most important side effects are those of impairment of growth and development, organ dysfunction, and induction of second primary malignancy. Overall, the risk of second malignant neoplasm in children with sarcomas of bone and soft tissue is approximately 2% to 5% at 10 and 15 years after radiation therapy.[61,62] However, this depends on age, dose of radiation therapy, use of chemotherapy, and underlying genetic abnormalities. Toxicity from treatment of the primary is site dependent and is discussed earlier for each primary site.

FUTURE DEVELOPMENTS

The results of previous and current IRS studies will continue to define subgroups of patients and a risk-based approach. For children who do well, the goal will continue to be to maintain excellent outcome while minimizing toxicity. For those who do less well, optimal therapy will continue to be defined. The indications for radiotherapy and radiotherapy dose also continue to be refined.

For children with low-risk disease, the goal will be to decrease the intensity of therapy and limit alkylating agents while maintaining the excellent outcome for this group. For intermediate-risk patients, new combinations of chemotherapy with topoisomerase I inhibitors will be tested. For high-risk disease alternating doublets of active agents will be tried.

Future developments in radiation therapy and local control include further defining the use of risk-adjusted radiotherapy recommendations; reduced radiotherapy doses; and response-based radiotherapy using post chemotherapy clinical, radiotherapy, and surgical evaluations. The radiotherapy volumes may be further defined and dependent on risk category and response. The use of preoperative radiation therapy for poor-prognosis group III lesions is also a possibility. The increased use of brachytherapy and highly conformal complex treatment planning and delivery techniques including IMRT, extracranial radiosurgery, and proton therapy may result in decreased short- and long-term treatment–related toxicity while potentially improving local control.

REFERENCES

1. Gurney JG, Severson RK, Davis S, et al: Incidence of cancer in children in United States. Cancer 75:2186, 1995.
2. Pratt CB, Pappo AS, Gieser P, et al: Role of adjuvant chemotherapy in the treatment of surgically resected pediatric nonrhab-

CHAPTER 66

PEDIATRIC SARCOMAS OF BONE

Andreas Schuck

INCIDENCE

Osteosarcoma occurs in 5.6 cases/million children per year.
Each year Ewing's sarcoma occurs in 2.8 cases/million children.

BIOLOGIC CHARACTERISTICS

Osteosarcoma: inactivation of retinoblastoma gene
Ewing's sarcoma: chromosomal translocation at t11;22 (q24;q12)

STAGING EVALUATION

Localized versus metastatic disease

PRIMARY THERAPY

Osteosarcoma: surgical resection, multiagent chemotherapy; 5-year survival, 60% to 70%
Ewing's sarcoma: surgery, radiation therapy, or both; neoadjuvant and adjuvant multiagent chemotherapy; 5-year survival, 60% to 70%

ADJUVANT THERAPY

Osteosarcoma: neoadjuvant and adjuvant multiagent chemotherapy
Ewing's sarcoma: neoadjuvant and adjuvant multiagent chemotherapy

LOCALLY ADVANCED DISEASE

Osteosarcoma: multiagent neoadjuvant and adjuvant chemotherapy, surgical resection of primary and limited metastatic disease; 5-year overall survival, 20% to 30%
Ewing's sarcoma: more aggressive multiagent neoadjuvant and adjuvant chemotherapy, radiation therapy, or surgery, or a combination, to primary and radiation therapy to metastatic disease; 5-year overall survival, 10% to 30%

PALLIATION

Chemotherapy, surgery, and for radiation therapy

Osteosarcoma and Ewing's sarcoma are the two most common malignant bone tumors in the pediatric and adolescent age groups. Although osteosarcoma occurs more frequently than Ewing's sarcoma, it is rarely treated with radiation therapy. Therefore, this section is devoted largely to the discussion of Ewing's sarcoma. Like all other pediatric malignancies, patients should be treated on protocol and in institutions familiar with, and experienced in, the treatment of childhood tumors.

ETIOLOGY AND EPIDEMIOLOGY

The incidence of Ewing's sarcoma is approximately 2.8 cases/million in children younger than age 15 years.[1] Generally, it occurs in the teenage years during the adolescent growth spurt.[2] However, the age of onset is variable; approximately 30% of cases occur in the first decade of life and 10% occur in the third decade. More males than females are affected. There is a predilection for whites in whom it is more frequent than among Asians. It rarely occurs in black children. The cause of Ewing's sarcoma is unknown, and it does not appear to be induced by any known agents.

Osteosarcoma also is primarily a disease of adolescents and young adults; a different type of osteosarcoma linked to Paget's disease occurs in older adults. This section focuses on osteosarcoma in the younger age group. There is limited understanding of the etiology of osteosarcoma. The peak incidence coincides with a period of rapid bone growth, suggesting a correlation with the evolution of osteosarcoma. Furthermore, it is known to be induced by radiation therapy, particularly in children with retinoblastoma or other genetic abnormalities.[3]

PATHOLOGY AND PATHWAY OF SPREAD

Ewing's sarcoma is an undifferentiated blue round cell tumor usually of the bone. Pathologically, it appears as a monomorphic pattern of densely packed, small round malignant cells with hyperchromatic nuclei and varying amounts of cytoplasm.[4] Immunohistochemistry studies reveal cell-surface glycoprotein p30/32 MIC2 (CD 99) and vimentin, HBA-71, and β_2-microglobulin positivity. Occasionally, cytokeratin and neuron-specific enolase (NSE) are positive. These studies can help differentiate Ewing's sarcoma from other small round cell malignancies of childhood. Approximately 87% of cases within the family of Ewing's tumor are Ewing's sarcoma of bone.[5] The remainder are peripheral primitive neuroectodermal tumor (PNET) or extraosseous Ewing's sarcoma further characterized in the next chapter.

Approximately 75% of patients with Ewing's sarcoma present with localized disease at diagnosis (Fig. 66-1). However, approximately 80% of children experience distant metastases if treated with only local therapy. This suggests that in most cases, there are unidentifiable micrometastases at diagnosis. The most common site of metastasis is the lung followed by bone. Other distant sites include bone marrow, soft tissue, and, rarely, liver or central nervous system (CNS) (see Fig. 66-1).

Osteosarcoma is derived from bone-forming mesenchyme and is described as a malignant sarcomatous stroma associated with the production of osteoid bone, the defining histopathologic feature.[4] The most common types in the pediatric population are the conventional osteosarcomas, including osteoblastic, chondroblastic, and fibroblastic types. Each type has varying amounts of osteoid formation and a

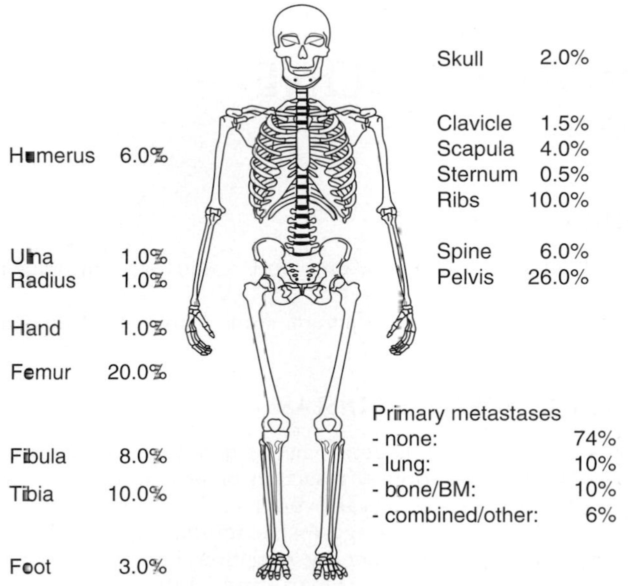

Figure 66-1 Distribution of primary sites and sites of metastases in Ewing's sarcoma. BM, bone marrow.

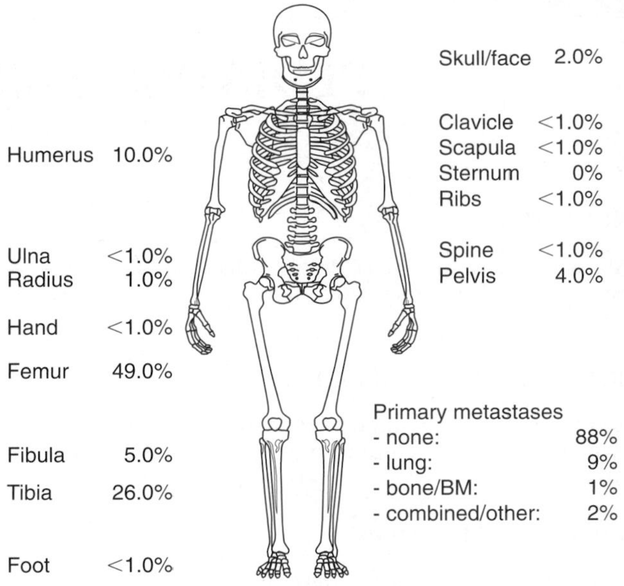

Figure 66-2 Distribution of primary sites and sites of metastases in osteosarcoma.

different predominant component. There is no difference in outcome or treatment recommendations among these different types. Other types of less common osteosarcomas include telangiectatic, small cell, juxtacortical, periosteal, and high-grade surface sarcomas.

Approximately 90% of children with osteosarcoma present with localized disease at diagnosis (Fig. 66-2). If treated to the primary only, roughly 90% will experience metastatic disease.[4]

BIOLOGIC CHARACTERISTICS AND MOLECULAR BIOLOGY

The histogenesis of Ewing's sarcoma has been controversial. It was first described as an endothelioma of the bone. It is now believed to have a neural origin, specifically from post-ganglionic, parasympathetic, primordial cells.[6,7] Previously, extraosseous Ewing's sarcoma and PNET were considered separate entities from Ewing's sarcoma of bone and were treated differently. However, now they are believed to be from the same family of tumors.[7] This is confirmed by their similar characteristics. Both exhibit identical chromosomal translocations, t11:22 (q24;q12); and more than 85% of patients share a common surface antigen MIC2.[8-10] Ewing's sarcoma, atypical Ewing's sarcoma, and PNET of bone exist in the spectrum within this family, from the most undifferentiated tumors to those with neural differentiation. PNET can be differentiated from Ewing's sarcoma by the presence of a globular growth pattern, NSE positivity, and Homer-Wright rosettes.

Osteosarcoma is associated with the inactivation of the retinoblastoma tumor suppressor gene (13q14), which occurs in approximately one-third of osteosarcoma cases.[11] Other genetic abnormalities include translocations, gene amplification, and abnormal p53 function.[12,13]

CLINICAL MANIFESTATIONS AND STAGING

Ewing's sarcoma patients present in general with localized pain, swelling, and a palpable mass. The frequency with which Ewing's sarcoma occurs within the different regions of the body is illustrated in Figure 66-1. In Ewing's sarcoma plain radiographs show a lytic, destructive lesion of the diaphysis with or without a soft tissue mass. Codman's triangle may form from the elevated periosteal reaction. An "onion skin" effect, derived from the development of parallel, multilaminar, periosteal reactions, is evident.

Osteosarcoma patients present with similar signs and symptoms: In general, localized pain, swelling, and a palpable mass. The frequency with which osteosarcoma occurs within the different regions of the body is illustrated in Figure 66-2. Plain radiographs on patients with osteosarcoma generally show sclerotic or lytic lesions of the metaphysis. Codman's triangle may form from the elevated periosteal reaction. In osteosarcoma periosteal new bone formation may be present, with the blastic component showing a bony sunburst pattern.

The evaluation for Ewing's sarcoma and osteosarcoma patients is similar.[14] A complete history and physical examination is performed, with particular attention to the duration of symptoms, presence of pain, difficulty of function, neurologic symptomatology, and location and size of mass. Routine blood work, urinalysis, bone scan, plain radiographs, computed tomography (CT), or magnetic resonance imaging (MRI) of the primary region, or a combination, are obtained to evaluate extent of disease. Chest radiograph and chest CT are obtained to rule out lung metastases. If the chest radiograph is negative and the CT scan is positive, an excision may be needed for accurate staging and treatment recommendations. If available, an ^{18}F-fluorodeoxyglucose positron emission tomography (FDG-PET) scan should be performed. Electrocardiogram and echocardiogram are included in the evaluation before chemotherapy is initiated. In the case of Ewing's sarcoma, a bone marrow biopsy is obtained. A summary of staging and follow-up investigations is given in Table 66-1.

A biopsy of the primary lesion should be obtained after complete evaluation, ideally by the surgeon who will perform the definitive resection. The biopsy should be placed carefully to avoid contamination of uninvolved areas and vital structures, as well as hematoma development. It should not

Table 66-1 Staging Investigations at Diagnosis in Osteosarcoma and Ewing's Sarcoma (ES)

Investigation	Diagnosis	Follow-Up
Radiograph in two planes, whole bone with adjacent joints	+	+
MRI and/or CT, affected bone(s) and adjacent joints	+	+
Biopsy: material for histology and molecular biology	+	
Thoracic CT (lung window)	+	+
Bone marrow biopsy and aspirates (in ES): microscopy (molecular biology still investigational)		
Whole-body ^{99m}Tc bone scan	+	+
FDG-PET	$+^1$	$+^1$

+, mandatory; $+^1$, indicated, if available; CT, computed tomography; MRI, magnetic resonance imaging; FDG-PET, ^{18}Fluorine-fluorodeoxyglucose positron emission tomography; ^{99m}Tc, 99m-technetium.

increase the extent of surgery or preclude limb-sparing procedure or sparing of a strip of skin outside the radiation port.

STAGING

Currently, there is no staging system for Ewing's sarcoma. Patients are classified as having either localized disease or metastatic disease and are treated accordingly. In osteosarcoma, available staging systems are those of the Musculoskeletal Tumor Society and lately of the International Union Against Cancer (UICC) and the American Joint Committee on Cancer (AJCC).[15,16]

The prognosis for patients with Ewing's sarcoma depends on a number of factors, the most important of which is presence or absence of metastatic disease. Other prognostic factors include lesion site and size.[17] Furthermore, histologic response to chemotherapy is a predictor of outcome. The prognostic features of osteosarcoma are similar: presence or absence of metastatic disease, tumor location, size, complete resection of primary, and response to adjuvant chemotherapy.[18-21]

TREATMENT OF EWING'S SARCOMA

Primary Therapy

Historically, patients with Ewing's sarcoma received treatment to the primary lesion only; cure rates were fewer than 20%. In the early 1960s, single-institution studies began to show improved outcome with the addition of adjuvant chemotherapy.[22-24] Today the standard treatment consists of local therapy and neoadjuvant and adjuvant polychemotherapy. Local therapy consists of surgery, radiotherapy, or a combination of both. Local therapy issues will be further discussed later in this chapter. Concerning systemic therapy, a number of randomized trials have been performed to determine the value of different drug combinations. The first Intergroup Ewing's Sarcoma Study (IESS) investigated the use of polychemotherapy from 1973 through 1978. Patients received radiation therapy to the primary lesion and were randomized among three adjuvant chemotherapy treatment arms: vincristine, actinomycin D, and cyclophosphamide (VAC); VAC plus doxorubicin (Adriamycin; VACAdr); or VAC plus bilateral pulmonary radiation therapy.[25] This study showed a significant improvement in all parameters with the addition of Adriamycin. Furthermore, VAC plus bilateral lung irradiation, although less effective than VACAdr, showed superior results to VAC alone. Thus Adriamycin was considered an essential drug in further trials. The importance of Adriamycin, as well as high initial treatment intensity, was further highlighted by a systematic meta-analysis of clinical trails by Smith and colleagues.[26] Besides the standard VACAdr regime, an additional benefit of the use of ifosfamide and etoposide has been discussed.

The third IESS investigated the addition of etoposide and ifosfamide to VACAdr, which at 5 years showed a statistically significant benefit to the addition of these two drugs.[27] In the European Cooperative Intergroup Ewing Sarcoma Study (EICESS) 92, the value of the single agents was evaluated. In standard-risk patients (localized disease and tumor volume of fewer than 100 mL), VACAdr was randomized against VAIA (ifosfamide instead of cyclophosphamide). There was no significant difference in event-free survival (EFS) between the groups. In high-risk patients (larger tumors or metastatic disease), VAIA was randomized against VAIA plus etoposide; again no significant difference in EFS was observed. A further treatment intensification strategy is the use of high-dose chemotherapy with autologous hematopoietic stem cell rescue. Because of its toxicity, this treatment is mainly used for very high-risk patients. In the ongoing Euro-Ewing 99 trial, in poor histologic responders the use of high-dose chemotherapy with busulfan is randomized against conventional therapy or, in metastatic patients with lung metastases only, against conventional chemotherapy and whole-lung irradiation with 15 Gy or 18 Gy, depending on the age of the patient.

A summary of results of different phase III trials is given in Table 66-2.

LOCALLY ADVANCED DISEASE AND PALLIATION

Children with metastatic Ewing's disease at diagnosis continue to have a poor outcome despite aggressive multiagent chemotherapy. The current overall approach in these patients is to intensify adjuvant and neoadjuvant chemotherapy. High-dose chemotherapy with busulfan or melphalan is used in the treatment of patients with bone metastases. Radiation therapy and sometimes surgery are used to treat the primary disease and sites of bone metastases. In patients with lung metastases only, the use of whole-lung irradiation has shown favorable results in the German Cooperative Study Group (CESS) and EICESS trials.[28] Radiation therapy can be used as a palliative local measure in patients in whom curative management fails.

LOCAL THERAPY

Local therapy is an essential modality in the treatment of Ewing's sarcoma. With systemic therapy alone, cure cannot be obtained. The modality of local therapy with best local control rates and better functional outcome has been a matter of debate for some time. Essentially, local therapy can be given with surgery alone, radiotherapy alone, or a combination of both, and either as preoperative or postoperative radiotherapy. To date, there has been no randomized trial comparing local therapy modalities and no such trial is expected in the next few years. From retrospective analyses of several groups, the impression has been that local control is improved when

Table 66-2 **Treatment Results in Selected Clinical Studies of Localized ESFT**

Study	References	Schedule	Patients	5-y EFS
IESS STUDIES				
IESS-I [1973-1978]	Nesbit, J Clin Oncol 8:1664, 1990	VAC VAC + WLI VACD	342	24% 44% 60%
IESS-II [1978-1982]	Burgert, J Clin Oncol 8:1514, 1990	VACD-HD VACD-MD	214	68% 48%
First POG–CCG (INT-0091) [1988-1993]	Grier, N Engl J Med 348:694, 2003	VACD VACD + IE	200 198	54% 69%
Second POG–CCG [1995-1998]	Granowetter, Med Pediatr Oncol 37:172, 2001 (abstr.)	VCD + IE 48 wk of SG VCD + IE 30 wk	492	75% (3 y) 76% (3 y)
MEMORIAL SLOAN-KETTERING CANCER CENTER STUDIES				
T2 [1970-1978]	Rosen, Cancer 41:888, 1978	VACD (adjuvant)	20	75%
P6 [1990-1995]	Kushner, J Clin Oncol 13:2796, 1995	HD-CVD + IE	36	77% (2 y)
P6 [1991-2001]	Kolb, J Clin Oncol 21:3423, 2003	HD-CVD + IE	68	Localized: 81% (4 y) Metastatic: 12% (4 y)
ST. JUDE STUDIES				
EW-79 [1978-1986]	Hayes, J Clin Oncol 7:208, 1989	VACD	52	82% <8 cm (3 y) 64% ≥8 cm (3 y)
EW-87 [1987-1991]	Meyer, J Clin Oncol 10:1737, 1992	Therapeutic window with IE	26	Clinical responses in 96%
EW-92 [1992-1996]	Marina, J Clin Oncol 17:180, 1999	VCDIE × 3 VCD/IE Intensification	34	78% (3 y)
UKCCSG/MRC STUDIES				
ET-1 [1978-1986]	Craft, Eur J Cancer 33:1061, 1997	VACD	120	41% Extr. 52% Axial 38% Pelvic 13%
ET-2 [1987-1993]	Craft, J Clin Oncol 16:3628, 1998	VAID	201	62% Extr. 73% Axial 55% Pelvic 41%
CESS STUDIES				
CESS-81 [1981-1985]	Jürgens, Cancer 61:23, 1988	VACD	93	<100 mL 80% ≥100 mL 31% (both 3 y) Viable tumor <10%: 79% >10%: 31% (both 3 y)
CESS-86 [1986-1991]	Paulussen, J Clin Oncol 19:1818, 2001	<100 mL (SR): VACD ≥100 mL (HR): VAID	301	52% (10 y) 51% (10 y)
EICESS STUDIES (CESS+UKCCSG)				
EICESS-92 [1992-1999]	EICESS group, personal communication, May 2004	SR: VAID/VACD HR: VAID/EVAID	155 326	68%/61% 51%/61%
ROI/Bologna, Italy				
REN-3 [1991-1997]	Bacci, Eur J Cancer 38:2243, 2002	VDC + VIA + IE	157	71%
SFOP/FRANCE				
EW-88 [1988-1991]	Oberlin, Br J Cancer 85:1646, 2001	VD + VD/VA	141	58%
SSG/SCANDINAVIA				
SSG IX [1990-1999]	Elomaa, Eur J Cancer 36:875, 2000	VID + PID	88	58% (metastases-free survival)

A, actinomycin D; C, cyclophosphamide; CCG, Children's Cancer Group; CESS-86,81, Cooperative Ewing's Sarcoma Study-86,81; D, doxorubicin; E, etoposide, Extr., extremities; EFS, event-free survival; EICESS-92, European Intergroup Cooperative Ewing's Sarcoma Study-92; ESFT, Ewing's sarcoma family of tumors; EW-79,87, Ewing Study-79,87; ET1,2, Ewing's tumor study 1,2; EW-88,92, Ewing Study-88,92; HD, high-dose; HR, high risk; I, ifosfamide; IESS, Intergroup Ewing's Sarcoma Study; MD, moderate-dose; MRC, Medical Research Council; NA, not available; n.s., not significant; P, cisplatinum; P6, P6 Protocol; POG, Pediatric Oncology Group; REN-3, REN-3 Study; ROI, Rizzoli Orthopedic Institute; SFOP, French Society of Pediatric Oncology; SR, standard risk; SSG IX, Scandinavian Sarcoma Group IX; T2, T2 Protocol; UKCCSG, United Kingdom Children's Cancer Study Group; V, vincristine; WLI, whole lung irradiation; wk, week; y, year.

surgery is possible.[29-32] These data are usually confounded by a selection bias favoring patients in whom surgery is possible. Several European and North American collaborative trials have been performed. Overall, local control rates range from 53% to 93% with the poorer results usually reported in the earlier series.[25,33-36]

Definitive Radiotherapy

Patients who receive radiotherapy as the only local therapy modality usually represent an unfavorably selected group of patients. They frequently present with large tumors, or tumors in unfavorable locations (e.g., vertebral tumors), or both, making radiotherapy difficult but surgery impossible. In a recent analysis of 1058 patients with localized Ewing's sarcoma treated in the EICESS trials, 266 patients had received radiotherapy alone for local treatment. Local or combined local and systemic failures in this subgroup occurred in 26% of patients, which was worse than the recurrence rate following surgery with or without radiotherapy (4%-10%).[31,32] It was impossible to define a subgroup of patients in whom the use of radiotherapy alone achieved the same local control rate as surgery. Even for the favorable subgroup of patients with small extremity tumors, local control with surgery was better than with definitive radiotherapy. In a recent analysis by Bacci and colleagues, these observations were confirmed in 136 patients with extremity tumors.[29] Therefore, when marginal or wide resection is possible, surgery should be performed.

Definitive radiotherapy is indicated when only an intralesional resection is possible. Debulking procedures do not improve local control and are associated with additional unnecessary morbidity. In the experience of the CESS and EICESS trials, patients with an intralesional resection followed by radiotherapy had the same local control rate as patients who had radiotherapy alone.[31,32]

Postoperative Radiotherapy

Postoperative radiotherapy is always indicated following intralesional resections. These debulking procedures are insufficient to obtain local control and should be avoided. In the EICESS trials local control with surgery alone was excellent in all patients with a wide resection according to the Enneking classification and with a good histologic response following initial chemotherapy (good histologic response: <10% viable tumor cells in the resected specimen).[37] Only one local failure in 101 patients occurred in this subgroup. Patients with wide resection and poor histologic response were at higher risk of local failure (12%). This local failure rate was improved with postoperative radiotherapy (6%).[31] There was also a trend to benefit with postoperative irradiation in patients who had a marginal resection. Other groups also observed a good local control rate with the use of combined surgery and radiotherapy in patients with high-risk features.[38]

Preoperative Radiotherapy

The systematic use of preoperative radiotherapy was incorporated into the EICESS 92 trial. The governing objective was to sterilize the tumor compartment before surgery and thus to potentially reduce the rate of dissemination during surgery. With growing experience with the use of preoperative radiotherapy, it was used in this trial when narrow resection margins were expected. More than 40% of the EICESS patients were treated with preoperative radiotherapy. However, in an analysis of the data of these 246 patients, a reduction in systemic failure could not be demonstrated.[31] Conversely, the local control rate following preoperative radiotherapy was excellent, with only 5% of the patients experiencing local or combined local and systemic failures.

When narrow resection margins at surgery are expected, preoperative radiotherapy is feasible and associated with excellent local control. Preoperative irradiation may increase the infection rate postoperatively and may also interfere with bony union.

TECHNIQUES OF IRRADIATION

Radiation Dose and Fractionation

To control Ewing's sarcoma, a radiation dose of more than 40 Gy is necessary. In the St. Jude's Children's Research Hospital's experience with lower-radiation doses, a high rate of local recurrence was observed.[35] Although a clear dose-response correlation at doses more than 40 Gy could not yet be established, for definitive radiotherapy, doses between 55 and 60 Gy are usually given. When surgery precedes or follows radiotherapy, the doses range between 45 and 55 Gy depending on the individual risk factors (i.e., resection margins and response).

Usually, conventional fractionation with daily fractions of 1.8 to 2 Gy is given. Hyperfractionated radiotherapy with twice-daily 1.6 Gy was also applied; after 22.4 Gy a 10-day break was scheduled to permit the administration of chemotherapy. There has been no difference in local control between the two different fractionation groups.[39]

Target Volume

In terms of volume, previous treatment recommendations were to include the entire bone. The Pediatric Oncology Group (POG) and other series confirmed that local failures occur generally within the high-dose radiation volume.[36] In a randomized trial, the treatment of the whole tumor-bearing compartment showed no better results than radiation to the tumor and an additional safety margin.[40] Therefore, the planning target volume is defined as the initial tumor extent on MRI with an additional longitudinal margin of at least 2 to 3 cm and lateral margins of 2 cm in long bones. If doses of more than 45 Gy are used, a shrinking field technique is applied. In patients with an axial tumor site, a minimum of a 2-cm safety margin around the initial tumor extent must be employed. In tumors protruding into preformed cavities (i.e., thorax, pelvis) without infiltration, the residual intracavitary tumor volume following chemotherapy is used for treatment planning. Surgically contaminated areas, scars, and drainage sites must be included in the radiation fields. Circumferential irradiation of extremities should be avoided to reduce the risk of lymphedema. In growing children growth plates must be considered. They should either be fully included in the radiation field, or they should not be included at all. A dose gradient through the epiphysis results in asymmetric growth and may lead to functional deficits. Similarly, vertebral bodies should either be fully included or spared from the radiation field. Three-dimensional conformal radiotherapy should be given in patients with Ewing's sarcoma. In selected cases, such as in vertebral tumors, intensity-modulated radiotherapy (IMRT) or proton therapy may be beneficial. Figures 66-3 and 66-4 show examples of treatment planning.

Radiation of Lung Metastases

Good treatment results in patients with lung metastases have been achieved using whole-lung irradiation.[28] In patients who obtained clinical complete remission in the lung and were treated with additional external-beam radiotherapy to both

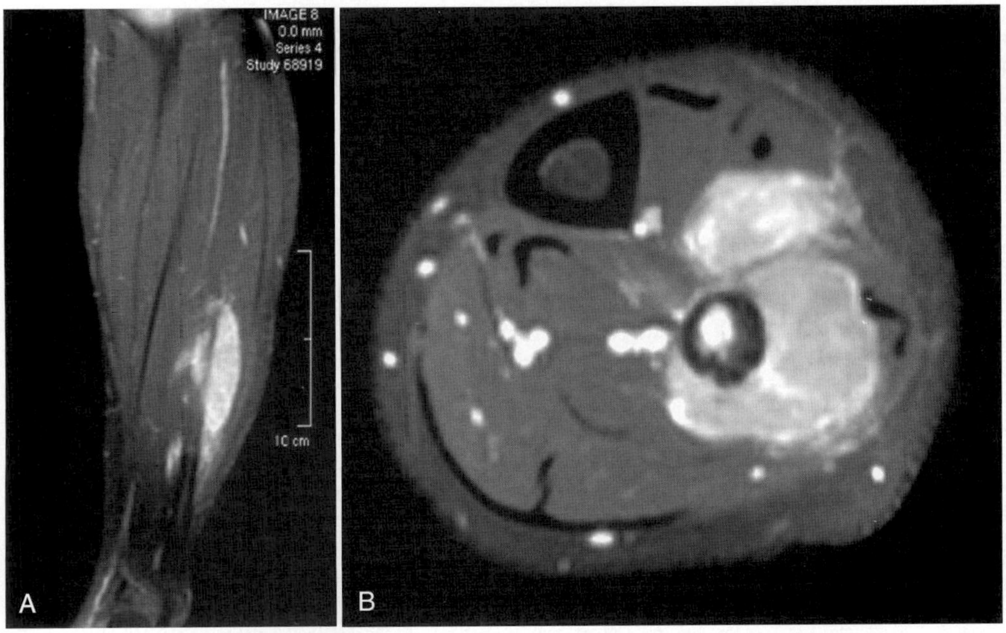

Figure 66-3 Pretreatment axial and coronal contrast enhanced T1 MRI of a Ewing's sarcoma of the fibula.

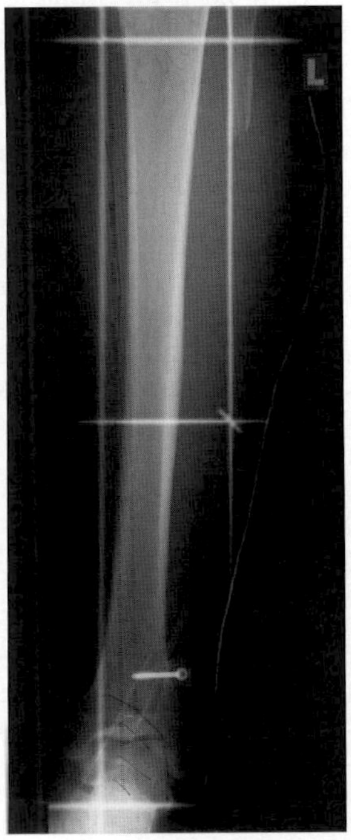

Figure 66-4 Radiation fields resulting from CT-based three-dimensional treatment planning following wide resection of the lower fibula with poor histologic response. The radiation portal covers the initial tumor extent with additional margins of at least 2 cm. Furthermore, lymphatic drainage is facilitated by avoiding circumferential radiotherapy. The scar (marked with radiopaque material) is included in the portals.

lungs, survival was improved compared to patients who received only chemotherapy. In an analysis of the EICESS 92 trial, patients with lung metastases who received whole-lung radiotherapy had an EFS of 47% at 5 years compared to 24% in patients without lung irradiation. The dose is 15 to 20 Gy in 1.5 Gy daily fractions. In a CT-based treatment plan, doses more than the prescribed dose in the lung should be avoided; without CT-based planning, the lung correction factor should be considered. The opposing radiation portals should include both lungs down to the recesses. Treatment in deep inspiration may help reduce the volume of irradiated liver, stomach, and upper kidneys. Adriamycin and actinomycin D must not be given during whole-lung radiotherapy because of the increased risk of pneumonitis; and actinomycin D should also be avoided after lung irradiation (risk of recall pneumonitis). Therefore lung radiotherapy is best given after completion of conventional chemotherapy. In the context of a busulfan-containing regimen, lung irradiation is obsolete.

Radiation of Bone Metastases

Radiotherapy may be indicated in patients presenting with bone metastases. When these are few, radiotherapy can be given to all initially involved sites with doses of approximately 50 Gy depending on surrounding critical structures. Irradiation of more than 50% of the estimated bone marrow volume can result in significant myelosuppression and accentuate the toxicity of chemotherapy. Therefore in patients presenting with multiple bone metastases, precluding irradiation of all sites, radiotherapy can be given to sites of residual tumor on imaging or PET scan. So far, however, there is no clinical data that proves the value of these approaches. Following high-dose busulfan therapy, two incidences of myelopathy have been reported with the application of 50 Gy in conventional fractionation to vertebral sites (personal communication). In this context a dose reduction is necessary.

TREATMENT OF OSTEOSARCOMA

Primary Therapy

The overall current recommended approach to treatment of osteosarcoma is surgical resection of the primary tumor either by amputation or a limb-sparing procedure. Local treatment is preceded by neoadjuvant chemotherapy and followed by postoperative chemotherapy. Radiation is used in patients in whom complete surgical resection cannot be obtained and, as palliation, in patients with inoperable metastases. Historically, patients with osteosarcoma were also treated with local therapy alone, either surgery or radiation therapy. Single-institution studies showed an improvement in overall survival among patients receiving adjuvant chemotherapy compared with historical controls.[20,41,42] Two prospective, randomized studies confirmed this: one at the University of California–Los Angeles and another national multi-institution study.[43,44] Currently, the initial chemotherapeutic agents used include methotrexate, cisplatin, Adriamycin, and ifosfamide. Patients with tumor necrosis greater than 90% have the best outcome.[19,20] If the primary tumor shows only minimal response to neoadjuvant chemotherapy, many believe the chemotherapy agents should be altered for the postoperative therapy; but this has not been proved. Currently, between 60% and 70% of patients with localized osteosarcoma are cured.

Locally Advanced Disease and Palliation

The overall approach to metastatic disease with osteosarcoma is with multiagent chemotherapy. The overall prognosis depends on location and number of metastases, complete surgical resection of all tumor, and response to chemotherapy.[45,46] Patients with lung-only metastasis or a limited number of metastases who can undergo complete surgical resection fare better; 3-year survival is approximately 50% compared with 20% to 30% for more advanced disease.

Radiation therapy to the lungs for metastases, when appropriate, can be given at a dose of 15 to 20 Gy to the whole lung. The use of whole-lung radiation therapy in the setting of metastatic disease is controversial. Whole-lung radiation therapy as prophylaxis against metastatic disease is also controversial and usually not recommended. European Organization for Research and Treatment of Cancer (EORTC) randomized trials showed that prophylactic whole-lung radiation therapy compared well with chemotherapy.[47] However, no benefit was shown in the United States.[48]

Radiation therapy may be incorporated in the treatment of osseous metastatic sites not amenable to surgical resection. In an analysis of the prognosis of relapsing patients treated in the Cooperative Osteosarcoma Study Group (COSS) trials, results were best when metastases could be surgically removed. Radiotherapy of inoperable sites, however, was associated with an improved survival compared to patients who received no local therapy.[49]

Within the last few years, the use of ^{153}Sm-EDTMP (^{153}Samarium ethylenediamine tetramethylene phosphonic acid) therapy has been investigated in unresectable osteosarcoma (primary and metastases). This therapeutic beta-emitting isotope that also emits a gamma-photon to permit imaging and dosimetry localizes to osteoblastic lesions with very high tumor/nontumor ratios.[50] Although it is not yet possible to make any definitive statements about the long-term efficacy of this treatment modality, a multimodal concept of high-activity ^{153}Sm-EDTMP in combination with external beam radiation, polychemotherapy, and autologous hematopoietic progenitor cell support for unresectable osteosarcoma seems to be promising.[51,52]

Local Therapy

Surgery is the mainstay of local treatment of osteosarcoma. Surgical resection is performed either by amputation or a limb-sparing approach and has a 5% local failure rate. Although not well studied and rarely used, the addition of radiation therapy in limb-sparing approaches is a possibility and can be considered in special circumstances. Osteosarcoma is usually considered as a radioresistant tumor. In vitro, it shows similar radiosensitivity to other human tumor cell lines.[53] Also, there have been case reports of patients with inoperable or residual tumor treated with radiation doses ranging between 50 Gy and 70 Gy who remained in continuous remission.[54] In a recent analysis of osteosarcoma patients refusing surgery but receiving systemic therapy and local irradiation, local progression-free survival at 5 years was 56%.[55] Survival was approximately 90% after 5 years in the subgroup of irradiated patients responding to chemotherapy. Therefore, although surgery is the local treatment of choice, cure can also be achieved with radiation in inoperable tumors or patients refusing surgery.

It is therefore reasonable to offer radiation therapy in the treatment of osteosarcoma for unresectable primaries or following incomplete resection, patients who refuse surgery, and unresectable metastatic tumor. It is recommended to treat the tumor to the highest tolerable dose based on the surrounding structures using a shrinking-field technique.

TREATMENT-PLANNING TECHNIQUE

The treatment-planning techniques used for osteosarcoma of the extremities and other sites are similar to those described for the treatment of Ewing's sarcoma.

FUTURE POSSIBILITIES AND CHALLENGES

Future challenges include maintaining good outcome in patients with localized disease while decreasing treatment toxicity and increasing organ functionality. For patients with metastatic disease and poor responders, the challenge is to improve outcome. Future possibilities include identifying new active agents.

New radiation therapy approaches to the treatment of pediatric bone sarcomas include the use of brachytherapy, intraoperative radiation therapy, neutrons, protons, and intensity modulation. Some of these modalities are currently under investigation and development.[56-58]

REFERENCES

1. Gurney J, Severson R, Davis S, et al: Incidence of cancer in children in United States. Cancer 75:2186, 1995.
2. Dorfman H, Czerniak B: Bone cancers. Cancer 75:203, 1995.
3. Newton WA Jr, Meadows AT, Shimada H, et al: Bone sarcomas as second malignant neoplasms following childhood cancer. Cancer 67:193, 1991.
4. Link M, Grier H, Donaldson S: Sarcomas of bone. *In* Fernbach D, Vietti T (eds): Clinical Pediatric Oncology. St. Louis, Mosby-Year Book, 1991, p 545.
5. Horowitz M, Malawer M, Woo S, et al: Ewing's sarcoma family of tumors: Ewing's sarcoma of bone and soft tissue and the peripheral primitive neuroectodermal tumors. *In* Pizzo P (ed): Pediatric Oncology. Philadelphia, Lippincott-Raven, 1997, p 831.
6. Thiele C: Biology of pediatric peripheral neuroectodermal tumors. Cancer Metastasis Rev 10:311, 1991.
7. Cavazzana AO, Miser JS, Jefferson J, et al: Experimental evidence for a neural origin of Ewing's sarcoma of bone. Am J Pathol 127:507, 1987.
8. Ambros IM, Ambros PF, Strehl S, et al: MIC2 is a specific marker for Ewing's sarcoma and peripheral primitive neuroectodermal tumors from MIC2 expression and specific chromosome aberration. Cancer 67:1886, 1991.
9. Zucman J, Delattre O, Desmaze C, et al: Cloning and characterization of the Ewing's sarcoma and peripheral neuroepithelioma t(11;22) translocation breakpoints. Genes Chromosomes Cancer 5:271, 1992.
10. Truc-Carl C, Aurias A, Mugneret F, et al: Chromosomes in Ewing's sarcoma: I. An evaluation of 85 cases of remarkable consistency of t(11;22)(q24;q12). Cancer Genet Cytogenet 32:229, 1988.

11. Friend SH, Bernards R, Rogelj S, et al: A human DNA segment with properties of the gene that predisposes to retinoblastoma and osteosarcoma. Nature 323:643, 1986.
12. Tebbi CK, Gaeta J: Osteosarcoma. Pediatr Ann 17:285, 1988.
13. Landanyi M, Cha C, Lewis R, et al: MDM gene amplification in metastatic osteosarcoma. Cancer Res 53:16, 1993.
14. Halperin E, Constine L, Tarbell N, et al: Osteosarcoma. *In* Pediatric Radiation Oncology, 3rd ed. New York, Raven Press 1997, pp 267-289.
15. Enneking WF: A system of staging musculoskeletal neoplasms. Clin Orthop Relat Res 204:9, 1986.
16. Sobin LH, Wittekind C (eds): TNM Classification of Malignant Tumours, 6th ed. London, Wiley, 2002.
17. Sauer R, Jurgens H, Burgers J, et al: Prognostic factors in the treatment of Ewing's sarcoma. Radiother Oncol 10:101, 1987.
18. Link MP, Goorin AM, Horowitz M, et al: Adjuvant chemotherapy of high-grade osteosarcoma of the extremity: updated results of the multi-institutional osteosarcoma study. Clin Orthop Relat Res 270:8, 1991.
19. Glasser D, Lane J, Huvos A, et al: Survival, prognosis and therapeutic response in osteogenic sarcoma. Cancer 69:698, 1991.
20. Myers PA, Heller G, Healey J, et al: Chemotherapy for nonmetastatic osteogenic sarcoma: the Memorial Sloan-Kettering experience. J Clin Oncol 10:5, 1992.
21. Bielack S, Kempf-Bielack B, Delling G, et al: Prognostic factors of high-grade osteosarcoma of the extremities or trunk. An analysis of 1702 patients treated on neoadjuvant Cooperative Osteosarcoma Study Group protocols. J Clin Oncol 20:776, 2002.
22. Hustu HO, Pinkel D, Pratt CB: Treatment of clinically localized Ewing's sarcoma with radiotherapy and combination chemotherapy. Cancer 30:1522, 1972.
23. Pomeroy TC, Johnson RE: Integrated therapy of Ewing's sarcoma. Front Radiat Ther Oncol 10:152, 1975.
24. Pomeroy TC, Johnson RE: Prognostic factors for survival in Ewing's sarcoma. AJR Am J Roentgenol 123:898, 1975.
25. Nesbit M, Gehan E, Burget E, et al: Multimodal therapy for the management of primary, nonmetastatic Ewing's sarcoma of bone: a long term follow up of the first intergroup study. J Clin Oncol 8:1664, 1990.
26. Smith MA, Ungerleider RS, Horowitz ME, Simon R: Influence of doxorubicin dose intensity on response and outcome for patients with osteogenic sarcoma and Ewing's sarcoma. J Natl Cancer Inst 83:1460, 1991.
27. Grier H, Krailo M, Link M, et al: Improved outcome in nonmetastatic Ewing's sarcoma (EWS) and PNET of bone with the addition of ifosfamide and etoposide + vincristine, Adriamycin, cyclophosphamide and actinomycin [Abstract]. Presented at the meeting of the American Society of Clinical Oncology, Dallas, TX, 1994.
28. Paulussen M, Ahrens S, Burdach S, et al: Primary metastatic (stage IV) Ewing tumor: survival analysis of 171 patients from the EICESS studies. Annals of Oncology 9:275,1998.
29. Bacci F, Ferrari S, Longhi A, et al: Role of surgery in local treatment of Ewing's sarcoma of the extremities in patients undergoing adjuvant and neoadjuvant chemotherapy. Oncol Rep 11:111, 2004.
30. Sailer S, Harmon D, Mankin H, et al: Ewing's sarcoma: surgical resection as a prognostic factor. Int J Radiat Oncol Biol Phys 15:43, 1988.
31. Schuck A, Ahrens S, Paulussen M, et al: Local therapy in localized Ewing tumors: results of 1058 patients treated in the CESS 81, CESS 86 and EICESS 92 trials. Int J Radiat Oncol Biol Phys 55:168, 2003.
32. Schuck A, Hofmann J, Rube C, et al: Radiotherapy in Ewing's sarcoma and PNET of the chest wall: results of the trials CESS 81, CESS 86 and EICESS 92. Int J Radiat Oncol Biol Phys 42:1001, 1998.
33. Burgert E, Nesbit M, Garnsey L, et al: Multimodal therapy for the management of nonpelvic, localized Ewing's sarcoma of bone: Intergroup Study IESS-II. J Clin Oncol 8:1514, 1990.
34. Craft A, Cotterill S, Malcolm A, et al: Ifosfamide-containing chemotherapy in Ewing's sarcoma: The Second United Kingdom Children's Cancer Study Group and the Medical Research Council Ewing's Tumor Study. J Clin Oncol 16:3628, 1998.
35. Arai Y, Kun LE, Brooks MT, et al: Ewing's sarcoma: local tumor control and patterns of failure following limited-volume radiation therapy. Int J Radiat Oncol 21:1501, 1991.
36. Donaldson S, Shuster J, Andreozzi C: The Pediatric Oncology Group (POG) experience in Ewing's sarcoma of bone. Med Pediatr Oncol 17:283, 1989.
37. Salzer-Kuntschik M, Delling G, Beron G, et al: Morphological grades of regression in osteosarcoma after polychemotherapy—study COSS 80. J Cancer Res Clin Oncol 106 Suppl:21, 1983.
38. Krasin M, Rodriguez-Galindo C, Davidoff A, et al: Efficacy of combined surgery and irradiation for localized Ewing's sarcoma family of tumors. Pediatr Blood Cancer 43:229, 2004.
39. Dunst J, Jurgens H, Sauer R, et al: Radiation therapy in Ewing's sarcoma: an update of the CESS 86 trial. Int J Radiat Oncol Biol Phys 32:919, 1995.
40. Donaldson S, Torrey M, Link A, et al: A multidisciplinary study investigating radiotherapy in Ewing's sarcoma: end results of POG #8346. Pediatric Oncology Group. Int J Radiat Oncol Biol Phys 42:125, 1998.
41. Suttow WW, Gehan EA, Dymen TPJ, et al: Multidrug adjuvant chemotherapy for osteosarcoma: interim report of the Southwest Oncology Group studies. Cancer Treat Rep 62:265, 1978.
42. Pratt C, Champion J, Fleming I, et al: Adjuvant chemotherapy for osteosarcoma of the extremity. Cancer 65:439, 1990.
43. Eilber F, Giuliano A, Edkardt J, et al: Adjuvant chemotherapy for osteosarcoma: a randomized prospective trial. J Clin Oncol 5:21, 1987.
44. Link M, Goorin A, Miser A, et al: The effect of adjuvant chemotherapy on relapse-free survival in patients with osteosarcoma of the extremity. N Engl J Med 314:1600, 1986.
45. Karger L, Zoubek A, Potschger U, et al: Primary metastatic osteosarcoma: presentation and outcome of patients treated on neoadjuvant Cooperative Osteosarcoma Study Group protocols. J Clin Oncol 21:2011, 2003.
46. Temeck B, Wexler L, Steinberg S, et al: Metastasectomy for sarcomatous pediatric histologies: results and prognostic factors [Abstract]. Ann Thorac Surg 59:1385, 1995.
47. Burgers JM, van Glabbeke M, Bussan A, et al: Osteosarcoma of the limbs. Report of the EORTC-SIOP 03 Trial 20781 investigating the value of adjuvant treatment with chemotherapy and/or prophylactic lung irradiation. Cancer 61:124, 1988.
48. Rab GY, Ivins JC, Childs CS Jr, et al: Elective whole lung irradiation in the treatment of osteogenic sarcoma. Cancer 38:939, 1976.
49. Kempf-Bielack B, Bielack S, Jürgens H, et al: Osteosarcoma relapse after combined modality therapy: an analysis of unselected patients in the Cooperative Osteosarcoma Study Group (COSS). J Clin Oncol 23:559, 2005.
50. Anderson PM, Wiseman GA, Dispenzieri A, et al: High dose samarium-153 ethylene diamine tetramethylene phosphonate: low toxicity of skeletal irradiation in patients with osteosarcoma and bone metastases. J Clin Oncol 20:189, 2002.
51. Franzius C, Bielack S, Flege S, et al: High-activity Samarium-153-EDTMP therapy followed by autologous peripheral blood stem cell support in unresectable osteosarcoma. Nuklearmedizin 40:215, 2001.
52. Franzius C, Schuck A, Bielack S: High-dose Samarium-153-Ethylene diamine tetramethylene phosphonate: low toxicity of skeletal irradiation in patients with osteosarcoma and bone metastases. J Clin Oncol 20:1953, 2002.
53. Phillips TL, Sheline GE: Radiation therapy of malignant bone tumors. Radiology 92:1537, 1969.
54. Sweetnam R: Osteosarcoma. Br Med J 2:536, 1979.
55. Machak GN, Tkachev SI, Solovyev YN, et al: Neoadjuvant chemotherapy and local radiotherapy for high grade osteosarcoma of the extremities. Mayo Clin Proc 78:147, 2003.
56. Yamamuro T, Kotoura Y: Intraoperative radiation therapy for osteosarcoma. *In* Humphrey G (ed): Osteosarcoma in Adolescents and Young Adults. Boston, Kluwer, 1993, p 178.
57. Chauvel P: Osteosarcomas and adult soft tissue sarcomas: is there a place for high LET radiation therapy? Ann Oncol 3:S107, 1992.
58. Carrie C, Breteau N, Negrier S, et al: The role of fast neutron therapy in unresectable pelvic osteosarcoma: preliminary report. Med Pediatr Oncol 22:355, 1994.

CHAPTER 67

WILMS' TUMOR

John A. Kalapurakal and Patrick R. M. Thomas

INCIDENCE

Cause unknown
Incidence: 8.1 per million children and 650 new cases each year
Median age: 3.5 years

HISTOLOGY

FH Wilms' tumor	87%
Anaplastic	5%
Clear cell sarcoma	3%
Rhabdoid tumor of the kidney	2%
Mesoblastic nephroma	2%
Renal cell carcinoma	<1%

BIOLOGIC CHARACTERISTICS

Two regulatory genes: *WT1* (11p13) and *WT2* (11p15) implicated in Wilms' tumor development. LOH at 1p and 16q are associated with higher relapse rates.
The COG study includes LOH results in addition to tumor stage and histology for tumor risk stratification.

STAGING EVALUATION

History, physical, complete blood counts, chemistry, urinalysis, chest x-ray, abdominal ultrasonogram, CT and/or MRI scans of the abdomen.

PRIMARY THERAPY

Surgical resection (nephrectomy and tumor staging) is primary therapy in the United States. Preoperative chemotherapy is routinely used in Europe.

ADJUVANT THERAPY

NWTSG studies show vincristine and dactinomycin result in excellent cure rates for Stage I and II patients. Irradiation and doxorubicin are added for Stage III and IV patients.
COG study intensifies chemotherapy for patients with LOH at 1p and 16q.
Chemotherapy is intensified for focal and diffuse anaplastic Wilms' tumor, Stage IV CCSK, and RTK.
Flank or abdominal irradiation dose is 10.8 Gy. Higher doses are recommended for Stage III anaplastic tumors and RTK.

RETRIEVAL THERAPY

According to original stage, prior treatment and sites of relapse
Therapy includes surgery, irradiation, and intensive multiagent chemotherapy with or without stem cell transplantation.

Wilms' tumor, or nephroblastoma, is the most common childhood renal tumor, accounting for about 6% of all pediatric malignant diseases.[1] It was first described in 1814, but Max Wilms in 1899 first identified the true nature of the condition as a neoplasm with mixed cellular elements.[2,3] His name, therefore, has become synonymous with nephroblastoma. The early advances in managing these small patients with huge tumors were made by surgeons, who reduced the operative mortality from 25% to the current rate of less than 1%. The survival of children with Wilms' tumor gradually increased concomitantly from less than 10% to about 50% by the 1940s and 1950s. It was at that time that the multimodality team approach to children with cancer was developed. Postoperative radiation therapy (RT) became routine after results from Boston Children's Hospital reported an increased potential of cure. The advent of effective chemotherapy (dactinomycin and vincristine) also had a major impact on the survival of these children.[4] The multidisciplinary management of Wilms' tumor has resulted in a striking improvement in survival. Thus, the grim outlook at the beginning of the 20th century of a 90% mortality rate has changed to a survival rate of approximately 90% at the dawn of the 21st century. Randomized clinical trials in North America under the aegis of the National Wilms' Tumor Study Group (NWTSG) and those in Europe, largely by the International Society of Pediatric Oncology (SIOP), have resulted in Wilms' tumor therapy becoming a paradigm for successful multidisciplinary interaction in the treatment of cancer. Successive NWTSG clinical trials have been based on postoperative therapies, whereas preoperative strategies have been the focus of SIOP investigators.[5,6]

The clinical risk factors such as tumor stage and histology were categorized so that treatment could be modulated in intensity according to risk groups, the objective being to achieve cure with minimum complications. As a result, children with low-risk tumors now receive minimal therapy, whereas those at high risk benefit from more intensive therapy. The modern survivors of Wilms' tumor enjoy a better quality of life owing to sequential reduction in the intensity of therapy.[7]

The renal tumor committee of the Children's Oncology Group (COG) has succeeded the NWTSG. All future Wilms' tumor studies will be conducted by the COG.

ETIOLOGY AND EPIDEMIOLOGY

The cause of Wilms' tumor is unknown. The peak incidence is between 3 and 4 years of age. Wilms' tumor may arise as sporadic or hereditary tumors, or in the setting of specific genetic disorders.[8] The overall annual incidence of Wilms' tumor is 8.1 per million children, and approximately 650 new cases can be expected each year in North America. Wilms' tumor is found more often in black children than in whites, with a ratio of

1.25:1. Girls are affected more than boys in the same ratio.[1] No environmental or other factors have been ascertained to explain these differences.

PREVENTION AND EARLY DETECTION

Prevention awaits an identified cause. However, congenital anomalies (aniridia, genitourinary malformations, hemihypertrophy, or signs of overgrowth) may be seen in 13% to 28% of children, depending on whether they have unilateral or bilateral disease.[9] The syndromes associated with the highest risk for developing Wilms' tumor include the syndrome of aniridia, genitourinary malformation, mental retardation (generally referred to as WAGR syndrome); the Beckwith-Wiedemann syndrome; and the Denys-Drash syndrome. These groups of higher risk children can be screened for the development of Wilms' tumor using ultrasonographic examinations of both kidneys every 3 months for the first 5 years of life and yearly thereafter.[8,10]

BIOLOGIC CHARACTERISTICS AND MOLECULAR BIOLOGY

The biologic characterization of Wilms' tumor has provided the foundation for our understanding of key concepts in cancer genetics, including the roles of tumor suppressor genes and relation of genomic imprinting in tumorigenesis. Although Wilms' tumor was one of the original examples in Knudson's two-hit model of cancer development, subsequent research has shown that multiple genes and several genetic events contribute to the formation of this malignant disorder.[11] The molecular changes that have been described in Wilms' tumor can be classified as primary events predisposing to the development of tumor or secondary events associated with tumor progression.

WT1

Initial insights into the molecular biology of Wilms' tumor were derived from the observation that in patients with WAGR syndrome the risk for developing the tumor is more than 30%. Cytogenetic analysis of individuals with this syndrome showed deletions at chromosome 11p13, which was later found to be the locus of a contiguous set of genes including *PAX6*, the gene causing aniridia, and *WT1*, one of the Wilms' tumor genes. The *WT1* gene encodes a transcription factor that is crucial to normal kidney and gonadal development.[8] The Denys-Drash syndrome, which is characterized by pseudohermaphroditism, glomerulopathy, renal failure, and a 95% chance of Wilms' tumor development, is caused by point mutations in the zinc-finger DNA-binding region of the *WT1* gene.[10] Although *WT1* has a clear role in tumorigenesis of Wilms' tumor in patients with the WAGR and Denys-Drash syndromes, only a minority of patients with sporadic Wilms' tumor carries *WT1* mutations in the germ line (<5%) or in tumor tissue (6%–18%).[8]

WT2

The Beckwith-Wiedemann syndrome is an overgrowth disorder manifested by large birth weight, macroglossia, organomegaly, hemihypertrophy, neonatal hypoglycemia, abdominal-wall defects, ear abnormalities, and predisposition to Wilms' tumor and other malignant disorders. Approximately 5% of individuals with this syndrome develop Wilms' tumor. Beckwith-Wiedemann syndrome maps to chromosome 11p15, a locus called WT2 because loss of heterozygosity (LOH) at this locus has been detected in Wilms' tumor.[12]

FWT1 and FWT2

Familial predisposition to Wilms' tumor is rare, affecting only 1.5% of patients with the tumor. Analysis of families has revealed familial Wilms' tumor (FWT) predisposition at FWT1 (17q) and FWT2 (19q) loci.[8]

Loss of Heterozygosity at 1p and 16q

Secondary genetic changes in Wilms' tumor have been reported in the *p53* gene and at chromosomes 1p and 16q.[13] One of the major goals of the recently concluded NWTS-5 trial was to prospectively analyze the prognostic significance of LOH at chromosomes 1p and 16q. A recent analysis of this data revealed that the relative risks (RR) for relapse for patients with stage I-IV favorable histology (FH) tumors with LOH stratified by stage were 1.77 for LOH 1p ($P < 0.01$) and 1.39 for LOH 16q ($P = 0.05$). When the effects of LOH for both 1p and 16q were considered jointly, the RR for relapse in stage I and II FH disease was 3.19 ($P < 0.01$), and for stage III and IV FH disease was 2.42 ($P = 0.02$). The RR for death for patients with stage I and II FH disease with LOH for both regions was 5.11 ($P < 0.01$), and for stage III and IV was 1.96 ($P = 0.27$).[14]

PATHOLOGY AND PATHWAYS OF SPREAD

Initially, most pediatric renal tumors were classified as Wilms' tumor, with either favorable or unfavorable histology. After careful histopathologic examination of all unfavorable histology tumors registered in the first two NWTSG studies, pathologists from the study group recognized that certain tumors represented separate disease entities. Therefore, from NWTS-3 onwards, clear-cell sarcoma of the kidney (CCSK) and rhabdoid tumor of the kidney (RTK) were excluded from Wilms' tumor trials, although the NWTSG continued to organize separate therapeutic trials for these disease entities.

Most Wilms' tumors are solitary lesions, although a substantial proportion are multifocal, with 6% involving both kidneys, and another 12% arising multifocally within a single kidney. The classic untreated Wilms' tumor consists of varying proportions of three (triphasic) cell types: blastemal, stromal, and epithelial, commonly recapitulating various stages of normal renal development (Fig. 67-1A,B). Less commonly, heterologous epithelial or stromal components are identified, including mucinous or squamous epithelium, skeletal muscle, cartilage, osteoid, or fat. Not all specimens are triphasic; biphasic, and monophasic patterns are frequently encountered. Approximately 87% of Wilms' tumors are of the FH subtype.[15,16]

The histologic feature of greatest clinical significance in untreated Wilms' tumor is anaplasia, which is defined by the presence of greatly enlarged polyploid nuclei (Fig. 67-1C,D). The frequency of anaplasia is approximately 5% and is correlated with the patient's age. It is rare in the first 2 years of life, but the frequency increases to approximately 13% in patients older than 5 years. It is far more frequent in black than in white patients and has been strongly linked with the presence of *p53* mutations.[17,18] Anaplasia is judged to be a marker of resistance to chemotherapy, but whether it also confers increased aggressiveness or tendency to disseminate still remains unclear. The distinction between focal and diffuse anaplastic tumors is prognostically significant.[19]

Further links between the histologic pattern and the clinical behavior of Wilms' tumor have long been sought. Blastemal-rich tumors tend to be extremely invasive and present at an advanced stage, although many respond well to chemotherapy. By contrast, predominantly epithelial and

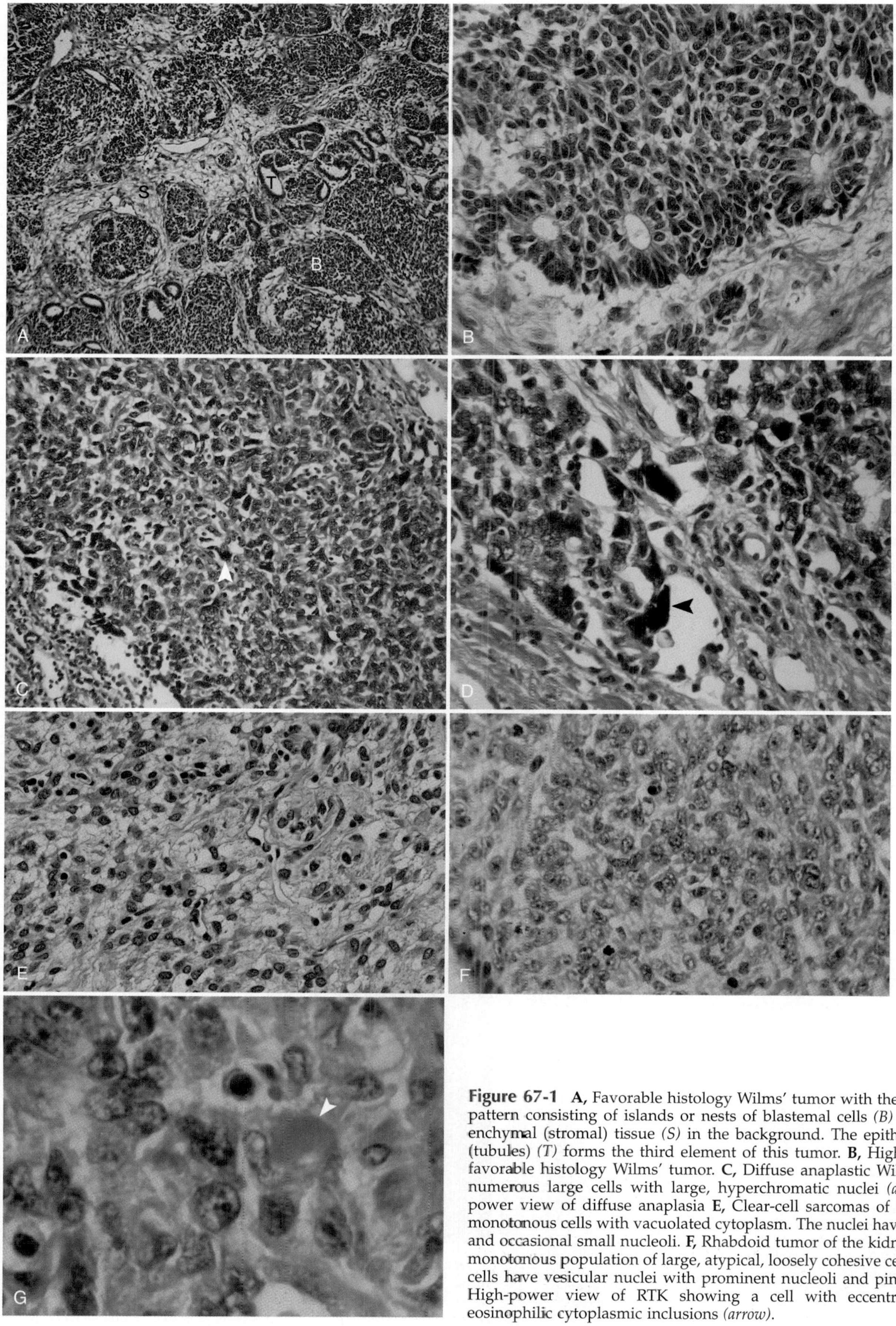

Figure 67-1 **A,** Favorable histology Wilms' tumor with the classic triphasic pattern consisting of islands or nests of blastemal cells *(B)* with loose mesenchymal (stromal) tissue *(S)* in the background. The epithelial component (tubules) *(T)* forms the third element of this tumor. **B,** High-power view of favorable histology Wilms' tumor. **C,** Diffuse anaplastic Wilms' tumor with numerous large cells with large, hyperchromatic nuclei *(arrow)*. **D,** High-power view of diffuse anaplasia **E,** Clear-cell sarcomas of the kidney with monotonous cells with vacuolated cytoplasm. The nuclei have fine chromatin and occasional small nucleoli. **F,** Rhabdoid tumor of the kidney (RTK) with a monotonous population of large, atypical, loosely cohesive cells. Many tumor cells have vesicular nuclei with prominent nucleoli and pink cytoplasm. **G,** High-power view of RTK showing a cell with eccentric nucleus and eosinophilic cytoplasmic inclusions *(arrow)*.

rhabdomyomatous Wilms' tumors are more likely to present at a low stage, reflecting less aggressiveness, yet many are resistant to chemotherapy. More recently, preliminary analysis of the group assigned no adjuvant chemotherapy in a trial of young children with small stage I tumors provides further support for the excellent prognosis of epithelial-differentiated Wilms' tumors.[20] Although much of the past success of the NWTSG has relied on the accurate histologic subclassification of Wilms' tumors into high-risk and low-risk types, further risk classification will probably depend on molecular genetic features.

The existence of precursor lesions called nephrogenic rests to Wilms' tumor has been recognized for many years. These lesions consist of abnormally persistent embryonal nephroblastic tissue with small clusters of blastemal cells, tubules, or stromal cells. Nephrogenic rests can be subclassified by their positions within the renal lobe and histologic appearance: perilobar nephrogenic rests are limited to the periphery of the renal cortex, and intralobar nephrogenic rests occur randomly throughout the renal lobe. The term nephroblastomatosis is used to refer to the presence of multiple nephrogenic rests. There are several possible fates for nephrogenic rests. Most become dormant or involute spontaneously and only a small number develop a clonal transformation into Wilms' tumor. The presence of nephrogenic rests within a kidney resected for a Wilms' tumor indicates the need for monitoring the contralateral kidney for tumor development, particularly in young infants.[21]

The other major cellular types of kidney tumors, their frequency expressed as a percentage of all childhood kidney tumors, and their patterns of spread and relapse (Table 67-1), are as follows:

1. Mesoblastic nephroma (2%). This is the most common renal tumor encountered in the first month of life, and the median age at presentation is 3 months. Hypercalcemia may be present. Local recurrence after surgery and distant metastases are rare. Children have excellent survival rates after surgery.[22]
2. Clear cell sarcoma (3%). Once considered a Wilms' tumor variant, it is now recognized as a separate entity. The tumor cells have poorly stained cytoplasm with cytoplasmic vacuolations (Fig. 67-1E). Bone metastases, rare in the other tumor types, may be observed in up to 23% of children with CCSK.[15,23]
3. Rhabdoid tumor of the kidney or malignant rhabdoid tumor (2%). This rare but extremely aggressive neoplasm predominantly affects infants, in whom hypercalcemia may also be present, as in mesoblastic nephroma. Rhabdoid cells are characterized by eosinophilic cytoplasm that contains hyaline globular inclusions (Fig. 67-1F,G). Metastases to the lung and infradiaphragmatic relapses are frequent.[15,16]
4. Renal cell carcinoma (< 1%). This type of carcinoma is rare in children. Its patterns of spread are the same as its adult counterpart (i.e., the lungs, lymph nodes, and bone).

Table 67-1 Relapse Patterns in Patients without Metastases at Diagnosis*

Site†	FH	Ana	CCSK	RTK	MN	RCC
Lung	66	40	19	54	—	50
Liver	10	20	4	12	—	—
Bone	1	4	50	4	—	33
Brain	—	—	19	12	—	—
Flank-abd	18	48	8	50	4	—
Kidney	10	—	—	—	—	—
Other	11	12	15	15	—	33

*Percentage of all relapsed patients in column.
†More than one site might have been involved.
abd, abdomen; Ana, anaplasia; CCSK, clear cell sarcoma of the kidney; FH, favorable histology; MN, mesoblastic nephroma; RCC, renal cell carcinoma; RTK, rhabdoid tumor of the kidney.
Adapted from D'Angio GJ, Rosenberg H, Sharples, K, et al: Imaging methods for primary renal tumors at childhood: costs versus benefits. Med Pediatr Oncol 21:205-212, 1993.

CLINICAL MANIFESTATIONS, PATIENT EVALUATIONS, AND STAGING

Children with Wilms' tumor do not show any tumor-specific symptoms. The most common presentation is with an asymptomatic abdominal mass, although about 33% of patients present with abdominal pain, anorexia, vomiting, malaise, or a combination of these symptoms. Physical examination reveals hypertension in about 25% of patients and congenital anomalies (aniridia, genitourinary malformations, hemihypertrophy, or signs of overgrowth) in 13% to 28% of children, depending on whether they have unilateral or bilateral disease. Up to 30% of patients have hematuria and less than 10% have coagulopathy.

The laboratory workup after physical examination should include complete blood counts, routine chemistries, and urinalysis, noting the presence or absence of protein, and white or red blood cells. Imaging studies before surgery are designed to establish the presence of a renal mass, a functioning normal contralateral kidney, patent renal vein and inferior vena cava free from thrombosis, and the presence or absence of metastases in the lungs. Diagnostic imaging studies include posteroanterior and lateral views of the chest, abdominal ultrasonography (particularly useful in the detection of tumor thrombosis), and CT or MRI scanning (Fig. 67-2). Chest radiograph or CT scan of the chest can be used to detect lung metastasis. The clinical significance of tumors that are detected by chest CT but not on chest radiographs remains unclear.[24,25] MRI scans of the abdomen can help to distinguish between nephrogenic rests and Wilms' tumor.[26] Postoperatively, when the histology is established, a bone scan and skeletal survey should be obtained for patients with CCSK and an MRI scan of the brain for those with RTK.

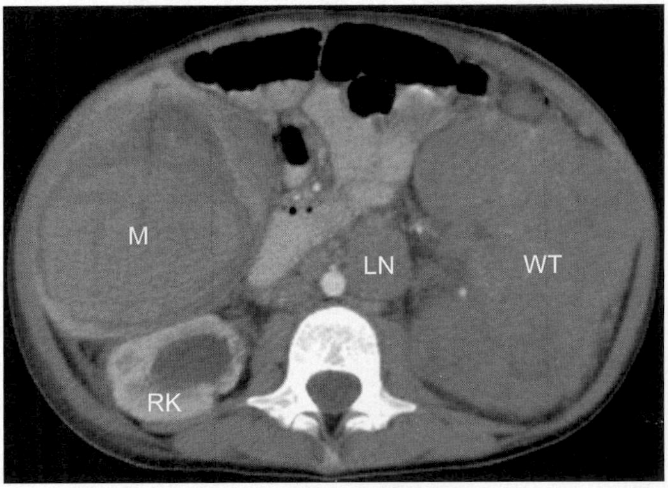

Figure 67-2 Abdominal CT scan of a 4-year-old girl with a large left-sided Wilms' tumor (*WT*) measuring 10.5 cm × 11 cm × 17 cm. The right kidney (*RK*) did not show any lesions. There were multiple enlarged para-aortic lymph nodes (*LN*) and liver metastases (*M*).

Staging

Wilms' tumors are staged on the basis of anatomic tumor extent, and therapy is currently based on stage and histology (Table 67-2).[27] Classifications based on tumor extent have evolved over the years. After analysis of the prognostic significance of several clinicopathologic factors in NWTS-1 and NWTS-2, the use of a grouping system was abandoned in favor of a staging system, which has been in use from NWTS-3 onward. Patients with lymph-node involvement, previously included with group II disease, are now classified as having stage III disease, and those with local tumor spill were moved from group III to stage II disease.[28] Refinements to the inclusion criteria for stages I and II disease were introduced in the NWTS-5 study. Criteria for stage I was refined to accommodate an important subset of WT that is being managed by nephrectomy alone. Prior to NWTS-5, the distinction between stages I and II in the renal sinus was established by the hilar plane, which was an imaginary plane connecting the most medial aspects of the upper and lower poles of the kidney. This criterion was difficult to apply because of tumor distortion, and thus the hilar plane criterion has been replaced with renal sinus vascular or lymphatic invasion. This definition includes not only the involvement of vessels within the hilar soft tissue, but also vessels located in the radial extensions of the renal sinus into the renal parenchyma.[29,30]

Table 67-2 **National Wilms' Tumor Study—Five Staging System**

Stage	Description
I	Tumor is confined to the kidney and is completely resected. The surface of the renal capsule is intact. Tumor was not ruptured before or during removal. There is no residual tumor apparent beyond the margins of resection. There is no tumor penetration of the renal capsule or involvement of renal sinus vessels.
II	Tumor extends beyond the kidney but is completely resected (negative margins and lymph nodes); at least one of the following may be present: Penetration of the renal capsule Invasion of the renal sinus vessels Biopsy of tumor before removal Spillage of tumor locally during removal
III	Residual nonhematogenous tumor is confined to the abdomen. Any one or more of the following may be present: Lymph nodes on biopsy are found to be involved in the hilum or periaortic chains. There has been diffuse peritoneal contamination by tumor such as by spillage of tumor beyond the flank before or during surgery or by tumor beyond the flank or by tumor growth that has penetrated through the peritoneal surface. Implants are found on the peritoneal surfaces. The tumor extends beyond the surgical margins either microscopically or grossly. The tumor is not completely excisable because of local infiltration into vital structures.
IV	Hematogenous metastases in the lung, liver, bone or brain. Lymph node metastasis beyond the abdomen.
V	Bilateral renal involvement is evident at diagnosis. An attempt should be made to stage each side according to the above criteria on the basis of extent of disease before biopsy.

PRIMARY THERAPY

Primary surgical resection of Wilms' tumor remains the standard initial therapy undertaken in North America. A transabdominal transperitoneal approach is recommended to provide adequate exposure for complete locoregional staging.[31] This procedure includes mobilization and inspection of the contralateral kidney to exclude bilateral disease before nephrectomy, if possible. It also permits inspection of hilar and regional nodes, which remain crucial factors in staging. Although suspicious lymph nodes are excised irrespective of location, a formal lymph-node dissection is not beneficial or recommended.

Most Wilms' tumors that appear to involve contiguous structures actually only compress or adhere to the adjacent organ without invasion. Therefore, radical en bloc resection in these tumors, which is associated with increased surgical complications, can be avoided. However, wedge resection of infiltrated structures such as the diaphragm, liver, or psoas muscle can be undertaken if all disease can be completely removed with little operative morbidity. This procedure is advantageous because the tumor can be downstaged to stage II and subsequent therapy reduced. Tumor extension into the renal vein and proximate inferior vena cava can, in most cases, be removed en bloc with the kidney. However, primary resection of extension into the inferior vena cava to the hepatic level or into the atrium is associated with higher operative morbidity. In these circumstances, preoperative chemotherapy decreases the size and extent of the tumor thrombus, facilitating subsequent excision.

Tumor spillage remains an important concept in the surgery of Wilms' tumor. Surgeons must be aware of any tumor-capsule violation with contamination of the peritoneal cavity during attempt at local tumor control. The accurate assessment of a local spill (stage II) from diffuse contamination (stage III) is difficult. Nevertheless, peritoneal soilage definitely increases the risk for local and abdominal recurrence, although current data suggest that overall survival is not adversely affected.[32]

Some tumors are initially judged to be unresectable or to pose too great a surgical risk because of massive size. In these cases, preoperative chemotherapy results in reduction of the tumor mass and generally renders it resectable.

RADIATION THERAPY

Flank/Abdominal Irradiation

Radiation therapy continues to play an important role in the management of Wilms' tumor. Successive NWTS trials have refined the indications for radiotherapy. In NWTS-1 and NWTS-2, an age-adjusted dose schedule was used for flank irradiation: 18 to 24 Gy for children younger than 18 months; 24 to 30 Gy for those aged 19 to 30 months; 30 to 35 Gy for those aged 31 to 40 months; and 35 to 40 Gy for children older than 40 months. The abdominal relapse rate was 3% to 5% for group II and III tumors, and there was no dose-response relation observed across these dose ranges.[33,34] NWTS-3 proved that radiotherapy could be avoided in children with stage II tumors if vincristine and dactinomycin were given. This study also showed that children with stage III favorable histology tumors who received 10.8 Gy and vincristine, dactinomycin, and doxorubicin had tumor control similar to that of those who received 20 Gy with vincristine and dactinomycin. This was an important finding because it eliminated the need for an age-adjusted dose schedule and significantly reduced the recommended dose of irradiation.[35]

NWTS-1, NWTS-2, and NWTS-3 showed that delay in initiating irradiation beyond 10 days was correlated with poor outcome.[33–35] The impact of RT delay on FH patients in NWTS-3 and NWTS-4 has been recently reported. In this report, an RT delay of more than 10 days did not significantly influence flank or abdominal tumor-recurrence rates. It is currently recommended that children with Wilms' tumor continue to be irradiated without undue delay (within 14 days of nephrectomy), to eliminate recurrence as a variable in the analyses of outcome in future Wilms' tumor clinical trials.[36]

In NWTS-4, the frequency of abdominal tumor recurrence in children with local tumor spillage and stage II tumors of all histologies was 16.5%. These children did not receive flank irradiation, in accordance with the revised guidelines in NWTS-4. Survival after local recurrence was poor, with only 43% surviving at 2 years. The incidence of tumor recurrence for patients with stage III tumors with local spill after irradiation was only 7.8%.[32]

Although diffuse anaplastic tumors are resistant to chemotherapy, and presumably relatively resistant to radiotherapy, these tumors have not shown a radiation dose response between 10.8 Gy and 40 Gy.[37] The optimum radiation dose for anaplastic Wilms' tumor and unfavorable histology tumors remains unknown. In NWTS-5, children with stage I focal and diffuse anaplasia were treated with two-drug chemotherapy (vincristine and dactinomycin) alone without flank irradiation. However, preliminary analysis revealed a low relapse-free survival rate of 64%.[66] Hence, in the COG study, flank irradiation (10.8 Gy) will be recommended for these tumors. The survival rates for children with stage III diffuse anaplastic tumors and rhabdoid tumors continue to be poor (Table 67-4). The COG study will test the value of a higher dose of irradiation (19.8 Gy) together with intensified chemotherapy (Tables 67-3 and 67-5). The COG protocol will also prospectively study whether flank irradiation could be avoided in children with stage I CCSK who have undergone lymph-node sampling and central pathology review (see Tables 67-3 and 67-5).

Whole Lung Irradiation (WLI)

In children with lung metastases detected on chest radiographs, WLI continues to be administered, leading to high cure rates. In NWTS-3, the 4-year relapse-free survival and overall survival were 72% and 78%, respectively, in children with favorable histology Wilms' tumor and lung metastases.[38] These results are superior to the survival rates reported by investigators from the United Kingdom Children's Cancer Study Group (UKCCSG) study in which all patients did not receive WLI.[39] In children with pulmonary metastases visible on CT scans but not chest radiographs, the role of WLI is unclear. In such patients treated on NWTS-3 and NWTS-4, the

Table 67-3 Irradiation Recommendations for the COG Renal Tumor Protocols

Tumor Stage/Histology	Irradiation (RT) Dose (Gy) and Fields
Stage I and II FH	No RT
Stage III FH, Stage I-III focal anaplasia, Stage I-II diffuse anaplasia, Stage I-III CCSK‡	10.8 Gy flank* RT
Stage III diffuse anaplasia, Stage I-III RTK	19.8 Gy (infants 10.8 Gy) flank* RT†
Stage IV (lung metastases, FH)	12 Gy (whole-lung irradiation in children who are not in complete remission at week 6 after induction chemotherapy)
Stage IV (lung metastases, UH)	12 Gy whole-lung irradiation regardless of chemotherapy response
Stage IV (brain metastases)	25.2 Gy (whole brain) + 10 Gy (local boost)
Stage IV (bone metastases)	25.2 Gy (tumor + 3-cm margin)
Lymph-node metastases not surgically resected	19.8 Gy
Relapsed Wilms' tumor (flank/abdomen)	12.6–18 Gy (<12 months of age) and 21.6 Gy in older children if previous radiation dose is ≤10.8 Gy. 9 Gy boost to gross residual tumor after surgery

*Whole-abdomen irradiation (WAI) is indicated when there is diffuse tumor spillage, intraperitoneal tumor rupture, peritoneal tumor seeding, and cytology-positive ascites. When WAI dose is >10.8 Gy, renal shielding is required to limit the dose to the remaining kidney to <15 Gy.

†A boost of 10.8 Gy is to be administered to areas of gross residual tumor after surgery.

‡Patients with stage I CCSK will not receive flank irradiation if lymph-node sampling and central pathologic review were performed.

CCSK, clear-cell sarcomas of the kidney; COG, Children's Oncology Group; FH, favorable histology; RTK, rhabdoid tumors of the kidney; UH, unfavorable histology.

Table 67-4 Long-Term Results of NWTS-3 and NWTS-4

Stage/Histology	Patients (*n*)	10-y Relapse-Free Survival (%)	10-y Overall Survival (%)
Stage I FH	1582	91.4	96.6
Stage II FH	1006	85.5	93.4
Stage III FH	1038	84.2	89.5
Stage IV FH	592	75.2	80.7
Stage V FH	344	65.1	77.9
All FH	4562	84.4	90.8
Clear-cell sarcoma	170	67.1	77.1
Stage II-III anaplasia	128	43.0	49.2
Stage IV anaplasia	55	18.2	18.2
Rhabdoid tumor	88	27.3	28.4

FH, favorable histology; NWTS, National Wilms' Tumor Study. NWTS unpublished data.

Table 67-5 **Children's Oncology Group (COG) Renal Tumor Protocol Schema**

Tumor Risk Classification	Multimodality Treatment
Very low risk favorable histology Wilms' tumor: <2 years, stage I FH, tumor weight <550 g	Nephrectomy without adjuvant therapy, only if central pathology review and lymph node sampling has been performed
Low risk favorable histology Wilms' tumor: ≥2 years, stage I FH, tumor weight ≥550g, Stage II FH without LOH of 1p and 16q	Nephrectomy, no RT, Regimen EE4A
Standard risk favorable histology Wilms' tumor:	
Stage I and II FH with LOH of 1p and 16q	Nephrectomy, Regimen DD4A
Stage III FH without LOH of 1p and 16q	Nephrectomy, RT, Regimen DD4A
High risk favorable histology Wilms' tumor:	
Stage III and IV FH with LOH of 1p and 16q, Stage IV FH slow/incomplete responders	Nephrectomy, RT, Regimen M, WLI
Stage IV FH: complete resolution of lung metastases at week 6 with regimen DD4A (rapid early responders)	Nephrectomy, RT, Regimen DD4A. No WLI
Stage I-III focal anaplasia Stage I diffuse anaplasia	Nephrectomy, RT, Regimen DD4A
Stage IV focal anaplasia Stage II-IV diffuse anaplasia Stage IV CCSK Stage I-IV RTK	Nephrectomy, RT, Regimen UH1
Stage I-III CCSK	Nephrectomy, RT, Regimen I

AMD, dactinomycin; CARBO, carboplatin; CCSK, clear cell sarcoma of kidney; CY, cyclophosphamide; DOX, doxorubicin; ETOP, etoposide; FH, favorable histology; RTK, rhabdoid tumor of kidney; VCR, vincristine; Regimen EE4A (VCR/AMD); RT, Regimen DD4A (VCR/AMD/ADR); Regimen M (VCR/AMD/ADR; CY/ETOP); Regimen I (VCR/DOX/CY; CY/ETOP); Regimen UH1 (CY/CARBO/ETOP; VCR/DOX/CY).

4-year, event-free survival with WLI was 89% compared to 80% with chemotherapy alone, a difference that was not significant.[40] The current COG protocol will recommend WLI based on the response of pulmonary metastatic lesions to one course of chemotherapy with vincristine, dactinomycin, and doxorubicin. Central radiology review of chest CT scans will be performed prior to and at week 6 after chemotherapy. WLI will be omitted only in patients who have achieved a complete response to chemotherapy on chest CT review at week 6. All other children will receive WLI (12 Gy).

The current irradiation recommendations of the renal tumors committee of COG are shown in Table 67-3. There are several differences in the current COG recommendations compared to NWTS-5: patients with local tumor spillage are upstaged to stage III; patients with stage I focal and diffuse anaplastic tumors will receive flank RT; the irradiation dosage for children with stage III diffuse anaplasia and stage I-III RTK will be increased to 19.8 Gy; in an effort to study if irradiation could be omitted in stage I CCSK, those who have undergone nodal sampling and central pathology review will not receive flank RT.

CHEMOTHERAPY

Chemotherapy and Combined-Modality Treatment

Single-agent chemotherapy has been used for Wilms' tumor since the 1950s, when both dactinomycin and vincristine were found to be active. The NWTS-1 showed that radiotherapy conferred no advantage in children younger than 24 months with group I tumors who also received 15 months of dactinomycin.[41] NWTS-2 showed that radiotherapy could be avoided in all children with group I Wilms' tumor if they received vincristine and dactinomycin.[42] The results of NWTS-3 proved that children with stage II tumors required only vincristine and dactinomycin without any irradiation. This study also demonstrated the interaction between chemotherapy and irradiation; that 10.8 Gy with three drugs (vincristine, dactinomycin, doxorubicin) was equivalent to 20 Gy with two drugs (vincristine, dactinomycin).[38] In NWTS-4, two overall questions were posed concerning duration of therapy (6 months vs. 15 months) and the fractionation of dactinomycin and doxorubicin (pulse-intensive, single-dose vs. 5-day course of dactinomycin or 3-day course of doxorubicin). Results have shown no advantage to prolonged therapy or divided doses, which actually proved to be more toxic; the consolidated 2-year, relapse-free rate and survival results were 90% and 97%, respectively, for the low- and high-risk patients (see Table 67-4). Thus, the shorter courses of the pulse-intensive regimens are now considered standard. This reduces patient clinic time and is more convenient and less costly for both parents and staff.[43]

Anaplastic Histology

The first NWTSG trial to stratify patients with anaplastic Wilms' tumor into a distinct treatment group was NWTS-3. On NWTS-3 and NWTS-4, patients received 15 months of vincristine, dactinomycin, and doxorubicin, and were randomized to receive cyclophosphamide. Patients with stages II-IV diffuse anaplastic tumors who were treated with cyclophosphamide had a significant improvement in 4-year, relapse-free survival rates (27% vs. 55%) (Table 67-4).[37] Patients with all stages of focal anaplastic histology or stage I diffuse anaplastic histology had excellent outcomes, regardless of treatment regimen.[37] Based on these results, NWTS-5 incorporated cyclophosphamide into the treatment plan for patients with stages II-IV diffuse anaplastic Wilms' tumor. These patients received regimen I, which consisted of vincristine/doxorubicin/cyclophosphamide alternating with cyclophosphamide/etoposide. The preliminary results of NWTS-5 indicate that the patient outcomes are similar to NWTS-4. The new COG protocol will evaluate whether a treatment regimen containing cyclophosphamide/carboplatin/etoposide alternating with vincristine/doxorubicin/cyclophosphamide (regimen UH1) will improve the event-free and overall survival of patients with stage II-IV diffuse anaplasia (see Table 67-5).

On NWTS-5, patients with stage I diffuse and focal anaplastic tumors were treated with regimen EE-4A (vincristine and dactinomycin). Preliminary analysis of these patients revealed an unexpectedly low relapse-free survival rate of 64%.[66] To improve upon these results, the COG study will recommend that patients with stage I focal and diffuse anaplastic disease be treated with regimen DD-4A (vincristine, dactinomycin, doxorubicin) and flank irradiation. Patients with stages II/III focal anaplasia will be treated likewise. However, the treatment of stage IV focal anaplasia will be intensified (regimen UH1) because of higher relapse rates with regimen DD-4A (see Table 67-5).

Clear-Cell Sarcoma of the Kidney

Data from NWTS 1-4 suggested that the addition of doxorubicin to the combination of vincristine and dactinomycin improved the relapse-free survival rates of patients with CCSK.[44,45] NWTS-3 demonstrated no improvement in outcomes of patients with CCSK with the addition of cyclophosphamide.[38] In NWTS-4, children with CCSK who received a longer course of chemotherapy with vincristine, dactinomycin, and doxorubicin (15 months) had better 8-year relapse-free survival rates of 88% compared to 61% after shorter course (6 months) chemotherapy. However, this did not lead to a difference in overall survival. The overall survival rates of CCSK patients treated on NWTS-4 was significantly superior to that of NWTS-3 (83% vs. 67%). The pulse-intensive chemotherapy administration of dactinomycin and doxorubicin in NWTS-4 is presumed to be one of the reasons for the improvement in outcomes (see Table 67-4).[46] Preliminary analysis of NWTS-5 has shown promising results with regimen I chemotherapy except for patients with stage IV disease (NWTS, unpublished data). Based on these results, the COG study will continue to treat patients with stages I-III CCSK on a version of regimen I. Patients with stage IV CCSK will be treated with regimen UH-1 (see Table 67-5).

Rhabdoid Tumor of the Kidney

Patients with RTK have been treated on NWTS trials with agents such as vincristine, dactinomycin, and doxorubicin, with or without cyclophosphamide. The outcomes attained with these agents have been consistently very poor (see Table 67-4).[38,47] To try to improve upon these results, NWTS-5 adopted a different treatment strategy consisting of carboplatin/etoposide alternating with cyclophosphamide. Preliminary analysis of patients treated with this regimen revealed a survival percentage of approximately 26%, which was not an improvement compared to previous studies, and thus the treatment arm was closed.[67] The COG protocol will evaluate whether a treatment regimen containing cyclophosphamide/carboplatin/etoposide alternating with vincristine/doxorubicin/cyclophosphamide improves the event-free and overall survival rates in these patients (see Table 67-5).

TREATMENT RESULTS

Treatment results are outlined in Table 67-4.

TECHNIQUES OF IRRADIATION

Parallel-opposed (AP-PA) treatment portals using 4-MV or 6-MV photons are recommended for flank, whole abdomen, and whole-lung irradiation. The details regarding the planning techniques and setup of these irradiation portals are shown and described in Figures 67-3 to 67-5. If the lungs and either flank or abdomen have to be treated simultaneously, it is preferred that they be included in one irradiation portal. However, if these two sites have to be treated sequentially, then appropriate field gap-calculations should be used for field matching, to avoid overlap between the two portals, particularly over critical structures such as the liver and kidney.

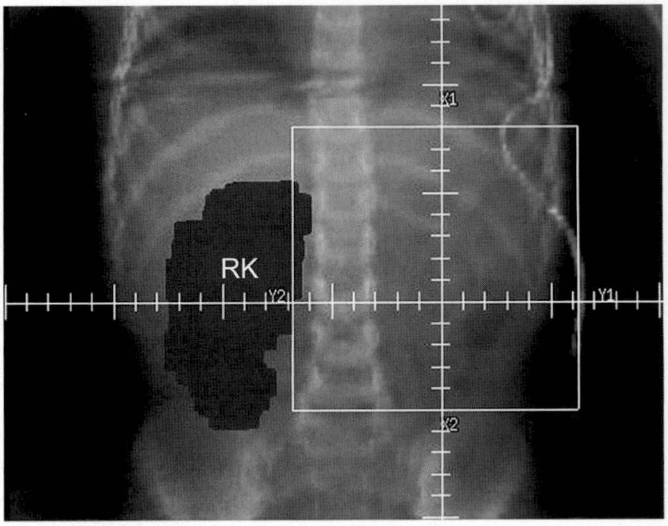

Figure 67-3 Anteroposterior (AP) left flank irradiation portal in a child with a stage III favorable histology Wilms' tumor. The superior and inferior field margins are placed approximately 1 cm from the preoperative renal tumor volume. The medial field margin should include the entire width of the vertebral body to irradiate the lymph nodes and avoid scoliosis. The outline of the normal right kidney *(RK)* is shown.

CURRENT CLINICAL RECOMMENDATIONS

Based on the results of NWTS-5, the new COG renal tumor protocol will use LOH at both 1p and 16q in addition to tumor stage and pathologic classification for defining tumor-risk groups and assigning risk-adapted therapy (see Table 67-5). The goals of therapy in the COG study are to reduce the incidence of treatment-related morbidity in low-risk groups who have good survival rates and increase treatment intensity in high-risk tumors to improve cure rates.

OTHER STUDIES

In addition to the NWTSG, there have been randomized studies managed by SIOP, evaluating preoperative therapy[48,49] and the UKCCSG.[39,50]

RETRIEVAL THERAPY

Children with relapsed favorable histology Wilms' tumor have a variable prognosis, depending on the site of relapse, the time from initial diagnosis to relapse, and their previous therapy. Favorable prognostic factors include no previous treatment with doxorubicin; relapse more than 12 months after diagnosis; and intra-abdominal relapse in a patient not previ-

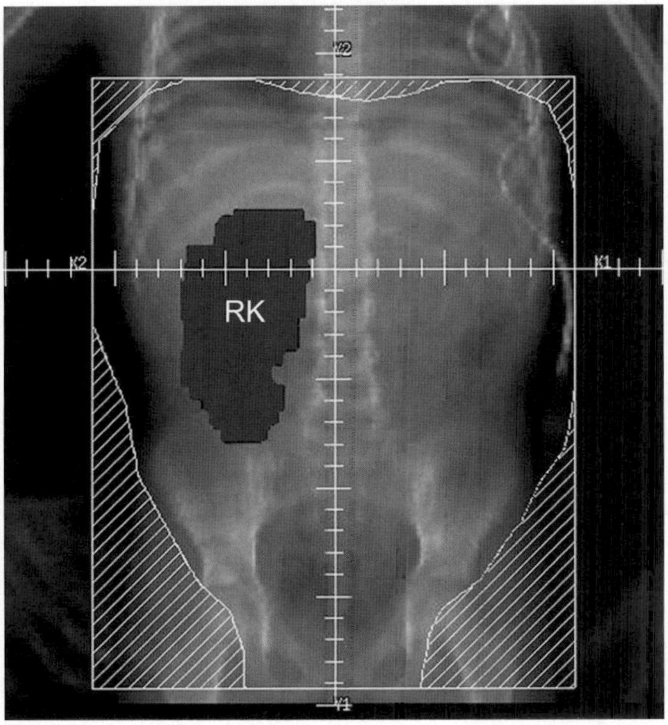

Figure 67-4 Anteroposterior (AP) whole abdomen irradiation portal. The upper margin of the abdominal field must include the diaphragm. The acetabulum and femoral head should be excluded from the irradiated volume to decrease the probability of slipped femoral epiphysis. The outline of the normal right kidney (*RK*) is shown.

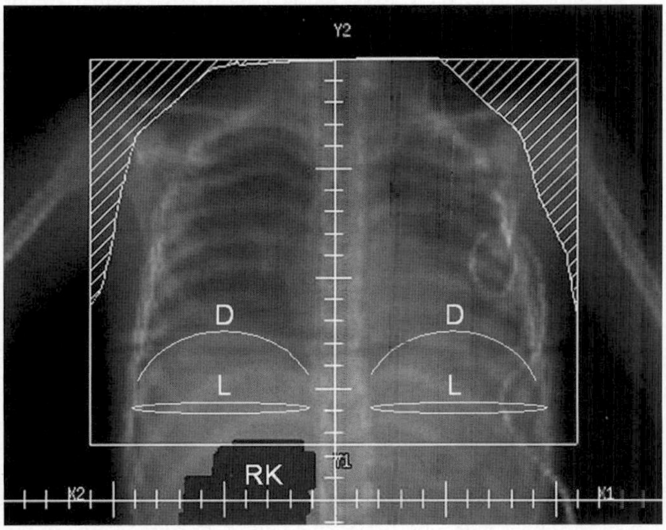

Figure 67-5 Anteroposterior (AP) whole-lung irradiation (WLI) portal. The dome of the diaphragm (*D*) and the lower extent (*L*) of the costophrenic angles at the lung bases are shown. A lateral radiograph of the chest at the time of simulation, or review of the sagittal and coronal images during CT simulation, is required to ascertain inclusion of the anterior and posterior costophrenic angles with a 1-cm margin at the inferior edge of the treatment volume. The outline of the normal right kidney (*RK*) is shown.

ously treated with abdominal irradiation.[51,52] Children in more favorable groups should be treated aggressively because they generally have a good response to retrieval therapy. Although surgical excision of pulmonary metastases does not improve outcome, surgical biopsy or excision should be performed to histologically confirm recurrent disease and, particularly in the case of intra-abdominal recurrence, to reduce the tumor burden prior to the initiation of RT and combination chemotherapy.[53] The optimal chemotherapy regimen has not been defined but should include doxorubicin, if not used previously. The combination of etoposide and carboplatin is active against recurrent Wilms' tumor.[54]

In children who previously have not received RT, the recommended flank radiation dose is 12.6 to 18 Gy (birth–12 months) and 21.6 Gy (13 months or older). Supplemental boost fields could be added for gross residual disease. In children who have been previously irradiated, the total nominal flank dose after retreatment should not exceed 30.6 Gy (<36 months of age) or 39.5 Gy in older children. The COG protocol will recommend postoperative irradiation for all children with abdominal relapse because these tumors are generally large and infiltrative, and surgical resection with negative margins is unlikely.

Patients who relapse after previous treatment with a regimen that included doxorubicin or who develop a recurrence in the abdomen (including liver) after previous irradiation have a poor prognosis.[51] Several reports have suggested that high-dose chemotherapy with stem cell rescue should be used in the management of those patients with adverse prognostic factors at the time of relapse, although the relative efficacy of this approach remains unproven. The reported event-free and overall survival rates range from 50% to 70% following intensive multiagent chemotherapy with or without stem cell transplantation.[52,55–58]

LATE EFFECTS

As the follow-up of successfully treated children increases, data are emerging on the late consequences of treatment. The types of late sequelae and their severity depend on the age and sex of the child, extent of surgery, chemotherapy drugs, and several radiation-related factors. The most common cause for renal failure in Wilms' tumor patients is bilateral nephrectomy, and the second leading cause is radiation-induced damage or surgical complications involving the remaining kidney. The frequency of renal failure in bilateral Wilms' tumor was 16.4% for NWTS-1 and NWTS-2, 9.9% for NWTS-3, and 3.8% for NWTS-4.[59] The incidence of scoliosis ranges from 40% to 60% with irradiation doses of 25 to 40 Gy. However, the rate of scoliosis should be low with the current doses of 10.8 Gy.[60,61] The cumulative frequency of congestive heart failure among patients on NWTS 1-4 was 4.4% at 20 years among patients treated initially with doxorubicin and 17.4% among patients treated with doxorubicin for a first or subsequent relapse. The factors that were significantly associated with the incidence of heart failure were female sex, cumulative doxorubicin dose, lung irradiation, and left-sided abdominal irradiation.[62] Women who are Wilms' tumor survivors could have adverse pregnancy outcomes such as malposition of the fetus and premature labor. Their offspring may be premature and of low birth weight, and have congenital malformations. These complication rates were more likely with higher doses of irradiation.[63,64] The cumulative 15-year risk of second malignant neoplasms (SMNs) was 1.6% among patients enrolled on the NWTS, after a mean follow up of 7.5 years per patient. Higher doses of abdominal irradiation and doxorubicin increased the risk of SMNs.[65]

REFERENCES

1. Gurney JG, Severson RK, Davis S, et al: Incidence of cancer in children in the United States: sex-, race-, and 1-year age-specific rates by histologic type. Cancer 75:2186-2195, 1995.
2. Rance TF: Case of fungus haematodes of the kidneys. Med Phys J 32:19, 1814.
3. Wilms M: Die Mischgeschwülste der Niere. Leipzig: Verlag von Arthur Georgi, 1899, pp 1-90.
4. Gross RE, Neuhauser BD: Treatment of mixed tumors of the kidney in childhood. Pediatrics 6:843-852, 1950.
5. National Wilms' Tumor Study Committee: Wilms' tumor: status report, 1990. J Clin Oncol 9:877-887, 1991.
6. Tournade MF, Com-Nougue C, Voûte PA, et al: Results of the Sixth International Society of Pediatric Oncology Wilms' tumor trial and study: A risk-adapted therapeutic approach in Wilms' tumor. J Clin Oncol 11:1014-1023, 1993.
7. Kalapurakal JA, Dome JS, Perlman EJ, et al: Management of Wilms' tumor: current practice and future goals. Lancet Oncol 5: 37-46, 2003.
8. Coppes MJ, Pritchard-Jones K: Principles of Wilms' tumor biology. Urol Clin North Am 27:423-433, 2000
9. Coppes MJ, de Kraker J, van Dijken PJ, et al: Bilateral Wilms' tumor: long-term survival and some epidemiological features. J Clin Oncol 7:310-315, 1989.
10. Little MH, Williamson KA, Mannens M, et al: Evidence that WT1 mutations in Denys-Drash syndrome patients may act in a dominant negative fashion. Hum Mol Genet 2:259-264, 1993.
11. Dome JS, Coppes MJ: Recent advances in Wilms' tumor genetics. Curr Opin Pediatr 14:5-11, 2002.
12. Koufos A, Grundy P, Morgan K, et al: Familial Wiedemann-Beckwith syndrome and a second Wilms' tumor locus both map to 11p15.5. Am J Hum Genet 44:711-719, 1989.
13. Grundy PE, Telzerow PE, Breslow N, et al: Loss of heterozygosity for chromosomes 16q and 1p in Wilms' tumors predicts an adverse outcome. Cancer Res 52:3094-3098, 1992.
14. Grundy PE, Breslow NE, Li S, et al: Loss of heterozygosity for chromosomes 1p and 16q is an adverse prognostic factor in favorable histology Wilms' tumor: a report from the National Wilms' Tumor Study Group. J Clin Oncol 23:7312-7321, 2005.
15. Beckwith JB, Palmer NF: Histopathology and prognosis of Wilms' tumor: results from the National Wilms' Tumor Study. Cancer 41:1937-1948, 1978.
16. Beckwith JB: Wilms' tumor and other renal tumors of childhood: a selective review from the National Wilms' Tumor Study Pathology Center. Hum Pathol 14:481-492, 1983.
17. Bonadio JR, Storer B, Norkool P, et al: Anaplastic Wilms' tumor: clinical and pathologic studies. J Clin Oncol 3:513-520, 1985.
18. Bardeesy N, Falkoff D, Petruzzi MJ, et al: Anaplastic Wilms' tumor, a subtype displaying poor prognosis, harbors p53 gene mutations. Nat Genet 7:91-97, 1994.
19. Faria P, Beckwith JB, Mishra K, et al: Focal versus diffuse anaplasia in Wilms' tumor—new definitions with prognostic significance: a report from the National Wilms' Tumor Study Group. Am J Surg Pathol 20:909-920, 1996.
20. Green DM, Breslow NE, Beckwith JB, et al: Treatment with nephrectomy only for small, stage I/favorable histology Wilms' tumor: a report from the National Wilms' Tumor Study Group. J Clin Oncol 19:3719-3721, 2001.
21. Beckwith JB: Precursor lesions of Wilms' tumor: clinical and biological implications. Med Pediatr Oncol 21:158-168, 1993.
22. Beckwith JB, Palmer NF: Wilms' tumor and other renal tumors in childhood. *In* Feingold M (ed): Pathology of Neoplasia in Children and Adolescents. Philadelphia, WB Saunders, 1986, pp 313-332.
23. Marsden HB, Lawler W, Kumar PM: Bone metastasizing renal tumor of childhood: morphological and clinical features and differences from Wilms' tumor. Cancer 42:1922-1928, 1978.
24. Owens CM, Veys PA, Pritchard J, et al: Role of chest computed tomography at diagnosis in the management of Wilms' tumor: a study by the United Kingdom Children's Cancer Study Group. J Clin Oncol 20:2768-2773, 2002.
25. Green DM: Use of chest computed tomography for staging and treatment of Wilms' tumor in children. J Clin Oncol 20:2763-2764, 2002.
26. Gylys-Morin V, Hoffer FA, Kozakewich H, et al: Wilms' tumor and nephroblastomatosis: imaging characteristics at gadolinium-enhanced MR imaging. Radiology 188:517-521, 1993.
27. National Wilms' Tumor Study Group: NWTS-5 protocol. Seattle, NWTSG, 1995.
28. Farewell VT, D'Angio GJ, Breslow NE, et al: Retrospective validation of a new staging system for Wilms' tumor. Cancer Clin Trials 4:167-171, 1981.
29. Beckwith JB: National Wilms' Tumor Study: an update for pathologists. Pediatr Dev Path 1:79-84, 1998.
30. Weeks DA, Beckwith JB, Luckey DW: Relapse-associated variables in stage I favorable histology Wilms' tumor. A report of the National Wilms' Tumor Study. Cancer 60:1204-1212, 1987.
31. Blakely ML, Ritchey ML: Controversies in the management of Wilms' tumor. Semin Pediatr Surg 10:127-131, 2001.
32. Shamberger RC, Guthrie KA, Ritchey ML, et al: Surgery-related factors and local recurrence of Wilms' tumor in National Wilms' Tumor Study-4. Ann Surg 229:292-297, 1999.
33. D'Angio GJ, Tefft M, Breslow NE, et al: Radiation therapy of Wilms' tumor: results according to dose, field, post-operative timing, and histology. Int J Radiat Oncol Biol Phys 4:769-780, 1978.
34. Thomas PRM, Tefft M, Farewell VT, et al: Abdominal relapses in irradiated Second National Wilms' Tumor Study patients. J Clin Oncol 2:1098-1101, 1984.
35. Thomas PRM, Tefft M, Compaan PJ, et al: Results of two radiotherapy randomizations in the Third National Wilms' Tumor Study (NWTS-3). Cancer 68:1703-1707, 1991.
36. Kalapurakal JA, Li SM, Breslow NE, et al: Influence of radiation therapy delay on abdominal tumor recurrence in patients with favorable histology Wilms' tumor treated on NWTS-3 and NWTS-4: a report from the National Wilms' Tumor Study Group. Int J Radiat Oncol Biol Phys 57:495-499, 2003.
37. Green DM, Breslow NE, Beckwith NE, et al: Treatment of children with stages II to IV anaplastic Wilms' tumor: a report from the National Wilms' Tumor Study Group. J Clin Oncol 12:2126-2131, 1994.
38. D'Angio GJ, Breslow N, Beckwith JB, et al: Treatment of Wilms' tumor: results of the Third National Wilms' Tumor Study. Cancer 64:349-360, 1989.
39. Pritchard J, Imeson J, Barnes J, et al: Results of the United Kingdom Children's Cancer Study Group First Wilms' Tumor Study. J Clin Oncol 13:124-133, 1995.
40. Meisel JA, Guthrie KA, Breslow NE, et al: Significance and management of computed tomography detected pulmonary nodules: a report from the National Wilms' Tumor Study Group. Int J Radiat Oncol Biol Phys 44:579-585, 1999.
41. D'Angio GJ, Evans AE, Breslow N, et al: The treatment of Wilms' tumor: results of the National Wilms' Tumor Study. Cancer 38:633-646, 1976.
42. D'Angio GJ, Evans A, Breslow N, et al: The treatment of Wilms tumor: results of the Second National Wilms' Tumor Study. Cancer 47:2302-2311, 1981.
43. Green DM, Breslow NE, Beckwith JB, et al: A comparison between single dose and divided dose administration of dactinomycin and doxorubicin. J Clin Oncol 16:237-245, 1998.
44. Green DM, Breslow NE, Beckwith JB, et al: Treatment of children with clear-cell sarcoma of the kidney: a report from the National Wilms' Tumor Study Group. J Clin Oncol 12:2132-2137, 1994.
45. Argani P, Perlman EJ, Breslow NE, et al: Clear cell sarcoma of the kidney: a review of 351 cases from the National Wilms' Tumor Study Group Pathology Center. Am J Surg Pathol 24:4-18, 2000.
46. Seibel N, Li S, Breslow NE, et al: Effect of duration of treatment on treatment outcome for patients with clear-cell sarcoma of the kidney: a report from the National Wilms' Tumor Study Group. J Clin Oncol 22:468-473, 2004.
47. Weeks DA, Beckwith B, Mierau GW, et al: Rhabdoid tumor of kidney. Am J Surg Pathol 13:439-458, 1989.
48. Graf N, Tournade MF, de Kraker J: The role of preoperative chemotherapy in the management of Wilms' tumor. The SIOP studies. Urol Clin North Am 27:443-454, 2000.
49. Tournade MF, Com-Nogue C, de Kraker J, et al: Optimal duration of preoperative therapy in unilateral and nonmetastatic Wilms' tumor in children older than 6 months: results of the Ninth Inter-

national Society of Pediatric Oncology Wilms' Tumor Trial and Study. J Clin Oncol 19:488-500, 2001.
50. Mitchell C, Jones PM, Kelsey A, et al: The treatment of Wilms' tumor: results of the United Kingdom Children's Cancer Study Group (UKCCSG) second Wilms' tumor study. Br J Cancer 83:602-608, 2000.
51. Grundy P, Breslow NE, Green DM, et al: Prognostic factors of children with recurrent Wilms' tumor: results from the second and third National Wilms' Tumor Study. J Clin Oncol 7:638-647, 1989.
52. Tannous R, Giller G, Holmes E, et al: Intensive therapy for high risk (HR) relapsed Wilms' tumor (WT). A CCG-4921/POG-9445 study report. Proc Am Soc Clin Oncol 19:588a, 2000.
53. Green DM, Breslow N, Li Y, et al: The role of surgical excision in the management of relapsed Wilms' tumor patients with pulmonary metastases. J Pediatr Surg 26:728-733, 1991.
54. Pein F, Tournade MF, Zucker J-M: Etoposide and carboplatin: a highly effective combination in relapsed or refractory Wilms' tumor. A phase II study by the French Society of Pediatric Oncology (SFOP). J Clin Oncol 12:931-936, 1994.
55. Garaventa A, Hartmann O, Bernard JL, et al: Autologous bone marrow transplantation for pediatric Wilms' tumor: the experience of the European Bone Marrow Transplantation Solid Tumor Registry. Med Pediatr Oncol 22:11-14, 1994.
56. Pein F, Michon J, Valteau-Couanet D, et al: High-dose melphalan, etoposide and carboplatin followed by autologous stem-cell rescue in pediatric high-risk recurrent Wilms' tumor: a French Society of Pediatric Oncology Study. J Clin Oncol 16:3295-3301, 1998.
57. Campbell AD, Cohn SL, Reynolds M, et al: Treatment of relapsed Wilms' tumor with high-dose therapy and autologous hematopoietic stem-cell rescue: the experience at Children's Memorial Hospital. J Clin Oncol 22:885-2890, 2004.
58. Kremens B, Gruhn B, Klingebiel T, et al: High-dose chemotherapy with autologous stem cell rescue in children with nephroblastoma. Bone Marrow Transplant 30:893-898, 2002.
59. Ritchey ML, Green DM, Thomas PRM, et al: Renal failure in Wilms' tumor patients: a report from the National Wilms' Tumor Study Group. Med Pediatr Oncol 26:75-80, 1996.
60. Paulino AC, Wen BC, Brown CK, et al: Late effects in children treated with radiation therapy for Wilms' tumor. Int J Radiat Oncol Biol Phys 19:488-500, 2000.
61. Thomas PRM, Griffith KD, Fineberg BB, et al: Late effects of treatment for Wilms' tumor. Int J Radiat Oncol Biol Phys 9:651-657, 1983.
62. Green DM, Grigoriev YA, Nan B, et al: Congestive heart failure after treatment for Wilms' tumor: a report from the National Wilms' Tumor Study Group. J Clin Oncol 19:1926-1934, 2001.
63. Green DM, Peabody EM, Nan B, et al: Pregnancy outcome after treatment for Wilms' tumor: a report from the National Wilms' Tumor Study Group. J Clin Oncol 20:2506-2513, 2002.
64. Kalapurakal JA, Peterson S, Peabody EM, et al: Pregnancy outcomes after abdominal irradiation that included or excluded the pelvis in childhood Wilms' tumor survivors: a report from the National Wilms' Tumor Study. Int J Radiat Oncol Biol Phys 58:1364-1368, 2004.
65. Breslow NE, Takashima JR, Whitton JA, et al: Second malignant neoplasms following treatment for Wilms' tumor: a report from the National Wilms' Tumor Study Group. J Clin Oncol 13:1851-1859, 1995.
66. Dome JS, Cotton CA, Perlman EJ, et al: Treatment of anaplastic histology Wilms' tumor: results from the fifth National Wilms' Tumor Study. J Clin Oncol (in press).
67. Tomlinson GE, Breslow NE, Dome J, et al: Rhabdoid tumor of the kidney in the National Wilms' Tumor Study: age at diagnosis as a prognostic factor. J Clin Oncol 23:7641-7645, 2005.

CHAPTER 68

RETINOBLASTOMA

Robert S. Lavey

INCIDENCE

Retinoblastoma is the most common intraocular tumor in children.

Approximately 250 cases of retinoblastoma are diagnosed annually in the United States.

Approximately 90% of cases of retinoblastoma are diagnosed before 5 years of age.

Between 7% and 10% of patients have positive family history for retinoblastoma.

BIOLOGIC CHARACTERISTICS

Poorly differentiated, malignant neuroectodermal tumor of the sensory retina.

Results from inactivation of both alleles of the *RB* tumor suppressor gene.

40% of patients have a heritable germ-line mutation associated with a high risk of additional malignancies.

STAGING EVALUATION

Perform visual acuity evaluation and ophthalmoscopic examination.

Perform ultrasound exam of orbits; if nondiagnostic, then perform computed tomography (CT) scan.

Perform magnetic resonance imaging (MRI) scan of the brain and orbits.

Examine the orbits under anesthesia with retinal imaging.

Conduct metastatic evaluation (bone scan, bone marrow aspirate and biopsy, and cerebrospinal fluid [CSF] evaluation) only if tumor extends outside the globe.

TREATMENT

Intraocular retinoblastoma
- 90% 5-year survival
- Group A—intraretinal tumors <3 mm in diameter located away from fovea and optic nerve
  - Treat with focal therapy (laser, cryotherapy, or radioactive plaque).
  - 99% of eyes preserved with excellent visual acuity.
- Group B—all other discrete intraretinal tumors
  - Treat with intravenous chemotherapy (IVC) and focal therapy.
  - Progressive disease treated with external beam radiation therapy (EBRT).
  - 95% of eyes preserved, acuity may be diminished if tumor near fovea or optic nerve.
- Group C—discrete local disease with minimal subretinal or vitreous seeding
  - Treat with IVC, intraocular chemotherapy, and focal therapy.
  - Progressive disease treated with EBRT.
  - 70% to 80% of eyes preserved without requiring enucleation.
- Group D—diffuse disease with significant subretinal or vitreous seeding
  - If unilateral disease, enucleate immediately.
  - Treat bilateral disease with IVC, intraocular chemotherapy, and focal therapy.
  - Progressive disease treated with EBRT.
  - 50% to 70% of eyes preserved without requiring enucleation.
- Group E—advanced intraocular disease
  - Generally enucleate immediately.
  - If both eyes Group D-E, give IVC and intraocular chemotherapy and consider EBRT for progressive disease; try to preserve eye with better vision.
  - <5% of eyes preserved.
- Enucleated globe with tumor involving cut end of optic nerve, extending into sclera, or both extensively invading choroid and extending along optic nerve beyond the lamina cribrosa.
- Adjuvant chemotherapy with or without EBRT given to decrease risk for metastasis.

Metastatic disease
- Myeloablative chemotherapy with local radiation therapy (RT) gives more than 50% relapse-free survival if central nervous system (CNS) is not involved.
- Probability of cure low if CNS is involved or standard-dose chemotherapy is used.

The entity of a discrete tumor arising from the retina was first reported by the Scottish surgeon James Waldrop in 1809.[1] The name *retinoblastoma* was first proposed more than 100 years later by the American ophthalmologist Frederick Verhoeff and adopted by the American Ophthalmological Society in 1926 in the belief that the tumor was derived from undifferentiated embryonic retinal cells called retinoblasts.[2] It is now known that retinoblastomas derive from cells of the immature neuroepithelial inner layer of the optic cup that have the potential to differentiate into rod and cone photoreceptors and Müller cells.[3] It is uncertain whether retinoblastomas arise from neuroblasts that are already committed to the cone lineage or from retinoblasts that are directed into the cone pathway after loss of the ability to differentiate along their appropriate lineage. Retinoblastoma has become the prototype for malignancies caused by the inactivation of a tumor suppressor gene.

EPIDEMIOLOGY

Retinoblastoma is the sixth most common solid tumor and the most common intraocular tumor in children. Including all age groups, retinoblastoma is the second most common malignant intraocular tumor after uveal melanoma. The number of new retinoblastoma cases reported annually is approximately 250 in the United States and 50 in the United Kingdom.[4] There are 10.6 cases of retinoblastoma per million children younger than 5 years of age, 1.5 cases per million children ages 5 to 9 years, and 0.3 case per million children 10 to 14 years of age.[5] The incidence does not differ by race, gender, or left or right eye in these countries. Almost 90% of all cases of retinoblastoma in the United States are diagnosed before the patient has reached the age of 5 years.[6,7] Retinoblastoma is seen rarely in children older than the age of 6 years, and very few occurrences of retinoblastoma have been reported in teenagers[8] or adults.[9]

Approximately 40% of patients have the heritable form of retinoblastoma[10] derived from germ line inactivation or deletion of the *RB* gene, discussed in detail in the Genetics section of this chapter. The inheritance of a single inactive allele of the *RB* gene confers the predisposition to cancer, but a second inactivating mutation must occur in at least one retinoblast cell for retinoblastoma to appear. Because the tumor requires inactivation of both copies of the *RB* gene, it is a recessive trait. However, the tumor appears to be dominant because so many retinoblasts are at risk that the probability that at least one will undergo the second mutation required to develop a tumor is more than 90%. As a result, 45% to 50% of children having one parent with heritable retinoblastoma develop retinoblastoma during their early childhood.[11] The median age at diagnosis of heritable retinoblastoma is less than 12 months.[12] The heritable form of retinoblastoma produces multiple tumors in both eyes in 85% of patients.[13] Only 7% to 10% of retinoblastoma patients have a positive family history for retinoblastoma, so 75% to 80% of heritable retinoblastoma cases result from a new germ line mutation, which is associated with advanced paternal age.[14] The incidence rate of heritable retinoblastoma around the world is remarkably constant, indicating that environmental influences play little role in the development of the hereditary form of retinoblastoma.[15]

Hereditary retinoblastoma patients have a cancer predisposition syndrome associated with a several hundredfold risk of developing an osteosarcoma, soft tissue sarcoma or other mesenchymal tumor through their teenage years, melanoma or brain tumor through middle age, and epithelial malignancy such as lung or bladder cancer in later life.[16,17] Between 2% and 8% of heritable retinoblastoma patients develop a midline intracranial tumor usually involving the pineal or suprasellar region that histologically resembles retinoblastoma and is usually characterized as a pinealoma, primitive neuroectodermal tumor (PNET), or trilateral retinoblastoma. This intracranial tumor is a primary cancer and not a metastasis from the retinoblastoma.[18,19] The intracranial tumor is diagnosed at a mean age of 23 months.[20] A congenital anomaly or mental retardation is found in fewer than 0.1% of heritable retinoblastoma patients.[21]

Approximately 60% of patients with retinoblastoma have the nonheritable, sporadic form of the disease. The sporadic form is far more common in developing tropical and subtropical regions of the world than in the developed countries, is the most common solid tumor of childhood in several underdeveloped countries, and has been associated with viral infection and a deficiency of fruit and vegetables in the maternal diet.[22] The median age at diagnosis of nonheritable retinoblastoma is approximately 24 months, significantly later in infancy than heritable cases.[23] Separate mutations inactivating each copy of the *RB* gene of a single retinal cell are required for these tumors to arise. Patients generally have unilateral disease and no increased risk for development of other malignancies.[24]

GENETICS

The *RB* gene was the first identified tumor suppressor gene. The *RB* pathway was the first, and remains one of the most important, tumor suppressor pathways to be elucidated in human cancer.[25] The *RB* gene encodes a 4.7 kilobase messenger RNA transcript that produces a protein of 110 kilodaltons and 928 amino acids. The Rb protein (Rb) regulates the expression of specific genes involved in cell division, differentiation, senescence, and apoptosis.[26]

The major cell-cycle function of Rb is to inhibit the transition of cells out of gap 1 (G_1) phase into S phase.[27] Rb inhibits cell division through its interactions with the E2F site of the promoter region of several genes essential for cell-cycle progression, including *c-Myc* and *c-Myb*. Most E2Fs have a transactivation domain that stimulates expression of genes containing E2F binding sites in their promoters. Rb binds E2F within the transactivation domain, thereby masking its activity.[28] Rb also has intrinsic transcriptional repressor activity and is able to block the expression of genes when brought to promoters by E2F.[29] Rb binds to and recruits promoter proteins that alter chromatin structure. Alteration of local chromatin structure into a restricted conformation prevents access by the transcriptional machinery, thereby inhibiting expression. Rb orchestrates the assembly of multiprotein complexes, which are then recruited to specific promoters by E2F, where they control access of the transcriptional machinery.

The *RB* gene was found on the long arm of chromosome 13 in band q14.[30] Introduction of a functional *RB* gene into retinoblastoma cells[31] and other *RB*-deficient tumors[32] suppresses the neoplastic phenotype, indicating that the gene product is a tumor suppressor. Fewer than 10% of retinoblastoma patients have a constitutional chromosome 13q abnormality (usually a deletion) that can be detected by karyotyping.[33] These extensive deletions can be associated with the *13q syndrome*, with features such as growth and mental retardation, facial dysmorphism, microcephaly, skeletal anomalies, and genitourinary abnormalities. Approximately 15% to 20% of germinal mutations are too small to detect by cytogenetics but can be detected with techniques for analyzing gross DNA rearrangements (e.g., Southern blot). The remaining 75% of *RB* gene mutations are small alterations involving one or a few nucleotides that can only be detected by high-resolution methods.[34]

Inactivation of the *RB* gene is both necessary and sufficient for the development of retinoblastoma.[35] Rb acts as a tumor suppressor by inhibiting proliferation and promoting differentiation of retinal progenitor cells.[36]

PATHOLOGY

Retinoblastoma is a poorly differentiated, malignant neuroectodermal tumor arising in the sensory retina. Its typical appearance is a chalky white with bright white calcific speckles interspersed throughout the tumor. Tumors may grow endophytically, exophytically, or in a diffusely infiltrative manner. Endophytic tumors grow from the retina into the vitreous chamber and may invade the anterior portion of the eye. Clusters of tumor cells may become detached and form floating tumor spheres called vitreous seeds. Exophytic tumors grow from the retina into the subretinal space, often causing serous detachment of the retina, and may extend into the choroid. Commonly, tumors demonstrate a combination of endophytic and exophytic growth. Diffusely infiltrative growth, which resembles inflammation throughout the retina and uveitis without a predominant mass, is often mistaken for benign disease. It is the least common pattern and usually presents unilaterally in children older than 4 years of age without a family history of retinoblastoma.

Histologically, the retinoblastoma tumor is soft and friable with large areas of necrosis containing multiple calcifications.

It is composed of uniform small, round, or polygonal cells with a large nucleus and scant cytoplasm. Mitotic and apoptotic cells are both common. Tumors may be largely undifferentiated or may form rosettes or fleurettes. Flexner-Wintersteiner rosettes are the most common and are characteristic of retinoblastoma. They consist of a radial arrangement of cuboidal or columnar cells surrounding an apical lumen with their nuclei positioned away from the lumen. Homer-Wright rosettes are also arranged radially but have cytoplasmic fibrils extending into the center rather than a lumen. Fleurettes are comprised of cells with abundant pale cytoplasm and small nuclei joined by cytoplasmic junctions creating the appearance of a bouquet of flowers.

NATURAL HISTORY AND CLINICAL PRESENTATION

Retinoblastoma tumors initially grow rapidly in the retina without an intrinsic blood supply. Continued growth of the tumor leads to detachment and destruction of the retina, vitreous, or subretinal hemorrhage; angle closure glaucoma from pressure of the tumor pushing the iris lens diaphragm forward; direct occlusion of the chamber angle by tumor cells or red blood cells; or proliferation of iris neovascularization to involve the anterior chamber angle. Eventually, the tumor fills the eye. Tumor cells can invade the optic nerve and grow posteriorly into the chiasm, subarachnoid space, and brain. Less commonly, the tumor will follow vessels and nerves that penetrate the sclera and expand as a mass lesion in the orbit.[37] Some tumors will spontaneously involute, activating a process that will result in phthisis. Once mutations occur (perhaps loss of the suppressor gene PNET) that allow them to grow without extracellular matrix anchorage dependence, the tumor may seed the low-oxygen, low-nutrient microenvironments of the vitreum and subretinal space. Early vitreous seeds are limited to a thickness of two tumor cells surrounding an inner core of necrotic oxygen-starved tumor. Advanced tumors can disseminate hematogenously to bone marrow, bone, and organs.

The most common presenting sign of retinoblastoma is leukocoria (*white pupil*) in one or both eyes, the replacement of the normal red reflex of the eye with a diffusely whitish appearing *cat's eye* pupil in flash photographs or in dim light. Leukocoria occurs when light entering the eye is reflected back out through the pupil by the yellow or yellow-white tumor. Retinoblastomas in the posterior pole of the globe that have reached 3 mm in basal diameter are sufficiently large to generate a leukocoria reflex. In a retrospective chart review of 1265 patients with retinoblastoma from New York Hospital, leukocoria was the presenting sign in 56% of cases.[38]

Strabismus is the second most common presenting sign, noted in 20% of patients seen at New York Hospital.[38] Strabismus occurs because of a loss of central vision with disruption of the fusional reflex. Neovascularization of the surface of the iris (rubeosis iridis) occurs in 17% of patients and can lead to spontaneous bleeding into the anterior chamber of the eye and change the color of the iris.[39] Other less-common signs and symptoms include a red, painful eye with glaucoma; cloudy cornea; decreased visual acuity; and an aseptic orbital cellulitis.

DIAGNOSIS AND EVALUATION

The visual acuity in each eye should be evaluated. Indirect ophthalmoscopic examination using a low light level with pupillary dilation reveals single or multiple white, cream-colored, or creamy-pink retinal masses projecting into the vitreous. Retinal detachment as well as vitreous hemorrhage or seeding may be seen. A B-scan ultrasound exam should be done to measure the height of each discrete tumor. Ultrasound is able to detect a tumor as small as 2 mm in diameter;[40] ultrasonography is almost as good as computed tomography (CT) in its ability to detect the presence of calcium within retinoblastoma tumors. If it shows the classic shadowing of intralesional calcium, a CT scan is not required. Retinoblastoma-simulating lesions causing ocular disruption or phthisis can also produce calcium, but their dystrophic calcifications are usually deposited along the lines of normal structures. If ultrasonography fails to demonstrate the presence of calcium, a CT scan should be performed. A CT scan is more sensitive for retinoblastoma than magnetic resonance imaging (MRI) because of its superiority in detecting calcification. Soft tissue components of retinoblastoma showed enhancement with contrast material in all cases.[41]

An MRI scan of the brain and orbits with gadolinium enhancement and fat suppression should be performed to distinguish retinoblastoma from similar-appearing lesions and to determine whether there is extraocular extension, infiltrative spread along the intracanalicular and cisternal portions of the optic nerve, subarachnoid seeding, involvement of the brain, or a synchronous midline tumor (trilateral retinoblastoma).[42] The use of fine-needle aspiration biopsy should be limited to those rare cases in which a diagnosis remains ambiguous after imaging studies and expert examination under anesthesia have been performed. The diagnostic accuracy of fine-needle aspirate in pediatric intraocular lesions is 95%.[43]

After imaging studies have been completed, an examination under anesthesia (EUA) of the anterior segment, iris, and vitreous cavity is performed. A hand-held slit-lamp evaluation of the anterior and posterior vitreous should be part of this examination, looking for the presence of vitreous seeding diffusely as well as locally over lesions. Intraocular pressure is important to document; an elevated tonometric pressure indicates a lesser chance for salvage of the eye. Retinal imaging is extremely useful in documenting the size and location of the tumors.

Evaluation for metastatic disease is only undertaken if clinical symptoms, examination, neuroimaging, or the pathology of an enucleated eye indicates that tumor has extended outside the globe. A complete metastatic evaluation includes lumbar puncture with examination of the cerebrospinal fluid, radionuclide bone scan, and bone marrow aspirate and biopsy.[44]

STAGING

The first staging system for retinoblastoma, published by Martin and Reese in 1942, established four categories of disease: unilateral tumors confined to the globe, bilateral tumors, recurrent or extraocular tumors, and metastatic tumors.[45] A more detailed staging system for intraocular disease (Table 68-1), published by Reese and Ellsworth in 1964, became the standard for decades.[46] The Reese-Ellsworth group classification system was designed to predict the likelihood of preserving vision following treatment with external beam radiation therapy (EBRT). Small anterior tumors are categorized as group III or group IV because they were not usually controlled by the lateral beam EBRT technique generally in use at that time; but they are quite responsive to modern EBRT techniques, cryotherapy, or a radioactive plaque. Any eye with vitreous seeding is categorized in group Vb (very unfavorable), although local vitreous seeding can often be successfully

Table 68-1 Reese-Ellsworth Classification for Conservative Treatment of Retinoblastoma

GROUP I VERY FAVORABLE
Solitary tumor, <4DD, at or behind the equator
Multiple tumors, none >4DD, all at or behind the equator
GROUP II FAVORABLE
Solitary tumor, 4-10DD, at or behind the equator
Multiple tumors, 4-10DD, behind the equator
GROUP III DOUBTFUL
Any lesion anterior to the equator
Solitary tumors, >10DD, behind the equator
GROUP IV UNFAVORABLE
Multiple tumors, some >10DD
Any lesion extending anteriorly to the ora serrata
GROUP V VERY UNFAVORABLE
Massive tumors involving more than half the retina
Vitreous seeding

DD, disk diameter.

treated with a radioactive plaque. The classification does not take into account retinal detachment or subretinal tumor seeding. Each is prognostic for vision preservation.

The International (or ABC) Classification for Intraocular Retinoblastoma (Table 68-2) was proposed by Murphree and Hungerford in 1994 to replace the Reese-Ellsworth system and has been adopted by the Children's Oncology Group. It is based on the natural history of retinoblastoma and on the likelihood of retaining vision in the affected eye when systemic chemotherapy is used as the primary treatment. Group A tumors are confined to the retina, small, and away from critical visual structures (optic nerve and fovea, the central portion of the retina). Group A eyes are virtually all preserved with excellent visual acuity. Group B tumors are also confined to the retina, but they are larger or located close to the fovea or optic nerve. Ninety-five percent of group B eyes are preserved, but visual acuity varies from 20/20 to 20/200 depending on tumor location. Group C and group D tumors have spread into the vitreous or subretinal space, locally for group C and diffusely for group D. Approximately 70% to 80% of group C and 50% to 70% of group D eyes are preserved. Group E eyes have been destroyed by the tumor, and only approximately 2% are salvaged. Staging systems that are prognostic for survival in patients with extraocular disease have been published.[47,48] Both schemes classify intraocular disease as stage I, orbital disease as stage II, intracranial metastasis as stage III, and hematogenous metastasis as stage IV.

Retinoblastoma itself causes few deaths in the developed world, because it is usually diagnosed prior to metastasizing and can be controlled locally. Although most deaths during the first 4 years after diagnosis are caused by metastatic disease, second malignant neoplasms in patients with heritable disease become the predominant cause of death beyond 5 years after diagnosis.[49] Patients with heritable retinoblastoma are no more likely to develop metastases than patients with the sporadic form of disease.[50] The 5-year cumulative survival rate was 91% in SEER (Surveillance, Epidemiology, and End Results) data from 1974 to 1985[5] and 87% to 97% in three modern, single-institution series,[40,100,109] a marked improvement from the 30% rate recorded in the 1930s.

Table 68-2 International (ABC) Classification for Intraocular Retinoblastoma

GROUP A SMALL INTRARETINAL TUMORS AWAY FROM FOVEOLA AND DISC
Small tumors confined to the retina
No tumor with greatest dimension >3 mm
No tumor <2DD (3mm) from fovea or 1DD (1.5 mm) from optic nerve
No vitreous seeding
No retinal detachment
GROUP B ALL REMAINING DISCRETE TUMORS CONFINED TO THE RETINA
Tumors confined to the retina not in group A
No subretinal or vitreous seeding
No subretinal fluid beyond 3 mm from the tumor
No retinal detachment >5 mm from tumor base
GROUP C DISCRETE LOCAL DISEASE WITH MINIMAL SUBRETINAL OR VITREOUS SEEDING
Local subretinal seeding <2DD (3 mm) from the tumor
Local fine vitreous seeding close to discrete tumor
No tumor masses, clump, or snowballs in vitreous or in the subretinal space
No retinal detachment >5 mm from tumor base
GROUP D DIFFUSE DISEASE WITH SIGNIFICANT VITREOUS OR SUBRETINAL SEEDING
Massive vitreous or subretinal seeding
Snowballs or tumor masses in the vitreous or subretinal space
Subretinal fluid involving up to total retinal detachment
GROUP E PRESENCE OF ANY ONE OR MORE OF THESE POOR PROGNOSIS FEATURES
Tumor touching the lens
Tumor anterior to anterior vitreous face involving ciliary body or anterior segment
Diffuse infiltrating retinoblastoma
Neovascular glaucoma
Opaque media from hemorrhage
Tumor necrosis with aseptic orbital cellulites
Phthisis bulbi

DD, disc diameter.

TREATMENT

Retinoblastoma therapy is undertaken with the goal of curing the patient while, if possible, preserving vision and minimizing adverse treatment effects. The probability of vision preservation is strongly associated with early detection and treatment. Because there are several effective treatments for nonmetastatic disease, the selection of chemotherapy, cryotherapy, radioactive plaque, and EBRT is based on need and their potential long-term complications. Enucleation is reserved for recurrent disease and eyes in which there is little chance for salvage of useful vision.

Enucleation

The first treatment described for retinoblastoma was enucleation in 1809.[1] Most retinoblastoma patients underwent enucleation of at least one eye in the 19th through mid-20th centuries. Salvage of the eye using radiation therapy (RT), cryotherapy, laser photocoagulation, thermotherapy, and chemotherapy has become increasingly more common over the past few decades.[51,52]

Enucleation is currently indicated in patients with unilateral disease and extensive vitreous or subretinal seeding in the affected eye (international classification group D or group E). In patients with bilateral groups A to D disease, enucleation is generally reserved for disease that cannot be controlled by chemotherapy and local treatment. Often, both eyes can be salvaged. If group E disease is present in one eye and group A disease in the other, after the group E eye is enucleated the group A eye is given local therapy. If group E disease is present in one eye and groups B, C, and D disease in the other, after the group E eye is enucleated the group B to D eye is given chemotherapy. Generally, enucleation should be done as soon as feasible to minimize the risk of tumor metastasis. However, if invasion of the group E tumor into the optic nerve is evident on MRI scan, enucleation of the group E eye should be delayed until after at least three cycles of chemotherapy. We have found no increased risk of perioperative complication in patients so treated. If there is nearly equally advanced disease in both eyes, it is reasonable to delay enucleation until the response to primary chemotherapy is evaluated in each eye. The eye that responds better to treatment is then salvaged. Although pathologic risk factors in the enucleation specimen may be obscured by pretreatment with chemotherapy, with this approach the child has already received the chemotherapy regimen that would be given if high-risk pathologic features were found on initial enucleation.

Enucleation involves careful removal of the intact eye after severing the rectus muscles without perforating or compressing the globe. A long segment of optic nerve, typically at least 10 to 15 mm, is removed together with the globe. Removal of less than 5 mm of optic nerve is associated with decreased survival.[53-55] An orbital implant is placed prior to surgical closure. Normal orbital growth is expected if a conically shaped implant as large as the orbit can accommodate is used.[56] Failure to replace the eye with a large orbital implant and failure to maintain the ocular prosthesis in position will result in orbital growth deficiency.[57,58] If the child has unilateral retinoblastoma, samples of fresh-frozen tumor and blood should be sent for *RB* gene testing. The tumor sample is necessary to determine whether the patient has heritable retinoblastoma, because the *RB* mutation will be evident in the blood of only 15% of these patients. The procedures of enucleation, implant placement, and tumor harvesting are described in detail elsewhere.[59]

The survival rate after enucleation alone was 86% for unilateral disease and 97% for bilateral disease confined to the globes.[60] The generally recognized risk period for extraocular recurrence of disease after enucleation is 12 to 18 months. In patients with heritable disease diagnosed before 12 months of age, an MRI of the brain should be obtained every 6 months until the patient has reached 3 years of age to screen for development of a midline PNET (trilateral retinoblastoma). Long-term complications of enucleation include extrusion of the implant because of inadequate surgical closure or conjunctival cysts and orbital growth deficiency associated with an insufficiently large implant or migration of the implant.

Chemotherapy

Chemotherapy is used for retinoblastoma in three basic situations: to produce regression of metastatic disease, to prevent recurrence or metastasis of locally advanced disease, or to locally contral intraocular disease.[61]

Metastatic Disease

Chemotherapy given in standard doses has been shown to produce short-term regression of metastatic disease but with a very low probability of cure.[62] The results of high-dose chemotherapy with autologous stem cell rescue are more promising among patients without central nervous system (CNS) involvement. A 67% 3-year relapse-free survival among 25 patients with high-risk or recurrent disease was reported. Seven of the eight relapses occurred in the CNS, indicating the need for agents with better CNS activity.[63] Intrathecal chemotherapy has not been effective.[64] The Children's Oncology Group is adopting high-dose chemotherapy with autologous stem cell rescue and consolidative EBRT for its current protocol for metastatic retinoblastoma based on several pilot studies.[63,65-67]

ENUCLEATED DISEASE AT ELEVATED RISK FOR DISTANT METASTASIS

Extensive research has addressed whether there are histopathologic features in the enucleated specimen prognostic for the development of metastatic disease. Tumors involving the cut end of the optic nerve of the sclera are generally treated with chemotherapy alone or followed by local EBRT. It is controversial whether tumor invasion along the optic nerve beyond the lamina cribrosa (the point of insertion of the meninges) without associated massive invasion of the choroid is a risk factor for metastasis, or whether adjuvant chemotherapy is indicated only if both postlaminar and choroidal invasion are present. Centers also differ on whether scleral involvement is an indication for chemotherapy. Patients with tumors involving only the choroid or the prelaminar portion of the optic nerve are not at elevated risk for metastasis.[68,69]

A retrospective review of patients observed or given 6 cycles of postenucleation chemotherapy (carboplatin, etoposide, and vincristine *or* cyclophosphamide, doxorubicin, and vincristine) found that the only factor associated with metastasis on multivariate analysis was optic nerve invasion. Among patients with massive choroidal or postlaminar optic nerve infiltration, 24% of those observed and 2% of those given chemotherapy developed metastases ($P = .02$).[70]

The value of adjuvant chemotherapy for patients who have undergone enucleation with high-risk features has not been demonstrated in a randomized trial. The only reported trial, conducted jointly by the Pediatric Oncology Group and Children's Cancer Study Group, was terminated in 1980 due to slow accrual and low incidence of disease recurrence. Of 54 patients with Reese-Ellsworth Group V unilateral retinoblastoma, recurrence was noted in only 11% of those randomized to observation and 7% of those randomized to chemotherapy following enucleation.[71]

Intraocular Disease

Chemotherapy largely replaced EBRT as a primary treatment for intraocular disease during the 1990s. This change was driven by the desire to avoid the long-term adverse effects of external beam irradiation. In London starting in 1989, eight cycles of carboplatin, etoposide, and vincristine (CEV) were given at 21-day intervals prior to 40 to 44 Gy of EBRT in an attempt to increase the probability of controlling locally advanced disease with vitreous seeding.[72] The observation that large tumors usually responded rapidly to chemotherapy soon led to the substitution of focal therapies for external beam irradiation. Chemotherapy was used to reduce large tumors to a size suitable for eradication by focal laser, cryotherapy, or both. Regardless of their response to chemotherapy, tumors will almost invariably recur if not treated with a focal therapy.

The Toronto group reported on 40 eyes in 31 patients with bilateral retinoblastoma treated primarily with chemotherapy and focal therapies between 1991 and 1996. After two chemotherapy cycles, residual potentially active tumors were treated focally by laser or cryotherapy. External beam irradiation was reserved for progressive disease not amenable to focal therapy. The actuarial relapse-free survival at a median follow-up of 2.7 years was 85% for all eyes. Relapse-free survival was 91% in the 28 newly diagnosed eyes compared to 70% in the 12 previously treated eyes. Only 5 of 40 eyes (13%) required RT or enucleation for tumor control.[73]

The Philadelphia group reported on 49 eyes, 45 with Reese-Ellsworth group V disease, in 30 patients treated in 1994 or 1995 with two cycles of CEV. Two weeks after the completion of chemotherapy, 54% of patients had complete responses and the remainder responded partially. Complete responders received no additional therapy, whereas the partial responders received focal therapy or external beam irradiation. The inadequacy of the two-cycle regimen is indicated by the finding of persistent or recurrent disease in 70% of patients on repeat examination 6 weeks after the completion of chemotherapy.[74] The number of CEV cycles was increased to 6 in 1995. Among 75 eyes in 47 patients followed for a median of 13 months, event-free survival was 74%. Focal therapy was given to 51 eyes (89%). Eighteen eyes (24%) required EBRT or enucleation. Of the 13 irradiated eyes, 7 were salvaged and the other 6 required enucleation for disease progression. Event-free survival was 100% for Reese-Ellsworth group I to III disease, approximately 80% for group IV disease, and approximately 25% for group V disease. No serious adverse effects were noted.[75] All these patients would have undergone EBRT or enucleation, or both, had chemotherapy not been given. The 5-year actuarial probability of receiving EBRT was 10% for 83 eyes with Reese-Ellsworth group I to IV disease and 47% for 75 eyes with group V disease. The 5-year actuarial probability of enucleation was 4% for 51 eyes with Reese-Ellsworth group I to III disease, 26% for 32 eyes with group IV disease, and 53% for 75 eyes with group V disease. Overall, 50% of patients underwent EBRT and/or enucleation. Among 128 eyes in 73 patients with bilateral disease, the 5-year actuarial probability of undergoing external beam irradiation was 28% and of being irradiated, enucleated, or both was 45%.[76] Independent prognostic factors for complete response to chemotherapy in 42 eyes treated in London were age older than 2 months, macular location, and sporadic presentation.[77] Several other centers have reported sizable series demonstrating the control of intraocular disease by chemotherapy combined with focal therapy, generally with better results in Reese-Ellsworth group I to III than group IV to V disease.[78-83]

Intraocular injection of carboplatin facilitates intensive exposure of tumor to the drug without systemic side effects.[84] A recent dose-escalation study at Children's Hospital Los Angeles found that 6 cycles of CEV with subtenon carboplatin and focal therapies controlled 2 of 3 (66%) International Classification group C, 11 or 19 (58%) group D, and 0 of 3 group E eyes with a median follow-up of 24 months. Three of the group D and two of the group E eyes with recurrent disease were salvaged by EBRT.

The most serious complication associated with chemotherapy in retinoblastoma patients is the development of acute myelogenous leukemia (AML). Twelve cases of AML have been identified in children following retinoblastoma, nine of them fatal. The current Children's Oncology Group protocol uses 6 cycles of vincristine and carboplatin without etoposide for children with International Classification group B disease. Patients with group C or D disease receive 6 cycles of CEV chemotherapy at 28-day intervals with subtenon carboplatin given prior to CEV during cycles 2 through 4. Focal laser or cryotherapy under anesthesia is initiated with the third course of chemotherapy. An evaluation under anesthesia (EUA) is performed on day 0 or 1 of each chemotherapy cycle and every 3 weeks thereafter until no active tumor is seen on a minimum of three consecutive examinations. The frequency of EUA is then reduced to every 2 to 3 months until age 3 years. After age 3 years, an EUA or indirect ophthalmoscopy followed by B-scan ultrasonography is conducted every 6 months until age 5 years, then annually. Any focal regrowth or edge recurrence is usually seen within 2 to 6 months, but intraocular recurrence has been found as late as 6 years after the completion of chemotherapy. Locally residual or recurrent tumors are treated with cryotherapy, laser therapy, or a radioactive episcleral plaque.

Focal Therapies

Laser or Thermotherapy

International Classification group A tumors posterior to the equator are usually controlled by transpupillary laser thermotherapy applied directly to their surface during EUA as sole treatment. In New York 86 of 91 (95%) of tumors with a base diameter of 2 mm or less were controlled with laser alone.[85] Laser is used on groups B to D posterior pole tumors after their volume is reduced by chemotherapy to coagulate the blood supply to the residual tumor and to produce hyperthermia in the surrounding tissue.

Complications of focal laser consolidation include burns of the iris at the pupillary margin and focal lens opacities, both of which are rare in experienced hands. The most significant long-term complication is decreased vision from retinal pigment epithelium scar migration in lesions near the foveola that are consolidated focally.

Cryotherapy

Successful treatment of a small retinoblastoma tumor by cryotherapy was first reported in 1967.[86] A single cryotherapy treatment generally destroys tumors as large as 2.5 mm in diameter and 1 mm in thickness located at or anterior to the equator and confined to the sensory retina. Tumors as large as 3.5 mm in diameter and 2.0 mm in thickness can be controlled using repeated cryotherapy treatments.[87] Cryotherapy is not the treatment of choice if vitreous seeding has occurred over a local lesion. Cryotherapy is not recommended for tumors posterior to the equator.

Episcleral Plaque Radiotherapy

Primary plaque RT may be the treatment of choice in isolated International Classification group B intraocular retinoblastoma located at or anterior to the equator. The use of plaques for posterior pole tumors is limited by permanent visual loss caused by a concentrated dose of radiation to the retina and optic nerve. Plaque therapy is appropriate for treatment of one or two moderate-sized tumors not adjacent to the optic disc or macula. Salvage plaque RT can control tumors that are residual or recurrent after chemotherapy, EBRT, laser therapy, and/or cryotherapy. Plaques direct the radiation focally to a retinoblastoma tumor, minimizing late radiation side effects on normal tissues. Advantages of plaque RT compared to EBRT are greater dose intensity of radiation to the tumor, shorter duration of treatment, and better localization of dose, resulting in fewer cataracts and minimal risk of bone hypoplasia and second malignancy induction.

The focal irradiation of retinoblastoma was first reported in 1929 and used radon seed implants.[88] A radium applicator for retinoblastoma was described in 1948.[89] It was superseded by the cobalt-60 (^{60}Co) plaque. ^{60}Co has been replaced by lower-energy isotopes that give markedly less radiation to the patient's normal periorbital tissues. Iodine-125 (^{125}I) emits energies of 27 to 35 keV and has a half-life of 60 days. Iridium-192 (^{192}Ir) emits energies of 295 to 612 keV and has a half-life of 74.5 days. Ruthenium-109 (^{109}Ru) is a beta emitter. ^{125}I and ^{109}Ru are of sufficiently low energy that the metal plaque containing them provides an effective shield against significant irradiation of the patient's periorbital bone and soft tissues and personnel caring for the patient.

The largest plaque experience in the treatment of retinoblastoma has been with ^{125}I, first reported in 1987.[90] The ^{125}I seeds are secured in a concave-shaped gold carrier. The conformality of the ^{125}I radiation dose distribution was improved in the 1990s by deepening the wells into which the ^{125}I seeds are inserted.[91] The wells in the plaque are differentially loaded to produce the dose distribution that best conforms to the shape, size, and location of the tumor. The number, strength, and position of seeds glued into wells are based on MRI, ultrasound, and photographic imaging of the eye. ^{125}I plaques may be used to treat tumors up to 10 mm in height and 16 mm in basal diameter. The tumor must be located at least 2 mm from the optic nerve, or the posterior edge of the plaque must be trimmed to shield the nerve, to avoid severe loss of vision.

Unlike ^{125}I, the ^{109}Ru plaque cannot be customized, because the isotope is an integral part of the plaque. The only choice with ^{109}Ru is the size of the plaque. Because ruthenium is a low-energy beta emitter, its use is restricted to lesions less than 6 mm high.[92] For small lesions, this low energy carries the advantage of less radiation dose to normal tissues and less shielding required than with ^{125}I. A second advantage of ^{109}Ru is that its long half-life allows the same plaque to be used continuously for up to 1 year.

Placement of the episcleral plaque is directed by the radiation dosimetry plan generated prior to the procedure and confirmation of the tumor anatomy by the surgeon at the beginning of the procedure. A margin of 1 to 2 mm surrounding the tumor base is incorporated into the treatment plan. The dosimetry plan indicates the position in clock hours of the center of the anterior edge of the plaque, the location of the plaque eyelets, and the distance those points are located posterior to the limbus. The center and edges of the lesion to be treated are identified by scleral indentation and marked with a surgical marking pen. A cold or dummy nonradioactive plaque identical in size and shape to the radioactive plaque is then secured with temporary nonabsorbable sutures and its location verified by scleral depression along the edges. After the correct position of the plaque is verified, the cold plaque is replaced by the radioactive plaque. The conjunctiva is closed with interrupted absorbable sutures. For ^{125}I plaques, a one-quarter-inch-thick sheet of lead is taped over the plaque for protection of the patient's caretakers. The lead shield is not necessary for ^{109}Ru plaques because of their lower energy.

The radiation dose is prescribed to the apex of the tumor as measured by ultrasound. If overlying local vitreous seeds are present, the seeds are included in the tumor thickness measurement. The thickness of the tumor is defined as the distance from the interior surface of the sclera to the apex of the tumor. The sclera is assumed to be 1 mm thick. The dose rate to the prescription point is usually in the range of 40 to 80 cGy per hour. The total dose prescribed to the tumor apex in primary plaque therapy is typically 40 Gy. If plaque therapy is given during or shortly after CEV chemotherapy, the dose should be reduced to 20 to 30 Gy.[77]

The experience of treating 208 retinoblastoma tumors in 141 patients using plaque RT in Philadelphia between 1976 and 1999 has been reviewed. The mean tumor size was 4.1 mm in height and 7.7 mm in base diameter. The radioisotope was ^{125}I in 86%, ^{60}Co in 8%, ^{192}Ir in 3%, and ^{109}Ru in 3% of the tumors. Plaques delivered radiation for a median of 54 hours. Recurrences were detected at a median of 4 months after treatment. The tumor control rate was 88% among the 60 tumors for which a plaque was used as primary therapy and 80% among the 148 tumors for which a plaque was used as secondary treatment after failure of another modality. The 1-year actuarial control rate was 92% for 30 tumors treated after other focal modalities, 92% for 30 tumors treated after chemotherapy, 75% for 64 tumors treated after external beam irradiation, and 66% for 27 tumors treated after both external beam irradiation and chemotherapy. Tumor control was also significantly associated with the prescribed dose. The clinical factors associated with tumor recurrence were increasing patient age and the presence of vitreous or subretinal seeds. The 5-year actuarial rates for individual complications were nonproliferative retinopathy in 27%, proliferative retinopathy in 15%, maculopathy in 25%, papillopathy in 26%, cataract in 31%, and glaucoma in 11% of eyes. Most cataracts and glaucoma cases developed in eyes that had previously received external beam irradiation and may have occurred without the plaque therapy. No cases of scleral necrosis were observed.[93]

St. Jude reported on 26 solitary tumors less than 7 mm in height and 19 mm in diameter treated with an ^{125}I plaque. The plaque was given as initial treatment to 5 of the tumors and as salvage following chemotherapy, external beam irradiation, or both, to the remaining 21 tumors. The median dose to the tumor apex or 5 mm, whichever depth was greater, was 44 Gy given at a median rate of 42 cGy per hour. Twenty-five of the 26 (95%) tumors remained under control at a median of 13 months after treatment. The one tumor that progressed was successfully controlled by a second plaque procedure.[94]

External Beam Radiation Therapy

Role

Successful treatment of bilateral retinoblastoma by EBRT was first reported in 1903.[95] EBRT was the treatment of choice for patients with bilateral disease whose tumors were not amenable to focal therapy during most of the 20th century. Among patients with bilaterally advanced disease, the eye with less chance of vision preservation was usually enucleated, and the eye with less-advanced disease was attempted to be salvaged with EBRT. The Reese-Ellsworth Classification system was developed to predict the probability of vision preservation using EBRT. Enucleation could be reserved for salvage of radiation failures. Although the efficacy of EBRT against retinoblastoma was not in doubt, its long-term side effects, particularly cataract development, midfacial hypoplasia, and induction of often-fatal malignancies, were of grave concern. Other major complications reported after EBRT are retinopathy, optic neuropathy, choroidal or vitreous hemorrhage, glaucoma, keratitis, dry eye, glaucoma, conjunctivitis, retinal or vitreous detachment, neurocognitive deficits, and growth hormone deficiency. In the 1990s, chemotherapy in conjunction with focal therapies began to supersede EBRT as the primary treatment option for most patients with International Classification group B to D disease. EBRT is now mainly used as secondary therapy to salvage chemoreduction and focal therapy failures, prevent recurrence of tumors involving the cut end of the optic nerve, and palliate or consolidate systemic therapy of metastatic disease.[96] The rate of tumor response to EBRT is slower than to chemotherapy. The response to chemotherapy occurs mostly during the first month and is close to reaching its maximum within 2 months after the start of treatment. Following RT, decrease in tumor volume continues beyond 6 months after treatment. By 1 year after treatment, both modalities produce a mean decrease in tumor volume of 90% to 95%.[97] Most tumor recurrences after EBRT are observed within 2 years, but recurrences requiring enucleation have been observed as late as 7 years after treatment.[98-100]

The main outcome measure of EBRT for intraocular retinoblastoma is control of disease in the eye without the need for enucleation. Many eyes in which there is recurrence of tumor after EBRT are salvaged with the focal therapies described earlier in this article. Despite the requirement for salvage treatment in approximately 45% to 60% of eyes, the goal of vision preservation is achieved in 70% to 90% of cases.[23,98,101-105] Cause-specific survival following external beam irradiation is 90% to 100% in most series.[98,102,103,106]

EBRT alone or followed by focal therapy preserves 80% to 100% of group I to III eyes.[98,101,107-111] Classification of an eye as *unfavorable* (group IV) or *very unfavorable* (group V) in the Reese-Ellsworth system does not indicate that the eye is unlikely to be preserved using EBRT. In Miami, 20 of 24 (83%) of eyes irradiated for group V disease were conserved.[112] Of 63 group Vb eyes treated in New York, 49% were controlled by EBRT alone, 81% were preserved at 1 year, and 53% were still intact 10 years after EBRT.[113] In London, enucleation was avoided by EBRT alone or followed by focal salvage therapy in 8 of 12 (67%) group IV and 19 of 29 (66%) group V eyes.[107,108] In Memphis, 3 of 3 group IV and 11 of 14 (79%) group V eyes were preserved by EBRT alone or followed by focal salvage therapy.[109,110]

Disease that progresses diffusely after chemotherapy and focal therapies can frequently be controlled by EBRT. Twenty-two of 32 (69%) eyes that failed chemoreduction and focal therapy were salvaged by EBRT alone (47%) or with additional focal therapy (22%) in Los Angeles with a median follow-up of 38 months. The median radiation dose was 45 Gy given in 1.8 or 2.0 Gy fractions. Eyes that could not be controlled with salvage EBRT were enucleated. It appears that attempted salvage with EBRT does not place the patient's life at risk, because none of the patients developed metastatic disease.[114] Secondary treatment for locally progressive disease after chemotherapy and focal therapies should include the entire retina. The entire vitreum is included in the target volume for patients with any history of significant vitreous seeding.

Techniques

Numerous techniques of delivering EBRT have been used. The optimal target volume for EBRT is the entire retina, because new tumors develop in previously uninvolved areas of the retina in 20% to 50% of eyes treated with focal therapies.[105,115-117] Through the 1970s the standard treatment technique was a single lateral D-shaped field 3 to 4 cm in length and width for treatment of one eye with the addition of an opposing field for treatment of both eyes. The straight anterior border of the field was positioned at the bony rim of the orbit to treat the portion of the retina and vitreum situated posterior to the equator. To avoid divergence anteriorly through the lens of either eye, the anterior half of the beam was blocked or the beam was angled a few degrees posteriorly.[103,106,108] The field extended posteriorly to include the proximal 10 mm of the optic nerve. In patients with unilateral disease, a superior oblique lateral beam can be used to exit through the contralateral maxilla instead of the contralateral eye and frontal lobe.[99] The rationale for the lateral-beam approach was to limit the radiation dose to the brain posterior to the orbit and to the germinative epithelial cells in the equatorial bow (located one-third to one-half of the distance from the anterior to the posterior surface) of the lens. Unfortunately, a laterally directed radiation beam that avoids the posterior surface of the lens inevitably underdoses the anterior retina. The retinal surface extends 1 to 3 mm anterior to the bony canthus and the equator to within 1 to 2 mm of the posterior surface of the lens. Multiple institutions reported a high incidence of new retinal tumor development in the underdosed portion of the retina at or anterior to the equator following lateral beam irradiation.[23,99,102,119]

The emergence of improved surgical techniques for aspiration of a subcapsular cataract with implantation of an intraocular posterior chamber lens[120,121] has led several institutions to question the wisdom of sacrificing full dosing of the retina and vitreum to avoid irradiating the lens.[23,96,101,109,122] Those in favor of whole-eye irradiation reason that the prolonged period before impairment of sight by a cataract prevents disuse amblyopia from occurring in the growing child.

While exposing the lens to the fully prescribed dose, a single anterior beam can partially spare the temporal bone in addition to providing fairly homogeneous coverage of the entire retina and vitreum. This results in less midfacial hypoplasia than lateral beam treatment.[109] Replacement of ^{60}Co with an electron beam markedly diminished the dose delivered to the brain posterior to the orbit using the anterior technique. Techniques using three-dimensional CT-based treatment planning have been developed to better conform the radiation dose to the globe, decreasing the dose to the bony orbit and surrounding soft tissues compared to an electron beam. At Hahnemann University Hospital, unilateral disease was treated with four noncoplanar fields covering the entire retina and the proximal 5 to 8 mm of optic nerve. Bilateral disease was treated with two anterior-oblique beams covering each globe together with two opposing lateral beams.[122] The dose distributions of four treatment techniques, anterior electron, anterior and lateral photon, and four anterior oblique beam nonaxial conformal or intensity modulated (IM), were compared for five retinoblastoma patients. The IM plan resulted in the smallest volume receiving more than 25% of the prescribed dose, followed by the 3-dimensional conformal, electron, and anterior-lateral pair plans.[96]

At Children's Hospital Los Angeles, eight noncoplanar anterior-oblique beams using step-and-shoot IMRT are used to treat either the globe or the entire retina with sparing of the lens along with the proximal 10 mm of optic nerve. The planning target volume includes a 3-mm margin beyond the gross target. This technique has been used to treat either one or both eyes. For eyes with a history of vitreous seeding, the planning target volume encompassing the retina and vitreum with a 3-mm margin includes the posterior lens. The planning target volume excludes the entire lens in eyes with no history of vitreous seeding, limiting the cumulative dose to the equatorial bow of the lens to less than 10 Gy. Taping the eyelids together during the entire period the patient is sedated helps prevent pain and photophobia from occurring during or within weeks after the completion of EBRT as a result of corneal dryness and abrasion. To minimize eye dryness in patients in whom the lacrimal gland and goblet cells are irradiated, we insert a plug in the medial nasolacrimal duct during the first week of EBRT. The procedures for IMRT planning and delivery at Children's Hospital Los Angeles are described in detail elsewhere in other publications.[122,124]

Dose and Fractionation

Standard EBRT dose schemes for the primary treatment for intraocular retinoblastoma deliver between 36 and 50 Gy in daily fractions of 1.5 to 2.0 Gy. Common fractionation schemes are 40 Gy in 20 fractions of 2.0 Gy or 45 Gy in 25 fractions of 1.8 Gy given 5 days per week. The chance of complications, but not of tumor control, is increased by using a total dose more than 50 Gy in 2.0 Gy fractions or a fraction size more than 2.5 Gy.[111,125] Coucke and colleagues estimated that the risk of developing retinopathy is 5% after receiving 42 Gy compared to 30% after 57 Gy in 2-Gy fractions. They also found a higher rate of retinopathy among patients treated with fraction sizes more than 2.5 Gy per day.[126] Enucleation was required because of radiation complications in 8 of 38 (21%) eyes given between 50 and 60 Gy over 3.5 to 6 weeks at Stanford.[106]

Second Malignant Neoplasms

Patients with the heritable form of retinoblastoma and carrying the *RB* gene mutation are at significantly increased risk for developing a variety of other malignant tumors, as discussed earlier. Treatment with EBRT further increases their risk of developing a second malignant neoplasm (SMN). The largest series consists of 1729 patients treated in New York or Boston between 1914 and 1984. A 2005 update of the series had an average follow-up of 25 years for patients with heritable disease and 30 years for patients with nonheritable disease. The actuarial rate of SMN within 50 years after retinoblastoma diagnosis was 36% (260 SMNs) among all patients with heritable disease compared to 6% (17 SMNs) among patients with nonheritable retinoblastoma. There were 19-fold more SMNs in heritable-disease patients than in the general population, compared to 1.2 times the expected SMN rate in nonheritable-disease patients. Among the patients with heritable disease, the SMN risk at 50 years was 38% for those who had received EBRT, compared to 21% for those who had not been irradiated. The excess rate of SMN compared to the general population was 22-fold for irradiated heritable-disease patients and 6.9-fold for unirradiated heritable-disease patients. The excess risk exceeded 100-fold for bone and soft tissue sarcomas (STSs) and tumors of the eye, orbit, and nasal cavity. The risk was increased 10- to 100-fold for pineoblastoma, melanoma, and tumors of the CNS, buccal cavity, and uterus. Among the unirradiated heritable-disease patients, the risk for both bone and STSs was also increased more than 20-fold, indicating a genetic link of sarcomas with the *RB* gene.[127]

An association between radiation dose and risk of sarcoma has been reported by several institutions. The SMN risk was significantly elevated at sites that received more than 50 Gy for retinoblastoma at the Institut Gustave Roussy.[128] Among the patients treated in Boston or New York, the relative risk for sarcoma was 1.9 after 5 to 9.9 Gy, 3.7 after 10 to 29.9 Gy, 4.5 after 30 to 59.9 Gy, and 10.7 after 60 Gy or more, compared to patients receiving 0 to 4.9 Gy.[24] An excess risk for osteosarcoma was noted among survivors of childhood cancer in general following a radiation dose greater than 10 Gy.[128-130] These groups did not find a significantly elevated risk from doses less than 10 Gy.[129-131] SMN risk is also associated with the volume of tissue exposed to a high-radiation dose in retinoblastoma patients.[24,132,133] A common parameter of proton- and conformal photon–EBRT planning is therefore to minimize the volume of bone and soft tissue that receives a dose greater than 10 Gy.

Data from two large series indicate that the excess SMN risk from EBRT occurs only in patients irradiated before the age of 1 year.[134,135]

Electrophilic chemotherapeutic agents such as carboplatin are independently associated with the development of sarcoma in survivors of childhood malignancies.[129-131]

Orbital and Midface Hypoplasia

The bony walls of the orbit grow rapidly during the first year of life. The orbit attains nearly 80% of its adult size by the age of 3 years. However, bones of the upper midface continue to enlarge until puberty.[136] In patients treated with lateral-beam EBRT for unilateral disease, the irradiated orbit and midface do not grow as large as the untreated side. Growth reduction is also commonly noted after enucleation, despite the insertion of an ocular prosthesis or implant. The mean volume of 35 orbits was identical several years following either enucleation or 44 to 54 Gy EBRT in Jerusalem. A 14% asymmetry was measured by CT scan of patients with unilateral disease at a mean of 47 months after either treatment.[137] There was also no significant difference in orbital growth among 18 bilateral disease patients in whom one eye was enucleated and the other orbit was irradiated at St. Jude.[57]

In retinoblastoma patients, diminished facial bone growth has been reported after radiation doses greater than 30 Gy.[138,139] The incidence of hypoplasia significantly increases following doses more than 35 Gy.[134] All 25 patients treated at St. Jude with more than 26 Gy when they were younger than 12 months of age developed hypoplasia.[109]

Retinal Changes

Visual acuity following EBRT can be very good, even after treatment of tumors in the macula.[140] Rod function is not significantly impaired by a fractionated radiation dose of 50 Gy. At a median of 15 years following EBRT for bilateral retinoblastoma, 81 of 99 patients had a visual acuity greater than 20/50, 28% of whom used a corrective lens.[141]

Retinopathy is caused by an occlusive microangiopathy manifested by microaneurysms, retinal and vitreous hemorrhages, and macular edema. The incidence of retinopathy after EBRT is associated with both total radiation dose and dose per fraction. Exposure to CEV chemotherapy prior to or during EBRT also increases the risk for retinopathy. Retinopathy developed in 5 of 11 (45%) eyes treated with EBRT during chemotherapy and 9 of 22 (41%) eyes treated with EBRT following chemotherapy compared with in 5 of 23 (22%) eyes treated with EBRT alone or preceding chemotherapy in Los Angeles.[114] Because of the high rate of retinopathy observed after exposure to 40 to 45 Gy for salvage of progressive disease after chemoreduction and focal therapy, the EBRT dose was reduced to 36 Gy in 18 fractions at Children's Hospital Los Angeles in 1999. Significant retinopathy has occurred to date in only 1 of 14 eyes treated with 36 Gy for salvage using IMRT.

An Experimental Model

A transgenic mouse-retinoblastoma model of heritable retinoblastoma may provide guidance for advances in EBRT. In this model system, the dose required to control 50% of eyes (TCD_{50}) was 45 Gy using 2.0 Gy fractions, given once daily compared to only 33 Gy using 1.2 Gy fractions, given twice daily.[142] Six subconjunctival injections of carboplatin given prior to the hyperfractionated EBRT further decreased the TCD_{50} to 14 Gy.[143] Animal models will be helpful in determining the optimal use and future role of EBRT.

105. Bedford MA, Bedotto D, Mac Faul PD: Retinoblastoma: A study of 139 cases. Br J Ophthal 55:19-27, 1971.
106. Egbert PR, Donaldson SS, Moazed K, Rosenthal R: Visual results and ocular complications following radiotherapy for retinoblastoma. Arch Ophthalmol 96:1826-1830, 1978.
107. Hungerford JL, Toma NMG, Plowman PN, et al: External beam radiotherapy for retinoblastoma:I: whole eye technique. Br J Ophthalmol 79:109-111, 1995.
108. Toma NMG, Hungerford JL, Plowman PN, et al: External beam radiotherapy for retinoblastoma: II. Lens sparing technique. Br J Ophthalmol 79:112-117, 1995.
109. Fontanesi J, Pratt CB, Kun LE, et al: Treatment outcome and dose-response relationship in infants younger than 1 year treated for retinoblastoma with primary irradiation. Med Pediatr Oncol 26:297-304, 1996.
110. Fontanesi J, Pratt CB, Hustu HO, et al: Use of irradiation for therapy of retinoblastoma in children older than 1 year old: The St. Jude Children's Research Hospital experience and review of literature. Med Pediatr Oncol 24:321-326, 1995.
111. Pradhan DG, Sandrige AL, Mullaney P, et al: Radiation therapy for retinoblastoma: A retrospective review of 120 patients. Int J Radiat Oncol Biol Phys 39:3-13, 1997.
112. Scott IU, Murray TG, Feuer WJ, et al: External beam radiotherapy in retinoblastoma. Arch Ophthalmol 117:766-770, 1999.
113. Abramson DH, Beaverson KL, Chang ST: Outcome following initial external beam radiotherapy in patients with Reese-Ellsworth group Vb retinoblastoma. Arch Ophthalmol 122:1316-1323, 2004.
114. Lavey RS, Perry DJ, Atchaneeyasakul L, et al: Salvage of recurrent retinoblastoma with radiation and/or chemotherapy: Tumor control and complications. Int J Radiat Oncol Biol Phys 45:406, 1999.
115. Abramson DH, Greenfield DS, Ellsworth RM: Bilateral retinoblastoma. Correlations between age at diagnosis and time course for new intraocular tumors. Ophthalmic Paediatr Genet 13:1-7, 1991.
116. Messmer, EP, Saverwein W, Heinrich T, et al: New and recurrent tumor foci following local treatment as well as external beam radiation in eyes of patients with hereditary retinoblastoma. Graefes Arch Clin Exp Ophthalmol 228:426-431, 1990.
117. Rosengren B, Tengroth B: Retinoblastoma treated with a ^{60}CO applicator. Acta Radiol Ther Phys Biol 16:110-116, 1977.
118. Cassady JR, Sagerman RH, Tretter P, Ellsworth RM: Radiation therapy in retinoblastoma. Radiology 93:405-409, 1996.
119. Weiss DR, Cassady JR, Peterson R: Retinoblastoma: A modification in radiation therapy technique. Radiology 114:705-708, 1975.
120. Portellos M, Buckley EG: Cataract surgery and intraocular lens implantation in patients with retinoblastoma. Arch Ophthalmol 116:449-452, 1998.
121. Shinha R, Titiyal JS, Sharma N, Vajpayee RB: Management of radiotherapy-induced cataracts in eyes with retinoblastoma. J Cataract Refract Surg 30:1145-1146, 2004.
122. Lavey RS, Olch AJ: Retinoblastoma. *In* Mundt AJ, Roeske JC (eds): Intensity Modulated Radiation Therapy: A Clinical Perspective. Hamilton, Ontario, BC Decker, 2005. pp. 579-583.
123. Freire JE, Brady LW, Shields JA, Shields CL: Eye and orbit. *In* Perez CA, Brady LW, Halperin EC, Schmidt-Ullrich RK (eds): Principles and Practice of Radiation Oncology. Philadelphia: Lippincott Williams & Wilkins, 2004, pp. 876-896.
124. Olch A, Lavey RS: A normal tissue sparing technique for the treatment of retinoblastoma using non-coplanar intensity modulated photon beams. Radiology (S1):550, 2004.
125. Schmid C, Coucke P, Balmer A, et al: Retinoblastoma: A retrospective study of external beam radiation at CHUV-Lausanne. Schweiz Med Wochenschr 1225:45, 1992.
126. Coucke PA, Schmid C, Balmer A, et al: Hypofractionation in retinoblastoma: An increased risk of retinopathy. Radiother Oncol 28:157-161, 1993.
127. Kleinerman RA, Tucker MA, Tarone RE, et al: Risk of new cancers after radiotherapy in long-term survivors of retinoblastoma: An extended follow-up. J Clin Oncol 23:2272-2279, 2005.
128. De Vathaire F, Francois P, Hill C, et al: Role of radiotherapy and chemotherapy in the risk of second malignant neoplasms after cancer in childhood. Br J Cancer 59:792-796, May 1989.
129. Tucker MA, D'Angio GJ, Boice JD Jr, et al: Bone sarcomas linked to radiotherapy and chemotherapy in children. N Engl J Med 317:588-593, 1987.
130. Hawkins MM, Wilson LMK, Burton HS, et al: Radiotherapy, alkylating agents, and risk of bone cancer after childhood cancer. J Natl Cancer Inst 88:270-278, 1996.
131. Le Vu B, De Vathaire F, Shamsaldin A, et al: Radiation dose, chemotherapy and risk of osteosarcoma after solid tumors during childhood. Int J Cancer 77:370-377, 1998.
132. Wenzel CT, Halperin EC, Fisher SR: Second malignant neoplasms of the head and neck in survivors of retinoblastoma. Ear Nose Throat J 80:109-112, 2001.
133. Abramson DH, Ellsworth RM, Kitchin FD, Tung G: Second nonocular tumors in retinoblastoma survivors. Are they radiation-induced? Ophthalmology 91:1351, 1984.
134. Abramson DH, Frank CM: Second nonocular tumors in survivors of bilateral retinoblastoma. Ophthalmology 105:573-580, 1998.
135. Moll AC, Imhof SM, Schouten-Van Meeteren AY, et al: Second primary tumors in hereditary retinoblastoma: A register-based study, 1945-1997. Ophthalmology 108:1109-1114, 2001.
136. Farkas LG, Posnick JC, Hreczko TM, Pron GE: Growth patterns in the orbital region: A morphometric study. Cleft Palate Craniofac J 29: 315-318, 1992.
137. Peylan-Ramu N, Bin-Nun A, Skleir-Levy M, et al: Orbital growth retardation in retinoblastoma survivors: Work in progress. Med Pediatr Oncol 37:465-470, 2001.
138. Kaste SC, Chen G, Fontanesi J, et al: Orbital development in long-term survivors of retinoblastoma. J Clin Oncol 15:1183-1189, 1997.
139. Peylan-Ramu N, Bin-Nun A, Skleir-Levy M, et al: Orbital growth retardation in retinoblastoma survivors: Work in progress. Med Pediatr Oncol 37:465- 470, 2001.
140. Abramson DH, Melson MR, Servodidio C: Visual fields in retinoblastoma survivors. Arch Ophthalmol 122:1324-1330, 2004.
141. Messmer EP, Fritze H, Mohr C, et al: Long-term treatment effects in patients with bilateral retinoblastoma: Ocular and mid-facial findings. Graefes Arch Clin Exp Ophthalmol 229:309, 1991.
142. Hayden BC, Murray TG, Cicciarelli N, et al: Hyperfractionated external beam radiation therapy in the treatment of murine transgenic retinoblastoma. Arch Ophthalmol 120:353-359, 2002.
143. Sobrin L, Hayden BC, Murray TG, et al: External beam radiation "salvage" therapy in transgenic murine retinoblastoma. Arch Ophthalmol 122:251–257, 2004.

CHAPTER 69

NEUROBLASTOMA

Suzanne Wolden

Neuroblastoma comprises a range of tumors (neuroblastoma, ganglioneuroblastoma, and ganglioneuroma) that arise from primitive adrenergic neuroblasts of neural crest tissue, typically in very young children. The clinical behavior and, therefore, therapy for neuroblastoma varies tremendously depending on an array of clinical and biologic characteristics. Although some tumors regress spontaneously, others are highly malignant and often fatal.

Significant progress in therapy has been made during the past several decades owing to an increased understanding of tumor behavior and effective risk-group stratification. Patients with low- and intermediate-risk tumors now have high survival rates with minimal intervention, and those with high-risk disease have improving survival as a result of intensive multimodality therapy.

Neuroblastoma is a fascinating and multifaceted disease. The investigation of biologic features of neuroblastoma and subsequent translation of these findings into effective therapy may serve as a model for other diseases.

ETIOLOGY AND EPIDEMIOLOGY

Neuroblastoma accounts for 8% to 10% of all childhood cancers, with approximately 650 cases diagnosed annually in the United States.[1] It is the most common extracranial solid tumor in children and the most common malignancy of infants. The median age at diagnosis is 17 months, and the male-to-female ratio is 1.1:1. Forty percent of patients are diagnosed at younger than 1 year of age, 89% are younger than 5 years of age, and 98% are younger than 10 years of age.[2]

Most primary neuroblastoma tumors occur in an anatomic distribution that is consistent with the location of neural crest tissue because the tumor arises from primitive adrenergic neuroblasts of neural crest tissue. The adrenal gland is the most common primary tumor site, accounting for 35% of cases overall. However, children younger than 1 year of age have a tumor arising from the adrenal gland in only 25% of cases. Other common sites include the low thoracic and abdominal paraspinal ganglia (30%) and posterior mediastinum (19%). Ganglia in the pelvic and cervical regions account for 2% to 3% of tumors, and in 1%, a primary site is never known.[3]

PREVENTION AND EARLY DETECTION

Because neuroblastomas frequently produce high levels of catecholamines that can be detected in the urine, mass screening for the disease in infants has been studied in a number of countries. Extensive trials in numerous countries have shown that tumors detected by screening tend to be extremely favorable. Unfortunately, screening has not had an impact on survival or early detection of high-risk neuroblastoma.[4]

The development and subsequent regression of clusters of neuroblastoma is a normal embryologic event, and the development of clinically detectable neuroblastoma appears to be a consequence of disruption of this process. Microscopic neuroblastoma-like nodules can frequently be found at autopsy in infants who die of unrelated causes.[5] Furthermore, clusters of cells consistent with neuroblastoma occur uniformly in the adrenal glands of all fetuses, peaking between 17 and 20 weeks of gestation, and then spontaneously regress by birth or in early infancy.[6]

The cause of neuroblastoma is not known in most cases. Prenatal or postnatal exposure to drugs, chemicals, or radiation has never been proven to be associated with an increased incidence of the disease.[2] A small fraction of neuroblastomas are considered familial neuroblastoma and are associated with a germline mutation. At least 20% of patients with familial neuroblastoma have bilateral or multifocal disease and tend to present at an earlier age.[7]

BIOLOGIC CHARACTERISTICS/ MOLECULAR BIOLOGY

Specific molecular characteristics of neuroblastoma have been well described and have a significant influence on prognosis and selection of therapy. Two of the most notable alterations are deletion of the short arm of chromosome 1 (1p) and *MYCN* (also known as N-*myc*) amplification. The former is thought to result in the loss of a tumor suppressor gene on 1p, whereas *MYCN* is a proto-oncogene found on the distal short arm of chromosome 2. There is a strong correlation between these genetic events, and both are found more commonly in advanced disease and are associated with a significantly worse prognosis.[8] *MYCN* amplification occurs in 25% of primary neuroblastomas overall but in only 5% to 10% in patients with low-stage and stage IVS disease and 30% to 40% in patients with advanced disease.[9]

Chromosomal ploidy or DNA index (DI) is another significant marker of prognosis that is particularly useful in infants younger than 18 months of age. Near-diploid or pseudodiploid tumors have near-normal nuclear DNA content but often have structural chromosomal abnormalities, including *MYCN* amplification. Hyperdiploid or near-triploid tumors typically lack *MYCN* amplification and 1p deletion and are more likely to have a favorable outcome.[10]

PATHOLOGY AND PATHWAYS OF SPREAD

Neuroblastoma is one of many small, round, blue-cell tumors of childhood but can be distinguished by staining for neuron-specific enolase, synaptophysin, and neurofilament. Electron microscopy can also be used and typically reveals neurosecretory granules that contain catecholamines, microfilaments, and parallel arrays of microtubules within the neuropil.[11] The characteristic histologic appearance is that of small, uniform cells containing dense, hyperchromatic nuclei and scant cytoplasm with neuropil. Homer-Wright pseudorosettes representing neuroblasts surrounding areas of eosinophilic neuropil are seen in up to 50% of cases.

Histologic subtypes represent different points along the maturation pathway and include (in order of increasing differentiation) neuroblastoma, ganglioneuroblastoma, and ganglioneuroma. Ganglioneuromas are considered benign and consist of mature ganglion cells, neuropil, and Schwann cells. Ganglioneuroblastomas have pathologic characteristics of both neuroblastoma and ganglioneuroma and have an intermediate behavior as well.

Table 69-1 The Shimada Pathologic Classification System

Prognosis	Schwann Cell Stroma	Age (yr)	Pattern	MKI*
Favorable	Rich	All	No nodular	—
	Poor	1.5–5	Differentiated	<100
	Poor	<1.5	—	<200
Unfavorable	Rich	All	Nodular	—
	Poor	>5	—	—
	Poor	1.5–5	Undifferentiated	—
	Poor	1.5–5	Differentiated	>100
	Poor	<1.5	—	>200

*MKI, mitosis–karyorrhexis index

Data from Shimada H, Chatten J, Newton WA Jr, et al: Histopathologic prognostic factors in neuroblastic tumors: definition of subtypes of ganglioneuroblastoma and an age-linked classification of neuroblastomas. J Natl Cancer Inst 73:405, 1984.

The Shimada system is the most widely used classification scheme and is outlined in Table 69-1. It is divided into favorable and unfavorable prognostic groups based on age, amount of Schwann cell stroma, nodular versus diffuse histologic pattern, degree of differentiation, and mitotic–karyorrhectic index. Other systems, including the Joshi system, also use characteristics to define favorable and unfavorable groups.[12] The International Neuroblastoma Pathology Committee classifies tumors according to the degree of differentiation toward ganglion cells, amount of Schwann cell stroma present, whether the tumor is nodular, degree of calcification, and the mitotic–karyorrhectic index.[3]

Neuroblastoma commonly spreads via lymphatics to regional lymph nodes, often in the para-aortic chain, and less commonly, to the next echelon of lymphatics, such as the left supraclavicular fossa (Virchow's node) in patients with abdominal tumors. Hematogenous spread often occurs to bone marrow, bone, and liver. Neuroblastoma appears to have a proclivity for the bones of the skull and especially the posterior orbit, which can cause the clinical presentation of "raccoon eyes" from periorbital ecchymosis. Lung and brain metastases are rare at presentation. However, with improvements in systemic therapy, isolated parenchymal brain metastases are beginning to occur in high-risk patients after apparent disease remission and require craniospinal radiotherapy because of a high risk of leptomeningeal dissemination (unpublished data from Memorial Sloan-Kettering Cancer Center).

CLINICAL MANIFESTATIONS/PATIENT EVALUATION/STAGING

The clinical presentation for neuroblastoma is highly variable because of the wide variety of disease sites. Primary tumor location and extent of disease vary with age. Most children (57%) younger than 1 year of age have local/regional disease at the time of diagnosis, whereas most children (81%) older than 1 year of age have disseminated disease. Children with abdominal tumors may present with abdominal pain, distention, or gastrointestinal disturbances. Many with disseminated disease present with bone pain, weight loss, fever, or failure to thrive. Paraneoplastic syndromes, such as opsomyoclonus (myoclonic jerking and random eye movement) are rare, occurring in less than 4% of patients. The catecholamines secreted from most neuroblastomas are not likely to cause hypertension, flushing, or tachycardia.

A plain radiograph of the chest or abdomen may show a soft tissue mass representing the primary tumor, and calcifications are present in 85% of tumors. Staging of neuroblastoma requires numerous imaging modalities. The primary tumor and regional lymph nodes should be imaged with computerized tomography (CT) or magnetic resonance imaging (MRI).[13,14] These studies should also be used to assess for metastases in the liver as well as spinal extension and resectability of the primary tumor. They may also be used to clarify the extent of bone metastases in specific locations, such as the skull.

Bone metastases may be determined with ^{99m}technetium (Tc) bone scan, meta-iodobenzylguanidine (MIBG) scan, and/or fluorodeoxyglucose positron emission tomography (FDG PET) scan. For high-risk patients, it may be worthwhile to perform all three studies because different forms of imaging may be more useful than others for different patients. MIBG is a sensitive and specific method (close to 90%) to assess the primary tumor and metastatic disease. A ^{99m}Tc bone scan is typically used for detection of bone metastases, even if MIBG studies are used.[15,16] Studies regarding the utility of FDG PET for neuroblastoma are ongoing. Complete staging includes two bilateral posterior iliac crest bone marrow aspirates and biopsies. A single positive result is sufficient for the documentation of bone marrow involvement.[17]

Because excess catecholamines are produced in most cases, urine catecholamines and their metabolites, specifically norepinephrine, vanillylmandelic acid (VMA), 3-methoxy-4-hydroxyphenylglycol (MHPG), and/or homovanillic acid (HVA) are typically measured. Urinary catecholamines are often given as ratios to urinary creatinine.[18]

Previous staging systems including the Evans and D'Angio classification,[19] historically used by the Children's Cancer Group (CCG) and a system formerly used by the Pediatric Oncology Group[20,21] have been replaced by the International Neuroblastoma Staging System (INSS) as the standard staging system. The INSS system is outlined in Table 69-2. To interpret the literature, it is necessary to make comparisons between the INSS and the two other staging systems, as differences can be significant. INSS stage 1 is similar to stages I and A. Stage 4 is essentially the same as stages IV and D, and stage 4S is the same as IVS and D-S. The greatest differences are in the middle stages (II and III; B and C). In the INSS system, stage 2 is divided into 2A (incompletely excised tumor) and 2B (ipsilateral lymph node involvement). The INSS has also formalized definitions of response to treatment in an attempt to facilitate cross-study comparisons.[17]

Current protocols for neuroblastoma are based on risk stratification. The proposed risk groups based on clinical and biologic features are outlined in Table 69-3. Survival varies from approximately 85% to 99% for low-risk patients to 20% to 40% for high-risk patients. Disease stage and patient age at diagnosis, as well as biologic characteristics (*MYCN*, ploidy), have major prognostic significance. A new histopathologic classification, the International Neuroblastoma Pathology Classification, based on the original Shimada system, is likely to become the new international standard.

Table 69-2 International Neuroblastoma Staging System

STAGE 1: Localized tumor with complete gross excision, with or without microscopic residual disease; representative ipsilateral lymph nodes negative for tumor (nodes adherent to and removed with the primary tumor may be positive).
STAGE 2A: Localized tumor with incomplete gross excision; representative nonadherent lymph nodes negative for tumor microscopically.
STAGE 2B: Localized tumor with or without complete gross excision, with ipsilateral, nonadherent lymph nodes positive for tumor. Enlarged contralateral lymph nodes must be negative microscopically.
STAGE 3: Unresectable unilateral tumor infiltrating across the midline,* with or without regional lymph node involvement; or localized unilateral tumor with contralateral regional lymph node involvement; or midline tumor with bilateral extension by infiltration (unresectable) or by lymph node involvement.
STAGE 4: Any primary tumor with dissemination to distant lymph nodes, bone, bone marrow, liver, skin, and/or other organs (except as defined in stage 4S).
STAGE 4S: Localized primary tumor (as defined for stage 1, 2A, or 2B), with dissemination limited to skin, liver, and/or bone marrow† (limited to infants <1 year of age).

*The midline is defined as the vertebral column. Tumors originating on one side and crossing the midline must infiltrate to or beyond the opposite side of the vertebral column.

†Marrow involvement in stage 4S should be minimal, that is, <10% of total nucleated cells identified as malignant on bone marrow biopsy or on marrow aspirate. More extensive marrow involvement would be considered to be stage 4. The MIBG scan (if performed) should be negative in the marrow.

Data from Brodeur GM, Seeger RC, Barrett A, et al: International criteria for diagnosis, staging and response to treatment in patients with neuroblastoma. J Clin Oncol 6:1874-1881, 1988; and Brodeur GM, Pritchard J, Berthold F, et al: Revisions in the international criteria neuroblastoma diagnosis, staging and response to treatment. J Clin Oncol 11:1466-1477, 1993.

PRIMARY THERAPY

The therapeutic approach for neuroblastoma varies tremendously, depending on risk group stratification. The available treatment modalities include surgery, chemotherapy, radiation therapy, and a number of newer experimental treatments such as radioimmunotherapy. The following is a discussion of therapy for low, intermediate, and high-risk disease, with an emphasis on the role of radiotherapy. A basic treatment algorithm for each risk group is shown in Figure 69-1.

Low Risk

Patients with low-risk neuroblastoma (see Table 69-3) can often be cured with surgery alone, even when only a partial resection is obtained. Adjuvant radiotherapy was used in the past for incompletely resected tumors, but has been shown to be unnecessary. Chemotherapy and radiotherapy are now reserved for progressive or recurrent disease. The CCG recently reported on the outcome of Evans stage I-II neuroblastoma treated with surgery as primary therapy. Event-free survival (EFS) and overall survival (OS) for all stage I patients were 93% and 99%, respectively, and for stage II patients were 81% and 98%, respectively. Additional therapy (radiation, surgery, and/or chemotherapy) was needed in only 10% of stage I patients and 20% of stage II patients.[22] *MYCN* amplification is rare in low-risk neuroblastoma and has not been shown to convey a worse prognosis in this group.[23] In the current Central Oncology Group (COG) protocol for low-risk neuroblastoma (#P9641), a dose of 21 Gy is recommended for stage I and II patients who require radiotherapy.

Most patients with stage 4S neuroblastoma are in the low-risk category. In spite of having disseminated disease on presentation (as defined in Table 69-2), spontaneous regression occurs frequently, and OS is excellent.[24] However, infants with rapidly progressive disease can suffer fatal respiratory compromise or bowel ischemia caused by severe hepatomegaly. Low-dose radiotherapy should be immediately considered for such patients. Treatment can be given efficiently, because simulation and anesthesia are not necessary; the liver generally fills the entire abdomen and can be seen on a port film, and the babies are young enough to be immobilized in a papoose. The typical fractionation schedule in this setting is 1.5 Gy for 3 fractions, which usually leads to rapid relief of symptoms.

Table 69-3 Proposed Neuroblastoma Risk Groups Based on Clinical and Biologic Tumor Features

INSS Stage	Low Risk	Intermediate Risk	High Risk
1	All	None	None
2A, 2B	Age <1 yr Age 1–21 yr; MYCN nonAMP* Age 1–21 yr; MYCN AMP; FH†	None	Age 1–21 yr; MYCN AMP; UH
3	None	Age <1 yr; MYCN nonAMP Age 1–21 yr; MYCN nonAMP; FH	Age 0–21 yr; MYCN AMP Age 1–21 yr; MYCN nonAMP; UH
4	None	Age <1 yr; MYCN nonAMP	Age <1 yr; MYCN AMP Age 1–21 yr
4S	MYCN nonAMP; FH; DI>1‡	MYCN nonAMP; UH	MYCN AMP MYCN nonAMP; DI = 1

*AMP, amplified; MYCN, amplification status; nonAMP, nonamplified.
†Histopathologic classification: FH, favorable; UH, unfavorable
‡Ploidy status: DI > 1, hyperdiploid; DI, 1 = diploid
Data from Brodeur G, Maris J: Neuroblastoma. *In* Pizzo P, Poplack D (eds): Principles and Practice of Pediatric Oncology, 4th ed. Philadelphia: Lippincott Williams & Wilkins, 2002, pp 895-937.

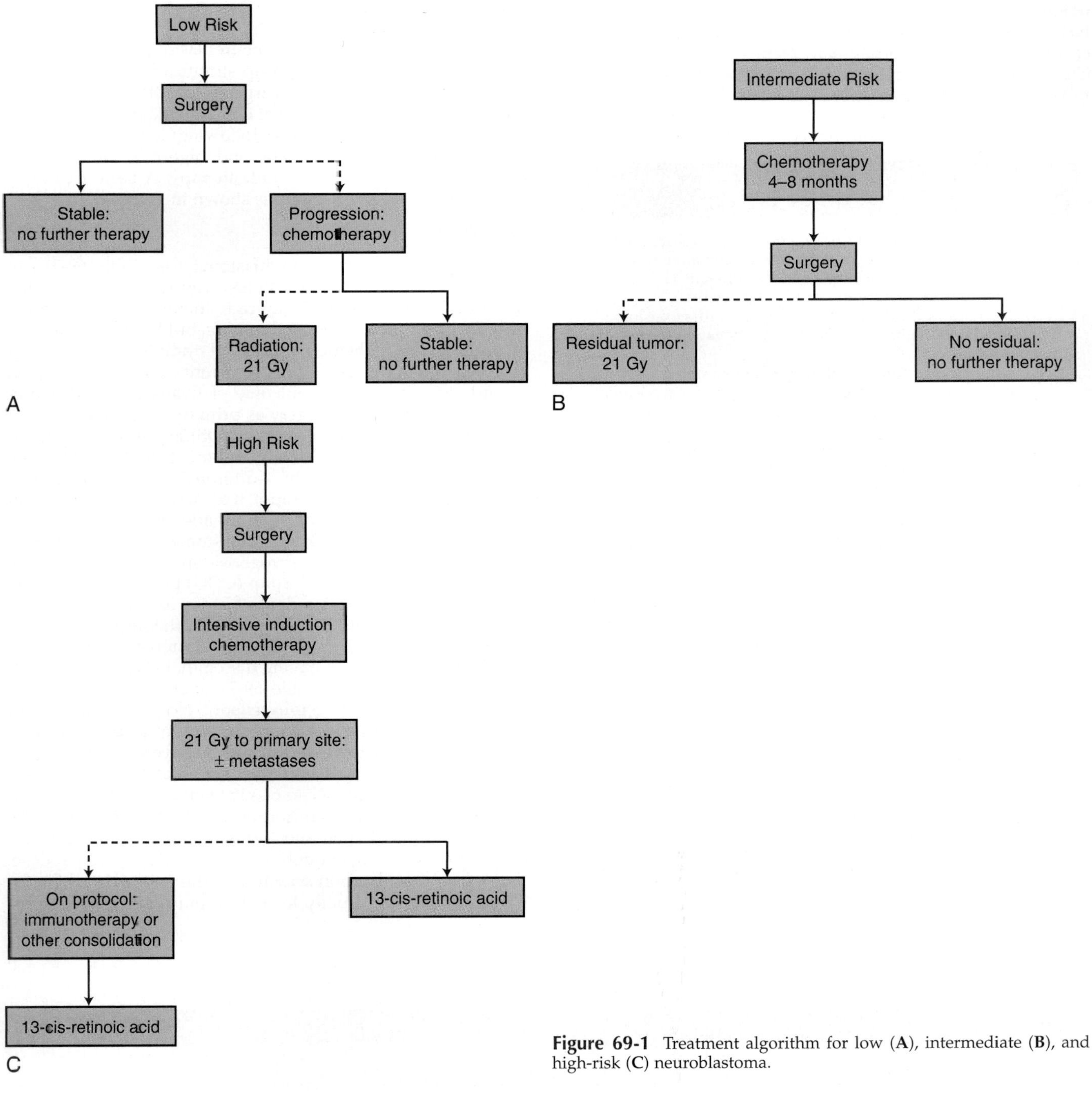

Figure 69-1 Treatment algorithm for low (**A**), intermediate (**B**), and high-risk (**C**) neuroblastoma.

The risk of long-term harm to the child from radiotherapy is very small because of the low dose.

Intermediate Risk

The current treatment approach for intermediate-risk patients (see Table 69-3) consists of surgery for the primary tumor as well as standard-dose, multi-agent chemotherapy for 4 to 8 months. An initial biopsy is always performed to obtain a diagnosis and to analyze biologic features. Definitive surgery may be delayed until after chemotherapy, which often makes the tumor more easily resectable. Survival for patients with intermediate risk disease has been reported to be 75% to 98%.

Older studies that addressed the use of radiation for intermediate risk patients have used a variety of outdated staging systems that make interpretation of the data very difficult. Analysis of CCG data for stage II disease showed a 6-year survival of 98% for those treated initially with surgery alone compared with 95% for those receiving radiation and/or chemotherapy.[25] Therefore, intermediate-risk stage 2 patients do not require radiation as part of their initial treatment.

For patients with stage 3 intermediate-risk neuroblastoma, the older literature supported the use of radiotherapy.[26] However, because of changes in the staging system with incorporation of biologic features as well as more sensitive diagnostic tools and more intensive chemotherapy, these findings may not be applicable to current management. Stage 3 patients with favorable biology who are treated with surgery and chemotherapy alone have excellent outcomes.

In the most recent COG study (#A3961), intermediate-risk patients undergo surgery as well as chemotherapy, consisting of cyclophosphamide, doxorubicin, carboplatin, and etoposide. The duration of chemotherapy is based on biologic risk factors for individual patients. Radiation therapy is indicated only for those with disease progression or persistent tumor after chemotherapy and second-look surgery.

High Risk

Although survival rates have improved for high-risk neuroblastoma with increasingly intensive therapy, considerable progress is still needed. Children older than 1 year of age with stage 4 disease who were enrolled in CCG studies from 1978 to 1985 had a 4-year survival of 9% compared to 30% for patients treated from 1991 to 1995.[27] The CCG completed a phase III trial that demonstrated that high-dose chemotherapy and radiation therapy followed by transplantation of autologous bone marrow is superior to conventional chemotherapy as consolidation in children with high-risk neuroblastoma with the 3-year EFS of 34% and 22%, respectively. In the same study, 3-year EFS for patients randomized to receive 13-*cis*-retinoic acid at the completion of cytotoxic therapy was 46% compared to 29% who received no further therapy.[28]

The current therapeutic approach for high-risk disease includes intensive induction chemotherapy, surgical resection of the primary tumor, and possible myeloablative consolidation therapy with stem cell rescue, followed by targeted therapy for residual disease. Patients who have a complete or very good partial response to induction chemotherapy enjoy a better prognosis.[29]

The COG currently recommends 21 Gy to the primary tumor site, regardless of the extent of surgical resection, as well as to sites of metastatic disease that display persistent MIBG avidity on the pretransplant scans. The ongoing N8 protocol for high-risk disease at Memorial Sloan-Kettering Cancer Center recommends the same dose of radiotherapy to sites of initial bulky metastases (>3 cm) in bone, lymph nodes, or other sites, even when the disease has resolved on post-therapy scans.

Evidence for the benefit of primary-site radiotherapy comes from single-institution trials such as those at Memorial Sloan-Kettering, where a total dose of 21 Gy is given in twice daily 1.5 Gy fractions. Among 99 patients treated with primary-site radiotherapy, the local failure rate was 10%.[30] Only seven of these patients had disease at the primary site at the time of irradiation and three of these had local recurrence, suggesting that 21 Gy is not an adequate dose for gross residual disease.

In spite of an improved outcome for patients with high-risk neuroblastoma who were treated with autologous transplantation, including 10 Gy total body irradiation (TBI), on the randomized CCG study 3891, local failure was a major component of unsuccessful treatment. The 5-year locoregional recurrence rate was 51% for patients who received continuation chemotherapy compared to 33% for patients who received transplantation. Patients with residual tumor at the primary site after chemotherapy and surgery received 10 Gy of local radiotherapy, whether or not they were randomized to receive TBI.[28]

Haas-Kogan and colleagues[31] examined the role of radiotherapy on local control in CCG 3891. It appears that both 10 Gy to the primary site as well as 10 Gy of TBI decreased the local recurrence rate. The largest benefit was seen when patients received both local radiotherapy and TBI, for a total dose of 20 Gy. Because radiotherapy was not randomized in this study, it is difficult to draw firm conclusions, yet these data, along with single-institution data, argue that primary-site radiotherapy improves outcomes in high-risk patients. Currently, the COG recommends 21.6 Gy in once-daily fractions of 1.8 Gy to the primary tumor site with myeloablative chemotherapy that does not include TBI. The ideal timing for radiotherapy is following myeloablative chemotherapy and resection, when the volume of disease is minimal. Although evidence suggests that 21 Gy is inadequate for gross residual disease, the optimal dose is not known, and studies to address this question are planned.

RECURRENT DISEASE AND PALLIATION

Current approaches for treating recurrent or refractory neuroblastoma include novel cytotoxic agents and targeted delivery of radionuclides, retinoids, and immunotherapy. Topotecan, paclitaxel, irinotecan, rebeccamycin, and oral etoposide are the most frequently investigated cytotoxic agents.[32–35] Radiotherapy plays an important role in palliation for neuroblastoma. Patients with incurable disease often live for an extended period of time. However, they often suffer severe pain and functional impairment from metastases, most commonly to bone. External beam radiotherapy is the most effective tool for managing painful metastases. Fractionation schemes depend on the site, field size, marrow reserves, and anticipated life span of the patient. A high-functioning child may benefit from 2 Gy fractions to 30 Gy whereas an end-stage patient may be better served by a single fraction of 7 Gy.

TECHNIQUES OF IRRADIATION

Radiation techniques depend on the site being treated. Most commonly, patients with high-risk disease have a primary tumor arising from the adrenal gland. Radiation volume for localized neuroblastoma is determined by the surgeon's operative findings and pre-surgical imaging studies. Margins and normal tissue-sparing parameters vary from protocol to protocol. Based on patterns of failure data, it is important to include the para-aortic lymph nodes in the radiation field.[36] CT planning is imperative to precisely delineate the target region as well as normal tissues, including the kidneys, liver, and, in some cases, ovaries. Treatment should encompass entire vertebral bodies to reduce the risk of scoliosis. Simple anterior and posterior beams, as demonstrated in Figure 69-2, are often the best solution, but intensity-modulated radiation therapy (IMRT) may be helpful if standard techniques do not provide adequate sparing of critical organs. Bone metastases are also often best treated with simple opposed beams. However, more sophisticated approaches, such as IMRT, may be needed when treating sites in the head and neck because of the complex anatomy and critical structures.

Neuroblastoma is common in very young children, necessitating the frequent use of anesthesia for radiation treatments. In this case, propofol is safe and well tolerated, even for twice-daily treatments.

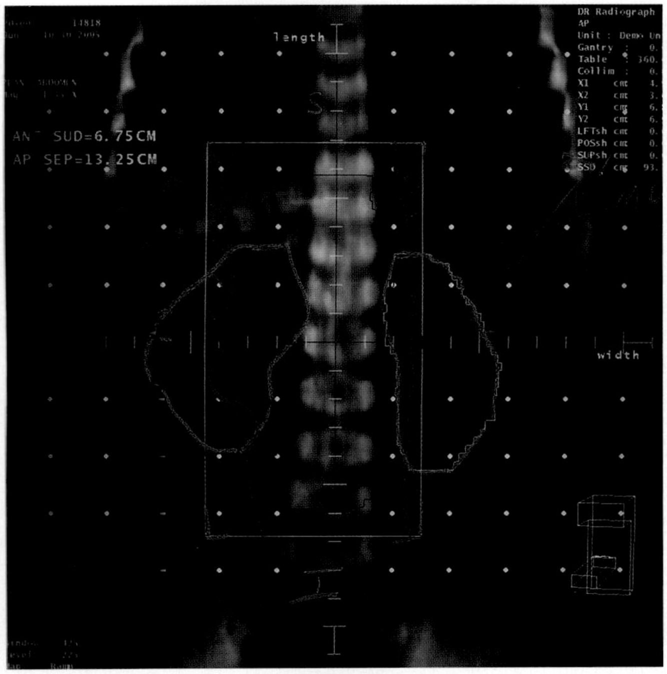

Figure 69-2 Typical anterior and posterior radiotherapy field for adrenal neuroblastoma. Generous coverage of para-aortic lymph nodes is recommended. Adequate kidney sparing is accomplished by treating post-chemotherapy tumor volume.

TREATMENT ALGORITHMS/CONTROVERSIES/PROBLEMS/CHALLENGES/FUTURE POSSIBILITIES/CLINICAL TRIALS

Intraoperative radiation therapy (IORT) has been studied as an alternative to external beam treatment. Haas-Kogan and colleagues[37] reported results for 23 patients, of whom 21 were high risk, and received IORT. Electron-beam energies ranged from 4 MeV to 16 MeV, and the median dose was 10 Gy (range 7–16 Gy). A gross total resection (GTR) was achieved in 18 patients, and of these, six experienced disease recurrence; two were locoregional recurrences. IORT was given to the 18 patients who had a GTR, and 14 of them were disease-free at the time of publication. Five patients had subtotal resections (STR), and all five recurred locally and died of their disease. IORT was well tolerated with a low risk of complications. The authors concluded that IORT for the primary tumor produced excellent local control after a GTR but was inadequate after an STR. IORT has also been used for re-irradiation of recurrent disease after previous external beam radiotherapy, again with positive results.[38]

I^{131} MIBG therapy is one example of targeted radiation. I^{131} MIBG is bound at the cell membrane and is actively transported into cells by most neuroblastoma tumors. Therapeutic use of I^{131} MIBG has been used in patients with unresectable disease with excellent results. Trials combining I^{131}MIBG with chemotherapy, surgery, and radiation therapy are currently in progress. In addition to 13-*cis*-retinoic acid, new retinoids are being developed to treat recurrent or refractory disease. Fenretinide is one such compound that induces apoptosis even in cells resistant to 13-*cis*-retinoic acid.[39] Immunotherapy, including anti-GD2 murine monoclonal antibodies (3F8 and GD2a), and the human-mouse chimeric monoclonal antibody ch14.18, are currently under investigation for their roles in recurrent and refractory disease as well as consolidation of initial therapy.[40,41]

Consideration for long-term complications is critical when treating neuroblastoma. Patients treated years ago with higher doses of radiotherapy frequently suffered from spinal deformities secondary to surgery and radiation.[42] Major orthopedic problems from radiotherapy still occur but are infrequent with a dose of 21 Gy. Symmetric treatment of vertebral bodies is recommended.

It is possible that the kidneys of infants and young children are more sensitive to radiotherapy than are those of adults and older children. Abnormal creatine clearance has been reported in infants with stage IVS disease who received 12.25 and 14 Gy.[43] As a general rule, it is desirable to limit as much of each kidney as possible to doses less than 15 to 18 Gy to prevent major impairment in renal function. One must also inform parents about the low risk of second malignancies.[44] A recent study of long-term survivors of high-risk neuroblastoma shows that the majority have late complications of therapy including hearing loss, hypothyroidism, ovarian failure, musculoskeletal abnormalities, and pulmonary dysfunction. However, most complications were considered to be of mild-to-moderate severity.[45] All members of multimodality teams that care for neuroblastoma patients must be mindful of late-effects and strive to minimize complications while ensuring the best chance for cure.

REFERENCES

1. Smith M, Ries L, Gurney J: Cancer incidence and survival among children and adolescents: United States SEER program 1975–1995. Bethesda, MD: National Cancer Institute, SEER program, 1999.
2. Brodeur G, Maris J: Neuroblastoma. *In* Pizzo P, Poplack D (eds): Principles and Practice of Pediatric Oncology, 4th ed. Philadelphia: Lippincott Williams and Wilkins, 2002, pp 895-937.
3. Halperin E, Constine L, Tarbell N, Kun L: Neuroblastoma. *In* Pediatric Radiation Oncology, 3rd ed. Philadelphia: Lippincott Williams and Wilkins, 1999, pp 163-203.
4. Schilling FH, Spix C, Berthold F, et al: Neuroblastoma screening at one year of age. N Engl J Med 346:1047-1053, 2002.
5. Beckwith J, Perrin E: In situ neuroblastomas: a contribution to the natural history of neural crest tumors. Am J Pathol 43:1089, 1963.
6. Ikeda Y, Lister J, Bouton JM, Buyukpamukcu M: Congenital neuroblastoma, neuroblastoma in situ, and the normal fetal development of the adrenal. J Pediatr Surg 16:636, 1981.
7. Kushner BH, Gilbert F, Helson L: Familial neuroblastoma: case reports, literature review, and etiologic considerations. Cancer 57:1887, 1986.
8. Fong CT, Dracopoli NC, White PS, et al: Loss of heterozygosity for the short arm of chromosome 1 in human neuroblastomas: correlation with N-myc amplification. Proc Natl Acad Sci U S A 86:3753, 1989.
9. Brodeur GM, Seeger RC, Schwab M, et al: Amplification of N-myc in untreated neuroblastomas correlates with advanced disease stage. Science 224:1121-1124, 1984.
10. Matthay KK: Neuroblastoma: biology and therapy. Oncology 11:1857-1866, 1997.
11. Delellis RA: The adrenal glands. *In* Sternbert SS (ed): Diagnostic Surgical Pathology, vol 1. New York: Raven Press, 1989, p 445.
12. Joshi V, Cantor A, Altshuler G, et al: Prognostic significance of histopathologic features of neuroblastoma: a grading system based on the review of 211 cases from the Pediatric Oncology Group (abstract). Proc Am Soc Clin Oncol 10:311, 1991.
13. Golding SJ, McElwain TJ, Husband JE: The role of computed tomography in the management of children with advanced neuroblastoma. Br J Radiol 57:661, 1984.
14. Fletcher BD, Kopiwoda SY, Strandjord SE, et al: Abdominal neuroblastoma: magnetic resonance imaging and tissue characterization. Radiology 155:699, 1985.
15. Heisel MA, Miller JH, Reid BS, et al: Radionuclide bone scan in neuroblastoma. Pediatrics 71:206, 1983.

16. Voute PA, Hoefnagel C, Marcuse HR, et al: Detection of neuroblastoma with [I-131]meta-iodobenzylguanidine. Prog Clin Biol Res 175:389-398, 1985.
17. Brodeur GM, Pritchard J, Berthold F, et al: Revisions in the international criteria neuroblastoma diagnosis, staging and response to treatment. J Clin Oncol 11:1466, 1993.
18. LaBrosse EH, Comay E, Bohuan C, et al. Catecholamine metabolism in neuroblastoma. J Natl Cancer Inst 57:633-643, 1976.
19. Evans AE, D'Angio G, Randolph J: A proposed staging for children with neuroblastoma. Children's Cancer Study Group A. Cancer 27:374, 1971.
20. Nitschke R, Smith EI, Shochat S, et al: Localized neuroblastoma treated by surgery. A Pediatric Oncology Group Study. J Clin Oncol. 6:1271, 1988.
21. Hayes FA, Green A, Hustu HO, et al: Surgicopathologic staging of neuroblastoma: prognostic significance of regional lymph node metastases. J Pediatr 102:59-62, 1983.
22. Perez CA, Matthay KK, Atkinson JB, et al: Biologic variables in the outcome of stages I and II neuroblastoma treated with surgery as primary therapy: a Children's Cancer Group study. J Clin Oncol 18:18-26, 2000.
23. Cohn SL, Look AT, Joshi VV, et al: Lack of correlation of N-myc gene amplification with prognosis in localized neuroblastoma: a Pediatric Oncology Group study. Cancer Res 55:721-726, 1995.
24. Nickerson HJ, Matthay KK, Seeger RC, et al: Favorable biology and outcome of stage IV-S neuroblastoma with supportive care or minimal therapy: a Children's Cancer Group Study. J Clin Oncol 18:477-486, 2000.
25. Matthay KK, Sather HN, Seeger RC, et al: Excellent outcome of stage II neuroblastoma is independent of residual disease and radiation therapy. J Clin Oncol 7:236-44, 1989.
26. Castleberry RP, Kun LE, Shuster JJ, et al: Radiotherapy improves the outlook for patients older than 1 year with Pediatric Oncology Group stage C neuroblastoma. J Clin Oncol 9:789-795, 1991.
27. Matthay KK, Lukens J, Stram D, et al: Improving survival from 1978-1995 using risk based treatment for neuroblastoma: Children's Cancer Group (CCG). Med Pediatr Oncol 27:220, 1996.
28. Matthay KK, Villablanca JG, Seeger RC, et al: Treatment of high-risk neuroblastoma with intensive chemotherapy, radiotherapy, autologous bone marrow transplantation, and 13-cis-retinoic acid. Children's Cancer Group. N Engl J Med 341:1165-1173, 1999.
29. Matthay KK, Castelberry RP: Treatment of advanced neuroblastoma: the U.S. experience. In Brodeur GM, Sawada T, Tsuchida Y, Voute PA (eds): Neuroblastoma. Amsterdam: Elsevier Science, 2000, pp 437-452.
30. Kushner BH, Wolden S, La Quaglia MP, et al: Hyperfractionated low-dose radiotherapy for high-risk neuroblastoma after intensive chemotherapy and surgery. J Clin Oncol 19:2821-2828, 2001.
31. Haas-Kogan DA, Swift PS, Selch M, et al: Impact of radiotherapy for high-risk neuroblastoma: a Children's Cancer Group study. Int J Radiat Oncol Biol Phys 56:28-39, 2003.
32. Saylors RL III, Stewart CF, Zamboni WC, et al: Phase I study of topotecan in combination with cyclophosphamide in pediatric patients with malignant solid tumors: a Pediatric Oncology Group Study. J Clin Oncol 16:945-952, 1989.
33. Furman WL, Stewart CF, Poquette CA, et al: Direct translation of a protracted irinotecan schedule from a xenograft model to a phase I trial in children. J Clin Oncol 17:1815-1824, 1999.
34. Weitman S, Moore R, Barrera H, et al: In vitro antitumor activity of rebeccamycin analog (NSC #655649) against pediatric solid tumors. J Pediatr Hematol Oncol 20:136-139, 1998.
35. Davidson A, Gowing R, Lowis S, et al: Phase II study of 21 day schedule oral etoposide in children. New Agents Group of the United Kingdom Children's Cancer Study Group (UKCCSG). Eur J Cancer 33:1816-1822, 1997.
36. Wolden SL, Gollamudi SV, Kushner BH, et al: Local control with multi-modality therapy for stage 4 neuroblastoma. Int J Radiat Oncol Biol Phys 46:969-974, 2000.
37. Haas-Kogan DA, Fisch BM, Wara WM, et al: Intraoperative radiation therapy for high-risk pediatric neuroblastoma. Int J Radiat Oncol Biol Phys 47:985-992, 2000.
38. Goodman KA, Wolden SL, LaQuaglia MP, et al: Intraoperative high-dose rate brachytherapy for pediatric solid tumors: a 10-year experience. Brachytherapy 2:139-146, 2003.
39. Matthay KK, DeSantes K, Hasegawa B, et al: Phase I dose escalation of I^{131} metaiodobenzylguanidine with autologous bone marrow support in refractory neuroblastoma. J Clin Oncol 16:229-236, 1998.
40. Yu AL, Batova A, Alvarada C, et al: Usefulness of a chimeric anti-GD2 (ch14.18) and GM-CSF for refractory neuroblastoma: a POG phase II study. Proc Am Soc Clin Oncol 16:513a, 1997.
41. Cheung NK, Kushner BH, Yeh SDJ, et al: 3F8 monoclonal antibody treatment of patients with stage 4 neuroblastoma: a phase II study. Int J Oncol 12:1299-1306, 1998.
42. Paulino AC, Mayr NA, Simon JH, et al: Locoregional control in infants with neuroblastoma: role of radiation therapy and late toxicity. Int J Radiat Oncol Biol Phys 52:1025-1031, 2002.
43. Peschel RE, Chen M, Seashore J: The treatment of massive hepatomegaly in stage IV-S neuroblastoma. Int J Radiat Oncol Biol Phys 7:549-553, 1981.
44. Kushner BH, Cheung NK, Kramer K, et al: Neuroblastoma and treatment-related myelodysplasia/leukemia: the Memorial Sloan-Kettering experience and a literature review. J Clin Oncol 16:3880-3889, 1998.
45. Laverdiere C, Cheung NK, Kushner BH, et al: Long-term complications in survivors of advanced stage neuroblastoma. Ped Blood and Cancer 45:324-332, 2005.

CHAPTER 70

PEDIATRIC LEUKEMIAS AND LYMPHOMAS

Karen J. Marcus

EPIDEMIOLOGY

Acute leukemias (ALL and AML) and lymphomas (Hodgkin's and non-Hodgkin's lymphomas) together represent approximately 40% of malignancies in children.

The annual incidence of new cases in the United States in children under 15 years is

ALL: 2500-3500
AML: 500
NHL: 500

BIOLOGY, CLASSIFICATION, AND STAGING

- ALL is classified by
  - immunophenotype: B-cell progenitor, T-cell progenitor, non-B, non-T
  - morphology, immunologic markers
  - cellular DNA content (ploidy)
  - cytogenetics (presence of specific translocations, trisomies, other chromosomal or genetic aberrations)
  - staging involves evaluation of bone marrow, cerebrospinal fluid, and evaluation of extramedullary sites.
- AML is classified according to the French-American-British morphology. Staging is as for ALL.
- NHL is classified by either the Revised European American Lymphoma (REAL) Classification or the World Health Organization (WHO) Classification of Tumors of the Haematopoietic and Lymphoid Tissues. The major subtypes are precursor B-cell lymphoblastic lymphoma, Burkitt's lymphoma, and diffuse large cell lymphoma. Large cell lymphomas can be of B-cell origin or T-cell origin and are subclassified as anaplastic or immunoblastic lymphoma.
  - Staging involves examination of bone marrow as well as radiographic and nuclear imaging for nodal and extranodal sites plus the cerebrospinal fluid.

THERAPY

- The primary treatment of leukemias and lymphomas includes systemic chemotherapy. The intensity of therapy for leukemia and the duration of therapy for lymphoma are determined by risk stratification according to biologic and clinical features.
- ALL therapy involves induction, intensification or consolidation, central nervous system therapy, and maintenance therapy.
- AML therapy includes induction chemotherapy based on FAB classification. Intensification or consolidation may be with bone marrow transplant.
- NHL therapy involves chemotherapy based on the biologic and clinical features of histologic subtype and clinical stage.

INDICATIONS FOR RADIATION THERAPY

- ALL
  - Cranial irradiation for central nervous system prophylaxis in high risk patients
  - Cranial irradiation for treatment of children with central nervous system involvement at diagnosis or relapse
  - Testicular irradiation for relapse in the testes
  - Total body irradiation as part of the myeloablative regimen in bone marrow transplantation
- AML
  - Primary use is total body irradiation for transplantation.
- NHL
  - Total body irradiation is part of the myeloablative regimen in bone marrow transplantation.

LATE SEQUELAE

- Neurocognitive
- Endocrinologic
- Growth
- Induction of secondary malignancies

TREATMENT OF RELAPSE AND PALLIATION

- Local radiotherapy can be used to palliate symptomatic recurrences in leukemias and lymphomas.
- Relapses in the testes and central nervous system are treated by intensive systemic chemotherapy with radiation therapy.
- Treatment of relapse often includes bone marrow transplantation with total body irradiation as part of the myeloablative regimen.

ACUTE LYMPHOBLASTIC LEUKEMIA

Acute lymphoblastic leukemia (ALL) is the most common malignancy in children, accounting for one fourth of all childhood cancers. The advances in the treatment of ALL since the 1940s represent one of the most tremendous success stories in modern medicine. The early successes resulted from the identification of single-agent chemotherapy and then the development of combination chemotherapy, recognition of the need for central nervous system preventive therapy, and maintenance chemotherapy. Concurrent with these developments, new understanding of immunophenotyping, molecular characterization, and treatment responses allowed the definition of risk groups to tailor therapy.

EPIDEMIOLOGY

ALL accounts for 75% of childhood leukemia and is diagnosed in approximately 2500 to 3000 children in the United States annually,[1,2] with a peak age incidence between 2 and 5 years. The incidence of ALL is higher among boys than girls. This difference is more pronounced in pubertal children[3] and particularly evident in cases of T-cell ALL. In the United States, ALL occurs more commonly among white children than among black children.[4]

ETIOLOGY

A single etiology of ALL has not been identified; however, several predisposing risk factors have been identified. These include genetics, environmental factors, viral infection, and immunodeficiency. Genetics appears to play a role in the cause of ALL in some children, as evidenced by the association between specific chromosomal abnormalities and childhood ALL. The most constitutional chromosomal abnormality associated with childhood leukemia is trisomy 21 or Down syndrome[5]; less common chromosomal abnormalities include Kleinfelter's syndrome and trisomy G syndrome.[6] Most cases of leukemia in children cannot be attributed to any known factors.

ALL is believed to develop from the malignant transformation of a single abnormal progenitor cell, which then expands indefinitely. In pediatric ALL, evidence suggests that it occurs in committed lymphoid precursors. In contrast, in Philadelphia chromosome–positive ALL and in pediatric acute myelogenous leukemia (AML), this event may occur earlier, as mutations are observed in multiple cell lineages.[7,8] The sequence of events resulting in malignant transformation is likely to be multifactorial. Leukemia can develop along any point in the normal stages of lymphoid development, which reflects the fact that ALL is a biologically heterogeneous disorder.

MOLECULAR BIOLOGY AND CLASSIFICATION

ALL has been classified according to morphologic, immunologic, cytogenetic, biochemical, and molecular genetic characteristics. The most widely accepted morphologic classification of ALL is that proposed by the French-American-British (FAB) Cooperative Working Group.[9,10] The FAB system defines three categories of lymphoblasts. L1 lymphoblasts are smaller, with scant cytoplasm and inconspicuous nucleoli. L2 lymphoblasts are larger, demonstrate marked heterogeneity in size, and contain prominent nucleoli and more abundant cytoplasm. L3 lymphoblasts are large, with more abundant, basophilic cytoplasm, and often have cytoplasmic vacuolation. The L3 lymphoblast is morphologically identical to the Burkitt's lymphoma cell. The morphologic classification, although useful in the past, is not currently a prognostic factor nor is it used in determining treatment.

IMMUNOPHENOTYPING

The immunobiologic studies of ALL cells indicate that leukemic transformation and clonal expansion occur at different stages of lymphocyte maturation. The use of monoclonal antibodies has classified leukemias; however, these monoclonal antibodies are not purely lineage specific and, therefore, the term "lineage associated" is used. In approximately 80% of cases of childhood ALL, the leukemia cells do not react with either T-cell or B-cell surface markers but are found to have the common ALL antigen (CALLA) CD10 on their cell surfaces.[11,12] These leukemic cells are actually of an early B-cell lineage. Approximately 15% of children will have ALL that is of T-cell origin, and a small percentage of children have mature B-cell ALL. Children with mature B-cell ALL have a poorer prognosis than those of earlier B lineage. Patients with B-cell precursor ALL whose lymphoblasts express CALLA or CD10 on their surfaces have a more favorable prognosis.[13,14] Those with expression of the stem cell antigen CD 34 (found on two thirds of B-cell precursor ALL) is also associated with a favorable prognosis.[15–17]

CYTOGENETICS

Advances in cytogenetics have led to an increasing understanding of the biology of ALL. Cytogenetic abnormalities identified in ALL include abnormalities in chromosomal number (ploidy) as well as those in chromosomal structure. Ploidy is determined either by counting the modal number of chromosomes in a preparation of a metaphase karyotype or by measuring DNA content by flow cytometry. Hyperdiploidy exists when there are more than 46 chromosomes. Most cases of ALL are diploid or hyperdiploid. Ploidy in childhood B-lineage leukemia has prognostic significance.[18-20] Children with higher ploidy, more than 50 chromosomes, have a better prognosis than children with 47 to 50 chromosomes; those with 56 to 67 chromosomes (higher hyperdiploid) have the best prognosis.[21-23] Those patients who have hyperdiploid leukemia also tend to have other favorable prognostic features. Prognostic features of childhood ALL are discussed later. The exception is the small subgroup of children with near tetraploid (82 to 84 chromosomes), who have a poorer prognosis.[21] Those with near-haploid ALL, 24 to 28 chromosomes, have the worst prognosis.[24,25]

Structural chromosomal abnormalities occur in ALL leukemia cells. The most common of these abnormalities are translocations. Translocations lead to alterations in the regulation of oncogenes. The activation of oncogenes and the loss of tumor suppressor genes are examples of the altered regulation believed to be involved in the evolution of leukemia. The most frequently identified translocation in ALL is the t(12;21) and leads to the TEL-AML 1 fusion protein. This occurs in 16% to 22% of cases and is associated with a favorable prognosis. In contrast, the t(8;14), t(9;22), t(4;11), and t(1;19) are all associated with early treatment failure.[20,26] The t(9;22)(q34;q11) results in the formation of the Ph chromosome. This translocation, found in 5% of childhood ALL, has the worst prognosis in pediatric ALL.[27,28] Children with Ph^+ ALL have a poor response to therapy, a lower induction rate, a higher frequency of involvement of the central nervous system, and a higher likelihood of early recurrence.[29,30]

Other unique chromosomal translocations have been observed in childhood ALL. The role of these and all translocations in the development of leukemia remains speculative. Some translocations that result in altered gene expression appear to confer a proliferative advantage for the leukemic cells. When patients with ALL are in remission, the cytogenetic abnormalities described earlier are not detectable. When relapse occurs, reappearance of the original cytogenetic abnormality confirms that there is a recurrence of the original leukemia.

PRESENTATION AND EVALUATION

The presenting signs and symptoms of ALL are related to the degree of bone marrow infiltration as well as the extent of extramedullary involvement. These can include fever, petechiae, lymphadenopathy, and bone pain. Hepatosplenomegaly is found in two thirds of patients. Children with T-cell ALL have some distinctive features. T-cell ALL more frequently occurs in older boys, presents with high initial white blood cell counts, and a mediastinal mass is often found at diagnosis. The definitive diagnosis is made by bone marrow aspirate, although a bone marrow biopsy may be required in some cases. This allows morphologic assessment,

Table 70-1 Initial Evaluation

History/physical examination
Laboratory studies
Bone marrow aspirate/biopsy*
CBC, differential
Coagulation profile
LDH
Uric acid
Electrolytes
Liver and renal function tests
Chest radiograph
Serum immunoglobulin
Varicella zoster titer
HIV test
PPD skin test
Urinalysis
Cultures
Echocardiogram
Cerebrospinal fluid examination†

*Bone marrow studies: morphology, cytogenetics, immunophenotype, cytochemistry

†Therapeutic lumbar puncture performed for diagnosis concurrent with administration of intrathecal chemotherapy.

CBC, complete blood count; LDH, lactic dehydrogenase; PPD, purified protein derivative.

immunophenotyping, karyotyping, and molecular evaluations such as reverse-transcriptase polymerase chain reaction (RT-PCR) and fluorescence in situ hybridization (FISH) for chromosomal characterization. At the time of initial diagnosis, the evaluation of patients includes cerebrospinal fluid (CSF) examination, uric acid levels, liver function tests, renal function, coagulation screening, chest radiograph, evaluation for infection, immunoglobulin levels, varicella/zoster titers, and echocardiogram (Table 70-1). Manifestations of central nervous system (CNS) involvement, such as headache, lethargy, papilloedema, and cranial neuropathies (most often the third, fourth, sixth, and seventh) are infrequently present at diagnosis. Involvement of the CNS at diagnosis is found in less than 5% of children with ALL.[31] CNS involvement is divided into three levels, based on the number of white blood cells (WBC) and the presence of lymphoblasts on the cytospin. CNS-1 is defined as no evidence of lymphoblasts in the CSF. CNS-2 is defined as fewer than five WBC per μL with blasts present in the cytospin, and CNS-3 is defined as five or more WBC per μL with blasts, or presence of cranial nerve palsy, in the cytospin.

PROGNOSTIC FACTORS

Several clinical and biologic factors determined at diagnosis have been identified and shown to have prognostic significance (Table 70-2). These prognostic factors are used to assign patients to risk strata that tailor the treatment. These factors have been integral in the development of all modern therapeutic trials. Although many of these factors have shown prognostic importance, not all are currently used to determine risk stratification. A presenting leukocyte count (WBC) of more than 50,000 is considered to be a high-risk feature, and a WBC of more than 100,000 is considered to be very high risk. Age at diagnosis of more than 10 years is considered high risk, and age under 1 year is a very high-risk feature. The presence of the Ph+ chromosome, T-cell immunophenotype, expression of myeloid antigens on the leukemic blast cells, and the presence of CNS disease at diagnosis are all considered high-risk features. Responses to treatment are also prognostic. These include the time to achieve remission, and the decrease in peripheral blast count following administration of steroids, where longer time to remission or poor response to initial steroids are associated with worse outcomes. All of the foregoing features are used in risk-group stratification and treatment recommendations. Other clinical and biologic features that have been associated with poorer outcomes but are not used for treatment stratification include male sex, non-white race, and an initial hemoglobin of >10 mg/dL.[32-36]

Table 70-2 Prognostic Factors in Acute Lymphoblastic Leukemia

Initial white blood cell count
Age at diagnosis
Sex
Race
Presence of mediastinal mass
Organomegaly/lymphadenopathy
Hemoglobin level
Platelet count
Cytogenetics/ploidy
Immunophenotype
French-American-British morphology
Expression of myeloid antigens on leukemic cells
Serum immunoglobulins
Nutritional status
Rapidity of response

Table 70-3 Uniform Age and White Blood Cell Count Criteria for B-Precursor Acute Lymphoblastic Leukemia Standard and High-Risk Cohorts *Adopted at the Cancer Treatment and Evaluation Program/National Cancer Institute Workshop*

Risk	Definition	4-Year Event-Free Survival (%)	B-Precursor Patients (%)
Standard	WBC count <50,000/μL Age 1.00–9.99 yr	80.3	68
High	WBC count ≥50,000/μL or Age ≥ 10.00 yr	63.9	32

WBC, white blood count.

From Smith M, Arthur D, Camitta B, et al: Uniform approach to risk classification and treatment assignment for children with acute lymphoblastic leukemia. J Clin Oncol 14:20, 1996. Reprinted from the American Society of Clinical Oncology.

As therapy for ALL has become more intensive and the outcomes have improved, many of these factors have lost statistical significance as prognostic factors. In addition, the definitions of high leukocyte counts and age varies among cooperative groups. To allow comparisons of results, the National Cancer Institute held a workshop to develop a uniform set of prognostic factors.[37] The age and white blood cell count criteria for childhood ALL agreed on at the Cancer Treatment and Evaluation Program/National Cancer Institute Workshop are shown in Table 70-3.

The presenting WBC (white blood cell count) and age at diagnosis are uniformly accepted as prognostic features. Children with the highest initial WBC have a poorer prognosis.[38,39] Infants younger than 1 year of age have the worst prognosis, and adolescents also have a poorer event-free survival (EFS) than younger children, except those younger than 1 year.[40,41] Children older than 10 years often have other poor risk features, including T-cell phenotype.[41] Infants with ALL have shown the worst outcome—EFS 10% to 20%.[40] Infants also have other poor risk features, including very high presenting WBC, presence of CNS leukemia, massive organomegaly, and poor day 14 response to induction chemotherapy.[40] Infant ALL has unique biologic features, including chromosomal abnormalities that are associated with a worse prognosis. Structural abnormalities of chromosome 11, such as rearrangement of band q23, within the malignant lymphoblastic lymphoma (*MLL*)/*ALL-1* gene, are often present.[42,43] The 4;11 translocation is commonly seen, and many have leukemia cells that co-express myeloid markers (CD15).[40,42,44] This finding suggests that infant ALL arises in a multipotent precursor cell. The immunophenotype of ALL has prognostic significance. In the past, children with T-cell ALL had a poorer survival compared to children with B-progenitor ALL; however, with intensified treatment, these patients fared as well as B-progenitor patients.[45] The rapidity of response to therapy has become a major prognostic indicator. The initial response as measured by the residual leukemia found in the bone marrow on day 14 of induction is an independent prognostic factor.[46,47]

TREATMENT

The foregoing prognostic indicators are used to stratify children with ALL into risk groups. The stratification is dependent on prompt, accurate evaluation and sophisticated techniques. To accomplish this, as well as to treat patients with the increased intensity of current therapy, evaluation and treatment is most appropriately carried out in recognized pediatric oncology centers. The treatments for the different risk groups vary in intensity and by institution. However, the framework for all risk groups includes four key elements: remission induction, CNS preventive therapy, consolidation, and maintenance (Fig. 70-1).

Induction treatment is designed to achieve complete remission, defined as no evidence of leukemia. Peripheral blood counts must be within the normal range, and the bone marrow must be of normal cellularity and contain less than 5% lymphoblasts. There should be no evidence of CNS disease on examination of the CSF, and there must be no extramedullary disease. Remission can be achieved in 85% of children with ALL using vincristine and a glucocorticoid; however, the addition of L-asparaginase and/or the addition of an anthracycline will improve the remission induction rate to 95%.[48]

The prevention of CNS disease is one of the major elements of successful ALL treatment. The approach to CNS prophylaxis has evolved over the decades since it was first incorporated into ALL therapy in the 1970s. Craniospinal irradiation and cranial irradiation plus intrathecal methotrexate reduced the relapse rate in the CNS from 50% to less than 10%.[49] To avoid the myelosuppression and the effects on spinal growth, intrathecal methotrexate was substituted for spinal irradiation as part of the standard CNS preventive therapy. Intrathecal therapy has been shown to successfully prevent CNS relapse in standard-risk patients and avoids the neurocognitive sequelae and secondary tumors that can result from cranial irradiation. Triple intrathecal chemotherapy in conjunction with intensive systemic therapy has provided adequate CNS prevention for children without high-risk features. Children with an increased risk for CNS relapse include those with other high-risk features, such as high initial white count, T-cell phenotype, very young age, t(4;11), the presence of the Ph^+, and lymphomatous presentation. For patients with these features, cranial irradiation is generally incorporated into the treatment protocol, with the exception of those with infant ALL, who are treated with very intensive chemotherapy to avoid the late sequelae of cranial irradiation in this age group. The CNS-directed therapy for CNS-3 patients is not preventive, but therapeutic. The techniques of cranial irradiation are discussed later.

Once complete remission has been achieved, consolidation and maintenance therapy are used to provide continued cytoreduction of the leukemic cell burden without permitting the emergence of drug-resistant clones. During the consolidation phase, intensified therapy is given once complete remission has been achieved. Intensification has improved the outcome for patients with high-risk disease.[50,51] The post-induction intensification therapy often includes L-asparaginase, and doxorubicin.[52,53] The chemotherapy drugs used for induction were not as effective for maintenance therapy. The most effective maintenance regimens use methotrexate and 6-mercaptopurine (6-MP), administered continuously.[54-57] Methotrexate is given intermittently, and 6-MP is given daily. Some protocols use intermittent pulses of vincristine and prednisone in addition to methotrexate and 6-MP.[58] The appropriate maintenance therapy differs according to the risk group, with more intensive therapy used for patients in higher risk groups.

INDICATIONS FOR RADIATION THERAPY

The role of radiation therapy in the treatment of childhood ALL has diminished in recent years. Improvements in the efficacy of chemotherapy administration and a clearer understanding of the prognostic factors have been responsible for this changing role. However, radiation therapy remains an important modality in ALL in specific situations. These include prophylactic cranial irradiation in select groups of high-risk patients, therapeutic central nervous system treatment for patients with meningeal leukemia, treatment of testicular disease, and total body irradiation for some patients for whom bone marrow transplant is recommended.

CNS prophylaxis for standard-risk patients is achieved with systemic and intrathecal chemotherapy without cranial irradiation. Children with high-risk features are at an increased risk for CNS relapse and are often treated with prophylactic cranial irradiation. These features include a presenting WBC count of 50,000 or greater; those with WBC counts over 100,000 are at particularly high risk for CNS relapse. Additional high-risk features that are indications on most treatment protocols for cranial irradiation are T-cell phenotype, Ph^+ ALL, and the presence of the (4;11) translocation. Infants younger than 1 year with 11q23 abnormalities are at very high risk for CNS relapse but, owing to their young age, are treated without cranial irradiation, using intensified chemotherapy to treat the CNS. The standard dose for high-risk ALL cranial prophylaxis has been 1800 cGy; however, published trials from the Berlin-Frankfurt-Munster group and ongoing open multi-institutional protocols have used 1200 cGy in patients with CNS-1 disease.[59]

Children who present with CNS-3 disease at diagnosis, regardless of the other features of their disease, are deemed high-risk and are considered to have meningeal leukemia. The treatment of these patients varies, and some protocols use craniospinal irradiation, or cranial irradiation in addition to intrathecal chemotherapy. Irradiation is not administered until the patient is in remission, including clearance of the spinal fluid. St Jude Children's Research Hospital administers

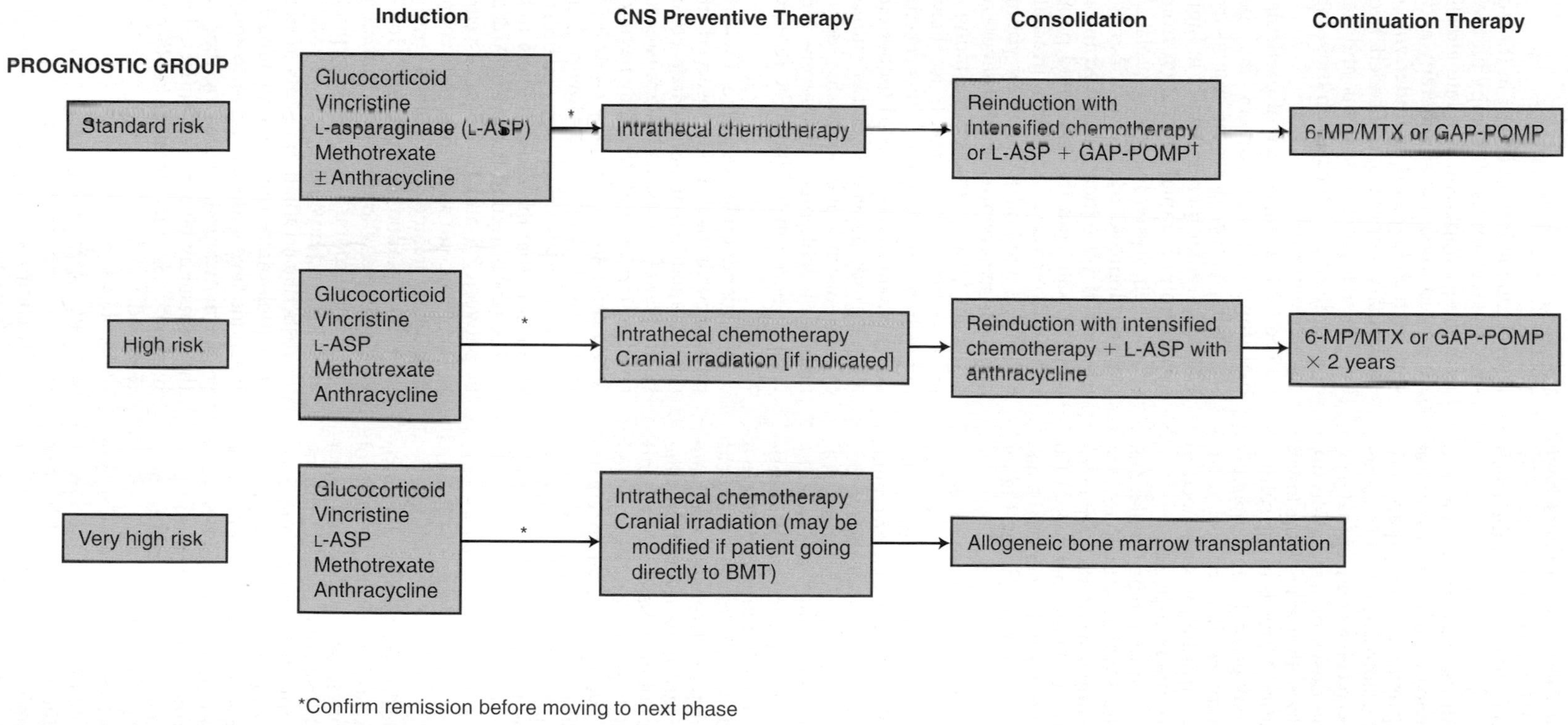

Figure 70-1 Treatment algorithm for acute lymphoblastic leukemia. BMT, bone marrow transplant; CNS, central nervous system; 6-MP, 6-mercaptopurine; MTX, methotrexate. GAP-POMP (GAP refers to the schedule of mercaptopurine administration given on 14 days of each 21-day cycle, thus a 7-day GAP) repeats a 3-week cycle until 2 years of continuous complete remission. Vincristine, prednisone, mercaptopurine, methotrexate; high-dose cycle; vincristine, mercaptopurine, high-dose intravenous and intrathecal methotrexate.

delayed craniospinal irradiation of 2400 cGy.[31] Others have used lower doses of cranial irradiation, such as 1800 cGy, administered during the reinduction phase early in the treatment course.[60]

Isolated CNS relapse is rare with the current approach to ALL treatment. The treatment depends on the time from first remission as well as the extent of previous CNS therapy. All patients need intensive systemic chemotherapy and intrathecal chemotherapy, and most will also receive craniospinal irradiation or cranial irradiation.[61] The doses of irradiation are 2400 to 3000 cGy to the cranial field with a somewhat lower dose, 1200 cGy to 1800 cGy, to the spine.[62] This is in the setting of CNS relapse, and some patients will go on to bone marrow transplantation (BMT) with total body irradiation. In that situation, the total dose of craniospinal irradiation may need to be modified depending on timing of the transplant.

Cranial nerve palsies can be seen in meningeal leukemia. Urgent radiotherapy to the base of the skull initially to reverse the palsy is often given, with full cranial irradiation given at the scheduled time for CNS treatment. Doses between 1000 and 1200 cGy are used. Although the use of higher doses has been reported, no dose-response was observed for higher doses.[63]

The technique for cranial irradiation must ensure coverage of the cranial meninges as well as other areas of potential access to CNS system, such as the cribriform plate; the posterior retina and posterior globe of the eye; the exit of cranial nerves III, IV, V, and VI; and the inferior extent of the temporal meninges. The cribriform plate should be identified, following the anterior clinoids anteriorly, and locating the superior orbital plate will assist in identification of the cribriform plate. The field extends to the C1-C2 interspace unless a clinical field arrangement is used, in which case the field would be brought to the C2-C3 interspace. To ensure adequate dose to the meninges, the entire calvarium is covered, and the energy should be 6 MeV or 4 MeV photons. Custom cerrobend blocks are used to shield normal tissues. Parallel-opposed lateral fields are used. Immobilization is critical to ensure precise treatment and reproducibility. Immobilization devices are recommended for this when possible. Sedation may be required for younger patients who are unable to fully cooperate.

TESTICULAR LEUKEMIA

Testicular involvement that is clinically apparent at diagnosis is infrequent; however, occult disease is found in 25% of boys.[64] Overt involvement is manifest as painless testicular enlargement that is often unilateral. Testicular biopsies during maintenance or at the conclusion of all therapy have been abandoned, as the biopsy results did not accurately predict eventual relapse.[65-67] Some protocols have used prophylactic bilateral testicular irradiation, although this approach has not been widely used because the current systemic therapy protocols have lessened the rate of testicular relapse and testicular irradiation causes permanent sterility.[68,69]

Testicular relapse occurs in less than 5% of cases in the current era of intensive therapy.[70,71] Both systemic therapy as well as local therapy, directed at the testes, are used to treat testicular relapse. Re-induction therapy is needed as well as CNS-directed treatment. Bilateral testicular irradiation is used in doses of 2400 to 2600 cGy in 200-cGy fractions.[72] The treatment is delivered with the child supine in the frog-leg position with the soles of the feet touching. The penis is taped or secured out of the radiation therapy field. Bolus may be needed to ensure adequate dose to the testes, or electrons can be used. The entire scrotal contents are irradiated.

LATE SEQUELAE

With dramatic improvement in the outcome of children with ALL, the late effects of therapy on the survivors have become increasingly apparent. The late effects are multifactorial and are related to both chemotherapy and radiotherapy and vary with each child, based on underlying clinical factors. A multidisciplinary approach is needed because the late sequelae involve many organ systems and vary in severity. The following discussion focuses on those late effects that are chiefly related to irradiation.

The CNS sequelae are of particular concern. Neurocognitive functional impairment has been observed in ALL survivors. Lower doses of cranial irradiation—for example, 1200 cGy rather than 1800 cGy in high-risk patients—and the elimination of cranial irradiation from standard-risk patients should help lessen the late sequelae. However, in a prospective, randomized trial comparing 1800 cGy with no cranial irradiation, all patients received intrathecal and intravenous methotrexate, and the irradiated patients had no worse neurocognitive effects.[73] Children irradiated when younger than 8 years of age and particularly younger than 5 years of age appear to experience the most severe neurocognitive sequelae. Leukoencephalopathy is devastating and fortunately uncommon in the current era. It is characterized by multifocal demyelination. Although this occurs most commonly in patients who have received higher cumulative doses of radiation therapy as well as higher cumulative doses of intrathecal and systemic methotrexate (such as those with recurrent meningeal leukemia), this severe form of neurotoxicity has been observed in children who received no cranial irradiation at all.[74,75]

Neuroendocrine sequelae involving the hypothalamic-pituitary axis have been observed in ALL survivors treated with cranial irradiation. Most commonly seen is growth hormone deficiency, which appears to be dose-related in that children treated with 1800 cGy have reduced growth hormone levels compared to healthy controls, but not as low as those treated with 2400 cGy.[76] However, growth delay and short stature have also been seen in unirradiated ALL survivors, suggesting that the cause is likely to be multifactorial.

The risk of second tumors in ALL survivors is estimated to be between 3% and 12%, 5 to 24 years following initial diagnosis.[77,78] Second solid tumors have most commonly occurred in patients treated with cranial irradiation and are within or near the radiation therapy field. However, there are reports of ALL patients who were not irradiated but developed secondary CNS tumors.[79] The most common hematopoietic tumors are AML and myelodysplastic syndrome.[77,78]

Testicular irradiation results in sterility. Some studies have shown elevated follicle-stimulating hormone and luteinizing hormone levels, decreased testosterone levels, and delays in sexual maturation, suggesting that the endocrine function of the testes may be adversely affected at doses of 2400 cGy and higher.[80,81] Supplemental or replacement androgens may be required.

ACUTE MYELOGENOUS LEUKEMIA

AML comprises a group of hematologic malignancies that arise from the precursors of the myeloid, monocytoid, erythroid, and megakaryocytic cell lineages. AML represents 15% to 25% of childhood leukemia but accounts for more than 30% of deaths from leukemia. The classification used in AML is the French-American-British (FAB) schema. The FAB classification defines seven subtypes of AML (M1 to M7), characterized by morphologic, histochemical, immunophenotypic, and cytoge-

Table 70-4 **Morphology of Acute Myelogenous Leukemia—French-American-British (FAB) System of Classification**

FAB Type	Name
M1	Acute myeloblastic: no maturation
M2	Acute myeloblastic with maturation
M3	Acute promyelocytic: hypergranular type
M3v	Acute promyelocytic: microgranular variant
M4	Acute myelomonocytic
M4Eo	Acute myelomonocytic with eosinophilia
M5a	Acute monocytic
M5b	Acute monocytic with differentiation
M6	Acute erythroleukemia
M7	Acute megakaryoblastic

netic features (Table 70-4). An M0 subtype has been used for an acute undifferentiated leukemia.[82]

Children with AML present with a broad range of signs and symptoms. Fever is present in one third of patients due to the release of pyrogens from leukemic cells or from macrophages and lymphocytes reacting to the proliferating leukemic blasts, or from secondary bacterial infections from neutropenia. Pallor, headache, tinnitus, fatigue, and congestive heart failure can be present if anemia is severe. Bleeding from thrombocytopenia or from disseminated intravascular coagulation (DIC) can occur. Bone pain is a frequent complaint. Hepatosplenomegaly, due to organ infiltration, is present is approximately 50% of children at diagnosis.

Treatment of AML involves, first, stabilization of the patient at diagnosis, and aggressive, supportive care to treat potential complications, such as DIC, infectious complications, tumor lysis syndrome, and hyperleukostasis. Induction of remission involves multiagent chemotherapy. Induction is followed by post-remission consolidation, intensification, CNS prophylaxis, and, in some studies, maintenance chemotherapy. Induction therapy for AML most commonly includes Ara-C (cytosine arabinoside) coupled with an anthracycline with or without additional agents such as etoposide, thioguanine, and dexamethasone.[83,84]

Post-remission intensification, particularly with increased dose-intensity of Ara-C, resulted in lower relapse rates and longer remission duration.[85,86] CNS prophylaxis, with intrathecal Ara-C and intrathecal methotrexate, is used for all patients. Children with the highest risk of a CNS relapse are those with M4 or M5 AML or with very high presenting peripheral blast counts. CNS relapse is generally followed by bone marrow relapse. With the use of prophylaxis in all patients with AML, the incidence of CNS relapse is 5%.[85,87]

Extramedullary disease besides the CNS can also occur, such as the development of chloromas, most commonly in M4 and M5 subtypes. There was no benefit to the use of local radiotherapy to treat chloromas, in addition to systemic therapy in children.[88] If a chloroma is causing significant morbidity, such as vision loss or spinal cord compression, radiation therapy is indicated.

Because the use of intensified chemotherapy has improved the EFS in children with AML, it has been questioned whether even greater dose-intensification, such as with myeloablative therapy and stem cell rescue, could improve the EFS even further. Randomized trials have shown that children with AML who undergo allogeneic stem cell transplants from HLA-matched siblings have an improved relapse-free survival.[89-95] For children with AML, allogeneic BMT from an HLA-matched family member provides the best overall survival. Total body irradiation is often used as a part of the myeloablative regimen for BMT.

NON-HODGKIN'S LYMPHOMA

Lymphomas in children are the third most common malignancy of childhood, superceded only by ALL and brain tumors. Hodgkin's disease is discussed separately. In children younger than 15 years, 60% of cases are non-Hodgkin's lymphoma (NHL). If one includes children up through age 18, Hodgkin's disease is slightly more frequent.[96] NHL is diagnosed annually in the United States in approximately 500 children. The median age at diagnosis is 10 years; NHL is less frequent in children younger than 3 years. There is no bimodal age distribution; the frequency increases with increasing age. For unknown reasons, NHL is more common in whites than in blacks, and two to three times more frequent in men than in women.[97] Specific populations at increased risk for developing NHL include children with congenital immunodeficiency disorders, such as Wiskott-Aldrich syndrome, ataxia-telangiectasia, and X-linked lymphoproliferative syndrome.[98]

In contrast to NHL in adults, NHLs in children are primarily aggressive, diffuse tumors, frequently with extranodal presentation. There are three main subtypes: Burkitt's, lymphoblastic, and large-cell lymphoma, shown in Table 70-5. The staging system used in childhood NHL is the Murphy/SJCRH staging system, which incorporates extent of disease and clinical patterns (Table 70-6).[99] Treatment of childhood NHL is based on the stage, immunophenotype, and histology.

Burkitt's lymphoma, or small noncleaved cell lymphoma, makes up 39% of childhood NHL and is of B-cell phenotype. These lymphomas present in the abdomen or in the head and neck. The epidemiology of Burkitt's lymphoma is of great interest due to its major differences in incidence and clinical features based on geography. For example, it is the most common childhood malignancy in equatorial Africa, yet is very rare in Japan.[100] In Africa, the endemic subtype occurs, and is characterized by younger age at diagnosis, and frequent involvement of the jaw, abdomen, orbit, and paraspinal area.[100] The sporadic subtype, which occurs in the United States and Western Europe, is characterized by older median age at diagnosis, and frequent involvement of the abdomen, nasopharynx, and bone marrow. There are cytogenetic differences that mirror the differences in the geographic distribution.[100] The association of Epstein-Barr virus (EBV) with Burkitt's lymphoma varies with geography; EBV is associated with the endemic (African) subtype.[100]

The treatment of Burkitt's lymphoma uses cyclophosphamide-based chemotherapy, with the addition of agents including vincristine, prednisone, doxorubicin, and methotrexate. Children with advanced-stage Burkitt's have an improved outcome with the addition of cytarabine or high-dose methotrexate. Children with bone marrow or CNS involvement have an improved outcome with more intensive regimens, resulting in an 85% EFS, even for advanced-stage patients.[101]

Lymphoblastic lymphomas make up approximately 29% of childhood non-Hodgkin's lymphomas. They share morphologic, immunophenotypic, and cytogenetic features with ALL. The distinction between leukemia and lymphoblastic lymphoma is considered by many to be arbitrary; however, there appear to be subtle differences in the molecular biology, cytogenetics, and immunophenotypic markers, suggesting that there may be some fundamental differences in the biology.[102]

Table 70-5 **Non-Hodgkin's Lymphomas in Children**

Subtype	Proportion of Cases (%)*	Phenotype	Common Site of Primary	Translocation
Burkitt's	39	B-cell	Abdomen or head/neck	t(8;14)(q24;q32) t(2;8)(p11;q24) t(8;22)(q24;q11)
Lymphoblastic	28	T-cell	Mediastinum or head/neck	t(1;14)(p32;q11) t(11;14)(p13;q11) t(11;14)(p15;q11) t(10;14)(p24;q11) t(7;19)(q35;p13) t(8;14)(q24;q11) t(1;7)(p34;q34)
Large-cell	26	B-cell, T-cell, indeterminate	Mediastinum, abdomen, head/neck, or skin	t(2;5)(p23;q35)

*Other histologies account for approximately 7%.[98]

Table 70-6 **Staging of Non-Hodgkin's Lymphoma in Children**

Stage I	Involvement of a single extranodal site or single anatomic nodal site, excluding the mediastinum or abdomen
Stage II	Involvement of a single extranodal site with regional nodal involvement
	Two or more nodal areas on the same side of the diaphragm
	Two extranodal sites with or without regional nodal involvement on the same side of the diaphragm
	A primary gastrointestinal tract tumor, usually ileocecal, with or without mesenteric node involvement that is completely resected
Stage III	Two single extranodal sites on opposite sides of the diaphragm
	Two or more nodal groups above and below the diaphragm
	All primary intrathoracic tumors
	All extensive (unresectable) intra-abdominal primary tumors
	All paraspinal or epidural tumors
Stage IV	Any of the above with initial involvement of the bone marrow, central nervous system, or both

When patients present with lymphoblastic lymphoma that appears to be localized to nodal or extranodal tissue, molecular evaluation of the bone marrow and peripheral blood usually demonstrates involvement with lymphoma. The St. Jude criteria defines ALL by the proportion of lymphoblasts in the bone marrow of greater than 25%, whereas some use 10% lymphoblasts in the marrow.[99] The distinction between lymphoma with marrow involvement and acute leukemia is often difficult. Immunophenotyping reveals only minor differences in antigen expression between B-cell and T-cell lymphoblastic lymphomas and ALL. Ninety percent of lymphoblastic lymphomas are of T-cell lineage, and 10% are of B-cell lineage.[103] The treatment of lymphoblastic lymphoma in children uses multi-agent chemotherapy using drugs similar to those used for ALL, including vincristine, prednisone, L-asparaginase, doxorubicin, cytarabine, cyclophosphamide, and high-dose methotrexate. Children with more advanced disease are often treated with high-risk ALL therapy.

Large cell lymphomas represent approximately 27% of childhood lymphomas. Anaplastic large-cell, diffuse large B-cell, and peripheral T-cell lymphomas comprise most pediatric large-cell lymphomas. Approximately 40% to 50% are anaplastic T-cell lymphomas, 30% to 40% are diffuse B-cell lymphomas, and the remainder are non-anaplastic peripheral T-cell lymphomas. Historically, the treatment of childhood NHL in the United States has been histology-based. However, there has been a shift toward using an immunophenotype-directed approach, which has been the standard practice in Europe for many years. With this approach, children with B-cell large-cell will be treated on regimens for Burkitt's lymphoma.

Anaplastic large-cell lymphomas are rare in very young children, but peak in adolescence. Seventy-five percent of these lymphomas have a characteristic chromosomal translocation, the t(2;5)(p23:q35).[104] The optimal approach for treatment of anaplastic NHL in children has not been established. A randomized comparison of ACOP versus APO (doxorubicin, vincristine, prednisone with or without cyclophosphamide) showed no significant difference in outcome.[105] Three-year EFS rates for children with advanced-stage disease are approximately 60% to 70%.[106]

The role of local radiation therapy in the management of NHL in children has been more limited due to the improved outcomes with more effective chemotherapy. A prospective, randomized trial evaluating the need for local radiation therapy in early-stage NHL found no benefit to the addition of local radiation therapy.[107] A second trial, built on the results of the first, confirmed this. Although children with primary lymphoma of bone were not randomized in the first trial and all received local radiotherapy, in the second trial, radiation therapy was not given, and there were no local relapses.[108] Based on these results, the current management of localized NHL of bone includes chemotherapy but does not use consolidative local radiation therapy. Children with advanced-stage lymphoma do not benefit from involved-field radiation therapy.[109]

Cranial irradiation as part of CNS prophylaxis in pediatric lymphoma has been eliminated, with the exception of children with advanced lymphoblastic lymphoma. Radiation therapy is used for relapse or refractory disease and as a palliative modality. Children with persistent disease following chemotherapy or who relapse are often considered for high-dose chemotherapy protocols with stem cell rescue if they have chemosensitive disease, and for these children, consolidative radiation therapy can be considered either prior to or following transplant. There are no prospective, randomized trials in pediatrics to confirm the benefit of this approach.

Urgent radiation therapy is rare; however, there are occasions when it is considered. Mediastinal masses in children can cause significant airway compromise or superior vena cava compression. If a tissue diagnosis cannot be established to allow administration of systemic therapy, urgent radiation therapy may be considered. It should be noted that if one treats empirically with systemic therapy for the most likely diagnosis, the correct treatment is given in most cases.[110] If radiation therapy is given, only a few fractions are needed to achieve stabilization and allow appropriate systemic therapy to be initiated once a histologic diagnosis is made.

Encouraging progress has been made in the treatment of childhood leukemias and lymphomas. However, many children continue to succumb to disease despite aggressive therapy, and many children experience significant treatment-related short- and long-term sequelae. Oncologists and radiation oncologists need to strive for improvements in treatment while minimizing the late effects of therapy. Continued research in the biology of these malignancies, coupled with a search for new biologic and clinical prognostic factors, will help to achieve this goal.

REFERENCES

1. Gurney J, Severson RK, Davis S, et al: Incidence of cancer in children in the United States: sex-, race-, and 1-year age-specific rates by histologic type. Cancer 75:2186, 1995.
2. Greenlee RT, Murray T, Bolden S, et al: Cancer Statistics, 2000. CA Cancer J Clin 50:7-34, 2000.
3. Fraumeni JF, Wagoner J: Changing sex differentials in leukemia. Public Health Rep 79:1093, 1974.
4. Pollock BH, DeBaun MR, Camitta BM, et al: Racial differences in the survival of childhood B-precursor acute lymphoblastic leukemia: a Pediatric Oncology Group study. J Clin Oncol 18:813-823, 2000.
5. Dordelmann M, Schrappe M, Reiter A, et al: Down's syndrome in childhood acute lymphoblastic leukemia: clinical characteristics and treatment outcome in four consecutive BFM trials. Berlin-Frankfurt-Munster Group. Leukemia 12:645-651, 1998.
6. Muts-Homshma S, Muller H, Geracost J: Klinefelter's syndrome and acute non-lymphocytic leukemia. Blut 44:15, 1981.
7. Schenk TM, Keyhani A, Bottcher S, et al: Multilineage involvement of Philadelphia chromosome positive acute lymphoblastic leukemia. Leukemia 12:666-674, 1998.
8. Kasprzyk A, Harrison CJ, Secker-Walker LM: Investigation of clonal involvement of myeloid cells in Philadelphia-positive and high hyperdiploid acute lymphoblastic leukemia (Published erratum appears in Leukemia 14:5,26, 2000). Leukemia 13:2000-2006, 1999.
9. Bennett JM, Catovsky D, Daniel MT, et al: Proposals for the classification of the acute leukaemias. French-American-British (FAB) co-operative group. Br J Haematol 33:451-458, 1976.
10. Bennett J, Catovsky D, Daniel MT: French-American-British (FAB) Cooperative Group: the morphological classification of acute leukemias—concordance among observers and clinical correlation. Br J Hematol 47:553, 1981.
11. Abshire TC, Buchanan GR, Jackson JF, et al: Morphologic, immunologic and cytogenetic studies in children with acute lymphoblastic leukemia at diagnosis and relapse: a Pediatric Oncology Group study. Leukemia 6:357-362, 1992.
12. Ludwig WD, Reiter A, Loffler H, et al: Immunophenotypic features of childhood and adult acute lymphoblastic leukemia (ALL): experience of the German Multicentre Trials ALL-BFM and GMALL. Leuk Lymphoma 13(Suppl 1):71-76, 1994.
13. Greaves MF, Janossy G, Peto J, et al: Immunologically defined sub-classes of acute lymphoblastic leukaemia in children: their relationship to presentation features and prognosis. Br J Haematol 48:179-197, 1981.
14. Crist W, Boyett J, Roper M, et al: Pre-B cell leukemia responds poorly to treatment: a Pediatric Oncology Group study. Blood 63:407-414, 1984.
15. Borowitz MJ, Shuster JJ, Civin CI, et al: CD34 expression is a favorable prognostic marker on B-precursor acute lymphocytic leukemia: a Pediatric Oncology Group study. J Clin Oncol 2:11A, 1989.
16. Borowitz MJ, Shuster JJ, Civin CI, et al: Prognostic significance of CD34 expression in childhood B-precursor acute lymphocytic leukemia: a Pediatric Oncology Group study. J Clin Oncol 8:1389-1398, 1990.
17. Uckun FM, Sather H, Gaynon P, et al: Prognostic significance of the CD10+CD19+CD34+ B-progenitor immunophenotype in children with acute lymphoblastic leukemia: a report from the Children's Cancer Group. Leuk Lymphoma 27:445-457, 1997.
18. Look AT, Roberson PK, Williams DL, et al: Prognostic importance of blast cell DNA content in childhood acute lymphoblastic leukemia. Blood 65:1079-1086, 1985.
19. Trueworthy R, Shuster J, Look T, et al: Ploidy of lymphoblasts is the strongest predictor of treatment outcome in B-progenitor cell acute lymphoblastic leukemia of childhood: a Pediatric Oncology Group study. J Clin Oncol 10:606-613, 1992.
20. Chromosomal abnormalities and their clinical significance in acute lymphoblastic leukemia. Third International Workshop on Chromosomes in Leukemia. Cancer Res 43:868-873, 1983.
21. Pui CH, Carroll AJ, Head D, et al: Near-triploid and near-tetraploid acute lymphoblastic leukemia of childhood. Blood 76:590-596, 1990.
22. Rubin CM, Le Beau MM: Cytogenetic abnormalities in childhood acute lymphoblastic leukemia. Am J Pediatr Hematol Oncol 13:202-216, 1991.
23. Heerema NA, Sather HN, Sensel MG, et al: Prognostic impact of trisomies of chromosomes 10, 17, and 5 among children with acute lymphoblastic leukemia and high hyperdiploidy (>50 chromosomes). J Clin Oncol 18:1876-1887, 2000.
24. Brodeur GM, Williams DL, Look AT, et al: Near-haploid acute lymphoblastic leukemia: a unique subgroup with a poor prognosis? Blood 58:14-19, 1981.
25. Heerema NA, Nachman JB, Sather HN, et al: Hypodiploidy with less than 45 chromosomes confers adverse risk in childhood acute lymphoblastic leukemia: a report from the Children's Cancer Group. Blood 94:4036-4045, 1999.
26. Bloomfield CD, Goldman AI, Alimena G, et al: Chromosomal abnormalities identify high-risk and low-risk patients with acute lymphoblastic leukemia. Blood 68:205-212, 1986.
27. Nowell P: Molecular monitoring of pre-B acute lymphocytic leukemia. J Clin Oncol 5:692, 1987.
28. Arico M, Valsecchi MG, Camitta B, et al: Outcome of treatment in children with Philadelphia chromosome-positive acute lymphoblastic leukemia. N Engl J Med 342:998-1006, 2000.
29. Ribeiro RC, Abromowitch M, Raimondi SC, et al: Clinical and biologic hallmarks of the Philadelphia chromosome in childhood acute lymphoblastic leukemia. Blood 70:948-953, 1987.
30. Roberts WM, Rivera GK, Raimondi SC, et al: Intensive chemotherapy for Philadelphia-chromosome-positive acute lymphoblastic leukemia. Lancet 343:331-332, 1994.
31. Bleyer WA: Central nervous system leukemia. Pediatr Clin North Am 35:789-814, 1988.
32. Lilleyman JS, Hann IM, Stevens RF, et al: Cytomorphology of childhood lymphoblastic leukaemia: a prospective study of 2000 patients. United Kingdom Medical Research Council's Working Party on Childhood Leukaemia. Br J Haematol 81:52-57, 1992.
33. Hurwitz CA, Mirro J Jr: Mixed-lineage leukemia and asynchronous antigen expression. Hematol Oncol Clin North Am 4:767-794, 1990.
34. Kalwinsky DK, Roberson P, Dahl G, et al: Clinical relevance of lymphoblast biological features in children with acute lymphoblastic leukemia. J Clin Oncol 3:477-484, 1985.

35. Revesz T, Banczur M, Gyodi E, et al: The association of HLA-DR5 antigen with longer survival in childhood leukaemia. Br J Haematol 48:508-510, 1981.
36. Ludwig WD, Theil E, Bartram CR, et al: Clinical importance of T-ALL subclassification according to thymic or rethymic maturation stage. Hamatol Bluttransfus 33:419-427, 1990.
37. Smith M, Arthur D, Camitta B, et al: Uniform approach to risk classification and treatment assignment for children with acute lymphoblastic leukemia. J Clin Oncol 14:18-24, 1996.
38. Simone JV, Verzosa MS, Rudy JA: Initial features and prognosis in 363 children with acute lymphocytic leukemia. Cancer 36:2099-2108, 1975.
39. Sather HN: Age at diagnosis in childhood acute lymphoblastic leukemia. Med Pediatr Oncol 14:166-172, 1986.
40. Reaman G, Zeltzer P, Bleyer WA, et al: Acute lymphoblastic leukemia in infants less than one year of age: a cumulative experience of the Children's Cancer Study Group. J Clin Oncol 3:1513-1521, 1985.
41. Crist W, Pullen J, Boyett J, et al: Acute lymphoid leukemia in adolescents: clinical and biologic features predict a poor prognosis—a Pediatric Oncology Group study. J Clin Oncol 6:34-43, 1988.
42. Ludwig WD, Bartram CR, Harbott J, et al: Phenotypic and genotypic heterogeneity in infant acute leukemia. I. Acute lymphoblastic leukemia. Leukemia 3:431-439, 1989.
43. Katz F, Malcolm S, Gibbons B, et al: Cellular and molecular studies on infant null acute lymphoblastic leukemia. Blood 71:1438-1447, 1988.
44. Katz F, Simpson E, Lam G, et al: Rearrangement of T-cell receptor and immunoglobulin heavy chain genes in childhood acute mixed lineage leukaemia. Leuk Res 12:955-960, 1988.
45. Goldberg JM, Silverman LB, Levy DE, et al: Childhood T-cell acute lymphoblastic leukemia: The Dana-Farber Cancer Institute Acute Lymphoblastic Leukemia Consortium Experience. J Clin Oncol 21:3616-3622, 2003.
46. Miller DR, Leikin S, Albo V, et al: Use of prognostic factors in improving the design and efficiency of clinical trials in childhood leukemia: Children's Cancer Study Group report. Cancer Treat Rep 64:381-392, 1980.
47. Miller DR, Coccia PF, Bleyer WA, et al: Early response to induction therapy as a predictor of disease-free survival and late recurrence of childhood acute lymphoblastic leukemia: a report from the Children's Cancer Study Group. J Clin Oncol 7:1807-1815, 1989.
48. Ortega JA, Nesbit ME Jr, Donaldson MH, et al: L-Asparaginase, vincristine, and prednisone for induction of first remission in acute lymphocytic leukemia. Cancer Res 37:535-540, 1977.
49. Aur RJ, Simone JV, Hustu HO, et al: Reduced pulsatile growth hormone secretion in children after therapy for acute lymphocytic leukemia. Cancer 29:381-391, 1972.
50. Rivera GK, Mauer AM: Controversies in the management of childhood acute lymphoblastic leukemia: treatment intensification, CNS leukemia, and prognostic factors. Semin Hematol 24:12-26, 1987.
51. Pui CH, Crist WM: Biology and treatment of acute lymphoblastic leukemia. J Pediatr 124:491-503, 1994.
52. Rivera GK, Raimondi SC, Hancock ML, et al: Improved outcome in childhood acute lymphoblastic leukaemia with reinforced early treatment and rotational combination chemotherapy. Lancet 337:61-66, 1991.
53. Schorin MA, Blattner S, Gelber RD, et al: Treatment of childhood acute lymphoblastic leukemia: results of Dana-Farber Cancer Institute/Children's Hospital Acute Lymphoblastic Leukemia Consortium Protocol 85-01. J Clin Oncol 12:740-747, 1994.
54. Aur RJ, Simone JV, Verzosa MS, et al: Childhood acute lymphocytic leukemia: study VIII. Cancer 42:2123-2134, 1978.
55. Mauer AM, Simone JV: The current status of the treatment of childhood acute lymphoblastic leukemia. Cancer Treat Rev 3:17-41, 1976.
56. Holland JF, Glidewell O: Chemotherapy of acute lymphocytic leukemia of childhood. Cancer 30:1480-1487, 1972.
57. Frei E III: Acute leukemia in children. Model for the development of scientific methodology for clinical therapeutic research in cancer. Cancer 53:2013-2025, 1984.
58. Bleyer WA, Sather HN, Nickerson HJ, et al: Monthly pulses of vincristine and prednisone prevent bone marrow and testicular relapse in low-risk childhood acute lymphoblastic leukemia: a report of the CCG-161 study by the Children's Cancer Study Group. J Clin Oncol 9:1012-1021, 1991.
59. Schrappe M, Reiter A, Henze G, et al: Prevention of CNS recurrence in childhood ALL: Results with reduced radiotherapy combined with CNS-directed chemotherapy in four consecutive ALL-BFM trials. Klin Paediatr 210:192-199, 1998.
60. Reiter A, Schrappe M, Ludwig WD, et al: Chemotherapy in 998 unselected childhood acute lymphoblastic leukemia patients. Results and conclusions of the multicenter trial ALL-BFM 86. Blood 84:3122-3133, 1994.
61. Winick NJ, Smith SD, Shuster J, et al: Treatment of CNS relapse in children with acute lymphoblastic leukemia: a Pediatric Oncology Group study. J Clin Oncol 11:271-278, 1993.
62. Bleyer WA, Poplack DG: Prophylaxis and treatment of leukemia in the central nervous system and other sanctuaries. Semin Oncol 12:131-148, 1989.
63. Ha CS, Chung WK, Koller CA, Cox JD: Role of radiation therapy to the brain in leukemic patients with cranial nerve palsies in the absence of radiologic findings. Leuk Lymphoma 32:497-503, 1999.
64. Kim TH, Hargreaves HK, Brynes RK, et al: Pretreatment testicular biopsy in childhood acute lymphocytic leukaemia. Lancet 2:657-658, 1981.
65. Nachman J, Plamer NF, Sather HN, et al: Open-wedge testicular biopsy in childhood acute lymphoblastic leukemia after two years of maintenance therapy: diagnostic accuracy and influence on outcome—a report from Children's Cancer Study Group. Blood 75:1051-1055, 1990.
66. Pui CH, Dahl GV, Bowman WP, et al: Elective testicular biopsy during chemotherapy for childhood leukaemia is of no clinical value. Lancet 2:410-412, 1985.
67. Kim TH, Hargreaves HK, Chan WC, et al: Sequential testicular biopsies in childhood acute lymphocytic leukemia. Cancer 57:1038-1041, 1986.
68. Kay H, Rankin A: Testicular irradiation in leukaemia (letter). Lancet 2:1115, 1981.
69. Nesbit ME, Sather H, Robinson LL, et al: Sanctuary therapy: a randomized trial of 724 children with previously untreated acute lymphoblastic leukemia: a report from Children's Cancer Study Group. Cancer Res 42:674-680, 1982.
70. Cap J, Foltinova A, Misikova Z: Prognostic significance of testicular relapse in boys with acute lymphoblastic leukemia. Neoplasma 39:115-118, 1992.
71. Dordelmann M, Reiter A, Zimmermann M, et al: Intermediate dose methotrexate is as effective as high dose methotrexate in preventing isolated testicular relapse in childhood acute lymphoblastic leukemia. J Pediatr Hematol Oncol 20:444-450, 1998.
72. Mirro J Jr, Wharam MD, Keizer H, et al: Testicular leukemic relapse: rate of regression and persistent disease after radiation therapy. J Pediatr 99:439-440, 1981.
73. Waber DP, Shapiro BL, Carpentieri SC, et al: Excellent therapeutic efficacy and minimal late neurotoxicity in children treated with 18 Grays of cranial radiation therapy for high-risk acute lymphoblastic leukemia: a 7-year follow-up study of the Dana-Farber Cancer Institute Consortium Protocol 87-01. Cancer 92:15-22, 2001.
74. Laxmi SN, Takahashi S, Matsumoto K, et al: Treatment-related disseminated necrotizing leukoencephalopathy with characteristic contrast enhancement of the white matter. Radiat Med 14:303-307, 1996.
75. Rubinstein LJ, Herman MM, Long TF, et al: Disseminated necrotizing leukoencephalopathy: a complication of treated central nervous system leukemia and lymphoma. Cancer 35:291-305, 1975.
76. Stubberfield TG, Byrne GC, Jones TW: Growth and growth hormone secretion after treatment for acute lymphoblastic leukemia in childhood. 18-Gy versus 24-Gy cranial irradiation. J Pediatr Hematol Oncol 17:167-171, 1995.
77. Neglia JP, Meadows AT, Robison LL, et al: Second neoplasms after acute lymphoblastic leukemia in childhood. N Engl J Med 325:1330-1336, 1991.

78. Kimball Dalton VM, Gelber RD, Li F, et al: Second malignancies in patients treated for childhood acute lymphoblastic leukemia. J Clin Oncol 16:2848-2853, 1998.
79. Nygaard R, Garwicz S, Haldorsen T, et al: Second malignant neoplasms in patients treated for childhood leukemia. A population-based cohort study from the Nordic countries. The Nordic Society of Pediatric Oncology and Hematology (NOPHO). Acta Paediatr Scand 80:1220-1228, 1991.
80. Blatt J, Serhins RJ, Niebruge D, et al: Leydig cell function in boys following treatment for testicular relapse of acute lymphoblastic leukemia. J Clin Oncol 3:1227-1231, 1985.
81. Brauner R, Czernichow P, Cramer P, et al: Leydig-cell function in children after direct testicular irradiation for acute lymphoblastic leukemia. N Engl J Med 309:25-28, 1983.
82. Bennett JM, Catovsky D, Daniel MT, et al: Proposal for the recognition of minimally differentiated acute myeloid leukaemia (AML-MO). Br J Haematol 78:325-329, 1991.
83. Woods WG, Kobrinsky N, Buckley J, et al: Intensively timed induction therapy followed by autologous or allogeneic bone marrow transplantation for children with acute myeloid leukemia or myelodysplastic syndrome: a Children's Cancer Group pilot study. J Clin Oncol 11:1448-1457, 1993.
84. Woods WG, Neudorf S, Gold S, et al: A comparison of allogeneic bone marrow transplantation, autologous bone marrow transplantation, and aggressive chemotherapy in children with acute myeloid leukemia in remission: a report from the Children's Cancer Group. Blood 97:56-62, 2001.
85. Creutzig U, Ritter J, Schellong G: Identification of two risk groups in childhood acute myelogenous leukemia after therapy intensification in study AML-BFM-83 as compared with study AML-BFM-78. AML-BFM Study Group. Blood 75:1932-1940, 1990.
86. Ravendranath Y, Steuber CP, Krischer J, et al: High-dose cytarabine for intensification of early therapy of childhood acute myeloid leukemia: a Pediatric Oncology Group study. J Clin Oncol 9:572-580, 1991.
87. Woods WG, Kobrinsky N, Buckley JD, et al: Timed-sequential induction therapy improves postremission outcome in acute myeloid leukemia: a report from the Children's Cancer Group. Blood 87:4979-4989, 1996.
88. Dusenbery K, Arthur D, Howells W, et al: Granulocytic sarcomas (chloromas) in pediatric patients with newly diagnosed acute myeloid leukemia. Proc Am Soc Clin Oncol 15:369A, 1996.
89. Dahl GV, Kalwinsky DK, Mirro J, et al: Allogeneic bone marrow transplantation in a program of intensive sequential chemotherapy for children and young adults with acute nonlymphocytic leukemia in first remission. J Clin Oncol 8:295-303, 1990.
90. Cassileth PA, Harrington DP, Appelbaum FR, et al: Chemotherapy compared with autologous or allogeneic bone marrow transplantation in the management of acute myeloid leukemia in first remission. N Engl J Med 339:1649-1656, 1998.
91. Appelbaum FR: Allogeneic hematopoietic stem cell transplantation for acute leukemia. Semin Oncol 24:114-123, 1997.
92. Dinndorf P, Bunin N: Bone marrow transplantation for children with acute myelogenous leukemia. J Pediatr Hematol Oncol 17:211-224, 1995.
93. Frassoni F, Labopin M, Gluckman E, et al: Results of allogeneic bone marrow transplantation for acute leukemia have improved in Europe with time—a report of the acute leukemia working party of the European group for blood and marrow transplantation (EBMT). Bone Marrow Transplant 17:13-18, 1996.
94. Graus F, Saiz A, Sierra J, et al: Neurologic complications of autologous and allogeneic bone marrow transplantation in patients with leukemia: a comparative study. Neurology 46:1004-1009, 1996.
95. Zittoun R, Suciu S, Watson M, et al: Quality of life in patients with acute myelogenous leukemia in prolonged first complete remission after bone marrow transplantation (allogeneic or autologous) or chemotherapy: a cross-sectional study of the EORTC-GIMEMA AML 8A trial. Bone Marrow Transplant 20:307-315, 1997.
96. Ries LAG, Miller BA, Hankey BF, et al: SEER cancer statistics review. 1973-1991, Bethesda, MD: National Institutes of Health, 1994.
97. Gurney JG, Severson RK, Davis S, Robinson LL: Incidence of cancer in children in the United States: sex-, race-, and 1-year age-specific rates by histologic type. Cancer 75:2186-2195, 1995.
98. Sandlund JT, Downing JR, Crist WM: Non-Hodgkin's lymphoma in childhood. N Eng J Med 334:1238-1248, 1996.
99. Murphy SB: Classification, staging, and end results of treatment of childhood non-Hodgkin's lymphoma: Dissimilarities from lymphomas in adults. Semin Oncol 7:332, 1980.
100. Magrath IT, Bhati K. Pathogenesis of small noncleaved cell lymphomas (Burkitt's lymphoma). *In* Magrath IT (ed): The non-Hodgkin's lymphomas. London: Arnold, 1997, pp 385-409.
101. Patte C, Auperin A, Michon J, et al: The Société Française d'Oncologie Pédiatrique LMB89 protocol: highly effective multiagent chemotherapy tailored to the tumor burden and initial response in 561 unselected children with B-cell lymphomas and L3 leukemia. Blood 97:3370-3379, 2001.
102. Harris NL, Jaffe ES, Stein H, et al: A revised European-American classification of lymphoid neoplasms: a proposal from the International Lymphoma Study Group. Blood 84:1361-1392, 1994.
103. Bernard A, Bounsell II, Reinherz EL, et al: Cell surface characterization of malignant T cells from lymphoblastic lymphoma using monoclonal antibodies. Evidence for phenotypic differences between malignant T cells from patients with acute lymphoblastic leukemia and lymphoblastic lymphoma. Blood 57:1105, 1981.
104. Kaneko Y, Frizzera G, Edamura S, et al: A novel translocation, t(2;5)(p23;q35), in childhood phagocytic large T-cell lymphoma mimicking malignant histiocytosis. Blood 73:806-813, 1989.
105. Hutchison RE, Berard CW, Shuster JJ, et al: B-cell lineage confers a favorable outcome among children and adolescents with large-cell lymphoma. A Pediatric Oncology Group Study. J Clin Oncol 13:2023-2032, 1995.
106. Murphy SB: Pediatric lymphomas: recent advances and commentary on K_i-positive anaplastic large-cell lymphomas of childhood. Ann Oncol 5:S31-S33, 1994.
107. Link MP, Shuster JJ, Donaldson SS, et al: Treatment of children and young adults with early-stage non-Hodgkin's lymphoma. N Engl J Med 337:1259-1266, 1997.
108. Suryanarayan K, Shuster JJ, Donaldson SS, et al: Treatment of localized primary non-Hodgkin's lymphoma of bone in children: a Pediatric Oncology Group study. J Clin Oncol 17:456-459, 1999.
109. Murphy SB, Hustu HO: A randomized trial of combined modality therapy of childhood non-Hodgkin's lymphoma. Cancer 45:630-637, 1980.
110. Loeffler JS, Leopold KA, Recht A, et al: Emergency prebiopsy radiation for mediastinal masses: impact on subsequent pathologic diagnosis and outcome. J Clin Oncol 4:716-721, 1986.

CHAPTER 71

PEDIATRIC HODGKIN'S LYMPHOMA

Melissa M. Hudson and Louis S. Constine

EPIDEMIOLOGY

Pediatric Hodgkin's lymphoma presenting in childhood and adolescence exhibits distinct epidemiologic features in relation to geographic distribution, gender, association with Epstein-Barr virus (EBV), and histologic subtype. For example, the incidence for children (in contrast to adults) is relatively higher in developing countries and in men; the nodular lymphocyte predominant subtype is also more frequent.

BIOLOGIC CHARACTERISTICS

Activation of EBV may play a role in the development of Hodgkin's lymphoma, with incidence varying by age, sex, ethnicity, histologic subtype, and regional economic level. The association is greater in populations of lower socioeconomic status, cases of mixed cellularity subtype, and cases occurring in children (or the elderly).

STAGING EVALUATION

Staging evaluation should include history and physical examination; complete blood count; blood chemistries; upright posteroanterior and lateral thoracic radiographs; computed tomography (CT) of the neck, chest, abdomen, and pelvis; functional nuclear imaging studies (Gallium-67 [^{67}Ga] or ^{18}fluoro-2-deoxyglucose [FDG] positron emission tomography [PET]); and bone marrow biopsies in selected patients with clinical stage III to IV disease or B symptoms. Staging laparotomy is rarely appropriate. Two thirds of children are stage I or II, and one third have B symptoms.

PRIMARY THERAPY

Contemporary treatment for children and adolescents with Hodgkin's lymphoma involves a risk-adapted approach based on the patient's presenting features at diagnosis. Factors in the risk assessment include the presence of B symptoms, mediastinal and peripheral lymph-node bulk, extranodal extension of disease to contiguous structures, number of involved nodal regions, Ann Arbor stage, and gender. Treatment of localized favorable disease most commonly uses ABVD (Adriamycin [doxorubicin], bleomycin, vinblastine, and dacarbazine) or derivative chemotherapy. Combinations derived from both ABVD and MOPP (nitrogen mustard, vincristine, procarbazine, and prednisone) still provide the most effective chemotherapy strategies for children and adolescents with intermediate- or high-risk disease presentations. In most effective regimens, low-dose radiation therapy (RT) is administered following chemotherapy to areas of bulk disease, or nodes involved at diagnosis. However, treatment with chemotherapy alone yields excellent results in subgroups of children with early-stage, favorable Hodgkin's lymphoma. Cure rates range from 85% to 100% in patients with localized favorable disease and 70% to 90% in those with advanced or unfavorable disease. Identification of prognostic features of patients who require radiation to optimize disease control is a focus of many ongoing pediatric trials.

TOXICITY

Children have a relatively increased risk, compared with adults, for cardiopulmonary compromise, musculoskeletal development because of RT, and subsequent malignant neoplasms. Consequently, treatment approaches are devised to minimize these risks.

Optimal treatment for pediatric Hodgkin's lymphoma achieves cure without long-term morbidity. In the past, treatment approaches were similar for adults and children; but irradiation of large volumes to high dose in physically immature children produced unacceptable musculoskeletal hypoplasia and cardiovascular dysfunction and increased the risk of subsequent malignancies. These concerns motivated the development of combined-modality therapy regimens in which cycles of chemotherapy replaced a portion of the radiation therapy (RT) in laparotomy-staged children.[1-6] Concurrent with advances in diagnostic imaging technology, investigators eventually abandoned surgical staging after demonstrating efficacy of the combined-modality treatment approach. In time, risk-adapted trials evolved that prescribed fewer cycles of multiagent chemotherapy and lower radiation doses and treatment volumes for patients with favorable clinical presentations. Definition of the risk groups for disease stratification can vary in different trials and has changed with therapeutic advances. In some trials gender-related predispositions also influence the treatment algorithm. For example, following cumulative doses of alkylating agent chemotherapy used in primary treatment regimens, boys exhibit a greater sensitivity to gonadal toxicity compared to girls, who generally maintain ovarian function unless chemotherapy is combined with abdominopelvic radiation.[7] Conversely, young women treated with thoracic radiation during puberty have a markedly increased risk of a breast cancer that is not observed in their male counterparts; but current approaches with more restricted radiation volumes are decreasing this risk.[8] Because of the spectrum of prognostic factors in pediatric Hodgkin's lymphoma, and the unique developmental and gender-related predispositions to therapy effects, no single treatment method is ideal for all patients. Contemporary treatment for children and adolescents with Hodgkin's lymphoma uses a risk-adapted approach that considers presenting risk features at diagnosis. Therapy duration and intensity are selected to maintain long-term remission with minimal treatment-related morbidity.

ETIOLOGY AND EPIDEMIOLOGY

Pediatric Hodgkin's lymphoma exhibits distinctive epidemiologic features. The childhood form, which presents in patients younger than 15 years of age, is associated with a marked male predominance, increasing family size, and decreasing socioeconomic status.[9,10] In developed countries Hodgkin's lymphoma is rarely diagnosed in children younger than 5 years of age. The young adult form, which presents in patients ages 15 to 34 years, is associated with a higher socioeconomic status in industrialized countries. Overall, the incidence is highest in developed countries (North America and Europe) and very rare in Asian populations; in childhood, however, some developing regions have relatively higher incidences.[11] In adolescents, the incidence between men and women is roughly equal, and most older adolescent patients are white. The risk for young adult Hodgkin's lymphoma decreases significantly with increased sibship size and birth order.[12,13] Specifically, the risk of Hodgkin's lymphoma in young adults is lower in individuals with multiple older, but not younger, siblings. Histologic subtypes also vary by age at presentation. Mixed cellularity subtype is more common in childhood Hodgkin's lymphoma, whereas nodular sclerosing subtype is more frequently observed in affluent societies.

Pediatric Hodgkin's lymphoma exhibits epidemiologic features similar to that seen with paralytic poliomyelitis. Delayed exposure to an infectious agent might increase the risk of the young adult form of Hodgkin's lymphoma, whereas early and intense exposure to an infectious agent might increase the risk for the childhood form of Hodgkin's lymphoma.[13] However, recent data also support an association between nursery school or daycare attendance and reduced risk of Hodgkin's lymphoma among young adults, supporting a model in which childhood exposure to common infections promotes maturation of cellular immunity.[14] The presence of high-antibody titers to Epstein-Barr virus (EBV), in situ hybridization evidence of EBV genomes in Reed-Sternberg cells, and EBV early RNA 1 and 2 (EBER1 and EBER2) sequences provide evidence that enhanced activation of EBV may play a role in the development of Hodgkin's lymphoma.[15,16] The incidence of EBV-associated Hodgkin's lymphoma varies by age, sex, ethnicity, histologic subtype, and regional economic level.[17,18] More specifically, an association with EBV is greater in populations of lower socioeconomic status, cases of mixed cellularity Hodgkin's lymphoma, and cases occurring in children or the elderly.[15]

BIOLOGIC CHARACTERISTICS/MOLECULAR BIOLOGY *(Refer to Adult Chapter)*

PATHOLOGY AND PATHWAYS OF SPREAD

The pathologic features of Hodgkin's lymphoma are similar in adults and children; however, the distribution of the histologic subtypes defined by the World Health Organization (WHO) may vary by age at presentation.[19] Nodular lymphocyte-predominant Hodgkin's lymphoma makes up almost 10% of pediatric cases. This histologic subtype usually presents as clinically localized disease and is more common among male and younger patients. Affecting approximately 70% of adolescents and children, nodular sclerosing Hodgkin's lymphoma represents the most common histologic subtype in pediatric cases.[20] Nodular sclerosing Hodgkin's lymphoma most commonly involves the lower cervical, supraclavicular, and mediastinal lymph nodes. The bulky growth of some involved nodal regions (particularly in the mediastinum) may be associated with persistent radiographic abnormalities even when the patient has fully responded to therapy. Mixed-cellularity Hodgkin's lymphoma is observed in approximately 15% of patients, is more common in children aged 10 years or younger, and more frequently presents as advanced disease with extranodal involvement.[20] Finally, lymphocyte-depleted Hodgkin's lymphoma is rare in children but relatively more common in patients infected with human immunodeficiency virus (HIV).[21] Lymphocyte-depleted disease in the HIV-positive patients is often associated with EBV. Lymphocyte-rich classical Hodgkin's lymphoma makes up approximately 5% of all Hodgkin's lymphoma and closely overlaps with the nodular lymphocyte-predominant (LP) subtype in presenting clinical features and prognosis.[22] The median age at presentation is, however, higher than for the latter (32 years); and there is a slightly higher incidence of mediastinal involvement and stage III disease at presentation.[23]

CLINICAL MANIFESTATIONS, PATIENT EVALUATION, AND STAGING

Clinical Manifestations

Pediatric patients most commonly present with painless cervical or supraclavicular lymphadenopathy. Mediastinal lymphadenopathy occurs in up to 66% of patients and may be associated with a nonproductive cough or other symptoms of tracheal or bronchial compression. Axillary or inguinal lymphadenopathy is less frequently seen as the first presenting sign. Primary infradiaphragmatic disease is rare in pediatric patients and occurs in fewer than 5% of cases. Splenic involvement occurs in 30% to 40% of pediatric patients with Hodgkin's lymphoma, whereas hepatic involvement is exceedingly rare. The pulmonary parenchyma, chest wall, pleura, and pericardium are the most commonly involved extranodal sites of disease. Bone marrow involvement at the time of initial presentation of Hodgkin's lymphoma is also uncommon in children. Approximately 65% of children have stage I and II disease and 35% have stage III and IV disease (Table 71-1).

Nonspecific systemic symptoms are often associated with lymphadenopathy and may include fatigue, anorexia, mild weight loss, and pruritus. The prognostically significant constitutional or *B* symptoms that are included in the staging assignment are unexplained fever with temperatures taken orally that are higher than 38°C, unexplained weight loss of 10% within 6 months preceding diagnosis, and drenching night sweats. B symptoms occur in approximately 33% of patients (see Table 71-1). Laboratory changes observed at presentation are nonspecific but may provide clues about the extent of disease. Hematologic abnormalities may include anemia, neutrophilic leukocytosis, lymphopenia, eosinophilia, and monocytosis. Anemia may be associated with the presence of advanced disease and may result from impaired mobilization of iron stores or less commonly from hemolysis. Several autoimmune disorders have been reported in patients with Hodgkin's lymphoma including nephrotic syndrome, autoimmune hemolytic anemia, autoimmune neutropenia, and immune thrombocytopenia. These conditions typically remit as the lymphoma is responding to therapy. Several acute phase reactants including erythrocyte sedimentation rate, serum copper, ferritin, and C-reactive protein levels may be elevated at diagnosis and useful in follow-up evaluations.

Patient Evaluation

Posteroanterior and lateral thoracic radiographs should be performed as soon as Hodgkin's lymphoma becomes part of the differential diagnosis to assess mediastinal involvement,

Table 71-1 Pediatric Hodgkin's Lymphoma: Demographic and Clinical Characteristics at Presentation

	CHILDREN*,† (%) 1985	ADULTS† (%) 1912
TOTAL PATIENTS		
<10 y	360 (18.1)	
≥10 y	1625 (81.9)	1912 (100.0)
GENDER		
Male	1100 (55.4)	1147 (60.0)
Female	885 (44.6)	765 (40.0)
HISTOLOGY		
Lymphocyte predominant	192 (9.7)	96 (5.0)
Lymphocyte depleted	—	115 (6.0)
Mixed cellularity	307 (15.5)	325 (17.0)
Nodular sclerosing	1431 (72.1)	1377 (72.0)
Not classified	55 (2.8)	
B SYMPTOMS		
Present	564 (28.4)	612 (32.0)
Absent	1421 (71.6)	1300 (68.0)
STAGE‡		
I	229 (11.5)	210 (11.0)
II	1078 (54.3)	899 (47.0)
III	391 (19.7)	593 (31.0)
IV	287 (14.5)	210 (11.0)

*Data taken from Ruhl et al.[28] and Nachman et al.[29]
†Data taken from Cleary et al.[111]
‡Data derived from both pathologically and clinically staged patients.
y, year.

airway patency, and other intrathoracic structures. This is particularly important if sedation is planned for diagnostic procedures. An excisional lymph node biopsy is the preferred diagnostic procedure, because it permits evaluation of the malignant Hodgkin's Reed-Sternberg cells within the background of characteristic architectural changes of the specific histologic subtypes. All nodal regions, including Waldeyer's ring, should be assessed by careful physical examination. An upright chest radiograph should be obtained to assess mediastinal bulk that is defined by mediastinal lymphadenopathy measuring 33% or more of the maximum intrathoracic cavity. Computed tomography (CT) is most frequently used to evaluate the nodal regions in the neck, axilla, thoracic and abdominal cavities, and pelvis. Administration of both oral and intravenous contrast agents is required for CT to accurately distinguish lymphadenopathy from other infradiaphragmatic structures. Organ size is an unreliable indicator of lymphomatous involvement in the liver or spleen, because tumor deposits may be less than 1 cm in diameter and not visualized by diagnostic imaging modalities. Increased size of either organ can, of course, be caused by nonmalignant causes. The presence of hypodense lesions by CT and/or abnormal functional avidity by gallium or positron emission tomography (PET) provides stronger evidence of tumor infiltration in these organs, though is not unequivocal.

Functional nuclear-imaging studies are appropriately used in patients with Hodgkin's lymphoma as a diagnostic and monitoring modality. Gallium-67 (^{67}Ga) is useful in the evaluation of supradiaphragmatic Hodgkin's lymphoma, but its low resolution and physiologic biodistribution limit evaluation of the abdominal and pelvic lymph nodes. PET scanning uses uptake of the radioactive glucose analogue, ^{18}fluoro-2-deoxyglucose (FDG) as a correlate of tumor activity. Compared to gallium scanning, PET has a higher resolution, better dosimetry, less intestinal activity, and the potential for quantifying activity. Fused positron emission tomography/computed tomography (PET-CT) offers the advantage of integrating functional and anatomic tumor characteristics. Residual or persistent gallium or FDG avidity appears to be useful in predicting prognosis and the need for additional therapy in post-treatment evaluation.[24-26] Because extranodal disease involving the bones and bone marrow is relatively uncommon in children, these staging evaluations can be omitted in patients presenting with localized and asymptomatic disease. A technetium-99 bone scan with corresponding plain radiographs of abnormal areas should be reserved for the child who has bone pain, a serum alkaline-phosphatase concentration elevated beyond that expected for age, or extranodal disease identified by other staging evaluations. A bone marrow biopsy should be performed in any patient with clinical stage III or IV disease or B symptoms. Because the pattern of infiltration in the bone marrow may be diffuse or focal and is often accompanied by reversible marrow fibrosis, a bone marrow aspirate alone is inadequate to assess the marrow for disease.

Staging

Physical examination and diagnostic imaging evaluations are used in pediatric patients to designate a clinical stage according to the Ann Arbor staging system.[27] In the past, pathologic staging, based on the findings of a staging laparotomy, including splenectomy, was routinely used to assess infradiaphragmatic disease. The increasing use of systemic therapy in children and the development of more accurate diagnostic imaging modalities eventually led to the routine use of clinical staging and abandonment of surgical staging. Currently, surgical staging, most typically nodal sampling without splenectomy, is pursued only if the anticipated findings will significantly alter the treatment plan.

PRIMARY THERAPY

Risk-Adapted Treatment Approach

Contemporary treatment for children and adolescents with Hodgkin's lymphoma involves a risk-adapted approach based on the patient's presenting features at diagnosis.[28-35] Factors included in the risk assessment may vary across studies; but they most often include the presence of *B* symptoms, mediastinal and peripheral lymph node bulk, extranodal extension of disease to contiguous structures, number of involved nodal regions, Ann Arbor stage, and gender. A favorable clinical presentation is typically characterized because of localized (stage I/II) nodal involvement in the absence of B symptoms and nodal bulk. Mediastinal bulk (see "Patient Evaluation") is designated when the ratio of the maximum measurement of the mediastinal mass to intrathoracic cavity on an upright chest radiograph is 33% or more. The definition of peripheral lymph node bulk has also varied across studies from 4 cm to 10 cm. Fewer than three or four involved nodal regions are considered favorable. In some risk-adapted treatment protocols, patients with localized disease presenting with unfavorable features are designated intermediate in risk and treated similarly to those with advanced-stage disease; whereas in others a therapy intermediate in intensity is prescribed. The criteria for unfavorable clinical presentations has also differed among studies, but most often it is comprised of the presence of B symptoms, bulky lymphadenopathy, hilar lymphadenopathy, more than 3 to 4 involved nodal regions, extranodal extension to contiguous structures, or advanced-stage (IIIB-IV) disease. The results of recent trials indicate that children and adolescents with early-stage or favorable presentations of Hodgkin's lymphoma are excellent candidates for reduced therapy.[28,29,32,33] Ongoing trials are evaluating whether intensification of therapy improves outcomes in patients with intermediate- and high-risk presentations.

Although not widely used to guide therapy assignment in pediatric trials, other factors such as gender, age at diagnosis, and histology are most definitely considered in individual patients. The trials organized by the German-Austrian Pediatric Oncology Group (GPOH) have been unique in their aims to prospectively evaluate gender-based therapy.[28] Long-term follow-up of the GPOH 90 and 95 studies demonstrate that the substitution of etoposide for procarbazine in the vincristine, prednisone, procarbazine, and doxorubicin (OPPA) regimen does not compromise disease-free survival and provides less potential risk for gonadal toxicity.[28,34] Although age at presentation has not been used as a criterion to assign therapy in prospective trials, reports describing outcomes after treatment with chemotherapy alone stress the benefits of this approach in younger children at higher risk of radiation-related toxicity.[29,31] Lastly, anecdotal reports of excellent outcome in patients with completely resected nodular lymphocyte–predominant disease have motivated the development of a Children's Oncology Group trial targeting this diagnostic subtype.[34,36,37] Patients with completely resected disease will be enrolled for observation alone; patients with localized, persistent disease will have brief combination chemotherapy with cyclophosphamide, vincristine, doxorubicin, and prednisone. A summary of trials in children with early- and advanced-stage Hodgkin's lymphoma is provided in Tables 71-2 and 71-3.

Chemotherapy Regimens and Radiation Therapy

MOPP and Derivative Chemotherapy

The prototype alkylator combination that provided the first effective systemic therapy for Hodgkin's lymphoma was nitrogen mustard, vincristine, procarbazine and prednisone (MOPP).[38] Follow-up studies of MOPP-treated survivors confirmed that secondary acute myeloid leukemia (s-AML) and infertility resulted from the alkylating agents in the regimen and exhibited a dose-dependent relationship.[39] Subsequently, investigators developed a variety of MOPP-derivative regimens in an effort to reduce the risk of secondary leukemogenesis and gonadal toxicity.

The risk of secondary leukemia following alkylating agent chemotherapy peaks in frequency in the first 5 to 10 years after treatment and plateaus to less than 2% after 10 years from diagnosis.[40] Older age at treatment, history of splenectomy, presentation with advanced disease, treatment with high cumulative doses of alkylating agents, and history of relapse have been reported to predispose to this complication.[40-45] Some alkylating agents are more potent leukemogens than others; the 15-year cumulative incidence of s-AML is 4% to 8% after MOPP-based therapy compared to less than 1% with cyclophosphamide, Oncovin (vincristine), procarbazine, prednisone (COPP)-based therapy that substitutes cyclophosphamide for nitrogen mustard.[46] Pediatric protocols that limit the total dose of alkylating agents or substitute other less-leukemogenic drugs, such as cyclophosphamide, for mechlorethamine, have been associated with very low incidence rates of s-AML.[46]

Gonadal injury is common in pediatric patients treated with MOPP and its derivative combinations. Azoospermia is typically irreversible in men treated with six or more cycles of MOPP-like therapy.[39,47] However, germ cell function may be preserved if treatment is limited to no more than three cycles of alkylator therapy.[48] In contrast, most young women will maintain or resume menses after a temporary period of amenorrhea following treatment including alkylating agents.[47] Ovarian transposition and shielding reduces the incidence of gonadal injury in young women requiring pelvic radiation, but these patients will experience a higher risk of premature menopause.

ABVD and Derivative Chemotherapy

The Adriamycin (doxorubicin), bleomycin, vinblastine, and dacarbazine (ABVD) combination provided a systemic therapy that produced superior disease-free survival compared to MOPP and was not associated with an excess risk of secondary leukemia or infertility.[4,49] However, follow-up of patients treated with the ABVD regimen established its association with cardiopulmonary toxicity that was enhanced with the addition of thoracic radiation.[4] Many ABVD derivatives soon followed, aiming to reduce the risk of these sequelae.

Anthracycline agents are an important component of chemotherapy regimens for children with Hodgkin's lymphoma because of their significant lympholytic effects. In adults the cumulative incidence of cardiomyopathy increases significantly after anthracycline exceeds 550 mg/m^2; children may be at increased risk of cardiac dysfunction at lower cumulative doses.[50-52] Other risk factors for anthracycline toxicity identified in studies of childhood leukemia survivors include younger age at treatment (especially younger than 5 years old) and female gender. Combination treatment with chest radiation or other cardiotoxic agents such as amsacrine or cyclophosphamide may also enhance risk of cardiac dysfunction.[52-56] Because treatment protocols for pediatric Hodgkin's lymphoma frequently include chest radiation or other chemotherapeutic agents with potential cardiotoxicity, most regimens limit doses of anthracycline agents to fewer than 200 mg/m^2, particularly for patients with favorable-risk disease presentations.

Bleomycin in the ABVD regimen increases the risk of pulmonary toxicity most commonly manifested as pulmonary fibrosis and chronic pneumonitis.[57] Thoracic radiation may augment this risk. Patients at highest risk of pulmonary complications are those treated with cumulative bleomycin doses exceeding 400 U/m^2, which far exceed doses used in pediatric regimens for Hodgkin's lymphoma. Contemporary protocols use bleomycin doses in the range of 60 to 100 U/m^2; these cumulative exposures are usually associated with asymptomatic pulmonary restriction and diffusion deficits in long-term survivors, some of which will improve over time.[58,59] Serial monitoring of pulmonary function during therapy and withholding bleomycin doses in patients exhibiting significant declines in pulmonary function (20% or more from baseline) may reduce the risk of further pulmonary injury and does not appear to compromise disease control.[60]

Chemotherapy Combinations Including Etoposide

Etoposide has been increasingly incorporated into treatment regimens for pediatric Hodgkin's lymphoma over the last few decades. This agent is used in risk-adapted regimens for favorable patients as an effective alternative to alkylating agents in an effort to reduce gonadal toxicity.[30,33,35,61,62] Etoposide has been added to alkylating and anthracycline chemotherapy in regimens for advanced and unfavorable patients to enhance treatment response. Treatment with topoisomerase-II inhibitors like etoposide and doxorubicin produces an excess risk

Table 71-2 Treatment Results for Early Pediatric Hodgkin's Lymphoma

Reference	Group or Institution	Number of Patients	Stage	Chemotherapy	Radiation (Gy), Field	SURVIVAL (%) DFS, EFS, or RFS	Overall	Follow-up Interval (y)
COMBINED MODALITY TRIALS								
Dörffel, 2003[34]	GPOH-HD 95	408	I-IIA	2 OPPA/OEPA	20-35, IF for PR;	94.0	97.0 (all)	7.5
		269	II_EA, IIB, IIIA	2 OPPA/OEPA + 2 COPP	no RT if CR	87.0		
Shankar, 1997[87]	Royal Marsden	125	II	6-10 ChlVPP	35, IF	85.0	92.0	10.0
Shankar et al., 1998[61]	Royal Marsden	46	I-III	8 VEEP	30-35, IF	82.0	93.0	5.0
Landman-Parker	SFOP	171	I-II	4 VBVP, good responders	20, IF	91.0	97.5	5.0
et al., 2000[33]	MDH-90	27	I-II	4VBVP + 1-2 OPPA, poor responders	20, IF	78.0		5.0
Hudson et al., 1993[60]	St. Jude	58	CS II/III	4-5 COP(P)/3-4 ABVD	20, IF	96.0/97.0	96.0/100.0	5.0
Hunger, 1997[85]	Stanford	44	CS/PSI-III	3 MOPP/3 ABVD	15-25.5, IF	100.0	100.0	10.0
Donaldson et al., 2002[32]	Stanford/St. Jude/ Dana Farber Consortium	110	CS I/II†	4 VAMP	15-25.5, IF	93.0	99.0	5.0
Hudson, 2004[84]	Stanford/St. Jude/ Dana Farber Consortium	77	I	3 VAMP/3 COP (2 cycles/RT/2 cycles/ RT/2 cycles/ RT)	15, IF for CR; 25.5,	100.0	92.7 (all)	5.8
			II		IF for PR	78.4		
Nachman et al., 2002[29]	USA-CCG	294	CS IA/B, IIA*	4 COPP/ABV	21, IF	97.0	100.0	3.0
CHEMOTHERAPY ALONE TRIALS								
Lobo-Sanahuja et al., 1994[72]	Costa Rica	52	CS IA-IIIA	6 CVPP	None	90.0	100.0	5.0
Sackmann-Muriel	GATLA	10	CS IA, IIA	3 CVPP	None	86.0		6.7
et al., 1997[62]		16	CS IB, IIB	6 CVPP	None	87.0		6.7
Nachman et al., 2002[29]	USA-CCG	106	CS IA/B, IIA†	4 COPP/ABV	None	91.0	100.0	3.0

*Without adverse features.

†With adverse features.

(Adverse disease features comprise one or more of the following: hilar adenopathy; involvement of >4 nodal regions; mediastinal tumor with diameter ≥ one-third of the chest diameter; node or nodal aggregate with a diameter > 10 cm.)

ABVD, Adriamycin (doxorubicin), bleomycin, vinblastine, and dacarbazine; CCG, Children's Cancer Group; ChlVPP, chlorambucil, vinblastine, procarbazine, and prednisolone; COP, cyclophosphamide, Oncovin (vincristine), and procarbazine; COPP, cyclophosphamide, Oncovin (vincristine), prednisone, and procarbazine; COPP/ABV, cyclophosphamide, Oncovin (vincristine), procarbazine, prednisone/Adriamycin (doxorubicin), bleomycin, and vinblastine; CR, complete response; CS, clinical stage; DFS, disease-free survival; EFS, event-free survival; IF, involved field; GATLA, Grupo Argentino de Tratamiento de Leucemia Aguda; GPOH-HD, German-Austrian Pediatric Oncology Group-Hodgkin's disease; MOPP, mechlorethamine, vincristine, procarbazine, and prednisone; OEPA, Oncovin (vincristine), etoposide, prednisone, and Adriamycin (doxorubicin); OPPA, Oncovin (vincristine), procarbazine, prednisolone, and Adriamycin (doxorubicin); PR, partial response; PS, pathologic stage; R, regional; RFS, relapse-free survival; RT, radiation therapy; SFOP, French Society of Pediatric Oncology; VAMP, vinblastine, doxorubicin, methotrexate, and prednisone; VBVP, vinblastine, bleomycin, etoposide, and prednisone; VEEP, vincristine, etoposide, epirubicin, and prednisolone; y, year.

Table 71-3 Treatment Results for Advanced Pediatric Hodgkin's Lymphoma

Reference	Group or Institution	Number of Patients	Stage	Chemotherapy	Radiation (Gy), Field	Survival (%) DFS, EFS, or RFS	Survival (%) Overall	Follow-up Interval (y)
COMBINED MODALITY TRIALS								
Dörffel, 2003[34]	GPOH-HD 95	341	II_EA, III_EA/B, IIIB, IVA/B	2 OPPA/OEPA + 4 COPP	20-35, IF for PR; no RT if CR	83	97 (all)	7.5
Mauch, 1983[86]	Joint Center/Harvard	83	IA-IIIB	6 MOPP	25-40	77	95	11
Shankar, 1997[87]	Royal Marsden	80	III	6-10 ChlVPP	35, IF	73	84	10
		27	IV	6-10 ChlVPP	35, IF	38	71	
Hudson, 1993[60]	St. Jude	27	CS IV	4-5 COP(P)/3-4 ABVD	20 Gy, IF	85	86	5
Hunger, 1997[85]	Stanford	13	III-IV	3 MOPP/3 ABVD	15-25.5, IF	69	85	10
Friedmann, 2002[30]	Stanford/St. Jude/ Dana Farber Consortium	56	CS I/II bulky (n = 26), CS III/IV (n = 30)	6 VEPA	15-25.5, IF	67.8	81.9	5
Hudson, 2004[84]	Stanford/St. Jude/ Dana Farber Consortium	82	III	3 VAMP/ 3 COP (followed by consolidative RT)	15, IF for CR; 25.5, IF for PR/NR	68.9	92.7 (all)	5.8
			IV			68.5		
Fryer, 1990[4]	USA-CCG	64	PS III-IV	12 ABVD	21, R	87	89	3
Weiner, 1997[2]	USA-POG	80	CS/PS IIB, $IIIA_2$, IIIB, IV	4 MOPP/4 ABVD	21, EF	80	87	5
Nachman, 2002[29]	USA-CCG	394	CS I/II*, CS IIB,	6 COPP/ABV	21, IF	87	95	3
		141	CS III	COPP/ABV + CHOP + Ara-C/ VP-16	21, IF	90	100	
			CS IV					
CHEMOTHERAPY ALONE TRIALS								
Atra, 2002[31]	UKCCSG	67	CS IV	6-8 ChlVPP	None	55.2	80.8	5
Ekert, 1988[68]	Australia/New Zealand	53	CS IV	6-8 MOPP or 6 ChlVPP	None	92	94	4
Ekert, 1999[83]	Australia/New Zealand	53	CS I-IV	5-6 VEEP	None	78	92	5
Sripada, 1995[88]	Madras, India	43	CS IIB-IVB	6 COPP/ABV	None	90		5
Van den Berg, 1997[73]	The Netherlands	21	CS I-IV (<4 cm node)	6 MOPP	None	91	100	5
		17		6 ABVD		70	94	
		21	CS I-IV	3 MOPP/3 ABVD		91	91	
Hutchinson, 1998[6]	USA-CCG	57	PS III/IV	6 MOPP/6 ABVD	None	77	84	4
Nachman, 2002[29]	USA-CCG	394	CS I/II*, CS IIB, CS III	6 COPP/ABV	None	83	100	3
		141	CS IV	COPP/ABV + CHOP + Ara-C/VP-16	None	81	94	
Weiner, 1997[2]	USA-POG	81	CS IIB, III_2A, IIIB, IV	4 MOPP/ 4 ABVD	None	79	96	5

*With adverse features.

(Adverse disease features comprise one or more of the following: hilar adenopathy; involvement of >4 nodal regions; mediastinal tumor with diameter ≥ one-third of the chest diameter; node or nodal aggregate with a diameter > 10 cm.)

ABVD, Adriamycin (doxorubicin), bleomycin, vinblastine, and dacarbazine; ara-C, Arabinosylcytosine; CCG, Children's Cancer Group; ChlVPP, chlorambucil, vinblastine, procarbazine, and prednisolone; CHOP, cyclophosphamide, Adriamycin (doxorubicin), Oncovin (vincristine), and prednisone; COP, cyclophosphamide, Oncovin (vincristine), and prednisone; COP(P), cyclophosphamide, Oncovin (vincristine), prednisone, and procarbazine; COPP/ABV, cyclophosphamide, Oncovin (vincristine), procarbazine, prednisone/Adriamycin (doxorubicin), bleomycin, and vinblastine; CR, complete response; CS, clinical stage; CVPP, cyclophosphamide, vinblastine, procarbazine, and prednisone; DFS, disease-free survival; EF, extended field; EFS, event-free survival; GPOH-HD, German-Austrian Pediatric Oncology Group-Hodgkin's disease; IF, involved field; MOPP, mechlorethamine, vincristine, procarbazine, and prednisone; NR, no response; OEPA, Oncovin (vincristine), etoposide, prednisone, and Adriamycin (doxorubicin); OPPA, Oncovin (vincristine), procarbazine, prednisolone and Adriamycin (doxorubicin); POG, Pediatric Oncology Group; PR, partial response; PS, pathologic stage; R, regional; RFS, relapse-free survival; RT, radiation therapy; UKCCSG, United Kingdom Children Cancer Study Group; VEEP, vincristine, etoposide, epirubicin, and prednisolone; VEPA, vinblastine, etoposide, prednisone, and Adriamycin (doxorubicin); y, year.

of s-AML that differs in epidemiology and biology from alkylator-related s-AML.[63] s-AML that occurs in association with topoisomerase-II inhibitors is characterized by a brief time of onset from primary diagnosis, absence of a preceding myelodysplastic phase, monoblastic and myelomonoblastic histology, and translocations involving the *MLL* gene at chromosome band 11q23. Studies of childhood leukemia patients suggest that intermittent weekly or twice weekly dosing schedules may result in transforming mutations of myeloid progenitor cells by epipodophyllotoxins.[64] A relationship between leukemogenic activity and cumulative epipodophyllotoxin dose could not be established in an evaluation of s-AML cases developing in patients treated with multiagent chemotherapy regimens including epipodophyllotoxins, alkylating agents, doxorubicin, and dactinomycin for pediatric solid tumors.[63] However, the risk of s-AML following treatment with regimens that restricted etoposide doses to 5.0 gm/m^2 or less did not exceed that associated with other agents used in solid tumor regimens.[63] In general, these data support the relative safety of using limited doses of etoposide, but reports of s-AML in patients receiving etoposide for treatment of favorable pediatric Hodgkin's lymphoma raise concerns about whether this agent should be avoided in favorable disease presentations.[33]

Radiotherapy Considerations

The curability of pediatric Hodgkin's lymphoma and the vulnerability of the developing child to both radiation and chemotherapy are critical issues in appropriately integrating radiation into the complex treatment algorithms currently used. Most newly diagnosed children will be treated with risk-adapted chemotherapy alone or combined-modality therapy including low-dose, involved-field radiation. Full-dose, extended-field RT using techniques that are standard for adults has essentially been abandoned because of concerns primarily relating to growth inhibition, cardiac toxicity, and second malignant neoplasms. Historically, the results of treatment with RT alone were superior at institutions that treated many Hodgkin's lymphoma patients. Although different institutions and radiation oncologists may use slightly different treatment techniques, underlying principles and, in fact, most of the technical details remain constant.[65] Because most children are treated on institutional (or multi-institutional) studies, the radiation oncologist should confirm all aspects of the diagnostic workup and staging; and they must also understand study requirements to deliver appropriate radiation. In a recent review of the DAL-HD-90 trial (German-Austrian pediatric multicenter trial), up-front centralized patient review entered into the study altered the treatment approach in a large number of children.[66]

Volume

Most children with Hodgkin's lymphoma are treated with combined chemotherapy and low-dose involved-field radiation. Meticulously and judiciously designed fields are necessary for maximum success in terms of both disease control and minimal tissue damage. The definitions of such fields depend on the anatomy of the region in terms of lymph node distribution, patterns of disease extension into regional areas, and consideration for match-line problems should disease recur. Involved fields typically should include not just the identifiably abnormal lymph nodes, but the entire lymph node region containing the involved nodes (Table 71-4). The traditional definitions of lymph node regions can be helpful, but are not necessarily sufficient. For example, the cervical and supraclavicular lymph nodes are generally treated when abnormal nodes are located anywhere within this area; this is consistent with the anatomic definition of lymph node regions used for staging purposes. However, the hila are usually irradiated when the mediastinum is involved, despite the fact that the hila and mediastinum are separate lymph node regions. Similarly, the supraclavicular fossa (SCV) is often treated when the axilla or the mediastinum is involved, and the ipsilateral external iliac nodes are often treated when the inguinal nodes are involved. However, in both situations take care to shield relevant normal tissues to the degree possible, such as the breast in the former situation and ovaries in the latter. Moreover, the decision to treat the axilla or mediastinum without the SCV, and the inguinal nodes without the iliacs, might be appropriate depending on the size and distribution of involved nodes at presentation. In a very young child (younger than age 5 years), consideration may be given to treating bilateral areas (e.g., both sides of the neck) to avoid growth asymmetry. However, this is less of a concern with low-radiation doses, and unilateral fields are usually appropriate if the disease is unilateral. Efforts to exclude unnecessary normal tissues are always important, such as breast tissue in a child with isolated mediastinal disease and no axillary involvement.

Table 71-4 **Involved Field Radiation Guidelines**

Involved Node(s)	Radiation Field
Cervical	Neck and infraclavicular/supraclavicular†
Supraclavicular	Neck and infraclavicular/supraclavicular ± axilla
Axilla	Axilla ± infraclavicular/supraclavicular
Mediastinum	Mediastinum, hila, infraclavicular/supraclavicular*†
Hila	Hila, mediastinum
Spleen	Spleen ± para-aortics
Para-aortics	Para-aortics ± spleen
Iliac	Iliacs, inguinal, femoral
Inguinal	External iliac, inguinal, femoral
Femoral	External iliac, inguinal, femoral

*Prechemotherapy volume is treated except for lateral borders of the mediastinal field, which is postchemotherapy.

†Upper cervical region not treated if supraclavicular involvement is extension of the mediastinal disease.

Treatment of *involved supradiaphragmatic fields* or a *mantle field* requires precision because of the distribution of lymph nodes and the critical adjacent normal tissues. These fields can be simulated with the arms up over the head or down with hands on the hips. The former pulls the axillary lymph nodes away from the lungs, allowing greater lung shielding. However, the axillary lymph nodes then move into the vicinity of the humeral heads, which should be blocked in growing children. Thus the position chosen involves weighing concerns regarding lymph nodes, lung, and humeral heads. Attempts should be made to exclude or position breast tissue under the lung and axillary blocking.

When the decision is made to include some or all of a critical organ in the radiation field, such as liver, kidney, or heart, normal tissue constraints, depending on the chemotherapy used and patient age, are critical. Thus the width of a mediastinal field is generally based on the postchemotherapy residual disease, whereas the cephalad-caudad dimension respects the original disease extent. As previously stated, humeral head blocks are appropriate unless bulky axillary adenopathy is thereby shielded. Laryngeal and occipital blocks are also used unless disease is located in the vicinity of these structures; these blocks can be placed at the beginning of treatment or after some portion of it. Depending on the response of the disease to chemotherapy and the dose administered, field reductions may be possible. The entire heart or lungs are rarely treated above doses of 10 to 16 Gy, depending on the distribution of disease and chemotherapy used. Specific treatment decisions are protocol dependent because some children treated for advanced-stage Hodgkin's disease will receive RT only to areas of initial bulk disease or postchemotherapy residual disease. However, this approach remains investigational and involved-field radiation therapy (IFRT) may remain the appropriate treatment.

When treating the *subdiaphragmatic region*, a treatment-planning CT or diagnostic information obtained from the CT or MRI helps draw the blocks. When treating the *pelvis*, special attention must be given to the ovaries and testes. The ovaries should be relocated, and marked with surgical clips, laterally along the iliac wings or centrally behind the uterus. In this manner appropriate shielding may be used. The testes receive 5% to 10% of the administered pelvic dose, which is sufficient to cause transient or permanent azoospermia, depending on the total pelvic dose. The greatest shielding can be afforded to the testes if the patient is placed in a frog-legged position with an individually constructed testes shield. If multileaf collimation is available, the multileaf can be placed over the testes, additionally decreasing the transmitted dose. Clearly, careful planning and judgment are necessary.

As previously stated, RT for unfavorable and advanced Hodgkin's lymphoma is variable and protocol dependent. Although IFRT remains the standard when patients are treated with combined-modality therapy, restricting RT to areas of initial bulk disease (generally defined as 5 cm or more at the time of disease presentation) or postchemotherapy residual disease (generally defined as 2 cm or more, or residual PET avidity) is under investigation.

Dose

In the setting of combined therapy, certainly the intensity of the chemotherapy is important to consider in the choice of the radiation dose and volume. However, doses of 15 to 25 Gy are typical with shrinking fields and boosts individualized. In the tables summarizing recent clinical trials for early- and advanced-stage Hodgkin's lymphoma (see Tables 71-2 and 71-3), the radiation doses selected to complement the chemotherapy regimen are provided. In general, doses of more than 25 Gy are uncommon in the pediatric setting. Of interest in this regard is the recently analyzed DAL-HD-90 trial, in which doses of 20 to 25 Gy were administered in combination with vincristine, prednisone, procarbazine, and doxorubicin (OPPA) or OEPA, with or without COPP. The radiation doses administered were 20 to 25 Gy, with a local boost of 5 to 10 Gy for insufficient remission following chemotherapy. Tumor burden, indicated by bulky disease or number of involved nodes, proved not to be prognostically significant because of the relatively high doses used for bulk disease.[67] Most current treatment approaches for children would not include radiation doses of this magnitude.

Treatment Approaches

Chemotherapy Alone versus Combined with Radiation Therapy

Non–cross-resistant combination chemotherapy alone is well established as an effective modality for the treatment of pediatric Hodgkin's lymphoma.[1,2,31,62,68-73] This treatment approach eliminates the risk of radiation-induced growth complications, thyroid and cardiopulmonary dysfunction, and solid tumor carcinogenesis. However, the higher-cumulative doses of anthracyclines, alkylating agents, and bleomycin chemotherapy increase the risk of cardiopulmonary toxicity, infertility, and leukemogenesis and may be less effective as combined-modality therapy for treatment of bulky nodal disease. Chemotherapy alone trials have been limited by their small numbers of patients, nonrandom treatment assignments, lack of long-term follow-up related to disease control, and late-treatment sequelae. Despite these deficiencies, identification of clinical factors predicting an optimal outcome following treatment with chemotherapy alone remains an important objective of many ongoing trials because of the desire to avoid late radiation sequelae.

Investigators from North American pediatric cooperative groups have undertaken three longitudinal controlled trials to evaluate chemotherapy see alone versus combined-modality therapy in pediatric Hodgkin's lymphoma.[2,6,29] The first two trials failed to show a statistically significant advantage in event-free survival or overall survival with the addition of RT to non–cross-resistant chemotherapy. The Children's Cancer Group compared 12 cycles of alternating MOPP/ABVD to 6 cycles of ABVD plus low-dose (21 Gy) radiation.[6] Event-free and overall survival suggested a survival advantage for the combined-modality group (90% 4-year event-free survival) over the chemotherapy-alone group (84% 4-year event-free survival), but this difference was statistically insignificant. In a Pediatric Oncology Group trial, adding low-dose radiation to four cycles of alternating MOPP and ABVD chemotherapy did not improve disease-free or overall survival.[2] However, statistical and quality-assurance issues produced problems with interpretation of these data. Unfortunately, the findings of both studies are irrelevant to present-day investigators because the treatments evaluated included the more leukemogenic MOPP-based therapy and an excessive number of treatment cycles.

Using a more contemporary regimen, the Children's Cancer Group compared chemotherapy alone with the COPP/ABV hybrid to combined modality therapy including low-dose, involved-field radiation.[29] Clinical risk features including the presence of B symptoms, hilar lymphadenopathy, mediastinal and peripheral lymph node bulk, and the number of involved nodal regions determined treatment assignment. Patients who achieved a complete response to chemotherapy were eligible to be randomized to receive low-dose, involved-field radiation or no further therapy. The trial was prematurely terminated because patients treated with chemotherapy alone had a significantly higher number of relapses. The difference in outcome was most marked for stage IV patients in whom combined-modality therapy produced a 3-year 90% event-free survival compared to 81% in those randomized to receive chemotherapy alone.

In a nonrandomized trial that omitted radiation for patients achieving a complete remission with chemotherapy, German-Austrian pediatric oncology investigators reported a similar advantage for patients treated with radiation consolidation following combination chemotherapy in the recent GPOG-HD 95 trial.[34] In this study patients treated with RT after partial response to combination chemotherapy had a superior relapse-free survival (93%) compared to those who achieved a complete response with chemotherapy alone (89%). The difference in outcomes for patients treated with combined modality therapy versus chemotherapy alone was significant for patients treated for advanced- and intermediate-risk disease but not early-stage disease.

Overall, the results of chemotherapy-alone investigations support the efficacy of this treatment approach in children with early-stage favorable Hodgkin's lymphoma, and current trials are in process to confirm this. Subgroups of children with early-stage unfavorable Hodgkin's disease may also be appropriate for chemotherapy alone, but the standard of practice continues to include consolidative radiation. However, the results of recent trials suggest that children with advanced and unfavorable symptomatic or bulky disease, or both, at presentation may have better outcomes using a combined-modality approach. Identification of prognostic features of patients who require radiation to optimize disease control is a focus of many ongoing pediatric trials.

TREATMENT OF RELAPSED AND REFRACTORY DISEASE

The generally excellent outcome in pediatric Hodgkin's lymphoma has limited opportunities to evaluate salvage therapy programs. Most relapses in patients with Hodgkin's lymphoma occur within the first 3 years, but some patients may relapse as long as 10 years after initial diagnosis. Treatment and prognosis after relapse depend on the primary therapy and duration of remission (time of relapse). Retreatment with conventional multiagent chemotherapy and RT may salvage 40% to 50% of children relapsing after a sustained remission (1 year or longer); but adverse effects of treatment, including second malignancies, may reduce ultimate survival.[74-76] Patients who develop refractory disease during or within 1 year after completing therapy respond poorly to conventional salvage therapy, as do patients with multiple relapses. These high-risk patients have a better chance of achieving a durable remission if they are consolidated with myeloablative therapy followed by hematopoietic stem cell transplantation (HSCT). Overall survival rates in children and adolescents with relapsed Hodgkin's lymphoma treated with this approach range from 30% to 60%. Because of the higher transplant-related mortality associated with allogeneic transplantation, autologous HSCT is preferred for patients with relapsed Hodgkin's lymphoma. However, recent investigations of reduced-intensity allogeneic transplantation have demonstrated acceptable rates of transplant-related mortality.[77,78] Nonmyeloablative conditioning regimens most often use fludarabine or low-dose total-body irradiation to provide a nontoxic immunosuppression and establish a graft-versus-lymphoma effect. Information about treatment outcomes using this approach is limited to reports of small, heterogeneous, adult-patient cohorts treated with a variety of conditioning regimens. Longer follow-up is needed to establish the efficacy of this approach.

IFRT to sites of recurrent disease should be considered in the setting of HSCT. In a Stanford report, patients with stages I to III disease at relapse who received autologous bone marrow transplantation (AuBMT) and IFRT had a 3-year freedom from relapse of 100% and overall survival of 85%, compared with 67% and 60%, respectively, for patients not receiving IFRT.[79] For patients not previously irradiated, IFRT was associated with an improved freedom from relapse of 85% and overall survival of 93%, in contrast to 57% and 55%, respectively, for those previously irradiated. Morbidity was similar to those not irradiated, although RT may have contributed to the peritransplant death of two patients. Central issues relating to the use of IFRT are the dose, target volume, and timing with respect to the transplant. RT doses are generally 15 to 25 Gy, in 1.5- to 2.0-Gy fractions. This variation relates to potential normal tissue toxicity as well as the consideration for higher-radiation doses in patients with an identifiable tumor that demonstrates radiation responsiveness. Radiation volume can vary and include treatment to all sites of initial disease, recurrent disease, persistent disease following salvage chemotherapy, persistent disease following the preparative regimen for transplant, or all nodal sites. Unless protocol-specific therapy is directed, individual considerations for such decision-making are necessary at this time. IFRT can be administered prior to the high-dose chemotherapy program to place patients in a minimal disease state. RT can also be administered after the high-dose chemotherapy program to decrease the potential for disease progression elsewhere during the time RT is being administered, and RT-related peritransplant morbidity such as esophagitis, pneumonitis, cardiomyopathy, and veno-occlusive disease. Possible disadvantages of this approach include the loss of the pretransplant cytoreductive effect and the theoretical carcinogenic effect of RT on the newly proliferating hematopoietic system.

Treatment Algorithms

Table 71-5 summarizes recommendations for risk-adapted treatment approaches. Because patients with localized favorable disease presentations can achieve long-term disease-free survival using regimens that do not contain alkylators, ABVD or derivative chemotherapy is preferred for this group.[32,33,80,81] However, alkylating agents or etoposide can be added to the regimen without compromising disease outcome if the investigator prefers to restrict anthracycline chemotherapy exposure to preserve cardiac function.[28,29,82] Combined-modality treatment approaches including low-dose IFRT have produced excellent results in children with favorable localized disease and reduce cumulative chemotherapy doses.

Combinations derived from both ABVD and MOPP still provide the most effective chemotherapy strategies for children and adolescents with intermediate- or high-risk disease presentations.[28,29] In most regimens reporting good long-term outcomes, low-dose RT is administered following chemotherapy to areas of bulk disease, or nodes involved at diagnosis. In contrast to treatment regimens used for adults with advanced or unfavorable Hodgkin's lymphoma that commonly prescribe six cycles of ABVD, an alkylating agent regimen is most often alternated with ABVD or similar hybrid therapy in an effort to reduce potential cardiopulmonary toxicity in pediatric patients. Attempts to completely omit alkylating agents in these high-risk groups have resulted in unsatisfactory outcomes, as have protocols prescribing ABVD or derivative chemotherapy alone.[30,83] Chemotherapy administration may be according to a conventional twice-monthly schedule or compacted into a weekly schedule. Advantages of the compacted schedule included enhanced dose-intensity, which may reduce the development of resistant disease. Long-term follow-up is required to establish the superiority of this approach over conventional dosing schedules.

Table 71-5 Recommendations for Treatment Approach in Pediatric Hodgkin's Lymphoma

Clinical Presentation	Stage	Recommended Treatment Approach
EARLY <3-4 nodal regions; no B symptoms, bulk, or extranodal extension from contiguous nodal disease	IA, IIA	**RECOMMENDED THERAPY** 2-4 cycles non–cross-resistant chemotherapy without alkylators plus low-dose IFR (15-25 Gy)
		OTHER CONSIDERATIONS 6 cycles non–cross-resistant chemotherapy alone
		IN CLINICAL TRIAL SETTING ONLY 4 cycles of chemotherapy alone
INTERMEDIATE ≥3-4 nodal regions; bulky lymphadenopathy (mediastinal ratio ≥ 33%; peripheral lymph node mass ≥6-10 cm)	IA, IIA, IIB*	**RECOMMENDED THERAPY** 4-6 cycles (3-5 compacted, dose-intensive cycles) non–cross-resistant chemotherapy plus low-dose IFR (15-25 Gy)
	IIIA	**OTHER CONSIDERATIONS** 6-8 cycles (5 compacted, dose-intensive cycles) non–cross-resistant chemotherapy alone
ADVANCED Stage II patients with fever or weight loss; any patient with advanced stage	IIB* IIIB IV	**RECOMMENDED THERAPY** 6-8 cycles (5-6 compacted, dose-intensive cycles) of non–cross-resistant chemotherapy plus low-dose IFR (15-25 Gy)
		OTHER CONSIDERATIONS 8 cycles (6-7 compacted, dose-intensive cycles) non–cross-resistant chemotherapy alone

*Stage IIB patients have been variably treated as intermediate or unfavorable risk. Some studies use associated factors, e.g., weight loss, bulk disease, extranodal extension, for further risk stratification.

IFR, involved-field radiation.

REFERENCES

1. Weiner MA, Leventhal BG, Marcus R, et al: Intensive chemotherapy and low-dose radiotherapy for the treatment of advanced-stage Hodgkin's disease in pediatric patients: A Pediatric Oncology Group study. J Clin Oncol 9(9):1591-1598, 1991.
2. Weiner MA, Leventhal B, Brecher ML, et al: Randomized study of intensive MOPP-ABVD with or without low-dose total-nodal radiation therapy in the treatment of stages IIB, IIIA2, IIIB, and IV Hodgkin's disease in pediatric patients: A Pediatric Oncology Group study. J Clin Oncol 15(8):2769-2779, 1997.
3. Donaldson SS, Link MP: Combined modality treatment with low-dose radiation and MOPP chemotherapy for children with Hodgkin's disease. J Clin Oncol 5(5):742-749, 1987.
4. Fryer CJ, Hutchinson RJ, Krailo M, et al: Efficacy and toxicity of 12 courses of ABVD chemotherapy followed by low-dose regional radiation in advanced Hodgkin's disease in children: A report from the Children's Cancer Study Group. J Clin Oncol 8(12):1971-1980, 1990.
5. Gehan EA, Sullivan MP, Fuller LM, et al: The intergroup Hodgkin's disease in children. A study of stages I and II. Cancer 65(6):1429-1437, 1990.
6. Hutchinson RJ, Fryer CJ, Davis PC, et al: MOPP or radiation in addition to ABVD in the treatment of pathologically staged advanced Hodgkin's disease in children: Results of the Children's Cancer Group Phase III Trial. J Clin Oncol 16(3):897-906, 1998.
7. Bramswig JH, Heimes U, Heiermann E, et al: The effects of different cumulative doses of chemotherapy on testicular function. Results in 75 patients treated for Hodgkin's disease during childhood or adolescence. Cancer 65(6):1298-1302, 1990.
8. Travis LB, Hill DA, Dores GM, et al: Breast cancer following radiotherapy and chemotherapy among young women with Hodgkin disease. JAMA 290(4):465-475, 2003.
9. Grufferman S, Delzell E: Epidemiology of Hodgkin's disease. Epidemiol Rev 6:76-106, 1984.
10. Spitz MR, Sider JG, Johnson CC, et al: Ethnic patterns of Hodgkin's disease incidence among children and adolescents in the United States, 1973-82. J Natl Cancer Inst 76(2):235-239, 1986.
11. Parkin DM, Bray F, Ferlay J, Pisani P: Global cancer statistics, 2002. CA Cancer J Clin 55(2):74-108, 2005.
12. Westergaard T, Melbye M, Pedersen JB, et al: Birth order, sibship size and risk of Hodgkin's disease in children and young adults: A population-based study of 31 million person-years. Int J Cancer 72(6):977-981, 1997.
13. Chang ET, Montgomery SM, Richiardi L, et al: Number of siblings and risk of Hodgkin's lymphoma. Cancer Epidemiol Biomarkers Prev 13(7):1236-1243, 2004.
14. Chang ET, Zheng T, Weir EG, et al: Childhood social environment and Hodgkin's lymphoma: New findings from a population-based case-control study. Cancer Epidemiol Biomarkers Prev 13(8):1361-1370, 2004.
15. Weiss LM, Movahed LA, Warnke RA, Sklar J: Detection of Epstein-Barr viral genomes in Reed-Sternberg cells of Hodgkin's disease. N Engl J Med 320(8):502-506, 1989.
16. Wu TC, Mann RB, Charache P, et al: Detection of EBV gene expression in Reed-Sternberg cells of Hodgkin's disease. Int J Cancer 46(5):801-804, 1990.
17. Glaser SL, Lin RJ, Stewart SL, et al: Epstein-Barr virus-associated Hodgkin's disease: Epidemiologic characteristics in international data. Int J Cancer 70(4):375-382, 1997.
18. Weinreb M, Day PJ, Niggli F, et al: The role of Epstein-Barr virus in Hodgkin's disease from different geographical areas. Arch Dis Child 74(1):27-31, 1996.
19. Stein H, Delsol G, Pileri S, et al: Hodgkin Lymphoma. *In* Jaffe ES, Harris NL, Stein H, Vardiman JW (eds): World Health Organization Classification of Tumors. Tumors of Hematopoietic and Lymphoid Tissues. Lyon, France, IARC Press; 2001, pp 237-253.
20. Donaldson SS, Hudson M, Oberlin O, et al: Pediatric Hodgkin's disease. *In* Mauch PM, Armitage JO, Diehl V, et al (eds): Hodgkin's Disease. Philadelphia: Lippincott Williams & Wilkins; 1999, pp 531-605.
21. Uccini S, Monardo F, Stoppacciaro A, et al: High frequency of Epstein-Barr virus genome detection in Hodgkin's disease of HIV-positive patients. Int J Cancer 46(4):581-585, 1990.
22. Anagnostopoulos I, Hansmann ML, Franssila K, et al: European Task Force on Lymphoma project on lymphocyte predominant

Hodgkin disease: Histologic and immunohistologic analysis of submitted cases reveals 2 types of Hodgkin disease with a nodular growth pattern and abundant lymphocytes. Blood. 96(5):1889-1899, 2000.
23. Diehl V, Sextro M, Franklin J, et al: Clinical presentation, course, and prognostic factors in lymphocyte-predominant Hodgkin's disease and lymphocyte-rich classical Hodgkin's disease: Report from the European Task Force on Lymphoma Project on Lymphocyte-Predominant Hodgkin's Disease. J Clin Oncol 17(3):776-783, 1999.
24. Weiner M, Leventhal B, Cantor A, et al: Gallium-67 scans as an adjunct to computed tomography scans for the assessment of a residual mediastinal mass in pediatric patients with Hodgkin's disease. A Pediatric Oncology Group study. Cancer 68(11):2478-2480, 1991.
25. Jerusalem G, Beguin Y, Fassotte MF, et al: Whole-body positron emission tomography using 18F-fluorodeoxyglucose for post-treatment evaluation in Hodgkin's disease and non-Hodgkin's lymphoma has higher diagnostic and prognostic value than classical computed tomography scan imaging. Blood 94(2):429-433, 1999.
26. Friedberg JW, Fischman A, Neuberg D, et al: FDG-PET is superior to gallium scintigraphy in staging and more sensitive in the follow-up of patients with de novo Hodgkin lymphoma: A blinded comparison. Leuk Lymphoma 45(1):85-92, 2004.
27. Carbone PP, Kaplan HS, Musshoff K, Smithers DW, Tubiana M: Report of the Committee on Hodgkin's Disease Staging Classification. Cancer Res Nov 31(11):1860-1861, 1971.
28. Ruhl U, Albrecht M, Dieckmann K, et al: Response-adapted radiotherapy in the treatment of pediatric Hodgkin's disease: An interim report at 5 years of the German GPOH-HD 95 trial. Int J Radiat Oncol Biol Phys 51(5):1209-1218, 2001.
29. Nachman JB, Sposto R, Herzog P, et al: Randomized comparison of low-dose involved-field radiotherapy and no radiotherapy for children with Hodgkin's disease who achieve a complete response to chemotherapy. J Clin Oncol 20(18):3765-3771, 2002.
30. Friedmann AM, Hudson MM, Weinstein HJ, et al: Treatment of unfavorable childhood Hodgkin's disease with VEPA and low-dose, involved-field radiation. J Clin Oncol 20(14):3088-3094, 2002.
31. Atra A, Higgs E, Capra M, et al: ChlVPP chemotherapy in children with stage IV Hodgkin's disease: Results of the UKCCSG HD 8201 and HD 9201 studies. Br J Haematol 119(3):647-651, 2002.
32. Donaldson SS, Hudson MM, Lamborn KR, et al: VAMP and low-dose, involved-field radiation for children and adolescents with favorable, early-stage Hodgkin's disease: Results of a prospective clinical trial. J Clin Oncol 20(14):3081-3087, 2002.
33. Landman-Parker J, Pacquement H, Leblanc T, et al: Localized childhood Hodgkin's disease: Response-adapted chemotherapy with etoposide, bleomycin, vinblastine, and prednisone before low-dose radiation therapy—results of the French Society of Pediatric Oncology Study MDH90. J Clin Oncol 18(7):1500-1507, 2000.
34. Dorffel W, Luders H, Ruhl U, et al: Preliminary results of the multicenter trial GPOH-HD 95 for the treatment of Hodgkin's disease in children and adolescents: Analysis and outlook. Klin Padiatr 215(3):139-145, 2003.
35. Schellong G, Potter R, Bramswig J, et al: High cure rates and reduced long-term toxicity in pediatric Hodgkin's disease: the German-Austrian multicenter trial DAL-HD-90. The German-Austrian Pediatric Hodgkin's Disease Study Group. J Clin Oncol 17(12):3736-3744, 1999.
36. Murphy SB, Morgan ER, Katzenstein HM, Kletzel M: Results of little or no treatment for lymphocyte-predominant Hodgkin disease in children and adolescents. J Pediatr Hematol Oncol 25(9):684-687, 2003.
37. Pellegrino B, Terrier-Lacombe MJ, Oberlin O, et al: Lymphocyte-predominant Hodgkin's Lymphoma in children: Therapeutic abstention after initial lymph node resection—A study of the French Society of Pediatric Oncology. J Clin Oncol 21(15):2948-2952, 2003.
38. De Vita VTJ, Canellos G, Moxley J: A decade of combination chemotherapy of advanced Hodgkin's disease. Cancer 30:1495-1504, 1972.
39. Longo DL, Young RC, Wesley M, et al: Twenty years of MOPP therapy for Hodgkin's disease. J Clin Oncol 4(9):1295-1306, 1986.
40. Bhatia S, Robison LL, Oberlin O, et al: Breast cancer and other second neoplasms after childhood Hodgkin's disease. N Engl J Med 334(12):745-751, 1996.
41. Metayer C, Lynch CF, Clarke EA, et al: Second cancers among long-term survivors of Hodgkin's disease diagnosed in childhood and adolescence. J Clin Oncol 18(12):2435-2443, 2000.
42. Sankila R, Garwicz S, Olsen JH, et al: Risk of subsequent malignant neoplasms among 1,641 Hodgkin's disease patients diagnosed in childhood and adolescence: A population-based cohort study in the five Nordic countries. Association of the Nordic Cancer Registries and the Nordic Society of Pediatric Hematology and Oncology. J Clin Oncol 14(5):1442-1446, 1996.
43. Swerdlow AJ, Barber JA, Hudson GV, et al: Risk of second malignancy after Hodgkin's disease in a collaborative British cohort: The relation to age at treatment. J Clin Oncol 18(3):498-509, 2000.
44. van Leeuwen FE, Klokman WJ, Veer MB, et al: Long-term risk of second malignancy in survivors of Hodgkin's disease treated during adolescence or young adulthood. J Clin Oncol 18(3):487-497, 2000.
45. Bhatia S, Yasui Y, Robison LL, et al: High risk of subsequent neoplasms continues with extended follow-up of childhood Hodgkin's disease: Report from the Late Effects Study Group. J Clin Oncol 21(23):4386-4394, 2003.
46. Schellong G, Riepenhausen M, Creutzig U, et al: Low risk of secondary leukemias after chemotherapy without mechlorethamine in childhood Hodgkin's disease. German-Austrian Pediatric Hodgkin's Disease Group. J Clin Oncol 15(6):2247-2253, 1997.
47. Horning SJ, Hoppe RT, Kaplan HS, Rosenberg SA: Female reproductive potential after treatment for Hodgkin's disease. N Engl J Med 304(23):1377-1382, 1981.
48. da Cunha MF, Meistrich ML, Fuller LM, et al: Recovery of spermatogenesis after treatment for Hodgkin's disease: Limiting dose of MOPP chemotherapy. J Clin Oncol 2(6):571-577, 1984.
49. Bonadonna G, Valagussa P, Santoro A: Alternating non-cross-resistant combination chemotherapy or MOPP in stage IV Hodgkin's disease. A report of 8-year results. Ann Intern Med 104(6):739-746, 1986.
50. Keefe DL. Anthracycline-induced cardiomyopathy. Semin Oncol 28(4 Suppl 12):2-7, 2001.
51. Lipshultz SE, Colan SD, Gelber RD, et al: Late cardiac effects of doxorubicin therapy for acute lymphoblastic leukemia in childhood. N Engl J Med 324(12):808-815, 1991.
52. Lipshultz SE, Lipsitz SR, Mone SM, et al: Female sex and drug dose as risk factors for late cardiotoxic effects of doxorubicin therapy for childhood cancer. N Engl J Med 332(26):1738-1743, 1995.
53. Krischer JP, Epstein S, Cuthbertson DD, et al: Clinical cardiotoxicity following anthracycline treatment for childhood cancer: The Pediatric Oncology Group experience. J Clin Oncol 15(4):1544-1552, 1997.
54. Adams MJ, Hardenbergh PH, Constine LS, Lipshultz SE: Radiation-associated cardiovascular disease. Crit Rev Oncol Hematol 45(1):55-75, 2003.
55. Green DM, Gingell RL, Pearce J, et al: The effect of mediastinal irradiation on cardiac function of patients treated during childhood and adolescence for Hodgkin's disease. J Clin Oncol 5(2):239-245, 1987.
56. Hancock SL, Donaldson SS, Hoppe RT: Cardiac disease following treatment of Hodgkin's disease in children and adolescents. J Clin Oncol 11(7):1208-1215, 1993.
57. Kreisman H, Wolkove N: Pulmonary toxicity of antineoplastic therapy. Semin Oncol 19(5):508-520, 1992.
58. Marina NM, Greenwald CA, Fairclough DL, et al: Serial pulmonary function studies in children treated for newly diagnosed Hodgkin's disease with mantle radiotherapy plus cycles of cyclophosphamide, vincristine, and procarbazine alternating with cycles of doxorubicin, bleomycin, vinblastine, and dacarbazine. Cancer 75(7):1706-1711, 1995.
59. Mefferd JM, Donaldson SS, Link MP: Pediatric Hodgkin's disease: Pulmonary, cardiac, and thyroid function following combined modality therapy. Int J Radiat Oncol Biol Phys 16(3):679-685, 1989.
60. Hudson MM, Greenwald C, Thompson E, et al: Efficacy and toxicity of multiagent chemotherapy and low-dose involved-field

radiotherapy in children and adolescents with Hodgkin's disease. J Clin Oncol 11(1):100-108, 1993.
61. Shankar AG, Ashley S, Atra A, et al: A limited role for VEEP (vincristine, etoposide, epirubicin, prednisolone) chemotherapy in childhood Hodgkin's disease. Eur J Cancer 34(13):2058-2063, 1998.
62. Sackmann-Muriel F, Zubizarreta P, Gallo G, et al: Hodgkin disease in children: Results of a prospective randomized trial in a single institution in Argentina. Med Pediatr Oncol 29(6):544-552, 1997.
63. Smith MA, Rubinstein L, Anderson JR, et al: Secondary leukemia or myelodysplastic syndrome after treatment with epipodophyllotoxins. J Clin Oncol 17(2):569-577, 1999.
64. Pui CH, Ribeiro RC, Hancock ML, et al: Acute myeloid leukemia in children treated with epipodophyllotoxins for acute lymphoblastic leukemia. N Engl J Med 325(24):1682-1687, 1991.
65. Kaplan H: Hodgkin's Disease. Harvard University Press, 1980.
66. Dieckmann K, Potter R, Wagner W, et al: Up-front centralized data review and individualized treatment proposals in a multicenter pediatric Hodgkin's disease trial with 71 participating hospitals: The experience of the German-Austrian Pediatric Multicenter Trial DAL-HD-90. Radiother Oncol 62(2):191-200, 2002.
67. Dieckmann K, Potter R, Hofmann J, et al: Does bulky disease at diagnosis influence outcome in childhood Hodgkin's disease and require higher radiation doses? Results from the German-Austrian Pediatric Multicenter Trial DAL-HD-90. Int J Radiat Oncol Biol Phys 56(3):644-652, 2003.
68. Ekert H, Waters KD, Smith PJ, et al: Treatment with MOPP or ChlVPP chemotherapy only for all stages of childhood Hodgkin's disease. J Clin Oncol 6(12):1845-1850, 1988.
69. Baez F, Ocampo E, Conter V, et al: Treatment of childhood Hodgkin's disease with COPP or COPP-ABV (hybrid) without radiotherapy in Nicaragua. Ann Oncol 8(3):247-250, 1997.
70. Behrendt H, Brinkhuis M, Van Leeuwen EF: Treatment of childhood Hodgkin's disease with ABVD without radiotherapy. Med Pediatr Oncol 26(4):244-248, 1996.
71. Ekert H: Treatment of childhood Hodgkin's disease. J Clin Oncol 9(3):528-529, 1991.
72. Lobo-Sanahuja F, Garcia I, Barrantes JC, et al: Pediatric Hodgkin's disease in Costa Rica: Twelve years' experience of primary treatment by chemotherapy alone, without staging laparotomy. Med Pediatr Oncol 22(6):398-403, 1994.
73. van den Berg H, Stuve W, Behrendt H: Treatment of Hodgkin's disease in children with alternating mechlorethamine, vincristine, procarbazine, and prednisone (MOPP) and adriamycin, bleomycin, vinblastine, and dacarbazine (ABVD) courses without radiotherapy. Med Pediatr Oncol 29(1):23-27, 1997.
74. Williams CD, Goldstone AH, Pearce R, et al: Autologous bone marrow transplantation for pediatric Hodgkin's disease: A case-matched comparison with adult patients by the European Bone Marrow Transplant Group Lymphoma Registry. J Clin Oncol 11(11):2243-2249; 1993.
75. Lieskovsky YE, Donaldson SS, Torres MA, et al: High-dose therapy and autologous hematopoietic stem-cell transplantation for recurrent or refractory pediatric Hodgkin's disease: results and prognostic indices. J Clin Oncol 22:4532-4540, 2004.
76. Baker KS, Gordon BG, Gross TG, et al: Autologous hematopoietic stem-cell transplantation for relapsed or refractory Hodgkin's disease in children and adolescents. J Clin Oncol 17(3):825-831, 1999.
77. Carella AM, Cavaliere M, Lerma E, et al: Autografting followed by nonmyeloablative immunosuppressive chemotherapy and allogeneic peripheral-blood hematopoietic stem-cell transplantation as treatment of resistant Hodgkin's disease and non-Hodgkin's lymphoma. J Clin Oncol 18(23):3918-3924, 2000.
78. Robinson SP, Goldstone AH, Mackinnon S, et al: Chemoresistant or aggressive lymphoma predicts for a poor outcome following reduced-intensity allogeneic progenitor cell transplantation: an analysis from the Lymphoma Working Party of the European Group for Blood and Bone Marrow Transplantation. Blood 100(13):4310-4316, 2002.
79. Poen JC, Hoppe RT, Horning SJ: High-dose therapy and autologous bone marrow transplantation for relapsed/refractory Hodgkin's disease: The impact of involved field radiotherapy on patterns of failure and survival. Int J Radiat Oncol Biol Phys 36(1):3-12, 1996.
80. Oberlin O, Leverger G, Pacquement H, et al: Low-dose radiation therapy and reduced chemotherapy in childhood Hodgkin's disease: The experience of the French Society of Pediatric Oncology. J Clin Oncol 10(10):1602-1608, 1992.
81. Vecchi V, Pileri S, Burnelli R, et al: Treatment of pediatric Hodgkin disease tailored to stage, mediastinal mass, and age. An Italian (AIEOP) multicenter study on 215 patients. Cancer 72(6):2049-2057, 1993.
82. Schellong G: Treatment of children and adolescents with Hodgkin's disease: the experience of the German-Austrian Paediatric Study Group. Baillieres Clin Haematol 9(3):619-634, 1996.
83. Ekert H, Toogood I, Downie P, et al: High incidence of treatment failure with vincristine, etoposide, epirubicin, and prednisolone chemotherapy with successful salvage in childhood Hodgkin disease. Med Pediatr Oncol 32(4):255-258, 1999.
84. Hudson MM, Krasin M, Link MP, et al: Risk-adapted, combined-modality therapy with VAMP/COP and response-based, involved-field radiation for unfavorable pediatric Hodgkin's disease. J Clin Oncol 22(22):4541–4550, 2004.
85. Hunger SP, Link MP, Donaldson SS: ABVD/MOPP and low-dose involved-field radiotherapy in pediatric Hodgkin's disease: the Stanford experience. J Clin Oncol 12(10):2160-2166, 1994.
86. Mauch PM, Weinstein H, Botnick L, et al: An evaluation of long-term survival and treatment complications in children with Hodgkin's disease. Cancer 51(5):925-932, 1983.
87. Shankar AG, Ashley S, Radford M, et al: Does histology influence outcome in childhood Hodgkin's disease? Results from the United Kingdom Children's Cancer Study Group. J Clin Oncol 15(7):2622-2630, 1997.
88. Sripada PV, Tenali SG, Vasudevan M, et al: Hybrid (COPP/ABV) Therapy in childhood Hodgkin's disease: a study of 53 cases during 1989-1993 at the Cancer Institute Madras, India. Pediatr Hematol Oncol 12:333-341, 1995.

CHAPTER 72

RARE PEDIATRIC TUMORS

Ori Shokek and Moody D. Wharam, Jr.

LANGERHANS CELL HISTIOCYTOSIS

LCH is a monoclonal proliferation of Langerhans cells.

Children younger than 5 years are most commonly affected.

Extent of disease and age are prognostically important. Single-system disease (most commonly osseous) is favorable. Patients with multisystem disease fare less well. Children younger than age 2 years with multisystem disease and organ dysfunction fare poorly.

Staging evaluation is partly determined by presentation but at a minimum consists of routine laboratory studies; skeletal survey or bone scintigraphy, or both; and axial imaging of involved sites.

Treatment is heterogeneous and determined by disease extent. Radiotherapy is used for skeletal lesions that are recurrent, painful, anatomically not amenable to other local treatments, or at risk for fracture. A radiotherapy dose response has not been observed, and major series have reported treatment of osseous lesions using 3 to 15 Gy.

Diabetes insipidus (DI) is a manifestation attributed to pituitary or hypothalamic involvement. The observed benefit of pituitary-hypothalamic irradiation has been limited to patients treated within days of symptom onset.

NASOPHARYNGEAL CARCINOMA

Compared with nasopharyngeal carcinoma in adults, the disease in children in both endemic and nonendemic geographic regions is almost always of the World Heath Organization types II or III histologies and is almost always associated with Epstein-Barr virus infection.

Children ages 10 to 15 years are most commonly affected, and there is a moderate male predominance.

Staging evaluation consists of routine blood work; fiberoptic examination of the nasopharynx; axial imaging of local disease and of the neck and supraclavicular fossae; metastatic workup of the lungs, liver, and bones; dental assessment and prophylaxis; baseline endocrinologic assessment; and baseline audiologic assessment.

Locoregional disease usually presents at advanced stages. Treatment consists of primary radiotherapy, usually with chemotherapy. The optimal timing of chemotherapy is uncertain, but clinical trials have shown excellent outcome with neoadjuvant chemotherapy. Concurrent chemoradiotherapy is being investigated, paralleling trends in the treatment of adult nasopharyngeal carcinoma.

Total doses more than 60 Gy are associated with improved disease control.

JUVENILE NASOPHARYNGEAL ANGIOFIBROMA

Nasopharyngeal angiofibroma is characterized by irregular vascular channels within a fibrous stroma. It is uncertain if the entity represents a hamartomatous process, a pathologic or reactive vascular proliferation, or a true neoplasm. Hormonal mechanisms of tumorigenesis have been proposed as well.

Adolescent males are predominantly affected. The disease is almost never seen in females.

The tumor arises in the nasopharynx and can be locally aggressive. Metastasis is not described. Staging evaluation consists of fiberoptic examination of the nasopharynx and axial imaging of the head and neck.

Treatment of resectable disease is surgical. Radiotherapy is generally reserved for locally advanced or recurrent tumors. Excellent disease control is achieved with 30 to 40 Gy.

PLEUROPULMONARY BLASTOMA

Pleuropulmonary blastoma is a dysembryonic neoplasm that arises as intrapulmonary, pleural-based, mediastinal disease, or all three.

Children younger than age 5 years are most commonly affected.

There are three histologic types: Type I is cystic and carries a favorable prognosis. Type II is cystic and solid and carries an intermediate prognosis. Type III is solid and clinically unfavorable.

Staging evaluation consists of chest computed tomography (CT) plus, for patients with type II and type III disease, abdominal CT, head magnetic resonance imaging (MRI), and bone scintigraphy.

Treatment varies by histologic type. Type I disease is usually resected, and chemotherapy is given adjuvantly. Type II and type III tumors are less frequently resectable, and neoadjuvant chemotherapy may facilitate surgery. Radiotherapy is individualized and should be considered for sites of known residual disease after surgery and for pleural contamination. Local and hemithorax radiation fields are used. Even with total doses approaching normal tissue tolerance, reported local control rates are suboptimal.

EXTRARENAL WILMS' TUMOR

Extrarenal Wilms' tumor (EWT) is histologically similar to renal Wilms' tumor. It is seen most commonly in or close to genitourinary sites, and it is thought to arise from ectopic metanephric blastema.

Children younger than age 5 years are most commonly affected.

Primary treatment consists of surgery and chemotherapy, but optimal management is uncertain because of the scarcity of clinical data. It is reasonable to consider the stage-by-stage recommendations established for renal Wilms' tumor.

LANGERHANS CELL HISTIOCYTOSIS

The varied presentations of Langerhans cell histiocytosis (LCH) in children and adults require treatment of varied intensity, with radiotherapy employed only in select situations. The indications for radiotherapy are grounded in an understanding of etiology, pathology, nomenclature, epidemiology, clinical stratification, and treatment.

LCH derives its name from its lesional cells. Langerhans cells are dendritic antigen-presenting cells normally found in the skin, squamous mucosal epithelium, spleen, and lymphatic system. At skin and mucosal sites, they attack and digest bacteria, then travel to lymphoid organs to interact with immune system cells to stimulate cell-mediated and humoral immunity.[1] Langerhans cells are characterized by Birbeck granules on electron microscopy. The Birbeck granule protein langerin has been identified,[2] and immunohistochemical staining for both langerin and glycoprotein CD1a is used to establish the diagnosis.

The etiology and pathogenesis of LCH are not known. Clonality[3] supports LCH as neoplastic, but immunologic dysfunction has been proposed as a primary etiology, and associations with certain human leukocyte antigen (HLA) phenotypes are reported.[4,5] An association with human herpes virus (HHV-6) has been established,[6] but causation has not been demonstrated.

The nomenclature of LCH was formalized by the Writing Group of the Histiocyte Society (1987) and revised jointly by the Reclassification Working Group of the Histiocyte Society and the World Health Organization (WHO) Committee on Histiocytic/Reticulum Cell Proliferations (1997). Varied syndromes, which had names now clinically obsolete, reflected the different clinical manifestations of LCH. These syndromes included eosinophilic granuloma of bone, Letterer-Siwe disease, Hand-Schüller-Christian syndrome, Hashimoto-Pritzker syndrome (self-healing histiocytosis), pure cutaneous histiocytosis, Langerhans-cell granulomatosis, and nonlipid reticuloendotheliosis. Before Langerhans cells were recognized as the lesional histiocytes, these related syndromes were grouped under the umbrella term *histiocytosis* X. Other histiocytic disorders, not generally encountered by radiation oncologists and considered separate from LCH, include isolated pulmonary–Langerhans cell disease of adults[7,8] and certain non–Langerhans cell histiocytoses.[7,9]

Clinical Stratification

Two important prognostic features of LCH at presentation are extent of disease and age. Single-system disease, which usually involves bone, skin, or lymph nodes, has a good prognosis and requires minimal treatment. Patients with multisystem disease fare less well. Very young children (younger than age 2 years) with multisystem disease and resultant organ dysfunction (hematopoietic, hepatic, and pulmonary) fare especially poorly.[10-13] Modern clinical stratification[7] is based on disease extent: single-system disease involving a single site; single-system disease involving multiple sites; and multisystem disease with or without organ dysfunction.

The French Langerhans' Cell Histiocytosis Study Group[14] reported 348 cases of LCH diagnosed between 1983 and 1993 at 32 centers. The observed annual incidence was .45 cases per 10,000 children ages 0 to 15 years and 1.25 per 10,000 children ages 0 to 2 years. The median age at diagnosis was 30 months, and 56% were male. At presentation, 31% had single-system unifocal or bifocal bone involvement, 19% had single-system multifocal bone involvement, 39% had multisystem disease without organ dysfunction, and 11% had multisystem disease with organ dysfunction. The DAL-HX83/90 studies representing the combined German, Austrian, Dutch, and Swiss experience registered 275 patients, of whom 178 (65%) had single-system disease.[15] Of the 178 patients, 155 had bone disease (unifocal in 121, multifocal in 34), 19 had skin disease, and 4 had lymph node disease. Median age was 7 years, 3 months for patients with unifocal bone disease; 3 years, 11 months for patients with multifocal bone disease; 1 month for those with skin disease; and 3 years, 11 months for those with lymph node disease. Of patients with single-system bone disease, 40% had skull lesions, 18% spine, 17% lower extremities, 10% pelvis, 8% upper extremities, and 7% thoracic bones, with similar patterns in patients with unifocal and multifocal bone disease.

Staging Workup

In addition to routine laboratory studies, LCH patients require a skeletal survey or bone scintigraphy, or both. Patients with polyuria and polydipsia need prompt urine osmolarity and water deprivation testing and cranial magnetic resonance imaging (MRI) to assess for diabetes insipidus (DI) secondary to pituitary or hypothalamic involvement, or both. Dental abnormalities secondary to bone involvement require dental radiographs. Pulmonary involvement is evaluated with computed tomography (CT) and pulmonary function testing.[15,16]

There are conflicting data for the utility of skeletal survey versus bone scintigraphy. In DAL-HX83/90, 125 patients had both types of skeletal imaging. Of 222 bone lesions, 97% were detected by plain radiographs, compared to 82% on bone scintigraphy; and only 2% were seen on scintigraphy but not on radiographs.[15] Another study comparing the utility of these two modalities suggested a need for both.[17] In patients with skeletal disease, CT will delineate the extent of osseous destruction and any soft tissue involvement; and MRI demonstrates marrow involvement and, in skull lesions, extension into dura and brain.[16]

Treatment and Outcome

Skeletal Disease

Skeletal LCH lesions, either in single-system or multisystem disease, can present with pain or a palpable mass. Symptoms may include fracture, motion deficit, peripheral nerve palsy, exophthalmos, otitis media, tooth loss, or hearing impairment. Alternatively, skeletal lesions may also be discovered incidentally during initial staging workup or later in the course of the disease.[15]

For single-system monostotic LCH, curettage at the time of obtaining diagnostic material is often sufficient for treatment. Pediatric Oncology Group (POG) study 8047[18] was a prospective trial for patients with single-system unifocal or bifocal bone disease. Open biopsy of all lesions was recommended. If two lesions were present, both lesions would be biopsied, but only one would be surgically treated (with curettage or excision) to determine the benefit of surgical treatment compared with biopsy. Patients experiencing recurrence would be randomized to receive either 3 Gy in two fractions or 6 Gy in four fractions. Twenty-three patients were analyzed. Good local control with curettage and excision was demonstrated, but the utility of biopsy alone and optimal radiation dose were not determined. There were two patients with bifocal disease in whom the second lesions were neither curettaged nor biopsied. One of the second lesions healed spontaneously, and the other was irradiated 8 weeks after surgery because of pain. Three lesions progressed and were irradiated. Two of the lesions that progressed were the only site of disease progression. With a median follow-up interval of 3 years,

9 months, 2 of the 21 patients with unifocal disease developed disease at new sites, and both recurrences resolved without therapy.

Good local control is reported with curettage, excision, biopsy alone, intralesional steroid injection, or radiotherapy.[15,19-23] Because of concern regarding late effects, radiotherapy is usually not favored when other treatment modalities are feasible. Historically, indications for irradiation of bony lesions have included recurrence or failure to heal following surgical treatment, anatomic sites for which surgical intervention is difficult or dangerous, pain, and risk of bone collapse.[18] When radiotherapy is used, low doses are sufficient. The University of California, Los Angeles (UCLA) experience with radiotherapeutic management showed long-term control of 35 of 40 bone lesions (88%), with no difference in dose between controlled (median 9 Gy, range 6 to 15 Gy) and recurrent (median 10 Gy, range 8 to 15 Gy) lesions.[21] Whether lower doses are efficacious is uncertain (Fig. 72-1).

Single-system multifocal bone disease may be treated with chemotherapy,[15] and good outcomes are also reported with systemic steroids[10] or nonsteroidal anti-inflammatory drugs (e.g., indomethacin).[24] Thirty-four patients treated on DAL-HX83/90 enjoyed excellent outcome with multiagent chemotherapy; six patients experienced reactivation of skeletal disease, and only one developed extraskeletal disease in the form of CNS involvement with DI. No deaths were observed.[15]

Skeletal lesions have a relatively long healing time. Alexander described 38 lesions in 18 patients. The shortest interval required for healing was 5 months, and 14 months was the average interval.[23] Womer described 42 lesions in 21

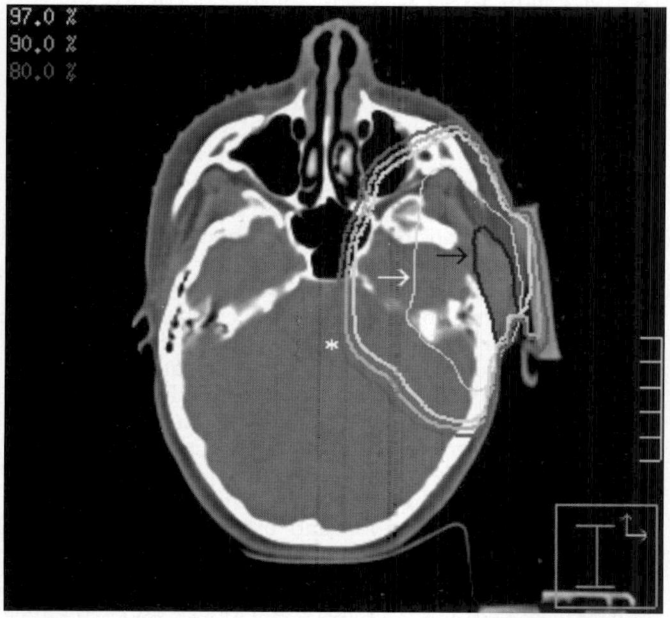

Figure 72-1 A simulation CT image shows the gross and clinical tumor volumes (*black and white arrows, respectively*) and isodose lines (*asterisk*) of a 27-year-old woman who presented with single-system monostotic LCH of the left squamosal temporal bone. Cranial MRI showed an enhancing soft tissue mass arising in the left squamosal temporal bone, extending laterally into the subcutaneous tissue and medially into the intracranial compartment with mass effect on the left temporal lobe. The patient was treated with 3D conformal radiotherapy to 10 Gy in four fractions, prescribed to the 97% isodose line. The left temporal lesion remains controlled at nearly 4 years. 3D, three-dimensional; CT, computed tomography; LCH, Langerhans-cell histiocytosis; MRI, magnetic resonance imaging.

patients, variably treated with biopsy alone, curettage, radiotherapy (2 to 12 Gy), or various chemotherapy regimens. The median time to radiographically partial and complete healing was 3 and 12 months, with no difference by type of therapy.[19]

Nonskeletal Single-System Disease

Cutaneous LCH often simulates seborrheic dermatitis with irritation, erythema, and scaling in the scalp and groin, occasionally with petechial hemorrhages. Skin is second only to bone as a site of single-system disease but is rare. In a report of 19 patients with single-system skin disease treated with local means (excision) or systemic therapy (steroids, vinblastine, mercaptopurine) or both, 11 patients responded to initial therapy and became permanently disease-free, 4 developed multifocal skin disease, and 4 developed multisystem disease, with 1 death.[15]

Topical mechlorethamine (nitrogen mustard) is currently considered first-line therapy.[25] Sheehan reported complete healing of skin lesions using topical mechlorethamine in 14 of 16 children with multisystem disease.[26] Topical or systemic steroids, psoralen/UVA light (PUVA), oral trimethoprim-sulfamethoxazole, and oral thalidomide have been used in cutaneous LCH when topical mechlorethamine has failed. Radiotherapy is rarely used.[25]

Single-system lymph node disease is even more rare than single-system skin disease. Four patients, all with neck nodes, were treated on DAL-HX83/90 with surgical excision and remained disease-free.[15]

Multisystem Disease

Multisystem disease is treated with systemic cytotoxics. Representative studies demonstrating modern therapy and outcomes include AIEOP-CNR-H.X '83,[12] DAL-HX83,[13] LCH-I,[11] and LCH-II.[27] Long-term overall survival (OS) for patients with favorable disease ranged between 93% and 100%, whereas it ranged between 46% and 62% for those with unfavorable disease. All studies considered patients presenting with organ dysfunction to have unfavorable disease; a second criterion used by LCH-I and LCH-II was age younger than 2 years.

Diabetes Insipidus

DI is a well-recognized manifestation of LCH attributed to involvement of the posterior pituitary or hypothalamus or both.[28] It is seen most often in patients with multisystem disease and those with proptosis[29] or other cranial sites of involvement (skull, dental, otic).[28] A prevalence of up to 50% has been reported.[30] The French Langerhans' Cell Histiocytosis Study Group reported DI in 18% of 348 patients whose median follow-up was 36 months.[14] The prevalence of DI in the DAL-HX83 study was 10%.[30] DI may precede or follow the diagnosis of LCH: Of the 19 patients on DAL-HX83 with DI seen at any time, 8 patients had DI at or as long as 4 years before diagnosis, and the remainder developed DI after diagnosis at a median interval of 3 years, 4 months (ranging from 13 months to 5 years). All but 1 of the patients who developed DI had disseminated disease at presentation.

Historically, patients who benefited from hypothalamic-pituitary irradiation (HPI) for DI were treated within days of symptom onset.[31] Similar observations have been made in recently reported series. Minehan[32] reported the Mayo Clinic experience with 47 patients with DI, treated between 1950 and 1989. Ten (36%) of 28 evaluable patients who received HPI responded to treatment: A complete response (CR), defined as discontinuation of vasopressin or radiographic normalization, was observed in six patients. A partial response (PR), defined as a reduction in vasopressin dose or radiographic improvement, was observed in four. Five of the six complete responders were irradiated within 14 days of the diagnosis of DI, whereas only 1 of 14 patients treated after 14 days obtained a CR. A dose response was not observed: The mean dose in the responding and nonresponding patients was 11.2 and 10 Gy. None of 17 patients managed without HPI responded. Additional endocrine abnormalities were observed (growth hormone deficiency in eight patients, panhypopituitarism in six) and were more common among the patients who received radiotherapy compared with those who did not (43% versus 12%). Rosenzweig[28] reported the Joint Center/Massachusetts General Hospital experience with 17 patients with DI treated between 1975 and 1992. Fourteen patients received HPI. Two patients had a CR, defined as no need for vasopressin. Both patients had an incomplete vasopressin deficiency at diagnosis, suggesting early disease. Both received radiotherapy within 3 days of symptom onset, compared with a median interval of 30 days for the entire cohort. One of the responding patients received 8 Gy, and the other showed a partial response after an initial 6 Gy and a complete response after an additional 12 Gy. The 12 irradiated patients who did not respond received 6 to 18 Gy. Two patients (14%) developed panhypopituitarism after receiving HPI. None of three patients managed without HPI responded.

NASOPHARYNGEAL CARCINOMA

Epidemiology and Etiology

Pediatric nasopharyngeal carcinoma (NPC) has a median age at presentation of 12 to 15 years. The male-to-female ratio is between 1.7:1 and 3.2:1.[33-39] In the National Cancer Data Base, pediatric cases in the United States made up 2.8% of total NPC cases between 1985 and 1994.[40]

WHO histologic classification defines three major subtypes: keratinizing squamous carcinomas (type I), nonkeratinizing carcinomas (type II), and undifferentiated carcinomas (type III). Reactive lymphoid infiltrates are often seen in association with type III tumors (*lymphoepitheliomas*) and sometimes with type II.[41]

Adult NPC is endemic in Southern China, Southeast Asia, the Mediterranean basin, and Alaska[42]; and in these regions, it usually consists of type II or type III tumors, the latter being the more common. In contrast, type I tumors are rare, making up less than 5% of endemic adult cohorts.[43-50] The histologic distribution in nonendemic adult cohorts in the Western world is notable for a higher proportion of type I tumors. The epidemiologic study from the National Cancer Data Base reported type I tumors in 75% of patients,[40] and the American Intergroup 0099 study reported type I tumors in 24% of patients.[51]

An association between Epstein-Barr virus (EBV) infection and NPC is observed in patients with type II and type III tumors, and this association appears causative: EBV DNA is detectable in nearly all adult NPC patients in endemic regions but not in their healthy controls,[52,53] matched plasma and tumor samples are genotypically concordant, and there is a strong correlation between plasma EBV DNA levels and treatment outcome.[52] The association between EBV infection and NPC is infrequently observed in patients with type I tumors, but patients with type II or type III tumors even in nonendemic adult cohorts appear to exhibit the association. For example, in a study of 151 American NPC patients, elevated anti-EBV titers were detected in 85% of those with type II and type III tumors but in only 16% of those with type I tumors.[54]

Unlike adult patients, pediatric patients in both endemic and nonendemic regions almost always have type II or type III tumors[34-39] and most have EBV infection. Eight of eight patients tested on the German-Austrian Pediatric Oncology Group (GPOH) NPC-1 study were positive for Epstein-Barr virus-encoded ribonucleic acid (EBER).[36] Eleven of eleven patients tested on POG 9486 were serologically positive.[38] Nine of 11 patients in POG's Rare Tumor Registry tested positive by in situ hybridization for EBV DNA in tumor samples.[55] Compared with type I tumors, type II and type III tumors are more radiosensitive, and higher locoregional control is generally observed in adult patients with type II and type III tumors,[57] with distant relapse as the major pattern of failure.[43-51] The implications of adult clinical trials for pediatric patients are discussed in the following text.

Recent investigations reveal additional molecular differences between adult and pediatric NPC. One study found a significantly higher rate of *c-Kit* positivity in pediatric patients compared with adults (88% versus 28%). This study also observed, among its pediatric cohort, a trend toward decreased recurrence when comparing *c-Kit*–positive to *c-Kit*–negative patients.[58]

Presentation, Staging, and Workup

Palpable neck adenopathy is a typical presenting sign in pediatric NPC. Common symptoms include nasal obstruction, bleeding, and discharge, as well as otalgia, otitis, and hearing loss. Symptoms of locally advanced disease may include trismus, ptosis, ophthalmoplegia, visual loss, and dysgeusia.[42] Hypertrophic pulmonary osteoarthropathy and the syndrome of inappropriate secretion of antidiuretic hormone have been reported as paraneoplastic syndromes.[59,60]

The AJCC staging system employed for adult NPC is used also for children (see Chapter 30). Most pediatric patients present with advanced-stage disease. Among 33 patients treated at Memorial Sloan-Kettering Cancer Center, 29 had stage III to IVB disease[34]; among 22 patients treated on the multi-institutional GPOH NPC-1 study, 1 had stage II disease, 11 had stage III disease, and 10 had stage IV disease.[35,36] Distant disease at presentation is uncommon: 4 (5%) of the 81 patients in the Mumbai, India, series[39] presented with distant disease, with skeletal metastases in all 4 patients, pulmonary metastases in 2, hepatic metastases in 2, bone marrow involvement in 2, and skin involvement in 1.

Clinical evaluation should include fiberoptic examination of the nasopharynx. Imaging studies to evaluate local disease include MRI for soft tissue extent and CT to assess bone erosion. These studies should cover the neck and supraclavicular fossae. Metastatic workup of the lungs, liver, and bones employs routine blood work and imaging studies. CT is commonly used. Positron emission tomography (PET) scanning may be useful, but its utility is not fully defined. Some authors recommend CSF cytology for patients with skull base erosion and bone marrow aspiration and biopsy for patients with advanced disease.[42] Dental evaluation and prophylaxis are important. Given the anticipated need for irradiation of the skull base, baseline endocrinologic and audiologic evaluations are required. Before treatment, myringotomy tubes may be required. A feeding gastrostomy tube should be considered.

Treatment

As in adults, the primary tumor is unresectable. Initial surgical management is usually limited to biopsy; and radiotherapy, alone or in combination with chemotherapy, is the mainstay of management. Neck dissection may be appropriate when there are persistent neck nodes following locoregional treatment and in cases of isolated neck recurrence.[42]

Chemoradiotherapy in Adults

Modern randomized trials have suggested modestly better outcome with chemoradiotherapy than with radiotherapy alone, but the optimal timing of chemotherapy and radiotherapy is not yet certain. In the United States, the 1998 report of Intergroup trial 0099[51] has established radiotherapy with concurrent and adjuvant chemotherapy as the standard of care (see Chapter 30).[61]

The progression-free survival in the radiotherapy alone arm of Intergroup study 0099 (24% at 3 years) was lower than expected. In 10 other randomized trials[43-50,62,63] published in the last two decades, failure outcome with radiotherapy alone, reported heterogeneously as disease-free, relapse-free, progression-free, or failure-free survival, was as low as 42% at 3 years[43] and as high as 72% at 2 years.[49] It is important to note that all but 1 of these 10 trials treated cohorts with less than 5% type I tumors; the one exception is a multi-institutional Italian trial (Rossi, 1988),[62] in which 28% of patients were reported to have tumors of squamous histology, and still its radiotherapy alone arm enjoyed a 4-year relapse-free survival of 56%. For these reasons, it is uncertain that the magnitude of benefit of concurrent chemoradiotherapy observed in Intergroup 0099 should be expected in cohorts where type I tumors are rare,[61,63] namely, adults in endemic regions and children.

Table 72-1 summarizes the findings of Intergroup trial 0099 and of the 10 other trials. Three trials (Chan, 2002[47]; Kwong, 2004[63]; and Lin, 2003[48]) tested radiotherapy alone or with concurrent chemoradiotherapy. Significant improvement in OS and failure outcome was observed in only one trial[48]; interestingly, its patient population had a 3:1 distribution of type II to type III tumors, the reverse of what is usually observed in endemic areas. A recently published meta-analysis[64] comparing radiotherapy alone or with variably timed chemotherapy demonstrated an absolute OS benefit to chemotherapy of 4% at 5 years, corresponding to a hazard ratio of 0.82 ($p = .01$). The largest effect was found for concurrent chemotherapy, with an OS benefit of 20% at 5 years, corresponding to a hazard ratio of .48 ($p = .004$). The meta-analysis consisted of 10 of the 11 trials discussed earlier; Kwong, 2004[63] was published shortly after the meta-analysis and was not included.

Chemoradiotherapy in Children

Comparisons of radiotherapy alone to chemoradiotherapy in pediatric NPC are limited to retrospective data. Wolden and colleagues described the outcome of pediatric NPC patients treated from 1971 to 1998 at Memorial Sloan-Kettering Cancer Center.[34] Thirty-three patients were treated, 20 with combined radiotherapy and chemotherapy, and 13 with radiotherapy alone, with no apparent difference in stage grouping between the two groups. Two chemotherapy regimens were used: The first regimen, given to 12 patients, consisted of dactinomycin, cyclophosphamide, bleomycin, vincristine, methotrexate, and doxorubicin, with two cycles given before radiotherapy and four cycles after; the second regimen, given to 8 patients, consisted of two cycles of cisplatin concurrently with radiotherapy followed by three cycles of cisplatin and 5-fluorouracil. Radiotherapy was given to 25 patients in once-daily fractions of 1.8 to 2.0 Gy and to 8 patients using a concomitant boost technique (1.8 Gy each day initially, followed by 1.8 Gy to the large field plus a 1.6 Gy boost field at least 6 hours apart). The median radiotherapy dose was 66 Gy to the primary tumor and involved nodes and 50 Gy to the uninvolved cervical and supraclavicular regions. With a median follow-up interval of 8.4 years for surviving patients, the actuarial 10-year OS was 58%. Seven patients experienced local failure as part of initial relapse. Six of these seven failed distantly as well. No patient experienced regional failure without local failure. An advantage to chemotherapy was observed in terms of 10-year OS and freedom from distant metastases at 10 years (76% versus 36%, $p < .05$; and 84% versus 43%, $p = .01$) but not significantly in terms of locoregional control (84% versus 65%, $p = .25$), and no difference was observed between the two chemotherapy regimens used. In another report, radiotherapy was given in standard fractionation to 65 to 70 Gy to the primary and involved nodes and to 45 to 50 Gy to the uninvolved neck and supraclavicular regions. Three cohorts were described: 23 patients treated with radiotherapy alone, 13 with adjuvant chemotherapy, and 12 with neoadjuvant chemotherapy. Chemotherapy consisted of various combinations of cisplatin, bleomycin, epirubicin, 5-fluorouracil, and cyclophosphamide. The report suggested that the choice of treatment was largely based on the time period during which a given patient was treated. Of 21 relapses among the entire group, 9 occurred at locoregional sites only, 2 occurred at locoregional and distant sites, and 10 occurred at distant sites only. Actuarial outcomes were reported at 5 years for the first two cohorts and at 3 years for the third, as follows: locoregional control was 52%, 71%, and 89%; failure-free survival was 47%, 54%, and 72%; and OS was 46%, 58%, and 76%. OS was not significantly different among the three treatment cohorts ($p > .05$); significance was not stated with regard to locoregional control or failure-free survival.[35]

Several pediatric NPC protocols have employed neoadjuvant chemotherapy, often with lower total radiotherapy doses than those used in adult NPC, nevertheless showing good survival outcomes and excellent locoregional control. The St. Jude NPC-1 study accrued 21 patients age 10 to 17 years with advanced disease (T3-4 and/or N1-3, M0). They were treated with four cycles, given every 3 to 4 weeks, of methotrexate, cisplatin, 5-fluorouracil, and leucovorin. This induction regimen was followed by once-daily irradiation. The primary received 60 to 74 Gy, with brachytherapy boosting given to the primary of four patients; involved lymph node regions received 60 to 70 Gy. All 21 patients achieved complete remission. With a median follow-up of 41 months, no locoregional failures were observed, and distant failure was observed in only one patient.[37]

Based on the encouraging results of NPC-1, the POG opened protocol 9486 in 1996. The protocol intended to accrue two groups of patients: those with stage I to II disease (stratum 01) and those with stage III to IV disease (stratum 02). The protocol called for radiotherapy alone for the early-stage patients, whereas advanced-stage patients would be treated with neoadjuvant chemotherapy similar to NPC-1 (four 3-week cycles of methotrexate, cisplatin, 5-fluorouracil, and leucovorin) followed by radiotherapy. On either stratum, the dose to involved sites (primary or involved nodes) was 61.2 Gy (except the posterior neck, which received 55.8 Gy), and the uninvolved neck received 50.4 Gy. Of 17 eligible patients who enrolled, only 1 had early-stage disease; the remaining 16 patients had advanced disease. Response at the end of treatment was complete in 11 patients and partial in 4, with a single patient having progressive disease at the primary and nodal sites. The latter patient died of disease. No patients relapsed locally, but three patients who had achieved a complete response to protocol therapy failed distantly. The 4-year event-free survival (EFS) and OS were 77% and 75%, respectively.[38] The multi-institutional GPOH NPC-1 study showed similar results using a similar treatment regimen.[36]

Combined-modality regimens incorporating concurrent chemotherapy have not been widely adopted in the treatment

Table 72-1 Randomized Trials of Radiotherapy Versus Chemoradiotherapy in Adults

	Treatment Arms	Outcome		Pattern of Failure*			
		3-y PFS	**3-y OS**	**T Locoreg**	**Iso Dist**		
Al-Sarraf et al, 1998[51]	RT alone	24%	47%	41%	20%		
	RT with conc. CDDP & adj. CDDP + 5FU	69%	78%	14%	9%		
		$p < .001$	$p = .005$				
		2-y PFS		**Locoreg**	**Dist**		
Chan et al, 2002[47]	RT alone	69%		8%	26%		
	RT with conc. CDDP	76%		7%	21%		
		$p = .10$					
		3-y FFS	**3-y OS**	**3-y Locoreg**	**3-y Dist**		
Kwong et al, 2004[63‡]	RT alone	58%	77%	28%	29%		
	RT with conc. uracil + tegafur	69%	87%	20%	15%		
		$p = .14$	$p = .06$	$p = .39$	$p = .026$		
		5-y PFS	**5-y OS**	**T Local**	**T Reg**	**T Dist**	
Lin et al, 2003[48]	RT alone	53%	54%	24%	6%	29%	
	RT with conc. CDDP + 5FU	72%	72%	9%	3%	19%	
		$p = .001$	$p = .002$	$p = .001$	$p = .16$	$p = .045$	
		Failure with Median Follow-up of 49 Mo		**T Locoreg**	**Reg Only**	**Dist**	
VUMCA I, 1996[44]	RT alone	55%		18%	4%	32%	
	RT with neoadj. bleomycin + epirubicin + CDDP	33%		11%	4%	18%	
		$p < .01$					
		3-y RFS	**3-y OS**	**Local**	**Reg**	**Dist**	**Multiple**
Chua et al, 1998[43]	RT alone	42%	71%	18%	12%	25%	1.3%
	RT with neoadj. CDDP + epirubicin	48%	78%	14%	9%	20%	1.5%
		$p = .45$	$p = .57$	$p = .35$	$p = .38$	$p = .27$	$p = .65$
		5-y RFS	**5-y OS**	**5-y Frdm from Local Rec**	**5-y Frdm from Dist Rec**		
Ma et al, 2001[46]	RT alone	49%	56%	74%	75%		
	RT with neoadj. CDDP + bleomycin + 5FU	59%	63%	82%	79%		
		$p = .05$	$p = .11$	$p = .04$	$p = .40$		
		5-y DFS	**5-y OS**	**5-y Locoreg RFS†, MFS†**	**5-y Dist**		
Hareyama et al, 2002[45]	RT alone	43%	48%	68%	56%		
	RT with neoadj. CDDP + 5FU	55%	60%	65%	74%		
		†	†				
		4-y RFS	**4-y OS**	**T Locoreg**	**Iso Dist**		
Rossi et al, 1988[62]	RT alone	56%	67%	27%	14%		
	RT with adj. vincristine + cyclophosphamide + doxorubicin	58%	59%	24%	15%		
		$p = .45$	$p = .13$				
		5-y RFS	**5-y OS**	**T Local**	**Iso Dist**		
Chi et al, 2002[50]	RT alone	50%	61%	21%	26%		
	RT with adj. CDDP + 5FU + leucovorin	54%	55%	10%	17%		
		$p = .38$	$p = .50$				
		2-y DFS	**2-y OS**	**Iso Locoreg**	**Locoreg + Dist**	**Iso Locoreg**	
Chan et al, 1995[49]	RT alone	72%	81%	10%	5%	18%	
	RT with neoadj. & adj. CDDP + 5FU	68%	80%	14%	3%	27%	
		$p = .29$	$p = .45$	p value using Fisher's exact test for the comparison of relapse pattern between the two treatment arms = .86.			

*Actual incidences are reported in most trials, except where actuarial rates are indicated by the time interval for those rates. Actuarial rates may not necessarily denote site of *first* failure. Statistical significance is noted by p values where available.

†Difference stated to be nonsignificant, but p values not reported.

‡Results of secondary randomization regarding adjuvant chemotherapy are not shown but are discussed in the text.

adj., adjuvant; CDDP, cisplatin; conc., concurrent; DFS, disease-free survival; Dist, distant; 5FU, 5-fluorouracil; FFS, failure-free survival; Frdm, freedom; Iso, isolated; Locoreg, locoregional; MFS, metastasis-free survival; Mo, month; neoadj., neoadjuvant; OS, overall survival, PFS, progression-free survival; Rec, recurrence; reg, regional; RFS, recurrence-free survival; RT, radiotherapy; T, total; y, year.

of pediatric NPC, generally because of concern regarding acute and late toxicities. The Children's Oncology Group's ARAR 0331 protocol is open and tests radiotherapy with neoadjuvant and concurrent chemotherapy for patients with stage IIb to IV disease. Neoadjuvant chemotherapy consists of three cycles of cisplatin and 5-fluorouracil, and cisplatin alone is given during radiotherapy. Radiotherapy dose (61.2 to 70.2 Gy) is based on response to neoadjuvant chemotherapy. Radiotherapy alone (70.2 Gy) is given to patients presenting with stage I and IIa disease. Amifostine is used in both strata, with the objective of decreasing xerostomia.

Dose-Response and Techniques

Whereas some older pediatric data had not demonstrated improved disease control with higher radiation doses,[65] more recent series suggest a benefit to a total dose exceeding 60 Gy. Radiotherapy dose more than 60 Gy in Wolden's cohort provided significantly higher 10-year locoregional control (93% versus 60%, $p < .03$), and there was a nearly significant benefit in terms of progression-free survival and OS (80% versus 48%, $p = .06$; 76% versus 36%, $p = .08$).[2] Similar observations have been made by other investigators.[35,39,66]

The Institut Gustave Roussy experience reported in abstract form in 2004[33] describes outcome with radiation dose adapted to response to neoadjuvant chemotherapy. Seventy-four evaluable patients received multiagent, cisplatin-based chemotherapy. Low-dose radiotherapy (50 Gy) was given to 40 patients who achieved a good response, whereas the rest received high-dose radiotherapy (65 to 70 Gy). Complete response at the completion of therapy was observed in 66 patients. With a median follow-up of 10 years, locoregional failures were observed in 8 patients and distant failures in 18. Locoregional failure did not differ significantly between the low- and high-dose groups. EFS and OS at 5 years were 64% and 68%, said to be significantly better in the low-dose group.

Radiotherapy field design in pediatric NPC follows that of adults[42] and is discussed in Chapter 30. In children, it is particularly important to minimize dose, when possible, to the middle ear, temporomandibular joint, and larynx.

Late Effects

Late effects of treatment for pediatric NPC are significant. The relatively long follow-up interval for the Memorial Sloan-Kettering Cancer Center cohort (8.4 years for surviving patients) allowed the authors to provide a detailed description of late effects.[34] Of the 33 patients, 32 were treated with conventional or three-dimensional conformal radiotherapy, and 1 patient was treated with intensity-modulated radiotherapy. All patients had moderate to severe xerostomia; and, despite fluoride therapy and expert dental care for most patients, one third developed dental problems requiring intervention. Significant neck fibrosis and muscle atrophy were seen in 61%. Chronic serous otitis media occurred in 18% and was treated with myringotomy tube placement. Elevated thyroid-stimulating hormone (TSH) levels were seen in 12%; all cases were subclinical yet treated with thyroid hormone replacement. Mild facial bone hypoplasia was apparent in 9%. Significant trismus was seen in 9% and optic neuropathy in one patient. Mild osteoradionecrosis was observed in a single patient who was irradiated to 60 Gy and treated with the neoadjuvant and adjuvant doxorubicin-based regimen. Hearing deficits were mentioned as additional potential complications but not directly observed. Salivary gland tumors were observed as second malignancies in two patients; one underwent a resection and had remained disease-free at 4 years posttreatment, whereas the other died of disease. Overall, the 10-year actuarial rate of grade 3 to 4 complications was 24%. When this rate was analyzed by treatment variables, neither the use of chemotherapy nor radiation dose were predictive for adverse sequelae, whereas a trend was observed favoring three-dimensional conformal and intensity-modulated radiotherapy over conventional treatment (0% versus 28%, $p = .3$).

JUVENILE NASOPHARYNGEAL ANGIOFIBROMA

Epidemiology, Pathology, and Etiology

Juvenile nasopharyngeal angiofibroma (JNA) typically arises during adolescence with median age 13 to 18 years and male gender predilection, with females rarely encountered.[67-73] It is characterized by irregular vascular channels within a fibrous stroma.[71] Its etiology is uncertain. Some authors believe the tumor is a vascular hamartoma or a pathologic and reactive proliferation of vessels,[72] whereas others view it as truly neoplastic.[71] Recent observations support the latter hypothesis. For example, citing the observed 25-fold incidence of JNA in patients with familial adenomatous polyposis (FAP) versus the general population, a study examined aberrations in the adenomatous polyposis coli (APC)/β-catenin pathway of sporadic JNA cases. Nuclear β-catenin accumulation was diffusely present in the stromal cells but not in the endothelial cells of all 16 examined cases. Further, clonal, activating alterations were detected in the β-catenin oncogene in the tumors of 12 of 16 cases but in none of the corresponding normal nasopharyngeal tissue from these patients. Based on this evidence, the authors concluded that the stromal cells are the neoplastic cells of JNA and that the genetic aberrations are somatic.[71] Given that the overwhelming majority of JNA patients are peripubertal males, hormonal mechanisms of tumorigenesis have been explored. JNA samples are variably positive for androgen, estrogen, and progesterone receptors,[74-79] and some series have described tumor responses to the testosterone receptor blocker flutamide.[80]

Presentation and Staging

JNA frequently exhibits locally aggressive behavior evidenced by bony erosion and infiltration of local structures. The tumor typically arises in the posterolateral wall of the roof of the nasal cavity and grows within the nasopharynx and nasal cavity. It may extend to involve a variety of local sites including the sphenoid and ethmoid sinuses, pterygopalatine fossa, and sphenopalatine foramen. It may further extend to involve intracranial structures including the sella turcica, cavernous sinus, and orbit. Presenting symptoms reflect disease extent and include nasal obstruction, snoring, epistaxis, cheek swelling, headache, proptosis, visual changes, and cranial nerve palsies.[69,81,82]

A number of staging systems have been proposed. They are generally illustrative of local extent, and some specifically incorporate bone invasion.[83,84] Two representative systems are summarized in Table 72-2.

Because the literature is limited to small retrospective series, it is difficult to estimate the proportion of patients presenting within each stage. A representative surgical series consisted of four patients with Fisch stage I disease, 16 with stage II, eight with stage III, and two with stage IV,[70] whereas a radiotherapy series described a distribution weighted more heavily toward advanced stages (5 patients with Chandler stage III and 10 with stage IV).[68] The difference in stage distribution between these surgical and radiotherapy series is evident in other series.[68,73,85,86]

Table 72-2 **Juvenile Nasopharyngeal Angiofibroma Staging Systems**

	Fisch[83]	Chandler[84]
Stage I	Tumor limited to the nasopharynx and nasal cavity, without bone destruction.	Tumor confined to the nasopharynx.
Stage II	Tumor invades the pterygomaxillary fossa, maxillary, ethmoid, and/or sphenoid sinuses, with bone destruction.	Tumor extends into the nasal cavity and/or sphenoid sinus.
Stage III	Tumor invades the infratemporal fossa, orbit, and/or parasellar region, remaining lateral to the cavernous sinus.	Tumor extends into the antrum, ethmoid sinus, pterygomaxillary fossa, infratemporal fossa, orbit, and/or cheek.
Stage IV	Tumor with massive invasion of the cavernous sinus, the optic chiasmal region, and/or the pituitary fossa.	Tumor extends into the cranial cavity.

Treatment

Resection is considered the treatment of choice, especially for less-advanced tumors. A variety of standard surgical approaches are recognized. Endoscopic approaches are being more widely adapted. With a mean follow-up interval of 23 months in one series,[70] six local recurrences were observed; five occurred among the 15 patients treated with the standard approaches, whereas only one occurred among the 15 treated endoscopically (most with early-stage disease). Recurrent tumors were salvaged surgically or with embolization or both, and the authors stated that all patients were without disease. Similar or higher rates of local control with surgery have been documented in other modern series.[73,85,86]

A significant risk of surgery is operative hemorrhage, because of the highly vascular structure of JNA. Preoperative arterial embolization is part of standard management[70] and has been shown to decrease operative blood loss.[87,88] It has been employed also with the goal of decreasing local recurrence, but this has not been consistently achieved.[73,87,89]

Radiotherapy has been a primary modality in the management of JNA for decades, and publications from the 1970s and 1980s document good local control relative to surgically treated patients.[90,91] For example, Cummings' series of 55 patients described long-term local control of 80% using 30 to 35 Gy, and salvage using surgery or a second course of radiotherapy ultimately controlled all patients.[91]

The largest recent radiotherapy reports were published by UCLA[69] and by the University of Florida.[68] Twenty-seven UCLA patients were treated from 1960 to 2000 with primary radiotherapy. One hundred and two additional patients during that time interval were treated surgically at UCLA. The majority of the radiotherapy patients (23/27) had intracranial extension, and the four remaining patients had tumors deemed unresectable because of proximity to the optic nerve or because they received significant vascular supply from the internal carotid artery. Until 1985 radiotherapy dose ranged from 30 to 55 Gy, and thereafter it was reduced to 36 to 40 Gy. With an average follow-up interval of 6 years, local recurrence was observed in four patients (15%) whose primary treatment was 30 to 40 Gy. The time to recurrence ranged from 2 to 5 years. Salvage therapy consisted of reirradiation using 20 to 36 Gy for two patients and surgery for two patients. With a follow-up interval of 2 to 7 years after salvage therapy, one of the patients who was salvaged surgically experienced a second recurrence 1 year later; he was reirradiated to 45 Gy and, with another 7 years of follow-up, remained disease-free. The Florida series consisted of 15 patients who had radiotherapy from 1975 to 1996 as either primary treatment (6/15) or salvage for recurrent disease after surgery (9/15). Five patients had Chandler stage III disease, and 10 had stage IV disease. Radiotherapy dose ranged from 30 to 35 Gy. With a minimum follow-up interval of 2.5 years, local recurrence was observed in two patients (15%) at 26 and 38 months after radiotherapy. Surgical salvage was successful in both patients, and ultimate local control for the entire cohort was 100%.

Tumor response to radiotherapy takes months. Lee and colleagues observed that 9 of 11 patients followed radiographically continued to have abnormal findings 6 months after radiotherapy, and 7 continued to display radiographic abnormalities after 2 years. Asymptomatic, stable radiographic abnormalities were not considered to represent evidence of recurrent or persistent disease.[69] Reddy and colleagues also observed slow regression but noted complete response by physical examination in all 13 patients in whom the tumor was controlled after radiotherapy. The median time to CR among these 13 patients was 13 months, with a range of 1 to 39 months. The two patients who did not achieve a CR were those who ultimately developed a local recurrence.[68] These observations are in general agreement with those of Cummings two decades earlier, who noted the disappearance of visible abnormalities in 50% of irradiated patients at 12 months and in 90% at 36 months.[91] Epistaxis is a common presenting symptom of JNA. Lee and colleagues reported that epistaxis resolved in all 13 irradiated patients by completion of radiotherapy.[69]

Late Effects of Radiotherapy

The moderate radiotherapy doses used for JNA and the complications of surgery in patients with advanced stages of disease lend support to the use of radiotherapy.[69] Nevertheless, late effects of radiotherapy may be significant. In the 27 primarily irradiated patients at UCLA, panhypopituitarism was observed in one patient (at 4 years), growth retardation was noted in another (at 6 years), and cataract was observed in two patients (at 3 and 7 years). One additional patient experienced temporal lobe necrosis and severe keratopathy and endophthalmitis at 10 years, requiring evisceration of the eye; however, he had undergone primary radiotherapy to 30 Gy, salvage intracranial surgery for local recurrence, and reirradiation to an additional 45 Gy for a second local recurrence.[69] In the 15 University of Florida patients irradiated primarily or for recurrent disease after initial surgery, cataracts were observed in 3 patients (at 5 to 10 years) who had a tumor that invaded the orbit, in-field basal cell carcinoma in one patient (after 14 years), and delayed transient CNS syndrome in 1 patient.[68] Radiation-induced neoplasms are of concern in the pediatric population. In Cummings' 55 irradiated patients, two developed second malignant neoplasms (thyroid carcinoma at 14 years after radiotherapy and basal cell carcinoma at 13 years),[91] and various case reports are summarized in the paper by Lee and colleagues.[69]

Radiotherapy Techniques

Historically, radiotherapy techniques have consisted of parallel-opposed fields with or without a third anteroposterior field.[68] Modern CT planning and intensity-modulated radiotherapy allows additional conformality and complexity of beam arrangements.

PLEUROPULMONARY BLASTOMA

Pleuropulmonary blastoma (PPB) is a rare pediatric tumor of young children. It presents as an intrapulmonary, pleural-based, or mediastinal neoplasm, or as all three (Fig. 72-2). It was formally described in 1988 by Manivel[92] as a dysembryonic tumor composed of "small primitive cells with blastomatous qualities separated by an uncommitted stroma," deemed distinct from pulmonary blastoma in adults by virtue of its variable intrathoracic location, primitive embryonic-like blastema and stroma, absence of a carcinomatous component, and potential differentiation toward a number of sarcoma histologies (commonly rhabdomyosarcoma, chondrosarcoma, or liposarcoma).

The family history in one fourth of PPB patients is positive for various neoplasms or dysplasias, or both, including PPB, pulmonary cysts, cystic nephromas, sarcomas, medulloblastomas, thyroid neoplasias and dysplasias, malignant germ cell tumors, Hodgkin's disease, leukemia, and Langerhans-cell histiocytosis.[93] PPB may arise within preexisting benign cystic lung lesions (e.g., congenital cystic adenomatoid malformation and acquired bronchopulmonary dysplasia), and this association is seen in at least one fifth of cases.[94-96]

The pathologic classification of PPB is based on gross and microscopic morphology and divides the tumor into three

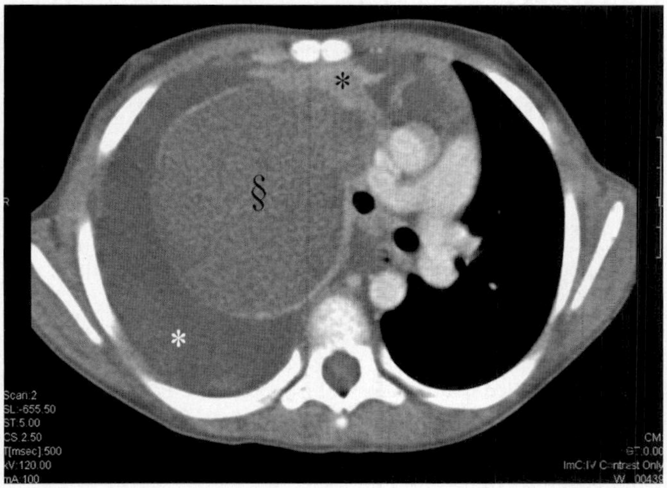

Figure 72-2 CT at presentation of a 3-year-old girl with type III PPB demonstrated an encapsulated hypodense 9 × 9 × 6 cm lesion (§) arising in the right upper lobe, abutting the mediastinum with resultant leftward shift. Compressed lung anteriorly (*black asterisk*) and inhomogeneous pleural fluid (*white asterisk*) were seen. CT, computed tomography; PPB, pleuropulmonary blastoma. (Courtesy of Melissa R. Spevak, MD.)

types: type I, comprising approximately 15% of cases, is purely cystic in appearance; type II, comprising 40% to 45%, is cystic and solid; and type III, comprising 40%, is entirely solid. The morphologic classification is biologically valid: In a report from the Pleuropulmonary Blastoma Registry (a Children's Oncology Group affiliate), median age was significantly different (9, 31, and 42 months; range, 0 to 37, 6 to 64, and 1 to 147 months), and survival at 75 months was 84%, 51%, and 44%.[97]

A PPB Registry report published by Priest in 1997 described important clinical features of PPB.[96] Among the 50 patients, presenting symptoms included respiratory distress (n = 21), fever (n = 16), chest or abdominal pain (n = 13), cough (n = 13), anorexia (n = 6), and malaise (n = 5). Pneumonia, suspected clinically or radiographically or both, was evident in 15 patients, and a pneumothorax was noted in 5 patients. The parietal pleura was involved in 20 cases. Pleural effusions were noted in 21 patients, but malignant cytology was found in only 2 of 12 cases. Mediastinal extension was seen in 11 cases. Metastatic disease at diagnosis was observed in only 1 patient (involving an ovary). Among this variably treated cohort, 25 patients experienced recurrent disease. Recurrence was local in 19. Distant sites included the contralateral chest (n = 2), CNS (n = 11), bone (n = 6), adrenal gland (n = 1), and liver (n = 1). Nodal dissemination to the hila or mediastinum, or both, was not observed.

Guidelines for staging evaluation and treatment are available at the PPB Registry's web site (http://www.ppbregistry.org). Chest CT should be performed in all patients. Abdominal CT, head MRI, and bone scan are performed routinely in those with type II or type III disease.

For type I PPB, maximal surgical excision is recommended, followed by adjuvant chemotherapy with vincristine, actinomycin D, and cyclophosphamide.[97] The recommendation regarding maximal surgery is empirical, because univariate analysis of Priest's 50-patient cohort did not show a correlation between extent of surgery and survival.[96] Other data support the use of chemotherapy. A review of 33 type I patients (27 Registry, 6 in the literature) demonstrated recurrence in none of 15 who received adjuvant chemotherapy but in 7 of 18 treated with surgery alone; all recurrent lesions had morphologically progressed to type II or type III lesions, and the authors stated that salvage was poor.[97] For type II and type III PPB, vincristine, actinomycin D, and cyclophosphamide are alternated with cisplatin and doxorubicin.[97] Type II and type III PPB are less easily resectable,[96] and preoperative chemotherapy is recommended.[97]

PPB Registry recommendations suggest that radiotherapy be individualized but state that it should be "strongly considered for sites of known residual disease after surgery" (http://ppbregistry.org, February 2005). Data regarding the utility of radiotherapy are lacking. Among Priest's 50 patients, 16 received radiotherapy: The more aggressive morphologic types frequently presented with extensive intrathoracic involvement, including widespread pleural contamination; and patients with type III PPB were more likely to have received radiotherapy (59%) than those with type II (17%) or type I (0%) tumors (p = .004). Eleven received focal external beam irradiation, 15 received hemithorax irradiation, and 2 received intracavitary ^{32}P. Half (8/16) of the irradiated patients recurred (in-field in 5/8). Focal external beam treatment doses ranged up to 55 Gy. Hemithorax doses ranged for most patients between 9 Gy and 14 Gy.[96] A report of intraoperative high dose rate brachytherapy for gross intrathoracic disease in two patients revealed that one failed locally and distantly and died, and the other experienced long-term control.[98]

EXTRARENAL WILMS' TUMOR

Extrarenal Wilms' tumor (EWT) is a rare but well-documented entity. It is histologically similar to renal Wilms' tumor (WT) but may contain teratomatous elements. It is thought to arise from ectopic metanephric blastema.[99] This is supported by the close proximity of the urogenital ridge and mesonephron during embryologic development and by the observation that EWT commonly arises in or close to the spermatic cord, epididymis, uterus, or cervix.[100] The etiology of EWT is unknown, but the association between EWT and horseshoe kidney further supports defective embryogenesis.[101,102] The finding of *WT1* messenger RNA (mRNA) expression in two of eight EWT cases suggests a genetic similarity between EWT and WT.[103]

Symptoms at presentation vary with the primary site. There are no distinguishing imaging characteristics, and the diagnosis can only be made histologically.[99,100]

The EWT literature is typically case reports of one or a few patients; however, a study published in 1991 provided data on 34 patients,[100] most of whom were previously reported. Most were young children, but four were young and middle-aged adults (median age, 3.6 years; range, 2 months to 56 years). The anatomic location was retroperitoneal in 13 patients and inguinal in 10; other sites included the scrotum, supratesticular area, endocervix, uterus, adnexa, vagina, sacrococcyx, and chest wall. Disease was localized in all but one patient who had both regional and distant spread at presentation. Primary treatment was usually surgery and chemotherapy, and 11 patients also received radiotherapy. OS at 2 years was 82%. Chemotherapy agents typically used for WT appeared to be equally effective for EWT, and the authors noted that chemotherapy indications should be the same as for comparable-stage WT. Radiotherapy recommendations were less certain. Of the 34 patients, 9 failed, 3 locally. Radiotherapy was given as part of primary treatment to two of the three patients. Doses of 20 Gy to 50 Gy were used, and the authors acknowledged that most patients were treated before the National Wilms' Tumor Studies (NWTS) showed the efficacy of lower doses.

Coppes and others suggest that radiotherapy should be limited to patients with postoperative unresectable gross residual disease and for metastatic disease.[100,104] Alternatively, some have suggested that stage III WT guidelines be applied to all EWT.[99] If WT and EWT are considered biologically similar, it is reasonable to consider the stage-by-stage recommendations outlined in a number of key WT studies: NWTS-1 and NWTS-2 demonstrated no need for radiotherapy in patients with tumor limited to the kidney and completely resected (then-termed group I, now stage I).[105,106] In NWTS-3, favorable histology (FH) patients with stage II disease (tumor completely removed but with evidence of extracapsular extension, renal vessel infiltration/thrombus, prior biopsy, or local spillage) were randomized to 20 Gy or no adjuvant radiotherapy, showing no difference in survival; and FH patients with stage III disease (positive surgical margins, regional nodal involvement, peritoneal implants, or diffuse peritoneal contamination) were randomized to 20 Gy or 10 Gy, with an additional 10 Gy permitted as a local boost to gross residual disease, likewise showing no difference in survival.[107] Currently, in NWTS-5, patients with stage III FH, stage IV FH with abdominal stage III, and stage II to IV anaplastic WT receive 10 Gy to their abdominal disease (given as 10.8 Gy in six fractions or 10.5 Gy in seven fractions).[108] Histologic subtypes have not been consistently analyzed in the EWT literature.[100] In the absence of data to inform the timing of radiotherapy for EWT, the NWTS guidelines should be respected. This applies also to the EWT patient with pulmonary metastases.

REFERENCES

Langerhans Cell Histiocytosis

1. Banchereau J, Steinman RM: Dendritic cells and the control of immunity. Nature 392:245-252, 1998.
2. Valladeau J, Ravel O, Dezutter-Dambuyant C, et al: Langerin, a novel C-type lectin specific to Langerhans cells, is an endocytic receptor that induces the formation of Birbeck granules. Immunity 12:71-81, 2000.
3. Willman CL, Busque L, Griffith BB, et al: Langerhans'-cell histiocytosis (histiocytosis X)—a clonal proliferative disease. N Engl J Med 331:154-160, 1994.
4. McClain KL, Laud P, Wu WS, et al: Langerhans cell histiocytosis patients have HLA Cw7 and DR4 types associated with specific clinical presentations and no increased frequency in polymorphisms of the tumor necrosis factor alpha promoter. Med Pediatr Oncol 41:502-507, 2003.
5. Bernstrand C, Carstensen H, Jakobsen B, et al: Immunogenetic heterogeneity in single-system and multisystem langerhans cell histiocytosis. Pediatr Res 54:30-36, 2003.
6. Glotzbecker MP, Carpentieri DF, Dormans JP: Langerhans cell histiocytosis: A primary viral infection of bone? Human herpes virus 6 latent protein detected in lymphocytes from tissue of children. J Pediatr Orthop 24:123-129, 2004.
7. Favara BE, Feller AC, Pauli M, et al: Contemporary classification of histiocytic disorders. The WHO Committee on Histiocytic/Reticulum Cell Proliferations. Reclassification Working Group of the Histiocyte Society. Med Pediatr Oncol 29:157-166, 1997.
8. Yousem SA, Colby TV, Chen YY, et al: Pulmonary Langerhans' cell histiocytosis: Molecular analysis of clonality. Am J Surg Pathol 25:630-636, 2001.
9. Histiocytosis syndromes in children. Writing Group of the Histiocyte Society. Lancet 1:208-209, 1987.
10. Broadbent V, Gadner H: Current therapy for Langerhans cell histiocytosis. Hematol Oncol Clin North Am 12:327-338, 1998.
11. Gadner H, Grois N, Arico M, et al: A randomized trial of treatment for multisystem Langerhans' cell histiocytosis. J Pediatr 138:728-734, 2001.
12. Ceci A, de Terlizzi M, Colella R, et al: Langerhans cell histiocytosis in childhood: Results from the Italian Cooperative AIEOP-CNR-H.X '83 study. Med Pediatr Oncol 21:259-264, 1993.
13. Gadner H, Heitger A, Grois N, et al: Treatment strategy for disseminated Langerhans cell histiocytosis. DAL HX-83 Study Group. Med Pediatr Oncol 23:72-80, 1994.
14. A multicentre retrospective survey of Langerhans' cell histiocytosis: 348 cases observed between 1983 and 1993. The French Langerhans' Cell Histiocytosis Study Group. Arch Dis Child 75:17-24, 1996.
15. Titgemeyer C, Grois N, Minkov M, et al: Pattern and course of single-system disease in Langerhans cell histiocytosis data from the DAL-HX 83- and 90-study. Med Pediatr Oncol 37:108-114, 2001.
16. Azouz EM, Saigal G, Rodriguez MM, et al: Langerhans' cell histiocytosis: Pathology, imaging and treatment of skeletal involvement. Pediatr Radiol 35:103-115, 2005.
17. Van Nieuwenhuyse JP, Clapuyt P, Malghem J, et al: Radiographic skeletal survey and radionuclide bone scan in Langerhans cell histiocytosis of bone. Pediatr Radiol 26:734-738, 1996.
18. Berry DH, Gresik M, Maybee D, et al: Histiocytosis X in bone only. Med Pediatr Oncol 18:292-294, 1990.
19. Womer RB, Raney RB, Jr., D'Angio GJ: Healing rates of treated and untreated bone lesions in histiocytosis X. Pediatrics 76:286-288, 1985.
20. Egeler RM, Thompson RC, Jr., Voute PA, et al: Intralesional infiltration of corticosteroids in localized Langerhans' cell histiocytosis. J Pediatr Orthop 12:811-814, 1992.
21. Selch MT, Parker RG: Radiation therapy in the management of Langerhans cell histiocytosis. Med Pediatr Oncol 18:97-102, 1990.
22. el-Sayed S, Brewin TB: Histiocytosis X: Does radiotherapy still have a role? Clin Oncol (R Coll Radiol) 4:27-31, 1992.
23. Alexander JE, Seibert JJ, Berry DH, et al: Prognostic factors for healing of bone lesions in histiocytosis X. Pediatr Radiol 18:326-332, 1988.

24. Munn SE, Olliver L, Broadbent V, et al: Use of indomethacin in Langerhans cell histiocytosis. Med Pediatr Oncol 32:247-249, 1999.
25. Chu T: Langerhans cell histiocytosis. Australas J Dermatol 42:237-242, 2001.
26. Sheehan MP, Atherton DJ, Broadbent V, et al: Topical nitrogen mustard: An effective treatment for cutaneous Langerhans cell histiocytosis. J Pediatr 119:317-321, 1991.
27. Minkov M, Grois N, Arico M, et al: Preliminary results of the LCH-II clinical trial of the Histiocyte Society. Med Pediatr Oncol 41:263, 2003.
28. Rosenzweig KE, Arceci RJ, Tarbell NJ: Diabetes insipidus secondary to Langerhans' cell histiocytosis: Is radiation therapy indicated? Med Pediatr Oncol 29:36-40, 1997.
29. Dunger DB, Broadbent V, Yeoman E, et al: The frequency and natural history of diabetes insipidus in children with Langerhans-cell histiocytosis. N Engl J Med 321:1157-1162, 1989.
30. Grois N, Flucher-Wolfram B, Heitger A, et al: Diabetes insipidus in Langerhans cell histiocytosis: Results from the DAL-HX 83 study. Med Pediatr Oncol 24:248-256, 1995.
31. Greenberger JS, Cassady JR, Jaffe N, et al: Radiation therapy in patients with histiocytosis: Management of diabetes insipidus and bone lesions. Int J Radiat Oncol Biol Phys 5:1749-1755, 1979.
32. Minehan KJ, Chen MG, Zimmerman D, et al: Radiation therapy for diabetes insipidus caused by Langerhans cell histiocytosis. Int J Radiat Oncol Biol Phys 23:519-524, 1992.

Nasopharyngeal Carcinoma

33. Habrand J, Guillot Valls D, Petras S, et al: Carcinoma of the nasopharynx in children and adolescents treated with initial chemotherapy (CT) followed by adapted doses of radiotherapy (RT). Int J Radiat Oncol Biol Phys 60:S247, 2004.
34. Wolden SL, Steinherz PG, Kraus DH, et al: Improved long-term survival with combined modality therapy for pediatric nasopharynx cancer. Int J Radiat Oncol Biol Phys 46:859-864, 2000.
35. Ayan I, Altun M: Nasopharyngeal carcinoma in children: Retrospective review of 50 patients. Int J Radiat Oncol Biol Phys 35:485-492, 1996.
36. Mertens R, Granzen B, Lassay L, et al: Nasopharyngeal carcinoma in childhood and adolescence: Concept and preliminary results of the cooperative GPOH study NPC-91. Gesellschaft fur Padiatrische Onkologie und Hamatologie. Cancer 80:951-959, 1997.
37. Douglass EC, Fontanesi J, Ribeiro RC, et al: Improved long-term disease-free survival in nasopharyngeal carcinoma (NPC) in childhood and adolescence: A multi-institution treatment protocol [abstract]. J Clin Oncol 15:1470, 1996.
38. Rodriguez-Galindo C, Wofford M, Castleberry RP, et al: Preradiation chemotherapy with methotrexate, cisplatin, 5-fluorouracil, and leucovorin for pediatric nasopharyngeal carcinoma. Cancer 103:850-857, 2005.
39. Laskar S, Sanghavi V, Muckaden MA, et al: Nasopharyngeal carcinoma in children: Ten years' experience at the Tata Memorial Hospital, Mumbai. Int J Radiat Oncol Biol Phys 58:189-195, 2004.
40. Marks JE, Phillips JL, Menck HR: The National Cancer Data Base report on the relationship of race and national origin to the histology of nasopharyngeal carcinoma. Cancer 83:582-588, 1998.
41. Greene FL, Page DL, Fleming ID, et al: AJCC Cancer Staging Manual, 6th ed. New York, Springer-Verlag, 2002.
42. Ayan I, Kaytan E, Ayan N: Childhood nasopharyngeal carcinoma: From biology to treatment. Lancet Oncol 4:13-21, 2003.
43. Chua DT, Sham JS, Choy D, et al: Preliminary report of the Asian-Oceanian Clinical Oncology Association randomized trial comparing cisplatin and epirubicin followed by radiotherapy versus radiotherapy alone in the treatment of patients with locoregionally advanced nasopharyngeal carcinoma. Asian-Oceanian Clinical Oncology Association Nasopharynx Cancer Study Group. Cancer 83:2270-2283, 1998.
44. International Nasopharynx Cancer Study Group: Preliminary results of a randomized trial comparing neoadjuvant chemotherapy (cisplatin, epirubicin, bleomycin) plus radiotherapy vs. radiotherapy alone in stage IV(> or = N2, M0) undifferentiated nasopharyngeal carcinoma: A positive effect on progression-free survival. VUMCA I trial. Int J Radiat Oncol Biol Phys 35:463-469, 1996.
45. Hareyama M, Sakata K, Shirato H, et al: A prospective, randomized trial comparing neoadjuvant chemotherapy with radiotherapy alone in patients with advanced nasopharyngeal carcinoma. Cancer 94:2217-2223, 2002.
46. Ma J, Mai HQ, Hong MH, et al: Results of a prospective randomized trial comparing neoadjuvant chemotherapy plus radiotherapy with radiotherapy alone in patients with locoregionally advanced nasopharyngeal carcinoma. J Clin Oncol 19:1350-1357, 2001.
47. Chan AT, Teo PM, Ngan RK, et al: Concurrent chemotherapy-radiotherapy compared with radiotherapy alone in locoregionally advanced nasopharyngeal carcinoma: Progression-free survival analysis of a phase III randomized trial. J Clin Oncol 20:2038-2044, 2002.
48. Lin JC, Jan JS, Hsu CY, et al: Phase III study of concurrent chemoradiotherapy versus radiotherapy alone for advanced nasopharyngeal carcinoma: Positive effect on overall and progression-free survival. J Clin Oncol 21:631-637, 2003.
49. Chan AT, Teo PM, Leung TW, et al: A prospective randomized study of chemotherapy adjunctive to definitive radiotherapy in advanced nasopharyngeal carcinoma. Int J Radiat Oncol Biol Phys 33:569-577, 1995.
50. Chi KH, Chang YC, Guo WY, et al: A phase III study of adjuvant chemotherapy in advanced nasopharyngeal carcinoma patients. Int J Radiat Oncol Biol Phys 52:1238-1244, 2002.
51. Al-Sarraf M, LeBlanc M, Giri PG, et al: Chemoradiotherapy versus radiotherapy in patients with advanced nasopharyngeal cancer: Phase III randomized Intergroup study 0099. J Clin Oncol 16:1310-1317, 1998.
52. Lin JC, Wang WY, Chen KY, et al: Quantification of plasma Epstein-Barr virus DNA in patients with advanced nasopharyngeal carcinoma. N Engl J Med 350:2461-2470, 2004.
53. Feinmesser R, Miyazaki I, Cheung R, et al: Diagnosis of nasopharyngeal carcinoma by DNA amplification of tissue obtained by fine-needle aspiration. N Engl J Med 326:17-21, 1992.
54. Neel HB III, Pearson GR, Weiland LH, et al: Application of Epstein-Barr virus serology to the diagnosis and staging of North American patients with nasopharyngeal carcinoma. Otolaryngol Head Neck Surg 91:255-262, 1983.
55. Hawkins EP, Krischer JP, Smith BE, et al: Nasopharyngeal carcinoma in children—A retrospective review and demonstration of Epstein-Barr viral genomes in tumor cell cytoplasm: A report of the Pediatric Oncology Group. Hum Pathol 21:805-810, 1990.
56. Naegele RF, Champion J, Murphy S, et al: Nasopharyngeal carcinoma in American children: Epstein-Barr virus-specific antibody titers and prognosis. Int J Cancer 29:209-212, 1982.
57. Sanguineti G, Geara FB, Garden AS, et al: Carcinoma of the nasopharynx treated by radiotherapy alone: Determinants of local and regional control. Int J Radiat Oncol Biol Phys 37:985-996, 1997.
58. Bar-Sela G, Arush MW, Sabo E, et al: Pediatric nasopharyngeal carcinoma: Better prognosis and increased c-Kit expression as compared to adults. Pediatr Blood Cancer 45:291-297, 2005.
59. Ellouz R, Cammoun M, Attia RB, et al: Nasopharyngeal carcinoma in children and adolescents in Tunisia: Clinical aspects and the paraneoplastic syndrome. IARC Sci Publ, 115-129, 1978.
60. Krmar RT, Ferraris JR, Ruiz SE, et al: Syndrome of inappropriate secretion of antidiuretic hormone in nasopharynx carcinoma. Pediatr Nephrol 11:502-503, 1997.
61. Cooper JS, Lee H, Torrey M, et al: Improved outcome secondary to concurrent chemoradiotherapy for advanced carcinoma of the nasopharynx: Preliminary corroboration of the intergroup experience. Int J Radiat Oncol Biol Phys 47:861-866, 2000.
62. Rossi A, Molinari R, Boracchi P, et al: Adjuvant chemotherapy with vincristine, cyclophosphamide, and doxorubicin after radiotherapy in local-regional nasopharyngeal cancer: results of a 4-year multicenter randomized study. J Clin Oncol 6:1401-1410, 1988.
63. Kwong DL, Sham JS, Au GK, et al: Concurrent and adjuvant chemotherapy for nasopharyngeal carcinoma: A factorial study. J Clin Oncol 22:2643-2653, 2004.

64. Langendijk JA, Leemans Ch R, Buter J, et al: The additional value of chemotherapy to radiotherapy in locally advanced nasopharyngeal carcinoma: A meta-analysis of the published literature. J Clin Oncol 22:4604-4612, 2004.
65. Jenkin RD, Anderson JR, Jereb B, et al: Nasopharyngeal carcinoma—A retrospective review of patients less than thirty years of age: A report of Children's Cancer Study Group. Cancer 47:360-366, 1981.
66. Onal C, Ozyar E: In regard to Laskar et al: Nasopharyngeal carcinoma in children: Ten years' experience at the Tata Memorial Hospital, Mumbai (Int J Radiat Oncol Biol Phys 58:189-195, 2004). Int J Radiat Oncol Biol Phys 60:686, 2004 (author reply).

Juvenile Nasopharyngeal Angiofibroma

67. Kania RE, Sauvaget E, Guichard JP, et al: Early postoperative CT scanning for juvenile nasopharyngeal angiofibroma: Detection of residual disease. AJNR Am J Neuroradiol 26:82-88, 2005.
68. Reddy KA, Mendenhall WM, Amdur RJ, et al: Long-term results of radiation therapy for juvenile nasopharyngeal angiofibroma. Am J Otolaryngol 22:172-175, 2001.
69. Lee JT, Chen P, Safa A, et al: The role of radiation in the treatment of advanced juvenile angiofibroma. Laryngoscope 112: 1213-1220, 2002.
70. Mann WJ, Jecker P, Amedee RG: Juvenile angiofibromas: Changing surgical concept over the last 20 years. Laryngoscope 114:291-293, 2004.
71. Abraham SC, Montgomery EA, Giardiello FM, et al: Frequent beta-catenin mutations in juvenile nasopharyngeal angiofibromas. Am J Pathol 158:1073-1078, 2001.
72. Liang J, Yi Z, Liang P: The nature of juvenile nasopharyngeal angiofibroma. Otolaryngol Head Neck Surg 123:475-481, 2000.
73. Petruson K, Rodriguez-Catarino M, Petruson B, et al: Juvenile nasopharyngeal angiofibroma: Long-term results in preoperative embolized and non-embolized patients. Acta Otolaryngol 122:96-100, 2002.
74. Farag MM, Ghanimah SE, Ragaie A, et al: Hormonal receptors in juvenile nasopharyngeal angiofibroma. Laryngoscope 97:208-211, 1987.
75. Hwang HC, Mills SE, Patterson K, et al: Expression of androgen receptors in nasopharyngeal angiofibroma: an immunohistochemical study of 24 cases. Mod Pathol 11:1122-1126, 1998.
76. Kruk-Zagajewska A, Piatkowski K, Thielemann A: Value of free testosterone and estrogen-progesterone receptor concentration in juvenile patients with angiofibroma [in Polish]. Otolaryngol Pol 56:561-565, 2002.
77. Kumagami H: Sex hormones in juvenile nasopharyngeal angiofibroma tissue. Auris Nasus Larynx 20:131-135, 1993.
78. Gatalica Z: Immunohistochemical analysis of steroid hormone receptors in nasopharyngeal angiofibromas. Cancer Lett 127:89-93, 1998.
79. Kumagami H: Testosterone and estradiol in juvenile nasopharyngeal angiofibroma tissue. Acta Otolaryngol 111:569-573, 1991.
80. Gates GA, Rice DH, Koopmann CF Jr, et al: Flutamide-induced regression of angiofibroma. Laryngoscope 102:641-644, 1992.
81. Cruz AA, Atique JM, Melo-Filho FV, et al: Orbital involvement in juvenile nasopharyngeal angiofibroma: Prevalence and treatment. Ophthal Plast Reconstr Surg 20:296-300, 2004.
82. Sennes LU, Butugan O, Sanchez TG, et al: Juvenile nasopharyngeal angiofibroma: The routes of invasion. Rhinology 41:235-240, 2003.
83. Fisch U: The infratemporal fossa approach for nasopharyngeal tumors. Laryngoscope 93:36-44, 1983.
84. Chandler JR, Goulding R, Moskowitz L, et al: Nasopharyngeal angiofibromas: Staging and management. Ann Otol Rhinol Laryngol 93:322-329, 1984.
85. Nicolai P, Berlucchi M, Tomenzoli D, et al: Endoscopic surgery for juvenile angiofibroma: When and how. Laryngoscope 113: 775-782, 2003.
86. Onerci TM, Yucel OT, Ogretmenoglu O: Endoscopic surgery in treatment of juvenile nasopharyngeal angiofibroma. Int J Pediatr Otorhinolaryngol 67:1219-1225, 2003.
87. Siniluoto TM, Luotonen JP, Tikkakoski TA, et al: Value of preoperative embolization in surgery for nasopharyngeal angiofibroma. J Laryngol Otol 107:514-521, 1993.
88. Li JR, Qian J, Shan XZ, et al: Evaluation of the effectiveness of preoperative embolization in surgery for nasopharyngeal angiofibroma. Eur Arch Otorhinolaryngol 255:430-432, 1998.
89. McCombe A, Lund VJ, Howard DJ: Recurrence in juvenile angiofibroma. Rhinology 28:97-102, 1990.
90. Jereb B, Anggard A, Baryd I: Juvenile nasopharyngeal angiofibroma. A clinical study of 69 cases. Acta Radiol Ther Phys Biol 9:302-310, 1970.
91. Cummings BJ, Blend R, Keane T, et al: Primary radiation therapy for juvenile nasopharyngeal angiofibroma. Laryngoscope 94: 1599-1605, 1984.

Pleuropulmonary Blastoma

92. Manivel JC, Priest JR, Watterson J, et al: Pleuropulmonary blastoma. The so-called pulmonary blastoma of childhood. Cancer 62:1516-1526, 1988.
93. Priest JR, Watterson J, Strong L, et al: Pleuropulmonary blastoma: A marker for familial disease. J Pediatr 128:220-224, 1996.
94. Tagge EP, Mulvihill D, Chandler JC, et al: Childhood pleuropulmonary blastoma: Caution against nonoperative management of congenital lung cysts. J Pediatr Surg 31:187-189; discussion 190, 1996.
95. Lopez-Andreu JA, Ferris-Tortajada J, Gomez J: Pleuropulmonary blastoma and congenital cystic malformations. J Pediatr 129:773-775, 1996.
96. Priest JR, McDermott MB, Bhatia S, et al: Pleuropulmonary blastoma: A clinicopathologic study of 50 cases. Cancer 80:147-161, 1997.
97. Hill DA: USCAP Specialty Conference: Case 1-Type I Pleuropulmonary Blastoma. Pediatr Dev Pathol 8:77-84, 2005.
98. Nag S, Tippin D, Ruymann FB: Intraoperative high-dose-rate brachytherapy for the treatment of pediatric tumors: The Ohio State University experience. Int J Radiat Oncol Biol Phys 51:729-735, 2001.

Extrarenal Wilms' Tumor

99. Arda IS, Tuzun M, Demirhan B, et al: Lumbosacral extrarenal Wilms' tumour: A case report and literature review. Eur J Pediatr 160:617-619, 2001.
100. Coppes MJ, Wilson PC, Weitzman S: Extrarenal Wilms' tumor: Staging, treatment, and prognosis. J Clin Oncol 9:167-174, 1991.
101. Fernandes ET, Kumar M, Douglass EC, et al: Extrarenal Wilms' tumor. J Pediatr Surg 24:483-485, 1989.
102. Kapur VK, Sakalkale RP, Samuel KV, et al: Association of extrarenal Wilms' tumor with a horseshoe kidney. J Pediatr Surg 33:935-937, 1998.
103. Roberts DJ, Haber D, Sklar J, et al: Extrarenal Wilms' tumors. A study of their relationship with classical renal Wilms' tumor using expression of WT1 as a molecular marker. Lab Invest 68:528-536, 1993.
104. McAlpine J, Azodi M, O'Malley D, et al: Extrarenal Wilms' tumor of the uterine corpus. Gynecol Oncol 96:892-896, 2005.
105. D'Angio GJ, Evans AE, Breslow N, et al: The treatment of Wilms' tumor: Results of the national Wilms' tumor study. Cancer 38:633-646, 1976.
106. D'Angio GJ, Evans A, Breslow N, et al: The treatment of Wilms' tumor: Results of the Second National Wilms' Tumor Study. Cancer 47:2302-2311, 1981.
107. D'Angio GJ, Breslow N, Beckwith JB, et al: Treatment of Wilms' tumor: Results of the Third National Wilms' Tumor Study. Cancer 64:349-360, 1989.
108. Thomas PR: Wilms' Tumor: Changing role of radiation therapy. Semin Radiat Oncol 7:204-211, 1997.

PART J

LYMPHOMA AND HEMATOLOGIC MALIGNANCIES

Overview

Andrea K. Ng and Peter Mauch

BASIC ISSUES IN LYMPHOMA

Recently our understanding of the molecular basis of various lymphoid malignancies has grown, which has improved our ability to diagnose, stage, treat, and follow up on affected patients. The current pathologic classification incorporates molecular characteristics, in addition to morphologic and clinical features in identifying distinctive subtypes of disease entities.[1,2] Advances in DNA microarray techniques allow improved prognostic classification of patients and provide the opportunity to develop molecularly targeted therapy for specific disease types.[3-7] More accurate staging is now available through modern medical imaging techniques and the increasing experience with functional imaging.[8-12]

We have seen significant changes in the treatment of lymphoid malignancies. For diseases in which a high cure rate has already been achieved, the emphasis is now on treatment reduction. Meanwhile, more dose-dense and dose-intense treatment[13-15] and incorporation of targeted therapy including novel agents against molecular targets or pathways, immunotherapy, and radioimmunotherapy are being used in diseases in which the cure rate is still suboptimal.[16] As treatment becomes more successful and as more patients are cured, there has been growing attention on late effects of therapy.[17-19] Efforts to reduce late effects, through treatment modification, early detection, risk reduction, and prevention of late complications, are mostly focused on survivors of Hodgkin's disease. This may serve as a useful model for the follow-up care of other lymphoma patients as cure rates improve, to further improve the survival and quality of life of patients who have been cured of lymphoid malignancies.

PATHOLOGIC CLASSIFICATION

The classification of lymphoid malignancies has evolved over the past century. Earlier lymphoma classification relied mainly on subtleties of morphology, cell lineage and differentiation, clinical survival data, or all of these. In 1994, the International Lymphoma Study Group published the Revised European-American Lymphoma (REAL) classification of tumors of hematopoietic and lymphatic tissues, which was later modified and updated in the World Health Organization (WHO) project.[1,2] The REAL-WHO classification, unlike prior classifications, combined information on morphology, immunophenotype, genetic features, and clinical features to define individual disease entity. It is comprised of a list of diseases that includes Hodgkin's lymphoma, non-Hodgkin's lymphomas, lymphoid leukemias, and plasma cell neoplasms. Despite its seeming complexity, its clinical practicality has been supported by the fact that most cases could be classified into one of the disease categories; an excellent interobserver reproducibility has been demonstrated; and the disease entities in the classification were indeed clinically distinctive, both at initial presentation and in treatment outcome.

Modern pathologic classification allows researchers, pathologists, and clinicians to have a common language in defining, diagnosing, and treating different disease types. It is anticipated that with the rapid progress in the field of genetic analysis, continued updating and revisions of any current classification will be necessary. Advances in the field may provide additional markers for classification and identify new categories of disease that are not currently recognized.

MOLECULAR BASIS OF LYMPHOID MALIGNANCIES

Exciting progress has occurred in the field of molecular biology in lymphoid malignancies in recent years. Emerging data are now available on the origin of the malignant cells of Hodgkin's disease, the Hodgkin Reed-Sternberg cells, and the molecular events that lead to the malignant transformation.[20-22] The nuclear factor-κ-B (NF-κB) pathway has been implicated to play an important role in the pathogenesis of Hodgkin's disease,[23,24] and continued research in the area may provide new therapeutic targets for the disease.

Researchers have used complementary DNA (cDNA) microarray techniques to identify molecular prognostic factors for lymphoma.[3-5,7] For diffuse large B-cell lymphoma (DLBCL), using transcriptional profiling, subtypes of disease with distinct clinical outcome have been identified.[3-5] Genes that have been implicated in predicting treatment outcome included ones that regulate molecular signaling pathways and apoptotic response to treatment.[4,5] Recent studies using similar techniques also showed that the tumor microenvironment and host inflammatory response may play a key role in identifying subgroups of patients with differing prognosis in both follicular lymphoma and DLBCL.[7,25] Although not yet put into clinical practice, molecular prognostic factors promise to further improve risk stratification, and more importantly, provide molecular insights into the clinical heterogeneity of the disease, and may help with the design of therapy targeted to specific molecular pathways.

STAGING

Improvement in imaging techniques had led to the modification of the original Ann Arbor staging classification for lymphoma, allowing incorporation of computed tomography scan results in assessing disease extent.[26] Functional imaging is increasingly used as part of the initial staging. A growing body of literature describes using positron emission tomography (PET) scanning for initial staging and restaging of patients with lymphoma.[8-12,27] Its use has been shown to alter initial management plans.[8,27] The sensitivity and specificity vary depending on the histologic subtypes,[9] and its role must be better defined for individual subtypes of lymphoid malignancies. There is also a need to standardize the imaging techniques, quality, and interpretation criteria of the nuclear medicine studies.

Accurate staging serves a number of important purposes in the management of lymphoma patients. It provides prognostic information and allows uniform reporting and interpretation of clinical trial results. Most importantly, it guides treatment decisions. In general, the role of radiation therapy (RT) is largely limited to patients with early-stage disease. Furthermore, in patients with indolent, early-stage lymphoma, RT alone may have a curative role.

TREATMENT

The following text summarizes the major treatment-related issues, with a focus on the role of RT, for the four types of lymphoid malignancies: Hodgkin's lymphoma, non-Hodgkin's lymphoma, mycosis fungoides, and plasma cell neoplasms.

Hodgkin's Disease

Stages I and II Hodgkin's Disease

Historically, RT alone has been the mainstay of treatment for early-stage Hodgkin's disease. With the availability of more effective and less toxic chemotherapy, the current standard treatment for early-stage Hodgkin's disease is combined-modality therapy. Advantages of combined-modality therapy over RT alone include the significantly higher disease-free survival that has been demonstrated in several randomized trials and the avoidance of large-field RT.[28-30] It also eliminates the need to perform staging laparotomy to select pathologically staged, early-stage patients for RT alone.

As discussed, one of the main challenges in the management of patients with early-stage Hodgkin's disease is to minimize treatment-related late complications while preserving the excellent disease-control rate. Strategies to reduce treatment, from the RT standpoint, include the use of smaller treatment field, lower radiation doses, or elimination of RT.

Current data suggest that involved-field RT is adequate when given as part of combined-modality therapy.[31,32] Whether the radiation treatment field can be further reduced to include only the initially involved node(s) rather than treating the entire nodal region is unclear, and more data are needed to determine if the *involved field* can safely be redefined to include a more restricted area. Lower doses of RT have been successfully employed in the pediatric population.[33-35] It is quite possible that in the near future, when current ongoing trial results on adult early-stage patients become available, doses lower than 30 Gy may prove to be adequate for patients with favorable-prognosis disease.

Six randomized trials have been performed examining whether RT can be safely omitted,[36-41] four of which included only early-stage patients,[36,39-41] and two included patients of all stages.[37,38] The study design, patient population, chemotherapy, and RT employed varied among the trials. All but one trial, which was underpowered,[39] showed a significant disease- or event-free survival benefit with the addition of RT. The chemotherapy-alone arm was closed in two of the trials because of the high number of relapses.[37,41] Based on these results, combined-modality therapy remains the standard of treatment in patients with early-stage disease.

Stages III and IV

The current standard of chemotherapy for advanced-stage Hodgkin's disease is the ABVD regimen (Adriamycin [doxorubicin], bleomycin, vinblastine, and dacarbazine). However, there have been recent promising data on more dose-dense and dose-intense regimens, including the dose-escalated BEACOPP (bleomycin, etoposide, doxorubicin, cyclophosphamide, vincristine, procarbazine, and prednisone) and Stanford V.[13,14] Both regimens are currently being compared to ABVD in multi-institutional randomized trials conducted in Europe and the United States.

The role of RT in patients with advanced-stage Hodgkin's disease is limited. Most randomized trials do not show a significant benefit with the addition of RT to chemotherapy.[42-47] However, there are subgroups of patients who may benefit from consolidative RT, namely, patients who failed to achieve a complete response to chemotherapy and those with bulky disease at presentation.[43,47] Of note, in the Stanford V regimen RT is given to patients with tumor bulk 5 cm or larger, macroscopic splenic disease, or both, which accounts for approximately 90% of the patients.[13] The integral role of the RT in this treatment program was shown in an Italian trial in which the Stanford V arm did much more poorly than expected,[48] which was probably because RT was not delivered as specified by the Stanford V treatment program.

The use of functional imaging results at the end of chemotherapy to identify candidates for consolidative RT is currently being explored in one of the ongoing German Hodgkin's Study Group trials, in which RT is given only to patients with persistently postchemotherapy PET-positive disease. Such response-adapted therapy is also undergoing tests in the pediatric population and may have a future role in early-stage patients as well.[34,35]

Nodular Lymphocyte-Predominant Hodgkin's Disease

Nodular lymphocyte-predominant Hodgkin's disease (NLPHD) is a disease entity distinct from classical Hodgkin's disease based on its morphologic, immunophenotypic, and clinical characteristics.[2,49] Most cases of NLPHD present with stages I or II disease. Because of its rarity, currently no standard treatment is available for the disease. RT alone to a regional field may be potentially curative. Patients with additional relapses tend to remain responsive to further therapy. These patients are more likely to die from treatment-related causes than from the lymphoma, which argues for limiting treatment up front because of the indolent nature of the disease.[50,51]

Non-Hodgkin's Lymphoma

Non-Hodgkin's lymphoma is a heterogeneous disease. The two most common histologic subtypes are DLBCL and follicular lymphoma, accounting for 75% of all cases of non-Hodgkin's lymphoma. The role of RT in both of these subtypes is mostly limited to patients with early-stage disease. Marginal-zone lymphoma or mucosa-associated lymphoid tumor (MALT) is another subtype of non-Hodgkin's lymphoma, which is highly responsive to RT; and in patients who present with localized, early-stage disease, RT alone may be curative.

DIFFUSE LARGE B-CELL LYMPHOMA

Two cooperative groups in the United States, the Southwest Oncology Group (SWOG) and the Eastern Cooperative Oncology Group (ECOG), have each published results of their prospective randomized trial investigating the role of RT in limited-stage DLBCL after CHOP (cyclophosphamide, Adriamycin [doxorubicin], vincristine, and prednisone) chemotherapy in early-stage aggressive lymphoma.[52,53] The two trials differed in the patient inclusion criteria: the ECOG study included less favorable patients.[53] For example, patients with bulky stage II disease were included in the ECOG trial but excluded in the SWOG trial,[52] and the SWOG study had a higher percentage of patients with extranodal disease. The trial designs were also different in that the SWOG study compared an abbreviated course of chemotherapy followed by RT with a longer course of chemotherapy alone, whereas the ECOG study compared the same chemotherapy with or without additional RT. In the ECOG study, only patients who achieved complete response were randomized, and all patients with a partial response received RT.

Five-year published results of the SWOG study showed a significant disease-free survival benefit in the combined-modality therapy arm, but the differences were no longer significant with longer follow-up, because of later relapses in patients in the combined-modality therapy arm.[54] On subgroup analysis, however, patients with a stage-modified International Prognostic Index (IPI) score of 0 (younger than age 60 years, nonbulky stage I, normal lactate dehydrogenase [LDH], ECOG performance status <2) had a 5-year overall survival of 94% when treated with three cycles of CHOP followed by RT. The results suggested that in patients with very limited DLBCL, three cycles of chemotherapy followed by RT is the treatment of choice given its excellent results and the low associated morbidity. In patients with unfavorable features, RT cannot replace inadequate chemotherapy, and more effective systemic therapy is needed in these patients. The SWOG trial, which used the same chemotherapy in both arms, showed a significant disease-free survival benefit in the combined-modality therapy arm, with no significant difference in overall survival. Patients with a partial response had an excellent 6-year failure-free survival of 63%, which was attributed to the fact that these patients all received consolidative RT.

Two other trials conducted by the Groupe d'Etude des Lymphomes de l'Adulte (GELA),[55,56] published only in abstract forms, also compared chemotherapy alone with combined-modality therapy. The trial that was limited to patients age 60 years or younger compared the aggressive combination chemotherapy regimen ACVBP (doxorubicin, cyclophosphamide, vincristine, bleomycin, and prednisone induction) at 2-week intervals, followed by high-dose methotrexate, etoposide, and cytarabine consolidation, with three cycles of CHOP followed by involved-field RT.[55] The finding of a significantly higher disease-free survival in the chemotherapy-alone arm in this trial is in line with the results of the SWOG trial, highlighting that the addition of RT cannot make up for inadequate chemotherapy. In the GELA trial on patients older than 60 years,[56] patients were treated with four cycles of CHOP with or without RT. No significant differences in event-free survival or overall survival were detected at 5 years in this study. A remarkably high 5-year disease-free survival of 69% was achieved with four cycles of CHOP alone. Published results of these two GELA trials, when available, will provide additional information on the role of RT in early-stage aggressive lymphoma.

FOLLICULAR LYMPHOMA

Approximately 20% to 25% of patients with follicular lymphoma present with stages I to II disease. A number of retrospective series show that RT alone is curative in approximately 35% to 40% of cases.[57-64] Median doses of 36 to 40 Gy resulted in control rates of 90% to 95%. Relapses beyond 10 years are uncommon, accounting for fewer than 5% of cases. In most of the series, the radiation fields varied over time, with larger fields employed in the earlier years, and more limited fields in patients treated in the modern era. Because more than half of the patients with stages I to II disease will eventually relapse, the use of involved- or regional-field RT preserves the ability to effectively treat patients with recurrent disease, or those who transform to a higher-grade histology.

Less data are available on the role of RT in advanced-stage follicular lymphoma. Several small series, which include stage III patients, have reported results on the use of *central* or *comprehensive* lymphoid irradiation, with 10- to 15-year disease-free survival of 30% to 40%.[65-67] Molecular complete responses, assessed by polymerase chain reaction techniques, have also been demonstrated after the treatment.[68] This approach of wide-field RT, however, is not widely accepted because of concerns with long-term toxicity from the treatment for an indolent disease and the ability to deliver effective salvage therapy at the time of relapse.

MUCOSA-ASSOCIATED LYMPHOID TUMOR LYMPHOMA

Marginal zone B-cell lymphoma, or MALT lymphoma, accounts for approximately 8% to 10% of non-Hodgkin's lymphoma. Most cases are localized at presentation and tend to remain localized for long periods of time. This subtype of lymphoma is highly responsive to RT. Doses of roughly 30 Gy to involved nodal regions or extranodal sites will yield a local control rate of close to 100%, with a chance of long-term cure in approximately 75% of the patients.[69-72] Relapses tend to occur at other extranodal sites where MALT lymphomas tend to occur or in a nonirradiated contralateral paired organ. The likelihood of achieving a second remission in patients with limited relapses remains excellent with further local RT.

Mycosis Fungoides

Mycosis fungoides is the most common type of cutaneous T-cell lymphoma. It is nonetheless a rare disease, with approximately 1400 new cases in the United States each year. Many challenges exist for its management, including difficulty in establishing a diagnosis because of the often nonspecific clinical presentation and controversies in the pathologic diagnostic criteria.[73-75] A number of topical, skin-directed therapy options are available for patients with more limited-stage disease,[76-80] and various systemic therapy options,[81-85] including novel biologic agents, are available for patients with more extensive involvement. However, because of the rarity of the disease, there is a paucity of prospective randomized data in identifying the best treatment approach.

RT represents one of the most effective modalities for the treatment of mycosis fungoides. Fractionated doses of 30 to 36 Gy are associated with a high rate of durable response.[86-91] Local-field RT is reserved in patients who present with stage IA, unifocal disease or with closely clustered lesions that can be encompassed within an en face electron-beam treatment field.[92] It has a palliative role in patients with localized symptomatic skin lesions that are refractory to systemic treatment.[93,94] In patients with bulky nodal or visceral involvement, local photon-beam therapy can also provide effective palliation.

In most other cases of mycosis fungoides, total-skin electron beam therapy (TSEBT) is the mainstay of treatment.[86-89,95,96] Depending on the disease stage and extent of involvement, TSEBT can be given alone as first-line treatment, or in conjunction with other systemic agents.[76,77] It can be given as second-line therapy in patients who have failed other modalities of therapy. However, the optimal treatment combination and timing of treatment are still unknown at this time.

The establishment and maintenance of a TSEBT program requires substantial resources, including dedicated space and equipment, physics and dosimetric support, and experienced radiation oncologists and nursing staff.[97] An adequate patient population is also needed to justify and sustain the program. As a result, only a limited number of centers in North America provide TSEBT.

The delivery of TSEBT is associated with a number of technical and patient management challenges.[95-98] According to the European Organization for Research and Treatment of Cancer (EORTC) TSEBT consensus statement,[95] a total dose of 31 to 36 Gy to the skin surface with a resulting minimum dose of 26 Gy at the 80% isodose line is recommended. Furthermore, to ensure that the epidermis and dermis fall within the high-dose region, the 80% isodose line should be at 4 mm or deeper to the skin surface. Areas that tend to be underdosed, including the scalp, perineum, and the soles of the feet require extra-boost dose, whereas areas that tend to be overexposed or are vulnerable, such as eyes, hands and fingernails, and ankles, need appropriate shielding. Patients who require TSEBT often need to travel long distances to centers that provide the treatment; or they must stay at temporary accommodations close to the treatment centers for a period that can span from 2 to 3 months. Patients treated with TSEBT can experience significant acute toxicities that need to be closely monitored and dealt with.[95,97,99] Especially in patients with advanced disease with immune suppression, cutaneous and systemic infectious complications potentially are life-threatening and need to be promptly addressed. Despite the challenges associated with the delivery of TSEBT, it has well-established effectiveness, both in the primary setting and in patients who failed other modalities, and can also provide effective palliation when given a second or even third time to a lower dose.[93,94]

Multiple Myeloma and Plasma Cell Malignancies

The role of RT is limited to only a number of specific scenarios in the management of plasma cell malignancies. In patients with solitary plasmacytoma of the bone, local RT to doses of 45 to 50 Gy can provide effective local control of 90% or higher.[100-103] However, approximately half of the patients will progress to multiple myeloma at 10 years, and by 15 years most will develop multiple myeloma. Unlike solitary plasmacytoma of the bone, extraosseous solitary plasmacytoma is associated with a lower risk of progression to multiple myeloma and has a more favorable disease-free survival.[103-105] Most series employ doses of 45 to 50 Gy, which yield local control rates of 85% to 90%.

Multiple myeloma at this time is an incurable disease. Autologous stem cell transplantation produces a higher response rate and prolongs survival, but it is not curative.[106] Earlier preparative regimens mostly contained total body irradiation (TBI); but more recent data indicate that TBI contributes to increased toxicity, without improving disease control, in part because of the reduced salvage potential.[107] The current role of RT in the management of multiple myeloma is therefore largely limited to palliation, in patients with painful bony lesions, nerve root or cord compression, or lytic lesions in a weight-bearing bone at risk for pathologic fractures. Kyphoplasty in conjunction with RT for patients with compression fracture of the vertebral bodies may provide more immediate and effective palliation.[108] Fractionation schemes of 30 Gy in 10 fractions or other biological equivalent doses are recommended, because lower doses are associated with less-durable palliation, and retreatment is often significantly less effective.[109] In the delivery of palliative RT, especially to the vertebral bodies, one must be mindful of allowing room for future TBI in patients who are candidates for transplantation. However, this consideration may now be irrelevant given that most current preparative regimens for multiple myeloma no longer contain TBI.

REFERENCES

1. Harris NL, Jaffe ES, Stein H, et al: A revised European-American classification of lymphoid neoplasms: A proposal from the International Lymphoma Study Group. Blood 84:1361-1392, 1994.
2. Harris NL, Jaffe ES, Diebold J, et al: World Health Organization classification of neoplastic diseases of the hematopoietic and lymphoid tissues: Report of the Clinical Advisory Committee meeting—Airlie House, Virginia, November 1997. J Clin Oncol 17:3835-3849, 1999.
3. Alizadeh AA, Eisen MB, Davis RE, et al: Distinct types of diffuse large B-cell lymphoma identified by gene expression profiling. Nature 403:503-511, 2000.
4. Rosenwald A, Wright G, Chan WC, et al: The use of molecular profiling to predict survival after chemotherapy for diffuse large-B-cell lymphoma. N Engl J Med 346:1937-1947, 2002.
5. Shipp MA, Ross KN, Tamayo P, et al: Diffuse large B-cell lymphoma outcome prediction by gene-expression profiling and supervised machine learning. Nat Med 8:68-74, 2002.
6. Savage KJ, Monti S, Kutok JL, et al: The molecular signature of mediastinal large B-cell lymphoma differs from that of other diffuse large B-cell lymphomas and shares features with classical Hodgkin lymphoma. Blood 102:3871-3879, 2003.
7. Dave SS, Wright G, Tan B, et al: Prediction of survival in follicular lymphoma based on molecular features of tumor-infiltrating immune cells. N Engl J Med 351:2159-2169, 2004.
8. Sasaki M, Kuwabara Y, Koga H, et al: Clinical impact of whole body FDG-PET on the staging and therapeutic decision making for malignant lymphoma. Ann Nucl Med 16:337-345, 2002.
9. Elstrom R, Guan L, Baker G, et al: Utility of FDG-PET scanning in lymphoma by WHO classification. Blood 101:3875-3876, 2003.
10. Friedberg JW, Fischman A, Neuberg D, et al: FDG-PET is superior to gallium scintigraphy in staging and more sensitive in the follow-up of patients with de novo Hodgkin lymphoma: A blinded comparison. Leuk Lymphoma 45:85-92, 2004.
11. Israel O, Keidar Z, Bar-Shalom R: Positron emission tomography in the evaluation of lymphoma. Semin Nucl Med 34:166-179, 2004.
12. Kumar R, Maillard I, Schuster SJ, et al: Utility of fluorodeoxyglucose-PET imaging in the management of patients with Hodgkin's and non-Hodgkin's lymphomas. Radiol Clin North Am 42:1083-1100, viii, 2004.
13. Horning SJ, Hoppe RT, Breslin S, et al: Stanford V and radiotherapy for locally extensive and advanced Hodgkin's disease: mature results of a prospective clinical trial. J Clin Oncol 20:630-637, 2002.
14. Diehl V, Franklin J, Pfreundschuh M, et al: Standard and increased-dose BEACOPP chemotherapy compared with COPP-ABVD for advanced Hodgkin's disease. N Engl J Med 348:2386-2395, 2003.
15. Tilly H, Lepage E, Coiffier B, et al: Intensive conventional chemotherapy (ACVBP regimen) compared with standard CHOP for poor-prognosis aggressive non-Hodgkin lymphoma. Blood 102:4284-4289, 2003.
16. Coiffier B, Lepage E, Briere J, et al: CHOP chemotherapy plus rituximab compared with CHOP alone in elderly patients with diffuse large-B-cell lymphoma. N Engl J Med 346:235-242, 2002.
17. Donaldson SS, Hancock SL, Hoppe RT: The Janeway lecture. Hodgkin's disease—finding the balance between cure and late effects. Cancer J Sci Am 5:325-333, 1999.

18. Robison LL, Bhatia S: Late-effects among survivors of leukaemia and lymphoma during childhood and adolescence. Br J Haematol 122:345-359, 2003.
19. Ng AK, Mauch PM: Late complications of therapy of Hodgkin's disease: Prevention and management. Curr Hematol Rep 3:27-33, 2004.
20. Rajewsky K, Kanzler H, Hansmann ML, et al: Normal and malignant B-cell development with special reference to Hodgkin's disease. Ann Oncol 8(Suppl 2):79-81, 1997.
21. Marafioti T, Hummel M, Foss HD, et al: Hodgkin and Reed-Sternberg cells represent an expansion of a single clone originating from a germinal center B-cell with functional immunoglobulin gene rearrangements but defective immunoglobulin transcription. Blood 95:1443-1450, 2000.
22. Stein H, Marafioti T, Foss HD, et al: Down-regulation of BOB.1/OBF.1 and Oct2 in classical Hodgkin disease but not in lymphocyte predominant Hodgkin disease correlates with immunoglobulin transcription. Blood 97:496-501, 2001.
23. Hinz M, Lemke P, Anagnostopoulos I, et al: Nuclear factor κB-dependent gene expression profiling of Hodgkin's disease tumor cells, pathogenetic significance, and link to constitutive signal transducer and activator of transcription 5a activity. J Exp Med 196:605-617, 2002.
24. Bargou RC, Emmerich F, Krappmann D, et al: Constitutive nuclear factor-κB-RelA activation is required for proliferation and survival of Hodgkin's disease tumor cells. J Clin Invest 100:2961-2969, 1997.
25. Monti S, Savage KJ, Kutok JL, et al: Molecular profiling of diffuse large B-cell lymphoma identifies robust subtypes including one characterized by host inflammatory response. Blood 105:1851-1861, 2005.
26. Lister TA, Crowther D, Sutcliffe SB, et al: Report of a committee convened to discuss the evaluation and staging of patients with Hodgkin's disease: Cotswolds meeting. J Clin Oncol 7:1630-1636, 1989.
27. Lee YK, Cook G, Flower MA, et al: Addition of 18F-FDG-PET scans to radiotherapy planning of thoracic lymphoma. Radiother Oncol 73:277-283, 2004.
28. Hagenbeek A, Eghbali H, Fermé C, et al: Three cycles of MOPP/ABV hybrid and involved-field irradiation is more effective than subtotal nodal irradiation in favorable supradiaphragmatic clinical stages I-II Hodgkin's disease: Preliminary results of the EORTC-GELA H8-F randomized trial in 543 patients. Blood 96:576a, 2000.
29. Press OW, LeBlanc M, Lichter AS, et al: Phase III randomized intergroup trial of subtotal lymphoid irradiation versus doxorubicin, vinblastine, and subtotal lymphoid irradiation for stage IA to IIA Hodgkin's disease. J Clin Oncol 19:4238-4244, 2001.
30. Sieber M, Franklin J, Tesch H, et al: Two cycles of ABVD plus extended field radiotherapy is superior to radiotherapy alone in early stage Hodgkin's disease: Results of the German Hodgkin's Lymphoma Study Group (GHSG) Trial HD7. Blood 100:A341, 2002.
31. Engert A, Schiller P, Josting A, et al: Involved-field radiotherapy is equally effective and less toxic compared with extended-field radiotherapy after four cycles of chemotherapy in patients with early-stage unfavorable Hodgkin's lymphoma: Results of the HD8 trial of the German Hodgkin's Lymphoma Study Group. J Clin Oncol 21:3601-3608, 2003.
32. Bonadonna G, Bonfante V, Viviani S, et al: ABVD plus subtotal nodal versus involved-field radiotherapy in early-stage Hodgkin's disease: long-term results. J Clin Oncol 22:2835-2841, 2004.
33. Donaldson SS, Hudson MM, Lamborn KR, et al: VAMP and low-dose, involved-field radiation for children and adolescents with favorable, early-stage Hodgkin's disease: Results of a prospective clinical trial. J Clin Oncol 20:3081-3087, 2002.
34. Landman-Parker J, Pacquement H, Leblanc T, et al: Localized childhood Hodgkin's disease: Response-adapted chemotherapy with etoposide, bleomycin, vinblastine, and prednisone before low-dose radiation therapy—results of the French Society of Pediatric Oncology Study MDH90. J Clin Oncol 18:1500-1507, 2000.
35. Ruhl U, Albrecht M, Dieckmann K, et al: Response-adapted radiotherapy in the treatment of pediatric Hodgkin's disease: an interim report at 5 years of the German GPOH-HD 95 trial. Int J Radiat Oncol Biol Phys 51:1209-1218, 2001.
36. Pavlovsky S, Maschio M, Santarelli MT, et al: Randomized trial of chemotherapy versus chemotherapy plus radiotherapy for stage I-II Hodgkin's disease. J Natl Cancer Inst 80:1466-1473, 1988.
37. Nachman JB, Sposto R, Herzog P, et al: Randomized comparison of low-dose involved-field radiotherapy and no radiotherapy for children with Hodgkin's disease who achieve a complete response to chemotherapy. J Clin Oncol 20:3765-3771, 2002.
38. Laskar S, Gupta T, Vimal S, et al: Consolidation radiation after complete remission in Hodgkin's disease following six cycles of doxorubicin, bleomycin, vinblastine, and dacarbazine chemotherapy: is there a need? J Clin Oncol 22:62-68, 2004.
39. Straus DJ, Portlock CS, Qin J, et al: Results of a prospective randomized clinical trial of doxorubicin, bleomycin, vinblastine and dacarbazine (ABVD) followed by radiation therapy (RT) versus ABVD alone for stages I, II and IIIA nonbulky Hodgkin's disease. Blood 104(12):3483-3489, 2004.
40. Meyer R, Gospodarowicz M, Connors J, et al: A Randomized Phase III Comparison of Single-Modality ABVD with a Strategy that Includes Radiation Therapy in Patients with Early-Stage Hodgkin's Disease: The HD-6 Trial of the National Cancer Institute of Canada Clinical Trials Group (Eastern Cooperative Oncology Group Trial JHD06). Blood 102:A81, 2003.
41. Thomas J: Six cycles of EBVP followed by 36 Gy involved-field irradiation vs. no irradiation in favourable supradiaphragmatic clinical stage I-II Hodgkin's Lymphoma: the EORTC-GELA strategy in 771 patients. Eur J Haematol 73:E0, 2004.
42. Pavlovsky S, Santarelli MT, Muriel FS, et al: Randomized trial of chemotherapy versus chemotherapy plus radiotherapy for stage III-IV A & B Hodgkin's disease. Ann Oncol 3:533-537, 1992.
43. Fabian CJ, Mansfield CM, Dahlberg S, et al: Low-dose involved field radiation after chemotherapy in advanced Hodgkin disease. A Southwest Oncology Group randomized study. Ann Intern Med 120:903-912, 1994.
44. Diehl V, Loeffler M, Pfreundschuh M, et al: Further chemotherapy versus low-dose involved-field radiotherapy as consolidation of complete remission after six cycles of alternating chemotherapy in patients with advanced Hodgkin's disease. German Hodgkin's Study Group (GHSG). Ann Oncol 6:901-910, 1995.
45. Loeffler M, Brosteanu O, Hasenclever D, et al: Meta-analysis of chemotherapy versus combined modality treatment trials in Hodgkin's disease. International Database on Hodgkin's Disease Overview Study Group. J Clin Oncol 16:818-829, 1998.
46. Ferme C, Sebban C, Hennequin C, et al: Comparison of chemotherapy to radiotherapy as consolidation of complete or good partial response after six cycles of chemotherapy for patients with advanced Hodgkin's disease: Results of the Groupe d'Etudes des Lymphomes de l'Adulte H89 trial. Blood 95:2246-2252, 2000.
47. Aleman BM, Raemaekers JM, Tirelli U, et al: Involved-field radiotherapy for advanced Hodgkin's lymphoma. N Engl J Med 348:2396-2406, 2003.
48. Chisesi T, Federico M, Levis A, et al: ABVD versus Stanford V versus MEC in unfavourable Hodgkin's lymphoma: Results of a randomised trial. Ann Oncol 13 (Suppl 1):102-106, 2002.
49. Anagnostopoulos I, Hansmann ML, Franssila K, et al: European Task Force on Lymphoma project on lymphocyte predominance Hodgkin disease: Histologic and immunohistologic analysis of submitted cases reveals 2 types of Hodgkin disease with a nodular growth pattern and abundant lymphocytes. Blood 96:1889-1899, 2000.
50. Bodis S, Kraus MD, Pinkus G, et al: Clinical presentation and outcome in lymphocyte-predominant Hodgkin's disease. J Clin Oncol 15:3060-3066, 1997.
51. Diehl V, Sextro M, Franklin J, et al: Clinical presentation, course, and prognostic factors in lymphocyte-predominant Hodgkin's disease and lymphocyte-rich classical Hodgkin's disease: Report from the European Task Force on Lymphoma Project on

Lymphocyte-Predominant Hodgkin's Disease. J Clin Oncol 17:776-783, 1999.
52. Miller TP, Dahlberg S, Cassady JR, et al: Chemotherapy alone compared with chemotherapy plus radiotherapy for localized intermediate- and high-grade non-Hodgkin's lymphoma. N Engl J Med 339:21-26, 1998.
53. Horning SJ, Weller E, Kim K, et al: Chemotherapy with or without radiotherapy in limited-stage diffuse aggressive non-Hodgkin's lymphoma: Eastern Cooperative Oncology Group study 1484. J Clin Oncol 22:3032-3038, 2004.
54. Miller T, Leblanc M, Spier C, et al: CHOP Alone Compared to CHOP Plus Radiotherapy for Early Stage Aggressive Non-Hodgkin's Lymphomas: update of the Southwest Oncology Group (SWOG) Randomized Trial. Blood 98:3024a, 2001.
55. Reyes F, Lepage E, Munck J, et al: Chemotherapy alone with the ACVBP regimen is superior to three cycles of CHOP plus radiotherapy for treatment of low risk localized aggressive lymphoma: the LNH93-1 GELA study. Blood 100:93a, 2003.
56. Fillet G, Bonnet C, Mounier N, et al: Radiotherapy is unnecessary in elderly patients with localized aggressive non-Hodgkin's lymphoma: results of the GELA LNH 93-4 Study. Blood 100:92a, 2003.
57. Soubeyran P, Eghbali H, Bonichon F, et al: Localized follicular lymphomas: prognosis and survival of stages I and II in a retrospective series of 103 patients. Radiother Oncol 13:91-98, 1988.
58. Taylor RE, Allan SG, McIntyre MA, et al: Low grade stage I and II non-Hodgkin's lymphoma: results of treatment and relapse pattern following therapy. Clin Radiol 39:287-290, 1988.
59. Lawrence TS, Urba WJ, Steinberg SM, et al: Retrospective analysis of stage I and II indolent lymphomas at the National Cancer Institute. Int J Radiat Oncol Biol Phys 14:417-424, 1988.
60. Vaughan Hudson B, Vaughan Hudson G, MacLennan KA, et al: Clinical stage 1 non-Hodgkin's lymphoma: long-term follow-up of patients treated by the British National Lymphoma Investigation with radiotherapy alone as initial therapy. Br J Cancer 69:1088-1093, 1994.
61. Pendlebury S, el Awadi M, Ashley S, et al: Radiotherapy results in early stage low grade nodal non-Hodgkin's lymphoma. Radiother Oncol 36:167-171, 1995.
62. Mac Manus MP, Hoppe RT: Is radiotherapy curative for stage I and II low-grade follicular lymphoma? Results of a long-term follow-up study of patients treated at Stanford University. J Clin Oncol 14:1282-1290, 1996.
63. Gospodarowicz M, Lippuner T, Pintilie M: Stage I and II follicular lymphoma: long-term outcome and pattern of failure following treatment with involved-field radiation therapy alone. Int J Radiat Oncol Biol Phys 45:217a, 1999.
64. Wilder RB, Jones D, Tucker SL, et al: Long-term results with radiotherapy for Stage I-II follicular lymphomas. Int J Radiat Oncol Biol Phys 51:1219-1227, 2001.
65. Jacobs JP, Murray KJ, Schultz CJ, et al: Central lymphatic irradiation for stage III nodular malignant lymphoma: long-term results. J Clin Oncol 11:233-238, 1993.
66. De Los Santos JF, Mendenhall NP, Lynch JW Jr: Is comprehensive lymphatic irradiation for low-grade non-Hodgkin's lymphoma curative therapy? Long-term experience at a single institution. Int J Radiat Oncol Biol Phys 38:3-8, 1997.
67. Ha CS, Kong JS, Tucker SL, et al: Central lymphatic irradiation for stage I-III follicular lymphoma: report from a single-institutional prospective study. Int J Radiat Oncol Biol Phys 57:316-320, 2003.
68. Ha CS, Tucker SL, Lee MS, et al: The significance of molecular response of follicular lymphoma to central lymphatic irradiation as measured by polymerase chain reaction for t(14;18)(q32;q21). Int J Radiat Oncol Biol Phys 49:727-732, 2001.
69. Schechter NR, Portlock CS, Yahalom J: Treatment of mucosa-associated lymphoid tissue lymphoma of the stomach with radiation alone. J Clin Oncol 16:1916-1921, 1998.
70. Fung CY, Grossbard ML, Linggood RM, et al: Mucosa-associated lymphoid tissue lymphoma of the stomach: long term outcome after local treatment. Cancer 85:9-17, 1999.
71. Tsang RW, Gospodarowicz MK, Pintilie M, et al: Stage I and II MALT lymphoma: Results of treatment with radiotherapy. Int J Radiat Oncol Biol Phys 50:1258-1264, 2001.
72. Hitchcock S, Ng AK, Fisher DC, et al: Treatment outcome of mucosa-associated lymphoid tissue/marginal zone non-Hodgkin's lymphoma. Int J Radiat Oncol Biol Phys 52:1058-1066, 2002.
73. Sander CA, Flaig MJ, Kaudewitz P, et al: The revised European-American Classification of Lymphoid Neoplasms (REAL): A preferred approach for the classification of cutaneous lymphomas. Am J Dermatopathol 21:274-278, 1999.
74. Knobler R, Burg G, Whittaker S, et al: EORTC cutaneous lymphoma task force. European Organisation for Research and Treatment of Cancer. Eur J Cancer 38(Suppl 4):S60-S64, 2002.
75. Willemze R, Jaffe ES, Burg G, et al: WHO-EORTC classification for cutaneous lymphomas. Blood 105:3768-3785, 2005.
76. Quiros PA, Jones GW, Kacinski BM, et al: Total skin electron beam therapy followed by adjuvant psoralen/ultraviolet-A light in the management of patients with T1 and T2 cutaneous T-cell lymphoma (mycosis fungoides). Int J Radiat Oncol Biol Phys 38:1027-1035, 1997.
77. Chinn DM, Chow S, Kim YH, et al: Total skin electron beam therapy with or without adjuvant topical nitrogen mustard or nitrogen mustard alone as initial treatment of T2 and T3 mycosis fungoides. Int J Radiat Oncol Biol Phys 43:951-958, 1999.
78. Esteve E, Bagot M, Joly P, et al: A prospective study of cutaneous intolerance to topical mechlorethamine therapy in patients with cutaneous T-cell lymphomas. French Study Group of Cutaneous Lymphomas. Arch Dermatol 135:1349-1353, 1999.
79. Breneman D, Duvic M, Kuzel T, et al: Phase 1 and 2 trial of bexarotene gel for skin-directed treatment of patients with cutaneous T-cell lymphoma. Arch Dermatol 138:325-332, 2002.
80. British Photodermatology Group guidelines for PUVA. Br J Dermatol 130:246-255, 1994.
81. Thomsen K, Hammar H, Molin L, et al: Retinoids plus PUVA (RePUVA) and PUVA in mycosis fungoides, plaque stage. A report from the Scandinavian Mycosis Fungoides Group. Acta Derm Venereol 69:536-538, 1989.
82. Heald P, Rook A, Perez M, et al: Treatment of erythrodermic cutaneous T-cell lymphoma with extracorporeal photochemotherapy. J Am Acad Dermatol 27:427-433, 1992.
83. Jumbou O, N'Guyen JM, Tessier MH, et al: Long-term follow-up in 51 patients with mycosis fungoides and Sezary syndrome treated by interferon-alfa. Br J Dermatol 140:427-431, 1999.
84. Duvic M, Martin AG, Kim Y, et al: Phase 2 and 3 clinical trial of oral bexarotene (Targretin capsules) for the treatment of refractory or persistent early-stage cutaneous T-cell lymphoma. Arch Dermatol 137:581-593, 2001.
85. Olsen E, Duvic M, Frankel A, et al: Pivotal phase III trial of two dose levels of denileukin diftitox for the treatment of cutaneous T-cell lymphoma. J Clin Oncol 19:376-388, 2001.
86. Hoppe RT: Total skin electron beam therapy in the management of mycosis fungoides. Front Radiat Ther Oncol 25:80-89; discussion 132-133, 1991.
87. Strohl RA: The role of total skin electron beam radiation therapy in the management of mycosis fungoides. Dermatol Nurs 6:191-194, 196, 220, 1994.
88. Kirova YM, Piedbois Y, Haddad E, et al: Radiotherapy in the management of mycosis fungoides: Indications, results, prognosis. Twenty years experience. Radiother Oncol 51:147-151, 1999.
89. Maingon P, Truc G, Dalac S, et al: Radiotherapy of advanced mycosis fungoides: Indications and results of total skin electron beam and photon beam irradiation. Radiother Oncol 54:73-78, 2000.
90. Hagedorn M, Hasche E, Kober B, et al: [Long term results of total skin electron beam therapy (TSEBT) in the treatment of mycosis fungoides]. Hautarzt 54:256-264, 2003.
91. Ysebaert L, Truc G, Dalac S, et al: Ultimate results of radiation therapy for T1-T2 mycosis fungoides (including reirradiation). Int J Radiat Oncol Biol Phys 58:1128-1134, 2004.
92. Wilson LD, Kacinski BM, Jones GW: Local superficial radiotherapy in the management of minimal stage IA cutaneous T-cell lymphoma (Mycosis Fungoides). Int J Radiat Oncol Biol Phys 40:109-115, 1998.

93. Wilson LD, Quiros PA, Kolenik SA, et al: Additional courses of total skin electron beam therapy in the treatment of patients with recurrent cutaneous T-cell lymphoma. J Am Acad Dermatol 35:69-73, 1996.
94. Becker M, Hoppe RT, Knox SJ: Multiple courses of high-dose total skin electron beam therapy in the management of mycosis fungoides. Int J Radiat Oncol Biol Phys 32:1445-1449, 1995.
95. Jones GW, Kacinski BM, Wilson LD, et al: Total skin electron radiation in the management of mycosis fungoides: Consensus of the European Organization for Research and Treatment of Cancer (EORTC) Cutaneous Lymphoma Project Group. J Am Acad Dermatol 47:364-370, 2002.
96. Rampino M, Ragona R, Monetti U, et al: Total skin electron beam therapy in mycosis fungoides. Our experience from 1985 to 1999. Radiol Med (Torino) 103:108-114, 2002.
97. Jones GW, Hoppe RT, Glatstein E: Electron beam treatment for cutaneous T-cell lymphoma. Hematol Oncol Clin North Am 9:1057-1076, 1995.
98. Chen Z, Agostinelli AG, Wilson LD, et al: Matching the dosimetry characteristics of a dual-field Stanford technique to a customized single-field Stanford technique for total skin electron therapy. Int J Radiat Oncol Biol Phys 59:872-885, 2004.
99. Desai KR, Pezner RD, Lipsett JA, et al: Total skin electron irradiation for mycosis fungoides: Relationship between acute toxicities and measured dose at different anatomic sites. Int J Radiat Oncol Biol Phys 15:641-645, 1988.
100. Frassica DA, Frassica FJ, Schray MF, et al: Solitary plasmacytoma of bone: Mayo Clinic experience. Int J Radiat Oncol Biol Phys 16:43-48, 1989.
101. Dimopoulos MA, Goldstein J, Fuller L, et al: Curability of solitary bone plasmacytoma. J Clin Oncol 10:587-590, 1992.
102. Liebross RH, Ha CS, Cox JD, et al: Solitary bone plasmacytoma: Outcome and prognostic factors following radiotherapy. Int J Radiat Oncol Biol Phys 41:1063-1067, 1998.
103. Liebross RH, Ha CS, Cox JD, et al: Clinical course of solitary extramedullary plasmacytoma. Radiother Oncol 52:245-249, 1999.
104. Wax MK, Yun KJ, Omar RA: Extramedullary plasmacytomas of the head and neck. Otolaryngol Head Neck Surg 109:877-885, 1993.
105. Michalaki VJ, Hall J, Henk JM, et al: Definitive radiotherapy for extramedullary plasmacytomas of the head and neck. Br J Radiol 76:738-741, 2003.
106. Kyle RA: The role of high-dose chemotherapy in the treatment of multiple myeloma: A controversy. Ann Oncol 11(Suppl 1):55-58, 2000.
107. Moreau P, Facon T, Attal M, et al: Comparison of 200 mg/m(2) melphalan and 8 Gy total body irradiation plus 140 mg/m(2) melphalan as conditioning regimens for peripheral blood stem cell transplantation in patients with newly diagnosed multiple myeloma: Final analysis of the Intergroupe Francophone du Myelome 9502 randomized trial. Blood 99:731-735, 2002.
108. Dudeney S, Lieberman IH, Reinhardt MK, et al: Kyphoplasty in the treatment of osteolytic vertebral compression fractures as a result of multiple myeloma. J Clin Oncol 20:2382-2387, 2002.
109. Adamietz IA, Schober C, Schulte RW, et al: Palliative radiotherapy in plasma cell myeloma. Radiother Oncol 20:111-116, 1991.

CHAPTER 73

HODGKIN'S DISEASE

Andrea K. Ng, Lawrence Weiss, and Arnold Freedman

INCIDENCE

Each year 7500 to 8000 new cases of Hodgkin's disease occur in the United States.

BIOLOGIC CHARACTERISTICS

Hodgkin and Reed-Sternberg (HRS) cells are the malignant cells in Hodgkin's disease.

Increasing epidemiologic and molecular evidence support that a combination of genetic susceptibility, immune response impairment, and exposure to specific infectious agents may play a central role in the pathogenesis of the disease.

PATHOLOGY

Classical Hodgkin's disease ($CD15^+$, $CD30^+$, $CD45^-$) four subtypes: nodular sclerosis, lymphocyte predominant, mixed cellularity, and lymphocyte depleted

Nodular lymphocyte-predominant Hodgkin's disease (NLPHD) ($CD45^+$, $CD20^+$, $CD\ 15^-$, $CD\ 30^-$)

STAGING EVALUATION

History and physical examination focusing on constitutional symptoms, nodal involvement, and organomegaly

Complete blood count, erythrocyte sedimentation rate, and serum albumin

Computed tomography (CT) of chest, abdomen, and pelvis

Positron emission tomography

Bone marrow biopsy if constitutional symptoms present and/or advanced-stage disease

THERAPY IN EARLY-STAGE DISEASE

Standard therapy is combined-modality therapy with four to six cycles of Adriamycin (doxorubicin), bleomycin, vinblastine, and dacarbazine (ABVD) followed by involved-field radiation therapy (IFRT), with 5-year disease-free survival of approximately 90%.

Abbreviated regimens in patients with unfavorable prognostic features (bulky disease, four or more sites of disease, presence of constitutional symptoms) should be avoided.

Given the lack of data supporting its efficacy, chemotherapy alone should be restricted to the setting of a clinical trial.

THERAPY IN ADVANCED-STAGE DISEASE

Standard therapy is chemotherapy alone with ABVD, with 5-year disease-free survival of approximately 70% to 80%.

Alternatives to ABVD, including dose-escalated BEACOPP and Stanford V, have shown promising results, and are currently being compared against ABVD in ongoing randomized trials.

There may be a role for consolidative radiation therapy (RT) in selected cases, including initial bulky disease or lack of complete response to chemotherapy.

SALVAGE THERAPY

High-dose therapy with autologous bone marrow or stem cell transplantation (SCT) is the salvage therapy of choice in patients who are refractory to, or relapsed after, a short initial remission to chemotherapy.

Selected patients may be candidates for conventional dose salvage therapy, namely, patients with limited nodal relapse, absence of constitutional symptoms, and long remission duration.

PALLIATION

RT is an effective form of palliative treatment in patients with significant local symptoms.

Single- and multiagent regimens have also been shown to provide effective palliation.

Hodgkin's disease was first described by the British physician Thomas Hodgkin in 1832, when he reported six cases of pathologic enlargement of lymph nodes and spleen at Guy's Hospital.[1] Attempts to treat the disease using various chemical or surgical means were unsuccessful until around the turn of the century, when the effectiveness of x-rays in shrinking the disease was first demonstrated. Only crude, low-energy radiograph equipment was available at the time, which merely allowed the temporary reduction of the enlarged lymph nodes. The development of kilovoltage equipment in the 1920s and the subsequent pioneering work of Gilbert, a Swiss radiotherapist, paved the way for the definitive treatment of patients with Hodgkin's disease.[2] Vera Peters at Ontario Institute of Radiotherapy first reported the curability of early-stage Hodgkin's disease in 1950 using high doses of fractionated radiation therapy (RT).[3] The availability of modern, high-energy RT equipment in the late 1950s and early 1960s allowed the delivery of higher doses of radiation to deep-seated tumor with less limitations by reactions in the superficial tissues. The introduction of effective combination chemotherapy further improved the treatment outcome of Hodgkin's disease, especially in patients with unfavorable prognostic features or advanced-stage disease.[4] Over the last three decades, continued improvements in RT techniques allowing more uniform and better-targeted dose delivery, development of more effective and less toxic multiagent chemotherapy regimens, advances in radiographic imaging technology, and the refinement of prognostic factors that allow better tailoring of treatments, previously fatal Hodgkin's disease has now become one of the most curable forms of malignancy.

ETIOLOGY AND EPIDEMIOLOGY

Hodgkin's disease is a relatively uncommon neoplasm, with approximately 7500 to 8000 new cases in the United

States each year, representing less than 1% of all cancer diagnoses.[5] The incidence, age, and gender distribution of Hodgkin's disease vary depending on the geographic location. The age-incidence curve in developed countries is characterized by a bimodal distribution.[6,7] There is an initial peak in young adults at around age 25 years and a second peak occurring at age 60 to 70 years, in which a male predominance is observed. Most cases seen in young adulthood are of nodular sclerosis (NS) histology, and many of the factors that have been associated with the development of Hodgkin's disease in these patients appeared to be a reflection of delayed exposure to infectious agents or higher socioeconomic status, or both. These include early birth order, small sibship size, growing up in single-family houses, few playmates, and high parental education.[8-10] In contrast, in economically disadvantaged parts of the world, Hodgkin's disease is relatively rare among young adults.[7] Mixed cellularity (MC) is the predominant histologic subtype in developing countries, with an initial peak in childhood for boys and a late peak in older patients.

The etiology of Hodgkin's disease is an unresolved issue but is likely to be complex and may vary depending on the different subtypes. A combination of genetic susceptibility, immune-response impairment, and environmental exposures, especially specific infectious agents, are likely to play a central role in the pathogenesis of the disease.

Several of the epidemiologic and clinical features of the disease are suggestive of infectious causes, and there has been increasing evidence that Epstein-Barr virus (EBV) may be involved in the pathogenesis of Hodgkin's disease in at least a subset of cases. Patients with a history of infectious mononucleosis, in which EBV is the causative agent, are at an approximately threefold increased risk for Hodgkin's disease.[7,11,12] Elevated levels of the IgG and IgA immunoglobulins against the EBV capsid antigen have been demonstrated months to years before clinical Hodgkin's development.[13,14] In approximately one third to half of cases of classical Hodgkin's disease occurring in Western populations, monoclonal EBV genome can be detected in the Reed-Sternberg cells.[15,16] EBV positivity is predominantly associated with the MC subtype,[17] which is more common among young children and older adults, and is less-frequently associated with NS cases seen mostly in young adults in the developed world.

The observation of familial aggregation of cases of Hodgkin's disease suggests that genetic susceptibility as well as environmental exposure may contribute to the development of Hodgkin's disease. A fivefold increased risk has been demonstrated in first-degree relatives, and siblings of young adults with Hodgkin's disease have a sevenfold increased risk.[18] The excess risk appears to be more pronounced in same-sex siblings, which may be related to more shared environmental exposure.[19] In a twin study of young adults with Hodgkin's disease, monozygotic twins of patients had an almost 100-fold increased risk,[20] whereas no increased risk for dizygotic twins was observed, supporting the contribution of heritable factors to the development of the disease. In particular, follow-up twin studies have suggested that persons with genetically determined lower interleukin-6 (IL-6) levels may be less susceptible to young adult Hodgkin's lymphoma.[21] Finally, a number of specific human-leukocyte antigen (HLA) haplotypes are identified as associated with an increased risk of Hodgkin's disease.[22-24] Because immune response is genetically determined by the HLA type, patients with these HLA haplotypes may have increased susceptibility to certain infections, which in turn leads to increased Hodgkin's disease risk.

BIOLOGIC CHARACTERISTICS/ MOLECULAR BIOLOGY

The malignant cells in Hodgkin's disease, Hodgkin and Reed-Sternberg (HRS) cells, are large, uni- or multinucleated cells that make up less than 1% of the cells present in the tissue sample, with the majority of the tumor consisting of a variety of nonneoplastic inflammatory cells and fibrosis. Significant advances have been made in recent years in the elucidation of the origin of HRS cells and the identification of events underlying the malignant transformation.

Results of molecular single-cell studies have shown that in more than 90% of cases, HRS cells have monoclonal immunoglobulin gene rearrangements that are characteristic of mature B lymphocytes, and somatically mutated *VH* genes that are specific markers for germinal-center B cells and their descendants, supporting a germinal center or postgerminal center B-cell origin.[25,26] However, unlike normal B cells that have undergone successful maturation through the germinal cells, HRS cells characteristically show absence of immunoglobulin gene expression. This has been attributed to mutations in the coding or regulatory regions,[27] lack of expression of transcription factors responsible for activation of the promoters and enhancers,[28,29] and, more recently, epigenetic silencing of the immunoglobulin heavy-chain transcription.[30] Despite their inability to express immunoglobulin receptors, HRS cells are resistant to apoptosis, which normally removes immunoglobulin-negative B cells that have traversed the germinal center.

There is increasing evidence connecting the prevention of apoptosis and survival of HRS cells to the activation of the nuclear factor kappa-B (NF-κB) transcription factor-signaling pathway. The first evidence supporting a role of NF-κB was from the demonstration of constitutive expression of NF-κB in several Hodgkin's disease–derived cell lines as well as in primary HRS cells from a patient.[31] Hodgkin's lymphoma cells depleted of constitutive NF-κB revealed strongly impaired tumor growth in severe combined immunodeficient mice.[32] The suppression of NF-κB activity in Hodgkin's disease cell lines significantly reduces the growth and increases the rate of apoptosis of the HRS cells.[33,34] The cause of the constitutive activation of NF-κB has not been determined, but mutations in NF-κB inhibitors have been identified in a subset of cases of Hodgkin's disease.[35]

Molecular-profiling experiments using Hodgkin's disease–derived cell lines with suppressed and unsuppressed NF-κB activity have been performed to better understand the NF-κB signaling pathway and identify its target genes. One regulator of apoptosis expressed in dependence of NF-κB is *cIAP2*, a direct inhibitor of caspase 3, suggesting that HRS cells are protected from caspase-3–induced apoptosis by *cIAP2*.[36] Another NF-κB–dependent regulator of apoptosis is CD95, which is upregulated in HRS cells. However, unlike the other NF-κB–dependent regulators, CD95 is known to trigger rather than prevent apoptosis. Recent data indicate that the resistance of HRS cells to CD95-mediated apoptotic cell death is caused by functional inhibition of death receptor pathways by cellular FADD (FAS-associating protein with death domain)-like IL1B-converting enzyme inhibitory proteins (c-FLIP), which is one of the most strongly NF-κ–regulated genes.[37] Suppression experiments with downregulation of c-FLIP dramatically induces apoptosis in HRS cell lines.

The contribution of NF-κB signaling to the development of Hodgkin's disease is further supported by recent epidemiologic data showing that regular aspirin use is associated with reduced risk of developing Hodgkin's disease, presumably through inhibition of NF-κB transcription.[38] Continued efforts in the elucidation of the NF-κB pathway in the pathogenesis of Hodgkin's disease may have important therapeutic implications through pharmacologic downregulation of NF-κB activity and its target genes and increasing the susceptibility of HRS to apoptosis.

PATHOLOGY

Since the 1930s, a number of pathologic classification systems for Hodgkin's disease have been developed. The Rye classification system, introduced at a conference in Rye, New York, in 1966, divided cases of Hodgkin's disease into lymphocyte predominance (LP), NS, MC, and lymphocyte depletion (LD).[39] This system was widely adopted in the next 25 years and was subsequently modified in the Revised European-American Lymphoma (REAL) classification and later in the World Health Organization (WHO) classification (Table 73-1).[40,41] In the current classification system, Hodgkin's disease is specifically recognized as a lymphoma. Based on morphologic, immunophenotypical, and clinical characteristics, it is divided into two distinct entities: classical Hodgkin's disease and nodular lymphocyte predominant Hodgkin's disease (NLPHD). Table 73-2 compares the morphologic and immunophenotypical features of the malignant cells of these two entities. The diagnosis of Hodgkin's disease is based on morphologic assessment with identification of HRS cells or their variants, along with immunohistochemical studies.

Table 73-1 The World Health Organization Histologic Classification of Hodgkin's Lymphoma[41]

Nodular Lymphocyte Predominant Hodgkin's Lymphoma (NLPHL)

Classical Hodgkin's lymphoma (CHL)
Nodular sclerosis classical Hodgkin's lymphoma (NSHL)
Mixed cellularity classical Hodgkin's lymphoma (MCHL)
Lymphocyte rich classical Hodgkin's lymphoma (LRCHL)
Lymphocyte-depleted classical Hodgkin's lymphoma (LDHL)

Table 73-2 Comparison of Morphologic and Immunophenotypical Characteristics of the Malignant Cells of Classical Hodgkin's Disease and NLPHD

	Classical Hodgkin's Disease (HRS cells)	NLPHD (L/H cells)
Nuclei	Mono- and multinucleated, mono- and multilobulated	Mononucleated, multilobulated
Nucleoli	Large	Multiple, small
CD30	+	–
CD15	+*	–
CD45	–	+
CD20	–*	+
CD79a	–*	+

*In most cases.
HRS, Hodgkin and Reed-Sternberg; L/H, lymphocytic/histiocytic; NLPHD, nodular lymphocyte predominant Hodgkin's lymphoma.

Classical Hodgkin's Disease

In the majority of cases of the HRS of classical Hodgkin's disease, most markers for B cells or T cells, as well as leukocyte common antigen (CD45) are absent, whereas a number of antigens including CD30 and CD15, which are not usually expressed by normal B cells or T cells, can be detected. The immunophenotypical and genetic features of the malignant cells of the four histologic subtypes of classical Hodgkin's disease are similar. However, the four subtypes vary in the morphology of the HRS cells, nature of the surrounding reactive cells, association with EBV, and clinical characteristics.

The NS subtype accounts for approximately 70% of classical Hodgkin's disease, affecting predominantly young adults. Morphologically, it is characterized by the presence of one or more sclerotic bands radiating from a thickened lymph node capsule. The British National Lymphoma Investigation subclassified NS Hodgkin's disease into two grades based on the percentage of nodules showing lymphocyte depletion or increased number of anaplastic-appearing Hodgkin's cells.[42,43] However, the prognostic value of this grading system with modern therapy is unclear.

The MC subtype is more frequently seen in developing countries, accounting for more than half of the cases, whereas in the more developed parts of the world, it makes up approximately 25% of classical Hodgkin's disease. Morphologically, HRS cells are seen scattered in a diffuse inflammatory background with the absence of nodular sclerosing fibrosis. In contrast to the NS and lymphocyte-rich classical Hodgkin's disease (LRCHD), EBV positivity is much more frequent in the MC subtype.[17]

LRCHD accounts for approximately 5% of classical Hodgkin's disease, has a male predominance, and has older median age at presentation. It is characterized by a background infiltrate of small, mature, predominantly B lymphocytes with rare HRS and variants. It can resemble NLPHD morphologically, and immunohistochemical studies of the malignant cells are essential to make the distinction.[44]

The LD subtype has an increased number of HRS and is depleted in lymphocytes. Many cases that were previously classified as LD Hodgkin's disease are now determined to be anaplastic or large-cell non-Hodgkin's lymphoma based on immunohistochemical studies.[45] Reliable clinical data on this subtype is limited given its rarity and uncertainty concerning its diagnosis.

Nodular Lymphocyte Predominant Hodgkin's Disease

NLPHD makes up 5% of Hodgkin's lymphoma. The malignant cells of NLPHD are the lymphocytic/histiocytic (L/H) cells, or both, which are also known as popcorn cells, because of their characteristic appearance. Unlike classical Hodgkin's disease, the neoplastic cells of NLPHD typically lack the expression of CD15 and CD30 markers but are consistently CD20 and CD45 positive.[44] A nodular pattern usually completely or partially replaces the lymph node. The nodules tend to be large and closely packed, and the L/H cells are typically seen within or around the nodules. There are usually large numbers of CD57 positive small lymphocytes in the nodules, often with ringing around the L/H cells. In approximately 3% to 5% of cases, transformation to diffuse large B-cell lymphoma has been reported.[46]

CLINICAL MANIFESTATIONS/PATIENT EVALUATION/STAGING

Patterns of Disease Involvement

Hodgkin's disease typically begins at a single site within the lymphatic system, and spreads to contiguous nodal regions in an orderly fashion.[2,47] The pattern of disease involvement of contiguous sites was demonstrated in a study in which the sites of disease involvement were carefully documented in 100 consecutive Hodgkin's disease patients who underwent staging laparotomy.[47] In another study on 719 surgically staged patients, the pattern of disease involvement was found to vary depending on the histologic subtype.[47] Patients with NS histology typically had disease limited to above the diaphragm and had mediastinal involvement, whereas patients with LP Hodgkin's disease had predominantly peripheral nodal presentation. Liver involvement was rare, almost always occurred only in the presence of splenic involvement, and was mostly seen in patients with MC or LD histology.

Clinical Presentation

The most common clinical presentation of Hodgkin's disease is nontender lymphadenopathy, mostly in the cervical nodal chain, occurring in approximately 70% of cases. Axillary or inguinal adenopathy are less frequently reported, found in approximately 15% and 10% of patients, respectively. Another common presentation is mediastinal adenopathy detected on radiographic imaging. In cases of large mediastinal adenopathy, patients may occasionally present with local symptoms including shortness of breath, chest pain, cough, or superior vena cava syndrome. Rarely, patients may present with an enlarging anterior chest wall mass caused by local extension.

Patients may also present exclusively with constitutional symptoms in the absence of any physical findings. These symptoms, also known as B symptoms, include fever, unexplained weight loss, and drenching night sweats. Severe, generalized pruritus, not classified as a B symptom, is noted in approximately 10% to 15% of patients and has been associated with a poorer prognosis.[48] Alcohol-induced pain, typically at the site of lymphadenopathy or bony involvement, can be a presenting symptom in some patients.[49]

Staging System

The Ann Arbor staging classification (Table 73-3), developed in 1971, is a four-stage system formulated to provide prognostic information and to guide therapeutic decisions. However, it does not reflect other important prognostic factors such as bulky disease or multiple sites of involvement.[50] The availability of improved imaging techniques has also changed its applicability. At a 1988 meeting in the Cotswolds, England, revisions were made to the Ann Arbor staging system (Table 73-4).[51] Main changes include the following: (1) Allowed the use of CT scanning to assess disease involvement below the diaphragm. (2) For stage II disease the number of anatomic nodal sites was indicated by a subscript, such as stage II_3. (3) For stage III disease upper- and lower-abdominal involvement was subdivided as III_1 and III_2, respectively. (4) Bulky disease was denoted by X, defined as more than 1/3 widening of the mediastinum at T5-6 level or more than 10-cm maximum dimension of the nodal mass. (5) Unconfirmed/uncertain complete remission (CRu) was introduced to denote presence of residual imaging abnormality but absence of pathologically confirmed residual disease.

Table 73-3 Ann Arbor Staging Classification

Stage	Definitions
Stage I	Involvement of single lymph node region (I) or of single extralymphatic organ or site (I_E)
Stage II	Involvement of two or more lymph node regions on the same side of the diaphragm alone (II) or with involvement of limited, contiguous extralymphatic organ or tissue (II_E)
Stage III	Involvement of lymph node regions on both sides of the diaphragm (III) which may include the spleen (III_S) or limited, contiguous extralymphatic organ or site (III_E) or both (III_{SE})
Stage IV	Diffuse or disseminated foci of involvement of one or more extralymphatic organs or tissues, with or without associated lymphatic involvement

The absence or presence of fever, night sweats, and/or unexplained weight loss of 10% or more of body weight in the 6 months preceding admission are to be denoted in all cases by the suffix letters A or B, respectively. The CS denotes the stage as determined by all diagnostic examinations and a single biopsy only. If a second biopsy of any kind has been obtained, whether negative or positive, the term PS is used.

CS, clinical stage; PS, pathologic stage.

Table 73-4 The Cotswolds Staging Classification for Hodgkin's Disease

Stage	Definitions
Stage I	Involvement of a single lymph node region or lymphoid structure (e.g. spleen, thymus, Waldeyer's ring) or involvement of a single extralymphatic site (I_E).
Stage II	Involvement of two or more lymph node regions on the same side of the diaphragm (hilar nodes, when involved on both sides, constitute stage II disease); localized contiguous involvement of only one extranodal organ or site and lymph node region(s) on the same side of the diaphragm (II_E). The number of anatomic regions involved should be indicated by a suffix (e.g., II_3).
Stage III	Involvement of lymph node regions on both sides of the diaphragm (III), which may also be accompanied by involvement of the spleen (III_S) or by localized contiguous involvement of only one extranodal organ site (III_E) or both (III_{SE}). III_1: With or without involvement of splenic, hilar, celiac, or portal nodes. III_2: With involvement of para-aortic, iliac, and mesenteric nodes.
Stage IV	Diffuse or disseminated involvement of one or more extranodal organs or tissues, with or without associated lymph node involvement.

The absence or presence of fever, night sweats, and /or unexplained weight loss of 10% or more of body weight in the 6 months preceding admission is to be denoted in all cases by the suffix letters A or B. The clinical stage (CS) denotes the stage as determined by all diagnostic examinations and a single biopsy only. If a second biopsy of any kind has been obtained, whether negative or positive, the term pathologic stage (PS) is used.

Patient Evaluation and Staging Workup

An adequate surgical biopsy for pathologic assessment by an experienced hematopathologist is essential in the initial diagnosis of Hodgkin's disease. All patients must undergo a careful history and physical examination. Particular attention should be placed on the presence and duration of constitutional symptoms, as well as other symptoms that may be indicative of extent and bulkiness of local disease. On physical examination all nodal groups should be thoroughly palpated with clear documentation of the extent of disease involvement. The extent of neck disease is of particular importance because it may have implications for the superior border of the radiation field after a complete response to chemotherapy. Baseline blood work, some of which has been shown to have prognostic value in patients with Hodgkin's disease, should be obtained. These include complete blood count with differential, sedimentation rate, and serum albumin. Radiographic staging studies include a posteroanterior and lateral chest radiograph with measurement of the tumor mass: thoracic ratio at either T5-6 or at the diaphragm, and CT scan of the chest, abdomen, and pelvis. In review of the chest CT, in addition to evaluating the extent of mediastinal disease, any axillary involvement, pericardial nodal involvement, or chest wall invasion should be noted, because they will affect the radiation field design at the end of the chemotherapy. Baseline nuclear medicine imaging studies are also routinely performed, and most centers are now replacing gallium scintigraphy with ^{18}F-fluorodeoxyglucose positron emission tomographic (FDG-PET) scanning, which is more sensitive both in the initial staging and follow-up of Hodgkin's disease patients.[52-54] The performance of bone marrow biopsy should be limited to patients with advanced-stage disease or in those with constitutional symptoms given the low yield in patients with early-stage, favorable-prognosis disease of less than 1%.[55,56] The recommended patient evaluation and staging studies for newly diagnosed Hodgkin's disease are listed in Table 73-5.

Table 73-5 Patient Evaluation and Staging

HISTORY
Constitutional symptoms
Symptoms that may be indicative of extent and bulk of local disease, such as pulmonary symptoms, swelling, pain
PHYSICAL EXAMINATION
Careful palpation of all nodal groups
Palpate for organomegaly
RADIOGRAPHIC STAGING
CT scans of neck/chest/abdomen/pelvis
Nuclear medicine imaging (PET scan)
PATHOLOGIC EVALUATION
Excisional biopsy depending on location of disease
Bone marrow biopsy only in patients with advanced stage disease and/or constitutional symptoms
BLOOD WORK
CBC with differential
ESR
Serum albumin
PRETREATMENT BASELINE EVALUATION
Patients receiving Adriamycin: baseline MUGA scan
Patients receiving bleomycin: baseline pulmonary function tests

CBC, complete blood count; CT, computed tomography; ESR, erythrocyte sedimentation rate; MUGA, multigated acquisition scan; PET, positron emission tomography.

Surgical staging, developed in the 1960s, involved laparotomy, splenectomy and liver and multiple lymph node biopsies.[57] The rationale for performing staging laparotomy was to determine the extent of disease below the diaphragm and identify patients who may be candidates for RT alone after confirming absence of disease in the abdomen. The performance of staging laparotomy has largely been eliminated in current clinical practice since the introduction of more effective and less toxic combination chemotherapy for Hodgkin's disease. Furthermore, a randomized study conducted by the European Organization for Research and Treatment of Cancer (EORTC) failed to show a survival benefit of pathologic staging over clinical staging.[58]

PRIMARY THERAPY FOR EARLY-STAGE HODGKIN'S DISEASE

Early-stage Hodgkin's disease comprises approximately 60% of all cases of Hodgkin's disease. Historically, the primary therapy for early-stage Hodgkin's disease had been extended-field radiation therapy (EFRT) alone, with addition of chemotherapy in the presence of unfavorable prognostic factors such as large mediastinal adenopathy, constitutional symptoms, high number of involved sites, and/or elevated sedimentation rate. Since the introduction of the ABVD regimen (Adriamycin [doxorubicin], bleomycin, vinblastine, and dacarbazine), a more effective and less toxic combination chemotherapy regimen than MOPP (mechlorethamine, vincristine, procarbazine, prednisone), there has been a shift to the use of combined-modality therapy in early-stage patients, which yields long-term cure rates of 80% to 90%. Randomized studies have shown a significantly higher freedom-from-treatment failure (FFTF) with combined-modality therapy than with RT alone.[59-61] Furthermore, the addition of chemotherapy to RT allows the use of more limited radiation treatment fields.

Because of the excellent survival in this relatively young group of patients, late effects of therapy have been increasingly recognized.[62-65] Most of the current trials on early-stage Hodgkin's disease focus on treatment reduction and modification. In these trials, patients are stratified into risk groups for tailored therapy. Examples of various prognostic classification systems used by cooperative groups are shown in Table 73-6.

The key questions addressed by the trials on the use of combined-modality therapy for early-stage Hodgkin's disease included the following: (1) What is the optimal combination chemotherapy regimen? (2) How many cycles of chemotherapy are needed? (3) What are the appropriate radiation field size and dose? (4) Can RT be eliminated?

Optimal Combination Chemotherapy Regimen

Investigators have explored alternatives or modification of the ABVD regimen to limit toxicity in favorable patients or to improve efficacy in unfavorable patients. Examples include VBM (vinblastine, bleomycin, and methotrexate),[66-69] MVP (methotrexate, vinblastine, and prednisone),[67] VAPEC-B (doxorubicin, cyclophosphamide, etoposide, vincristine, bleomycin, and prednisolone),[70] AV (doxorubicin and vinblastine),[61] NOVP (mitoxantrone, vincristine, vinblastine, and prednisone)[71], and EBVP II (epirubicin, bleomycin, vinblastine, and prednisone) administered monthly.[72,73] The Stanford V regimen (nitrogen mustard, Adriamycin, vincristine, vinblastine, etoposide, bleomycin, and prednisone, followed by RT to initial nodal involvement in selected cases), a short but intensive 12-week regimen, was originally developed for

Table 73-6 The Prognostic Classification Systems for Clinical Staging of I-II Hodgkin's Disease

Institution	Prognostic Classification
EORTC	**Unfavorable Prognosis** *Presence of **any** one of the following:* Age >50 y No B symptoms with ESR ≥50 B symptoms with ESR ≥30 ≥4 sites of involvement Bulky mediastinal involvement **Favorable Prognosis** Absence of *all* of the factors in the unfavorable prognosis group
GHSG	**Unfavorable Prognosis** *Presence of **any** one of the following:* Elevated ESR (≥50 mm without or ≥30 mm with B symptoms) ≥3 sites of involvement Extranodal involvement Large mediastinal mass **Favorable Prognosis** Absence of *all* of the factors in the unfavorable prognosis group
NCIC (excluded patients with bulky disease)	**Low Risk** *Presence of **all** of the following:* LP/NS Age <40 y ESR <50 <3 sites of involvement **High risk** All other patients

EORTC, European Organization for Research and Treatment of Cancer; ESR, erythrocyte sedimentation rate; GHSG, German Hodgkin Study Group; LP, lymphocyte predominance; NCIC, National Cancer Institute of Canada; NS, nodular sclerosis; y, year.

patients with advanced-stage disease or bulky, early-stage disease.[74,75] A modified 8-week regimen is being investigated in nonbulky, clinical stage (CS) I to IIA patients, and in the most recent version (Stanford V-C) the nitrogen mustard is replaced by cyclophosphamide and the radiation dose is reduced from 30 Gy to 20 Gy. Most of these regimens showed promising results at least in patients with favorable-prognosis disease, with relapse-free survival rates of approximately 90%. However, only retrospective or prospective single-arm data are available. The German Hodgkin Study Group (GHSG) 13 trial is a newly opened 4-arm study comparing two cycles of ABVD, AVD, ABV, and AV, all followed by 30 Gy of involved-field irradiation in CS I to II patients without risk factors. The results of this trial will provide information on whether individual drugs can be eliminated from the ABVD regimen in this patient population.

Attempts to use less intensive chemotherapy in patients with unfavorable-prognosis disease have been disappointing. In the EORTC H7U study, comparing unfavorable-prognosis CS I to II patients treated with six cycles of EBVP II and involved-field irradiation versus six cycles of MOPP/ABV and involved-field irradiation, the 6-year event-free survival (EFS) was significantly lower in the EBVP II arm (68% versus 90%, $P < .0001$). To improve the treatment outcome in patients with unfavorable features, ongoing trials are exploring whether these patients may benefit from the BEACOPP regimen (bleomycin, etoposide, doxorubicin, cyclophosphamide, vincristine, procarbazine, and prednisone), originally developed for patients with advanced-stage disease. Both the EORTC H9U and the GHSG HD11 studies are comparing four to six cycles of ABVD with four cycles of BEACOPP-baseline, followed by involved-field irradiation to 20 to 30 Gy. Preliminary results of the GHSG HD11 trial showed no significant FFTF and overall survival differences between BEACOPP and ABVD nor between the 20 Gy and 30 Gy arm at a median follow-up of 2 years.[76] However, the 2-year failure-free survival (FFS) of approximately 90% was considered unacceptable, and this prompted the GHSG to incorporate dose-escalated BEACOPP into the treatment scheme in the current GHSG HD14 trial. In this trial patients with CS I to II disease with risk factors are randomized to four cycles of ABVD versus two cycles of dose-escalated BEACOPP and two cycles of ABVD, followed by involved-field irradiation to 30 Gy.

Optimal Duration of Chemotherapy

Whether the number of cycles of chemotherapy can be shortened in patients with favorable-prognosis disease was addressed by the GHSG HD10 trial, in which CS I to II patients without risk factors were randomized to four cycles or two cycles of ABVD, followed by 30 Gy or 20 Gy of involved-field irradiation.[77] At a median follow-up of 28 months, the 2-year FFTF was 96.6% and the 2-year overall survival was 98.5%, with no significant differences between the four arms. In patients with unfavorable-prognosis disease, the optimal number of cycles of chemotherapy was one of the study questions in two successive EORTC trials using different chemotherapy regimens. In the EORTC H8U trial patients were randomized to six cycles of MOPP/ABV followed by involved-field irradiation, four cycles of MOPP/ABV followed by involved-field irradiation or four cycles of MOPP/ABV followed by EFRT.[78] At a median follow-up of 39 months, the FFS rates were 89%, 92%, and 92%, respectively ($p = .32$); and the overall survival rates were 90%, 94%, and 92%, respectively ($p = .19$). In the EORTC H9U trial randomizing patients to six cycles of ABVD, four cycles of ABVD, or four cycles of BEACOPP, all followed by involved-field irradiation, the most recent interim analysis showed 4-year EFS and overall survival of 90% and 94%, respectively (no arm comparison provided). Longer follow-up time is needed, however, to determine whether two cycles and four cycles of chemotherapy may be adequate for patients with favorable- and unfavorable-prognosis disease, respectively, when given in conjunction with RT.

Optimal Radiation Field Size

The available data addressing the issue of whether smaller fields can be employed as part of combined-modality therapy had been evaluated largely in patients with unfavorable-prognosis disease, but the results should be applicable to patients with favorable-prognosis disease as well. As described previously, two of the three arms in the EORTC H8U trial compared four cycles of MOPP/ABV followed by either involved-field irradiation or EFRT, and no significant differences in failure-free or overall survival were detected at a median follow-up of 39 months. In the GHSG HD8 trial 1204 patients with CS I to II Hodgkin's disease with adverse factors were randomized to receive two cycles of COPP (cyclophosphamide, vincristine, procarbazine, and prednisone) and ABVD followed by EFRT or involved-field radiotherapy (IFRT).[79] At a median follow-up time of 54 months, the 5-year FFTF rates of the two arms were 86% and 84%, respectively (p = .56), and the 5-year overall survival rates were 91% and 92%, respectively (p = .24). Patients on the extended-field arm were significantly more likely to experience acute side effects including leukopenia, thrombocytopenia, nausea, gastrointestinal toxicity, and pharyngeal toxicity. A higher risk of second malignancy was also observed in the extended-field arm compared with the involved-field arm (4.5% versus 2.8%), although the difference was not statistically significant. In an Italian trial, 136 patients with CS I unfavorable and CS IIA favorable and unfavorable Hodgkin's disease received four cycles of ABVD followed by either subtotal nodal irradiation or IFRT.[80] At a median follow-up of 116 months, the 12-year freedom from progression of the two arms was 93% and 94%, respectively, and the 12-year overall survival rates were 96% and 94%, respectively. Three cases of second malignancies were reported, all of which were in the EFRT arm.

Optimal Radiation Dose

The appropriate radiation dose after chemotherapy in early-stage Hodgkin's disease is currently being explored by two trials. The EORTC H9F trial is a three-arm trial in which all patients receive six cycles of EBVP II.[73] After a complete response, patients were randomized to receive no further treatment, 36 Gy, or 20 Gy of IFRT. Patients with a partial response all received 36 Gy of involved-field irradiation with or without a 4-Gy boost. In an interim analysis on 771 patients, the chemotherapy alone arm was closed because of lower-than-expected EFS (discussed in the following text). The 4-year EFS of all patients in this trial was 80% and the 4-year overall survival was 98%. However, comparison results of the three arms are not yet available. The GHSG HD10 and HD11 trials on low-risk and high-risk early-stage patients, respectively, showed no differences between 20 Gy versus 30 Gy of IFRT.[77] However, both trials only had 2-year results, and additional follow-up is needed to establish the safety of 20 Gy of radiation treatment.

Chemotherapy Alone for Early-Stage Hodgkin's Disease

Because of the well-documented late effects of radiotherapy for Hodgkin's disease, based largely on patients treated with RT alone with larger treatment fields and higher doses of radiation than currently employed, investigators have explored the option of eliminating RT and treating patients with early-stage disease with chemotherapy alone. Table 73-7 summarizes the six randomized trials that compared combined-modality therapy with chemotherapy alone.[73,81-85] These trials varied in the study design, patient population, types of chemotherapy, and radiation fields employed. The findings and the limitations of each of the trials are discussed in the following text.

Pavlovsky and colleagues from the Grupo Argentino de Tratamiento de la Leucemia Aguda (GATLA) randomized 277 patients with CS I to II Hodgkin's disease to receive six monthly cycles of MOPP variant CVPP (cyclophosphamide, vinblastine, procarbazine, and prednisone), followed by IFRT to 30 Gy, versus six cycles of CVPP alone.[81] At 84 months, the disease-free survival (DFS) of the combined-modality–therapy arm was significantly higher than that of the chemotherapy-alone arm (71% versus 62%, p = .01). On subgroup analysis, the difference between the two arms were highly significant among patients with unfavorable features (older than age 45 years, more than 2 sites, or bulky disease), with DFS of 75% in the combined-modality–therapy arm versus 34% in the chemotherapy-alone arm (p = .001). Among favorable patients the difference in DFS was insignificant (77% versus 70%). The main limitation of this study is the inferior chemotherapy regimen used, which likely explained the poor treatment outcome, especially for the unfavorable patients treated with chemotherapy alone. In addition, 45% of patients in this trial were children younger than age 16 years. The results therefore may not be entirely applicable to the adult population.

The Children's Cancer Group (CCG) conducted a randomized trial on patients younger than age 21 years comparing low-dose IFRT and no RT after a complete response to chemotherapy.[82] Sixty-eight percent had CS I to II disease. Patients were stratified into three risk groups based on CS and presence of adverse factors. On an as-treated analysis, the 3-year EFS of the chemotherapy-alone arm was 85%, which was significantly lower than that of the combined-modality–therapy arm of 93% (p = .0024). The randomization was stopped on the recommendation of the Data Monitoring Committee because of a significantly higher number of relapses on the no-RT arm. Of note, among the 34 relapses with known sites of relapse in the chemotherapy-alone arm, 29 were exclusively in the original sites of disease, 3 were in both previously involved and new sites, and only 2 were exclusively in new sites. However, as in the previous study, the relevance of the results of this pediatric trial to adult patients is unclear. Moreover, the follow-up is relatively short in this study.

Laskar and colleagues reported results of a randomized trial from Tata Memorial Hospital comparing six cycles of ABVD with or without IFRT.[83] Only patients who achieved a complete response to the chemotherapy were randomized. Patients of all stages were included, and 55% had CS I to II disease. Significant differences in 6-year EFS (88% versus 76%, p = .01) and overall survival (100% versus 89%, p = .002) were observed, favoring the combined-modality–therapy arm. This is the only trial that demonstrated a survival benefit with the addition of RT. This study is limited by the high proportion of pediatric patients, with 46% younger than age 15 years. Also, the generalizability of the results to cases seen in the Western world is unclear, because 71% of cases were of mixed-cellularity histology, reflecting the high proportion of EBV-related cases in developing countries.

In a Memorial Sloan-Kettering Cancer Center trial, patients with nonbulky CS IA to IIB and CS IIIA were randomized to six cycles of ABVD with or without RT. The target accrual was 90 patients per arm.[84] After 152 patients were accrued at 10 years, the trial was closed because of slow accrual. No significant differences in freedom from progression (86% versus 81%) and overall survival (97% versus 90%) were found at a median follow-up of 60 months. Seven of the eight relapses in the chemotherapy-alone arm were in initially involved nodal sites. This trial, however, was underpowered to determine if the two treatment approaches are truly equivalent. Furthermore, care should be taken in the interpretation of long-term toxicity data when they become available because the majority of patients randomized to receive RT were treated with EFRT.

In a randomized trial conducted by the National Cancer Institute of Canada (NCIC) and Eastern Cooperative Oncology Group (ECOG), patients with nonbulky CS I to II disease were stratified into low-risk (LP/NS, age <40 years, erythrocyte sedimentation [ESR] <50, and <3 sites of disease) and high-risk groups.[85] Low-risk patients were randomized to EFRT versus four to six cycles of ABVD, and high-risk patients were randomized to two cycles of ABVD followed by RT versus

Table 73-7 **Randomized Trials Comparing Combined-Modality Therapy with Chemotherapy Alone in Early-Stage Hodgkin's Disease**

Institution	No.	Patient Population	Treatment Arms	Median Follow-Up	RESULTS Combined *Modality Therapy*	*Chemotherapy Alone*
GATLA[81]	277	CS I-II (Included patients with unfavorable factors: age >45 y, >2 sites or bulky disease) 45% < 16 y	CVPP × 6 → 30 Gy IFRT / No RT	84 mo	DFS: 71% OS: 89% Favorable group: DFS: 77% OS: 92% Unfavorable group: DFS: 75% OS: 84%	62% (*p* = .01) 82% 70% 91% 34% (*p* = .001) 66%
CCG[82]	829	Group 1: CS I-II without adverse factors* and without B Sx in CS II Group 2: CS I-II with adverse factors and CS III Group 3: CS IV	Group 1: COPP/ABV × 4 Group 2: COPP/ABV × 6 Group 3: intensive multidrug chemotherapy with GCSF support If CR → 21 Gy IFRT / No RT If PR → 21 Gy IFRT	Not reported	Intent to treat: 3-y EFS: 92% As treated: 3-y EFS: 93% 3-y OS: 98%	 87% (*p* = .057) 85% (*p* = .0024) 99% Arm closed
Tata Memorial Hospital[83]	251	CS I-IV (55% CS I-II, 46% age <15 y, 71% MC histology, 15% bulky disease)	ABVD × 6 If CR → RT[†] / No RT	63 mo	8-y EFS: 88% 8-y OS: 100%	76% (*p* = .01) 89% (*p* = .002)
MSKCC[84]	152	CS IA-IIB, CS IIIA (bulky disease excluded)	ABVD × 6 → RT[‡] / No RT	60 mo	5-y FFP: 86% 5-y OS: 97%	81% (*p* = .61) 90% (*p* = .08)
NCIC/ECOG[85]	399	CS I-IIA (bulky disease excluded) Low risk: LP/NS, age <40, ESR <50 and <3 sites High risk: all other	Low risk: STNI / ABVD × 4-6 High risk: ABVD × 2 + STNI / ABVD × 4-6	4.2 y	(Low risk: STNI; High risk: CMT) 5-y PFS: 93% 5-y EFS: 88% 5-y OS: 94%	 87% (*p* = .006) 86% (*p* = .06) 96% (*p* = .42)
EORTC H9F[73]	771	CS I-II, favorable-prognosis	EBVP II × 6 If CR → 36 Gy IFRT / 20 Gy IFRT / No RT If PR → 36 Gy IFRT ± 4 Gy	29 mo	Not separately reported	>20% cumulative proportion of adverse events Arm closed

*Adverse factors: hilar disease, >4 sites, LMA, or bulky disease >10 cm.
†IFRT 30 + 10 Gy boost for early-stage and EFRT 25 + 10-Gy boost for advanced-stage.
‡Modified EFRT in 83% of patients (91% received 36 Gy).
ABV, Adriamycin (doxorubicin), bleomycin, and vinblastine; ABVD, Adriamycin (doxorubicin), bleomycin, vinblastine, and dacarbazine; CCG, Children's Cancer Group; CMT, combined-modality therapy; COPP, cyclophosphamide, vincristine, procarbazine, and prednisone; CR, complete response; CS, clinical stage; CVPP, cyclophosphamide, vinblastine, procarbazine, and prednisone; DFS, disease-free survival; EBVP II, epirubicin, bleomycin, vinblastine, and prednisone; ECOG, Eastern Cooperative Oncology Group; EFRT, extended-field radiation therapy; EFS, event-free survival; EORTC, European Organization for Research and Treatment of Cancer; FFP, freedom from progression; GATLA, Grupo Argentino de Tratamiento de Leucemia Aguda; GCSF, granulocyte colony-stimulating factor; IFRT, involved-field radiation therapy; mo, month; MC, mixed cellularity; MSKCC, Memorial Sloan-Kettering Cancer Center; NCIC, National Cancer Institute of Canada; OS, overall survival; PFS, progression-free survival; PR, partial response; RT, radiation therapy; Sx, symptom; STNI, subtotal nodal irradiation; y, year.

four to six cycles of ABVD. At a median follow-up of 4.2 years, patients treated with chemotherapy alone had a significantly inferior 5-year progression-free survival of 87% versus 93% in patients treated with either EFRT or combined-modality therapy (*p* = .006). There were no significant differences in overall survival. In examining the results of this trial, it needs to be taken into consideration that the *standard arm* in the low-risk group was EFRT, which was shown to be inferior to combined-modality therapy in several randomized trials even among favorable patients and is currently no longer viewed as standard treatment. Furthermore, as in the Memorial Sloan-Kettering Cancer Center trial, most patients assigned to receive RT were treated with EFRT, which will likely have significant contribution to late effects.

The final trial is the EORTC H8F trial, which randomized CS I to II, favorable-prognosis patients after a complete response to six cycles of EBVP II to the following three arms: 36 Gy, 20 Gy of IFRT, or no further treatment.[73] Results comparing the arms are not yet available, but at the most recent interim analysis, the chemotherapy alone was closed because of higher than expected number of relapses. The main criticism of this study is the inadequate chemotherapy employed. However, this study was restricted to selected patients with favorable features, and the EBVP II regimen was chosen because its efficacy in combination with IFRT had been proved in the earlier EORTC H7F trial.

Recommendation on Treatment for Early-Stage Hodgkin's Disease

Combined-modality therapy with four to six cycles of ABVD chemotherapy followed by IFRT should be considered the standard therapy for early-stage Hodgkin's disease at this time. Longer follow-up is needed from trial results to determine whether individual drugs can be eliminated from the ABVD regimen in patients with favorable-prognosis disease. The use of abbreviated regimens in patients with unfavorable prognostic features is not recommended, and ongoing trials are addressing whether these patients may benefit from more aggressive chemotherapy. There appears to be adequate data to suggest that the use of IFRT after chemotherapy does not compromise disease control and is associated with less acute toxicity, but longer follow-up time is needed to assess its impact on late effects. Additional treatment reductions, including further lowering the number of cycles of chemotherapy, eliminating specific drugs, or further reducing the radiation dose, are currently being studied in favorable-prognosis patients, and answers will likely be available in the near future. The inferior FFS associated with chemotherapy alone compared with combined-modality therapy as demonstrated in several randomized trials suggests that chemotherapy alone for early-stage disease should be restricted to clinical trial participants who will be closely monitored.

PRIMARY TREATMENT FOR ADVANCED-STAGE HODGKIN'S DISEASE

The introduction of the combination chemotherapy regimen, MOPP, in the mid-1960s substantially improved the curability of patients with advanced-stage Hodgkin's disease.[4] The ABVD regimen was initially introduced as a form of second-line therapy in patients who had a poor response to, or relapse after, MOPP chemotherapy.[86] Its role as primary treatment in newly diagnosed patients was subsequently substantiated by several randomized trials in advanced-stage patients, showing that ABVD-containing regimens are associated with a higher FFS than MOPP.[87-89] To test the Goldie-Coldman hypothesis, investigators have also explored whether regimens containing both MOPP and ABVD are superior to ABVD alone. Results of an Intergroup randomized trial comparing MOPP/ABV hybrid versus ABVD in advanced-stage Hodgkin's disease showed that the addition of MOPP to ABVD did not confer any therapeutic benefit, but it did add to treatment-related toxicity.[90] ABVD is significantly less myelosuppressive, and it also does not carry the risk of gonadal dysfunction and leukemogenesis.

Hasenclever and Diehl developed a prognostic scoring system using data from more than 5000 patients with advanced-stage Hodgkin's disease, mostly treated with doxorubicin-based combination chemotherapy.[91] Seven factors were found to have similar independent prognostic value in predicting freedom from progression and overall survival. These included hypoalbuminemia (<4 g/dL), anemia (<10.5 g/dL), male sex, age 45 years or older, stage IV disease, leukocytosis (>15,000/mm^3), and lymphocytopenia (<600 mm^3, <8% of the white-cell count, or both). The freedom from progression at 5 years ranged from 49% in patients with five or more of the factors to 84% in patients without any of the factors (Table 73-8). However, patients with five or more of the adverse factors account for only 7% of the study population. This prognostic scoring system has been widely used in trials for patient selection and patient stratification, and it may also have a role in guiding tailored therapy based on relapse risk in advanced-stage patients.

Alternatives to ABVD

With six to eight cycles of ABVD, patients with advanced-stage disease have a long-term FFS of 60% to 65% and overall survival of 70% to 75%. To further improve treatment results, research institutions have developed dose-escalated or dose-dense regimens, or both, for advanced-stage Hodgkin's disease. Summarized in the following text are key regimens that have shown promising results.

The Stanford V regimen is a 12-week, seven-drug regimen that is administered weekly (Table 73-9).[92] It contains lower cumulative doses of mechlorethamine, Adriamycin, and bleomycin than MOPP and ABVD, respectively, to limit leukemogenesis, sterility, and cardiac and pulmonary toxicity.

Table 73-8 The International Prognostic Scoring System for Advanced-Stage Hodgkin's Disease

Prognostic Score	5-Year Freedom from Progression	5-Year Overall Survival
0	84%	89%
1	77%	90%
2	67%	81%
3	60%	78%
4	51%	61%
>5	42%	56%

Each of the following factors carries a score of 1: hypoalbuminemia, anemia, male sex, age ≥45 y, stage IV disease, leukocytosis, and lymphocytopenia.
y, year.

Table 73-9 Schedule of the Stanford V Regimen

Drug	Dose (mg/m^2)	WEEK 1	2	3	4	5	6	7	8	9	10	11	12
Mechlorethamine	6.0	X	—	—	—	X	—	—	—	X	—	—	—
Doxorubicin	25.0	X	—	X	—	X	—	X	—	X	—	X	—
Vinblastine	6.0	X	—	X	—	X	—	X	—	X	—	X	—
Vincristine	1.4	—	X	—	X	—	X	—	X	—	X	—	X
Bleomycin	5.0	—	X	—	X	—	X	—	X	—	X	—	X
Etoposide	60.0	—	—	XX	—	—	—	XX	—	—	—	XX	—
Prednisone qod	40.0	X	X	X	X	X	X	X	X	X	X	X	X

Patients with initial bulky disease (≥5 cm) received involved-field radiation therapy to 36 Gy.

Patients with initial disease of 5 cm or larger or macroscopic splenic disease, or both, which account for approximately 90% of the patients, receive 36 Gy of IFRT 2 weeks after the chemotherapy. In their most recent report on 142 patients with stage III or IV or locally extensive mediastinal stage I or II Hodgkin's disease, a 5-year freedom from progression and overall survival of 89% and 96%, respectively, were achieved.[92] No secondary leukemia was observed at a median follow-up of 5.4 years, but one case of acute leukemia was reported in an earlier ECOG pilot study using the same regimen on 45 patients.[93] The importance of RT as part of Stanford V was highlighted by a multi-institutional randomized trial from Italy.[94] In this study 355 patients with bulky stage II or advanced-stage Hodgkin's disease were randomized to receive Stanford V, MEC (mitoxantrone, etoposide, and Ara-C) hybrid, and ABVD. Among the 275 evaluable patients, the 3-year relapse-free survival of patients on the Stanford V arm was 75.7%, which was significantly lower than that of patients treated with MEC hybrid and ABVD, which were 94.9% and 91.5%, respectively ($p = .01$). The inferior outcome with Stanford V in the Italian trial was attributed to the fact that RT was given only at the discretion of the treating physician rather than according to the Stanford V guidelines, and as such, only 65% of patients underwent RT. An Intergroup trial comparing ABVD and Stanford V in patients with locally extensive and advanced-stage Hodgkin's disease is currently ongoing in the United States, and the results will establish how Stanford V, when delivered as originally designed, compares with the current gold-standard of ABVD.

GHSG developed a dose-escalated BEACOPP regimen (Table 73-10), which showed significantly superior survival outcome compared with conventional-dose regimens in the GHSG HD9 study.[95] In this three-armed trial, 1201 eligible patients with stage IIB, IIIA, IIIB, and IV were randomized to eight cycles of COPP-ABVD, baseline-dose BEACOPP, or increased-dose BEACOPP. The 5-year freedom-from-relapse rate was significantly higher in the dose-escalated BEACOPP arm than the baseline-dose BEACOPP and COPP-ABVD arms (87%, 76%, and 60%, $p < .001$). The corresponding 5-year overall survival rates were 91%, 88%, and 83%, $p = .002$. However, patients treated with dose-escalated BEACOPP were significantly more likely to develop grades 3 and 4 hematologic toxicity. Furthermore, an actuarial risk of secondary leukemia of 2.4% was observed, which was significantly higher than the other two arms.

In an attempt to reduce treatment-related toxicity, the GHSG is investigating the efficacy of modified versions of the BEACOPP regimen. Sieber and colleagues reported results of a pilot study on a 14-day variant of the BEACOPP in patients with bulky stage IIB or stage III to IV disease.[96] Baseline doses of chemotherapy were used, but the cycles were repeated every 2 weeks instead of every 3 weeks. RT was given to 70% of patients, all of whom had initial disease of more than 5 cm. Short-term results at a median follow-up time of 34 months showed a promising FFTF of 90% and survival of 97%. The acute toxicity was comparable to baseline-dose BEACOPP given every 3 weeks; and to date, no cases of secondary leukemia were observed. The ongoing GHSG HD12 trial is exploring another strategy of chemotherapy de-escalation.[76] Patients with bulky stage IIB and stages III to IV disease were randomized to receive eight cycles of dose-escalated BEACOPP with or without RT, versus four cycles of escalated and four cycles of baseline BEACOPP with or without RT. Preliminary results at a median follow-up of 30 months showed no differences between the four arms. In the GHSG HD15 trial, patients with bulky stage II and stage III to IV disease are randomized to receive eight cycles of dose-escalated BEACOPP and six cycles of dose-escalated BEACOPP, versus eight cycles of BEACOPP-14. RT is only administered in selected cases, an approach that will be discussed in the following section. Results of this trial are not yet available. Currently, a randomized multicenter trial comparing four cycles of dose-escalated followed by four cycles of baseline-dose BEACOPP versus eight cycles of ABVD is being conducted in patients with stage III to IV disease (EORTC 20012).

Another approach that has been tested to further improve treatment outcome in patients with advanced-stage disease is to include gemcitabine, an agent that has shown activity against relapsed or refractory Hodgkin's disease, into the treatment program.[97] The regimen of ABVG, substituting dacarbazine with gemcitabine, was tested in a phase I study in patients with advanced-stage disease.[98] However, the trial was closed early because of lower-than-expected progression-free survival and increased pulmonary toxicity. Similarly, the GHSG substituted gemcitabine for etoposide in a trial testing the BAGCOPP regimen (bleomycin, doxorubicin, cyclophosphamide, vincristine, procarbazine, prednisone, gemcitabine).[99] This trial was also terminated prematurely because of an unexpectedly high rate of acute pulmonary toxicity, which was attributed to the concurrent exposure to bleomycin and gemcitabine. The conclusion was therefore made by both groups that this drug combination should be avoided because of the excessive pulmonary toxicity.

The Role of Radiation Therapy in Advanced-Stage Hodgkin's Disease

The rationale for the addition of RT to combination chemotherapy in advanced-stage Hodgkin's disease is based

Table 73-10 Schedule for the Dose-Escalated BEACOPP

		Days													
Drug	Dose (mg/m²)	1	2	3	4	5	6	7	8	9	10	11	12	13	14
Bleomycin	10.0	—	—	—	—	—	—	—	X	—	—	—	—	—	—
Etoposide	100.0	X	X	X	—	—	—	—	—	—	—	—	—	—	—
Doxorubicin	35.0	X	—	—	—	—	—	—	—	—	—	—	—	—	—
Cyclophosphamide	1200.0	X	—	—	—	—	—	—	—	—	—	—	—	—	—
Vincristine	1.4	—	—	—	—	—	—	—	X	—	—	—	—	—	—
Procarbazine	100.0	X	X	X	X	X	X	X	—	—	—	—	—	—	—
Prednisone	40.0	X	X	X	X	X	X	X	X	X	X	X	X	X	X

The regimen is repeated on day 22 for a total of eight cycles; filgrastim from day 8 of each cycle until the leukocyte count returned to normal; radiation therapy given for bulky disease of >5 cm.

on the patterns of failure after chemotherapy, in which the majority of relapses are at the site of initial disease.[100,101] A number of randomized trials have been performed addressing the role of consolidative RT after chemotherapy in advanced-stage Hodgkin's disease.[102-107] The International Database on Hodgkin's Disease Overview Study Group conducted a meta-analysis comparing combined-modality therapy with chemotherapy alone.[108] Eight trials of *additional design* evaluated the benefit of additional RT after the same chemotherapy. The results showed a significant improvement in tumor control rate of 11% with the addition of RT ($p = .0001$), but no survival advantage was demonstrated. The benefit of RT was more pronounced in patients with stage I to III disease, mediastinal involvement, NS, or LP histology. Eight trials of *parallel design* compared combined-modality therapy versus substituting RT with further chemotherapy; and a significant survival benefit of 8% with additional chemotherapy was shown ($p = .045$), suggesting that RT cannot replace inadequate chemotherapy. The results of this study must be interpreted with caution because of inherent problems associated with a meta-analysis. It combines trials with varying patient populations (age, presence or absence of specific risk factors), randomization criteria (upfront or only after a complete response), protocol adherence, types of chemotherapy, and RT fields and dose.

A closer examination of individual trials may provide helpful information especially on subset of patients who may benefit from the addition of RT. Summarized in Table 73-11 are some of the more recent randomized studies comparing chemotherapy with or without RT in advanced-stage Hodgkin's disease.[102-107] Several of the trials showed a DFS benefit with the addition of RT, whereas most do not show a survival benefit. The previously described study from Tata Memorial Hospital, which included patients of all stages, is the only study that showed a significant survival benefit of combined-modality therapy over chemotherapy alone.[83] On subgroup analysis, the benefit was more pronounced for patients with advanced-stage disease. The 8-year overall survival for patients with stage III to IV disease was 80% in the chemotherapy-alone arm versus 100% in the combined-modality arm (p = .006). Other subgroups that appeared to especially benefit from RT in this trial included patients with B symptoms and patients' age less than 15.

In the randomized trial conducted by Southwest Oncology Group (SWOG),[102] patients who achieved a complete remission were randomized to 20 Gy of RT to sites of initial disease versus no further treatment. Although no differences in relapse-free and overall survival were detected for the overall group, patients with nodular sclerosis histology or bulky disease (defined as >6 cm), or both, had significant relapse-free survival benefit with the addition of RT. The 5-year relapse-free survival for patients with nodular sclerosis histology randomized to RT was 77% compared with 56% for those randomized to no further treatment ($p = .01$). For patients with bulky disease and nodular sclerosis histology, the 5-year remission duration estimates with and without RT were 76% and 46%, respectively ($p = .006$).

In the EORTC trial, as in the SWOG study, only patients who had a complete response were randomized to receive either RT or no further treatment.[107] The authors also separately reported results of the 250 patients with a partial response who all went on to receive 30 Gy of consolidative RT with or without additional boost. The 5-year relapse-free survival rates were 79% and 87%, respectively, which were comparable to the treatment results of patients who had a complete response, leading to the conclusion that patients with a partial response after chemotherapy may benefit from RT. In this study at a median follow-up of 79 months, second malignancy data, mostly acute leukemia, was also reported. The 5-year cumulative risk of second malignancy was significantly higher in the 172 patients randomized to RT than the 161 patients randomized to no RT (7.8% and 4.0%, $p = 0.05$). However, among the 250 patients with a partial response who all received RT to a higher dose compared to the randomized patients, the 5-year cumulative risk of second malignancy was only 3.2%; and the reason for the discrepancy is not entirely clear. Finally, longer follow-up time is needed to determine the solid tumor risk.

As previously described, one of the study questions of the GHSG HD12 study is the role of RT in advanced-stage Hodgkin's disease.[76] Preliminary results showed no difference in treatment outcome with or without RT after either eight cycles of dose-escalated BEACOPP or four cycles of escalated and four cycles of baseline BEACOPP at a median follow-up of 30 months. In the GHSG HD15 trial described earlier, comparing eight cycles of dose-escalated BEACOPP and six cycles of dose-escalated BEACOPP, versus eight cycles of BEACOPP-14, patients with a complete response or with residual disease of less than 2.5 cm do not receive RT. Patients with residual disease of 2.5 cm or greater undergo PET scanning; and if positive, 30Gy of IFRT is given. Using these criteria, approximately 10% of patients are receiving RT on this trial. Results of this study, when available, will provide information on the usefulness of functional imaging postchemotherapy in guiding the decision on consolidative RT.

Optimal Radiation Field Size and Dose

Limited data are available on the appropriate radiation treatment field and optimal dose after chemotherapy in advanced-stage Hodgkin's disease. In many of the trials, the radiation field encompassed at least all initially involved sites. For instance, in the EORTC trial, the protocol mandated that both the spleen and the paraaortic nodes be included in the treatment field even if only one of the sites was involved.[107] Patients also received low-dose whole-lung or whole-liver irradiation if disease were initially present at these sites. Although referred to as *involved field,* patients can be treated to a large volume because of their disease extent. Other groups have restricted the radiation treatment field to initially bulky sites. In both the Stanford V and BEACOPP regimens, only sites that were initially 5 cm or greater were included in the radiation field.[92,95] Whether it is necessary to include all initially involved sites is not clear, and the optimal field size likely depends on the effectiveness of the systemic therapy in eradicating small volumes of disease.

The radiation dose employed in various trials on advanced-stage Hodgkin's disease also varied. Randomized data on the optimal dose specifically on patients with advanced-stage disease are unavailable. The GHSG combined data from two of the randomized trials on patients with stages I to III disease, with or without bulk, and found no differences in FFTF and overall survival between 20 Gy, 30 Gy, and 40 Gy of consolidative RT.[104] Early results from the GHSG HD11, which included intermediate-stage patients, also showed no differences between 20Gy and 30Gy of RT after either BEACOPP or ABVD.[77]

Recommendation on Treatment of Advanced-Stage Hodgkin's Disease

Presently, ABVD remains the regimen with the most reliable long-term results, and six to eight cycles of ABVD is still considered by most as the standard therapy for advanced-stage

Table 73-11 Randomized Trials Comparing Combined-Modality Therapy and Chemotherapy Alone in Advanced-Stage Hodgkin's Disease

Institution	Number	Patient Population	Treatment Arms	Median Follow-up	RESULTS *Combined-Modality Therapy*	*Chemotherapy Alone*
SWOG[102]	278	Stage III-IV	MOP-BAP × 6; If CR → 20 Gy RT / No RT	8 y	5-yRFS: 74% 5-y OS: 86%	66% ($p > .2$) 79% ($p > .2$)
GHSG [103]	288	Stage III-IV	COPP/ABVD × 6; If CR → 20 Gy RT / COPP/ABVD × 2		5-y RFS: 76% 5-y OS: 92%	79% (p = ns) 96% (p = ns)
GATLA[106]	151	Stage III-IV	CVPP × 3 → CVPP × 3 (total 6) / 30 Gy RT CVPP × 3	7 y	7-y FFS: 45% 7-y OS: 71%	21% ($p = .0016$) 58 ($p = .15$)
GELA[105]	559	Stage IIB-IV	MOPP/ABV × 6 → STNI / MOPP/ABV × 2 ABVPP × 6, if CR ≥ 75% PR → STNI / ABVPP × 2	48 m	MOPP/ABV + RT: 5-y DFS: 82% ABVPP + RT 5-y DFS: 75% MOPP/ABV + RT: 5-y OS: 88% ABVPP + RT: 5-y OS: 78%	MOPP/ABV alone 80% ABVPP alone 68% MOPP/ABV alone 85% ABVPP alone 94%
EORTC[107]	421 (333 randomized)	Stage III-IV (excluded stage IIIAs)	MOPP-ABV × 6-8; If CR → 24 Gy RT / No RT; If PR → 30 Gy RT	79 m	5-y EFS: 84% 5-y OS: 79% If PR: 5-y EFS: 79% 5-y OS: 87%	91% ($p = .35$) 85% ($p = .07$)
GHSG[76]	1396	Bulky Stage II, Stage III-IV	esc.BEA × 8 → RT to bulky sites / No RT esc.BEA × 4/BE × 4 → RT to bulky sites / No RT	30 m	No difference in FFTF and OS, no arm comparison provided	

ABVD, Adriamycin (doxorubicin), bleomycin, vinblastine, and dacarbazine; ABVPP, doxorubicin, bleomycin, vinblastine, procarbazine, and prednisone; BEA, bleomycin, etoposide, Adriamycin (doxorubicin); COPP, cyclophosphamide, vincristine, procarbazine, and prednisone; CR, complete response; CVPP, cyclophosphamide, vinblastine, procarbazine, and prednisone; DFS, disease-free survival; EFS, event-free survival; EORTC, European Organization for Research and Treatment of Cancer; FFTF, freedom-from-treatment failure; GATLA, Grupo Argentino de Tratamiento de Leucemia Aguda; GELA, Groupe d'Etude des Lymphomes de l'Adulte; GHSG, German Hodgkin Study Group; m, month; MOPP, mechlorethamine, vincristine, procarbazine, and prednisone; OS, overall survival; PR, partial response; RFS, relapse-free survival; RT, radiation therapy; STNI, subtotal nodal irradiation; SWOG, Southwest Oncology Group; y, year.

Hodgkin's disease. The other promising regimens, Stanford V and variants of BEACOPP, are currently being compared against ABVD in large multicenter trials conducted in North America (ECOG 2496) and Europe (EORTC 20012), respectively.

Available data do not support the routine addition of RT after chemotherapy in patients with advanced-stage disease. However, in selected case scenarios, including initial bulky disease or lack of complete response to chemotherapy, RT should be considered. Although no randomized data exist that directly address the appropriate volume of irradiation, based on the known patterns of relapse of the disease, a treatment field encompassing all initially involved sites is logical, and doses of as low as 20 Gy may be adequate. However, in treatment programs with more dose-intense or dose-dense chemotherapeutic regimens, the radiation fields have been limited to initial bulky sites, which did not appear to compromise disease control. In this setting of more restricted radiation fields, higher doses of 30-36 Gy have been employed.[92,95]

PRIMARY TREATMENT FOR NODULAR LYMPHOCYTE PREDOMINANT HODGKIN'S DISEASE

In the REAL and WHO classification systems, NLPHD is classified as a distinct entity based on morphologic and immunophenotypical features.[40,41] Clinically, it is characterized by a male predominance; older age at diagnosis of 30 to 50 years; peripheral nodal presentation seldom with mediastinal, liver, spleen, or bone marrow involvement; predominantly early-stage disease; an indolent clinical course; and late, multiple relapses.[44,109-111] Because of its rarity, constituting only approximately 5% of all cases of Hodgkin's disease, no clear standard therapy for this form of the disease has been established. Management recommendations include watch and wait,[110] surgery alone,[112] RT with or without chemotherapy,[109-111,113] and immunotherapy.[114] Observations have been made that ABVD may not be as effective in patients with NLPHD, and alkylating agent–containing regimens may be a better choice when chemotherapy is indicated.[109] Because

NLPHD is rarely fatal, and the main causes of death in these patients are treatment-related rather than disease-related,[109,110] it is sensible to choose a modality with well-established effectiveness while limiting the overall treatment exposure of these patients. In patients with early-stage NLPHD, to avoid exposure to alkylating agents, one reasonable treatment option is regional-field radiation therapy. In patients with neck or axillary involvement, the mediastinum, which is rarely involved, can be blocked, thereby avoiding exposure of the lungs and heart to radiation. Relapses occur in 20% to 25% of patients, but patients tend to remain responsive to further therapy despite multiple relapses.[110] Because of the small number of available cases, collaborative efforts among multiple large institutions are essential to provide answers on the optimal treatment for this disease entity.

REFRACTORY/RECURRENT DISEASE

Hodgkin's disease is one of the few malignancies in which patients with relapsed disease still enjoy a reasonable chance of long-term cure. Relapsed disease is defined as disease progression after a complete response to primary treatment, whereas refractory disease refers to progression of disease during primary treatment or biopsy-proven persistence despite primary treatment. The management approach for patients with relapsed or refractory disease depends primarily on the initial treatment exposure.

Recurrent Disease after Radiation Therapy Alone

Table 73-12 summarizes a series reporting on salvage outcome using conventional-dose chemotherapy with or without irradiation on patients with relapsed Hodgkin's disease after initial RT.[115-120] The long-term freedom from additional relapses ranges from 55% to 80%, which compares favorably with patients with newly diagnosed advanced-stage Hodgkin's disease treated with initial chemotherapy. This suggests that prior exposure to RT does not lead to resistance to, or compromise the ability to deliver effective doses of, chemotherapy.

Several prognostic factors have been identified for salvage outcome in patients who relapsed after RT alone. These include age at diagnosis,[116-120] histology,[117,118] extranodal relapse,[119] relapse stage,[116] treatment era,[120] type of systemic salvage regimen,[115] and the addition of RT to the salvage treatment.[117] However, age at diagnosis is the only factor that has consistently shown significant influence on salvage outcome in all studies. This suggests that one of the key contributing factors to the overall inferior prognosis in older patients with newly diagnosed Hodgkin's disease is likely their lower probability of successful salvage after relapse.

Patients treated with RT alone are rarely encountered nowadays for reasons outlined earlier. Although RT is associated with a higher relapse rate than combined-modality therapy, the chance of successful salvage without having to resort to high-dose therapy with stem-cell rescue is excellent in these patients. This is a factor that is worth taking into consideration when deciding on initial treatment for newly diagnosed patients.

Primary Refractory Disease or Recurrent Disease after Chemotherapy

The standard salvage therapy for patients who are refractory, or relapsed after a short initial remission to chemotherapy, is high-dose therapy with autologous bone marrow or stem cell transplantation (SCT). A considerable amount of pilot, phase II, and retrospective data on the use of autologous transplantation in relapsed or refractory Hodgkin's disease show excellent results, with EFS rates ranging from 35% to 60% at 5 years.[121-128] However, the results must be interpreted with caution because of patient selection biases. One key factor that influences outcome is chemosensitivity to second-line cytoreductive chemotherapy prior to the high-dose therapy and transplantation.[122-128] Other factors that have been shown to be of prognostic significance include duration of complete response to initial treatment,[123] extranodal disease,[123,124] constitutional symptoms,[123,125,128] or bulky disease.[122] A study from the University of Nebraska found that the seven-factor prognostic score developed by the International Prognostic Factors Project for advanced-stage Hodgkin's disease was also predictive of outcome of patients with relapsed or refractory Hodgkin's disease who underwent autologous, hematopoietic SCT.[129] Patients with scores of 0 to 1, 2 to 3, or more than 4 had 10-year EFS of 38%, 23%, and 7%, respectively.

Two randomized trials have been conducted comparing high-dose therapy with bone marrow or hematopoietic stem cell rescue versus conventional-dose chemotherapy as salvage for patients with refractory or relapsed Hodgkin's disease after chemotherapy. The British National Lymphoma Investigation group prospectively randomized 40 patients to either high-dose BEAM regimen (carmustine, etoposide, cytarabine, melphalan) followed by autologous bone marrow transplantation or mini-BEAM.[130] The inclusion criteria lacked complete response after MOPP or similar regimen, or relapsed disease either within 1 year, or failure after two or more chemotherapy regimens. At a median follow-up of 34 months, 3-year

Table 73-12 Series on Conventional-Dose Salvage for Relapse after Radiation Therapy Alone

Authors	No.	RFS, FFSR, CSS	OS	Comments
Santoro et al[115]	122	7-y RFS: 81.2%	7-y OS: 80.5%	Doxorubicin-containing salvage regimen
		7-y RFS: 54.3%	7-y OS: 44.4%	MOPP salvage
Roach et al[116]	109	10-y FFSR: 57.0%	10-y OS: 57.0%	
Healey et al[117]	110	10-y FFSR: 58.0%	10-y OS: 62.0%	
Specht et al[118]	681	10-y CSS: 70.0%	10-y OS: 58.0%	Initial PS I-II
Horwich et al[119]	473	10-y CSS: 63.0%	10-y OS: 50.0%	Initial CS I-II
Ng et al[120]	157	10-y FFSR: 58.0%	10-y OS: 46.0%	Initial diagnosis before 1980
		10-y FFSR: 70.0%	10-y OS: 89.0%	Initial diagnosis after 1980

CS, clinical stage; CSS, cause-specific survival; FFSR, freedom from second relapse; MOPP, mechlorethamine, vincristine, procarbazine, and prednisone; OS, overall survival; PS, pathologic stage; RFS, relapse-free survival; y, year.

actuarial EFS of the two arms was 53% and 10%, respectively ($p = .025$) and progression-free survival were 88% and 35%, respectively ($p = .005$), favoring the high-dose therapy arm. The GHSG conducted a similar study comparing high-dose BEAM followed by autologous SCT and dexamethasone with conventional-dose BEAM.[131] Only patients with chemosensitive disease were included in the trial. At a median follow-up of 39 months, the FFTF of the two arms were 55% and 34%, respectively ($p = .019$). Significant survival differences were not detected in either of the two trials, however.

Role of Radiation Therapy before or after High-Dose Therapy

Further relapses after high-dose therapy tend to occur at sites of initial relapsed disease. The role of IFRT given either before or after high-dose therapy has not been addressed prospectively by randomized trials, but two retrospective studies indicated that the addition of RT may contribute to improved outcome, despite the fact that patients who received RT had worse prognostic factors such as bulky disease or chemotherapy refractory disease. In one study from Stanford, subgroups of patients who significantly benefited from IFRT given either before or after the transplantation included patients with relapsed stage I to III disease and patients who did not receive prior RT.[132] In a study from University of Chicago, the use of IFRT in conjunction with high-dose therapy significantly improved local control of all sites of disease.[133] Patients with persistent disease following high-dose therapy had significantly improved progression-free survival (40% versus 12.1%, $p = .04$).

The optimal temporal relationship between RT and high-dose therapy is unclear. In patients with persistent disease after cytoreductive chemotherapy, RT given prior to transplantation can allow further disease debulking. Furthermore, irradiation pretransplantation avoids exposure of newly engrafted stem cells to radiation, which may increase the risk of myelodysplasia and leukemia. This is especially relevant in patients with pelvic disease requiring RT to a large volume of bone marrow. In these patients, stem cell mobilization or bone marrow harvest should be performed before initiation of pelvic irradiation. Delivery of RT prior to transplantation, however, can increase peritransplant morbidity such as pneumonitis and veno-occlusive disease. Also, there is a risk of systemic disease progression during the time of the RT with the delay of the high-dose therapy.

Limited Relapse after Chemotherapy

A small proportion of patients who relapsed after chemotherapy can be successfully salvaged with conventional-dose salvage chemotherapy or RT, or both. A number of series showed that in selected patients with favorable features, a salvage rate as high as 80% can be achieved without exposing patients to high-dose therapy.[134-137] Potential candidates for conventional-dose salvage therapy include patients with initial remission duration of 1 year or longer, limited nodal relapse without extranodal disease, and absence of constitutional symptoms at relapse. In one series of 28 patients with limited nodal relapse after chemotherapy, the combination of salvage chemotherapy and RT yielded significantly superior outcome than RT alone.[136] In patients who received combined-modality salvage therapy, the 7-year freedom from further relapse was 93% and the overall survival was 85%, whereas the corresponding actuarial estimates in patients treated with RT alone were significantly lower at 36% ($p = .002$) and 36% ($p = .03$), respectively.

Given the finite risk of early mortality associated with high-dose therapy and autologous transplantation, and the acute toxicity and long-term risk of myelodysplasia and acute leukemia associated with the procedure,[138] in carefully selected patients with favorable criteria at relapse, salvage with conventional-dose therapy while reserving high-dose therapy with stem cell rescue for subsequent relapses should be strongly considered.

PALLIATION

The prognosis is generally poor in patients with relapsed disease after SCT, or in patients with refractory disease and multiple relapses who are not candidates for high-dose salvage therapy. Weekly low-dose vinblastine provides significant palliation in these patients with a response rate of approximately 60% and prolonged remission is seen in some patients.[139] Gemcitabine is another promising agent that has a response rate of approximately 50% despite multiple courses of prior therapy.[140] Even more encouraging results have been demonstrated when gemcitabine is given in conjunction with other agents. In a trial conducted by the NCIC evaluating the treatment combination consisting of gemcitabine, cisplatin, and dexamethasone administered on an outpatient basis, the regimen was well-tolerated and an overall response rate of 70% was achieved.[97]

RT can also be an effective form of palliation for Hodgkin's disease. Examples include bulky mediastinal disease resulting in respiratory compromise or superior vena cava syndrome, bulky abdominal or pelvic disease causing local obstruction, painful bony lesions, spinal cord compression, and nerve root impingement causing neurologic compromise and pain. Despite refractoriness to chemotherapy, the disease can remain responsive to RT and significant symptom relief can be achieved with modest doses of RT. For patients with a relatively short life expectancy, a more rapid fractionation scheme with larger fraction sizes can be considered. In patients with symptomatic disease in close proximity to prior-radiation treatment fields, recent advances in radiation technology allow the delivery of adequate doses to local sites without exceeding normal tissue tolerance (discussed in the following text).

TECHNIQUES OF IRRADIATION

RT is one of the most effective modalities for the treatment of Hodgkin's disease. However, RT alone using large treatment fields is rarely employed nowadays because of its long-term toxicity and the availability of effective and less toxic combination chemotherapy regimens. Most patients with Hodgkin's disease are now treated with a combined-modality approach, with limitation of the radiation treatment field to an involved field. Currently, the involved field is the minimum radiation field size used for the treatment of early-stage disease, but further limiting the treatment field to the involved lymph node only is currently being investigated. The following section describes radiation fields that have been used in the treatment of Hodgkin's disease.

Mantle Field

The mantle field has been the most frequently used treatment field in RT for Hodgkin's disease. The nodal groups encompassed by a mantle field include the bilateral cervical and supraclavicular, submental, bilateral axillary, mediastinal, and bilateral hilar nodes. An anteroposterior field arrangement with equal weighting is used. The typical superior border is at the level of the superior external auditory meatus with hyperextension of the neck to limit the exit dose from the posterior field. The inferior border is at least 5 cm below the carina to ensure adequate coverage of the subcarinal nodes and the hila. However, the inferior border may need to be lowered in patients with significant inferior extension of disease or pericardial nodal involvement. Careful review of the prechemotherapy staging scans is crucial in accurately determining the appropriate inferior field border, allowing a 2-cm margin below the inferior-most extent of disease. The lateral extent of the treatment field also needs to be extended in the presence of chest wall invasion at presentation, in which case the initial extent of chest wall disease needs to be included in the treatment field. The size of a mantle field can be large, and there can be significant dose inhomogeneity because of varying separation of a patient's upper body and the irregularly contoured lung blocks that affect the scatter doses to different areas within the field.[141] Simple ways used to reduce hot spots in the neck and axillary region and to avoid underdosing of the lower mediastinum include the use of extended source-to-surface distance, compensators, or *field-within-field* technique of shrinking the field after a specific number of monitor units have been delivered for each fraction of treatment. Shown in Figure 73-1 is an example of using the field-within-field technique in a patient treated to the bilateral neck, mediastinum, and ipsilateral axilla.

Most patients do not have involvement of all the sites covered by a full mantle field and modifications may be made based on the initial extent of disease for an involved-field design. For example, the axilla can be excluded from the treatment field in patients without axillary involvement. This allows sparing of a considerable amount of breast tissue and is of special relevance in young women who are at increased risk for breast cancer after RT for Hodgkin's disease. Also, although the cervical and supraclavicular nodes are part of a single nodal group, in patients with clearly documented limitation of disease to the supraclavicular region by nuclear imaging studies, reducing the superior border of the radiation field to the level of larynx can be considered. This may help limit the degree of acute oropharyngeal mucosal toxicity and salivary gland dysfunction.

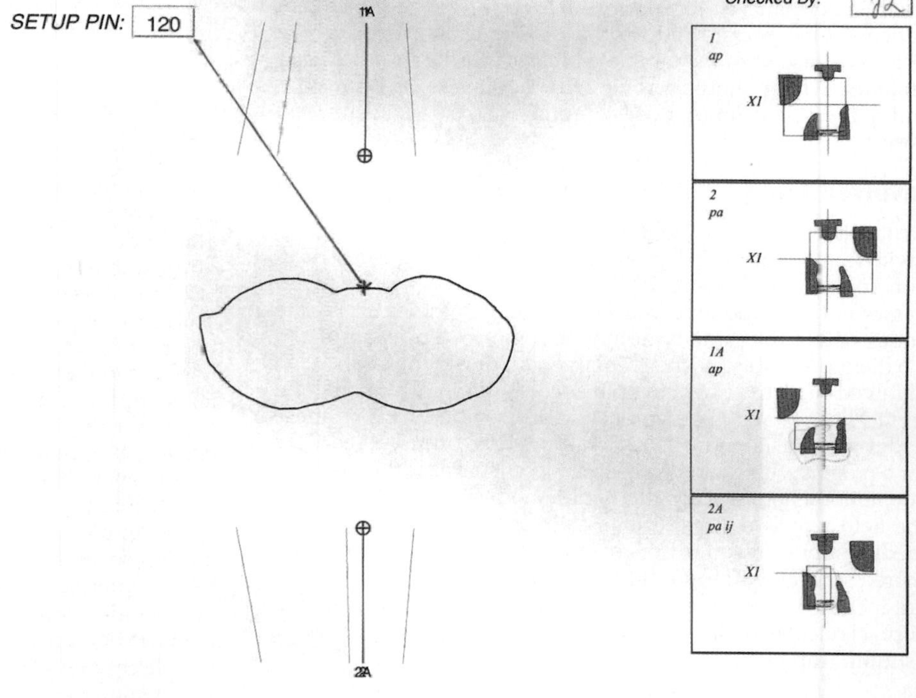
Set-Up Diagram

Longwood Radiation Oncology Center

Name: [redacted] **Therapy Number:** A047301 *Planned By:* jkt *Checked By:* JL

SETUP PIN: 120

Tumor dose per session: *180.0 cGy* *Patient Supine* *Machine: BWH 6Ex*

Date: *11-24-2004 11:34 AM* *Single Course* *Photon Energy: 6 MV*

	Name	MV	X1	X2	Y1	Y2	X x Y	Wdg	Blk	G	C	T	MU
1	ap	6	18.9	7.5	13.0	11.0	**26.4 x 24.0**	None	crbd	0	0	0	171
1A	ap ij	6	13.0	7.5	13.0	-2.0	**20.5 x 11.0**	None	crbd	0	0	0	19
2	pa	6	7.5	18.9	13.0	11.0	**26.4 x 24.0**	None	crbd	180	0	0	158
2A	pa ij	6	7.5	2.5	13.0	3.0	**10.0 x 16.0**	None	crbd	180	0	0	15

Figure 73-1 Field-within-field technique to improve dose homogeneity. Set-up diagram of a patient with bilateral neck, right axillary, and mediastinal involvement. The anterior field was treated to 171 MU, after which the IJs were closed to a more restricted field off the areas of hotspots for the remaining 19 MU; the posterior field was treated to 158 MU, after which the IJs were closed to a more restricted field for the remaining 15 MU. Graphic plan of the coronal view shows the isodose distribution using this technique. IJ, independent jaw; MU, monitor units.

Paraaortic (Parasplenic) Field

The paraaortic field with or without the spleen was, in the past, frequently given along with the mantle field as part of subtotal nodal irradiation. Matching techniques to avoid overlap between the two treatment fields have been well-described,[142] but they are more of historical interest because of the rare use of subtotal nodal irradiation nowadays. The field encompasses the entire paraaortic nodal chain and extends down to the level of the L4 vertebral body. The superior border is typically matched to the inferior border of the mantle field. The spleen or the splenic pedicle, depending on whether or not a staging laparotomy has been performed, is also included.

Inverted-Y Field

The inverted-Y field is mostly used in patients with infradiaphragmatic presentation, which accounts for less than 10% of Hodgkin's disease. Nodal groups included in this treatment field are the paraaortic, bilateral iliac, and bilateral inguinal-femoral nodes. In women of childbearing age who wish to preserve fertility, the ovaries can be transposed to an extrapelvic site outside of the radiation field, either laterally or medially behind the uterus under the central block. The effectiveness of oophoropexy in preserving the ovarian function of women undergoing pelvic irradiation, however, is controversial, and varying success rates have been reported.[143-145] In men receiving irradiation to the iliac and inguinal femoral nodal region, the testes may receive 3% of the prescribed dose from the primary beam through the blocks, which are of a thickness calculated to reduce the transmitted beam by 5 half-values. Along with the scatter dose, the dose received by the testes may result in permanent azoospermia in a significant proportion of patients. One way to reduce the primary-beam dose to the testes is to use both the template blocks and the multileaf collimators, which should provide 10 half-layers of protection and reduce the primary dose component to 0.01% of the total dose.

Involved Field

To facilitate radiation field design, the lymphatic system is divided into lymph node regions, based on the Rye classification for staging (Figure 73-2).[146] An involved field encompasses not only the involved nodes but also the other lymph nodes within the same lymph node region.[147] For example, in a patient presenting with an enlarged cervical lymph node, an involved-field treatment would include the entire ipsilateral cervical chain and the supraclavicular region, because these nodes are considered one region. Similarly, an involved field for a patient with groin disease would encompass the inguinal and femoral nodes. In a patient with mediastinal involvement, the field would cover the mediastinal, hilar, subcarinal, and medial supraclavicular nodes. Although the hilar nodes are scored separately traditionally, the hilar and subcarinal nodes are included in the mediastinal field. In addition, the medial supraclavicular nodes are included to cover the upper mediastinum (top of T1).

Utility of New Technology in Radiation Therapy

There have been significant advances in radiation planning and treatment delivery in recent years, including the use of PET-CT fusion to more accurately delineate the target volume, and the use of intensity-modulated radiation therapy (IMRT) to allow more conformal therapy. These techniques are increasingly adopted in the radiation treatment of a number of disease sites. However, they are currently not routinely incorporated into the treatment of patients with Hodgkin's disease for various reasons. First, most patients with Hodgkin's disease receive combined-modality therapy, and the radiation treatment field is based on the postchemotherapy volume. Most patients do not have FDG-avid disease at the end of the chemotherapy prior to the RT. Moreover, as previously described, an involved field includes an entire nodal group, rather than the lymph node that was initially FDG avid. Also, the doses used in the treatment of Hodgkin's disease rarely exceed 36 to 40 Gy, and as such, highly conformal therapy to spare normal tissue may not be as essential. Finally, there is the theoretical concern that with IMRT and multiple fields approach, the low doses of radiation to a large volume of normal tissue may increase the long-term second malignancy risk in these young patients.

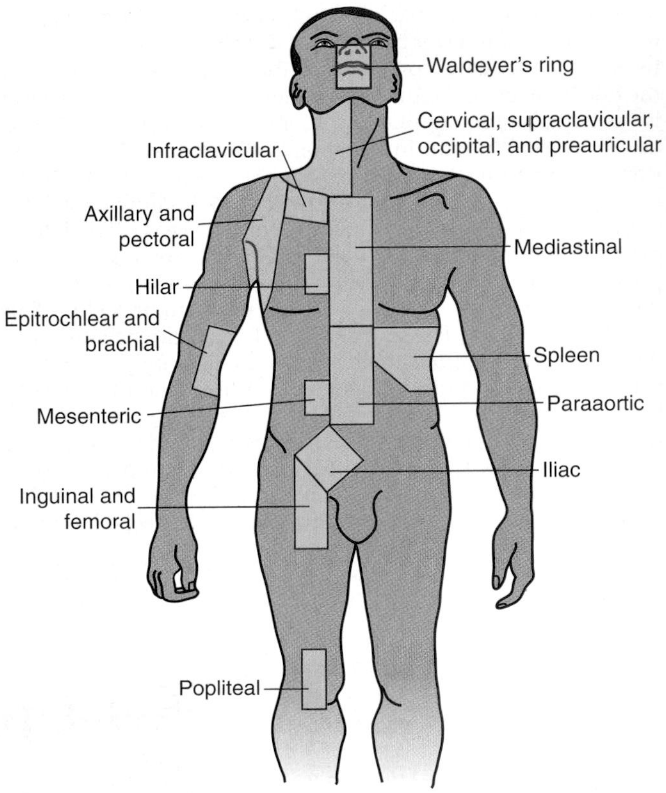

Figure 73-2 The anatomic definitions of separate lymph node regions based on the Rye classification for staging.

However, there are selected case scenarios in which these new techniques may be useful in Hodgkin's disease RT. One example is in patients with significant lateral extension of disease along the chest wall. Treatment with a traditional anteroposterior/posteroanterior (AP/PA) approach will include a large amount of lung in the treatment field. The use of IMRT conforming to the irregular shape of the chest wall disease encasing the lungs may be of value in this situation. Another example is in patients with recurrent disease in close proximity to a previously treated site, in which further radiation treatment may exceed tolerance of nearby normal structure. Shown in Figure 73-3 is the graphic plan of a patient who had previously received bilateral neck irradiation and now had in-field recurrence in the paracervical spinal region. Further RT was limited by the cord tolerance, but with IMRT an adequate dose was delivered to the area of recurrent disease while limiting the spinal cord dose to less than 10 Gy. In both scenarios, the use of PET-CT fusion in the planning

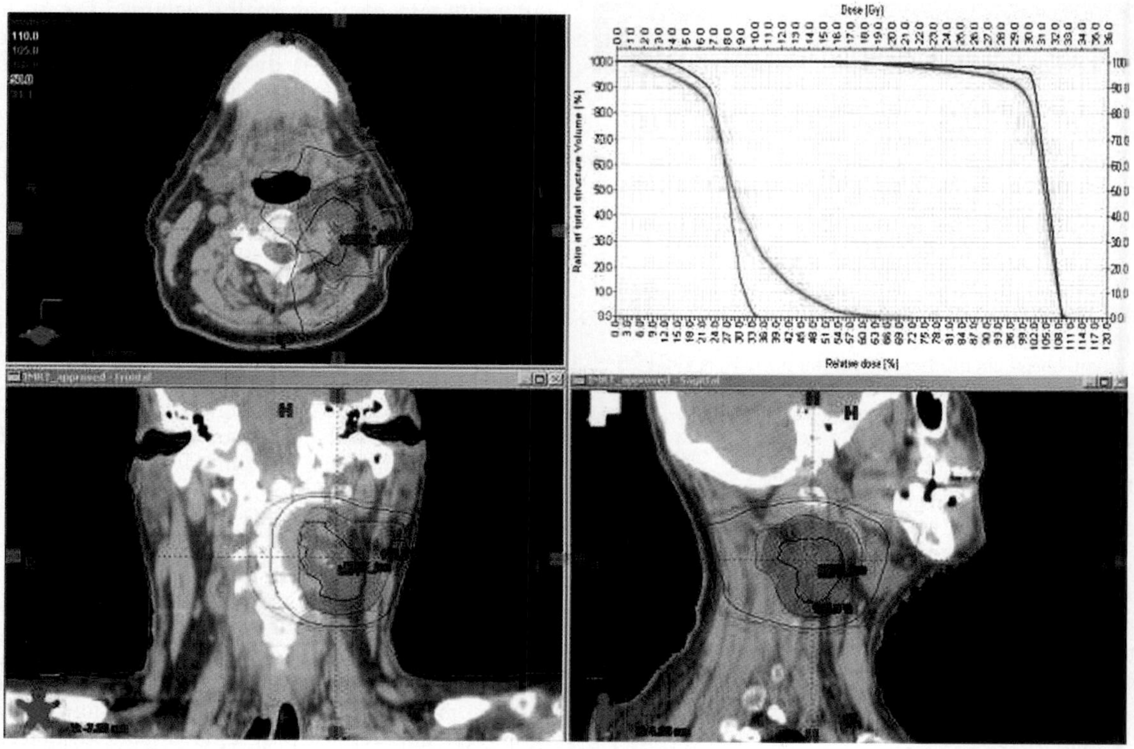

Figure 73-3 Graphic plan and DVH of retreatment to the paracervical spine region using IMRT technique. The sparing of the spinal cord is shown in the graphic plan of the axial cut. The spinal cord DVH (*brown*) shows that the maximum cord dose is limited to 10 Gy, whereas the target volume received is around 30 Gy. DVH, dose-volume histogram; IMRT, intensity-modulated radiation therapy.

process can further help in accurately determining the target. With highly conformal therapy, applying novel techniques to improve immobilization and reproducibility of treatment setup are crucial. Thermoplastic immobilization devices can be useful for treatment to the head and neck region and the upper mediastinum. Respiratory gating techniques may also be valuable, especially when treating sites that are subject to the effect of diaphragmatic motion, such as pericardial nodes, spleen, or stomach.

TREATMENT ALGORITHM, CHALLENGES, AND FUTURE DIRECTIONS

Treatment Algorithm

The treatment algorithm for patients with early- and advanced-stage Hodgkin's disease is outlined in Table 73-13 and Table 73-14, respectively. For patients with unfavorable-prognosis disease or advanced-stage disease, the challenge remains further improving the cure of Hodgkin's disease. More effective multiagent chemotherapy regimens are being developed and tested in clinical trials. In addition to traditional chemotherapy, other promising approaches include the use of targeted immunotherapy, which may serve as an adjunct to chemotherapy,[114,148,149] and myeloablative or nonmyeloablative allogeneic SCT in which the graft-versus-Hodgkin's lymphoma effect may provide therapeutic benefits in patients with chemotherapy refractory disease.[150,151] In patients with early-stage disease without unfavorable features, cure rates of more than 90% have been achieved. The key challenge in the management of these patients is to identify ways to limit late effects of Hodgkin's disease therapy; as multiple studies have demonstrated over time, there is a significantly increased risk of mortality from causes other than Hodgkin's disease, with second malignancies and cardiac disease being the two leading problems.

Table 73-13 Treatment Algorithm for Patients with Early-Stage Hodgkin's Disease

CLASSICAL HODGKIN'S DISEASE, FAVORABLE PROGNOSIS
Four cycles of ABVD (restaging PET/CT scan after two to three cycles and at the end of chemotherapy)
Involved-field radiation therapy 3 to 4 weeks postchemotherapy to 30 Gy to 36 Gy
CLASSICAL HODGKIN'S DISEASE, UNFAVORABLE PROGNOSIS
Six cycles of ABVD (restaging PET/CT after 3 cycles and at the end of chemotherapy)
IFRT 3 to 4 weeks postchemotherapy to 30 Gy to 36 Gy
NODULAR LYMPHOCYTE PREDOMINANT HODGKIN'S DISEASE
Regional-field radiation therapy alone to 30 Gy to 36 Gy

ABVD, Adriamycin (doxorubicin), bleomycin, vinblastine, and dacarbazine; CT, computed tomography; IFRT, involved-field radiation therapy; PET, positron emission tomography.

Second Malignancies

Second malignancy after Hodgkin's disease was first recognized as a problem in the early 1970s. Multiple early studies reported an increased risk of acute leukemia, which has a shorter latency, is associated with the use of alkylating

Table 73-14 Treatment Algorithm for Patients with Advanced-Stage Hodgkin's Disease

CLASSICAL HODGKIN'S DISEASE
Six cycles of ABVD (restaging PET/CT after three cycles and at the end of chemotherapy)
Other regimens, depending on institutional experience, include Stanford V and dose-escalated BEACOPP
Consolidative radiation therapy to 30 to 36 Gy to sites of initial bulky disease (>5 cm) or without complete response to chemotherapy
NODULAR LYMPHOCYTE PREDOMINANT HODGKIN'S DISEASE
Alkylating agent–based chemotherapy regimen, such as ChlVPP

ABVD, Adriamycin (doxorubicin), bleomycin, vinblastine, and dacarbazine; BEACOPP, bleomycin, etoposide, doxorubicin, cyclophosphamide, vincristine, procarbazine, and prednisone; ChlVPP, chlorambucil, vinblastine, procarbazine, and prednisolone; CT, computed tomography; PET, positron emission tomography.

chemotherapy, and has an extremely poor prognosis. In more recent years, solid tumors, often taking 15 or more years to develop, have emerged as the most significant subtype of second malignancy, accounting for up to 75% to 85% of cases.[152-155] Increasing attention is being directed to the more common individual tumor types, including lung cancer[156] and breast cancer.[159-161]

Radiation exposure has clearly been identified as a risk factor for solid tumors after Hodgkin's disease, with most solid tumors arising either within or at the edges of prior radiation fields. In addition, results of several retrospective studies suggested that smaller field size is associated with a lower risk.[154,162,163] Several recent case-control studies carefully looked at the dose-response relationship in the development of breast cancer and lung cancer,[161,164,165] all of which showed a significant trend of increasing risk of tumor development with increasing radiation dose.

The contribution of chemotherapy alone to the risk of solid tumor is more difficult to ascertain because in most available studies, the number of patients treated with chemotherapy alone was too low to allow for any meaningful conclusions. Two studies have shown that chemotherapy alone, using predominantly alkylating agent–based chemotherapy, was associated with a significantly increased risk of lung cancer.[152,156,158] However, studies on breast cancer after Hodgkin's disease have demonstrated a significant decreased risk of breast cancer after alkylating chemotherapy exposure,[161,164] which was attributed to the protective effect of chemotherapy-induced premature menopause against breast cancer development.

Other nontreatment-related risk factors that have been identified include younger age at RT for subsequent breast cancer development,[152-154,166] as well as tobacco use, which has a multiplicative effect on lung cancer risk with Hodgkin's disease therapy exposure.[157,158,165]

These data on second-malignancy risks and risk factors highlight the importance of current efforts to reduce treatment, especially in patients with early-stage, favorable-prognosis Hodgkin's disease. The results also have important implications for follow-up, early-detection, and cancer prevention strategies in these patients.

Cardiovascular Disease

A wide spectrum of radiation-induced cardiovascular disease has been identified, including pericardial disease, coronary artery disease, cardiomyopathy, valvular disease, arrhythmia, and autonomic dysfunction.[167-171] Among these cardiac abnormalities, coronary artery disease is the major contributor to the excess risk of cardiac mortality, accounting for two thirds of all cases of fatal cardiac events in survivors of Hodgkin's disease. Multiple studies show an association between mediastinal irradiation and risk of fatal cardiovascular complications, predominantly in the form of acute myocardial infarctions.[170-172] Significant dose-response relationships have also been demonstrated. In addition, emerging data are available showing the contribution of traditional cardiac risk factors to the risk of cardiac disease after Hodgkin's disease.[173,174] Because of the increased risk of cardiac morbidity and mortality with time after Hodgkin's disease therapy, investigators have explored the role of cardiac screening in long-term survivors of Hodgkin's disease.[175] However, the specific types of tests to be performed, timing, and frequency are unclear and must be refined and tailored to individual patients.

Strategies to Reduce Late Effects and Future Directions

Strategies include (1) treatment reduction, which is currently being investigated by ongoing prospective trials; (2) continued long-term follow-up of treated patients to better understand the patterns, temporal trend, and risk factors for the late effects; and (3) development of prevention, early-detection, and early-intervention programs for patients determined to be at high risk for late complications. Finally, the pathogenesis and biology of Hodgkin's disease are currently being actively explored.[32,33,37] Further understanding the molecular mechanism in the development of Hodgkin's disease may provide new targets in the treatment of the disease. In addition to potentially improving cure rate, targeted therapy may reduce the need to use traditional cytotoxic therapy, thereby reducing treatment-related late complications.

REFERENCES

1. Hodgkin T: On some morbid experiences of the absorbent glands and spleen. Med Chir Trans 17:69-97, 1832.
2. Gilbert R: Radiotherapy in Hodgkin's disease (malignant granulomatosis); anatomic and clinical foundations; governing principles, results. Am J Roentgenol 41:198-241, 1939.
3. Peters M: A study in survivals in Hodgkin's disease treated radiologically. Am J Roentgenol 63:299-311, 1950.
4. DeVita V, Serpick A, Carbone P: Combination chemotherapy in the treatment of advanced Hodgkin's disease. Ann Intern Med 73:881-895, 1970.
5. Gloeckler Ries LA, Reichman ME, Lewis DR, et al: Cancer survival and incidence from the Surveillance, Epidemiology, and End Results (SEER) program. Oncologist 8:541-552, 2003.
6. Macmahon B: Epidemiological evidence of the nature of Hodgkin's disease. Cancer 10:1045-1054, 1957.
7. Grufferman S, Delzell E: Epidemiology of Hodgkin's disease. Epidemiol Rev 6:76-106, 1984.
8. Serraino D, Franceschi S, Talamini R, et al: Socio-economic indicators, infectious diseases and Hodgkin's disease. Int J Cancer 47:352-357, 1991.
9. Westergaard T, Melbye M, Pedersen JB, et al: Birth order, sibship size and risk of Hodgkin's disease in children and young adults: A population-based study of 31 million person-years. Int J Cancer 72:977-981, 1997.
10. Chang ET, Zheng T, Weir EG, et al: Childhood social environment and Hodgkin's lymphoma: New findings from a population-based case-control study. Cancer Epidemiol Biomarkers Prev 13:1361-1370, 2004.
11. Miller RW, Beebe GW: Infectious mononucleosis and the empirical risk of cancer. J Natl Cancer Inst 50:315-321, 1973.

12. Kvale G, Hoiby EA, Pedersen E: Hodgkin's disease in patients with previous infectious mononucleosis. Int J Cancer 23:593-597, 1979.
13. Mueller N, Evans A, Harris NL, et al: Hodgkin's disease and Epstein-Barr virus. Altered antibody pattern before diagnosis. N Engl J Med 320:689-695, 1989.
14. Mueller N, Mohar A, Evans A, et al: Epstein-Barr virus antibody patterns preceding the diagnosis of non-Hodgkin's lymphoma. Int J Cancer 49:387-393, 1991.
15. Weiss LM, Movahed LA, Warnke RA, et al: Detection of Epstein-Barr viral genomes in Reed-Sternberg cells of Hodgkin's disease. N Engl J Med 320:502-506, 1989.
16. Wu TC, Mann RB, Charache P, et al: Detection of EBV gene expression in Reed-Sternberg cells of Hodgkin's disease. Int J Cancer 46:801-804, 1990.
17. Glaser SL, Lin RJ, Stewart SL, et al: Epstein-Barr virus-associated Hodgkin's disease: Epidemiologic characteristics in international data. Int J Cancer 70:375-382, 1997.
18. Grufferman S, Cole P, Smith PG, et al: Hodgkin's disease in siblings. N Engl J Med 296:248-250, 1977.
19. Grufferman S, Barton JW III, Eby NL: Increased sex concordance of sibling pairs with Behçet's disease, Hodgkin's disease, multiple sclerosis, and sarcoidosis. Am J Epidemiol 126:365-369, 1987.
20. Mack TM, Cozen W, Shibata DK, et al: Concordance for Hodgkin's disease in identical twins suggesting genetic susceptibility to the young-adult form of the disease. N Engl J Med 332:413-418, 1995.
21. Cozen W, Gill PS, Ingles SA, et al: IL-6 levels and genotype are associated with risk of young adult Hodgkin lymphoma. Blood 103:3216-3221, 2004.
22. Hors J, Dausset J: HLA and susceptibility to Hodgkin's disease. Immunol Rev 70:167-192, 1983.
23. Oza AM, Tonks S, Lim J, et al: A clinical and epidemiological study of human leukocyte antigen-DPB alleles in Hodgkin's disease. Cancer Res 54:5101-5105, 1994.
24. Staratschek-Jox A, Shugart YY, Strom SS, et al: Genetic susceptibility to Hodgkin's lymphoma and to secondary cancer: Workshop report. Ann Oncol 13(Suppl 1):30-33, 2002.
25. Kanzler H, Kuppers R, Hansmann ML, et al: Hodgkin and Reed-Sternberg cells in Hodgkin's disease represent the outgrowth of a dominant tumor clone derived from (crippled) germinal center B cells. J Exp Med 184:1495-1505, 1996.
26. Marafioti T, Hummel M, Foss HD, et al: Hodgkin and Reed-Sternberg cells represent an expansion of a single clone originating from a germinal center B-cell with functional immunoglobulin gene rearrangements but defective immunoglobulin transcription. Blood 95:1443-1450, 2000.
27. Rajewsky K, Kanzler H, Hansmann ML, et al: Normal and malignant B-cell development with special reference to Hodgkin's disease. Ann Oncol 8(Suppl 2):79-81, 1997.
28. Stein H, Marafioti T, Foss HD, et al: Down-regulation of BOB.1/OBF.1 and Oct2 in classical Hodgkin disease but not in lymphocyte predominant Hodgkin disease correlates with immunoglobulin transcription. Blood 97:496-501, 2001.
29. Theil J, Laumen H, Marafioti T, et al: Defective octamer-dependent transcription is responsible for silenced immunoglobulin transcription in Reed-Sternberg cells. Blood 97:3191-3196, 2001.
30. Ushmorov A, Ritz O, Hummel M, et al: Epigenetic silencing of the immunoglobulin heavy chain gene in classical Hodgkin lymphoma-derived cell lines contributes to the loss of immunoglobulin expression. Blood 104:3326-3334, 2004.
31. Bargou RC, Leng C, Krappmann D, et al: High-level nuclear NF-κB and Oct-2 is a common feature of cultured Hodgkin/Reed-Sternberg cells. Blood 87:4340-4347, 1996.
32. Bargou RC, Emmerich F, Krappmann D, et al: Constitutive nuclear factor-κB-RelA activation is required for proliferation and survival of Hodgkin's disease tumor cells. J Clin Invest 100:2961-2969, 1997.
33. Hinz M, Loser P, Mathas S, et al: Constitutive NF-κB maintains high expression of a characteristic gene network, including CD40, CD86, and a set of antiapoptotic genes in Hodgkin/Reed-Sternberg cells. Blood 97:2798-2807, 2001.
34. Hinz M, Lemke P, Anagnostopoulos I, et al: Nuclear factor κB-dependent gene expression profiling of Hodgkin's disease tumor cells, pathogenetic significance, and link to constitutive signal transducer and activator of transcription 5a activity. J Exp Med 196:605-617, 2002.
35. Emmerich F, Theurich S, Hummel M, et al: Inactivating I κB ε mutations in Hodgkin/Reed-Sternberg cells. J Pathol 201(3):413-420, 2003.
36. Diehl V, Stein H, Hummel M, et al: Hodgkin's lymphoma: Biology and treatment strategies for primary, refractory, and relapsed disease. Am Soc Hematol Educ Program 225-247, 2003.
37. Mathas S, Lietz A, Anagnostopoulos I, et al: c-FLIP mediates resistance of Hodgkin/Reed-Sternberg cells to death receptor-induced apoptosis. J Exp Med 199:1041-1052, 2004.
38. Chang ET, Zheng T, Weir EG, et al: Aspirin and the risk of Hodgkin's lymphoma in a population-based case-control study. J Natl Cancer Inst 96:305-315, 2004.
39. Lukes RJ, Craver LF, Hall TC, et al: Report of the nomenclature committee. Cancer Res 26:1311, 1966.
40. Harris NL, Jaffe ES, Stein H, et al: A revised European-American classification of lymphoid neoplasms: A proposal from the International Lymphoma Study Group. Blood 84:1361-1392, 1994.
41. Harris NL, Jaffe ES, Diebold J, et al: World Health Organization classification of neoplastic diseases of the hematopoietic and lymphoid tissues: Report of the Clinical Advisory Committee meeting—Airlie House, Virginia, November 1997. J Clin Oncol 17:3835-3849, 1999.
42. Bennett MH, MacLennan KA, Easterling MJ, et al: The prognostic significance of cellular subtypes in nodular sclerosing Hodgkin's disease: An analysis of 271 non-laparotomised cases (BNLI report no. 22). Clin Radiol 34:497-501, 1983.
43. MacLennan KA, Bennett MH, Vaughan Hudson B, et al: Diagnosis and grading of nodular sclerosing Hodgkin's disease: A study of 2190 patients. Int Rev Exp Pathol 33:27-51, 1992.
44. Anagnostopoulos I, Hansmann ML, Franssila K, et al: European Task Force on Lymphoma project on lymphocyte predominance Hodgkin disease: Histologic and immunohistologic analysis of submitted cases reveals 2 types of Hodgkin disease with a nodular growth pattern and abundant lymphocytes. Blood 96:1889-1899, 2000.
45. Kant JA, Hubbard SM, Longo DL, et al: The pathologic and clinical heterogeneity of lymphocyte-depleted Hodgkin's disease. J Clin Oncol 4:284-294, 1986.
46. Miettinen M, Franssila KO, Saxen E: Hodgkin's disease, lymphocytic predominance nodular. Increased risk for subsequent non-Hodgkin's lymphomas. Cancer 51:2293-2300, 1983.
47. Rosenberg SA, Kaplan HS: Evidence for an orderly progression in the spread of Hodgkin's disease. Cancer Res 26:1225-1231, 1966.
48. Gobbi PG, Cavalli C, Gendarini A, et al: Reevaluation of prognostic significance of symptoms in Hodgkin's disease. Cancer 56:2874-2880, 1985.
49. Atkinson K, Austin DE, McElwain TJ, et al: Alcohol pain in Hodgkin's disease. Cancer 37:895-899, 1976.
50. Carbone PP, Kaplan HS, Musshoff K, et al: Report of the Committee on Hodgkin's Disease Staging Classification. Cancer Res 31:1860-1861, 1971.
51. Lister TA, Crowther D, Sutcliffe SB, et al: Report of a committee convened to discuss the evaluation and staging of patients with Hodgkin's disease: Cotswolds meeting. J Clin Oncol 7:1630-1636, 1989.
52. Elstrom R, Guan L, Baker G, et al: Utility of FDG-PET scanning in lymphoma by WHO classification. Blood 101:3875-3876, 2003.
53. Friedberg JW, Fischman A, Neuberg D, et al: FDG-PET is superior to gallium scintigraphy in staging and more sensitive in the follow-up of patients with de novo Hodgkin lymphoma: A blinded comparison. Leuk Lymphoma 45:85-92, 2004.
54. Naumann R, Beuthien-Baumann B, Reiss A, et al: Substantial impact of FDG PET imaging on the therapy decision in patients with early-stage Hodgkin's lymphoma. Br J Cancer 90:620-625, 2004.
55. Macintyre EA, Vaughan Hudson B, Linch DC, et al: The value of staging bone marrow trephine biopsy in Hodgkin's disease. Eur J Haematol 39:66-70, 1987.

56. Gomez-Almaguer D, Ruiz-Arguelles GJ, Lopez-Martínez B, et al: Role of bone marrow examination in staging Hodgkin's disease: experience in Mexico. Clin Lab Haematol 24:221-223, 2002.
57. Glatstein E, Guernsey JM, Rosenberg SA, et al: The value of laparotomy and splenectomy in the staging of Hodgkin's disease. Cancer 24:709-718, 1969.
58. Carde P, Hagenbeek A, Hayat M, et al: Clinical staging versus laparotomy and combined modality with MOPP versus ABVD in early-stage Hodgkin's disease: The H6 twin randomized trials from the European Organization for Research and Treatment of Cancer Lymphoma Cooperative Group. J Clin Oncol 11:2258-2272, 1993.
59. Sieber M, Franklin J, Tesch H, et al: Two cycles ABVD plus extended field radiotherapy is superior to radiotherapy alone in early stage Hodgkin's disease: Results of the German Hodgkin's Lymphoma Study Group (GHSG) Trial HD7. Blood 100:A341, 2002.
60. Hagenbeek A, Eghbali H, Fermé C, et al: Three cycles of MOPP/ABV hybrid and involved-field irradiation is more effective than subtotal nodal irradiation in favorable supradiaphragmatic clinical stages I-II Hodgkin's disease: Preliminary results of the EORTC-GELA H8-F randomized trial in 543 patients. Blood 96, 2000.
61. Press OW, LeBlanc M, Lichter AS, et al: Phase III randomized intergroup trial of subtotal lymphoid irradiation versus doxorubicin, vinblastine, and subtotal lymphoid irradiation for stage IA to IIA Hodgkin's disease. J Clin Oncol 19:4238-4244, 2001.
62. van Rijswijk RE, Verbeek J, Haanen C, et al: Major complications and causes of death in patients treated for Hodgkin's disease. J Clin Oncol 5:1624-1633, 1987.
63. Cosset JM, Henry-Amar M, Meerwaldt JH: Long-term toxicity of early stages of Hodgkin's disease therapy: The EORTC experience. EORTC Lymphoma Cooperative Group. Ann Oncol 2(Suppl 2):77-82, 1991.
64. Hoppe RT: Hodgkin's disease: Complications of therapy and excess mortality. Ann Oncol 8:115-118, 1997.
65. Ng AK, Bernardo MP, Weller E, et al: Long-term survival and competing causes of death in patients with early-stage Hodgkin's disease treated at age 50 or younger. J Clin Oncol 20:2101-2108, 2002.
66. Horning SJ, Hoppe RT, Mason J, et al: Stanford-Kaiser Permanente G1 study for clinical stage I to IIA Hodgkin's disease: Subtotal lymphoid irradiation versus vinblastine, methotrexate, and bleomycin chemotherapy and regional irradiation. J Clin Oncol 15:1736-1744, 1997.
67. Moody AM, Pratt J, Hudson GV, et al: British National Lymphoma Investigation: Pilot studies of neoadjuvant chemotherapy in clinical stage Ia and IIa Hodgkin's disease. Clin Oncol (R Coll Radiol) 13:262-268, 2001.
68. Martinelli G, Cocorocchio E, Saletti PC, et al: Efficacy of vinblastine, bleomycin, methotrexate (VBM) combination chemotherapy with involved field radiotherapy in early stage (I-IIA) Hodgkin disease patients. Leuk Lymphoma 44:1919-1923, 2003.
69. Gobbi PG, Broglia C, Merli F, et al: Vinblastine, bleomycin, and methotrexate chemotherapy plus irradiation for patients with early-stage, favorable Hodgkin lymphoma: The experience of the Gruppo Italiano Studio Linfomi. Cancer 98:2393-2401, 2003.
70. Radford JA, Williams MV, Hancock BW, et al: Minimal initial chemotherapy plus involved field radiotherapy (RT) vs. mantle field RT for clinical stage IA/IIA supradiaphragmatic Hodgkin's disease (HD). Results of the UK Lymphoma Group LY07 Trial. Eur J Haematol 73:E08a, 2004.
71. Tormo M, Terol MJ, Marugan I, et al: Treatment of stage I and II Hodgkin's disease with NOVP (mitoxantrone, vincristine, vinblastine, prednisone) and radiotherapy. Leuk Lymphoma 34:137-142, 1999.
72. Noordijk EM, Carde P, Hagenbeek A, et al: Combination of radiotherapy is advisable in all patients with clinical stage I-II Hodgkin's disease: Six-year results of EORTC-GPMC controlled clinical trials H7-VF, H7-F and H7-U. Int J Radiat Oncol Biol Phys 39:173a, 1997.
73. Thomas J: Six cycles of EBVP followed by 36Gy involved-field irradiation vs. no irradiation in favourable supradiaphragmatic clinical stage I-II Hodgkin's Lymphoma: The EORTC-GELA strategy in 771 patients. Eur J Haematol 73:E0, 2004.
74. Horning SJ, Rosenberg SA, Hoppe RT: Brief chemotherapy (Stanford V) and adjuvant radiotherapy for bulky or advanced Hodgkin's disease: An update. Ann Oncol 7:105-108, 1996.
75. Horning SJ, Williams J, Bartlett NL, et al: Assessment of the Stanford V regimen and consolidative radiotherapy for bulky and advanced Hodgkin's disease: Eastern Cooperative Oncology Group pilot study E1492. J Clin Oncol 18:972-980, 2000.
76. Diehl V, Brilliant C, Franklin J, et al: BEACOPP chemotherapy for advanced Hodgkin's disease: Results of further analysis of the HD9- and HD12- trials of the German Hodgkin Study Group (GHSG). Blood 104:91a, 2004.
77. Diehl V, Brilliant C, Engert A, et al: Reduction of combined modality treatment intensity in early stage Hodgkin's lymphoma, interim analysis of HD10 trial of GHSG. Eur J Haematol 73:E03a, 2004.
78. Ferme C, Eghbali H, Hagenbeek A, et al: MOPP/ABV hybrid and irradiation in unfavorable supradiaphragmatic clinical stages I-II Hodgkin s disease: Comparison of three treatment modalities. Preliminary results of the EORTC-GELA H8-U randomized trial in 995 patients. Blood 96:576a, 2000.
79. Engert A, Schiller P, Josting A, et al: Involved-field radiotherapy is equally effective and less toxic compared with extended-field radiotherapy after four cycles of chemotherapy in patients with early-stage unfavorable Hodgkin's lymphoma: Results of the HD8 trial of the German Hodgkin's Lymphoma Study Group. J Clin Oncol 21:3601-3608, 2003.
80. Bonadonna G, Bonfante V, Viviani S, et al: ABVD plus subtotal nodal versus involved-field radiotherapy in early-stage Hodgkin's disease: Long-term results. J Clin Oncol 22:2835-2841, 2004.
81. Pavlovsky S, Maschio M, Santarelli MT, et al: Randomized trial of chemotherapy versus chemotherapy plus radiotherapy for stage I-II Hodgkin's disease. J Natl Cancer Inst 80:1466-1473, 1988.
82. Nachman JB, Sposto R, Herzog P, et al: Randomized comparison of low-dose involved-field radiotherapy and no radiotherapy for children with Hodgkin's disease who achieve a complete response to chemotherapy. J Clin Oncol 20:3765-3771, 2002.
83. Laskar S, Gupta T, Vimal S, et al: Consolidation radiation after complete remission in Hodgkin's disease following six cycles of doxorubicin, bleomycin, vinblastine, and dacarbazine chemotherapy: Is there a need? J Clin Oncol 22:62-68, 2004.
84. Straus DJ, Portlock CS, Qin J, et al: Results of a prospective randomized clinical trial of doxorubicin, bleomycin, vinblastine and dacarbazine (ABVD) followed by radiation therapy (RT) versus ABVD alone for stages I, II and IIIA nonbulky Hodgkin's disease. Blood 104(12):3483-3489, 2004.
85. Meyer R, Gospodarowicz M, Connors J, et al: A randomized phase III comparison of single-modality ABVD with a strategy that includes radiation therapy in patients with early-stage Hodgkin's disease: The HD-6 trial of the National Cancer Institute of Canada Clinical Trials Group (Eastern Cooperative Oncology Group Trial JHD06). Blood 102:A81, 2003.
86. Santoro A, Bonadonna G, Bonfante V, et al: Alternating drug combinations in the treatment of advanced Hodgkin's disease. N Engl J Med 306:770-775, 1982.
87. Santoro A, Bonadonna G, Valagussa P, et al: Long-term results of combined chemotherapy-radiotherapy approach in Hodgkin's disease: Superiority of ABVD plus radiotherapy versus MOPP plus radiotherapy. J Clin Oncol 5:27-37, 1987.
88. Somers R, Carde P, Henry-Amar M, et al: A randomized study in stage IIIB and IV Hodgkin's disease comparing eight courses of MOPP versus an alteration of MOPP with ABVD: A European Organization for Research and Treatment of Cancer Lymphoma Cooperative Group and Groupe Pierre-et-Marie-Curie controlled clinical trial. J Clin Oncol 12:279-287, 1994.
89. Canellos GP, Anderson JR, Propert KJ, et al: Chemotherapy of advanced Hodgkin's disease with MOPP, ABVD, or MOPP alternating with ABVD. N Engl J Med 327:1478-1484, 1992.
90. Duggan DB, Petroni GR, Johnson JL, et al: Randomized comparison of ABVD and MOPP/ABV hybrid for the treatment of

advanced Hodgkin's disease: Report of an intergroup trial. J Clin Oncol 21:607-614, 2003.
91. Hasenclever D, Diehl V: A prognostic score for advanced Hodgkin's disease. International Prognostic Factors Project on Advanced Hodgkin's Disease. N Engl J Med 339:1506-1514, 1998.
92. Horning SJ, Hoppe RT, Breslin S, et al: Stanford V and radiotherapy for locally extensive and advanced Hodgkin's disease: Mature results of a prospective clinical trial. J Clin Oncol 20:630-637, 2002.
93. Horning SJ, Williams J, Bartlett NL, et al: Assessment of the Stanford V regimen and consolidative radiotherapy for bulky and advanced Hodgkin's disease: Eastern Cooperative Oncology Group pilot study E1492. J Clin Oncol 18:972-980, 2000.
94. Chisesi T, Federico M, Levis A, et al: ABVD versus Stanford V versus MEC in unfavourable Hodgkin's lymphoma: Results of a randomised trial. Ann Oncol 13(Suppl 1):102-106, 2002.
95. Diehl V, Franklin J, Pfreundschuh M, et al: Standard and increased-dose BEACOPP chemotherapy compared with COPP-ABVD for advanced Hodgkin's disease. N Engl J Med 348:2386-2395, 2003.
96. Sieber M, Bredenfeld H, Josting A, et al: 14-day variant of the bleomycin, etoposide, doxorubicin, cyclophosphamide, vincristine, procarbazine, and prednisone regimen in advanced-stage Hodgkin's lymphoma: Results of a pilot study of the German Hodgkin's Lymphoma Study Group. J Clin Oncol 21:1734-1739, 2003.
97. Baetz T, Belch A, Couban S, et al: Gemcitabine, dexamethasone and cisplatin is an active and non-toxic chemotherapy regimen in relapsed or refractory Hodgkin's disease: A phase II study by the National Cancer Institute of Canada Clinical Trials Group. Ann Oncol 14:1762-1767, 2003.
98. Friedberg JW, Neuberg D, Kim H, et al: Gemcitabine added to doxorubicin, bleomycin, and vinblastine for the treatment of de novo Hodgkin disease: Unacceptable acute pulmonary toxicity. Cancer 98:978-982, 2003.
99. Bredenfeld H, Franklin J, Nogova L, et al: Severe pulmonary toxicity in patients with advanced-stage Hodgkin's disease treated with a modified bleomycin, doxorubicin, cyclophosphamide, vincristine, procarbazine, prednisone, and gemcitabine (BEACOPP) regimen is probably related to the combination of gemcitabine and bleomycin: A report of the German Hodgkin's Lymphoma Study Group. J Clin Oncol 22:2424-2429, 2004.
100. Brizel DM, Winer EP, Prosnitz LR, et al: Improved survival in advanced Hodgkin's disease with the use of combined modality therapy. Int J Radiat Oncol Biol Phys 19:535-542, 1990.
101. Yahalom J, Ryu J, Straus DJ, et al: Impact of adjuvant radiation on the patterns and rate of relapse in advanced-stage Hodgkin's disease treated with alternating chemotherapy combinations. J Clin Oncol 9:2193-2201, 1991.
102. Fabian CJ, Mansfield CM, Dahlberg S, et al: Low-dose involved field radiation after chemotherapy in advanced Hodgkin disease. A Southwest Oncology Group randomized study. Ann Intern Med 120:903-912, 1994.
103. Diehl V, Loeffler M, Pfreundschuh M, et al: Further chemotherapy versus low-dose involved-field radiotherapy as consolidation of complete remission after six cycles of alternating chemotherapy in patients with advanced Hodgkin's disease. German Hodgkin's Study Group (GHSG). Ann Oncol 6:901-910, 1995.
104. Loeffler M, Diehl V, Pfreundschuh M, et al: Dose-response relationship of complementary radiotherapy following four cycles of combination chemotherapy in intermediate-stage Hodgkin's disease. J Clin Oncol 15:2275-2287, 1997.
105. Ferme C, Sebban C, Hennequin C, et al: Comparison of chemotherapy to radiotherapy as consolidation of complete or good partial response after six cycles of chemotherapy for patients with advanced Hodgkin's disease: Results of the Groupe d'Etudes des Lymphomes de l'Adulte H89 trial. Blood 95:2246-2252, 2000.
106. Pavlovsky S, Santarelli MT, Muriel FS, et al: Randomized trial of chemotherapy versus chemotherapy plus radiotherapy for stage III-IV A & B Hodgkin's disease. Ann Oncol 3:533-537, 1992.
107. Aleman BM, Raemaekers JM, Tirelli U, et al: Involved-field radiotherapy for advanced Hodgkin's lymphoma. N Engl J Med 348:2396-2406, 2003.
108. Loeffler M, Brosteanu O, Hasenclever D, et al: Meta-analysis of chemotherapy versus combined modality treatment trials in Hodgkin's disease. International Database on Hodgkin's Disease Overview Study Group. J Clin Oncol 16:818-829, 1998.
109. Bodis S, Kraus MD, Pinkus G, et al: Clinical presentation and outcome in lymphocyte-predominant Hodgkin's disease. J Clin Oncol 15:3060-3066, 1997.
110. Diehl V, Sextro M, Franklin J, et al: Clinical presentation, course, and prognostic factors in lymphocyte-predominant Hodgkin's disease and lymphocyte-rich classical Hodgkin's disease: Report from the European Task Force on Lymphoma Project on Lymphocyte-Predominant Hodgkin's Disease. J Clin Oncol 17:776-783, 1999.
111. Feugier P, Labouyrie E, Djeridane M, et al: Comparison of initial characteristics and long-term outcome of patients with lymphocyte-predominant Hodgkin lymphoma and classical Hodgkin lymphoma at clinical stages IA and IIA prospectively treated by brief anthracycline-based chemotherapies plus extended high-dose irradiation. Blood 104:2675-2681, 2004.
112. Pellegrino B, Terrier-Lacombe MJ, Oberlin O, et al: Lymphocyte-predominant Hodgkin's lymphoma in children: Therapeutic abstention after initial lymph node resection—A study of the French Society of Pediatric Oncology. J Clin Oncol 21:2948-2952, 2003.
113. Wilder RB, Schlembach PJ, Jones D, et al: European Organization for Research and Treatment of Cancer and Groupe d'Etudes des Lymphomes de l'Adulte very favorable and favorable, lymphocyte-predominant Hodgkin disease. Cancer 94:1731-1738, 2002.
114. Ekstrand BC, Lucas JB, Horwitz SM, et al: Rituximab in lymphocyte-predominant Hodgkin disease: Results of a phase 2 trial. Blood 101:4285-4289, 2003.
115. Santoro A, Viviani S, Villarreal CJ, et al: Salvage chemotherapy in Hodgkin's disease irradiation failures: Superiority of doxorubicin-containing regimens over MOPP. Cancer Treat Rep 70:343-348, 1986.
116. Roach M III, Brophy N, Cox R, et al: Prognostic factors for patients relapsing after radiotherapy for early-stage Hodgkin's disease. J Clin Oncol 8:623-629, 1990.
117. Healey EA, Tarbell NJ, Kalish LA, et al: Prognostic factors for patients with Hodgkin disease in first relapse. Cancer 71:2613-2620, 1993.
118. Specht L, Horwich A, Ashley S: Salvage of relapse of patients with Hodgkin's disease in clinical stages I or II who were staged with laparotomy and initially treated with radiotherapy alone. A report from the international database on Hodgkin's disease. Int J Radiat Oncol Biol Phys 30:805-811, 1994.
119. Horwich A, Specht L, Ashley S: Survival analysis of patients with clinical stages I or II Hodgkin's disease who have relapsed after initial treatment with radiotherapy alone. Eur J Cancer 33:848-853, 1997.
120. Ng AK, Li S, Neuberg D, et al: Comparison of MOPP versus ABVD as salvage therapy in patients who relapse after radiation therapy alone for Hodgkin's disease. Ann Oncol 15:270-275, 2004.
121. Yahalom J, Gulati SC, Toia M, et al: Accelerated hyperfractionated total-lymphoid irradiation, high-dose chemotherapy, and autologous bone marrow transplantation for refractory and relapsing patients with Hodgkin's disease. J Clin Oncol 11:1062-1070, 1993.
122. Crump M, Smith AM, Brandwein J, et al: High-dose etoposide and melphalan, and autologous bone marrow transplantation for patients with advanced Hodgkin's disease: Importance of disease status at transplant. J Clin Oncol 11:704-711, 1993.
123. Reece DE, Connors JM, Spinelli JJ, et al: Intensive therapy with cyclophosphamide, carmustine, etoposide ± cisplatin, and autologous bone marrow transplantation for Hodgkin's disease in first relapse after combination chemotherapy. Blood 83:1193-1199, 1994.
124. Wheeler C, Eickhoff C, Elias A, et al: High-dose cyclophosphamide, carmustine, and etoposide with autologous transplantation in Hodgkin's disease: A prognostic model for treatment outcomes. Biol Blood Marrow Transplant 3:98-106, 1997.

125. Horning SJ, Chao NJ, Negrin RS, et al: High-dose therapy and autologous hematopoietic progenitor cell transplantation for recurrent or refractory Hodgkin's disease: Analysis of the Stanford University results and prognostic indices. Blood 89:801-813, 1997.
126. Sureda A, Arranz R, Iriondo A, et al: Autologous stem-cell transplantation for Hodgkin's disease: Results and prognostic factors in 494 patients from the Grupo Español de Linfomas/Transplante Autologo de Medula Osea Spanish Cooperative Group. J Clin Oncol 19:1395-1404, 2001.
127. Lazarus HM, Loberiza FR Jr, Zhang MJ, et al: Autotransplants for Hodgkin's disease in first relapse or second remission: A report from the autologous blood and marrow transplant registry (ABMTR). Bone Marrow Transplant 27:387-396, 2001.
128. Ferme C, Mounier N, Divine M, et al: Intensive salvage therapy with high-dose chemotherapy for patients with advanced Hodgkin's disease in relapse or failure after initial chemotherapy: Results of the Groupe d'Etudes des Lymphomes de l'Adulte H89 Trial. J Clin Oncol 20:467-475, 2002.
129. Bierman PJ, Lynch JC, Bociek RG, et al: The International Prognostic Factors Project score for advanced Hodgkin's disease is useful for predicting outcome of autologous hematopoietic stem cell transplantation. Ann Oncol 13:1370-1377, 2002.
130. Linch DC, Winfield D, Goldstone AH, et al: Dose intensification with autologous bone-marrow transplantation in relapsed and resistant Hodgkin's disease: Results of a BNLI randomised trial. Lancet 341:1051-1054, 1993.
131. Schmitz N, Pfistner B, Sextro M, et al: Aggressive conventional chemotherapy compared with high-dose chemotherapy with autologous hemopoietic stem-cell transplantation for relapsed chemosensitive Hodgkin's disease: A randomised trial. Lancet 359:2065-2071, 2002.
132. Poen JC, Hoppe RT, Horning SJ: High-dose therapy and autologous bone marrow transplantation for relapsed/refractory Hodgkin's disease: The impact of involved field radiotherapy on patterns of failure and survival. Int J Radiat Oncol Biol Phys 36:3-12, 1996.
133. Mundt AJ, Sibley G, Williams S, et al: Patterns of failure following high-dose chemotherapy and autologous bone marrow transplantation with involved field radiotherapy for relapsed/refractory Hodgkin's disease. Int J Radiat Oncol Biol Phys 33:261-270, 1995.
134. Roach M III, Kapp DS, Rosenberg SA, et al: Radiotherapy with curative intent: An option in selected patients relapsing after chemotherapy for advanced Hodgkin's disease. J Clin Oncol 5:550-555, 1987.
135. Brada M, Eeles R, Ashley S, et al: Salvage radiotherapy in recurrent Hodgkin's disease. Ann Oncol 3:131-135, 1992.
136. Uematsu M, Tarbell NJ, Silver B, et al: Wide-field radiation therapy with or without chemotherapy for patients with Hodgkin disease in relapse after initial combination chemotherapy. Cancer 72:207-212, 1993.
137. Wirth A, Corry J, Laidlaw C, et al: Salvage radiotherapy for Hodgkin's disease following chemotherapy failure. Int J Radiat Oncol Biol Phys 39:599-607, 1997.
138. Josting A, Wiedenmann S, Franklin J, et al: Secondary myeloid leukemia and myelodysplastic syndromes in patients treated for Hodgkin's disease: A report from the German Hodgkin's Lymphoma Study Group. J Clin Oncol 21:3440-3446, 2003.
139. Little R, Wittes RE, Longo DL, et al: Vinblastine for recurrent Hodgkin's disease following autologous bone marrow transplant. J Clin Oncol 16:584-588, 1998.
140. Zinzani PL, Bendandi M, Stefoni V, et al: Value of gemcitabine treatment in heavily pretreated Hodgkin's disease patients. Haematologica 85:926-929, 2000.
141. Miller R, Geijn J, Raubitschek A, et al: Dosimetric considerations in treating mediastinal disease with mantle fields: Characterization of the dose under mantle blocks. Int J Radiat Oncol Biol Phys 32:1083-1095, 1995.
142. Lutz WR, Larsen RD: Technique to match mantle and para-aortic fields. Int J Radiat Oncol Biol Phys 9:1753-1756, 1983.
143. Hunter MC, Glees JP, Gazet JC: Oophoropexy and ovarian function in the treatment of Hodgkin's disease. Clin Radiol 31:21-26, 1980.
144. Gabriel DA, Bernard SA, Lambert J, et al: Oophoropexy and the management of Hodgkin's disease. A reevaluation of the risks and benefits. Arch Surg 121:1083-1085, 1986.
145. Williams RS, Littell RD, Mendenhall NP: Laparoscopic oophoropexy and ovarian function in the treatment of Hodgkin disease. Cancer 86:2138-2142, 1999.
146. Lukes RJ, Carver LF, Hall TC, et al: Report of the nomenclature committee in symposium: Obstacles to the control of Hodgkin's disease. Cancer Res 26:1311, 1966.
147. Yahalom J, Mauch P: The involved field is back: Issues in delineating the radiation field in Hodgkin's disease. Ann Oncol 13(Suppl 1):79-83, 2002.
148. Borchmann P, Schnell R, Fuss I, et al: Phase I trial of the novel bispecific molecule H22xKi-4 in patients with refractory Hodgkin lymphoma. Blood 100:3101-3107, 2002.
149. Schnell R, Borchmann P, Staak JO, et al: Clinical evaluation of ricin A-chain immunotoxins in patients with Hodgkin's lymphoma. Ann Oncol 14:729-736, 2003.
150. Cooney JP, Stiff PJ, Toor AA, et al: BEAM allogeneic transplantation for patients with Hodgkin's disease who relapse after autologous transplantation is safe and effective. Biol Blood Marrow Transplant 9:177-182, 2003.
151. Ruiz-Arguelles GJ, Lopez-Martinez B, Lopez-Ariza B: Successful allogeneic stem cell transplantation with nonmyeloablative conditioning in patients with relapsed Hodgkin's disease following autologous stem cell transplantation. Arch Med Res 34:242-245, 2003.
152. Swerdlow AJ, Barber JA, Hudson GV, et al: Risk of second malignancy after Hodgkin's disease in a collaborative British cohort: the relation to age at treatment. J Clin Oncol 18:498-509, 2000.
153. van Leeuwen FE, Klokman WJ, Veer MB, et al: Long-term risk of second malignancy in survivors of Hodgkin's disease treated during adolescence or young adulthood. J Clin Oncol 18:487-497, 2000.
154. Ng AK, Bernardo MV, Weller E, et al: Second malignancy after Hodgkin disease treated with radiation therapy with or without chemotherapy: Long-term risks and risk factors. Blood 100:1989-1996, 2002.
155. Cellai E, Magrini SM, Masala G, et al: The risk of second malignant tumors and its consequences for the overall survival of Hodgkin's disease patients and for the choice of their treatment at presentation: Analysis of a series of 1524 cases consecutively treated at the Florence University Hospital. Int J Radiat Oncol Biol Phys 49:1327-1337, 2001.
156. Kaldor JM, Day NE, Bell J, et al: Lung cancer following Hodgkin's disease: A case-control study. Int J Cancer 52:677-681, 1992.
157. van Leeuwen FE, Klokman WJ, Stovall M, et al: Roles of radiotherapy and smoking in lung cancer following Hodgkin's disease. J Natl Cancer Inst 87:1530-1537, 1995.
158. Swerdlow AJ, Schoemaker MJ, Allerton R, et al: Lung cancer after Hodgkin's disease: a nested case-control study of the relation to treatment. J Clin Oncol 19:1610-1618, 2001.
159. Yahalom J, Petrek JA, Biddinger PW, et al: Breast cancer in patients irradiated for Hodgkin's disease: A clinical and pathologic analysis of 45 events in 37 patients. J Clin Oncol 10:1674-1681, 1992.
160. Hancock SL, Tucker MA, Hoppe RT: Breast cancer after treatment of Hodgkin's disease. J Natl Cancer Inst 85:25-31, 1993.
161. Travis LB, Hill DA, Dores GM, et al: Breast cancer following radiotherapy and chemotherapy among young women with Hodgkin disease. JAMA 290:465-475, 2003.
162. Biti G, Cellai E, Magrini SM, et al: Second solid tumors and leukemia after treatment for Hodgkin's disease: An analysis of 1121 patients from a single institution. Int J Radiat Oncol Biol Phys 29:25-31, 1994.
163. Henry-Amar M: Second cancer after the treatment for Hodgkin's disease: a report from the International Database on Hodgkin's Disease. Ann Oncol 3(Suppl 4):117-128, 1992.
164. van Leeuwen FE, Klokman WJ, Stovall M, et al: Roles of radiation dose, chemotherapy, and hormonal factors in breast cancer following Hodgkin's disease. J Natl Cancer Inst 95:971-980, 2003.

165. Travis LB, Gospodarowicz M, Curtis RE, et al: Lung cancer following chemotherapy and radiotherapy for Hodgkin's disease. J Natl Cancer Inst 94:182-192, 2002.
166. Cuttuli B, Borel C, Dhermain F, et al: Breast cancer occurred after treatment for Hodgkin's disease: Analysis of 133 cases. Radiother Oncol 59:247-255, 2001.
167. Maunoury C, Pierga JY, Valette H, et al: Myocardial perfusion damage after mediastinal irradiation for Hodgkin's disease: A thallium-201 single photon emission tomography study. Eur J Nucl Med 19:871-873, 1992.
168. Glanzmann C, Huguenin P, Lutolf UM, et al: Cardiac lesions after mediastinal irradiation for Hodgkin's disease. Radiother Oncol 30:43-54, 1994.
169. Benoff LJ, Schweitzer P: Radiation therapy-induced cardiac injury. Am Heart J 129:1193-1196, 1995.
170. Cosset JM, Henry-Amar M, Pellae-Cosset B, et al: Pericarditis and myocardial infarctions after Hodgkin's disease therapy. Int J Radiat Oncol Biol Phys 21:447-449, 1991.
171. Boivin JF, Hutchison GB, Lubin JH, et al: Coronary artery disease mortality in patients treated for Hodgkin's disease. Cancer 69:1241-1247, 1992.
172. Hancock SL, Tucker MA, Hoppe RT: Factors affecting late mortality from heart disease after treatment of Hodgkin's disease. JAMA 270:1949-1955, 1993.
173. Hull MC, Morris CG, Pepine CJ, et al: Valvular dysfunction and carotid, subclavian, and coronary artery disease in survivors of Hodgkin lymphoma treated with radiation therapy. JAMA 290:2831-2837, 2003.
174. Strasser JF, Li S, Neuberg D, et al: Late cardiac toxicity after mediastinal radiation therapy for Hodgkin's disease. Int J Radiat Oncol Biol Phys 60:S217, 2004.
175. Heidenreich PA, Hancock SL, Lee BK, et al: Asymptomatic cardiac disease following mediastinal irradiation. J Am Coll Cardiol 42:743-749, 2003.

CHAPTER 74

NON-HODGKIN'S LYMPHOMA

Richard W. Tsang and Mary K. Gospodarowicz

EPIDEMIOLOGY/INCIDENCE

An estimated 54,370 new cases of non-Hodgkin's lymphoma (NHL) arise each year, and it causes 19,410 deaths in the United States.

The incidence is increasing in many countries, including the United States.

The most common types of NHL are diffuse large B-cell (≈30%) and follicular lymphoma (≈25%).

The etiology is uncertain, but immunosuppression and infectious agents—including Epstein-Barr virus (EBV), human T-cell lymphotropic virus I (HTLV-1), and *Helicobacter pylori*—contribute.

BIOLOGIC CHARACTERISTICS

Lymphomas are a diverse group of diseases clinically, pathologically, and genetically.

Prognosis relates to histologic subtype, age, extent of disease, and treatment.

STAGING EVALUATION

Pathologic diagnosis by experienced hematopathologist.

History and physical examination; blood count; lactate dehydrogenase (LDH); bone marrow biopsy; computed tomography (CT) of the neck, thorax, abdomen, and pelvis, ^{18}F-fluorodeoxyglucose positron emission tomography (FDG-PET), or gallium scan.

PRIMARY THERAPY

Stages I and II follicular and marginal-zone lymphomas are treated with involved-field radiation therapy (IFRT), expecting a more than 95% local control rate and 50% long-term disease-free survival. Stages III and IV follicular and marginal-zone lymphomas are not cured with currently available therapy; but chemotherapy and radiation therapy (RT) are effective in controlling the disease.

Stages I and II diffuse large B-cell lymphoma and other aggressive histology subtypes are treated with combined-modality therapy (CMT), expecting a cure in 60% to 80% of patients depending on age and tumor burden. Stages III and IV diffuse large B-cell lymphoma and other aggressive histology subtypes are treated primarily with doxorubicin-based chemotherapy.

SALVAGE THERAPY

Diffuse large B-cell lymphoma and other aggressive histology lymphomas refractory to chemotherapy or relapsing after previous complete response is treated with high-dose chemotherapy and autologous stem cell transplantation (ASCT) when possible. Patients with bulky disease or incomplete response to salvage chemotherapy receive local RT to sites of disease as planned-combined salvage treatment. RT may be delivered before or after bone marrow transplantation (BMT). Patients so treated have a cure rate of 20% to 40%.

PALLIATION

Palliative low-dose RT for follicular and marginal-zone lymphomas often provides local control and relief of symptoms. Diffuse large cell lymphomas are less responsive to RT, particularly if the disease is bulky and resistant to chemotherapy. Doses of more than 35 Gy may be required to have a better chance of local control and symptom relief.

The term *non-Hodgkin's lymphoma* (NHL) encompasses a heterogeneous group of neoplasms of the lymphoid system. The common factor is the malignant cell, a lymphocyte. Beyond that, malignant lymphomas differ in their etiology, pathogenesis, genetics, clinical manifestations, patterns of spread, response to treatment, and survival. Both incidence and mortality of NHL are increasing worldwide. The increased incidence has been related to environmental factors including occupational exposures and human immunodeficiency virus (HIV) infection. The most prevalent lymphomas in North America are of B-cell origin with follicular lymphomas and diffuse large B-cell lymphomas. Lymphomas presenting in extranodal sites account for 20% to 45% of all cases. Primary extranodal lymphomas with their propensity to present with localized disease are of special interest to radiation oncologists.

The management of NHL is primarily influenced by histology and stage. Radiation therapy (RT) achieves local tumor control and is curative for those with truly localized disease. Chemotherapy is required to control generalized disease, both occult and clinically apparent. Although RT has traditionally been the treatment of choice for localized disease and remains the principal treatment modality for localized indolent lymphomas (follicular lymphoma and mucosa-associated lymphoid tissue [MALT] lymphoma), combined-modality therapy (CMT) is the current standard approach for patients with localized large cell lymphomas. Chemotherapy has the potential to cure patients with large cell lymphomas and high-grade lymphomas but not indolent lymphomas. The management of patients with indolent lymphomas is a challenge, given that most patients present with generalized disease, and there currently exists no curative systemic therapy.

ETIOLOGY AND EPIDEMIOLOGY

The incidence of NHLs has been increasing worldwide,[1-4] including in North America.[5,6] In 2006 the American Cancer Society estimated that 58,870 new cases were diagnosed and 18,840 deaths occurred in the United States.[7] In many developed countries, there is evidence for a 2% to 4% per year rise in the incidence of NHL over the last four decades. This increase is more marked for older persons. In the United States the incidence has doubled between 1950 and 1980, from 5.9 to 13.7 per 100,000 persons per year,[8] but the annual rise in incidence rate had slowed to 1% to 2% in the 1990s.[6] Some of the increase has been because of increase in immunosuppression (human immunodeficiency virus [HIV] infection and iatrogenic), spread of infectious agents such as human T-cell lymphotropic virus type 1 (HTLV-1) and Epstein-Barr virus (EBV), increased use of chemicals, and increased case-finding because of improved pathologic diagnosis.[9] However, these factors do not explain the magnitude of the rise in incidence. A possible role of ultraviolet rays in sunlight as a ubiquitous immunosuppressive factor has been refuted.[10]

The epidemiology of certain histologic subtypes of lymphomas follows distinct patterns related to the epidemiology of the putative causative agent and any environmental cofactors. The classical example is Burkitt's lymphoma in Africa, with the endemic role of EBV and the contribution of immunosuppression because of malaria infection.[11,12] Similarly, EBV related T/natural killer (T/NK) cell lymphoma of the nasal region is more frequent in oriental populations of south Asia[13-16] and Peru.[17] Adult T-cell leukemia or lymphoma caused by HTLV-1 is endemic in the Caribbean and southern Japan.[18] The frequency of HIV-related lymphomas is proportional to the HIV infection rate in the population, explaining the observation of high incidence rates in large urban cities, and a role of Kaposi sarcoma–associated herpes virus.[19] MALT lymphomas of the stomach are seen more frequently in regions where *Helicobacter pylori* infection is endemic.[20]

Despite an increasing body of knowledge on the genetic and phenotypic events underlying the development and progression of NHL, the causative agent has not been identified in most cases. The putative causative agents and associated conditions with a predisposition for the development of NHL are listed in Table 74-1. Changes in the immune state, either immunosuppression or autoimmune disease, with immune stimulation can predispose to NHL. The immunosuppression can be primary, that is, inherited (severe combined immunodeficiency syndrome), secondary to retrovirus infection (HIV), or iatrogenic (following solid organ or bone marrow transplantation [BMT]).[21] Patients with the acquired immunodeficiency syndrome (AIDS) have a lymphoma prevalence rate of 4.3%.[22] The incidence of NHL in HIV-positive individuals has declined since the late 1990s, because of highly effective antiretroviral therapy.[23,24] NHLs arising in patients with AIDS are heterogeneous with respect to clinical presentation. Infectious agents other than EBV are possible, as human herpes simplex virus sequences have been implicated in primary effusion lymphomas seen infrequently in patients with AIDS.[19,25] Chronic antigenic stimulation, as seen in Sjögren's syndrome,[26] Hashimoto's thyroiditis,[27] rheumatoid arthritis,[28] and celiac disease,[29] is also associated with an increased risk of NHL.

Infectious agents have been shown to be etiologic factors in NHL, such as *H. pylori* in gastric MALT lymphomas[30,31] and more recently *Chlamydia psittaci* in ocular adnexal lymphomas.[32] Viruses have been implicated, and the two most closely linked are EBV[12,33] and the HTLV-1. HTLV-1 carriers have a 2% cumulative risk of developing adult T-cell leukemia/lymphoma and is a major public health problem in some parts of the world where the seropositivity rate is high.[34,35] A previous diagnosis of Hodgkin's lymphoma has also been suggested as a risk factor for the subsequent development of NHL,[36] possibly related to underlying immunosuppression.

Epidemiologic studies suggest an association with environmental factors including industrial chemicals,[37] rural residence possibly linking to use of pesticides or other agricultural chemicals,[38] and diet.[39,40] The association with use of hair dyes is controversial.[41,42] A small excess risk was also found in atomic bomb survivors for males but not for females,[43] whereas minimal or no risk was found for diagnostic radiograph exposure[44] and localized radiation for benign disease.[45]

Table 74-1 Causative Agents and Associated Conditions with a Predisposition to the Development of Non-Hodgkin's Lymphoma

CONGENITAL IMMUNODEFICIENCY
Severe combined immunodeficiencies
Ataxia-telangiectasia
ACQUIRED IMMUNODEFICIENCY
Organ or hematopoietic stem cell transplantation
HIV infection
AUTOIMMUNE DISORDERS
Sjögren's syndrome
Hashimoto's thyroiditis
Nontropical sprue
Rheumatoid arthritis
VIRAL AGENTS
Epstein-Barr virus
HTLV-1
Herpes virus type 8
Hepatitis C
BACTERIAL
Helicobacter pylori
Chlamydia psittaci
Borrelia burgdorferi
DRUGS
Alkylating agents
Other immunosuppressive drugs
PESTICIDES
Phenoxyl herbicides
Organophosphate insecticides
Fungicides
SOLVENTS AND OTHER CHEMICALS
Benzene
Trichloroethylene
Hair dyes
DIET
N-nitroso compounds
Fat

HTLV-1, human T-cell lymphotropic virus I.

PREVENTION AND EARLY DETECTION

With a better definition of environmental causative factors for NHL, it is expected that preventive strategies will be developed. For adult T-cell leukemia/lymphoma, initiatives are being implemented to reduce the disease burden in susceptible populations, the most important being the control of breast feeding to prevent maternal-fetal transmission of the HTLV-1 virus. Other promising areas of prevention currently include heightened awareness of potentially toxic agents and the development of improved products with less carcinogenic potential (chemicals and hair dyes). Assays of genomic instability that aim to identify persons at high risk of developing lymphoid malignancies are under investigation.[46] For viral agents the development of vaccines is possible.[47] For organ transplantation, avoidance of transplanting an EBV-positive donor organ into a EBV-negative recipient should reduce the risk of posttransplant NHL. Cytotoxic T-cell infusion therapy has also been shown to have a beneficial effect for allogeneic transplant recipients.[48,49] For persons infected with HIV, effective combination antiviral treatments have contributed to a decreased incidence of lymphomas.[23,24] The detection and eradication of *H. pylori* infection in the stomach is an important strategy with potential to control or prevent MALT lymphoma[50-52] and its transformation. As additional microorganisms and viruses other than the ones mentioned here are being discovered to play critical roles in the pathogenesis of some lymphomas,[19,32] prevention and early treatment strategies will become increasingly important.

BIOLOGIC CHARACTERISTICS AND PATHOLOGY

Previous classifications of NHLs were derived from morphologic observations stressing architectural change in relation to normal lymph node and cytologic appearances.[53,54] More recently, concepts emphasizing lineage, function, and differentiation using phenotypic and molecular techniques were introduced, resulting in a Revised European American Lymphoma (REAL) classification in 1994,[55] and the World Health Organization (WHO) classification in 2001,[56] shown in Table 74-2. The WHO classification recognized three major categories of lymphoid malignancies: B-cell, T-cell, and Hodgkin's lymphoma. The emphasis was on identification and characterization of unique clinical-pathologic diseases with currently available techniques.

The diagnosis of the new pathologic and clinical entities continues to be based on morphology but is assisted by immunophenotyping and genotyping. The relevance of immunophenotype has been evaluated in a retrospective review of 560 cases treated on clinical trials at the M. D. Anderson Hospital between 1984 and 1995.[57] The M. D. Anderson Hospital experience established T-cell phenotype as an adverse prognostic factor independent of other factors including the International Prognostic Index (IPI), and the M. D. Anderson prognostic tumor score. A clinical evaluation of the REAL classification has been performed using a cohort of 1403 previously untreated patients seen between 1988 and 1990 at several major lymphoma treatment centers and cooperative clinical trials groups.[58] In this study the diagnostic accuracy for individual lymphoma entities was at least 85%, and the reproducibility of diagnosis was 85%. Immunophenotyping improved the diagnostic accuracy by 10% to 45% in a number of major histologic types.

The most common lymphoma entities were diffuse large cell lymphoma (DLCL) (31%) and follicular lymphoma (22%). MALT–marginal zone lymphoma constituted 7.6% of cases, peripheral T-cell lymphomas made up 7%, small B-lymphocytic represented 6.7%, mantle cell 6%, anaplastic large T/null cell constituted 2.4%, primary mediastinal large B-cell made up 2.4%, and high-grade non-Burkitt and Burkitt accounted for fewer than 3% of cases. To elucidate age-related differences in NHL, Carbone and colleagues have evaluated 950 consecutive HIV-negative adult patients seen in Aviano, Italy, between 1988 and 1995.[59] They observed that the incidence of follicular lymphomas increased with age, the intermediate-grade lymphomas were more frequent in elderly, and the high-grade lymphomas showed a significant downward trend with age. An excess of T-cell lymphoma was seen in patients younger than 35 years of age.

Surface marker studies provide an objective basis for difficult morphologic problems (Table 74-3). The lineage of the B-cell lymphomas is confirmed by pan B-cell markers (CD22, CD19, CD20). T-cell lineage is evident from the presence of T-cell markers (CD3, CD2, CD7), and T-cell subset from CD4 and CD8 analysis. Among indolent lymphomas, the CD5+, CD10–, CD23+ phenotype is characteristic of small lymphocytic lymphoma (chronic lymphocytic leukemia); and the CD5–, CD10+, CD23± phenotype is characteristic of follicular lymphoma and the CD5–, CD10–, CD23– phenotype of MALT lymphoma (see Table 74-3). The CD5+, CD10–, CD23– phenotype is characteristic of mantle cell lymphoma. Among T-cell lymphomas the CD30+ phenotype is characteristic of anaplastic large cell lymphoma (Fig. 74-1), whereas CD56+ is associated with extranodal T/NK lymphoma of nasal type. Although surface marker analysis enhances the accuracy of the diagnosis, few surface marker characteristics are totally lineage specific. Ancillary cytologic and histologic techniques used to establish proliferative activity include labelling index, mitotic index, S-phase fraction,[60,61] and Ki-67 antigen stain-

Table 74-2 World Health Organization Classification

B-CELL NEOPLASMS
Peripheral B-cell Neoplasms
Precursor B lymphoblastic leukemia/lymphoma
Mature B-cell Neoplasms
CLL/small lymphocytic lymphoma
B-cell prolymphocytic leukemia
Lymphoplasmacytic lymphoma
Splenic marginal zone lymphoma
Extranodal marginal zone B-cell lymphoma of MALT (MALT-lymphoma)
Nodal marginal zone lymphoma
Follicular lymphoma
Mantle cell lymphoma
Diffuse large B-cell lymphoma
Mediastinal (thymic) large B-cell lymphoma
Intravascular large B-cell lymphoma
Primary effusion lymphoma
Burkitt lymphoma/leukemia
Hairy cell leukemia
Plasma cell myeloma
Solitary plasmacytoma of bone
B-cell proliferations of uncertain malignant potential
Lymphomatoid granulomatosis
Posttransplant lymphoproliferative disorder, polymorphic
T-CELL AND NK-CELL NEOPLASMS
Precursor T-cell Neoplasms
Precursor T-cell lymphoblastic leukemia/lymphoma
Blastic NK cell lymphoma
Mature T-cell and NK-cell Neoplasms
T-cell prolymphocytic leukemia
T-cell large granular lymphocytic leukemia
Aggressive NK-cell leukemia
Adult T-cell leukemia/lymphoma
Extranodal NK/T-cell lymphoma, nasal type
Enteropathy-type T-cell lymphoma
Hepatosplenic T-cell lymphoma
Subcutaneous panniculitis-like T-cell lymphoma
Mycosis fungoides and Sézary syndrome
Primary cutaneous anaplastic large cell lymphoma
Peripheral T-cell lymphoma, unspecified
Angioimmunoblastic T-cell lymphoma
Anaplastic large cell lymphoma
T-Cell Proliferation of Uncertain Malignant Potential
Lymphomatoid papulosis

CLL, chronic lymphocytic leukemia; MALT, mucosa-associated lymphoid tissue; NK, natural killer.

Table 74-3 **Phenotypic Characteristics of Non-Hodgkin's Lymphoma**

Lymphoma Type	Characteristic CD Antigen Profile
B-cell markers	CD19, CD20, CD22
T-cell markers	CD2, CD3, CD4, CD7, CD8
Anaplastic large cell lymphoma	CD30+ (Ki-1 antigen)
Small lymphocytic lymphoma (B-CLL)	CD5+, CD10–, CD23+, B cell markers
Follicular lymphoma	CD5–, CD10+, CD23±, CD43–, B-cell markers
Marginal-zone (MALT) lymphoma	CD5–, CD10–, CD23–, B cell markers
Mantle cell lymphoma	CD5+, CD10±, CD23–, CD43+, B-cell markers

B-CLL, B-cell chronic lymphocytic leukemia; MALT, mucosa-associated lymphoid tissue

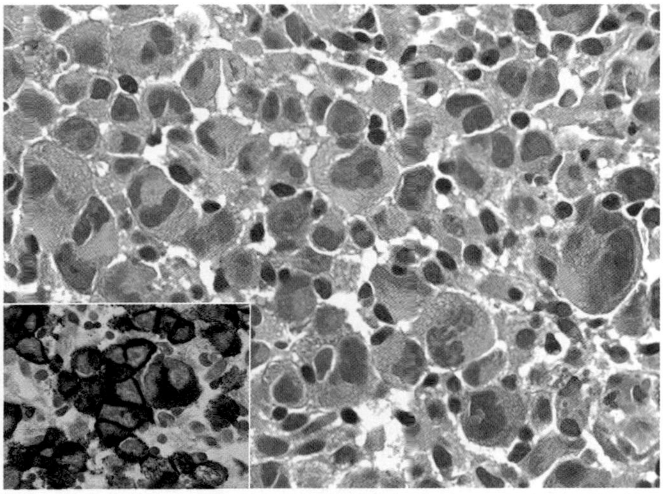

Figure 74-1 Anaplastic large cell lymphoma of lymph node (hematoxylin and eosin stained section). The lymphoma cells are intensely CD30 immunoreactive (*inset*). (Courtesy of Dr. Bruce Patterson, Princess Margaret Hospital, Toronto.)

ing.[62,63] There is strong evidence that S-phase fraction correlates with histologic type, grade, and survival, independent of other clinical prognostic factors.[60,61]

The most common types of NHL seen in North America are diffuse large B-cell lymphoma (DLBCL) and the follicular lymphoma (FL), and the management of lymphomas is based largely on experience with these two disease entities. The propensity for indolent lymphomas to transform to large cell lymphomas has been well documented,[64,65] but our knowledge of factors leading to transformations is limited. Recent studies have implicated alterations in normal p53 function as the factor leading to transformation.[66,67] The more common new entities in the WHO classification include mantle cell lymphoma and various T-cell lymphomas.

Mantle Cell Lymphoma

Mantle cell lymphoma occurs in older adults and commonly presents with generalized disease with spleen, bone marrow, and gastrointestinal tract involvement. Circulating lymphoma cells are frequently found in the blood. It is associated with a characteristic immunophenotype (CD5+, CD10±, and CD23–) and genotype with t(11;14) translocation and *BCL1* (cyclin D1/*CCND1*) gene overexpression.[68-72] Currently this disease is not curable with chemotherapy and a median survival for patients with generalized disease is 3 to 5 years, but early use of high-dose therapy is promising.[73,74] Expression of a microarray gene profile characterized by high proliferation confers a worse prognosis.[75] Localized mantle cell lymphoma is uncommon, and there is little information on response to therapy and curability. Small data sets suggest that the survival of patients with localized mantle cell lymphoma is better than those with advanced disease and that RT has an important role.[72,76]

T-Cell Lymphoma

Peripheral T-cell lymphomas are a heterogeneous group of T-cell neoplasms, more common in Asia,[77,78] usually affecting adults, and commonly widespread at presentation. An aggressive clinical course is typical; and although potentially curable, many T-cell lymphomas are resistant to current chemotherapy regimens. *TCR* (T-cell antigen receptor) gene rearrangements may be identified but are not mandatory for diagnosis. Specific subtypes of T-cell lymphoma to consider include extranodal NK/T-cell lymphoma of nasal type and enteropathy-type T-cell lymphoma, previously called malignant histiocytosis of the intestine. This disease usually involves the jejunum, and in approximately 50% of cases it is associated with a history of gluten-sensitive enteropathy (enteropathy-associated T-cell lymphoma [EATL]).[79,80] Most EATLs express the HML-1 (human mucosal lymphocyte-1) antigen, supporting an origin from the intraepithelial T-cells of MALT. EATLs are high-grade pleomorphic large cell lymphomas associated with a very poor prognosis. The entity of NK/T-cell lymphoma of nasal type includes disorders previously known as lethal midline granuloma and nasal T-cell lymphoma. It is characterized by an angiocentric and angioinvasive infiltrate[13,56,81] (Fig. 74-2), with CD56+ (T/NK cell) immunophenotype, and are characteristically EBV-positive (EBV+). This disease responds poorly to chemotherapy and usually follows an aggressive course.[13,15,81,82] Other rare presenting sites may include skin, lung, testis, and central nervous system.

The WHO classification, although aimed to classify distinct disease entities and acknowledges the uniqueness of certain presentations (e.g., the T-cell lymphomas cited previously), generally neglects to consider the presenting site of the lymphoma. Recent evidence strongly suggests that the presenting site is an important factor for primary extranodal lymphomas. Examples include different etiology for MALT lymphoma arising in different sites, which is associated with differences in relapse rate.[83] Similar histology lymphomas may have distinct outcomes, such as DLCL involving the brain (poor prognosis) versus stomach or Waldeyer's ring structures (good prognosis).[84] With further understanding of the etiology and pathogenesis of lymphomas, future modifications to classification of these diseases are expected.

MOLECULAR BIOLOGY

The various pathologic subtypes of NHL are characterized by distinctive nonrandom genetic alterations. The categories of molecular lesions include chromosomal translocations with activation of oncogene as the most commonly observed abnormality (e.g., *BCL2* in follicular lymphomas), oncogenic viruses (e.g., EBV and HTLV-1), and inactivation of tumor suppression gene by chromosome mutation or deletions (e.g., *p53*). Some of the well-characterized genetic lesions with their

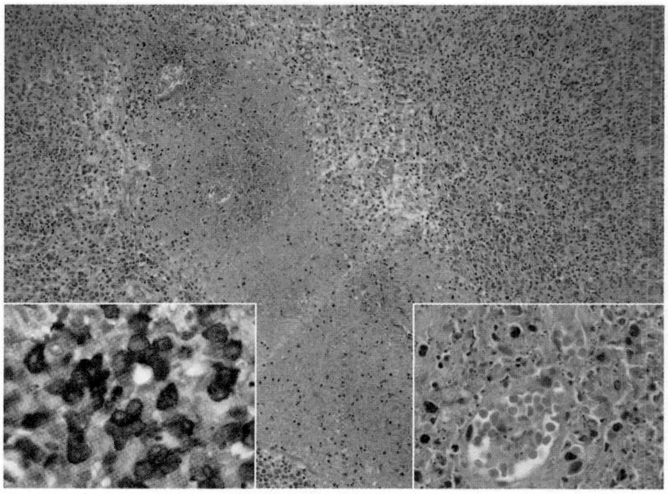

A

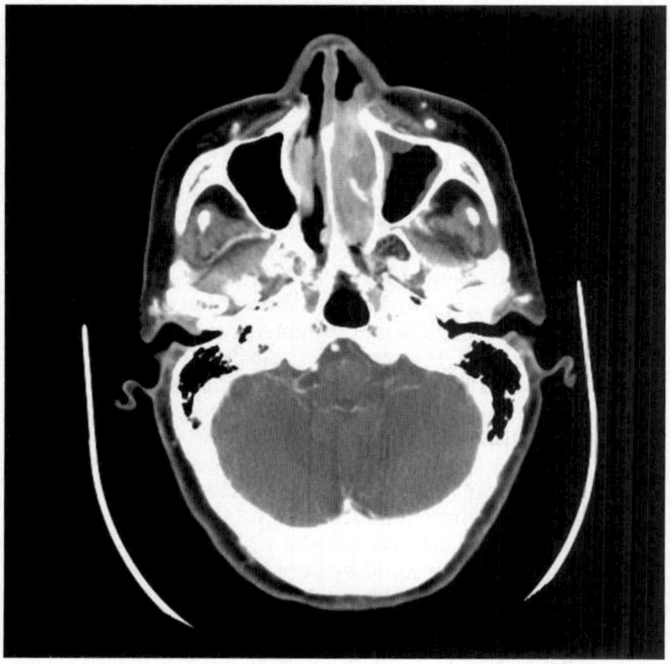

B

Figure 74-2 **A,** Photomicrograph of an extranodal NK/T-cell lymphoma, nasal type (hematoxylin and eosin stained section). There is abundant necrosis, and the lymphoma cells have an angiocentric and angioinvasive growth pattern (*inset right lower corner*). The lymphoma cells are immunoreactive for EBV latent membrane protein (*inset left lower corner*). **B,** Extranodal NK/T-cell lymphoma, nasal type. Axial CT scan showing involvement of the left nasal cavity. CT, computed tomography; EBV, Epstein-Barr virus; NK, natural killer. (**A,** Courtesy of Dr. Bruce Patterson, Princess Margaret Hospital, Toronto.)

corresponding pathologic subtype are presented in Table 74-4. Many of the genetic lesions involve the translocation of an oncogene to a juxtaposition of the immunoglobulin gene (in B-cell) or T-cell receptor gene (in T-cell). Locations of breakpoints usually occur at the joining (J) or switch (S) sequences involved in antigen receptor gene rearrangement as part of normal lymphoid development to produce antigenic variation. The causes of these translocations are largely unknown, but once established these lesions appear to be highly specific for the type of malignant lymphoma that they characterize.

BCL2

The t(14;18)(q32;q21) translocation involving *BCL2* is the most common chromosome translocation in NHL. *BCL2* encodes a 26-kd membrane protein that controls and prevents cellular apoptosis. The gene is translocated to a J segment of the *IGH* gene on chromosome 14, giving rise to deregulation of *BCL2*, with the result being the inhibition of apoptosis of B-cells. This lesion is present in more than 90% of follicular lymphomas and in transformed follicular lymphomas.[85] In the latter situation additional genetic lesions are acquired (*p53* mutation, deletion of chromosome 6q27, *MYC*), in parallel with more rapid growth and an aggressive clinical course. The *p53* mutation is associated with a poor survival rate in aggressive B-cell lymphomas, independent of the predictive effects of the IPI.[67] The t(14;18) translocation is also found in 20% of de novo DLBCL and appears to be an unfavorable prognostic factor.

BCL1

The t(11;14)(q13;q32) translocation is found in 70% of mantle cell lymphomas.[70,71,86] *BCL1*, also known as *PRAD1* (now designated *CCND1*), encodes for cyclin D1 that regulates cell cycle progression. This lesion appears to be highly specific for mantle cell lymphoma, with the translocation of *BCL1* on chromosome 11 to *IGH* gene on chromosome 14, making it an extremely useful adjunct to immunophenotyping in distinguishing mantle cell lymphoma from other types of lymphomas.

BCL6

The *BCL6* gene located on 3q27 is translocated in 40% of diffuse large B-cell lymphomas.[87,88] Reciprocal translocations can involve a number of other chromosomal locations, including 14q32 (*IGH*), 2p11 (*IGK*) and so forth, all juxtaposing to 3q27.[89] *BCL6* is thought to mediate the DNA-binding activity of a number of zinc-finger transcription factors, and characterizes the germinal center B-cell gene signature in microarray studies.[90] The presence of the *BCL6* translocation in DLBCL carries a favorable prognosis, in comparison with those carrying *BCL2* who have a worse outcome, whereas those with neither translocation have an intermediate prognosis.[87]

BCL8

The *BCL8* gene, located on chromosome 15, has recently been cloned.[91] It has been documented that 3% to 4% of DLCLs carry a t(14;15)(q32;q11-13) translocation. *BCL8* is not expressed in normal lymphoid cells, but it is found in human testes and prostate.

MYC

The *MYC* oncogene, located on chromosome 8q24, regulates cellular proliferation and differentiation. Its translocation is seen in 100% of Burkitt's lymphomas typically to chromosome 14q32 (*IGH*), less commonly to 2p11 (*IGK*) and 22q11 (Igλ). EBV infection is responsible for and can be documented in almost all cases of endemic Burkitt's lymphoma and approximately 30% of the sporadic cases.[89,92] Aberrations of 8q24 can also be seen in follicular lymphoma, DLBCL, and mantle cell lymphoma and is characterized by transformation or progression of the disease, generally denoting a poor prognosis.[93,94]

Table 74-4 **Common Genetic Alterations in Non-Hodgkin's Lymphoma**

Oncogene	Translocation	Gene Product	Cellular Activity	Disease
BCL1	t(11;14)(q13;q32)	Cyclin D1	G_1/S progression suppression	Mantle cell (> 90%)
BCL2	t(14;18)(q32;q11)	BCL-2	of apoptosis	Follicular (~85%) DLBCL (~30%)
BCL3	t(14;19)(q32;q13)	?	Transcription repressor	Atypical CLL ALL
BCL3	17q2	?	?	Transformed follicular
BCL6	3q27	BCL-6	Zinc finger transcription factor	Diffuse large cell
c-MYC	8q24	c-MYC	Transcription activation, cell cycle control	Burkitt's ?transformed NHL
p53	17p	p53	Tumor suppressor	Transformed NHL
ALK/NPM	t(2;5)(p23;q35)	Anaplastic lymphoma kinase	Tyrosine kinase	T-anaplastic large cell
LYT10	10q24	?	Transcription factor	Cutaneous T-cell lymphoma (~15%)
PAX5	t(9;14)(p13;q32)	BSAP	Transcription factor	Lymphoplasmacytoid lymphoma
BCL8	t(14;15)(q32;q11-13)	?	Protein kinase A	Diffuse large cell (~4%)
MALT1	t(11;18)(q21;q21) t(14;18)(q32;q21)	API2-MALT1 fusion transcript	Activates NF-κB Deregulation MALT1	MALT (30%—site dependent) MALT (~10%)
BCL10	t(1;14)(p22;q32)	BCL-10	Proapoptotic	MALT (<4%)

ALL, acute lymphoblastic leukemia; BCL, B-cell lymphoma; BSAP, B-cell specific activator protein; CLL, chronic lymphocytic leukemia; DLBCL, diffuse large B-cell lymphoma; MALT, mucosa-associated lymphoid tissue; NF-κB, nuclear factor-κB; NHL, non-Hodgkin's lymphoma; ?, unknown.

Other Chromosome Translocations

The t(2;5)(p23;q35) translocation characterizes anaplastic large cell lymphomas of T-cell origin. This translocation involves the fusion of the *NPM* (nucleophosmin) gene on 5q35 and the *ALK* (anaplastic lymphoma kinase) gene on 2p23.[95] Studies also indicate that lymphoplasmacytoid lymphoma (LPL), including Waldenström's macroglobulinemia (when associated with monoclonal immunoglobulin M [IgM] paraprotein), is associated with a t(9;14)(p13;q32) translocation. The oncogene involved is the *PAX5* gene, which encodes a B-cell transcription factor controlling B-cell proliferation and differentiation.[96,97] In approximately 15% of cutaneous T-cell lymphomas (CTCLs), rearrangement of the *NFKB2/LYT10* gene is found.[98] In MALT lymphomas characteristic genetic abnormalities can include trisomy 3,[31,99] and chromosomal translocations t(11;18)(q21;q21),[100-103] t(1;14)(p22;q32),[104] and t(14;18)(q32;q21) (see Table 74-4).[105]

Microarray Gene Profiling Studies

Gene-expression studies are increasingly used to characterize lymphomas and the most studied is DLBCL, which is a genetically heterogeneous disease. Microarray analysis of cDNA (the *lymphochip*, National Cancer Institute [NCI], Bethesda), using hierarchical clustering techniques, initially classified DLBCL into two groups.[106] One expressed *germinal center B-cell–like* genes (GCB signature), such as *A-myb, LMO2, JNK3, CD10, BCL6, CREL,* and *BCL2*; whereas the other expressed *activated B-cell–like* genes (ABC signature), such as *CCND2, IRF4, FLIP, NF-κB,* and *CD44*. In a preliminary study of 38 patients, the clinical outcome following standard treatment with anthracycline-based chemotherapy showed a 5-year survival for the GCB group of 76%, compared with the ABC group of 16%.[106] In a larger study with 240 patients, where GCB accounted for 48% of DLBCL, ABC made up 30%, and a third subgroup termed *type 3* represented 22%,[90] the prognostic significance of genotyping was confirmed. The 5-year survival rates for the three groups were GCB, 60%; ABC, 35%; type 3, 39%. Further, additional distinct gene signatures were identified with prognostic significance: MLC class II signature (good prognosis), lymph node signature (good prognosis), and proliferation signature (poor prognosis). Based on a selection of the most prognostic genes, either a larger series of 17 genes,[90] or condensing further to 3 immunostains for *CD10, BCL6* and *MUM-1*,[107] studies have shown that gene expression profiling provides additional prognostic information in addition to the clinical IPI scores.[90,107] Additional studies using oligonucleotide microarrays and a different analysis technique have also successfully identified two categories of patients with very different survival rates (70% versus 12%) in DLBCL.[108]

The microarray assays are not widely available and are treated as an experimental technology. However, they helped identify genes that are likely to be prognostic and therefore when in everyday use could be very helpful to the clinician in discerning prognostic information. An example is the recent finding that two GCB signature genes, *BCL6* and *CD10*, when demonstrated positive on staining were associated with a high overall survival (OS), in contrast to *MUM-1* and *CCND2* with expressions associated with poor survival.[107] However, caution is required in interpreting and correlating studies of gene expression with that of protein overexpression, because the latter can be a posttranslational event and may not directly correlate with gene overexpression. An example is the finding of BCL2 protein overexpression having a negative impact on clinical outcome,[109] whereas *BCL2* gene expression is characteristic of the GCB signature and connotes a favorable prognosis.[90,110]

Other examples of microarray studies discovering significant findings correlating with clinical outcome include primary mediastinal B-cell lymphomas,[111] mantle cell lymphoma,[75] and follicular lymphoma.[112] In the case of follicular lymphoma, it is interesting that the gene signature of the nonmalignant infiltrating immune cells, rather than the malignant cells, had the prognostic effect.[112] It is likely that within the next decade, most lymphomas will have their distinct genetic signatures identified. In addition to its usefulness in obtaining an accurate diagnosis and enhancing prognostication, these techniques could also be helpful in the study of minimal residual disease, such as the detection of a small number of morphologically normal but genetically monoclonal population of malignant cells. The most important aspect of this evolving field is the insight provided into the molecular events underlying malignant transformation, cell cycle regulation, signal transduction, and cell death. Characterization of these mechanisms opens up the potential for novel therapeutic strategies, for example targeting small molecules such as NF-κB.[113]

CLINICAL MANIFESTATIONS, PATIENT EVALUATION, AND STAGING CLASSIFICATION

Clinical Manifestations

Presenting signs and symptoms of NHL are highly variable. The most common presentation is with an asymptomatic lymph node enlargement. Peripheral lymph node involvement, although rare (epitrochlear, popliteal, etc.), is most common in indolent lymphomas and is common in generalized disease. Small, nonprogressive, waxing and waning lymph node enlargement is characteristic of indolent lymphomas. Lack of progressive enlargement of lymph nodes may lead to a delay in diagnosis. The most common presenting sites of nodal lymphomas are neck, inguinal, and abdominal lymph nodes. Mediastinal lymph node involvement is less common than in Hodgkin's lymphoma, except for primary mediastinal (thymic) lymphoma. Some patients present with systemic symptoms of fever, weight loss, and, less frequently, night sweats, usually heralding the presence of more advanced disease.

In primary extranodal lymphomas, presenting symptoms depend on the site of origin and do not differ significantly from symptoms of other malignancies affecting a specific organ. Occasionally, the clinical appearance of a lymphomatous lesion may not be characteristic of a malignancy and may mimic benign inflammatory lesions. Careful histopathologic examination, therefore, is extremely important in arriving at an early diagnosis. Characteristically, gastric lymphomas present with symptoms of peptic ulcer, bowel lymphomas with intestinal obstruction, or diarrhea, whereas primary bone lymphoma present with pain. Primary lymphomas with diffuse involvement of an organ (e.g., liver, spleen, bone marrow) rather than a distinct tumor are particularly difficult to diagnose and are often diagnosed with advanced disease. Tumor bulk at presentation is also related to primary site. Usually primary lymphomas of skin or orbital structures are visible and therefore diagnosed early; extradural lymphomas develop symptoms early and present with small bulk disease. In contrast, gastrointestinal lymphomas with nonspecific symptoms, and thyroid lymphomas (especially if associated with preexisting goiter) often present with bulky disease. In the absence of nodal involvement, lymphoma is often not suspected or distinguished clinically from carcinoma; therefore, immunophenotypic and histochemical analyses are particularly important.

Patient Evaluation

The goal of evaluation is to determine disease extent, determine its anatomic distribution, and ascertain normal organ and immune function relevant to the choice of therapy. With the diverse presentation of lymphomas, it is difficult to have a uniform set of investigations for every patient,[114] but the following recommended procedures serve as minimum investigations (Table 74-5). Additional tests may be necessary based on such factors as the presenting complaint, the subtype of lymphoma, and predilection of organ involvement (e.g., brain and cerebrospinal fluid [CSF]).

Table 74-5 Diagnostic Workup for Non-Hodgkin's Lymphoma

GENERAL
History, including systemic symptoms (unexplained fever, night sweats, weight loss > 10% of body weight), risk factors for HIV infection
Physical examination: special attention to lymphatic sites, organomegaly
For palpable lymph nodes: note and record number, size, location, shape, texture, and mobility
Mirror examination of larynx and pharynx if clinically indicated
SPECIAL TESTS
Standard
Bone marrow biopsy (minimum unilateral iliac crest)
Review of slides by expert hematopathologist
Cytologic evaluation, if any effusion present
Lumbar puncture to examine cerebrospinal fluid for parameningeal sites, testes, extradural presentations, or when clinically indicated
IMAGING STUDIES
Standard
CT scans of neck, thorax, abdomen, and pelvis
Gallium scan or FDG-PET
Complementary
Upper GI or small bowel series when clinically indicated
CT scan of brain when clinically indicated
Bone scan if clinically indicated
MRI if clinically indicated
LABORATORY STUDIES
Standard
CBC (including platelet count, reticulocyte count), blood chemistries (including BUN, creatinine, uric acid levels)
LDH, bilirubin, transaminases, alkaline phosphatase
Complementary
Erythrocyte sedimentation rate
Serum electrophoresis
HIV serology when clinically indicated

BUN, blood urea nitrogen; CBC, complete blood (cell) count; CT, computed tomography; FDG-PET, ^{18}F-fluorodeoxyglucose positron emission tomography; GI, gastrointestinal; LDH, lactate dehydrogenase; MRI, magnetic resonance imaging.

History and Physical Examination

A complete history with attention to duration of symptoms and rate of lymph node enlargement should be obtained. Constitutional symptoms (fever, night sweats, and unexplained weight loss) as well as performance status should be documented. Risk factors for lymphoma, particularly immunosuppressive conditions including risk factors for HIV infection, immunosuppressive therapy, and the presence of autoimmune diseases, should also be documented. Physical examination should include the lymphoid system, including, where relevant, Waldeyer's ring structures. The location and size of lymph node masses should be documented. This is especially important for the subsequent determination of RT target volume because following chemotherapy, no gross disease may be present at the time of radiation treatment planning.

Pathologic Diagnosis

Histologic confirmation of the diagnosis by an experienced hematopathologist is mandatory. Inadequate specimens should prompt the consideration of repeat biopsy with attention to obtaining fresh tissue for immunophenotypic and cytogenetic studies. A diagnosis can also be established solely on the basis of a fine needle aspirate of a tumor mass.[115,116]

Laboratory Tests

Minimum laboratory tests include a complete blood count, lactate dehydrogenase (LDH), bilirubin, transaminases, and creatinine level. An HIV serology test should be performed when risk factors of HIV infection are present, or in high-grade lymphomas, even if there are no obvious risk factors. A unilateral bone marrow biopsy should be done. CSF cytology is performed in patients with risk factors for leptomeningeal spread, i.e., bone marrow or peripheral blood involvement; high-grade lymphoma; HIV infection; and lymphoma presenting in brain, testes, epidural space, eye, or paranasal sinuses.

Imaging Studies

Computed tomography (CT) of the neck, thorax, abdomen, and pelvis are the minimum standard. The radiographic assessment of the extent of extranodal involvement is of particular importance in the planning of RT, because 50% of localized lymphomas occur in extranodal sites. Other radiographs should be obtained based on the actual or suspected organ involved. Bipedal lymphangiogram is associated with significant false-positive and false-negative rates and in today's practice is no longer used.[114,117,118] Magnetic resonance imaging (MRI) is indicated in delineating areas of suspected involvement of bone or CNS, such as spinal cord and epidural space, brain stem, base of skull and cavernous sinuses, and leptomeninges. MRI of the spinal column is very sensitive for detection of bone marrow involvement.[119] The role of routine MRI scans for the thorax, abdomen, and pelvis has not been established. Bone scans are not recommended as routine tests except in patients with bone pain or those presenting with localized bone lymphoma. A total body ^{67}Gallium (^{67}Ga) scan or a ^{18}F-fluorodeoxyglucose positron emission tomography (FDG-PET) scan is useful staging procedure and also serves as a follow-up test to document response to therapy. ^{67}Ga scintigraphy has 76% to 100% sensitivity and 75% to 96% specificity to determine if a residual mass represents residual cancer or only fibrosis and necrosis.[120] The sensitivity of ^{67}Ga scan for diagnosis of recurrence is 95%, and the specificity is 89%.[120] Patients with persistently positive gallium scans after 1 to 3 courses of chemotherapy have lower disease-free rates than those who became gallium negative.[121,122] FDG-PET scan is replacing ^{67}Ga scans in clinical practice, and one nonrandomized study comparing the two imaging modalities in terms of sensitivity concluded that FDG-PET is more disease-site sensitive than ^{67}Ga (100% versus 71.5%).[123] Other investigators have made similar conclusions from studies of small numbers of patients.[124,125] Whole-body FDG-PET has a high predictive value for differentiating active from necrotic residual masses in lymphomas.[126-128] Emerging evidence also suggests that persistent FDG-PET activity after 1 to 3 cycles of chemotherapy confers a worse prognosis.[129-131]

Staging Classification

The American Joint Committee on Cancer and the International Union Against Cancer have endorsed the use of the Ann Arbor classification for staging of NHL. The Ann Arbor staging classification has been used for more than 20 years.[132,133] In the Ann Arbor system, Waldeyer's ring, thymus, spleen, appendix, and Peyer's patches of the small intestine are considered lymphatic tissues; and involvement of these areas does not constitute an "E" lesion, originally defined as extralymphatic involvement. However, because of the unique pathologic and clinical characteristics of primary lymphoma affecting these organs, most clinicians consider them separate clinical entities and report their involvement as extranodal presentation. The Ann Arbor classification differentiates locoregional from widespread lymphoma and documents anatomic extent of disease and B symptoms, but it is not optimal for describing the extent of local disease, invasion of adjacent organs, tumor bulk, or multiple sites of involvement within one organ, such as skin and the gastrointestinal tract. Several modifications to the Ann Arbor classification have been proposed in the past. In head and neck lymphoma, the size of the primary tumor has been classified according to the tumor, node, metastasis (TNM) classification for squamous cell carcinoma of that region.[134] In gastric lymphoma, substaging of stage I to reflect the depth of the stomach wall penetration has been suggested. These proposals reflect local tumor bulk but do not add substantially to the overall value of staging classification. In stage II disease, distinction of involvement of the immediate nodal region (II_1) versus more extensive regional lymph node involvement (II_2) has been found to have prognostic significance in primary gastrointestinal lymphomas.[135,136] Currently, the Ann Arbor staging classification supplemented by description of prognostic factors including tumor bulk, hematologic and biochemical parameters, sites of involvement, and pathology, remains as the basis for patient assessment.

PROGNOSTIC FACTORS

Although the anatomic extent of disease reflected by Ann Arbor stage is an important prognostic factor, many other factors are known to influence the outcome in patients with NHL. They include histologic type, phenotype (B-cell versus T-cell),[77,78] tumor bulk,[137,138] number of involved nodal regions and extranodal sites, and proliferation indices (S-phase fraction, Ki-67 antigen)[62,63,139] as well as age, gender, and performance status (Table 74-6).[140] Prognostic factors related to tumor

Table 74-6 Prognostic Factors in Non-Hodgkin's Lymphoma

Factor	Favorable	Adverse
Histologic type	Low-grade MALT	Diffuse large cell Mantle cell
Immunophenotype	B-cell	T-cell, NK-cell
Tumor bulk	<5 cm	>10 cm
Ann Arbor stage	I, II	III, IV
Symptoms	Asymptomatic	B-symptoms
Proliferative indices	S-phase fraction <5% Ki-67 <80%	High % S-phase Ki-67 >80%
Age	<60 years	≥60 years
LDH	Normal level	Abnormal level
β_2 microglobulin	Normal level	High level
HLA-DR expression	Present	Absent
CD44 expression	Low	High
BCL2 protein	High	Low
BCL6 rearrangement	Present	Absent
Site of extranodal presentation	Orbit, skin, tonsil	Brain, testis

HLA, human-leukocyte antigen; LDH, lactate dehydrogenase; MALT, mucosa-associated lymphoid tissue; NK, natural killer.

Table 74-7 **International Prognostic Index for Non-Hodgkin's Lymphomas**

Risk Factors	Unfavorable Feature	Risk Group	Number of Risk Factors	5-y Survival (%)
Age	>60 y	Low	0 or 1	73
LDH	>1 × normal	Low-intermediate	2	51
Performance status*	2-4	High-intermediate	3	43
Stage (Ann Arbor)	III-IV	High	4 or 5	26
Extranodal involvement	>1 site			

*Eastern Cooperative Oncology Group Classification.
LDH, lactate dehydrogenase; y, year.

bulk and extent of disease include hemoglobin and albumin levels, LDH, erythrocyte sedimentation rate (ESR), β_2-microglobulin level, and interleukin 6 levels.[141-145] IPI was derived from patients treated with doxorubicin-based chemotherapy in phase II and III trials. Based on factors identified in multivariate analysis, the IPI is based on patient's age, serum LDH, performance status, and number of involved extranodal sites (Table 74-7).[145] Patients are grouped according to the number of adverse factors, for example, age older than 60 years, stage III or IV, abnormal LDH level, performance status greater than 1, and more than one involved extranodal site. Patients in the low-risk group (0 to 1 adverse factors) treated with doxorubicin-based chemotherapy ± RT had a 73% 5-year survival, those in low intermediate group (two adverse factors) had a 51% 5-year survival, patients in the high intermediate group (three adverse factors) had a 43% 5-year survival, and those in high-risk group (four or five adverse factors) had a 26% 5-year survival.[145] A similar pattern of decreasing survival with an increasing number of adverse factors was observed in younger patients. The validity of the IPI has been confirmed in a population of patients with T-cell lymphomas.[146] The IPI was less useful in indolent lymphomas,[147] and a different index has been proposed—the follicular lymphoma IPI (FLIPI).[148] The FLIPI is based on the following adverse prognostic factors: age older than 60 years, stage III or IV, abnormal LDH level, five or more involved nodal areas, and hemoglobin less than 120 g/L.[148] Other prognostic factors include high expression of CD44 cell surface adhesion molecule,[149] expression of HLA-DR, presence of BCL6 rearrangement, high levels of BCL2 protein secretion,[109] survivin expression,[150] and *p53* mutation.[67] The prognostic significance of gene profiling with microarray studies have been discussed previously. In addition to the genetic and phenotypic factors, the presenting site of lymphoma has prognostic implications; for example, lymphoma presenting in testis, ovary, eye, central nervous system, and liver has a particularly adverse prognosis, whereas orbital and skin lymphomas generally have a good prognosis.

PRINCIPLES OF MANAGEMENT

Almost all patients with localized NHL are treated with curative intent. A palliative approach is used only when, because of the condition of the patient or the extent or location of the disease, a radical course of treatment carries no chance of cure. Knowledge of histology, extent, and pattern of disease is essential to select the appropriate therapeutic strategy. Local radiation is routinely used, both for cure and local control. However, the recognition of the high risk for occult distant disease mandates the use of chemotherapy in most cases. The main modalities used in treatment programs for NHL are chemotherapy and RT, but surgery is used in diagnosis and management of selected cases. For localized disease the initial decision for patients treated with curative intent is the use of a combined-modality approach—chemotherapy and RT, or a local treatment alone with RT. The choice is predicated on the inherent risk of occult distant disease, availability of curative chemotherapy, and the potential need for local control. Patients with advance disease (stages III and IV) are mainly treated with chemotherapy alone.

Radiation Therapy

The aim of RT is to deliver an adequate dose of radiation to the target volume to ensure a high rate of local control. The design for a proper course of RT must take into account the extent of disease, the appropriate margins, routes of lymphatic and possible extranodal spread, and the radiation tolerance of normal tissues and organs. Dose fractionation parameters must assure local control with acceptable acute and long-term toxicity. The technique should guarantee reproducibility of treatment on a daily basis. Custom-designed fields should be used to conform to the target volume while keeping the volume of irradiated normal tissues to a minimum. The use of CT simulation with delineation of target volumes (gross tumor volume, clinical target volume [CTV], and planning target volume [PTV]), as well as dosimetric evaluation in three dimensions is the standard for most indications.

RT techniques and prescriptions are discussed in detail later in this chapter. It is important to note that when RT follows chemotherapy in CMT protocols, RT is usually started 4 to 6 weeks following the last course of chemotherapy to allow recovery of blood counts and to minimize the drug-radiation sensitization effect. McManus and colleagues documented an increased risk of RT treatment interruption because of both thrombocytopenia and neutropenia with concurrent chemotherapy.[151]

Chemotherapy

Frequently used chemotherapy regimens for NHL are listed in Table 74-8. These include single agents used for indolent lymphoma, anthracycline-containing regimens potentially curative for diffuse large cell B-cell (e.g., CHOP-(R) [cyclophosphamide, Adriamycin (doxorubicin), Oncovin (vincristine), and prednisone]-rituximab) or T-cell lymphomas, and regimens used for patients with recurrent disease. For high-grade lymphoblastic and Burkitt's lymphomas, dose-intensive protocols are used with concurrent intrathecal chemotherapy for CNS prophylaxis.[152,153] In combined-modality approach for localized disease, it is useful to deliver the chemotherapy first to promptly treat potential systemic microscopic disease and reduce the bulk of the known local disease. In this setting, the goal of chemotherapy is to facilitate a response but not necessarily obtain a complete response at the

Table 74-8 Common Chemotherapy Regimens for Non-Hodgkin's Lymphoma

Indolent Lymphoma	Histologically aggressive Lymphoma	Salvage Therapy
Chlorambucil ± prednisone	CHOP-(R)	DHAP
CVP-(R)	cyclophosphamide	dexamethasone
cyclophosphamide	doxorubicin	cytarabine (araC)
vincristine	vincristine	cisplatin
prednisone	prednisone	ESHAP
(rituximab)	(rituximab)	etoposide
CHOP or CHOP-(R) (see next column)	MACOP-B	methylprednisolone
Fludarabine	methotrexate with folinic acid rescue	cytarabine
FCM-(R)	doxorubicin	cisplatin
fludarabine	cyclophosphamide	mini-BEAM
cyclophosphamide	vincristine	BCNU
mitoxantrone	bleomycin	etoposide
(rituximab)	prednisone	cytarabine (araC)
2-Chlorodeoxyadenosine (2-CDA)	m-BACOD	melphalan
Tositumomab (Bexxar) and ^{131}Iodine	methotrexate with folinic acid rescue	ICE
Tositumomab	bleomycin	ifosfamide
^{90}Yttrium-ibritumomab Tiuxetan	doxorubicin	carboplatin
(Zevalin)	cyclophosphamide	etoposide
	vincristine	GDP
	dexamethasone	gemcitabine
	ProMACE-CytaBOM	dexamethasone
	cyclophosphamide	cisplatin
	doxorubicin	
	etoposide	
	prednisone	
	cytarabine	
	bleomycin	
	vincristine	
	methotrexate with folinic acid rescue	

local site. Quite often, residual thickening or a minimal mass of tissue remains by palpation or imaging, which should not deter the clinician from proceeding with the original RT plan.

The common acute but reversible toxicity of chemotherapy includes nausea and vomiting, alopecia, mucositis, fatigue, pancytopenia with risk of infection and bleeding, and any organ-specific toxicity such as neuropathy for vinca alkaloids, diabetes for glucocorticoids, and pneumonitis for bleomycin. Rituximab may cause infusion-related side effects such as fever, chills, and rigors, which can be avoided with a slower infusion rate. Advances in supportive care (e.g., antiemetic drug and growth factor support) have alleviated many of these acute side effects. Severe long-term toxicity is infrequent but may include gonadal damage particularly in males, cardiomyopathy (with doxorubicin), pulmonary fibrosis (with bleomycin or methotrexate), neurotoxicity (with vinca alkaloids or cisplatin), and impairment of hematopoietic reserve (with alkylating drugs).

Surgery

The principal role for surgery is to establish the diagnosis of lymphoma. It is important to be aware of requirements for optimal pathology interpretation, which include immunophenotypic and molecular studies. Special fixative and fresh tissue is commonly required and it is important to alert the surgeon of a probable diagnosis of lymphoma if at all possible. The therapeutic role of surgery is not well defined. Case series reports have identified a small proportion of patients with stage I nodal or extranodal lymphomas that have been cured with surgery alone. Although surgery can provide excellent local control in select extranodal sites, cure is infrequent because of a high likelihood of microscopic residual disease. The need for the use of chemotherapy, RT, or both is generally not diminished following surgical excision of lymphoma. Therefore aggressive surgical procedures that compromise function or cosmesis should be avoided. For example, radical neck dissection is not required for lymphoma presenting in the neck, total parotidectomy with possible risk to the facial nerve is not indicated for parotid lymphoma, mastectomy is not indicated for a breast lymphoma, and cystectomy is not required to cure bladder lymphoma. Situations where surgery is a potentially good treatment option for local control include possibly partial gastrectomy for localized gastric lymphoma and orchiectomy for testis lymphoma.

MANAGEMENT OF LOCALIZED (STAGES I AND II) DISEASE

Small Lymphocytic Lymphoma and Follicular Lymphoma, Grades 1 and 2

Stages I and II presentations account for 20% to 30% of indolent lymphomas.[154] With the availability of sensitive techniques to detect subclinical disease (e.g., *BCL2* by PCR), some patients with stage I or II disease may have a clonal population of B cells identified in the peripheral blood, bone marrow, or both.[155] However, the clinical significance of this finding with respect to the clinical outcome in patients treated with local therapy is unknown. Localized RT produces excellent local disease control (more than 95%), and a freedom from relapse rate of 50% at 10 years. Data from Stanford University,[156,157] Princess Margaret Hospital (PMH),[158-160] M. D. Anderson Hospital,[161-163] the British National Lymphoma Investigation (BNLI),[164] and St. Bartholomew's Hospital in London[165] documented comparable results with more than 90% local control and 10-year relapse-free rates of approxi-

Table 74-9 Localized (Stages I-II) Follicular Lymphoma, Treatment Results with Radiation Therapy ± Chemotherapy

First Author (y)	Institution	Number of Patients	Treatment	Freedom from Relapse (10-y)	Overall Survival (10-y)
Soubeyran, et al., 1988[166]	Fondation Bergonié, France	103	RT ± CT	49%*	56%
Kelsey, et al., 1994[169]	British National Lymphoma Investigation	148	RT + CT	42%	42%
		(RCT)	RT	33%	52%
Vaughan Hudson, et al., 1994[164]	British National Lymphoma Investigation	208	RT	47%	64%
Mac Manus, et al., 1996[156]	Stanford	177	RT	44%	64%
Seymour, et al., 2003[171]	M. D. Anderson Cancer Center	83	RT + CT	72%	80%
Petersen, et al., 2004[160]	Princess Margaret Hospital, Canada	460	RT	51%	62%

*Relapse-free survival rate.
CT, chemotherapy; RCT, randomized controlled trial; RT, radiation therapy; y, year.

mately 50% with overall survival rates (OSRs) of 70%. A number of representative single institution results published in the last decade are summarized in Table 74-9. At Stanford, the use of extended-field (EF), subtotal, or total lymphoid irradiation gave a higher relapse-free rate of 67% at 10 years, compared to 36% for patients treated to only one side of the diaphragm.[156] However, the OSR was similar.[156]

Prognostic factors predictive of a high risk of relapse included age, extent of disease as reflected by stage, systemic symptoms, and tumor bulk.[156,159,166] Follicular-mixed cell histology is also an adverse factor for relapse.[156] The addition of chemotherapy (e.g., CVP) tested in several randomized trials in the 1970s did not confer an OS advantage.[167-170] Phase II trials of patients with poor prognostic factors (constitutional symptoms, high LDH, follicular large cell histology) treated with CMT (e.g., CHOP-bleomycin) documented 10-year failure-free rate and OSRs of 73% and 82% respectively, suggesting benefit for CMT.[171] With no definitive data showing a survival advantage with CMT, involved-field radiation therapy (IFRT) is currently the preferred therapy in this group of patients. Given the benefits of adding rituximab to either CVP (cyclophosphamide, vincristine, and prednisone) or CHOP in stages III and IV patients, it is important to study if rituximab-containing combinations, with or without RT, may yield better results compared with RT alone. A study of selected stages I to II patients who were observed with no initial treatment showed that 38% required therapy after a median of 86 months.[172] However, a policy of observation is not appropriate for all patients because a plateau in the disease-free survival curve for the radiation-treated patients beyond 15 years has been observed suggesting that a proportion of patients are cured.[156,160]

There is marked variation in RT practice for localized indolent lymphoma.[114,173] RT target volume varies widely.[156,174,175] Extensive radiation has potential to compromise bone marrow reserve, is associated with immunosuppression and a higher risk of secondary solid tumors. IFRT is currently considered as the standard approach. With moderate doses of radiation (30 to 35 Gy, over a 4-week period), the local control rate is more than 95%. Relapse at unirradiated sites occurs in more than 50% of patients. Treatment at the time of recurrence requires chemotherapy, but RT is also very useful in selected cases. High response rates are observed even with a low total dose of 4 Gy (2 Gy × 2).[176-178] Because of the indolent nature of these lymphomas, long-term follow-up is required to test the effects of any new treatment approaches on survival. The relative rarity of localized disease, the long follow-up required, and competing mortality from unrelated causes form significant barriers to the conduct of clinical trials in this disease.

Marginal Zone Lymphoma, Mucosa-Associated Lymphoid Tissue Type

MALT lymphomas are usually indolent B-cell tumors, presenting with stages I to II disease in 70% to 90% of cases. They are characterized by infiltration of mucosa, lymphoepithelial lesions, and clonal proliferation of centrocyte-like B-cells.[31,56,179,180] MALT lymphomas arise most commonly in the stomach, orbit, thyroid, salivary glands, breast, lung, skin, and bladder.[31] The etiology of gastric MALT lymphoma is linked to infection with *H. pylori*. Recent data indicate an association of *C. psittaci* with orbital adnexal MALT lymphoma.[32] Cutaneous MALT lymphoma has been associated with *Borrelia burgdorferi* infection in Europe[181] but not in the United States.[182,183] Although the majority of patients with gastric MALT lymphoma respond to antibiotics therapy, the t(11;18)(q21;q21) translocation has been reported to associate with resistance to *H. pylori* therapy.[184,185] The fact that this translocation is also found in MALT lymphoma arising from nongastric sites such as lung and orbit[100] suggests a common genetic mechanism in the development of disease in these sites for some patients. IFRT with doses of 25 to 35 Gy results in more than 95% local control and a significant proportion of patients may be cured.[83,186,187] Although MALT lymphomas are usually indolent, transformation into aggressive large cell lymphomas occurs. Current experience with MALT lymphomas shows a tendency to localized disease and cure with local therapy.[83,188] The nodal counterpart of MALT, also known as monocytoid B-cell lymphoma, occurs in an older age group and is similar morphologically and immunologically to MALT lymphoma.[189]

Large Cell Lymphomas (Diffuse Large B-cell Lymphoma)

The treatment of localized large cell lymphomas has evolved from the use of RT alone to the routine use of CMT. The best results with RT alone were obtained in small trials that included meticulously staged patients with favorable prognostic factors.[190,191] Pathologic stage I patients have 10-year relapse-free rates of approximately 90% with RT alone.[190,191] Similarly, stage IA or IIA patients with favorable clinical attributes treated with RT alone to a dose of 35 Gy achieved a 77% relapse-free rate at 10 years.[192] In the early 1980s, several phase III trials showed the superiority of chemotherapy and radiation.[167,168] CMT became the standard approach, with the administration of three to eight courses of doxorubicin-containing chemotherapy followed by IFRT. Brief chemotherapy with three courses of CHOP followed by radiation (30 Gy or equivalent) produces excellent results in patients with nonbulky (<10 cm) stages I to II with 10-year progression-free survival (PFS) of 74% and OS of 63% after a median follow-up of 7.3 years.[193] Other investigators achieved similar results with four to six cycles of CHOP and RT,[194,195] alternating CHVP with RT,[196] or four cycles of ProMACE (prednisone, methotrexate, doxorubicin, cyclophosphamide, and etoposide)-MOPP (mechlorethamine, vincristine, procarbazine, and prednisone) and RT.[197] Representative CMT results published in the last decade are presented in Table 74-10. With the success of chemotherapy in advanced NHL, the role of routine radiotherapy in localized disease was questioned and trials of chemotherapy alone for localized nonbulky DLCLs have been conducted.

The results of two large phase III trials testing chemotherapy alone versus CMT are shown in Table 74-11. In the Eastern Cooperative Oncology Group (ECOG) trial (E1484), 345 patients with stages I and II disease (including bulky tumors) were treated with eight courses of CHOP chemotherapy and randomized to receive consolidation IFRT or no further treatment.[198] For those with complete response randomized to RT, the dose was 30 Gy, whereas all partial response patients received 40 Gy. With an intent-to-treat analysis, the 6-year disease-free survival was 53% in the CHOP arm and 69% in the CMT arm ($p = 0.05$). The OS at 6 years was 67% for CHOP alone and 79% for CMT ($p = 0.23$).[198] Patients with a partial response to CHOP received RT; their 6-year failure-free survival was 63%, similar to those achieving a complete response to CHOP. This trial confirmed the benefit of IFRT in patients who received CHOP chemotherapy in terms of disease control. However, no OS benefit was evident in this trial, but the trial had inadequate power to detect a clinically important (10%) survival difference.

The SWOG trial included 401 stages I and II nonbulky (tumor mass <10-cm maximum diameter) patients and compared treatment with eight courses of CHOP versus three courses of CHOP followed by IFRT.[199] The radiation dose was 40 Gy with a boost to 50 Gy for partial responders to three courses of CHOP. Patients treated with CMT had a superior 5-year PFS (PFS: 77% versus 64%, $p = 0.03$) and OSRs (82% versus 72%, $p = 0.02$).[199] The adverse risk factors included stage II disease, older than age 60 years, increased LDH, and ECOG performance status of greater than 1. This raised a concern that patients with adverse prognostic factors might have had inadequate chemotherapy in the CMT arm. The decision to use fewer than six courses of chemotherapy should be based on known prognostic factors that predict for tumor burden.[143,145,199,200] We currently recommend that patients without unfavorable risk factors (i.e., nonbulky disease, nodal stage I, normal LDH, no B symptoms, and good performance status) be treated with three courses of CHOP followed by IFRT. Patients with one or more risk factors should be approached with a longer course of chemotherapy (six cycles) and IFRT. Rituximab should be used in combination with CHOP for DLBCL in view of the beneficial results obtained in patients with stages III and IV disease.[201]

The general principles of RT in CMT protocols is to use IFRT, to a dose of 30 to 35 Gy over 3 to 4 weeks. Additional phase III trials from the French cooperative group Groupe d'Etude des Lymphomes de l'Adulte (GELA) have been reported.[202,203] A benefit for CMT was not demonstrated when compared to chemotherapy alone. The GELA LNH 93-4 trial studied patients older than age 60 years, with zero IPI factors,

Table 74-10 Localized (Stages I and II) Histologically Aggressive Lymphoma, Treatment Results with Combined-Modality Therapy

First Author (y)	Institution	Number of Patients	Treatment	Progression-Free Survival (5-y)	Overall Survival (5-y)
Cosset, et al., 1991[196]	IGR, France	55 (Bulk ≥ 5 cm)	CHVP + RT	68%*	69%
Tondini, et al., 1993[194]	Milan	183	CHOP × 4 + RT	83%	83%
Osterman, 1996[501]	Umea/Lund,	50 (stage I)	CHOP + RT	81%	74% – RS
Munck, 1996[502]	IGR, France	96 (Bulk > 5 cm)	CHVP + RT	71%†	77%
Villikka, 1997[503]	Helsinki University	76 (stage I)	various CT ± RT	87%	82%
Donato, 1998[504]	La Sapienza, Rome	39	various CT + RT	65%†	68%
van der Maazen, et al., 1998[195]	Nijmegen, Netherlands	94 (stage I)	CHOP + RT	83%*/10 y	70%/10 y
Zinzani, 2001[505]	Bologna, Italy	118	MACOP-B ± RT	78%/14 y	69%/14 y)
Shenkier, 2001[193]	Vancouver	308	CHOP × 3 + RT	81% 74%/10 y	80% 63%/10 y
Miller, 2004[506]	SWOG-0014	62 (1 risk factor)	CHOP-R × 3 + RT	94%/2 y	95%/2 y

*Freedom from relapse rate
†Disease-free survival rate
CHOP, cyclophosphamide, Adriamycin (doxorubicin), Oncovin (vincristine), and prednisone; CHOP-R, cyclophosphamide, Adriamycin (doxorubicin), Oncovin (vincristine), prednisone and rituximab; CHVP, cyclophosphamide, doxorubicin, VM26 (teniposide), prednisone; CT, computed tomography; IGR, Institut Gustave Roussy; MACOP-B, Adriamycin, cyclophosphamide, vincristine, methotrexate, bleomycin and prednisolone; RS, relative survival; RT, radiation therapy; SWOG, Southwest Oncology Group; y, year.

Table 74-11 **Localized (Stages I-II) Aggressive Lymphoma, Randomized Clinical Trials of Combined-Modality Treatment versus Radiation Treatment, and Combined-Modality Treatment versus Chemotherapy**

Author	Institution	Number of Patients	Treatment	5-y PFS	5-y Survival
Monfardini, et al., 1980[167]	Istituto Nazionale Tumori, Milan	37 31	RT (40 Gy-50 Gy) RT + CVP × 6	45% 76% *p* = .007	52% 80% *p* = .09
Nissen, et al., 1983[168]	Finsen Institute, Denmark	22 34	RT (37 Gy-43 Gy) RT + COP	15/22 relapsed 4/34 relapsed *p* < .001	13/22 died 3/34 died *p* < .01
Yahalom, et al., 1993[170]	MSKCC, New York	14 12	RT (30 Gy-55 Gy) RT + CHOP x 6	20% (7 y) 86% (7 y) *p* = .004	47% (7 y) 92% (7 y) *p* = .08
Miller, et al., 1998[199]	SWOG 8736‡	200 201	CHOP × 3 + RT (40 Gy-55 Gy) CHOP x 8	77% 64% *p* = .02	82% 72% *p* = .02
Horning, et al., 2004[198]	ECOG E1484†	103 112	CHOP × 8 + RT (30 Gy-40 Gy) CHOP × 8	69% (6 y)* 53% (6 y)* *p* = .05	79% (6 y) 67% (6 y) *p* = .23
Fillet, et al., 2002[203]	GELA, Europe LNH 93-4 Interim results	Total: 455 Age > 60 IPI 0	CHOP × 4 + RT (40 Gy) CHOP × 4	64% 69% *p* = .4	70% 78% p = .2
Reyes, et al., 2005[202]	GELA, Europe LNH 93-1 (Age 16-60 y IPI score 0)	329 318	CHOP × 3 + RT (40 Gy) ACVBP × 3 + CT consolidation	74% 82% *p* < .001	81% 90% *p* = .001

*Disease-free survival rate.
†Excluded stage I non-bulky patients,
‡Excluded stage II with tumor bulk ≥ 10 cm.
ACVCP, doxorubicin, cyclophosphamide, vincristine, bleomycin and prednisone induction; CHOP, cyclophosphamide, Adriamycin (doxorubicin), Oncovin (vincristine), and prednisone; CT, computed tomography; CVP, cyclophosphamide, vincristine, and prednisone; ECOG, Eastern Cooperative Oncology Group; GELA, Groupe d'Etude des Lymphomes de l'Adulte; IPI, International Prognostic Index; LNH, Lymphoma non-Hodgkin's; MSKCC, Memorial Sloan-Kettering Cancer Center; PFS, progression-free survival; RT, radiation therapy; SWOG, Southwest Oncology Group.

and compared CHOP × 4 versus CHOP × 4 + RT.[203] It might well be that four cycles of CHOP is inadequate therapy for this group of patients and the addition of RT cannot compensate for suboptimal chemotherapy. The GELA LNH 93-1 trial showed that for patients younger than the age of 60 years, an intensive chemotherapy regimen (ACVBP [doxorubicin, cyclophosphamide, vincristine, bleomycin and prednisone induction] followed by sequential consolidation treatments) gave more favorable event-free survival and OS when compared with CHOP × 3 + RT.[202] Whether the addition of RT is beneficial to chemotherapy alone when regimens more intensive than CHOP (e.g., CHOP + rituximab, or the ACVBP regimen) are used awaits further testing in phase III trials. A trial of high-dose chemotherapy included high-risk stages I and II patients but did not show superiority for the early use of autologous bone marrow transplantation (AuBMT).[204,205] At present, intensive therapy with hematopoietic stem cell support is not routinely indicated for stages I and II disease unless the disease is resistant to initial chemotherapy and radiation.

Other Histologic Subtypes

Less common, but distinct clinicopathologic entities including peripheral T-cell lymphoma, anaplastic large cell lymphoma, and mantle cell lymphoma may present with localized disease. At present, the treatment strategies for these entities are similar to large cell lymphomas, with the use of CMT. In a study of a small number of patients with stages I to II mantle cell lymphoma, the use of RT-containing regimen was associated with an improved disease control and survival.[76] As the knowledge regarding their clinical behavior, genetic origin, and etiology evolve, innovative therapy will become available for these specific diseases over the next decade.

Very Aggressive Lymphomas (Lymphoblastic Lymphoma, Burkitt's Lymphoma)

Very aggressive lymphomas, such as lymphoblastic and Burkitt's lymphomas, usually present with advanced-stage disease. Infrequently, localized presentations occur and the treatment in such cases is similar to that for advanced stage disease. Chemotherapy protocols with high-dose intensity including CNS prophylaxis are required for best results. Commonly used regimens are described by Magrath[206] and Bernstein[207] for Burkitt's lymphoma, and Coleman[152] for lymphoblastic lymphomas. CNS prophylaxis including intrathecal chemotherapy, with or without cranial radiation, is a common element for these protocols. After a complete response is obtained, high-dose chemotherapy with bone marrow support may be considered as a consolidation treatment.[208,209]

MANAGEMENT OF ADVANCED (STAGES III AND IV) DISEASE

Follicular Lymphomas

The advanced-stage follicular lymphomas are not cured with current approaches. For asymptomatic patients observation may be appropriate.[210,211] Symptomatic patients require chemotherapy to induce CR, and RT is reserved for control of local symptoms. In the Stanford report, initially observed patients required treatment after a median interval of 3 years. Their OS was 73% at 10 years.[210] Spontaneous regression of disease lasting a median of 13 months was observed in 23% of cases. Histologic transformation to a more aggressive histology (usually DLBCL) occurred in 60% at 6 years in one series,[64] and 31% at 10 years in another.[65] Deferred therapy tested in a randomized study showed no detrimental effect on survival (78% versus 70% for early treatment, $p = .24$).[212]

Selected stage III patients have been managed with total lymphoid irradiation (TLI). At Stanford, 66 patients treated between 1961 and 1982 (minimum 35 Gy or, for whole body, maximum of 1.5 Gy) had a 40% 10-year freedom-from-relapse rate and a 50% survival rate.[213] Other series report similar results.[155,174,175] All available data indicate a high probability of disease control within radiation fields. However, with the long natural history of this disease and the selection of patients submitted to protocol treatment, it is difficult to ascertain whether extensive lymphatic irradiation improves survival or results in cure. Other strategies for the treatment of indolent lymphoma include total body irradiation (TBI),[214-216] α–interferon,[212,217] purine analogues,[218,219] rituximab-chemotherapy combinations,[63,220-222] radioimmunotherapy,[223-226] and high-dose chemotherapy with RT and autologous hematopoietic stem cell transplantation.[227-230] Favorable responses have been documented for each of these approaches, but no firm evidence for cure has been evident. A meta-analysis of trials using α-interferon concluded that when used at a dose of at least 5 mU (or ≥36 mU/month) in combination with relatively intensive chemotherapy, improvement in survival and remission duration was seen.[217]

Large Cell Lymphomas

CHOP alone results in a complete response rates of 50% to 55% and long-term cure rates of 30% to 35%.[231] For DLBCL, the most common histologically aggressive lymphoma, the CHOP-rituximab regimen is currently considered as the standard chemotherapy for advanced (stages III and IV) disease. The addition of rituximab to CHOP results in improved PFS and OS in patients aged 60 years or older,[201] and in patients younger than 60 years with low-risk IPI.[232]

To date, *adjuvant* RT following a complete response to chemotherapy has not been shown to improve the OS in advanced stage NHL.[233,234] On the premise that bulky sites of lymphoma are more difficult to control with chemotherapy alone, some centers selectively administer adjuvant RT to initially bulky sites following complete or incomplete response to chemotherapy.[235,236] A randomized trial of 88 patients from Mexico given RT to sites of initial tumor bulk (defined as more than 10 cm) following complete response to chemotherapy suggested an improved 5-year DFS (72% with RT versus 35% without RT, $p < .01$) and OS (81% with RT versus 55% without RT, $p < .01$).[237] Confirmatory trials are required before this strategy can be routinely recommended. However, adjuvant RT is often useful to prevent local relapse in sanctuary sites. RT to the uninvolved testis in primary testicular lymphoma prevents relapse in the contralateral testicle.[238] Cranial irradiation is used to prevent CNS relapse in high-risk cases, but the value of cranial RT in patients treated with intrathecal chemotherapy has not been confirmed in a randomized trial. In addition RT has value as a palliative modality and is discussed in the following text.

Because of the suboptimal results of the CHOP regimen in patients with advanced stage lymphomas and the lack of survival advantage for higher dose-intensity approaches, which are nonmyeloablative, early high-dose therapy with BMT was tested in patients with adverse prognostic factors. Verdonck and colleagues treated patients with three courses of CHOP and randomized those with partial response to ABMT conditioned with cyclophosphamide and TBI versus additional five courses of CHOP chemotherapy. There were no significant differences in DFS or OS.[239] Similarly, an Italian trial of stages I to IV patients with partial response to the initial chemotherapy treated with dexamethasone, ARAC, cisplatin (DHAP) or ABMT showed no significant benefit for the BMT arm.[240] RT (36 Gy) was used in 52% of patients treated with DHAP and in 73% of patients with ABMT. A randomized study by Gianni and colleagues examined the role of high-dose sequential chemotherapy followed by autologous BMT as primary initial therapy.[241] This was compared to the standard chemotherapy with MACOP-B (Adriamycin, cyclophosphamide, vincristine, methotrexate, bleomycin and prednisolone) in 98 patients with bulky (>10 cm) stages I and II and stages III and IV disease. RT to sites of tumor bulk was part of the protocol for both treatment arms. TBI (12.5 Gy in 5 fractions) was initially used for the BMT arm but was later discontinued because of excessive toxicity. In this trial, the BMT group had a superior 7-year event-free survival (76%, versus 49% for MACOP-B, $p = 0.004$), but the difference in the OS was not statistically significant (81% versus 55%, $p = .09$). A multicenter French study by GELA randomized patients in complete remission (CR) to sequential consolidation chemotherapy (LNH 84) versus ABMT. No advantage was shown for DFS or OS.[204] However, a reanalysis of this trial with inclusion of a larger number of subsequently treated patients (LNH 87-2) showed an improved 5-year DFS (59% versus 39%, $p = 0.01$), and OS (65% versus 52%, $p = 0.06$) for ABMT, in the high-intermediate and high-risk subgroups.[205,242,243]

A subsequent GELA protocol (LNH 93-3) in high-risk and high–intermediate-risk patients showed a worse outcome for the autologous stem cell transplant arm.[244] The GELA trials did not use RT, despite the inclusion of stages I and II patients (some with bulky disease), which accounted for 30% to 40% of the patients studied.[204,205] At this time, early BMT as part of initial therapy cannot be considered standard,[245-248] and its use in high-risk cases requires further investigation.

Other Histologic Subtypes

Distinct clinicopathologic entities such as peripheral T-cell lymphoma, anaplastic large cell lymphoma, and mantle cell lymphoma are currently treated similarly as DLCLs. Because standard chemotherapy results in a low cure rate for mantle cell lymphomas,[68,69,72] new approaches have been advocated, including the incorporation of rituximab,[249] new drugs,[250,251] and autologous[73,252-254] or allogeneic[255,256] stem cell transplantation.

Assessment of Response and Follow-up

Cure requires the ability to eradicate disease, therefore the key is to attain complete remission with the initial treatment plan. In patients treated with RT alone, response is usually assessed 4 to 6 weeks following the completion of therapy. Because the RT dose fractionation schedule is determined prior to treatment and is usually based on information regarding dose response relationship and tolerance of tissues within the treatment volume, the presence of residual disease at the end of the treatment course is not an indication for additional RT. The assessment of response includes examination of the organ of presentation, repeat imaging studies if indicated, and a general examination to rule out disease progression. In patients treated with chemotherapy or CMT, where chemotherapy is used first, the response is assessed following one or two courses of chemotherapy and every 1 to 2 months thereafter. Chemotherapy is usually continued for two courses beyond attainment of complete remission. Gallium-67 (^{67}Ga) and PET scanning is useful in determining completeness of response, as discussed earlier. However, it must be emphasized that FDG-PET cannot detect residual microscopic disease reliably.[257] For cases where the standard therapy is CMT, a negative PET following chemotherapy does not imply that RT can be safely omitted.[257] Although most recurrences in patients with aggressive lymphoma occur within 2 to 3 years following the diagnosis, late relapse occurs. Accordingly, prolonged follow-up is indicated. Some tumor locations pose special problems in follow-up assessment. For example, primary bone lymphoma often has persisting radiologic and MRI abnormalities following treatment, and bone scan will show changes that cannot distinguish active disease from bone healing and remodelling. Residual mediastinal abnormalities are common, particularly if a bulky mass was present prior to treatment. Resolution of gallium avidity is helpful in such cases. PET scanning is useful in distinguishing viable lymphoma from fibrosis.

Salvage Therapy and the Role of Radiation Therapy

For patients with relapsed or chemotherapy-refractory large cell lymphoma, RT alone is rarely curative. However, in highly selected cases, durable long-term control of disease can be achieved with salvage RT.[258] Conventional salvage chemotherapy also has a very low curative potential. Common salvage regimens include DHAP,[259-261] mini-BEAM (carmustine, etoposide, cytarabine, and melphalan),[262] ESHAP (etoposide, methylprednisolone, cytarabine, and cisplatin),[263] ICE (ifosfamide, carboplatin, and etoposide) ± rituximab,[264,265] and GDP (gemcitabine, dexamethasone, and cisplatin)[266] (see Table 74-8). For patients with chemotherapy-sensitive disease, high-dose therapy followed by hematopoietic stem cell rescue is beneficial.[253,263,267-271] A phase III trial (PARMA) tested the role of high-dose therapy in 109 patients. Those demonstrating a response to two cycles of DHAP chemotherapy were randomized to four further courses of DHAP, versus a conditioning regimen of BEAC followed by ABMT. The 5-year event-free and OS rates for the transplant arm were 46% and 53%, versus 12% (p = .001) and 32% (p = .038) for the conventional DHAP arm, respectively.[260] RT to a dose of 26 Gy in 20 fractions was given twice daily, as a protocol treatment for patients with tumor bulk greater than 5 cm at the time of relapse in the transplant arm, and to 35 Gy in 20 fractions in the conventional chemotherapy arm. There was a trend favoring the RT patients with a lower relapse rate in the transplant group (8/22 RT patients relapsed versus 18/33 nonradiated patients relapsed, p = .19), and no obvious difference in the conventional chemotherapy group (10/12 RT patients relapsed, versus 35/42 nonradiated patients relapsed). Although this trial was not designed to examine the role of radiation in the salvage setting, it lends support to the use of RT for bulky disease when incorporated into a salvage treatment plan that includes high-dose therapy. The role of RT in bulky disease following partial response to salvage chemotherapy deserves further study in a randomized trial in patients undergoing hematopoietic stem cell transplant. Until such evidence is available, we recommend routine RT to sites of bulky disease, in sequence with salvage chemotherapy, and also RT to sites of incomplete response to chemotherapy.[253,272-275] Moderate doses of 30 to 35 Gy should be the goal, with individualization of the treatment plan in regard to the exact target volume (IFRT is preferred); the timing of RT in relation to chemotherapy and transplant should facilitate collection and harvesting stem cells and minimize treatment-related toxicity. For example, if large RT fields are required, RT should be given after stem cell harvesting and preferably pretransplant. Thoracic RT that will include significant volumes of lung tissue is less risky if given after transplantation.[276,277] In general, the principles of RT should be to treat the most likely site of relapse or progressive disease. The decision to treat with RT is influenced by the distribution and location of the disease. The spinal cord may be more radiation-sensitive in the post-transplant setting, because there are two case reports of radiation myelopathy with conventional fractionated doses of 40 to 45 Gy.[278,279]

Total Body Irradiation

The use of TBI as part of the conditioning regimen before hematopoietic stem cell transplant for lymphomas is premised on its successful role in the treatment of acute leukemias.[280] Although TBI is given for both tumor cell kill and immunosuppressive effects to prevent graft rejection in allogeneic transplants for leukemia,[280] its rationale in autologous transplant for lymphoma is mainly for tumor cell kill. The role of TBI in addition to myeloablative doses of chemotherapy in the autologous transplant setting has not been formally tested in a phase III trial. Therefore the use of TBI in intensive therapy regimens has been largely dictated by the local experience of the transplant center, and the availability of TBI. TBI appears to be more commonly used in North America[267,269,277,281] than in Europe.[204,282,283] RT fractionation allows the delivery of a higher total dose with less toxicity,[284,285] in comparison with single dose where 6 Gy (uncorrected for lung density) is associated with a significant risk of radiation pneumonitis.[286,287] The total dose for TBI is limited to 12 to 14 Gy in 1.5 to 2 Gy fractions delivered twice or three times a day. The addition of TBI to chemotherapy conditioning undoubtedly contributes to acute morbidity and the risk of posttransplant complications,[241,288,289] unless the dose-intensity of chemotherapy is adjusted. Previous IFRT, particularly to the thorax given just before BMT, is a risk factor for increased mortality.[269,274,275,277,290] A French study found impaired long-term platelet count recovery in patients conditioned with TBI.[291] In Toronto aggressive histology lymphomas were transplanted with high-dose melphalan and etoposide without TBI, whereas transformed indolent lymphomas receive TBI (12 Gy in 6 fractions) in addition. The 4-year PFS rates—49% in aggressive histology and 40% in transformed lymphoma—are not significantly different regardless of the use of TBI.[268] However, TBI in patients older than age 60 years resulted in a high incidence of pulmonary complications.[292]

The European BMT Working Party experience with indolent lymphomas showed no difference in PFS with or without TBI in the conditioning regimen.[283] Therefore it remains unclear whether the therapeutic ratio of TBI is favorable enough in the transplant setting to be used routinely outside of a trial. Innovative approaches using radioimmunotherapy to more selectively deliver targeted radiation in the salvage setting before BMT are under investigation. Preliminary results of anti-CD20 conjugated with ^{131}iodine (tositumomab) given in myeloablative doses followed by ABMT have produced encouraging results by the Seattle Group.[293] In a dose escalation study that delivered up to 27.25 Gy to dose-limiting normal organs, 16 out of 19 treated patients achieved complete responses.[294]

MANAGEMENT OF PRIMARY EXTRANODAL LYMPHOMAS

For a designation of primary extranodal lymphoma, in the context of gastrointestinal lymphoma Dawson and colleagues proposed that a patient had to present with main disease manifestation in an extranodal site and may only have had regional lymph node involvement, with no peripheral lymph node involvement and no liver or spleen involvement.[295] Later these criteria were relaxed to allow for contiguous involvement of organs including liver and spleen, and allowed for distant nodal disease providing that the extranodal lesion was the presenting site and constituted the predominant disease bulk.[296] Primary extranodal lymphomas account for approximately 25% to 45% of all lymphomas.[5,84,140,297,298] The most common is skin lymphoma, with the majority of them being T-cell histology.[5] For B-cell histology the most common are gastric lymphoma, Waldeyer's ring lymphoma (tonsil lymphoma being most frequent),[84] and brain. Others include intestinal, lung, orbital adnexa, bone, extradural, thyroid, testis, and other less common sites such as paranasal sinuses, breast, bladder, and the like. Many have unique clinical characteristics. Because of the propensity of extranodal lymphomas to be truly localized, they have special importance to the radiation oncologist.

Gastric Lymphoma

Mucosa-Associated Lymphoid Tissue Lymphoma

Permanent regression of primary low grade B-cell gastric MALT lymphoma following treatment with antibiotics indicates that eradication of *H. pylori* is sufficient therapy for most patients with *H. pylori*–associated MALT lymphoma of the stomach.[31,50,51,185,299-301] Depending on the strictness of the response criteria, complete response rates of 50% to 95% have been reported. Recommended anti-*Helicobacter* triple drug therapy includes a proton pump inhibitor (or ranitidine bismuth citrate), clarithromycin, and amoxicillin (or metronidazole).[302,303] The expected rates of eradication of *Helicobacter* are more than 90%.[52,303] Although eradication of *H. pylori* may be seen soon after the completion of drug therapy, disappearance of lymphoma usually takes several months and delays up to 18 months to histologic complete response have been documented. Molecular markers t(11;18)(q21;q21) and trisomy 3 predict for antibiotic resistance.[184,304,305] The t(11;18)(q21;q21) translocation has been found in high frequency in gastric MALT lymphoma not associated with *H. pylori*.[306] The presence of these markers or lack of response to antibiotic therapy are two main indications to treat with definitive RT. Patients with asymptomatic minimal residual disease can have an indolent course and not require further treatment,[307] particularly if elderly or infirm. The results of treatment with RT are excellent. In a small prospective series, Schechter and colleagues documented a 100% complete response rate following RT to a median dose of 30 Gy (28.5 Gy to 43.5 Gy). At a median follow-up of 27 months, no failures were observed.[308] Other investigators[83,309] documented similar results. A dose of 30 Gy appears adequate. Another approach to the management of antibiotic-refractory gastric MALT lymphoma involves the use of chlorambucil alone,[310] rituximab,[311-313] or combination chemotherapy.[314] Regardless of the choice of treatment, the disease is generally indolent biologically.[301] Further phase II and phase III clinical trials are required to define the optimal management for this disease.

Diffuse Large Cell Lymphoma

In the past most patients with gastric lymphoma were diagnosed at surgery, and treatment for diffuse large B-cell lymphoma included surgical resection with postoperative RT or postoperative chemotherapy. In the last two decades, nonsurgical approaches with primary chemotherapy followed by RT produced similar results.[315-320] At the PMH, patients with stages IA and IIA gastric lymphoma treated with complete gross surgical resection, and low-dose (20 Gy to 25 Gy) postoperative RT had an 86% 10 year relapse-free survival.[318,321] D'Amore reviewed the Danish Lymphoma Study Group experience and found that patients with gastric lymphoma who received RT as part of their therapy had a reduced relative risk of relapse to 0.3.[136] Others have shown good results in patients with complete resection of tumor followed by full-course chemotherapy alone.[322]

The current standard of therapy is stomach preservation with combined CHOP chemotherapy (and rituximab) and RT. Patients with *H. pylori* infection should also receive antibiotics to eradicate this infection.[323,324] Chemotherapy alone, with rituximab (without routine RT) is curative in a substantial proportion of patients with DLBCL,[324,325] but the data are not mature enough to safely delete RT at this time. Moderate dose RT (30 to 40 Gy) will produce high local control rates.

Intestinal Lymphoma

Primary small bowel lymphoma is more common than large bowel or rectal lymphoma. Distinct histologic presentations include MALT lymphoma, DLBCL, enteropathy-associated T-cell lymphoma (EATL), mantle cell lymphoma, follicular lymphoma, and immunoproliferative small intestinal disease (IPSID). Intestinal lymphoma is commonly diagnosed at laparotomy and surgical resection is standard. In advanced disease where resection is not technically feasible, treatment is made up of anthracycline-based chemotherapy followed, in some cases, by RT. Indolent intestinal lymphoma may be treated with surgical resection followed by adjuvant whole abdominal RT (20 to 25-Gy in 1 to 1.25-Gy daily fractions). In aggressive histology lymphoma surgery followed by chemotherapy is recommended. If a short course of chemotherapy is used, whole abdominal RT is added. In patients where complete tumor resection is not feasible, chemotherapy followed by RT is recommended.[158,321] In the absence of randomized trials, the optimal treatment strategy is controversial. The outcomes reported in the literature vary depending on the extent of disease and histology. In a large series of intestinal lymphomas, Domizio documented a 75% 5-year survival for patients with indolent B-cell lymphomas and only a 25% 5-year survival for those with T-cell tumors.[326] The poor outcome of patients with intestinal T-cell lymphoma has also been documented by multiple investigators.[136,327-329] Prognostic factors in primary intestinal lymphoma include, besides phenotype, age, performance status, B-symptoms, and mesenteric lymph node involvement (stage II disease).[136,327-329]

IPSID, alpha-heavy chain disease, and Mediterranean lymphoma all refer to various manifestations of a B-cell lymphoma of MALT type affecting the small intestine.[330,331] It is chiefly observed in the Middle East and Africa. Patients present with poor performance status and severe malabsorption and frequently cannot tolerate standard therapy. Several authors have reported that treatment with the tetracycline group of antibiotics[332] or *H. pylori* eradication[333] can produce clinical, histologic, and immunologic remissions. Remissions have also been described following chemotherapy.[334] The role of RT and surgical resection in IPSID remains to be defined. Historically, IPSID is a highly lethal disease with survival rates as low as 23% at 5 years.[335] Patients with resectable stages I and II_1 disease have a 5-year survival of 40% to 47% compared with 0% to 25% for unresectable or stage II_2 disease. Fortunately, there appears to be a decrease in the incidence of this disease associated with improvements in sanitation and health facilities in some parts of the world.[336]

Rectal presentations are less common than other sites in the lower intestinal tract. Aggressive histology lymphoma is the most common, although lower grade lymphomas also occur.[337,338] Treatment usually includes chemotherapy and RT (35 Gy in 1.5- to 2-Gy daily fractions) for patients presenting with bulky lesions or aggressive histology lymphoma, or both. IFRT alone (30 Gy in 1.5- to 1.75-Gy daily fractions) has been successful in providing long-term disease control for MALT lymphoma of the rectum.[188]

Waldeyer's Ring Lymphomas

Traditionally, local RT alone was used with high local control rates with moderate doses (35 to 50 Gy). Most failures occurred distant to the radiation field. Currently, CMT is the standard approach and results in local control rates in excess of 80% and survival rates of 60% to 75% depending on the bulk and nodal extent of the presenting lesion.[84,137,339,340] Location of disease in the tonsil only is a favorable prognostic attribute.[340] A prospective randomized trial by Aviles and colleagues demonstrated the superiority of CMT in this disease with 5-year failure free survival rates of 48% for RT alone, 45% for CT alone, and 83% for CMT ($p < .001$), and established CMT as the standard therapeutic approach.[341]

Paranasal Sinuses and Nasal Lymphoma

Paranasal sinus lymphoma occurs more commonly in males and in patients older than 50 years. Important differences in clinical features, phenotypic and genotypic characteristics, and prognosis are apparent between disease occurring in Western[134,342] and Asian populations.[13,81] Common presenting features include painless nasal obstruction, nasal discharge or bleeding, facial swelling, or palatal lesions with dental impacts. Involvement of the orbit can cause epiphora, proptosis, or diplopia. Tumors are most commonly of diffuse, large B-cell type. In Asians, a destructive, erosive lesion is a characteristic presentation and T/NK-cell tumors predominate and show the characteristic features of angioinvasion, necrosis, and epitheliotropism. Indolent lymphomas are rare. The nasal type of CD56-positive T/NK-cell lymphoma is a distinct clinical-pathologic entity associated with the EBV.[13,56] Tumors with an identical phenotype and genotype can occur rarely in other extranodal sites, usually in the skin, subcutis, gastrointestinal tract, and testis.[56] For diffuse large B-cell lymphomas, the current practice of CMT yields overall 5-year survival rates of 60% to 75%.[81,134] In T/NK-cell disease the Asian experience with stages I and II presentations are disappointing, with a response rate to doxorubicin-containing chemotherapy of less than 50%, and 5-year survival of 30% to 70%.[343-346] The early use of RT to a higher dose of 45 to 50 Gy appears to be important for optimal local control.[14,347] For patients who responded favorably to initial treatment, the use of consolidation therapy with high-dose chemotherapy and autologous stem cell transplantation appears to result in prolonged remissions.[82]

Salivary Gland Lymphomas

The parotid gland is the most common presenting site. An increased risk is seen in patients with Sjögren's syndrome.[348,349] Myoepithelial sialoadenitis (MESA) characteristic of Sjögren's syndrome is a part of the spectrum of salivary gland MALT lymphoma. These lymphomas generally follow an indolent course and tend to remain localized for prolonged periods of time. Radiation offers excellent local control, with a complete remission rate of 100% and 5-year survival of 90%,[350] and no advantage for chemotherapy. Equally good results with local therapy were obtained by other investigators.[83,351] Therefore, there is no role for chemotherapy in the management of indolent tumors, but CMT using an anthracycline-based regimen is standard for transformed aggressive histology lesions.

Thyroid Lymphomas

Women are affected more commonly than men and the median age of presentation is more than 60 years. Patients often present with a rapidly enlarging, bulky neck mass causing local aerodigestive obstructive symptoms. Primary thyroid lymphoma occurs most frequently in patients with Hashimoto's thyroiditis.[27,352] MALT lymphomas are common and have a better prognosis than non-MALT tumors.[353] Surgery is a diagnostic procedure, and thyroidectomy is not indicated for clinically evident lymphoma diagnosed by fine-needle or core biopsy.[354] CMT has become the standard treatment approach for diffuse large B-cell lymphomas. With chemotherapy and locoregional RT (35 to 40 Gy), local control is achieved in the majority of patients,[355] and survival and relapse-free survival should exceed 75%.[356-358] For localized MALT or follicular lymphomas, RT alone is appropriate therapy with a local control rate of more than 95% expected.[83] Adequately treated MALT lymphoma of the thyroid rarely relapses systemically.[83,359]

Orbital Lymphomas

Orbital lymphomas are commonly seen in elderly patients with a median age in the sixth decade. These tumors arise in superficial tissues including the conjunctiva and eyelids, or in deep tissues including the lacrimal gland and retrobulbar tissues. MALT lymphoma is most often seen in the conjunctiva, whereas retro-orbital presentations are associated with diffuse large cell histology[360] but are less common.[361] Treatment is directed to cure, while preserving vision and the integrity of the orbit. Orbital lesions are easily controlled with low doses of RT (25 to 30 Gy in 10 to 20 daily fractions), with local control rate of 95% or more.[83,187,362-365] Higher doses are not required, and their use results in increased acute and long-term morbidity. The whole orbit should be treated.[366] Conjunctival MALT lymphoma treated with surgical excision has only been occasionally observed to regress spontaneously.[367] For DLBCL, 3 to 6 cycles of chemotherapy followed by RT to a dose of 30 to 35 Gy in 1.5- to 1.75-Gy daily fractions is recommended. The overall actuarial 10-year survival rates are 75% to 80%. These excellent survival rates are in part because of a predominance of indolent histology. The risk of locoregional failure is extremely low. Contralateral orbit involvement is common either synchronously or metachronously. Distant failure rates vary from 20% to 50%; but as in other cases of indolent lymphoma, prolonged survival is observed.[83,359,368] In patients with bulky tumors, where the cornea cannot be protected, RT alone may result in severe radiation complications. In such cases, chemotherapy alone or CMT is preferable.

Testicular Lymphomas

In contrast to germ cell tumors, primary testis lymphoma affects mostly men older than 50 years. Staging assessment is focused on identification of para-aortic lymph node involvement and distant spread, particularly the CNS. Initial therapy invariably involves orchiectomy. Almost all testicular lymphomas are diffuse large B-cell lymphomas. Reported overall 5-year survival rates range from 16% to 65% with median survivals of 12 to 24 months.[238,369-371] Distant failures were commonly observed. In the International Extranodal Lymphoma Study Group (IELSG) study of 373 patients 57% had stage I and 21% had stage II disease.[238] Median PFS was 4 years. High risk of CNS relapse was observed with an actuarial risk of 34% at 10 years.[238] CNS relapse has been documented despite the use of chemotherapy.[371-373] Other sites of relapse involve extranodal organs including skin, pleura, Waldeyer's ring, lung, liver, spleen, bone, and bone marrow. Failure in the contralateral testis is well documented and occurs in 15% of patients at 3 years, rising to an actuarial risk of 42% at 15 years.[238] Scrotal irradiation with moderate doses (25 to 30 Gy in 10 to 15 daily fractions) reduces this risk to less than 10%.[238] Doxorubicin-based chemotherapy improves survival of patients with localized testicular lymphoma.[238] A clear pattern of failure in the CNS warrants a recommendation for routine CNS prophylaxis with intrathecal chemotherapy, and the IELSG data suggest that a combination of systemic and intrathecal therapy, with scrotal RT was associated with an improved outcome.[238]

Bladder Lymphomas

Primary NHL of the urinary bladder is rare. Published case reports indicate that primary lymphoma of the bladder occurs mostly in the sixth and seventh decades of life and is more common in women. MALT lymphomas have been observed and the prognosis is favorable.[83,374,375] Large cell lymphomas have also been described. The prognosis is related to histologic type and extent of tumor.[376] As in other extranodal lymphomas, indolent lymphomas are managed with RT alone, but aggressive lymphomas are treated with CMT. Several reports suggest that primary lymphoma of the bladder is associated with a favorable prognosis.[375,377,378] Long-term survival historically has been observed in approximately 40% to 50% of patients.

Female Genital Tract Lymphomas

Ovarian Lymphomas

Lymphoma of the ovary is rare as a primary presentation, but Burkitt's lymphoma has a predilection to involve the ovary.[379] The disease is commonly bilateral and often bulky. A 2- and 5-year OS of 42% and 24% have been cited, respectively.[380] Because ovarian lymphomas are most commonly of aggressive histology, the initial treatment approach should include CMT. Burkitt's lymphoma is managed primarily with chemotherapy alone.

Lymphoma of the Uterus, Cervix Uteri, and Vagina

The standard therapy for patients with stage IE lesions has usually included RT with or without surgery. However, there is no evidence that radical resection is necessary. RT alone for localized indolent histology tumors offers a very high probability of local control; CMT is appropriate for aggressive histology tumors.[381,382] Given the impact of RT on ovarian function in those in the reproductive age range, the use of chemotherapy alone has been recommended with some clinical justification. A 5-year OSR of 73% is quoted by Harris and Scully[383] with a 89% 5-year survival for patients with stage IE disease.

Breast Lymphoma

Breast lymphoma affecting young women tends to be associated with pregnancy and lactation and is an aggressive histology lymphoma sometimes presenting with bilateral disease diffusely involving both breasts. In contrast, the disease affecting older women tends to present with discrete masses, commonly unilateral. Reports in the literature suggest synchronous bilateral involvement in up to 13% of cases and metachronous contralateral involvement in 7% of cases. The most common histologic type is diffuse large B-cell lymphoma. Indolent histology lymphomas are less common and if observed usually consist of secondary involvement from systemic disease.[384] MALT lymphoma affecting the breast is rare but has been reported.[385] Mastectomy is not recommended and the breast is preserved in the majority of cases. RT results in excellent local control, especially in patients presenting without bulky disease or those with indolent histology. The OS of patients treated with local treatment methods ranges from 40% to 66% at 5 to 10 years.[386-389] The local control rates in patients treated with RT alone range from 75% to 78%.[386,390] Isolated CNS relapses have been reported. Similarly, late failure in the contralateral breast may occur following therapy of unilateral primary breast lymphoma. CMT is recommended for aggressive lymphomas,[391,392] whereas patients with indolent lymphoma can be successfully treated with RT alone. CNS prophylaxis with intrathecal chemotherapy should be given to all patients with very aggressive histology, including Burkitt's or Burkitt-like lymphomas.

Bone Lymphoma

With RT alone, 5- and 10-year OSRs of 58% and 53% have been reported for solitary bone lesions. Key issues relating to local control are the intramedullary and soft tissue extent of disease in relation to RT volume. MRI is particularly important in revealing extension of disease in the bone and soft tissues. Treatment approaches using RT have given high levels of local control (85%), but unacceptable rates of local or marginal failure (20%) probably related to underestimation of tumor extent and bulk, and systemic failure rates approaching 50% were reported. Therefore patients with localized lymphoma of bone should be treated with CMT comprising initial anthracycline-based chemotherapy and IFRT. There is no indication for CNS prophylaxis. With CT and RT the OSR and relapse-free rates should exceed 70% to 80% at 5 years.[393-397]

Lung Lymphoma

Three broad categories of lymphoma of the lung are recognized: (1) indolent B-cell histology, MALT or follicular lymphoma; (2) aggressive histology, usually a diffuse, large cell B-cell type; and (3) rare T-cell lymphomas usually occurring as part of a more widespread angiocentric and angiodestructive systemic process. Imaging usually shows multiple lesions, either nodules or masslike consolidation.[398] Initial treatment may involve surgical resection; however, given current less invasive alternatives to establish a diagnosis, there is no indication for radical resection because it does not improve outcome. Indolent lymphomas are the most common,[399,400] and the disease is usually responsive to both chemotherapy[401] and RT[83]; but low tolerance of lung to RT limits its applicability to treatment of only part of the lung. Prolonged survival is commonly observed, with a 94% OS at 5 years and a median survival not reached at 10 years.[402] The prognosis is clearly not as good for aggressive histology even when treated with chemotherapy, or CMT with survival rates of 47% at 5 years,[403] and median survivals of 3 years. Systemic progression is common and relapse-free rates of approximately 40% to 50% are expected. T-cell lymphomas have a poor prognosis with a 50% mortality at 2 years even with CMT.

Primary Central Nervous System Lymphoma

The most common site of primary central nervous system lymphoma (PCNSL) is the brain.[404] Primary leptomeningeal lymphoma, without parenchymal brain disease, accounts for only 7% of PCNSL. Primary spinal cord lymphoma is less common.[405] The eye, a direct extension of the CNS, is another site of PCNSL. Aggressive histology B-cell lymphomas are most common. T-cell lymphomas have been reported but are exceedingly rare, with a prognosis similar to the B-cell lymphoma.[406]

Lymphoma of the Brain

Most patients present with symptoms of headache and raised intracranial pressure. Lesions are often multifocal or diffuse and are periventricular with easy access to the CSF. The incidence of meningeal seeding varies from 7.6% to 69% when a vigorous search is conducted.[407,408] Systemic lymphoma is apparent in only 7% to 8% of autopsied patients. The diagnosis has to be confirmed histologically, but it is suspected based on characteristic CT or MRI appearances of the tumor. A diffuse contrast enhancement of tumor on both CT and MRI is typical, but a small proportion of patients have nonenhancing lesions. Conventional treatment consists of whole brain irradiation and corticosteroids. Primary brain lymphoma is extremely sensitive to RT and corticosteroids, producing a rapid symptomatic response. The recommended doses are 40 to 50 Gy to the whole brain in 1.8- to 2.0-Gy fractions. Performance status, age, and solitary tumor are the most important prognostic factors. The median survival has been reported to be 12 to 18 months with 2- and 5-year survival rates of 28% and 3% to 4%, respectively.[409-411] Given the initial good responses obtained with radiation, and that the pathology is not different from that of DLCLs of nodal origin, the poor survival rate of primary brain lymphomas remains largely unexplained.

In the PMH experience with RT alone, patients with Karnofsky Performance Status (KPS) score greater than 60 had an actuarial 5-year survival of 56%, versus 10% for those with KPS less than 60; whereas survival was 42% for those younger than age 60 years, versus 9% for those older than 60 years of age; for solitary lesions the survival was 30% versus 15% for multiple lesions.[411] The IELSG study of 378 patients identified five independent poor prognostic factors for OS: age older than 60 years, a ECOG performance status 2 or higher, elevated LDH level, elevated CSF protein level, and involvement of deep brain structures.[412] Patients with 0 to 1 of these factors had a 2-year survival of 80%, 2 to 3 factors have 48%, dropping to 15% for those with 4 to 5 factors.[412] These factors remain prognostic when the analysis was restricted to patients treated with intravenous methotrexate.

Because of poor results with RT alone and concerns regarding radiation neurotoxicity,[413,414] chemotherapy has become the initial standard treatment. In the 1990s several reports suggested improved median survivals for patients receiving chemotherapy followed by planned RT or RT at progression.[415-420] However, there are no randomized trials proving the benefit of CMT. In fact, a policy change from an RT approach to initial chemotherapy consisting of methotrexate did not result in an improvement in survival for an unselected population of 122 patients in the province of British Columbia in Canada, in which up to one third of patients did not receive potentially curative therapy.[421] Despite this, protocols using strategies with high-dose methotrexate, in various combinations with carmustine, procarbazine, vincristine, and dexamethasone have produced impressive results with or without RT, and with mild to moderate late neurologic toxicity.[415,417,418,422] Neuwelt observed a median survival of 44.5 months in chemotherapy-treated patients, but only 17.8 months in those treated with RT alone.[415] The group at Memorial Hospital used methotrexate (3 g/m^2), procarbazine, and vincristine followed by RT of 45 Gy in 52 patients and reported a median survival of 60 months.[417] Other chemotherapy approaches included very high dose of methotrexate (7 g/m^2) alone and deferred RT, and such treatment in 23 patients achieved an overall response rate of 74%, but only 52% had complete response.[419] For patients failing chemotherapy, RT as salvage therapy remained useful, with a response rate of 74%.[423]

These reports show that PCNSL is a chemosensitive disease, but the optimal approach has not yet been clearly defined. The use of intrathecal chemotherapy appears unnecessary, particularly if intravenous methotrexate is employed.[412] Long-term treatment–related neurologic toxicity is a major problem. In a series from the Memorial Hospital, about one third of PCNSL survivors developed dementia; and those older than 60 years and who receive whole brain RT are at increased risk.[413,424] Further refinements of treatment protocols for primary brain lymphoma are needed. Temozolomide has promising activity[425] and is being examined in ongoing clinical trials.

Ocular Lymphoma

Two patterns of intraocular involvement occur: lymphoma involving the optic nerve, retina, and vitreous, commonly associated with CNS involvement; and lymphoma involving the uveal tract (choroid, ciliary body, and iris), associated with visceral involvement.[426] The diagnosis can be confused with an inflammatory syndrome of uveitis and vitreitis or glaucoma.[427] Bilateral involvement is common, but symptoms will usually affect one eye earlier than the other. CSF cytology and imaging of both eyes and brain with MRI or CT is required to delineate local disease extent. Most cases are of the diffuse large cell type. Both B- and T-cell phenotypes have been reported.[426] Treatment results are poor, with a high risk of progression to the CNS,[428,429] and long-term disease control is unusual. RT provides only temporary palliation. Reported survivals range from 6 to 18 months[430] to 60 months,[428] with the prognosis similar to primary CNS lymphoma.[431] There are reports of response with high-dose intravenous Ara-C or methotrexate.[431,432]

Extradural Lymphoma

Primary extradural lymphoma presents commonly with pain, and progressive neurologic deficit or spinal cord compression. The presence of spinal cord compression constitutes a medical emergency. Histologic diagnosis is imperative and surgical biopsy and decompression are the first steps in management. The main objectives of surgery include adequate decompression of the spinal cord and removal of tissue appropriate for histologic diagnosis. Postoperative therapy has historically involved RT to the affected area of the spine. The RT volume should take into account the presence of paraspinal mass or regional lymph node involvement. RT alone results in excellent local disease control; but as with other localized aggressive histology lymphomas, it is associated with a 40% to 50% distant failure. The use of chemotherapy following surgery and RT is associated with a reduced distant failure rate and an improved survival. In the PMH experience the 5-year survival of patients treated with RT alone was 33% compared with 86% for those treated with CMT. Although the traditional approach is to deliver RT before chemotherapy, this may not be the most optimal sequence. Eeles and colleagues documented that the use of chemotherapy followed by RT does not compromise neurologic function, as compared to that achieved when RT is followed by chemotherapy.[433,434] The overall neurologic prognosis for recovery is excellent even in patients who were initially severely paretic.[435,436] A controversial aspect of the management of primary extradural lymphoma relates to the use of CNS prophylaxis. In the PMH experience isolated CNS relapse in patients treated without CNS prophylaxis was rare.[434]

Cutaneous Lymphomas

Histopathologic classification for cutaneous lymphomas has been proposed by a joint WHO-EORTC effort, describing clinical-pathologic disease entities unique to the skin.[437] Primary lymphomas of the skin can be divided into three broad categories:

1. Cutaneous B-cell lymphomas (CBCLs—25%), including indolent histologies with follicular center lymphoma and marginal-zone (MALT), and the clinically aggressive: diffuse large B-cell lymphoma, leg type, or other location.
2. CTCLs of indolent clinical behavior (70%): mycosis fungoides and its variants, primary cutaneous anaplastic large cell lymphoma (C-ALCL), lymphomatoid papulosis, and other rare types (e.g., subcutaneous panniculitis-like T-cell lymphoma).
3. CTCL of aggressive clinical behavior (<10%): Sézary syndrome, peripheral T-cell lymphoma, and several rare entities such as NK cell lymphoma of nasal type.

Diffuse large B-cell lymphomas commonly occur in the legs of elderly patients, are clinically aggressive, and have an estimated 5-year disease-specific survival of 55%.[437-442] CMT is the standard as in DLBCL of other sites. In contrast, primary cutaneous follicular center lymphomas are usually confined to the head and neck region or the trunk, with 5-year survival of more than 95%.[437,438] Unlike nodal follicular lymphoma, BCL2 protein expression and t(14;18) translocation are infrequent.[437,443,444] MALT lymphomas are indolent, respond well to local therapy, and have excellent prognosis.[437,445] Infection with *B. burgdorferi* has been implicated in the pathogenesis of CBCL,[181,446] although a study of 38 cases conducted in the United States did not demonstrate such an association,[182] and another study showed no geographic correlation between the incidence of Lyme disease with CBCL.[183] RT is a preferred treatment modality with very high local control rates (85% to 100%) and favorable survival.[447,448] Following local therapy, the relapse rate is high, frequently with new skin lesions, but death from indolent CBCL is uncommon.[437]

Mycosis fungoides is the most common type of CTCL of indolent clinical behavior, and is discussed elsewhere (Chapter 76). The other indolent CTCL is primary C-ALCL, characterized by CD30+ positivity, but is distinct from the nodal type of ALCL.[56,437] In contrast to nodal ALCL, most C-ALCL does not stain for the ALK protein and is also negative for the t(2;5) translocation.[437] In patients with a solitary nodule, or localized skin disease, RT is the treatment of choice. These lymphomas can relapse in the skin, but generally have a favorable prognosis,[449] with 5-year survival of 95%.[437] In a Dutch study of 79 patients, only 16% of patients have a systemic relapse of lymphoma 10 years after initial treatment.[449] Lymphomatoid papulosis is a related condition, also CD30+, and has an indolent course with spontaneously remitting disease.[449] Cytotoxic treatment is usually not necessary and life expectancy is not adversely affected, but infrequently the disease can progress to other types of T-cell lymphomas.

Other aggressive types of CTCL represent an extremely heterogeneous group and most are characterized as peripheral T-cell lymphomas—unspecified further in the WHO classification.[56] Some have morphologic and phenotypic characteristics of NK/T-cell lymphoma of nasal type,[450] and other rare entities include the aggressive CD8+ T-cell lymphoma, and gamma-delta T-cell lymphoma. Most are negative for CD30 and have a poor prognosis, with an estimated 5-year survival of 15% to 20%.[437,438]

Mediastinal (Thymic) Large Cell Lymphoma

Several clinicopathologic features have distinguished primary mediastinal (thymic) large B-cell lymphoma from nodal DLBCL lymphoma. The disease typically presents in females (female-to-male ratio of 3:1) in the fourth or fifth decade of life, as a rapidly growing invasive tumor with contiguous spread into mediastinal tissues. Pleural and pericardial invasion with effusion and B symptoms are common and 30% to 40% of patients have superior vena caval obstruction at diagnosis. The lesions are frequently bulky (65% being >10-cm diameter), and involve the thymus. Sufficient tissue for phenotypic and genotypic studies is mandatory because the differential diagnosis includes Hodgkin's lymphoma, lymphoblastic lymphoma, thymoma, germinoma/teratoma, and Castleman's disease. Tumors often have moderate to marked sclerosis. The outcome for patients treated with CHOP-based chemotherapy or CMT is equivalent to other diffuse large B-cell lymphomas of equivalent stage, for example, CR rates of 70% to 80% and 5-year survival of 60% to 80%.[154,451,452] Chemotherapy regimens more intensive than CHOP, e.g., MACOP-B, or high-dose therapy with stem cell transplantation, have been reported in retrospective studies to give improved results with 10-year OS ranging from 70% to 77%.[452-454] Occasionally these tumors have demonstrated marked chemoresistance and radioresistance. Factors determining outcome include bulk (>10 cm), the use of CMT,[453,454] and stage.

RADIATION THERAPY FOR PALLIATION

In the context of recurrent lymphomas, patients are encountered in whom no curative therapy is available. Radiation is an extremely effective modality in providing symptom relief and local control. Palliative RT has been underused in lymphoma because of a variety of other systemic treatment options. The following are situations where palliative RT should be considered: (1) stages III and IV indolent histology lymphoma, with localized bulky disease; (2) relapsed or primary refractory NHL, any stage, with predominant localized disease, ineligible for intensive therapy because of old age, poor tolerance to chemotherapy, or chemotherapy resistance; (3) relapse of lymphoma postautologous or allogeneic BMT; (4) localized HIV-related lymphoma in patients unsuitable for chemotherapy. When palliative RT is considered, it is important to establish the goal of therapy. Distinction should be made between attempts to achieve a prolonged local control of disease, for example radical RT given for local control in a noncurative situation, or RT given purely for the relief of symptoms. This decision is usually based on the clinical condition of the patient; the location, size, and distribution of disease; and the life expectancy of the patient. Radical RT for local control is not infrequently required for selected patients with chemotherapy-refractory aggressive histology lymphomas where the disease is predominantly localized. In these situations, if normal tissue tolerance allows, it is desirable to deliver full-dose RT with 30 to 40 Gy in 10 to 20 fractions over 2 to 4 weeks. For rapidly progressive disease, accelerated fractionation should be considered, to 35 to 40 Gy in 20 to 30 fractions over 2 to 3 weeks, depending on volume and normal tissue tolerance. Accelerated hyperfractionation was reported to be more effective than conventional fractionation in Burkitt's lymphomas,[455] but there are only few reports of the use of altered fractionation regimens. Concomitant chemotherapy and RT to 40 Gy for chemorefractory bulky lymphoma was administered in a phase II study of 21 patients and yielded a response rate of 70%; majority were partial responses.[456] When radiation is given for relief of disease-related symptoms, a short course of higher dose-per-fraction therapy can be used as dictated by individual circumstance. Acceptable regimens include 20 Gy in 5 fractions over 1 week, 25 to 30 Gy in 10 to 12 fractions over 2 weeks, or 12 to 16 Gy in 2 fractions over 1 week.

For indolent lymphomas, excellent palliative responses to very low doses of radiation, such as 4 Gy given in 2 fractions, have been observed.[176,178,457] This was explained by the predominant mode of tumor cell death being largely mediated by apoptosis.[458] Response rates of 90% have been obtained in selected patients with this approach.[176,178,457] These results are similar with the historical response rates of 71% to 83% for TBI doses of 150 to 220 cGy (10 to 15 cGy per fraction, 2 to 3 fractions per week) given over several weeks.[214-216]

RADIATION THERAPY TECHNIQUES AND PRESCRIPTION DEFINITIONS

Because of the wide distribution of lymphoid tissues in the body, the technical aspects for planning of RT for lymphomas are highly dependent on the location and extent of the target volume. Examples of the commonly used techniques and selected issues that require special attention are discussed in the following text. In most cases, established techniques for other cancers presenting in the same sites can be adapted for treatment of lymphomas. In general, proper planning involves the appropriate use of immobilization devices, simulation, CT-assisted tumor localization and planning, localization of adjacent normal tissues, custom-designed beam modifying devices, and computerized calculation of isodose distributions. The goal of these steps is to achieve dose uniformity in the target volume to within ±5% of the prescribed dose as specified by International Commission on Radiation Units and Measurements (ICRU) Report 24[459] and ICRU Report 62,[460] while minimizing RT dose to normal tissues. Intensity-modulated radiation therapy (IMRT) will gain increasing importance to reduce any morbidity because of the exposure of organs at risk located adjacent to the target volume, particularly in instances of repeat course of RT for relapsed disease.[461] The support of allied health care disciplines including dental, nutritional, physiotherapy, social, and psychology services is essential to good patient care.

The common terms used to describe the extent of RT are involved field (IF), EF, and total lymphoid (or nodal) irradiation (TLI or TNI). The use of these terms varies considerably in the literature.[114] Generally, IF defines RT to the clinically involved region, with or without the first echelon adjacent lymph node region uninvolved by disease. EF defines RT to include the adjacent first echelon and the second echelon adjacent lymph node regions. The definitions and examples of IFRT and extended-field radiation therapy (EFRT) volumes are given in Table 74-12 and Table 74-13. In general, IFRT coverage implies that the CTV includes the whole nodal region as defined by Kaplan and Rosenberg.[462,463] A unilateral cervical IFRT is illustrated in Figure 74-3. With the routine use of CMT in the management of localized aggressive lymphoma, there has not been a trial to address whether whole nodal region coverage is still required, or whether a more limited coverage of the initially involved tumor mass with a margin will suffice. Total lymphoid RT implies treatment to all the major lymphoid regions, with the mantle and the inverted Y fields, with or without Waldeyer's ring fields. Its use at present is uncommon in NHL.

The dose of RT required to achieve local control varies depending on histologic type and tumor bulk. Follicular lymphoma and MALT lymphoma are more responsive to RT, and a dose of 30 Gy delivered in 15 to 20 fractions over 3 to 4 weeks results in local control rates in excess of 95%. For small cutaneous or orbital lesions RT doses of 25 Gy are sufficient to achieve 90% to 95% local control. Large cell lymphomas are less sensitive and require doses from 35 to 45 Gy. For low-bulk disease treated with full courses of chemotherapy, excellent

Table 74-12 Examples of Involved-Field Radiation Therapy*†

Involved by Disease	Radiation Field Coverage	Comment
Right neck node(s)	Entire right neck (see Fig. 74-3)	Stage I
Left neck node(s)	Entire right and left neck	Coverage uninvolved left neck
Bilateral neck nodes	Right and left neck nodes, and superior mediastinum (see Fig. 74-6)	Stage II
Right axillary node(s)	Right axilla	Stage I
Superior mediastinal lymphadenopathy	Mediastinum, both lung hila, subcarinal nodes, both supraclavicular fossa	Stage I
Right inguinal node(s)	Right inguinal-femoral, and right external iliac nodes (see Fig. 74-8)	Stage I
Right parotid gland	Right and left parotid glands, right and left neck nodes	Stage IE
Thyroid gland	Right and left neck, thyroid, superior mediastinum (see Fig. 74-6)	Stage IE
Stomach	Entire stomach, perigastric and celiac lymph nodes	Stage IE
Right humerus	Right humerus and right axilla	Stage IE, bone
Left maxillary sinus	Left maxillary sinus and nasal cavity	Stage IE, maxillary sinus

*The radiation coverage indicated here is not necessarily the recommended coverage for the involved field but is merely cited as an example of what would be regarded as the involved-field based on our definition provided in the table.

†Radiation defined by IF (nodal): the clinically involved nodal region ± the uninvolved adjacent nodal region(s); IF (extranodal site): the clinically involved tissue/organ, ± the uninvolved adjacent drainage lymph node region.

Table 74-13 Examples of Extended-Field Radiation Therapy*†

Involved by Disease	Radiation Field Coverage	Comment
Right neck node(s)	Mantle	Stage I
Right axillary node(s)	Right and left axilla, right and left neck, superior mediastinum	Left neck and left axilla coverage is beyond adjacent nodal region
Bilateral neck nodes	Mantle	Hilar and subcarinal coverage is beyond the adjacent nodal region
Single right inguinal node	Inverted Y	Left inguinal, left pelvic, and paraaortic coverage is beyond adjacent nodal region
Small bowel	Whole abdomen	

*The radiation coverage indicated here is not necessarily the recommended coverage for the extended-field, but is merely cited as an example of what would be regarded as the extended-field based on our definition provided in the table.

†Radiation therapy defined by EF: the clinically involved nodal region, the uninvolved adjacent nodal region(s), and uninvolved nodal region(s) beyond the adjacent nodal region.

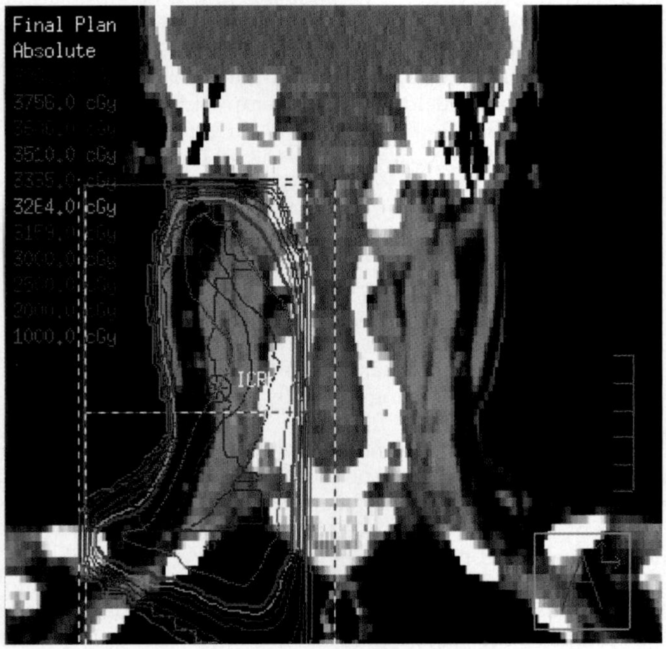

Figure 74-3 IFRT of left cervical lymph node region. Isodose distribution with AP/PA opposing fields using 6 MV photons. AP/PA, anteroposterior/posteroanterior; IFRT, involved-field radiation therapy.

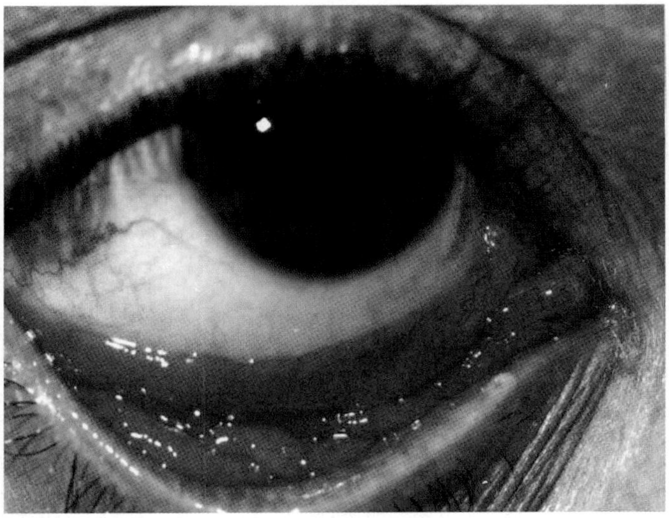

Figure 74-4 Extranodal marginal zone lymphoma of MALT type, involving the conjunctiva. The characteristic salmon-pink infiltration is seen most easily by pulling the lower eyelid downward. MALT, mucosa-associated lymphoid tissue.

local control rates are obtained with 30 Gy,[198] whereas for bulky lymphomas treated with CMT, a minimum dose of 35 Gy is required. Some centers routinely administer doses of 40 Gy,[464] or up to 45 to 50 Gy in the combined-modality setting.[114] There are no randomized trials designed to determine the optimal dose of RT, and the practice has developed based on institutional experience,[114] but higher doses are difficult to justify with excellent local control reported in patients who are in CR after chemotherapy.

In CMT protocols where chemotherapy is given before RT, there may be no abnormality or minimal residual disease at the time of RT planning. Therefore, in the determination of the target volume following chemotherapy, a decision must either cover the initial extent of disease or the post-chemotherapy nodal area, which can be normal or consist of minimal residual abnormalities. In general, if the disease displaced normal tissues without infiltration into surrounding extranodal tissues and there was a good response to chemotherapy, the radiation fields need not cover the entire initial extent of the tumor volume. An example is a bulky mediastinal mass that did not infiltrate lung tissue and has reduced in size following chemotherapy, where the RT plan need only cover the postchemotherapy abnormality. If, however, the disease was infiltrative initially into adjacent normal tissue, regression of the tumor mass still leaves microscopic residual disease in the infiltrated tissue and consideration must be given to adequately cover initial disease extent. An example would be bone lymphoma where the RT volume following a good response to chemotherapy should include the prechemotherapy extent of disease.

Orbital Lymphomas

Primary orbital lymphomas are highly curable with RT. Doses of 20 to 25 Gy results in excellent local control rates of more than 95%.[83,363,366] For anterior orbital lesions in the conjunctiva (Fig. 74-4), a direct anterior beam with orthovoltage (250 kv), telecobalt, or 4 to 6 MV photons can be used. Alternatively, an anterior electron beam can be used if the lesion is superficial and there is a desire to spare the posterior orbital structures. A small lead shield suspended in front of the lens can reduce the lens dose to less than 5% to 10%.[465] For unilateral retrobulbar lesions, a two-field technique with

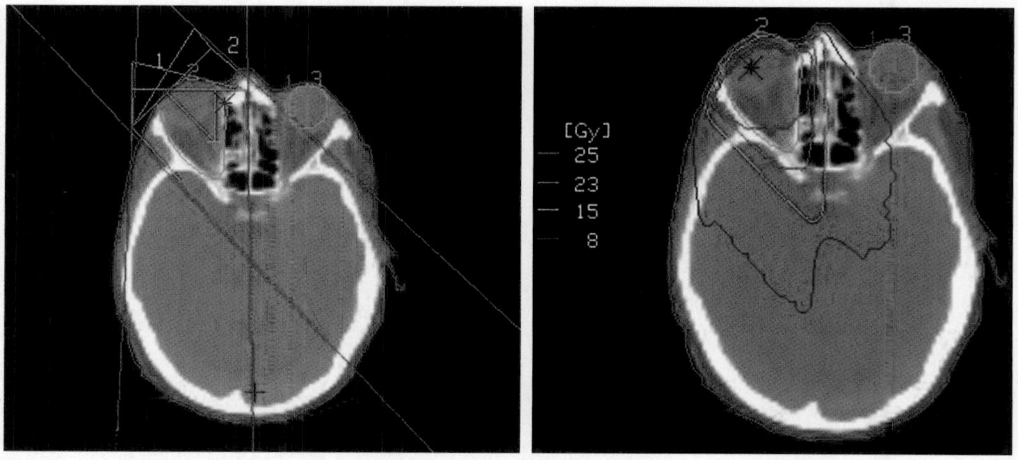

Figure 74-5 Orbital MALT lymphoma, two-field wedged pair technique treating the whole orbit (6 MV photons). MALT, mucosa-associated lymphoid tissue.

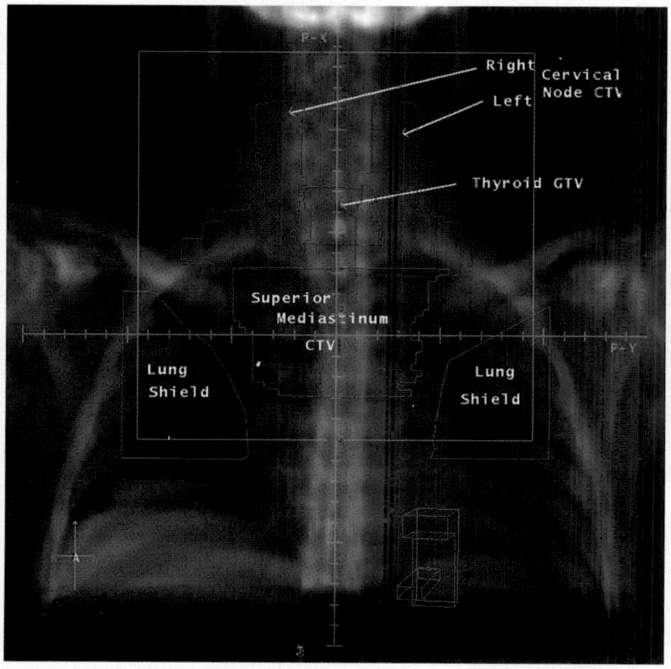

Figure 74-6 A modified mantle field encompassing bilateral cervical and superior mediastinal lymph nodes, with shielding for the lungs.

an anterior and a oblique wedged-field using 4 to 6 MV photons usually produces a satisfactory result (Fig. 74-5). Again, shielding for the lens can be placed for both fields to spare the lens. Lens dose of more than 2 to 3 Gy (single fraction) or more than 12 Gy fractionated (fraction size 1.5 to 2 Gy) may lead to cataract formation.[466] Damage to the bony orbit, retina, optic nerve, and soft tissues should not be seen with doses of less than 40 Gy.[456] However, some dryness of the eye because of lacrimal gland effects can be observed because the tolerance dose of the lacrimal gland is 40 Gy in 20 fractions.[467]

Thyroid Lymphoma

The RT target volume includes the thyroid bed, bilateral cervical, and superior mediastinal lymph nodes. A modified mantle field will cover this volume with sparing of the axilla, pericardium, and minimize lung exposure (Fig. 74-6). With the patient in the supine position with the neck extended, the upper field border is at the tip of the mastoid bone, and the lower border just below tracheal bifurcation. The lateral borders should ensure adequate clearance of the neck at the supraclavicular fossa. Customized shields for the lungs are necessary. As in the mantle technique, because the field shape and surface contours are irregular, nonuniformity of dose should be corrected with an attenuator. For a euthyroid patient, thyroid doses of 35 to 40 Gy for Hodgkin's lymphoma results in a 47% risk of overt or subclinical hypothyroidism at 27 years after treatment.[468] Other abnormalities such as nodular thyroid disease, goiter, and thyroid cancer are also lifetime risks.[469,470]

Waldeyer's Ring and Salivary Gland

A typical field arrangement for tonsillar lymphoma is shown in Figure 74-7. The target volume includes bilateral tonsillar fossa, nasopharynx, posterior tongue, and bilateral cervical (posterior neck nodes, jugular chain, and supraclavicular fossa). This can be accomplished with a four-field asymmetric collimator technique with two parallel-opposed lateral fields matching to two anterior-posterior fields to treat the lower neck, using one isocenter as reference, or with IMRT (see Fig. 74-7). The inferior jaws (y-axis) are closed to the level of the central axis for the lateral fields, and the superior jaws (y-axis) are closed to the central axis for the anterior-posterior fields to create a perfect geometric match. The location of the match is chosen to be above the level of the shoulder, preferably above the level of the larynx so that the anterior-posterior fields can be shielded centrally to avoid unnecessary exposure to the larynx, trachea, esophagus, and spinal cord. Acute morbidity of irradiation to doses of 35 to 40 Gy includes xerostomia, loss of taste, and mucositis, which are usually mild to moderate in degree. Because the treatment includes most of the salivary glands, a degree of permanent xerostomia can be seen, being manifested in decreased saliva flow rates on stimulation.[471] The severity of xerostomia is dependent on the total dose and the volume of salivary gland irradiated.[472] Emami and colleagues estimated that the TD 5/5 for salivary gland function is 32 Gy and the TD 50/5 is 46 Gy.[473] Therefore, careful planning of radiation fields should minimize this complication, and consideration given to spare salivary gland tissue as much as possible without compromise of cure. For example, a stage IE DLCL involving a unilateral parotid gland treated with chemotherapy can be spared the irradiation of the contralateral parotid gland. An ipsilateral technique, with lateral high-energy electrons, is often adequate for this purpose. Radiation

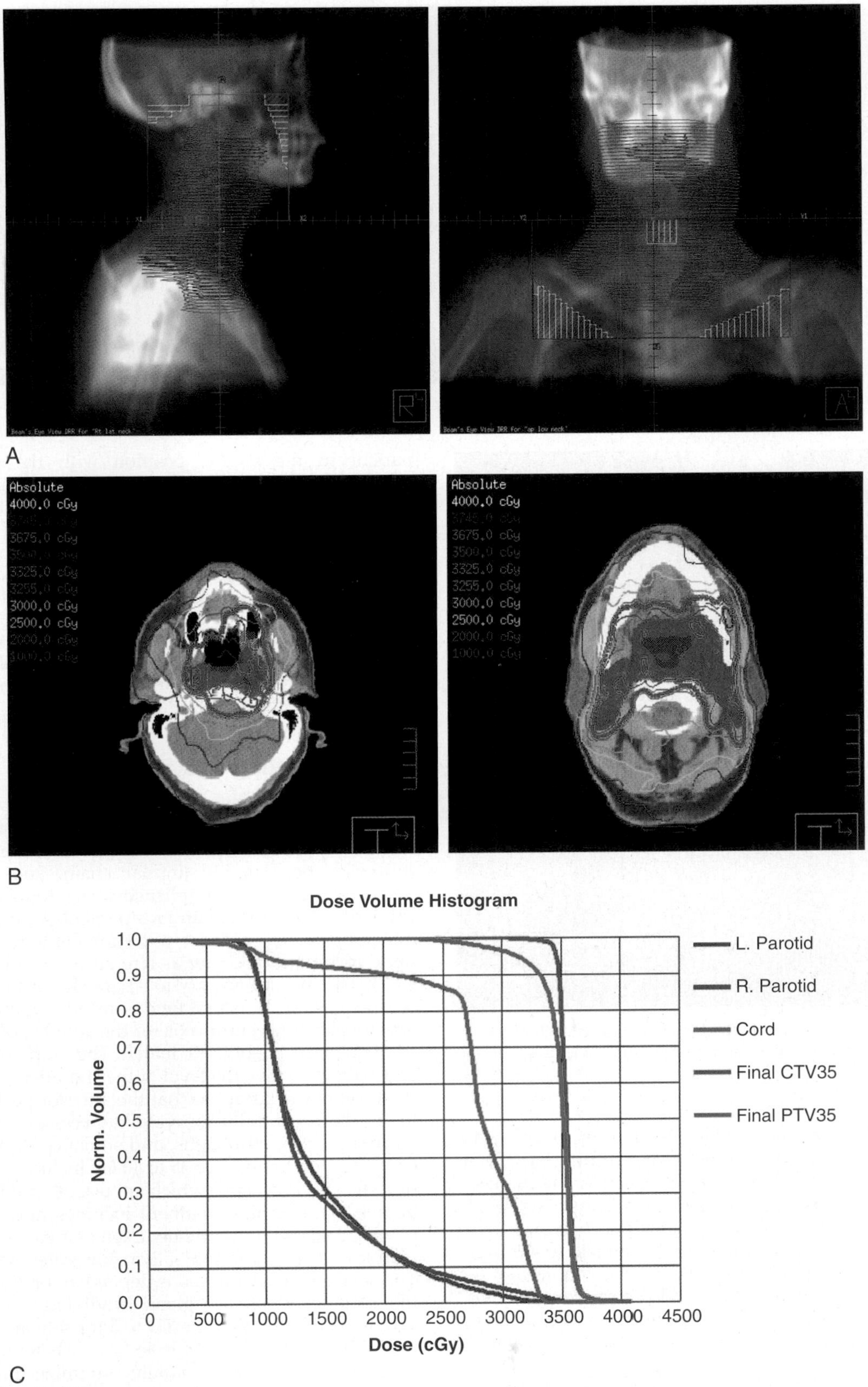

Figure 74-7 **A**, Four-field asymmetric technique with lateral opposing fields to the Waldeyer's ring structures and upper cervical lymph nodes, with a geometrically perfect match to AP/PA opposing fields for the lower neck (6 MV photons). Midline shielding is placed at the junction to avoid overdose to spinal cord. This treatment plan delivers full dose to much of the parotid salivary glands. **B**, IMRT technique for Waldeyer's ring structures and upper cervical lymph nodes, prescribed dose 35 Gy in 20 fractions, aiming to spare the parotid glands. **C**, Dose volume histogram for IMRT treatment plan to Waldeyer's ring (B); note that the V_{15} and V_{20} for parotid glands are 30% and 15%, respectively. AP/PA, anteroposterior/posteroanterior; IMRT, intensity-modulated radiation therapy.

doses of 35 to 40 Gy given in 1.8 to 2-Gy fractions are within the tolerance of all the other critical head and neck tissues such as the spinal cord, neurovascular structures, larynx, trachea, esophagus, and soft tissues.

Radiation to Thoracic Structures

Common techniques include the mantle, the modified mantle as described earlier, and IF to the mediastinum. Because of the irregular field arrangement and contour variation, care is required to ensure dose uniformity with the use of attenuators. Customized shielding blocks are mandatory for the protection of lung and cardiac tissues. The $TD_{5/5}$ for 20 fractions of whole lung radiation was 26.5 Gy (TD_{50} 30.5 Gy) from pediatric series of patients irradiated for Wilms' tumor.[474] Partial lung irradiation with fractionated doses have been studied by Mah and associates, using radiographic changes as the end-point.[475] A steep dose response relationship was found, where the TD_5 was 24.7 Gy, increasing to 33.9 Gy for TD_{50}, and to 43.5 Gy for TD_{95}, normalized to 15 fractions. Many chemotherapy drugs potentiate the effects of RT on lung tissue, such as bleomycin, cyclophosphamide, and doxorubicin.[476] Symptomatic pneumonitis occurs in 5% to 10% of patients treated for lymphoma.[474] Use of optimal dose-fractionation parameters, careful treatment planning with evaluation of DVH and mean doses to the lungs,[477-479] and allowing a 3 to 4 week interval between chemotherapy and RT should minimize the incidence of symptomatic radiation pneumonitis. IMRT offers improved sparing of organs at risk in selected patients and is particularly important for retreatment of relapsed disease.[461]

Information on the cardiac tolerance to irradiation has been largely based on patients treated for Hodgkin's lymphoma. The $TD_{5/5}$ for 50% to 60% inclusion of the heart is 40 Gy in 16 fractions.[480] The commonest syndrome is delayed pericarditis with pancarditis occurring after much higher doses.[480,481] Late effects include coronary artery disease, cardiomyopathy, and myocardial infarction.[482-484] As for lung tissue, careful treatment planning with maximum cardiac shielding (subcarinal area and the left ventricle), and the avoidance of dose per fraction more than 2 Gy should minimize the risk of pericarditis.[485] The potential cardiotoxic effects of doxorubicin can also be additive to the long-term damaging effects of radiation on the heart.

Gastric Lymphoma and Issues Relating to Abdominal Irradiation

In planning radiation directed to intraabdominal structures, the radiation tolerance of the liver ($TD_{5/5}$:25 Gy, whole organ), bowel (small bowel, 20 cm × 20 cm fields, $TD_{5/5}$:45 Gy), spinal cord ($TD_{5/5}$:50 Gy), and kidneys ($TD_{5/5}$:20 Gy) must be respected.[486-488] CT planning is extremely helpful, and the principle and technique similar to that used for gastric carcinoma can be adapted for use. The intention here is to deliver a tumor dose of 35 Gy to the entire stomach and limit the total dose to both kidneys to less than 20 Gy, while keeping a significant volume of liver to low doses. With fractionated doses of 35 to 40 Gy, major serious complications to the bowel are uncommon. In most instances, the RT toxicity can be reduced by using 3D conformal technique to minimize the dose to the liver and the kidneys. For example, the CTV can be separated into *superior* (treated with anteroposterior/posteroanterior [AP/PA] fields) and *inferior* (treated with an AP and two wedged-laterals) volumes, with a common isocenter at the junction. The AP field is common to both volumes. The photon beams are applied using 6/18 MV for the AP/PA fields and 18 MV for lateral fields. The PTV margin is defined using 4D CT or fluoroscopy to allow for breathing and setup variation.

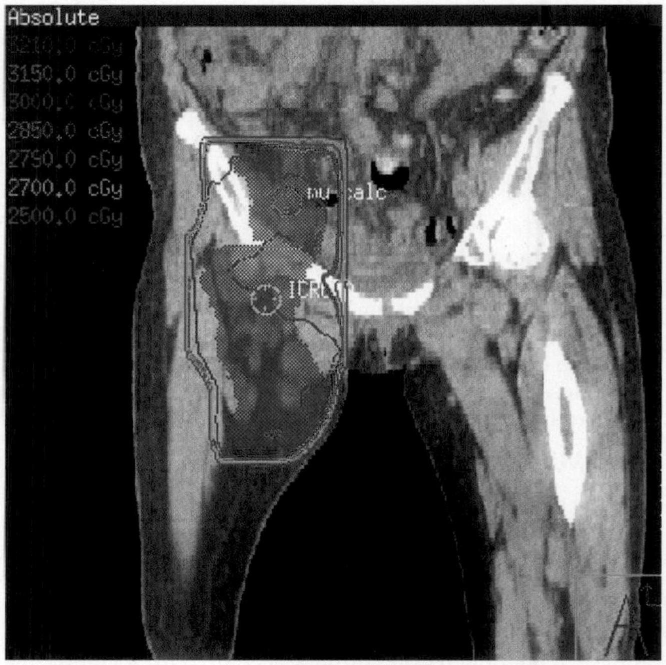

Figure 74-8 IFRT for right inguinal femoral lymph nodes, with AP/PA opposing fields (6 MV photons), with coverage of the ipsilateral external iliac lymph nodes. AP/PA, anteroposterior/posteroanterior; IFRT, involved-field radiation therapy.

Pelvic Radiation and Effects on the Reproductive System

Because radiation for lymphomas frequently involves large fields (e.g., inverted Y, whole pelvis, or hemi-pelvis), treatment planning must address effects of direct as well as scatter radiation to the genital organs. For example, the inverted Y field directly exposes the ovaries, and doses of 20 to 24 Gy will invariably produce ovarian ablation, with loss of hormonal function resulting in menopause and sterility.[489] Therefore, treatment planning for pelvic lymph node RT should spare one ovary if possible, with ultrasound or CT guidance to locate the ovary (e.g., hemi-pelvic radiation for stage I inguinal lymphoma, see Fig. 74-8). When bilateral pelvic irradiation is inevitable, the use of surgical oophoropexy with transposition of one ovary to the lateral abdomen and marking it with surgical clips to ensure exclusion from the radiation fields should be considered. However, this procedure alone can produce infertility because of interference with the vascular supply of the transposed ovary. Successful pregnancies with this approach have been reported in Hodgkin's lymphoma patients.[490,491] In males, direct radiation to the testes generally occurs in the CMT of primary testes lymphoma, or for testicular relapse of lymphoma where chemotherapy does not have full effect for this sanctuary site. Treatment planning is clinical and simulation of the field is not required. A direct anterior field with 4 to 6 MV photons with a visual check to encompass all scrotal contents is usually adequate. Because the germinal epithelium of the testes is extremely radiosensitive, where doses as low as 15 cGy can produce transient oligospermia,[492] and doses of 4 to 6 Gy can result in permanent azoospermia, infertility is always a consequence of scrotal irradiation.

Sperm banking should be considered before commencing therapy, preferably before chemotherapy. However, Leydig cell function with testosterone production can be preserved after doses of 30 to 35 Gy,[493] but dysfunction as manifested in a rise in LH and FSH levels can be seen even for lower doses of 5 to 6 Gy.[493] Based on a review of the literature, Izard concluded that approximately 50% of males receiving 14 Gy in fractionated doses will have an abnormal LH, whereas 33 Gy is required to see an abnormal testosterone level in 50%.[494]

Indirect (i.e., scatter) radiation to the testes is also a special consideration when planning fields close to the scrotum, particularly if the field size is large. The scatter dose is mainly a function of distance from the field edge, where gonadal doses of less than 5% are usually achieved with a distance from the field edge of 10 cm or more, for a field size of 25 cm^2.[493] The scatter dose can be reduced further by shielding with a leaded box directly applied to the scrotum.[495]

Bone Marrow

With the more frequent use of CMT and BMT in the treatment of lymphomas, radiation is frequently required in patients who had extensive previous chemotherapy or who had undergone BMT. Hematopoietic reserve may be significantly compromised in these patients, increasing the risk of radiation-induced myelosuppression.[496] This is particularly a problem where the treatment field encompasses a significant proportion of the bone marrow (e.g., mantle or inverted Y techniques, cranial-spinal radiation). The use of granulocyte-colony stimulating factor (G-CSF) has been shown to ameliorate neutropenia.[151,497,498] The optimal timing and dose-schedule has not been determined, but a dose of 5 µg/kg/day for 3 injections given when the leukocyte count was lower than 2.5 $\times 10^9$ L was reported to be successful[497] in minimizing treatment interruptions. However, G-CSF does not correct thrombocytopenia, which is likely to be a limiting factor once neutropenia is reversed. Although platelet transfusions can be performed for platelet counts of less than 10 to 20 $\times 10^9$ L, or for active bleeding, there is a risk of rendering patients platelet-transfusion dependent for prolonged periods of time, particularly when RT is given in the post-ABMT setting. A study from the Royal Marsden Hospital showed that a pretreatment platelet count of less than 100 $\times 10^9$ L was predictive of severe thrombocytopenia with RT given post-BMT.[496] It is possible that platelet growth factors (thrombopoietin) will become clinically available within the next few years[499] and its use may avert radiation induced thrombocytopenia. Anemia, if present, is usually not a dose-limiting problem and red cell transfusions can be given as required. Erythropoietin therapy, in conjunction with oral ferrous sulfate, increases hemoglobin level for patients undergoing RT.[500]

UNRESOLVED ISSUES IN THE RT MANAGEMENT OF MALIGNANT LYMPHOMAS

The efficacy of RT in achieving local disease control has been accepted for many years. With excellent local control rates, attention has been focused on the optimization of chemotherapy. Rituximab is an important component of systemic therapy in DLBCL. Therefore the questions of optimal RT target volume or the optimal dose-fractionation schemes have not been prospectively tested in randomized trials. This is most evident in the management of DLCL with CMT, where the RT dose varies from 30 to 50 Gy, depending on the center rather than disease characteristics.[114] Similarly the RT volume can vary from IF, with or without inclusion of adjacent first echelon nodes, to extended fields.[114] Currently, there are few phase III trials that address RT-related issues in the management of NHL. Some of the controversies in the RT management of the NHL are as follows:

1. The management of follicular lymphomas: The role of IF versus extended field RT in the management of localized follicular lymphomas is controversial. Current ability to identify homogeneous patient group with the use of genotyping and assessment of minimal residual disease (*BCL2* by PCR) opens the opportunity to study systemic RIT in this disease. The use of CMT in localized stages of the disease requires phase III trials.
2. Optimal RT dose-fractionation, and CTV in combined-modality protocols: Excellent results are obtained with doses ranging from 30 to 50 Gy. Trials are required to address the issue of whether 30 Gy is optimal for patients who completely responded to chemotherapy, and whether the IFRT CTV should encompass the whole nodal region.
3. Role of RT in stages I to II diffuse large B-cell lymphomas: Chemotherapy alone has been shown to cure a substantial proportion of patients with localized DLBCL. Whether RT offers additional benefit when a chemotherapy regimen more intensive than CHOP is used (e.g., the GELA protocol with ACVBP—doxorubicin, cyclophosphamide, vindesine, bleomycin, and prednisone, followed by high-dose methotrexate with leucovorin, etoposide, ifosfamide, and cytarabine), or when rituximab is added—has not been addressed in a phase III study.
4. Optimal RT in the setting of high-dose chemotherapy and stem cell support: The role of IFRT or total body radiation in the setting of BMT requires further refinement. This relates to the indications, selection of patients for therapy, dose-fractionation parameters, and the timing with chemotherapy and BMT.

NHLs represent a heterogeneous group of diseases that may affect any part of the body. They are characterized by a tendency to present as or progress to generalized disease. Therefore optimal systemic therapy is paramount. However, lymphomas are also characterized by a high degree of radioresponsiveness and therefore RT is an important modality in controlling these malignancies (Fig. 74-9). Recent progress in biology and histopathology as well as cytogenetic techniques have allowed us to study homogeneous patient populations and provide an opportunity for reassessing the role of RT in their management. Late effects of treatment manifesting as normal tissue toxicity and especially second cancers are continuing concerns following curative therapy. Attention to late morbidity while we devise treatments to improve the cure rate remains an important goal.

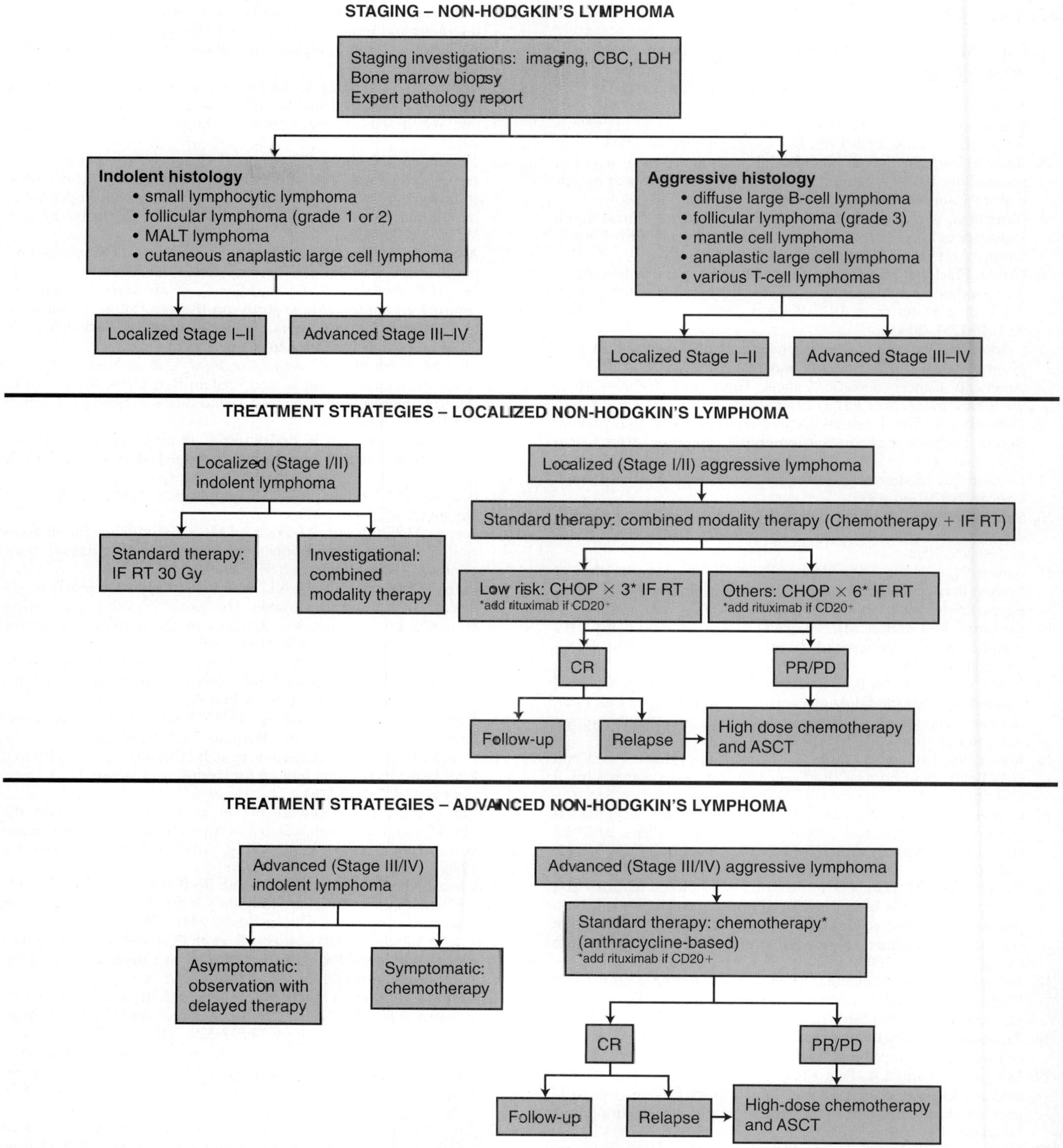

Figure 74-9 Approach to the patient with newly diagnosed NHL. ASCT, autologous stem cell transplantation; CBC, complete blood count; CHOP, cyclophosphamide, Adriamycin (doxorubicin), Oncovin (vincristine), and prednisone; CR, complete response; IFRT, involved-field radiation therapy; LDH, lactate dehydrogenase; MALT, mucosa-associated lymphoid tissue; PR, partial response.

REFERENCES

1. Carli PM, Boutron MC, Maynadie M, et al: Increase in the incidence of non-Hodgkin's lymphomas: evidence for a recent sharp increase in France independent of AIDS. Br J Cancer 70:713-715, 1994.
2. Dal Maso L, Franceschi S, Polesel J, et al: Risk of cancer in persons with AIDS in Italy, 1985-1998. Br J Cancer 89:94-100, 2003.
3. Seow A, Lee J, Sng I, et al: Non-Hodgkin's lymphoma in an Asian population: 1968-1992 time trends and ethnic differences in Singapore. Cancer 77:1899-1904, 1996.
4. Morgan G, Vornanen M, Puitinen J, et al: Changing trends in the incidence of non-Hodgkin's lymphoma in Europe Biomed Study Group. Ann Oncol 8(Suppl 2):49-54, 1997.
5. Groves FD, Linet MS, Travis LB, et al: Cancer surveillance series: Non-Hodgkin's lymphoma incidence by histologic subtype in the United States from 1978 through 1995. J Natl Cancer Inst 92:1240-1251, 2000.
6. Clarke CA, Glaser SL: Changing incidence of non-Hodgkin lymphomas in the United States. Cancer 94:2015-2023, 2002.
7. American Cancer Society: Cancer Facts and Figures. 2006. www.cancer.org/docroot/STT/stt_o.asp.
8. Weisenburger DD: Epidemiology of non-Hodgkin's lymphoma: Recent findings regarding an emerging epidemic. Ann Oncol 1:19-24, 1994.
9. Greiner TC, Medeiros LJ, Jaffe ES: Non-Hodgkin's lymphoma. Cancer 75:370-380, 1995.
10. Smedby KE, Hjalgrim H, Melbye M, et al: Ultraviolet radiation exposure and risk of malignant lymphomas. J Natl Cancer Inst 97:199-209, 2005.
11. Anwar N, Kingma DW, Bloch AR, et al: The investigation of Epstein-Barr viral sequences in 41 cases of Burkitt's lymphoma from Egypt: Epidemiologic correlations. Cancer 76:1245-1252, 1995.
12. Rochford R, Cannon MJ, Moormann AM: Endemic Burkitt's lymphoma: A polymicrobial disease? Nat Rev Microbiol 3:182-187, 2005.
13. Jaffe ES, Chan JK, Su IJ, et al: Report of the Workshop on Nasal and Related Extranodal Angiocentric T/Natural Killer Cell Lymphomas. Definitions, differential diagnosis, and epidemiology. Am J Surg Pathol 20:103-111, 1996.
14. Koom WS, Chung EJ, Yang WI, et al: Angiocentric T-cell and NK/T-cell lymphomas: Radiotherapeutic viewpoints. Int J Radiat Oncol Biol Phys 59:1127-1137, 2004.
15. Cheung MM, Chan JK, Lau WH, et al: Early stage nasal NK/T-cell lymphoma: Clinical outcome, prognostic factors, and the effect of treatment modality. Int J Radiat Oncol Biol Phys 54:182-190, 2002.
16. Au WY, Ma SY, Chim CS, et al: Clinicopathologic features and treatment outcome of mature T-cell and natural killer-cell lymphomas diagnosed according to the World Health Organization classification scheme: A single center experience of 10 years. Ann Oncol 16:206-214, 2005.
17. Arber DA, Weiss LM, Albujar PF, et al: Nasal lymphomas in Peru. High incidence of T-cell immunophenotype and Epstein-Barr virus infection. Am J Surg Pathol 17:392-399, 1993.
18. Takatsuki K: Kenneth MacGredie memorial lectureship. Adult T-cell leukemia/lymphoma. Leukemia 11(Suppl 3):54-56, 1997.
19. Deloose ST, Smit LA, Pals FT, et al: High incidence of Kaposi sarcoma-associated herpesvirus infection in HIV-related solid immunoblastic/plasmablastic diffuse large B-cell lymphoma. Leukemia 19(5):851-855, 2005.
20. Doglioni C, Wotherspoon AC, Moschini A, et al: High incidence of primary gastric lymphoma in northeastern Italy. Lancet 339:834-835, 1992.
21. Opelz G, Henderson R: Incidence of non-Hodgkin lymphoma in kidney and heart transplant recipients. Lancet 342:1514-1516, 1993.
22. Cote TR, Biggar RJ, Rosenberg PS, et al: Non-Hodgkin's lymphoma among people with AIDS: incidence, presentation and public health burden. AIDS/Cancer Study Group. Int J Cancer 73:645-650, 1997.
23. Bhaskaran K, Brettle R, Porter K, et al: Systemic non-Hodgkin lymphoma in individuals with known dates of HIV seroconversion: Incidence and predictors. AIDS 18:673-681, 2004.
24. Stebbing J, Gazzard B, Mandalia S, et al: Antiretroviral treatment regimens and immune parameters in the prevention of systemic AIDS-related non-Hodgkin's lymphoma. J Clin Oncol 22:2177-2183, 2004.
25. Cesarman E, Chang Y, Moore PS, et al: Kaposi's sarcoma-associated herpesvirus-like DNA sequences in AIDS-related body-cavity-based lymphomas. N Engl J Med 332:1186-1191, 1995.
26. Tzioufas AG, Boumba DS, Skopouli FN, et al: Mixed monoclonal cryoglobulinemia and monoclonal rheumatoid factor cross-reactive idiotypes as predictive factors for the development of lymphoma in primary Sjogren's syndrome. Arthritis Rheum 39:767-772, 1996.
27. Aozasa K: Hashimoto's thyroiditis as a risk factor of thyroid lymphoma. Acta Pathologica Japonica 40:459-468, 1990.
28. Tennis P, Andrews E, Bombardier C, et al: Record linkage to conduct an epidemiologic study on the association of rheumatoid arthritis and lymphoma in the Province of Saskatchewan, Canada. J Clin Epidemiol 46:685-695, 1993
29. Ilyas M, Niedobitek G, Agathanggelou A, et al: Non-Hodgkin's lymphoma, coeliac disease, and Epstein-Barr virus: A study of 13 cases of enteropathy-associated T- and B-cell lymphoma. J Pathol 177:115-122, 1995.
30. Parsonnet J, Hansen S, Rodriguez L, et al: Helicobacter pylori infection and gastric lymphoma. N Engl J Med 330:1267-1271, 1994.
31. Isaacson PG: Update on MALT lymphomas. Best Pract Res Clin Haematol 18:57-68, 2005.
32. Ferreri AJ, Guidoboni M, Ponzoni M, et al: Evidence for an association between Chlamydia psittaci and ocular adnexal lymphomas. J Natl Cancer Inst 96:586-594, 2004.
33. Jaffe ES, Diebold J, Harris NL, et al: Burkitt's lymphoma: A single disease with multiple variants. The World Health Organization classification of neoplastic diseases of the hematopoietic and lymphoid tissues. Blood 93:1124, 1999.
34. Cleghorn FR, Manns A, Falk R, et al: Effect of human T-lymphotropic virus type I infection on non-Hodgkin's lymphoma incidence. J Natl Cancer Inst 87:1009-1014, 1995.
35. Nicot C: Current views in HTLV-I-associated adult T-cell leukemia/lymphoma. Am J Hematol 78:232-239, 2005.
36. Prosper F, Robledo C, Cuesta B, et al: Incidence of non-Hodgkin's lymphoma in patients treated for Hodgkin's disease. Leuk Lymphoma 12:457-462, 1994.
37. Blair A, Linos A, Stewart PA, et al: Evaluation of risks for non-Hodgkin's lymphoma by occupation and industry exposures from a case-control study. Am J Ind Med 23:301-312, 1993.
38. Cantor KP, Blair A, Everett G, et al: Pesticides and other agricultural risk factors for non-Hodgkin's lymphoma among men in Iowa and Minnesota. Cancer Res 52:2447-2455, 1992.
39. Zheng T, Holford TR, Leaderer B, et al: Diet and nutrient intakes and risk of non-Hodgkin's lymphoma in Connecticut women. Am J Epidemiol 159:454-466, 2004.
40. Chang ET, Ekstrom Smedby K, Zhang SM, et al: Dietary factors and risk of non-Hodgkin lymphoma in men and women. Cancer Epidemiol Biomarkers Prev 14:512-520, 2005.
41. Correa A, Jackson L, Mohan A, et al: Use of hair dyes, hematopoietic neoplasms, and lymphomas: a literature review. II. Lymphomas and multiple myeloma. Cancer Invest 18:467-479, 2000.
42. Tavani A, Negri E, Franceschi S, et al: Hair dye use and risk of lymphoid neoplasms and soft tissue sarcomas. Int J Cancer 113:629-631, 2005.
43. Preston DL, Kusumi S, Tomonaga M, et al: Cancer incidence in atomic bomb survivors. Part III. Leukemia, lymphoma and multiple myeloma, 1950-1987. [Erratum in Radiat Res 139(1):129, 1994.] Radiat Res 137:S68-S97, 1994.
44. Boice JD Jr, Morin MM, Glass AG, et al: Diagnostic x-ray procedures and risk of leukemia, lymphoma, and multiple myeloma. [Erratum in JAMA 265(21):2810, 1991.] JAMA 265:1290-1294, 1991.
45. Inskip PD, Kleinerman RA, Stovall M, et al: Leukemia, lymphoma, and multiple myeloma after pelvic radiotherapy for benign disease. Radiation Res 135:108-124, 1993.

46. Kirsch IR, Lipkowitz S: A measure of genomic instability and its relevance to lymphomagenesis. Cancer Research 52:5545s-5546s, 1992.
47. Morgan AJ: Epstein-Barr virus vaccines. Vaccine 10:563-571, 1992.
48. Rooney CM, Smith CA, Ng CY, et al: Infusion of cytotoxic T-cells for the prevention and treatment of Epstein-Barr virus-induced lymphoma in allogeneic transplant recipients. Blood 92:1549-1555, 1998.
49. Savoldo B, Heslop HE, Rooney CM: The use of cytotoxic t cells for the prevention and treatment of Epstein-Barr virus induced lymphoma in transplant recipients. Leuk Lymphoma 39:455-464, 2000.
50. Fischbach W, Goebeler-Kolve ME, Dragosics B, et al: Long term outcome of patients with gastric marginal zone B-cell lymphoma of mucosa associated lymphoid tissue (MALT) following exclusive Helicobacter pylori eradication therapy: experience from a large prospective series. Gut 53:34-37, 2004.
51. Zucca E, Bertoni F, Roggero E, et al: The gastric marginal zone B-cell lymphoma of MALT type. Blood 96:410-419, 2000.
52. Marshall BJ, Windsor HM: The relation of Helicobacter pylori to gastric adenocarcinoma and lymphoma: pathophysiology, epidemiology, screening, clinical presentation, treatment, and prevention. Med Clin North Am 89:313-344, viii, 2005.
53. Rappaport H: Tumor of the hematopoietic system. Washington, DC, Armed Forces Institute of Pathology, 1966.
54. Stansfeld AG, Diebold J, Noel H, et al: Updated Kiel classification for lymphomas. Lancet 1:292-293, 1988.
55. Harris N, Jaffe ES, Stein H, et al: A revised European-American classification of lymphoid neoplasms: A proposal from the International Lymphoma Study Group. Blood 84:1361-1392, 1994.
56. Jaffe ES, Harris NL, Stein H, et al: Pathology and genetics of tumours of hematopoietic and lymphoid tissues, in Kleihues P, Sobin LH (eds): World Health Organization Classification of Tumours. Lyon, France, IARC Press, 2001.
57. Melnyk A, Rodriguez A, Pugh WC, et al: Evaluation of the Revised European-American Lymphoma classification confirms the clinical relevance of immunophenotype in 560 cases of aggressive non-Hodgkin's lymphoma. Blood 89:4514-4520, 1997.
58. The Non-Hodgkin's Lymphoma Classification Project: A clinical evaluation of the International Lymphoma Study Group classification of non-Hodgkin's lymphoma. Blood 89:3909-3918, 1997.
59. Carbone A, Franceschi S, Gloghini A, et al: Pathological and immunophenotypic features of adult non-Hodgkin's lymphomas by age group. Hum Pathol 28:580-587, 1997.
60. Rehn S, Glimelius B, Strang P, et al: Prognostic significance of flow cytometry studies in B-cell non-Hodgkin lymphoma. Hematol Oncol 8:1-12, 1990.
61. Joensuu H, Klemi PJ, Söderström KO, et al: Comparison of S-phase fraction, working formulation, and Kiel classification in non-Hodgkin's lymphoma. Cancer 68:1564-1571, 1991.
62. Miller TP, Grogan TM, Dahlberg S, et al: Prognostic significance of the Ki-67-associated proliferative antigen in aggressive Non-Hodgkin's lymphomas: A prospective Southwest Oncology Group trial. Blood 6:1460-1466, 1994.
63. Saito B, Shiozawa E, Yamochi-Onizuka T, et al: Efficacy of rituximab plus chemotherapy in follicular lymphoma depends on Ki-67 expression. Pathol Int 54:667-674, 2004.
64. Acker B, Hoppe RT, Colby TV, et al: Histologic conversion in the non-Hodgkin's lymphomas. J Clin Oncol 1:11-16, 1983.
65. Bastion Y, Sebban C, Berger F, et al: Incidence, predictive factors, and outcome of lymphoma transformation in follicular lymphoma patients. J Clin Oncol 15:1587-1594, 1997.
66. Symmans WF, Katz RL, Ordonez NG, et al: Transformation of follicular lymphoma. Expression of p53 and BCL-2 oncoprotein, apoptosis and cell proliferation. Acta Cytologica 39:673-682, 1995.
67. Ichikawa A, Kinoshita T, Watanabe T, et al: Mutations of the p53 gene as a prognostic factor in aggressive B-cell lymphoma. N Engl J Med 337:529-534, 1997.
68. Zucca E, Stein H, Coiffier B: European Lymphoma Task Force (ELTF): Report of the workshop on Mantle Cell Lymphoma (MCL). Ann Oncol 5:507-511, 1994.
69. Fisher RI, Dahlberg S, Nathwani BN, et al: A clinical analysis of two indolent lymphoma entities: mantle cell lymphoma and marginal zone lymphoma (including the mucosa-associated lymphoid tissue and monocytoid B-cell subcategories): A Southwest Oncology Group study. Blood 85:1075-1082, 1995.
70. Pittaluga S, Wlodarska I, Stul MS, et al: Mantle cell lymphoma: A clinicopathological study of 55 cases. Histopathology 26:17-24, 1995.
71. Segal GH, Masih AS, Fox AC, et al: CD5-expressing B-cell non-Hodgkin's lymphomas with bcl-1 gene rearrangement have a relatively homogeneous immunophenotype and are associated with an overall poor prognosis. Blood 85:1570-1579, 1995.
72. Velders GA, Kluin-Nelemans JC, De Boer CJ, et al: Mantle-cell lymphoma: A population-based clinical study. J Clin Oncol 14:1269-1274, 1996.
73. Mangel J, Leitch HA, Connors JM, et al: Intensive chemotherapy and autologous stem-cell transplantation plus rituximab is superior to conventional chemotherapy for newly diagnosed advanced stage mantle-cell lymphoma: A matched pair analysis. Ann Oncol 15:283-290, 2004.
74. Dreyling M, Lenz G, Hoster E, et al: Early consolidation by myeloablative radiochemotherapy followed by autologous stem cell transplantation in first remission significantly prolongs progression-free survival in mantle cell lymphoma—Results of a prospective randomized trial of the European MCL network. Blood 105(7):2677-2684, 2005.
75. Rosenwald A, Wright G, Wiestner A, et al: The proliferation gene expression signature is a quantitative integrator of oncogenic events that predicts survival in mantle cell lymphoma. Cancer Cell 3:185-197, 2003.
76. Leitch HA, Gascoyne RD, Chhanabhai M, et al: Limited-stage mantle-cell lymphoma. Ann Oncol 14:1555-1561, 2003.
77. Rudiger T, Weisenburger DD, Anderson JR, et al: Peripheral T-cell lymphoma (excluding anaplastic large-cell lymphoma): Results from the Non-Hodgkin's Lymphoma Classification Project. Ann Oncol 13:140-149, 2002.
78. Liang R, Todd D, Ho FC: Aggressive non-Hodgkin's lymphoma: T-cell versus B-cell. Hematol Oncol 14:1-6, 1996.
79. Isaacson PG, O'Connor NTJ, Spencer J, et al: Malignant histiocytosis of the intestine: A T-cell lymphoma. Lancet 2:688-691, 1985.
80. Spencer J, Cerf-Bensussan N, Jarry A, et al: Enteropathy associated T-cell lymphoma (malignant histiocytosis of the intestine) is recognized by a monoclonal antibody (HML-1) that defines a membrane molecule on mucosal lymphocytes. Am J Pathol 132:1-5, 1988.
81. Kim GE, Koom WS, Yang WI, et al: Clinical relevance of three subtypes of primary sinonasal lymphoma characterized by immunophenotypic analysis. Head Neck 26:584-593, 2004.
82. Au WY, Lie AK, Liang R, et al: Autologous stem cell transplantation for nasal NK/T-cell lymphoma: A progress report on its value. Ann Oncol 14:1673-1676, 2003.
83. Tsang RW, Gospodarowicz MK, Pintilie M, et al: Localized mucosa-associated lymphoid tissue lymphoma treated with radiation therapy has excellent clinical outcome. J Clin Oncol 21:4157-4164, 2003.
84. Lopez-Guillermo A, Colomo L, Jimenez M, et al: Diffuse large B-cell lymphoma: Clinicobiological characterization and outcome according to the nodal or extranodal primary origin. J Clin Oncol 23(12):2797-2780, 2005.
85. Dalla-Favera R, Ye BH, Lo Coco F, et al: Identification of genetic lesions associated with diffuse large-cell lymphoma. Ann Oncol 1:55-60, 1994.
86. Weisenburger DD, Armitage JO: Mantle cell lymphoma—an entity comes of age. Blood 87:4483-4494, 1996.
87. Offit K, Lo Coco F, Louie D, et al: Rearrangement of the bcl-6 gene as a prognostic marker in diffuse large cell lymphoma. N Engl J Med 331:74-80, 1994.
88. Kramer MH, Hermans J, Wijburg E, et al: Clinical relevance of BCL2, BCL6, and MYC rearrangements in diffuse large B-cell lymphoma. Blood 92:3152-3162, 1998.
89. Gaidano G, Dalla-Favera R: Molecular biology of lymphomas, *In* DeVita Jr VT, Hellman S, Rosenberg SA (eds): Principles and Practice of Oncology. Lymphomas, 5th ed. Philadelphia, Lippincott-Raven, 1997, pp 2131-2145.

90. Rosenwald A, Wright G, Chan WC, et al: The use of molecular profiling to predict survival after chemotherapy for diffuse large-B-cell lymphoma. N Engl J Med 346:1937-1947, 2002.
91. Dyomin VG, Rao PH, Dalla-Favera R, et al: BCL8, a novel gene involved in translocations affecting band 15q11-13 in diffuse large-cell lymphoma. Proc Natl Acad Sci U S A 94:5728-5732, 1997.
92. Magrath IT: African Burkitt's lymphoma. History, biology, clinical features, and treatment. Am J Ped Hematol Oncol 13:222-246, 1991.
93. Au WY, Horsman DE, Gascoyne RD, et al: The spectrum of lymphoma with 8q24 aberrations: A clinical, pathological and cytogenetic study of 87 consecutive cases. Leuk Lymphoma 45:519-528, 2004.
94. Knezevich S, Ludkovski O, Salski C, et al: Concurrent translocation of BCL2 and MYC with a single immunoglobulin locus in high-grade B-cell lymphomas. Leukemia 19:659-663, 2005.
95. Morris SW, Kirstein MN, Valentine MB, et al: Fusion of a kinase gene, ALK, to a nucleolar protein gene, NPM, in non-Hodgkin's lymphoma. Science 263:1281-1284, 1994.
96. Iida S, Rao P, Butler M, et al: Chromosomal translocation (9;14)(p13;q32) associated with lymphocytic lymphoma. Blood 86(Suppl 1):430a, 1995.
97. Baker SJ, Reddy EP: Role of E2A and PAX5/BSAP transcription factors. Oncogene 11:413-426, 1995.
98. Neri A, Fracchiolla NS, Rosceti E, et al: Molecular analysis of cutaneous B- and T-cell lymphomas. Blood 86:3160-3172, 1995.
99. Wotherspoon AC, Finn TM, Isaacson PG: Trisomy 3 in low-grade B-cell lymphomas of mucosa-associated lymphoid tissue. Blood 85:2000-2004, 1995.
100. Ye H, Liu H, Attygalle A, et al: Variable frequencies of t(11;18)(q21;q21) in MALT lymphomas of different sites: Significant association with CagA strains of H. pylori in gastric MALT lymphoma. Blood 102:1012-1018, 2003.
101. Morgan JA, Yin Y, Borowsky AD, et al: Breakpoints of the t(11;18)(q21;q21) in mucosa-associated lymphoid tissue (MALT) lymphoma lie within or near the previously undescribed gene MALT1 in chromosome 18. Cancer Res 59:6205-6213, 1999.
102. Remstein ED, James CD, Kurtin PJ: Incidence and subtype specificity of API2-MALT1 fusion translocations in extranodal, nodal, and splenic marginal zone lymphomas. Am J Pathol 156:1183-1188, 2000.
103. Auer IA, Gascoyne RD, Connors JM, et al: t(11;18)(q21;q21) is the most common translocation in Malt lymphomas. Ann Oncol 8:979-985, 1997.
104. Du MQ, Peng H, Liu H, et al: BCL10 gene mutation in lymphoma. Blood 95:3885-3890, 2000.
105. Streubel B, Lamprecht A, Dierlamm J, et al: T(14;18)(q32;q21) involving IGH and MALT1 is a frequent chromosomal aberration in MALT lymphoma. Blood 101:2335-2339, 2003.
106. Alizadeh AA, Eisen MB, Davis RE, et al: Distinct types of diffuse large B-cell lymphoma identified by gene expression profiling. Nature 403:503-511, 2000.
107. Hans CP, Weisenburger DD, Greiner TC, et al: Confirmation of the molecular classification of diffuse large B-cell lymphoma by immunohistochemistry using a tissue microarray. Blood 103:275-282, 2004.
108. Shipp MA, Ross KN, Tamayo P, et al: Diffuse large B-cell lymphoma outcome prediction by gene-expression profiling and supervised machine learning. Nat Med 8:68-74, 2002.
109. Gascoyne RD, Adomat SA, Krajewski S, et al: Prognostic significance of Bcl-2 protein expression and Bcl-2 gene rearrangement in diffuse aggressive non-Hodgkin's lymphoma. Blood 90:244-251, 1997.
110. Iqbal J, Sanger WG, Horsman DE, et al: BCL2 translocation defines a unique tumor subset within the germinal center B-cell-like diffuse large B-cell lymphoma. Am J Pathol 165:159-166, 2004.
111. Rosenwald A, Wright G, Leroy K, et al: Molecular diagnosis of primary mediastinal B cell lymphoma identifies a clinically favorable subgroup of diffuse large B cell lymphoma related to Hodgkin lymphoma. J Exp Med 198:851-862, 2003.
112. Dave SS, Wright G, Tan B, et al: Prediction of survival in follicular lymphoma based on molecular features of tumor-infiltrating immune cells. N Engl J Med 351:2159-2169, 2004.
113. Lam LT, Davis RE, Pierce J, et al: Small molecule inhibitors of IκB kinase are selectively toxic for subgroups of diffuse large B-cell lymphoma defined by gene expression profiling. Clin Cancer Res 11:28-40, 2005.
114. Tsang RW, Gospodarowicz MK, O'Sullivan B: Staging and management of localized non-Hodgkin's lymphomas: Variations among experts in radiation oncology. Int J Radiat Oncol Biol Phys 52:643-651, 2002.
115. Saddik M, Dabbagh L, Mourad WA: Ex vivo fine-needle aspiration cytology and flow cytometric phenotyping in the diagnosis of lymphoproliferative disorders: A proposed algorithm for maximum resource utilization. Diagn Cytopathol 16:126-131, 1997.
116. Schmitz L, Beneke J, Kubic V: Diagnosis of small non-cleaved cell lymphoma by fine needle aspiration utilizing cytomorphologic features combined with cytogenetic analysis. Acta Cytol 41:759-764, 1997.
117. Castellino RA, Hilton S, O'Brien JP, et al: Non-Hodgkin lymphoma: Contribution of chest CT in the initial staging evaluation. Radiology 199:129-132, 1996.
118. North LB, Wallace S, Lindell MM, et al: Lymphography for staging lymphomas: Is it still a useful procedure? AJR Am J Roentgenol 161:867-869, 1993.
119. Tardivon AA, Vanel D, Munck J-N, et al: Magnetic resonance imaging of the bone marrow in lymphomas and leukemias. Leuk Lymphoma 25:55-68, 1997.
120. Front D, Bar-Shalom R, Israel O: The continuing clinical role of gallium 67 scintigraphy in the age of receptor imaging. Semin Nucl Med 27:68-74, 1997.
121. Front D, Bar-Shalom R, Mor M, et al: Aggressive non-Hodgkin lymphoma: Early prediction of outcome with 67Ga scintigraphy. Radiology 214:253-257, 2000.
122. Janicek M, Kaplan W, Neuberg D, et al: Early restaging gallium scans predict outcome in poor-prognosis patients with aggressive non-Hodgkin's lymphoma treated with high-dose CHOP chemotherapy. J Clin Oncol 15:1631-1637, 1997.
123. Kostakoglu L, Leonard JP, Kuji I, et al: Comparison of fluorine-18 fluorodeoxyglucose positron emission tomography and Ga-67 scintigraphy in evaluation of lymphoma. Cancer 94:879-888, 2002.
124. Shen YY, Kao A, Yen RF: Comparison of 18F-fluoro-2-deoxyglucose positron emission tomography and gallium-67 citrate scintigraphy for detecting malignant lymphoma. Oncol Rep 9:321-325, 2002.
125. Van Den Bossche B, Lambert B, De Winter F, et al: 18FDG PET versus high-dose 67Ga scintigraphy for restaging and treatment follow-up of lymphoma patients. Nucl Med Commun 23:1079-1083, 2002.
126. de Wit M, Bumann D, Beyer W, et al: Whole-body positron emission tomography (PET) for diagnosis of residual mass in patients with lymphoma. Ann Oncol 8(Suppl 1):57-60, 1997.
127. Weihrauch MR, Re D, Scheidhauer K, et al: Thoracic positron emission tomography using 18F-fluorodeoxyglucose for the evaluation of residual mediastinal Hodgkin disease. Blood 98:2930-2934, 2001.
128. Naumann R, Vaic A, Beuthien-Baumann B, et al: Prognostic value of positron emission tomography in the evaluation of post-treatment residual mass in patients with Hodgkin's disease and non-Hodgkin's lymphoma. Br J Haematol 115:793-800, 2001.
129. Kostakoglu L, Coleman M, Leonard JP, et al: PET predicts prognosis after 1 cycle of chemotherapy in aggressive lymphoma and Hodgkin's disease. J Nucl Med 43:1018-1027, 2002.
130. Schot B, van Imhoff G, Pruim J, et al: Predictive value of early 18F-fluoro-deoxyglucose positron emission tomography in chemosensitive relapsed lymphoma. Br J Haematol 123:282-287, 2003.
131. Spaepen K, Stroobants S, Dupont P, et al: Prognostic value of positron emission tomography (PET) with fluorine-18 fluorodeoxyglucose ([18F]FDG) after first-line chemotherapy in non-Hodgkin's lymphoma: is [18F]FDG-PET a valid alternative to conventional diagnostic methods? J Clin Oncol 19:414-419, 2001.

132. Fleming ID, Cooper JS, Henson DE, et al: AJCC Cancer Staging Manual, 5th ed. Philadelphia, Lippincott-Raven, 1997.
133. UICC: TNM Classification of Malignant Tumours, 6th ed. New York, Wiley-Liss, 2002.
134. Logston M, Ha C, Kavadi V, et al: Lymphoma of the nasal cavity and paranasal sinuses. Cancer 80:477-488, 1997.
135. Rohatiner A, d'Amore F, Coiffier B, et al: Report on a workshop convened to discuss the pathological and staging classifications of gastrointestinal tract lymphoma. Ann Oncol 5:397-400, 1994.
136. d'Amore F, Brincker M, Gronbaek K, et al: Non-Hodgkin's lymphoma of the gastrointestinal tract: a population-based analysis of incidence, geographic distribution, clinicopathologic presentation features, and prognosis. J Clin Oncol 12:1673-1684, 1994
137. Oguchi M, Ikeda H, Isobe K, et al: Tumor bulk as a prognostic factor for the management of localized aggressive non-Hodgkin's lymphoma: A survey of the Japan Lymphoma Radiation Therapy Group. Int J Radiat Oncol Biol Phys 48:161-168, 2000.
138. Wilder RB, Rodriguez MA, Ha CS, et al: Bulky disease is an adverse prognostic factor in patients treated with chemotherapy comprised of cyclophosphamide, doxorubicin, vincristine, and prednisone with or without radiotherapy for aggressive lymphoma. Cancer 91:2440-2446, 2001.
139. Tsutsui K, Shibamoto Y, Yamabe H, et al: A radiotherapeutic experience for localized extranodal non-Hodgkin's lymphoma: Prognostic factors and re-evaluation of treatment modality. Radiother Oncol 21:83-90, 1991.
140. d'Amore F, Christensen BE, Brincker H, et al: Clinicopathological features and prognostic factors in extranodal non-Hodgkin lymphomas. Danish LYFO Study Group. Eur J Cancer 27:1201-1208, 1991.
141. Mackintosh JF, Cowan RA, Jones M, et al: Prognostic factors in stage I and II high and intermediate grade non-Hodgkin's lymphoma. Eur J Cancer Clin Oncol 24:1617-1622, 1988.
142. Seymour JF, Talpaz M, Cabanillas F, et al: Serum interleukin-6 levels correlate with prognosis in diffuse large-cell lymphoma. J Clin Oncol 13:575-582, 1995.
143. Sutcliffe SB, Gospodarowicz MK, Bergsagel DE, et al: Prognostic groups for management of localized Hodgkin's disease. J Clin Oncol 3:393-401, 1985.
144. Velasquez WS, Fuller LM, Jagannath S, et al: Stages I and II diffuse large cell lymphomas: Prognostic factors and long-term results with CHOP-bleo and radiotherapy. Blood 77:942-947, 1991.
145. The International non-Hodgkin's Lymphoma Prognostic Factors Project: A predictive model for aggressive Non-Hodgkin's lymphoma. N Engl J Med 329:987-994, 1993.
146. Ansell SM, Habermann TM, Kurtin PJ, et al: Predictive capacity of the International Prognostic Factor Index in patients with peripheral T-cell lymphoma. J Clin Oncol 15:2296-2301, 1997.
147. Lopez-Guillermo A, Montserrat E, Bosch F, et al: Applicability of the International Index for aggressive lymphomas to patients with low-grade lymphoma. J Clin Oncol 12:1343-1348, 1994.
148. Solal-Celigny P, Roy P, Colombat P, et al: Follicular lymphoma international prognostic index. Blood 104:1258-1265, 2004.
149. Horst E, Meijer CJ, Radaszkiewicz T, et al: Adhesion molecules in the prognosis of diffuse large-cell lymphoma: Expression of a lymphocyte homing receptor (CD44), LFA-1 (CD11a/18), and ICAM-1 (CD54). Leukemia 4:595-599, 1990.
150. Adida C, Haioun C, Gaulard P, et al: Prognostic significance of survivin expression in diffuse large B-cell lymphomas. Blood 96:1921-1925, 2000.
151. Mac Manus M, Lamborn K, Khan W, et al: Radiotherapy-associated neutropenia and thrombocytopenia: Analysis of risk factors and development of a predictive model. Blood 89:2303-2310, 1997.
152. Coleman CN, Picozzi Jr VJ, Cox RS, et al: Treatment of lymphoblastic lymphoma in adults. J Clin Oncol 4:1628-1637, 1986.
153. Magrath IT, Haddy TB, Adde MA: Treatment of patients with high grade Non-Hodgkin's lymphomas and central nervous system involvement: Is radiation an essential component of therapy? Leuk Lymphoma 21:99-105, 1996.
154. Armitage JO, Weisenburger DD: New approach to classifying non-Hodgkin's lymphomas: clinical features of the major histologic subtypes. Non-Hodgkin's Lymphoma Classification Project. J Clin Oncol 16:2780-2795, 1998.
155. Ha CS, Cabanillas F, Lee M-S, et al: Serial determination of the bcl-2 gene in the bone marrow and peripheral blood after central lymphatic irradiation for stages I-III follicular lymphoma: A preliminary report. Clin Cancer Res 3:215-219, 1997.
156. Mac Manus M, Hoppe RT: Is radiotherapy curative for stage I and II low-grade follicular lymphoma? Results of a long-term follow-up study of patients treated at Stanford University. J Clin Oncol 14:1282-1290, 1996.
157. Parayani S, Hoppe RT, Burke JS, et al: Extralymphatic involvement in diffuse Non-Hodgkin's lymphoma. J Clin Oncol 1:682-688, 1983.
158. Gospodarowicz M, Bush R, Brown T, et al: Curability of gastrointestinal lymphoma with combined surgery and radiation. Int J Rad Oncol Biol Phys 9:3-9, 1983.
159. Gospodarowicz MK, Bush RS, Brown TC, et al: Prognostic factors in nodular lymphomas: A multivariate analysis based on the Princess Margaret experience. Int J Radiat Oncol Biol Phys 10:489-497, 1984.
160. Petersen PM, Gospodarowicz M, Tsang R, et al: Long-term outcome in stage I and II follicular lymphoma following treatment with involved field radiation therapy alone. J Clin Oncol 22(14S):563, 2004.
161. McLaughlin P, Fuller L, Redman J, et al: Stage I-II low-grade lymphomas: A prospective trial of combination chemotherapy and radiotherapy. Ann Oncol 2:137-140, 1991.
162. McLaughlin P, Seymour J, Fuller L, et al: Combined modality therapy for stage I-II MALT lymphoma and mantle cell lymphoma. Ann Oncol 7:211-213, 1996.
163. Besa PC, McLaughlin PW, Cox JD, et al: Long term assessment of patterns of treatment failure and survival in patients with stage I or II follicular lymphoma. Cancer 75:2361-2367, 1995.
164. Vaughan Hudson B, Vaughan Hudson G, MacLennan KA, et al: Clinical stage 1 non-Hodgkin's lymphoma: Long-term follow-up of patients treated by the British National Lymphoma Investigation with radiotherapy alone as initial therapy. Br J Cancer 69:1088-1093, 1994.
165. Richards MA, Gregory WM, Hall PA, et al: Management of localized non-Hodgkin's lymphoma: The experience at St. Bartholomew's Hospital 1972-1985. Hematol Oncol 7:1-18, 1989.
166. Soubeyran P, Eghbali H, Bonichon F, et al: Localized follicular lymphomas: Prognosis and survival of stages I and II in a retrospective series of 103 patients. Radiother Oncol 13:91-98, 1988.
167. Monfardini S, Banfi A, Bonadonna G, et al: Improved 5 year survival after combined radiotherapy—Chemotherapy for stage I and II non-Hodgkin's lymphoma. Int J Radiat Oncol Biol Phys 6:125-134, 1980.
168. Nissen NI, Ersboll J, Hansen HS, et al: A randomized study of radiotherapy versus radiotherapy plus chemotherapy in Stage I-II Non-Hodgkin's Lymphomas. Cancer 52:1-7, 1983.
169. Kelsey SM, Newland AC, Hudson GV, et al: A British National Lymphoma Investigation randomised trial of single agent chlorambucil plus radiotherapy versus radiotherapy alone in low grade, localised non-Hodgkin's lymphoma. Med Oncol 11:19-25, 1994.
170. Yahalom J, Varsos G, Fuks Z, et al: Adjuvant cyclophosphamide, doxorubicin, vincristine, and prednisone chemotherapy after radiation therapy in stage I low-grade and intermediate-grade non-Hodgkin lymphoma. Results of a prospective randomized study. Cancer 71:2342-2350, 1993.
171. Seymour JF, Pro B, Fuller LM, et al: Long-term follow-up of a prospective study of combined modality therapy for stage I-II indolent non-Hodgkin's lymphoma. J Clin Oncol 21:2115-2122, 2003.
172. Advani R, Rosenberg SA, Horning SJ: Stage I and II follicular non-Hodgkin's lymphoma: Long-term follow-up of no initial therapy. J Clin Oncol 22:1454-1459, 2004.
173. Stuschke M, Hoederath A, Sack H, et al: Extended field and total central lymphatic radiotherapy in the treatment of early stage lymph node centroblastic-centrocytic lymphomas: Results of a prospective multicenter study. Study Group NHL-fruhe Stadien. Cancer 80:2273-2284, 1997.

174. De Los Santos JF, Mendenhall NP, Lynch JW: Is comprehensive lymphatic irradiation for low-grade Non-Hodgkin's lymphoma curative therapy? Long-term experience at a single institution. Int J Radiat Oncol Biol Phys 38:3-8, 1997.
175. Ha CS, Kong JS, Tucker SL, et al: Central lymphatic irradiation for stage I-III follicular lymphoma: report from a single-institutional prospective study. Int J Radiat Oncol Biol Phys 57:316-320, 2003.
176. Johannsson J, Specht L, Mejer J, et al: Phase II study of palliative low-dose local radiotherapy in disseminated indolent non-Hodgkin's lymphoma and chronic lymphocytic leukemia. Int J Radiat Oncol Biol Phys 54:1466-1470, 2002.
177. Haas RL, Girinsky T: HOVON 47/EORTC 20013: chlorambucil vs 2 × 2 Gy involved field radiotherapy in stage III/IV previously untreated follicular lymphoma patients. Ann Hematol 82:458-462, 2003.
178. Haas RL, Poortmans P, de Jong D, et al: High response rates and lasting remissions after low-dose involved field radiotherapy in indolent lymphomas. J Clin Oncol 21:2474-2480, 2003.
179. Isaacson P: The MALT lymphoma concept updated. Ann Oncol 6:319-320, 1995
180. Harris NL, Isaacson PG: What are the criteria for distinguishing MALT from non-MALT lymphoma at extranodal sites? Am J Clin Pathol 111:S126-S132, 1999.
181. Cerroni L, Zochling N, Putz B, et al: Infection by Borrelia burgdorferi and cutaneous B-cell lymphoma. J Cutan Pathol 24:457-461, 1997.
182. Wood GS, Kamath NV, Guitart J, et al: Absence of Borrelia burgdorferi DNA in cutaneous B-cell lymphomas from the United States. J Cutan Pathol 28:502-750, 2001.
183. Munksgaard L, Frisch M, Melbye M, et al: Incidence patterns of Lyme disease and cutaneous B-cell non-Hodgkin's lymphoma in the United States. Dermatology 201:351-352, 2000.
184. Liu H, Ruskon-Fourmestraux A, Lavergne-Slove A, et al: Resistance of t(11;18) positive gastric mucosa-associated lymphoid tissue lymphoma to Helicobacter pylori eradication therapy. Lancet 357:39-40, 2001.
185. Inagaki H, Nakamura T, Li C, et al: Gastric MALT lymphomas are divided into three groups based on responsiveness to Helicobacter pylori eradication and detection of API2-MALT1 fusion. Am J Surg Pathol 28:1560-1567, 2004.
186. Hitchcock S, Ng AK, Fisher DC, et al: Treatment outcome of mucosa-associated lymphoid tissue/marginal zone non-Hodgkin's lymphoma. Int J Radiat Oncol Biol Phys 52:1058-1066, 2002.
187. Le QT, Eulau SM, George TI, et al: Primary radiotherapy for localized orbital MALT lymphoma. Int J Radiat Oncol Biol Phys 52:657-663, 2002.
188. Tsang RW, Gospodarowicz MK, Pintilie M, et al: Stage I and II malt lymphoma: Results of treatment with radiotherapy. Int J Radiat Oncol Biol Phys 50:1258-1264, 2001.
189. Nizze H, Cogliatti SB, von Schilling C, et al: Monocytoid B-cell lymphoma: Morphologic variants and relationship to low grade B-cell lymphoma of the mucosa-associated lymphoid tissue. Histopathology 22:409-414, 1991
190. Hallahan DE, Farah R, Vokes EE, et al: The patterns of failure in patients with pathological stage I and II diffuse histiocytic lymphoma treated with radiation therapy alone. Int J Radiat Oncol Biol Phys 17:767-771, 1989.
191. Hoppe RT: The role of radiation therapy in the management of the Non-Hodgkin's lymphomas. Cancer 55:2176-2183, 1985.
192. Sutcliffe SB, Gospodarowicz MK, Bush RS, et al: Role of radiation therapy in localized non-Hodgkin's lymphoma. Radiother Oncol 4:211-223, 1985.
193. Shenkier TN, Voss N, Fairey R, et al: Brief chemotherapy and involved-region irradiation for limited-stage diffuse large-cell lymphoma: An 18-year experience from the British Columbia Cancer Agency. J Clin Oncol 20:197-204, 2002.
194. Tondini C, Zanini M, Lombardi F, et al: Combined modality treatment with primary CHOP chemotherapy followed by locoregional irradiation in stage I and II histologically aggressive non-Hodgkin's lymphomas. J Clin Oncol 11:720-725, 1993.
195. van der Maazen RW, Noordijk EM, Thomas J, et al: Combined modality treatment is the treatment of choice for stage I/IE intermediate and high grade non-Hodgkin's lymphomas. Radiother Oncol 49:1-7, 1998.
196. Cosset JM, Henry-Amar M, Vuong T, et al: Alternating chemotherapy and radiotherapy combination for bulky stage I and II intermediate and high grade non-Hodgkin lymphoma: An update. Radiother Oncol 20:30-37, 1991.
197. Longo DL, Glatstein E, Duffey PL, et al: Treatment of localized aggressive lymphomas with combination chemotherapy followed by involved-field radiation therapy. J Clin Oncol 7:1295-1302, 1989.
198. Horning SJ, Weller E, Kim K, et al: Chemotherapy with or without radiotherapy in limited-stage diffuse aggressive non-Hodgkin's lymphoma: Eastern Cooperative Oncology Group Study 1484. J Clin Oncol 22(15):3032-3038, 2004.
199. Miller T, Dahlberg S, Cassady J, et al: Chemotherapy alone compared with chemotherapy plus radiotherapy for localized intermediate- and high-grade non-Hodgkin's lymphoma. N Engl J Med 339:21-26, 1998.
200. Kaminski MS, Coleman CN, Colby TV, et al: Factors predicting survival in adults with stage I and II large-cell lymphoma treated with primary radiation therapy. Ann Intern Med 104:747-756, 1986.
201. Coiffier B, Lepage E, Briere J, et al: CHOP chemotherapy plus rituximab compared with CHOP alone in elderly patients with diffuse large-B-cell lymphoma. N Engl J Med 346:235-242, 2002.
202. Reyes F, Lepage E, Ganem G, et al: ACVBP versus CHOP plus radiotherapy for localized aggressive lymphoma. N Engl J Med 352:1197-1205, 2005.
203. Fillet G, Bonnet N, Mounier N, et al: Radiotherapy is unnecessary in elderly patients with localized aggressive non-Hodgkin's lymphoma: Results of the GELA LNH 93-4 study [abstract]. Blood 100:92a, 337, 2002.
204. Haioun C, Lepage E, Gisselbrecht C, et al: Comparison of autologous bone marrow transplantation with sequential chemotherapy for intermediate-grade and high-grade non-Hodgkin's lymphoma in first complete remission: A study of 464 patients. J Clin Oncol 12:2543-2551, 1994.
205. Haioun C, Lepage E, Gisselbrecht C, et al: Benefit of autologous bone marrow transplantation over sequential chemotherapy in poor-risk aggressive non-Hodgkin's lymphoma: updated results of the prospective study LNH87-2. Groupe d'Etude des Lymphomes de l'Adulte. J Clin Oncol 15:1131-1137, 1997.
206. Magrath I, Adde M, Shad A, et al: Adults and children with small non-cleaved-cell lymphoma have a similar excellent outcome when treated with the same chemotherapy regimen. J Clin Oncol 14:925-934, 1996.
207. Bernstein JI, Coleman CN, Strickler JG, et al: Combined modality therapy for adults with small noncleaved cell lymphoma (Burkitt's and non-Burkitt's type). J Clin Oncol 4:847-858, 1986.
208. Milpied N, Ifrah N, Kuentz M, et al: Bone marrow transplantation for adult poor prognosis lymphoblastic lymphoma in first complete remission. Br J Haematol 73:82-87, 1989.
209. Troussard X, Leblong V, Kuentz M, et al: Allogeneic bone marrow transplantation in adults with Burkitt's lymphoma or acute lymphoblastic leukemia in first complete remission. J Clin Oncol 8:809-812, 1990.
210. Horning SJ, Rosenberg SA: The natural history of initially untreated low-grade Non-Hodgkin's lymphoma. N Engl J Med 311:1471-1475, 1984.
211. Lister TA, Coiffier B, Armitage JO: Non-Hodgkin's lymphoma. In: Abeloff MD, Armitage JO, Niederhuber JE, et al (eds): Clinical Oncology, 3rd ed. Philadelphia, Elsevier Churchill Livingstone, 2004, pp 3015-3076.
212. Brice P, Bastion Y, Lepage E, et al: Comparison in low-tumor-burden follicular lymphomas between an initial no-treatment policy, prednimustine, or interferon alfa: a randomized study from the Groupe d'Etude des Lymphomes Folliculaires. Groupe d'Etude des Lymphomes de l'Adulte. J Clin Oncol 15:1110-1117, 1997.
213. Paryani SB, Hoppe RT, Cox RS, et al: The role of radiation therapy in the management of stage III follicular lymphomas. J Clin Oncol 2:841-848, 1984.
214. Hoppe RT, Kushlan P, Kaplan HS, et al: The treatment of advanced stage favorable histology non-Hodgkin's lymphoma:

a preliminary report of a randomized trial comparing single agent chemotherapy, combination chemotherapy, and whole body irradiation. Blood 58:592-598, 1981.
215. Qasim MM: Total body irradiation as a primary therapy in non-Hodgkin's lymphoma. Clin Radiol 30:287-286, 1979.
216. Roncadin M, Arcicasa M, Zagonel V, et al: Total body irradiation and prednimustine in chronic lymphocytic leukemia and low grade non-Hodgkin's lymphoma. Cancer 74:978-984, 1994.
217. Rohatiner AZ, Gregory WM, Peterson B, et al: Meta-analysis to evaluate the role of interferon in follicular lymphoma. J Clin Oncol 23:2215-2223, 2005.
218. Hochster HS, Kim K, Green MD, et al: Activity of fludarabine in previously treated non-Hodgkin's low-grade lymphoma: Results of an Eastern Cooperative Oncology Group study. J Clin Oncol 10:28-32, 1992.
219. Kay AC, Saven A, Carrera CJ, et al: 2-Chlorodeoxyadenosine treatment of low-grade lymphomas. J Clin Oncol 10:371-377, 1992.
220. Czuczman MS, Koryzna A, Mohr A, et al: Rituximab in combination with fludarabine chemotherapy in low-grade or follicular lymphoma. J Clin Oncol 23:694-704, 2005.
221. Coiffier B, Haioun C, Ketterer N, et al: Rituximab (anti-CD20 monoclonal antibody) for the treatment of patients with relapsing or refractory aggressive lymphoma: A multicenter phase II study. Blood 92:1927-1932, 1998.
222. Marcus R, Imrie K, Belch A, et al: CVP chemotherapy plus rituximab compared with CVP as first-line treatment for advanced follicular lymphoma. Blood 105:1417-1423, 2005.
223. Press OW, Eary J, Appelbaum FR, et al: A phase II trial of 131I-B1(anti-CD20) antibody therapy with autologous stem cell transplantation for relapsed B cell lymphomas. Lancet 346:336-340, 1995.
224. Kaminski MS, Zelenetz AD, Press OW, et al: Pivotal study of iodine I 131 tositumomab for chemotherapy-refractory low-grade or transformed low-grade B-cell non-Hodgkin's lymphomas. J Clin Oncol 19:3918-3928, 2001.
225. Kaminski MS, Tuck M, Estes J, et al: 131I-tositumomab therapy as initial treatment for follicular lymphoma. N Engl J Med 352:441-449, 2005.
226. Witzig TE, Gordon LI, Cabanillas F, et al: Randomized controlled trial of yttrium-90-labeled ibritumomab tiuxetan radioimmunotherapy versus rituximab immunotherapy for patients with relapsed or refractory low-grade, follicular, or transformed B-cell non-Hodgkin's lymphoma. J Clin Oncol 20:2453-2463, 2002.
227. Cao TM, Horning S, Negrin RS, et al: High-dose therapy and autologous hematopoietic-cell transplantation for follicular lymphoma beyond first remission: The Stanford University experience. Biol Blood Marrow Transplant 7:294-301, 2001.
228. Freedman AS, Gribben JG, Neuberg D, et al: High-dose therapy and autologous bone marrow transplantation in patients with follicular lymphoma during first remission. Blood 88:2780-2786, 1996.
229. Williams CD, Harrison CN, Lister TA, et al: High-dose therapy and autologous stem-cell support for chemosensitive transformed low-grade follicular non-Hodgkin's lymphoma: A case-matched study from the European Bone Marrow Transplant Registry. J Clin Oncol 19:727-735, 2001.
230. Schouten HC, Qian W, Kvaloy S, et al: High-dose therapy improves progression-free survival and survival in relapsed follicular non-Hodgkin's lymphoma: Results from the randomized European CUP trial. J Clin Oncol 21:3918-3927, 2003.
231. Fisher R, Gaynor E, Dahlberg S, et al: Comparison of a standard regimen (CHOP) with three intensive chemotherapy regimens for advanced non-Hodgkin's lymphoma. N Engl J Med 328:1002-1006, 1993.
232. Pfreundschuh M, Trumper L, Gill D, et al: First analysis of the completed Mabthera International (MInT) trial in young patients with low-risk diffuse large B-cell lymphoma (DLBCL): Addition of rituximab to a CHOP-like regimen significantly improves outcome of all patients with the identification of a very favorable subgroup with IPI=0 and no bulky disease [abstract 157]. Blood 104:48a, 2004.
233. Shipp MA, Klatt MM, Yeap B, et al: Patterns of relapse in large-cell lymphoma patients with bulk disease: Implications for the use of adjuvant radiation therapy. J Clin Oncol 7:613-618, 1989.
234. Velasquez W, Fuller LM, Oh KK, et al: Combined modality therapy in Stage III and Stage IIIE diffuse large cell lymphomas. Cancer 53:1478-1483, 1984.
235. Ferreri AJ, Dell'Oro S, Reni M, et al: Consolidation radiotherapy to bulky or semibulky lesions in the management of stage III-IV diffuse large B cell lymphomas. Oncology 58:219-226, 2000.
236. Schlembach PJ, Wilder RB, Tucker SL, et al: Impact of involved field radiotherapy after CHOP-based chemotherapy on stage III-IV, intermediate grade and large-cell immunoblastic lymphomas. Int J Radiat Oncol Biol Phys 48:1107-1110, 2000.
237. Aviles A, Delgado S, Nambo MJ, et al: Adjuvant radiotherapy to sites of previous bulky disease in patients stage IV diffuse large cell lymphoma. Int J Radiat Oncol Biol Phys 30:799-803, 1994.
238. Zucca E, Conconi A, Mughal TI, et al: Patterns of outcome and prognostic factors in primary large-cell lymphoma of the testis in a survey by the International Extranodal Lymphoma Study Group. J Clin Oncol 21:20-27, 2003.
239. Verdonck L, van Putten, WLJ, Hagenbeek, A, et al: Comparison of CHOP chemotherapy with autologous bone marrow transplantation for slowly responding patients with aggressive non-Hodgkin's lymphoma. N Engl J Med 332:1045-1051, 1995.
240. Martelli M, Vignetti M, Zinzani PL, et al: High-dose chemotherapy followed by autologous bone marrow transplantation versus dexamethasone, cisplatin, and cytarabine in aggressive non-Hodgkin's lymphoma with partial response to front-line chemotherapy. J Clin Oncol 14:534-542, 1996.
241. Gianni AM, Bregni M, Siena S, et al: High-dose chemotherapy and autologous bone marrow transplantation compared with MACOP-B in aggressive B-cell lymphoma. N Engl J Med 336:1290-1297, 1997.
242. Haioun C, Lepage E, Gisselbrecht C, et al: Autologous bone marrow transplantation (ABMT) versus sequential chemotherapy for aggressive non-Hodgkin's lymphoma (NHL) in first complete remission (CR): A study of 541 patients (LNH87-2 protocol). Ann Oncol 7(Suppl 3):24, 1996.
243. Haioun C, Lepage E, Gisselbrecht C, et al: Survival benefit of high-dose therapy in poor-risk aggressive non-Hodgkin's lymphoma: Final analysis of the prospective LNH87-2 protocol—A Groupe d'Etude des Lymphomes de l'Adulte study. J Clin Oncol 18:3025-3030, 2000.
244. Gisselbrecht C, Lepage E, Molina T, et al: Shortened first-line high-dose chemotherapy for patients with poor-prognosis aggressive lymphoma. J Clin Oncol 20:2472-2479, 2002.
245. Martelli M, Gherlinzoni F, De Renzo A, et al: Early autologous stem-cell transplantation versus conventional chemotherapy as front-line therapy in high-risk, aggressive non-Hodgkin's lymphoma: An Italian multicenter randomized trial. J Clin Oncol 21:1255-1262, 2003.
246. Santini G, Salvagno L, Leoni P, et al: VACOP-B versus VACOP-B plus autologous bone marrow transplantation for advanced diffuse non-Hodgkin's lymphoma: Results of a prospective randomized trial by the non-Hodgkin's Lymphoma Cooperative Study Group. J Clin Oncol 16:2796-2802, 1998.
247. Kluin-Nelemans HC, Zagonel V, Anastasopoulou A, et al: Standard chemotherapy with or without high-dose chemotherapy for aggressive non-Hodgkin's lymphoma: Randomized phase III EORTC study. J Natl Cancer Inst 93:22-30, 2001.
248. Kaiser U, Uebelacker I, Abel U, et al: Randomized study to evaluate the use of high-dose therapy as part of primary treatment for "aggressive" lymphoma. J Clin Oncol 20:4413-4419, 2002.
249. Lenz G, Dreyling M, Hoster E, et al: Immunochemotherapy with rituximab and cyclophosphamide, doxorubicin, vincristine, and prednisone significantly improves response and time to treatment failure, but not long-term outcome in patients with previously untreated mantle cell lymphoma: Results of a prospective randomized trial of the German Low Grade Lymphoma Study Group (GLSG). J Clin Oncol 23:1984-1992, 2005.
250. O'Connor OA, Wright J, Moskowitz C, et al: Phase II clinical experience with the novel proteasome inhibitor bortezomib in patients with indolent non-Hodgkin's lymphoma and mantle cell lymphoma. J Clin Oncol 23:676-684, 2005.

251. Kouroukis CT, Belch A, Crump M, et al: Flavopiridol in untreated or relapsed mantle-cell lymphoma: results of a phase II study of the National Cancer Institute of Canada Clinical Trials Group. J Clin Oncol 21:1740-1745, 2003.
252. Brugger W, Hirsch J, Grunebach F, et al: Rituximab consolidation after high-dose chemotherapy and autologous blood stem cell transplantation in follicular and mantle cell lymphoma: a prospective, multicenter phase II study. Ann Oncol 15:1691-1698, 2004.
253. Rapoport AP, Meisenberg B, Sarkodee-Adoo C, et al: Autotransplantation for advanced lymphoma and Hodgkin's disease followed by post-transplant rituxan/GM-CSF or radiotherapy and consolidation chemotherapy. Bone Marrow Transplant 29:303-312, 2002.
254. Vose JM, Bierman PJ, Weisenburger DD, et al: Autologous hematopoietic stem cell transplantation for mantle cell lymphoma. Biol Blood Marrow Transplant 6:640-645, 2000.
255. Rifkind J, Mollee P, Messner H, et al: Allogeneic stem cell transplantation for mantle cell lymphoma—Does it deserve a better look? Leuk Lymphoma 46:217-223, 2005.
256. Maris MB, Sandmaier BM, Storer BE, et al: Allogeneic hematopoietic cell transplantation after fludarabine and 2 Gy total body irradiation for relapsed and refractory mantle cell lymphoma. Blood 104:3535-4352, 2004.
257. Lavely WC, Delbeke D, Greer JP, et al: FDG PET in the follow-up management of patients with newly diagnosed Hodgkin and non-Hodgkin lymphoma after first-line chemotherapy. Int J Radiat Oncol Biol Phys 57:307-315, 2003.
258. Kirkove C, Timothy AR: Radiotherapy as salvage treatment in patients with Hodgkin's disease or non-Hodgkin's lymphoma relapsing after initial chemotherapy. Hematol Oncol 9:163-167, 1991.
259. Press O, Livingston R, Mortimer J, et al: Treatment of relapsed non-Hodgkin's lymphoma with dexamethasone, high-dose cytarabine, and cisplatin before marrow transplantation. J Clin Oncol 9:423-431, 1991.
260. Philip T, Guglielmi C, Hagenbeek A, et al: Autologous bone marrow transplantation as compared with salvage chemotherapy in relapses of chemotherapy-sensitive non-Hodgkin's lymphoma. N Engl J Med 333:1540-1545, 1995.
261. Lefrere F, Delmer A, Suzan F, et al: Sequential chemotherapy by CHOP and DHAP regimens followed by high-dose therapy with stem cell transplantation induces a high rate of complete response and improves event-free survival in mantle cell lymphoma: A prospective study. Leukemia 16:587-593, 2002.
262. Stewart AK, Brandwein JM, Sutcliffe SB, et al: Mini-beam as salvage chemotherapy for refractory Hodgkin's disease and non-Hodgkin's lymphoma. Leuk Lymphoma 5:111-115, 1991.
263. Velasquez WS, McLaughlin P, Tucker S, et al: ESHAP—an effective chemotherapy regimen in refractory and relapsing lymphoma: A 4-year follow-up study. J Clin Oncol 12:1169-1176, 1994.
264. Moskowitz CH, Bertino JR, Glassman JR, et al: Ifosfamide, carboplatin, and etoposide: a highly effective cytoreduction and peripheral-blood progenitor-cell mobilization regimen for transplant-eligible patients with non-Hodgkin's lymphoma. J Clin Oncol 17:3776-3785, 1999.
265. Kewalramani T, Zelenetz AD, Nimer SD, et al: Rituximab and ICE as second-line therapy before autologous stem cell transplantation for relapsed or primary refractory diffuse large B-cell lymphoma. Blood 103:3684-3688, 2004.
266. Crump M, Baetz T, Couban S, et al: Gemcitabine, dexamethasone, and cisplatin in patients with recurrent or refractory aggressive histology B-cell non-Hodgkin lymphoma: a Phase II study by the National Cancer Institute of Canada Clinical Trials Group (NCIC-CTG). Cancer 101:1835-1842, 2004.
267. Horning SJ, Negrin RS, Chao NJ, et al: Fractionated total-body irradiation, etoposide, and cyclophosphamide plus autografting in Hodgkin's disease and non-Hodgkin's lymphoma. J Clin Oncol 12:2552-2558, 1994.
268. Prince HM, Imrie K, Crump M, et al: The role of intensive therapy and autologous blood and marrow transplantation for chemotherapy-sensitive relapsed and primary refractory non-Hodgkin's lymphoma: Identification of major prognostic groups. Br J Haematol 92:880-889, 1996.
269. Gulati S, Yahalom J, Acaba L, et al: Treatment of patients with relapsed and resistant non-Hodgkin's lymphoma using total body irradiation, etoposide, and cyclophosphamide and autologous bone marrow transplantation. J Clin Oncol 10:936-941, 1992.
270. Weaver CH, Petersen FB, Appelbaum FR, et al: High-dose fractionated total-body irradiation, etoposide, and cyclophosphamide followed by autologous stem-cell support in patients with malignant lymphoma. J Clin Oncol 12:2559-2566, 1994.
271. Shipp MA, Abeloff MD, Antman KH, et al: International Consensus Conference on High-Dose Therapy with Hematopoietic Stem Cell Transplantation in Aggressive Non-Hodgkin's Lymphomas: Report of the jury. J Clin Oncol 17:423-429, 1999.
272. Song DY, Jones RJ, Welsh JS, et al: Phase I study of escalating doses of low-dose-rate, locoregional irradiation preceding Cytoxan-TBI for patients with chemotherapy-resistant non-Hodgkin's or Hodgkin's lymphoma. Int J Radiat Oncol Biol Phys 57:166-171, 2003.
273. Dawson LA, Saito NG, Ratanatharathorn V, et al: Phase I study of involved-field radiotherapy preceding autologous stem cell transplantation for patients with high-risk lymphoma or Hodgkin's disease. Int J Radiat Oncol Biol Phys 59:208-218, 2004.
274. Friedberg JW, Neuberg D, Monson E, et al: The impact of external beam radiation therapy prior to autologous bone marrow transplantation in patients with non-Hodgkin's lymphoma. Biol Blood Marrow Transplant 7:446-453, 2001.
275. Wadhwa P, Shina DC, Schenkein D, et al: Should involved-field radiation therapy be used as an adjunct to lymphoma autotransplantation? Bone Marrow Transplant 29:183-189, 2002.
276. Tsang RW, Gospodarowicz MK, Sutcliffe SB, et al: Thoracic radiation therapy before autologous bone marrow transplantation in relapsed or refractory Hodgkin's disease. PMH Lymphoma Group, and the Toronto Autologous BMT Group. Eur J Cancer 35:73-78, 1999.
277. Emmanouilides C, Asuncion DJ, Wolf C, et al: Localized radiation increases morbidity and mortality after TBI-containing autologous stem cell transplantation in patients with lymphoma. Bone Marrow Transplant 32:863-867, 2003.
278. Schwartz DL, Schechter GP, Seltzer S, et al: Radiation myelitis following allogeneic stem cell transplantation and consolidation radiotherapy for non-Hodgkin's lymphoma. Bone Marrow Transplant 26:1355-1359, 2000.
279. Chao MW, Wirth A, Ryan G, et al: Radiation myelopathy following transplantation and radiotherapy for non-Hodgkin's lymphoma. Int J Radiat Oncol Biol Phys 41:1057-1061, 1998.
280. Gale RP, Butturini A, Bortin MM: What does total body irradiation do in bone marrow transplants for leukemia? Int J Radiat Oncol Biol Phys 20:631-634, 1991.
281. Freedman AS, Takvorian T, Anderson KC, et al: Autologous bone marrow transplantation in B-cell non-Hodgkin's lymphoma: Very low treatment-related mortality in 100 patients in sensitive relapse. J Clin Oncol 8:784-791, 1990.
282. Pettengell R, Radford JA, Morgenstern GR, et al: Survival benefit from high-dose therapy with autologous blood progenitor-cell transplantation in poor-prognosis non-Hodgkin's lymphoma. J Clin Oncol 14:586-592, 1996.
283. Schouten HC, Colombat P, Verdonck LF, et al: Autologous bone marrow transplantation for low-grade non-Hodgkin's lymphoma: The European Bone Marrow Transplant Group experience. Ann Oncol 5(Suppl 2):S147-S149, 1994.
284. Cosset JM, Girinsky T, Malaise E, et al: Clinical basis for TBI fractionation. Radiother Oncol Suppl. 1:60-67, 1990.
285. Cosset JM, Baume D, Pico JL, et al: Single dose versus hyperfractionated total body irradiation before allogeneic bone marrow transplantation: A non-randomized comparative study of 54 patients at the Institut Gustave-Roussy. Radiother Oncol 15:151-160, 1989.
286. Morgan TL, Falk PM, Kogut N, et al: A comparison of single dose and fractionated total body irradiation on the development of pneumonitis following bone marrow transplantation. Int J Radiat Oncol Biol Phys 36:61-66, 1996.
287. van Dyk J, Keane TJ, Kan S, et al: Radiation pneumonitis following large single dose irradiation: A re-evaluation based on absolute dose to lung. Int J Radiat Oncol Biol Phys 7:461-467, 1981.

288. Chen CI, Abraham R, Tsang R, et al: Radiation-associated pneumonitis following autologous stem cell transplantation: Predictive factors, disease characteristics and treatment outcomes. Bone Marrow Transplant 27:177-182, 2001.
289. Jules-Elysee K, Stover DE, Yahalom J, et al: Pulmonary complications in lymphoma patients treated with high-dose therapy and autologous bone marrow transplantation. Am Rev Respir Dis 146:485-491, 1992.
290. Appelbaum FR, Sullivan KM, Buckner D, et al: Treatment of malignant lymphoma in 100 patients with chemotherapy, total body irradiation, and marrow transplantation. J Clin Oncol 5:1340-1347, 1987.
291. Brice P, Marolleau JP, Pautier P, et al: Hematologic recovery and survival of lymphoma patients after autologous stem-cell transplantation: Comparison of bone marrow and peripheral blood progenitor cells. Leuk Lymphoma 22:449-456, 1996.
292. Chen CI, Crump M, Tsang R, et al: Autotransplants for histologically transformed follicular non-Hodgkin's lymphoma. Br J Haematol 113:202-208, 2001.
293. Press OW, Eary JF, Gooley T, et al: A phase I/II trial of iodine-131-tositumomab (anti-CD20), etoposide, cyclophosphamide, and autologous stem cell transplantation for relapsed B-cell lymphomas. Blood 96:2934-2942, 2000.
294. Press OW, Eary J, Appelbaum FR, et al: Radiolabeled antibody therapy of B cell lymphomas with autologous bone marrow support. N Engl J Med 324:1219-1224, 1993.
295. Dawson I, Cornes J, Morson B: Primary malignant lymphoid tumours of the intestinal tract: report of 37 cases with a study of factors influencing prognosis. Brit J Surg 49:80-89, 1961.
296. Lewin K, Ranchod M, Dorfman R: Lymphomas of the gastrointestinal tract: A study of 117 cases presenting with gastrointestinal disease. Cancer 42:693-707, 1978.
297. Economopoulos T, Asprou N, Stathakis N, et al: Primary extranodal non-Hodgkin's lymphoma in adults: Clinicopathological and survival characteristics. Leuk Lymphoma 21:131-136, 1996.
298. Newton R, Ferlay J, Beral V, et al: The epidemiology of non-Hodgkin's lymphoma: comparison of nodal and extra-nodal sites. Int J Cancer 72:923-930, 1997.
299. Bayerdorffer E, Neubauer A, Rudolph B, et al: Regression of primary gastric lymphoma of mucosa-associated lymphoid tissue type after cure of Helicobacter pylori infection. MALT Lymphoma Study Group. Lancet 345:1591-1594, 1995.
300. Savio A, Zamboni G, Capelli P, et al: Relapse of low-grade gastric MALT lymphoma after Helicobacter pylori eradication: true relapse or persistence? Long-term post-treatment follow-up of a multicenter trial in the north-east of Italy and evaluation of the diagnostic protocol's adequacy. Recent Results Cancer Res 156:116-124, 2000.
301. Pinotti G, Zucca E, Roggero E, et al: Clinical features, treatment and outcome in a series of 93 patients with low-grade gastric MALT lymphoma. Leuk Lymphoma 26:527-537, 1997.
302. Veldhuyzen van Zanten SJ, Sherman PM, Hunt RH: Helicobacter pylori: new developments and treatments. CMAJ 156:1565-1574, 1997.
303. Malfertheiner P, Megraud F, O'Morain C, et al: Current concepts in the management of Helicobacter pylori infection—the Maastricht 2-2000 Consensus Report. Aliment Pharmacol Ther 16:167-180, 2002.
304. Liu H, Ye H, Ruskone-Fourmestraux A, et al: T(11;18) is a marker for all stage gastric MALT lymphomas that will not respond to H. pylori eradication. Gastroenterology 122:1286-1294, 2002.
305. Taji S, Nomura K, Matsumoto Y, et al: Trisomy 3 may predict a poor response of gastric MALT lymphoma to Helicobacter pylori eradication therapy. World J Gastroenterol 11:89-93, 2005.
306. Ye H, Liu H, Raderer M, et al: High incidence of t(11;18)(q21;q21) in Helicobacter pylori-negative gastric MALT lymphoma. Blood 101:2547-2550, 2003.
307. Fischbach W, Goebeler-Kolve M, Starostik P, et al: Minimal residual low-grade gastric MALT-type lymphoma after eradication of Helicobacter pylori. Lancet 360:547-548, 2002.
308. Schechter NR, Portlock CS, Yahalom J: Treatment of mucosa-associated lymphoid tissue lymphoma of the stomach with radiation alone. J Clin Oncol 16:1916-1921, 1998.
309. Fung CY, Grossbard ML, Linggood RM, et al: Mucosa-associated lymphoid tissue lymphoma of the stomach: Long term outcome after local treatment. Cancer 85:9-17, 1999.
310. Bertoni F, Conconi A, Capella C, et al: Molecular follow-up in gastric mucosa-associated lymphoid tissue lymphomas: Early analysis of the LY03 cooperative trial. Blood 99:2541-2544, 2002.
311. Martinelli G, Laszlo D, Ferreri AJ, et al: Clinical activity of rituximab in gastric marginal zone non-Hodgkin's lymphoma resistant to or not eligible for anti-Helicobacter pylori therapy. J Clin Oncol 23:1979-1983, 2005.
312. Conconi A, Martinelli G, Thieblemont C, et al: Clinical activity of rituximab in extranodal marginal zone B-cell lymphoma of MALT type. Blood 102:2741-2745, 2003.
313. Raderer M, Jager G, Brugger S, et al: Rituximab for treatment of advanced extranodal marginal zone B cell lymphoma of the mucosa-associated lymphoid tissue lymphoma. Oncology 65:306-310, 2003.
314. Wohrer S, Drach J, Hejna M, et al: Treatment of extranodal marginal zone B-cell lymphoma of mucosa-associated lymphoid tissue (MALT lymphoma) with mitoxantrone, chlorambucil and prednisone (MCP). Ann Oncol 14:1758-1761, 2003.
315. Koch P, Grothaus-Pinke B, Hiddemann W, et al: Primary lymphoma of the stomach: three-year results of a prospective multicenter study. The German Multicenter Study Group on GI-NHL. Ann Oncol 8(Suppl 1):85-88, 1997.
316. Koch P, del Valle F, Berdel WE, et al: Primary gastrointestinal non-Hodgkin's lymphoma: II. Combined surgical and conservative or conservative management only in localized gastric lymphoma—results of the prospective German Multicenter Study GIT NHL 01/92. J Clin Oncol 19:3874-3883, 2001.
317. Koch P, del Valle F, Berdel WE, et al: Primary gastrointestinal non-Hodgkin's lymphoma: I. Anatomic and histologic distribution, clinical features, and survival data of 371 patients registered in the German Multicenter Study GIT NHL 01/92. J Clin Oncol 19:3861-3873, 2001.
318. Gospodarowicz MK, Pintilie M, Tsang R, et al: Primary gastric lymphoma: brief overview of the recent Princess Margaret Hospital experience. Recent Results Cancer Res 156:108-115, 2000.
319. Maor MH, Velasquez WS, Fuller LM, et al: Stomach conservation in stages IE and IIE gastric non-Hodgkin's lymphoma. J Clin Oncol 8:266-271, 1990.
320. Aviles A, Nambo MJ, Neri N, et al: The role of surgery in primary gastric lymphoma: results of a controlled clinical trial. Ann Surg 240:44-50, 2004.
321. Gospodarowicz MK, Sutcliffe SB, Clark RM, et al: Outcome analysis of localized gastrointestinal lymphoma treated with surgery and postoperative radiation. Int J Radiat Oncol Biol Phys 19:1351-1355, 1990.
322. Shepherd FA, Evans WK, Kutas G, et al: Chemotherapy following surgery for stages IE and IIE non-Hodgkin's lymphoma of the gastrointestinal tract. J Clin Oncol 6:253-260, 1988.
323. Chen LT, Lin JT, Shyu RY, et al: Prospective study of Helicobacter pylori eradication therapy in stage I(E) high-grade mucosa-associated lymphoid tissue lymphoma of the stomach. J Clin Oncol 19:4245-4251, 2001.
324. Raderer M, Chott A, Drach J, et al: Chemotherapy for management of localised high-grade gastric B-cell lymphoma: How much is necessary? Ann Oncol 13:1094-1098, 2002.
325. Binn M, Ruskone-Fourmestraux A, Lepage E, et al: Surgical resection plus chemotherapy versus chemotherapy alone: Comparison of two strategies to treat diffuse large B-cell gastric lymphoma. Ann Oncol 14:1751-1757, 2003.
326. Domizio P, Owen RA, Shepherd NA, et al: Primary lymphoma of the small intestine: A clinicopathological study of 119 cases. Am J Surg Pathol 17:429-442, 1993.
327. Morton JE, Leyland MJ, Vaughan Hudson G, et al: Primary gastrointestinal non-Hodgkin's lymphoma: A review of 175 British National Lymphoma Investigation cases. Br J Cancer 67:776-782, 1993.
328. Daum S, Ullrich R, Heise W, et al: Intestinal non-Hodgkin's lymphoma: A multicenter prospective clinical study from the German Study Group on Intestinal non-Hodgkin's Lymphoma. J Clin Oncol 21:2740-2746, 2003.

329. Gale J, Simmonds PD, Mead GM, et al: Enteropathy-type intestinal T-cell lymphoma: clinical features and treatment of 31 patients in a single center. J Clin Oncol 18:795-803, 2000.
330. Haber DA, Mayer RJ: Primary gastrointestinal lymphoma. Sem Oncol 15:154-169, 1988.
331. Isaacson PG: Gastrointestinal lymphomas of T- and B-cell types. Mod Pathol 12:151-158, 1999.
332. Al-Saleem T, Al-Mondhiry H: Immunoproliferative small intestinal disease (IPSID): A model for mature B-cell neoplasms. Blood 105:2274-2280, 2005.
333. Fischbach W, Tacke W, Greiner A, et al: Regression of immunoproliferative small intestinal disease after eradication of Helicobacter pylori. Lancet 349:31-32, 1997.
334. Akbulut H, Soykan I, Yakaryilmaz F, et al: Five-year results of the treatment of 23 patients with immunoproliferative small intestinal disease: A Turkish experience. Cancer 80:8-14, 1997.
335. Al-Bahrani Z, Al-Mohindry H, Bakir F, et al: Clinical and pathologic subtypes of primary intestinal lymphoma: Experience with 132 patients over a 14-year period. Cancer 52:1666-1672, 1983.
336. Lankarani KB, Masoompour SM, Masoompour MB, et al: Changing epidemiology of IPSID in Southern Iran. Gut 54:311-312, 2005.
337. Orita M, Yamashita K, Okino M, et al: A case of MALT (mucosa-associated lymphoid tissue) lymphoma occurring in the rectum. Hepatogastroenterology 46:2352-2354, 1999.
338. Aosaza K, Ohsawa M, Soma T, et al: Malignant lymphoma of the rectum. Jpn J Clin Oncol 20:380-386, 1990.
339. Liang R, Ng RP, Todd D, et al: Management of Stage I-II diffuse aggressive non-Hodgkin's lymphoma of Waldeyer's ring: Combined modality therapy versus radiotherapy alone. Hematol Oncol 5:223-230, 1987.
340. Ezzat AA, Ibrahim EM, El Weshi AN, et al: Localized non-Hodgkin's lymphoma of Waldeyer's ring: Clinical features, management, and prognosis of 130 adult patients. Head Neck 23:547-558, 2001.
341. Aviles A, Delgado S, Ruiz H, et al: Treatment of non-Hodgkin's lymphoma of Waldeyer's ring: Radiotherapy versus chemotherapy versus combined therapy. Eur J Cancer, Oral Oncol 32B:19-23, 1996.
342. Abbondanzo SL, Wenig BM: Non-Hodgkin's lymphoma of the sinonasal tract. A clinicopathologic and immunophenotypic study of 120 cases. Cancer 75:1281-1291, 1995.
343. Cheung MM, Chan JK, Lau WH, et al: Primary non-Hodgkin's lymphoma of the nose and nasopharynx: clinical features, tumor immunophenotype, and treatment outcome in 113 patients. J Clin Oncol 16:70-77, 1998.
344. Kim WS, Song SY, Ahn YC, et al: CHOP followed by involved field radiation: is it optimal for localized nasal natural killer/T-cell lymphoma? Ann Oncol 12:349-352, 2001.
345. Kim K, Chie EK, Kim CW, et al: Treatment outcome of angiocentric T-cell and NK/T-cell lymphoma, nasal type: Radiotherapy versus chemoradiotherapy. Jpn J Clin Oncol 35:1-5, 2005.
346. Li CC, Tien HF, Tang JL, et al: Treatment outcome and pattern of failure in 77 patients with sinonasal natural killer/T-cell or T-cell lymphoma. Cancer 100:366-375, 2004.
347. You JY, Chi KH, Yang MH, et al: Radiation therapy versus chemotherapy as initial treatment for localized nasal natural killer (NK)/T-cell lymphoma: A single institute survey in Taiwan. Ann Oncol 15:618-625, 2004.
348. Pariente D, Anaya JM, Combe B, et al: Non-Hodgkin's lymphoma associated with primary Sjogren's syndrome. Eur J Med 1:337-342, 1992.
349. Royer B, Cazals-Hatem D, Sibilia J, et al: Lymphomas in patients with Sjögren's syndrome are marginal zone B-cell neoplasms, arise in diverse extranodal and nodal sites, and are not associated with viruses. Blood 90:766-775, 1997.
350. Aviles A, Delgado S, Huerta-Guzman J: Marginal zone B cell lymphoma of the parotid glands: results of a randomised trial comparing radiotherapy to combined therapy. Eur J Cancer. Part B, Oral Oncology 6:420-422, 1996.
351. Olivier KR, Brown PD, Stafford SL, et al: Efficacy and treatment-related toxicity of radiotherapy for early-stage primary non-Hodgkin lymphoma of the parotid gland. Int J Radiat Oncol Biol Phys 60:1510-1514, 2004.
352. Thieblemont C, Mayer A, Dumontet C, et al: Primary thyroid lymphoma is a heterogeneous disease. J Clin Endocrinol Metab 87:105-111, 2002.
353. Laing RW, Hoskin P, Hudson BV, et al: The significance of MALT histology in thyroid lymphoma: A review of patients from the BNLI and Royal Marsden Hospital. Clin Oncol 6:300-304, 1994.
354. Cha C, Chen H, Westra WH, et al: Primary thyroid lymphoma: Can the diagnosis be made solely by fine-needle aspiration? Ann Surg Oncol 9:298-302, 2002.
355. DiBiase SJ, Grigsby PW, Guo C, et al: Outcome analysis for stage IE and IIE thyroid lymphoma. Am J Clin Oncol 27:178-184, 2004.
356. Tsang R, Gospodarowicz MK, Sutcliffe SB, et al: Non-Hodgkin's lymphoma of the thyroid gland: Prognostic factors and treatment outcome. Int J Radiat Oncol Biol Phys 27:599-604, 1993.
357. Belal AA, Allam A, Kandil A, et al: Primary thyroid lymphoma: A retrospective analysis of prognostic factors and treatment outcome for localized intermediate and high grade lymphoma. Am J Clin Oncol 24:299-305, 2001.
358. Ha CS, Shadle KM, Medeiros LJ, et al: Localized non-Hodgkin lymphoma involving the thyroid gland. Cancer 91:629-635, 2001.
359. Thieblemont C, Bastion Y, Berger F, et al: Mucosa-associated lymphoid tissue gastrointestinal and nongastrointestinal lymphoma behavior: Analysis of 108 patients. J Clin Oncol 15:1624-1630, 1997.
360. Hardman-Lea S, Kerr-Muir M, Wotherspoon AC, et al: Mucosal-associated lymphoid tissue lymphoma of the conjunctiva. Arch Ophthalmol 112:1207-1212, 1994.
361. Stafford SL, Kozelsky TF, Garrity JA, et al: Orbital lymphoma: Radiotherapy outcome and complications. Radiother Oncol 59:139-144, 2001.
362. Pelloski CE, Wilder RB, Ha CS, et al: Clinical stage IEA-IIEA orbital lymphomas: outcomes in the era of modern staging and treatment. Radiother Oncol 59:145-151, 2001.
363. Uno T, Isobe K, Shikama N, et al: Radiotherapy for extranodal, marginal zone, B-cell lymphoma of mucosa-associated lymphoid tissue originating in the ocular adnexa: a multiinstitutional, retrospective review of 50 patients. Cancer 98:865-871, 2003.
364. Fung CY, Tarbell NJ, Lucarelli MJ, et al: Ocular adnexal lymphoma: clinical behavior of distinct World Health Organization classification subtypes. Int J Radiat Oncol Biol Phys 57:1382-1391, 2003.
365. Agulnik M, Tsang R, Baker MA, et al: Malignant lymphoma of mucosa-associated lymphoid tissue of the lacrimal gland: Case report and review of literature. Am J Clin Oncol 24:67-70, 2001.
366. Pfeffer MR, Rabin T, Tsvang L, et al: Orbital lymphoma: Is it necessary to treat the entire orbit? Int J Radiat Oncol Biol Phys 60:527-530, 2004.
367. Matsuo T, Yoshino T: Long-term follow-up results of observation or radiation for conjunctival malignant lymphoma. Ophthalmology 111:1233-1237, 2004.
368. Zinzani PL, Magagnoli M, Galieni P, et al: Nongastrointestinal low-grade mucosa-associated lymphoid tissue lymphoma: analysis of 75 patients. J Clin Oncol 17:1254-1258, 1999.
369. Touroutoglou N, Dimopoulos MA, Younes A, et al: Testicular lymphoma: Late relapses and poor outcome despite doxorubicin-based therapy. J Clin Oncol 13:1361-1367, 1995.
370. Linassier C, Desablens B, Lefrancq T, et al: Stage I-IIE primary non-Hodgkin's lymphoma of the testis: Results of a prospective trial by the GOELAMS Study Group. Clin Lymphoma 3:167-172, 2002.
371. Crellin AM, Hudson BV, Bennett MH, et al: Non-Hodgkin's lymphoma of the testis. Radiother Oncol 27:99-106, 1993.
372. Zietman AL, Coen JJ, Ferry JA, et al: The management and outcome of stage IAE non-Hodgkin's lymphoma of the testis. J Urol 155:943-946, 1996.
373. Zouhair A, Weber D, Belkacemi Y, et al: Outcome and patterns of failure in testicular lymphoma: a multicenter Rare Cancer Network study. Int J Radiat Oncol Biol Phys 52:652-656, 2002.
374. Abraham N Jr, Maher TJ, Hutchison RE: Extra-nodal monocytoid B-cell lymphoma of the urinary bladder. Mod Pathol 6:145-149, 1993.
375. Al-Maghrabi J, Kamel-Reid S, Jewett M, et al: Primary low-grade B-cell lymphoma of mucosa-associated lymphoid tissue

type arising in the urinary bladder: Report of 4 cases with molecular genetic analysis. Arch Pathol Lab Med 125:332-336, 2001.
376. Melekos MD, Matsouka P, Fokaefs E, et al: Primary non-Hodgkin's lymphoma of the urinary bladder. Eur Urol 21:85-88, 1992.
377. Ohsawa M, Aozasa K, Horiuchi K, et al: Malignant lymphoma of bladder. Report of three cases and review of the literature. Cancer 72:1969-1974, 1993.
378. Bates AW, Norton AJ, Baithun SI: Malignant lymphoma of the urinary bladder: A clinicopathological study of 11 cases. J Clin Pathol 53:458-461, 2000.
379. Dimopoulos MA, Daliani D, Pugh W, et al: Primary ovarian non-Hodgkin's lymphoma: outcome after treatment with combination chemotherapy. Gynecol Oncol 64:446-450, 1997.
380. Osborne BM, Robboy SJ: Lymphomas or leukemia presenting as ovarian tumors: An analysis of 42 cases. Cancer 52:1933-1943, 1983.
381. Stroh EL, Besa PC, Cox JD, et al: Treatment of patients with lymphomas of the uterus or cervix with combination chemotherapy and radiation therapy. Cancer 75:2392-2399, 1995.
382. Vang R, Medeiros LJ, Ha CS, et al: Non-Hodgkin's lymphomas involving the uterus: A clinicopathologic analysis of 26 cases. Mod Pathol 13:19-28, 2000.
383. Harris NL, Scully RE: Malignant lymphoma and granulocytic sarcoma of the uterus and vagina. A clinicopathologic analysis of 27 cases. Cancer 53:2530-2545, 1984.
384. Domchek SM, Hecht JL, Fleming MD, et al: Lymphomas of the breast: Primary and secondary involvement. Cancer 94:6-13, 2002.
385. Gopal S, Awasthi S, Elghetany MT: Bilateral breast MALT lymphoma: A case report and review of the literature. Ann Hematol 79:86-99, 2000.
386. Liu FF, Clark RM: Primary lymphoma of the breast. Clin Radiol 37:567-570, 1986
387. Giardini R, Piccolo C, Rilke F: Primary non-Hodgkin's lymphomas of the female breast. Cancer 69:725-735, 1992.
388. Hugh JC, Jackson FI, Hanson J, et al: Primary breast lymphoma: An immunohistologic study of 20 new cases. Cancer 66:2602-2611, 1990.
389. Jeon HJ, Akagi T, Hoshida Y, et al: Primary non-Hodgkin malignant lymphoma of the breast. An immunohistochemical study of seven patients and literature review of 152 patients with breast lymphoma in Japan. Cancer 70:2451-2459, 1992.
390. DeBlasio D, McCormick B, Straus D, et al: Definitive irradiation for localized non-Hodgkin's lymphoma of breast. Int J Radiat Oncol Biol Phys 17:843-846, 1989.
391. Abbondanzo SL, Seidman JD, Lefkowitz M, et al: Primary diffuse large B-cell lymphoma of the breast. A clinicopathologic study of 31 cases. Pathol Res Pract 192:37-43, 1996.
392. Wong WW, Schild SE, Halyard MY, et al: Primary non-Hodgkin lymphoma of the breast: The Mayo Clinic Experience. J Surg Oncol 80:19-25; discussion 26, 2002.
393. Dubey P, Ha CS, Besa PC, et al: Localized primary malignant lymphoma of bone. Int J Radiat Oncol Biol Phys 37:1087-1093, 1997.
394. Fairbanks RK, Bonner JA, Inwards CY, et al: Treatment of stage IE primary lymphoma of bone. Int J Radiat Oncol Biol Phys 28:363-372, 1994.
395. Rathmell AJ, Gospodarowicz MK, Sutcliffe SB, et al: Localised lymphoma of bone: prognostic factors and treatment recommendations. The Princess Margaret Hospital Lymphoma Group. Br J Cancer 66:603-606, 1992.
396. Christie DR, Barton MB, Bryant G, et al: Osteolymphoma (primary bone lymphoma): an Australian review of 70 cases. Australasian Radiation Oncology Lymphoma Group (AROLG). Aust N Z J Med 29:214-219, 1999.
397. Barbieri E, Cammelli S, Mauro F, et al: Primary non-Hodgkin's lymphoma of the bone: treatment and analysis of prognostic factors for Stage I and Stage II. Int J Radiat Oncol Biol Phys 59:760-764, 2004.
398. King LJ, Padley SP, Wotherspoon AC, et al: Pulmonary MALT lymphoma: Imaging findings in 24 cases. Eur Radiol 10:1932-1938, 2000.
399. Ferraro P, Trastek VF, Adlakha H, et al: Primary non-Hodgkin's lymphoma of the lung. Ann Thorac Surg 69:993-997, 2000.
400. Kurtin PJ, Myers JL, Adlakha H, et al: Pathologic and clinical features of primary pulmonary extranodal marginal zone B-cell lymphoma of MALT type. Am J Surg Pathol 25:997-1008, 2001.
401. Zinzani PL, Tani M, Gabriele A, et al: Extranodal marginal zone B-cell lymphoma of MALT-type of the lung: Single-center experience with 12 patients. Leuk Lymphoma 44:821-824, 2003.
402. Cordier JF, Chailleux E, Lauque D, et al: Primary pulmonary lymphomas. A clinical study of 70 cases in nonimmunocompromised patients. Chest 103:201-208, 1993.
403. Kennedy JL, Nathwani BN, Burke JS, et al: Pulmonary lymphomas and their pulmonary lymphoid lesions: A clinic's pathologic and immunologic study of 64 patients. Cancer 56:539-552, 1985.
404. DeAngelis LM: Current management of primary central nervous system lymphoma. Oncology 9:63-71, 1995.
405. Cappellani G, Giuffre F, Tropea R, et al: Primary spinal epidural lymphomas. Report of ten cases. J Neurosurg Sci 30:147-151, 1986.
406. Shenkier TN, Blay JY, O'Neill BP, et al: Primary CNS lymphoma of T-cell origin: A descriptive analysis from the International Primary CNS Lymphoma Collaborative Group. J Clin Oncol 23:2233-2239, 2005.
407. Lachance DH, Brizel DM, Gockerman JP, et al: Cyclophosphamide, doxorubicin, vincristine, and prednisone for primary central nervous system lymphoma: Short-duration response and multifocal intracerebral recurrence preceding radiotherapy. Neurology 44:1721-1727, 1994.
408. DeAngelis LM, Yahalom J, Heinemann MH, et al: Primary CNS lymphoma: Combined treatment with chemotherapy and radiotherapy. Neurology 40:80-86, 1990.
409. Krogh-Jensen M, d'Amore F, Jensen MK, et al: Incidence, clinicopathological features and outcome of primary central nervous system lymphomas. Population-based data from a Danish lymphoma registry. Danish Lymphoma Study Group, LYFO. Ann Oncol 5:349-354, 1994.
410. Nelson DF, Martz KL, Bonner H, et al: Non-Hodgkin's lymphoma of the brain: Can high dose, large volume radiation therapy improve survival? Report on a prospective trial by the Radiation Therapy Oncology Group (RTOG): RTOG 8315. Int J Radiat Oncol Biol Phys 23:9-17, 1992.
411. Laperriere NJ, Cerezo L, Milosevic MF, et al: Primary lymphoma of brain: Results of management of a modern cohort with radiation therapy. Radiother Oncol 43:247-252, 1997.
412. Ferreri AJ, Blay JY, Reni M, et al: Prognostic scoring system for primary CNS lymphomas: The International Extranodal Lymphoma Study Group experience. J Clin Oncol 21:266-272, 2003.
413. Correa DD, DeAngelis LM, Shi W, et al: Cognitive functions in survivors of primary central nervous system lymphoma. Neurology 62:548-555, 2004.
414. Lai R, Abrey LE, Rosenblum MK, et al: Treatment-induced leukoencephalopathy in primary CNS lymphoma: A clinical and autopsy study. Neurology 62:451-456, 2004.
415. Neuwelt EA, Goldman DL, Dahlborg SA, et al: Primary CNS lymphoma treated with osmotic blood-brain barrier disruption: Prologned survival and preservation of cognitive function. J Clin Oncol 9:1580-1590, 1991.
416. DeAngelis LM, Yahalom J, Thaler HT, et al: Combined modality therapy for primary CNS lymphoma. J Clin Oncol 10:635-643, 1992.
417. Abrey LE, Yahalom J, DeAngelis LM: Treatment for primary CNS lymphoma: The next step. J Clin Oncol 18:3144-3150, 2000.
418. Korfel A, Martus P, Nowrousian MR, et al: Response to chemotherapy and treating institution predict survival in primary central nervous system lymphoma. Br J Haematol 128:177-183, 2005.
419. Batchelor T, Carson K, O'Neill A, et al: Treatment of primary CNS lymphoma with methotrexate and deferred radiotherapy: A report of NABTT 96-07. J Clin Oncol 21:1044-1049, 2003.
420. DeAngelis LM, Seiferheld W, Schold SC, et al: Combination chemotherapy and radiotherapy for primary central nervous system lymphoma: Radiation Therapy Oncology Group Study 93-10. J Clin Oncol 20:4643-4648, 2002.

421. Shenkier TN, Voss N, Chhanabhai M, et al: The treatment of primary central nervous system lymphoma in 122 immunocompetent patients. Cancer 103:1008-1017, 2005.
422. Ferreri AJ, Reni M, Bolognesi A, et al: Combined therapy for primary central nervous system lymphoma in immunocompetent patients. Eur J Cancer 12:2008-2012, 1995.
423. Nguyen PL, Chakravarti A, Finkelstein DM, et al: Results of whole-brain radiation as salvage of methotrexate failure for immunocompetent patients with primary CNS lymphoma. J Clin Oncol 23:1507-1513, 2005.
424. Abrey LE, DeAngelis LM, Yahalom J: Long-term survival in primary CNS lymphoma. J Clin Oncol 16:859-863, 1998.
425. Reni M, Mason W, Zaja F, et al: Salvage chemotherapy with temozolomide in primary CNS lymphomas: Preliminary results of a phase II trial. Eur J Cancer 40:1682-1688, 2004.
426. Qualman SJ, Mendelsohn G, B MR, et al: Intraocular lymphoma: Natural history based on a clinicopathologic study of eight cases and review of the literature. Cancer 52:878-886, 1983.
427. Corriveau C, Easterbrook M, Payne DG: Intraocular lymphoma and the masquerade syndrome. Can J Ophthalmol 21:144-149, 1986.
428. Hormigo A, Abrey L, Heinemann MH, et al: Ocular presentation of primary central nervous system lymphoma: Diagnosis and treatment. Br J Haematol 126:202-208, 2004.
429. Verbraeken HE, Hanssens M, Priem H, et al: Ocular non-Hodgkin's lymphoma: A clinical study of nine cases. Br J Ophthalmol 81:31-36, 1997.
430. Trudeau M, Shepherd FA, Blackstein ME, et al: Intraocular lymphoma: Report of three cases and review of the literature. Am J Clin Oncol 11:126-130, 1988.
431. Ferreri AJ, Blay JY, Reni M, et al: Relevance of intraocular involvement in the management of primary central nervous system lymphomas. Ann Oncol 13:531-538, 2002.
432. Strauchen JA, Dalton J, Friedman AH: Chemotherapy in the management of intraocular lymphoma. Cancer 63:1918-1921, 1989.
433. Eeles RA, O'Brien P, Horwich A, et al: Non-Hodgkin's lymphoma presenting with extradural spinal cord compression: Functional outcome and survival. Br J Cancer 63:126-129, 1991.
434. Rathmell AJ, Gospodarowicz MK, Sutcliffe SB, et al: Localized extradural lymphoma: Survival, relapse pattern and functional outcome. The Princess Margaret Hospital Lymphoma Group. Radiother Oncol 24:14-20, 1992.
435. McDonald AC, Nicoll JA, Rampling RP: Non-Hodgkin's lymphoma presenting with spinal cord compression: A clinicopathological review of 25 cases. Eur J Cancer 36:207-213, 2000.
436. Perry JR, Deodhare SS, Bilbao JM, et al: The significance of spinal cord compression as the initial manifestation of lymphoma. Neurosurgery 32:157-162, 1993.
437. Willemze R, Jaffe ES, Burg G, et al: WHO-EORTC classification for cutaneous lymphomas. Blood 105:3768-3785, 2005.
438. Willemze R, Kerl H, Sterry W, et al: EORTC classification for primary cutaneous lymphomas: A proposal from the Cutaneous Lymphoma Study Group of the European Organization for Research and Treatment of Cancer. Blood 90:354-371, 1997.
439. Bekkenk MW, Vermeer MH, Geerts ML, et al: Treatment of multifocal primary cutaneous B-cell lymphoma: A clinical follow-up study of 29 patients. J Clin Oncol 17:2471-2478, 1999.
440. Vermeer MH, Geelen FA, van Haselen CW, et al: Primary cutaneous large B-cell lymphomas of the legs. A distinct type of cutaneous B-cell lymphoma with an intermediate prognosis. Dutch Cutaneous Lymphoma Working Group. Arch Dermatol 132:1304-1308, 1996.
441. Grange F, Petrella T, Beylot-Barry M, et al: Bcl-2 protein expression is the strongest independent prognostic factor of survival in primary cutaneous large B-cell lymphomas. Blood 103:3662-3668, 2004.
442. Grange F, Bekkenk MW, Wechsler J, et al: Prognostic factors in primary cutaneous large B-cell lymphomas: A European multicenter study. J Clin Oncol 19:3602-3610, 2001.
443. Cerroni L, Arzberger E, Putz B, et al: Primary cutaneous follicle center cell lymphoma with follicular growth pattern. Blood 95:3922-3928, 2000.
444. Goodlad JR, Krajewski AS, Batstone PJ, et al: Primary cutaneous follicular lymphoma: A clinicopathologic and molecular study of 16 cases in support of a distinct entity. Am J Surg Pathol 26:733-741, 2002.
445. Cerroni L, Signoretti S, Hofler G, et al: Primary cutaneous marginal zone B-cell lymphoma: A recently described entity of low-grade malignant cutaneous B-cell lymphoma. Am J Surg Pathol 21:1307-1315, 1997.
446. Roggero E, Zucca E, Mainetti C, et al: Eradication of Borrelia burgdorferi infection in primary marginal zone B-cell lymphoma of the skin. Hum Pathol 31:263-268, 2000.
447. Kurtin PJ, DiCaudo DJ, Habermann TM, et al: Primary cutaneous large cell lymphomas. Morphologic, immunophenotypic, and clinical features of 20 cases. Am J Surg Pathol 18:1183-1191, 1994.
448. Rijlaarsdam JU, Toonstra J, Meijer O, et al: Treatment of primary cutaneous B-cell lymphomas of follicle center cell origin: A clinical follow-up study of 55 patients treated with radiotherapy or polychemotherapy. J Clin Oncol 14:549-555, 1996.
449. Bekkenk MW, Geelen FA, van Voorst Vader PC, et al: Primary and secondary cutaneous CD30+ lymphoproliferative disorders: A report from the Dutch Cutaneous Lymphoma Group on the long-term follow-up data of 219 patients and guidelines for diagnosis and treatment. Blood 95:3653-3661, 2000.
450. Mraz-Gernhard S, Natkunam Y, Hoppe RT, et al: Natural killer/natural killer-like T-cell lymphoma, CD56+, presenting in the skin: An increasingly recognized entity with an aggressive course. J Clin Oncol 19:2179-2188, 2001.
451. Nguyen LN, Ha CS, Hess M, et al: The outcome of combined-modality treatments for stage I and II primary large B-cell lymphoma of the mediastinum. Int J Radiat Oncol Biol Phys 47:1281-1285, 2000.
452. Aviles A, Garcia EL, Fernandez R, et al: Combined therapy in the treatment of primary mediastinal B-cell lymphoma: Conventional versus escalated chemotherapy. Ann Hematol 81:368-373, 2002.
453. Zinzani PL, Martelli M, Bertini M, et al: Induction chemotherapy strategies for primary mediastinal large B-cell lymphoma with sclerosis: A retrospective multinational study on 426 previously untreated patients. Haematologica 87:1258-1264, 2002.
454. Todeschini G, Secchi S, Morra E, et al: Primary mediastinal large B-cell lymphoma (PMLBCL): Long-term results from a retrospective multicentre Italian experience in 138 patients treated with CHOP or MACOP-B/VACOP-B. Br J Cancer 90:372-376, 2004.
455. Norin T, Onyango J: Radiotherapy in Burkitt's lymphoma. Int J Radiat Oncol Biol Phys 2:399-406, 1977.
456. Girinsky T, Lapusan S, Ribrag V, et al: Phase II study of concomitant chemoradiotherapy in bulky refractory or chemoresistant relapsed lymphomas. Int J Radiat Oncol Biol Phys 61:476-479, 2005.
457. Sawyer EJ, Timothy AR: Low dose palliative radiotherapy in low grade non-Hodgkin's lymphoma. Radiother Oncol 42:49-51, 1997.
458. Haas RL, de Jong D, Valdes Olmos RA, et al: In vivo imaging of radiation-induced apoptosis in follicular lymphoma patients. Int J Radiat Oncol Biol Phys 59:782-787, 2004.
459. International Commission on Radiation Units and Measurements: ICRU Report 24: Determination of absorbed dose in a patient irradiated by beams of X or gamma rays in radiotherapy procedures. Bethesda, International Commission on Radiation Units and Measurements, 1976. www.icru.org/pubs.htm.
460. International Commission on Radiation Units and Measurements: ICRU Report 62: Prescribing, Recording and Reporting Photon Beam Therapy (Supplement to ICRU Report 50). Bethesda, International Commission on Radiation Units and Measurements, 1999. www.icru.org/pubs.htm.
461. Goodman KA, Toner S, Hunt M, et al: Intensity-modulated radiotherapy for lymphoma involving the mediastinum. Int J Radiat Oncol Biol Phys 62:198-206, 2005.
462. Kaplan HS, Rosenberg SA: The treatment of Hodgkin's disease. Med Clin North Am 50:1591-1610, 1966.
463. Fuks Z, Kaplan HS: Recurrence rates following radiation therapy of nodular and diffuse malignant lymphomas. Radiology 108:675-684, 1973.

464. Fuller LM, Krasin MJ, Velasquez WS, et al: Significance of tumor size and radiation dose to local control in stage I-III diffuse large cell lymphoma treated with chop-bleo and radiation. Int J Radiat Oncol Biol Phys 31:3-11, 1995.
465. Dunbar SF, Linggood RM, Doppke KP, et al: Conjunctival lymphoma: Results and treatment with a single anterior electron field. A lens sparing approach. Int J Radiat Oncol Biol Phys 19:249-257, 1990.
466. Gordan KB, Char DH, Sagerman RH: Late effects of radiation on the eye and ocular adnexa. Int J Radiat Oncol Biol Phys 31:1123-1139, 1995.
467. Bessell EM, Henk JM, Wright JE, et al: Orbital and conjunctival lymphoma treatment and prognosis. Radiother Oncol 13:237-244, 1988.
468. Hancock SL, Cox RS, McDougall IR: Thyroid diseases after treatment of Hodgkin's disease. N Engl J Med 325:599-605, 1991.
469. Jereczek-Fossa BA, Alterio D, Jassem J, et al: Radiotherapy-induced thyroid disorders. Cancer Treat Rev 30:369-384, 2004.
470. Hancock SL, McDougall IR, Constine LS: Thyroid abnormalities after therapeutic external radiation. Int J Radiat Oncol Biol Phys 31:1165-1170, 1995.
471. Liu RP, Fleming TJ, Toth BB, et al: Salivary flow rates in patients with head and neck cancer 0.5 to 25 years after radiotherapy. Oral Surg Oral Med Oral Pathol 70:724-729, 1990.
472. Cooper JS, Fu K, Marks J, et al: Late effects of radiation therapy in the head and neck region. Int J Radiat Oncol Biol Phys 31:1141-1164, 1995.
473. Emami B, Lyman J, Brown A, et al: Tolerance of normal tissue to therapeutic irradiation. Int J Radiat Oncol Biol Phys 21:109-122, 1991.
474. McDonald S, Rubin P, Phillips TL, et al: Injury to the lung from cancer therapy: clinical syndromes, measurable endpoints, and potential scoring systems. Int J Radiat Oncol Biol Phys 31:1187-1203, 1995.
475. Mah K, Van Dyk J, Keane T, et al: Acute radiation-induced pulmonary damage: a clinical study on the response to fractionated radiation therapy. Int J Radiat Oncol Biol Phys 13:179-188, 1987.
476. Mah K, Keane TJ, Van Dyk J, et al: Quantitative effect of combined chemotherapy and fractionated radiotherapy on the incidence of radiation-induced lung damage: A prospective clinical study. Int J Radiat Oncol Biol Phys 28:563-574, 1994.
477. Fay M, Tan A, Fisher R, et al: Dose-volume histogram analysis as predictor of radiation pneumonitis in primary lung cancer patients treated with radiotherapy. Int J Radiat Oncol Biol Phys 61:1355-1363, 2005.
478. Rodrigues G, Lock M, D'Souza D, et al: Prediction of radiation pneumonitis by dose-volume histogram parameters in lung cancer—A systematic review. Radiother Oncol 71:127-138, 2004
479. Graham MV, Purdy JA, Emami B, et al: Clinical dose-volume histogram analysis for pneumonitis after 3D treatment for non-small cell lung cancer (NSCLC). Int J Radiat Oncol Biol Phys 45:323-329, 1999.
480. Fajardo LP: Cardiovascular System, Pathology of Radiation Injury. New York, Masson, 1982, pp 15-33.
481. Stewart JS, Fajardo LF, Gillette SM, et al: Radiation injury to the heart. Int J Radiat Oncol Biol Phys 31:1205-1211, 1995.
482. Hull MC, Morris CG, Pepine CJ, et al: Valvular dysfunction and carotid, subclavian, and coronary artery disease in survivors of Hodgkin lymphoma treated with radiation therapy. JAMA 290:2831-2837, 2003.
483. Heidenreich PA, Hancock SL, Lee BK, et al: Asymptomatic cardiac disease following mediastinal irradiation. J Am Coll Cardiol 42:743-749, 2003.
484. Eriksson F, Gagliardi G, Liedberg A, et al: Long-term cardiac mortality following radiation therapy for Hodgkin's disease: Analysis with the relative seriality model. Radiother Oncol 55:153-162, 2000.
485. Cosset JM, Henry-Amar M, Pellar-Cosset B, et al: Pericarditis and myocardial infarction after Hodgkin's disease therapy. Int J Radiat Oncol Biol Phys 21:447-449, 1991.
486. Coia LR, Myerson RJ, Tepper JE: Late effects of radiation therapy on the gastrointestinal tract. Int J Radiat Oncol Biol Phys 31:1213-1236, 1995.
487. Cassady JR: Clinical radiation nephropathy. Int J Radiat Oncol Biol Phys 31:1249-1256, 1995.
488. Lawrence TS, Robertson JM, Anscher MS, et al: Hepatic toxicity resulting from cancer treatment. Int J Radiat Oncol Biol Phys 31:1237-1248, 1995.
489. Grigsby PW, Russell A, Bruner D, et al: Late injury of cancer therapy on the female reproductive tract. Int J Radiat Oncol Biol Phys 31:1281-1299, 1995.
490. Williams RS, Littell RD, Mendenhall NP: Laparoscopic oophoropexy and ovarian function in the treatment of Hodgkin disease. Cancer 86:2138-2142, 1999.
491. Classe JM, Mahe M, Moreau P, et al: Ovarian transposition by laparoscopy before radiotherapy in the treatment of Hodgkin's disease. Cancer 83:1420-1424, 1998.
492. Rowley MJ, Leach DR, Warner GA, et al: Effect of graded doses of ionizing radiation on the human testis. Radiat Res 59:665-677, 1974.
493. Shapiro E, Kinsella TJ, Makuch RW, et al: Effects of fractionated irradiation on endocrine aspects of testicular function. J Clin Oncol 3:1232-1239, 1985.
494. Izard MA: Leydig cell function and radiation: A review of the literature. Radiother Oncol 34:1-8, 1995.
495. Fraass BA, Kinsella TJ, Harrington FS, et al: Peripheral dose to the testes: The design and clinical use of a practical and effective gonadal shield. Int J Radiat Oncol Biol Phys 11:609-615, 1985.
496. Price A, Cunningham D, Horwich A, et al: Haematological toxicity of radiotherapy following high-dose chemotherapy and autologous bone marrow transplantation in patients with recurrent Hodgkin's disease. Eur J Cancer 30A:903-907, 1994.
497. Adamietz IA, Rosskopf B, Dapper FD, et al: Comparison of two strategies for the treatment of radiogenic leukopenia using granulocyte colony stimulating factor. Int J Radiat Oncol Biol Phys 35:61-67, 1996.
498. Knox SJ, Fowler S, Marquez C, et al: Effect of filgrastim (G-CSF) in Hodgkin's disease patients treated with radiation therapy. Int J Radiat Oncol Biol Phys 28:445-450, 1994.
499. Vadhan-Raj S, Murray LJ, Bueso-Ramos C, et al: Stimulation of megakaryocyte and platelet production by a single dose of recombinant human throbopoietin in patients with cancer. Ann Intern Med 126:673-681, 1997.
500. Lavey RS, Dempsey WH: Erythropoietin increases hemoglobin in cancer patients during radiation therapy. Int J Radiat Oncol Biol Phys 27:1147-1152, 1993.
501. Osterman B, Cavallin-Stahl E, Hagberg H, et al: High-grade non-Hodgkin's lymphoma stage I: A retrospective study of treatment, outcome and prognostic factors in 213 patients. Acta Oncol 35:171-177, 1996.
502. Munck JN, Dhermain F, Koscielny S, et al: Alternating chemotherapy and radiotherapy for limited-stage intermediate and high-grade non-Hodgkin's lymphomas: long-term results for 96 patients with tumors >5 cm. Ann Oncol 7:925-931, 1996.
503. Villikka K, Muhonen T, Ristamaki R, et al: Stage I non-Hodgkin's lymphoma treated with doxorubicin-containing chemotherapy with or without radiotherapy. Acta Oncol 36:619-624, 1997.
504. Donato V, Iacari V, Zurlo A, et al: Radiation therapy and chemotherapy in the treatment of head and neck extranodal non-Hodgkin's lymphoma in early stage with a high grade of malignancy. Anticancer Res 18:547-554, 1998.
505. Zinzani PL, Stefoni V, Tani M, et al: MACOP-B regimen followed by involved-field radiation therapy in early-stage aggressive non-Hodgkin's lymphoma patients: 14-year update results. Leuk Lymphoma 42:989-995, 2001.
506. Miller T, Unger J, Spier C, et al: Effect of adding rituximab to three cycles of CHOP plus involved field radiotherapy for limited stage aggressive diffuse large B-cell lymphoma (SWOG-0014) (Abstract 158). Blood 104:48a-49a, 2004.

CHAPTER 75

MULTIPLE MYELOMA AND OTHER PLASMA CELL NEOPLASMS

Morie A. Gertz and Michael G. Chen

INCIDENCE AND EPIDEMIOLOGY

More than 15,000 new cases of multiple myeloma (MM) are diagnosed annually in the United States.

MM accounts for 1.1% of all new cancers and 2% of cancer-related deaths.

The rate in blacks is twice that in whites (9.3/100,000 population per year).

Agricultural workers have a higher risk than other occupational groups.

ETIOLOGY AND BIOLOGIC CHARACTERISTICS

The etiology remains unknown.

This hematologic malignancy with mature plasma cell morphology evolves from a cell late in B-cell development.

No distinctive cytogenetic or molecular abnormalities are identified.

Interleukin-6 is an essential cytokine in the growth and pathogenesis of MM.

STAGING EVALUATION AND PROGNOSTIC FACTORS

Diagnostic criteria for MM include an increased number of monoclonal plasma cells in bone marrow, monoclonal protein in serum or urine, and lytic bone lesions.

Prognostic factors of most importance for MM are increased β_2-microglobulin level, decreased serum albumin level, and elevated plasma cell labeling index.

PRIMARY THERAPY AND RESULTS

Treatment of patients with symptomatic disease is indicated, excluding those with monoclonal gammopathy of undetermined significance or "smoldering" MM.

Standard therapy is now defined in light of the patient's candidacy for high-dose therapy with stem cell transplantation. Median survival for patients who receive transplants is 60 months.

Higher response rates, but no differences in overall survival, are seen with combinations of conventional-dose alkylating agents. A survival advantage of approximately 1 year has been shown for patients' receiving high-dose therapy in two prospective randomized studies.

For solitary plasmacytoma of bone and extramedullary plasmacytoma, radiotherapy is the treatment of choice, with effective local control but high rates of progression to MM. Magnetic resonance imaging may help to predict which patients are at higher risk of subsequent progression to MM.

The role of allogeneic bone marrow transplantation after reduced-intensity conditioning is being investigated as a strategy for long-term disease control.

TREATMENT OF PRIMARY REFRACTORY AND RELAPSING MYELOMA

Second- or third-line chemotherapy is standard therapy.

Localized radiotherapy is useful in palliation of painful or life-threatening disease. Hemibody irradiation can be used occasionally for pain palliation of extensive disease.

ADJUVANT THERAPY

Adjuvant therapy has no role in plasma cell disorders.

Central to an understanding of the role of radiotherapy in the treatment of multiple myeloma (MM) and solitary plasmacytoma of bone (SPB) is an appreciation of the place of these diseases in the larger category of the monoclonal gammopathies, also referred to as *paraproteinemias* or *dysproteinemias*. Monoclonal gammopathies are a group of diseases characterized by the proliferation of a clone of plasma cells, which produce an electrophoretically and immunologically homogeneous protein usually referred to as *monoclonal protein, M protein, M component*, or *paraprotein*. The distribution of monoclonal proteins found in patients at Mayo Clinic is shown in Figure 75-1. The diagnoses associated with detection of monoclonal gammopathy are depicted in Figure 75-2. Differentiation of monoclonal gammopathy of undetermined significance (MGUS) from MM and SPB is important to selection of appropriate therapy and is discussed later in this chapter. Most of this chapter is devoted to MM and its treatment, with an emphasis on radiotherapeutic applications.

The term *multiple myeloma* denotes the neoplasia that results when a clonal population of plasma cells undergoes unrestrained growth within the bone marrow cavity. The progressive proliferation of plasma cells results in marrow replacement with normochromic or slightly macrocytic anemia. Direct infiltration of the overlying bony cortex by the malignant cells causes lytic bone disease, osteoporosis, and compression fractures of the spine. In addition, the production of a monoclonal light chain in the urine can result in a severe toxic response in renal tubules, with renal failure on the basis of myeloma cast nephropathy.

ETIOLOGY AND EPIDEMIOLOGY

An estimated 15,270 new cases of MM occurred in the United States in 2004, representing 1.1% of all new cases of cancer. MM accounts for 13.4% of all hematologic malignancies diagnosed in the United States, 19% of all deaths resulting from

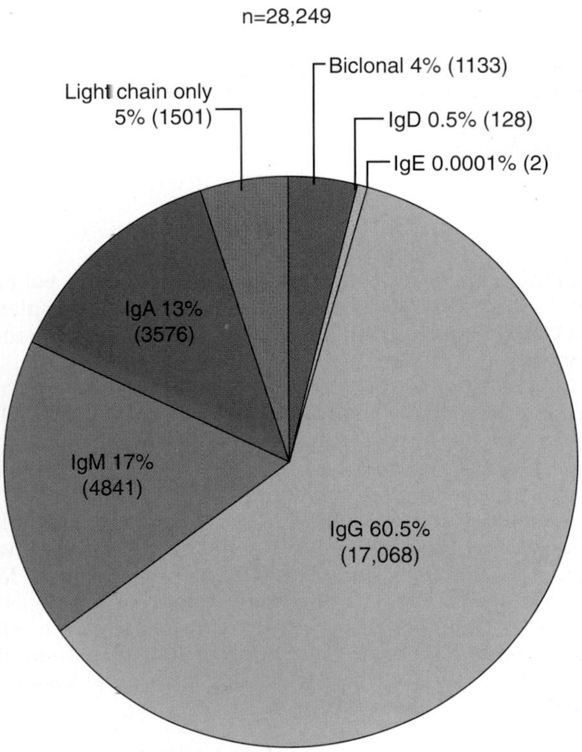

Figure 75-1 Distribution of monoclonal serum proteins determined by serum immunoelectrophoresis in patients with monoclonal gammopathies at Mayo Clinic over a 40-year period.

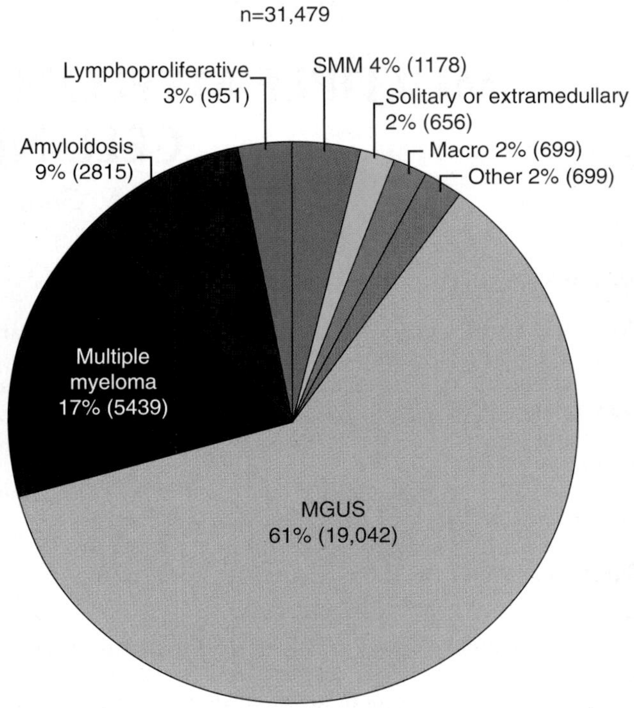

Figure 75-2 Distribution of clinical diagnoses in patients with a serum monoclonal protein detected at Mayo Clinic over a 40-year period. Macro, macroglobulinemia; MGUS, monoclonal gammopathy of undetermined significance; SMM, smoldering multiple myeloma.

hematologic malignancies, and 2% of all cancer deaths. The overall incidence of MM is comparable to that of cervical cancer, and it is one fourth as common as non-Hodgkin's lymphoma. MM is more prevalent in U.S. blacks, representing 2.7% of cancer deaths, and the ninth most common cause of death from cancer in U.S. blacks. Survival rates in black patients with MM are similar to those in white patients.[1] MM is an uncommon malignancy in the Pacific rim.

The male-to-female ratio for the disease is 1.13:1. The 5-year survival rate for MM was 24% from 1974 to 1976 and 32% from 1992 to 1999 ($P < 0.05$). In the prechemotherapy era, 5-year survival of MM patients was 12%.[2]

The average age of patients presenting with MM is approximately 63 years; however, 0.3% of patients are younger than 30 years.[3] In Olmsted County, Minnesota, the overall incidence of MM is 4.3 cases per 100,000 population per year. The rate increases with age, although no significant change in age-adjusted incidence occurred between 1945 and 2001.[4]

Radiation has been linked to the pathogenesis of MM, but radiation exposure is found in only approximately 1% of patients. In the Hiroshima and Nagasaki tumor registries, no evidence indicated an excess risk for MM.[5] The risk for MM has been inversely associated with socioeconomic status, with a 63% higher risk in the lowest quartile compared with the highest quartile of socioeconomic status.[6]

Data regarding the role of antigenic stimulation are conflicting.[7] Several studies have demonstrated an increased prevalence of MM in persons exposed to diesel exhaust,[8] gasoline,[9,10] and fuel oil.[11] Epidemiologic studies in the United States have demonstrated associations between MM and agricultural workers.[12] In France, farmers have an adjusted mortality increase of 60% because of MM.[13] Other occupational groups associated with the development of MM include miners,[14] workers exposed to wood dust,[15] and sheet metal workers.[16] No increased risk has been seen in cigarette smokers.[17,18] Higher rates are reported in obese patients.[19] One recent exhaustive study suggested no relationship between diesel exhaust and MM,[20] but exposure to the chemical alachlor, a commonly used pesticide, demonstrated an increasing trend for incidence of lymphohematopoietic cancers associated with lifetime exposure to the pesticide. The risk for MM gave a rate ratio of 5.66 in the highest exposure category.[21]

The etiology of MM remains unknown. Studies of cytogenetic abnormalities in MM demonstrate no consistent chromosome break point that identifies the majority of patients. Cytogenetic abnormalities, however, are least frequent in patients with MGUS, and an increase in frequency is seen as this condition evolves into MM untreated and MM relapsed. MM probably originates from a germinal center B cell of the lymph node. Receptors allow these cells to migrate from the lymph node to the bone marrow.

Myeloma plasma cells express several adhesion molecules, including neural cell adhesion molecule (NCAM).[22] Adhesion molecules are involved in homing of plasma cells to bone marrow. Although MM is a neoplasm of end-stage plasma cells, most investigators believe myeloma stem cells exist as a self-renewing population derived from an earlier compartment. The identity of the cells responsible for the initiation and maintenance of MM remains unclear. Circulating B cells clonally related to MM plasma cells have been reported in some patients with myeloma. Recent data suggest that myeloma stem cells are $CD138^-$ B cells, whereas the terminally differentiated plasma cell is consistently $CD138^+$. These $CD138^-$ B cells can replicate and differentiate into the malignant CD138+ plasma cells.[23] Overexpression of Bcl-2 protein has been seen in clinical myeloma and myeloma cell lines. Cytokines, including tumor necrosis factor (TNF)-α, interleukin (IL)-1, and IL-6, play an essential role in the biology of the malignancy as well as in mediating the bony manifestations of the disease. Both IL-6 and Bcl-2 have been shown to prevent apoptosis, and IL-6 has been implicated as an essential growth factor in MM.[24] IL-6 appears to be the most important cytokine mediating MM-induced bone resorption.[25]

PATHOLOGY

The morphology of the plasma cell in MM is relevant prognostically (Fig. 75-3). Immature and plasmablastic plasma cells are associated with a poor prognosis. When 3% of the plasma cells in the bone marrow are indistinguishable from lymphoblasts, this has been defined as *plasmablastic myeloma* and is associated with a higher prevalence of renal insufficiency and bone disease.[26] In one study, the median survival of patients with the plasmablastic subtype of myeloma was 2 months. Other prognostic features seen on evaluation of the bone marrow biopsy specimen include marked dysplasia, number of mitoses per high-power field, and packing of the bone marrow by tumor.[27] Electron microscopic analysis of myeloma cells demonstrating nuclear cytoplasmic asynchrony has been associated with a poor prognosis. Ultrastructural analysis and nuclear maturity of myeloma cells are relevant prognostically.[28]

MM is distinct in that the bone marrow is involved in virtually all patients, yet the peripheral blood shows large numbers of circulating cells in only a few patients. The confinement of plasma cells to the bone marrow probably is mediated by cellular contact between the myeloma cell and marrow stroma. Investigations on adhesion molecules in bone marrow myeloma cells have demonstrated strong expression of N-CAM (CD56). This adhesion receptor is not present on normal bone marrow plasma cells.[29] Adhesion can be important in IL-6–mediated tumor growth.[30] When serum levels of NCAM were measured, levels were higher in patients with MM than in those with MGUS.[31] Higher levels of NCAM were seen in patients with high tumor burdens. Serum NCAM levels were associated with poor survival.

Expression of the antiapoptotic gene *BCL2* may mediate chemoresistance. Cell lines with upregulated *BCL2* expression were resistant to doxorubicin.[32] Myeloma cell lines incubated with an antisense oligonucleotide to Bcl-2 restore chemotherapy sensitivity.[33,34] Gene-mediating multidrug resistance codes for a glycoprotein molecule called *P170.* P170 appears to enhance an efflux pump, reducing intracellular accumulation of chemotherapeutic agents such as vincristine and doxorubicin. P170 expression can be assayed immunocytochemically.[35] The percentage of cells that are positive for the multidrug resistance gene depends on previous exposure to chemotherapy, with higher proportions of cells expressing P170 glycoprotein with successive exposures to chemotherapy. By inhibiting this efflux pump, higher intracellular levels of chemotherapy are achieved. The potential exists to reduce resistance to second-line therapies in MM.[36]

Sensitive techniques have been able to demonstrate circulating cells belonging to the malignant clone in MM. Circulating plasma cells have been detected by immunofluorescence microscopy, three-color flow cytometry, and allele-specific oligonucleotide polymerase chain reaction (PCR) analysis. With the last technique, circulating cells were found in 13 of 15 patients with MM.[37] Clonally rearranged cells can be detected in the stem cell harvest of patients with MM who are being considered for bone marrow transplantation (BMT). Of 32 leukaphereses, 14 were contaminated with clonally rearranged cells.[38] With a PCR-based method using clone-specific immunoglobulin (Ig) heavy-chain gene sequences, seven of seven patients with MM had tumor cells in all peripheral blood samples.[39] The presence of peripheral blood monoclonal plasma cells predicts survival in MM as well as relapse-free and overall survival in patients who are candidates for BMT.[40] Myeloma cell precursors circulate as primitive cells and differentiate into plasma cells in the presence of TNF-α and IL-4.[41]

IL-6 appears to be the major growth factor for human myeloma cells in vitro. In advanced MM, cell growth totally depends on IL-6 in more than 95% of patients.[42] Dexamethasone-mediated death of myeloma cells can be reversed by concomitant IL-6 therapy.[43] Monoclonal antibodies directed against the soluble IL-6 receptor inhibit the growth of human myeloma cell lines and may offer therapeutic benefit.[44] Mice that are incapable of producing IL-6 are completely resistant to plasma cell tumor development.[45] IL-6 receptor antagonists inhibit cell growth because they are proapoptotic factors in IL-6–dependent myeloma cell lines.[46]

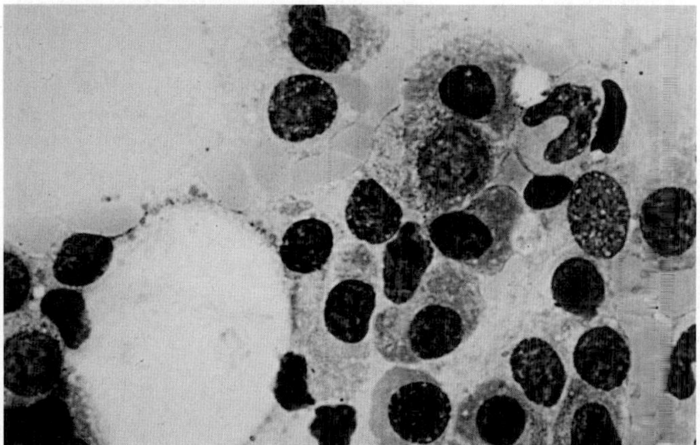

Figure 75-3 Bone marrow diagnostic for multiple myeloma. (Wright stain; original magnification ×1000.)

MOLECULAR GENETICS

Studies on genes in MM cells have led to insights regarding the precursor cells of MM and its pathogenesis. Ectopic expression of *BCL2* can lead to progression of disease by preventing apoptosis of myeloma cells. High-level expression of *BCL2* suppresses apoptotic death in myeloma cell lines.[47] Higher expression levels of the *BCL2*-related gene *BCLXL* are observed in apoptosis-resistant myeloma cell lines.[48,49]

Expression of c-*MYC* was studied in 180 patients with MM. Expression of c-*MYC* correlated with the grade of malignancy. This finding suggests that c-*MYC* could be involved in myeloma mutagenesis.[50] High levels of c-*MYC* transcripts and protein could regulate myeloma cell proliferation and apoptotic death by controlling p53 expression.[51] Aberrant translational control of c-*MYC* may contribute to myeloma pathogenesis.[52] The oncogene *MYC* has also been implicated in the molecular alterations that occur when MGUS progresses to MM.[53]

In a study of 45 patients with MM, point mutation of the *p53* gene was detected in only 1 patient.[54] In a second study of

52 patients, *p53* mutations found in 13% were associated with more advanced myeloma.[55] *p53* has a limited role in the disease.[56] *p53* events are related to the terminal phases of the disease.[57]

Abnormalities of the retinoblastoma gene (*RB*) were sought in 35 myeloma patients. Absent or reduced expression was found in four patients (11%). This finding was associated with advanced disease and refractoriness to treatment.[58] Phosphorylated *RB* is expressed constitutively in MM cells, promoting myeloma cell growth.[59] Deletion of *RB* was found in more than 50% of patients with MM by fluorescence in situ hybridization (FISH); *RB* deletion can result in deregulation of IL-6 expression and expansion of IL-6–dependent myeloma clones.[60]

Mutations of *RAS* are more prevalent in MM than in other lymphoid malignancies. In a study using genomic DNA in 128 patients, *RAS* mutations were far more common in patients with aggressive plasma cell leukemias (30%) than in MM patients (9%). The *RAS* mutations appear to represent a late molecular lesion in the process of myeloma evolution.[61] When levels of *RAS* were studied in 160 patients with newly diagnosed MM, the median survival for patients with mutations of N-*RAS* was no different from that of patients with no *RAS* mutations. However, patients with K-*RAS* mutations had significantly higher tumor burdens at diagnosis and a median survival of 2 years versus 3.7 years for those who did not have K-*RAS* mutations. The *RAS* mutations do appear to have an independent impact on the median survival of patients with MM.[62]

IgH rearrangements can be found in 75% of patients.[63] Dysregulation of cyclin D_1 can be detected in 30% of MM tumors. Cell lines that overexpress cyclin D_1 have a translocation detectable into a gamma switch region that suggests an error in VDJ recombination.[64] V_H analysis of the clonal cells in MGUS showed much lower mutation frequencies than in MM.[65] In myeloma, no V_H gene intraclonal diversity is noted, and no evidence indicates V_H gene somatic mutation over the course of the disease. This finding strongly implies that the malignant clone in MM evolves from a cell late in B-cell development.[66,67] The clonogenic cell in MM likely originates from a preswitched but somatically mutated B cell.[68–71] Genetic studies have demonstrated that the progression of MM from plateau phase to relapse does not involve a new B-cell clone, and progression beyond the plateau phase is not due to clonal succession.[72] Advances using molecular probes for FISH have demonstrated aneuploid chromosomes where conventional cytogenetics are normal. Chromosome 13 abnormalities have been associated with an unfavorable prognosis in patients with myeloma. When patients with newly diagnosed MM were studied for deletion of chromosome 13 on bone marrow plasma cells using interphase FISH, a deletion of chromosome 13 was found in 54% of patients. These patients were less likely to respond to therapy and had a significantly shorter median overall survival.[73] The translocation t(11;14) results in upregulation of cyclin D_1 and is the most common translocation detected in patients with MM. Sixteen percent of patients carry the t(11;14) and had better survival and response to therapy.[74] Immunoglobulin heavy-chain translocations are seen in 60% of patients, and these translocations are more likely to be nonhyperdiploid. Conversely, 88% of patients with hypodiploidy carry the IgH translocation.[75] Patients with light-chain myeloma never display a functional immunoglobulin heavy-chain recombination. Most patients with light-chain myeloma have one immunoglobulin heavy-chain allele with a germline configuration. The second allele is usually involved in an illegitimate recombination. Light-chain myeloma may be due to the absence of legitimate immunoglobulin heavy-chain rearrangement at the DNA level.[76]

CLINICAL MANIFESTATIONS AND PATIENT EVALUATION

Multiple Myeloma and Monoclonal Gammopathy of Undetermined Significance

The key to early detection of MM is recognizing the associated clinical syndromes and presentations and permitting appropriate diagnostic tests to be performed. The clinician must order electrophoresis of serum and of urine for all patients who present with normochromic normocytic or slightly macrocytic anemia.[77] In MM, the degree of anemia is often modest (hemoglobin in the range of 11 to 12 g/dL). Electrophoresis of serum and urine can often obviate needless diagnostic investigations for gastrointestinal tract blood loss or other invasive techniques. In a patient who has any degree of unexplained renal insufficiency (i.e., a nonhypertensive, nondiabetic patient), urine immunoelectrophoresis often leads to recognition of myeloma cast nephropathy.

The most common problem is dealing with patients who present with bone pain. Radiographs of the spine in patients with MM frequently show osteoporosis and compression fractures. It is virtually impossible to distinguish the compression fractures associated with MM from those seen in patients with senile osteoporosis (Fig. 75-4). Spine radiographs poorly demonstrate the small lytic lesions frequently responsible for collapse of these vertebrae. All patients with back or rib pain, even with no malignant features on radiographs, should have

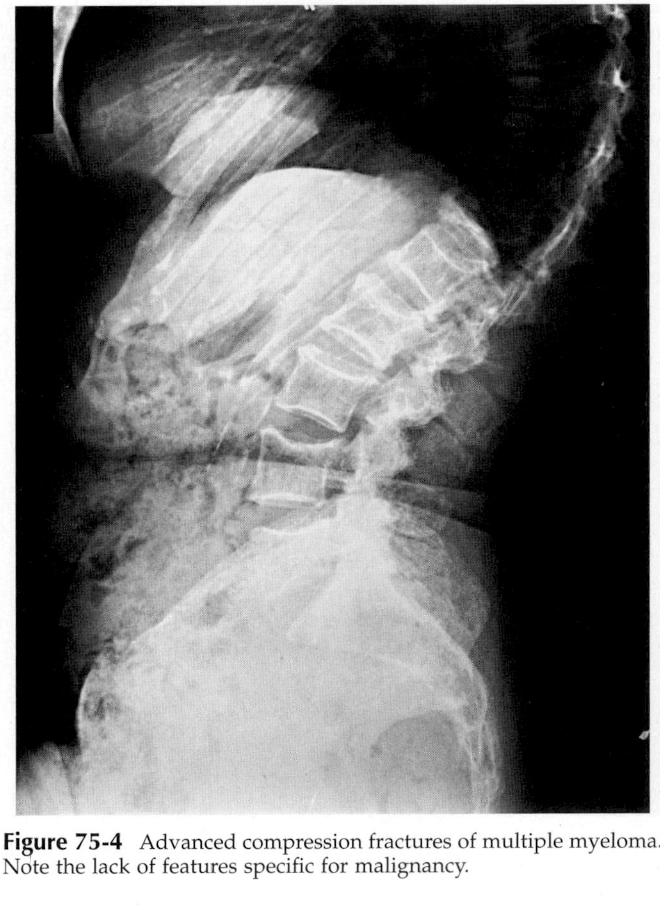

Figure 75-4 Advanced compression fractures of multiple myeloma. Note the lack of features specific for malignancy.

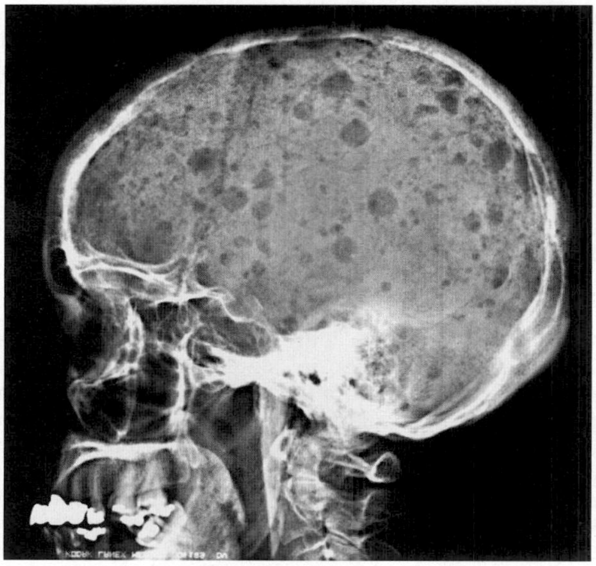

Figure 75-5 Calvarial radiograph from a patient with multiple myeloma.

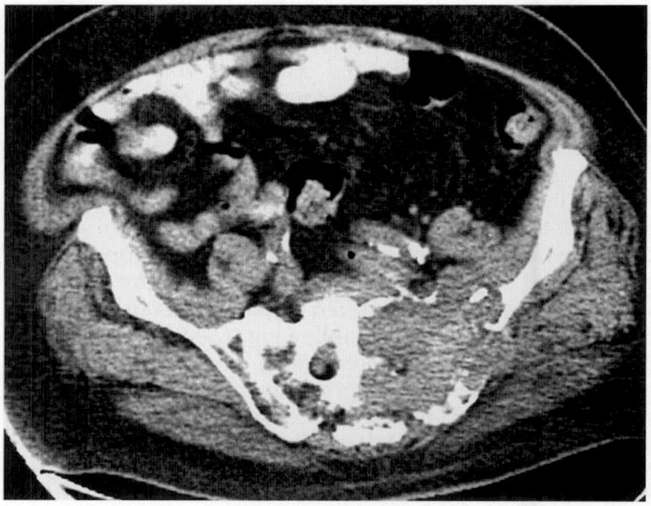

Figure 75-6 Diagnostic computed tomographic scan of pelvic plasmacytoma. Plain radiographs revealed only rarefaction and were not diagnostic.

electrophoresis of serum and urine. If a monoclonal protein is found, radiographs of the entire skeleton often demonstrate lytic lesions in the calvaria, pelvis, and long bones of the humerus and femur (Fig. 75-5).

Assessment of bone disease initially requires a radiographic bone survey. Because the lesions of MM are primarily lytic lesions with little evidence of bony repair, radionuclide bone scans tend to be an inferior approach to the detection of these bony lesions. In difficult cases in which osteoporosis and monoclonal gammopathy are found with no other changes, computed tomography (CT) scan or magnetic resonance imaging (MRI) of the spine and pelvis can be valuable in detecting clear-cut evidence of neoplasia (Fig. 75-6).[78] Moreover, MRI can be valuable in monitoring the response to treatment in patients who have small or no measurable monoclonal proteins.[79] Positron emission tomography (PET) may be useful in MM, as the lytic lesions are PET avid. When 66 patients were studied with PET and compared with CT and MRI, negative PET findings reliably predicted stable MGUS.[80] All patients with active myeloma had focal or diffusely positive scans, four of whom had negative full radiographic bone surveys. Extramedullary uptake was detected by PET in 23% of relapsing patients. PET also tracks response, showing a decline in lesion metabolic activity with successful intervention.[81] It is more sensitive than other imaging techniques, and it can find additional lesions in a third of patients, which affected therapeutic decision-making for a quarter of these patients.[82] A recent study has suggested that sestamibi PET scanning is more sensitive than fluorine deoxyglucose PET scanning.[83]

In our experience, many physicians neglect to perform electrophoresis studies in patients presenting with back pain or osteoporosis, an oversight that can delay a diagnosis of MM. The need for screening electrophoresis cannot be overemphasized. In one study, 29 of 219 patients presenting with unexplained osteoporosis and pain had monoclonal proteins, leading to further investigation.[84] The most common reason for a delayed diagnosis of MM is the simple finding that MM was not included in the differential diagnosis.[85]

A second clinical problem is distinguishing MGUS from overt MM. In MGUS, the patient is expected to be asymptomatic, without evidence of anemia, hypercalcemia, or renal insufficiency. The patient should have no complaints of rib or back pain. In general, a bone marrow study or routine radiographic bone survey is not indicated in MGUS if the monoclonal component is less than 2.5 g/dL. In the absence of symptoms and with a low monoclonal protein value, regular monitoring of the level of the monoclonal protein should suffice. Monoclonal gammopathies are present in nearly 3% of patients older than 70 years, and a routine bone marrow examination would result in an additional million bone-marrow studies to assess these asymptomatic persons. Patients with monoclonal gammopathies, however, should be monitored indefinitely, because the risk for transformation to a malignant plasma-proliferative process is approximately 1% per year.[86] The risk for transformation is predicted by the initial size of the M-protein peak. Patients with low monoclonal protein levels, 0.5 g/dL or less, had a 6% risk for developing MM at 10 years compared with 11% risk at 10 years for those with a 1.5-g/dL peak and 24% risk at 10 years for those with a 2.5-g/dL peak.[87]

The frequency of monitoring patients with MGUS depends on risk factors identified at initial evaluation. Certainly, patients with monoclonal gammopathy (M-protein level greater than 3 g/dL) require more frequent assessment than those who have an M-protein spike of only 1 g/dL. In addition, patients who are being observed because of small, asymptomatic lytic bone lesions (indolent myeloma) are at much higher risk for early progression to overt MM.[88] For most patients, annual assessment suffices.

Solitary Plasmacytoma

Localized plasmacytomas are rare diseases that account for less than 10% of all plasma cell neoplasms. Similar to MM but without infiltration of the bone marrow, these neoplasms are composed of sheets of plasma cells involving bone or soft tissue.[89–91] When the lesion is isolated in bone, the disorder is called *solitary plasmacytoma of bone* (SPB) or *solitary myeloma of bone*. When in soft tissues, the lesion is called *extramedullary plasmacytoma* (EMP) and is found in the head and neck 80% of the time.

SPBs are found predominantly in men (male-to-female ratio of 2:1) and at a median age of 55 years. SPBs are slightly more common than EMPs and occur at a younger age than MM.[92–106] More than half the patients with SPB present with bone pain in the axial skeleton, and the disorder predominantly involves the vertebral column. This condition can cause symptoms of radiculopathy or myelopathy from nerve root or spinal cord compression. Ganjoo and Malpas[89] summarized pooled data from more than 250 patients in 14 series on the sites of presentation of SPB in the axial and appendicular skeleton and on the incidence of spinal lesions by site in the spine. After reviewing the often disparate literature on SPB, these authors suggested the following essential criteria for a diagnosis of SPB: solitary bone lesion on skeletal survey, histologic proof of plasmacytoma by biopsy, less than 5% plasma cells on marrow aspirate, and absence of other major criteria for the diagnosis of MM (anemia, hypercalcemia, impaired renal function, presence of monoclonal protein). Advances in diagnostic imaging (MRI and PET) have facilitated exclusion of patients with early systemic MM by increasing the sensitivity of detection of occult bone marrow abnormalities in patients originally referred with a diagnosis of SPB[78] or EMP.[107] Current diagnostic criteria for SPB require biopsy-proven monoclonal plasmacytoma of bone in a single site only. MRI and/or PET imaging, if performed, must be negative outside the primary site. The primary lesion may be associated with a low serum or urine M-protein component. "Low" is defined as serum IgG of less than 3.5 g/dL, IgM of less than 2 g/dL, and a urine monoclonal protein level of less than 1 g/dL, and the bone marrow must contain less than 10% monoclonal plasma cells, and no other myeloma-related organ dysfunction is found.[108]

EMPs are primary soft tissue plasma cell tumors with a predisposition for the head and neck.[109–121] EMPs also can occur in a wide variety of other tissues, such as in the gastrointestinal tract, skin, lung, lymph nodes, spleen, genitourinary tract, and breast, but these sites are rare.[90] In the head and neck, the upper respiratory tract (including the paranasal sinuses) is the most frequently affected. This pattern of occurrence shows some similarity to the distribution of mucosa-associated lymphoid tissue (MALT) and MALT-type lymphomas in these sites. Predominance of IgA monoclonal proteins in EMP has been reported.[122] EMP and SPB share a similar slight male predominance and a younger mean age at diagnosis than MM. Criteria for diagnosis of EMP are similar to those for SPB and include careful histopathologic differentiation from other benign processes and poorly differentiated neoplasms and radiographic exclusion (MRI or PET imaging) of occult lesions in bone marrow and other noncontiguous sites.

A variant of MM sometimes associated with a solitary or limited number of sclerotic bone lesions is *osteosclerotic myeloma,* or the *POEMS syndrome* (*p*olyneuropathy, *o*rganomegaly, *e*ndocrinopathy, *M* protein, and *s*kin changes).[123–130] This condition is also referred to in the literature as *Crowe-Fukase* or *Takatsuki's disease.*[125,127] Waldenström[128] considered the essential features of the syndrome to be a triad of polyneuropathy, osteosclerosis, and a monoclonal component with lambda chains. Similar to SPB, the bone marrow in patients with POEMS syndrome usually contains less than 5% plasma cells, and hypercalcemia and renal insufficiency occur rarely. A monoclonal protein is found in the serum in most cases, but the level is rarely higher than 3 g/dL. Most of the patients have a lambda monoclonal protein, and Bence Jones proteinuria is infrequent.

Confirmation of the diagnosis of POEMS syndrome rests on identification of monoclonal plasma cells in the biopsy specimen from an osteosclerotic lesion. This variant form of plasma cell neoplasm is relevant to this discussion because more than half the patients with this syndrome respond to local radiotherapy to a dominant sclerotic bone lesion with substantial improvement of the neuropathy.[124,126] In patients with widespread osteosclerotic lesions, chemotherapy has been used, although the use of neurotoxic drugs may be contraindicated.

Stem cell transplantation has been used successfully for the management of POEMS syndrome in patients for whom radiotherapy was unsuccessful.[131]

Staging of Multiple Myeloma

Classification of patients with MM by stage is important. Comparison of outcomes in single-arm studies of MM depends on patient selection and case mix. Therefore, ensuring that patients have comparable severity of disease is important when comparing the outcomes of various studies. In addition, stage may be useful in selecting patients with unfavorable outcomes for more intensive therapies. Conversely, patients who are at a low stage and whose prognosis is good may be candidates for less intensive therapies and may achieve outcomes similar to those of aggressively treated patients.

The most common staging system in clinical use is that of Durie and Salmon (Table 75-1). This system has several problems, and in some studies, it has been shown to be not particularly predictive of survival.[132,133] One problem with the Durie-Salmon staging system is that the criteria for stage I MM in this scheme are also consistent with smoldering MM and indolent MM, which do not require any form of therapy. In most clinical therapy studies, no more than 10% of patients have stage I disease, and many studies exclude patients with stage I from participation. The second difficulty is the subjective nature of interpretation of advanced lytic lesions to distinguish stage II from stage III. No specific well-defined criteria exist to ensure that all institutions use the same

Table 75-1 Durie-Salmon Staging

Stage	Durie-Salmon Staging Criteria
I	All of these required: hemoglobin > 10 g/dL, Ca^{2+} < 10.5 mg/dL, IgG < 5 g/dL or IgA < 3 g/dL, and light-chain loss < 4 g/d
	No lytic bone lesions
II	Not fitting stage I or III
III	Any 1 of the following: hemoglobin < 8.5 g/dL, Ca^{2+} >12 mg/dL, IgG > 7 g/dL, IgA >5 g/dL, or light-chain loss > 12 g/d
	Advanced lytic lesions
A	Creatinine < 2 mg/dL
B	Creatinine ≥ 2 mg/dL
Stage	**Durie-Salmon Plus Criteria**
I	MGUS: M-protein spike <3 g/dL and marrow plasma cells <10%
A	Indolent or smoldering MM: M-protein spike ≥3 g/dL or marrow plasma cells ≥10%; solitary plasmacytoma permitted
B	<5 Focal lesions or mild diffuse disease
II	5–20 Focal lesions or moderate diffuse disease
III	>20 Focal lesions
A	Creatinine <2 mg/dL and no extramedullary disease
B	Creatinine ≥2 mg/dL or extramedullary disease

MGUS, monoclonal gammopathy of undetermined significance; MM, multiple myeloma.

Table 75-2 United Kingdom Medical Research Council Staging System (1980)

Stage	Criteria
A	All required: urea ≤8 mmol/L, hemoglobin ≥10.0 g/dL, and PS 0 or 1
B	Neither A nor C
C	Any 1 required: hemoglobin <7.5 g/dL, urea >10 mmol/L, or PS > 1

PS, performance status.

Table 75-3 International Myeloma Working Group Stages

Stage	Criteria
I	β_2-microglobulin < 3.5 µg/mL and albumin ≥3.5 g/dL
II	β_2-microglobulin < 3.5 µg/mL and albumin <3.5 g/dL or β_2-microglobulin = 3.5 – 5.5 µg/mL
III	β_2-microglobulin ≥ 5.5 µg/mL

Table 75-4 Greipp Staging System

Stage	Criteria
I	S-phase bone marrow plasma cells <0.8% and β_2-microglobulin <2.7 µg/mL
II	Only 1 of 2 stage I criteria abnormal
III	S-phase cells ≥0.8% and β_2-microglobulin ≥2.7 µg/mL

definition of advanced MM. Finally, the system does not adequately incorporate impairment of renal function, which is a strong prognostic factor in virtually all studies, and it adds A and B criteria for creatinine, which fundamentally increases the number of stages to 5: I, IIA, IIB, IIIA, and IIIB.

Due to the limitations of the Durie-Salmon staging system, a Durie-Salmon Plus staging system has been developed. It includes stage I for MGUS. Stage IA MM is now smoldering or indolent MM. These stage I or IA patients may have a single plasmacytoma or limited disease by imaging. Stage IB myeloma must have less than five focal lesions or mild diffuse disease; stage II must have 5 to 20 focal lesions with moderate diffuse disease; and stage III must have more than 20 focal lesions with severe diffuse disease. In addition, the IIIA and IIIB criteria have been revised. In addition to lower creatinine, stage IIIA patients must have no extramedullary disease. Patients who have extramedullary disease are classified as stage IIIB.

In several studies, the Medical Research Council of the United Kingdom staging system has provided better prognostic distinction. The staging system is given in Table 75-2. It has the advantage of including three easily measurable variables that are highly reproducible among laboratories. This system, however, excludes some of the newest prognostic factors, which appear to be the most powerful predictors of outcomes. In most recent studies, the most powerful variable in predicting ultimate outcome is the serum level of β_2-microglobulin, which appears to be an excellent measure of total tumor burden.[134] This finding has been incorporated into a staging system looking at β_2-microglobulin and C-reactive protein, with C-reactive protein measured as a surrogate for IL-6 activity.[135]

Two simpler staging systems have more recently been proposed. The Southwest Oncology Group (SWOG) has proposed a staging system based on serum albumin and β_2-microglobulin levels. The most widely accepted is the International Myeloma Working Group staging system, where stage III myeloma is a β_2-microglobulin level higher than 5.5 µg/mL. Stage I includes patients with a β_2-microglobulin level that is less than 3.5 µg/mL and a serum albumin level that is less than 3.5 g/dL, and stage II includes all patients who do not fit stage I or stage III. This easy-to-remember staging system divides patients into three groups of virtually equal size, was based on data derived from more than 11,000 patients, and only lacks sufficient numbers of patients who had cytogenetic studies performed to determine its role in staging (Table 75-3).

Measurement of the number of S-phase plasma cells by flow cytometry or by immunofluorescence provides insight into the kinetics of the myeloma cell and has been shown to be a powerful predictor of outcome.[136] Greipp and colleagues[137] combined the serum β_2-microglobulin and the percentage of S-phase cells measured by immunofluorescence microscopy (labeling index) to derive the staging system detailed in Table 75-4. This system has the advantage of having only two variables for stratification. One disadvantage is that the technique to measure the percentage of S-phase plasma cells is not widely available. These staging systems reflect the types of studies necessary to evaluate patients with myeloma, and a recommended minimum evaluation is given in Table 75-5.

Table 75-5 Required Testing to Evaluate Multiple Myeloma

Category	Test
Blood	Complete blood cell count
	Na^+
	K^+
	Ca^{2+}
	Alkaline phosphatase
	Aspartate aminotransferase
	Uric acid
	Creatinine
	Immunofixation of serum
	Serum protein electrophoresis, including albumin[138]
	Lactate dehydrogenase
	C-reactive protein
	β_2-microglobulin
	Analysis for circulating plasma cells[40] (flow cytometry $CD38^+$ or immunofluorescence microscopy κ,λ)
Urine	Urine protein electrophoresis
	Urine immunofixation
	Creatinine clearance
Radiography	Bone survey to include all bones
	Chest radiograph
Miscellaneous	Electrocardiogram
	Bone marrow aspirate biopsy and % S-phase measure[137]

Response is generally assessed by the reduction in monoclonal protein; a reduction of 25% to 50% would be considered a minor response and 50% to 99% an objective response. Complete eradication of the monoclonal protein in the serum and in the urine with less than 5% plasma cells in the bone marrow would be considered a complete response.[138] Patients who either did not have a bone marrow test performed or whose monoclonal protein was no longer visible but detectable by immunofixation are considered to have a near-complete response. A review of 1500 myeloma patients enrolled in SWOG studies evaluated the outcomes for patients and 6- and 12-month landmarks and demonstrated that the median survivals were not different for those who had a greater than 50% response compared with those who had a greater than 75% response versus nonresponders, in the absence of disease progression. This suggests that, with standard-dose therapy, the magnitude of response does not predict survival, and, therefore, the goal of therapy should be stabilization of disease rather than the degree of M-protein reduction.[139] In recipients of autologous transplants, however, a complete response predicts improved outcome after transplantation.[140]

PRIMARY THERAPY FOR MULTIPLE MYELOMA

The treatment of MM is reserved for patients who are symptomatic. Because of the incurable nature of MM, asymptomatic patients (i.e., those with indolent MM and smoldering MM) are monitored on a regular basis until symptoms develop. Early therapeutic intervention for asymptomatic patients has not been demonstrated to improve survival in this illness. Therefore, patients who fulfill the criteria for smoldering MM or indolent MM are observed without treatment.[141] This rationale resembles the treatment philosophy in patients with asymptomatic chronic lymphocytic leukemia or advanced low-grade lymphoma. Both disorders are considered incurable and are slowly progressive.

Most patients with MM have symptomatic disease at diagnosis and require cytotoxic therapy. Specific indications for treatment include an increasing level of M protein in serum or urine, decreasing concentration of hemoglobin, increasing concentration of calcium and creatinine, lytic bone lesions, and EMP. Chemotherapy is the standard initial treatment for symptomatic MM. At presentation, palliative irradiation is often used at sites of painful disease that is refractory to analgesics. However, this treatment could delay the institution of chemotherapy.

MM was the first malignant disease in which a reliable tumor marker was recognized. The monoclonal protein found in the serum or in the urine, a direct product of plasma cell production, provides an excellent way to monitor a patient's total tumor burden. All monitoring schemes categorize responsiveness or progression of the disease not by the status of the bone marrow, but rather by the percentage of change in the monoclonal protein during and after therapy. Serial measurements provide the most direct method for disease assessment. Only 3% of patients with MM do not have a monoclonal protein in the serum or urine. Two thirds of these patients will have a measurable free light chain in the serum by nephelometry. Moreover, the short half-life of free light chains in the serum makes them suitable to assess response early in the course of therapy.[142,143]

Role of Chemotherapy

In 1962, the Southwest Cancer Chemotherapy Study Group first established melphalan (L-phenylalanine mustard) as an active drug in the therapy of MM.[144] This was followed by the report of the Midwest Cooperative Chemotherapy Group on the efficacy of cyclophosphamide.[145] The combination of melphalan and prednisone has been standard therapy of myeloma worldwide for the past three decades.[146,147] It produces an objective response rate in 50% to 60% of patients, with median response and survival durations of 20 and 35 months, respectively. However, this chemotherapy regimen rarely results in lasting complete remission. In an effort to improve on these results, many clinical trials have used other combinations of chemotherapeutic drugs, such as the M2 protocol (vincristine, carmustine, melphalan, cyclophosphamide, and prednisone) from Memorial Sloan-Kettering Cancer Center in New York,[148] with varying degrees of success. A meta-analysis of many combination chemotherapy programs compared with a melphalan-prednisone regimen was reported by Gregory and coworkers.[149] They concluded that a melphalan-prednisone regimen is superior for patients with an intrinsically good prognosis and inferior for those patients with a poor prognosis.

The Eastern Cooperative Oncology Group compared a melphalan-prednisone regimen with the M2 protocol. Patients were followed for more than 10 years. Overall survival was not significantly different for the two groups (27 and 29 months, respectively; $P = 0.3$). Objective responses were seen more commonly with M2 (72%) than with the melphalan-prednisone regimen (51%), but this difference did not translate into improved survival.[150]

In a SWOG-sponsored study,[151] patients were randomly assigned to one of three chemotherapy regimens. The most important variable contributing to higher response rates and improved survival was the dose of glucocorticoids used. Their standard therapy of vincristine, melphalan, cyclophosphamide, and prednisone (VMCP) alternating with vincristine, carmustine (BCNU), doxorubicin (Adriamycin), and prednisone (VBAP) was less important than the intensity of glucocorticoid therapy and provision of this maintenance therapy. In this study, interferon played only a small role and did not prolong relapse-free or overall survival. For patients who are not candidates for stem cell transplantation, melphalan and prednisone should still be considered standard therapy.

The Italian Multiple Myeloma Study Group[152] recently reported the use of oral melphalan and prednisone combined with thalidomide for previously untreated patients. These patients were considered unsuitable for stem cell transplantation. All were older than 60 years, with a median age of 72 years. A complete response or near-complete response occurred in 45%, a greater than 90% reduction in the M-protein level occurred in an additional 12%, and 50% to 89% had a reduction of 36%, giving an overall response rate of 93%, which is certainly comparable with the results after stem cell transplantation. It was well tolerated. The most serious adverse effect was deep vein thrombosis. The complete response rate of 42% compares well with those seen after transplantation and may be an exciting step forward for patients who are not eligible to receive a transplant.

For patients who are resistant to melphalan and prednisone or who respond but subsequently have a relapse while still receiving therapy, salvage regimens are based on high-dose dexamethasone and include a combination of thalidomide and dexamethasone, thalidomide alone, bortezomib alone, and combinations of agents. However, once primary chemotherapy resistance develops, even a dexamethasone-based regimen results in few responses of short duration. Of 47 patients with strictly defined refractory or relapsing disease, the response rate to the combination of vincristine, doxorubicin (Adriamycin), and dexamethasone (VAD) was only 28%. The median response duration was 3.6 months, and the median overall survival was 8.3 months. The toxic effects related to dexamethasone were substantial, with 33 life-threatening toxic reactions recorded in 52 evaluable patients. Five treatment-related deaths occurred.[153]

In an attempt to reduce the toxicity of the VAD regimen and to reduce the reliance on an indwelling central venous catheter, we have studied high-dose methylprednisolone in a similar group. The response rates were comparable (35%), with median survival of 19 months for patients responsive to treatment. The toxicity of methylprednisolone is less than that of dexamethasone.[154] VAD therapy has not been shown to be superior to alkylating agent–based regimens in previously untreated patients. Untreated patients were randomly assigned to four different treatment groups: melphalan and prednisone, melphalan and dexamethasone, dexamethasone, and dexamethasone and interferon. The survival in all four groups was identical, and the results were consistent with the fact that treatment with melphalan and prednisone remains the gold standard for older patients with MM. Dexamethasone-based regimens did not improve overall survival.[155] The prognosis for relapsed MM is poor. When 578 patients with newly diagnosed MM were assessed, the overall survival at 1, 2, and 5 years was 72%, 55%, and 22%, respectively, and the median overall survival was 28.4 months. After first relapse, the median overall survival was 17.1 months, and the duration of response decreased consistently with each successive regimen, suggesting evolution of drug-resistant subclones as well as an increased proliferative rate of the myeloma cells. The median survival of patients who experienced relapse after initial treatment and received salvage therapy was 1.5 years.[156]

The use of autologous stem cells as part of management is considered the standard of care. In one prospective randomized study,[157] the probability of event-free survival for 5 years was 28% in the transplant group and 10% in the conventional-dose group. The estimated rate of survival for 5 years was 52% in the high-dose group and 12% in the conventional-dose group (P = .03). Bladé and associates[158] analyzed the survival of patients eligible for BMT but who were treated conventionally. The median survival of this group was also 5 years. We have found that dose-intensive chemotherapy followed by BMT can overcome drug resistance and produce responses in refractory and heavily pretreated patients.[159] The UK Medical Research Council, in a prospective randomized study, demonstrated higher rates of complete response, 44% versus 8% with conventional therapy, and an improved overall survival of 54.1 versus 42.3 months.[160] A sample algorithm for the treatment of patients with newly diagnosed MM is given in Figure 75-7.

If autologous BMT is considered for primary therapy or eventually as therapy for relapsing or refractory disease after standard chemotherapy, we have found it essential to avoid melphalan and prednisone for induction, which can deplete hematopoietic stem cells in the peripheral blood or bone marrow.[161,162] Pretransplant induction regimens include dexamethasone; thalidomide and dexamethasone[163]; doxorubicin, vincristine, and dexamethasone[164,165]; vincristine, doxorubicin, and methylprednisolone[166]; and a regimen of dexamethasone and thalidomide combined with cytotoxic chemotherapy (cisplatin, doxorubicin, and cyclophosphamide) as induction therapy.[167]

Newer supportive modalities are useful in the management of patients with MM. Although chemotherapy can destroy the malignant clone and may prevent progression of bony disease, it does not lead to remineralization or recalcification of previously involved bone. Monthly infusions of pamidronate and zoledronic acid[168,169] for 9 consecutive months reduced the proportion of patients who had any skeletal events from 41% to 24%. Patients who received pamidronate had significant decreases in bone pain and improved quality of life.[170] Pamidronate (90 mg/mo) or zoledronic acid (4 mg/mo) has a significant palliative effect in patients with bone pain secondary to metastasis. Best results were obtained in patients with osteolytic bone disease.[171]

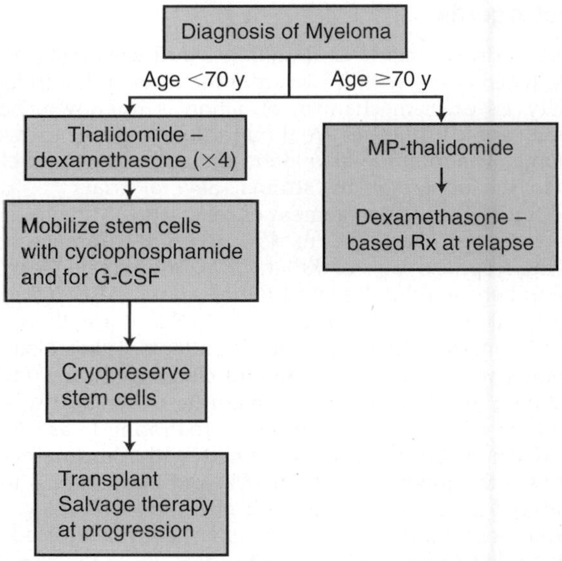

Figure 75-7 Algorithm for treatment of newly diagnosed multiple myeloma. G-CSF, granulocyte colony-stimulating factor; MP, melphalan and prednisone.

Bisphosphonates act by inhibiting bone resorption. They have a major effect on osteoclasts and reduce bone-resorbing cytokine production. They have limited bioavailability and achieve the highest concentrations when administered parenterally. Zoledronic acid has an in vivo potency 100,000 times that of etidronate, and it is 100 times more potent than the bisphosphonate most commonly administered orally, alendronate. These agents reduce the frequency of skeletal-related events, including the need for radiation for bone pain, pathologic fracture, and spinal cord compression. Zoledronic acid consistently reduces the incidence of all types of skeletal-related events from 1.39 events per year with pamidronate to 1.04 with zoledronic acid. The toxic effects of zoledronic acid include an increase in the serum creatinine level, proteinuria, and osteonecrosis of the jaw. Vertebroplasty is high-pressure injection of low-viscosity material into the vertebral body, designed to stabilize painful vertebral compression fractures. It can be done on an outpatient basis by an interventional radiologist. Its risks include leak of the material and potential encroachment on a nerve root. The anemia of MM is often not improved with the institution of systemic therapy. We have found that erythropoietin in a dose of 150 U/kg given three times per week results in a 2-g increase in the hemoglobin concentration in nearly half the patients treated. This often can obviate the need for supportive transfusion and can be a useful adjunct in the treatment of patients with MM.[172] Darbepoetin has recently been introduced for the treatment of the anemia of MM. Its usual dose is 200 μg every 2 weeks.[173]

Novel Agents

Thalidomide was used as a sedative and antiemetic in the 1950s, when it was withdrawn from the market due to teratogenicity. Its exact mechanism of action is unknown, but its antiangiogenic properties are thought to inhibit the growth of myeloma. Thalidomide also alters the adhesion of myeloma cells to the bone-marrow stroma. Several trials[174,175] using thalidomide in the management of relapsed MM have shown response rates from 30% to 45%, with the largest trial[176] showing response rates of 30% to 37%. There is no clear relationship between the dose and the response. Although doses of up to 800 mg have been used, 50 to 200 mg is the typical dose for long-term management of patients. It has also been combined with dexamethasone and clarithromycin,[174] which has shown an increase in response rate in newly untreated patients to 66%. The toxic effects of thalidomide are severe, and, when thalidomide is combined with dexamethasone, deep vein thrombosis results in 16% and grade 3 or 4 toxicities in 44% of patients. Although effective, it is toxic. New immunomodulatory agents in development for reduced toxicity include CC-5013 (Revlimid). Studies on its salvage effect in patients with myeloma have demonstrated activity,[177] and studies combining CC-5013 with dexamethasone in newly diagnosed, previously untreated MM are under way.

Bortezomib represents a new class of anticancer compounds, the proteasome inhibitors. These drugs induce cell death by blocking degradation of apoptotic molecules that are normally catabolized via proteasome proteolysis. They inhibit nuclear factor (NF)-κB activation by stopping the cleavage of its bound suppressor. Increased NF-κB activity has been described[178] in myeloma cells and correlates with resistance to treatment. Proteasome inhibitors seem to overcome chemotherapy resistance.[179] A recent phase 3 study[180] of bortezomib with dexamethasone suggested that the time to progression was shorter in the bortezomib group. Combinations using standard chemotherapeutics with bortezomib may have higher response rates in myeloma than bortezomib as a single agent.[181] Bortezomib produces a response in approximately one third of patients with relapsed MM; its primary toxic effects are both thrombocytopenia and peripheral neuropathy.[182]

Role of Radiotherapy

Since the advent of chemotherapy in the late 1960s, radiotherapy has played a more adjunctive role in the treatment of MM. With the exception of its primary use in the treatment of localized plasma cell disease (e.g., SPB and EMP) and occasionally more disseminated disease such as osteosclerotic myeloma (POEMS syndrome), radiotherapy is now used more frequently for relief of impending spinal compression or nerve root compression, prevention of pathologic fracture in weight-bearing bones, and immediate palliation of pain, usually osseous in origin, than as primary therapy for untreated disease. The efficacy of conventional megavoltage radiotherapy for these indications is well documented.[183–186] After pathologic fracture of weight-bearing bones and orthopedic stabilization by pinning, arthroplasty, or rod placement, it has been customary to administer radiotherapy to the operative bed after surgical healing has occurred. Lately, in many instances, it has been our practice not to use adjunctive irradiation if the patient is to receive chemotherapy for MM, because of the comparable efficacy of chemotherapy in destroying residual disease.

In the prechemotherapy era, megafield irradiation techniques were developed, notably by the group at the Memorial Hospital in New York using the Heublein method[187] and by Fitzpatrick and Rider[188] at the Princess Margaret Hospital in Toronto. The Memorial group used total-body irradiation (TBI), and the Princess Margaret group used hemibody irradiation (HBI) to treat disease on presentation and in later years for palliation of chemotherapy-refractory disease. Holder[189] reported considerable pain palliation in one of the earliest series of patients with MM who were treated with TBI.

Bergsagel[190] proposed a theoretical framework for the use of TBI given as sequential HBI in the treatment of MM, and hypothesized a three-log tumor cell kill with a 10-Gy total-body dose. This concept was based on in vivo radiosensitivity of a mouse plasma cell tumor, assayed for surviving fraction of tumor stem cells by an in vitro cell-cloning technique, and on clinical studies in a patient with multiple plasmacytomas of the skin. A D_0 value of approximately 1.1 Gy was determined from the dose-response data. Glück and coworkers[191] reported radiosensitivity studies on seven clonogenic human myeloma cell lines and found different radiosensitivities, depending on dose fractionation and dose rate. In his seminal article, Bergsagel also proposed autologous BMT with density gradient–separated marrow stem cells harvested from the patient with MM before BMT. TBI was an integral part of the preparative regimen for BMT because of the relative radiosensitivity of the myeloma cell. More recently, use of TBI for BMT has superseded sequential HBI in the treatment of relapsing or refractory MM.

Because of the toxicity of TBI, HBI was largely used in the late 1970s and in the 1980s for the treatment of recurrent and refractory MM.[192–201] Usually, it involved sequential single-fraction irradiation of the lower hemibody followed by upper hemibody treatment, allowing a rest period between treatments to permit reseeding of the irradiated bone marrow by circulating hematopoietic stem cells from the shielded marrow. Relief of bone pain could be achieved in most patients.[192] In other reports,[200,201] a 40% to 60% decrease in M protein and an average 50% decrease in total body myeloma cell mass were demonstrated. More than 50% of these chemotherapy-refractory patients responded by these objective and subjective criteria. However, little impact on remission status and overall survival was noted.

The toxicities of HBI for patients with MM, particularly hematologic toxicity, are addressed in several of these reports.[196,197,199,201] These effects place serious limitations on the use of HBI in nontransplant settings. The poor hematologic tolerance can be attributed to patient factors (age, heavy pretreatment, poor performance status) and the nature of the disease itself. Reports from France[199] and the United Kingdom[202] summarize current trials on the use of HBI in MM. However, with the exception of a brief preliminary report from South Africa,[203] a direct prospective comparison of HBI with chemotherapy in a large multicenter trial has not been done. Except for these reports, the use of HBI as primary treatment for untreated or refractory MM has declined in the past decade.

Using a similar rationale, namely, systemic radiotherapy as consolidation after chemotherapy for patients with untreated MM, the Northern California Oncology Group[204] initiated a phase 2/3 trial in 72 patients with previously untreated, high-tumor-burden stage III MM who first received induction chemotherapy with VMCP. This was to be followed by sequential HBI (lower hemibody first), and, finally, by eight cycles of consolidation VMCP. Nineteen of the 40 patients who received induction chemotherapy and HBI developed grade 4 hematologic toxicity, eight with long-standing neutropenia or thrombocytopenia. Although feasibility could be demonstrated, the data suggested no added survival advantage for this program. Finally, SWOG[205] performed a randomized trial comparing additional VMCP chemotherapy with sequential HBI in a group of 180 responders to two-drug combination chemotherapies (VMCP and VBAP) that are not cross-resistant. These investigators found that additional chemotherapy was superior to sequential HBI for remission consolidation. The authors also stated that the findings did not support the use of HBI in nonresponding patients with MM.[205]

Role of Blood and Bone Marrow Transplantation in Untreated or Recurrent and Refractory Multiple Myeloma

Despite the demonstrated sensitivity of the myeloma cell to chemotherapy and radiotherapy, lasting complete remission with these therapies is rare, and MM remains uniformly fatal, with a 10-year survival of 3%. Irrespective of an initial 65% response rate to standard dexamethasone-based therapy, all patients eventually have a relapse and die of their disease.

One of the more promising concepts in chemotherapy in recent years has been the dose-escalation hypothesis, one of the best applications of which was the intravenous administration of high-dose melphalan by McElwain and Powles[206] in the treatment of MM. They reported substantially increased complete remission rates in patients receiving higher than conventional doses of melphalan for primary or refractory MM. This pioneering work led to trials of melphalan and other alkylating agents in high doses, with or without TBI, followed by hematopoietic rescue using transplanted blood- or bone marrow–derived hematopoietic stem cells to offset the considerable hematologic toxicity of the high-dose chemotherapy and TBI. Because this subject has been extensively reviewed[207,208] and is discussed elsewhere in this book, it is only summarized here, with an emphasis on the role of TBI as part of the preparative regimen for BMT and on the possible use of conventional radiotherapy in pretransplantation or posttransplantation consolidation.

The earliest BMT trials in MM used rationale and methods proven in the treatment of acute and chronic leukemia: total ablation of the disease in the bone marrow by preparative regimens using high-dose chemotherapy and TBI followed by grafting healthy marrow from syngeneic (identical twin)[209–212] or allogeneic (HLA-matched sibling) donors.[213–217] The centers most closely identified with these efforts are the group at the University of Washington[211,212] and the European Group for Bone Marrow Transplant (EGBMT).[216,217] Both syngeneic BMT and allogeneic BMT have the advantage of total replacement of the diseased bone marrow by healthy tissue. In addition, allogeneic BMT has the theoretical advantage of a graft-versus-myeloma effect, which is supported by certain publications.[218–220] As with allogeneic BMT for other hematologic diseases, however, finding suitable HLA-matched sibling donors may be difficult, and because of the older age of patients with MM (median age of 52 years for allogeneic BMT), morbidity and mortality from graft-versus-host disease may be enhanced.

Because the curative potential of allogeneic transplantation lies in the graft-versus-myeloma effect, attempts to reduce the toxicity associated with allotransplantation have led to reduced-intensity conditioning followed by donor infusion of allogeneic cells. A trial[221] combined autologous stem cell transplantation with reduced-intensity conditioning allogeneic transplantation to initially reduce tumor burden to the level where allogeneic immunocompetent cells would have an opportunity to destroy residual disease. Fifty-four patients, whose median age was 52 years, underwent autologous transplantation after conditioning with melphalan, 200 mg/m^2, followed a median of 62 days later by reduced-intensity conditioning with 2 Gy of TBI and postgrafting immunosuppression with mycophenolate and cyclosporine. Most patients did not require hospitalization. Sustained engraftment was uniform, and after 552 days, the overall survival was 78%; 38% developed acute graft-versus-host disease, and 46% had chronic graft-versus-host disease necessitating therapy. Fifty-seven percent of the patients achieved complete responses, and 26% had partial responses, for an overall response rate of 83%. This two-step approach is now the subject of a national phase 3 clinical trial of tandem autotransplants compared to a single autologous stem cell transplant followed by reduced-intensity conditioning allogeneic transplantation.[221]

The results of syngeneic BMT are only anecdotal because of the relative rarity of an identical twin match and the uncommonness of the disease. In the pioneering Columbia University report,[209] the patient had a relapse after 2 years, but 2 years later, at the time of the report, the patient was alive with chemotherapy-controlled disease. In 162 patients who had allogeneic BMT for MM, the EGBMT[216] reported 32% survival at 4 years and 28% at 7 years. In the 72 patients (44%) who achieved complete remission after BMT, overall progression-free survival was 34% at 6 years. However, only nine patients remained in complete remission more than 4 years after allogeneic BMT. With allogeneic BMT, some of the decreased survival can be attributed to peritransplantation mortality, approaching 40% in some series, because of graft-versus-host disease and other complications of the procedure itself. This has also been the experience in a large national trial (S9321)[222] that reported treatment-related mortality of 40% and a median survival of 18 months.

Because of these difficulties with allogeneic BMT, autologous peripheral blood stem cell transplantation and reduced-intensity conditioning allogeneic BMT have become the more common procedures in the treatment of untreated, refractory, or recurrent MM. Applicability to older patients (upper age limit of 75 years in many centers) without the need for a matched donor and with less risk for transplant-related mortality (less than 3% in larger centers) has made this procedure accessible to more patients with MM. The disadvantages of autologous BMT in this bone-marrow malignancy include the difficulty of removing tumor cells from the transplanted peripheral blood or marrow and the lack of a potential graft-versus-myeloma effect. Purging of the apheresis product to remove any malignant cells has been attempted using in vivo immunotoxins, in vitro chemotherapy, and positive selection for CD34 stem cells. Prospective studies have failed to show an improvement in overall or disease-free survival. Purging is not routinely used.[223,224]

Mohrbacher and Anderson[207] comprehensively reviewed the autologous BMT and peripheral blood stem cell transplantation experiences at centers in Europe and the United States. Several thousand patients have been treated on various protocols, including those with newly diagnosed, relapsed, sensitive, or primary resistant disease. After autologous BMT, approximately 25% to 40% of the patients achieved complete remission, with median duration of responses of 24 to 36 months. Patients with sensitive disease and those who were less heavily pretreated had more favorable outcomes, as has been the experience with transplantation for other hematologic malignancies.

It has recently been demonstrated in a prospective, randomized study[225] that sequential tandem autologous transplantation produces superior survival compared with single stem cell transplantation. Drawbacks of this study included conditioning that does not conform to current standards, and the fact that the single-transplant group achieved a median survival of only 48 months, which is shorter than survival in many other reported studies.[225] The second transplantation is normally completed within 6 months of the first.[226] A recent prospective randomized study[227] of patients aged 50 to 70 years has demonstrated a survival advantage associated with tandem transplantation. One hundred ninety-four patients were randomly assigned to receive melphalan and prednisone chemotherapy or to undergo tandem transplantation with a reduced dose of melphalan at 100 mg/m^2. The response rate was higher with the myeloablative therapy, and the transplant group had increased event-free survival and overall survival. When analysis was limited to patients aged 65 to 70 years, the overall survival medians were 37 months for the group that received melphalan and prednisone and 58 months for the group that received melphalan, 100 mg/m^2. Tandem low-dose melphalan and transplantation improved the response rate and event-free and overall survival, specifically in those aged 65 to 70 years.[227]

TECHNIQUES OF IRRADIATION: VOLUME, DOSES, AND RESULTS

Primary Radiotherapy for Solitary Plasmacytoma of Bone

Although some authors recommend that treatment portals for SPB include the entire involved bone with 2- to 3-cm margins to encompass the entire medullary cavity of the bone, other reports recommend radiation fields encompassing only the primary lesion, with generous margins encompassing the osseous lesion and any soft tissue extensions of tumor. CT or MRI may be particularly helpful in delineating extraosseous extensions of tumor into adjacent soft tissue, particularly in spinal and pelvic bone presentations of SPB. Similar portals would be designed for each of the more infrequent multiple plasmacytomas seen in the occasional indolent presentations of MM and osteosclerotic myeloma with associated POEMS syndrome.

Several reports of SPB series[97,99,102,103,105,106] recommend dosages of radiation of at least 40 Gy in 4 weeks, preferably 45 to 50 Gy in 4½ to 5 weeks, if allowable by normal tissue tolerances. Mill and collaborators[95,183,228] reviewed radiation dose levels for local disease control at their institution and summarized results from other centers in the United States and the United Kingdom. Similar results were also reported from Mayo Clinic by Frassica and coworkers[99] and from France by Bataille and Sany.[97] In the Mayo Clinic series, no patient receiving 45 Gy or more of conventionally fractionated radiotherapy for SPB had local treatment failure. As in other disease sites, precise definition of a radiation dose-response relationship from these retrospective studies is difficult, but the preponderance of data suggests that higher doses and treatment with curative intent can lead to cure.

Bataille and Sany[97] and Dimopoulos and coworkers[229] reviewed radiotherapy results from their centers and from the literature on 114 and 138 patients with SPB, respectively, and found a low rate (11% and 4%, respectively) of local disease recurrence after radiotherapy. Subsequent analyses of the M. D. Anderson Cancer Center data by Liebross and coworkers[105] and by Wilder and associates[106] showed that patients with persistence of M protein for more than 1 year after radiotherapy progressed to MM within 2.2 years of treatment. Those patients with myeloma protein that disappeared after radiotherapy had a high likelihood of cure. Data from these and other series are summarized in Table 75-6. Overall, the rate of progression to MM by 10 years was 44% to 54%, with most SPB patients eventually developing MM. Several of the reports suggested a higher rate of progression in patients with SPB and detectable myeloma protein at presentation. Electrophoresis, immunoelectrophoresis, and immunofixation of serum and urine are essential tests to follow patients with SPB to detect disease progression. In series from Mayo Clinic[99] and M. D. Anderson Cancer Center,[229] approximately one third of the patients remained free of disease at 10 years, with a median time to relapse of 2 years. Relapses many years later were not uncommon. All the patients in the University of Florida study by Bolek and coworkers[104] eventually developed MM by 15 years. In general, median overall survival for patients with SPB exceeds 10 years, possibly because of lower tumor burden and slower tumor kinetics compared with patients with MM.

Primary Radiotherapy for Extramedullary Plasmacytoma

EMPs are plasmacytomas arising outside the bone marrow, commonly with a predilection for the upper aerodigestive passages and sharing some of the features of non-Hodgkin's lymphoma occurring in the head and neck. The nasopharynx, tonsils, maxillary sinus, nasal vestibule, and trachea are the most frequent sites of disease at presentation. Regional cervical lymph nodes may be involved in 10% to 15% of cases, and a patient presents occasionally with nodal metastasis and no detectable primary site. Treatment volume and technique are similar to those for radiotherapy for the more common tumors in these sites and should include draining lymph nodes, as recommended by Knowling and coworkers[115] and by Mayr and coworkers.[100]

Mill and coworkers suggested no apparent difference in the dose responsiveness of EMP and SPB in an early dose-response analysis,[95] as well as in a later update of the world literature.[228] Knowling and colleagues[115] at the Princess Margaret Hospital in Toronto reported that radiotherapy was unsuccessful in five of their 25 patients with EMP: one developed a single bony lesion, two progressed to MM, and two developed multiple EMP. In this Canadian series, the most

Table 75-6 Clinical Outcome of Patients with Solitary Plasmacytomas Treated with Radiotherapy Alone

Variable	Bataille and Sany[97]	Knowling et al[115]	Frassica et al[99]	Holland et al[102]	Dimopoulos et al[103]	Bolek et al[104]
Patients (n)	18	25	46	32	45	27
Median age (y)	51	50	56	60	53	55
Myeloma protein (%)	33	24	54	NA	58	52
Local recurrence (%)	11	8	11	6	4	4
Progression to myeloma (%)	44	48	54	53	46	54
10-y disease-free survival (%)	15	16	25	56	42	55
Median survival (y)	NA	7	8	4	13	10

NA, not available.

Table 75-7 **Clinical Outcome of Patients with Extramedullary Plasmacytomas Treated with Radiotherapy and Surgery**

Variable	Corwin and Lindberg[92]	Knowling et al[115]	Mayr et al[100]	Soesan et al[119]*	Holland et al[102]	Tesei et al[121]
Patients (n)	12	25	13	25	14	22
Median age (y)	59	59	61	46	58	NA
Myeloma protein (%)	NA	24	NA	16	NA	NA
Local recurrence (%)	17	8	15	12	7	9
Progression to myeloma (%)	17	8	23	NA	36	14
5-y disease-free survival (%)	NA	71	58	48	64	92
Median survival (y)	10	8	6	10	5	NA

*Only stages I and II patients. Ten stage III patients in the original series were not analyzed.
NA, not available.

common dose fractionation was 35 Gy in 15 fractions up to 45 Gy in 15 to 24 fractions. Table 75-7 summarizes six series of patients with EMP who were treated mostly by radiotherapy and surgery. Local disease recurrence after radiotherapy was marginally higher than in SPB series (see Table 75-6), but progression to MM occurred at a much lower rate, as first noted by Corwin and Lindberg.[92] Because of this lower conversion to MM, disease-free survival is superior to survival in patients with SPB.

The clinical behavior of EMP suggests a plasmacytic disorder that is distinct from SPB and MM and a need for aggressive therapy directed at a potentially more curable group of patients. Some authors have recommended higher doses of radiation on the basis of data suggesting a higher local relapse rate for EMP. Wiltshaw[90] reported 34% local disease recurrence in a group of 53 patients with EMP in published series and 21% in her own series. Soesan and colleagues[119] retrospectively analyzed 35 patients with EMP and recommended adjuvant alkylating chemotherapy for patients with early-stage disease. However, the role of adjunctive chemotherapy remains controversial. Plowman[91] suggested that adjuvant chemotherapy is not of convincing benefit and that interferon-α after radiotherapy or concurrent with radiotherapy could be considered.

Radiotherapy for Multiple Myeloma with Palliative Intent

Radiotherapy has long been recognized as a prompt and highly effective modality in the palliation of painful bony lesions and mass effects from soft tissue extensions and plasmacytomas of MM. Reports summarizing the radiotherapeutic experiences at several centers worldwide document the efficacy of radiotherapy in the control of lytic bone lesions and in reversing the morbidity of spinal cord and nerve root compression.[95,183–186] For the usual axial skeleton presentations in patients with MM, with or without spinal cord or nerve root impingement, most centers deliver 30 Gy in 10 fractions or 40 to 45 Gy in 4 to 4½ weeks to the lesions with generous margins. For vertebral body presentations, this requires treatment of one or two vertebral bodies above and below the involved vertebra and inclusion of the transverse processes of the vertebrae. Traditional plain bone radiography often suffices, but MRI and CT of the affected bone and soft tissue disease often can enhance the accuracy of the fields to allow inclusion of all the diseased tissue and to detect nearby subclinical involvement as well.[229]

For patients who present with spinal cord or nerve root compromise, either by direct extension from an involved vertebra or by extradural deposits of MM generally behind the spinal cord, some controversy exists on the necessity for surgical decompression.[230–233] Jacobs and coworkers[234] argued for surgical decompression and postoperative radiotherapy as both a diagnostic test (if first site of disease) and a therapeutic maneuver, and they presented evidence to support a better outcome with a combined-modality approach. In contrast, a larger series from Australia by Wallington and colleagues[235] showed no added efficacy for surgical decompression by χ^2 analysis, but their analysis included patients with lymphoma and those with MM. In their study, a total radiation dose of 40 Gy or more was associated with achievement of local disease control.

The University of Arizona group[236,237] has been a proponent of lower radiation doses in the treatment of MM, a concept popularized many years ago by the Columbia University group[238] and often used at some centers for palliating bone metastases from other malignancies as well as for MM. Leigh and Shimm[237] suggested that a total dose of 10 Gy with a mean fraction size of 3.1 Gy provides durable symptom relief in most patients and that no increase in response frequency occurs with doses greater than 15 Gy. These investigators argued that initial low-dose irradiation allows later retreatment at similar doses and decreases toxicity.

These ideas were challenged by Adamietz and colleagues[185] in their series of 70 patients with MM who were treated with chemotherapy combined with or followed by local irradiation for painful lesions. These investigators presented evidence of a decreased response rate (complete pain relief at the irradiated site) with subsequent treatments, especially if a low-dose strategy was used, with no response by the third course of treatment to the same site.

The Hannover group[185] also presented provocative results that the local response rate was 80% in patients receiving irradiation during melphalan and prednisone chemotherapy, and this palliative effect lasted 32 months. However, if irradiation was given without systemic therapy, the local response rate was 40% and lasted 25 months. These investigators suggested enhanced efficacy for concurrent therapy or that the group treated with irradiation alone was treated at a time of resistant disease. The University of Arizona group[237] was not able to substantiate these findings on the efficacy of concurrent treatment, but they suggested that 97% of their patients with MM were pretreated extensively with chemotherapy, whereas 47% of the German patients had not yet received chemotherapy.

Another rationale for low-dose palliative radiotherapy is that it does not preempt the later use of TBI as part of the preparative regimen for allogeneic or autologous BMT.

However, even doses in the range of 20- to 25-Gy conventional fractionation to limited fields over the spinal cord, for example, added to 12-Gy TBI (possibly equivalent to 30-Gy conventional radiotherapy), raise some concerns about the tolerance of these critical structures. Our practice has been to shield those segments of spinal cord during some or all of the TBI, so as not to exceed these tolerances. This is done knowing that this shielding may protect residual MM in the shielded areas.

Systemic Radiotherapy: Total-Body Irradiation and Hemibody Irradiation

Until recently, many of the preparative regimens for allogeneic and autologous BMT for MM included bone marrow–ablative TBI and dose-intensive chemotherapy, often melphalan or other alkylating agents. The TBI dose was usually 12 Gy delivered as 2 Gy twice daily for 3 days, allowing at least 6 hours between fractions and given at low dose rates of 0.05 to 0.15 Gy per minute. Because of alleged toxic effects of radiation, the Arkansas group[222] has changed the dose fractionation in a current SWOG MM transplant trial to 12 Gy in eight fractions over 4 days (1.5 Gy twice daily) at low dose rates. The M. D. Anderson group[208] has used 8.5-Gy TBI given as 1.7 Gy twice daily in five fractions over 2½ days.

Early in 2002, Moreau and colleagues[239] reported the results of the Intergroupe Francophone du Myelome 9502 randomized trial comparing two commonly used conditioning regimens: melphalan alone (200 mg/m^2) versus melphalan (140 mg/m^2) plus 8-Gy TBI. The study involved 282 evaluable patients with newly diagnosed MM, mostly stage III, treated with VAD induction and autologous stem cell transplantation. They concluded that melphalan alone was less toxic (hematologic toxicity, severe mucositis) than melphalan plus TBI, and the median duration of event-free survival was similar. The 45-month survival was superior in the melphalan-alone group, attributable in part to better salvage regimens after relapse. This study and others have been influential in shifting most myeloma transplant centers away from bone marrow–ablative, TBI-containing preparative regimens to programs using drugs alone, at least before autologous transplantation.

Some of the current investigational trials of nonmyeloablative allogeneic transplantation (mini-allotransplantation) for refractory or relapsing MM are evaluating single-dose TBI, usually 2 Gy delivered in one fraction, combined with various chemotherapy regimens. Many of these trials have reported only minor acute treatment-related toxicities and faster hematopoietic engraftment. This approach shows promise, as reviewed earlier, because of potential allograft-versus-myeloma effects.

As with autologous blood stem cell transplantation and BMT for Hodgkin's and non-Hodgkin's lymphoma, consolidation radiotherapy before or after transplantation to sites of bulky bone or extramedullary disease has been used, notably at the Dana Farber Cancer Institute in Boston.[240,241] These investigators favor pretransplantation radiotherapy to achieve maximum cytoreduction before transplantation. Unlike the experience in patients with lymphomas, the propensity to relapse in sites of bulky disease in MM has not been studied extensively. Tsang and coworkers[242] at the Princess Margaret Hospital have recently reviewed and updated their experience, previously reported by Knowling and colleagues[115] on solitary plasmacytomas (SPB and EMP). They found that tumors less than 5 cm in bulk treated with a median dose of 35 Gy were well controlled, but that large tumor bulk locally (≥5 cm) predicted local failure. Because TBI may also be used as part of the conditioning regimen before transplantation, combined doses from consolidation radiotherapy and TBI should be monitored carefully, so that the radiation tolerances of sensitive organs such as spinal cord, brain, lung, and gastrointestinal tract are not exceeded.

The doses, techniques, and dose fractionations for TBI and HBI are reviewed in the preceding sections and in other chapters in this book (see the chapters on bone marrow and stem cell transplantation and radiation techniques).The contribution of radiation dose to the considerable risk of secondary hematologic malignancy (acute leukemia) from alkylating chemotherapy is not known, possibly because of the incurability of MM and the limited life span of the average patient with MM.

FUTURE DIRECTIONS

Advances in our ability to treat MM and other monoclonal gammopathies depend ultimately on understanding the etiology and pathogenesis of these diseases. In the past decade, interest has been renewed in the molecular and cellular biology of the myeloma clone, and provocative findings on the oncogenesis of MM have been reported. However, the cause of these diseases remains elusive, as does the identity of the myeloma precursor cell itself.

Advances in the clinical staging of MM, particularly with respect to prognostic factors such as clinical laboratory parameters, are allowing more rational decisions on appropriate therapy. This work continues in MM centers and in cooperative cancer groups worldwide. Although progress has been made in the therapeutic management of MM in the past 30 years, particularly with the introduction of chemotherapy and promising results from transplant studies, curative therapy for all plasmacytomas and for MM remains to be defined. We believe that radiotherapy combined with drugs continues to be an important modality in the treatment of MM. Much research remains to be done in finding the right schedules for transplantation, the best sources of hematopoietic stem cells, and optimal preparative regimens for transplantation.

Promising work is being reported on the use of radioimmunoconjugates, immunotoxins, and monoclonal antibodies directed against the myeloma cell. The combination of these modalities with high-dose intensive therapies is being explored in MM and in other hematologic malignancies. A signal advance in the palliative treatment of the debilitating bone manifestations of MM has been the use of bisphosphonate compounds such as pamidronate and zoledronic acid. Advances in our knowledge of osteoclast-osteoblast biology should allow other improvements in these therapies.

Until better therapies emerge based on an understanding of the basic biology of MM, clinical research in the next decade will continue to focus on more effective and less toxic drug and radiotherapy regimens. The need to find new therapeutic approaches to treat this disease remains one of the daunting challenges in oncology today.

REFERENCES

1. Modiano MR, Villar-Werstler P, Crowley J, et al: Evaluation of race as a prognostic factor in multiple myeloma: an ancillary of Southwest Oncology Group Study 8229. J Clin Oncol 14:974-977, 1996.
2. Jemal A, Tiwari RC, Murray T, et al: American Cancer Society: Cancer statistics, 2004. CA Cancer J Clin 54:8-29, 2004.
3. Bladé J, Kyle RA, Greipp PR: Multiple myeloma in patients younger than 30 years: report of 10 cases and review of the literature. Arch Intern Med 156:1463-1468, 1996.

4. Kyle RA, Therneau TM, Rajkumar SV, et al: Incidence of multiple myeloma in Olmsted County, Minnesota: trend over 6 decades. Cancer 101:2667-2674, 2004.
5. Preston DL, Kusumi S, Tomonaga M, et al: Cancer incidence in atomic bomb survivors. Part III. Leukemia, lymphoma and multiple myeloma, 1950-1987. Radiat Res 137(Suppl):S68-S97, 1994.
6. Koessel SL, Theis MK, Vaughan TL, et al: Socioeconomic status and the incidence of multiple myeloma. Epidemiology 7:4-8, 1996.
7. Lewis DR, Pottern LM, Brown LM, et al: Multiple myeloma among blacks and whites in the United States: the role of chronic antigenic stimulation. Cancer Causes Control 5:529-539, 1994.
8. Hansen ES: A follow-up study on the mortality of truck drivers. Am J Ind Med 23:811-821, 1993.
9. Heineman EF, Olsen JH, Pottern LM, et al: Occupational risk factors for multiple myeloma among Danish men. Cancer Causes Control 3:555-568, 1992.
10. Infante PF: State of the science on the carcinogenicity of gasoline with particular reference to cohort mortality study results. Environ Health Perspect 101(Suppl 6):105-109, 1993.
11. Semenciw RM, Morrison HI, Riedel D, et al: Multiple myeloma mortality and agricultural practices in the Prairie provinces of Canada. J Occup Med 35:557-561, 1993.
12. Demers PA, Vaughan TL, Koepsell TD, et al: A case-control study of multiple myeloma and occupation. Am J Ind Med 23:629-639, 1993.
13. Viel JF, Richardson ST: Lymphoma, multiple myeloma and leukaemia among French farmers in relation to pesticide exposure. Soc Sci Med 37:771-777, 1993.
14. Strom SS, Spitz MR, Cech IM, et al: Excess leukemia and multiple myeloma in a mining county in northeast Texas. Tex Med 90:55-59, 1994.
15. Demers PA, Boffetta P, Kogevinas M, et al: Pooled reanalysis of cancer mortality among five cohorts of workers in wood-related industries. Scand J Work Environ Health 21:179-190, 1995.
16. Fritschi L, Siemiatycki J: Lymphoma, myeloma and occupation: results of a case-control study. Int J Cancer 67:498-503, 1996.
17. Friedman GD: Cigarette smoking, leukemia, and multiple myeloma. Ann Epidemiol 3:425-428, 1993.
18. Brown LM, Everett GD, Gibson R, et al: Smoking and risk of non-Hodgkin's lymphoma and multiple myeloma. Cancer Causes Control 3:49-55, 1992.
19. Friedman GD, Herrinton LJ: Obesity and multiple myeloma. Cancer Causes Control 5:479-483, 1994.
20. Wong O: Is there a causal relationship between exposure to diesel exhaust and multiple myeloma? Toxicol Rev 22:91-102, 2003.
21. Lee WJ, Hoppin JA, Blair A, et al: Cancer incidence among pesticide applicators exposed to alachlor in the Agricultural Health Study. Am J Epidemiol 159:373-380, 2004.
22. Van Riet I, Bakkus M, De Greef C, et al: Homing mechanisms in the etiopathogenesis of multiple myeloma. Stem Cells 13(Suppl 2):22-27, 1995.
23. Matsui W, Huff CA, Wang Q, et al: Characterization of clonogenic multiple myeloma cells. Blood 103:2332-2336, 2004. Epub Nov 20, 2003.
24. Niesvizky R, Siegel D, Michaeli J: Biology and treatment of multiple myeloma. Blood Rev 7:24-33, 1993.
25. Bataille R, Chappard D, Klein B: The critical role of interleukin-6, interleukin-1B and macrophage colony-stimulating factor in the pathogenesis of bone lesions in multiple myeloma. Int J Clin Lab Res 21:283-287, 1992.
26. Murakami H, Nemoto K, Sawamura M, et al: Prognostic relevance of morphological classification in multiple myeloma. Acta Haematol 87:113-117, 1992.
27. Sukpanichnant S, Cousar JB, Leelasiri A, et al: Diagnostic criteria and histologic grading in multiple myeloma: histologic and immunohistologic analysis of 176 cases with clinical correlation. Hum Pathol 25:308-318, 1994.
28. Kurabayashi H, Kubota K, Shirakura T, et al: Prediction of prognosis by electron microscopic analysis of myeloma cells. Ann Hematol 73:169-173, 1996.
29. Van Riet I, Van Camp B: The involvement of adhesion molecules in the biology of multiple myeloma. Leuk Lymphoma 9:441-452, 1993.
30. Kim I, Uchiyama H, Chauhan D, et al: Cell surface expression and functional significance of adhesion molecules on human myeloma-derived cell lines. Br J Haematol 87:483-493, 1994.
31. Smith SR, Auerbach B, Morgan L: Serum neural cell adhesion molecule in multiple myeloma and other plasma cell disorders. Br J Haematol 92:67-70, 1996.
32. Tu Y, Xu FH, Liu J, et al: Upregulated expression of *BCL-2* in multiple myeloma cells induced by exposure to doxorubicin, etoposide, and hydrogen peroxide. Blood 88:1805-1812, 1996.
33. van de Donk NW, de Weerdt O, Veth G, et al: G3139, a Bcl-2 antisense oligodeoxynucleotide, induces clinical responses in VAD refractory myeloma. Leukemia 18:1078-1084, 2004.
34. Liu Q, Gazitt Y: Potentiation of dexamethasone-, paclitaxel-, and Ad-p53-induced apoptosis by Bcl-2 antisense oligodeoxynucleotides in drug-resistant multiple myeloma cells. Blood 101:4105-4114, 2003. Epub Jan 09, 2003.
35. Patriarca F, Melli C, Damiani D, et al: Plasma cell P170 expression and response to treatment in multiple myeloma. Haematologica 81:232-237, 1996.
36. Sonneveld P, Marie JP, Huisman C, et al: Reversal of multidrug resistance by SDZ PSC 833, combined with VAD (vincristine, doxorubicin, dexamethasone) in refractory multiple myeloma: a phase I study. Leukemia 10:1741-1750, 1996.
37. Billadeau D, Van Ness B, Kimlinger T, et al: Clonal circulating cells are common in plasma cell proliferative disorders: a comparison of monoclonal gammopathy of undetermined significance, smoldering multiple myeloma, and active myeloma. Blood 88:289-296, 1996.
38. Bird JM, Bloxham D, Samson D, et al: Molecular detection of clonally rearranged cells in peripheral blood progenitor cell harvests from multiple myeloma patients. Br J Haematol 88:110-116, 1994.
39. Corradini P, Voena C, Omede P, et al: Detection of circulating tumor cells in multiple myeloma by a PCR-based method. Leukemia 7:1879-1882, 1993.
40. Witzig TE, Gertz MA, Lust JA, et al: Peripheral blood monoclonal plasma cells as a predictor of survival in patients with multiple myeloma. Blood 88:1780-1787, 1996.
41. Sawamura M, Murakami H, Tamura J, et al: Tumour necrosis factor-alpha and interleukin 4 promote the differentiation of myeloma cell precursors in multiple myeloma. Br J Haematol 88:17-23, 1994.
42. Zhang XG, Bataille R, Widjenes J, et al: Interleukin-6 dependence of advanced malignant plasma cell dyscrasias. Cancer 69:1373-1376, 1992.
43. Hardin J, MacLeod S, Grigorieva I, et al: Interleukin-6 prevents dexamethasone-induced myeloma cell death. Blood 84:3063-3070, 1994.
44. Halimi H, Eisenstein M, Oh JW, et al: Epitope peptides from interleukin-6 receptor which inhibit the growth of human myeloma cells. Eur Cytokine Netw 6:135-143, 1995.
45. Hilbert DM, Kopf M, Mock BA, et al: Interleukin 6 is essential for in vivo development of B lineage neoplasms. J Exp Med 182:243-248, 1995.
46. Demartis A, Bernassola F, Savino R, et al: Interleukin 6 receptor superantagonists are potent inducers of human multiple myeloma cell death. Cancer Res 56:4213-4218, 1996.
47. Schwarze MM, Hawley RG: Prevention of myeloma cell apoptosis by ectopic *bcl-2* expression or interleukin 6-mediated up-regulation of *bcl-xL*. Cancer Res 55:2262-2265, 1995.
48. Massaia M, Borrione P, Attisano C, et al: Dysregulated *Fas* and *Bcl-2* expression leading to enhanced apoptosis in T cells of multiple myeloma patients. Blood 85:3679-3687, 1995.
49. Gauthier ER, Piche L, Lemieux G, et al: Role of *bcl-X(L)* in the control of apoptosis in murine myeloma cells. Cancer Res 56:1451-1456, 1996.
50. Skopelitou A, Hadjiyannakis M, Tsenga A, et al: Expression of C-*myc* p62 oncoprotein in multiple myeloma: an immunohistochemical study of 180 cases. Anticancer Res 13:1091-1095, 1993.
51. Epstein J, Hoover R, Kornbluth J, et al: Biological aspects of multiple myeloma. Baillieres Clin Haematol 8:721-734, 1995.
52. Paulin FE, West MJ, Sullivan NF, et al: Aberrant translational control of the c-*myc* gene in multiple myeloma. Oncogene 13:505-513, 1996.

53. Gernone A, Dammacco F: Molecular alterations of IL-6R, lck and *c-myc* genes in transforming monoclonal gammopathies of undetermined significance. Br J Haematol 93:623-631, 1996.
54. Yasuga Y, Hirosawa S, Yamamoto K, et al: N-*ras* and p53 gene mutations are very rare events in multiple myeloma. Int J Hematol 62:91-97, 1995.
55. Neri A, Baldini L, Trecca D, et al: p53 gene mutations in multiple myeloma are associated with advanced forms of malignancy. Blood 81:128-135, 1993.
56. Preudhomme C, Facon T, Zandecki M, et al: Rare occurrence of *p53* gene mutations in multiple myeloma. Br J Haematol 81:440-443, 1992.
57. Portier M, Moles JP, Mazars GR, et al: p53 and RAS gene mutations in multiple myeloma. Oncogene 7:2539-2543, 1992.
58. Zandecki M, Facon T, Preudhomme C, et al: The retinoblastoma gene (RB-1) status in multiple myeloma: a report on 35 cases. Leuk Lymphoma 18:497-503, 1995.
59. Urashima M, Ogata A, Chauhan D, et al: Interleukin-6 promotes multiple myeloma cell growth via phosphorylation of retinoblastoma protein. Blood 88:2219-2227, 1996.
60. Dao DD, Sawyer JR, Epstein J, et al: Deletion of the retinoblastoma gene in multiple myeloma. Leukemia 8:1280-1284, 1994.
61. Corradini P, Ladetto M, Voena C, et al: Mutational activation of N- and K-*ras* oncogenes in plasma cell dyscrasias. Blood 81:2708-2713, 1993.
62. Liu P, Leong T, Quam L, et al: Activating mutations of N- and K-*ras* in multiple myeloma show different clinical associations: analysis of the Eastern Cooperative Oncology Group Phase III Trial. Blood 88:2699-2706, 1996.
63. Owen RG, Johnson RJ, Rawstron AC, et al: Assessment of IgH PCR strategies in multiple myeloma. J Clin Pathol 49:672-675, 1996.
64. Chesi M, Bergsagel PL, Brents LA, et al: Dysregulation of cyclin D1 by translocation into an IgH gamma switch region in two multiple myeloma cell lines. Blood 88:674-681, 1996.
65. Sahota SS, Leo R, Hamblin TJ, et al: Ig VH gene mutational patterns indicate different tumor cell status in human myeloma and monoclonal gammopathy of undetermined significance. Blood 87:746-755, 1996.
66. Vescio RA, Cao J, Hong CH, et al: Myeloma Ig heavy chain V region sequences reveal prior antigenic selection and marked somatic mutation but no intraclonal diversity. J Immunol 155:2487-2497, 1995.
67. Berenson JR, Vescio RA, Hong CH, et al: Multiple myeloma clones are derived from a cell late in B lymphoid development. Curr Top Microbiol Immunol 194:25-33, 1995.
68. Bakkus MH, Van Riet I, Van Camp B, et al: Evidence that the clonogenic cell in multiple myeloma originates from a pre-switched but somatically mutated B cell. Br J Haematol 87:68-74, 1994.
69. Corradini P, Boccadoro M, Voena C, et al: Evidence for a bone marrow B cell transcribing malignant plasma cell VDJ joined to C mu sequence in immunoglobulin (IgG)- and IgA-secreting multiple myelomas. J Exp Med 178:1091-1096, 1993.
70. Palumbo A, Battaglio S, Astolfi M, et al: Multiple independent immunoglobulin class-switch recombinations occurring within the same clone in myeloma. Br J Haematol 82:676-680, 1992.
71. Kiyoi H, Naito K, Ohno R, et al: Comparable gene structure of the immunoglobulin heavy chain variable region between multiple myeloma and normal bone marrow lymphocytes. Leukemia 10:1804-1812, 1996.
72. Ralph QM, Brisco MJ, Joshua DE, et al: Advancement of multiple myeloma from diagnosis through plateau phase to progression does not involve a new B-cell clone: evidence from the Ig heavy chain gene. Blood 82:202-206, 1993.
73. Fonseca R, Harrington D, Oken MM, et al: Biological and prognostic significance of interphase fluorescence in situ hybridization detection of chromosome 13 abnormalities (delta13) in multiple myeloma: an Eastern Cooperative Oncology Group study. Cancer Res 62:715-720, 2002.
74. Fonseca R, Blood EA, Oken MM, et al: Myeloma and the t(11;14)(q13;q32): evidence for a biologically defined unique subset of patients. Blood 99:3735-3741, 2002.
75. Fonseca R, Debes-Marun CS, Picken EB, et al: The recurrent IgH translocations are highly associated with nonhyperdiploid variant multiple myeloma. Blood 102:2562-2567, 2003. Epub Jun 12, 2003.
76. Magrangeas F, Cormier ML, Descamps G, et al: Light-chain only multiple myeloma is due to the absence of functional (productive) rearrangement of the IgH gene at the DNA level. Blood 103:3869-3875, 2004. Epub Jan 8, 2004.
77. Hata H, Matsuzaki H, Yoshida M, et al: Red blood cell volume (MCV) as a new prognostic factor of multiple myeloma [letter]. Eur J Haematol 54:57-58, 1995.
78. Tertti R, Alanen A, Remes K: The value of magnetic resonance imaging in screening myeloma lesions of the lumbar spine. Br J Haematol 91:658-660, 1995.
79. Moulopoulos LA, Dimopoulos MA, Alexanian R, et al: Multiple myeloma: MR patterns of response to treatment. Radiology 193:441-446, 1994.
80. Durie BG, Waxman AD, D'Agnolo A, et al: Whole-body (18)F-FDG PET identifies high-risk myeloma. J Nucl Med 43:1457-1463, 2002.
81. Jadvar H, Conti PS: Diagnostic utility of FDG PET in multiple myeloma. Skeletal Radiol 31:690-694, 2002. Epub Sep 26, 2002.
82. Schirrmeister H, Buck AK, Bergmann L, et al: Positron emission tomography (PET) for staging of solitary plasmacytoma. Cancer Biother Radiopharm 18:841-845, 2003.
83. Mileshkin L, Blum R, Seymour JF, et al: A comparison of fluorine-18 fluoro-deoxyglucose PET and technetium-99m sestamibi in assessing patients with multiple myeloma. Eur J Haematol 72:32-37, 2004.
84. Pandey J, Kothari SY, Lata K, et al: A simple screening procedure for detection of infraclinical cases of multiple myeloma. Indian J Pathol Microbiol 36:453-457, 1993.
85. Ong F, Hermans J, Noordijk EM, et al: Presenting signs and symptoms in multiple myeloma: high percentages of stage III among patients without apparent myeloma-associated symptoms. Ann Hematol 70:149-152, 1995.
86. Ucci G, Riccardi A, Luoni R, et al: Cooperative Group for the Study and Treatment of Multiple Myeloma: Presenting features of monoclonal gammopathies: an analysis of 684 newly diagnosed cases. J Intern Med 234:165-173, 1993.
87. Kyle RA, Therneau TM, Rajkumar SV, et al: A long-term study of prognosis in monoclonal gammopathy of undetermined significance. N Engl J Med 346:564-569, 2002.
88. Dimopoulos MA, Moulopoulos A, Smith T, et al: Risk of disease progression in asymptomatic multiple myeloma. Am J Med 94:57-61, 1993.
89. Ganjoo RK, Malpas JS: Plasmacytoma. *In* Malpas JS, Bergsagel DE, Kyle RA (eds): Myeloma: Biology and Management. Oxford, Oxford University Press, 1995, pp 463-476.
90. Wiltshaw E: The natural history of extramedullary plasmacytoma and its relation to solitary myeloma of bone and myelomatosis. Medicine (Baltimore) 55:217-238, 1976.
91. Plowman PN: Radiotherapy of myeloma. *In* Malpas JS, Bergsagel DE, Kyle RA (eds): Myeloma: Biology and Management. Oxford, Oxford University Press, 1995, pp 314-321.
92. Corwin J, Lindberg RD: Solitary plasmacytoma of bone vs. extramedullary plasmacytoma and their relationship to multiple myeloma. Cancer 43:1007-1013, 1979.
93. Woodruff RK, Malpas JS, White FE: Solitary plasmacytoma. II: Solitary plasmacytoma of bone. Cancer 43:2344-2347, 1979.
94. Tong D, Griffin TW, Laramore GE, et al: Solitary plasmacytoma of bone and soft tissues. Radiology 135:195-198, 1980.
95. Mill WB, Griffith R: The role of radiation therapy in the management of plasma cell tumors. Cancer 45:647-652, 1980.
96. Mendenhall CM, Thar TL, Million RR: Solitary plasmacytoma of bone and soft tissue. Int J Radiat Oncol Biol Phys 6:1497-1501, 1980.
97. Bataille R, Sany J: Solitary myeloma: clinical and prognostic features of a review of 114 cases. Cancer 48:845-851, 1981.
98. Chak LY, Cox RS, Bostwick DG, et al: Solitary plasmacytoma of bone: treatment, progression, and survival. J Clin Oncol 5:1811-1815, 1987.

99. Frassica DA, Frassica FJ, Schray MF, et al: Solitary plasmacytoma of bone: Mayo Clinic experience. Int J Radiat Oncol Biol Phys 16:43-48, 1989.
100. Mayr NA, Wen BC, Hussey DH, et al: The role of radiation therapy in the treatment of solitary plasmacytomas. Radiother Oncol 17:293-303, 1990.
101. Brinch L, Hannisdal E, Abrahamsen AF, et al: Extramedullary plasmacytomas and solitary plasma cell tumours of bone. Eur J Haematol 44:132-135, 1990.
102. Holland J, Trenkner DA, Wasserman TH, et al: Plasmacytoma: treatment results and conversion to myeloma. Cancer 69:1513-1517, 1992.
103. Dimopoulos MA, Goldstein J, Fuller L, et al: Curability of solitary bone plasmacytoma. J Clin Oncol 10:587-590, 1992.
104. Bolek TW, Marcus RB, Mendenhall NP: Solitary plasmacytoma of bone and soft tissue. Int J Radiat Oncol Biol Phys 36:329-333, 1996.
105. Liebross RH, Ha CS, Cox JD, et al: Solitary bone plasmacytoma: outcome and prognostic factors following radiotherapy. Int J Radiat Oncol Biol Phys 41:1063-1067, 1998.
106. Wilder RB, Ha CS, Cox JD, et al: Persistence of myeloma protein for more than one year after radiotherapy is an adverse prognostic factor in solitary plasmacytoma of bone. Cancer 94:1532-1537, 2002.
107. Kato T, Tsukamoto E, Nishioka T, et al: Early detection of bone marrow involvement in extramedullary plasmacytoma by whole-body F-18 FDG positron emission tomography. Clin Nucl Med 25:870-873, 2000.
108. Durie BG, Kyle RA, Belch A, et al: Scientific Advisors of the International Myeloma Foundation: Myeloma management guidelines: a consensus report from the Scientific Advisors of the International Myeloma Foundation. Hematol J 4:379-398, 2003. Erratum in: Hematol J 5:285, 2004.
109. Kotner LM, Wang CC: Plasmacytoma of the upper air and food passages. Cancer 30:414-418, 1972.
110. Pahor AL: Extramedullary plasmacytoma of the head and neck, parotid and submandibular salivary glands. J Laryngol Otol 91:241-258, 1977.
111. Woodruff RK, Whittle JM, Malpas JS: Solitary plasmacytoma. I: Extramedullary soft tissue plasmacytoma. Cancer 43:2340-2343, 1979.
112. Harwood AR, Knowling MA, Bergsagel DE: Radiotherapy of extramedullary plasmacytoma of the head and neck. Clin Radiol 32:31-36, 1981.
113. Bush SE, Goffinet DR, Bagshaw MA: Extramedullary plasmacytoma of the head and neck. Radiology 140:801-805, 1981.
114. Kapadia SB, Desai U, Cheng VS: Extramedullary plasmacytoma of the head and neck: a clinicopathologic study of 20 cases. Medicine (Baltimore) 61:317-329, 1982.
115. Knowling MA, Harwood AR, Bergsagel DE: Comparison of extramedullary plasmacytomas with solitary and multiple plasma cell tumors of bone. J Clin Oncol 1:255-262, 1983.
116. Batsakis JG: Pathology consultation: plasma cell tumors of the head and neck. Ann Otol Rhinol Laryngol 92:311-313, 1983.
117. Gaffney CC, Dawes PJ, Jackson D: Plasmacytoma of the head and neck. Clin Radiol 38:385-388, 1987.
118. Kerr PD, Dort JC: Primary extramedullary plasmacytoma of the salivary glands. J Laryngol Otol 105:687-692, 1991.
119. Soesan M, Paccagnella A, Chiarion-Sileni V, et al: Extramedullary plasmacytoma: clinical behaviour and response to treatment. Ann Oncol 3:51-57, 1992.
120. Wax MK, Yun KJ, Omar RA: Extramedullary plasmacytomas of the head and neck. Otolaryngol Head Neck Surg 109:877-885, 1993.
121. Tesei F, Caliceti U, Sorrenti G, et al: Extramedullary plasmacytoma (EMP) of the head and neck: a series of 22 cases [Italian]. Acta Otorhinolaryngol Ital 15:437-442, 1995.
122. Papadimitriou CS, Schwarze EW: Extramedullary nongastrointestinal plasmacytoma: an immunohistochemical study of sixteen cases. Pathol Res Pract 176:306-312, 1983.
123. Bardwick PA, Zvaifler NJ, Gill GN, et al: Plasma cell dyscrasia with polyneuropathy, organomegaly, endocrinopathy, M protein, and skin changes: the POEMS syndrome. Report on two cases and a review of the literature. Medicine (Baltimore) 59:311-322, 1980.
124. Delauche MC, Clauvel JP, Seligmann M: Peripheral neuropathy and plasma cell neoplasias: a report of 10 cases. Br J Haematol 48:383-392, 1981.
125. Takatsuki K, Sanada I: Plasma cell dyscrasia with polyneuropathy and endocrine disorder: clinical and laboratory features of 109 reported cases. Jpn J Clin Oncol 13:543-555, 1983.
126. Kelly JJ Jr, Kyle RA, Miles JM, et al: Osteosclerotic myeloma and peripheral neuropathy. Neurology 33:202-210, 1983.
127. Nakanishi T, Sobue I, Toyokura Y, et al: The Crow-Fukase syndrome: a study of 102 cases in Japan. Neurology 34:712-720, 1984.
128. Waldenström JG: POEMS: a multifactorial syndrome [editorial]. Haematologica 77:197-203, 1992.
129. Miralles GD, O'Fallon JR, Talley NJ: Plasma-cell dyscrasia with polyneuropathy: the spectrum of POEMS syndrome. N Engl J Med 327:1919-1923, 1992.
130. Soubrier MJ, Dubost JJ, Sauvezie BJ: French Study Group on POEMS Syndrome: POEMS syndrome: a study of 25 cases and a review of the literature. Am J Med 97:543-553, 1994.
131. Dispenzieri A, Gertz MA: Treatment of POEMS syndrome. Curr Treat Options Oncol 5:249-257, 2004.
132. Kropff M, Leo E, Steinfurth G, et al: DNA-image cytometry and clinical staging systems in multiple myeloma. Anticancer Res 14:2183-2188, 1994.
133. Ong F, Hermans J, Noordijk EM, et al: Is the Durie and Salmon diagnostic classification system for plasma cell dyscrasias still the best choice? Application of three classification systems to a large population-based registry of paraproteinemia and multiple myeloma. Ann Hematol 70:19-24, 1995.
134. Bauduer F, Troussard X, Delmer A: Prognostic factors in multiple myeloma. Review of the literature [French]. Bull Cancer (Paris) 80:1035-1042, 1993.
135. Bataille R, Boccadoro M, Klein B, et al: C-reactive protein and beta-2 microglobulin produce a simple and powerful myeloma staging system. Blood 80:733-737, 1992.
136. San Miguel JF, Garcia-Sanz R, Gonzalez M, et al: A new staging system for multiple myeloma based on the number of S-phase plasma cells. Blood 85:448-455, 1995.
137. Greipp PR, Lust JA, O'Fallon WM, et al: Plasma cell labeling index and beta 2-microglobulin predict survival independent of thymidine kinase and C-reactive protein in multiple myeloma. Blood 81:3382-3387, 1993.
138. Pasqualetti P, Collacciani A, Maccarone C, et al: Prognostic factors in multiple myeloma: selection using Cox's proportional hazard model. Biomed Pharmacother 50:29-35, 1996.
139. Durie BG, Jacobson J, Barlogie B, et al: Magnitude of response with myeloma frontline therapy does not predict outcome: importance of time to progression in Southwest Oncology Group chemotherapy trials. J Clin Oncol 22:1857-1863, 2004. Epub Apr 26, 2004.
140. Rajkumar SV, Fonseca R, Dispenzieri A, et al: Effect of complete response on outcome following autologous stem cell transplantation for myeloma. Bone Marrow Transplant 26:979-983, 2000.
141. Kyle RA: Monoclonal gammopathy of undetermined significance and solitary plasmacytoma: implications for progression to overt multiple myeloma. Hematol Oncol Clin North Am 11:71-87, 1997.
142. Katzmann JA, Clark RJ, Abraham RS, et al: Serum reference intervals and diagnostic ranges for free kappa and free lambda immunoglobulin light chains: relative sensitivity for detection of monoclonal light chains. Clin Chem 48:1437-1444, 2002.
143. Mead GP, Carr-Smith HD, Drayson MT, et al: Serum free light chains for monitoring multiple myeloma. Br J Haematol 126:348-354, 2004.
144. Bergsagel DE, Sprague CC, Austin C, et al: Evaluation of new chemotherapeutic agents in the treatment of multiple myeloma. IV. L-phenylalanine mustard (NSC-8806). Cancer Chemother Rep 21:87-99, 1962.
145. Korst DR, Clifford GO, Fowler WM, et al: Multiple myeloma. II. Analysis of cyclophosphamide therapy in 165 patients. JAMA 189:758-762, 1964.

146. Alexanian R, Haut A, Khan AU, et al: Treatment for multiple myeloma. Combination chemotherapy with different melphalan dose regimens. JAMA 208:1680-1685, 1969.
147. Alexanian R, Bonnet J, Gehan E, et al: Combination chemotherapy for multiple myeloma. Cancer 30:382-389, 1972.
148. Case DC Jr, Lee DJ III, Clarkson BD: Improved survival times in multiple myeloma treated with melphalan, prednisone, cyclophosphamide, vincristine and BCNU: M-2 protocol. Am J Med 63:897-903, 1977.
149. Gregory WM, Richards MA, Malpas JS: Combination chemotherapy versus melphalan and prednisolone in the treatment of multiple myeloma: an overview of published trials. J Clin Oncol 10:334-342, 1992.
150. Oken MM, Harrington DP, Abramson N, et al: Comparison of melphalan and prednisone with vincristine, carmustine, melphalan, cyclophosphamide, and prednisone in the treatment of multiple myeloma: results of Eastern Cooperative Oncology Group Study E2479. Cancer 79:1561-1567, 1997.
151. Salmon SE, Crowley JJ, Grogan TM, et al: Combination chemotherapy, glucocorticoids, and interferon alfa in the treatment of multiple myeloma: a Southwest Oncology Group study. J Clin Oncol 12:2405-2414, 1994.
152. Palumbo A, Bertola A, Musto P, et al: Oral melphalan, prednisone and thalidomide for newly diagnosed myeloma patients [abstract]. J Clin Oncol 22(Suppl):569s, 2004.
153. Gertz MA, Kalish LA, Kyle RA, et al: an Eastern Cooperative Oncology Group study: Phase III study comparing vincristine, doxorubicin (Adriamycin), and dexamethasone (VAD) chemotherapy with VAD plus recombinant interferon alfa-2 in refractory or relapsed multiple myeloma. Am J Clin Oncol 18:475-480, 1995.
154. Gertz MA, Garton JP, Greipp PR, et al: A phase II study of high-dose methylprednisolone in refractory or relapsed multiple myeloma. Leukemia 9:2115-2118, 1995.
155. Facon T, Mary JY, Attal M, et al: Melphalan-prednisone versus dexamethasone-based regimens for newly diagnosed myeloma patients aged 65-75 years. Final analysis of the IFM 95-01 trial on 489 patients [abstract]. Blood 102 (11 Pt 2):147a, 2003.
156. Kumar SK, Therneau TM, Gertz MA, et al: Clinical course of patients with relapsed multiple myeloma. Mayo Clin Proc 79:867-874, 2004.
157. Attal M, Harousseau JL, Stoppa AM, et al: Intergroupe Francophone du Myelome: A prospective, randomized trial of autologous bone marrow transplantation and chemotherapy in multiple myeloma. N Engl J Med 335:91-97, 1996.
158. Bladé J, San Miguel JF, Fontanillas M, et al: Survival of multiple myeloma patients who are potential candidates for early high-dose therapy intensification/autotransplantation and who were conventionally treated. J Clin Oncol 14:2167-2173, 1996.
159. Gertz MA, Pineda AA, Chen MG, et al: Refractory and relapsing multiple myeloma treated by blood stem cell transplantation. Am J Med Sci 309:152-161, 1995.
160. Child JA, Morgan GJ, Davies FE, et al: Medical Research Council Adult Leukaemia Working Party: High-dose chemotherapy with hematopoietic stem-cell rescue for multiple myeloma. N Engl J Med 348:1875-1883, 2003.
161. Barlogie B, Smith L, Alexanian R: Effective treatment of advanced multiple myeloma refractory to alkylating agents. N Engl J Med 310:1353-1356, 1984.
162. Gertz MA, Lacy MQ, Inwards DJ, et al: Factors influencing platelet recovery after blood cell transplantation in multiple myeloma. Bone Marrow Transplant 20:375-380, 1997.
163. Rajkumar SV, Hayman S, Gertz MA, et al: Combination therapy with thalidomide plus dexamethasone for newly diagnosed myeloma. J Clin Oncol 20:4319-4323, 2002.
164. Zervas K, Dimopoulos MA, Hatzicharissi E, et al: Greek Myeloma Study Group: Primary treatment of multiple myeloma with thalidomide, vincristine, liposomal doxorubicin and dexamethasone (T-VAD doxil): a phase II multicenter study. Ann Oncol 15:134-138, 2004.
165. Hussein M: Pegylated liposomal doxorubicin, vincristine, and reduced-dose dexamethasone as first-line therapy for multiple myeloma. Clin Lymphoma 4(Suppl 1):S18-S22, 2003.
166. Raje N, Powles R, Kulkarni S, et al: A comparison of vincristine and doxorubicin infusional chemotherapy with methylprednisolone (VAMP) with the addition of weekly cyclophosphamide (C-VAMP) as induction treatment followed by autografting in previously untreated myeloma. Br J Haematol 97:153-160, 1997.
167. Lee CK, Barlogie B, Munshi N, et al: DTPACE: an effective, novel combination chemotherapy with thalidomide for previously treated patients with myeloma. J Clin Oncol 21:2732-2739, 2003.
168. Rosen LS, Gordon D, Kaminski M, et al: Long-term efficacy and safety of zoledronic acid compared with pamidronate disodium in the treatment of skeletal complications in patients with advanced multiple myeloma or breast carcinoma: a randomized, double-blind, multicenter, comparative trial. Cancer 98:1735-1744, 2003.
169. Berenson JR: Advances in the biology and treatment of myeloma bone disease. Semin Oncol 29 Suppl 17:11-16, 2002.
170. Berenson JR, Lichtenstein A, Porter L, et al: Myeloma Aredia Study Group: Efficacy of pamidronate in reducing skeletal events in patients with advanced multiple myeloma. N Engl J Med 334:488-493, 1996.
171. Thurlimann B, Morant R, Jungi WF, et al: Pamidronate for pain control in patients with malignant osteolytic bone disease: a prospective dose-effect study. Support Care Cancer 2:61-65, 1994.
172. Garton JP, Gertz MA, Witzig TE, et al: Epoetin alfa for the treatment of the anemia of multiple myeloma: a prospective, randomized, placebo-controlled, double-blind trial. Arch Intern Med 155:2069-2074, 1995.
173. Hedenus M, Adriansson M, San Miguel J, et al: Darbepoetin Alfa 20000161 Study Group: Efficacy and safety of darbepoetin alfa in anaemic patients with lymphoproliferative malignancies: a randomized, double-blind, placebo-controlled study. Br J Haematol 122:394-403, 2003.
174. Coleman M, Leonard J, Lyons L, et al: BLT-D (clarithromycin [Biaxin], low-dose thalidomide, and dexamethasone) for the treatment of myeloma and Waldenström's macroglobulinemia. Leuk Lymphoma 43:1777-1782, 2002.
175. Bartlett JB, Dredge K, Dalgleish AG: The evolution of thalidomide and its IMiD derivatives as anticancer agents. Nat Rev Cancer 4:314-322, 2004.
176. Singhal S, Mehta J, Desikan R, et al: Antitumor activity of thalidomide in refractory multiple myeloma. N Engl J Med 341:1565-1571, 1999. Erratum in: N Engl J Med 342:364, 2000.
177. Dredge K, Dalgleish AG, Marriott JB: Thalidomide analogs as emerging anti-cancer drugs. Anticancer Drugs 14:331-335, 2003.
178. Berenson JR, Ma HM, Vescio R: The role of nuclear factor-κB in the biology and treatment of multiple myeloma. Semin Oncol 28:626-633, 2001.
179. Richardson PG, Hideshima T, Mitsiades C, et al: Proteasome inhibition in hematologic malignancies. Ann Med 36:304-314, 2004.
180. Richardson P, Sonneveld P, Schuster M, et al: Bortezomib demonstrates superior efficacy to high-dose dexamethasone in relapsed multiple myeloma: final report of the APEX study [abstract]. Blood 104:100a, 2004.
181. Orlowski RZ: Bortezomib and its role in the management of patients with multiple myeloma. Expert Rev Anticancer Ther 4:171-179, 2004.
182. Kane RC, Bross PF, Farrell AT, et al: U.S. FDA approval for the treatment of multiple myeloma progressing on prior therapy. Oncologist 8:508-513, 2003.
183. Mill WB: Radiation therapy in multiple myeloma. Radiology 115:175-178, 1975.
184. Bosch A, Frias Z: Radiotherapy in the treatment of multiple myeloma. Int J Radiat Oncol Biol Phys 15:1363-1369, 1988.
185. Adamietz IA, Schober C, Schulte RW, et al: Palliative radiotherapy in plasma cell myeloma. Radiother Oncol 20:111-116, 1991.
186. Leigh BR, Kurtts TA, Mack CF, et al: Radiation therapy for the palliation of multiple myeloma. Int J Radiat Oncol Biol Phys 25:801-804, 1993.
187. Medinger FG, Craver LF: Total body irradiation, with review of cases. Am J Roentgenol 48:651-657, 1942.
188. Fitzpatrick PJ, Rider WD: Half body radiotherapy. Int J Radiat Oncol Biol Phys 1:197-207, 1976.
189. Holder DL: Total-body irradiation in multiple myeloma. Radiology 84:83-86, 1965.

190. Bergsagel DE: Total body irradiation for myelomatosis. Br Med J 2:325, 1971.
191. Glück S, Van Dyk J, Messner HA: Radiosensitivity of human clonogenic myeloma cells and normal bone marrow precursors: effect of different dose rates and fractionation. Int J Radiat Oncol Biol Phys 28:877-882, 1994.
192. Jaffe JP, Bosch A, Raich PC: Sequential hemi-body radiotherapy in advanced multiple myeloma. Cancer 43:124-128, 1979.
193. Rowland CG: Single fraction half body radiation therapy. Clin Radiol 30:1-3, 1979.
194. Coleman M, Saletan S, Wolf D, et al: Whole bone marrow irradiation for the treatment of multiple myeloma. Cancer 49:1328-1333, 1982.
195. Rowland CG, Garrett MJ, Crowley FA: Half body radiation in plasma cell myeloma. Clin Radiol 34:507-510, 1983.
196. Rostom AY, O'Cathail SM, Folkes A: Systemic irradiation in multiple myeloma: a report on nineteen cases. Br J Haematol 58:423-431, 1984.
197. Thomas PJ, Daban A, Bontoux D: Double hemibody irradiation in chemotherapy-resistant multiple myeloma. Cancer Treat Rep 68:1173-1175, 1984.
198. Tobias JS, Richards JD, Blackman GM, et al: Hemibody irradiation in multiple myeloma. Radiother Oncol 3:11-16, 1985.
199. Troussard X, Roussel A, Reman O, et al: Hemibody irradiation in stage III multiple myeloma: results of 20 patients. Nouv Rev Fr Hematol 30:213-218, 1988.
200. Jacobs P, le Roux I, King HS: Sequential half-body irradiation as salvage therapy in chemotherapy-resistant multiple myeloma. Am J Clin Oncol 11:104-109, 1988.
201. Singer CR, Tobias JS, Giles F, et al: Hemibody irradiation: an effective second-line therapy in drug-resistant multiple myeloma. Cancer 63:2446-2451, 1989.
202. Giles FJ, McSweeney EN, Richards JD, et al: Prospective randomised study of double hemi-body irradiation with and without subsequent maintenance recombinant alpha 2b interferon on survival in patients with relapsed multiple myeloma. Eur J Cancer 28A:1392-1395, 1992.
203. Jacobs P, Johnson C, le Roux I: Half-body irradiation in multiple myeloma [letter]. S Afr Med J 85:1308, 1995.
204. MacKenzie MR, Wold H, George C, et al: Consolidation hemibody radiotherapy following induction combination chemotherapy in high-tumor-burden multiple myeloma. J Clin Oncol 10:1769-1774, 1992.
205. Salmon SE, Tesh D, Crowley J, et al: Chemotherapy is superior to sequential hemibody irradiation for remission consolidation in multiple myeloma: a Southwest Oncology Group study. J Clin Oncol 8:1575-1584, 1990.
206. McElwain TJ, Powles RL: High-dose intravenous melphalan for plasma-cell leukaemia and myeloma. Lancet 2:822-824, 1983.
207. Mohrbacher A, Anderson KC: Bone marrow transplantation in multiple myeloma. *In* Malpas JS, Bergsagel DE, Kyle RA (eds): Myeloma: Biology and Management. Oxford, Oxford University Press, 1995, pp 322-352.
208. Vesole DH, Jagannath S, Tricot G, et al: Autologous bone marrow and peripheral blood stem cell transplantation in multiple myeloma. Cancer Invest 14:378-391, 1996.
209. Osserman EF, DiRe LB, DiRe J, et al: Identical twin marrow transplantation in multiple myeloma. Acta Haematol 68:215-223, 1982.
210. Wolff SN, McCurley TL, Giannone L: High-dose chemoradiotherapy with syngeneic bone marrow transplantation for multiple myeloma: a case report and literature review. Am J Hematol 26:191-198, 1987.
211. Buckner CD, Fefer A, Bensinger WI, et al: Marrow transplantation for malignant plasma cell disorders: summary of the Seattle experience. Eur J Haematol Suppl 51:186-190, 1989.
212. Bensinger WI, Demirer T, Buckner CD, et al: Syngeneic marrow transplantation in patients with multiple myeloma. Bone Marrow Transplant 18:527-531, 1996.
213. Bensinger WI, Buckner CD, Gahrton G: Allogeneic stem cell transplantation for multiple myeloma. Hematol Oncol Clin North Am 11:147-157, 1997.
214. Bensinger WI, Buckner CD, Anasetti C, et al: Allogeneic marrow transplantation for multiple myeloma: an analysis of risk factors on outcome. Blood 88:2787-2793, 1996.
215. Bensinger WI, Buckner CD, Clift RA, et al: Phase I study of busulfan and cyclophosphamide in preparation for allogeneic marrow transplant for patients with multiple myeloma. J Clin Oncol 10:1492-1497, 1992.
216. Gahrton G, Tura S, Ljungman P, et al: European Group for Bone Marrow Transplantation: Allogeneic bone marrow transplantation in multiple myeloma. N Engl J Med 325:1267-1273, 1991.
217. Gahrton G, Tura S, Ljungman P, et al: Prognostic factors in allogeneic bone marrow transplantation for multiple myeloma. J Clin Oncol 13:1312-1322, 1995.
218. Tricot G, Vesole DH, Jagannath S, et al: Graft-versus-myeloma effect: proof of principle. Blood 87:1196-1198, 1996.
219. Verdonck LF, Lokhorst HM, Dekker AW, et al: Graft-versus-myeloma effect in two cases. Lancet 347:800-801, 1996.
220. Aschan J, Lonnqvist B, Ringden O, et al: Graft-versus-myeloma effect (letter). Lancet 348:346, 1996.
221. Maloney DG, Molina AJ, Sahebi F, et al: Allografting with non-myeloablative conditioning following cytoreductive autografts for the treatment of patients with multiple myeloma. Blood 102:3447-3454, 2003. Epub Jul 10, 2003.
222. Barlogie B, Kyle R, Anderson K, et al: Comparable survival in multiple myeloma (MM) with high dose therapy (HDT) employing MEL 140 mg/m^2 + TBI 12 Gy autotransplants versus standard dose therapy with VBMCP and no benefit from interferon (IFN) maintenance: results of intergroup trial S9321 [abstract]. Blood 102:42a, 2003.
223. Stewart AK, Vescio R, Schiller G, et al: Purging of autologous peripheral-blood stem cells using CD34 selection does not improve overall or progression-free survival after high-dose chemotherapy for multiple myeloma: results of a multicenter randomized controlled trial. J Clin Oncol 19:3771-3779, 2001.
224. Vescio R, Schiller G, Stewart AK, et al: Multicenter phase III trial to evaluate CD34(+) selected versus unselected autologous peripheral blood progenitor cell transplantation in multiple myeloma. Blood 93:1858-1868, 1999.
225. Attal M, Harousseau JL, Facon T, et al: Intergroupe Francophone du Myelome: Single versus double autologous stem-cell transplantation for multiple myeloma. N Engl J Med 349:2495-2502, 2003. (Erratum in: N Engl J Med 350:2628, 2004.)
226. Morris C, Iacobelli S, Brand R, et al: Chronic Leukaemia Working Party Myeloma Subcommittee, European Group for Blood and Marrow Transplantation: Benefit and timing of second transplantations in multiple myeloma: clinical findings and methodological limitations in a European Group for Blood and Marrow Transplantation registry study. J Clin Oncol 22:1674-1681, 2004. Epub Mar 22, 2004.
227. Palumbo A, Bringhen S, Petrucci MT, et al: Intermediate-dose melphalan improves survival of myeloma patients aged 50 to 70: results of a randomized controlled trial. Blood 104:3052-3057, 2004. Epub Jul 20, 2004.
228. Mill WB, Wasserman TH: Multiple myeloma and plasmacytomas. *In* Perez CA, Brady LW (eds): Principles and Practice of Radiation Oncology. Philadelphia, JB Lippincott Company, 1987, pp 1086-1100.
229. Dimopoulos MA, Moulopoulos A, Delasalle K, et al: Solitary plasmacytoma of bone and asymptomatic multiple myeloma. Hematol Oncol Clin North Am 6:359-369, 1992.
230. Philips ED, el-Mahdi AM, Humphrey RL, et al: The effect of the radiation treatment on the polyneuropathy of multiple myeloma. J Can Assoc Radiol 23:103-106, 1972.
231. Garland LH, Kennedy BR: Roentgen treatment of multiple myeloma. Radiology 50:297, 1948.
232. Garrett MJ: Spinal myeloma and cord compression: diagnosis and management. Clin Radiol 21:42-46, 1970.
233. Benson WJ, Scarffe JH, Todd ID, et al: Spinal-cord compression in myeloma. Br Med J 1:1541-1544, 1979.
234. Jacobs P, King HS, Le Roux I, et al: Extradural spinal myeloma and emergency neurosurgery [letter]. S Afr Med J 77:316-318, 1990.
235. Wallington M, Mendis S, Premawardhana U, et al: Local control and survival in spinal cord compression from lymphoma and myeloma. Radiother Oncol 42:43-47, 1997.
236. Salmon SE, Cassady JR: Plasma cell neoplasms. *In* DeVita VT Jr, Hellman S, Rosenberg SA (eds): Cancer: Principles & Practice of

Oncology, 4th ed. Philadelphia, JB Lippincott Company, 1993, pp 1853-1895.
237. Leigh BR, Shimm DS: Response to Drs. Adamietz and Böttcher [letter]. Int J Radiat Oncol Biol Phys 29:221, 1994.
238. Farhangi M, Osserman EF: The treatment of multiple myeloma. Semin Hematol 10:149-161, 1973.
239. Moreau P, Facon T, Attal M, et al: Intergroupe Francophone du Myelome: Comparison of 200 mg/m^2 melphalan and 8 Gy total body irradiation plus 140 mg/m^2 melphalan as conditioning regimens for peripheral blood stem cell transplantation in patients with newly diagnosed multiple myeloma: final analysis of the Intergroupe Francophone du Myelome 9502 randomized trial. Blood 99:731-735, 2002.
240. Anderson KC, Barut BA, Ritz J, et al: Monoclonal antibody-purged autologous bone marrow transplantation therapy for multiple myeloma. Blood 77:712-720, 1991.
241. Anderson KC, Andersen J, Soiffer R, et al: Monoclonal antibody-purged bone marrow transplantation therapy for multiple myeloma. Blood 82:2568-2576, 1993.
242. Tsang RW, Gospodarowicz MK, Pintilie M, et al: Solitary plasmacytoma treated with radiotherapy: impact of tumor size on outcome. Int J Radiat Oncol Biol Phys 50:113-120, 2001.

CHAPTER 76

MYCOSIS FUNGOIDES

Benjamin D. Smith, Glenn Jones, and Lynn D. Wilson

INCIDENCE

- Five cases per million, 1400 cases per year in the United States

BIOLOGIC CHARACTERISTICS

- Indolent malignancy of skin-homing $CD4^+$ T-cells
- Classic immunophenotype: $CD2^+$, $CD3^+$, $CD4^+$, $CD5^+$, $CD45RO^+$, CLA^+ (cutaneous lymphoid antigen), $CD8^-$, $CD30^-$
- Early stage is limited to skin and associated with epidermotropism. In advanced stages, epidermotropism is lost and malignant cells invade nodes, blood, and viscera.

STAGING EVALUATION

- TNM staging is based on percentage of cutaneous involvement and nature of lesions
- History and physical examination
- Skin biopsy with immunophenotyping and PCR for T-cell receptor gene rearrangement
- Complete blood count with manual differential and chemistries

  In those with suspected stage IIB–IV disease, check LDH, soluble interleukin-2 receptor, peripheral blood flow cytometry, and peripheral blood T-cell receptor gene rearrangement
- Chest radiograph for all patients

  Computed tomography for stage IIA–IV

PRIMARY THERAPY AND RESULTS

- Skin-directed therapies include radiation, psoralen and ultraviolet A (PUVA), narrow band ultraviolet B, mechlorethamine, carmustine, steroids, and topical bexarotene.
- Total skin electron beam therapy (TSEBT) monotherapy produces 10-year, relapse-free survival of approximately 50% for Stage IA disease. TSEBT monotherapy is rarely curative for patients with more advanced disease.
- TSEBT provides rapid and effective palliation, with complete response rates of 95% for T1, 90% for T2, 60% for T3, and 75% for T4.
- Systemic therapies include interferon-α, retinoids, bexarotene, extracorporeal photochemotherapy, denileukin diftitox, nucleoside analogues, and cytotoxic chemotherapy.

ADJUVANT THERAPY

- For T1 and T2 disease, retrospective experiences suggest that TSEBT followed by adjuvant PUVA or mechlorethamine may improve disease-free survival.
- For T3 or T4 disease, retrospective experiences suggest that TSEBT followed by adjuvant extracorporeal photopheresis may cause specific survival.

LOCALLY ADVANCED DISEASE

- TSEBT is effective for most cutaneous lesions.
- Traditional multiagent systemic chemotherapy does not enhance survival but may produce palliation.
- Allogeneic bone marrow transplant with a preparative regimen that includes total body irradiation is a promising new approach for young patients with a good performance status.

PALLIATION

- Most patients require therapy to relieve cutaneous symptoms.
- All of the skin-directed therapies produce substantial palliation.
- Novel biologic agents such as bexarotene and denileukin diftitox have efficacy in disease refractory to standard treatments.
- Photon radiation is effective for palliation of visceral and nodal disease.

Mycosis fungoides (MF) is a low-grade, non-Hodgkin's lymphoma caused by skin-homing $CD4^+$ T-cells that form cutaneous patches, plaques, and tumors.[1,2] MF was initially described in 1806 when Alibert described a patient with cutaneous tumors that he attributed to yaws. Although initially called pian fungoides, he later changed the name to mycosis fungoides.[3] In 1938, Sézary and Bouvrain described a leukemic variant called the Sézary syndrome (SS),[4] and Lutzner and Jordan[5] elucidated the ultrastructure of the Sézary cell in 1968. The term *cutaneous T-cell lymphoma* (CTCL) was introduced by Edelson in 1975 and encompasses a variety of cutaneous lymphoproliferative disorders, including MF/SS, adult T-cell leukemia/lymphoma, primary cutaneous $CD30^+$ anaplastic lymphoma, lymphomatoid papulosis, pagetoid reticulosis, and others.[6] In clinical practice, the terms MF and CTCL are often used interchangeably; however, such usage is incorrect.[7] MF constitutes only 50% of all CTCLs and the clinical history and therapy for each subtype of CTCL are different.[2]

Mycosis fungoides is a challenging disorder from all perspectives. Despite improving molecular techniques, diagnosis early in the course of disease is often difficult due to the nonspecific nature of skin lesions and the numerous benign dermatoses that may mimic MF. Once a diagnosis has been correctly established, the optimal initial treatment strategy often remains unclear, given heterogeneity of clinical presentations and limited data from controlled studies. Although radiotherapy is the most effective single agent in the treatment of MF,[8] total skin electron beam therapy (TSEBT) is not readily available at many centers. In this chapter, we provide a summary of the clinically relevant aspects of MF and describe the role and techniques of radiotherapy in patient management.

EPIDEMIOLOGY AND ETIOLOGY

MF primarily affects adults older than age 40, with incidence rates peaking in the eighth decade. The incidence of MF doubled from the early 1970s through the early 1980s[9] but then stabilized at 5 per million, resulting in approximately 1400 cases per year in the United States (Fig. 76-1).[10-13] In contrast, the incidence of non-MF CTCLs increased rapidly between 1991 and 1994 and then plateaued at a rate of 3 per million (see Fig. 76-1). The relative survival for all patients with MF/SS reported by the Surveillance, Epidemiology, and End Results (SEER) program is 75% at 10 years and 64% at 20 years (Fig. 76-2).[10,11] The 5-year relative survival of MF has improved over time, rising from 72% for those diagnosed between 1973 and 1977 to 86% for those diagnosed between 1993 and 1996 (Fig. 76-3).[14,15]

With the exception of black race (2.0:1) and male gender (2.2:1), risk factors for the development of MF remain highly speculative.[9] Although numerous etiologic agents, including exposure to pesticides, industrial occupation, exposure to radiation, tobacco use, and alcohol consumption, have been investigated, no consistent causative factors have been identified.[16] High rates of seropositivity for both cytomegalovirus[17] and human T-cell lymphotrophic virus type I[18,19] have been reported, but these studies await further corroboration before a causal relationship can be inferred.[20-22]

The precise etiology of MF remains unclear. The observation that MF is more common in blacks and tends to present in sun-shielded areas (i.e., "bathing trunk" distribution) suggests that actinic exposure may be protective. Sun exposure may mediate its protective effect by exerting a cytotoxic effect on the epidermal antigen-presenting dendritic cell, also known as the Langerhans cell. This cell presents antigens to the malignant CD4+ T cells of MF and may stimulate their growth. The histologic evidence for this interaction is Pautrier's microabscess, an intraepidermal collection of malignant CD4+ T cells clustered around an antigen-presenting dendritic cell. This finding is considered pathognomonic for MF. Therefore, some investigators have postulated that MF is an antigen-driven malignancy, although a specific antigen has yet to be identified.[23]

PREVENTION AND EARLY DETECTION

No agents have been identified that will prevent the development of MF. However, early diagnosis is critical, as local therapy directed against unilesional MF is highly curative.[24-26] The most typical presentation of early disease—an erythematous patch with scale arising in a sun-shielded area—may be confused with a number of benign dermatoses, including atopic dermatitis, psoriasis, and tinea corporis.[27] At this early stage, most of the lymphocytes noted on histopathology represent reactive inflammatory cells rather than the malignant clone.[28] As a result, the histopathology of early MF mimics numerous benign inflammatory conditions,[28,29] and a rapid and correct histologic diagnosis is not always possible. In this setting, molecular studies such as polymerase chain reaction (PCR) for the T-cell receptor will identify a clonal T-cell population in 50% to 80% of patients who ultimately develop overt histologic evidence of MF.[30,31]

BIOLOGIC CHARACTERISTICS/MOLECULAR BIOLOGY

A malignant clone in patch-plaque MF bears the immunophenotype of activated, skin-homing CD4+ helper T cells.[23] When a naïve T cell identifies its cognate antigen in a skin-draining lymph node, activation occurs, and the T cell begins to express cutaneous lymphocyte antigen (CLA) and CC chemokine receptor 4 (CCR4). As these activated T cells pass through the capillaries of inflamed skin, CLA and CCR4 bind to their respective ligands on the dermal capillaries, resulting in extravasation of the activated T cells into the dermal connective tissue. Once outside the circulation, activated T cells migrate to the epidermis and interact with antigen-presenting dendritic (Langerhans) cells (Fig. 76-4).

Clinically, progression of MF is associated with loss of epidermotropism and increasing tumor burden. Molecular studies have shown that progression of MF is associated with *p53* mutation,[32] numerous chromosomal rearrangements,[33] and microsatellite instability.[34] In addition, the malignant cells in MF develop mechanisms to escape destruction by the host immune system. For example, although benign activated T

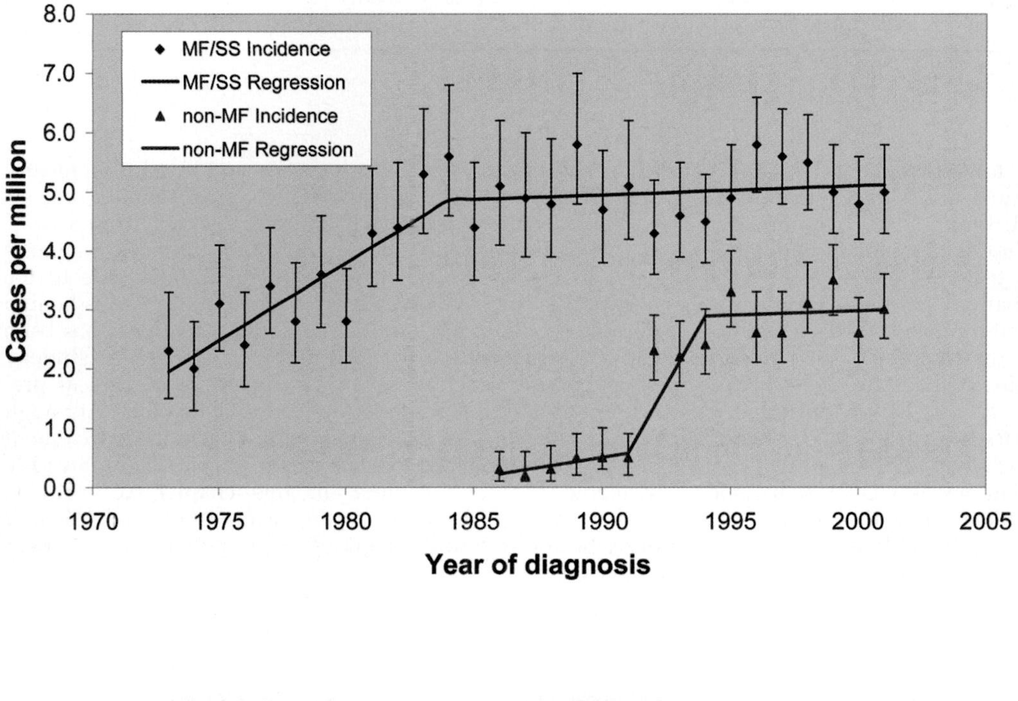

Figure 76-1 The incidence of Mycosis Fungoides/Sézary Syndrome (MF/SS) and non-MF cutaneous T-cell lymphoma (CTCL) reported by the National Cancer Institute's Surveillance, Epidemiology, and End Results (SEER) program between 1973 and 2001. (Data from Surveillance, Epidemiology, and End Results [SEER] Program [*www.seer.cancer.gov*] SEER*Stat Database: Incidence—SEER 11 Regs + AK Public-Use, Nov 2003 Sub (1973-2001 varying), National Cancer Institute, DCCPS, Surveillance Research Program, Cancer Statistics Branch, released April 2004, based on the November 2003 submission; Surveillance Research Program, National Cancer Institute SEER*Stat software [*www.seer.cancer.gov/seerstat*] version 5.2.2.)

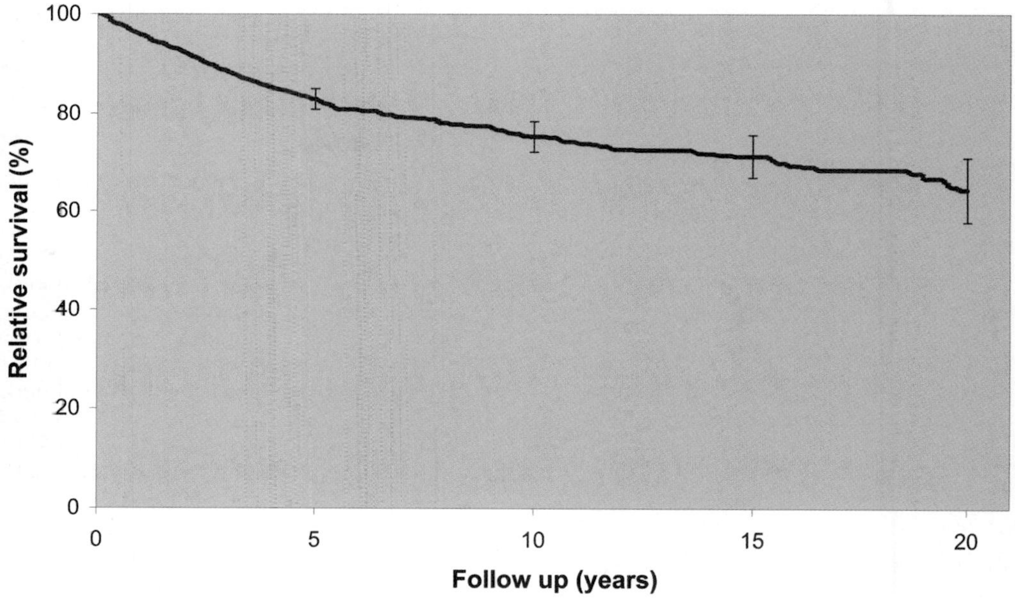

Figure 76-2 Relative survival of all patients (N = 2830) diagnosed with Mycosis Fungoides/Sézary Syndrome (MF/SS) reported by the National Cancer Institute's Surveillance, Epidemiology, and End Results program.[10,11] Relative survival is defined as the survival of a population of interest divided by the survival of an age-, sex-, race-, and year of diagnosis-matched control population. It therefore approximates the cause-specific survival.

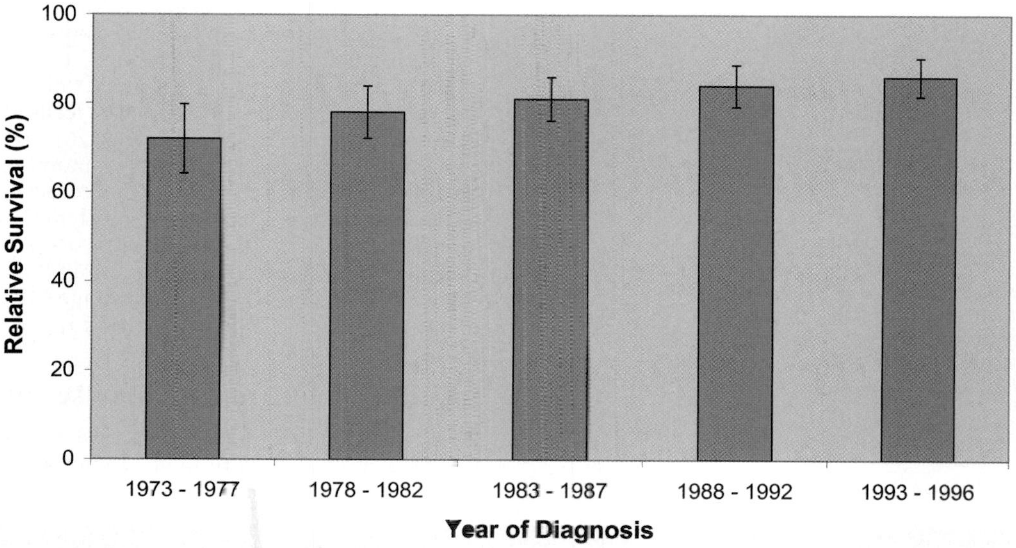

Figure 76-3 Five-year relative survival grouped by year of diagnosis for all patients diagnosed with Mycosis Fungoides/Sézary Syndrome (MF/SS) reported by the National Cancer Institute's Surveillance, Epidemiology, and End Results program. (Data from Surveillance, Epidemiology, and End Results [SEER] Program [*www.seer.cancer.gov*] SEER*Stat Database: Incidence—SEER 11 Regs + AK Public-Use, Nov 2003 Sub [1973-2001 varying], National Cancer Institute, DCCPS, Surveillance Research Program, Cancer Statistics Branch, released April 2004, based on the November 2003 submission; Surveillance Research Program, National Cancer Institute SEER*Stat software [*www.seer.cancer.gov/seerstat*] version 5.2.2.)

cells are eliminated by fas/fas-ligand–mediated apoptosis, the malignant T cells of MF evade fas-mediated apoptosis via fas downregulation, mutation, or alternative splicing.[35]

As a malignancy of the immune system, MF results in substantial alteration of host immunity with consequent increased risk of infection[36] and, possibly, second malignancy.[37] For example, in patients with Sézary syndrome, the absolute number of normal circulating T cells often drops dramatically, reaching levels typically only seen in AIDS.[38] In addition, malignant $CD4^+$ T cells produce large amounts of interleukin (IL)-10 and transforming growth factor (TGF)-β, resulting in further suppression of cell-mediated immunity.[39,40] The malignant cells of MF also produce large amounts of soluble IL-2 receptor, which can inactivate IL-2,[41] a cytokine needed to promote normal T-cell activation. Additionally, the malignant cells of Sézary syndrome can elaborate large amounts of IL-4 and IL-5, producing a syndrome characterized by atopy and eosinophilia.[40]

PATHOLOGY AND PATHWAYS OF SPREAD

The diagnosis of mycosis fungoides remains challenging, even for the experienced clinician and dermatopathologist, due to both the absence of a diagnostic gold standard and the number of benign inflammatory dermatoses that may mimic MF, particularly in its early stages. Currently, diagnosis relies on integrating clinical presentation with histopathologic, immunophenotypic, and genotypic data. A comparison of the

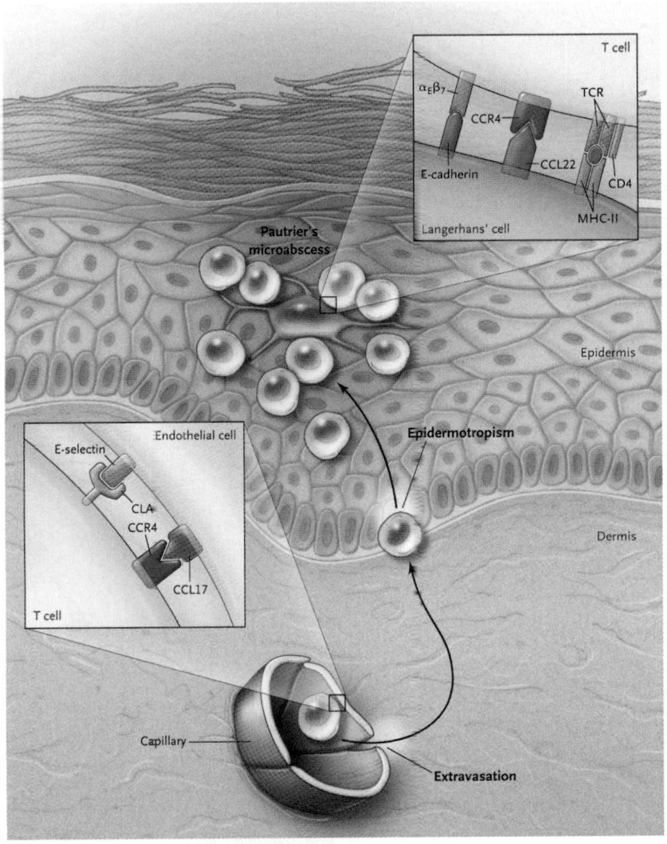

Figure 76-4 Activated skin-homing T cells extravasate through the dermal capillaries due to interactions of cutaneous lymphocyte antigen (CLA) and chemokine receptor 4 (CCR4) with their respective ligands on the dermal capillaries, E-selectin, and chemokine ligand 17 (CCL17). T cells then migrate to the epidermis and interact with antigen-presenting dendritic cells. (From Girardi M, Heald PW, Wilson LD: Medical progress: the pathogenesis of mycosis fungoides. N Engl J Med 350:1978-1988, 2004. Copyright © 2004 Massachusetts Medical Society.)

European Organization for the Research and Treatment of Cancer (EORTC) and World Health Organization (WHO) classifications of CTCLs is presented in Table 76-1.

Histopathology

The most striking finding of early MF is profound epidermotropism, characterized by lymphocytes clustered along the basement membrane of the epidermis (Fig. 76-5A and B).[42] Microdissection studies have shown that virtually all of the lymphocytes in the epidermis belong to the malignant clone, whereas most dermal lymphocytes are reactive.[43,44]

Several microscopic findings help to discriminate early MF from benign inflammatory mimics. For example, an EORTC study reported that identification of epidermal lymphocytes with extremely convoluted, medium-large (7-9 μm) nuclei enabled correct diagnosis of MF with 100% sensitivity and 92% specificity (Fig. 76-5B).[29] In contrast, a study from Stanford University found that intraepidermal atypical lymphocytes surrounded by a clear halo (an artifact of fixation) were the most robust indicators of MF in a multivariate model.[45] Another finding, Pautrier's microabscess, is considered pathognomonic, but is seen in less than 20% of early lesions (Fig. 76-5D).[45] Efforts are currently underway to establish a grading system to standardize pathology reporting and improve diagnostic accuracy.[28,46]

As MF progresses from patch to plaque stage, the lymphoid infiltrate increases in density and begins to invade the deeper reticular dermis (Fig. 76-5C). Furthermore, due to the increased burden of neoplastic cells, findings such as Pautrier's microabscesses (see Fig. 76-5D), haloed lymphocytes, and convoluted nuclei are more readily identified, resulting in improved diagnostic accuracy. Tumor formation results from vertical growth of the lymphoid infiltrate, and may be associated with complete loss of epidermotropism and sparing of the upper papillary dermis (Fig. 76-5E). Erythrodermic MF often resembles patch-stage MF, although epidermotropism may be more subtle, and neoplastic cells may be quite sparse.[47]

Immunophenotyping of Skin Lesions

Assessment of T-cell marker expression within the lymphoid infiltrate provides additional information that helps to

Table 76-1 Classification of Cutaneous T-Cell Lymphomas

Type of Disease	EORTC Classification	WHO Classification
Indolent	Mycosis fungoides	Mycosis fungoides
	Mycosis fungoides and follicular mucinosis	Mycosis fungoides-associated follicular mucinosis
	Pagetoid reticulosis	Pagetoid reticulosis
	Large cell cutaneous T-cell lymphoma, CD30-positive	Primary cutaneous anaplastic large cell lymphoma
	Anaplastic	
	Immunoblastic	
	Pleomorphic	
	Lymphomatoid papulosis	Lymphomatoid papulosis
Aggressive	Sézary syndrome	Sézary syndrome
	Large cell cutaneous T-cell lymphoma, CD30-negative	Peripheral T-cell lymphoma, not otherwise specified
	Immunoblastic	
	Pleomorphic	
Provisional	Granulomatous slack skin	Granulomatous slack skin
	Cutaneous T-cell lymphoma, pleomorphic, small-to-medium size	Peripheral T-cell lymphoma, not otherwise specified
	Subcutaneous panniculitis-like T-cell lymphoma	Subcutaneous panniculitis-like T-cell lymphoma

Adapted from Sander CA, Flaig MJ, Jaffe ES: Cutaneous manifestations of lymphoma: a clinical guide based on the WHO classification. Clin Lymphoma 2:86-100; discussion 101-102, 2001; Willemze R, Kerl H, Sterry W, et al: EORTC classification for primary cutaneous lymphomas: a proposal from the Cutaneous Lymphoma Study Group of the European Organization for Research and Treatment of Cancer. Blood 90:354-371, 1997.

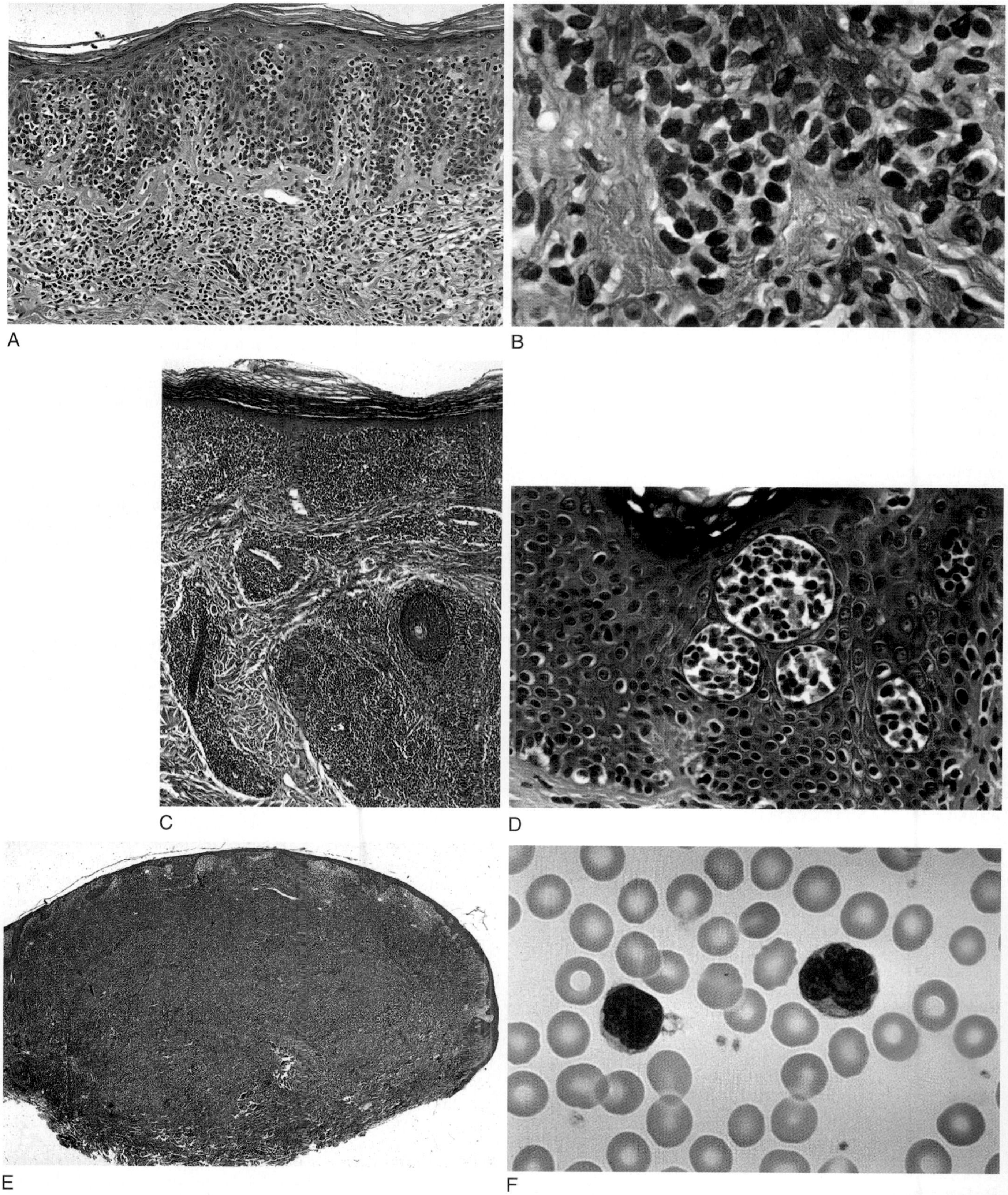

Figure 76-5 **A,** Advanced patch-stage lesion of mycosis fungoides (MF) exhibiting abundant lymphocytes within the basal layer of the epidermis, associated with an underlying band-like lymphocytic infiltrate and papillary dermal fibrosis. **B,** Advanced patch-stage lesion of MF exhibiting enlarged, convoluted lymphocytes within the epidermis. The lymphocyte cell size approximates the width of keratinocyte nuclei. **C,** Plaque-stage MF shows, in addition, involvement of the reticular dermis. **D,** Pautrier's microabscesses are well-defined aggregates of lymphocytes within the epidermis, which are strongly indicative of MF. **E,** In tumor stage MF, the dermis is distended by the lymphocytic infiltrate. Epidermotropic capacity is often lost. **F,** Sézary cells, such as the cell at the right, are enlarged circulating lymphocytes that exhibit cerebriform nuclear convolutions. (Photos and legend courtesy of Earl Glusac, MD; Reprinted with permission from Figure 5 in Smith BD, Wilson LD: Management of mycosis fungoides. Part 1. Diagnosis, staging, and prognosis. Oncology 17:1281-1288, 2003.)

establish a diagnosis of MF. The hallmark of MF is expression of CD4, the marker of mature helper T cells. A typical immunophenotype for MF is CD2$^+$ (pan T cell), CD3$^+$ (pan T cell), CD4$^+$ (helper T cell), CD5$^+$ (pan T cell), CD45RO$^+$ (memory T cell), CLA$^+$, CD8$^-$ (cytotoxic T cell), CD30$^-$ (activated T cell).[48] Although many benign dermatoses express a similar immunophenotype, two markers, CD7 and Leu-8, are often underexpressed in MF and may be helpful in distinguishing between MF and benign mimics. Finally, rare cases of apparently classic MF that are CD4$^-$, but CD3$^+$ and CD8$^+$, have been reported.[49]

T-Cell Receptor Gene Rearrangement

Clonal T-cell receptor gene rearrangements are frequently identified in MF skin lesions and may help to differentiate between early MF patches and benign mimics. Clinical data indicate that PCR will identify a dominant clonal T-cell receptor-γ rearrangement in 63% to 90% of skin biopsies that show definite histologic evidence of MF.[50,51] Furthermore, PCR identifies a clonal T-cell population in 50% to 80% of histologically borderline biopsies obtained from patients who subsequently develop classic MF.[30,31] In contrast, T-cell clonality occurs in only 6% to 24% of benign dermatoses that contain a lymphoid infiltrate.[50,51] These observations suggest that identification of a clonal T-cell population should always be considered in light of the clinical and histologic context, and may help to confirm a diagnosis of MF when already suspected on these grounds.

Transformation to Large Cell Histology

Transformation to a large cell variant occurs in up to 39% of patients initially diagnosed with MF.[52] Histologic diagnosis of transformation requires large cells (≥4 times the size of a small lymphocyte) comprising > 25% of the lymphoid infiltrate or forming microscopic nodules.[53] Transformation is associated with expression of CD30 in 30% of cases and expression of CD20 in 45% of cases. Transformed MF is typically aggressive, with clinical behavior similar to high-grade lymphoma.

CLINICAL MANIFESTATIONS

According to the EORTC classification of cutaneous lymphomas, the term mycosis fungoides should be reserved for those CD4$^+$ cutaneous lymphomas that are "characterized by the subsequent evolution of patches to more infiltrated plaques and eventually tumors."[2] Over time, MF may spread to involve lymph nodes, blood, bone marrow, and visceral organs. Symptoms may vary by degree of involvement, but weight loss, night sweats, and fever are uncommon unless infection is present.

Premycotic Phase

Early MF typically begins with mildly erythematous, slightly scaling, annular or arcuate macules that classically involve sun-shielded areas (Fig. 76-6A). These lesions may wax and wane for years before histologic findings show definitive evidence of MF.

Patch Phase

In this stage, patches lose their predilection for sun-shielded areas and may become eczematous, hypopigmented, or hyperpigmented. The trunk, pelvis, and proximal extremities are most commonly involved. Histologic features consistent with MF may now be discernible.

Plaque Phase

If untreated, some patches will progress to form more generalized, deeply infiltrative, scaling plaques that often have well-demarcated, palpable borders and may exhibit central clearance and arcuate morphology (Fig. 76-6B). Associated findings include hyperkeratosis of the palms and soles and fissures.

Tumor Phase

More than 80% of tumors emerge in the setting of established patch-plaque MF (Fig. 76-6C). The most common sites of tumor involvement include the face, digits, and perineum. Tumors frequently ulcerate and are prone to infection.

Tumeur d'Emblée

The term tumeur d'emblée refers to the rare patient who presents with tumors that arise in the absence of antecedent skin lesions; some cases may be more appropriately classified as CD30$^-$ cutaneous large T-cell lymphoma rather than mycosis fungoides.[54] The clinical course may be more aggressive than patients with classic MF.

Erythroderma

Erythroderma is defined as greater than 80% body surface involvement with confluent patches and/or plaques. It is associated with intense pruritus, hyperkeratosis of the palms and soles, skin atrophy, and lichenification (Fig. 76-6D). Erythroderma may arise de novo or from progression of patch/plaque MF.

Lymph Nodes

Lymph node involvement is present in 15% of newly diagnosed patients and is associated with advanced cutaneous disease.[55] Nodes are typically non-tender, mobile, and measure from 1 to 4 cm. Bulky adenopathy is uncommon.

Internal Organs

Visceral involvement is typically seen only in patients with advanced cutaneous disease, nodal disease, and blood involvement. The most common sites include the lungs, central nervous system, oral cavity, and oropharynx,[55] although MF has been observed in other sites such as the breast, thyroid, and pancreas. Visceral involvement is often subclinical and does not routinely precipitate death. Bone marrow involvement at initial staging has been reported in 6% to 28% of patients, and is also associated with advanced skin and nodal disease.[56,57]

Sézary Syndrome

SS is defined as erythroderma plus evidence of malignant circulating T cells that satisfy any of the five criteria listed in Table 76-2.[58] For the purposes of these criteria, the Sézary cell is defined as "any atypical lymphocyte with [a] moderately to highly enfolded or grooved nucleus"[58] (see Fig. 76-5F). Clinical findings may include edema and tumorous involvement of the face leading to leonine facies, severe fissures of the palms and soles, intense pruritus, and cutaneous pain.

Currently, no consensus has emerged regarding the pathologic link between MF and SS. However, some clinical observations help to elucidate the relationship between these two disorders. SS usually arises de novo without antecedent MF. Rarely, MF will evolve to an erythrodermic stage with concomitant hematologic findings that satisfy a diagnosis of SS; these cases should be considered "SS preceded by MF." Most patients with a history of MF who develop erythroderma do

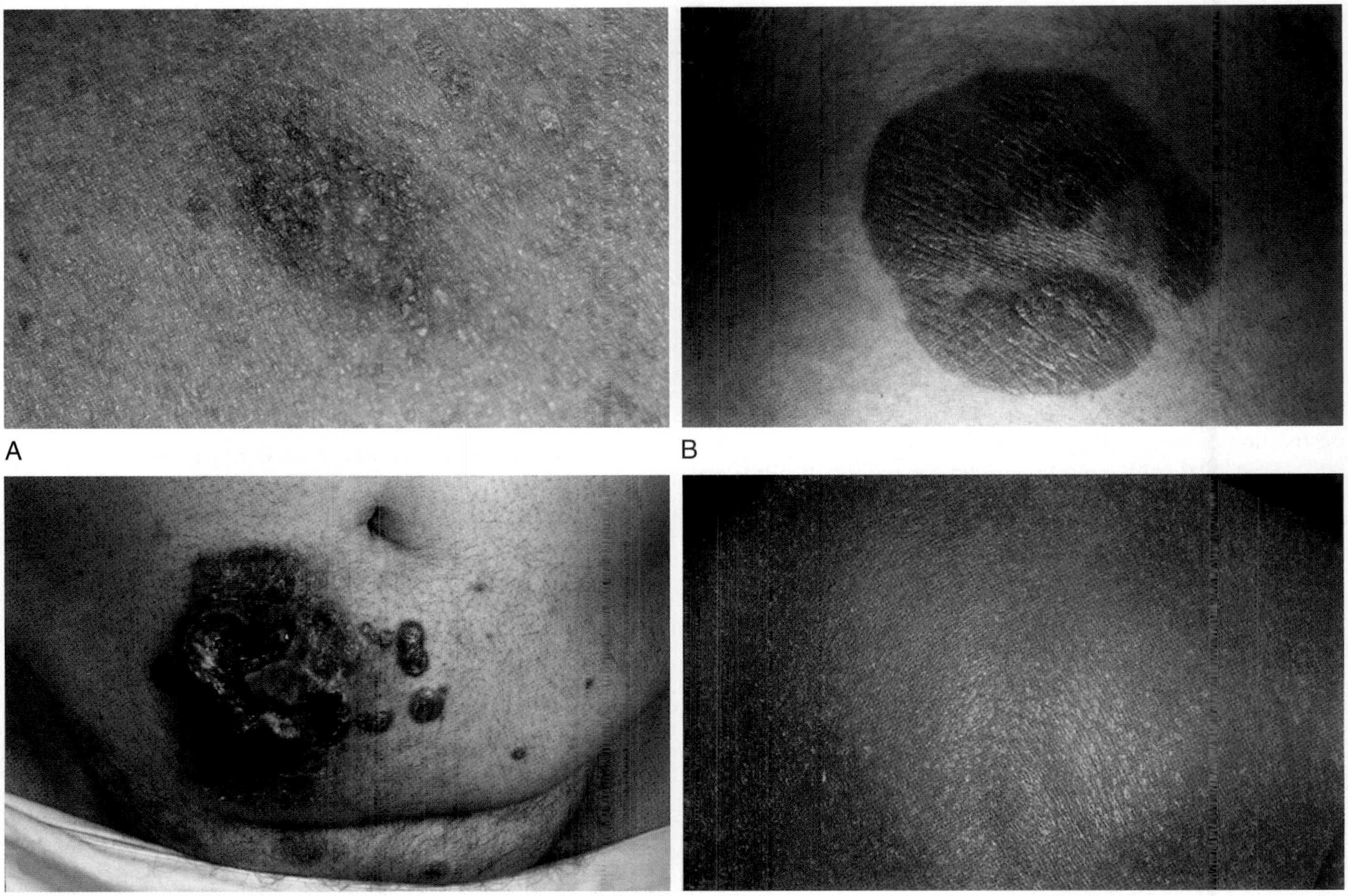

A B C D

Figure 76-6 **A,** Typical early patch with erythema and mild scale. **B,** Typical plaque, with raised, palpable borders, central clearing, and overlying scale. **C,** Large tumor with necrosis and ulceration. **D,** Generalized erythroderma. (Reprinted with permission from Figure 1 in Smith BD, Wilson LD: Management of mycosis fungoides. Part 1. Diagnosis, staging, and prognosis. Oncology 17:1281-1288, 2003.)

Table 76-2 Proposed Hematologic Criteria for the Diagnosis of Sézary Syndrome

Absolute Sézary cell count ≥ 1000 cells/µL.
CD4/CD8 ratio ≥ 10 due to an increase in $CD3^+$ or $CD4^+$ cells by flow cytometry.
Aberrant expression of pan–T-cell markers (CD2, CD3, CD4, CD5) by flow cytometry. Deficient CD7 expression on T cells (or expanded $CD4^+$, $CD7^-$ cells ≥ 40%) is a tentative criterion.
Increased lymphocyte count with T-cell clone in blood identified by Southern blot or polymerase chain reaction.
A chromosomally abnormal T-cell clone.

Adapted from Vonderheid EC, Bernengo MG, Burg G, et al: Update on erythrodermic cutaneous T-cell lymphoma: report of the International Society for Cutaneous Lymphomas. J Am Acad Dermatol 46:95-106, 2002.

not meet hematologic criteria for SS, and are therefore considered erythrodermic MF.

VARIANTS OF MYCOSIS FUNGOIDES

The progression from subtle patches to indurated plaques, cutaneous tumors, and erythroderma represents classic, so-called "Alibert-Bazin," mycosis fungoides. According to the EORTC classification, variants such as bullous and hyperpigmented or hypopigmented MF manifest similar clinical behavior and should not be considered separately from classic MF.[2] Several variants sharing some clinical and pathologic features with MF have been described.

Mycosis Fungoides–Associated Follicular Mucinosis

Patients with MF-associated follicular mucinosis present with follicular papules, comedo-like lesions, milia-like lesions, patches, and plaques, all of which may produce alopecia.[1] Although it typically involves the head and neck, any skin site may be affected.[2] Pathologically, atypical lymphocytes invade follicles and deposit acid mucopolysaccharides in the pilosebaceous units. Cases without mucin deposition have been reported as follicular or pilotropic MF.[59] Follicular mucinosis tends to be refractory to topical treatments, such as psoralen plus ultraviolet A (PUVA) and nitrogen mustard, and risk of relapse in these patients after treatment with TSEBT is higher compared to other patients without a history of follicular mucinosis.[60] Systemic retinoids are considered the treatment of choice, and 5-year survival is approximately 70%.[2]

Pagetoid Reticulosis/Woringer-Kolopp Disease

Pagetoid reticulosis, also known as Woringer-Kolopp disease, typically presents as slow-growing, hyperkeratotic or psoriasiform, localized patch or plaque involving a distal extremity. Pathologically, an abundant epidermotropic infiltrate composed of atypical large lymphocytes is noted, along with pagetoid spread of individual lymphocytes interspersed among keratinocytes. Benign-appearing small lymphocytes are found in the upper dermis.[1] The prognosis for localized pagetoid reticulosis is excellent with either surgery or radiotherapy, and disease-related deaths have not been reported.[2] Ketron-Goodman type is a disseminated, more aggressive cutaneous lymphoproliferative disorder that histologically resembles localized pagetoid reticulosis.

Granulomatous Slack Skin

This rare variant presents with lax skin in the axillae, neck, breasts, and inguinal regions. Histologic features include epithelioid or giant cell dermal granulomas and associated destruction of elastin fibers.[2] Notably, Hodgkin's disease has been associated with granulomatous slack skin in approximately one third of reported cases.[61] Due to its rarity, optimal treatment has not been established.

RELATED CUTANEOUS T-CELL LYMPHOPROLIFERATIVE DISORDERS

In addition to MF and its variants, several other distinct cutaneous T-cell lymphoproliferative disorders have been described. Their clinical and pathologic features and optimal therapy is briefly reviewed in the following.

Primary Cutaneous Anaplastic Large Cell Lymphoma/CD30$^+$ Large Cell CTCL

This entity typically presents as a red or flesh-colored nodule or tumor that frequently ulcerates. Histopathology shows sheets of CD30$^+$ large lymphocytes without epidermotropism. In contrast to systemic CD30$^+$ anaplastic large cell lymphoma, overexpression of anaplastic lymphoma kinase (ALK) is not found in primary cutaneous CD30$^+$ large cell lymphoma. Patients with localized disease are typically treated with radiotherapy alone, and prognosis is excellent with a 5-year survival of 90%.[2,62]

Lymphomatoid Papulosis

Lymphomatoid papulosis (LyP) presents with grouped erythematous or violaceous papules and/or nodules at different stages of development. Lesions typically resolve spontaneously within 2 to 8 weeks, but scarring is common.[63] Three different histologic subtypes have been described, with types A and C consisting of malignant CD30$^+$ T cells, often with an extensive inflammatory infiltrate, and type B simulating classic plaque-stage MF. For type C lesions, discrimination between LyP and CD30$^+$ large cell lymphoma may be difficult on histologic grounds, and assessment of the clinical context may be required to ensure the proper diagnosis.[2] Although cytologically malignant, it should be emphasized that LyP is clinically benign, with a 5-year survival of 100%.[2,62] Thus, neither aggressive chemotherapy nor radiotherapy is indicated.[64] Treatment options include PUVA or low-dose methotrexate, but neither is considered curative. In the long term, at least 15% to 20% of patients with LyP develop a second malignancy, most commonly MF, CD30$^+$ large cell lymphoma, or Hodgkin's disease.[64,65] In patients undergoing TSEBT for MF, a history of LyP increases the risk of relapse.[60]

Adult T-Cell Lymphoma/Leukemia

Adult T-cell lymphoma/leukemia (ATLL) develops in 2% to 4% of individuals infected with human T-cell lymphotrophic virus type I (HTLV-I), a retrovirus endemic in southern Japan and the Caribbean.[1,63,66,67] Skin findings are present in up to 60% of patients with ATLL, and they strongly resemble those of MF, including plaques, tumors, and erythroderma. The characteristic immunophenotype is CD2$^+$ CD3$^+$ CD4$^+$ CD5$^+$ CD7$^-$ CD8$^-$ and the malignant cells strongly express the high affinity IL-2 receptor (CD25, CD122, and CD132). Clinical features vary from an acute form presenting with B symptoms, hypercalcemia, metabolic bone disease, hepatosplenomegaly, generalized adenopathy, and leukemic infiltration to a smoldering or chronic form presenting with skin infiltration and little or no systemic involvement. Although patients often respond to conventional chemotherapy, long-term survival is rare. Newer promising agents include denileukin diftitox[68] and interferon-α in combination with zidovudine.[69]

CD30$^-$ Large Cutaneous T-Cell Lymphoma

This entity, which is a subset of peripheral T-cell lymphoma not otherwise specified in the WHO classification,[1] often presents with disseminated, rapidly growing plaques, nodules, or tumors. Histologically, CD30$^-$ large T-cell lymphoma resembles MF undergoing large cell transformation. Thus, inquiry into a previous history of indolent patches or plaques is important to discriminate between these two entities. Although combination chemotherapy is recommended, 5-year survival is poor at approximately 15%.[2]

Subcutaneous Panniculitis-Like T-Cell Lymphoma

Subcutaneous panniculitis-like T-cell lymphoma is a malignancy of CD8$^+$ T lymphocytes that typically presents with subcutaneous nodules or plaques involving the legs or trunk and associated B symptoms. Although some cases have an indolent course, many cases are fatal, particularly when associated with hemophagocytic syndrome. Treatment for indolent disease is often observation, and treatment for advanced disease includes combination chemotherapy and possibly cyclosporine.[1,2]

PROGNOSIS AND STAGING

The American Joint Committee on Cancer (AJCC) staging system for MF identifies extent and character of skin lesions, extracutaneous disease, and leukemic transformation as the major predictors of poor prognosis (Tables 76-3 and 76-4).[70] Shortcomings of this system include: 1) difficulty in assigning T stage for patients who fall on the border between T1 and T2; 2) failure to discriminate between the prognosis of patients with extensive patches as compared to extensive plaques; 3) similarity in prognosis between patients with tumors and erythroderma; 4) the questionable prognostic relevance of enlarged, pathologically uninvolved lymph nodes; and 5) the rarity of the N2 descriptor, as biopsies of nonpalpable lymph nodes are seldom performed.[71,72]

Data from a cohort of 468 patients with newly diagnosed MF evaluated at Stanford University are presented in Table 76-5.[55] More than 60% of patients presented with patches and/or plaques without nodal or visceral disease. Such patients rarely developed disseminated disease, even at 20 years of follow-up. In contrast, 50% to 60% of patients presenting with tumors or erythroderma develop extracutaneous disease.

Data from Stanford showed that patients with limited patches and plaques (stage IA, T1 N0 M0) experience 10-year survival similar to a matched control population. In contrast, median survival for patients with extensive patches and plaques (T2), tumors (T3), and erythroderma (T4), was 11, 3.2, and 4.6 years, respectively.[73] Patients with either pathologically documented lymph node involvement or visceral involvement experienced a median survival of approximately one year.[55]

A multi-institutional study showed that survival is also related to the pattern and extent of lymph node involvement.[74] For example, partial or complete effacement of nodal architecture by malignant lymphocytes conferred a median survival of 2.3 years. In contrast, lymph nodes with aggregates of atypical lymphocytes but preserved nodal architecture resulted in a median survival of 6 years, and lymph nodes with only dermatopathic changes or few atypical lymphocytes resulted in a median survival of 9 years.

Other factors that may herald a poor prognosis include: age ≥60,[75] elevated lactate dehydrogenase (LDH),[75] elevated soluble IL-2 receptor levels,[41] a low percentage of $CD8^+$ tumor-infiltrating lymphocytes,[76] extent of skin involvement in those with T3 disease,[77] T-cell clonality within the cutaneous infiltrate detected by PCR,[78,79] an identical T-cell clone in the skin and peripheral blood,[80] and T-cell clonality in dermatopathic lymph nodes.[81]

The AJCC also included a blood descriptor, B0 versus B1, to document the absence or presence of more than 1000 Sézary cells ($CD4^+$, $CD7^-$) per μL. Among patients with erythroderma, the presence of B1 disease is a significant, independent predictor of survival, doubling the risk of death.[82]

For those patients with transformation to a large cell variant of MF, median survival ranges from 19 to 36 months.[52,53] Factors predictive of poor survival after transformation include short interval between diagnosis of MF and transformation (<2 y), and the presence of stage IIB-IV disease.[52]

Table 76-3 TNM(B) Classification for Mycosis Fungoides *Adapted from the Sixth edition of the AJCC Cancer Staging Manual*[70]

- T1—Patches and/or plaques involving < 10% body surface area
- T2—Patches and/or plaques involving ≥ 10% body surface area
- T3—One or more cutaneous tumors
- T4—Generalized erythroderma
- N0—Lymph nodes clinically uninvolved
- N1—Lymph nodes clinically enlarged but histologically uninvolved
- N2—Lymph nodes clinically non-palpable but histologically involved
- N3—Lymph nodes clinically enlarged and histologically involved
- M0—No visceral disease present
- M1—Visceral disease present
- B0—No circulating atypical cells (<1000 Sézary cells [$CD4^+$ $CD7^-$]/μL)
- B1—Circulating atypical cells present (≥1000 Sézary cells [$CD4^+$ $CD7^-$]/μL)

Adapted from Greene FL, Page DL, Fleming ID, et al: AJCC Cancer Staging Handbook, 6th ed. New York, Springer, 2002.

Table 76-4 Staging Classification for Mycosis Fungoides

IA	T1	N0	M0
IB	T2	N0	M0
IIA	T1-2	N1	M0
IIB	T3	N0-1	M0
IIIA	T4	N0	M0
IIIB	T4	N1	M0
IVA	T1-4	N2-3	M0
IVB	T1-4	N0-3	M1

The B descriptor is not considered in stage classification

Adapted from Greene FL, Page DL, Fleming ID, et al: AJCC Cancer Staging Handbook, 6th ed. New York, Springer, 2002.

PATIENT EVALUATION

History

All patients should have a thorough history performed by the evaluating dermatologists, radiation oncologists, and any other consultants (Table 76-6). Careful attention should be given to the duration, change in appearance, and distribution of the eruption according to the patient. Inquiry related to a history of pruritus, pain, exfoliation, fissures, bullae, and perineal discomfort should be made. Previous diagnostic considerations, procedures, and therapies should be recorded in detail to establish temporal relationships. The clinical interview, along with the examination, are the two most important aspects of the workup, as they can help exclude other diagnoses and establish whether the narrative and findings are consistent with a diagnosis of MF.

Physical Examination

All patients should undergo a complete physical examination with special attention to the skin surface, lymph nodes, and abdomen. Specific notations should be made of the number, location, character, and distribution of cutaneous lesions. The percentage of cutaneous involvement should also be

Table 76-5 Initial Stage and Natural History of 463 Patients with Mycosis Fungoides Evaluated at Stanford University at the Time of Initial Diagnosis

	T stage at initial presentation (%)	Percentage with nodal or visceral involvement on initial diagnosis as a function of T stage	Percentage developing nodal or visceral involvement over 20 years as a function of T stage
T1	28	0	0
T2	36	2	10
T3	20	13	36
T4	16	25	41

Data from de Coninck EC, Kim YH, Varghese A, et al: Clinical characteristics and outcome of patients with extracutaneous mycosis fungoides. J Clin Oncol 19:779-784, 2001.

Table 76-6 Recommended Workup for Patients with Suspected Mycosis Fungoides

History and physical examination with attention to skin, lymph nodes, liver, and spleen
Skin biopsy with attention to
- Histology
  - Epidermal lymphocytes with medium-large, extremely convoluted nuclei
  - Haloed epidermal lymphocytes
  - Pautrier's microabscesses
- Immunophenotype
  - Classically $CD2^+$ $CD3^+$ $CD4^+$ $CD5^+$ $CD45RO^+$ $CD8^-$ $CD30^-$
  - Rarely $CD4^-$ $CD3^+$ $CD8^+$
- PCR for T-cell receptor gene rearrangement

Biopsy of enlarged lymph nodes with attention to
- Histology, both number of atypical lymphocytes and disruption of nodal architecture
- In dermatopathic nodes, consider PCR for T-cell clonality and immunophenotyping to rule out occult involvement

Evaluation of blood
- CBC with manual differential, liver function tests, and serum chemistries for all patients
- In those with suspected stage IIB-IV disease
  - LDH, soluble interleukin-2 receptor
  - Flow cytometry for CD2, CD3, CD4, CD5, CD7, CD8, CD20, CD45RO
  - PCR for T-cell receptor gene rearrangement

Imaging
- Posteroanterior and lateral chest radiograph for stages IA-IB
- Computed tomography of chest, abdomen, and pelvis for suspected stage IIA-IV

CBC, complete blood count; LDH, lactate dehydrogenase; PCR, polymerase chain reaction.

quantified. Other non-MF cutaneous findings, such as previous excision sites, pigmented lesions, or any findings consistent with other skin malignancy, should be noted. Adenopathy should be carefully documented with respect to location, size, consistency, mobility, and discomfort on palpation. Photographs of the skin for baseline documentation should be considered.

Diagnostic Testing

Pathology

A minimum of two biopsies of involved skin should be performed for hematoxylin and eosin evaluation. Material for immunophenotyping and T-cell receptor gene rearrangement should be obtained. Excisional biopsy of adenopathy is recommended, and tissue should be submitted for the same pathologic studies. Needle aspiration of nodes is not recommended.

Routine bone marrow examination is generally unnecessary, but may be considered in patients with blood or other visceral involvement. Bone marrow involvement at initial staging has been reported in 6% to 28% of patients, and is associated with advanced skin and nodal disease.[56,57] However, there is no evidence to suggest that marrow involvement is an independent predictor of outcome.[57,75] Furthermore, although a clonal T-cell population within the marrow is identified in 75% of patients with identical skin and peripheral blood T-cell clones, this finding does not appear to alter prognosis.[56]

Hematology and Chemistry

A complete blood count including differential and smear in addition to serum chemistries (to include renal and hepatic function) should be obtained prior to initiation of therapy. For patients with stage IIB-IV disease, serum levels of soluble IL-2 receptor and LDH reflect overall tumor burden and can be used to assess response to therapy.

A thorough examination of the peripheral blood for evidence of malignant T cells is indicated for those with stage IIB-IV MF, and may be considered for those with stage IA-IIA. Peripheral blood flow cytometry should be performed to assess expression of CD2, CD3, CD4, CD5, CD7, CD8, CD20, and CD45RO. Findings suggestive of blood involvement include an elevated CD4:CD8 ratio (normal range 0.5-3.5), or an expanded population of $CD4^+CD7^-$ or $CD45RO^+$ lymphocytes.[58] If initially abnormal, findings on peripheral blood flow cytometry should be followed to assess response to therapy. If flow cytometry is unremarkable, peripheral blood PCR for T-cell receptor gene rearrangement should be considered. PCR reveals a clonal T-cell population identical to that found in the cutaneous infiltrate in 40% of patients with erythroderma and 14% of patients with patches, plaques, or tumors.[50]

Diagnostic Imaging

Chest radiography should be completed for all patients via posteroanterior and lateral views. Computed tomography of the chest, abdomen, and pelvis may be obtained for patients with tumors, erythroderma, or nodal involvement but is not necessary for those with stage IA or IB, given the low yield.[83] Lymphangiography and ultrasonography of the abdomen and pelvis are optional. Positron emission tomography (PET) is currently performed in some centers.

PRIMARY THERAPY

Because MF is a disease of *cutaneous* (i.e., skin-homing) lymphocytes, therapy is quite distinct from that of nodal lymphomas. For patients with disease limited to the skin, topical therapy alone produces high rates of remission and even cure. Topical therapies include mechlorethamine (nitrogen mustard), carmustine (BCNU), steroids, bexarotene gel, PUVA, ultraviolet B (UVB), and either localized or total skin electron radiotherapy. For patients with localized unilesional MF, topical therapies alone produce long-term, disease-free survival rates in excess of 85%.[24-26] For those with more than one patch or plaque but with less than 10% body surface area involvement (T1 N0 and T1 N1), topical therapies alone produce long-term, disease-free survival rates ranging from 30% to 50%. For patients with more extensive patches or plaques, topical therapies may produce remission, but long-term cure is unlikely. Such patients should receive intensive topical therapy to induce a complete remission followed by less intensive adjuvant topical therapy to sustain a remission.[84,85]

Those with tumors or erythroderma experience severe cutaneous symptoms and are at high risk for extracutaneous dissemination. Of all the topical therapies, TSEBT is associated with the highest rates of complete response for this patient subgroup.[85-87] Therefore, it is recommended that TSEBT be administered to induce cutaneous remission and that adjuvant systemic and/or topical therapy be administered to sustain remission. Systemic therapies include interferon, retinoids, oral bexarotene, denileukin diftitox, extracorporeal photochemotherapy (photopheresis), and cytotoxic chemotherapy.

In the following section, we first discuss all nonradiation topical therapies and then discuss the various systemic therapies. Finally, we discuss the clinical data for radiation and compare this to clinical data for various topical and systemic therapies to develop evidence-based guidelines for the treatment of MF.

SKIN-DIRECTED THERAPY

Mechlorethamine

Topical mechlorethamine hydrochloride (HN2), also known as nitrogen mustard, is an alkylating agent with proven activity in the treatment of MF patches and plaques. Mechlorethamine is typically applied daily and continued for at least 6 months after complete response.[71] Cutaneous intolerance, manifested by erythema and pruritus, occurs in approximately 50% of patients treated with aqueous HN2,[88] but is reduced to less than 10% in patients treated with HN2 dissolved in ointment such as Aquaphor.[71] Other cutaneous side effects of HN2 may include xerosis, hyperpigmentation, and, rarely, bullous reactions, urticaria, and Stevens-Johnson syndrome.[88] Bone marrow suppression is not observed due to minimal systemic absorption. The carcinogenicity of HN2 remains debated, as one series reported no increased risk for secondary skin cancers in patients treated with HN2 monotherapy,[71] whereas another series reported an eight-fold increase in the risk for non-melanoma skin cancers attributable to HN2 monotherapy.[89] HN2 may also potentiate the carcinogenicity of other topical therapies, such as total skin radiation or PUVA.[90]

Carmustine

Topical BCNU is another alkylating agent with activity in MF. Due to systemic absorption that may produce bone marrow suppression, the drug should be applied to no more than 10% of the body surface area, duration of treatment should be limited to 4 months, and complete blood counts should be monitored. Cutaneous hypersensitivity is uncommon (7% in one series) but chronic skin telangiectasis and hyperpigmentation may occur.[91]

Topical Steroids

High potency topical glucocorticoids are an important component in the treatment of MF due to their ability to alleviate cutaneous symptoms and induce lesion regression. Typically, steroids are applied to active lesions only, as widespread application can induce reversible depression of serum cortisol in 10% to 15% of patients.[92] Persistent application can lead to skin atrophy.

Topical Rexinoids

Bexarotene belongs to a new class of agents called rexinoids that bind to the retinoid X receptor, resulting in transcription of various genes that control cellular differentiation and proliferation.[93] Topical bexarotene gel was recently approved after phase I/II trials demonstrated a 44% to 54% response rate in refractory cutaneous MF.[94,95] Most patients develop an irritant dermatitis and thus require close observation and dose titration. Due to its irritant effects, bexarotene gel is not indicated for patients with more than 15% body surface area involvement. As with systemic retinoids, bexarotene in both its topical and systemic forms should be avoided in pregnant women due to possible teratogenicity.

Psoralen Plus Ultraviolet A and Ultraviolet B

Ultraviolet light used in the treatment of MF includes UVB (wavelength 320 nm to 290 nm), narrow band UVB (wavelength 311 nm), or PUVA (wavelength 400 to 320 nm). Because UVB has limited penetration, its efficacy is limited to thin patches. PUVA penetrates more deeply and will effectively treat some plaque lesions. PUVA requires ingestion of a photochemotherapeutic agent, 8-methoxypsoralen, prior to UVA exposure. UVA activates 8-methoxypsoralen, resulting in DNA cross-linking and apoptotic cell death.[96]

Both PUVA and UVB are initially administered 2 to 3 days a week as the light-dose is gradually increased. Once a complete response has been achieved, treatment frequency may be gradually reduced to once every 2 to 4 weeks. Ultraviolet treatments may be continued on a maintenance basis for several years, provided the patient remains in complete response with treatment administered once every 4 to 8 weeks.

Acute side effects of PUVA and UVB include skin erythema that may be painful, hyperpigmentation, xerosis, pruritus, and blistering. Eye goggles are used to decrease the risk for cataract formation. One side effect unique to PUVA is nausea and vomiting after ingestion of 8-methoxypsoralen (8-MOP). This may be avoided by substituting 8-MOP with either a topical "psoralen bath" or 5-methoxypsoralen, a non-emetogenic analogue that is currently available in Europe.[97] Long-term toxicity includes photoaging and increased risk for melanoma and non-melanoma skin cancers.[98,99]

SYSTEMIC THERAPY

Interferon

Interferon-α-2a (IFN-α) is an effective agent, particularly for patch and plaque disease, likely due to a direct antitumor effect and/or immunomodulation.[100] IFN-α has been used alone[100,101] or in combination with retinoids, PUVA,[102-104] and extracorporeal photopheresis.[105] To date, no randomized trials have compared IFN-α plus another therapy with IFN-α alone, although one prospective trial showed a benefit from combining IFN-α with PUVA as compared to IFN-α plus a retinoid.[106] Toxicity may include flulike symptoms, psychiatric disturbances including depression and confusion, elevated transaminases, leukopenia, thrombocytopenia, proteinuria, and myelopathy.[103,104] Despite these side effects, in a recent phase II trial of IFN-α and PUVA, only 8% of patients withdrew as a result of toxicity.[104]

Retinoids

Oral retinoids such as isotretinoin and acitretin influence cellular differentiation and may be particularly beneficial in the treatment of MF-associated follicular mucinosis. Retinoids can be safely combined with other therapies such as PUVA,[107] IFN-α, and TSEBT.[108] Side effects include photosensitivity, xerosis, myalgias, arthralgias, headaches, impaired night vision, corneal opacities, teratogenicity, elevated transaminases, hyperlipidemia, and pancreatitis.[73]

Rexinoids

Oral bexarotene has been approved by the U.S. Food and Drug Administration for use in all stages of treatment refractory MF.[109,110] Preliminary data suggest that bexarotene can be combined safely with other therapies including PUVA, extracorporeal photopheresis, IFN-α, and HN2.

Hypertriglyceridemia, the most common adverse event, occurs in 80% of treated patients and may result in reversible pancreatitis if triglyceride levels exceed 800 mg/dL.[93] Therefore, atorvastatin or fenofibrate should be initiated if triglyceride levels exceed 350 mg/dL. Gemfibrozil increases serum bexarotene concentrations, resulting in a paradoxical elevation of triglycerides, and should therefore be avoided.[93] Another side effect, central hypothyroidism, affects approximately 75% of patients but responds well to levothyroxine and resolves when treatment is discontinued.[93] Patients taking bexarotene therefore require monitoring of estimated free thyroxine, as levels of thyroid-stimulating hormone (TSH) will always be low. Other side effects include self-limited headaches, mild neutropenia, mild transaminase elevations, skin peeling, and pruritus. In the phase II-III trial of oral bexarotene for advanced, refractory cutaneous T-cell lymphoma, only 10% of patients receiving the optimal dose withdrew as a result of an adverse event.[109]

Denileukin Diftitox

Denileukin diftitox is a recombinant fusion protein that contains portions of IL-2 and diphtheria toxin and has proven activity in refractory MF, stages IB to IVA.[111] It selectively targets T cells that express the high affinity IL-2 receptor (a complex of CD25, CD122, and CD132), resulting in endocytosis of diphtheria toxin, inhibition of protein synthesis, and cell death. Accordingly, in the phase III clinical trial leading to its approval, only patients with neoplastic T cells expressing the high affinity IL-2 receptor were included. Denileukin diftitox is typically administered by a 30-minute venous infusion given on 5 consecutive days and repeated every 3 weeks for up to eight cycles.

Toxicities were commonly encountered in the phase III clinical trial of denileukin diftitox. Acute hypersensitivity reactions, including dyspnea, back pain, hypotension, and chest pain, occurred in 60% of patients. Furthermore, a vascular leak syndrome characterized by hypotension, hypoalbuminemia, and edema was encountered in 25% of patients. Other toxicities may include constitutional symptoms, thrombotic events, infections, transaminase elevations, renal impairment, and lymphopenia. In total, 21% of the patients in this trial withdrew due to adverse events.[111] Subsequent investigations have suggested that pretreatment with corticosteroids substantially reduces the risk for acute toxicity.[112]

Extracorporeal Photochemotherapy

Extracorporeal photochemotherapy (EP), also known as photopheresis, is a novel immune therapy that has shown activity in the treatment of erythrodermic MF.[96,113] Peripheral blood leukocytes are harvested by leukapheresis, mixed with 8-methoxypsoralen, exposed to 2 joules/cm^2 of ultraviolet A, and then reinfused into the patient. This results in DNA cross-linking and gradual apoptotic death of the circulating MF cells that were exposed to PUVA. For unclear reasons, monocytes are resistant to the apoptotic effects of EP, but instead are stimulated to become immature antigen-presenting dendritic cells due to the physical process of leukapheresis. Therefore, once treated, leukocytes are reinfused into the bloodstream, and activated dendritic cells may phagocytose remnants of the apoptotic MF cells, present their antigens on major histocompatibility class I, and stimulate expansion of anti-tumor CD8$^+$ T cells.[114]

EP is typically administered on 2 consecutive days every 4 weeks, although the frequency may be increased in patients with extensive disease.[115] For patients who achieve a complete response, therapy should be maintained for approximately 6 months and then gradually tapered. In general, EP is well tolerated, although hypotension, arrhythmias, and heart failure may occur due to fluid shifts. Therefore, patients with a history of cardiac disease require close monitoring.[113] EP has been safely combined with IFN-α and TSEBT.[105,116,117]

Chemotherapy

Systemic chemotherapy is typically reserved for refractory cutaneous disease, visceral disease, or large cell transformation. Chemotherapy is not typically used in the initial management of patients with MF, as a randomized phase III trial comparing concurrent TSEBT and systemic chemotherapy to sequential topical therapy failed to show an improvement in disease-free or overall survival.[118]

For patients who may benefit from chemotherapy, two main strategies exist. The first relies on oral agents such as methotrexate,[119] etoposide, or chlorambucil. This strategy avoids the need for central venous lines, which are associated with a high risk for infection due to frequent bacteremia caused by open skin lesions. The second strategy relies on intravenously administered chemotherapy. One exciting new prospect is pegylated liposomal doxorubicin, an agent that tends to remain intravascular but will extravasate into the inflamed lesional skin of MF. A pilot study conducted on 34 patients with CTCL reported complete response in 15, partial response in 15, and six severe adverse events.[120] Attention has also been focused on purine analogues such as fludarabine, 2′-deoxycoformycin, and 2-chlorodeoxyadenosine. However, clinical trials of these agents have produced response rates ranging from only 28% to 51% and have documented substantial toxicity, including myelosuppression, infection, and pulmonary dysfunction.[121-124] Other agents with activity in MF include the lipophilic antifolate trimetrexate[125]; 5-fluorouracil; cyclophosphamide, doxorubicin, vincristine, and prednisone (CHOP)[126]; cisplatin; etoposide; bleomycin; vinblastine; and gemcitabine.[127]

High-Dose Chemotherapy with Autologous or Allogeneic Bone Marrow Transplant

Limited experience has been reported using high-dose chemotherapy with either autologous or allogeneic transplant in the treatment of advanced, refractory MF. Autologous stem cell rescue has resulted in several complete responses; however, 15 of the 17 patients reported in the literature relapsed within 1 year.[128-130] In contrast, myeloablative chemotherapy with allogeneic bone marrow transplant (BMT) may result in prolonged disease-free survival. One series of three patients treated with cytoreductive chemotherapy and total body irradiation found that two of the three patients remained disease-free at 4.5 years and 15 months after transplant. The third patient recurred after allogeneic transplant but developed a second complete response upon withdrawal of prophylactic cyclosporine, suggesting a graft-versus-tumor effect.[131,132] Nonmyeloablative, so-called mini-allo transplants, have also been reported, with one series reporting clearance of clonal T cells and durable complete remissions in three of three patients, although one died from infectious complications.[133] Collectively, these experiences suggest that allogeneic BMT may be potentially curative and should be considered for younger patients with good performance status.

RADIOTHERAPY

Radiation is the most effective single modality in the treatment of MF[8] and plays an important role in the treatment of localized or disseminated cutaneous disease and in the palliation of nodal and visceral metastases.

Dose

A dose response has been reported both for radiation of single MF lesions and for TSEBT. For example, in a study of 110 lesions from 14 patients with at least 1 year of follow-up, Cotter and colleagues[134] reported an infield recurrence rate of 42% for those treated to a total dose of 10 Gy, 32% for 10.01 to 20 Gy, 21% for 20.01 to 30 Gy, and 0% for >30 Gy. In a study of 30 lesions from patients with stage IA MF treated with localized radiotherapy, Wilson and coworkers[25] reported local failure in 20% (4/20) treated with 20 Gy, compared with 0% (0/10) treated with >20 Gy. Kim and colleagues[135] treated different lesions from the same patient with various total doses and fraction sizes, finding that division of the total dose into two fractions separated by 1 or 7 days did not alter local control. This suggests that the malignant cells of MF have minimal ability to execute sublethal damage repair and provides justification for using low daily fraction sizes to minimize normal tissue toxicity without sacrificing local control. Collectively, these experiences demonstrate that curative treatment of localized MF requires total doses of at least 20 Gy and perhaps up to 30 Gy. To spare normal tissue toxicity and to ensure that patients can receive TSEBT in the future, a fraction size of 1.2 to 2.0 Gy is recommended.

A dose-response relationship has also been demonstrated with TSEBT. A meta-analysis of published results reported greater rates of complete remission when using greater prescribed doses and more penetrating electrons.[86] Historically, the Stanford University experience with 176 patients undergoing TSEBT from 1958 to 1975 revealed that complete response rates increased with total dose: 18% for 8 to 9.9 Gy, 55% for 10 to 19.9 Gy, 66% for 20 to 24.9 Gy, 75% for 25 to 29.9 Gy, and 94% for 30 to 36 Gy.[136] Similarly, patients treated with higher doses experienced improved overall survival, regardless of T stage. The experience at Hamilton Regional Cancer Center between 1977 and 1992 further supported the importance of high-dose TSEBT. From 1977 to 1980, 25 consecutive patients received 30 Gy TSEBT. From 1980 to 1992, 121 consecutive patients received 35 Gy TSEBT.[137] Treatment with high-dose TSEBT was an independent predictor of response, with a complete response rate of 64% for the 30 Gy group and 85% for the 36 Gy group. Given these data, the European Organization for the Research and Treatment of Cancer (EORTC) consensus statement recommended that modern TSEBT deliver a total dose of 31 to 36 Gy to the skin surface to produce a dose of 26 Gy at a depth of 4 mm in truncal skin along the central axis.[138]

Clinical Results—Limited Superficial Radiotherapy

Approximately 5% of patients with stage IA disease present with a single skin lesion, or with two or three lesions in close proximity, such that all clinically apparent disease can be encompassed by either one field or several abutting fields.[25] Radiotherapy is the treatment of choice in this situation. Results from three institutions have reported long-term disease-free survival in excess of 85%.[25,26,139] Wilson and coworkers[25] published a series of 21 patients with minimal stage IA disease managed with local, superficial radiotherapy. Ten were treated with 100 to 280 Kv and 11 with 4 to 12 MeV electrons with appropriate bolus. The median dose was 20 Gy, and 17 of 21 received ≥20 Gy. With a median follow up of 36 months, the rate of complete clinical remission was 97%, and the long-term, disease-free survival was 91% among patients receiving 20 Gy. Similarly, Micaily and others[26] reported an 86% 10-year disease-free survival in 18 patients with unilesional MF treated with localized radiotherapy to a median dose of 30.6 Gy. In summary, radiotherapy for unilesional stage IA disease is an excellent first-line therapy given minor acute and chronic toxicities and excellent long-term results. Because very few patients with two to four lesions have been reported in the literature, optimal treatment for this subgroup remains unclear. While some advocate limited superficial radiotherapy, others advocate a strategy such as TSEBT or PUVA to treat all skin surfaces.

CLINICAL RESULTS—TOTAL SKIN ELECTRON BEAM THERAPY

Limited Patches and/or Plaques: T1 N0 M0 (IA) and T1 N1 M0 (IIA)

Initial treatment options for patients with patches and/or plaques involving less than 10% body surface area include topical mechlorethamine, topical carmustine, phototherapy, bexarotene gel, and TSEBT. Currently, no randomized data exist to support selection of a radiation-based strategy over another topical strategy for this patient population. Although single-institution experiences suggest that patients managed with TSEBT may experience superior complete response rates and relapse-free survival, there is little strong evidence to suggest that this will translate into improved overall survival.

For example, patients with T1 disease treated with modern TSEBT experience a complete response rate of at least 90%[86,140] (Table 76-7), compared with a complete response rate of 65% to 70% for topical mechlorethamine.[71,89] Furthermore, 10-year relapse-free survival is approximately 50% for TSEBT[141]

Table 76-7 **Newly Diagnosed Patch Plaque Mycosis Fungoides Managed at Hamilton, Ontario***

	Stage IA				Stage IB			
Number receiving TSEB without adjuvant therapy	n = 143				n = 79			
Rate of complete remission	95%				89%			
Years of follow-up	2.5	5	10	15	2.5	5	10	15
Progression-free experience	62%	50%	40%	40%	44%	22%	12%	12%
Time to second progression[141]	94%	82%	66%	61%	88%	69%	49%	39%
Cause-specific survival (death from mycosis fungoides)	100%	99%	99%	96%	100%	98%	91%	91%
Overall survival (death from any cause)	99%	94%	89%	76%	99%	91%	80%	75%
Number receiving:								
TSEB with 60 sessions adjuvant PUVA	n = 11				n = 21			
Progression-free experience	100%	N/A	N/A	N/A	89%	N/A	N/A	N/A

*This table contains data from Hamilton updated through 2004 and representative of the results of TSEBT as first-line therapy for stage IA and IB. Results shown for 222 patients receiving TSEBT alone document high rates of complete remission. For those who fail TSEBT, limited second-line therapies[141] may produce prolonged remissions, as indicated by the time to second progression outcome measure. Results shown for 32 patients receiving TSEBT plus adjuvant PUVA indicate that PUVA significantly improves progression-free survival ($P = 0.03$), with follow-up under 5 years as of 2004.[141]

TSEBT, total skin electron beam therapy.

compared with 34% for mechlorethamine.[71] However, in this group of patients whose long-term survival is similar to healthy controls, initial treatment with TSEBT has not been associated with an overall survival advantage.[140] The administration of TSEBT for patients with stage IA MF remains controversial, and although some reserve TSEBT for those refractory to standard therapies, others recommend TSEBT as first-line therapy for even paucilesional stage IA disease.

Other first-line therapies for T1 MF include phototherapy and carmustine. For patients with limited patches, UVB therapy results in a complete response rate of approximately 80% with a median response duration of 2 years.[142,143] PUVA is appropriate for both patches and plaques, producing complete response rates of at least 80%. Although relapse is common, most patients will respond to additional PUVA.[144,145] Similar to mechlorethamine, topical BCNU produced a complete response rate of 86%, partial response rate of 12%, and 5-year relapse-free survival of 35%.[91]

For T1 disease that recurs after mechlorethamine, BCNU, UVB, or PUVA, retreatment with these agents may result in another response. Other options for recurrent or refractory T1 disease include TSEBT,[138] class I steroids (complete response 63%, partial response 31%),[92] interferon-α monotherapy (complete response 50%, partial response 35%),[100] topical bexarotene (complete response 21%, partial response 42%),[94] and oral bexarotene (complete response 7%, partial response 47%).[110]

For patients who recur after initial treatment with TSEBT, relapse is typically limited to <5% of the skin surface. Salvage treatments including spot radiation, topical steroids, mechlorethamine, or PUVA have all resulted in prolonged second remissions. For example, data from Hamilton showed that 70% of patients were free of disease 15 years after first-line TSEBT and second-line salvage treatments as needed.[141]

Extensive Patches and/or Plaques: T2 N0 M0 (IB) and T2 N1 M0 (IIa)

For patients in this group with either severe cutaneous symptoms or deeply infiltrative plaques, we favor TSEBT as initial treatment due to superior response rates that produce rapid palliation. For example, complete response rates for T2 disease range from 76% to 90% (see Table 76-7), compared with a complete response rate of 34% for topical mechlorethamine.[71,85,138] Adjuvant therapy following TSEBT is crucial for patients with T2 disease, as 10-year relapse-free survival is only 10% in those treated with TSEBT alone.[141] Retrospective data from Yale University found that patients receiving adjuvant PUVA experienced a 5-year disease-free survival of 85% versus 50% for those not receiving adjuvant PUVA.[84] A prospective pilot study at Hamilton documented a similar benefit (see Table 76-7). Retrospective data from Stanford University showed that patients treated with TSEBT and adjuvant topical mechlorethamine experienced 10-year relapse-free survival of approximately 40% compared to 10% with TSEBT alone.[85]

Patients with T2 disease who are relatively asymptomatic can receive treatment similar to that recommended for T1 disease. Again, topical mechlorethamine is a reasonable choice for these patients, resulting in a complete response rate of 34%, partial response rate of 38%, and 10-year relapse-free survival rate of 20%.[71] Similarly, BCNU produced a complete response rate of 47%, partial response rate of 37%, and 5-year relapse-free survival rate of 10%.[91] Topical corticosteroids may also be helpful for patients with extensive patches, with data suggesting a complete response rate of 25% and partial response rate of 57%.[92]

As an alternative to topical chemotherapy, topical phototherapy may be considered for extensive patch/plaque disease. UVB should be reserved for extensive patch disease only, due to its superficial penetration. In contrast, PUVA may be considered for patients with patches or thin plaques and has resulted in complete response rates of 60% to 100%.[92,144,145] Phase II trials suggest promising improvements in both complete response rate and duration of remission when adding IFN-α to PUVA for the treatment of T2 disease.[103,104,106]

Cutaneous Tumors: T3 N0-1 M0 (IIB)

Radiotherapy is an important treatment modality for cutaneous tumors due to its ability to treat the full thickness of deeply infiltrative lesions. For the rare patient with asymptomatic tumors involving less than 10% of the skin, either topical HN2 with local radiotherapy or TSEBT are reasonable first-line treatment options, with both producing a similar 5-year overall survival of approximately 50%.[85] However, most patients with T3 disease present with extensive, symptomatic tumors. Such patients often benefit from TSEBT as a first-line, palliative treatment, due to a superior complete response rate as compared with topical HN2 plus localized radiotherapy, 44% to 54% versus 8%.[85,86]

Adjuvant therapy should be strongly considered for patients who achieve a complete response to TSEBT. Retrospective data suggest that adjuvant topical mechlorethamine may improve the duration of response, resulting in 5-year relapse-free survival of 55% compared to 30% with TSEBT alone.[85] Adjuvant photopheresis is another reasonable option, with retrospective data reporting 5-year overall survival of 100% for patients receiving this modality compared with 50% in patients who did not receive adjuvant therapy.[116] Other adjuvant therapies worthy of consideration include IFN-α, bexarotene, and denileukin diftitox.[146]

Erythroderma: T4 N0-1 M0 (III)

TSEBT is an appropriate initial therapy for erythrodermic MF due to its ability to produce a rapid and sustained response, thereby ameliorating the severe cutaneous symptoms experienced by such patients. Retrospective data indicate that TSEBT monotherapy produced a 100% complete response rate and 5-year progression-free survival of 69% for patients with T4 N0 M0 B0 MF.[87] However, when including those with blood or visceral involvement, the complete response rate dropped to 74%, and only 36% remained progression-free at 5 years. Patients with erythroderma and blood or visceral involvement may benefit from adjuvant photopheresis, as retrospective data suggest that such treatment improves 2-year cause-specific survival from 69% without EP to 100% with EP.[117]

For patients without access to TSEBT, several other topical treatment options exist. For example, a series of 10 patients treated with PUVA reported a complete response rate of 70% and median progression-free survival of 5 months.[147] Although not studied in a randomized setting, prospective phase II experiences suggested that addition of IFN-α to PUVA may improve the duration of response.[102-104] Another option for T4 disease is photopheresis monotherapy, as 80% of patients will experience at least some cutaneous improvement.[96] Patients with a normal peripheral blood CD4/CD8 ratio appear more likely to respond.[115]

Total Skin Electron Therapy—Toxicity

TSEBT is generally well-tolerated, and toxicity is minimized by using low daily fraction sizes[148] and a shielding regimen that reduces the dose to eyes, ears, lips, hands, and feet. Common acute toxicities from TSEBT include pruritus, dry desquamation, erythema, alopecia, xerosis, bullae of the feet, edema of the hands and feet, hypohidrosis (diminished perspiration),[149] and loss of fingernails and toenails.[141,150] Rare acute side effects include gynecomastia in men, mild epistaxis, and mild parotiditis.[141] Because of the superficial penetration of electrons, patients do not experience gastrointestinal or hematologic toxicities. In general, TSEBT does not cause serious long-term complications,[151] although permanent nail dystrophy, xerosis, telangiectasias, partial scalp alopecia, and fingertip dysesthesias have been described.[138] Second cutaneous malignancies, including squamous cell carcinoma, basal cell carcinoma, and malignant melanoma, have been observed in patients treated with TSEBT, particularly in those exposed to multiple therapies that are themselves known to be mutagenic, such as PUVA and mechlorethamine.[90]

FOLLOW-UP

Follow-up after definitive treatment for MF is best carried out by a multidisciplinary team with expertise in CTCL. Because most patients managed with TSEBT now receive adjuvant treatment, they remain in close contact with their dermatologists every 1 to 3 months for many years. Biopsy of clinically borderline or suspicious lesions is important to document relapse and to rule out transformation to a large cell variant. In addition, close surveillance is required to detect treatment-related skin cancers and ensure that appropriate therapy is initiated promptly. Patients with an elevated CD4:CD8 ratio, LDH, or soluble IL-2 receptor level at initial diagnosis should have these values followed closely to determine response to therapy.

LOCALLY ADVANCED DISEASE AND PALLIATION

Young patients with locally advanced disease and a good performance status should be treated with curative intent. Although still experimental, limited experience suggests that allogeneic BMT should be strongly considered.[132,133,152] However, for most patients whose age or performance status preclude allogeneic transplant, treatment options include novel biologic agents, cytotoxic chemotherapy, and radiation. For example, oral bexarotene has shown efficacy in patients with relapsed or refractory MF, producing an overall response rate of 57% for stage IIB, 32% for stage III, 44% for stage IVA, and 40% for stage IVB.[109] Another option, denileukin diftitox, resulted in an overall response rate of 30% for patients with treatment-refractory stage IB-IVA disease.[111] Systemic chemotherapy should also be considered and may result in complete response rates of 20% to 60%.[126]

Radiotherapy plays an important role in the palliation of both cutaneous and extracutaneous disease. For those patients with extensive skin disease recurrent after TSEBT, a second course of TSEBT may produce substantial palliation with acceptable toxicity. At Yale University, 14 patients have received two courses of TSEBT and five have received three courses of TSEBT.[153] The median dose was 36 Gy for the first course, 18 Gy for the second, and 12 Gy for the third. After the second course, 86% achieved a complete response with a median disease-free interval of 11.5 months. In a similar experience from Stanford University, 15 patients received a second course of TSEBT to a median dose of 23 Gy.[154] The complete response rate was 40%, and the partial response rate was 60%. Toxicity was limited to xerosis, telangiectasias, pigment changes, and alopecia. Criteria for re-treatment include complete response to the initial course, an extended disease-free interval after the initial course, diffuse cutaneous involvement at relapse, and failure of other modalities.

Finally, patients with symptomatic nodal or visceral disease often benefit from a course of palliative megavoltage radiotherapy to a total dose of 20 to 30 Gy delivered in 2 to 3 Gy fractions.

TECHNIQUES OF IRRADIATION

Historical Development

Localized radiation was first used to treat MF in 1902, shortly after the discovery of x rays.[155] In 1939, Summerville reported treatment of extensive cutaneous MF with an "x-ray bath" of kilovoltage photons delivered with two large fields.[156] A total air exposure of 900 roentgen delivered in daily fractions of 10 roentgen produced a complete response. In 1945, Levin and Behrman proposed that the total air exposure at the skin surface should be 600 to 800 roentgen for patches or plaques and 1000 to 1600 roentgen for tumors.[157]

The development of TSEBT began in the early 1950s. Trump and colleagues[158] at the Massachusetts Institute of Technology used a Van de Graaff generator to produce a vertically oriented, stationary beam of 2.5 MeV electrons incident on a motorized couch. By placing the patient in the prone, supine, and lateral decubitus positions and translating the couch through the electron beam, all skin surfaces could receive a meaningful dose. This treatment approach produced complete responses in two patients with extensive MF. In 1960, Stanford University reported the first method for linear accelerator-based TSEBT.[159] With a patient standing 10 feet from the end of the accelerator, two fields were treated, one directed above the patient's head and a second directed below the patient's feet. This approach is known as the dual-field technique. In addition, patients were treated in two positions with respect to the accelerator: anteroposterior and posteroanterior. Over time, it became clear that increasing the number of treatment positions improved dose homogeneity in the lateral dimension.[160,161] Ultimately, Stanford adopted a six-treatment position technique in which patients stand in six different orientations with respect to the accelerator: anteroposterior, posteroanterior, right and left anterior oblique, and right and left posterior oblique.[162] Although commonly called the "six-field" technique, it should be remembered that two fields are actually treated for each of the six treatment positions.

The first clinical results of TSEBT were published in 1962 by a group from St. John's Hospital for Diseases of the Skin in London.[163] Using the dual-field, four-treatment position technique developed at Stanford, all five patients treated for MF experienced "very good" responses at total doses ranging from 12 to 18 Gy. However, four of five patients relapsed within 8 months and disease was difficult to control in the axillae and perineum due to underdosing. In 1971, Stanford University reported 107 patients with MF who received TSEBT between 1957 and 1968.[162] Using a variety of doses, they produced a 52% complete response rate. In addition, among patients with localized patches or plaques, 30% experienced long-term disease-free survival, providing the first evidence that MF could actually be cured.

Target Volumes

The target volume for patients with patch/plaque disease should include the epidermis and dermis.[86] The thickness of the epidermis varies from 0.05 to 0.50 mm and is greatest in the distal extremities. The thickness of the dermis varies from 1 to 4 mm and is greatest in the hands and feet. Therefore, the thickness of the skin varies from a minimum of approximately

2 mm on the trunk to a maximum of about 4.5 mm at the hands and soles of the feet.[86] As a result, the EORTC TSEBT consensus statement recommends that the 80% isodose line should be ≥4 mm deep to the skin surface to ensure that the epidermis and dermis fall within the high dose region. Due to their thickness, the deep margin of cutaneous tumors is often underdosed when treated with TSEBT alone and may require supplemental boosts with appropriately selected electrons or photons to ensure adequate dose delivery at depth.

Limited Superficial Radiotherapy

Minimal stage IA disease should be treated with a single radiation field where possible, although abutting fields may be required at a convex surface such as the scalp, an axillary fold, breast, hand, or foot. The junction of abutting fields should be shifted during the course of treatment to improve homogeneity. Field margins can be limited by lead cut-out to only 1 to 2 cm beyond the visible (or palpable) clinical lesion. Electrons of 6 to 16 MeV energy with appropriate bolus material are sufficient, and the dose should be approximately 30 Gy with the expectation of cure. One or several fields of 6 to 16 MeV electrons can also be used to encompass the limited volumes required to palliate symptomatic skin lesions, including most tumor nodules and skin ulcers. Although a single dose of 4 to 8 Gy may produce a complete response and full symptom relief, a fractionated dose of at least 20 Gy is more likely to achieve a complete and durable clinical remission.[25,86,134] Whether irradiating a limited region of the skin for cure or for palliation, dose prescriptions should specify conventional or lower doses per fraction (e.g., 1.2-2.0 Gy) and the total dose should be limited (e.g., 20-30 Gy). This preserves as much radiation tolerance of the skin as possible and enables future delivery of local radiotherapy or TSEBT without moderate-to-severe toxicities. Furthermore, in situations of co-existing cancer diagnoses (e.g., Hodgkin's, breast, prostate or rectal cancers), radiation treatments for those diagnoses must be carefully planned to minimize the superficial skin exposure to preserve the option of TSEBT in the future.

Node, Viscera, and Blood Radiotherapy

Nodal regions (e.g., axillary and inguinal) and some visceral organs (e.g., lungs, larynx, and brain) can be encompassed using standard beam arrangements and energies. Prescriptions are typically 20 to 30 Gy in 10 to 20 fractions over 2 to 4 weeks.

Several experiences using TSEBT in combination with either low-dose total body irradiation[164] or total nodal irradiation[165,166] have been reported. However, such treatment may increase the risk of secondary malignancies or myelodysplastic syndrome[166] and has not demonstrated superiority over conventional systemic agents. For patients undergoing allogeneic bone marrow transplantation, incorporation of total body irradiation in the preparative regimen may be beneficial.[132] A dose of 12 to 15 Gy in 6 to 10 fractions is recommended; single fractions are discouraged because of a lower therapeutic ratio.

TSEBT delivers a total dose to the blood and marrow of approximately 0.4 Gy in 30 or more fractions over 6 to 14 weeks. In general, hematologic values remain normal during a course of TSEBT. However, for those with Sézary syndrome, the number of circulating Sézary cells may fall by 50% to 95% and, in rare instances, may remain in a sustained remission.

Modern TSEBT

Technical advances since the initial Stanford and St. John's publications have included dose escalation to 35 to 36 Gy, improvements in shielding, and integration of boost treatments to underdosed regions, culminating in the publication of a consensus statement from the EORTC regarding appropriate techniques for TSEBT (Table 76-8).[138]

Table 76-8 EORTC Guidelines for Total Skin Electron Beam Therapy

- Dose inhomogeneity in air at treatment distance should be <10% within vertical and lateral dimensions
- 80% isodose line should be ≥ 4 mm deep to the skin surface to ensure that the epidermis and dermis fall within the high-dose region.
- 80% isodose line should receive a minimum total dose of 26 Gy.
- 20% isodose line should be < 20 mm from the skin surface to minimize dose to underlying structures
- 30 to 36 fractions should be used to minimize acute side effects.
- Total dose to bone marrow from photon contamination should be less than 0.7 Gy
- Patch treatments should be used to underdosed areas, such as the perineum, scalp, and soles of feet.
- Internal and external eye shields should be used to ensure that the dose to the globe is not more than 15% of the prescribed skin surface dose

Adapted from Jones GW, Kacinski BM, Wilson LD, et al: Total skin electron radiation in the management of mycosis fungoides: Consensus of the European Organization for Research and Treatment of Cancer (EORTC) Cutaneous Lymphoma Project Group. J Am Acad Dermatol 47:364-370, 2002.

The method of TSEBT used clinically at Yale achieves these objectives with a 6 MeV modern linear accelerator using the dual-field, six-treatment position technique. The patient stands 3.8 meters from the accelerator head, which rotates 17.5 degrees above and below horizontal to produce the dual fields. A 3.2 mm Lexan polycarbonate screen is placed in front of the patient and serves to attenuate and scatter the incident electrons, resulting in an electron energy of 3.9 MeV at the skin surface (Fig. 76-7). A total of six treatment positions are designated: anteroposterior, right and left anterior oblique, posteroanterior, and right and left posterior oblique (Fig. 76-8). These positions maximize skin unfolding, thereby improving dose homogeneity in the lateral dimension. Each position is treated with two fields, an upper field and a lower field, to maximize dose homogeneity in the vertical dimension. On treatment day one, the anteroposterior, right posterior oblique, and left posterior oblique positions are treated. On treatment day two, the posteroanterior, right anterior oblique, and left anterior oblique positions are treated with the same dose. Over the course of a 2-day treatment cycle, a patient will receive 2 Gy to the entire skin surface. This pattern continues, with patients receiving treatment 4 days a week for a total of 9 weeks, thereby delivering a total dose of 36 Gy to the skin surface (Table 76-9).

This technique places the dose maximum at 1 mm, the 80% isodose line at 6 mm, and the 20% isodose line at 12 mm,[167] thus satisfying the EORTC criteria for TSEBT.[141] Photon contamination due to bremsstrahlung scattering in the machine head, intervening air, scatterers or degraders, and patient, is acceptable at 1.2%. A comparison of the depth-dose curves for a single anteroposterior treatment position and for all six treatment positions is presented graphically in Figure 76-9 and by film dosimetry in Figure 76-10.[167] Using six treatment positions shifts the isodose curve toward the skin surface due to the obliquity of the incident electrons.

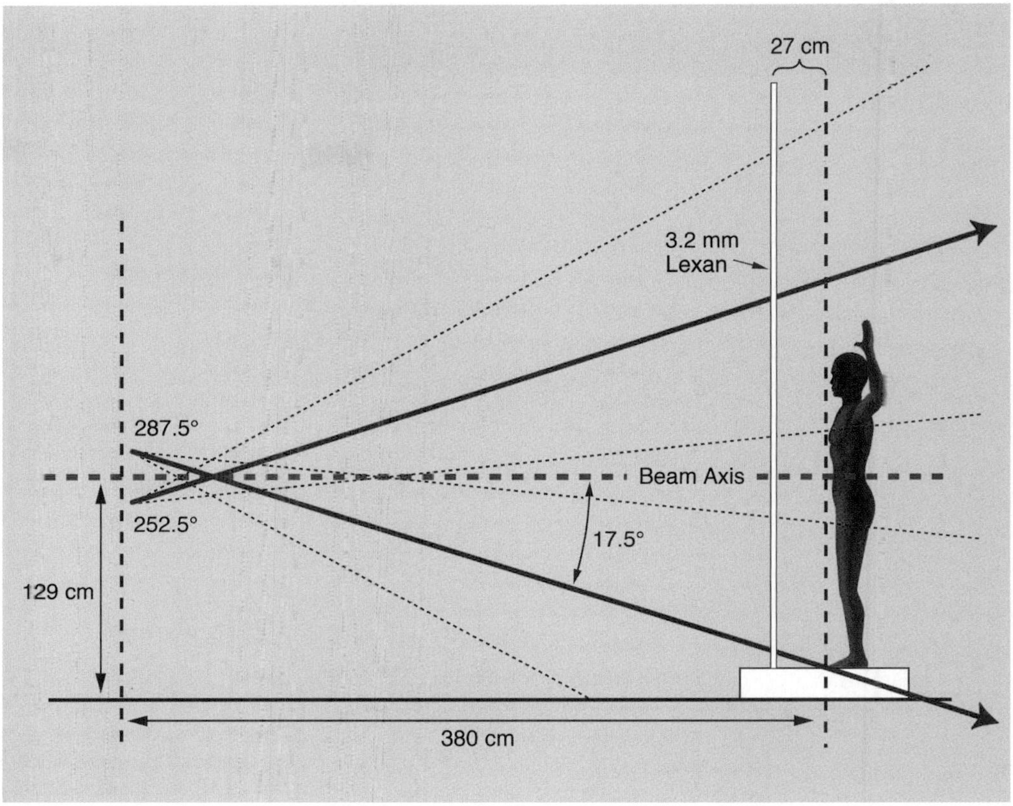

Figure 76-7 Geometry of dual-field total skin electron beam technique

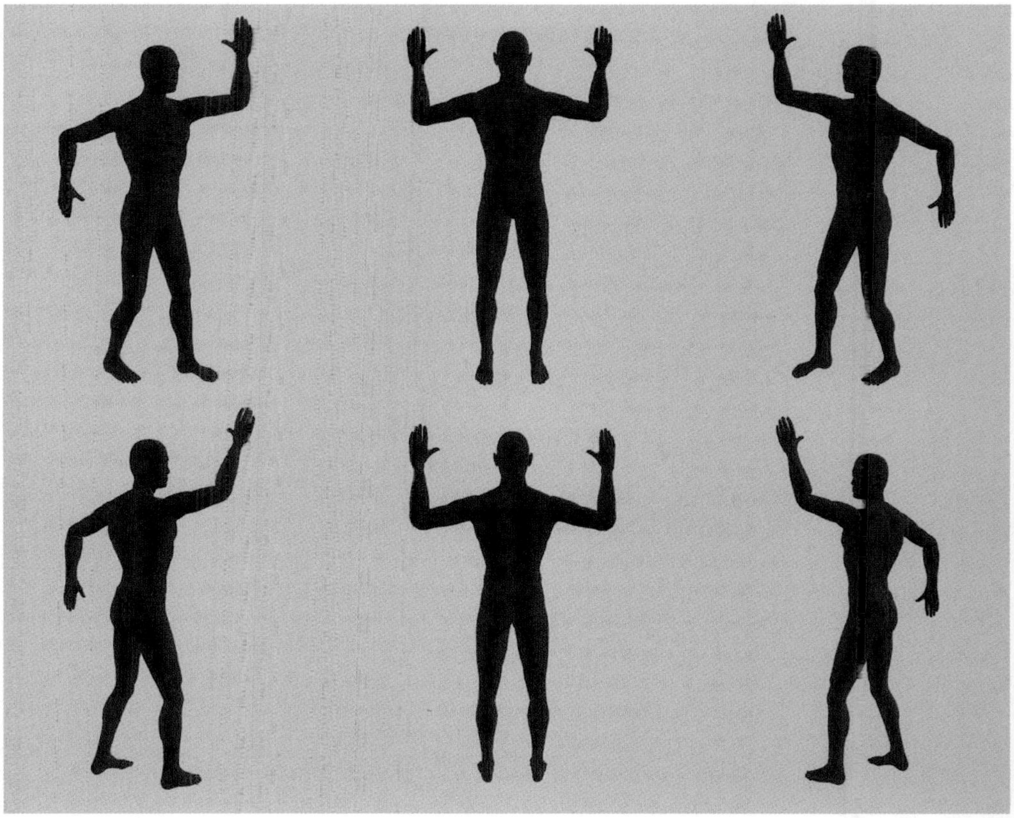

Figure 76-8 Treatment positions used in total skin electron beam therapy. Top row (*from left to right*): right anterior oblique, anteroposterior, and left anterior oblique treatment positions. Bottom row (*from left to right*): right posterior oblique, posteroanterior, and left posterior oblique treatment positions. (Reprinted with permission from Figure 1 in Smith BD, Wilson LD: Management of mycosis fungoides: Part 2. Treatment. Oncology 17:1419-1433, 2003.)

Table 76-9 Treatment Protocol at Yale-New Haven Hostpital

TREATMENT CYCLE	
Day 1	AP, RPO, LPO treatment positions
Day 2	PA, RAO, LAO treatment positions
DOSE	
Dose per cycle	2 Gy
Cycles per week	2
Total cycles	18
Total dose	36 Gy
BOOSTS	
Perineum	100 cGy/d, first 9 and last 9 treatment days
Soles of feet	100 cGy/d, first 7 and last 7 treatment days
BLOCKING	
External eye shields	First 11 cycles
Internal eye shields	Last 7 cycles
Lip shield	Cycles 1–4
Lead mitt for hands	Every other cycle
Fingernail shield	Every other cycle, alternating with mitts
Foot block	Cycles 1–3, 5, 7, 9, 11, 13, 15, 17, 18
Testicular shield	Used with perineal boost only

AP, anteroposterior; LAO, left anterior oblique; LPO, left posterior oblique; PA, posteroanterior; RAO, right anterior oblique; RPO, right posterior oblique.

Data from Chen Z, Agostinelli AG, Wilson LD, et al: Matching the dosimetry characteristics of a dual-field Stanford technique to a customized single-field Stanford technique for total skin electron therapy. Int J Radiat Oncol Biol Phys 59:872-885, 2004.

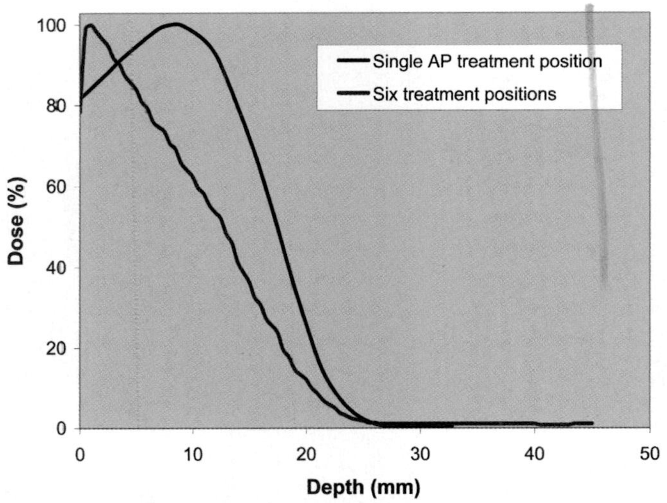

Figure 76-9 Depth dose curves for dual-field total skin electron beam therapy (TSEBT). *Blue line:* Depth dose curve for an anteroposterior dual-field 4 MeV electron beam incident on polystyrene, a tissue-equivalent material. Note that the surface receives approximately 80%, and that the maximum dose is deposited 8 mm from the surface. *Red line:* Depth dose curve for dual-field, six treatment position, standard TSEBT. Due to multiple beams entering the skin surface at oblique angles, the dose delivered to the skin surface rises dramatically, and drops to 80% by 8 mm.

(Graph courtesy of Zhe Chen, PhD; adapted with permission from Figures 6 and 11 in Chen Z, Agostinelli AG, Wilson LD, et al: Matching the dosimetry characteristics of a dual-field Stanford technique to a customized single-field Stanford technique for total skin electron therapy. Int J Radiat Oncol Biol Phys 59:872-885, 2004.)

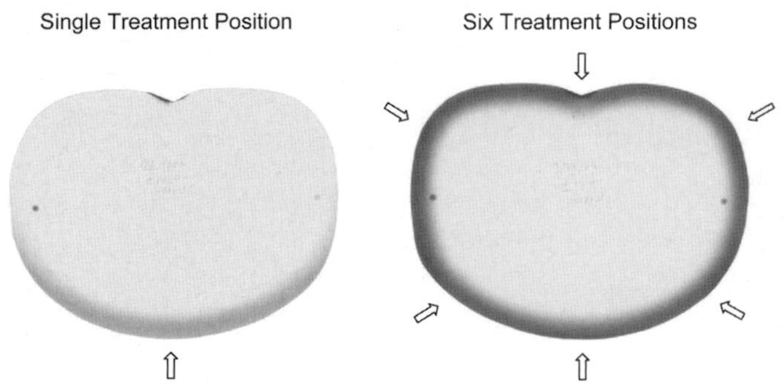

Figure 76-10 Axial film dosimetry for single treatment position and six treatment position techniques. The dark region is proportional to the electron dose delivered to the film. (Adapted with permission from Figure 5 in Chen Z, Agostinelli AG, Wilson LD, et al: Matching the dosimetry characteristics of a dual-field Stanford technique to a customized single-field Stanford technique for total skin electron therapy. Int J Radiat Oncol Biol Phys 59:872-885, 2004.)

Due to shielding inherent to these treatment positions, the soles of feet, perineum, and scalp are underdosed and always require supplemental treatment. 120 kV, HVL 4.2 mm Al, can be used to deliver patch treatments to the soles of feet (14 Gy, 14 fractions, treatment days 1-7 and 30-36) and perineum (18 Gy, 18 fractions, treatment days 1-9 and 28-36). The scalp dose can be supplemented with either orthovoltage patches (6-20 Gy over 1-3 weeks) or with an electron reflector mounted above the patient's head[168] (see Table 76-9). Other areas of potential underdosing include the ventral penis, the upper medial thighs, inframammary folds, folds under any pannus, and the lateral and flatter regions of the face and trunk. Supplemental patch fields, as guided by in vivo dosimetry or clinical suspicion, are appropriate for these regions, to ensure that the surface dose is at least 50% of the prescribed TSEBT dose.[169,170] When determining the total dose given in patch treatments, doses to areas such as the feet and perineum may be reduced as clinically indicated to enhance patient tolerance, provided such areas are uninvolved.

The hands, wrists, ears, ankles, and dorsal penis may be overdosed due to a variety of factors including tissue heterogeneity (e.g., bone), high convexity, and overlap between more than three of the six primary fields.[86] Thus, these regions should be shielded for a certain proportion of the treatments to reduce the total dose to 36 Gy or less. Detailed dosimetric measurements are typically required to determine the most appropriate shielding regimen for a particular treatment arrangement and patient geometry (see Table 76-9). Lead, bags containing rice, and plywood boards are appropriate methods of shielding. The eyes can be shielded with a combination of external eye shields and lead internal eye shields.[171] Although internal eye shields may cause conjunctival irritation and corneal abrasions, the risk is usually less than 1%.[141] The shielding regimen used at our institution and the resulting doses to various anatomic structures are presented in Tables 76-9 and 76-10.

Because many tumors have a thickness greater than 6 mm, TSEBT alone may result in significant underdosing. As a result, for patients with bleeding, weeping, or painful tumors at presentation, an initial or concurrent boost of 10 Gy in five fractions with either 6 to 16 MeV electrons or orthovoltage photons has been effective. In addition, asymptomatic plaques and tumors that persist at the end of treatment receive a similar boost to ensure adequate dose delivery at depth.

Table 76-10 **Dose to Anatomic Sites Using in vivo TLD Dosimetry**

	Dose Per 2-Day TSEBT Treatment Cycle*		Total Dose with Blocking and Boosts	
	Gy	*Percentage*	*Gy*	*Percentage*
Central axis	2.0	100	36	100
Top of head	2.3	115	41.4	115
Forehead	2.4	118	42.5	118
Eye	0.1	12	2.2	6
Eyelid	—	—	24.5	68
Lips	—	—	30	83
Posterior neck	2.1	104	37.4	104
Shoulder	1.7	87	31.3	87
Axilla	2.2	109	39.2	109
Hand	1.6	82	15.6	43
Mid-back	2.0	100	36	100
Umbilicus	2.1	104	37.4	104
Flank	2.0	99	35.6	99
Lateral thigh	1.9	95	34.2	95
Perineum	0.6	31	29	81
Top of feet	2.3	117	28.5	79
Soles of feet	0	0	14	39

*Dose using dual-field, six treatment position setup with scalp electron reflector and eye shields.
—, Not reported; TLD, thermal luminescent detector.
Data from Chen Z, Agostinelli AG, Wilson LD, et al: Matching the dosimetry characteristics of a dual-field Stanford technique to a customized single-field Stanford technique for total skin electron therapy. Int J Radiat Oncol Biol Phys 59:872-885, 2004.

OTHER RADIATION MANAGEMENT ISSUES

Cutaneous symptoms, including xerosis, pruritus, and pain from fissures or ulceration, are often severe and should be managed aggressively with topical steroids, emollients, oral antihistamines, and aggressive wound care with nonocclusive dressings.[73] Acute skin toxicity from TSEBT usually responds to the above measures, although treatment breaks of 1 to 2 weeks may occasionally be required.[172] Large bullae that develop during TSEBT should be lanced under sterile conditions and require nonocclusive dressings until they re-epithelialize.

As previously discussed, patients with advanced MF may experience a profound degree of immunosuppression. As a result, cutaneous and systemic infections are an important cause of morbidity and mortality. The most common infections include cellulitis due to *Staphylococcus aureus* or β-hemolytic streptococci, cutaneous herpes simplex or herpes zoster (both of which may disseminate cutaneously), bacteremia (most commonly with *S. aureus*), and bacterial pneumonia.[36] Signs and symptoms of such infections should be evaluated promptly and treated aggressively. Independent of MF, TSEBT also suppresses cutaneous immunity, likely due to destruction of normal skin-homing lymphocytes and epidermal antigen-presenting dendritic cells. Therefore, any new eruption that develops during the course of TSEBT should be evaluated promptly, as disseminated cutaneous bacterial, fungal, and viral infections are not uncommon[173] (Fig. 76-11).

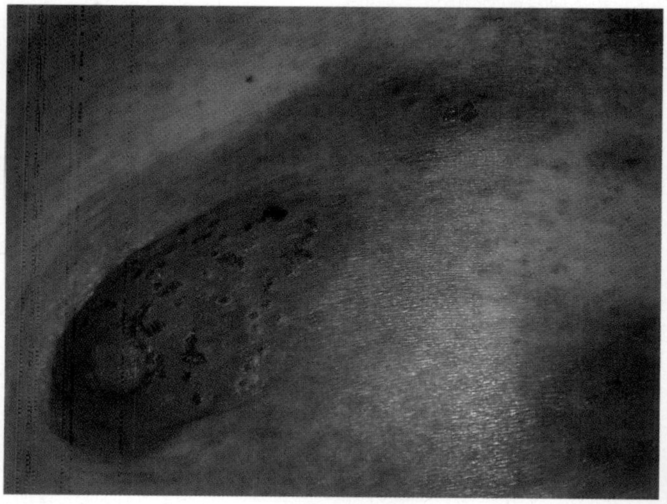

Figure 76-11 Disseminated herpes simplex during the course of total skin electron beam therapy (TSEBT). Patient developed a disseminated, pustular eruption shortly after beginning TSEBT. Numerous pustules were noted throughout the body, but all were localized to preexisting MF patches and plaques. Direct fluorescent antibody testing was positive for herpes simplex. (From Smith BD, Son CB, Wilson LD: Disseminated herpes simplex after total skin electron beam radiotherapy for mycosis fungoides. J R Soc Med 96:500-501, 2003.)

TREATMENT ALGORITHM, CONTROVERSIES, PROBLEMS, CHALLENGES, AND FUTURE POSSIBILITIES

A treatment algorithm for newly diagnosed and recurrent MF is presented in Table 76-11.[174] Multiple treatment options are listed, reflecting different institutional preferences and the paucity of randomized trials comparing different treatment modalities. A major challenge is the need for prospective randomized trials to compare radiation-based and non-radiation–based approaches to initial treatment. Adequately powered trials are problematic given the rarity of MF and difficulty in accruing patients. Thus, in the absence of randomized data, treatment will continue to be guided by institutional expertise and patient preference.

Table 76-11 **Treatment Recommendations by Stage**

Stage	Initial Treatment	Treatment for Relapsed or Refractory Disease
Unilesional patch *T1 N0 M0 (Stage IA)*	Localized, superficial radiotherapy Topical BCNU Topical HN_2 Topical bexarotene PUVA UVB	Same as initial treatment
Limited patch-plaque *T1 N0-1 M0 (Stage IA)*	Topical HN_2 Topical BCNU PUVA UVB (if only patches) Topical bexarotene TSEBT ± PUVA or HN_2	Same as initial treatment TSEBT Topical or oral bexarotene Interferon-α alone PUVA + interferon-α Topical corticosteroids
Extensive patch-plaque Symptoms controlled Minimal plaque thickness *T2 N0-1 M0 (Stage IA,IIA)*	Topical HN_2 Topical BCNU PUVA ± interferon-α UVB (if only patches) TSEBT + adjuvant PUVA or HN_2	Same as initial treatment TSEBT Topical or oral bexarotene Interferon-α alone Topical corticosteroids
Extensive patch-plaque Symptomatic Indurated plaques *T2 N0-1 M0 (Stage IB,IIA)*	TSEBT + adjuvant PUVA or HN_2	Topical HN_2 Topical BCNU PUVA + interferon-α Topical or oral bexarotene Topical corticosteroids Repeat TSEBT
Cutaneous tumors *T3 N0-1 M0 (Stage IIB)*	TSEBT + adjuvant HN_2 or photopheresis Bexarotene Denileukin diftitox	Topical HN_2 and local radiotherapy Oral bexarotene Denileukin diftitox Systemic chemotherapy Repeat TSEBT
Erythroderma *T4 N0-1 M0 (Stage III)*	TSEBT + adjuvant photopheresis PUVA + interferon-α Photopheresis alone Interferon-α	Methotrexate Oral bexarotene Denileukin diftitox Gemcitabine Fludarabine ± interferon-α Pentostatin ± interferon-α 2-chlorodeoxyadenosine Standard B-cell lymphoma chemotherapy Repeat TSEBT Allogeneic transplant
Nodal or visceral disease *Stage IV*	Clinical trial Allogeneic transplant Methotrexate TSEBT Topical HN_2 Topical BCNU PUVA + interferon-α Topical corticosteroids Localized, superficial radiotherapy	Same as initial treatment Systemic chemotherapy as listed
Transformed to large cell variant	Same as stage IV Consider rituximab if $CD20^+$ Trimetrexate Allogeneic transplant	Same as stage IV

BCNU, bischloroethylnitrosurea; HN_2, mechlorethamine; PUVA, psoralen plus ultraviolet A; TSEBT, total skin electron beam therapy; UVB, ultraviolet B.

Adapted with permission from Smith BD, Wilson LD: Management of mycosis fungoides: Part 2. Treatment. Oncology (Huntingt) 17:1419-1433, 2003 (Table 2).

The clinical management of patients with MF is complex and typically requires an interdisciplinary team approach that attends to the patient as a whole. Most patients require a fairly detailed understanding of the disease, its implications and risks, and all treatment options. Most patients are seeking a cure, which for some is unrealistic. Improvements in quality of life are possible, regardless of presenting stage. The relative contributions of various factors in determining quality of life have not been systematically explored. However, clinical experience indicates that the most salient factors are: controlling symptoms; achieving remission regardless of previous clinical trajectory; using treatments that are efficient and of limited duration (to be less disruptive to lifestyle and personal circumstances over the long term); addressing any anxiety and depression; and providing sustained and reliable support and expertise that extends into years and even decades of follow-up.

Many biologic and clinical questions pertaining to the pathophysiology and treatment of MF remain unanswered. For example, it is unclear whether the development of MF is initially driven by a specific exogenous antigen or by random mutational events occurring in activated T cells. In addition, the molecular factors that influence disease progression and response to various treatment modalities are just beginning to be elucidated. Clinically, the staging system requires major revision, and more studies with homogeneous patient populations are required to evaluate putative prognostic factors.

The future will likely bring additional novel systemic therapies for MF. For example, biologic and immunologic agents including monoclonal antibodies directed against CD4 and CD52 (alemtuzumab, Campath-1H), topical tazorotene (a novel retinoid), IL-2, IL-12, and individualized dendritic cell-based tumor vaccines are under investigation and may continue to improve the treatment of recurrent or refractory disease.[175,176] Strategies for integrating novel biologics with standard therapies such as TSEBT are needed to maximize the benefits of each. For those with advanced disease, a combination of TSEBT to induce cutaneous remission and biologic therapy to induce systemic remission shows the greatest promise for providing long-term disease control.

REFERENCES

1. Sander CA, Flaig MJ, Jaffe ES: Cutaneous manifestations of lymphoma: a clinical guide based on the WHO classification. Clin Lymphoma 2:86-100; discussion 101-102, 2001.
2. Willemze R, Kerl H, Sterry W, et al: EORTC classification for primary cutaneous lymphomas: a proposal from the Cutaneous Lymphoma Study Group of the European Organization for Research and Treatment of Cancer. Blood 90:354-371, 1997.
3. Alibert JLM: Tableau du Pian Fungoide Description des Maladies de la Peau, Observées à l'Hôpital Saint-Louis et Exposition des meilleurs Méthodes Suivies pour leur Traitement. Paris, Barrois L'Aine & Fils, 1806.
4. Sezary A, Bouvrain Y: Erythrodermie avec presence de cellules monstreuses dans derme et sang circulant. Bull Soc Fr Dermatol Syph 45:254-260, 1938.
5. Lutzner MA, Jordan HW: The ultrastructure of an abnormal cell in Sezary's syndrome. Blood 31:719-726, 1968.
6. Edelson RL, Berger CL, Raafat J, et al: Karyotype studies of cutaneous T cell lymphoma: evidence for clonal origin. J Invest Dermatol 73:548-550, 1979.
7. Jones GW, Thorson B: Cutaneous T-cell lymphoma (mycosis fungoides). Lancet 348:130-131, 1996.
8. Hoppe RT: Mycosis fungoides: radiation therapy. Dermatol Ther 16:347-354, 2003.
9. Weinstock MA, Horm JW: Mycosis fungoides in the United States. Increasing incidence and descriptive epidemiology. JAMA 260:42-46, 1988.
10. Surveillance, Epidemiology, and End Results (SEER) Program (*www.seer.cancer.gov*) SEER*Stat Database: Incidence—SEER 11 Regs + AK Public-Use, Nov 2003 Sub (1973-2001 varying), National Cancer Institute, DCCPS, Surveillance Research Program, Cancer Statistics Branch, released April 2004, based on the November 2003 submission.
11. Surveillance Research Program, National Cancer Institute SEER*Stat software (*www.seer.cancer.gov/seerstat*) version 5.2.2.
12. Kim HJ, Fay MP, Feuer EJ, Midthune DN: Permutation tests for joinpoint regression with applications to cancer rates. Stat Med 19:335-351, 2000; correction 20:655, 2001.
13. Joinpoint Regression Program, Version 2.7. September 2003; National Cancer Institute.
14. Weinstock MA, Reynes JF: The changing survival of patients with mycosis fungoides: a population- based assessment of trends in the United States. Cancer 85:208-212, 1999.
15. Weinstock MA, Gardstein B: Twenty-year trends in the reported incidence of mycosis fungoides and associated mortality. Am J Public Health 89:1240-1244, 1999.
16. Morales Suarez-Varela MM, Llopis Gonzalez A, Marquina Vila A, et al: Mycosis fungoides: review of epidemiological observations. Dermatology 201:21-28, 2000.
17. Herne KL, Talpur R, Breuer-McHam J, et al: Cytomegalovirus seropositivity is significantly associated with mycosis fungoides and Sezary syndrome. Blood 101:2132-2136, 2003.
18. Pancake BA, Wassef EH, Zucker-Franklin D: Demonstration of antibodies to human T-cell lymphotropic virus-I tax in patients with the cutaneous T-cell lymphoma, mycosis fungoides, who are seronegative for antibodies to the structural proteins of the virus. Blood 88:3004-3009, 1996.
19. Shohat M, Hodak E, Hannig H, et al: Evidence for the cofactor role of human T-cell lymphotropic virus type 1 in mycosis fungoides and Sezary syndrome. Br J Dermatol 141:44-49, 1999.
20. Wood GS, Salvekar A, Schaffer J, et al: Evidence against a role for human T-cell lymphotrophic virus type I (HTLV-I) in the pathogenesis of American cutaneous T-cell lymphoma. J Invest Dermatol 107:301-307, 1996.
21. Li G, Vowels BR, Benoit BM, et al: Failure to detect human T-lymphotropic virus type-I proviral DNA in cell lines and tissues from patients with cutaneous T-cell lymphoma. J Invest Dermatol 107:308-313, 1996.
22. Boni R, Davis-Daneshfar A, Burg G, et al: No detection of HTLV-I proviral DNA in lesional skin biopsies from Swiss and German patients with cutaneous T-cell lymphoma. Br J Dermatol 134:282-284, 1996.
23. Girardi M, Heald PW, Wilson LD: The pathogenesis of mycosis fungoides. N Engl J Med 350:1978-1988, 2004.
24. Heald PW, Glusac EJ: Unilesional cutaneous T-cell lymphoma: clinical features, therapy, and follow-up of 10 patients with a treatment-responsive mycosis fungoides variant. J Am Acad Dermatol 42:283-285, 2000.
25. Wilson LD, Kacinski BM, Jones GW: Local superficial radiotherapy in the management of minimal stage IA cutaneous T-cell lymphoma (Mycosis Fungoides). Int J Radiat Oncol Biol Phys 40:109-115, 1998.
26. Micaily B, Miyamoto C, Kantor G, et al: Radiotherapy for unilesional mycosis fungoides. Int J Radiat Oncol Biol Phys 42:361-364, 1998.
27. Zackheim HS, McCalmont TH: Mycosis fungoides: the great imitator. J Am Acad Dermatol 47:914-918, 2002.
28. Glusac EJ: Of cells and architecture: new approaches to old criteria in mycosis fungoides. J Cutan Pathol 28:169-173, 2001.
29. Santucci M, Biggeri A, Feller AC, et al: Efficacy of histologic criteria for diagnosing early mycosis fungoides: an EORTC cutaneous lymphoma study group investigation. European Organization for Research and Treatment of Cancer. Am J Surg Pathol 24:40-50, 2000.
30. Ashton-Key M, Diss TC, Du MQ, et al: The value of the polymerase chain reaction in the diagnosis of cutaneous T-cell infiltrates. Am J Surg Pathol 21:743-747, 1997.
31. Dadej K, Gaboury L, Lamarre L, et al: The value of clonality in the diagnosis and follow-up of patients with cutaneous T-cell infiltrates. Diagn Mol Pathol 10:78-88, 2001.
32. Li G, Chooback L, Wolfe JT, et al: Overexpression of p53 protein in cutaneous T cell lymphoma: relationship to large cell transformation and disease progression. J Invest Dermatol 110:767-770, 1998.
33. Mao X, Lillington D, Scarisbrick JJ, et al: Molecular cytogenetic analysis of cutaneous T-cell lymphomas: identification of common genetic alterations in Sezary syndrome and mycosis fungoides. Br J Dermatol 147:464-475, 2002.
34. Scarisbrick JJ, Mitchell TJ, Calonje E, et al: Microsatellite instability is associated with hypermethylation of the hMLH1 gene and reduced gene expression in mycosis fungoides. J Invest Dermatol 121:894-901, 2003.

35. van Doorn R, Dijkman R, Vermeer MH, et al: A novel splice variant of the Fas gene in patients with cutaneous T-cell lymphoma. Cancer Res 62:5389-5392, 2002.
36. Axelrod PI, Lorber B, Vonderheid EC: Infections complicating mycosis fungoides and Sezary syndrome. JAMA 267:1354-1358, 1992.
37. Kantor AF, Curtis RE, Vonderheid EC, et al: Risk of second malignancy after cutaneous T-cell lymphoma. Cancer 63:1612-1615, 1989.
38. Heald P, Yan SL, Edelson R: Profound deficiency in normal circulating T cells in erythrodermic cutaneous T-cell lymphoma. Arch Dermatol 130:198-203, 1994.
39. Bagot M, Nikolova M, Schirm-Chabanette F, et al: Crosstalk between tumor T lymphocytes and reactive T lymphocytes in cutaneous T cell lymphomas. Ann N Y Acad Sci 941:31-38, 2001.
40. Saed G, Fivenson DP, Naidu Y, et al: Mycosis fungoides exhibits a Th1-type cell-mediated cytokine profile whereas Sezary syndrome expresses a Th2-type profile. J Invest Dermatol 103:29-33, 1994.
41. Wasik MA, Vonderheid EC, Bigler RD, et al: Increased serum concentration of the soluble interleukin-2 receptor in cutaneous T-cell lymphoma. Clinical and prognostic implications. Arch Dermatol 132:42-47, 1996.
42. Smith BD, Wilson LD: Management of mycosis fungoides. Part 1. Diagnosis, staging, and prognosis. Oncology (Huntingt) 17:1281-1288, 2003.
43. Yazdi AS, Medeiros LJ, Puchta U, et al: Improved detection of clonality in cutaneous T-cell lymphomas using laser capture microdissection. J Cutan Pathol 30:486-491, 2003.
44. Gellrich S, Lukowsky A, Schilling T, et al: Microanatomical compartments of clonal and reactive T cells in mycosis fungoides: molecular demonstration by single cell polymerase chain reaction of T cell receptor gene rearrangements. J Invest Dermatol 115:620-624, 2000.
45. Smoller BR, Bishop K, Glusac E, et al: Reassessment of histologic parameters in the diagnosis of mycosis fungoides. Am J Surg Pathol 19:1423-1430, 1995.
46. Guitart J, Kennedy J, Ronan S, et al: Histologic criteria for the diagnosis of mycosis fungoides: proposal for a grading system to standardize pathology reporting. J Cutan Pathol 28:174-183, 2001.
47. Kohler S, Kim YH, Smoller BR: Histologic criteria for the diagnosis of erythrodermic mycosis fungoides and Sezary syndrome: a critical reappraisal. J Cutan Pathol 24:292-297, 1997.
48. Fung MA, Murphy MJ, Hoss DM, et al: Practical evaluation and management of cutaneous lymphoma. J Am Acad Dermatol 46:325-357, 2002.
49. Lu D, Patel KA, Duvic M, et al: Clinical and pathological spectrum of CD8-positive cutaneous T-cell lymphomas. J Cutan Pathol 29:465-472, 2002.
50. Delfau-Larue MH, Laroche L, Wechsler J, et al: Diagnostic value of dominant T-cell clones in peripheral blood in 363 patients presenting consecutively with a clinical suspicion of cutaneous lymphoma. Blood 96:2987-2992, 2000.
51. Wood GS, Tung RM, Haeffner AC, et al: Detection of clonal T-cell receptor gamma gene rearrangements in early mycosis fungoides/Sezary syndrome by polymerase chain reaction and denaturing gradient gel electrophoresis (PCR/DGGE). J Invest Dermatol 103:34-41, 1994.
52. Diamandidou E, Colome-Grimmer M, Fayad L, et al: Transformation of mycosis fungoides/Sezary syndrome: clinical characteristics and prognosis. Blood 92:1150-1159, 1998.
53. Vergier B, de Muret A, Beylot-Barry M, et al: Transformation of mycosis fungoides: clinicopathological and prognostic features of 45 cases. French Study Group of Cutaneous Lymphomas. Blood 95:2212-2218, 2000.
54. O'Quinn RP, Zic JA, Boyd AS: Mycosis fungoides d'emblee: CD30-negative cutaneous large T-cell lymphoma. J Am Acad Dermatol 43:861-863, 2000.
55. de Coninck EC, Kim YH, Varghese A, et al: Clinical characteristics and outcome of patients with extracutaneous mycosis fungoides. J Clin Oncol 19:779-784, 2001.
56. Sibaud V, Beylot-Barry M, Thiebaut R, et al: Bone marrow histopathologic and molecular staging in epidermotropic T-cell lymphomas. Am J Clin Pathol 119:414-423, 2003.
57. Graham SJ, Sharpe RW, Steinberg SM, et al: Prognostic implications of a bone marrow histopathologic classification system in mycosis fungoides and the Sezary syndrome. Cancer 72:726-734, 1993.
58. Vonderheid EC, Bernengo MG, Burg G, et al: Update on erythrodermic cutaneous T-cell lymphoma: report of the International Society for Cutaneous Lymphomas. J Am Acad Dermatol 46:95-106, 2002.
59. Vergier B, Beylot-Barry M, Beylot C, et al: Pilotropic cutaneous T-cell lymphoma without mucinosis. A variant of mycosis fungoides? French Study Group of Cutaneous Lymphomas. Arch Dermatol 132:683-687, 1996.
60. Wilson LD, Cooper DL, Goodrich AL, et al: Impact of non-CTCL dermatologic diagnoses and adjuvant therapies on cutaneous T-cell lymphoma patients treated with total skin electron beam radiation therapy. Int J Radiat Oncol Biol Phys 28:829-837, 1994.
61. LeBoit PE: Granulomatous slack skin. Dermatol Clin 12:375-389, 1994.
62. Liu HL, Hoppe RT, Kohler S, et al: CD30+ cutaneous lymphoproliferative disorders: the Stanford experience in lymphomatoid papulosis and primary cutaneous anaplastic large cell lymphoma. J Am Acad Dermatol 49:1049-1058, 2003.
63. Siegel RS, Pandolfino T, Guitart J, et al: Primary cutaneous T-cell lymphoma: review and current concepts. J Clin Oncol 18:2908-2925, 2000.
64. Cabanillas F, Armitage J, Pugh WC, et al: Lymphomatoid papulosis: a T-cell dyscrasia with a propensity to transform into malignant lymphoma. Ann Intern Med 122:210-217, 1995.
65. Beljaards RC, Willemze R: The prognosis of patients with lymphomatoid papulosis associated with malignant lymphomas. Br J Dermatol 126:596-602, 1992.
66. Bunn PA, Jr., Schechter GP, Jaffe E, et al: Clinical course of retrovirus-associated adult T-cell lymphoma in the United States. N Engl J Med 309:257-264, 1983.
67. Hollsberg P, Hafler DA: Seminars in medicine of the Beth Israel Hospital, Boston. Pathogenesis of diseases induced by human lymphotropic virus type I infection. N Engl J Med 328:1173-1182, 1993.
68. Di Venuti G, Nawgiri R, Foss F: Denileukin diftitox and hyper-CVAD in the treatment of human T-cell lymphotropic virus 1-associated acute T-cell leukemia/lymphoma. Clin Lymphoma 4:176-178, 2003.
69. Hermine O, Bouscary D, Gessain A, et al: Brief report: treatment of adult T-cell leukemia-lymphoma with zidovudine and interferon alfa. N Engl J Med 332:1749-1751, 1995.
70. Greene FL, Page DL, Fleming ID, et al: AJCC Cancer Staging Handbook, 6th ed. New York, Springer, 2002.
71. Kim YH, Martinez G, Varghese A, et al: Topical nitrogen mustard in the management of mycosis fungoides: update of the Stanford experience. Arch Dermatol 139:165-173, 2003.
72. Kashani-Sabet M, McMillan A, Zackheim HS: A modified staging classification for cutaneous T-cell lymphoma. J Am Acad Dermatol 45:700-706, 2001.
73. Kim YH, Hoppe RT: Mycosis fungoides and the Sezary syndrome. Semin Oncol 26:276-289, 1999.
74. Vonderheid EC, Diamond LW, van Vloten WA, et al: Lymph node classification systems in cutaneous T-cell lymphoma. Evidence for the utility of the Working Formulation of Non-Hodgkin's Lymphomas for Clinical Usage. Cancer 73:207-218, 1994.
75. Diamandidou E, Colome M, Fayad L, et al: Prognostic factor analysis in mycosis fungoides/Sezary syndrome. J Am Acad Dermatol 40:914-924, 1999.
76. Hoppe RT, Medeiros LJ, Warnke RA, et al: CD8-positive tumor-infiltrating lymphocytes influence the long-term survival of patients with mycosis fungoides. J Am Acad Dermatol 32:448-453, 1995.
77. Quiros PA, Kacinski BM, Wilson LD: Extent of skin involvement as a prognostic indicator of disease free and overall survival of patients with T3 cutaneous T-cell lymphoma treated with total skin electron beam radiation therapy. Cancer 77:1912-1917, 1996.
78. Delfau-Larue MH, Dalac S, Lepage E, et al: Prognostic significance of a polymerase chain reaction-detectable dominant T-lymphocyte clone in cutaneous lesions of patients with mycosis fungoides. Blood 92:3376-3380, 1998.

79. Guitart J, Camisa C, Ehrlich M, et al: Long-term implications of T-cell receptor gene rearrangement analysis by Southern blot in patients with cutaneous T-cell lymphoma. J Am Acad Dermatol 48:775-779, 2003.
80. Beylot-Barry M, Sibaud V, Thiebaut R, et al: Evidence that an identical T cell clone in skin and peripheral blood lymphocytes is an independent prognostic factor in primary cutaneous T cell lymphomas. J Invest Dermatol 117:920-926, 2001.
81. Bakels V, Van Oostveen JW, Geerts ML, et al: Diagnostic and prognostic significance of clonal T-cell receptor beta gene rearrangements in lymph nodes of patients with mycosis fungoides. J Pathol 170:249-255, 1993.
82. Kim YH, Bishop K, Varghese A, et al: Prognostic factors in erythrodermic mycosis fungoides and the Sezary syndrome. Arch Dermatol 131:1003-1008, 1995.
83. Bass JC, Korobkin MT, Cooper KD, et al: Cutaneous T-cell lymphoma: CT in evaluation and staging. Radiology 186:273-278, 1993.
84. Quiros PA, Jones GW, Kacinski BM, et al: Total skin electron beam therapy followed by adjuvant psoralen/ultraviolet-A light in the management of patients with T1 and T2 cutaneous T-cell lymphoma (mycosis fungoides). Int J Radiat Oncol Biol Phys 38:1027-1035, 1997.
85. Chinn DM, Chow S, Kim YH, et al: Total skin electron beam therapy with or without adjuvant topical nitrogen mustard or nitrogen mustard alone as initial treatment of T2 and T3 mycosis fungoides. Int J Radiat Oncol Biol Phys 43:951-958, 1999.
86. Jones GW, Hoppe RT, Glatstein E: Electron beam treatment for cutaneous T-cell lymphoma. Hematol Oncol Clin North Am 9:1057-1076, 1995.
87. Jones GW, Rosenthal D, Wilson LD: Total skin electron radiation for patients with erythrodermic cutaneous T-cell lymphoma (mycosis fungoides and the Sezary syndrome). Cancer 85:1985-1995, 1999.
88. Esteve E, Bagot M, Joly P, et al: A prospective study of cutaneous intolerance to topical mechlorethamine therapy in patients with cutaneous T-cell lymphomas. French Study Group of Cutaneous Lymphomas. Arch Dermatol 135:1349-1353, 1999.
89. Vonderheid EC, Tan ET, Kantor AF, et al: Long-term efficacy, curative potential, and carcinogenicity of topical mechlorethamine chemotherapy in cutaneous T cell lymphoma. J Am Acad Dermatol 20:416-428, 1989.
90. Licata AG, Wilson LD, Braverman IM, et al: Malignant melanoma and other second cutaneous malignancies in cutaneous T-cell lymphoma. The influence of additional therapy after total skin electron beam radiation. Arch Dermatol 131:432-435, 1995.
91. Zackheim HS, Epstein EH, Jr., Crain WR: Topical carmustine (BCNU) for cutaneous T cell lymphoma: a 15-year experience in 143 patients. J Am Acad Dermatol 22:802-810, 1990.
92. Zackheim HS, Kashani-Sabet M, Amin S: Topical corticosteroids for mycosis fungoides. Experience in 79 patients. Arch Dermatol 134:949-954, 1998.
93. Talpur R, Ward S, Apisarnthanarax N, et al: Optimizing bexarotene therapy for cutaneous T-cell lymphoma. J Am Acad Dermatol 47:672-684, 2002.
94. Breneman D, Duvic M, Kuzel T, et al: Phase 1 and 2 trial of bexarotene gel for skin-directed treatment of patients with cutaneous T-cell lymphoma. Arch Dermatol 138:325-332, 2002.
95. Heald P, Mehlmauer M, Martin AG, et al: Topical bexarotene therapy for patients with refractory or persistent early-stage cutaneous T-cell lymphoma: results of the phase III clinical trial. J Am Acad Dermatol 49:801-815, 2003.
96. Edelson R, Berger C, Gasparro F, et al: Treatment of cutaneous T-cell lymphoma by extracorporeal photochemotherapy. Preliminary results. N Engl J Med 316:297-303, 1987.
97. British Photodermatology Group guidelines for PUVA. Br J Dermatol 130:246-255, 1994.
98. Young AR: Carcinogenicity of UVB phototherapy assessed. Lancet 345:1431-1432, 1995.
99. Abel EA, Sendagorta E, Hoppe RT: Cutaneous malignancies and metastatic squamous cell carcinoma following topical therapies for mycosis fungoides. J Am Acad Dermatol 14:1029-1038, 1986.
100. Ross C, Tingsgaard P, Jorgensen H, et al: Interferon treatment of cutaneous T-cell lymphoma. Eur J Haematol 51:63-72, 1993.
101. Jumbou O, N'Guyen JM, Tessier MH, et al: Long-term follow-up in 51 patients with mycosis fungoides and Sezary syndrome treated by interferon-alfa. Br J Dermatol 140:427-431, 1999.
102. Roenigk HH, Jr., Kuzel TM, Skoutelis AP, et al: Photochemotherapy alone or combined with interferon alpha-2a in the treatment of cutaneous T-cell lymphoma. J Invest Dermatol 95:198S-205S, 1990.
103. Kuzel TM, Roenigk HH, Jr., Samuelson E, et al: Effectiveness of interferon alfa-2a combined with phototherapy for mycosis fungoides and the Sezary syndrome. J Clin Oncol 13:257-263, 1995.
104. Chiarion-Sileni V, Bononi A, Fornasa CV, et al: Phase II trial of interferon-alpha-2a plus psolaren with ultraviolet light A in patients with cutaneous T-cell lymphoma. Cancer 95:569-575, 2002.
105. Wollina U, Looks A, Meyer J, et al: Treatment of stage II cutaneous T-cell lymphoma with interferon alfa-2a and extracorporeal photochemotherapy: a prospective controlled trial. J Am Acad Dermatol 44:253-260, 2001.
106. Stadler R, Otte HG, Luger T, et al: Prospective randomized multicenter clinical trial on the use of interferon-2a plus acitretin versus interferon-2a plus PUVA in patients with cutaneous T-cell lymphoma stages I and II. Blood 92:3578-3581, 1998.
107. Thomsen K, Hammar H, Molin L, et al: Retinoids plus PUVA (RePUVA) and PUVA in mycosis fungoides, plaque stage. A report from the Scandinavian Mycosis Fungoides Group. Acta Derm Venereol 69:536-538, 1989.
108. Jones G, McLean J, Rosenthal D, et al: Combined treatment with oral etretinate and electron beam therapy in patients with cutaneous T-cell lymphoma (mycosis fungoides and Sezary syndrome). J Am Acad Dermatol 26:960-967, 1992.
109. Duvic M, Hymes K, Heald P, et al: Bexarotene is effective and safe for treatment of refractory advanced-stage cutaneous T-cell lymphoma: multinational phase II-III trial results. J Clin Oncol 19:2456-2471, 2001.
110. Duvic M, Martin AG, Kim Y, et al: Phase 2 and 3 clinical trial of oral bexarotene (Targretin capsules) for the treatment of refractory or persistent early-stage cutaneous T-cell lymphoma. Arch Dermatol 137:581-593, 2001.
111. Olsen E, Duvic M, Frankel A, et al: Pivotal phase III trial of two dose levels of denileukin diftitox for the treatment of cutaneous T-cell lymphoma. J Clin Oncol 19:376-388, 2001.
112. Foss FM, Bacha P, Osann KE, et al: Biological correlates of acute hypersensitivity events with DAB(389)IL-2 (denileukin diftitox, ONTAK) in cutaneous T-cell lymphoma: decreased frequency and severity with steroid premedication. Clin Lymphoma 1:298-302, 2001.
113. Lim HW, Edelson RL: Photopheresis for the treatment of cutaneous T-cell lymphoma. Hematol Oncol Clin North Am 9:1117-1126, 1995.
114. Berger CL, Hanlon D, Kanada D, et al: Transimmunization, a novel approach for tumor immunotherapy. Transfus Apheresis Sci 26:205-216, 2002.
115. Heald P, Rook A, Perez M, et al: Treatment of erythrodermic cutaneous T-cell lymphoma with extracorporeal photochemotherapy. J Am Acad Dermatol 27:427-433, 1992.
116. Wilson LD, Licata AL, Braverman IM, et al: Systemic chemotherapy and extracorporeal photochemotherapy for T3 and T4 cutaneous T-cell lymphoma patients who have achieved a complete response to total skin electron beam therapy. Int J Radiat Oncol Biol Phys 32:987-995, 1995.
117. Wilson LD, Jones GW, Kim D, et al: Experience with total skin electron beam therapy in combination with extracorporeal photopheresis in the management of patients with erythrodermic (T4) mycosis fungoides. J Am Acad Dermatol 43:54-60, 2000.
118. Kaye FJ, Bunn PA, Jr., Steinberg SM, et al: A randomized trial comparing combination electron-beam radiation and chemotherapy with topical therapy in the initial treatment of mycosis fungoides. N Engl J Med 321:1784-1790, 1989.
119. Zackheim HS, Kashani-Sabet M, Hwang ST: Low-dose methotrexate to treat erythrodermic cutaneous T-cell lymphoma:

results in twenty-nine patients. J Am Acad Dermatol 34:626-631, 1996.
120. Wollina U, Dummer R, Brockmeyer NH, et al: Multicenter study of pegylated liposomal doxorubicin in patients with cutaneous T-cell lymphoma. Cancer 98:993-1001, 2003.
121. Foss FM, Ihde DC, Linnoila IR, et al: Phase II trial of fludarabine phosphate and interferon alfa-2a in advanced mycosis fungoides/Sezary syndrome. J Clin Oncol 12:2051-2059, 1994.
122. Foss FM, Ihde DC, Breneman DL, et al: Phase II study of pentostatin and intermittent high-dose recombinant interferon alfa-2a in advanced mycosis fungoides/Sezary syndrome. J Clin Oncol 10:1907-1913, 1992.
123. Greiner D, Olsen EA, Petroni G: Pentostatin (2′-deoxycoformycin) in the treatment of cutaneous T-cell lymphoma. J Am Acad Dermatol 36:950-955, 1997.
124. Kuzel TM, Hurria A, Samuelson E, et al: Phase II trial of 2-chlorodeoxyadenosine for the treatment of cutaneous T-cell lymphoma. Blood 87:906-911, 1996.
125. Sarris AH, Phan A, Duvic M, et al: Trimetrexate in relapsed T-cell lymphoma with skin involvement. J Clin Oncol 20:2876-2880, 2002.
126. Rosen ST, Foss FM: Chemotherapy for mycosis fungoides and the Sezary syndrome. Hematol Oncol Clin North Am 9:1109-1116, 1995.
127. Zinzani PL, Baliva G, Magagnoli M, et al: Gemcitabine treatment in pretreated cutaneous T-cell lymphoma: experience in 44 patients. J Clin Oncol 18:2603-2606, 2000.
128. Bigler RD, Crilley P, Micaily B, et al: Autologous bone marrow transplantation for advanced stage mycosis fungoides. Bone Marrow Transplant 7:133-137, 1991.
129. Russell-Jones R, Child F, Olavarria E, et al: Autologous peripheral blood stem cell transplantation in tumor-stage mycosis fungoides: predictors of disease-free survival. Ann N Y Acad Sci 941:147-154, 2001.
130. Sterling JC, Marcus R, Burrows NP, et al: Erythrodermic mycosis fungoides treated with total body irradiation and autologous bone marrow transplantation. Clin Exp Dermatol 20:73-75, 1995.
131. Burt RK, Guitart J, Traynor A, et al: Allogeneic hematopoietic stem cell transplantation for advanced mycosis fungoides: evidence of a graft-versus-tumor effect. Bone Marrow Transplant 25:111-113, 2000.
132. Guitart J, Wickless SC, Oyama Y, et al: Long-term remission after allogeneic hematopoietic stem cell transplantation for refractory cutaneous T-cell lymphoma. Arch Dermatol 138:1359-1365, 2002.
133. Soligo D, Ibatici A, Berti E, et al: Treatment of advanced mycosis fungoides by allogeneic stem-cell transplantation with a nonmyeloablative regimen. Bone Marrow Transplant 31:663-666, 2003.
134. Cotter GW, Baglan RJ, Wasserman TH, et al: Palliative radiation treatment of cutaneous mycosis fungoides—a dose response. Int J Radiat Oncol Biol Phys 9:1477-1480, 1983.
135. Kim JH, Nisce LZ, D'Anglo GJ: Dose-time fractionation study in patients with mycosis fungoides and lymphoma cutis. Radiology 119:439-442, 1976.
136. Hoppe RT, Fuks Z, Bagshaw MA: The rationale for curative radiotherapy in mycosis fungoides. Int J Radiat Oncol Biol Phys 2:843-851, 1977.
137. Jones GW, Tadros A, Hodson DI, et al: Prognosis with newly diagnosed mycosis fungoides after total skin electron radiation of 30 or 35 Gy. Int J Radiat Oncol Biol Phys 28:839-845, 1994.
138. Jones GW, Kacinski BM, Wilson LD, et al: Total skin electron radiation in the management of mycosis fungoides: Consensus of the European Organization for Research and Treatment of Cancer (EORTC) Cutaneous Lymphoma Project Group. J Am Acad Dermatol 47:364-370, 2002.
139. Wong R, Jones G, Farrar N, et al: Local superficial radiotherapy (LSRT) for newly diagnosed stage IA patch-plaque mycosis fungoides (MF) with only one, two, or three presenting lesions. Int J Radiat Oncol Biol Phys 57(Suppl 1):S289-S290, 2003.
140. Kim YH, Jensen RA, Watanabe GL, et al: Clinical stage IA (limited patch and plaque) mycosis fungoides. A long-term outcome analysis. Arch Dermatol 132:1309-1313, 1996.
141. Jones G, Wilson LD, Fox-Goguen L: Total skin electron beam radiotherapy for patients who have mycosis fungoides. Hematol Oncol Clin North Am 17:1421-1434, 2003.
142. Ramsay DL, Lish KM, Yalowitz CB, et al: Ultraviolet-B phototherapy for early-stage cutaneous T-cell lymphoma. Arch Dermatol 128:931-933, 1992.
143. Diederen PV, van Weelden H, Sanders CJ, et al: Narrowband UVB and psoralen-UVA in the treatment of early-stage mycosis fungoides: a retrospective study. J Am Acad Dermatol 48:215-219, 2003.
144. Herrmann JJ, Roenigk HH, Jr., Hurria A, et al: Treatment of mycosis fungoides with photochemotherapy (PUVA): long-term follow-up. J Am Acad Dermatol 33:234-242, 1995.
145. Honigsmann H, Brenner W, Rauschmeier W, et al: Photochemotherapy for cutaneous T cell lymphoma. A follow-up study. J Am Acad Dermatol 10:238-245, 1984.
146. Rook AH, Kuzel TM, Olsen EA: Cytokine therapy of cutaneous T-cell lymphoma: interferons, interleukin-12, and interleukin-2. Hematol Oncol Clin North Am 17:1435-1448, ix, 2003.
147. Abel EA, Sendagorta E, Hoppe RT, et al: PUVA treatment of erythrodermic and plaque-type mycosis fungoides. Ten-year follow-up study. Arch Dermatol 123:897-901, 1987.
148. Rosenblatt E, Kuten A, Leviov M, et al: Total skin electron irradiation in mycosis fungoides dose and fractionation considerations. Leuk Lymphoma 30:143-151, 1998.
149. Price NM: Electron beam therapy. Its effect on eccrine gland function in mycosis fungoides patients. Arch Dermatol 115:1068-1070, 1979.
150. Desai KR, Pezner RD, Lipsett JA, et al: Total skin electron irradiation for mycosis fungoides: relationship between acute toxicities and measured dose at different anatomic sites. Int J Radiat Oncol Biol Phys 15:641-645, 1988.
151. Price NM: Radiation dermatitis following electron beam therapy. An evaluation of patients ten years after total skin irradiation for mycosis fungoides. Arch Dermatol 114:63-66, 1978.
152. Masood N, Russell KJ, Olerud JE, et al: Induction of complete remission of advanced stage mycosis fungoides by allogeneic hematopoietic stem cell transplantation. J Am Acad Dermatol 47:140-145, 2002.
153. Wilson LD, Quiros PA, Kolenik SA, et al: Additional courses of total skin electron beam therapy in the treatment of patients with recurrent cutaneous T-cell lymphoma. J Am Acad Dermatol 35:69-73, 1996.
154. Becker M, Hoppe RT, Knox SJ: Multiple courses of high-dose total skin electron beam therapy in the management of mycosis fungoides. Int J Radiat Oncol Biol Phys 32:1445-1449, 1995.
155. Scholtz W: Ueber den Einfluess def Rontgenstrahlen auf die Haut in gesundem und krankem Zustande. Arch Dermatol Syph 59:421-449, 1902.
156. Sommerville J: Mycosis fungoides treated with general x-ray "bath." Br J Dermatol Syph 51:323-324, 1939.
157. Levin OL, Behrman HT: Roentgen ray therapy of mycosis fungoides. Arch Dermatol Syph 51:307-308, 1945.
158. Trump G, Wright KA, Evans WW, et al: High energy electrons for the treatment of extensive superficial malignant lesions. Am J Roentgenol Rad Ther 69:623-629, 1953.
159. Karzmark CJ, Loevinger R, Steele RE, et al: A technique for large-field, superficial electron therapy. Radiology 74:633-643, 1960.
160. Page V, Gardner A, Karzmark CJ: Patient dosimetry in the electron treatment of large superficial lesions. Radiology 94:635-641, 1970.
161. Bjarngard BE, Chen GT, Piontek RW, et al: Analysis of dose distributions in whole body superficial electron therapy. Int J Radiat Oncol Biol Phys 2:319-324, 1977.
162. Fuks Z, Bagshaw MA: Total-skin electron treatment of mycosis fungoides. Radiology 100:145-150, 1971.
163. Szur L, Silvester JA, Bewley DK: Treatment of the whole body surface with electrons. Lancet 1:1373-1377, 1962.
164. Halberg FE, Fu KK, Weaver KA, et al: Combined total body X-ray irradiation and total skin electron beam radiotherapy with an improved technique for mycosis fungoides. Int J Radiat Oncol Biol Phys 17:427-432, 1989.

165. Micaily B, Vonderheid EC, Brady LW, et al: Total skin electron beam and total nodal irradiation for treatment of patients with cutaneous T-cell lymphoma. Int J Radiat Oncol Biol Phys 11:1111-1115, 1985.
166. Micaily B, Campbell O, Moser C, et al: Total skin electron beam and total nodal irradiation of cutaneous T-cell lymphoma. Int J Radiat Oncol Biol Phys 20:809-813, 1991.
167. Chen Z, Agostinelli AG, Wilson LD, et al: Matching the dosimetry characteristics of a dual-field Stanford technique to a customized single-field Stanford technique for total skin electron therapy. Int J Radiat Oncol Biol Phys 59:872-885, 2004.
168. Peters VG: Use of an electron reflector to improve dose uniformity at the vertex during total skin electron therapy. Int J Radiat Oncol Biol Phys 46:1065-1069, 2000.
169. Gamble LM, Farrell TJ, Jones GW, et al: Composite depth dose measurement for total skin electron (TSE) treatments using radiochromic film. Phys Med Biol 48:891-898, 2003.
170. Anacak Y, Arican Z, Bar-Deroma R, et al: Total skin electron irradiation: evaluation of dose uniformity throughout the skin surface. Med Dosim 28:31-34, 2003.
171. Asbell SO, Siu J, Lightfoot DA, et al: Individualized eye shields for use in electron beam therapy as well as low-energy photon irradiation. Int J Radiat Oncol Biol Phys 6:519-521, 1980.
172. Reavely MM, Wilson LD: Total skin electron beam therapy and cutaneous T-cell lymphoma: a clinical guide for patients and staff. Dermatol Nurs 16:36, 39, 57, 2004.
173. Smith BD, Son CB, Wilson LD: Disseminated herpes simplex after total skin electron beam radiotherapy for mycosis fungoides. J R Soc Med 96:500-501, 2003.
174. Smith BD, Wilson LD: Management of mycosis fungoides: Part 2. Treatment. Oncology (Huntingt) 17:1419-1428; discussion 1430, 1433, 2003.
175. Duvic M, Edelson R: Cutaneous T-cell lymphoma. J Am Acad Dermatol 51:S43-45, 2004.
176. Apisarnthanarax N, Talpur R, Duvic M: Treatment of cutaneous T cell lymphoma: current status and future directions. Am J Clin Dermatol 3:193-215, 2002.

INDEX

Note: *Page numbers followed by f refer to figures; page numbers followed by t refer to tables.*

A

C

D

E

F

G

H

I

J

K

L

N

O

P

Q

R

S

T

U

V

W

X

Y

Z